Laboratory Parameter	SI	Conventional (C)	Conversion Factor (CF) CF × C = SI
Glucose, plasma			
Overnight fast, normal	4.2–6.4 mmol/L	75–115 mg/dL	0.05551
Overnight fast, diabetes mellitus			
National Diabetes Data Group	>7.8 mmol/L	>140 mg/dL	0.05551
American Diabetes Association	>7.0 mmol/L	>126 mg/dL	0.05551
72-h fast, normal men	>2.8 mmol/L	>50 mg/dL	0.05551
72-h fast, normal women	>2.2 mmol/L	>40 mg/dL	0.05551
Glucose Tolerance Test, 2-h postprandial plasma glucose			
Normal	<7.8 mmol/L	<140 mg/dL	0.05551
Impaired glucose tolerance	7.8–11.1 mmol/L	140–200 mg/dL	0.05551
Diabetes mellitus	>11.1 mmol/L	>200 mg/dL	0.05551
Gonadal Steroids, plasma			
Androstenedione			
Women	3.5–7.0 nmol/L	1–2 ng/mL	3.492
Men	3.0–5.0 nmol/L	0.8–1.3 ng/mL	3.492
Dihydrotestosterone			
Women	0.17–1 nmol/L	0.05–3 ng/mL	3.467
Men	0.87–2.6 nmol/L	0.25–0.75 ng/mL	3.467
Estradiol			
Women, basal	70–220 pmol/L	20–60 pg/mL	3.671
Women, ovulatory surge	>740 pmol/L	>200 pg/mL	3.671
Men	<180 pmol/L	<50 pg/mL	3.671
Progesterone			
Women, luteal phase	6–64 nmol/L	2–20 ng/mL	3.180
Women, follicular phase	<6 nmol/L	<2 ng/mL	3.180
Men	<6 nmol/L	<2 ng/mL	3.180
Testosterone			
Women	<3.5 nmol/L	<1 ng/mL	4.467
Men	10–35 nmol/L	3–10 ng/mL	4.467
Gonadotropins, plasma			
Follicle-Stimulating Hormone (FSH)			
Women, basal	1.4–9.6 IU/L	1.4–9.6 mIU/mL	—
Women, ovulatory surge	2.3–21 IU/L	2.3–21 mIU/mL	—
Women, postmenopausal	34–96 IU/L	34–96 mIU/mL	—
Men	0.9–15 IU/L	0.9–15 mIU/mL	—
Luteinizing Hormone (LH)			
Women, basal	0.8–26 IU/L	0.8–26 mIU/mL	—
Women, ovulatory surge	25–57 IU/L	25–57 mIU/mL	—
Women, postmenopausal	40–104 IU/L	40–104 mIU/mL	—
Men	1.3–13 IU/L	1.3–13 mIU/mL	—
Growth Hormone (GH), plasma			
After 100 g glucose orally	<2 μg/L	<2 ng/mL	—
After insulin-induced hypoglycemia	>9 μg/L	>9 ng/mL	—
Human Chorionic Gonadotropin β Subunit (β-hCG), plasma			
Men and nonpregnant women	<3 IU/L	<3 mIU/mL	—
β-Hydroxybutyrate, plasma	<300 μmol/L	<3 mg/dL	96.05
Insulin, plasma			
Fasting	35–145 pmol/L	5–20 uU/mL	7.175
During hypoglycemia (plasma glucose <2.8 nmol/L <50 mg/mL)	<35 pmol/L	<5 uU/mL	7.175
Insulin C Peptide, plasma	0.5–2 μg/L	0.5–2 pg/mL	—
Insulin-Like Growth Factor I (IGF-I, Somatomedin-C)			
Women	0.45–2.2 kU/L	0.45–2.2 U/mL	—
Men	0.34–1.9 kU/L	0.34–1.9 U/mL	—
Lactate, plasma	0.56–2.2 mmol/L	5–20 mg/dL	0.111
Magnesium, serum	0.8–1.30 mmol/L	1.8–3.0 mg/dL	0.4114
Osmolality, plasma	285–295 mmol/kg	285–295 mOsmol/L	—
Oxytocin, plasma			
Random	1–4 pmol/L	1.25–5 ng/L	0.80
Women, ovulatory surge	4–8 pmol/L	5–10 ng/L	0.80
Parathyroid Hormone, serum (**Intact PTH** using IRMA assay)	10–65 ng/L	10–65 pg/mL	—
Phosphorus, inorganic, serum	1–1.5 mmol/L	3.0–4.5 mg/dL	0.3229
Prolactin, serum			
Nonpregnant women and men	2–15 μg/L	2–15 ng/mL	—
Pyruvate, plasma	39–102 μmol/L	0.3–0.9 mg/dL	0.01129
Renin Activity, plasma, normal-sodium intake			
Supine	3.2±1 μg/L/h	3.2±1 ng/mL/h	—
Standing	9.3±4.3 μg/L/h	9.3±4.3 ng/mL/h	—
Sodium, serum	136–145 mmol/L	136–145 mEq/L	—
Thyroid Function Tests			
Free thyroxine estimate	9–26 pmol/L	0.7–2.0 ng/dL	12.87
Radioactive iodine uptake, 24 h	0.05–0.30	5–30%	—
Resin T_3 uptake, serum	0.25–0.35	25–35%	—
Reverse triiodothyronine (rT_3), serum	0.15–0.61 nmol/L	10–40 ng/dL	0.01536
Thyroid hormone–binding ratio (THBR)	0.85–1.10	85–110%	—
Thyrotropin (TSH), serum	0.5–5 mU/L	0.5–5 μU/mL	—
Thyroxine (T_4), serum	64–154 nmol/L	5–12 μg/dL	12.87
Triiodothyronine (T_3), serum	1.1–2.9 nmol/L	70–190 ng/dL	0.01536
Triglycerides, plasma	<1.80 mmol/L	<160 mg/dL	0.01129
Vitamin D, see Calciferols			

WILLIAMS TEXTBOOK OF
ENDOCRINOLOGY

9th Edition

Jean D. Wilson, M.D.

Charles Cameron Sprague Distinguished Chair
  and Clinical Professor of Internal Medicine
The University of Texas Southwestern Medical Center
Dallas, Texas

Daniel W. Foster, M.D.

Donald W. Seldin Distinguished Chair
  and Chairman of Internal Medicine
The University of Texas Southwestern Medical Center
Dallas, Texas

Henry M. Kronenberg, M.D.

Professor of Medicine
Harvard Medical School
Chief, Endocrine Unit
Massachusetts General Hospital
Boston, Massachusetts

P. Reed Larsen, M.D.

Professor of Medicine
Harvard Medical School
Chief, Thyroid Division
  and Senior Physician, Brigham and Women's Hospital
Boston, Massachusetts

W.B. SAUNDERS COMPANY

A Division of Harcourt Brace & Company

Philadelphia • London • Toronto • Montreal • Sydney • Tokyo

W.B. SAUNDERS COMPANY
A Division of Harcourt Brace & Company

The Curtis Center
Independence Square West
Philadelphia, Pennsylvania 19106

Library of Congress Cataloging-in-Publication Data

Williams textbook of endocrinology.—9th ed. / edited by Jean D. Wilson . . . [et al.]

p.   cm.

Includes index.

ISBN 0–7216–6152–1

I. Williams, Robert Hardin.   II. Wilson, Jean D.
  [DNLM: 1. Endocrine Glands.   2. Endocrine Diseases.
  WK 100 W721 1998]

RC648.T46 1998   616.4—dc20

DNLM/DLC   96–41440

WILLIAMS TEXTBOOK OF ENDOCRINOLOGY   ISBN 0–7216–6152–1

Printed in the United States of America.

Last digit is the print number: 9   8   7   6   5   4   3   2

CONTRIBUTORS

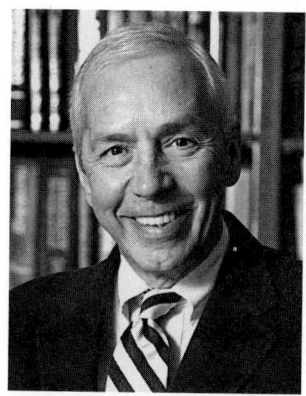

Thomas E. Andreoli

The Nolan Chair in Internal Medicine, Professor and Chairman of Internal Medicine, University of Arkansas College of Medicine, Little Rock

Posterior Pituitary and Water Metabolism

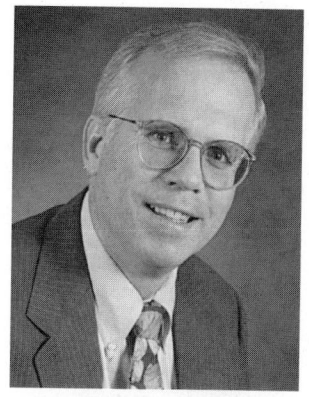

Lowell B. Anthony

Associate Professor of Medicine, Louisiana State University School of Medicine, New Orleans

Disorders of Vasodilator Hormones: Carcinoid Syndrome and Mastocytosis

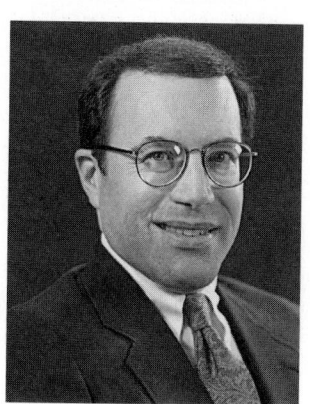

Andrew Arnold

Associate Professor of Medicine, Harvard Medical School; Physician, Massachusetts General Hospital, Boston

Pathogenesis of Endocrine Tumors

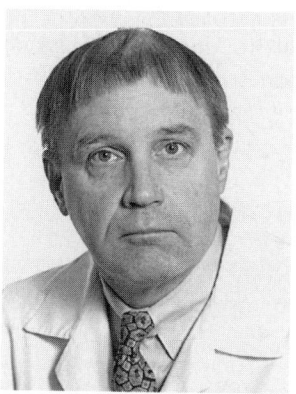

John P. Atkinson

Professor of Medicine and Molecular Microbiology, Washington University School of Medicine, St. Louis

Autoimmunity and the Endocrine System

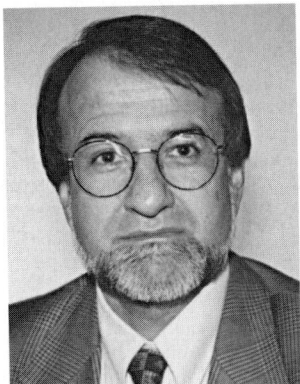

Daniel G. Bichet

Professor of Medicine, University of Montreal Faculty of Medicine, Montreal, Quebec, Canada

Posterior Pituitary and Water Metabolism

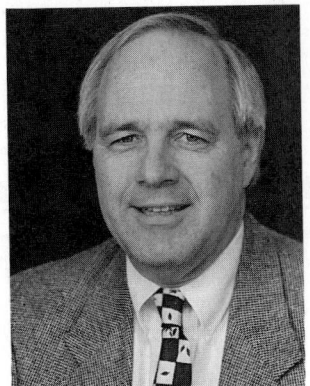

F. Richard Bringhurst

Associate Professor of Medicine, Harvard Medical School; Physician, Massachusetts General Hospital, Boston

Hormones and Disorders of Mineral Metabolism

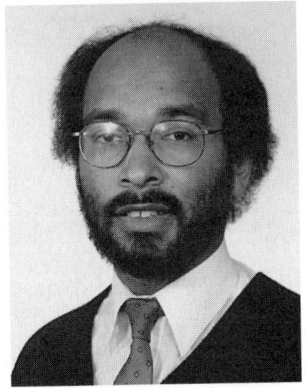

Emery N. Brown

Assistant Professor of Anesthesia, Harvard Medical School; Assistant in Anesthesia, Massachusetts General Hospital, Boston

Measurement of Hormones

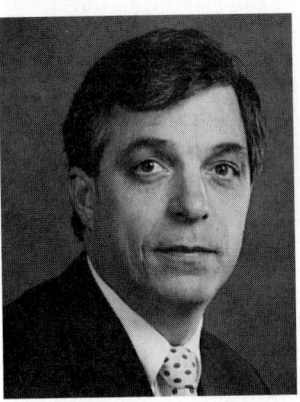

Bruce R. Carr

Paul C. MacDonald Professor of Obstetrics and Gynecology, The University of Texas Southwestern Medical Center, Dallas

Disorders of the Ovaries and Female Reproductive Tract; Fertility Control and Its Complications

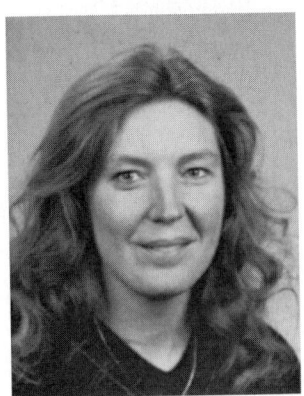

M. Linette Casey

Associate Professor of Biochemistry and of Obstetrics and Gynecology, The University of Texas Southwestern Medical Center, Dallas

Endocrine Changes of Pregnancy

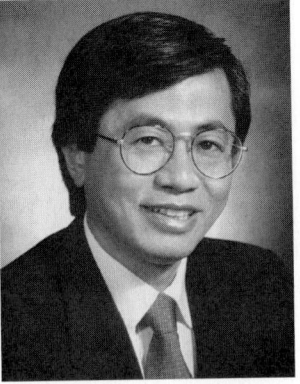

William W. Chin

Professor of Medicine, Harvard Medical School; Chief, Division of Genetics, and Senior Physician, Brigham and Women's Hospital, Boston

Mechanism of Action of Hormones That Act at the Cell Surface

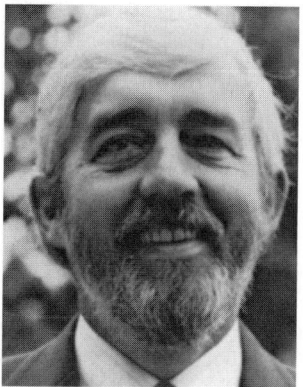

James H. Clark

Professor Emeritus of Cell Biology, Baylor College of Medicine, Houston

Mechanisms of Action of Hormones That Act as Transcription-Regulatory Factors

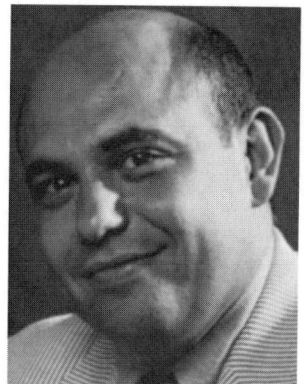

Felix A. Conte

Professor of Pediatrics, University of California, San Francisco

Disorders of Sex Differentiation

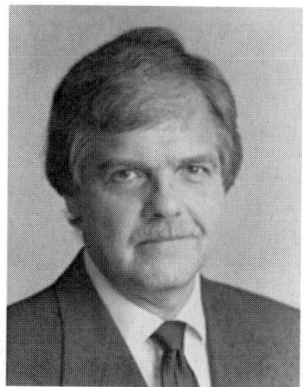

Philip E. Cryer

Irene E. and Michael M. Karl Professor of Medicine, Washington University School of Medicine, St. Louis

Glucose Homeostasis and Hypoglycemia

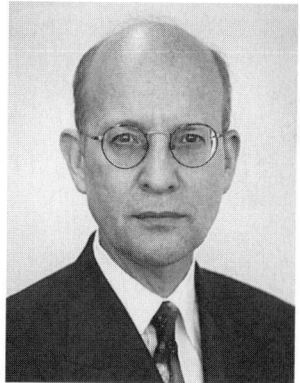

Terry F. Davies

Florence and Theodore Baumritter Professor of Medicine, Mount Sinai School of Medicine, New York

The Thyroid Gland

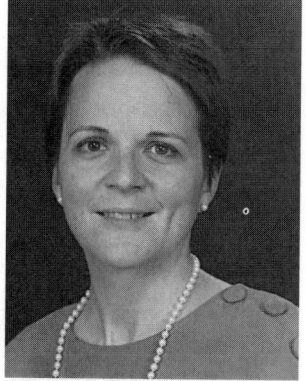

Marie B. Demay

Assistant Professor of Medicine, Harvard Medical School; Assistant Physician, Massachusetts General Hospital, Boston

Hormones and Disorders of Mineral Metabolism

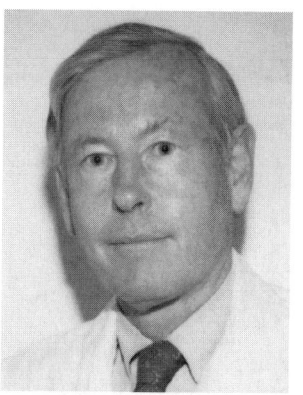

Robert G. Dluhy

Associate Professor of Medicine, Harvard Medical School; Senior Physician, Brigham and Women's Hospital, Boston

Endocrine Hypertension

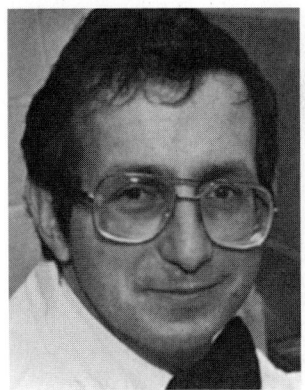

George S. Eisenbarth

Professor of Pediatrics, Medicine, and Immunology, University of Colorado School of Medicine, Denver

Immunoendocrinopathy Syndromes

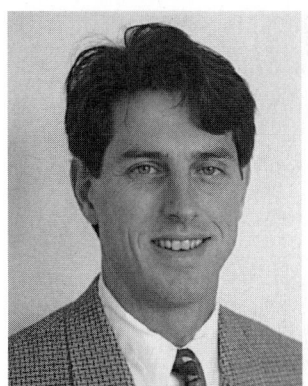

Robert V. Farese, Jr.

Professor of Pathology and Medicine, Gladstone Institute of Cardiovascular Disease, University of California, San Francisco

Disorders of Lipid Metabolism

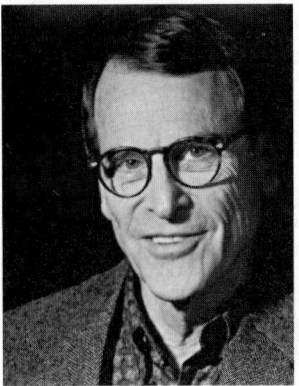

Delbert A. Fisher

Professor Emeritus of Pediatrics and Internal Medicine, University of California, Los Angeles, School of Medicine, Los Angeles; Chief Scientific Officer, Quest Diagnostics-Nichols Institute, San Juan Capistrano, CA

Endocrinology of Fetal Development

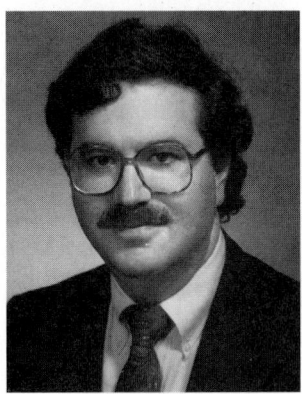

Jeffrey S. Flier

Professor of Medicine, Harvard Medical School; Physician, Beth Israel Deaconess Medical Center, Boston

Eating Disorders: Obesity, Anorexia Nervosa, and Bulimia Nervosa

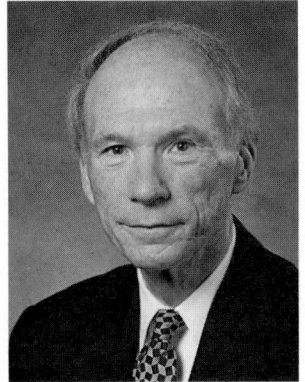

Daniel W. Foster

Donald W. Seldin Distinguished Chair and Chairman of Internal Medicine, The University of Texas Southwestern Medical School, Dallas

Principles of Endocrinology; Diabetes Mellitus; Eating Disorders: Obesity, Anorexia Nervosa, and Bulimia Nervosa

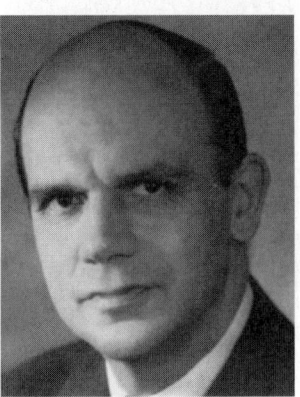

Andrew G. Frantz

Professor of Medicine, Columbia University College of Physicians and Surgeons, New York

Endocrine Disorders of the Breast

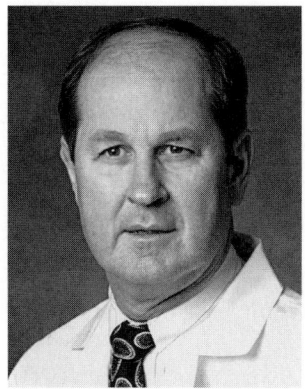

Robert F. Gagel

Professor of Medicine, University of Texas M.D. Anderson Cancer Center, Houston

Multiple Endocrine Neoplasia

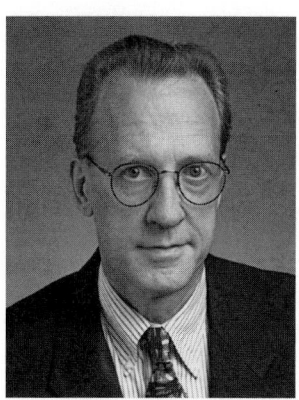

James E. Griffin

Diana and Richard C. Strauss Professor in Biomedical Research and Professor of Internal Medicine, The University of Texas Southwestern Medical Center, Dallas

Disorders of the Testes and the Male Reproductive Tract;
Fertility Control and Its Complications

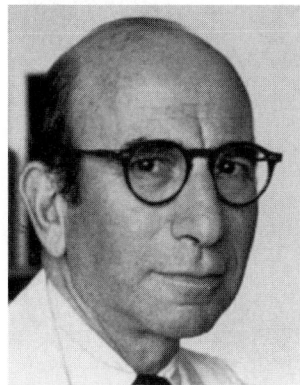

Melvin M. Grumbach

Edward B. Shaw Professor of Pediatrics, University of California, San Francisco

Disorders of Sex Differentiation; Puberty: Ontogeny,
Neuroendocrinology, Physiology, and Disorders

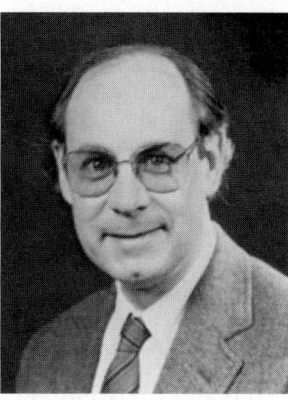

Joel F. Habener

Professor of Medicine, Harvard Medical School; Associate Physician, Massachusetts General Hospital, Boston

Genetic Control of Hormone Formation

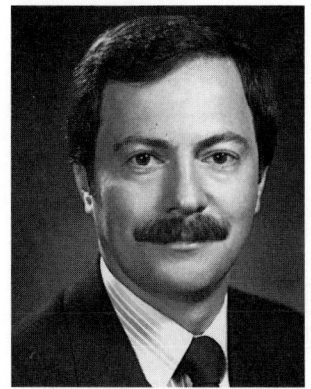

Ian D. Hay

Professor of Medicine, Mayo Medical School, Rochester, MN

The Thyroid Gland

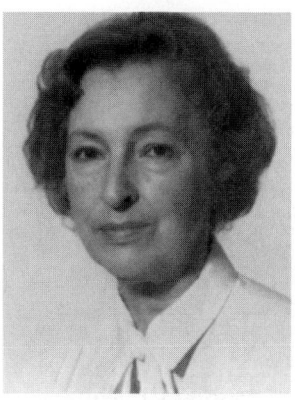

Eva Horvath

Associate Professor of Pathology, University of Toronto Faculty of Medicine, Toronto, Ontario, Canada

The Anterior Pituitary

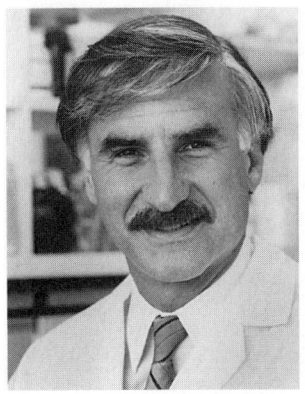

C. Ronald Kahn

Mary K. Iacocca Professor of Medicine, Harvard Medical School; Director, Elliott P. Joslin Research Laboratory, Boston

Mechanism of Action of Hormones That Act at the Cell Surface

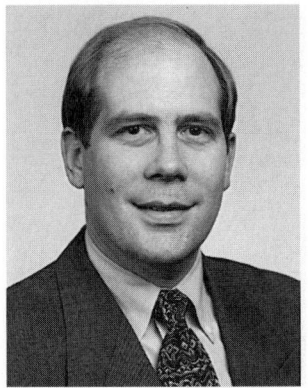

David R. Karp

Assistant Professor of Internal Medicine, The University of Texas Southwestern Medical Center, Dallas

Autoimmunity and the Endocrine System

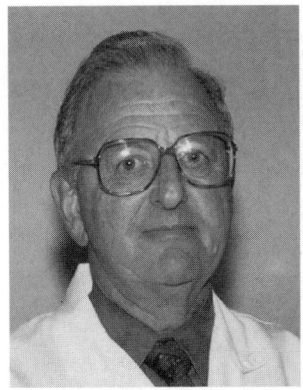

Stanley G. Korenman

Professor of Medicine and Associate Dean, University of California, Los Angeles, School of Medicine, Los Angeles

Sexual Function and Dysfunction

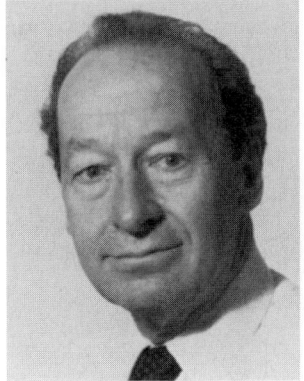

Kalman Kovacs

Professor of Pathology, University of Toronto Faculty of Medicine, Toronto, Ontario, Canada

The Anterior Pituitary

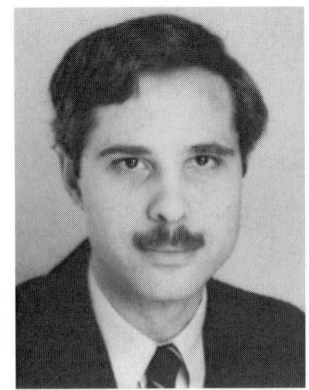

William J. Kovacs

Associate Professor of Medicine, Vanderbilt University School of Medicine, Nashville

The Adrenal Cortex

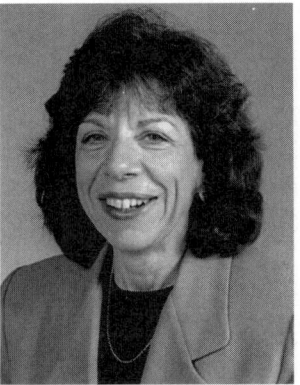

Barbara E. Kream

Professor of Medicine, University of Connecticut Health Center, Farmington

Metabolic Bone Disease

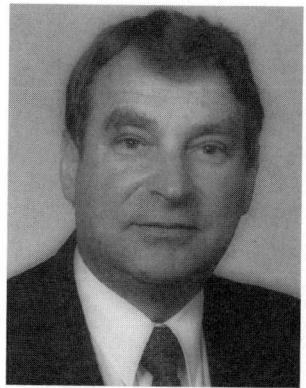

Guenther J. Krejs

Professor and Chairman of Internal Medicine, Karl Franzens University, Graz, Austria

Non–Insulin-Secreting Tumors of the Gastroenteropancreatic System

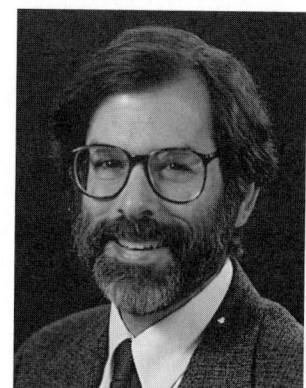

Henry M. Kronenberg

Professor of Medicine, Harvard Medical School; Chief, Endocrine Unit, Massachusetts General Hospital, Boston

Principles of Endocrinology; Hormones and Disorders of Mineral Metabolism

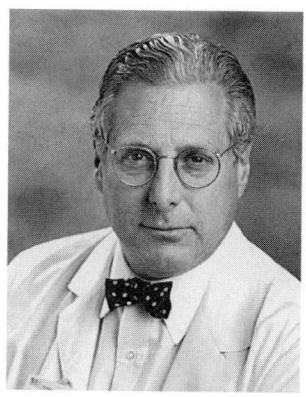

Lewis Landsberg

Irving S. Cutter Professor and Chairman of Medicine, Northwestern University Medical School, Chicago

Catecholamines and the Adrenal Medulla

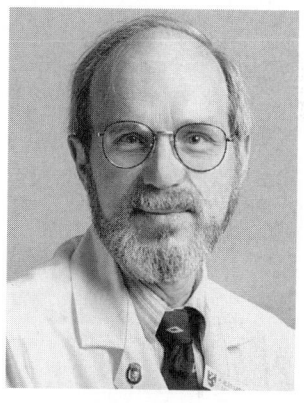

P. Reed Larsen

Professor of Medicine, Harvard Medical School; Chief, Thyroid Division, and Senior Physician, Brigham and Women's Hospital, Boston

Principles of Endocrinology; The Thyroid Gland

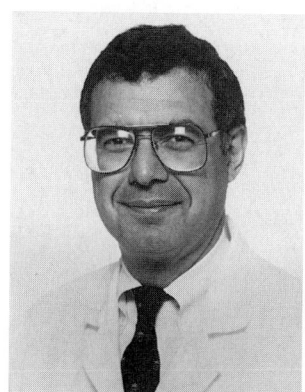

Edward R. Laws, Jr.

Professor of Neurosurgery and Internal Medicine, University of Virginia School of Medicine, Charlottesville

The Anterior Pituitary

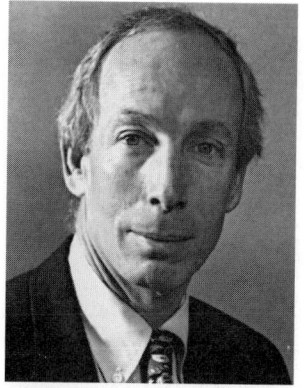

Marc E. Lippman

Professor of Medicine and Pharmacology and Director, Lombardi Cancer Center, Georgetown University Medical School, Washington, DC

Endocrine-Responsive Cancer

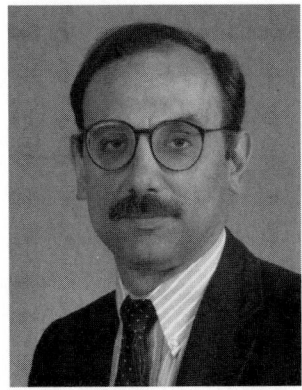

Joseph A. Lorenzo

Professor of Clinical Medicine, University of Connecticut Health Center, Farmington

Metabolic Bone Disease

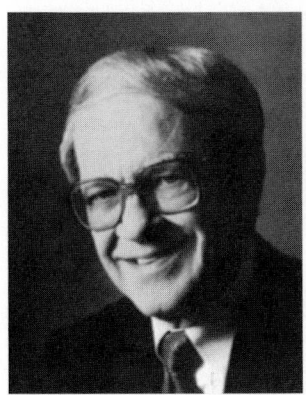

Paul C. MacDonald†

Professor of Obstetrics and Gynecology, Director, Cecil H. and Ida Green Center for Reproductive Biology Sciences, The University of Texas Southwestern Medical Center, Dallas

Endocrine Changes of Pregnancy

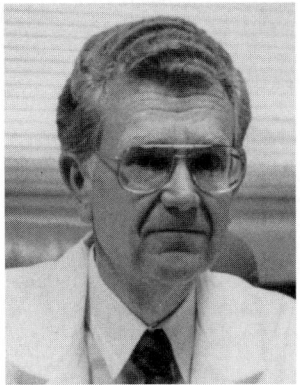

Robert W. Mahley

Professor of Pathology and Medicine and Director, Gladstone Institute of Cardiovascular Disease, University of California, San Francisco

Disorders of Lipid Metabolism

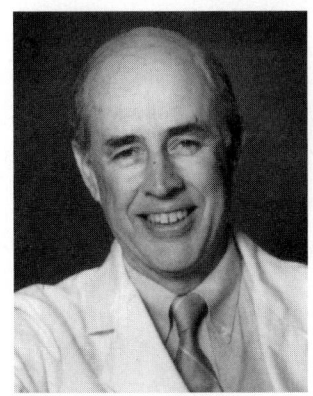

John A. Oates

The Thomas F. Frist, Sr., Professor of Medicine and Pharmacology, Vanderbilt University School of Medicine, Nashville

Disorders of Vasodilator Hormones: Carcinoid Syndrome and Mastocytosis

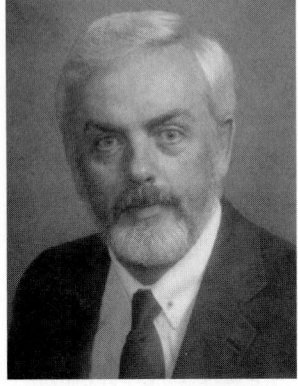

Bert W. O'Malley

Professor and Chairman of Cell Biology, Baylor College of Medicine, Houston

Mechanisms of Action of Hormones That Act as Transcription-Regulatory Factors

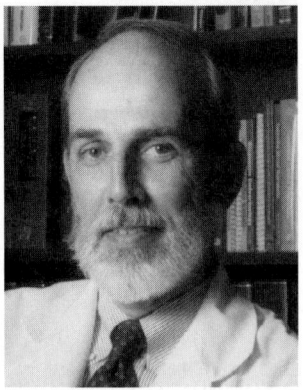

David N. Orth

Professor of Medicine, Vanderbilt University School of Medicine, Nashville

The Adrenal Cortex

†Deceased.

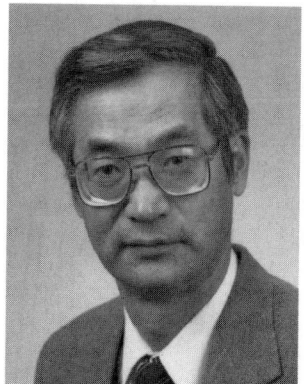

Charles Y. C. Pak
Robert T. Hayes Distinguished Chair in Mineral Metabolism Research and Professor of Internal Medicine, The University of Texas Southwestern Medical Center, Dallas
Kidney Stones

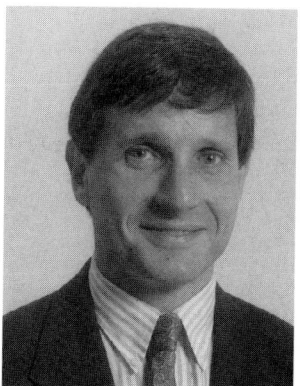

Kenneth S. Polonsky
Professor of Medicine, University of Chicago Medical Center, Chicago
Glucose Homeostasis and Hypoglycemia

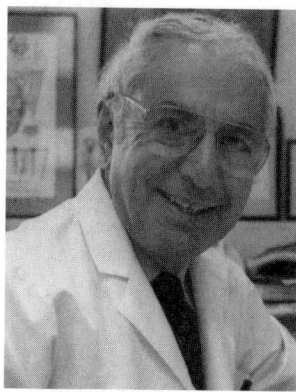

Lawrence G. Raisz
Professor of Medicine, University of Connecticut Health Center, Farmington
Metabolic Bone Disease

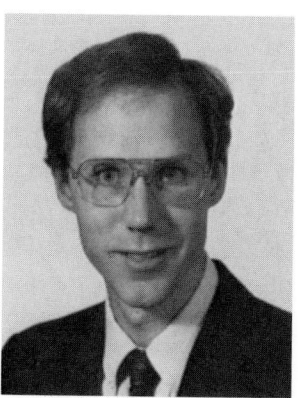

W. Brian Reeves
Associate Professor of Internal Medicine, University of Arkansas College of Medicine, Little Rock
Posterior Pituitary and Water Metabolism

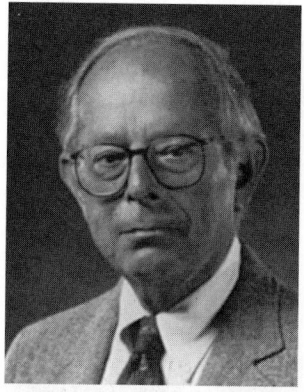

Seymour Reichlin
Research Professor of Medicine, University of Arizona College of Medicine, Tucson
Neuroendocrinology

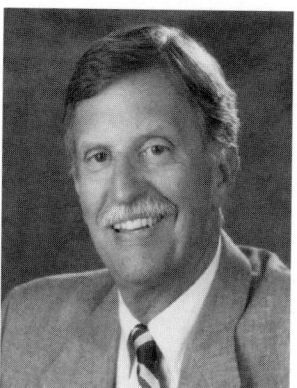

Edward O. Reiter
Professor of Pediatrics, Tufts University School of Medicine; Chairman of Pediatrics, Baystate Medical Center Children's Hospital, Springfield, MA
Normal and Aberrant Growth

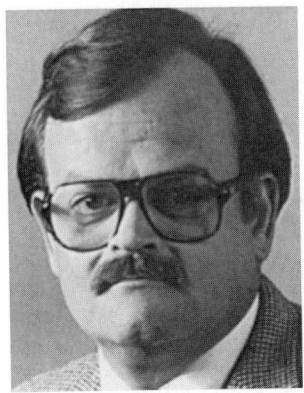

L. Jackson Roberts II

Professor of Pharmacology and Medicine, Vanderbilt University School of Medicine, Nashville

Disorders of Vasodilator Hormones: Carcinoid Syndrome and Mastocytosis

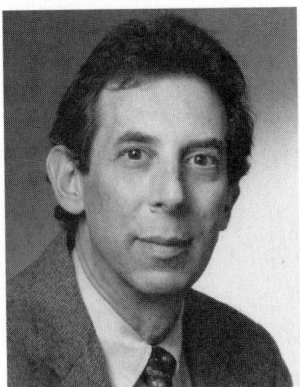

Ron G. Rosenfeld

Professor and Chairman of Pediatrics, Oregon Health Sciences University, Portland

Normal and Aberrant Growth

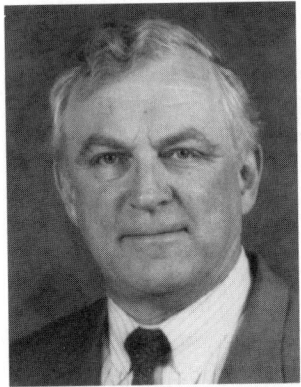

William T. Schrader

Vice President for Endocrine Research, Ligand Pharmaceuticals, La Jolla, CA

Mechanisms of Action of Hormones That Act as Transcription-Regulatory Factors

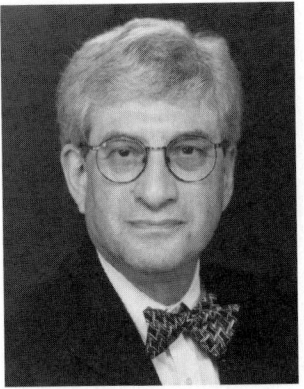

Gino V. Segre

Associate Professor of Medicine, Harvard Medical School; Associate Physician, Massachusetts General Hospital, Boston

Measurement of Hormones

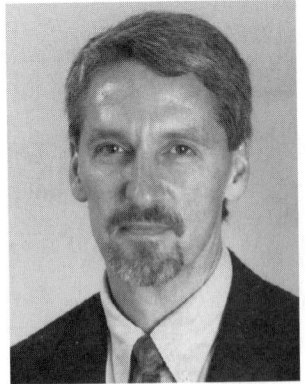

Robert J. Smith

Associate Professor of Medicine, Harvard Medical School; Elliott P. Joslin Research Laboratory, Boston

Mechanism of Action of Hormones That Act at the Cell Surface

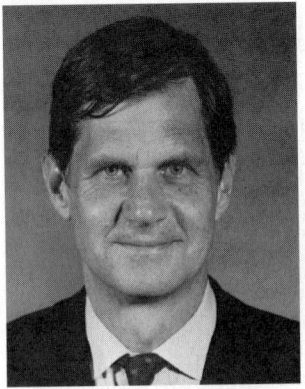

Gordon J. Strewler

Professor of Medicine, Harvard Medical School, Boston; Chairman of Medicine, Brockton/West Roxbury Veterans Administration Medical Center, West Roxbury, MA

Humoral Manifestations of Malignancy

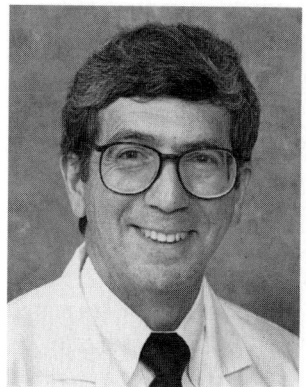

Dennis M. Styne

Professor and Chairman of Pediatrics, University of California, Davis

Puberty: Ontogeny, Neuroendocrinology, Physiology, and Disorders

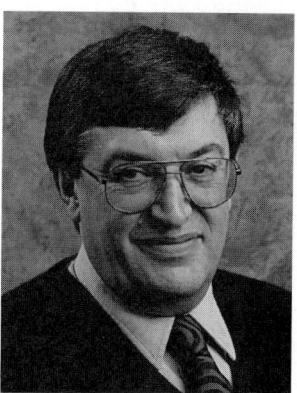

Michael O. Thorner

Kenneth R. Crispell Professor and Chairman of Internal Medicine, University of Virginia School of Medicine, Charlottesville

The Anterior Pituitary

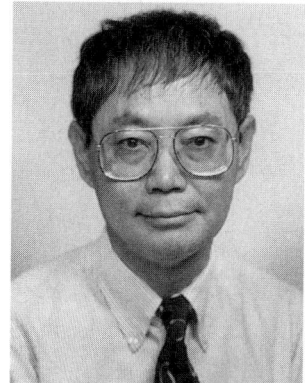

Ming-Jer Tsai

Professor of Cell Biology, Baylor College of Medicine, Houston

Mechanisms of Action of Hormones That Act as Transcription-Regulatory Factors

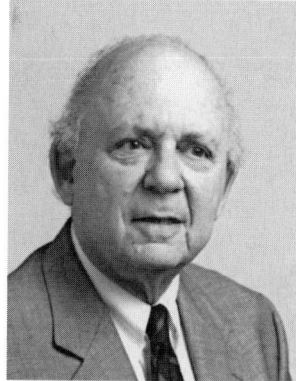

Roger H. Unger

Touchstone West Distinguished Chair in Diabetes and Professor of Internal Medicine, The University of Texas Southwestern Medical Center, Dallas

Diabetes Mellitus

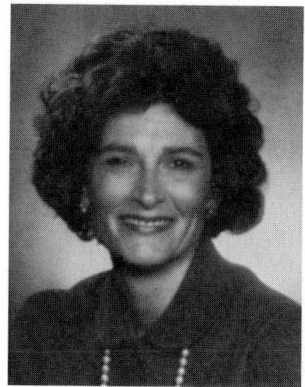

Mary Lee Vance

Professor of Medicine and Neurosurgery, University of Virginia Health Sciences Center, Charlottesville

The Anterior Pituitary

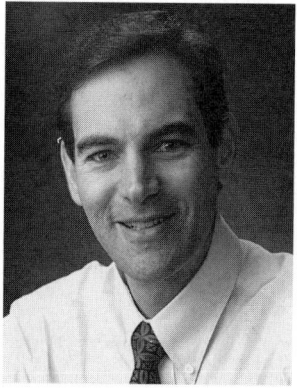

Charles F. Verge

Lecturer in Pediatrics, University of New South Wales, Sydney, Australia

Immunoendocrinopathy Syndromes

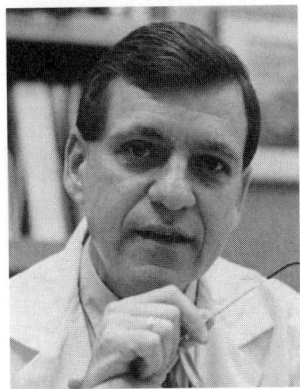

Karl H. Weisgraber

Professor of Pathology and Associate Director, Gladstone Institute of Cardiovascular Disease, University of California, San Francisco

Disorders of Lipid Metabolism

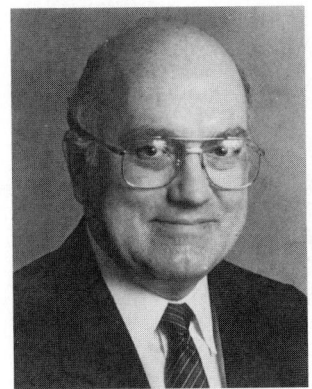

Gordon H. Williams

Professor of Medicine, Harvard Medical School; Senior Physician, Brigham and Women's Hospital, Boston

Endocrine Hypertension

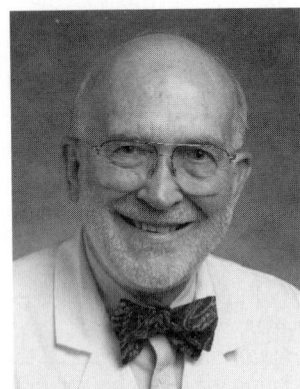

Jean D. Wilson

Charles Cameron Sprague Distinguished Chair in Biomedical Research and Clinical Professor of Internal Medicine, The University of Texas Southwestern Medical Center, Dallas

Principles of Endocrinology; Disorders of the Testes and the Male Reproductive Tract; Endocrine Disorders of the Breast

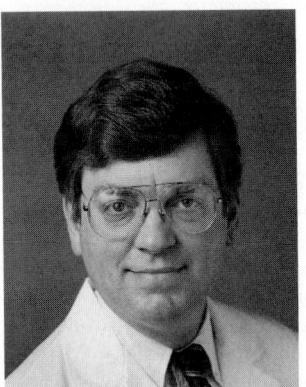

James B. Young

Professor of Medicine, Northwestern University Medical School, Chicago

Catecholamines and the Adrenal Medulla

PREFACE

Williams Textbook of Endocrinology is designed to serve as a bridge between basic science and clinical endocrinology. This aim was clearly formulated in the preface to the first edition:

> *The rapidity and extent of advances in endocrinology have made it increasingly difficult for the student and physician to take full advantage of information available for the understanding, diagnosis, and treatment of clinical disorders. It is the realization of these difficulties that prompted the writing of this book. The main objective is to provide a condensed and authoritative discussion of the management of clinical endocrinopathies, based upon the application of fundamental information obtained from chemical and physiologic investigations.*

The pace of change in endocrinology has accelerated since the publication of the eighth edition. In particular, advances in molecular genetics, including the application of gene knockout and site-directed mutagenesis, have provided new insights into endocrine pathology, and developments in immunology have radically transformed our understanding of hormone action (and interaction) and disease development. Indeed, the borders between endocrinology, neurophysiology, and immunology have become blurred with the recognition of the multiple interactions between the cellular mediators of these systems. At the same time, technological changes in clinical medicine, including development of new assay procedures, genetic screening, and improved imaging capabilities, provide extended power for diagnosis and have caused a shift of emphasis from therapy to the prevention of disease.

The ninth edition of *Williams Textbook of Endocrinology* has been extensively revised to reflect the rapid change in endocrine science. Molecular genetics, cell biology, and molecular biology are integrated throughout. New chapters have been added on the pathogenesis of endocrine tumors and on autoimmunity, and nine chapters have new authors. In this endeavor we are pleased to welcome two new editors, Henry M. Kronenberg and P. Reed Larsen, each a distinguished scientist and clinician who has contributed in the overall planning and has authored a major chapter.

A distinctive feature of this book from its first appearance has been the fact that the contributors are at the forefronts of their disciplines, thereby ensuring the freshness of each edition. This continues to be true. Those who wrote in previous editions have devoted an immense effort to updating chapters, and the new authors have expended an equal or greater effort in formulating new chapters. Neither task is easy, and to our authors we say thank you.

We have again utilized a dual system of laboratory units, first listing values according to the Système International (SI), the system utilized in most medical journals and in hospital laboratories in many countries, followed in parentheses by the conventional values used in hospitals in the United States and some other places. In most instances, converting from SI to conventional units is straightforward, but in some instances values can be expressed in more than one way in both systems. It is imperative that each reader consult his or her laboratory for normal values. Readers must be alert to units, not only in our textbook, but also in clinical practice.

The ninth edition of *Williams Textbook of Endocrinology* could not have been edited without the dedicated help of the coworkers in our offices—Christy K. Gonzales, Carol Hendry, Daryl Webster, and Ann Marie Thompson. We also acknowledge the special contributions made by Richard Zorab, Leslie E. Hoeltzel, and Gina Scala at the W.B. Saunders Company. Their attention to detail and dedication to excellence have made a major impact on the book.

THE EDITORS

CONTENTS

Color plates are located between pages 875 and 877

Section 1

HORMONES AND HORMONE ACTION

PRINCIPLES OF ENDOCRINOLOGY

Jean D. Wilson, Daniel W. Foster, Henry Kronenberg, and P. Reed Larsen

The capacity of specialized tissues to function in an integrated fashion in intact organisms is made possible in large part by three systems of extracellular communication: (1) the nervous system, which transmits electrochemical signals as two-way traffic between the brain and peripheral tissues or between tissues in reflex circuits; (2) the endocrine system, which releases chemical mediators termed *hormones* into the circulation for action away from their sites of origin; and (3) the immune system, which protects the organism against external (bacteria, viruses, fungi) and internal (malignancy) threats. The distinctive features of the endocrine system were delineated by Starling in the Croonian Lectures for 1905, in which he described separate endocrine and neurogenic control mechanisms for the regulation of gastric function.[1] *Endocrinology* was defined as that branch of biologic science that is concerned with the actions of hormones and the organs in which the hormones are formed. Its boundaries included study of the anatomy and physiological function of the major endocrine organs, the secretory products of these organs, the mechanisms of hormone action, and the clinical manifestations of hormone dysfunction. Shortly thereafter it became apparent that there is no sharp distinction between the endocrine and the nervous systems. The nervous system liberates chemical agents that can act as local mediators or gain access to the circulation and act as circulating hormones. Conversely hormones of several types also serve as neurogenic mediators within the central nervous system (CNS). Furthermore, at the

level of the hypothalamus and the pituitary there is anatomic linkage between the nervous and the endocrine systems that serves to integrate the two into one functional control unit (see Chapter 8). The traditional definition of endocrinology has become even more blurred by the recognition that circulating hormones can also have local or autocrine effects in the cells in which they are synthesized, such as locally formed estrogen in the CNS and local conversion of thyroxine (T_4) to triiodothyronine (T_3) in the pituitary, CNS, and brown fat. Alternatively locally formed hormones can diffuse into adjacent or nearby cells to exert paracrine effects, such as the role of testosterone in regulating spermatogenesis, the effects of cortisol on the adrenal medulla, and the regulation of glucagon secretion by insulin.

The immune system was long considered to function autonomously but is now recognized as a regulated system, subject to both endocrine and neural control. In turn the immune system exerts a reciprocal controlling effect on neuroendocrine systems (see Chapter 7).[2] The immune system is also involved in the pathogenesis of endocrine disease by means of humoral and cell-mediated immunity and the release of powerful cytokines. For example, the suppression of the thyroid axis during systemic illness may be conditioned by the secretion of interleukins such as interleukin-6, which suppresses the hypothalamic-pituitary axis and inhibits the peripheral conversion of T_4 to T_3.

An evolutionary perspective is useful for understanding

the probable origin of the endocrine system. Single-cell yeast triggers mating responses by secreting peptides that activate G protein–linked receptors on nearby cells. In fruit flies the differentiation of retinal cells is controlled by receptors of the tyrosine kinase family and intracellular enzyme cascades that resemble those involved in the response to insulin; steroid hormones in flies likewise act through receptors of the thyroid-retinoid-steroid hormone class. Activin and folliculostatin act in the vertebrate embryo to control early steps in embryonic development. Almost certainly the hormone-receptor systems of higher organisms evolved as minor variations of ancient autocrine and paracrine mechanisms for cell-to-cell signaling in primitive organisms. The fundamental unity of the endocrine, neural, and immune systems is the consequence of the common evolutionary origins of these systems.

For these reasons there is a certain artificiality in attempting to define a specific arena of knowledge as endocrinology. Nevertheless, certain features serve to unify the discipline. First, regardless of their sites of action or the complexity of interactions among the various control systems, the central focus of endocrinology is on hormones. Second, the synthesis and secretion of hormones are controlled by similar types of regulatory mechanisms; namely, feedback control in which the level of the hormone signals the need for more or less hormone production. Third, there is a tight coupling between the basic science of endocrinology and clinical medicine. Clinical phenomena are frequently of fundamental importance to the basic science, and virtually all advances in the basic science of endocrinology have clinical ramifications.

FUNCTION OF HORMONES

Hormonal function involves four broad domains: (1) reproduction; (2) growth and development; (3) maintenance of the internal environment; and (4) production, utilization, and storage of energy (Fig. 1–1).

Reproduction

Hormones not only regulate gametogenesis but also control the dimorphic anatomic, functional, and behavioral development of males and females that is essential for sexual reproduction. It is of particular interest in this regard that no exclusive male or female hormones have been identified. All hormones characterized to date are present in both sexes, and both sexes have receptor mechanisms that allow response to all hormones. Sexual dimorphism is the result of differences in the amounts of individual hormones and differences in their patterns of secretion, rather than in their presence or absence. It follows that sexual reproduction requires a precise genetic programming that allows for the synthesis of an appropriate enzyme complement in the ovary or testis that in turn

catalyzes the formation of appropriate amounts of hormones at the critical stages of life.

Growth and Development

Endocrine control is fundamental for growth and development and involves the interaction of hormones of all classes—peptide, steroid, catecholamine, and thyroid. Although hormones are necessary for normal growth and development, it is of equal importance that they also regulate the limitation of growth. For example, if closure of the epiphyses does not occur, skeletal growth continues indefinitely. Hormones influence growth in several ways. Some appear to regulate common mediators. Thyroid hormone, for example, is required for the induction of the formation of insulin-like growth factors or somatomedins by growth hormone. Others have direct effects on the growth of specific tissues. Bone maturation of the untreated congenitally hypothyroid infant is arrested with the bone age fixed at the time at which hypothyroidism occurs. In later childhood one of the earliest symptoms suggesting the presence of hypothyroidism is growth retardation. The critical role played by thyroid hormone in the development of the CNS leads to one of the most classic clinical manifestations of fetal and neonatal thyroid hormone deficiency. The term *cretin* refers to the clinical syndrome of mental retardation and various other CNS abnormalities in iodine-deficient areas of the world (see Chapter 11), which is one of the most dramatic examples of the multipotential effects of a hormone in clinical medicine.[3]

Maintenance of the Internal Environment

Hormones are critical to the maintenance of the internal environment so as to sustain the structure and function of cells. In this regard they regulate the volume and electrolyte content of body fluids; blood pressure and heart rate; acid-base balance; body temperature; and the mass of bone, muscle, and fat. These homeostatic mechanisms not only operate on a minute-to-minute basis but also make possible the adaptation to extreme environmental change.

Energy Production, Utilization, and Storage

Hormones are the pre-eminent mediators of substrate flux and of the utilization of food for energy production or storage. In the anabolic state after a meal, the excess fuel is stored as glycogen and fat under the influence of insulin. In the catabolic state that occurs postprandially or after prolonged fasting, glucagon and other counterregulatory hormones guarantee the availability of substrate for energy production by inducing glycogen breakdown and mobilizing amino acids and free fatty acids for gluconeogenesis and ketogenesis, respectively. Oxidation of fatty acids and ketones maintains the plasma glucose level in a safe range to protect CNS function, and food intake is regulated by leptin secreted from adipocytes. The rate of oxygen consumption, termed the *basal metabolic rate*, is determined by the level of thyroid hormone. Although no longer used, measurement of the basal metabolic rate was one of the earliest diagnostic tests for establishing the presence of thyroid dysfunction. It remains one of the most specific means of demonstrating whether a patient is responsive to thyroid hormone at a cellular level under circumstances in which the hypothalamic-pituitary axis is unresponsive, such as in generalized resistance to thyroid hormone.[4]

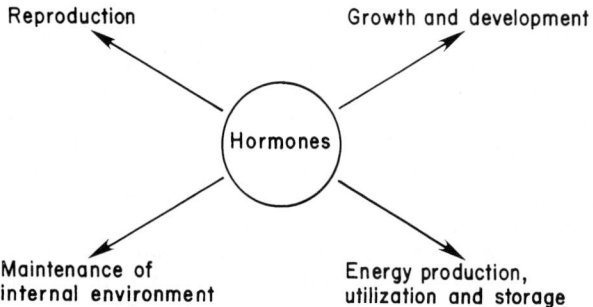

Figure 1–1. The four primary arenas of hormone action.

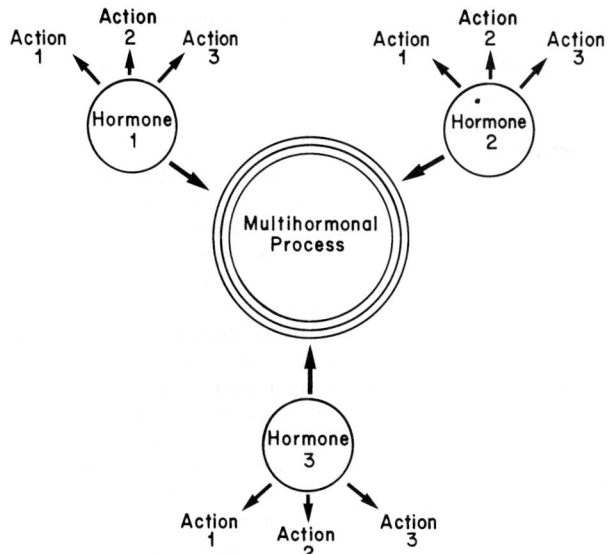

Figure 1–2. Actions of hormones. A single hormone may act independently or in concert with other hormones. For example, in this scheme the multihormone process might be maintenance of the plasma glucose level, hormone 1 being insulin; hormone 2, glucagon; and hormone 3, epinephrine. Each hormone may also act to control or influence more than one process.

INTERACTION OF HORMONES

The effects of hormones are complex (see Chapters 4 and 5). A single hormone can have different effects in various tissues and different effects in the same tissue at different times of life. Similarly, some biologic processes are under the control of single hormones, whereas others require complex interactions among several hormones (Fig. 1–2).

One Hormone, Multiple Actions

An example of a hormone with multiple effects is testosterone. Its actions include fusion of the labioscrotal folds in the male embryo during embryogenesis, induction of male differentiation of the wolffian ducts, regression of the embryonic breast (in some species), growth of the male urogenital tract, control of spermatogenesis, growth of beard and body hair, retention of nitrogen and promotion of muscle growth, control of erythropoietin synthesis, temporal regression of scalp hair, growth of the sebaceous glands and regulation of sebum production, development of prostatic hyperplasia in aging males of several species, secretion of the ejaculate, virilization of the hypothalamus, and many aspects of sexually dimorphic behavior. It was originally believed that testosterone exerted these effects by different mechanisms, but it is now clear that diverse effects can be modulated by a common mechanism. Most actions of testosterone can be explained by binding of the hormone (or its active metabolite dihydrotestosterone) to a specific receptor protein and attachment of the hormone-receptor complex to binding sites in the chromosomes in target tissues to control the synthesis of mRNAs. The diverse effects of hormones are largely due not to different mechanisms of action but rather to the fact that at different stages of development cells are programmed to respond to the hormone-receptor complex in different ways. On occasion hormone effects can be due to cross-talk among receptors. Some actions of testosterone, for example, are due to its binding to the estradiol receptor and hence to its effects as an antiestrogen; and at high concentrations testosterone may exert anabolic effects by binding to the glucocorticoid recep-

tor, thus blocking the catabolic effects of glucocorticoids. Still other hormonal effects may be indirect. Testosterone, for example, enhances erythropoietin formation, which stimulates erythropoiesis and causes the differences in hemoglobin concentration between men and women. Receptors for thyroid hormones are present in most cells, and thousands of genes are under the control of thyroid hormones.[5] Although the binding of T_3 to its nuclear receptor (TR) initiates these events, the subsequent consequences of this interaction differ in different cells. The presence of two genes that encode two different TRs (TRαβ) and the presence of multiple splice products of these genes provide a further level of specificity within target tissues. Again the complexity of the CNS comes to mind; for example in mice genetically engineered not to produce TRβ, the early development of the cochlear apparatus is deranged, whereas development of the remainder of the CNS is relatively intact.[6, 7] A similar pattern in which diverse effects can result from a single mode of action is characteristic of most hormones, including peptides that act at the cell surface.

One Function, Multiple Hormones

It is commonplace to think of hormones and their actions in isolation, but virtually all physiological processes under endocrine regulation are influenced by more than one hormone. A classic example is maintenance of the plasma glucose level within a narrow range so as to be high enough to prevent dysfunction of the CNS on the one hand and low enough to prevent the detrimental effects of hyperglycemia on the other (see Chapter 20). Such regulation could not be accomplished smoothly by a single hormone, no matter how powerful. Control of plasma glucose levels at the upper boundary of normality is primarily exerted by insulin, which modulates hepatic glucose production and enhances glucose transport into cells for both utilization and storage, thereby protecting against hyperglycemia. When plasma glucose levels fall toward or below the normal range, the major glucose-elevating hormone is glucagon, which stimulates glucose production in the liver by means of glycogen breakdown and enhances gluconeogenesis, thus protecting the CNS. Because hypoglycemia is a greater risk to life than hyperglycemia, additional glucose-raising hormones are released as the plasma glucose level falls to dangerous levels: epinephrine, norepinephrine, cortisol, and growth hormone. Thus at least six hormones participate in maintaining a physiological level of plasma glucose. Furthermore additional hormones influence the process indirectly: thyroid hormones, which influence appetite; somatostatin (somatotropin release-inhibiting factor [SRIF]), which blocks the release of insulin and glucagon and slows nutrient absorption from the gut; and glucose-dependent insulinotropic peptide (GIP, gastric inhibitory peptide) and glicentin (glucagon-like peptide), which enhance insulin release in response to glucose absorption. Another example of multiple hormonal control is lactation, which involves (at a minimum) prolactin, placental lactogen, glucocorticoids, growth hormone, thyroid hormone, estrogen, progesterone, and oxytocin (see Chapter 17).

The existence of such complex control mechanisms has two major implications. First, there can be a remarkable degree of fine-tuning: blood glucose levels can be maintained within normal limits under nutritional conditions that vary in the extreme. Second, complex control mechanisms provide an additional level of safety for protecting vital functions in that alternative mechanisms can take over when one hormone in the series is deficient (a fail-safe mechanism). Even for processes that are under predominant control by one hormonal system, other hormones commonly play permissive roles. For example the differentiation and growth of the male external genitalia is mediated predominantly by dihydrotestosterone, but growth hormone and T_4 are also essential for normal development of the genitalia during postnatal life.

CHEMICAL NATURE OF HORMONES

Hormones fall into two chemical categories. The majority are peptides or amino acid derivatives, a category that includes complex polypeptides (luteinizing hormone [LH], human chorionic gonadotropin [hCG]), intermediate-sized peptides (insulin and glucagon), small peptides (thyrotropin-releasing hormone [TRH]), dipeptides (T_4 and T_3), and derivatives of single amino acids (catecholamines, serotonin, and histamine). The remainder are steroid derivatives of cholesterol that are of two types: (1) those with an intact steroid nucleus (adrenal and gonadal steroids) and (2) those in which the B ring of the steroid has been cleaved (vitamin D and its various metabolites).

The existence of diverse structures for chemical mediation implies that the mechanisms for chemical control must have evolved over a long time. However, there is no fixed relationship between hormones in primitive species and those in more advanced species. In some cases, such as estrogen and thyroid hormone, identical hormones are present in species from the most primitive vertebrates to mammals. Furthermore, the characteristics of the hypothalamic-pituitary axis are similar, and the activating and inactivating enzymes for thyroid hormones are highly conserved across species.[8, 9] Conversely, the steroid hormone ecdysone of insects has no known counterpart in humans. Structural homology between different hormones (e.g., between prolactin, placental lactogen, and growth hormone) or between hormone receptors (e.g., between the receptors for prolactin and growth hormone) allow some deductions to be drawn regarding patterns of evolution.

Regardless of chemical structure or how they evolved, all hormones share certain characteristics. First, they are present in the circulation at low concentration. The plasma levels of steroid and thyroid hormones range between picomolar and micromolar, whereas that for peptide hormones is generally between 1 pmol/L and 1 μmol/L. Second, because they are present in such small amounts, hormones must be directed to sites of action by specific mechanisms, commonly by specific receptors in target tissues that recognize and bind the hormone with high affinity. There is considerable variability in the distribution of receptors; the insulin receptor is present in virtually all tissues, whereas the mineralocorticoid receptor has a more limited distribution. Although receptors are essential for hormone response, some tissues possess receptors but lack other molecules necessary for hormone response. For example, insulin receptors are present on erythrocytes, but the red blood cell does not exhibit typical insulin responses. It is generally true, nevertheless, that the principal target organs for a given hormone contain the largest complement of receptor molecules; and, as a consequence, the concentration of hormones in target tissues can be higher than that in the circulation.

Another mechanism by which hormones can be directed to specific target tissues is by delivery within a restricted circulation. The liver is a major target tissue for insulin not because of unique receptor content but because the amount delivered to hepatic tissue through the portal circulation is higher than that reaching extrahepatic tissues through the systemic circulation. The same is true for the delivery of the various releasing hormones from the hypothalamus to the pituitary through the hypophyseal-portal system and for the delivery of hormones from the adrenal cortex to the adrenal medulla. Because of dilution and the rapid clearance of these hormones from the systemic circulation, the concentrations in the circu-lation-restricted sites are higher than those achieved systemically.

A third means of targeting is by direct diffusion to adjacent sites. For example testosterone synthesized in the Leydig cells of the testes both is released into plasma and diffuses into the adjacent spermatogenic tubule to achieve the high level of the hormone necessary for promoting spermatogenesis.

A fourth mechanism is local formation of hormone within a tissue from circulating precursors. One example is the formation of dihydrotestosterone from testosterone within androgen target tissues such as prostate. Similarly estradiol can be formed from circulating androgenic precursors in target tissues such as brain. With respect to thyroid hormone, tissues such as brain, pituitary, and brown fat synthesize the active thyroid hormone T_3 by local deiodination of T_4.[10] This is especially critical for the brain because circulating T_3 does not readily cross the blood-brain barrier. Local synthesis is also used to advantage in the pituitary, where the hypothalamic-pituitary axis can respond to circulating T_4 by virtue of the action of a specific deiodinase that is a highly efficient activator of the prohormone T_4.[11] This system also permits facultative local activation of thyroid hormone such as occurs in brown adipose tissue in the neonate.[12] In summary, the hormone action in specific tissues can be focused or amplified by several mechanisms.

The concept of a target tissue, important as it is, should not be exaggerated. Consider, for example, insulin. By most criteria the major sites of insulin action are liver, muscle, and adipose tissue. However insulin has distinct or permissive effects in many tissues or systems, including the pancreas, kidneys, brain, lungs, immune system, platelets, nervous system, and bone. The same type of gradation is true for the action of many, probably most, hormones. Thus the "targeting" of hormone action may primarily influence the magnitude of hormonal response rather than determine whether a response will occur. In rigorous terms the all-or-none concept of a target tissue should be replaced by quantitative assessments; that is, whether a tissue is a major or a minor site of hormone action.

HORMONE SYNTHESIS, STORAGE, AND RELEASE

With one major exception, the synthetic mechanisms that result in hormone formation are not unique. Peptide hormones are synthesized by the same biochemical pathways as other proteins and are subsequently processed by cleavage or chemical modification to form the active molecules. The initial product is often a large molecule that is progressively shortened in distinct steps (e.g., pre-proparathyroid hormone → proparathyroid hormone → parathyroid hormone [PTH]) (see Chapters 2 and 24). Steroid hormones and catecholamines are synthesized from smaller precursor molecules. Cholesterol, the parent molecule for steroid hormones, is modified by sequential hydroxylations and cleavages of carbon-carbon bonds to form the end products. For many years it was assumed that endocrine organs possessed unique enzymatic capacities that allowed these synthetic reactions to take place, but, in fact, the synthesis of some hormones can occur in diverse tissues. Glucagon is formed in the wall of the gastrointestinal tract as well as in the pancreas. Many peptide hormones are formed in the CNS, the pituitary, and the gastrointestinal tract; indeed hCG appears to be synthesized in almost every tissue of the body. Even when hormones cannot be synthesized de novo in a tissue, they may be formed by transformation reactions. Estrogen, for example, can be formed from testosterone and androstenedione in ovary, brain, adipocytes, and hair follicles. Synthesis of the active forms of vitamin D is even more complicated. The prohormone 7-dehydrocholesterol, or provitamin D_3, is synthesized in the skin and is converted there to vitamin D, which enters the circulation and is then sequentially hydroxylated in the liver (25-hydroxyvitamin D) and the kidney (1,25-dihydroxyvitamin D).

The formation of thyroid hormone is distinctive in the sense that it appears to be restricted to thyroid cells and involves unique reactions. Thyroid hormone is 65% iodine by weight, and, because iodine is a trace element, specific concentrating processes in the thyroid cells provide adequate quantities of iodine for hormone synthesis. Indeed, the evolution of vertebrates to a terrestrial existence made iodine availability even more critical, and iodine deficiency is the most common endocrine disease, affecting the health of at least 250 million people in iodine-deficient areas of the world.[13] Not only does iodine have to be concentrated over 100-fold from the plasma, but also it has to be oxidized and attached to specific tyrosine residues in thyroglobulin, a protein with a molecular weight of 660,000 that contains four potential T_4 molecules.

A second trace element, selenium, is also essential to thyroid hormone physiology. Selenium is present in the deiodinases as selenocysteine, which is encoded by the codon U-G-A, which in most mRNAs acts as a stop translation signal. Thus synthesis of the deiodinases requires a distinct synthetic pathway in which the stop codon function of U-G-A is suppressed (see Chapter 11). Selenium, like iodine, is deficient in many areas of the world, including parts of China, New Zealand, Finland, and Africa. The requirement for both iodine and selenium makes thyroid hormone synthesis the most precariously balanced endocrine system in vertebrates.

Three fundamental characteristics distinguish endocrine organs from nonendocrine tissues that happen to make hormones. First, the rates of synthesis are generally greater in the endocrine organs. Thus the placenta produces much more hCG per unit weight than does liver or testis. Second, there is appropriate processing machinery to complete conversion of prohormones to hormones. Pro-opiomelanocortin, for example, is efficiently converted to corticotropin in the pituitary but not in the brain. The third characteristic is that endocrine glands contain mechanisms for the regulated release of the hormone into the circulation, usually from specialized vesicles.

The rate of hormone release from an endocrine organ is limited ultimately by the rate of its synthesis. Most tropic hormones and regulatory factors act by controlling the rate of hormone synthesis, although there are exceptions (e.g., thyrotropin enhances T_4 release before enhancing T_4 synthesis). In most instances only limited quantities of hormones are stored within the body. For example the content of testosterone in the testes is so small that the total amount must turn over several times each day to account for the daily production rate in normal men. The storage of reserves of peptide hormones in the pancreas and the pituitary serves a critical function in emergencies and periods of stress but only for short periods. Continuous synthesis and turnover of hormones is the usual state. Two exceptions to the generalization that storage is limited are T_4 and 1,25-dihydroxyvitamin D. In both instances precursor forms of the actual hormone (thyroglobulin and either 7-dehydrocholesterol or cholecalciferol) are stored in large amounts and serve as reservoirs for hormone formation in times of need. The consequence is to provide a safeguard against long periods of iodine deficiency or the absence of sunlight, respectively. The 5 mg of thyroid hormone stored in the normal thyroid is sufficient to last about 2 mo; and if the stored hormone is released abruptly, as in subacute thyroiditis, hyperthyroidism can result. For most hormones, however, no such long-term safeguards exist.

TRANSPORT

Water-soluble hormones are transported in plasma in solution and require no specific transport mechanism. Hormones insoluble in water require carrier mechanisms; namely, transport proteins. Because in most instances only the free or unbound hormone enters cells, the transport proteins act as reservoirs so that bound hormone is in dynamic equilibrium with a small amount of free hormone in the plasma. As unbound hormone enters cells it is replaced by hormone newly released from the carrier protein. This process ensures that all cells have access to even the most insoluble hormones.[13] Transport proteins are of two types. Albumin and transthyretin (formerly termed *prealbumin*) bind many small ligands and act as general transport molecules. The specific transport proteins—thyroxine-binding globulin (TBG), testosterone-binding globulin (TeBG, also called sex hormone–binding globulin [SHBG]), and corticosteroid-binding globulin (CBG)—possess binding sites of high affinity and resemble intracellular receptor proteins in their specificities and affinities of binding.

These specific transport systems are nonexclusive in the sense that alternative systems can function in their absence. Thus in hereditary deficiency of TBG, thyroid hormones are transported adequately by albumin and transthyretin. Likewise in analbuminemia hormones can be carried by other proteins. No situation is known in which transport of hormones ceases or in which abnormal transport by itself causes disease.

Transport proteins for hormones have several common features. First, they have a profound effect on clearance rates for hormones. In general the greater the capacity for high-affinity binding of a hormone the slower is the clearance rate.[13] This phenomenon occurs because the rate of metabolic clearance (usually by the liver or kidneys) is determined by the level of free hormone. Women, for example, have higher levels of TeBG and clear hormones that are tightly bound to this protein (testosterone and dihydrotestosterone) about half as rapidly as in men.[14] Second, the transport proteins have binding capacities that are higher than the physiological concentrations of the hormones that they bind. This difference means that when hormones are overproduced or administered in pharmacologic quantities for therapy, enormous amounts can be delivered to tissues. Third, because the rate of hormone production is ultimately determined by the level of free hormone, synthesis can be adjusted appropriately to compensate for changes in the concentration of the transport proteins. As a consequence the increases or decreases in the amounts of transport protein have little effect on endocrine control mechanisms in the steady state, although they may cause diagnostic confusion by altering hormone levels in plasma. To illustrate, an increase in the level of CBG is followed by a transient decrease in the level of free cortisol, which in turn is followed by an increase in cortisol production until CBG is saturated sufficiently for the free hormone level to approximate normal. It follows that changes in transport proteins cause pathologic endocrine states only if the regulatory feedback systems are impaired, which basically means that the endocrine system is abnormal. The most common clinical problem involving transport proteins has to do with the increases in TBG that accompany estrogen therapy or pregnancy.

The mechanism of hormone transport across cell membranes is not well understood. In the case of peptide hormones that act by means of cell-surface receptors, the hormone-receptor complexes can be internalized by endocytosis.[15] The internalization process may serve primarily to deliver the hormones to intracellular sites of degradation and hence function as a termination signal to limit hormone action. In the case of hormones with cytosolic receptors, hormone that is bound to plasma transport proteins may be selectively transported across the membranes of some cells, but under most circumstances free hormone diffuses passively across cell membranes down activity gradients.[14] The presence of intracellular proteins that bind the hormones keeps the intracellular concentration of the free hormone low and thus favors the diffusion process.

FEEDBACK RELATIONSHIPS

The distinguishing characteristic of endocrine systems is the feedback control of hormone production. The paradigm for feedback control is the interaction of the pituitary gland with the thyroid, adrenals, and gonads. Hormones produced in peripheral endocrine organs feed back on the hypothalamic-pituitary system, thus regulating the production of the tropic hormones that control the peripheral endocrine glands (Fig. 1–3). Virtually all hormones are under feedback control, some by the peripheral hormones themselves (androgens, glucocorticoids, thyroid hormones), some by cations (calcium on PTH secretion), some by metabolites (glucose on insulin and glucagon), some by other hormones (somatostatin on insulin and glucagon), and some by osmolality or extracellular fluid volume (vasopressin, renin, and aldosterone).

The feedback relationship is the reason that simultaneous assessment of hormone/effector pairs is frequently necessary for assessment of hormone status (Fig. 1–4). The plasma insulin level must be interpreted in terms of the plasma glucose level in a simultaneously drawn sample. Thyrotropin levels

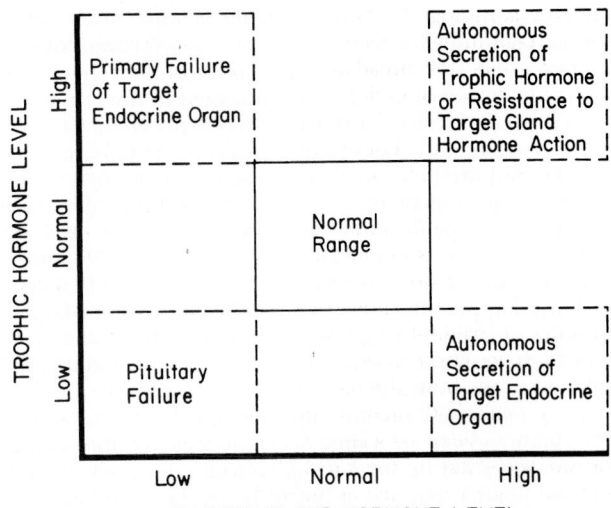

Figure 1–4. Alteration in trophic and target organ hormone pairs and their interpretation (e.g., TSH and thyroxine). (Adapted from Hershman JM. Endocrine Pathophysiology: A Patient-Oriented Approach. 2nd ed. Philadelphia: Lea & Febiger, 1982.)

may be interpretable only in terms of the serum T_4 level, and the immunometric assay of thyrotropin provides information as to whether the hypothyroid individual is adequately, inadequately, or overtreated with levothyroxine. The feedback relation is also the basis for most dynamic tests of endocrine function. Disturbances in feedback are almost invariably involved in the pathophysiology of endocrine disease. This phenomenon is so pervasive in endocrinology that it can be argued that feedback control, rather than the hormones themselves, is the unifying feature of the endocrine system. Feedback control is not always operative, however. For example estrogen production in men and testosterone production in women are not regulated in this manner. In both situations gonadotropin production is controlled by the predominant steroids (testosterone in men and estradiol and progesterone in women). Estrogens in men are synthesized predominantly in extraglandular tissue from circulating androgens, and under physiological conditions the amounts of estrogen formed do not influence the secretion of LH and instead are determined by the level of circulating precursor androgens available and of aromatase in extraglandular tissues. Androgens are formed in women in the ovary under the control of LH but do not appear to participate in the regulation of LH secretion. In these two situations considerable variability can occur in the formation (and action) of the hormones without altering gonadotropin production. Feedback mechanisms also do not appear to be fully operative in the control of placental hormone secretion; the production of these hormones is programmed to supply temporary needs but is not subject to ordinary moment-to-moment regulatory control. Finally, so-called ectopic hormone production is rarely under feedback control regardless of whether it is derived from a tumor or from nontumorous tissue. Renin production by the uterus, for example, does not respond to volume expansion or contraction.

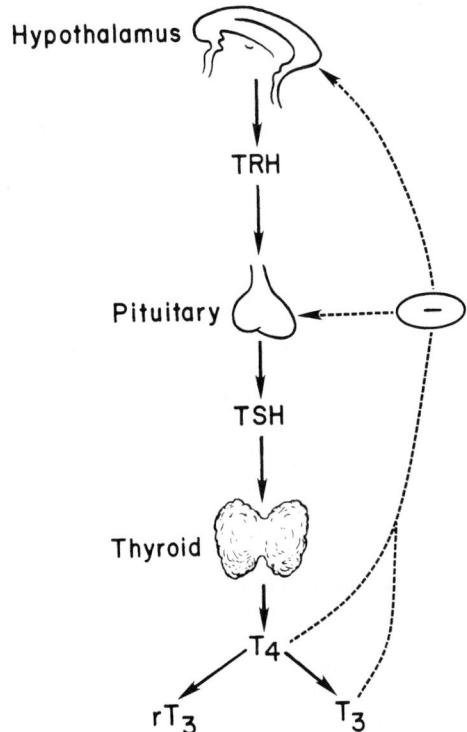

Figure 1–3. A classic feedback system: control of thyroid hormone release. When thyroid hormone levels are inadequate, the repressive effect of triiodothyronine (T_3) and thyroxine (T_4) on the hypothalamus and pituitary is removed. Thyrotropin-releasing hormone (TRH) release stimulates thyrotropin (TSH), which in turn activates thyroxine synthesis in the thyroid gland. When triiodothyronine and thyroxine levels are adequate, inhibition of release of thyrotropin-releasing hormone and thyrotropin occurs. Conversion of thyroxine, a prohormone, to triiodothyronine is probably also regulated.

BIORHYTHMS

Rhythms in the release of hormones constitute a common feature of almost all endocrine systems, and disturbance in the normal operation of cyclic release is a common cause of endocrine pathology.[16] These rhythms can vary over minutes to hours (the pulsatile secretion of LH, thyrotropin, and testosterone), days (the circadian variability in cortisol secretion), weeks (the menstrual cycle), or even longer periods (seasonal variability in T_4 levels). Patterns of release may also differ at different stages of life. For example the sleep-associated surges of gonadotropin secretion that herald the onset of puberty differ from the rhythms of gonadotropin release in adult life. Cyclic or pulsatile variations in hormone concentrations related to alterations in release are more apparent when the half-life of the hormone is short. Insulin, for example, with a half-life of 5 to 6 min, shows extreme variations in concentration, whereas insulin-like growth factors (somatomedins) have a slow turnover and consequently have almost constant values in plasma throughout the day.

Hormonal rhythmicity is caused by a variety of factors. Some, such as sleep-associated alterations and stimulation of prolactin secretion by the suckling reflex, are due to neurogenic factors. Others, such as the circadian variability in glucocorticoid production, are controlled by environmental signals acting through uncertain mechanisms. The menstrual cycle is the result of a complex interplay between positive and negative feedback systems.

One of the most remarkable endocrine rhythms is that involved in the pulsatile secretion of hormones from the pituitary and the ensuing pulsatile release of hormones from the endocrine glands, such as the system linking luteinizing hormone–releasing hormone (LHRH), LH, and testosterone. In simplistic terms such oscillations are initiated in the synchronous discharge of an ultradian pacemaker in the arcuate nucleus and the ensuing release of LHRH from LHRH-containing neurons. In the steady state such cyclic fluctuation of hormone levels in blood also requires inertia or time delay in the negative feedback system that controls its operation.[17] Inertia is the time required for a signal to pass along the whole of the feedback loop. If, for example, the synthesis of testosterone requires x seconds, an increase in LH levels cannot be followed by an increase in testosterone production for x seconds. The resulting oscillation becomes magnified by the time required for plasma testosterone to influence LH production. At a minimum, then, the magnitude of the oscillations is a function of the pacemaker itself, the half-life of the effectors in plasma, and the inertia built into the system. Such oscillations may be fundamental to the operation of feedback systems; indeed, the administration of LHRH by a constant infusion rather than in a pulsatile fashion results in inhibition rather than enhancement of LH secretion.[18, 19] Furthermore the frequency of pulsatile stimulation may alter the ratios of the gonadotropins released from the pituitary.[20] The mechanisms by which the endocrine biorhythms operate, the reasons why attenuation does not occur in the steady state, and the physiological (and pathologic) ramifications of these rhythms are poorly understood.

ENDOCRINE PATHOLOGY

Endocrine disorders can be divided into seven broad categories: (1) subnormal hormone production, (2) hormone overproduction, (3) production of abnormal hormone, (4) disorders of hormone receptors, (5) abnormalities of hormone transport or metabolism, (6) multiple hormone abnormalities, and (7) benign and malignant tumors that produce hormones. There is considerable overlap among these groups. For example, because of enzyme deficiency, impaired hormone production can lead to increased synthesis of another hormone, as in the overproduction of adrenal androgen in patients with cortisol deficiency due to CYP21 (21-hydroxylase)

deficiency. Hormone overproduction can also be secondary to impaired hormone action (and consequently to failure of feedback) in the hormone resistance states. Finally, hormone overproduction, hormone underproduction, and resistance to hormone action may occur at different times in the course of a disease in a single individual, as frequently occurs with insulin in patients with non–insulin-dependent diabetes mellitus and obesity. Nevertheless a categorization based on the fundamental defect is a useful way to approach endocrine pathology.

Subnormal Hormone Production

Impairment of hormone production can have several causes. Absence or malformation of endocrine organs can be due to defects in embryogenesis, as in the sublingual thyroid and in gonadal dysgenesis. Alternatively, the endocrine organ may develop but lack some enzyme essential for hormone synthesis, as in some forms of congenital goiter and in the various types of congenital adrenal hyperplasia. More commonly, a normal endocrine gland is destroyed by a secondary process. Such processes can include granulomatous or infectious agents, as in tuberculosis of the adrenals; infarction, as in the postpartum necrosis of the pituitary that leads to Sheehan's syndrome; autoimmune disorders as in Hashimoto's thyroiditis; chemical exposure as in testicular damage due to cancer chemotherapy; or a variety of forms of physical damage, including radiation, surgical extirpation, and thermal injuries. Despite the multiple etiologies now recognized for hormone underproduction, the cause in many instances remains unknown. A common example is primary hypothyroidism without goiter, in which no evidence may exist for an autoimmune mechanism. In general the effects of hormone deficiency are well understood because it is possible to reproduce and study the manifestations of deficiency by removal or ablation of the appropriate endocrine organ in experimental animals.

Hormone Excess

Hormone overproduction is less well understood than is hormone deficiency because fewer animal models exist for such disorders. Furthermore, hormone overproduction tends to cause severe disease because there are few effective means of counteracting persistent hormone excess. Causes are diverse. Tumors, either benign or malignant, can affect an endocrine gland, as in Cushing's syndrome arising from a carcinoma or an adenoma of the adrenal cortex. Tumors of nonendocrine tissues can secrete hormones such as corticotropin or hCG that drive target glands to hypersecrete and cause disease. The homeostatic mechanisms that control normal hormone secretion can be set at an abnormal level, as in Cushing's disease with bilateral adrenal hyperplasia caused by corticotropin-secreting pituitary microadenomas. Hyperplasia and autonomous tumor formation in some instances form a continuum; for example prolonged hyperplasia of the parathyroid glands in renal insufficiency can lead eventually to autonomous hyperparathyroidism or even adenoma formation. In Graves' disease there is no down-regulation of the thyrotropin or thyroid hormone receptors because thyroid hormone does not feed back at this level on its own synthesis or its action. It appears that most of the defense mechanisms in vertebrates are designed to defend against deficiencies of the various hormones. The lack of defense mechanisms against hormone excess is especially disadvantageous in the face of hormone overproduction. It is of interest that manifestations of hyperfunction do not occur for all hormones; no syndrome of testosterone excess in males has been characterized.

Production of Abnormal Hormones

Most pathologic states involve the excess or deficiency of otherwise normal hormones, but in some circumstances abnormal hormones are produced. A single-gene mutation may alter both structure and function. Thus a mild form of diabetes mellitus is caused by an abnormal insulin molecule as the result of missense mutations that cause single amino acid substitutions in the molecule; such abnormal insulins do not bind well to the insulin receptor and are relatively ineffective.[21] Occasionally immunoglobulins function as hormones, as in the thyroid-stimulating immunoglobulins that cause hyperthyroidism (see Chapter 11) and the antibodies to the insulin receptor that can sometimes mimic the action of insulin (see Chapter 21). In other cases hormone precursors or incompletely processed peptide hormones may be released into the circulation; this situation is common in hormone production by many malignancies (see Chapter 36). Finally, more than one gene specifies the structures for some hormones, some of which are not expressed normally but can be expressed in pathologic states (see Chapter 2).

Disorders of Hormone Receptors

Disorders of hormone receptors can result in either loss of function or gain of function. Hormone resistance, which is defined as a defect in the capacity of normal target tissues to respond to a hormone, was first recognized by Albright and colleagues in their characterization of pseudohypoparathyroidism in 1942.[22] That disorder is now known to result from several hereditary defects, the most common of which resides in the G protein in cell membranes ($G\alpha_s$) that activates the catalytic subunit of adenylate cyclase after binding of PTH to its receptor (see Chapter 24). Syndromes of resistance have been described for many hormones, most commonly due to abnormalities in cell-surface and intracellular receptors but on occasion due to the result of defects in hormone metabolism within cells or abnormalities in other steps in hormone action.[23] Studies of the hereditary resistance syndromes (e.g., androgen resistance in the testicular feminization syndrome, thyroid hormone resistance in families with mutations in the ligand-binding domain of the TRβ) and of acquired hormone resistance (e.g., insulin resistance of obesity) have been of particular importance in establishing the role of receptors in normal hormone action and in the pathogenesis of disease. A common feature of such resistance is the presence of a normal or an elevated level of the hormone in the circulation. This increase is the consequence of the fact that most hormone production is under some type of regulatory feedback control, and failure of hormone action leads to increased hormone production. Because partial defects can be compensated for by an increased hormone concentration and have little clinical consequence, hormone resistance may go unrecognized. It should be suspected whenever hormone levels are inappropriately high in the presence of either no abnormality or evidence of hormone deficiency.

Hereditary resistance to hormones that are essential for life (e.g., cortisol and corticotropin) is inevitably partial because severe or complete defects in the action of these hormones would be lethal. Fetuses with profound defects in these receptors are probably eliminated as stillbirths or abortions. When severe defects exist (e.g., the absence of functional androgen receptor in complete testicular feminization), it can be assumed that the hormone is not essential for the life of the individual.

It is useful to consider hormone resistance as prereceptor, receptor, or postreceptor. More than one kind of resistance can be present, as with the insulin resistance of obesity, which has both receptor and postreceptor components. Prereceptor resistance is usually due to abnormal hormones or to antibodies to hormones. Abnormalities of receptors themselves can be either hereditary or acquired. Postreceptor hormone resistance is the category least well understood. In the case of hormones of the steroid/thyroid class, the general outline by which postreceptor action is mediated is clear, namely, through binding of the hormone-receptor complex to specific nucleotide sequences in the regulatory regions of genes called regulatory elements.[24] Similarly, in the case of the hormones that act by means of the G proteins, the intracellular cascade of reactions that follow hormone binding is understood in considerable detail.[25] In the case of other hormones such as insulin, the postreceptor events involved in hormone action are less clear, but mutations of the human insulin receptor have provided insight into the sequence of events after insulin binds to its receptor.[26] Elucidation of the mechanisms of postreceptor hormone resistance will constitute a major advance in physiology and medicine.

The fact that mutations of receptors can also cause gain of function was first recognized when it was established that the premature puberty in boys with the syndrome of testotoxicosis is due to mutations in the LH receptor that cause it to function autonomously in the absence of LH.[27] Interestingly, the loss of function mutations in the same gene causes the syndrome of LH resistance, a disorder that resembles testicular feminization.[28] Another type of gain of function mutation occurs in prostate cancer in which somatic mutations that cause single amino acid substitutions in the hormone-binding domain of the androgen receptor can cause loss of specificity or promiscuity of hormone action in which the receptor can respond to hormones that would ordinarily be ineffective.[29] Families have been described in which hyperthyroidism is due to gain of function mutations in the thyrotropin receptor, and increased sensitivity to thyrotropin may be involved in the pathogenesis of autonomous thyroid nodules. Still other gain of function mutations are involved in the pathogenesis of endocrine tumors (see Chapter 6).

Abnormalities of Hormone Transport or Metabolism

Under ordinary circumstances abnormalities of hormone transport or metabolism do not cause endocrine pathology. For example, in two extreme situations—hereditary absence of thyroid-binding globulin and cirrhosis of the liver with a markedly diminished rate of cortisol catabolism—no endocrine pathology results because feedback control mechanisms compensate for the defects. Hormone production is controlled by the level of free hormone and consequently can be adjusted up or down as required. Abnormalities of transport and metabolism can cause deviation of laboratory parameters from normal but usually do not cause either hyperfunction or hypofunction. The important point is to recognize that unusual hormonal values do not necessarily imply functional abnormality. Under some circumstances, however, such abnormalities may cause pathology. For example, administration of physiologic replacement doses of glucocorticoid to an individual with cirrhosis of the liver can cause florid Cushing's syndrome, because free hormone levels are elevated in the presence of a decreased rate of steroid catabolism. The effect is equivalent to unregulated entry of hormones into the circulation, as would occur with Cushing's disease. Defects of hormone metabolism are more likely to cause endocrine pathology than are defects in transport because of the existence of alternative mechanisms of transport, but defects in transport can complicate endocrine pharmacology. For example, in a subject with a low thyroxine-binding globulin, administration of sufficient quantities of levothyroxine to raise the thyroid hormone level into the normal range causes hyperthyroidism.

Multiple Hormone Abnormalities

The original paradigm for disorders involving multiple hormones is hypopituitarism, but disorders are now characterized that involve hyperfunction (the multiple endocrine neoplasia syndromes; see Chapter 32) or mixed patterns of hyperfunction and hypofunction of various endocrine glands (the polyglandular autoimmune syndromes; see Chapter 33). These inherited syndromes are of importance out of all proportion to their frequency for two reasons. First, it is mandatory after the diagnosis is made to evaluate patients periodically for involvement of additional endocrine glands and to evaluate relatives at risk before the appearance of serious manifestations of the disorders. Second, analysis of the mechanisms by which these relatively rare single-gene defects predispose individuals to the development of these disorders has provided insight into the pathogenesis of more common endocrine diseases. Many instances of medullary carcinoma of the thyroid, for example, involve somatic mutations of the same gene responsible for the hereditary tumors in multiple endocrine neoplasia type 2.

Tumors of Endocrine Glands

Tumors of endocrine glands may be functional or nonfunctional (see Chapter 6). Functional tumors such as pheochromocytoma or adrenocortical adenomas produce dramatic clinical syndromes. However, the most common endocrine tumors, namely, those of thyroid epithelium, are largely nonfunctional. A major clinical challenge is to identify the 5% of patients with malignant thyroid nodules from the 95% with benign tumors. Although it is possible to take advantage of certain aspects of endocrine physiology in the evaluation of such tumors (e.g., the demonstration of the presence or absence of iodine-concentrating capacity or of thyroid hormone overproduction), the problem is most efficiently diagnosed by evaluation of the histologic characteristics of the tumor cells. With both thyroid and adrenal tumors the endocrinologist assumes the role of oncologist in that many of the therapies for endocrine tumors require the manipulation and monitoring of the hypothalamic-pituitary target organ axis to suppress tumor growth or the administration of agents to interfere with hormone synthesis, as in adrenal carcinoma or tumors that produce corticotropin-releasing hormone.

ASSESSMENT OF ENDOCRINE FUNCTION

Measurement of Hormones

The development of techniques for the measurement of hormones in biologic fluids made it possible to assess endocrine function in quantitative terms, and most endocrine disorders can be diagnosed by measurements of hormone levels in plasma or urine (see Chapter 3). Measurement of individual hormones, however, does not always allow separation of the normal and the abnormal; for example, when the range of normal values is very broad or early in the development of endocrine pathology when the deviation from normal is slight. In some circumstances, serial hormone measurements over time may provide diagnostic insight, as in the repeated measurement of calcium levels and of PTH in subjects with suspected hyperparathyroidism or of urine-free cortisol in patients with cyclical Cushing's disease. Furthermore, assessment of diurnal and sleep-related changes in hormone release may provide unique insight into the endocrine status, such as documentation of nocturnal surges of LH secretion as an indication that puberty has commenced in a boy or documentation of the loss of a normal diurnal rhythm of cortisol secretion as an early manifestation of Cushing's disease.

Measurement of both arms of a hormone feedback system (e.g., T_4 and thyrotropin, calcium and PTH, testosterone and LH) can provide insight not available from individual values (see Fig. 1–4). Indeed, this principle is key to the assessment of endocrine status. The remarkable utility of immunometric assays for thyrotropin in diagnosing thyroid hormone excess or deficiency has already been mentioned. The most critical aspect of this test is that it obviates problems associated with the broad normal range for total and even free thyroid hormone levels in that it provides an independent assessment of whether a given thyroid hormone level is appropriate for that patient. Nonetheless, establishing that the thyrotropin level is abnormal does *not* complete the evaluation of the patient with thyroid dysfunction. The target hormone must also be measured because in some circumstances thyrotropin levels can be abnormal in the absence of permanent thyroid dysfunction (see Chapter 11). Likewise, a high normal serum PTH level in a patient with a simultaneous serum calcium value of 2.9 mmol/L (12 mg/dL) has a different implication than that of the same PTH value and a serum calcium concentration in the midnormal range. Furthermore, the measurement of appropriate hormone pairs can frequently provide etiologic information; for example in pointing to pituitary failure as compared with primary failure of peripheral endocrine organs or suggesting the presence of hormone resistance or of gain of function mutations in hormone receptors. Feedback control is altered by a variety of stresses, such as malnutrition and concurrent illness, and early in the course of disorders such as Cushing's disease assessment of hormone pairs may not provide adequate information.

Dynamic Endocrine Testing

Dynamic tests involving the stimulation or suppression of hormone production can provide critical insight into hormone pathology. For example the fact that the urine can be maximally concentrated with water deprivation implies that the osmolality-sensing mechanism in the hypothalamus, the secretion of vasopressin, the vasopressin receptor, and the postreceptor events in the formation of a concentrated urine all are normal. *Stimulation tests* are used when hypofunction is suspected and are designed to assess the reserve capacity to form and secrete hormone. Such tests usually involve either the administration of an exogenous trophic hormone such as thyrotropin or hCG or stimulation of the endogenous production of a hormone (metyrapone to stimulate corticotropin secretion or hypoglycemia to enhance growth hormone secretion). *Suppression tests* are used when endocrine hyperfunction is suspected and are designed to determine whether negative-feedback control is intact, as in the administration of glucocorticoids to inhibit corticotropin secretion in suspected Cushing's syndrome or in the administration of glucose in suspected acromegaly.

These dynamic tests are particularly useful for detecting subtle endocrine dysfunction and for localizing the site of the defect, for example in a subject with documented Cushing's syndrome. The central problem in their interpretation, however, is that the range of normal responses has not been adequately defined either in suitable numbers of normal control subjects or in patients with concurrent diseases, particularly in the presence of coexisting endocrine disorders, other medical disorders, or psychiatric disease. Furthermore, drugs of a variety of types may interfere with dynamic testing, as illustrated by the fact that glucocorticoids inhibit and estrogens enhance the response of growth hormone to most stimuli. Finally, even when a dynamic abnormality is documented, such information provides no insight into the natural history of the disorder.

SUMMARY

In this brief introduction we have attempted to outline some of the principles of endocrinology that are covered much more extensively in the remainder of the book. Our purpose has been to show that endocrinology is in many ways an orderly clinical discipline, by which we mean that the general principles are usually informative whether applied to normal physiology or to endocrine disease.

REFERENCES

1. Starling EH. The Croonian Lectures on the chemical correlation of the functions of the body. Lancet 1905; 2:339–341, 423–425, 501–503, 579–583.
2. Bateman A, Singh A, Kral T, et al. The immune-hypothalamic-pituitary-adrenal axis. Endocr Rev 1989; 10:92–111.
3. Delange F. The disorders induced by iodine deficiency. Thyroid 1994; 4:107–128.
4. Refetoff S, Weiss RE, Usala SJ, et al. The syndromes of resistance to thyroid hormone: update 1994. Endocr Rev 1994; 3:336–342.
5. Brown DD, Wang Z, Kanamori A, et al. Amphibian metamorphosis: a complex program of gene expression changes controlled by thyroid hormone. Recent Prog Horm Res 1995; 50:309–315.
6. Forrest D, Erway LC, Ng L, et al. Thyroid hormone receptor beta is essential for development of auditory function. Nat Genet 1996; 13:354–357.
7. Forrest D, Golarai G, Connor J, et al. Genetic analysis of thyroid hormone receptors in development and disease. Recent Prog Horm Res 1996; 51:1–22.
8. Croteau W, Davey JC, Galton VA, et al. Cloning of the mammalian type II iodothyronine deiodinase: a selenoprotein differentially expressed and regulated in human and rat brain and other tissues. J Clin Invest 1996; 98:405–417.
9. Davey JC, Becker KB, Schneider MJ, et al. Cloning of a cDNA for the type II iodothyronine deiodinase. J Biol Chem 1995; 270:26786–26789.
10. Larsen PR, Silva JE, Kaplan MM. Relationships between circulating and intracellular thyroid hormones: physiological and clinical implications. Endocr Rev 1981; 2:87–102.
11. Larsen PR. Thyroid-pituitary interactions: feedback regulation of thyrotropin secretion by thyroid hormones. N Engl J Med 1982; 306:23.
12. Silva JE, Larsen PR. Adrenergic activation of triiodothyronine production in brown adipose tissue. Nature 1983; 305:712–713.
13. Mendel CM. The free hormone hypothesis: a physiologically based mathematical model. Endocr Rev 1989; 10:232–274.
14. Rosner W. The functions of corticosteroid-binding globulin and sex hormone-binding globulin: recent advances. Endocr Rev 1990; 11:80–91.
15. Goldstein JL, Anderson RGW, Brown MS. Coated pits, coated vesicles, and receptor-mediated endocytosis. Nature 1979; 279:679–685.
16. Van Cauter E, Aschoff J. Endocrine and other biological rhythms. In: DeGroot LJ, et al., eds. Endocrinology. 2nd ed. Vol 3. Philadelphia: WB Saunders, 1989: 2658–2705.
17. Burgi HI. General aspects of endocrinology. In: Labhart A, ed. Clinical Endocrinology Theory and Practice. New York: Springer-Verlag, 1974: 1–23.
18. Wickings EJ, Zaidi P, Brabant G, et al. Stimulation of pituitary and testicular functions with LH-RH agonist or pulsatile LH-RH treatment in the rhesus monkey during the non-breeding season. J Reprod Fertil 1981; 63:129–136.
19. Akhtar FB, Marshall GR, Wickings EJ, et al. Reversible induction of azoospermia in rhesus monkey by constant infusion of a gonadotropin-releasing hormone agonist using osmotic minipumps. J Clin Endocrinol Metab 1983; 56:534–540.
20. Gross KM, Matsumoto AM, Southworth MB, et al. The pattern of luteinizing hormone releasing hormone (LHRH) administration controls the relative secretion of follicle stimulating hormone (FSH) and luteinizing hormone (LH) in man. Clin Res 1984; 32:74A.
21. Haneda M, Chan SJ, Kwok SCM, et al. Studies on mutant human insulin genes: identification and sequence analysis of a gene encoding (Ser^{b24}) insulin. Proc Natl Acad Sci USA 1983; 80:6366–6370.
22. Albright F, Burnett CH, Smith PH, et al. Pseudohypoparathyroidism: an example of Seabright's bantam syndrome. Endocrinology 1942; 30:922–932.
23. Verhoeven GFM, Wilson JD. The syndromes of primary hormone resistance. Metabolism 1979; 28:253–289.
24. Carson-Jurica MA, Schrader WT, O'Malley BW. Steroid receptor family: structure and functions. Endocr Rev 1990; 11:201–220.
25. Gilman AG. G proteins: transducers of receptor-generated signals. Annu Rev Biochem 1987; 56:615–649.
26. Kahn CR, Goldstein BJ. Molecular defects in insulin action. Science 1989; 245:13.
27. Laue L, Chan WY, Hsueh AJW, et al. Genetic heterogeneity of constitutively activating mutations of the human luteinizing hormone receptor in familial male precocious puberty. Proc Natl Acad Sci USA 1995; 92:1906–1910.
28. Latronico AC, Anasti J, Arnhold IJP, et al. Testicular and ovarian resistance to luteinizing hormone caused by inactivating mutations of the luteinizing hormone receptor gene. N Engl J Med 1996; 334:507–508.
29. Taplin M-E, Bubley GJ, Shuster TD, et al. Mutation of the androgen-receptor gene in metastatic androgen-independent prostate cancer. N Engl J Med 1995; 332:1393–1398.

2

GENETIC CONTROL OF HORMONE FORMATION

Joel F. Habener

INTRODUCTION

The polypeptide hormones constitute a critically important and diverse set of regulatory molecules that convey specific information among cells and organs. This type of molecular communication arose early in the development of life and evolved into a complex system for the control of growth, development, and reproduction and for the maintenance of metabolic homeostasis. These hormones consist of approximately 200 or more small proteins ranging from as few as three amino acids, e.g., thyrotropin-releasing hormone (TRH) to 192 amino acids (e.g., growth hormone). In a broader sense these polypeptides function both as hormones whose actions are mediated on distant organs by way of their transport through the bloodstream and as local cell-to-cell communicators (Fig. 2–1). This latter function of the polypeptide hormones is exemplified by their elaboration and secretion within neurons of the central, autonomic, and peripheral nervous systems, where they act as neurotransmitters (see Chapter 8). The multiple functions of the polypeptide hormone genes have aroused great interest in the mechanisms of their synthesis and release.

The purpose of this chapter is to review the structures, diversity, and mechanisms that govern the expression of genes encoding peptide hormones. The synthesis of nonpeptide hormones such as catecholamines, thyroid hormones, and steroid hormones involves the action of multiple enzymes, and hence

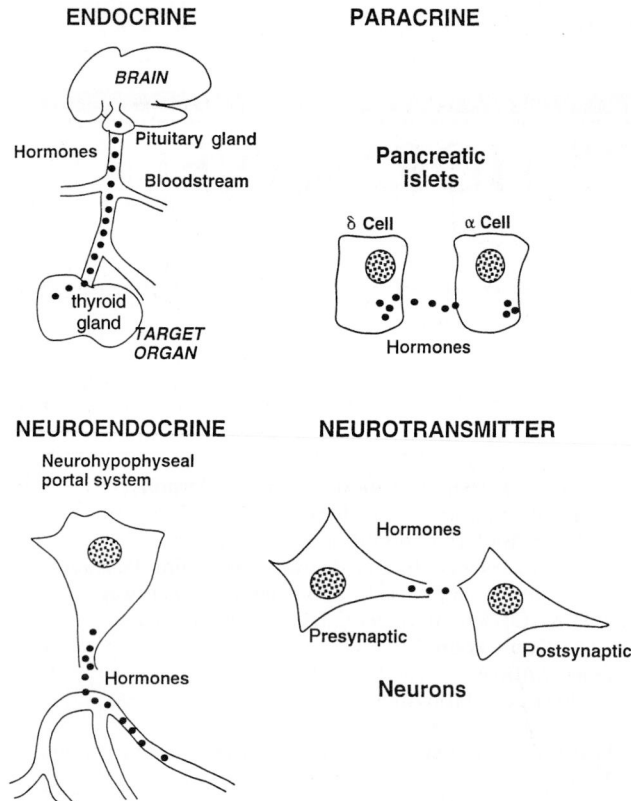

Figure 2–1. Different modes of utilization of polypeptide hormones in the expression of their biologic actions. The peptide hormones are expressed in at least four ways in fulfilling their functions as cellular messenger molecules: (1) endocrine mode, for purposes of communication among organs, e.g. pituitary-thyroid axis; (2) paracrine mode, for communication among adjacent cells, often located within endocrine organs; (3) neuroendocrine mode, for synthesis and release of peptides from specialized peptidergic neurons for action on distant organs via the bloodstream, e.g., neuroendocrine peptides of the hypothalamus; and (4) neurotransmitter mode, for action of peptides in concert with classic amino acid–derived aminergic transmitters in the neuronal communication network. Identical polypeptides are often utilized in the nervous system both as neuroendocrine hormones and as neurotransmitters. In some instances the identical gene product is used in all four modes of expression.

the expression of multiple genes, and is discussed in the individual chapters devoted to such hormones.

DEVELOPMENT OF MOLECULAR ENDOCRINOLOGY AS A DISCIPLINE

The modern era in this field was inaugurated in the early 1950s with the determination by Popenoe and du Vigneaud[2] (and their co-workers) of the amino acid sequences of vasopressin and oxytocin. In ensuing years the amino acid sequences of approximately 200 different polypeptide hormones and regulatory polypeptides were established. A major breakthrough for studies of physiological and cellular endocrine regulation came with the application of the principle of the radioimmunoassay.[3] Exploitation of this technique provided insight into the workings of endocrine control mechanisms under physiological and pathologic circumstances in vivo. The availability of both natural and synthetic peptides in homogeneous form led to the synthesis of numerous analogues that proved useful as potent hormone agonists and antagonists and led to the identification of hormone receptors.

Development of recombinant DNA technology resulted in an acceleration of studies of cellular control mechanisms.

The initial successful cloning of the cDNAs for insulin[4] and growth hormone[5] established that the genetic engineering of recombinant DNA molecules can be utilized to determine the structures of proteins by way of decoding the nucleotide sequences. It is also possible with this technique to remove a segment of genetic material from its normal context and replicate it in the form of plasmids or phages within host bacteria, yeasts, or insect cells in high yields; this segment can then be reintroduced into a variety of cultured cells or into the germ line of mice (transgenic mice), where it can be studied and manipulated under controlled circumstances. It is now possible to target the insertion of expressible genes into predetermined sites in the genes of culture cells and mice and also to ablate and/or replace specific genes by targeted DNA recombination in embryonal stem cells (targeted gene knockouts or replacement).

To a large extent the techniques of gene cloning have altered the approaches to the analysis of the structure and function of polypeptide hormones. Instead of isolating minuscule amounts of peptide from large amounts of tissue and analyzing amino acid sequences, it is now possible to obtain DNA templates from the messenger RNAs (mRNAs) encoding the polypeptides. Recombinant DNA molecules prepared from these RNA templates can be cloned and amplified, thereby producing large amounts of DNA for nucleotide sequencing and deduction of the amino acid sequences. Genes have now been cloned for approximately 200 hormonal regulatory peptides, many of which are present in only trace amounts in the tissues in which they originate.

The expansion of technology for DNA sequencing,[6, 7] and the combined efforts of the laboratories participating in the Human Genome Project make it likely that the primary structure of the human genome may be known by the year 2002 or 2003.[8, 9] The goals are to establish a linkage map of the genome, a map of expressed genes, and finally the complete nucleotide sequence of the entire human genome. Determination of the structure of genes, however, provides only the foundation of information about the control of gene expression.

EVOLUTION OF PEPTIDE HORMONES AND THEIR FUNCTIONS

Peptide hormones arose early in evolution. Indeed polypeptides structurally similar to mammalian peptides are present in lower vertebrates, insects, yeasts, and bacteria.[10] For example the α-factor (mating pheromone) of yeast is similar in structure to mammalian luteinizing hormone-releasing hormone (LHRH; also called gonadotropin-releasing hormone [GnRH]).[11] Other such examples include glucagon-like immunoreactivity in the corpus cardiacum of the tobacco hornworm; vasoactive intestinal peptide (VIP), and pancreatic polypeptide-like substances in the earthworm; and cholecystokinin, neurotensin, and substance P in coelenterates (hydra and sea anemone). Insulin, corticotropin (adrenocorticotropin [ACTH]), and somatostatin (somatotropin release-inhibiting factor [SRIF]) are present in ciliated protozoa (*Tetrahymena*) and in various strains of *Escherichia coli*. Thus the genes encoding polypeptide hormones and regulatory peptides evolved early and initially functioned in cell-to-cell communication to cope with nourishment, growth, development, and reproduction. As a circulatory system developed to connect individual organs, similar, if not identical, gene products became circulating hormones. Perhaps as a consequence of the development of the blood-brain barrier, the local cell-to-cell regulatory functions of the polypeptides in the brain may have been maintained apart from the endocrine functions of the peptides in the rest of the body. The peptidergic neurons that populate the hypothalamus may represent a transition between the cell-to-cell communication and the organ-to-organ regulatory functions of the peptides.

The known regulatory peptides number in the hundreds, and additional peptide hormones will be found in the isolation of substances responsible for specific biologic activities or by the decoding of gene sequences. A typical mammalian cell expresses genes encoding between 5000 and 10,000 different proteins, and in all differentiated cells the repertoire of expressed genes that encode proteins is probably somewhere around 50,000 to 100,000. By searching for similarities among approximately 2,000 known protein sequences, Doolittle[12] estimated that there may be as few as 500 to 1000 fundamental proteins, each probably distinct with regard to its functional properties. For example one may envision distinct amino acid sequences that are specific for binding sites of cellular receptors, chelation of heavy-metal ions, expression of proteolytic activity, structural components of membranes, enzymatic hydrolysis of ATP, and DNA-binding domains. The findings that the coding sequences of genes are separated into blocks in the DNA (exons) by intervening DNA sequences (introns), and that the exons appear to constitute distinct functional domains, lend credence to the belief that specific protein-encoding gene segments have functions that have remained essentially unchanged throughout evolution, presumably because of the selective advantages of these functions to survival.

STEPS IN THE EXPRESSION OF A PROTEIN-ENCODING GENE

Several steps are involved in the transfer of information encoded in the polynucleotide language of DNA to the poly-amino acid language of biologically active proteins, and any one or more of these steps can serve as control points in the regulation of gene expression (Fig. 2–2):

1. Rearrangements and transpositions of DNA segments. These processes occur in evolution, with the exception that such somatic gene rearrangements in the immunoglobulin genes take place during the lifetime of an individual.

2. Transcription. Synthesis of RNA results in the formation of RNA copies of the two gene alleles and is catalyzed by RNA polymerase II–associated transcription factors.

3. Post-transcriptional processing. Specific modifications of RNA include the formation of mRNA from the precursor RNA by way of excision of introns and rejoining of exons and modifications of the 3′ end of the RNA by polyadenylation and of the 5′ end by addition of 7-methylguanine "caps."

4. Translation. Amino acids are assembled by base pairing of the nucleotide triplets (anticodons) of the specific "carrier" aminoacylated tRNAs to the corresponding codons of the mRNA bound to polyribosomes and are polymerized into the polypeptide chains.

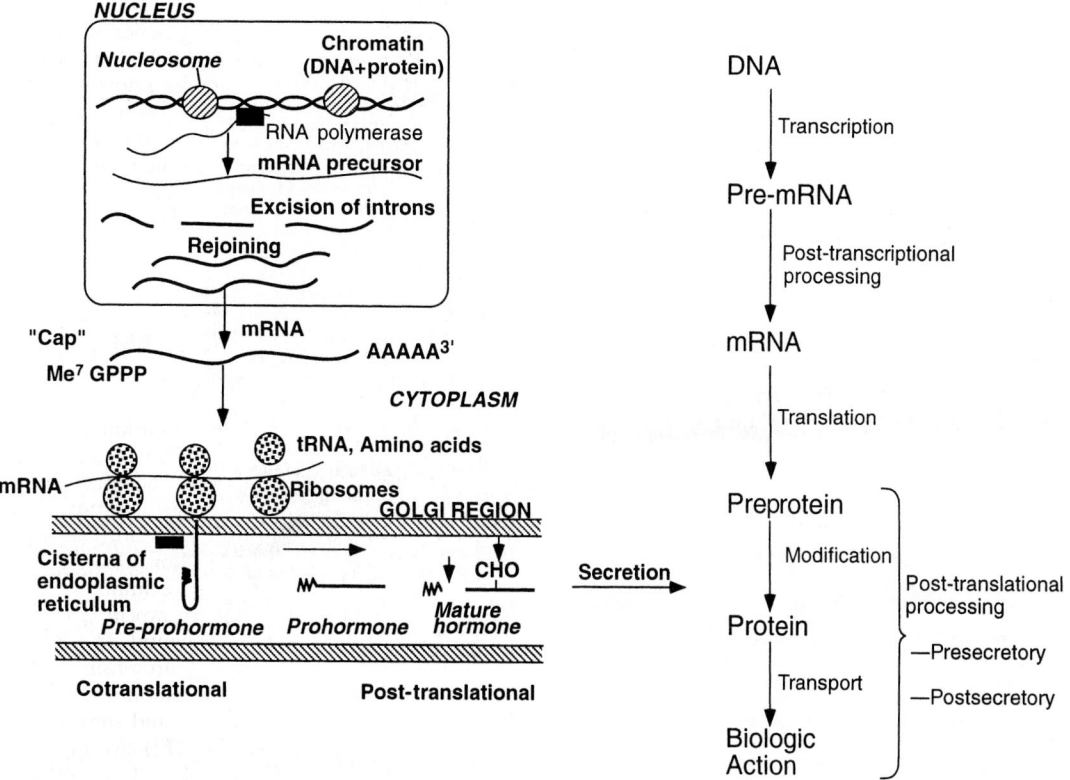

Figure 2–2. Steps in the cellular synthesis of polypeptide hormones. The steps that take place within the nucleus include transcription of genetic information into an mRNA precursor (pre-mRNA) followed by post-transcriptional processing, which includes RNA cleavage, excision of introns, and rejoining of exons, resulting in formation of mRNA. Ends of mRNA are modified by addition of methylguanosine caps at the 5′ end and addition of poly(A) tracts at the 3′ ends. The cytoplasmic mRNA is assembled with ribosomes. Amino acids, carried by aminoacylated transfer RNAs (tRNAs), are then polymerized into a polypeptide chain. The final step in protein synthesis is that of post-translational processing. These processes take place both during growth of the nascent polypeptide chain (cotranslational) and after release of the completed chain (post-translational), and they include proteolytic cleavages of polypeptide chain (conversion of pre-prohormones or prohormones to hormones), derivatizations of amino acids (e.g., glycosylation, phosphorylation), and cross-linking and assembly of the polypeptide chain into its conformed structure. The diagram depicts post-translational synthesis and processing of a typical secreted polypeptide, which requires vectorial, or unidirectional, transport of the polypeptide chain across the membrane bilayer of the endoplasmic reticulum, thus resulting in sequestration of the polypeptide in the cisterna of the endoplasmic reticulum, a first step in the export process of proteins destined for secretion from the cell (see Fig. 2–6). Most translational processing occurs within the cell as depicted (presecretory), and in some instances outside the cell, during which time further proteolytic cleavages or modifications of the protein may take place (postsecretory). CHO, carbohydrate.

5. Post-translational processing and modification. The final steps in protein synthesis may involve one or more cleavages of peptide bonds, which result in the conversion of biosynthetic precursors (prohormones) to intermediate or final forms of the protein; derivatization of amino acids (e.g., glycosylation, phosphorylation, acetylation, myristoylation); and the folding of the processed polypeptide chain into its native conformation.

Each step in gene expression requires the integration of enzymatic and other biochemical reactions that provide high fidelity in the reproduction of the encoded information and provide control points for the expression of the specific cell phenotypes.

The post-translational processing of proteins enhances diversity in gene expression through the modifications of the protein. Although the functional information contained in a protein is ultimately encoded in the primary amino acid sequence, the actual biologic activities are a consequence of the higher-ordered secondary, tertiary, and quaternary structures of the polypeptide or polypeptides. Given the wide range of possible modifications of the amino acids, such as glycosylation, phosphorylation, acetylation, and sulfation,[13] any one of which may affect the conformation or function of the protein, a single gene may ultimately encode a wide variety of specific proteins as a result of post-translational processes.

Polypeptide hormones are synthesized in the form of larger precursors that convey specific properties to the peptide (Fig. 2–3), including (1) directing intracellular trafficking, by which the cell distinguishes among specific classes of proteins and directs them to specific sites within the cell; and (2) the generation of multiple biologic activities from a common genetically encoded protein by regulated or cell-specific variations in the post-translational modifications (Fig. 2–4).[14]

All the peptide hormones and regulatory peptides studied thus far contain signal (leader) sequences at the amino termini; these hydrophobic sequences recognize specific sites on the membranes of the rough endoplasmic reticulum that direct the transport of nascent polypeptides into the secretory pathway of the cell (see Figs. 2–2 and 2–3).[14] The consequence

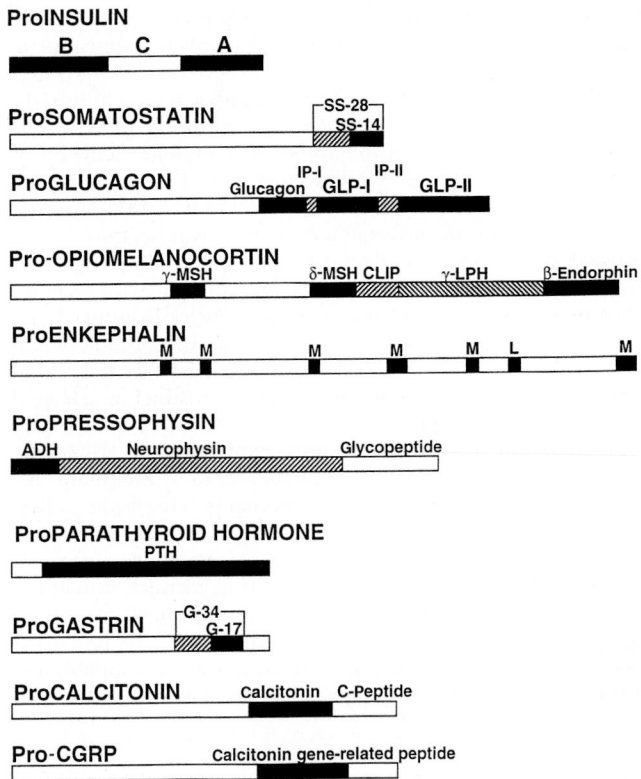

Figure 2–4. Diagrammatic illustration of primary structures of several prohormones. Darkly shaded regions of prohormones denote regions of sequence that constitute known biologically active peptides after their post-translational cleavage from prohormones. Sequences indicated by hatching denote regions of precursor that alter biologic specificity of that region of precursor. For example, the precursor contains the sequence of γ-melanocyte-stimulating hormone (γ-MSH), but when the latter is covalently attached to the clip peptide, it constitutes corticotropin (ACTH). Somatostatin-28 (SS-28) is an NH₂-terminally extended form of somatostatin-14 (SS-14) that has a higher potency than has somatostatin-14 on certain receptors. The neurophysin sequence linked to the COOH terminus of vasopressin (ADH) functions as a carrier protein for hormone during its transport down the axon of neurons in which it is synthesized. Precursor proenkephalin represents a polyprotein that contains multiple similar peptides within its sequence, either met-enkephalin (M) or leu-enkephalin (L). Procalcitonin and procalcitonin gene-related product (CGRP) share identical NH₂-terminal sequences but differ in their COOH-terminal regions as a result of alternative splicing during the post-transcriptional processing of the RNA precursor. GLP, glucagon-like peptide; IP, intervening peptide; γ-LPH, γ-lipotropin.

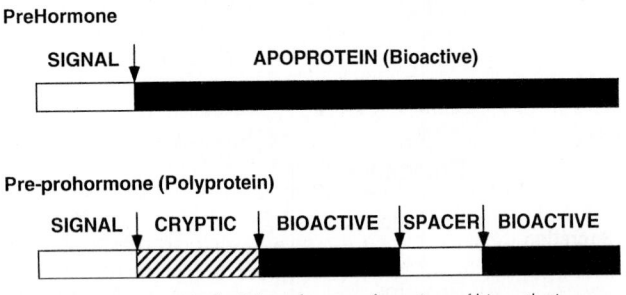

Figure 2–3. Diagrammatic depiction of two configurations of biosynthetic precursors of polypeptide hormones. Diagrams represent polypeptide backbones of protein sequences encoded in mRNA. One form of precursor consists of the NH₂-terminal signal, or presequence, followed by the apoprotein portion of the polypeptide that needs no further proteolytic processing for activity. A second form of precursor is a pre-prohormone that consists of the NH₂-terminal signal sequence followed by a polyprotein, or prohormone, sequence consisting of two or more peptide domains linked together that are subsequently liberated by cleavages during post-translational processing of the prohormone. The reason for synthesis of polypeptide hormones in the form of precursors is only partly understood. Clearly, NH₂-terminal signal sequences function in the early stages of transport of polypeptide into the secretory pathway. Prohormones, or polyproteins, often serve to provide a source of multiple bioactive peptides (see Fig. 2–4). However, many prohormones contain peptide sequences that are removed by cleavage and have no known biologic activity, and they are referred to as cryptic peptides. Other peptides may serve as spacer sequences between two bioactive peptides, e.g., the C peptide of proinsulin. In instances in which a bioactive peptide is located at the COOH terminus of the prohormone, the NH₂-terminal prohormone sequence may simply facilitate cotranslational translocation of polypeptide in endoplasmic reticulum (see Fig. 2–6).

of the specialized signal sequences of the precursor proteins is that proteins destined for secretion are selected from a great many other cellular proteins for sequestration and subsequent packaging into secretory granules and export from the cell.

Furthermore most, if not all, of the smaller hormones and regulatory peptides are produced as a consequence of post-translational cleavages of the precursors within the Golgi complex of secretory cells.

SUBCELLULAR STRUCTURE OF CELLS THAT SECRETE PROTEIN HORMONES

Secretory cells contain an abundance of endoplasmic reticulum, Golgi complexes, and secretory granules[5] (Fig. 2–5). The proteins that are to be secreted from the cells are transferred during their synthesis into the subcellular organelles that transport the proteins to the plasma membrane.

Protein secretion begins with translation of the mRNA on the rough endoplasmic reticulum, which consists of polyribosomes attached to elaborate membranous saccules that con-

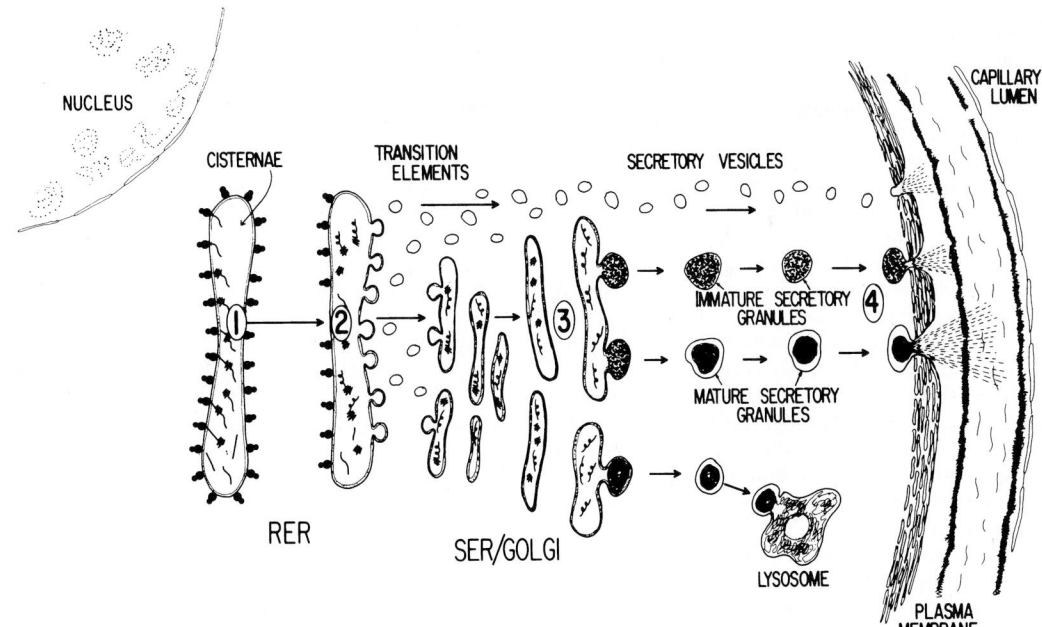

Figure 2–5. Schematic representation of subcellular organelles involved in the transport and secretion of polypeptide hormones or other secreted proteins within a protein-secreting cell. (1) Synthesis of proteins on polyribosomes attached to endoplasmic reticulum (RER), and vectorial discharge of proteins through the membrane into the cisterna. (2) Formation of shuttling vesicles (transition elements) from endoplasmic reticulum followed by their transport to and incorporation by the Golgi complex. (3) Formation of secretory granules in the Golgi complex. (4) Transport of secretory granules to the plasma membrane, fusion with the plasma membrane, and exocytosis resulting in the release of granule contents into the extracellular space. Note that secretion may occur via transport of secretory vesicles and immature granules, as well as mature granules. Some granules are taken up and hydrolyzed by lysosomes (crinophagy). RER, rough endoplasmic reticulum; SER, smooth endoplasmic reticulum; Golgi, Golgi complex. (From Habener JF. Hormone biosynthesis and secretion. In: Felig P, Baxter JD, Broadus AE, et al, eds. Endocrinology and Metabolism. New York: McGraw-Hill, 1981: 29–59. Copyright © 1981 by McGraw-Hill, Inc. Used by permission of McGraw-Hill Book Company.)

tain cavities (cisternae). The newly synthesized, nascent proteins are discharged into the cisternae by transport across the lipid bilayer of the membrane, and within the cisternae proteins are carried to the Golgi complex by mechanisms that are incompletely understood. The proteins gain access to the Golgi complex either by direct transfer from the cisternae, which are in continuity with the membranous channels of the Golgi complex, or by way of shuttling vesicles known as transition elements (see Fig. 2–5). Different secretory cells use one or the other of these two mechanisms for transport of protein from the rough endoplasmic reticulum to the Golgi complex. Within the Golgi complex the proteins are packaged into secretory vesicles or immature secretory granules. Immature granules undergo maturation through condensation of the proteinaceous material and application of a second membrane around the initial Golgi membrane. On receiving the appropriate extracellular stimuli, the granules migrate to the cell surface and fuse to become continuous with the plasma membrane, releasing the proteins into the extracellular space by exocytosis.

The second pathway of intracellular transport and secretion involves the transport of proteins contained within secretory vesicles and immature secretory granules (see Fig. 2–5). Although the use of this alternative vesicle-mediated transport pathway remains to be demonstrated conclusively (it is generally considered to be a constitutive, or unregulated, pathway), different extracellular stimuli may modulate hormone secretion differently, depending on the pathway of secretion. For example in the parathyroid gland[16] and in a pituitary cell line derived from corticotropic cells (AtT-20), newly synthesized hormone is released more rapidly than is hormone synthesized earlier. These findings suggest that the newly synthesized hormone may be transported by way of a vesicle-mediated pathway without incorporation into mature storage granules.

INTRACELLULAR SEGREGATION AND TRANSPORT OF POLYPEPTIDE HORMONES

Specific amino acid sequences encoded in the proteins serve as directional signals in the sorting of proteins within subcellular organelles.[14, 17] A typical eucaryotic cell synthesizes an estimated 5000 different proteins, using a common pool of polyribosomes.[18] However, each of the different proteins is directed to the appropriate location within the cell, where its biologic function is expressed. For example proteins can be transported into mitochondria, membranes, the nucleus, or other subcellular organelles to serve as regulatory proteins, enzymes, or structural proteins. A subset of proteins is exported from the cell, e.g., immunoglobulins, serum albumin, blood coagulation factors, and protein and polypeptide hormones. This directional transport of proteins involves informational signals that reside wholly or in part within the primary structure or in the conformational properties of the protein. Consequently post-translational modifications may alter protein function.

Signal Hypothesis

Initial clues to the processes that result in the specific transport of exported proteins into the secretory pathway (reviewed in reference 14) came from determinations of the amino acid sequences of the proteins synthesized by the cell-free translation of mRNAs encoding secreted polypeptides.[19] With the possible exception of the egg white protein ovalbumin,[20] all secretory proteins are synthesized as precursors extended at the NH_2 termini by sequences of 15 to 30 amino acids termed signal or leader sequences. When secretory polypeptides are translated in cell-free systems containing cellular membranes, the signal sequences are not present on the translated proteins, indicating that the leader sequences were cleaved in the presence of microsomal membranes.[19] These observations led to the deduction that the signal sequence is required for transport of the protein across the membrane of the endoplasmic reticulum. On emergence of the signal sequence from the large ribosomal subunit, the ribosomal complex makes contact with the membrane, resulting in translocation of the nascent polypeptide across the endoplasmic reticulum membrane into the cisterna as the first step in the transport of the polypeptide within the secretory pathway (Fig. 2–6).

Because the processing activity of intact cells can be reproduced with microsomal membranes, it was possible to extract components from the microsomal membranes and conduct cell-free translation experiments to identify the macromolecules responsible for processing of the precursor and for translocation.[21] The endoplasmic reticulum and the cytoplasm contain a signal recognition particle complex that consists of six different proteins and a 7S RNA.[21, 22] This complex binds to the polyribosomes involved in the translation of appropriate mRNAs when the NH₂-terminal signal sequence first emerges from the large subunit of the ribosome. The interaction of the signal recognition particle with the signal sequence and the polyribosome arrests further translation of mRNA. The nascent protein remains in a state of arrested translation until it binds to a high-affinity binding protein on the endoplasmic reticulum, the signal recognition particle receptor, or docking protein.[22] On interaction with the specific docking protein the translational block is released, and protein synthesis resumes.

The protein is then transferred across the membrane of the endoplasmic reticulum, presumably through a proteinaceous tunnel. At some point, near the termination of synthesis of the polypeptide chain, the NH₂-terminal signal sequence is cleaved from the polypeptide, presumably by a specific peptidase located on the cisternal surface of the endoplasmic reticulum membrane. The removal of the hydrophobic signal sequence frees the protein (prohormone) so that it may assume its characteristic secondary structure during transport through the endoplasmic reticulum and the Golgi apparatus.

This sequence in the transport of specific polypeptides ensures optimal processing of secretory proteins, even when synthesis commences on free ribosomes. The presence of a cytoplasmic form of the signal recognition particle complex that blocks translation guarantees that the synthesis of the presecretory proteins is not completed in the cytoplasm; the efficient transfer of proteins occurs only after the contact has been made with the specific receptor or docking protein on the membrane. Identification of the signal recognition particle and the docking protein does not explain the mode of translocation of the nascent polypeptide chain across the membrane bilayer. Further studies are necessary to identify the macromolecules responsible for the transport process.

Cellular Processing of Prohormones

The signal sequences of prehormones and pre-prohormones are involved in the transport of these molecules, but the function of the intermediate hormone precursors (prohormones) is not fully understood. The conversion of prohor-

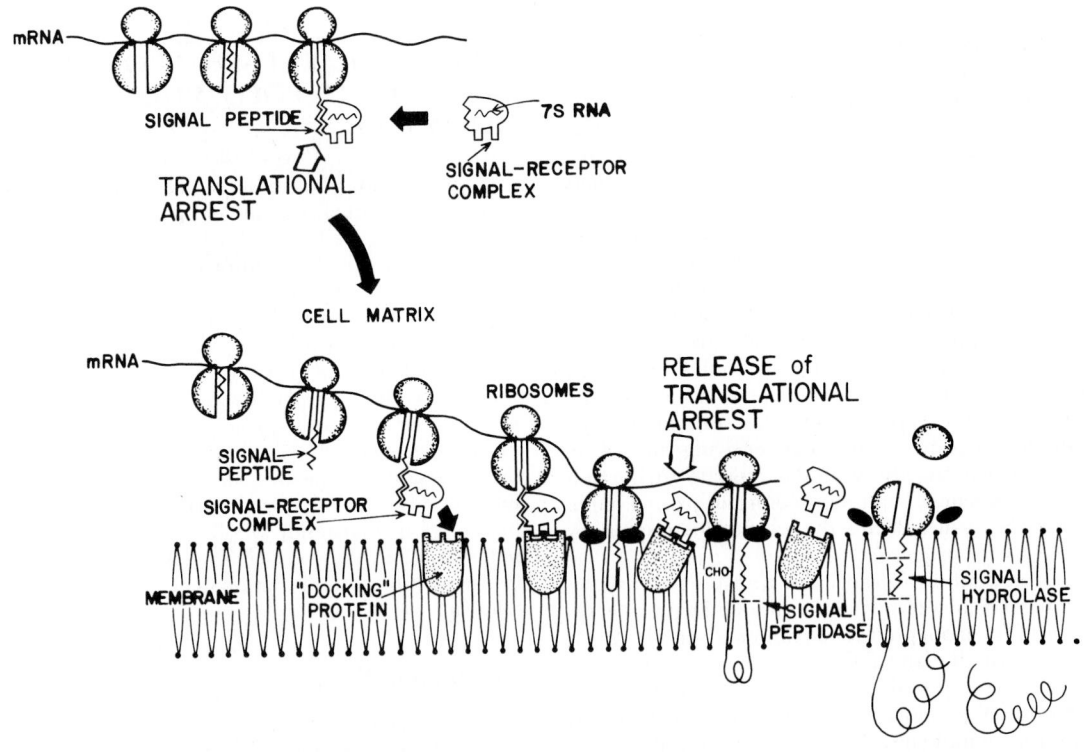

Figure 2–6. Diagram depicting cellular events in the initial stages of synthesis of a polypeptide hormone according to the signal hypothesis. In this schema a signal recognition particle, consisting of a complex of six proteins and an RNA (7S RNA), interacts with the NH₂-terminal signal peptide of the nascent polypeptide chain after approximately 70 amino acids are polymerized, which results in the arrest of further growth of the polypeptide chain. The complex of the signal recognition particle and the polyribosome nascent chain remains in a state of translational arrest until it recognizes and binds to a docking protein, which is a receptor protein located on the cytoplasmic face of the endoplasmic reticular membrane. This interaction of the signal recognition particle complex with the docking protein releases the translational block, and protein synthesis resumes. The nascent polypeptide chain is discharged across the membrane bilayer into the cisterna of the endoplasmic reticulum and is released from the signal peptide by cleavage with a signal peptidase located in the cisternal face of the membrane. In this model the signal peptide is cleaved from the polypeptide chain by signal peptidase before the chain is completed (cotranslational cleavage). The configuration of the polypeptide during transport across the membrane and the forces and mechanisms responsible for its translocation are unknown. The loop, or hairpin, configuration of the chain that is shown is an arbitrary model; other models are equally possible.

mones to their final products begins in the Golgi apparatus, and the time that elapses between the synthesis of pre-preparathyroid hormone and the first appearance of parathyroid hormone correlates closely with the time required for radioautographic grains to reach the Golgi apparatus.[23] Similarly the conversion of proinsulin to insulin takes place about an hour after the synthesis of proinsulin is completed and occurs during the transport within the secretory granule.[24] The conversion of prohormones to hormones can also be blocked by inhibitors of cellular energy production such as antimycin A and dinitrophenol[25] and by drugs that interfere with the functions of microtubules (vinblastine, colchicine).[26] Thus the translocation of the prohormone from the rough endoplasmic reticulum to the Golgi complex requires energy and probably involves microtubules.

There is no evidence that sequences specific to the prohormone per se are involved in the transport of the prohormones from the rough endoplasmic reticulum to the Golgi apparatus or that they are involved in the packaging of the hormone in the vesicles or granules. Indeed many secretory proteins (including growth hormone, prolactin, and albumin) do not have intermediate precursors (see Fig. 2–3). Size constraints may determine whether an intermediate form exists. When the bioactivity of peptides resides at the COOH termini of the precursors (e.g., somatostatin, calcitonin, and gastrin), NH$_2$-terminal extensions may be required to provide sufficient "spacer" sequence to allow the signal sequence on the growing nascent polypeptide chain to emerge from the large ribosome subunit for interaction with the signal recognition particle and to provide adequate length to span the large ribosomal subunit and the membrane of the endoplasmic reticulum during transport of the nascent polypeptide across the membrane (see Fig. 2–6). When the final hormonal product is 100 amino acids long or longer (e.g., growth hormone, prolactin, or the α and β subunits of the glycoprotein hormones), there may be no requirement for a prohormone intermediate.

Unlike the situation with prehormones, in which the amino acids at the cleavage site between the signal sequence and the remainder of the molecule (hormone or prohormone) vary from one hormone to the next, the prohormone intermediates are cleaved uniformly at sites of the basic amino acids lysine or arginine, or both, usually two to three in tandem, by endopeptidases with trypsin-like activities. The cDNA encoding a calcium-dependent serine protease involved in the processing of proinsulin to insulin was cloned from an insulinoma.[27] This prohormone-converting enzyme, designated PC1, is a member of a family of at least five such enzymes. The best studied are PC2 and PC1/3, which cleave proinsulin between the alpha chain/C peptide and beta chain/C peptide, respectively. The targeted disruption of the PC2 gene in mice causes incomplete processing of proinsulin, leaving the alpha chain and C peptide intact (D.F. Steiner, personal communication). Proglucagon in the pancreas also remains incompletely processed, indicating that PC2 is also required for the formation of glucagon.

After endopeptidase cleavage the remaining basic residues are removed by exopeptidases that resemble carboxypeptidase B. Amidation of the COOH-terminal residue of the peptide hormone appears to enhance stability by conferring resistance to carboxypeptidase, and specific amidation enzymes in the Golgi complex work in concert with the cleavage enzymes to modify the COOH terminal of the bioactive peptides.[28]

All proproteins and prohormones are probably cleaved by common enzymatic processes within the Golgi complex. The significance of a general cleavage process of prohormones remains unknown, as does the reason for the existence of prohormone intermediates in some but not all secretory proteins. As indicated earlier, precursor peptides removed from the prohormones may have unrecognized intrinsic biologic activities.

PROCESSES OF HORMONE SECRETION

Extracellular stimuli that change homeostatic balance control the secretion of polypeptide hormones, and the hormones released act on the respective target organs to reestablish homeostasis (Fig. 2–7). Endocrine systems typically consist of closed-loop feedback mechanisms such that, if hormones from organ A stimulate organ B, organ B in turn secretes hormones that inhibit the secretion of hormones from organ A (see Chapter 1). The concerted actions of both positive and negative hormonal influences thereby maintain homeostasis. For example an increase in the concentration of plasma electrolytes due to dehydration stimulates the release of vasopressin (AVP, also called antidiuretic hormone [ADH]) in the neural lobe of the pituitary, and vasopressin in turn acts on the kidney to increase the reabsorption of water from the renal tubule, thereby readjusting serum electrolyte concentrations toward normal levels. Likewise the release of parathyroid hormone in response to a fall in blood calcium level stimulates bone and kidney to promote return of calcium levels to normal, and corticotropin secretion by the anterior pituitary stimulates the adrenal cortex to secrete cortisol, which in turn feeds back to suppress further pituitary secretion of corticotropin. In some instances endocrine regulation

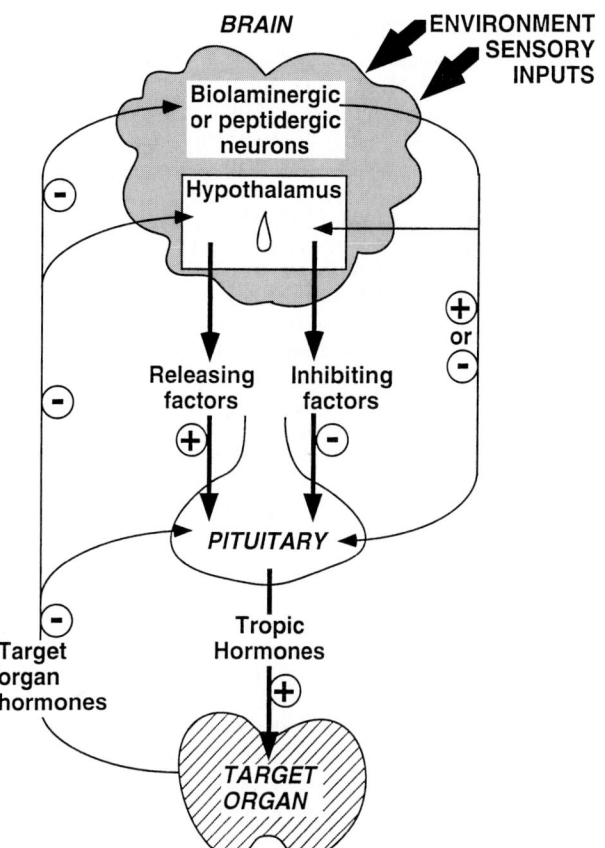

Figure 2–7. Regulatory feedback loops of the hypothalamic–pituitary–target organ axis. Being a combination of both stimulatory and inhibitory factors, hormones often act in concert to maintain homeostatic balance in the setting of physiological or pathophysiological perturbations. The concerted actions of hormones typically establish closed feedback loops by stimulatory and inhibitory effects coupled to maintain homeostasis.

involves the responses of several endocrine glands and their respective target organs. After a meal a dozen or more hormones are released as a result of gastric distention, variations in the pH of the contents of the stomach and duodenum, and increased concentrations of glucose, fatty acids, and amino acids in the blood. The rise in plasma glucose and amino acid levels stimulates the release of insulin and suppresses the release of glucagon from the pancreas. Both effects promote the net uptake of glucose by the liver; insulin increases cellular transport and uptake of glucose, and the lower blood levels of glucagon decrease the outflow of glucose because of diminished rates of glycogenolysis and gluconeogenesis.

STRUCTURE OF A GENE ENCODING A POLYPEPTIDE HORMONE

At least three features of gene structure are important to understanding the expression of peptide-encoding genes. First sequences of all the known biologic peptides are contained within larger precursors that often encode for additional peptides, many of which have unknown biologic activity. Second the coding regions of genes (exons) are interrupted by sequences (introns) that are transcribed but subsequently cleaved from the initial RNA transcripts during nuclear processing and assembly into specific mRNAs. Third specific regulatory sequences in the regions of DNA flanking the 5' ends of structural genes constitute targets for the interactions of DNA-binding proteins that regulate the expression of the gene.

The DNA of higher organisms is wound into a tightly packed chromosomal structure in association with proteins organized into elements called nucleosomes.[29] Nucleosomes contain four or five different histone subunits that form a core structure about which approximately 140 base pairs of genomic DNA are wound. The nucleosomes are arranged as beads on a string, and coils of nucleosomes form the fundamental organizational units of the chromosome. Nucleosomes serve several purposes. They enable a large amount of DNA (approximately 2×10^9 pairs) of the genome to be compacted into a small volume, and they may be involved in the replication of DNA and gene transcription. In addition to histones other proteins are associated with DNA, and the structure may provide specific recognition sites for regulatory proteins and enzymes involved in DNA replication, rearrangements of DNA segments, and gene expression.

The topography of a typical protein-encoding gene consists of two functional units: (1) a transcriptional region and (2) a promoter or regulatory region (Fig. 2–8).

Transcriptional Regions

The transcriptional unit is the segment of gene that is transcribed into a mRNA precursor. Note that the nucleotide thymidine (T) in DNA is transcribed as uridine (U) in RNA. The coding sequence of the gene consists of the exon sequences that are spliced from the primary transcript during the post-transcriptional processing of the precursor RNA; these exons contain the code for the mRNA sequence that is translated into protein and for untranslated sequences at the 5'- and 3'-flanking regions. The 5' sequence begins typically with a methylated guanine residue known as the cap site. The 3'-untranslated region contains within it a short sequence, AATAAA, that signals the site of cleavage of the 3' end of the RNA and the addition of a poly(A) tract of 100 to 200 nucleotides beginning approximately 20 bases from the AATAAA sequence. Although the functions of these modifications of

the ends of mRNAs are not completely understood, they appear to enhance stability, perhaps by providing resistance to degradation by exonucleases.

Likewise the enzymatic splicing mechanisms that excise intron sequences and rejoin exon sequences are incompletely understood. Short "consensus" sequences of nucleotides reside at the splice junctions, e.g., the bases GT and AG at the 5' and 3' ends of the introns, respectively, are highly conserved. Additional loosely conserved nucleotides flank these dinucleotides.[30] A population of small nuclear RNAs, known as the U1 RNAs, contain short nucleotide sequences that are complementary to the splice junctions. These small RNAs may serve as templates that base-pair with the splice junctions and provide secondary structure for specific endonucleolytic cleavages.[31] The RNAs exist as a complex with distinct proteins that harbor endonuclease and ligase activities and form small nuclear ribosomal particles (snRNPs). Designated aggregates of different snRNPs form spliceosomes. Spliceosomes recognize and bind to GT/AG nucleotide sequence motifs at the exon-intron boundaries and to special sequence motifs in the adjoining intron, resulting in the formation of a lariat-like loop of the intronic sequence. The spliceosome then cleaves out the intronic sequence and ligates (joins) the exons together to produce the functional mRNA. Alternative exon splicing of pre-mRNAs is an important step in the developmental and metabolic regulation of expression of these genes (discussed further later).

The protein-coding sequence of the mRNA begins with the codon AUG for methionine and ends with the codon immediately preceding one of the three nonsense, or stop, codons (UGA, UAA, and UAG).

Exon Recognition in RNA Splicing

High precision and accuracy in the splicing out of introns and the knitting together of exons is essential for normal function. A single base error, if it occurred, would alter the reading frame of the mRNA that encodes the protein and cause the synthesis of an aberrant protein product. In addition the splicing apparatus must recognize small exons embedded in a sea of intronic sequences. The average size of exons in primates is 120 to 130 nucleotides, usually ranging from approximately 50 to 300, although exons as small as 3 to 7 nucleotides can occur.[32] In contrast, introns are typically several kilobases in length and can be up to 100 kilobases.

One mechanism for explaining the accuracy of splicing is known as "exon definition."[32] This model proposes that the splicing machinery searches or scans the pre-mRNA for two closely spaced splice sites in an exonic polarity. When the pair of splice sites is encountered, the exon is defined by the binding of U1 and U2 type snRNPs and associated splicing factors that make up the spliceosome. Once the exon is thereby defined, the spliceosome apparatus juxtaposes the two exons, cleaves out the intron, and joins the exons together. The critical importance of the splicing of pre-mRNAs in the context of alternative exon splicing is discussed later in this chapter.

Regulatory Regions

The regulatory sequences in the 5' sequences upstream from structural genes are termed promoters and enhancers (see Fig. 2–8). These sequences can be divided into at least four groups with respect to their functions and distances from the transcriptional initiation site. The sequence TATAA (TATA, or Goldberg-Hogness box) is present within 25 to 30 nucleotides upstream from the point of transcriptional initiation. The integrity of the TATA sequence is required for ensuring the accuracy of initiation of transcription at a particu-

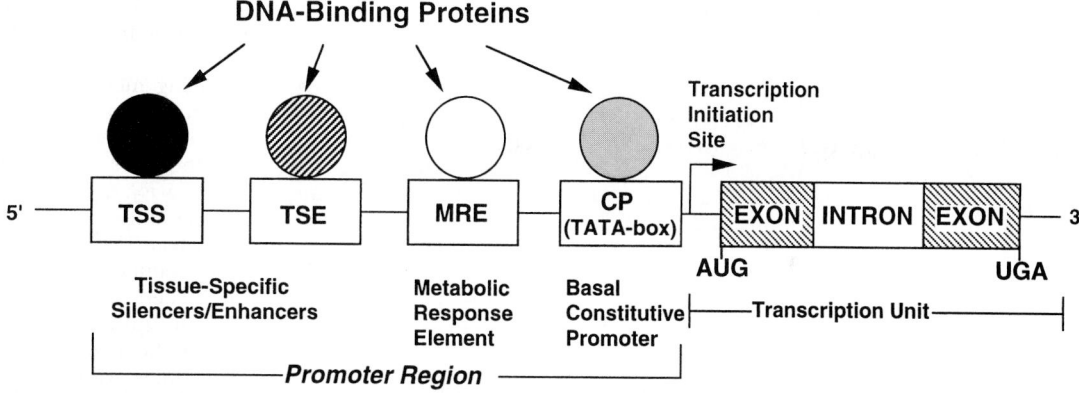

Figure 2–8. Diagrammatic structure of a "consensus" gene encoding a prototypical polypeptide hormone. Such a gene typically consists of a promoter region and a transcription unit. The transcription unit is the region of DNA composed of exons and introns that is transcribed into a mRNA precursor. Transcription begins at the cap site sequence in DNA and extends several hundred bases beyond the poly(A) addition site in the 3' region. During post-transcriptional processing of the RNA precursor, the 5' end of mRNA is capped by addition of methylguanosine residues. The transcript is then cleaved at the poly(A) addition site approximately 20 bases 3' to the AATAAA signal sequence, and the poly(A) tract is added to the 3' end of the RNA. Introns are cleaved from the RNA precursor, and exons are joined together. Dinucleotides GT and AG are invariably found at the 5' and 3' ends of introns. Translation of mRNA invariably starts with the codon ATG for methionine. Translation is terminated when the polyribosome reaches the stop codons TGA, TAA, or TAG. The promoter region of the gene located 5' to the cap site contains numerous short regulatory DNA sequences that are targets for interactions with specific DNA-binding proteins. These sequences consist of the basal constitutive promoter (TATA box), metabolic response elements that modulate transcription, e.g., in response to cAMP, steroid hormone receptors, and thyroid hormone receptors, as well as tissue-specific enhancers and silencers that permit or prevent transcription of the gene, respectively. The enhancer and silencer elements direct expression of specific subsets of genes to cells of a given phenotype. Whether a gene will or will not be expressed in a particular cellular phenotype depends on complex interactions of the various DNA-binding proteins among themselves and, most important, with the TATA box proteins of the basal constitutive promoter.

lar site. The TATA box binds a complex of several proteins, including RNA polymerase II. The proteins, referred to as TATA box transcription factors (TFs), number six or more basal factors (IIA, IIB, IID, IIE, IIF, IIH) and, along with RNA polymerase II, form the general or basal transcriptional machinery required for the initiation of RNA synthesis.[33, 34]

These factors contain multiple subunits and are essential for transcription to occur. However, a key factor is TFIID, which consists of the TATA-binding protein (TBP) and at least 12 associated proteins known as TBP-associated factors (TAFs), designated by their apparent molecular weights.[33, 34] TBP binds directly to the TATA box sequence, straddling the sequence like a saddle, and causing an acute bend in the DNA.[35] The TAFs associate on the surface of TBP along with the other TFII factors. TFIIA and TFIIB associate with the stirrups of the TBP saddle. The binding of TBP alone to the TATA box supports basal transcription, and the regulation of the rates of transcription (up or down) requires the presence of TAFs. The TAFs serve as coactivators or co-repressors for enhancer or silencer-binding proteins, activators or repressors, respectively. The example shown (Fig. 2–9) depicts the cAMP response element–binding protein (CREB) bound to the cAMP-response element (CRE).[36] On phosphorylation by cAMP-dependent protein kinase A, phosphoCREB recruits the co-activator CREB-binding protein (CBP). CBP "couples" with the TBP-associated factors, resulting in a marked enhancement of rates of gene transcription.

Several of the TAFs have strong homologies in tertiary structures with histones. For example, TAF40 and TAF60 resemble histones H4 and H3, respectively.[37] These findings suggest that the TFIID complex of TBP and the various TAFs constitutes an elaborate nucleosome in which the composition of subunits depends on the makeup of a specific promoter. That is, promoters of individual genes contain multiple enhancers (and silencers) that bind specific activators or repressors, respectively, which in turn recruit specific coactivators that, in the appropriate combination, generate either productive or nonproductive transcriptional complexes with the basal transcriptional machinery. Such a model implies that the TAFs and other components of the basal machinery may be rate-limiting within a given cell, resulting in a "competition" of various gene promoters for these factors. In such a situation,

genes whose promoters are in a favorable context to recruit coactivators efficiently are transcribed more efficiently than other genes with less favorable promoter contexts.

A series of sequences upstream from the TATA sequence that serve as amplifiers of the transcriptional response include CCAAT or CCGCCC, which bind the transcription factors CTF or SV40 protein 1 (SP-1), respectively. Located farther upstream are sequences that function either as tissue- or cell-specific enhancers or suppressors and/or as metabolic response elements. The tissue-specific elements confer latent transcriptional inducibility to a gene but require stimulation by a metabolic response element or elements. The metabolic response elements are the key sequences involved in the up- or down-regulation of transcription and are targets for the binding of "fourth messengers," DNA-binding proteins whose binding and transcriptional *trans*-activation activities are regulated by second messengers such as cAMP-dependent protein kinase, diacylglycerol-dependent protein kinase C, calcium/calmodulin-dependent protein kinase, and steroid hormone- or thyroid hormone–bound receptors (see later section on coupling of effector action to cellular responses). Specific sequence elements have been identified that bind cAMP-regulated proteins such as the CREB, and the proteins JUN and FOS bind to the tetradecanoyl phorbol acetate response element.[36, 38] Similarly, elements have been identified that bind receptors for the steroid and thyroid hormones and for retinoic acid. The cell-specific enhancer and metabolic response functions often are co-localized within the same short DNA sequence or element. Combinations of elements with their cognate DNA-binding proteins usually work in synergy to generate a large transcriptionally productive complex involving interactions with the TATA box factors of the basal promoter (see Fig. 2–9). The identification of regulatory DNA elements and the cloning of the genes that encode DNA-binding proteins will lead to a better understanding of gene control mechanisms.

Introns and Exons

Genes encoding proteins and ribosomal RNAs in eucaryotes are interrupted by intervening DNA sequences (introns) that separate them into coding blocks (exons).[39] In bacterial

Basal transcriptional complex

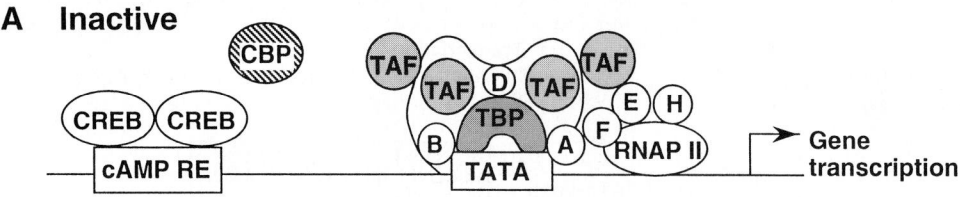

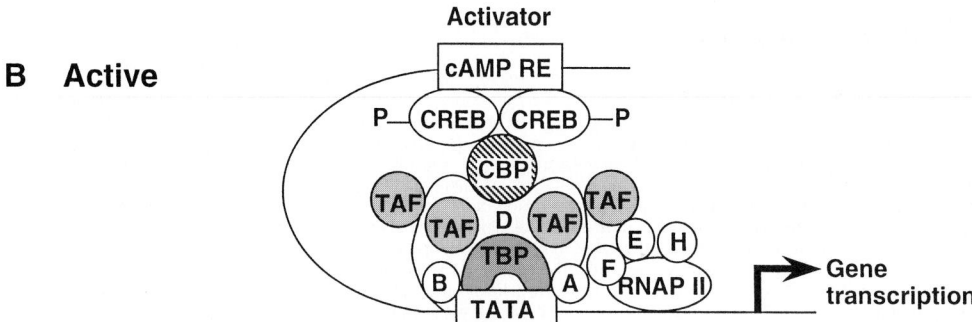

Figure 2–9. Diagrammatic depiction of the basal transcriptional proteins of the constitutive promoter (TATA box). *A*, In the absence of protein binding to enhancer or metabolic response, e.g., the cAMP response element (CRE), the basal rate of transcription mediated by the TATA box factors TFIIA to F and RNA polymerase II (RNAP II) is low. TBP is the TATA box–binding protein subunit of TFIID, which consists of a complex of TBP with several TBP-associated proteins (TAFs). *B*, When specific proteins such as cAMP response element–binding proteins (CREBs) bind to the cAMP response element (cAMP-RE), the basal transcription complex is activated, which initiates the synthesis of mRNA. One mechanism proposed is that the DNA segment containing the activator protein bound to the enhancer (CREB bound to the cAMP-RE) loops around, recruits a specific coactivator such as CREB-binding protein (CBP) and couples productively to the basal transcriptional complex. (Adapted from O'Malley BW. The steroid receptor superfamily: more excitement predicted for the future. Mol Endocrinol 1990; 4:363–369. © The Endocrine Society.)

genes, in contrast, the nucleotide sequences of the chromosomal genes match the corresponding sequences in the mRNAs. Interruption of the continuity of genetic information appears to be unique to nucleated cells. The reasons for such interruption are not completely understood, but introns appear to separate exons into functional domains with respect to the proteins that they encode. An example is the gene for proglucagon, the precursor of glucagon, in which five introns separate six exons, three of which encode glucagon and the two glucagon-related peptides contained within the precursor (Fig. 2–10).[40] A second example is the growth hormone gene, which is divided into five exons by four introns that separate the promoter region of the gene from the protein-coding region and divide the latter into three segments, two coding for the growth-promoting activity of the hormone and the third for its metabolic functions.[41] As a general rule the genes for the precursors of hormones and regulatory peptides contain introns at or about the region where the signal peptides

join the apoproteins or prohormones, thus separating the signal sequences from the components that function as hormones or peptides.

The finding that the transcripts of genes consist of a mosaic of introns and exons explains two aspects of the genetic structure. Intron-coded sequences in transcripts account for a large part of the heterogeneous nuclear RNA in eucaryotic cells. Introns also explain the extra DNA that is present in the genomes of higher cells, the "selfish DNA" that is replicated but has no recognized function. Only 5 to 10% of eucaryotic DNA provides coding sequences for proteins and RNAs. Another 10 to 15%, about which little is known, appears to contain highly reiterated sequences, called repetitive DNA, scattered throughout the genome. Thus approximately 70 to 80% of DNA sequences are without known function. On average the intron sequences contain about 10 times the amount of DNA that is present in the exons.

Several functions have been proposed for this organiza-

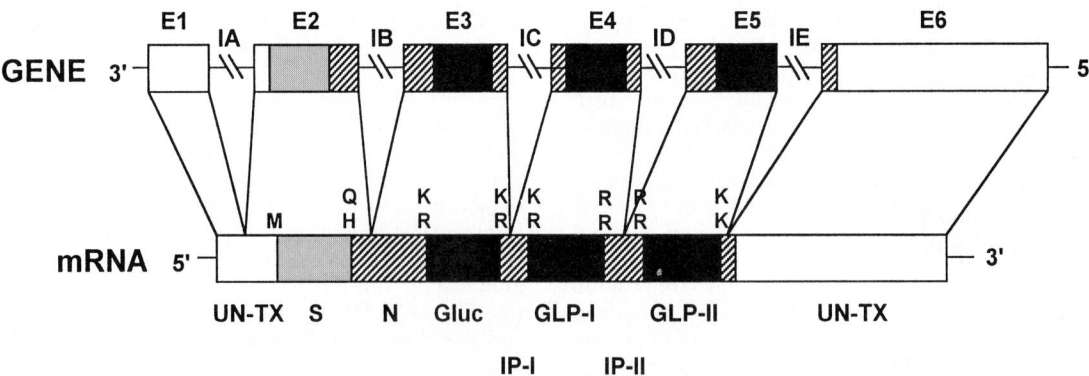

Figure 2–10. Diagram of the pancreatic glucagon gene and its encoded mRNA (cDNA). The glucagon gene is an example of a gene in which exons precisely encode separate functional domains. The gene consists of six exons (E1–E6) and five introns (1A–1E). mRNA encoding pre-proglucagon, the protein precursor of glucagon, consists of 10 specific regions: from left to right, a 5′-untranslated sequence (UN-TX, unshaded); a signal sequence (S, stippled); an NH₂-terminal extension sequence (N, hatched); glucagon (GLUC, shaded); a first intervening peptide (IP-I, hatched); a first glucagon-like peptide (GLP-I, shaded); a second intervening peptide (IP-II, hatched); a second glucagon-like peptide (GLP-II, shaded); a dilysyl dipeptide (hatched) after the GLP-II sequence; and an untranslated region (UN-TX, unshaded). Exons from left to right encode the 5′-untranslated region; signal sequence; glucagon; GLP-I; GLP-II; and 3′-untranslated sequence. Letters shown above the mRNA denote amino acids located at positions in pre-proglucagon that are cleaved during cellular processing of precursor. Q, glutamine; H, histidine; K, lysine; R, arginine. M denotes the amino acid methionine, which marks the initiation of translation of mRNA into pre-proglucagon.

tion.[39, 42] Topographic separations of exons encoding specific functions may reflect the evolutionary processes of genetic recombination. The result of such recombination is the bringing together, within a single gene, of multiple functional components that are widely distributed within the genome and the eventual creation of chimeric proteins with new functions. The existence of specific functional coding blocks of DNA separated by noncoding DNA sequences allows recombination to take place anywhere within the intron DNA without interruption of the reading frames of the exons, because the intron RNA is eventually excised.

Introns may have additional roles. Not only can specific recombinations between introns bring exons together into new transcriptional units to make special differentiated products, but also the utilization of new splicing patterns could create new gene products. For example differentiation could be influenced by the appearance of a new splicing enzyme that utilizes existing intron sequences to make new exons, thereby providing additional coding information for new proteins. Introns may also serve as a repository for DNA sequences that serve as control, or regulatory, sequences. In fact a glucocorticoid response element that regulates expression of the rat growth hormone gene resides within the second intron of that gene. Clearly the genome is in a dynamic state of rearrangement.

Transposable DNA elements (transposons) are present in higher organisms as well as plants.[43] Genetic rearrangement occurs by recombination and by transposition of sequences via extrachromosomal mechanisms.[44] For example pseudogenes, which are derived from the transcripts of expressed genes, are located throughout the genome.[45] These pseudogenes, although not functionally expressed, are believed to be derived from reverse transcription of RNA transcripts into DNA with reinsertion of the DNA back into the genome. Such a mechanism could provide a means of amplifying specific functional DNA sequences such as protein-encoding and protein-regulatory segments.

The functions of introns in the evolutionary process may explain their absence in procaryotes. It is tempting to speculate that procaryotes represent an end product in the evolutionary process. At one time the genomes of microorganisms may have contained introns, but as the organisms became highly differentiated the genomes reached an end point in evolution, becoming "frozen" after they had arranged themselves to provide the highest benefit to the organism. Subsequently the introns were simply lost because they afforded no further benefit. Similar reasoning may explain the low frequency of introns in yeasts, which are highly differentiated eucaryotes. To obtain additional genetic information, bacteria and yeasts would have to rely on the acquisition of extra chromosomal DNA sequences in the form of viruses or plasmids. This hypothetical argument may explain the occasional exceptions to the "one exon, one function" rule in mammalian cells. The genes that encode some peptide hormones are not interrupted by introns in a manner that corresponds to the separation of the functional components of the precursor. Notable in this regard is the precursor pro-opiomelanocortin, from which the peptides corticotropin, α-MSH, and β-endorphin are cleaved during the post-translational processing of the precursor. The protein-coding region of the pro-opiomelanocortin gene is devoid of introns. Likewise no introns interrupt the protein-coding region of the gene for the proenkephalin precursor, which contains seven copies of the enkephalin sequences. It is possible that in the past introns separated each of these coding domains and were lost during the course of evolution. A precedent for the selective loss of introns appears to be exemplified by the rat insulin genes. The rat genome harbors two nonallelic insulin genes: one contains two introns, and the other a single intron. The most likely explanation is that an ancestral gene containing two introns was duplicated, and one of the introns was eliminated sometime thereafter.

In summary the role of introns in evolution and in the control of gene expression remains to be fully determined. Understanding the regulation of intron and exon splicing during development will provide insight into the evolution and functions of genes.

REGULATION OF GENE EXPRESSION

The regulation of expression of genes encoding polypeptide hormones can take place at one or more levels (Fig. 2–11):[46, 47] (1) DNA synthesis (cell growth and division), (2) RNA transcription, (3) post-transcriptional processing of mRNA, (4) translation, and (5) post-translational processing. In different endocrine cells regulation of production of a hormone can occur at different levels (see also later section on generation of biologic diversification).

Levels of Gene Control

Newly synthesized prolactin transcripts are formed within minutes after exposure of a prolactin-secreting cell line to TRH,[48] whereas cortisol stimulates growth hormone synthesis over a period of 1 to 2 h in both somatotropic cell lines and pituitary slices by increasing the rates of gene transcription and by enhancement of the stability of mRNA.[49, 50] In contrast, regulation of proinsulin biosynthesis takes place primarily at the level of translation;[51, 52] within minutes after raising the plasma glucose level, the rate of proinsulin biosynthesis increases 5- to 10-fold as the result of enhancement of the initiation of translation of proinsulin mRNA. Rapid metabolic regulation at the level of post-transcriptional processing of mRNA precursors is not clearly established, but alternative exon-splicing plays a major role in mRNA formation during development (see section on generation of biologic diversification). For example the primary RNA transcripts derived from the calcitonin gene are alternatively spliced to provide two or more tissue-specific mRNAs that encode chimeric protein precursors with both common and different amino acid sequences, suggesting that the processing of the calcitonin gene transcripts may be regulated. The regulation of the biosynthesis of parathyroid hormone by calcium takes place principally at the levels of DNA synthesis and cell division. Stimulation of the parathyroid gland by lowering calcium levels appears to have little effect on the rates of RNA synthesis but leads to hyperplasia of the gland.[53] In addition hypocalcemia causes a decrease in intracellular turnover of parathyroid hormone.

In many instances the regulation of gene expression fulfills the secretory and biosynthetic needs of the endocrine organ. For example after a meal there is an immediate requirement for insulin release. Because this release depletes insulin stores in the pancreatic beta cells within a few minutes, increased translational efficiency of preformed proinsulin mRNA rapidly provides additional hormone. In contrast the release of parathyroid hormone remains almost constant at all times, and small fluctuations in the secretion rate are adequate to maintain the levels of serum ionized calcium within a narrow range, under physiological conditions. However, prolonged hypocalcemia, as in chronic renal failure, results in marked hyperplasia; low levels of ionized calcium can thus be considered a "growth factor" for the parathyroid glands.[53]

Despite tissue-specific differences in the processing of prohormones, alterations in the rates of conversion of a prohormone to a hormone under physiological circumstances have not been identified as a point of cellular control. Gluco-

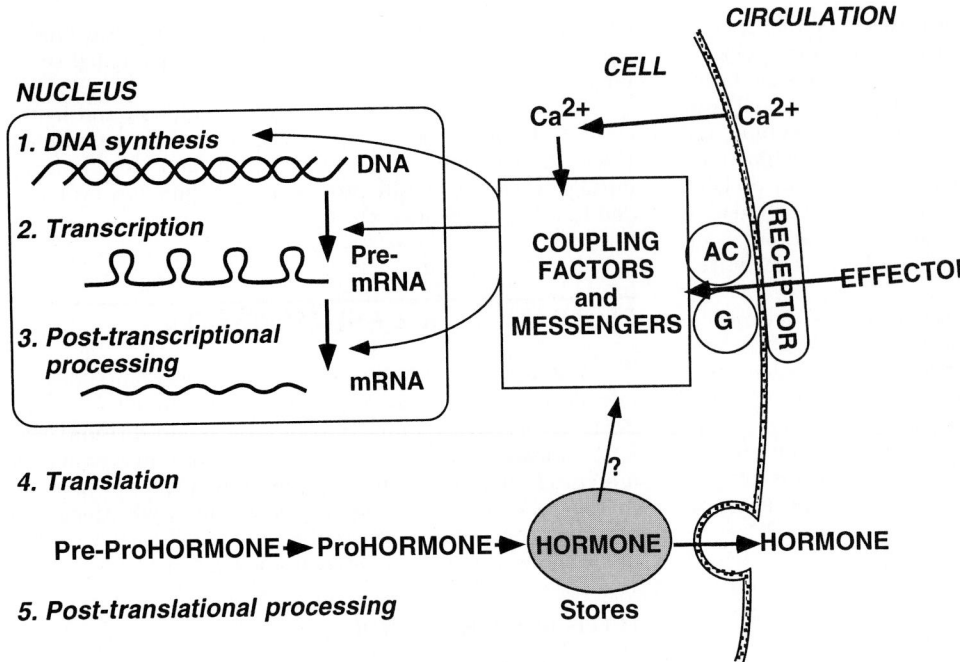

Figure 2–11. Diagram of an endocrine cell showing potential control points for regulation of gene expression in hormone production. Specific effector substances bind either to plasma membrane receptors (peptide effectors) or to cytosolic or nuclear receptors (steroids), which leads to the initiation of a series of events that couple the effector signal with gene expression. In the illustration shown, peptide effector-receptor complex interactions act initially via activation of adenylate cyclase (AC) coupled with a GTP-binding protein. Coupling factors and substances such as glucose, cAMP, and cations activate protein kinases (PK), resulting in a series of phosphorylations of macromolecules. As discussed in the text, specific effectors for various endocrine cells appear to act at one or more of the indicated five levels of gene expression, with the possible exception of post-translational processing of prohormones, for which no definite examples of metabolic regulation have yet been found.

corticoids, however, appear to regulate the post-translational processing and compartmentalization of murine mammary tumor virus protein in hepatic carcinoma cells.[54] At least two post-translational processes in production of viral proteins are regulated by glucocorticoids, one controlling glycoprotein processing by modification of carbohydrate residues and the other involved in phosphorylation of the proteins.[54] Thus glucocorticoids control both the transcription of the mammary tumor virus gene and the processing of the mammary tumor virus proteins.

Coupling of Hormone Secretion to Gene Regulation

The biosynthetic processes must be coupled in some manner with the secretory processes of endocrine cells. Synthesis of new hormone is required to replace that which is released, and, conversely, synthesis of new hormone must also decrease to prevent overloading of the cell with hormone when secretory demands decrease. Little is known about the cellular mechanisms that link secretory events to biosynthetic events, i.e., whether the extracellular stimulatory factors that regulate rates of secretion also directly affect rates of hormone biosynthesis, or whether the process of secretion somehow provides regulatory signals that are transmitted to the steps in biosynthesis. As indicated earlier, the coupling of secretory and biosynthetic activities in a particular endocrine gland may depend to a large degree on the amount of hormone that is stored. A gland with large stores of hormone can meet secretory demands for a longer time than a gland with a smaller store. Most endocrine cells store hormone to some extent, as evidenced by the presence of secretory granules. Such a storage system has probably evolved to provide a reservoir of hormone to meet secretory demands over a very short time.

Cis and Trans Mechanisms of Gene Regulation

Certain genes or sets of genes are expressed only in specific tissues. Two mechanisms have been proposed for differential gene expression: *cis* and *trans* mechanisms (Fig. 2–

12). In the simpler *cis* mechanism, a specific signaling factor interacts with a sensor-receptor region of the gene to activate transcription of the structural gene. The *cis* mechanism is assumed to work by causing structural or conformational change in the chromatin.

The *trans* mechanism requires that the presence of a diffusible intermediary product of a regulatory gene activates transcription of a second gene. In this model the intracellular signal interacts with the sensor region of a regulatory gene, resulting in the transcription of an RNA from an associated integrator gene (acting in *cis*). The RNA either serves as a template encoding a protein that in turn interacts with the activator receptor responsible for initiating transcription of the producer gene or serves directly as an activator RNA. As discussed earlier, many integrator genes encode DNA-binding proteins, which in turn interact with DNA control elements of genes. The *cis* and *trans* models are depicted in Figure 2–12. The concept that repetitive *cis* recognition sequences might provide the structural basis for the coordinate induction of unlinked structural genes arose from the observation that some DNA sequences exist in multiple copies in the eucaryotic genome.[55, 56] For example the so-called Alu sequences, which consist of homologous segments of approximately 300 bases, are present in 300,000 to 500,000 copies scattered throughout the human genome,[57] and many or all repeated sequences have or had the capacity to transpose during evolution.[58] One mechanism for the evolution of new gene products is the diffusion of transposable *cis* regulatory sequences within the genome.[39, 59, 60] One can envision that transposable DNA sequence elements could occasionally carry with them and deposit specific control sequences in the right genomic environment, which would result in the expression of specific gene functions.

Although the functions for the Alu sequences are not known, the DNA-binding proteins that regulate the expression of genes are themselves encoded by superfamilies of sequence-related genes. So in essence, the hypothesis set forth by Britten and Davidson has proved to be correct: the genes encoding the DNA-binding proteins are the integrator genes, and the genes encoding other cellular proteins are the producer genes. The sensor and the activator receptors are similar; they respond alike to the interactions of DNA-binding proteins. This circumstance raises interesting questions regarding how

A   Cis

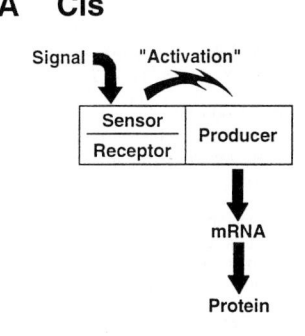

B   Trans

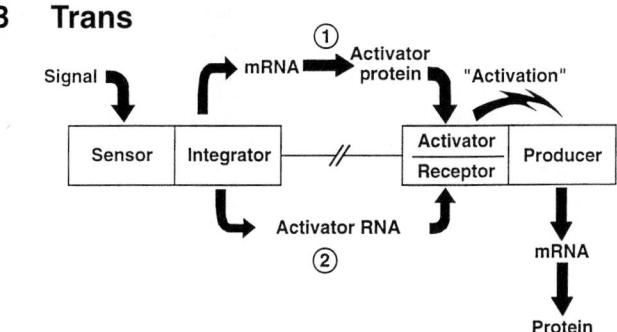

Figure 2–12. Historical depiction of *cis* (A) and *trans* (B) models for activation of gene expression. In both models the specific intracellular signal interacts with a sensor-receptor on the gene. In the *cis* model, the sensor-receptor (activator) is adjacent to the producer gene, which is the transcriptional unit, leading to production of mRNA and protein. In the *trans* model, the sensor is separated from the activator-receptor, which is adjacent to the producer gene, and the activator substance, originating from the sensor, acts in *trans* by transport to the activator receptor. This activator substance may be either an RNA molecule or a protein activator translated from RNA. Activator binds or otherwise interacts with an activator-receptor sequence on the gene, which results in initiation of transcription. Experimental evidence has now established that activation of most, if not all, genes involves *trans*-acting regulatory activators, DNA-binding proteins referred to as transcription factors.

so many genes all can be regulated by DNA-binding proteins, whose genes in turn are regulated by binding proteins, and so on. If there were an open-ended cascade of unique DNA-binding protein genes, the DNA sequences required to encode the proteins would predictably exceed the amount of functional DNA in the genome. The situation poses an apparent dilemma akin to that faced by immunologists a number of years ago in attempting to understand how the repertoire of some 10^6 different antibody proteins (preimmune repertoire) could be expressed when the total number of unique expressed genes in animal cells was estimated to be less than 10^5. The generation of antibody diversity turned out to depend on somatic recombination and mutation, i.e., gene rearrangement and point mutations followed by clonal selection of antibody-producing lymphocytes in response to a challenge by a specific antigen. The generation of diversity in the regulation of gene expression by DNA-binding proteins likewise almost certainly involves a combinatorial process. As envisioned this process is not gene rearrangement but involves the formation of unique proteins at the various levels of gene expression (multiple-related genes, alternative patterns of RNA splicing, post-translational modifications) (see later under section on generation of biologic diversification), limited but distinct permissiveness in the formation of active protein dimers, and assembly of unique combinations of multiple protein-DNA interactions.

Autoregulation of Genes Encoding Transcription Factors

The promoters of genes encoding transcription factors appear to be autoregulated by their own encoded proteins.

Such autoregulation is necessitated by the economy placed on the size of the genome. If transcription factor genes all required unique transcription factors for their expression, the number of genes coding transcription factors alone would be endless. Examples of positive autoregulation include CREB,[61] JUN,[62] and Pit-1,[63] which up-regulate their respective genes. Negative autoregulation is observed with the cAMP response element modulator (CREM) inducible cAMP early response (ICER) repressor, which down-regulates its own promoter.[64]

Autoregulation combined with the interactions (both positive and negative) of the 2000 or so distinct existent transcription factors may account for the complex orchestration of gene expression.

Repression of Transcription

Repression of transcription is a critical process so as to restrict expression to only a subset of genes in any given cell phenotype and to prevent expression in an incorrect cell type even though the activators are present in the cell (reviewed in reference 65). Of the approximately 100,000 different genes expressed in the human genome, only 5000 or so are ever expressed in a given cell type. Thus, 95% of genes that are capable of expression are maintained in a transcriptionally silent state (Fig. 2–13). One mechanism of repression is that of competition between an activator and a weak activator for

Competition
(Repressor lacking trans-activation domain (TAD) competes with activator for binding to a tissue-specific enhancer site)

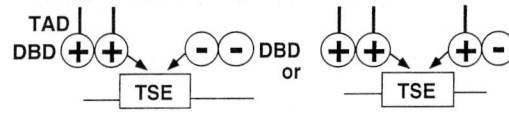

Sequestration
(Repressor prevents activator from binding to DNA)

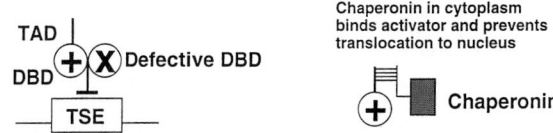

Quenching / tethering
(Repressor interferes with the activity of DNA-bound activator)

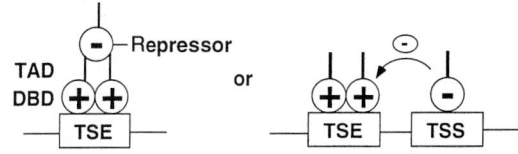

Active
(Direct interactive interference with the basal transcriptional machinery)

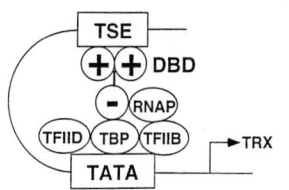

Figure 2–13. Mechanisms of transcriptional repression. It is generally considered that at least four mechanisms of transcriptional repression exist: competition, sequestration, quenching or tethering, and active. Examples of these mechanisms are given in the text. Transcriptional activators are designated by the (+) and repressors by the (−). The transcription factors are presumed to bind to DNA as dimers in the illustrations. TAD and DBD designate *trans*-activation and DNA-binding domains of the transcription factors, respectively. TSE and TSS indicate tissue-specific enhancers or silencers, respectively.

binding to a common DNA element. For proteins that bind to DNA as dimers, such as the basic region–leucine zipper (bZIP) proteins, a heterodimer between a strong and a weak activator may dampen transcription. Examples of competition repression are represented by the truncated repressor isoforms of the bZIP activators CREB, CREM, CCAAT/enhancer binding protein (C/EBPα), and C/EBPβ.

Another mechanism of repression involves sequestration in which the repressor binds to the activator and prevents it from binding to DNA or prevents translocation from the cytoplasm to the nucleus.[65] Id, the dominant negative regulators of the activator MyoD in muscle development and C/EBP homologous protein (CHOP) CHOP/GADD-153, the negative regulator of C/EBP activators, are examples of repressors that have defective DNA-binding domains, dimerize with activators, and prevent the heterodimer from binding to DNA.[66] Examples of repression by sequestration of activators in the cytoplasm are NFκB, sterol response element binding protein (SREBP), nuclear factor activating transcription (NFAT), and the glucocorticoid receptor (GR). These activators are bound to cytoplasmic chaperonin proteins that serve as anchors. When the cell receives the appropriate signals such as the activation of a protein kinase, phosphatase, or protease, the activator is released from the chaperonin or anchor. For example, phosphorylation of IkB, the chaperonin inhibitor of NFκB, releases NFκB from IkB and allows it to be translocated to the nucleus. Dephosphorylation of NFAT by the phosphatase calcineurin releases it for nuclear translocation. The SREBP is released from its anchorage in the cytoplasm by proteolytic cleavages. The unoccupied GR is bound to the cytoplasmic heat shock protein 90 and is released by binding of glucocorticoids to GR.

A third form of repression is quenching or tethering.[65] The repressor binds to the activator, thereby masking its *trans*-activational capabilities. The repressor may or may not contact the DNA adjacent to the activator binding site. The mechanism of inhibition is believed to be one of interference with the ability of the activator to couple to coactivators such as one or more of the TAFs discussed earlier. An example of quenching is that of interaction of GR with members of the bZIP FOS and JUN family of transcription factors that constitute the AP-1 complex. On so-called "simple" DNA elements, GR is an activator of transcription, on so-called composite elements such as those that exist in the promoter of the proliferin gene, GR acts as a repressor of transcription by either binding next to the AP-1 factors or tethering to AP-1 factors bound to the composite element and thereby quenching activation by AP-1.[67]

Repressors that operate by competition and quenching mechanisms are highly specialized to repress a particular type of activator on a specified DNA element. Thus they do not interfere globally with the multiple enhancers that typically reside in the promoter of a gene. These types of repressors function by modulating levels of gene transcription.

A fourth type of repression, active repression, inhibits all transcription from a gene, regardless of the kinds and numbers of enhancers present.[67] Active repression inhibits basal transcription and is believed to involve some form of direct interference with the basal transcription factors and the various essential coactivating TAFs. The process of active repression also implies that only a single repressor binding site or "silencer" element need exist, located anywhere in the promoter of the gene, to shut down all transcriptional activity from a gene.

Tissue-Specific Gene Expression

In one cell type expression of a single gene may account for a large fraction of the total protein synthesis, and in another cell type expression of the same gene may be undetectable. The chromatin is more loosely arranged in genes that are capable of expression than in those same genes in a tissue in which they are never expressed. Thus the DNA of expressed genes is more susceptible to cleavage by DNase than is the same DNA in tissues in which the genes are quiescent.[68] This looseness may facilitate access of RNA polymerase to the gene for transcription. In addition inactive genes appear to have a higher content of methylated cytosine residues than do the same genes in tissues in which they are expressed.[69]

Determinants for the tissue-specific transcriptional expression of genes exist in control sequences that usually reside within 1000 base pairs of the 5′-flanking region of the transcriptional sequence. Eucaryotic enhancer sequences were first described for immunoglobulin genes, a finding that extended the description of enhancer control elements in viral genomes.[70] However the first clear characterization of the properties of these elements came from studies of two model genes, insulin and chymotrypsin, which are expressed in the endocrine and exocrine pancreas, respectively.[71] Recombinant DNA techniques were used to link 5′-flanking regions of the insulin and chymotrypsin genes to the coding sequence of a reporter gene (chloramphenicol acetyltransferase). Expression of the reporter gene serves as an assay for activity of the gene control regions in the 5′-flanking sequences. When the recombinant insulin gene was introduced into pancreatic beta cells, chloramphenicol transferase was expressed. When the insulin recombinant gene was placed in pancreatic exocrine cells, chloramphenicol acetyltransferase was not expressed. The reverse was true for the chymotrypsin recombinant gene, namely expression occurred in the exocrine cell but not in the beta cell. These observations have profound implications for understanding the nature of control elements in the tissue-specific expression of genes. The specific and restricted expression of genes in a cell-specific manner is determined by the assembly of specific combinations of DNA-binding proteins on a predetermined array of control elements of the promoter regions of genes so as to create a transcriptionally active complex of proteins that includes the components of the general or basal transcriptional apparatus (TATA box factors).

Transcription Factors Important in Developmental Organogenesis in Endocrine Systems

Transcription factors that are critical for organogenesis include the homeodomain proteins[72] and the nuclear receptor proteins.[73–75] The family of homeotic selector or homeodomain proteins is highly conserved throughout the animal kingdom, from flies to humans. The spatial and temporal expression of these proteins and the target genes that they activate determine the orderly development of specific tissues, limbs, and organs. Likewise the actions of nuclear receptors for steroid and thyroid hormones and retinoic acid are critical for normal development to occur. Mutations that impair these essential transcription factors result in the loss or impairment of development of a specific organ or organs. Examples of impaired organogenesis attributable to mutations in essential transcription factors include partial anterior pituitary agenesis (Pit-1), adrenal and gonadal agenesis (SF-1, DAX-1), and pancreatic agenesis (IDX-1).

Partial Pituitary Agenesis

The transcription factor Pit-1 is a POU-homeodomain protein[76] that serves to activate the promoters of the genes for growth hormone, prolactin, and thyrotropin, or thyroid-stimulating hormone β (*TSH*β), in the anterior pituitary soma-totropes, lactotropes, and thyrotropes, respectively. Pit-1 is also the major enhancer activating factor for the promoter of the growth hormone–releasing hormone receptor gene.[77] Mutations in Pit-1 that impair its DNA-binding and transcriptional activation functions are responsible for the phenotype of the Jackson and Snell dwarf mice.[76] Mutations in the human gene encoding Pit-1 have been described in patients with hereditary anterior pituitary deficiency in which there is no production of growth hormone, prolactin, or thyrotropin, resulting in growth impairment and mental deficiency.[78] Production of the other hormones of the anterior pituitary gland, corticotropin and the gonadotropins LH and follicle-stimulating hormone (FSH), is unaffected.[78] In the human Pit-1 mutations, Pit-1 can bind to its cognate DNA control elements but is defective in activating gene transcription. Furthermore the mutated Pit-1 acts as a dominant negative inhibitor of the normal Pit-1 formed by the unaffected allele.

Pancreatic Agenesis

The homeodomain protein *i*slet *d*uodenum homeobox-1, or IDX-1 (*s*omatostatin *t*ranscription *f*actor-1 [STF-1], insulin promoter factor-1 [IPF-1]), appears to be responsible for the development and growth of the pancreas, and targeted disruption of the IDX-1 gene in mice causes pancreatic agenesis.[79] A child born without a pancreas was homozygous for inactivating mutations in the IDX-1 gene,[80] and the parents and their ancestors who are heterozygous for the affected allele have a high incidence of maturity-onset (type II) diabetes mellitus, suggesting that a decrease in gene dosage of IDX-1 may predispose to the development of diabetes. The possibility that a mutated IDX-1 allele may be one of several "diabetes genes" is supported by the observations that IDX-1, in concert with the helix-loop-helix transcription factors E47 and beta-2, appears to up-regulate the transcription of the insulin gene.[81]

Agenesis of the Adrenal Gland and Gonads

Two transcription factors are critical for the development of the adrenal gland, gonads, pituitary gonadotropes, and the ventral medial hypothalamus, namely SF-1 (steroidogenic factor-1)[82] and DAX-1 (*D*osage-sensitive sex reversal, *A*drenal hypoplasia congenita, *X*-chromosome).[83] SF-1 binds to half-sites of estrogen response elements that bind estrogen receptors in the promoters of genes. DAX-1 binds to retinoic acid receptor (RAR)–binding sites in promoters and inhibits RAR actions. The targeted disruption of SF-1 in mice causes adrenal and gonadal agenesis.[82] In addition pituitary gonadotropes are absent, and the ventral medial hypothalamus is severely underdeveloped.

X-linked adrenal hypoplasia congenita (AHC) is recognized as an X-linked, developmental disorder of the human adrenal gland that is lethal if untreated. The gene responsible for AHC encodes DAX-1, a member of the nuclear receptor proteins related to RAR (*R*etinoic *A*cid *R*eceptor).[83] Inactivating mutations identified in the DAX-1 gene result in the syndrome of AHC and hypogonadotrophic hypogonadism.

Coupling of Effector Action to Cellular Response

The induction and suppression of genes within a specific tissue occur in the minute-to-minute and day-to-day regulation of rates of production of the specific proteins produced by the cells, such as in the production of polypeptide hormones in response to extracellular stimuli.

At least two classes of macromolecules, phosphoproteins, and steroid hormone receptors, appear to be involved in the physiological regulation of hormone gene expression. These macromolecules mediate the actions of peptide and steroid hormones, respectively. Peptide ligands bind to receptor complexes on the plasma membrane, which results in hydrolysis of phosphatidylinositol, mobilization of calcium, formation of phosphorylated nucleotide intermediates, activation of protein kinases, and phosphorylation of specific regulatory proteins, such as transcription factors.[84] The hydrophobic composition of steroids allows them to diffuse through the plasma membrane, bind to specific receptor proteins, and interact with other macromolecules in the nucleus, including specific domains near the gene that is activated (see Chapter 3).[73, 74] Calcium and phosphorylated nucleotides such as cAMP, ATP, and GTP appear to have important functions in secretory processes. In particular, fluxes of calcium to and from the extracellular fluid into the cell and to and from intracellular organelles (e.g., mitochondria) into the cytosol are closely coupled to secretion.[85]

Signal Transduction Pathways

The signaling pathways that involve protein phosphorylations are multiple and complex. They typically consist of sequential phosphorylations and dephosphorylations of molecules referred to as protein kinase or phosphatase cascades.[86] These cascades are initiated by hormones that bind to and activate receptors on the surface of cells and that enhance the generation of small second messenger molecules such as cAMP, diacylglycerol (DAG), or calcium ions. These second messengers then activate protein kinases that phosphorylate and thereby activate key target proteins, such as by transcription factors that control gene expression (or repression) (Fig. 2–14). As discussed earlier, one group of transcription factors, the DNA-binding proteins, interacts with cAMP-responsive and phorbol ester–responsive DNA elements to stimulate gene transcription in the cAMP–protein kinase A, diacylglycerol–protein kinase C, and calcium-calmodulin signal transduction pathways (see Fig. 2–14). These proteins bind to the DNA in the form of heterodimers or homodimers via a coiled helical structure termed the leucine zipper motif.[36] Phosphorylation of these proteins may modulate the dimerization, DNA recognition and binding, and transcriptional transactivation activities by changing their conformations and capacities to interact with coactivator proteins such as the CREB-binding protein and the components of the basal transcriptional machinery, thereby allowing for RNA polymerase to initiate gene transcription.[87]

Generally the second messengers activate kinases that phosphorylate serine and/or threonine residues on proteins, whereas the receptor kinases phosphorylate tyrosine residues.[86, 88] Examples of receptor tyrosine kinases are receptors for insulin, IGF, EGF, PDGF, leptin (the obesity hormone), and cytokines. Although the different signal transduction pathways are described as more or less distinct for semantic purposes, there is in fact considerable cross-talk among the different pathways. Understanding the complex interactions among different signal transduction pathways in endocrine systems is a major challenge. The growth factor and cytokine receptors are similar in some respects and differ in others. For example phosphorylation of transcription factors by growth factors occurs on both serine/threonine and tyrosine residues,[88] whereas phosphorylation activated by cytokines through the JAK/STAT pathway appears to occur exclusively on tyrosine residues.[89]

Cyclic AMP–Dependent Signaling Pathway

Cyclic AMP is a common second messenger in the protein phosphorylation mechanism (Fig. 2–15).[36, 90] In this model the

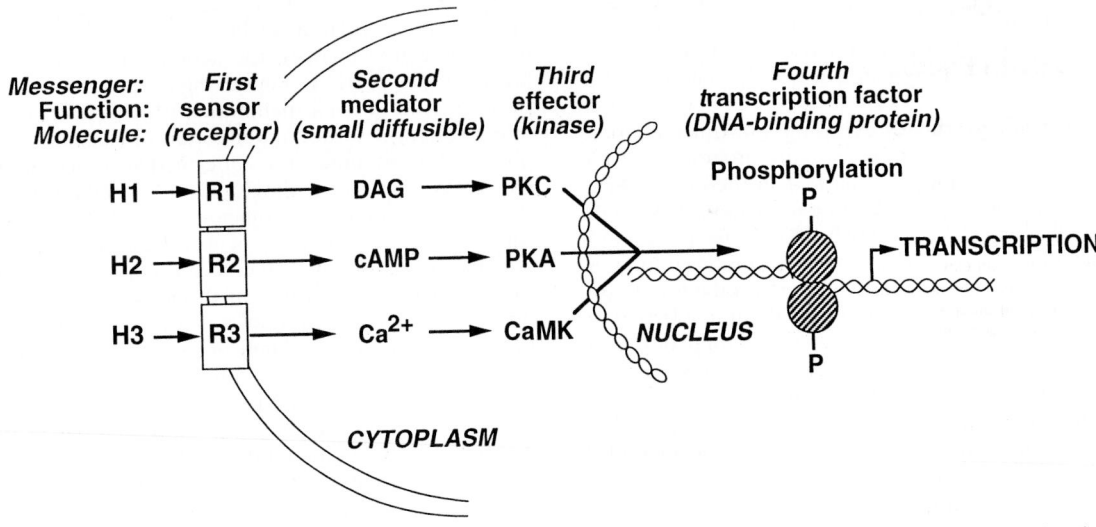

Figure 2–14. Diagram showing three cell-surface receptor-coupled signal transduction pathways involved in the activation of a superfamily of nuclear transcription factors. Peptide hormone molecules (H_1, H_2, H_3) interact with sensor receptors (R_1, R_2, and R_3) coupled to either the diacylglycerol (DAG)–protein kinase C (PKC), the cAMP–protein kinase A (PKA), or the calcium-calmodulin pathways in which small diffusible second messenger molecules are generated (DAG, cAMP, Ca^{2+}). The third messengers or effector protein kinases are generated and phosphorylate transcription factors such as members of the CREB/ATF and JUN/AP-1 families of DNA-binding proteins to modulate DNA-binding affinities and/or transcriptional activation. The various proteins bind as dimers determined by a poorly understood code that is not promiscuous inasmuch as only certain homodimer or heterodimer combinations are permissible.

stimulatory factor (ligand) interacts with a receptor in the plasma membrane and activates adenylate cyclase, enhancing the generation of cAMP, which in turn converts an inactive form of a protein kinase to an active form by way of dissociation of a regulatory (R) subunit from the active catalytic (C) subunit. The protein kinase (active subunit) catalyzes the phosphorylation of certain intracellular proteins that function in gene activation and inactivation. As indicated earlier, one example of phosphorylated intermediates in the activation of gene expression is the stimulation of the transcription of the prolactin gene by TRH.[48] The exact mechanisms by which phosphoproteins activate gene transcription are unknown.

Growth Factor/Mitogen-Activated Signaling Pathways

The signaling cascades referred to as mitogen-activated protein (MAP) kinase pathways that are activated by growth

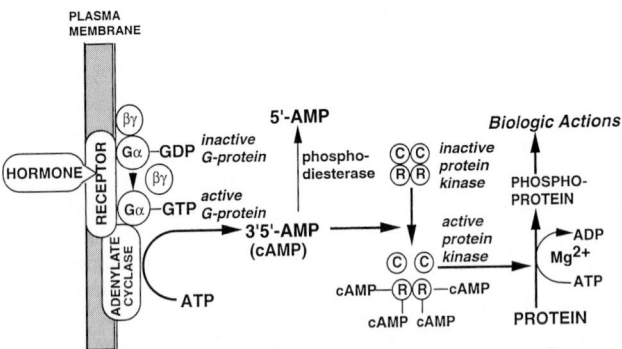

Figure 2–15. Proposed cellular mechanism through which a peptide hormone effector might activate gene expression of an endocrine cell. In the model shown, binding of peptide hormone to plasma membrane receptor activates GTP-binding proteins by converting GDP to GTP on the α subunit (Gα), resulting in dissociation of the β and γ subunits (Gβ and Gγ). GTP-Gα then activates adenylate cyclase, which leads to formation of 3′,5′-cAMP and a cascade of reactions, resulting in conversion of inactive cAMP-dependent protein kinase A to the active kinase by dissociation of the inhibitory (regulatory) subunits from the active catalytic subunit. The active kinase (C) then enters the nucleus and phosphorylates specific proteins. The presumed final active product in this cascade of reactions is a phosphoprotein that interacts with regulatory sites on the gene, thereby activating gene transcription and expression. C and R refer to catalytic and regulatory (cAMP-receptor) subunits of protein kinase, respectively.

factor hormones involve several protein kinases (at least four), in which sequential phosphorylations lead to the activation of nuclear transcription factors and stimulation of gene transcription (Fig. 2–16).[88] Three distinct MAP kinase pathways have been identified: ERK, Jnk/SAPK, and P38/HOG-1, and the kinases in each pathway are present in different isoforms.[88] By successive phosphorylations, the receptor tyrosine kinase activates a MAP kinase kinase kinase that activates a MAP kinase kinase that activates a MAP kinase. The nomenclature is ERK (extracellular signal–regulated kinase) for the MAP kinase, MEK (MAP/ERK kinase) for the MAP kinase kinase, and MEKK for the MAP kinase kinase kinase (Fig. 2–16).

Ligand activation of receptor tyrosine kinases by autophosphorylation recruits adaptor proteins such as Grb2. These proteins bind to phosphotyrosine substrates in the receptors formed by the autophosphorylation of the receptor and recruit guanine nucleotide exchange factors that nucleotidylate small G proteins such as RAS (convert RAS-GDP to RAS-GTP). The GTP-bound form of RAS binds the MEKK, thereby targeting it to the plasma membrane and increasing MEKK protein kinase activity. MEKK then phosphorylates and activates MEK, which in turn phosphorylates and activates ERK (the MAP kinase) (Fig. 2–17A). The three related but distinct MAP kinase cascades are illustrated in Figure 2–17. The NH$_2$-terminal JUN kinase (JNK) and HOG-1/p38 pathways differ from the ERK pathway in that they are preferentially activated by stress rather than by mitogens.

Cytokine-Activated JAK/STAT Signaling Pathway

The JAK/STAT pathway involves a family of soluble tyrosine kinases known as the Janus kinases (JAK) that activate transcription factors designated STATS for "signal transduction activating transcription."[89] More than 30 different cytokine polypeptides activate the JAK/STAT pathway, including the interferons, at least 15 interleukins, growth hormone, prolactin, tissue necrosis factor α (TNF α), and leptin.[89] The cytokine receptors are tyrosine kinases. After ligand-mediated assembly of the receptors, the JAKs become phosphorylated on tyrosine residues and are thereby activated as tyrosine kinases (see Fig. 2–17B). The intracellular cytoplasmic domain of the receptor kinase is then phosphorylated on tyrosine

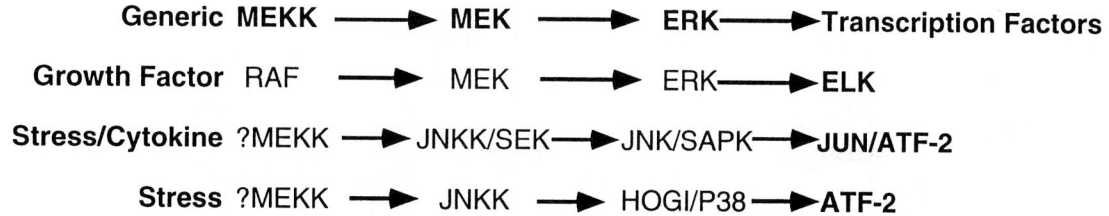

Generic	MEKK →	MEK →	ERK →	Transcription Factors
Growth Factor	RAF →	MEK →	ERK →	**ELK**
Stress/Cytokine	?MEKK →	JNKK/SEK →	JNK/SAPK →	**JUN/ATF-2**
Stress	?MEKK →	JNKK →	HOGI/P38 →	**ATF-2**

Figure 2–16. Mitogen-activated signal transduction pathways. Growth factors and cytokines activate an important family of signal transduction pathways involving protein kinase cascades, resulting in the activation of transcription factors and resultant stimulation of gene transcription. The "generic" pathway is shown at the top, followed by three distinct pathways currently under investigation. The binding of a hormone or cytokine to a receptor tyrosine kinase represents the first protein kinase in the cascade. This results in the activation of a second kinase MEKK (*M*itogen and *E*xtracellular signal-regulated *K*inase *K*inase), which activates a MEK, which in turn activates ERK (*E*xtracellular signals *R*egulated *K*inase) and the phosphorylation and activation of a key transcription factor. Although for semantic purposes the three pathways are considered separately, there appears to be considerable cross-talk among the pathways activated by growth factor hormones, cytokines, or cellular stress.

residues providing binding sites for the SH2 domains on the STATs, latent cytoplasmic transcription factors. The STATs attached to the receptors are phosphorylated by the activated JAKs. The STATs then dimerize, translocate to the nucleus, and regulate gene transcription by binding to specific DNA sites in the promoters of target genes.[89] At least four distinct Janus kinases and six STATs appear to have cell-type specificity of expression and specific ligand-responsive activation.[89] Additional STAT isotype homodimers and heterodimers recognize specific enhancer elements in the promoter regions of target genes.

Although the various signal transduction pathways are discussed individually, considerable cross-talk appears to exist among these pathways, both at the levels of the kinase and phosphatase signaling cascades and in the different families of transcription factors involved. For example the CREB is activated by phosphorylation via at least three signaling pathways (Fig. 2–18). A single serine residue in the P-box required for activation of CREB can, in certain cell types and in certain conditions, be phosphorylated by the cAMP-dependent pro-

tein kinase A, calcium calmodulin–dependent kinase, or the CREB kinase termed RSK-2 kinase.[36, 91] These kinases represent the terminal kinases in their respective pathways.

In the regulation of gene expression by steroid hormones (e.g., regulation of corticotropin secretion in the pituitary by cortisol), the steroids penetrate the plasma membrane and bind to specific receptors located in the cytoplasm, and the hormone-receptor complexes attach to specific target sites on the chromatin (Fig. 2–19).[73–75] (see Chapter 4). The interaction of the hormone with the receptor causes dissociation of the receptor from a complex of proteins that includes the 90-kd heat shock protein (hsp90). The hormone-receptor complexes interact with the chromatin-bound receptors and either enhance or inhibit transcription of genes.[75] The *cis*-acting DNA-regulatory elements that bind the receptors for steroid and thyroid hormones, retinoic acids, and vitamin D have been identified, and the structures of the receptors have been determined by cDNA cloning. The *cis* elements consist of typically short sequences of 15 to 20 base pairs that have a dyadic symmetry, so-called palindromic sequences; i.e., the ends of

A Mitogen-Activated Pathway

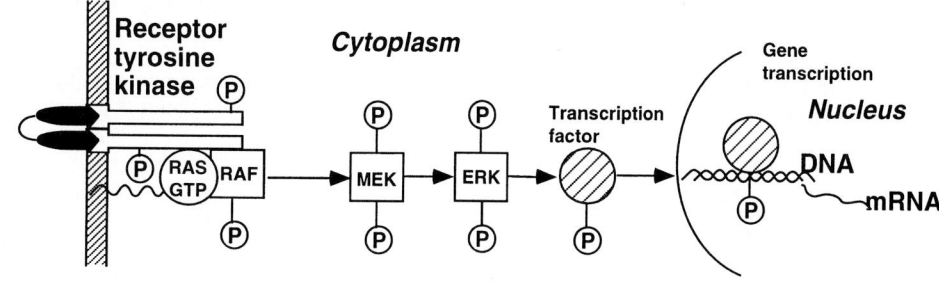

Figure 2–17. *A,* Diagram depicting a prototypical growth factor, mitogen-activated signaling pathway. The receptor tyrosine kinase is autophosphorylated on binding a hormone or cytokine, recruits RAS, a membrane-bound small G protein, phosphorylates RAF, a MEKK (see Fig. 2–16) resulting in the sequential activations of the protein kinases MEK and ERK, and finally phosphorylation of the transcription factor. *B,* Depiction of a prototypical JAK/STAT signal transduction pathway. In this model autophosphorylation of the receptor tyrosine kinase by binding a cytokine recruits a Janus kinase (JAK), which is phosphorylated and thereby activated. JAK then phosphorylates one or more of the STAT transcription factors (*S*ignal *T*ransduction *A*ctivating *T*ranscription). The phosphorylation of STATs causes them to dimerize and translocate to the nucleus, where they bind specific DNA elements called GAS elements (*G*ene-*A*ctivating *S*equences).

B Cytokine-Activated Pathway

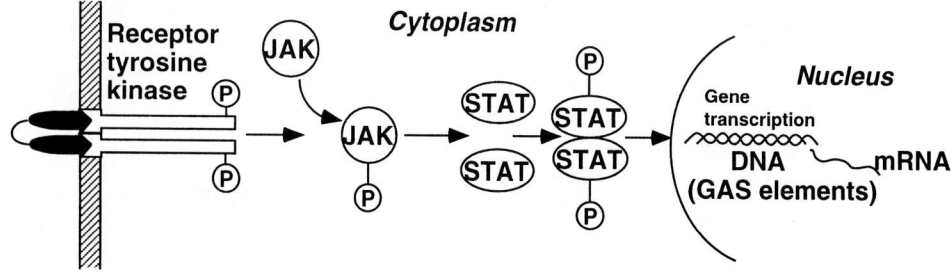

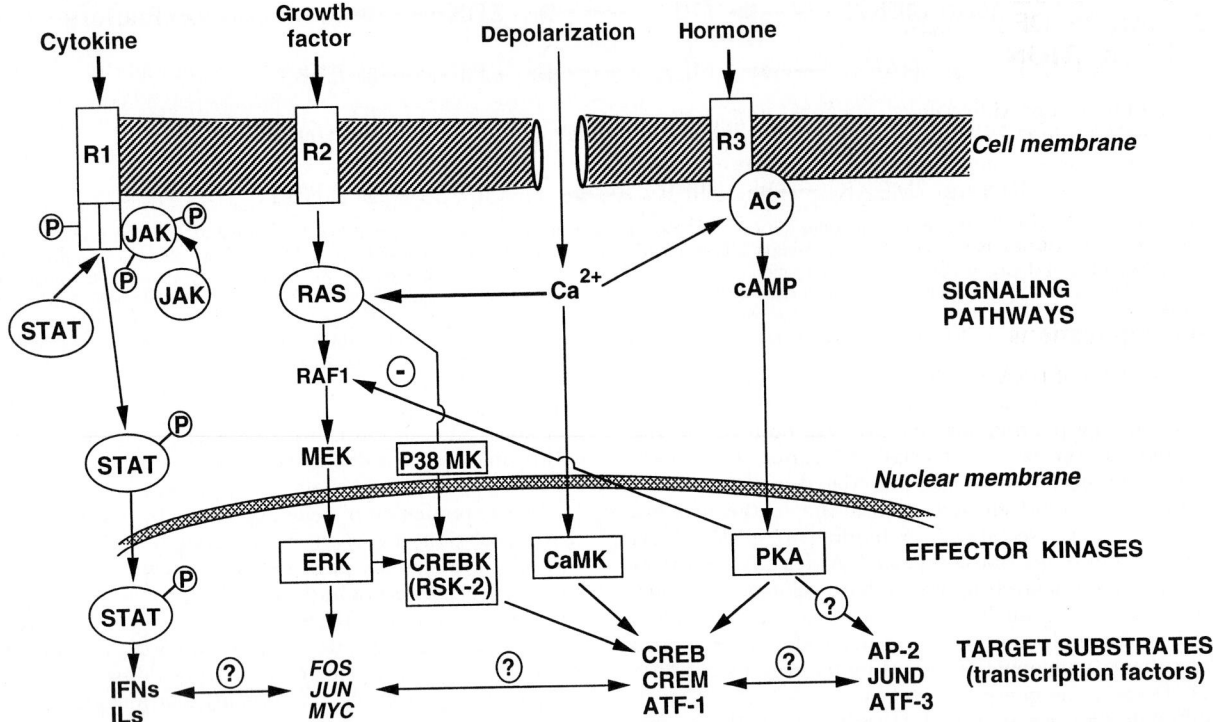

Figure 2–18. Example of complex cross-talk among signaling pathways convergent on the activation of specific transcription factors. Current evidence suggests that the transcription factor CREB is activated not only by phosphorylation by cAMP-dependent kinase (PKA) but also by phosphorylation directed by the calcium-calmodulin kinase (CaMK), growth factor/mitogen-activated (RAS), and stress-activated P38 kinase pathways. The latter two pathways activate CREB kinases (CREBK), one of which is RSK2.

the sequences contain several bases that are complementary to each other and form a potential stem-loop structure. These palindromic sequences are characteristic of control sequences in many eucaryotic genes. Subtle substitution changes of two to three base pairs within these elements can change binding specificities for a given receptor, e.g., from binding a glucocorticoid receptor to an estrogen receptor. Serial repetitive arrays of these elements on a gene promoter give multiplicative, synergistic responses, a circumstance that probably reflects the cooperative protein-protein interactions among the receptors occupying the DNA-binding sites.

The receptors contain distinct DNA-binding and ligand-binding domains.[73–75] The DNA-binding domains comprise metal-binding sites, so-called zinc fingers that chelate zinc atoms and result in the formation of a higher-ordered helical structure that is important for binding to the DNA elements. In a manner not yet completely understood, the ligand-binding domains mediate the transcriptional *trans*-activation functions of the receptors in conjunction with the zinc finger region. Occupancy of the receptor by ligand is believed to lead to an allosteric conformational change in the receptor, thereby resulting in the formation of a transcriptionally competent protein capable of interacting with the hormone response elements.

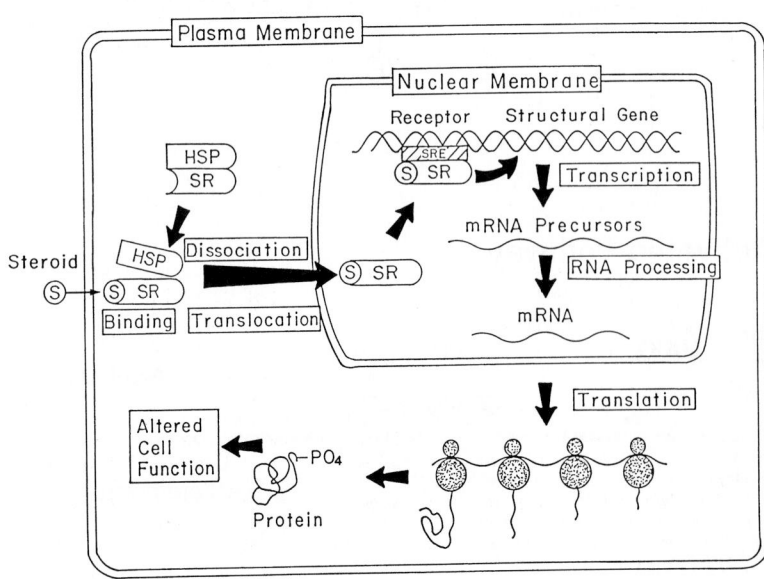

Figure 2–19. Proposed mechanism of action of steroids (glucocorticoids, estrogens, and progesterone) in activation of specific gene transcription. In this model the steroid (S) readily diffuses across the plasma membrane and binds to a cytosolic receptor (SR). In the absence of steroid, the receptor resides in the cytoplasm as an inactive complex with heat shock protein (hsp). When the steroid binds to the receptor, the hsp dissociates from it. The steroid-receptor complex is translocated to the nucleus, where it binds to a chromatin receptor consisting of the steroid receptor response DNA element (SRE), thereby activating the transcription of specific genes involved in steroid hormone action. RNA transcripts are translated into proteins that mediate changes in cell function. Some evidence suggests an alternative model in which steroid receptor resides in the nucleus and not in the cytoplasm. In this model, presumably, steroid diffuses through the cytoplasm into the nucleoplasm, where it binds to the receptor before gene activation occurs. (Adapted from Chan L, O'Malley BW. Mechanism of action of the sex steroid hormones. Reprinted by permission of The New England Journal of Medicine 1976; 294:1322–1328, 1372–1382, 1429–1437.)

GENERATION OF BIOLOGIC DIVERSIFICATION

In addition to providing control points for the regulation of gene expression, the various steps involved in gene expression can serve as a means for diversification of information stored in the gene (Fig. 2–20). These steps include the following: (1) gene duplication and copy number, (2) transcription, (3) post-transcriptional RNA processing, (4) translation, and (5) post-translational processing.

Gene Duplications

At the level of DNA, diversification of genetic information comes about by way of gene duplication and amplification. Many of the polypeptide hormones are derived from families of multiple, structurally related genes. Examples include the growth hormone family, consisting of growth hormone, prolactin, and placental lactogen; the glucagon family, consisting of glucagon, VIP, secretin, gastric-inhibitory peptide, and GHRH; and the glycoprotein hormones, thyrotropin, LH, FSH, and human chorionic gonadotropin (hCG). A remarkable example of gene amplifications is the extraordinarily large number of genes encoding the pheromone and odorant receptors.[92, 93] As many as 1000 such receptor genes may exist in mouse and rat genomes, each receptive to a particular odorant ligand. Over the course of evolution an ancestral gene encoding a prototypical polypeptide representative of each of these families was duplicated one or more times, and through mutation and selection the progeny proteins of the ancestral gene assumed different biologic functions. As discussed earlier the structural organization of the genome of higher animals lends itself to recombination, resulting in rearrangement of transcriptional units and regulatory sequences.[60]

One hypothesis for explaining the mechanisms by which new genetic information may arise suggests that mutations are introduced into DNA via RNA intermediates.[94] This hypothesis is based on two lines of evidence. First the error frequency in DNA replication in mammalian eucaryotes is approximately one incorrect base incorporated for every 10^9 to 10^{11} bases, whereas the error rate in RNA synthesis is on the order of one incorrect base for every 10^3 to 10^4 bases. This difference is due to the fact that proofreading enzymes correct misincorporated bases during DNA synthesis, whereas RNA synthesis has no such correction mechanism. Second the mammalian genome contains large numbers of pseudogenes that appear to consist of DNAs complementary in sequence to mRNAs (cDNAs) and that are partially mutated duplicates of structural genes, many of which lack introns and have 3'-poly(A) tracts. Their resemblance to mRNAs suggests that they have been reverse-transcribed from mRNA back into DNA and then reinserted into the genome. Such pseudogenes, or "processed" genes, have been observed for the alpha chain of hemoglobin, immunoglobulins, α-tubulin, and β-tubulin. Perhaps as much as 20% of the mammalian genome originated as RNA that was reverse-transcribed back to DNA,[60] implying that a reintegration event must have occurred in the germ line for about 10% of genes within the last 10 to 20 million years. In evolutionary terms this is a relatively high rate of introduction of new genetic information.

Transcription

Another way of creating diversity in expression is by providing genes with alternative promoters (reviewed in reference

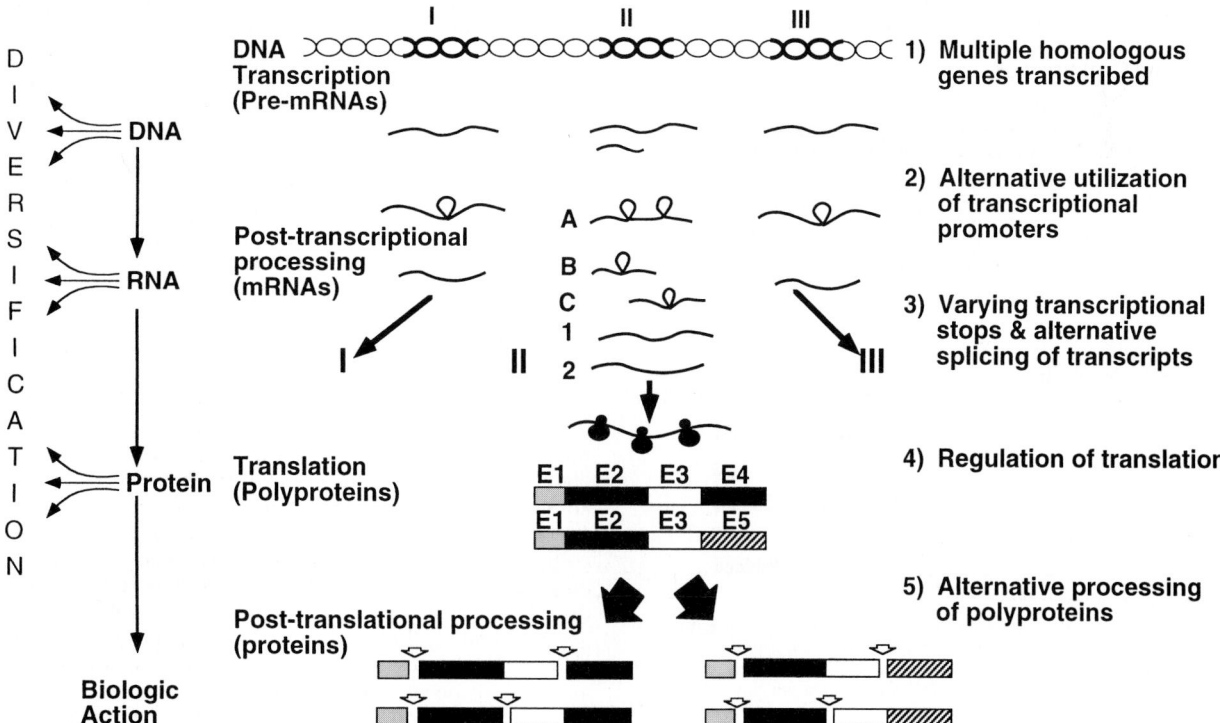

Figure 2–20. Schema indicating levels in expression of genetic information at which diversification of information encoded in a gene may take place. The three major levels of genetic diversification are (1) gene duplication, a process that occurs in terms of evolutionary time; (2) variation in the processing of RNA precursors, which results in formation of two or more mRNAs by way of alternative pathways of splicing of transcript (see Figs. 2–19 and 2–20); and (3) use of alternative patterns in processing of protein biosynthetic precursors (polyproteins, or prohormones). These three levels in gene expression provide a means for diversification of gene expression at levels of DNA, RNA, or protein. One or more of a combination of these processes leads to formation of a final biologically active peptide or hormone. In the diagram, loops depicted in transcripts denote introns; in diagrammatic structures of proteins, the stippled, shaded, and unshaded areas denote exons. SP, signal peptide. See text for details.

95) and by utilizing a large array of *cis*-regulatory elements in the promoters regulated by transcription factors.

Alternative Promoters

Many of the genes encoding hormones and their receptors utilize more than one promoter during development and/or when expressed in different tissue types. The employment of alternative promoters results in the formation of multiple transcripts that differ at their 5′ ends (Fig. 2–21). Multiple promoters provide flexibility in the control of expression of the genes; for example expression of genes in different tissues or in different developmental stages may require different combinations of tissue-specific transcription factors. Such

a circumstance enables the genes in different cell types to respond to different signal transduction systems or genes in the same cell type to respond to different signal transduction systems. A single promoter may not be adequate to respond to a complex array of transcription factors and a changing environment of cellular signals.

Alternative promoters in genes can be organized in different patterns (Fig. 2–21). The most common site is within the 5′ noncoding or leader exons, and the utilization of different promoters in the 5′ untranslated region of the gene, often accompanied by alternative exon splicing, results in the formation of mRNAs with different 5′ sequences. The utilization of alternative promoters in 5′ leader exons can generate diversity in several different ways, including the developmental stage-specific and temporal expression of genes, the tissue specificity of expression, the levels of expression, the responsivity of gene expression to specific metabolic signals, the stability of the mRNAs, the efficiencies of translation, and the structures of the amino termini of proteins encoded by the genes.[95]

Genes that use alternative 5′ leader promoters during development include those that encode insulin-like growth factor I (IGF-I), IGF-II, the retinoic acid receptors, and glucokinase, all of which are regulated by multiple promoters in embryonic and adult tissues and are subject to developmental and tissue-specific regulation.[95] During fetal development, promoters P2, P3, and P4 of the *IGF2* gene are active in the liver. These promoters are shut off after birth, at which time the P1 promoter is activated. The P1 and P2 promoters of the *IGF1* gene respond differently to growth hormone: P2 in liver is responsive to growth hormone, whereas P1 in muscle is not. The retinoic acid receptor exists in three isoforms (RARα, β, and γ), encoded by separate genes that give rise to at least 17 different mRNAs generated by a combination of multiple promoters and alternative splicing.[96] The RAR isoforms appear to differ in their specificity for retinoic acid–responsive promoters, in their affinities for ligands, and in their *trans*-activating capabilities. The different RAR isoforms are expressed at different times in different tissues during development, and these different RAR isoforms may provide a means of producing diverse cellular responses to a single ligand, retinoic acid.[96]

Glucokinase illustrates the alternative use of 5′ leader promoters that have different metabolic responsiveness.[95] Expression of glucokinase in pancreatic beta cells and some other neuroendocrine cells utilizes an upstream promoter (1β), whereas in liver a promoter (IL) 26 kb downstream of the 1β promoter is used exclusively. In beta cells expression of the glucokinase gene is apparently not responsive to hormones, whereas the liver IL promoter is up-regulated by insulin and down-regulated by glucagon.

In the case of the α-amylase gene alternative promoters in the 5′ noncoding exons are expressed in two different tissues and have different strengths of expression.[95] A strong upstream promoter directs expression within the parotid gland, in contrast to the weak expression in liver directed by an alternative downstream promoter.

Examples of the alternative usage of promoters in the coding regions of genes are the progesterone receptor (PR) and the CREM. In both, different protein isoforms are produced that have markedly different functional activities. The genes encoding the chicken and human progesterone receptors (hPRs) express two isoforms of the receptor (isoforms A and B).[97] In isoform A, translation is initiated at a methionine residue 164 amino acids downstream from the methionine that initiates the translation of the longer form B. Analyses of the mechanisms responsible for the synthesis of two different isoforms revealed that two promoters exist in the hPR gene: one upstream of the 5′ leader exon and the other in the first coding exon. Both hPR isoforms equivalently activate a canonical PRE; isoform B is more efficient than A at activating

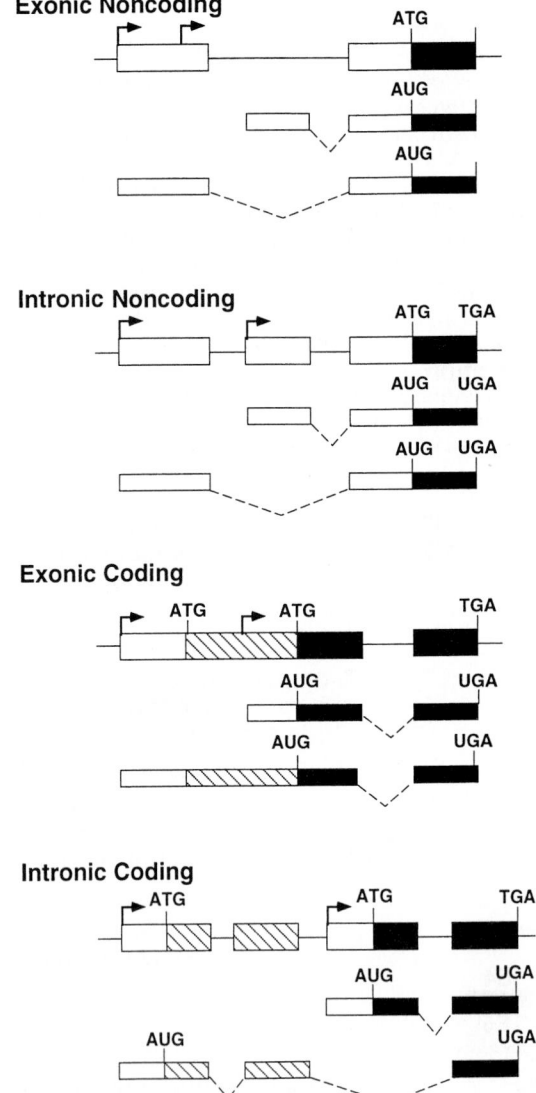

Exonic Noncoding

Intronic Noncoding

Exonic Coding

Intronic Coding

Figure 2–21. Utilization of alternative promoters in the expression of genes as a means of generating biologic diversification of gene expression. The use of alternative promoters allows a gene to be expressed in a variety of unique contexts that alter the properties of the mRNA that is expressed. Such alternative promoter usage may render the mRNA more or less stable, affect translational efficiencies, or switch the translation of one protein isoform to another. The use of alternative promoters in genes characteristically occurs during development, or after development is completed, to designate tissue-specific patterns of expression of the gene. Exons are shown as boxes, in which the protein-coding regions are shaded. Introns are designated by horizontal lines. Dashed lines indicate introns that are spliced out. (Adapted from Ayoubi TAY, Van De Ven WJM. Regulation of gene expression by alternative promoters. FASEB J 1996; 10:453–460, with permission.)

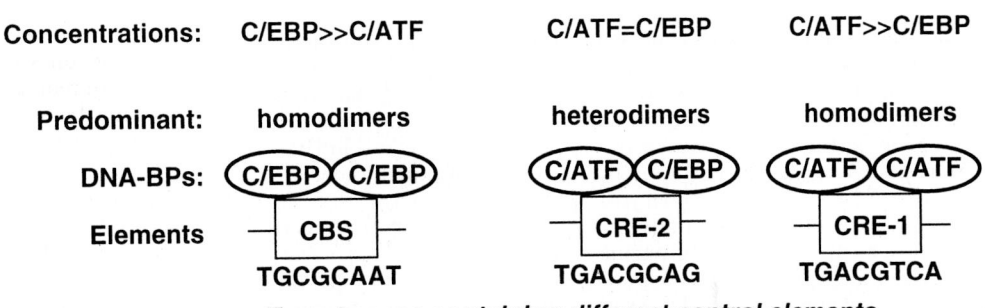

Figure 2–22. Illustration of how DNA-binding site preferences are determined by relative nuclear concentrations of C/EBP and C/ATF. When C/EBP levels exceed those of C/ATF, formation of C/EBP homodimers is favored, which preferentially bind CCAAT box–like DNA sequences (CBS). When C/ATF levels are greater than those of C/EBP, C/ATF homodimers are favored, which bind symmetrical CRE sequences (e.g., CRE-1 of the rat proenkephalin gene promoter). At intermediate concentrations C/ATF and C/EBP heterodimers are formed that preferentially bind asymmetrical CRE-like sequences (e.g., CRE-2 of the rat proenkephalin gene). BP, binding protein.

the PRE in the mouse mammary tumor virus promoter, whereas isoform A, but not B, activates transcription from the ovalbumin promoter.[97]

The utilization of an alternative intronic promoter within the protein coding sequence of a gene is exemplified by the CREM gene.[64] The CREM gene employs a constitutively active, unregulated promoter (P1) that encodes predominantly activator forms of CREM and an internal promoter (P2) located in the fourth intron that is regulated by cAMP signaling and that encodes a repressor isoform, ICER.

Diversity of Transcription Factors

Another mechanism of creating diversity at the level of gene transcription is the interplay of multiple transcription factors on *cis*-regulatory sequences. The promoters of typical genes may contain 20 or 30 or more *cis*-acting control elements, either enhancers or silencers. These control elements may respond to ubiquitous transcription factors found in all cell types and to cell type–specific factors. Different patterns of gene expression can be affected by several different mechanisms acting in concert. The spacing, relative locations, and juxtapositioning of control elements with respect to each other and to the basal transcriptional machinery can also influence levels of expression. Transcription factors often act in the form of dimers or higher oligomers with factors of the same or different classes. A given transcription factor may act as either an activator or a repressor as a consequence of the aforementioned circumstances. The ambient levels of transcription factors in the nucleus in conjunction with their relative DNA-binding affinities and *trans*-activation potencies may determine the levels of expression of genes.

Examples of diversity at the level of pairing of transcription factors are the so-called bZIP proteins C/ATF and C/EBPα (Fig. 2–22). C/ATF is a member of the ATF/CREB family of factors and is expressed during the activation of stress-induced signaling pathways.[98] C/EBPα is expressed during terminal differentiation. Homodimers of C/ATF and of C/EBP typically bind to symmetrical CREs and CCAAT boxes, respectively. However, C/ATF and C/EBP can form heterodimers and bind neither to symmetrical CREs nor to CCAAT boxes but instead bind to asymmetrical CREs. DNA-binding and *trans*-activational activities of transcription factors can also depend on the state of their phosphorylation. As discussed earlier complex signal transduction pathways within cells can be brought into play by environmental influences.

Post-transcriptional Processing (Alternative Exon Splicing)

Identification of the exon/intron structure of transcriptional units encoding polypeptide hormones and other pro-

teins raised the possibility that the use of alternative pathways in RNA splicing could provide distinct molecules. Alternative splicing occurs by two distinct mechanisms, exon skipping or intron slippage (Fig. 2–23). There are many examples of the use of both mechanisms to generate diversity in endocrine systems. Genes encoding prohormones in which the pre-mRNAs are alternatively spliced by exon skipping or switching are procalcitonin/CGRP, prosubstance P/K, and the prokininogens. Alternative processing of the RNA transcribed from the calcitonin gene results in production of different mRNAs in neural tissues and the thyroid.[99] The mRNA in the C cells of the thyroid encodes a precursor to calcitonin, whereas the mRNA in the neural tissues generates a neuropeptide known as the calcitonin gene-related peptide, which may function in the perception of pain, appetite control, and modulation of the autonomic and endocrine systems. The RNA precursor that encodes substance P can be spliced in at least two ways.[100] One pattern results in the mRNA that encodes both substance P and substance K in a common protein precursor. Other mRNAs are apparently spliced so as to exclude the coding

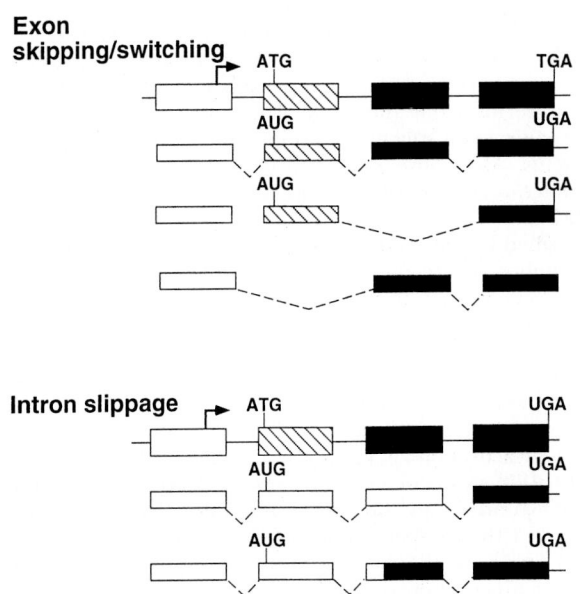

Figure 2–23. Alternative exon splicing provides a means of generating biologic diversification of gene expression. Mechanisms of exon skipping or switching and intron slippage are frequently utilized in the alternative processing of pre-mRNAs to provide unique mRNAs and encoded proteins during development and in a tissue-specific pattern of expression in the fully differentiated tissues or organs. Exons are shown as boxes with protein-coding regions shaded to designate the origin of protein isoforms. Introns are depicted as horizontal lines. Dashed lines denote spliced-out introns (and exons).

sequence for substance K. Another RNA-splicing pattern occurs in the processing of transcripts arising from the gene encoding bradykinin.[101] High- and low-molecular-weight kininogens are translated from mRNAs that differ by the alternative use of 3'-end exons encoding the COOH termini of the prohormones, a situation similar to that in the transcription of the calcitonin gene.

Other examples of genetic diversification arise from flexibility in the intron slippage splicing of coding regions, which allows an array of coding sequences (exons) to be put together in a number of possible useful combinations. For example the coding sequences of the growth hormone, LH/hCG,[102] and leptin receptors[103] can be brought together in two different ways, one including, the other excluding, an exon specifying the transmembrane spanning domains that anchor the receptors to the surface of cells. If mRNA splicing excludes the anchor's peptide sequence, the protein is secreted rather than inserted into the membrane.

The pituitary adenylate cyclase activating peptide (PACAP) receptor is an example of alternative exon splicing that alters the function of a receptor.[104] PACAP is a member of the glucagon-related superfamily of peptide hormones that is expressed in the pituitary, brain, intestine, pancreas, and many other organs. It shares homology with VIP, which is also expressed in intestines and pancreas and which like PACAP binds to at least three distinct receptors. Two small exons designated "hip" and "hop" are alternatively spliced singly or together within the mRNA that encodes the cytoplasmic loop of the receptor. As a consequence of the alternative exon splicing, the coupling to the GTP-binding proteins G_s and C_q is altered, switching from activation of the cAMP signaling to activation of phosphoinositol signaling pathways. The physiological significance of this exon switching is unclear. Such switching may play a role in the function of the gene during development.

Lopez[105] described 44 transcription factors belonging to 14 different families in which alternative splicing creates different isoforms, many of which are repressors because of impairment of dimerization, DNA-binding, or *trans*-activation. Examples of alternative exon skipping in transcription factors are the CREB and the CREM proteins.[36, 64] The CREB and CREM genes consist of 12 or more exons, many of which are alternatively spliced. These genes encode activator or repressor isoforms from the same gene during development by alternative exon splicing of the pre-mRNAs that encode these proteins. Alternative exon splicing of the CREB pre-mRNA activates an alternative internal start site for translation of the CREB mRNA.[106] The expression of the CREM gene is also diversified by alternative exon splicing during development.[64] In addition to the alternative utilization of an internal cAMP-responsive promoter to encode the self-regulated repressor, ICER, multiple exons that comprise *trans*-activation domains of CREM and two exons encoding the DNA-binding domain are spliced in and out during the maturation of germ cells in the rat and mouse testis. The role of the two DNA-binding domains of CREM is unknown. However, CREM isoforms lacking *trans*-activation sequences are potent repressors of CREB and CREM. A major switch from CREM repressors (isoforms CREMα and β) to the CREM activators (CREMτ isoforms) occurs in the midpachytene phase of spermatocyte development by way of the splicing in of two exons encoding glutamine-rich activation domains. An additional alternative exon splicing occurs later in the maturation of spermatids in which all *trans*-activation exons, including those encoding the glutamine-rich sequences and the kinase-inducible domain (P-box), are deleted.[107] An example of alternative splicing by the intron slippage mechanism occurs in the transcription factor ERB-Aα.[64] The NH₂-terminal segment of the thyroid hormone receptor activator isoform ERB-Aα1 contains the DNA-binding domain, and the ligand-binding domain is at the COOH terminus. Alternative spicing of the pre-mRNA generates two different transcripts, α2 and α3, which encode ERB-A isoforms with truncated (α3) or frame-shifted (α2) proteins that are unable to bind the thyroid hormone ligand. These COOH-terminally altered isoforms of ERB-A repress the activator form α1.

FOS-B is a member of the AP-1 complex family of immediate early genes that is activated by protein kinase C. Alternative splicing by deletion of 140 bp in the 3' sequence of the mRNA shifts the reading frame and the termination of translation.[64] The truncated FOS-B formed by the excision of the coding intron is a repressor of FOS/JUN AP-1 complexes.

Translation

Translation provides a fourth level for the creation of diversity of gene expression. The rate of translational initiation can be regulated as illustrated by the proinsulin and prohormone convertase mRNAs in which translation is augmented by glucose and cAMP. Molecular diversity of translation is generated by the utilization of alternative translation initiation (start) codons (methionine codons, AUGs). Translational initiation involves the assembly of the 40S ribosome subunit on the 5' methylguanosine cap of the mRNA,[108] and the ribosome subunit scans 5' to 3' along the mRNA until it encounters an AUG sequence in a context of surrounding nucleotides favorable for the initiation of protein synthesis. The subunit then pauses and recruits the 80S subunit plus other translational initiation factors to begin the polymerization of amino acids. The use of an alternative downstream start codon for translation can occur by mechanisms of loose scanning or reinitiation (Fig. 2–24).[109] Loose scanning is believed to occur when the 5' most AUG codon is not in a strongly favorable context and allows the 40S to continue scanning until it encounters another AUG downstream. Thus by the loose scanning mechanism both start codons are used, and the mRNA is monocistronic. In contrast, translational reinitiation involves the termination of translation, and its reinitiation at a downstream start codon. Thus two proteins are encoded from the same mRNA by a start and stop mechanism, and the mRNA is considered to be polycistronic. Translational reinitiation can occur either by continued scanning of the same 40S ribosomal subunit after termination of translation followed by reinitiation, as in loose scanning, or by complete dissociation of the ribosomal subunits at the time of termination followed by reassembly of a new ribosome at a downstream start codon referred to as an internal ribosomal entry site (IRES). Such

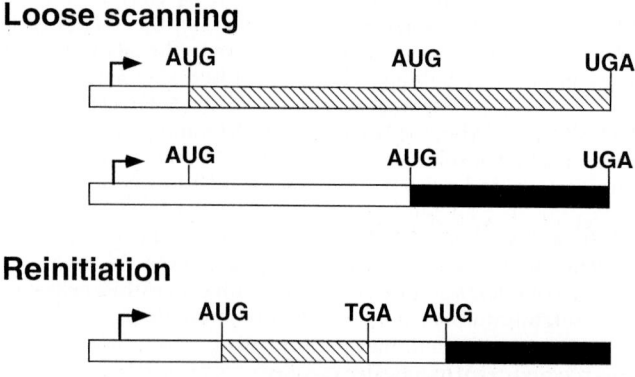

Loose scanning

Reinitiation

Figure 2–24. Alternative AUG translational initiation codons are used to change the coding sequences of mRNAs so as to encode different protein isoforms. The two mechanisms illustrated involve loose scanning and reinitiation of translation. The proteins encoded by the mRNAs are shown as filled or cross-linked boxes. See text for detailed description.

utilization of alternative translation start codons occurs in mRNAs encoding certain classes of transcription factors illustrated by the bZIP proteins CREB, CREM, and certain of the C/EBPs, the C/EBPα and C/EBPβ isoforms. In these DNA-binding proteins the alternative use of internal start codons results in a switch from activators to repressors.

The CREB gene uses translational reinitiation by the somewhat novel mechanism of alternative exon switching during spermatogenesis.[107] At developmental stages XII to XIV of the seminiferous tubule of the rat, an exon (exon W) is spliced into the CREB mRNA. Exon W introduces an inframe stop codon, thereby terminating translation approximately 40 amino acids upstream of the DNA-binding domain.[106, 110] The termination of translation then permits reinitiation of translation of each of two downstream start codons, resulting in the synthesis of two repressor or inhibitor isoforms of CREB known as I-CREBs that are powerful dominant negative inhibitors of activator forms of CREB and CREM, because they consist of the DNA-binding domain devoid of any trans-activation domains.[106, 107, 110] The function, if any, of the amino terminal truncated protein containing the activation domains devoid of the DNA-binding domain is unknown. The alternative splicing of exon W in the CREB pre-mRNA may serve to interrupt a forward positive-feedback loop during spermatogenesis. As discussed earlier the transcription of the CREB gene is up-regulated by cAMP signaling via CREB interactions with CREs located in the promoter. Spermatogenesis in the rat and mouse takes place in 12-d cycles in which the germ cells, arranged in cell association stages within the seminiferous epithelium, undergo progressive waves of development. Cyclic AMP levels in the seminiferous tubules rise and fall dramatically over the 12-d cycle. As a consequence the autoactivation of the expression of the CREB genes (mRNA and protein levels) rises and falls coincident with the changes in cAMP levels owing to positive autoregulation. The switching of exon W causes a change in the product of the CREB gene from activators to repressors (I-CREBs), further ensuring that the CREB gene is repressed as the levels of cAMP fall. The cyclical increases and decreases in the expression of the CREB gene may control the cyclical expression of key cAMP-responsive target genes required for spermatogenesis. This proposed function of CREB in spermatogenesis is supported by the finding that a targeted disruption (knockout) of the expression of the CREB gene in mice causes infertility in the male mice that survive (many die soon after birth owing to failure of the lungs to inflate); infertility is characterized by an arrest of spermatogenesis at the midpachytene stage (stages V to VI).[111]

CREM, C/EBPα, and C/EBPβ mRNAs also utilize alternative downstream start codons to synthesize repressors during development. These repressors consist of the DNA-binding domains and lack trans-activation domains, similar to the I-CREBs. The CREM repressor (S-CREM) is expressed during brain development.[64] The C/EBPα30 and C/EBPα20 isoforms are expressed during the differentiation of adipocytes, and the C/EBP repressor (LIP) is expressed during the development of the liver.[64]

Post-translational Processing

Diversification of biologic information can also occur during post-translational processing of proteins. Many precursors of polypeptide hormones, particularly those encoding small peptides, contain multiple peptides that are cleaved during post-translational processing. Other polyprotein precursors, however, contain several copies of the same peptide, as illustrated by the precursors of the TRH[112] and the α-mating factor of yeast,[113] each of which contains four copies of the respective peptide. Polyproteins that contain different peptides include proenkephalins,[114] pro-opiomelanocortin,[115] and proglucagon.[116]

In many instances biologic diversification at the level of post-translational processing occurs in a tissue-specific manner. The processing of pro-opiomelanocortin differs markedly in the anterior and intermediate lobes of the pituitary.[117] In the anterior pituitary the primary peptide products are corticotropin and β-endorphin, whereas in the intermediate lobe a primary product is α-MSH. The smaller peptides can be further modified by acetylation and phosphorylation of amino acid residues. Likewise the processing of proglucagon differs in the pancreatic alpha cells and in the intestinal L cells (Fig. 2–25).[40] In the pancreatic alpha cells the predominant bioactive product of the processing of proglucagon is glucagon itself; the glucagon-like peptides are not processed efficiently from proglucagon in the alpha cells and are biologically inactive because of NH₂-terminal and COOH-terminal extensions. On the other hand, in the intestinal L cell the glucagon immunoreactive product is glicentin, which consists of the NH₂-terminal extension of the proglucagon plus glucagon and the small COOH-terminal peptide known as intervening peptide I. Glicentin has no glucagon-like biologic activity, but glucagon-like peptide I in its shortened form of 31 amino acids, GLP-I(7–37) is released from the intestines into the bloodstream and is the intestinal "incretin" factor that augments the release of insulin from pancreatic beta cells in response to food intake.[118]

This potential for diversification of biologic information by the alternative pathways of gene expression is further amplified by the fact that these pathways can occur in multiple combinations.

RECOMBINANT DNA TECHNIQUES

The two major breakthroughs that made the development of DNA technology possible were the discoveries of reverse transcriptase[119, 120] and restriction endonucleases.[121] Reverse transcriptase in tumor viruses allows the virus to make DNA copies of the RNA templates. This enzyme makes it possible to synthesize DNA from mRNA, an essential step in the preparation of recombinant DNA for purposes of cloning. Restriction endonucleases cleave DNA at specific sequences, generally of four to six base pairs. Each restriction endonuclease is specific for a given sequence of nucleotides; these enzymes make it possible to cleave DNA reproducibly and predictably at specific sites, a property that is critical for the engineering of DNA segments.

In practice the analysis of a particular gene is begun by first preparing and cloning cDNAs from mRNAs of a particular cell (Fig. 2–26).[122–126] The cDNAs are inserted into bacterial plasmids that have been cleaved at a single site with a restriction endonuclease. Vectors that are commonly used are derivatives of the plasmid pBR322, which was engineered specifically for the purposes of cloning DNA fragments (see Fig. 2–26). The cleavage site is located within the gene that confers resistance to the antibiotic ampicillin. The plasmid also carries a gene for resistance to tetracycline. Thus bacteria containing the plasmids can be selected by their resistance to tetracycline; those specifically containing DNA inserts can be selected by their sensitivity to ampicillin because the ampicillinase gene is inactivated by the inserted foreign DNA. The recombinant plasmids containing DNA sequences that are complementary to the specific mRNAs of interest are identified by hybridizing recombinant plasmids to the initial mRNA preparations used in the cloning. The hybrid-selected mRNA is subsequently eluted and translated in a cell-free system appropriate for the protein under study.[127] Alternatively, specific inhibition of the

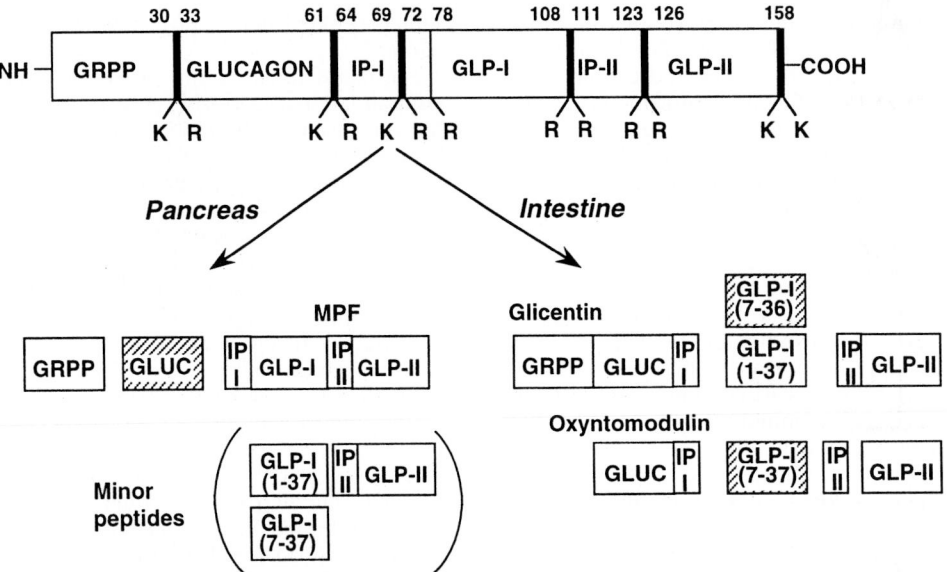

Figure 2–25. Alternative pathways of processing of proglucagon in gut and pancreatic islets. Pathways shown on the left and the right represent predicted patterns of processing of proglucagon in pancreatic islets and intestine, respectively. Processing of proglucagon occurs at pairs of basic amino acids, lysine (K) and arginine (R). In intestine the major glucagon-containing peptide is glicentin, which consists of glucagon in covalent linkages with NH_2-terminal and short COOH-terminal extensions, glucagon-related polypeptide (GRPP), and intervening peptide I (IP-I). Although not proved, it is likely that the two glucagon-related peptides, glucagon-like peptide I (GLP-I) in various forms and glucagon-like peptide II (GLP-II), are the major biologically active peptides liberated in the gut by processing of proglucagon. In pancreatic islets the major glucagon peptide is glucagon itself. The COOH-terminal peptides resulting from cleavages that liberate glucagon are not further processed efficiently to glucagon-related peptides but rather remain as a major proglucagon fragment (MPF).

translation of a mRNA can be used to identify the DNA of interest: DNA that is complementary to the mRNA being translated will bind the RNA, thus precluding translation and causing a reduced amount of the protein being synthesized.[128]

The ability to prepare DNA by reverse transcription of mRNA was important because there are more copies of mRNA in cells than there are genes that encode particular polypeptides. Usually cells contain only two copies of the gene, whereas 10,000 to 100,000 copies of the mRNA may be present in cells in which the gene is expressed. Hence it is easier to isolate recombinant DNAs by reverse transcription of RNA templates from these cells than to isolate specific gene sequences.

The cloning of genomic DNA is similar to the cloning of cDNA, except that the genomic sequences are longer and that different cloning vectors are required. Derivatives of the bacteriophage λ can accommodate DNA fragments of from 10 to 20 kb, and certain hybrids of bacteriophages and plasmids (cosmids) can accommodate inserts of DNA of up to 40 to 50 kb. Moreover yeast artificial chromosome (YAC) libraries can harbor segments of chromosomes up to several megabases.

Recombinant cDNAs are valuable for determination of the protein-encoding nucleotide sequences and as hybridization probes to measure cellular levels of mRNAs, mRNA precursors, and the numbers of gene copies in the DNA. The latter measurements require the separation of the cellular RNA or of restriction endonuclease digests of genomic DNA on agarose gels, followed by transfer of the polynucleotide fragments to nitrocellulose filters and hybridization with ^{32}P-labeled cDNA probes. These procedures are known as Northern (RNA) and Southern (DNA) transfer, respectively. It is sometimes possible to hybridize labeled probes directly to tissue slices or to spreads of metaphase chromosomes. For example cDNA encoding pro-opiomelanocortin, the precursor to corticotropin, localizes to specific neurons that contain pro-opiomelanocortin mRNA when hybridized to histologic sections of the medial basal hypothalamus of rats.[129] Similarly the human insulin gene maps to the distal end of the short arm of chromosome 11 by hybridization of mitotic chromo-

some preparations from cultured human lymphocytes with a labeled recombinant plasmid encoding pre-proinsulin.[130] These powerful techniques make it possible to analyze individual cells for expression of specific genes.

The rapid amplification of specific DNA sequences (the polymerase chain reaction[131, 132]) makes it possible to amplify DNA sequences from 50 to several thousand base pairs over a million-fold in just a few hours by using an automated thermal cycler. The technique is so sensitive that a DNA from a single cell can be amplified.[132] The applications of this technique are diverse. Not only is it possible to amplify and clone rare sequences for research purposes, but the technique is applicable to medical diagnosis and forensic science. Scarce viruses can be detected in a drop of serum or urine or a single white blood cell. Genotyping can be done from a blood or semen stain, saliva, or a single hair. Paradoxically, the exquisite sensitivity of the polymerase chain reaction opens the possibility of producing false-positive results by even minute contaminations of the samples being tested. Thus extreme precautions must be taken to avoid the introduction of contaminants.

APPLICATIONS OF SOMATIC CELL GENETICS AND GENE TRANSFER TECHNIQUES TO ANALYSIS OF GENE CONTROL

It is difficult to apply classic mammalian genetics to the analysis of genetic control and development because many mutations that affect the developmental process and the regulation of genes are lethal and, as such, are difficult to propagate. Specifically engineered genes can now be introduced into the genomes of cultured cell lines and into the germ cells of animals (transgenic animals) for study of the regulation of genes that determine development and cellular differentiation. For example in transgenic animals tissue-specific promoters can be used to misdirect the expression of specific genes

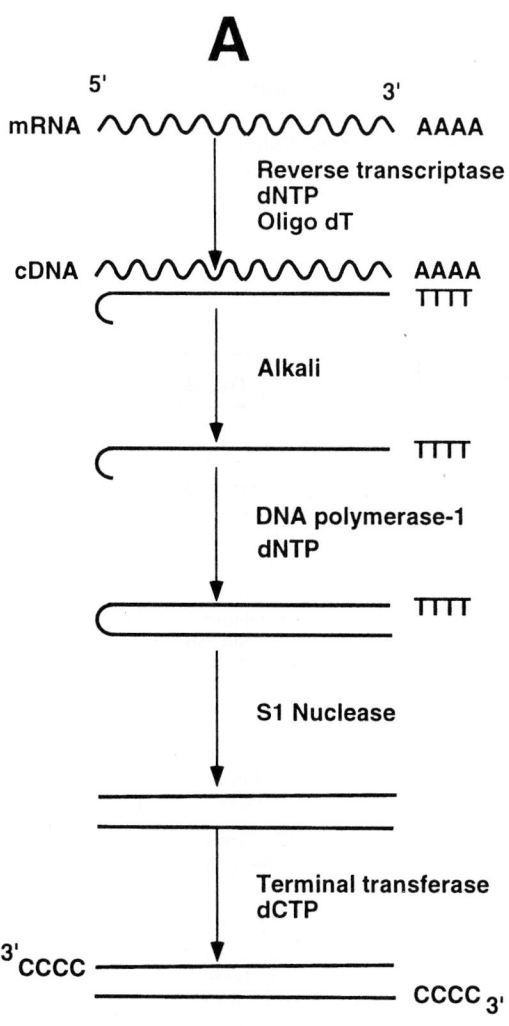

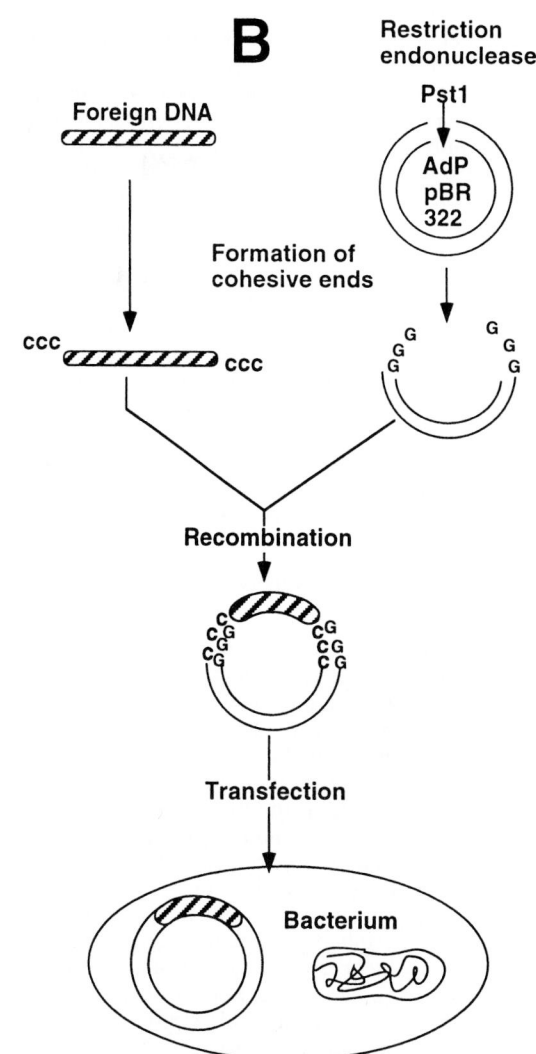

Figure 2–26. An approach used in the construction and molecular cloning of recombinant DNA. *A,* Preparation of double-stranded DNA from an mRNA template. The enzyme reverse transcriptase is used to reverse-transcribe a single-stranded DNA copy complementary to the mRNA primed with an oligonucleotide of polydeoxythymidylic acid hybridized to the poly(A) tract at the 3′ end of mRNA. A complementary copy of the DNA strand is then prepared with DNA polymerase. Ends of double-stranded DNA are made flush by cleavage with the enzyme S1 nuclease, and homopolymer extensions of deoxycytidine are synthesized on 3′ ends of DNA with the enzyme terminal transferase. Oligo(dC) homopolymer extensions form sticky ends for purposes of insertion of DNA into a linearized plasmid on which complementary oligo(dG) homopolymer extensions have been synthesized. *B,* Insertion of foreign DNA into a bacterial plasmid for molecular cloning. A bacterial plasmid, typically pBR322 that has been specifically engineered for purposes of cloning DNA, is linearized by cleavage with restriction endonuclease Pst 1. Poly(dG) homopolymer extensions are synthesized onto 3′ ends of plasmid DNA. Foreign DNA with complementary poly(dC) homopolymer extensions is hybridized to and inserted into the plasmid. Recombinant plasmid DNA is transfected into susceptible host strains of bacteria in which plasmid replicates apart from bacterial chromosomal DNA. Bacteria are then grown on a plate containing tetracycline. Colonies that are resistant to tetracycline are tested for sensitivity to ampicillin. Because native plasmids contain genes encoding resistance to both tetracycline and ampicillin, and the gene encoding resistance to ampicillin is inactivated by insertion of a foreign DNA at the Pst 1 site, bacterial colonies harboring plasmids with DNA inserts are resistant to tetracycline and sensitive to ampicillin. Subsequent screening of tetracycline-resistant, ampicillin-sensitive clones containing specific DNA-inserted sequences is carried out by either DNA hybridization with labeled DNA probes or by other techniques, such as hybridization arrest and cell-free translation.

to tissues in which they are foreign and to analyze the consequences of such expression on development and function. Likewise tissue-specific promoters can be used to direct expression of transcriptional reporter genes to investigate promoter function in embryos or tissue slices in situ. Genes can also be disrupted or replaced by techniques of homologous recombination.

Several methods are available for the introduction of genetic material into mammalian cells in culture:[133] (1) fusion of two somatic cells to create hybridomas; (2) gene transfer by DNA-mediated endocytosis; (3) transfection of cells with recombinant retroviruses or adenoviruses containing covalently linked foreign DNA; (4) microinjection of genes into cell nuclei; and (5) implantation into the mouse uterus of blastocysts that have been injected with embryonic stem cells

in which a gene of interest has been disrupted or replaced by targeted homologous recombination for the production of so-called knockout mice.

Somatic Cell Fusion

Two distinct somatic cell lines can be fused by incubation with a fusion-promoting agent such as inactivated Sendai virus or polyethylene glycol. The cells may be derived from different species of animals, e.g., human and mouse. Initially a fused cell has two nuclei, each containing the chromosomes of one of the parent cells. In the course of cell division the nuclear membranes disintegrate, and a single nucleus forms (heterokaryon) that contains chromosomes from both parent cells and that expresses certain genes from both parents. Appropriate genetic markers can be used to select hybrid cells from parental cells. The large multiple genomes of the hybrids are unstable, and chromosomes are typically lost during successive cell divisions. Eventually, stable clones are isolated, each containing only one or a few chromosomes from one of the parental cell lines. One advantage of the hybridomas is that libraries of hybrid cells can be selected that contain a single chromosome from one animal species. For example by cytologic procedures the 24 human chromosomes (22 autosomal pairs plus X and Y chromosomes) can be identified and distinguished from the chromosomes of other species. Cell lines containing these chromosomes can be used to map the presence of particular genes, and the combination of somatic cell fusion with gene hybridization makes it possible to detect genes genotypically and phenotypically. For example the human genes for growth hormone, human placental lactogen (hPL, also called chorionic somatomammotropin), and a third growth hormone–like protein are on chromosome 17,[134] and the gene for human prolactin is on chromosome 6.[135]

Direct Transfer of Genes into Cells

DNA fragments carrying single genes can be inserted into living mammalian cells by endocytosis. In this procedure a purified DNA fragment carrying the desired gene is in particles with carrier DNA and calcium phosphate that bind to the plasma membrane and enter cells by endocytosis. Studies of gene function and regulation can be performed in cells transiently transfected for 24 to 96 h. The transfected DNA forms circular episomes within the nucleus and is subjected to regulatory influences that can mimic the regulation of the endogenous chromosomal gene. To facilitate studies of gene regulation, the regulatory sequences of interest can be linked in *cis* to convenient "reporter" functions, such as the enzymes bacterial chloramphenicol acetyltransferase, alkaline phosphatase, or firefly luciferase. These enzymes are (1) stable in the host cells; (2) foreign (exogenous) to the host cells, i.e., have no endogenous activity; and (3) readily measured by simple assays. Many different DNAs can be cotransfected simultaneously. For example a *trans* expression vector encoding a transcription factor, such as one encoding the glucocorticoid receptor,[136] can be cotransfected with a *cis* element reporter vector containing the glucocorticoid response element. Thereby it is possible by mutational analyses to map regions of the expressed proteins that are important for transcriptional activation, binding of ligands, or phosphorylation.

Although many (1 to 10%) of the cultured cells transiently take up DNA, in a small fraction of cells, approximately 1 to 100 per million, the foreign DNA becomes integrated into the chromosomal DNA of the host cell, and forms a stable cell line. The transferred genes are integrated into one or a few sites in the host chromosomes; several copies of the gene may be integrated into one site. The cells expressing the foreign gene can be selected with markers cointroduced with the foreign gene, e.g., a gene encoding a protein that inactivates neomycin. Cells containing the gene for neomycin resistance grow in the presence of neomycin, which kills cells not expressing neomycin resistance.

Another method for introducing specific genes into the genome is to prepare recombinant DNAs between the gene of interest and the genomes of a virus such as simian virus.[137] After several cell divisions in the presence of the virus, the recombinant particles become integrated into the host chromosome and carry the foreign DNA along with them.

An alternative technique of gene transfer is that of microinjection. With fine microcapillary pipettes, DNA solutions can be injected directly into the nucleus of a recipient cell. Several hundred copies of a DNA fragment may be introduced into each nucleus, and an expert operator can inject solution into 500 to 1000 cells/h. The advantage of the microinjection technique is that DNA fragments, which usually ligate to form chain-like concatamers, are rapidly integrated into the host chromosomes. The efficiency of cellular transformation with this technique is higher than that with the calcium phosphate procedure. In some instances up to 20% of microinjected cells form stable transformants.

Transgenic Mice

The technique of microinjection has also been used to insert genetic material into one-cell mammalian embryos that are then allowed to develop (Fig. 2–27).[138] This approach allows analysis of gene regulation during development of a complex organism. DNA is injected into the male pronucleus of fertilized mouse ova, and the ova is then inserted into the reproductive tract of pseudopregnant foster mothers. The transgenic animals that develop from this procedure contain the foreign DNA integrated into one or more of the host chromosomes at an early stage of embryo development. As a consequence the foreign DNA is generally transmitted to the germ line, and the foreign genes may be expressed. Because the foreign DNA is injected at the one-cell stage, there is a good chance that the DNA will be distributed among all the progeny cells as development proceeds. More than half of postinjection embryos are viable, and of these approximately 10% carry the foreign genes.

With this procedure genes encoding growth hormone,[139] somatostatin,[140] and vasopressin[141] have been introduced into the germ lines of mice and expressed at high levels in most of the tissues analyzed. Transgenic animals with high levels of growth hormone in plasma grew two to three times faster than normal littermates. Transgenic animals expressing the foreign somatostatin and vasopressin genes showed few phenotypic changes even when levels of bioactive hormones in the plasma were 100 to 200 times above normal. The absence of demonstrable phenotypic changes in these transgenic animals may be a consequence of down-regulation or uncoupling of receptors for the hormone in target organs.

Transgenic approaches can also be used to prevent the development of the lineage of a particular cell phenotype or to impair the expression of a selected gene. The practical implications of this technology are discussed later.

Targeted Disruption or Replacement of Genes (Knockout Mice)

Methods for targeted disruption or replacement of genes utilize homologous recombination in cultured pluripotential embryonic stem cells, which are then injected into mouse blastocysts and implanted into the uteri of pseudopregnant mice[142, 143] (Fig. 2–27). Because the embryonic stem cells are injected into multicellular 3½-d blastocysts, many of the offspring are mosaics, but some are germline heterozygous for the recombined gene. First filial (F_1) generation mice are then bred to homozygosity so as to manifest the phenotype of the gene knockout. Using this approach, several hundred knockout mice have been created. Many of these mice are models for human genetic disorders, including pancreatic agenesis (homeodomain protein IDX-1), familial hypocalciuric hypercalcemia (calcium receptor), intrauterine growth retardation (IGF-II receptor), salt-sensitive hypertension (atrial natriuretic peptide), and obesity (β_3-adrenergic receptor).

"Targeted transgenesis" combines the targeted homologous recombination in embryonic stem cells with gain-of-function transgenic approaches.[144] This methodology allows for targeted integration of a single copy transgene to a single desired locus in the genome, thereby avoiding problems of random and multiple copy integrations that may compromise

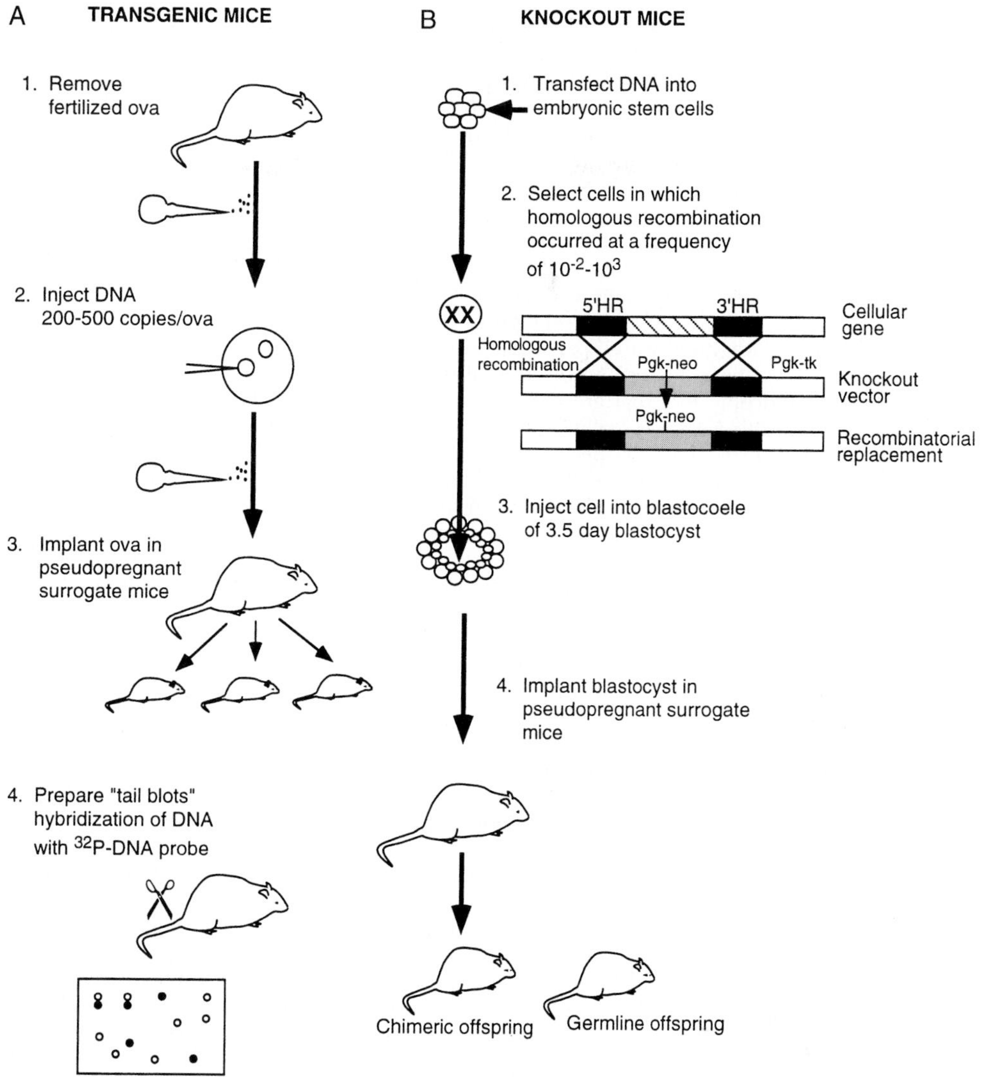

A   TRANSGENIC MICE

1. Remove fertilized ova

2. Inject DNA 200-500 copies/ova

3. Implant ova in pseudopregnant surrogate mice

4. Prepare "tail blots" hybridization of DNA with ^{32}P-DNA probe

Figure 2–27. Approaches for *(A)* the integration of foreign genes into the germ line of mice, and *(B)* to disrupt or knockout a specific gene. *A,* DNA containing a specific foreign gene is microinjected into the male pronucleus of fertilized ova obtained from the oviduct of a mouse. Ova are then implanted into the uterus of pseudopregnant surrogate mothers. Progeny are analyzed for the presence of foreign genes by hybridization with a ^{32}P-labeled DNA probe and DNA prepared from a piece of tail of a mouse that has been immobilized on a nitrocellulose filter (tail blots). *B,* To create a knockout of a gene pluripotential embryonic stem (ES) cells are used in vitro to introduce an engineered plasmid DNA sequence that will recombine with a homologous gene that is targeted. The recombination excises a portion of the gene in the ES cells, rendering it inactive (no longer expressible). ES cells in which the homologous recombination occurred successfully are selected by a combined positive-negative drug selection. The engineered ES cells are injected into the blastocoele of 3½-d blastocysts that are then implanted into the uterus of pseudopregnant mice. The offspring are both chimeric and germ line for expression of the knockout gene and must be crossbred to homozygosity for the genotype of a complete knockout of the gene that is targeted for disruption.

B   KNOCKOUT MICE

1. Transfect DNA into embryonic stem cells

2. Select cells in which homologous recombination occurred at a frequency of 10^{-2}-10^3

5'HR   3'HR   Cellular gene

Homologous recombination   Pgk-neo   Pgk-tk   Knockout vector

Pgk-neo   Recombinatorial replacement

3. Inject cell into blastocoele of 3.5 day blastocyst

4. Implant blastocyst in pseudopregnant surrogate mice

Chimeric offspring   Germline offspring

---

faithful expression of the transgene in the conventional approach.

Conditional Expression or Disruption of Targeted Genes

Although targeted transgenesis using chosen site integration and targeted disruption of genes is useful in functional analyses of genes, there is a need to be able to induce or to inhibit expression of transgenes conditionally. Two approaches to achieve conditional gene inactivation have been developed, the Cre recombinase-loxP system[145, 146] and the reverse tetracycline–inducible *trans*-activator system.[147, 148]

POTENTIAL APPLICATIONS OF RECOMBINANT DNA TECHNOLOGY AND MOLECULAR GENETICS TO DIAGNOSIS AND TREATMENT OF ENDOCRINE DISEASES

The availability of recombinant molecular probes has led to the detection of mutations, gene deletions, and insertions by the use of either allele-specific probes (point mutations) or restriction fragment length polymorphisms as genetic markers of disease. The fact that foreign genes can be expressed in microorganisms (bacteria and yeasts) and mammalian cells makes it possible to produce large amounts of specific gene products such as polypeptide hormones for use in therapy for endocrine deficiency diseases. As indicated earlier the development of techniques for stable integration of foreign genes into cultured cells and into germ lines of experimental animals raises the possibility of correcting defective genes by the introduction of correct genes.

Detection of Specific Genetic Defects by Molecular Probe Hybridization

Restriction fragment length polymorphisms arise as a fortuitous consequence of individual variations in normal (or abnormal) DNA sequences.[149] These variations, most often point mutations (base substitutions), are detectable because they either generate or eradicate specific sites that are cleaved by restriction endonucleases. Therefore the restriction endonuclease fragments generated by enzymatic cleavage from the two alleles differ in length. Because fragments of different length can be separated by agarose gel electrophoresis and detected with specific DNA probes, it is possible to determine which form of a polymorphic sequence is carried by any individual and through any family. The frequency of nucleotide site polymorphisms in the population is estimated to be 0.03 to 1%.[149, 150] Thus a nucleotide in a given position in the genome differs among individuals on the average every 100 to 3000 base pairs. Therefore the probability is 0.1 to 4.0% that a restriction endonuclease fragment defined by an enzyme recognizing a four-base sequence will differ in size. These restriction fragment length polymorphisms can be assayed in individuals. Because restriction fragment length polymorphisms are inherited as simple mendelian traits, relationships can be established by pedigree analysis. Evaluation of many DNA marker loci allows recognition of well-spaced, highly polymorphic genetic markers and a correlation of the cosegregation of a specific fragment with a particular disease state. Large pedigrees must be analyzed, however, to find at least one or more polymorphic loci that are close enough to the gene responsible for the disease to be informative. The advantage of this technique is that no specific gene isolation is required, and the restriction fragment length polymorphisms can be random sequences, functionally unrelated and physically distant from the DNA encoding the locus responsible for the particular disease. To ensure cosegregation of the marker locus with the disease locus, the loci should be located no more than 20 million base pairs apart on the genome. This methodology has been used to isolate the (defective) genes responsible for chronic granulomatous disease, muscular dystrophy, and cystic fibrosis and to identify polymorphic loci linked to Huntington's disease (chorea).[151]

The use of restriction fragment length polymorphisms offers great potential in the future for the diagnosis of many hereditary endocrine diseases such as polyglandular endocrinopathy, the multiple endocrine neoplasia syndromes, and non–insulin-dependent (type II) diabetes mellitus.[152–154]

A second use of recombinant DNA techniques in detection of defective genes is the application of small, synthetic oligonucleotide probes to detect known point mutations in specific genes. Defective gene expression is often a consequence of a single point mutation in the transcriptional unit. Many of these change a codon and cause a substitution of an amino acid in the encoded protein. The fact that substitution of a single base can lead to profound changes was demonstrated as early as 1959 when Ingram[155] showed that a single amino acid change altered the phenotype of persons with sickle cell anemia. More than 130 separate point mutations have now been identified in the globin genes, all of which result in a defect in gene transcription or a defect in hemoglobin function.[156] Each of these disorders can be identified by hybridization-blotting techniques that utilize small oligonucleotide probes. Such techniques can be applied to any situation in which a specific base mutation is recognized.

The technique of oligonucleotide probe hybridization is probably applicable to certain genetically determined endocrine disorders. At least three point mutations have been identified in the coding region of the insulin gene. Two of these mutations, one resulting in a glycine instead of a phenylalanine[157] and another in a serine instead of a phenylalanine,[158] are in the region of the beta chain containing the phenylalanine at position 24, an amino acid that is critically important to receptor binding. These substitutions thus provide an explanation for the diabetes mellitus in these two kindreds. The third point mutation is in the codon for arginine at position 65 of the proinsulin gene.[159] This substitution blocks conversion of proinsulin to insulin and results in impairment of production of biologically active insulin at the level of post-translational processing of proinsulin.

The application of the polymerase chain reaction for the rapid amplification of DNA sequences has enabled the identification of the genetic defects in vitamin D receptors[160] and thyroid hormone receptors[161] in patients with syndromes of vitamin D and thyroid hormone resistance, respectively.

After the target gene sequence is identified, the genetic locus of concern can be analyzed by amplification and sequencing of DNA from as little as 1 mL of blood. The power of this technique for the amplification and analysis of DNA opens the way for genetic screening of the population.

Gene Therapy

The success of future gene therapy strategies depends on the development of methods to deliver foreign genes effectively into humans by approaches that are minimally invasive. Much work is centered on developing virus-based vectors, such as recombinant adenoviruses and retroviruses, that can package and deliver foreign genes to cells after simply injecting the vectors into an animal.[162] Obstacles that must first be overcome before such an approach is feasible include successful targeting of recombinant virus to the desired cell phenotype and effective means of preventing the virus from destroying the host cells, and/or mounting immune responses.

As described earlier, foreign genes can be introduced and expressed in cultured cells and laboratory animals. It is now feasible to introduce genes encoding hormones into animals. For example the fact that the integration of the growth hormone gene into the germ line of mice results in marked acceleration of growth suggests a practical means for accelerating the growth of livestock.[139] The benefit would accrue from shorter production time and possibly from increased efficiency in food utilization. Furthermore valuable hormones might be commercially produced by extraction from the blood of the animal expressing the specific hormone genes.

Before gene transfer experiments can be undertaken in humans, it will be necessary to obtain additional information about the regulation of the expression of genes. Because the expression of genes encoding polypeptide hormones is characteristically regulated by products of target organs of the hormone, it will be desirable if not essential to include the regulatory elements along with the transcriptional units in the genes that are transferred and to target integration of the genes into a region of genome where no deleterious consequences would occur. For example it would be important not to interrupt or inactivate a gene that has essential biologic functions or to activate otherwise quiescent genes such as proto-oncogenes.

I am indebted to the members of the laboratory, whose forbearance and helpful discussions of this chapter were invaluable. I thank Townley Budde for help in the preparation of the manuscript. J.F.H. is an Investigator with the Howard Hughes Medical Institute.

REFERENCES

1. Watson JD, Crick FHC. Molecular structure of nucleic acids. Nature 1953; 171:737–738.
2. Popenoe EA, du Vigneaud V. A partial sequence of amino acids in performic acid–oxidized vasopressin. J Biol Chem 1954; 206:353–360.
3. Yalow RS. Radioimmunoassay: a probe for the fine structure of biologic systems. Science 1978; 200:1236–1245.
4. Ullrich A, Shine J, Chirgwin J, et al. Rat insulin genes: construction of plasmids containing the coding sequences. Science 1977; 196:1313–1319.
5. Seeburg PH, Shine J, Martial JA, et al. Nucleotide sequence and amplification in bacteria of structural gene for rat growth hormone. Nature 1977; 270:486–490.
6. Gilbert W. DNA sequencing and gene structure. Science 1981; 214:1305–1312.
7. Sanger F. Determination of nucleotide sequences in DNA. Science 1981; 214:1205–1210.
8. Collins FS. Ahead of schedule and under budget: the genome project passes its fifth birthday. Proc Natl Acad Sci USA 1995; 92:10821–10823.
9. Guyer MS and Collins FS. How is the human genome project doing, and what have we learned so far? Proc Natl Acad Sci USA 1995; 92:10841–10848.
10. Roth J, LeRoith D, Shiloach J, et al. The evolutionary origins of hormones, neurotransmitters, and other extracellular chemical messengers. N Engl J Med 1982; 306:523–527.

11. Loumaye E, Thorner J, Catt KJ. Yeast mating pheromone activates mammalian gonadotrophs: evolutionary conservation of a reproductive hormone? Science 1982; 218:1323–1325.

12. Doolittle RF. Similar amino acid sequences: chance or common ancestry? Science 1981; 214:149–159.

13. Uy R, Wold F. Post-translational covalent modification of proteins. Science 1977; 198:890–896.

14. Lingappa VR. Intracellular traffic of newly synthesized proteins. J Clin Invest 1989; 83:739–751.

15. Palade G. Intracellular aspects of the process of protein synthesis. Science 1975; 189:347–358.

16. Morrissey JJ, Cohn DV. Regulation of secretion of parahormone and secretory protein-I from separate intracellular pools by calcium, dibutyryl cyclic AMP, and *l*-isoproterenol. J Cell Biol 1979; 82:93–102.

17. Blobel G. Intracellular protein topogenesis. Proc Natl Acad Sci USA 1980; 77:1496–1500.

18. Lehninger AL. Biochemistry. 2nd ed. New York: Worth, 1975.

19. Blobel G, Dobberstein B. Transfer of proteins across membranes. II. Reconstitution of functional rough microsomes from heterologous components. J Cell Biol 1975; 67:852–862.

20. Palmiter RD, Gagnon J, Walsh KA. Ovalbumin: a secreted protein without a transient hydrophobic leader sequence. Proc Natl Acad Sci USA 1978; 75:94–98.

21. Walter P, Blobel F. Signal recognition particle contains a 7S RNA essential for protein translocation across the endoplasmic reticulum. Nature 1982; 299:691–698.

22. Meyer DI, Krause E, Dobberstein B. Secretory protein translocation across membranes: the role of the "docking protein." Nature 1982; 297:647–650.

23. Habener JF, Amherdt M, Ravazzola M, et al. Parathyroid hormone biosynthesis. J Cell Biol 1979; 80:715–731.

24. Orci L, Like AA, Amherdt M, et al. Monolayer cell culture of neonatal rat pancreas: an ultrastructural and biochemical study of functioning endocrine cells. J Ultrastruct Res 1973; 43:270–297.

25. Chu LLH, MacGregor RR, Cohn DV. Energy-dependent intracellular translocation of proparathormone. J Cell Biol 1977; 72:1–10.

26. Kemper B, Habener JF, Rich A, et al. Microtubules and the intracellular conversion of proparathyroid hormone to parathyroid hormone. Endocrinology 1975; 96:903–912.

27. Smeekens SP, Steiner DF. Identification of a human insulinoma cDNA encoding a novel mammalian protein structurally related to the yeast dibasic processing protease Kex2. J Biol Chem 1990; 265:2997–3000.

28. Bradbury AF, Finnie MDA, Smyth DG. Mechanism of C-terminal amide formation by pituitary enzymes. Nature 1982; 298:686–688.

29. Kornberg RD, Klug A. The nucleosome. Sci Am 1981; 244:52–64.

30. Sharp PA. Speculations on RNA processing. Cell 1981; 23:643–646.

31. Rogers J, Wall R. A mechanism for RNA splicing. Proc Natl Acad Sci USA 1980; 77:1877–1879.

32. Berget SM. Exon recognition in vertebrate splicing. J Biol Chem 1995; 270:2411–2414.

33. Tjian R. Molecular machines that control genes. Sci Am 1995; 54–61.

34. Buratowski S. Mechanisms of gene activation. Science 1995; 270:1773–1774.

35. Burley SK. Picking up the TAB. Nature 1996; 381:112–113.

36. Habener JF, Miller CP, Vallejo M. Cyclic AMP-dependent regulation of gene transcription by CREB and CREM. Vitam Horm 1995; 51:1–57.

37. Burley SK, Xie X, Clark KL, et al. Histone-like transcription factors in eukaryotes. Curr Opin Struct Biol 1997; 7:94–102.

38. Curran T, Franza RB Jr. Fos and Jun: the AP-1 connection. Cell 1988; 55:395–397.

39. Crick F. Split genes and RNA splicing. Science 1979; 204:264–271.

40. Mojsov S, Heinrich G, Wilson IB, et al. Preproglucagon gene expression in pancreas and intestine diversifies at the level of post-translational processing. J Biol Chem 1986; 261:11880–11889.

41. Miller W, Eberhardt NL. Structure and evolution of the growth hormone gene family. Endocr Rev 1983; 4:97–130.

42. Gilbert W. Why genes in pieces? Nature 1978; 271:501.

43. McClintock B. Genes and mutations. Cold Spring Harb Symp Quant Biol 1951; 16:13–47.

44. Calos MP, Miller JH. Transposable elements. Cell 1980; 20:579–595.

45. Hollis GF, Hieter PA, McBride OW, et al. Processed genes: a dispersed human immunoglobulin gene bearing evidence of RNA-type processing. Nature 1982; 296:321–325.

46. Darnell JE. Variety in the level of gene control in eukaryotic cells. Nature 1982; 297:365–371.

47. Brown DD. Gene expression in eukaryotes. Science 1981; 211:667–674.

48. Murdoch GH, Franco R, Evans RM, et al. Polypeptide hormone regulation of gene expression. J Biol Chem 1983; 258:15329–15335.

49. Wegnez M, Schachter BS, Baxter JD, et al. Hormonal regulation of growth hormone mRNA. DNA 1982; 1:145–153.

50. Baxter JD, Ivarie RD. Regulation of gene expression by glucocorticoid hormones: studies of receptors and responses in cultured cells. Receptors Horm Action 1978; 2:251–284.

51. Itoh N, Okamoto H. Translational control of proinsulin synthesis by glucose. Nature 1980; 283:100–102.

52. Skelly RH, Schuppin GT, Ishihara H, et al. Glucose-regulated translational control of proinsulin biosynthesis with that of the proinsulin endopeptidases PC2 and PC3 in the insulin-producing MIN6 cell line. Diabetes 1996; 45:37–43.

53. Habener JF. Regulation of parathyroid hormone secretion and biosynthesis. Annu Rev Physiol 1981; 43:211–223.

54. Firestone GI, Farhang P, Yamamoto KR. Glucocorticoid regulation of protein processing and compartmentalization. Nature 1982; 300:221–225.

55. Britten RF, Davidson EH. Gene regulation for higher cells: a theory. Science 1969; 165:349–357.

56. Davidson EH, Britten RF. Regulation of gene expression: possible role of repetitive sequences. Science 1979; 204:1052–1059.

57. Schmidt CW, Jelinek WR. The Alu family of dispersed repetitive sequences. Science 1982; 216:1065–1070.

58. Sharp PA. Conversion of RNA to DNA in mammals: Alu-like elements and pseudogenes. Nature 1983; 301:471–472.

59. Davidson EH, Jacobs HT, Britten RJ. Very short repeats and coordinate induction of genes. Nature 1983; 301:468–470.

60. Dover G. Molecular drive: a cohesive mode of species evolution. Nature 1982; 299:111–117.

61. Meyer TE, Waeber G, Lin J, et al. The promoter of the gene encoding cAMP-response element binding protein CREB contains cAMP response elements: evidence for positive autoregulation of gene transcription. Endocrinology 1993; 132:770–780.

62. Hattori K, Angel P, Le Beau MM, et al. Structure and chromosomal localization of the functional intronless human JUN protooncogene. Proc Natl Acad Sci USA 1988; 85:9148–9152.

63. Chen R, Inhraham HA, Treacy MN, et al. Autoregulation of pit-1 gene expression mediated by two *cis*-active promoter elements. Nature 1990; 346:583–586.

64. Foulkes NS, Sassone-Corsi P. More is better: activators and repressors from the same gene. Cell 1992; 68:411–414.

65. Johnson AD. The price of repression. Cell 1995; 81:655–658.

66. Ron D, Habener JF. CHOP, a novel developmentally regulated nuclear protein that dimerizes with transcription factors C/EBP and LAP and functions as a dominant-negative inhibitor of gene transcription. Genes Dev 1992; 6:439–453.

67. Starr DB, Matsui W, Thomas JR, et al. Intracellular receptors use a common mechanism to interpret signaling information at response elements. Genes Dev 1996; 10:1271–1283.

68. Wu C, Gilbert W. Tissue-specific exposure of chromatin structure at the 5′ terminus of the preproinsulin II gene. Proc Natl Acad Sci USA 1981; 78:1577–1580.

69. Razin A, Riggs AD. DNA methylation and gene function. Science 1980; 210:604–610.

70. Marx JL. Immunoglobulin genes have enhancers. Science 1983; 221:735–757.

71. Walker MD, Edlund T, Boulet AM, et al. Cell-specific expression controlled by the 5′-flanking region of insulin and chymotrypsin genes. Nature 1983; 306:557–561.

72. Krumlauf R. Hox genes in vertebrate development. Cell 1996; 78:191–201.

73. Beato M. Gene regulation by steroid hormones. Cell 1989; 56:335–344.

74. O'Malley B. The steroid receptor superfamily: more excitement predicted for the future. Mol Endocrinol 1990; 4:363–369.

75. Evans RM. The steroid and thyroid hormone receptor superfamily. Science 1988; 240:889–896.

76. Rosenfeld MG. POU-domain transcription factors: pou-er-ful developmental regulators. Genes Dev 1991; 5:897–907.

77. Lin C, Lin S-C, Chang C-P, et al. Pit-1–dependent expression of the receptor for growth hormone–releasing factor mediates pituitary cell growth. Nature 1992; 360:765–768.

78. Latchman DS. Transcription-factor mutations and disease. N Engl J Med 1996; 334:28–33.

79. Jonsson J, Carlsson L, Edlund T, et al. Insulin-promoter-factor 1 is required for pancreas development in mice. Nature 1994; 371:606–609.

80. Stoffers DA, Zinkin NT, Stanojevic V, et al. Pancreatic agenesis attributable to a single nucleotide deletion in the human *IPF1* gene coding sequence. Nat Genet 1997; 15:106–110.

81. Peers B, Leonard J, Sharma S, et al. Insulin expression in pancreatic islet cells relies on cooperative interactions between the helix loop helix factor E47 and the homeobox factor STF-1. Mol Endocrinol 1994; 8:1798–1806.

82. Luo X, Ikeda Y, Parker KL. A cell-specific nuclear receptor is essential for adrenal and gonadal development and sexual differentiation. Cell 1994; 77:481–490.

83. Zanaria E, Muscatelli F, Bardoni B, et al. An unusual member of the nuclear hormone receptor superfamily responsible for X-linked adrenal hypoplasia congenita. Nature 1994; 372:635–641.

84. Cohen P. The role of protein phosphorylation in neural and hormonal control of cellular activity. Nature 1982; 296:613–620.

85. Rubin RP. The role of calcium in the release of neurotransmitter substances and hormones. Pharmacol Rev 1970; 22:389–428.

86. Hill CS, Treisman R. Transcriptional regulation by extracellular signals: mechanisms and specificity. Cell 1995; 80:199–211.

87. Janknecht R, Hunter T. A growing coactivator network. Nature 1996; 383:22–23.

88. Cobb MH, Goldsmith EJ. How MAP kinases are regulated. J Biol Chem 1995; 270:14843–14846.

89. Schindler C, Darnell JE Jr. Transcriptional responses to polypeptide ligands: the JAK-STAT pathway. Annu Rev Biochem 1995; 64:621–651.
90. Habener JF. Cyclic AMP second messenger signaling pathway. In: DeGroot LJ, et al, eds. Endocrinology. 3rd ed. Vol 1. WB Saunders, 1995: 77–92.
91. Xing J, Ginty DD, Greenberg ME. Coupling of the RAS-MAPK pathway to gene activation by RSK2, a growth factor–regulated CREB kinase. Science 1996; 273:959–963.
92. Axel R. The molecular logic of smell. Sci Am 1995; 273:154–159.
93. Dulac C, Axel R. A novel family of genes encoding putative pheromone receptors in mammals. Cell 1995; 83:195–206.
94. Reanney D. Genetic noise in evolution. Nature 1984; 307:318–319.
95. Ayoubi TAY, Van De Ven WJM. Regulation of gene expression by alternative promoters. FASEB J 1996; 10:453–460.
96. Leid M, Kastner P, Chambon P. Multiplicity generates diversity in the retinoic acid signaling pathways. Trends Biochem Sci 1992; 17:427–433.
97. Kastner P, Krust A, Turcotte B, et al. Two distinct estrogen-regulated promoters generate transcripts encoding the two functionally different human progesterone receptor forms A and B. EMBO J 1990; 9:1603–1614.
98. Vallejo M, Ron D, Miller CP, et al. C/ATF, a novel member of the activating transcription factor family of DNA-binding proteins dimerizes with CAAT/enhancer binding proteins and directs their binding to cAMP response elements. Proc Natl Acad Sci USA 1993; 90:4679–4683.
99. Rosenfeld MG, Mermod JJ, Amara SG, et al. Production of a novel neuropeptide encoded by the calcitonin gene via tissue-specific RNA processing. Nature 1983; 304:129–135.
100. Nawa H, Hirose T, Takashima H, et al. Nucleotide sequences of cloned cDNAs for two types of bovine brain substance P precursor. Nature 1983; 306:32–36.
101. Kitamura N, Takagaki Y, Furuto S, et al. A single gene for bovine high molecular weight and low molecular weight kininogens. Nature 1983; 305:545–549.
102. Segaloff DL, Ascoli M. The lutropin/choriogonadotropin receptor . . . 4 years later. Endoc Rev 1993; 14:324–347.
103. Lee G-H, Proenca R, Montez JM, et al. Abnormal splicing of the leptin receptor in diabetic mice. Nature 1996; 379:632–635.
104. Rawlings SR. PACAP, PACAP receptors, and intracellular signaling. Mol Cell Endocrinol 1994; 101:C5–C9.
105. López AJ. Developmental role of transcription factor isoforms generated by alternative splicing. Dev Biol 1995; 172:396–411.
106. Walker WH, Girardet C, Habener JF. An alternatively spliced, polycistronic mRNA controls a switch from activator to repressor isoforms of transcription factor CREB during spermatogenesis. J Biol Chem 1996; 271:20145–20158.
107. Walker WH, Sanborn BM, Habener JF. An isoform of transcription factor CREM expressed during spermatogenesis lacks the phosphorylation domain and represses cAMP-induced transcription. Proc Natl Acad Sci USA 1994; 91:12423–12427.
108. Dreyfuss G, Hentze M, Lamond AI, et al. From transcript to protein. Cell 1996; 85:963–972.
109. Kozak M. The scanning model for translation: an update. J Cell Biol 1989; 108:229–241.
110. Walker WH, Habener JF. Role of transcription factors CREB and CREM in cAMP-induced regulation of transcription during spermatogenesis. Trends Endocrinol Metab 1996; 4:133–138.
111. Blendy JA, Kaestner KH, Schmid W, et al. Targeting of the CREB gene leads to up-regulation of a novel CREB mRNA isoform. EMBO J 1996; 15:1098–1106.
112. Lechan RM, Wu P, Jackson IMD, et al. Thyrotropin-releasing hormone precursor: characterization in rat brain. Science 1986; 231:159–161.
113. Kurjan J, Herskowitz I. Structure of a yeast pheromone gene (MF): a putative factor precursor contains four tandem copies of mature factor. Cell 1982; 30:933–943.
114. Noda M, Teranishi Y, Yakahashi T, et al. Isolation and structural organization of the human preproenkephalin gene. Nature 1982; 297:431–434.
115. Nakanishi S, Inoue A, Kita T, et al. Nucleotide sequence of cloned cDNA for bovine corticotropin-β-lipotropin precursor. Nature 1979; 278:423–427.
116. Heinrich G, Gros P, Lund PK, et al. Pre-proglucagon messenger RNA: nucleotide and encoded amino acid sequences of the rat pancreatic cDNA. Endocrinology 1984; 115:2176–2181.
117. Zakarian S, Smyth DG. β-Endorphin is processed differently in specific regions of rat pituitary and brain. Nature 1982; 296:250–252.
118. Mojsov S, Weir GC, Habener JF. Insulinotropin: glucagon-like peptide I(7–37) coencoded in the glucagon gene is a potent stimulator of insulin release in perfused rat pancreas. J Clin Invest 1987; 79:616–619.
119. Baltimore D. Viruses, polymerases, and cancers. Science 1976; 192:632–636.
120. Temin HM. The DNA provirus hypothesis. Science 1976; 192:1075–1080.
121. Nathans D, Smith HO. Restriction endonucleases in the analysis and restructuring of DNA molecules. Annu Rev Biochem 1975; 44:273–293.
122. Motulsky AG. Impact of genetic manipulation on society and medicine. Science 1983; 219:135–140.
123. Wu R, ed. Recombinant DNA (part A). Methods Enzymol 1979; 68:1–555.
124. Wu R, Grossman L, Moldave K, eds. Recombinant DNA (part B). Methods Enzymol 1983; 100:1–540.
125. Wu R, Grossman L, Moldave K, eds. Recombinant DNA (part C). Methods Enzymol 1983; 101:1–746.
126. Maniatis T, Fritsch EF, Sambrook J. Molecular Cloning: A Laboratory Manual. Plainview, NY: Cold Spring Harbor Laboratory, 1996.
127. Riccardi RP, Miller JS, Roberts BE. Purification and mapping of specific mRNAs by hybridization-selection and cell-free translation. Proc Natl Acad Sci USA 1979; 76:4927–4931.
128. Chin WW, Kronenberg HM, Dee PC, et al. Nucleotide sequence of mRNA encoding the pre-alpha-subunit of mouse thyrotropin. Proc Natl Acad Sci USA 1981; 78:5329–5333.
129. Gee CE, Chen CL, Roberts JL, et al. Identification of proopiomelanocortin neurones in rat hypothalamus by in situ cDNA-mRNA hybridization. Nature 1983; 306:374–376.
130. Harper ME, Ullrich A, Saunders GF. Localization of the human insulin gene to the distal end of the short arm of chromosome II. Proc Natl Acad Sci USA 1981; 78:4458–4460.
131. Frohman MA, Dush MK, Martin GR. Rapid production of full-length cDNAs from rare transcripts: amplification using a single gene-specific oligonucleotide primer. Proc Natl Acad Sci USA 1988; 85:8998–9002.
132. Eisenstein BI. The polymerase chain reaction: a new method of using molecular genetics for medical diagnosis. N Engl J Med 1990; 322:178–183.
133. Ruddle FH. Applications of somatic cell genetics and gene transfer techniques for the analysis of genetic control and development. In: Schmitt FO, Bird ST, Bloom FE, eds. Molecular Genetic Neuroscience. New York: Raven, 1982:63–72.
134. Owerbach D, Rutter WJ, Martial JA, et al. Genes for growth hormone, chorionic somatomammotropin, and growth hormone–like gene on chromosome 17 in humans. Science 1980; 209:289–292.
135. Owerbach D, Rutter WJ, Cooke NE, et al. The prolactin gene is located on chromosome 6 in humans. Science 1981; 212:815–816.
136. Gonzalez GA, Montminy MR. Cyclic AMP stimulates somatostatin gene transcription by phosphorylation of CREB at serine 133. Cell 1989; 59:675–680.
137. Berg P. Dissections and reconstructions of genes and chromosomes. Science 1981; 213:296–303.
138. Brinster RL, Chen HY, Trumbauer M, et al. Somatic expression of herpes thymidine kinase in mice following injection of a fusion gene into eggs. Cell 1981; 27:223–231.
139. Palmiter RD, Brinster RL, Hammer RE, et al. Dramatic growth of mice that developed from eggs microinjected with metallothionein–growth hormone fusion genes. Nature 1982; 300:611–615.
140. Low MJ, Goodman RH, Brinster RL, et al. Tissue-specific post-translational processing of rat pre-prosomatostatin encoded by a metallothionein-somatostatin fusion gene expressed in transgenic mice. Cell 1985; 41:211–219.
141. Habener JF, Cwikel BJ, Hermann H, et al. Transgenic mice express a vasopressin-metallothionein fusion gene in the magnocellular neurons of the brain and manifest a syndrome of mild nephrogenic diabetes insipidus. J Biol Chem 1989; 264:18844–18852.
142. Bronson SK, Smithies O. Altering mice by homologous recombination using embryonic stem cells. J Biol Chem 1994; 29:7155–27158.
143. Majzoub JA, Muglia LJ. Molecular medicine: knockout mice. N Engl J Med 1996; 334:904–907.
144. Jasin M, Moynahan ME, Richardson C. Targeted transgenesis. Proc Natl Acad Sci USA 1996; 93:8804–8808.
145. Barinaga M. Knockout mice: round two. Science 1994; 265:26–28.
146. Rajewsky K, Gu H, Kühn R, et al. Molecular medicine in genetically engineered animals: conditional gene targeting. J Clin Invest 1996; 98:600–603.
147. Gossen M, Freundlieb S, Bender G, et al. Transcriptional activation by tetracyclines in mammalian cells. Science 1995; 268:1766–1769.
148. Kistner A, Gossen M, Zimmermann F, et al. Doxycycline-mediated quantitative and tissue-specific control of gene expression in transgenic mice. Proc Natl Acad Sci USA 1996; 93:10933–10938.
149. Bostein D, White RL, Skolnick M, et al. Construction of a genetic linkage map in man using restriction fragment length polymorphisms. Am J Hum Genet 1980; 32:314–331.
150. McConkey EH. Molecular evolution, intracellular organization, and the quinary structure of proteins. Proc Natl Acad Sci USA 1982; 79:3236–3240.
151. Gusella JF, Wexler NS, Conneally PM. A polymorphic DNA marker genetically linked to Huntington's disease. Nature 1983; 306:234–237.
152. Bell GI, Selby MJ, Rutter WJ. The highly polymorphic region near the human insulin gene is composed of simple tandemly repeating sequences. Nature 1982; 295:31–35.
153. Rotwein PS, Chirgwin J, Provincer M, et al. Polymorphism in the 5'-flanking region of the human insulin gene: a genetic marker for noninsulin-dependent diabetes. N Engl J Med 1983; 308:65–71.
154. Bell GI, Horita S, Karam JH. A polymorphic locus near the human insulin gene is associated with insulin-dependent diabetes mellitus. Diabetes 1984; 33:176–183.
155. Ingram VM. Abnormal haemoglobins III. The chemical difference between normal and sickle cell haemoglobins. Biochim Biophys Acta 1959; 36:402–411.
156. Treisman R, Orkin SH, Maniatis T. Specific transcription and RNA splicing defects in five cloned β-thalassaemia genes. Nature 1983; 302:591–596.

157. Kwok SCM, Steiner DF, Rubenstein AH, et al. Identification of a point mutation in the human insulin gene giving rise to a structurally abnormal insulin (insulin Chicago). Diabetes 1983; 32:872–875.

158. Haneda M, Chan SJ, Kwok SCM, et al. Studies on mutant human insulin genes: identification and sequence analysis of a gene encoding [Ser824]insulin. Proc Natl Acad Sci USA 1983; 80:6366–6370.

159. Robbins DC, Blix PM, Rubenstein AH, et al. A human proinsulin variant at arginine 65. Nature 1981; 291:679–681.

160. Hughes MR, Malloy PJ, Kieback DG, et al. Point mutations in the human vitamin D receptor gene associated with hypocalcemic rickets. Science 1988; 242:1702–1705.

161. Usala SJ, Tennyson GE, Bale AE, et al. A base mutation of the c-erb A beta thyroid hormone receptor in a kindred with generalized thyroid hormone resistance: molecular heterogeneity in two other kindreds. J Clin Invest 1990; 85:93–100.

162. Gu H, Marth JD, Orban PC, et al. Deletion of a DNA polymerase β gene segment in T cells using cell type-specific gene targeting. Science 1994; 265:103–106.

GENERAL READING

Alberts B, Bray D, Lewis J, et al. Molecular Biology of the Cell. 2nd ed. New York: Garland, 1989.

Antonarakis SE. Diagnosis of genetic disorders at the DNA level. N Engl J Med 1989; 320:153–163 (erratum: 1989; 321:56).

Darnell J, Lodish H, Baltimore D. Molecular Cell Biology. New York: WH Freeman, 1986.

Habener JF, ed. Molecular Cloning of Hormone Genes. Clifton, NJ: Humana, 1987.

Lewin B. Genes IV. 4th ed. New York: John Wiley & Sons, 1990.

Maniatis T, Goodbourn S, Fischer JA. Regulation of inducible and tissue-specific gene expression. Science 1987; 236:1237–1244.

Mitchell PJ, Tjian R. Transcriptional regulation in mammalian cells by sequence-specific DNA binding proteins. Science 1989; 245:371–378.

Ptashne M. How eukaryotic transcriptional activators work. Nature 1988; 335:683–689.

Walson JD, Tooze J, Kurtz DT. Recombinant DNA: A Short Course. New York: WH Freeman, 1983.

3

MEASUREMENT OF HORMONES

Gino V. Segre and Emery N. Brown

INTRODUCTION

The diagnosis of endocrine disorders and the understanding of how hormones regulate physiological processes entered a new era when methods were developed to measure hormones in blood. Prior to the 1960s hormones were usually determined by cumbersome in vivo bioassays. Such assays were based on the response of target tissues to injected test material, such as chorionic gonadotropin bioassays based on increases in ovarian weight in immature rats[1] or luteinizing hormone bioassays based on increases in the weight of the rat prostate gland.[2] Subsequent in vitro hormone assays relied on principles of competitive binding in which the capacity of a hormone in a test sample to compete with radiolabeled hormone for binding to *naturally occurring* binding proteins was measured, and its concentration was estimated by comparing the reduced binding of the radioligand in the presence of hormone in the test sample with binding of the radioligand in the presence of various concentrations of hormone standards under identical conditions. Since few naturally occurring, high-affinity binding proteins are available, this approach had severe limitations.

The breakthrough in the assay of hormones at low concentration came from the work of Berson and Yalow, who recognized that antibodies could serve as hormone (or analyte)-specific, high-affinity binding proteins.[3–7] (*Analyte*, or *ligand*, is a general term that refers to the substance being measured, regardless of its chemical nature.) Since antibodies can be generated to bind virtually any molecule, the use of antibodies in competitive protein-binding assays transformed endocrinology and several other disciplines into quantitative disciplines. The immunogen can be natural or synthetic, or it can function as a hapten after suitable modification. The full

potential of antibody-based competitive protein-binding assays (radioimmunoassays [RIAs]) could not have been realized, however, without the availability of highly pure hormones for radiolabeling (so-called "tracer") and the development of methods for introducing radioactive iodine into these molecules without impairing their capacity to bind to the antibodies.[8, 9] Over the last decades the menu of tests has grown exponentially as solid-phase peptide synthesis and improved chemical technologies have made hormones, hormonal fragments, and hormonal analogues widely available. Radioreceptor assays (RRAs) and bioassays continue to be important for some purposes. First, the measurements of some hormones, such as 1,25-dihydroxycholecalciferol, continue to rely on binding of this active metabolite of vitamin D to nuclear receptors.[10, 11] Second, hormonal fragments or mutant hormones that lack biologic activity may cross-react with authentic hormones when measured by immunoassay, thus providing potentially misleading information that can be clarified by using RRAs and bioassays.[12–14] Third, standards of hormone activity usually are based on measuring the hormone's biologic potency, rather than its immunoreactivity. Fourth, RRAs and bioassays make it possible to characterize the properties of synthetic hormone fragments, chemically modified hormones, and newly discovered hormones. For most clinical purposes, however, RRAs and bioassays lack the precision, specificity, sensitivity, and speed desirable for routine use. Moreover, many RRAs and bioassays are expensive and labor-intensive.

The first three sections of this chapter describe the principles that underlie RIAs, immunometric assays (both *immunoradiometric assays* (IRMAs) and *immunochemiluminometric assays* [ICMAs]), and RRAs. Those seeking more information, especially concerning technical aspects of immunoassays, are referred to texts edited by Berson and Yalow,[15] and Edwards.[16]

The fourth section describes select examples of bioassays. Section five summarizes the criteria for validation of these assays, and the last section deals with traditional and novel statistical procedures used in the reduction and analysis of immunoassay data. Indeed, understanding the procedures by which hormone assays are validated and analyzed is of increasing importance to clinicians as more and more assays are performed by large commercial reference laboratories or by local laboratories that use manufactured kits. On the one hand, many commercial vendors have conducted extensive performance evaluations that establish accurate normal ranges and limitations of immunoassays, and the high quality of reagents and instrumentation now available has enhanced the quality of many clinical assays and makes it possible to compare results from different laboratories with more confidence. On the negative side, however, consultation between the clinician and the laboratory is sometimes more remote because the technical pitfalls of an assay may not be understood by those performing the test locally. In addition, "in-house" correlations of assay results with clinical diagnoses are seldom performed independently. Consequently, despite the availability of improved tests, clinical decision-making still requires the physician to understand basic assay principles, the limitations and validation of each assay, and the statistical methods used to analyze samples. The clinician should be able to ask critical and sophisticated questions of the laboratory director or commercial vendors concerning the parameters of specific assays. Only with such knowledge can the hormone measurements be integrated optimally with the history, physical examination, and other laboratory data.

RADIOIMMUNOASSAYS (RIAs)

RIAs rely on the availability of hormones of sufficiently high purity for labeling with radioisotopes, an adequate, although not necessarily highly purified, supply of hormone for use as immunogen and standard, and antibodies that recognize epitopes in the hormone with high sensitivity and specificity. Most clinical RIAs use polyclonal antiserum rather than monoclonal antibodies, because the myriad of antibodies in antisera are likely to include one or more high-affinity antibodies. In contrast, the likelihood of producing a monoclonal antibody of sufficiently high affinity to be clinically useful is relatively low. Monoclonal antibodies to a specific hormone, however, are more likely to be specific.

RIAs obey the principles of competitive protein-binding assays (Fig. 3–1). The analyte concentration is determined by first measuring the lowered binding of highly purified, radiolabeled "tracer" hormone by analyte in the unknown sample. The concentration of the analyte in the sample is then estimated by comparing the number of counts bound to the antiserum in the presence of the unknown with those bound in the presence of the standard preparation, or

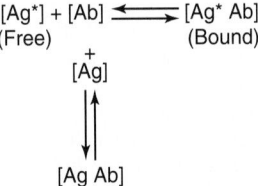

Figure 3–1. Radioimmunoassays and radioreceptor assays are governed by the laws of mass action, in which labeled and unlabeled analyte compete for the limited number of binding sites on either the antiserum or the receptor, respectively. Asterisk (*) indicates the "reporter," usually radioiodine.

"calibrator," at multiple concentrations. Since the amount of serum or plasma added to the assay influences binding of the radioligand to the antiserum, the standards should be assayed under conditions that mimic the conditions used to assay the unknown sample, including the addition of hormone-free serum or plasma or another protein carrier to the standards. With increasing concentration of the analyte or standard, less of the radiolabeled hormone is bound to the antiserum. Assay sensitivity depends on the affinity of antibodies in the antiserum and on the specific activity of the tracer hormone.

Although many immunization protocols have been proposed for making antisera, few have been tested systematically. Usually, after the initial immunization, a booster dose is given a few months later. Generally, titers and/or affinities of antibodies increase after the booster dose, although there is no close relationship between the titer and the affinity.[7] From personal experience and from the experience of others, higher affinity antibodies within the antiserum may be "selected" by the animal's immune system as long as 6 to 18 mo after the initial immunization. Since this feature is not widely recognized, immunization programs often are discontinued prematurely. Since RIAs are most sensitive when the concentration of antibodies is limited, low-affinity antibodies in the antiserum are of little practical significance; high-affinity antibodies determine the sensitivity of the assay. However, cross-reactivity between the immunogen and other molecules is more likely with polyclonal antiserum, because one or more of the high-affinity antibodies generated may recognize epitopes shared by related hormones. The usual high degree of antibody specificity makes this a relatively unusual event, however. Because of the competitive nature of the reaction, RIAs use a relatively small mass of high-affinity antibodies, so that even small animals, i.e., guinea pigs and rabbits, may produce sufficient antiserum to measure the analyte in millions of samples. The mass of tracer to be used is decided empirically. Since the mass of the tracer limits the assay's sensitivity, low amounts need to be used when the concentration of the unlabeled analyte to be measured is low. Low temperature incubation conditions, generally 4°C, also improve sensitivity. If, however, assay sensitivity is not an issue, higher concentrations of antiserum, larger amounts of tracer, and higher incubation temperatures allow the reaction to proceed more rapidly.

Of the methods available for introducing radioactive iodide into the ligand,[7–9] adaptations of the chloramine-T method, originally developed by Hunter and Greenwood, are most widely used.[7, 8] The chloramine-T methods and most other iodination techniques oxidize methionine residues within peptides. This oxidation often renders the peptide biologically inactive, an issue crucial for RRAs, but one that is not necessarily important for RIAs. Labeling of the radioligand at more than a single site obviously increases its specific activity but with the risk of further altering its structure and thereby lowering its immunoreactivity. Although the introduction of only one radioiodine atom per molecule of ligand is generally recommended, the optimal conditions for labeling usually are determined empirically. Reverse-phase high-performance liquid chromatography (HPLC) is usually employed to separate radioligands that bind to the antiserum from unlabeled hormone, free iodide, and radiolabeled hormone that binds inefficiently to the antiserum (so-called "damaged" hormone).

In a typical RIA, fixed amounts of radioactive tracer and antiserum are added simultaneously to tubes that contain standard or unknown mixtures. Specific protocols can be tailored to fit the clinical needs of the assay. Incubation of the samples at 4°C increases sensitivity, as noted previously, partly owing to reduced degradation of the components of the assay by enzymes in the sample. Sensitivity may be enhanced by allowing standard or test sample to preincubate with the antiserum for an empirically determined period of time, before the addition of tracer (so-called "nonequilibrium" assays).[7] Techniques that have been used to separate antibody-bound (usually designated "B") from free unbound tracer (usually designated "F") include precipitation of antigen-antibody complexes with a second antibody directed against the analyte-specific, first antibody. Nonimmune serum from the same species as the first antibody usually is added to ensure complete precipitation of antibody-antigen complexes. Although the second-antibody technique is perhaps least subject to artifact, it is more expensive than other options. Addition of aqueous polyethylene glycol is an alternative for precipitating antigen-antibody complexes and often is used together with the second-antibody method to hasten precipitation and lower the amount of second antibody necessary.[17] Separation of bound from free fractions can also be achieved by adsorbing unbound tracer to a solid-phase matrix, such as charcoal or cellulose,[18, 19] separating antibody-bound tracer from unbound tracer by centrifugation, decanting the supernatant fractions, and assaying one or both fractions for radioactivity. The high reproducibility of robotic instruments for delivering precise volumes of reagents and for aspirating the supernatant make it necessary to collect and count only the precipitant. Total binding, binding in the absence of added hormone (so-called Bo), is estimated in replicates, generally placed at the beginning and end of each assay; some assays are sufficiently stable to use "historical" calibrators, that is, standard curves that are established at weekly or monthly intervals. When the concentration of a specific analyte is too low to be measured by these conventional methods, samples can be adsorbed to a resin, such as cartridges of octadecylsilyl (C18 Sep-Pak cartridges),[20] and eluted in a smaller volume for subsequent assay. Since techniques that involve concentration or extraction of the sample invariably introduce additional error into hormone estimates, the clinician should know when these methods are used and the extent to which they affect the precision of the measurement.

The data can be expressed in several ways. For example, they can be expressed as a ratio of bound counts to free counts (B/F), as a ratio of bound counts in the presence of the sample/total counts bound to the antiserum in the absence of added hormone (B/T), or as a percentage of bound counts in the presence of the sample/counts bound in the absence of added hormone $\times$ 100 (B/Bo). As discussed in greater detail below, the number of replicates necessary for estimating hormone concentrations accurately is continuously being reduced, both because of the improved precision of mechanical pipetting techniques and because market pressures have led many commercial vendors to perform singlicate determinations. While this practice is acceptable with certain assays, the physician must ask for quality-ensurance data to support these abbreviated protocols. Logarithmic, semilogarithmic, or Log/Logit transformation of the data often yields a linear relationship between analyte concentration and B/Bo, a desirable characteristic, especially in the era when computers capable of fitting data to curvilinear functions were not available for routine use.

IMMUNORADIOMETRIC ASSAYS (IRMAs) AND IMMUNOCHEMILUMINOMETRIC ASSAYS (ICMAs)

Immunometric assays are the method of choice for measuring most hormones, especially peptides and proteins.[21] Un-like RIAs, IRMAs use saturating concentrations of two or more antisera that recognize noncompeting epitopes present in the analyte. The principles that underlie IRMAs and ICMAs are the same, except that the signals detected differ. In IRMAs the reporter antiserum is labeled with radioiodine, whereas in ICMAs it is coupled to a chemical reagent that emits a particular wavelength of light when activated. ICMAs most commonly use acridinium esters, although other luminescent compounds, such as luminol and isoluminol, have been used successfully.[22–25] The signal generated in ICMAs is measured in a few seconds with a luminometer, shortening the time required for the procedure. ICMAs are at least as sensitive as IRMAs, have more rapid turnaround time, and avoid both the hazard of radiation exposure and the cost of radioisotope disposal. Both types of immunometric assays require immobilization to a solid-phase matrix of "capture" antibodies in sufficient excess to bind all the analyte in an unknown sample. A second antiserum containing antibodies that do not compete with the first antiserum for binding to the analyte is labeled to high specific-activity and is then added in solution to the assay. The reporter-antiserum binds to the analyte, which has been immobilized by its binding to the first antiserum (Fig. 3–2). Since IRMAs and ICMAs do not require antiserum with as high an affinity for the ligand as do RIAs, many immunometric assays use monoclonal antibodies that can be produced in limitless quantities. Alternatively, large animals, such as sheep and goats, from whom large volumes of serum can be harvested, can be immunized. The antiserum to be labeled must be free from extraneous protein, and antibodies are usually purified and selected by affinity chromatography, in which the desired peptide fragment is covalently coupled to a solid-phase matrix. After the antiserum is incubated with the resin, the bound antiserum is eluted with dilute acid or a chaotropic

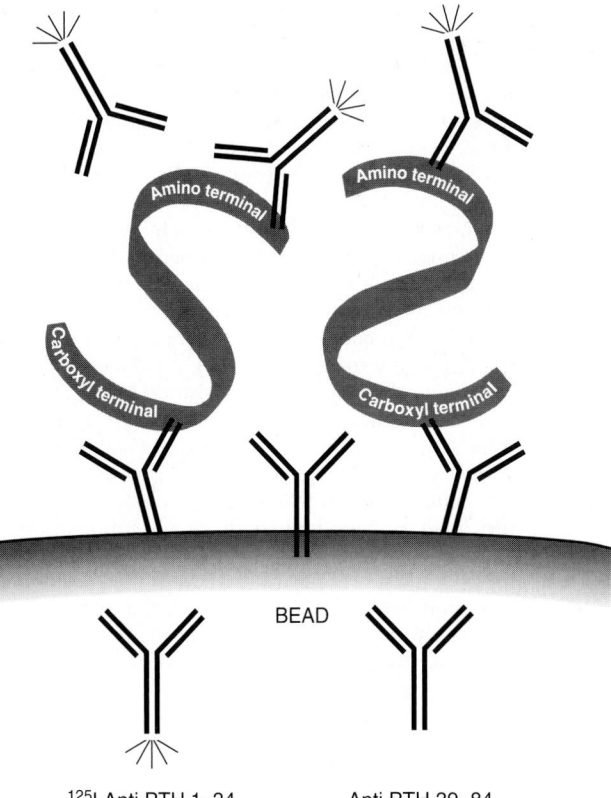

Figure 3–2. A schematic representation of an immunoradiometric assay (IRMA) or immunochemiluminometric assay (ICMA) for measuring immunoreactive PTH. See text for details.

agent to yield immunoglobulins that recognize an epitope or epitopes present in the fragment.[26] The capture antiserum also is usually affinity-purified, although a lower degree of purity is acceptable, because the coupling of extraneous proteins to the solid-phase matrix usually does not affect the assay. In fact, the saturation of "free" sites on the affinity matrix usually lowers nonspecific binding of the reporter antiserum.

Antiserum can be immobilized by simple adherence to the support or covalently coupled after the resin has been activated. The antiserum can also be biotinylated and then bound to a matrix to which avidin has been covalently coupled, or it can be bound to the matrix by a second antibody that recognizes the immunoglobulins from the animal species that generated the analyte-specific, first antiserum. Immobilized capture antiserum is exposed to the test sample or to dilutions of the standard under conditions that are empirically determined. The reporter antiserum can be added after an interval to allow the analyte first to be captured, but adding it at the same time as the sample or standard usually has no ill effects on assay performance. The unknown analyte or standard functions as a bridge from the solid-phase matrix to the reporter antiserum. Since the analyte is the limiting factor in the reaction, the amount of soluble, reporter antiserum bound to the solid-phase matrix is a function of the analyte concentration.

Many solid-phase matrices are suitable as long as the amount of capture antiserum bound to the matrix is rigorously controlled. In one format, capture antiserum is immobilized to 8-mm plastic beads, which facilitates washing, and separation of bound from free reporter antiserum without centrifugation.[27] The surface area to which the capture antiserum can bind on a single large bead is much smaller, however, than the surface area to which it can bind on many small beads that occupy a similar volume. Since the binding reactions proceed at a rate that is partially determined by the concentration of the capture antiserum, the assay kinetics are more rapid when many small beads and, therefore, higher antiserum concentrations are used. On the other hand, immobilizing the capture antiserum on small beads requires that the same amount of capture antiserum be dispensed to each tube; the suspension of beads must, therefore, be thoroughly homogeneous. Another approach is to use paramagnetic particles to which avidin is bound. One antiserum is then biotinylated, and an antiserum that does not compete with the first is labeled with a reporter. The reporter antiserum binds to the paramagnetic particle only when the analyte binds to both antisera, and the amount of bound reporter increases as a function of the analyte concentration. Separation of immobilized reporter-antiserum from soluble, free reporter antiserum is achieved magnetically without centrifugation.[25]

Immunometric assays have several advantages over RIAs. They are more specific for the analyte, because signal generation depends on the ability of the analyte to bind simultaneously two different antisera with recognition for different epitopes of the analyte. The large size of immunoglobulins, relative to that of most analytes, allows the reporter antiserum to be labeled to high specific activity, whereas the sensitivities of RIAs are limited by the mass of the labeled analyte. Moreover, radiolabeled antiserum is more stable than labeled peptide tracers, "nonspecific serum effects" are less troublesome, and nonspecific binding of the reporter antiserum to the matrix is minimal, provided that unreacted sites on the resin or beads are blocked. The useful range of the standard curve is perhaps 5- to 100-fold greater than those of most RIAs, especially RIAs designed to measure analytes at low concentrations, so that fewer samples need to be reassayed at higher dilution. Last, immunometric assays are more precise and easier to perform than RIAs because immobilization of the reporter to the solid-phase matrix facilitates washing and separation of bound from free reporter antiserum.

The speed with which IRMAs and ICMAs can be performed has been utilized to advantage in the operating room. Surgeons are frequently confronted with the dilemma of whether more extensive neck exploration is necessary to identify additional parathyroid glands, after the first diseased gland has been removed. Because of the rapid disappearance of intact parathyroid hormone (PTH) from blood, PTH levels in samples collected 15 min after the gland is removed will be reduced more than 60% as compared with preoperative levels if only a single adenoma is involved. Values will remain high, however, if there is multigland involvement. When the temperature at which PTH is measured in either an IRMA or an ICMA is raised from 4°C to room temperature, PTH levels can be available within 20 min after a blood sample has been collected. The assay loses some of its sensitivity at room temperature, but it can readily distinguish high levels from normal or low hormone concentrations.[28, 29]

RADIORECEPTOR ASSAYS (RRAs)

Radioreceptor assays (RRAs) measure the interaction of a ligand with a biological receptor that mediates the actions of the hormone. These ligands may be agonists, partial agonists, competitive antagonists, or "inverse agonists."[30] Whereas the specificity of immunoassays is determined by certain epitopes recognized by the antiserum, the specificity in RRAs depends on the biologic activity of the analytes. Both immunoassays and RRAs have limitations, although these differ; neither is necessarily "more specific" than the other.

Like RIAs, RRAs are competitive binding assays in which receptors rather than antibodies function as the binding protein. Target tissues or cells usually serve as the receptor source. Clonal cell lines, which are relatively easy to maintain compared with primary cell cultures, have been widely used to characterize the properties of receptors. Generally, the biochemical characteristics of receptors on clonal cell and primary cell cultures are the same, provided that they are derived from the same tissue source. However, pharmacologic, physiological, and regulatory properties vary among clonal cells, even among those from the same source. Fibroblasts and circulating white blood cells express a variety of receptors[31–33] and have the advantage that they can be readily obtained. The receptors in classic target cells and nontarget cells are usually identical. For protein and peptide hormone assays, radioiodinated tracers of high-specific activity are prepared. Radioiodination can impair the bioactivity of the radioligand, presumably because oxidation modifies the structures. Suitable radioligands can be prepared by two approaches. The first involves "gently" labeling the peptide with chloramine T or lactoperoxidase, for example, and separating radiolabeled hormone that binds with high affinity, from unlabeled hormone and other reactants by HPLC. Another approach, extensively used in studies of PTH receptors, is to iodinate an oxidation-resistant, synthetic analogue of PTH in which methionine residues have been replaced with the sterically similar, non-natural amino acid norleucine.[34, 35]

As with RIAs, the interaction between the hormone and its receptor is governed largely by the laws of mass action in which the affinity of the receptors for the ligand determines its binding. Certain features, however, distinguish RRAs from RIAs. For example, agonist occupancy of receptors that signal through guanyl-nucleotide regulatory proteins (G proteins) induces a conformational change in the G protein, which promotes GTP binding to a site that previously was occupied with GDP. This, in turn, accelerates the dissociation of the receptor-bound ligand and, thus, lowers the receptor's affinity for the ligand. A single receptor species thus may have both high- and low-affinity forms and cannot be readily distinguished from two or more receptors with differing affinities for the ligand, unless the cloned cDNAs for receptors are expressed in reporter cells that do not express endogenous receptors for the test compound. Occupancy of a single receptor species with a "pure" antagonist, in contrast, does not activate the G protein, and thus the antagonist has only a single binding kinetic with its cognate receptor. In membrane preparations, the system can sometimes be stabilized either by depleting the preparation of GTP by repetitive washing or by constitutively occupying the GTP-binding site using nonhydrolyzable forms of GTP, such as GTPγS. Such approaches, however, cannot be applied to RRAs with intact cells.

There are many examples of "negative" cooperativity in ligand binding to receptors, as well as a few examples of "positive" cooperativity.[31, 36, 37] Negative cooperativity refers to the phenomenon that increasing receptor occupancy results in more rapid dissociation of bound hormone. When analyzed by the Scatchard formula, the plot of B/F versus concentration of bound hormone is curvilinear and is bowed downward (Fig. 3–3). "Positive" cooperativity occurs when dissociation of bound hormone is progressively retarded by increasing concentrations of bound hormone. When this occurs, Scatchard analysis also is curvilinear, but the curve is bowed upward (Fig. 3–3). Of course, without studies of cloned receptors, neither negative nor positive cooperativity can be distinguished from the possibility that the cells or membranes under study express more than one receptor with differing affinities for the ligand.

With a few exceptions, RRAs have not been widely used clinically, although their impact on our understanding of hormone action has been enormous. RRAs using nuclear receptors for 1,25-dihydroxyvitamin D are the most routinely performed of these assays.[10, 11] Usually, RRAs are less sensitive than either immunoassays or cell- or plasma membrane–based bioassays that measure amplified responses to ligand binding such as hormone-stimulated cAMP or "downstream" responses such as luteinizing hormone (LH)–stimulated testosterone synthesis by Leydig cells.[38] The poor sensitivity of RRAs often requires extraction or concentration of the sample prior to assay, invariably lowering the precision of the measurement. Furthermore, RRAs for peptide hormones generally use partially purified preparations of plasma membranes, which frequently contain enzymes that degrade either receptor and/or the radioligand. Consequently, enzyme inhibitors and low-temperature incubation conditions are routinely used in RRAs.

RRAs have been used to measure autoantibodies to hormone receptors, such as those that bind to receptors for thyroid-stimulating hormone (TSH) and insulin.[39–41] In these situations, they have provided insight into the pathophysiology of certain disease states. RRAs can also be used to measure hormonally active substances, such as dexamethasone or other steroids, for which no immunoassay exists.[42] Autoantibodies that bind to TSH receptors can either stimulate or inhibit TSH action, properties that can be sorted by measuring the capacity of the unknown sample to increase cAMP or to inhibit the TSH-stimulated cAMP response in cells. Although a cultured rat thyroid cell line (FTRL-5) has been used,[43] the cloning of the cDNA for the TSH receptor has led to the development of in vitro assays that use recombinant receptors.[44]

The measurement of immunoglobulins that interact with the TSH receptor is important in selected clinical situations. TSH-like bioactivity measurements can be useful in the differential diagnosis of exophthalmos, particularly if it is unilateral,[45] of pretibial myxedema, and when the diagnosis of the underlying hyperthyroidism is uncertain; autoantibodies are present in the blood of the vast majority of patients with Graves' disease but are not usually detectable in those with toxic nodular goiter.[46] Measurement of these autoantibodies is also useful in the perinatal setting; high levels of maternal thyroid-stimulating autoantibodies define fetuses at greater risk for developing neonatal thyrotoxicosis, and serial measurements of thyroid-stimulating antibodies may help distinguish intrinsic Graves' disease in the infant, in which the autoantibody levels persist, from transient thyrotoxicosis due to passive transfer of maternal autoantibodies, in which they progressively decline.[47–49]

Similarly, RRAs are one of several methods for detecting autoantibodies that interact with the insulin receptor and that can cause either hypoglycemia or hyperglycemia and insulin resistance.[50, 51] Most insulin-treated patients develop antibodies to insulin, even when human insulin is administered. These antibodies can cause severe insulin resistance, although usually they do not interfere with clinical management. In patients with profound insulin resistance, however, it is sometimes useful to distinguish antibodies to heterologous insulin from autoantibodies to the receptor. An assay to detect autoantibodies to the insulin receptor uses a small concentration of ^{125}I-insulin incubated with a detergent-solubilized tissue, such as placenta, that contains insulin receptors. The receptor-insulin complex serves as the tracer, and the antireceptor antibody immunoprecipitates the ligand-receptor complex.[52] An alternative strategy uses radioiodinated, purified insulin receptors.[53]

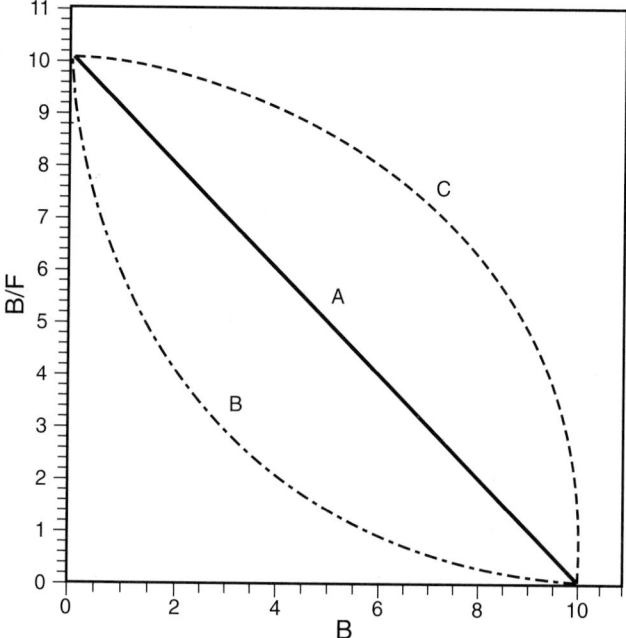

Figure 3–3. Schematic representation of a Scatchard analysis of radioligand binding to a single species of receptor. The same number of receptors is present in A, B, and C. A, When initial binding events do not influence the affinity of the receptor. B, When ligand bound to the receptor dissociates faster as a function of increasing receptor occupancy; the downward curve represents both competition and negative cooperativity. C, When ligand bound to the receptor dissociates slower as a function of increasing receptor occupancy; the upward curve represents both competition and positive cooperativity.

OTHER FUNCTIONAL HORMONE BIOASSAYS

General Considerations

These assays generally measure a second messenger, such as cAMP, whose level is increased by a particular hormone, or in the case of inhibitors of hormone action the assays are used to assess the capacity of a patient sample to inhibit agonist-stimulated cAMP accumulation. More commonly, however, the assays measure a downstream response: a highly-sensitive in vitro bioassay for follicle-stimulating hormone (FSH), for example, is based on FSH-stimulated steroidogenesis in granulosa cells,[54] and the most sensitive available assay for LH is based on measuring androgen synthesis in dispersed Leydig cells.[38] Other assays that measure hormone-specific cAMP generation, such as that for PTH, have been reported but are seldom used clinically.[55, 56]

Ratios of Biologically Active and Immunoreactive Hormones

The simultaneous measurement of bioactivity and immunoreactivity of LH and TSH has shown *qualitative differences* in the hormone that may relate to physiological processes. As discussed in Chapters 9 and 16, LH secretion is pulsatile. The ratio of bioactive LH, as determined by androgen synthesis in Leydig cells, and immunoreactive LH, the "B/I ratio," varies from 2 to 4 at the nadir of the serum LH pulsation, to values of 4 to 6 with LH peaks.[57] Postmenopausal women and patients with gonadal dysgenesis have higher B/I ratios of LH than normally cycling women, and estrogen treatment restores this ratio toward normal.[58] B/I ratios of TSH also vary. Generally, the TSH-stimulated cAMP accumulation by rat thyroid cells has been compared with immunoreactive TSH. Decreased B/I ratios have been reported in patients with hypothalamic hypothyroidism,[59, 60] whereas B/I ratios are high in hyperthyroid patients with TSH-producing tumors.[61, 62] In vitro, TRH stimulation of rat pituitary explants decreases the B/I ratio of TSH.[63] The biochemical explanations for these differences are not clear, but post-translation modifications, such as the state of hormone glycosylation, are thought to play a role.[64]

ASSAY VALIDATION

General Considerations

In vivo bioassays are subject to a variety of factors that do not influence in vitro tests. When using in vivo tests, it is necessary to consider hormonal clearance mechanisms and secondary effects induced by injection of the test substance, which may, in turn, influence the response being measured. For example, TSH, LH, and FSH are cleared from the circulation far more rapidly when they are administered in their glycosylated form than when they are deglycosylated, although the two forms bind their cognate receptors and activate effector pathways equally in vitro. Also, in vivo, the hypoglycemic effects of insulin are influenced by "counterregulatory" changes in glucagon, catecholamine, and growth hormone secretion that tend to elevate blood glucose. Therefore, although in vivo bioassays are useful in many circumstances, they are subject to variables that usually can only be imprecisely controlled.

Although in vitro assays are easier to control than in vivo assays, they are subject to variables that influence their performance, depending on the inherent properties of the specific test. Immunoassays, for example, are usually unaffected by biologic variability of the hormone or by the presence of unrelated substances that may influence the actions of the hormone. However, since relatively short linear peptide segments commonly constitute the major epitopes recognized by antibodies in the immunoassay, such antibodies also may bind to molecules that share a common epitope, such as precursor forms and hormonal fragments that may be present in blood or other biologic fluids. As discussed later, different hormones also may share common epitopes. RRAs, on the other hand, cannot distinguish between related compounds that bind to the same receptor but do not have the same immunologic properties. Also, RRAs usually do not distinguish receptor agonists from receptor antagonists, although these different properties can be resolved by measuring effector or other downstream responses.

The validity of any assay procedure requires that varying known concentrations of the analyte be accurately measured when they are added to the fluid, usually serum or plasma. Traditionally, the second requirement was that the hormone should not be detectable in body fluids after the gland that secretes it has been extirpated. Many current assays, however, measure paracrine, autocrine, or juxtacrine factors, in addition to traditional hormones. Since these factors, as well as certain hormones, are synthesized at multiple sites, it is usually not possible to fulfill this criterion, except in mice, where genes encoding peptides and proteins can be deleted genetically by homologous recombination.

Validation of immunologic assays or bioassays also requires that the apparent hormone concentration be independent of the dilution at which it is measured and that the concentration of the hormone in the unknown sample decrease with a dilution curve that is superimposable on the dilution curve of the standard over a reasonably wide concentration range. The sample and standard are said to be "immunochemically identical," when this criterion is met in an immunoassay. Although different RIAs may be specific for a particular hormone, immunochemical identity may be present with one assay, but not with another assay (Fig. 3–4). Meeting this criterion means only that the analyte can be measured reliably, but it does not mean that the standard and the analyte are *chemically identical*. In the past, the choice of appropriate standards was a serious issue. Hormones generally were extracted and partially purified from animal glands or the standards were based on dilutions of plasma from patients with high blood levels. Many of these problems have been solved now that purified human hormones or their fragments can be synthesized by solid-phase protein chemistry or by the expression of cloned cDNAs. Similar qualifications apply to bioassays, since intact hormone and its fragments may have identical biologic properties in a given assay but differ chemically (see later).

IRMAs and ICMAs can give artifactually low results, if the amount of immobilized capture antiserum is insufficient to scavenge all the analyte in the sample that is recognized by the reporter antiserum. When the excess analyte remains in solution, it binds the reporter antiserum, thus precluding the binding of the reporter antiserum to the immobilized antiserum-analyte complex. Dose-dilutions of such samples depict a "hook" in which, with decreasing volume of sample, bound reporter-antiserum levels increase before decreasing along a dilution curve parallel to that of the standard. The authors have observed this phenomenon in blood from a few cancer patients with ectopic corticotropin production and in patients with parathyroid carcinoma, all of whom had extraordinarily high hormone levels. Therefore, when the clinical presentation predicts a very high level of hormone but the IRMA or ICMA result is unexpectedly low, the clinician should ask for the sample to be measured at multiple dilutions.

A "hook" phenomenon in RIAs appears to be the result of positive cooperativity; when tracer is incubated with low concentrations of unlabeled analyte, binding to the antiserum increases, in a dose-dependent manner, above that observed in the absence of competing unlabeled analyte. Further increases in the concentration of unlabeled analyte result in a decrease in radioligand binding.[65]

Even though standard and sample may not have identical

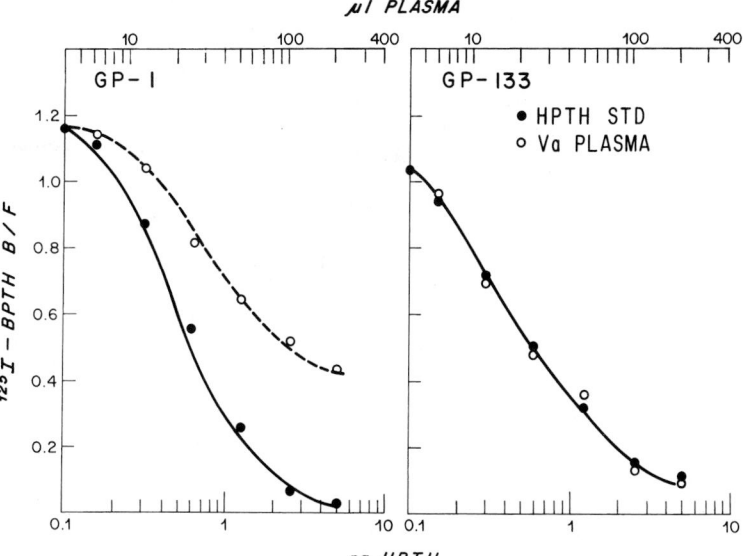

Figure 3–4. Immunoreactivity of plasma parathyroid hormone (PTH) as detected by two antisera to PTH, GP-1 and GP-133. The dose-dilution curve of venous plasma (○--○) differed from that of purified human PTH (●-●) (HPTH) when assayed with GP-1 (*left panel*) but was indistinguishable from the human PTH when the same sample was assayed with GP-133 (*right panel*). The latter is an example of immunochemical identity.

properties in a given immunoassay or bioassay, the assay may, nonetheless, provide a "rough" estimate of hormone concentration that is useful clinically. The ultimate criteria by which any assay should be judged in the clinical setting is its usefulness for establishing a particular diagnosis and for differentiating among various diseases whose presentations are clinically similar. The suitability of any specific assays for research, obviously, depends on the specific disease or physiological process under study.

Assay Conditions and Sample Preparation

Many hormones are degraded by enzymes in blood and other biologic fluids. Degradation of hormone at any step prior to the time that samples are added to the assay, such as during collection and processing of the sample, is generally assessed by assaying recovery of known hormone concentrations, when they are processed under conditions that mimic those of the test samples. In theory, it may only be necessary that test samples and standards be degraded identically during the assay procedure to permit accurate quantification (unless degradation is complete). Practically, every effort to prevent degradation should be explored. Low temperature increases the sensitivity of immunoassays and RRAs, in part by slowing the rate at which components in the assay are degraded and in part by their influence on analyte-antibody and analyte-receptor interactions. Enzyme inhibitors, such as EDTA (ethylenediaminetetraacetic acid) and trypsin inhibitors, are routinely added. Degradation of the tracers, samples, and receptors generally is more substantial than degradation of antiserum. The most reliable method for assessing tracer degradation is to compare binding of the tracer to the antiserum (or receptor) under the usual incubation conditions with rebinding of the same tracer after it has been incubated under conditions that mimic as closely as possible those used to assay test samples. Sample stability is particularly critical, because many steps are involved in collection, processing, and storing. Short-term sample stability is determined usually by assaying replicates stored for short periods of time under various conditions, i.e., room temperature, 4°C, frozen, and after several freeze-thaw cycles. Samples also should be stored frozen at −20°C and −80°C and assayed at intervals up to 6 to 12 mo or longer to determine their long-term stability. Optimal patient care requires that the physician know these parameters, know that blood samples are collected in tubes containing the appropriate enzyme inhibitors to block hormone degradation, and be certain that samples have been processed appropriately.

Cross-Reactivity of Hormones

Conditions that interfere nonspecifically with the chemical reaction can usually be avoided. For an assay to measure a specific analyte accurately, however, issues relating to cross-reactivity also must be addressed. The use and limitations of heterologous hormone and plasma standards were discussed earlier. Blood or tissue extracts, however, may contain different hormones that cross-react immunologically. In some instances the dose-dilution curve of the test sample differs from the standard and thus provides a clue to the presence of chemically distinct molecules in the sample. Plasma obtained from pregnant women, for example, contains placental lactogen, that has epitopes that resemble those of growth hormone and that partially cross-react in some assays.[66] Some peptides are products of the same gene and share amino acid sequence overlap, although their biologic functions are quite different. For example, the proopiomelanocortin gene encodes corticotropin, melanocyte-stimulating hormone (MSH), and lipotropin, all three of which may cross-react in some assays.[67] Other hormones, such as gastrin and cholecystokinin, are encoded by different genes but have the same C-terminal pentapeptide and cross-react in some assays. Similarly, some peptides have identical properties in an RRA and in some other bioassays, although they are chemically and immunochemically distinct. PTH and PTH-related peptide are indistinguishable by RRAs, by bioassay for cAMP production, and by some other assays of downstream responses; they share limited NH_2-terminal sequence homology, but no immunoassays, to date, recognize both peptides.[68–70] Also, transforming growth factor α (TGF α) and epidermal growth factor (EGF) bind with similar affinities to the same receptor, and biologic responses caused by these two peptides are usually similar,[71, 72] but they share little sequence homology and do not immunologically cross-react.

Heterogeneity of Hormones in Blood

The measurement of peptide hormones is often complicated by the presence of closely related peptides in the circulation. These forms may be precursors or hormonal fragments with varying degrees of biologic activity. For example, proinsulin levels are low in normal subjects but usually exceed the concentration of insulin in plasma from patients with insulinomas.[73, 74] Since insulin assays usually do not distinguish between these two peptides, accurate assessment of proinsulin levels requires the use of an immunoassay that recognizes determinants in the connecting or C-peptide that links insulin's alpha and beta chains.

In some instances the concentration of the form of the hormone that is thought to be the principal biologic species, in fact, constitutes only a small portion of the total plasma immunoreactive hormone, even in normal subjects. Berson and Yalow first showed that PTH in plasma is immunochemically different from hormone extracted from the gland when assayed with one antiserum but identical when assayed with a second antiserum.[75] Subsequent studies showed that 50 to 70% of the immunoreactive PTH in the blood of normal subjects consists of fragments that lack about one third of the NH$_2$-terminal portion of the PTH sequence (Fig. 3–5).[12] Consequently, these fragments cannot be biologically active. Moreover, intact hormone is cleared rapidly from the blood by both hepatic and renal mechanisms, whereas the mid-COOH-terminal fragments are cleared mainly by the kidneys.[76, 77] Therefore, mid-COOH-terminal fragments constitute more than 95% of the circulating immunoreactive PTH in patients with severe renal insufficiency, when assayed by COOH-terminal or "midregion" PTH assays. Nearly all early PTH RIAs used antiserum that recognized epitopes common to intact hormone and these mid-COOH-terminal fragments, because the high levels of these PTH fragments made it relatively easy to measure immunoreactive PTH in blood; assays with antiserum that recognized epitopes in the NH$_2$-terminal sequence must be more sensitive by an order of magnitude to be clinically useful.[78, 79]

The heterogeneity of PTH in blood results both from secretion of hormonal fragments by the parathyroid glands and from postsecretory metabolism of the intact hormone,[12, 76, 80–84] mostly by enzymes in Kupffer cells that line hepatic sinusoids.[85] Since NH$_2$-terminal PTH fragments do not normally circulate, NH$_2$-terminal assays provide the required specificity for measuring intact hormone, but none were sensitive enough to measure PTH in the blood of all normal subjects.[79] An IRMA that was highly specific for intact PTH was then developed in collaborative studies between the Nichols Institute and the authors' laboratory.[27] This assay readily detects PTH in all normal subjects. An antiserum to the COOH-terminal portion of the PTH molecule was used to capture PTH from the sample, and the analyte was then detected with a radioiodinated NH$_2$-terminal antiserum. This assay and similar two-site assays subsequently developed by others distinguish all patients with hypercalcemia due to malignancy and other hypercalcemic states from those with hyperparathyroidism and separate nearly all patients with hypoparathyroidism and hyperparathyroidism from normal subjects. Additionally, with assays that recognize intact PTH, it became possible to predict the development of osteodystrophy that occurs commonly in patients with end-stage renal disease, a prediction not possible with midregion or COOH-terminal PTH assays.[86–88]

STATISTICAL PROCEDURES FOR IMMUNOASSAY DATA-REDUCTION

General Considerations

To appreciate how the reliability of assay analyses is established, it is useful to review the basic concepts that underlie the statistical data-reduction procedures used in immunoassays. These same concepts, with some modifications, also apply to RRAs and bioassays. Data-reduction is the process through which a biochemical measurement made in an immunoassay is converted into a quantitative estimate of an analyte. For most immunoassays performed on automated analyzers, data-reduction is performed by prepackaged software that is incorporated into the analyzer and is not generally directly accessible to the physician. Nonetheless, to have confidence in the measurement and to avoid assigning undue importance to small changes in hormone concentration, the physician should understand the computations that the software is performing. The data-reduction process is described in four stages: calibration, measurement, quality control, and the definition of the minimal detectable concentration for the assay.

Calibration

Calibration is the process by which a dose-response relation is established between prescribed standard concentrations, or calibrators, of the assay analyte and their responses, or measured signals.[89] The calibrators contain known concentrations of the analyte that span the range believed to be medically or biologically important. Until recently, a calibration was performed with each run or batch of experimental samples to be analyzed. The calibration consisted of two to three replicates of each of 5 to 9 concentrations of the standard. Given the increasing reliability of new automated analyzers, some calibrations are currently performed with only

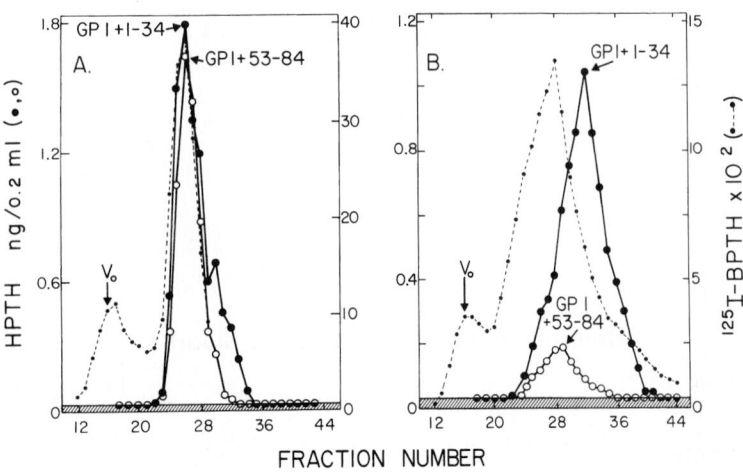

Figure 3–5. Comparison of immunoreactive parathyroid hormone (PTH) in fractions after gel filtration on Bio-Gel P-10 of plasma from the parathyroid vein *(A)* and from the peripheral circulation *(B)* from the same patient with primary hyperparathyroidism. Samples were assayed using antiserum GP-1, which was modified to recognize epitopes in the COOH-terminal portion of the PTH molecule by incubating it with excess concentrations of PTH(1–34) to block recognition by antibodies recognizing this portion of the sequence (GP-1 + 1–34, ●—●). Alternatively, GP-1 incubated with excess concentrations of PTH(53–84) recognizes epitopes present within the NH$_2$-terminal portion of the sequence (GP-1 + 53–84, ○—○). Radioiodinated bovine PTH was cochromatographed as a marker for the elution position of intact hormone (●--●). V$_o$ marks the void volume of the column. The cross-hatched areas represent the detection limits of the RIAs. (Redrawn from Segre GV, Habener JF, Powell P, et al. Parathyroid hormone in human plasma: immunochemical characterization and biological implications. J Clin Invest 1972; 51:3163–3172. By copyright permission of the American Society for Clinical Investigation.)

FRACTION NUMBER

one replicate of each calibrator, and computation of the dose-response curve may be repeated only once a day or once a month. The dose-response relation has been estimated by a variety of statistical procedures. The non–model-based procedures include hand-drawn curves and interpolating splines. Interpolating splines are mathematical procedures for computing the smoothest curve connecting a set of experimental data whose measurement error is small. They do not alter the data but simply connect the experimental points. Many kinds of current immunoassay data-reduction software use interpolating splines. The model-based procedures assume that the dose-response relation obeys a specific functional equation and then use formal statistical procedures, such as nonlinear least squares or maximum likelihood, to fit this equation to the set of calibrators and their responses.[90] The four-parameter logistic equation and modifications of it are the most widely used model-based calibration procedures, because they have been shown empirically to describe well the dose-response curve for a wide range of immunoassay systems. The four-parameter logistic equation is

$$y = \frac{a - d}{1 + \left(\dfrac{x}{c}\right)^{\mathrm{b}}} + d$$

where y is the measured level, a is the measured level at the zero dose for RIAs or high dose for IRMAs, b is the slope of the equation on the log scale, c is the EC_{50}, the concentration corresponding to 50% specific binding, d is the measured level at the high dose for RIAs or zero dose for IRMAs, and x is the calibrator concentration (Fig. 3–6).

Measurement

Measurement is the process by which the concentration of the analyte in a sample specimen is determined. The dose-response curve is the principal tool used to quantify or measure the analyte. In this context, the *dose* is the concentration of analyte in the sample specimen, and the *response* is the quantitative signal generated in the assay in response to a given dose. It is crucial that the dose-response curve describe

a monotonic relation between analyte and response. That is, one analyte concentration corresponds to one and only one response value. Hence, given the dose-response curve and the assay's response to a sample specimen, it is possible to determine the concentration of the analyte in the specimen by finding the analyte value on the dose-response curve that corresponds to that response. (The possible *hook* effects described earlier, which may be present at low analyte levels in RIAs and at high analyte levels in IRMAs, illustrate the importance of this criterion.) This procedure is termed backfitting. If replicates of the specimen have been measured in the assay, the measured concentration is reported as the average of the backfitted values. The average and standard deviations of the estimate are used to compute the specimen's coefficient-of-variation (CV), the ratio of the standard deviation to the average. If replicates of a given calibrator are assayed and used to compute average and standard deviations of the estimate, the resultant CV is the intra-assay CV at that dose. The interassay CV at a specified dose is obtained by computing the mean and standard deviations between assays. What constitutes an unacceptable CV depends on the specific assay, the dose-range of interest, and how the results influence clinical decision-making. The value of 20% is often used empirically, as the upper limit of acceptable interassay CVs. The increased reliability of automated analyzers, the rising cost of assaying large numbers of samples, and the desire to reduce radioactive wastes have made assaying only one replicate of a sample specimen an increasingly common practice.

Quality Control

Quality control, the process through which an immunoassay's reproducibility and sensitivity are verified to be within previously defined limits,[91] is accomplished by measuring two or three specified samples of known concentrations with each assay calibration or during certain times in routine assay experiments. The choice of the appropriate control concentrations is important; they are usually selected to represent low, middle, and high ranges of the assay. When the assay is first established, acceptable variation in measuring these controls, or control limits, is determined for each concentration. These limits are defined empirically by choosing at least 20 consecutive assays during which it is considered to have performed "in control." The most common practice for monitoring assay quality is to chart the assayed values of the control specimens over time and to use the control limits along with various statistical criteria to detect both systematic and random errors and to determine when the assay is *out-of-control*. Commonly used control charts include the Levey-Jennings, the Cumulative Sum (CUSUM), and the Westgard Multi-rule charts. The Levey-Jennings system is most sensitive to random errors, CUSUM systems are most sensitive to systematic errors, and the Westgard Multi-rule system detects both.

The quality-control analysis applied to the controls helps ensure that the reported assay results are accurate by comparing control results with guidelines based on previous assay runs in which the performance was considered acceptable. While the quality control of the assay is generally assessed by charting the performance of the control specimens, the calibrators also play an indirect role in evaluating quality control. For example, if sufficient numbers of the measured calibrator concentrations are inconsistent with their expected concentrations, the quality of the assay is considered poor, and it generally is repeated. In the same way, the control specimens are used indirectly to calibrate the assay, since, if a significant number of the controls do not agree with their intended concentrations, the calibration is considered to be in error, and the assay is repeated. The frequency with which a quality-control analysis is undertaken varies, depending on

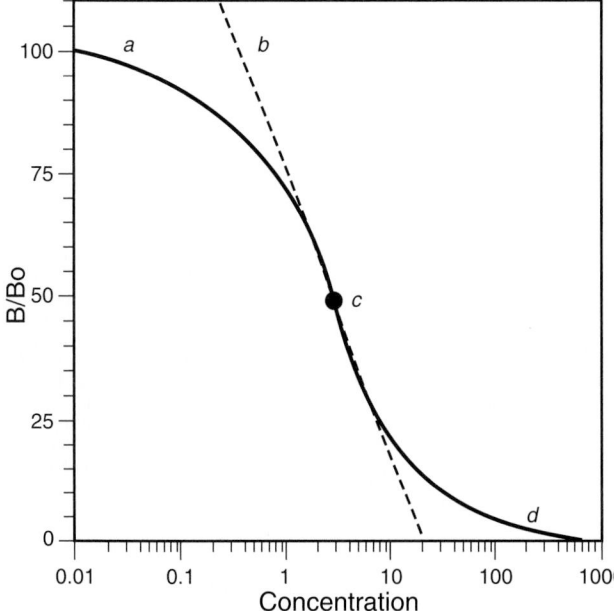

Figure 3–6. A four-parameter logistic-equation dose-response curve for a radioimmunoassay. See text for details.

the analyte being measured, the perceived reliability of the assay system, costs, and the medical or scientific importance of the reported results.

Minimal Detectable Concentration (MDC)

Definition of the minimal detectable concentration (MDC) for each immunoassay is essential for detecting disease states associated with low analyte concentrations; a common example is the use of low TSH levels to define hyperthyroidism and excess thyroid hormone replacement. It also is a criterion for developing a new assay and the property most often reported when comparing the performance of different assays for the same analyte. The MDC is usually determined when the assay is first established in a special calibration analysis; the dose-response curve is estimated with an excess of calibrator replicates; for example, 8 to 20 *zero-dose* calibrators, in which no analyte is added, and two or more replicates of each non-blank calibrator. Both the zero-dose and the standard calibrators are in the same medium (i.e, serum or buffer), and the medium should resemble that of the clinical test samples as closely as possible. These conditions differ from the immunoassay calibration used in the performance of routine assays, in which the dose-response curve is estimated with at most two replicates of each calibrator and in which an MDC is not usually determined or is estimated with only a few zero-dose replicates.

Several mathematical formulations of the MDC have been proposed[5, 92-94]; three of them are derived from the work of Currie and are used routinely in immunoassay data-reduction computations: they are the *critical limit*, the *detection limit*, and the *determination limit*.[92] The *critical limit* is the upper confidence limit of the zero-dose calibrator. In statistical terms it is termed an upper 1-α confidence limit, with an α chosen to be either 0.025 or 0.05. Thus, the level of confidence associated with this limit is 0.975 or 0.95, respectively. The critical limit sets a cutoff at which it can be concluded that an analyte has been detected and is not zero with probability 1-α. The quantity α defines the probability of a type I error, the probability of classifying a truly zero measurement as detectable. One way of understanding the critical-limit definition is to imagine assaying 1000 zero-dose calibrators. Even though none contains analyte, the assay will measure a small positive quantity

in some of the samples. A histogram consisting of all measured concentrations gives an empirical determination of the uncertainty in the zero-blank calibrator. The histogram's total area is 1, which is the sum of the areas in each group, or *bin*, in the histogram. Dividing the number of samples in each bin by 1000 gives a normalized histogram, or probability density (Fig. 3–7). If α is set to 0.025, the critical limit becomes the 975th largest measured value; 25 values are larger than the critical limit. In terms of the probability density, there is a 0.025 probability of a truly blank value being larger than the critical limit.

The *detection limit* defines the analyte concentration that has the critical limit as its 1-β lower confidence limit. Like α, β is also typically set to either 0.025 or 0.05. This MDC definition defines a cutoff level such that analyte concentrations beyond this value may be reported as reliably detected, where *reliably detected* means with a probability of at least 0.975 or 0.95. The probability β is the likelihood of a type II error; it represents the probability of classifying a truly nonzero measurement as undetectable. The detection limit can be thought of as being determined in the same way as the critical limit except, instead of measuring blank calibrators, 1000 measurements are performed on each of several analyte concentrations close to zero. Because the assay is not a perfect procedure, the 1000 measurements of a given concentration will fall in a range centered around the true value. The set of measurements for each concentration can again be converted into a normalized histogram, or probability density. If β is set at 0.05, for example, the detection limit is the concentration whose 50th largest measurement equals the critical limit (see Fig. 3–7). The detection limit is more conservative than the critical limit, since it considers both type I and type II errors. In practice, the critical and detection limits are determined with 20 to 50 replicates—not 1000.

The critical limit and the detection limit provide *qualitative definitions* of the minimal detection concept, since neither assigns a level of precision to its MDC estimate. On the other hand, the *determination limit*, also termed the *limit of quantitation*, is the smallest analyte concentration that can be measured *quantitatively* with a specified level of precision, where the level of precision is defined in terms of a coefficient of variation (CV). A CV of 20% or less is frequently used in this definition, although a smaller or larger CV may be more appropriate, depending on the specific application of the assay.

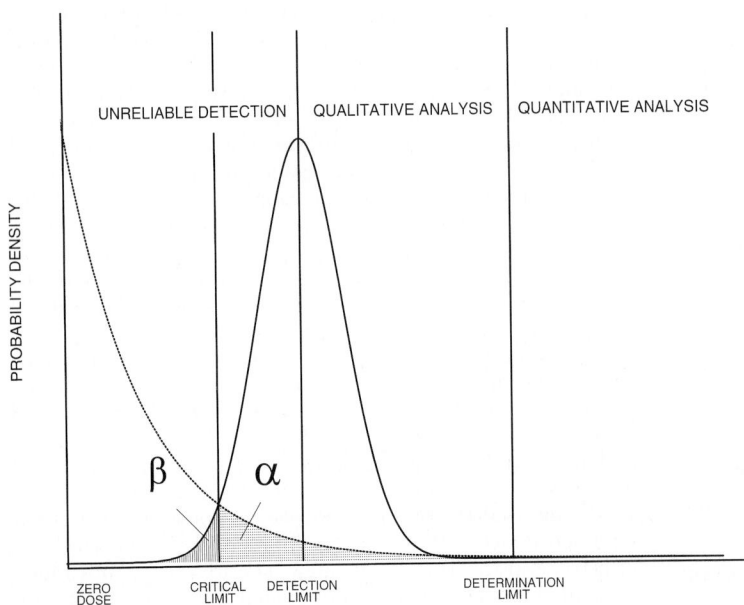

Figure 3–7. The relationship between the *critical limit,* the *detection limit,* and the *determination limit* as defined by Currie.[92] These three definitions separate the neighborhood near the zero point into three analytic zones, which from left to right are the regions of (1) unreliable detection, (2) qualitative analysis, and (3) quantitative analysis. The *detection limit* defines the border between region 1 and region 2, whereas the *determination limit* the border between region 2 and region 3. The curve on the left represents measurements of a zero-dose calibrator, the curve on the right represents measurements of a low-dose calibrator. Alpha (α) is the probability of classifying a truly zero measurement as detectable (type I error). Beta (β) is the probability of classifying a truly nonzero measurement as undetectable (type II error).

These three definitions separate the neighborhood near zero into three analytic zones: the regions of (1) unreliable detection, (2) qualitative analysis, and (3) quantitative analysis (see Fig. 3–7). The detection limit defines the border between region 1 and region 2, whereas the determination limit the border between region 2 and region 3. The critical limit lies within the region of unreliable detection because it does not consider type II error. Therefore, it can give a misleading MDC estimate. Nevertheless, it is the most commonly used MDC definition, because it is the simplest to compute and because it represents the lowest legitimate estimate of the MDC.[95] It is crucial to recognize, however, that calibrations are not conducted with large numbers of replicates in routine immunoassays; at most, two or three replicates of each calibrator and, at most, two zero calibrators are typically used. Hence, the MDC that is determined as part of the special calibration analysis when an assay is established is an overly optimistic estimate of the MDC for an assay performed under *routine conditions*.

Application of Bayes' Rule to the Reduction of Immunoassay Data

Immunoassay data can also be reduced, based on Bayes' rule.[96] Bayes' rule computes the probability of one event, given that another event has occurred. The principal advantage of Bayes' rule is that it makes error computations an explicit part of each specimen measurement, including those assayed as singlicates and it provides a MDC definition that can be computed from any assay calibration experiment that includes a zero-dose calibrator. The detection limit defined by this approach is higher than the critical limit described in the previous section. The use of Bayes' rule is especially appropriate for immunoassay data-reduction analyses, because it acknowledges that one or at most a few calibrators are routinely assayed at each dose. Since the Bayesian approach allows data that are collected routinely in the clinical laboratory to be interpreted with statistical rigor, its application can improve the calibration and quality control components of the data-reduction process and help resolve some of the ambiguities in the definition and determination of the MDC.

REFERENCES

1. Steelman SM, Pohley FM. Assay of follicle-stimulating hormone based on the augmentation with human chorionic gonadotropin. Endocrinology 1953; 53:604–616.
2. Greep RO, van Dyke HB, Chow BF. Use of the anterior lobe of the prostate gland in the assay of metakentrin. Proc Soc Exp Biol Med 1941; 46:644–649.
3. Yalow RS, Berson SA. Assay of plasma insulin in human subjects by immunological methods. Nature 1959; 184:1648–1649.
4. Yalow RS, Berson SA. Immunoassay of endogenous plasma insulin in man. J Clin Invest 1960; 39:1157–1175.
5. Yalow RS, Berson SA. Special problems in the radioimmunoassay of small polypeptides. In: Margoulies M, ed. Protein and Polypeptide Hormones. Amsterdam: Excerpta Medica, 1969: 71–76.
6. Yalow RS. Radioimmunoassay methodology: application to problems of heterogeneity of peptide hormones. Pharmacol Rev 1973; 25:161–178.
7. Berson SA, Yalow RS. General radioimmunoassay. In: Berson SA, Yalow RS, eds. Methods in Investigative and Diagnostic Endocrinology. Amsterdam: North Holland, 1973: 84–120.
8. Hunter WM, Greenwood FC. Preparation of iodine-131 labelled human growth hormone of high specific activity. Nature 1962; 194:495–496.
9. Bolton AE, Hunter WM. The labelling of proteins to high specific radioactivities by conjugation to a ^{125}I-containing acylating agent. Biochem J 1973; 133:529–538.
10. Eisman JA, Hamstra AJ, Kream BE, et al. A sensitive, precise, and convenient method for determination of 1,25-dihydroxyvitamin D in human plasma. Arch Biochem Biophys 1976; 176:235–243.
11. Eisman JA, Hamstra AJ, Kream BE, et al. 1,25-Dihydroxyvitamin D in biological fluids: a simplified and sensitive assay. Science 1976; 193:1021–1023.
12. Segre GV, Habener JF, Powell D, et al. Parathyroid hormone in human plasma: immunochemical characterization and biological implications. J Clin Invest 1972; 51:3163–3172.
13. Given BD, Mako ME, Tager HS, et al. Diabetes due to secretion of an abnormal insulin. N Engl J Med 1980; 302:129–135.
14. Shoelson S, Haneda M, Blix P, et al. Three mutant insulins in man. Nature 1983; 302:540–543.
15. Berson SA, Yalow RS. Methods in Investigative and Diagnostic Endocrinology. Amsterdam: North Holland, 1973.
16. Edwards R. Immunoassays. In Rickwood D, Hames BD, series eds. Essential Data Series. New York: John Wiley & Sons, 1996.
17. Desbuquois B, Aurbach GD. Use of polyethylene glycol to separate free and antibody-bound peptide hormones in radioimmunoassays. J Clin Endocrinol Metab 1971; 33:732–738.
18. Yalow RS, Berson SA. Separation techniques—antigen adsorption. In Berson SA, Yalow RS, eds. Methods in Investigative and Diagnostic Endocrinology. Part I. Amsterdam: North Holland, 1973: 120–125.
19. Yalow RS. Radioimmunoassays of hormones. In: Wilson JD, Foster DW, eds. Williams Textbook of Endocrinology. Philadelphia: WB Saunders, 1992: 1635–1645.
20. Eng J, Yalow RS. Evidence against extrapancreatic insulin synthesis. Proc Natl Acad Sci USA 1981; 78:4576–4578.
21. Segre GV. Advances in techniques for measurement of parathyroid hormone: current applications in clinical medicine and directions for future research. Trends Endocrinol Metab 1990; 1:243–247.
22. Kricka LJ. Chemiluminescent and bioluminescent techniques. Clin Chem 1991; 37:1472–1481.
23. Klee GG, Preissner CM, Schryver PG, et al. Multisite immunochemiluminometric assay for simultaneously measuring whole-molecule and amino-terminal fragments of human parathyrin. Clin Chem 1992; 38:628–635.
24. Rongen HA, Hoetelmans RM, Bult A, et al. Chemiluminescence and immunoassays. J Pharm Biomed Anal 1994; 12:433–462.
25. Piran U, Riordan WJ, Livshin LA. New noncompetitive immunoassays of small analytes. Clin Chem 1995; 41:986–990.
26. Hage DS, Taylor B, Schryver P, et al. Use of affinity chromatography in developing acridinium ester–labeled antibodies for the immunoassay of parathyrin. Clin Chem 1991; 37:117–118.
27. Nussbaum SR, Zahradnik RJ, Lavigne JR, et al. Highly sensitive two-site immunoradiometric assay of parathyrin and its clinical utility in evaluating patients with hypercalcemia. Clin Chem 1987; 33:1364–1367.
28. Nussbaum SR, Thompson AR, Hutcheson KA, et al. Intraoperative measurement of parathyroid hormone in the surgical management of hyperparathyroidism. Surgery 1988; 104:1121.
29. Irvin GL III, Deriso GT III. A new, practical intraoperative parathyroid hormone assay. Am J Surg 1994; 168:466–468.
30. Black JW, Shankey NP. Inverse agonists exposed. Nature 1995; 374:214–215.
31. Roth J, Kahn CR, Lesniak MA, et al. Receptors for insulin, NSILA-s, and growth hormone: applications to disease states in man. Recent Prog Horm Res 1975; 31:95–139.
32. Lesniak MA, Roth J. Regulation of receptor concentration by homologous hormone: effect of human growth hormone on its receptor in IM-9 lymphocytes. J Biol Chem 1976; 251:3720–3729.
33. Yamamoto I, Potts JT Jr, Segre GV. Circulating bovine lymphocytes contain receptors for parathyroid hormone. J Clin Invest 1983; 71:404–407.
34. Segre GV, Rosenblatt M, Reiner BL, et al. Characterization of parathyroid hormone receptors in canine renal cortical plasma membranes using a radioiodinated sulfur-free hormone analogue: correlation of binding with adenylate cyclase activity. J Biol Chem 1979; 254:6980–6986.
35. Yamamoto I, Bringhurst FR, Potts JT Jr, et al. Properties of parathyroid hormone receptors on circulating bovine lymphocytes. J Bone Min Res 1988; 3:289–295.
36. De Meyts P, Roth J, Neville DM Jr, et al. Insulin interactions with its receptors: experimental evidence for negative cooperativity. Biochem Biophys Res Commun 1973; 55:154–161.
37. Eastman RC, Lesniak MA, Roth J, et al. Regulation of receptor by homologous hormone enhances sensitivity and broadens scope of radioreceptor assay for human growth hormone. J Clin Endocrinol Metab 1979; 49:262–268.
38. Dufau ML, Pock R, Neubauer A, et al. In vitro bioassay of LH in human serum: the interstitial cell testosterone (RICT) assay. J Clin Endocrinol Metab 1976; 42:958–969.
39. Flier JS, Kahn CR, Roth J, et al. Antibodies that impair insulin receptor binding in an unusual diabetic syndrome with severe insulin resistance. Science 1975; 190:63–65.
40. Smith BR, Hall R. Thyroid-stimulating immunoglobins in Graves' disease. Lancet 1974; 2:427–431.
41. Manley SW, Bourbe JR, Hauber RW. The thyrotropin receptor in guinea pig thyroid homogenate: interaction with the long-acting thyroid stimulator. J Endocrinol 1974; 61:437–445.
42. Lan NC, Baxter JD. A radioreceptor assay for direct measurement of plasma free glucocorticoid activity. J Clin Endocrinol Metab 1982; 55:516–523.
43. Ambesi-Impiombato FS, Parks LAM, Coon HG. Culture of hormone-dependent epithelial cells from rat thyroids. Proc Natl Acad Sci USA 1980; 77:3455–3459.
44. Filetti S, Foti D, Costante G, et al. Recombinant human thyrotropin receptors in a radioreceptor assay for the measurement of TSH receptor antibodies. J Clin Endocrinol Metab 1991; 72:1096–1101.
45. Grove AS Jr. Evaluation of exophthalmos. N Engl J Med 1975; 292:1005–1013.

46. Zakarija M, McKenzie JM, Banovac K. Clinical significance of assay of thyroid-stimulating antibody in Graves' disease. Ann Intern Med 1980; 93:28–32.

47. Sunshine P, Kusumoto H, Kriss JP. Survival time of circulating long-acting thyroid stimulator in neonatal thyrotoxicosis: implications for diagnosis and therapy of the disorder. Pediatrics 1965; 36:869–876.

48. Teng CS, Tong TC, Hutchison JH, et al. Thyroid-stimulating immunoglobulins in neonatal Graves' disease. Arch Dis Child 1980; 55:894–895.

49. Mackenzie JM, Zakarija M. Fetal and neonatal hyper- and hypothyroidism due to maternal TSH receptor antibodies. Thyroid 1992; 2:155–159.

50. Taylor SI, Grunberger G, Marcus-Samuels B, et al. Hypoglycemia associated with antibodies to the insulin receptor. N Engl J Med 1982; 307:1422–1426.

51. Dons RF, Havlik R, Taylor SI, et al. Clinical disorders associated with autoantibodies to the insulin receptor. J Clin Invest 1983; 72:1072–1080.

52. Harrison LC, Flier JS, Itin A, et al. Radioimmunoassay of the insulin receptor: a new probe of receptor structure and function. Science 1979; 203:544–547.

53. Boden G, Fujita-Yamaguchi Y, Shimoyama R, et al. Nonbinding inhibitors antiinsulin receptor antibodies: a new type of autoantibodies in human disease. J Clin Invest 1988; 81:1971–1978.

54. Wang C. Bioassays of follicle-stimulating hormone. Endocrin Rev 1988; 9:374–377.

55. Nissenson RA, Abbott SR, Teitelbaum AP. Endogenous biologically active parathyroid hormone measurement by a guanyl nucleotide amplified renal adenylate cyclase assay. J Clin Endocrinol Metab 1981; 52:840.

56. Klee GG, Preissner CM, Schloegel IW, et al. Bioassay of parathyrin: analytic characteristics and clinical performance in patients with hypercalcemia. Clin Chem 1988; 34:482.

57. Dufau ML, Beitins IZ, McArthur JW, et al. Effects of luteinizing hormone–releasing hormone (LHRH) upon bioactive and immunoactive serum LH levels in normal subjects. J Clin Endocrinol Metab 1976; 43:658–667.

58. Lucky AW, Rebar RW, Rosenfeld RL, et al. Reduction of the potency of luteinizing hormone by estrogen. N Engl J Med 1979; 300:1034–1036.

59. Faglia G, Bitensky L, Pinchera A, et al. Thyrotropin secretion in patients with central hypothyroidism: evidence for reduced biological activity of immunoreactive thyrotropin. J Clin Endocrinol Metab 1979; 48:989–998.

60. Beck-Peccoz P, Amr S, Menezes-Ferreira MM, et al. Decreased receptor binding of biologically inactive thyrotropin-releasing hormone in central hypothyroidism. N Engl J Med 1985; 312:1085–1090.

61. Nissim M, Lee KO, Petrick PA, et al. A sensitive TSH bioassay based on iodide uptake in FRTL-5 thyroid cells: comparison with the adenosine 3′, 5′-monophosphate response to human serum TSH and enyzmatically deglycosylated bovine and human TSH. Endocrinology 1987; 121:1278–1287.

62. Beck-Peccoz P, Piscitelli G, Amr S, et al. Endocrine, biochemical, and morphological studies of pituitary adenoma secreting GH, TSH and alpha-subunit: evidence for secretion of TSH with increased bioactivity. J Clin Endocrinol Metab 1986; 62:704–711.

63. Gesundheit N, Fink DL, Silverman LA, et al. Effect of thyrotropin-releasing hormone on the carbohydrate structure of secreted mouse thyrotropin: analysis by lectin chromatography. J Biol Chem 1987; 262:5197–5203.

64. Amr S, Meneses-Ferreira M, Shinohigashi Y, et al. Activities of deglycosylated thyrotropin at the thyroid membrane receptor–adenylate cyclase system. J Endocrinol Invest 1985; 8:537–541.

65. Weintraub BD, Rosen SW, McCammon JA, et al. Apparent cooperativity in radioimmunoassay of human chorionic gonadotropin. Endocrinology 1973; 92:1250–1255.

66. Greenwood FC, Hunter WM, Klopper A. Assay of human growth hormone in pregnancy at parturition and in lactation: detection of a growth hormone–like substance from the placenta. Br Med J 1964; 1:22–24.

67. Cretien M. Lipotropins. In: Berson SA, Yalow RS, eds. Methods in Investigative and Diagnostic Endocrinology. Part II. Amsterdam: North-Holland, 1973: 617–632.

68. Pandian MR, Morgan CH, Carlton E, et al. An immunoradiometric assay for parathyroid hormone–related peptide and its clinical application in the differential diagnosis of hypercalcemia. Clin Chem 1992; 38:282–289.

69. Segre GV. Receptors for parathyroid hormone and parathyroid hormone–related protein. In: Bilezikian JP, Marcus R, Levine MA, eds. The Parathyroids. New York: Raven, 1994; 213–228.

70. Segre GV. Receptors for parathyroid hormone and parathyroid hormone–related protein. In: Bilezikian JP, Raisz L, Rodan GA, eds. Principles of Bone Biology. San Diego, CA: Academic Press, 1996; 377–403.

71. Derynck R. Transforming growth factor-alpha. Cell 1988; 54:593–595.

72. Derynck R. The physiology of transforming growth factor-alpha. Adv Cancer Res 1992; 58:27–52.

73. Goldsmith SJ, Yalow RS, Berson SA. Significance of plasma insulin Sephadex fractions. Diabetes 1969; 18:834–839.

74. Gabbay KH, Bergenstal RM, Wolff J, et al. Familial hyperproinsulinemia: partial characterization of circulating proinsulin-like material. Proc Natl Acad Sci USA 1979; 76:2881–2885.

75. Berson SA, Yalow RS. Immunochemical heterogeneity of parathyroid hormone in plasma. J Clin Endocrinol 1968; 28:1037–1047.

76. Martin KJ, Hruska KA, Freitag JJ, et al. The peripheral metabolism of parathyroid hormone. N Engl J Med 1979; 301:1092–1098.

77. Segre GV, D'Amour P, Hultman A, et al. Effects of hepatectomy, nephrectomy, and nephrectomy/uremia on the metabolism of parathyroid hormone in the rat. J Clin Invest 1981; 67:439–448.

78. Segre GV, Tregear GW, Potts JT Jr. Development and application of sequence-specific radioimmunoassays for analysis of the metabolism of parathyroid hormone. In: O'Malley BW, Hardman JG, eds. Methods in Enzymology. Vol 37. New York: Academic Press, 1975: 38–66.

79. Segre GV. Amino-terminal radioimmunoassays for human parathyroid hormone. In: Cohn DV, Fugita T, Potts JT Jr, et al, eds. Endocrine Control of Bone and Calcium Metabolism (Proceedings of the Ninth Conference on Calcium-Regulating Hormones, Kobe, Japan, October 1983). Amsterdam: Excerpta Medica, 1984: 17–20.

80. Silverman R, Yalow RS. Heterogeneity of parathyroid hormone: clinical and physiological implications. J Clin Invest 1973; 52:1958–1971.

81. Segre GV, Niall HD, Habener JF, et al. Metabolism of parathyroid hormone: physiological and clinical significance. Am J Med 1974; 56:774–784.

82. Segre GV, Niall HD, Sauer RT, et al. Edman degradation of radioiodinated parathyroid hormone: application to sequence analysis and *in vivo* metabolism. Biochemistry 1977; 16:2417–2427.

83. Flueck J, DiBella FB, Edis AJ, et al. Immunoheterogeneity of parathyroid hormone in venous effluent serum from hyperfunctioning parathyroid glands. J Clin Invest 1977; 60:1367–1375.

84. Mayer GP, Keaton JA, Hurst JG, et al. Effects of plasma calcium concentration on the relative proportion of hormone and carboxyl fragments in parathyroid venous blood. Endocrinology 1979; 104:1778–1784.

85. Segre GV, Perkins AS, Witters LA, et al. Metabolism of parathyroid hormone by isolated rat Kupffer cells and hepatocytes. J Clin Invest 1981; 67:449–457.

86. Quarles LD, Lobaugh B, Murphy G. Intact parathyroid hormone overestimates the presence and severity of parathyroid-mediated osseous abnormalities in uremia. J Clin Endocrinol Metab 1992; 75:145–150.

87. Sherrard DJ, Hercz G, Pei Y, et al. The spectrum of bone disease in end-stage renal failure: an evolving disorder. Kidney Int 1993; 43:436–442.

88. Hercz G, Pei Y, Greenwood C, et al. Aplastic osteodystrophy without aluminum: the role of "suppressed" parathyroid function. Kidney Int 1993; 44:860–866.

89. Maciel RJ. Standard curve fitting in immunodiagnostics: a primer. J Clin Immunoassay 1985; 8:98–106.

90. O'Connel M, Belanger BA, Haaland PD. Calibration and assay development using the four-parameter logistic model. Chemometrics and Intelligent Laboratory Systems 1993; 20:97–114.

91. Westgard JO, Klee GG. Performance characteristics of a control procedure. In: Tietz NW, ed. Clinical Chemistry. Philadelphia, WB Saunders, 1986: 435–458.

92. Currie LA. Limits for qualitative detection and quantitative determination. Anal Chem 1968; 40:586–593.

93. Ekins R, Newman B. Theoretical aspects of saturation analysis. Acta Endocrinol Suppl 1970; 147:11–30.

94. Chan DW. General principles of immunoassay. In: Chan DW, Perlstein MT, eds. Immunoassay: A Practical Guide. San Diego, CA: Academic Press, 1987; 10–11.

95. Feldkamp CS. Evaluation and clinical validation of immunoassays. In: Nakamura RM, Kasahara Y, Richnitz GA, eds. Immunochemical Assays and Biosensor Technology for the 1990's. Washington, DC: American Society of Microbiology, 1992: 96.

96. Brown EN, McDermott T, Block KJ, et al. Defining the smallest analyte concentration an immunoassay can measure. Clin Chem 1996; 42:893–903.

4

MECHANISMS OF ACTION OF HORMONES THAT ACT AS TRANSCRIPTION-REGULATORY FACTORS

Ming-Jer Tsai, James H. Clark, William T. Schrader, and Bert W. O'Malley

INTRODUCTION

Steroid hormones, 1,25-dihydroxycholecalciferol, thyroid hormone, and retinoic acid act via remarkably similar mechanisms at multiple levels of biologic organization to produce the same general effects, i.e., the induction of RNA and protein synthesis. Therefore, this chapter presents a generalized model of their actions at the molecular and cellular levels.

Steroid hormones enter most cells by diffusion, although in some cases active uptake or export may be involved (Fig. 4–1). In target cells (i.e., cells sensitive to hormone), the steroid binds to receptors, proteins that have specific binding sites for the hormone and are located in both the cytoplasm and the nucleus. Binding of the steroid to its receptor mole-

cule produces conformational (allosteric) changes that result in the formation of an "activated" or "transformed" receptor-steroid complex that has a high affinity for DNA-binding sites. It was originally thought that the activation or transformation step occurs in the cytoplasm, but the process may also occur in the nuclear compartment (see Fig. 4–1). The binding of the receptor-hormone complex to regulatory elements usually results in activation of a nearby gene or genes, i.e., transcription of the gene by RNA polymerase to produce messenger RNA (mRNA). The mRNA is translated on cytoplasmic ribosomes to produce the appropriate protein, which alters cell function, growth, or differentiation. In some cases receptor-DNA interaction serves to inhibit rather than activate gene transcription.

Once the receptor-hormone complex has interacted with

Molecular Pathway of Steroid Hormone Action

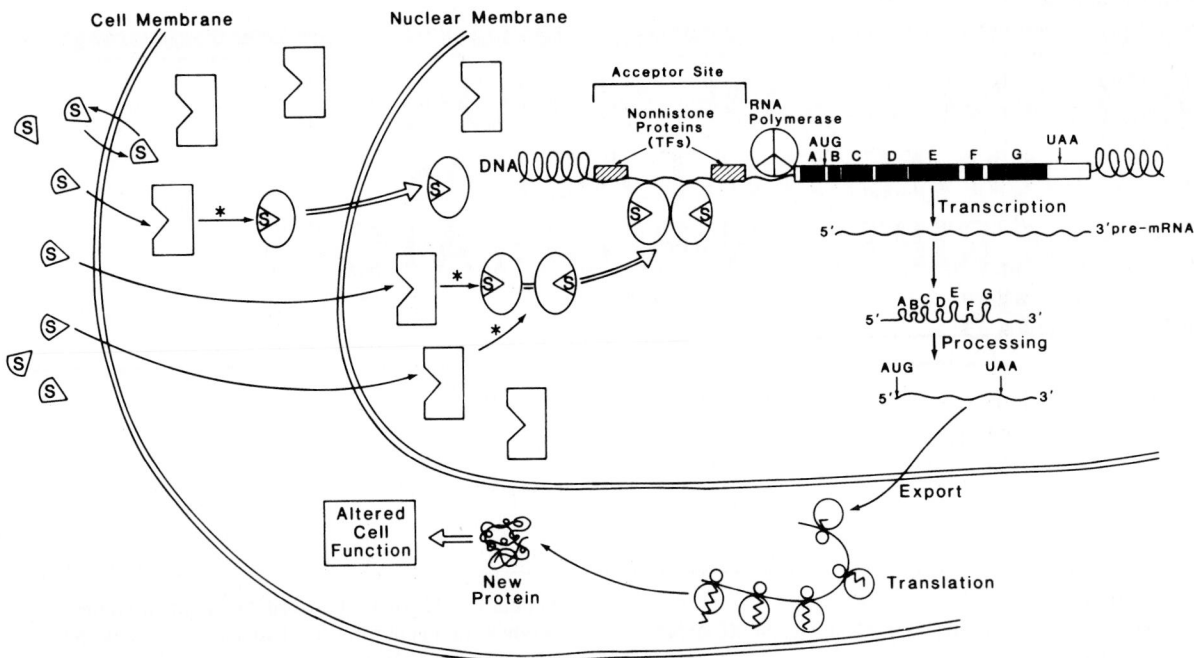

Figure 4–1. A complete understanding of the relationship between steroid receptor binding and the mechanism of hormone action depends on valid characterization and accurate measurement of steroid receptors.[1] In this section the criteria for and methods by which characterization and measurement can be accomplished are described to provide the necessary background for the discussions presented later in the chapter.

DNA, the receptor undergoes changes that are not well understood but that result in the dissociation of the hormone and receptor (recycling) and elimination of the steroid from the cell. These steps convert the receptor to a form that can subsequently bind hormone again and recycle. The steroid may be metabolized to forms that do not bind tightly to the receptor and hence diffuse out of the cell.

STEROID RECEPTORS: DEFINITION AND MEASUREMENT

A complete understanding of the mechanism of hormone action depends on a comprehension of steroid receptors.[1]

Receptor Criteria

FINITE BINDING CAPACITY. The biologic response to steroid hormones is a saturable phenomenon, and it follows that there should be a finite number of receptor sites per cell. Demonstration that the hormone-binding system under study can be saturated is usually accomplished by exposing the receptor to various concentrations of radioactive steroid and subsequently measuring the amount of bound or free steroid, or both, after equilibrium is achieved. This process would be simple if there existed only a single class of binding sites for a given steroid; however, this is seldom the case. Most tissues have multiple binding components, each with its own affinity and capacity for the steroid under study. These complexities are discussed further in the following sections.

HIGH AFFINITY. Steroid hormones should possess a high affinity for their respective receptors because the circulating levels of steroid usually range from 0.1 to 10 nmol/L; e.g., the hormone should have an affinity for the receptor that is in the range of these blood levels; otherwise, physiological

responses would not occur. These considerations are true for a variety of receptors but do not preclude receptor C-ligand interactions of weaker affinity if blood or tissue levels of steroids or receptors are elevated.

STEROID SPECIFICITY. Generally speaking, receptors display high specificities of binding for a specific hormone or class of hormones. This specificity enables a target cell to respond to a hormonal signal without interference from other signals. Thus, hormones of the same class, their agonists, and their antagonists should compete for binding to a given class of receptor and should not bind to other receptor systems. Nevertheless, receptors do not display absolute stereospecificity; that is, the binding site on the receptor has a limited capacity for recognition and differentiation of different ligands. This point will be discussed in more detail later.

TISSUE OR CELLULAR SPECIFICITY. Most steroid hormones produce cell types or tissues. It follows that receptors should exist in these cell types, and not necessarily in others. For instance, only certain tissues are stimulated by gonadal steroids, and these tissues are referred to as target organs, e.g., the uterus, vagina, brain, and mammary gland in the case of estrogen receptor. The amount of estrogen receptor in these tissues is higher per unit mass than in nontarget tissues such as diaphragm and spleen.

CORRELATION WITH BIOLOGIC RESPONSE. Implicit in all studies of receptors that bind steroid hormones and meet the foregoing criteria is the assumption that this binding results in a biologic response. Thus, binding of hormone to receptors must precede or accompany tissue responses, and the extent of response should be related to receptor occupancy. This criterion, the demonstration of receptor-dependent hormonal response, is often difficult to document.

Analysis of Single-Component Systems

In most cases steroid receptors exist in the presence of other binding molecules that complicate the analysis of receptor binding. However, for the purpose of illustration, we shall consider a system that contains only one receptor site. In such a system, the total amount of receptor (R_t) is determined under equilibrium conditions by adding steroid (S) until saturation or near-saturation is obtained (Fig. 4–2). The amount of bound ligand (RS) is related to the amount of free ligand or ligands and of total receptor (R_t) and the dissociation constant (K_d) of the receptor-ligand complex in the following way:

$$[RS] = \frac{[R_t][S]}{K_d + [S]}$$

This formulation of rapid-equilibrium kinetics is employed in the derivation of the Michaelis-Menten equation and applies equally to ligand binding under equilibrium conditions. As steroid is added to the system, the receptor sites become saturated. The actual point of saturation is equal to the number of receptor sites (n) or R_t. The dissociation constant (K_d) is the concentration of steroid at which 50% of the receptor sites are bound. This value in Figure 4–2 is 1 nmol/L. Although one can make reasonable estimates of R_t and K_d from saturation plots, these parameters should be obtained by Scatchard analysis,[2] as shown in Figure 4–2B.

Analysis of Multiple-Component Systems

The simple system described in the preceding section does not exist unless the receptor has been purified and has only one class of binding sites. Additional binding sites are usually present and complicate the measurement of receptors.

SPECIFIC AND NONSPECIFIC BINDING. As discussed earlier, the binding of a ligand to its receptor is stereospecific and thus is defined as specific. Nonspecific binding is the result of the ligand binding to nonreceptor sites, which are usually of low affinity and high capacity relative to the receptor. The total amount of steroid bound in such a system (RS + NS) is the sum of that bound to receptor sites (RS) and that bound to nonspecific sites (NS; Fig. 4–3A).

The data from Figure 4–3A are plotted according to the method of Scatchard in Figure 4–3B. The RS/S ratio is a curvilinear function of the amount of ligand bound (RS). This curve represents the summation of specific and nonspecific components, both of which are plotted individually as well and appear as linear functions in this graph. These components can be resolved with the use of competitive inhibitors or by geometric fitting procedures, described later.

A direct assessment of the amounts of specific and non-specific binding can be made with the use of competitive inhibition of labeled-steroid binding by nonlabeled steroid. In practice the receptor is exposed to multiple concentrations

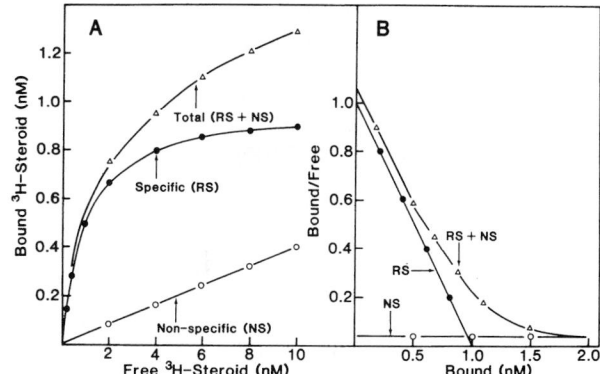

Figure 4–3. Saturation (A) and Scatchard (B) analyses of specific and nonspecific binding.

of radioactive steroid in the presence or absence of excess nonradioactive steroid (see Fig. 4–3A). The line designated as RS + NS represents the amount of ^{3}H-labeled ligand that is bound to both receptor (or "specific") sites and nonspecific sites and thus contains both saturable and nonsaturable components. Nonspecific binding sites (NS) are measured as the radioactive steroid bound in the presence of excess unlabeled competitive ligand. The competing nonlabeled ligand occupies essentially all high-affinity receptor sites but does not interfere appreciably with the binding of ^{3}H-labeled ligand to nonspecific sites. Receptor sites are estimated by subtracting NS from RS + NS. The number of receptor sites and the K_d can be determined from a direct plot of these data (see Fig. 4–3B).

The use of inhibition to determine receptor-binding parameters is based on the assumption that the nonlabeled steroid is a competitive inhibitor; e.g., when the nonlabeled ligand is identical to the radioactive ligand. In some cases, however, it is necessary to use a nonidentical inhibitor, and the assumption of competitive inhibition must be verified. To establish the validity of competitive inhibition to determine receptor parameters, it must be established that nonspecific binding sites are of low affinity and high capacity relative to the receptor system by demonstrating a straight line for nonspecific binding (see Fig. 4–3A) or by Scatchard analysis.

For receptor assays, the use of the term nonspecific to describe nonreceptor binding is adequate. However, nonspecific actually means nondisplaceable by a competitive steroid in the concentration range of ^{3}H-labeled steroid used in the assay.

COMPETITIVE INHIBITION OF RECEPTOR BINDING. To use the displacement method for the measurement of receptor parameters, the inhibition must be due to competitive inhibition. Inhibition of steroid binding to receptor sites may occur by either competitive or noncompetitive means; i.e., by mechanisms that involve mutually exclusive binding of ligands (competitive) or by inactivation (either reversible or irreversible) of the ligand-binding capacity of the receptor (noncompetitive). Competitive inhibitors decrease steroid binding to receptor sites by combining with the receptor in such a manner that the labeled steroid can no longer be bound—as when ligand and inhibitor compete for the same or adjacent and overlapping sites (Fig. 4–4). Note that increasing the concentration of inhibitor alters the apparent K_d for the receptor-steroid complex but does not change the number of binding sites.

In contrast with the effects of a competitive inhibitor on binding parameters, noncompetitive inhibitors do not alter the apparent K_d of the interaction but decrease the apparent number of receptor sites (Fig. 4–5). Thus, the demonstration

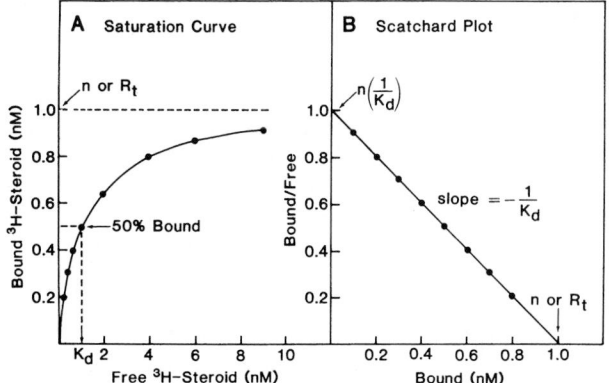

Figure 4–2. Saturation and Scatchard analyses of receptor steroid binding (n or R_t, number of receptor sites; K_d, dissociation constant).

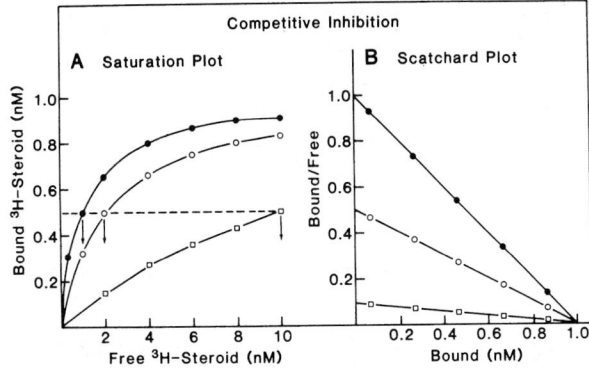

Figure 4–4. Competitive inhibition of receptor binding. ●, no competing steroid added; ○, competing steroid added at a concentration of 1 nmol/L; □, competing steroid added at a concentration of 10 nmol/L; dashed line in *A* marks point at which 50% of total specific binding is achieved; arrow indicates apparent shift in K_d.

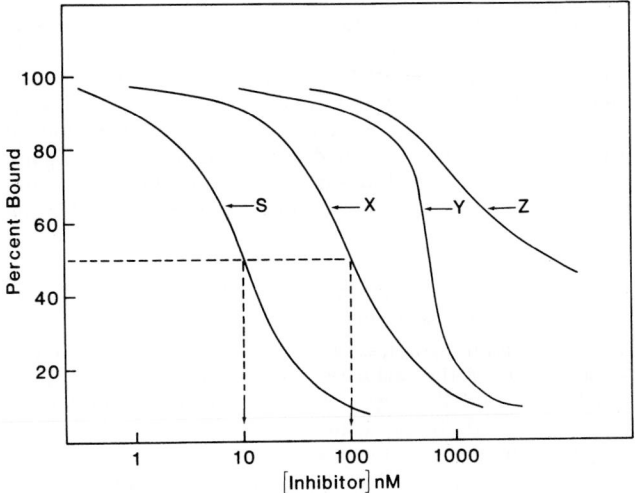

Figure 4–6. Competitive inhibition analysis and relative binding affinity. Concentrations of receptor and ³H-labeled steroid are 1 nmol/L and 10 nmol/L, respectively. S, steroid identical to the ³H-labeled steroid; X, steroid with a relative affinity of 0.1; Y and Z, noncompetitive inhibitors. Horizontal dashed line indicates point of 50% inhibition; vertical dashed lines indicate concentration of competing steroid that inhibits 50% of binding of ³H-labeled steroid to receptor.

of suppression of ³H-labeled steroid binding to receptors is not sufficient to establish competitive inhibition. Noncompetitive inhibition may occur for many reasons. For example, the inhibitor may precipitate or denature the receptor or its active site; alternatively, the inhibitor may bind to a second site on the receptor and, in so doing, alter the active site of the receptor.

Another technique for studying the specificity and binding affinity of steroid receptors is to keep the concentration of ³H-labeled steroid constant and to vary the concentration of inhibiting steroid (Fig. 4–6). The relative binding affinity (RBA) is determined by comparing the point at which 50% inhibition is observed for S (the nonlabeled steroid that is identical to the ³H-labeled steroid) and for X (the test compound). In the experiment shown, 50% inhibition occurs for S at 10 nmol/L and for X at 0.1 μmol/L; therefore, the relative affinity of the receptor for X is 0.1 of that for S. The determination of the RBA is valid only when the slopes of the two curves are parallel, as is the case for S and X in Figure 4–6. If the slopes are not parallel, as shown for compounds Y and Z, the RBA cannot be assessed because inhibition is occurring by a noncompetitive mechanism and will have to be assessed by the methods shown in Figures 4–4 and 4–5.

ASSOCIATION AND DISSOCIATION OF RECEPTOR-STEROID COMPLEXES. The equilibrium constant (K_d) for receptor-steroid binding is a function of the rate of association (on reaction) and the rate of dissociation (off reaction). Receptor sites that bind hormone at a high rate and release it at a low rate have high affinities. The rate of association can be assessed by exposing the receptor to labeled hormone and

measuring the amount of hormone bound as a function of time. The rate of dissociation is measured by adding a large excess of nonlabeled hormone to solution containing labeled hormone-receptor complexes. The excess nonlabeled hormone blocks reassociation of labeled hormone with the receptor during the dissociation process. Aliquots of the mixture are removed and assayed for the amount of unbound labeled hormone as a function of time. A single semilogarithmic plot of this value versus time yields a straight line whose slope is the rate constant for dissociation. The half-life of the complex can be determined as the time needed for the concentration of free hormone to double in value. Active steroids are usually characterized by long half-lives of the receptor-steroid complex.

MULTIPLE SPECIFIC COMPONENTS. Many receptor systems contain two or more specific sites that bind the same steroid with high affinities. In the examples shown in Figures 4–7 and 4–8, the nonspecific binding component has been eliminated for convenience and will be discussed later. The saturation curves do not appear by casual inspection to be composed of two binding components, but the Scatchard analyses (see Figs. 4–7*B* and 4–8*B*) demonstrate their presence. The usual saturation analysis might include only the lower

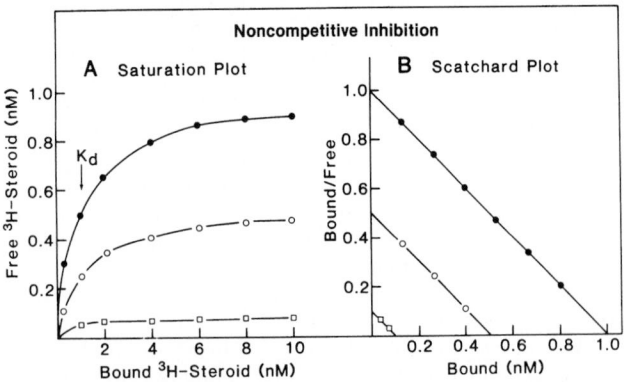

Figure 4–5. Noncompetitive inhibition of receptor binding. ●, no inhibitors added; ○, inhibitor added at 1 nmol/L; □, inhibitor added at 10 nmol/L.

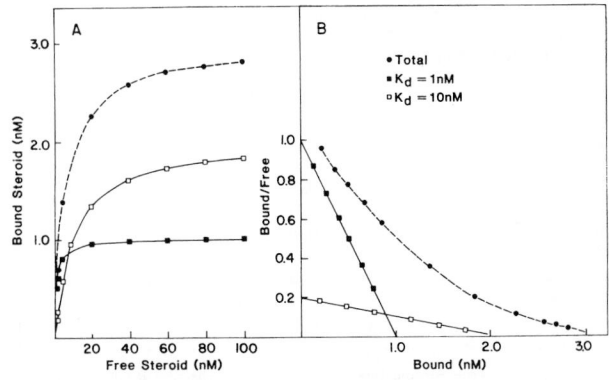

Figure 4–7. Saturation (*A*) and Scatchard (*B*) analyses of two specific binding sites of identical concentrations but different affinities. ●, total specific binding; ■, specific binding related to binding site with K_d of 10^{-9} M; □, specific binding related to binding site with K_d of 10^{-8} M.

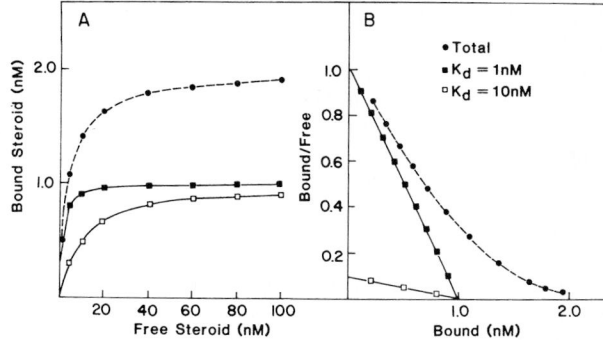

Figure 4–8. Saturation *(A)* and Scatchard *(B)* analyses of two specific binding sites of dissimilar concentrations and affinities. ●, total specific binding; ■, specific binding related to binding site with K_d of 10^{-9}M and concentration of 1 nmol/L; □, specific binding related to binding site with K_d of 10^{-8}M and concentration of 2 nmol/L.

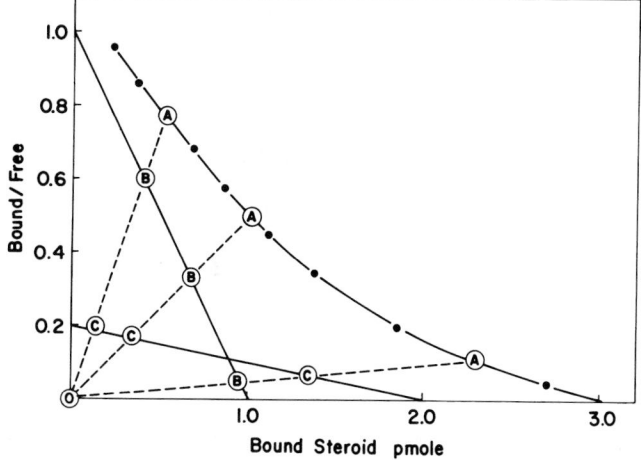

Figure 4–10. Resolution of two binding sites by vectorial analysis of a curved Scatchard plot. Each point A of the Scatchard plot is the vectorial sum of points B and C for each of the binding components *(solid straight lines)*. These two linear components can be resolved by adjusting their slopes until OC + OB = A for all dashed lines drawn from the origin (O) to points A on the Scatchard plot.

range of ligand concentration, and extrapolation of an apparent straight line would yield an improper estimate of the number of binding sites. In addition, it would be concluded falsely that only one specific binding component was present. Errors of this type are more exaggerated when the binding component with lower affinity is in excess over the higher-affinity component (see Fig. 4–7). In such cases, binding analyses at low concentrations of ligand lead to overestimation of the number of sites and underestimation of binding affinity.

In the example shown in Figure 4–9, two different types of specific binding are represented: one that displays the usual saturation curve, a rectangular hyperbola, and a second that is represented by a sigmoid function.[3] These two sites yield a Scatchard plot with linear (type I) and curvilinear (type II) components. When such complex curves are present, the failure to perform complete saturation analysis or direct extrapolation of the linear portion of the Scatchard plot results in overestimation of the first site. In addition, the false conclusion would be drawn that only a single specific binding component exists. The curvilinear portion of the curve is often mistakenly considered to be a straight line and is equated to nonspecific binding or binding of no significance. It should be noted that the nonspecific binding component in these analyses has been subtracted and is not shown in Figure 4–9.

RESOLVING MIXED BINDING SYSTEMS. The ideal way of resolving complex binding systems such as those just discussed is physical purification of the various components so that each can be studied as an isolated system. However, such purification is usually not feasible because of the limited quantities of tissue available. In the simplest case, the system is

composed of one specific or saturable component and one nonspecific component (as in Fig. 4–3), and competitive inhibition can be used to determine these components. In addition, graphic analysis of curvilinear Scatchard plots can be used to resolve curved plots into two straight lines, which, when summed point by point in a vectorial manner, reproduce the original curve. The data in Figure 4–10 are identical to those in Figure 4–8. Note that sections contributed by two independent components must sum to the curve. The data from routine steroid-binding studies are limited, and the Scatchard curves are usually determined imprecisely, so the resolution of more than two components is not possible by this method.

Analytic methods employing geometric or parametric procedures, such as those discussed earlier, are useful. However, complete and detailed steroid-binding data frequently cannot be obtained because of limitations in biologic material, and other methods must be utilized.

Differential inhibition of ligand binding has been employed to analyze several mixed systems. The use of [³H]-estradiol and diethylstilbestrol (DES) for the assay of estrogen receptors in the presence of α-fetoprotein (α-FP) is a good example. α-Fetoprotein is present in large quantities in the neonatal rat and has an affinity for estradiol ($K_d = 10^{-9}$ to 10^{-10} M) similar to that of the receptor. The amount of receptor is measured by taking advantage of the fact that DES binds with low affinity to α-FP but competes effectively with [³H]estradiol for estrogen receptor binding sites. Thus, the binding of labeled estradiol to R can be determined by subtracting the amount of [³H]estradiol bound in the presence of DES from the amount bound in the absence of DES.

In some receptor systems, it is possible to eliminate one of the binding components and measure the receptor without interference. For instance, the addition of a reducing agent, such as dithiothreitol, to nuclear exchange assays causes the disappearance of type II estrogen receptor binding sites and permits independent assessment of the estrogen receptor type I site (see Fig. 4–9 for representative plot of these two types of sites, and reference 3 for details).

Exchange Assays

Most biologic systems contain receptors that are bound to ligand and receptors that are not bound to ligand (unoccupied). The measurement of both forms is obligatory to pro-

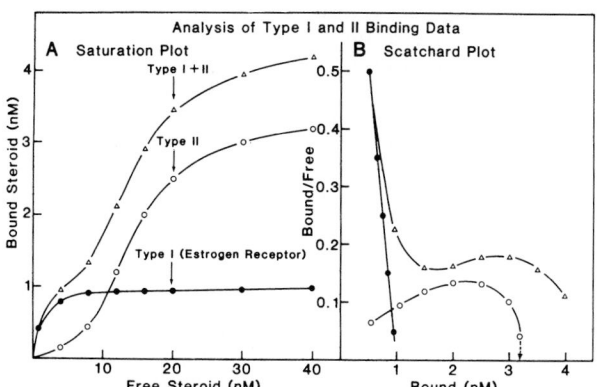

Figure 4–9. Saturation and Scatchard analyses of type I and II binding sites. △, total specific binding; ●, binding related to type I site (estrogen receptor); ○, specific binding related to type II sites; arrow in *B* indicates number of type II sites.

Exchange Assay and Receptor Measurement

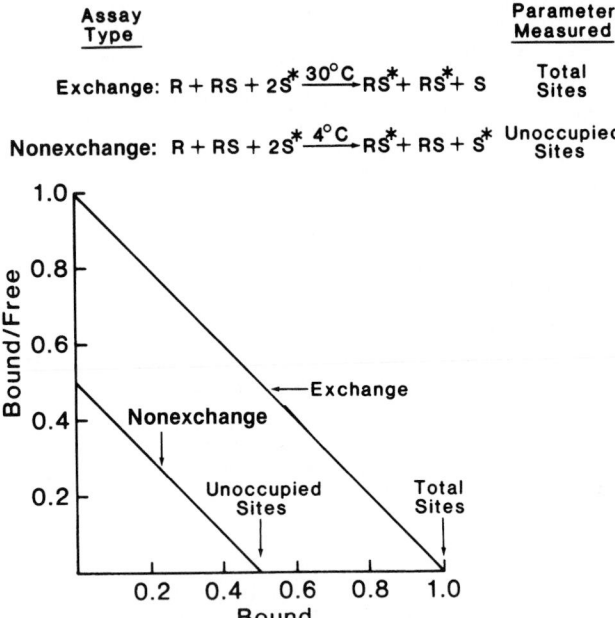

Assay Type		Parameter Measured
Exchange:	$R + RS + 2S^* \xrightarrow{30°C} RS^* + RS^* + S$	Total Sites
Nonexchange:	$R + RS + 2S^* \xrightarrow{4°C} RS^* + RS + S^*$	Unoccupied Sites

Figure 4–11. Determination of receptor binding by exchange and nonexchange assays. Results of these two procedures are plotted by the Scatchard method in the lower portion of the figure. R, unoccupied receptor sites; RS, occupied receptor sites; S*, ^{3}H-labeled steroid; RS*, receptor–^{3}H-labeled steroid complex.

vide insight into receptor physiology. Exchange assays for the assessment of occupancy state involve dissociation of the endogenous steroid from occupied receptor sites and association of a labeled steroid.

As an example, in the estradiol exchange assay[4, 5] the cytosolic or nuclear fraction to be assayed is warmed to 30°C for 30 min in the presence of varying concentrations of [^{3}H]-estradiol. At this temperature, endogenous (nonlabeled) steroid dissociates from occupied sites (RS; Fig. 4–11), and the added labeled steroid (S) is exchanged. Unoccupied sites (R) will also be bound by the labeled steroid. The resulting complexes (RS) can then be analyzed by Scatchard plots (see Fig. 4–11). Nonexchange receptor methods that detect only unoccupied sites underestimate the total amount of receptor present; in this example, the number of sites is one half of that observed with the exchange method.

BIOCHEMISTRY AND MOLECULAR BIOLOGY OF STEROID RECEPTORS

Introduction

Steroid receptors constitute a class of ligand-activated transcription factors that includes, among others, the thyroid hormone and vitamin D receptors.[6–9] All of the known steroid receptors have been cloned: progesterone receptors,[10–12] estrogen receptors,[13, 14] androgen receptors,[15, 16] glucocorticoid receptors,[17–19] mineralocorticoid receptors,[20, 21] thyroid hormone receptors,[7, 22, 23] retinoic acid receptors,[24–27] retinoid X (9-*cis*-retinoic acid) receptor,[28, 29] and vitamin D$_3$ receptors,[30–32] (for a review see references 7, 33, and 34). Steroid receptors mediate the vast majority of known activities of steroid hormones.

CONTROL OF FUNCTIONAL RECEPTOR ACTIVITY. Receptor proteins, like other regulatory proteins and enzymes, may exist in both active and inactive states, and factors that

affect receptor activity influence hormone responsiveness. Steroid hormone receptors are phosphorylated,[35, 36] and dephosphorylation of the glucocorticoid receptor appears to destroy a functional hormone-binding site. Readdition of ATP in the presence of protein kinase restores the site. This reversible activation-deactivation reaction occurs in living cells. For example, in primary culture mouse thymus cells lose glucocorticoid receptor when intracellular ATP pools are depleted (as by uncouplers of oxidative phosphorylation or by oxygen deprivation) and regain receptor activity when ATP is replenished. The extent to which this type of regulation occurs in normal tissues is not known. Evidence from antibody assays for receptor proteins suggests that the intracellular pool of inactive receptor is small.

Hormones themselves influence effective receptor levels by three mechanisms. The first, called down-regulation, is a reduction in receptor level after hormone treatment. For example, uterine progesterone receptor levels decrease within 1 h after administration of progesterone to rabbits. A second means of regulation is augmentation of the receptor level. In castrated rats, estrogen administration increases estrogen receptor levels in the uterus, generally between 12 and 24 h after injection. Similarly, estradiol administration increases progesterone receptor levels over the same time frame. In both of these examples, it is assumed that de novo receptor synthesis is increased, although other possibilities such as activation may be involved in some circumstances. Finally, the hormone can alter the ligand-binding site. The binding of estradiol-17β to its receptor in rat uterus promotes receptor dimerization or aggregation and increases the half-life of the hormone-receptor complexes.

STRUCTURAL ORGANIZATION OF RECEPTOR PROTEINS. Steroid receptors are present in small amounts in cells, ranging from about 0.001% (aldosterone receptors) to 0.1% (progesterone receptors) of soluble cell protein. Thus, their purification for structural studies has been difficult, and yields are small, typically around 1 μg of pure receptor/kg of starting tissue. Receptor proteins for most steroid hormones have now been purified to apparent homogeneity from target tissues, but receptors overexpressed in bacteria,[37, 38] yeast,[39, 40] insect,[41–43] and mammalian cells[44] are also being studied.

The structural features of the steroid receptors are highly conserved (Fig. 4–12). The N-terminal A/B domain contains activation function domain I (AF1). The C domain contains four cysteines that form two type II zinc fingers; it is responsible for DNA binding and dimerization. The C domain is followed by a less conserved D domain, also called the hinge region. At the C-terminal end is the E domain, which is responsible for ligand binding and contains the major dimerization domain and a second activation function domain (AF2). In addition, this domain may also have the ability to silence basal promoter activity. Some of the receptors have an additional F domain of unknown function.[9] The three principal regions of consensus homology are referred to as regions I, II, and III (see Fig. 4–12).[45] Region I is the most highly conserved and is a cysteine-rich DNA-binding domain. Regions II and III are less highly conserved. These structural similarities suggest that the steroid receptor superfamily represents an old family of regulatable transcription factors. Perhaps the early forms of these receptors were regulated by intracellular metabolic ligands in an intracrine fashion.[34] Some of the receptors may have lost their ligand-binding ability, such as the receptor for ERBA,[46] whereas others acquired ligand specificity for steroids, thyroid hormones, retinoic acid, and other unidentified ligands. Low-stringency Southern blot hybridization analysis with the DNA-binding domain of the glucocorticoid receptor suggests the existence of an abundance of related receptor proteins.[47, 48]

In fact, the steroid receptor superfamily of related genes

The Steroid Receptor Supergene Family
Homology of Consensus Domains

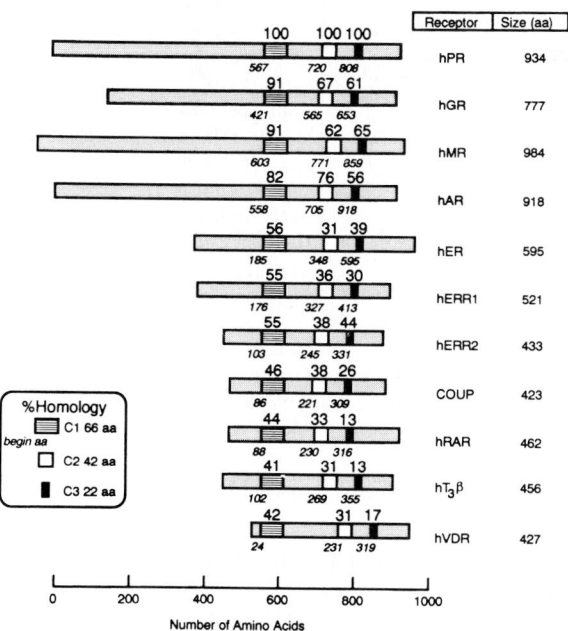

Figure 4–12. Homology of the steroid receptor supergene family. There are three regions of homology, referred to as regions I, II, and III. Region I has been identified as the DNA-binding domain. The functional significance of the homologies in regions II and III remains to be determined.

binding regions (95% and 90%, respectively). This striking conservation suggests that both might be regulated by the same or a similar ligand.

Steroid Receptor Gene Family

Before the steroid receptors were cloned, it was established chemically that they are organized into functional domains. Proteolytic cleavage analysis first revealed receptor fragments in which DNA-binding activity was separated from steroid binding[65, 66] and the various domains have now been identified more precisely.[67–72]

DNA Sequences Mediating Steroid Hormone Regulation of Genes

Most steroid-regulated genes share one important structural feature: steroid receptor binding sites termed *steroid re-*

is large. After elucidation of the receptors for the more traditional members of this family (adrenal steroids, gonadal steroids, thyroid hormone, vitamin D₃, and retinoic acid), a large number of receptor isotypes or variants were discovered (see Fig. 4–13).[7] More than 50 orphan receptors in search of a function and a ligand exist according to present estimates. Because they were cloned by cDNA cross-hybridization screening using cDNA probes, we have few clues as to their cellular roles in most cases, but there is some information suggesting possible roles in development and physiology.[49–53] Among the orphan receptors are ERR1, ERR2, TR2, NUR77, COUP-TFI, AND COUP-TFII.[45, 47, 54–59] COUP-TFs bind upstream of several hormone-regulated genes and participate in their regulation. The chicken ovalbumin gene, for example, contains within its upstream promoter the DNA sequence GTGTCAAAGGT-CAAA, termed the chicken ovalbumin upstream promoter (COUP) element. COUP-transcription factor (COUP-TF) is a DNA-binding protein that binds to the COUP sequence[60, 61] and is found in HeLa, chicken oviduct, HIT, and many other cell types.[60–63] The DNA-binding domain of COUP-TFI is a 66-amino-acid zinc finger motif in which all 20 invariant amino acids of the receptor superfamily are conserved, and 11 of 12 conserved residues are identical.[45] Several genes belonging to this subfamily have been isolated.[49] There are two COUP-TF genes (COUP-TFI and TFII) in mammals and three genes each for *Xenopus* and zebrafish. These genes are highly conserved in the DNA-binding domains (>94% amino acid identity) and the putative ligand-binding domains (>90% amino acid identity). They may play roles in neurogenesis, organogenesis, and cell fate determination (for review see reference 49).

A *Drosophila* homologue of COUP-TF, the *seven up* gene,[64] is required for photoreceptor cell formation during eye development. The *Drosophila seven up* gene and human COUP-TFI are virtually identical in the DNA-binding and putative ligand-

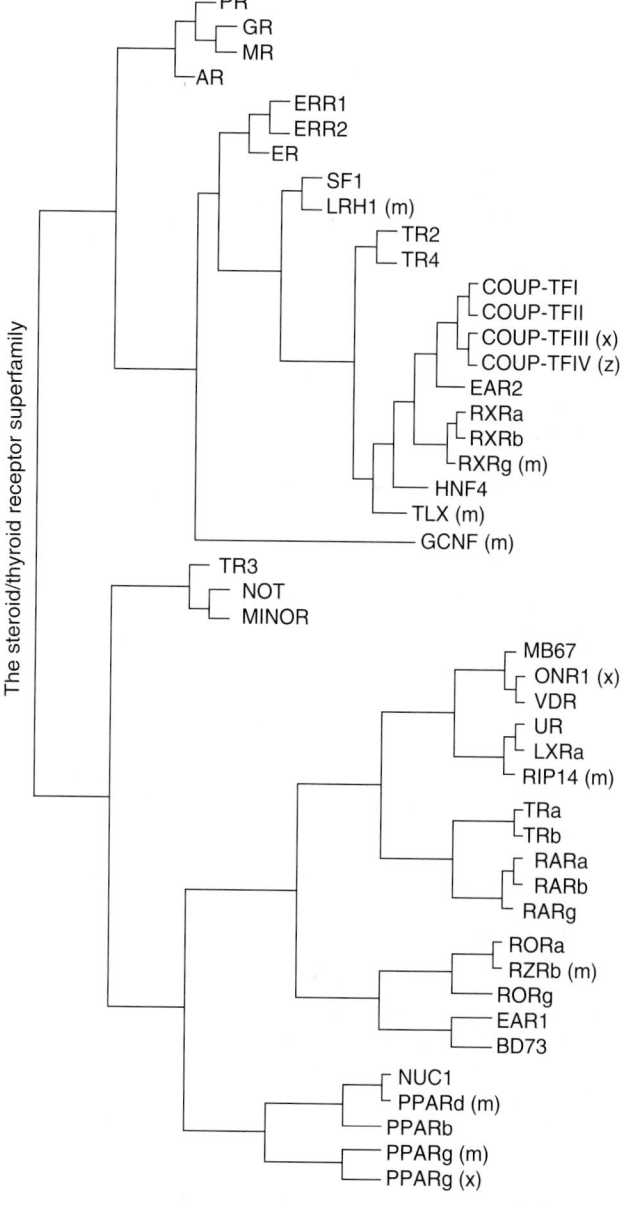

Figure 4–13. Evolutionary tree for the vertebrate steroid hormone–thyroid hormone receptor superfamily. Where it is possible, human genes and their names are used in this evolutionary tree. If human genes are not available, mouse (m), *Xenopus* (x) and zebrafish (z) genes are used, as indicated in the parentheses.

Class	Receptor	P Box	D BOX	SRE
I	GR,PR,MR,AR	GSCKV	AGRND ASRND	→GGTACA N3 TGTTCT←
II	ER	EDCKV	PATNQ	→GGTCA N3 TGACC←
IIIa	TRα,TRβ	EGCKG	KYDSC KYEGK	→AGGTCA N4 AGGTCA→ →AGGTCA N2 AGGTCA→
IIIb	RARα,β,γ	EGCKG	NRDKN	→AGGTCA N5 AGGTCA→ →AGGTCA N2 AGGTCA→ →AGGTCA N7 AGGTCA→
IIIc	RXRα,β,γ	EGCKG	RDNKD	→AGGTCA N2 AGGTCA→
IIId	VDR	EGCKG	PFNGD	→AGGTCA N3 AGGTCA→

Figure 4–14. The SREs of the various steroid hormone receptors.

sponse elements (SREs). SREs have the characteristics of enhancer elements.[73] They are independent of position and orientation, and their presence has a profound effect on transcriptional activity when stimulated by hormone.[74, 75]

Receptor interactions with specific DNA sequences have been investigated in several ways. DNA sequences of potential interest are defined by deletion studies and gene transfection into cells in culture or by studies of receptor-DNA interaction, such as gel mobility shift assays. SREs have been described for each of the known ligand-activated nuclear receptors (Fig. 4–14). SREs are characterized by imperfect hexanucleotide palindromes separated by spacer nucleotides, suggesting that receptors bind these sequences as dimers.[76] The gonadal and adrenal steroid receptors (class A) have a trinucleotide spacer, and the thyroid hormone–retinoic acid–vitamin D_3 receptor family (class B) has a less stringent spacing requirement. The latter receptors vary from having no spacers to as many as six nucleotides separating the palindromic half-sites. Negatively regulated steroid response elements (nSREs) appear to be SREs that, on binding a steroid receptor, force it into a sterically inactive complex to prevent the formation of an active transcription complex or antagonize other activator-dependent transcription (for a review see references 77 to 80).

The first SREs identified were the glucocorticoid response elements (GREs) of the mouse mammary tumor virus (MMTV) long terminal repeat[81–83] and of the chick lysozyme gene.[84] As more GREs were discovered,[85–87] it became apparent that the same sequences that confer steroid responsiveness onto glucocorticoids could also function as response elements for progesterone,[88, 89] mineralocorticoids,[20] and androgens,[90, 91] but not estrogen.[92] The estrogen response element 80 (ERE80)[93] is similar to, but structurally distinct from, the canonical GRE.[94] The consensus is that ERE is more closely related to the thyroid hormone response element (TRE) except that it is in a palindromic structure.[95] For the peroxisome proliferator–activated receptor (PPAR), retinoid X receptor (RXR), vitamin D receptor (VDR), retinoic acid receptor (RAR), and thyroid hormone receptor (TR), the SREs consist of an AGGTCA direct repeat. However, the number of nucleotides in the spacer between these two AGGTCA sequences is different for different SREs (see Fig. 4–14). One class of orphan receptors, such as nerve growth factor 1B (NGF1B), binds to a DNA response element consisting of only one AGGTCA sequence with a few additional nucleotides 5′ of it (for a review see reference 96). COUP-TF response element also has a structure similar to that of class B receptors except that it can bind to any AGGTCA direct repeat or an inverted repeat with a wide range of nucleotides in the spacer, anywhere between 0 and 10 nucleotides.[97] This promiscuous binding allows it to compete with other class B receptors that bind to AGGTCA direct repeats. Indeed, cotransfection experiments indicate that the COUP-TF response element inhibits the activity of RXR, VDR, RAR, and TR.[97]

Organization of Functional Elements in Receptors

ORGANIZATION OF THE HORMONE-BINDING DOMAIN. The hormone-binding domains for RXR, RAR, and TRα, as determined by x-ray crystallography,[98–100] have a similar structure that consists of a series of antiparallel alpha-helices interspersed with short beta strands to form a hydrophobic ligand-binding pocket (as shown in Figure 4–15A; see color section between pages 875 and 877). The major difference in the occupied RARγ and TRα compared with the unoccupied RXRα is the carboxyl H12 (helix 12) alpha-helix, which contains the AF2 transcriptional activation domain. In the occupied receptors, this helix folds back toward the ligand-binding core to cover the ligand entry site. This ligand-induced conformational change is necessary for the receptor to become active (for a review see reference 9).

The dimerization interface for the RXRα has also been defined by analysis of the crystal structure.[98] Instead of the heptad repeat region proposed to be important for dimer formation, helix 10 (H10) plays a major part in the homodimerization. The dimerization interface is formed in part by H9 and by the loop between H7 and H8. In this way, the two monomers form a symmetrical dimer with a mirror image. The amino acids important for interaction with hormone were defined by testing a large number of steroid analogues for a particular class of receptor.

The hormone-binding site is a hydrophobic pocket that binds the steroid A ring with precision and the D ring with somewhat broader flexibility. Substituents at the latter end are also recognized. For example, progesterone and testosterone differ only at the D ring, but the two receptors are selective for the proper hormone.

The importance of amino acids in the ligand-binding domain has been defined by insertional mutagenesis studies,[101, 102] which revealed that mutations in roughly the last 200 to 250 amino acids of the glucocorticoid and progesterone receptors abolish steroid-binding activity. Certain amino acids in this region play a central role in hormone binding. Analysis of the crystal structures of liganded TRα and RARγ provided additional information as to which amino acids interact with triiodothyronine (T_3) or retinoic acid; most of the alpha-helices, beta-turn, and loop regions are important in the contact between ligands and receptors. Both van der Waals contacts and hydrogen bonds stabilize the ligand-binding pocket. Some of the amino acids that interact with ligand in the crystal structure were also identified by mutational analysis.[99]

RECEPTOR DNA-BINDING DOMAIN. Sequence analysis

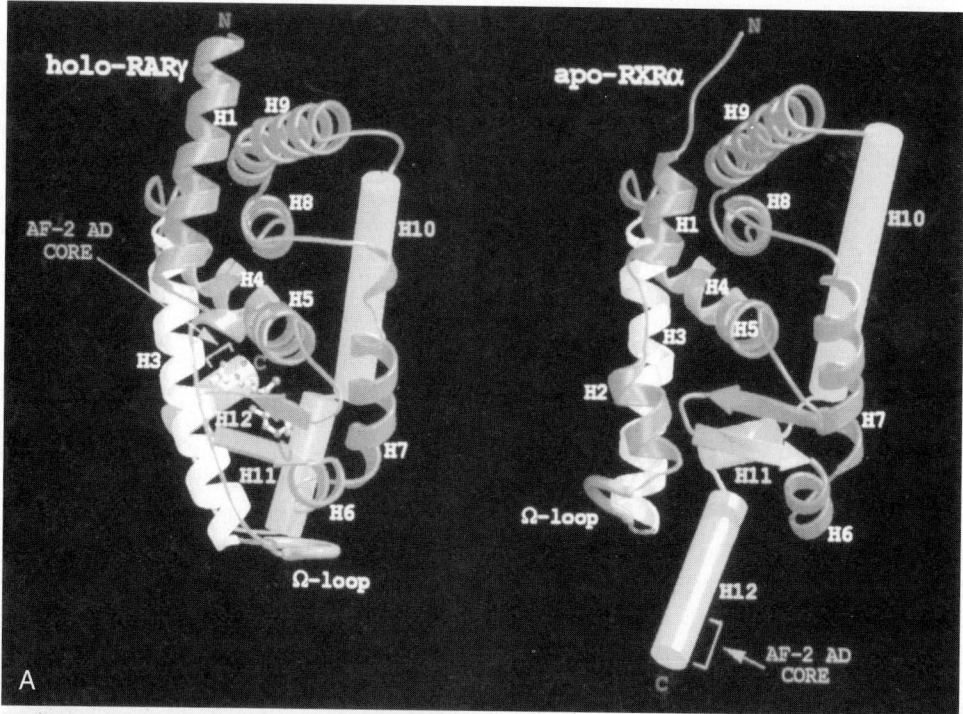

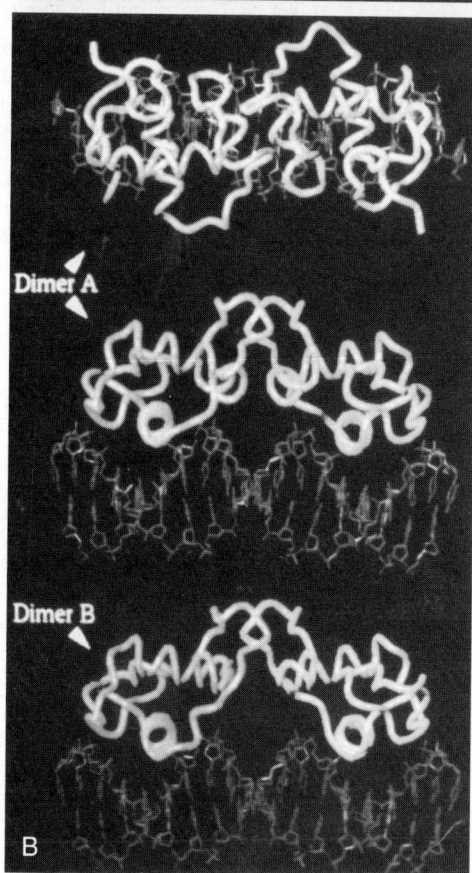

Figure 4–15. *A,* Structure of the ligand-binding domain of RXR (without ligand) and RAR bound to its ligand. *B,* Crystal structure of the DNA-binding domain of ER binding to its response element (see color section between pages 875 and 877). (*A* reprinted with permission from Renaud JP, Rochel M, Ruff V, et al. Crystal structure of the RAR-gamma ligand-binding domain bound to all-trans retinoic acid. Nature 1995; 378:681–689. Copyright 1995 Macmillan Magazines Ltd. *B* from Schwabe JWR, Chapman L, Finch JT, et al. The crystal structure of the estrogen receptor DNA-binding domain bound to DNA: how receptors discriminate between their response elements. Cell 1993; 75:567–578. Copyright 1993, Cell Press.)

suggested that the 66- to 68-amino-acids of region I encode the DNA-binding domain,[102–104] but direct evidence was not obtained until receptor chimeras were constructed in which the 66-amino-acid DNA-binding domain of the human glucocorticoid receptor was inserted in place of the homologous sequence of the human estrogen receptor.[25, 105, 106] This estrogen receptor–glucocorticoid receptor chimera was stimulated

by estrogen to activate a glucocorticoid-responsive reporter gene but was unable to stimulate an estrogen-inducible gene; e.g., this domain contains the information necessary for the sequence-specific recognition of target DNA (Fig. 4–16). Nine invariant cysteine residues have the potential to coordinate Zn^{2+} in a structure analogous to that of the protein transcription factor TFIIIA.[107] The technique of EXAFS (extended x-

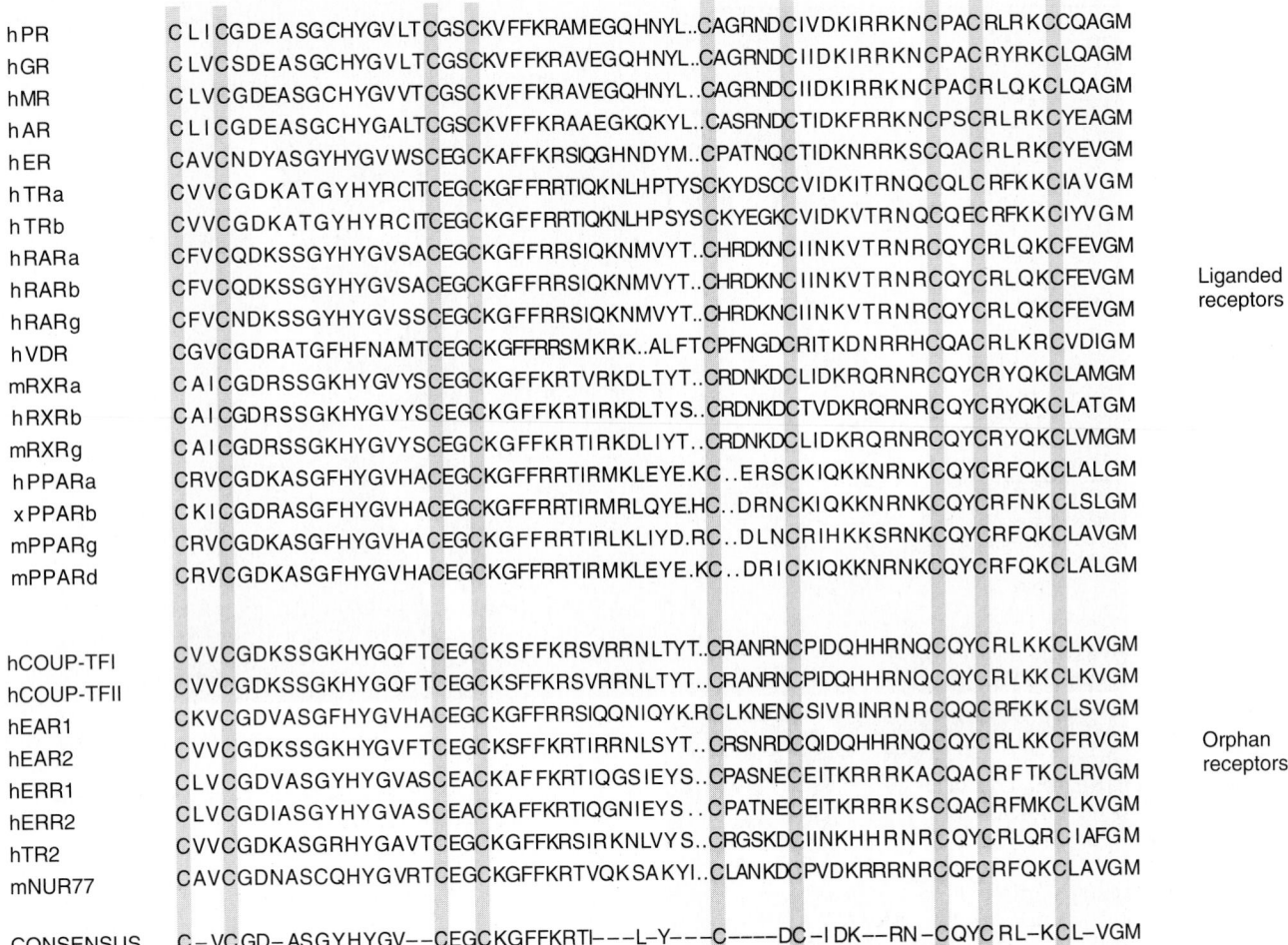

Figure 4–16. Sequence alignment of the DNA-binding domain of the various steroid receptors. There are nine invariant cysteines, which form the basis of two zinc coordinating finger structures.

ray absorption fine structure) spectroscopy has demonstrated that a tetrahedral arrangement of four cysteines coordinate Zn^{2+} or Cd^{2+} in the glucocorticoid receptor.[108] Titration experiments indicate that Zn^{2+} is required for maintenance of the DNA-binding activity.[109] This finding predicts the occurrence of two fingers (see Fig. 4–16), separated by a linker region of 15 to 17 amino acids. Unlike TFIIIA, which coordinates Zn^{2+} by a pair of cysteines and a pair of histidines (type I), steroid receptors coordinate Zn^{2+} only with cysteines (type II). Substitution of cysteine pairs with histidine pairs inactivates DNA binding,[110] and nonpaired substitution of cysteines with histidines partially inactivates DNA binding.[111] The ninth highly conserved cysteine is not essential for DNA binding, eliminating the possibility of an alternative finger structure involving this cysteine. For some steroid receptors, the two Zn^{2+} fingers are encoded by separate introns[111–115]; the two fingers are sufficiently different in structure that if they arose by duplication, they have since subsequently diverged considerably.

To determine the structural features of the Zn^{2+} fingers that determine DNA-binding specificity (for a review see reference 116), the approach was analogous to that of studies of the interaction of the lac repressor with the lac operator,[117] namely, the generation of "change-of-specificity" mutations. Studies in which individual fingers of the estrogen and glucocorticoid receptors were swapped[118] indicated that the first finger is largely responsible for DNA-binding specificity. A number of large-scale point mutation projects were initiated

independently to identify which of the amino acids of the two zinc fingers determines target gene specificity,[119–121] and a representative set of such mutations is shown in Figure 4–17. In the experiment shown, human glucocorticoid receptor was converted to a "promiscuous receptor" that activated both glucocorticoid responsive (GRE) and estrogen response elements (ERE) by a single Gly-to-Glu conversion in the second "knuckle" of the first finger (experiment 2). An additional conversion of the adjacent Ser to a Gly produced a hybrid receptor that activated a GRE reporter construct only weakly while activating the ERE reporter strongly (experiment 3). Almost complete conversion of glucocorticoid receptor to estrogen receptor was accomplished by changing a Phe to a Gly. The amino acids responsible for this change in specificity are located in the proximal portion of the first finger, and this region is referred to as a P box (see Fig. 4–14). To complete the change in specificity from a glucocorticoid receptor to an estrogen receptor, additional conversions (not shown) were necessary in the first knuckle of the distal finger, the D box (see Fig. 4–14).

These experiments identified two different classes of steroid receptor DNA-binding fingers (see Fig. 4–14). The two major classes of receptors differ primarily in the three variant amino acids of the P box. The first class (the glucocorticoid, progesterone, mineralocorticoid, and androgen receptors) is capable of stimulating the same steroid response element as discussed earlier. The second class of receptors has similar P boxes but divergent D boxes. In this formulation, the estrogen

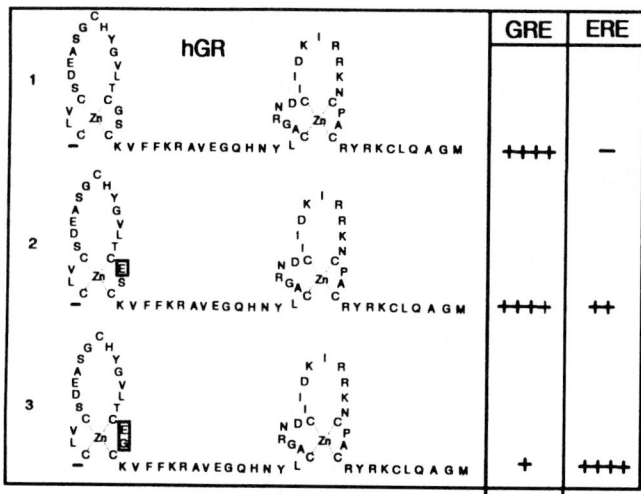

Figure 4–17. Summary of change-of-specificity studies. Boxed residues represent mutations to the wild-type receptor. Such experiments have defined two regions of the receptors that are largely responsible for sequence specificity.

receptor is related to the thyroid hormone, retinoic acid, and vitamin D receptors. This interpretation fits with the observation mentioned above that the ERE, retinoic acid response element (RARE), and vitamin D response element (VDRE) have the same DNA recognition sequence of AGG-TCA repeats except that the ERE is a palindromic repeat with a trinucleotide spacer, whereas the other response elements are direct repeats with different numbers of nucleotide spacers. Although certain receptors may recognize the same or similar response elements within a class, there are differences in the DNA-binding affinities and subtle differences in the interaction with target DNA.[122–124] These differences emphasize the role of additional sequences in the zinc fingers in determining the outcome of receptor-DNA interactions.

Magnetic resonance imaging and crystal structures of DNA-binding domains have been determined for several receptors (see Fig. 4–15B).[125–128] These structures confirm earlier deductions that the DNA-binding domains contain two modules, each coordinating one zinc molecule. In addition, the P box amino acids in the first module form a helix that interacts with the major groove of the recognition sequence. The second module, containing the second zinc molecule, is important for dimerization of two receptor DNA-binding domains by their D boxes and for phosphate contacts.

TRANSCRIPTION ACTIVATION REGIONS. The ultimate function of receptors, the modulation of transcription, has been analyzed with the use of receptor-deficient cell lines into which expression vectors are introduced. These vectors contain complementary DNAs (cDNAs) encoding steroid receptors and a target sequence containing specific response elements linked to a gene whose product is readily assayable, such as chloramphenicol acetyltransferase and luciferase. Mutations that involve conserved cysteines in the C region cause loss of glucocorticoid receptor trans-activation.[111] The rat glucocorticoid receptor contains an 86-amino-acid region including the DNA-binding region that is sufficient to mediate gene activation in stably and transiently transfected cells.[129] Similar findings have been reported for the human glucocorticoid[130] and progesterone[131] receptors. For several receptors, deletion of amino acids in the NH2 terminus results in reduced activation capacity.[11, 106, 130–132] Thus, both NH2-terminal and COOH-terminal regions are involved in transcriptional activation.

Since DNA binding is necessary for the receptor to activate its target gene, it is difficult to separate the gene activation and DNA-binding functions of receptor molecules. However,

functional hybrid proteins composed of the DNA-binding domains from unrelated transcription factors linked to receptor hormone-binding domains allow analysis of activation potential independent of receptor DNA-binding activity. A transactivation domain is defined as a portion of the protein that, when combined with DNA-binding activity, increases transcriptional initiation.[133–135] Chimeric proteins containing the hormone-binding domain of the human estrogen or glucocorticoid receptor and the DNA-binding domain of the yeast transcription factor GAL4, which itself has no intrinsic activation function, exhibited hormone-dependent activation of a GAL4-responsive reporter gene.[136] These results indicate that an activation domain is present in the hormone-binding region of the estrogen and glucocorticoid receptors. This transactivation domain in the human glucocorticoid receptor is in a 30-amino-acid region (tau2; amino acids 526 to 556) downstream of the DNA-binding domain.[137] A second transactivation domain (tau1; 185 amino acids in length—amino acids 77 to 262) is present in the NH2-terminal region of the protein. Both sequences appear to function independently of their position in the molecule and are acidic in character. In the rat glucocorticoid receptor, an enhancer region, enh2[138] is present between amino acids 237 and 318 and is not analogous in sequence to the enhancer region defined for the estrogen receptor.[139] Thus, receptors contain two or more activation domains (Fig. 4–18).

The chicken and human progesterone receptors provide a unique system in which to analyze the function of the NH2 terminus of the protein because the A forms of these receptors lack more than 100 amino acids found in the NH2 terminus of the B protein, including an acidic region. The chicken receptor A (but not the B receptor) activated transcription from the ovalbumin promoter, whereas both proteins activated transcription from a reporter plasmid containing a GRE or progesterone response element (PRE) fused to the thymidine kinase promoter and the chloramphenicol acetyltransferase gene.[140, 141] The lack of activation of ovalbumin gene by the B receptor was further investigated with the use of a chimera of the human estrogen receptor and the NH2-terminal 128 amino acids of the progesterone receptor B. This fusion protein did not induce ovalbumin gene transcription, whereas the estrogen receptor alone did.[141] The A form of the progesterone receptor (PR) can antagonize the function of many other steroid receptors, including that of ER and PR-B, suggesting an inhibitory role for the NH2-terminal domain of PR-A that is independent of DNA-binding specificity. In addition, the N-terminal region of receptors may help determine gene specificity.

Regulatory elements do not exist as isolated pieces of DNA in vivo but are arranged in complex chromatin structures. It is probable that to achieve appropriate gene activation, receptors must interact with other transcription factors and with structural components of chromatin. Current evidence suggests that steroid receptors interact with factors that

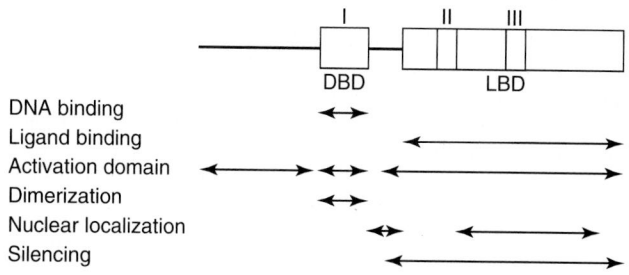

Figure 4–18. Steroid receptor functional domains. Horizontal bars below each receptor schematic show boundaries of the receptor required for retention of the function.

allow the chromatin remodeling (or nucleosome removal) required for gene activation.

Interactions of Receptors with Other Proteins

RECEPTOR DIMERIZATION. Dimerization of the estrogen receptor[142, 143] is believed to facilitate the binding of the estrogen-receptor complexes to target DNA enhancer sequences.[144] However, receptor monomers are equally capable of binding to nonspecific DNA sequences, such as calf thymus DNA.[145] The function of receptor dimer-DNA complexes was demonstrated by mixing experiments with receptor mutants of various sizes.[146, 147] However, because the end point of the assays was based on DNA-binding activity, it was unclear from these experiments whether the receptors dimerized before binding DNA or bound cooperatively on a DNA template, but the stoichiometry of receptor protein molecules to DNA is 2:1.[129] The fact that glutaraldehyde cross-linking, which stabilizes receptor monomers as dimers, had no effect on the apparent Stokes radius determined by gel filtration suggests that the glucocorticoid receptor is a homodimer in the absence of binding DNA. More direct evidence for receptor dimerization in the absence of DNA was obtained for the progesterone receptors by both chemical cross-linking and nondenaturing gradient gel electrophoresis.[148]

The dimerization domains have been identified by mutational analysis and by crystal structure analysis, as discussed earlier. A weak dimerization domain in the DNA-binding domain may involve the first zinc finger, the second zinc finger, or sequences downstream of the second zinc finger. The second and stronger dimerization domain is localized in the ligand-binding domain in the helix H10, H9 regions of the RXRα (see Fig. 4–15A). Dimerization requires hydrophobic interaction of these helices.[98–100]

INTERACTIONS WITH NONRECEPTOR PROTEINS. Certain steroid receptors bind to a 90-kd heat shock protein called hsp90. This molecule is a component of the heterodimeric untransformed 8S receptor complex for the progesterone, glucocorticoid, estrogen, and androgen receptors (see references 149 to 151 and references therein). Hsp90 is a protein found in high abundance (1 to 2% of cytosolic proteins[152, 153]). Pulse-chase experiments in tissue culture cells revealed that there is a time lag between the synthesis of hsp90 and the association with the glucocorticoid receptor.[154] Moreover, chemical cross-linking of the receptors in intact cells resulted in covalent association of hsp90.[155] When a steroid receptor is complexed to hsp90, the complex is unable to bind to calf thymus DNA, but binding of the steroid ligand, high salt concentrations, high temperature, and various other treatments facilitate the dissociation of the complex. Removal of hsp90, however, does not convert the receptor from an inactive to an active molecule.[156, 157] Instead, binding of hsp90 stablizes the glucocorticoid receptor in a form that is able to bind to its ligand with high affinity.[157, 158]

Deletion mutagenesis mapping studies performed on the glucocorticoid and progesterone receptors[159, 160] have localized the hsp90 interaction site to a fairly large COOH-terminal region that includes part of the steroid-binding domain. Interestingly, small deletions created throughout this entire region do not disrupt the formation of the hsp90-receptor complex.[160] Thus, the receptor may have multiple hsp90 contact sites. Antibodies directed against peptide fragments within the DNA-binding domain[161, 162] and the linker region[163] do not bind to the receptor-hsp90 complex.

Additional proteins associate with the untransformed receptor complex. A 56-kd protein, p56, is associated with the progesterone, estrogen, androgen, and glucocorticoid receptors.[164] It appears that p56 is an intranuclear phosphoprotein.[165]

Hsp70, a highly conserved protein in all cells from bacteria to higher eucaryotes, is normally found in the cytoplasm, but under conditions of stress it is concentrated in the nucleus of the cell, where it activates certain target genes in the heat shock response.[167] Unlike hsp90, hsp70 binds ATP and may be a member of the energy-dependent chaperonin class of proteins that are thought to be involved in protein folding[168] and in the transport of proteins to the nucleus. Although salt and heat treatment do not dissociate hsp70 from the progesterone receptor, high concentrations of ATP do cause dissociation.[166] The role, if any, of hsp70 in mediating receptor function is unknown.

RECEPTOR ACTIVITY MODIFICATIONS BY PHOSPHORYLATION. All steroid receptors studied to date are phosphoproteins, and post-translational modification is a potential pathway for control of hormone action. However, the functional significance of receptor phosphorylation has yet to be determined.

Phosphorylation has been implicated in the hormone-binding capacity of the androgen,[169] estrogen,[170] and glucocorticoid[171] receptors. The binding of androgen by the androgen receptor[172] and of estrogen by the estrogen receptor[173] are enhanced by the presence of phosphotyrosine.[173] Moreover, treatment of estrogen receptor synthesized in vitro with a purified tyrosine kinase increases the hormone-binding capacity from 1 and 4% to nearly maximal levels.[174] Other work has shown no evidence for the importance of this pathway. The progesterone receptor appears to be phosphorylated exclusively on serine residues,[175] and the phosphorylated amino acids in the glucocorticoid receptor are 89% phosphoserine and 11% phosphotyrosine.[176] Thus, it is not clear that the phosphorylation-dependent hormone binding of the estrogen and androgen receptors can be extended to all steroid receptors.

Hormone-dependent phosphorylation of the steroid receptors results in a characteristic decrease of electrophoretic mobility.[177] The human progesterone B receptor in cells in culture has a nascent molecular mass of 114 kd. About 6 to 10 h after hormone treatment of the cells, the receptor undergoes a phosphorylation that results in increased apparent molecular masses of 117 and 120 kd,[178] but the phosphorylation maturation does not appear to be necessary for hormone-binding activity.[179] Similarly, hormone-induced phosphorylation of purified progesterone receptor has no effect on the binding affinity for DNA.[180] In contrast, other studies of hormone-dependent receptor processing have indicated that crude preparations of the progesterone receptor from cells treated with hormone have an enhanced affinity for DNA.[181, 182] Because similar hormone treatments increase the phosphorylation of the progesterone[183–185] and glucocorticoid[186] receptors, phosphorylation may regulate aspects of DNA binding or transcriptional activation, or both, by steroid receptors.[187] However, mutation of the phosphorylated serine or threonine residues of some receptors does not affect receptor activity.[188] Nevertheless, phosphorylation may still be important for efficient *trans*-activation in special situations, such as ligand-independent or growth factor–dependent receptor activity.[189, 190]

Receptor Localization in the Cell

ANTIBODIES TO RECEPTOR PROTEINS. Monoclonal and polyclonal antibodies that recognize specific receptors for each steroid do not cross-react with receptors for different hormones. However, some monoclonal antibodies are reactive against the same receptor from other species. Thus, the proteins are distinctly different for each hormone but are conserved to some degree from birds to mammals. Receptor antibodies have been used to develop sensitive assays not dependent on hormone binding.

IMMUNOCYTOCHEMISTRY. In broken cell preparations glucocorticoid, progesterone, and estrogen receptors are present in cellular cytosols in the absence of hormone, whereas after hormone treatment receptors are extractable only at high salt levels, suggesting that cytoplasmic receptors bind hormone and rapidly translocate into the nucleus.[191–193] With the production of specific antireceptor antibodies and the development of immunocytochemical techniques, progesterone, estrogen, and androgen receptors are located primarily in the nucleus in the absence of hormone treatment.[194, 195] Nevertheless, several studies revealed immunoreactive glucocorticoid receptors in the cytoplasm of cells[196–199] in which progesterone receptor was exclusively nuclear. Glucocorticoid receptor–galactosidase fusion proteins are almost exclusively cytoplasmic in the absence of dexamethasone but become nuclear with the addition of hormone.[200] The presence of detectable cytoplasmic glucocorticoid receptor may be due to diffusion of the receptor from the nucleus in the absence of hormone.[201] The rate of diffusion of glucocorticoid receptor from liver nuclei of adrenalectomized rats is higher in the presence of dexamethasone than in its absence and is higher than the diffusion rate of progesterone receptor. These data suggest that glucocorticoid receptors are primarily nuclear regardless of the hormonal state. It is clear, however, that all receptors reside in the nucleus after hormone administration.

Nuclear localization of proteins occurs by two mechanisms: diffusion of proteins through the nuclear membrane and interaction of proteins with the nuclear pore, a process mediated by a translocation signal in the protein.[202] In the former case, the exclusion limit for spherical proteins is a molecular mass of 67 kd,[203] although the elliptical shape of steroid receptors[204] might facilitate diffusion despite larger size.

Amino acid sequences that bear strong homology to the nuclear translocation signal of simian virus 40 T antigen[205, 206] are located on the COOH-terminal side of the DNA-binding region in several receptors (Fig. 4–19). Nearly identical sequences are found in the glucocorticoid, progesterone, androgen, and mineralocorticoid receptors from various species. In contrast, sequences in this region of the estrogen, vitamin D, thyroid hormone, and retinoic acid receptors do not exhibit strong homology to the T antigen nuclear localization signal. Vitamin D and thyroid hormone receptors are tightly associated with the nucleus even in the absence of hormone and

TABLE 4–1. Induction of Ovalbumin mRNA During Acute Estrogen Administration*

Hormonal Status	Number of Ovalbumin mRNA Molecules/Cell
Withdrawn	4
0.5 h × DES	9
1 h × DES	50
4 h × DES	2300
8 h × DES	5100
29 h × DES	17,000
7 d × DES	43,000
Egg-laying hen	147,000

*Chicks were treated with DES for 10 d and then withdrawn from hormone for 11 or 12 d. The animals were then injected with a single dose of DES for the times indicated. Molecules of ovalbumin mRNA per cell were calculated from cDNA hybridization data.

Reprinted with permission from Harris SE, Rosen JM, Means AR, et al. Use of a specific probe for ovalbumin mRNA to quantitate estrogen-induced gene transcripts. Biochemistry 1975; 14:2072. Copyright 1975 American Chemical Society.

thus may differ from the larger receptors in their subcellular localization mechanisms.[207–209]

Receptor sequences in rabbit progesterone[210] and rat glucocorticoid receptors have been shown to function as nuclear translocation signals by analyses of deletion mutants.[200, 211] In addition to the constitutive nuclear localization signal, a hormone-dependent nuclear localization signal is present in the hormone-binding domain of the progesterone receptor.[210] The primary signal for nuclear localization of rat glucocorticoid receptor deletion mutants is located in the steroid-binding domain of the molecule and is unrelated to sequences found in T antigen.[7, 70]

HORMONAL CONTROL OF GENE EXPRESSION

Hormone Effects on Protein and RNA Synthesis

Hormones regulate growth, differentiation, and metabolic activity in most tissues. The regulation of protein synthesis is the principal action of steroid hormones, although certain functions are exceptions to this rule. Because RNAs play a central role in the control of protein synthesis, a large body of experimental evidence accumulated, suggesting that animal hormones also regulate the amount of cell enzymes and secretory proteins via RNA mediators,[211–213] and it soon became apparent that steroid hormones exert a qualitative influence on DNA transcription.[214]

REGULATION OF MESSENGER RNA LEVELS. The synthesis of ovalbumin in the chicken oviduct is dependent on prior administration of estrogen.[213, 215–218] After purification of the ovalbumin mRNA to near-homogeneity, a radioactive cDNA probe was utilized to quantify the number of ovalbumin mRNA molecules per cell (Table 4–1). In the absence of hormone, oviduct cells contain less than five copies of ovalbumin mRNA, and within 4 h of DES administration the mRNA reaches levels greater than 2000 molecules per cell; by 24 h the level approaches 20,000 molecules per cell. The accumulation curves are consistent with an enhancement of ovalbumin gene transcription.

"Nuclear Localization" Sequences of the Steroid Receptors and SV40 T antigen

Protein	1st. AA	Sequence							
SV40 T Ag.		P	K	K	K	R	K	V	
GR	491	R	K	T	K	K	K	I	K
MR	673	R	K	S	K	K	L	G	K
AR	628	R	K	L	K	K	L	G	N
PR	637	R	K	F	K	K	F	N	K
ER	256	R	K	D	R	R	G	G	R
T₃Rβ	179	K	R	L	A	K	R	K	L
RAR	162	R	K	A	H	Q	E	T	F
VDR	102	R	K	R	E	M	I	L	L

Figure 4–19. Nuclear localization sequences determined by comparison with a known sequence of this type present in simian virus 40 (SV40).

HORMONES INCREASE THE RATE OF MESSENGER RNA SYNTHESIS

In certain cases, however, steroid hormones can decrease the turnover of mRNA and documentation that ovalbumin

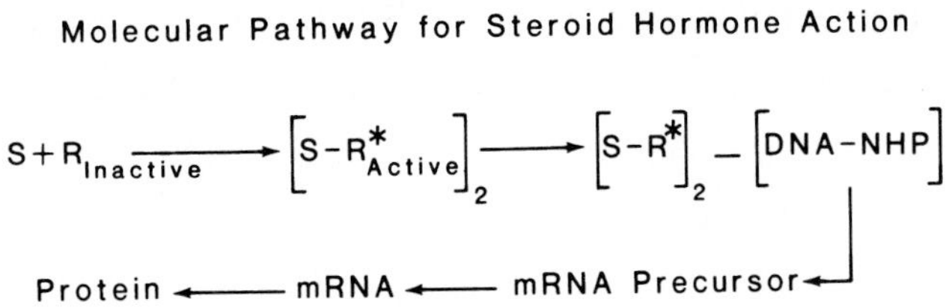

Molecular Pathway for Steroid Hormone Action

$$S + R_{Inactive} \longrightarrow \left[S\text{-}R^{*}_{Active} \right]_2 \longrightarrow \left[S\text{-}R^{*} \right]_2 - \left[DNA\text{-}NHP \right]$$

$$\text{Protein} \longleftarrow \text{mRNA} \longleftarrow \text{mRNA Precursor} \longleftarrow$$

Figure 4–20. Steroid hormone (S) enters the cell and binds to an inactive receptor (Rinactive) in the nucleus (or cytoplasm). The receptor is activated and binds to nuclear DNA as a dimer. This activated dimer complex binds upstream of genes to regulatory sites (DNA-NHP) composed of DNA and nonhistone chromosomal protein (NHP). This interaction leads to synthesis of mRNA precursor, which is processed to mature mRNA before exiting the nucleus. The mRNA is then transported to the cytoplasm, where it is translated on polysomes to produce the induced protein.

mRNA synthesis is increased required analysis of pulse-labeled RNA obtained in nuclear run-off assays.

Chick oviduct nuclei obtained before and after hormonal stimulation of target cells were incubated with radioactive precursors to RNA, and the labeled RNA was hybridized to ovalbumin cDNA or to ovalbumin gene fragments. In the absence of hormone, no synthesis of radiolabeled mRNA was detected, but within 1 h after the exposure of cells to steroid hormones synthesis was induced.[216, 219] The intracellular concentration of MMTV RNA in liver cells exposed to glucocorticoids increased 100-fold.[220-222] The rate of MMTV gene transcription is nearly maximal within 15 min of exposure to dexamethasone. These results were subsequently confirmed for the actions of steroid hormones on the synthesis of a variety of mRNAs in other systems[223-228] (Fig. 4–20). Not all steroid responses at the level of DNA are inductive. For example, glucocorticoid inhibits the synthesis of pro-opiomelanocortin mRNA and prolactin mRNA and inhibits thymus cell function. Nevertheless, the major effect of steroid hormones is to induce the accumulation of specific mRNAs in target cells, and for the most part the effect is at the level of gene transcription.

HORMONES REGULATE MESSENGER RNA STABILITY

Differential stability is a fundamental property of mRNAs and proteins.[229] The average half-lives of most eucaryotic mRNAs range from 8 to 20 h; the average half-life for protein is about 48 to 72 h. More labile mRNAs contain structural features that make them susceptible to nuclease degradation; one common feature of labile mRNAs consists of uridine residues interspersed with occasional adenine residues, denoted by $(U)_nA$, usually in 3'-nontranslated regions of unstable mRNAs, that are thought to be sites of attack for endonucleases. Deletion of these residues stabilizes the mRNA.[230] In addition to their effects on gene transcription, hormones can stabilize mRNA and protein products emanating from their target genes. This is a powerful combination in that a five-fold increase in transcription, a five-fold increase in the half-life of mRNA, and a five-fold increase in protein half-life can result in a 125-fold increase in the protein product of that gene. In the absence of steroid hormone, vitellogenin mRNA in the liver of *Xenopus* has a half-life of 16 h, and in the presence of estrogen its half-life is 500 h[231]; the half-life of total mRNA in these cells is unaffected by hormone.[230] The stabilization is dependent on the presence of estrogen-receptor complex, suggesting that mRNA stabilization occurs via a receptor-dependent process.

Gene Structure and Evolution

The fact that most genes are split into pieces and the protein-coding information is assembled at the RNA level changed our concepts about the evolution of proteins.[232-235]

GENE STRUCTURE. In eucaryotic cells, the DNA regions that correspond to sequences expressed in mature mRNA are referred to as *structural sequences* or *exons*.[236, 237] Exons include both the coding regions that are translated into protein and the nontranslated regions that appear in the mature mRNA. The regions of DNA that lie between the exons are called *intervening sequences* or *introns*. The gene is thus an alternating series of exons and introns, the introns being eliminated from the mature cytoplasmic RNA by splicing reactions within the nucleus (Fig. 4–21).

The majority of eucaryotic structural genes contain intervening sequences ranging from as few as one (an insulin gene) to as many as 50 (a collagen gene).[233, 234, 238, 239] Only a limited number of genes, such as those coding for the histones and for adrenergic receptors, are devoid of intervening sequences.

INTRONS. Introns vary from as few as 50 bases to 10,000 bases or more. Introns occur in both the coding region and the untranslated parts of the ultimate mRNA. Introns for the most part differ in sequence except that there is an absolute requirement for a GT at the 5' end and an AG at the 3' end of all intron sequences. The intron sequences are generally pyrimidine rich, especially at the 3' end. The combined length of the introns is usually greater than that of the exons, causing the gene to occupy much more genomic DNA than the coding capacity would require. In other words, genes are not exact structural counterparts of their mRNAs. Introns are a feature of eucaryotic organisms and are not found in bacteria.[234, 236]

GENE EVOLUTION. Introns have been postulated to function as (1) protective elements that prevent recombination by unequal crossing over between closely related genes, (2) adventitious structural elements reminiscent of random insertions in DNA by transposition, (3) regulatory elements that control either the production of biologically active mRNA or its export to the cytoplasm, or (4) remnants of the evolutionary construction of genes. The evolutionary hypothesis is now generally accepted.

A hypothesis for the probable origin of intervening sequences is shown in Figure 4–22. The open boxes represent coding regions of DNA (exons), and the thin solid lines represent either introns or flanking DNA sequences. Panel I shows gene assembly from diverse exon elements without the benefit of introns, and panel II represents the alternative method of gene assembly in which introns are generated. Genes probably evolved by the assembly of blocks of coding sequences during DNA recombination. Panel I shows the problem inherent in the assembly of complex genes from diverse exon segments. The recombination must occur at precise sites at either end of the exon. Otherwise, the reading frame of the resulting mRNA would be altered and the functional integrity of the resulting polypeptide might be destroyed. Because recombina-

Structure of a Simple Eucaryotic Gene

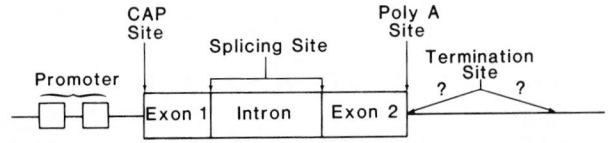

Figure 4–21. Most genes are composed of exons (structural sequences retained in mature mRNA) and introns (intervening sequences removed during splicing of pre-mRNA). Transcription begins at CAP site and ends at poly(A) site. The exact point of termination is variable among genes. Initiation of transcription by RNA polymerase is controlled at the promoter region.

An Evolutionary Hypothesis for the Origin of Intervening Sequences

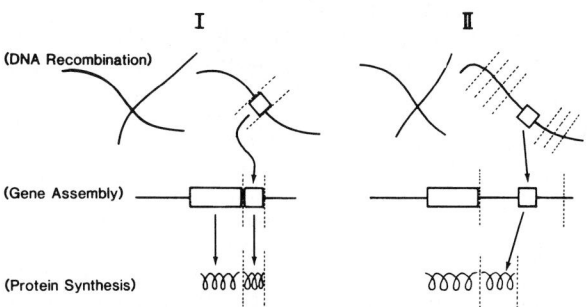

Figure 4–22. Column I depicts gene assembly from diverse exon elements in a manner that would not account for introns. Column II represents a more likely method of gene assembly that accounts for the generation of introns. See text for details.

Evolution of a Multidomain Secretory Protein

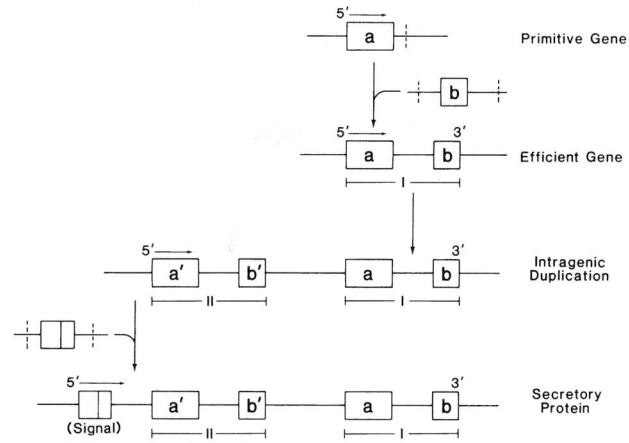

Figure 4–23. A primitive gene (exon a) evolves by a recombination event, which brings a new exon (b) into the gene unit. At this point the gene is composed of two exons and one intron. An intragenic duplication event occurs, probably by unequal crossing over, followed by addition of a final exon, which acts as a signal sequence for secretion. The final gene unit contains five exons and four introns.

tion is random, a requirement for absolute precision in breakage (or excision) of the segments of DNA to be reassembled makes the event an occurrence of low probability and would greatly lengthen evolutionary process. Panel II depicts the same event as it is now thought to have occurred, leading to the development of complex eucaryotic genes. Recombination, to bring together the diverse exon segments, could occur at any one of numerous sites in the flanking DNA sequence on either side of the exon sequences. This model greatly facilitates evolution because the probability of occurrence is orders of magnitude greater than that for the model depicted in panel I. In this manner, eucaryotes have a faster genetic development per unit time. The creation of intervening sequences between the two exons poses no problem, provided that an early mechanism existed (or developed) for splicing these introns out of the primary RNA transcripts. Such RNA-splicing enzymes do exist, and introns do not provide a barrier to functional gene expression.

Introns provide two additional evolutionary advantages to the organism. Recombination of exons from separate genes permits the rapid assembly of new combinations of coding sequences, which, if they provided a selective advantage to the organism, could be held constant. In addition, homologous recombination is facilitated by the extra length of the intron existing between exon units, allowing proteins to duplicate their own exons and grow in length. These concepts explain the fact that introns define separate functional domains for a number of proteins, such as immunoglobulins, myoglobin, ovomucoid, globin, glyceraldehyde-phosphate dehydrogenase, proinsulin, and α-fetoprotein.

A theoretical example of the evolution of a complex gene coding for a secretory protein is shown in Figure 4–23. In an early stage of evolution, a primitive gene existed that coded for a functionally inefficient protein a. A second exon coding for a peptide b that complemented peptide a was brought into the genetic unit via recombination. Because peptide b provided peptide a with increased functional efficiency, the recombination was stabilized by positive selection. With time, an intragenic duplication of the gene occurred via unequal crossing over to provide exons a' and b'. This led to a larger, even more efficient protein, and the duplication was stabilized. This event provided additional evolutionary flexibility because exons a' and b' were now free to undergo small "trial mutations" without disrupting the basic function of exons a and b, thereby eventually providing a broader range of activity for the gene product as a whole. Finally, to provide advantageous secretory capacity for the protein, a "signal" exon was acquired by a fortuitous but stabilized recombination event. The final gene structure (see Fig. 4–23) is common among structural genes. The question arises of how the splicing reac-

tion evolved. It appears that the earliest RNA molecules were capable of self-splicing; that is, no enzyme protein was required for removal of introns or nonsense sequences.[240] This reaction of RNA catalysis is inefficient, and with time the evolution of enzyme-RNA complexes termed spliceosomes improved the accuracy and efficiency of this process. These complexes are located in the nuclear compartment.

Processing of Messenger RNA Precursors

During the transcription reaction, the entire gene (exons plus introns) is transcribed 5' to 3' (left to right, Fig. 4–24) as one high-molecular-weight RNA that exactly represents the genetic sequence. This form of RNA is inactive biologically for the production of protein. For translation to take place the introns must be removed to produce the smaller biologically active cytoplasmic mRNA, consisting of contiguous exons joined together in the order in which they are represented in DNA. This means that colinearity of gene and protein exists between the individual exons and the corresponding parts of the protein chain.[241–247]

Transcription of the Natural Ovomucoid Gene

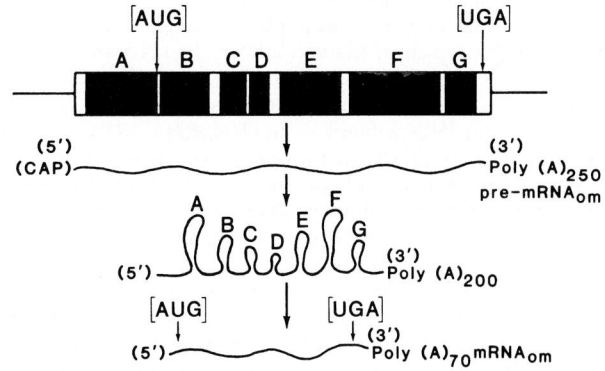

Figure 4–24. Ovomucoid gene of chicken contains eight exons and seven introns. The primary transcript contains a continuous RNA copy of the entire gene. It receives a CAP at the 5' end, and poly(A) is added to the 3' end. It attaches to nuclear matrix, where a complex splicing enzyme system removes all intron sequences (labeled A to G). When transcript is free from introns, it detaches from matrix and is transported to cytoplasm, where it can be translated.

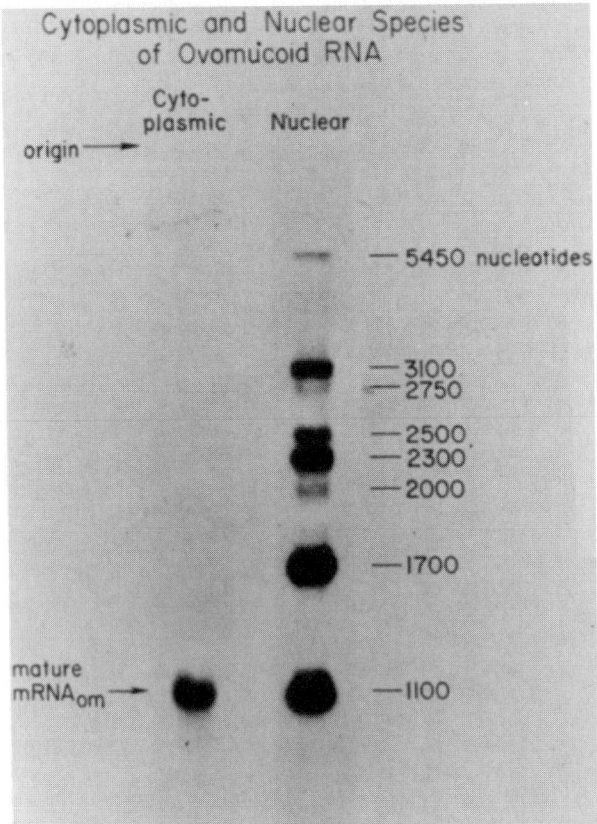

Figure 4–25. Northern blot hybridization to detect mRNA precursors. RNA has been extracted from cytoplasm and from purified nuclei of oviduct cells. RNA is separated according to size on a denaturing gel, and ovomucoid RNA is detected by hybridizing to a [³²P]ovomucoid DNA probe. Cells were washed and subjected to autoradiography. Film shows dark bands in all regions where ovomucoid RNA exists. As shown, cytoplasm contains only mature mRNA devoid of introns. In contrast, nucleus contains high-molecular-weight species of ovomucoid RNA, representing primary transcript (5450 nucleotides) and various processing intermediates.

PRECURSOR MESSENGER RNA. The enzymatic splicing of the primary transcript (pre-mRNA) requires two independent steps: (1) excision of the intron and (2) ligation of the adjacent exons to form an uninterrupted coding sequence. When cytoplasmic and nuclear RNA is extracted from a chick oviduct, electrophoresed on denaturing gels, and hybridized to a cloned [³²P] cDNA segment of ovomucoid, the results shown in Figure 4–25 are obtained. In the cytoplasm, a single ovomucoid mRNA species of 1100 nucleotides (NT) represents biologically active, mature mRNA. In contrast, nuclear RNA contains a series of discrete bands, suggesting that splicing occurs via a sequential pathway rather than in a random manner.[248] The largest band of nuclear RNA (5450 nucleotides) [NT] corresponds to the size of the gene, represents the primary transcript, and contains the RNA complement of eight exons and seven introns. The smaller band is again the mature mRNA devoid of introns. In between, each band represents a specific precursor intermediate from which some introns have been removed. For instance, the 1700 NT intermediate contains only one remaining intron of 600 NT (see Fig. 4–25). The probable explanation is that the conformation of RNA influences the accessibility of the splicing junctions to the enzyme.[245–250]

The excision of introns in pre-mRNA is enzymatically complex, requiring small nuclear RNAs (snRNA: U1, U2, U4, U5, and U6) and more than 30 precursor RNA-processing (PRP) proteins.[251] In addition, three short sequences in the intron of pre-mRNA are essential: 5′ splice site, 3′ splice site, and A branch point which is usually 15 to 40 NT upstream from the 3′ splice site. The splicing process starts first with the pairing of U2-snRNA (in ribonucleoprotein complex, or snRNP, form) to the intron of the 5′ splice site. Next U2-snRNA (also in snRNP form) interacts with the branch point. Subsequent association of U1- and U2-snRNAs brings 5′ and 3′ splicing sites into proximity. Finally, a preformed, U4-U5-U6-snRNP complex joins the splicing complex to form the final spliceosome that performs the splicing reaction, consisting of two *trans*-esterifications. First, the branch point A forms a lariat intermediate with a 5′ splicing guanine and releases the 5′ exon; subsequently, the 5′ exon replaces the 3′ intron and releases the intron in a lariat structure. In this way, the 5′ exon is ligated to the 3′ exon as the intron sequence is spliced out.

The splicing of pre-mRNA may be a rate-limiting step for mRNA generation and could be a control site for regulating mRNA levels, but hormones do not appear to regulate mRNA levels by influencing processing of mRNA precursors. The existence of introns and the requirement for their removal have provided insight into the pathogenesis of genetic diseases. Gene mutations occurring in the middle of individual introns are generally without effect, because the introns are not part of the mRNA, whereas mutations in intron sequences immediately adjacent to the intron-exon junctions or branching site interfere with splicing and create inactive mRNAs containing a residual intron. A number of examples of such mutations have been reported in diseases such as human thalassemias. In addition, differential splicing (exon inclusion) plays a major role in gene expression during development, such as in sex determination in *Drosophila*.[43]

MATURE CYTOPLASMIC MESSENGER RNA. A typical structure of an eucaryotic mRNA is shown in Figure 4–26. The CAP site is defined by the first nucleotide (+1) of the mRNA precursor (and consequently the mature mRNA), which is generally a purine followed by a pyrimidine. Shortly after synthesis of pre-mRNA, a hypermethylated pyrophosphate containing nucleotide (guanine) is added to the structural nucleotides (e.g., N_1, N_2) so that a final average 5′ end of an mRNA molecule can be represented as $M^7G(5')ppp(5')N_1mp-N_2p$, with M representing the methyl groups. The CAP site is often followed by an untranslated leader region, followed by a ribosome-binding site that includes the initiation codon (AUG or GUG) for translation. If the mRNA codes for a secreted protein, the subsequent region contains a signal sequence that codes for a short processed peptide (15 to 30 amino acids) and provides the means of attachment for ribosomes translating the mRNA to the intracisternal membranes as a complex. In this manner, secreted proteins can be channeled into the appropriate cytoplasmic compartments and membranes. The coding sequence is followed by a termination codon (UAA, UAG, and UGA), which ends protein synthesis and releases the mRNA from ribosomes. The termination codon is followed by an untranslated region that is variable in size and sequence among mRNAs.[234, 235] The 3′ terminus contains a sequence of 30 to

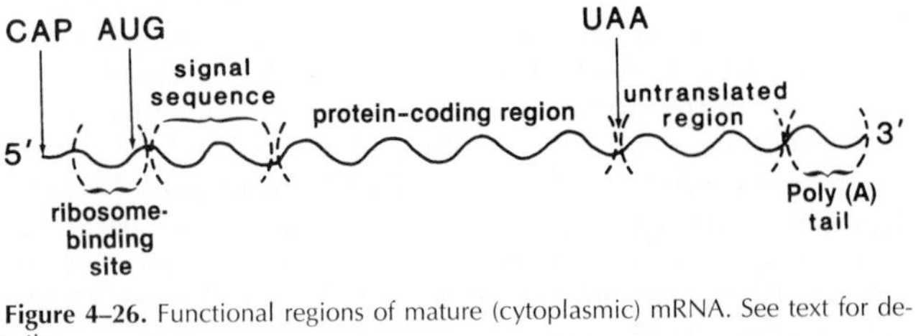

CAP AUG
signal sequence
protein-coding region
UAA
untranslated region
5′
ribosome-binding site
Poly (A) tail
3′

Figure 4–26. Functional regions of mature (cytoplasmic) mRNA. See text for details.

150 or more adenylic acid residues. The poly(A) sequence is not coded in the DNA but is added in the nucleus after transcription; it may aid in stabilization or export, or both, of the mRNA to the cytoplasm. The hexanucleotide AAUAAA at the 3'-untranslated sequences of all mRNAs about 25 nucleotides before the poly(A) tail appears to act as a polyadenylation signal for the poly(A) polymerase. Transcription does not always end at the last nucleotide of the last exon; in certain cases gene transcription may terminate thousands of nucleotides downstream from the exon terminus. In each case, however, the extra nucleotides are removed in concert with the addition of poly(A) to the last nucleotide of the terminal exon. Although termination of transcription and addition of poly(A) are potential regulatory sites for gene expression, there is no evidence for such control of eucaryotic genes to date.

Organization of Eucaryotic Chromosomes

Each human cell contains 3×10^9 base pairs of DNA that encode about 100,000 functional genes. This extraordinary length of DNA fits into the nucleus of a cell whose diameter may be only 6 μm. In addition, most (90%) of the DNA in most cells is not called into action for cellular functions. For these reasons it seems logical for the cell to package most of its DNA into inaccessible structures so that the length of the DNA is reduced and unexpressed genes are inaccessible to transcription factors and RNA polymerase. Genes and segments of DNA expressed in the lifetime of a given cell must be in more accessible structures.[252–257]

HIGHER-ORDER STRUCTURE. The organization of eucaryotic DNA is illustrated in Figure 4–27. Free DNA has a fiber diameter of approximately 2 nm. The ratio of the length of DNA to the length of the unit that contains it can be normalized to a value of one. Because an extremely high packing ratio for the genetic material must be reached, the DNA is packaged in a hierarchy of structures. Eucaryotic chromosomes are formed by the interaction between DNA and the

five basic histones (H1, H2A, H2B, H3, and H4).[254, 258, 259] All the histones except H1 interact directly with DNA to form a first-level organization of particles in chromatin, the histone octamer, which combines with about 200 base pairs of DNA to form bead-like structures (nucleosomes) along the DNA, increasing the fiber width to 10 nm and creating a length compaction ratio of 6 (see Fig. 4–27). The DNA is wound around the outside of the core histone particles and may be available to interact with regulatory proteins or RNA polymerase. This nucleosomal level of organization is now supercoiled on itself into a structure referred to as a solenoid.[260, 261] Histone H1 plays a critical role in linking the nucleosomal strands to produce the solenoid. The fiber now becomes thicker (30 nm), and the length compaction ratio reaches approximately 40.

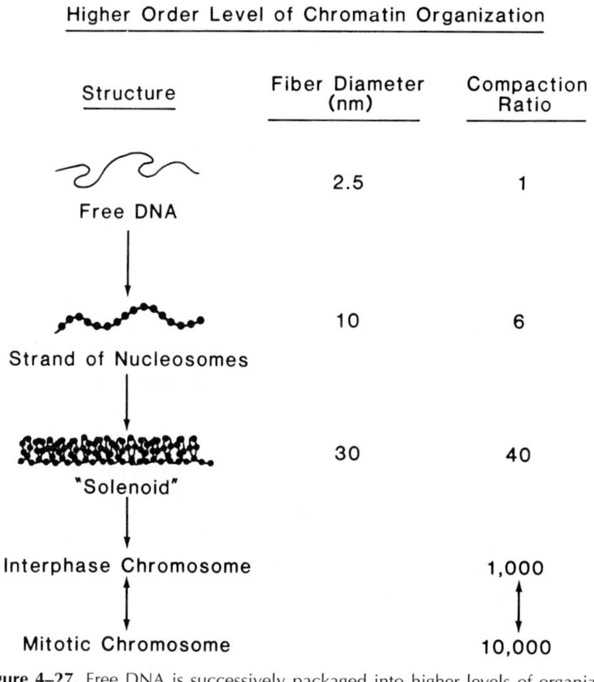

The final structural organization of chromatin is believed to involve a further supercoiling of the solenoid to achieve a final length compaction ratio of approximately 1000 in interphase chromosomes. The mitotic chromosomes are packaged even more tightly to a length compaction ratio of approximately 10,000. Nonhistone proteins involved in chromosomal organization include all of the proteins necessary for replicating and transcribing DNA and the enzymes involved in structural and covalent modifications or degradations.[261, 262] Most important are the regulatory proteins, which play an important role in determining the appropriate structures for gene expression and in controlling the initiation of transcription.[257, 262, 263]

ACTIVE DOMAINS IN CHROMOSOMES. Expressible genes are packaged into chromatin differently than the regions of the DNA that are not expressed.[262, 264, 265] Genes that are transcriptionally active or that have the potential for expression in response to appropriate inducers are more susceptible to cleavage by nucleases. Such genes include globin, ovalbumin, vitellogenin, insulin, immunoglobulin, histone, and a variety of integrated genes for viral proteins. It is thought that nuclease sensitivity is due to accessibility to the enzyme because the DNA exists in a more unraveled or "open" superstructure. Acquisition of a nuclease-sensitive state appears to be a general prerequisite for eucaryotic gene expression. The borders of nuclease sensitivity around expressible genes can be defined with cloned DNA fragments as specific hybridization probes,[262] and the DNase I–sensitive conformation extends beyond the boundaries of the transcription units of genes into the sequences that flank the 5' and 3' ends of the genes.

DNase I sensitivity appears to reflect a more accessible chromatin structure that correlates with the capacity of a cell to express the gene in question. This property appears to be a necessary but not sufficient step in gene transcription[265, 266] (Fig. 4–28). In the chicken, these chromosomal DNase I–sensitive domains range in size from 20 kb for the glyceraldehyde-phosphate dehydrogenase gene to more than 100 kb for the three members of the ovalbumin gene family. The domain containing the constitutive glyceraldehyde-phosphate dehydrogenase gene is sensitive to DNase I in all cells because it is expressed in all cells. For hormone-regulatable genes such as the ovalbumin gene family, the genes are sensitive to DNase I only in the oviduct target cells in which these genes are expressed. Furthermore, when the transcription of ovalbumin X and Y genes is eliminated by the withdrawal of hormone from estrogen-stimulated chickens, the entire domain remains in a DNase I–sensitive configuration. For this reason DNase I–sensitive domains may provide the chromosomal structural capacity required for gene expression, and they appear to be determined during differentiation because they are cell specific and contain many of the potentially expressible genes of that cell type (see Fig. 4–28).

Dominant control sequences at the borders of these do-

Higher Order Level of Chromatin Organization

Structure	Fiber Diameter (nm)	Compaction Ratio
Free DNA	2.5	1
Strand of Nucleosomes	10	6
"Solenoid"	30	40
Interphase Chromosome		1,000
Mitotic Chromosome		10,000

Figure 4–27. Free DNA is successively packaged into higher levels of organization by complex supercoiling. At each level, the length of the DNA is reduced by a factor approximating the compaction ratio. This packaging is due primarily to interactions with histones.

Relationship Between Cell Differentiation and DNase I Sensitivity of Tissue-Specific Genes – A Working Model

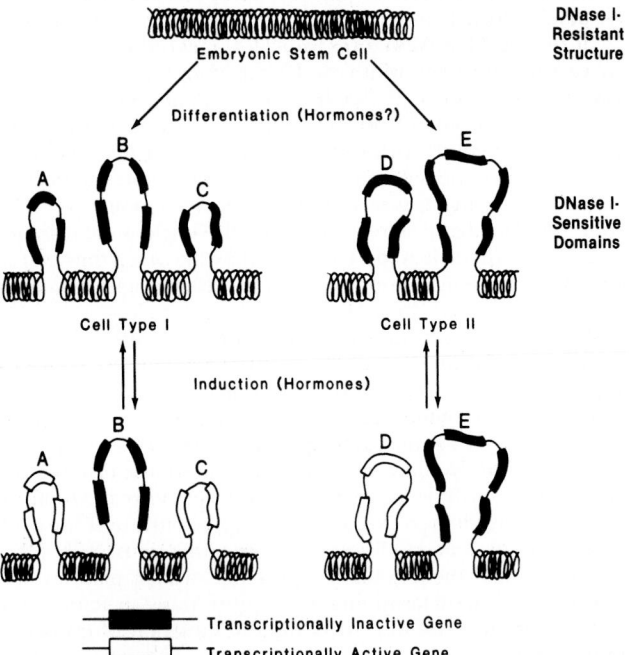

Figure 4–28. At early stages of differentiation, much of the DNA is packaged into higher-order structure with histones and is unavailable to interact with either biochemical probes, such as DNase I, or regulatory molecules, such as steroid receptors and RNA polymerase. During differentiation, regions of genomic DNA that contain potentially expressible genes are converted to "open" or uncoiled structures, which are now accessible to regulatory molecules and RNA polymerase. This structure is necessary but not sufficient for expression. Hormone-receptor complexes now bind to these regions and activate the genes.

mains are thought to maintain the domain structure, perhaps by binding proteins and preventing the packaging of the DNA into the solenoid structure that represses the included genes.[267] Such sequences are likely to be composed of enhancers that bind transcription factors and prevent the folding and packaging of protein-free DNA by histones at the time of DNA replication. In other words, all genes that are capable of transcription in a given cell must be contained within these accessible regions of chromatin at the time of terminal differentiation. The domains are both tissue specific and irreversible. The DNA that is not in these domains appears to be packaged into inaccessible chromatin structure by histones and is unavailable for subsequent interactions with regulatory molecules (see Fig. 4–28).[265, 266]

NUCLEAR MATRIX. The nuclear matrix is a dense fibrillar network of proteins that lies within the nuclear membrane.[268] This structure acts as a framework, or skeleton, for many nuclear processes and may connect with cytoskeleton proteins. The structure of the matrix is not yet understood, although it is composed of a large number of different proteins. The chromatin itself is intermittently attached to the nuclear matrix, and the primary RNA transcripts of genes probably attach to it soon after or even during transcription. RNA processing also may take place on the matrix (Fig. 4–29).[268] After repeated low-salt and high-salt (2 mol/L NaCl) extraction of nuclei, approximately 10 to 15% of the nuclear proteins remain.[268, 269] The dehistonized and uncoiled DNA is attached to the residual protein matrix in short regions interspersed with unattached "loops" of DNA that average 30 to 100 kb in length (not shown in Fig. 4–29). If the dehistonized and unattached DNA in the loops is digested with a site-specific restriction endonuclease, 85% of the DNA can be released

from the preparation. The residual matrix-bound 15% of DNA can be purified and analyzed for the presence of specific sequences.

In the chicken, actively transcribed genes are located in the residual matrix-bound DNA.[269, 270] Genes not expressed are in the released DNA fraction after restriction enzyme treatment because they are not attached to the matrix. Hormone-regulatable genes such as the ovalbumin gene become attached to matrix during hormonal stimulation. In contrast, when hormone is withdrawn and ovalbumin gene transcription ceases, the gene is no longer attached to the matrix. Constitutively expressed genes are generally attached to the matrix, and the attachment is independent of the absolute rate of transcription. This correlation between the transcription of genes and their association with the nuclear matrix indicates that the nuclear matrix is a likely site for cellular DNA transcription. Such attachment to the matrix could either facilitate transcription of DNA by RNA polymerase or be a concomitant of transcription. Steroid hormone–receptor complexes are associated with the nuclear matrix, and on hormonal withdrawal, the receptors dissociate with the nuclear matrix.

STRUCTURAL REQUIREMENTS FOR GENE EXPRESSION. The cellular forces involved in steroid hormone induction of transcription are summarized in Figure 4–30:

1. The steroid receptor is activated by hormone, dimerizes, and binds DNA. The receptor is the obligatory and active intermediate required for steroid hormone action and acts as a transducer to transfer the informational signal inherent in a steroid hormone molecule to the regulatable target gene. Steroid hormone receptors are members of a larger, incompletely defined class of nuclear transcription factors.

2. The primary sequence of the gene to be expressed contains not only the inherited structural code for the protein but also distinct promoter and enhancer elements, both of which bind transcription factors and receptors and determine the maximal rate of hormone-induced gene expression. An enhancer element is the cognate DNA-binding site for the receptor dimer. After the receptor binds to the DNA response element, coregulator proteins (coactivators or corepressors) then assemble at the receptor via protein-protein interactions, to form the final active complex.

3. Inducible genes are contained within large structurally

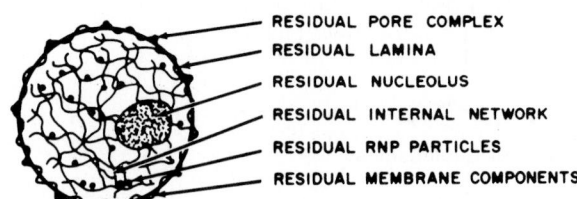

- LIPID FREE
- REPRESENTS ONLY 10% OF TOTAL NUCLEAR PROTEINS. CONTAINS RELATED PROTEINS
- SITE OF ATTACHMENTS OF DNA LOOPS
- CONTAINS FIXED SITES FOR DNA SYNTHESIS
- ASSOCIATED WITH HnRNA
- SPECIFIC BINDING OF HORMONES
- PROTEINS PHOSPHORYLATED
- MAY HAVE DYNAMIC PROPERTIES

Figure 4–29. Major structural features of nuclear matrix. (Courtesy of Dr. Donald S. Coffey, Johns Hopkins School of Medicine.)

Determinants for Hormonal Induction of Gene Expression

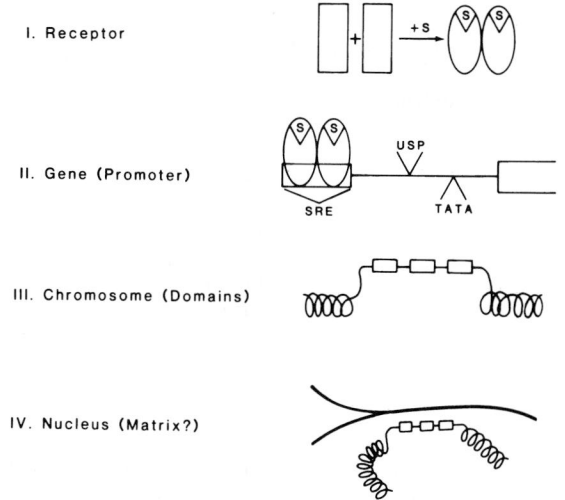

Figure 4–30. Major structural levels of control are (I) steroid-receptor interaction; (II) regulatory sequences around (or in) structural genes; (III) chromosomal structure, including "expressible domains"; and (IV) interactions of chromosomal genes with nuclear matrix.

distinct (DNase I–sensitive) domains that constitute an index of molecular differentiation and probably maintain the capacity of genes to respond to inductive influences.

4. The chromatin itself is attached to the nuclear matrix, so the actively expressed regions of these domains appear to be more firmly bound and perhaps more easily transcribed by the nuclear transcription apparatus.

Additional potentially important levels of substructure include modification of primary DNA sequence (e.g., methylation and Z-DNA, a left-handed coil of DNA)[271] and chromatin fine structure (nuclease hypersensitivity).[263, 272]

Regulatory Elements Located Adjacent to Genes

The initiation of gene transcription requires the formation of a complex between RNA polymerase and DNA at a site that surrounds the first base to be transcribed into RNA. The amount of RNA polymerase in eucaryotic cells is small, ranging from 5×10^4 to 10^5 molecules per cell. Since 10^4 genes may be expressed in a given cell type, the genes are in competition for RNA polymerase and must attract the enzyme to their respective regulatory regions to be transcribed, the promoter-enhancer region. This region may include the DNA sequence that is stably bound in the initiation complex and sequences whose recognition is necessary but that are not an integral part of the stable binding site (Fig. 4–31). The promoter appears to regulate the rate and accuracy of transcription. Additional regulatory elements adjacent to the promoter region may act as enhancers to activate or "silence" functional

promoters. Hormone control elements are one class of regulator elements.[273–278]

PROMOTERS. The basic promoter for eucaryotic genes transcribed by RNA polymerase II consists of two main parts (see Fig. 4–31). Beginning at -30 nucleotides (30 bases upstream) before the start site of transcription, the core promoter is a 7 base pair AT-rich sequence called the TATA box. A consensus sequence for all TATA boxes can be described as TATAT/AAT/A. The TATA box may contain either an A or a T in positions 5 and 7, and a G-C pair may be present within the box. Changing only one interior nucleotide pair in the sequence to a GC residue eliminates 80% of the transcription from that gene.[279] Many promoters also have an initiator sequence, Inr, which also can direct RNA polymerase to a correct initiation site.[280] An Inr can exist either alone in a promoter or with a TATA box. For promoters that do not contain either a TATA box or an initiator, transcriptional initiation usually occurs in several different sites. Many of the "housekeeping gene" promoters belong to this class. At approximately 80 nucleotides upstream of the structural gene an additional sequence that has been conserved in some promoters is referred to as an upstream promoter element and is thought to modify the basal rate of transcription of a given promoter (see Fig. 4–31). In this case, the proximal (TATA box) and more distal elements of the promoter function as a unit to regulate transcription.[281]

ENHANCERS AND SILENCERS. Enhancer elements are short (about 15 base pairs) DNA sequences that increase the rate of transcription of adjacent genes. They are usually located in the 5′-flanking region of eucaryotic genes but are largely position and orientation independent (see Fig. 4–31). Genes that are expressed at high levels may have multiple enhancers. In contrast, silencers are *cis* elements that act to decrease or silence transcription of genes in the absence of positive regulation (see Fig. 4–31). Both enhancer and silencer elements are activated by regulatory factors that bind to the core recognition sequences.[282] Enhancers can either be regulatable or nonregulatable (see Fig. 4–31), and in relation to endocrinology they can be viewed as steroid hormone–regulatable or steroid hormone–independent enhancers. The steroid hormone–regulatable enhancer (SRE) is activated when it is bound by hormone-receptor complexes.[82, 94, 283] Steroid hormone–independent enhancers interact with other *trans*-acting factors.

Each type of steroid receptor has an affinity for its cognate SRE sequence that is approximately 1000 times greater than the affinity for nonspecific DNA sequences. The high affinity is a dominant force in the protein's ability to find these small (15 base pair) SRE regulatory sequences among the 3 billion base pairs of DNA in the human genome. The SRE is composed of two half-sites, each of which binds one molecule of steroid receptor.[146, 147, 284] Optimal stability seems to be provided when a second dimer binds to another nearby enhancer and the two dimers touch each other. Two SREs have a much greater effect ($>$10-fold) on gene expression than does one; in this case $1 + 1 = 10$, not 2. If the two SREs are located at a distance from one another, the DNA may bend so that the receptor dimers come into proximity and couple (Fig. 4–32). This type of "protein-protein touching" seems to be a general mechanism by which gene expression is stimulated. Many of the principles involved in protein-protein contacts for *trans*-factor function in microorganisms and yeast appear to hold for animal cells as well.[285] In some cases, synergism occurs not by cooperative binding of *trans*-activators to their response elements but by interaction of the two *trans*-activators with different target sites (proteins) in the transcriptional machinery to enhance transcription.

One mechanism by which steroid hormones occasionally inhibit gene transcription might be occupation of an SRE by

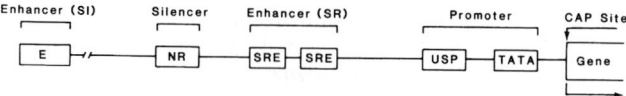

Figure 4–31. Typical combination of regulatory elements for a tightly controlled gene. CAP site is located at $+1$ base pair in the gene. Promoter is usually located within -100 base pairs upstream from the gene. Enhancers, of which SREs are one type, may be located anywhere surrounding the gene (or within an intron). Silencers or negative regulators (NR) are also position independent, as are steroid-independent (SI) enhancers.

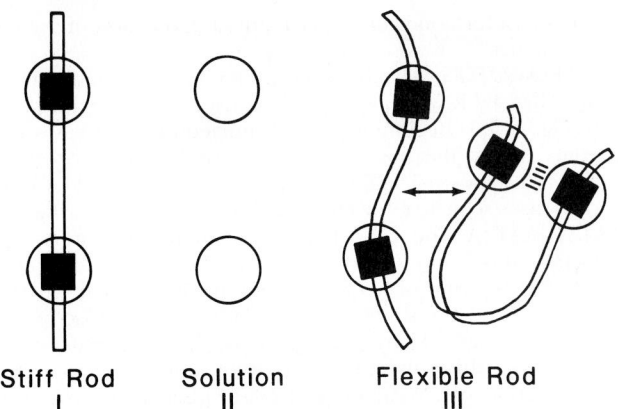

Stiff Rod
I

Solution
II

Flexible Rod
III

Figure 4–32. Schematic model for protein-protein interactions between transcription factors. Proteins bound to separate sites on a stiff rod are unable to interact (I). Proteins can interact in solution, depending on their concentration and diffusion rates (II). Proteins bound to sites on a flexible rod can fold back (looping out intervening DNA) and form a stable protein-protein complex (III). At low concentrations of DNA-binding protein, reaction III is most advantageous. Genomic DNA is a flexible rod.

a receptor dimer that interferes with binding of a promoter *trans*-factor required for gene expression (Fig. 4–33).[79, 286] Such protein-protein interference could occur whenever a negative regulatory factor binds within the transcriptional control region and interferes with the coupling of positive regulatory factors. Silencing often requires the recruitment of corepressor proteins that can directly silence the promoter complex. Such mechanisms would allow cells to use the same regulatory protein to stimulate transcription of some genes and to down-regulate the expression of other genes. The pattern of expression would be determined by the architecture of the sequences in the 5′-flanking sequence of the genes (see Fig. 4–33).

COMBINATIONS OF *CIS* ELEMENTS PROVIDE TRANSCRIPTIONAL SPECIFICITY. A typical array of regulatory components for a steroid hormone–regulated gene is shown at

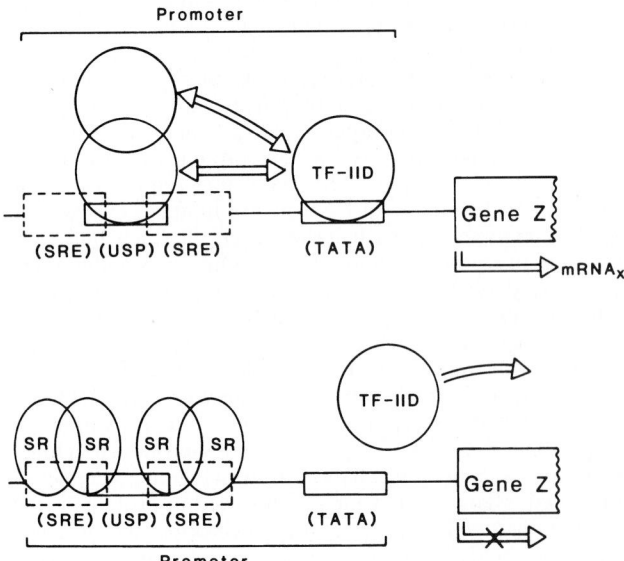

Figure 4–33. A hypothesis for down-regulation of gene transcription mediated by steroid receptors. A protein complex binds to an upstream promoter (USP) and activates transcription via interactions with TATA proteins (e.g., TFIID). In this region of the transcription unit, SREs overlap with the USP site. Consequently, when steroid receptors bind to the SREs, they displace the USP complex and thereby remove the USP-mediated stabilization of TATA proteins, shutting down transcription.

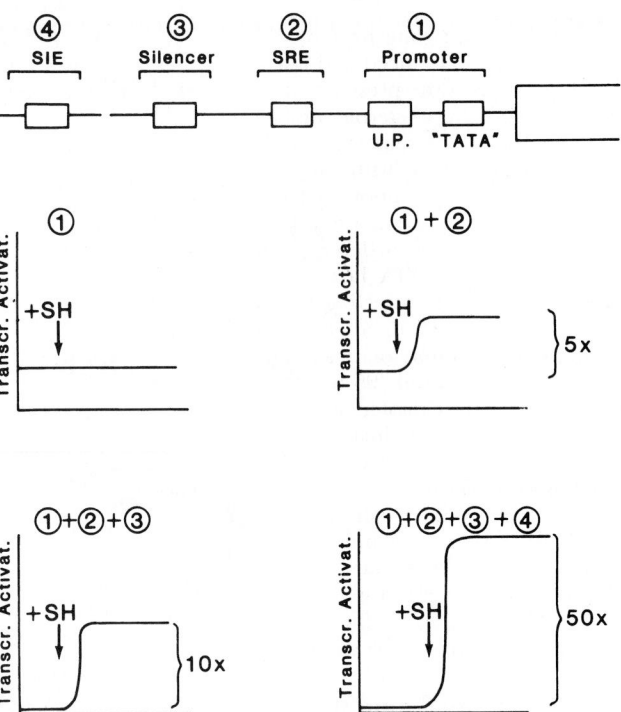

Figure 4–34. Evolution of a tightly controlled gene with a marked inductive response to steroid hormones (SH). See text for explanation.

the top of Figure 4–34. The structural gene contains the information transcribed into mRNA and later into the protein product of the gene. The mRNA is not synthesized, however, unless the regulatory elements of the gene are intact and "activated." These elements are located near the beginning (5′ end) of the gene; they are termed *cis* elements because they are linked to the same strand of DNA (gene unit). The *cis* elements that regulate expression of steroid-controlled genes are classified into four main groups: (1) promoters, (2) steroid-responsive enhancers, (3) silencers, and (4) steroid-independent enhancers (see Fig. 4–34). In the presence of a promoter, a gene is transcribed at a constant (constitutive) rate (see Fig. 4–34, *panel 1*). If the promoter is "strong," the rate of transcription is high; if the promoter is "weak," expression is low. In this case, the transcription of the gene is not controlled by steroid hormones. In contrast, the presence of a nearby SRE (enhancer) subjects the gene to control by steroid hormones (see Fig. 4–34, *panel 2*). For example, hormone stimulation might increase the rate of transcription fivefold over the basal level. If a silencer element is next added to the regulatory cassette, the basal level is decreased to near zero, but the maximal level after hormone stimulation is unaltered (see Fig. 4–34, *panel 3*). Finally, the addition of one or more steroid-independent enhancers leads to synergistic increases in the level of expression in response to hormone (see Fig. 4–34, *panel 4*) but does not influence the basal level of transcription in the absence of hormone. Such combinations of regulatory *cis* elements have been assembled around genes over thousands of millions of years of evolution.

Assembly of these elements occurs by random DNA recombination, and retention occurs by positive evolutionary selection. That is, when a *cis* element "jumps" into the vicinity of a gene, it is retained in the gene's regulatory cassette if it provides a selective advantage for the cell's function and survival. The presence in a given gene of multiple similar or identical copies of each type of *cis* element would magnify each type of response. The ovalbumin gene of the chicken is an example of the type of gene portrayed in Figure 4–34, panel 4. It has a strong promoter, is silent in the absence of hormone, and is induced to high expression by steroid hormones because of the presence of a particularly efficient combination of SREs and steroid-independent enhancers.

The regulatory sequences around eucaryotic promoters have been delineated with two methodologies. The first involves in vitro transcription of cloned gene fragments in the presence of RNA polymerase and crude cellular transcription factors, for example, in determining the nucleotide requirements within the TATA box. Promoter functions also have been studied by transfecting cloned genes back into cells in culture and studying their expression in vivo. In typical experiments, deletion of upstream 5'-flanking sequences to position -95 (i.e., only 95 base pairs are retained) generally has no effect on promoter function; deletion to -75 reduces transcription to approximately 50% of the control level; and deletion to -50 reduces the level to about 5%, because only the TATA element remains. Finally, animals infected with transgenes carrying specific DNA sequences have been used to determine promoter and enhancer elements. In this case, deletions and other mutations are introduced into the flanking regulatory regions of genes. The modified genes are then introduced into animals in which developmental and tissue-specific expression can be studied.

Models for Regulating the Expression of Gene Sets

Hormonal regulation of gene expression at the level of DNA transcription, originally shown for the regulation of genes for egg-white proteins by gonadal steroids and regulation of viral (MMTV) gene expression by glucocorticoids, is now accepted for all ligand-dependent regulation of members of the steroid, thyroid hormone, vitamin receptor superfamily. It is possible to distinguish at least five potential control points. These sequential steps can be separately defined as (1) structural activation of genes, (2) initiation of transcription, (3) precursor mRNA processing and export to cytoplasm, (4) translation of mRNA, and (5) degradation of mRNA and protein. At present there is good evidence for the existence of control at steps 1, 2, and 5 but little evidence for selective control by hormones at steps 3 and 4. Of perhaps equal interest for future investigation is the question of how gene expression is coordinated among different loci of the genome. Coordinately expressed genes involved in specific cell functions are often distributed at distant loci throughout the genome. Major remaining questions are how each cell activates the appropriate set of genes to produce its phenotype and how the appropriate gene sets are coordinately regulated to produce a given function. In addition, the regulatory element associated with each gene is subjected to multiple controls.

In eucaryotes each gene has its own control element that can be activated when complexed with its cognate *trans*-acting factor. Common control of genes that are unrelated and have evolved separately from each other could be due to a translocation event in which the hormone control elements of genes are duplicated and distributed to the transcription units of other genes.

Consider the example shown in Figure 4–35. Two genes, X and Y, exist on separate chromosomes. Each gene has its own promoter element (p) and one or more control elements. Gene X is under control of inducers a and b, and gene Y is under control of inducer c; a, b, and c could represent the binding sites for receptors for different steroid hormones. As evolution proceeds to stage 2, the DNA sequence containing the a element undergoes a translocation so that a replicate copy is now located in the 5'-flanking region of gene Y. Thus, gene Y now comes under control of receptors for both hormones a and c. When genomic translocations and recombina-

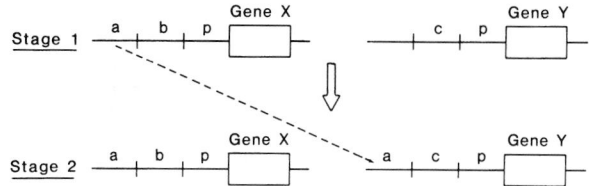

Evolution of Co-ordinate Gene Control

Figure 4–35. In an early stage of evolution (stage 1), gene X is under control of hormones because it contains regulatory sites (a and b) that interact with receptors for hormones and allow the promoter (p) to function. Gene Y is under constitutive synthesis (c). At stage 2, hormone control element a has been duplicated in the genome and has been translocated to the 5'-flanking region of gene Y. This translocation now brings gene Y under hormonal control by virtue of its proximity to the promoter of gene Y. In this manner a group of genes located anywhere on the genome can be brought under control of a single regulatory molecule. See text for details.

tions lead to some selective advantage for the organism, the genomic rearrangement is "locked in" and becomes permanent. In this way, a single hormone can control any gene that contains a copy of the appropriate control element. Also, a single gene may have acquired the appropriate control elements for a number of different hormone receptors. All the genes containing a common control element for hormone a would be coordinately activated in response to the same hormonal stimulus (see Fig. 4–35). The overall result is that multiple genes are expressed coordinately under the direction of a common regulatory element.

Such genes might specify proteins with related functions, such as the set of enzymes in a metabolic pathway. An example of both coordinate control and multihormonal control is chicken oviduct system. The genes for ovalbumin, ovomucoid, conalbumin, and lysozyme all are under coordinate control of estrogen. This could be accomplished easily if each gene had at least one copy of a common control element to make it responsive to estrogen.[265, 277]

Trans-Acting Factors and Gene Expression

In addition to appropriate *cis* elements near eucaryotic genes, a cell must also contain appropriate *trans*-acting factors to bind to the *cis* elements and control transcription. Multiple individual factors usually must bind simultaneously within the 5'-flanking region of genes for optimal transcriptional regulation to occur. For example, a given gene may have five *cis* elements that bind a total of 10 to 20 different *trans*-acting factors. Multimeric protein complexes form at each DNA element; in a manner that is not clearly understood at present, an appropriate mixture of *trans*-acting factors provides an "activation surface" or alters chromatin structure in such a way that recruitment of RNA polymerase to that gene occurs and initiation of transcription ensues.[285] Genes are in competition for a limited amount of RNA polymerase, and the genes with the most effective and most stable array of factors are transcribed repetitively and at a high rate. Transcription can be subdivided into four general steps: (1) a "template commitment" step during which transcription factors bind and form a stable complex with DNA, (2) a step in which a preinitiation complex (rapid-start complex) is formed that poises factors and RNA polymerase for RNA synthesis when ribonucleotide substrates are provided, (3) initiation of transcription, and (4) elongation of RNA chains and termination of transcription.

***TRANS*-ACTIVATION OF THE PROXIMAL PROMOTER (TATA BOX).** Multiple general transcription factors, TFIID, IIA, IIB, IIE, IIF, and IIH, and RNA polymerase II, bind to the promoter region and are required for initiation of transcrip-

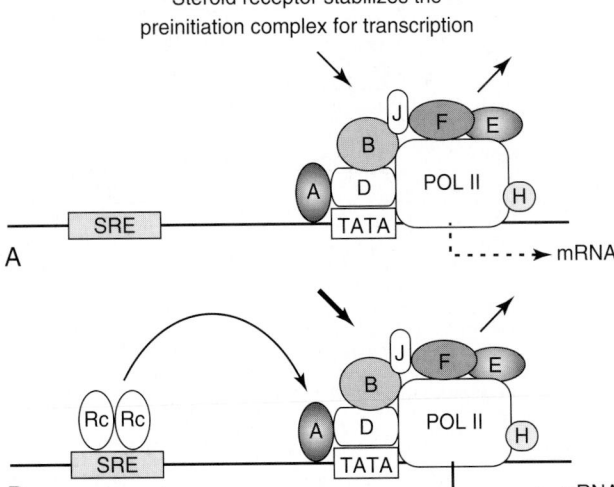

Steroid receptor stabilizes the
preinitiation complex for transcription

Figure 4–36. Steroid receptor stabilizes the preinitiation complex for transcription. Steroid receptors act by stabilizing the preinitiation complex formed at the proximal promoter (TATA box). A reversible association of general transcription factors, TFIIA, IIB, IID, IIH, and IIJ, Pol II (polymerase), and IIE/F, is shown schematically *(A)*. Only when all factors are present can Pol II initiate RNA synthesis. When upstream SREs are occupied by receptor dimers, the resulting tight-binding tetramer of receptor exerts a stabilizing effect on proximal promoter factors to generate a committed complex that allows Pol II to effect rapid-start RNA synthesis *(B)*. This stabilization by receptor promotes repeated initiations of transcription.

tion.[287–290] The primary DNA-binding protein required to form this complex is TFIID.[291] Each transcription factor may contain subunits. For example, TFIID is composed of at least eight different proteins. The TATA-binding protein (TBP) is a DNA sequence-specific binding protein that acts as a tether for the TBP-associated factors (TAFs). TFIIA binds and stabilizes TFIID and TFIIB, and RNA polymerase is brought into the complex. TFIIE and TFIIF then bind with RNA polymerase and promote initiation of transcription (Fig. 4–36). Transcription occurs only when this complex of proteins is in residence at the TATA box. Because these factors are in short supply in eukaryotic nuclei and bind with RNA polymerase only weakly to the TATA element, help in recruitment and stabilization of these factors at the TATA element must be provided by factors bound to other upstream elements.

UPSTREAM PROMOTER FACTORS. The upstream (distal) promoter (USP) is located near the TATA box and is heterogeneous in structure. Each type (e.g., CAAT box, SP1 site, and COUP box) binds a selected subset of factors. Once bound to the USP site, these factors recruit and stabilize TATA factors to promote transcription initiation by polymerase. Adenovirus major late transcription factor and ATF (HeLa cell transformation factor) protein both bind to upstream sequences, stabilize TFIID, or TFIIB, and enhance TATA-dependent transcription.[292–296] Little functional difference exists between an upstream promoter and an enhancer.

ENHANCER FACTORS. Again, a wide variety of enhancer elements bind various transcription factors to enhance transcription. Because these elements may be located at great distances (e.g., about 2000 base pairs) from the promoter, they must somehow fold back and interact with promoter factors by "looping out" of the intervening DNA so that the proteins touch each other.[275] One of the best-studied groups of enhancer regulatory proteins is the steroid receptor superfamily. These powerful *trans*-activators of gene expression provide a good model for mechanistic studies of enhancer function. Steroid receptors bind at upstream enhancer elements and recruit or stabilize the assembly of general transcription factors (GTFs) at the promoter (TATA box) (Fig. 4–36). This

basic function is coordinated by receptor-associated coregulator proteins.

COREGULATORS FOR NUCLEAR RECEPTORS. Although steroid hormone receptors may directly contact the core transcriptional machinery, the major transcriptional impact may come by interaction with coregulator proteins that bind to the receptors at SREs and bridge to the transcriptional machinery. The coregulators are divided into two coactivators that enhance gene activation and corepressors that silence genes. Coregulators usually interact directly with receptors in a ligand-dependent manner. For example, SRC-1 binds agonist-occupied receptors, but not unoccupied or antagonist-occupied receptors,[297] enhances the transcriptional activity of many steroid receptors more than 10-fold, and can reverse receptor-receptor squelching in cell transfection studies. Another common eucaryotic coactivator protein is CREB-binding protein.

In contrast, corepressors bind select unoccupied (or antagonist-occupied) receptors to silence their activity.[298, 299] At present, two corepressors have been described, nuclear receptor corepressor (N-CoR) and silencing mediator for retinoid and thyroid hormone receptors (SMRT), both of which act in concert with unoccupied thyroid hormone receptor and retinoic acid receptor to silence certain nuclear genes.[298, 299]

At present, the downstream targets within the promoter complex are unknown for any coregulators. Coregulator proteins vary in concentration and at different stages of development, thereby contributing to tissue-specific hormone response. The concentrations of receptor and coactivator determine the quantitative response to hormone: [hormone-receptor] × [coactivator] = gene activation. The model presented in Figure 4–37 summarizes our current thinking on this subject.

Molecular Mechanism of Steroid Receptor Action

The pathway of steroid receptor action has been known since the early 1970s (Fig. 4–38). Additional insight into the mechanism or mechanisms of receptor action, however, has come from in vitro studies of receptor function in a cell-free (reconstituted) transcription system.[9, 300–302]

ROLE OF STEROID RECEPTOR IN *TRANS*-ACTIVATION OF TARGET GENES. Hormone-dependent transcription of the vitellogenin gene was first observed in homogenates of *Xenopus* nuclei,[303] and bacterially expressed truncated glucocorticoid receptor fragments[301] and native progesterone receptor[300, 304] were shown to enhance RNA synthesis in in vitro transcription assays. As expected, enhancement of transcription by progesterone-receptor complexes requires the presence of PREs in the template[300] and is inhibited by addition of competitor DNA containing PREs, and test constructs containing two PREs yield 30-fold induction of levels of transcription in the presence of progesterone receptor.

In the presence of transcription factors provided by HeLa cell extracts, progesterone receptor directs the formation of a stable preinitiation complex at the promoter (see Fig. 4–36).[300] In separate studies, receptors were shown to interact with proteins at the USP site, which in turn may interact with and stabilize factors at the TATA box, suggesting that enhancer-binding proteins may interact with transcription factors to recruit and stabilize the preinitiation complexes at proximal promoters and thus enhance the initiation of transcription. Investigations with other steroid receptors (e.g., glucocorticoid and estrogen) indicate that this may be a general mechanism by which steroid receptors regulate the expression of target genes.[305, 306]

MULTIPLE HORMONE RESPONSE ELEMENTS MEDIATE TRANSCRIPTION SYNERGISTICALLY. SREs are often found in multiple copies in the 5'-flanking regions of hormone-

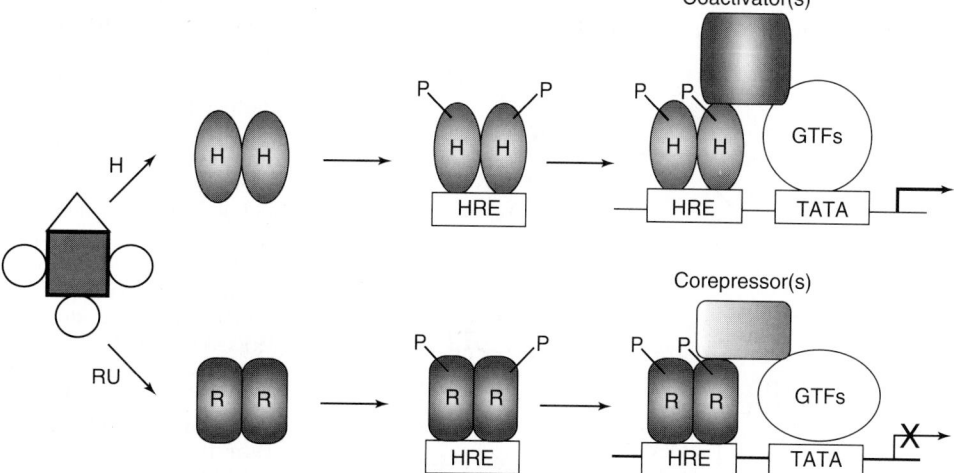

Figure 4–37. Involvement of coactivator and corepressor on *trans*-activation and repression by the steroid hormone receptor.

responsive genes.[93, 124, 304, 307, 308] Deletion or mutation of one of two SREs decreases the inducibility of target genes, suggesting that the SREs cooperate synergistically. One copy of PRE enhanced receptor-dependent transcription fourfold, and two copies enhanced transcription 30-fold.[300, 309] Similar cooperative interactions have been observed between glucocorticoid receptors,[310] heat shock transcription factors,[311] and OCT2 factors.[312] Synergism can also occur with heterologous response elements, such as between GRE and nuclear factor 1 (NF1) in the promoter region of MMTV,[313] and GRE and a CACA promoter element. Synergism appears to be dependent both on cooperative binding of *trans*-activators and on overall conformation. High levels of gene induction can also be achieved by placing a combination of heterologous elements, such as EREs and PREs, upstream of a promoter. This synergistic induction is due not to cooperative binding of receptors but to interactions between different activation domains in the heterologous receptor complex. These results demonstrate that complex regulation of eucaryotic gene expression can be acquired by assembling unique subsets of *cis* elements. Expression of a given gene can be regulated over a wide range through either (1) cooperative binding or (2) cooperative interactions of specific activation domains with other transcription factors at target genes.

ROLE OF LIGAND IN STEROID RECEPTOR FUNCTION.

Steroid receptor–mediated induction of target gene expression in vivo is dependent on the presence and concentration of steroid hormone.[6, 314, 315] Consistent with this model, RNase-hypersensitive sites, which correlate with the state of expression of hormone-responsive genes, can be detected in and around the SREs in the presence of the cognate hormone.[316] Receptor binds to the PRE/GRE element of the tyrosine aminotransferase gene only in the presence of hormone.[317] Furthermore, estrogen[147, 318, 319] or progesterone[181] receptors in nuclear extracts bind to their respective SRE elements in DNA only when the extracts are prepared from hormone-treated cells. Likewise in nuclear extracts from T47D cells ligand-free progesterone receptors do not bind to PRE sites and do not enhance transcription of PRE-containing test genes except when progesterone is added (see Fig. 4–38).[156, 320] In contrast, in in vitro transcription experiments, purified progesterone receptors bind and function to enhance the expression of PRE-containing target genes in a hormone-independent manner.

High-salt extraction and ATP treatment of receptor converts the unliganded progesterone receptor to a 4S form, which does not contain hsp90, 70- or 59-kd proteins and is still inactive in the cell-free transcription assay. Addition of

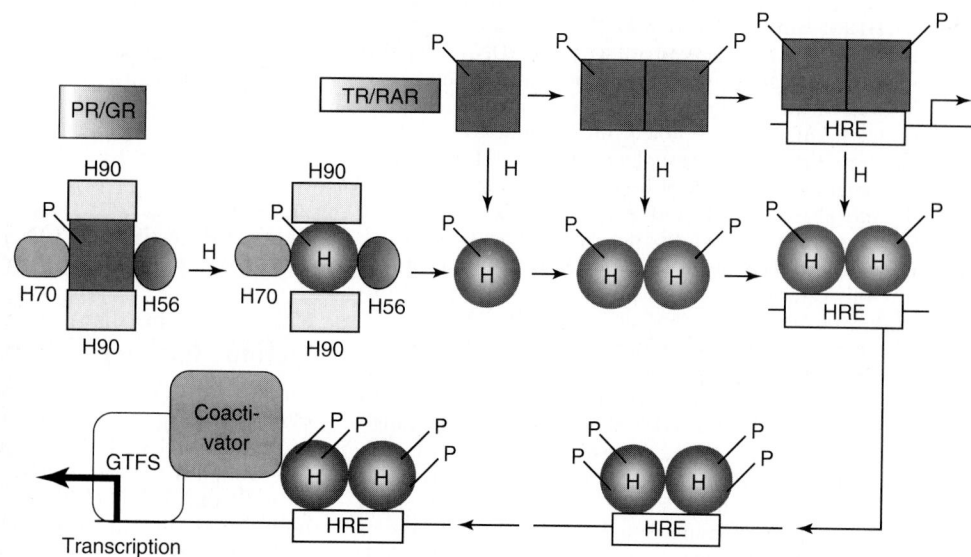

Figure 4–38. Model for hormone-dependent activation of the steroid–thyroid hormone receptor family. Before binding hormone the inactive receptor is complexed with heat shock proteins (e.g., hsp90, hsp70, and p59). Hormone induces dissociation of all heat shock proteins, including hsp70, from receptor and induces a conformational (allosteric) change in the molecule. After dimerization, DNA binding, and phosphorylation, the receptor activates the target gene, leading to a high output of mRNA (see text for detailed description of this model). (Modified and redrawn from Tsai MJ, O'Malley BW. Molecular mechanisms of action of steroid/thyroid receptor superfamily members. Annu Rev Biochem 1994; 63:451–486. Reproduced with permission from Annual Review of Biochemistry, © 1994, by Annual Reviews, Inc.)

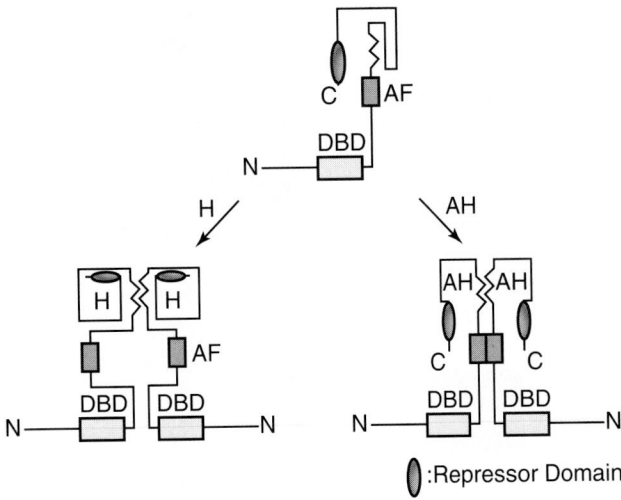

:Repressor Domain

Figure 4–39. Model for the mechanism of steroid hormone action. In the absence of hormone, the dimerization function is not available; thus the receptor cannot bind to DNA with high affinity. On binding agonist or antagonist, the dimerization domain is exposed; this exposure facilitates the dimerization of receptor and thus the DNA binding. The difference between agonist and antagonist bound receptors is the C-terminal repressor domain where it is available when it is bound by antagonists but is not available when it is bound by agonists. For a more detailed description, see text. (Modified and redrawn from Tsai MJ, O'Malley BW. Molecular mechanisms of action of steroid/thyroid receptor superfamily members. Annu Rev Biochem 1994; 63:457–486. Reproduced with permission from the Annual Review of Biochemistry, ©, 1994, by Annual Reviews, Inc.)

progesterone, however, converts heat shock protein–free receptor into a form able to activate PRE-dependent transcription. The receptor must assume the appropriate "active conformation" to interact with and stabilize requisite promoter factors (Fig. 4–39). These results are consistent with the observations that neither thyroid hormone receptors nor vitamin D receptors are associated with heat shock protein in their native unliganded state but are still inactive.

The molecular mechanism by which a steroidal ligand transforms the receptor to an active form has been studied for the progesterone receptor and for other receptors (for a review see reference 9) using a variety of techniques, including protease probing of structural changes in the receptor, in vitro transcription, mutational analysis, mobility shift assay for DNA binding, and monclonal antibody probing. After ligand-induced conformational change and release of heat shock proteins, the receptor can dimerize, bind to its DNA response element (HRE), and undergo phosphorylation by a DNA-dependent kinase. Once bound to its target DNA site, the receptor activates target genes by interacting with other coactivators and transcription factors to initiate transcription.

Conversion of the receptor from an inactive form to an active form has been investigated by protease digestion, mutational analysis, and study of the crystal structure (see Fig. 4–39). In the absence of ligand, the progesterone receptor ligand-binding domain is believed to exist in a loose structure that is easily digested by protease, especially in the C-terminal region. At this C-terminal region progesterone receptor contains a repressor domain (R) and an activation domain (AF). In the absence of ligand, the dimerization domain either is blocked or is not in a proper conformation so that the PR cannot dimerize and bind to its response element with high affinity. On binding ligand (H), a conformational change allows formation of a dimerized PR, which can bind PRE with high affinity and contains exposed activator functions (AF). An additional conformational change in the C-terminal region disrupts the repressor domain function, and the receptor is free to trans-activate target genes. When occupied by antihor-

mones (AH) the inactive conformation of the receptor is stabilized, and the association of DNA-bound receptor with corepressors is favored. This model is supported by crystal structure analyses of RXR, RAR, and TR, which confirms the conformational difference in the C-terminal region between liganded and unliganded receptors.[98–100] Finally, our preliminary results suggest the presence of a cellular corepressor that interacts with the C terminus of the progesterone receptor and actively represses the trans-activation function of the progesterone receptor bound to DNA. This corepressor-progesterone receptor interaction may be stabilized when an antiprogestagen (e.g., mifepristone) occupies the receptor.

In summary, steroid-activated receptor dimers bind to SREs and stabilize transcription factors bound at the distal and proximal promoter elements. The binding of receptor tetramers to two SREs is most efficient in this process. When these transcription factors are bound stably, they recruit coactivator proteins, which attract RNA polymerase to that gene, resulting in a high rate of transcription (see Fig. 4–38).

Ligand-Independent Activation of Steroid Receptors

In addition to a possible synergistic effect of phosphorylation and ligand-dependent activation of receptor,[321] agents such as 8-Br-cAMP and okadaic acid that stimulate intracellular phosphorylation pathways can also activate receptors in the "absence" of ligand.[321] Dopamine[322, 323] and inducers of cAMP[324, 325] activate certain steroid receptors. Indeed dopamine can activate chicken progesterone and human receptors in the absence of ligand by events mediated by dopamine D₁ receptors. Glucocorticoid and mineralocorticoid receptor subtypes were not activated.[323] Pure hormone antagonists (e.g., ICI 164,384) prevent this activation.[323, 326] Dopamine requires an intact progesterone receptor for its effect on sexual behavior in the rat.[327]

Growth factors also appear capable of activating certain steroid receptors, particularly the human estrogen receptor. In cultured cells, insulin-like growth factor I (IGF-I), epidermal growth factor (EGF), and transforming growth factor α (TGF-α) stimulate transcription of estrogen target genes by activating human estrogen receptor in a ligand-independent fashion.[324, 328, 329] As an in vivo corollary, EGF, acting via its membrane receptor, causes uterine growth in ovariectomized mice that is similar to that caused by estrogen itself.[326] In fact EGF acts via its membrane receptor to drive unoccupied estrogen receptor to its nuclear form and turn on estrogen target genes in mice; this effect of EGF can also be blocked by administration of a pure antiestrogen.[328, 330]

This cross-talk between membrane receptors and intracellular receptor pathways has exciting biologic implications. Perhaps the concept of activation of intracellular receptors should be expanded to include activation from cell membrane sites.

PHYSIOLOGICAL CONSIDERATIONS IN STEROID HORMONE ACTION

Role of Metabolism and Transport in Steroid Hormone Action

STEROID TRANSPORT IN THE BLOOD. The delivery of steroids to target tissues is accomplished by the blood, which transports steroids in both bound and unbound (free) states. The unbound steroid is generally considered to be the active or available form of the hormone; however, the uptake of bound steroid may play an important role in some cell types,[331] and uptake of hormone is influenced by target organ transit time and the rate of intracapillary dissociation of bound hormone.[332, 333] The affinity of blood transport proteins for steroids varies from weak ($K_d = 10^{-3}$ M) to strong (10^{-10} to 10^{-8} M). One such binding molecule is the sex hormone–binding globulin (SHBG; or testosterone-binding globulin TeBG) that binds testosterone and estradiol with equal affinity ($K_d = 10^{-10}$ M).[334] A protein that binds estrogens—but not androgens—is α-FP, which is present in both the pregnant and the neonatal rat. During the neonatal and prepubertal life of the rat, α-FP levels gradually decrease from high values in the newborn to low values just before and after puberty.[335] Therefore, the quantity of free gonadal steroid gradually increases as the concentration of α-FP decreases. In this manner increasing concentrations of steroid are available for cellular interactions. These observations have led several investigators to suggest that α-FP plays a protective role in the fetus and neonate and may be involved in the onset of puberty.

Corticosteroid-binding globulin (CBG) is also of special interest and importance.[336] CBG binds glucocorticoids and progesterone with a K_d of 10^{-7} to 10^{-6} M at 37°C and therefore may be important in the control of free hormone. CBG may influence the action of adrenocortical steroids by targeting these hormones to specific organs where CBG is recognized and accumulated.[331]

Binders of gonadal steroids that do not demonstrate pharmacospecificity or stereospecificity may play important roles in steroid hormone physiology. Serum albumin has a relatively weak affinity for estrogen ($K_d = 10^{-4}$ to 10^{-5} M) but is a significant estrogen binder[336] and plays a major role in testosterone transport (see Chapter 16).

METABOLISM AND STEROID BINDING. The quantity of steroid available in vivo for receptor binding depends not only on transport relationships but also on the rate of metabolism and excretion of the hormone. A hormone with a high affinity for its receptor and thus with a predicted high potency also may have a high metabolic clearance rate. Hence, the exposure time of the hormone to a target cell is short, and the potency may be blunted. This phenomenon is exemplified by the weak estrogenic potency of estriol after a single injection.[337] The anticipated potency would be 0.1 that of estradiol if estrogenic potency were dependent solely on the affinity of the estrogen receptor for the hormone. However, uterine growth after administration is far greater for estradiol than for estriol, partly because estriol is cleared from the blood more rapidly. Conversely, a hormone with a low metabolic clearance rate and a relatively low affinity may display unexpectedly high biologic activity. This is the case for the long-acting estrogen agonists-antagonists tamoxifen and clomiphene. The affinity of the estrogen receptor for these drugs is only 1/20 to 1/30 that for estradiol, but their effects are long-lasting because of the long half-life of these drugs. Therefore, their biologic effectiveness is greater than predicted by the binding affinities.

The actions of estrogen receptor and progesterone receptor do not usually depend on the metabolic conversion of these steroids to active forms.[338, 339] Therefore, once receptor-steroid binding has occurred as a result of steroid entry into the cell, the receptor-steroid complex is functionally active. Metabolism is important in some cases; for instance, the conversion of testosterone to 5α-dihydrotestosterone (5α-DHT) is a requirement for androgen action in some tissues. In addition, the aromatization of testosterone to estradiol is required for masculinization of the central nervous system. Estradiol and estrone undergo extensive interconversion in human endometrium, where the conversion of estradiol to estrone may be a mechanism for lowering the level of estradiol in the tissue and thereby controlling the level of functional estrogen-receptor complexes in cells. This metabolism may also be involved in the dissociation of receptor-hormone complex

from nuclear-binding sites. Progesterone is rapidly converted to 5α-pregnane-3,20-dione in the chick oviduct.[340] This steroid competes effectively with progesterone for binding to the progesterone receptor and is as potent as progesterone in the stimulation of avidin synthesis. 5α-Pregnane-3,20-dione is also capable of stimulating luteinizing hormone (LH) release in the rat and hamster. However, this compound is not active as a uterotropic agent, which correlates with its lack of binding to the progesterone receptor in the rat uterus. Thus the metabolism of progesterone to 5α-pregnane-3,20-dione and other inactive metabolites in the uterus may reduce the effectiveness of progesterone, thereby providing yet another control mechanism for hormone-induced responses.

Target Organ Responses to Steroid Hormones

Steroid hormones interact to control many metabolic and biosynthetic events in virtually every tissue and organ in the body. All these responses appear to be regulated by the binding of steroids to their respective receptors.

ESTROGEN AND PROGESTERONE ACTIONS. Estrogen and progesterone control the growth, development, and physiology of the female reproductive tract and other organ systems.

Uterus: Early and Late Uterotropic Responses. Many hormones induce early responses within minutes after hormone exposure[341] and later effects that culminate in cellular hypertrophy and hyperplasia (true growth). For example, estrogen and other growth-promoting hormones cause biphasic pleiotropic response patterns (reviewed by Tata[342]). Uterotropic responses to estrogen can be classified according to their time of appearance and functional relationship (Tables 4–2 and 4–3). Early responses include hyperemia, calcium influx, histamine release, eosinophil infiltration, increased DNA and protein precursor uptake, and enhanced glucose oxidation. Early responses also include increased synthesis of RNA and protein, which eventually cause the uterus to grow. However, as discussed later, the stimulation of these biosynthetic events is not necessarily obligatory in the stimulation of uterine growth. Late responses, some of which are simply extensions of those begun during the early period, include increased and sustained RNA and protein synthesis. This biosynthetic activity results in cellular hypertrophy and DNA synthesis and hyperplasia that eventuate in true growth of the uterus. Obviously, true growth requires an environment in which substrate avail-

TABLE 4–2. Early Uterotropic Responses to Estrogen

Supportive or Metabolic

Hyperemia
Histamine mobilization
Eosinophil infiltration
Water imbibition
Albumin accumulation
Increased electrolyte levels
Lysosome labilization
Increased cyclic nucleotide and prostaglandin levels and associated enzyme activation
Increased glucose metabolism and associated enzyme activity
Increased uptake of RNA
Calcium influx
Ornithine decarboxylase

Biosynthetic

Increased lipid synthesis
Increased activity of RNA
Synthesis of the induced protein and its mRNA
Increased synthesis of glucose-6-phosphate dehydrogenase
Increased chromatin template activity and RNA polymerase initiation sites
Increased synthesis of histone and nonhistone proteins

TABLE 4–3. Late Uterotropic Responses to Estrogen

Supportive or Metabolic

Many of the functions that are listed in Table 4–2 continue for many hours after estrogen administration

Biosynthetic

Increased general and specific protein and RNA synthesis
Continued stimulation of RNA polymerase activity
DNA synthetics and mitosis
Cellular hypertrophy and hyperplasia
Increased synthesis of or changes in histone and nonhistone proteins

ability is optimal, as provided by the increased blood flow and other supportive events listed in Tables 4–2 and 4–3.

Rapid elevations in cyclic AMP levels are demonstrable after estrogen treatment in the uterus, and cyclic AMP may mediate a subset of estradiol effects.[343] Estrogen treatment in vivo and in vitro also stimulates cyclic GMP accumulation in the rat uterus,[344] a response that appears to depend on RNA and protein synthesis. Estrogen causes eosinophils to be attracted to uterine capillaries and migrate into the extracellular spaces of the uterus, where they release hydrolytic enzymes that depolymerize the uterine ground substance. Eosinophils may also cause mast cells to release histamine, and this release, coupled with the hydrolysis of mucopolysaccharides, increases vascular permeability and creates an osmotic environment that favors water imbibition and precursor uptake.[345]

Uterine growth may be promoted by estrogen-induced histamine release that causes increased capillary permeability and hyperemia,[346] but these events are probably not primary in the growth process. Eosinophil infiltration and its attendant responses can be blocked with glucocorticoids without any significant effect on DNA, RNA, and protein synthesis in the uterus.[347] Early uterotropic responses induced by estradiol in rats are not blocked by nafoxidine, an antiestrogen that blocks late responses.[348] Estrogen-induced uterine growth is independent of cyclic AMP, prostaglandins, and β-adrenergic action[349] and independent of ornithine decarboxylase.[350]

Furthermore, estriol causes transient nuclear binding of the estrogen receptor and stimulates all the early uterotropic responses but does not stimulate uterine hyperplasia and growth.[341, 351, 352] Estriol apparently fails in this regard because it does not occupy the estrogen receptor long enough to maintain the biosynthetic events that culminate in cell proliferation and growth. Thus, the early uterotropic responses are supportive but are not obligatory for the stimulation of uterine hypertrophy and hyperplasia.

The sustained stimulation of RNA and protein synthesis that culminates in cell proliferation appears to require occupancy of 10 to 20% of nuclear estrogen receptors for more than 4 to 6 h[341, 353] (Fig. 4–40). Long-term occupancy of estrogen receptors also promotes mRNA stability and continued synthesis of several proteins[354, 355] and is associated with an increase in the number of nuclear type II estrogen-binding sites, which correlates with the late uterotropic growth.[356]

It follows that examination of initial binding interactions of hormone-receptor complexes with acceptor sites provides limited information about physiological events necessary to elicit growth responses. Also, the minimal number of receptor sites appears to involve only 10 to 20% of the total number of receptors available.

Progesterone modifies the growth and metabolic activity of the uterus. Progesterone inhibits further endometrial proliferation induced by estrogen and converts the endometrium to the secretory type. The endometrial glands become irregular and convoluted, the glycogen content of the epithelium increases, and the stroma becomes edematous. In this progestational or secretory state, the endometrium is ready for implantation of the blastocyst and the subsequent maintenance of pregnancy. The functions of progesterone require a prior increase in receptor levels by estrogen. Progesterone in turn decreases the levels of estrogen receptor and progesterone receptor (termed down-regulation).

Some of the actions of ovarian steroids may be indirect. For example, a factor from the pituitary may be involved in the growth response of the oviduct and uterus to estradiol,[357, 358] but it is likely that the role of the pituitary in uterus growth is permissive, namely that pituitary hormones maintain the integrity of the metablic machinery.[359]

It also has been proposed that the liver acts as an intermediary in the stimulation by estrogen of the quail oviduct,[360] but not the rat uterus.[361] It has also been proposed that estrogens stimulate the synthesis of peptide growth factors that act as mitogens on estrogen-responsive cells.[362] There is evidence for a paracrine function of uterine stromal tissue on the epithelium of this organ.[363] Epidermal growth factor (EGF) and its receptor are present in the uterus of several species and in the mammary gland of the mouse.[364, 365] Known to be mitogenic in many cell types, EGF is capable of activating the estrogen

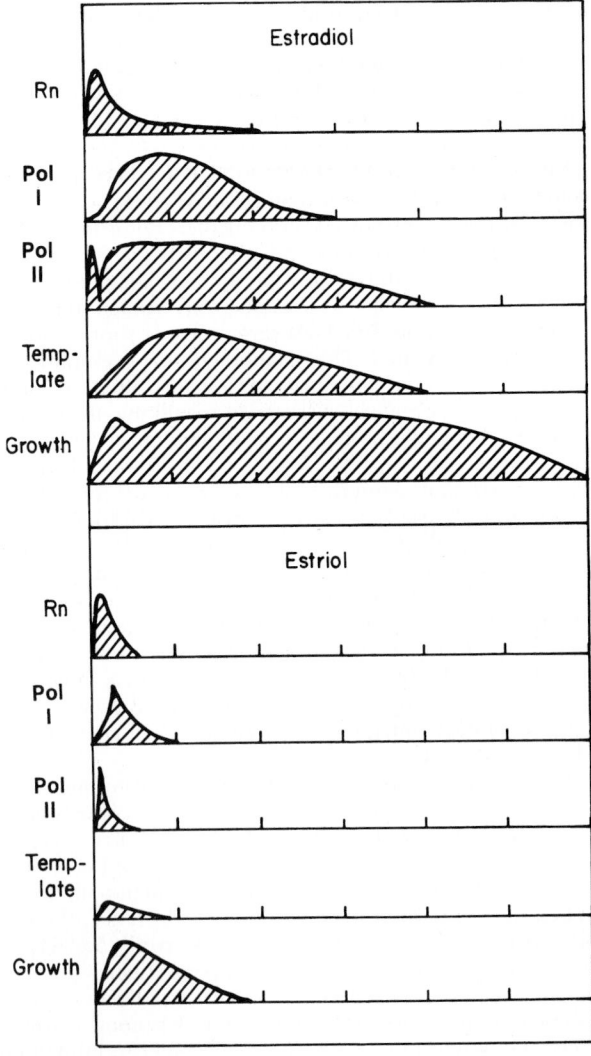

Figure 4–40. Effects of estradiol and estriol on estrogen receptor binding and uterotropic responses. Hormones were injected at time zero in equal quantities (1 μg), and the following responses were monitored as a function of time (each interval on the x axis equals 12 h): quantity of estrogen-receptor complexes in nucleus (Rn), RNA polymerase I activity (Pol I), RNA polymerase II activity (Pol II), chromatin template activity (Template), and uterine net weight (Growth).

receptor in a ligand-independent fashion via an undefined phosphorylation cascade.

Local application of estrogen to the vagina causes cellular proliferation and cornification that cannot be explained by systemic absorption.[366] It seems probable that ovarian steroids act via cellular receptors to stimulate cellular growth directly as well as by elevating the local production of growth factors that may act on the same or adjacent cells.

Chick Oviduct. Estrogen causes the growth and differentiation of the immature chick oviduct, as shown diagrammatically in Figure 4–41.[226, 362] These processes include the stimulation of epithelial cells to invaginate and form the tubular glands, which constitute 90% of the cell population of the mature oviduct and synthesize ovalbumin, conalbumin, lysozyme, ovomucoid, and various other egg white proteins. The initial stimulation of protein synthesis and growth of the oviduct is caused exclusively by estrogen; however, if the estrogen is withdrawn from the animal, secondary administration of estrogen, progesterone, or glucocorticoid results in a resumption of egg-white protein synthesis. Why nonestrogenic hormones can function during secondary but not during primary stimulation is not known.

Liver. Estrogen controls the synthesis of different liver proteins in different species. In birds and amphibians, estrogen stimulates the synthesis of large quantities of vitellogenin and very-low-density lipoproteins that are carried by the blood and deposited in the developing oocytes as yolk.[367] The binding of the estrogen-receptor complexes to nuclear sites in avian liver is different from that in the uterus. The cytosol of chicken liver contains few, if any, detectable receptor sites, and the appearance of nuclear-bound hormone-receptor complexes after estrogen exposure results from activation of receptor sites or de novo synthesis; it is assumed that receptor synthesis is involved.

Control of Steroid Receptor Concentrations

The intracellular concentration of steroid receptors is an important determinant of hormone response, and several interacting factors control steroid receptor levels (Fig. 4–42). The receptor-steroid (RS) complex may stimulate mRNA transcription and enhance the synthesis of new receptor molecules. The RS complex may be reutilized either by being converted to a nonbinding form that is subsequently activated to a binding form or by being recycled directly as an activated binding form. Alternatively, the receptor may undergo degradation to an inactive form (R'). Associated with each of these

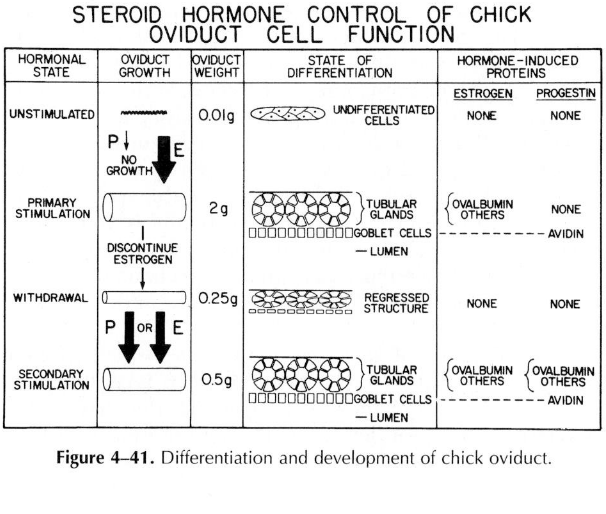

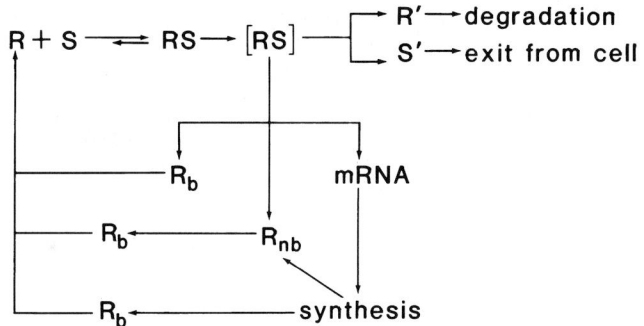

Figure 4–42. Pathways for receptor regulation.

receptor pathways is the loss or elimination of the steroid from the cell (S').

ESTROGEN RECEPTOR CONCENTRATION. Estrogen-responsive cells in the uterus of a castrated rat maintain levels of receptor that enable it to respond to administered estrogen. This basal level of receptor is probably controlled by constitutive synthesis of the receptor. Thus estrogen target tissues in both male and female animals can usually detect and respond to estrogens.[368–370]

Although estrogen target cells maintain a constitutive level of cytosolic receptor, receptor levels are influenced by endogenous and exogenous steroids. As pointed out earlier, an injection of estradiol causes a rapid depletion of cytosolic receptors, which bind tightly in the nucleus as estrogen-receptor complexes. This binding is followed by replenishment of cytosolic receptor by the reactivation or reutilization of nuclear-bound receptor and the de novo synthesis of new receptor molecules. In tissues that do not grow in response to hormone, replenishment may involve only reactivation or recycling.[371, 372]

A nonbinding form of the estrogen receptor in the chick oviduct can be reactivated.[373] Addition of ATP or ADP to the nonbinding form converts it to the binding form, but how these interconversions are related to replenishment of the estrogen receptors is not known.

In tissues that grow in response to hormone stimulation, such as uterus, vagina, and mammary gland, both reactivation and synthesis may be involved in the replenishment process, and synthesis of additional receptor molecules is required in cells that undergo division to maintain a constant amount of receptor per cell. Cells that grow in size and do not divide may also require receptor synthesis to prevent dilution brought about by cellular hypertrophy. Kassis and Gorski[374] demonstrated that reutilization or recycling of the estrogen receptor can occur when short-acting estrogens cause nuclear accumulation.

The replenishment of cytosolic receptors after hormone-induced depletion is important in determining the ability of the uterus to respond to hormone stimulation. Within the first 6 h after an injection of estradiol, when little replenishment has taken place, a second injection of estradiol does not enhance uterotropic responses above those obtained with the first injection.[375] A second injection at 12 h, however, when cytosolic receptors are replenished, causes enhanced uterotropic responses.

CONTROL OF THE PROGESTERONE RECEPTOR BY ESTROGEN. The uterus is relatively insensitive to progesterone until after exposure to estrogen. For example, progesterone treatment does not produce a secretory uterine epithelium in the nonestrogenized uterus[374]; however, after estrogen priming, progesterone treatment has dramatic effects on the production of secretory responses.[376] Several studies have shown that estrogen priming stimulates the synthesis of the progeste-

STEROID HORMONE CONTROL OF CHICK OVIDUCT CELL FUNCTION

HORMONAL STATE	OVIDUCT GROWTH	OVIDUCT WEIGHT	STATE OF DIFFERENTIATION	HORMONE-INDUCED PROTEINS	
				ESTROGEN	PROGESTIN
UNSTIMULATED	P↓ ↑E NO GROWTH	0.01g	UNDIFFERENTIATED CELLS	NONE	NONE
PRIMARY STIMULATION	DISCONTINUE ESTROGEN	2g	TUBULAR GLANDS GOBLET CELLS — LUMEN	OVALBUMIN OTHERS	NONE AVIDIN
WITHDRAWAL	P OR E	0.25g	REGRESSED STRUCTURE	NONE	NONE
SECONDARY STIMULATION		0.5g	TUBULAR GLANDS GOBLET CELLS — LUMEN	OVALBUMIN OTHERS	OVALBUMIN OTHERS AVIDIN

Figure 4–41. Differentiation and development of chick oviduct.

rone receptor, thereby enhancing the ability of the uterus to respond to progesterone.[14] These effects occur in both the endometrium and the myometrium of the guinea pig uterus[377] and in the neurons of the hypothalamus.[378]

EFFECTS OF PROGESTERONE ON THE PROGESTERONE RECEPTOR. Progesterone decreases the quantity of cytosolic progesterone receptor in the guinea pig uterus by decreasing the rate of progesterone receptor gene transcription.[379–381] This decreased transcription, coupled with the fact that the mRNA for progesterone receptor is short-lived, causes a rapid decline in receptor levels.[382] If rats are maintained on estrogen, however, progesterone receptor levels do not decrease after progesterone administration. Progesterone may suppress the synthesis of its own receptor by desensitizing the uterus to estrogen. The level of cytosolic progesterone receptor correlates with the ability of the uterus to respond to progesterone. When cytosolic progesterone receptor levels are low, an injection of progesterone has no antagonistic effect on estrogen-induced early uterotropic events. Thus the ability of the uterus to respond to progesterone depends on the presence of its receptor.

CONTROL OF THE ESTROGEN RECEPTOR BY PROGESTERONE. The action of progesterone on the estrogen-primed uterus is often considered to be antagonistic to estrogen but probably should be viewed as a modifier of estrogen action. Nevertheless, progesterone reduces the ability of estrogens to cause uterine growth and vaginal cornification.[359, 383] Progesterone does not interfere with the initial binding of estradiol to the cytosolic estrogen receptor or with the nuclear binding of the estradiol-receptor complex but does decrease the level of cytosolic estrogen receptor.[384] This decrease in estrogen receptor level correlates with a decreased ability of estradiol to stimulate uterine growth.[385] In addition, progesterone reduces the level of nuclear-bound estrogen-receptor complexes in the hamster uterus.[386, 387] This reduction in nuclear estrogen-receptor complexes may be due to the induction of an estrogen receptor–regulatory factor[388] involved in the dephosphorylation-inactivation mechanisms.[389] With continued estrogen administration, progesterone causes a temporary reduction in the level of nuclear estrogen-receptor complexes, followed by a return to elevated levels.[390]

NONRECEPTOR BINDING PROTEINS. Several nonreceptor proteins that bind estrogen and progesterone are found in both cytosolic and nuclear fractions.

Cytosolic Nonreceptor Binding Sites. The cytosol from immature rat uteri contains type II estrogen-binding sites with a sedimentation coefficient of 4S on density gradients, but these binding proteins do not undergo translocation to the nucleus.[391, 392] Type II sites have a lower affinity ($K_d \sim 20$ nM) than that of the receptor ($K_d \sim 1$ nM), but the number of type II sites may exceed that of type I sites. Type II sites display stereospecificity for binding estrogen and are present in other estrogen targets, such as the vagina, mouse and human mammary tumors, MCF-7 cells, rabbit endometrial cells, and müllerian ducts of the chick embryo. Similar binding sites have been observed in the prostate,[393, 394] seminal vesicle,[395] and rabbit corpus luteum,[396] so the presence of secondary binding sites for estrogenic hormones appears to be a general phenomenon.

Although the function of type II sites is not known, their presence complicates the interpretation of receptor assays based on binding technologies. The number of these sites may range from 2 to 10 times the amount of estrogen receptor, and as the quantity of type II sites increases, the error introduced in the estimation of the K_d and of the number of type I sites increases. This problem has been discussed in detail by Clark and Peck.[1, 341]

Hypothalamic-Pituitary Interactions

Receptors for steroid hormones are found in various specific loci in the brain that are known to be associated with the actions of steroid hormones[1, 397]; e.g., gonadotropes contain estrogen receptors, and corticotropes contain glucocorticoid receptors. Thus the brain contains response systems for steroid hormones. The steroid receptors in brain and pituitary tissue are similar to those in other tissues and are thought to act via the same mechanisms. Steroids stimulate the synthesis of brain proteins thought to be involved in the control of gonadotropin secretion by the pituitary.

Estrogen stimulates the synthesis of progesterone receptors in the hypothalamus, as in other target tissues, and this increase in progesterone receptor levels appears to be required for sexual behavior during the estrous cycle. Thus steroid hormones interact with the hypothalamic-pituitary system to control ovulation and reproductive behavior.

Some responses to steroid hormones in the brain occur rapidly and are postulated to result from steroid-membrane interactions, rather than from stimulation of gene transcription.[398] Diencephalic neuronal discharge rates increase within seconds after iontophoretic administration of estradiol-17β-hemisuccinate. Likewise, cortisol administration alters the response of hypothalamic neurons acutely, and the release of corticotropin-releasing hormone is rapidly inhibited by application of glucocorticoids to hypothalamic fragments or synaptosomes in vitro.

Steroid Receptors and the Female Reproductive Cycle

RECEPTOR BINDING IN THE OVARY. The ovary is responsive to exogenous estrogens. Estradiol treatment of the hypophysectomized rat does not increase the number of follicle-stimulating hormone (FSH) receptors per granulosa cell but does increase the number of estradiol receptors.[399] Estrogen also increases the number of granulosa cells and hence increases the amount of FSH receptors in the ovary. Both hormones, in concert, increase the LH receptor levels of granulosa cells and sensitize these cells to the ovulatory effect of LH. Luteinizing hormone in turn increases progesterone receptor levels in granulosa cells. Follicular atresia is associated with the loss of receptors for estrogen, FSH, and LH.

STEROID RECEPTORS IN THE UTERUS. The concentration of nuclear estrogen receptor in the uterus correlates with the level of estrogen in the blood of the rat.[400] The number of nuclear complexes is at a minimum during estrus and metestrus (1000 sites per cell), increases between metestrus and diestrus (3500 sites per cell), and reaches a maximum at proestrus (5000 sites per cell). Uterine weight, protein content, and the ratio of protein to DNA are higher in proestrus than in metestrus or diestrus, suggesting that protein synthesis in the uterus fluctuates throughout the estrous cycle. Thus maximal estrogenic responses are accompanied by peak concentrations of nuclear estrogen-receptor complexes in the proestrus uterus. Similar observations have been made in the oviduct and uterus in the cat, in which the amount of nuclear-bound estrogen in both organs correlates with ciliation and cell height in the oviduct during the estrous cycle.

The level of cytosolic progesterone receptor varies during the estrous cycle in all species, and estrogen appears to control its synthesis. During the follicular phase of the cycle, the level of cytosolic progesterone receptor is relatively low, and as estrogen blood levels increase, the amount of progesterone receptor increases, an increase that is probably a requisite for progesterone action during pregnancy and during the luteal phase.

Elevated levels of serum progesterone deplete cytosolic progesterone receptors and enhance nuclear receptor-progesterone complexes, but there is an eventual decrease in total progesterone receptor levels after progesterone administration. Likewise, cytosolic progesterone receptor levels increase before the preovulatory peak in plasma progesterone receptor synthesis and decrease in association with the high levels of progesterone during the luteal phase. The receptor level also remains low during pregnancy in the guinea pig. Similar changes occur during the estrous cycle in the hamster, rat, mouse, and human.

The decrease in progesterone receptor level under the influence of elevated progesterone levels in the blood is due to an actual decrease in the total number of receptors; i.e., progesterone, via its inhibition of estrogen receptor synthesis, probably suppresses the synthesis of its own receptor. Alternatively, this decrease may result from a combination of low estrogen levels and a change in the relative abundance of receptors among specific cell types.

PREGNANCY AND LACTATION. *Uterus.* Blood levels of estradiol are transiently elevated between days 1 and 4 of pregnancy in the rat. At this time the quantity of nuclear estrogen complexes in the uterus increases (days 2 and 3 of the implantation period) and then decreases (on day 4). These data suggest that elevated blood levels of estradiol cause nuclear accumulation of the hormone-receptor complex, which in turn may stimulate the events that lead to blastocyst implantation. The reduction of estrogen receptor levels may be linked to rising progesterone levels at this time.

The amount of cytosolic progesterone receptor gradually increases during pregnancy in the rat to high levels, whereas nuclear levels of receptor accumulate and then decrease just before parturition. The number of cytoplasmic sites available for nuclear binding is large compared with the quantity of nuclear sites measured. The reason for this distribution is not clear because blood levels of progesterone are high during pregnancy. Either all the receptor sites are not measured in these studies or the metabolic conversion of progesterone to 5α-reduced steroids results in apparent discrepancies. The ability of the rat uterus to form 5 α-pregnane-3,20-dione and 3α-hydroxy-5α-pregnan-20-one increases substantially between days 11 and 21 of pregnancy so even though blood levels of progesterone are high at these times, tissue levels may be low. This metabolic sequence could produce a cellular environment wherein the tissue level of progesterone is gradually lowered during pregnancy, and hence fewer estrogen-receptor complexes are formed. Elevated levels of cytoplasmic progesterone receptor during the last few days of pregnancy in the rat could be due to increased levels of estrogen at this time. The decrease in nuclear levels of progesterone receptor before birth is probably an important mechanism for decreasing the control of the uterus by progesterone and increasing its sensitivity to estrogen and may contribute to the onset of parturition.

Progesterone receptors during pregnancy also have been studied in guinea pig, hamster, and mouse. In contrast to the results for the rat, levels of cytosolic progesterone receptor either change little, as in the mouse, or are depressed, as in the guinea pig. Additional work is required to understand these species differences.

Corpus Luteum. The corpus luteum of the rabbit requires estrogen for its maintenance and contains cytosolic estrogen receptors similar to those in other tissues.[401] The level of nuclear-bound estrogen-receptor complexes in the corpus luteum of the rat increases between days 2 and 12 of pregnancy and then gradually decreases, despite the continuing elevated levels of estrogen. However, blood levels do not necessarily reflect the concentration of estrogen in the corpus luteum, and administration of estradiol to hypophysectomized pregnant rats maintains cytosolic estrogen receptors in luteal tissue.

Mammary Gland. The mammary gland is a target organ for several hormones, and steroids stimulate the development and growth of this tissue. During pregnancy, the levels of estrogen receptor increase,[402] apparently under the control of prolactin.

In the lactating rat, the level of cytoplasmic estrogen receptor increases dramatically,[403] whereas nuclear estrogen-receptor complexes remain low throughout lactation because blood estrogen levels are low. The elevation of cytoplasmic receptor number in lactating tissue does not depend on the presence of the ovary. While estrogen receptors control ductal proliferation, progesterone receptors contribute to duct branching and to alveolar proliferation.[404]

Placenta. Estrogen receptors are present in the rat.[405] The basal zone of the rat placenta contains large numbers of cytosolic estrogen receptors (30,000 per cell on day 9 of pregnancy), while levels of nuclear receptor are low (3400 per cell). This distribution of receptors is probably due to the low levels of estrogen in the blood at this time, but the reason for the high levels of cytoplasmic receptor in placenta during early pregnancy is unknown. By day 15 of pregnancy the levels of receptor decrease to 600 and 200 sites per cell for cytoplasmic and nuclear receptors, respectively; for the secretion of progesterone by trophoblastic giant cells may bring about this decline.

Receptors in Development and Aging

RECEPTORS AND DEVELOPMENT. Steroid receptors are present in their respective target organs before the maturation of the endocrine glands that secrete the effector hormones. In the guinea pig, estrogen receptors are present in the fetal uterus and are fully capable of responding to exogenous estrogen administration to the mother.[406] In the rat, which has a short gestational period, estrogen receptors appear in the uterus during the first 10 d of life.[407] The level of estrogen receptors in the uterus of the neonatal rat and fetal guinea pig is either equal to or greater than that in the adult animal. Estrogen receptors also appear during neonatal life in the hypothalamus and pituitary of the rat. The development of receptors in these tissues does not depend on steroid hormone stimulation but is a developmental feature of the reproductive target organs that prepares them to be target tissues for steroid hormones.

In contrast to the situation in the mammal, oviduct development in the chicken is dependent on the presence of estrogen. In most female birds, the right müllerian duct regresses, and the left duct develops into the oviduct and shell gland. The development of the left oviduct and regression of the right duct are estrogen dependent. The quantity of cytosolic receptors increases from day 8 to day 12 of embryonic development, and the quantity of nuclear estrogen-receptor complexes increases dramatically between days 10 and 18. This nuclear accumulation of receptor probably results from endogenous estrogens in the yolk.

RECEPTORS AND AGING. It has been proposed that aging might be caused by the reverse of development; i.e., receptors may decrease in numbers or affinity for their tropic hormones and thereby render systems less sensitive to hormonal stimulation and lead to decreased function and aging. Some support for this concept has been obtained from studies in the rat, which gradually loses its regular 4- to 5-d estrous cycle and enters a stage of persistent estrus at approximately 1 to 1.5 y of age.[408] This stage is usually followed by periods of persistent diestrus. During these periods the estrogen receptor concentration decreases, but there is no decrease in binding affinity. Thus receptor loss may be associated with aging, but whether it is a cause-effect relationship is unknown.

RECEPTOR ISOFORM INTERACTIONS. Most species, including humans, have two isoforms of the progesterone receptor, termed PR_B and PR_A. The larger, PR_B, form contains extra amino acids at the N terminus and is a strong positive stimulator of gene expression. The shorter, PR_A, form has a weaker stimulatory capacity for genes and appears to be able to antagonize gene stimulation by PR_B.[409, 410] The physiological usefulness of these isoforms is unclear at present, but the PR_B/PR_A ratio varies among tissues and at times during organ development.

STEROID HORMONE ANTAGONISM

Compounds that block the action of a steroid hormone are called antagonists or antihormones. Most act by binding to receptors and interfering with their normal function.

Antiestrogens

Antiestrogens can be divided into three groups: (1) short-acting antagonists, such as estriol; (2) long-acting antagonists, such as tamoxifen and clomiphene; and (3) physiological antagonists, such as progesterone, androgens, and glucocorticoids.

SHORT-ACTING ANTAGONISTS. Short-acting estrogens, such as estriol and estradiol-17α, are actually time-dependent mixed agonists-antagonists (Fig. 4–43). They stimulate early uterotropic responses but have little effect on true uterine hypertrophy and hyperplasia when injected in saline.[1, 411] This explains why they have no antagonistic action when examined by short-term uterotropic assays but display partial antagonism when long-term uterine growth assays are used. This dichotomy may be understood by examining the idealized data shown in Figure 4–44. The response patterns for estradiol and estriol at three dose levels are plotted as a function of time after a single injection. If uterotropic responses are measured at 6 h after an injection of either estradiol or estriol, they are identical (see Fig. 4–44B), and therefore no antagonism will be noted. However, measurements made at 24 h do show antagonism (see Fig. 4–44C) that results from the reduced capacity of estriol to stimulate true uterine growth. When estradiol and estriol are administered simultaneously the overall uterotropic effect of estradiol is reduced at 24 h.

The short-acting agonists do cause nuclear binding of the

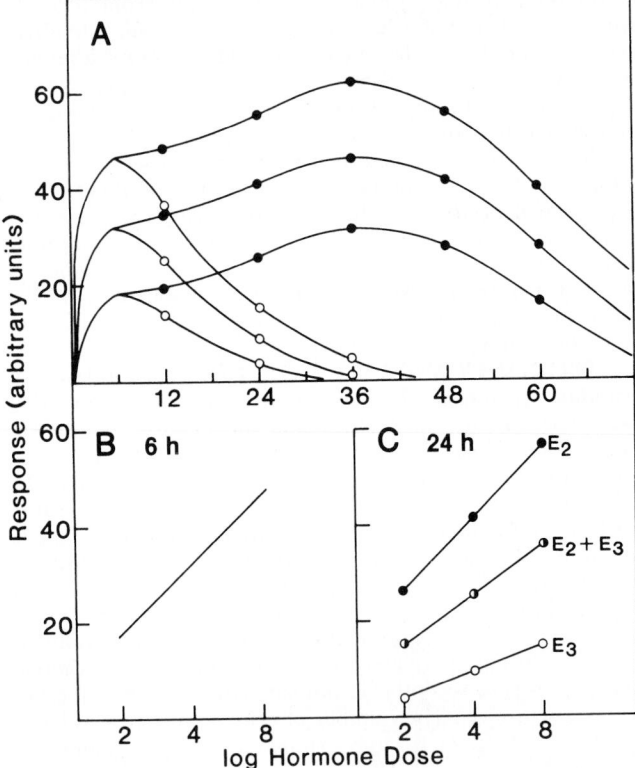

Figure 4–44. Effects of long-acting and short-acting estrogens on the uterotropic response in the rat. The uterotropic response (growth) in *A* is measured as a function of time after an injection of three dose levels of estradiol (●) or estriol (○). Identical dose response at 6 h for both hormones is shown in *B*. Dose-response curves at 24 h for estradiol (E_2), estriol (E_3), and a combination of these hormones are shown in *C*.

hormone-receptor complex and thus are able to stimulate early uterotropic events. However, they are unable to maintain the receptor in the nucleus for a sufficient period of time to cause uterine growth. The antagonistic actions of these compounds result from competition between estradiol-receptor and estriol-receptor complexes for functional nuclear sites. When short-acting estrogens are administered via a pellet implant to cause continuous release of hormones and continuous occupancy of the receptor, no antagonism is observed. Thus the biologic response with short-acting estrogens is dependent on the conditions of administration and is the consequence of receptor occupancy.

Why short-acting estrogens occupy nuclear-bound receptors for short periods after an injection is not completely clear. The rate of dissociation of estriol from the receptor is higher than that of estradiol,[412] leading to the suggestion that this difference in dissociation rate accounts for short-term nuclear retention.[413] Estriol is also cleared from the body more rapidly than is estradiol.[414] It is also possible that estriol-receptor complexes dissociate from their nuclear binding sites more rapidly than do estradiol-receptor complexes, resulting in faster turnover or processing of receptor and loss of hormone from the tissues.

LONG-ACTING ANTAGONISTS. Triphenylethylene derivatives, such as tamoxifen and clomiphene (Fig. 4–45), are mixed agonists-antagonists of estrogen action.[415] An agonist stimulates a response (Fig. 4–46A), whereas an antagonist inhibits the action of an agonist. A mixed agonist-antagonist partially inhibits the action of an agonist but partially mimics the response of the agonist. The degree of agonist or antagonist activity depends on the species, organ, tissue, or cell type that is being examined and on the end-point assay chosen.

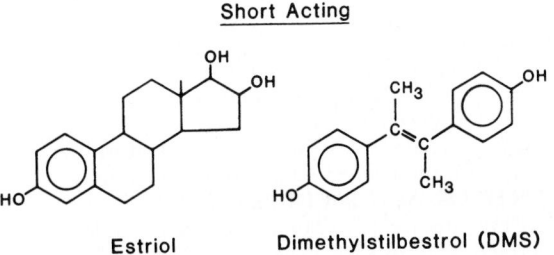

Figure 4–43. Chemical structures of long-acting and short-acting estrogens.

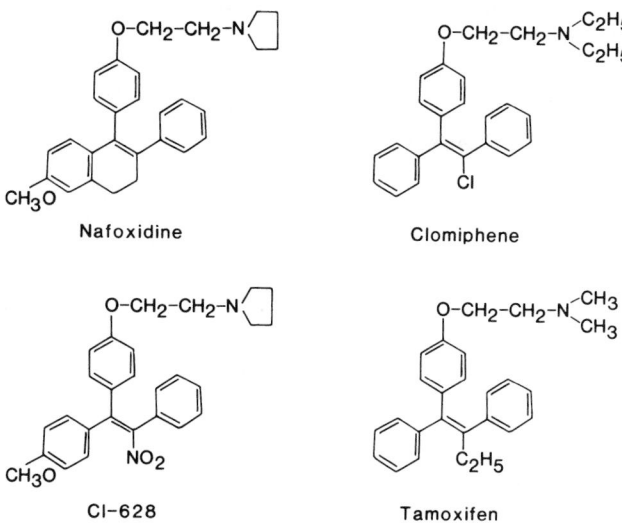

Figure 4–45. Antiestrogens of the triphenylethylene type.

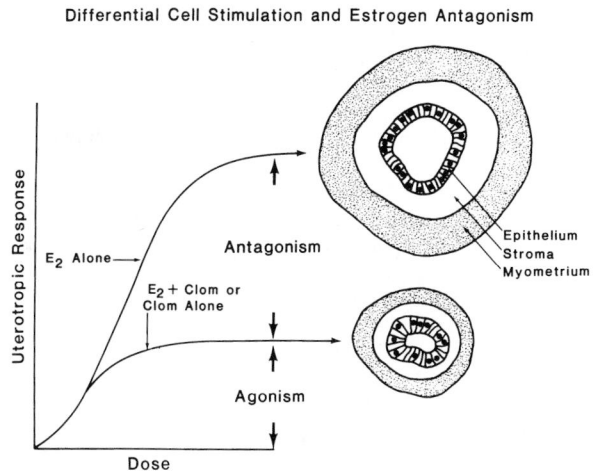

Figure 4–47. The agonistic and antagonistic effects of estradiol and clomiphene on uterine growth and histology. E_2, estradiol; Clom, clomiphene.

Clomiphene and tamoxifen cause growth of the rat uterus when administered alone but inhibit the growth-promoting effects of estradiol when given simultaneously (Fig. 4–47). The drugs stimulate hypertrophy of the epithelial cells of the endometrium but have little effect on the stromal or myometrial compartments, whereas estradiol stimulates cellular hypertrophy and hyperplasia in all three tissue layers and thus produces a larger uterus than clomiphene alone. The inhibition of estradiol action on uterine growth results from the antagonism of growth in the stromal and myometrial compartments. Therefore, triphenylethylene drugs are estrogen agonists in the epithelial cells and estrogen antagonists in other uterine cells.

The mechanisms by which long-acting estrogen antagonists block estrogen action in some cell types, yet stimulate estrogen responses in others, are not fully understood. However, these drugs bind to the estrogen receptor and cause nuclear accumulation of drug-receptor complexes. This accumulation is accompanied by long-term depletion of cytosolic receptors and altered nuclear processing of the drug-receptor complex.

Differences have been reported in the physiocochemical characteristics of antiestrogen-receptor and estradiol-receptor complexes.[318, 416–422] Agonists and antagonists induce different conformations in the receptor that may account for their differences in activity. Pure estrogen antagonists appear to drive the receptor into an inactive form while mixed antagonists-agonists induce intermediate conformations between wholly active and inactive states. These intermediate conformations have intermediate affinities for coactivators and corepressors. If a given cell has a higher concentration of the appropriate coactivator, the mixed antagonist would be more prone to exert an agonist effect in that tissue. The opposite would occur if the cell had a higher concentration of corepressor, thereby providing a potential basis for tissue-selective effects of such ligands.[423]

Understanding the mechanism of action of long-acting agonists-antagonists is complicated further by interspecies variation. In contrast to the mixed agonistic-antagonistic functions in the rat, these compounds are estrogenic in the adult mouse, with little if any antiestrogenic activity.[424] In the chick oviduct and liver, however, these compounds are estrogen antagonists and have virtually no detectable agonist activity.[367, 425] However, tamoxifen, when administered with progesterone, induces cytodifferentiation of oviduct tubular gland cells and stimulates the synthesis of conalbumin and ovalbumin, whereas tamoxifen alone has no effect. The interactions that bring about these effects are also likely to be explained by the mechanism discussed earlier. In primates, clomiphene and tamoxifen are primarily antiestrogenic.[426, 427] Different species manifest a broad spectrum of agonistic-antagonistic responses to nonsteroidal antiestrogens (for reviews see references 426 and 428).

These species differences in response to nonsteroidal antiestrogens essentially disappear in cell culture. Tamoxifen and 4-hydroxytamoxifen block the estrogen-stimulated increases in several specific proteins in MCF-7 cells and have no agonistic activity.[429] Tamoxifen and nafoxidine inhibit [³H] thymidine incorporation and DNA polymerase activity and reduce cell number in MCF-7 cell cultures.[430] Estrogen-stimulated prolactin synthesis is inhibited by tamoxifen, and no agonistic effect is seen with the drug alone.[431, 432]

Drugs may act in part via indirect mechanisms that do not involve the estrogen receptor at all. Triphenylethylene antiestrogen binding sites (TABSs) that bind tamoxifen and clomiphene with high affinity ($K_d \sim 10^{-9}$ M) are present in estrogen target and nontarget tissues.[433, 434] In addition, somewhat similar sites with lower affinity ($K_d \sim 10^{-8}$ M) are associated with low-density lipoprotein (LDL) in rat serum.[435] Other compounds, such as chlorpomazine, ketocholesterol, and cholesterol, have a reduced affinity.[436]

The subcellular localization of TABS appears to vary with species or cell type or both. TABSs have been characterized in

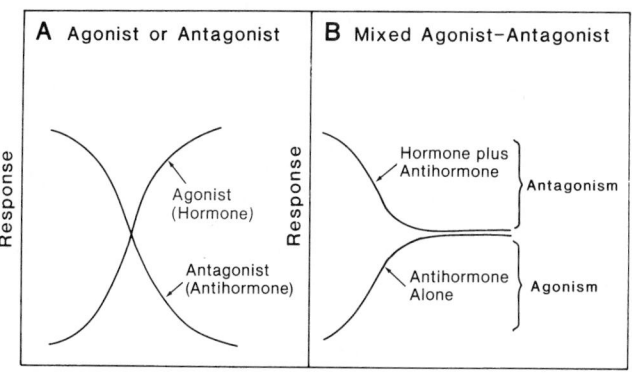

Figure 4–46. Effects of agonists, antagonists, and mixed agonists-antagonists on response.

the cytosol of the chick oviduct, guinea pig and rat uterus, human mammary carcinoma, and nontarget human tissues.[437–439] Cytosolic and nuclear localization has been reported in the guinea pig uterus,[438] and the level of these sites may be modulated by estradiol and progesterone.[435, 440] Nuclear localization also occurs in human breast cancer tissue and in chicken and rat liver.

The functions of TABSs have not been defined. The estrogenic and antiestrogenic properties of nonsteroidal antiestrogens correlate with their relative binding affinities for the estrogen receptor and not for TABS,[441] and the *cis* and *trans* isomers of clomiphene bind to TABS with similar affinities but have dissimilar agonist-antagonist profiles. Tamoxifen resistance has been described in a line of MCF-7 breast cancer cells that contained extremely low levels of TABS and normal levels of estrogen receptor, but there was no relation between the levels of TABS and tamoxifen sensitivity.[441]

PURE ANTIESTROGENS. Another class of drugs appear to be pure antagonists.[442] ICI 164384 is a 7α-alkylamide analogue of estradiol that lacks agonist activity for uterine growth in both rats and mice and does not induce the progesterone receptor in the immature rat. ICI 164384 binds to the estrogen receptor with an affinity similar to that of estradiol, but its ability to inhibit estrogen-induced mRNA synthesis is 50- to 150-fold less than predicted.[442] Similar discrepancies have been noted for tamoxifen and hydroxytamoxifen[443] and may result from a differential ability of these compounds to enter cells or from binding interactions with nonreceptor proteins. ICI 164384 decreases the affinity of estrogen receptor binding to EREs and increases the degradation rate of the estrogen receptor.[444, 445]

PHYSIOLOGICAL ESTROGEN ANTAGONISTS. Other hormones alter the actions of estrogen at the cellular level and modify estrogen-directed functions.

Progesterone. Progesterone probably should be referred to as a modifier of estrogen action rather than an antagonist, but progesterone reduces the ability of estrogens to cause uterine growth and vaginal cornification. This modification of estrogen action involves receptor mechanisms that have been discussed previously under the section on control of steroid receptor concentration, specifically decreases in the number of cytosolic and nuclear-bound estrogen-receptor complexes.[446]

Most of the studies of the effects of progesterone on estrogen receptor levels have been done under nonphysiological circumstances. However, in the studies of Brenner and colleagues[447] physiological conditions were maintained by creating artificial menstrual cycles in ovariectomized rhesus monkeys. Cytosolic estrogen receptor levels were elevated during the first half of the cycle and decreased during the second half, suggesting that progesterone lowers cytosolic estrogen receptor levels even when estradiol is present. In pig endometrium, progesterone induces estrogen sulfotransferase, an enzyme that inactivates estradiol, thus interfering with the estrogen-dependent replenishment of the estrogen receptor.[448] Therefore, progesterone acts by several mechanisms to decrease the level of estrogen receptor and reduce the response to estrogen.

Progesterone also decreases the number of nuclear type II estrogen-binding sites by a mechanism that does not appear to be related to effects on estrogen receptor levels. The inhibitory effects of progesterone do appear to be mediated by the progesterone receptor.

Antiprogestagens

Some progesterone derivatives have antagonistic properties. Mifepristone (RU 486) interrupts the luteal phase of the menstrual cycle and terminates pregnancy in women[449] and induces early onset of vaginal bleeding when administered during the luteal phase to cycling monkeys.[320, 450] Such actions are due to a direct antagonistic effect of mifepristone at the receptor level in the uterine endometrium. This compound binds to progesterone receptors in the rabbit uterus and to glucocorticoid receptors in the thymus, where it acts as an antiglucocorticoid. In T47D cells mifepristone binds to the progesterone receptor and inhibits cellular proliferation, as does RU 5020 (promegestone), a synthetic progestagen.[451] Thus mifepristone is an agonist by this criterion, but it does antagonize the stimulation of insulin receptors by promegestone. Agonistic properties also have been observed in T47D cells, which grow in response to mifepristone.[452] Therefore, in T47D cells mifepristone manifests mixed agonistic-antagonistic properties.

Mifepristone binds well to all mammalian progesterone receptors except those of the hamster,[453] a species in which the drug has no antiprogestational effects. Progesterone receptors from the chick oviduct display a low affinity for mifepristone. Reduced affinity in the chicken and loss of affinity in the hamster are due to structural differences in the receptors in these species.

The mechanism by which mifepristone exerts its antagonistic activity does not involve any differences in activation and transformation of the drug-receptor complex.[320, 420] Both progesterone and mifepristone form complexes that bind to hormone response elements in a qualitatively and quantitatively similar manner. The only difference appears to be in the sedimentation and gel retardation characteristics of the two receptor-hormone response element complexes. Thus the binding of the mifepristone-receptor complex to hormone response elements probably results in a conformation that is different from that of the receptor-progesterone complex. Studies involving protease digestion and antibody epitope recognition indicate that progesterone agonists and antagonists impart different conformational changes to the progesterone receptor.[422, 454] Progesterone agonists induce a conformation resistant to the protease digestion or recognition by an antibody to the last 14 amino acids of the C-terminal tail of the receptor. In contrast, the C-terminal end of the antagonist-bound receptor is sensitive to protease digestion and is available for antibody recognition. Mutational analysis indicates that there is a repressor domain in the C-terminal end. When receptor is bound by an agonist the repressor domain is not available on the surface of the molecule and presumably is not active, and the receptor can activate transcription (see Fig. 4–38). In contrast, when receptor is bound by an antagonist, the repressor domain is freely available to inhibit transcription. Thus, inability of the antagonist to activate the receptor appears due to the induction of a conformation that cannot counteract the receptor's repressor function.

As pointed out earlier, the actions of anti–steroid hormone drugs in vitro are not necessarily identical to their actions in vivo. More work in vivo is needed on this important class of antiprogestagens before definitive statements can be made regarding their mechanism of action and their true pharmacologic and physiological effects.

An inhibitor of progesterone-receptor binding in the cytosol of rat placenta is a macromolecule that decreases the affinity of the receptor for progesterone but has no effect on the number of receptor sites.[455] Inhibitory activity in trophoblast cytosol is greatest on days 9 and 12 of pregnancy and decreases so that it is no longer detectable by day 18; this coincides with a sharp decrease in progesterone receptor concentration.

CLINICAL AND BIOMEDICAL CONSIDERATIONS

Major improvements in our knowledge of the mode of action of the gonadal steroids are important to the understanding of medical pharmacology, physiology, pathology, diagnosis, and therapy.

Pharmacologic Concepts

Hormone antagonists have played an important part in the elucidation of the mechanism of action of steroids. Conversely, understanding of the basic biochemical actions of hormones makes it possible to postulate and document the existence of several types of hormonal antagonists. Any agent that interferes with steroid hormone action may do so through one of the following mechanisms: (1) depletion or downregulation of the specific steroid hormone receptor, (2) inhibition of the nuclear binding or alteration of the conformation of the steroid hormone-receptor DNA complex, (3) interference with receptor coupling to coactivator proteins at the target gene binding site, (4) perturbation of the receptor cycle, and (5) inhibition of steroid hormone–induced gene transcription by other or indirect mechanisms.

Pathologic and Diagnostic Considerations

Molecular studies of steroid hormone action have provided an understanding of many endocrine syndromes that were previously perplexing from a pathogenetic and diagnostic point of view and have suggested treatments for some of these diseases. These disorders are discussed in detail in the following chapters of this book.

GENERAL COMMENTS ON MOLECULAR GENETICS AND HORMONE RESISTANCE DISEASE

Elucidation of the pathophysiology of steroid hormone resistance syndromes has provided insight into the normal pathway of nuclear receptor action. Each new type of hormone resistance that is recognized and each new mutation that is uncovered behind that process provide an opportunity for defining the nature of a specific reaction essential for the action of the hormone. How does the receptor affinity for DNA affect transcriptional regulation? How does ligand binding alter receptor conformation and activity at the genome? What additional functional domains and requisite trans-acting factors are yet to be defined for the receptor molecule? How do coregulator proteins (coactivators and corepressors) interact with receptors and transduce stimuli to the core transcriptional machinery? Site-directed point mutagenesis of the various receptors has provided many clues to amino acids that contribute significantly to receptor function. The interpretation of such studies has, in many instances, been difficult because of limitations in the cotransfection assay. In this assay, the receptors are expressed in heterologous cells together with a steroid response element linked to a reporter gene, such as the chloramphenicol acetyltransferase or luciferase gene. Most of the structure-function conclusions drawn from these studies have relied on this method of measuring receptor activity, but significant differences exist between cotransfected and endogenous genes. For instance, cotransfected genes exist as episomes and are unlikely to exist in a native chromatin structure. Furthermore, transfection efficiencies are low, so only a fraction of the cells acquire the DNA. Because receptors are often overexpressed in this subpopulation of cells, transfected cells may contain wild-type or mutant receptors in vast excess over the levels that occur naturally. Although this type of assay should reflect the gross functional state of the nascent mutagenized protein, more subtle assessments regarding functionality may be difficult to make.

Gene deletion ("knock-out") experiments in mice using homologous recombination technology are useful adjuncts to standard transgenic technology to advance our understanding of the biology of steroid receptor superfamily members. The advancement of in vitro technologies for receptor crystallization and x-ray diffraction and nuclear magnetic resonance analysis constitute a formidable technology to employ in receptor mechanism studies.

Finally, characterization of the increasing numbers of patients with steroid-resistant disorders should provide important insight into how these proteins function in target cells. In contrast to random in vitro mutagenesis, studies of genetic diseases of hormone resistance in humans and animals permit the investigation of subtle mutations that impair function under physiological conditions in vivo. The mutational experiments of nature are invaluable in understanding human disease conditions and normal physiological processes. Continued study of the mutations that cause tissue resistance to hormones will improve our knowledge of the mechanisms by which these receptors regulate cellular transcription.

REFERENCES

1. Clark JH, Peck EJ, Jr. Female sex steroids, receptors and function. In: Gross F, Labhart A, Lipsett MB, et al, eds. Heidelberg: Springer-Verlag, 1993: 31–68.
2. Scatchard G. The attractions of proteins for small molecules and ions. Ann NY Acad Sci 1949; 51:660–672.
3. Markaverich BM, Williams M, Upchurch S, et al. Heterogeneity of nuclear estrogen-binding sites in the rat uterus: a simple method for the quantitation of type I and II sites by [³H]estradiol exchange. Endocrinology 1981; 109:62–68.
4. Anderson JN, Clark JH, Peck EJ. Estrogen and nuclear binding sites: determination of specific sites by [³H]estradiol exchange. Biochem J 1972; 126:561–567.
5. Katzenellenbogen J, Johnson HJ, Carlson KE. Studies on the uterine cytoplasmic estrogen binding protein, thermal stability and ligand dissociation rate: an assay of empty and filled sites by exchange. Biochemistry 1973; 12:4092–4099.
6. Beato M. Gene regulation by steroid hormones. Cell 1989; 56:335–344.
7. Evans RM. The steroid and thyroid hormone receptor superfamily. Science 1988; 240:889–895.
8. O'Malley BW. The steroid receptor superfamily: more excitement predicted for the future. Mol Endocrinol 1990; 4:363–369.
9. Tsai MJ, O'Malley BW. Molecular mechanisms of action of steroid/thyroid receptor superfamily members. Annu Rev Biochem 1994; 63:451–486.
10. Conneely OM, Sullivan WP, Toft DO, et al. Molecular cloning of the chicken progesterone receptor. Science 1986; 233:767–770.
11. Gronemeyer H, Turcotte B, Quirin-Stricker C, et al. The chicken progesterone receptor: sequence, expression and functional analysis. EMBO J 1987; 6:3985–3994.
12. Misrahi M, Atger M, D'Auriol L, et al. Complete amino acid sequence of the human progesterone receptor deduced from cloned cDNA. Biochem Biophys Res Commun 1987; 143:740–748.
13. Koike S, Sakai M, Muramatsu M. Molecular cloning and characterization of rat estrogen receptor cDNA. Nucleic Acids Res 1987; 15:2499–2513.
14. Walter P, Green S, Krust A, et al. Cloning of the human estrogen receptor cDNA. Proc Natl Acad Sci USA 1985; 82:7889–7893.
15. Chang C, Kokontis J, Liao S. Molecular cloning of human and rat complementary DNA encoding androgen receptors. Science 1988; 240:324–327.
16. Lubahn DB, Joseph DR, Sullivan PM, et al. Cloning of the human androgen receptor cDNA and localization to the X-chromosome. Science 1988; 340:327–330.
17. Hollenberg SM, Weinberger C, Ong ES, et al. Primary structure and expression of a functional human glucocorticoid receptor cDNA. Nature 1985; 318:635–641.
18. Miesfeld R, Rusconi S, Godowski PJ, et al. Genetic complementation of a glucocorticoid receptor deficiency by expression of cloned receptor cDNA. Cell 1986; 46:389–399.
19. Murray JC, Smith RF, Ardinger HA, et al. RFLP for the glucocorticoid receptor (GRL) located at 5q11-5q13. Nucleic Acids Res 1987; 15:6765.
20. Arriza JL, Weinberger C, Cerelli G, et al. Cloning of human mineralocorticoid receptor complementary DNA: structural and functional kinship with the glucocorticoid receptor. Science 1987; 237:268–275.
21. Patel PD, Sherman TG, Goldman DJ, et al. Molecular cloning of a mineralocorticoid (type I) receptor complementary DNA from rat hippocampus. Mol Endocrinol 1989; 3:1877–1885.
22. Thompson CC, Weinberger C, thyroid hormone receptor expressed in the mammalian central nervous system. Science 1987; 237:1610–1614.

23. Benbrook D, Pfahl M. A novel thyroid hormone receptor encoded by a cDNA clone from a human testis library. Science 1987; 238:788–791.

24. Giguere V, Ong ES, Segui P, et al. Identification of a receptor for the morphogen retinoic acid. Nature 1987; 330:624–629.

25. Petkovich M, Brand NJ, Krust A, et al. A human retinoic acid receptor which belongs to the family of nuclear receptors. Nature 1987; 330:444–450.

26. Zelent A, Krust A, Petkovich M, et al. Cloning of murine alpha and beta retinoic acid receptors and a novel receptor gamma predominantly expressed in skin. Nature 1989; 339:714–717.

27. Krust A, Kastner P, Petkovich M, et al. A third retinoic acid receptor. Proc Natl Acad Sci USA 1989; 86:5310–5314.

28. Mangelsdorf DJ, Ong ES, Dyck JA, et al. Nuclear receptor that identifies a novel retinoic acid response pathway. Nature 1990; 345:224–229.

29. Mangelsdorf DJ, Borgmeyer U, Heyman RA, et al. Characterization of three RXR genes that mediate the action of 9-*cis*-retinoic acid. Genes Dev 1992; 6:329–344.

30. Hughes MR, Malloy PJ, Kieback DG, et al. Point mutations in the human vitamin D receptor gene cause hypocalcemic rickets. Science 1988; 242:1702–1705.

31. McDonnell DP, Mangelsdorf DJ, Pike WJ, et al. Molecular cloning of complementary DNA encoding the avian receptor for vitamin D. Science 1987; 235:1214–1217.

32. Baker AR, McDonnell DP, Hughes MR, et al. Cloning and expression of full-length cDNA encoding human vitamin D receptor. Proc Natl Acad Sci USA 1988; 85:3294–3298.

33. Green S, Chambon P. Carcinogenesis: a superfamily of potentially oncogenic hormone receptors. Nature 1986; 324:615–617.

34. O'Malley BW. Did eucaryotic steroid receptors evolve from intracrine gene regulators? Endocrinology 1989; 125:1119–1120 (editorial).

35. Mendel DB, Orti E, Smith LI, et al. Evidence for a glucocorticoid receptor cycle and nuclear dephosphorylation of the steroid-binding protein. Prog Clin Biol Res 1990; 322:97–117.

36. Orti E, Mendel DB, Smith LI, et al. A dynamic model of glucocorticoid receptor phosphorylation and cycling in intact cells. J Steroid Biochem 1989; 34:85–96.

37. Bonifer C, Dahlman K, Stromstedt PE, et al. DNA binding of glucocorticoid receptor protein A fusion proteins expressed in *E. coli*. J Steroid Biochem 1989; 32:5–11.

38. Power RF, Conneely OM, McDonnell DP, et al. High level expression of a truncated chicken progesterone receptor in *Escherichia coli*. J Biol Chem 1990; 265:1419–1424.

39. Mak P, McDonnell DP, Weigel NL, et al. Expression of functional chicken progesterone receptors in yeast. J Biol Chem 1989; 264:21613–21618.

40. Metzger D, White JH, Chambon P. The human oestrogene receptor functions in yeast. Nature 1988; 334:31–36.

41. Beekman JM, Cooney AJ, Elliston JF, et al. A rapid one-step method to purify baculovirus-expressed human estrogen receptor to be used in the analysis of the oxytocin promoter. Gene 1994; 146:285–289.

42. Srinivasan G, Thompson EB. Overexpression of full-length human glucocorticoid receptor in Spodoptera frugiperda cells using the baculovirus expression vector system. Mol Endocrinol 1990; 4:209–216.

43. Valcarcel J, Singh R, Zamore PD, et al. The protein Sex-lethal antagonizes the splicing factor U2AF to regulate alternative splicing of transformer pre-mRNA. Nature 1993; 362:171–175.

44. Webb P, Lopez GN, Greene GL, et al. The limits of the cellular capacity to mediate an estrogen response. Mol Endocrinol 1992; 6:157–167.

45. Wang LH, Tsai SY, Cook RG, et al. COUP transcription factor is a member of the steroid receptor superfamily. Nature 1989; 340:163–166.

46. Debuire B, Henry C, Benaissa M, et al. Sequencing the erbA gene of avian erythroblastosis virus reveals a new type of oncogene. Science 1984; 224:1456–1459.

47. Giguere V, Yang N, Segui P, et al. Identification of a new class of steroid hormone receptors. Nature 1988; 331:91–94.

48. Watson MA, Milbrandt J. The NGFI-B gene, a transcriptionally inducible member of the steroid receptor gene superfamily: genomic structure and expression in rat brain after seizure induction. Mol Cell Biol 1989; 9:4213–4219.

49. Qiu YH, Tsai SY, Tsai MJ. COUP-TF: an orphan member of the steroid/thyroid hormone receptor superfamily. Trends Endocrinol Metab 1994; 5:234–239.

50. Luo X, Ikeda Y, Parker KL. A cell-specific nuclear receptor is essential for adrenal and gonadal development and sexual differentiation. Cell 1994; 77:481–490.

51. Tontonoz P, Hu E, Graves RA, et al. mPPAR gamma 2: tissue-specific regulator of an adipocyte enhancer. Genes Dev 1994; 8:1224–1234.

52. Lee SST, Pineau T, Drago J, et al. Targeted disruption of the alpha isoform of the peroxisome proliferator-activated receptor gene in mice results in abolishment of the pleiotropic effects of peroxisome proliferators. Mol Cell Biol 1995; 15:3012–3022.

53. Conneely OM, O'Malley BW. Orphan receptors: structure and function relationships. In: Tsai MJ, O'Malley BW, eds. Mechanism of Steroid Hormone Regulation of Gene Transcription. Austin: RG Landes, 1994; 111–133

54. Chang CS, Kokontis J. Identification of a new member of the steroid receptor superfamily by cloning and sequence analysis. Biochem Biophys Res Commun 1988; 155:971–977.

55. Hazel TG, Nathans D, Lau LF. A gene inducible by serum growth factors encodes a member of the steroid and thyroid hormone receptor superfamily. Proc Natl Acad Sci USA 1988; 85:8444–8448.

56. Milbrandt J. Nerve growth factor induces a gene homologous to the glucocorticoid receptor gene. Neuron 1988; 1:183–188.

57. Miyajima N, Kadowaki Y, Fukushige SI, et al. Identification of two novel members of erbA superfamily by molecular cloning: the gene products of the two are highly related to each other. Nucleic Acids Res 1988; 16:11057–11066.

58. Wang LH, Ing NH, Tsai SY, et al. The COUP-TFs compose a family of functionally related transcription factors. Gene Expr 1991; 1:207–216.

59. Ladias JAA, Karathanasis SK. Regulation of the apolipoprotein A1 gene by ARP-1, a novel member of the steroid receptor superfamily. Science 1991; 251:561–565.

60. Bagchi MK, Tsai SY, Tsai MJ, et al. Purification and characterization of chicken ovalbumin gene upstream promoter transcription factor from homologous oviduct cells. Mol Cell Biol 1987; 7:4151–4158.

61. Wang LH, Tsai SY, Sagami I, et al. Purification and characterization of chicken ovalbumin upstream promoter transcription factor from HeLa cells. J Biol Chem 1987; 262:16080–16086.

62. Sagami I, Tsai SY, Wang H, et al. Identification of two factors required for transcription of the ovalbumin gene. Mol Cell Biol 1986; 6:4259–4267.

63. Hwung YP, Crowe DT, Wang LH, et al. The COUP transcription factor binds to an upstream promoter element of the rat insulin II gene. Mol Cell Biol 1988; 8:2070–2077.

64. Mlodzik M, Hiromi Y, Weber U, et al. The Drosophila seven-up gene, a member of the steroid receptor gene superfamily, controls photoreceptor cell fates. Cell 1990; 60:211–224.

65. Vedeckis WV, Schrader WT, and O'Malley BW. Progesterone-binding components of chick oviduct: analysis of receptor structure by limited proteolysis. Biochemistry 1980; 2:343–349.

66. de Boer W, Bolt J, Kuiper GG, et al. Analysis of steroid- and DNA-binding domains of the calf uterine androgen receptor by limited proteolysis. J Steroid Biochem 1987; 28:9–19.

67. Rusconi S, Yamamoto KR. Functional dissection of the hormone and DNA binding activities of the glucocorticoid receptor. EMBO J 1987; 6:1309–1315.

68. Green S, Kumar V, Krust A, et al. Structural and functional domains of the estrogen receptor. Cold Spring Harbor Symp Quant Biol 1986; 51(pt 2):751–758.

69. Carlstedt-Duke J, Stromstedt P-E, Wrange O, et al. Domain structure of the glucocorticoid receptor protein. Proc Natl Acad Sci USA 1987; 84:4437–4440.

70. Maxwell BL, McDonnell DP, Conneely OM, et al. Structural organization and regulation of the chicken estrogen receptor. Mol Endocrinol 1987; 1:25–35.

71. White R, Lees JA, Needham M, et al. Structural organization and expression of the mouse estrogen receptor. Mol Endocrinol 1987; 1:735–744.

72. Haussler MR, Mangelsdorf DJ, Komm BS, et al. Molecular biology of the vitamin D hormone. Recent Prog Horm Res 1988; 44:263–305.

73. Maniatis T, Goodbourn S, Fischer JA. Regulation of inducible and tissue-specific gene expression. Science 1987; 236:1237–1245.

74. Chandler VL, Maler BA, Yamamoto KR. DNA sequences bound specifically by glucocorticoid receptor in vitro render a heterologous promoter hormone responsive in vivo. Cell 1983; 33:489–499.

75. Ponta H, Kennedy N, Skroch P, et al. Hormonal response region of the mouse mammary tumor virus long terminal repeat can be dissociated from the proviral promoter and has enhancer properties. Proc Natl Acad Sci USA 1985; 84:1020–1024.

76. Chalepakis G, Postma JPM, Beato M. A model for hormone receptor binding to the mouse mammary tumor virus regulatory element based on hydroxyl radical footprinting. Nucleic Acids Res 1988; 16:10237–10247.

77. Shieh S, Tsai M-J. Cell-specific and ubiquitous factors are responsible for the enhancer activity of the rat insulin II gene. J Biol Chem 1991; 266:16708–16714.

78. Drouin J, Charron J, Gagner JP, et al. Pro-opiomelanocortin gene: a model for negative regulation of transcription by glucocorticoids. J Cell Biochem 1987; 35:293–304.

79. Akerblom IE, Slater EP, Beato M, et al. Negative regulation by glucocorticoids through interference with a cAMP-responsive enhancer. Science 1988; 241:350–353.

80. Sakai D, Helms S, Carlstedt-Duke J, et al. Hormone-mediated repression: a negative glucocorticoid response element from the bovine prolactin gene. Genes Dev 1988; 2:1144–1154.

81. Payvar F, Wrange O, Carlstedt-Duke J, et al. Purified glucocorticoid receptors bind selectively in vitro to a cloned DNA fragment whose transcription is regulated by glucocorticoids in vivo. Proc Natl Acad Sci USA 1981; 78:6628–6632.

82. Scheidereit C, Geisse S, Westphal HM, et al. The glucocorticoid receptor binds to defined nucleotide sequences near the promoter of mouse mammary tumor virus. Nature 1983; 304:749–752.

83. Bronnegard M, Poellinger L, Okret S, et al. Characterization and sequence-specific binding to mouse mammary tumor virus DNA of purified activated human glucocorticoid receptor. Biochemistry 1987; 26:1697–1704.

84. Renkawitz R, Schutz G, von der Ahe D, et al. Sequences in the promoter region of the chicken lysozyme gene required for steroid regulation and receptor binding. Cell 1984; 37:503–510.

85. Struhe U, Klock G, Schutz G. A DNA sequence of 15 base pairs is sufficient to mediate both glucocorticoid and progesterone induction of gene expression. Proc Natl Acad Sci USA 1987; 84:7871–7875.

86. Danesch U, Gloss B, Schmid W, et al. Glucocorticoid induction of the rat tryptophan oxygenase gene is mediated by two widely separated glucocorticoid-responsive elements. EMBO J 1987; 6:625–630.

87. Scheidereit C, Westphal HM, Carlson C, et al. Molecular model of the interaction between the glucocorticoid receptor and the regulatory elements of inducible genes. DNA 1986; 5:383–391.

88. Cato ACB, Miksicek R, Schutz G, et al. The hormone regulatory element of mouse mammary tumor virus mediates progesterone induction. EMBO J 1986; 5:2237–2240.

89. von der Ahe D, Janich S, Schneider C, et al. Glucocorticoid and progesterone receptors bind to the same sites in two hormonally regulated promoters. Nature 1985; 313:706–709.

90. Parker MG, Webb P, Needham M, et al. Identification of androgen response elements in mouse mammary tumor virus and rat prostate C3 gene. J Cell Biochem 1987; 35:285–292.

91. Ham J, Thomson A, Needham M, et al. Characterization of response elements for androgen, glucocorticoids and progestins in mouse mammary tumor virus. Nucleic Acids Res 1988; 16:5263–5277.

92. Otten AD, Sanders MM, McKnight GS. The MMTV LTR promoter is induced by progesterone and dihydrotestosterone but not by estrogen. Mol Endocrinol 1988; 2:143–147.

93. Klein-Hitpass L, Tsai SY, Greene GL, et al. Specific binding of estrogen receptor to the estrogen response element. Mol Cell Biol 1989; 9:43–49.

94. Klock G, Strahle U, Schutz G. Oestrogen and glucocorticoid responsive elements are closely related but distinct. Nature 1987; 329:734–736.

95. Baniahmad C, Baniahmad A, O'Malley BW. A rapid method combining a functional test of fusion proteins in vivo and their purification. Biotechniques 1994; 16:194–196.

96. Cooney AJ, Tsai SY. Nuclear receptor-DNA interactions. In: Tsai M-J, O'Malley BW, eds. Mechanism of Steroid Hormone Regulation of Gene Transcription. Austin: RG Landes, 1994.

97. Cooney AJ, Tsai SY, O'Malley BW, et al. Chicken ovalbumin upstream promoter transcription factor (COUP-TF) dimer binds to different GGTCA response elements, allowing COUP-TF to repress hormonal induction of the vitamin D₃, thyroid hormone and retinoic acid receptors. Mol Cell Biol 1992; 12:4153–4163.

98. Bourguet W, Ruff M, Chambon P, et al. Crystal structure of the ligand-binding domain of the human nuclear receptor RXR-alpha. Nature 1995; 375:377–382.

99. Renaud J-P, Rochel N, Ruff M, et al. Crystal structure of the RAR-gamma ligand-binding domain bound to all-*trans* retinoic acid. Nature 1995; 378:681–689.

100. Wagner RL, Apriletti JW, McGrath ME, et al. A structural role for hormone in the thyroid hormone receptor. Nature 1995; 378:690–696.

101. Giguere V, Hollenberg SM, Rosenfeld MG, et al. Functional domains of the human glucocorticoid receptor. Cell 1986; 46:645–652.

102. Conneely OM, Dobson AD, Carson MA, et al. Structure-function relationships of the chicken progesterone receptor. Biochem Soc Trans 1988; 16:683–687.

103. Kumar V, Green S, Staub A, et al. Localization of the oestradiol-binding and putative DNA-binding domains of the human oestrogen receptor. EMBO J 1986; 5:2231–2236.

104. Weinberger C, Hollenberg SM, Rosenfeld MG, et al. Domain structure of human glucocorticoid receptor and its relationship to the v-erbA oncogene product. Nature 1985; 318:670–672.

105. Green S, Chambon P. Oestradial induction of a glucocorticoid-responsive gene by a chimaeric receptor. Nature 1987; 325:75–78.

106. Kumar V, Green S, Stack G, et al. Functional domains of the human estrogen receptor. Cell 1987; 51:941–951.

107. Miller J, McLachlan AD, Klug A. Repetitive zinc-binding domains in the protein transcription factor IIIA from Xenopus oocytes. EMBO J 1985; 4:1609–1614.

108. Freedman LP, Luisi BF, Korszun ZR, et al. The function and structure of the metal coordination sites within the glucocorticoid receptor DNA binding domain. Nature 1988; 334:543–546.

109. Medici N, Minucci S, Nigro V, et al. Metal binding sites of the estradiol receptor from calf uterus and their possible role in the regulation of receptor function. Biochemistry 1989; 28:212–219.

110. Green S, Chambon P. Chimeric receptors used to probe the DNA-binding domain of the estrogen and glucocorticoid receptors. Cancer Res 1989; 49:2282s–2285s.

111. Severne Y, Wieland S, Schaffner W, et al. Metal binding "finger" structures in the glucocorticoid receptor defined by site-directed mutagenesis. EMBO J 1988; 7:2503–2508.

112. Huckaby CS, Conneely OM, Beattie WG, et al. Structure of the chromosomal chicken progesterone receptor gene. Proc Natl Acad Sci USA 1987; 84:8380–8384.

113. Misrahi M, Loosfelt H, Atger M, et al. Organization of the entire rabbit progesterone receptor mRNA and of the promoter and 5′ flanking region of the gene. Nucleic Acids Res 1988; 16:5459–5472.

114. Ponglikitmongkol M, Green S, Chambon P. Genomic organization of the human estrogen receptor gene. EMBO J 1988; 7:3385–3388.

115. Green S, Chambon P. Nuclear receptors enhance our understanding of transcription regulation. Trends Genet 1988; 4:309–314.

116. Berg JM. DNA binding specificity of steroid receptors. Cell 1989; 57:1065–1068.

117. Lehming N, Sartorius J, Oehler S, et al. Recognition helices of lac and lambda repressor are oriented in opposite directions and recognize similar DNA sequences. Proc Natl Acad Sci USA 1988; 85:7947–7951.

118. Green S, Kumar V, Theulaz I, et al. The N-terminal DNA-binding "zinc finger" of the oestrogen and glucocorticoid receptors determines target gene specificity. EMBO J 1988; 7:3037–3044.

119. Mader S, Kumar V, deVerneuil H, et al. Three amino acids of the oestrogen receptor are essential to its ability to distinguish an oestrogen from a glucocorticoid-responsive element. Nature 1989; 338:271–274.

120. Danielsen M, Hinck L, Ringold GM. Two amino acids within the knuckle of the first zinc finger specify DNA response element activation by the glucocorticoid receptor. Cell 1989; 57:1131–1132.

121. Umesono K, Evans RM. Determinants of target gene specificity for steroid/thyroid hormone receptors. Cell 1989; 57:1139–1146.

122. von der Ahe D, Renoir M, Buchou T, et al. Receptors of glucocorticosteroid and progesterone recognize distinct feature of a DNA regulatory element. Proc Natl Acad Sci USA 1986; 83:2817–2821.

123. Gowland PL, Buetti E. Mutations in the hormone regulatory element of mouse mammary tumor virus differentially affect the response to progestins, androgens, and glucocorticoids. Mol Cell Biol 1989; 9:3999–4008.

124. Chalepakis G, Arnemann J, Slater EP, et al. Differential gene activation by glucocorticoids and progestins through the hormone regulatory element of the mouse mammary tumor virus. Cell 1988; 53:371–382.

125. Luisi BF, Xu WX, Otwinowski Z, et al. Crystallographic analysis of the interaction of the glucocorticoid receptor with DNA. Nature 1991; 352:497–505.

126. Hard T, Kellenbach E, Boelens R, et al. Solution structure of the glucocorticoid receptor DNA-binding domain. Science 1990; 249:157–160.

127. Lee MS, Kliewer SA, Provencal J, et al. Structure of the retinoid X receptor alpha DNA binding domain: a helix required for homodimeric DNA binding. Science 1993; 260:1117–1121.

128. Li E, Sucov HM, Lee K, et al. Normal development and growth of mice carrying a targeted disruption of the alpha1 retinoic acid receptor gene. Proc Natl Acad Sci USA 1993; 90:1590–1594.

129. Wrange O, Erikson P, Perlmann T. The purified activated glucocorticoid receptor is a homodimer. J Biol Chem 1989; 64:5253–5259.

130. Hollenberg SM, Giguere V, Sequi P, et al. Colocalization of DNA-binding and transcriptional activation functions in the glucocorticoid receptor. Cell 1987; 49:39–46.

131. Rossini GP, Wikstrom AC, Gustafsson JA. Glucocorticoid receptor complexes are associated with small RNA in vitro. J Steroid Biochem 1989; 32:633–641.

132. Danielsen M, Northrop JP, Ringold GM. The mouse glucocorticoid receptor: mapping of functional domains by cloning, sequencing and expression of wild-type and mutant receptor proteins. EMBO J 1986; 5:2513–2522.

133. Guarente L. UASs and enhancers: common mechanism of transcriptional activation in yeast and mammals. Cell 1988; 52:303–305.

134. Sigler PB. Transcriptional activation: acid blobs and negative noodles. Nature 1988; 333:210–212.

135. Ptashne M. How eukaryotic transcriptional activators work. Nature 1988; 335:683–689.

136. Webster NJG, Green S, Jin J, et al. The hormone-binding domains of the estrogen and glucocorticoid receptors contain an inducible transcription activation function. Cell 1988; 54:199–207.

137. Hollenberg SM, Evans RM. Multiple and cooperative *trans*-activation domains of the human glucocorticoid receptor. Cell 1988; 55:899–906.

138. Godowski PJ, Picard D, Yamamoto KR. Signal transduction and transcriptional regulation by glucocorticoid receptor-LexA fusion proteins. Science 1988; 241:812–816.

139. Danielian PS, White R, Lees JA, et al. Identification of a conserved region required for hormone-dependent transcriptional activation by steroid hormone receptors. EMBO J 1992; 11:1025–1033.

140. Tora L, Gronemeyer H, Turcotte B, et al. The N-terminal region of the chicken progesterone receptor specifies target gene activation. Nature 1988; 333:185–188.

141. Conneely OM, Kettelberger DM, Tsai M-J, et al. Promoter-specific activating domains of the chicken progesterone receptor. In: Roy AK, Clark JH, eds. Gene Regulation by Steroid Hormones IV. New York, Springer-Verlag, 1989; 220–223.

142. Weichman BM, Notides AC. Estradiol-binding kinetics of the activated and nonactivated estrogen receptor. J Biol Chem 1977; 252:8856–8862.

143. Gordon MS, Notides AC. Computer modeling of estradiol interactions with the estrogen receptor. J Steroid Biochem 1986; 25:177–181.

144. Eriksson P, Wrange O. Protein-protein contacts in the glucocorticoid receptor homodimer influence its DNA binding properties. J Biol Chem 1996; 265:3535–3542.

145. de Boer W, Bolt J. Transformation (4S-5S) of the nuclear estrogen receptor is reversible, but not accompanied by a change in the affinity for DNA. J Steroid Biochem 1988; 31:931–937.

146. Tsai SY, Carlstedt-Duke J, Weigel NL, et al. Molecular interactions of steroid hormone receptor with its enhancer element: evidence for receptor dimer formation. Cell 1988; 55:361–369.

147. Kumar V, Chambon P. The estrogen receptor binds tightly to its response element as a ligand-induced homodimer. Cell 1988; 55:145–156.

148. Rodriguez R, Weigel NL, O'Malley BW, et al. Dimerization of the chicken progesterone receptor in vitro can occur in the absence of hormone and DNA. Mol Endocrinol 1990; 4:1782–1790.

149. Joab I, Radanyi C, Renoir M, et al. Common non-hormone binding component in non-transformed chick oviduct receptors of four steroid hormones. Nature 1984; 308:850–853.

150. Aranyi P, Radanyi C, Renoir M, et al. Covalent stabilization of the nontransformed chick oviduct cytosol progesterone receptor by chemical cross-linking. Biochemistry 1988; 27:1330–1336.

151. Baulieu EE. Steroid hormone antagonists at the receptor level: a role for the heatshock protein mw 90,000 (hsp90). J Cell Biochem 1987; 35:161–174.

152. Craig EA. The heat shock response. CRC Crit Rev Biochem 1985; 18:239–280.

153. Riehl RM, Sullivan WP, Vroman BT, et al. Immunological evidence that the nonhormone binding component of avian steroid receptors exists in a wide range of tissues and species. Biochemistry 1985; 24:6586–6591.

154. Howard KJ, Distelhorst CW. Evidence for intracellular association of the glucocorticoid receptor with the 90-kda heat shock protein. J Biol Chem 1988; 263:3474–3481.

155. Rexin M, Busch W, Gehring U. Chemical cross-linking of heteromeric glucocorticoid receptors. Biochemistry 1988; 27:5593–5601.

156. Bagchi MK, Tsai SY, Tsai MJ, et al. Progesterone enhances target gene transcription by receptor free of heat shock proteins hsp 90, hsp 56 and hsp 70. Mol Cell Biol 1991; 11:4998–5004.

157. Picard D, Khursheed B, Garabedian MJ, et al. Signal transduction by steroid receptors: reduced levels of hsp90 compromise receptor action in vivo. Nature 1990; 348:166–168.

158. Smith DF, Toft DO. Steroid receptors and their associated proteins. Mol Endocrinol 1993; 7:4–11.

159. Pratt WB, Jolly DJ, Pratt DV, et al. A region in the steroid binding domain determines formation of the non-DNA binding GS glucocorticoid receptor complex. J Biol Chem 1988; 263:267–273.

160. Carson-Jurica MA, Lee AT, Dobson ADW, et al. Interaction of the chicken progesterone receptor with HSP-90. J Steroid Biochem 1990; 34:1–14.

161. Smith DF, McCormick DJ, Toft DO. Studies with antibodies against the conserved cysteine region of progesterone receptor. J Steroid Biochem 1988; 30:1–7.

162. Smith DF, Lubahn DB, McCormick DJ, et al. The production of antibodies against the conserved cysteine region of steroid receptors and their use in characterizing the avian progesterone receptor. Endocrinology 1988; 122:2816–2825.

163. Weigel NL, Schrader WT, O'Malley BW. Antibodies to chicken progesterone receptor peptide 523-536 recognize a site exposed in receptor-deoxyribonucleic acid complexes but not in receptor-heat shock protein-90 complexes. Endocrinology 1989; 125:2494–2501.

164. Tai PKK, Maeda Y, Nakao K, et al. A 59 kilodalton protein associated with progestin, estrogen, androgen and glucocorticoid receptors. Biochem J 1986; 25:5269–5275.

165. Gasc JM, Renoir JM, Faber LE, et al. Nuclear localization of 2 steroid receptor-associated proteins, hsp90 and p59. Exp Cell Res 1990; 186:362–367.

166. Kost SL, Smith DF, Sullivan WP, et al. Binding of heatshock protein to the avian progesterone receptor. Mol Cell Biol 1989; 9:3829–3832.

167. Velazquez JM, Lindquist S. hsp70: Nuclear concentration during environmental stress and cytoplasmic storage during recovery. Cell 1984; 36:655–662.

168. Cheng MY, Hartl FU, Martin J, et al. Mitochondrial heat shock protein hsp60 is essential for assembly of proteins imported into yeast mitochondria. Nature 1989; 337:620–625.

169. Liao S, Rossini GP, Hiipakka RA. Factors that can control the interaction of the androgen-receptor complex with the genomic structure in the prostate. In: Bresciani F, ed. Perspectives in Steroid Receptor Research. New York: Raven Press, 1980:99–112.

170. Auricchio F, Migliaccio A, Castoria G, et al. Direct evidence of in vivo phosphorylation-dephosphorylation of the estradiol-17(beta) receptor: role of Ca²⁺-calmodulin in the activation of hormone binding sites. J Steroid Biochem 1984; 20:31–35.

171. Grandics P, Miller A, Schmidt TJ, et al. Phosphorylation in vivo of rat hepatic glucocorticoid receptor. Biochem Biophys Res Commun 1984; 120:59–65.

172. Golsteyn EJ, Graham JS, Goren HJ, et al. Phosphorylation status of nuclear and cytosolic androgen receptors in the rat ventral prostate. Prostate 1989; 14:91–101.

173. Auricchio F, Migliaccio A, Castoria G, et al. Phosphorylation of estradiol receptor on tyrosine and interaction of estradiol and glucocorticoid receptors with antiphosphotyrosine antibodies. Adv Exp Med Biol 1988; 231:519–539.

174. Migliaccio A, DiDomenico M, Green S, et al. Phosphorylation on tyrosine of in vitro synthesized human estrogen receptor activates its hormone binding. Mol Endocrinol 1989; 3:1061–1069.

175. Sheridan PL, Evans RM, Horwitz KB. Phosphotryptic peptide analysis of human progesterone receptors: new phosphorylated sites formed in nuclei after hormone treatment. J Biol Chem 1989; 264:6520–6528.

176. Rao KV, Fox CF. Epidermal growth factor stimulates tyrosine phosphorylation of human glucocorticoid receptor in cultured cells. Biochem Biophys Res Commun 1987; 144:512–519.

177. Logeat F, LeCunff M, Pamphile R, et al. The nuclear-bound form of the progesterone receptor is generated through a hormone-dependent phosphorylation. Biochem Biophys Res Commun 1985; 131:421–427.

178. Horwitz KB, Alexander PS. In situ photolinked nuclear progesterone receptors of human breast cancer cells: subunit molecular weights after transformation and translocation. Endocrinology 1983; 113:2195–2201.

179. Sheridan PL, Francis MD, Horwitz KB. Synthesis of human progesterone receptor in T47D cells. Nascent A- and B-receptors are active without a phosphorylation-dependent post-translational maturation step. J Biol Chem 1989; 264:7054–7058.

180. Bailly A, LePage C, Rauch M, et al. Sequence-specific DNA binding of the progesterone receptor to the uteroglobin gene: effects of hormone, antihormone and receptor phosphorylation. EMBO J 1986; 5:3235–3241.

181. Edwards DP, Kuhnel B, Estes PA, et al. Human progesterone receptor binding to mouse tumor virus deoxynucleic acid: dependence on hormone and nonreceptor nuclear factor(s). Mol Endocrinol 1989; 3:381–391.

182. Denner LA, Weigel NL, Schrader WT, et al. Hormone-dependent regulation of chicken progesterone receptor deoxyribonucleic binding and phosphorylation. Endocrinology 1989; 125:3051–3058.

183. Sullivan WP, Madden B, McCormick DJ, et al. Hormone-dependent phosphorylation of the avian progesterone receptor. J Biol Chem 1988; 263:14717–14723.

184. Sullivan WP, Smith DF, Beito TG, et al. Hormone-dependent processing of the avian progesterone receptor. J Cell Biochem 1988; 36:103–119.

185. Denner LA, Bingman WE, Greene GL, et al. Phosphorylation of the chicken progesterone receptor. J Steroid Biochem 1987; 27:235–243.

186. Hoeck W, Rusconi S, Groner B. Hormone-dependent phosphorylation of the glucocorticoid receptor occurs mainly in the amino-terminal transactivation domain. J Biol Chem 1989; 264:14396–14402.

187. Sheridan PL, Krett NL, Gordon JA, et al. Human progesterone receptor transformation and nuclear down-regulation are independent of phosphorylation. Mol Endocrinol 1988; 2:1329–1342.

188. Weigel NL, Denner LA, Poletti A, et al. Phosphorylation/dephosphorylation regulates the activity of progesterone receptors. Adv Prot Phosphatases 1993; 7:237–269.

189. Weigel NL. Receptor phosphorylation. In: Tsai MJ, O'Malley BW, eds. Mechanism of Steroid Hormone Regulation of Gene Transcription. Austin: RG Landes, 1994: 93–110.

190. Kato S, Endoh H, Masuhiro Y, et al. Activation of the estrogen receptor through phosphorylation by mitogen-activated protein kinase. Science 1995; 270:1491–1494.

191. Gorski J, Toft DO, Shyamala G, et al. Hormone receptors: studies on the interaction of estrogen with the uterus. Recent Prog Horm Res 1968; 24:45–80.

192. Jensen EV, Suzuki T, Kawashima T, et al. A two-step mechanism for the interaction of estrogen with the rat uterus. Proc Natl Acad Sci USA 1968; 59:632–638.

193. Siiteri PK, Schwarz BE, Moriyama I, et al. Estrogen binding in the rat and human. Adv Exp Med Biol 1973; 36:97–112.

194. Perrot-Applanat M, Groyer-Picard M-T, Lorenzo F, et al. Immunocytochemical study with monoclonal antibodies to progesterone receptor in human breast tumors. Cancer Res 1987; 47:2652–2661.

195. King WJ, Greene GL. Monoclonal antibodies localize oestrogen receptor in the nuclei of target cells. Nature 1984; 307:745–747.

196. Wikstrom AC, Bakke O, Okret S, et al. Intracellular localization of the glucocorticoid receptor: evidence for cytoplasmic and nuclear localization. Endocrinology 1987; 120:1232–1242.

197. Fuxe K, Harfstrand A, Agnati LF, et al. Immunocytochemical studies on the localization of glucocorticoid receptor immunoreactive nerve cells in the lower brain stem and spinal cord of the male rat using a monoclonal antibody against rat liver glucocorticoid receptor. Neuroscience 1985; 60:1–6.

198. Antakly T, Thompson EB, O'Donnell D. Demonstration of the intracellular localization and up-regulation of glucocorticoid receptor by in situ hybridization and immunocytochemistry. Cancer Res 1989; 49:2230s–2234s.

199. Qi M, Hamilton BJ, DeFranco D. v-mos oncoproteins affect the nuclear retention and re-utilization of glucocorticoid receptors. Mol Endocrinol 1989; 3:1279–1288.

200. Picard D, Yamamoto KR. Two signals mediate hormone-dependent nuclear localization of the glucocorticoid receptor. EMBO J 1987; 6:3333–3340.

201. Gasc JM, Delahaye F, Baulieu EE. Compared intracellular localization of the glucocorticosteroid and progesterone receptors: an immunocytochemical study. Exp Cell Res 1989; 181:492–504.

202. Dingwall C, Laskey RA. Protein import into the cell nucleus. Annu Rev Biol 1986; 2:367–390.

203. Paine PL, Moore LC, Horowitz SB. Nuclear envelope permeability. Nature 1975; 254:109–114.

204. Sherman MR, Corvol PL, O'Malley BW. Progesterone-binding components of chick oviduct. J Biol Chem 1970; 245:6085–6096.

205. Kalderon D, Roberts BL, Richardson WD, et al. A short amino acid sequence able to specify nuclear location. Cell 1984; 39:499–509.

206. Lanford RE, Kanda P, Kennedy RC. Induction of nuclear transport with a synthetic peptide homologous to the SV40 antigen transport signal. Cell 1986; 46:575–582.

207. Clemens TL, Garrett KP, Zhou XY, et al. Immunocytochemical localization of the 1,25-dihydroxyvitamin D₃ receptor in target cells. Endocrinology 1988; 122:1224–1230.

208. Oppenheimer JH. Thyroid hormone action at the cellular level. Science 1979; 203:971–979.

209. Walters MR, Hunziker W, Norman AW. 1,25-Dihydroxyvitamin D_3 receptors: intermediates between triiodothyronine and steroid receptors. Trends Biochem Sci 1981; 6:268–271.

210. Guiochon-Mantel A, Loosfelt H, Lescop P, et al. Mechanisms of nuclear localization of the progesterone receptor: evidence for interaction between monomers. Cell 1989; 57:1147–1154.

211. Gorski J, Noteboom WD, Nicollette JA. Estrogen control of the synthesis of RNA and protein in the uterus. J Cell Comp Physiol 1965; 66:91.

212. Hastie ND, Bishop JO. The expression of three abundance classes of mRNA in mouse tissues. Cell 1976; 9:761–774.

213. Means AR, Comstock JP, Rosenfeld GC, et al. Ovalbumin messenger RNA of chick oviduct: partial characterization, estrogen dependence and translation in vitro. Proc Natl Acad Sci USA 1972; 69:1146–1150.

214. O'Malley BW, McGuire WL, Middleton PA. Altered gene expression during differentiation: population changes in hybridizable RNA after stimulation of the chick oviduct with oestrogen. Nature 1968; 218:1249.

215. Chan L, O'Malley BW. Mechanism of action of the sex steroid hormones. N Engl J Med 1976; 294:1322–1328.

216. LeMeur M, Glanville N, Mandel JL, et al. The ovalbumin gene family: hormonal control of X and Y gene transcription and mRNA accumulation. Cell 1981; 23:561–571.

217. McKnight GS, Palmiter RD. Transcriptional regulation of the ovalbumin and conalbumin genes by steroid hormones in chick oviduct. J Biol Chem 1979; 254:9050–9058.

218. Rhoads RE, McKnight GS, Schimke RT. Synthesis of ovalbumin in a rabbit reticulocyte cell-free system programmed with hen oviduct ribonucleic acid. J Biol Chem 1971; 246:7407–7410.

219. Swaneck GE, Nordstrom JL, Kreuzaler R, et al. Effect of estrogen on gene expression in chicken oviduct: evidence for transcriptional control of ovalbumin gene. Proc Natl Acad Sci USA 1979; 76:1049–1053.

220. Ringold GM, Yamamoto KR, Bishop JM, et al. Glucocorticoid-stimulated accumulation of mouse mammary tumor virus RNA: increased rate of synthesis of viral RNA. Proc Natl Acad Sci USA 1977; 74:2879–2883.

221. Parks WP, Scolnick EM, Kozikowski EH. Dexamethasone stimulation of murine mammary tumor virus expression: a tissue culture source of virus. Science 1974; 184:158–160.

222. Ringold G, Lasfargues EY, Bishop JM, et al. Production of mouse mammary tumor virus by cultured cells in the absence and presence of hormones: assay by molecular hybridization. Virology 1975; 65:135–147.

223. Tomkins GM, Gelehrter TD, Granner D, et al. Control of specific gene expression in higher organisms. Science 1969; 166:1474–1478.

224. Anderson JE. The effect of steroid hormones on gene transcription. In: Goldberger RF, Yamamoto KR, eds. Biological Regulation and Development. New York: Plenum, 1984: 169–212.

225. O'Malley BW, Means AR. Female steroid hormones and target cell nuclei. Science 1974; 183:610–620.

226. O'Malley BW, McGuire WL, Kohler PO, et al. Studies on the mechanism of steroid hormone regulation of synthesis of specific proteins. Recent Prog Horm Res 1969; 25:105–160.

227. Roy AK, Clark JH. Gene Regulation by Steroid Hormones II. New York: Springer-Verlag, 1983.

228. Spindler SR, Mellon SH, Baxter JD. Growth hormone gene transcription is regulated by thyroid and glucocorticoid hormones in cultured rat pituitary tumor cells. J Biol Chem 1982; 257:11627–11632.

229. Hargrove JL, Schmidt FH. The role of mRNA and protein stability in gene expression. FASEB J 1989; 3:2360–2370.

230. Shapiro DJ, Blume JE, Nielsen DA. Regulation of messenger RNA stability in eukaryotic cells. Bioessays 1987; 6:221–226.

231. Brock ML, Shapiro DJ. Estrogen stabilizes vitellogenin mRNA against degradation. Cell 1983; 34:207–214.

232. Alberts B, Bray D, Lewis J, et al. Molecular Biology of the Cell. New York: Garland, 1983.

233. Brown DD. Proceedings of ICN-UCLA Symposia on Molecular Cellular Biology. New York: Academic, 1981.

234. Lewin B. Genes. New York: Wiley, 1983.

235. May LL. Genetics: A Molecular Approach. New York: Macmillan, 1981.

236. Breathnack R, Chambon P. Organization and expression of eukaryotic split genes coding for proteins. Annu Rev Biochem 1981; 50:349–383.

237. O'Malley BW, Stein JP, Means AR. The evaluation of a complex eucaryotic gene. Metabolism 1982; 31:646–653.

238. Axel R, Maniatis T, Fox CF. Eucaryotic Gene Regulation. New York: Academic, 1979.

239. Gilbert W. Introns and exons: playgrounds of evolution. In: Axel R, Maniatis T, Fox M, eds. Eucaryotic Gene Regulation. New York: Academic Press, 1979: 1–12.

240. Cech TR. RNA as an enzyme. Sci Am 1986; 255:64–75.

241. Padgett RA, Grabowski PJ, Konarska MM, et al. Splicing of messenger RNA precursors. Annu Rev Biochem 1986; 55:1119–1150.

242. Crick F. Split genes and RNA splicing. Science 1979; 204:264–271.

243. Darnell JE, Jr. Variety in the level of gene control in eucaryotic cells. Nature 1982; 297:365–371.

244. Darnell JE, Jr. Transcription units for mRNA production in eucaryotic cells and their DNA viruses. Prog Nucleic Acids Res Mol Biol 1979; 22:327–353.

245. Lewin B. Eucaryotic genomes. New York: John Wiley & Sons, 1980.

246. Perry RP. Processing of RNA. Annu Rev Biochem 1976; 45:605–629.

247. Ziff EB. Transcription and RNA processing by the DNA tumor viruses. Nature 1980; 287:491–499.

248. Tsai MJ, Ting AC, Nordstrom JL, et al. Processing of high-molecular-weight ovalbumin and ovomucoid precursor RNAs to messenger RNA. Cell 1980; 22:219–230.

249. Perry RP. RNA processing comes of age. J Cell Biol 1981; 91:28s–38s.

250. Tilghman SM, Curtis PJ, Tiemeier DC, et al. The intervening sequence of a mouse beta-globin gene is transcribed within the 15S beta-globin mRNA precursor. Proc Natl Acad Sci USA 1978; 1309–1313.

251. Moore MJ, Query CC, Sharp PA. Splicing of precursors to mRNA by the spliceosome. In: Gesteland RF, Atkins JF, eds. The RNA World. Plainview, NY: Cold Spring Harbor Laboratory Press, 1993: 303–357.

252. Fawcett DW. The Cell. Philadelphia: WB Saunders, 1981: 266–302.

253. Kornberg RD. Structure of chromatin. Annu Rev Biochem 1977; 46:931–954.

254. Kornberg RD, Klug A. The nucleosome. Sci Am 1981; 244:52–64.

255. Miller OL. The nucleolus, chromosomes, and visualization of genetic activity. J Cell Biol 1981; 91: 15S–27S.

256. Watson JD. Molecular Biology of the Gene. 3rd ed. Menlo Park, NJ: WA Benjamin, 1976.

257. Weisbrod S. Active chromatin (a review). Nature 1982; 297:289–295.

258. Klug A, Rhodes D, Smith J, et al. A low-resolution structure for the histone core of the nucleosome. Nature 1980; 287:509–516.

259. Laskey RA, Earnshaw WC. Nucleosome assembly. Nature 1980; 286:763–767.

260. McGhee JD, Rau DC, Charney E, et al. Orientation of the nucleosome within the higher order structure of chromatin. Cell 1980; 22:87–96.

261. McGhee JD, Felsenfeld G. Nucleosome structure. Annu Rev Biochem 1980; 49:1115–1156.

262. Weintraub H, Groudine M. Chromosomal subunits in active genes have an altered conformation. Science 1976; 193:848–856.

263. Elgin SCR. DNase I–hypersensitive sites of chromatin. Cell 1981; 27:413–415.

264. Lamb MM, Daneholt B. Characterization of active transcription units in Balbiani rings of Chronomus tentans. Cell 1979; 17:835–848.

265. Lawson GM, Knoll BJ, March CJ, et al. Definition of 5′ and 3′ structure boundaries of the chromatin domain containing the ovalbumin multigene family. J Biol Chem 1982; 257:1501–1507.

266. O'Malley BW, ed. Proceedings of UCLA Symposia on Molecular and Cellular Biology. XXVI. New York: Academic, 1982: 507.

267. Grosveld F, van Assendelft GB, Greaves DR, et al. Position-independent, high-level expression of the human beta-globin gene in transgenic mice. Cell 1987; 51:975–985.

268. Barrack ER, Coffey DS. Biological properties of the nuclear matrix: steroid hormone binding. Recent Prog Horm Res 1982; 28:133–195.

269. Ciejek EM, Tsai M-J, O'Malley BW. Actively transcribed genes are associated with the nuclear matrix. Nature 1983; 306:607–609.

270. Robinson SI, Nelkin BD, Vogelstein B. The ovalbumin gene is associated with the nuclear matrix of chicken oviduct cells. Cell 1982; 28:99–106.

271. Zubay G. Biochemistry. Reading MA: Addison-Wesley, 1983.

272. Razin A, Riggs AD. DNA methylation and gene function. Science 1980; 210:604–609.

273. Ptashne M, Jeffrey A, Johnson AD, et al. How the (lambda) repressor and Cro work. Cell 1980; 19:1–11.

274. Brown DD. Gene expression in eucaryotes. Science 1981; 211:667–674.

275. McKnight SL, Gavis ER, Kingsbury R. Analysis of transcriptional regulatory signals of the HSV-thymidine kinase gene: identification of an upstream control region. Cell 1981; 25:385–398.

276. McKnight SL, Kingsbury R. Transcriptional control signals of a eucaryotic protein-coding gene. Science 1982; 217:316–324.

277. Ptashne M, Gilbert W. Genetic repressors. Sci Am 1970; 222:36–44.

278. Rodriguez RL, Chamberlin MJ. Promoters: Structure and Function. New York: Praeger, 1982.

279. Corden J, Wasylyk B, Buchwalder A, et al. Promoter sequences of eukaryotic protein-coding genes. Science 1980; 209:1406–1414.

280. Smale ST, Baltimore D. The "initiator" as a transcription control element. Cell 1989; 57:103–113.

281. Serfling E, Jasin M, Schaffner W. Enhancers and eukaryotic gene transcription. Trends Genet 1985; 1:224–230.

282. Darnell J, Lodish H, Baltimore D. Molecular Cell Biology. New York: Scientific American Books, 1990.

283. Payvar F, DeFranco DB, Firestone GL, et al. Sequence-specific binding of glucocorticoid receptor to MTV-DNA at sites within and upstream of the transcribed region. Cell 1983; 35:381–392.

284. Tsai SY, Tsai M-J, O'Malley BW. Cooperative binding of steroid hormone receptors contributes to transcriptional synergism at target enhancer elements. Cell 1989; 57:443–448.

285. Ptashne M. How gene activators work. Sci Am 1989; 260:40–47.

286. Charron J, Drouin J. Glucocorticoid inhibition of transcription from episomal pro-opiomelanocortin gene promoter. Proc Natl Acad Sci USA 1986; 83:8903–8904.

287. McKnight SL, Lane MD, Gluecksohnwaelsch S. Is CCAAT enhancer-binding protein a central regulator of energy metabolism? Genes Dev 1989; 3:2021–2024.

288. Hawley DK, Roeder RG. Separation and partial characterization of three

function steps in transcription initiation by human RNA polymerase II. J Biol Chem 1985; 260:8163–8172.

289. Reinberg D, Horikoshi M, Roeder RG. Factors involved in specific transcription by mammalian RNA polymerase II. J Biol Chem 1987; 262:3322–3330.

290. Buratowski S, Hahn S, Guarente L, et al. Five intermediate complexes in transcription initiation by RNA polymerase II. Cell 1989; 56:549–561.

291. Van Dyke MW, Sawadogo M, Roeder RG. Stability of transcription complexes on class II genes. Mol Cell Biol 1989; 9:342–344.

292. Sawadogo M, Roeder RG. Interaction of a gene-specific transcription factor with the adenovirus major late promoter upstream of the TATA box region. Cell 1985; 43:165–175.

293. Hai TW, Horikoshi M, Roeder RG, et al. Analysis of the role of the transcription factor ATF in the assembly of a functional preinitiation complex. Cell 1988; 54:1043–1051.

294. Horikoshi M, Hai T, Lin YS, et al. Transcription factor ATF interacts with the TATA factor to facilitate establishment of a preinitiation complex. Cell 1988; 54:1033–1042.

295. Lin YS, Green MR. Mechanism of activation of an acidic transcriptional activator in vitro. Cell 1991; 64:971–981.

296. Sundseth R, Hansen U. Activation of RNA polymerase II transcription by the specific DNA-binding protein LSF. J Biol Chem 1992; 267:7845.

297. Onate SA, Tsai SY, Tsai M-J, et al. Sequence and characterization of a coactivator for the steroid hormone receptor superfamily. Science 1995; 270:1354–1357.

298. Chen JD, Evans RM. A transcriptional co-repressor that interacts with nuclear hormone receptors. Nature 1995; 377:454–457.

299. Horlein AJ, Naar AM, Heinzel T, et al. Ligand-independent repression by the thyroid hormone receptor mediated by a nuclear receptor co-repressor. Nature 1995; 377:397–404.

300. Klein-Hitpass L, Tsai SY, Weigel NL, et al. The progesterone receptor stimulates cell-free transcription by enhancing the formation of a stable preinitiation complex. Cell 1990; 60:247–257.

301. Freedman LP, Yoshinaga SK, Vanderbilt JN, et al. In vitro transcription enhancement by purified derivatives of the glucocorticoid receptor. Science 1989; 245:298–301.

302. Bagchi M. Mechanisms of target gene activation by steroid hormone receptors: insights from cell-free transcription system. In: Tsai M-J, O'Malley BW, eds. Mechanism of Steroid Hormone Regulation of Gene Transcription. Austin: RG Landes, 1994: 60–70.

303. Corthesy B, Hipskind R, Theulaz I, et al. Estrogen-dependent in vitro transcription from the vitellogenin promoter in liver nuclear extracts. Science 1988; 239:1137–1139.

304. Bagchi MK, Tsai SY, Weigel NL, et al. Regulation of in vitro transcription by progesterone receptor: characterization and kinetic studies. J Biol Chem 1990; 265:5129–5134.

305. Tsai SY, Srinivasan G, Allan GF, et al. Recombinant human glucocorticoid receptor induces transcription of hormone response genes in vitro. J Biol Chem 1990; 265:17055–17061.

306. Elliston JF, Fawell SE, Klein-Hitpass L, et al. Mechanism of estrogen receptor–dependent transcription in a cell-free system. Mol Cell Biol 1990; 10:6607–6612.

307. Glass CK, Holloway JM, Devary OV, et al. The thyroid hormone receptor binds with opposite transcriptional effects to a common sequence motif in thyroid hormone and estrogen response elements. Cell 1988; 54:313–323.

308. Jantzen K, Fritton HP, Igo-Kemenes T, et al. Partial overlapping of binding sequences for steroid hormone receptors and DNase I hypersensitive sites in the rabbit uteroglobin gene region. Nucleic Acids Res 1987; 15:4535–4552.

309. Allan GF, Ing NH, Tsai SY, et al. Synergism between steroid response and promoter elements during cell-free transcription. J Biol Chem 1991; 266:5905–5910.

310. Schmid W, Strahle U, Schutz G, et al. Glucocorticoid receptor binds cooperatively to adjacent recognition sites. EMBO J 1989; 8:2257–2263.

311. Topol J, Ruden DM, Parker CS. Synergistic action of the glucocorticoid receptor with transcription factors. Cell 1985; 42:527–537.

312. Poellinger L, Yoza BK, Roeder RG. Functional cooperativity between protein molecules bound at two distinct sequence elements of the immunoglobulin heavy chain promoter. Nature 1989; 337:573–576.

313. Schule R, Muller M, Kaltschmidt C, et al. Many transcription factors interact synergistically with steroid receptors. Science 1988; 242:1418–1420.

314. O'Malley BW, Roop DR, Lai EC, et al. The ovalbumin gene: organization, structure, transcription and regulation. Recent Prog Horm Res 1979; 35:1–42.

315. Yamamoto KR. Steroid regulated transcription of specific genes and gene networks. Annu Rev Genet 1985; 19:209–252.

316. Fritton HP, Igo-Kemenes TI, Nowock J, et al. Alternative sets of DNase I–hypersensitive sites characterize the various functional states of the chicken lysozyme gene. Nature 1984; 311:163–165.

317. Becker PB, Gloss B, Schmid W, et al. In vivo protein-DNA interactions in a glucocorticoid response element require the presence of the hormone. Nature 1986; 324:686–688.

318. Beekman JM, Allan GF, Tsai SY, et al. Transcriptional activation by the estrogen receptor requires a conformational change in the ligand binding domain. Mol Endocrinol 1993; 7:1266–1274.

319. Brown M, Sharp PA. Human estrogen receptor forms multiple protein DNA complexes. J Biol Chem 1990; 265:11238–11243.

320. Bagchi MK, Tsai SY, Tsai M-J, et al. Identification of a functional intermediate in receptor activation in progesterone-dependent cell-free transcription. Nature 1990; 345:547–550.

321. Denner LA, Weigel NL, Maxwell BL, et al. Regulation of progesterone receptor–mediated transcription by phosphorylation. Science 1990; 250:1740–1743.

322. Power RF, Lydon JP, Conneely OM, et al. Dopamine activation of an orphan member of the steroid receptor superfamily. Science 1991; 252:1546–1548.

323. Power RF, Mani SK, Codina J, et al. Dopaminergic and ligand-independent activation of steroid hormone receptors. Science 1991; 254:1636–1639.

324. Aronica SM, Katzenellenbogen BS. Stimulation of estrogen receptor–mediated transcription and alteration in the phosphorylation state of the rat uterine estrogen receptor by estrogen, cyclic adenosine monophosphate, and insulin-like growth factor-1. Mol Endocrinol 1993; 7:743–752.

325. Ignar-Trowbridge DM, Nelson KG, Bidwell MC, et al. Coupling of dual signaling pathways: epidermal growth factor action involves the estrogen receptor. Proc Natl Acad Sci USA 1992; 89:4658–4662.

326. Smith CL, Conneely OM, O'Malley BW. Modulation of the ligand-independent activation of the human estrogen receptor by hormone and antihormone. Proc Natl Acad Sci USA 1993; 90:6120–6124.

327. Mani SK, Allen JM, Clark JH, et al. Convergent pathways for steroid hormone– and neurotransmitter-induced rat sexual behavior. Science 1994; 265:1246–1249.

328. Smith CL, Conneely OM, O'Malley BW. Estrogen receptor activation by ligand-dependent and ligand-independent pathways. In: Moudgil VK, ed. Boston: Birkhauser, Inc., 1993: 333–356.

329. Ignar-Trowbridge DM, Teng CT, Ross KA, et al. Peptide growth factors elicit estrogen receptor–dependent transcriptional activation of an estrogen-responsive element. Mol Endocrinol 1993; 7:992–998.

330. Nelson KG, Takahashi T, Bossert NL, et al. Epidermal growth factor replaces estrogen in the stimulation of female genital-tract growth and differentiation. Proc Natl Acad Sci USA 1991; 88:21–25.

331. Siiteri PK, Mura JT, Hammond GL, et al. The serum transport of steroid hormones. Recent Prog Horm Res 1982; 38:457–510.

332. Pardridge WM. Transport of protein-bound hormones into tissues in vivo. Endocrine Rev 1981; 2:102–123.

333. Ekins R, Edwards P, Sinha A. Organ-specific regulation of hormone efflux from tissue capillaries: a physiological role of hormone binding proteins? Steroids 1988; 52:369–370.

334. Soloff MS, Creange JE, Potts GO. Unique estrogen-binding properties of rat pregnancy plasma. Endocrinology 1971; 88:427–432.

335. Raynaud JP. Influence of rat estradiol binding plasma protein (EBP) on uterotrophic activity. Steroids 1973; 21:249–258.

336. Westphal U. Steroid-Protein Interactions. New York: Springer-Verlag, 1971.

337. Anderson JN, Peck EJ Jr, and Clark JH. Nuclear receptor estrogen complex: in vivo and in vitro binding of estradiol and estriol as influenced by serum albumin. J Steroid Biochem 1974; 5:103–107.

338. Sanger F, Nicklen S, Coulson AR. DNA sequencing with chain-terminating inhibitors. Proc Natl Acad Sci USA 1977; 74:5463–5467.

339. Schrader WT, Toft DO, O'Malley BW. Progesterone binding protein of chick oviduct. VI. Interaction of purified progesterone receptor components with nuclear constituents. J Biol Chem 1972; 247:2401–2407.

340. O'Malley BW, Strott CA. The mechanism of action of progesterone. In: Greep RO, Astwood EB, eds. Handbook of Physiology, Section 7: Endocrinology. Washington, DC: American Physiology Society, 591–602.

341. Clark JH and Peck EJ Jr. Steroid hormone receptors: basic principles and measurement. In: O'Malley BW, Birnbaumer L, eds. Receptors and Hormone Action. New York: Academic, 1977: 383–410.

342. Tata JR. The action of growth and developmental hormones: evolutionary aspects. In: Goldberger RF, Yamamoto KR, eds. Biological Regulation and Development. New York: Plenum, 1984: 1–58.

343. Szego CM, Davis JS. Adenosine 3′5′-monophosphate in rat uterus: acute elevation by estrogen. Proc Natl Acad Sci USA 1967; 58:1711–1718.

344. Flandroy L, Fastrez-Boute A, Galand P. Oestrogen-induced changes in uterine cGMP: relationship with other parameters of hormonal stimulation. Arch Int Physiol Biochim 1976; 84:1072–1078.

345. Tchernitchin A, Tchernitchin X. Characterization of the estrogen receptors in the uterine and blood eosinophil leukocytes. Experientia 1977; 32:1240–1242.

346. Szego CM, Lawson DA. Influence of histamine on uterine metabolism: stimulation of incorporation of radioactivity from amino acids into protein, lipid and purines. Endocrinology 1973; 74:372–381.

347. Tchernitchin A, Roorijck J, Tchernitchin X, et al. Effects of cortisol on uterine eosinophilia and other oestrogenic responses. Mol Cell Endocrinol 1976; 2:331–337.

348. Galand P, Mairesse N, Roorijck J, et al. Differential blockade of estrogen-induced uterine responses by the antiestrogen nafoxidine. J Steroid Biochem 1983; 19:1259–1263.

349. Zor U, Koch Y, Lamprecht SA, et al. Mechanism of oestradiol action on the rat uterus: independence of cyclic AMP, prostaglandin E₂ and beta-adrenergic mediation. J Endocrinol 1973; 58:525–533.

350. Rorke EA, Katzenellenbogen BS, Dissociated regulation of growth and ornithine decarboxylase activity by estrogen in the rat uterus. Biochem Biophys Res Commun 1984; 122:1186–1193.

351. Anderson JN, Peck EJ Jr., and Clark JH. Estrogen-induced uterine re-

sponses and growth: relationship to receptor estrogen binding by uterine nuclei. Endocrinology 1975; 96:160–167.

352. Harris J, Gorski J. Evidence for a discontinuous requirement for estrogen in stimulation of deoxyribonucleic acid synthesis in the immature rat uterus. Endocrinology 1978; 103:240–245.

353. Anderson JN, Clark JH, and Peck EJ Jr. The relationship between nuclear receptor estrogen binding and uterotrophic responses. Biochem Biophys Res Commun 1972; 48:1460–1468.

354. Guyette WA, Matusik RJ, Rosen JM. Prolactin-mediated transcriptional and post-transcriptional control of casein gene expression. Cell 1979; 17:1013–1023.

355. Palmiter RD. Quantitation of parameters that determine the rate of ovalbumin synthesis. Cell 1975; 4:189–197.

356. Markaverich BM, Clark JH. Two binding sites for estradiol in rat uterine nuclei: relationship to uterotrophic response. Endocrinology 1979; 105:1458–1462.

357. Kirkland JL, Gardner RM, Ireland JS. The effect of hypophysectomy on the uterine response to estradiol. Endocrinology 1977; 101:403–410.

358. Sonnenschein C, Soto AM. Pituitary uterotrophic effect in the estrogen-dependent growth of the rat uterus. J Steroid Biochem 1978; 9:533–537.

359. Huggins C, Jensen EV. The depression of estrone-induced uterine growth by phenolic estrogens with oxygenated functions at positions 6 or 16: the impeded estrogens. J Exp Med 1955; 102:334–346.

360. Laugier C, Pageaux JF, Soto AM, et al. Mechanisms of estrogen action: indirect effect of estradiol on proliferation of quail oviduct cells. Proc Natl Acad Sci USA 1983; 80:1621–1625.

361. Schatz R, Soto AM, Sonnenschein C. Estrogen-induced cell multiplication: direct or indirect effect on rat uterine cells? Endocrinology 1984; 115:501–506.

362. Sirbasku DA, Benson RH. Estrogen-inducible growth factors that may act as mediators (estromedins) of estrogen-promoted tumor cell growth. Cold Spring Harb Conf Cell Prolif 1988; 6:477–497.

363. Cunha GR, Chung LW, Shannon JM, et al. Hormone-induced morphogenesis and growth role of mesenchymal-epithelial interactions. Recent Prog Horm Res 1983; 39:559–598.

364. Edery M, Pang K, Larson L, et al. Epidermal growth factor receptor levels in mouse mammary glands in various physiological states. Endocrinology 1985; 117:405–411.

365. Mukku VR, Stancel GM. Receptors of epidermal growth factor in the rat uterus. Endocrinology 1985; 117:149–154.

366. Robson JM, Adler J. Site of action of oestrogens. Nature 1940; 212:146–160.

367. Snow LD, Eriksson H, Hardin JW, et al. Nuclear estrogen receptor in the avian liver: correlation with biologic response. Steroid Biochem 1978; 9:1017–1026.

368. Anderson JN, Peck EJ, Clark JH. Nuclear receptor estrogen complex: accumulation, retention and localization in the hypothalamus and pituitary. Endocrinology 1973; 93:711–717.

369. Cidlowski JA, Muldoon TG. Sex-related differences in the regulation of cytoplasmic estrogen receptor levels in responsive tissues of the rat. Endocrinology 1976; 94:833–841.

370. Clark JH, Campbell PS, and Peck EJ Jr. Receptor estrogen complex in the nuclear fraction of the pituitary and hypothalamus of male and female immature rats. Neuroendocrinology 1972; 77:218–228.

371. Munck A, Wira C, Young DA, et al. Glucocorticoid-receptor complexes and the earliest steps in the action of glucocorticoids on thymus cells. J Steroid Biochem 1972; 3:567–578.

372. Rousseau GG, Baxter JD, Higgins SJ, et al. Steroid-induced nuclear binding of glucocorticoid receptors in intact hepatoma cells. J Mol Biol 1973; 79:539–554.

373. Raymoure WJ, McNaught RW, Smith RG. Reversible activation of non–steroid-binding oestrogen receptor. Nature 1985; 314:745–747.

374. Kassis JA, Gorski J. Estrogen receptor replenishment: evidence for receptor recycling. J Biol Chem 1984; 256:7380–7382.

375. Anderson JN, Peck EJ Jr, Clark JH. Nuclear receptor estradiol complex: a requirement for uterotropic responses. Endocrinology 1974; 95:174–178.

376. Reynolds SRM. Determinants of uterine growth and activity. Physiol Rev 1951; 31:244–273.

377. Thi MT, Baulieu EE, Milgrom E. Comparison of the characteristics and of the hormonal control of endometrial and myometrial progesterone receptors. J Endocrinol 1975; 66:349–356.

378. McEwen BS. Gonadal steroid receptors in neuroendocrine tissues. In: O'Malley BW, Birnbaumer, L, eds. New York: Academic, 1983: 353–400.

379. Milgrom E, Atger M, Baulieu EE. Progesterone in uterus and plasma. IV. Progesterone receptors in guinea pig uterus cytosol. Steroids 1970; 16:741–764.

380. Freifeld ML, Feil PD, Bardin CW. The in vivo regulation of the progesterone "receptor" in guinea pig uterus: dependence on estrogen and progesterone. Steroids 1974; 23:93–103.

381. Milgrom E, Thi L, Atger M, et al. Mechanisms regulating the concentration and the conformation of progesterone receptors in the uterus. J Biol Chem 1973; 248:6366–6377.

382. Alexander IE, Clarke CL, Shine J, et al. Progestin inhibition of progesterone receptor gene expression in human breast cancer cells. Mol Endocrinol 1989; 3:1377–1386.

383. Lerner LJ. Hormone antagonists: inhibitors of specific activities of estrogen and androgen. Recent Prog Horm Res 1964; 20:435–490.

384. Hsueh AJ, Peck EJ Jr, Clark JH. Control of uterine estrogen receptor levels by progesterone. Endocrinology 1976; 98:438–444.

385. Hsueh AJ, Peck EJ Jr, Clark JH. Progesterone antagonism of the oestrogen receptor and oestrogen-induced uterine growth. Nature 1975; 254:337–339.

386. Okulicz WC, Evans RW, Leavitt WW. Progesterone regulation of estrogen receptor in the rat uterus: a primary inhibitory influence on the nuclear fraction. Steroids 1981; 37:463–470.

387. Okulicz WC, Evans RW, Leavitt WW. Progesterone regulation of the occupied form of nuclear estrogen receptor. Science 1981; 213:1503–1505.

388. MacDonald RG, Okulicz WC, Leavitt WW. Progesterone-induced inactivation of nuclear estrogen receptor in the hamster uterus is mediated by acid phosphatase. Biochem Biophys Res Commun 1982; 104:570–576.

389. Auricchio F, Migliaccio A, Castoria G, et al. ATP-dependent enzyme-activating hormone binding of estradiol receptor. Biochem Biophys Res Commun 1981; 101:1171–1178.

390. Okulicz WC. Temporal limitation of progesterone inhibition of occupied nuclear estrogen receptor retention in the rat uterus. Endocrine Soc 1985; 81 (abstract).

391. Eriksson H, Upchurch S, Hardin JW, et al. Heterogeneity of estrogen receptors in the cytosol and nuclear fractions of the rat uterus. Biochem Biophys Res Commun 1978; 81:1–7.

392. Clark JH, Hardin JW, Upchurch S, et al. Heterogeneity of estrogen binding sites in the cytosol of the rat uterus. J Biol Chem 1978; 253:433–437.

393. Ekman P, Barrack ER, Greene GL, et al. Estrogen receptors in human prostate: evidence for multiple binding sites. J Clin Endocrinol Metab 1983; 57:166–176.

394. Swaneck GE, Alvarez JM, Sufrin G. Multiple species of estrogen binding sites in the nuclear fraction of the rat prostate. Biochem Biophys Res Commun 1982; 106:1441–1447.

395. Weinberger MJ. Heterogeneity and distribution of estrogen binding sites in guinea pig seminal vesicle. J Steroid Biochem 1984; 20:1327–1332.

396. Yuh KC, Keyes PL. Properties of nuclear and cytoplasmic estrogen receptor in the rabbit corpus luteum: evidence for translocation. Endocrinology 1979; 105:690–696.

397. Pfaff DW, McEwen BS. Actions of estrogen and progestins on nerve cells. Science 1981; 219:808–814.

398. Rousseau GG, Baxter JD. Glucocorticoid receptors. In: Baxter JD, Rousseau GG, eds. Glucorticoid Hormone Action. New York: Springer-Verlag, 1979: 49–77.

399. Richards JS. Content of nuclear estradiol receptor complex in rat corpora lutea during pregnancy: relationship to estrogen concentration and cytosol receptor availability. Endocrinology 1975; 96:227–230.

400. Clark JH, Anderson J, Peck EJ Jr. Receptor estrogen complex in the nuclear fraction of the rat uterus during the estrous cycle. Science 1972; 176:528.

401. Scott RS, Rennie PI. An estrogen receptor in the corpora lutea of the pseudopregnant rabbit. Endocrinology 1971; 89:297–301.

402. Muldoon TG. Mouse mammary tissue estrogen receptors: ontogeny and molecular heterogeneity. In: Hamilton TH, Clark JH, Sadler W, eds. Ontogeny of Receptors and Reproductive Hormone Action. New York: Raven, 1979: 212–236.

403. Hseuh AJW, Peck EJ Jr, Clark JH. Oestrogen receptors in the mammary gland of the lactating rat. J Endocrinol 1973; 58:503–511.

404. Lydon JP, DeMayo FJ, Funk CR, et al. Mice lacking progesterone receptor exhibit pleiotropic reproductive abnormalities. Genes Dev 1995; 9:2226–2278.

405. McCormack SA, Glasser SR. Ontogeny and regulation of a rat placental estrogen receptor. Endocrinology 1978; 102:273–280.

406. Pasqualini JR, Sumida C, Gelly C, et al. Specific [³H]estradiol binding in the fetal uterus and testis of the guinea pig: quantitative evolution of [³H]estradiol receptors in the different fetal tissues (kidney, lung, uterus and testis) during fetal development. J Steroid Biochem 1976; 7:1031–1038.

407. Clark JH, Gorski J. Ontogeny of the estrogen receptor during early uterine development. Science 1970; 169:76–86.

408. Roth GS, Hess GD. Changes in the mechanism of hormone and neurotransmitter action during aging: current status of the role of receptor and post-receptor alterations. Mech Ageing Dev 1982; 20:175–194.

409. Gould MN, Grau DR, Seidman LA, et al. Interspecies comparison of human and rat mammary epithelial cell–mediated mutagenesis by polycyclic aromatic hydrocarbons. Cancer Res 1986; 46:4942–4945.

410. Tung L, Mohamed MK, Hoeffler JP, et al. Antagonist-occupied human progesterone B-receptors activate transcription without binding to progesterone response elements and are dominantly inhibited by A-receptors. Mol Endocrinol 1993; 7:1256–1265.

411. Clark JH, Markaverich BM. The agonistic and antagonistic effects of short-acting estrogens. Pharmacol Ther 1982; 21:429–453.

412. Brecher PI, Wotix HH. Stereospecificity of the uterine nuclear hormone receptors. Proc Soc Exp Biol Med 1968; 128:470–473.

413. Bouton M, Raynaud JP. The relevance of interaction kinetics in determining biological responses to estrogens. Endocrinology 1979; 105:509–515.

414. Jensen EV, Jacobson HI, Flesher JW, et al. Estrogen Receptors in Target Tissues. New York: Academic Press, 1966: 133–156.

415. Clark JH, Markaverich BM. The agonistic-antagonistic properties of clomiphene. Pharmacol Ther 1966; 15:467–519.

416. Tate AC, Greene GL, Desombre ER, et al. Differences between estrogen- and antiestrogen-estrogen receptor complexes from human breast tumors

identified with an antibody raised against the estrogen receptor. Cancer Res 1984; 44:1012–1018.

417. Tate AC, Jordan VC. Nuclear [³H]4-hydroxytamoxifen (4-OHTAM)- and [³H]estradiol (E₂)-estrogen receptor complexes in the MCF-7 breast cancer and GH3 pituitary tumor cell lines. Mol Cell Endocrinol 1984; 36:211–219.

418. Lees JA, Fawell SE, Parker MG. Identification of two transactivation domains in the mouse oestrogen receptor. Nucleic Acids Res 1989; 17:5477–5487.

419. Sabbah M, Gouilleux F, Sola B, et al. Structural differences between the hormone and antihormone estrogen receptor complexes bound to the hormone response element. Proc Natl Acad Sci USA 1991; 88:390–394.

420. El-Ashry D, Onate SA, Nordeen SK, et al. Human progesterone receptor complexed with the antagonist RU486 binds to hormone response elements in a structurally altered form. Mol Endocrinol 1989; 3:1545–1558.

421. Fritsch M, Leary CM, Furlow JD, et al. A ligand-induced conformational change in the estrogen receptor is localized in the steroid binding domain. Biochemistry 1992; 31:5303–5311.

422. Weigel NL, Beck CA, Estes PA, et al. Ligands induce conformational changes in the carboxyl-terminus of progesterone receptors which are detected by a site-directed antipeptide monoclonal antibody. Mol Endocrinol 1992; 6:1585–1597.

423. Katzenellenbogen JA, O'Malley BW, Katzenellenbogen BS. Tripartite steroid hormone receptor pharmacology: interaction with multiple effector sites as a basis for the cell- and promotor-specific action of these hormones. Mol Endocrinol 1996; 10:119–131.

424. Terenius L. Structure-activity relationships of anti-oestrogens with regard to interaction with 17β-oestradiol in the mouse uterus and vagina. Acta Endocrinol 1971; 66:431–447.

425. Binart N, Catelli MH, Geynet C, et al. Monohydroxytamoxifen: an antiestrogen with high affinity for the chick oviduct oestrogen receptor. Biochem Biophys Res Commun 1979; 91:812–818.

426. Clark JH, Markaverich BM. Agonist and antagonist properties of clomiphene: a review. Pharmacol Ther 1982; 15:467–519.

427. Natrajan PK, Greenblat RB. Clomiphene Citrate: Induction of Ovulation. Philadelphia: Lea & Febiger, 1979; 35–76.

428. Furr BJA, Jordan VC. The pharmacology and clinical uses of tamoxifen. Pharmacol Ther 1984; 25:127–205.

429. Westley BR, Rochefort H. Estradiol-induced proteins in the MCF-7 human breast cancer cell line. Biochem Biophys Res Commun 1979; 90:410–416.

430. Coezy E, Borgna JL, Rochefort H. Tamoxifen and metabolites in MCF-7 cells: correlations between binding to estrogen and cell growth inhibition. Cancer Res 1982; 42:317–323.

431. Lieberman ME, Gorski J, Jordan VC. An estrogen receptor model to describe the regulation of prolactin synthesis by antiestrogens in vitro. J Biol Chem 1983; 258:4741–4745.

432. Lieberman ME, Jordan VC, Fritsch M, et al. Direct and reversible inhibition of estradiol-stimulated prolactin synthesis by antiestrogen in vitro. J Biol Chem 1983; 258:4734–4740.

433. Sutherland RL. Estrogen antagonists in chick oviduct: antagonist activity of eight synthetic triphenylethylene derivatives and their interactions with cytoplasmic and nuclear estrogen receptors. Endocrinology 1981; 109:2061–2068.

434. Sutherland RL, Murphy LC, SanFoo M, et al. High affinity anti-oestrogen binding site distinct from the oestrogen receptor. Nature 1980; 288:273–275.

435. Winneker RC, Clark JH. Estrogen stimulation of the antiestrogen specific binding site in rat uterus and liver. Endocrinology 1983; 112:1910–1915.

436. Murphy PR, Breckenridge WC, Lazier CB. Binding of oxygenerated choles-terol metabolites to antiestrogen binding sites from chicken liver. Biochem Biophys Res Commun 1985; 127:786–792.

437. Faye JC, Lasserre B, Bayard F. Antiestrogen specific, high-affinity saturable binding sites in rat uterine cytosol. Biochem Biophys Res Commun 1980; 93:1225–1231.

438. Gulino A, Pasqualini JR. Heterogeneity of binding sites for tamoxifen and tamoxifen derivatives in estrogen target and nontarget fetal organs of guinea pig. Cancer Res 1982; 42:1913–1921.

439. Kon OL. An antiestrogen-binding protein in human tissues. J Biol Chem 1983; 258:3173–3177.

440. Guilino A, Pasqualini JR. Modulation of tamoxifen specific binding sites and estrogen receptors by estradiol and progesterone in the neonatal uterus of guinea pig. Endocrinology 1983; 112:1870–1873.

441. Miller MA, Katzenellenbogen BS. Characterization and quantitation of antiestrogen binding sites in estrogen receptor-positive and -negative human breast cancer cell lines. Cancer Res 1983; 43:3094–3100.

442. Wiseman LR, Wakeling AE, May FB, et al. Effects of the antioestrogen, ICI 164, 384 on oestrogen-induced RNAs in MCF-7 cells. J Steroid Biochem 1989; 33:1–6.

443. May FB, Westley BR. Effects of tamoxifen and 4-hydroxytamoxifen on the pNR-1 and pNR-2 estrogen-regulated RNAs in human breast cancer cells. J Biol Chem 1987; 262:15894–15899.

444. Arbuckle NP, Dauvois S, Parker MG. Effects of antioestrogens on the DNA binding activity of oestrogen receptors in vitro. Nucleic Acids Res 1992; 20:3839–3844.

445. Reese JC, Katzenellenbogen BS. Examination of the DNA-binding ability of estrogen receptor in whole cells: implications for hormone-independent transactivation and the actions of antiestrogens. Mol Cell Biol 1992; 12:4531–4538.

446. Clark JH, Paszko Z, Peck EJ Jr. Nuclear binding and retention of the receptor estrogen complex: relation to the agonistic and antagonistic properties of estriol. Endocrinology 1977; 100:91–96.

447. Brenner RM, Resko JA, West NB. Cyclic changes in oviductal morphology and residual cytoplasmic estradiol binding capacity induced by sequential estradiol-progesterone treatment of spayed rhesus monkeys. Endocrinology 1974; 95:1094–1104.

448. Saunders DE, Lozon MM, Corombos JD, et al. Role of porcine endometrial estrogen sulfotransferase in progesterone-mediated down-regulation of estrogen receptors. J Steroid Biochem 1989; 32:749–757.

449. Herrmann W, Wyss F, Riondel A, et al. The effects of an antiprogesterone steroid in women: interruption of the menstrual cycle and of early pregnancy. 1982; CR Seances Acad Sci 294:933–938.

450. Asch RH, Rojas FJ. The effects of RU486 on the luteal phase of the rhesus monkey. J Steroid Biochem 1985; 22:227–230.

451. Horwitz KB. The antiprogestin RW 38486: receptor-mediated progestin versus antiprogestin actions screened in estrogen-insensitive T47D human breast cancer cells. Endocrinology 1985; 116:2236–2245.

452. Bowden RT, Hissom JR, Moore MR. Growth stimulation of T47D human breast cancer cells by anti-progestin RU486. Endocrinology 1989; 14:2642–2644.

453. Gray OG, Leavitt WW. RU486 is not an antiprogestin in the hamster. J Steroid Biochem 1987; 28:493–497.

454. Allan GF, Leng XH, Tsai SY, et al. Hormone and antihormone induce distinct conformational changes which are central to steroid receptor activation. J Biol Chem 1992; 267:19513–19520.

455. Olge FF. Kinetic and physiochemical characteristics of an endogenous inhibitor to progesterone-receptor binding in rat placenta cytosol. Biochem J 1981; 199:371–381.

MECHANISM OF ACTION OF HORMONES THAT ACT AT THE CELL SURFACE

C. Ronald Kahn, Robert J. Smith, and William W. Chin

INTRODUCTION

Hormone Systems and Intercellular Communication

Multicellular organisms depend on communication among cells for regulation of metabolic processes, control of cell growth and differentiation, and integration of physiological function. Cell-to-cell communication is mediated, in large part, by the action of molecules in the endocrine, paracrine, autocrine, and neurotransmitter systems. The primary signals of cellular communication are hormones and growth factors. These signaling molecules can be divided chemically into peptides, amino acids and their derivatives (including iodothyronines), steroids, prostaglandins and prostacyclins, and catecholamines.

Humans and higher mammals produce more than 100 different hormones, each of which is capable of interacting with one or more of the cell types distributed in tissues throughout the body. The specificity of informational transfer between cells is governed not only by the capacity of each target cell to respond to some of these hormones and not to

others but also by the concentration of the hormone and the space of distribution of the active substance. Some hormones act on cells located at a distance (endocrine effect), whereas other hormones and growth factors act on adjacent cells (paracrine effect) or on the secretory cell itself (autocrine effect). Many neurotransmitters and hormones acting by paracrine or autocrine mechanisms are theoretically capable of stimulating multiple tissues, but their action is limited by the fact that the concentration of hormone required for biologic response is achieved only within the limited space of a synapse or on cells adjacent to the same extracellular space.

The major factor determining the tissue response to a hormone is the presence of a cellular receptor for the hormone and the postreceptor machinery to which that receptor is coupled. Each receptor serves two critical functions: (1) recognition of the hormone as an entity distinct from all of the other substances present in blood or extracellular fluid, a recognition that is accomplished by specific, high-affinity binding; and (2) transformation of the binding interaction into a signal that modifies cellular metabolism and/or growth. For steroid hormones and iodothyronines, the receptors and initial sites of action are intracellular, i.e., in the cytoplasm or nucleus of the cell. For peptide hormones, growth factors, neurotransmitters, and prostaglandins, the receptors are on the plasma membrane of the cell, and thus the initial interaction is extracellular. Although many concepts of hormone action are similar for these two broad classes of hormones, this chapter focuses on the mechanism of action of hormones that act at the cell surface and the nature of some of the proteins involved in this action. The mechanism of action of steroid and thyroid hormones is discussed in Chapter 4.

Development of the Receptor Concept

The concept that cells possess specific receptors for hormones and other molecules derives from pharmacologic studies on the actions of toxins and drugs[1, 2] prior to the development of the concept of the endocrine system. These early investigators concluded that certain agents have a specificity of action that is governed by the presence of specific "receptive substances," i.e., receptors on or in the target cell. This idea was quickly adopted by pharmacologists as a model for understanding the effects of drugs, but early attempts to demonstrate receptors for hormones were largely inconclusive.

The first convincing evidence that some hormones act via surface membrane receptors came from indirect studies. In one, it was shown that treatment of cells with antibodies to peptide hormones, such as thyrotropin (thyroid-stimulating hormone [TSH]) and insulin, can reverse the actions of these hormones, a finding consistent with the idea that the hormone was on the cell surface and accessible to the antibody.[3] By contrast, antibodies to steroid hormones do not block hormone actions once initiated, because the steroid hormone had entered the cell to interact with its receptor and was inaccessible. Similar conclusions were reached by experiments demonstrating that peptide hormones can remain active after being covalently coupled to large polymeric beads that prevented their entrance into the cell,[4, 5] and by experiments demonstrating that membrane receptors could be digested by enzymatic treatment of intact cells with proteases.[6] Most important, however, Sutherland and other researchers proposed the *second-messenger concept of hormone action*.[7–9] In this scheme, the hormone is the first messenger of intercellular communication and is secreted into the bloodstream, where it is free to interact with membrane receptors on target cells. This interaction results in generation of a second, intracellular messenger that mediates the hormone's effects on intracellular enzymes, gene expression, and even on the cell membrane itself (Fig. 5–1). Although the second messenger was originally conceived of as a small organic molecule, such as cyclic AMP (cAMP), cyclic GMP (cGMP), or an inositol phosphate, second messengers can also be ions, such as calcium or hydrogen, or

enzymes such as protein kinases, which modify intracellular proteins by phosphorylation. This model of a hormone binding to its membrane receptor, transmembrane signal transduction, and generation of one or more intracellular signals is the paradigm on which current concepts of peptide hormone and neurotransmitter action are built.

The Whole Body Picture

Although the details of the mechanism of peptide hormone action have been characterized at the cellular and molecular levels, it is important to keep in mind the physiological nature of hormone action. The distribution and fate of a hormone in intact animals can be visualized after the administration of radiolabeled hormones followed by dissection of the target organs or autoradiography[10, 11] or by the use of noninvasive techniques such as external scintillation scanning with high-energy gamma emitters such as radioactive iodine (^{123}I)[12, 13] or photoemission tomography.[14]

An example of the analysis of the biokinetics of insulin in a human by scintillation scanning is illustrated in Figure 5–2 (see color section between pages 875 and 877). Within 1 to 3 minutes of intravenous administration, insulin distributes in the intravascular space and is seen in the blood pool, as exemplified by the heart. The hormone is rapidly cleared from the bloodstream and within 5 minutes is bound to receptors on target tissues, including liver, muscle, and adipose tissue. Some uptake of hormone and degradation fragments also occurs in nontarget tissues, such as kidney and spleen, through receptor-independent mechanisms. By 15 minutes, most of the insulin is bound, internalized, and degraded. At 30 minutes after the injection, only minimal amounts of degradation fragments of the hormone are detectable in kidney and bladder.

In contrast to these distribution kinetics, there is usually a lag in both the onset and the offset of hormone action. This delay is determined by the time required for distribution of the hormone; by the time required for the hormone to exit the vascular space and to enter the extracellular fluid space, where it may interact with its target tissues; by the time required to bind to receptors; and by the half-life of the proteins or other secondary mediators of hormone action generated by the initial signal.[15–17] These kinetic factors may play an important role in determining the exact course of hormone action and whether there is a positive or negative signal. For example, some hormones, such as luteinizing hormone–releasing hormone (LHRH, also called gonadotropin-releasing hormone [GnRH]), exert their maximal effect when released in a pulsatile fashion and produce desensitization when continuously secreted.[18] When hormones are given therapeuti-

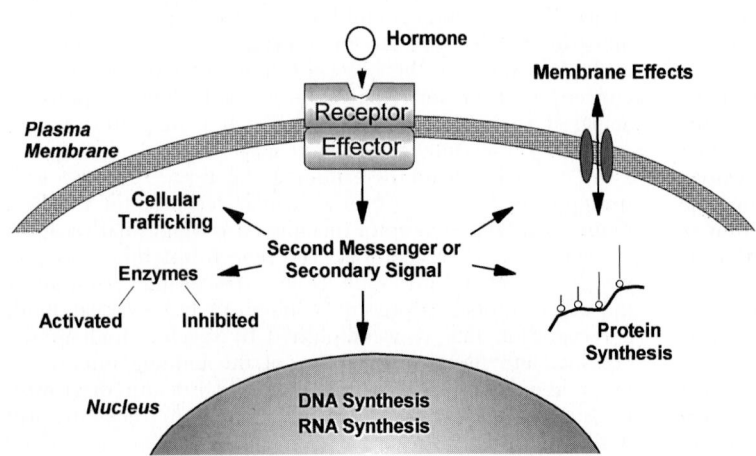

Figure 5–1. *A general model for the action of peptide hormones, catecholamines, and other membrane-active hormones. The hormone in the extracellular fluid interacts with the receptor and activates an associated effector system (which may or may not be in the same molecule). This activation results in generation of an intracellular signal or second messenger that, through a variety of common and branched pathways, produces the final effects of the hormone on metabolic enzyme activity, protein synthesis, membrane transport, cellular trafficking, DNA and RNA synthesis, and cellular growth and differentiation.*

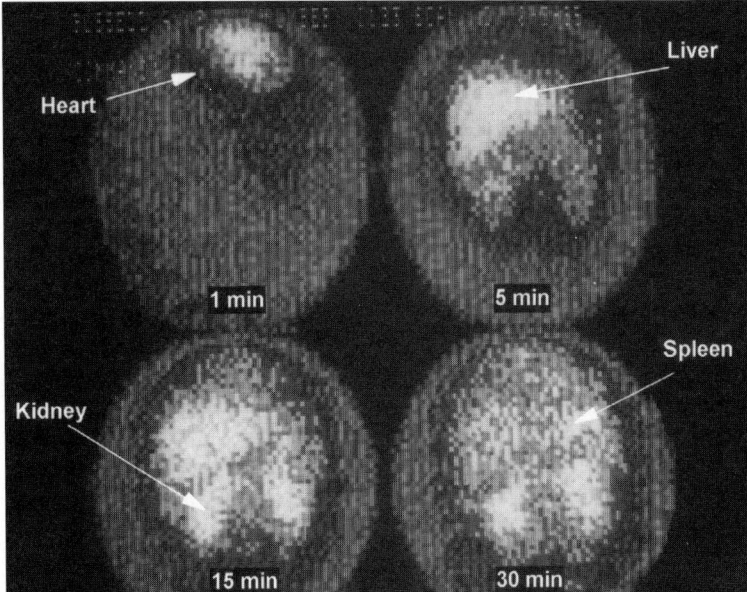

Figure 5–2. Scintiscans obtained 3 min *(upper left)*, 10 min *(upper right)*, 20 min *(lower left)*, and 30 min *(lower right)* after antecubital vein injection of 0.84 mCi of labeled insulin into a normal female volunteer (age 25, weight 63 kg, height 168 cm). Studies of insulin receptors in vivo using ^{131}I-insulin and scintillation scanning. L, liver; RK, right kidney; LK, left kidney; Sp, spleen. (See color section between pages 875 and 877.)

cally, one must also recognize that differences in kinetics can result from absorption from subcutaneous depots or other sites and from whether the hormone first enters into the portal circulation, the peripheral circulation, or some other extravascular space.

PROPERTIES OF THE HORMONE-RECEPTOR INTERACTION

Direct Studies of Membrane Receptors

Direct studies of the peptide hormone receptor interaction were first achieved with angiotensin[19] and corticotropin (ACTH, adrenocorticotropin)[20] and, soon after, with insulin[4, 21] and glucagon.[22] Binding studies have now been performed for virtually all of the peptide hormones, neurotransmitters, and many prostaglandins.

For in vitro binding studies, a radioactively labeled hormone—usually with ^{125}I or tritium (^{3}H)—is incubated with isolated intact cells or cell membranes that possess the receptor in the presence or absence of unlabeled hormone until equilibrium is obtained.[23–26] The receptor-bound hormone is then separated from the free hormone by centrifugation, precipitation, or some other method. The percentage of hormone bound to the receptor is then determined by counting the radioactive tracer in a gamma or scintillation counter. Unlabeled hormone competes with the labeled hormone for binding to the receptor, allowing a competition, or inhibition, curve to be produced (Fig. 5–3). The tracer that remains bound in the presence of a large excess of unlabeled hormone is considered to be nonspecific. In some cases it is necessary to use hormone analogues for binding studies, particularly if the native hormone is difficult to label radioactively, has a low affinity for the receptor, or is easily degraded. For some receptors, especially neurotransmitter receptors, receptor antagonists are used as the labeled ligand, since the antagonist binds to the receptor with higher affinity and specificity than the normal agonist.[27, 28] Antireceptor antibodies have also been used as ligands for receptor detection.[29–32] Such antibodies often recognize domains of the receptor distinct from the hormone-binding domain and thus allow detection of receptors with altered regions of ligand binding. Such assays are particularly valuable in assessing possible receptor alterations in disease[30] and in studies of receptor expression using flow cytometric analysis.[29, 33]

Although the principle of radioreceptor assay is similar to that of radioimmunoassay (see Chapter 3), there are several important differences. First, the interaction of hormone and receptor requires biologic specificity (rather than immunologic specificity), and it is critical that the hormone is labeled in a manner that does not alter its integrity or bioactivity. Second, because the receptors are part of a cell membrane, the receptor is usually in a particulate form, rather than in aqueous solution. Alternatively, the receptors may be solubilized by detergent treatment, so that the properties of hormone-receptor interaction can be studied in solution.

Hormone-Receptor Interaction

For most hormones of this class, the interaction between the hormone and the receptor is rapid and reversible,[23, 26, 34]

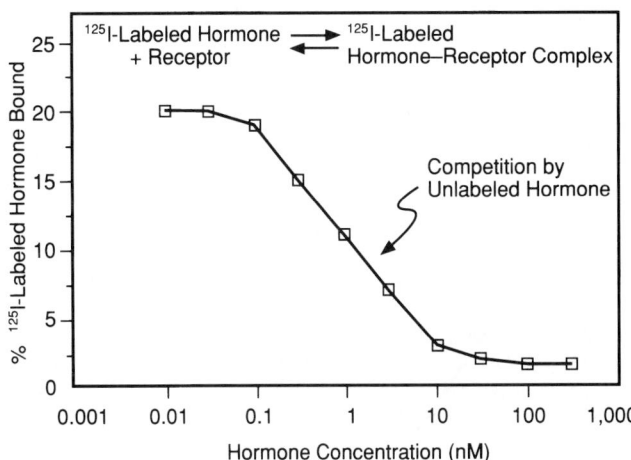

Figure 5–3. A typical hormone-binding study. ^{125}I-labeled hormone is incubated with receptor and increasing concentrations of unlabeled hormone. After separation of bound and free hormone, the percentage of bound ^{125}I is calculated and plotted against the total hormone concentration (labeled plus unlabeled hormone). The result is a competition (or inhibition) curve. Note that even at extremely high concentrations, there is some binding of hormone. This binding is considered to be nonspecific and is subtracted from the total to give the specific binding.

$$H + R \underset{k_R}{\overset{k_F}{\rightleftharpoons}} HR$$

Hormone-Receptor
Equilibrium Reaction

$$K_{eq} = \frac{[HR]}{[H]\,[R]} = \frac{k_F}{k_R}$$

Equilibrium
Equation

$$\frac{[HR]}{[H]} = K\,[R]$$

Rearranged Equilibrium
Equation

$$\frac{[HR]}{[H]} = K\,(R_0 - HR) = K\,[R_0] - K\,[HR]$$

$$\frac{B}{F} = K\,[R_0] - K\,(B)$$

Scatchard
Equation

Figure 5–4. Analysis of hormone-receptor interactions: deriving the Scatchard equation. This analysis assumes a simple bimolecular interaction with a monomer hormone, a monomeric receptor, and no cooperative interactions. Often the system is more complex, with two or more classes of receptors that differ in affinity or that exhibit cooperative interactions.

H = free hormone concentration

R = free receptor concentration

HR = concentration of hormone-receptor complexes

k_F = forward reaction rate

k_R = reverse reaction rate

K_{eq} = equilibrium constant

R_0 = total receptor concentration

B = amount of hormone bound

F = amount of hormone free

---

allowing rapid initiation and rapid termination of hormone action. The number of receptors for a given hormone on any cell type varies from zero to more than 1 million. Although the number of receptors is usually highest on the known target cells for hormone action, nontarget cells may also possess receptors. For example, insulin receptors are present in relatively high concentration not only on liver, muscle, and fat cells but also on lymphocytes, gonadal cells, and even brain cells.[35] Similarly, TSH receptors are found on both thyroid cells and adipocytes,[36] and prolactin receptors are present on mammary cells, hepatocytes, and some lymphoid cells.[37, 38] The presence of receptors for a hormone on a nontarget cell may reflect the fact that the tissue possesses some previously

unrecognized action of the hormone or indicates that the hormone has a role in the cell in some earlier state of development.

RECEPTOR AFFINITY. Hormones bind to their receptors with high affinity and specificity. Because most peptide hormones are present in the circulation at picomolar (10^{-12} M) to nanomolar (10^{-9} M) concentrations, receptors must have appropriately high affinities (10^{-12} to 10^{-8} M^{-1}) to achieve significant binding at physiological levels. Receptor affinity may be calculated from the kinetics of association and dissociation, or from equilibrium binding data (Fig. 5–4). The most common method of analysis is the Scatchard plot. In this method, the bound/free ratio of hormone at equilibrium is

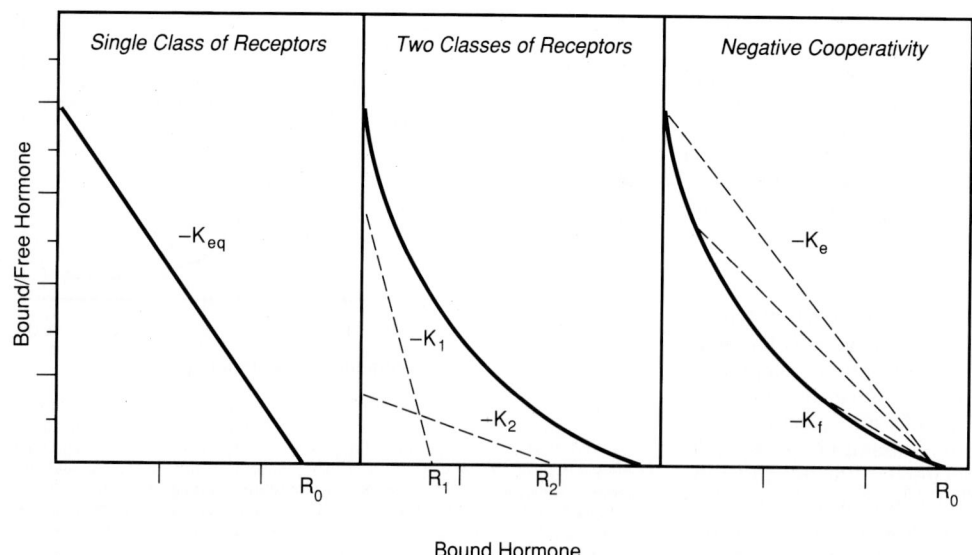

Figure 5–5. Scatchard analysis of hormone-receptor interaction. When the bound/free ratio is plotted against the bound hormone for a single class of noninteractive sites (an ideal bimolecular reversible reaction), a straight line is obtained *(left)*. The slope of the line is the negative value of the equilibrium constant ($-K_{eq}$), and the intercept on the abscissa is the total receptor concentration (R_0). Curvilinear Scatchard plots may arise as the result of two classes of sites *(middle)* or the presence of negative cooperativity *(right)*. In the two-class model, the curve is the sum of two straight lines representing a high-affinity, low-capacity site (K_1, R_1) and a low-affinity, high-capacity site (K_2, R_2). In the negative cooperativity model, there is a single class of interactive sites. The total receptor concentration is R_0. The high-affinity state is K_e (the affinity of the empty receptor). As the sites are filled, the affinity falls, eventually reaching a low-affinity state K_{fl} (the affinity of the filled receptor).

plotted against the total hormone bound.[24, 39] If the hormone is a monomer (most are) and if there is a single class of noninteracting receptor sites, the Scatchard plot results in a straight line (Fig. 5–5, *left panel*). The slope of the line represents the negative value of the equilibrium binding constant, $-K_{eq}$, and the intercept on the abscissa corresponds to the total receptor concentration, R_0. Many receptors exhibit two classes of binding sites of differing affinity and capacity, e.g., a high-affinity low-capacity site and a low-affinity high-capacity site, resulting in a curvilinear Scatchard plot (see Fig. 5–5, *center panel*). A curvilinear Scatchard plot and complex kinetics of interaction more commonly occur if there are interactions between receptors resulting in positive or negative cooperativity[24, 40–43] (see Fig. 5–5, *right panel*).

RECEPTOR SPECIFICITY. The most characteristic and essential feature of the hormone-receptor interaction is the specificity of binding. At the first level, specificity means that each hormone binds to its specific receptor, e.g., glucagon binds only to glucagon receptors, insulin to insulin receptors. At a more subtle level, specificity implies that a hormone and its derivatives bind to their receptor with an affinity that is directly related to its bioactivity (Fig. 5–6). Human insulin is about 50 times as potent in stimulating the metabolism of

isolated fat cells as human proinsulin and binds to the insulin receptor with 50 times the affinity of proinsulin.[21] Insulin-like growth factor I (IGF-I, also called somatomedin-C) has an even lower affinity for the insulin receptor and even lower insulin-like activity. Most of the differences in potency of hormone analogues and derivatives are due to differences in binding affinity to the receptor. Hormones may also differ in their ability to initiate signal transduction after binding, i.e., their intrinsic activity, although this is less common. Competitive antagonists are ligands that bind to the receptor with high affinity but have no intrinsic activity. Some weak agonists can act as antagonists under certain conditions.

The structural features of hormones that define receptor affinity and intrinsic activity are only partially understood. For some simple peptide hormones such as corticotropin, glucagon, angiotensin, and many gastrointestinal hormones, such as cholecystokinin and gastrin, the binding affinities and intrinsic activities appear to be governed by small linear domains of the molecule.[18, 44–46] For these molecules, it is usually possible to produce peptide fragments that retain bioactivity and competitive antagonists that bind to the receptor but lack intrinsic activity. For hormones with complex three-dimensional structures, such as insulin, IGF-I, and growth hormone

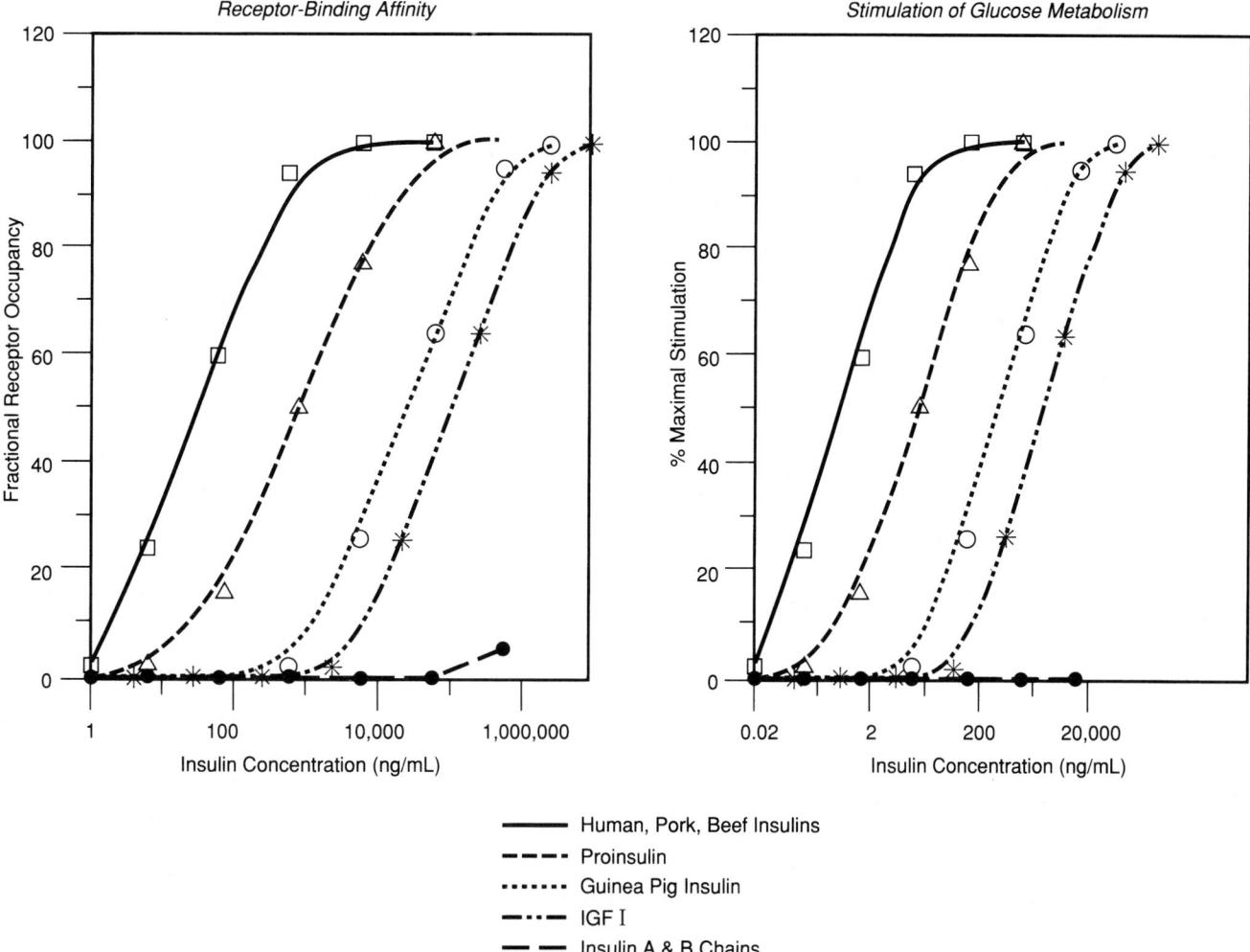

Figure 5–6. Correlation between binding and bioactivity. *Left Panel,* The binding of a series of insulin analogues to the receptor in rat liver plasma membranes. *Right Panel,* The ability of the same analogues to stimulate glucose metabolism in isolated adipocytes. Note the almost perfect correlation between receptor affinity *(left)* and relative bioactivity *(right)*. Also, note that the bioactivity scale reflects increased insulin sensitivity because of the presence of spare receptors. IGF-I, insulin-like growth factor I. To convert insulin values from nanograms per milliliter to picomoles per liter, multiply by 1.722×10^5. (Adapted from Freychet P, Roth J, Neville DM Jr. Insulin receptors in the liver: specific binding of [^{125}I]-insulin to the plasma membrane and its relation to insulin bioactivity. Proc Natl Acad Sci USA 1971; 68:1833–1837, with permission.)

(GH), the ligand binding and activity domains overlap and are formed by residues from different parts of the molecule that come together as the molecule folds to form a bioactive surface.[47, 48] For this latter more complex class of hormones, production of smaller active "molecular cores" or competitive antagonists at the receptor level is difficult, if not impossible.

Structure of Membrane Receptors

The interaction of ligand with its cognate membrane receptor is the first step in transduction of the hormonal signals from outside of the cell to the inside, where it can modulate function.[49–52] As noted earlier, the receptor plays two roles in this transduction process: (1) binding the extracellular signaling molecule or hormone that is present in minute amounts at the cell surface with both high affinity and specificity; and (2) relaying the information inherent in this ligand-binding event to sites within the cell. Because the members of the hormone superfamily include small molecules such as catecholamines and neuropeptides and large glycoprotein hormones (i.e., TSH and gonadotropins), the binding domains of the receptors must vary to accommodate this range of ligands. Likewise, the signal produced by hormone binding is transduced intracellularly via multiple effector pathways that include cAMP, cGMP, arachidonic acid, inositol triphosphate, Ca^{2+}, and other ions as second messengers and are produced by enzymes (e.g., adenylate and guanylate cyclases, and phospholipases A_2 and C) and ion channels. In many cases, the hormone-receptor complexes do not interface directly with these effectors but rather act via an intermediate modulating signal transducer, such as guanine nucleotide–binding proteins (G proteins). This large number of receptors and effector components produce intracellular signals that are receptor-specific and usually result in signal amplification and divergence into multiple secondary and tertiary effects and may allow for interactions between related pathways.

The structures of many membrane receptors have been elucidated.[45, 53–55] Most often this has involved the isolation of the membrane receptors using classic biochemical techniques, followed by partial amino acid sequence analysis. From these, oligonucleotide probes have been prepared and used to screen specific libraries for cDNAs encoding the membrane receptor proteins.[56, 57] Expression cloning has also allowed the identification, isolation, and characterization of cDNAs and

genes encoding functional membrane receptors.[55, 58] Such studies have revealed four common motifs for the structure of membrane receptors: seven transmembrane G protein–coupled receptors, receptor-type ion channels, single transmembrane receptors that possess intrinsic enzyme activities, and transmembrane receptors that interact with other cellular proteins with enzyme activity (Fig. 5–7 and Table 5–1).

RECEPTOR MOTIFS. The largest family of membrane receptors uses G proteins to couple to specific intracellular effector systems, such as the adenylate cyclase or phosphatidylinositol turnover pathways. Its members include α- and β-adrenergic, dopaminergic, serotoninergic, muscarinic cholinergic, and peptidergic receptors and the receptor for sensing extracellular calcium ions.[55, 56, 59–62] These receptors characteristically contain seven transmembrane domains and, like most membrane receptors, have one or more sites of extracellular glycosylation. Each transmembrane domain consists of 20 to 30 hydrophobic amino acid residues in an alpha-helical structure and is long enough (approximately 30 nm) to span the lipid membrane bilayer. The seven transmembrane domains are connected by three extracellular and three intracellular hydrophilic loops. Most possess a cytoplasmic tail that contains potential serine phosphorylation sites that may be targets for regulation of receptor activity. Seven transmembrane receptors for peptide hormones usually have a large NH_2-terminal extension that participates in ligand binding.[55, 57]

Another class of receptors represent the ligand-gated ion channels, of which there are two subtypes.[63–72] One subtype includes the nicotinic acetylcholine, γ-aminobutyric acid (GABA), glycine, and kainate receptors, all of which possess four transmembrane spanning domains.[63, 73] The other includes the ligand-gated ion channels that encode specific conduits for sodium, calcium, and potassium cations and are composed of multiple subunits, each containing six transmembrane spanning domains that form homomultimers or heteromultimers.[65, 66, 70–72]

A third class of membrane receptors contains the effector activity, such as tyrosine or serine kinase activity, as an intrinsic part of the structure.[74–76] The best characterized of these receptors are the protein tyrosine kinases, as typified by the receptors for insulin, IGF-I, epidermal growth factor (EGF), and platelet-derived growth factor (PDGF) receptors. Each of these membrane receptors contains an extracellular ligand-binding domain, a single transmembrane spanning domain,

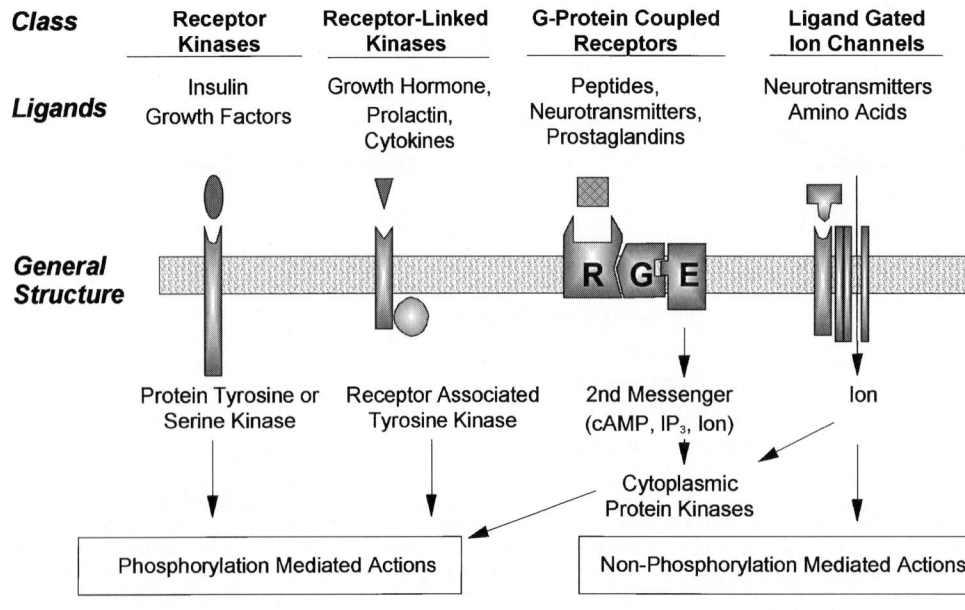

Figure 5–7. Four major classes of membrane receptors exist for hormones and neurotransmitters. Many growth factors, including insulin, bind to cell-surface receptors that act as protein tyrosine kinases stimulating the phosphorylation of proteins on tyrosine residues. Growth hormone, prolactin, and many cytokines act on receptors that associate with cytoplasmic tyrosine kinases. A third class of agonists binds to receptors (R) that are coupled to separate effector (E) molecules by G proteins (G). Effectors may be enzymes that produce second messengers that, in turn, can activate distinct protein (generally serine/threonine) kinases. The fourth major class of receptors includes ligand-gated ion channels. Some of these are self-contained, as illustrated on the right. In others, the receptor and the ion channel are coupled by G proteins, as shown in the center.

TABLE 5–1. Classification of Hormone Receptors and Effectors

Adenylate Cyclase

Corticotropin
β-Adrenergic catecholamines
Luteinizing hormone and human chorionic gonadotropin
Follicle-stimulating hormone
Glucagon
Prostaglandins
Parathyroid hormone
Thyrotropin (thyroid-stimulating hormone [TSH])
α-Adrenergic (inhibition)
Somatostatin (inhibition)

Guanylate Cyclase

Atrial natriuretic peptide (ANP, also called atrial natriuretic factor)

Receptor Protein Tyrosine Kinases

Insulin
Insulin-like growth factor (somatomedin-C)
Epidermal growth factor
Colony-stimulating factor 1
Fibroblast growth factor

Receptor-Associated Tyrosine Kinases

Growth hormone
Prolactin
Erythropoietin
Interleukins
Nerve growth factor
T-cell receptor

Phosphoinositol Turnover and Calcium Flux

Acetylcholine receptor (muscarinic)
α-Adrenergic catecholamines
Angiotensin (also activates tyrosine kinases)
Luteinizing hormone–releasing hormone
Thyrotropin-releasing hormone
Vasopressin

Ion Channels

Acetylcholine receptor (nicotinic)
γ-Aminobutyric acid

and an intracellular kinase domain. Some, such as the insulin and IGF-I receptors, are linked by disulfide bonds to form dimers.

Finally, the membrane receptors for GH, prolactin, granulocyte-macrophage colony-stimulating factor (GM-CSF), cytokines (interleukin-2 [IL-2], IL-4, IL-6, and IL-7), and leptin[77–79] are similar in structure to the receptor kinases and contain a single transmembrane spanning domain. Although they have no intrinsic enzymatic activity, they interact with other membrane or cytoplasmic proteins that possess tyrosine kinase activity, one of the best characterized of which is the Janus kinase (JAK) family of kinases.[80, 81] Several members of this receptor family may also be expressed as circulating, non–membrane-associated forms, as a result of alternative splicing of an exon encoding the membrane-spanning domain.[82] These circulating receptor forms act as serum-binding proteins for these ligands.

All four classes of membrane-associated hormone receptors possess multiple functional domains. These domains have been defined by in vitro mutagenesis and by the creation of chimeric receptors that possess specific domains derived from different receptors and are known to include regions that bind ligand, interact with effector systems, either indirectly (i.e., via G proteins) or directly (ligand-coupled ion channels), possess inherent enzyme activity (i.e., tyrosine kinases), determine membrane localization and internalization, and are involved in desensitization of signaling.

Receptors can also be viewed as having several distinct structural domains. The NH_2 terminus of the receptor protein is usually extracytoplasmic and contains one or more domains that interact with the hormonal ligands.[56, 57] These regions are

often glycosylated, have complex disulfide linkages, may have sites of fatty acid acylation, and may contain sulfate and phosphate groups.

The "center" of the receptor consists of one to seven transmembrane spanning domains. In addition to serving as anchors to the membrane, the transmembrane domains may play roles in both signal transduction and, in the case of G protein–coupled receptors, may also be involved in the interaction with ligands. For example, the fourth transmembrane spanning domain of the type 2 β-adrenergic receptor is critical for interactions with agonists.[83] In the adrenergic receptor, the intracytoplasmic loops also serve as the site of interaction with the G proteins.[84]

The COOH-terminal domain is intracellular and is usually the effector domain of the receptor, as in the case of the tyrosine kinases, or interacts with intracellular effector molecules serving this function. This domain may also play a role in internalization and/or modulation of receptor activity, i.e., desensitization. The ability of receptors to bind to different ligands and to transduce specific signals resides in structural subtleties of the specific domains and the complex pathways of effector interaction. More detailed discussion of receptor structure-function relationships appears in the section on receptor-effector systems.

Families of Membrane Receptors

Although an essential feature of specificity of signaling requires that hormones have distinct receptor sites on the membrane and separate pathways of action, many hormones belong to families of peptides that have overlapping structural features and/or biologic activities. Examples include the prolactin, GH, and placental lactogen family of hormones; the insulin and IGF family; the families of secretin-like and gastrin-like gastrointestinal hormones; LH and human chorionic gonadotropin (hCG); and corticotropin, melanocyte-stimulating hormone, and other derivatives of pro-opiomelanocortin. Many of these families of hormones are related evolutionarily and are derived from identical precursors; however, the physiological roles of the various members of these families may be quite different and, in some cases, even opposing in nature.

In most cases, related hormones interact with families of related receptors. For example, the prolactin and GH receptors have an overall sequence identity of approximately 30%, with four highly homologous regions in the extracellular domain and one in the cytoplasmic domain.[82, 85, 86] The receptors for insulin and IGF-I are virtually identical in overall structure and have about 80% sequence identity throughout their length.[87, 88]

Structural similarities of hormone receptors may extend beyond the families of hormones with which they interact and include the use of similar effector pathways. The receptors for insulin, IGF-I, EGF, and PDGF have homologous intracellular tyrosine kinase domains that possess the enzymatic activity required for signal transduction but different extracellular domains for ligand binding. Likewise, receptors that act through G proteins have similar overall structure with seven transmembrane segments, although the ligands they bind are quite different, ranging from large glycoproteins, such as LH and hCG, to small organic molecules, such as catecholamines, and ions such as Ca^{2+}. In the case of receptors coupled to G proteins, although the intermediate signal transduction mechanisms are similar, the final effectors and effects of the hormones are quite different.

There are some exceptions to the general rule that homologous hormones have structurally related receptors. For example, IGF-II is a peptide growth factor with a structure closely related to that of insulin and IGF-I, but the primary receptor for IGF-II is a large single-chain polypeptide that bears no resemblance to the tetrameric receptors for IGF-I and insulin.[89] Furthermore, unlike the receptors for IGF-I and insulin, the IGF-II receptor has no intrinsic tyrosine kinase activity, nor is it phosphorylated on tyrosine residues. In fact, the IGF-II receptor is a receptor of a class very different from the insulin and IGF-I receptors, possessing two functional binding sites—one for IGF-II and one for glycoproteins containing mannose-6-phosphate. Although some studies suggest that it has a role in IGF-II signaling, the primary function of the IGF-II/mannose-6-phosphate receptor appears to be the transport of both of these ligands to lysosomes for degradation.

A single hormone or neurotransmitter may also interact with more than one receptor that differs in structure. Acetylcholine binds to a nicotinic receptor composed of four different subunits that form an ion channel and a muscarinic, seven transmembrane receptor coupled to phospholipid turnover through a G protein. In addition, many neurotransmitter receptors and some peptide hormone receptors are present as multiple, closely related receptor isotypes that may be products of distinct genes and have ligand-binding sites that differ slightly in affinity for the various related ligand agonists and antagonists.[84]

The physiological and pathological significance of families of related hormones and receptors is evidenced, for example, by the almost interchangeable biologic effects of LH and hCG and by the similar effects of GH and prolactin on breast tissue. Other examples of overlapping hormone action include circumstances in which one hormone is elevated to pathologically high levels and mimics the action of another hormone by binding to its receptor with a low affinity, a phenomenon termed *specificity spillover* (see the section on membrane receptor and disease).

LIFE CYCLE OF THE HORMONE-RECEPTOR COMPLEX

Biosynthesis and Turnover of Membrane Receptors

Like all components of the cell, membrane receptors are in a constant state of turnover. Receptor synthesis begins on the rough endoplasmic reticulum (ER), where proteins destined for the plasma membrane are sorted from other proteins by the presence of a signal sequence and other conformational determinants.[90–92] The ER also provides a form of quality control, sorting out incompletely folded or misfolded proteins, unassembled protein subunits, and proteins whose transport is post-translationally regulated. The immature receptors then pass through the Golgi complex, where they are modified by glycosylation, fatty acid acylation, disulfide bond formation, and, in some cases, cleavage into subunits. The mature receptors are inserted into the plasma membrane by a poorly understood process that probably involves fusion of vesicles from the Golgi complex with the plasma membrane.

After the receptors are inserted into the plasma membrane, they are available for ligand binding and signal transduction. Under ordinary circumstances, the half-time for receptor synthesis matches the half-time for degradation so that the total receptor pool remains constant. Alterations in synthesis or degradation rate can result in changes in receptor number and altered biologic response. The most common of these is the ability of many peptide hormones to accelerate degradation of their own receptors, leading to down-regulation of receptor number. Such changes may play a critical role under certain conditions.

Receptor Aggregation and Internalization

In the basal state, most hormone receptors are distributed diffusely over the surface of the cell. After binding hormones, receptors tend to aggregate.[34, 93, 94] The initial aggregates are small (most likely dimers) and may be important in signal generation (see later). Larger aggregates are eventually formed and undergo internalization. For most receptors, internalization occurs through specialized regions of the membrane called coated pits, which are lined on the intracellular surface with the protein clathrin.[95] The coated pits invaginate and pinch off to form endosomal vesicles, which are surrounded by a cage-like structure formed by clathrin (Fig. 5–8). Eventually these receptor-containing endosomes, or receptosomes, are acidified and fuse with lysosomes. In this acidic environment the ligand usually dissociates from the receptor and undergoes degradation, and the receptor is recycled to the cell surface, where it is again available for hormone binding.[96–98] A receptor may make 50 or more cycles into the cell and back to the surface membrane before it undergoes degradation. Thus, whereas the hormone is degraded in minutes, the half-time for degradation of receptors varies from a few hours to about a day.

For some receptors, internalization may contribute to the hormone signaling process. The tyrosine kinase activity of insulin receptors on internalized endosomes is actually higher than that at the plasma membrane, and many of the receptor substrates are located in the cytoplasm or on internal membranes.[99] Likewise, mutations that impair internalization of the angiotensin II receptor fail to activate phospholipase C normally.[100] This point, however, remains controversial, since most mutant receptors with defective internalization appear to signal normally.

Aggregation and internalization are common features of ligand-receptor interactions and occur for a variety of membrane receptors, including hormone receptors, immunoglobulin receptors, and nutrient receptors. Indeed, internalization, rather than cellular signaling, is the primary function of nutrient receptors, such as the low-density lipoprotein, cyanocobalamin, and transferrin receptors[101, 102] (Table 5–2). The degree of internalization appears to be governed by factors intrinsic and extrinsic to the receptor itself. Low-density lipoprotein (LDL) and other nutrient receptors are preferentially localized in coated pits (which favors internalization), whereas most hormone receptors are distributed over the surface of the cell and localize in coated pits only after ligand binding. In addition, some receptors possess a specific amino acid sequence (glutamine-proline-X-tyrosine, where X is any amino acid) that is located in the region of the protein just inside the cell membrane. This forms a beta-turn that seems to be critical for internalization.[103] For some receptors, covalent modification by enzymes, such as phosphorylation on threonine, serine, and tyrosine residues, may also play a role in stimulating internalization.[104]

HORMONE DEGRADATION AND HORMONE TRANSPORT. Hormone degradation may occur via receptor-mediated and receptor-independent mechanisms. Receptor-mediated degradation is a by-product of internalization and occurs when the hormone is released in the strong degradative environment of the lysosome. Receptor-independent mechanisms include degradation by circulating proteases and degradation by membrane-associated enzymes distinct from the receptor. The extent to which receptor-mediated and receptor-independent pathways play a role in degradation varies from hormone to hormone. For insulin the majority of degradation is receptor-mediated, whereas for glucagon, circulating and receptor-independent membrane proteases appear to be more significant.[105, 106] In specialized cells such as endothelial cells the receptor internalization process may be modified and

BIOSYNTHESIS AND TURNOVER OF
HORMONE RECEPTORS

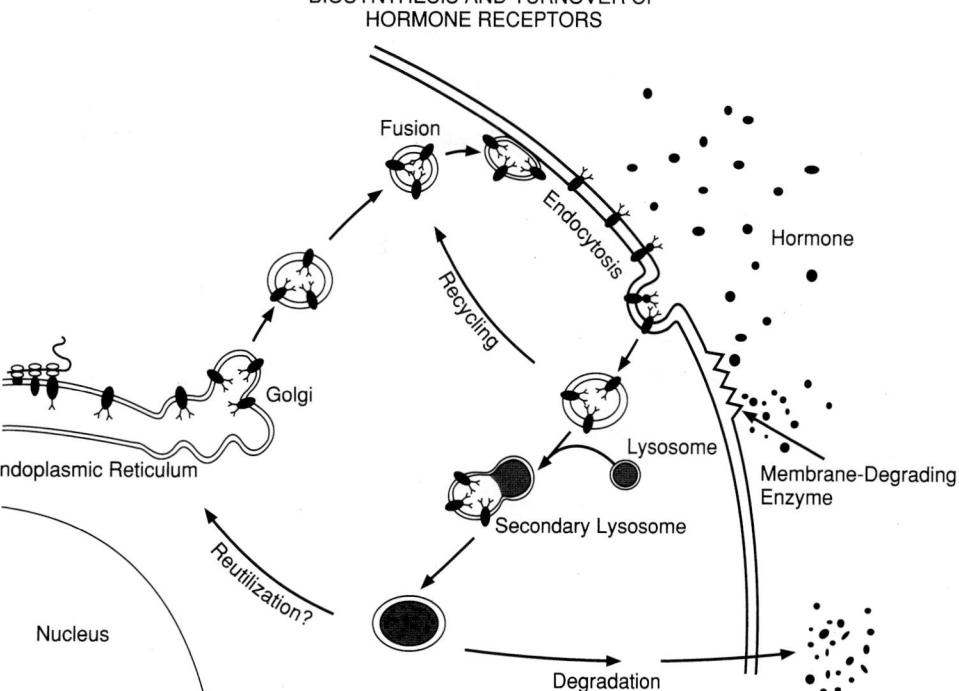

Figure 5–8. A general model for the life cycle of the hormone receptor. Membrane receptors are synthesized in the rough endoplasmic reticulum, glycosylated in the Golgi apparatus, and inserted into the membrane, probably by a process involving membrane fusion. After binding the hormone, the receptors aggregate and are internalized by either coated or noncoated pits. The endosome containing the hormone-receptor complex may fuse with lysosomes, resulting in degradation of both the hormone and the receptor, or, more likely, the hormone is degraded and the receptor recycles to the membrane.

used to carry the hormone across the vascular barrier to the extracellular space.[107, 108] This transendothelial transport may be important in bringing the hormone to the receptor on the target cell, because in many tissues the capillary network possesses tight junctions that block access of the hormone to the target cell.[109] In the endothelial cell during the process of transcytosis, there is little or no fusion of the endosomes bearing the hormone-receptor complex with lysosomes and thus little or no degradation. The exact mechanisms that govern the fate of internalized hormones, receptor recycling, and transendothelial transport are the subject of much current research.

MEMBRANE-LIPIDS, RECEPTOR AGGREGATION, AND CELLULAR SIGNALING. Peptide hormone receptors on the cell surface are integrated into the phospholipid bilayer of the plasma membrane, and this lipid environment may influence hormone action. Although the membrane limits the movement of receptors to a two-dimensional, rather than three-dimensional space, in general the transmembrane domain of receptors is alpha-helical and allows free mobility of the receptor in the lipid environment.[110, 111] In addition, the membrane lipid serves as a barrier between the ligand-binding domain outside the cell and the signal transduction domain in the membranous or intracellular portions of the receptor.

TABLE 5–2. Classification of Receptors by Mechanisms of Internalization

	Class I	Class II
Ligand	Peptide hormones, neurotransmitters	Nutrients (e.g., low-density lipoproteins, transferrin)
Internalization		
Rate	Low	High
Mechanism	Ligand stimulated	Constitutive
Primary function	Signaling	Internalization
Membrane localization	Diffuse or microvilli	Coated pits

After ligand binding the receptors aggregate or cluster.[34, 112, 113] This microaggregation or dimerization may play a critical role in receptor signaling, as evidenced by the fact that divalent antireceptor antibodies that bind to and cross-link receptors often mimic hormone action, whereas monovalent antibodies that bind to receptors, but cause no aggregation, do not [113, 114] (Fig. 5–9A and B). Although hormones in the circulation generally exist as monomers, most hormonal ligands also induce receptor dimerization or aggregation by two potential mechanisms. First, many receptors undergo some type of conformational change after ligand binding, a change that may be important in both receptor aggregation and cell signaling. Monomeric hormones may also interact with the extracellular domains of two separate receptors, thus facilitating receptor dimerization,[115] as was first demonstrated at a crystallographic level for the GH receptor interaction (see Figure 5–9C; see color section between pages 875 and 877) and has been suggested for other receptors by functional studies. Thus, peptide hormones and their receptors may have two distinct domains of interaction. The primary interaction usually involves the higher affinity interaction between one surface of the peptide hormone and its receptor. This interaction is then followed by a second between the opposite surface of the peptide hormone and an adjacent receptor. In some cases, such as for GH, only one hormone molecule is involved in bridging the two receptors. In other cases (e.g., insulin), two hormone molecules bridge the receptors by mutually complementary interactions between primary and secondary binding domains on the receptor.[116] This process of bivalent binding by a monomeric ligand results in a higher affinity of interaction and provides a mechanism for receptor cross-linking and induction of conformational change.

Because many membrane receptors require aggregation for normal signaling, diseases that result in simultaneous production of abnormal and normal receptors, such as a heterozygous genetic defect in which one allele codes for a mutant receptor and the other allele codes for a normal receptor, may produce profound alterations in signaling as the result of

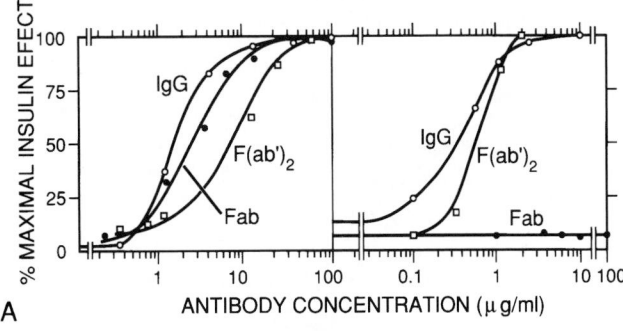

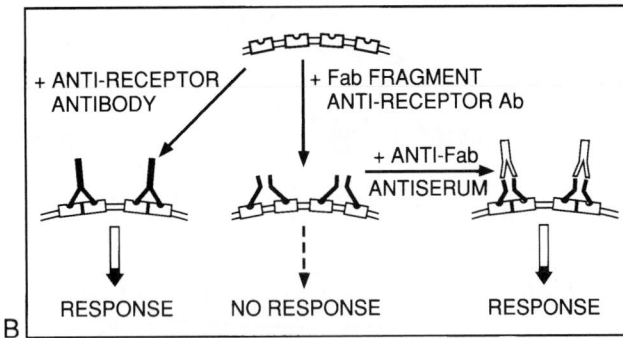

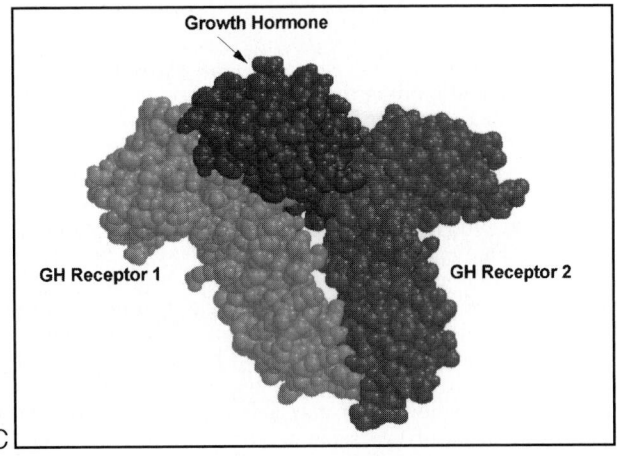

Figure 5–9. *A,* The role of valence in the binding of antibodies to the insulin receptor. *Left,* Inhibition of ^{125}I-labeled insulin binding to isolated adipocytes by antireceptor immunoglobulin F(ab')₂, and Fab. *Right,* Ability of the same preparations to stimulate glucose oxidation in these cells. Note that both monovalent (Fab) and bivalent [F(ab')₂ and immunoglobulin G] antibodies inhibit insulin binding, but only bivalent antibodies mimic insulin action. This is depicted schematically in *B.* These data, and other data indicating that hormones also stimulate receptor aggregation, have suggested an important role for receptor aggregation in cellular signaling. *C,* X-ray crystallographic model of a single growth hormone molecule binding to the extracellular domain of two adjacent growth hormone receptors (see color section between pages 875 and 877). (*A* and *B* from Kahn CR, Baird KL, Jarrett DB, et al. Direct demonstration that receptor cross-linking or aggregation is important in insulin action. Proc Natl Acad Sci USA 1978; 75:4209–4213, with permission. *C,* Data from Cunningham BC, Ultsch M, de Vos AM, et al. Science 1991; 254:821–825.)

dimerization between normal and mutant receptors.[117] Alterations in the physical properties of the plasma membrane, such as a change in phospholipid content or lipid saturation, can also augment or inhibit receptor mobility and aggregation. It is not surprising therefore that alterations in membrane lipid composition affect receptor binding and transmembrane signaling in cells in tissue culture.[118, 119] The pathophysiological significance of similar alterations in human disease, however, has not been fully explored.

GENERATION, INTEGRATION, AND CONTROL OF RECEPTOR SIGNALS

Signal Amplification and the Relationship Between Receptor Occupancy and Bioeffect

Because the concentration of peptide hormones in the circulation is usually between 10^{-12} and 10^{-9} M, target cells must not only recognize a hormone with high affinity and specificity but also amplify the hormone signal to regulate cellular metabolic processes that operate on substrates in the millimolar (10^{-3} M) concentration range. This process of amplification occurs at both the receptor and the postreceptor levels.

SPARE RECEPTORS AND COUPLING. At the level of the receptor, many peptide hormones produce a maximal biologic response when only a fraction of the total cell-surface receptors are occupied (Fig. 5–10). For example, insulin stimulation of glucose transport in adipocytes is maximal when only about 2% of all insulin receptors are occupied.[120, 121] Similar observations have been made for the actions of corticotropin (ACTH) on glucocorticoid production in the adrenal and gonadotropins on steroidogenesis in the ovary and testis.[122] This phenomenon has given rise to the concept of *spare receptors,* implying that the maximal hormonal response occurs when fewer than 100% of receptors are occupied. This does not mean, however, that some receptors are active and others inactive. Rather it appears that all receptors are active, but occupancy of only a small fraction is sufficient to produce the final bioeffect. In some cases maximal hormonal response occurs with as few as 50 to 100 receptors occupied, even though the cell has tens or hundreds of thousands of receptors for the hormone in question.

A second, more subtle difference between receptor occupancy and hormone action is *nonlinear coupling.* This implies that the half-maximal effect occurs with less than 50% of the occupancy required for a maximal effect. Nonlinear coupling and spare receptors often exist together, resulting in very sensitive dose-response curves for hormone action.

Receptor occupancy and signal generation play important physiological roles both in the kinetics of hormone action and in the potential for regulation in disease states. Because the affinity of most receptors for their hormonal ligands is relatively low, considering the circulating concentration of the hormone, the binding of the hormone to its receptor would be slow if it were not for the high number of receptors on the cell surface. The excess receptors increase the forward reaction rate, especially at low hormone concentrations, so that hormone binding and signal activation are rapid. Conversely, as the concentration of hormone in the blood begins to fall, the occupation of spare receptors by the hormone may allow the signal to persist beyond the circulating half-life of the hormone.

Similar types of signal amplification occur at postreceptor steps in the hormone action pathway.[122] For example, hormones that act through stimulation of adenylate cyclase and accumulation of cAMP usually produce more cAMP than is required for maximal activation of cAMP-dependent protein kinase. Likewise, cAMP-dependent protein kinase is usually activated beyond the level required for maximal substrate phosphorylation. Thus, a series of increasingly sensitive dose-response curves amplifies the hormone signal at each step in the action pathway (see Fig. 5–10*B*).

HORMONE-RESISTANT STATES. In a system with no spare receptors and no postreceptor amplification, a 50% decrease in receptor number or a 50% decrease in any postreceptor step would result in a 50% decrease in the final biologic

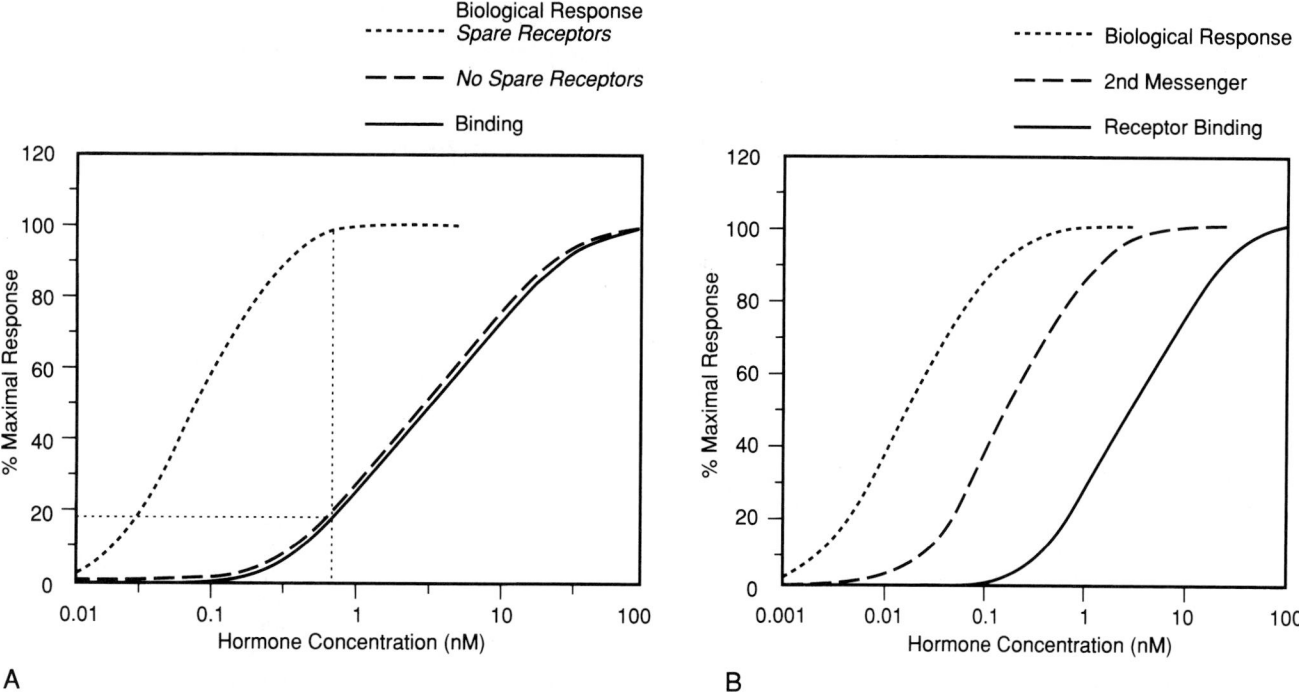

Figure 5–10. Correlation between hormone binding and biologic response. *A,* Effect of spare receptors for amplifying signal. The solid line represents a hormone binding to its receptor. The dashed line indicates a biologic response in which there are no spare receptors. The dotted line indicates a response for which there are spare receptors. In the last case, the maximal biologic response occurs with less than 20% receptor occupancy. *B,* Amplification of hormonal signaling. When it is possible to measure intermediate steps in hormonal signaling, there is often progressive signal amplification as one goes from receptor binding to second messenger to final biologic response.

response. By contrast, in a system with many spare receptors, a 50% fall in receptor number produces only a small rightward shift in the dose-response curve for hormone action and no change in the maximal response. A decrease in maximal response occurs only when receptor concentration falls to very low levels (Fig. 5–11).

Thus, analysis of the relationship between hormone concentration and hormone action in a pathologic state can provide insight into the site of the altered hormone response (Fig. 5–12). Hormone-resistant states in which there is only decreased sensitivity to the hormone, i.e., a rightward shift in the dose-response curve with no change in maximal response,[123] implies a defect at a step that is not rate-limiting. In cells with spare receptors this defect is often a decrease in the number of receptors. Decreased sensitivity may also be at a postreceptor step involved in amplification. In both of these states of decreased sensitivity, increasing the hormone concentration overcomes the resistance and eventually produces a normal biologic response. In some states of hormone resistance, there is a decrease in the maximal response, i.e., decreased responsiveness, with or without a concomitant decrease in sensitivity. Decreased responsiveness implies a defect at some rate-limiting step in the hormone action pathway. Usually, but not always, this is a postreceptor site. In such states, increasing hormone concentrations produces increasing bioresponse only up to a point, and the maximal response is never normal.

Integration and Control of Hormone Signals

The classic concept that a single hormone acts on a single type of receptor to produce a single type of postreceptor signal and biologic response is no longer valid. At every step in the pathway there is an opportunity for divergence of the

signal and for interaction between the primary signal and other signaling pathways. These may amplify or attenuate the action of the hormone (Fig. 5–13). Peptide hormones that interact with families of related hormone receptors may produce several independent but interrelated signals. Some receptor systems also interact with several different types of second messenger systems. For example, angiotensin II acts through a G protein–coupled receptor to stimulate both phosphoinositide turnover and calcium flux.[124] The same receptor also activates cytoplasmic tyrosine kinases, through an undefined mechanism, resulting in stimulation of tyrosine phosphorylation of several proteins and activation of the downstream signals associated with SRC homology-2 (SH2) domain proteins binding to these phosphotyrosine substrates. Likewise, even the apparently self-contained tyrosine kinase receptors (the insulin, IGF-I, EGF, PDGF, and CSF-1 receptors) may produce multiple postreceptor signals. Although the exact mechanism of such divergent effects remains unknown, these findings clearly indicate the complexity of the signaling pathway. Superimposed on these divergent signals, each individual pathway may contain multiple levels of both positive and negative feedback.

Interaction between different hormones and their signaling pathways may take a variety of forms. At the simplest level, these may represent synergistic or antagonistic effects of two hormones on a single effector system or enzyme, such as the interplay between insulin and glucagon on glycogenolysis and glycogen synthesis. Such interactions may occur via heterologous receptor regulation or via interaction of postreceptor signals. At a more subtle level, one branch of the signal pathway for a hormone may synergize with a pathway of action of another hormone, while other divergent branches of these pathways may antagonize one another. In its entirety, the endocrine signaling system comprises a series of convergent and divergent pathways interacting through feedback control to maintain a delicate homeostatic balance.

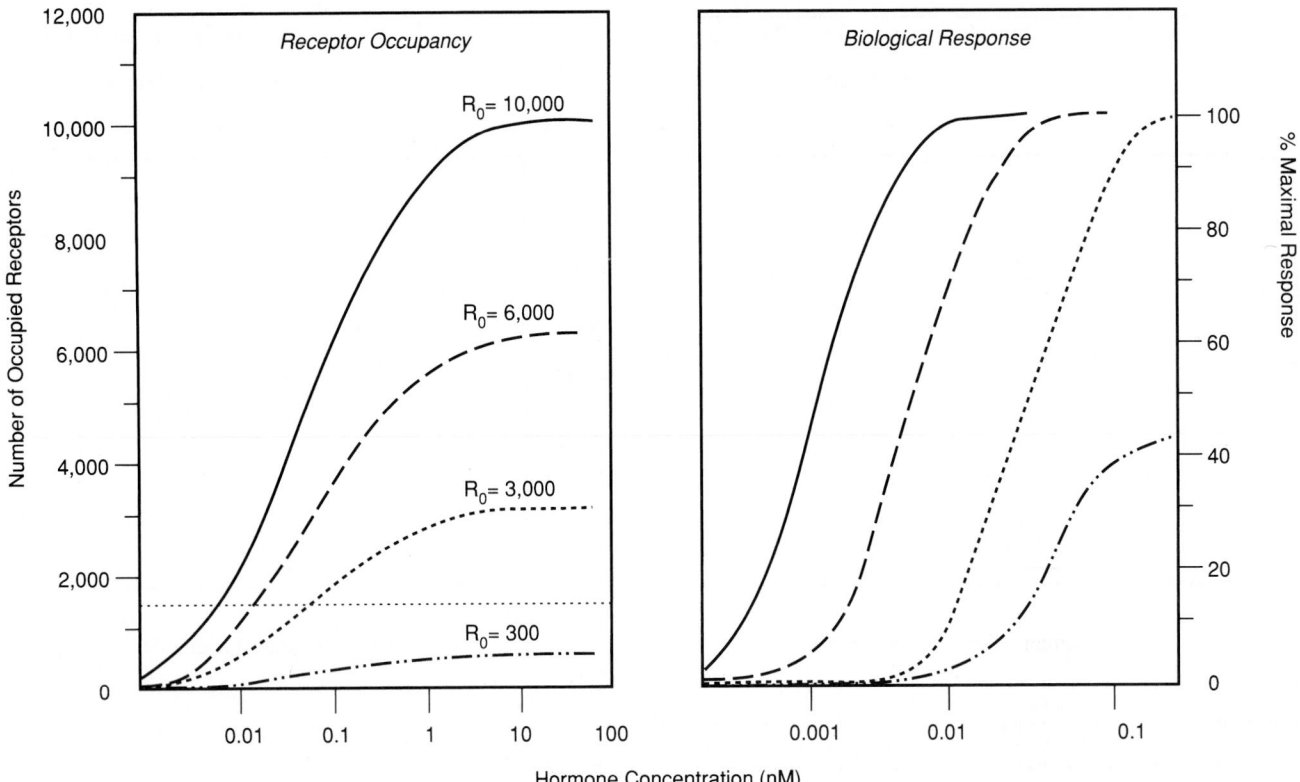

Figure 5–11. Effect of spare receptors on signaling after a loss of receptors. The original curve *(solid line)* represents the binding curve and biologic response curve for $K_d = 0.1$, total receptor sites = 10,000 per cell, and a capacity of cell to respond to 10,000 occupied receptors. When only the number of receptor sites per cell is reduced, there is at each hormone concentration a proportional reduction in the concentration of the hormone-receptor complex and in biologic response and a shift in the dose-response curve to the right. Because only about 18% receptor occupancy is needed to achieve a maximal response, this maximal response is reduced only when the total receptor concentration R_0 falls below 1800.

RECEPTOR REGULATION AND MECHANISMS OF DESENSITIZATION

Homologous Receptor Regulation

To achieve the precise balance of hormone signals that characterizes normal endocrine homeostasis, multiple regulatory factors modulate each step of hormone action. Physiological and pathologic factors alter hormone binding affinity, receptor number, signal transmission ability of membrane receptors, and postreceptor steps in hormone action and thus play a role in normal physiology and in disease (Table 5–3). This regulation of receptor binding and signaling may serve to desensitize or hypersensitize a hormone response. The regulatory mechanism can be classified by the site of regulation—i.e., factors that alter receptor binding versus factors that affect receptor or postreceptor signaling—and by the nature of the regulatory factor—*homologous regulation* referring

TABLE 5–3. Mechanisms of Regulation of Hormone Receptors and Their Signals

Hormone binding
Receptor concentration
    Down-regulation
    Up-regulation
Receptor signaling
    Receptor phosphorylation
    Altered membrane lipids
    Interaction with nonreceptor proteins
    Conformational changes
Postreceptor alterations

to effects of the hormone itself and *heterologous regulation* related to effects of other hormones or drugs.

Hormone binding increases the rate of internalization of many polypeptide hormone and growth factor receptors,[101, 125, 126] and this *ligand-induced internalization* increases the fraction of receptors inside the cell and accelerates receptor degradation.[127–131] The net result is a *down-regulation* of the total number of receptors and a decrease in the number of receptors available to bind hormone on the cell surface.[132, 133] This type of negative homologous regulation may function as a simple negative-feedback loop that reduces receptor concentration when hormone concentrations are chronically elevated, thus protecting the cell against excessive hormone action. The regulation process is often imperfect, however, in that a small increase in hormone concentration produces a relatively large amount of down-regulation, thus leading to a hormone-resistant state. For example, in obesity and in type II diabetes mellitus, hyperinsulinemia leads to down-regulation of the insulin receptor and contributes to insulin resistance.

Although most hormones cause down-regulation of their receptors, in some circumstances hormones can act as positive homologous regulators. For example, when liver cells are exposed to prolactin, receptor synthesis is stimulated, and the consequent increase in receptor number is not offset by receptor down-regulation.[134] The net result is a positive feedback loop leading to enhanced cellular responsiveness to the hormone.

In addition to regulating the number of cell surface receptors in target cells, hormone binding can initiate other forms of homologous regulation at the receptor level, the postreceptor level, or both. For example, hormone-induced

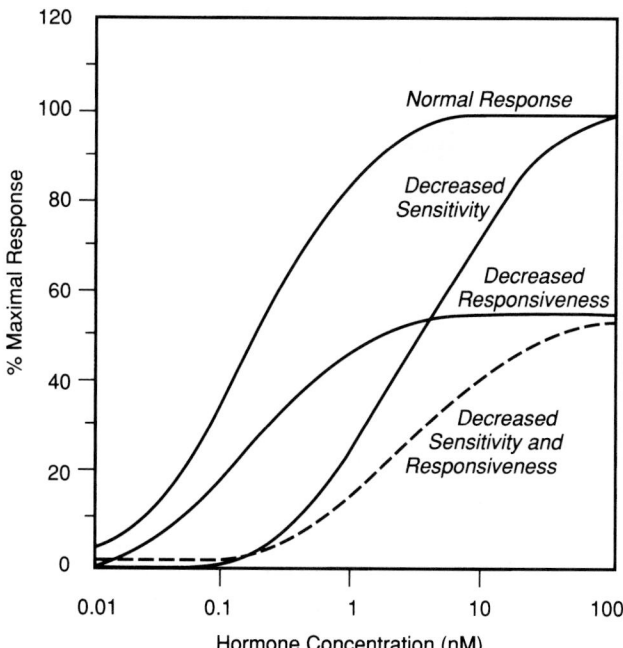

Figure 5–12. Types of resistance to hormone action. In hormone-resistant states, there may be a rightward shift of the dose-response curve (decreased sensitivity), a decrease in maximal response (decreased responsiveness), or a combination of the two. Decreased sensitivity indicates a defect at a non–rate-limiting step (often the receptor), whereas decreased responsiveness indicates a defect at a rate-limiting step (usually postreceptor). (Adapted from Kahn CR. Insulin resistance, insulin insensitivity and insulin unresponsiveness: a necessary distinction. Metabolism 1978; 27[Suppl 2]:1893–1902, with permission.)

to the inner surface of the plasma membrane via a geranylgeranyl isoprenyl lipid-anchoring group in a favored position for phosphorylation of the receptor. The receptor is phosphorylated on multiple serine residues by the kinase; this leads to the coupling of the protein β-arrestin to the receptor; and β-arrestin inhibits further G protein association with the receptor.

The overall result of this elaborate homologous regulatory scheme is rapid desensitization of β-adrenergic receptors following their initial hormone-induced activation. Although receptor phosphorylation has a negative regulatory effect on β-adrenergic receptor signaling, hormone-induced phosphorylation of other receptors can have a positive effect on signaling. For example, insulin binding also results in phosphorylation of its receptor. In this case, however, phosphorylation of specific receptor tyrosine residues is a direct action of the protein kinase intrinsic to the insulin receptor, resulting in enhanced insulin receptor kinase activity toward cellular substrates and potentiation of insulin action.[136, 137]

Heterologous Receptor Regulation

Positive heterologous regulation also plays an essential role in the complex interactions characteristic of endocrine regulation. Follicle-stimulating hormone (FSH) stimulates the production of LH receptors in the ovary, which leads to normal maturation of the ovum.[138] Prolactin also potentiates LH action in the Leydig cell, in part, by increasing the number of LH receptors.[139] Thyroid hormone augments the expression of β-adrenergic receptors, accounting for some of the findings of a hyperadrenergic state in hyperthyroid patients.[140] Estrogens cause an increase in the number of oxytocin receptors in the uterus[141] and also augment the effect of prolactin to increase expression of prolactin receptor number in mammary tissues.[142] Negative heterologous regulation also occurs. Stimulation of protein kinase C by adrenergic agents alters insulin receptor signaling and down-regulates the EGF receptor.[143] Down-regulation of the EGF receptor also occurs after stimulation of cells by PDGF through protein kinase C–independent mechanisms.[144] Some hormones exert both positive and negative effects by acting at different points in the hormone action cascade and thus produce complex effects. Glucocorticoids, for example, lower the binding affinity of insulin receptors in adipose tissue but increase receptor expression at a transcriptional level in lymphoid tissue.[145, 146] Glucocorticoids also increase the synthesis of many insulin counterregulatory enzymes at the transcriptional level.[147] A variety of other factors, including membrane lipid composition, the state of cell growth and differentiation, drugs, and

activation of G protein–coupled receptors leads to desensitization within seconds to minutes, despite the continued presence of hormone and cell surface receptors.[59, 135] The mechanism of this type of homologous receptor desensitization, which was first elucidated in studies on β-adrenergic receptors, is illustrated in Figure 5–14.[59] After hormone binding, the activated receptor associates with specific heterotrimeric G proteins that mediate hormone signaling through their subsequent interaction with intracellular second messengers; e.g., activating adenylate (adenylyl) cyclase and thus stimulating the formation of cAMP. As part of this signaling reaction, the G protein dissociates into a G_α monomer and a $G_{\beta\gamma}$ heterodimer. The free βγ heterodimer rapidly associates with a cytosolic protein kinase (β-adrenergic receptor kinase in this example), serving both to activate the kinase and to localize it

Figure 5–13. Interaction between hormone-signaling pathways. *Left,* A simple (idealized) signal response system, which rarely exists in nature. Most signaling pathways contain a multitude of divergent and convergent pathways, positive- and negative-feedback loops, and other interactions *(right).*

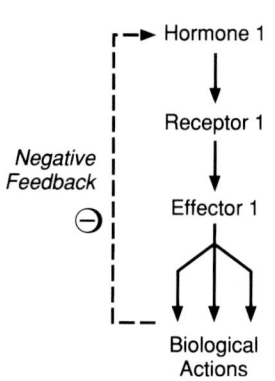

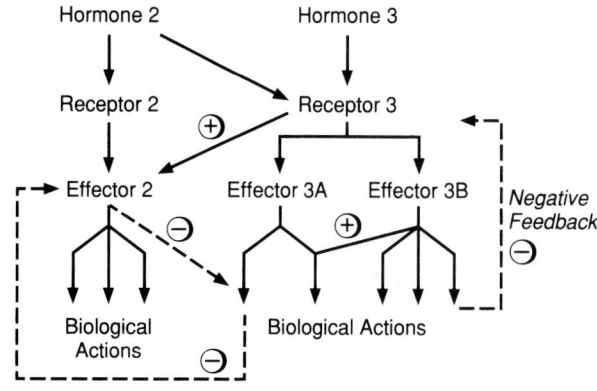

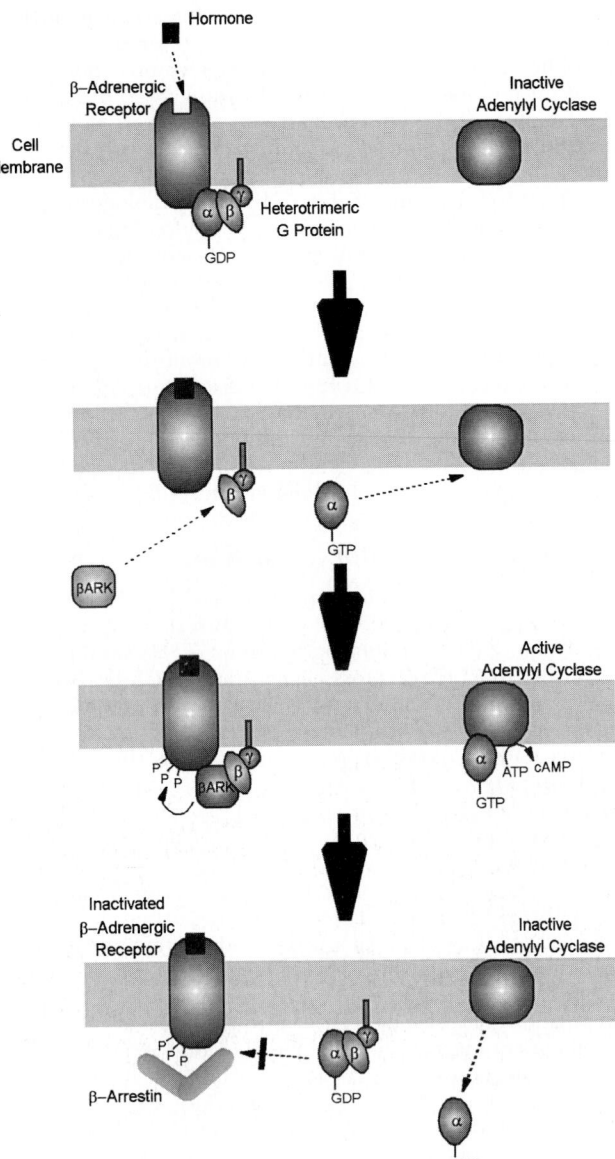

Figure 5–14. Proposed mechanism for ligand-induced desensitization of the β-adrenergic receptor. Hormone binding leads to GTP loading of receptor-associated heterotrimeric G protein α subunit, which subsequently dissociates and activates adenylate (adenylyl) cyclase. The remaining βγ dimer associates with β-adrenergic receptor kinase (βARK), which then phosphorylates the receptor. This leads to binding of β-arrestin to the receptor, which blocks further G protein association and thus prevents continued signaling.

viral infection, may also alter receptor binding and signal transduction properties (Table 5–4). Although knowledge of receptor regulation is still incomplete, signal transduction in the endocrine system is regulated as much at the level of the target cell as by alterations in hormone levels.

CELLULAR MECHANISMS OF PEPTIDE HORMONE ACTION

Protein Phosphorylation in Hormone Action

The actions of peptide hormones, whether mediated by cell-surface receptors that possess intrinsic enzyme or ion

TABLE 5–4. Factors Affecting Receptor Concentration or Affinity and Postreceptor Signaling

Homologous hormone
Heterologous hormones
Ions and other small molecules
Drugs
Membrane lipid composition
Cell growth and differentiation
Viral infection
Antibodies to the receptor
Covalent modifications (e.g., phosphorylation, glycosylation)

channel activities or linked via a G protein to the generation of cAMP or some other form of second messenger, ultimately are coupled to the metabolic machinery of the cell. This process occurs by mechanisms that include modification of enzymes or proteins critical to intracellular pathways, stimulation of transport processes, or regulation of transcription of genes encoding proteins involved in the hormone action cascade. One of the most important regulatory mechanisms involves the covalent, reversible modification of proteins through transfer of phosphate groups from ATP to specific hydroxy amino acids—usually serine, but sometimes threonine or tyrosine (Fig. 5–15A). Protein modification by phosphorylation and dephosphorylation of serine residues often represents a final step in the transmission of peptide hormone signals. Many key regulatory enzymes exist in alternative phosphorylated and dephosphorylated states that differ markedly in their catalytic activity (Table 5–5). In some cases, phosphorylation activates the enzyme; in others, it inactivates the enzyme. The level of enzyme phosphorylation is determined by the activities of two types of enzymes: protein kinases that catalyze phosphorylation and phosphoprotein phosphatases that catalyze dephosphorylation (see Fig. 5–15B). Specific kinases and phosphatases may be limited in their actions to a single target enzyme or may act on multiple regulatory proteins.

SERINE PHOSPHORYLATION PATHWAYS. Serine phosphorylation control mechanisms are involved in the actions of cAMP-dependent protein kinase, calmodulin-sensitive pathways, protein kinase C–mediated actions, and many other regulatory processes.[148] The control of a single biologic response can involve modification of rates of both phosphorylation and dephosphorylation reactions, as a consequence of the interrelated effects of multiple hormones. In the glycogen pathway, for example, insulin and epinephrine have opposite actions on the net flux of glucose into and out of glycogen through hormone-specific effects on the same phosphorylation/dephosphorylation reactions (Fig. 5–16).[149] Stimulation by insulin of the phosphorylation of a serine residue at a location designated site 1 in the G subunit of protein phosphatase-1 increases the activity of protein phosphatase-1, which then dephosphorylates both glycogen synthase and glycogen phosphorylase, leading to their activation and deactivation, respectively. The result is increased glycogen synthesis

TABLE 5–5. Selected Enzymes and Proteins Regulated by Phosphorylation and Dephosphorylation

Activation by Phosphorylation	Inhibition by Phosphorylation
Phosphorylase kinase	Glycogen synthase
Glycogen phosphorylase	Pyruvate kinase
Triglyceride lipase	β-Adrenergic receptor
ATP citrate lyase	Insulin receptor (serine or threonine)
Ribosomal S6 kinase	
Insulin receptor (tyrosine)	

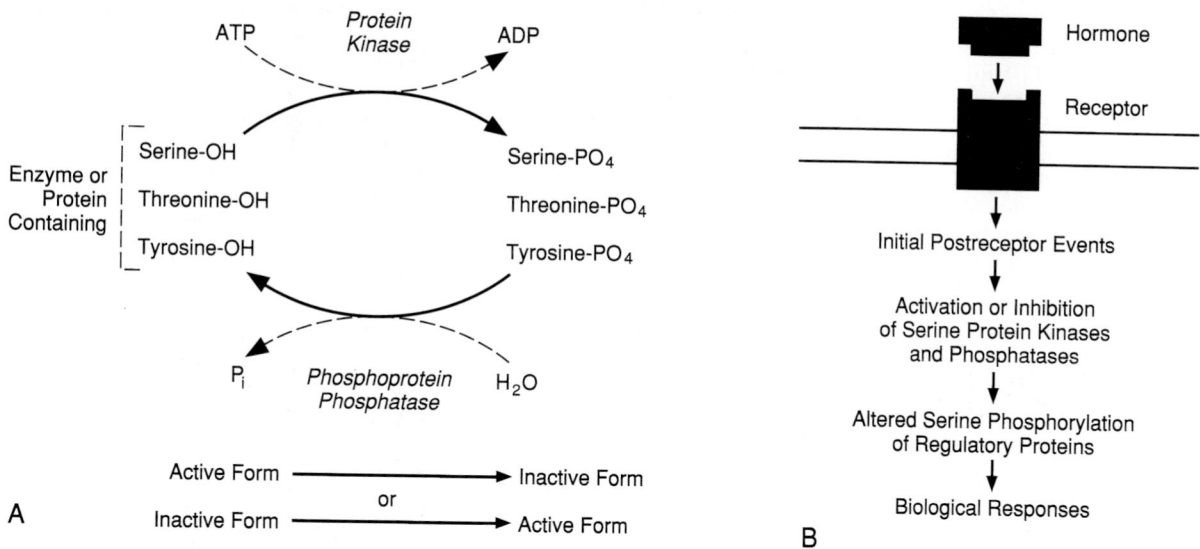

Figure 5–15. *A*, Regulation of enzymes and other proteins by phosphorylation and dephosphorylation. In phosphorylation of a protein, a protein kinase stimulates the transfer of a phosphate group from ATP to a hydroxyl group on the side chain of a serine, threonine, or tyrosine residue. The phosphate group can be removed by the action of phosphoprotein phosphatases. This process usually results in conversion of an active protein or enzyme to an inactive form, or vice versa (see Table 5–5). *B*, Role of phosphorylation and dephosphorylation of serine in mediating the effects of peptide hormones in metabolic pathways.

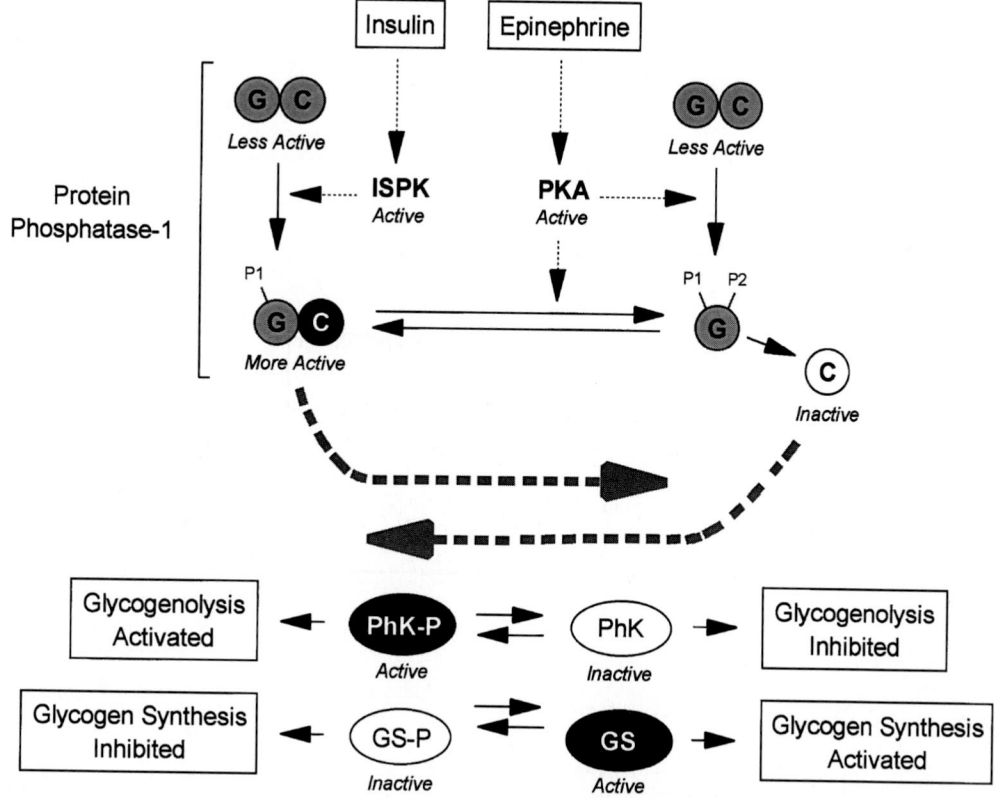

Figure 5–16. Regulation of glycogen metabolism by insulin and epinephrine through oppositely directed effects on protein phosphatase-1. Insulin stimulates one or more insulin-dependent protein kinases (ISPK), which activate protein phosphatase-1 as a consequence of serine phosphorylation at site 1 in its regulatory G subunit. Inhibition of phosphorylase kinase (PhK) and stimulation of glycogen synthase (GS) by subsequent protein phosphatase-1–mediated dephosphorylation result in net glycogen synthesis. Epinephrine stimulates protein kinase A (PKA), which phosphorylates a serine residue at site 2 in the G subunit of protein phosphatase-1. This leads to inactivation of protein phosphatase-1 through dissociation of its catalytic C subunit, accumulation of PhK and GS in phosphorylated forms, and consequent net glycogen breakdown. (Redrawn from Cohen P. Dissection of the protein phosphorylation cascades involved in insulin and growth factor action. Biochem Soc Trans 1993; 21:555–567; and from Cohen P. Signal integration at the level of protein kinases, protein phosphatases and their substrates. Trends Biochem Sci 1992; 17:408–413, with permission from Elsevier Science.)

and decreased glycogen breakdown. Epinephrine, by contrast, initiates a series of cellular signaling events that lead to the activation of cAMP-dependent protein kinase, which phosphorylates a different serine residue (site 2) in the G subunit of protein phosphatase-1. This causes the dissociation of the G subunit from the enzyme, the release of protein phosphatase-1 from glycogen, decreased dephosphorylation of glycogen synthase and glycogen phosphorylase, and a resulting increase in net glycogen breakdown. The site 2 inhibitory effect overcomes the site 1 activating effect when both serines are phosphorylated, thus explaining the fact that epinephrine can stimulate net glycogenolysis even in the presence of insulin.

The cAMP-dependent protein kinase involved in the epinephrine signaling pathway is a particularly important serine kinase that is involved in the actions of many members of the large G protein–coupled receptor family.[150] Its activity is regulated by the second messenger molecule cAMP, which is formed intracellularly in response to activation of the integral membrane enzyme adenylate (adenylyl) cyclase, as shown in Figure 5–17. Following hormone binding, G protein–coupled receptors associate with heterotrimeric G proteins, and the resulting complex activates or inhibits the adenylate cyclase enzyme, depending on receptor coupling with G_s or G_i proteins, respectively. Activation of adenylate cyclase leads to

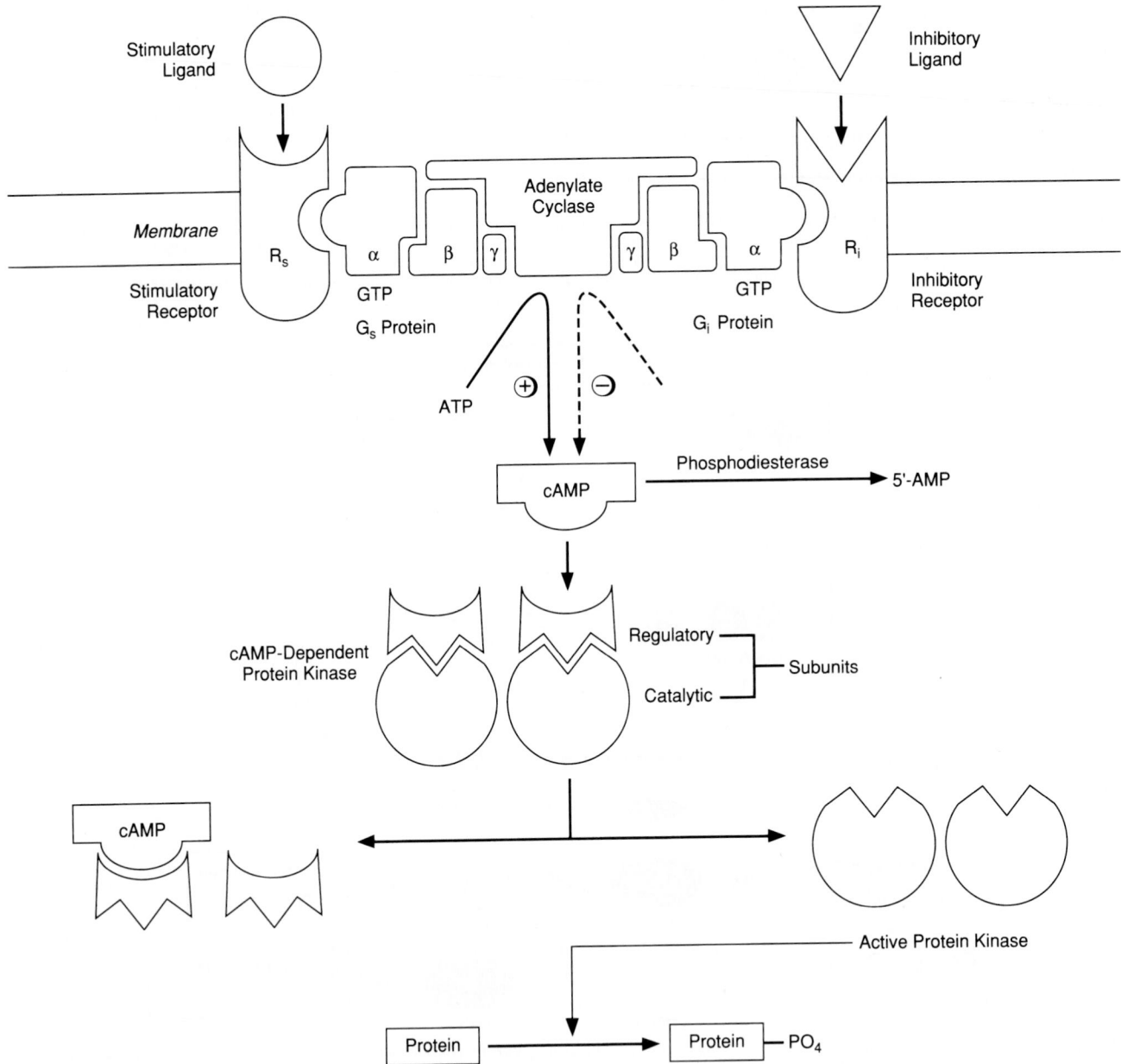

Figure 5–17. Schematic depiction of the adenylate cyclase system. Stimulatory ligands (H_s) and inhibitory ligands (H_i) interact with their respective receptors (R_s and R_i). The H_s-R_s complex then activates adenylate cyclase via interaction with the regulatory coupling protein G_s. In the process G_s binds GTP and hydrolyzes it to GDP. The H_i-R_i complex inhibits adenylate cyclase via a homologous regulatory protein G_i. When the catalytic component of adenylate cyclase is activated, ATP is converted to cAMP, which in turn activates cAMP-dependent protein kinase and results in substrate phosphorylation. cAMP-dependent protein kinases consist of four subunits, two catalytic subunits (C) and a dimer regulatory subunit (R-R), which can bind two molecules of cAMP. When cAMP binds to the regulatory dimer of the holoenzyme, the two catalytic subunits are released and become fully active. With removal of cAMP, the regulatory dimer reassociates with catalytic subunits, inactivating the latter. Recent data indicate that a total of four cAMP molecules bind to the regulatory dimer.

Note that R is widely used as an abbreviation for receptor as well as for regulatory components, especially for the regulatory component of cAMP-dependent protein kinases. Also note that C is widely used as an abbreviation for a catalytic component of an enzyme, especially for adenylate cyclase and cAMP-dependent protein kinase.

rapid formation of cAMP from ATP. In a concentration-dependent manner, cAMP then forms a complex with the regulatory subunit of cAMP-dependent protein kinase, leading to the release of free, active subunits of the enzyme.

TYROSINE PHOSPHORYLATION IN RECEPTOR SIGNALING. Many peptide hormone and growth factor receptors contain an intrinsic tyrosine kinase activity that is activated by hormone binding. These include, for example, receptors for insulin, IGF-I, EGF, PDGF, nerve growth factor, and fibroblast growth factor (FGF).[74, 151–154] Growth hormone receptors and various cytokine receptors do not contain an intrinsic kinase activity but activate nonreceptor tyrosine kinases within the cell.[155, 156] The activation of these receptor and nonreceptor tyrosine kinases is followed by autophosphorylation (usually via a *trans* interaction between two kinase molecules) and the tyrosine phosphorylation of other proteins within the cell.[157, 158] It was initially thought that the signaling by tyrosine kinases involves the tyrosine phosphorylation and activation of serine-threonine kinases or phosphatases. This would provide a direct connection between receptors that activate tyrosine kinases and the elaborate serine-threonine kinase regulatory pathways noted earlier. However, it now clear that phosphotyrosine residues in receptors and nonreceptor proteins most often function as specific docking sites that bind with high affinity to modular domains in other proteins, including SH2 and phosphotyrosine binding (PTB) domains.[158–160] These hormone-induced protein interactions sometimes lead to stimulation of catalytic activity in the associated protein or, alternatively, activate cellular signaling responses by initiating the assembly of multiple proteins into a catalytically active complex.[161] The major goals of current studies are to establish how hormone-stimulated tyrosine phosphorylation leads to divergent responses arising from a single hormone, specific responses to different tyrosine kinase receptors, and interactions between different hormone signaling pathways.

Regulation of Membrane Transport

Many peptide hormones regulate the interaction of the cell with its environment by governing the movement of nutrients and ions into and out of the cell. The control of ion transport may be directly affected by receptors that act as ligand-gated ion channels, whereas the control of influx of nutrients, such as glucose and amino acids, involves actions of the hormones on specific transport systems for these molecules (Fig. 5–18).

AMINO ACID TRANSPORT. At least five different carrier systems for amino acids are present in the plasma membrane of mammalian cells,[162, 163] each of which depends on the function of a specific transport protein that recognizes a group of closely related amino acids. Most of these amino acid transporters function as cotransport systems, or symports, that transport Na^+ together with the amino acid. Not all amino acid transport systems are hormonally regulated. The neutral amino acid transport system, which shows preference for alanine, glycine, and proline, termed system A, is the most active of the hormonally regulated systems and responds to insulin, glucagon, and glucocorticoids, and to other peptide hormones.[162, 164]

The regulatory effects of different hormones on amino acid transport in differentiated tissues appear to be determined, in large part, by tissue-specific expression of hormone receptors. Thus, amino acid transport is increased by corticotropin in adrenal tissue, by glucagon in the liver, by LH in the ovary, and by insulin in muscle, liver, fat, and a number of other tissues. Although the exact steps involved in hormone stimulation of transport remain uncertain, the effect does not appear to be direct. There is usually a lag of 5 to 15 min

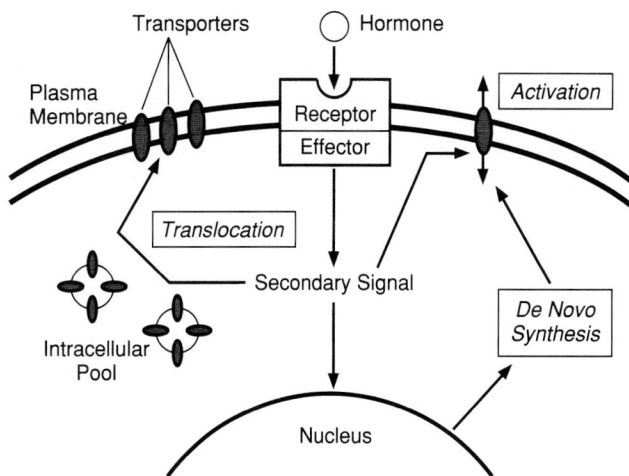

Figure 5–18. Possible mechanisms of hormone stimulation of membrane transport. Hormones act on amino acid and glucose transport by a number of mechanisms, which include de novo synthesis, activation, and translocation of transporters from an intracellular pool to the plasma membrane.

between hormone administration and the increase in transport, and the cell is then committed to the increase in transport for a period of time, even if the hormone is removed.[165] For hormones known to act via cAMP, the stimulation of transport can be mimicked in isolated cells by cAMP analogues.

As with many other hormone actions, there is nonlinear coupling between receptor occupancy and transport activation, so that half the maximum response may be observed with 5 to 20% receptor occupancy. In most cases the increase in transport activity is associated with an increase in the V_{max} of the transporter. Possible mechanisms for this increase in V_{max} include de novo synthesis of the transporter molecules, post-translational conversion of inactive transporters to an active form, translocation of transporters from an intracellular pool to a membrane pool, or some effect secondary to an increase in membrane potential that might secondarily increase transport as a result of the dependence of these systems on the cotransport of sodium ions (see Fig. 5–8). Although the characterization of amino acid transporter proteins has progressed slowly, the cDNAs that encode several transporters have been cloned. The availability of cDNAs corresponding to additional transporters should make it possible to define the molecular basis of amino acid transport regulation by cell surface receptors.[163, 166]

GLUCOSE TRANSPORT. Hormone regulation of sugar transport, especially glucose transport, is an important action of insulin.[167, 168] Seven mammalian glucose transporter genes have been identified by cDNA cloning and sequencing.[167, 169] All of the transporters are proteins of 45 to 50 kd and possess 12 membrane-spanning domains. One (SGLT1) is a Na^+, glucose cotransporter involved in the active transport of glucose by intestinal epithelium and renal tubular cells; four transporters (GLUT1 to GLUT4) are involved in Na^+-independent facilitative diffusion of glucose into cells. GLUT5 appears to preferentially transport fructose, and the role of GLUT7 as a mediator of glucose flux across endoplasmic reticulum membrane is being investigated. A cDNA designated GLUT6 represents a pseudogene.

The vast majority of studies on hormonal regulation of glucose transporters have focused on GLUT1 and GLUT4.[168] GLUT1 is the most widely distributed of the transporter isoforms and is expressed in many fetal and adult mammalian tissues. The protein is abundant in most cultured cells, and the quantity of GLUT1 in various cultured cells is increased by multiple hormones, including thyroid hormone, insulin,

IGF-I, PDGF, FGF, GH, and transforming growth factor β. GLUT4 has a more limited tissue distribution, with abundant expression only in skeletal muscle, cardiac muscle, and adipose tissue. GLUT4 is of great importance, however, because it is the principal insulin-regulated glucose transporter. Changes in GLUT4 in response to insulin are a significant determinant of overall glucose uptake and plasma glucose concentrations.[169–172]

Insulin stimulation of glucose transport by GLUT4 appears to involve a unique translocation mechanism.[173] Under basal conditions, most GLUT4 transporters are in an intracellular pool associated with microsomal membranes. Insulin causes a rapid movement of these transporters to the plasma membrane, where they take up glucose from the extracellular milieu. Although the major effects of insulin on glucose transport can be explained by this translocation mechanism, the transporters may also be activated so that each transporter can take up more glucose, especially in response to other stimulators of transport. Insulin also stimulates translocation of IGF-II receptors and LDL receptors to the plasma membrane, where they then participate in the uptake of the IGF-II and lipoproteins, respectively.

Regulation of Gene Expression by Membrane Receptors

In addition to the modulation of phosphorylation of key proteins and enzymes, cytoskeleton assembly, transport, and other phenomena, binding of peptide hormones to membrane receptors may influence the regulation of gene expression.[174, 175] The best-characterized examples of such messengers/transcription factors are the cAMP response element–binding protein (CREB)[176] and c-*jun*/c-*fos*, which appear to mediate protein kinase C action.[177]

A general scheme for peptide hormone regulation of gene expression is shown in Figure 5–19. In this model, the interaction of hormone, receptor, and effector results in stimulation of a cytoplasmic or receptor-associated protein kinase, such as cAMP kinase, protein kinase C, or Janus (JAK) protein tyrosine kinases. These kinases, or other downstream kinases, phosphorylate regulatory proteins capable of entering the nucleus and binding to specific DNA sequences in the control regions (generally the 5′-flanking sequences) of the gene to be regulated. This sequence or hormone-response element (HRE) is generally only 6 to 10 nucleotides long but may be duplicated to allow binding of the regulatory protein as a dimer. Such HREs are members of a family of DNA sequences known as enhancers, which may be both orientation- and position-independent. They bind nuclear transcription factors and modulate the overall rate of gene transcription. Binding of the regulatory protein to the HRE results in an increase or a decrease in transcription of the regulated gene and a consequent increase or decrease in levels of its respective messenger RNA (mRNA) and protein products. Peptide hormones may also regulate gene expression by influencing mRNA translation, mRNA half-life or stability, and protein processing and/or degradation.

cAMP REGULATION OF GENE EXPRESSION. A palindromic octamer DNA sequence TGACGTCA (cAMP-response element, or CRE) is present in the 5′ region of several cAMP-responsive genes, including those encoding somatostatin (somatotropin release–inhibiting factor, or SRIF), phosphoenolpyruvate carboxykinase, vasoactive intestinal peptide, and the α subunit of the glycoprotein hormones.[178] This sequence mediates cAMP stimulation of gene expression in the presence of either a homologous or a heterologous promoter. A 43-kd protein in the nuclei of cells that are responsive to cAMP binds to the CRE with high affinity. This protein has been termed the *cAMP-response element–binding protein (CREB)*.

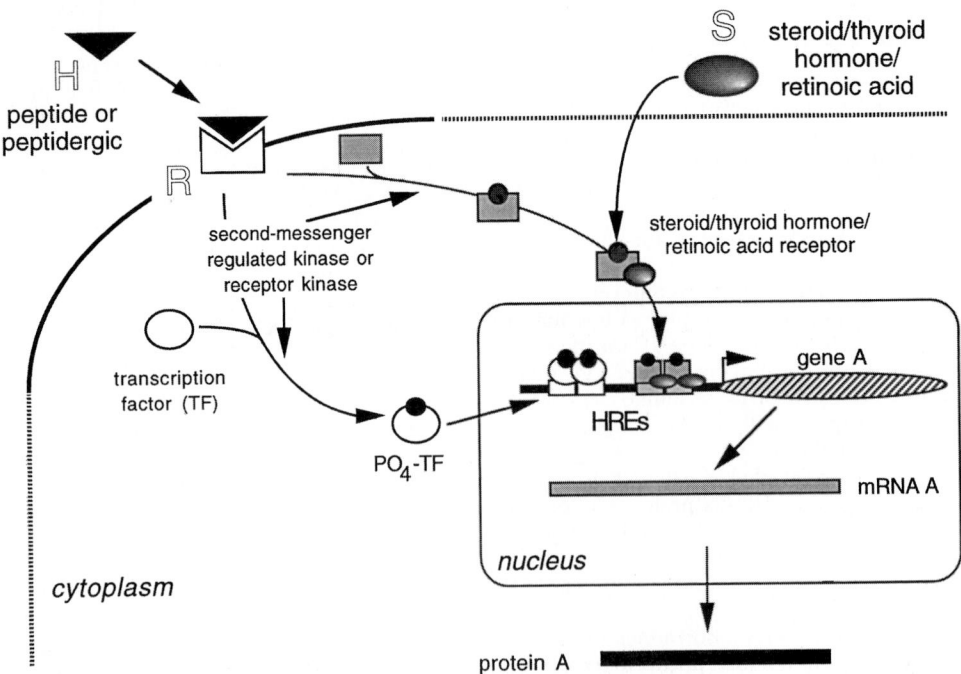

Figure 5–19. General scheme of peptide hormone regulation of gene expression. Interaction of a peptide or peptidergic hormone (H) with its target cell surface receptor (R) results ultimately in the production of second messengers or an activated receptor kinase. These molecules may, in turn, activate other cytoplasmic kinases that can phosphorylate transcription factors (TFs). Such modified TFs (PO₄-TFs) can then act in the nucleus to modulate gene expression by binding to hormone response elements (HREs) in gene regulatory regions, often by dimers, as shown. Alterations of gene A transcription may lead to changes in steady-state levels of corresponding mRNA A and protein A. Steroid/thyroid hormones and retinoic acids (S) act by binding to ligand-regulated transcription factors, known as nuclear steroid/thyroid hormone/retinoic acid receptors, that act at different HREs. This figure depicts the ability of cell surface receptors to modify the response of these nuclear receptors by a post-translational or phosphorylation event. In this fashion, molecular cross-talk may be achieved via hormone systems that have fundamental differences in modes of action.

cDNAs encoding CREB and a CREB-like protein in rats and humans provide some insights into the nature of these proteins.[176, 179] CREB is a protein of 341 amino acids that contains three functional regions: (1) a *trans*-activation domain with a number of potential phosphorylation sites; (2) a DNA-binding domain with a high content of basic amino acid residues; and (3) a "leucine zipper" dimerization domain (Fig. 5–20).

Phosphorylation of CREB at Ser-133 by the catalytic subunit of cAMP-dependent protein kinase results in a more than 10-fold increase in CRE-dependent transcription without an apparent effect on DNA affinity. Although both monomer and dimer forms bind to the CRE, only the dimer appears to possess transcriptional activity.

The DNA-binding domain of CREB involves a stretch of basic amino acids located near its COOH terminus that shares some sequence similarity with the cellular proto-oncogene *c-jun*. This proto-oncogene also contains a leucine zipper dimerization domain, which suggests the possibility that CREB can form heterodimers with the proto-oncogenes containing a similar domain, such as *c-fos* and *c-jun*, leading to coordinate regulation of gene expression and additional level of complexity in the cAMP regulation pathway.

A nuclear protein with a molecular weight of 265 kd (CREB binding protein [CREB-BP]) interacts with phosphorylated CREB. CREB-BP and a related factor, p300, are coactivators that bridge DNA-bound phosphorylated CREB with the basal transcription machinery. CREB-BP, which possesses domains that permit association with other transcription factors in addition to phosphorylated CREB, and a bromodomain region that may be responsible for its *trans*-activational activity, is required for cAMP-regulated gene expression. Nuclear receptors such as glucocorticoid and retinoic acid receptors also interact directly with CREB-BP, an association that is also important in their transcriptional activities. Thus, CREB-BP (p300) may serve as a cointegrator molecule to facilitate cross-talk between the CREB and nuclear receptor–mediated signaling systems.[180]

PROTEIN KINASE C AND AP-1. Another transcriptional factor involved in the regulation of gene expression by peptide hormones is activation protein-1 (AP-1). AP-1 can interact with the heptamer sequence TGACTCA in phorbol ester/protein kinase C–regulated genes.[181] This sequence is similar to the CRE except for the absence of a central G protein residue. The product of the photo-oncogene *c-jun* and a related protein in yeast called GCN4 are the major components of AP-1. The photo-oncogene *c-jun* is a transcription factor that contains a DNA-binding domain with basic amino acid residues and a leucine zipper dimerization domain similar to those described for CREB (see Fig. 5–20). Another nuclear transcription factor that interacts at the AP-1 site is *c-fos*. The photo-oncogene *c-fos* is a member of the family of early response genes activated in the conversion of quiescent serum-starved 3T3 fibroblasts to growing cells. However, *c-fos* can bind efficiently to DNA only in the presence of *c-jun*. Hence, only the heterodimer, and not the *c-fos* homodimer, can stimulate transcription. Furthermore, the *c-fos/c-jun* heterodimer has higher affinity for the AP-1–regulatory sites than the *c-jun* homodimer. Thus, hormones that stimulate protein kinase C affect gene expression indirectly by phosphorylating, and hence activating, *c-jun* and other proteins, in analogy to the regulation of CREB by protein kinase A.

OTHER HORMONE-REGULATED TRANSCRIPTION FACTORS. Additional nuclear protein factors are targets for cellular kinases in the membrane receptor-signaling pathway. Activated cytokine and GH/prolactin receptors associate with a family of cytoplasmic tyrosine kinases known as JAKs. The target of JAK is a family of transcription factors called signal transducers and activators of transcription (STAT).[182, 183] There are at least six members of the STAT family, each of which contains an SH2 domain that is important for recruitment to the activated cytokine receptor, phosphorylation by JAK, and formation of biologically active STAT homodimers and heterodimers on cytokine/GH/prolactin response elements. Other DNA-binding factors will certainly be discovered to play intricate and interactive roles in the regulation of gene expression. For example, insulin regulates the expression of a number of genes at the transcriptional level, but the insulin response element in DNA and its regulatory protein or proteins have not yet been well defined (reviewed in reference 147). Also, TGFβ signaling likely involves multiple transcription factors.[184]

Some of these peptide hormone–regulatory factors, such as CREB, CREB-BP, *c-jun*, and *c-fos*, are also involved in interactions with nuclear ligand-regulated receptors, including the vitamin A (retinoic acid) and vitamin D receptors.[185] These complex associations form the basis for molecular cross-talk

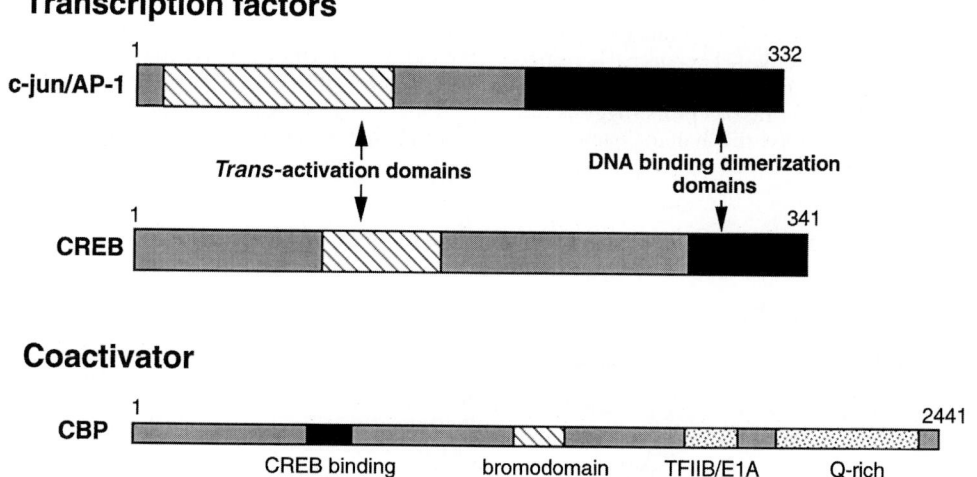

Figure 5–20. Schematic diagram of transcription factors and a coactivator that mediate peptide hormone signal transduction. These proteins act via the cAMP and Ca²⁺ protein kinase C pathways, i.e., CREB and *c-jun*/AP-1, respectively. In addition, the major coactivator of the cAMP system that interacts with phosphorylated CREB, namely, CREB binding protein (CBP), is shown. Among the transcription factors, NH₂-terminal *trans*-activation domains, often with multiple phosphorylation sites, and COOH-terminal DNA-binding domains, and with leucine zipper dimerization motifs, are depicted. In CBP, the CREB binding or interacting site and a putative *trans*-activation region, bromodomain, are shown. Other features include a TFIIB/E1A interaction site and a glutamine-rich (Q-rich) region. The sizes of these proteins, in amino acid residues, are shown.

between nuclear receptors and transcription factors regulated by cell surface receptors. Yet another avenue for cross-talk is illustrated in Figure 5–19. The activities of nuclear receptors are regulated by their cognate ligands, steroid/thyroid hormones, and retinoic acid. They may be further modified by the actions of cytoplasmic kinases activated by ligand-regulated plasma membrane receptors.

Receptors Linked to Adenylate Cyclase

cAMP-LINKED RECEPTORS. cAMP is the prototypical second messenger. Intracellular levels of cAMP are determined, in large part, by ligand-receptor interactions, a process that involves the interaction of three cellular components near the plasma membrane: the ligand receptor, a signal transducer (G protein), and the effector enzyme (adenylate cyclase)[186–194] (Figs. 5–17 and 5–21). In vitro reconstitution studies with purified receptors, G proteins, and adenylate cyclase introduced into phospholipid vesicles have shown that these three components are sufficient for ligand stimulation of cAMP production. In this fashion, the cAMP second messenger is produced by the interaction of three *functional cassettes*. Signal diversity, as well as specificity, is governed primarily by heterogeneity in each of the components, i.e., the existence of multiple receptors, G proteins, and effector adenylate cyclases.

Studies of adrenergic receptors have provided insight into the mechanisms of linkage of receptors to G proteins and adenylate cyclase.[84] Different adrenergic receptors can either stimulate or inhibit adenylate cyclase. Interaction of the β_1 and β_2 subtypes with their cognate ligands results in increased cAMP levels, whereas α_2-adrenergic receptor-ligand interaction decreases cAMP levels. The cloning of the adrenergic receptor cDNAs and genes has provided valuable information about their amino acid structures and have suggested possible mechanisms for specificity of action (Fig. 5–22).

The adrenergic receptors share considerable protein sequence homology.[84, 195] Each is a single polypeptide chain with an approximate molecular size of 64 to 80 kd, and each shares sequence homology with the visual pigment receptor rhodopsin. The human β_1- and β_2-adrenergic receptors are 477 and 413 amino acid residues in size, respectively. Functional domains of the receptors have been identified by utilizing in vitro mutagenesis and reconstitution experiments. On the basis of the deduced protein sequence, the β-adrenergic receptor appears to possess seven hydrophobic, alpha-helical regions that correspond to the seven transmembrane domains, similar to those previously seen in rhodopsin. In the human β_1- and β_2-receptors, the sequences of these domains are more conserved than is the overall molecule (71 versus 54%, respectively). Comparison of transmembrane domains between β-adrenergic and muscarinic cholinergic receptors suggests that the most conserved regions involve the half of each alpha

helix closest to the cytoplasm. The great variability in the helices near the external (extracytoplasmic) region among different receptors suggests a role in ligand binding.

The identification of functional domains among the adrenergic receptors has been facilitated by the ability to produce chimeric receptor forms by combining various regions of the different adrenergic receptor subtypes. For example, although ligands interact with transmembrane regions 2 to 7, adrenergic agonist specificity is determined primarily by transmembrane region 4. In contrast, antagonist interactions may involve transmembrane regions 6 and 7.[83] The NH$_2$ terminus, COOH terminus, and the large third intracytoplasmic domain are not involved in ligand interactions, as shown by deletion-mutagenesis and protease digestion studies. Thus, the catecholamine appears to interact with its receptor primarily via a pocket formed by the transmembrane domains as they appear at the extracytoplasmic face.

An equally important domain for this class of receptors is the region required for G protein coupling. This domain appears to be located in the second and third cytoplasmic loops and in the COOH-terminal tail of the receptor. Still another domain mediates receptor desensitization, a process in which effector response is rapidly decreased after exposure of receptor to agonist. In the adrenergic receptor system, homologous desensitization (see earlier) requires the cytoplasmic enzymes cAMP-dependent protein kinase and β-adrenergic receptor kinase to phosphorylate serine/threonine kinase targets in regions of the COOH-terminal tail or the third cytoplasmic loop of the receptor to uncouple the receptor from its associated G protein.[196, 197] A molecule known as β-arrestin may further modulate the interaction between the β-adrenergic receptor and β-adrenergic receptor kinase.[197] All of the genes that encode adrenergic receptors lack introns within the protein coding regions. This lack is somewhat surprising in view of the domain organization, because in many eucaryotic genes exons encode specific functional domains.

G PROTEINS. The G proteins are the critical signal transducers between the receptor and the effector in the plasma membrane, both topologically and functionally (see Figs. 5–17 and 5–21). The G protein family is extensive, with more than 50 members described to date. These proteins share structural homology and the ability to bind GDP and GTP with relatively high affinity. The G proteins can be divided into two groups based on molecular size. Smaller G proteins (20 to 25 kd in size) are present in both higher and lower eucaryotes.[60] The best-characterized protein in this class is the p21 or *ras* protooncogene. Larger G proteins (80 to 90 kd in size) are more relevant to hormone action pathways. The latter share structural homology with a number of regulators of protein synthesis, including elongation factor Tu.

High-molecular-weight G proteins exist as heterotrimers

G-protein-coupled 7-membrane-spanning receptor

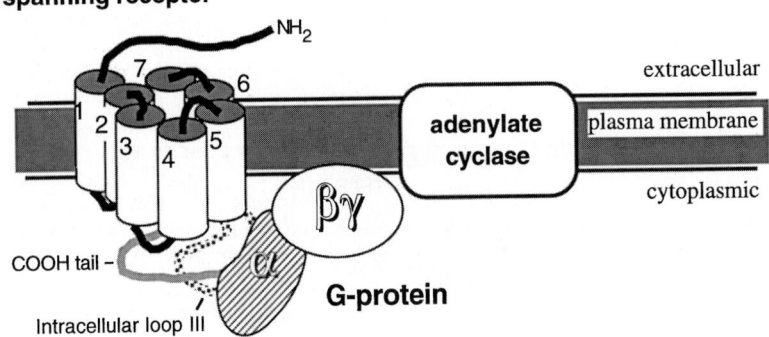

Figure 5–21. Schematic diagram of the locations of the G protein–coupled seven membrane-spanning receptor, G protein ($\alpha\beta\gamma$ heterotrimer), and adenylate cyclase within the plasma membrane. The G protein interacts with the receptor largely via the intracellular loop III and the COOH tail.

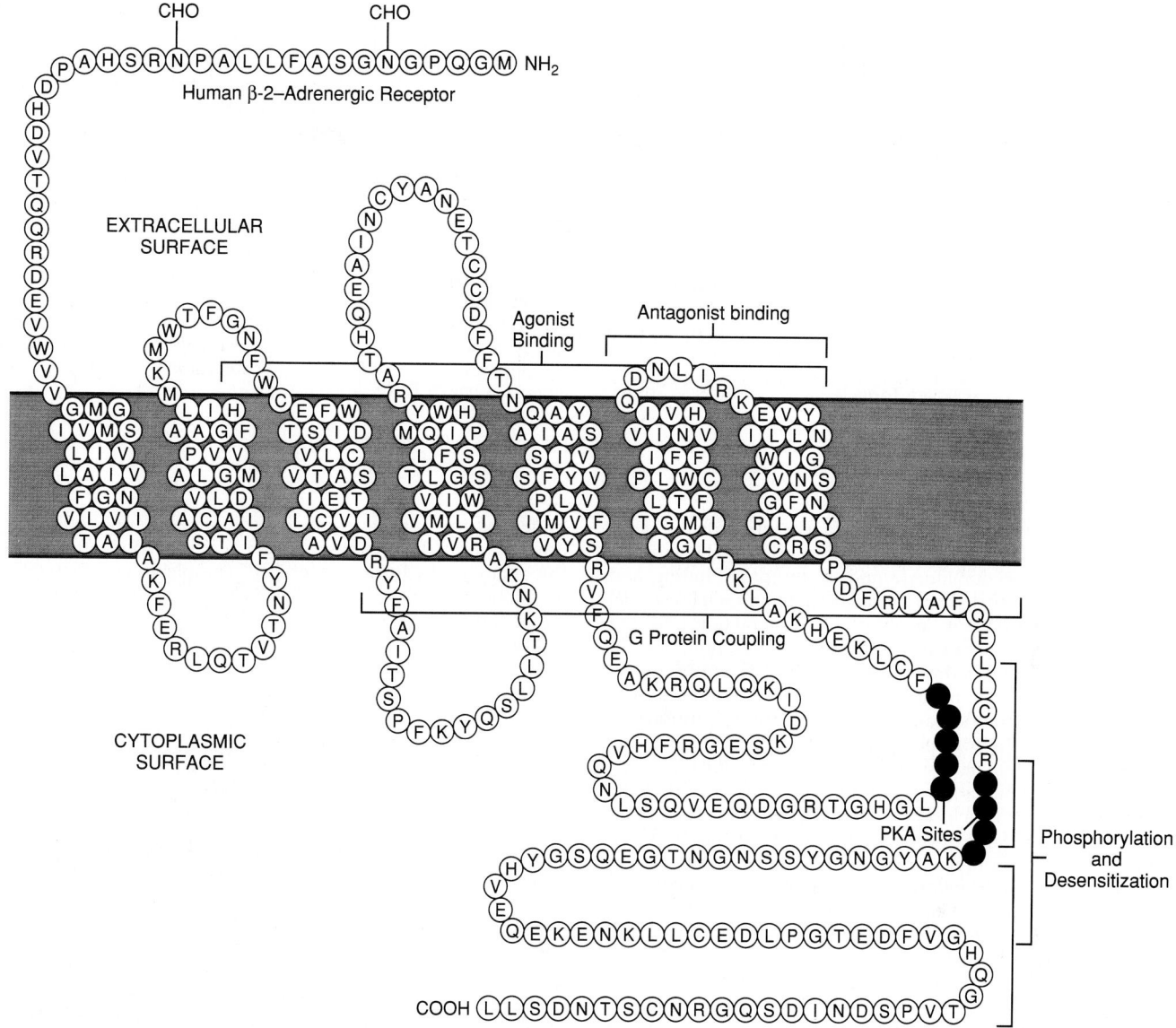

Figure 5–22. Structure of the β₂-adrenergic receptor. A model of the human β₂-adrenergic receptor, based on its deduced amino acid sequence, is shown. The CHO indicates probable glycosylation sites in the extracellular domain of the receptor. The residues indicated in the shaded circles represent probable phosphorylation (by protein kinase A [PKA]) sites in the intracellular domain of the receptor. The clusters of residues between the two horizontal lines delimiting the plasma membrane represent hydrophobic, alpha-helical membrane-spanning domains. Domains of putative agonist and antagonist binding, G protein coupling, and phosphorylation (involved in desensitization) are shown. (Modified with permission from Dohlman HG, Caron MG, Lefkowitz RJ. A family of receptors coupled to guanine nucleotide regulatory proteins. Biochemistry 1987; 26:2657–2664. Copyright 1987 American Chemical Society.)

consisting of three different subunits: α, β, and γ[191–194, 198–201] (Fig. 5–23). The α subunits are activated by binding GTP in the presence of Mg^{2+}, which facilitates the interaction with an appropriate effector system such as adenylate cyclase. The βγ subunits are not easily dissociable from each other and serve as a dimer that can function by interacting with the α subunit or by itself. Multiple G proteins may serve different signal transduction functions. For example, the ability of the adrenergic receptor subtypes to stimulate or decrease cAMP production resides in the interaction of β₁- and β₂-adrenergic receptors with stimulatory G proteins (Gs) and of α₂-adrenergic receptor with inhibitory G proteins (Gi). G proteins are located near the plasma membrane, with the precise interaction of the trimer with the lipid bilayer not well known. The α subunits are more variable in structure than the βγ subunits (Table 5–6). At least 16 genes encoding the α subunit, and more than 20 α subunit proteins have been elucidated. These α subunits show considerable structural homology and have

molecular sizes that range from 39 to 52 kd. There are four αs (α(s1–4)) subunits derived from the alternative splicing of exon 3 in the αs gene. This splicing results in long and short forms that differ by 15 amino acid residues. The long form has a lower affinity and faster dissociation rate for GDP than the short form, which suggests functional heterogeneity among G proteins derived from these different αs variants. The αi subunit exists in at least three forms, each derived from a different gene. When present in the αβγ heterotrimer, αi results in a G protein that mediates the inhibition of adenylate cyclase. αi may also couple some receptors to K^+ and Ca^{2+} channels. Other α subunits include αo, derived largely from brain, αt or α-transducin found in association with the visual pigment rhodopsin, and other less well characterized forms. αs is present in nearly all cells, but not all αi subunits are present in every cell.

Again, the molecular cloning of the α subunit cDNAs and crystallographic data provide insight into the domain

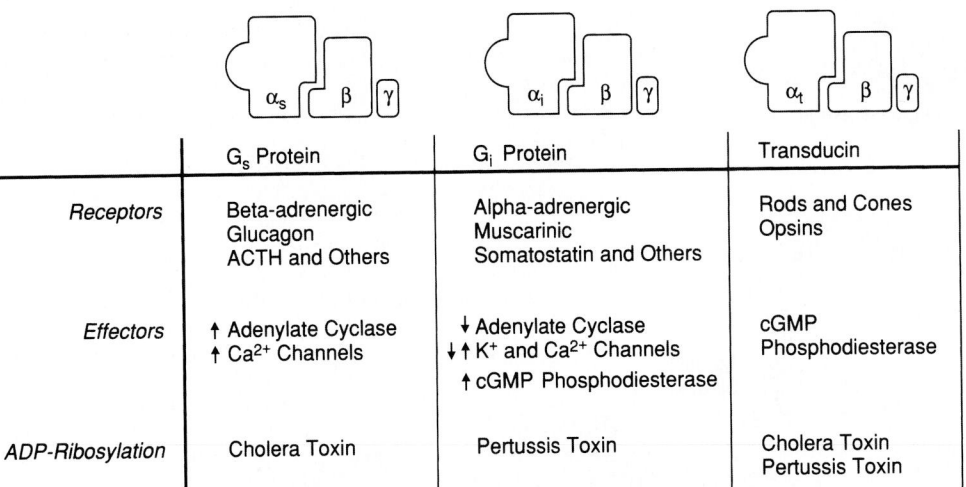

	G_s Protein	G_i Protein	Transducin
Receptors	Beta-adrenergic Glucagon ACTH and Others	Alpha-adrenergic Muscarinic Somatostatin and Others	Rods and Cones Opsins
Effectors	↑ Adenylate Cyclase ↑ Ca^{2+} Channels	↓ Adenylate Cyclase ↓↑ K^+ and Ca^{2+} Channels ↑ cGMP Phosphodiesterase	cGMP Phosphodiesterase
ADP-Ribosylation	Cholera Toxin	Pertussis Toxin	Cholera Toxin Pertussis Toxin

Figure 5–23. Structure and properties of G proteins and transducin. Heterotrimeric subunits are α, β, and γ.

organization of G protein subunits. Each α subunit has at least five domains including (1) a Mg^{2+}-dependent GTP binding site, (2) a GTPase domain, (3 and 4) receptor binding and effector interaction domains located in the COOH-terminal end,[202] and (5) a domain involved in βγ interaction near the NH_2-terminal region. In some cultured cell lines, mutations in the COOH-terminal end of the α subunit of G_s cause uncoupling of the receptors from the G proteins.[203] Additional evidence regarding the domain involved in receptor interaction comes from the ability of pertussis toxin to ADP-ribosylate the $α_s$ subunit on a cysteine residue located in the COOH-terminal end of the molecule and to uncouple $α_i$, $α_o$, and $α_t$ from the receptors. Similar conclusions have been reached from analyses of $α_s/α_i$ chimeras. Also, it should be noted that different α isoforms possess different intrinsic GTPase activities.

The β subunit is found in five homologous forms (53 to 90% similarity) with molecular sizes of 35 to 39 kd.[191, 192, 198, 204] The γ subunits are more heterogeneous, with seven isoforms and apparent molecular sizes of 6 to 18 kd.[191, 192, 198] The β and γ subunits are usually observed in tight association, with formation of a βγ dimer. However, there may be limited interactions of different γ subunit isoforms with a specific β subunit, and vice versa. Both β and γ subunits can also apparently function as homodimers rather than heterodimers, as

TABLE 5–6. Selected Features of G Protein Subunit Structure and Function

Subunit	Feature
α subunits	Are unique for each G protein >20 isoforms in 4 major classes Are 39–52 kd Bind guanine nucleotides and possess intrinsic GTPase activity Are substrates for bacterial toxin ADP-ribosylation Bind to receptors, effectors, and β/γ complex
β subunits	5 homologous (53–90%) isoforms Are 35–39 kd Bind tightly, but not covalently, to the γ subunit
γ subunits	Dissimilar subunits 7 isoforms Are small (about 6–8 kd) May be involved in G protein membrane attachment
β/γ complex	Binds to the α subunit May function as inhibitor of G protein activation, as well as direct activator Is probably required for G protein–receptor interaction, but not for α/effector interaction

evidenced from studies with yeast mutants lacking one or the other subunit. The βγ subunits are required for regulation of the α subunit by hormone-receptor complexes and may serve to anchor the G proteins to plasma membranes via lipid modifications. Furthermore, the high affinity of βγ for α indicates that this dimer may also inhibit the action of α subunits. This suggests a potential regulatory role of the βγ dimer in addition to its direct regulation of effector molecules.

Other features of the G proteins include the existence of factors that modify their activities and the subcellular compartmentalization of certain G proteins along with their receptors and effectors. These observations suggest yet additional layers of regulatory control that may serve important physiological roles.

ACTIVATION OF ADENYLATE CYCLASE. The general mechanism of G protein–linked hormone activation of adenylate cyclase is well understood[198, 204, 205] (Fig. 5–24). In the absence of ligand, the hormone receptor interacts directly with the heterotrimer G protein. Note that either α or βγ can bind to the receptor, but the interaction of the GDP-bound α is increased by the presence of βγ. In this state the rate of GDP dissociation from the α subunit is low and limits GTPase activity of the G protein complex. The presence of the hormone ligand causes formation of the hormone-receptor complex, which in turn promotes GDP dissociation from the α subunit of the heterotrimer and allows intracellular GTP to bind to the α subunit. This binding results in (1) dissociation of the α subunit from receptor and βγ; (2) lowering of the affinity of the receptor for the ligand; (3) production of an activated α subunit that can interact with an effector molecule such as adenylate cyclase; and (4) induction of the inherent GTPase activity in the α subunit. Like many signaling events, the presence of ligand causes a rapid but short-lived intracellular response. The increased ability of the "activated" α subunit to break down GTP and thus to increase GDP/GTP ratios gradually favors GDP rather than GTP binding to the G protein complex and attenuates the activation process. Thus, a G protein signal transduction cycle can be produced and regulated. It should be stressed that the rate of GTP hydrolysis may greatly affect the longevity of the α and βγ responses.

While the role of the α subunit in this signal transduction process is well known, the role of the βγ dimer was established subsequently. At first, it was believed that the key role of βγ was largely a regulatory one involving the inhibition of $α_s$ activity. In this model, G_i inhibits adenylate cyclase by providing excess βγ subunits, which then rapidly bind the relatively small amounts of $α_s$ within a cell to limit stimulatory activity. By this indirect mechanism, effector activity is inhibited by the

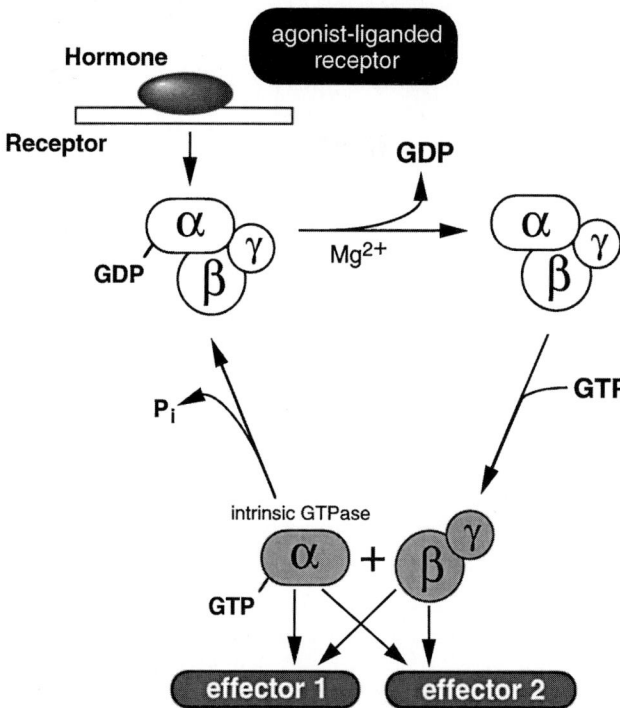

Figure 5–24. G protein signal transduction. In the absence of ligand binding to the receptor, the heterotrimer G protein (αβγ) binds GDP via its α subunit but apparently without interaction with receptor effectors. Formation of the hormone-receptor or agonist-liganded receptor complex results in interaction of the receptor and G protein, and subsequent replacement of GDP with GTP in the presence of Mg^{2+}. At this point, the GTP-bound activated α subunit dissociates from the βγ subunit. Then either one or both contact effectors (effector 1, effector 2, etc.) and modulate their activities. Simultaneously, the intrinsic GTPase activity of the α subunit hydrolyzes GTP to GDP, which terminates peptide hormone signaling.

hormone-receptor complex. On the contrary, it was shown that the βγ dimer, in the absence of α, could either directly or indirectly (via stimulation of phospholipase A_2) activate the M-type potassium channel in the heart.[191] In addition, a yeast mutant lacking the α subunit responds to yeast mating factor (a cAMP-linked response), suggesting that βγ serves a stimulatory role with respect to this effector system.[191] Subsequently, βγ has been shown to possess multiple independent activities. βγ can stimulate effectors such as type II and IV adenylate cyclases, phospholipase Cβ (PLCβ), β-adrenergic receptor kinase, and phosphoinositide 3-kinase (PI 3-kinase). It may also inhibit the activity of type I adenylate cyclase. Further, βγ can activate the MAP kinase/growth factor pathway via *ras*, a function that illustrates the potential for signal cross-talk at the level of G protein subunits. Finally, as noted later, different forms of adenylate cyclase may be selectively and differentially regulated by α and/or βγ subunits.

The "activated" α subunit modulates the activity of adenylate cyclase, the ultimate effector enzyme in this system. Adenylate cyclase is an integral membrane glycoprotein present in all tissues as a single polypeptide possessing 12 transmembrane domains and an apoprotein of about 124 kd size.[206] Adenylate cyclase is present in at least 10 isoforms that bear approximately 60% similarity.[207] Each isoform has a unique tissue distribution. As a result, type I and VIII enzymes are found solely in neurons, while others are more widely expressed. Interaction with activated $α_s$ or the diterpene forskolin augments enzyme activity, with rapid conversion of ATP to cAMP. The cAMP, in turn, reacts with cAMP-dependent protein kinase (kinase A), a tetramer containing two each of the regulatory and catalytic subunits (see Fig. 5–17). In the absence of cAMP, regulatory subunits prevent activation of

the catalytic subunit. However, in the presence of cAMP, the regulatory subunits dissociate from the catalytic subunit, which unmasks its enzyme activity. This kinase then may phosphorylate other proteins within the cell to produce secondary and tertiary messengers.

A special feature of this signal transduction system is the heterogeneity of structure and function allowed by the cassette design (see Figs. 5–7, 5–17, and 5–21). For example, as noted, multiple G proteins may interact with a single receptor-hormone complex to activate or inhibit different effector systems in response to a single agonist, as illustrated in Figure 5–13. Similarly, multiple receptors may interact with a single G protein. Thus, flexibility of interaction at the receptor–G protein and G protein–effector interfaces results in a complex regulatory network. For example, the β-adrenergic receptor, in reconstitution studies, can activate either G_s and G_i, and G_s can interact with both adenylate cyclase and ion channels in atrial tissues. Because various G proteins are expressed in a tissue-specific fashion and because their levels may be hormonally regulated, these pathways can be regulated at every step, both physiologically and pathologically.

Another important feature of this signal transduction system is its ability to amplify signals. Because activation of G proteins results in dissociation of the G proteins from bound complexes, a single hormone-receptor complex can activate multiple G proteins. For instance, in the β-adrenergic receptor system, one agonist-receptor complex can activate up to 20 G proteins (Fig. 5–25). Similarly, light activation of rhodopsin can cause a 1000-fold increase in the stimulation of G_t.

EFFECTS OF BACTERIAL TOXINS ON G PROTEINS. Two bacterial toxins interact with G proteins and alter cellular cAMP levels[198] (Table 5–7). Pertussis toxin (derived from *Bordetella pertussis*) causes ADP-ribosylation of $α_i$, $α_o$, and $α_t$ at a cysteine residue near the COOH-terminal end. This reaction uncouples receptor from G_i, constitutively activates adenylate cyclase, and increases cellular cAMP levels. Inhibition of G_i may account for the pertussis-associated increase in sensitivity to histamines and for pertussis-associated hypoglycemia by blocking the inhibitory effect of α-adrenergic influences on histamine-mediated pathways and insulin secretion.

Cholera toxin, by comparison, ADP-ribosylates $α_s$ at an internal arginine residue, which results in a decreased α association with βγ and effective stabilization of $α_s$ in the GDP-bound conformation. The final result is an inhibition of GTPase activity, prolonged ability of $α_s$ to stimulate effector systems, and increased cAMP levels. The severe diarrhea that is characteristic of infection with *Vibrio cholerae* and the analogous symptoms produced by some toxin-producing strains of *Escherichia coli* are thought to be due to continuous activation of the adenylate cyclase. The interdiction of GTP hydrolysis in a number of hormone systems by the use of a nonhydrolyzable

TABLE 5–7. Interaction of Bacterial Toxins with G Proteins and Cyclase Systems

Parameter	Cholera Toxin	Pertussis Toxin
Cellular receptor	Gangliosides	?
G protein target for ADP-ribosylation	$α_s$, $α_{olf}$	$α_i$, $α_t$, $α_o$
Effects		
G proteins	Activates G_s	Inactivates G_i, G_o
cAMP	Increases	Variable increases
Final biologic effects	Increased ion flux in gastrointestinal tract	Increases insulin secretion and lipolysis; bronchoconstriction, decreased neutrophil response

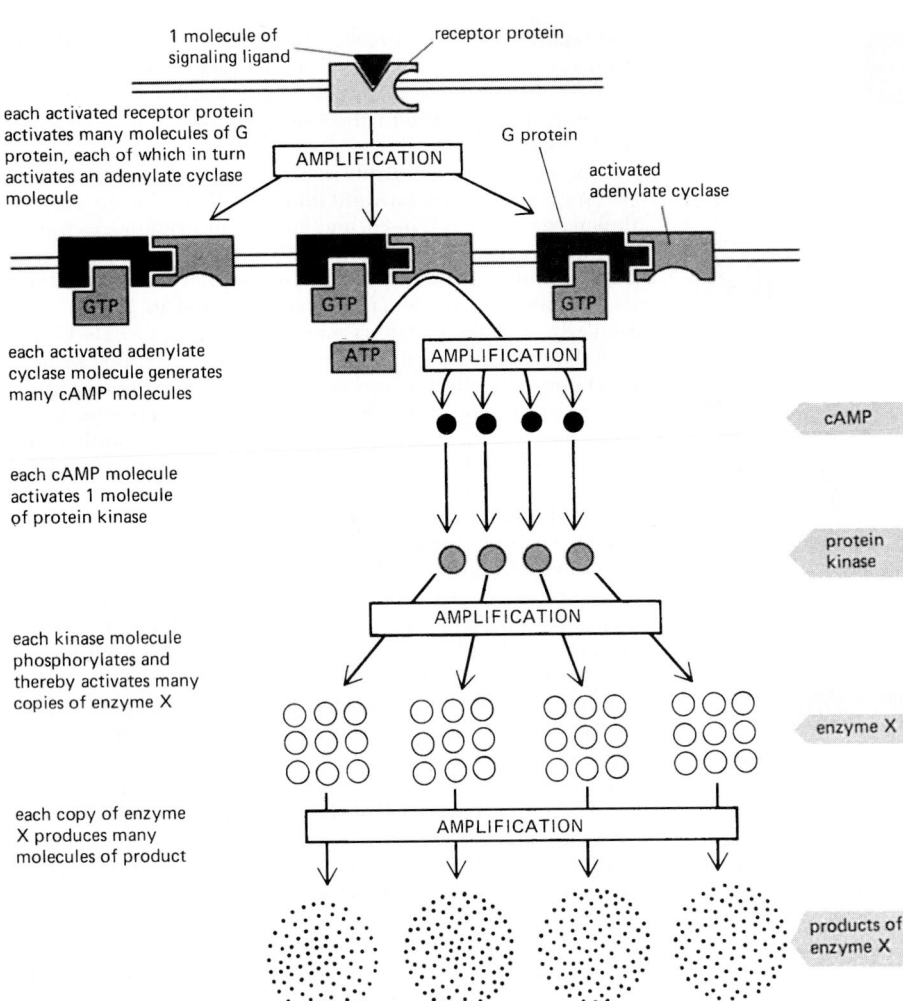

each activated receptor protein activates many molecules of G protein, each of which in turn activates an adenylate cyclase molecule

each activated adenylate cyclase molecule generates many cAMP molecules

each cAMP molecule activates 1 molecule of protein kinase

each kinase molecule phosphorylates and thereby activates many copies of enzyme X

each copy of enzyme X produces many molecules of product

Figure 5–25. Amplification of cellular signaling after stimulation of a cAMP-linked receptor. (From Alberts B, Bray D, Lewis J, et al. Molecular Biology of the Cell. New York: Garland, 1983: 750, with permission.)

GTP analogue or aluminum fluoride causes persistent G protein activation and ligand-receptor dissociation.

Receptor Tyrosine Kinases

GENERAL STRUCTURAL FEATURES. The function of receptors as direct catalysts of phosphorylation reactions became a subject of intense investigation after the recognition that several receptors contain an intrinsic hormone-stimulated tyrosine kinase activity. The first such evidence came from studies of the EGF receptor.[208–210] EGF binding activates a receptor-associated protein kinase that differed from most known cellular protein kinases in that it phosphorylated proteins on tyrosine rather than serine residues. This tyrosine protein kinase activity was similar to several oncogene-associated tyrosine kinase activities and was ultimately shown to be intrinsic to the EGF receptor. Multiple other peptide hormone receptors also contain hormone-activated tyrosine kinase activities. These include receptors for insulin,[211–213] IGF-I,[213, 214] PDGF,[215, 216] colony-stimulating factor-1 (CSF-1),[217, 218] and FGF[219] (see Table 5–1). Although there now are more than 50 known receptors and oncogene products with tyrosine kinase activity, the total cellular content of tyrosine phosphoproteins is much lower than that of serine phosphoproteins, representing less than 1% of all protein phosphorylation in the cell under normal conditions.

Based on comparisons of their individual protein structures, the tyrosine kinase–containing peptide hormone receptors have been divided into multiple classes, three of which

are illustrated in Figure 5–26.[76, 220–222] The insulin and IGF-I receptors are the most complex, with a heterotetrameric structure consisting of two α and two β subunits joined by disulfide cross-bridges. The α subunits are entirely extracellular and contain a cysteine-rich region that is believed to be involved in hormone binding. The β subunits possess an extracellular domain, a transmembrane domain, and an intracellular domain that contains an ATP-binding site and a catalytic kinase domain. The α and β subunits are synthesized as part of a single precursor molecule that undergoes proteolytic processing to form the two subunits in a manner analogous to synthesis of insulin from proinsulin.[223]

A second class is represented by the EGF receptor, which differs from insulin and IGF-I receptors in that the domains for hormone binding and tyrosine kinase are contained in a single transmembrane protein chain that exists in the membrane as a monomer.[210] The configurations of the ATP-binding site and the tyrosine kinase domain are similar to those of the insulin and IGF-I receptors, and cysteine-rich domains appear to be important for hormone binding, although these domains exist in two interrupted regions in the EGF receptor. The EGF receptor appears to be inactive in the monomeric form, and transmission of the hormone signal requires the dimerization of receptors.[224] In this dimerized state, the EGF receptor resembles the insulin and IGF-I receptors, except that the two receptor halves are noncovalently, rather than covalently, associated.

PDGF receptors define a group of tyrosine kinase receptors that contain binding and tyrosine kinase domains in a

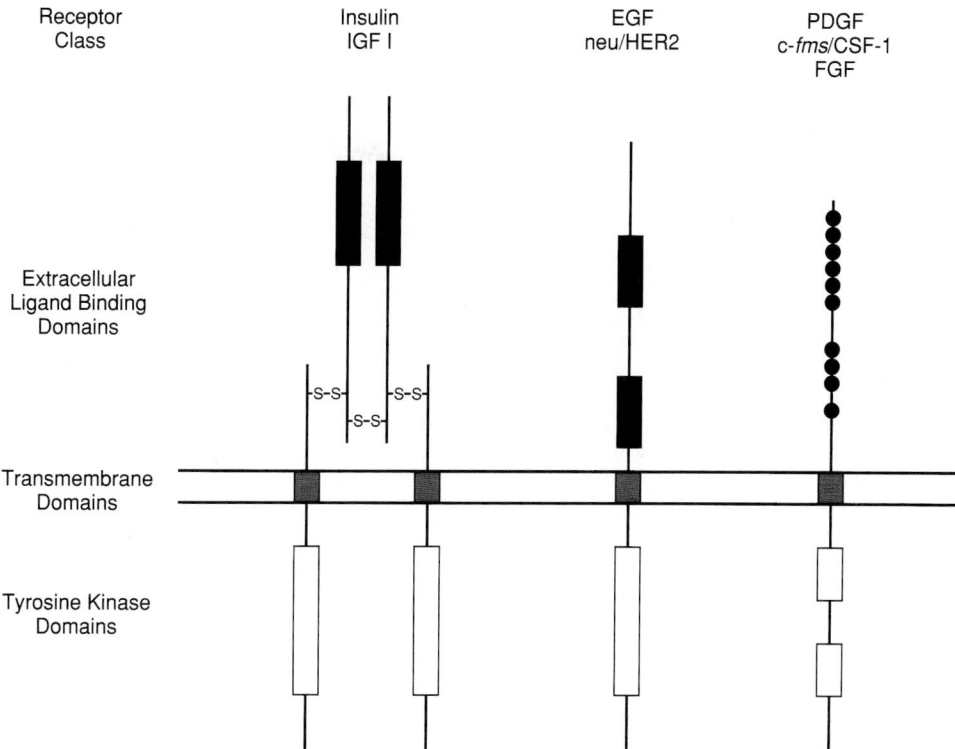

Figure 5–26. Structural features of different subclasses of tyrosine kinase receptors. The black rectangles represent cysteine-rich repeat regions and the circles represent conserved cysteine residues. Disulfide bonds in these regions are thought to have an important role in establishing the structure of the hormone-binding site. The white rectangles represent the tyrosine kinase domain, which is an interrupted sequence in PDGF and related receptors.

single peptide chain but have a cysteine-rich extracellular structure that is thought to form IgG-like repeats. In addition, the tyrosine kinase domain is interrupted by about 100 amino acids that are unrelated to other tyrosine kinases.[215–220] As with the EGF receptor, the monomeric PDGF receptor is inactive, and full ligand-induced activation requires receptor dimerization. The significance of the structural similarities and differences among these and other classes of tyrosine kinase receptors is not fully understood, but the structural features of each receptor class probably have importance in regard to both receptor evolution and function.

INVOLVEMENT OF RECEPTOR TYROSINE KINASE ACTIVITY IN HORMONE ACTION. For each receptor of this type, the tyrosine kinase activity is the only known intrinsic catalytic activity. The enzyme is activated immediately after hormone binding, as evidenced by rapid receptor autophosphorylation, which is initiated within seconds and is maximal within several minutes. Although the molecular events that lead from tyrosine phosphorylation to hormone action have been only partially defined, the tyrosine kinase activity mediates some or all of the actions of the hormones.

The insulin receptor is an example of a tyrosine kinase receptor that mediates hormone action. With the isolation of cDNA for the insulin receptor, it became possible to modify individual regions of the receptor by site-directed mutagenesis. The resulting mutant receptors can then be expressed by the process of transfection at high levels in cells that normally have few insulin receptors, and the consequences of the receptor mutation on hormone action can be studied. When normal insulin receptors are overexpressed in Chinese hamster ovary cells, which have low numbers of endogenous insulin receptors, insulin can be shown to stimulate a number of biologic responses (Fig. 5–27). If the transfected insulin receptors are mutated at the site of ATP binding, they retain insulin-binding activity but lack tyrosine kinase activity and fail to stimulate biologic actions including glucose uptake, ribosomal protein S6 activation, glycogen synthesis, and DNA synthesis.[225, 226] Likewise, replacement of one or more of the

tyrosine autophosphorylation sites in the β subunit with phenylalanine residues by site-directed mutagenesis prevents autophosphorylation in this region and impairs the effects of insulin on tyrosine kinase activity and biologic responses.[217, 227, 228] Similarly, when monoclonal antibodies to the kinase domain of the insulin receptor are microinjected into cells, the effects of insulin on the receptor tyrosine kinase activity and the biologic responses to insulin are decreased.[229]

Additional evidence for the role of the kinase in hormone

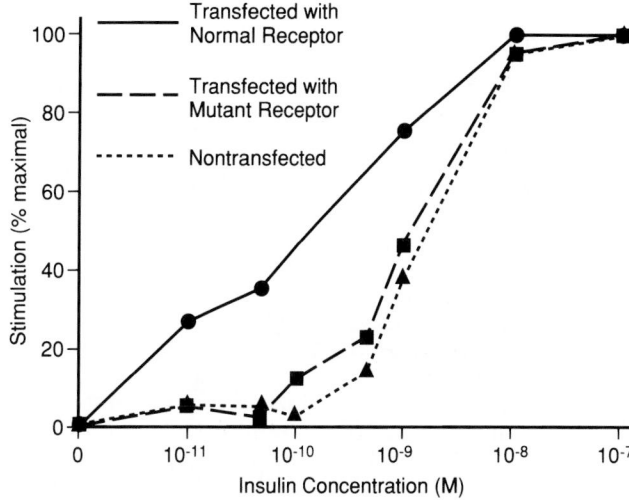

Figure 5–27. Effect of insulin on thymidine incorporation into DNA (DNA synthesis) in Chinese hamster ovary (CHO-K1) fibroblasts transfected with normal human insulin receptors or mutant insulin receptors with alanine substituted for lysine in the region of ATP binding (amino acid 1018). The nontransfected CHO cells have a much lower number of insulin receptors than either of the transfectants. (Adapted from Chou CK, Dull TJ, Russel DS, et al. Human insulin receptors mutated at the ATP-binding site lack protein tyrosine kinase activity and fail to mediate postreceptor effects of insulin. J Biol Chem 1987; 262:1842–1847, with permission.)

action has come from studies of signaling under physiological and pathologic conditions. In some patients with the type A syndrome of insulin resistance,[230] insulin binding is normal, but there is a marked decrease in receptor tyrosine kinase activity and in receptor autophosphorylation (Fig. 5–28).[231, 232] Similarly, in type II diabetes mellitus, insulin resistance is associated with decreased receptor tyrosine kinase activity.[233–235] Taken together, these observations suggest that insulin-stimulated tyrosine kinase activity and receptor autophosphorylation are necessary for insulin action. Other tyrosine kinase receptors, such as the EGF,[125, 236, 237] PDGF,[238] and CSF-1 receptors,[239] have similar associations between active receptor tyrosine kinases and hormone action.

Peptide hormones bind to the extracellular portions of transmembrane receptors, and the extracellular binding domains are responsible for both the affinity and the specificity of the receptors. This selective binding mechanism appears to be adequate under most circumstances to ensure specificity of hormone action, e.g., preventing insulin from activating EGF-sensitive pathways. Despite the similar structural and catalytic properties of the intracellular receptor tyrosine kinases, specificity of hormone action may also be determined by differences in structure of the intracellular domains. It is possible to create receptors with the extracellular binding domain of one receptor and the intracellular tyrosine kinase of a different receptor by combining portions of the cDNAs for the two different receptors and then expressing the *chimeric receptors* in transfected cells.[240] By this method receptors have been constructed that contain the extracellular domain of the insulin receptor and the intracellular tyrosine kinase domain of the EGF receptor or the tyrosine kinase of the oncogene v-*ros*[241] (Fig. 5–29). The chimeric receptors bind insulin with high affinity, and insulin is able to activate the v-*ros* or EGF kinase domains. In contrast to cells transfected with intact insulin receptors, however, insulin does not stimulate glucose uptake or DNA synthesis but, instead, produces EGF-like effects via the insulin-EGF receptor chimera. Thus, activation of intracellular tyrosine kinase activity is not sufficient to produce hormone-specific cellular responses. The specific actions of a

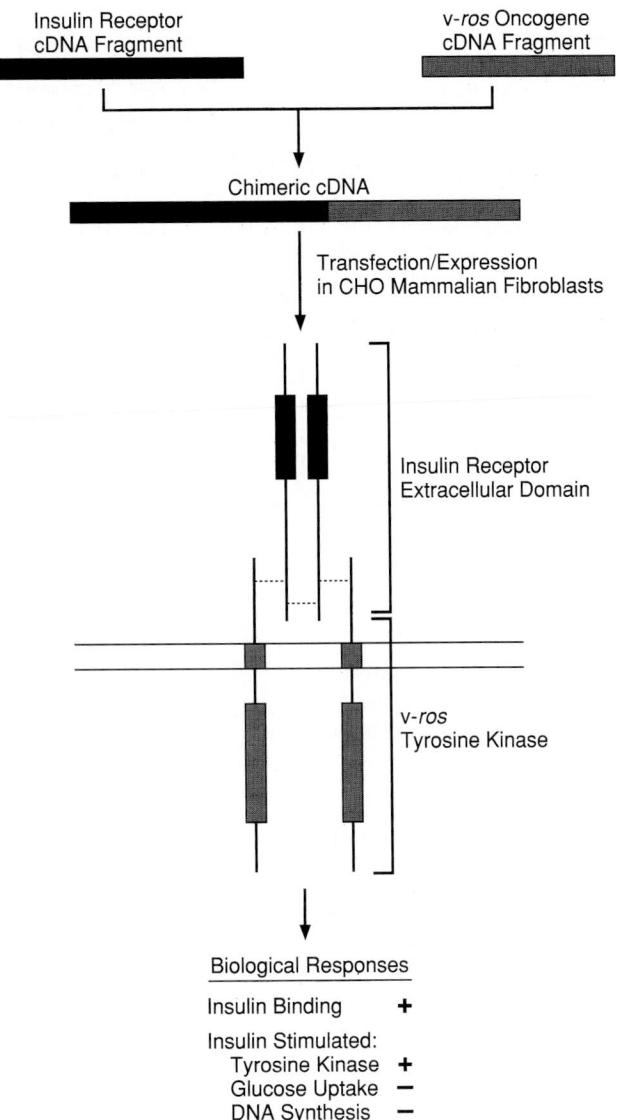

Figure 5–29. Use of chimeric receptor constructs to investigate the role of specific receptor domains in mediating hormone action. A hybrid receptor cDNA can be created by combining a fragment of the insulin receptor cDNA corresponding to the α subunit and extracellular portion of the β subunit with cDNA corresponding to the transmembrane and intracellular domains of the v-*ros* oncogene. When expressed in mammalian cells (e.g., Chinese hamster ovary [CHO] fibroblasts), the resulting hybrid receptor binds insulin with high affinity and undergoes insulin-stimulated autophosphorylation. Although the receptor tyrosine kinase has thus been activated, insulin-stimulated glucose uptake and DNA synthesis are not observed. See text for further details.

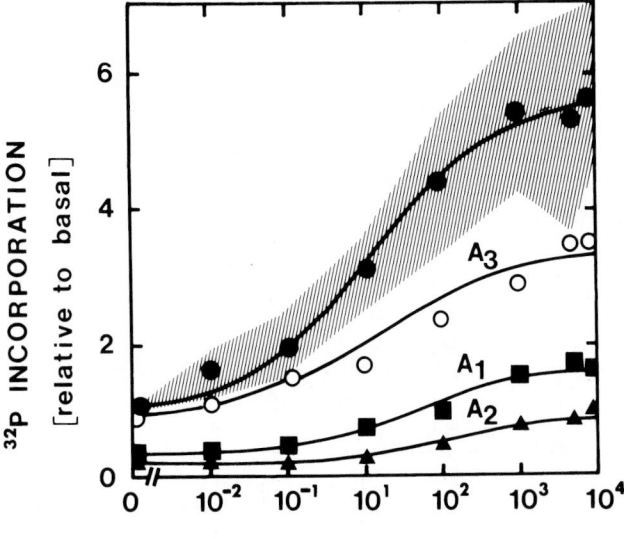

Figure 5–28. Insulin stimulation of phosphorylation of isolated erythrocyte insulin receptors from normal control subjects (shaded area) and three patients with type A syndrome of insulin resistance. (Adapted from Grigorescu F, Flier JS, Kahn CR. Defect in insulin receptor phosphorylation in erythrocytes and fibroblasts associated with severe insulin resistance. J Biol Chem 1984; 259:15003–15006, with permission.)

hormone are determined by both its capacity to bind to its own receptors and the individual intracellular structures of those receptors.

REGULATION OF RECEPTOR TYROSINE KINASE ACTIVITY. For each of the known tyrosine kinase peptide hormone receptors, the earliest intracellular events after hormone binding are increased tyrosine kinase catalytic activity and autophosphorylation of the receptor. The tyrosine kinase receptors behave like classic allosteric enzymes in which the primary role of the domain or subunit for ligand binding is to suppress the kinase activity intrinsic to the intracellular domain. In the case of the insulin receptor, the α subunit may be viewed as the ligand-binding regulatory subunit and the β subunit as the catalytic kinase subunit, in analogy with cAMP-dependent protein kinase, discussed earlier in this chapter. Ligand binding to the receptor or removal of the ligand-binding domain by proteolysis or in vitro mutagenesis results in activation of the kinase. It is not clear exactly how the binding of hormone to an extracellular portion of the receptor results in derepression of the tyrosine kinase, since the receptor remains intact. However, the derepression probably results from a binding-induced conformational change in the receptor and/or from receptor-receptor aggregation. In the case of the insulin receptor, hormone binding leads to changes in accessibility of the receptor to chemicals and enzymes and to changes in chromatographic properties that can be best explained by a shift in conformation.[242, 243]

REGULATION BY MULTISITE PHOSPHORYLATION. For all of the receptors that have been studied, autophosphorylation occurs on multiple tyrosine residues.[220] The functional significance of these phosphorylation sites has been only partially defined, but the autophosphorylation of certain residues can have a positive or a negative regulatory effect on the tyrosine kinase catalytic activity. For example, autophosphorylation of tyrosine residues within the tyrosine kinase domain of the insulin receptor both increases and stabilizes the kinase so that catalytic activity is retained even after dissociation of the bound hormone.[136, 137] Analogous tyrosine residues in the EGF receptor are not phosphorylated, but autophosphorylation at a site within the COOH-terminal tail of the receptor increases kinase activity.[244] Specific structural features of each receptor kinase and specific aspects of the autophosphorylation may be important in establishing distinct hormone signals generated by different receptors. Mutation of the insulin receptor at Tyr-1146 alters the growth-stimulating potential of the receptor but not its metabolic activity,[245] whereas mutation of Tyr-1150 and Tyr-1151 produces the opposite effect.[228] Deletion of the intervening sequence in the kinase domain of the PDGF receptor alters its ability to stimulate mitogenesis but not its acute effects on phosphatidylinositol turnover or ion influx.[238] Studies with several different tyrosine kinase receptors have shown that hormone binding and tyrosine kinase activation require the association of αβ dimers into tetramers[246, 247] or the formation of dimers in the case of monomeric receptors.[248] This may be important, in part, as a mechanism that promotes interchain autophosphorylation and thus has a role in the amplification of hormone signaling.

Several tyrosine kinase receptors are phosphorylated not only on tyrosine residues but also on serine and threonine residues by cellular kinases extrinsic to the receptor. The extent of receptor serine phosphorylation appears to be modulated, and this phosphorylation may decrease tyrosine autophosphorylation and the tyrosine kinase activity of the receptors. For example, protein kinase C phosphorylates the EGF receptor on serine residues and decreases EGF-stimulated tyrosine kinase activity.[249] The insulin receptor is also phosphorylated on serine residues in response to phorbol esters, presumably through phorbol-activated protein kinase C activity. As with the EGF receptor, serine phosphorylation of the insulin receptor decreases tyrosine kinase activity and decreases insulin action.[250] Prolonged stimulation with insulin itself, in addition to its effects on tyrosine autophosphorylation, leads to increased serine phosphorylation of the insulin receptor,[251, 252] and this serine phosphorylation may have a role in modulating or turning off insulin action. As with the β-adrenergic receptor kinase, a specific insulin receptor–associated serine kinase may be present,[253] although such an enzyme has not been well characterized. It is interesting to note that insulin-stimulated serine phosphorylation of insulin receptors does not occur in cells transfected with mutant receptors that cannot undergo tyrosine autophosphorylation.[254] Thus, the normal insulin-signaling pathway must be intact to allow insulin stimulation of serine phosphorylation.

In addition to the role of serine phosphorylation in recep-

tor regulation, the COOH-terminal tail of the insulin receptor β subunit may regulate receptor signaling by folding into the catalytic site and thus blocking receptor tyrosine kinase activity.[220] It is speculated that phosphorylation of tyrosine residues in the COOH terminus may cause the molecule to unfold, thus increasing the susceptibility of the catalytic region to activating tyrosine phosphorylation and also increasing the access of substrates. A regulatory response of this type would provide a mechanism for decreasing basal kinase activity and make possible a greater increase in signaling with hormone activation. Figure 5–30 summarizes some of these modulators of insulin receptor kinase activity. Similar mechanisms have been suggested for the EGF receptor. Other possible modulators include proteins and peptides within the cell that may modify hormone responsiveness by either activating or inhibiting receptor tyrosine kinase activity.

SIGNAL TRANSDUCTION BY RECEPTOR TYROSINE KINASES. A characteristic of receptor tyrosine kinases is their capacity to activate multiple responses within individual target cells. For example, insulin receptors initiate cellular responses that include such diverse effects as the stimulation of glucose transport, glycolysis, glycogen synthesis, triglyceride synthesis, protein synthesis, and DNA synthesis. The pleiotropic actions of insulin receptors and a similar multiplicity of responses induced by other receptor tyrosine kinases derive from the capacity of a single type of receptor to initiate cellular responses through several different mechanisms. In addition to catalyzing receptor autophosphorylation, receptor tyrosine kinases may phosphorylate nonreceptor proteins in cells that, through activation or inactivation, transmit the hormone signal to the cellular machinery (Fig. 5–31A).[255] These substrates for receptor kinases may exert actions in the cytoplasm, or they may translocate to the nucleus and exert effects on gene expression. Autophosphorylated tyrosine residues within the receptors not only function in the regulation of receptor kinase activity as discussed earlier but also serve as docking sites that bind SH2 and PTB domains of cytosolic signaling

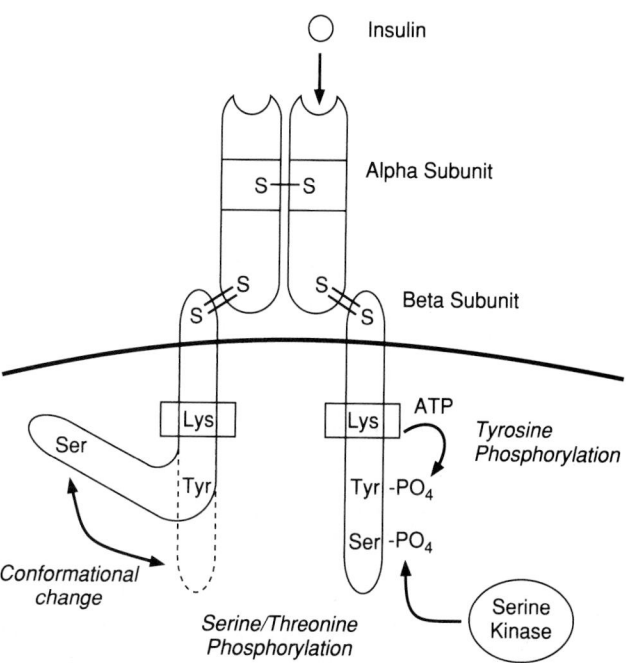

Figure 5–30. Potential mechanisms for modulation of insulin receptor kinase activity. These mechanisms include tyrosine autophosphorylation, which is stimulatory; serine/threonine phosphorylation by protein kinase C and cAMP kinase, which is inhibitory; and conformational changes, which could produce positive or negative effects.

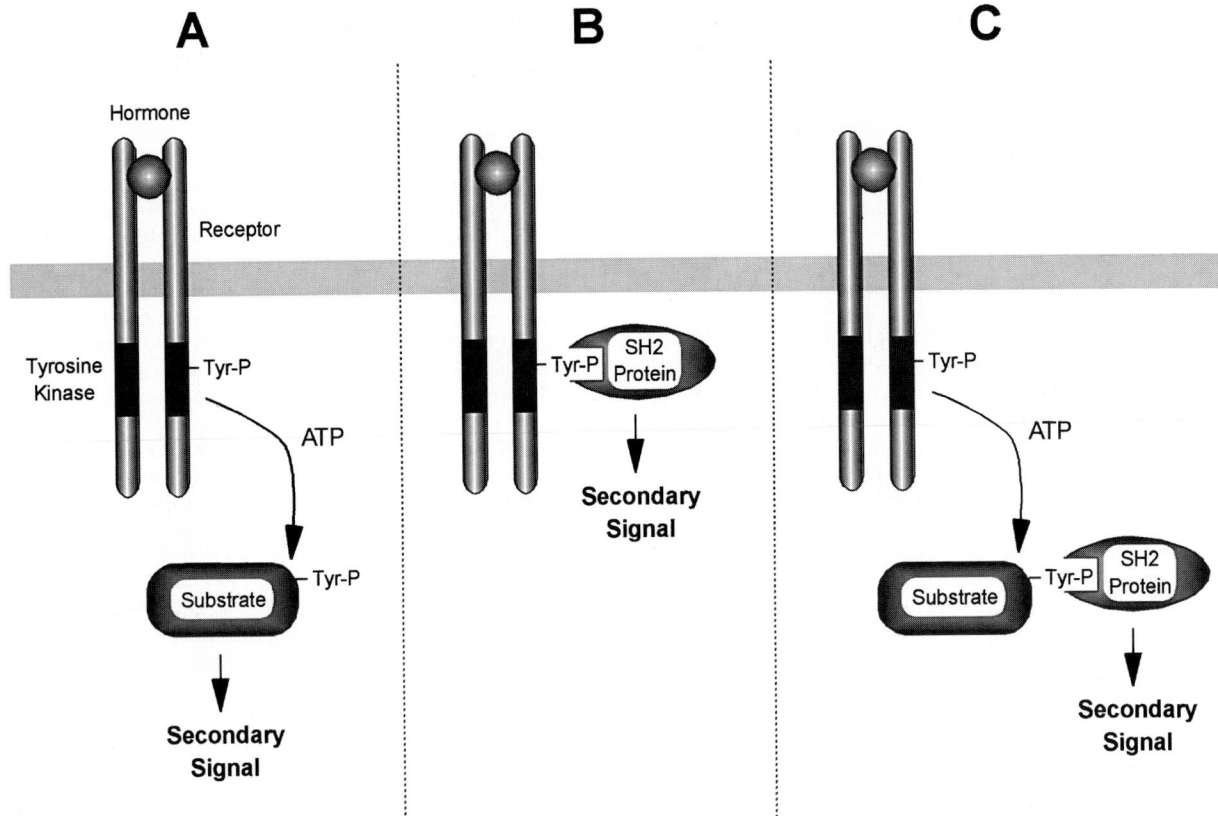

Figure 5–31. Three mechanisms of signal transduction by receptor tyrosine kinases. *A,* Tyrosine phosphorylation leads to activation or inactivation of nonreceptor substrate proteins and consequent signal transmission. *B,* Tyrosine phosphorylated residues in the receptors form docking sites for nonreceptor proteins (e.g., via phosphotyrosine-binding SH2 domains), which are activated by receptor binding. *C,* Receptors phosphorylate tyrosine residues in nonreceptor proteins, which form regulatory docking sites for additional proteins containing phosphotyrosine-binding domains.

molecules (see Fig. 5–31*B*).[256] Interactions of this type between receptors and other proteins, which represent a major initial signaling mechanism for EGF, PDGF, FGF, CSF-1, and other receptor tyrosine kinases, occur only when tyrosine is in a phosphorylated state and thus provide an important functional link between hormone binding, receptor autophosphorylation, and postreceptor signaling. In the case of insulin and IGF-I receptors, specific cellular substrates for the receptor tyrosine kinases appear to serve the same function as autophosphorylation sites in other receptor tyrosine kinases. Nonreceptor proteins, including insulin receptor substrate-1 (IRS1)[257, 258] and IRS2[259] are phosphorylated on multiple tyrosine residues by activated receptors and then function as docking proteins that initiate cellular signaling responses by forming complexes with SH2 domain-containing proteins (see Fig. 5–31*C*).

The presence of multiple tyrosine phosphorylation sites in tyrosine kinase receptors and in proteins such as IRS1 allows for specific interactions with a number of different SH2 domain-containing proteins. For example, the EGF receptor contains five tyrosine residues in the intracellular COOH-terminal tail of the receptor that undergo hormone-stimulated phosphorylation,[157] and each phosphotyrosine residue interacts specifically with SH2 domain-containing regulatory molecules.[158, 260] In the docking protein IRS1, there are 14 potential tyrosine phosphorylation sites, eight of which have surrounding sequence characteristic of residues that bind SH2 domains.[257] X-ray crystallographic structures have now been obtained for a number of SH2 domains complexed with specific phosphopeptides, and this has provided insight into the structural basis for interactions of individual SH2 domains with phosphotyrosine and other amino acids surrounding the

tyrosine residue.[261–265] As a general principle, SH2 domains interact with phosphotyrosine residues contained in the sequence Tyr-hydrophobic-X-hydrophobic, where position X can be occupied by a number of different amino acids (Fig. 5–32). Other amino acids located near the tyrosine residue in individual peptide sequences also interact with structural elements in SH2 domains, such that there is considerable specificity of interaction between proteins containing different SH2 domains and distinct phosphopeptide binding sites. As illustrated for the IRS1 protein in Figure 5–33, multiple phosphotyrosine

Phosphotyrosine Binding Motif

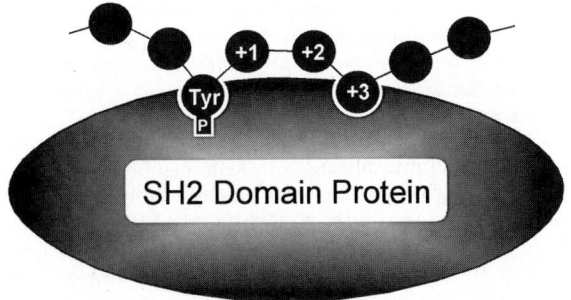

Figure 5–32. Interaction between a phosphotyrosine protein sequence and a protein SH2 domain. High-affinity interaction requires phosphorylation of the tyrosine residue. Specificity of interaction between protein pairs (e.g., between individual receptors and SH2 domain-containing proteins) is provided by additional requirements for certain amino acids at positions +1 and +3 (often Met or branched-chain amino acids), as well as less important contributions to binding from amino acids at other positions relative to the tyrosine residue.

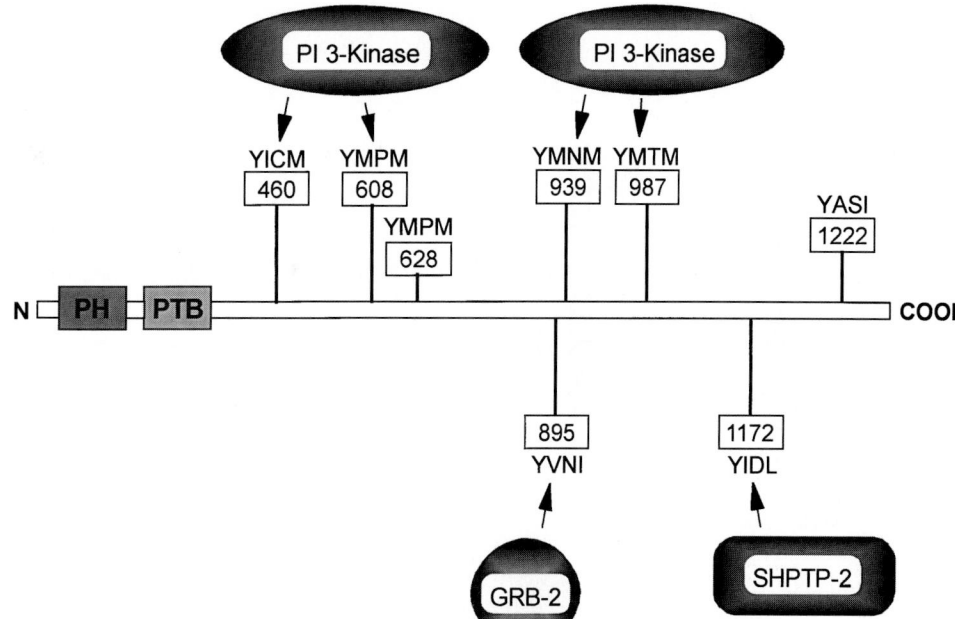

Figure 5–33. Potential tyrosine phosphorylation sites in IRS1. Favored interaction sites are shown for phosphatidylinositide 3-kinase (PI 3-kinase), SH protein phosphatase-2 (SHPTP-2), and growth factor receptor–bound protein-2 (Grb-2).

docking residues provide sites for high-affinity interaction with different SH2 domain-containing signaling proteins.[258] This provides a mechanism for transmitting the hormonal signal from a single receptor to a branching network of cellular response pathways. Docking proteins such as IRS-1 and receptors that contain multiple tyrosine phosphorylation sites have the capacity to bind simultaneously more than one SH2 domain-containing protein. It is likely that competition or steric hindrance between sites can play a role in normal and pathologic regulation of specific hormone signaling responses.

Binding of SH2 domain-containing proteins to receptor autophosphorylation sites or to phosphotyrosine residues in proteins such as IRS1 initiates signaling events through mechanisms that include conformational change in the associated molecule that alters its activity, or localization of the interacting protein to the region of the plasma membrane where it can activate a response. As an example of conformation-mediated signaling, the regulatory subunit of the enzyme phosphatidylinositide 3-kinase (PI 3-kinase) contains two SH2 domains that associate with two phosphotyrosine binding sites on IRS1 or similar phosphotyrosine sequences in receptor tyrosine kinases (Fig. 5–34).[266, 267] This interaction leads to a conformational change that activates the associated catalytic subunit of PI 3-kinase. The resulting production of 3-phosphoinositides by PI 3-kinase then activates pathways that lead to cellular responses such as increased glucose uptake. The IRS1/PI 3-kinase complex may function not only in activating the PI 3-kinase enzyme but also in localizing PI 3-kinase to specific target regions within the cell.[268]

Activation of the Ras pathway by the protein Grb2 represents an example of localization-mediated signaling. The Grb2 protein lacks intrinsic catalytic activity and is thought to function as an *adapter* that links and localizes other proteins into an active signaling complex.[269] As shown in Figure 5–35, Grb2 exists in a complex with the guanine nucleotide-exchange factor Sos through the association of proline-rich regions in Sos with two SH3 domains in Grb2. Activation of receptor tyrosine kinases leads to the tyrosine phosphorylation of the substrate protein Shc, which then forms a complex with Grb2-Sos by binding to the SH2 domain of Grb2.[270] Through mechanisms that are not yet fully defined, Shc is thought to function by localizing Grb2-Sos to the region of the plasma membrane,

where Sos can catalyze GDP-GTP exchange from the membrane-anchored Ras protein.[271] In the insulin and IGF-I signaling pathways, the IRS1 protein may have a similar capacity to localize the Grb2-Sos complex and catalyze Ras GDP-GTP exchange.[271] Ras-GTP then activates Raf kinase, and this initiates a kinase cascade with the sequential phosphorylation of mitogen-activated protein (MAP) kinase-kinase, MAP kinase, p90RSK (receptor-activated signal kinase) and, ultimately, growth and metabolic responses in the cell.[272–274] Since each step in the kinase cascade illustrated in Figure 5–35 represents an enzyme-catalyzed reaction, this mechanism for transmitting a hormone signal to the cellular machinery has the capacity to provide both a high degree of specificity and exponential amplification of the initial signal triggered by hormone binding.

POSSIBLE MEDIATORS OF RECEPTOR KINASE SYSTEMS. In addition to regulation of cellular metabolism by tyrosine phosphorylation, insulin and other growth factors may control synthesis of second messengers that could mediate some hormone actions on intracellular enzymes. Some of these mediators are members of the inositol phosphate family, discussed later. In addition, insulin may cause activation of a phosphatidylinositol-glycan–specific phospholipase C (reviewed in reference 275). This phospholipase is thought to hydrolyze a membrane-associated substrate to produce the phosphatidylinositol-glycan and 1,2-diacylglycerol (DAG), which then modulates the activities of several intracellular enzymes. Because these products are apparently released outside the cell, they may be taken up back into cells to exert their effects. Although this hypothesis is interesting, the structure and activities of these mediators have not been confirmed. Thus their role in insulin action remains to be defined.

RECEPTORS THAT ACTIVATE INTRACELLULAR TYROSINE KINASES. The cytokine receptor family includes more than 25 different transmembrane receptor proteins that lack intrinsic tyrosine kinase activity but have the capacity to activate various intracellular tyrosine kinases following hormone binding.[78] These include receptors for GH, prolactin, interleukins, interferons, and a number of growth factors, such as erythropoietin, thrombopoietin, granulocyte colony-stimulating factor, granulocyte-macrocyte colony-stimulating factor, and leukemia inhibitory factor. All members of the large fam-

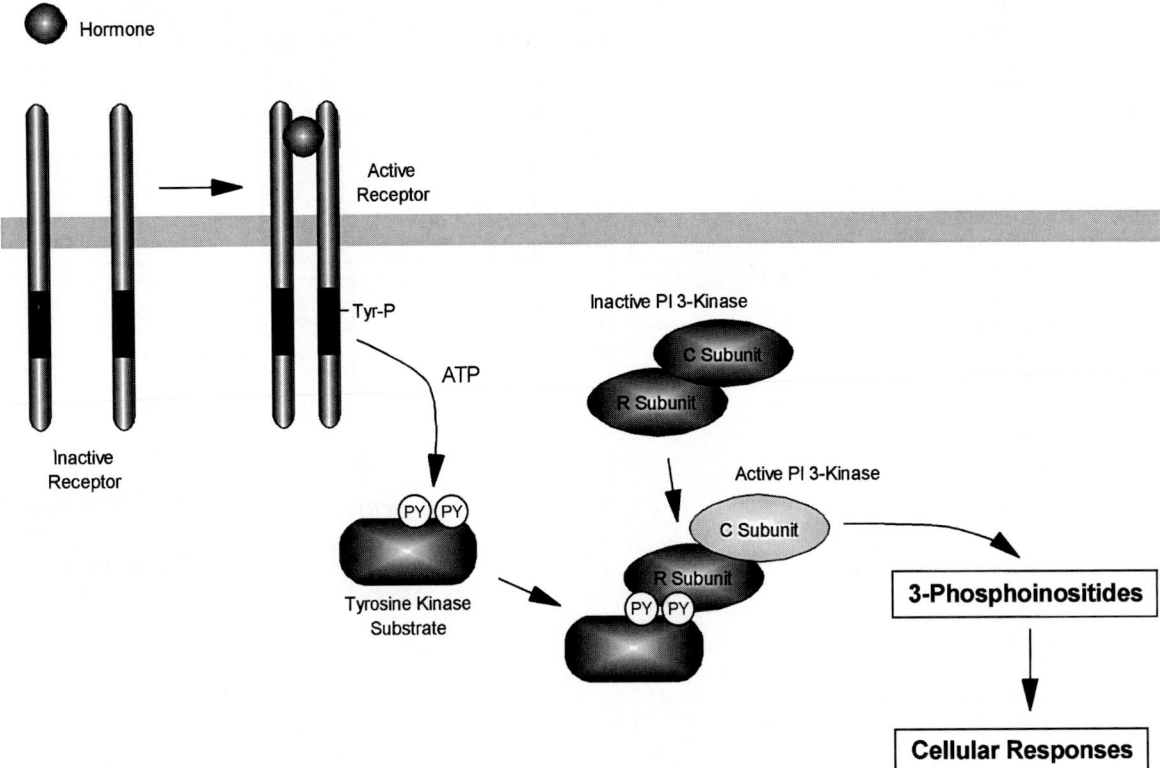

Figure 5–34. Activation of phosphoinositide (PI) 3-kinase by receptor tyrosine kinases. Two SH2 domains in the regulatory subunit of PI 3-kinase associate with tyrosine residues that are phosphorylated in response to hormone-stimulated activation of the receptor kinase domain. The PI 3-kinase regulatory subunit may associate with a docking protein (as illustrated) or with autophosphorylation sites on the receptor itself. This leads to a conformational change and activation of the catalytic subunit of PI 3-kinase.

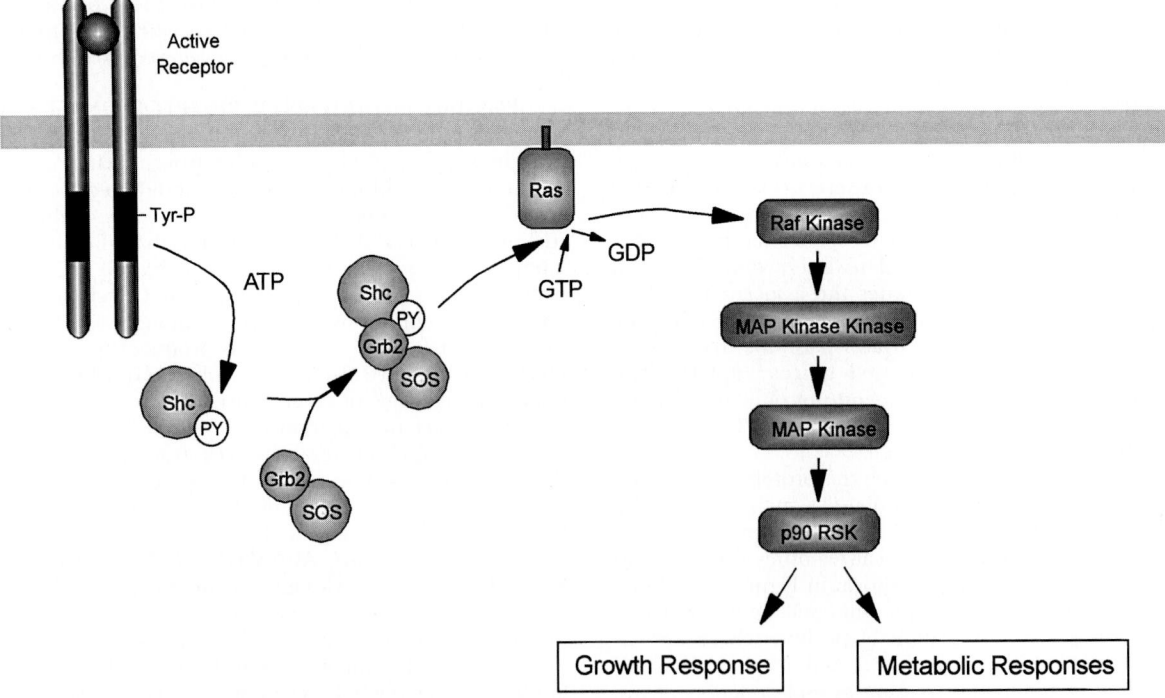

Figure 5–35. Activation of the Ras-MAP kinase pathway by receptor tyrosine kinases. Tyrosine phosphorylation of the Shc protein leads to its association with the adapter protein Grb2 and consequent localization of the Grb2-Sos complex to the region of membrane-anchored Ras. Sos catalyzes Ras GTP-GDP exchange, Ras activates the Raf kinase, and this leads to an activating phosphorylation cascade, as illustrated.

ily of cytokine receptors, which have only limited sequence similarity but are thought to derive from a common ancestral gene, lack a consensus intracellular catalytic domain. Although the signaling mechanism of each of these receptors has unique characteristics, an important component of signaling by all of the cytokine family of receptors appears to involve the ligand-induced activation of various members of the JAK family of intracellular tyrosine kinases[276–278] and the subsequent activation of members of a family of transcription factors that couple ligand binding to the activation of gene expression and thus have been designated *signal transducers and activators of transcription* (STATs).[279]

The mechanism through which GH receptors activate the JAK/STAT signaling pathway is illustrated in Figure 5–36.[82] Analysis of the co-crystal structure of human GH with its receptor has shown that a single GH molecule forms a complex with two GH receptors.[280] JAK2 becomes associated with the intracellular region of the dimerized GH receptor,[281] and, presumably through a conformational change induced by the receptors, the JAK2 tyrosine kinase is activated.[277] JAK2 becomes autophosphorylated, possibly through a *trans* mechanism involving two JAK2 molecules, and the JAK2 tyrosine kinase also phosphorylates specific tyrosine residues in the GH receptor.[82] The function of GH receptor phosphorylation has not yet been defined. Based on the occurrence of association motifs in JAK2, it is likely that the SH2 domains of STAT proteins interact directly with JAK2 and thus bring the STAT proteins into proximity so that they can be phosphorylated by the JAK2 tyrosine kinase.[82] The STAT proteins subsequently dissociate, possibly as a consequence of conformational change induced by their tyrosine phosphorylation, and form dimers through the association of the SH2 domain and phosphotyrosine of one STAT protein with the complementary phosphotyrosine and SH2 domain of another STAT protein.[282] The STAT dimer then translocates to the nucleus, where it binds to specific target sequences in various genes, such as c-*fos*, and activates transcription.[81, 283] Although GH receptor–activated JAK2 can phosphorylate multiple STAT proteins, including STATs 1, 3, and 5, specific phosphorylation of STAT5 occurs in response to GH.[284] It is likely that specificity in the activation of different members of the JAK family of

tyrosine kinases (JAK1, 2, and 3) by various cytokine receptors and their consequent phosphorylation of specific STAT proteins plays a role in establishing distinct cellular responses to different cytokines. STAT-independent pathways may be involved in signaling by cytokine receptors. For example, GH and all other members of the cytokine hormone family except for IL-4 have the capacity to activate the pathway leading from Ras to MAP kinase via the Shc/Grb2/Sos cascade, discussed earlier.[285] The physiological importance of the activation of multiple cell-signaling intermediates, including the STAT proteins, MAP kinase, and other proteins such as IRS1,[286] by GH and other cytokine receptors has not yet been established. This is an important area of current investigation, since these same intermediates are shared by a diverse array of hormones with distinct physiological functions.

Receptors Associated with Guanylate Cyclase

The effects of several agonists are mediated by cGMP,[287] including atrial natriuretic peptides (ANP), guanylin, sea urchin sperm proteins (resact and speract), and free radical nitric oxide (NO). ANP is expressed in the heart, whereas its related natriuretic peptides (BNP and CNP) are more widely distributed. ANP can initiate a hypotensive effect in the whole animal by increasing vascular smooth muscle relaxation and renal sodium loss. Guanylin is produced by epithelial lining cells of the intestinal mucosa, where it plays a role in salt and water homeostasis in the intestine. Resact and speract moderate sperm-egg interactions in the sea urchin. NO is synthesized from L-arginine by the action of constitutive and inducible NO synthases and is induced in various tissues by cytokines and endotoxins.[288] Among the established roles of NO, the most prominent action is vascular smooth muscle relaxation.

GUANYLATE CYCLASE. ANP, guanylin, and the sea urchin sperm proteins increase cGMP levels in the target cell by activating guanylate cyclase (GC) via direct binding of its membrane-associated forms (mGC). In contrast, NO, and possibly carbon monoxide (CO), initiate their actions by interacting with a soluble form of GC (sGC). GC catalyzes the formation cGMP from GTP, in analogy with adenylate cy-

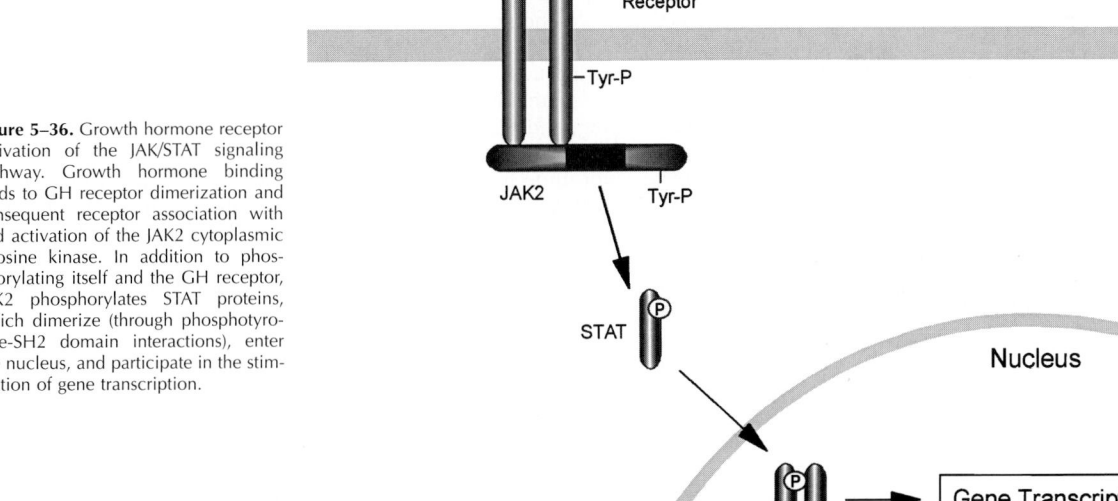

Figure 5–36. Growth hormone receptor activation of the JAK/STAT signaling pathway. Growth hormone binding leads to GH receptor dimerization and consequent receptor association with and activation of the JAK2 cytoplasmic tyrosine kinase. In addition to phosphorylating itself and the GH receptor, JAK2 phosphorylates STAT proteins, which dimerize (through phosphotyrosine-SH2 domain interactions), enter the nucleus, and participate in the stimulation of gene transcription.

clase.[289] Like the tyrosine and serine/threonine kinases, and unlike adenylate cyclase, GCs may directly serve both receptor and effector functions.

The deduced amino acid sequence of guanylate cyclase subunits derived from cloned cDNAs predicts a single transmembrane domain, similar to that of the tyrosine kinases. The COOH-terminal domain is intracellular and is highly conserved in sea urchins and mammals. In contrast, the extracellular domain is variable, contains the NH_2 terminus, and may serve as a ligand-binding domain. Further studies have shown that membrane-bound GC is likely a homotetramer composed of subunits available in six isoforms. There are combinations of these mGC isoforms that dictate preference for specific ligands such as ANP/BNP versus CNP. On the other hand, the soluble GC that is observed in most cell types of the cardiovascular system is a heterodimer consisting of α and β subunits. Integral to the sGC is a heme prosthetic group that is essential for interaction of the enzyme with NO and CO. Rat brain mGC, expressed in mammalian cells by DNA transfection, binds to and is activated by ANPs.

cGMP AS A SECOND MESSENGER. The cGMP generated by the guanylate cyclase enzymes can activate cGMP-dependent protein kinases (cGMP-PK), stimulate the actions of specific phosphodiesterases which in turn inactivate cGMP and cAMP, "cross-activate" the cAMP-dependent protein kinases, and control cation channels in the heart and kidney. The cGMP-PKs have a number of functions, including (1) relaxation of smooth muscle, (2) inhibition of platelet activation, (3) reduced endothelial permeability, and (4) augmented negative inotropic cardiac affect.

In summary, the membrane and soluble forms of GC serve as both receptor and effector. As such, this signaling system constitutes another example of a receptor, like the tyrosine and serine/threonine kinase receptors, that can catalyze the production of a second messenger without the interposition of other regulatory intermediates.

Receptors and Phosphatidylinositol Turnover

A number of hormones and ligands mediate their cellular actions via calcium ions and DAG as second messengers[290–295] (see Table 5–1). The second messengers, in turn, modulate the activity of protein kinases that are regulated by calcium binding–regulatory protein (e.g., calmodulin) or by DAG. These enzymes phosphorylate specific intracellular proteins, which results in further hormone action. Examples of hormones using this signaling system in specific tissues include α_1-adrenergic and muscarinic cholinergic agents, vasopressin (V_1), histamine (H_1), cholecystokinin, LHRH, thyrotropin-releasing hormone, angiotensin II, and oxytocin.

ROLE OF G PROTEINS. In general, the various hormone ligands that stimulate phosphoinositide turnover interact with the receptors that activate G proteins, as described for adenylate cyclase.[296–299] These G proteins, however, are coupled to phospholipase C activity,[290, 291, 293–295] an enzyme that fosters the conversion of membrane-bound phosphatidylinositol 4,5-bisphosphate to the second messenger form, inositol 1,4,5-trisphosphate (IP_3) (see Fig. 5–36). The PLC isozymes are grouped into three major classes: PLCβ, γ, and δ.[300] Each PLC is represented by a single polypeptide. PLCβ is activated by either α or $\beta\gamma$ G protein subunits, whereas PLCγ is associated with receptor tyrosine kinases via multiple SH2 and SH3 domains. It is also clear that different PLC isozymes may interact with specific activated G proteins or phosphorylated receptors.

IP_3 interacts with an IP_3 receptor on intracellular calcium-containing stores (Fig. 5–37). Evidence that G proteins are coupled to receptors involved in changes in calcium and DAG levels comes from various types of evidence, including the fact

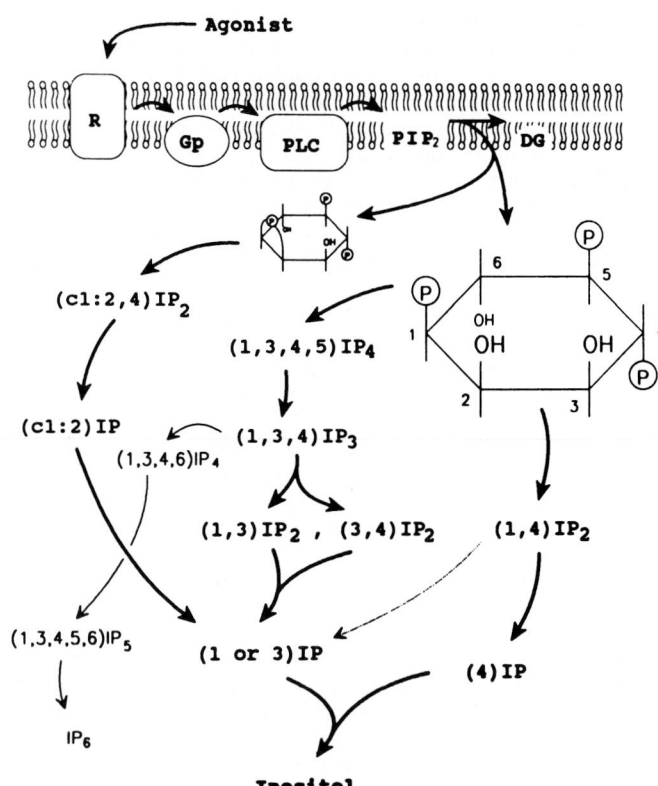

Figure 5–37. Pathways in the synthesis and metabolism of phosphatidylinositol. Ligand-receptor (R) interaction results in the activation of phospholipase C (PLC) via a G protein (Gp). Phospholipase C hydrolyzes membrane-bound phosphatidylinositol 4,5-bisphosphate (PIP_2) and active second messengers, inositol 1,4,5-trisphosphate (IP_3) and diacylglycerol (DG). Known metabolic pathways of IP_3 are shown. (From Putney JW Jr, Takemura H, Hughes AR, et al. How do inositol phosphates regulate calcium signaling? FASEB J 1989; 3:1899–1905, with permission.)

that pertussis toxin blocks calcium activation in mast cells and neutrophils. In addition, aluminum fluoride, which activates G proteins, increases IP_3 formation. Several hormones coupled to this pathway, such as thyrotropin-releasing hormone and vasopressin, also increase GTP hydrolysis, and a nonhydrolyzable analogue of GTP (GTPγS) decreases agonist binding to receptors for α_1-adrenergic agents, muscarinic nicotinic agonists, and angiotensin II.

The products of other PI kinases, including PI 3K, PI 4K, PI 4–P 5K, and PI 3–P 4K, are also lipid second messengers.[301] In particular, the products of PI 3K action such as PI 3-P, may mediate mitogenesis, reversal of apoptosis, vesicular trafficking, and regulation of the cytoskeleton. PI 3K interacts directly with growth factor receptors. Finally, the ubiquitous phosphoinositide transfer protein (PITP) serves a critical role in intracellular signaling by binding phosphoinositides in the cytoplasm and ensuring the presence of high levels of substrate for the glycolipid pathway.[298, 302]

EFFECTS OF INTRACELLULAR CALCIUM. The hormones that regulate phosphatidylinositol turnover also regulate intracellular calcium levels.[290, 291, 293–295, 303, 304] Calcium inside cells is maintained at a concentration of approximately 0.1 nM, whereas extracellular calcium levels are about 1 μM. Thus, there is a 10,000-fold concentration gradient across the two sides of the cell's plasma membrane. This gradient is maintained by a number of plasma membrane–based calcium pumps, channels, and transporters that are largely either voltage gated or ligand regulatable (see Fig. 5–37). There is also an internal releasable calcium pool in an intracellular nonmitochondrial, non–endoplasmic reticulum compartment.

This compartment involves small membrane vesicles termed *calciosomes* that are similar to those in the sarcoplasmic reticulum of muscle. This internal releasable pool of calcium is the major means by which IP_3 regulates cytoplasmic calcium levels. About 50% of the calcium in this compartment is releasable on IP_3 stimulation; other mediators of calcium release are cyclic ADP ribose and calcium itself. Indeed, the IP_3 response is maximally sensitive to calcium concentrations of 0.1 to 0.3 μM but is inhibited by higher levels. The intracellular IP_3 generated by interactions of ligand, membrane, receptor, and G protein induces this calcium release by binding to an IP_3 receptor (a homotetramer with a subunit size of 260 kd) in the calciosome.[305, 306] The IP_3 receptor and calcium channel activities may reside in the same protein, indicating that the IP_3 receptor is a gated ion channel. Multiple IP_3 receptor isoforms have been identified, each with different tissue distributions.

One of the cardinal features of cellular calcium release is its transient nature, which is properly called "pulses" or "bursts." Superimposition of these bursts leads to an intracellular Ca^{2+} wave. In addition to transient increases in intracellular calcium levels induced by IP_3, calcium waves initiated by the IP_3 interaction may be further propagated by a calcium-sensitive, IP_3-insensitive calcium pool[307] (see Fig. 5–37). The action of IP_3 is attenuated by metabolism of IP_3 to an inactive inositol bisphosphate (see Fig. 5–36). IP_3 may also be converted to inositol 1,3,4,5-tetrakisphosphate via the action of IP_3 kinase, which phosphorylates IP_3 in the presence of ATP. Inositol 1,3,4,5-tetrakisphosphate, however, may not be inactive and may serve to augment the effect of IP_3 by increasing the transfer of calcium among intracellular pools.[308] Thus avenues for both augmentation and reduction in signal activity are inherent in the phosphatidylinositol turnover pathway. Another mechanism that mediates increased calcium release from intracellular pools in muscle involves another gated ion channel, which is called the "ryanodine" receptor (Fig. 5–38).

CALCIUM-DEPENDENT KINASE. Ultimately both the inositol phosphate derivatives and calcium interact with specific protein kinases and mediate phosphorylation-dependent actions.[253] Calcium/calmodulin-dependent protein kinases exist in at least five forms in mammalian systems[309] and serve to mediate calcium-dependent changes in kinase activity.

The action of phospholipase C on phosphatidylinositol 4,5-bisphosphate also results in the production of DAG, which activates protein kinase C.[295, 310] Like the tumor-promoting phorbol esters, DAG augments the ability of protein kinase C to bind calcium and phosphatidylserine and thus allows activation of the enzyme at low intracellular calcium levels.[311] Calcium further augments the ability of DAG to activate protein kinase C, perhaps by altering the specificity of phospholipase C to cleave phosphatidylinositol monophosphate, as well as phosphatidylinositol 4,5-bisphosphate, thereby increasing the production of DAG. In addition, calcium may sensitize protein kinase C to DAG activation. The protein kinase C then continues to phosphorylate other intracellular proteins in a fashion similar to calcium/calmodulin-dependent protein kinases. Together these act on a wide variety of metabolic pathways in both the cytosol and the nucleus.

PROTEIN KINASE C. Part of the diversity of this pathway comes from the fact that protein kinase C is not a single enzyme but a family of related isozymes.[300] The enzymes are approximately 80 kd in size and are encoded by more than seven different genes.[312, 313] Furthermore, alternative splicing may result in even greater complexity of these forms. These protein kinase C isozymes are expressed in a tissue-specific fashion and thus may play a role in the differential effects of DAG stimulation of protein kinase C in different tissues. The three major groups of protein kinase C are termed conventional (α, βI, βII, γ), novel (δ, ϵ, σ, μ), or atypical (ζ, λ). However, the interactions of DAG with each protein kinase C are variable. For example, DAG stimulates all conventional

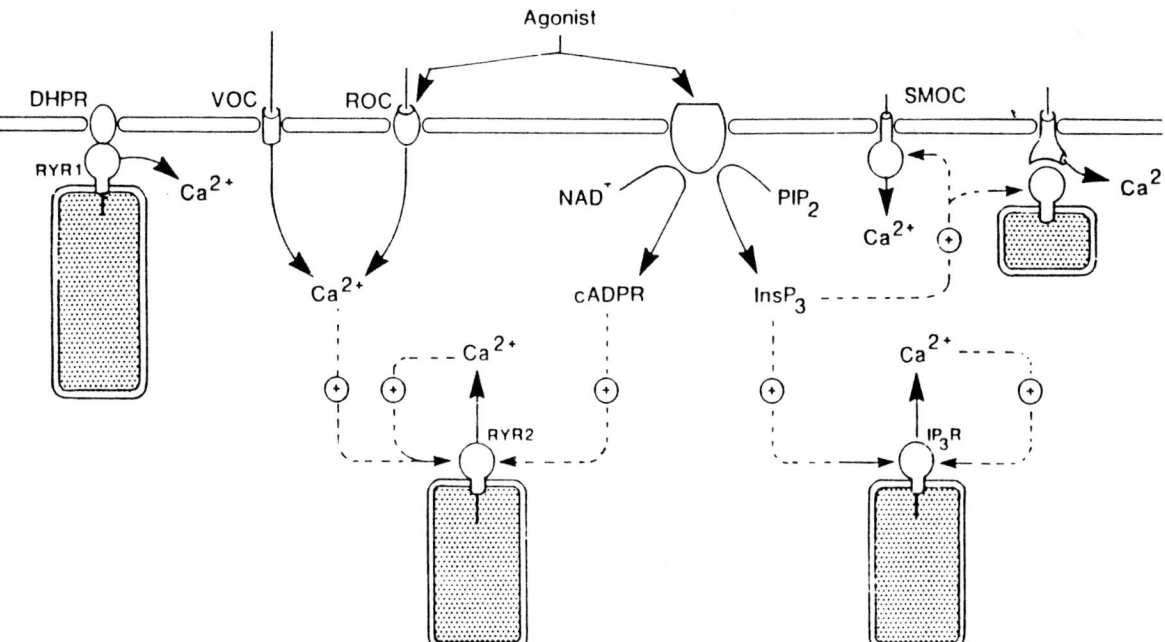

CALCIUM SIGNALLING

Figure 5–38. Calcium signaling. Intracytoplasmic calcium is derived from extracellular and internal sources. The entry of calcium from extracellular sources is mediated via voltage-operated channels (VOC), receptor-operated channels (ROC), or second messenger–operated channels (SMOC). Internal sources of calcium are regulated by ryanodine (RYR) and $InsP_3$ receptors (IP_3R). There are two major ryanodine receptors, RYR1 in skeletal muscle and RYR2 in heart muscle. Further, RYR in nonmuscle cells may be regulated by cyclic ADP ribose (cADPR). Note that both cADPR and $InsP_3$ may serve to sensitize RYR and IP_3R to the effects of ambient Ca^{2+} to stimulate further calcium release from calciosomes. (From Berridge MJ. The biology and medicine of calcium signalling. Mol Cell Endocrinol 1994; 98:119–124, with permission.)

and most novel forms of protein kinase C, but not the atypical enzymes.

Protein kinase C may also be stimulated by substances other than DAG, including unsaturated fatty acids, such as arachidonic acid, which is derived from the breakdown of phosphatidylcholine, and related compounds via the phospholipase A_2–phosphatidylcholine system, again providing a mechanism for interaction between different signaling pathways.

Activation of protein kinase C by DAG may also help intracellular calcium levels return to normal by stimulating calcium pump activity and/or by decreasing IP_3 production. Another interesting aspect of IP_3 and DAG interactions involves the ability of membrane potential changes within cells to alter IP_3 metabolism.[295, 310] Furthermore, stimulation of IP_3 can augment cAMP generation via adenylate cyclase–linked receptors, and vice versa. Also, the activity of DAG can be attenuated by the conversion of DAG to phosphatidate via DAG kinase. This interaction results in the resynthesis of phosphatidylinositols and a reduction in intracellular protein kinase C activity. Like protein kinase C, DAG kinase is 80 kd in size and possesses an ATP-binding site and two cysteine-rich zinc finger–like motifs.[314] It also contains two motifs that are typical of calcium-binding proteins, called EF hand motifs. DAG kinase activity is increased in the presence of calcium. A number of protein tyrosine kinases may also stimulate phosphatidylinositol kinase activity, which leads to activation of the calcium-DAG pathway.

Receptors and Ion Channels

Ion channels including those that control potassium, sodium, calcium, and chloride fluxes at the plasma membrane level can be regulated by charge gradients across the cell membrane, i.e., voltage gated, or by binding of hormones and neurotransmitters to the channel or associated receptors, i.e., ligand gated.[315–318] The ligand-gated ion changes occur in a distinct class of membrane receptors and may or may not require G proteins for signal transduction. The ligand-gated ion channels include the nicotinic cholinergic, $GABA_a$, glycine, glutamate, and kainic acid receptors.

The best studied of the ligand-gated ion channels is the nicotinic cholinergic receptor, which was first described in *Torpedo california*.[319] This receptor consists of five glycosylated subunits, two of which are identical (Fig. 5–39). The interaction of nicotinic cholineric agonists with the receptor activates a cation channel inherent in the receptor structure. The subunits of the nicotinic cholinergic receptor are encoded by separate genes. The molecular sizes of the α, β, γ, and δ subunits are 40, 48, 58, and 64 kd, respectively. Each receptor subunit possesses a high degree of sequence homology, including four transmembrane spanning domains. The second transmembrane spanning domain may form the lining for the ion pore. As a pentameric complex, the $\alpha_2\beta\gamma\delta$ ligand-gated ion channel has a molecular size of approximately 250 kd. Each receptor requires two agonist molecules, each binding to an α subunit, to induce a rapid conductance change.

The basic subunit structures of the other known ligand-gated ion channels are similar to that of the nicotinic receptor. The α subunits of the $GABA_a$ receptor have 75% homology to the acetylcholine receptor, and the α, β, γ, and δ subunits are 30 to 40% homologous. In addition, the $GABA_a$ subunit shares 35% homology with the similar subunit of the glycine receptor. Thus, the ligand-gated ion channels appear to be derived from a common ancestral gene.

Each subunit of the ligand-gated channel receptors contains an extensive extracellular NH_2-terminal domain with multiple sites of glycosylation. This structure is similar to that in a number of G protein–linked receptors. There is a large intracytoplasmic loop located between transmembrane regions 3 and 4 that contains multiple potential sites for phosphorylation, suggesting a role for regulation by cellular protein kinases. The COOH terminus of most subunits is short and is located in the cytoplasmic space.

In some ligand-gated ion channels G proteins act as signal

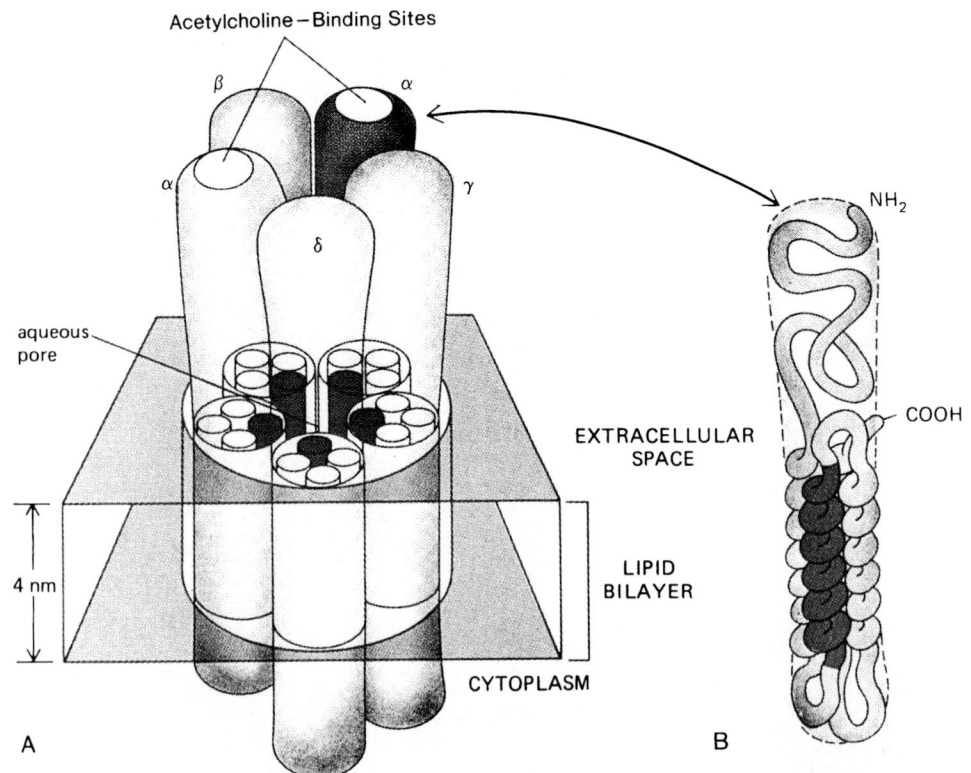

Figure 5–39. Schematic diagram of the nicotinic acetylcholine receptor. *A*, The receptor is composed of five subunits arranged in a pentagonal array to form the aqueous pore. The two α subunits interact with ligand. *B*, Each subunit contains alpha-helical regions that span the plasma membrane with four hydrophobic domains. In addition, there is along NH_2-terminal extracellular region, and one of the transmembrane regions in each subunit serves to line the pore.

transducers.[296, 316, 320–322] For instance, the muscarinic cholinergic–regulated potassium channel and the β-adrenergic–gated L-type calcium channel in the heart probably involve the participation of βγ and α_s G proteins, respectively.[323]

Receptors and Lipid Second Messengers

Lipid second messengers in addition to DAG are involved in signal transduction. Two major sources of lipid second messengers are glycerolipids and sphingolipids.[324, 325]

GLYCEROLIPIDS. With phosphatidylinositol (4,5)-bisphosphate [PI(4,5)P$_2$] as a substrate, PI 3 kinase action yields phosphatidylinositol (3,4,5)-P$_3$ [PI(3,4,5)P$_3$] which is known to activate specific protein kinase Cs (PKCs). In the previous section, we have already considered the action of phosphatidylinositol-phospholipase C (PI-PLC) on phosphatidylinositol (4,5)-bisphosphate to yield inositol trisphosphate [inositol (1,4,5)-P$_3$] and diacylglycerol (DAG). IP$_3$ and DAG activate calcium release from calciosomes via interaction with the IP$_3$ receptor and activation of a family of PKCs, respectively.

Using phosphatidylcholine as a substrate, a number of phospholipases, including phosphatidylcholine-PLC, PLD, and PLA$_2$, produce DAG, phosphatidic acid, and lysophosphatidylcholine and arachidonate, respectively. These putative lipid second messengers then activate different subsets of protein kinase Cs. Arachidonate may also activate PLCγ and sphingomyelinase in addition to PKCs.

SPHINGOLIPIDS. Interleukin-1β (IL-1β), nerve growth factor (NGF), tumor necrosis factor α (TNFα), vitamin D, ionizing radiation, and the cytokine Fas can increase the levels of the putative lipid second messenger ceramide. Ceramide is produced by the enzymatic cleavage of sphingomyelin by sphingomyelinase to yield ceramide and phosphocholine. Sphingomyelinase is present in the plasma membranes of all higher eucaryotic cells.

Ceramide exerts a number of actions. They include the activation of ceramide-associated protein kinase (CAPK), ceramide-activated protein phosphatase IIA (CAPP), a putative G-nucleotide exchange factor, Vav, and PKCζ, an atypical PK, acting as a direct target. CAPK is 90 kd in size, membrane limited, and a member of the serine/threonine protein kinase family. CAPP is a member of the PP2A family of serine/threonine protein phosphatases that exist as heterotrimers. One function of CAPK may be to phosphorylate important signaling proteins such as Raf-1 in the mitogenic signal pathway. Further, sphingolipid metabolism yields sphingosine-1-phosphate (SPP), which may also serve as a lipid second messenger.

Importantly, both glycerolipid and sphingolipid second messengers may be involved in molecular cross-talk. For example, DAG may be antiapoptotic, whereas ceramide may promote apoptosis. Such antagonism may be typical of the effects of such lipid second messengers.

MEMBRANE RECEPTORS AND DISEASE

The number and affinity of peptide hormone receptors and the postbinding steps in hormone action have important roles in coordinating receptor activity with the overall metabolic state of the cell and in limiting hormone action. In a variety of pathologic states, alterations in receptor expression, hormone binding, or signal transduction can cause changes in hormone responsiveness that cause or contribute to the disease. Disease states may be characterized by decreased receptor signaling (hormone resistance) or by increased receptor signaling (constitutively active receptors). Different types of receptor abnormalities that can lead to significant clinical disorders are summarized in Table 5–8. These include genetic defects in receptors or their associated effector molecules, disturbances in receptor regulation, specificity spillover leading to cross-signaling between different hormones and receptors, and antireceptor antibodies that have effects on receptor function. Examples of each of these types of receptor abnormalities and the mechanisms through which they cause disease are briefly discussed in the following sections.

Genetic Defects in Receptors

An understanding of receptor mutations and the mechanisms through which they cause human disease is expanding as a consequence of the cloning of cDNAs encoding many receptors and the elements of their signaling cascades and the development of new methods for studying the structure and function of human genes. As an area of endocrine investigation, the study of receptor mutations has led to the redefinition of many disease states. In some instances, clinical disorders previously thought to result from a uniform disease process have been shown to represent a common pathway of expression of multiple genetic defects. In other instances, apparently diverse disorders have been shown to develop from a common receptor mechanism or from different degrees of altered function in a single receptor. A summary of many currently known receptor genetic defects and their consequent clinical disorders is presented in Table 5–9.

INSULIN RECEPTOR MUTATIONS. (See also Chapter 21.) At least three syndromes of severe insulin resistance appear to result from genetic defects in the insulin receptor or insulin action pathways. These disorders include the type A syndrome of insulin resistance, leprechaunism, and lipoatrophic diabetes mellitus (Table 5–10). In addition to decreased insulin responsiveness and glucose intolerance or overt diabetes, these syndromes share a number of common features, including variable degrees of acanthosis nigricans and hyperandrogenism. With the development of new techniques for molecular cloning, specific defects in insulin receptors now have been defined in many of these patients.

Type A Syndrome. The type A syndrome is characterized by extreme insulin resistance, acanthosis nigricans, and hyperandrogenism occurring in the absence of obesity or lipoatrophy.[230] It is distinguished from type B insulin resistance by a lack of antibodies to the insulin receptor or other evidence of autoimmune disease. Even before the identification of specific molecular defects in patients with type A insulin resistance, biochemical evidence indicated that this group of disorders is heterogeneous. Patients usually have a decreased number of insulin receptors, presumably as a result of a defect in receptor biosynthesis.[230, 326] In some individuals, however, receptor levels are normal, and receptor tyrosine kinase activity is decreased[231, 232, 327] (see Fig. 5–28). In others, an abnormal, unprocessed insulin receptor is present.[328] Even in patients with decreased receptor number, insulin receptor mRNA levels varied from markedly decreased to normal.[326] It is now clear that this heterogeneity is due to different mutations in the insulin receptor gene.

Many insulin receptor mutations have been described, a few of which are summarized in Figure 5–40. In one patient a genetic recombination event appears to have occurred, with a

---

TABLE 5–8. Types of Receptor Abnormalities Associated with Human Disease

Genetic defects in receptors or effector molecules
Disordered receptor regulation
Specificity spillover
Antireceptor antibodies

TABLE 5–9. Genetic Defects in Membrane Receptors

Receptor	Effect of Mutation	Clinical Disorder
Insulin	Inhibiting	Insulin resistance
		Leprechaunism
		Lipoatrophic diabetes (total lipodystrophy)
Growth hormone	Inhibiting	Laron-type dwarfism
TSH	Activating, somatic	Solitary toxic thyroid adenoma
	Activating, germ line	Toxic thyroid hyperplasia
	Inhibiting	TSH resistance
LH/hCG	Activating	Male-limited precocious puberty
	Inhibiting	Male pseudohermaphroditism
PTH/PTHrP	Activating	Jansen-type metaphyseal chondrodysplasia (metaphyseal dysostosis)
Vasopressin V_2	Inhibiting	Congenital nephrogenic diabetes insipidus
ACTH (corticotropin)	Inhibiting	Congenital isolated glucocorticoid deficiency
MSH	Activating or inhibiting	Coat color variation in mammals
Extracellular calcium-sensing	Inhibiting	Familial hypercalcemic hypercalciuria (heterozygote)
		Neonatal severe hyperparathyroidism (homozygote)

hCG, human chorionic gonadotropin; LH, luteinizing hormone; MSH, melanocyte-stimulating hormone; PTH, parathyroid hormone; PTHrP, parathyroid hormone–related protein; TSH, thyroid-stimulating hormone.

resulting loss of the tyrosine kinase domain of the insulin receptor in one of the two alleles.[329] In another patient a point mutation resulted in the substitution of valine for glycine in a critical part of the ATP-binding site of the receptor β subunit[330]; this mutation produces a marked decrease in tyrosine kinase activity of the receptor.[330] Both of these patients also have decreased receptor number, which suggests that there may be an abnormality in the second insulin receptor allele or a suppressive effect of the mutant receptor on normal receptor expression. In a third patient, a point mutation converted the sequence of the proreceptor cleavage site from Arg-Lys-Arg-Arg to Arg-Lys-Arg-Ser,[328, 331] resulting in the accumulation of unprocessed receptor. The proreceptor binds insulin ineffectively and has reduced insulin-stimulated kinase activity. Many additional mutations have been demonstrated in the insulin receptors of patients with the type A syndrome of insulin resistance, and it is also likely that some patients have defects in nonreceptor proteins in the insulin action pathway that modify either receptor function or postreceptor signaling pathways.

Leprechaunism. The syndrome of leprechaunism is also probably heterogeneous in origin. In addition to insulin resistance and other features shared with patients with the type A syndrome (see Table 5–10), patients with leprechaunism have intrauterine and neonatal growth retardation and a clinical course complicated by fasting hypoglycemia that is frequently fatal within the first year of life.[332] In one of these patients, insulin resistance was due to compound heterozygous mutations of the insulin receptor alleles.[333] In one allele a missense mutation converts Lys-460 to Glu-460 in the receptor α subunit, and in the second allele a nonsense mutation in the α subunit leads to chain termination.

The specific mechanisms through which mutations in the insulin receptor lead to all of the features of the leprechaun

TABLE 5–10. Clinical Syndromes of Extreme Insulin Resistance That Result From Genetic Defects in the Insulin Receptor or Insulin Action Pathways

Syndrome	Clinical Features
Type A syndrome	Glucose intolerance, acanthosis nigricans, hyperandrogenism
Lipoatrophic diabetes	Glucose intolerance, atrophy of subcutaneous fat, hypertriglyceridemia, acanthosis nigricans, hyperandrogenism
Leprechaunism	Intrauterine growth retardation, "leprechaun" facies, paradoxical fasting hypoglycemia, mild hirsutism, hyperandrogenism

phenotype still are not understood. The marked growth retardation in these patients suggests that both growth and metabolic regulatory pathways are affected by the genetic defects. In some patients the responses to IGF-I, EGF, and other growth factors are decreased, which suggests a defect in a common postreceptor pathway.[334] Alternatively, abnormal insulin receptors may somehow interact with other receptors and modulate their function.[335, 336] It is certain that additional genetic defects will be defined in patients with type A insulin resistance, leprechaunism, and also lipoatrophic diabetes. An understanding of such specific genetic abnormalities will provide insights into normal receptor and postreceptor events in insulin action, in addition to explaining the basis for these rare disorders.

GROWTH HORMONE (GH) RECEPTOR MUTATIONS. (See also Chapter 30.) The syndrome of Laron-type dwarfism, alternatively designated the Laron syndrome or primary GH insensitivity, is characterized by decreased somatic growth evident from the first months of life and clinical features similar to those in patients with isolated GH deficiency.[337, 338] In contrast to GH-deficient patients, however, circulating levels of GH are elevated, and the GH-dependent somatomedin IGF-I appears to be deficient.[339] The GH molecule itself is normal, which is consistent with molecular defects in GH receptors or in more downstream elements in the GH signaling pathway.[340, 341] In most affected subjects GH receptors are markedly deficient,[342] and levels of the circulating GH binding protein that is thought to be derived from cell-surface receptors also are decreased.[343] A number of mutations of the GH receptor recently have been defined in the Laron syndrome,[344, 345] and it is certain that additional mutations will be identified. The GH receptor mutations described to date involve the extracellular domain of the receptor. Most result in decreased receptor expression or decreased GH binding, although one mutation (Arg-152–His substitution) described in two unrelated families is characterized by normal GH binding but a failure of receptors to dimerize after hormone binding.[346] The lack of GH signal transmission and profound growth failure in affected patients with this mutation supports the concept of an important role for ligand-induced receptor dimerization in GH signal transduction.[280] The lack of mutations in the GH receptor intracellular domain in patients with the Laron syndrome thus far studied may indicate that significant regions of the intracellular domain are not required for signal transduction. Alternatively, mutations in the intracellular domain of the GH receptor may interfere with the signal transduction pathway shared with other ligand-receptor systems[82, 156] and thus produce a phenotype distinct from Laron dwarfism.

Mutation				Effect	Syndrome

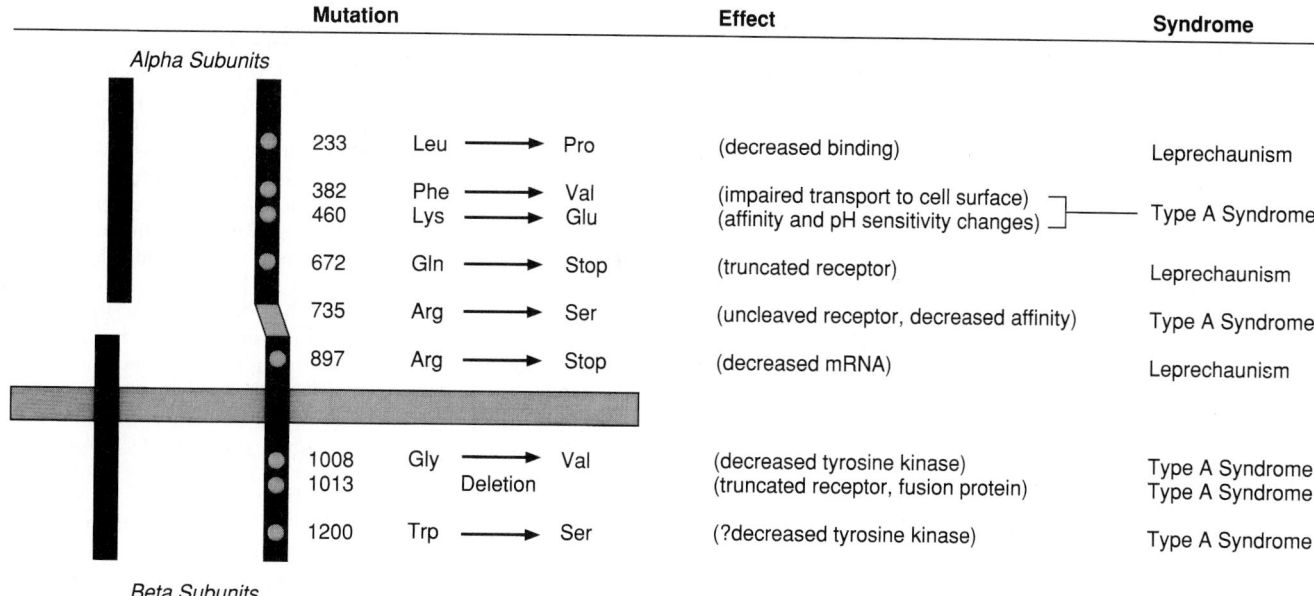

Alpha Subunits					
233	Leu	→	Pro	(decreased binding)	Leprechaunism
382	Phe	→	Val	(impaired transport to cell surface)	Type A Syndrome
460	Lys	→	Glu	(affinity and pH sensitivity changes)	
672	Gln	→	Stop	(truncated receptor)	Leprechaunism
735	Arg	→	Ser	(uncleaved receptor, decreased affinity)	Type A Syndrome
897	Arg	→	Stop	(decreased mRNA)	Leprechaunism
1008	Gly	→	Val	(decreased tyrosine kinase)	Type A Syndrome
1013		Deletion		(truncated receptor, fusion protein)	Type A Syndrome
1200	Trp	→	Ser	(?decreased tyrosine kinase)	Type A Syndrome
Beta Subunits					

Figure 5–40. Mutations in the insulin receptor associated with clinical syndromes of insulin resistance. Note that the two mutations Val-382 and Glu-460 occur in a single patient (compound heterozygote). See text for further description.

THYROTROPIN (TSH) RECEPTOR MUTATIONS. (See also Chapter 11.) The TSH receptor, a member of the large family of seven transmembrane segment G protein–coupled receptors, is localized in the basolateral membrane of thyroid follicular cells, where it mediates the effects of TSH on thyroid function and growth. A number of mutations in the TSH receptor gene have been defined that generate a constitutively active receptor and result in disorders of thyroid overgrowth.[347, 348] As described earlier in this chapter, the activation and inactivation of signaling by G proteins involves a coordinated receptor coupling and uncoupling of these proteins. Mutations in certain receptor structural regions can alter this protein coupling so that the G protein is locked into an active GTP-bound form. Activating somatic cell mutations of this type in the TSH receptor gene of thyroid follicular cells appear to be the major cause of solitary toxic thyroid adenomas. At this time, it is not known whether multinodular goiter results from a higher frequency of occurrence of multiple mutations similar to those described for solitary adenomas in the chronically overstimulated thyroid. When activating TSH receptor mutations occur in germline cells, hereditary or sporadic toxic thyroid hyperplasia develops.[349, 350] In contrast to Graves' disease (see Chapter 11), which is autoimmune in origin, toxic thyroid hyperplasia consequent to TSH receptor mutations is not associated with ophthalmopathy, thyroid-stimulating antibodies, or lymphocytic infiltration of the thyroid. Since the two disorders differ in prognosis and treatment approach, it is important to consider these clinical distinctions when one evaluates patients with thyrotoxicosis and a diffusely enlarged thyroid.

In addition to activating mutations that lead to thyrotoxicosis, it can be anticipated that mutations in some regions of the TSH receptor should impair receptor activity and cause hypothyroidism. Indeed, several individuals in one family have been described with mutations in both TSH receptor alleles, TSH resistance, elevated TSH levels, and a compensated euthyroid state.[351] Further studies on patients with congenital hypothyroidism ultimately may lead to the definition of additional gene defects that impair function sufficiently to prevent compensation via increased TSH production.

LUTEINIZING HORMONE/HUMAN CHORIONIC GONADOTROPIN (LH/hCG) RECEPTOR MUTATIONS. (See also Chapters 29 and 31.) The LH/hCG receptor is a G protein–coupled receptor for which activating and inhibiting mutations have been defined. Several mutations in this receptor gene result in constitutive G protein (G$_s$) activation and a resulting increase in cAMP levels in receptor-expressing cells in the absence of hormone.[352, 353] All mutations of this type described to date cause single amino acid substitutions in the regions of either the sixth transmembrane segment or the third cytoplasmic loop of the receptor, indicating that these domains are likely to have critical roles in stabilizing the receptor/G protein complex. Constitutive increase in cAMP levels as a consequence of such mutations in the LH/hCG receptors results in increased testosterone synthesis in testicular Leydig cells despite low gonadotropin levels and leads to the clinical syndrome of familial male-limited precocious puberty (also called testotoxicosis).[354] Affected patients typically present between ages 1 and 4 with signs of rapid virilization, and growth acceleration. Ultimately, as a consequence of premature epiphyseal closure, the adult stature is reduced. This disorder exhibits an autosomal dominant pattern of inheritance, consistent with a subset of mutant LH/hCG receptors encoded by a single defective allele that causes overstimulation of Leydig cells and increased testosterone production. Whereas LH alone activates steroidogenesis in Leydig cells, both LH and FSH are required to activate ovarian steroidogenesis, and female carriers of a mutant LH/hCG gene do not develop precocious puberty.

In addition to activating mutations of the LH/hCG receptor, inactivating mutations have been described also commonly involving the sixth transmembrane domain.[355] Although the mutant receptors bind LH normally, this does not lead to an increase in cellular cAMP, presumably as a consequence of defective interaction between the receptor and G proteins. Since undifferentiated Leydig cells require LH for proliferation and differentiation, 46,XY males with these mutations have a primary failure of testicular development in utero. As a consequence, they have the syndrome of male pseudohermaphroditism, characterized by female-appearing external genitalia in a 46,XY male (see Chapter 29). In contrast to activating mutations of the LH/hCG receptor, which produce male-limited precocious puberty when present as single alleles, inactivating mutations must affect both alleles (homozygotes or compound heterozygotes) to prevent compensation by a single normal allele. Homozygous females with inactivating LH/hCG receptor mutations have primary amenorrhea with ovarian resistance to LH.[355] This disturbance of phenotype in women is mild, because functional ovarian LH receptors are not required for early ovarian development but are required for a normal menstrual cycle.

OTHER RECEPTOR MUTATIONS. For other hormone receptors, similar complex relationships between gene sequence abnormalities, receptor function, and disease have been defined (see Table 5–9). Activating mutations of the parathyroid hormone/parathyroid hormone–related peptide (PTH/PTHrP) receptor gene lead to the clinical consequences expected in a state of excess PTH receptor signaling, including hypercalcemia and hypophosphatemia.[356, 357] These individuals also develop a form of short-limbed dwarfism (designated Jansen-type metaphyseal chondrodysplasia), consistent with a previously suspected but unproven role for PTHrP in bone elongation and ossification via interaction with the PTH/PTHrP receptor (see Chapter 27). Inactivating mutations in the vasopressin V2 receptor cause congenital nephrogenic diabetes insipidus,[358, 359] a disorder with an X-linked recessive pattern of inheritance, reflecting the X chromosome location of the V2 receptor gene (see Chapter 10). Inactivating mutations in the ACTH receptor gene cause the syndrome of hereditary glucocorticoid deficiency.[360]

Mutations in the extracellular calcium-sensing receptor cause familial hypercalciuric hypercalcemia in heterozygotes and a more severe disorder with a distinct phenotype, neonatal severe hyperparathyroidism, in homozygotes.[361] For several other receptors, mutations have been demonstrated in non-human mammalian species, although alterations in gene structure that cause a characteristic phenotype or disease in humans have not yet been identified. For example, MSH receptor mutations are known to be responsible for coat color differences in some animals[362]; however, the effects of MSH receptor mutations in humans are unknown. Genetic defects have also been described for receptors that are homologous to hormone receptors, but do not interact with true hormonal ligands. These include the G protein–coupled photoreceptor rhodopsin, which, when inactivated by mutation, leads to forms of retinitis pigmentosa.[363]

Genetic Defects in Postreceptor Signaling Pathway Intermediates

It can be anticipated that many mutations in genes encoding proteins that function as intermediates in postreceptor signaling pathways will also be shown to have important roles in producing endocrine disease. Several mutations of this type have been defined for the small GTP-binding proteins that link G protein–coupled receptors to cellular pathways (Table 5–11). The best characterized disorder resulting from this kind of mutation is pseudohypoparathyroidism type Ia, an inherited disease with PTH resistance and osteodystrophy.[364] At that time, Fuller Albright hypothesized that pseudohypo-

parathyroidism is the result of target organ unresponsiveness to hormone, even though cell-surface receptors and effector systems had not yet been identified for any hormone.[364] It is now known that patients with pseudohypoparathyroidism type Ia have inactivating mutations in the $G_{\alpha s}$ GTP-binding protein.[365, 366] Consistent with the involvement of individual G proteins in mediating the actions of multiple different receptors, these patients also have resistance to the action of PTH and may have evidence of other endocrine deficiency disorders, including hypothyroidism, amenorrhea, and infertility.[366]

Activating mutations of the $G_{\alpha s}$ GTP-binding protein produce disorders of excessive growth in many endocrine tissues (see Chapter 6). A single allele with an activating mutation in $G_{\alpha s}$ (heterozygote) has potent enough effects on endocrine cell growth to produce pathologically significant overgrowth, and clinical disorders resulting from these types of mutations are relatively common. In one study activating $G_{\alpha s}$ mutations were found in 18 (43%) of 42 pituitary adenomas examined.[367] Similar $G_{\alpha s}$ mutations, through their occurrence in somatic cells of different endocrine tissues, can cause thyroid and adrenal adenomas, and $G_{\alpha i}$ mutations have been associated with adrenal and ovarian adenomas.[367] Furthermore, as many as 10% of thyroid carcinomas may have mutations in the $G_{\alpha s}$ gene.[368, 369] Thus, G protein mutations appear to have important roles in causing malignant as well as benign endocrine tumors.

Receptor Regulation and Desensitization in Disease

Both the number and the affinity of peptide hormone receptors, as well as postbinding steps in hormone action, are regulated by physiological factors. Disturbances in these normal regulatory responses of receptors can lead to abnormalities in hormone responsiveness that cause or contribute to clinical disorders. Most disease states of this type are characterized by decreased hormone action or hormone resistance, rather than increased hormone responsiveness. Because physiological and pathologic insulin receptor regulation has been extensively studied, it will be reviewed as a model system that is representative of peptide hormone receptors in general.

The pathways involved in regulation of insulin receptors have been discussed in the foregoing sections of this chapter. The cell-surface receptor number is down-regulated in response to extracellular insulin, apparently as a result of the internalization of insulin-receptor complexes, with subsequent degradation to some degree of both insulin and the receptor.[128, 132] The binding affinity of the insulin receptor is affected by many factors, including extracellular insulin,[132] other hormones such as glucocorticoids,[370] fasting,[371] exercise,[372] and diet composition[373] (see Table 5–4). In contrast to changes in receptor number, which appear to derive from modifications in the normal pathways of receptor synthesis and degradation, the molecular mechanisms that cause altered binding affinity are less well defined. Binding affinity of the insulin receptor is inversely related to plasma membrane fluidity,[374] and some of the regulation of binding affinity may result from altered physical properties of the membrane.[375] Even less is known about insulin receptor regulation at the postbinding level, although serine phosphorylation and possibly other modifications in the receptor may alter tyrosine kinase activity, as discussed earlier in this chapter.

OBESITY. Insulin resistance is common in obesity[376] and appears to result from alterations in both receptor number and postbinding receptor activity.[377–381] Lower numbers of insulin-binding sites are present in monocytes and adipocytes from obese patients and in a variety of animal models of obesity.[378, 379] Characteristically, circulating insulin levels are elevated and correlate inversely with insulin receptor num-

TABLE 5–11. Genetic Defects in Receptor-Coupled G Proteins

G Protein	Effect of Mutation	Clinical Disorder
$G_{\alpha s}$	Inhibiting	Pseudohypoparathyroidism Ia
	Activating	Multitissue, somatic: McCune-Albright syndrome
		Pituitary, somatic: adenomas
		Thyroid, somatic: adenomas, carcinomas
		Adrenal, somatic: adenomas
$G_{\alpha i}$	Activating	Adrenal, somatic: adenomas
		Ovary, somatic: adenomas

Figure 5–41. Insulin binding to receptors on cells of obese patients. *Left,* Circulating monocytes. *Right,* Adipocytes. For each graph, four obese patients were selected to show a range of findings. The upper curve in each represents an obese patient who was indistinguishable from normal; these patients had normal receptors, normal levels of plasma insulin, and normal sensitivity to insulin. The two middle curves in each graph show a moderate decrease in receptor concentration, which was associated with moderate hyperinsulinemia and insulin resistance. The lower curve in each graph shows a more severe deficiency of insulin receptors in a patient who had more severe hyperinsulinemia and insulin resistance. Dietary treatment (600 kcal/d) for several weeks (not shown) is associated with restoration of receptor concentration to normal (or near-normal) levels. To convert insulin values from nanograms per milliliter to picomoles per liter, multiply by 1.722×10^5. (From Bar RS, Harrison LC, Muggeo M, et al. Regulation of insulin receptors in normal and abnormal physiology in humans. Adv Intern Med 1978; 24:23–52, with permission.)

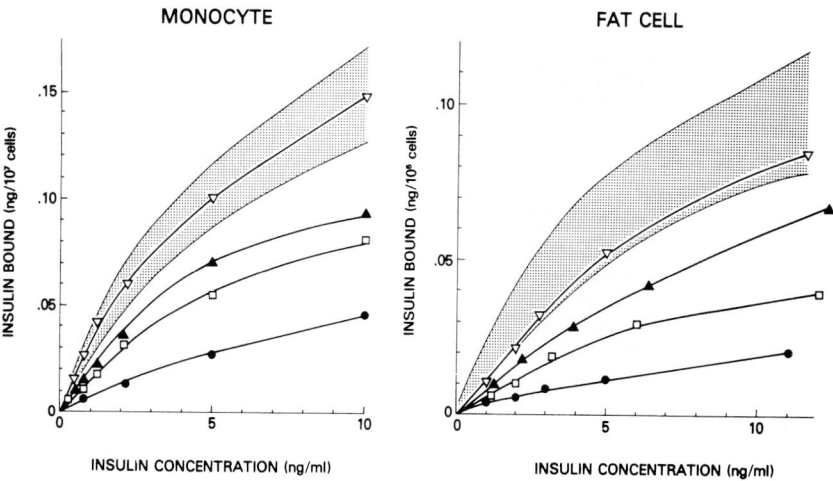

ber[371] (Fig. 5–41). If insulin levels are lowered, for example by diet or drugs that interfere with insulin secretion, the receptor number returns to normal even though the degree of obesity may not be significantly changed.[380] This suggests that the decreased number of insulin receptors in insulin-resistant obese patients may result from the effects of excess insulin on normal pathways of receptor down-regulation. In addition, coexistent postbinding defects in insulin action have been demonstrated in euglycemic clamp studies.[382, 383] These defects may have their basis in postbinding pathways of receptor signaling or in true postreceptor sites, such as in the glucose transport system. The observation that insulin receptor number can be restored to normal if insulin levels are decreased in obese patients suggests that the changes in receptor number are secondary to the insulin resistance, and not a primary causal factor. Possibly, postbinding alterations in insulin action in obesity initiate resistance to the hormone, insulin levels rise as a compensatory response, and this increase results in a decrease in insulin receptor number and more profound insulin resistance.

TYPE II DIABETES MELLITUS. (See also Chapter 21.) Type II diabetes mellitus is characterized by resistance to insulin in both obese and nonobese individuals.[381] Many type II diabetics have low levels of insulin by the time the disease is fully manifested, but some patients have elevated insulin levels in association with glucose intolerance, presumably reflecting partial compensation for insulin resistance. The cellular abnormalities associated with insulin resistance of type II diabetes in patients with elevated insulin levels are similar to those in obesity, with both decreased receptor number and impaired postbinding insulin action.[382, 383] In patients who do not have elevated insulin levels, receptor number is not markedly decreased, and insulin resistance appears to result primarily from postbinding abnormalities. Because the majority of type II diabetics are obese, the common occurrence of insulin resistance is not unexpected, and similar underlying abnormalities may exist in both obesity and type II diabetes mellitus. This parallel with obesity cannot explain all insulin resistance in type II diabetes, however, because nonobese diabetics may also be insulin resistant.[381] Independent of obesity, defects in insulin action in type II diabetes may result from decreased receptor tyrosine kinase activity (Fig. 5–42) and from defects in postreceptor steps in insulin action.[384–387] Thus, the insulin resistance of type II diabetes mellitus is due to multiple alterations in hormone action pathways. Which, if any, of these alterations is primary remains to be determined. With the exception of insulin-resistant states associated with antireceptor antibodies (see later), most other acquired disorders of insulin responsiveness appear to be explained by alterations

in postreceptor pathways with or without some alteration in receptor function. These other disorders include states of glucocorticoid excess,[388–390] GH excess,[391] uremia,[392] and diabetic ketoacidosis.[393] For a more complete discussion, the reader is referred to Chapter 21.

Specificity Spillover Syndromes

Peptide hormone receptors provide mechanisms for transduction of hormone signals and also for specificity of biologic responses through the high-affinity binding of the respective hormones. Because the receptors mediate the interactions with intracellular pathways, under most circumstances the receptor plays a more important role than does the hormone in determining the pattern of biologic responses. As evident from the foregoing sections of this chapter, receptors for different hormones and the peptide hormones themselves can be classified into families with structural similarities that reflect evolution from common ancestral molecules. These

INSULIN RECEPTOR KINASE IN NIDDM

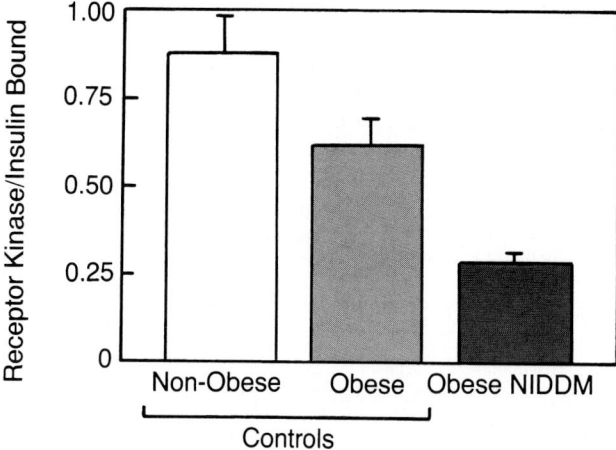

Figure 5–42. Insulin receptor tyrosine kinase activity in liver biopsy specimens from normal and obese humans and those with type II diabetes mellitus (Obese NIDDM). The data are expressed as kinase activity per insulin bound to correct for the decrease in receptor number. Note that kinase activity is still decreased in type II diabetes even allowing for this change. (From Caro JF, Ittoop O, Pories WJ, et al. Studies on the mechanism of insulin resistance in the liver from humans with noninsulin-dependent diabetes. Reproduced from the Journal of Clinical Investigation, 1986, vol. 78, pp. 249–258 by copyright permission of the American Society of Clinical Investigation.)

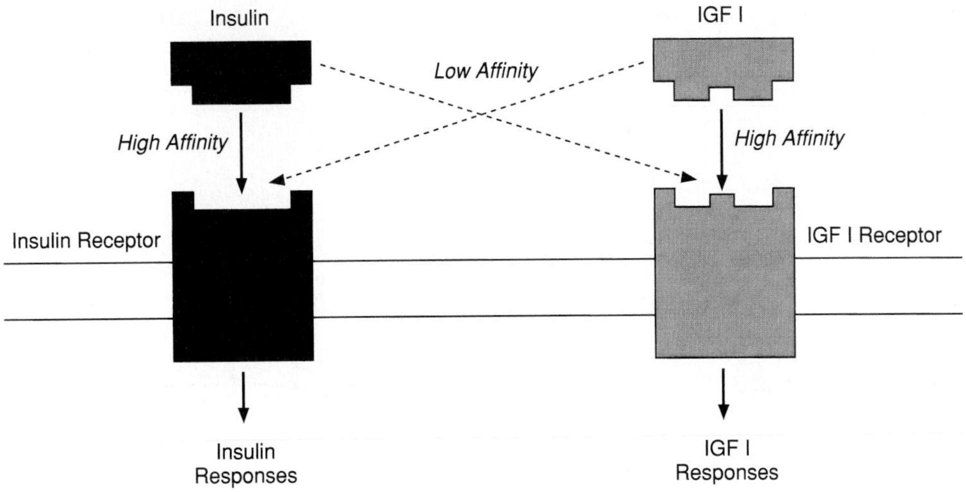

Figure 5–43. Specificity spillover between insulin and IGF-I. Each hormone binds to and activates the specific receptor for the other with approximately 10-fold lower potency than its own homologous receptor.

structural homologies can result in the binding of a given hormone to the receptors for another hormone, albeit with lower affinity. This crossover of hormone binding is illustrated for insulin, IGF-I, and their respective receptors in Figure 5–43. In diseases in which there are elevated hormone levels, syndromes of specificity spillover can result from the activation of receptors for one hormone via low-affinity binding of another hormone.[394]

Several examples of specificity spillover syndromes are described in Table 5–12. In acromegaly, high levels of GH lead to abnormal tissue growth through the activation of GH receptors. In a significant number of patients, however, there is also evidence of excess prolactin activity, as evidenced by galactorrhea, amenorrhea, and infertility. In some individuals, these changes are associated with concurrent elevations of both GH and prolactin levels; in others prolactin levels are normal, and the apparent hyperprolactinemia syndrome is best explained by binding of GH to prolactin receptors.[395] Similar hormone-receptor cross-reactivity appears to explain the occurrence of hyperthyroidism in some patients with trophoblastic tumors[396, 397] that produce large quantities of chorionic gonadotropin, which can bind with low affinity to the TSH receptor. In some patients with trophoblastic tumors, variant forms of chorionic gonadotropin are produced that exhibit even greater affinity for TSH receptors than does the chorionic gonadotropin of normal pregnancy, and this may lead to even more marked hyperthyroidism.[398] Nonpancreatic neoplasms that produce large quantities of IGF-II can lead to

significant specificity spillover and hypoglycemia, although it is not clear whether this results from the binding of IGF-II to insulin receptors, to IGF-I receptors, or to both.[399–401] Other disorders that may be due to specificity spillover include the hyperandrogenism of certain forms of severe insulin resistance (cross-reactivity of insulin with ovarian IGF-I receptors)[402] and possibly macrosomia in infants of diabetic mothers (insulin cross-reactivity with IGF-I receptors in somatic tissues).[403]

Antireceptor Antibodies

Immunologic abnormalities are associated with a broad spectrum of endocrine disorders (see Chapters 7 and 33). Antibodies against endocrine tissue components have been demonstrated in type I diabetes mellitus,[404] adrenal insufficiency,[405] Hashimoto's thyroiditis,[406, 407] and some forms of gonadal insufficiency.[407, 408] These antibodies provide valuable clues to the existence of specific endocrine disorders, often before hormone deficiency can be detected, but in most cases the role of specific antibodies in endocrine tissue destruction has not been clearly established. Thus, it is not certain whether specific anti–endocrine tissue antibodies are markers of disease or whether they have a pathogenetic role.

In a subgroup of autoimmune endocrine disorders, antireceptor antibodies play an important role in the development of clinical states of deficient or excess hormone action.[408] Disorders resulting from antireceptor antibodies have been described for peptide hormone receptors (insulin, TSH), for β-adrenergic receptors, and for neurotransmitter receptors (acetylcholine), as summarized in Table 5–13. Although the basis for the antireceptor endocrine disorders has not been defined, it is likely related to some alteration in specific immune response genes, because some patients exhibit more than one type of autoimmune disease.

INSULIN RECEPTOR ANTIBODIES. Antibodies to the insulin receptor were first identified in patients with severe insulin resistance and additional clinical findings termed the type B syndrome of insulin resistance.[230, 409] This syndrome is characterized by glucose intolerance and diabetes mellitus, insulin levels 10 to 100 times higher than normal in both basal and stimulated states, and resistance to injected insulin. In addition, these patients usually have a skin disorder, termed acanthosis nigricans, in which there is dermal thickening and hyperpigmentation in the axillae and skinfolds in other body regions. Patients with type B insulin resistance typically are middle-aged women with other evidence of autoimmune disease that may include alopecia, vitiligo, Raynaud's phenomenon, arthralgias and arthritis, splenomegaly, elevated levels of

TABLE 5–12. Specificity Spillover Syndromes Involving Peptide Hormones

Hormone	Cross-Reacting Receptor	Clinical Syndrome
Growth hormone	Prolactin	Galactorrhea with acromegaly
Insulin	IGF-I (in ovary)	Hyperandrogenism with insulin resistance
Insulin	IGF-I (?)	Macrosomia in newborn of diabetic mother
IGF-II	Insulin and/or IGF-I	Tumor hypoglycemia
ACTH	MSH	Hyperpigmentation in primary adrenal insufficiency
Human chorionic gonadotropin	TSH	Hyperthyroidism with trophoblastic tumors

ACTH, adrenocorticotropic hormone; IGF, insulin-like growth factor; MSH, melanocyte-stimulating hormone; TSH, thyroid-stimulating hormone;

TABLE 5–13. Hormone-Receptor Signal Transduction and Oncogenes*

Proto-oncogene	Hormone/Receptor Analogue	Location	Function
ERBB	EGF-R	Transmembrane	Tyrosine kinase
NEU/HER2	EGF-R	Transmembrane	Tyrosine kinase
FMS	GM-CSF-R	Transmembrane	Tyrosine kinase
RET	GDNF-R	Transmembrane	Tyrosine kinase
SRC	pp60	Membrane-associated	Tyrosine kinase
RAS	p21	Membrane-associated	Small GTP-binding protein
RAF	—	Cytoplasmic	Signaling kinase
SIS	PDGFβ	Cytoplasmic, ? secreted	Growth factor
INT2	FGF	Cytoplasmic, ? secreted	Growth factor
ERBA	T$_3$-R	Nuclear	Transcription factor
JUN	AP-1	Nuclear	Transcription factor
FOS	Heterodimer with JUN	Nuclear	Transcription factor

*Proto-oncogenes related to the signal transduction pathway are listed.
R, receptor; EGF, epidermal growth factor; GM-CSF, granulocyte-macrophage colony-stimulating factor; GDNF, glial-derived neurotrophic factor; PDGF, platelet-derived growth factor; FGF, fibroblast growth factor; T$_3$, triiodothyronine.

antinuclear and anti-DNA antibodies, and elevated erythrocyte sedimentation rate.

Most patients have high levels of polyclonal immunoglobulin antibodies that bind to the insulin receptor and block hormone binding. Studies in vitro have shown that antibody binding to the receptor is followed initially by metabolic effects that mimic the response to insulin binding.[113, 410, 411] Subsequently the antibodies appear to induce receptor internalization, down-regulation, and postbinding desensitization, thus resulting in hormone unresponsiveness. A chronic down-regulated and desensitized state appears to predominate in vivo and thus causes the insulin resistance.

The investigation of antibody-receptor interactions in type B insulin resistance provided insight into normal mechanisms of receptor activation. These antibodies mimic hormone effects only when present in a bivalent form.[113] Monovalent (Fab) antibody fragments, which have only a single antigen-binding site, bind to receptors and block hormone binding but do not stimulate postreceptor responses. This finding confirmed the important role of receptor-receptor interactions in the initiation of cellular responses. In some patients, anti-insulin receptor antibodies cause excess receptor stimulation and hypoglycemia, rather than insulin resistance.[411, 412] Hypoglycemia can be present initially or can evolve in the course of a disease that begins with insulin resistance. The spectrum of clinical findings from insulin resistance to hypoglycemia reflects the properties of specific antibodies that are predominant at a given point in time.

Anti-insulin receptor antibodies have also been described in some patients with new-onset type I diabetes mellitus.[413] In this case, the antibodies may occur as an anti-idiotype response to anti-insulin antibodies in the circulation. These antireceptor antibodies are of low titer and probably play no clinically significant role.

TSH RECEPTOR ANTIBODIES. The most common endocrine disorder in which antireceptor antibodies play an important role is Graves' disease (see Chapter 11). As part of an autoimmune process, patients with Graves' disease have circulating antibodies that recognize diverse thyroid cell surface antigens and in many cases stimulate cell growth and thyroid hormone synthesis and release.[414] An enigmatic serum factor termed *long-acting thyroid stimulator,* or LATS, was originally described in patients with Graves' disease[415] and is now known to consist of various anti-TSH receptor and antithyroid antibodies. Stimulatory activity of these LATS immunoglobulins results, in most patients, from the interaction of the immunoglobulin with the TSH receptor or with cell-surface gangliosides closely associated with the receptor.[416, 417] In contrast to anti-insulin receptor antibodies, which usually lead to insulin resistance, anti-TSH receptor antibodies usually activate the receptor and thus contribute to the thyrotoxicosis of Graves' disease (Fig. 5–44). In occasional patients, anti-TSH receptor antibodies block rather than stimulate the receptor and lead to hypothyroidism.

In the course of disease in a single patient, the nature of receptor antibodies in the circulating pool can shift from stimulatory to inhibitory and back to stimulatory.[418] This change in activity results from the expression of antibodies that recognize different domains of the receptors and may ultimately give insight into the mechanism of receptor signaling. Because the antireceptor antibodies block hormone binding, receptor activation must result directly from antibody binding.

Anti-TSH receptor antibodies are important not only in explaining the pathogenesis of hyperthyroidism in Graves' disease but also in monitoring the response to therapy.[419, 420] Treatment with antithyroid drugs (propylthiouracil or methimazole) frequently induces a remission, and high anti-TSH receptor antibody levels are a good predictor of relapse in these patients and thus can be followed periodically to assess the status of the remission and the requirement for continued therapy.

RECEPTORS AND ONCOGENES

Specific genes play roles in the initiation and maintenance of the malignant state. Studies of genes in oncogenic viruses and in the DNA of some tumor cells that can transform normal fibroblasts have led to the identification and characterization of *oncogenes.*[421] More than 50 different oncogenes have been described. Oncogenes usually have cellular counterparts that play key roles in normal growth control and differentiation and are termed cellular or *proto-oncogenes.*[421] It is likely that certain viruses have developed the capacity to transform cells by virtue of acquiring a proto-oncogene.

A major challenge in modern biology is the determination of the molecular mechanisms that lead to tumorigenesis.[422] For example, a proto-oncogene under the control of viral elements may be abnormally regulated, leading to abnormal levels of the corresponding protein product and ultimate cellular dysfunction. Alternatively, mutations of the proto-oncogene could result in altered function of the encoded protein.

In view of the critical role of membrane receptors in the regulation of cellular activities, including growth and development, it is not surprising that proto-oncogenes may encode

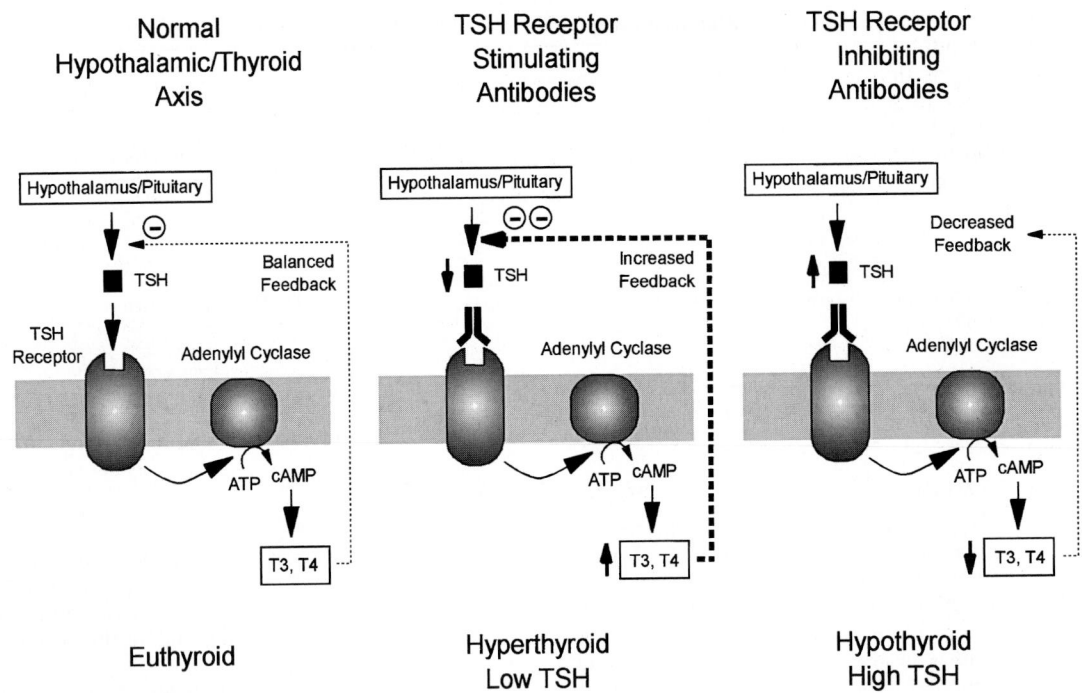

Figure 5–44. TSH receptor stimulation of T_3 and T_4 production in normal persons and patients with antireceptor antibodies in Graves' disease. *Left Panel,* In the normal individual, negative feedback by thyroid hormones at the hypothalamus and pituitary controls TSH production and ensures a euthyroid state. *Middle Panel,* Most often in patients with Graves' disease, antireceptor antibodies activate the TSH receptor and lead to hyperthyroidism as a consequence of continued T_3 and T_4 production despite feedback inhibited (low) TSH levels. *Right Panel,* A minority of patients have TSH receptor inhibiting antibodies, which lead to hypothyroidism and prevent TSH from stimulating the receptor despite high TSH levels resulting from the lack of feedback inhibition by thyroid hormones.

important components of the receptor signal-transduction pathway.[423, 424] Table 5–12 illustrates the diversity of proto-oncogenes that may be involved in cellular signaling. Some encode receptors with intrinsic kinase activity, while others are GTP-binding proteins that may be membrane associated.[425] Several encoded proteins are located in the cytoplasm and possess tyrosine or serine/threonine kinase functions or may be secreted as autocrine or paracrine factors. Last, proto-oncogenes can encode nuclear proteins, some of which may exhibit transcriptional activity.

An example of a proto-oncogene that serves a receptor function is the EGF receptor.[424, 425] The EGF receptor is a single polypeptide with one transmembrane domain, an extracellular ligand-binding region, and tyrosine kinase activity. EGF mediates a potent mitogenic response in appropriate cells, and uncontrolled EGF activity can result in abnormal cell growth. The avian erythroblastosis virus, which can transform erythroid and fibroblast cells, contains a viral oncogene, v-*erb* B. v-*erb* B encodes a form of EGF receptor that is truncated both in the NH_2-terminal, extracellular domain and in the COOH-terminal, cytoplasmic tail and is active in the *absence* of the ligand. Constitutive action of EGF receptor apparently contributes to cellular transformation. Another key example is the *ret* proto-oncogene, which is a receptor tyrosine kinase with glial-derived neurotrophic factor (GDNF) as its natural ligand. Specific mutations in *ret* are etiologic in multiple endocrine neoplasia type 2[426, 427] (see Chapter 32).

Two key types of proto-oncogenes encode products that are membrane associated: one is *src*, which encodes a tyrosine kinase function, and the other is *ras*, which is a member of the low-molecular-weight GTP-binding protein family.[428, 429] Mutants of *ras* often possess altered intrinsic GTPase activity and participate in tumorigenesis, either alone or in concert with other oncogenes. These *ras* forms may malfunction by being maintained in the GTP-bound, active state. Several GH-producing pituitary tumors harbor a defect in the α_s subunit

of the G protein,[430] and a number of adrenal and ovarian malignancies contain an abnormal α_i subunit.[367]

Yet other proto-oncogenes may encode growth factors or other secretagogues that can influence cell growth and differentiation. As an example, v-*sis* encodes the β subunit of PDGF. This subunit may form an active dimer that can stimulate cell growth.[431, 432] Similarly, *int*-2 and KS-*hst* encode growth factors in the fibroblast growth factor family. Alternatively, proto-oncogenes may encode cytosolic proteins with kinase properties. For example, *raf*-1 encodes a serine/threonine kinase activity located in the cytoplasm. However, its physiological function is unclear.[433]

A number of nuclear proteins, some capable of binding specific DNA sequences, are also proto-oncogenes. These transcription regulatory proteins are critical for the distal part of the hormone signaling pathway. Some early growth response genes such as *jun* and *fos* appear to bind specific, hormone-dependent, enhancer DNA sequences in gene-regulatory regions (AP-1 sites).[434] Another major example is *ERBA*, the second gene in the avian erythroblastosis virus and one that collaborates with v-*erb* B. c-*erb* A encodes the thyroid hormone receptor α isoform, and is a member of a large family of ligand-dependent transcription factors that include the steroid hormone retinoic acid and vitamin D receptors[175] (see Chapter 4). v-*erb* A is a mutant *erb* A whose gene product cannot bind thyroid hormone. As such, it may function to repress thyroid hormone action via dimerization with wild-type thyroid hormone receptors. Such novel activity may represent an example of dominant negative regulation by oncogene products.[435]

Finally, fusion of normal and malignant cells occasionally extinguishes the malignant phenotype, suggesting the existence of an "oncogene" that results in tumorigenic activity only in the absence of its expression. The best-studied example of recessive oncogenes is the retinoblastoma (Rb) gene.[436] The absence of both Rb genes in a particular somatic cell increases its susceptibility to transformation. The Rb gene product is a 105-kd nuclear DNA-binding protein that probably participates in the regulation of the cell cycle. Furthermore, the action of the oncogenes in several well-known DNA tumor viruses may be manifest by the ability of their products to counteract Rb function by direct binding. It is expected that many other cellular oncogenes encode factors that participate in cellular signaling.

REFERENCES

1. Langley JN. On nerve endings and on special excitable substances. Proc R Soc Lond 1906; 78:170–194.
2. Ehrlich P. The Collected Papers of P. Ehrlich. Oxford: Pergamon, 1956: 183–194.
3. Pastan I, Roth J, Macchia V. Binding of hormone to tissue: the first step in polypeptide hormone action. Proc Natl Acad Sci USA 1996; 56:1802–1809.
4. Cuatrecasas P. Interaction of insulin with the cell membrane: the primary action of insulin. Proc Natl Acad Sci USA 1969; 63:450–454.
5. Schimmer BP, Ueda K, Sato GH. Site of action of adrenocroticotropic hormone (ACTH) in adrenal cell cultures. Biochem Biophys Res Commun 1968; 32:806–810.
6. Kono T. Destruction of insulin effector system of adipose tissue cells by proteolytic enzymes. J Biol Chem 1969; 244:1772–1778.
7. Sutherland EW. Studies on the mechanism of hormone action (Nobel lecture). Science 1972; 177:401–408.
8. Ross EM, Gilman AG. Biochemical properties of hormone-sensitive adenylate cyclase. Annu Rev Biochem 1980; 49:533–564.
9. Auerbach GD. Polypeptide and amine hormone regulation of adenylate cyclase. Annu Rev Physiol 1982; 44:653–666.
10. Zeleznik AJ, Roth J. Demonstration of the insulin receptor in vivo in rabbits and its possible role as a reservoir for the plasma hormone. J Clin Invest 1978; 61:1363–1367.
11. Rouleau MF, Mitchell J, Goltzman D. In vivo distribution of parathyroid hormone receptors in bone: evidence that a predominant osseous target cell is not the mature osteoblast. Endocrinology 1986; 123:187–191.
12. Sodoyez JC, Sodoyez-Goffaux F, Guillaume M, et al. ^{125}I-insulin metabolism in normal rats and humans: external detection by a scintillation camera. Science 1983; 219:865–868.
13. Haldemann AR, Rosler H, Barth A, et al. Somatostatin receptor scintigraphy in central nervous system tumors: role of blood-brain barrier permeability. J Nucl Med 1995; 36:403–410.
14. Eckelman WC, Reba RC, Rzeszotarski WJ, et al. External imaging of cerebral muscarinic acetylcholine receptors. Science 1984; 223:291–293.
15. Bergman RN. Toward physiological understanding of glucose tolerance. Diabetes 1989; 38:1512–1527.
16. Castillo C, Bogardus C, Bergman R, et al. Interstitial insulin concentrations determine glucose uptake rates but not insulin resistance in lean and obese men. J Clin Invest 1994; 93:10–16.
17. Miles PD, Levisetti M, Reichart DR, et al. Kinetics of insulin action in vivo: identification of rate-limiting steps. Diabetes 1995; 44:947–953.
18. Conn PM, Crowley WF Jr. Gonadotropin-releasing hormone and its analogs. Annu Rev Med 1994; 45:391–405.
19. Lin SY, Goodfriend TL. Angiotensin receptors. Am J Physiol 1970; 218:1319–1328.
20. Lefkowitz RJ, Roth J, Pricer W, et al. ACTH receptors in the adrenal: specific binding of ACTH-^{125}I and the relation to adenyl cyclase. Proc Natl Acad Sci USA 1970; 65:745–752.
21. Freychet P, Roth J, Neville DM Jr. Insulin receptors in the liver: specific binding of [^{125}I] insulin to the plasma membrane and its relation to insulin bioactivity. Proc Natl Acad Sci USA 1971; 68:1833–1837.
22. Rodbell M, Krans HMJ, Pohl SL, et al. The glucagon-sensitive adenyl cyclase system in plasma membranes of rat liver. III. Binding of glucagon: method of assay and specificity. J Biol Chem 1971; 246:1861–1871.
23. Hollenberg MD, Nexo E. Receptors and Recognition. London: Chapman & Hall, 1981: 1–31.
24. Rovati GE, Rodbard D, Munson PJ. DESIGN: Computerized optimization of experimental design for estimating Kd and Bmax in ligand binding experiments. I. Homologous and heterologous binding to one or two classes of sites. Anal Biochem 1988; 174:636–649.
25. Kahn CR, Harrison LC, eds. Insulin Receptors, Parts A and B. New York: Alan R. Liss, 1988.
26. Posner B. Polypeptide Hormone Receptors. New York: Marcel Dekker, 1985.
27. Matozaki T, Goke B, Tsunoda Y, et al. Two functionally distinct cholecystokinin receptors show different modes of action on Ca^{2+} mobilization and phospholipid hydrolysis in isolated rat pancreatic acini: studies using a new cholecystokinin analog JMV-180. J Biol Chem 1990; 265:6247–6254.
28. Pitschner HF, Schlepper M, Schulte B, et al. Selective antagonists reveal different functions of M cholinoreceptor subtypes in humans. Trends Pharmacol Sci Suppl 1989; 92–96.
29. Maron R, Taylor SI, Jackson R, et al. Analysis of insulin receptors on human lymphoblastoid cell lines by flow cytometry. Diabetologia 1984; 27:118–120.
30. Katoh M, Raguet S, Zachwieja J, et al. Hepatic prolactin receptors in the rat: characterization using monoclonal antireceptor antibodies. Endocrinology 1987; 120:739–749.
31. Gagnerault MC, Postel-Vinay MC, Dardenne M. Expression of growth hormone receptors in murine lymphoid cells analyzed by flow cytofluorometry. Endocrinology 1996; 137:1719–1726.
32. Alonso-Whipple C, Couet ML, Doss R, et al. Epitope mapping of human luteinizing hormone using monoclonal antibodies. Endocrinology 1988; 123:1854–1860.
33. Bandyopadhyay G, Standaert ML, Zhao L, et al. Activation of protein kinase C (α, β, and zeta) by insulin in 3T3/L1 cells: transfection studies suggest a role for PKC-zeta in glucose transport. J Biol Chem 1997; 272:2551–2558.
34. Gertler A, Grosclaude J, Strasburger CJ, et al. Real-time kinetic measurements of the interactions between lactogenic hormones and prolactin-receptor extracellular domains from several species support the model of hormone-induced transient receptor dimerization. J Biol Chem 1996; 271:24482–24491.
35. LeRoith D, Lowe WL Jr, Shemer J, et al. Development of brain insulin receptors. Int J Biochem 1988; 20:225–230.
36. Konishi J, Iida Y, Kasagi K, et al. Adipocyte TSH receptor–related antibodies in Graves' disease detected by immunoprecipitation. Endocrinol Jpn 1982; 29:219–226.
37. Boutin JM, Edery M, Shirota M, et al. Identification of a cDNA encoding a long form of prolactin receptor in human hepatoma and breast cancer cells. Mol Endocrinol 1989; 3:1455–1461.
38. Leite-De-Moares MC, Touraine P, Kelly PA, et al. Prolactin receptor expression in lymphocytes from patients with hyperprolactinemia or acromegaly. J Endocrinol 1995; 147:353–359.
39. Scatchard G. The attraction of proteins for small molecules and ions. Ann NY Acad Sci 1949; 51:660–672.
40. Kahn CR, Freychet P, Neville DM Jr, et al. Quantitative aspects of the insulin receptor interaction in liver plasma membranes. J Biol Chem 1974; 249:2249–2257.
41. Boeyaems JM, Dumont JE. The two-step model of ligand-receptor interaction. Mol Cell Endocrinol 1977; 7:33–47.
42. DeLean A, Robard D. Kinetics of cooperative binding. In: O'Brien J, ed. The Receptor. New York: Plenum, 1979: 143–192.
43. Burgaud JL, Baserga R. Intracellular transactivation of the insulin-like growth factor 1 receptor by an epidermal growth factor receptor. Exp Cell Res 1996; 223:412–419.
44. Rorstad OP, Wanke T, Coy DH, et al. Selectivity of binding of peptide analogs to vascular receptors for vasoactive intestinal peptide. Mol Pharmacol 1990; 37:971–977.
45. Schimmer BP. The 1994 Upjohn Award Lecture: molecular and genetic approaches to the study of signal transduction in the adrenal cortex. Can J Physiol Pharmacol 1995; 73:1097–1107.
46. Matozaki T, Martinez J, Williams JA. A new CCK analogue differentiates two functionally distinct CCK receptors in rat and mouse pancreatic acini. Am J Physiol 1989; 257:G594–G600.
47. Blundell T, Wood S. The conformation, flexibility, and dynamics of polypeptide hormones. Annu Rev Biochem 1982; 51:123–154.
48. De Meyts P, Urso B, Christoffersen C, et al. Mechanism of insulin and IGF-I receptor activation and signal transduction specificity. Ann NY Acad Sci 1995; 766:388–401.
49. Raymond JR, Hnatowich M, Lefkowitz RJ, et al. Adrenergic receptors: models for regulation of signal transduction processes. Hypertension 1990; 15:119–131.
50. Muldoon TG, Evans AC Jr. Hormones and their receptors. Arch Intern Med 1988; 148:961–967.
51. Yip CC. Cell-membrane hormone receptors: some perspectives on their structure and function relationship. Biochem Cell Biol 1988; 66:549–556.
52. Mitchell RH. How do receptors at the cell surface send signals to the cell interior? BMJ 1987; 295:1320–1323.
53. De Meyts P, Christoffersen CT, Urso B, et al. Role of the time factor in signaling specificity: application to mitogenic and metabolic signaling by the insulin and insulin-like growth factor-I receptor tyrosine kinases. Metabolism 1995; 44:1–11.
54. Hollenberg MD. Structure-activity relationships for transmembrane signaling: the receptor's turn. FASEB J 1991; 5:178–186.
55. Gershengorn MC. Thyrotropin-releasing hormone receptor: cloning and regulation of its expression. Recent Prog Horm Res 1993; 48:341–363.
56. McFarland KC, Sprengel R, Phillips HS, et al. Lutropin-choriogonadotropin receptor: an unusual member of the G protein–coupled receptor family. Science 1989; 245:494–499.
57. Loosfelt H, Misrahi M, Atger M, et al. Cloning and sequencing of porcine LH-hCG receptor cDNA: variants lacking transmembrane domain. Science 1989; 245:525–528.
58. Masu Y, Nakayama K, Tamaki H, et al. cDNA cloning of bovine substance-K receptor through oocyte expression system. Nature 1987; 329:836–838.
59. Lefkowitz RJ. G protein–coupled receptor kinases. Cell 1993; 74:409–412.
60. Strader CD, Sigal IS, Dixon RA. Genetic approaches to the determination of structure-function relationships of G protein–coupled receptors. Trends Pharmacol Sci 1989; 10:346–340.
61. Strader CD, Fong TM, Graziano MP, et al. The family of G-protein–coupled receptors. FASEB J 1995; 9:745–754.

62. Brown EM, Segre GV, Goldring SR. Serpentine receptors for parathyroid hormone, calcitonin, and extracellular calcium ions. Baillieres Clin Endocrinol Metab 1996; 10:123–161.

63. Dingledine R, Myers SJ, Nicholas RA. Molecular biology of mammalian amino acid receptors. FASEB J 1990; 4:2636–2645.

64. Jan LY, Jan YN. Voltage-sensitive ion channels. Cell 1989; 56:13–25.

65. Bolton TB, Beech DJ, Komori S. Voltage- and receptor-gated channels. Prog Clin Biol Res 1990; 327:229–243.

66. Marsh D. Peptide models for membrane channels. Biochem J 1996; 315:345–361.

67. Jones SV. Muscarinic receptor subtypes: modulation of ion channels. Life Sci 1995; 52:457–464.

68. Johnston GA. GABAA receptor pharmacology. Pharmacol Ther 1996; 68:173–198.

69. Baez M, Kursar JD, Helton LA, et al. Molecular biology of serotonin receptors. Obesity Res 1995; 3(Suppl 4):441S–447S.

70. Dani JA, Mayer ML. Structure and function of glutamate and nicotinic acetylcholine receptors. Curr Opin Neurobiol 1995; 5:310–317.

71. Pin JP, Duvoisin R. The metabotropic glutamate receptors: structure and functions. Neuropharmacology 1995; 34:1–26.

72. Catterall WA. Structure and function of voltage-sensitive ion channels. Science 1988; 242:50–61.

73. Schimerlick MI. Structure and regulation of muscarinic receptors. Annu Rev Physiol 1989; 51:217–227.

74. Ullrich A, Schlessinger J. Receptor tyrosine kinase family. Cell 1990; 61:200–203.

75. White MF, Kahn CR. The insulin signaling system. J Biol Chem 1994; 269:1–4.

76. Fantl WJ, Johnson DE, Williams LT. Signalling by receptor tyrosine kinases. Annu Rev Biochem 1993; 62:453–481.

77. Goodwin RG, Friend D, Ziegler SF. Cloning of the human and murine interleukin-7 receptors: demonstration of a soluble form and homology to a new receptor superfamily. Cell 1990; 60:941–951.

78. Finidori J, Kelly PA. Cytokine receptor signalling through two novel families of transducer molecules: Janus kinases, and signal transducers and activators of transcription. J Endocrinol 1995; 147:11–23.

79. Chua SC Jr, Chung WK, Wu-Peng XS, et al. Phenotypes of mouse diabetes and rat fatty due to mutations in the OB (leptin) receptor. Science 1996; 271:994–996.

80. Ihle JN, Witthuhn BA, Quelle FW, et al. Signaling by the cytokine receptor superfamily: JAKs and STATs. Trends Biochem Sci 1994; 19:222–227.

81. Schindler C, Darnell JE Jr. Transcriptional responses to polypeptide ligands: the JAK-STAT pathway. Annu Rev Biochem 1995; 64:621–651.

82. Carter-Su C, Schwartz J, Smit LS. Molecular mechanism of growth hormone action. Annu Rev Physiol 1996; 58:187–207.

83. Frielle T, Daniel KW, Caron MG. Structural basis of β-adrenergic receptor subtype specificity studied with chimeric β₁/β₂-adrenergic receptors. Proc Natl Acad Sci USA 1988; 85:9494–9498.

84. O'Dowd BR, Lefkowitz RJ, Caron MG. Structure of the adrenergic and related receptors. Annu Rev Neurosci 1989; 12:67–83.

85. Leite-De-Moares MC, Touraine P, Gagnerault MC, et al. Prolactin receptors and the immune system. Ann Endocrinol (Paris) 1995; 56:567–570.

86. Boutin JM, Jolicoeur C, Okamura H, et al. Cloning and expression of the rat prolactin receptor, a member of the growth hormone/prolactin receptor gene family. Cell 1988; 53:69–77.

87. De Meyts P. The structural basis of insulin and insulin-like growth factor-I receptor binding and negative co-operativity, and its relevance to mitogenic versus metabolic signalling. Diabetologia 1994; 37:S135–S148.

88. Rechler MM, Nisley SP. The nature and regulation of receptors for insulin-like growth factors. Annu Rev Physiol 1985; 47:425–552.

89. Morgan DO, Edman JC, Standring DN, et al. Insulin-like growth factor II receptor as a multifunctional binding protein. Nature 1987; 329:301–307.

90. Goldstein JL, Brown MS. Regulation of low-density lipoprotein receptors: implications for pathogenesis and therapy of hypercholesterolemia and atherosclerosis. Circulation 1987; 76:504–507.

91. Hedo JA, Kahn CR, Hayoshi M, et al. Biosynthesis and glycosylation of the insulin receptor: evidence for a single polypeptide precursor of the two major subunits. J Biol Chem 1983; 258:10020–10026.

92. Knutson VP, Ronnett GV, Lane MD. The effects of cycloheximide and chloroquine on insulin receptor metabolism: differential effects on receptor recycling and inactivation and insulin degradation. J Biol Chem 1985; 260:14180–14188.

93. Weidner KM, Hartmann G, Sachs M, et al. Properties and functions of scatter factor/hepatocyte growth factor and its receptor c-Met. Am J Respir Cell Mol Biol 1993; 8:229–237.

94. Carpentier JL, Fehlmann M, Van Obberghen E, et al. Redistribution of ¹²⁵I-insulin on the surface of rat hepatocytes: as a function of dissociation time. Diabetes 1985; 34:1002–1007.

95. Pearse BMF, Bretscher MS. Membrane recycling by coated vesicles. Annu Rev Biochem 1981; 50:85–101.

96. Ascoli M. Lysosomal accumulation of the hormone-receptor complex during receptor-mediated endocytosis of human choriogonadotropin. J Cell Biol 1984; 99:1242–1250.

97. Opresko LK, Chang CP, Will BH, et al. Endocytosis and lysosomal targeting of epidermal growth factor receptors are mediated by distinct sequences independent of the tyrosine kinase domain. J Biol Chem 1995; 270:4325–4333.

98. Marshall S. Kinetics of insulin receptor internalization and recycling in adipocytes: shunting of receptors to a degradative pathway by inhibitors of recycling. J Biol Chem 1985; 260:4136–4144.

99. Khan MN, Baquiran GB, Brule C, et al. Internalization and activation of the rat liver insulin receptor kinase in vivo. J Cell Biol 1989; 264:12931–12940.

100. Thomas WG, Baker KM, Motel TJ, et al. Angiotensin II receptor endocytosis involves two distinct regions of the cytoplasmic tail. J Biol Chem 1995; 270:22153–22159.

101. Goldstein JL, Anderson RG, Brown MS. Receptor-mediated endocytosis and the cellular uptake of low-density lipoprotein. Ciba Found Symp 1982; 92:77–95.

102. Jing S, Spencer T, Miller K, et al. Role of the human transferrin receptor cytoplasmic domain in endocytosis: localization of a specific signal sequence for internalization. J Cell Biol 1990; 110:283–294.

103. Chen WJ, Goldstein JL, Brown MS. NPXY, a sequence often found in cytoplasmic tails, is required for coated pit-mediated internalization of the low-density lipoprotein receptor. J Biol Chem 1990; 265:3116–3123.

104. Sorkin A, Waters C, Overholser KA, et al. Multiple autophosphorylation site mutations of the epidermal growth factor receptor: analysis of kinase activity and endocytosis. J Biol Chem 1991; 266:8355–8362.

105. Duckworth WC. Insulin degradation: mechanisms, products and significance. Endocrinol Rev 1988; 9:319–345.

106. Tsubouchi H, Miyazaki H, Gohda E, et al. Degradation of [¹²⁵I] iodoglucagon by normal rat plasma in radioimmunoassay mixture containing aprotinin and its prevention by p-chloromercuriphenyl sulfonate and leupeptin. Endocrinology 1986; 119:1137–1145.

107. King GL, Johnson SM. Receptor-mediated transport of insulin across endothelial cells. Science 1985; 227:865–869.

108. Dernovsek KD, Bar RS, Ginsberg BH, et al. Rapid transport of biologically intact insulin through cultured endothelial cells. J Clin Endocrinol Metab 1984; 58:761–765.

109. Bergman RN, Steil GM, Bradley DC, et al. Modeling of insulin action in vivo. Annu Rev Physiol 1992; 54:861–883.

110. Jacobson K, Ishihara A, Inman R. Lateral diffusion of proteins in membranes. Annu Rev Physiol 1987; 49:167–175.

111. Goncalves E, Yamada K, Thatte HS, et al. Optimizing transmembrane domain helicity accelerates insulin receptor internalization and lateral mobility. Proc Natl Acad Sci USA 1993; 90:5762–5766.

112. Schechter Y, Hernaez L, Schlessinger J, et al. Local aggregation of hormone-receptor complexes is required activation by epidermal growth factor. Nature 1979; 838:835–838.

113. Kahn CR, Baird KL, Jarrett DB, et al. Direct demonstration that receptor cross-linking or aggregation is important in insulin action. Proc Natl Acad Sci USA 1978; 75:4209–4213.

114. Ishizaka T, Ishizaka K. Triggering of histamine release from rat mast cells by divalent antibodies against IgE-receptors. J Immunol 1978; 120:800–805.

115. Cunningham BC, Ultsch M, de Vos AM, et al. Dimerization of the extracellular domain of the human growth hormone receptor by a single hormone molecule. Science 1992; 254:821–825.

116. De Meyts P. The structural basis of insulin and insulin-like growth factor-I receptor binding and negative cooperativity, and its relevance to mitogenic versus metabolic signaling. Diabetologia 1995; 37:s135–s148.

117. Chang PY, Goodyear LJ, Benecke H, et al. Impaired insulin signaling in skeletal muscles from transgenic mice expressing kinase-deficient insulin receptors. J Biol Chem 1995; 270:12593–12600.

118. Simon I, Brown TJ, Ginsberg BH. Modification of membrane physical properties, biological response and insulin binding in Friend cells by low serum concentration. Biochim Biophys Acta 1987; 896:165–172.

119. Field CJ, Ryan EA, Thomson AB, et al. Diet fat composition alters membrane phospholipid composition, insulin binding, and glucose metabolism in adipocytes from control and diabetic animals. J Biol Chem 1990; 265:11143–11150.

120. Kono T, Barham FW. The relationship between the insulin-binding capacity of fat cells and the cellular response to insulin: studies with intact and trypsin-treated fat cells. J Biol Chem 1971; 246:6210–6216.

121. Gliemann J, Gammeltoft S, Vinten J. Time course of insulin receptor binding and insulin-induced lipogenesis in isolated rat fat cells. J Biol Chem 1975; 250:3368–3374.

122. Dufau ML. Endocrine regulation and communicating functions of the Leydig cell. Annu Rev Physiol 1988; 85:8032–8036.

123. Kahn CR. Insulin resistance, insulin insensitivity, and insulin unresponsiveness: a necessary distinction. Metabolism 1978; 27:1893–1902.

124. Huckle WR, Earp HS. Regulation of cell proliferation and growth by angiotensin II. Prog Growth Factor Res 1994; 5:177–194.

125. Glenney JR Jr, Chen WS, Lazar CS, et al. Ligand-induced endocytosis of the EGF receptor is blocked by mutational inactivation and by microinjection of anti-phosphotyrosine antibodies. Cell 1988; 52:675–684.

126. Posner BI, Khan MN, Kay DG, et al. Internalization of hormone receptor complexes: route and significance. Adv Exp Med Biol 1986; 205:185–201.

127. Kasuga M, Kahn CR, Hedo JA, et al. Insulin-induced receptor loss in cultured human lymphocytes is due to accelerated receptor degradation. Proc Natl Acad Sci USA 1981; 78:6917–6921.

128. Ronnett GV, Knutson VP, Lane MD. Insulin-induced down-regulation of insulin receptors in 3T3-L1 adipocytes. J Biol Chem 1982; 257:4285–4291.

129. Hartzell HC, Frambrough DM. Acetylcholine receptor production and

incorporation into membranes of developing muscle fibers. Dev Biol 1973; 30:153–165.

130. Bockaert J, Roy C, Rajerison R, et al. Specific binding of [³H] lysine-vasopressin to pig kidney plasma membranes: relationship of receptor occupancy to adenylate cyclase activation. J Biol Chem 1973; 248:5922–5931.

131. Hinkle PM, Tashijian AH Jr. Thyrotropin-releasing hormone regulates the number of its own receptors in GH₃ strain of pituitary cells in culture. Biochemistry 1975; 14:3845–3851.

132. Gavin JR III, Roth J, Neville DM Jr, et al. Insulin-dependent regulation of insulin-receptor concentration. Proc Natl Acad Sci USA 1974; 71:84–88.

133. Hauger RL, Aguilera G, Catt KJ. Angiotensin II regulates its receptor sites in the adrenal glomerulosa zone. Nature 1978; 271:176–177.

134. Posner BI, Kelley PA, Friesen HG. Prolactin receptor in rat liver: possible induction by prolactin. Science 1978; 188:57–59.

135. Premont RT, Inglese J, Lefkowitz RJ. Protein kinases that phosphorylate activated G protein–coupled vectors. FASEB J 1995; 9:175–182.

136. White MF, Shoelson SE, Keutmann H, et al. A cascade of tyrosine autophosphorylation in the β-subunit activates the insulin receptor. J Biol Chem 1988; 263:2969–2980.

137. Rosen OM, Herrera R, Olowe Y, et al. Phosphorylation activates the insulin receptor tyrosine protein kinase. Proc Natl Acad Sci USA 1983; 80:3237–3240.

138. Nimrod A, Tsafriri A, Linder HR. In vitro induction of binding sites for HCG in rat granulosa cells by FSH. Nature 1977; 267:632–633.

139. Williams LT, Lefkowitz RJ, Hathaway DR, et al. Thyroid hormone regulation of beta-adrenergic receptor number. J Biol Chem 1977; 252:2787–2789.

140. Hammond HK, White FC, Buxton IL, et al. Increased myocardial beta-receptors and adrenergic responses in hyperthyroid pigs. Am J Physiol 1987; 252:H283–H290.

141. Soloff M. Uterine receptor for oxytocin: effects of estrogen. Biochem Biophys Res Commun 1975; 65:205–212.

142. Posner BI, Kelley PA, Friesen HG. Induction of lactogenic receptor in rat liver: influence of estrogen and the pituitary. Proc Natl Acad Sci USA 1974; 71:2407–2410.

143. Zachary I, Sinnett-Smith SW, Rozengart E. Early events elicited by bombesin and structurally related peptides in quiescent Swiss 3T3 cells. I. Activation of protein kinase C and inhibition of epidermal growth factor binding. J Cell Biol 1986; 102:2211–2222.

144. Wrann M, Fox CF, Ross R. Modulation of epidermal growth factor receptors on 3T3 cells by platelet-derived growth factor. Science 1980; 210:1363–1365.

145. Goldfine ID, Kahn CR, Neville DM Jr, et al. Decreased binding of insulin to its receptors in rats with hormone-induced insulin resistance. Biochem Biophys Res Commun 1973; 53:852–857.

146. McDonald AR, Goldfine IG. Glucocorticoid regulation of insulin receptor gene transcription in IM-9 cultured lymphocytes. J Clin Invest 1988; 81:499–504.

147. O'Brien RM, Granner DK. PEPCK gene as model of inhibitory effects of insulin on gene expression. Diabetes Care 1990; 13:327–339.

148. Cohen P. The role of protein phosphorylation in the hormonal control of enzyme activity. Eur J Biochem 1985; 151:439–448.

149. Dent P, Lavoinne A, Nakielny S, et al. The molecular mechanisms by which insulin stimulates glycogen synthesis in mammalian skeletal muscle. Nature 1990; 348:302–307.

150. Bandyopadhyay D, Kusari A, Kenner KA, et al. Protein-tyrosine phosphatase 1B complexes with the insulin receptor in vivo and is tyrosine-phosphorylated in the presence of insulin. J Biol Chem 1997; 272:1639–1645.

151. Yarden Y, Ullrich A. Molecular analysis of signal transduction by growth factors. Biochemistry 1988; 27:3113.

152. Kim Y, Nakajima R, Matsuo T, et al. Gene expression of insulin signal-transduction pathway intermediates is lower in rats fed a beef tallow diet than rats fed a safflower oil diet. Metabolism 1996; 45:1080–1088.

153. Pazin MJ, Williams LT. Triggering signaling cascades by receptor tyrosine kinases. Trends Biochem Sci 1992; 17:374–378.

154. Carpenter G. Receptors for epidermal growth factor and other polypeptide mitogens. Annu Rev Biochem 1987; 56:881–914.

155. Smit LS, Meyer DJ, Billestrup N, et al. The role of the growth hormone (GH) receptor and JAK1 and JAK2 kinases in the activation of Stats 1, 3, and 5 by GH. Mol Endocrinol 1996; 10:519–533.

156. Ihle JN. Signaling by the cytokine receptor superfamily. Trends Endocrinol Metab 1994; 5:137–143.

157. Hone J, Accili D, Psiachou H, et al. Homozygosity for a null allele of the insulin receptor gene in a patient with leprechaunism. Hum Mutat 1995; 6:17–22.

158. Fantl WJ, Escobedo JA, Martin GA, et al. Distinct phosphotyrosines on a growth factor receptor bind to specific molecules that mediate different signalling pathways. Cell 1992; 69:413–423.

159. Myers MG Jr, White MF. The new elements in insulin signaling: insulin receptor substrate-1 and proteins with SH2 domains. Diabetes 1993; 42:643–650.

160. Pawson T, Gish GD. SH2 and SH3 domains: from structure to function. Cell 1992; 71:359–362.

161. Pawson T. Protein modules and signalling networks. Nature 1995; 373:573–580.

162. Shotwell MA, Kilberg MS, Oxender DL. The regulation of neutral amino acid transport in mammalian cells. Biochem Biophys Acta 1983; 737:267–284.

163. McGivan JD, Pastor-Anglada M. Regulatory and molecular aspects of mammalian amino acid transport. Biochem J 1994; 299:321–334.

164. Cariappa R, Kilberg MS. Hormone-induced system A amino acid transport activity in rat liver plasma membrane and Golgi vesicles. J Biol Chem 1990; 265:1470–1475.

165. Fehlmann M, LeCam A, Freychet P. Insulin and glucagon stimulation of amino acid transport in isolated rat hepatocytes. J Biol Chem 1979; 254:10431–10437.

166. Liao K, Lane MD. Expression of a novel insulin-activated amino acid transporter gene during differentiation of 3T3-L1 preadipocytes into adipocytes. Biochem Biophys Res Commun 1995; 208:1008–1015.

167. Levine R, Goldstein MS. On the mechanism of action of insulin. Recent Prog Horm Res 1955; 11:343–380.

168. Hayes N, Biswas C, Strout HV, et al. Activation by protein synthesis inhibitors of glucose transport into L6 muscle cells. Biochem Biophys Res Commun 1993; 190:881–887.

169. Fukumoto H, Seino S, Imura H, et al. Sequence, tissue distribution, and chromosomal localization of mRNA encoding a human glucose transporter-like protein. Proc Natl Acad Sci USA 1988; 85:5434–5438.

170. Birnbaum MB. Identification of a novel gene encoding an insulin-responsive glucose transport protein. Cell 1989; 57:305–315.

171. Charron MJ, Brosius FC, Alper SL, et al. A glucose transport protein expressed predominantly in insulin-responsive tissues. Proc Natl Acad Sci USA 1989; 86:2535–2539.

172. James DE, Brown R, Navarro J, et al. Insulin-regulatable tissues express a unique insulin-sensitive glucose transport protein. Nature 1988; 333:183–185.

173. Simpson IA, Cushman SW. Hormonal regulation of mammalian glucose transport. Annu Rev Biochem 1986; 55:1059–1089.

174. Johnson PF, McKnight SL. Eukaryotic transcriptional regulatory proteins. Annu Rev Biochem 1989; 58:1059–1089.

175. Evans RM. The steroid and thyroid hormone receptor superfamily. Science 1992; 240:889–895.

176. Montminy MR, Gonzalez GA, Yamamoto KK. Regulation of cAMP inducible genes by CREB. Trends Neurosci 1990; 18:184–188.

177. Angel P, Allegretto EA, Okino ST, et al. Oncogene jun encodes a sequence-specific trans-activator similar to AP-1. Nature 1988; 332:166–169.

178. Montminy MR, Sevarino KA, Wagner JA, et al. Identification of a cyclic-AMP responsive element within the rat somatostatin gene. Proc Natl Acad Sci USA 1986; 83:6682–6686.

179. Hoeffler JP, Meyer TE, Yun Y, et al. Cyclic AMP-responsive DNA-binding protein: structure based on a cloned placental cDNA. Science 1988; 242:1430–1432.

180. Kamei Y, Xu L, Heinzel T, et al. A CBP integrator complex mediates transcriptional activation and AP-1 inhibition. Cell 1996; 85:403–414.

181. Angel P, Imagawa M, Chiu R, et al. Phorbol ester–inducible genes contain a common cis element recognized by a TPA-modulated trans-acting factor. Cell 1987; 49:729–739.

182. Ihle JN. STATs: signal transducers and activators of transcription. Cell 1996; 84:331–334.

183. Leung S, Li X, Stark GR. STATs find that hanging together can be stimulating. Science 1996; 273:750–751.

184. Massague J. TGFβ signaling: receptors, transducers, and MAD proteins. Cell 1996; 85:947–950.

185. Schule R, Umesono K, Mangelsdorf DJ, et al. Jun-Fos and receptors for vitamins A and D recognize a common response element in the human osteocalcin gene. Cell 1990; 61:497–504.

186. Robishaw JD, Foster KA. Role of G proteins in the regulation of the cardiovascular system. Annu Rev Physiol 1989; 51:229–244.

187. Firtel RA, van Haastert PJ, Kimmel AR, et al. G protein–linked signal transduction pathways in development: dictyostelium as an experimental system. Cell 1989; 58:235–239.

188. Johnson GL, Dhanasekaran N. The G-protein family and their interaction with receptors. Endocr Rev 1989; 10:317–331.

189. Lochrie MA, Simon MI. G protein multiplicity in eukaryotic signal transduction systems. Biochemistry 1988; 27:4957–4965.

190. Gilman AG. The Albert Lasker Medical Awards: G proteins and regulation of adenylyl cyclase. JAMA 1989; 262:1819–1825.

191. Neer EJ, Clapham DE. Roles of G protein subunits in transmembrane signaling. Nature 1988; 333:129–134.

192. Ross EM. Signal sorting and amplification through G protein–coupled receptors. Neuron 1989; 3:141–152.

193. Birnbaumer L, Codina J, Mattera R, et al. Signal transduction by G proteins. Kidney Int Suppl 1987; 23:S14–S42.

194. Spiegel AM. Signal transduction by guanine nucleotide binding proteins. Mol Cell Endocrinol 1987; 49:1–16.

195. Caron MG. The guanine nucleotide regulatory protein-coupled receptors for nucleosides, nucleotides, amino acids and amine neurotransmitters. Curr Opin Cell Biol 1989; 1:159–166.

196. Benovic JL, Bouvier M, Caron MG, Lefkowitz RJ. Regulation of adenylyl cyclase–coupled beta and adrenergic receptors. Annu Rev Cell Biol 1988; 4:405–420.

197. Hausdorff WP, Caron MG, Lefkowitz RJ. Turning off the signal: desensitiza-

tion of beta-adrenergic receptor function [published erratum appears in FASEB J 1990 Sep; 4(12):3049]. FASEB J 1990; 4:2881–2889.

198. Casey PJ, Gilman AG. G protein involvement in receptor-effector coupling. J Biol Chem 1988; 263:2577–2580.

199. Gilman AG. G Proteins: Transducers of receptor-generated signals. Annu Rev Biochem 1987; 56:615–649.

200. Casey PJ, Graziano MP, Freissmuth M, Gilman AG. Role of G proteins in transmembrane signaling. Cold Spring Harbor Symp Quant Biol 1988; 53:203–208.

201. Freissmuth M, Casey PJ, Gilman AG. G proteins control diverse pathways of transmembrane signaling. FASEB J 1989; 3:2125–2131.

202. Masters SB, Sullivan KA, Miller RT, et al. Carboxyl terminal domain of Gs alpha specifies coupling of receptors to stimulation of adenylyl cyclase. Science 1988; 241:448–451.

203. Gupta SK, Diez E, Heasley LE, et al. A G protein mutant that inhibits thrombin and purinergic receptor activation of phospholipase A$_2$. Science 1990; 249:662–666.

204. Neer EJ. Heterotrimeric G proteins: organizers of transmembrane signals. Cell 1995; 80:249–257.

205. Limbird LE. Receptors linked to inhibition of adenylate cyclase: additional signaling mechanisms. FASEB J 1988; 2:2686–2695.

206. Salter RS, Krinks MH, Klee CB, et al. Calmodulin activates the isolated catalytic unit of brain adenylate cyclase. J Biol Chem 1981; 256:9830–9833.

207. Sunahara R, Dessauer C, Gilma A. Complexity and diversity of mammalian adenylyl cyclases. Annu Rev Pharmacol Toxicol 1996; 36:461–480.

208. Ushiro H, Cohen S. Identification of phosphotyrosine as a product of epidermal growth factor–activated protein kinase in A-431 cell membranes. J Biol Chem 1980; 255:8363–8365.

209. Hunter T, Cooper JA. Tyrosine protein kinases and their substrates: an overview. Adv Cyclic Nucleotide Protein Phosphorylation Res 1984; 17:443–455.

210. Ullrich A, Coussens L, Hayflick JS, et al. Human epidermal growth factor receptor cDNA sequence and aberrant expression of the amplified gene in A431 epidermoid carcinoma cells. Nature 1984; 309:418–425.

211. Kasuga M, Karlsson FA, Kahn CR. Insulin stimulates the phosphorylation of the 95,000-dalton subunit of its own receptor. Science 1982; 215:185–187.

212. Ullrich A, Bell JR, Chen EY, et al. Human insulin receptor and its relationship to the tyrosine kinase family of oncogenes. Nature 1985; 313:756–761.

213. Jacobs S, Kull FC, Earp HS, et al. Somatomedin-C stimulates the phosphorylation of the beta-subunit of its own receptor. J Biol Chem 1983; 258:9581–9584.

214. Ullrich A, Gray A, Tam AW, et al. Insulin-like growth factor I receptor primary structure: comparison with insulin receptor suggests structural determinants that define functional specificity. EMBO J 1986; 5:2503–2512.

215. Escobedo JA, Navankasattusas S, Cousens LS, et al. A common PDGF receptor is activated by homodimeric A and B forms of PDGF. Science 1988; 240:1532–1534.

216. Yarden Y, Escobedo JA, Kuang WJ, et al. Structure of the receptor for platelet-derived growth factor helps define a family of closely related growth factor receptors. Nature 1986; 323:226–232.

217. Cunningham BC, Wells JA. High-resolution epitope mapping of hGH-receptor interactions by alanine-scanning mutagenesis. Science 1989; 244:1081–1085.

218. Coussens L, Van Beveren C, Smith D, et al. Structural alteration of viral homologue of receptor proto-oncogene fms at carboxyl terminus. Nature 1986; 320:277–280.

219. Lee PL, Johnson DE, Cousens LS, et al. Purification and complementary DNA cloning of a receptor for basic fibroblast growth factor. Science 1989; 245:57–60.

220. Yarden Y, Ullrich A. Growth factor receptor tyrosine kinases. Annu Rev Biochem 1988; 57:443–478.

221. Ullrich A, Schlessinger J. Signal transduction by receptors with tyrosine kinase activity. Cell 1990; 61:203–212.

222. Schlessinger J, Ullrich A. Growth factor signaling by receptor tyrosine kinases. Neuron 1992; 9:383–391.

223. Olson TS, Bamberger MJ, Lane MD. Post-translational changes in tertiary and quaternary structure of the insulin prereceptor: correlation with acquisition of function. J Biol Chem 1988; 263:7342–7351.

224. Schlessinger J. The epidermal growth factor receptor as a multifunctional allosteric protein. Biochemistry 1988; 27:3119–3123.

225. Chou CK, Dull TJ, Russell DS, et al. Human insulin receptors mutated at the ATP-binding site lack protein tyrosine kinase activity and fail to mediate postreceptor effects of insulin. J Biol Chem 1987; 262:1842–1847.

226. Ebina Y, Araki E, Taira M, et al. Replacement of lysine residue 1030 in the putative ATP-binding region of the insulin receptor abolishes insulin- and antibody-stimulated glucose uptake and receptor kinase activity. Proc Natl Acad Sci USA 1987; 84:704–708.

227. Kim Y, Iwashita S, Tamura T, et al. Effect of a high-fat diet on the gene expression of pancreatic GLUT2 and glucokinase in rats. Biochem Biophys Res Commun 1995; 208:1092–1098.

228. Ellis L, Clauser E, Morgan DO, et al. Replacement of insulin receptor tyrosine residues 1162 and 1163 compromises insulin-stimulated kinase activity and uptake of 2-deoxyglucose. Cell 1986; 45:721–732.

229. Morgan DO, Roth RA. Acute insulin action requires insulin receptor kinase activity: introduction of an inhibitory monoclonal antibody into

mammalian cells blocks the rapid effects of insulin. Proc Natl Acad Sci USA 1987; 84:41–45.

230. Kahn CR, Flier JS, Bar RS, et al. The syndromes of insulin resistance and acanthosis nigricans: insulin receptor disorders in man. N Engl J Med 1976; 294:739–745.

231. Chardin P. Small GTP-binding proteins of the ras family: a conserved functional mechanism? Cancer Cells 1991; 3:117–126.

232. Grigorescu F, Flier JS, Kahn CR. Defect in insulin receptor phosphorylation in erythrocytes and fibroblasts associated with severe insulin resistance. J Biol Chem 1984; 259:15003–15006.

233. Kadowaki T, Kasuga M, Akanuma Y, et al. Decreased autophosphorylation of the insulin receptor-kinase in streptozotocin-diabetic rats. J Biol Chem 1984; 259:14208–14216.

234. Freidenberg GR, Henry RR, Klein HH, et al. Decreased kinase activity of insulin receptors from adipocytes of non–insulin-dependent diabetic subjects. J Clin Invest 1987; 79:240–250.

235. Comi RJ, Grunberger G, Gorden P. Relationship of insulin binding and insulin-stimulated tyrosine kinase activity is altered in type II diabetes. J Clin Invest 1987; 79:453–462.

236. Honegger AM, Dull TJ, Felder S, et al. Point mutation at the ATP binding site of EGF receptor abolishes protein-tyrosine kinase activity and alters cellular routing. Cell 1987; 51:199–209.

237. Honegger AM, Szapary D, Schmidt A, et al. A mutant epidermal growth factor receptor with defective tyrosine kinase is unable to stimulate proto-oncogene DNA synthesis. Mol Cell Biol 1987; 7:4568–4571.

238. Escobedo JA, Barr PJ, Williams LT. Role of tyrosine kinase and membrane-spanning domains in signal transduction by the platelet-derived growth factor receptor. Mol Cell Biol 1989; 8:5126–5131.

239. Roussel MF, Downing JR, Rettenmier CW, et al. A point mutation in the extracellular domain of the human CSF-1 receptor (c-fms proto-oncogene product) activates its transforming potential. Cell 1988; 55:979–988.

240. Riedel H, Dull TJ, Schlessinger J, et al. A: Cytoplasmic domains determine signal specificity, cellular characteristics, and influence ligand binding of epidermal factor and insulin receptors. EMBO J 1989; 8:2943–2954.

241. Ellis L, Morgan DO, Clauser E, et al. Mechanisms of receptor-mediated transmembrane communication. Cold Spring Harbor Symp Quant Biol 1986; 51:773–784.

242. Pilch PF, Czech MP. Hormone binding alters the conformation of the insulin receptor. Science 1980; 210:1152–1153.

243. Maturo JM III, Hollenberg MD, Aglio LS. Insulin receptor: insulin-modulated interconversion between distinct molecular forms involving disulfide-sulfhydryl exchange. Biochemistry 1983; 22:2579–2586.

244. Bertics PJ, Gill GN. Self-phosphorylation enhances the protein-tyrosine kinase activity of the epidermal growth factor receptor. J Biol Chem 1985; 260:14642–14647.

245. Wilden PA, Backer JM, Kahn CR, et al. The insulin receptor with phenylalanine replacing tyrosine-1146 provides evidence for separate signals regulating cellular metabolism and growth. Proc Natl Acad Sci USA 1990; 87:3358–3362.

246. Boni-Schnetzler M, Kaligian A, Del Vecchio RL, et al. Ligand-dependent intersubunit association within the insulin receptor complex activates its intrinsic kinase activity. J Biol Chem 1988; 263:6822–6828.

247. Sweet LJ, Morrison BD, Wilden PA, et al. Insulin-dependent intermolecular subunit communication between isolated alpha beta heterodimeric insulin receptor complexes. J Biol Chem 1987; 262:16730–16738.

248. Axelrod D, Ravdin P, Koppel DE, et al. Lateral motion of fluorescently labeled acetylcholine membranes of developing muscle fibers. Proc Natl Acad Sci USA 1976; 73:4594–4598.

249. Cochet C, Gill GN, Meisenhelder J, et al. C-kinase phosphorylates the epidermal growth factor receptor and reduces its epidermal growth factor–stimulated tyrosine protein kinase activity. J Biol Chem 1984; 259:2553–2558.

250. Takayama S, White MF, Lauris V, et al. Phorbol esters modulate insulin receptor phosphorylation and insulin action in hepatoma cells. Proc Natl Acad Sci USA 1984; 81:7797–7801.

251. Gazzano H, Kowalski A, Fehlmann M, et al. Two different protein kinase activities are associated with the insulin receptor. Biochem J 1983; 216:575–582.

252. White MF, Takayama S, Kahn CR. Differences in the sites of phosphorylation of the insulin receptor in vivo and in vitro. J Biol Chem 1985; 260:9470–9478.

253. Smith DM, King MJ, Sale GJ. Two systems in vitro that show insulin-stimulated serine kinase activity towards the insulin receptor. Biochem J 1988; 250:509–519.

254. Russell DS, Gherzi R, Johnson EJ, et al. The protein-tyrosine kinase activity of the insulin receptor is necessary for insulin-mediated receptor down-regulation. J Biol Chem 1987; 262:11833–11840.

255. Wahl MI, Jones GA, Nishibe S, et al. Growth factor stimulation of phospholipase C-γl activity: comparative properties of control and activated enzymes. J Biol Chem 1992; 267:10447–10456.

256. Koch CA, Anderson DJ, Moran MF, et al. SH2 and SH3 domains: elements that control interactions of cytoplasmic signaling proteins. Science 1991; 252:668–674.

257. Margolis B, Lax I, Kris R, et al. All autophosphorylation sites of epidermal growth factor (EGF) receptor and HER2/neu are located in their carboxyl-terminal tails. J Biol Chem 1989; 264:10667–10671.

258. Myers MG Jr, Sun XJ, White MF. The IRS-1 signaling system. Trends Biochem Sci 1994; 19:289–294.

259. Sun XJ, Wang LM, Zhang Y, et al. Role of IRS-2 in insulin and cytokine signalling. Nature 1995; 377:173–177.

260. Ruff Jamison S, McGlade J, Pawson T, et al. Epidermal growth factor stimulates the tyrosine phosphorylation of SHC in the mouse. J Biol Chem 1993; 268:7610–7612.

261. Waksman G, Kominos D, Robertson SC, et al. Crystal structure of the phosphotyrosine recognition domain SH2 of v-src complexed with tyrosine-phosphorylated peptides. Nature 1992; 358:646–653.

262. Musacchio A, Noble M, Pauptit R, et al. Crystal structure of a Src-homology 3 (SH3) domain. Nature 1992; 359:851–855.

263. Booker GW, Breeze AL, Downing AK, et al. Structure of an SH2 domain of the p85α subunit of phosphatidylinositol-3 OH-kinase. Nature 1992; 358:684–687.

264. Eck MJ, Shoelson SE, Harrison SC. Recognition of a high-affinity phospho-tyrosyl peptide by the Src homology-2 domain of p56lck. Nature 1993; 362:87–91.

265. Waksman G, Shoelson SE, Pant N, et al. Binding of a high affinity phospho-tyrosyl peptide to the Src SH2 domain: crystal structures of the complexed and peptide-free forms. Cell 1993; 72:779–790.

266. Backer JM, Myers MG Jr, Shoelson SE, et al. Phosphatidylinositol 3'-kinase is activated by association with IRS-1 during insulin stimulation. EMBO J 1992; 11:3469–3479.

267. Yonezawa K, Ueda H, Hara K, et al. Insulin-dependent formation of a complex containing an 85-kDa subunit of phosphatidylinositol 3-kinase and tyrosine-phosphorylated insulin receptor substrate 1. J Biol Chem 1992; 267:25958–25966.

268. Heller-Harrison RA, Morin M, Czech M. Insulin regulation of membrane-associated insulin receptor substrate 1. J Biol Chem 1995; 270:24442–24450.

269. Lowenstein EJ, Daly RJ, Batzer AG, et al. The SH2 and SH3 domain-containing proteins GRB2 links receptor tyrosine kinases to ras signaling. Cell 1992; 70:431–442.

270. Pelicci G, Lanfrancone L, Grignani F, et al. A novel transforming protein (SHC) with an SH2 domain is implicated in mitogenic signal transduction. Cell 1992; 70:93–104.

271. Skolnik EY, Batzer AG, Li N, et al. The function of GRB2 in linking the insulin receptor to ras signaling pathways. Science 1993; 260:1953–1955.

272. Wood KW, Sarnecki C, Roberts TM, et al. ras mediates nerve growth factor receptor modulation of three signal-transducing protein kinases: MAP kinase, Raf-1, and RSK. Cell 1992; 68:1041–1050.

273. Ahn NG, Seger R, Bratlien RL, et al. Multiple components in an epidermal growth factor–stimulated protein kinase cascade: in vitro activation of a myelin basic protein/microtubule–associated protein 2 kinase. J Biol Chem 1991; 266:4220–4227.

274. Leevers SJ, Marshall CJ. Activation of extracellular signal–regulated kinase, ERK2, by p21ras oncoprotein. EMBO J 1992; 11:569–574.

275. Low MG, Saltiel AR. Structural and functional roles of glycosyl-phosphati-dylinositol in membranes. Science 1988; 239:268–275.

276. Wilks AF, Harpur AG, Kurban RR, et al. Two novel protein-tyrosine kinases, each with a second phosphotransferase-related catalytic domain define a new class of protein kinase. Mol Cell Biol 1991; 11:2057–2065.

277. Argetsinger LS, Campbell GS, Yang X, et al. Identification of JAK2 as a growth hormone receptor–associated tyrosine kinase. Cell 1993; 74:237–244.

278. Miyazaki T, Kawahara A, Fujii H, et al. Functional activation of Jak1 and Jak3 by selective association with IL-2 receptor subunits. Science 1994; 266:1045–1047.

279. Shual K, Ziemiecki A, Wilks AF, et al. Polypeptide signalling to the nucleus through tyrosine phosphorylation of Jak and Stat proteins. Nature 1993; 366:580–582.

280. de Vos AM, Ultsch M, Kossiakoff AA. Human growth hormone and extracellular domain of its receptor: crystal structure of the complex. Science 1992; 255:306–312.

281. VanderKuur JA, Wang X, Zhang L, et al. Domains of the growth hormone receptor required for association and activation of JAK2 tyrosine kinase. J Biol Chem 1994; 269:21709–21717.

282. Greenlund AC, Farrar MA, Viviano BL, et al. Ligand-induced IFN gamma receptor tyrosine phosphorylation couples the receptor to its signal transduction system (p91). EMBO J 1994; 13:1591–1600.

283. Darnell JE Jr, Kerr IM, Stark GR. Jak-STAT pathways and transcriptional activation in response to IFNs and other extracellular signaling proteins. Science 1994; 264:1415–1421.

284. Chow JC, Ling PR, Qu Z, et al. Growth hormone stimulates tyrosine phosphorylation of JAK2 and STAT5, but not insulin receptor substrate-1 or SHC proteins in liver and skeletal muscle of normal rats in vivo. Endocrinology 1996; 137:2880–2886.

285. Campbell GS, Miyaska T, Pang L, et al. Stimulation by growth hormone of MAP kinase activity in 3T3-F442A fibroblasts. J Biol Chem 1992; 267:6074–6080.

286. Argetsinger LS, Hsu GW, Myers MG Jr, et al. Growth hormone, interferon-gamma, and leukemia inhibitory factor promoted tyrosyl phosphorylation of insulin receptor substrate-1. J Biol Chem 1995; 270:14685–14692.

287. Vaandrager A, de Jonge H. Signaling by cGMP-dependent protein kinases. Mol Cell Biochem 1996; 157:23–30.

288. Laskin J, Heck D, Laskin D. Multifunctional role of nitric oxide in inflammation. Trends Endocrinol Metab 1994; 5:377–382.

289. Schulz S, Chinkers M, Garbers DL. The guanylate cyclase/receptor family of proteins. FASEB J 1989; 3:2026–2035.

290. Hokin LE. Receptors and phosphoinositide-generated second messengers. Annu Rev Biochem 1985; 54:202–235.

291. Catt KJ, Balla T. Phosphoinositide metabolism and hormone action. Annu Rev Med 1989; 40:487–509.

292. Williamson JR, Monck JR. Hormone effects on cellular Ca²⁺ fluxes. Annu Rev Physiol 1989; 51:107–124.

293. Exton JH. Signaling through phosphatidylcholine breakdown. J Biol Chem 1990; 265:1–4.

294. Putney JW Jr. Formation and actions of calcium-mobilizing messenger, inositol 1,4,5-trisphosphate. Am J Physiol 1987; 252:G149–G157.

295. Berridge MJ. Inositol trisphosphate and diacylglycerol: two interacting second messengers. Annu Rev Biochem 1987; 56:159–193.

296. Brown AM, Yatani A, Imoto Y, et al. Direct G-protein regulation of Ca²⁺ channels. Ann NY Acad Sci 1989; 560:373–386.

297. Birnbaumer L, Brown AM. G proteins and the mechanism of action of hormones, neurotransmitters, and autocrine and paracrine regulatory factors. Am Rev Respir Dis 1990; 141:S106–S114.

298. Liscovitch M, Cantley LC. Signal transduction and membrane traffic: the PITP/phosphoinositide connection. Cell 1995; 81:659–662.

299. Majerus P, Ross T, Cunningham T, et al. Recent insights in phosphatidyl-inositol signaling. Cell 1990; 63:459–465.

300. Jaken S. Protein kinase C isozymes and substrates. Curr Opin Cell Biol 1996; 8:168–173.

301. Carpenter CL, Cantley LC. Phosphoinositide kinases. Curr Opin Cell Biol 1996; 8:153–158.

302. Huisamen B, Lochner A. Inositolpolyphosphates and their binding proteins—a short review. Mol Cell Biochem 1996; 157:229–232.

303. Bootman M, Berridge MJ. The elemental principles of calcium signaling. Cell 1995; 83:675–678.

304. Petersen OH. New aspects of cytosolic calcium signaling. News Physiol Sci 1996; 11:13–17.

305. Supattapone S, Worley PF, Baraban JM, et al. Solubilization, purification, and characterization of an inositol trisphosphate receptor. J Biol Chem 1988; 263:1530–1534.

306. Joseph S. The inositol trisphosphate receptor family. Cell Signal 1996; 6:1–7.

307. Putney JW Jr. The molecular heterogeneity of protein kinase C and its implications for cellular regulation. Nature 1988; 334:661–665.

308. Morris AP, Gallacher DV, Irvine RF, et al. Synergism of inositol trisphosphate and tetrakisphosphate in activating Ca²⁺-dependent K⁺ channels. Nature 1987; 330:653–655.

309. Hanks SK, Quin AM, Hunter T. The protein kinase family: conserved features and deduced phylogeny of the catalytic domain. Science 1990; 241:42–52.

310. Bell RM. Protein kinase C activation by diacylglycerol second messengers. Cell 1986; 45:631–632.

311. Nishizuka Y. The molecular heterogeneity of protein kinase C and its implications for cellular regulation. Nature 1988; 334:661–665.

312. Panayotou G, Waterfield MD. Cell surface receptors for polypeptide hormones, growth factors and neuropeptides. Curr Opin Cell Biol 1989; 1:167–176.

313. Blackshear PJ, Nairn AC, Kuo JF. Protein kinases 988: a current perspective. FASEB J 1988; 2:2957–2969.

314. Sakane F, Yamada K, Kanoh H, et al. Porcine diacylglycerol kinase sequence has zinc finger and E-F hand motifs. Nature 1990; 344:345–348.

315. Rosenthal W, Hischeler J, Trautwein W, et al: Receptor and G protein-mediated modulations of voltage-dependent calcium channels. Cold Spring Harb Symp Quant Biol 1988; 53:247–254.

316. Rosenthal W, Hescheler J, Trautwein W, et al. Control of voltage-dependent Ca²⁺ channels by G protein–coupled receptors. FASEB J 1988; 2:2784–2790.

317. Levitan ES, Schofield PR, Burt DR, et al. Structural and functional basis for GABAA receptor heterogeneity. Nature 1988; 335:76–79.

318. Birnbaumer L, Codina J, Yatani A, et al. Molecular basis of regulation of ionic channels by G proteins. Recent Prog Horm Res 1989; 45:121–206.

319. Changeux JP: The acetylcholine receptor: its molecular biology and biotechnological prospects. Bioessays 1989; 10:48–54.

320. Kurachi Y. Regulation of G protein–gated K⁺ channels. News Physiol Sci 1989; 4:158–161.

321. Meldolesi J, Pozzan T. Pathways of Ca²⁺ influx at the plasma membrane: voltage-, receptor-, and second messenger-operated channels. Exp Cell Res 1987; 171:271–283.

322. Hallam TJ, Rink TJ. Receptor-mediated Ca²⁺ entry: diversity of function and mechanism. Trends Pharmacol Sci 1989; 10:8–10.

323. Wickman K, Clapham DE. Ion channel regulation by G proteins. Physiol Rev 1995; 75:865–885.

324. Liscovitch M, Cantley LC. Lipid second messengers. Cell 1994; 77:329–334.

325. Spiegel S, Foster D, Kolesnick R. Signal transduction through lipid second messengers. Curr Opin Cell Biol 1996; 8:159–167.

326. Taylor SI. Insulin action and inaction. Clin Res 1986; 35:459–472.

327. Fukushima N, Matsuura N, Nohara Y, et al. A case of insulin resistance associated with acanthosis nigricans. Tohoku J Exp Med 1984; 144:129–138.

328. Yoshimasa Y, Seino S, Whittaker J, et al. Insulin-resistant diabetes due to a point mutation that prevents insulin proreceptor processing. Science 1988; 240:784–787.

329. Taira M, Hashimoto N, Shimada F, et al. Human diabetes associated with a deletion of the tyrosine kinase domain of the insulin receptor. Science 1989; 245:63–66.

330. Odawara M, Kadowaki T, Yamamoto R, et al. Human diabetes associated with a mutation in the tyrosine kinase domain of the insulin receptor. Science 1989; 245:66–68.

331. Kobayashi M, Sasaoka T, Takata Y, et al. Insulin resistance by unprocessed insulin proreceptors point mutation at the cleavage site. Biochem Biophys Res Commun 1988; 153:657–663.

332. Schilling EE, Rechler MM, Grunfeld C, et al. Primary defect of insulin receptors in skin fibroblasts cultured from an infant with leprechaunism and insulin resistance. Proc Natl Acad Sci USA 1979; 76:5877–5881.

333. Kadowaki T, Bevins CL, Cama A, et al. Two mutant alleles of the insulin receptor gene in a patient with extreme insulin resistance. Science 1988; 240:787–790.

334. Kaplowitz PB, D'Ercole AJ. Fibroblasts from a patient with leprechaunism are resistant to insulin, epidermal growth factor, and somatomedin C. J Clin Endocrinol Metab 1982; 55:741–748.

335. Beguinot F, Smith RJ, Kahn CR, et al. Phosphorylation of insulin-like growth factor I receptor by insulin receptor tyrosine kinase in intact cultured skeletal muscle cells. Biochemistry 1988; 27:3222–3228.

336. Moxham CP, Duronio V, Jacobs S. Insulin-like growth factor I receptor β-subunit heterogeneity: evidence for hybrid tetramers composed of insulin-like growth factor I and insulin receptor heterodimers. J Biol Chem 1989; 264:13238–13244.

337. Laron Z, Pertzelan A, Karp M. Pituitary dwarfism with high serum levels of growth hormone: a new inborn error of metabolism? Isr J Med Sci 1966; 2:152–155.

338. Laron Z, Pertzelan A, Karp M. Pituitary dwarfism with high serum levels of growth hormone. Isr J Med Sci 1968; 4:883–894.

339. Daughaday WH, Laron Z, Pertzelan A, et al. Defective sulfation factor generation: a possible etiological link in dwarfism. Trans Assoc Am Physicians 1969; 82:129–138.

340. Laron Z, Kowadlo-Sibergeld A, Eshet R, et al. Growth hormone resistance. Ann Clin Res 1980; 12:269–277.

341. Elders MJ, Garland JT, Daughaday WH, et al. Laron's dwarfism: studies on the nature of the defect. J Pediatr 1973; 83:253–263.

342. Eshet R, Laron Z, Pertzelan A, et al. Defect of human growth hormone receptors in the liver of two patients with Laron-type dwarfism. Isr J Med Sci 1984; 20:8–11.

343. Daughaday WH, Trivedi B. Absence of serum growth hormone binding protein in patients with growth hormone receptor deficiency (Laron dwarfism). Proc Natl Acad Sci USA 1987; 84:4636–4640.

344. Bennett PH. Epidemiology of diabetes mellitus. In: Rifkin H, Porte D Jr, eds. Diabetes Mellitus. New York: Elsevier, 1990:357–377.

345. Coleman DL. Effects of parabiosis of obese with diabetic and normal mice. Diabetologia 1973; 4:294–298.

346. Yalow RS, Berson SA. Immunoassay of endogenous plasma insulin in man. J Clin Invest 1960; 39:1157–1175.

347. Van Sande J, Parma J, Tonacchera M, et al. Genetic basis of endocrine disease: somatic and germline mutations of the TSH receptor gene in thyroid diseases. J CLin Endocrinol Metab 1995; 80:2577–2585.

348. Haffner SM, Stern MP, Hazuda HP, et al. Increased insulin concentrations in nondiabetic offspring of diabetic parents. N Engl J Med 1988; 319:1297–1301.

349. Himsworth HP. The syndrome of diabetes mellitus and its cause. Lancet 1949; 2:465–472.

350. Otonkosi T, Mally MI, Hayek A. Opposite effects of β-cell differentiation and growth on *reg* gene expression in human fetal pancreatic cells. Diabetologia 1994; 43:1164–1166.

351. Goodyear LJ, Giorgino F, Balon TW, et al. Effects of contractile activity on tyrosine phosphoproteins and phosphatidylinositol 3-kinase activity in rat skeletal muscle. Am J Physiol 1995; 268:E987–E995.

352. Rothenberg PL, Willison LD, Simon J, et al. Glucose-induced insulin receptor tyrosine phosphorylation in insulin-secreting B-cells. Diabetes 1995; 44:802–809.

353. McGrew MJ, Bogdanova N, Hasegawa K, et al. Distinct gene expression patterns in skeletal and cardiac muscle are dependent on common regulatory sequences in the MLC1/3 locus. Mol Cell Biol 1996; 16:4524–4534.

354. Mitch WE, Jurkovitz C, England BK. Mechanisms that cause protein and amino acid catabolism in uremia. Am J Kidney Dis 1993; 21:91–95.

355. Latronico AC, Anasti J, Arnhold IJP, et al. Brief report: testicular and ovarian resistance to luteinizing hormone caused by inactivating mutations of the luteinizing hormone–receptor gene. N Engl J Med 1986; 334:507–512.

356. Schipani E, Kruse K, Jüppner H. A constitutively active mutant PTH-PTHrP receptor in Jansen-type metaphyseal chondrodysplasia. Science 1995; 268:98–100.

357. Schipani E, Langman CB, Parfitt AM, et al. Constitutively activated receptors for parathyroid hormone and parathyroid hormone–related peptide in Jansen's metaphyseal chrondrodysplasia. N Engl J Med 1996; 335:708–714.

358. Rosenthal W, Seibold A, Antaramian A, et al. Molecular identification of the gene responsible for congenital nephrogenic diabetes insipidus. Nature 1992; 359:233–235.

359. Merendino JJ Jr, Spiegel AM, Crawford JD, et al. Brief report: a mutation in the vasopressin V2-receptor gene in a kindred with X-linked nephrogenic diabetes insipidus. N Engl J Med 1997; 328:1538–1541.

360. Tsigos C, Arai K, Hung W, et al. Hereditary isolated glucocorticoid deficiency is associated with abnormalities of the adrenocorticotropin receptor gene. J Clin Invest 1993; 92:2458–2461.

361. Pollak MR, Brown EM, Chou YHW, et al. Mutations in the human Ca^{2+}-sensing receptor gene cause familial hypocalciuric hypercalcemia and neonatal severe hyperparathyroidism. Cell 1993; 75:1297–1303.

362. Robbins LS, Nadeau JH, Johnson KR, et al. Pigmentation phenotypes of variant extension locus alleles result from point mutations that alter MSH receptor function. Cell 1993; 72:827–834.

363. Sung CH, Schneider BG, Agarwal N, et al. Functional heterogeneity of mutant rhodopsins responsible for autosomal dominant retinits pigmentosa. Proc Natl Acad Sci USA 1991; 88:8840–8844.

364. Albright F, Burnett C, Smith PH. Pseudohypoparathyroidism: an example of "Seabright-Bantam" syndrome. Endocrinology 1942; 30:922–932.

365. Billestrup N, Nielsen JH. The stimulatory effect of growth hormone, prolactin, and placental lactogen on B-cell proliferation is not mediated by insulin-like growth factor-1. Endocrinology 1991; 129:883–888.

366. Antonetti DA, Algenstaedt P, Kahn CR. Insulin receptor substrate 1 binds two novel splice variants of the regulatory subunit of phosphatidylinositol 3-kinase in muscle and brain. Mol Cell Biol 1996; 16:2195–2203.

367. Lyons J, Landis CA, Harsh G, et al. Two G protein oncogenes in human endocrine tumors. Science 1990; 249:655–659.

368. Harris RB, Martin RJ. Site of action of putative lipostatic factor: food intake and peripheral pentose shunt activity. Am J Physiol 1990; 259:R45–R52.

369. Brown EJ, Schreiber SL. A signaling pathway to translational control. Cell 1996; 86:517–520.

370. Grunfeld C, Baird KL, Van Obberghen E, et al. Glucocorticoid-induced insulin resistance in vitro: evidence for both receptor and post-receptor defects. Endocrinology 1981; 109:1723–1730.

371. Bar RS, Gorden P, Roth J, et al. Fluctuations in the affinity and concentration of insulin receptors on circulating monocytes of obese patients: effects of starvation, refeeding and dieting. J Clin Invest 1976; 58:1123–1135.

372. Pedersen O, Beck-Nielsen H, Heding L. Increased insulin receptors after exercise in patients with insulin-dependent diabetes mellitus. N Engl J Med 1980; 302:886–892.

373. Kolterman OG, Greenfield M, Reaven GM, et al. Effect of a high carbohydrate diet on insulin binding to adipocytes and on insulin action in vivo in man. Diabetes 1979; 28:731–736.

374. Ginsberg BH, Brown TJ, Simon I, et al. Effect of the membrane lipid environment on the properties of insulin receptors. Diabetes 1981; 30:773–780.

375. Trivier E, De Cesare D, Jacquot S, et al. Mutations in the kinase Rsk-2 associated with Coffin-Lowry syndrome. Nature 1997; 384:567–570.

376. Rabinowitz D. Some endocrine and metabolic aspects of obesity. Annu Rev Med 1970; 21:241–258.

377. Truglia JA, Livingston JN, Lockwood DH. Insulin resistance: receptor and post-binding defects in human obesity and non–insulin-dependent diabetes mellitus. Am J Med 1985; 79:13–22.

378. Archer JA, Gorden P, Roth J. Defect in insulin binding to receptors in obese man: amelioration with caloric restriction. J Clin Invest 1975; 55:166–174.

379. Adamo M, LeRoith D, Simon J, et al. Effect of altered nutritional states on insulin receptors. Annu Rev Nutr 1988; 8:144–166.

380. Wigand JP, Blackard WG. Down-regulation of insulin receptors in obese man. Diabetes 1979; 28:287–291.

381. Reaven GM. Insulin-independent diabetes mellitus: metabolic characteristics. Metabolism 1980; 29:445–454.

382. Olefsky JM, Reaven GM. Insulin binding in diabetes: relationships with plasma insulin levels and insulin sensitivity. Diabetes 1977; 26:680–688.

383. Kolterman OG, Gray RS, Griffin J, et al. Receptor and postreceptor defects contribute to the insulin resistance in noninsulin-dependent diabetes mellitus. J Clin Invest 1981; 68:957–969.

384. Freidenberg GR, Reichart DR, Olefsky JM, et al. Reversibility of defective adipocyte insulin receptor kinase activity in non–insulin-dependent diabetes mellitus: effect of weight loss. J Clin Invest 1988; 82:1398–1406.

385. Caro JF, Ittoop O, Pories WJ, et al. Studies on the mechanism of insulin resistance in the liver from humans with noninsulin-dependent diabetes. J Clin Invest 1986; 78:249–258.

386. Arner P, Pollare T, Lithell H, et al. Defective insulin receptor tyrosine kinase in human skeletal muscle in obesity and Type II (noninsulin-dependent) diabetes mellitus. Diabetologia 1987; 30:437–440.

387. Haring HU, Obermaier-Kusser B. Insulin receptor kinase defects in insulin-resistant tissues and their role in the pathogenesis of NIDDM. Diabetes Metab Rev 1989; 5:431–441.

388. Truglia JA, Hayes GR, Lockwood DH. Intact adipocyte insulin-receptor phosphorylation and in vitro tyrosine kinase activity in animal models of insulin resistance. Diabetes 1988; 37:147–153.

389. Karasik A, Kahn CR. Dexamethasone-induced changes in phosphorylation of the insulin and epidermal growth factor receptors and their substrates in intact rat hepatocytes. Endocrinology 1988; 123:2214–2222.

390. Block NE, Buse MG. Effects of hypercortisolemia and diabetes on skeletal

muscle insulin receptor function in vitro and in vivo. Am J Physiol 1989; 256:E39–E48.

391. Hansen I, Tsalikian E, Beaufrere B, et al. Insulin resistance in acromegaly: defects in both hepatic and extrahepatic insulin action. Am J Physiol 1986; 250:E269–E273.

392. Cecchin F, Ittoop O, Sinha MK, et al. Insulin resistance in uremia: insulin receptor kinase activity in liver and muscle from chronic uremic rats. Am J Physiol 1988; 254:E394–E401.

393. van Putten JP, Wieringa T, Krans HM. Low pH and ketoacids induce insulin receptor binding and postbinding alterations in cultured 3T3 adipocytes. Diabetes 1985; 34:744–750.

394. Fradkin JE, Eastman RC, Lesniak MA, et al. Specificity spillover at the hormone receptor—exploring its role in human disease. N Engl J Med 1989; 320:640–645.

395. dePablo F, Eastman RC, Roth J, et al. Plasma prolactin in acromegaly before and after treatment. J Clin Endocrinol Metab 1981; 53:344–352.

396. Carayon P, Lefort G, Nisula BC. Interaction of human chorionic gonadotropin and human lutenizing hormone with human thyroid membranes. Endocrinology 1980; 106:1907–1916.

397. Nisula BC, Taliadouros GS, Carayon P. Primary and secondary biologic activities intrinsic to the human chorionic gonadotropin molecule. In: Segal SJ, ed. Chorionic Gonadotropin. New York: Plenum, 1980: 17–35.

398. Mann KP, Schneider N, Hoermann R. Thyrotropic activity of acidic isoelectric variants of human chorionic gonadotropin from trophoblastic tumors. Endocrinology 1986; 118:1558–1566.

399. Gorden P, Hendricks CM, Kahn CR, et al. Hypoglycemia associated with non–islet-cell tumors and insulin-like growth factors. N Engl J Med 1981; 305:1452–1455.

400. Hyodo T, Megyesi K, Kahn CR, et al. Adrenocortical carcinoma and hypoglycemia: evidence for production of non-suppressible insulin-like activity by the tumor. J Clin Endocrinol Metab 1977; 44:1175–1184.

401. Daughaday WH, Emanuele MA, Brooks MH, et al. Synthesis and secretion of insulin-like growth factor II by a leiomyosarcoma with associated hypoglycemia. N Engl J Med 1988; 319:1434–1440.

402. Taylor SI, Dons RF, Hernandez ER, et al. Insulin resistance associated with androgen excess in women with autoantibodies to the insulin receptor. Ann Intern Med 1982; 97:851–855.

403. Milner RDG, Hill DJ. Fetal growth control: the role of insulin and related peptides. Clin Endocrinol 1984; 21:415–433.

404. Wilson K, Eisenbarth GS. Immunopathogenesis and immunotherapy of type I diabetes. Annu Rev Med 1990; 41:497–508.

405. Neufeld M, Maclaren NK, Blizzard RM. Two types of autoimmune Addison's disease associated with different polyglandular autoimmune (PGA) syndromes. Medicine 1981; 60:355–362.

406. Dussault JH, Rousseau F. Immunologically mediated hypothyroidism. Endocrinol Metab Clin North Am 1987; 16:417–429.

407. Neufeld M, Maclaren NK, Blizzard RM. Autoimmune polyglandular syndromes. Pediatr Ann 1980; 9:154–162.

408. Blecher M. Receptors, antibodies, and disease. Clin Chem 1984; 30:1137–1156.

409. Flier JS, Kahn CR, Roth J, et al. Antibodies that impair insulin receptor binding in an unusual diabetic syndrome with severe insulin resistance. Science 1975; 190:63–65.

410. Grunfeld C, Van Obberghen E, Karlsson FA, et al. Antibody-induced desensitization of the insulin receptor: studies of the mechanism of desensitization in 3T3-L1 fatty fibroblasts. J Clin Invest 1980; 66:1124–1134.

411. Flier JS, Bar RS, Muggeo M, et al. The evolving clinical course of patients with insulin receptor antibodies: spontaneous remission or receptor proliferation with hypoglycemia. J Clin Endocrinol Metab 1978; 47:985–995.

412. Kolterman OG. Longitudinal evaluation of the effects of sulfonylurea therapy in subjects with type II diabetes mellitus. Am J Med 1985; 79:23–33.

413. Elias D, Maron R, Cohen IR, et al. Mouse antibodies to the insulin receptor developing spontaneously as anti-idiotypes. J Biol Chem 1984; 259:6416–6419.

414. Smith BR, McLachlan SM, Furmaniak J. Autoantibodies to the thyrotropin receptor. Endocr Rev 1988; 9:106–121.

415. Adams DD. The presence of an abnormal thyroid-stimulating hormone in the serum of some tyrotoxic patients. J Clin Endocrinol Metab 1958; 18:699–712.

416. Beckner SK, Brady RO, Fishman PH. Reevaluation of the role of gangliosides in the binding and action of thyrotropin. Proc Natl Acad Sci USA 1981; 78:4848–4852.

417. Yavin E, Yavin Z, Schneider MD, et al. Monoclonal antibodies to the thyrotropin receptor: implications for receptor structure and the action of autoantibodies to Graves' disease. Proc Natl Acad Sci USA 1981; 78:3180–3184.

418. Furmaniak J, Nakajima Y, Hashim FA, et al. The TSH receptor: structure and interaction with autoantibodies in thyroid disease. Acta Endocrinol Suppl 1987; 281:157–165.

419. Madec AM, Laurent MC, Lorcy Y, et al. Thyroid-stimulating antibodies: an aid to the strategy of treatment of Graves' disease? Clin Endocrinol 1984; 21:247–255.

420. Rapoport B, Greenspan FS, Filetti S, et al. Clinical experience with a human thyroid cell bioassay for thyroid-stimulating immunoglobulin. J Clin Endocrinol Metab 1984; 58:332–338.

421. Bishop JM. The molecular genetics of cancer. Science 1987; 235:305–311.

422. Krontiris T. Oncogenes. Mol Med 1995; 333:303–306.

423. Hunter T. The functions of oncogene products. Prog Clin Biol Res 1989; 288:25–34.

424. Bishop J, Capobianco A, Doyle HJ, et al. Proto-oncogenes and plasticity in cell signaling. Cold Spring Harbor Symp Quant Biol 1994; 59:165–171.

425. Sharif M, Sasakawa N, Hanley M. Malignant transformation by G protein–coupled hormone receptors. Mol Cell Endocrinol 1994; 100:115–119.

426. Trupp M, Arenas E, Fainzilber M, et al. Functional receptor for GDNF encoded by the c-ret proto-oncogene. Nature 1996; 381:785–789.

427. Treanor J, Goodman LJ, deSauvage F, et al. Characterization of a multicomponent receptor for GDNF. Nature 1996; 382:80–83.

428. McCormick F. ras GTPase activating protein: signal transmitter and signal terminator. Cell 1989; 56:5–8.

429. Burgoyne RD. Small GTP-binding proteins. Trends Biochem Sci 1989; 14:394–396.

430. Landis CA, Masters SB, Spada A, et al. GTPase inhibiting mutations activate the α chain of Gs and stimulate adenyl cyclase in human pituitary tumors. Nature 1989; 340:692–696.

431. Williams LT. Signal transduction by the platelet-derived growth factor receptor. Science 1989; 243:1564–1570.

432. Doolittle RF, Hunkapiller MW, Hood LE. Simian sarcoma virus onc gene, v-sis, is derived from the gene (or genes) encoding a platelet-derived growth factor. Science 1983; 221:275–277.

433. Morrison DK, Kaplan DR, Escobedo JA, et al. Direct activation of the serine/threonine kinase activity of Raf-1 through tyrosine phosphorylation by the PDGF β-receptor. Cell 1989; 58:649–657.

434. Kouzarides T, Ziff E. Leucine zippers of fos, jun, and GCN4 dictate dimerization specificity and thereby control DNA binding. Nature 1989; 340:568–571.

435. Damm K, Thompson CC, Evans RM. Protein encoded by v-erbA functions as a thyroid-hormone receptor antagonist. Nature 1989; 399:593–597.

436. Weinberg RA. Oncogenes, antioncogenes and the molecular basis of multistep carcinogenesis. Cancer Res 1989; 49:3713–3721.

437. Chen D, Van Horn DJ, White MF, et al. Insulin receptor substrate 1 rescues insulin action in CHO cells expressing mutant insulin receptors that lack a juxtamembrane NPXY motif. Mol Cell Biol 1995; 15:4711–4717.

438. Cohen P. Dissection of the protein phosphorylation cascades involved in insulin and growth factor action. Biochem Soc Trans 1993; 21:555–567.

439. Cohen P. Signal integration at the level of protein kinases, protein phosphatases and their substrates. Trends Biochem Sci 1992; 17:408–413.

6

PATHOGENESIS OF ENDOCRINE TUMORS

Andrew Arnold

INTRODUCTION

A great deal is now known about the mechanisms underlying human tumorigenesis in general and about neoplasia of the endocrine glands in particular. The application of general principles of neoplasia to endocrine tumors has been a productive area of research and is now being translated into clinical applications. Endocrine tumorigenesis also involves some special, if not unique, features that must be considered in understanding the pathogenesis of endocrine tumors. The aim of this chapter is to present the general principles of neoplasia as a framework through which current knowledge about and future advances in endocrine tumorigenesis can be understood.

MOLECULAR TUMOR BIOLOGY

Both inherited tumor predisposition syndromes and the more common noninherited ("sporadic") forms of neoplasia are genetic diseases in the sense that highly specific forms of damage to DNA that result in deregulation of the genes that control cell growth are central causes of tumor development. As a general rule, damage to one such gene is not sufficient to confer a neoplastic phenotype on a cell; instead, multiple mutations accumulate over time. Inherited tumor syndromes constitute a special case in which mutation of one key gene is already present in each somatic cell at birth.

Clonality

Concepts of Clonality and Clonal Evolution

All cancers and many benign hypercellular expansions are monoclonal; that is, they are composed of cells that are the descendants of a single clonal progenitor cell in which the accumulation of a sufficient number of DNA alterations (and, perhaps, other epigenetic damage that does not actually change the DNA) caused a selective advantage. Over time this selective advantage, manifested as an increase in proliferative capacity, a decrease in the normal cell death rate, or both, leads to the development of a neoplasm. The monoclonality of tumors implies that the necessary accumulation of mutations occurs only rarely in the large population of cells in a tissue. Viewed in another way, the identification of a specific monoclonal (also called clonal) change in DNA, found in all or most of the cells of a neoplasm but not in that individual's constitutional DNA (e.g., obtained from adjacent normal tissue or leukocytes), indicates that this DNA alteration had been advantageous in the accelerated evolutionary process that is oncogenesis. Such a DNA lesion, especially if it recurs in other tumors of the same type, is therefore likely to contribute to tumor development. In fact, one of the strongest types of evidence to implicate a given gene as a driving force in tumorigenesis is the demonstration of clonal DNA changes within or near that gene. This situation contrasts with the one in which an increase or a decrease in the expression (RNA or protein levels) of a particular gene occurs in a tumor; such changes can be secondary consequences of tumor-related processes and may or may not themselves contribute to the neoplastic phenotype.

An original clonal progenitor or transformed cell does not necessarily contain all the genetic lesions that are ultimately present in the mature, clinically apparent tumor. A continuing process of "clonal evolution" may result in the development of additional DNA damage that provides an incremental selective advantage to the single tumor cell in which it occurs. Over time, the progeny of this cell may become the dominant clonal population. The percentage of neoplastic cells in the final tumor that contain such a "later" mutation may vary markedly and depends on factors such as the duration of the mutation's existence and the relative rates of proliferation and death of the various cell populations.

Endocrine tumors are often sufficiently differentiated to express the hormonal activity characteristic of the corresponding normal cell type, but the hormonal function of the tumor is typically regulated in an abnormal fashion. It is important to understand that the genes that cause tumors of endocrine tissues do so only because of their effects on cell proliferation and accumulation. Such genes need not influence hormonal function. Furthermore, a mutant gene that alters hormonal function but confers no selective growth advantage will not be tumorigenic. Nevertheless, the frequent coexistence of growth deregulation and hormonal hyperfunction in endocrine tumors does indicate that the tumor-causing genes may directly or indirectly alter hormone control pathways. In certain instances, such as a mutation affecting the alpha subunit of stimulatory G protein ($G_{\alpha s}$) in growth hormone–producing and thyroid adenomas, a single mutant gene can directly contribute to both cell proliferation and hormonal hyperfunction. In general, however, the relationship between hypercellularity due to clonally selected mutant genes and hormonal hyperfunction is poorly understood.

Hyperplasia Versus Neoplasia

Not all hypercellular expansions are monoclonal. For instance, the generalized proliferative response of all cells of a tissue to an extrinsic stimulus yields a polyclonal expansion, examples of which include the hyperthyroidism of Graves' disease and the early, reversible secondary hyperparathyroidism in states of chronic hypocalcemia. Such polyclonal expansions represent biologic hyperplasia, whereas any monoclonal growth (benign or malignant) is a true neoplasm. Analyses of tumor clonality have been used to distinguish between these types of tumorigenic mechanisms. Nevertheless, the genesis of some tumors may involve both types of processes. For example, a generalized stimulus to polyclonal hyperplasia can, by increasing the chances of mitosis-related DNA damage in one cell, foster the emergence of a monoclonal population capable of eventually overwhelming or replacing its hyperplastic neighbors.

The clinical and histopathologic use of the term *hyperplasia* does not necessarily correspond with the biologic meaning described earlier, a situation that has engendered much confusion. For example, the usual tumors responsible for primary hyperparathyroidism have been clinicopathologically classified as adenomas when a single gland is abnormal, and as hyperplasia when the individual patient has multiple hypercellular glands. No histopathologic criteria can reliably predict whether a single or multiple glands are involved on the basis of analysis of only one such gland. Not only are clinical adenomas monoclonal neoplasms,[1] but many parathyroid glands from patients with multigland "hyperplasia" are also monoclonal.[2] It is therefore important to ensure that the terms used in the description of endocrine tumorigenesis be clearly defined.

Examination of Clonality to Provide Insights into Tumor Pathogenesis

The clonal status of a cellular proliferation is of fundamental importance in deciphering its pathogenesis; thus, endocrine tumors have been studied to determine whether the expansion is monoclonal or polyclonal. One way of determining that a tumor is monoclonal is to identify a DNA or chromosomal lesion that, because of its tumor-specificity and presence in all or most of the neoplastic cells, directly defines the expansion as monoclonal. Examples of cytogenetically defined clonal abnormalities are chromosome translocations such as

the t(9;22) Philadelphia chromosome in chronic myelogenous leukemia and the t(14;18) translocation in follicular lymphoma. The use of classic cytogenetics is technically more difficult in solid tumors than in hematopoietic tumors, because hematopoietic cells divide in culture much more readily and yield excellent metaphase chromosomal spreads. Endocrine tumors are difficult to culture and to analyze cytogenetically. Fortunately, improved methods for the cytogenetic and "molecular cytogenetic" study of tumors, including fluorescence in situ hybridization (FISH), comparative genomic hybridization, and chromosome painting, promise to open up new avenues for the detection of clonal chromosomal lesions in endocrine tumors.[3–5]

Examples of monoclonal abnormalities defined by molecular methods in endocrine neoplasia include $G_{\alpha s}$ gene mutations in growth hormone–producing pituitary tumors,[6] TSH (thyrotropin) receptor gene mutations in thyroid tumors,[7] and *PRAD1*/cyclin D1 gene rearrangements in parathyroid adenomas.[8] Identification of tumor-specific changes such as deletions of DNA markers in particular regions of the tumor genome also serves as evidence of monoclonality, even though the specific genes affected by such deletions may not be known.[9–14]

Indirect methods can determine the clonal status of tumors without the necessity of identifying the specific genes or chromosomal regions that are clonally mutated and involved in tumorigenesis. These methods have generally exploited the phenomenon of random X-chromosome inactivation (the Lyon phenomenon) in women.[15] Random X-chromosome inactivation occurs early in female embryonic development, in all somatic cells. In any cell, the choice of which X chromosome will be inactivated is random, but once that choice is made, the decision is faithfully transmitted to all progeny of that cell (Fig. 6–1A). Usually, therefore, the maternally derived X chromosome will be inactive in about 50% of the cells in a normal tissue, and the paternally derived X chromosome will be inactive in about 50%. Polyclonal growth, representing a generalized expansion of many or all original cells within a tissue, maintains the relatively even mix of active maternal and paternal X chromosomes characteristic of the normal tissues. In contrast, the neoplastic cells within a monoclonal tumor are derived from a single progenitor and all should reflect the identical X-chromosome pattern, with either the maternal or the paternal X chromosome uniformly inactivated (see Fig. 6–1A).

A unifying feature of methods based on the analysis of X-chromosome inactivation to determine the clonal status of a tumor is the use of a normally occurring variant, or polymorphism, at the genetic or protein level, to distinguish between a woman's two X chromosomes. The other step in these methods involves assaying some property that reflects the state of X-chromosome inactivation imposed on the tumor cell chromosomes at the polymorphic site. Assays to reflect X-chromosome inactivation status include assessment of gene expression (RNA or protein levels) or regional DNA methylation.

A polymorphism in glucose-6-phosphate dehydrogenase (G6PD) was the first to be used in X-chromomsome–inactivational analyses of tumor clonality.[16] However, the disadvantage of the G6PD system is that only a small minority of women are heterozygous for electrophoretically distinguishable isoforms of this X chromosome–encoded enzyme. Thus, most tumors were unsuitable for clonal analysis. Furthermore, the method failed to detect the monoclonality of certain tumors,[1, 17, 18] perhaps because of differences in the level of G6PD expression in tumor cells compared with "contaminating" admixed normal cells within the analyzed samples.

DNA polymorphisms are now preferentially used for clonal analyses to distinguish between the two X chromo-

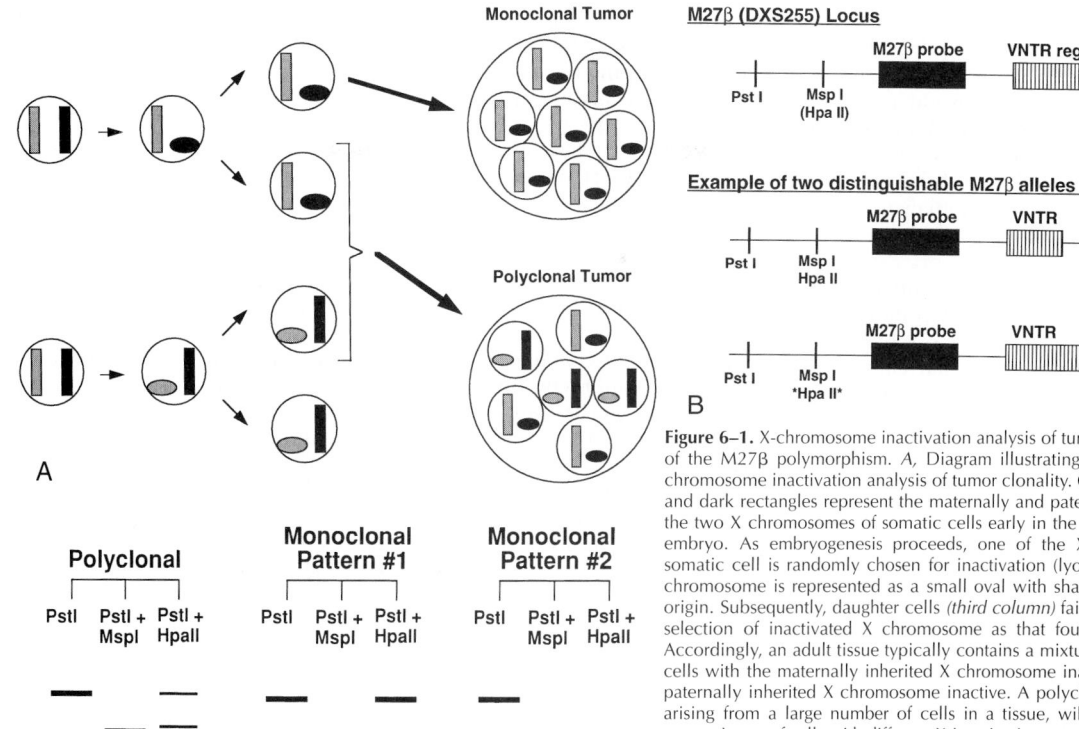

M27β (DXS255) Locus

Example of two distinguishable M27β alleles in an individual

A

Polyclonal   **Monoclonal Pattern #1**   **Monoclonal Pattern #2**

C

Figure 6–1. X-chromosome inactivation analysis of tumor clonality with the use of the M27β polymorphism. *A,* Diagram illustrating general principles of X-chromosome inactivation analysis of tumor clonality. On the left, lightly shaded and dark rectangles represent the maternally and paternally inherited copies of the two X chromosomes of somatic cells early in the development of a female embryo. As embryogenesis proceeds, one of the X chromosomes in each somatic cell is randomly chosen for inactivation (lyonization); the inactivated chromosome is represented as a small oval with shading corresponding to its origin. Subsequently, daughter cells *(third column)* faithfully maintain the same selection of inactivated X chromosome as that found in their parent cells. Accordingly, an adult tissue typically contains a mixture of approximately 50% cells with the maternally inherited X chromosome inactive, and 50% with the paternally inherited X chromosome inactive. A polyclonal tumor *(lower right),* arising from a large number of cells in a tissue, will maintain this relatively even mixture of cells with different X-inactivation patterns. A monoclonal tumor *(upper right),* derived from a single somatic cell, will have a uniform pattern of X-chromosome inactivation in all cells. *B,* Partial restriction endonuclease map of the M27β locus (DXS255), and an example of two distinguishable M27β alleles. The variable number of tandem repeat (VNTR, minisatellite) region, which is highly variable in its length from person to person, is shown in stripes. A 2.5 kb DNA fragment used as the hybridization probe is shown as a solid rectangle. Cleavage sites for restriction enzyme Pst I flank the locus. The enzyme Msp I cleaves the sequence CCGG whether or not the internal cytosine is methylated. In contrast, the enzyme Hpa II cleaves this sequence only if the internal cytosine is unmethylated. The diagrammed Msp I/Hpa II site actually represents a 270 base pair region containing three such sites, two of which vary in their methylation status in accord with location on the active versus the inactive X chromosome.[20] In the example of two distinguishable alleles, variation in size of the minisatellite repeat region (VNTR) causes a difference in the size of the Pst I restriction fragment detectable by hybridization to the labeled M27β probe. If an individual with these two alleles had a monoclonal tumor, in which the larger allele was uniformly associated with the active X chromosome, the Msp I/Hpa II site of this allele would be consistently methylated and, therefore, resistant to cleavage by Hpa II *(asterisks).* The resulting Southern blot pattern would correspond to monoclonal pattern No. 1 in *C. C,* Schematic diagram of prototypical Southern blot hybridization patterns for X-inactivation analysis using M27β. A monoclonal tumor can exhibit only one of the two monoclonal patterns shown. The Pst I + Msp I control digestion is useful for marking the sizes of fully cleaved alleles. (From Arnold A, Brown MF, Urena P, et al. Monoclonality of parathyroid tumors in chronic renal failure and in primary parathyroid hyperplasia. J Clin Invest 1995; 95:2047–2053. By copyright permission of The American Society for Clinical Investigation.)

somes. High rates of heterozygosity make it possible to analyze most tumors. Some multiallelic polymorphisms, based on differences in the number of highly repeated sequence units in a genomic location, are heterozygous in more than 90% of women, and a large number of DNA polymorphisms have been described on the X chromosome (and on all chromosomes). Most, however, cannot currently be used in clonality studies because they have not been characterized for detectable changes that correlate with the state of activity of the X chromosome on which an allele resides. Some of the X-linked polymorphisms that have been valuable in clonal analyses of human tumors include restriction fragment length polymorphisms (RFLPs) in the *HPRT* and *PGK* gene regions,[19] a minisatellite repeat (>10 nucleotide core repeated unit) region called M27β or DXS255,[2, 20] and a microsatellite repeat (<10 nucleotide core repeated unit) locus within the androgen receptor gene.[21, 22]

Changes in DNA methylation in the vicinity of certain polymorphic sites on the X chromosome correlate with the activity of that X chromosome and are useful in clonal analyses. Methylation of specific cytosine nucleotides is an epigenetic process that is faithfully replicated from a given cell to its progeny, and this process may have a role in maintaining the activity status of the particular X chromosome. Methylation at certain specific sites may be easily detected through the action of "methylation-sensitive" restriction endonucle-

ases, which cleave when their target sites are unmethylated but cannot do so when a methyl group is present. One cannot predict how or whether X-chromosome inactivation will affect the methylation of a particular nucleotide in or near a gene; correlations must be established separately for individual genomic sites. For example, a useful restriction site in the *HPRT* region is consistently methylated when on the active X chromosome and unmethylated when on the inactive X chromosome; the opposite pattern is observed for an informative site in the *PGK* region. Despite the need for such empirical validation, the use of DNA methylation as a surrogate marker for the status of X-chromosome activity has major advantages in clonality studies and eliminates the vulnerability of the assay to the vagaries of gene expression in tumor cells.

The analysis of clonality in endocrine tumors has yielded important insights. For example, the fact that most ACTH (corticotropin)-producing pituitary tumors are monoclonal showed that Cushing's disease could not be explained solely by a generalized hypothalamic stimulation of corticotrophs.[23, 24] Typical parathyroid adenomas are also monoclonal outgrowths[1, 10, 12–14] and are not, as previously suggested, asymmetrical forms of multiglandular hyperplasia.[17, 18] Most solitary thyroid nodules are monoclonal, which might have been expected, but so are some nodules within multinodular goiters.[25]

Figure 6–1*B* and *C* illustrates the methodology used in a study of X-chromosome inactivation in the pathogenesis of refractory secondary (or tertiary) hyperparathyroidism in patients with uremia. Because of multigland involvement, it has been assumed that this disease predominantly involves polyclonal (non-neoplastic) cellular proliferations, but the clonality of these "hyperplastic" tumors had not been comprehensively assessed. Clonality was examined with the M27β (DXS255) DNA polymorphism; 64% of informative patients with renal failure undergoing hemodialysis and with refractory hyperparathyroidism harbored at least one monoclonal parathyroid tumor, and 63% of all tumors examined had monoclonal X-inactivation patterns.[2] One often-overlooked pitfall in the interpretation of any X-inactivation analysis must be emphasized: polyclonal patterns cannot be interpreted definitively. For example, admixed normal cells or tumor-specific aberrancies in DNA methylation could obscure the detection of a monoclonal cell population. Thus, the true extent of monoclonality in severe secondary or tertiary hyperparathyroidism could be even higher (but not lower) than demonstrated. These unexpected results indicate that monoclonal parathyroid neoplasms are common in uremic refractory hyperparathyroidism and raise the possibility that autonomous parathyroid function in this disorder is due to the outgrowth of true neoplasms, presumably on a background of pre-existing (and more reversible) polyclonal parathyroid hyperplasia.

Predisposing Influences

Both environmental and genetic factors can contribute to the risk of developing a particular type of tumor over a lifetime. In highly penetrant inherited syndromes the genetic predisposition is overriding, but in most instances the intimate relation between environmental and genetic factors makes the traditional "nature versus nurture" question difficult to assess.

An often overlooked genetic component to tumor predisposition is sex. However, the specific mechanisms by which sex influences the risk of endocrine tumors such as thyroid cancer, parathyroid adenoma, and adrenal cancer are not well understood. Additional genetic variables, which may be frequent in the population, also influence the chance of tumor development. For example, two independent studies have shown that one allele of a common nucleotide polymorphism within the vitamin D receptor gene is overrepresented in women with primary hyperparathyroidism.[26, 27] It is possible that this hyperparathyroidism-associated allele may yield fewer vitamin D receptors[28] than the other common allele and thereby confer less of an antiproliferative effect on parathyroid cells, subtly but significantly increasing the lifetime risk of parathyroid neoplasia.

An important environmental factor in endocrine tumorigenesis is ionizing radiation. Both thyroid and parathyroid tumors have been linked to prior head and neck irradiation in a dose-dependent fashion.[29, 30] While the latency period for tumor development after radiation exposure in the United States is quite long, childhood thyroid cancer is already being observed with increased frequency in the aftermath of the 1986 Chernobyl nuclear accident.[31, 32] Whether such heightened susceptibility is solely a function of age and amount of exposure or relates in part to other factors, such as iodine deficiency in the region, has not been established but highlights the point that tumor predisposition and development can be influenced by complex interacting factors.

Oncogenes and Tumor Suppressor Genes

Two broad categories of genes are implicated in the excessive cell proliferation and other properties that results in the outgrowth and evolution of a neoplastic clone. An *oncogene* carries a "gain-of-function" mutation in its regulatory or coding region that results in deregulation of its normal product or in the formation of an abnormal protein product. Typically, only one mutated allele need be present for an oncogene to exert its tumorigenic action. The normal, unmutated version of an oncogene is called a proto-oncogene. Proto-oncogenes may be converted to oncogenes by various molecular genetic mechanisms, such as fusion of part of its coding region with that of another gene, chromosomal translocations or inversions that alter its regulatory environment, and point mutations.

A *tumor suppressor gene*, in contrast, normally acts to restrain cell proliferation or other aspects of the malignant phenotype. This restraint can directly control proliferation, for example by regulating the cell cycle, or affect proliferation indirectly, for example by maintaining genomic stability. Thus, the definition of a tumor suppressor gene is not restrictive as to its specific cellular function. Tumors are provoked by inactivating or "loss-of-function" mutations in such genes; the most common inactivating mechanisms are gene deletion and point mutations. Typically, both alleles of a tumor suppressor gene must be inactivated to eliminate the functional protein product and to contribute to tumorigenesis. The existence of a critical tumor suppressor gene is often inferred from the frequent finding that a particular subchromosomal stretch of DNA is clonally lost in a particular tumor type. The deletion typically involves only one of a gene's two alleles. Because such deletions are often large, the case that the correct tumor suppressor gene has been found can be made most convincingly when the nondeleted allele of the gene is shown to harbor another clonal inactivating lesion, such as a coding region mutation or microdeletion.

Some oncogenes or tumor suppressor genes contribute to tumors of only one or a few cell types, whereas other genes are involved in many different types of tumors. No single gene is always involved in the development of most types of tumors, and different combinations of mutated genes may have similar cellular and clinical consequences (genetic heterogeneity). Finally, genetic "hits" affecting multiple oncogenes and tumor suppressor genes within a single cell appear to be required if that cell is to become neoplastic. Thus, in most instances no single activated oncogene or inactivated tumor suppressor gene is necessary or sufficient for the development of tumors.

Mutational Mechanisms: Replication-Dependent Versus Time-Dependent

Tumors may acquire mutations that in themselves increase the rate at which new mutations develop at other sites in the genome. Many tumor biologists have commented on the apparently excessive number of genetic changes observed in individual cancers relative to measured rates of mutation in normal cells. Genetic changes are usually considered to occur or to be "fixed" during DNA replication or mitosis.[33] However, some mutations may be time-dependent rather than replication-dependent, meaning that they can arise even in the absence of cell proliferation.[33, 34] One mechanism by which somatic mutations may occur would be by a defect in postreplication mismatch repair, the pathway responsible for removing and correcting mismatched base pairs in DNA.[34] At least one form of inherited genetic instability can result from inactivation of "mutator" genes in the mismatch repair system, *hMSH2* or *hMLH1*, for example.[35] Such mutational mechanisms might be quite important in benign or slow-growing endocrine tumors that derive from slowly proliferating normal tissues.

SOMATIC GENETIC ALTERATIONS IN ENDOCRINE TUMORS: EXAMPLES

Neoplasia is, in large part, a genetic disease in which most of the critical DNA damage occurs somatically, rather than being inherited ("germline"). Somatic alterations of both oncogenes and tumor suppressor genes are implicated in endocrine tumorigenesis, and a few illustrative examples will be discussed.

TSH Receptor and $G_{\alpha s}$ in Toxic Thyroid Adenomas

The fact that solitary toxic thyroid adenomas often contain somatic mutations in different genes whose products are functionally interrelated highlights the point that heterogeneous genetic lesions can converge on common pathways to predispose to neoplasia. Solitary toxic thyroid adenomas are characterized by autonomous (TSH-independent) hyperfunction and growth. Because TSH is normally a stimulus to both functional activity and growth of thyroid cells, toxic adenomas behave as though they are stimulated by TSH chronically and inappropriately, and somatic mutations within the TSH receptor itself that lead to TSH-independent (constitutive) activation of the receptor are clonal lesions in a subset of toxic adenomas.[7, 36] Thus, the TSH receptor is a proto-oncogene that can be activated by a variety of point mutations.[7] Analysis of how these point mutations mimic the effects of TSH binding has provided insight into the mechanism of activation of G protein–coupled receptors.

The TSH receptor is a member of the large family of G protein–coupled receptors, and its major actions on thyrocyte proliferation and differentiated function are mediated through the cyclic AMP signaling pathway. The predominant G protein involved in transducing the stimulatory effect of the receptor on adenylyl cyclase is $G_{\alpha s}$. $G_{\alpha s}$ is also a proto-oncogene and has undergone clonally selected, activating point mutation in 25 to 30% of toxic thyroid adenomas.[9, 37] $G_{\alpha s}$ genes bearing such gain-of-function mutations have been termed *gsp* oncogenes, and are also present in some growth hormone–secreting pituitary tumors.[6] Not surprisingly, these pituitary tumors demonstrate constitutive activation of the cyclic AMP pathway, a prime mediator of proliferation and hormonal function in the somatotroph. In this context it is instructive to raise the example of McCune-Albright syndrome (see Chapter 31), in which activating $G_{\alpha s}$ mutations are present in multiple tissues of a given patient owing to mutation early in embryonic development and subsequent genetic mosaicism. Hyperthyroidism and acromegaly are among the characteristic components of this syndrome.

Cyclin D1 (PRAD1) in Hyperparathyroidism and General Oncology

Another illustrative example is that of the cyclin D1, or *PRAD1*, oncogene. Unlike many endocrine tumor–associated oncogenes, *PRAD1* is also frequently involved in nonendocrine tumors. Interestingly, this gene, now appreciated to be of central importance to molecular oncology and to normal cellular physiology, was discovered in the molecular dissection of an endocrine tumor.

Many human oncogenes were discovered because they are adjacent to nonrandom chromosome breakpoints in tumors. Chromosome breaks and rearrangements probably occur frequently in normal cells but are recognized only when they happen to result in deregulation of the expression of a growth-related gene and confer a selective advantage on the cell. *PRAD1* was identified as the putative oncogene adjacent to one such breakpoint on chromosome 11 in a subset of parathyroid adenomas (Fig. 6–2).[8, 38–40] On the 11q13 side of the inversion breakpoint, the promoter and coding exons of the *PRAD1* gene remain in contiguity with each other. Across the

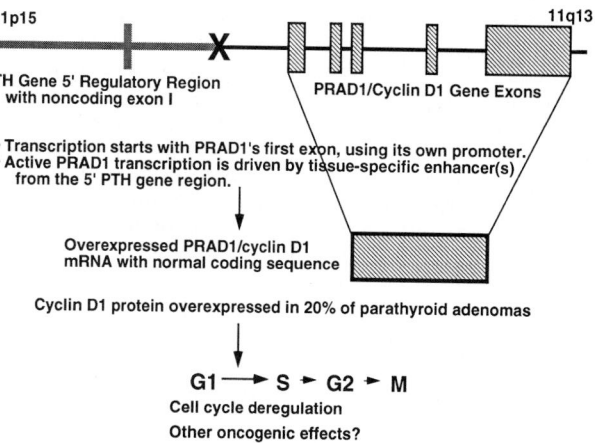

Figure 6–2. Diagram of the molecular structure of the PTH-PRAD1 DNA rearrangement in a subset of parathyroid adenomas and its functional consequences. Dark "X" represents the chromosome breakpoint between the *PTH* gene regulatory region, plus *PTH* noncoding exon 1 *(solid light vertical bar)* and part of its first intron, from 11p15 *(left)*, and the intact promoter and 5 exons of the *PRAD1* (cyclin D1) gene from 11q13. *PRAD1* gene transcription proceeds in a left-to-right direction, as drawn. (Modified from Arnold A. Genetic basis of endocrine disease 5: molecular genetics of parathyroid gland neoplasia. J Clin Endocrinol Metab 1993;77:1108–12. © 1993, The Endocrine Society.)

breakpoint are regulatory sequences from the upstream region of the parathyroid hormone *(PTH)* gene on 11p15 that normally function to enhance *PTH* gene transcription in the presence of parathyroid tissue–specific signals (likely to be DNA binding proteins found in the nucleus). Such transcriptional enhancer sequences are capable of acting over distances of many kilobases to enhance transcription, and *PRAD1* (cyclin D1) transcription is increased in these tumors.[41] While the variability in potential breakpoint sites makes it difficult to determine the true incidence of such rearrangements, cyclin D1 protein levels are elevated in about 20% of parathyroid adenomas.[42] In a broader context, the tissue-specific enhancer-driven expression of cyclin D1 in parathyroid tumors is analogous to the activation of oncogenes such as *BCL2* or *MYC* in B-cell lymphomas.[40] In these tumors chromosomal rearrangements lead to a juxtaposition of immunoglobulin gene enhancer elements and the oncogene, which is thereby inappropriately activated.

The PRAD1 gene product is structurally related to the cyclin family of proteins, which controls the cell cycle. However, prior to discovery of *PRAD1*, no mammalian cyclins were known to participate in the control of the critical transition from G_1 to S phase; this checkpoint would be an appropriate site for attack by an oncogenic protein because movement into S phase commits a cell to the remainder of the cycle and another mitosis.[43–45] It is now established that cyclin D1 is a "G_1 cyclin" that functions to push the cell toward or through this key juncture.[44]

Cyclins are regulatory subunits of holoenzymes whose catalytic subunits are cyclin-dependent kinases, or CDKs. The major kinase partner for cyclin D1 appears to be CDK4 and, in some cell types, CDK6. Natural inhibitors of CDK function also exist, and $p16^{INK4a}$ is recognized as a key inhibitor of cyclin D-CDK4/6 complexes. Thus, inactivation of p16 might be expected to be as oncogenic as cyclin D1 overexpression, and p16 is, indeed, a tumor suppressor gene in familial melanoma and several types of sporadic human tumors.[45] Interestingly, inactivating mutations of p16 are uncommon, if they occur at all, in parathyroid adenomas.[46] Hence, the cellular consequences of p16 loss and cyclin D1 activation may not precisely overlap.

The significance of *PRAD1* in human neoplasia extends

far beyond its involvement in endocrine tumors. It is the long-sought "*BCL1*" oncogene that is deregulated by the characteristic t(11;14) translocation in mantle cell or centrocytic B-cell lymphomas.[40] As such, assessment of cyclin D1 expression is useful in the molecular diagnosis of B-cell neoplasia. In addition, cyclin D1/*PRAD1* is a key oncogene in breast cancer, squamous cell cancer of the head and neck, esophageal cancer, and a variety of other tumors.[40] Cyclin D1 and other members of its oncogenic pathway or pathways may serve as targets for development of antineoplastic therapies.

RET Gene Rearrangements in Papillary Thyroid Cancer

Activating mutations of the *RET* proto-oncogene are responsible for multiple endocrine neoplasia type 2 (see Chapter 32), but this gene is also involved in human disease through another mechanism: clonal somatic rearrangements of this gene are found in about 25% of papillary thyroid cancers, but not in other types of thyroid (or nonthyroidal) cancer.[47–49]

RET encodes a member of the receptor tyrosine kinase superfamily, and one endogenous ligand that binds to and activates RET is the glial-cell-line–derived neurotrophic factor (GDNF).[50, 51] Normally, *RET* acts mainly during embryogenesis, with expression in cells derived from the neural crest and in the developing central and peripheral nervous systems and kidney.[49, 52] Inactivating germline mutations of *RET* are a cause of Hirschsprung's disease, in which parasympathetic ganglia fail to migrate properly in the gastrointestinal tract (see Chapter 32).

Receptor tyrosine kinases (RTKs) such as RET dimerize as a consequence of ligand binding. Dimerization then leads to autophosphorylation of the receptor, and the phosphorylated receptor can bind and/or phosphorylate other molecules in a signaling cascade.[53] The RET protein, like other RTKs, has extracellular, transmembrane, and intracellular (tyrosine kinase) domains (Fig. 6–3). The papillary cancer–specific *RET* rearrangements described to date involve a chromosomal break that fuses the intracellular tyrosine kinase domain-encoding portion of the *RET* gene to one of three alternative partners.[49] The *RET* fusion partner gene segment provides a new promoter that is constitutively active in thyroid cells and encodes a new in-frame N terminus for the oncoprotein (see Fig. 6–3). The three different *RET* fusion oncogenes have been termed *RET-PTC1*, *RET-PTC2*, and *RET-PTC3*; the corresponding fusion partner genes are *H4*, *R1α*, and *ELE1*.[49] The N termini of these fusion oncoproteins allow for dimerization and activation of the RET tyrosine kinase, bypassing the usual requirement for ligand binding.

The specificity of these *RET* fusion oncogenes for papil-lary-type thyroid cancer is not well understood. It would appear that only this thyroid cell type has the propensity for production of such fusions or that only this cell has the molecular machinery capable of responding to this form of RET kinase activation. Alternatively, development of a papillary cancer may be an inevitable response to the occurrence of the *RET* rearrangement early in the life of a thyroidal neoplasm.

Finally, the *RET* proto-oncogene and its fusion partners might be especially susceptible to breakage and fusion as a consequence of ionizing radiation. More than 60% of papillary cancers that have developed in young people exposed to the nuclear fallout from the Chernobyl reactor contain *RET-PTC* fusion oncogenes.[54]

GERMLINE MUTATIONS PREDISPOSING TO ENDOCRINE NEOPLASIA: EXAMPLES

Patients who develop a particular tumor on the basis of a strong inherited predisposition typically constitute only a minority of patients with that tumor. Nonetheless, the lessons learned from identifying the molecular basis of inherited tumor predisposition are important, both clinically and from a fundamental biologic perspective. In addition, some genes in which germline mutations cause rare genetic syndromes have subsequently been found to be somatically mutated in the more common, sporadic occurrences of the same tumors.

Germline mutations that predispose to neoplasia can occur in either proto-oncogenes or tumor suppressor genes; in other words, mutations that cause inherited tumor syndromes can be of either the gain-of-function or the loss-of-function type. However, most germline mutations identified to date are inactivating mutations, thus identifying the affected genes as tumor suppressors, by definition. A few genes responsible for heritable endocrine neoplasia syndromes have been discovered, and others are still being sought.

RET Mutations in MEN 2

Multiple endocrine neoplasia type 2 (MEN 2) is a collection of three syndromes, MEN 2A, familial medullary thyroid cancer (FMTC), and MEN 2B, which are discussed in more detail in Chapter 32. All are autosomal dominant syndromes in which the most consistent feature is predisposition to medullary thyroid cancer. Genetic linkage analysis demonstrated that the *MEN2* gene or genes must lie near the centromere on chromosome 10, and an evaluation of candidate genes known to map to this region led to the identification of germline *RET* point mutations that cosegregated with the

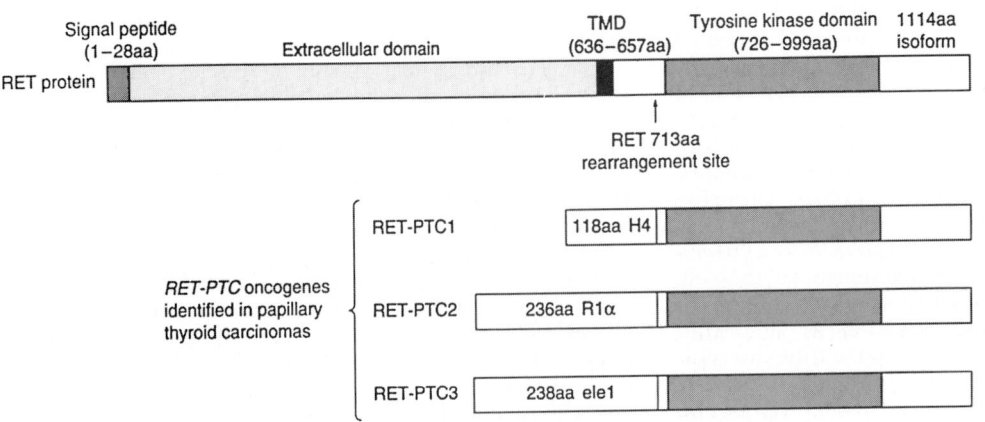

Figure 6–3. Schematic representation of the normal RET protein (*upper*) and the oncoproteins created by the *RET-PTC* oncogenes in papillary thyroid cancer (*lower*). aa, amino acid; TMD, transmembrane domain. For each rearranged oncoprotein, the number of N-terminal amino acids contributed by the specified partner gene is shown, fused to the tyrosine kinase domain and C terminus of *RET*. (From Pasini B, Ceccherini I, Romeo G. RET mutations in human disease. Trends Genet 1996; 12:138–144, with permission. Copyright 1996, Elsevier Science.)

disease.[55] The existence of de novo *RET* mutations in patients with an MEN2 phenotype but a negative family history, and the demonstration that the *MEN2*-associated mutations activate *RET* as a transforming oncogene,[56] further helped establish that germline *RET* mutations are the predominant cause of MEN 2.[49, 55] Only a few codons (for cysteine residues in the extracellular domain) harbor the *RET* mutations in almost all MEN-2A and most FMTC patients, and only a single codon (for a conserved threonine within the tyrosine kinase domain's catalytic core) is mutated in virtually all patients with MEN 2B. This molecular specificity contrasts with the many ways in which tumor suppressor genes are typically found to be inactivated, and provided the first clue that *RET* mutations in MEN 2 are activating mutations. In fact, MEN 2 was the first inherited human tumor syndrome found to be due to an activated, oncogene in the germline, and only one other such example has been reported to date, an activating germline point mutation of CDK4 in some melanoma-prone families.[57] The limited number of locations for *RET* mutations in MEN 2 makes it relatively easy to detect the mutations and make the molecular diagnosis. This methodology is available commercially.

At a time when the general concept of germline DNA testing for cancer predisposition has been enveloped in controversy, MEN 2 has provided the best example in oncology for the efficacy of molecular diagnosis in mainstream clinical management. Specific features not often present in other cancer predispositions that have contributed to the impact of the molecular diagnosis of MEN 2 include (1) the high penetrance of a life-threatening cancer (MTC), (2) the ease and accuracy of DNA diagnosis (better than previously available pentagastrin testing), and (3) the availability of a lifesaving intervention (thyroidectomy) without major risk.

As alluded to earlier, somatic *RET* mutations (much more often of the MEN-2B type than the MEN-2A type) are also present in a minority of sporadic MTCs and pheochromocytomas,[55] but not in primary hyperparathyroidism.[58, 59]

It is important to recognize that, in MEN 2, the germline *RET* mutation is present in all somatic cells of the affected individual. However, the MEN 2-related tumors are not, strictly speaking, inherited but develop from a hyperplastic endocrine cell mass into clonal neoplasms over time. The monoclonality of the MTCs and pheochromocytomas in MEN 2[60, 61] indicates that somatic molecular mutations, probably affecting several oncogenes or tumor suppressor genes, or both, must occur in a single cell and act in concert with the inherited germline *RET* mutation for the neoplasms to emerge. In fact, several such clonal somatic molecular lesions, including allelic deletions on chromosomes 1, 3, 11, 17, and 22, have been found in MEN 2-associated tumors,[62–65] pointing to the genomic locations of important but unidentified putative tumor suppressor genes.

MEN1 Tumor Suppressor Gene

Multiple endocrine neoplasia type 1 (MEN 1) is a familial predisposition to tumors of the parathyroid glands, anterior pituitary, pancreatic islets, and duodenum. Carcinoid tumors, thyroid and adrenal adenomas, and lipomas also occur more frequently in this disorder. This syndrome is discussed extensively in Chapter 32. MEN 1 is inherited in an autosomal dominant pattern, indicating that a single mutant gene is responsible for transmitting the tumor predisposition. Genetic linkage analysis has implicated a region on the long arm of chromosome 11 (11q13) as the site of the *MEN1* gene (i.e., the site of the normal gene whose mutant form causes MEN 1).[66] However, this target region on 11q13 contains a large number of genes, and no candidate gene has as yet been confirmed to be the actual *MEN1* gene. Hence, the mecha-

nisms by which the genetic defect in MEN 1 leads to tumor formation are not well understood.

Despite this ignorance, considerable evidence indicates that the *MEN1* gene is a tumor suppressor gene. One of the two cellular copies of the *MEN1*-linked chromosomal region is frequently found to be somatically and clonally deleted in parathyroid and pancreatic tumor tissues from patients with MEN 1.[10, 11, 67, 68] Importantly, when the parental origin of the deleted allele could be identified, it always derived from the parent unaffected by MEN 1. Thus, patients with MEN 1 are believed to have inherited one inactivated copy of the critical gene from the affected parent, and the remaining normal copy becomes somatically inactivated, often by a large regional deletion, in a clonal progenitor cell from which the tumor will emerge. Because the germline-affected *MEN1* chromosomal region appears to be grossly intact, it is likely that germline mutations in the *MEN1* gene are small deletions or point mutations that will require sequencing of DNA for detection.

After the somatic deletion on 11q13 has occurred, a parathyroid or an islet cell, for example, would be devoid of the normal tumor suppressor function of the *MEN1* gene and could thereby acquire a selective advantage over its neighbors. The high incidence of endocrine tumors in MEN 1 (which demonstrates almost 100% penetrance) implies that somatic inactivation of the remaining normal gene copy is a common development in endocrine tissue. It does not mean, however, that loss of function in both MEN-1 alleles is *sufficient* for tumorigenesis, and additional cooperating oncogenic lesions may be needed. This concept is consistent with the finding that patients identified by linkage analysis as constitutionally homozygous for the mutant *MEN1* gene do not exhibit more severe or accelerated endocrine tumor development.[69]

Allelic losses of DNA markers on 11q13, centered on the *MEN1* critical region, are found in sporadically occurring tumors of the MEN-1 types, most commonly in about 25% of parathyroid adenomas.[70] Thus, the *MEN1* tumor suppressor gene may also be the target of somatic inactivating lesions in sporadic endocrine tumors.

CONCLUSION

Genetic paradigms that originated in the study of malignant neoplasia are useful in the molecular dissection of endocrine tumors, including common benign endocrine tumors. Identification of clonally selected mutations in oncogenes and tumor suppressor genes has opened the door to understanding the control of growth in endocrine tissues. Furthermore, the fact that these genetic alterations can affect endocrine cell function as well as cell number may be exploited in devising medical therapies in the future.

REFERENCES

1. Arnold A, Staunton CE, Kim HG, et al. Monoclonality and abnormal parathyroid hormone genes in parathyroid adenomas. N Engl J Med 1988; 318:658–662.
2. Arnold A, Brown MF, Urena P, et al. Monoclonality of parathyroid tumors in chronic renal failure and in primary parathyroid hyperplasia. J Clin Invest 1995; 95:2047–2053.
3. Kallioniemi A, Kallioniemi O-P, Sudar D, et al. Comparative genomic hybridization for molecular cytogenetic analysis of solid tumors. Science 1992; 258:818–821.
4. Speicher MR, Ballard SG, Ward DC. Karyotyping human chromosomes by combinatorial multi-fluor FISH. Nat Genet 1996; 12:368–375.
5. LeBeau MM. One FISH, two FISH, red FISH, blue FISH. Nat Genet 1996; 12:341–344.
6. Shimon I, Melmed S. Growth hormone- and GHRH-producing tumors. In: Arnold A, ed. Endocrine Neoplasms. Norwell, MA: Kluwer Academic (in press).
7. van Sande J, Parma J, Tonacchera M, et al. Genetic basis of endocrine

disease: somatic and germline mutations of the TSH receptor gene in thyroid diseases. J Clin Endocrinol Metab 1995; 80:2577–2585.

8. Arnold A. Genetic basis of endocrine disease 5: molecular genetics of parathyroid gland neoplasia. J Clin Endocrinol Metab 1993; 77:1108–1112.

9. Fagin JA. Genetic basis of endocrine disease 3: molecular defects in thyroid gland neoplasia. J Clin Endocrinol Metab 1992; 75:1398–1400.

10. Friedman E, Sakaguchi K, Bale AE, et al. Clonality of parathyroid tumors in familial multiple endocrine neoplasia type 1. N Engl J Med 1989; 321:213–218.

11. Byström C, Larsson C, Blomberg C, et al. Localization of the MEN1 gene to a small region within chromosome 11q13 by deletion mapping in tumors. Proc Natl Acad Sci USA 1990; 87:1968–1972.

12. Arnold A, Kim HG. Clonal loss of one chromosome 11 in a parathyroid adenoma. J Clin Endocrinol Metab 1989; 69:496–499.

13. Cryns VL, Yi SM, Tahara H, et al. Frequent loss of chromosome arm 1p DNA in parathyroid adenomas. Genes Chromosomes Cancer 1995; 13:9–17.

14. Tahara H, Smith AP, Gaz RD, et al. Genomic localization of novel candidate tumor suppressor gene loci in human parathyroid adenomas. Cancer Res 1996; 56:599–605.

15. Lyon M. Gene action in the X-chromosome of the mouse. Nature 1961; 190:372–373.

16. Fialkow PJ. Clonal origin of human tumors. Biochim Biophys Acta 1976; 458:283–321.

17. Fialkow PJ, Jackson CE, Block MA, et al. Multicellular origin of parathyroid "adenomas." N Engl J Med 1977; 297:696–698.

18. Jackson CE, Cerny JC, Block MA, et al. Probable clonal origin of aldosteronomas versus multicellular origin of parathyroid "adenomas." Surgery 1982; 92:875–879.

19. Vogelstein B, Fearon ER, Hamilton SR, et al. Clonal analysis using recombinant DNA probes from the X-chromosome. Cancer Res 1987; 47:4806–4813.

20. Fey MF, Peter H-J, Hinds HL, et al. Clonal analysis of human tumors with M27β, a highly informative polymorphic X chromosomal probe. J Clin Invest 1992; 89:1438–1444.

21. Willman CL, Busque L, Griffith BB, et al. Langerhans'-cell histiocytosis (histiocytosis X): a clonal proliferative disease. N Engl J Med 1994; 331:154–160.

22. Busque L, Zhu J, DeHart D, et al. An expression-based clonality assay at the human androgen receptor locus (HUMARA) on chromosome X. Nucleic Acids Res 1994; 22:697–698.

23. Biller BMK, Alexander JM, Zervas NT, et al. Clonal origins of adrenocorticotropin-secreting pituitary tissue in Cushing's disease. J Clin Endocrinol Metab 1992; 75:1303–1309.

24. Gicquel C, Le Bouc Y, Luton J-P, et al. Monoclonality of corticotroph macroadenomas in Cushing's disease. J Clin Endocrinol Metab 1992; 75:472–475.

25. Namba H, Matsuo K, Fagin J. Clonal composition of benign and malignant human thyroid tumors. J Clin Invest 1990; 86:120–125.

26. Carling T, Kindmark A, Hellman P, et al. Vitamin D receptor genotypes in primary hyperparathyroidism. Nat Med 1995; 1:1309–1311.

27. Mitlak B, Smith AP, Arnold A. Association of a polymorphic allele of the vitamin D receptor gene with primary hyperparathyroidism in women and men. J Bone Miner Res 1996; 11(Suppl. 1):S489.

28. Morrison NA, Qi JC, Tokita A, et al. Prediction of bone density from vitamin D receptor alleles. Nature 1994; 367:284–287.

29. Schneider AB, Fogelfeld L. Radiation-induced endocrine tumors. In: Arnold A, ed. Endocrine Neoplasms. Norwell, MA: Kluwer Academic (in press).

30. Schneider AB, Ron E, Lubin J, et al. Dose-response relationships for radiation-induced thyroid cancer and thyroid nodules: evidence for the prolonged effects of radiation on the thyroid. J Clin Endocrinol Metab 1993; 77:362–369.

31. Nikiforov Y, Gnepp DR, Fagin JA. Thyroid lesions in children and adolescents after the Chernobyl disaster: implications for the study of radiation tumorigenesis. J Clin Endocrinol Metab 1996; 81:9–14.

32. Williams D. Thyroid cancer and the Chernobyl accident. J Clin Endocrinol Metab 1996; 81:6–8.

33. Strauss B. The origin of point mutation in human tumor cells. Cancer Res 1992; 52:249–253.

34. MacPhee D. Mismatch repair, somatic mutations, and the origins of cancer. Cancer Res 1995; 55:5489–5492.

35. Loeb L. Microsatellite instability: marker of a mutator phenotype in cancer. Cancer Res 1994; 54:5059–5063.

36. Russo D, Arturi F, Suarez HG, et al. Thyrotropin receptor gene alterations in thyroid hyperfunctioning adenomas. J Clin Endocrinol Metab 1996; 81:1548–1551.

37. Lyons J, Landis C, Harsh G, et al. Two G protein oncogenes in human endocrine tumors. Science 1990; 249:655–659.

38. Arnold A, Kim HG, Gaz RD, et al. Molecular cloning and chromosomal mapping of DNA rearranged with the parathyroid hormone gene in a parathyroid adenoma. J Clin Invest 1989; 83:2034–2040.

39. Motokura T, Bloom T, Kim HG, et al. A novel cyclin encoded by a bcl1-linked candidate oncogene. Nature 1991; 350:512–515.

40. Arnold A. The cyclin D1/PRAD1 oncogene in human neoplasia. J Investig Med 1995; 43:543–549.

41. Rosenberg CL, Kim HG, Shows TB, et al. Rearrangement and overexpression of D11S287E, a candidate oncogene on chromosome 11q13 in benign parathyroid tumors. Oncogene 1991; 6:449–453.

42. Hsi E, Zukerberg L, Yang W-I, et al. Cyclin D1/PRAD1 expression in parathyroid adenomas: an immunohistochemical study. J Clin Endocrinol Metab 1996; 81:1736–1739.

43. Hosokawa Y, Arnold A. Cyclin D1/PRAD1 as a central target in oncogenesis. J Lab Clin Med 1996; 127:246–252.

44. Sherr CJ. G₁ phase progression: cycling on cue. Cell 1994; 79:551–555.

45. Hunter T, Pines J. Cyclins and cancer II: cyclin D and CDK inhibitors come of age. Cell 1994; 79:573–582.

46. Tahara H, Smith A, Gaz R, et al. Loss of chromosome arm 9p DNA and analysis of the p16 and p15 cyclin-dependent kinase inhibitor genes in human parathyroid adenomas. J Clin Endocrinol Metab (in press).

47. Santoro M, Carlomagno F, Hay ID, et al. Ret oncogene activation in human thyroid neoplasms is restricted to the papillary cancer subtype. J Clin Invest 1992; 89:1517–1522.

48. Santoro M, Sabino N, Ishizaka Y, et al. Involvement of RET oncogene in human tumours: specificity of RET activation to thyroid tumours. Br J Cancer 1993; 68:460–464.

49. Pasini B, Ceccherini I, Romeo G. RET mutations in human disease. Trends Genet 1996; 12:138–144.

50. Trupp M, Arenas E, Fainzilber M, et al. Functional receptor for GDNF encoded by the c-ret proto-oncogene. Nature 1996; 381:785–789.

51. Durbec P, Marcos-Gutierrez CV, Kilkenny C, et al. GDNF signalling through the RET receptor tyrosine kinase. Nature 1996; 381:789–793.

52. Schuchardt A, D'Agati V, Larsson-Blomberg L, et al. Defects in the kidney and enteric nervous system of mice lacking the tyrosine kinase receptor RET. Nature 1994; 367:380–383.

53. Fantl W, Johnson D, Williams L. Signalling by receptor tyrosine kinases. Annu Rev Biochem 1993; 62:453–481.

54. Fugazzola L, Pilotti S, Pinchera A, et al. Oncogenic rearrangements of the RET proto-oncogene in papillary thyroid carcinomas in children exposed to the Chernobyl nuclear accident. Cancer Res 1995; 55:5617–5620.

55. Mulligan LM, Ponder BAJ. Genetic basis of endocrine disease: multiple endocrine neoplasia type 2. J Clin Endocrinol Metab 1995; 80:1989–1995.

56. Santoro M, Carlomagno F, Romano A, et al. Activation of RET as a dominant transforming gene by germline mutations of MEN2A and MEN2B. Science 1995; 2647:381–383.

57. Zuo L, Weger J, Yang Q, et al. Germline mutations in the p16^INK4a binding domain of CDK4 in familial melanoma. Nat Genet 1996; 12:97–99.

58. Pausova Z, Soliman E, Amizuka N, et al. Role of the RET proto-oncogene in sporadic hyperparathyroidism and in hyperparathyroidism of multiple endocrine neoplasia type 2. J Clin Endocrinol Metab 1996; 81:2711–2718.

59. Padberg B, Schroder S, Jochum W, et al. Absence of RET proto-oncogene point mutations in sporadic hyperplastic and neoplastic lesions of the parathyroid gland. Am J Pathol 1995; 147:1600–1607.

60. Baylin S, Gann D, Hsu S. Clonal origin of inherited medullary thyroid carcinoma and pheochromocytoma. Science 1976; 193:321–323.

61. Baylin S, Hsu S, Gann D, et al. Inherited medullary thyroid carcinoma: the result of a final monoclonal mutation imposed on one of multiple clones of susceptible cells. Science 1978; 199:429–431.

62. Mathew C, Smith B, Thorpe K, et al. Deletion of genes on chromosome 1 in endocrine neoplasia. Nature 1987; 328:524–526.

63. Khosla S, Patel V, Hay I, et al. Loss of heterozygosity suggests multiple genetic alterations in pheochromocytomas and medullary thyroid carcinomas. J Clin Invest 1991; 87:1691–1699.

64. Moley J, Brother M, Fong C-T, et al. Consistent association of 1p loss of heterozygosity with pheochromocytomas from patients with multiple endocrine neoplasia type 2 syndromes. Cancer Res 1992; 52:770–774.

65. Mulligan L, Gardner E, Smith B, et al. Genetic events in tumour initiation and progression in multiple endocrine neoplasia type 2. Genes Chromosomes Cancer 1993; 6:166–177.

66. Larsson C, Skogseid B, Oberg K, et al. Multiple endocrine neoplasia type I gene maps to chromosome 11 and is lost in insulinoma. Nature 1988; 332:85–87.

67. Thakker RV, Bouloux P, Wooding C, et al. Association of parathyroid tumors in multiple endocrine neoplasia type 1 with loss of alleles on chromosome 11. N Engl J Med 1989; 321:218–224.

68. Bale A, Norton J, Wong E, et al. Allelic loss on chromosome 11 in hereditary and sporadic tumors related to familial multiple endocrine neoplasia type 1. Cancer Res 1991; 51:1154–1157.

69. Brandi M, Weber G, Svensson A, et al. Homozygotes for the autosomal dominant neoplasia syndrome (MEN 1). Am J Hum Genet 1993; 53:1167–1172.

70. Friedman E, De Marco L, Gejman PV, et al. Allelic loss from chromosome 11 in parathyroid tumors. Cancer Res 1992; 52:6804–6809.

7

AUTOIMMUNITY AND THE ENDOCRINE SYSTEM

David R. Karp and John P. Atkinson

The hallmark of the adaptive immune system is its exquisite specificity. Both cellular and humoral immune responses are capable of recognizing the millions of different foreign antigens that are part of microbial pathogens. However, many similar antigens already exist within the host. The immune system must be able to identify and destroy infectious agents and to ignore self-antigens. This ability to discriminate self from nonself is critical. The mechanisms that control it are operative at multiple levels of the immune response. When these controls break down, a pathologic immune response, or autoimmunity, occurs. This chapter provides a basic overview of the mechanisms responsible for the generation and maintenance of immunologic nonresponsiveness to self-antigens and of the mechanisms that produce disruption of this control, leading to autoimmune disease.

GENERATION OF SPECIFICITY

The ability to recognize specific antigens results from the generation of diverse populations of T and B lymphocytes. These two mononuclear cells constitute the bulk of the adaptive immune system. T cells recognize foreign antigens displayed on the surface of host cells (see later) and subsequently proliferate and differentiate into cytotoxic T cells, killing the infected host cells, or into helper T cells, secreting cytokines that promote inflammatory and antibody responses. Helper T cells are further subdivided by the pattern of cytokines they secrete, a feature that may determine whether a protective immune response becomes autoimmune. B cells can recognize both soluble and cell-associated antigens, independent of the antigen processing required for T-cell recognition. Activated B cells secrete antibodies that neutralize infectious microorganisms, target them for uptake via polymorphonuclear leukocytes or monocytes (opsonization), and activate the complement system.

Although T and B cells have different functions, the mechanisms that generate diversity and specificity are similar. On T cells the antigen is recognized by a heterodimeric cell surface protein termed the T-cell receptor (TCR). On B cells, surface immunoglobulin (sIg) plays this role. sIg is a transmembrane form of the antibody that is secreted by the activated B cell. TCR and sIg have analogous structures. Most TCRs consist of single alpha and beta chains linked by disulfide bonds. Immunoglobulin molecules consist of two pairs of heavy and light chains. Each heavy and light chain pair forms an antigen-binding domain. The two heavy chains are disulfide bonded as well, so that every immunoglobulin molecule is capable of binding two identical antigens. Each polypeptide chain of the TCR or immunoglobulin is composed of constant and variable regions. The constant regions anchor the proteins to the cell surface and interact with other proteins involved with transmembrane signaling and lymphocyte activation. In the case of antibody molecules, the constant region also determines the isotype (IgM, IgG, IgA, or IgE) of the secreted protein and interacts with other cell surface molecules, such as immunoglobulin receptors, and with proteins of the complement system.

The variable portions of the TCR and of immunoglobulins are responsible for the diversity and specificity of the immune response and are unique to each cell. The process that generates this diversity is termed somatic recombination. During lymphocyte development regions of genomic DNA are recombined to generate novel sequences. In general, a region of DNA coding for most of the TCR or immunoglobulin variable region, termed the V region, is first recombined with a smaller region of DNA, termed the joining (J) region. The genes for the immunoglobulin heavy chain and the TCR beta chain also contain diversity (D) segments that recombine between the V and the J regions. Although these recombination events are highly regulated, they are imprecise. At each step, one or a few nucleotides can be randomly removed or inserted at the junction. These events have the effect of increasing the diversity of recombined genes and the possibility of generating

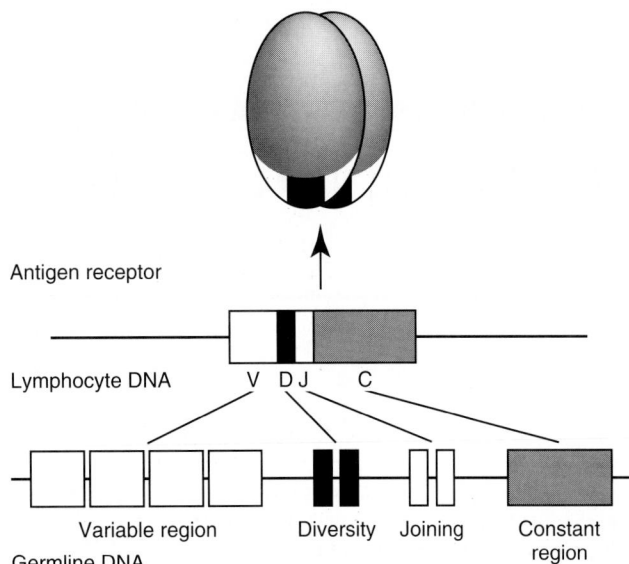

Figure 7–1. Generation of diverse antigen receptors. Both immunoglobulin and T-cell receptor (TCR) diversity are derived from the combination of different genetic elements. Germline genes for variable (V) portions of the antibody or TCR proteins recombine in lymphocytes with DNA coding for diversity (D), junctional (J), and constant (C) portions of the molecule. Depending on the locus, tens to hundreds of variable genes can be used. D regions are not present in every molecule. The joining of DNA in the lymphocyte is not perfect, leading to additional protein sequences not predicted by the germline DNA. In the antigen receptor, the variable regions of the TCR alpha and beta chains or immunoglobulin heavy and light chains combine to form a single antigen recognition unit.

out-of-frame sequences that do not produce functional proteins. Finally, the recombined variable region consisting of V, D (if present), and J segments is recombined to the appropriate constant region.

Enormous diversity is generated by this system. The number of V genes varies with the TCR or immunoglobulin chain studied, ranging from fewer than 10 to several hundred (Fig. 7–1). In general, fewer than six D or J regions are present in each genetic locus. When the number of possible V regions is combined with the number of J and D regions and with the random insertion or deletion of nucleotides, it has been estimated that over 10^{14} different TCRs or immunoglobulin molecules can be generated.[1] Thus, the chances of any two lymphocytes having identical receptors is infinitely small. The large number of potential receptors guarantees that a response to nearly any antigenic stimulus can occur. Since many of these antigen receptors recognize self-antigens, the immune system must exercise tight control to prevent autoimmunity.

RECOGNITION OF ANTIGENS

The most striking difference between immunoglobulin molecules and the TCR is in the nature of the antigen recognized by each. Antibodies bind to the antigen alone, which can be an intact protein, peptide, lipid, carbohydrate, or nucleic acid. Typically a small number (fewer than 20) of amino acid residues in a protein antigen contact a similar number of residues in the antibody molecule. The portion of the antibody that is involved in binding antigen is formed by juxtaposition of the variable portions of both the heavy and the light chains. The attraction of antigen to antibody includes hydrogen bonding, electrostatic interactions, van der Waals forces, and hydrophobic interactions. The form of the antigen can be variable. Some antibodies recognize complex epitopes

consisting of combinations of polypeptide chains or require specific secondary or tertiary peptide structure for recognition. Other antibodies recognize linear epitopes of a protein regardless of their conformation. In addition, antibodies are multivalent. IgG is the prototype of monomeric immunoglobulin and consists of two identical heavy chains and two identical light chains creating two separate antigen-binding domains. In milk and other secretions IgA is a dimer or trimer. IgM is a pentamer capable of binding as many as 10 antigenic molecules, a property that allows for an increase in the avidity of binding and for formation of cross-linked lattices of antigen-antibody complexes. Such complexes facilitate the clearance of microorganisms from the circulation and the activation of complement. Inappropriately handled immune complexes are pathogenic in autoimmune disorders, such as systemic lupus erythematosus, in which deposition of the complexes in the kidney leads to glomerulonephritis.

Unlike antibodies, TCRs do not recognize antigen alone. Instead they recognize antigen in the context of protein products of the major histocompatibility complex (MHC). The MHC is a region of tightly linked, highly polymorphic genes that were originally defined by their control of graft rejection between individuals of the same species. Genes within this region also control a variety of immune responses. In mice and guinea pigs, for example, MHC genes determine whether antibodies to certain protein antigens are made, and in humans these genes control the immune response after bone marrow transplantation (graft-versus-host disease). Finally, MHC molecules that stimulate T-cell responses to foreign antigen determine which T cells respond and shape the outcome of that response.

In the 1960s several different genetic loci were discovered within the MHC. Some loci control skin graft rejection and the immune response to viral infections. The immune responses controlled by these genes are made up largely of cytotoxic T lymphocytes, and the proteins encoded by these genes are termed class I MHC molecules. Other genes in the MHC control responses to soluble or particulate antigens that do not infect the cell. These responses are characterized by helper T cells and antibody production, and the proteins encoded by these genes are termed MHC class II molecules.

Structure of MHC Molecules

MHC class I molecules consist of a 44-kilodalton (kd) heavy chain encoded by genes in the MHC and a 12-kd light chain, termed β_2-microglobulin, that is not MHC-encoded. All the interindividual variation is found in the heavy chain. In humans, the predominant class I molecules are the products of the approximately 50 *HLA-A* alleles, 100 *HLA-B* alleles, and 50 *HLA-C* alleles.[2] Class I molecules are expressed on all nucleated cells and have certain key features. The extracellular portion of the molecule has three domains of approximately 90 amino acids each; the first two, termed $\alpha 1$ and $\alpha 2$, are most distal from the membrane and contain the polymorphic residues that define different class I alleles. The membrane proximal domain, $\alpha 3$, varies from isotype to isotype (i.e., between HLA-A and HLA-B) but is essentially constant within a given isotype. Class I molecules have transmembrane domains of approximately 25 amino acids and small intracytoplasmic tails of approximately 30 residues.

Analysis of class I molecules by x-ray crystallography revealed a novel structure for the $\alpha 1$ and $\alpha 2$ domains.[3–6] These domains interact to form a peptide-binding region consisting of a "floor" made up of eight beta strands overlaid by two alpha-helical regions that form the "walls" of the binding groove. The first crystals of these proteins contained additional electron density in this region, representing a mixture of naturally occurring bound peptides. The physical proper-

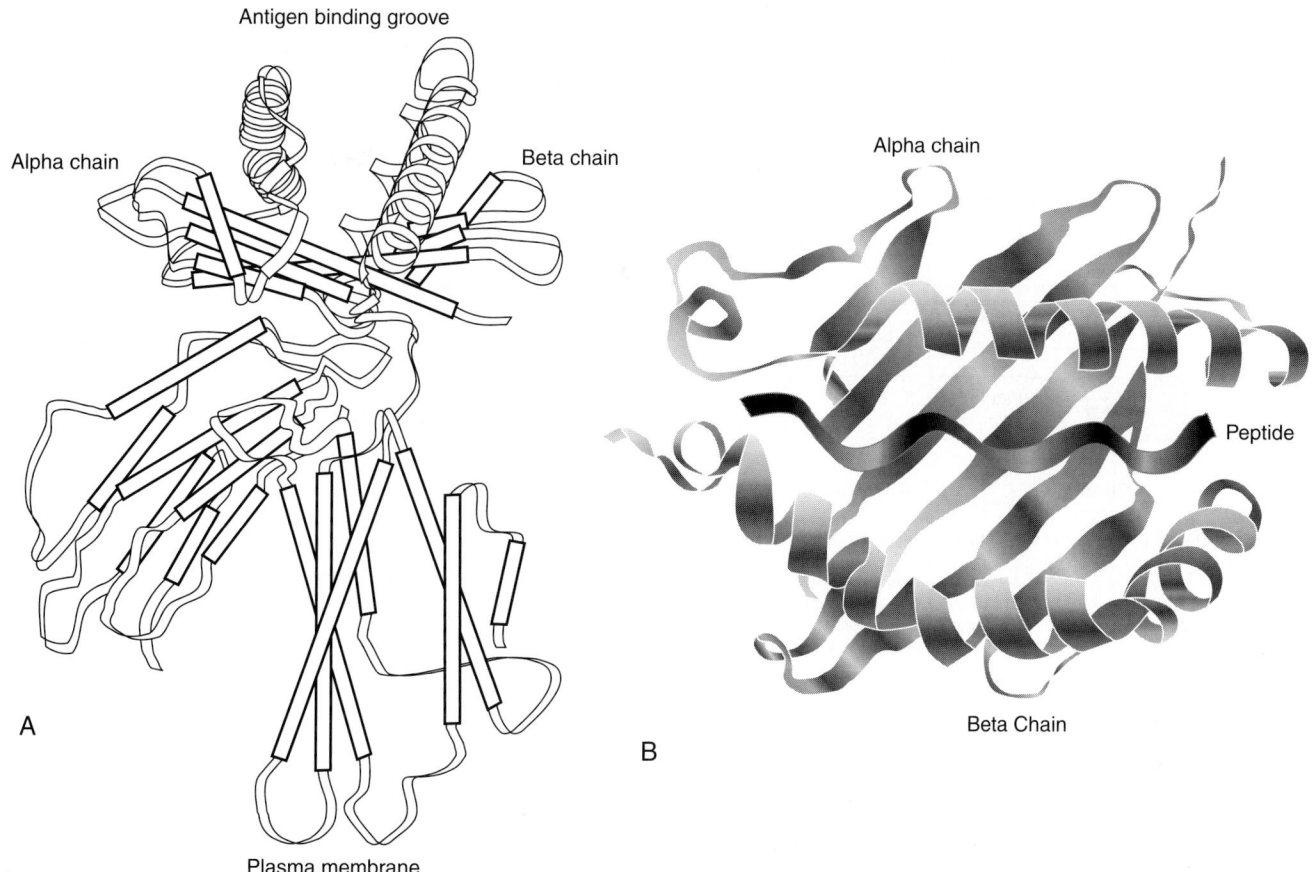

Figure 7–2. Three-dimensional structure of an MHC molecule. A representation of HLA-DR1 based on x-ray crystallographic data[9] is shown. The structure of MHC class I molecules is similar, with β_2-microglobulin replacing one of the membrane proximal domains. *A*, Side view of the HLA-DR1 molecule looking down the antigen-binding groove located in the membrane distal portion of the molecule. *B*, Top view of HLA-DR1 showing the position of an antigenic peptide bound between the helices of the alpha and beta polypeptide chains. Only the antigen-binding portion of the molecule is shown for clarity.

ties of class I molecules dictate that peptides that bind to these regions be of a certain length and chemical composition,[7, 8] with most naturally occurring class I–binding peptides being 9 to 11 amino acids in length. The binding peptides are anchored in the class I peptide groove by chemical interactions at the amino and carboxyl termini and by interactions between amino acid side chains along the length of the peptide and amino acids that form "pockets" along the floor and sides of the MHC groove. The differences among class I molecules determine the size and chemical composition of these pockets. That is, some can accommodate aromatic or aliphatic amino acids, while others prefer charged residues. Thus, class I alleles from different individuals can bind and present dissimilar sets of peptides derived from the same antigen. One possible explanation for the association of certain class I alleles with particular autoimmune disorders is that viral peptides selected and bound to class I in those individuals resemble self-antigens (see later).

Class II proteins are composed of two polypeptide subunits, each encoded by MHC genes. The alpha chain is approximately 33 kd, and the beta chain is approximately 29 kd in size. These polypeptides associate noncovalently to form a cell surface heterodimer. In humans three forms of class II molecules are expressed at the cell surface: HLA-DR, HLA-DQ, and HLA-DP. Unlike class I, class II molecules are expressed on a restricted subset of cells, primarily B lymphocytes, monocytes, macrophages, and dendritic cells. These cells are termed "professional antigen-presenting cells" owing to their expression of both class I and class II molecules.

The structure of MHC class II molecules is similar to that of class I molecules[9] (Fig. 7–2). The two membrane distal regions of the alpha and beta chains fold to form a peptide-binding groove, and the membrane proximal regions are typical immunoglobulin-like domains. Like class I molecules, class II molecules have transmembrane and small intracytoplasmic domains. The ends of the groove are open in class II, accommodating peptides that can be 10 to 30 residues long, extending over the ends of the MHC molecule. As in class I, the peptides bind in an extended conformation, but the binding pockets of class II have less stringent requirements and make many contacts with the conserved atoms of the polypeptide backbone.[10] While individual alleles of class II have different capabilities to bind certain peptides, one peptide may bind to many different class II alleles.[11]

Antigen Presentation

Different mechanisms control peptide association with class I and class II MHC molecules. The peptides presented to class I molecules are derived largely from endogenously synthesized proteins that have been degraded in the cytosol.[12] One mechanism for this degradation involves a large (approximately 650 kd) protein complex termed the proteosome, a barrel-shaped structure containing several different proteolytic enzymes (Fig. 7–3). Cytosolic proteins slated for degradation are cleaved into small peptides that are transported into the endoplasmic reticulum by a heterodimeric protein located in the endoplasmic reticulum membrane. The genes encoding the transporter proteins (TAP-1 and TAP-2, for transporter of antigenic peptides) and genes for two subunits of the proteo-

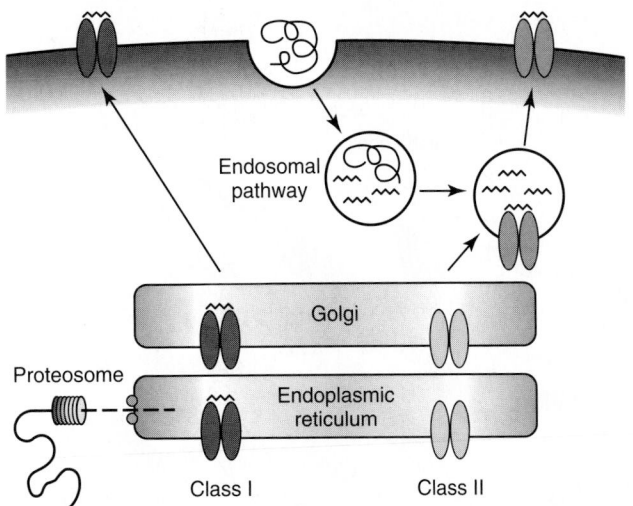

Figure 7–3. Schematic of antigen presentation. In general, cytosolic proteins are degraded by the proteosome complex and enter the endoplasmic reticulum through the TAP transporters. There the peptides bind to newly synthesized MHC class I molecules and travel to the cell surface. MHC class II molecules do not encounter antigenic peptides until they reach the endosomal pathway, where they generally bind fragments of extracellular proteins.

Endosomal pathway

Golgi

Proteosome

Endoplasmic reticulum

Class I   Class II

some reside in the MHC. These genes are polymorphic, although to a much lesser degree than the MHC class I or class II molecules. Thus, the expression of proteins required for degradation of viral proteins and for the transport and binding of antigenic peptide products is controlled by one region of the genome.

As mentioned earlier, peptides that associate with class II molecules are derived mainly from exogenous proteins that have been phagocytosed or taken up by receptor-mediated mechanisms.[13] Once inside the cell, the proteins are taken to vesicular organelles of the endosome-lysosome system, which contain proteases that degrade the proteins to small peptides. Meanwhile, newly synthesized class II molecules are also directed from the endoplasmic reticulum, through the Golgi apparatus to vesicles of the endosomal pathway. Early during biosynthesis, the alpha and beta chains of class II molecules associate with another polypeptide, the invariant chain. This nonpolymorphic transmembrane protein helps direct class II molecules to the endosomal pathway and prevents class II molecules from being loaded with self-peptides. In the endosome the invariant chain itself is degraded, and the peptides derived from antigenic proteins bind to the class II molecules. The peptide-MHC complexes then are directed to the cell surface. There are several exceptions to the paradigm that endogenous antigens are presented by class I and that exogenous antigens are presented by class II molecules. When exogenous antigens enter the cell and are released directly into the cytoplasm, they can be presented by class I. Conversely, certain viral infections can generate cytoplasmic proteins that enter the endosomal pathway and are presented by class II. In brief, redundancy in antigen presentation ensures a maximal immune response but may predispose to improper regulation and autoimmunity.

In accordance with early genetic studies, the pattern of antigen presentation determines the nature of the T-cell response. Peptides derived from exogenous antigens, primarily viral proteins in infected cells, are presented on MHC class I molecules. These peptide-MHC complexes are recognized mainly by T cells that express the CD8 co-receptor (CD8[+]) and have cytolytic activity. The interaction of polymorphic residues in the TCR with the amino acids at the peptide-MHC

surface leads to activation of cellular processes within the T cell, but the nature of the most proximal events that signal T-cell activation is not known. The activation of CD8[+] T cells leads to the elaboration of cytolytic enzymes and proteins and causes death of the infected antigen-presenting cell and elimination of the virus. When antigens are presented in the context of class II MHC molecules, they activate CD4[+] helper T cells that then synthesize and secrete low-molecular-weight proteins termed cytokines. These cytokines act locally to stimulate B cells to differentiate and secrete antibodies, and they promote phagocytosis and destruction of antigens by macrophages. In this way, the antigen stimulates an immune response to eliminate the pathogen that produced it. In other words, the response to an intracellular pathogen such as an infectious virus is the killing of the infected cells, and the response to soluble antigens such as bacteria and extracellular virus is directed toward a B-cell activation and antibody production.

TOLERANCE TO SELF-ANTIGENS

The enormous diversity in the repertoire of antibodies and TCRs ensures the availability of B and T lymphocytes that recognize self-antigens. Such self-reactive cells are either eliminated or inactivated by a process known as induction of tolerance. Loss of tolerance to self-antigens is thought to be central to the development of autoimmune diseases. Tolerance is not inherited but can develop either at an immature stage of development (in the bone marrow or thymus) or in mature peripheral lymphocytes. Immature lymphocytes must be "educated" not to respond to self-antigens, and a characteristic feature of tolerance induction is that all T or B cells go through a developmental stage when exposure to antigen results in deletion or inactivation rather than proliferation or activation. During this time, the immature cells are exposed to self-proteins or peptides, allowing only non–self-reactive cells to mature. The cells that encounter self-antigens can be removed by several means, including clonal deletion, usually by a process of cell death termed apoptosis, which involves degradation of DNA, nuclear fragmentation, and cell shrinkage. Potentially self-reactive cells can also become nonreactive (clonal anergy), particularly if they encounter antigens on nontraditional antigen-presenting cells that lack co-stimulatory molecules (see later). Some potentially self-reactive cells mature but do not proliferate or respond to self-antigens. This phenomenon, termed "clonal ignorance,"[14] is poorly understood but may be involved in autoimmunity. Ignorant cells can circulate until activated by a process other than direct contact with the antigen. Once activated, they recognize self-antigen and mount a pathologic response. Specific examples of clonal ignorance and autoimmunity are given later.

Most T lymphocytes lose their ability to react with self-antigens as they mature in the thymus (Fig. 7–4). When T-cell precursors leave the bone marrow and emigrate to the thymus, they do not express either the TCR or the two major co-receptor molecules, CD4 and CD8. CD4 and CD8 are cell surface glycoproteins associated with the TCR on mature T lymphocytes. In the periphery, T cells that express the αβ TCR also express either CD4 or CD8 but not both. These co-receptors serve two major functions in mature cells. First, they bind to nonpolymorphic regions of MHC molecules; CD8 interacts with amino acids in the α3 (membrane proximal) domain of class I molecules, and CD4 binds to residues in the β2 domain of class II molecules. This binding strengthens the interaction between the T cell and the antigen-presenting cell, increasing the likelihood that signaling via the TCR complex will occur. Second, the intracytoplasmic domains of CD4 and

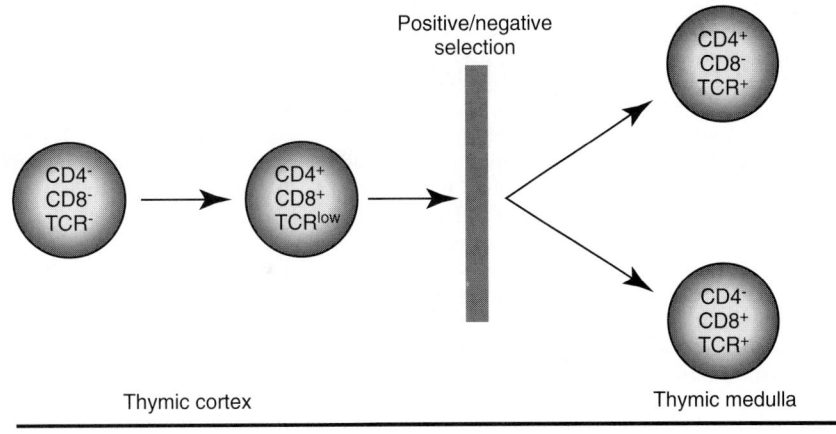

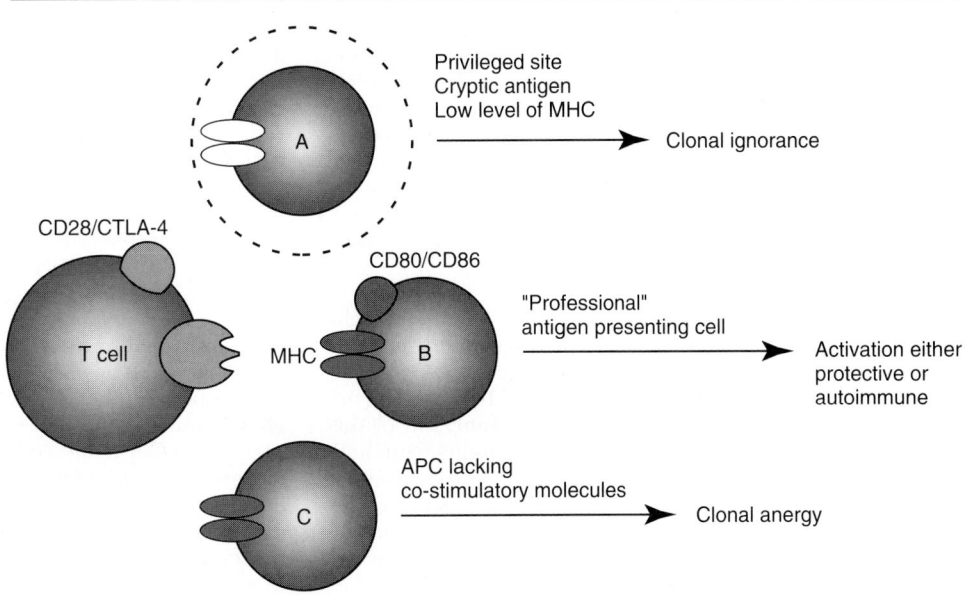

Figure 7–4. Mechanisms of T-cell tolerance. *Upper Panel,* "Central" tolerance is generated in the thymus. Bone marrow–derived precursors enter the thymic cortex, where they begin to express both CD4 and CD8 molecules as well as unique T-cell receptors. At a critical stage, thymocytes that can recognize self-MHC molecules are expanded (positive selection). Those that recognize self-MHC and self-peptides too strongly die by apoptosis (negative selection). At this stage expression of either CD4 or CD8 is lost. *Lower Panel,* "Peripheral" tolerance can be due to unavailability of the relevant antigen-presenting cell (A) or to expression of MHC and peptide on nonprofessional antigen-presenting cells (C). When cells express MHC molecules and co-stimulatory molecules, as well as sufficient amounts of antigenic peptide, T-cell activation occurs (B).

CD8 are associated with the lymphocyte-specific protein tyrosine kinase, lck. On interaction of the CD4 or CD8 molecule with class II or class I molecules, respectively, the lck molecule is activated and phosphorylates other proteins associated with the TCR, beginning the chain of events associated with T-cell activation. During T-cell development in the thymic cortex, immature thymocytes express both CD4 and CD8 simultaneously, and TCR surface expression begins at a low level. In a process known as positive selection, cells that express TCRs that recognize self-MHC expressed on thymic epithelium continue to mature. Cells that cannot recognize self-MHC are not stimulated and die, whereas cells that express a TCR that recognizes class I MHC lose CD4 expression and express CD8 only and cells with TCRs that recognize class II lose expression of CD8. The interaction with self-MHC is absolutely crucial for positive selection to occur. In mice genetically engineered to lack expression of either class I or class II molecules, the numbers of mature CD8 or CD4 single-positive T cells in the periphery are nearly zero. In normal animals thymocytes positive either for CD8 or CD4 migrate to the thymic medulla, where they encounter bone marrow–derived antigen-presenting cells that express self-peptides. Those immature thymocytes with TCRs that recognize self-peptides with sufficiently high affinity are activated to undergo apoptosis and die. Thus, the generation of the full repertoire of mature cells involves selection of cells capable of recognizing peptides in the context of self-MHC and elimination of those with a high probability of self-reactivity.

Self-reactive T cells are also regulated outside the thymus. T cells require at least two signals for activation. The first is recognition by the TCR of the peptide-MHC complex, which provides the T cell with its specificity. The second signal is provided by the interaction of T-cell proteins with "co-stimulatory" molecules on the antigen-presenting cell. A pair of related molecules, CD28 and CTLA-4, interact with the proteins B7-1 and B7-2 on the surface of antigen-presenting cells such as monocytes, dendritic cells, and B cells. When both signals are delivered to the T cell through the TCR and CD28, full activation occurs, as indicated by the expression of the interleukin-2 gene or by cell proliferation. Without the second (CD28) signal, TCR stimulation causes anergy, as when peptides are presented by cells that express class II molecules (but not protein B7-1 or B7-2) as a result of exposure to inflammatory cytokines. In vitro, anergic T cells are incapable of responding to peptide presented by fully competent antigen-presenting cells. As a consequence, continuous exposure of peripheral T cells to self-peptides presented on cells lacking co-stimulatory molecules effectively eliminates them from the repertoire. However, alterations in the expression of co-stimulatory molecules and activation of tolerant T-cell clones can occur during protective immune responses. In the response to an infection, cytokines such as IL-2, IL-4, and interferon γ are produced locally. If the activated T cells then encounter competent antigen-presenting cells that express cognate self-antigen, further T-cell activation can occur with potentially pathogenic consequences.

B-cell tolerance to self-antigens has been studied in transgenic animals.[15] In mice that express a transgenic immunoglobulin heavy and light chain that recognizes hen egg lysozyme (HEL), nearly all B cells express the anti-HEL antibody on their surface, and high titers of anti-HEL are present in the serum. These mice were mated with mice that express a transgene for the HEL protein and that have B cells that express a normal repertoire of antibodies; the offspring have normal numbers of B cells, but the B cells have reduced levels of IgM anti-HEL on their surfaces. There is no anti-HEL antibody in the serum, nor could it be induced by HEL immunization. However, if the B cells are transferred to normal (nontransgenic) mice, they gradually regain the ability to respond to HEL as a foreign protein. In this model, tolerance is caused by clonal anergy. By varying the form of the transgenic HEL protein, different degrees of anergy could be induced. High-level expression of a membrane-bound form of HEL resulted in deletion of HEL-reactive B cells. In the normal state B-cell tolerance is mainly a function of T-cell tolerance and the lack of T-cell help for self-antigens. Clonal anergy or deletion of B cells is most important for tolerance to T-independent antigens such as blood group glycoproteins.

MECHANISMS OF AUTOIMMUNITY

By definition, autoimmunity is due to the failure of mechanisms that control recognition of and reactivity to self-antigens. Autoimmunity can result from the failure of T-cell tolerance, the failure of B-cell tolerance, or a dysregulation of natural immunity. Most of the steps in the regulation of the immune system have been examined in both spontaneous and induced models of autoimmunity, but there is no instance where all the cellular or molecular events leading up to the autoimmune state are known. The postulated mechanisms of autoimmunity are extrapolated from knowledge of the means by which diversity, self-recognition, and tolerance occur in the immune system.

Molecular Mimicry

One hypothesis regarding the cause of autoimmunity is molecular mimicry; namely, the mounting of a protective immune response to a microbial pathogen that contains antigens similar to host antigens. Such antigens can be proteins, carbohydrates, or lipids. B cells that respond to these antigens can make antibodies that bind to host tissues. This type of molecular mimicry can be thought of as cross-reactivity at the level of antibody-antigen interactions, rather than as failure of lymphocyte tolerance. This antibody response is fostered if there is also a T-cell response to a cross-reactive epitope. In this case, T-cell reactivity would have to overcome tolerance to the self-protein, if it existed. Most cross-reactive antigen receptors are of low avidity and are functionally unimportant, but in the course of infections, higher avidity receptors may emerge, with the potential for tissue damage. The control of such pathologic T- and B-cell clones is a critical feature in the development of autoimmunity.

Cross-reactivity between microbial and self-structures is well documented. Perhaps the best studied is the relationship between antistreptococcal antibodies and the nonsuppurative consequences of rheumatic fever. Antibodies to several streptococcal polysaccharides and glycoproteins have been shown to bind to human cardiac, vascular, articular, and neuronal tissues.[16, 17] Immunoglobulin specific for the type-specific M protein cross-reacts with cardiac actin and myosin, chondrocytes, cartilage, and synovium.[18] Myocarditis is another cardiac disorder of molecular mimicry; infection with coxsackievirus B

predisposes to chronic myocarditis, when high titers of antiviral antibodies bind to myocyte antigens and elicit pathologic effects. In a mouse model for myocarditis, antibodies to viral capsid proteins exhibit cardiac pathogenicity.[19] The antiviral antibodies bound to both human and mouse cardiac myosin and caused an inflammatory reaction. These antibodies probably arose from B cells that originally secreted low-affinity IgM that cross-reacts with both viral and cardiac proteins. When the titer and affinity of these antibodies are low, the individual is tolerant to their effects, but with infection the titers and affinity of these antibodies increase. Depending on the pathogen, a single infection may produce pathogenic antibodies, while for others repeated infection is necessary. Tissue damage resulting from the protective immune response releases these antigens to stimulate the cross-reactive B cells and enhance the affinity and titer of the cross-reactive antibodies.

The self-peptides that bind to various MHC molecules and have the potential of stimulating T cells have been identified by eluting and sequencing the peptides from purified MHC proteins.[20] Comparison of these sequences with large protein databases has demonstrated that many proteins are potentially cross-reactive with microbial proteins.[21] In some cases, synthetic peptides corresponding to the microbial epitopes can activate T cells specific for both the microbial proteins and the self-antigens. One group of microbial proteins associated with cellular autoimmunity are the heat shock proteins (hsps), which are highly conserved throughout evolution. By their ubiquitous nature peptides derived from hsps frequently bind to MHC molecules that can be the targets of T cells activated by microbial hsp. For example, T cells reactive to mycobacterial hsp65 are demonstrable in nonobese diabetic (NOD) mice at the onset of inflammation of the pancreatic islets.[22–24] T-cell clones isolated from such mice can transfer diabetes, even to mice not prone to the disorder, indicating that this response is not causal and not just the passive consequence of autoimmunity. However, immunity to some hsps can be protective and can play a major role in the response to a variety of pathogens.[25] Such immune responses become pathogenic for uncertain reasons, possibly because of disturbance of the balance between cytokine effects and the type of T-cell response at the site of inflammation.[26]

A somewhat different form of molecular mimicry has been utilized in the development of experimental models of autoimmunity. For example, in experimental autoimmune encephalomyelitis (EAE), a rodent model for multiple sclerosis (MS), mice or rats are immunized with bovine myelin basic protein (MBP), a candidate autoantigen in MS, and an adjuvant (to hyperstimulate the immune system). Under these conditions, humoral and cellular responses to bovine MBP cause cross-reactive immune responses that target self-MBP and other neuronal antigens. The resulting neurologic disease can resemble MS in many ways, including demyelination and a relapsing-remitting course. Again, T-cell clones have been isolated that are specific for several particular peptide epitopes and can transfer disease. These encephalitogenic clones have some features in common, particularly usage of the same TCR αβ family. Other model systems based on the immunization of animals with foreign protein and adjuvant include immunization with acetylcholine receptor to cause myasthenia gravis and immunization with collagen to cause a chronic synovitis resembling rheumatoid arthritis (RA). While these models do not tell us how idiopathic autoimmunity occurs, they demonstrate that the mature T-cell repertoire can contain cells with pathologic self-reactivities. The antigens that correspond to these T cells are not encountered normally, either because they exist in "immunologically privileged sites" such as the cornea and the central nervous system or because they are not processed by antigen-presenting cells under normal circumstances. During acute inflammation from whatever cause, these barriers between lymphocytes and their targets are broken, causing pathologic immune responses that can include more inflammation and chronic autoimmune states. These models make it possible to examine the potential roles of such factors as TCRs, self-antigens, MHC molecules, and cytokines under controlled circumstances and have led to the development of therapeutic strategies directed at blocking one or more components of the autoimmune response.

Molecular mimicry is probably not rare. Even though B and T cells that are highly reactive for self-antigens are normally down-regulated, significant numbers of receptors are likely to be present for almost all microbial antigens that are cross-reactive with some host structure. Depending on the tissue, a significant immune response to self may be tolerated. For example, myocarditis resulting from streptococcal infection can be transient and of little functional significance, but damage to heart valves can cause permanent scarring and clinical morbidity. Thus, molecular mimicry may be necessary but not necessarily sufficient for development of autoimmune disease. It is the control and effect of the antiself response that is important.

Enhanced Antigenicity of Self-Proteins

Several features of the tolerance to self-antigens are important for molecular mimicry. First, T-cell deletion or tolerance is not 100% effective, as indicated by the fact that some circulating T cells are capable of responding to many self-antigens when assayed in vitro. These T cells are "ignorant" of their cognate self-antigens because they are not effective, either because the antigens are located in an anatomically sequestered site (the cornea or the central nervous system) or because the antigenic epitopes of self-antigens are hidden within proteins and are not normally degraded or processed to the active form. Until some event exposes these antigens to the autoreactive T cells, the autoimmune potential is masked. The event that exposes these autoantigens to the immune system includes inflammation in which vascular permeability is increased, there is an influx of cells capable of antigen presentation, and tissue destruction exposes proteins, nucleic acids, and carbohydrates that interact with B cells or are processed and presented to T cells. Cytokines released in the initial immune response cause up-regulation of MHC molecules and augmentation of antigen processing. This mechanism would explain the responses to intracellular antigens such as double-stranded DNA and ribonucleoprotein in systemic lupus erythematosus.

Alternatively, B cells that respond to an infectious agent can produce antigen receptors (IgM) that cross-react with intact self-protein. The self-protein is internalized and degraded, and the peptide fragments are presented by the B cell. Some of these peptides stimulate autoreactive T cells and promote a vigorous antiself response. This concept of the "cryptic self" has been documented in experimental systems. For example, mice immunized with a combination of human and mouse cytochrome c develop autoreactive T cells specific for the mouse protein. This reactivity is the result of B cells that cross-react with both types of cytochrome and present mouse cytochrome peptides to naive T cells.

Furthermore, the protein epitopes that initiate an autoimmune response may not be the same as those that perpetuate it. In the autoimmune encephalomyelitis model, mice that are immunized to one peptide derived from MBP eventually develop T-cell responses to additional parts of the same molecule and to other proteins in the central nervous system.[27] This process, known as "epitope spreading," is presumed to result from inflammation, enhanced antigen processing, and B-cell activation, as described earlier. A similar series of events occurs in the NOD mouse in which T cells become autoreactive to a series of self-proteins in a defined sequence prior to the onset of diabetes. The first such autoreactive T cells recognize a specific region of the protein glutamic acid decarboxylase (GAD65), but with time T cells recognize additional regions of GAD65 and eventually recognize antigens such as hsps, carboxypeptidase H, and insulin.[28, 29] This phenomenon probably occurs in human autoimmune diseases and will complicate the design of specific therapies. Furthermore, if in a disease such as RA symptoms do not occur until a polyclonal response has developed, it will be difficult to determine which self-antigen started the autoimmune response.

Errors in the Maintenance of Tolerance

The generation and maintenance of self-tolerance requires the recognition of self-antigens by developing T and B lymphocytes and the elimination of such lymphocytes. At several stages of the lymphocyte life span, cell death is necessary for controlling the immune response: when self-antigens are recognized in the thymus, when antigens are recognized in the absence of appropriate co-stimulatory molecules, and when signals are delivered through molecules other than the antigen receptors. In these instances, the cells undergo "programmed cell death," termed apoptosis. In contrast to cell necrosis caused by thermal or chemical injury, apoptosis requires active participation by the dying cell. Cells undergoing apoptosis shrink, and DNA is cleaved by endonucleases. Failure of cells to undergo apoptosis leads to polyclonal lymphocyte activation and generation of autoreactive cells, as has been demonstrated in mouse models of autoimmune disease. The primary signal for a cell to undergo apoptosis is ligation of the cell surface molecule, Fas. Fas is a member of the tumor necrosis factor (TNF) receptor family, and the Fas ligand (FasL) resembles the TNF molecule. Binding of Fas to antibody or FasL induces cell death in lymphocytes and other cells. Mice carrying mutations that impair Fas or FasL develop lymphadenopathy and splenomegaly and develop high titers of IgM and IgG antibodies, including autoantibodies such as anti-DNA and rheumatoid factor.[30] Under certain circumstances, these mutations lead to a lupus-like illness characterized by fatal nephritis and inflammatory arthritis in which the control of activated lymphocytes in the periphery is severely impaired. Since Fas and FasL are normally up-regulated by cell activation, it is possible that in normal mice T cells activated by self-antigens are in close proximity, signal each other through Fas, and induce mutual apoptosis; this mechanism would be lacking in mice with mutations of Fas or FasL, leading to uncontrolled lymphocyte proliferation.[31, 32] Patients with defective expression of Fas have a syndrome that resembles the mouse disorder, namely a lymphoproliferative disorder with or without autoimmune pancytopenia.[33] Interestingly, these patients have an increased percentage of CD4$^-$/CD8$^-$ T cells in peripheral blood, suggesting that Fas does not play a major in negative selection but instead controls peripheral responses. Finally, there has been one report of patients with systemic lupus erythematosus with increased levels of a soluble form of Fas that was able to block apoptosis and produce features of autoimmunity when injected into mice.[34] It is attractive to hypothesize that patients with systemic lupus erythematosus or other systemic autoimmune diseases have genetic or acquired defects in Fas-mediated apoptosis and are therefore unable to regulate activation of self-reactive lymphocytes completely. A better understanding of the regulation and action of Fas and FasL may provide important information about the pathogenesis of autoimmunity.

Immunoregulatory Disturbances

The type of protective immune response is not simply a question of whether cytotoxic or helper T cells respond to antigen presented in the context of self-MHC but is also influenced by the fact that there are different types of helper T cells. T helper 1 (T_H1) cells and T helper 2 (T_H2) cells may respond to the same antigen but have different functional phenotypes and different effects.[35] T_H1 and T_H2 cell phenotypes have been best characterized in the mouse and are defined by the pattern of cytokines secreted on activation.[35] T_H1 cells secrete IL-2, interferon γ, and TNF to cause a delayed-type hypersensitivity response with macrophage activation and to stimulate the production of a subset of IgG antibodies. T_H2 cells secrete IL-4, IL-5, IL-6, IL-10, and IL-13, cytokines that promote B cell responses such as the switching of immunoglobulin production to other IgG subtypes and to IgE. A third class of cells, T_H0, secretes both types of cytokines and is thought to be the precursor of the other two T_H types. The generalization is that T_H1 cells regulate cell-mediated immunity and that T_H2 cells modulate humoral immunity. Although most information about T_H1 and T_H2 cells comes from animal studies, such helper T-cell subsets almost certainly exist in humans and may influence the outcome of an immune response.

T_H1 and T_H2 cells also regulate each other. The cytokine IL-12 is produced by antigen-presenting cells and induces the differentiation of naive T cells into T_H1 cells. The interferon γ produced by T_H1 cells prevents the development of T_H2 cells.[36] Likewise, the production by T_H2 cells of IL-4, IL-10, and IL-13 inhibits T_H1 proliferation and induces additional T_H2 response. The T-cell response in mice can be driven along T_H1 or T_H2 lines by the administration of cytokines or anticytokine antibodies or by disruption of cytokine genes. Alteration of the balance between T_H1 and T_H2 cells can affect the outcome of infections that require one type of response or the other.[37, 38]

The type of T helper response that occurs to self-antigens may also be important for the development of autoimmunity. For example, in experimental autoimmune encephalomyelitis, the central nervous system lesions resemble delayed-type hypersensitivity reactions characteristic of T_H1 cells; namely, the lesions stain for T_H1–type cytokines but not for T_H2–type cytokines.[39, 40] Transfer of T_H1 cells specific for MBP-derived peptides can induce the disease, whereas transfer of T_H2 cells with the same specificity does not. Furthermore, a switch to a T_H2 type of response may occur as the animals spontaneously recover, suggesting that the sequence of T-cell activation in an immune response controls potential autoreactive T cells.

T_H1 cells also appear to play the predominant pathogenic role in insulin-dependent diabetes mellitus (IDDM) and autoimmune arthritis in mice. Female, NOD mice spontaneously develop diabetes during the first 6 months of life. T cells, particularly T_H1 cells, are the first cells that infiltrate the islets of Langerhans in these animals,[41] and antibodies to interferon γ, a T_H1 cytokine, can prevent the onset of diabetes.[42, 43] Similarly, administration of IL-4, a T_H2 cytokine that blocks T_H1 development, prevents diabetes in these animals.[44] Local effects, including production of nitric oxide in response to infection, and genetic parameters can influence the relative levels of T_H1 and T_H2 cells. In mice, autoimmune arthritis can be induced by immunization with type II collagen and a suitable adjuvant. When adjuvant is replaced by the administration of IL-12 for 5 days prior to collagen injection, the mice develop an erosive polyarthritis and secrete high levels of interferon γ and IgG.[45] Taken together, these data suggest that T_H1 responses may be necessary for protective immunity, particularly against intracellular organisms, but that persistence of such a response may be detrimental to the host. The development of a T_H2 response to the same antigen can control the immune response and lead to lifelong immunity. Protocols designed to enhance the T_H2 response are being evaluated in patients with autoimmune diseases, including

immunization with high doses of antigen, immunization with mutant antigenic peptides, and oral administration of antigen.

GENETICS OF AUTOIMMUNITY AND THE ROLE OF THE MHC

Hereditary factors play an important role in autoimmune disease, as indicated by the fact that the concordance rate is 30 to 50% for identical twins developing autoimmune syndromes. Some of the genes most strongly associated with autoimmunity have been identified, but there is no known determinant that can predict with certainty the onset or severity of disease. The pathogenesis of these disorders almost certainly involves heredity, environmental factors, and the nature of the immune response.

The MHC plays a central role in the genetics of autoimmunity. This is due in part to the relative ease with which these polymorphic loci can be analyzed and in part to the role that MHC gene products play in the generation of the mature T-cell repertoire and in antigen presentation. Other genetic loci are implicated in autoimmunity as well. For example, polymorphisms in specific genes can be detected as the result of the analysis of families with multiple affected individuals in more than one generation utilizing the restriction fragment length polymorphism (RFLP) techniques. Total genomic DNA is digested with various restriction endonucleases to produce fragments of discrete size that can be separated by electrophoresis and transferred to a two-dimensional membrane. The presence of fragments corresponding to specific genes is determined by Southern hybridization. In this technique, a short piece of cloned DNA that contains a sequence specific for the gene in question is labeled with a radionuclide or other tracer and allowed to anneal or hybridize to the membrane under carefully controlled conditions in which the probe will bind tightly only to those DNA fragments containing the gene in question. Their position can be recorded on x-ray film or by other means, and different alleles of each locus can be assigned on the basis of fragment size and correlated with the presence or absence of disease in individual family members. With the use of this technique, many genes have been linked to autoimmune syndromes. In RA, for example, restriction fragment analysis identified an association with the MHC and with genes that encode the TCR and immunoglobulin heavy chain.

More sophisticated genetic analyses are now being employed to locate genes involved in autoimmune conditions such as RA and systemic lupus erythematosus. In this way it is hoped that self-antigens that either shape the T-cell repertoire or act as targets of autoimmune T cells can be identified.

Many autoimmune disorders are linked to certain MHC haplotypes. In most cases, the linkage is strongest for specific alleles of one MHC protein (Table 7–1). The association of a particular HLA molecule with an autoimmune disease is usually expressed as the relative risk; i.e., the ratio of the prevalence of the disease in persons with the HLA allele in question to the prevalence in those without that HLA type. A relative risk greater than 1.0 implies a positive association between HLA and the disease; a risk less than 1.0 implies a negative or protective effect. The absolute value of the relative risk varies widely, underscoring the fact that additional genes and environmental influences contribute to the development of disease. However, a very high relative risk may imply a direct role for the HLA molecule in the development of autoimmunity, as illustrated by ankylosing spondylitis (AS), an inflammatory arthritis of the axial skeleton. The *HLA-B27* allele is present in 95% of whites with AS in the United States, whereas its prevalence in the general white population is only 8%. In

TABLE 7–1. Linkage of Human Leukocyte Antigens to Immunologic Diseases

Disease	HLA Allele	Relative Risk*
Rheumatoid arthritis	DR4 (certain sub-types)	6
Insulin-dependent diabetes mellitus	DR3	5
	DR4	6–7
	DR3/DR4	20
	DR3, DQw8/DQw2	30
	DR2	0.25
Pemphigus vulgaris	DR4	24
Chronic active hepatitis	DR3	14
Sjögren's syndrome	DR3	10
Celiac disease	DR3	12
Ankylosing spondylitis	B27	90

*Relative risk is the incidence of the disease or condition in persons carrying a particular HLA allele compared to the incidence in those not carrying that allele.

Adapted from Abbas AK, Lichtman AH, Pober JS. Cellular and Molecular Immunology. 2nd ed. Philadelphia: WB Saunders, 1994: 388, with permission.

blacks in the United States, the *HLA-B27* allele is present in 2% of the general population but is found in 50% of patients with AS. These findings impart a relative risk of developing this disorder of 25 to 90 for persons carrying the *HLA-B27* allele. HLA-B27 also occurs more frequently in some related conditions, such as psoriatic arthritis and the arthritis that occurs after enteric or genitourinary infections. However, fewer than 20% of persons who carry the *HLA-B27* allele ever develop any of these disorders, implicating non-HLA genes and environmental factors in the pathogenesis. Evidence for a direct role of HLA-B27 in the development of AS and related autoimmune disorders comes from the study of a rat that carried genes encoding the human HLA-B27 heavy chain and human β_2-microglobulin as transgenes.[46] Offspring that express high levels of HLA-B27 molecules develop an autoimmune disorder with features similar to AS and psoriatic arthritis, including, in addition to arthritis, inflammatory lesions of the skin and toenails, synovitis of the axial skeleton, and inflammatory lesions of the gut and genitourinary tract. These latter findings may point to an immune reaction against an enteric pathogen that triggers autoreactive lymphocytes or that is the harbinger of a response to a microbial antigen that spreads to the joints and other connective tissues. Many questions still need to be answered about the HLA-B27 transgenic rat model for AS.

Many early associations of autoimmune diseases with MHC haplotypes focused on *HLA-DR* alleles because these haplotypes were the easiest to determine. More detailed molecular typing of families with autoimmune diseases has shown that some strong associations are with alleles that are in dysequilibrium with *HLA-DR*. One example is IDDM, discussed later. In other diseases, the ability to determine the actual DNA sequence of particular *HLA-DR* alleles has refined the association between HLA and autoimmunity. In RA, the prevalence of the *HLA-DR4* allele was determined serologically, particularly in whites,[47] whereas it is now apparent with molecular techniques that these HLA-DR4 molecules are in fact heterogeneous. Although the DR alpha chain is nonpolymorphic, different DR4 beta chains define DR4 subtypes, only some of which are associated with RA.[48, 49] Comparison of their sequences reveals a common motif in the alpha-helical portion of the HLA-DR beta chain, a region that contains residues important for the binding of antigenic peptides. The HLA-DR beta sequences associated with RA may more efficiently bind and present a microbial peptide that cross-reacts with self-antigens. Alternatively, this sequence motif may affect the negative selection of potentially autoreactive T-cell clones in the thymus, in which case HLA-DR molecules that lack the RA sequence would present particular self-peptides that delete the

autoreactive T cells. These T cells would be less effectively eliminated by interaction with cells bearing the RA sequence. Another possibility is that these putative self-peptides presented by RA-associated HLA-DR4 molecules could activate regulatory T cells in the periphery. Individuals who lack the RA-associated HLA-DR molecules would be able to present certain self-antigens or microbial antigens to activate T cells whose effect is to down-modulate an autoimmune response. The RA-associated HLA-DR molecules would be less able to activate these "suppressor" T cells and allow pathogenic T-cell responses to proceed.

By serologic techniques, a strong association has been found between HLA-DR3 and/or HLA-DR4 and development of IDDM.[48] The strongest association is with certain HLA-DQ beta chains. Specifically, patients with IDDM more commonly have the neutral amino acids alanine, valine, or serine at position 57 at the end of the peptide-binding cleft. The acidic residue, aspartic acid, occurs more often in control subjects and less commonly in IDDM patients. The NOD mouse, which spontaneously develops diabetes mellitus, has a serine at position 57 of the IA beta chain, which is homologous to HLA-DQ. Strains of mice that do not develop diabetes usually have aspartate at this position. When an IA beta transgene that codes for a protein with aspartic acid at position 57 is introduced into NOD mice, the incidence of spontaneous diabetes is reduced. As in RA, the binding of certain peptides by these HLA-DQ or IA molecules probably influences the expression of an autoimmune T-cell repertoire. HLA-DQ molecules that have aspartate at position 57 either delete autoreactive T cells more effectively in the thymus or activate protective T cells more efficiently in the periphery.

While these associations between RA and diabetes mellitus and particular HLA-DR or HLA-DQ protein sequences provide strong evidence for a direct role in disease causation, they do not explain the entire association between the MHC and autoimmunity. First, the prevalence of different HLA alleles differs among ethnic groups, and the risk factors do not always correlate in different populations. Although the HLA-DR4 sequence is more prevalent in whites with RA, it is not overexpressed in blacks in the United States, whereas the disease appears clinically to be the same in both ethnic groups. No association between a particular HLA-DR sequence and RA has been found in blacks. Likewise, in Japan, patients with IDDM frequently have an HLA-DQ molecule with aspartate at residue 57 of the beta chain. If the role of MHC in the etiology of autoimmunity is to present peptides to either pathogenic or protective T cells, then different HLA alleles must perform this function in different populations. Whether these different HLA molecules all present the same disease-associated peptide or whether many different peptides are presented by each allele to produce the same disease is not known. Finally, different MHC molecules may cooperate to make an individual resistant or susceptible to autoimmune disease. Half of the patients with IDDM are heterozygous for *HLA-DR3* and *HLA-DR4*, while only *HLA-DR4* is linked to the disease-associated DQ molecule. Therefore, other peptides must be presented by DR3 or a molecule linked to DR3 in combination with DQ for disease to occur. In mice susceptible to autoimmune arthritis induced by immunization with type II collagen, certain IA alleles actually bind a peptide derived from collagen. This peptide is presumed to play a role in the pathogenesis of this disease, because the injection of this antigen into neonatal mice renders them resistant to experimental arthritis induced by whole collagen immunizations as adults. Mice from this arthritis-prone strain that carry a transgene that expresses an IE molecule (equivalent to the human HLA-DR) from an arthritis-resistant strain have a lower incidence and severity of arthritis caused by collagen immunization. This suggests that the IE (DR) molecule may be responsible for either deletion of arthritogenic T-cell clones or activation of protective T cells. Only when one disease-promoting MHC molecule is present and another disease-protecting molecule is absent is there a high likelihood of autoimmunity. This would explain why only a fraction of the population expressing one particular HLA allele get a particular disease.

Another potential role for the MHC in the development of autoimmunity is through other genes within or linked to the MHC. Within the MHC are many other genes, including genes for lymphotoxin, TNF α, components of the proteosome, peptide transporters, the steroid 21-hydroxylase (CYP21) for glucocorticoid synthesis, and several complement proteins. Although each of these is a candidate susceptibility gene for autoimmunity, their role has been difficult to study, owing in large part to the infrequency of polymorphisms in these genes compared to the class I and class II genes. For example, there are several alleles of the genes coding for the peptide transporters (TAP genes) necessary for class I–restricted antigen presentation, some of which transport different peptides. If certain of these TAP transporters allow pathogenic peptides to enter the endoplasmic reticulum with greater efficiency than others, it could predispose to disease by any of the mechanisms discussed earlier in the setting of the correct *HLA-A* or *HLA-B* alleles. This concept has been difficult to test experimentally. Also, the small number of recombination events between the TAP genes and the *HLA-A, HLA-B,* and *HLA-C* genes makes it difficult to distinguish between true association and linkage dysequilibrium.

Genes for proteins in the classic and alternative pathways of complement activation found in the MHC include genes for the homologous proteins, C2 and factor B, and the duplicated genes for C4 (*C4A* and *C4B*). Homozygous deletion of both the *C2* genes or of one or both *C4* genes is commonly associated with the development of systemic lupus erythematosus or a lupus-like syndrome. Even a partial deficiency of C2 or C4 may lower the effectiveness of elimination of viral or bacterial antigens,[50] and with inefficient complement activation microbial products could be inefficiently presented, presented in an atypical location, or allowed to persist indefinitely. This may allow the exposure of tolerant T cells to potentially cross-reactive proteins for a critical period of time. After this exposure, tolerance would be broken, and the pathogenic T-cell clones would expand and react with host antigens. Since many complement deficiencies are genetically linked to one or another class I or class II allele, this may explain some of the HLA associations seen. For example, the predilection of individuals who are heterozygous for DR3 and DR4 to develop IDDM may reflect an interaction between the complement system and class II proteins. HLA-DR3 is in linkage dysequilibrium with genetic absence of one of the *C4* genes. HLA-DR4 is linked to the IDDM-prone DQ molecule. With a relatively inefficient complement system, viral or bacterial antigens are not cleared appropriately and might be presented in high enough concentration by HLA-DQ to stimulate autoreactive T cells. While such a scheme remains to be proved, it illustrates the fact that the pathogenesis of autoimmune diseases involves multiple interacting gene products, even though all of them may be linked to one region of the MHC. Finally, deficiency of complement proteins may be part of the pathogenesis of autoimmunity regardless of MHC association. Deficiency of proteins such as C4, which is encoded within the MHC, and C1, which is not, both are associated with lupus, and linkage analysis of C4-deficient patients indicates that the association is strongest with the complement proteins, not MHC class I or class II molecules.[51] The meaning of this linkage is unknown, but it implies that the opsonization, clearance, and appropriate presentation of environmental and infectious antigens is essential if untoward immune responses are to be avoided.

CONCLUSION

It is clear that autoimmunity does not involve a single disease mechanism. Tolerance to self-antigens is dependent on genetics of the TCR loci, the polymorphic proteins encoded by the MHC, and anatomic and functional sequestration of self-antigens. Development of autoimmunity is the result of the interaction of many gene products, only some of which are understood, with environmental factors, presumably infectious agents. The multifactorial nature of the disorders commonly regarded as "autoimmune" lends a certain imprecision to their study. For example, nearly half of the juvenile RA cases in certain geographic areas are due to a response to spirochetal antigens in the synovium, i.e., Lyme disease. This raises the possibility that other disorders considered to be autoimmune, such as RA, inflammatory bowel disease, interstitial lung disease, and IDDM, will turn out to be infectious in origin. These may be chronic infections such as hepatitis B and C, or transient infections in which organ-specific inflammation occurs long after the infection has been eliminated. In some cases, adaptive immunity, i.e., the response of mature T and B cells, will be at fault. In others, a breakdown of "innate" immunity, such as the complement system, natural killer cells, macrophage or granulocyte activity, and the function of the epithelium, could be crucial in determining whether an immune response is perpetuated as autoimmunity.

The relationship of gender to autoimmunity has not been dealt with here. There is no theory of autoimmunity that adequately accounts for the marked sex differences among the presumed autoimmune syndromes. In systemic lupus erythematosus, the male-to-female ratio in patients is 1 to 10, whereas Reiter's syndrome and AS occur predominantly in men. Other disorders such as Graves' disease also display strong sex differences. Although different effects of androgens and estrogens can be demonstrated on cells of the immune system in the laboratory, it has not been demonstrated how this relates to observed gender biases.

A more precise understanding of the pathogenesis of autoimmunity will derive from several areas. First, there must be increased insight into how the immune system responds to microbial antigens, both nonpathogenic organisms encountered on a day-to-day basis and those bacterial and viral infections that may challenge the balance of self-tolerance versus recognition of nonself. Second, the immune response is under precise control. Experimental models will provide data on the nature of the interaction between different T-cell subsets, B cells, and antigen-presenting cells. Third, molecular genetic studies, including the Human Genome Project, will make it possible to map the numerous genes responsible for autoimmune reactions. Together, these approaches will provide insight into the etiology, progression, and control of these disorders.

REFERENCES

1. Davis MM, Bjorkman PJ. T-cell antigen receptor genes and T-cell recognition. Nature 1988; 334:395–402.
2. Bodmer JG, Marsh SGE, Albert ED, et al. Nomenclature for factors of the HLA system, 1994. Tissue Antigens 1994; 44:1–18.
3. Bjorkman PJ, Saper MA, Samraoui B, et al. Structure of the human class I histocompatibility antigen, HLA-A2. Nature 1987; 329:506–512.
4. Madden DR, Gorga JC, Strominger JL, et al. The structure of HLA-B27 reveals nonamer self-peptides bound in an extended conformation. Nature 1991; 353:321–325.
5. Madden DR, Gorga JC, Strominger JL, et al. The three-dimensional structure of HLA-B27 at 2.1 Å resolution suggests a general mechanism for tight peptide binding to MHC. Cell 1992; 70:1035–1048.
6. Guo HC, Jardetzky TS, Garrett TP, et al. Different length peptides bind to HLA-Aw68 similarly at their ends but bulge out in the middle. Nature 1992; 360:364–366.
7. Garrett TP, Saper MA, Bjorkman PJ, et al. Specificity pockets for the side chains of peptide antigens in HLA-Aw68. Nature 1989; 342:692–696.

8. Guo HC, Madden DR, Silver ML, et al. Comparison of the P2 specificity pocket in three human histocompatibility antigens: HLA-A*6801, HLA-A*0201, and HLA-B*2705. Proc Natl Acad Sci USA 1993; 90:8053–8057.

9. Jardetzky TS, Brown JH, Gorga JC, et al. Three-dimensional structure of a human class II histocompatibility molecule complexed with superantigen. Nature 1994; 368:711–718.

10. Madden DR. The three-dimensional structure of peptide-MHC complexes. Annu Rev Immunol 1995; 13:587–622.

11. Busch R, Strang G, Howland K, et al. Degenerate binding of immunogenic peptides to HLA-DR proteins on B cell surfaces. Int Immunol 1990; 2 (in press).

12. Germain RN, Margulies DH. The biochemistry and cell biology of antigen processing and presentation. Annu Rev Immunol 1993; 11:403–450.

13. Cresswell P. Assembly, transport, and function of MHC class II molecules. Annu Rev Immunol 1994; 12:259–293.

14. Theofilopoulos AN. The basis of autoimmunity. Part I: Mechanisms of aberrant self-recognition. Immunol Today 1995; 16:90–98.

15. Goodnow CC. Transgenic mice and analysis of B-cell tolerance. Annu Rev Immunol 1992; 10:489–518.

16. Goldstein I, Rebeyrotte P, Parlebas J, et al. Isolation from heart valves of glycopeptides which share immunological properties with *Streptococcus haemolyticus* group A polysaccharides. Nature 1968; 219:866–868.

17. Husby G, van de Rijn I, Zabriskie JB, et al. Antibodies reacting with cytoplasm of subthalamic and caudate nuclei neurons in chorea and acute rheumatic fever. J Exp Med 1976; 144:1094–1110.

18. Dale JB, Beachey EH. Epitopes of streptococcal M proteins shared with cardiac myosin. J Exp Med 1985; 162:583–591.

19. Gauntt CJ, Arizpe HM, Higdon AL, et al. Molecular mimicry, anti-coxsackievirus B3 neutralizing monoclonal antibodies, and myocarditis. J Immunol 1995; 154:2983–2995.

20. Rammensee HG, Friede T, Stevanoviic S. MHC ligands and peptide motifs: first listing. Immunogenetics 1995; 41:178–228.

21. Behar SM, Porcelli SA. Mechanisms of autoimmune disease induction: the role of the immune response to microbial pathogens. Arthritis Rheum 1995; 38:458–476.

22. Brudzynski K, Martinez V, Gupta RS. Secretory granule autoantigen in insulin-dependent diabetes mellitus is related to 62 kDa heat-shock protein (hsp60). J Autoimmun 1992; 5:453–463.

23. Brudzynski K. Insulitis-caused redistribution of heat-shock protein HSP60 inside beta-cells correlates with induction of HSP60 autoantibodies. Diabetes 1993; 42:908–913.

24. Elias D, Markovits D, Reshef T, et al. Induction and therapy of autoimmune diabetes in the non-obese diabetic (NOD/Lt) mouse by a 65-kDa heat shock protein. Proc Natl Acad Sci USA 1990; 87:1576–1580.

25. DeNagel DC, Pierce SK. Heat shock proteins in immune responses. Crit Rev Immunol 1993; 13:71–81.

26. Res P, Thole J, de Vries R. Heat-shock proteins and autoimmunity in humans. Springer Semin Immunopathol 1991; 13:81–98.

27. Lehmann PV, Forsthuber T, Miller A, et al. Spreading of T-cell autoimmunity to cryptic determinants of an autoantigen. Nature 1992; 358:155–157.

28. Kaufman DL, Clare-Salzler M, Tian J, et al. Spontaneous loss of T-cell tolerance to glutamic acid decarboxylase in murine insulin-dependent diabetes. Nature 1993; 366:69–72.

29. Tisch R, Yang XD, Singer SM, et al. Immune response to glutamic acid decarboxylase correlates with insulitis in non-obese diabetic mice. Nature 1993; 366:72–75.

30. Nagata S, Suda T. Fas and Fas ligand: *lpr* and *gld* mutations. Immunol Today 1995; 16:39–42.

31. Sidman CL, Marshall JD, Von Boehmer H. Transgenic T cell receptor interactions in the lymphoproliferative and autoimmune syndromes of lpr and gld mutant mice. Eur J Immunol 1992; 22:499–504.

32. Singer GG, Abbas AK. The fas antigen is involved in peripheral but not thymic deletion of T lymphocytes in T cell receptor transgenic mice. Immunity 1994; 1:365–371.

33. Rieux-Laucat F, Le Diest F, Hivroz C, et al. Mutations in fas associated with human lymphoproliferative syndrome and autoimmunity. Science 1995; 268:1347–1349.

34. Cheng J, Zhou T, Liu C, et al. Protection from Fas-mediated apoptosis by a soluble form of the Fas molecule. Science 1994; 263:1759–1762.

35. Paul WE, Seder RA. Lymphocyte responses and cytokines. Cell 1994; 76:241–251.

36. Wynn T, Jankovic D, Hieny S, et al. IL-12 exacerbates rather than suppresses T helper 2–dependent pathology in the absence of endogenous IFN-gamma. J Immunol 1995; 154:3999–4009.

37. Sher A, Coffman RL. Regulation of immunity to parasites by T cells and T cell–derived cytokines. Annu Rev Immunol 1992; 10:385–409.

38. Wynn T, Jankovic D, Hieny S, et al. IL-12 enhances vaccine-induced immunity to *Schistosoma mansoni* in mice and decreases T helper 2 cytokine expression, IgE production, and tissue eosinophilia. J Immunol 1995; 154:4701–4709.

39. Merrill JE, Kono DH, Clayton J, et al. Inflammatory leukocytes and cytokines in the peptide-induced disease of experimental allergic encephalomyelitis in SJL and B10.PL mice. Proc Natl Acad Sci USA 1992; 89:574–578.

40. Khoury SJ, Hancock WW, Weiner HL. Oral tolerance to myelin basic protein and natural recovery from experimental autoimmune encephalomyelitis are associated with downregulation of inflammatory cytokines and differential upregulation of transforming growth factor beta, interleukin 4, and prostaglandin E expression in the brain. J Exp Med 1992; 176:1355–1364.

41. Shehadeh NN, LaRosa F, Lafferty KJ. Altered cytokine activity in adjuvant inhibition of autoimmune diabetes. J Autoimmun 1993; 6:291–300.

42. Debray-Sachs M, Carnaud C, Boitard C, et al. Prevention of diabetes in NOD mice treated with antibody to murine IFN gamma. J Autoimmun 1991; 4:237–248.

43. Campbell IL, Kay TW, Oxbrow L, et al. Essential role for interferon-gamma and interleukin-6 in autoimmune insulin-dependent diabetes in NOD/Wehi mice. J Clin Invest 1991; 87:739–742.

44. Rapoport MJ, Jaramillo A, Zipris D, et al. Interleukin 4 reverses T cell proliferative unresponsiveness and prevents the onset of diabetes in non-obese diabetic mice. J Exp Med 1993; 178:87–99.

45. Germann T, Szeliga J, Hess H, et al. Administration of interleukin 12 in combination with type II collagen induces severe arthritis in DBA/1 mice. Proc Natl Acad Sci USA 1995; 92:4823–4827.

46. Hammer RE, Maika SA, Richardson JA, et al. Spontaneous inflammatory disease in transgenic rats expressing HLA-B27 and human beta 2m: An animal model of HLA-B37–associated human disorders. Cell 1990; 63:1099–1112.

47. Stastny P. Association of the B-cell alloantigen DRw4 with rheumatoid arthritis. N Engl J Med 1978; 298:869–871.

48. Nepom GT, Erlich H. MHC class-II molecules and autoimmunity. Annu Rev Immunol 1991; 9:493–525.

49. Winchester R. The molecular basis of susceptibility to rheumatoid arthritis. Adv Immunol 1994; 56:389–466.

50. Atkinson JP. Some thoughts on autoimmunity. Arthritis Rheum 1995; 38:301–305.

51. Howard PF, Hochberg MC, Bias WB, et al. Relationship between C4 null genes, HLA-D region antigens, and genetic susceptibility to systemic lupus erythematosus in Caucasian and Black Americans. Am J Med 1986; 81:187–193.

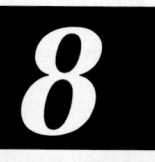

NEUROENDOCRINOLOGY

Seymour Reichlin

INTRODUCTION

Homeostasis, growth, development, and reproduction are regulated by the interactions of the endocrine and nervous systems: almost all endocrine secretions are controlled directly or indirectly by the brain, and virtually all hormones influence brain activity. Neurons provide an organized network of point-to-point connections as the basic unit of the nervous system. The basic unit of the endocrine system is the secretory cell, which provides its regulatory influence through the circulation. Nerve cells and endocrine cells have many attributes in common. Nerve cells have a secretory function and the capac-

ity to propagate action potentials, and endocrine cells have electric potentials as well as a secretory capacity. Neurons, in common with endocrine glands, activate target cells through chemical mediators that react with specific cell receptors.[1] Many peptides and neurotransmitters in nerve cells are identical with those secreted by endocrine glands and regulatory epithelial cells of the gastrointestinal tract.[2] Some of these regulatory molecules and their receptors are found in organisms as primitive as unicellular protozoa[3, 4]; during evolution they have been adapted for use as intercellular signaling messengers.[4, 5]

The field of *neuroendocrinology,* traditionally defined as the study of the relation between the nervous system and the

165

endocrine system, now includes the study of the secretions of the nervous system, regardless of whether they enter the bloodstream or act locally.[6, 7] The specificity of the action of hormones is endowed by the presence of receptors on target tissues, whereas neuronal specificity comes from both receptor distribution and anatomic connections (sometimes referred to as "hard wiring").

The immune system is the third integrative system maintaining homeostasis. Neural and endocrine factors influence the immune response, and in turn cytokines—the secretions of lymphocytes, monocytes, and vascular elements—modulate both neural and endocrine functions. The immune system is a communication network that recognizes foreign antigens such as bacterial toxins and fungi and secretes signaling peptides (cytokines) that regulate brain, endocrine, and immunocyte function.[8] Virtually all endocrine changes involved in the adaptation to stress, the maintenance of homeostasis, and the regulation of reproduction are integrated with specific behaviors.

This chapter deals with the neural control of the endocrine system and with the endocrine control of neural function, specifically the secretions of the brain and the interactions among brain, endocrine, and immune systems. It also reviews the pathophysiology of disorders in neural regulation of endocrine secretion. Some of these topics are considered in other chapters as well: the anterior pituitary in Chapter 9; the adrenal medulla and the sympathetic nervous system in Chapter 13; the reproductive system in Chapters 15, 16, and 17; the role of the neurohypophysis in water balance in Chapter 10; and the immunologic basis of endocrine disease in Chapters 7 and 31. The development of neuroendocrinology has been the subject of reviews,[9–18] textbooks, monographs, and review volumes.[19–32]

NEURAL CONTROL OF GLANDULAR SECRETION

There are several types of secretory cells: *exocrine cells,* which release their products to the exterior of the body or into a lumen that communicates with the exterior; *endocrine cells,* which secrete their products into the circulation; *neurohormonal cells,* which are nerve cells that release their products into the general circulation; *paracrine cells,* which influence adjacent cells by their secretions; and *autocrine cells,* which influence their own function by their own secretions. Exocrine cells are controlled by *secretomotor fibers*; pituitary-dependent target glands are controlled by the hypothalamic *neurosecretory fibers*; and neurosecretory cells in turn are regulated by *neurotransmitters* and hormones. Lymphocytes and macrophages do not receive a direct nerve supply but possess receptors for many hormones and neurotransmitters, and the organs responsible for their generation, differentiation, and degradation (bone marrow, thymus, lymph nodes, and spleen) are innervated by autonomic nerve fibers.

Secretomotor Control

Secretomotor fibers that terminate on cell membranes in synapses regulate the flow of saliva, tears, sweat, sebum, gastric acid, pepsin, and other digestive enzymes as well as the secretion of epinephrine from the adrenal medulla, melatonin from the pineal gland, renin from renal juxtaglomerular cells, and insulin and glucagon from pancreatic islet cells. As components of the sympathetic and parasympathetic nervous systems, secretomotor fibers are regulated by the central nervous system. Secretomotor control traditionally has been attributed

to the release at nerve endings of norepinephrine (sympathetic nerves) and acetylcholine (cholinergic nerves); however, neuropeptide transmitters usually are also present in the same fibers that contain catecholamines and acetylcholine, and the effects of nerve stimulation are often due to the synergistic action of more than one transmitter.[33–36] For example parasympathetic neuronal control of the parotid gland is mediated both by acetylcholine and vasoactive intestinal peptide (VIP). Stimulation of the nerve supply to the parotid (the chorda tympani) releases both factors. Acetylcholine stimulates secretion of enzyme-rich saliva, whereas VIP by itself has little effect on salivary production but enhances parotid blood flow. When administered together, VIP and acetylcholine cause a greater increase in salivary secretion than that caused by acetylcholine alone.[37] In target cells, secretomotor effects usually interact with circulating hormones or cytokines. For example in the pancreatic islet cells insulin secretion is stimulated by high glucose levels and by glucagon-like peptide and is inhibited by norepinephrine released from secretomotor nerve endings.

Preganglionic cholinergic sympathetic fibers that terminate in sympathetic ganglia contain active peptides such as VIP. Co-localization of two or more kinds of neurotransmitters and neuropeptides also occurs in neurons of the central nervous system. The details of co-localization are discussed later.

Neurosecretion

The concept of *neurosecretion* was elucidated by Ernst Scharrer and colleagues in the 1930s on the basis of the morphologic study of the hypothalamus of fish and mammals. They recognized that the secretions of the neural lobe originated in the hypothalamus,[39] a concept supported by the discovery of axoplasmic flow (the transport of cytoplasm and organelles from the body of the nerve cell to the axon terminus)[40–42] and by the demonstration that secretions of the neurohypophysis accumulate proximal to the site of section or ligation of the pituitary stalk.

The mammalian neurohypophysis is a typical neurosecretory gland. Secretions such as vasopressin (arginine vasopressin [AVP], also called antidiuretic hormone [ADH]) and oxytocin are formed in cells in the hypothalamus, transported to the neural lobe by axoplasmic flow, and released into the blood as hormones to regulate organ function at remote sites. Because analogous neurons can terminate in synapses on other neurons *within* the neuraxis, the concept of neurosecretion now includes the release of any neuronal secretory product from a nerve ending; the secretion can serve as either a neurotransmitter or a neuromodulator (Fig. 8–1).[43] Neurotransmitters are released into the synaptic cleft and stimulate (or inhibit) postsynaptic neurons. The distinction between a neurotransmitter and a neuromodulator is not absolute, but neuromodulators tend to have a longer latency before response and a longer duration of action and function to modify the responsiveness of the target neuron to one or more neurotransmitters.[43] Because communication within the nervous system is almost exclusively through chemical messengers, neurosecretion is fundamental to all neurons. The route that is taken by the secretory product of an axon and its site of action depend on its anatomic relationships to other structures.

The presence of endogenous opioids in pain pathways and the widespread distribution of peptidergic neuron systems outside the hypothalamus indicate that many brain functions are modulated by neurosecretions of specific neurons.[44] The secretory products of *peptidergic neurons* are synthesized on the endoplasmic reticulum, packaged into granules in the Golgi apparatus, and transported by axoplasmic flow to nerve endings (Fig. 8–2). Release occurs by reverse pinocytosis in re-

SUPRAOPTICOHYPOPHYSEAL

RELEASES VASOPRESSIN (AVP) AND OXYTOCIN INTO THE PERIPHERAL CIRCULATION.

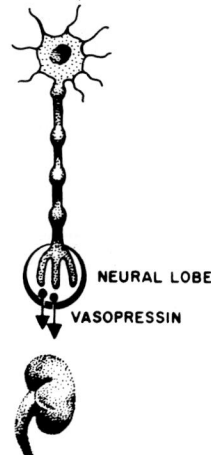

NEURAL LOBE

VASOPRESSIN

HYPOPHYSEOTROPIC

RELEASES HYPOPHYSEOTROPIC HORMONES INTO INTERSTITIAL SPACE OF MEDIAN EMINENCE OF HYPOTHALAMUS, THENCE THE RELEASING FACTORS REACH THE PITUITARY VIA THE HYPOPHYSEAL-PORTAL VESSELS.

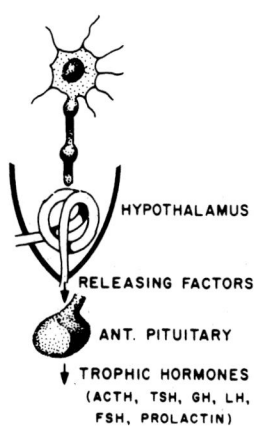

HYPOTHALAMUS

RELEASING FACTORS

ANT. PITUITARY

TROPHIC HORMONES
(ACTH, TSH, GH, LH, FSH, PROLACTIN)

NEUROMODULATORS

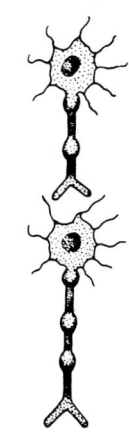

Figure 8–1. Three types of neurosecretory cells. *Left,* A supraopticohypophyseal cell that secretes vasopressin (AVP). The cell body, which is located in the hypothalamus, projects its neuronal process into the neural lobe, and neurohormone is released from nerve endings. Similar peptidergic neurons are located in the medial basal hypothalamus *(center).* Neurohormones in this case are released into the specialized blood supply to the pituitary to regulate its secretion. Although the distance involved is small, the secretion can be termed a *neurohormone* because it enters the circulating blood. Similar in plan are neurosecretory neurons that terminate in relation to another neuron *(right).* Such neurosecretions may serve as neurotransmitters or neuromodulators. ACTH, corticotropin; TSH, thyrotropin; GH, growth hormone; LH, luteinizing hormone; FSH, follicle-stimulating hormone.

Figure 8–2. Neurobiologic features of the peptidergic neuron. Neurosecretory neurons can be regarded as having secretory functions that are in many ways analogous to those of glandular cells. A secretory product, which is formed on the endoplasmic reticulum under the direction of mRNA, is packaged in granules and transported along the axon by axoplasmic flow to reach nerve terminals, where the granules are released. Virtually all neurons carry out similar functions: some secrete neurotransmitters, such as acetylcholine or norepinephrine; others, such as motor nerves, secrete acetylcholine and myotropic factors. In all neurons there is a constant orthograde (forward) flow of cytoplasm and formed elements such as mitochondria. Retrograde flow also takes place to bring substances that enter nerve endings back to the body of the cell. In typical neurotransmitter neurons the neurotransmitters are synthesized by enzymes and are packaged into secretory granules. These granules are transported in a manner similar to that of neuropeptide-containing granules. In many neurons cosecretion of one or two peptides may occur in association with secretion of a classic neurotransmitter. (From Reichlin S. Summarizing comments. In: Gotto AM Jr, Peck EJ Jr, Boyd AE III, et al, eds. Brain Peptides: A New Endocrinology. New York: Elsevier/North-Holland, 1979: 379–403, with permission.)

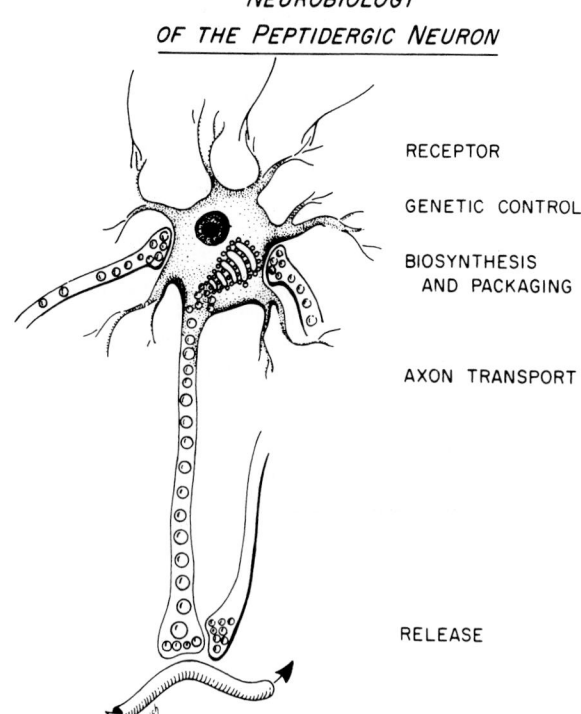

NEUROBIOLOGY OF THE PEPTIDERGIC NEURON

RECEPTOR

GENETIC CONTROL

BIOSYNTHESIS AND PACKAGING

AXON TRANSPORT

RELEASE

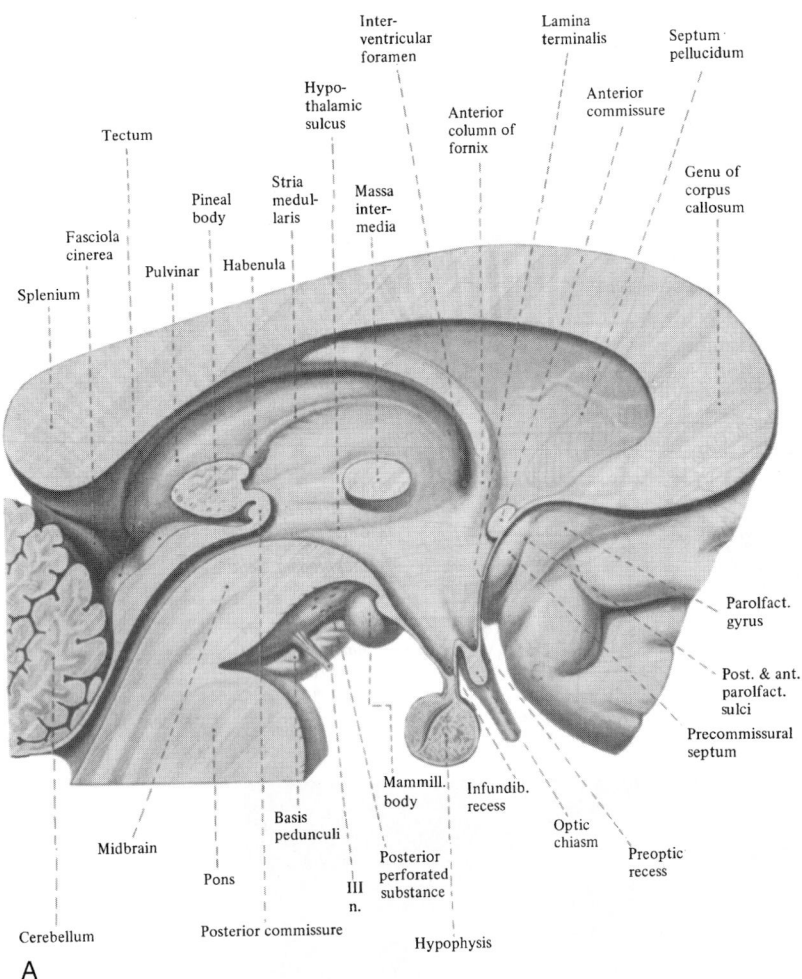

Figure 8–6. *A,* Midsagittal view of the human brain showing the hypothalamus and neighboring structures.

A

(which forms the base of the third ventricle) is shaped like a funnel (Fig. 8–6). The base of the hypothalamus forms a mound called the *tuber cinereum,* the central region of which—*the median eminence of the tuber cinereum*—gives rise to the pituitary stalk. A delicate extension of anterior pituitary tissue termed the *pars tuberalis* extends forward to envelop the tuber cinereum. Covering the surface of the median eminence is a capillary plexus derived from the superior hypophyseal branches of the carotid artery. The superficial plexus gives rise to hairpin-like capillary loops that penetrate the median eminence to provide contact with nerve endings and the interstitial space of the median eminence. Blood from this capillary plexus is collected into *portal veins* that enter the vascular pool of the pituitary. The vascular complex in the base of the hypothalamus and its "arteriolized" venous drainage to the pituitary compose a circulatory system analogous to the portal vein system of the liver, which is termed the *hypophyseal-portal circulation.* This dense collection of blood

vessels ramifies in the superficial layers of the base of the brain to form a small but conspicuous structure (see later).

Neurohypophysis

ANATOMY. The neural lobe develops embryologically as a down-growth from the ventral diencephalon. It is composed of dilated terminals of two major hypothalamic nerve tracts, capillaries, and supportive, glia-like nonsecreting cells (termed *pituicytes*). Unlike most brain capillaries, which form a barrier to diffusion (the blood-brain barrier), neural lobe capillaries resemble those of other endocrine glands in being fenestrated and thus permitting diffusion of secretions into the circulation.[59, 60]

The major nerve tracts of the neurohypophysis arise from relatively large-celled (*magnicellular*) paired nuclei: the supraoptic nucleus is located above the optic tract, and the paraventricular nucleus is located on each side of the third

TABLE 8–1. Sequences of the Principal Peptides of the Neurohypophysis

	1 2 3 4 5 6 7 8 9	1 2 3 4 5 6 7 8 9
Mammals (except pig)	Cys-Tyr-Ile-Gln-Asn-Cys-Pro-Leu-Gly-NH₂ Oxytocin	Cys-Tyr-Phe-Gln-Asn-Cys-Pro-Arg-Gly-NH₂ Arginine vasopressin
Pig	Cys-Tyr-Ile-Gln-Asn-Cys-Pro-Leu-Gly-NH₂ Oxytocin	Cys-Tyr-Phe-Gln-Asn-Cys-Pro-Lys-Gly-NH₂ Lysine vasopressin
Birds, reptiles, amphibians, lungfishes	Cys-Tyr-Ile-Gln-Asn-Cys-Pro-Ile-Gly-NH₂ Mesotocin	Cys-Tyr-Ile-Gln-Asn-Cys-Pro-Arg-Gly-NH₂ Vasotocin
Bony fishes (palcopteryglans and neopteryglans)	Cys-Tyr-Ile-Ser-Asn-Cys-Pro-Ile-Gly-NH₂ Isotocin	Cys-Tyr-Ile-Gln-Asn-Cys-Pro-Arg-Gly-NH₂ Vasotocin

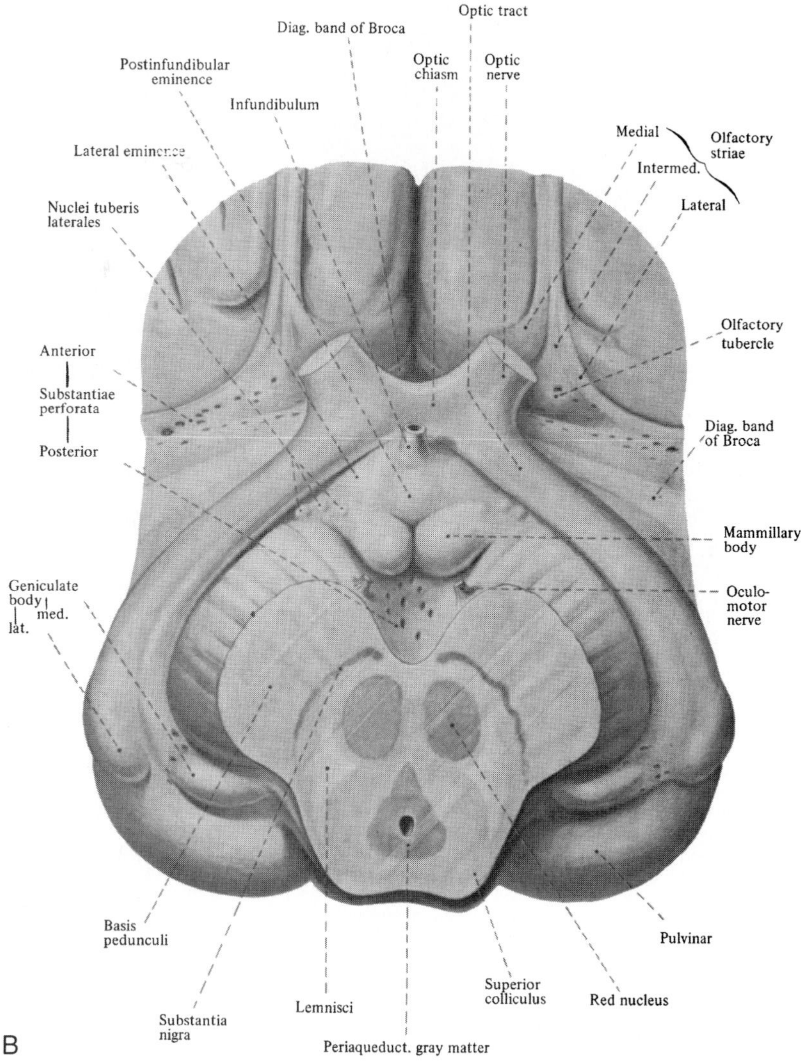

Optic tract

Diag. band of Broca

Optic chiasm

Optic nerve

Postinfundibular eminence

Infundibulum

Medial

Intermed.

Olfactory striae

Lateral emincnce

Lateral

Nuclei tuberis laterales

Olfactory tubercle

Anterior

Substantiae perforata

Posterior

Diag. band of Broca

Mammillary body

Geniculate body med. lat.

Oculo-motor nerve

Basis pedunculi

Pulvinar

Substantia nigra

Lemnisci

Superior colliculus

Red nucleus

Periaqueduct. gray matter

B

Figure 8–6 *Continued B,* Base of the human brain, showing the hypothalamus and neighboring structures. Several landmarks outline the hypothalamus on gross inspection. It is bounded anteriorly by the optic chiasm, laterally by the sulci formed with the temporal lobes, and posteriorly by the mamillary bodies (in which the mamillary nuclei are located). Dorsally, the hypothalamus is delineated from the thalamus by the hypothalamic sulcus. The smooth, rounded base of the hypothalamus is the tuber cinereum; the pituitary stalk descends from its central region, which is termed the *median eminence.* The median eminence stands out from the rest of the tuber cinereum because of its dense vascularity, which is formed by the primary plexus of the hypophyseal-portal system. The long portal veins run along the ventral surface of the pituitary stalk. (From Nauta WJ, Haymaker W. Hypothalamic nuclei and fiber connections. In: Haymaker W, Anderson E, Nauta WJ, eds. The Hypothalamus. Springfield, IL: Charles C Thomas, 1969: 136–209, with permission.)

ventricle (Figs. 8–7 and 8–8). Both tracts are unmyelinated and descend through the infundibulum and neural stalk to terminate in the neural lobe. Their principal secretions are AVP, which regulates water conservation by the kidney, and oxytocin, which acts on breast and uterus (Table 8–1). Some of the fibers terminate in the median eminence and participate in regulation of the anterior lobe.[58-63]

Vasopressin-containing (*vasopressinergic*) fibers are distributed widely within the neuraxis and neural lobe,[60, 64] where they function to regulate water conservation. Some paraventricular vasopressinergic neurons project to the choroid plexus of the lateral ventricles and modulate water and salt exchange

between the brain and the cerebrospinal fluid (CSF).[65] They also project to brain regions involved in emotion and memory. Within the brain stem they end in the sensory nuclei of the vagus and glossopharyngeal nerves to convey information about blood pressure and blood volume. Within the spinal cord they terminate on cells of the autonomic nervous system that are involved in the regulation of blood pressure. Central fibers of these vasopressinergic and oxytocinergic pathways function independently of those that innervate the neurohypophysis. For example central vasopressin levels exhibit a circadian rhythm independent of the state of hydration,[66] whereas peripheral vasopressin levels, which reflect the secre-

Figure 8–7. Course of the neurosecretory substance from the hypothalamic cell body along the neural stalk to the neurohypophysis. This diagram illustrates the concept of cell body formation of oxytocin and AVP and passage of the material down the stalk to a storage site in the neural lobe. Localized accumulations of prohormone form swellings along the axon. (From Bargmann W, Scharrer E. The site of origin of the hormones of the posterior pituitary. Z Zellforsch Mikrosk Anat 1951; 39:255–259, with permission.)

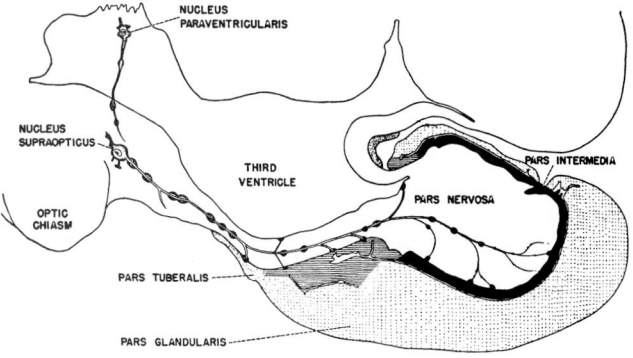

NUCLEUS PARAVENTRICULARIS

NUCLEUS SUPRAOPTICUS

OPTIC CHIASM

THIRD VENTRICLE

PARS INTERMEDIA

PARS NERVOSA

PARS TUBERALIS

PARS GLANDULARIS

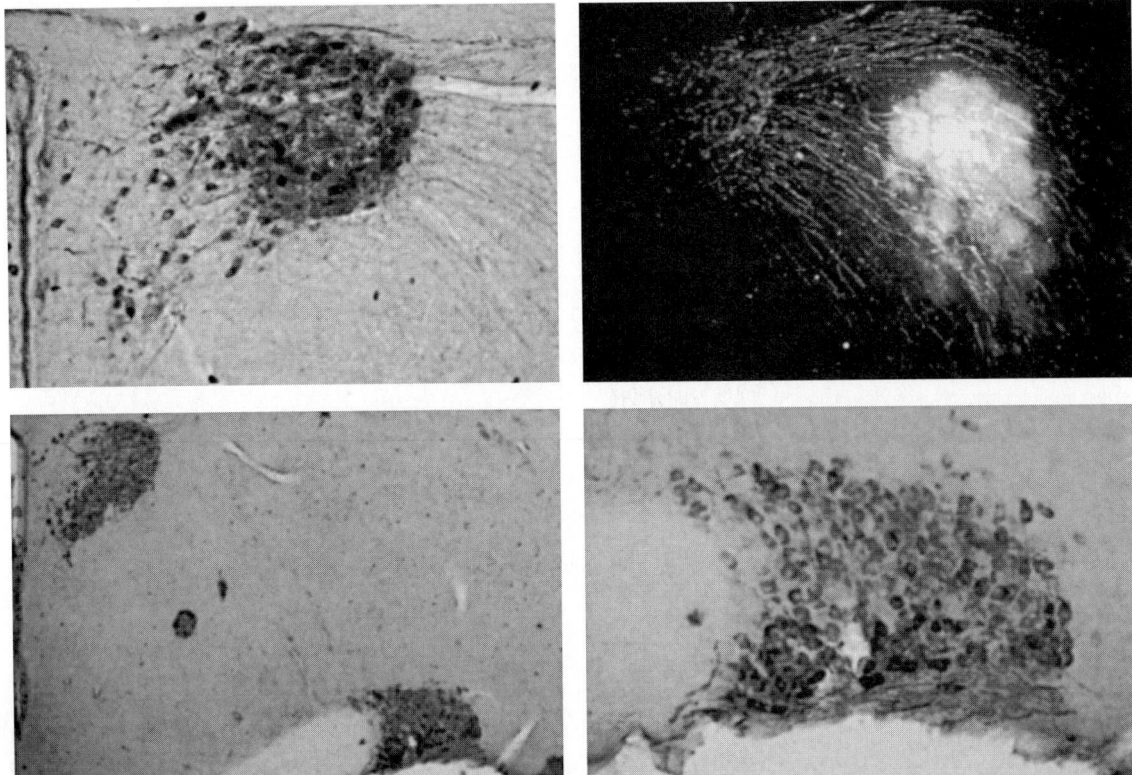

Figure 8–8. Photomicrographs of coronal sections of rat hypothalamus immunostained with antibodies to AVP and oxytocin to show the paraventricular and supraoptic nuclei. *Lower left,* Both nuclei are immunostained, the paraventricular nucleus forming a wing-like structure lateral to the third ventricle and the supraoptic nucleus in this level appearing at the extreme lateral margin of the optic tract. *Upper left,* Higher magnification of the paraventricular nucleus. AVP-staining neurons form a central core in the lateral magnicellular group rimmed by oxytocin-containing neurons. *Lower right,* Higher magnification of the supraoptic nucleus. AVP-containing neurons (staining darker) are more concentrated in the ventral part of the nucleus at this level. *Upper right,* Darkfield photomicrograph of the paraventricular nucleus reacted only with monoclonal antibody specific to AVP. Numerous beaded axonal fibers project laterally from cell bodies through and around the fornix, which shows here as a white mass in the lateral hypothalamus. (Photographs by Alfred T. Lamme, FBPA. Illustrations published with permission of Plenum Publishing Corporation. From Zimmerman EA, Hou-Yu A, Nilaver G, et al. Anatomy of pituitary and extrapituitary vasopressin secretory systems. In: Reichlin S, ed. The Neurohypophysis: Physiological and Clinical Aspects. New York: Plenum, 1984:5–33.)

tion of the neurohypophysis, do not follow a circadian pattern and are controlled by blood volume and plasma osmolarity. Oxytocin levels in CSF are also dissociated from blood levels.[67]

Vasopressin and oxytocin are synthesized in separate populations of supraoptic and paraventricular neurons, but subpopulations of each type contain additional neuropeptides and neurotransmitters under certain circumstances such as after intracerebroventricular administration of colchicine, which impairs axoplasmic flow, or after dehydration, which activates both vasopressinergic and oxytocinergic neurons. mRNA for both oxytocin and vasopressin is demonstrable in the supraoptic nuclei in salt-loaded rats.[63] Vasopressinergic neurons (Table 8–2) contain many neurotransmitters and neuropeptides, including tyrosine hydroxylase (a marker of catecholamine synthesis), galanin (GAL), dynorphin (DYN), leu-enkephalin (Leu-ENK), peptide PHI, cholecystokinin (CCK), and thyrotropin-releasing hormone (TRH). Oxytocin-containing neurons co-express many of the same peptides.[63] Other neurons that terminate in the neural lobe contain TRH, corticotropin-releasing hormone (CRH), vasoactive intestinal polypeptide (VIP), somatostatin (also called somatotropin release-inhibiting factor [SRIF]), luteinizing hormone–releasing hormone (LHRH, also called gonadotropin-releasing hormone, GnRH), and neurotensin (NT).[63] The co-localization of vasopressin and CRH is important because they act synergistically to promote the release of corticotropin (see later).

Although the magnicellular neurons of the paraventricular nucleus stand out most strikingly on histologic study, the small-celled component (parvicellular nucleus) is equally important because it regulates the secretion of thyrotropin (also called thyroid-stimulating hormone [TSH]), corticotropin (also called adrenocorticotropin, adrenocorticotropic hormone [ACTH]), and prolactin (see later), and because it exerts a major effect on eating behavior. Paraventricular cells receive neuronal projections directly and indirectly from higher centers of the brain; from visceral centers that sense blood volume, blood glucose level, blood pressure, and peptides derived from fat cells; and from regions that determine circadian rhythms. These inputs involve an array of neuropeptides and neurotransmitters (see Table 8–2). The parvicellular component of the paraventricular nucleus (the head nucleus of the neuroendocrine system) modulates the secretion of anterior lobe hormones and integrates them with other neurally driven homeostatic functions.

HORMONES OF THE NEUROHYPOPHYSIS. Vasopressin and oxytocin, the principal hormones of the neural lobe, have antidiuretic (water-conserving) and oxytocic (uterus-contracting) activities. Both hormones are nonapeptides, i.e., they contain nine amino acids, and both have a Cys-Cys bridge in the 1-6 position (see Table 8–1). Most submammalian vertebrates have only one neurohypophyseal peptide, arginine vasotocin,[68] the phylogenetic precursor of oxytocin and vasopressin. A single amino acid change in vasotocin in position 8 (arginine to leucine) gives rise to oxytocin, and a single amino acid change in position 3 (leucine to phenylalanine) gives rise to vasopressin. The prohormones for oxytocin and vasopressin also share extensive homology, reinforcing the concept that the two peptides originated from a common gene.[69] Mammals, except for the pig, have identical vasopressins; in porcine vasopressin, arginine in position 9 is replaced by lysine. Vaso-

TABLE 8–2. Neuroactive Materials in the Paraventricular Nucleus and the Arcuate Nucleus

Paraventricular Nucleus

Magnicellular Division

Angiotensin II
Cholecystokinin
Glucagon
Oxytocin
Peptide 7B2
Proenkephalin B (dynorphin, rimorphin, α-neoendorphin)
Vasopressin
Nitric oxide (NO)

Parvicellular Division

γ-Aminobutyric acid (GABA)
Angiotensin II
Atrial natriuretic factor
Cholecystokinin
Corticotropin-releasing hormone
Dopamine
Follicle-stimulating hormone–releasing factor
Galanin
Glucagon
Neuropeptide Y
Neurotensin
Peptide 7B2
Proenkephalin A (met-enkephalin, leu-enkephalin, BAM 22P, metorphamide, met-enkephalin-Arg^6-Phe^7, met-enkephalin-Arg^6-Gly^7-Leu^8)

Parvicellular Division Continued

Somatostatin
Thyrotropin-releasing hormone (TRH)
Vasopressin
Interleukin-1 (IL-1)
Vasoactive intestinal peptide (VIP)–peptide-histidine-isoleucine (PHI)
Nitric oxide

Arcuate Nucleus

Acetylcholine (?)
γ-Aminobutyric acid
Dopamine
Galanin
Growth hormone–releasing hormone (GHRH)
Luteinizing hormone–releasing hormone (LHRH)
Neuropeptide Y
Neurotensin
Pancreatic polypeptide
Proenkephalin A
Prolactin
Melanocortins (corticotropin, α-melanocyte-stimulating hormone [α-MSH], γ-melanocyte-stimulating hormone [γ-MSH])
Endogenous opioids (β-endorphin, β-lipotropin [β-LPH])
Somatostatin
Substance P

Modified from Lechan RM. Neuroendocrinology of pituitary hormone regulation. Endocrinol Metab Clin North Am 1987; 16:475–502.

pressin possesses minimal oxytocic activity, and oxytocin exhibits slight antidiuretic activity. Three vasopressin receptors (V_{1A}, V_{1B}, V_2) and one oxytocin receptor have been characterized (Table 8–3).[70] Each is a seven-membrane spanning protein and each binds to both vasopressin and oxytocin. Analysis of the gene encoding the vasopressin receptor has revealed several different mutations in families with vasopressin-resistant diabetes insipidus (DI) (see later and Chapter 10).

Vasopressin and oxytocin are found in the neurohypophysis in association with peptides termed *neurophysins*, which are now recognized to be components of the respective prohormones propressophysin and prooxyphysin (Fig. 8–9).[71–73] Neurophysins are secreted together with vasopressin and oxytocin.[74]

In one form of congenital DI in the rat the vasopressin molecule is abnormal because of a homozygous mutation that causes a frame shift during transcription of the prohormone.[73] As of 1995 six different mutations (deletions or substitutions) in the human vasopressin gene had been identified in nine separate families with central DI,[75, 76] all but one in the neurophysin moiety and the other in the signal peptide of the prohormone. An unexplained aspect of the human disorder is that it is inherited as an autosomal dominant trait and may occur later in life. Because a defect in only one allele is responsible for the disease, the presence of abnormal neurophysin may lead to progressive cell damage. The genetics of DI are considered further in Chapter 10.

REGULATION OF VASOPRESSIN SECRETION. As outlined earlier, vasopressin and its related neurophysin (neurophysin II) and oxytocin and its related neurophysin (neurophysin I) are synthesized as prohormones in the supraoptic and paraventricular neurons (see Fig. 8–8). The prohormones are transported in membrane-bound vesicles through the axons to the neural lobe, where they are stored and later released. Processing of the prohormone to the secreted products vasopressin, oxytocin, and the two neurophysins takes place in the vesicles during the course of transport. Nerve action potentials arising in the cell body are propagated along the axon and trigger the secretion of the neurohypophyseal hormones and neurophysins in a fixed ratio.

Neurotransmitters and Hormonal Control. Neurohypophyseal function is directly controlled by cholinergic and nor-

adrenergic afferent fibers,[61, 77] several neuropeptides, glucocorticoids, and estrogens. Acetylcholine stimulates the release of vasopressin through a nicotinic cholinergic receptor (see Table 8–3) (the mechanism by which nicotine acts as an antidiuretic). Acetylcholine also stimulates oxytocin secretion. Adrenergic influences, in contrast, inhibit oxytocin secretion through β-adrenergic receptors. Stress-induced inhibition of

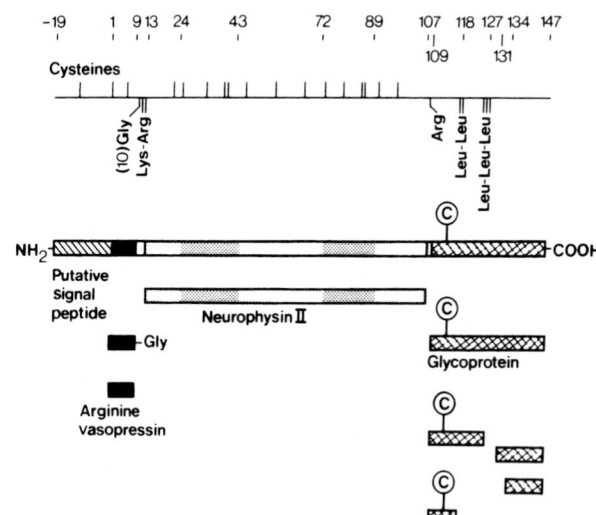

Figure 8–9. Schematic representation of the structure of bovine AVP–neurophysin II precursor, based on recombinant DNA analysis. Sequence coding for AVP is located immediately after the signal peptide, followed by sequence coding for neurophysin II. Following the neurophysin region is a glycoprotein segment. The top line illustrates the amino acid number. The second line from the top shows the crucial amino acid sequence at which post-translational processing of the peptide takes place in secretory granules. The indication of glycine in position 10 is a characteristic extension in peptide hormones that contain a terminal amide. Glycine is exchanged for NH$_2$ during processing. Lys-Arg sequences at positions 11 and 12 are typical enzymatic cleavage sites, as is Arg in position 107. In the neurohypophyseal system, the entire prohormone is packaged in secretory granules and is processed during axoplasmic transport. AVP (a nonapeptide) is secreted in equimolar amounts as neurophysin II. (From Land H, Schültz G, Schmale H, et al. Nucleotide sequence of cloned cDNA encoding bovine arginine vasopressin–neurophysin II precursor. Reprinted by permission from Nature, Vol. 295, pp. 299–303. Copyright © 1982 Macmillan Journals Ltd.)

TABLE 8–3. Receptors for Neurotransmitters and Neuropeptides Involved in Hypothalamic-Pituitary Control*

Classic Neurotransmitters

Group	Name	General Structure Transmembrane Sequences	Mode of Action
Biogenic amines			
α_{1A}-Adrenoreceptors	α_{1A}	7	$G_{q/11}$
	α_{1B}	7	$G_{q/11}$
	α_{1D}	7	$G_{q/11}$
α_{2A}-Adrenoreceptors	α_{2A}	7	$G_{i/o}$
	α_{2B}	7	$G_{i/o}$
	α_{2C}	7	$G_{i/o}$
β-Adrenoreceptors	β_1	7	G_s
	β_2	7	G_s
	β_3	7	G_s
Serotonin (5-OH-tryptamine)	$5\text{-}HT_{1A}$	7	$G_{i/o}$
	$5\text{-}HT_{1B}$	7	$G_{i/o}$
	$5\text{-}HT_{1D}$	7	$G_{i/o}$
	$5\text{-}HT_{1E}$	7	$G_{i/o}$
	$5\text{-}HT_{2A}$	7	$G_{q/11}$
	$5\text{-}HT_{2B}$	7	$G_{q/11}$
	$5\text{-}HT_{2C}$	7	$G_{q/11}$
	$5\text{-}HT_3$	4	Cation channel
	$5\text{-}HT_4$	7	G_s
Dopamine	D_1	7	G_s
	D_2	7	$G_{i/o}$
	D_3	7	$G_{i/o}$
	D_4	7	$G_{i/o}$
	D_5	7	G_s
Histamine	H_1	7	$G_{q/11}$
	H_2	7	G_s
	H_3	?	?
Acetylcholine			
Muscarinic	M_1	7	$G_{q/11}$
	M_2	7	$G_{i/o}$
	M_3	7	$G_{q/11}$
	M_4	7	$G_{i/o}$
	M_5	7	$G_{q/11}$
Nicotinic	Muscle	4 Multiunit	Na/K/Ca
	Ganglionic	4 Multiunit	Na/K/Ca
	Central nervous system	4 Multiunit	Na/K/Ca
Excitatory Amino Acids (Glutamate)			
Ionotropic	NMDA	Multiunit ?4TM	Na/K/Ca
	AMPA	?	Na/K/Ca
	Kainate	?	Na/K/Ca
Metabotropic	$mGlu_1$	7	$G_{q/11}$
	$mGlu_2$	7	$G_{i/o}$
	$mGlu_3$	7	$G_{i/o}$
	$mGlu_4$	7	$G_{i/o}$
	$mGlu_5$	7	$G_{q/11}$
	$mGlu_6$	7	$G_{i/o}$
	$mGlu_7$	7	$G_{i/o}$
Inhibitory Amino Acid (γ-Aminobutyric Acid [GABA])	$GABA_A$	Multiunit	Internal Cl
	$GABA_B$	?	$G_{i/o}$

Neuropeptides

Group	Name	General Structure Transmembrane Sequences	Mode of Action
Neurohypophyseal hormones			
Vasopressin	V_{1A}	7	$G_{q/11}$
	V_{1B}	7	$G_{q/11}$
	V_2	7	G_s
Oxytocin	OT	7	$G_{q/11}$
Hypophysiotropic hormones			
TRH	TRH	7	$G_{q/11}$
GHRH	GHRH	7	G_s
LHRH	LHRH	7	$G_{q/11}$
CRH	CRH	7	G_s
Somatostatin	SST_1	7	$G_{i/o}$
	SST_{2A}	7	$G_{i/o}$
	SST_{2B}	7	$G_{i/o}$
	SST_3	7	$G_{i/o}$
	SST_4	7	$G_{i/o}$
	SST_5	7	$G_{i/o}$
Endogenous opioid peptides			
	μ	7	$G_{i/o}$
	δ	7	$G_{i/o}$
	κ	7	$G_{i/o}$
Melanocortins	MC_1	7	G_s
	MC_2 (corticotropin)	7	G_s
	MC_3		
	MC_4	7	G_s
	MC_5	7	G_s
		7	G_s
Gut-brain peptides			
Tachykinins			
Substance P	NK_1	7	$G_{i/o}$
Substance K	NK_2	7	$G_{i/o}$
Neurokinin B	NK_3	7	$G_{i/o}$
Neurotensin	NT	7	$G_{q/11}$
VIP	VIP_1	7	G_s
	VIP_2	7	G_s
PACAP	PACAP	7	G_s
Galanin	G	7	$G_{i/o}$
Cholecystokinin	CCK_A	7	$G_{q/11}$
	CCK_B (gastrin receptor)	7	$G_{q/11}$
Neuropeptide Y	Y_1	7	$G_{i/o}$
	Y_2	7	$G_{i/o}$
Vasoactive peptides			
Angiotensin	AT_1	7	$G_{q/11}$
	AT_2	7	cGMP
Atrial natriuretic peptide	ANP_A	1	cGMP
	ANP_B	1	cGMP
Endothelin	ET_A	7	$G_{q/11}$
	ET_B	7	$G_{q/11}$

*Receptors cited are human, or rat if human not available.

NMDA, N-methyl-D-aspartate; AMPA, α-amino-3-hydroxy-5-methyl-4-isoxazdeproprionic acid; TRH, thyrotropin-releasing hormone; GHRH, growth hormone–releasing hormone; LHRH, luteinizing hormone–releasing hormone; CRH, corticotropin-releasing hormone; NT, neurotensin; VIP, vasoactive peptide; PACAP, pituitary adenylate cyclase activating peptide; cGMP, cyclic guanosine monophosphate.

cGMP: Guanylate cyclase activity intrinsic to the receptor.

$G_{i/o}$: Receptor coupled to the $G_{i/o}$ family. Opens K^+ channel, closes Ca^{2+} channel, inhibits adenylate cyclase.

$G_{q/11}$: Receptor coupled to the $G_{q/11}$ family. Stimulates phosphoinositol cascade.

G_s: Receptor coupled to the G_s family. Stimulates adenylate cyclase and increases intracellular cAMP.

Some receptors have intrinsic tyrosine phosphorylase activity, others have intrinsic tyrosine hydroxylase activity. The former stimulate phosphorylation of tyrosine kinases; the latter stimulate breakdown of tyrosine kinase.

The designation of functional type is oversimplified. Many examples can be cited in which receptor activation can stimulate both adenylate cyclase and phosphoinositide turnover.

Adapted from Watson S, Girdlestone D. Receptor and channel nomenclature supplement. Trends Pharmacol Sci 1995; (Suppl 16):1–73, with permission.

the milk let-down reflex results from β-adrenergic inhibition of oxytocin release. AVP secretion is also inhibited by β-adrenergic fibers.

These neurons are also influenced by several peptides. Angiotensin II releases AVP[78] and stimulates thirst.[79] Atrial natriuretic peptide (ANP) inhibits AVP release and blocks the effects of angiotensin II and hypertonic saline on AVP release and on drinking behavior (see later).[80] Neurohypophyseal neurons are also stimulated by endogenous opioids (endorphins).[81] The antidiuretic action of morphine is due to the release of AVP, an effect that can be duplicated by intracerebroventricular administration of β-endorphin. A role for endorphins in the regulation of AVP secretion is supported by the fact that naloxone, an opiate antagonist, can reverse inappropriate AVP secretion in some situations.[82] Studies with opioid receptor antagonists suggest that "acute hypovolemia affects vasopressin secretion by influencing two opposing pathways with different opioidergic components."[83] The dominant stimulatory pathway is mediated in part by endogenous opioids acting at k_2- or k_3-receptors; the weaker inhibitory effect is mediated by μ- or k_1-receptors. Oxytocin-secreting neurons are innervated by a specialized brain stem pathway that uses inhibin B as a neurotransmitter.[84]

Vasopressin release is stimulated by agents that increase local concentrations of NO in the hypothalamus,[85] and blockade of NO synthesis blocks vasopressin release induced by acetylcholine and by the inflammatory cytokine interleukin-2 (IL-2).[86] The enzyme that synthesizes NO (NO synthase) is expressed in oxytocic, and not in vasopressinergic neurons in the magnicellular nuclei.[87] This finding could account for "cross-talk" between the oxytocin and the vasopressinergic neurons through a paracrine mechanism.

IL-1, IL-2, and IL-6 are inflammatory cytokines that induce vasopressin release. Their effects may be mediated by induction of the synthesis of NO and prostaglandin by glial cells in the hypothalamus.

Glucocorticoids, estrogens, and thyroid hormone play important physiological roles in neurohypophyseal function, and magnicellular neurons express specific nuclear receptors for these hormones.

In adrenal insufficiency vasopressinergic neurons are activated, as documented by increased concentrations of mRNA coding for vasopressin,[88] increased blood levels of vasopressin,[89] and a changed set point for osmotic control. This change in set point results in inappropriate secretion of vasopressin (syndrome of inappropriate ADH secretion [SIADH]) in adrenal insufficiency, a state reversed by glucocorticoid treatment (see later).

Estrogens activate oxytocinergic neurons, as evidenced by increased blood levels of oxytocin-related neurophysin,[90] increased oxytocin gene expression in humans,[91] and increased levels of oxytocin and vasopressin gene expression during pregnancy in the rat.[92] Magnicellular neurons also contain thyroid hormone receptor α,[93] possibly explaining the SIADH of severe hypothyroidism.

Osmolar Control. The most important factors that regulate vasopressin secretion are plasma osmolality and "effective" circulating blood volume. Blood pressure, nausea, and emotional stress also influence its release.[61, 82, 94–98] (also see Chapter 10). Maintenance of normal osmolality in blood is the major homeostatic function of the neurohypophysis. Indeed, blood osmolality is kept within a narrow range (±1.8%), the mean set point of plasma osmolality normally being about 282 mmol/L. Infusion of hypertonic saline sufficient to increase osmolality to about 287 mmol/L, a level termed the *osmotic threshold*,[94–96] triggers vasopressin secretion. Above this value vasopressin secretion increases rapidly and progressively with increasing plasma osmolality (Fig. 8–10). In contrast, water loading inhibits the release of vasopressin and

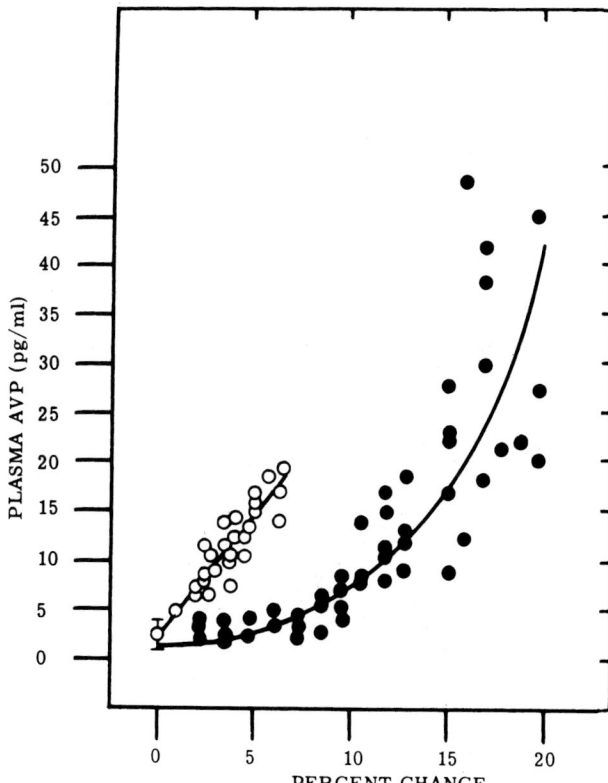

Figure 8–10. Relationship of plasma AVP level to the percent *increase* in blood osmolality (○) or *decrease* in blood volume (●) in conscious rats. Plasma AVP level is a linear function of osmolality and a curvilinear function of blood volume; virtually no change in AVP is detectable until there has been a 10 to 15% fall in blood volume. To convert AVP values to picomoles per liter, multiply by 0.92. (From Dunn FL, Brennan TJ, Nelson AE, et al. The role of blood osmolality and volume in regulating vasopressin secretion in the rat. Reproduced from the Journal of Clinical Investigation, 1973, vol. 52, pp. 3212–3219 by copyright permission of the American Society for Clinical Investigation.)

suppresses the synthesis of vasopressin as evidenced by reduced levels of vasopressin mRNA.

Osmosensitive structures are located in the neurons of the neurohypophysis and in the structures that surround the third ventricle (Fig. 8–11).[97, 98] Osmotic shifts change the volume of magnicellular neurons, which, by altering the stretching of the cell membrane, changes "mechanosensitive cationic channels" and triggers electrical activity.[97, 98] Oxytocinergic neurons in the magnicellular system are also volume sensitive. Other, possibly more important osmoreceptors are located in the anterior wall of the third ventricle in specialized periventricular structures (discussed further in the section on circumventricular organs) that project neurons to the vasopressin-secreting system.[98, 99] Peripheral osmoreceptors in the hepatoportal vessels also respond to osmotic changes and send signals via the afferent vagus to brain stem nuclei, which in turn communicate with the vasopressinergic system. Osmoreceptive function is integrated with sensors of sodium concentration (in the subfornical organ [SFO] of the third ventricle [see later]) and with volume receptors in peripheral vessels.

The fact that vasopressin secretion is influenced through multiple reflex pathways probably explains why some patients with hypothalamic disease lose osmoreceptor control of vasopressin secretion but retain some regulatory responses such as those to cholinergic stimuli. In other patients osmoreceptor control of vasopressin can be retained, whereas the thirst sensation is lost. Separate populations of osmoreceptor, vasopressin-secreting, and thirst-generating neurons may exist, although with some overlap in distribution.

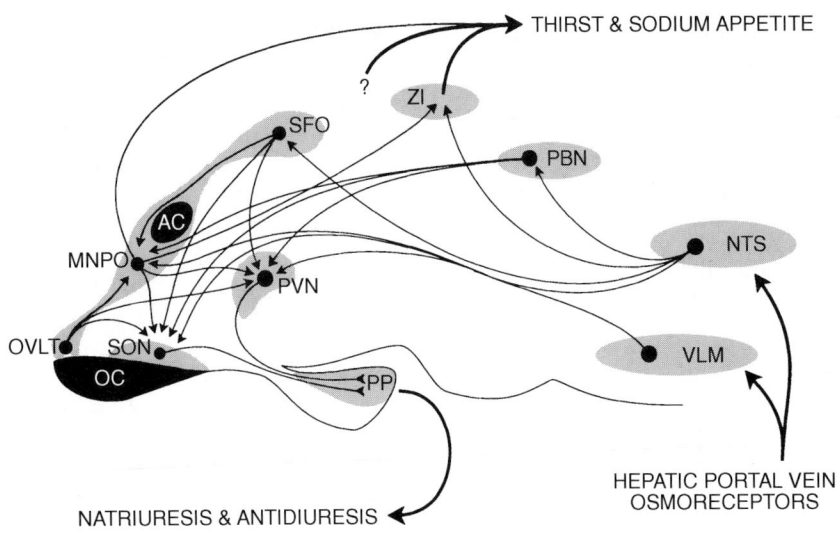

Figure 8–11. Schematic illustration of selected neural pathways involved in osmoregulation. Peripheral neural pathways include hepatic portal vein osmoreceptors that project by vagal afferents to the nucleus of the tractus solitarius (NTS) and the ventrolateral medulla (VLM). Osmoreceptor cells in several periventricular organs (subfornical organ [SFO], median preoptic nucleus in the subcommissural region [MNPO], organum vasculosum of the lamina terminalis [OVLT]) project neurons to the supraoptic nucleus (SON) and the paraventricular nucleus (PVN), which regulate vasopressin secretion, thirst, and sodium appetite. In addition, the SON and PVN nuclei possess intrinsic osmoreceptor capacity. AC, anterior commissure; OC, optic chiasm; PBN, parabrachial nucleus; PP, posterior pituitary; ZI, zona incerta. (From Bourque CW, Oliet SHR, Richard D. Osmoreceptors, osmoreception, and osmoregulation. Front Neuroendocrinol 1994; 15:231–274, with permission.)

Volume Control. Change in volume (as contrasted with change in osmolality) must be relatively large to trigger vasopressin release. For example, phlebotomy that reduces blood volume by 6 to 9% or the assumption of the upright posture that reduces central blood volume by 10 to 15% has no effect on vasopressin release.[95] Conversely a change in blood volume of more than 10%, as produced by the combination of phlebotomy and the assumption of the erect position, brings about vasopressin release. Under usual conditions, plasma osmolality is the prime determinant of vasopressin secretion, but severe volume depletion can override the osmoreceptor control. With less severe volume change, osmotic control is precise, but there is a shift of the osmotic set point so that a lower osmotic threshold is required to trigger vasopressin secretion in the volume-depleted state.

As noted earlier, adrenal insufficiency lowers the set point and thereby induces a relative increase in vasopressin secretion,[100] which contributes to the low serum sodium level in both primary and secondary adrenal insufficiency.[101] Glucocorticoids inhibit vasopressin secretion by impairing vasopressin gene transcription,[102] and glucocorticoid deficiency increases vasopressin mRNA.[89]

Receptors for volume control are located in the left atrium and in the baroreceptors of the carotid sinus and perhaps elsewhere. Volume depletion that is insufficient to lower blood pressure can activate the atrial receptors, whereas depletion that is sufficient to cause hypotension is required to mobilize baroreceptor reflexes.[103]

Neural impulses from volume and blood pressure sensors reach the brain stem via cranial nerve afferents that terminate in the midbrain, ascend through multisynaptic pathways, and impinge on the nuclei of the neurohypophyseal system.

Atrial Natriuretic Peptides. The left atrium exerts *endocrine control* of blood volume that is distinct from the role of the left atrial *volume receptors*. A family of muscle peptides with potent natriuretic activity, termed *atrial natriuretic peptides* (also called *atrial peptides* or *atriopeptins*), is part of a homeostatic feedback mechanism for regulation of intravascular volume.[80, 104, 105] Expansion of the left atrium stimulates muscle stretch receptors, leading to exocytosis of atrial natriuretic peptide–containing secretory granules from atrial myocytes into the blood. Atrial natriuretic peptide then acts on the kidney tubule to increase sodium excretion and thereby reduce circulating blood volume.

In the brain atrial natriuretic peptide[105] is located in areas involved in the regulation of blood volume through changes in drinking behavior[106] and vasopressin secretion.[107] Atrial na-

triuretic peptide and its receptor are present in the anterior tip of the third ventricle in the region of the SFO (see later in the section on periventricular organs), where angiotensin II receptors are also located.[108] Atrial natriuretic peptide and angiotensin II interact in the regulation of water intake and vasopressin secretion. Injections of atrial natriuretic peptide in the subfornical region inhibit vasopressin release and inhibit drinking in normal animals and in animals in whom drinking and vasopressin release have been stimulated by angiotensin II (Fig. 8–12).

The SFO, like other periventricular organs, lacks a blood-brain barrier. Atrial natriuretic peptide is also present in the neural pathways that connect peripheral volume receptors to the hypothalamus. Thus the peripheral and central atrial natriuretic peptide systems are integrated for the maintenance of blood volume homeostasis.[109, 110] A distinctive atrial natriuretic–like peptide is present in pig brain (*brain natriuretic peptide*).[111] Different genes encode atrial natriuretic peptide receptors in brain and kidney. Atrial natriuretic peptide is present in many neuronal endings in the median eminence.

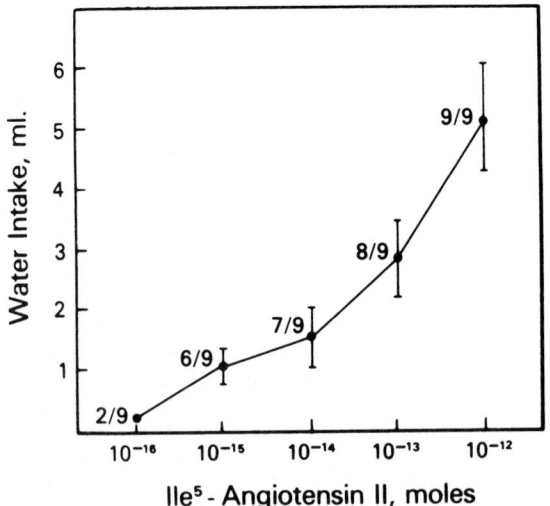

Figure 8–12. Dose-response curve of drinking produced by injection of angiotensin II directly into the subfornical organ, a structure located in the dorsal anterior wall of the third ventricle. (From Simpson J, Epstein JN, Camardo JS Jr. The localization of receptors for the dipsogenic action of angiotensin II in the subfornical organ of rat. J Comp Physiol Psychol 1978; 92:581–608. Copyright 1978 by the American Psychological Association. Reprinted by permission.)

It stimulates the formation of cyclic guanosine monophosphate in isolated pituitary cells and is synthesized in a subpopulation of anterior pituitary cells.

Relation Between Vasopressin Secretion and Drinking Behavior. Drinking behavior, like AVP secretion, is regulated by plasma osmolality and circulating blood volume, integrated by hypothalamic mechanisms, and designed to maintain the constancy of the internal milieu.[78, 79, 92, 93, 106, 107, 123–125] The sensation of thirst (in contrast to the sensation of a dry mouth) results in a signal arising from the hypothalamus. Thirst can be generated by severe hemorrhage or by inducing local hyperosmolality in the hypothalamus with injections of hypertonic saline. The thirst mechanism is integrated with the vasopressin-controlling mechanism; both are activated by osmoreceptors in the hypothalamus and periventricular organs and by peripheral volume receptors. Drinking behavior and AVP release can be activated by intrahypothalamic administration of acetylcholine analogues, suggesting that a common pathway mediates the two functions. The hypothalamic angiotensin II system may also be important in AVP regulation, as it is in drinking behavior. All of the biochemical components and enzyme systems for the formation of angiotensin II are present in the hypothalamus, and angiotensin II–containing neurons[79, 106] and angiotensin II receptors[108] are located in the region. Angiotensin II–containing neurons project from periventricular neurons in the anterior hypothalamus (SFO) to the paraventricular nucleus.

In humans, both shock and severe renovascular hypertension increase blood levels of angiotensin II and cause both increased drinking and increased vasopressin release. These effects are probably mediated by angiotensin II, because injection of angiotensin II into the third ventricle of the rat stimulates drinking and because drinking by dehydrated rats is blocked by local administration of the angiotensin II receptor antagonist saralasin.

Stress and Nausea. Pain and other incidental stresses rarely influence plasma AVP concentrations.[95] Nevertheless the influence of "higher" centers on AVP secretion can be demonstrated by induction of diuresis or antidiuresis through hypnotic suggestion in humans and by the abnormalities in water balance manifested by patients with anorexia nervosa[112] and psychosis.[113]

Nausea has a marked effect on vasopressin secretion, presumably by reflex stimulation from the medullary vomiting center (area postrema), which is responsive to chemical signals from drugs and toxins. The secretion of vasopressin is affected by inputs from various parts of the "visceral brain" and the reticular activating system, both regions involved in maintenance of consciousness and in emotional expression.

Inappropriate Vasopressin Secretion (Syndrome of Inappropriate Secretion of Antidiuretic Hormone [SIADH]). SIADH can be due to ectopic hormone secretion by malignancies of several kinds[96] (see Chapter 36), to adrenal or thyroid deficiency (see earlier), and to drugs that stimulate vasopressinergic neurons such as the opiates (see earlier and Chapter 10). SIADH can also be caused by stroke, intraventricular hemorrhage, or massive brain destruction.[96]

Neurogenic SIADH is probably due to loss of normal tonic inhibitory influences on the neurohypophyseal neurons and suggests a "release" phenomenon. Experimentally induced lesions of the anterior margins of the supraoptic nucleus increase neuronal activity in the supraopticohypophyseal pathway and give rise to inappropriate vasopressin release.[114] Inappropriate secretion of vasopressin also occurs in patients with anorexia nervosa[112] and in patients with schizophrenia.[113]

Extrahypothalamic Functions of Vasopressin. Central vasopressinergic fibers (and receptors) that are independent of the neurohypophysis are present in the cerebral cortex, limbic system, and brain vascular tissues.[60, 65, 115] Vasopressin has elec-

trophysiological effects on brain cells,[116] and in the choroid plexus regulates water and salt transport between the blood and the CSF.[65, 117]

Vasopressin also affects cognitive function.[118–120] Hypophysectomized rats lose their capacity to learn and remember, and intracerebral or systemic injection of vasopressin restores learning and memory in rats with DI; similarly injection of corticotropin, certain corticotropin analogues that lack the capacity to stimulate the adrenal cortex, or certain enkephalin-related peptides can also restore learning ability. In contrast, administration of antivasopressin antiserum impairs learning in the rat. Studies of the effects of corticotropin-related peptides on human memory are conflicting,[120] but vasopressin and certain vasopressin analogues that have no antidiuretic action are said to improve long-term memory in the elderly.[119] Nevertheless the significance of a central vasopressinergic system for memory consolidation is uncertain. Most of the work in animals has used pain-aversive conditioning and may not represent all types of learning. Hypophysectomy, the model associated with abnormal memory function, does not affect the concentration of vasopressin or of corticotropin-related peptides in the brain, both of which are present in extensive intrinsic neuronal networks. Furthermore the blood-brain barrier excludes entry of all but minute amounts of peptide,[121, 123] and systemic administration of corticotropin-related peptides does not affect the concentration of intrinsic brain peptides.[122, 123] Indeed vasopressin may act centrally by way of peripheral receptors that sense blood volume or osmolarity,[124] both of which are influenced by systemic injection of vasopressin.

REGULATION OF OXYTOCIN SECRETION

Milk Let-Down Reflex. With suckling, milk appears at the nipple after a delay of half a minute or so, a response termed milk *let-down*.[125–127] The stimulus of suckling initiates a neurogenic reflex beginning in afferent nerve endings in the nipple and conducted through the spinal cord, the midbrain, and the hypothalamus to trigger release of oxytocin from the neurohypophysis (Fig. 8–13). Neurotransmitters involved in this phenomenon include stimulatory inputs from cholinergic and α-adrenergic fibers[127] and from an inhibin-containing peptidergic neuronal pathway that conducts impulses from the midbrain.[84] Inhibition is induced by β-adrenergic fibers and endogenous opioids. In the breast oxytocin causes contraction of the myoepithelial cells that encircle mammary acini, thereby expelling the milk into the milk ducts and thence into the nipple. In the absence of this reflex contraction milk cannot be obtained, even from a full breast. The milk let-down reflex is accompanied by changes in hypothalamic neuronal function and can be blocked by specific neural lesions and by certain types of neural stimuli. In cows the let-down reflex can be abolished by a strange or threatening environment. Pain or fright inhibits milk let-down in the rabbit through adrenergic (presumably β-adrenergic) stimulation. In humans milk let-down occurs in response to suckling and can be conditioned by the crying of a hungry infant. Milk let-down is inhibited by emotional stress and can be triggered by sexual excitement and orgasm. Oxytocin has been administered therapeutically to some women with failure of normal milk let-down, but most women with DI nurse normally.[128]

Oxytocin in large doses can trigger prolactin release in animals, but its role as a prolactin "releasing factor" is unclear (see later in the section on prolactin regulation).

Oxytocin in Labor. Oxytocin is a potent stimulator of uterine contraction and is administered to induce labor and manage obstetric hemorrhage. However, its physiological role in the initiation and maintenance of normal labor in humans has not been established (see Chapter 27).[126–130] During pregnancy high levels of progesterone suppress uterine muscle excitability, expression of the oxytocin receptor, and respon-

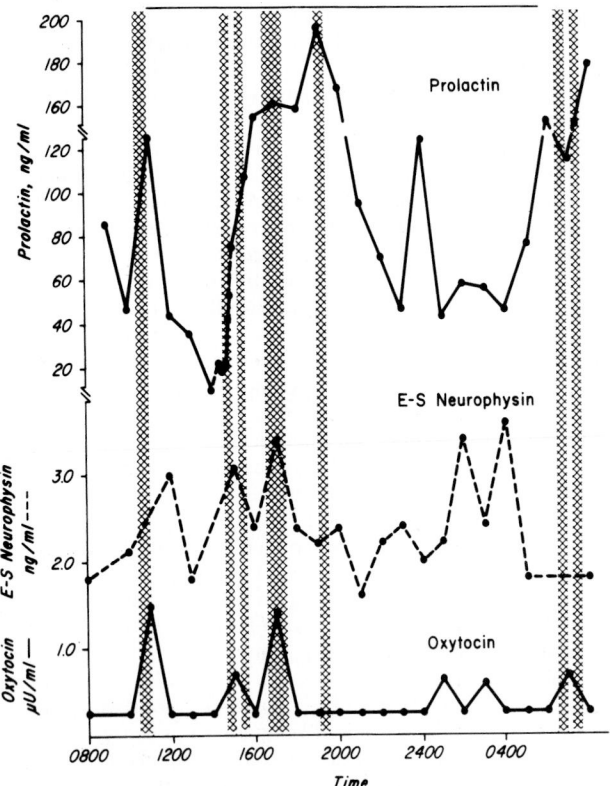

Figure 8–13. Patterns of release of prolactin, oxytocin, and oxytocin-related neurophysin (estrogen-stimulated neurophysin [ESN]) in a postpartum woman. Each vertical bar corresponds to a suckling episode. Neurophysin release parallels oxytocin release. Some episodes of hormone release, at night, are spontaneous and unrelated to nursing. (From Stern J, D'Amico J, Robinson AG, et al, unpublished.)

Human studies for defining the role of oxytocin in labor are limited, but in guinea pigs (who resemble humans in the mechanism of labor) oxytocin antagonists delay the onset and intensity of the expulsive phase and normal progress of labor.[130] It is perhaps of greater importance that there is a dramatic increase in oxytocin receptors in the uterus at term[129] and that oxytocin is secreted by the fetal chorion in the pregnant uterus at term,[134] findings that suggest a paracrine control system for initiating labor.

Intermediate Lobe

The intermediate lobe of the pituitary is derived embryologically from the posterior wall of Rathke's pouch and is well developed in most vertebrates, including the human fetus. In adults, however, the intermediate lobe decreases in size during the first two decades of life, leaving a small number of pro-opiomelanocortin (POMC)-synthesizing cells along the border of the anterior and neural lobes.[58, 135] In the adult it is referred to as "zona intermedia" rather than "pars intermedia." However, the α-melanocyte-stimulating hormone (α-MSH) found in some anterior pituitary cells (which has been taken to be a marker of the intermediate lobe) may actually be the product of anterior lobe corticotropin cells, so the existence of even a rudimentary functional intermediate lobe in the human must be questioned.[135]

In amphibians the intermediate lobe regulates secretion of MSH.[136, 137] MSH increases skin pigmentation by stimulating the dispersion of melanin granules in melanocytes; this function is the basis of environmentally adaptive pigmentation in frogs and salamanders. In rodents the intermediate lobe is innervated by a dopamine-secreting neural pathway from the hypothalamus (*tuberoinfundibular*) that tonically suppresses MSH secretion.[138] Hypertrophy of the intermediate lobe follows pituitary stalk section.

Melanocyte-Stimulating Hormones (MSH, Melanocortins)

The major MSH of the intermediate lobe, α-MSH, is synthesized as part of the large prohormone POMC, which is also the precursor of corticotropin, β-lipotropin (β-LPH), and β-endorphin in the anterior pituitary and of a number of corticotropin-related peptides in hypothalamic neurons (Fig. 8–14) (see Chapter 9).[139–141] Although the prohormone sequence is identical in the anterior lobe, intermediate lobe,

siveness to oxytocin. In the human (and guinea pig) a fall in progesterone triggers the onset of labor, but not by stimulating secretion of oxytocin.[126, 130] After labor begins, however, maternal oxytocin secretion, triggered by reflexes arising from the contracting uterus, increases and reaches a maximum at the time of delivery.[126] Women with DI have relatively normal pregnancies and delivery,[128, 131, 132] but oxytocin may be secreted normally in DI.[131, 132] In one woman with established oxytocin deficiency labor was reportedly normal.[133]

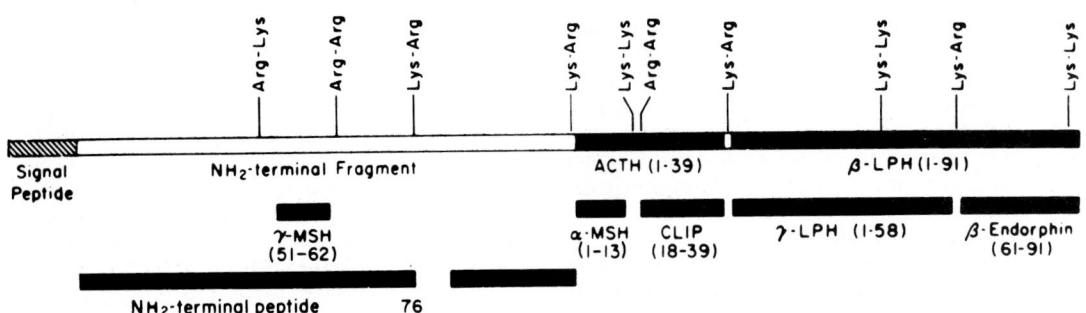

Figure 8–14. Organization of POMC, the precursor hormone of corticotropin (ACTH on figure), β-LPH, and related peptides. The precursor protein contains a leader sequence (signal peptide), followed by a long fragment that includes sequence 51–62 corresponding to γ-MSH. This fragment is cleaved at Lys-Arg bonds to form corticotropin 1–39, which in turn includes the sequences for α-MSH (corticotropin 1–13) and corticotropin-like intermediate lobe peptide (CLIP) (corticotropin 18–39), and a sequence corresponding to β-LPH (1–91) that includes γ-LPH 1–58), and β-endorphin (61–91). The β-endorphin sequence also includes a sequence corresponding to met-enkephalin (see also Fig. 8–40 for a more detailed description of met-enkephalin, which makes up the first five amino acids of β-endorphin 61–91). As outlined by Krieger[141] the precursor molecule in the anterior lobe of the pituitary is processed predominantly to corticotropin and β-LPH. In the intermediate pituitary lobe (in the rat), corticotropin and β-LPH are further processed to α-MSH and a β-endorphin–like material. In all extrapituitary tissues, post-translational processing of the prohormone resembles that in the intermediate lobe. Hypothalamic processing is similar but not identical to that in the intermediate lobe. In the latter, β-endorphin and α-MSH are present predominantly in their acetylated forms. β-LPH, β-lipotropin; γ-MSH; γ-melanocyte–stimulating hormone; α-MSH, α-melanocyte–stimulating hormone; γ-LPH, γ-lipotropin.

and hypothalamic neurons, the formation of the active hormones in these sites differs owing to variations in post-translational processing. In the intermediate lobe the initial proteolytic cleavages appear to be the same as those in anterior pituitary corticotropes, but most β-LPH is processed to γ-LPH and β-endorphin. The latter is converted to a variety of endorphin-related products that are not detectable in the anterior lobe, and corticotropin is broken down to form α-MSH and a fragment corresponding to corticotropin 18–39 (designated corticotropin-like intermediate lobe peptide [CLIP]). Many of the peptides are acetylated. In addition, POMC in the intermediate lobe is regulated primarily by dopamine and serotonin, whereas POMC gene expression in the anterior lobe is regulated by glucocorticoids[140, 141] and CRH[142] (see later).[159] Peptides with sequences resembling α-MSH (including corticotropin) are called *melanocortins* and are capable of binding to melanocortin receptors (see later). MSH-secreting neurons in the brain are regulated differently from those in the intermediate lobe. The central melanocortin neural system is discussed later in the section on regulation of tuberohypophyseal neurons. MSH may also be a prolactin-releasing factor (PRF) (see later in the section on prolactin regulation).

Intermediate lobe POMC cells may give rise to basophilic adenomas that cause Cushing's disease in humans, as also appears to be the case in dogs and horses.[143–145] The biologic behavior of such tumors is more aggressive than that of tumors of anterior lobe corticotropes.

Hypophyseotropic Neuronal System: Median Eminence and Tuberoinfundibular and Tuberohypophyseal Neurons

ANATOMY. The median eminence of the hypothalamus is the site at which anterior pituitary–regulating hypothalamic neurons release their secretions into the capillaries of the primary plexus of the hypophyseal-portal system (Figs. 8–15 to 8–23).[10, 18, 29, 56, 57, 146–166] The median eminence has three components: *neural,* consisting of nerve terminals and neurons in passage; *vascular,* consisting of the primary capillary plexus and the portal veins; and *epithelial,* consisting of the pars tuberalis of the anterior pituitary gland. Special features include densely packed nerve endings, capillaries with conspicuous perivascular spaces and fenestrations, supporting cells, and ependymal cells. One variety of ependymal cell, the tanycyte, traverses the median eminence from the lumen of the third ventricle to the outer mantle plexus. Nerve endings in the median eminence are the terminals of the *tuberohypophyseal* neurons, which arise chiefly in the mediobasal hypothalamus and include fibers from the supraoptico- and paraventricular magnicellular neurons.

Two types of tuberohypophyseal neurons project to the median eminence: peptide secreting (peptidergic) (e.g., TRH, LHRH, and somatostatin) and bioaminergic, the most important of which are dopaminergic. Some peptides in nerve endings are not released into the hypophyseal-portal circulation[153] but instead function to regulate the secretion of other nerve terminals (see later).

The anatomic relationships of nerve endings, basement membranes, interstitial spaces, fenestrated (windowed) capillary endothelia, and glia in the median eminence are similar to those in the neural lobe. As in the case of the neurohypophysis, the release of neuropeptides is stimulated by depolarization and neuromediators that lead to increased uptake of Ca^{2+}. Secretion at median eminence terminals is analogous to that in the neurohypophysis. The large contact area of the perivascular space and the special vessels in this region, whose fenestrations are similar to those of capillaries in ordinary endocrine glands, account for the fact that in contrast to

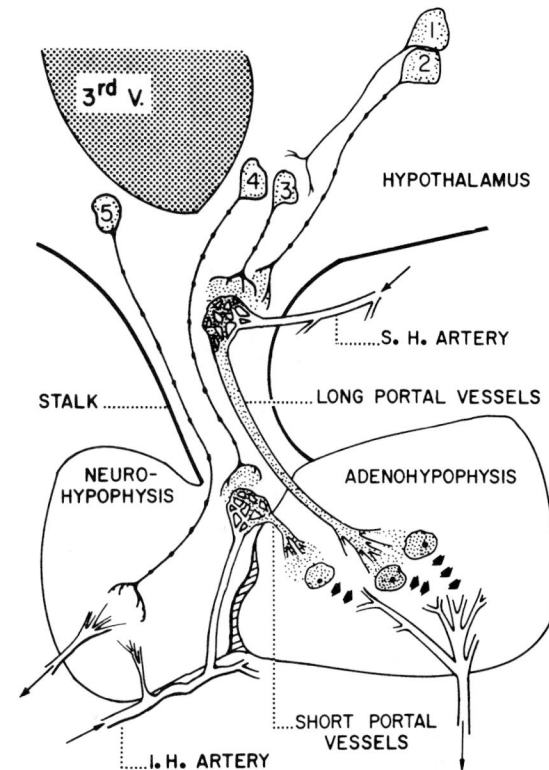

Figure 8–15. Neural control of the pituitary gland. This figure summarizes the types of neural input into pituitary regulation. Neuron 5 represents the peptidergic neurons of the supraopticohypophyseal and paraventriculohypophyseal tracts with hormone-producing cell bodies in the hypothalamus and nerve terminals in the neural lobe. Neurons 4 and 3 are the neurons of the tuberoinfundibular tract that secrete the hypophyseotropic hormones into the substance of the median eminence in anatomic relationship to the primary plexus. Neuron 1 represents a monoaminergic neuron ending in relation to the cell body of the peptidergic neuron. Neuron 2 represents a monoaminergic neuron ending on terminals of the peptidergic neuron to give axoaxonic transmission. Neurons 1 and 2 are the functional links between the remainder of the brain and the peptidergic neuron. Not shown are the fibers of the tuberohypophyseal tract. In certain animal species (but not in humans) these fibers arise in the arcuate nucleus of the hypothalamus and terminate on the cells of the intermediate lobe. In adult humans the intermediate lobe is vestigial. (From Gay VL. The hypothalamus: physiology and clinical use of releasing factors. Fertil Steril 23:51, 1972. Reproduced with permission of the publisher, The American Fertility Society.)

most of the brain, the neurohypophysis (including the median eminence) is permeable to molecules such as thyroxine (T_4) and growth hormone (GH). No synapses have been identified in the median eminence; hence these structures can be regarded as "presynaptic."[155]

The special structure of the median eminence thus allows the feedback effects of pituitary and pituitary–target gland hormones. However, the median eminence is not the only region of the hypothalamus where neuroactive substances interact. Throughout the regulatory areas of the hypothalamus hypophyseotropic neurons are innervated by neurons that secrete neurotransmitters and regulatory neuropeptides. These local feedback circuits interact with neurons projecting from other parts of the brain and with circulating hormones.[152]

Non-neuronal supporting cells in the hypothalamus also play a dynamic role in hypophyseotropic regulation. For example nerve terminals in the neurohypophysis are enveloped by glia (in the neural lobe they are called pituicytes); when the gland is inactive they surround the nerve endings, whereas the nerve ending is exposed when vasopressin secretion is enhanced as in states of dehydration. Within the median eminence, LHRH nerve endings are enveloped by the special-

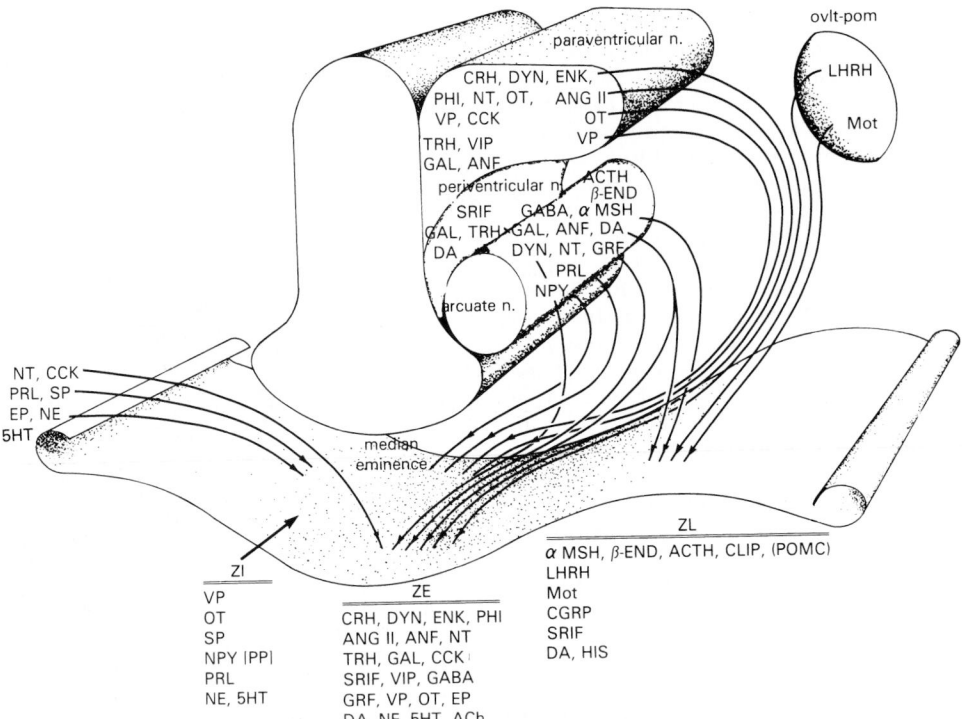

Figure 8–16. Diagrammatic representation of a number of peptides and neurotransmitters that terminate in the median eminence, together with their origin. ACh, acetylcholine; ACTH, corticotropin; ANF, atrial natriuretic peptide; ANG II, angiotensin II; CCK, cholecystokinin; CGRP, calcitonin gene-related peptide; CLIP, corticotropin-like intermediate lobe peptide; CRH, corticotropin-releasing hormone; DA, dopamine; DYN, dynorphin; β-END, β-endorphin; ENK, enkephalin; EP, epinephrine; 5HT, 5-hydroxytryptamine; GABA, γ-aminobutyric acid; GAL, galanin; GRF, growth hormone-releasing hormone; HIS, histamine; LHRH, luteinizing hormone–releasing hormone; Mot, motilin; α-MSH, α-melanocyte–stimulating hormone; n., nucleus; NE, norepinephrine; NPY, neuropeptide Y; NT, neurotensin; OT, oxytocin; ovlt-pom, organum vasculosum of the lamina terminalis–preoptic medial nucleus; PHI, peptide-histidine-isoleucine; POMC, pro-opiomelanocortin; PRL, prolactin; SP, substance P; SRIF, somatostatin; TRH, thyrotropin-releasing hormone; VIP, vasoactive intestinal peptide; VP, vasopressin; ZE, zona exterior; ZI, zona interior; ZL, zona lateralis. (From Jacobowitz DM. Multifactorial control of pituitary hormone secretion: the "wheels" of the brain. Synapse 1988; 2:186–192, with permission.)

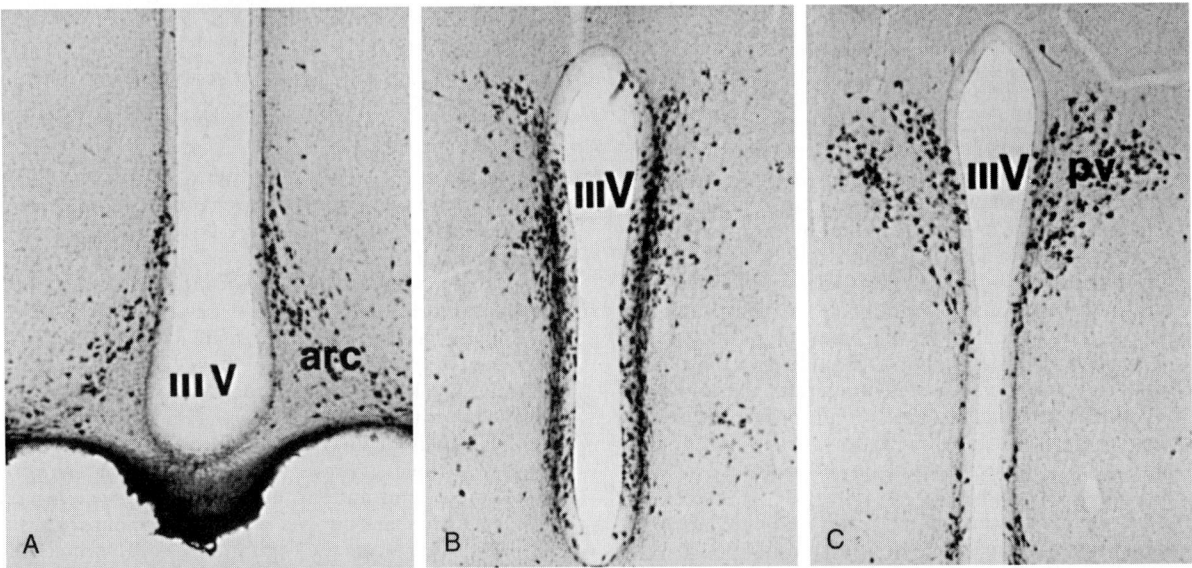

Figure 8–17. The tuberoinfundibular neuron system revealed by retrograde transport of wheat germ agglutinin. The location of cell bodies of neurons projecting to the median eminence of the hypothalamus can be traced (as in this study by Lechan and colleagues[158]) by injecting a small tracer dose of wheat germ agglutinin into the median eminence of the rat (A). Tracer, which is a lectin, binds to carbohydrate groups on nerve endings, is taken up into the cell by endocytosis, and is transported in retrograde fashion to be localized in cell bodies. Principal groups are the arcuate nucleus (arc), periventricular nucleus (which forms a feltwork of fibers and cells around the third ventricle) (IIIV) (B), and the small cell division of the paraventricular nucleus (C) (pv). Note that the distribution of cell bodies in the paraventricular nucleus differs somewhat from that shown for the neurohypophyseal peptides (see Fig. 8–8). Those projecting to the neural lobe are larger, are located laterally in the nucleus, and do not contain the retrograde tracer that was injected into the median eminence. (From Lechan RM, Nestler JL, Jacobson S. The tuberoinfundibular system of the rat as demonstrated by immunohistochemical localization of retrogradely transported wheat germ agglutinin [WGA] from the median eminence. Brain Res 1982; 245:1–15.)

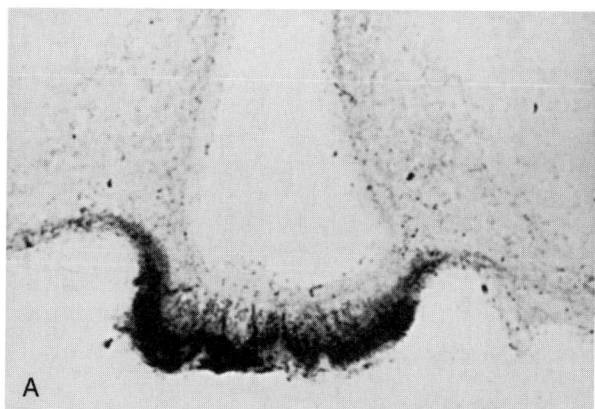

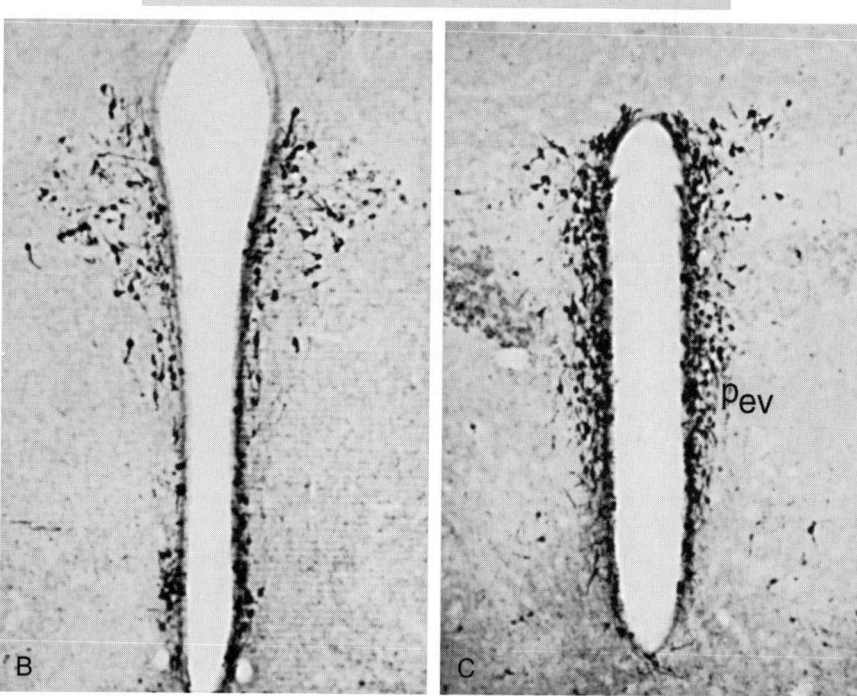

Figure 8–18. *A,* External median eminence of the rat, showing immunoreactive somatostatin in nerve terminals. *B,* Periventricular plexus (Pev) of somatostatin-containing cells in the anterior hypothalamus of the rat. The distribution corresponds well with the location of the periventricular plexus that contains retrogradely transported wheat germ agglutinin (see Fig. 8–17). *C,* The medial division of the paraventricular nucleus contains many somatostatin-positive cells. Note again the close similarity of these cells to those that project to the median eminence (see Fig. 8–17). (*A* courtesy of Dr. Ronald M. Lechan. From Lechan RM, Goodman RH, Rosenblatt M, et al. Prosomatostatin-specific antigen in rat brain: localization by immunocytochemical staining with an antiserum to a synthetic sequence of preprosomatostatin. Proc Natl Acad Sci USA 1983; 80:2780–2784, with permission.)

ized ependyma called *tanycytes,* which also cover or uncover neurons with changes in functional status. Hypothalamic astrocytes (a form of supporting glia) express somatostatin when exposed to the inflammatory cytokine IL-1. Astrocytes also secrete glutamate and NO, which are both excitatory neurotransmitters. Thus, supporting elements, with their own sets of receptors, can change the neuroregulatory milieu within the hypothalamus and median eminence.

Although most axons of the supraopticohypophyseal and paraventriculohypophyseal tracts pass *through* the median eminence on their way from cells of origin in the hypothalamus to their termination in the neural lobe, some paraventricular neurons project to the median eminence and play regulatory roles for corticotropin and prolactin (PRL) secretion.

The blood vessels in the primary plexus vary among species. In humans the capillaries penetrate the infundibulum and stalk to form loops and complex spiral structures termed *gomitoli.* Arterioles of the stalk and median eminence in humans have highly muscular walls, suggesting that hemodynamic changes in these vessels might affect pituitary function. Reflex constriction of these vessels after postpartum hemorrhage might be a factor in the genesis of pituitary infarction.

Blood reaches the plexus of the median eminence and upper stalk by way of the superior hypophyseal branch of the internal carotid artery (see Fig. 8–22). This plexus is drained by the long portal veins that run along the stalk and drain into the pituitary sinusoids. The capillary plexus in the lower portion of the stalk is supplied by the inferior hypophyseal artery and is drained by short portal veins that enter the pituitary almost directly. Blood flow in the long portal vessels is predominantly from the hypothalamus to the pituitary, but reverse flow from the pituitary to the median eminence may also occur by way of the short portal vessels that drain both the anterior and the posterior pituitary.[18, 156] However, any reverse flow of blood from the pituitary to the brain is minor.[56, 157]

The third component of the median eminence, the pars tuberalis, is a thin glandular sheath around the infundibulum and pituitary stalk. In some animals the epithelial component may make up as much as 10% of the total glandular tissue of the pituitary and contains pituitary tropic hormones including luteinizing hormone (LH) and thyrotropin. A physiological function of the pars tuberalis has not been established, but the fact that melatonin receptors are present suggests that it may influence pituitary function.

The cells of origin of the pituitary regulatory peptides have a distinct anatomic distribution, but all converge on the median eminence where they come into contact with the capillaries of the hypophyseal-portal plexus (see Figs. 8–18 to 8–21).[146–154, 158–166]

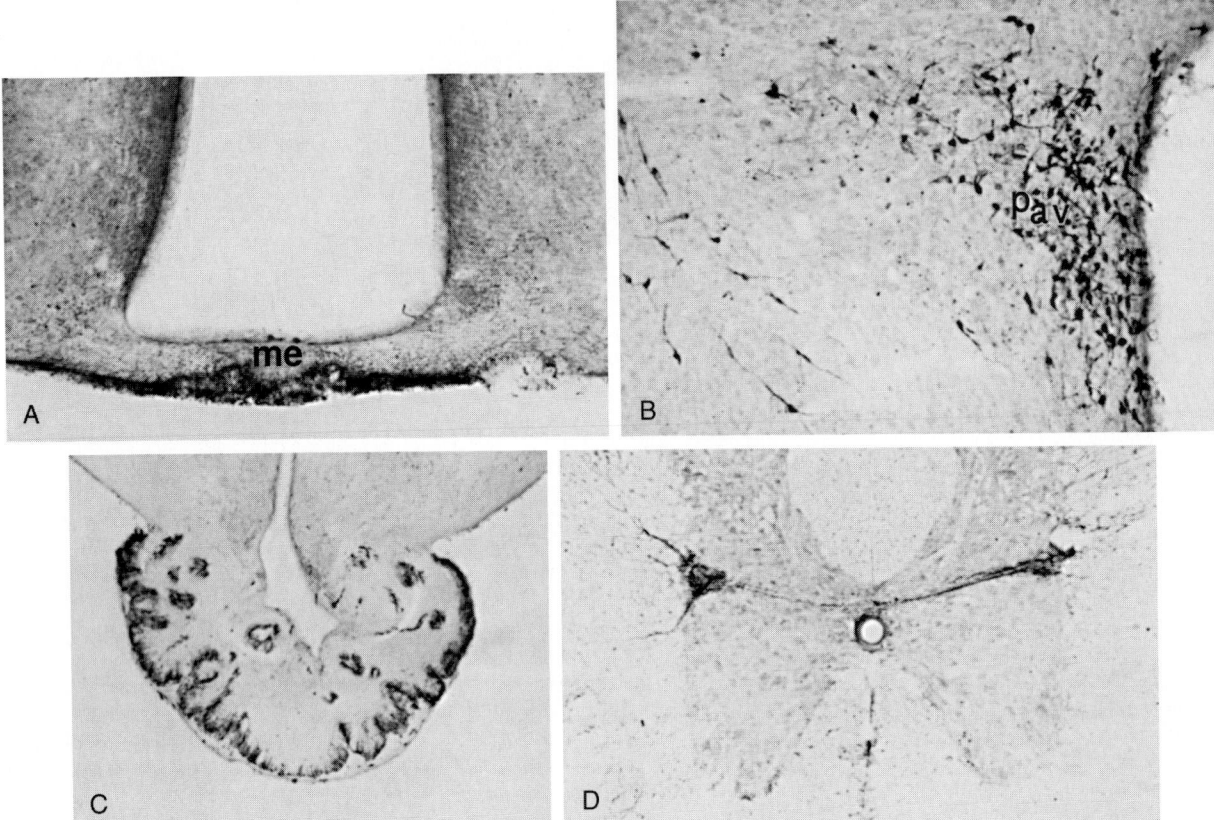

Figure 8–19. *A,* Distribution of thyrotropin-releasing hormone (TRH) immunoreactivity in the stalk–median eminence (me) of the rat. *B,* TRH-immunoreactive cell bodies in the medial division of the paraventricular nucleus (Pav) of the rat. *C,* TRH-immunoreactive nerve endings in the median eminence of the rhesus monkey. *D,* Transverse section of the upper thoracic spinal cord of the rat showing the distribution of TRH-immunoreactive fibers terminating in the intermediolateral column (site of the preganglionic sympathetic nervous system). (All figures courtesy of Dr. Ronald M. Lechan. *A* and *B* from Lechan RM, Jackson IM. Immunohistochemical localization of thyrotropin-releasing hormone in the rat hypothalamus and pituitary. Endocrinology 1982; 111:55–65. © 1982, The Endocrine Society. *C* from Lechan R, Lin HD, Ling N, et al. Distribution of immunoreactive growth hormone releasing factor [1–44]NH₂ in the tuberoinfundibular system of the rhesus monkey. Brain Res 1984; 309:55–61. *D* from Jackson IM. Thyrotropin-releasing hormone. Reprinted, by permission of the New England Journal of Medicine 306; 145–155, 1982.)

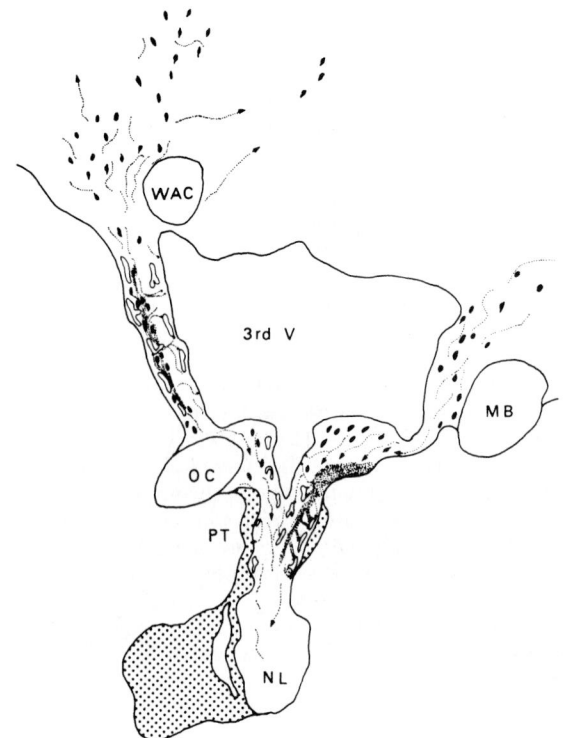

Figure 8–20. Distribution of cell bodies and fiber trajectories containing immunoreactive luteinizing hormone–releasing hormone (LHRH) in the human fetus. Note the heavy concentration in the septum and preoptic area and anterior commissure. PT, pars tuberalis; NL, neural lobe; OC, optic chiasm; MB, mamillary body; WAC, anterior commissure. (From Bugnon C, Bloch H, Lenys D, et al. Cytoimmunochemical study of the LHRH neurons in humans during fetal life. In: Scott DE, Kozlowski GP, Weindl A, eds. Neural Hormones and Reproduction. Basel: S. Karger, 1978: 183–196, with permission.)

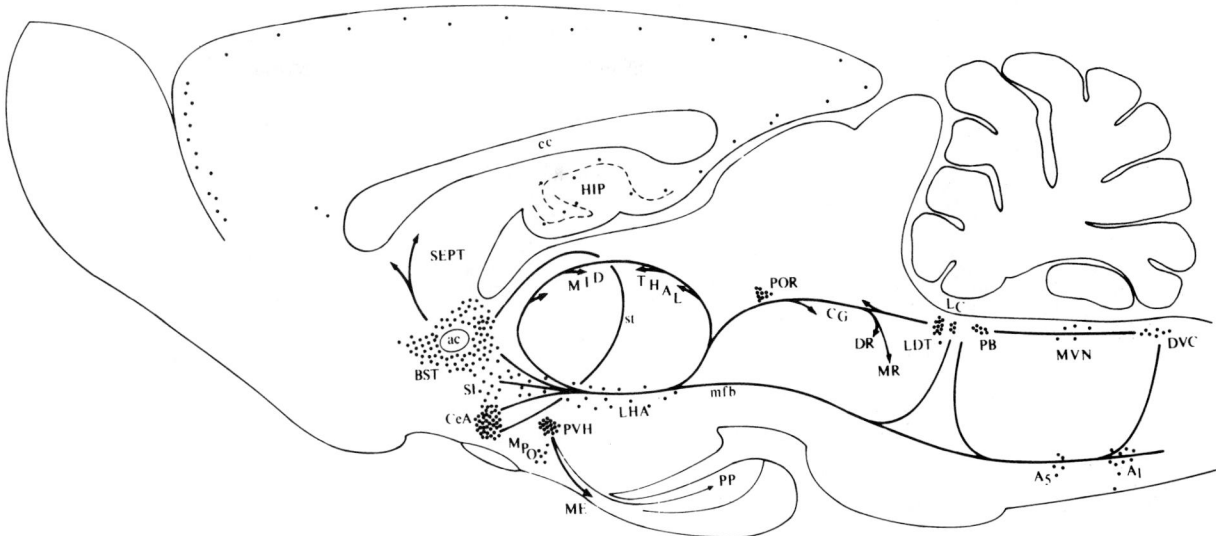

Figure 8–21. Major corticotropin-releasing hormone (CRH)-immunoreactive cells in the rat brain. The principal fibers regulating the anterior pituitary are shown as arising from the paraventricular nucleus (PVH), but there is an extensive distribution elsewhere, especially around the hypothalamus. A₁, noradrenergic cell group 1; A₅, noradrenergic cell group 5; ac, anterior commissure; BST, bed nucleus of the stria terminalis; cc, corpus callosum; CeA, central nucleus amygdala; CG, central gray; DR, dorsal raphe; DVC, dorsal vagal complex; HIP, hippocampus; LC, locus coeruleus; LDT, laterodorsal tegmental nucleus; LHA, lateral hypothalamic area; ME, median eminence; MID THAL, midline thalamic nuclei; mfb, medial forebrain bundle; MPO, medial preoptic area; MR, medial raphe; MVN, medial vestibular nucleus; PB, parabrachial nucleus; POR, perioculomotor nucleus; PP, posterior pituitary; PVH, periventricular nucleus; SEPT, septal region; SI, substantia innominata; st, stria. (From Swanson LW, Sawchenko PE, Rivier J, et al. Organization of ovine corticotropin-releasing factor immunoreactive cells and fibers in the rat brain: an immunohistochemical study. Neuroendocrinology 1983; 36:165–186.)

Figure 8–22. In this drawing of a pituitary vascular cast, the posterior portion of the infundibulum has been removed. The arrows demonstrate the potential efferent routes from the neurohypophysis: (1) portal vessels may convey blood to the adenohypophysis; (2) confluent pituitary veins may carry blood to the cavernous sinus; (3) blood may flow from the infundibulum to the hypothalamus via connecting capillaries; (4) tanycytes may transport some substances into the ventricle; (5) substances may leak through the endothelial fenestrations of portal vessels into the subarachnoid space; (6) certain hypophyseal arteries may, under certain conditions, serve as efferent vascular channels; and (7) retrograde axonal flow may carry substances from the neurohypophysis to the hypothalamus. Five of these routes are directed toward the brain. Follow-up studies indicate that in sheep there is little or no significant retrograde flow of blood above the median eminence. (From Bergland RM, Page RB. Can the pituitary secrete directly to the brain? [affirmative anatomical evidence]. Endocrinology 102, 1325–1338, 1978, © by The Endocrine Society.)

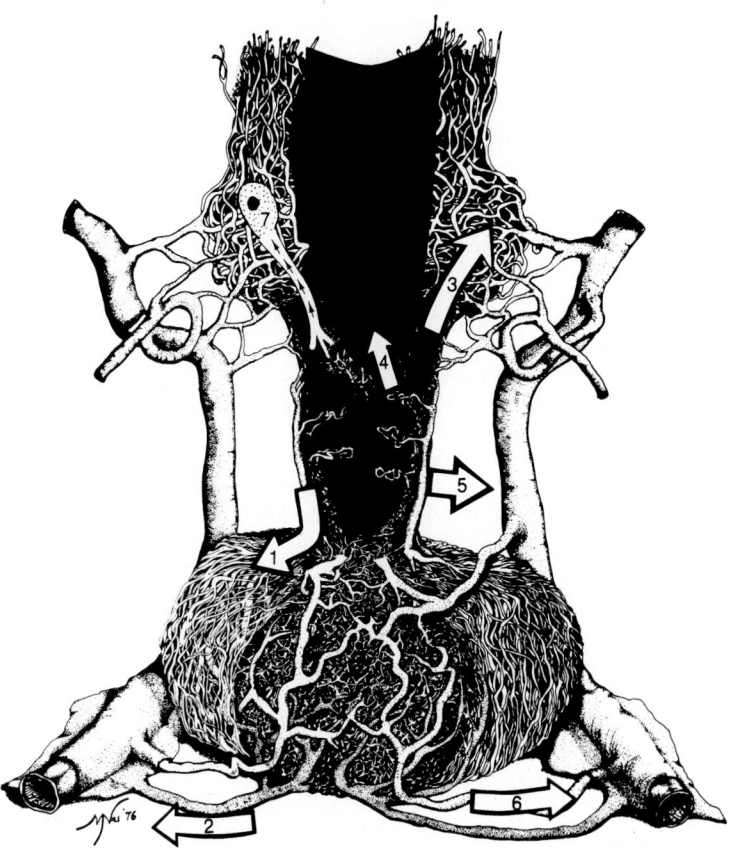

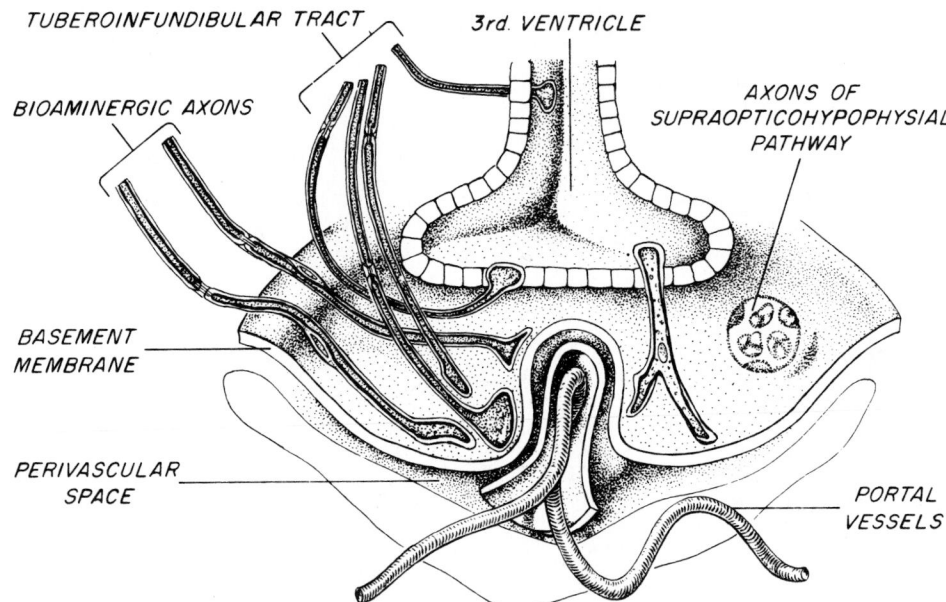

Figure 8–23. Diagram of anatomic relationships of important secretory structures in the median eminence, visualized as if one were looking rostrally at a cut section. The interstitial space in which all the nerve endings terminate is a free pool without a blood-brain barrier. It is separated from the lumen of the third ventricle by ependyma, whose tight junctions prevent direct diffusion from the medial eminence to the third ventricle lumen. Tuberoinfundibular neurons—some peptidergic, some bioaminergic—end in the interstitial space; many, but not all, end directly on capillary loops. Few if any true axoaxonic synapses are found here. Stretching between the lumen and the outer third of the median eminence are tanycytes, which are specialized cells that may have transport functions. The supraopticohypophyseal pathway is shown as a cut section of fibers in passage, but it should be recognized that some of the neurohypophyseal neurons end in the median eminence.

PORTAL VESSEL–CHEMOTRANSMITTER CONTROL. The hypophyseal–portal vessel–chemotransmitter hypothesis of pituitary control provides an explanation of how the anterior pituitary gland, which is devoid of secretomotor nerve fibers, is influenced by the nervous system.[167–170] Validation of the concept has come from the chemical identification of hypothalamic hormones, the demonstration of their presence in neuronal pathways projecting to the median eminence, and the documentation of their presence in blood collected from the hypophyseal-portal veins.

Hypophyseotropic Hormones of the Hypothalamus

The search for hypothalamic neurohormones with anterior pituitary–regulating properties focused on extracts of stalk median eminence neural lobe and hypothalamus.[171] Such hypophyseotropic materials were called *releasing factors* after the initial designation of corticotropin-releasing factor (now known as CRH). This factor was first extracted from neural lobe or hypothalamic tissues that stimulated the release of corticotropin from pituitary fragments maintained in organ culture.[171] In current usage, the term *releasing factor* is applied to hypothalamic substances of unknown chemical nature, whereas substances with established chemical identity are referred to as *releasing hormones*. The first hypophyseotropic hormone to be chemically defined was TRH.[172, 173]

All of the hypothalamic pituitary-regulating hormones are peptides with the exception of dopamine, which is a biogenic amine that is the principal prolactin-inhibiting factor (PIF) (Table 8–4). All are now available for human investigation and treatment, and therapeutic analogues have been synthesized for dopamine, LHRH, and somatostatin.

In addition to regulating hormone release, the hypophyseotropic factors control pituitary cell differentiation and proliferation and hormone synthesis. Somatostatin and dopamine are inhibitory and some act on more than one pituitary hormone. For example TRH is a potent releaser of PRL and of thyrotropin and under some circumstances releases corticotropin and GH. LHRH releases both LH and follicle-stimulating hormone (FSH). Somatostatin inhibits the secretion of GH, thyrotropin, and a wide variety of nonpituitary hormones. The principal inhibitor of PRL secretion, dopamine, also inhibits secretion of thyrotropin, gonadotropin and, under certain conditions, GH. Dual control is exerted by the interaction of inhibitory and stimulatory hypothalamic hormones. For example somatostatin interacts with growth hormone–releasing hormone (GHRH) and TRH to control secretion of GH and thyrotropin, respectively, and dopamine interacts with PRFs to regulate PRL secretion. Some hypothalamic hormones act synergistically, e.g., in regulating the secretion of corticotropin by CRH, vasopressin, and epinephrine (derived from the general circulation).

Secretion of the releasing hormones in turn is regulated

TABLE 8–4. Structural Formulas of Principal Human Hypothalamic Peptides Directly Related to Pituitary Secretion

Vasopressin

Cys-Tyr-Phe-Gln-Asn-Cys-Pro-Arg-Gly-NH$_2$ (MW = 1084.38)

Oxytocin

Cys-Tyr-Ile-Gln-Asn-Cys-Pro-Leu-Gly-NH$_2$ (MW = 1007.35)

Thyrotropin-Releasing Hormone

pGlu-His-Pro-NH$_2$ (MW = 362.42)

Luteinizing Hormone–Releasing Hormone (Gonadotropin-Releasing Hormone)

pGlu-His-Trp-Ser-Tyr-Gly-Leu-Arg-Pro-Gly-NH$_2$ (MW = 1182.39)

Corticotropin-Releasing Hormone (Human, Rat)

Ser-Glu-Glu-Pro-Pro-Ile-Ser-Leu-Asp-Leu-Thr-Phe-His-Leu-Leu-Arg-Glu-Val-Leu-Glu-Met-Ala-Arg-Ala-Glu-Gln-Leu-Ala-Gln-Gln-Ala-His-Ser-Asn-Arg-Lys-Leu-Met-Glu-Ile-Ile-NH$_2$ (MW = 4758.14)

Growth Hormone–Releasing Hormone (GHRH 1–40, 1–44-NH$_2$, Human)

Tyr-Ala-Asp-Ala-Ile-Phe-Thr-Asn-Ser-Tyr-Arg-Lys-Val-Leu-Gly-Gln-Leu-Ser-Ala-Arg-Lys-Leu-Leu-Gln-Asp-Ile-Met-Ser-Arg-Gln-Gln-Gly-Glu-Ser-Asn-Gln-Glu-Arg-Gly-Ala (MW = 4544.73), [-Arg-Ala-Arg-Leu-NH$_2$] (MW = 5040.4)

Somatostatin

Ala-Gly-Cys-Lys-Asn-Phe-Phe-Trp-Lys-Thr-Phe-Thr-Ser-Cys (MW = 1638.12)

Somatostatin-28

Ser-Ala-Asn-Ser-Asn-Pro-Ala-Met-Ala-Pro-Arg-Glu-Arg-Lys-Ala-Gly-Cys-Lys-Asn-Phe-Phe-Trp-Lys-Thr-Phe-Thr-Ser-Cys (MW = 3149.00)

Somatostatin-28 (1–12)

Ser-Ala-Asn-Ser-Asn-Pro-Ala-Met-Ala-Pro-Arg-Glu (MW = 1244.49)

Vasoactive Intestinal Peptide (Human, Pig, Rat)

His-Ser-Asp-Ala-Val-Phe-Thr-Asp-Asn-Tyr-Thr-Arg-Leu-Arg-Lys-Gln-Met-Ala-Val-Lys-Lys-Tyr-Leu-Asn-Ser-Ile-Leu-Asn-NH$_2$ (MW = 3326.26)

MW, molecular weight.

c DNA

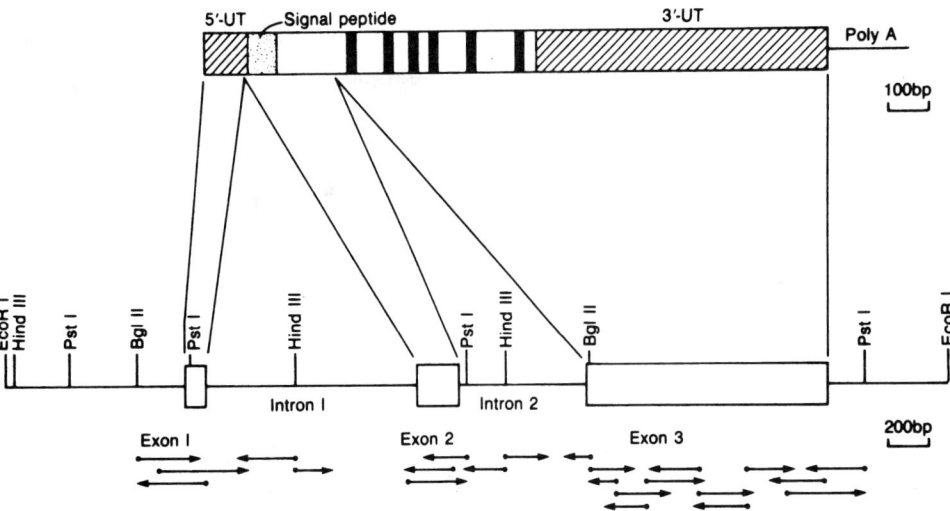

Genomic DNA

Figure 8–24. Structure of human *TRH* gene, showing six repeating codons for the TRH sequence. (From Yamada M, Radovick S, Wondisford FE, et al. Cloning and structure of human genomic DNA and hypothalamic cDNA encoding human preprothyrotropin-releasing hormone. Mol Endocrinol 1990; 4:551–556, with permission.)

by neurotransmitters and neuropeptides that interact with hormones such as glucocorticoids, gonadal steroids, and thyroid hormone. Control is also exerted by anterior pituitary hormones (short-loop feedback control) and hypophyseotropic factors themselves (ultrashort-loop feedback control).

The distribution of the hypophyseotropic hormones is not limited to the hypothalamus. Most are also found in extrahypothalamic regions of the brain and in other organs where they may have functions (e.g., effects on behavior or homeostasis) unrelated to pituitary regulation.

Thyrotropin-Releasing Hormone

CHEMISTRY AND EVOLUTION. TRH is a tripeptide, pyroGlu-His-Pro-NH$_2$.[174, 175] An intact amide and the cyclized glutamic acid terminus are essential for activity.[176, 178] TRH is synthesized as part of a large prohormone that contains five repeating sequences in the rat[178, 179] and six in the human (Fig. 8–24).[180] The prohormone undergoes extensive post-translational processing, including enzymatic cleavage, cyclization of NH$_2$-terminal glutamic acid, and exchange of an amide for the COOH-terminal glycine (see Fig. 8–24).

Although the TRH tripeptide is the only established hormone encoded within its large prohormone, other sequences may have biologic function: TRH mRNA and TRH prohormone are present in several types of neurons that do not express TRH[152, 181]; the sequence prepro-TRH(160–169), which is presumably released during precursor enzymatic processing, potentiates the thyrotropin-releasing effects of TRH[182]; and the message for the prepro-TRH(178–199) sequence, when expressed in a corticotropin-secreting cell line, inhibits corticotropin release.[183]

The concentration of TRH in neural tissues outside the hypothalamus is increased in lower animals so that in the frog, for example, the level in the extrahypothalamic brain is half that in the hypothalamus.[184] In some species of frogs TRH concentrations in skin are higher than those in the hypothalamus, an association presumed to be related to the embryologic origin of both skin and brain from neuroectoderm. TRH is present in primitive vertebrates (the larval form of the lamprey), in *Amphioxus* (a provertebrate), and in nerve ganglia of the snail. Since the lamprey probably does not synthesize thyrotropin and since *Amphioxus* and snails lack a pituitary

gland, the TRH molecule probably developed originally as a primitive neurosecretion before the evolution of thyrotropin, and the pituitary "co-opted" TRH as its regulatory hormone.[184] The increasing specialization of regulatory factors as the phylogenetic scale is ascended is a general feature of the evolution of neuropeptides and neurotransmitters.

EFFECTS ON THE PITUITARY GLAND AND MECHANISM OF ACTION. After intravenous injection of TRH in humans, serum thyrotropin levels rise within a few minutes (Fig. 8–25),[185–187] followed by a rise in serum triiodothyronine (T$_3$) levels; there is an increase in T$_4$ release as well, but a

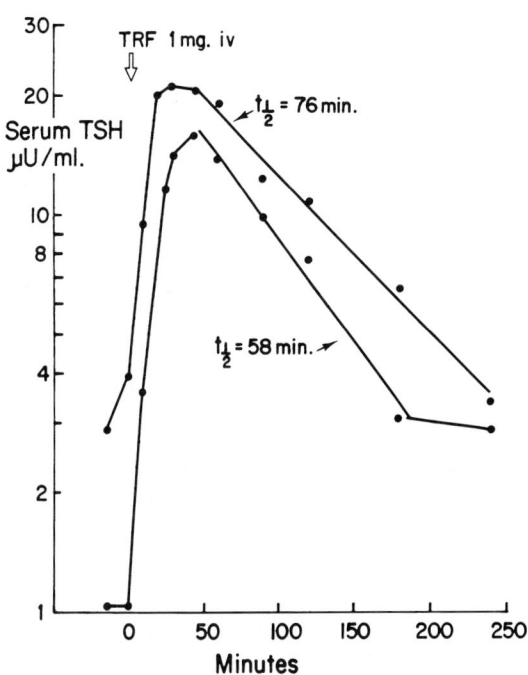

Figure 8–25. Effect of intravenous injection of TRH on serum thyrotropin levels in humans. TRF, thyrotropin-releasing hormone; TSH, thyrotropin. (From Hershman JM, Pittman JA Jr. Control of thyrotropin secretion in man. N Engl J Med 1971; 285:997–1006. Reprinted by permission of The New England Journal of Medicine, with permission.)

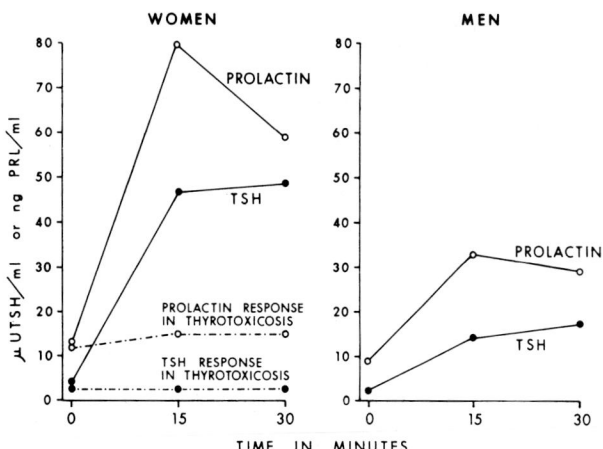

Figure 8–26. Prolactin (PRL) and thyrotropin (TSH on figure) secretory responses to intravenous injection of 800 μg of TRH in humans. This figure shows that TRH induces discharge of both PRL and thyrotropin, that the effect in females is greater than that in males (presumably owing to estrogen sensitization of the pituitary), and that thyrotoxicosis inhibits the response of both PRL and thyrotropin to TRH. An inhibitory effect on the TRH response is noted at the upper limit of the normal range of thyroid hormone levels and is a sensitive test of minor degrees of thyroid hormone excess. Although TRH is a potent prolactin-releasing factor (PRF), there is evidence that there is another PRF physiologically connected to PRL regulation. (Replotted from data of Bowers S, Friesen HG, Hwang P, et al. Prolactin and thyrotropin release in man by synthetic pyrogluta-mylhistidyl-prolinamide. Biochem Biophys Res Commun 1971; 45:1033–1041, with permission.)

change in blood levels of T_4 usually is not demonstrable because the pool of circulating T_4 (most of which is bound to carrier proteins) is so large. The clinical applications of TRH testing are covered later in this chapter and in Chapter 11. TRH action on the pituitary is blocked by previous treatment with thyroid hormone, which is a crucial element in feedback control of pituitary thyrotropin secretion.

As noted earlier, TRH is a potent PRF (Fig. 8–26).[185–187] The time course of response of blood PRL levels to TRH, the dose-response characteristics, and the suppression by thyroid hormone pretreatment (all of which parallel changes in thyrotropin secretion) suggest that TRH may be involved in the regulation of PRL secretion. Moreover TRH is present in the hypophyseal-portal blood of lactating rats.[188] However it is unlikely to be a physiological regulator of PRL secretion[189, 190] because the PRL response to nursing in humans is unaccompanied by changes in plasma thyrotropin levels.[190] Nevertheless TRH may occasionally cause hyperprolactinemia (with or without galactorrhea) in patients with hypothyroidism.

In normal individuals TRH has no influence on the secretion of pituitary hormones other than thyrotropin and PRL, but it enhances the release of hGH in acromegaly and of corticotropin in some patients with Cushing's disease. Furthermore prolonged stimulation of the *normal* pituitary with GHRH can sensitize it to the hGH-releasing effects of TRH.[191, 192] TRH also causes the release of hGH in some patients with uremia, hepatic disease, anorexia nervosa, and psychotic depression[187] and in children with hypothyroidism. TRH inhibits sleep-induced hGH release through its actions in the central nervous system (see later in the section on extrapituitary actions of TRH).

Stimulatory effects of TRH are initiated by binding of the peptide to specific receptors on the plasma membrane of the thyrotrope.[193, 194] Neither thyroid hormone nor somatostatin, both of which antagonize the effects of TRH, interfere with its binding. TRH was originally thought to activate membrane adenylate cyclase to stimulate formation of cAMP,[187, 195] and cAMP in turn was thought to stimulate thyrotropin secretion. However, cAMP does not increase under all conditions of TRH-induced thyrotropin release,[196] and it is now clear that

TRH action is mediated mainly through hydrolysis of phosphatidylinositol, with phosphorylation of key protein kinases and an increase in intracellular free Ca^{2+} as the crucial step in postreceptor activation (see Chapter 5).[196–198] TRH effects can be mimicked by exposure to a Ca^{2+} ionophore and are partially abolished by a Ca^{2+}-free medium. TRH stimulates the formation of mRNAs coding for thyrotropin[199] and PRL,[200] thus confirming that this peptide is trophic as well as a releasing factor. The mechanism of action of TRH on tissues other than the pituitary, in particular the nervous system, has not been elucidated.

TRH is degraded to acid TRH and to the dipeptide histidylprolineamide that cyclizes nonenzymatically to histidylproline diketopiperazine (cyclic His-Pro).[201] Acid TRH has some behavioral effects in rats that are similar to those of TRH but no other proven actions. Cyclic His-Pro is reported to act as a PRF and to have other neural effects, including reversal of ethanol-induced sleep (TRH is also effective in this system), elevation of brain cyclic guanosine monophosphate levels, an increase in stereotypical behavior, modification of body temperature, and inhibition of eating behavior. Some of the effects of TRH may be mediated through cyclic His-Pro, but the fact that cyclic His-Pro is abundant in some areas and is not proportional to the amount of TRH suggests that the peptide may not be derived solely from TRH.[179, 203]

EXTRAHYPOTHALAMIC DISTRIBUTION AND FUNCTION. TRH is present in virtually all parts of the brain: cerebral cortex, circumventricular structures, neurohypophysis, pineal gland, and spinal cord (see Fig. 8–19).[152, 187, 202, 204–206] TRH is also found in pancreatic islet cells and in the gastrointestinal tract.[207] Although it exists in low concentration, the total amount in extrahypothalamic tissues exceeds the amount in the hypothalamus.

The extensive extrahypothalamic distribution of TRH, its localization in nerve endings, and the presence of TRH receptors in brain tissue suggest that TRH serves as a neurotransmitter or neuromodulator outside the hypothalamus. Neural effects of TRH are summarized in Table 8–5. TRH is a general stimulant[187, 208–210] and induces hyperthermia on intracerebroventricular injection, suggesting a role in central thermoregulation.

CLINICAL APPLICATIONS. The use of TRH for the diag-

TABLE 8–5. Central Nervous System–Mediated Actions of Thyrotropin-Releasing Hormone

Increases spontaneous motor activity
Alters sleep patterns
Produces anorexia
Inhibits conditioned avoidance behavior
Causes head-to-tail rotation
Opposes actions of barbiturates on sleeping time, hypothermia, lethality
Opposes actions of ethanol, chloral hydrate, chlorpromazine, and diazepam on sleeping time and hypothermia
Enhances convulsion time and lethality of strychnine
Increases motor activity in morphine-treated animals
Potentiates levodopa-pargyline effects
Ameliorates human behavioral disorders?
Causes central inhibition of morphine-mediated secretion of GH and PRL
Alters brain cell membrane electric activity
Increases norepinephrine turnover
Releases norepinephrine and dopamine from synaptosomal preparations
Enhances disappearance of norepinephrine from nerve terminals
Potentiates excitatory actions of acetylcholine on cerebral cortical neurons
Increases blood pressure
Protects against spinal shock
Improves motor function in lower motor neuron disease (amyotrophic lateral sclerosis)

GH, growth hormone; PRL, prolactin.
Modified from Vale W, Rivier C, Brown M. Regulatory peptides of the hypothalamus. Annu Rev Physiol 1977; 39:437–527. Reproduced, with permission, from the Annual Review of Physiology, Vol. 39, © 1977 by Annual Reviews Inc.

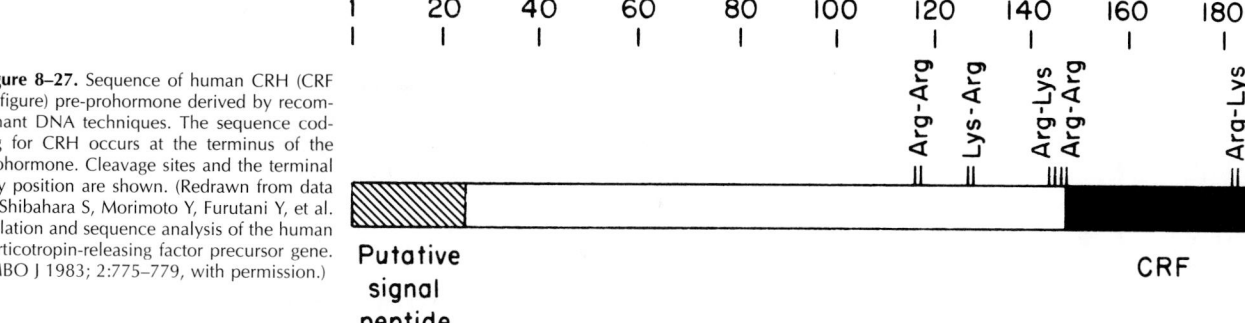

Figure 8–27. Sequence of human CRH (CRF in figure) pre-prohormone derived by recombinant DNA techniques. The sequence coding for CRH occurs at the terminus of the prohormone. Cleavage sites and the terminal Gly position are shown. (Redrawn from data of Shibahara S, Morimoto Y, Furutani Y, et al. Isolation and sequence analysis of the human corticotropin-releasing factor precursor gene. EMBO J 1983; 2:775–779, with permission.)

nosis of hyperthyroidism is less common since the development of ultrasensitive assays for TSH[187] (see Chapter 11); its use to discriminate between hypothalamic and pituitary causes of thyrotropin deficiency has also declined because of the test's poor specificity,[187, 212] but the application of ultrasensitive assays in conjunction with the TRH test has not been fully evaluated.[211] TRH testing also is not of value in the differential diagnosis of causes of hyperprolactinemia[213] but is useful for the demonstration of residual abnormal somatotropin-secreting cells in acromegalic patients who release hGH in response to TRH prior to treatment.

In some studies a beneficial effect of TRH has been reported in depressed patients, but most studies have found no value in treatment.[214] Although a role for TRH in depression is not established, many depressed patients have a blunted thyrotropin response to TRH, and changes in TRH responsiveness correlate with clinical course.[214] The mechanism by which blunting occurs is unknown.[215]

TRH has been proposed as a treatment for women with threatened premature labor to stimulate the production of lung surfactant in the preterm fetus. Despite encouraging results in early studies a large scale trial failed to show improvement in the survival of babies so treated.[216]

TRH has been evaluated for the treatment of spinal muscle atrophy and amyotrophic lateral sclerosis; transient improvement in strength was reported in both disorders[217–220] but the combined experience at many centers using a variety of treatment protocols including long-term intrathecal administration failed to confirm efficacy.[220–222] TRH administration also reduces the severity of experimentally induced spinal and ischemic shock,[223, 224] but no clinically useful therapeutic approaches have resulted from this line of research. TRH has been proposed to be an analeptic agent. Sleeping or drug-sedated animals are awakened by the administration of TRH,[225] TRH reportedly reversed sedative effects of ethanol in the human,[226] and TRH is said to have awakened a patient with a profound sleep disorder caused by a hypothalamic and midbrain eosinophilic granuloma.[227]

Corticotropin-Releasing Hormone

CHEMISTRY AND EVOLUTION. In 1955 Saffran and colleagues showed that the addition of an extract of neurohypophysis to pituitary incubates led to the release of corticotropin and coined the term *corticotropin-releasing factor.*[228] Simultaneously, Guillemin and Rosenberg showed that the addition of hypothalamic fragments to cultures of anterior pituitaries stimulated corticotropin secretion.[229] In 1981 the chemical structure of this factor, now designated CRH, was identified in ovine hypothalamic tissue, and the biologically active peptide was synthesized.[142, 230] Human CRH 1-41-NH$_2$[144, 232, 233] (see Table 8–4) differs from the ovine sequence by seven amino acids. Rat and human CRH are identical.

As with other neuropeptides CRH is synthesized as part of a prohormone and undergoes enzymatic modification to the amidated form (Fig. 8–27).[233] Mammalian CRH shares sequence homology with several peptides in lower animals, including sauvagine (derived from the skin of a certain species of frog), urotensin (the secretion of the caudal gland of a fish), and fish diuretic hormone; they are all potent releasers of corticotropin.[142, 230, 234, 235] A peptide in rat brain is homologous to both sauvagine and CRH and is even more potent as a corticotropin-releasing hormone than is CRH; this peptide, designated *urocortin,* binds to the type 2 CRH receptor. Its distribution in the brain and gastrointestinal tract suggests that it is involved in a wider range of nonpituitary functions than is CRH itself.[235]

The structure-function activities of CRH have received much attention because of the importance of developing agonist and antagonist analogues. The NH$_2$ terminus is not essential for action but removal of the terminal amide reduces activity.[142] Several potent antagonists have been synthesized.[236]

EFFECTS ON THE PITUITARY AND MECHANISM OF ACTION. The administration of CRH injection to humans causes a prompt release of corticotropin into the blood, followed by the secretion of cortisol (Fig. 8–28) and other adrenal steroids including aldosterone.[230–233, 237–239] Most studies have used ovine CRH, which is more potent and longer acting than human CRH, but human and porcine CRH appear to have equal diagnostic value.[232] The effect of CRH is specific to corticotropin release and is inhibited by glucocorticoids.

CRH acts by binding to specific receptors.[240–244] In the rat one form of the receptor is present in brain and another form is expressed in peripheral sites.[244] The human *pituitary* CRH receptor is 97% homologous at the amino acid level with the rat *brain* receptor and is a member of the receptor family that binds calcitonin, VIP, and GHRH and activates adenylate cyclase. The concentration of cAMP in the tissue is increased in parallel with the biologic effects and is reduced by glucocorticoids. The rate of transcription of the mRNA that encodes the corticotropin prohormone POMC is also enhanced by CRH, indicating that CRH is a trophic factor as well as a releasing hormone.

Detailed studies of the interaction of CRH with other hypothalamic factors that have CRH activity have helped clarify the neural control of corticotropin secretion in stress (discussed later).

CORTICOTROPIN–RELEASING HORMONE BINDING PROTEIN. Among hypophyseotropic factors, CRH is the only one for which a specific binding protein (in addition to the receptor) exists in tissue or blood. The first clue to the existence of a CRH-binding protein was the finding that high levels of immunoreactive CRH (equivalent to the concentration in hypophyseal-portal blood) are present in the circulation during the second and third trimesters of human pregnancy without activating the pituitary-adrenal axis.[245] The placenta is the principal source of pregnancy-related CRH-binding protein. Human and rat CRH-binding proteins are

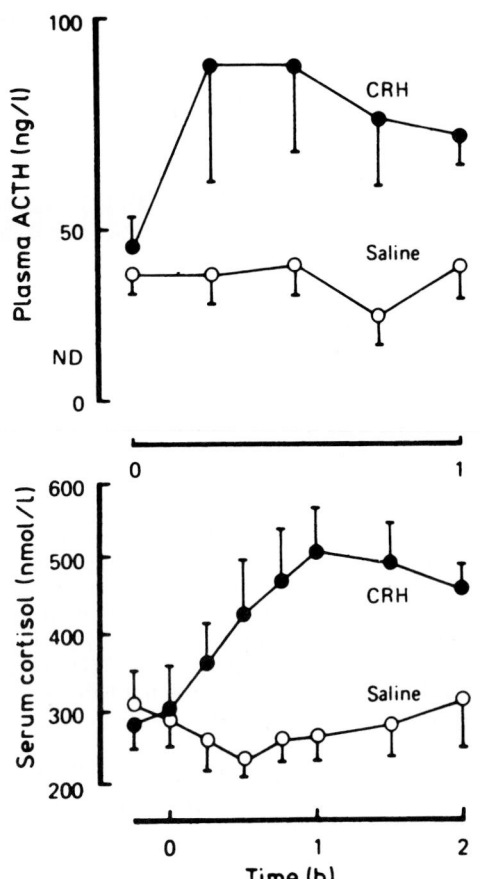

Figure 8–28. Changes in plasma levels of corticotropin and serum levels of cortisol after intravenous injection of CRH (●) in a group of six normal men. The initial prompt response in corticotropin is followed by a somewhat delayed secondary change in cortisol. Also shown are stable control periods (○). To convert corticotropin values to picomoles per liter, multiply by 0.2202. To convert cortisol values to millimoles per liter, multiply by 27.59. (From Grossman A, Kruseman ACN, Perry L, et al. New hypothalamic hormone, corticotropin-releasing factor, specifically stimulates the release of adrenocorticotropic hormone and cortisol in man. Lancet 1982; 1:921–922, with permission.)

homologous (85% amino acid identity), but in the rat the protein is expressed only in brain.[246] The binding protein is species specific; bovine CRH, which is almost identical in sequence to rat-human CRH, has a lower affinity of binding to the human binding protein.

The functional significance of the CRH-binding protein is not fully understood. CRH-binding protein does not bind to the CRH receptor but does inhibit CRH action. For this reason CRH-binding protein probably acts to modulate CRH actions at the cellular level. Corticotrope cells in the anterior pituitary have membrane CRH receptors and intracellular CRH-binding protein; conceivably the binding protein acts to sequestrate or terminate the action of membrane-bound CRH. CRH-binding protein is present in many regions of the central nervous system, including cells that synthesize CRH and cells that receive innervation from CRH-containing neurons.[246] The anatomic distribution of the protein, the variability of its location in relation to the presence of CRH, and its relative sparseness in the CRH tuberohypophyseal neuronal system suggest a control system that is as yet poorly understood.

EXTRAHYPOTHALAMIC FUNCTIONS. In the brain CRH is distributed widely outside of tuberoinfundibular cells[163]—namely, the hypothalamus, the cerebral cortex, the limbic system, and the spinal cord. This localization is believed to be the basis of neural effects that include increased sympathetic nervous system activity, release of norepinephrine and epi-

nephrine, hyperglycemia, hypertension, tachycardia, suppression of the hypothalamic component of gonadotropin regulation, suppression of GH secretion, inhibition of eating, and general arousal.[247–249] The physiological and behavioral responses induced by central injections of CRH in rats and monkeys suggest that many responses to stress, including psychological changes and dysphoria, are mediated by central CRH pathways.[247]

CRH is also found in the lung, liver, and gastrointestinal tract. In activated lymphocytes it is a proinflammatory peptide.[250]

CLINICAL APPLICATIONS. Corticotrope response to CRH is reduced or abolished by glucocorticoids. The CRH test is therefore valuable in differentiating hypercortisolism due to primary adrenocortical disease from that due to excessive corticotropin secretion (Fig. 8–29).[231, 232, 237–239] With corticotropin excess (as in corticotropin-secreting pituitary adenomas) corticotropin responses to CRH are enhanced. Long-term infusion of CRH leads to persistent elevation of plasma corticotropin and cortisol and reduced response to bolus injections of CRH, a pattern of response similar to that observed in approximately half of patients with depressive disorder.[238, 239] CRH has no established therapeutic role.

Growth Hormone–Releasing Hormone

CHEMISTRY AND EVOLUTION. Evidence for neural control of GH secretion came from studies of its regulation in animals with lesions of the hypothalamus and from the demonstration that hypothalamic extracts stimulate the release of GH from the pituitary.[251] When it was shown that GH is released episodically, follows a circadian rhythm, responds rapidly to stress, and is blocked by pituitary stalk section, the concept of neural control of GH secretion became a certainty.[251] However it was only with the discovery of the paraneoplastic syndrome of ectopic GHRH secretion by pancreatic adenomas in humans that sufficient starting material became available for sequencing (see Table 8–4).[252, 253] The term *somatocrinin* was proposed to replace the term GHRH[254] but has not been widely accepted.

Three molecular forms of GHRH occur in human tumors: GHRH 1–44-NH$_2$, GHRH 1–40-OH, and GHRH 1–37-OH (Fig. 8–30).[254, 255] Identical sequences are found in the hypothalamus. As with other neuropeptides the various forms of GHRH arise from post-translational modification of the prohormone.[256] The NH$_2$-terminal tyrosine of GHRH is essential for action; all three forms of GHRH in the hypothalamus are biologically active. In humans the two larger forms are equipotent and the smaller is less active. Fragments as short as 1–29-NH$_2$ are active, but GHRH 1–27-NH$_2$ is inactive. As is the case of LHRH, there are species differences among GHRHs; the peptides from seven species range in sequence homology with the human, from 93% in the pig to 67% in the rat.[257]

Ectopic secretion of GHRH is a rare cause of acromegaly in that fewer than 1% of patients with acromegaly have elevated serum levels of GHRH (see Chapter 9).[258] Approximately 20% of pancreatic adenomas and 5% of carcinoid tumors contain immunoreactive GHRH, but most are clinically silent.[259, 260]

EFFECTS ON THE PITUITARY AND MECHANISM OF ACTION. The administration of GHRH to individuals with normal pituitaries causes a prompt increase in serum hGH, followed by a rapid return to basal levels (Fig. 8–31).[257, 262, 263] Sustained infusions of GHRH over several hours cause a *decrease* in hGH levels, suggesting that GHRH, like LHRH, depends on pulsatile secretion for its physiological effect. Administration of GHRH in repeated boluses stimulates the formation of hGH and insulin-like growth factor I (IGF-I, also called soma-

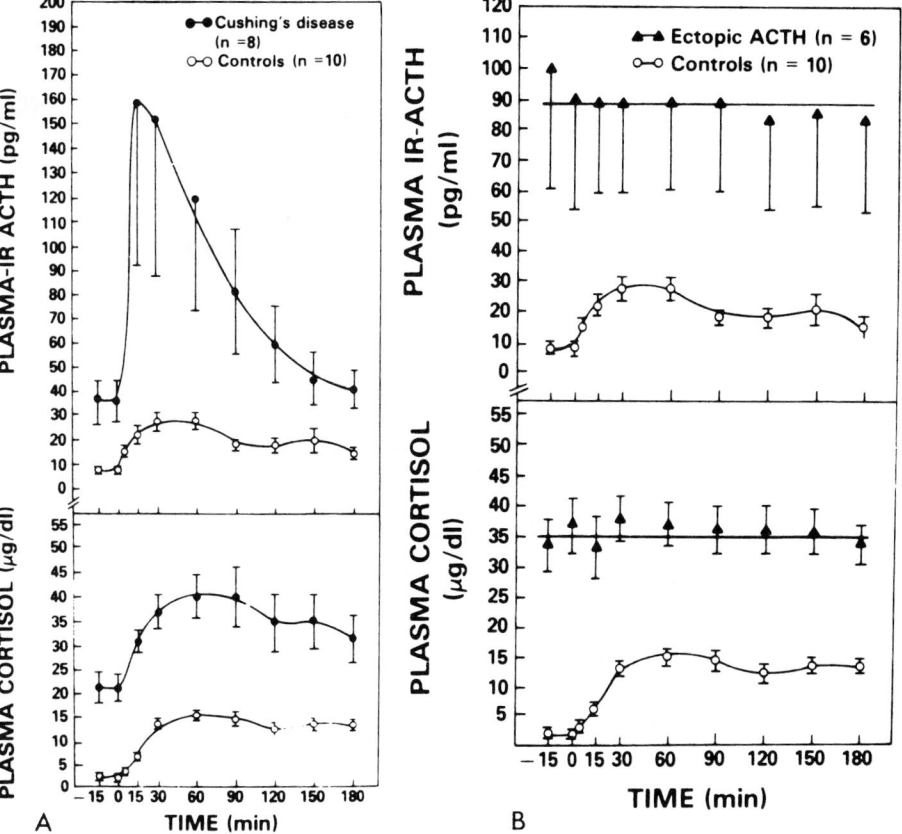

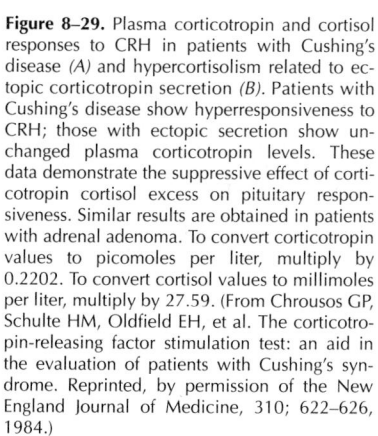

Figure 8–29. Plasma corticotropin and cortisol responses to CRH in patients with Cushing's disease *(A)* and hypercortisolism related to ectopic corticotropin secretion *(B)*. Patients with Cushing's disease show hyperresponsiveness to CRH; those with ectopic secretion show unchanged plasma corticotropin levels. These data demonstrate the suppressive effect of corticotropin cortisol excess on pituitary responsiveness. Similar results are obtained in patients with adrenal adenoma. To convert corticotropin values to picomoles per liter, multiply by 0.2202. To convert cortisol values to millimoles per liter, multiply by 27.59. (From Chrousos GP, Schulte HM, Oldfield EH, et al. The corticotropin-releasing factor stimulation test: an aid in the evaluation of patients with Cushing's syndrome. Reprinted, by permission of the New England Journal of Medicine, 310; 622–626, 1984.)

tomedin-C) so that it is potentially useful for the treatment of hGH deficiency due to hypothalamic disorders.[257, 263]

The effects of a single injection of GHRH are almost completely specific for GH secretion except for a minimal increase in PRL levels seen in some studies.[262, 263] GHRH has no effect on gut peptide hormones.[261] The response to GHRH is influenced by gonadal steroid hormones (enhanced by estrogen administration), by obesity (blunted by body weight 15% over ideal body weight), and by nutrition (enhanced by starvation).

The GHRH receptor is a member of a family of G protein–coupled receptors that include receptors for VIP, pituitary adenylate cyclase activating peptide, secretin, glucagon, calcitonin, parathyroid hormone, and gastric inhibitory polypeptide.[257, 264] GHRH activates cAMP by binding to a stimulatory G protein (G_s), which activates adenylate cyclase, in-

creases intracellular free Ca^{2+}, releases preformed GH, and stimulates GH mRNA transcription and new GH synthesis (see Chapter 9).[257, 265] GHRH may also influence phospholipid metabolism but not by the classic polyphosphoinositide hydrolysis.

The effects of GHRH are blocked by somatostatin and enhanced by glucocorticoids[266] and estrogen. Transgenic mice expressing GHRH cDNA coupled to a suitable promoter acquire somatotrope hyperplasia,[267] confirming the growth-stimulating effect of this factor on the pituitary.

GHRH has few known *extrapituitary* functions. The most important may be its activity as a sleep regulator.[268] The administration of GHRH or of the GH-releasing hexapeptide to rats and humans induces sleep.[269] Neutralization of endogenous GHRH reduces sleep.[268] It is therefore possible that both sleep and sleep-induced GH secretion, characteristic of normal cir-

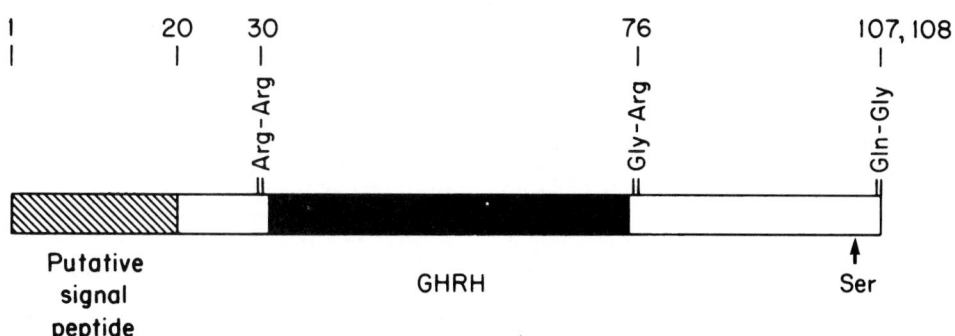

Figure 8–30. Diagram of the amino acid sequence of human growth hormone–releasing hormone (GHRH) derived by recombinant techniques from a pancreatic adenoma of a patient who had acromegaly related to ectopic secretion of GHRH. Following a signal sequence and an intervening sequence is the region coding for GHRH 1–44, followed by a glycine that will be exchanged for NH_2 during post-translational processing. In the particular tumor studied, two different prohormones were identified, one with 107 amino acids and the other with 108. (Drawn from data of Gubler U, Monahan JJ, Lomedico PT, et al. Cloning and sequence analysis of cDNA for the precursor of human growth hormone–releasing factor, somatocrinin. Proc Natl Acad Sci USA 1983; 80:4311–4314, with permission.)

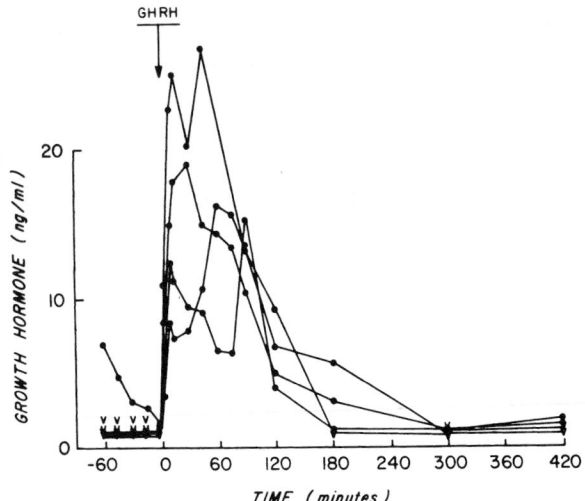

EFFECT OF GHRH ON GH SECRETION IN NORMAL ADULTS

Figure 8–31. Response of normal men to GHRH administered by intravenous injection. Note the prompt release of hGH, followed by a rather prolonged fall in hormone level, in some cases associated with a double peak. (From Thorner MO, Rivier J, Speiss J, et al. Human pancreatic growth-hormone–releasing factor selectively stimulates growth-hormone secretion in man. Lancet 1983; 1:24–28, with permission.)

cadian rhythms of GH, are due to circadian changes in central GHRH secretion.

Additional factors that induce sleep include the inflammatory cytokines, IL-1, IL-6, tumor necrosis factor α),[268] VIP and PRL,[270] the delta sleep peptide,[271, 272] muramyl peptides derived from gut bacteria,[273] and a class of sleep-inducing fatty acid primary amides.[274]

GROWTH HORMONE–RELEASING PEPTIDES. In studies of the opioid control of GH secretion, several peptide analogues of met-enkephalin were found to be potent releasers of GH. The first is the GH-releasing hexapeptide hexarelin (GHRP-6, His-D-Trp-Ala-Trp-D-Phe-Lys-NH$_2$).[275–278] Even more potent analogues have been developed. These compounds are active when administered by intranasal and oral routes, are more potent on a weight basis than GHRH itself, are more effective in vivo than in vitro, are more effective in the presence of GHRH and are almost ineffective in the absence of GHRH, do not bind to the GHRH or the somatostatin receptor, and do not act by suppressing somatostatin secretion or by activating adenylate cyclase in the pituitary (as is the case for GHRH). Patients with hypothalamic disease leading to GHRH deficiency have low or no response to hexarelin.[278–280] Unique binding sites for these compounds are present in both the hypothalamus and pituitary. Structural modeling studies of hexarelin led to the development of several nonpeptide GH-releasing compounds (L-692,429, L-692,585) that appear to have the same mechanism of action on GH secretion.[281]

CLINICAL APPLICATIONS. GHRH stimulates growth in children with intact pituitaries, but the optimal dosage, route, and frequency of administration, as well as possible usefulness via the nasal route, have not been determined.[257, 262, 263] As of June 1996 it has not been approved by the Food and Drug Administration (FDA) for routine therapy. The availability of biosynthetic hGH (which requires less frequent injections) and the development of peptide and nonpeptide hGH releasers that may be active by mouth or nasal spray (see earlier) have reduced enthusiasm for the clinical use of GHRH or its analogues. GHRH is not useful for the differential diagnosis of hypothalamic and pituitary causes of GH deficiency.

Because hGH secretion declines in aging men and women ("*somatopause*"),[282] hGH responses to GHRH have been as-

sessed in such individuals. Most studies report decreased responses, but in others no age-related changes have been seen.[282] In such studies it is important to exclude obesity and estrogen status as confounding factors. As noted earlier, patients with hypothalamic deficiency of GHRH (Fig. 8–32) respond to GHRH, as do most patients with acromegaly who may be hyperresponsive.[262, 263, 283]

Somatostatin

CHEMISTRY AND EVOLUTION. During efforts to isolate GHRH from hypothalamic extracts a factor was discovered that inhibited GH release from pituitary in vitro.[284] At about the same time a factor was described in pancreatic islet extracts that inhibited insulin secretion.[285] In retrospect these biologic activities proved to be due to somatostatin, which was isolated and sequenced by Brazeau and colleagues in 1973.[286] The work in this area and its clinical application have been summarized.[287–292]

The term *somatostatin* was originally applied to a cyclic peptide containing 14 amino acids (somatostatin-14; see Table 8–4). Subsequently a second form, N-extended somatostatin-28, was identified as a secretory product. Somatostatin-14 is identical with the terminal 14 amino acids of somatostatin-28, and they are derived by independent cleavage of the prohormone by specific enzymes.[290, 293–295]

Somatostatin-14 is the predominant form in the brain (including the hypothalamus), whereas somatostatin-28 is the major form in the gastrointestinal tract, especially the colon. The name somatostatin is descriptively inaccurate because the molecule also inhibits thyrotropin secretion and has nonpituitary roles including activity as a *neurotransmitter* or *neuromodulator* in the central and peripheral nervous systems and as a gut and pancreas regulatory peptide. As a pituitary regulator somatostatin is a true *neurohormone*, i.e., a neuronal secretory

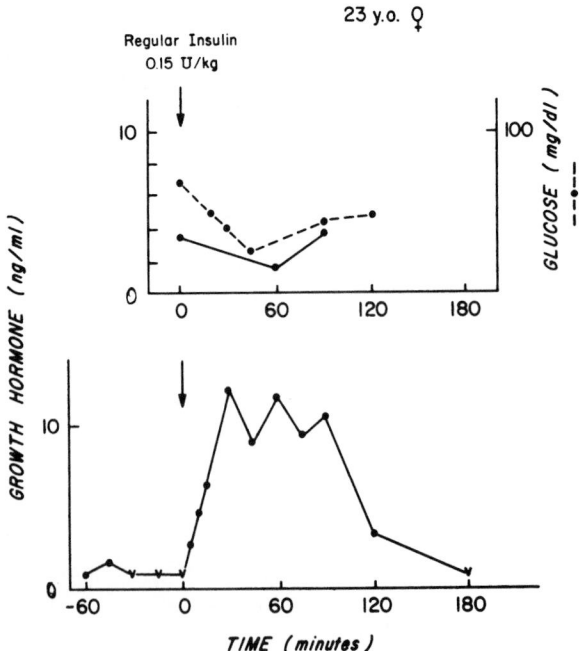

Figure 8–32. Responses of hGH to GHRH in a patient with hypothalamic hGH failure related to eosinophilic granuloma of the hypothalamus, and comparison with the response to insulin-induced hypoglycemia. This figure illustrates the failure of the hGH response to a physiological stimulus involving the hypothalamus (*top*) and the normal response to direct pituitary stimulation (*bottom*). GHRH was given as a bolus (*arrow, bottom*). To convert glucose values to millimoles per liter, multiply by 0.055510. (From J Goldman, ME Molitch, S Reichlin, unpublished, 1984.)

RAT SOMATOSTATIN GENE

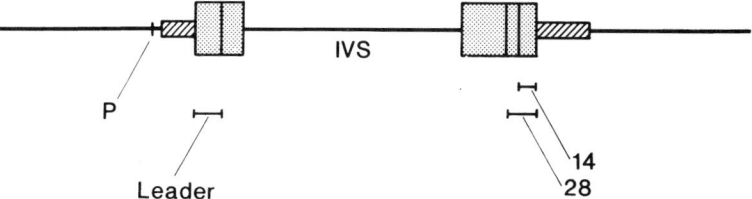

Figure 8–33. Diagram of gene sequence coding for somatostatin in the rat, which was characterized from recombinant bacteriophage libraries prepared from rat liver DNA. IVS, intervening sequence; P, promoter. (From Montminy MR, Goodman RH, Horovitch SJ, et al. Primary structure of the gene encoding rat preprosomatostatin. Proc Natl Acad Sci USA 1984; 81:3337–3340, with permission.)

product that enters the blood (hypophyseal-portal circulation) to affect cell function at remote sites. In the gut somatostatin is present in both the myenteric plexus (where it acts as a *neurotransmitter*) and in epithelial cells where it influences the function of adjacent cells as a *paracrine* secretion. Somatostatin also exerts paracrine control in the pancreas. In pancreas and gut somatostatin can influence its own secretion (an *autocrine* function). Gut exocrine secretion can be modulated by intraluminal action so that it is also a *lumone*. Because of its wide distribution, broad spectrum of regulatory effects, and evolutionary history, this peptide can be regarded as an archetype gut-brain peptide.

The genes that encode somatostatin in humans[293] and rats[294] and a number of other species (Fig. 8–33) exhibit striking sequence homology, even in primitive fish.[287, 290] Somatostatin appeared early in evolutionary history as evidenced by its presence in the protozoan *Tetrahymena pyriformis*[3, 4] and in the sea squirt, a primitive invertebrate. During evolution the amino acid sequence of somatostatin-14 has undergone little change, mammalian somatostatin and one of the two anglerfish somatostatins being identical. The other regions of somatostatin-28 also show considerable sequence homology. Conservation of sequence is a strong argument for an important function of somatostatin throughout evolution (as is also true for its receptors; see later).

One somatostatin gene is present in the human, and tissue-specific processing determines whether the 14- or 28-amino-acid form will be present.[290] At least seven genes for somatostatin are found in animal kingdoms; in anglerfish, e.g., two genes encode the two somatostatins. The genes are relatively simple and many of the control elements have been defined.[296, 297] "Minisomatostatins" have been developed for therapy and for radioisotope-based external imaging.[289, 290, 298, 299]

The function of somatostatin in GH and thyrotropin regulation, in the extrahypothalamic brain, and in therapy are considered here and in Chapter 9. Its function in pancreatic islet cell regulation is described in Chapter 21, and the manifestations of somatostatin excess as in somatostatinoma are described in Chapter 34.

EFFECTS ON PITUITARY AND MECHANISM OF ACTION. In the pituitary somatostatin inhibits secretion of GH and thyrotropin and, under certain conditions, of PRL and corticotropin as well. It exerts inhibitory effects on virtually all endocrine and exocrine secretions of the pancreas, gut, and gallbladder (Table 8–6). Somatostatin inhibits secretion by the salivary glands and, under some conditions, the secretion of parathyroid hormone and calcitonin. Somatostatin blocks hormone release in many endocrine-secreting tumors, including insulinomas, glucagonomas, VIPomas, carcinoid tumors, and some gastrinomas.

Five somatostatin receptor subtypes have been identified by gene cloning techniques, and one is expressed in two forms; all are homologous.[300, 301] Subtypes are important because they tend to be tissue specific, differ in the mechanism of intracellular action, differ in their effects on cell function, bind to specific somatostatin analogues differently, and are encoded by genes on different chromosomes. Certain of these differences have important implications for the use of somatostatin analogues in therapy and in diagnostic imaging.

All receptor subtypes are coupled to G proteins, all have seven-transmembrane spanning sequences, and all bind relatively well to somatostatin-14. Conversely, somatostatin-28 binds less tightly than does somatostatin-14 to receptors 1, 2, and 3 and binds extremely tightly to receptor 5. Octreotide, a somatostatin analogue, binds moderately well to the type 2 (A and B) and type 5 receptors and poorly to types 1 and 4. These differences account for the fact that octreotide is effective in inhibiting GH secretion in acromegaly and can be used in radiolabeled form to image pituitary tumors. The pituitary expresses all types of somatostatin receptors, whereas the pancreas contains only type 2 receptors; octreotide is a more potent inhibitor of GH secretion than of insulin secretion. As a consequence, glucose intolerance is not a problem with octreotide use.

Binding of somatostatin to its receptor leads to activation of one or more cell membrane–bound inhibitory G proteins, which in turn lower cellular cAMP and in addition reduce intracellular free Ca^{2+} concentrations through effects on the voltage-sensitive (L-type) Ca^{2+} channel.[302, 303] The effects of lowered cAMP can only partially account for the observed effects of somatostatin because this peptide also blocks the effects of cAMP-induced secretion and thus acts "downstream" from cAMP. It is more likely that changes in Ca^{2+} concentration are the crucial determinants of somatostatin action in blocking the secretion and synthesis of cellular proteins. The lowering of the Ca^{2+} level is not a direct effect but is probably secondary to an increase in K^+ conductance and membrane hyperpolarization.[300]

The ability of somatostatin to inhibit the growth of normal and some neoplastic cell lines has been attributed to a

TABLE 8–6. Biologic Actions of Somatostatin Outside the Central Nervous System

Inhibits Hormone Secretion by	Inhibits Other Gastrointestinal Actions
Pituitary gland	Gastric acid secretion
Thyrotropin, GH	Gastric secretion
Gastrointestinal tract	Gastric emptying
Gastrin	Pancreatic bicarbonate secretion
Secretin	Pancreatic enzyme secretion
Gastrointestinal polypeptide	Intestinal absorption
Motilin	Gastrointestinal blood flow
Glicentin (enteroglucagon)	AVP-stimulated water transport
VIP	Bile flow
Pancreas	
Insulin	
Glucagon	
Somatostatin	
Genitourinary tract	
Renin	

GH, growth hormone; AVP, arginine vasopressin; VIP, vasoactive intestinal peptide.

TABLE 8–7. Therapeutic Uses of the Long-Acting Somatostatin Analogue Octreotide

Neuroendocrine tumor hyperfunction
  VIPoma*
  Carcinoid tumors*
  Glucagonoma
  Insulinoma
  Nisidioblastosis
  GHRHomas (ectopic GHRH)
  Gastrinoma†
Pituitary tumor
  Somatotropinoma (acromegaly)
  Thyrotropinoma
Gut disease
  Diarrhea
    Diabetic neuropathy
    Ileostomy
    Idiopathic diarrhea of childhood
    AIDS associated
  Pancreatic fistula
  Bleeding esophageal varices, bleeding peptic ulcer†
Postural hypotension
Miscellaneous
  Migraine headache
  Psoriasis
  ?Meningioma

* Approved for use in the United States by the Food and Drug Administration in 1989.
† H₂ blockers are superior or equivalent.
VIP, vasoactive intestinal peptide; GHRH, growth hormone–releasing hormone.

third mechanism of action, namely, inhibition of the protein tyrosine phosphatase that is bound to the somatostatin receptor.[304, 305] The significance of this effect lies in the fact that tyrosine phosphatases catalyze the dephosphorylation of phosphotyrosines, a family of cell-activating proteins. Somatostatin has other antineoplastic effects, including inhibition of circulating growth factors (GH, IGF-I), inhibition of expression of receptors for growth factors such as epidermal growth factor, and inhibition of tumor angiogenesis factors.[305]

CLINICAL APPLICATIONS OF SOMATOSTATIN ANALOGUES. The potential therapeutic usefulness of somatostatin has generated much effort to synthesize analogues that resist degradation and have a longer duration of action than the few minutes characteristic of native peptide. A number of such analogues have been studied in clinical trials[289, 290, 292, 306] (see Chapters 9 and 34) and others are in trial. The actions of octreotide illustrate the general potential of somatostatin in therapy (Table 8–7; also see Table 8–6). It controls excess secretion of GH in acromegaly in most patients and shrinks tumors in about one third and is useful in the management of many forms of diarrhea (acting on salt and water excretion

mechanisms in the gut). Octreotide has been used to reduce external secretions in pancreatic fistulae (thus permitting healing) and to treat functioning neuroendocrine tumors, including VIPoma, carcinoid, glucagonoma, and insulinoma. It is seldom of use for the treatment of gastrinoma. A decrease in blood flow to the gastrointestinal tract is the basis of its use in bleeding esophageal varices and peptic ulcers and in the treatment of postprandial orthostatic hypotension.[307]

The only major undesirable side effect of the drug is reduction of bile production and of gallbladder contractility, leading to "sludging" of bile and an increased incidence of gallstones. Less significant side effects are due to impaired fat digestion and abdominal discomfort.

Somatostatin analogues labeled with a radioactive tracer have been used as external imaging agents. A technetium-labeled analogue of octreotide has been approved for clinical use in the United States and several other countries (Fig. 8–34).[299, 308–310] The majority of neuroendocrine tumors and many pituitary tumors that express somatostatin receptors are visualized by external imaging techniques after administration of this agent; a variety of nonendocrine tumors and inflammatory lesions are also visualized, all of which have in common the expression of somatostatin receptors. Such tumors include non–small cell cancer of the lung (100%), meningioma (100%), breast cancer (74%), and astrocytomas (67%).[299] Exocrine pancreatic tumors do not bind somatostatin. Because activated T cells of the immune system display somatostatin receptors (see later in the section on neuroendocrine-immune interaction), inflammatory lesions that take up the tracer include sarcoidosis, Wegener's granulomatosis, tuberculosis, and many cases of Hodgkin's disease and non-Hodgkin's lymphoma.[299] Although the tracer lacks specificity in differential diagnosis, its ability to identify the *presence* of abnormality and the extent of the lesion provides important information for management, including tumor staging. The use of a small handheld radiation detector in the operating room makes it possible to ensure the completeness of removal of medullary thyroid carcinoma metastases.[311] Finally, theoretical calculations suggest that radiolabeled somatostatin analogues might deliver a tumoricidal radiotherapeutic dose to some tumors.

Prolactin-Regulating Factors

DOPAMINE. In contrast to the secretion of other pituitary hormones, the secretion of PRL is *increased* in the absence of hypothalamic influences, and extracts of whole hypothalamus inhibit PRL release in vitro.[312] This bioactivity was termed *PIF (prolactin-inhibiting factor)*. Dopamine, the most important PIF,

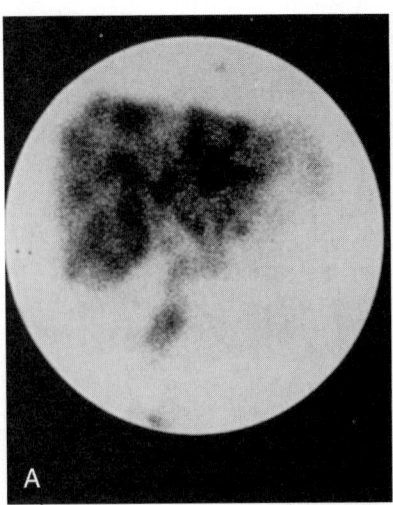
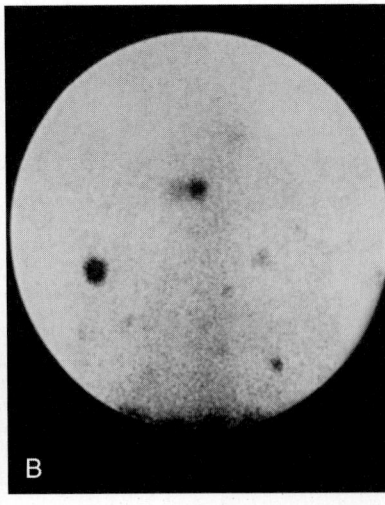

Figure 8–34. The use of indium III–labeled diethylenetriamine-penta-acetic acid (DTPA)–octreotide (radioactive somatostatin analogue) and external imaging techniques to localize a carcinoid tumor expressing somatostatin receptors. Pictures were taken 24 h after administration of labeled tracer. *A*, Anterior view of the abdomen showing metastases in an enlarged liver and the primary carcinoid tumor in the wall of the jejunum of a patient with severe flushing and diarrhea. *B*, Posterior view of the chest and neck showing a metastasis in a lymph node on the left side of the neck and multiple metastases in the ribs and pleura. (Reprinted, with permission. Lamberts SWJ, Krenning EP, Reubi J-C. The role of somatostatin and its analogs in the diagnosis and treatment of tumors. Endocrine Rev 1991; 12:450–482. © 1991, The Endocrine Society.)

is the secretory product of tuberoinfundibular dopaminergic pathways and is present in hypophyseal–portal vessel blood in sufficient concentration to inhibit PRL release.[184, 313–315] γ-Aminobutyric acid (GABA), a constituent of hypothalamic extracts, is a less potent PIF, and the known PRL inhibitory functions of the hypothalamus may be mediated almost exclusively by dopamine.

After administration of dopamine or levodopa (which is converted to dopamine in peripheral tissues and brain) or synthetic dopamine agonists such as bromocriptine, PRL levels drop sharply in normal and hyperprolactinemic individuals. Thyrotropin secretion is also inhibited by dopamine.

Dopamine suppresses virtually all aspects of PRL synthesis and secretion.[313–318] It acts on the lactotrope via the D_2 subtype dopamine receptor[318] to inhibit release and biosynthesis of PRL, to inhibit DNA synthesis and cell division, and to bring about the loss of stored PRL in granules by stimulating *crinophagy* (autodigestion of secretory product). Dopamine inhibits formation of cAMP (a stimulator of PRL secretion), synthesis of phosphoinositol, phospholipid turnover, and release of arachidonic acid. These actions are responsible for the therapeutic effect of dopamine agonists such as bromocriptine in hyperprolactinemic states.

PROLACTIN-RELEASING FACTORS. Although tonic suppression of PRL release by dopamine is the dominant effect of the hypothalamus on PRL secretion, a number of stimuli promote PRL release, not merely by disinhibition of PIF effects but by causing release of one or more PRFs.[166, 189, 319–324] The most important of the putative PRFs are TRH, vasopressin, VIP, oxytocin, and PHI-27 (peptide-histidine-isoleucine-27), but the endogenous opioids, bombesin, substance P, melatonin, bradykinin, epidermal growth factor, fibroblast growth factors, gastrin, and acetylcholine also can trigger PRL release. An uncharacterized neurointermediate lobe factor or factors may be important also (see later).[319, 321, 322]

As described earlier, administration of TRH stimulates PRL release with the same dose-response characteristics as for thyrotropin release. TRH secretion into the hypophyseal-portal blood supply is increased by nipple stimulation in rats, and in some experiments the administration of anti-TRH antisera partially blocks suckling-induced PRL release. However suckling is not believed to release thyrotropin in humans.

Vasopressin also stimulates PRL release and cannot be excluded as a physiological PRF. It is present in hypophyseal-portal blood and is released during stress and shock, as is PRL.

The addition of VIP to the pituitary stimulates PRL secretion. Concentrations of VIP in hypophyseal-portal blood are sufficient to produce effects in vivo, and its release is stimulated by serotonin, an agent that increases PRL secretion. Moreover, the administration of anti-VIP antiserum to rats blocks stress-induced PRL release and reduces the elevated PRL levels of nursing mothers.[323] Another candidate PRF is PHI, a peptide that releases PRL,[324] is co-localized with CRH in paraventricular neurons,[166] and is presumed to be released by the same stimuli that release corticotropin, such as stress.

PHI is structurally homologous with VIP and is synthesized as part of the VIP prohormone.

Suckling-induced PRL release (in the rat) is mediated in part by the neurointermediate lobe. Removal of this structure blocks suckling-induced PRL release, and exposure of the anterior pituitary to intermediate lobe extracts (devoid of VIP, AVP, and other known PRFs) stimulates PRL secretion.[319, 321] At least two kinds of PRF activity have been isolated from intermediate lobe tumors of the mouse.[322] However the relevance of the neurointermediate lobe for PRL regulation in primates (including the human) is not clear because this structure exists in only a rudimentary form if at all in primates (see earlier).

MELANOCYTE-STIMULATING HORMONE RELEASE-INHIBITING FACTOR. Dopamine also inhibits intermediate lobe synthesis of α-MSH, a product of processing of the corticotropin precursor POMC (see earlier in the section on the intermediate lobe and also Chapter 9). In the study of anterior pituitary control it was assumed that MSH secretion is controlled by hypothalamic factors analogous to those that regulate anterior pituitary hormones. One hypothalamic peptide, Pro-Leu-Gly-NH₂ (so-called MSH release-inhibiting factor [MIF], an enzymatic degradation product of oxytocin), is a potent inhibitor of MSH secretion.[136, 137] MIF is no longer considered to be an important MSH regulator,[325, 326] but its function is not understood.

α-MSH is probably more important as a centrally active neuropeptide than as a pituitary hormone. It is synthesized in the hypothalamus, and MSH receptors (MSHRs) are widely distributed in the brain (see later in the section on central peptidergic pathways).

Luteinizing Hormone–Releasing Hormone

CHEMISTRY AND EVOLUTION. Intense efforts to identify the nature of the activity in hypothalamic extracts that promotes release of LH by the pituitary[327, 328] culminated in the isolation of a decapeptide, LHRH[329] (see Table 8–4). LHRH, like other neuropeptides, is synthesized as part of a large prohormone that is cleaved enzymatically and further modified within secretory granules (Fig. 8–35).[330, 331]

Some workers believe that two different hypothalamic factors regulate the secretion of gonadotropins, one stimulating LH secretion and the other stimulating the release of FSH.[332, 333] Others[334–336] believe that all situations in which secretion of LH and FSH are dissociated can be explained by differences in the way in which the two types of gonadotropin-secreting cells respond to secretory patterns of LHRH, by the gonadal steroid milieu, and by the effects of inhibin, a peptide secretion of the gonads that selectively inhibits FSH secretion.[337] The rate at which LHRH pulses are administered alters the pattern of LH and FSH secretion, fast frequencies increasing secretion of both LH and FSH, slower frequencies increasing FSH relative to LH, and constant infusions suppressing secretion of both LH and FSH.[338] The administration of anti-

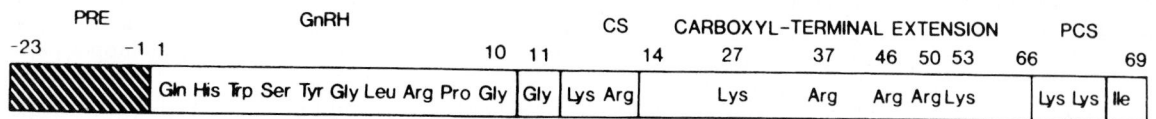

Figure 8–35. Schematic diagram of the structure of the precursor of human placental LHRH (GnRH in figure), as determined by nucleic acid sequencing of the corresponding cDNA (Seeburg and Adelman[330]). The precursor consists of a signal sequence (PRE) of 23 amino acids followed immediately by the LHRH decapeptide sequence. Cleavage of the signal peptide reveals an NH₂-terminal Gln, which cyclizes (enzymatically or spontaneously) to pyroGlu. The LHRH sequence is followed by a Gly, which is the donor for the COCH-terminal amide of LHRH, and Lys-Arg, which is a conventional dibasic amino acid cleavage site (CS). Immediately following the processing site is a 56-amino-acid peptide sequence (14–69) designated GAP (gonadotropin-releasing hormone–associated peptide), which has been reported to have effects on PRL secretion, although these results are controversial. A second potential dibasic cleavage site (PCS) and single amino acid putative cleavage sites are also shown. Of these, Arg-16 is a favored site. (From Miller RP, King JA. Structural and functional evolution of gonadotropin-releasing hormone. Int Rev Cytol 1987; 106:149–182, with permission.)

sera against LHRH inhibits the secretion of both LH and FSH. Male and female gonadal function can be restored in patients with hypothalamic LHRH deficiency by administering LHRH only in appropriate doses in a pulsatile manner. For these reasons, the view that there is only one hormone that releases gonadotropin is widely held.

Seven different forms of LHRH have been demonstrated in different species. All are 10-amino-acid–containing peptides (decapeptides) and all have at least 50% homology with mammalian LHRH.[339] All forms have identical pyro-Glu amino and Gly amide carboxy terminal structures, testifying to the functional importance of both the size and the termini in the evolution of these peptides in all vertebrate species—including the jawless fish, the lamprey—thought to have evolved more than 500 million years ago. LHRH may have an even more ancient origin; some strains of yeast, a unicellular eucaryote, secrete *mating factor* α, which acts as a pheromone regulating sexual reproduction. Mating factor α, a linear peptide of 13 amino acids, 5 of which are identical with amino acids of human LHRH,[340] binds to rat pituitary LHRH receptors, and releases LH.[339, 340]

Among vertebrates the two most common LHRHs are mammalian LHRH (mLHRH), the form found in the hypothalamus of higher vertebrates, and chicken LHRH (cLHRH), which has a glycine for arginine substitution in the 8 position. Genes that code for LHRH have been characterized in humans, rats, and two species of salmon. As with other regulatory peptides, the nucleotide sequences encoding the functional peptide are highly homologous, but the intervening sequences show wide divergence.[339] Response elements for at least three nuclear regulatory steroids—retinoic acid, estrogen, and thyroid hormone—are found in the gene. Deletion of this gene in a mutant strain of mice leads to hypogonadism.[338]

The prohormone contains a 56-amino-acid sequence that is cleaved from the rest of the molecule by enzymatic processing in the LHRH-expressing cells. This peptide[330, 331] has no known function; the fact that its sequence, in contrast to that of LHRH decapeptide, is variable among species suggests that it is unlikely to be hormonally important.

EMBRYOGENESIS. Unlike other hypophyseotropic neurons LHRH-expressing neurons differentiate in early fetal life *outside* the brain in the olfactory placode, a patch of epithelium in the nasal region that also gives rise to olfactory receptors and is innervated by the terminalis and vomeronasal nerves.[341–343] LHRH neurons then migrate into the olfactory lobe to reach their final destination in the preoptic hypothalamus and medial basal hypothalamus with projections to the median eminence, where they become adorned by an elaborate array of afferent neurons. Crucial to the targeting process through the nasal septum and cribriform plate is the presence of neural and glial elements that form a "scaffold" through which the cells are conducted and a specific adhesion molecule, "neural cell adhesion molecule," that appears to direct tracking.

The circuitous route by which LHRH neurons take up their place within the central nervous system and the complex anatomic and regional targeting mechanism can go awry during development, as illustrated by the human disorder hypogonadotropic hypogonadism (see Chapter 29). In an aborted fetus with this disorder the LHRH immunoreactive cells were absent from their normal place in the brain and were clustered in the nose on either side of the midline below the cribriform plate.[344] The responsible gene encodes a protein of the fibronectin family that is involved in neurotaxis (see later in the section on hypophyseotropic hormone deficiency).

Transplantation of LHRH neurons into the preoptic hypothalamus of adult mice with congenital defects in the biosynthesis of LHRH repairs the defect sufficiently to support reproductive function.[345]

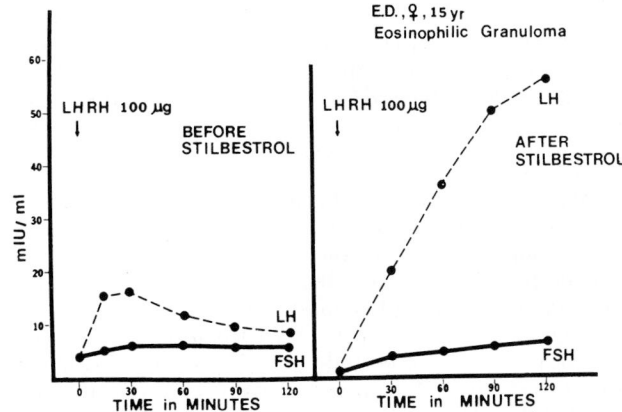

Figure 8–36. Gonadotropin secretory response to an LHRH bolus injection (100 µg) in a patient with hypothalamic hypopituitarism. Note that the luteinizing hormone (LH) response is greater than the follicle-stimulating hormone (FSH) response and that the peak response is somewhat delayed. After estrogen treatment, there was marked sensitization of the LH response, which is characteristic of the "positive" feedback effect of estrogens on hypothalamic-pituitary gonadotropin secretion. (From Reichlin S. Regulation of the endocrine hypothalamus. Med Clin North Am 1978; 62:235–250, with permission.)

EFFECTS ON THE PITUITARY AND MECHANISM OF ACTION. A single intravenous injection of LHRH causes a dose-related increase of LH and FSH levels in all vertebrate species (Fig. 8–36).[335, 346–349] The onset of FSH release after a single bolus injection is delayed in comparison with that of LH, and the values peak at 10 to 30 min after injection. The response is influenced by previous LHRH exposure, the gonadal steroid milieu, gender, the stage of sexual maturation, and the timing of administration of the hormone. Sustained high levels of LHRH suppress LH and FSH secretion; a normal pattern can be restored by intermittent injections.

LHRH action is initiated by binding to specific cell surface receptors,[350–353] leading to activation of a specific G protein ($G_{q/11}$), stimulation of multiple phospholipase activities in the plasma membrane, differential modulation of inositol-1,4,5-triphosphate and diacylglycerol signals, and cytoplasmic calcium response.[353] Increased synthesis and release of gonadotropins follow exposure to LHRH. Estrogens (which sensitize the pituitary to LHRH) increase, and androgens decrease, the number of LHRH receptors. The reduced number of receptors resulting from constant infusion of LHRH or from the use of superagonists probably explains the reduced secretion of gonadotropins that follows such treatment. These changes in receptor number are the basis of agonist treatment of precocious puberty and prostate cancer and of agonist-induced blockade of ovulation.[351, 353]

LHRH receptors are also present in the ovary and testis of the rat[354] and in the human ovary.[355] Although LHRH stimulates the release of steroid hormones from isolated rat ovaries[354] it is doubtful that circulating LHRH has a role in gonadal function because its concentration in blood is so low.

EXTRAHYPOTHALAMIC DISTRIBUTION AND FUNCTION. Most of the LHRH in mammalian brain is in the hypothalamus and related neural structures, but it is also found in the limbic system, including the hippocampus, cingulate cortex, and olfactory bulb,[355] structures that are responsible for emotional expression. LHRH has been implicated in sexual drive in rats[356] but not in monkeys[357] and probably not in humans.[358] An LHRH-like peptide in frog sympathetic ganglia is thought to be a neurotransmitter.[359] LHRH is present in the human amygdala and in the hindbrain and spinal cord of animals. LHRH is expressed in the placenta[330, 360] and stimulates placental secretion of chorionic gonadotropin.[360] Other potential sites of action correspond to the distribution of LHRH receptors and include human ovary, prostate, testis, and lymphocytes. LHRH is secreted into human milk[361] and LHRH receptors are present in human breast tissue and in at least one breast cancer cell line. A variety of functions have been attributed to LHRH. For example salmon LHRH is a GHRH, and in amphibians LHRH is a neurotransmitter in the autonomic nervous system.

CLINICAL APPLICATIONS. Under appropriately defined conditions, LHRH can induce spermatogenesis and normal testosterone production in men with hypothalamic hypogonadotropic hypogonadism, ovulation in women with hypothalamic amenorrhea,[335] and puberty in both boys and girls with delayed or arrested puberty.[346-348, 362, 363] High-potency LHRH analogues can suppress gonadal function in patients with precocious puberty[364] and in normal men[365, 366] and women.[367] The role of LHRH in gonadotropin regulation is discussed later.

The potential usefulness of LHRH as a contraceptive, as a regulator of gonadal function, and for the treatment of abnormal sexual development has led to the synthesis of analogues with either agonist or antagonist properties.[347-349] For example, the insertion of D-amino acids at sites that are normally cleaved by proteases markedly prolongs activity. Two general types of analogues are now available: "superagonists" that have prolonged action and antagonists that bind to LHRH receptors and block hormone action. Because the pattern of delivery of LHRH determines its effects on the pituitary, superagonists can inhibit gonadotropin secretion, as do true antagonists (see Chapters 15 and 16).

REGULATION OF SECRETION OF TUBEROHYPOPHYSEAL NEURONS

As outlined in previous sections, the tuberohypophyseal neurons are acted on by neurotransmitters; by the feedback effects of hormones secreted by target glands, such as the gonadal steroids, thyroid hormone, and cortisol; by pituitary peptide hormones (short-loop feedback control); by bioaminergic neurons from the brain stem; and by neuropeptide modulators. The secretion of specific releasing hormones is also regulated by local feedback circuits in which the hypophyseotropic hormone acts to regulate its own or neighboring neurons ("ultrashort-loop feedback control").

Few areas in neurobiology have seen such dramatic increases in knowledge as have those dealing with the identification of neurotransmitters and neuropeptides and their anatomic distribution, molecular structure, distribution and structure of receptors, mode of regulation, and mechanisms of action.[368-371] Neurotransmitters fall into several classes, each with its own mode of biosynthesis, anatomic distribution, and regulatory systems (see Table 8–3).[372-378] They include acetylcholine, the biogenic amines (dopamine, epinephrine, norepinephrine, serotonin, histamine), excitatory amino neurotransmitters (glutamate, glycine, aspartic acid, taurine), the inhibitory amino acid γ-aminobutyric acid (GABA), neuropeptides (now numbering 50 or more), gaseous neurotransmitters (NO, carbon monoxide), and miscellaneous neurotransmitters that include adenosine, cytokines (IL-1, IL-6, tumor necrosis factor [TNF]), endogenous cannabinoid or cannabinoids, benzodiazepines, sulfonylurea-like compounds, and neurotropic growth factors (nerve growth factor, brain growth factor, activins).[379] Through this repertoire of regulatory factors the hypothalamic-pituitary axis is integrated with behavioral changes and is enabled to respond to homeostatic and regulatory challenges.

TABLE 8–8. Summary of Function of Central Catecholaminergic Neurons and Sites of Action of Neuropharmacologic Agents

Step 1:	Uptake of amino acids into aminergic neurons: tyrosine, precursor of dopamine, norepinephrine, epinephrine
Drug:	No drug is known to interfere with tyrosine uptake.
Step 2:	Enzymatic synthesis
	Tyrosine is hydroxylated by tyrosine hydroxylase to form levodopa. Levodopa is decarboxylated to form dopamine, which in turn is hydroxylated to form norepinephrine. Norepinephrine is methylated to form epinephrine.
Drug:	α-Methyltyrosine blocks levodopa synthesis. Disulfiram (Antabuse) blocks dopamine conversion to norepinephrine.
Step 3:	Storage phase
	Norepinephrine, dopamine, and epinephrine are stored in specific granules within nerve terminals.
Drug:	Reserpine blocks storage of norepinephrine, dopamine, and epinephrine.
Step 4:	Release of preformed granules
	In response to neuronal depolarization, granules are extruded from nerve ending.
Drug:	Amphetamines may act, at least in part, on the release of norepinephrine.
Step 5:	Interaction of catecholamine with receptor located on postsynaptic neuron
	Extruded bioamine binds to specific receptors.
Drug:	Noradrenergic effects are duplicated by α-receptor agonist clonidine, β-receptor agonist isoproterenol; α-receptors are blocked by phentolamine, β-receptors by propranolol. Dopamine effects are duplicated by agonists apomorphine and bromocriptine and are blocked by antagonists phenothiazines and pimozide.
Step 6:	Reuptake process
	After release of preformed hormone, free neurotransmitter in synaptic cleft that has not reacted with receptor is taken up into presynaptic nerve ending.
Drug:	Cocaine and tricyclic antidepressants make norepinephrine more available by blocking reuptake.
Step 7:	Degradation of neurotransmitter and dopamine
	Norepinephrine bound to postsynaptic membranes or free in the presynaptic nerve ending is destroyed by the enzyme monoamine oxidase.
	The enzyme catechol O-methyltransferase is also responsible for inactivating these amines.
Drug:	Monoamine oxidase inhibitors (pargyline, isocarboxazid, tranylcypromine) make more neurotransmitter available to the postsynaptic cell.

Adapted from Cooper JR, Bloom FE, Roth RH. The Biochemical Basis of Neuropharmacology. 3rd ed. New York: Oxford University Press, 1978 and Martin JB, Reichlin S, eds. Clinical Neuroendocrinology. 2nd ed. Philadelphia: FA Davis, 1987, with permission.

Biogenic Amines

The function of central biogenic secreting neurons and the sites of action of some neuropharmacologic agents are summarized in Table 8–8, the overall effects of these agents on pituitary function are summarized in Table 8–9, and the classification is summarized in Table 8–3.

DOPAMINE. The dopamine-containing fibers concerned with pituitary regulation arise chiefly in the arcuate nucleus of the hypothalamus (Fig. 8–37) and project to the median eminence (tuberoinfundibular pathway) where dopamine enters portal vessel blood and, in species such as the rat, also the intermediate lobe of the pituitary (tuberohypophyseal pathway). Tuberoinfundibular and tuberohypophyseal dopaminergic cells make up only a small fraction of central dopaminergic pathways. Dopaminergic fibers that project to the basal ganglia (nigrostriatal pathway) are involved in extrapyramidal control; deficits in this system give rise to Parkinson's disease. Dopaminergic fibers directed to the cerebral cortex and limbic system (mesolimbic-cortical pathways) influence behavior and affect; dysfunction of these fibers may be a cause of schizophrenia.

Tuberoinfundibular neurons do not possess dopamine receptors (in contrast to the other dopaminergic neurons of

TABLE 8–9. Neurotransmitters and Pituitary Hormone Secretion

Hypothalamic-Pituitary Axis	E	α_1	α_2	β_1	β_2	NF	Dopamine	5-Hydroxytryptamine	Acetylcholine	H₁	H₂
CRH-ACTH	—	(↑)	(→)*	(→)	(→)	—	↑	↑	↑?	(↑)	—
GHRH-somatostatin–growth hormone	↑†	—	(↑)	(↓)	—	↑	↑‡	↑§	↑	(↑↓)	↑
GnRH-FSH-LH	—	(→)	(→)	—	—	—	→	—	↑↓	—	—
PIF-PRF-prolactin	—	—	(→↓)¶	—	—	—	↓↓‖	↑	→↓	(→)	—
TRH-TSH	—	—	(→)	(→)	(→)	—	↓‖	→↓	—	(→)	—

Key to symbols: →, no effect; ↑, stimulation; ↓, inhibition; —, action not ascertained; ?, action still questionable. The effect of activation of subtypes is indicated with parentheses.
* Inhibition in depressed patients.
† In combination with propranolol.
‡ Inhibitory to acromegaly and in vitro.
§ Inhibition of the GnRH-induced LH rise.
¶ Inhibition in children.
‖ TRH-induced rise; hypothyroid subjects.
CRH, corticotropin-releasing hormone; ACTH, adrenocorticotropic hormone (corticotropin); GHRH, growth hormone–releasing hormone; GnRH, gonadotropin-releasing hormone (luteinizing hormone–releasing hormone); LH, luteinizing hormone; PIF, prolactin-inhibiting factor; PRF, prolactin-releasing factor; TRH, thyrotropin-releasing hormone; TSH, thyroid-stimulating hormone (thyrotropin).
Modified from Müller EE. Brain messengers and the pituitary gland. In: Delbecco R, ed. Encyclopedia of Human Biology. Vol 2. San Diego, Academic Press, 1991, pp 11–28; and reprinted from Müller EE. Role of neurotransmitters and neuromodulators in the control of anterior pituitary hormone secretion. In: DeGroot LJ, ed. Endocrinology. 3rd ed. Philadelphia, WB Saunders, 1995:178–191, with permission.

the brain) and therefore they are not subject to presynaptic inhibition by dopamine or affected by drugs that block presynaptic dopamine uptake. This group of neurons, however, unlike those in other parts of the brain, express PRL receptors and thereby participate in the short-loop feedback control of PRL secretion by PRL.[138] Hence the effects of dopamine agonist and antagonist drugs on the pituitary and the brain depend on the receptor specificity of the drug, its ability to cross the blood-brain barrier, and its direct effects on the pituitary as contrasted with the central control of hypophyseotropic factors.[380]

Five different dopamine receptors have been identified in both the rat and human; all are G protein–coupled seven-membrane spanning molecules that modulate the activity of adenylate cyclase, phosphoinositol hydrolysis, and intracellular free Ca^{2+}.[381] The type 2 dopamine receptor predominates in the pituitary and its overall effect is to suppress the synthesis and secretion of PRL, thyrotropin, and GH.

NOREPINEPHRINE AND EPINEPHRINE. Almost all noradrenergic cells originate from the midbrain (locus coeruleus and adjacent regions) and project to the forebrain (including the cerebral cortex), the hypothalamus, the limbic system, the brain stem, and the spinal cord (see Fig. 8–37).[382, 383] The components that regulate the anterior pituitary project either to the median eminence (where they come into contact with nerve endings of the tuberoinfundibular system) or to the tuberoinfundibular cell bodies. Other central noradrenergic fibers are distributed to other regions of the brain and play essential roles in visceral homeostasis and adaptive behaviors, regulation of sleep, appetite, eating, blood pressure, and control of spontaneous physical activity. Several of the pathways are activated by physiological stimuli, but the diffuseness of the central noradrenergic pathways makes it difficult to localize the sites of such functions.

Of the central pathways concerned with biogenic amines those in which epinephrine is a neurotransmitter are among the least plentiful.[384] Like the noradrenergic system, cell bodies of origin in the midbrain have an extensive distribution, including the hypothalamus and the median eminence. Certain aspects of GH secretion depend on this neurotransmitter.[376]

SEROTONIN. Almost all the neurons that synthesize serotonin (5-hydroxytryptamine [5-HT]) originate from the raphe nuclei in the midbrain (see Fig. 8–37)[383, 385–387] and ascend to innervate virtually all parts of the forebrain and diencephalon. Serotoninergic fibers involved in pituitary control terminate in several sites of the hypothalamus, including the paraventricular nucleus, the median eminence, and the lumen of the third ventricle itself. Raphe nuclei also project downward into the brain stem and spinal cord.[385, 387] Some of these cells contain both peptide neurotransmitters and serotonin. For example many downstream projecting fibers contain both TRH and serotonin and form extensive projections to the intermediolateral column of the spinal cord (the site of origin of the sympathetic nerves) and to the motor horn cells of the ventral spinal cord.[387] Other serotoninergic fibers contain both

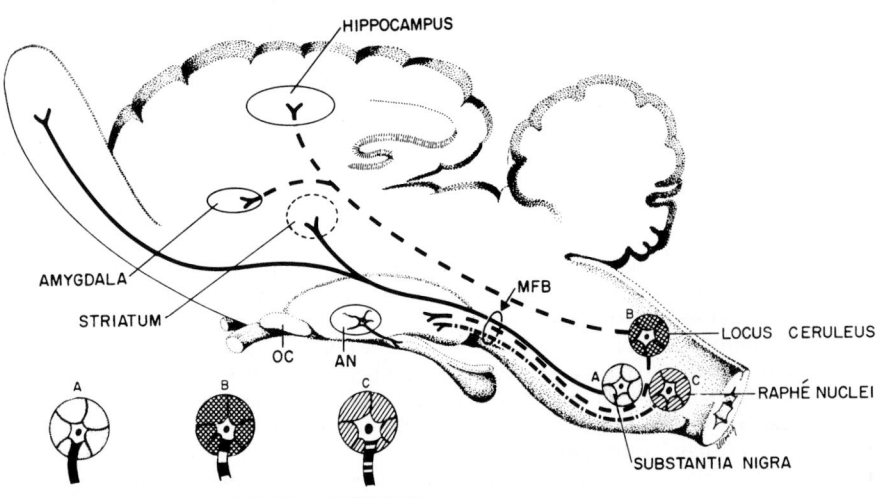

Figure 8–37. Simplified diagram showing the major distribution of the ascending monoaminergic pathways in mammalian brain. The principal source of all three major biogenic amines in the brain is the nuclei in the brain stem: the locus coeruleus, the source of most noradrenergic fibers; the raphe nucleus, the source of most serotoninergic fibers; and the substantia nigra, the source of most dopaminergic fibers. An important dopaminergic pathway arises in the arcuate nucleus of the hypothalamus and is the principal source of dopamine to the hypophyseal circulation. Epinephrinergic fibers arise from the region of the locus coeruleus in a pattern similar to that of norepinephrine. OC, optic chiasm; AN, arcuate nucleus; MFB, medial forebrain bundle. (From Martin JB, Reichlin S, Brown GM. Hypothalamic control of anterior pituitary secretion. In: Clinical Neuroendocrinology. Philadelphia: FA Davis, 1977:13–44.)

substance P and enkephalin.[383] Different serotonin receptors exhibit selective distributions and have different patterns of binding, response, and sensitivity to serotonin and its agonists and antagonists. At least seven types of serotonin receptors have been characterized, and two or more variants are recognized for types 1, 2, and 5.[388] All are G protein–coupled receptors with seven-membrane spanning domains.

HISTAMINE. Histamine-secreting neurons arising in the posterior hypothalamus in the tuberomammillary region project to the hypothalamus and in particular to the magnicellular and parvicellular nuclei.[389] Histaminergic neurons play an important role in the control of the neurohypophysis: dehydration activates the central histaminergic system; intrahypothalamic injection of histamine activates vasopressinergic neurons; and blockade of histamine synthesis reduces vasopressin responses to dehydration.[390] Histamine stimulates corticotropin release by activating CRH-containing neurons and activates cells that secrete oxytocin and other cells in the paraventricular and arcuate nuclei. This may be the mechanism by which histamine stimulates PRL and GH release.

Histamine receptors have been classified into two main groups, H_1 and H_2 receptors, which contain seven-transmembrane spanning domains. H_1 receptors mediate allergic response in the periphery, drowsiness, and neuroendocrine control.[378] H_2 receptors control gastrointestinal secretory activity.

In addition to its presence in nerve endings of histaminergic pathways, hypothalamic histamine is also derived from mast cells in regions in which there is no blood-brain barrier.[391] Because mast cells are regulated by cytokines and toxins they provide a pathway by which systemic inflammatory mediators can activate central histamine responsive neurons. Hypothalamic mast cells are also influenced by environmental stimuli and by gonadal steroids and may play a role in anterior pituitary regulation.[391a]

Acetylcholine

Vasopressin, corticotropin, and GH secretion are under cholinergic control, as is the suprachiasmatic (SC) nucleus. The location of the cholinergic cells that control hypophyseotropic neurons is not known with certainty, but there is an extensive projection of such neurons from the basal forebrain and midbrain to the SC nucleus.[392] A cholinergic pathway that arises in the nucleus basalis of the forebrain is distributed to the hippocampus. Loss of these neurons is a hallmark of Alzheimer's disease.[393]

Two classes of acetylcholine receptors exhibit different properties: "muscarinic," so named because they respond to the mushroom-derived toxin muscarine, and "nicotinic," because they are activated by nicotine. Five different "muscarinic"-type receptors, designated M_1 to M_5, contain seven-transmembrane spanning domains and are coupled to G proteins.[394] M receptors are involved in regulation of the pituitary and in the control of visceral function (stomach, small bowel, external secretions of the pancreas, islet cells of the pancreas). Several types of pituitary cells display muscarinic receptors and acetylcholine itself is synthesized in the pituitary.[395] The presence of acetylcholine receptors and of cells that secrete acetylcholine within the pituitary suggests an autocrine-paracrine mechanism.

"Nicotinic"-type receptors mediate muscular contraction through neuromuscular synaptic endings and mediate sympathetic nervous activity through postsynaptic receptors in the autonomic nervous system and in several central nervous system structures. Nicotinic receptors contain multiple subunits; at least eight different subunits have been characterized and all contain four-transmembrane spanning domains.[396] Acetylcholine-responsive cells, containing both muscarinic and nicotinic receptors, are found throughout the brain, including the hypothalamus.[397]

Amino Acids

EXCITATORY AMINO ACIDS. Excitatory amino acids (glutamate, aspartate, glycine) and the inhibitory GABA are important synaptic regulators. Glutamate can stimulate neurons so intensely that they are killed (by elevated intracellular free Ca^{2+} caused by membrane depolarization).[398] Early postnatal exposure to glutamate in rodents and primates causes neuronal destruction in the hypothalamus[399] in which most cells in the medial basal hypothalamus are destroyed, leading to hypothalamic hyperphagia, loss of spontaneous ovulation, and impaired secretion of GH. Glutamate plays an important role in the anoxic damage of the nervous system. Glutamate, GABA, and other amino acids are found in many important hypothalamic nuclei involved in anterior and posterior pituitary regulation.[399–404] As with other central neurotransmitters they are packaged and released in secretory granules and bind to glutamate receptors on postganglionic cells.

The two classes of glutamate receptors are those whose structure includes a cation-specific channel, the *ionotropic* receptors, and those that are G protein–coupled, the *metabotropic* receptors.[403] Ionotropic receptors control neuron excitability and fall into distinct types: NMDA (*N*-methyl-D-aspartate), AMPA (α-amino-3-hydroxy-5-methyl-4-isoxazolepropionic acid), and kainate.[405] NMDA receptors are also activated by glycine and serine. These receptors are relatively large, contain four- (or possibly five-) transmembrane domains, and are assembled from a repertoire of 16 different channel subunits in various combinations to form ion channels with different binding and transport capacities.[405] At least seven different metabotropic glutamate receptors have been characterized; all are G protein–coupled proteins containing seven-transmembrane domains. Their role in pituitary control, if any, is less well understood.

All regions of the hypothalamus and preoptic area express all three types of ionotropic receptor but they are present in low concentration only in the pituitary, indicating that glutamate acts mainly within the hypothalamus to regulate pituitary function.

INHIBITORY AMINO ACIDS. GABA and glycine are the principal inhibitory amino acid neurotransmitters.[401, 402, 406, 407] GABA is secreted by many neurons in the hypothalamus and elsewhere and plays an important role in brain function. The organization of the two known GABA receptors is extremely complex, involving interactions among at least three linked subunits.[406, 407] One is a Cl^- channel that controls membrane polarization. The benzodiazepine and barbiturate receptors on a subunit of the GABA receptor (GABA$_A$) function to potentiate GABA effects. GABA receptors are also present in the pituitary where they inhibit PRL release. GABA (along with barbiturates and benzodiazepines) inhibits virtually all tuberohypophyseal neurons, including those containing somatostatin and CRH.

Peptides

Tuberohypophyseal neurons of the hypothalamus are also controlled by peptide-secreting neurons (Table 8–10).[378, 408–412] These neurons arise in cell nuclei within the hypothalamus, are components of local collateral feedback control circuits, or are projections from the brain stem or elsewhere in the brain. Central neuropeptides are usually co-contained with other neurotransmitters (with which they may be synergistic). Some of the same neuropeptides involved in regulation *within* the hypothalamus are co-expressed within the pituitary where they may influence secretion by *paracrine* or *autocrine* mecha-

TABLE 8–10. Effect of Neuropeptides and Cytokines on Anterior Pituitary Hormone Secretion

Effects of Neuropeptides on the Hypothalamus

Peptide (Dosage)	Corticotropin	Prolactin	Growth Hormone	Thyrotropin	Follicle-Stimulating Hormone	Luteinizing Hormone
Substance P (μg)	NT	+?	−?	0	0	+
Neurotensin (μg)	NT	−, +	+	0	0	+?
Vasoactive intestinal peptide (ng)	NT	+	+	0	0	+
Gastric inhibitory polypeptide (μg)	NT	0	+	0	−	0
Motilin (μg)	NT	NT	−	NT	NT	NT
Galanin (ng)	0	+	+	0	0	0
Cholecystokinin (ng)	+	+	+	−	0	−
Angiotensin II (μg)	+	−	−	0	NT	+
Neuropeptide Y (ng)	+	0	−	0	+	+
Bombesin (ng)	NT	+	+	0	0	0
Calcitonin (μg)	+	−?	−	NT	NT	NT
IL-1α (ng)	+	0	NT	NT	0	−
IL-1β (ng)	+	0	−	−	NT	−

Effects of Neuropeptides on the Pituitary

Peptide (Dosage)	Corticotropin	Prolactin	Growth Hormone	Thyrotropin	Follicle-Stimulating Hormone	Luteinizing Hormone
Substance P (ng)	NT	+	0	0	−	−
Neurotensin (ng)	NT	+	0	+?	0	0
Vasoactive intestinal peptide (μg)	+	+	+	0	0	0
Peptide histidine isoleucine amide (μg)	NT	+	+	NT	NT	NT
Gastric inhibitory polypeptide (μg)	NT	NT	−	NT	+	+
Motilin (μg)	NT	NT	+	NT	NT	NT
Galanin (ng)	NT	0	0	NT	NT	NT
Cholecystokinin (μg)	0	+	0	0	0	0
Angiotensin II (ng)	+	+	0	0	NT	0
Neuropeptide Y (μg)	NT	NT	−	NT	+	+
Bombesin (ng)	NT	+	+	NT	NT	NT
Calcitonin (μg)	NT	+	0	−	NT	−
IL-1α (μg)	+,0	0	0	0	−	NT	NT
IL-1β (μg)	+	0	0	−	NT	NT

NT, not tested; +, stimulation; −, inhibition; 0, no effect; ?, controversial endings; IL, interleukin.

Findings should not be taken as fully valid under physiological conditions because of uncertainty about the physiological significance of concentrations tested and specific details of the test assays.

Modified from McCann SM. The role of several hypothalamic peptides in the control of anterior pituitary secretion. In: Müller EE, MacLeod RM, eds. Neuroendocrine Perspectives. Vol 1. New York: Elsevier Biomedical, 1982: 1–22; and reprinted from Müller EE. Role of neurotransmitters and neuromodulators in the control of anterior pituitary hormone secretion. In: DeGroot LJ, ed. Endocrinology. 3rd ed. Philadelphia: WB Saunders, 1995: 178–191, with permission.

nisms (see Chapter 9).[413] Examples include VIP (which is enhanced in thyrotrope cells of the pituitary and in parvicellular cells of the hypothalamus by hypothyroidism), substance P, and NT. Whether expressed by pituitary cells or not, many centrally active neuropeptides influence anterior pituitary cells directly.

A variety of peptides are distributed in parts of the central nervous system outside the pituitary-regulatory areas (Fig. 8–38). They influence behavior, homeostasis, pain perception, memory, learning, eating and drinking, body temperature, and sleep. More than 50 different peptides have been localized to specific neurons (see Tables 8–2 to 8–4).[6, 7] Because neuropeptides are formed as part of larger prohormones and are processed by enzymatic cleavage, many peptides of uncertain function are formed in the course of post-translational processing. The possibility that some may be important is suggested by the fact that POMC and procalcitonin give rise to more than one active hormone. The most abundant peptides in the brain are neuropeptide Y, CCK, VIP, and somatostatin. Peptides were historically given "trivial" names based on a biologic activity. A systematic method of naming peptides designates them by the first and last amino acid (in the single-letter code) and the number of amino acids. For example PHI-27 (peptide-histidine-isoleucine-27) is the peptide cosecreted with VIP.

Some peptides in long tracts and in local circuit neurons may act as neuromodulators, i.e., factors that modulate neuronal responses to neurotransmitters (see earlier discussion of secretomotor control and co-localization). Some neurons also interact with peptides, such as cytokines, derived from supportive glia (see later in the section on neuroendocrine-immune interaction) and with growth factors such as brain growth factor and nerve growth factor

ENDORPHINS AND ENDOGENOUS OPIOIDS. Central opioidergic neurons play an important role in the regulation of the anterior and posterior pituitary and in visceral functions such as pain, sleep, appetite, thirst, and sex drive. Administration of morphine or its analogues causes release of GH and PRL and inhibition of the release of gonadotropins and thyrotropin.[378, 408–411] Naloxone, an opiate antagonist, can reinitiate menses in some women with hypothalamic amenorrhea, suggesting that excess opioids play a role in the regulation of LHRH secretion. GH release that is induced by exercise and arginine is blunted by naloxone, whereas hypoglycemia-induced GH release is not. Morphine induces AVP release and in one study naloxone reversed SIADH, which suggests that this disorder could be brought about by excessive secretion of endogenous opioids in the neurohypophyseal system.[82]

Endorphin designates a class of endogenous morphine-like substances in the brain.[414, 415] *Endogenous opioid* is now used to describe any peptide with morphine-like activity. The search for these compounds was initiated when it was established that morphine and its analogues bind to specific receptors in the brain and in peripheral target tissues. The concept that the presence of a specific receptor in the brain is a marker of an endogenous ligand led to the discovery of other endogenous mediators such as digitalis-like compounds,[416] endogenous benzodiazepines, and endogenous cannabinoids.[417]

The pentapeptides met-enkephalin and leu-enkephalin were the first endogenous opioids to be isolated from brain.[414]

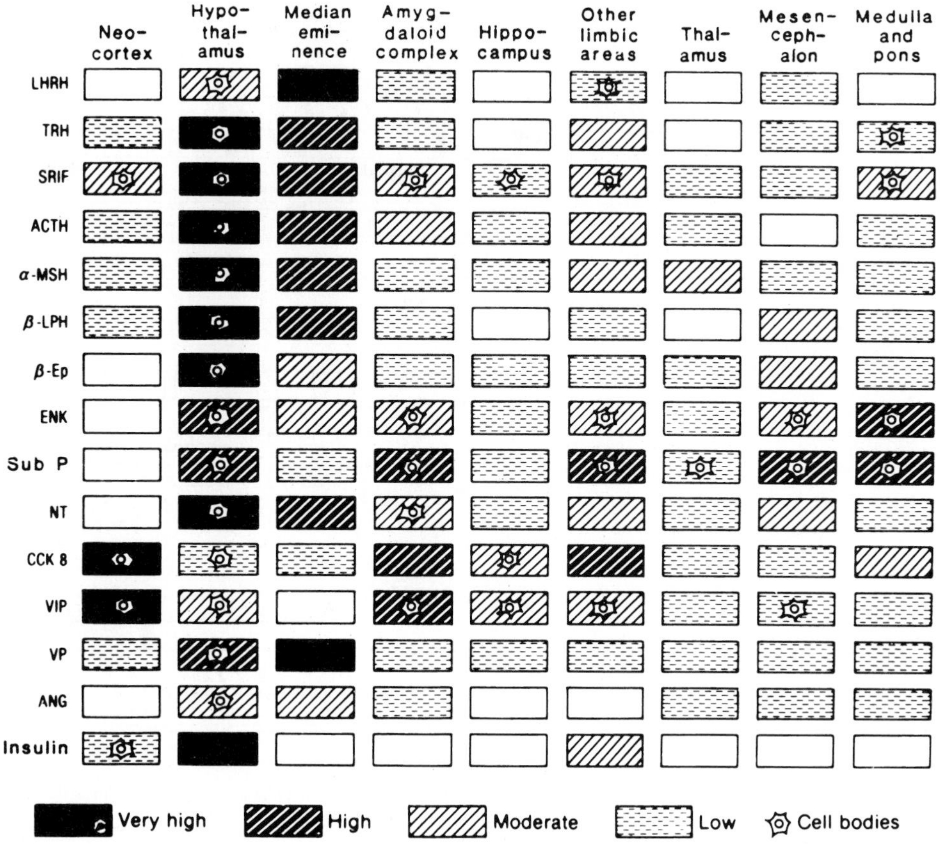

	Neo-cortex	Hypo-thalamus	Median emi-nence	Amyg-daloid complex	Hippo-campus	Other limbic areas	Thal-amus	Mesen-ceph-alon	Medulla and pons
LHRH		High ◉	Very high	Moderate		Low ◉		Low	Low
TRH	Low	Very high ◉	High	Low		Moderate		Low	Low ◉
SRIF	High ◉	Very high ◉	High	High ◉	Low ◉	High ◉		High	High ◉
ACTH	Low	Very high ◉	Moderate	High	Low	Low		Low	
α-MSH	Low	Very high ◉	High	Low	Low	Moderate	Moderate	Moderate	Moderate
β-LPH	Low	Very high ◉	Moderate	Low	Low	Low	Low	Low	Low
β-Ep		Very high ◉	Moderate	Low	Low	Low	Low	Low	Low
ENK	Low	High ◉	High	High ◉	Low	High ◉	Low	High ◉	High ◉
Sub P		High ◉	High	Moderate	Low	High ◉	Moderate ◉	High ◉	High ◉
NT		Very high ◉	High	High	Low ◉	Moderate	Low	Moderate	Moderate
CCK 8	Very high ◉	Moderate ◉	Low	High	High ◉	High	High ◉	Low	Low
VIP	Very high ◉	High ◉	Moderate	High	High ◉	High ◉	Moderate ◉	Low	Low
VP	Low	High ◉	Very high	Low	Low	Low	Low	Low	Low
ANG		High ◉	High	Low	Low	Low		Low	Low
Insulin	Low ◉	Very high				Low	Moderate		

■ Very high   ▨ High   ▧ Moderate   ░ Low   ◉ Cell bodies

Figure 8–38. Regional distribution of neuropeptides in the mammalian central nervous system. This compilation is intended to show the selectivity of some peptides, which presumably is related to specific functions. The hypothalamus contains the highest concentrations of most peptides, with the exception of cholecystokinin (CCK) and vasoactive intestinal peptide (VIP). Not shown is the distribution of peptide Y, which is present in the cortex in the highest concentration of any peptide. LHRH, luteinizing hormone–releasing hormone; TRH, thyrotropin-releasing hormone; SRIF, somatostatin; ACTH, corticotropin; MSH, melanocyte-stimulating hormone; LPH, lipotropin; Ep, endogenous pyrogen; ENK, enkephalin; Sub P, substance P; NT, neurotensin; VP, vasopressin; ANG, angiotensin. (From Krieger DT. Brain peptides: what, where, and why? Science 1983; 222:975–985. Copyright 1983 by the American Association for the Advancement of Science.)

[415, 418, 419] The amino acid sequence of met-enkephalin is identical with a sequence in β-LPH, a hormone that had been isolated previously from the pituitary (Fig. 8–39; also see Fig. 8–14).[420] β-LPH is the prohormone of several endogenous opioids, the most potent of which is designated β-endorphin.[418–421] β-LPH also includes a sequence corresponding to α-MSH and β-MSH binds to receptors distinct from the opioid receptors (see later).

β-LPH, the several enkephalins and endorphins, β-MSH molecule are synthesized together with corticotropin in the large prohormone POMC. Corticotropin is the final product in the anterior pituitary and larger forms are end products in

neurons and the intermediate lobe. α-MSH is the principal secretory peptide in the intermediate lobe of some species and in some neurons (see later).

Leu-enkephalin in brain (and in the adrenal medulla) can arise from three different prohormone precursors: POMC (see earlier), pre-proenkephalin A,[422] and pre-proenkephalin B (Fig. 8–40).[423] Pre-proenkephalin A contains four base sequences coding for met-enkephalin and one coding for leu-enkephalin. This same prohormone also contains sequences that encode opioids containing the enkephalin sequence. Pre-proenkephalin B codes for leu-enkephalin and other opioids including dynorphin and β-neoendorphin (see Fig. 8–40).[424]

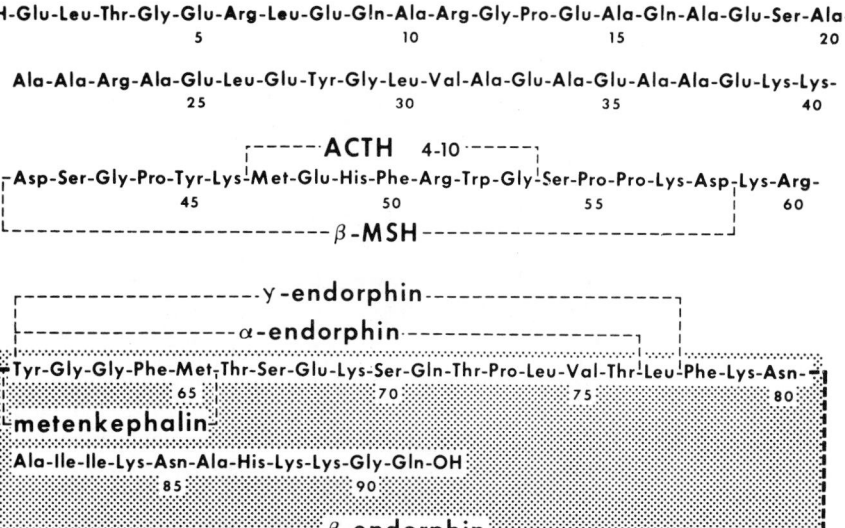

H-Glu-Leu-Thr-Gly-Glu-Arg-Leu-Glu-Gln-Ala-Arg-Gly-Pro-Glu-Ala-Gln-Ala-Glu-Ser-Ala-
5   10   15   20

Ala-Ala-Arg-Ala-Glu-Leu-Glu-Tyr-Gly-Leu-Val-Ala-Glu-Ala-Glu-Ala-Ala-Glu-Lys-Lys-
25   30   35   40

┌------ ACTH 4-10 ------┐
Asp-Ser-Gly-Pro-Tyr-Lys-Met-Glu-His-Phe-Arg-Trp-Gly-Ser-Pro-Pro-Lys-Asp-Lys-Arg-
45   50   55   60
└------------------ β-MSH ------------------┘

┌------------------ γ-endorphin ------------------┐
┌------------ α-endorphin ------------┐
Tyr-Gly-Gly-Phe-Met-Thr-Ser-Glu-Lys-Ser-Gln-Thr-Pro-Leu-Val-Thr-Leu-Phe-Lys-Asn-
65   70   75   80
metenkephalin

Ala-Ile-Ile-Lys-Asn-Ala-His-Lys-Lys-Gly-Gln-OH
85   90
β-endorphin

Figure 8–39. Homologies in structures of sheep β-LPH with corticotropin fragment (4–10), β-MSH (41–58), met-enkephalin (61–65), α-endorphin (61–76), γ-endorphin (61–77), and β-endorphin (61–91). ACTH, corticotropin; β-MSH, β-melanocyte–stimulating hormone. (From Martin JB, Reichlin S, Brown GM. Effects of hormones on the brain. In: Clinical Neuroendocrinology. Philadelphia: FA Davis, 1977: 275–303, with permssion.)

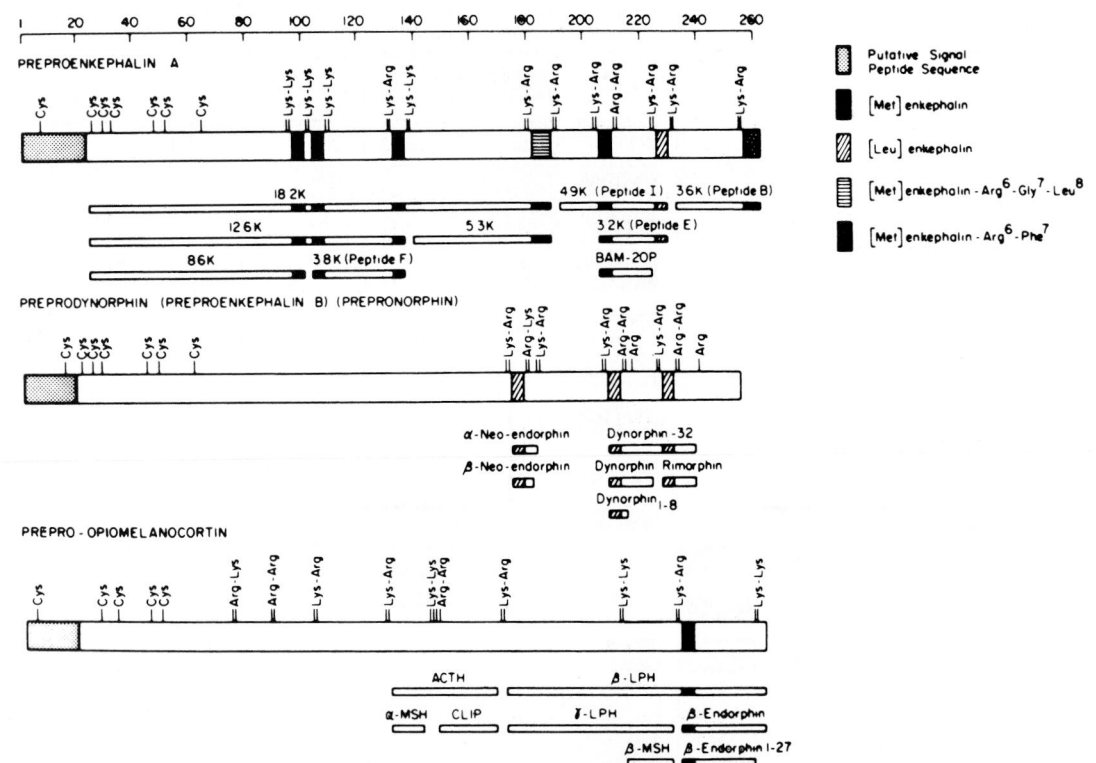

Figure 8–40. Biologic relationship between the three prohormones coding for enkephalins. Met-enkephalin is derived from pro-opiomelanocortin (POMC) (where it is represented by a single sequence) and from pre-proenkephalin A (where it is represented by four sequences). Leu-enkephalin is not part of the POMC prohormone but is represented as a single sequence in pre-proenkephalin A and as three sequences in pre-proenkephalin B. Various enkephalin-containing fragments, larger than the enkephalin pentapeptides, are also formed from the prohormone; some, such as dynorphin, have even higher opioid potency than do the enkephalins. ACTH, corticotropin; β-LPH, β-lipotropin; α-MSH, α-melanocyte–stimulating hormone; CLIP, corticotropin-like intermediate lobe peptide; γ-LPH, γ-lipotropin; β-MSH, β-melanocyte–stimulating hormone. (Courtesy of D.T. Krieger. From Krieger DT. The multiple faces of pro-opiomelanocortin, a prototype precursor molecule. Clin Res 1983; 31:342–353.)

Several of these are much more potent as opioids than the enkephalins.

Leu-enkephalin and met-enkephalin thus arise from three different prohormones (POMC and the two proenkephalins) and are present in functionally distinct neurons in the brain and in cells of the pituitary and the adrenal medulla. It appears that all three arise from a single ancestral gene.

The endorphin nociceptin appears to *increase* rather than decrease pain and may be involved in stimulating pain pathways and other visceral and neuroendocrine reactions.[425] Rich concentrations of enkephalin and opiate receptors in the hypothalamus and in the locus coeruleus may enhance the release of PRL and GH and suppress thyrotropin and gonadotropin release. The anatomic localization within the hypothalamus of various subtypes of opioid receptor is schematized in Figure 8–41.

In the gut the wide distribution of enkephalins in neurons and in secretory cells and the presence of opiate receptors in the intestine suggest a role for endogenous opioids in the regulation of intestinal function. Enkephalins are present in

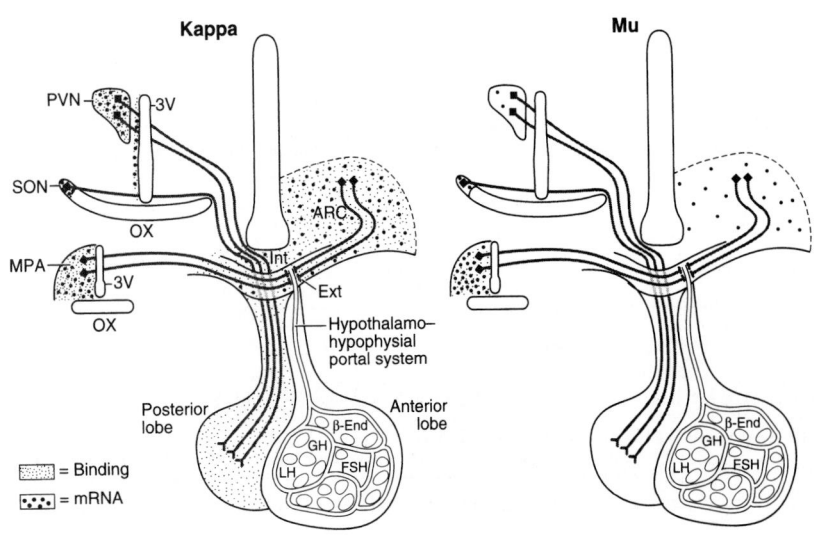

Figure 8–41. Opioid-receptor mRNA expression in the rat central nervous system: anatomic and functional implications. (From Mansour A, Fox CA, Akil H, et al. Opioid receptor mRNA expression in the rat CNS. Trends Neurosci 1995; 18:22–29, with permission.)

TABLE 8–11. Various Classes of Opioid Receptors, Principal Tissues, Principal Endogenous Ligands, and Relationship to Naloxone Antagonism

	Mu	Delta	Kappa	Epsilon	Sigma
Bioassay	Guinea pig ileum	Mouse vas deferens	Rabbit vas deferens	Rat vas deferens	—
Naloxone antagonism	Sensitive	Resistant	Resistant	Sensitive	Highly resistant
Probable endogenous ligand	? Endorphin	Met/leu-enkephalin	Dynorphin	Endorphin	?
Principal location	Periaqueductal gray	Limbic system	Substantia nigra	?	?
	Hypothalamus	Basal ganglia	Posterior pituitary		

From Grossman A. Brain opiates and neuroendocrine function. Clin Endocrinol Metab 1983; 12:725–746, with permission.

catecholaminergic neurons not only in the sympathetic nervous system but also in the carotid body and the adrenal medulla, where they are located in the same secretory granules that contain epinephrine. They are synthesized and secreted by pheochromocytomas. Endorphins are present in the pineal gland, kidney, eye, and placenta.

Three main classes of opioid receptors, μ, δ, κ, have been characterized (Table 8–11; also see Fig. 8–41).[426] They are homologous, G protein–linked seven-membrane spanning proteins. Hyperstimulation of the μ-opiate receptor is believed to cause tolerance (and withdrawal symptoms) by activating cAMP in neurons of the central catecholamine pathway.[427]

MELANOCORTINS. In the intermediate lobe α-MSH and N-acetyl β-endorphin are the principal products of POMC processing, and in the brain a number of the products include α-MSH and β-endorphin. Melanocortinergic neuronal cells arise mainly in the hypothalamus (arcuate nucleus) and brain stem (nucleus of the solitary tract) and project to most regions of the brain.

In the frog and chameleon α-MSH regulates melanocyte function and thus controls skin color.[136, 428] In these species adaptation of skin color to the environment is the result of a visual-neuroendocrine reflex mediated by the *stimulating* effects of α-MSH interacting with the *inhibitory* effects of melatonin, a secretion of the pineal gland. α-MSH induces dispersion of melanin pigment–containing granules through active changes in the cytoskeleton and stimulates growth and proliferation of melanocytes and the synthesis of melanin. In contrast, melatonin lightens skin by contracting the cytoskeleton fibers (on which melanin granules are bound) and concentrating melanin into dense clumps. In humans, injections of α-MSH or potent analogues of the hormone lead to increased skin pigmentation.[428, 429] Hyperpigmentation in primary adrenal sufficiency and Cushing's disease is due to the melanocortin-stimulating properties of corticotropin, the first 13 amino acids of which correspond to α-MSH.

α-MSH may also be a neurotransmitter or neuromodulator.[430] Centrally administered α-MSH exerts antipyretic (antifever) action in animals given pyrogens, in keeping with the distribution of MSH-containing neurons and melanocortin receptors in the preoptic area of the hypothalamus, a region known to contain thermoreceptors.[428, 431] Other neural effects of MSH are summarized in Table 8–12. In immunocompetent cells MSH exerts anti-inflammatory effects (see later in the section on neuroendocrine-immune interaction).[432, 433]

Five MSHRs, designated 1 to 5, have been identified.[433–437] MSHR-1 is the principal receptor of MSH in melanocytes and melanoma. MSHR-2 is the corticotropin receptor in the adrenal cortex. MSHR-3, MSHR-4, and MSHR-5 are present in the brain; MSHR-3 is localized in the arcuate nucleus and a few other regions, and MSHR-4 is widely distributed in the hypothalamus in regions that regulate anterior pituitary function. These receptors are G protein–coupled, contain seven-membrane spanning domains, and act through cAMP, inositol-phospholipid turnover, and (in melanocytes) tyrosinase.

Gaseous Neurotransmitters: Nitric Oxide and Carbon Monoxide

NO, formed from arginine by the action of two different NO synthases, functions as a neurotransmitter, as a regulator of arteriolar contractility, and as an inflammatory cytokine.[51–53] Within the central nervous system, NO is excitatory, synergizes with the excitatory amino acid glutamate, and in high concentrations is neurotoxic. In the pituitary NO is secreted by gonadotropes and by supporting (folliculostellate) cells in which it acts by a paracrine mechanism.[438]

NO is involved in secretion of LHRH,[439, 440] gonadotropin,[438–440] CRH,[441, 442] GH,[443] and PRL.[444] It influences sex drive in the rat[445] and possibly the human, and is mainly responsible for the vasodilation in the corpora cavernosa that results in penile erection.[446] NO thus plays a role at virtually every level of sexual function—sex drive, LHRH regulation, paracrine control of LH and FSH, and erectile function.

Carbon monoxide, formed by heme oxygenase, is an inhibitory neurotransmitter[54] involved in the regulation of CRH.[447, 448]

FEEDBACK CONCEPTS IN NEUROENDOCRINOLOGY

A simplified account of feedback control as it relates to neuroendocrine regulation is presented in this section.[448–451]

TABLE 8–12. Central Actions of Melanocortins

Neuroendocrine

Inhibits secretion of PRL and LH
Inhibits IL-1–induced hypothalamic-pituitary-adrenal activation
Stimulates GH secretion

Thermoregulatory

Antipyretic
Induces hypothermia

Behavioral

Stimulates grooming, sex behaviors
Stimulates learning, attention, motivation, arousal

Cardiovascular

Pressor
Increases cerebral blood flow

Neurotropic

Promotes functional recovery from brain lesions
Promotes neurite outgrowth

Melanocortin-Opiate Interactions

Inhibits morphine-induced analgesia, tolerance, dependence
Induces hyperalgesia
Inhibits β-endorphin–induced suppression of sex behavior
Inhibits β-endorphin–induced suppression of stimulation of PRL
Inhibits β-endorphin–induced suppression of LH

Melanocortin-Catecholamine Interaction

Modulates synthesis and release of dopamine and norepinephrine

LH, luteinizing hormone; GH, growth hormone; PRL, prolactin.
Courtesy of Dr. Jeffrey B. Tatro.

Hormonal systems form part of a feedback loop in which the *controlled variable* (generally the blood hormone level or some biochemical surrogate of the hormone) determines the rate of secretion of the hormone. In *negative feedback* systems the controlled variable inhibits hormone output, and in *positive feedback* control systems the controlled variable increases hormone secretion. Both negative and positive endocrine feedback control systems can be part of a *closed loop* in which regulation is entirely restricted to the interacting regulatory glands or an *open loop* in which the nervous system influences the feedback loop. All pituitary feedback systems have nervous system inputs that either alter the *set point* of the feedback control system or introduce *open-loop* elements that can influence or override the closed-loop control elements.

In *engineering* formulations of feedback, three controlled variables can be identified: a *sensing* element that detects the concentration of the controlled variable; a *reference input* that defines the proper control levels; and an *error signal* that determines the output of the system. The reference input is the set point of the system.

Hormonal feedback control systems resemble engineering systems in that the concentration of the hormone in the blood (or some function of the hormone) regulates the output of the controlling gland. Hormonal feedback differs from engineering systems in that the sensor element and the reference input element are not readily distinguishable. The set point of the controlled variable is determined by a complex cascade beginning with the kinetics of binding to a receptor and the activities of successive intermediate messengers. Sophisticated models incorporating control elements, compartmental analysis, and hormone production and clearance rates have been developed for many systems.

ENDOCRINE RHYTHMS

Virtually all functions of living animals (regardless of their position on the evolutionary scale) are subject to periodic or cyclic changes, many of which are influenced mainly by the nervous system (see Table 8–13 for definitions).[452–455] Most periodic changes are *free-running*, i.e., they are intrinsic to the organism independent of the environment and are driven by a biologic "clock."

Most free-running rhythms can be coordinated (*entrained*) by external signals (*cues*), such as light-dark changes, cycles of the lunar periods, or the ratio of the length of day to the

length of night. External signals of this type (*zeitgeber* or time givers) do not bring about the rhythm but provide the synchronizing time cue. Many endogenous rhythms have a period of approximately 24 h (*circadian* [around a day] or *diurnal* rhythms). Circadian changes follow an intrinsic program that is "about" 24 h long, whereas diurnal rhythms can be either circadian or dependent on shifts in light and dark.[455] Rhythms that occur more frequently than once a day are *ultradian*. *Infradian* rhythms have a period longer than 1 d, as in the approximately 28-d human menstrual cycle and the yearly breeding patterns of some animals.

Most endocrine rhythms are circadian.[455] The secretion of GH and PRL is maximal shortly after an individual has gone to sleep and that of cortisol is maximal between 2 and 4 AM. Thyrotropin secretion is lowest in the morning between 9 AM and 12 noon and maximal between 8 PM and midnight. Gonadotropin secretion in adolescents is increased at night.[453]

Superimposed on the circadian cycle are ultradian bursts of hormone secretion. Gonadotropin secretion during adolescence is characterized by rapid, high-amplitude pulsations at night, whereas in sexually mature individuals secretory episodes are lower in amplitude and occur throughout the 24 h.[453] GH, corticotropin,[455] and PRL[456] are also secreted in brief, fairly regular pulses. The short-term fluctuations in hormonal secretion have important functional significance. In the case of gonadotropins the normal endogenous rhythm of pituitary secretion reflects the pulsatile release of LHRH. The period of approximately 90 min between the peak of pulses corresponds to the optimal timing to induce maximal pituitary stimulation. Episodic secretion of GH also enhances its biopotency, but for many rhythms the function is not clear.

Most homeostatic activities are also rhythmic, including body temperature, water balance, blood volume, sleep, and activity.

Assessment of endocrine function must take into account the variability of hormone levels in the blood, and appropriately obtained samples at different times of day or night may provide useful dynamic indicators of hypothalamic-pituitary function. For example the loss of diurnal rhythm of GH and corticotropin secretion may be an early sign of hypothalamic dysfunction. Furthermore the optimal timing for the administration of glucocorticoids to suppress corticotropin secretion (as in therapy for congenital adrenal hyperplasia) must take into account the varying suppressibility of the pituitary at different times of day.

The best understood neural structures responsible for circadian rhythms are the suprachiasmatic (SC) nuclei, paired structures in the anterior hypothalamus above the optic chiasm.[448, 452] Individual cells of the SC nuclei possess an intrinsic capacity to oscillate in a circadian pattern,[457] and the nucleus is organized to permit many reciprocal neuron-neuron interactions through direct synaptic contacts. It is especially rich in neuropeptides, including somatostatin, VIP, neuropeptide Y, and NT, and microinjections of neuropeptide Y into the SC nucleus resets the timing cycle of some circadian rhythms in hamsters.[458] The SC nucleus also responds to the pineal hormone melatonin through melatonin receptors.[459, 460]

The SC nucleus receives neuronal input from many parts of the brain and from a direct projection from the retina that is distinct from the visual pathway—the retinohypothalamic pathway, which is the route by which the nucleus is cued by light-dark changes.[452] Anatomic dissociation of pathways subserving subjective visual and nonvisual stimulation explains the finding that circadian hormonal rhythms in some blind individuals are entrained to the light-dark cycle.[461]

Circadian rhythms during fetal life are regulated by maternal circadian rhythms.[462] Circadian changes can be detected 2 to 3 d before birth, and SC nuclei from fetuses of this age display spontaneous rhythmicity in vitro. Maternal regulation

TABLE 8–13. Terms Used to Describe Cyclic Endocrine Phenomena

Period:	length of the cycle
Circadian:	around a day
Diurnal:	exactly a day
Ultradian:	less than a day, i.e., minutes or hours
Infradian:	longer than a day, i.e., month or year
Mean:	arithmetic mean of all values within a cycle
Range:	difference between the highest and lowest values
Nadir:	minimal level (inferred from mathematical curve fitting calculations)
Acrophase:	time of maximal levels (inferred from curve fitting)
Zeitgeber:	"time-giver" (German), the external cue, usually the light-dark cycle that synchronizes endogenous rhythms
Entrainment:	the process by which an endogenous rhythm is regulated by a zeitgeber
Phase-shift:	induced change in an endogenous rhythm
Intrinsic clock:	neural structures that possess intrinsic capacity for spontaneous rhythms; for circadian rhythms these are located in the suprachiasmatic nucleus

Adapted from Van Cauter E, Turek FW. Endocrine and other biological rhythms. In: DeGroot LJ, ed. Endocrinology. 3rd ed. Philadelphia: WB Saunders, 1995: 2497–2548, with permission.

of fetal circadian rhythms may be mediated by circulating melatonin or by cyclic changes in the food intake of the mother.

Metabolic changes in the SC nucleus, such as an increased uptake of 2-deoxyglucose and an increased level of VIP, accompany circadian rhythms. This nucleus projects to the pineal gland by way of the autonomic nervous system (see later in the section on the pineal gland) and regulates its activity.

In addition to determining patterns of pituitary secretion, the circadian "pacemaker" influences many homeostatic functions. In humans the alteration of sleep brought about by jet lag and by working night shifts has profound effects on the sense of well-being and efficiency[463] and may be a factor in the pathogenesis of seasonal affective disorder (SAD), a disorder characterized by depression in winter when days are short and levels of illumination are low.[464] Seasonal affective disorder has been treated by manipulating the light-dark cycle.[464]

The timing of the circadian pacemaker can be shifted in humans by the administration of triazolam, a short-acting benzodiazepine,[465] or melatonin or by altered patterns of intense illumination.[463]

NEUROENDOCRINE CONTROL OF INDIVIDUAL PITUITARY HORMONES

Thyrotropin

The secretion of thyrotropin is regulated by two interacting elements: negative feedback by thyroid hormone and open-loop neural control by hypothalamic hypophyseotropic factors (Fig. 8–42). Thyrotropin secretion is also modified by other hormones, including estrogens, glucocorticoids, and possibly GH and is inhibited by cytokines in the pituitary and hypothalamus. Aspects of the pituitary-thyroid axis are also considered in Chapter 11.[152, 187, 466–470]

FEEDBACK CONTROL: PITUITARY-THYROID AXIS. In the context of a *feedback system* the level of thyroid hormone in blood or of its unbound fraction is the controlled variable and the "set point" is the normal resting level of plasma thyroid hormone. Secretion of thyrotropin is inversely regulated by the level of thyroid hormone so that deviations from the set point of control lead to appropriate changes in the rate of thyrotropin secretion (Fig. 8–43). Factors that determine the rate of thyrotropin secretion required to maintain a given level of thyroid hormone include the rate at which thyrotropin and thyroid hormone disappear from the blood (turnover rate) and the rate by which T_4 is converted to its more active form T_3.

Thyroid hormones act on both the pituitary and the hypothalamus. Feedback control of the pituitary by thyroid hormone is remarkably precise. The administration of small doses of T_3 and T_4 inhibits the thyrotropin response to TRH,[471] and barely detectable *decreases* in plasma thyroid hormone levels are sufficient to sensitize the pituitary to TRH.[472] TRH stimulates thyrotropin secretion within a few minutes through its action on a membrane receptor, whereas thyroid hormone actions, mediated by intranuclear receptors, require several hours to take effect (see Chapter 11).

The secretion of hypothalamic TRH is also regulated by thyroid hormone feedback. Systemic injections of T_3[473] or implantations of tiny T_3 pellets in the paraventricular nucleus of hypothyroid rats[474] (Fig. 8–44) reduce the concentration of TRH mRNA and TRH prohormone in TRH-secreting cells. Thyroid hormone also suppresses TRH secretion into hypophyseal-portal blood in sheep.[475]

T_4 in the blood gains access to TRH-secreting neurons in the hypothalamus by way of the CSF. The hormone is taken

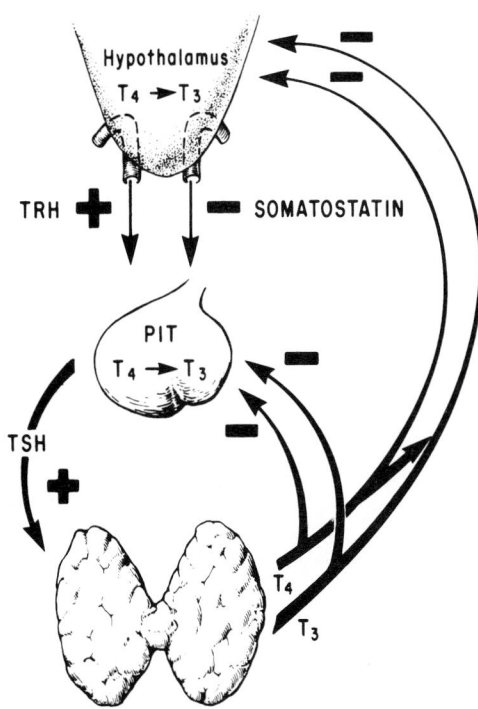

HYPOTHALAMIC – PITUITARY – THYROID AXIS

Figure 8–42. Hypothalamic-pituitary-thyroid axis. Thyrotropin from the pituitary stimulates the secretion of both T_4 and T_3 which act at the pituitary level to control secretion of thyrotropin by a negative feedback mechanism. In addition, T_4 is degraded to the much more potent T_3 within the pituitary by a monoiodinase. Secretion of thyrotropin is stimulated by TRH from the hypothalamus and is inhibited by somatostatin and to a lesser extent by dopamine. Hypothalamic factors thus interact at the pituitary level to determine the secretion rate. Thyroid hormone acts at the hypothalamus to stimulate secretion of somatostatin (this stimulating effect acts as a negative signal to the pituitary). The effect of thyroid hormones on secretion of TRH has not been determined precisely. Finally, within the hypothalamus, T_4 is also degraded to T_3, and this degradation may play a role in feedback control. T_3, triiodothyronine; T_4, thyroxine; TRH, thyrotropin-releasing hormone; PIT, pituitary; TSH, thyrotropin.

up by epithelial cells of the choroid plexus of the lateral ventricle of the brain, bound within the cell to locally produced transthyretin (T_4-binding prealbumin), and then secreted across the blood-brain barrier.[476] Within the brain, T_4 is converted to T_3 by type II deiodinase, and T_3 interacts with subtypes of the thyroid hormone receptor, $TR\alpha_1$, $TR\beta_1$, and $TR\beta_2$ in the paraventricular nucleus and other brain cells (see Chapter 11).[477] Thereby the set point of the pituitary-thyroid axis is determined by thyroid hormone levels within the brain.[478] T_3 in the circulation is not transported into brain in this manner but presumably gains access to the paraventricular TRH neurons across the blood-brain barrier. The brain T_4 transport and deiodinase system account for the fact that higher blood levels of T_3 are required to suppress pituitary-thyroid function after administration of T_3 than after administration of T_4.[478]

Transthyretin is present in the brain of early reptiles and in addition is synthesized by the liver in warm-blooded animals.[476] During embryogenesis in mammals transthyretin is first detected when the blood-brain barrier appears, ensuring thyroid hormone access to the developing nervous system.

NEURAL CONTROL. The hypothalamus determines the set point of feedback control around which the usual feedback regulatory responses are elicited. Lesions of the thyrotropic area lower basal thyroid hormone levels and make the pituitary more sensitive to inhibition by thyroid hormone,[466] and high doses of TRH raise thyrotropin and thyroid hormone

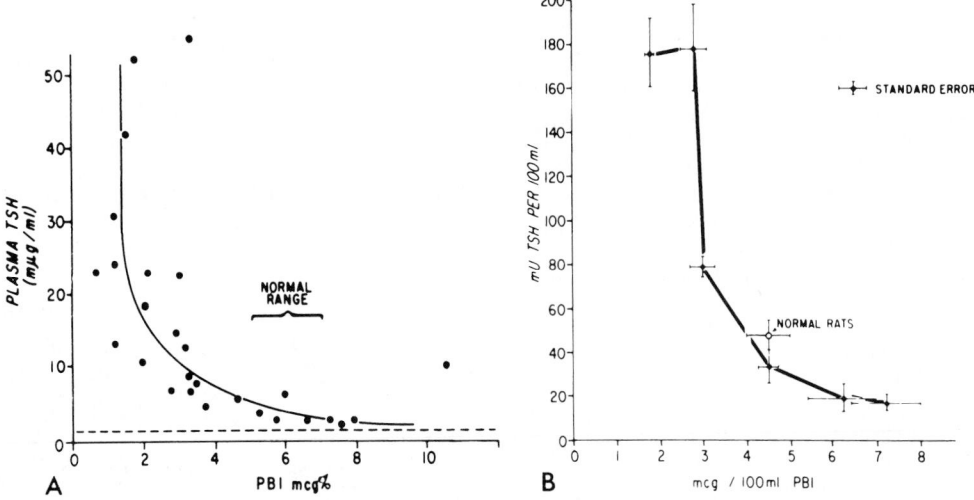

Figure 8–43. The relationship between plasma thyrotropin levels and thyroid hormone as determined by plasma protein-bound iodine (PBI) measurements in humans and rats. These curves illustrate, in the human (A) and the rat (B), that plasma thyrotropin levels are a curvilinear function of plasma thyroid hormone level. Human studies were carried out by giving myxedematous patients successive increments of thyrotropin T_4 at approximately 10-d intervals. Each point represents simultaneous measurements of plasma PBI and plasma TSH at various times in the six patients studied. The rat studies were performed by treating thyroidectomized animals with various doses of T_4 for 2 wk before assay of plasma thyrotropin and plasma PBI. These curves illustrate that the secretion of TSH is regulated over the entire range of thyroid hormone levels. At the normal set point for T_4, the small changes above and below the control level are followed by appropriate increases or decreases in plasma thyrotropin. TSH, thyrotropin; T_4, thyroxine. (A from S Reichlin, RD Utiger. Regulation of the pituitary thyroid axis in man: relationship of TSH concentration to concentration of free and total thyroxine in plasma. J Clin Endocrinol Metab 27, 251–255, 1967, © by The Endocrine Society. B from Reichlin S, Martin JB, Boshans RL, et al. Measurement of TSH in plasma and pituitary of the rat by a radioimmunoassay utilizing bovine TSH: effect of thyroidectomy or thyroxine administration on plasma TSH levels. Endocrinology 87, 1022–1031, 1970, © by The Endocrine Society.)

levels.[479] Synthesis of TRH in the paraventricular nuclei is regulated by feedback actions of thyroid hormones.[480] The hypothalamus can override normal feedback control through an open-loop mechanism. For example cold exposure causes a sharp increase in thyrotropin release in animals[481, 482] and in human newborns.[483] Circadian changes in thyrotropin secretion are another example of brain-directed changes in the set point of feedback control, but if thyroid hormone levels are sufficiently elevated, as in hyperthyroidism, TRH cannot overcome the inhibition.

Hypothalamic regulation of thyrotropin secretion is also influenced by two inhibitory factors, somatostatin and dopamine.[469, 484, 485] Antisomatostatin antibodies increase basal thyrotropin levels and potentiate the response to stimuli that normally induce thyrotropin release in the rat, such as cold exposure and TRH administration.[484, 485] Thyroid hormone in turn inhibits the release of somatostatin,[486] implying coordinated, reciprocal regulation of TRH and somatostatin by thyroid hormone. GH stimulates hypothalamic somatostatin synthesis[487] and can inhibit thyrotropin secretion. The role of somatostatin in the regulation of thyrotropin secretion in humans is uncertain.

Dopamine has modest effects on thyrotropin secretion, and blockade of dopamine receptors (in the human) stimulates thyrotropin secretion slightly.[469] Changes in the metabolism of thyroid hormone also influence T_3 homeostasis within the brain. In states of thyroid hormone deficiency brain T_3 levels are maintained by an increase in the deiodinase that converts T_4 to T_3.[488]

TRH neurons that regulate thyrotropin secretion are innervated by stimulatory and inhibitory neurofibers that arise from the brain, including brain stem, forebrain, neighboring cells in the paraventricular nucleus, and recurrent collaterals of TRH neurons (Table 8–14).[152] The physiological significance of these different neurotransmitters, their hierarchies of control, and their modes of integration with one another are not fully understood. In addition to the direct effects on TRH-secreting neurons, thyroid hormone also influences the secretion of many of the central neurotransmitters.[152]

The catecholamines are the best understood neurotransmitters affecting TRH. Cold exposure acting through peripheral cold receptors activates the central ascending catecholaminergic system. Norepinephrine (and epinephrine) bind to α_1- and α_2-receptors and activate adenylate cyclase with the formation of cAMP.[489]

TRH-secreting neurons in other parts of the central nervous system differ from TRH-secreting neurons of the paraventricular nucleus that regulate thyrotropin secretion in that they are not inhibited by thyroid hormone and are not involved in pituitary regulation. Pituitary-regulating TRH-secreting neurons are localized in the paraventricular nucleus. The supraoptic area is the site of temperature-sensitive neurons that mediate body temperature. Local cooling of the preoptic area mobilizes heat defense mechanisms: shivering, catecholamine discharge from the adrenal medulla and sympathetic nervous system, peripheral vasoconstriction, increased eating, and thyrotropin release.[466, 490] Local heating of this region inhibits heat conservation mechanisms and suppresses thyrotropin release. The increased secretion of thyrotropin after exposure of animals to a cold environment is brought about by release of TRH[481] secondary to signals from temperature receptors in the skin. TRH, acting as a central neurotransmitter in the preoptic region, increases body temperature.[490]

Central TRH pathways that arise in the midbrain (raphe nuclei) project to the spinal cord and target cells of the sympathetic nervous system in the intermediolateral column and ventral motor horn. Catecholamines are important determinants of heat production, especially in animals with brown fat such as the rat. TRH thus appears to influence body heat homeostasis at three levels: as a neurohormone that releases thyrotropin to activate the thyroid gland, as a central temperature-regulating neurotransmitter in the hypothalamus, and as a central transmitter in the brain stem and the spinal cord that regulates sympathetic nerve activity.

The pineal gland is reported to inhibit thyroid function in some[491] but not all[492] studies. The pineal gland contains TRH and in the frog its content changes with the season and with light and dark cycles independently of hypothalamic

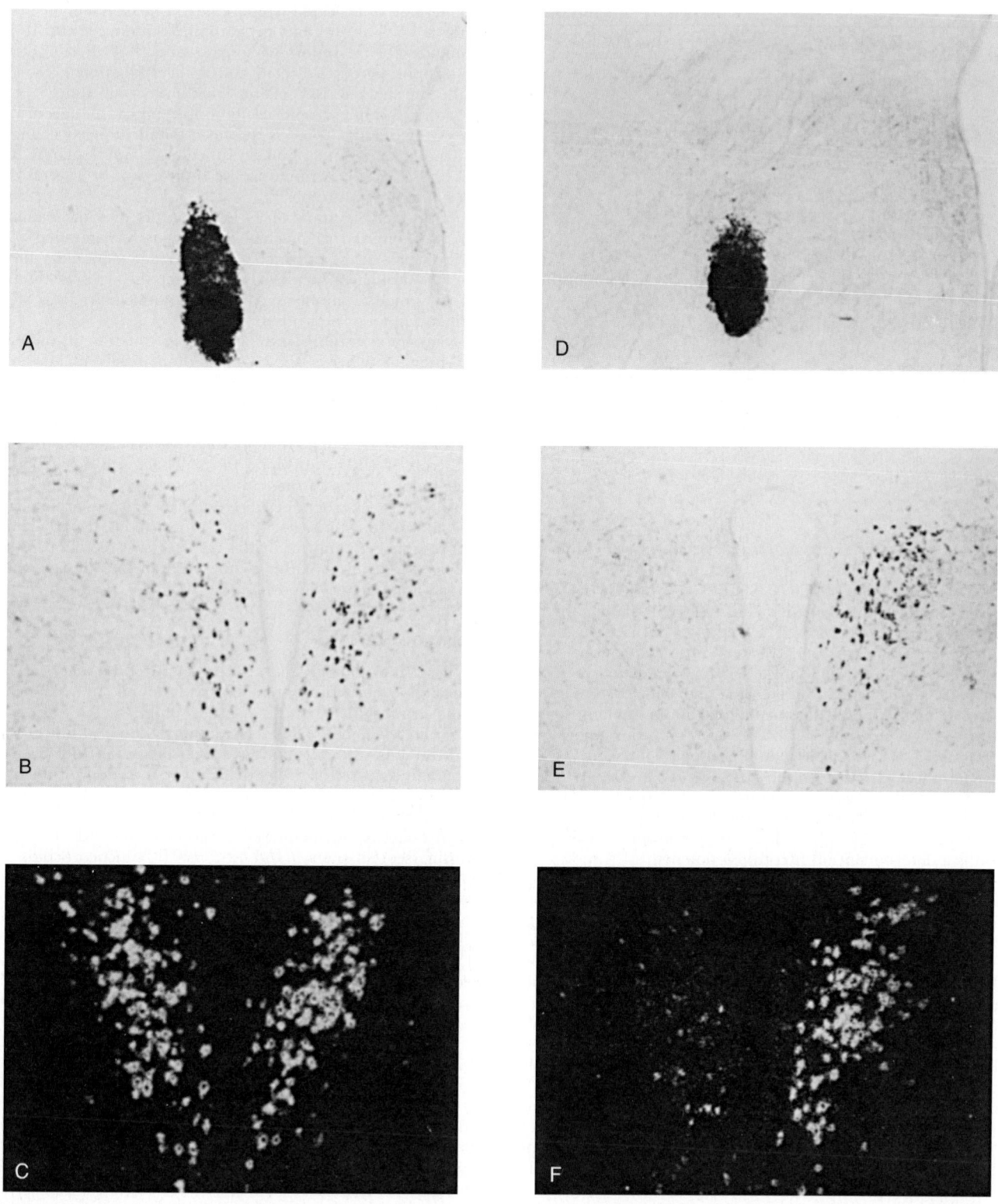

Figure 8–44. Direct effects of T$_3$ on TRH synthesis in the rat hypothalamic paraventricular nucleus (parvicellular division) were shown in this experiment by immunohistochemical detection of pre-proTRH (25–50) and of proTRH mRNA (by in situ hybridization) after implantation of a pellet of either T$_3$ *(D)* or inactive diiodotyrosine (T$_2$) as a control *(A)*. The T$_2$ pellet had no effect on the concentration of pre-proTRH *(B)* or on the concentration of proTRH mRNA *(C)*. In contrast, both the TRH prohormone *(E)* and the proTRH mRNA *(F)* concentrations were markedly reduced. These studies indicate that thyroid hormone regulates the hypothalamic component of the pituitary-thyroid axis, as well as the pituitary thyrotrop itself. Original magnification × 40 in *A* and *D;* × 79 in *B, C, E,* and *F.* (Photographs courtesy of Dr. RM Lechan. From Dyess EM, Segarson TP, Liposits Z, et al. Triiodothyronine exerts direct cell-specific regulation of thyrotropin-releasing hormone gene expression in the hypothalamic paraventricular nucleus. Endocrinology 123, 2291–2297, 1988, © by The Endocrine Society.)

TABLE 8–14. Neurotransmitters and Other Neuromediators That Innervate or Regulate Thyrotropin-Releasing Hormone–Secreting Neurons

Name	Functional Effect
Presence Proved by Histologic Procedures	
Norepinephrine	↑
Epinephrine	↑
Serotonin	↑, ↓
Neuropeptide Y	? ↓
Somatostatin	↓
Melanocortin	? ↓
Endorphins and enkephalins	↓
Neurotensin	? ↓
VIP	? ↑
TRH	? ↓
Presence Proved by Pharmacologic Techniques	
Dopamine	↑
Histamine	↑, ↓
GABA	↓
GHRH	↓
Interleukin-1	↓

↑, increase; ↓, inhibits; ↓, ↑, can either inhibit or stimulate depending on experimental situation; ?, effect probable, but data not entirely convincing.

VIP, vasoactive intestinal peptide; TRH, thyrotropin-releasing hormone; GABA, γ-aminobutyric acid; GHRH, growth hormone–releasing hormone.

Adapted from Toni R, Lechan RM. Neuroendocrine regulation of thyrotropin-releasing hormone (TRH) in the tuberoinfundibular system. J Endocrinol Invest 1993; 16:715–753, with permission.

thyrotropin.[493] The extrapyramidal system is also a regulatory area.[152, 466, 468]

FACTORS INFLUENCING SECRETION OF THYROTROPIN. In addition to feedback control by circulating thyroid hormone levels, thyrotropin secretion is influenced by an intrinsic circadian rhythm, cold exposure, starvation, stress, and inflammation, which are all changes mediated by tuberoinfundibular cells that secrete TRH and somatostatin.

Circadian Rhythm. Plasma thyrotropin in humans is characterized by a circadian periodicity, with a maximum between 9 PM and 5 AM and a minimum between 4 PM and 7 PM.[494] Smaller ultradian thyrotropin peaks occur every 90 to 180 min,[592] probably because of bursts of TRH release from the hypothalamus, and are physiologically important in controlling the synthesis and glycosylation of thyrotropin.[495] Glycosylation is a determinant of thyrotropin potency.

External cold exposure activates, and high ambient temperature inhibits, the pituitary-thyroid axis in animals[482] and analogous changes occur in humans under certain conditions. Exposure of infants to cold at the time of delivery causes an increase in blood thyrotropin levels, possibly because of alterations in the turnover and degradation of the thyroid hormones.[483] Blood thyroid hormone levels are higher in the winter than in the summer in individuals in cold climates[496] but not in other climates.[483] However it is difficult to document that changes in environmental or body temperature in adults influence thyrotropin secretion. For example exposure to cold ambient temperature or central hypothalamic cooling does not modify thyrotropin levels in young men.[497] Behavioral changes, activation of the sympathetic nervous system, and shivering appear to be more important in temperature regulation in adults than is the thyroid response.[482]

Stress is another determinant of thyrotropin secretion.[466, 468] Stress inhibits the release of thyrotropin, and in the rat this effect is in part due to release of somatostatin,[498] possibly the consequence of increased central CRH.[499] In humans physical stress also inhibits thyrotropin release, as indicated by the finding that in the euthyroid sick syndrome low T_3 and T_4 do not cause compensatory increases in thyrotropin secretion as would occur in normal individuals.[500–502]

The molecular basis of infection- or inflammation-induced thyrotropin suppression is now established: sterile abscesses or the injection of IL-1β (endogenous pyrogen, a secretory peptide of activated lymphocytes)[503] or of tumor necrosis factor α (TNF α) inhibits thyrotropin secretion,[573] and IL-1β stimulates the secretion of somatostatin.[505] TNF α inhibits thyrotropin secretion directly and induces functional changes in the rat characteristic of the "sick euthyroid" state.[504] It is likely that the thyrotropin inhibition in animal models of the sick euthyroid syndrome is due to cytokine-induced changes in hypothalamic and pituitary function.[506] Interleukin-6 and IL-1 and TNF α contribute to the suppression of TSH in the sick euthyroid syndrome.[507]

Transient elevation of T_4 levels occurs in some patients who are admitted to psychiatric hospitals,[468] suggesting that psychological stress can increase hypothalamic-pituitary function. Psychological factors generally act through the limbic system, which is connected to the hypothalamus by a well-defined system of neurons.[508]

Starvation inhibits pituitary-thyroid function in animals and humans. This is shown most dramatically in anorexia nervosa in which low blood levels of T_3 are present in the face of inappropriately low levels of thyrotropin. Low T_3 levels are a consequence of a reduced rate of T_4 secretion and a reduced rate of conversion of T_4 to T_3 in the periphery. Reduced levels of thyroid hormone in blood normally activate the hypothalamic-pituitary axis through the negative feedback loop, but in starvation neuroendocrine response fails to occur. The mechanism by which starvation brings about hypothalamic suppression is unknown; in the rat excessive secretion of somatostatin occurs, but this is not likely in the human when starvation increases blood hGH.

Corticotropin

Corticotropin secretion is regulated by the feedback action of glucocorticoids interacting with neural control mechanisms (Fig. 8–45).[509–512]

FEEDBACK CONTROL. The administration of glucocorticoids inhibits corticotropin secretion; removal of the adrenals (or administration of drugs that impair secretion of glucorticoids) leads to increased corticotropin release. The set point of pituitary feedback is determined by the hypothalamus acting through hypothalamic releasing hormones CRH and vasopressin (see Chapters 9 and 12).[142, 509–519] Glucocorticoids act on both the pituitary corticotropes and the hypothalamic neurons that secrete CRH and vasopressin. These regulatory actions are analogous to the control of the pituitary-thyroid axis. A still higher level of feedback control is exerted by glucocorticoid-responsive neurons in the hippocampus that project to the hypothalamus and affect the activity of CRH hypophyseotropic neurons and in turn determine the set point of pituitary responsiveness to glucocorticoids.[513]

Glucocorticoids are lipid soluble and enter the brain through the blood-brain barrier.[514] In brain and pituitary they can bind to two receptors, type I (the *mineralocorticoid* receptor, so named because it binds aldosterone and glucocorticoids with high affinity) and type II (*glucocorticoid* receptor, which has a low affinity for mineralocorticoids).[513, 514–519] Glucocorticoid action involves binding of the steroid-receptor complex to regulator sequences in the genome.[515] Type I receptors are saturated by basal levels of glucocorticoids, whereas type II receptors are not saturated under basal conditions but approach saturation during peak phases of the circadian rhythm and during stress. These differences and differences in regional distribution within the brain suggest that type I receptors determine basal activity of the hypothalamic-pituitary axis and that type II receptors mediate stress responses.

In the pituitary glucocorticoids inhibit secretion of corticotropin and the synthesis of POMC mRNA; in the hypothala-

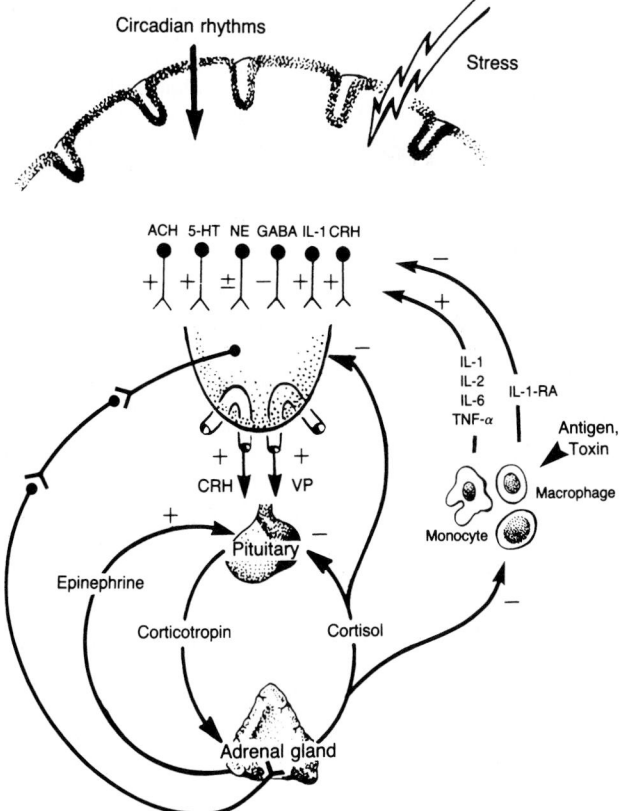

Figure 8–45. Schematic outline of function of the hypothalamic-pituitary-adrenal axis and its relationship to the peripheral immune system. The system includes two negative feedback loops: one in which glucocorticoids feed back on the brain and pituitary to control the output of corticotropin, and the other in which cytokines produced by immunocompetent cells act on the hypothalamus to regulate the output of glucocorticoids. In addition an open loop element of control is diagrammed. Corticotropin stimulates the adrenal cortex to release cortisol, which in turn exerts a direct negative feedback effect on the anterior pituitary. Secretion of corticotropin is stimulated by hypothalamic CRH and by vasopressin (VP); the release and synthesis of both regulatory peptides are inhibited by the feedback effects of glucocorticoids. Stress-induced epinephrine potentiates the effects of vasopressin and CRH. Within the hypothalamus, the secretion of CRH and vasopressin is regulated by neurotransmitters, the most important of which are portrayed here (see text). Excitatory effects are exerted by acetylcholine (ACH) and serotonin (5HT), and inhibitory effects are exerted by γ-aminobutyric acid (GABA). Norepinephrine (NE) is generally stimulatory, but the effect depends on the receptor being activated. Activated immunocytes—lymphocytes, monocytes, macrophages, endothelial cells, and Kupffer's cells—release acute-phase cytokines (interleukin-1β [IL-1β]; IL-2; IL-6; tumor necrosis factor α [TNF-α]) in response to antigens and toxins. These circulating toxins act on the hypothalamus to stimulate the release of CRH and vasopressin.[971] (From Reichlin S. Neuroendocrine-immune interactions. N Engl J Med 1993; 329:1246–1253. Copyright 1993, Massachusetts Medical Society.)

mus the secretion of CRH and vasopressin and the synthesis of their respective mRNAs is inhibited.[509, 511, 513–515, 517] Neuron membrane excitability and ion transport properties are suppressed by changes in glucocorticoid-directed synthesis of intracellular protein. Glucocorticoids may also act directly on neuronal cell membranes to change corticotropin secretion rapidly.[520]

Glucocorticoids block stress-induced corticotropin release. The latency of the inhibitory effect is so short (less than 30 min)[512] that it is possible that gene regulation is not the sole basis of the response. Long-term suppression (more than 1 h) clearly acts through genomic mechanisms.

Glucocorticoid receptors are also found outside the hypothalamus in the septum and amygdala,[513, 514, 519] structures that are involved in the emotional changes in hypercortisolism and hypocortisolism. Hippocampal neurons are damaged by

prolonged elevation of glucocorticoids during prolonged stress.[513]

NEURAL CONTROL. The set point of plasma cortisol feedback is determined by the central nervous system through modulation of CRH and vasopressin release. In the presence of high CRH levels, high concentrations of cortisol are required to inhibit corticotropin secretion. In contrast when CRH secretion is low (as in the late afternoon or in individuals with hypothalamic lesions), the controlling mechanism is highly susceptible to steroid suppression. The brain thus determines the set point of the "adrenostats" both in the pituitary and in the brain.

Unlike thyrotropin, which becomes completely unresponsive to TRH if thyroid hormone levels are sufficiently high, severe neurogenic stress and large amounts of CRH can break through the feedback inhibition by glucocorticoids. "Short-loop" feedback is exerted on corticotropin secretion by corticotropin itself. Administration of corticotropin to adrenalectomized animals maintained on a fixed dose of glucocorticoid suppresses corticotropin secretion[521]; i.e., corticotropin inhibits its own secretion, an effect mediated at the level of the hypothalamus.

Disconnection of the pituitary from the hypothalamus in several species leads to increased basal levels of corticotropin, and certain responses to physical stress (in contrast to psychological stress) are retained in such animals. These observations have led several investigators to postulate the existence of a *corticotropin inhibitory factor* analogous to dopamine in the control of PRL secretion and to somatostatin in the control of GH secretion.[522] Candidate hypothalamic peptides to inhibit corticotropin release at the level of the pituitary include atrial natriuretic peptide, activins and inhibins, melanin-concentrating hormone (in fish),[523] and sequence 178–199 of the TRH prohormone.[183] No consensus has been reached about this issue.

CRH-secreting neurons involved in anterior pituitary regulation arise in the parvicellular portion of the paraventricular nucleus and project to the median eminence (see Fig. 8–21). AVP, which is synergistic with CRH in stimulating corticotropin release,[142, 509–511, 527] is present in about 50% of CRH neurons. In some forms of stress, such as circulatory shock, corticotropin release is triggered mainly by AVP secretion. CRH and AVP are secreted into the hypophyseal-portal circulation in a pulsatile manner; changes in AVP are actually much larger than those of CRH.[522] These ultradian rhythms are responsible for the ultradian rhythms of corticotropin release. Similarly circadian rhythms of corticotropin are induced by rhythmic hypothalamic secretion. Important excitatory inputs come from the SC nucleus (the regulator of circadian rhythms), the amygdala (a way station of the limbic system, an element of the "emotional" brain), the raphe nuclei of the brain stem (site of origin of the serotonergic system), and the locus coeruleus of the brain stem, (site of origin of ascending noradrenergic fibers). Inhibitory inputs on CRH secretion arise in the hippocampus and in the locus coeruleus of the midbrain.[524–526] These anatomic inputs are neurotransmitter coded (Table 8–15), the most important excitatory influences being cholinergic, serotoninergic, β-noradrenergic, and neuropeptide Y–ergic.[527, 528] CRH neurons are also activated by prostaglandin E₂ and by cytokines IL-1, IL-2, IL-6, and TNF.[529] The principal inhibitory influences are mediated by neuropeptide Y and NO (see Table 8–15).[532] Acute administration of morphine stimulates the release of corticotropin, and chronic administration of morphine blocks corticotropin release induced by a variety of stresses.[530]

Pathways to the hypothalamus are to a degree stimulus specific and to some extent coded pharmacologically. For example hypoglycemia acts on hypothalamic glucoreceptors to cause release of vasopressin, histamine induces hypotension

TABLE 8–15. Effect of Various Neurotransmitters and Neuropeptides on Corticotropin-Releasing Hormone

Excitatory	Inhibitory	No Effect
Noradrenaline (β)	GABA	MCH
Serotonin	Opioids (μ, κ)	EGF
Acetylcholine (M)	ANP	NGF
Neuropeptide Y	Substance P	Melatonin
Interleukin-1β	Nitric oxide	EAA
Angiotensin II		

GABA, γ-aminobutyric acid; MCH, melanin-concentrating hormone; ANP, atrial natriuretic peptide; EGF, epidermal growth factor; NGF, nerve growth factor; EAA, excitatory amino acids; M, muscarinic receptor.

From Grossman A, Costa A. The regulation of hypothalamic CRH: impact of *in vitro* studies on the central control of the stress response. Funct Neurol 1993; 8:325–334, with permission.

(which presumably acts on vascular stretch receptors but also acts directly on CRH-secreting neurons), and IL-1 acts directly on CRH neurons or by inducing prostaglandins as intermediate mediators.[528] Endotoxin-induced CRH release may be mediated by reflexes arising in the stomach and transmitted by afferent fibers of the vagus nerve that synapse in the nucleus of the tractus solitarius and then project to the paraventricular nucleus.[531]

CRH, through its actions as a corticotropin regulator and a centrally active neurotransmitter, may be an integrative stress response mediator. Intrahypothalamic injection of CRH in rats[247] and monkeys[532] induces a characteristic behavior suggesting emotional distress, inhibits secretion of gonadotropin[533] and GH, and activates the sympathetic nervous system.

FACTORS INFLUENCING SECRETION OF CORTICOTROPIN

Circadian Rhythms. Levels of corticotropin and cortisol (in humans) peak in the early morning, fall during the day to reach a nadir at about midnight, and begin to rise between 1 AM and 4 AM.[455] Within the circadian cycle approximately 15 to 18 pulses of corticotropin can be discerned, the height of which varies with the time of day. The set point of feedback control by glucocorticoids also varies in a circadian pattern. Corticotropin secretion is driven by CRH rhythms and reflects changes in endogenous activity of the SC nucleus and possibly other parts of the brain. Pituitary-adrenal rhythms are entrained to the light-dark cycle and can be changed over several days by exposure to an altered light schedule.

External Stimuli and Response to Stress. Physical stressors that influence adrenocortical function include hypoglycemia, pain, restraint, trauma, burns, bone fracture, shock, exercise, infection, surgery, electroshock therapy, toxins, histamine, and inflammatory cytokines. Severe pain and anticipation of conflict, embarrassment, or failure are of particular importance. Emotional stress–induced corticotropin release in the human occurs when coping mechanisms fail or when sudden unexpected stress occurs. Many patients with depressive disorders have chronically high levels of glucocorticoids, retention of the normal circadian rhythm but at a higher set point, and resistance to glucocorticoid suppression, which are all postulated to be due to chronic hypersecretion of CRH.[509, 534]

Growth Hormone

GH secretion is regulated by hypothalamic GHRH and somatostatin interacting with circulating hormones at the level of both the pituitary and the hypothalamus (Fig. 8–46).[251]

FEEDBACK CONTROL. Feedback control of GH release is mediated by GH itself and its target secretion IGF-I.[535–537] Direct GH effects on the hypothalamus act by short-loop feedback, whereas those involving IGF-I (which is synthesized in the liver under the control of GH) are long-loop systems analogous to the pituitary-thyroid and pituitary-adrenal axes.

Control of GH secretion thus includes two closed-loop systems (GH and IGF-1) and one open-loop regulatory system (neural).

GH secretion is inhibited by the feedback effects of GH itself and by IGF-I.[536, 537] In the hypothalamus both GH and IGF-I increase the secretion of somatostatin and inhibit the release of GHRH.[538] In the pituitary IGF-I (but not GH) inhibits the stimulating effect of GHRH. The feedback effects of IGF-I account for the fact that in conditions in which circulating levels of IGF-I are low, such as anorexia nervosa,[539] kwashiorkor,[540] and Laron dwarfism (the result of a defect in the GH receptor),[541] blood GH levels are elevated.

NEURAL CONTROL. The predominant hypothalamic influence on GH release is stimulatory so that section of the pituitary stalk or lesions of the basal hypothalamus cause reduction of basal and induced GH release. When the somatostatinergic component is inactivated (e.g., by antisomatostatin antibody injection in rats), basal GH levels and GH responses to the usual provocative stimuli are enhanced.[542, 543]

GHRH-containing nerve fibers arise principally from the arcuate and ventromedial nuclei.[29, 57, 542] Somatostatin-containing nerve fibers that inhibit GH secretion are located mainly in the anterior hypothalamic periventricular system.[57, 160, 161] The systems that regulate GHRH and somatostatin release receive a variety of neural inputs (Figs. 8–47 and 8–48). Those from the hippocampus (presumably linked to the sleep

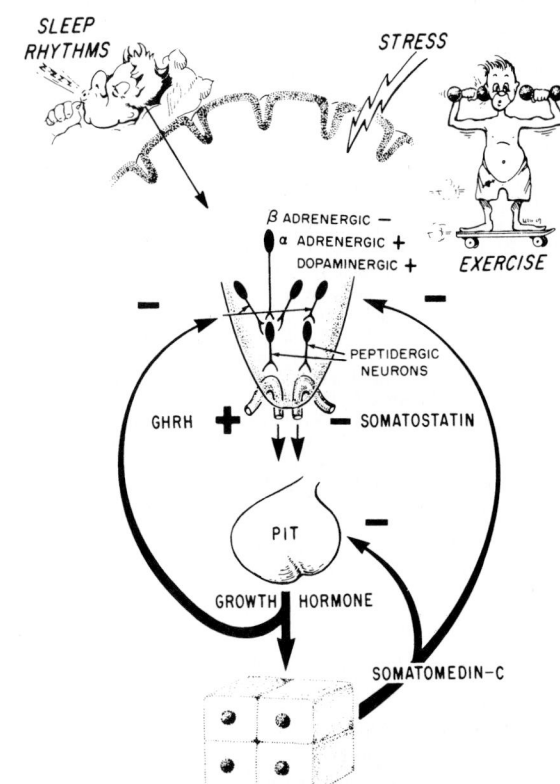

Figure 8–46. Regulation of GH secretion. GH secretion by the pituitary (PIT) is stimulated by GHRH and is inhibited by somatostatin. Negative-feedback control of the pituitary is exerted at the pituitary level by insulin-like growth factor 1 (IGF1), which also acts on the hypothalamus to stimulate secretion of somatostatin. On the basis of indirect pharmacologic data, it appears that release of GHRH is stimulated by acetylcholine and α-adrenergic and dopaminergic stimuli and is inhibited by β-adrenergic stimuli. Secretion of somatostatin, studied by direct assay in vitro, is stimulated by acetylcholine and VIP and is inhibited by GABA. Secretion of GH is modified by endogenous sleep rhythms, by stress, and by exercise. GHRH, growth hormone–releasing hormone.

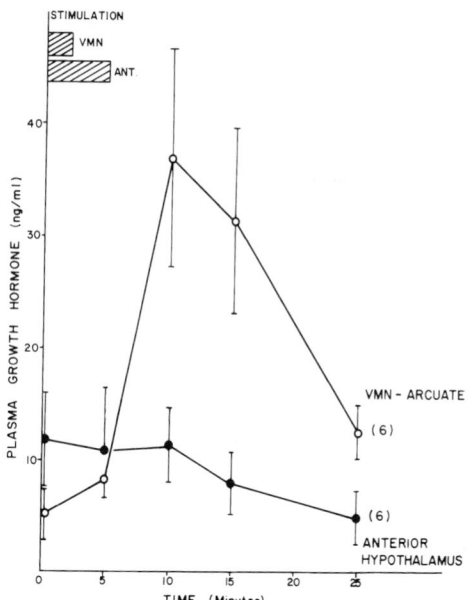

Figure 8–47. Effect on plasma GH level of electric stimulation of the ventromedial hypothalamic nucleus (VMN) of the rat. This figure shows the marked increase in plasma GH levels that follows electric stimulation of this nucleus. The ventromedial nucleus and ventral-basal hypothalamus are the only regions of the hypothalamus that are capable of this response, although certain extrahypothalamic sites may also cause this change. Note the short latent period of the response. The ventromedial nucleus is also important in that it has an effect on insulin secretion and satiety sensation and is the site of glucoreceptors. (From Martin JB. Plasma growth hormone [GH] response to hypothalamic or extrahypothalamic electric stimulation. Endocrinology 91, 107–115, 1972, © by The Endocrine Society.)

cycle) are excitatory, whereas those from the amygdaloid nuclei can be excitatory (basolateral amygdala) and inhibitory (corticomedial amygdala).[542, 543] As a part of the visceral brain involved in emotion and response to stress, the amygdala is probably involved in stress-induced GH release. Inhibitory inputs activate somatostatin release through the anterior hypothalamus, whereas the stimulatory pathways involve both ventromedial and arcuate nuclei.

The ventromedial nucleus is the site of glucose receptors capable of influencing insulin secretion and GH release, and it generates satiety signals through the paraventricular nucleus.[544] Insulin and somatostatin receptors and insulin-sensitive nerve pathways are located in this region.

Both GHRH and somatostatin are regulated by central neurotransmitters and neuropeptides such as dopamine.[545] The GH regulatory system receives impulses from dopaminergic, noradrenergic, adrenergic, serotoninergic, histaminergic, and cholinergic fibers. Control by the hippocampus and the amygdala is mediated by aminergic systems. Dopamine stimulates GHRH secretion by direct action on neuronal dopamine receptors and by stimulation of α-adrenergic receptors after conversion to norepinephrine. Norepinephrine and serotonin are potent stimulators of GH release. Epinephrine may also play a role in the control of GH secretion.[376] GH release is blunted by α-adrenergic blockers[282, 378, 546, 547] and is stimulated by β₂-adrenergic agonists such as clonidine.[548] This agent is used to test hGH reserve in children[548] and has been tried in the treatment of neuroendocrine hGH dysfunction.[549, 550]

It was long believed that cholinergic pathways do not influence GH secretion,[547] but in fact acetylcholine may be an important regulator of GH secretion. Blockade of acetylcholinergic muscarinic receptors reduces or abolishes GH secretory responses to glucagon and arginine,[551] morphine,[552] exercise,[553] and GHRH.[554–556] In contrast, drugs that potentiate

cholinergic transmission increase basal GH levels and enhance GH response to GHRH in normal individuals[557] or in subjects with obesity[557–559] or Cushing's disease.[560] In vitro acetylcholine inhibits somatostatin release from hypothalamic fragments,[561] and acetylcholine can act directly on the pituitary to inhibit GH release. The fact that some pituitary cells secrete acetylcholine suggests the operation of a paracrine cholinergic control system within the pituitary.[562] Cholinergic blockade with the muscarinic receptor antagonist pirenzepine reduces the GH excess of patients with poorly controlled diabetes mellitus.[563, 564]

Neurotransmitters may be specific for different physiological stimuli of GH secretion. For example sleep-induced GH release is mediated by serotoninergic fibers and possibly by cholinergic fibers. Spontaneous endogenous ultradian rhythmic discharge of GH is blocked by drugs that inhibit epinephrine synthesis, and α-adrenergic receptors are involved in the enhancement of GH by hypoglycemia and exercise.

Administration of morphine or injection of β-endorphin into the third ventricle[408–411] stimulates GH release, probably by activation of the GHRH neuronal system. Other peptides that simulate GH release are VIP, NT, and galanin.[565] Because VIP[566] and galanin[567] are intrinsic to the pituitary, both paracrine and neuroendocrine effects are probably mediated by these peptides. The injection of substance P into the third ventricle inhibits GH release by inducing somatostatin secretion. TRH has paradoxical effects on GH secretion; namely, it inhibits GH release when introduced directly into the brain, and systemic injection of TRH into humans inhibits the secretory surge of GH during sleep.[568] Likewise central TRH pathways generally inhibit GH secretion. Under several circumstances, however, such as malnutrition and acromegaly, TRH acts on the pituitary to stimulate GH secretion. When deprived of hypothalamic influences the pituitary somatotroph cell expresses and secretes TRH.[569]

FACTORS INFLUENCING SECRETION OF GROWTH HORMONE

Circadian Rhythm. Under basal conditions GH levels are low most of the time, with an ultradian rhythm of secretion of

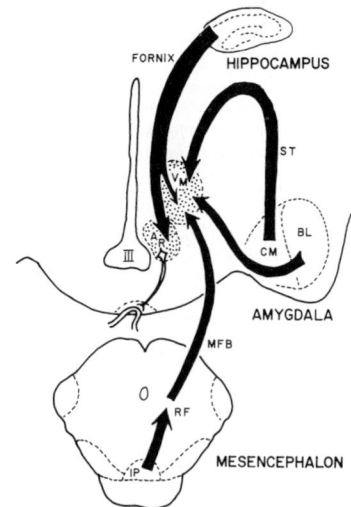

Figure 8–48. Neural pathways involved in GH regulation. This diagram illustrates the varied pathways by which impulses from the limbic system (visceral brain) ultimately impinge on the ventromedial nucleus, which in turn is capable of stimulating GH release through the mediation of GHRH. Pharmacologic blocking studies show that the pathways between the extrahypothalamic regions and the ventromedial nucleus are catecholaminergic, whereas those between the ventromedial nucleus and the stalk–median eminence region are not catecholaminergic. AR, arcuate nucleus; BL, basolateral nucleus; CM, corticomedial; IP, interpeduncular; MFB, medial forebrain bundle; RF, reticular formation; ST, stria terminalis; VM, ventromedial nucleus; III, third ventricle. (From Martin JB. Plasma growth hormone [GH] response to hypothalamic or extrahypothalamic electric stimulation. Endocrinology 91, 107–115, 1972, © by The Endocrine Society.)

about 13 pulses per 24 h.[570] Pulses occur almost uniformly with the first phase of slow-wave sleep[455, 570] Large pulses can also occur at random throughout the day and night unrelated to any identifiable extrinsic or internal event. These functional changes in GH secretion are determined by the central nervous system acting through the hypothalamus.

External and Metabolic Signals. Secretion of GH is modified by age, metabolic status, external stimuli, endogenous neural rhythms, and the feedback effects of GH acting through control of the production of IGF-I and somatostatin (Table 8–16; also see Fig. 8–46).[251, 262, 263, 571] Aging and obesity cause decreased GH secretion. Levels of GH are maximal during adolescence and decline gradually with age. By age 60 more than a third of men are functionally GH deficient, a state termed *somatopause*.[287] Obesity (as little as 15% above ideal body weight) also impairs spontaneous and induced hGH secretion.

Important triggers of GH release include the normal decrease in blood glucose level after intake of a carbohydrate-rich meal, absolute hypoglycemia, exercise, physical and emo-

tional stress, and high intake of protein (mediated by amino acids). GH secretion is enhanced by estrogen,[268] progesterone, testosterone, and thyroid hormone and is suppressed by glucocorticoids. The inhibitory effects of glucocorticoids are mediated at the level of the hypothalamus because they enhance the response of the pituitary to GHRH,[572] and glucocorticoid receptors are present in hypothalamic neurons that secrete somatostatin and GHRH.[573] Gonadal steroids and thyroid hormone[574] stimulate GH synthesis by interacting with regulatory sequences in the GH gene.

The paradoxical release of GH that follows glucose injection in some patients with optic nerve glioma (a lesion compressing the anterior hypothalamus) or metabolic encephalopathy, including uremia and hepatic coma, may be due to inactivation of the somatostatinergic inhibition. IL-1 can inhibit or stimulate GH secretion in the rat depending on dose,[575, 576] whereas in the human endotoxin and inflammatory cytokines stimulate hGH release.

Prolactin Regulation

Secretion of PRL, like that of other anterior pituitary hormones, is regulated by hormonal feedback and neural influences from the hypothalamus.[312–314, 319, 577–581] Feedback is exerted by PRL itself at the level of the hypothalamus. PRL secretion is stimulated by several external signals including suckling, mating, emotional and physical stress, and the sleep cycle (Table 8–17).[654–666] Secretion of PRL is also influenced by estrogens (Fig. 8–49) and by paracrine regulators within the pituitary such as VIP.

FEEDBACK CONTROL. Negative feedback control of PRL secretion is mediated by the interaction of PRL with PRL receptors in the tuberoinfundibular dopamine-secreting neurons of the arcuate nucleus, which increase the output and turnover of dopamine.[138]

NEURAL CONTROL. The predominant effect of the hypothalamus on PRL secretion is tonic suppression, which is mediated by regulatory hormones synthesized by tuberohypophyseal neurons. The set point of regulation is determined by dopamine (the principal PRL inhibitory factor); isolation of the pituitary (stalk section, transplantation or in vitro culture) or administration of dopamine receptor antagonists increases basal PRL secretion.

Several factors increase PRL release: stress, suckling, circadian rhythms, and, in some animals, mating and preovulatory neural signals. The effects of stress are probably mediated by VIP and PHI because immunoneutralization of these peptides blocks stress-induced PRL release in the rat. The effects of suckling may be mediated through a different neuronal pathway because treatment with anti-VIP and anti-PHI antibodies has only modest effects, whereas posterior lobectomy (in the rat) blocks suckling-induced PRL release. The posterior lobe secretes several peptides with PRL-releasing activity, including oxytocin, vasopressin, and TRH. However PRF activity in neural lobe extracts is probably due to an as yet uncharacterized factor arising from melanotropic cells of the intermediate lobe.[318] Mating in rats induces PRL secretion,[580] an effect mediated by both oxytocin and VIP.

Secretion of dopamine and PRFs is controlled by influences impinging on the hypothalamus. Central dopaminergic pathways inhibit PRL release, whereas central serotoninergic pathways are excitatory. Endorphinergic pathways stimulate PRL release, as do CCK, NT, and angiotensin II (see Table 8–10).[580]

The PRL regulatory system and its bioaminergic control have been scrutinized in detail because of the frequent occurrence of syndromes of PRL hypersecretion (see Chapters 9 and 17). Both the pituitary and hypothalamus have dopamine receptors and unfortunately the response to dopamine recep-

TABLE 8–16. Factors That Change Growth Hormone Secretion in Primates

Physiological	Hormones and Neurotransmitters	Pathologic
	Stimulatory Factors	
Episodic, spontaneous release	Insulin hypoglycemia	Acromegaly
Exercise	2-Deoxyglucose	TRH
Stress	Amino acid infusions, e.g.,	LHRH
Physical	Arginine	Glucose
Psychological	Leucine	Arginine
Sleep	Lysine	Interleukins 1, 2, 6
Postprandial glucose decline	Small peptides	Protein depletion
	GHRH	Fasting and starvation
	AVP	Anorexia nervosa
	α-MSH	
	ACTH 1–24 (corticotropin)	
	Glucagon	
	Galanin	
	Monoaminergic stimuli	
	Epinephrine, α-receptor stimulation	
	Levodopa	
	Apomorphine	
	Bromocriptine	
	Clonidine	
	5-Hydroxytryptophan	
	Fusaric acid (dopamine β-hydroxylase inhibitor)	
	Propranolol	
	Melatonin	
	Nonpeptide hormones	
	Estrogens	
	Diethylstilbestrol	
	Potassium infusion	
	Dibutyryl cAMP	
	Inhibitory Factors*†	
Postprandial hyperglycemia	Somatostatin	Acromegaly
Elevated free fatty acid levels	Melatonin	Levodopa
Elevated GH levels	Serotonin antagonists	Apomorphine
	Methylsergide	Phentolamine
	Cyproheptadine	Bromocriptine
	Phentolamine	Hyperthyroidism
	Chlorpromazine	Hypothyroidism
	Morphine	
	Cosyntropin	
	Progesterone	
	Theophylline	

*In many instances, the inhibition can be demonstrated only as a suppression of GH release induced by a pharmacologic stimulus.

†Modified from Martin JB, Brazeau P, Tannenbaum GS, et al. Neuroendocrine organization of growth hormone regulation. In: Reichlin S, Baldessarini RJ, Martin JB, eds. The Hypothalamus. Vol 56. New York: Raven, 1978: 329–357.

TRH, thyrotropin-releasing hormone; LHRH, luteinizing hormone–releasing hormone; GHRH, growth hormone–releasing hormone; AVP, arginine vasopressin; α-MSH, α-melanocyte-stimulating hormone; ACTH, adrenocorticotropic hormone; GH, growth hormone.

TABLE 8–17. Factors That Increase Serum Prolactin Levels in Humans

Physiological	Pathologic	Pharmacologic
Pregnancy	PRL-secreting pituitary tumors	TRH
Postpartum states	Hypothalamic-pituitary disorders	Psychotropic drugs
Non-nursing mothers (days 1–7)	("Functional"?)	Phenothiazines
Nursing mothers after suckling	Tumors (craniopharyngioma), metastases	Reserpine
Nipple stimulation (males and females)	Histiocytosis X	Oral contraceptives
Coitus (some subjects)	Inflammation-sarcoidosis	Estrogen therapy
Stress	Pituitary stalk section	Methyldopa
Exercise	Hypothyroidism	
Neonatal period (2–3 mo)	Renal failure	
Sleep		

PRL, prolactin; TRH, thyrotropin-releasing hormone.
Modified from Martin JB, Reichlin S. Clinical Neuroendocrinology. 2nd ed. Philadelphia: FA Davis, 1987: 45–63, with permission.

tor stimulation and blockade does not distinguish between central and peripheral actions of the drug.[581–587] Many commonly used neuroleptic drugs influence PRL secretion. Reserpine (a catecholamine depletor) and phenothiazines such as chlorpromazine and haloperidol enhance PRL release by disinhibition of dopamine action on the pituitary, and the PRL response is an excellent predictor of the antipsychotic effects of phenothiazines.[588] The major antipsychotic neuroleptic agents act on brain dopamine receptors in the mesolimbic system and in the pituitary-regulating tuberoinfundibular system. Consequently treatment of such patients with dopamine agonists such as bromocriptine can reverse the psychiatric benefits of such drugs. Bromocriptine rarely induces schizophrenia in individuals with no history of mental disorder.[589]

External and internal stimuli that modify PRL release

converge on the tuberohypophyseal neurons that secrete PIFs and PRFs. Pathways involved in the suckling reflex arise in nerves innervating the nipple, enter the spinal cord by way of spinal afferent neurons, ascend the spinal cord through spinothalamic tracts to the midbrain, and enter the hypothalamus by way of the median forebrain bundle. In most of the pathway neurons regulating the oxytocin-dependent milk let-down response (see earlier in the section on oxytocin) accompany those involved in PRL regulation and then separate at the level of the paraventricular nuclei. The suckling reflex brings about a release of PRFs and an inhibition of PIF activity.

FACTORS INFLUENCING SECRETION

Circadian Rhythm. PRL is detectable in plasma at all times during the day but exhibits a circadian rhythm with peak values in the early morning hours. Values are not closely correlated with other hormonal circadian rhythms, suggesting a distinct pathway of control.[455] Nursing mothers retain the nocturnal PRL surge, which begins from a higher basal level.[456]

External Stimuli. The suckling stimulus is the most important physiological regulator of PRL secretion. Within a few minutes of nipple stimulation, PRL levels rise and remain elevated for 10 to 20 min. This reflex is distinct from the milk let-down, which involves oxytocin release from the neurohypophysis and contraction of mammary alveolar myoepithelial cells (see earlier in the section on oxytocin). These reflexes provide a mechanism by which the infant regulates both the production and the delivery of milk. The nocturnal rise in PRL secretion in nursing women and in non-nursing women may have evolved as a mechanism of milk maintenance during prolonged nonsuckling periods at night.[590]

The evolution of these infant and maternal behaviors and their neuroendocrine components are essential to the survival of mammals. The PRL secretory and gonadotropin inhibitory responses to breast stimulation have major implications for human ecology. In some societies lactation-induced suppression of ovulation is the principal means by which pregnancies are spaced.[591] Inhibition of gonadotropins by suckling is mediated by the feedback effects of high PRL levels and by a non-PRL pathway as well.[592] External factors that influence PRL release include physical and emotional stress, exercise,[577, 578] and food ingestion.[593]

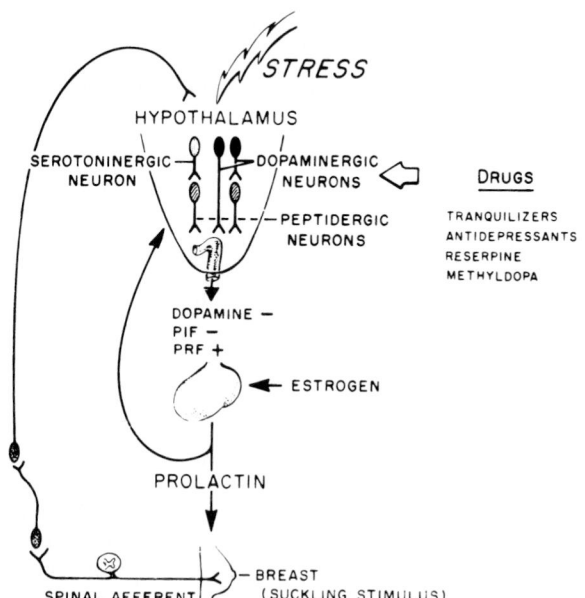

Figure 8–49. Hypothalamic regulation of PRL secretion. The predominant effect of the hypothalamus is inhibitory, an effect mediated principally by dopamine secreted by the tuberohypophyseal dopaminergic neuron system. One or more PRFs probably mediate acute release of PRL as in suckling and stress. There are several candidate PRFs, including TRH, VIP, oxytocin, and an as yet unknown intermediate lobe factor. PRF is controlled by serotonin. Estrogen sensitizes the pituitary to release PRL, which feeds back on the pituitary to regulate its own secretion (short-loop feedback) and also influences gonadotropin secretion by suppressing the release of LHRH. Short-loop feedback is probably mediated indirectly by modifications of hypothalamic catecholamine secretion and turnover. PIF, prolactin-inhibiting factor; PRF, prolactin-releasing factor.

Neuroendocrine Aspects of Sexual Function

Every component of reproductive activity in vertebrates depends on an interplay between neural and endocrine events.[579, 594–606] In addition to the regulation of pituitary-gonadal function, the integration of reproductive behavior, and the production of reproductive cycles, the nervous system determines the timing of the onset of puberty,[607–609] regulates the initiation and maintenance of lactation, and controls parenting behavior. Mating behavior in rodents is determined by hormones, but a role for gonadal steroids in gender identity in humans is not established.

FEEDBACK CONTROL. Pituitary function is regulated by the feedback effects of gonadal hormones on the pituitary and the hypothalamus (Figs. 8–50 and 8–51). All gonadal steroids—estrogens, progestogens, and androgens—bind to receptors in the pituitary to influence gonadotropin secretion. Steroid receptors in brain cells are involved in regulation of sexual behavior, control of LHRH secretion, and differentiation of the brain.[610–615] Steroid receptors also are found on glial supporting cells and in ependyma (cells lining the ventricles). As in the case of the thyroid and the adrenal cortex, neuroendocrine regulation of the gonads involves both closed-loop negative feedback by gonadal hormones (steroids and peptides) and open-loop components of neural control. Un-

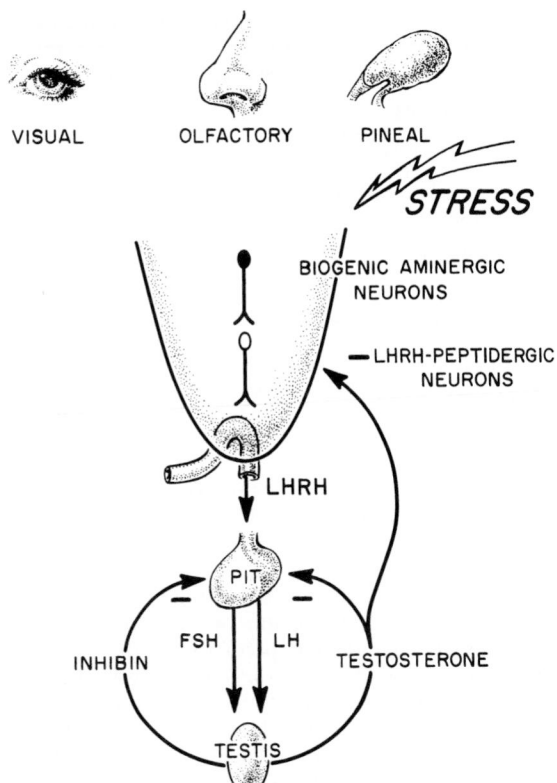

Figure 8–51. Regulation of gonadotropin secretion in the human male. Schematic diagram of gonadotropin control system in the male, showing the interaction of neural and hormonal feedback controls. The pituitary and testis are connected by a negative feedback link. Secretion of testosterone by the testis is stimulated by LH, whereas maturation and growth of the tubule cells are stimulated by FSH. The secretion of testosterone in turn inhibits the secretion of LH and FSH. It is likely that the major target of negative feedback is the hypothalamus; testosterone administration in humans does not interfere with the effectiveness of LHRH (pituitary sensitivity is relatively unaltered). A peptide secretion of the testis, inhibin, which is secreted by tubular epithelium, exerts a direct inhibitory effect on FSH secretion. Many different neurotransmitters regulate LHRH neurons. Some are excitatory (norepinephrine, neurokinin); others are inhibitory such as the endorphins and IL-1β. Testosterone negative feedback is exerted on neurons that project to the LHRH neurons, and not on the LHRH neurons themselves. Through this system a wide variety of impulses can be exerted on reproductive function. Visual influences include light-induced changes in seasonal breeders such as domestic cattle, deer, and birds. Olfactory signals in male rats influence gonadal function. The pineal gland in many species of animals inhibits gonadotropin secretion by direct effects of pineal secretions on either the hypothalamus or the pituitary. The role of the pineal gland in human reproduction control has not been established. LHRH, luteinizing hormone–releasing hormone; PIT, pituitary; FSH, follicle-stimulating hormone; LH, luteinizing hormone. (From Martin JB, Reichlin S, Brown GM. Neuroendocrinology of reproduction. In: Clinical Neuroendocrinology. Philadelphia: FA Davis, 1977: 93–128, with permission.)

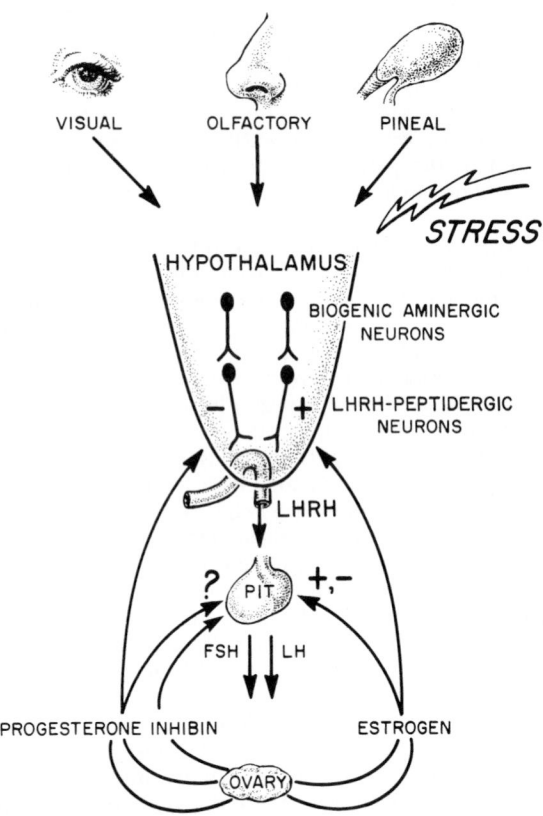

Figure 8–50. Regulation of gonadotropin secretion in the human female. Schematic diagram of gonadotropin control systems in the female, showing the interactions of neural and hormonal feedback controls. The development of the ovarian follicle is largely under the control of FSH. Ovulation is brought about by LH. Estrogenic hormones have complex effects on the feedback control mechanism of LH and FSH secretion. Depending on dose, time course, and previous hormonal status, estrogens can either inhibit or stimulate the secretion of LH through both negative and positive feedback controls. Progesterone also can either stimulate or inhibit LHRH secretion, depending on the setting in which it is given, but its effects at the pituitary level are relatively insignificant. Many different neurotransmitters regulate LHRH neurons. Some are excitatory (norepinephrine, neurokinin); others are inhibitory such as the endorphins and inflammatory cytokines. Estrogen negative feedback is exerted on neurons that project to the LHRH neurons, and not on the LHRH neurons themselves. Visual stimuli in many lower animals can influence the onset of sexual function (as in seasonal breeders). Olfactory signals through pheromones influence estrous cycles in many rodents and may do so in women as well. Pineal factors in lower animals delay the onset of puberty. LHRH, luteinizing hormone–releasing hormone; PIT, pituitary; FSH, follicle-stimulating hormone; LH, luteinizing hormone. (From Martin JB, Reichlin S, Brown GM. Neuroendocrinology of reproduction. In: Clinical Neuroendocrinology. Philadelphia: FA Davis, 1977: 93–128, with permission.)

like other feedback control systems, estrogens exert both negative and positive feedback effects (Fig. 8–52).

NEGATIVE FEEDBACK BY STEROIDS AND INHIBIN. In the presence of a normally functioning hypothalamus, LH and FSH secretion by the pituitaries of both sexes is suppressed by constant doses of estrogens and androgens and is increased after castration (or administration of antiestrogenic or antiandrogenic drugs) (Fig. 8–53). Negative feedback effects are mediated at the level of both the pituitary and the brain. If hypothalamic control is inactivated (e.g., by destruction of the medial basal hypothalamus or pituitary stalk section), basal gonadotropin secretion falls and the hypersecretory response to castration is blunted or abolished. Thus a functioning hypothalamus is necessary for normal pituitary response to gonadectomy. In castrated animals LHRH secretion is increased,[613] demonstrating that the hypothalamus or neurons projecting to the hypothalamus, or both, are targets of gonadal steroids.

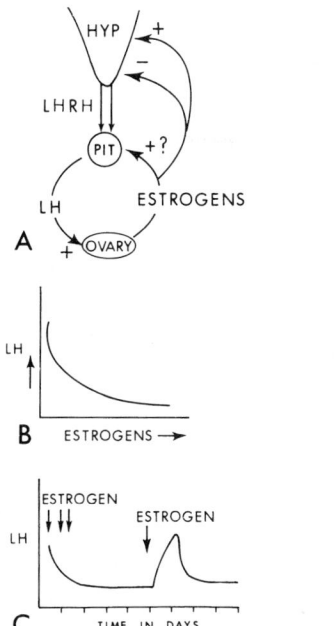

Figure 8–52. Pituitary-gonadal axis in the female: closed-loop negative feedback system with positive feedback elements and open-loop neural transients. *A,* Negative feedback. The level of estrogen in plasma controls LH secretion. When plasma estrogen levels are elevated, LH secretion is inhibited. When plasma estrogen levels are low, secretion of LH is enhanced *(B).* The precise target for estrogen in bringing out this negative inhibition is still not firmly established, but most work indicates that the effect is mediated at the hypothalamic level (here designated as a [−]), presumably through inhibition of the secretion of LHRH. *C,* Positive feedback. Estrogen transients (such as occur after administration of estrogens in animals or humans and in the spontaneous phases of the estrous cycle) are capable of stimulating the release of LH. The site of action of the positive hormone transient has not been fully established, but is probably a group of ascending catecholamine fibers arising in the locus coeruleus of the midbrain or cell bodies of adjacent hypothalamic neurokin-β peptidergic fibers, both of which display estrogen receptors. Although estrogen is shown here as both a positive and a negative stimulator, progesterone can also stimulate release of LHRH and is synergistic with estrogen in inhibiting LH secretion. There is evidence that the positive feedback element is exerted at the level of the pituitary (by sensitizing the LH-releasing mechanism to estrogen) and may be exerted at the hypothalamic level. In addition, the secretion of LHRH by the hypothalamus is subject to open-loop neural transients, such as sexual stimulation, which in some species, including humans, can alter LH secretion. HYP, hypothalamus; LHRH, luteinizing hormone–releasing hormone; PIT, pituitary; LH, luteinizing hormone.

LHRH neurons do not contain estrogen receptors, however, but are regulated by afferent signals from estrogen-sensitive neurons in the adjacent hypothalamus[614] or in the ascending catecholaminergic brain stem neurons.[611]

Suppression of pituitary secretion by gonadal steroids involves both neural and pituitary targets, is gender specific, and is influenced by both dosage and time-dependent variables. In women with normal menstrual cycles administration of physiological doses of estrogens suppresses basal levels of both LH and FSH. For the first 1 to 3 d after initiation of treatment pituitary responsiveness to LHRH is reduced, indicating that the suppressive effects of estrogen involve the pituitary.[616] The secretion of FSH is more sensitive to inhibition by estrogen than is the secretion of LH.[615] After approximately 3 d (and despite the fact that basal levels of LH and FSH remain depressed) the pituitary becomes *sensitized* to LHRH. In men treated with estrogens the plasma levels of LH and FSH are also reduced; in contrast to women, however, the response to LHRH remains suppressed.[616] Evidence that estrogen acts in the brains of women is the finding that expression of mRNA for LHRH in the hypothalamus in postmenopausal women is increased.[614] Testosterone treatment in men causes a fall in basal gonadotropin secretion unassociated

with a change in pituitary response to LHRH.[616] These findings imply that testosterone-negative feedback involves the hypothalamus, but long-term administration of estrogens or testosterone to men or women lowers gonadotropin secretion and suppresses pituitary response to LHRH, indicating a long-term effect on the pituitary.

Negative feedback, directed mainly at the pituitary FSH-secreting cell, is also exerted by inhibins, which are peptide hormones synthesized by germinal cells of the ovary and the testis.[337, 617] When germinal activity is low (as in normal prepubertal children) or if germinal epithelium is destroyed by chemotherapy, plasma FSH levels are disproportionately elevated and the FSH secretory response to LHRH is exaggerated (see Chapter 13). PRL also inhibits LHRH secretion[618] and causes the amenorrhea of hyperprolactinemia. Additional factors that inhibit gonadotropin release include dopamine, which directly inhibits LHRH release[618]; endogenous opioids; neuropeptide Y; CRH[619]; vasopressin; and inflammatory cytokines.[601]

A few neurons in the hypothalamus secrete LH[620] or PRL[621] but it is not known whether these neurons perform a specific function. Gonadotropins may also act directly on the hypothalamus to modulate gonadotropin secretion (short-loop feedback)[622] and LHRH may control its own secretion (ultrashort-loop feedback).[622]

POSITIVE FEEDBACK BY ESTROGENS: MIDCYCLE OVULATORY SURGE. The characteristic surge of gonadotropin secretion in adult women at midcycle (and in subhuman primates and other species) that induces ovulation is brought about by the sequential secretion of estrogen and progesterone.[600–602, 623] Both steroid hormones are secreted just before ovulation by the developing ovum, thereby signaling the hypothalamic-pituitary complex that it is ready to receive the LH ovulatory stimulatory signal. The neuroendocrine mechanisms by which estrogens and progesterone act as *positive*-feedback signals to induce the ovulatory surge are considered later in the section on neural control.

NEURAL CONTROL, THE "LHRH PACEMAKER." Imposed on the steroid regulatory inputs from the gonads are neural influences on the secretion of LHRH derived from several parts of the brain, an intrinsic "pulse generator" in the arcuate nucleus,[599] and perceptual links to the environment—odors via the olfactory bulb projections, circadian rhythms mediated via pineal secretion of melatonin, inputs from the limbic system that mediate emotional responses, and in some species reflexes from the genitalia.

Neural control of LHRH secretion is mediated by signals from four classes of neurotransmitters: bioamines, neuropeptides, excitatory amino acids, and gaseous neurotransmitters[373–375, 579, 596, 598, 601] Excitatory factors include norepinephrine acting through β₁-receptors,[579, 597, 601] neuropeptide Y, galanin, NT, substance P and other tachykinins,[600, 601] glutamic acid,[600] NO,[439, 440, 601] transforming growth factor α,[624] and prostaglandin E₂. Under appropriate conditions any of these factors can release LHRH; pharmacologic blockade of any single factor can block or reduce the LHRH ovulatory surge.

LHRH neurons also receive important inhibitory neural signals that mediate stress-induced inhibition of gonadotropin secretion. Central opioidergic neurons tonically suppress LHRH secretion except during the ovulatory surge when they are disinhibited.[601, 625] LHRH secretion is also reduced by CRH, vasopressin, and inflammatory cytokines (see earlier). The mechanism by which preovulatory secretion of estrogen and progesterone triggers the midcycle surge of gonadotropins is not well understood. In all species gonadotropin responsiveness to LHRH is increased at midcycle either because of sensitization of pituitary gonadotropes by estrogens or because of stimulation of LHRH secretion, or both, which in turn upregulates LHRH receptors. LHRH secretion is enhanced at

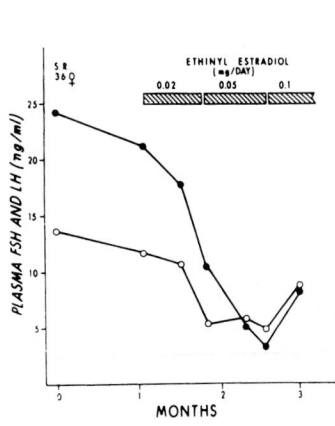

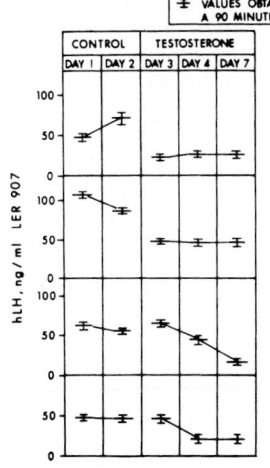

Figure 8–53. Inhibitory effects of gonadal steroids on LH secretion. Administration of estrogen to hypogonadal (menopausal) women *(left)* or of testosterone to men *(right)* results in a fall in the plasma LH level, which demonstrates negative feedback control. To convert LH values to international units per liter, multiply by 0.664. To convert FSH values to international units per liter, multiply by 0.002. *Left* (●) FSH; (○) LH. LH, luteinizing hormone; FSH, follicle-stimulating hormone. (*Left* from Schalch DS. Gonadotropin secretion in the human. In: Mack HC, Sherman AE, eds. Neuroendocrinology of Human Reproduction. Springfield, IL: Charles C Thomas, 1971: 127–145.)

midcycle in rodents and rhesus monkeys.[626] Since LHRH neurons do not have estrogen receptors, enhanced LHRH secretion is not caused by a direct action of estrogens on these cells. Rather estrogens act through cells that have estrogen receptors such as ascending noradrenergic fibers from the locus coeruleus in the brain stem and neurokininergic fibers that arise in the hypothalamus.[614]

It has not been possible to determine whether LHRH secretion in women is enhanced at midcycle, although indirect studies suggest that it is not. However increased LHRH secretion is not essential for the production of an ovulatory gonadotropin surge. In women who have a defect in LHRH secretion caused by lesions of the hypothalamus or pituitary stalk or who have Kallman's syndrome (Fig. 8–54)[627, 628] and in rhesus monkeys with hypothalamic lesions that impair LHRH input to the median eminence,[594, 598, 599, 628, 629] the injection of LHRH in a pulsatile manner approximating the normal 90-min ultradian rhythm restores menstrual cycles, ovulation, and fertility even if the LHRH is injected at the same frequency and intensity throughout the cycle.

In the rhesus monkey LHRH neurons display an intrinsic rhythm approximating the normal ultradian rhythm of LH secretion, a phenomenon termed the *LHRH pulse generator.* To account for the cyclic nature of midcycle ovulation Knobil proposed that the timing of the monthly ovulatory surge is driven by the ovary via secretions that cyclically increase the sensitivity of the pituitary gonadotrophs to endogenous LHRH.[594, 599, 611, 629] This view is compatible with the fact that abnormalities of ovulation can be induced by any interference with the normal intrinsic hypothalamic cyclic patterns or dysfunction of the pituitary or ovaries.

The rhythmic nature of the LHRH pulse generator is regulated by the hormonal milieu.[629] Testosterone slows the rate of discharge, which is the main mechanism by which testosterone inhibits gonadotropin release.[630] Progesterone also slows the pacemaker, whereas estrogen has no effect on the pacemaker.

THE FEMALE BRAIN. The capacity to develop an increase in LH secretion, i.e., the positive feedback response, is characteristic of females of all species. In rodents the response of the pituitary and hypothalamus in females to estrogens is prevented if the newborn is exposed to androgens during a critical developmental period (in rats this period extends from birth to the fifth postnatal day).[605, 631] In addition the ability to display adult female patterns of sexual behavior at maturity is lost, even when normal female hormonal balance is restored in adult life. These observations have led to the concept that differentiation of the "male" and "female" brain is deter-

mined by the hormonal milieu at a critical developmental stage, a concept supported by the finding of anatomic differences between male and female brains, particularly in the hypothalamus and spinal cord,[631] and by the fact that transplantation of the preoptic regions of the hypothalamus from neonatally androgenized rats into the preoptic region of neonatal females leads to male mating behavior.[632]

Hormonal "imprinting" is thought to be of minimal importance in human gender role behavior[633–635] but there are male-female differences in human brains.[631, 636–639] Brain nuclei that exhibit sexual differences in humans[636] include the "sexually dimorphic nucleus" of the hypothalamus,[637] the anterior commissure,[638] and the "bed nuclei of the stria terminalis" (Fig. 8–55).[639] Certain behaviors, mathematical ability, and the incidence of left-handedness and dyslexia[639] are also sex related.[633]

Attempts to link morphologic differences to differences in human sexual behavior have been made; e.g., the bed nucleus of the stria terminalis is said to be "feminine" in male-to-female transsexuals[639] and the sexually dimorphic nucleus[637] and anterior commissure[638] are reported to be typically "feminine" in male homosexuals. The extent to which these changes are primary (and thus indicative of underlying biologic differences) is unresolved. As noted earlier, pituitary regulation in men differs from that in women in that short-term estrogen administration in men does not sensitize the pituitary to LHRH.[616, 634]

These minor sex differences in the human notwithstanding, gender differences in gonadotropin regulation are not due to fundamental differences in hypothalamic function. Men and women display spontaneous LH and FSH ultradian rhythms of approximately the same duration[627, 629]; this pacemaker rhythm is slowed in both sexes by the administration of testosterone or progesterone.[630] In the absence of the testes, male monkeys release LH and FSH when given an estrogen pulse[481–483] and exposing female humans and monkeys to masculinizing doses of androgen in utero does not influence later menstrual cycling.[634] Although administration of gonadal steroids prenatally may influence certain behaviors, the pattern of gonadotropin regulation in the higher primates is different than it is in rats and mice.

CIRCADIAN RHYTHMS. In prepubertal children gonadotropins and gonadal steroids are secreted but at a low level.[640] As puberty progresses patterns of circadian and ultradian rhythms of gonadotropin (and gonadal steroid) secretion are characteristic of the stage of puberty.[453] In adult men and women an approximately 90-min ultradian rhythm is present, with larger bursts of gonadotropin secretion during sleep than

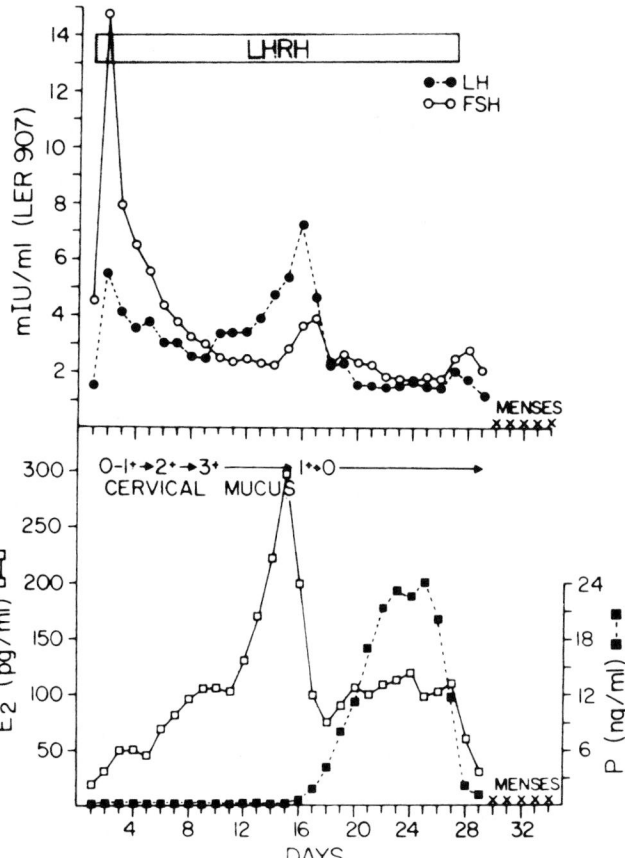

Figure 8–54. In this patient with hypothalamic LHRH deficiency related to Kallmann's syndrome, pulsatile administration of synthetic LHRH (by means of a programmed pump) stimulated ovulation. Shown are the blood levels of LH and FSH (demonstrating a normal ovulatory surge), a normal preovulatory estradiol (E_2) surge, and a normal postovulation rise in serum progesterone (P) level. Ultrasound examination was reported to demonstrate a single follicle in the right ovary on day 13 of treatment. This study demonstrates that the normal sequence of hormone secretion, including typical patterns for gonadotropins and ovarian hormones, can be induced by the administration of constant amounts of LHRH in a pulsatile fashion. To convert estradiol values to picomoles per liter, multiply by 3.671. To convert progesterone values to nanomoles per liter, multiply by 3.180. See Figure 8–53 for conversions of FSH and LH values. LH, luteinizing hormone; FSH, follicle-stimulating hormone. (From Crowley WF Jr, McArthur JW. Stimulation of the normal menstrual cycle of Kallman's syndrome by pulsatile administration of luteinizing hormone–releasing hormone [LHRH]. J Clin Endocrinol Metab, 51, 173–175, 1980, © by The Endocrine Society.)

during the day.[455] When neural control of gonadotropin regulation is perturbed, e.g., after stress, the amplitude of pulses is initially reduced first and, if severe, ultradian cyclic rhythm may be lost completely. If stress occurs prior to puberty (as in psychosocial dwarfism or competitive athletic training), puberty may be delayed indefinitely.

CONTROL OF THE TIMING OF PUBERTY. Long before the onset of puberty the pituitary and gonads are capable of being stimulated, and in girls estrogen is secreted at low levels.[640] Puberty does not begin, however, until the onset of pulsatile LHRH secretion by the hypothalamus. Other maturational brain changes include an increase in intellectual capacity and alterations in behavior and personality.[607–609, 641] Analysis of patients with hypothalamic disease[642] and studies of the effects of destruction of various parts of the brain in animals have shown that certain regions of the hypothalamus tonically inhibit gonadotropin secretion before puberty. The fundamental change during puberty has long been thought to be due to a reduction in tonic hypothalamic inhibition of LHRH release.

An alternative view has been proposed to explain the timing of puberty and the induction of puberty by brain lesions. Hypothalamic lesions that cause puberty induce the production of transforming growth factor α by astrocytes,[643] and transforming growth factor α acts through a paracrine mechanism to induce the secretion of prostaglandin E_2, which in turn acts on cells that project to the LHRH system.[643] Likewise an increase in hypothalamic transforming growth factor α is detectable at the time of the first estrous cycle in the normal rat[644] and rhesus monkey.[645]

In the presence of low LHRH secretion in prepubertal children the pituitary is exquisitely sensitive to suppression by the negative feedback effects of gonadal steroids. Before puberty only the negative feedback effect of gonadal steroids can be demonstrated; positive feedback in the female is demonstrable only after puberty is advanced.[607–609, 613, 641] The onset of puberty is influenced by both genetic and environmental factors. An important trigger for puberty is related to fat mass.[646–649] Moderately obese girls have an earlier puberty than do girls of normal weight, and individuals with malnutrition fail to develop normal pituitary-ovarian function. A decrease in body fat mass may be responsible for gonadal suppression in women with anorexia nervosa and for its return with refeeding. One hypothesis to explain the relation between fat mass and menstruation is that fat cells (in a state of high fat storage) secrete a neuroregulatory hormone into the blood, analogous to the appetite-regulating fat cell–derived protein hormone *leptin*.

EFFECT OF GONADAL STEROIDS ON THE BRAIN. Behavioral effects of gonadal steroids are mediated through re-

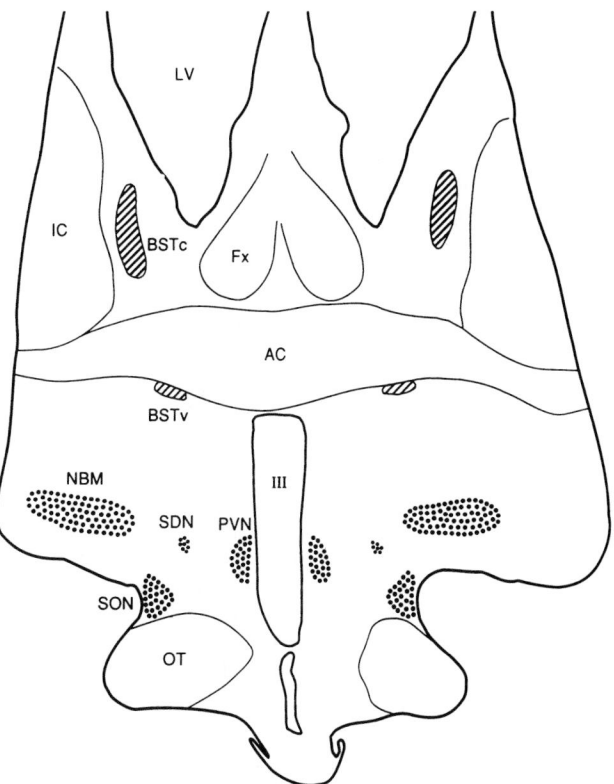

Figure 8–55. This diagram of a schematic frontal section of the human hypothalamus illustrates the location of the bed nucleus of the stria terminalis (BST), which is reported to be larger in men than in women. III, third ventricle; AC, anterior commissure; BSTc and BSTv, central and ventral subdivisions of the BST; FX, fornix; IC, internal capsule; LV, lateral ventricle; NBM, nucleus basalis of Meynert; OT, optic tract; PVN, paraventricular nucleus; SDN, sexually dimorphic nucleus; SON, supraoptic nucleus. (From Zhou JN, Hofman MA, Gooren LJG, et al. A sex difference in the human brain and its relation to transsexuality. Nature 1995; 378:68–70, with permission.)

ceptors in the brain.[604, 606, 650] After castration female cats will not mate and the genital tract becomes atrophic, both effects being reversible by estrogen treatment. That the effect of estrogen on behavior is mediated centrally is shown by the finding that tiny implants of estrogen in the hypothalamus restore normal sexual behavior without reversing the atrophic genital changes.[651] Estrogen receptors are present in the hypothalamus.[652] Generation of sex drive by a neural signal from an estrogen receptor within the hypothalamus of responsive animals is analogous to the generation of hunger by hypoglycemia and of thirst by hyperosmolarity.

In the hypothalamus progesterone decreases the rate of spontaneous firing and elevates the threshold of excitability to reflex stimulation from the uterine cervix. Progesterone in humans also raises body temperature and is responsible for the postovulatory rise in basal body temperature at ovulation. Spontaneous and pharmacologically induced contractions of the uterus are also inhibited by progesterone. In addition to genomic actions of steroid-receptor complexes, both estrogens and progesterones influence membrane excitability directly.

PHEROMONES AND SEXUAL FUNCTION. The female dog in heat emits a scent that is attractive to male dogs. This phenomenon is an example of a response mediated by a *pheromone*, a chemical substance secreted by one animal that causes behavioral or hormonal changes in another animal of the species.[653, 654] In nonvertebrates such as moths pheromones released by females are potent sex attractants that can be perceived by males over great distances.

Pheromone regulation of sex behavior is striking in rodents. In the female mouse gonadotropin secretion is altered by the presence of males. For example when housed in cages without males, female mice have irregular and prolonged estrous cycles, whereas on the third night after contact with the male estrous behavior and mating occur. This response can also be induced by exposing females to bedding contaminated with male urine. Female mouse urine contains a factor that stimulates LH release when applied to the vomeronasal organ of male mice.[655] Furthermore female mice mated with familiar males may abort if exposed to the urine of a strange male. Female rats deprived of their olfactory bulbs do not build nests or retrieve their young. The vaginal discharge of the hamster and rat contains a 17-kd protein termed *aphrodisin* that elicits copulatory behavior in the male.[656] In monkeys the fatty acids *(copulins)* formed in the vagina at estrus as a consequence of hormonally altered bacterial flora arouse grooming behavior in the male.[657]

Two primary classes of pheromones have been defined.[653] The *releasing* or *signaling* pheromones induce particular behaviors or changes in behavior pattern and include pheromones used in territorial marking, those eliciting or inhibiting agonist responses, those serving for sexual recognition and attraction, and those maintaining contact between mothers and young. The *priming* pheromones induce changes in endocrine or neuroendocrine activity in the partner, such as alterations of estrous cycle; induce puberty; induce alterations in the maintenance of pregnancy; or induce nursing behavior.

Little is known about the role of pheromones in human sexual activity. One proposed pheromone function in the human is the synchronization of menstrual cycles of college roommates and close friends,[658] but social interactions, common meal time, and similar activity patterns may be synchronizing signals. Subsequent studies have raised questions about the consistency of the synchronizing response and the role of pheromones in its induction.[659]

Two testicular steroids are responsible for the sex attractant properties of the urine of male pigs, androstenol, which has a musk-like odor, and androsterone, which smells like urine. Both steroids are also present in urine, plasma, sweat, and saliva of men and women and may arise from peripheral conversion of precursor steroids[660] or from skin bacteria.[661] Women unknowingly exposed to androstenol vapor reportedly exhibited increased socialization with men (but not with other women); exposed men showed no differences in social behavior.[662]

PINEAL GLAND

The pineal gland is derived embryologically from ependymal cells of the roof of the third ventricle and is the largest and most complex of the periventricular organs, weighing 0.10 to 0.18 g in humans.[663, 664] Unlike the periventricular organs embedded in the wall of the third ventricle of the brain, the pineal gland is attached to the roof of the third ventricle by a non-neural stalk and is separated from the aqueduct of Sylvius (which connects the third to the fourth ventricle) by the relatively thin tectal plate. The pineal gland is a secretory organ, synthesizes several active substances, and is occasionally the site of disease.

Pineal gland cells have ultrastructural features suggesting neurosecretory function.[665, 666] In fish and Amphibia the pineal gland is a light-sensitive structure; in higher vertebrates light-receptive function has disappeared (except for the residual expression of some retinal chemical markers) and the secretory activities are dominant. In species in which it is a light-sensitive organ the pineal gland is connected to the roof of the brain (epithalamus) by sensory nerves, but direct nerve connection to the brain is lost in mammals and is replaced by a postganglionic sympathetic nerve supply from the superior cervical ganglia.[452, 664–666] Preganglionic fibers in the superior sympathetic chain in the lateral cell column of the spinal cord are regulated by descending nerve impulses, some of which arise from the SC nucleus above the optic chiasm (see earlier in the section on endocrine rhythms). The SC nucleus receives a direct nerve input from the retina by a nonvisual pathway, the retinohypothalamic tract, that conveys information about light and dark independent of conscious perception. This neural pathway is the route through which external light regulates pineal gland activity. In the absence of light input pineal gland rhythms persist (driven by the SC nucleus pacemaker) but are not entrained to the external light-dark cycle.

Sympathetic nerve innervation to the pineal gland consists of noradrenergic fibers that end in the interstitial space of the gland or on the plasma membrane of pinealocytes.[452, 664–666] The endothelium of the pineal gland is fenestrated, thereby permitting the entry and exit of large molecules to the interstitial space of the gland. In this regard the pineal gland resembles other periventricular organs in not having a blood-brain barrier. Neuroendocrine functions of the pineal gland parenchymal cells are regulated by β-adrenergic receptors, and section of the sympathetic innervation or use of β-adrenergic antagonists inhibits pineal gland function.[667–670]

PHYSIOLOGICAL FUNCTION OF THE PINEAL GLAND. In rodents light-regulated gonadotropin secretion and timing of puberty are mediated by the pineal gland.[670, 671] For example extirpation of the pineal gland leads to precocious puberty and reverses the gonadal involution that follows exposure to constant darkness or shortened photoperiods in rats and hamsters.[671] If male rats are blinded or exposed to constant darkness testicular weight and testosterone levels decline; in female rats gonadotropin secretion and ovarian growth are impaired by blindness. These effects are reversed by pinealectomy, suggesting that darkness generates an inhibitory pineal gland signal. Melatonin appears to be the most important mediator of this effect (see later in the section on secretions of the pineal gland).

In the human altered environmental lighting (which in-

Tryptophan

5-Hydroxytryptophan

Serotonin

N-Acetylserotonin

Melatonin

Figure 8–56. Biosynthesis of melatonin from tryptophan in the pineal gland. Step 1 is catalyzed by tryptophan hydroxylase; step 2 by aromatic-L-amino acid decarboxylase; step 3 by N-acetylating enzyme; and step 4 by hydroxyindole-O-methyltransferase. (From Wurtman RJ, Axelrod J, Kelly DE, eds. Biochemistry of the pineal gland. In: The Pineal. New York: Academic, 1968: 47–75.)

fluences melatonin secretion by the pineal gland) and melatonin administration can "reset" the cycling mechanism of the SC nucleus, an area rich in melatonin receptors (see earlier in the section on endocrine rhythms). Nevertheless a role for the pineal gland in human puberty is not established. Indeed most pineal tumors cause precocious puberty not by changes in melatonin secretion but by paraneoplastic expression of human chorionic gonadotropin (see later).[672, 673] The pineal gland reaches adult size by 1 year of age and does not grow further.[674] Blood levels of melatonin (the principal secretion of the pineal gland) gradually fall from infancy through senescence.[675] On the basis of animal work it would be anticipated that if melatonin suppresses the onset of human puberty, levels in blood would fall with the onset of puberty. In some[676] but not all[677–684] studies melatonin secretion fell as anticipated, but it is possible that the decline in melatonin levels at puberty is *secondary* to gonadal steroid secretion. For example in one study of delayed puberty the excretion of melatonin in urine fell when puberty was initiated by treatment with LHRH,[685] and in another study the melatonin secretory profile did not correlate with age or stage of puberty[683] or adrenarche.[686] Changes in PRL, GH, adrenal, and thyroid function have been observed inconsistently after pinealectomy in animals.[687]

SECRETIONS OF THE PINEAL GLAND: MELATONIN. The pineal gland contains melatonin and other related indolamines, biogenic amines (norepinephrine, serotonin, histamine, dopamine, and octopamine), and peptides (LHRH, TRH, somatostatin, and the oxytocin analogue vasotocin).[688, 689] The pineal gland also contains the inhibitory neurotransmitter GABA, a protein that resembles neurophysin, and a protein termed *epiphysin.* Other uncharacterized peptides

may mediate the gonadotropin inhibitory actions of the pineal gland.

Melatonin was discovered as the result of an effort to isolate the pineal gland factor that causes lightening of amphibian skin. Melatonin is synthesized from tryptophan (Fig. 8–56)[664, 668–690]; the conversion of serotonin to N-acetylserotonin is the rate-limiting step.[668] The enzyme that performs the final synthetic reaction, hydroxyindole-O-methyltransferase, is also present in the retina, the harderian glands (orbital glands of unknown function in rodents), and red blood cells. The extent to which nonpineal sources contribute to melatonin blood levels is unknown but melatonin excretion persists at about 25% of basal levels after pinealectomy.

During the night (with lights off) melatonin secretion is highest (Fig. 8–57), the content of melatonin in the pineal gland is high, the level of the precursor serotonin is low, and the level of N-acetyltransferase (and its mRNA) is high.[668] Levels of N-acetyltransferase and its mRNA increase 25- to 100-fold or more within a few minutes of light deprivation.[668] Administration of β-adrenergic blocking agents or exposure to light causes a sharp decline in enzyme activity (half-life of 3.5 min). β-Adrenergic activation is mediated by cAMP.[668, 690]

FACTORS THAT INFLUENCE PINEAL GLAND SECRETION. Activation of the sympathetic nervous system increases the concentration of melatonin-synthesizing enzymes in the pineal gland and enhances melatonin secretion. Administration of levodopa, a precursor of dopamine, also increases melatonin synthesis in rats.

Melatonin is released into blood almost immediately after exposure to darkness and disappears on exposure to light (see Fig. 8–57).[670, 681, 691, 692] Occasional bursts of secretion are

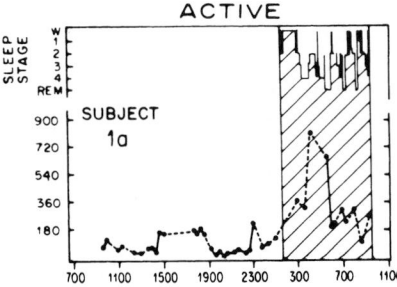
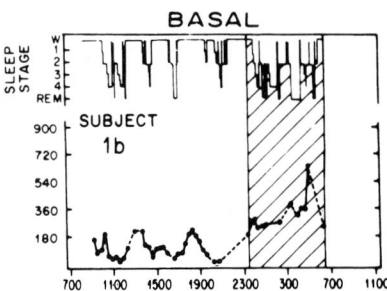

Figure 8–57. Pattern of melatonin secretion in a normal subject when active and at rest. The condition of lights off *(striped area)* brought about a release of melatonin. Note also that spontaneous release of melatonin also takes place. To convert melatonin values to picomoles per liter, multiply by 4.5. (From Weinberg U, D'Eletto RD, Weitzman ED, et al. Circulating melatonin in man: episodic secretion throughout the light-dark cycle. J Clin Endocrinol Metab, 48, 114–118, 1979, © by The Endocrine Society.)

unrelated to changes in lighting or stress.[692] The rhythm in melatonin excretion in urine can be entrained by the light-dark cycle and by sleep, diet, and activity.[670] Characteristic rhythms are unaffected by sleep deprivation or short-term exposure to sustained light.

The route by which melatonin reaches the pituitary and hypothalamus (its targets) is not known with certainty. Anatomic study of the mammalian pineal gland led Kappers and colleagues[666] to conclude that all secretions must leave by way of venous drainage into the peripheral circulation. They pointed out that there is no direct conduit from the pineal gland to the third ventricle and that the pineal gland, although partially located in the subarachnoid space, has a fairly thick capsule that would not favor direct subarachnoid release. However anatomic differences exist among species. In calves and children the level of melatonin in CSF is higher than that in blood, but in adult humans and monkeys the reverse is true, suggesting that in adults melatonin enters the CSF from blood.[693] The different levels may be due to the distribution of a melatonin-binding protein, whose level is higher in blood than in CSF.

Melatonin probably acts on both the hypothalamus and the pituitary to inhibit gonadotropin secretion.[694] Melatonin receptors are dense in two areas of the brain—the SC nucleus and the pars tuberalis of the pituitary.[695, 696] Since the SC nucleus regulates pineal gland secretion of melatonin and other circadian rhythms, the presence of melatonin receptors suggests that it is a site of negative feedback regulation of the pineal gland, as well as being the intrinsic circadian pacemaker.

The function of melatonin receptors in the pars tuberalis is unknown. This structure is the upward extension of the anterior pituitary and envelops the median eminence of the hypothalamus with a thin mantle of poorly differentiated cells that are chiefly gonadotropes and thyrotropes. Melatonin could act in this area to influence the release of hypophyseotropic hormones from nerve endings or the blood flow through the hypophyseal-portal blood vessels.

Serotonin is synthesized in pineal parenchymal cells and is taken up by sympathetic nerve endings in the gland along with dopamine and norepinephrine.[667–669] The role of these and other biologic mediators in the pineal gland is unknown. It is also unknown whether TRH, somatostatin, and LHRH, which are present in the pineal gland of some species, are secreted by this structure into the blood.

MELATONIN THERAPY IN HUMANS. Melatonin has become the focus of attention of the general public through books and the mass media[697–700] and is now available without a physician's prescription in the United States in pharmacies and health food stores. The interest in melatonin is based on some known effects in the human and on findings in rodents that suggest that it may have salutary effects on aging, cancer, cardiovascular disease, and immune function.

The best established use of melatonin is to "reset" the circadian clock and reduce sleep and behavioral disorders after jet travel across time zones (so-called jet lag) and in shift workers.[670, 697–699, 701–703] Melatonin can shift circadian phases; administration in the morning on awakening causes a delay in phase and in the afternoon causes a phase advance.[701–703] The most commonly prescribed schedule to prevent jet lag is to take melatonin shortly before bedtime in the new time zone.[698, 699] Seasonal affective disorder, thought to be caused by inappropriate timing of the day-night cycle, has been treated with melatonin and with artificial light.[703] Melatonin is also used for impaired sleep because it is said to induce sleep without altering the normal sleep structure.

On the basis of animal studies other potential uses of melatonin include reduction in the growth of mammary tumors in vivo and in vitro, potentiation of cancer chemotherapy,[697–699, 704, 705] prolongation of life,[706] and enhanced immune function.[707, 708] Melatonin levels are said to be low in depressed patients. Melatonin is a potent scavenger of free radicals in vitro,[708] and it has been suggested that the hormone has a physiological role in preventing the damaging effects of free radicals.[709] However it is unlikely that the levels of melatonin in blood[709] are sufficient to protect against oxidative damage.[710] The claim for life prolongation was based on studies in a mouse strain deficient in melatonin, whereas mice with normal pineal glands were not benefited.[710, 711] In the absence of controlled studies, it is not possible to judge the validity of these suggestions, other than its effects on sleep. It is regrettable that this hormone is being advocated for clinical use without adequate supporting studies.[710, 711]

CALCIFICATION OF THE PINEAL GLAND. Prior to the advent of computed tomography and magnetic resonance imaging, the calcified pineal gland was useful as a marker of the midline of the brain (and hence as a clue to space-occupying lesions) because it is readily visualized on conventional skull radiographs.[712] Calcification begins early in childhood and becomes increasingly evident in the second decade of life.[712] The prevalence of calcification is different among racial groups. An apatite form of calcium phosphate crystals is laid down in a matrix of ground substance secreted by pinealocytes to form nodules termed *acervuli*, and section of the nerves to the pineal gland of the hamster reduces the growth rate of acervuli.[671] Calcification has no known effect on pineal gland function, as inferred from the fact that the concentrations of characteristic pineal gland enzymes (hydroxyindole-*O*-methyltransferase, monoamine oxidase, and histamine *N*-methyltransferase) are relatively constant throughout life.

CIRCUMVENTRICULAR ORGANS

Ependymal cells that form a cuboidal, usually ciliated epithelium line the ventricles of the brain and the central canal of the spinal cord. In several regions of the third and fourth ventricles, the simple single-layered lining is modified into secretory structures that take up marker dyes from the blood (Fig. 8–58).[713–716] These regions are endowed with a wide variety of receptors on nerve endings that can respond to signals in blood such as osmolar state, sodium concentration, angiotensin II levels, bacterial toxins, and circulating cytokines. Through neuronal projections from the circumventricular organs to hypothalamic nuclei such signals can elicit appropriate homeostatic responses by the pituitary, autonomic nervous system, and central nervous system. Despite their contiguity with the ventricles the periventricular organs do not permit direct passage of large molecules into the ventricular space from which they are separated by tight junctions. Rather they constitute a specialized region within the brain in which circulating regulatory molecules can come into contact with sensory nerves that project to the hypothalamus. This unique communicative capacity has led to their designation as the "windows of the brain."

Periventricular organs of the third ventricle include the subcommissural organ (SCO), the SFO, the organum vasculosum of the lamina terminalis (OVLT), and the specialized ependyma of the median eminence (previously discussed as a component of the hypophyseal-pituitary control system). Another periventricular organ, the area postrema, is located at the posterior margin of the roof of the fourth ventricle. The pineal gland (see earlier) may be considered a periventricular organ because it is derived embryologically from ependymal cells; in some species it is embedded in the roof of the third ventricle; and in some primitive organisms it can sense light and influence brain function.

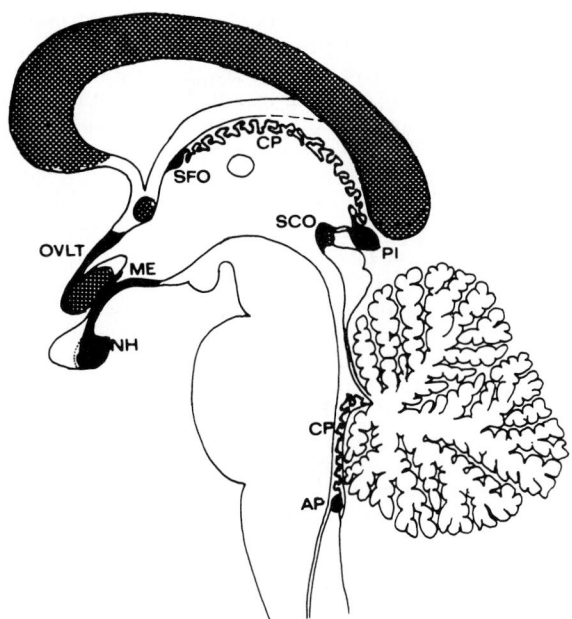

Figure 8–58. Median sagittal section through the human brain to show the circumventricular organs *(black)*. AP, area postrema; ME, median eminence; NH, neurohypophysis; OVLT, organum vasculosum of the lamina terminalis; PI, pineal body; SFO, subfornical organ; SCO, subcommissural organ; CP, choroid plexus. (From Weindl A. Neuroendocrine aspects of circumventricular organs. In: Ganong WF, Martini L, eds. Frontiers in Neuroendocrinology. Vol 3. New York: Oxford University Press, 1973: 3–32.)

SUBCOMMISSURAL ORGAN. The SCO is a collection of columnar cells in the roof of the third ventricle at the point at which the aqueduct between the third and fourth ventricles begins.[713, 717, 718] This region is beneath the habenular commissure (hence its name) and is adjacent to the pineal gland recess. Cells of the SCO differ from other ependymal cells in being taller and containing glycoprotein-rich secretory granules. On release into the ventricle the glycoproteins form cord-like structures in some species (Reissner's fibers) that are extruded through the aqueduct, the fourth ventricle, and the spinal cord lumen to terminate in the caudal spinal canal.[717, 718] In humans intracellular secretory granules are identifiable in the SCO, but the Reissner's fiber is absent. The SCO secretion in humans is therefore presumed to be more soluble and to be absorbed directly from the CSF. Little is known about the function of the SCO or the Reissner's fiber. It may promote downward transport of CSF.[719] Unlike other circumventricular neurons, the SCO has no direct nerve supply.

SUBFORNICAL ORGAN. The SFO contains both neurosecretory neurons and modified ependymal cells[713, 714, 720–722] and is located at the junction between the *lamina terminalis* and the *tela choroidea* of the third ventricle. Its name is derived from its location under the anterior fornices (see Fig 8–58). The neurons of the SFO receive cholinergic innervation from the midbrain and contain angiotensin II, atrial natriuretic peptide,[723] and neurosecretory granules whose intensity is modified by anesthesia, stress, hyperosmotic challenge, alcohol injection, and estrogen administration. The SFO plays an important role in salt and water regulation. Injection of angiotensin II or hypertonic saline into the SFO leads to release of vasopressin and stimulation of drinking, and the effects of angiotensin II are potentiated by saline. The endothelium of this region contains the enzyme that converts angiotensin I to angiotensin II, and local neurons contain mRNA coding for angiotensinogen, the precursor to angiotensin I.[722] Angiotensinergic neurons project to the paraventricular nucleus thereby providing a neural pathway by which stimuli

arising in the SFO can regulate vasopressin secretion. The SFO regulates and integrates drinking and vasopressin release in the defense of serum osmolality.

ORGANUM VASCULOSUM OF THE LAMINA TERMINALIS. The OVLT (supraoptic crest) lies in the midline of the lamina terminalis (anterior wall) of the third ventricle between the anterior commissure and the optic chiasm (see Fig. 8–58).[713–716] Its external surface is in contact with the CSF of the prechiasmatic cistern and its internal surface is in contact with the CSF of the brain. Large molecules are prevented from passing between the SFO from the CSF by tight junctions between the ependymal cells. The SFO has arterial and venous circulations independent of those in other circumventricular organs. Large molecules readily penetrate the OVLT, indicating that the blood-brain barrier is absent here. The OVLT is innervated by nerve endings containing LHRH, somatostatin, angiotensin, and neurophysin. The OVLT in the rat contains estrogen receptors and the application of estrogen or electric stimulation at this site is capable of stimulating ovulation through LHRH-containing neurons that project to the median eminence. Injection of LHRH in the same area increases sexual drive in hypophysectomized and normal rats, suggesting that the region regulates sexual behavior in the rat. Its function in primates is unknown.

The OVLT is involved in the response to bacterial toxin and inflammatory cytokines (see later in the section on neuroendocrine-immune interactions). Intravenous injection of *Escherichia coli* endotoxin or IL-1 activates the cells of the OVLT, including the lining endothelial cells,[724–726] and induces formation of prostaglandin E_2, IL-6, and TNF α, which are released into the anterior tip of the third ventricle in close contact with thermoregulatory cells to cause fever.[724, 725] Neuronal inputs from the OVLT and from the induced cytokines in the CSF activate CRH and vasopressinergic and oxytocinergic neurons thereby leading to release of corticotropin and vasopressin.

AREA POSTREMA. The area postrema is located at the caudal end of the floor of the fourth ventricle (see Fig. 8–58), lies over the sensory nucleus of the vagus (termed the *nucleus of the tractus solitarius* [NTS]), and projects neurons to the hypothalamus and other parts of the brain.[713–716, 727] The area postrema contains osmoreceptors and vasopressin receptors and influences thirst and vasopressin secretion through projections to the hypothalamus. It has the unique capacity to detect foreign substances that enter the blood and to induce vomiting through a dopaminergic neural pathway.[727] This chemosensory capacity permits the detection and expulsion of potentially harmful substances.

The area postrema lies immediately above the sensory nucleus of the vagus (NTS) with which it has extensive neuronal interactions. The NTS receives vagal afferents from peripheral receptors that sense blood pressure and circulating blood volume and project signals to hypothalamic nuclei to modulate autonomic nervous system control of the heart and blood vessels, peripheral secretion of angiotensin, and release of CRH and vasopressin. The NTS is also involved in the activation of the pituitary and neurohypophysis after the administration of endotoxin.[726] The central sensory function of the area postrema is complemented by sensory receptors in visceral organs. Intraperitoneal administration of endotoxin or IL-1 in rats triggers release of corticotropin and vasopressin, development of fever, and a syndrome ("sickness behavior") that includes decreased spontaneous activity, decreased eating, and a lowered pain threshold (hyperalgesia). These changes are prevented by section of the vagus nerve, indicating that they are reflex responses to impulses reaching the NTS. Vagal afferent nerve endings do not contain IL-1 receptors; rather a specialized group of small chemosensory structures, the *vagal paraganglia* (anatomically similar to the carotid body) are present in the hilum of the liver,[728, 729] display IL-1 receptors, and are innervated by vagal afferent fibers. These receptors sense the presence of inflammatory cytokines.

NEUROENDOCRINE DISEASE

Disease of the hypothalamus can cause pituitary dysfunction, abnormal mental function, disorders of behavior, and disturbances of visceral regulation.[23, 730–734] Destructive hypothalamic lesions cause pituitary insufficiency by damaging the tuberohypophyseal neurons or blood vessels in the median eminence.

Manifestations of pituitary insufficiency secondary to hypothalamic or pituitary stalk damage are not identical with those of pituitary insufficiency; namely hypothalamic injury causes decreased secretion of most pituitary hormones but can cause hypersecretion of hormones normally under inhibitory control by the hypothalamus, as in hypersecretion of PRL after damage to the pituitary stalk and precocious puberty caused by the loss of normal restraint over gonadotropin maturation. Impairment of inhibitory control of the neurohypophysis can lead to inappropriate vasopressin secretion (SIADH) (see earlier and Chapter 10). More subtle abnormalities in secretion can result from impairment of the control system. For example loss of the normal circadian rhythm of corticotropin secretion may occur before loss of pituitary-adrenal secretory reserve,[735] and responses to physiological stimuli may be paradoxical. Because hypophyseotropic hormone levels cannot be measured directly and because pituitary hormone secretion is regulated by complex, multilayered controls, assay of pituitary hormones in blood does not necessarily give a meaningful picture of events at hypothalamic and higher levels. Rarely tumors secrete excessive amounts of releasing hormones and cause hypersecretion of the pituitary.[733, 736]

In the diagnosis and treatment of suspected hypothalamic or pituitary disease four issues must be kept in mind: the extent of the lesion, the physiological impact, the specific cause, and the social-psychological setting. The etiology of hypothalamic disorders is summarized in Tables 8–18 and 8–19 and manifestations of hypothalamic disease are summarized in Table 8–20. As noted the age of the patient correlates with the cause of parasellar disease.

Disorders of the hypothalamic-pituitary unit can result from lesions at several levels. Defects can arise from destruction of the pituitary (as by tumor, infarct, inflammation, or autoimmune disease) or from a hereditary deficiency of a particular hormone as in rare cases of isolated FSH or GH deficiency. Selective loss of thyroid hormone receptors in the pituitary can give rise to increased thyrotropin secretion and thyrotoxicosis. Furthermore disorders can arise through disruption of the stalk–median eminence contact zone, the stalk itself, or the nerve terminals of the tuberohypophyseal system; such disruption occurs after surgical stalk section, with tumors involving the stalk, and in some inflammatory diseases. At a higher level tonic inhibitory and excitatory inputs can be lost as manifested by absence of circadian rhythms or the development of precocious puberty. Physical stress, cytokine products of inflammatory cells, toxins, and reflex inputs from peripheral homeostatic monitors also impinge on the tuber-

---

TABLE 8–18. Etiology of Hypothalamic Disease by Age

Premature Infants and Neonates

Intraventricular hemorrhage
Meningitis: bacterial
Tumors: glioma, hemangioma
Trauma
Hydrocephalus, kernicterus

1 mo–2 y

Tumors
   Glioma, especially optic glioma
   Histiocytosis X
   Hemangioma
Hydrocephalus
Meningitis
Familial disorders
   Laurence-Moon-Biedl syndrome
   Prader-Labhart-Willi syndrome

2–10 y

Neoplasms
   Craniopharyngioma
   Glioma, dysgerminoma, hamartoma, histiocytosis X, leukemia
   Ganglioneuroma, ependymoma, medulloblastoma
Meningitis
   Bacterial
   Tuberculous
Encephalitis
   Viral
   Exanthematous demyelinating
Familial
   Diabetes insipidus
Radiation therapy
Diabetic ketoacidosis

10–25 y

Tumors
   Craniopharyngioma
   Glioma, hamartoma, dysgerminoma
   Histiocytosis X, leukemia
   Dermoid, lipoma, neuroblastoma

10–25 y *Continued*

Trauma
Vascular
   Subarachnoid hemorrhage
   Aneurysm
   Arteriovenous malformation
Inflammatory disease
   Meningitis
   Encephalitis
   Sarcoidosis
   Tuberculosis
Structural brain defect
   Chronic hydrocephalus
   Increased intracranial pressure

25–50 y

Nutritional: Wernicke's disease
Tumors
   Glioma, lymphoma, meningioma
   Craniopharyngioma, pituitary tumors
   Angioma, plasmacytoma, colloid cysts
   Ependymoma, sarcoma, histiocytosis X
Inflammatory disease
   Sarcoidosis
   Tuberculosis, viral encephalitis
Subarachnoid hemorrhage, vascular aneurysm, arteriovenous malformation
Damage from pituitary radiation therapy

50 y and Older

Nutritional: Wernicke's disease
Tumors
   Sarcoma, glioblastoma, lymphoma
   Meningioma, colloid cysts, ependymoma, pituitary tumors
Vascular disease
   Infarct, subarachnoid hemorrhage
   Pituitary apoplexy
Inflammation: encephalitis, sarcoidosis, meningitis
Radiation therapy for nasopharyngeal carcinoma

Adapted from Plum F, Van Uitert R. Nonendocrine diseases and disorders of the hypothalamus. In: Reichlin S, Baldessarini RJ, Martin JB, eds. The Hypothalamus. Vol 56. New York: Raven, 1978: 415–473, with permission.

TABLE 8–19. Etiology of Endocrine Syndromes of Hypothalamic Origin

Hypophyseotropic Hormone Deficiency

Surgical pituitary stalk section
Basilar meningitis and granuloma, sarcoidosis, tuberculosis, sphenoid osteomyelitis, eosinophilic granuloma
Craniopharyngioma
Hypothalamic tumor
    Infundibuloma
    Teratoma (ectopic pinealoma)
    Neuroglial tumor, particularly astrocytoma
Maternal deprivation syndrome, psychosocial dwarfism
Isolated GHRH deficiency
Hypothalamic hypothyroidism
Panhypophyseotropic failure

Disorders of Regulation of Luteinizing Hormone–Releasing Hormone Secretion

Female
    Precocious puberty
    Delayed puberty
    Neurogenic amenorrhea
    Pseudocyesis
    Anorexia nervosa
    "Functional" amenorrhea
    "Functional" oligomenorrhea
    Drug-induced amenorrhea
Male
    Precocious puberty
    Fröhlich's syndrome
    Olfactory-genital dysplasia (Kallmann's syndrome)

Disorders of Regulation of Prolactin-Regulating Factors

Tumor
Sarcoidosis
Drug-induced
Reflex
Herpes zoster of chest wall
Post-thoracotomy
Nipple manipulation
Spinal cord tumor
"Psychogenic"
Hypothyroidism
Carbon dioxide narcosis

Disorders of Regulation of Corticotropin-Releasing Hormone

Paroxysmal corticotropin discharge (Wolff's syndrome)
Loss of circadian variation
Depression

GHRH, growth hormone–releasing hormone.

oinfundibular system. At the highest level of control, emotional stress and psychological disorders can activate the pituitary-adrenal stress response and suppress gonadotropin secretion (e.g., psychogenic amenorrhea) or inhibit GH secretion (e.g., psychosocial dwarfism) (see Chapter 30). Intrinsic disease of the anterior pituitary is reviewed in Chapter 9, and disturbances in neurohypophyseal function are discussed in Chapter 10. This chapter considers disease of the hypothalamic-pituitary unit.

Pituitary Isolation Syndrome

Destructive lesions of the pituitary stalk, as with head injury, surgical transection, tumor, or granuloma, produce a characteristic pattern of pituitary dysfunction. DI develops in approximately 80% of patients, depending on the level at which the stalk has been sectioned.[737] If the cut is close to the hypothalamus DI is almost always produced, whereas if the section is low on the stalk the incidence is less. The extent to which nerve terminals in the upper stalk are preserved determines the clinical course. The classic triphasic syndrome of initial polyuria followed by normal water control and then by vasopressin deficiency[739] over a period of 10 d to 1 wk is seen in about half the patients.[737, 738] The sequence is attributed to an initial loss of neurogenic control of the neural

lobe, followed by autolysis of the neural lobe with release of vasopressin into the circulation, and finally by complete loss of vasopressin. DI may develop after stalk injury without an overt transitional phase. Injury to the neurohypophysis or stalk, as during the course of surgical exploration of the pituitary, can sometimes give rise to transient SIADH. When DI occurs after head injury or operative trauma recovery can take place even after months or years. Sprouting of nerve terminals in the stump of the pituitary stalk may give rise to sufficient functioning tissue to maintain water balance. Full expression of polyuria requires adequate cortisol levels; if cortisol is deficient vasopressin deficiency may be present with only minimal polyuria. Glucocorticoid replacement restores full blown polyuria.

Although head injury, granulomas, and tumors are the most common causes of acquired DI, some cases develop in the absence of a clear-cut cause.[733, 740] Some cases may be due to autoimmune disease of the hypothalamus as suggested by the finding of autoantibodies to neurohypophyseal cells in a third of cases of "idiopathic DI" in one series.[741] Atrophy of the supraopticohypophyseal cells has rarely been observed at autopsy.[731, 783]

Congenital DI can be part of a hereditary disease. DI in the Brattleboro rat is due to an autosomal recessive genetic defect that impairs production of vasopressin but not of oxytocin.[73] In humans congenital DI can be due to mutations that alter either the vasopressin receptor or vasopressin itself.[75–77]

Menses cease after stalk section[742] and after hypophysectomy. Unlike the situation after hypophysectomy gonadotropins may be detectable in urine after stalk section. Plasma glucocorticoid levels and urinary excretion of cortisol and 17-hydroxycorticoids decline after hypophysectomy and stalk section, but the change is slower after stalk section.[743, 744] A transient increase in cortisol secretion after stalk section is believed to be due to release of preformed stores of corticotropin. The corticotropin response to the lowering of blood cortisol is markedly reduced, but release of corticotropin after stress may be normal,[745] possibly because of release of CRH from other parts of the brain. CRH is widely distributed in the brain and gastrointestinal tract (see earlier). Reduction in thyroid function after stalk section is similar to that seen with hypophysectomy.[746, 747] The fall in GH secretion is the most sensitive indication of damage to the stalk.[746]

Humans with stalk sections[748–750] or with tumors of the stalk region have consistent hyperprolactinemia and may have galactorrhea. PRL responses to hypoglycemia and to TRH are blunted[749] in part because of a loss of neural connections with the hypothalamus. PRL response to dopamine agonists and antagonists in the pituitary isolation syndrome are similar to those in patients with prolactinomas.[749] An incomplete pituitary isolation syndrome may occur with the empty sella syndrome,[751, 752] intrasellar cysts, or pituitary adenomas. Anterior

TABLE 8–20. Symptoms and Signs of Hypothalamic Disease*

Symptoms and Signs	No. of Cases
Sexual abnormalities (hypogonadism or precocious puberty)	43
Diabetes insipidus	21
Psychic disturbance	21
Obesity or hyperphagia	20
Somnolence	18
Emaciation, anorexia	15
Thermodysregulation	13
Sphincter disturbance	5

*From a review of 60 autopsy-proven cases.
Adapted from HG Bauer. Endocrine and other clinical manifestations of hypothalamic disease: a survey of 60 cases with autopsies. J Clin Endocrinol Metab, 14, 13–31, 1954, © by The Endocrine Society.

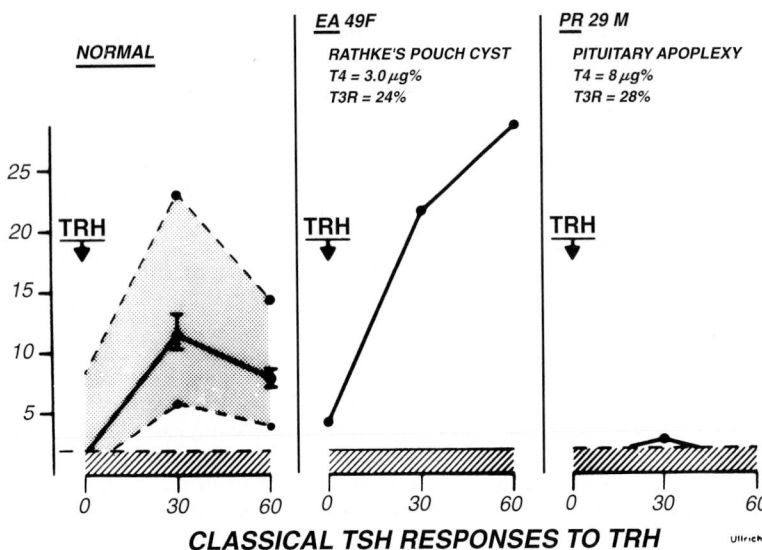

Figure 8–59. Typical pituitary response to TRH administration in patients with hypothalamic-pituitary disease that has caused hypothyroidism. If there is intrinsic pituitary damage, the response is abnormally low. If there is hypothalamic damage, the response is normal or exaggerated. It must be emphasized that some patients with hypothalamic disease may not respond to TRH and that some patients with pituitary disease may respond to TRH. TRH, thyrotropin-releasing hormone. (From Jackson IMD. Diagnostic tests for the evaluation of pituitary tumors. In: Jackson IMD, Reichlin S, eds. The Pituitary Adenoma. New York: Plenum, 1980: 219–238.)

pituitary failure after stalk section is in part due to loss of specific neural and vascular links to the hypothalamus and in part due to pituitary infarction.[753, 754]

Hypophyseotropic Hormone Deficiency

Selective pituitary failure can be due to a deficiency of specific pituitary cell types or a deficiency of one or more hypothalamic hormones. Deficiency of TRH secretion gives rise to hypothalamic hypothyroidism, also called tertiary hypothyroidism, which can occur in hypothalamic disease or as an isolated defect.[755–759] As a practical matter, hypothalamic and pituitary causes of thyrotropin deficiency are most readily distinguished by imaging methods. The TRH test for the differentiation of hypothalamic disease from pituitary disease, although theoretically reasonable, is of limited value. The typical pituitary response to TRH administration in patients with TRH deficiency is an enhanced and somewhat delayed peak (Fig. 8–59), whereas the response with pituitary failure is subnormal or absent.[755, 757] The hypothalamic type of response has been attributed to an associated GH deficiency that sensitizes the pituitary to TRH (possibly through suppression of somatostatin secretion),[758, 759] but GH also affects T_4 metabolism and may alter pituitary responses as well.[759] Deficient TRH secretion leads to altered thyrotropin synthesis by the pituitary, including impaired glycosylation. Poorly glycosylated thyrotropin has low biologic activity and dissociation of bioactive and immunoactive thyrotropin can lead to the apparent paradox of normal or elevated levels of thyrotropin in hypothalamic hypothyroidism.[756, 757] In practice the responses to TRH in hypothalamic and pituitary disease overlap so much that the response cannot be used for a differential diagnosis. Persistent failure to demonstrate responses to TRH is good evidence for the presence of intrinsic pituitary disease, but the presence of a response does not mean that the pituitary is normal.

Isolated LHRH deficiency is the most common hypophyseotropic hormone deficiency. In Kallmann's syndrome (gonadotropin deficiency commonly associated with hyposmia)[760, 761] hereditary agenesis of the olfactory lobe may be demonstrable by magnetic resonance imaging.[762] Defective development of the LHRH system is due to defective migration of the LHRH-containing neurons from the olfactory nasal epithelium in early embryologic life (see earlier in the section on LHRH).

Malformations of the midline structures, such as absence

of the septum pellucidum, can cause either hypogonadotropic hypogonadism[763] or, less commonly, precocious puberty.[764] The LHRH response test is of little value in hypothalamic hypogonadism.[765–767] Most patients with LHRH deficiency show little or no response to an initial test dose, but normal responses are seen after repeated injection (Fig. 8–60). This slow response has been attributed to down-regulation of LHRH receptors with prolonged LHRH deficiency. Furthermore with intrinsic pituitary disease the response to LHRH may be absent or normal. Consequently it is not possible to distinguish between hypothalamic and pituitary disease with a single injection of LHRH. Prolonged infusions or repeated administration of LHRH agonists may aid in the diagnosis.[767]

GHRH deficiency appears to be the cause of hGH deficiency in most patients with idiopathic dwarfism in keeping

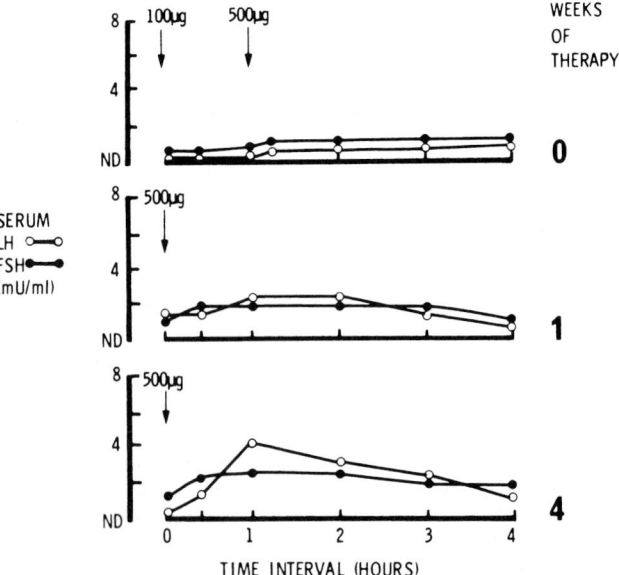

Figure 8–60. Demonstration of increasing responsiveness of gonadotropin secretion to LHRH after repeated administration of the hormone in a prepubertal boy with a craniopharyngioma. The hormone was given subcutaneously, 500 μg twice daily for 4 wk, and responsiveness was tested with intravenous doses. There was little or no response initially, but after a period of treatment, responsiveness gradually rose. (From Mortimer CH. Gonadotropin-releasing hormone. In: Martini L, Besser GM, eds. Clinical Neuroendocrinology. New York: Academic, 1977:213–236.)

with the fact that most children with idiopathic hypopituitarism have normal responses to TRH, LHRH, and GHRH,[768, 769] as do patients with hypothalamic disease of established cause.[770] In children with GHRH deficiency the response to the hGH-releasing hexapeptide is absent.[279, 280] Comparison of responses to GHRH with those to the hexapeptide may make it possible to differentiate between pituitary disease and GHRH deficiency. The latter is frequently associated with abnormal electroencephalograms, a history of birth trauma, and breech delivery.[771, 772] Furthermore, magnetic resonance imaging scans show that at least half of children with "idiopathic" hGH deficiency have evidence of a torn pituitary stalk,[772, 773] which is presumed evidence for birth trauma as the cause. hGH is the most vulnerable of the anterior pituitary hormones when the pituitary stalk is damaged. Midline hypothalamic defects, "septo-optic dysplasia," also lead to hGH deficiency.[774, 762]

Deficiency of PIF secretion leads to hyperprolactinemia.[749, 750, 775] PRL levels are also elevated by lesions that isolate the pituitary from the hypothalamus; values are usually less than 56 μg/L and rarely as high as 120 μg/L, but high levels have been reported with stalk compression.[750]

Adrenal insufficiency is a common manifestation of hypothalamic disease and is due to CRH deficiency[776] or isolated autoimmune destruction of adrenotropes.[777] The CRH stimulation test does not distinguish hypothalamic from pituitary failure as a cause of corticotropin deficiency.[778, 779]

Hypothalamic damage is common after radiation of the skull for neoplastic disease, and deficiency of GH and LHRH is the most common manifestation.[780, 781]

Hypophyseotropic Hormone Hypersecretion

Pituitary hypersecretion is occasionally caused by tumors of the hypothalamus.[733, 736] LHRH-secreting hamartomas can cause precocious puberty,[782] CRH-secreting gangliocytomas can cause Cushing's syndrome,[783, 784] and GHRH-secreting gangliocytomas of the hypothalamus can cause acromegaly.[785] Although they do not arise from the hypothalamus, paraneoplastic syndromes can also cause pituitary hypersecretion, as with CRH-secreting tumors[736] and GHRH-secreting tumors of the bronchi and pancreas.[191, 252, 253, 262] Bronchial carcinoids and pituitary islet cell tumors are the usual causes of this phenomenon.[736]

Neuroendocrine Disorders of Gonadotropin Regulation

PRECOCIOUS PUBERTY. The term *precocious puberty* is used when *normal* pituitary-gonadal function appears at an early age.[786, 787] This means the onset of androgen secretion and spermatogenesis before the age of 9 or 10 in boys and the onset of estrogen secretion and cyclic ovarian activity before age 8 in girls. True precocious puberty is due to disturbed central nervous system function, which may or may not have an identifiable structural basis. Pseudoprecocious puberty refers to premature sexual development resulting from excessive secretion of androgens, estrogens, or chorionic gonadotropin caused by tumors (both gonadal and extragonadal), administration of exogenous gonadal steroids, or genetically determined activation of gonadotropin receptors (see Chapter 31). Precocious puberty due to pineal gland disease and neurogenic causes is discussed in this chapter.

Idiopathic Sexual Precocity. Familial occurrence is uncommon but there is a hereditary form of idiopathic sexual precocity that is largely confined to males. In one study[771] girls with true precocity had a high incidence of abnormal

electroencephalograms and behavioral disturbances, suggesting the presence of brain damage. In another report idiopathic precocious puberty was unaccompanied by such changes.[787] The pathogenesis may be related to the rate of hypothalamic development. Many cases previously thought to be idiopathic are due to hypothalamic hamartomas. For example in the series of Pescovitz and co-workers[782] 14 of 95 cases in girls and 10 of 34 cases in boys were due to this disorder.

Neurogenic Precocious Puberty. Approximately two thirds of hypothalamic lesions that influence the timing of human puberty are located in the posterior hypothalamus,[642] but in the subset of patients who come to autopsy damage is extensive. Specific lesions known to cause precocity include craniopharyngioma (although delayed puberty is more common), astrocytoma, pineal tumors, encephalitis, miliary tuberculosis, tuberous sclerosis, the Sturge-Weber syndrome, porencephaly, craniostenosis, microcephaly, hydrocephalus, empty sella syndrome, and Tay-Sachs disease.

Hamartoma of the hypothalamus is an exception to the generalization that tumors of the brain cause precocious puberty by impairment of gonadotropin secretion (although hamartomas on occasion cause hypothalamic damage). A hamartoma is a tumor-like collection of normal looking nerve tissue lodged in an abnormal location. One type consists of an encapsulated nodule of nerve tissue attached to the posterior hypothalamus between the anterior portion of the mamillary body and the posterior region of the tuber cinereum.[787–792] The hypothalamic hamartoma grows into the cisternal space between the cerebral peduncles, adapts to the pyramidal shape of the cisterna, and may produce precocious puberty before other effects occur. Prior to the development of high-resolution scanning techniques[782, 791] this tumor was considered to be rare, but small ones can now be visualized. Miniature hamartomas of the tuber cinereum are common at autopsy. Precocious puberty occurs when the hamartoma makes connections with the median eminence and thus serves as an "accessory hypothalamus."[787–790] LHRH was found in the CSF of three such patients, raising the possibility that the tumors secrete LHRH,[787] and peptidergic nerves containing LHRH have been found in the tumors.[789, 790] Early pubertal development is probably due to unrestrained LHRH secretion. The hamartomas probably have an intrinsic "pulse generator" of LHRH secretion; pulsatility is required for stimulation of gonadotropin secretion, and isolated LHRH neurons possess intrinsic cyclic patterns of secretion (see earlier).

Manifestations of premature puberty in patients with hamartomas are similar to those of other cerebral causes of precocity. Hamartomas occur in both sexes and may be present as early as age 3 mo. In the past most cases were thought to be fatal by age 20, but many hamartomas cause no brain damage and need not be excised.[791] The interpeduncular fossa of the brain is difficult to approach and surgical experience is somewhat limited. Early in the course of illness epilepsy manifested as "brief, repetitive, stereotyped attacks of laughter"[792] may provide a clue to the disease. Late in the course hypothalamic damage can cause severe neurologic defects.

Hypothyroidism. Hypothyroidism can cause precocious puberty in girls that is reversible with thyroid therapy.[793, 794] Hyperprolactinemia and galactorrhea may be present. One possibility is that elevated thyrotropin levels (in children with thyroid failure) can cross-react with the FSH receptor.[795] Alternatively low levels of thyroid hormone might simultaneously activate release of LH, FSH, and thyrotropin.[793] A third possibility is that hypothyroidism causes hypothalamic encephalopathy that impairs the normal tonic suppression of gonadotropin release by the hypothalamus. The high PRL levels that sometimes accompany this disorder may be due to a deficiency

TABLE 8–21. Classification of Tumors of Pineal Region

A. Germ Cell Tumors

1. Germinoma
   a. Posterior third ventricle and pineal lesions
   b. Anterior third ventricle, suprasellar or intrasellar lesions
   c. Combined lesions in anterior and posterior third ventricle, apparently noncontiguous, with or without foci of cystic or solid teratoma
2. Teratoma
   a. Evidencing growth along two or three germ lines in varying degrees of differentiation
   b. Dermoid and epidermoid cysts with or without solid foci of teratoma
   c. Histologically malignant forms with or without differentiated foci of benign, solid, or cystic teratoma—teratocarcinoma, chorio-epithelioma, embryonal carcinoma (endodermal-sinus tumor or yolk-sac carcinoma), combinations of these with or without foci of germinoma, chemodectoma

B. Pineal Parenchymal Tumors

1. Pinealocytes
   a. Pineocytoma
   b. Pineoblastoma
   c. Ganglioglioma and chemodectoma
   d. Mixed forms exhibiting transitions between these
2. Glia
   a. Astrocytoma
   b. Ependymoma
   c. Mixed forms and other less frequent gliomas (e.g., glioblastoma, oligodendroglioma)

C. Tumors of Supporting or Adjacent Structures

1. Meningioma
2. Hemangiopericytoma

D. Non-neoplastic Conditions of Neurosurgical Importance

1. "Degenerative" cysts of pineal lined by fibrillary astrocytes
2. Arachnoid cysts
3. Cavernous hemangioma

From DeGirolami U. Pathology of tumors of the pineal region. In: Schmidek HH, ed. Pineal Tumors. New York: Masson, 1977: 1–19, with permission.

in PIF secretion, increased secretion of TRH, or increased sensitivity of the pituitary to TRH secretion.

Tumors of the Pineal Gland. Pineal gland tumors account for 0.2 to 1% of brain tumors in the United States and 4% of brain tumors in Japan.[796, 797] The various lesions in the pineal gland region are summarized in Table 8–21. *Pinealoma* refers to a tumor of the pineal parenchymal cell and can be a pineoblastoma or pineocytoma, depending on its degree of differentiation.[798] In one series only 9 of 53 pineal gland tumors were pinealomas.[799] The most common tumors of the pineal gland are germinomas (a form of teratoma), so designated because of their presumed origin in germ cells. Germinomas may also occur in the anterior hypothalamus or the floor of the third ventricle.[798] Identical tumors can be found in the testis and anterior mediastinum. Intracranial germinomas have a tendency to spread locally, infiltrate the hypothalamus, and metastasize to the spinal cord and CSF.[800–803] Extracranial metastases (to the skin, lung, or liver) are rare.[801] Teratomas derived from two or more germ cell layers also occur in the pineal region. Chorionic tissue in teratomas and germinomas may secrete human chorionic gonadotropin (hCG) in sufficient amounts to cause gonadal maturation,[804–808] and some of these tumors have histologic and functional characteristics of choriocarcinomas. A viral cause has been proposed.[809]

Precocious puberty is unusual in pineal gland disease. In one series of 65 pineal tumors no case of sexual precocity was noted.[810] In another study a third of subjects older than age 15 exhibited sexual precocity.[811] Neuroanatomic studies suggest that damage extends beyond the pineal region in cases of precocious puberty. Thus, precocious puberty in pineal disease is probably due to the pressure or destructive effects of tumor on the function of the adjacent hypothalamus or to the secretion of hCG. Most patients have other evidence of hypothalamic involvement such as DI, polyphagia, somnolence, obesity, or behavioral disturbance. Pineal gland tumors cause other endocrine abnormalities as well.[804, 812]

Pineal gland disease is an uncommon cause of true precocious puberty in boys. In one series of 11 patients 7 had detectable abnormalities in the brain but only 1 had a pineal gland disorder (a cyst).[813] Choriocarcinoma of the pineal gland is associated with high plasma levels of hCG.[800, 803–807] hCG can stimulate testosterone secretion from the testis but not estrogen secretion by the ovary and hence causes premature puberty almost exclusively in boys. The prevalence of elevated hCG levels in children with premature puberty due to tumors in the pineal region is unknown, but the fact that this phenomenon occurs further challenges the theory that nonparenchymal tumors cause precocious puberty by damaging the normal pineal gland.[814, 815]

Rarely pineal tumors cause *delayed* puberty; parenchymal tumors were responsible for 20 of 30 cases of hypogonadism associated with pineal tumors.[815] As yet no studies of gonadotropin inhibitory factors or circulating melatonin have been reported in such cases, but in two instances tumor tissue contained the enzymes necessary for melatonin synthesis.[816] In several animal species, melatonin inhibits gonadotropin secretion.

Manifestations of pituitary insufficiency, including DI, with tumors of the pineal region are probably the consequence of tumor-induced hypothalamic lesions. Germinomas of the floor of the third ventricle give rise to a characteristic clinical triad: DI, visual impairment, and hypopituitarism.[817] Tumors of identical morphologic structure may arise in the region of the pineal gland and tumors of the pineal gland can spread to the base of the brain. More than half of these germinomas can be diagnosed by measurements of hCG in CSF or blood.

Pinealomas cause a variety of neurologic syndromes[817] (Tables 8–22 and 8–23). Parinaud's syndrome, which consists of paralysis of upward gaze, pupillary areflexia (to light), paralysis of convergence, and a wide-based gait, occurs in about half of pinealomas. Gait disturbances can also occur because of brain stem or cerebellar compression.

Management of tumors in the pineal region is not straightforward. Operative mortality rates of 14 to 37% have been reported[818] but the rationale for an aggressive approach to the pineal region[819, 820] is based on the need for making a histologic diagnosis, the variety of lesions found in this region, the possibility of cure of an encapsulated lesion, and the effectiveness of chemotherapeutic agents for germinomas and choriocarcinoma. Stereotaxic biopsy of the pineal region provided diagnosis in 33 of 34 cases in one series.[820] In another series four of six pineal tumors were cured by microsurgical techniques.[821] More than 70% of tumors in the posterior third

TABLE 8–22. Pinealomas: Frequency (%) of Presenting Symptoms and Signs

1. Increased intracranial pressure	85
2. Spasticity	35
3. Ataxia	30
4. Parinaud's syndrome	25
5. Cerebellar-type nystagmus	25
6. Syncope	20
7. Vertigo	20
8. Cranial nerve palsy (other than cranial nerves VI, VIII)	20
9. Intention tremor	15
10. Scotoma	10
11. Tinnitus	10
12. Other	10

From Brady WL. The role of radiation therapy. In: Schmidek HH, ed. Pineal Tumors. New York: Masson, 1977: 99–113, with permission.

TABLE 8–23. Ocular Symptoms and Signs in 22 Cases of Pinealoma

Symptoms and Signs	No. of Patients
Symptoms	
Diplopia	7
"Blurred vision"	4
Reading difficulty	1
Signs	
Upward gaze palsy	12
Pupils: Areflexic to light, near response retained	13
Accommodative control disorder	3
Convergent-retraction nystagmus	10
Convergence paresis	3
Downward gaze palsy	0
Collier sign	0
Skew deviation	5
Third nerve palsy	0
Fourth nerve palsy (bilateral)	1
Sixth nerve palsy	3
Fundi: Normal	8
Papilledema	10
Optic atrophy	4
Vision: Reduced acuity	8
Vision fields: Normal	15
Constricted	3
Bitemporal	4

From Wray SH. The neuro-ophthalmic and neurologic manifestations of pinealomas. In: Schmidek HH, ed. Pineal Tumors. New York: Masson, 1977: 61–77, with permission.

ventricle are radiosensitive and respond to adequate radiation therapy within 3 to 6 mo.[822] Radiation therapy may be combined with shunting procedures when the tumor blocks the aqueduct of Sylvius and causes hydrocephalus. In contrast to previous recommendations,[823] a trial of radiation for diagnostic purposes is no longer advocated.[824]

Ectopic pinealomas in the chiasmal region generally should be explored surgically if hCG is not detected in CSF, the tumor should be debulked if possible, and a biopsy diagnosis should be made. This recommendation is based on the relative safety of these procedures and the fact that some lesions are not radiosensitive but are amenable to surgical removal. Germinomas are radiosensitive and potentially curable.[823, 825] The diagnosis may be made by cytologic study of CSF, by radioimmunoassay of CSF for hCG, or by radioimmunoassay of β-hCG levels. Documentation of a tumor by imaging techniques and the presence of hCG in CSF provides a diagnosis of germinoma and makes surgical biopsy unnecessary; this diagnosis is an indication for chemotherapy or radiation, or both. Clinical experience with chemotherapy for pineal region tumors is being accumulated.[826–828]

Approach to the Patient with Precocious Puberty. If mature germ cells are present in the child with precocious puberty the diagnosis is true, meaning neurogenic precocity, and if so the work-up is focused on the hypothalamic-pituitary system. If gonadal maturation has not occurred the disorder is due to abnormalities of the gonads or adrenals[829–831] (see Chapter 31).

Management of Sexual Precocity. Structural disease of the hypothalamus is treated by surgery or radiation, or both, when indicated. Idiopathic precocity is best treated with LHRH superagonists[832–834] and if these agents fail by inhibitors of gonadal steroid biosynthesis such as ketoconazole.[835] Precocious puberty is stressful to both the child and the parents and it is essential that psychological support is provided (see Chapter 31).[836–839]

PSYCHOGENIC AMENORRHEA. Menstrual cycles can cease in young nonpregnant women with no demonstrable abnormalities of the brain, pituitary, or ovary in several situations[840–844]: pseudocyesis (false pregnancy), anorexia nervosa, excessive exercise, psychogenic disorders, amenorrhea, and

hyperprolactinemic states (See Chapter 15). Psychogenic amenorrhea, the most common cause of secondary amenorrhea except for pregnancy, can occur with major psychopathology or minor psychic stress. It is often temporary. Psychogenic amenorrhea is probably mediated by excessive endogenous opioid activity because naloxone or naltrexone (opiate receptor blockers) can induce ovulation in some patients with this disorder.[842, 843]

Exercise amenorrhea may be a variant of psychogenic amenorrhea or may result from loss of body fat.[646–649] The syndrome is associated with intense and prolonged physical exertion such as running, swimming, or ballet dancing. Such women are always below ideal body weight and have low stores of fat. If this activity is begun before puberty normal sexual maturation can be delayed for many years. The mass of fat may be a regulator of gonadotropin secretion and dietary composition also may play a role. Exercise and psychogenic amenorrhea can have adverse effects because of the associated estrogen deficiency and accompanying osteopenia (also see Chapter 15).[845]

NEUROGENIC HYPOGONADISM IN MALES. A discussion of neurogenic hypogonadism in males should begin with an account of Fröhlich's syndrome (adiposogenital dystrophy), originally characterized as delayed puberty, hypogonadism, and obesity associated with a tumor that impinges on the hypothalamus.[846, 847] It was subsequently recognized that either hypothalamic or pituitary dysfunction can induce hypogonadism; the presence of obesity indicates that the appetite-regulating regions of the hypothalamus have been damaged. Several organic lesions of the hypothalamus can cause this disorder, including tumors, encephalitis, microcephaly, Friedreich's ataxia, and demyelinating diseases. However most males with delayed sexual development do not have serious neurologic conditions. Furthermore most obese boys with delayed sexual development have no structural damage to the hypothalamus but actually have *constitutional delayed puberty*, which is commonly associated with obesity. It is not known whether there is a functional disorder of the hypothalamus in this disorder.

An important cause of hypogonadotropic hypogonadism is Kallmann's syndrome, a disorder caused by failure of LHRH-containing neurons to migrate normally (see earlier in the section on LHRH and hypophyseotropic hormone deficiency). In adult men hypogonadism (including reduced spermatogenesis) can be induced by emotional stress[848] or severe exercise,[849] but this abnormality is seldom diagnosed because the symptoms are more subtle than menstrual cycle changes in similarly stressed women.[850] Acute physical stress can also decrease testosterone and gonadotropin levels.[850, 851] Excessive exercise in men can be associated with anorexia.[849] The combination of long hours of work, sleep deprivation, and stress may account for the finding that testosterone levels are low in male internal medicine residents[852] and in soldiers in training.[853] Spinal cord injury transiently lowers blood testosterone levels,[854] but in otherwise healthy paraplegic and quadriplegic men testosterone levels are normal.[854, 855] It is generally believed that psychosexual development of brain maturation depends on the presence of androgens and that hypogonadism in boys (regardless of cause) should be treated by the middle teen years (15 y at the latest).[856]

Neurogenic Disorders of Prolactin Regulation

Neurogenic causes of hyperprolactinemia include irritative lesions of the chest wall (herpes zoster, thoracotomy); excessive tactile stimulation of the nipple; and lesions within the spinal cord such as ependymoma (Table 8–24; also see Chapter 17). Prolonged mechanical stimulation of the nipples

TABLE 8–24. Differential Diagnosis of Galactorrhea or Hyperprolactinemia, or Both

A. Structural Hypothalamic Lesions with Damage to Ventral Hypothalamus or Pituitary Stalk

Craniopharyngioma	Metastatic neoplasms
Sarcoidosis	Rathke's pouch cyst
Encephalitis	Surgical stalk section
Radiation	Ectopic pinealoma
Head trauma	Histiocytosis X
Ectopic pinealoma	

B. Structural Pituitary Lesions

PRL-producing pituitary tumors	Pituitary angiosarcoma
Empty sella syndrome	Acromegaly
Combined PRL/GH-producing pituitary tumors	
Cushing's disease	

C. Drug-Induced Disorders

Prochlorperazine*	Trifluoperazine*	Sulpiride	Amphetamines
Chlorpromazine*	Thioridazine*	Fluphenazine	Amitriptyline
Cyproheptadine	Reserpine	Methyldopa	Pimozide
Metoclopramide	Prostaglandins	Estrogens	Androgens
Meprobamate			

D. Endocrine-Metabolic Disorders

Hypothyroidism (50% with myxedema have increased PRL but only 5% have galactorrhea, usually with amenorrhea)

Addison's disease	Nelson's syndrome	Sheehan's syndrome
Adrenocarcinoma	Adrenal hyperplasia	Diabetes mellitus
Liver disease	Chronic renal failure	

E. Irritative Lesions of Chest Wall

Herpes zoster	Thoracotomy	Thoracic burns
Tight garments	Mastectomy	Cystic breast disease
Chest trauma	Atopic dermatitis	Mammoplasty

F. Hypothalamic Biochemical Lesions with Presumed Decrease of Prolactin-Inhibiting Factor or Increase of Prolactin-Releasing Factor†

G. Other Described Causes

Pseudotumor cerebri	Syringomyelia	Pseudocyesis
Tabes dorsalis	Male hypogonadism	Pneumoencephalogram
Chorioepithelioma of testis	Stein-Leventhal syndrome	Intrauterine device use
Hysterectomy	Ovarian resection	
Dilatation and curettage	Neck surgery	

H. Lesions of Upper Spinal Cord

Extrinsic tumors	Cervical ependymoma

*Twenty-five percent of psychiatric patients taking phenothiazine derivatives have galactorrhea, but many have normal PRL levels; amenorrhea may also occur, and both may persist for several years after medication is stopped.

†Diagnosis of exclusion: patients may still have a biochemical and radiologically undetectable PRL-producing pituitary tumor that will become apparent only as time goes on.

PRL, prolactin; GH, growth hormone.

Compiled by Dr. Bruce Biller.

by suckling or the use of a breast pump can initiate lactation in some women who are not pregnant, and neurologic lesions that interrupt the hypothalamic-pituitary connection can cause hyperprolactinemia. Agents that block dopamine receptors (such as the phenothiazines) or prevent dopamine release (e.g., reserpine and methyldopa) must be excluded in all cases.

A third or more of hyperprolactinemic women have the disorder for many years and never manifest roentgenographic evidence of a pituitary adenoma.[582, 775] Moreover some patients with microprolactinoma have spontaneous remission of hyperprolactinemia over time,[755] suggesting that there may be "functional" factors in the pathogenesis. The role of psychogenic factors in the pathogenesis of hyperprolactinemia is in question.

Hyperprolactinemia also occurs after certain forms of epileptic seizures. In one series six of eight patients with temporal lobe seizures had a marked increase in PRL, whereas only one in eight frontal lobe seizures led to hyperprolactinemia.[857]

Because the nervous system exerts such profound effects on PRL secretion, patients with hyperprolactinemia (including those with adenomas) could have a deficit of PIF or an excess of PRF activity.[858] In studies of PRL secretion in patients apparently cured of hyperprolactinemia by removal of a pituitary microadenoma, regulatory abnormalities persisted in some[859] but not all patients.[755, 860] Persistence of regulatory abnormalities could be due to incomplete removal of tumor, abnormal function of the remaining part of the gland, or underlying hypothalamic abnormalities.

Neurogenic Disorders of Growth Hormone Secretion

HYPOTHALAMIC GROWTH FAILURE. Loss of the normal nocturnal increase in GH secretion and loss of GH secretory responses to provocative stimuli occur early in the course of hypothalamic disease and may be the most sensitive endocrine indicator of hypothalamic dysfunction. As noted earlier, anatomic malformations of midline cerebral structures are associated with abnormal GH secretion, presumably due to failure of the development of normal GH regulatory mechanisms. Such disorders include optic nerve dysplasia and midline prosencephalic malformations (absence of the septum pellucidum, abnormal third ventricle, and abnormal lamina terminalis). Idiopathic hypopituitarism with GH deficiency was considered earlier in this chapter.

Maternal Deprivation Syndrome and Psychosocial Dwarfism. Infant neglect or abuse can impair growth and cause failure to thrive (the maternal deprivation syndrome). Older children with growth failure in a setting of abuse or severe emotional disturbance (termed psychosocial dwarfism) may also show abnormal circadian rhythms and deficient hGH release after insulin-induced hypoglycemia or arginine infusion (See Chapter 30).[861–865] Deficiency in release of corticotropin and gonadotropins may also be present. This disorder is reversible by placing the child in a supportive milieu where growth and neuroendocrine hGH responses rapidly return to normal.[861, 865]

In rats the inhibitory effects of stress on GH secretion are blocked by treatment with antisera to somatostatin.[866] The extent to which an increase in somatostatin secretion is involved in the human response to deprivation is unknown. In the adult human, furthermore, physical or emotional stress usually causes an *increase* in hGH secretion.

Malnutrition interacts with psychological factors to cause growth failure in children with the maternal deprivation syndrome[863] and each case should be carefully evaluated from this point of view. Growth retardation in deprived children may also be a function of stress-induced sleep disturbance,[867] which can impair sleep-related hGH secretion. Higher cerebral functions are also impaired in children with the maternal deprivation syndrome.[868]

Neuroregulatory Growth Hormone Deficiency. The availability of biosynthetic hGH for treatment of short stature has brought into focus a group of patients who grow at low rates (below the third percentile) and have low levels of serum IGF-I but have a normal hGH secretory reserve. Studies of 24-h hGH secretion profiles indicate that many of these children do not have normal spontaneous hGH secretion (abnormal ultradian and circadian rhythms and decreased number or amplitude of secretory bursts, or both). These children may have a functional regulatory disturbance of the hypothalamus and appear to grow normally when given exogenous hGH.[869, 870]

There is considerable uncertainty about the criteria for the diagnosis of neuroregulatory hGH deficiency. Many normally growing children have profiles of hGH secretion that are indistinguishable from those in children with the postulated syndrome.[871] Patterns of hGH secretion do not predict which child will benefit from therapy and there is poor correlation between hGH secretion and growth. Further the results of repeated tests in children show considerable variability.[872] The prevalence of an hGH neuroregulatory deficiency syndrome is thus unclear and the decision to treat short children with hGH should be made cautiously.[873]

NEUROGENIC HYPERSECRETION OF GROWTH HORMONE

Diencephalic Cachexia. Children and infants with tumors in and around the third ventricle frequently become cachectic, which is often associated with elevated hGH levels and paradoxical GH secretory responses to glucose and insulin.[874, 875] GH hypersecretion may be due to a hypothalamic abnormality or to malnutrition. Deficits of pituitary-adrenal regulation are less common. A striking feature is the alert appearance and seeming euphoria despite the wasted state. A variety of associated neurologic abnormalities may be present (Table 8–25); the tumors that produce this syndrome are summarized in Table 8–26.[994]

Syndrome of Inappropriate Growth Hormone Hypersecretion. Apparently inappropriate hGH hypersecretion[570, 876] (the *syndrome of inappropriate somatotropin secretion*) occurs with uncontrolled diabetes mellitus, hepatic failure, uremia, anorexia nervosa, and protein-calorie malnutrition. Nutritional factors are probably important in this response because in normal persons obesity inhibits and fasting stimulates episodic GH hypersecretion.[877] In diabetes mellitus cholinergic blockers reverse the abnormality,[878] possibly by inhibiting hypothalamic somatostatin secretion (see earlier in the section on neurotransmitter regulation of GH). Loss of inhibition of GH secretion by IGF-I may also play a role because most disorders in which this syndrome occurs are associated with low IGF-I levels.

Role of the Hypothalamus in the Etiology of Acromegaly. The possible role of the hypothalamus in the pathogenesis of acromegaly has been the subject of studies and reviews (See Chapter 9.).[213, 879, 880] Although acromegaly can be caused by ectopic secretion of GHRH by pancreatic or other neuroendocrine tumors or by hypothalamic gangliocytoma,[785, 879–881] these disorders, with rare exceptions, cause pituitary hyperplasia rather than adenoma formation. Demonstration of monoclonality

TABLE 8–25. Clinical Features of Diencephalic Syndrome (Pooled Data of 67 Anatomically Defined Tumors)

Clinical Feature	%
Emaciation	100
Alert appearance	87
Increased vigor or hyperkinesis, or both	72
Vomiting	68
Euphoria	59
Pallor	55
Nystagmus	55
Irritability	32
Hydrocephalus*	33
Optic atrophy	24
Tremor	23
Sweating	15
Large hands, feet	5
Large genitalia	5
Polyuria	5
Papilledema	5
Positive pneumoencephalogram results	98
Endocrine anomalies†	90
CSF protein	64
CSF abnormal cells	23

*Hydrocephalus includes clinical plus pneumoencephalographic findings.
†Positive in 9 of 10 cases with adequately recorded investigation. (Occasionally, patients had electrolyte and blood pressure anomalies and eosinophilia.)
CSF, cerebrospinal fluid.
Modified from Burr IM, Slonim AE, Danish RK, et al. Diencephalic syndrome revisited. J Pediatr 1976; 88:439–444, with permission.

TABLE 8–26. Histology of Tumors Producing Diencephalic Syndrome

Tumor	No. of Patients
Gliomas	56
Astrocytoma	37
Not subclassified	10
Spongioblastoma	5
Astroblastoma	1
Oligodendroglioma	1
Mixed astrocytoma-spongioblastoma	1
Mixed astrocytoma-oligodendroglioma	1
Ependymoma	2
Ganglioglioma	1
Dysgerminoma	1
No histology	10

From Burr IM, Slonim AE, Danish RK, et al. Diencephalic syndrome revisited. J Pediatr 1976; 88:439–444, with permission.

in all adenomas and of mutations in hGH receptor–linked G_s proteins in about half of patients suggest that the disease begins as a clonal mutation and is intrinsic to the pituitary.

Neurogenic Disorders of Corticotropin Regulation

Hypothalamic CRH hypersecretion is the likely cause of sustained pituitary-adrenal hyperfunction in at least two situations: Cushing's syndrome caused by the rare CRH-secreting gangliocytomas of the hypothalamus[881] and severe depression.[882]

Severe depression is associated with pituitary-adrenal abnormalities, including inappropriately elevated corticotropin levels, abnormal cortisol circadian rhythms, and resistance to dexamethasone suppression.[882] The dexamethasone suppression test has in fact been used as an aid to diagnosis of depressive illness. Patients with depression also have diminished responses to CRH, suggesting that depressed individuals hypersecrete CRH.[238, 882]

Another syndrome of corticotropin hypersecretion has been described in one young man under the name of "periodic hypothalamic discharge" (Wolff's syndrome). The patient had a recurring cyclic disorder characterized by high fever, paroxysms of glucocorticoid hypersecretion, and electroencephalographic abnormalities.[883] On the other hand, most cases of Cushing's disease are not due to hypersecretion of CRH but are due to a primary pituitary clonal defect (see Chapters 9 and 12).[736, 880]

Nonendocrine Manifestations of Hypothalamic Disease

The hypothalamus is involved in the regulation of diverse functions and behaviors (Table 8–27).[9, 16, 23, 884–886] Psychological abnormalities in hypothalamic disease include antisocial behavior, attacks of rage, laughing, and crying; disturbed sleep patterns; excessive sexuality; and hallucinations. Both somnolence (with posterior lesions) and pathologic wakefulness (with anterior lesions) occur, as do bulimia and profound anorexia. The abnormal eating patterns are analogous to the syndromes of hyperphagia produced in rats by destruction of the ventromedial nucleus or of connections to the paraventricular nucleus.[884] Lateral hypothalamic damage causes profound anorexia.

Patients with hypothalamic damage may experience hyperthermia, hypothermia, unexplained fluctuations in body temperature, and poikilothermy. Disturbances of sweating, acrocyanosis, loss of sphincter control, and diencephalic epilepsy are occasional manifestations. Hypothalamic damage

TABLE 8–27. Neurologic Manifestations of Nonendocrine Hypothalamic Disease

Disorders of Temperature Regulation	Periodic Disease of Hypothalamic Origin
Hyperthermia	Diencephalic epilepsy
Hypothermia	Kleine-Levin syndrome
Poikilothermia	Periodic discharge syndrome of Wolff
Disorders of Food Intake	**Disorders of Autonomic Nervous System**
Hyperphagia (bulimia)	Pulmonary edema
Anorexia, aphagia	Cardiac arrhythmias
Disorders of Water Intake	Sphincter disturbance
Compulsive water drinking	**Hereditary Hypothalamic Disease**
Adipsia	Laurence-Moon-Biedl syndrome
Essential hypernatremia	**Miscellaneous**
Disorders of Sleep and Consciousness	Prader-Willi syndrome
Somnolence	Diencephalic syndrome of infancy
Sleep rhythm reversal	Cerebral gigantism
Akinetic mutism	
Coma	
Disorders of Psychic Function	
Rage behavior	
Hallucinations	

also causes loss of recent memory believed to be due to damage of the mamillothalamic pathways. Severe memory loss, obesity, and personality changes (apathy, loss of ability to concentrate, aggressive antisocial behavior, severe food craving, inability to work or attend school) may occur with suprasellar extension of pituitary tumors, hypothalamic radiation, or damage incurred from surgical removal of parasellar tumors. Hypothalamic tumors grow slowly and may reach a large size without producing much disturbance of behavior or visceral homeostasis, whereas surgery of limited extent can produce striking functional abnormalities. Presumably this is because slowly growing lesions permit compensatory responses to develop. These potential consequences should be weighed carefully with the neurosurgeon, patient, and patient's family in planning the therapeutic approach; these adverse effects have led to more conservative surgical guidelines for the treatment of craniopharyngioma.[887]

Glucocorticoid Effects on the Brain

Glucocorticoids affect behavior, emotional state, brain fluid compartmentalization, and aging of the brain. Glucocorticoid deficiency leads to anorexia, apathy, cognitive disorder, stupor, and coma. Excessive glucocorticoids can induce hyperphagia, pathologic insomnia, depression, and hallucinations. Glucocorticoid effects on cerebrovascular permeability and on choroidal transport of water and electrolytes are important in regulating CSF formation and brain volume. Steroid withdrawal, recovery from Cushing's syndrome, or adrenal deficiency, especially if it develops over a short period, can lead to cerebral edema in children.[888]

Hippocampal atrophy, as in Alzheimer's disease, is associated with a high blood cortisol level and an elevated set point of feedback control.[889] Hippocampal neurons are uniquely sensitive to glucocorticoids and can be damaged by associated stress. These effects are mediated by high intracellular Ca^{2+} and are potentiated by glutamate receptor excitotoxins.[890] Severe psychological stress and pain, as in survivors of concentration camps, may cause cerebral cortical atrophy, possibly related to damaging effects of glucocorticoids.

NEUROPEPTIDES IN VISCERAL AND METABOLIC REGULATION

Eating Behavior and Neuropeptides

Eating behavior is regulated by an interplay of metabolites in blood (including glucose, lipids, glycerol, and amino acids),

neural signals from the mouth and gastrointestinal tract, circulating hormones (glucocorticoids, estrogens, insulin), circulating and intrinsic neuropeptides, a hormone secreted by fat cells, and higher cerebral function.[891–894] These various regulators are integrated within the paraventricular nucleus of the hypothalamus. The ventromedial hypothalamus contains neurons that sense glucose levels (glucoreceptors) and influence activity of the sympathetic nervous system and eating. Chemoreceptors in the brain stem and gastrointestinal tract and liver[728, 729] can sense the presence of certain toxic substances and induce nausea and vomiting through afferent neural signals directed to the NTS, an afferent nucleus of the vagus nerve. The brain chemoreceptors are located in the area postrema, a structure in the floor of the fourth ventricle that lacks a blood-brain barrier and thereby can sense foreign, potentially toxic substances in blood.[727]

A number of gut-brain peptides can induce or suppress eating, acting through signals from the gastrointestinal tract or the paraventricular nucleus (Table 8–28). Several cytokines that circulate during inflammation and are induced within the brain by peripheral toxins (IL-1, IL-2, IL-6, and TNF α) are powerful appetite suppressors and cause the anorexia of inflammation.

Peptides regulate eating in several ways. CCK is released from the small bowel when food, especially lipid, enters the duodenum from the stomach. Administration of CCK to animals inhibits eating and induces the behaviors that accompany satiety.[895, 896] The two CCK systems (peripheral and central) are independent and act through different receptors[897] but each functions to reduce food intake. Within the range of peripheral CCK values observed after a meal, the effects are exerted both on the stomach and the brain. CCK receptors in circumferential muscular fibers in the pylorus have the ability to regulate the rate of gastric emptying.[897] Because CCK-induced satiety is blocked by vagotomy, the sense of satiety after peripheral CCK injection is probably induced by stimulating stomach stretch or afferent vagal CCK receptors.[898, 899]

CCK and other regulators of satiety influence meal size and the composition of food intake. Neuropeptide Y and its homologue peptide YY, e.g., enhance the amount and dura-

TABLE 8–28. Peptides, Hormones, and Neurotransmitters That Influence Eating Behavior

Stimulate Eating	Inhibit Eating
Neuropeptide Y (Y_1)*	Serotonin*
GABA (A)*	Cholecystokinin*
Norepinephrine ($α_2$)*	Dopamine (D_2)*
Glucocorticoid (type II)*	Insulin
Galanin†	TRH
Opioids†	Calcitonin
Aldosterone (type I)†	Bombesin
Opioids‡	VIP
GHRH‡	CRH
	Neurotensin
	CGRP
	Glucagon
	IL-1
	IL-2
	Tumor necrosis factor
	Prostaglandins
	Leptin

*Carbohydrate selective.
†Fat selective.
‡Protein selective.
Receptor type is shown in parentheses.
GABA, γ-aminobutyric acid; TRH, thyrotropin-releasing hormone; GHRH, growth hormone–releasing hormone; VIP, vasoactive intestinal peptide; CRH, corticotropin-releasing hormone; CGRP, calcitonin gene-related product.
Modified from Morley JE. Neuropeptide regulation of appetite and weight. Endocr Rev 1987; 8:256–287. © 1987, The Endocrine Society. Classification of nutrient specificity from Leibowitz SF. Neurochemical-neuroendocrine systems in the brain controlling macronutrient intake and metabolism. Trends Neurosci 1992; 15:491–497.

tion of carbohydrate intake and have little or no influence on protein or fat intake.[893, 900] Analogous effects are exerted by centrally acting norepinephrine (through the α_2-noradrenergic receptor) and GABA.[893] Fat intake, in contrast, is enhanced by centrally acting galanin and opioid peptides.[892, 893]

Although these complex neuroendocrine signaling pathways provide a basis for enhancing or terminating individual eating episodes, they do not explain the fact that over long periods most individuals maintain a stable body weight. Periods of forced starvation or forced feeding are followed by restoration to previous body weight. The *adipostat* hypothesis suggests that the brain can sense some measure of body fat mass, presumably through a neural signal.

The most likely fat depot–dependent appetite regulator is *leptin*,[894] a protein hormone secreted by fat cells at a rate determined by the degree of fat storage or synthesis. Fasting suppresses and feeding and insulin stimulate leptin synthesis.[901, 902] Leptin acts on the brain through a receptor[903] to suppress synthesis and secretion of neuropeptide Y, a potent stimulator of eating.[904] Obese humans have higher levels of leptin mRNA in fat tissue and elevated levels of the hormone in blood,[902] suggesting that in the human (in contrast to the mouse) obesity is due to a defective leptin receptor, a postreceptor defect, or a satiety signal overridden by other regulatory factors.[905]

In the regulation of eating, central and peripheral peptides interact with bioaminergic neurotransmitters such as dopamine and norepinephrine in the hypothalamus.[893] Anorexigenic drugs, such as amphetamines, act through these receptors. The multiple factors that influence eating and satiety—gut afferents, central and peripheral peptides, neurotransmitters, nutrients, psychological factors, nociceptive receptors, and steroid hormones—interact to govern behavior.

Drinking Behavior and Neuropeptides

Drinking behavior is a function of neural signals from volume receptors in the carotid sinus and left atrium, central receptors sensitive to changes in brain electrolytes and osmolality, and peripheral oropharyngeal sensors. As noted earlier in the section on neurohypophysis, osmosensitive structures are present in several periventricular organs, especially the OVLT and SFO. The best characterized of the water- and salt-regulating neuropeptides are AVP, angiotensin II, and the atrial natriuretic peptides.

Neurosteroids

Steroid hormones enter the brain by diffusion through lipid-rich membranes of the blood-brain barrier. Estradiol is formed in the brain from precursors such as testosterone,[906, 907] and dihydrotestosterone is formed in brain by the 5α-reduction of testosterone.[908] Steroids that arise de novo within the brain are called *neurosteroids*; the principal neurosteroids pregnenolone and dehydroepiandrosterone (DHEA)[909] are present in trace amounts in adrenalectomized and gonadectomized animals and in tissue or cell cultures of brain. Neurosteroids are synthesized mainly in oligodendroglia. Their function is unknown and it is not clear that they are actually secreted within the brain because their concentration in CSF approximates that of the free hormone in blood.[910] However, DHEA, formed from whatever mechanism, may play a role in brain function.[911] DHEA is an allosteric antagonist of the GABA receptor and can increase neuronal activity by blocking the inhibitory effects of GABA. In older men and women, in whom blood DHEA (of adrenocortical origin) has declined, restoration of blood levels to those of young adults is said to bring about a sense of increased well-being and euphoria.[912] These results have not been confirmed and it is too early to know whether neurosteroids and other hormones such as melatonin and GH, all of which decline with age, play a role in aging and merit consideration as "replacement" therapy.

NEUROENDOCRINE-IMMUNE INTERACTION

The immune system is a major adaptive system of animals, capable of recognizing foreign proteins, viruses, and bacteria as *nonself* and of mounting cellular reactions to defend the integrity of the host. Two general classes of cytokine responses by lymphocytes and monocytes are recognized—an acute response activated in the absence of prior exposure to antigen and a delayed response that depends on prior exposure to a specific antigen.[913]

Lymphocytes secrete immunoglobulins and lymphokines. Because some lymphokines are also secreted by other types of cells they have also been called cytokines. Lymphokines regulate differentiation, proliferation, and function of other lymphocytes and monocytes and exert diverse effects on many different tissues, including induction of fever, alteration of protein and lipid metabolism, and modulation of neuroendocrine function (see later).[913–918] Many endocrine and neural cells also synthesize cytokines that serve paracrine functions as diverse as activation or killing of cells. The endocrine disorders of autoimmunity disease are reviewed in Chapter 33. This section deals with the actions of cytokines in the neuroendocrine system.

The immune system is subject to neural and hormonal modulation; many of the same neuropeptides, protein hormones, and hormone receptors are expressed in nerve cells, endocrine cells, and lymphocytes, and the products of lymphocytes can influence neuroendocrine function.[8, 914–922] An emerging literature suggests that stress, both emotional and physical, can modulate the immune response, at least in part by neuroendocrine mechanisms.[917, 923, 924]

Neuroimmunology is the study of immune reactions involving the brain, nerves, and muscles, e.g., autoimmune allergic encephalitis, multiple sclerosis, and myasthenia gravis. In the past this term was also applied to the study of neural modulation of the immune response, but a more specific term for the interaction of nervous and immune systems is *neuroimmunomodulation*. To emphasize the role of neuroendocrine mechanisms, the term *neuroendocrine immunology* has been coined. This section considers the effects of lymphokines on neuroendocrine function, the effects of hormones and peptides on immune responses, and the hormones and neuropeptides produced by the immune system.

Effects of Cytokines on Neuroendocrine Function: The Acute-Phase Response

The acute immune cell response to foreign antigens is triggered within a few minutes of exposure, whereas the delayed response may take 1 wk to 10 d to develop.[913] An important generalizing concept, proposed by Blalock,[8] is that the peripheral pool of lymphocytes and monocytes serves as a sensing mechanism by which foreign substances are recognized and thereby mobilizes neuroendocrine adaptive responses. This has been referred to as *bidirectional communication* between immune system and brain.

On exposure to foreign molecules or the products of tissue injury, lymphocytes, monocytes, and other tissues secrete a variety of regulatory peptides whose function is to neutralize, inactivate, and sequester these invading substances (Table 8–29).[913–920] The acute-phase response mobilizes homeostatic

TABLE 8–29. Neuroendocrine Effects of Lymphokines and Monokines

Lymphokine-Monokine	Effect
IL-1	Causes fever
	Results in slow-wave sleep
	Causes CRH release
	Causes corticotropin and endorphin release
	Elevates glucocorticoid levels
	Stimulates GH and PRL (in humans)
	Inhibits thyrotropin release (in rats)
	Stimulates somatostatin secretion
	Inhibits TRH synthesis
	Stimulates AVP release
	Stimulates IL-6 production
IL-2	Stimulates release of corticotropin, glucocorticoids, PRL, and GH
	Stimulates synthesis of TNF and IL-1
IL-6	Stimulates release of corticotropin, glucocorticoids, GH, and PRL (present in folliculostellate pituitary cells)
TNF	Inhibits GH release (directly)
	Stimulates corticotropin adrenocortical secretion
	Inhibits thyrotropin, T_4, and T_3 secretion
	Inhibits thyroid response to thyrotropin
	Increases PRL release
IFN α or IFN β, or both	Induction of adrenal steroidogenesis
	Increases iodine uptake by thyroid cells
	Excites neurons
	Suppresses morphine withdrawal symptoms
	Causes catalepsy, analgesia
Thymosin	Elevates corticotropin and glucocorticoid levels

TNF, tumor necrosis factor; IFN α or IFN β, interferon-α or interferon-β; CRH, corticotropin-releasing hormone; GH, growth hormone; PRL, prolactin; TRH, thyrotropin-releasing hormone; AVP, arginine vasopressin; T_4, thyroxine; T_3, triiodothyronine.

Adapted from Blalock JE. A molecular basis for bidirectional communication between the immune and neuroendocrine systems. Physiol Rev 1989; 69:1–32, with permission.

mechanisms and initiates long-term adaptive immunity. Within a few minutes of an intravenous injection of the endotoxin of *E. coli*, lipopolysaccharide (LPS), e.g., there is an increase in the blood levels of several cytokines, TNF α,[916] IL-1β, IL-6, and IL-1β–receptor antagonist (Fig. 8–61). Among the important metabolic effects (see Table 8–29) are induction of negative nitrogen balance; inhibition of synthesis of liver proteins such as albumin, thyroid hormone-binding globulin, ceruloplasmin, and apolipoproteins; a decrease in circulating levels of iron and copper; and increased synthesis of other liver proteins, including fibrinogen, α_2-microglobulin, and amyloid precursor protein. Synthesis of triglyceride is inhibited and fat stores are mobilized through local lipolytic enzyme activation.

Systemic toxins and acute-phase cytokines change the set point of temperature regulation in the brain to cause fever, "sickness behavior" (inactivity, loss of interest, anorexia, and hyperalgesia), enhanced slow-wave sleep, and other behavioral disturbances ranging from malaise to delirium and coma.[925–927] The mechanism by which circulating cytokines and bacterial toxins change brain function has not been fully explained. Most workers believe that the blood-brain barrier excludes toxins and inflammatory cytokines from direct entry into the brain and that the effects are mediated at the brain surface (endothelia, periventricular organs [see earlier]) and visceral afferents from the vagus nerve (see earlier in the section on pituitary-adrenal regulation). Endothelial cells of the brain and ependyma-derived epithelia of the specialized periventricular organs synthesize and translocate a variety of molecules into brain, including inflammatory cytokines and small-molecular-weight second messengers including IL-1β, IL-6, TNF α, several prostaglandins, NO, and still other cytokines, some of which are neurotoxic. Within the brain these various cytokines can induce synthesis of other cytokines by astrocytes, microglia, tissue macrophages, resident basophils, and, to some extent, neurons themselves.

The flood of cytokines impinging on the brain causes

changes in the synthesis and release of several neurotransmitters and neuropeptides. Brain cytokine responses are both beneficial and destructive. Fever in some settings increases resistance to infection. The secretion of nerve growth factor, which exerts a beneficial effect on neuronal healing after brain injury, is enhanced by exposure to IL-1. However, excessive central brain cytokines lead to toxic levels of NO, potentiate excitotoxin effects of glutamate, and stimulate production of the Alzheimer protein precursor, which is toxic to neurons and exerts amnesic effects.

The cytokines have important neuroendocrine consequences, and altered hypothalamic-pituitary activity interacts with cytokine effects on individual endocrine organs. The following are additional cytokine effects on the endocrine system. Pituitary folliculostellate cells contain[928] and release IL-6[929] and NO.[438] One or more secretory cells of the pituitary contain IL-1β.[930] Furthermore neuronal pathways in the medial basal hypothalamus[923, 924] contain IL-1β, IL-6, and TNF,[724] and IL-6 is released from the hypothalamus after exposure to bacterial toxins.[933, 934] Thus the potential exists for regulation of anterior pituitary function via endocrine effects (circulating cytokines from activated lymphocytes), neuroendocrine effects (exerted by the hypothalamus through the classic tuberoinfundibular portal vessel system), and paracrine control within the pituitary itself.

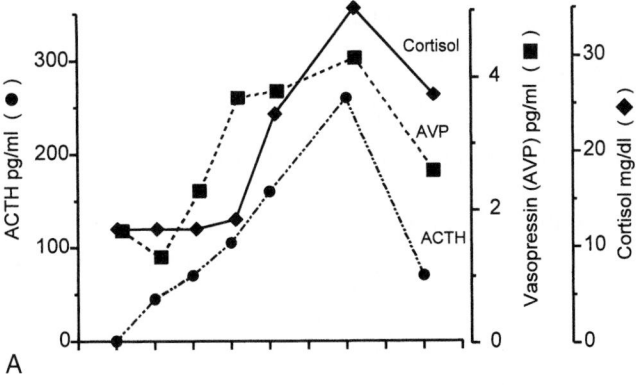

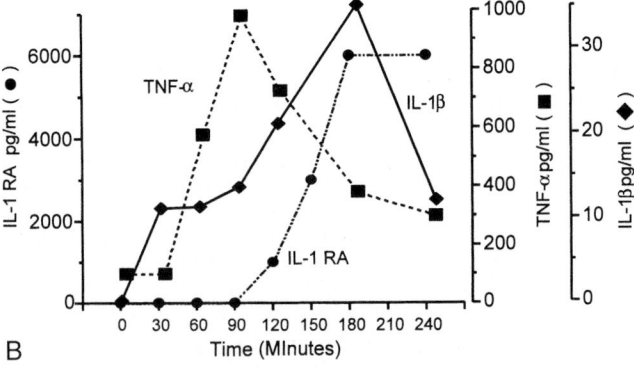

Figure 8–61. *A*, Effect of injection of *Escherichia coli* endotoxin (lipopolysaccharide) [LPS]) on circulating levels of corticotropin, vasopressin, and cortisol. *B*, Effect of injection of LPS on circulating levels of IL-1β; IL-1RA; and TNFα. AVP, vasopressin; ACTH, corticotropin; IL-1RA, interleukin-1 receptor antagonist; IL-1β, interleukin-1β; TNF-α, tumor necrosis factor α. (*A* redrawn from Michie HR, Majzoub JA, O'Dwyer ST, et al. Both cyclooxygenase-dependent and cyclogenase-independent pathways mediate the neuroendocrine response in humans. Surgery 1990; 108:254–259. *B* redrawn from Granowitz EV, Santos AA, Poutsiaka DD, et al. Production of interleukin-1-receptor antagonist during experimental endotoxaemia. Lancet 1991; 338: 1423–1424 © by the Lancet Ltd. 1991; and Michie HR, Manoque KR, Spriggs DR, et al. Detection of circulating tumor necrosis factor after endotoxin injection. N Engl J Med 1988; 318:1481–1486. Copyright 1988. Massachusetts Medical Society. All rights reserved.)

Cytokine-induced pituitary secretion has teleologic value as a host defense.[917, 918, 936] Pituitary-adrenal activation by toxin is the best understood of the endocrine interactions in the immune system. As noted earlier in the section on corticotropin regulation, release of CRH, vasopressin, and epinephrine leads to increased glucocorticoid secretion, which serves to modulate an inflammatory response that could be damaging to the host.[917, 935, 936] The major action of the cytokines is on the hypothalamic control element. Rats with congenital deficiency of CRH secretion (the Lewis rat) are vulnerable to hypersensitivity arthritis,[920] and patients with rheumatoid arthritis have a reduced pituitary-adrenal response to operative stress.[937]

The occurrence of SIADH in patients with pneumococcal pneumonia, pulmonary tuberculosis, and bronchiectasis is attributable to cytokine-induced release of vasopressin.[938] Inhibition of pituitary-thyroid function by inflammation is mediated by cytokines acting at multiple levels of the pituitary-thyroid axis, including peripheral thyroid hormone metabolism.[917, 925, 936] Conversion of T_4 to T_3 and the production of thyroid hormone–binding proteins are inhibited by several inflammatory cytokines, leading to the "sick euthyroid syndrome." At the level of the thyroid, synthesis of thyroid hormone, iodination of thyroglobulin, and responses to thyrotropin are all impaired, and the inappropriately low circulating thyrotropin levels are due to impaired pituitary responsiveness to TRH, impaired secretion of hypothalamic TRH, and enhanced hypothalamic secretion of somatostatin. Both the pituitary and the thyroid express IL-1 when exposed to circulating toxins, suggesting that paracrine-autocrine cytokine production also plays a role in local responses. In contrast to the pituitary-adrenal response to inflammation, which has homeostatic value, the benefit of induced hypothyroidism, if any, has not been demonstrated in the human[917] but is beneficial in rats with induced pneumonia.[939]

Pituitary-gonadal function is also impaired in inflammation through changes in the hypothalamus, pituitary, and gonads. The magnitude of LH and FSH pulses is reduced or suppressed completely, IL-1 is induced locally in both ovary and testis, and systemic and paracrine effects of IL-1 suppress synthesis and secretion of steroid hormones in both organs and reduce the response to gonadotropins. Loss of the normal LH and FSH ultradian rhythm is attributable to suppression of LHRH secretion by cytokine-stimulated secretion of hypothalamic CRH and vasopressin.[940, 941] No clear homeostatic benefit results from suppressed gonadal secretion in inflammatory illness, but this question has not been studied adequately.

In the human GH secretion is enhanced by inflammatory stimuli (and massive stresses like burns and surgery), whereas in the rat low concentrations of cytokines stimulate and high concentrations suppress GH secretion. These changes are brought about by altered secretion of GHRH and somatostatin. Elevated GH secretion may reduce the negative nitrogen balance of infection and other stresses and possibly stimulates lymphocyte-monocyte reactivity.

PRL secretion in humans and rats is enhanced by inflammation and by inflammatory cytokines but the mechanism of this response has not been elucidated. A homeostatic action of PRL has not been demonstrated but the effect of PRL as a lymphocyte-regulating hormone suggests that it may function to regulate immunocompetent cells (see later).

Neuroendocrine Regulation of the Immune Process

The nervous system can influence immune function through a number of routes[942]—hypothalamic-pituitary function; autonomic nervous system innervation of spleen, liver,

gut, and lymphoid organs[923, 924]; circulating catecholamines; sensory neuron peptides such as somatostatin and substance P; induction of fever; and changes in diet and activity. A less well-established route is the direct secretion into the blood of immune-regulating factors from the brain.[943]

The most important pituitary-dependent hormone that influences immune reactions is cortisol, which inhibits most aspects of the immune response, including proliferation of lymphocytes; production of immunoglobulins, cytokines, and the inflammatory mediators that follow antigen-antibody binding; and cellular toxicity including the production of inflammatory leukotrienes.[935] These inhibitory reactions form the basis of the anti-inflammatory actions of glucocorticoids (see Chapter 12) and occur within the range of values induced by stress or inflammation. The pituitary-adrenal response to stress may serve to modulate the intensity of the immune response and its inflammatory components, including changes in vascular tone and vascular permeability.[935] Loss of this function makes animals with adrenal insufficiency vulnerable to inflammation. The fact that the products of inflammation such as IL-1 can activate the hypothalamic-pituitary-adrenal axis (see earlier) suggests the operation of a negative feedback control loop to regulate the intensity of inflammation.[529] Because pituitary-adrenal function is almost completely controlled by the brain, this system is an excellent example of neuroimmunomodulation.

The physiological effects of other anterior pituitary hormones on the immune response are more subtle.[918] GH-deficient mice have thymic atrophy, involution of lymphatic tissue, and T-cell impairment, abnormalities that are reversible by GH treatment.[944] In addition, the decrease in GH secretion with aging may cause the decline in immune function with aging because thymic atrophy in the aged rat is reversed by GH treatment.[944, 945] PRL can also stimulate immune function.[946–950] Human T and B lymphocytes and some lymphoma cells contain membrane PRL receptors; the immunoincompetent state in hypophysectomized mice is corrected by PRL administration; antibodies to PRL inhibit lymphocyte proliferation in several cell lines; and cyclosporine, an immunosuppressant drug, blocks the lymphocyte-stimulating effects of PRL.[951] Lymphocyte PRL dependency may be a manifestation of a response to both pituitary PRL and an autocrine or paracrine system, because lymphocytes can also synthesize and secrete PRL.[8] The effects of hyperprolactinemia and of PRL suppression on human immune function have not been elucidated.

A role for gonadal function as a modulator of the immune process has been suspected because of the gender differences in the prevalence of the autoimmune diseases.[952] The sex ratio for Hashimoto's thyroiditis, e.g., is 25:1 in favor of women. Women with systemic lupus erythematosus who are given contraceptive steroids may show an exacerbation of disease,[952] and estradiol potentiates mitogen-induced B-cell stimulation in men.[953] Lymphocyte function varies during the menstrual cycle, T-lymphocyte function being reduced in the first half of the cycle.

Pituitary hormones that bind to receptors on lymphocytes include vasopressin, oxytocin, the endorphins, α-MSH, and LH.[8] Table 8–26 summarizes some of the immunoregulatory effects of these substances, some of which appear to act both centrally and peripherally in mediating responses to inflammation. Corticotropin, vasopressin, and α-MSH are inhibitors of pyrogen-induced fever[954]; nerve endings containing these peptides are localized in central temperature-regulating areas,[955] and in the periphery α-MSH counteracts several effects of IL-1 on monocyte and fibroblast function.[956–958]

Other neuropeptides that influence the immune response include substance P, somatostatin, CRH, and VIP. The concentrations required for biologic effect are seemingly too high to

TABLE 8–30. Immunoregulatory Effects of Several Hormones and Neuropeptides

Hormone-Neuropeptide	Effect
Corticotropin	Suppression of Ig and IFN-γ synthesis
	Augmentation of B-cell proliferation
	Suppression of IFN-γ–mediated macrophage activation
Glucocorticoids	Inhibition of all aspects of lymphokine synthesis and effects
Estrogens	Stimulation of a number of lymphocyte functions
GH	Enhancement of generation of T cells
PRL	Stimulation of thymulin secretion
	Stimulation of lymphocyte proliferation
Thyrotropin	Enhancement of Ig synthesis
hCG	Suppression of T_c and NK-cell activity
	Suppression of T-cell proliferation
	Suppression of mixed lymphocyte reactions
	Generation of T_s cells
α-Endorphin	Suppression of Ig synthesis and secretion
	Suppression of antigen-specific helper T cell
β-Endorphin	Enhancement of Ig and IFN-γ synthesis
	Modulation of T-cell proliferation
	Enhancement of generation of T_c cells
	Enhancement of NK-cell activity
	Chemotactic for monocytes and neutrophils
Leu- or met-enkephalin	Suppression of Ig synthesis
	Enhancement of IFN-γ synthesis
	Enhancement of NK-cell activity
	Chemotactic for monocytes
Substance P	Augmentation of T-cell proliferation
	Degranulation of mast cells and basophils
	Enhancement of macrophage phagocytosis
	Elicitation of O_2, H_2O_2, and thromboxane B_2 production
AVP and oxytocin	Replacement of IL-2 requirement for IFN-γ synthesis
Somatostatin	Suppression of histamine and leukotriene D_4 release from basophils
	Suppression of T-cell proliferation
VIP	Inhibition of mitogen-stimulated T cells through cAMP link
	Inhibition of release of T lymphocytes from popliteal nodes
	Inhibition of migration of T lymphocytes into mesenteric nodes
α-MSH	Suppression of IL-1–stimulated fever
	Suppression of monocyte secretion of IL-2
	Suppression of fibroblast production of prostaglandins
	Suppression of neutrophil migration

Ig, immunoglobulin; IFN-γ, interferon-γ; GH, growth hormone; PRL, prolactin; hCG, human chorionic gonadotropin; NK cells, natural killer T cells; T_s cells, T-suppressor cells; T_c cells, cytotoxic T cells; AVP, arginine vasopressin; VIP, vasoactive intestinal peptide; α-MSH, α-melanocyte–stimulating hormone.

Adapted from Blalock JE. A molecular basis for bidirectional communication between the immune and neuroendocrine systems. Physiol Rev 1989; 69:1–32, with permission.

be physiologically relevant, but these peptides may be released locally in high concentration from sensory nerve endings[959, 960] and from immunocompetent inflammatory cells.

Immunocompetent cells secrete many peptides and hormones (Table 8–30). Perhaps the best example of paracrine control of lymphocyte function by a secreted cytokine is that of CRH. Activated lymphocytes secrete CRH, and CRH in turn enhances lymphocyte activation.[250] CRH in inflammatory joint fluid of patients with rheumatoid arthritis is probably secreted by activated lymphocytes and monocytes.[250] Since CRH is an activating peptide and since CRH receptors are present on activated monocytes, this system could operate as a positive feedback system to increase the intensity of inflammation.

It has also been postulated that arthritis may be potentiated by substance P released from sensory neurons in the joint.[960] Substance P and its cosecreted peptide substance K (both derived from the same prohormone) have vasodilating properties and are mediators of the wheal-and-flare response to tissue injury.

Somatostatin can inhibit immunoglobulin E–dependent stimulation of basophils and the in vitro proliferation of T and B lymphocytes.[918, 961] VIP is generally an inhibitor of lymphocyte function and may act to restrict lymphocyte traffic through Peyer's patches in the gut.[962]

The secretion of pituitary hormones by lymphocytes is reportedly regulated by the same factors that regulate the pituitary. For example corticotropin secretion by lymphocytes is suppressed by glucocorticoids and stimulated by corticotropin-releasing factor; thyrotropin immunoreactivity of lymphocytes is stimulated by TRH and suppressed by thyroid hormone; and lymphocyte GH is stimulated by GHRH and suppressed by somatostatin.[8] The endocrine significance of hormone secretion by lymphocytes is uncertain. For example the claim that the lymphocytes of hypophysectomized mice infected with Newcastle virus can synthesize enough corticotropin to stimulate the adrenal cortex[963] has been criticized on methodologic grounds;[964] however, a case of Cushing's syndrome was apparently caused by excessive corticotropin secretion from a large inflammatory mass.[965] There is also controversy as to whether corticotropin receptors are present on lymphocytes.[966, 967]

Psychoneuroimmunology

Efforts to identify neural pathways of immune regulation were initiated because of evidence suggesting that psychological stress and depression can change human immune function,[923, 924, 968–970] that immune responses in animals can be conditioned in a classic pavlovian paradigm, and that neural lesions can inhibit various aspects of the immune response. These changes could affect immune surveillance and have implications for the course of cancer, for the course of acquired immunodeficiency syndrome (AIDS), and for the initiation or aggravation of autoimmune diseases, including those associated with the endocrine system such as Graves' disease and insulin-dependent diabetes mellitus. The extent to which such influences, if present, are mediated through known neuroendocrine pathways is unknown. Alternative regulatory pathways from the central nervous system to the immune system include the catecholamines (and cosecreted neuropeptides) of the autonomic nervous system that innervate lymph nodes, spleen, and thymus; adrenomedullary catecholamines; and the hormones that influence secretion of thymosin and other lymphocyte-regulating thymic hormones. Despite clear evidence that the nervous system can influence immune function through neural and neuroendocrine mechanisms, the role of these factors in human inflammatory disease remains to be defined.

REFERENCES

Introduction and Reviews

1. Snyder SH. Drug and neurotransmitter receptors in the brain. Science 1984; 224:22–31.
2. Brown JC. An overview of gastrointestinal endocrine physiology. Endocrinol Metab Clin North Am 1993; 22:719–730.
3. Roth J, LeRoith D, Shiloach J, et al. The evolutionary origins of hormones, neurotransmitters, and other extracellular chemical messengers. N Engl J Med 1982; 306:523–527.
4. Roth J, LeRoith D, Shiloach J, et al. Intercellular communication: an attempt at a unifying hypothesis. Clin Res 1983; 31:354–363.
5. Lauder JM. Neurotransmitters as growth regulatory signals: role of receptors and second messengers. Trends Neurosci 1993; 16:233–240.
6. Krieger DT, Martin JB. Brain peptides. N Engl J Med 1981; 304:876–885, 944–951.
7. Krieger DT. Brain peptides: what, where, and why? Science 1983; 222:975–985.
8. Blalock JE. A molecular basis for bidirectional communication between the immune and neuroendocrine systems. Physiol Rev 1989; 69:1–32.
9. The Hypothalamus. Proceedings of the Association for Research in Nervous and Mental Disease. New York: Hafner, 1940 (reprinted in 1966).

10. Harris GW. Neural control of the pituitary. Physiol Rev 1948; 28:139–179.
11. Friedgood HB. Neuroendocrinology. In: Williams RH, ed. Textbook of Endocrinology. 2nd ed. Philadelphia: WB Saunders, 1955.
12. Reichlin S. Medical progress. Neuroendocrinology. N Engl J Med 1963; 269:1246–1250, 1296–1303.
13. Szentágothai J, Flerkó B, Mess B. Hypothalamic Control of the Anterior Pituitary. New York: Grune & Stratton, 1968.
14. Heller H. History of neurohypophysial research. In: Greep RO, Astwood EB, Knobil E, et al, eds. Handbook of Physiology. Sect 7: Endocrinology. Vol IV. The Pituitary Gland and Its Neuroendocrine Control. Part 1. Washington, DC: American Physiological Society, 1974: 103–117.
15. Anderson E, Haymaker W. Breakthroughs in hypothalamic and pituitary research. Prog Brain Res 1974; 41:1–60.
16. Haymaker W, Anderson E, Nauta WJH. The Hypothalamus. Springfield, IL: Charles C Thomas, 1969.
17. Meites J, Donovan BT, McCann SM, eds. Pioneers in Neuroendocrinology. Vols I and II. New York: Plenum, Vol 1, 1975; Vol 2, 1978.
18. Flerkó B. The hypophysial portal circulation today. Neuroendocrinology 1980; 30:56–63.
19. Martini L, Ganong WF, eds. Neuroendocrinology. New York: Academic, Vol 1, 1966; Vol 2, 1967.
20. Martini L, Ganong WF, eds. Frontiers in Neuroendocrinology. New York: Oxford University Press, Vol 1 (Ganong, Martini), 1969; Vol 2 (Martini, Ganong), 1971; Vol 3 (Martini, Ganong), 1973; New York: Raven, Vol 4 (Martini, Ganong), 1976; Vol 5 (Ganong, Martini), 1978; Vol 6 (Martini, Ganong), 1980; Vol 7 (Martini, Ganong), 1982; Vol 8 (Martini, Ganong), 1984; Vol 9 (Martini, Ganong), 1986; Vol 10 (Martini, Ganong), 1988. (published as a quarterly journal beginning 1990)
21. Greep RO, Astwood EB, Knobil E, et al, eds. Handbook of Physiology. Sect 7: Endocrinology. Vol IV. The Pituitary Gland and Its Neuroendocrine Control. Part 1. Washington, DC: American Physiological Society, 1974.
22. Besser GM, Martini L, eds. Clinical Neuroendocrinology. New York: Academic, Vol I, 1977; Vol II, 1982.
23. Martin JB, Reichlin S, Brown GM. Clinical Neuroendocrinology. 2nd ed. Philadelphia: FA Davis, 1987.
24. Jeffcoate SL, Hutchinson JSM, eds. The Endocrine Hypothalamus. London: Academic, 1978.
25. Jackson IMD, Vale WW, eds. Extrapituitary functions of hypothalamic hormones. Fed Proc 1981; 49:2543–2544.
26. Krieger DT, Hughes JC, eds. Neuroendocrinology. Sunderland, MA: Sinauer Associates, 1980.
27. Müller EE, MacLeod RM, eds. Neuroendocrine Perspectives. Amsterdam: Elsevier Biomedical, Vol 1, 1982; Vol 2, 1983; Vol 3, 1984; Vol 4, 1985; Vol 5, 1986. New York: Springer-Verlag, Vol 6, 1987.
28. Nemeroff CB, Loosen PT. Handbook of Clinical Psychoneuroendocrinology. New York: Guilford, 1987.
29. Lechan RM. Neuroendocrinology of pituitary hormone regulation. Endocrinol Metab Clin North Am 1987; 16:475–501.
30. Veldhuis, JD, ed. Neuroendocrinology. Endocrinol Metab Clin No Am 1992; 21:767–950, 1993; 22:1–180.
31. Imura H, ed. The Pituitary Gland. 2nd ed. New York: Raven Press, 1994.
32. DeGroot LJ, ed. Endocrinology. 3rd ed. Philadelphia: WB Saunders, 1995.

Neural Control of Glandular Secretion

33. Schultzberg M, Hökfelt T, Lundberg JM. Peptide neurons in the autonomic nervous system. Adv Biochem Psychopharmacol 1980; 25:341–348.
34. Hökfelt T, Johansson O, Ljungdahl A, et al. Peptidergic neurons. Nature 1980; 284:515–521.
35. Hökfelt T, Lundberg JM, Schultzberg M, et al. Coexistence of peptides and putative transmitters in neurons. Adv Biochem Psychopharmacol 1980; 22:1–23.
36. Lundberg JM, Hökfelt T, Änggard A, et al. Organizational principles in the peripheral sympathetic nervous system: subdivision by coexisting peptides (somatostatin-, avian pancreatic polypeptide– and vasoactive intestinal polypeptide–like immunoreactive materials). Proc Natl Acad Sci USA 1982; 79:1303–1307.
37. Lundberg JM, Änggard A, Fahrenkrug J. Complementary role of vasoactive intestinal polypeptide (VIP) and acetylcholine for cat submandibular gland blood flow and secretion. Acta Physiol Scand 1982; 3:329–337.
38. Bern HA, Knowles FGW. Neurosecretion. In: Martini L, Ganong WF, eds. Neuroendocrinology. Vol 1. New York: Academic, 1966: 139–186.
39. Scharrer E, Scharrer B. Secretory cells within the hypothalamus. In: The Hypothalamus. Association for Research on Nervous and Mental Disease. New York: Hafner, 1940: 170–194.
40. Ochs S. Axoplasmic transport in peripheral nerve and hypothalamo-neurohypophyseal systems. In: Porter JC, ed. Hypothalamic Peptide Hormones and Pituitary Regulation. New York: Plenum, 1977: 13–40.
41. Pickering BT. The neurosecretory neurone: a model system for the study of secretion. Essays Biochem 1978; 14:45–81.
42. Livett BG. Axonal transport and neuronal dynamics: contributions to the study of neuronal connectivity. In: Porter R, ed. Neurophysiology II. Vol 10. Baltimore: University Park Press, 1976: 37–124.
43. Bloom FE. Contrasting principles of synaptic physiology: peptidergic and non-peptidergic neurons. In: Fuxe K, Hökfelt T, Luft R, eds. Central Regulation of the Endocrine System. New York: Plenum, 1979: 173–187.
44. Guillemin R. Peptides in the brain: the new endocrinology of the neuron (Nobel lecture).Science 1978; 202:390–402.
45. Trifaró J-M, Vitale ML. Cytoskeleton dynamics during neurotransmitter release. Trends Neurosci 1993; 16:466–472.
46. Hays RM, Franki N, Simon H, et al. Antidiuretic hormone and exocytosis: lessons from neurosecretion. Am J Physiol 1994; 267:C1507–C1524.
47. Greengard P, Valtorta F, Czernik AJ, et al. Synaptic vesicle phosphoproteins and regulation of synaptic function. Science 1993; 259:780–785.
48. Li C, Ullrich B, Zhang JZ, et al. Ca²⁺-dependent and -independent activities of neural and non-neural synaptotagmins. Nature 1995; 375:594–599.
49. Levi G, Raiteri M. Carrier-mediated release of neurotransmitters. Trends Neurosci 1993; 16:415–419.
50. Wurtman RJ, Anton-Tay F. The mammalian pineal as a neuroendocrine transducer. Recent Prog Horm Res 1969; 25:493–522.
51. Vincent SR, Hope BT. Neurons that say NO. Trends Neurosci 1992; 15:108–113.
52. Lowenstein CJ, Dinerman JL, Snyder SH. Nitric oxide: a physiologic messenger. Ann Intern Med 1994; 120:227–237.
53. Snyder SH. No endothelial NO. Nature 1995; 377:196–197.
54. Verma A, Hirsh DJ, Glatt CE, et al. Carbon monoxide: a putative neural messenger. Science 1993; 259:381–384.
55. Murphy S, Simmons ML, Agullo L, et al. Synthesis of nitric oxide in CNS glial cells. Trends Neurosci 1993; 16:323–328.

The Hypothalamic-Pituitary Unit

56. Page RB. The anatomy of the hypothalamo-hypophysial complex. In: Knobil E, Neill JD, eds. The Physiology of Reproduction. 2nd ed. New York: Raven, 1994: 1527–1619.
57. Halász B. Hypothalamo-anterior pituitary system and pituitary portal vessels. In: Imura H, ed. The Pituitary Gland. 2nd ed. New York: Raven, 1994: 1–28.
58. Wingstrand KG. Microscopic anatomy, nerve supply and blood supply of the pars intermedia. In: Harris GW, Donovan BT, eds. The Pituitary Gland. London: Butterworths, 1966: 1–27.

Neurohypophysis

59. Lederis K. Neurosecretion and the functional structure of the neurohypophysis. In: Greep RO, Astwood EB, Knobil E, et al, eds. Handbook of Physiology, Sect 7: Endocrinology. Vol IV. The Pituitary Gland and Its Neuroendocrine Control. Part 1. Washington, DC: American Physiological Society, 1974: 81–102.
60. Zimmerman EA, Hou-Yu A, Lilaver G, et al. Anatomy of pituitary and extrapituitary vasopressin secretory systems. In: Reichlin S, ed. The Neurohypophysis. New York: Plenum, 1984: 5–27.
61. Hayward JN. Functional and morphological aspects of hypothalamic neurons. Physiol Rev 1977; 57:574–658.
62. Mohr E, Bahnsen U, Kiessling C, et al. Expression of the vasopressin and oxytocin genes in rats occurs in mutually exclusive sets of hypothalamic neurons. FEBS Lett 1988; 242:144–148.
63. Meister B, Villar MJ, Ceccatelli S, et al. Comparative analysis on the localization of chemical messengers in magnocellular neurons of the hypothalamic supraoptic and paraventricular nuclei: an immunohistochemical study using experimental manipulations. Neuroscience 1990; 37:603–633.
64. Sofroniew MV, Weindl A. Extrahypothalamic neurophysin-containing perikarya, fiber pathways and the clusters in the rat brain. Endocrinology 1978; 102:334–337.
65. Raichle ME. Hypothesis: a central neuroendocrine system regulates brain ion homeostasis and volume. In: Martin JB, Reichlin S, Bick KL, eds. Neurosecretion and Brain Peptides. New York: Raven, 1981: 329–336.
66. Perlow MJ, Reppert SM, Artman HA, et al. Oxytocin, vasopressin, and estrogen-stimulated neurophysin: daily patterns of concentration in cerebrospinal fluid. Science 1982; 216:1416–1418.
67. Amico JA, Tenicela R, Johnston J, et al. A time dependent peak of oxytocin exists in the cerebrospinal fluid but not in the plasma of humans. J Clin Endocrinol Metab 1982; 57:947–951.
68. Acher R. Chemistry of neurohypophysial hormones: an example of molecular evolution. In: Greep RO, Astwood EB, Knobil E, et al, eds. Handbook of Physiology, Sect 7: Endocrinology. Vol IV. The Pituitary Gland and Its Neuroendocrine Control. Part 1. Washington, DC: American Physiological Society, 1974: 119–130.
69. Ruppert S, Scherer G, Schütz G. Recent gene conversion involving bovine vasopressin and oxytocin precursor genes suggested by nucleotide sequence. Nature 1984; 308:554–557.
70. Watson S, Girdlestone D. 1995 Receptor and ion channel nomenclature supplement. Trends Pharmacol Sci 1995; (Suppl 16):1–73.
71. Brownstein MJ, Russell JT, Gainer H. Synthesis, transport, and release of posterior pituitary hormones. Science 1980; 207:373–378.
72. Land H, Schutz G, Schmale H, et al. Nucleotide sequence of cloned cDNA encoding bovine arginine vasopressin–neurophysin II precursor. Nature 1982; 295:299–301.
73. Richter D. Molecular events in expression of vasopressin and oxytocin and their cognate receptors. Am J Physiol 1988; 255:(2 Pt 2):F207–219.
74. Robinson AG. The contribution of measured secretion of neurophysins to our understanding of neurohypophysial function. In: Reichlin S, ed. The Neurohypophysis. New York: Plenum, 1984: 65–93.

75. Hendy GN, Bichet DG. Diabetes insipidus. Baillieres Clin Endocrinol Metab 1995; 9:509–524.

76. Nagasaki H, Ito M, Yuasa H, et al. Two novel mutations in the coding region for neurophysin-II associated with familial central diabetes insipidus. J Clin Endocrinol Metab 1995; 80:1352–1356.

77. Sladek JR, Sladek GD. Neurological control of vasopressin release. Fed Proc 1985; 44:66–71.

78. Ramsey DJ. Effect of circulating angiotensin II on the brain. In: Ganong WF, Martini L, eds. Frontiers in Neuroendocrinology. Vol 7. New York: Raven, 1982: 263–286.

79. Ganten D, Fuxe K, Phillips MI, et al. The brain isorenin-angiotensin system: biochemistry, localization, and possible role in drinking and blood pressure regulation. In: Ganong WF, Martini L, eds. Frontiers in Neuroendocrinology. Vol 5. New York: Raven, 1978: 61–100.

80. Standaert DG, Needleman P, Saper CB. Atriopeptin: neuromediator in the central regulation of cardiovascular function. In: Martini L, Ganong WF, eds. Frontiers in Neuroendocrinology. Vol 10. New York: Raven, 1988: 63–78.

81. Mansour A, Fox CA, Akil H, et al. Opioid-receptor mRNA expression in the rat CNS: anatomic and functional implications. Trends Neurosci 1995; 18:22–29.

82. Miller M, Moses AM. Clinical states due to alteration of ADH release and action. In: Neurohypophysis. International Conference, Key Biscayne, FL, 1976. White Plains, NY: AJ Phiebig (Basel: S Karger), 1977: 153–166.

83. Iwasaki Y, Gaskill MB, Robertson GL. The effect of selective opioid antagonists on vasopressin secretion in the rat. Endocrinology 1994; 134:55–62.

84. Sawchenko PE, Plotsky PM, Pfeiffer SW, et al. Inhibin β in central neural pathways is involved in the control of oxytocin secretion. Nature 1988; 334:615–617.

85. Ota M, Crofton JT, Festavan GT, et al. Evidence that nitric oxide can act centrally to stimulate vasopressin release. Neuroendocrinology 1993; 57:955–959.

86. Raber J, Bloom FE. IL-2 induces vasopressin release from the hypothalamus and the amygdala: role of nitric oxide–mediated signaling. J Neurosci 1994; 14:6187–6195.

87. Miyagawa A, Okamura H, Ibata Y. Coexistence of oxytocin and NADPH-diaphorase in magnocellular neurons of the paraventricular and the supraoptic nuclei of the rat hypothalamus. Neurosci Lett 1994; 171:13–16.

88. Swanson LW, Simmons DM. Differential steroid hormone and neural influences on peptide mRNA levels in CRH cells of the paraventricular nucleus: a hybridization histochemical study in the rat. J Comp Neurol 1989; 285:413–435.

89. Aubry RH, Nankin HR, Moses AM, et al. Measurement of the osmotic threshold for vasopressin release in human subjects, and its modification by cortisol. J Clin Endocrinol Metab 1965; 25:1481–1492.

90. Amico JA, Hempel J. An oxytocin precursor intermediate circulates in the plasma of humans and rhesus monkeys administered estrogen. Neuroendocrinology 1990; 51:437–443.

91. Richard S, Zingg HH. The human oxytocin gene promoter is regulated by estrogens. J Biol Chem 1990; 265:6098–6103.

92. Van Tol HHM, Bolwerk ELM, Liu B, et al. Oxytocin and vasopressin gene expression in the hypothalamo-neurohypophyseal system of the rat during the estrous cycle, pregnancy, and lactation. Endocrinology 1988; 122:945–951.

93. Lopes da Silva S, vanHorssen AM, Chang C, et al. Expression of nuclear hormone receptors in the rat supraoptic nucleus. Endocrinology 1995; 136:2276–2283.

94. Moses AM. Diabetes insipidus and ADH regulation. In: Krieger DT, Hughes JC, eds. Neuroendocrinology. Sunderland, MA: Sinauer Associates, 1980: 141–148.

95. Robertson GL. The regulation of vasopressin function in health and disease. Recent Prog Horm Res 1977; 33:333–385.

96. Kovacs L, Robertson GL. Syndrome of inappropriate antidiuresis. Endocrinol Metab North Am 1992; 21:859–875.

97. Oliet SHR, Bourque CW. Osmoreception in magnocellular neurosecretory cells: from single channels to secretion. Trends Neurosci 1994; 17:340–344.

98. Bourque CW, Oliet SHR, Richard D. Osmoreceptors, osmoreception, and osmoregulation. Front Neuroendocrinol 1994; 15:231–274.

99. Verney EB. The antidiuretic hormone and the factors which determine its release. Proc R Soc Lond 1947; 135:23–106.

100. Aubry RH, Nankin HR, Moses AM, et al. Measurement of the osmotic threshold for vasopressin release in human subjects, and its modification by cortisol. J Clin Endocrinol Metab 1965; 25:1481–1492.

101. Oelkers W. Hyponatremia and inappropriate secretion of vasopressin (antidiuretic hormone) in patients with hypopituitarism. N Engl J Med 1989; 321:492–496.

102. Evans RM, Arriza JL. A molecular framework for the actions of glucocorticoid hormones in the nervous system. Neuron 1989; 2:1105–1112.

103. Share L. Vasopressin and cardiovascular regulation. Symposium. Fed Proc 1984; 43:78–106.

104. Laragh JH. Atrial natriuretic hormone, the renin-aldosterone axis, and blood pressure–electrolyte homeostasis. N Engl J Med 1985; 313:1330–1340.

105. Yeung VT, Lai CK, Cockram CS, et al. Atrial natriuretic peptide in the central nervous system. Neuroendocrinology 1991; 53:(Suppl 1):18–24.

106. Ohkubo H, Kageyama R, Ujihara M, et al. Cloning and sequence analysis of cDNA for rat angiotensinogen. Proc Natl Acad Sci USA 1983; 80:2196–2200.

107. Chang MS, Lowe DG, Lewis M, et al. Differential activation by atrial and brain natriuretic peptides of two different receptor guanylate cyclases. Nature 1989; 341:68–72.

108. Phillips MI, Felix D. Specific angiotensin II receptive neurons in the cat subfornical organ. Brain Res 1976; 109:531–540.

109. Fitzsimmons JT. Thirst. Physiol Rev 1972; 52:468–561.

110. Brody MJ, Johnson AK. Role of the anteroventral third ventricle region in fluid and electrolyte balance, arterial pressure regulation and hypertension. In: Martini L, Ganong WF, eds. Frontiers in Neuroendocrinology. Vol 6. New York: Raven, 1980: 249–292.

111. Sudoh T, Kangwa K, Minamino N, et al. A new natriuretic peptide in porcine brain. Nature 1988; 332:78–80.

112. Gold PW, Kaye W, Robertson GL, et al. Abnormalities in plasma and cerebrospinal-fluid arginine vasopressin in patients with anorexia nervosa. N Engl J Med 1983; 308:1117–1123.

113. Goldman MB, Luchins DJ, Robertson GL. Mechanisms of altered water metabolism in psychotic patients with polydipsia and hyponatremia. N Engl J Med 1988; 318:397–403.

114. Andersson B, Leksell LG, Lishajko F. Perturbations in fluid balance induced by medially placed forebrain lesions. Brain Res 1975; 99:261–275.

115. Ostrowski NL, Lolait SJ, Young WS 3rd. Cellular localization of vasopressin V1a receptor messenger ribonucleic acid in adult male rat brain, pineal, and brain vasculature. Endocrinology 1994; 135:1511–1528.

116. Dyball RE, Paterson AT. Neurohypophysial hormones and brain function: the neurophysiological effects of oxytocin and vasopressin. Pharmacol Ther 1983; 20:419–436.

117. Nilsson C, Lindvall-Axelsson M, Owman C. Neuroendocrine regulatory mechanisms in the choroid plexus-cerebrospinal fluid system. Brain Res Brain Res Rev 1992; 17:109–138.

Peptides in Memory and Learning

118. DeWeid D. Hormonal influences on motivation, learning, memory, and psychosis. In: Krieger DT, Hughes JC, eds. Neuroendocrinology. Sunderland, MA: Sinauer Associates, 1980: 194–205.

119. van Wiermsma Greidanus TB, van Raee JM, de Wied D. Vasopressin and memory. Pharmacol Ther 1983; 20:437–458.

120. Audibert A, Moeglen JM, Lancranjan I. Central effects of vasopressin in man. Int J Neurol 1980; 14:162–174.

121. Partridge WM, Frank HJL. Mechanisms of peptide transport from blood to brain. In: Müller EE, MacLeod RM, eds. Neuroendocrine Perspectives. Vol 2. Amsterdam: Elsevier Biomedical, 1983: 107–122.

122. Meisenberg G, Simmons WH. Minireview. Peptides and the blood-brain barrier. Life Sci 1983; 32:2611–2623.

123. Partridge WM. Receptor-mediated peptide transported through the blood-brain barrier. Endocr Rev 1986; 7:314–330.

124. Koob G, Bloom FE. Memory, learning, and adaptive behaviors. In: Krieger DT, Brownstein MJ, Martin JKB, eds. Brain Peptides. New York: John Wiley & Sons, 1983: 369–388.

Regulation of Oxytocin Secretion

125. Bissett GW. Milk ejection. In: Greep RO, Astwood EB, Knobil E, et al, eds. Handbook of Physiology. Sect 7: Endocrinology. Vol IV. The Pituitary Gland and Its Neuroendocrine Control. Part 1. Washington, DC: American Physiological Society, 1974: 493–520.

126. Chard T. Oxytocin. In: Martini L, Besser GM, eds. Clinical Neuroendocrinology. New York: Academic, 1977: 569–583.

127. Pickering BT. Oxytocin. In: DeGroot, LJ, ed. Endocrinology. 3rd ed. Philadelphia: WB Saunders, 1994: 421–431.

128. Amico JA. Diabetes insipidus and pregnancy. Front Horm Res 1985; 13:266–277.

129. Fuchs AR, Fuchs F, Husslein P, et al. Oxytocin receptors and human parturition: a dual role for oxytocin in the initiation of labor. Science 1982; 215:1396–1398.

130. Schellenberg J-C. The effect of oxytocin receptor blockade on parturition in guinea pigs. J Clin Invest 1995; 95:13–19.

131. Hime MC, Richardson JA. Diabetes insipidus and pregnancy. Case report, incidence and review of the literature. Obstet Gynecol Surv 1978; 33:375–379.

132. Shangold MM, Freeman R, Kumaresan P, et al. Plasma oxytocin concentrations in a pregnant woman with total vasopressin deficiency. Obstet Gynecol 1983; 61:662–667.

133. Cobo E, DeBernal M, Gaitan E. Low oxytocin secretion in diabetes insipidus associated with normal labor. Am J Obstet Gynecol 1972; 114:861–866.

134. Lefebre DL, Lariviere R, Zingg HH. Rat amnion: a novel site of oxytocin production. Biol Reprod 1993; 48:632–639.

Intermediate Lobe

135. Evans VR, Manning AB, Bernhard LH, et al. Alpha-melanocyte-stimulating hormone and N-acetyl-β-endorphin immunoreactivities are localized in the human pituitary but are not restricted to the zona intermedia. Endocrinology 1994; 134:97–106.

136. Kastin AJ, Viosca S, Schally AV. Regulation of melanocyte-stimulating hormone release. In: Greep RO, Astwood EB, Knobil E, et al, eds. Handbook of Physiology. Sect 7: Endocrinology. Vol IV. The Pituitary Gland and Its Neuroendocrine Control. Part 2. Washington, DC: American Physiological Society, 1974: 551–562.

137. Taleisnik S. Control of melanocyte-stimulating hormone (MSH) secretion. In: Jeffcoate SL, Hutchinson J, eds. The Endocrine Hypothalamus. New York: Academic, 1978: 421–438.

138. Moore KE, Johnston CA. The median eminence: aminergic control mechanisms. In: Müller EE, MacLeod RM, eds. Neuroendocrine Perspectives. Vol 1. Amsterdam: Elsevier Biomedical, 1982: 23–68.

139. Herbert E, Roberts J, Phillips M, et al. Biosynthesis, processing, and release of corticotropin, β-endorphin, and melanocyte-stimulating hormone in pituitary cell culture systems. In: Martini L, Ganong R, eds. Frontiers in Neuroendocrinology. Vol 6. New York: Raven, 1980: 67–102.

140. Roberts JL, Chen CLC, Eberwine JH, et al. Glucocorticoid regulation of proopiomelanocortin gene expression in rodent pituitary. Recent Prog Horm Res 1982; 38:227–256.

141. Krieger DT. The multiple faces of pro-opiomelanocortin, a prototype precursor molecule. Clin Res 1983; 31:342–353.

142. Vale W, Rivier C, Brown MR, et al. Chemical and biological characterization of corticotropin releasing factor. Recent Prog Horm Res 1983; 39:245–270.

143. Lamberts SWJ, DeLange SA, Stefanke SZ. Adrenocorticotropin-secreting pituitary adenomas originate from the anterior or the intermediate lobe in Cushing's disease: differences in the regulation of hormone secretion. J Clin Endocrinol Metab 1982; 54:286–291.

144. Krieger DT. Physiopathology of Cushing's disease. Endocr Rev 1983; 4:22–43.

145. Daughaday WH. Cushing's disease and basophilic microadenoma. N Engl J Med 1984; 310:919–929.

Hypophyseotropic Neuronal System

Median Eminence and Tuberoinfundibular and Tuberohypophyseal Neurons

146. Gay VL. The hypothalamus: physiology and clinical use of releasing factors. Fertil Steril 1972; 23:50–63.

147. Knigge KM, Silverman AJ. Anatomy of the endocrine hypothalamus. In: Greep RO, Astwood EB, Knobil E, et al, eds. Handbook of Physiology. Sect 7: Endocrinology. Vol IV. The Pituitary Gland and Its Neuroendocrine Control. Part 1. Washington, DC: American Physiological Society, 1974: 1–32.

148. Joseph SA, Knigge KN. The endocrine hypothalamus: recent anatomic studies. In: Reichlin S, Baldessarini RJ, Martin JB, eds. The Hypothalamus. Vol 56. New York: Raven, 1978: 15–47.

149. Hökfelt T, Elde R, Fuxe K, et al. Aminergic and peptidergic pathways in the nervous system with special reference to the hypothalamus. In: Reichlin S, Baldessarini RJ, Martin JB, eds. The Hypothalamus. Vol 56. New York: Raven, 1978: 69–135.

150. Jacobowitz DM. Multifactorial control of pituitary hormone secretion: the "wheels" of the brain. Synapse 1988; 2:186–192.

151. Swanson LW, Sawchenko PE. Hypothalamic integration: organization of the paraventricular and supraoptic nuclei. Annu Rev Neurosci 1983; 6:269–324.

152. Toni R, Lechan RM. Neuroendocrine regulation of thyrotropin-releasing hormone (TRH) in the tuberoinfundibular system. J Endocrinol Invest 1993; 16:715–753.

153. Clarke I, Jessop D, Millar R, et al. Many peptides that are present in the external zone of the median eminence are not secreted into the hypophysial portal blood of sheep. Neuroendocrinology 1993; 57:765–775.

154. Anthony EL, King JC, Stopa EG. Immunocytochemical localization of LHRH in the median eminence, infundibular stalk, and neurohypophysis. Evidence for multiple sites of releasing hormone secretion in humans and other mammals. Cell Tissue Res 1984; 236:5–14.

155. Negro-Vilar A. The median eminence as a model to study presynaptic regulation of neuropeptide release. Peptides 1982; 3:305–310.

156. Oliver C, Mical RS, Porter JC. Hypothalamic-pituitary vasculature: evidence for retrograde blood flow in the pituitary stalk. Endocrinology 1977; 101:598–604.

157. Page RB. Directional pituitary blood flow: a microcinephotographic study. Endocrinology 1983; 112:157–165.

158. Lechan RM, Nestler JL, Jacobson S. The tuberoinfundibular system of the rat as demonstrated by immunohistochemical localization of retrogradely transported wheat germ agglutinin (WGA) from the median eminence. Brain Res 1982; 245:1–15.

159. Lechan RM, Lin HD, Ling N, et al. Distribution of immunoreactive growth hormone releasing factor (1–44)NH₂ in the tuberoinfundibular system of the rhesus monkey. Brain Res 1984; 309:55–61.

160. Alpert LC, Brawer JR, Patel YC, et al. Somatostatinergic neurons in anterior hypothalamus: immunohistochemical localization. Endocrinology 1976; 98:255–258.

161. Krisch B. Hypothalamic and extrahypothalamic distribution of somatostatin-immunoreactive elements in the rat brain. Cell Tissue Res 1978; 195:499–513.

162. Bennett-Clarke C, Romagnano MA, Joseph SA. Distribution of somatostatin in the rat brain: telencephalon and diencephalon. Brain Res 1980; 188:473–486.

163. Swanson LW, Sawchenko PE, Rivier J, et al. Organization of ovine corticotropin-releasing factor immunoreactive cells and fibers in the rat brain: an immunohistochemical study. Neuroendocrinology 1983; 36:165–186.

164. Kahn D, Abrams GM, Zimmerman EA, et al. Neurotensin neurons in the rat hypothalamus: an immunohistochemical study. Endocrinology 1980; 107:47–54.

165. Vanderhaeghen JJ, Lotstra F, Demey J, et al. Immunohistochemical localization of cholecystokinin- and gastrin-like peptides in the brain and hypophysis of the rat. Proc Natl Acad Sci USA 1980; 77:1190–1194.

166. Hökfelt T, Fahrenkrug J, Tatemoto K, et al. The PHI (PHI-27)/corticotropin-releasing factor/enkephalin immunoreactive hypothalamic neuron: possible morphological basis for integrated control of prolactin, corticotropin, and growth hormone secretion. Proc Natl Acad Sci USA 1983; 80:895–898.

167. Hinsey JC, Markee JE. Pregnancy following bilateral section of the cervical sympathetic trunks in the rabbit. Proc Soc Exp Biol NY 1933; 31:270–271.

168. Friedgood HB. Studies on the sympathetic nervous control of the anterior hypophysis with special reference to a neuro-humoral mechanism. Symposium on endocrine glands. Harvard Tercentennial Celebration, 1936; reprinted in J Reprod Fertil 1970; 10:3–14.

169. Green JD, Harris GW. Neurovascular link between neurophysis and adenohypophysis. J Endocrinol 1947; 5:136–146.

170. Fink G. The development of the releasing factor concept. Clin Endocrinol 1976; 5:245s–260s.

Hypophyseotropic Hormones of the Hypothalamus

171. Saffran M. Chemistry of hypothalamic hypophysiotropic factors. In: Greep RO, Astwood EB, Knobil E, et al, eds. Handbook of Physiology. Sect 7: Endocrinology. Vol IV. The Pituitary Gland and Its Neuroendocrine Control. Part 2. Washington DC: American Physiological Society, 1974: 563–586.

Thyrotropin-Releasing Hormone

172. Wade N. The Nobel Duel. Garden City, NY: Anchor Press/Doubleday, 1981.

173. Reichlin S. TRH: historical aspects. Ann NY Acad Sci 1989; 553:1–6.

174. Bowers CY, Schally AV, Enzmann F, et al. Porcine thyrotropin releasing hormone is (pyro)Glu-His-Pro(NH₂). Endocrinology 1970; 86:1143–1153.

175. Burgus R, Dunn TF, Desiderio D, et al. Structure moléculaire du facteur hypothalamique hypophysiotrope TRF d'origine ovine: mise en évidence par spectrométrie de masse de la séquence PCA-His-Pro-NH₂. C R Acad Sci D 1969; 269:1870–1873.

176. Vale W, Rivier C, Brown M. Pharmacology of thyrotropin releasing factor (LRF) and somatostatin. In: Porter JC, ed. Hypothalamic Peptide Hormones and Pituitary Regulation. New York: Plenum, 1977: 123–156.

177. Sandow J, König W. Chemistry of the hypothalamic hormones. In: Jeffcoate SL, Hutchinson JS, eds. The Endocrine Hypothalamus. London: Academic, 1978: 150–212.

178. Lechan RM, Segerson TP. Pro-TRH gene expression and precursor peptides in rat brain. Observations by hybridization analysis and immunocytochemistry. Ann NY Acad Sci 1989; 553:29–59.

179. Lee SL, Stewart K, Goodman RH. Structure of the gene encoding rat thyrotropin releasing hormone. J Biol Chem 1988; 263:16604–16609.

180. Yamada M, Radovick S, Wondisford FE, et al. Cloning and structure of human genomic DNA and hypothalamic cDNA encoding human preprothyrotropin-releasing hormone. Mol Endocrinol 1990; 4:551–556.

181. Lechan RM, Snapper SC, Jackson IMD. Evidence that spinal cord TRH is independent of the paraventricular nucleus. Neurosci Lett 1983; 43:61–65.

182. Bulant M, Roussel J-P, Astier H, et al. Processing of thyrotropin releasing hormone prohormone (Pro-TRH) generates a biologically active peptide, prepro-TRH-(160–169) which regulates TRH-induced thyrotropin secretion. Proc Natl Acad Sci USA 1990; 87:4439–4443.

183. Redei E, Hilderbrand H, Aird F. Corticotropin release inhibiting factor is prepro-TRH 178–199. Endocrinology 1995; 136:3557–3563.

184. Jackson IMD, Reichlin S. Thyrotropin-releasing hormone (TRH): distribution in hypothalamic and extrahypothalamic brain tissues of mammalian and submammalian chordates. Endocrinology 1974; 95:854–862.

185. Bowers CY, Friesen HG, Hwang P, et al. Prolactin and thyrotropin release in man by synthetic pyroglutamyl-histidyl-prolinamide. Biochem Biophys Res Commun 1971; 45:1033–1041.

186. Snyder JJ, Jacobs LS, Rabello MM, et al. Diagnostic value of thyrotropin-releasing hormone in pituitary and hypothalamic disease: assessment of thyrotropin and prolactin in 100 patients. Ann Intern Med 1974; 81:751–757.

187. Jackson IMD. Thyrotropin-releasing hormone. N Engl J Med 1982; 306:145–155.

188. Fink G, Koch Y, Ben Aroya N, et al. Release of thyrotropin releasing hormone into hypophysial portal blood is high relative to other neuropeptides and may be related to prolactin secretion. Brain Res 1982; 243:186–189.

189. Reichlin S. Neuroendocrine regulation of prolactin secretion. Adv Biosci 1988; 69:277–292.

190. Gautvik KM, Tashjian AH Jr, Kourides IA, et al. Thyrotropin-releasing hormone is not the sole physiologic mediator of prolactin release during suckling. N Engl J Med 1974; 290:1162–1165.

191. Thorner MO, Perryman RL, Cronin MJ, et al. Somatotroph hyperplasia: successful treatment of acromegaly by removal of a pancreatic islet tumor secreting a growth hormone–releasing factor. J Clin Invest 1982; 70:965–977.

192. Borges JL, Uskavitch DR, Kaiser DL, et al. Human pancreatic growth hormone–releasing factor-40 (hpGRF-40) allows stimulation of GH release by TRH. Endocrinology 1983; 113:1519–1521.

193. Halpern J, Hinkle PM. Direct visualization of receptors for thyrotropin-releasing hormone with a fluorescein-labeled analog. Proc Natl Acad Sci USA 1981; 78:587–591.

194. Straub RE, Frech GC, Jobo RH, et al. Expression cloning of a cDNA encoding the mouse pituitary thyrotropin-releasing hormone receptor. Proc Natl Acad Sci USA 1990; 87:9514–9518.

195. Jun DS, Ahn SK, Yoon JH, et al. Involvement of a cAMP-responsive DNA element in mediating TRH responsiveness of the human thyrotropin alpha-subunit gene. Mol Endocrinol 1994; 8:528–536.

196. Heinflink M, Nussenzveig DR, Friedman AM, et al. Thyrotropin-releasing hormone receptor activation does not elevate intracellular cyclic adenosine 3′,5′-monophosphate in cells expressing high levels of receptors. J Clin Endocrinol Metab 1994; 79:650–652.

197. Tashjian AH Jr, Heslop JP, Berridge MJ. Subsecond and second changes in inositol polyphosphates in GH4C1 cells induced by thyrotropin-releasing hormone. Biochem J 1987; 243:305–308.

198. Winiger BP, Schlegel W. Rapid transient elevations of cytosolic calcium triggered by thyrotropin releasing hormone in individual cells of the pit line GH3B6. Biochem J 1988; 255:161–167.

199. Kim MK, McClaskey JH, Bodenner DL, et al. An AP-1 like factor and the pituitary specific factor Pit-1 are both necessary to mediate hormonal induction of human thyrotropin β gene expression. J Biol Chem 1993; 268:23366–23375.

200. Rosenfeld MG, Amara SG, Birnberg NC, et al. Prolactin and growth hormone gene expression as model systems for the characterization of neuroendocrine regulation. Recent Prog Horm Res 1983; 39:305–352.

201. Peterkofsky A, Battaini F, Koch Y, et al. Histidyl-proline diketopiperazine: its biological role as a regulatory peptide. Mol Cell Biochem 1982; 42:45–63.

202. Jackson IM, Adelman LS, Munsat TL, et al. Amyotrophic lateral sclerosis: thyrotropin-releasing hormone and cerebrospinal fluid. Neurology 1986; 36:1218–1223.

203. Myashita K, Murakami M, Yamada M, et al. Histidyl-proline diketopiperazine. Novel formation that does not originate from thyrotropin-releasing hormone. J Biol Chem 1993; 268:20863–20865.

204. Johannsson O, Hökfelt T, Pernow B, et al. Immunohistochemical support for three putative transmitters in one neuron: coexistence of 5-hydroxytryptamine, substance P, and thyrotropin-releasing hormone–like immunoreactivity in medullary neurons projecting to the spinal cord. Neuroscience 1981; 6:1857–1881.

205. Lechan RM, Snapper SC, Jacobson S, et al. The distribution of thyrotropin-releasing hormone (TRH) in the rhesus monkey spinal cord. Peptides 1984; 5(Suppl 1):185–194.

206. Lechan RM, Adelman LS, Forte S, et al. Organization of thyrotropin-releasing hormone (TRH) immunoreactivity in the human spinal cord. Soc Neurosci Abstr 1984; 431 (abstract).

207. Engler D, Scanlon MF, Jackson IMD. Thyrotropin releasing hormone in the systemic circulation of the neonatal rat is derived from the pancreas and other extraneural tissues. J Clin Invest 1981; 67:800–808.

208. Griffiths EC, Bennett GW, eds. Thyrotropin-Releasing Hormone. New York: Raven, 1983.

209. Jackson IMD, Metcalf G, eds. TRH. Ann NY Acad Sci 1989; 553:1–631.

210. Reichlin S. Neural functions of TRH. Acta Endocrinol 1986; 112:21–33.

211. Spencer CA, Schwartzbein D, Guttler RB, et al. Thyrotropin (TSH)-releasing hormone stimulation test responses employing third and fourth generation TSH assays. J Clin Endocrinol Metab 1993; 76:494–498.

212. Samuels HM, Ridgway EC. Central hypothyroidism. Endocrinol Metab Clin North Am 1992; 21:903–920.

213. Molitch ME. Pathogenesis of pituitary tumors. Endocrinol Metab Clin 1987; 16:503–527.

214. Loosen PT, Prange AJ Jr. The serum thyrotropin (TSH) response to thyrotropin-releasing hormone in psychiatric patients: a review. Am J Psychiatry 1982; 139:405–416.

215. Rubinow DR. Cerebrospinal fluid somatostatin and psychiatric illness. Biol Psychiatry 1986; 21:341–365.

216. ACTOBAT Study Group. Australian collaborative trial of antenatal thyrotropin-releasing hormone (ACTOBAT) for prevention of neonatal respiratory disease. Lancet 1995; 345:877–882.

217. Sobue I, Takayanagi T, Nakanishi T, et al. Controlled trial of thyrotropin-releasing hormone tartrate in ataxia of spinocerebellar degenerations. J Neurol Sci 1983; 61:235–248.

218. Engel WK, Siddique T, Nicoloff JT. Effect on weakness and spasticity in amyotrophic lateral sclerosis of thyrotropin-releasing hormone. Lancet 1983; 2:73–75.

219. Munsat TL, Lechan R, Taft JM, et al. TRH and diseases of the motor system. Ann NY Acad Sci 1989; 553:388–398.

220. Brooks BR. A summary of the current position of TRH in ALS therapy. Ann NY Acad Sci 1989; 553:431–461.

221. Askanas V, Engel WK, Eagelson K, et al. Influence of TRH and TRH analogues RGH-2202 and DN-1417 on cultured ventral spinal cord neurons. Ann NY Acad Sci 1989; 553:325–336.

222. Munsat TL, Taft J, Jackson IM, et al. Intrathecal thyrotropin-releasing hormone does not alter the progressive course of ALS: experience with an intrathecal drug delivery system. Neurology 1992; 42:1049–1053.

223. Holaday JW, Long JB, Martinez-Arizala A, et al. Effects of TRH in circulatory shock and central nervous system ischemia. Ann NY Acad Sci 1989; 445:370–379.

224. Faden AI, Jacobs TP, Holaday JW. Thyrotropin-releasing hormone improves neurologic recovery after spinal trauma in cats. N Engl J Med 1981; 305:1063–1067.

225. Breese GR, Cott JM, Cooper BR, et al. Effects of thyrotropin-releasing hormone (TRH) on the action of pentobarbital and other centrally acting drugs. J Pharmacol Exp Ther 1974; 193:11–22.

226. Knutsen H, Dolva LO, Skrede S, et al. Thyrotropin-releasing hormone antagonism of ethanol inebriation. Alcohol Clin Exp Res 1989; 13:365–370.

227. Griffing GT, Weiss SM, Bern M, et al. Thyrotropin (TRH) arousal and prolonged wakefulness in a hypersomnolent patient with histiocytosis-X. Clin Res 1989; 37:848A (abstract).

Corticotropin-Releasing Hormone

228. Saffran M, Schally AV, Benfey BG. Stimulation of the release of corticotropin from the adenohypophysis by a neurohypophysial factor. Endocrinology 1955; 57:439–444.

229. Guillemin R, Rosenberg B. Humoral hypothalamic control of anterior pituitary: study with combined tissue cultures. Endocrinology 1955; 57:599–607.

230. Speiss J, Rivier J, Rivier C, et al. Primary structure of corticotropin-releasing factor from ovine hypothalamus. Proc Natl Acad Sci USA 1981; 78:6517–6521.

231. Grossman A. Corticotropin-releasing hormone: basic physiology and clinical applications. In: DeGroot LJ, ed. Endocrinology. 3rd ed. Philadelphia: WB Saunders, 1995: 341–354.

232. Trainer PJ, Faria M, Newell-Price J, et al. A comparison of the effects of human and ovine corticotropin-releasing hormone on the pituitary-adrenal axis. J Clin Endocrinol Metab 1995; 80:412–417.

233. Shibahara S, Morimoto Y, Furutani Y, et al. Isolation and sequence analysis of the human corticotropin-releasing factor precursor gene. EMBO J 1983; 2:775–779.

234. Erspamer V, Melchiorri P. Actions of amphibian skin peptides on the central nervous system and the anterior pituitary. In: Müller EE, MacLeod RM, eds. Neuroendocrine Perspectives. Vol 2. Amsterdam: Elsevier Biomedical, 1983: 37–106.

235. Vaughan J, Donaldson C, Bittencourt J, et al. Urocortin, a mammalian neuropeptide related to fish urotensin I and to corticotropin-releasing factor. Nature 1995; 378:287–292.

236. Menzaghi F, Howard RL, Heinrichs SC, et al. Characterization of a novel and potent corticotropin-releasing factor antagonist in rats. J Pharmacol Exp Ther 1994; 269:564–572.

237. Müller OA, Stalla GK, von Werder K. Corticotropin releasing factor: a new tool for the differential diagnosis of Cushing's syndrome. J Clin Endocrinol Metab 1983; 57:227–229.

238. Chrousos GP, moderator. Clinical applications of corticotropin-releasing factor. Ann Intern Med 1985; 102:344–358.

239. Taylor AL, Fishman LM. Corticotropin-releasing hormone. N Engl J Med 1988; 319:213–222.

240. Wynn PC, Aguilera G, Morell J, et al. Properties and regulation of high-affinity pituitary receptors for corticotropin-releasing factor. Biochem Biophys Res Commun 1983; 110:602–608.

241. Leroux P, Pelletier G. Radioautographic study of binding and internalization of corticotropin-releasing factor by rat anterior pituitary corticotrophs. Endocrinology 1984; 114:14–21.

242. Chen R, Lewis KA, Perrin HM, et al. Expression cloning of a human corticotropin-releasing factor receptor. Proc Natl Acad Sci USA 1993; 90:8967–8971.

243. Perri MH, Donaldson CJ, Chen R, et al. Cloning and functional expression of a rat brain corticotropin releasing factor (CRF) receptor. Endocrinology 1993; 133:3058–3061.

244. Lovenberg TW, Chalmers DT, Liu C, et al. CRF_{2a} and CRF_{2b} receptor mRNAs are differentially distributed between the rat central nervous system and peripheral tissues. Endocrinology 1995; 136:4139–4142.

245. Linton EA, Wolfe CD, Behan DP, et al. Circulating corticotropin-releasing factor in pregnancy. Adv Exp Med Biol 1990; 274:147–164.

246. Potter E, Behan DP, Linton EA, et al. The central distribution of a corticotropin-releasing factor (CRF)-binding protein predicts multiple sites and modes of interaction with CRF. Proc Natl Acad Sci USA 1992; 89:4192–4196.

247. Sutton RE, Koob GF, LeMoal M, et al. Corticotropin releasing factor produces behavioral activation in rats. Nature 1982; 297:331–333.

248. Lenz HG. Extrapituitary effects of corticotropin-releasing factor. Horm Metab Res 1987; 16(Suppl):17–23.

249. Heilig M, Koob GF, Ekman R, et al. Corticotropin-releasing factor and

neuropeptide T: Role in emotional integration. Trends Neurosci 1994; 17:80–85.
250. Crofford LJ, Sano H, Karalis K, et al. Corticotropin-releasing hormone in synovial fluids and tissues of patients with rheumatoid arthritis and osteoarthritis. J Immunol 1993; 151:1587–1596.

Growth Hormone–Releasing Hormone

251. Reichlin S. Regulation of somatotrophic hormone secretion. In: Greep RO, Astwood EB, Knobil E, et al, eds. Handbook of Physiology. Sect 7: Endocrinology. Vol IV. The Pituitary Gland and Its Neuroendocrine Control. Washington, DC: American Physiological Society, 1974: 405–448.
252. Frohman LA, Szabo M, Berelowitz M, et al. Partial purification and characterization of a peptide with growth hormone–releasing activity from extrapituitary tumors in patients with acromegaly. J Clin Invest 1980; 65:43–54.
253. Thorner MO, Perryman RL, Cronin MJ, et al. Somatotroph hyperplasia. Successful treatment of acromegaly by removal of a pancreatic islet tumor secreting growth hormone–releasing factor. J Clin Invest 1982; 70:965–977.
254. Guillemin R, Brazeau P, Bohlen P, et al. Growth hormone–releasing factor from a human pancreatic tumor that caused acromegaly. Science 1981; 218:585–587.
255. Rivier J, Speiss J, Thorner M, et al. Characterisation of a growth hormone-releasing factor from a human pancreatic islet tumour. Nature 1982; 300:276–278.
256. Mayo KE, Vale W, Rivier J, et al. Expression-cloning and sequence of a cDNA encoding human growth hormone–releasing factor. Nature 1983; 306:86–88.
257. Cronin MJ, Thorner MO. Growth hormone–releasing hormone: basic physiology and clinical implications. In: DeGroot LJ, ed. Endocrinology. 3rd ed. Philadelphia: WB Saunders, 1995: 280–302.
258. Thorner MO, Frohman LA, Leong DA, et al. Extrahypothalamic growth hormone–releasing factor (GRF) is a rare cause of acromegaly: plasma GRF levels in 177 acromegalic patients. J Clin Endocrinol Metab 1984; 59:846–849.
259. Asa SL, Kovacs K, Thorner MO, et al. Immunohistological localization of growth hormone–releasing hormone in human tumors. J Clin Endocrinol Metab 1985; 60:423–427.
260. Dayal Y, Lin HD, Tallberg K, et al. Immunocytochemical demonstration of growth hormone–releasing factor in gastrointestinal and pancreatic endocrine tumors. Am J Clin Pathol 1986; 85:13–20.
261. Thorner MO, Rivier J, Spiess J. Human pancreatic growth hormone-releasing factor selectively stimulates growth hormone secretion in man. Lancet 1983; 1:24–28.
262. Frohman LA, Jansson JO. Growth hormone-releasing hormone. Endocr Rev 1986; 7:223–253.
263. Vance ML, Thorner MO. Some clinical considerations of growth hormone and growth hormone–releasing hormone. In: Martini L, Ganong WF, eds. Frontiers in Neuroendocrinology. Vol 10. New York: Raven, 1988: 279–294.
264. Usdin TB, Mezey É, Button DC, et al. Gastric inhibitory polypeptide receptor, a member of the secretin-vasoactive intestinal peptide receptor family, is widely distributed in peripheral organs and the brain. Endocrinology 1993; 133:2861–2870.
265. Barinaga M, Yamonoto G, Rivier C, et al. Transcriptional regulation of growth hormone gene expression by growth hormone–releasing factor. Nature 1983; 306:84–85.
266. Wehrenberg WB, Baird A, Ling N. Potent interaction between glucocorticoids and growth hormone–releasing factor in vivo. Science 1983; 221:556–558.
267. Mayo KE, Hammer RE, Swanson LW, et al. Dramatic pituitary hyperplasia in transgenic mice expressing a human growth hormone–releasing factor gene. Mol Endocrinol 1988; 2:606–612.
268. Krueger JM, Obel F Jr. Growth hormone–releasing hormone and interleukin-1 in sleep regulation. FASEB J 1993; 7:645–652.
269. Frieboes RM, Murck H, Maier P, et al. Growth hormone–releasing peptide-6 stimulates sleep, growth hormone, ACTH and cortisol release in normal man. Neuroendocrinology 1995; 61:584–589.
270. Obál F Jr, Payne L, Kacsoh B, et al. Involvement of prolactin in the REM sleep–promoting activity of systemic vasoactive intestinal peptide (VIP). Brain Res 1994; 645:143–149.
271. Schoenenberger GA, Maier PF, Tobler HJ, et al. The delta EEG (sleep)–inducing peptide (DSIP). XI. Amino-acid analysis, sequence, synthesis and activity of the nonapeptide. Pflugers Arch 1978; 376:119–129.
272. Borbely AA, Tobler I. Endogenous sleep-promoting substances and sleep regulation. Physiol Rev 1989; 69:605–670.
273. Krueger JM, Pappenheimer JR, Karnovsky ML. Sleep-promoting effects of muramyl peptides. Proc Natl Acad Sci USA 1982; 79:6102–6106.
274. Cravatt BF, Prospero-Garcia O, Siuzdak G, et al. Chemical characterization of a family of brain lipids that induce sleep. Science 1995; 268:1506–1509.
275. Bowers CY, Momany FA, Reynolds GA, et al. On the in vitro and in vivo activity of a new synthetic hexapeptide that acts on the pituitary to specifically release growth hormone. Endocrinology 1984; 114:1537–1545.
276. Bowers CY. GH releasing peptides. Structure and kinetics. J Pediatr Endocrinol 1993; 38:87–91.
277. Arimura A. Regulation of growth hormone secretion. In: Imura H, ed. The Pituitary Gland. 2nd ed. New York: Raven, 1994: 217–259.
278. Korbonits M, Grossman AB. Growth hormone–releasing peptide and its analogues. Trends Endocrinol Metab 1995; 6:43–49.
279. Loche S, Cambiaso P, Merola B, et al. The effect of hexarelin on growth hormone (GH) secretion in patients with GH deficiency. J Clin Endocrinol Metab 1995; 80:2692–2696.
280. Pombo M, Barreiro J, Pěnalva, A, et al. Absence of growth hormone (GH) secretion after the administration of either GH-releasing hormone (GHRH), GH-releasing peptide (GHRP-6) or GHRH plus GHRP-6 in children with neonatal pituitary stalk transection. J Clin Endocrinol Metab 1995; 80:3180–3184.
281. Cheng K, Chan WWS, Butler B, et al. Stimulation of growth hormone release from rat primary pituitary cells by L-692,429 a novel non-peptidyl GH secretogogue. Endocrinology 1992; 132:2729–2731.
282. Corpas E, Harman SM, Blackman MR. Human growth hormone and human aging. Endocr Rev 1993; 14:20–39.
283. Shibasaki T, Shizume K, Masuda A, et al. Plasma growth hormone response to growth hormone–releasing factor in acromegalic patients. J Clin Endocrinol Metab 1984; 58:215–217.

Somatostatin

284. Krulich L, Dhariwal AP, McCann SM. Stimulatory and inhibitory effects of purified hypothalamic extracts on growth hormone release from rat pituitary in vitro. Endocrinology 1968; 83:783–790.
285. Hellman B, Lernmark A. Inhibition of the in vitro secretion of insulin by an extract of pancreatic A₁ cells. Endocrinology 1969; 84:1484–1487.
286. Brazeau P, Vale W, Burgus R, et al. Hypothalamic polypeptide that inhibits the secretion of immunoreactive pituitary growth hormone. Science 1973; 179:77–79.
287. Reichlin S. Somatostatin. In: Krieger DT, Brownstein M, Martin JB, eds. Brain Peptides. New York: John Wiley & Sons, 1983: 711–752.
288. Reichlin S. Somatostatin. N Engl J Med 1983; 309:1495–1501, 1556–1563.
289. Gorden P, Comi RJ, Maton PM, et al. NIH conference: somatostatin and somatostatin analog (SMS 201–995) in treatment of hormone-secreting tumors of the pituitary and gastrointestinal tract and non-neoplastic diseases of the gut. Ann Intern Med 1989; 110:35–50.
290. Patel YC. General aspects of the biology and function of somatostatin. In: Thorner MO, Müller EE, eds. Basic and Clinical Aspects of Neuroscience. Vol 4. Berlin: Springer-Verlag, 1–16.
291. Chadwick DJ, Cardew G, eds. Somatostatin and its receptors. Ciba Found Symp 1995: 190.
292. Wass JAH. Somatostatin. In: DeGroot LJ, ed. Endocrinology. 3rd ed. Philadelphia: WB Saunders, 1995: 266–279.
293. Shen LP, Rutter WJ. Sequence of human somatostatin I gene. Science 1984; 224:168–171.
294. Montminy MR, Goodman RH, Horovitch SJ, et al. Primary structure of the gene encoding rat pre-prosomatostatin. Proc Natl Acad Sci USA 1984; 81:3337–3340.
295. Galanopoulou AS, Kent G, Rabbani SN, et al. Heterologous processing of prosomatostatin in constitutive and regulated secretory pathways. Putative role of the endoproteases furin, PC1, and PC2. J Biol Chem 1993; 268:6041–6049.
296. Montminy M, Brindle P, Arias J, et al. Regulation of somatostatin gene transcription by cAMP. Ciba Found Symp 1995: 190:20–25.
297. Kwok RP, Lundblad JR, Chrivia JC, et al. Nuclear protein CBP is a coactivator for the transcription factor CREB. Nature 1994; 370:223–226.
298. Lamberts SWJ. Non-pituitary actions of somatostatin: a review on the therapeutic role of SM 201–995 (Sandostatin). Acta Endocrinol 1986; 276(Suppl):41–55.
299. Krenning EP, Kwekkeboom DJ, Bakker WH, et al. Somatostatin receptor scintigraphy with [¹¹¹In-DTPA-d-Phe¹]- and [¹²³I-Tyr³]-octreatide: the Rotterdam experience with more than 1000 patients. Eur J Nucl Med 1993; 20:716–731.
300. Patel YC, Greenwood MT, Panetta R, et al. The somatostatin receptor family: a mini review. Life Sci 1995; 57:1249–1265 330.
301. Patel YC, Srikant CB. Subtype selectivity of peptide analogs for all five cloned human somatostatin receptors (hsstr 1–5). Endocrinology 1994; 135:2814–2817.
302. Schonbrunn A. Somatostatin action in pituitary cells involves two independent transduction mechanisms. Metabolism 1990; 39(Suppl 2):96–100.
303. Kleuss CS. Somatostatin modulates voltage-dependent Ca²⁺ channels in GH₃ cells via a specific G₀ splice variant. Ciba Found Symp 1995; 190:171–186.
304. Delesque N, Buscail L, Estève JP, et al. A tyrosine phosphate is associated with the somatostatin receptor. Ciba Found Symp 1995; 190:187–203.
305. Reubi J-C, Laissue JA. Multiple actions of somatostatin in neoplastic disease. Trends Pharmacol Sci 1995; 16:110–115.
306. O'Dorsio TM, ed. Sandostatin in the Treatment of GEP Endocrine Tumors. Berlin: Springer-Verlag, 1989.
307. Hoeldtke RD, Israel BC. Treatment of orthostatic hypotension with octreotide. J Clin Endocrinol Metab 1989; 68:1051–1059.
308. Lamberts SWJ, Bakker WH, Reubi JC, et al. Somatostatin receptor imaging in the localization of endocrine tumors. N Engl J Med 1990; 323:1246–1249.
309. Reichlin S. Clinical application of somatostatin receptor imaging. J Clin Endocrinol Metab 1990; 71:564–565.

310. Patel YC. Somatostatin-receptor imaging for the detection of tumors. N Engl J Med 1990; 323:1274–1276.
311. Schirmer WJ, O'Dorisio TM, Schirmer TP, et al. Intraoperative localization of neuroendocrine tumors with ^{125}I-TYR-octreotide and a hand-held gamma-detecting probe. Surgery 1993; 114:745–752.

Prolactin Regulatory Factors

312. Pasteels JL. Prolactin regulatory factors. Premiers résultats de culture combinée in vitro d'hypophyse et d'hypothalamus dans le but d'en apprecier la sécrétion de prolactine. C R Acad Sci (Paris) 1961; 253:3074–3075.
313. Neill JD. Prolactin: its secretion and control. In: Greep RO, Astwood EB, Knobil E, et al, eds. Handbook of Physiology. Sect 7: Endocrinology. Vol IV. The Pituitary Gland and Its Neuroendocrine Control. Part 2. Washington DC: American Physiological Society, 1974: 469–488.
314. MacLeod RM. Regulation of prolactin secretion. In: Martini L, Ganong WF, eds. Frontiers in Neuroendocrinology. Vol 4. New York: Raven, 1976: 169–194.
315. Neill JD. Neuroendocrine regulation of prolactin secretion. In: Martini L, Ganong WF, eds. Frontiers in Neuroendocrinology. Vol 6. New York: Raven, 1980: 129–155.
316. Cronin MJ. The role and direct measurement of the dopamine receptor(s). In: Müller EE, MacLeod RM, eds. Neuroendocrine Perspectives. Vol 1. Amsterdam: Elsevier Biomedical, 1982: 169–210.
317. Judd AM, Koike K, Schettini G, et al. Dopamine decreases prolactin secretion induced by increases in calcium mobilization in the 7315a pituitary tumor, but not the MtTW 15 pituitary tumor. In: MacLeod RM, Thorner MO, Scapagnini V, eds. Prolactin, Basis and Clinical Correlates. Padua: Livania, 1985: 205–212.
318. Senogles SE. The D2 dopamine receptor mediates inhibition of growth in GH4ZR7 cells: involvement of protein kinase-C epsilon. Endocrinology 1994; 134:783–789.
319. Ben-Jonathan N. Prolactin releasing and inhibiting factors in the posterior pituitary. In: Müller EE, MacLeod RM, eds. Neuroendocrine Perspectives. Vol 8. New York: Springer-Verlag, 1990: 1–38.
320. Arey BJ, Freeman ME. Oxytocin, vasoactive intestinal peptide and serotonin regulate the mating-induced surges of prolactin secretion in the rat. Endocrinology 1990; 126:279–284.
321. Ben-Jonathan N, Arbogast LA, Hyde JF. Neuroendocrine regulation of prolactin release. Prog Neurobiol 1989; 33:399–447.
322. Allen DL, Low MJ, Allen RG, et al. Identification of two classes of prolactin-releasing factors in intermediate lobe tumors from transgenic mice. Endocrinology 1995; 136:3093–3099.
323. Abe H, Engler D, Molitch ME, et al. Vasoactive intestinal peptide is a physiological mediator of prolactin release in the rat. Endocrinology 1985; 116:1383–1390.
324. Werner S, Hulting AL, Hökfelt T, et al. Effect of the peptide PHI-27 on prolactin release in vitro. Neuroendocrinology 1983; 37:476–478.
325. Sandman CA, Kastin AJ, Miller LH. Central nervous system actions of MSH and related pituitary peptides. In: Martini L, Besser GM, eds. Clinical Neuroendocrinology. New York: Academic, 1978: 443–469.
326. Ehrensing RH, Kastin AJ, Wurzlow GF, et al. Improvement in major depression after low subcutaneous doses of MIF-1. J Affective Disorders 1994; 31:227–233.

Luteinizing Hormone–Releasing Hormone

327. McCann SM, Taleisnik S, Friedman HM. LH-releasing activity in hypothalamic extracts. Proc Soc Exp Biol Med 1960; 104:432–434.
328. Campbell HJ, Feuer G, Harris GW. The effect of intrapituitary infusion of median eminence and other brain extracts on anterior pituitary gonadotrophic secretion. J Physiol (Lond) 1974; 170:474–486.
329. Matsuo H, Baba Y, Nair RMB, et al. Structure of the porcine LH- and FSH-releasing hormone. 1. The proposed amino acid sequence. Biochem Biophys Res Commun 1971; 43:1334–1339.
330. Seeburg PH, Adelman JP. Characterization of cDNA for precursor of human luteinizing hormone releasing hormone. Nature 1984; 311:666–668.
331. Seeburg PH, Mason AJ, Stewart TA, et al. The mammalian GnRH gene and its pivotal role in reproduction. Recent Prog Horm Res 1987; 43:690–698.
332. McCann SM, Mizunuma H, Samson WK. Differential hypothalamic control of FSH secretion: a review. Psychoneuroendocrinology 1983; 8:299–308.
333. Lumpkin MD, Moltz JH, Yu WH, et al. Purification of FSH-releasing factor: its dissimilarity from LHRH of mammalian, avian, and piscine origin. Brain Res Bull 1987; 18:175–178.
334. Wise PM, Rance N, Barr GD. Further evidence that luteinizing hormone–releasing hormone also is follicle-stimulating hormone–releasing hormone. Endocrinology 1979; 104:940–947.
335. Marshall LA, Monroe SE, Jaffe RB. Physiologic and therapeutic aspects of LHRH and its analogs. In: Martini L, Ganong WF, eds. Frontiers in Neuroendocrinology. Vol 10. New York: Raven, 1988: 239–278.
336. Sandow J. The regulation of LHRH action at the pituitary and gonadal receptor level: a review. Psychoneuroendocrinology 1983; 8:277–297.
337. Ying SY. Inhibins and activins. In: Martini L, Ganong WF, eds. Frontiers in Neuroendocrinology. Vol 10. New York: Raven, 1988: 167–184.
338. Marshall JC, Kelch RP. Gonadotropin-releasing hormone: role of pulsatile secretion in the regulation of reproduction. N Engl J Med 1986; 315:1459–1468.
339. Sherwood NM, Lovejoy DA, Coe IR. Origin of mammalian gonadotropin-releasing hormones. Endocr Rev 1993; 14:241–254.
340. Loumaye E, Thorner J, Catt KJ. Yeast mating pheromone activates mammalian gonadotrophs: evolutionary conservation of a reproductive hormone? Science 1982; 218:1323–1325.
341. Schwanzel-Fukuda M, Jorgenson KL, Bergen HT, et al. Biology of normal luteinizing hormone–releasing hormone neurons during and after their migration from olfactory placode. Endocr Rev 1992; 13:623–634.
342. Parhar L, Pfaff ED, Schwanzel-Fukuda M. Genes and behavior as studies through gonadotropin-releasing hormone (GnRH neurons: comparative and functional aspects). Cell Mol Neurobiol 1995; 15:107–116.
343. Silverman AJ, Livne I, Witkin JW. The gonadotropin-releasing hormone (GnRH), neuronal systems: immunocytochemistry and in situ hybridization. In: Knobil E, Neill JD, eds. The Physiology of Reproduction. 2nd ed. New York: Raven, 1994: 1683–1709.
344. Schwanzel-Fukuda M, Bick D, Pfaff DW. Luteinizing hormone–releasing hormone (LHRH)–expressing cells do not migrate normally in an inherited hypogonadal (Kallmann) syndrome. Mol Brain Res 1989; 6:311–326.
345. Miller GM, Silverman AJ, Rogers MC, et al. Neuromodulation of transplanted gonadotropin-releasing hormone neurons in male and female hypogonadal mice with preoptic area brain grafts. Biol Reprod 1995; 52:572–583.
346. Beiling CG, Wentz AC, eds. The LH-releasing hormone. New York: Masson Publishing, 1980.
347. Moghissi KS. Clinical applications of gonadotropin-releasing hormones in reproductive disorders. Endocrinol Metab Clin North Am 1992; 21:125–140.
348. Belchetz PE. Gonadotropin regulation and clinical applications of GnRH. Clin Endocrinol Metab 1983; 12:619–640.
349. Lincoln DW. Gonadotropin-releasing hormone (GnRH): basic physiology. In: DeGroot LJ, ed. Endocrinology. 3rd ed. Philadelphia: WB Saunders, 1994: 218–229.
350. Fan NC, Jeung E-B, Peng C, et al. The human gonadotropin-releasing hormone (GnRH) receptor gene: cloning, genomic organization and chromosomal assignment. Mol Cell Endocrinol 1994; 103:R1–R6.
351. Conn PM. The molecular basis of gonadotropin-releasing hormone action. Endocr Rev 1986; 7:3–10.
352. Stojilkovic SS, Reinhart J, Catt KJ. Gonadotropin-releasing hormone receptors: structure and signal transduction pathways. Endocr Rev 1994; 15:462–498.
353. Clayton RN, Catt KJ. Gonadotropin-releasing hormone receptors: characterization, physiological regulation, and relationship to reproductive function. Endocr Rev 1981; 2:186–209.
354. Popkin R, Fraser HM, Jonassen J. Stimulation of androstenedione and progesterone release by LHRH and LHRH agonist from isolated rat pre-ovulatory follicles. Mol Cell Endocrinol 1983; 29:169–179.
355. Hsueh AJW, Jones BC. Extrapituitary actions of gonadotropin-releasing hormone. Endocr Rev 1981; 2:437–461.
356. Moss RL. Actions of hypothalamic-hypophysiotropic hormones on the brain. Annu Rev Physiol 1979; 41:617–631.
357. Phoenix CH, Chambers KC. Sexual performance of old and young male rhesus macaques following treatment with GnRH. Physiol Behav 1990; 47:513–517.
358. Ehrensing RH, Kastin AJ, Schally AV. Behavioral and hormonal effects of prolonged high doses of LHRH in male impotency. Peptides 1981; 2(Suppl 1):115–121.
359. Kuffler SW, Sejnowski TJ. Peptidergic and muscarinic excitation at amphibian sympathetic synapses. J Physiol (Lond) 1983; 341:257–278.
360. Belisle S, Guevin JF, Bellabarba D, et al. Luteinizing-releasing hormone binds to enriched human placental membranes and stimulates in vitro the synthesis of bioactive human chorionic gonadotropin. J Clin Endocrinol Metab 1984; 59:119–126.
361. Amarant T, Fridkin M, Koch Y. Luteinizing hormone–releasing hormone and thyrotropin-releasing hormone in human and bovine milk. Eur J Biochem 1982; 127:647–650.
362. Hoffman AR, Crowley WF Jr. Induction of puberty in men by long-term pulsatile administration of low-dose gonadotropin-releasing hormone. N Engl J Med 1982; 307:1237–1241.
363. Stanhope R, Brook CGD, Pringle PJ, et al. Induction of puberty by pulsatile gonadotropin releasing hormone. Lancet 1987; 2:552–555.
364. Mansfield MJ, Beardsworth DE, Loughlin JS, et al. Long-term treatment of central precocious puberty with a long-acting analogue of luteinizing hormone-releasing hormone. N Engl J Med 1983; 309:1286–1290.
365. Borgmann V, Hardt W, Schmidt-Gollwitzer M, et al. Sustained suppression of testosterone production by the luteinising-hormone releasing-hormone agonist buserelin in patients with advanced prostate carcinoma. A new therapeutic approach? Lancet 1982; 1:1097–1099.
366. Labrie F, Dupont A, Belanger A, et al. New hormonal treatment in cancer of the prostate: combined administration of an LHRH agonist and an antiandrogen. J Steroid Biochem 1983; 19:999–1007.
367. Rabin D, McNeil LW. Pituitary and gonadal desensitization after continuous luteinizing hormone–releasing hormone infusion in normal females. J Clin Endocrinol Metab 1980; 51:873–876.

Regulation of Secretion of Tuberohypophyseal Neurons

368. Furness JB, Bornstein JC, Murphy R, et al. Roles of peptides in transmission in the enteric nervous system. Trends Neurosci 1992; 15:66–71.

369. Taubenhaus M, Soskin S. Release of lutenizing hormone from the anterior hypophysis by an acetylcholine-like substance from the hypothalamic region. Endocrinology 1941; 29:958–964.

370. Sawyer CH, Markee JE, Townsend BF. Cholinergic and adrenergic components in the neurohumoral control of the release of LH in the rabbit. Endocrinology 1949; 44:18–37.

371. Everett JW, Sawyer CH. A 24-hour periodicity in the "LH-release apparatus" of female rats, disclosed by barbiturate sedation. Endocrinology 1950; 47:198–218.

372. Palkovits M. Topography of chemically identified neurons in the central nervous system: progress in 1981–1983. In: Müller EE, MacLeod RM,, eds. Neuroendocrine Perspectives. Vol 3. Amsterdam: Elsevier Biomedical, 1984: 1–69.

373. Weiner RL, Ganong WF. Role of brain monoamines and histamine in regulation of anterior pituitary secretion. Physiol Rev 1978; 58:905–976.

374. Delitala G. Neurotransmitter control of anterior pituitary hormone secretion and its clinical implications in man. In: Besser GM, Martini L, eds. Clinical Neuroendocrinology. Vol II. New York: Academic, 1982: 68–139.

375. Barraclough CA, Wise PM. The role of catecholamines in the regulation of pituitary luteinizing and follicle-stimulating hormone secretion. Endocr Rev 1983; 4:91–119.

376. Terry LC. Neuropharmacologic regulation of anterior pituitary hormone secretion in man. In: Givens JR, ed. Hormone-Secreting Pituitary Tumors. Chicago: Year Book Medical, 1982: 27–44.

377. Iversen LL, Iversen SD, Snyder SH, eds. Chemical pathways in the brain. In: Handbook of Psychopharmacology. Vol 9. New York: Plenum, 1978.

378. Müller EE. Role of neurotransmitters and neuromodulators in the control of anterior pituitary hormone secretion. In: DeGroot LJ, ed. Endocrinology. 3rd ed. Philadelphia: WB Saunders, 1995: 178–191.

379. Meakin SO, Shooter EM. The nerve growth factor family of receptors. Trends Neurosci 1992; 15:323–331.

380. Thorner M. Is prolactin a marker for brain dopamine function? In: Brown GM, Koslow SH, Reichlin S, eds. Neuroendocrinology and Psychiatric Disorders. New York: Plenum, 1984: 55–66.

381. Seeman P, Van Tol HH. Dopamine receptor pharmacology. Trends Pharmacol Sci 1994: 15:264–270.

382. Moore RY, Bloom FE. Central catecholamine neuron systems. Anatomy and physiology of the norepinephrine and epinephrine systems. Annu Rev Neurosci 1979; 2:113–168.

383. Iversen LL, Iversen SD, Snyder SH, eds. Chemical pathways in the brain. In: Handbook of Psychopharmacology. Vol 9. New York: Plenum, 1978.

384. Swanson LW, Hartman BK. The central adrenergic system. An immuno-fluorescence study of the location of cell bodies and their efferent connections in the rat utilizing dopamine-β-hydroxylase as a marker. J Comp Neurol 1975; 163:467–505.

385. Bowker RM, Westlund KN, Sullivan MC, et al. Transmitters of the raphe-spinal complex: immunocytochemical studies. Peptides 1982; 3:291–298.

386. Steinbusch HW, Nieuwenhuys R. Distribution of serotonin-immunoreactivity in the central nervous system and pituitary of the rat with special references to the innervation of the hypothalamus. Adv Exp Med Biol 1981; 133:7–35.

387. Bowker RM, Westlund KN, Sullivan MC, et al. Descending serotonergic, peptidergic and cholinergic pathways from the raphé nuclei: a multiple transmitter complex. Brain Res 1983; 288:33–48.

388. Hoyer D, Clarke DE, Fozard JR, et al. International union of pharmacology classification of receptors for 5-hydroxytryptamine (serotonin). Pharmacol Rev 1994; 46:157–203.

389. Kjær A, Larsen PL, Knigge U, et al. Histamine stimulates c-fos expression in hypothalamic vasopressin-, oxytocin-, and corticotropin-releasing hormone-containing neurons. Endocrinology 1994; 134:482–491.

390. Kjær A, Larsen PJ, Knigge U, et al. Dehydration stimulates hypothalamic gene expression of histamine synthesis enzyme: importance for neuroendocrine regulation of vasopressin and oxytocin secretion. Endocrinology 1995; 136:2189–2197.

391. Theoharides T. Mast cells: the immune gate to the brain. Life Sci 1990; 46:607–617.

391a. Silver R, Silverman A-J, Vitkovic L, et al. Mast cells in the brain: evidence and functional significance. Trends Neurosci 1996; 19:25–31.

392. Bina KG, Rusak B, Semba K. Localization of cholinergic neurons in the forebrain and brainstem that project to the suprachiasmatic nucleus of the hypothalamus in rat. J Comp Neurol 1993; 335:295–307.

393. Sapolsky RM, Krey LC, McEwen BS. The neuroendocrinology of stress and aging: the glucocorticoid cascade hypothesis. Endocr Rev 1986; 7:284–301.

394. Wess J. Molecular basis of muscarinic acetylcholine receptor function. Trends Pharmacol Sci 1993; 14:308–313.

395. Carmeliet P, Denef C. Synthesis and release of acetylcholine by normal and tumoral pituitary corticotrophs. Endocrinology 1989; 124:2218–2227.

396. Lindstrom J, Schaeffer R, Whiting P. Molecular studies of the neuronal nicotinic acetylcholine receptor family. Mol Neurobiol 1987; 1:281–337.

397. Armstrong DM, Saper CB, Levey AI, et al. Distribution of cholinergic neurons in rat brain demonstrated by the immunocytochemical localization of choline acetyltransferase. J Comp Neurol 1983; 216:53–68.

398. Lipton SA, Rosenberg PA. Excitatory amino acids as a final common pathway for neurologic disorders. N Engl J Med 1994; 330:613–622.

399. Badger TM, Millard WJ, Martin JB, et al. Hypothalamic-pituitary function in adult rats treated neonatally with monosodium glutamate. Endocrinology 1982; 111:2031–2038.

400. Müller EE, Nistico G. Brain Messengers and the Pituitary. San Diego, CA: Academic, 1988.

401. Vincent SR, Hökfelt T, Wu JY. GABA neuron systems in hypothalamus and the pituitary gland. Neuroendocrinology 1982; 34:117–125.

402. Masotto C, Wisnewski G, Negro-Villar A. Different gamma-aminobutyric acid receptor subtypes are involved in the regulation of opiate-dependent and -independent luteinizing hormone–releasing hormone secretion. Endocrinology 1989; 125:548–553.

403. Brann DW, Mahesh VB. Excitatory amino acids: function and significance in reproduction and neuroendocrine regulation. Front Neuroendocrinol 1994; 15:3–49.

404. Meeker RB, Greenwood RS, Hayward JN. Glutamate receptors in the rat hypothalamus and pituitary. Endocrinology 1994; 134:621–629.

405. Seeburg PH. The molecular biology of mammalian glutamate receptor channels. Trends Neurosci 1993; 16:359–365.

406. Dunn SMJ. Molecular biology of the GABAA receptor. Int Rev Neurobiol 1994; 36:51–96.

407. Bowery NG. GABAB receptor pharmacology. Annu Rev Pharmacol Toxicol 1993; 33:109–147.

408. Clement-Jones V, Rees LH. Neuroendocrine correlates of the endorphins and enkephalin. In: Besser GM, Martini L, eds. Clinical Neuroendocrinology. Vol II. New York: Academic, 1982: 140–204.

409. McCann SM. The role of brain peptides in the control of anterior pituitary hormone secretion. In: Müller EE, MacLeod RM, eds. Neuroendocrine Perspectives. Vol 1. Amsterdam: Elsevier Biomedical, 1982: 1–22.

410. Grossman A. Brain opiates and neuroendocrine function. Clin Endocrinol Metab 1983; 12:725–746.

411. Morley JE. Neuroendocrine effects of endogenous opioid peptides in human subjects: a review. Psychoneuroendocrinology 1983; 8:361–379.

412. Harvey S, Fraser RA. Parathyroid hormone: neural and neuroendocrine perspectives. J Endocrinol 1993; 139:353–361.

413. Houben H, Denef C. Bioactive peptides in anterior pituitary cells. Peptides 1994; 15:547–582.

Endorphins and Endogenous Opioids

414. Kosterlitz HW. Endogenous opioid peptides: historical aspects. In: Hughes J, ed. Centrally Acting Peptides. Baltimore: University Park Press, 1978: 157.

415. Uhl GR, Childers SR, Snyder SH. Opioid peptides and the opiate receptor. Front Neuroendocrinol 1978; 5:289–328.

416. Ouabain: a new steroid hormone? Lancet 1995; 346:1381–1382 (editorial).

417. Mechoulam R, Hanus L, Martin BR. Search for endogenous ligands of the cannabinoid receptor. Biochem Pharmacol 1994; 48:1537–1544.

418. Krieger D. Endorphins and enkephalins. Disease of the Month 1982; 28:1–53.

419. Goodman RR, Fricker LD, Snyder SH. Enkephalins. In: Krieger DT, Brownstein MJ, Martin JB, eds. Brain Peptides. New York: John Wiley & Sons, 1983: 827–850.

420. Li CH, Barnafi L, Chrétien M, et al. Isolation and amino acid sequence of β-LPH from sheep pituitary glands. Nature 1975; 208:1093–1094.

421. Comb M, Seeburg PH, Adelman J, et al. Primary structure of the human met- and leu-enkephalin precursor and its mRNA. Nature 1982; 295:663–666.

422. Noda M, Teranishi Y, Takahashi H, et al. Isolation and structural organization of the human preproenkephalin gene. Nature 1982; 197:431–434.

423. Horikawa S, Takai T, Toyosato M, et al. Isolation and structural organization of the human preproenkephalin B gene. Nature 1983; 306:611–614.

424. Kakidani H, Furutani Y, Takahashi H, et al. Cloning and sequence analysis of cDNA for porcine β-neo-endorphin/dynorphin precursor. Nature 1982; 298:245–249.

425. Meunier J-C, Mollereau C, Toll L, et al. Isolation and structure of the endogenous agonist of opioid receptor–like ORL₁ receptor. Nature 1995; 377:532–535.

426. Reisine T, Bell GI. Molecular biology of opioid receptors. Trends Neurosci 1993; 16:506–510.

427. Hyman SE. Shaking out the cause of addiction. Science 1996; 273:611–612.

Melanocortins

428. Lerner AB. The discovery of the melanotropins: a history of pituitary endocrinology. Ann NY Acad Sci 1993; 680:1–12.

429. Levine N, Sheftel SN, Eytan T, et al. Induction of skin tanning by subcutaneous administration of a potent synthetic melanotropin. JAMA 1991; 266:2730–2736.

430. Krivoy WA, Guillemin R. On a possible role of β-melanocyte stimulating hormone (β-MSH) in the central nervous system of the mammalia: an effect of β-MSH in the spinal cord of the cat. Endocrinology 1960; 69:170–175.

431. Lipton JM, Clark WG. Neurotransmitters in temperature control. Annu Rev Physiol 1986; 48:613–623.

432. Catania A, Lipton JM. Alpha-melanocyte stimulating hormone in the modulation of host reactions. Endocr Rev 1993; 14:564–576.

433. Star RA, Rajora N, Huang J, et al. Evidence of autocrine modulation of macrophage nitric oxide synthase by alpha-melanocyte-stimulating hormone. Proc Natl Acad Sci USA 1995; 92:8016–8020.

434. Heterogeneity of brain melanocortin receptors suggested by differential ligand binding in situ. Brain Res 1994; 635:148–158.

435. Mountjoy KG, Mortrud MT, Low MJ, et al. Localization of the melanocortin-4 receptor (MC4-R) in neuroendocrine and autonomic control circuits in the brain. Mol Endocrinol 1994; 8:1298–1308.

436. Roselli-Rehfuss L, Mountjoy KG, Robbins LS, et al. Identification of a receptor for gamma melanotropin and other proopiomelanocortin peptides in the hypothalamus and limbic system. Proc Natl Acad Sci USA 1993; 90:8856–8860.

437. Mountjoy KG, Mortrud MT, Low MJ, et al. Localization of the melanocortin-4 receptor (MC4-R) in neuroendocrine and autonomic control circuits in the brain. Mol Endocrinol 1994; 8:1298–1308.

Gaseous Neurotransmitters: Nitric Oxide and Carbon Monoxide

438. Ceccatelli S, Hulting AL, Zhang X, et al. Nitric oxide synthesis in the rat anterior pituitary gland. Proc Natl Acad Sci USA 1993; 90:11,292–11,296.

439. Rettori V, Belkova N, Dees WL, et al. Role of nitric oxide in the control of luteinizing hormone–releasing hormone release *in vivo* and *in vitro*. Proc Natl Acad Sci USA 1993; 90:10130–10134.

440. Seilicovich A, Duvilanski BH, Pisera D, et al. Nitric oxide inhibits hypothalamic luteinizing hormone–releasing hormone release by releasing gamma-aminobutyric acid. Proc Natl Acad Sci USA 1995; 92:3421–3424.

441. Costa A, Trainer P, Besser M, et al. Nitric oxide modulates the release of corticotropin-releasing hormone from the rat hypothalamus in vitro. Brain Res 1993; 605:187–192.

442. Sandi C, Guaza C. Evidence for a role of nitric oxide in the corticotropin-releasing factor release induced by interleukin-1 beta. Eur J Pharmacol 1995; 274:17–23.

443. Kato M. Involvement of nitric oxide in growth hormone (GH)–releasing hormone–induced GH secretion in rat pituitary cells. Endocrinology 1992; 134:2133–2138.

444. Duvilanski BH, Zambruno C, Seilicovich A, et al. Role of nitric oxide in control of prolactin release by the adenohypophysis. Proc Natl Acad Sci USA 1995; 92:170–174.

445. Mani SK, Allen JM, Rettori V, et al. Nitric oxide mediates sexual behavior in female rats. Proc Natl Acad Sci USA 1994; 91:6468–6472.

446. Burnett AL. Role of nitric oxide in the physiology of erection. Biol Reprod 1995; 52:485–489.

447. Pozzoli G, Mancuso C, Mirtella A, et al. Carbon monoxide as a novel neuroendocrine modulator: inhibition of stimulated corticotropin-releasing hormone release from acute rat hypothalamic explants. Endocrinology 1994; 135:2314–2317.

448. Parkes D, Kasckoiw J, Vale W. Carbon monoxide modulates secretion of corticotropin-releasing factor from rat hypothalamic cell cultures. Brain Res 1994; 646:315–318.

Feedback Concepts in Neuroendocrinology

449. DiStefano JJ III, Stubberud AR, Williams IJ. Theory and Problems of Feedback and Control Systems. New York: Schaum Publishing, 1967.

450. Yates FE. Modeling periodicities in reproductive, adrenocortical and metabolic systems. In: Ferin M, Halberg F, Richart RM, et al, eds. Biorhythms and Human Reproduction. New York: John Wiley & Sons, 1974: 133–142.

451. Houk JC. Control strategies in physiological systems. FASEB J 1988; 2:97–107.

Endocrine Rhythms

452. Moore RY. The organization of the human circadian timing system. Prog Brain Res 1992; 93:101–115.

453. Boyar RM. Sleep-related endocrine rhythms. In: Reichlin S, Baldessarini RJ, Martin JB, eds. The Hypothalamus. Vol 56. New York: Raven, 1978: 373–386.

454. Chadwick DJ, Ackrill K. Circadian clocks and their adjustment. Ciba Found Symp 1995.

455. Van Cauter E, Turek FW. Endocrine and other biological rhythms. In: DeGroot LJ, ed. Endocrinology. 3rd ed. Philadelphia: WB Saunders, 1995: 2497–2548.

456. Stern JM, Reichlin S. Prolactin circadian rhythm persists throughout lactation in women. Neuroendocrinology 1990; 51:31–37.

457. Welsh DK, Logothetis DE, Meister M, et al. Individual neurons dissociated from rat suprachiasmatic nucleus express independently phased circadian firing rhythms. Neuron 1995; 14:697–706.

458. Albers HE, Ferris CF, Leeman SE, et al. Avian pancreatic polypeptide phase shifts hamster circadian rhythms when microinjected into the suprachiasmatic region. Science 1984; 223:833–835.

459. Weaver DR, Rivkees SA, Reppert SM. Localization and characterization of melatonin receptors in rodent brain by in vitro radioautography. J Neurosci 1989; 9:2581–2590.

460. Reppert SM, Weaver DR, Ebisawa T. Cloning and characterization of a mammalian melatonin receptor that mediates reproductive and circadian responses. Neuron 1994; 13:1177–1185.

461. Czeisler CA, Shanahan TL, Klerman EB. Suppression of melatonin secretion in some blind patients by exposure to bright light. N Engl J Med 1995; 332:54–55.

462. Reppert SM. Pre-natal development of a hypothalamic biological clock. In: Swaab DF, Hofman MA, Mirmiran M, et al, eds. Prog Brain Res 1992; 93:119–132.

463. Czeisler CA, Johnson MP, Duffy JF, et al: Exposure to bright light and darkness to treat physiologic maladaptation to night work. N Engl J Med 1990; 322:1253–1259.

464. Lewy AJ, Sack RI, Miller LS, et al. Anti-depressant and circadian phase shifting effects of light. Science 1987; 235:352–354.

465. Turek FW, Van Reeth O. Altering the mammalian circadian clock with the short-acting benzodiazepine, triazolam. Trends Neurosci 1988; 11:535–541.

Neuroendocrine Control of Individual Pituitary Hormones

Thyrotropin

466. Reichlin S. Control of thyrotropic hormone secretion. In: Martini L, Ganong WF, eds. Neuroendocrinology. Vol 1. New York: Academic, 1966: 445–536.

467. Reichlin S, Martin JB, Jackson IMD. Regulation of thyroid-stimulating hormone (TSH) secretion. In: Jeffcoate SL, Hutchinson JSM, eds. The Endocrine Hypothalamus. New York: Academic, 1978: 239–270.

468. Morley JE. Neuroendocrine control of thyrotropin secretion. Endocr Rev 1981; 2:396–436.

469. Scanlon MF, Hall R. Thyrotropin-releasing hormone: basic and clinical aspects. In: DeGroot LJ, ed. Endocrinology. 3rd ed. Philadelphia: WB Saunders, 1995: 208–217.

470. Wilber JF. Control of thyroid function: the hypothalamic-pituitary-thyroid axis. In: DeGroot LJ, ed. Endocrinology. 3rd ed. Philadelphia: WB Saunders, 1995: 602–616.

471. Snyder PJ, Utiger RD. Inhibition of thyrotropin response to thyrotropin releasing hormone by small quantities of thyroid hormones. J Clin Invest 1972; 51:2077–2084.

472. Vagenakis AG, Rapoport B, Azizi F, et al. Hyper-response to thyrotropin releasing hormone accompanying small decreases in serum thyroid hormone concentration. J Clin Invest 1974; 54:913–918.

473. Segerson TP, Kauer J, Wolfe HC, et al. Thyroid hormone regulates TRH biosynthesis in the paraventricular nucleus of the rat hypothalamus. Science 1987; 238:78–80.

474. Dyess EM, Segerson TP, Liposits Z, et al. Triiodothyronine exerts direct cell-specific regulation of thyrotropin-releasing hormone gene expression in the hypothalamic paraventricular nucleus. Endocrinology 1988; 123:2291–2297.

475. Dahl GE, Evans NP, Thrun LA, et al. A central negative feedback action of thyroid hormones on thyrotropin-releasing hormone secretion. Endocrinology 1994; 135:2392–2397.

476. Schreiber G, Southwell BR, Richardson SJ. Hormone delivery systems to the brain—transthyretin. Exp Clin Endocrinol 1995; 103:75–80.

477. Lechan RM, Qi Y, Jackson IM, et al. Identification of thyroid hormone receptor isoforms in thyrotropin-releasing hormone neurons of the hypothalamic paraventricular nucleus. Endocrinology 1994; 135:92–100.

478. Lechan RM, Kakucska I. Feedback regulation of thyrotropin-releasing hormone gene expression by thyroid hormone in the hypothalamic paraventricular nucleus. Ciba Found Symp 1992; 168:144–158.

479. Kaplan MM, Taft JA, Reichlin S, et al. Sustained rises in serum thyrotropin, thyroxine, and triiodothyronine during long term, continuous thyrotropin-releasing hormone treatment in patients with amyotrophic lateral sclerosis. J Clin Endocrinol Metab 1986; 63:808–814.

480. Kakucska I, Rand W, Lechan RM. Thyrotropin-releasing hormone gene expression in the hypothalamic paraventricular nucleus is dependent on feedback regulation by both triiodothyronine and thyroxine. Endocrinology 1992; 130:2845–2850.

481. Arancibia S, Tapai-Arancibia L, Assenmacher I, et al. Direct evidence of short-term cold-induced TRH release in the median eminence. Neuroendocrinology 1983; 37:225–228.

482. Galton VA. Environmental effects. In: Ingbar SH, Braverman LE, eds. Werner's the Thyroid. Philadelphia: JB Lippincott, 1986: 407–413.

483. Sack J, Fisher DA, Wang CC. Serum thyrotropin, prolactin and growth hormone levels during the early neonatal period in the human infant. J Pediatr 1976; 89:298–300.

484. Arimura A, Schally AV. Increases in basal and thyrotropin releasing hormone (TRH)–stimulated secretion of thyrotropin (TSH) by passive immunization with antiserum to somatostatin in rats. Endocrinology 1976; 98:1069–1072.

485. Ferland L, Labrie F, Jobin M, et al. Physiologic role of somatostatin in the control of growth hormone and thyrotropin secretion. Biochem Biophys Res Commun 1976; 68:149–151.

486. Berelowitz M, Maeda K, Harris S, et al. The effect of alterations in the pituitary-thyroid axis on hypothalamic content and in vitro release of somatostatin-like immunoreactivity. Endocrinology 1980; 107:24–29.

487. Rogers KV, Vician L, Steiner RA, et al. The effect of hypophysectomy and growth hormone administration on pre-prosomatostatin messenger

ribonucleic acid in the periventricular nucleus of the rat hypothalamus. Endocrinology 1988; 122:586–591.

488. Kaplan MM. The role of thyroid hormone deiodination in the regulation of hypothalamo-pituitary function. Neuroendocrinology 1984; 38:254–260.

489. Chrivia JC, Kwok RP, Lamb N, et al. Phosphorylated CREB binds specifically to the nuclear protein CBP. Nature 1993; 365:855–859.

490. Brown MR. Thermoregulation. In: Brownstein MJ, Martin JB, eds. Brain Peptides. New York: John Wiley & Sons, 1983: 301–314.

491. Relkin R. Pineal-hormonal interactions. In: Relkin R, ed. The Pineal Gland. New York: Elsevier Biomedical, 1983: 225–246.

492. Brammer GL, Morley JE, Geller E, et al. Hypothalamus-pituitary-thyroid axis interactions with pineal gland in the rat. Am J Physiol 1979; 236:E416–E420.

493. Jackson IMD, Sapirstein R, Reichlin S. Thyrotropin releasing hormone (TRH) in pineal and hypothalamus of the frog: effect of season and illumination. Endocrinology 1977; 100:97–100.

494. Brabant G, Prank K, Ranft U, et al. Physiological regulation of circadian and pulsatile thyrotropin secretion in normal man and woman. J Clin Endocrinol Metab 1990; 70:4403–4409.

495. Haisenleder DJ, Ortolano GA, Dalkin AC, et al. Differential actions of thyrotropin (TSH)-releasing hormone pulses in the expression of prolactin and TSH subunit messenger ribonucleic acid in rat pituitary cells *in vitro*. Endocrinology 1992; 130:2917–2923.

496. DuRuisseau J. Seasonal variation of PBI in healthy Montrealers. J Clin Endocrinol Metab 1965; 25:1513–1515.

497. Berg GR, Utiger RD, Schalch DS, et al. Effect of central cooling in man on pituitary-thyroid function and growth hormone secretion. J Appl Physiol 1966; 21:1791–1794.

498. Arimura A, Smith W, Schally AV. Blockade of the stress-induced decrease in blood GH by anti-somatostatin serum in rats. Endocrinology 1976; 98:540–543.

499. Peterfreund RA, Vale WW. Ovine corticotropin-releasing factor stimulates somatostatin secretion from cultured brain cells. Endocrinology 1983; 112:1275–1278.

500. Burger HG, Patel YC. TSH and TRH: their physiological regulation and the clinical applications of TRH. In: Martini L, Besser GM, eds. Clinical Neuroendocrinology. New York: Academic, 1977: 67–131.

501. Wartofsky L, Burman KD. Alterations in thyroid function in patients with systemic illness: the "euthyroid sick syndrome." Endocr Rev 1982; 3:164–217.

502. Peters JR, Foord SM, Diequez C, et al. TSH neuroregulation and alterations in disease states. Clin Endocrinol Metab 1983; 12:669–695.

503. Dubois JM, Dayer JM, Siegrist-Kaiser CA, et al. Human recombinant interleukin-1β decreases plasma thyroid hormone and thyroid stimulating hormone levels in rats. Endocrinology 1988; 123:2175–2181.

504. Pang XP, Hershman JM, Mirell CJ, et al. Impairment of hypothalamic-pituitary-thyroid function in rats treated with human recombinant tumor necrosis factor-alpha (cachectin). Endocrinology 1989; 125:76–84.

505. Scarborough DE, Lee SL, Dinarello CA, et al. Interleukin-1 beta stimulates somatostatin biosynthesis in primary cultures of fetal rat brain. Endocrinology 1989; 124:549–551.

506. Koenig J, Snow K, Clark B, et al. Intrinsic pituitary interleukin-1β is induced by bacterial lipopolysaccharide. Endocrinology 1990; 126:3053–3058.

507. Spath–Schwalbe E, Schrezenmeier H, Bornstein S, et al. Endocrine effects of recombinant interleukin 6 in man. Neuroendocrinology 1996; 63:237–243.

508. Palkovits M, Zaborsky L. Neural connections of the hypothalamus. In: Morgane PJ, Panksepp J, eds. Handbook of the Hypothalamus. New York: Marcel Dekker, 1979: 379–510.

Regulation of Hypothalamic-Pituitary-Adrenal Axis

509. Antoni FA. Hypothalamic control of adrenocorticotropin secretion: advances since the discovery of 41-residue corticotropin-releasing factor. Endocr Rev 1986; 7:351–378.

510. Grossman A. Corticotropin-releasing hormone: basic physiology and clinical applications. In: DeGroot L, ed. Endocrinology. 3rd ed. Philadelphia: WB Saunders, 1995: 341–354.

511. Imura H. Adrenocorticotropic hormone. In: DeGroot L, ed. Endocrinology. 3rd ed. Philadelphia: WB Saunders, 1995: 355–367.

512. Dallman MF, Akana SF, Levin N, et al. Corticosteroids and the control of function in the hypothalamo-pituitary-adrenal (HPA) axis. Ann NY Acad Sci 1994; 746:22–31.

513. Sapolsky RM, Krey LC, McEwen BS. The neuroendocrinology of stress and aging: the glucocorticoid cascade hypothesis. Endocr Rev 1986; 7:284–301.

514. deKloet ER, Oitzl MS, Joëls M. Functional implications of brain corticosteroid receptor diversity. Cell Mol Neurobiol 1993; 13:433–455.

515. Evans RM. The steroid and thyroid hormone receptor superfamily. Science 1988; 240:889–895.

516. Liposits ZS, Uht RM, Harrison RW, et al. Ultrastructural localization of glucocorticoid receptor (GR) in hypothalamic paraventricular neurons synthesizing corticotropin releasing factor (CRF). Histochemistry 1987; 87:407–412.

517. Joëls M, deKloet ER. Corticosteroid hormones: endocrine messengers in the brain. News Physiol Sci 1995; 10:71–76.

518. Arriza JL, Simerly RB, Swanson LW, et al. The neuronal mineralocorticoid receptor as a mediator of glucocorticoid response. Neuron 1988; 1:887–900.

519. Fuxe K, Wikstrom AC, Okret S, et al. Mapping of glucocorticoid receptor immunoreactive neurons in the rat tel- and diencephalon using a monoclonal antibody against rat liver glucocorticoid receptor. Endocrinology 1985; 117:1803–1812.

520. Hua SY, Chen YZ. Membrane receptor–mediated electrophysiological effects of glucocorticoid on mammalian neurons. Endocrinology 1989; 124:687–691.

521. Kitay JI, Holub N, Jailer JW. Inhibition of pituitary ACTH release: an extraadrenal action of exogenous ACTH. Endocrinology 1959; 64:475–482.

522. Engler D, Liu J-P, Clarke IJ, et al. Corticotropin-release inhibitory factor: evidence for dual stimulatory and inhibitory hypothalamic regulation over adrenocorticotropin secretion and biosynthesis. Trends Endocrinol Metab 1994; 5:272–283.

523. Jezová, Bartanusz V, Westergren I, et al. Rat melanin-concentrating hormone stimulates adrenocorticotropin secretion: evidence for a site of action in brain regions protected by the blood-brain barrier. Endocrinology 1992; 130:1024–1029.

524. Maran JW, Carlson DE, Grizzle WE, et al. Organization of the medial hypothalamus for control of adrenocorticotropin in the cat. Endocrinology 1978; 103:957–970.

525. Ward DG, Bolton MG, Gann DS. Inhibitory and facilitatory areas of the ventral midbrain mediating release of corticotropin in the cat. Endocrinology 1978; 102:1147–1154.

526. Carlson DE, Dornhorst A, Gann DS. Organization of the lateral hypothalamus for control of adrenocorticotropin release in the cat. Endocrinology 1980; 107:961–969.

527. Dornhorst A, Carlson DE, Seif SM, et al. Control of release of adrenocorticotropin and vasopressin by the supraoptic and paraventricular nuclei. Endocrinology 1981; 108:1420–1424.

528. Grossman A, Costa A. The regulation of hypothalamic CRH: impact of *in vitro* studies on the central control of the stress response. Funct Neurol 1993; 8:325–334.

529. Chrousos GP. The hypothalamic-pituitary-adrenal axis and immune-mediated inflammation. N Engl J Med 1995; 332:1351–1362.

530. Grossman A. Brain opiates and neuroendocrine function. Clin Endocrinol Metab 1983; 12:725–746.

531. Gaykema RPA, Dukstra I, Tilders FTH. Subdiaphragmatic vagotomy suppresses endotoxin-induced activation of hypothalamic corticotropin-releasing hormone neurons and ACTH secretion. Endocrinology 1995; 136:4717–4720.

532. Kalain NH. Behavioral effects of ovine corticotropin-releasing factor administered to rhesus monkeys. Fed Proc 1985; 44:249–253.

533. Rivier C, Rivier J, Vale W. Stress-induced inhibition of reproductive functions—role of endogenous corticotropin-releasing factor. Science 1986; 231:607–609.

534. Chrousos GP, moderator. Clinical applications of corticotropin-releasing factor. Ann Intern Med 1985; 102:344–358.

Growth Hormone Regulation

535. Brazeau P, Guillemin R, Ling N, et al. Somatomedin inhibition of the growth hormone secretion stimulated by the hypothalamic factor somatocrinin or the synthetic peptide hpGRF. C R Acad Sci III 1982; 295:651–654.

536. Berelowitz M, Szabo M, Frohman LA, et al. Somatomedin-C mediates growth hormone negative feedback by effects on both the hypothalamus and the pituitary. Science 1981; 212:1279–1281.

537. Abe H, Molitch ME, Van Wyk JJ, et al. Human growth hormone and somatomedin C suppress the spontaneous release of growth hormone in unanesthetized rats. Endocrinology 1983; 113:1319–1324.

538. Leshin LS, Barb CR, Kiser TE. Growth hormone–releasing hormone and somatostatin neurons within the porcine and bovine hypothalamus. Neuroendocrinology 1994; 59:251–264.

539. Vigersky RA, Loriaux DL, Anderson AE, et al. Anorexia nervosa: behavioral and hypothalamic aspects. Clin Endocrinol Metab 1976; 5:517–535.

540. Gunoz H, Neyz O, Sencer E, et al. Growth hormone secretion in protein energy malnutrition. Acta Paediatr Scand 1981; 70:521–526.

541. Underwood LE, Van Wyk JJ. Hormones in normal and aberrant growth. In: Williams RH, ed. Textbook of Endocrinology. 6th ed. Philadelphia: WB Saunders, 1981: 1149–1191.

542. Martin JB, Brazeau P, Tannenbaum GS. Neuroendocrine organization of growth hormone regulation. In: Reichlin S, Baldessarini RJ, Martin JB, eds. The Hypothalamus. Vol 56. New York: Raven, 1978: 329–357.

543. Martin JB. Regulation of growth hormone secretion. In: Raiti S, Tolman RA, eds. Human Growth Hormone. New York: Plenum, 1986: 303–324.

544. Frohman LA. Glucoregulation. In: Krieger DT, Brownstein MJ, Martin JB. Brain Peptides. New York: John Wiley & Sons, 1983: 281–300.

545. Boyd AE, Lebovitz HE, Pfeiffer JB. Stimulation of growth hormone secretion by L-dopa. N Engl J Med 1970; 283:1425–1429.

546. Casanueva FF. Physiology of growth hormone secretion and action. Endocrinol Metab Clin North Am 1992; 21:483–517.

547. Heidingsfelder S, Blackard WG. Adrenergic control mechanisms for growth hormone secretion. J Clin Invest 1968; 47:1407–1414.

548. Laron Z, Gil-Ad T, Topper E, et al. Oral dose of clonidine: an effective

screening test for growth hormone deficiency. Acta Paediatr 1982; 71:847–848.

549. Loche S, Lampis A, Cella SG, et al. Clonidine treatment in children with short stature. J Endocrinol Invest 1988; 11:763–767.

550. Pescovitz OH, Tan E. Lack of benefit of clonidine treatment for short stature in a double-blind, placebo-controlled trial. Lancet 1988; 2:874–877.

551. Delitala G, Frulio T, Pacifico A, et al. Participation of cholinergic muscarinic receptors in glucagon- and arginine-mediated growth hormone secretion in man. J Clin Endocrinol Metab 1982; 55:1231–1233.

552. Delitala G, Grossman A, Besser GM. Opiate peptides control growth hormone through a cholinergic mechanism in man. Clin Neuroendocrinol 1983; 18:401–405.

553. Massara G, Ghigo E, Demislis K, et al. Cholinergic involvement in the growth hormone releasing hormone–induced growth hormone release: studies in normal and acromegalic subjects. Neuroendocrinology 1986; 43:670–675.

554. Casanueva FF, Villanueva L, Diaz Y, et al. Atropine selectively blocks GHRH-induced GH secretion without altering LH, FSH, TSH, PRL and ACTH/cortisol secretion elicited by their specific hypothalamic releasing factors. Clin Endocrinol 1986; 25:319–323.

555. Massara F, Ghigo E, Goffi S, et al. Blockade of hp-GRF-40–induced GH release in normal men by a cholinergic muscarinic antagonist. J Clin Endocrinol Metab 1984; 59:1025–1026.

556. Casanueva FF, Villanueva L, Dieguez C, et al. Atropine blockade of growth hormone (GH)–releasing hormone–induced GH secretion in man is not exerted at pituitary level. J Clin Endocrinol Metab 1986; 62:186–191.

557. Cordido F, Dieguez C, Casanueva FF. Effect of central cholinergic neurotransmission enhancement by pyridostigmine on the growth hormone secretion elicited by clonidine, arginine, or hypoglycemia in normal and obese subjects. J Clin Endocrinol Metab 1990; 70:1361–1370.

558. Castro RC, Vieira JG, Chacra AR, et al. Pyridostigmine enhances, but does not normalize, the GH response to GH-releasing hormone in obese subjects. Acta Endocrinol 1990; 122:385–390.

559. Ghigo E, Mazza E, Corrias A, et al. Effect of cholinergic enhancement by pyridostigmine on growth hormone secretion in obese adults and children. Metabolism 1989; 38:631–633.

560. Leal-Cerro A, Pereira JL, Garcia-Luna PP, et al. Effect of enhancement of endogenous cholinergic tone with pyridostigmine on growth hormone responses to GH-releasing hormone in patients with Cushing's syndrome. Clin Endocrinol 1990; 33:291–295.

561. Richardson SB, Hollander CS, D'Eletto R, et al. Acetylcholine inhibits the release of somatostatin from rat hypothalamus in vitro. Endocrinology 1980; 107:122–129.

562. Carmeliet P, Denef C. Immunocytochemical and pharmacological evidence for an intrinsic cholinomimetic system modulating prolactin and growth hormone release in rat pituitary. Endocrinology 1988; 123:1128–1139.

563. Atiea JA, Creagh F, Page M, et al. Early morning hyperglycemia in insulin-dependent diabetes: acute and sustained effects of cholinergic blockage. J Clin Endocrinol Metab 1989; 69:390–395.

564. Ismail IS, Scanlon MF, Peters JR. Cholinergic control of growth hormone (GH) responses to GH-releasing hormone in insulin dependent diabetics: evidence for attenuated hypothalamic somatostatatinergic tone and decreased GH autofeedback. Clin Endocrinol 1993; 38:149–157.

565. Davis TM, Burrin JM, Bloom SR. Growth hormone (GH) release in response to GH-releasing hormone in man is 3-fold enhanced by galanin. J Clin Endocrinol Metab 1987; 65:1248–1252.

566. Lam KS, Lechan RM, Minamitani N, et al. Vasoactive intestinal peptide in the anterior pituitary is increased in hypothyroidism. Endocrinology 1989; 124:1077–1084.

567. Vrontakis ME, Yamamoto T, Schroedter IC, et al. Estrogen induction of galanin synthesis in the rat anterior pituitary gland demonstrated by in situ hybridization and immunohistochemistry. Neurosci Lett 1989; 100:59–64.

568. Chihara K, Kato Y, Maeda K, et al. Effects of thyrotropin-releasing hormone on sleep and sleep-related growth hormone release in normal subjects. J Sons Clin Endocrinol Metab 1977; 44:1094–1100.

569. Bruhn TO, Rondeel JM, Bolduc TG, et al. Thyrotropin-releasing hormone (TRH) gene expression in the anterior pituitary. I. Presence of pro-TRH messenger ribonucleic acid and pro-TRH-derived peptide in a subpopulation of somatotrophs. Endocrinology 1994; 134:815–820.

570. Winer LM, Shaw MA, Baumann G. Basal plasma growth hormone levels in man: new evidence for rhythmicity of growth hormone secretion. J Clin Endocrinol Metab 1990; 70:1678–1686.

571. Tannenbaum GS, Ling N. The interrelationship of growth hormone (GH)–releasing factor and somatostatin in generation of the ultradian rhythm of GH secretion. Endocrinology 1984; 115:1952–1957.

572. Wehrenberg WB, Baird A, Ling N. Potent interaction between glucocorticoids and growth hormone–releasing factor in vivo. Science 1983; 221:556–558.

573. Cintra A, Fuxe K, Solfrini V, et al. Central peptidergic neurons as targets for glucocorticoid action. Evidence for the presence of glycocorticoid receptor immunoreactivity in various types of classes of peptidergic neurons. J Steroid Biochem Mol Biol 1991; 40:93–103.

574. Hodin RA, Lazar MA, Wintman BI, et al. Identification of a thyroid hormone receptor that is pituitary-specific. Science 1989; 244:76–79.

575. Peisen JN, McDonnell KJ, Mulroney SE, et al. Endotoxin-induced suppression of the somatotropic axis is mediated by interleukin-1β and corticotro-

pin-releasing factor in the juvenile rat. Endocrinology 1995; 136:3378–3390.

576. Payne LC, Obal F Jr, Opp MR, et al. Stimulation and inhibition of growth hormone secretion by interleukin-1 beta: the involvement of growth hormone releasing hormone. Neuroendocrinology 1992; 56:118–123.

Prolactin Regulation

577. Reichlin S. Neuroendocrine regulation of prolactin secretion. Adv Biosci 1988; 69:277–292.

578. Ben-Jonathan N, Arbogast LA, Hyde JF. Neuroendocrine regulation of prolactin release. Prog Neurobiol 1989; 33:399–447.

579. Kordon C, Drouva SV, de la Escalera GM, et al. Role of classic and peptide neuromediators in the neuroendocrine regulation of luteinizing hormone and prolactin. In: Knobil E, Neill JD, eds. The Physiology of Reproduction. 2nd ed. New York: Raven, 1994: 1621–1681.

580. Gunnett JW, Freeman ME. The mating-induced release of prolactin: a unique neuroendocrine response. Endocr Rev 1983; 4:44–61.

581. Thorner MO. Prolactin: Clinical physiology and the significance and management of hyperprolactinemia. In: Martini L, Besser GM, eds. Clinical Neuroendocrinology. New York: Academic, 1977: 320–361.

582. Molitch ME, Reichlin S. Hyperprolactinemic disorders. Disease of the Month 1982; 28:1–58.

583. Müller EE, Genazzani AR, Murru S. Nomifensine: diagnostic test in hyperprolactinemic states. J Clin Endocrinol Metab 1978; 47:1352–1357.

584. Cocchi D, Locatelli V, Cella S, et al. Antidepressant drugs as a tool to investigate CNS–anterior pituitary interactions. Adv Biochem Psychopharmacol 1982; 32:317–328.

585. Webb CB, Thominet JL, Barowsky H, et al. Evidence for lactotroph dopamine resistance in idiopathic hyperprolactinemia. J Clin Endocrinol Metab 1983; 56:1089–1093.

586. Reichlin S, Molitch ME. Neuroendocrine aspects of pituitary adenoma. In: Camanni F, Müller EE, eds. Pituitary Hyperfunction: Physiopathology and Clinical Aspects. New York: Raven, 1984: 47–70.

587. Faglia G, Spada A, Moriondo P, et al. What is the role of dopamine in the pathogenesis of prolactinomas? In: Camanni F, Müller EE, eds. Pituitary Hyperfunction: Physiopathology and Clinical Aspects. New York: Raven, 1984: 279–288.

588. Creese I, Burt DR, Snyder SH. Dopamine receptor binding predicts clinical and pharmacological potencies of antischizophrenic drugs. Science 1976; 192:481–483.

589. Turner TH, Cookson JC, Wass JAH, et al. Psychotic reactions during treatment of pituitary tumours with dopamine agonists. Br Med J 1984; 289:1101–1103.

590. Samuels MH, Henry P, Kleinschmidt-Demasters B, et al. Pulsatile prolactin secretion in hyperprolactinemia due to presumed pituitary stalk interruption. J Clin Endocrinol Metab 1991; 73:1289–1293.

591. Short RV. Breast feeding. Sci Am 1984; 250:35–41.

592. Schallenberger E, Richardson DW, Knobil E. Role of prolactin in the lactational amenorrhea of the rhesus monkey (Macaca mulatta). Biol Reprod 1981; 25:370–374.

593. Ishizuka B, Quigley ME, Yen SSC. Pituitary hormone release in response to food ingestion: evidence for neuroendocrine signals from gut to brain. J Clin Endocrinol Metab 1957; 57:1111–1116.

Neuroendocrine Aspects of Sexual Function

594. Knobil E. The neuroendocrine control of the menstrual cycle. Recent Prog Horm Res 1980; 36:53–88.

595. Crowley WF Jr, Whitcomb RW, Jameson JL, et al. Neuroendocrine control of human reproduction in the male. Recent Prog Horm Res 1991; 47:27–62.

596. Shivers BD, Harlan RE, Pfaff DW. Reproduction: the central nervous system role of luteinizing hormone releasing hormone. In: Krieger DT, Brownstein MJ, Martin JB, eds. Brain Peptides. New York: John Wiley & Sons, 1983: 389–412.

597. Barraclough CA, Wise PM. The role of catecholamines in the regulation of pituitary luteinizing hormone and follicle-stimulating hormone secretion. Endocr Rev 1982; 3:91–119.

598. Adams JM, Taylor AE, Schoenfeld DA, et al. The midcycle gonadotropin surge in normal women occurs in the face of an unchanging gonadotropin-releasing hormone pulse frequency. J Clin Endocrinol Metab 1994; 79:858–864.

599. Knobil E. The GnRH pulse generator: past, present and future. In: Bouchard P, Caraty A, Coelingh Bennink HJT, et al, eds. GnRH, GnRH Analogs, Gonadotropins and Gonadal Peptides. London: Parthenon Publishing Group, 1992: 3–13.

600. Kalra SP, Mandatory neuropeptide-steroid signalling for the preovulatory luteinizing hormone-releasing hormone discharge. Endocr Rev 1993; 14:507–538.

601. Kalra SP, Kalra PS. Regulation of gonadotropin secretion. In: Imura H ed. The Pituitary Gland. 2nd ed. New York: Raven, 1994: 285–307.

602. Marshall JC. Hormonal regulation of the menstrual cycle and mechanisms of anovulation. In: Knobil E, Neill JD, eds. Physiology of Reproduction. 2nd ed. New York: Raven, 1994: 2046–2058.

603. Knobil E, Neill JD, eds. The Physiology of Reproduction. 2nd ed. New York: Raven, 1994.

604. Davidson JM. Hormones and sexual behaviour in the male. In: Krieger DT, Hughes JC, eds. Neuroendocrinology. Sunderland, MA: Sinauer Associates, 1980: 232–238.

605. Gorski RA. Sexual differentiation of the brain. In: Krieger DT, Hughes JC, eds. Neuroendocrinology. Sunderland, MA: Sinauer Associates, 1980: 215–222.

606. Michael RP. Hormones and sexual behavior in the female. In: Krieger DT, Hughes JC, eds. Neuroendocrinology. Sunderland, MA: Sinauer Associates, 1980: 223–232.

607. Donovan BT, van der Werff, ten Bosch JJ. Physiology of Puberty. Baltimore: Williams & Wilkins, 1965.

608. Ojeda SR, Andrews WW, Advis JP, et al. Recent advances in the endocrinology of puberty. Endocr Rev 1980; 1:228–257.

609. Styne DM, Grumbach MM. Puberty in the male and female: its physiology and disorders. In: Yen SSC, Jaffe RB, eds. Reproductive Endocrinology: Physiology, Pathophysiology and Clinical Management. 2nd ed. Philadelphia: WB Saunders, 1986: 313–384.

610. McEwen BS, Biegon A, Davis PG, et al. Steroid hormones: humoral signals which alter brain cell properties and functions. Recent Prog Horm Res 1982; 38:41–83.

611. Koch M, Ehret G. Immunocytochemical localization and quantitation of estrogen-binding cells in the male and female (virgin, pregnant, lactating) mouse brain. Brain Res 1989; 489:101–112.

612. Bauer-Dantoin AC, Weiss J, Jameson JL. Roles of estrogen, progesterone, and gonadotropin-releasing hormone (GnRH) in the control of pituitary GnRH receptor gene expression at the time of the preovulatory gonadotropin surges. Endocrinology 1995; 136:1014–1019.

613. Zoeller RT, Seeburg PH, Young WS 3rd. In situ hybridization histochemistry for messenger ribonucleic acid (mRNA) encoding gonadotropin-releasing hormone (GnRH): effect of estrogen on cellular levels of GnRH mRNA in female rat brain. Endocrinology 1988; 122:2570–2577.

614. Rance NE, Uswándi SV. Gonadotropin-releasing hormone gene expression is increased in the medial basal hypothalamus of postmenopausal women. J Clin Endocrinol Metab 1996; 81:3540–3546.

615. Marshall JC, Case GD, Valk TW, et al. Selective inhibition of follicle-stimulating hormone secretion by estradiol. Mechanism for modulation of gonadotropin responses to low dose pulses of gonadotropin-releasing hormone. J Clin Invest 1983; 71:248–257.

616. Seyler LE Jr, Graze K, Canalis E, et al. Effects of sex-steroid priming on pituitary responses to LH-RH. In: Beling CG, Wentz AC, eds. The LH-Releasing Hormone. New York: Masson, 1980: 87–112.

617. Ling N, Ueno N, Ying SY, et al. Inhibins and activins. Vitam Horm 1988; 44:1–46.

618. Evans WS, Cronin MJ, Thorner MO. Hypogonadism in hyperprolactinemia: proposed mechanisms. In: Ganong WF, Martini L, eds. Frontiers in Neuroendocrinology. Vol 7. New York: Raven, 1982: 77–122.

619. Rivier C, Rivier J, ValE W. Stress-induced inhibition of reproductive functions: role of endogenous corticotropin-releasing factor. Science 1989; 23:607–609.

620. Emanuele NV, Kostka D, Wallock L, et al. Hypothalamic luteinizing hormone increases dramatically following intracerebroventricular injection of colchicine. Neuroendocrinology 1985; 41:526–528.

621. Emanuele NV, Metcalfe L, Wallock L, et al. Hypothalamic prolactin: characterization by radioimmunoassay and bioassay and response to hypophysectomy and restraint stress. Neuroendocrinology 1986; 44:217–221.

622. Motta M, Piva F, Martini L. The hypothalamus as the center of endocrine feedback mechanisms. In: Martini L, Motta M, Fraschini F, eds. The Hypothalamus. New York: Academic, 1970: 463–490.

623. Woller MJ, Terasawa E. Changes in pulsatile release of neuropeptide-Y and luteinizing hormone (LH)–releasing hormone during the progesterone-induced LH surge in rhesus monkeys. Endocrinology 1994; 135:1679–1686.

624. Junier MP, Ma YJ, Costa ME, et al. Transforming growth factor alpha contributes to the mechanism by which hypothalamic injury induces precocious puberty. Proc Natl Acad Sci USA 1991; 88:9743–9747.

625. Quigley ME, Sheehan KL, Casper RF, et al. Evidence for an increased opioid inhibition of luteinizing hormone secretion in hyperprolactinemic patients with pituitary microadenoma. J Clin Endocrinol Metab 1980; 50:427–430.

626. Pau KY, Berria M, Hess DL, et al. Preovulatory gonadotropin-releasing hormone surge in ovarian intact rhesus macaques. Endocrinology 1993; 133:1650–1656.

627. Knobil E, Hotchkiss J. The menstrual cycle and its neuroendocrine control 1971–1984. In: Knobil E, Neill JD, eds. The Physiology of Reproduction. New York: Raven, 1988: 1143–1160.

628. Conn PM, Crowley WF Jr. Gonadotropin-releasing hormone and its analogs. Annu Rev Med 1994; 45:391–405.

629. Santoro N, Filicori M, Crowley WF Jr. Hypogonadotropic disorders in men and women: diagnosis and therapy with pulsatile gonadotropin-releasing hormone. Endocr Rev 1986; 17:11–23.

630. Spinder T, Spijkstra JJ, Gooren J, et al. Effects of long-term testosterone administration on gonadotropin secretion in agonadal female to male transsexuals compared with hypogonadal and normal women. J Clin Endocrinol Metab 1989; 68:200–207.

631. Gorski RA. Steroid-induced sexual characteristics in the brain. In: Müller EE, MacLeod RM, eds. Neuroendocrine Perspectives. Vol 2. Amsterdam: Elsevier Biomedical, 1983: 1–35.

632. Arendash GW, Gorski RA. Enhancement of sexual behavior in female rats by neonatal transplantation of brain tissue from males. Science 1982; 217:1276–1278.

633. Schumacher M, Legros JJ, Balthazart J. Steroid hormones, behavior, and sexual dimorphism in animals and men: the nature-nurture controversy. Exp Clin Endocrinol 1987; 90:129–156.

634. Gooren L. The neuroendocrine response of luteinizing hormone to estrogen administration in heterosexual, homosexual, and transsexual subjects. J Clin Endocrinol Metab 1986; 63:583–588.

635. Gooren LJG, Money J. Normal and abnormal sexual behavior In DeGroot LJ, ed. Endocrinology. 3rd ed. Philadelphia: WB Saunders, 1995: 1978–1992.

636. Madeira MD, Lieberman AR. Sexual dimorphism in the mammalian limbic system. Prog Neurobiol 1995; 45:275–333.

637. LeVay S. A difference in hypothalamic structure between heterosexual and homosexual men. Science 1991; 253:1034–1037.

638. Allen LS, Gorski RA. Sexual orientation and the size of the anterior commissure in the human brain. Proc Natl Acad Sci USA 1992; 89:7199–8202.

639. Zhou J-N, Hofman MA, Gooren LJG, et al. A sex difference in the human brain and its relation to transsexuality. Nature 1995; 378:68–70.

640. Klein KO, Baron J, Colli MJ, et al. Estrogen levels in childhood determined by an ultrasensitive recombinant cell bioassay. J Clin Invest 1994; 94:2475–2480.

641. Ojeda SR, Smith SS, Urbanski HF, et al. Onset of female puberty: underlying neuroendocrine mechanisms. In: Müller EE, MacLeod RM, eds. Neuroendocrine Perspectives. Vol 3. Amsterdam: Elsevier Biomedical 1984: 225–278.

642. Weinberger LM, Grant FC. Precocious puberty and tumors of the hypothalamus. Arch Intern Med 1941; 67:762–792.

643. Junier MP, Ma YJ, Costa ME, et al. Transforming growth factor alpha contributes to the mechanism by which hypothalamic injury induces precocious puberty. Proc Natl Acad Sci USA 1991; 88:9743–9747.

644. Ma YJ, Hill DF, Junier MP, et al. Expression of epidermal growth factor receptor changes in the hypothalamus during the onset of female puberty. Mol Cell Neurosci 1994; 5:246–262.

645. Ma YJ, Costa ME, Ojeda SR. Developmental expression of the genes encoding transforming growth factor alpha and its receptor in the hypothalamus of female rhesus macaques. Neuroendocrinology 1994; 60:346–359.

646. Frisch RE. Fatness, menarche, and female fertility. Perspect Biol Med 1985; 28:611–633.

647. Frisch RE. Body fat, menarche, fitness and fertility. Prog Reprod Biol Med 1990; 14:1–26.

648. McArthur JW, Beitins IZ, Bullen BA. Motility, nutrition and reproduction: recent clues to an ancient relationship. In: Givens JR, ed. The Hypothalamus. Chicago: Year Book Medical, 1984: 171–188.

649. Bates GW, Whitworth NS. Effects of body weight on female reproductive function. In: Givens JR, ed. The Hypothalamus. Chicago: Year Book Medical, 1984: 97–115.

Pheromones and Sexual Function

650. Crowley WR, Zemlan FP. The neurochemical control of mating behavior. In: Adler NT, ed. Neuroendocrinology of Reproduction. New York: Plenum, 1981: 451–484.

651. Rees HD, Switz GM, Michael RP. The estrogen-sensitive neural system in the brain of female cats. J Comp Neurol 1980; 193:789–804.

652. Michael RP, Bonsall RW, Rees HD. The nuclear accumulation of [³H] testosterone and [³H] estradiol in the brain of the female primate: evidence for the aromatization hypothesis. Endocrinology 1986; 118:1935–1944.

653. Leshner AI. Pheromonal and ultrasonic communication. In: An Introduction to Behavioral Endocrinology. New York: Oxford University Press, 1978: 114–145.

654. Aron C. Mechanisms of control of the reproduction function of olfactory stimuli in female mammals. Physiol Rev 1979; 59:229–284.

655. Singer AG, Clancy AN, Macrides F, et al. Chemical properties of a female mouse pheromone that stimulates gonadotropin secretion in males. Biol Reprod 1988; 38:193–199.

656. Magert HJ, Hadrys T, Cieslak A, et al. cDNA sequence and expression pattern of the putative pheromone carrier aphrodisin. Proc Natl Acad Sci USA 1995; 92:20910-20915.

657. Michael RP, Zumpe D. Influence of olfactory signals on the reproductive behaviour of social groups of rhesus monkeys (Macaca mulatta). J Endocrinol 1982; 95:189–205.

658. McClintock MK. Menstrual synchrony and suppression. Nature 1971; 229:244–245.

659. Weller L, Weller A. Menstrual synchrony: agenda for future research. Psychoneuroendocrinology 1995; 20:377–383.

660. Smals AG, Weusten JJ. 16-ene-steroids in the human testis. J Steroid Biochem Mol Biol 1991; 40:587–592.

661. Mallet AI, Holland KT, Rennie PJ, et al. Applications of gas chromatography–mass spectrometry in the study of androgen and odorous 16-androstene metabolism by human axillary bacteria. J Chromatogr 1991; 562:647–658.

662. Crowley JJ, Brooksbank BW. Human exposure to putative pheromones and

changes in aspects of social behaviour. J Steroid Biochem Mol Biol 1991; 39:647–659.

The Pineal Gland and Melatonin

663. Rolleston HD. The Endocrine Organs in Health and Disease with an Historical Review. New York: Oxford University Press, 1936: 452.

664. Wurtman RJ, Axelrod J, Kelly DE. The Pineal. New York: Academic, 1968.

665. Pévet P. Anatomy of the pineal gland of mammals. In: Relkin R, ed. The Pineal Gland. New York: Elsevier Biomedical, 1983: 1–76.

666. Kappers JA, Smith AR, De Vries RAC. The mammalian pineal gland and its control of hypothalamic activity. Prog Brain Res 1974; 41:149–174.

667. Wurtman RJ, Axelrod J. The pineal gland. Sci Am 1965; 213:50–60.

668. Klein DC. The pineal gland: a model of neuroendocrine regulation. In: Reichlin S, Baldessarini RJ, Martin JB, eds. The Hypothalamus. Vol 56. New York: Raven, 1978: 303–327.

669. Lewy AJ. Biochemistry and regulation of mammalian melatonin production. In: Relkin R, ed. The Pineal Gland. New York: Elsevier Biomedical, 1983: 77–128.

670. Arendt J. The pineal gland: basic physiology and clinical implications. In: DeGroot LJ, ed. Endocrinology. 3rd ed. Philadelphia: WB Saunders, 1995: 432–444.

671. Reiter RJ. The pineal and its hormones in the control of reproduction in mammals. Endocr Rev 1980; 1:109–131.

672. Moskowitz MA, Wurtman RJ. Pathological states involving the pineal. In: Martini L, Besser GM, eds. Clinical Neuroendocrinology. New York: Academic, 1977: 503–526.

673. Axelrod L. Endocrine dysfunction in patients with tumors of the pineal region. In: Schmidek HH, ed. Pineal Tumors. New York: Masson, 1977: 61–77.

674. Schmidt F, Penka B, Trauner M, et al. Lack of pineal growth during childhood. J Clin Endocrinol Metab 1995; 80:1221–1225.

675. Young IM, Francis PL, Leone AM, et al. Constant pineal output and increasing body mass account for declining melatonin levels during human growth and sexual maturation. J Pineal Res 1988; 5:71–85.

676. Waldhauser F, Weiszenbacher G, Frisch H, et al. Fall in nocturnal serum melatonin during prepuberty and pubescence. Lancet 1984; 1:362–365.

677. Waldhauser F, Boepple PA, Schemper M. Serum melatonin in central precocious puberty is lower than in age-matched prepubertal children. J Clin Endocrinol Metab 1991; 73:793–796.

677a. Luboshitzky R, Lavi S, Thuma I, et al. Increased nocturnal melatonin secretion in male patients with hypogonadotropic hypogonadism and delayed puberty. J Clin Endocrinol Metab 1995; 80:2144–2148.

678. Silman RE, Leone RM, Hooper RJ, et al. Melatonin, the pineal gland and human puberty. Nature 1979; 282:301–303.

679. Fevre M, Segel T, Marks JF, et al. LH and melatonin secretion patterns in pubertal boys. J Clin Endocrinol Metab 1978; 47:1383–1386.

680. Penny R. Melatonin excretion in normal males and females: increase during puberty. Metabolism 1982; 8:816–823.

681. Ehrenkranz JR, Tamarkin L, Comite F, et al. Daily rhythms of plasma melatonin in normal and precocious puberty. J Clin Endocrinol Metab 1982; 55:307–310.

682. Tetsuo M, Poth M, Markey SP. Melatonin metabolite excretion during childhood and puberty. J Clin Endocrinol Metab 1982; 55:311–313.

683. Cavallo A, Plasma melatonin rhythm in disorders of puberty; interactions of age and pubertal states. Horm Res 1991; 36:16–21.

684. Cavallo A, Richards GE, Smith ER. Relations between nocturnal melatonin profile and hormonal markers of puberty in humans. Horm Res 1992; 37:185–189.

685. Arendt J, Labib MH, Bojkowski C, et al. Rapid decrease in melatonin production during successful treatment of delayed puberty. Lancet 1989; 1:1326 (letter).

686. Cavallo A. Melatonin secretion during adrenarche in normal human puberty and in pubertal disorders. J Pineal Res 1992; 12:71–78.

687. Relkin R. Pineal-hormonal interactions. In: Relkin R, ed. The Pineal Gland. New York: Elsevier Biomedical, 1983: 225–246.

688. Blask DE, Vaughn MK, Reiter RJ. Pineal peptides and reproduction. In: Relkin R, ed. The Pineal Gland. New York: Elsevier Biomedical, 1983: 201–224.

689. Lerner AB, Case JD, Heinzelman RV. Structure of melatonin. J Am Chem Soc 1959; 81:6084–6085.

690. Coon SL, Roseboom PH, Baler R, et al. Pineal serotonin N-acetyltransferase: expression cloning and molecular analysis. Science 1995; 270:1681–1683.

691. Wetterberg L. Melatonin in humans: physiological and clinical studies. J Neural Transmission (Suppl) 1978; 13:289–310.

692. Weinberg U, D'Eletto RD, Weitzman ED, et al. Circulating melatonin in man: episodic secretion throughout the light-dark cycle. J Clin Endocrinol Metab 1979; 48:114–118.

693. Cardinali DP. Melatonin: a mammalian pineal hormone. Endocr Rev 1981; 2:327–346.

694. Martin JE, McKellar S, Klein DC. Melatonin inhibition of the in vivo pituitary response to luteinizing hormone–releasing hormone in the neonatal rat. Neuroendocrinology 1980; 31:13–17.

695. Weaver DR, Stehle JH, Stopa EG, et al. Melatonin receptors in human hypothalamus and pituitary: implications for circadian and reproductive responses to melatonin. J Clin Endocrinol Metab 1993; 76:295–301.

696. Reppert SM, Weaver DR, Ebisawa T. Cloning and characterization of a mammalian melatonin receptor that mediates reproductive and circadian responses. Neuron 1994; 13:1177–1185.

697. Pierpaoli W, Lesnikov VA. The pineal aging clock. Evidence, models, mechanisms, interventions. Ann NY Acad Sci 1994; 719:461–473.

698. Pierpaoli W, Regeleson W. The Melatonin Miracle. New York: Simon & Schuster, 1995.

699. Reiter RJ, Robinson J. Melatonin. New York: Bantam Books, 1995.

700. Cowley G. Melatonin Mania. Newsweek Nov 6 1995; 126:60.

701. Arendt J, Aldhous M, Marks V. Alleviation of jet lag by melatonin: preliminary results of controlled double blind trial. Br Med J 1986; 292:1170.

702. Brown GM. Light, melatonin and the sleep-wake cycle. J Psychiatry Neurosci 1994; 19:345–353.

703. Lewy AJ, Sack RL, Blood ML, et al. Melatonin marks circadian phase position and resets the endogenous circadian pacemaker in humans. Ciba Found Symp 1995; 183:303–317.

704. Hill SM, Blask DE. Effects of the pineal hormone melatonin on the proliferation and morphological characteristics of human breast cancer cells (MCF-7) in culture. Cancer Res 1988; 48:6121–6126.

705. Molis TM, Spriggs LL, Jupiter Y, et al. Melatonin modulation of estrogen-regulated proteins, growth factors, and proto-oncogenes in human breast cancer. J Pineal Res 1995; 18:93–103.

706. Pierpaoli WP, Regelson W. Pineal control of aging: effect of melatonin and pineal grafting on aging mice. Proc Natl Acad Sci USA 1994; 94:787–791.

707. Maestroni GJ. T-helper-2 lymphocytes as a peripheral target of melatonin. J Pineal Res 1995; 187:84–89.

708. Cagnoni ML, Lombardi A, Cerinic MM, et al. Melatonin for treatment of chronic refractory sarcoidosis. Lancet 1995; 346:1229–1230.

709. Reiter RJ. Oxidative processes and antioxidative defense mechanisms in the aging brain. FASEB J 1995; 9:526–533.

710. Reppert SM, Weaver DR. Melatonin madness. Cell 1995; 83:1059–1062.

711. Turek FW. Melatonin hype hard to swallow. Nature 96; 379:295–296.

712. Winkler P, Helmke K. Age-related incidence of pineal gland calcification in children: a roentgenological study of 1,044 skull films and a review of the literature. J Pineal Res 1987; 4:247–252.

713. McKinley MJ, McAllen RM, Mendelsohn FAO, et al. Circumventricular organs: neuroendocrine interfaces between the brain and the hemal milieu. Front Neuroendocrinol 1990; 11:91–127.

714. Weindl A, Sofroniew MV. Relation of neuropeptides to mammalian circumventricular organs. Adv Biochem Psychopharmacol 1981; 28:303–320.

715. Gross PM. Circumventricular organ capillaries. Prog Brain Res 1992; 91:219–233.

716. Johnson AK, Gross PM. Sensory circumventricular organs and brain homeostatic pathways. FASEB J 1993; 7:678–686.

717. Rodriguez EM, Oksche A, Hein S, et al. Cell biology of the subcommissural organ. Int Rev Cytol 1992; 135:39–121.

718. Losecke W, Naumann W, Sterba G. Preparation and discharge of secretion in the subcommissural organ of the rat. An electron-microscopic immunocytochemical study. Cell Tissue Res 1984; 235:201–206.

719. Cifuentes M, Rodriguez S, Perez J, et al. Decreased cerebrospinal fluid flow through the central canal of the spinal cord of rats immunologically deprived of Reissner's fibre. Exp Brain Res 1994; 98:431–440.

720. Akert K. The mammalian subfornical organ. J Neuro–Visceral Relations 1969; 31(Suppl 9):78–94.

721. Pickel VM, Chan J, Ganten D. Dual peroxidase and colloidal gold-labeling study of angiotensin converting enzyme and angiotensin-like immunoreactivity in the rat subfornical organ. J Neurosci 1986; 6:2457–2469.

722. Hellman W, Suzuki F, Ohkubo H, et al. Angiotensinogen gene expression in extrahepatic rat tissues: application of a solution hybridization assay. Naunyn Schmiedebergs Arch Pharmacol 1988; 338:327–331.

723. Standaert DG, Saper CB. Origin of the atriopeptin-like immunoreactive innervation of the paraventricular nucleus of the hypothalamus. J Neurosci 1988; 8:1940–1950.

724. Saper CB, Breder CD. The neurologic basis of fever. N Engl J Med 1994; 330:1880–1886.

725. Blatteis CM, Hales JR, McKinley MJ, et al. Role of the anteroventral third ventricle region in fever in sheep. Can J Physiol Pharmacol 1987; 65:1255–1260.

726. Sagar SM, Price KJ, Kasting NW, et al. Anatomic patterns of Fos immunostaining in rat brain following systemic endotoxin administration. Brain Res Bull 1995; 36:381–392.

727. Miller AD, Leslie RA. The area postrema and vomiting. Front Neuroendocrinol 1994; 15:301–320.

728. Watkins LR, Maier SF, Goehler LE. Cytokine-to-brain communication: a review & analysis of alternative mechanisms. Life Sci 1995; 57:1011–1026.

729. Kummer W, Neuhuber WL. Vagal paraganglia of the rat. J Electron Microsc (Tokyo) 1989; 12:343–355.

Neuroendocrine Disease

730. Riddoch G. Clinical aspects of hypothalamic disease. In: Le Gros Clark WE, Beattie J, Riddoch G, et al, eds. The Hypothalamus. Edinburgh: Oliver and Boyd, 1938: 101–130.

731. Daniel PM, Treip CS. The pathology of the hypothalamus. Clin Endocrinol Metab 1977; 6:3–19.

732. Plum F, Van Uitert R. Nonendocrine diseases and disorders of the hypothalamus. In: Reichlin S, Baldessarini RJ, Martin JB, eds. The Hypothalamus. Vol 56. New York: Raven, 1978: 415–473.

733. Scheithauer BW. The hypothalamus and neurohypophysis. In: Kovacs K, Asa SL, eds. Functional Endocrine Pathology. Boston: Blackwell Scientific, 1990: 170–244.

734. Swaab DF, Hofman MA, Lucassen PJ, et al. Functional neuroanatomy and neuropathology of the human hypothalamus. Anat Embryol 1993; 187:317–330.

735. Krieger DT, Glick S, Silverberg A, et al. A comparative study of endocrine tests in hypothalamic disease. Circadian periodicity of plasma 11-OHCS and growth hormone response to insulin hypoglycemia and metyrapone responsiveness. J Clin Endocrinol Metab 1968; 28:1589–1598.

736. Reichlin S. Functional aspects of endocrine neoplasms. In: Kovacs K, Asa SL, eds. Functional Endocrine Pathology. Boston: Blackwell Scientific, 1990: 898–913.

737. Randall RV, Clark EC, Dodge HW, et al. Polyuria after operation for tumors in the region of the hypophysis and hypothalamus. J Clin Endocrinol Metab 1960; 20:1614–1621.

738. Hollinshead WH. The interphase of diabetes insipidus. Mayo Clin Proc 1964; 39:92–100.

739. Fisher C, Ingram WR, Ranson SW. Diabetes Insipidus and the Neurohormonal Control of Water Balance. Ann Arbor, MI: Edwards Brothers, 1938.

740. Green JR, Buchan GC, Alvord EC Jr. Hereditary and idiopathic types of diabetes insipidus. Brain 1967; 90:707–714.

741. Scherbaum WA, Bottazzo GF. Autoantibodies to vasopressin cells in idiopathic diabetes insipidus: evidence for an autoimmune variant. Lancet 1983; 1:897–901.

742. Dugger GS, Van Wyk JJ, Newsome JF. The effect of pituitary-stalk section on thyroid function and gonadotropic-hormone secretion in women with mammary carcinoma. J Neurosurg 1962; 19:589–593.

743. Van Wyk JJ, Dugger GS, Newsome JF, et al. The effect of pituitary stalk section on the adrenal function of women with cancer of the breast. J Clin Endocrinol Metab 1960; 20:157–172.

744. Lipsett MB, West CD, MacLean JP, et al. Adrenal function after hypophysectomy in man. J Clin Endocrinol Metab 1957; 17:356–363.

745. Hökfelt T, Luft R. The effect of suprasellar tumours on the regulation of adrenocortical function. Acta Endocrinol 1959; 32:177.

746. Anthony GJ, Van Wyk JJ, French FS. Influence of pituitary stalk section on growth hormone, insulin and TSH secretion in women with metastatic breast cancer. J Clin Endocrinol Metab 1969; 29:1238–1250.

747. Li MC, Rall JE, MacLean JP, et al. Thyroid function following hypophysectomy in man. J Clin Endocrinol Metab 1955; 15:1228–1238.

748. Ehni G, Eckles NE. Interruption of the pituitary stalk in the patient with mammary cancer. J Neurosurg 1959; 16:628–652.

749. Molitch ME, Reichlin S. Hypothalamic hyperprolactinemia: neuroendocrine regulation in man. In: MacLeod RM, Thorner MO, Scapagnini V, eds. Prolactin, Basis and Clinical Correlates. Padua: Liviana, 1985: 709–719.

750. Smith MV, Laws ER Jr. Magnetic resonance imaging measurements of pituitary stalk compression and deviation in patients with nonprolactin-secreting intrasellar and parasellar tumors: lack of correlation with prolactin levels. Neurosurgery 1994; 34:834–839.

751. Haney AF, Kramer RS, Wiebe RH, et al. Hypothalamic-pituitary function and radiographic evaluation of women with hyperprolactinemia and an "empty" sella turcica. Am J Obstet Gynecol 1979; 134:917–924.

752. Cacciari E, Zucchini S, Abrosetto P, et al. Empty sella in children and adolescents with possible hypothalamic-pituitary disorders. J Clin Endocrinol Metab 1994; 78:767–771.

753. Adams JH, Daniel PM, Prichard MM. Some effects of transection of the pituitary stalk. Br Med J 1964; 2:1619–1625.

754. Adams JH, Daniel PM, Prichard MM. Transection of the pituitary stalk in man: anatomic changes in the pituitary glands of 21 patients. J Neurol Neurosurg Psychiatry 1966; 29:545–555.

Hypophyseotropic Hormone Deficiency

755. Lamberton RP, Jackson IMD. Investigation of hypothalamic-pituitary disease. Clin Endocrinol Metab 1983; 12:509–534.

756. Beck-Peccoz P, Amr S, Menezes-Ferriera M, et al. Decreased receptor binding of biologically inactive thyrotropin in central hypothyroidism. N Engl J Med 1985; 312:1085–1090.

757. Samuels MH, Ridgway EC. Central hypothyroidism. Endocrinol Metab Clin North Am 1992; 21:903–919.

758. Cobb WE, Reichlin S, Jackson IMD. Growth hormone secretory status is a determinant of the thyrotropin response to thyrotropin releasing hormone (TRH) in euthyroid patients with hypothalamic-pituitary disease. J Clin Endocrinol Metab 1981; 52:324–329.

759. Jorgensen JOL, Pederson SA, Laurberg P, et al. Effects of growth hormone therapy on thyroid function of growth hormone–deficient adults with and without concomitant thyroxine-substituted central hypothyroidism. J Clin Endocrinol Metab 1989; 69:1127–1132.

760. Crowley WF Jr, Jameson JL. Clinical counterpoint: gonadotropin-releasing hormone deficiency: perspectives from clinical investigation. Endocr Rev 1992; 13:635–640.

761. Santen RJ, Paulsen CA. Hypogonadotropic enuchoidism. I: Clinical study of the mode of inheritance. J Clin Endocrinol Metab 1973; 36:47–54.

762. Klinmuller D, Dewes W, Krahe T, et al. Magnetic resonance imaging of the brain in patients with anosmia and hypothalamic hypogonadism (Kallman's syndrome). J Clin Endocrinol Metab 1987; 65:581–584.

763. Krause Brucker W, Gardner DW. Optic nerve hypoplasia associated with absent septum pellucidum and hypopituitarism. Am J Ophthalmol 1980; 89:113–120.

764. Fitz CR. Holoprosencephaly and related entities. Neuroradiology 1983; 25:225–238.

765. Mortimer CH, Besser GH, McNeilly AS, et al. The luteinizing hormone and follicle stimulating hormone–releasing hormone test in patients with hypothalamic-pituitary-gonadal dysfunction. Br Med J 1974; 4:73–77.

766. Mortimer CH. Gonadotropin-releasing hormone. In: Martini L, Besser GM, eds. Clinical Neuroendocrinology. New York: Academic, 1977: 213–236.

767. Roth JC, Grumbach MM, Kaplan SL. Effect of synthetic luteinizing hormone–releasing factor on serum testosterone and gonadotropins in prepubertal, pubertal and adult males. J Clin Endocrinol Metab 1973; 37:680–686.

768. Costom BH, Grumbach MM, Kaplan SL. Effects of thyrotropin-releasing factor on serum thyroid stimulating hormone: an approach to distinguishing hypothalamic from pituitary forms of idiopathic hypopituitary dwarfism. J Clin Invest 1971; 50:2219–2225.

769. Schriock EA, Lustig RH, Rosenthal SM, et al. Effect of growth hormone (GH)–releasing hormone (GRH) on plasma GH in relation to magnitude and duration of GH deficiency in 26 children and adults with isolated GH deficiency or multiple pituitary hormone deficiencies: evidence for hypothalamic GRH deficiency. J Clin Endocrinol Metab 1984; 58:1043–1049.

770. Grossman A, Savage MO, Wass JA, et al. Growth-hormone–releasing factor in growth hormone deficiency: demonstration of a hypothalamic defect in growth hormone release. Lancet 1983; 2:137–138.

771. Liu N, Grumbach MM, de Napoli RA. Prevalence of electroencephalographic abnormalities in idiopathic precocious puberty and premature pubarche: bearing on pathogenesis and neuroendocrine regulation of puberty. J Clin Endocrinol Metab 1965; 25:1296–1308.

772. Kikuchi K, Fujisawa I, Momoi T, et al. Hypothalamic-pituitary function in growth hormone–deficient patients with pituitary stalk transection. J Clin Endocrinol Metab 1988; 67:817–823.

773. Triulzi F, Scotti G, di Natale B, et al. Evidence of a congenital midline brain anomaly in pituitary dwarfs: a magnetic resonance imaging study in 101 patients. Pediatrics 1994; 93:409–416.

774. Stewart C, Castro-Magana M, Sherman J, et al. Septo-optic dysplasia and median cleft face syndrome in a patient with isolated growth hormone deficiency and hyperprolactinemia. Am J Dis Child 1983; 137:484–487.

775. Molitch ME. Pathological hyperprolactinemia. Endocrinol Metab Clin North Am 1992; 21:877–901.

776. Stacpoole PW, Interland JW, Nicholson WE, et al. Isolated ACTH deficiency: a heterogeneous disorder. Critical review and report of four new cases. Medicine (Baltimore) 1982; 61:13–24.

777. Sauter NP, Toni R, McLaughlin CD, et al. Isolated adrenocorticotropin deficiency associated with an autoantibody to a corticotroph antigen that is not adrenocorticotropin or other proopiomelanocortin-derived peptides. J Clin Endocrinol Metab 1990; 70:1391–1397.

778. Schulte HM, Chrousos GP, Avgerinos P. The corticotropin releasing factor stimulation test: a possible aid in the evaluation of adrenal insufficiency. J Clin Endocrinol Metab 1984; 58:1064–1067.

779. Fukakta J, Shimuzu N, Imura H, et al. Human corticotropin–releasing hormone test in patients with hypothalamo-pituitary-adrenocortical disorders. Endocr J 1993; 40:597–606.

780. Brauner R, Rappaport R, Prevot C, et al. A prospective study of the development of growth hormone deficiency in children given cranial irradiation, and its relation to statural growth. J Clin Endocrinol Metab 1989; 68:346–351.

781. Ogilvy-Stuart AL, Wallace WH, Shalet SM. Radiation and neuroregulatory control of growth hormone secretion. Clin Endocrinol 1994; 41:163–168.

Hypophyseotropic Hormone Hypersecretion

782. Pescovitz OH, Comite F, Hench K, et al. The NIH experience with precocious puberty: diagnostic subgroups and response to short-term luteinizing hormone analogue therapy. J Pediatr 1986; 108:47–54.

783. Asa SL, Kovacs K, Tindall GT, et al. Cushing's disease associated with an intrasellar gangliocytoma producing corticotrophin-releasing factor. Ann Intern Med 1984; 101:789–793.

784. Hashimoto K, Suemaru S, Hattori T, et al. Multiple endocrine neoplasia with Cushing's syndrome due to paraganglioma producing corticotropin-releasing factor and adrenocorticotropin. Acta Endocrinol 1986; 113:189–195.

785. Asa SL, Scheithauer BW, Bilbao JM, et al. A case for hypothalamic acromegaly: a clinicopathological study of six patients with hypothalamic gangliocytomas producing growth hormone-releasing factor. J Clin Endocrinol Metab 1984; 58:796–803.

Neuroendocrine Disorders of Gonadotropin Regulation

786. Wilkins L. The Diagnosis and Treatment of Endocrine Disorders in Childhood and Adolescence. 3rd ed. Springfield, IL: Charles C Thomas, 1965.
787. Bierich JR. Sexual precocity. J Clin Endocrinol Metab 1975; 4:107–142.
788. Richter RB. True hamartoma of the hypothalamus associated with pubertas praecox. J Neuropathol 1951; 10:368.
789. Judge DM, Kulin HE, Page R, et al. Hypothalamic hamartoma. A source of luteinizing-hormone–releasing factor in precocious puberty. N Engl J Med 1977; 296:7–10.
790. Hochman HI, Judge DM, Reichlin S. Precocious puberty and hypothalamic hamartoma. Pediatrics 1981; 67:236–244.
791. Comite F, Pescovitz OH, Rieth KG, et al. Luteinizing hormone–releasing hormone analog treatment of boys with hypothalamic hamartoma and true precocious puberty. J Clin Endocrinol Metab 1984; 59:888–892.
792. Berkovic SF, Andermann F, Melanson D, et al. Hypothalamic hamartomas and ictal laughter: evolution of a characteristic epileptic syndrome and diagnostic value of magnetic resonance imaging. Ann Neurol 1988; 23:429–439.
793. Van Wyk JJ, Grumbach MM. Syndrome of precocious menstruation and galactorrhea in juvenile hypothyroidism; an example of hormonal overlap in pituitary feedback. J Pediatr 1960; 57:416–435.
794. Wood LC, Olichney M, Locke H, et al. Syndrome of juvenile hypothyroidism associated with advanced sexual development: report of two new cases and comment on the management of an associated ovarian mass. J Clin Endocrinol Metab 1965; 25:1289–1295.
795. Anasti JN, Flack MR, Froehlich J, et al. A potential novel mechanism for precocious puberty in juvenile hypothyroidism. J Clin Endocrinol Metab 1995; 80:276–279.

Pineal Tumors

796. Moskowitz MA, Wurtman RJ. Pathological states involving the pineal. In: Martini L, Besser GM, eds. Clinical Neuroendocrinology. New York: Academic, 1977: 503–526.
797. DeGirolami U. Pathology of tumors of the pineal region. In: Schmidek HH, ed. Pineal Tumors. New York: Masson, 1977: 1–19.
798. Russell DS, Rubinstein LJ. Pathology of Tumours of the Nervous System. 5th ed. Baltimore: Williams & Wilkins, 1989: 380–394.
799. DeGirolami U, Schmidek HH. Clinicopathological study of 53 tumors of the pineal region. J Neurosurg 1973; 39:455–462.
800. Bagshawe KD, Harland S. Immunodiagnosis and monitoring of gonadotropin-producing metastases in the central nervous system. Cancer 1976; 38:112–118.
801. Tompkins VN, Haymaker W, Campbell EH. Metastatic pineal tumors. J Neurosurg 1950; 7:159–160.
802. Castleman B, McNeely BU. Case 25-1971 (germinoma). Case records of the Massachusetts General Hospital. N Engl J Med 1971; 284:1427–1434.
803. Spiegel AM, DiChiro G, Gorden P, et al. Diagnosis of radiosensitive hypothalamic tumors without craniotomy. Endocrine and neuroradiologic studies of intracranial atypical teratomas. Ann Intern Med 1976; 85:290–293.
804. Axelrod L. Endocrine dysfunction in patients with tumors of the pineal region. In: Schmidek HH, ed. Pineal Tumors. New York: Masson, 1977: 61–77.
805. Giovannelli G. Pineal region tumors: endocrinological aspects. Childs Brain 1982; 9:267–273.
806. Ahmed SR, Shalet SM, Price DA, et al. Human chorionic gonadotropin secreting pineal germinoma and precocious puberty. Arch Dis Child 1983; 58:743–745.
807. Sklar CA, Conte FA, Kaplan SL, et al. Human chorionic gonadotropin-secreting pineal tumor: relation to pathogenesis and sex limitation of sexual precocity. J Clin Endocrinol Metab 1981; 53:656–660.
808. Kubo O, Yamasaki N, Kamjo Y, et al. Human chorionic gonadotropin produced by ectopic pinealoma in a girl with precocious puberty. J Neurosurg 1977; 47:101–105.
809. Kurmado K, Mori W. Virus-like particles in human pinealoma. Acta Neuropathol (Berl) 1976; 37:273–276.
810. Ringertz N, Nordestam H, Flyger G. Tumors of the pineal region. J Neuropathol 1954; 13:540–561.
811. Bing JF, Globus JH, Simon H. Pubertas praecox: a survey of the reported cases and verified anatomic findings. Mt Sinai J Med NY 1938; 4:935–965.
812. Sklar CA, Grumbach MM, Kaplan SL, et al. Hormonal and metabolic abnormalities associated with central nervous system germinoma in children and adolescents and the effect of therapy: report of 10 patients. J Clin Endocrinol Metab 1981; 52:9–16.
813. Kornreich L, Horev G, Blaser S, et al. Central precocious puberty: evaluation by neuroimaging. Pediatr Radiol 1995; 25:7–11.
814. Kitay JI. Pineal lesions and precocious puberty: a review. J Clin Endocrinol Metab 1954; 14:622–625.
815. Kitay JI, Altschule MD. The Pineal Gland. Cambridge, MA: Harvard University Press, 1954.
816. Wurtman RJ, Kammer H. Melatonin synthesis by an ectopic pinealoma. N Engl J Med 1966; 274:1233–1237.
817. Wray SH. The neuro-ophthalmic and neurologic manifestations of pinealomas. In: Schmidek HH, ed. Pineal Tumors. New York: Masson, 1977: 61–77.
818. Schmidek HH. Surgical management of pineal region tumors. In: Schmidek HH, ed. Pineal Tumors. New York: Masson, 1977: 99–113.
819. Stein BM. Supracerebellar-infratentorial approach to pineal tumors. Surg Neurol 1979; 11:331–337.
820. Popovic EA, Kelly PJ. Stereotactic procedures for lesions of the pineal region. Mayo Clinic Proc 1993; 68:965–970.
821. Neuwelt EA, Glasberg M, Frenkel E, et al. Malignant pineal region tumors. A clinico-pathological study. J Neurosurg 1979; 51:597–607.
822. Brady LW. The role of radiation therapy. In: Schmidek HH, ed. Pineal Tumors. New York: Masson, 1977: 99–113.
823. Takeuchi J, Handa H, Nagata I. Suprasellar germinoma. J Neurosurg 1978; 49:41–48.
824. Baumgartner JE, Edwards MS. Pineal tumors. Neurosurg Clin North Am 1992; 3:853–862.
825. Rubin P, Kramer S. Ectopic pinealoma: a radiocurable neuroendocrinologic entity. Radiology 1965; 85:512–523.
826. Calaminus G, Bamberg M, Baranzelli MC, et al. Intracranial germ cell tumors: a comprehensive update of the European data. Neuropediatrics 1994; 25:26–32.
827. Jakacki RI, Zeltzer PM, Boyett JM, et al. Survival and prognostic factors following radiation and/or chemotherapy for primitive neuroectodermal tumors of the pineal region in infants and children: a report of the Children's Cancer Group. J Clin Oncol 1995; 13:1377–1383.
828. Herrman HD, Westphal M, Winkler K, et al. Treatment of nongerminomatous germ-cell tumors of the pineal region. Neurosurgery 1994; 324:524–529.
829. Wilson BE, Netzloff ML. Primary testicular abnormalities causing precocious puberty. Leydig cell tumor, Leydig cell hyperplasia, and adrenal rest tumor. Ann Clin Lab Sci 1983; 13:315–320.
830. Rosenthal SM, Grumbach MM, Kaplan SL. Gonadotropin-independent familial sexual precocity with premature Leydig and germinal cell maturation (familial testotoxicosis): effect of a potent luteinizing hormone-releasing factor agonist and medroxyprogesterone acetate therapy in four cases. J Clin Endocrinol Metab 1983; 57:571–579.
831. Kawate N, Kletter GB, Wilson BE, et al. Identification of constitutively activating mutation of the luteinizing hormone receptor in a family with male limited gonadotrophin independent precocious puberty (testotoxicosis). J Med Genet 1995; 32:553–554.
832. Mansfield MJ, Beardsworth DE, Loughlin JS, et al. Long-term treatment of central precocious puberty with a long-acting analogue of luteinizing hormone releasing hormone. N Engl J Med 1983; 309:1286–1290.
833. Pasul D, Conte FA, Grumbach MM, et al. Long-term effect of gonadotropin-releasing hormone agonist therapy on final and near-final height in 26 children with true precocious puberty treated at a median age of less than 5 years. J Clin Endocrinol Metab 1995; 80:546–551.
834. Shankar RR, Pescovitz OH. Precocious puberty. Adv Endocrinol Metab 1995; 6:55–89.
835. Holland FJ, Fishman L, Bailey JD, et al. Ketoconazole in the management of precocious puberty not responsive to LHRH-analogue therapy. N Engl J Med 1985; 312:1023–1028.
836. Money J, Hampson JG. Idiopathic sexual precocity in the male. Management: report of a case. Psychosom Med 1955; 17:1–15.
837. Money J, Alexander D. Psychosexual development and absence of homosexuality in males with precocious puberty. J Nerv Ment Dis 1969; 148:111–123.
838. Ehrhardt AA, Meyer-Bahlburg HFL. Psychologic correlates of abnormal pubertal development. Clin Endocrinol Metab 1975; 4:207–222.
839. Hampson JG, Money J. Idiopathic sexual precocity in the female. Report of 3 cases. Psychosom Med 1955; 17:16–35.

Psychogenic Amenorrhea

840. Ihalainen O. Psychosomatic aspects of amenorrhoea. Acta Psychiatr Scand 1975; 262(Suppl):1–139.
841. Barnea ER, Naftolin F, Tolis G, et al. Hypothalamic amenorrhea syndromes. In: Givens JR, ed. The Hypothalamus. Chicago: Year Book Medical, 1984: 147–170.
842. Khoury SA, Reame NE, Kelch RP, et al. Diurnal patterns of pulsatile luteinizing hormone secretion in hypothalamic amenorrhea: reproducibility and responses to opiate blockade and an alpha-2-adrenergic agonist. J Clin Endocrinol Metab 1987; 64:755–762.
843. Yen SSC. Female hypogonadotropic hypogonadism: Hypothalamic amenorrhea syndrome. Endocrinol Metab Clin North Am 1993; 22:29–58.
844. Rebar RW. Effects of exercise on reproductive function in females. In: Givens JR, ed. The Hypothalamus. Chicago: Year Book Medical, 1984: 245–262.
845. Biller BM, Coughlin JF, Saxe V, et al. Osteopenia in women with hypothalamic amenorrhea: a prospective study. Obstet Gynecol 1991; 78:996–1001.

Hypothalamic Hypogonadism in Men

846. Reichlin S. Introduction. In: Reichlin S, Baldessarini RJ, Martin JB, eds. The Hypothalamus. Vol 56. New York: Raven, 1978: 1–14.
847. Reichlin S. Overview of the anatomic and physiologic basis of anterior pituitary regulation. In: Tolis G, Labrie F, Martin JB, et al, eds. Clinical Neuroendocrinology. New York: Raven, 1979: 1–14.
848. Kreuz LE, Rose RM, Jennings JR, et al. Suppression of plasma testosterone levels and psychological stress. Arch Gen Psychiatry 1972; 26:479–482.

849. Yates A, Leehey K, Shisslak CM. Running—an analogue of anorexia? N Engl J Med 1983; 308:251–255.

850. Whitcomb RW, Crowley WF Jr. Male hypogonadotropic hypogonadism. Endocrinol Metab Clin North Am 1993; 22:125–143.

851. Spratt DT, Cox P, Orav J, et al. Reproductive axis suppression in acute illness is related to disease severity. J Clin Endocrinol Metab 1993; 76:1548–1554.

852. Singer F, Zumoff B. Subnormal serum testosterone levels in male internal medicine residents. Steroids 1992; 57:86–89.

853. Opstad K. Circadian rhythm of hormones is extinguished during prolonged physical stress, sleep and energy deficiency in young men. Eur J Endocrinol 1994; 131:56–66.

854. Young RJ, Strachan RK, Seth J, et al. Is testicular endocrine function abnormal in young men with spinal cord injuries? Clin Endocrinol 1982; 3:303–306.

855. Cortes-Gallegos V, Castaneda G, Alonso R, et al. Diurnal variations of pituitary and testicular hormones in paraplegic men. Arch Androl 1982; 8:221–226.

856. Huffer V, Scott WH, Connor TB, et al. Psychological studies of adult male patients with sexual infantilism before and after androgen therapy. Ann Intern Med 1964; 61:255–268.

857. Meierkord, H, Shorvon S, Lightman S, et al. Comparison of the effects of frontal and temporal lobe partial seizures on prolactin levels. Arch Neurol 1992; 49:225–230.

Neurogenic Disorders of Prolactin Regulation

858. Reichlin J, Molitch M. Neuroendocrine aspect of pituitary adenoma. In: Cammanni F, Muller EE, eds. Pituitary Hyperfunction: Physiopathology and Clinical Aspects. New York: Raven, 1984: 47–70.

859. Tucker HS, Lankford HV, Gardner DF, et al. Persistent defect in regulation of prolactin secretion after successful pituitary tumor removal in women with galactorrhea-amenorrhea syndrome. J Clin Endocrinol Metab 1980; 51:968–971.

860. Barbarino A, Marinis LDE, Menini E, et al. Pre- and postoperative pituitary function tests in patients with prolactin-secreting pituitary adenoma. In: Camanni F, Müller EE, eds. Pituitary Hyperfunction: Physiopathology and Clinical Aspects. New York: Raven, 1984: 333–342.

Neurogenic Disorders of Growth Hormone Secretion

861. Powell GF, Brasel JA, Blizzard RM. Emotional deprivation and growth retardation simulating idiopathic hypopituitarism. II. Endocrinologic evaluation of the syndrome. N Engl J Med 1967; 267:1279–1283.

862. Krieger L, Mellinger RC. Pituitary function in the deprivation syndrome. J Pediatr 1971; 79:216–225.

863. Whitten CF, Petit MG. Evidence that growth failure from maternal deprivation is secondary to undereating. JAMA 1969; 209:1675–1682.

864. Underwood LE, Van Wyk JJ. Hormones in normal aberrant growth. In: Williams RH, ed. Textbook of Endocrinology. 6th ed. Philadelphia: WB Saunders, 1981: 1149–1191.

865. Albanese A, Hamill G, Jones J, et al. Reversibility of physiological growth hormone secretion in children with psychosocial dwarfism. Clin Endocrinol 1994; 40:687–692.

866. Tannenbaum GS, Epelbaum J, Colle E, et al. Antiserum to somatostatin reverses starvation-induced inhibition of growth hormone but not insulin secretion. Endocrinology 1978; 102:1909–1914.

867. Wolff G, Money J. Relationship between sleep and growth in patients with reversible somatotropin deficiency (psychosocial dwarfism). Psychol Med 1973; 3:18–27.

868. Money J, Annecillo C, Kelley JF. Growth of intelligence: failure and catchup associated respectively with abuse and rescue in the syndrome of abuse dwarfism. Psychoneuroendocrinology 1983; 8:309–319.

869. Bercu BB, Shulman D, Root AW, et al. Growth hormone (GH) provocative testing frequently does not reflect endogenous GH secretion. J Clin Endocrinol Metab 1986; 63:709–716 (erratum 1987; 64:382).

870. Bercu BB, Diamond FB Jr. Growth hormone neurosecretory dysfunction. Clin Endocrinol Metab 1986; 15:537–590.

871. Lin TH, Kirkland RT, Sherman BM, et al. Growth hormone testing in short children and their response to growth hormone therapy. J Pediatr 1989; 115:57–63.

872. Cacciari E, Tassoni P, Cicognani A, et al. Value and limits of pharmacological and physiological tests to diagnose growth hormone (GH) deficiency and predict therapy response: first and second retesting during replacement therapy of patients defined as GH deficient. J Clin Endocrinol Metab 1994; 79:1663–1669.

873. Grumbach MM. Growth hormone therapy and the short end of the stick (editorial). N Engl J Med 1988; 319:238–241.

874. Burr IM, Slonim AE, Danish RK, et al. Diencephalic syndrome revisited. J Pediatr 1976; 88:439–444.

875. Drop SL, Guyda HJ, Colle E. Inappropriate growth hormone release in the diencephalic syndrome of childhood: case report and 4 year endocrinological follow-up. Clin Endocrinol 1980; 13:181–187.

876. Reichlin S. Neuroregulatory abnormalities of growth hormone secretion. In: Müller EE, Cocchi D, Locatelli V, eds. Advances in Growth Hormone and Growth Factor Research. Rome: Pythagora, 1989: 445–464.

877. Ho KY, Veldhuis JD, Johnson ML, et al. Fasting enhances growth hormone secretion and amplifies the complex rhythms of growth hormone secretion in man. J Clin Invest 1988; 81:968–975.

878. Atiea JA, Cregagh F, Page M, et al. Early-morning hyperglycemia in IDDM. Acute effects of cholinergic blockade. Diabetes Care 1989; 12:443–448.

879. Molitch M. Pathogenesis of pituitary tumors. Endocrinol Metab Clin North Am 1987; 16:503–528.

880. Faglia G, Spada A, Ambrosi B, et al. What's the role of the hypothalamus in pituitary adenoma formation? In: Melmed S, Robbins RJ, eds. Molecular and Clinical Advances in Pituitary Disorders. Boston: Blackwell Scientific, 1991: 213–228.

881. Saeger W, Puchner MJ, Ludecke DK. Combined sellar gangliocytoma and pituitary adenoma in acromegaly or Cushing's disease. A report of 3 cases. Virchows Arch 1994: 425:93–99.

Neurogenic Disorders of Corticotropin Regulation

882. Gold PW, Goodwin FK, Chrousos GP. Clinical and biochemical manifestations of depression. Relation to the neurobiology of stress. N Engl J Med 1988; 319:348–353, 413–420.

883. Wolff SM, Adler RC, Buskirk ER, et al. A syndrome of periodic hypothalamic discharge. Am J Med 1964; 36:956–967.

Nonendocrine Manifestations of Hypothalamic Disease

884. Plum FC, Uitert RV. Nonendocrine diseases and disorders of the hypothalamus. In: Reichlin S, Baldessarini RJ, Martin JB, eds. The Hypothalamus. Vol 56. New York: Raven, 1978: 415–474.

885. Krieger DT. The hypothalamus and neuroendocrine pathology. In: Krieger DT, Hughes JC, eds. Neuroendocrinology. Sunderland, MA: Sinauer Associates, 1980: 13–22.

886. Morgane PJ, Panksepp J. The Handbook of the Hypothalamus. Behavioral Studies of the Hypothalamus. Vol 3, Parts A and B. New York: Marcel Dekker, 1980, 1981.

887. Fischer EG, Welch K, Belli JA, et al. Treatment of craniopharyngiomas in children. J Neurosurg 1985; 62:496–501.

Glucocorticoid Effects on the Brain

888. Green M. Benign intracranial hypertension (pseudotumor cerebri). Pediatr Clin North Am 1967; 14:819–830.

889. Sapolsky RM, Plotsky PM. Hypercorticolism and its possible neural bases. Biol Psychiatry 1990; 27:937–952.

890. Sapolsky R. Stress, the Aging Brain and the Mechanisms of Neuron Death. Cambridge: MIT Press, 1992.

Eating Behavior and Neuropeptides

891. Schneider BS, Friedman JM, Hirsch J. Feeding behavior. In: Krieger DT, Brownstein MJ, Martin JB, eds. Brain Peptides. New York: John Wiley & Sons, 1983: 251–279.

892. Morley JE. Neuropeptide regulation of appetite and weight. Endocr Rev 1987; 8:256–287.

893. Leibowitz SF. Neurochemical-neuroendocrine systems in the brain controlling macronutrient intake and metabolism. Trends Neurosci 1992; 15:491–497.

894. Zhang Y, Proenca A, Maffei M, et al. Positional cloning of the mouse obese gene and its human homologue. Nature 1994; 372:425–434.

895. Smith GP, Gibbs J, Jerome C, et al. The satiety effect of cholecystokinin: a progress report. Peptides 1981; 2:57–59.

896. Baile CA, Della-Fera MA, McLaughlin CL. Hormones and feed intake. Proc Nutr Soc 1983; 42:113–127.

897. McHugh PR. The control of gastric emptying. J Auton Nerv Syst 1983; 9:221–231.

898. Smith GT, Moran TH, Coyle JT, et al. Anatomic localization of cholecystokinin receptors to the pyloric sphincter. Am J Physiol 1984; 246:R127–R130.

899. Dourish CT, Rycroft W, Iversen SD. Postponement of satiety by blockade of brain cholecystokinin (CCK-B) receptors. Science 1989; 245:1509–1511.

900. Stanley BG, Kyrkouli SE, Lampert S, et al. Neuropeptide Y chronically injected into the hypothalamus: a powerful neurochemical inducer of hyperphagia and obesity. Peptides 1986; 7:1189–1192.

901. Saladin R, De Vos P, Guerre-Millo M, et al. Transient increase in obese gene expression after food intake or insulin administration. Nature 1995; 377:527–529.

902. Considine RV, Sinha MK, Heiman ML. Serum immunoreactive leptin concentrations in normal-weight and obese persons. N Engl J Med 1996; 334:292–295.

903. Tartaglia LA, Dembski M, Weng X, et al. Identification and expression cloning of a leptin receptor, OB-R. Cell 1995; 83:1263–1271.

904. Stephens TW, Basinski M, Bristow PK, et al. The role of neuropeptide Y in the antiobesity action of the obesity gene product. Nature 1995; 377:530–532.

905. Rohner-Jeanrenaud F, Jeanrenaud B. Obesity, leptin and the brain. N Engl J Med 1996; 334:324–325.

Neurosteroids and Steroid Metabolism in Brain

906. McClusky NJ, Walters MJ, Clark ASD, et al. Aromatase in the cerebral cortex, hippocampus, and mid-brain: ontogeny and developmental implications. Mol Cell Neurosci 1994; 5:691–698.

907. Shinoda K. Sex-steroid receptor mechanism related to neuronal aromatase and the stigmoid body. Horm Behav 1994; 28:545–555.

908. Martini L. The 5α-reduction of testosterone in the neuroendocrine structures: biochemical and physiological implications. Endocr Rev 1983; 4:1–25.

909. Baulieu EE, Robel P. Neurosteroids: a new brain function? J Steroid Biochem Mol Biol 1990; 37:395–403.

910. Schwarz S, Pohl P. Steroid hormones and steroid hormone binding globulins in cerebrospinal fluid studied in individuals with intact and with disturbed blood-cerebrospinal fluid barrier. Neuroendocrinology 1992; 55:174–182.

911. Paul SM, Purdy RH. Neuroactive steroids. FASEB J 1992; 6:2311–2322.

912. Morales AJ, Nolan JJ, Nelson JC, et al. Effects of replacement dose of dehydroepiandrosterone in men and women of advancing age. J Clin Endocrinol Metab 1994; 78:1360–1367.

Neuroendocrine-Immune Interaction

913. Paul WE, ed. Fundamental Immunology. New York: Raven, 1989.

914. Dinarello CA, Mier JW. Lymphokines. N Engl J Med 1987; 317:940–945.

915. Dinarello CA. Biology of interleukin 1. FASEB J 1988; 2:108–115.

916. DiNarello CA. The biological properties of interleukin-1. Eur Cytokine Netw 1994; 5:517–531.

917. Reichlin S. Neuroendocrine-immune interactions. N Engl J Med 1993; 329:1246–1253.

918. Reichlin S. Endocrine-immune interaction. In: DeGroot, LJ, ed. Endocrinology. 3rd ed. Philadelphia: WB Saunders, 1995: 2964–2989.

919. Tracey KJ, Lowry SF, Cerami A. Cachectin: a hormone that triggers acute shock and chronic cachexia. J Infect Dis 1988; 157:413–420.

920. Wilder RL. Neuroendocrine-immune system interactions and autoimmunity. Annu Rev Immunol 1995; 13:307–338.

921. Goetzl EJ, Sreedharan SP, Harkonen WS. Pathogenetic roles of neuroimmunologic mediators. Immunol Allergy Clin North Am 1988; 8:183–200.

922. Payan DG, McGillis JP, Goetzl EJ. Neuroimmunology. Adv Immunol 1986; 39:299–323.

923. Ader R, ed. Psychoneuroimmunology. New York: Academic, 1981.

924. Ader R, Felten DL, Cohen N. Psychoneuroimmunology. 2nd ed. San Diego: Academic, 1991.

925. Bartfai T, Ottoson D, eds. Neuro-immunology of Fever. Oxford: Pergamon Press, 1992.

926. Hopkins SJ, Rothwell NJ. Cytokines and the nervous system. I: Expression and recognition. Trends Neurosci 1995; 18:83–88.

927. Rothwell NJ, Hopkins SJ. Cytokines and the nervous system II: actions and mechanisms of action. Trends Neurosci 1995; 18:130–136.

928. Vankelecom H, Carmeliet P, Van Damme J, et al. Production of interleukin-6 by folliculo-stellate cells of the anterior pituitary gland in a histiotypic cell aggregate culture system. Neuroendocrinology 1989; 49:102–106.

929. Romero LI, Lechan RM, Clark BD, et al. IL-1 receptor antagonist inhibits hIL-1β but not bacterial lipopolysaccharide (LPS) stimulated IL-6 secretion by rat anterior pituitary cells. 72nd Annual Meeting of The Endocrine Society, Washington, DC. June 19–22, 1991.

930. Koenig JI, Snowe K, Clark BD, et al. Intrinsic pituitary interleukin 1-β is induced by bacterial lipopolysaccharide. Endocrinology 1990; 126:3053–3058.

931. Breder CD, Dinarello CD, Saper CB. Interleukin-1 immunoreactive innervation of the human hypothalamus. Science 1988; 240:321–324.

932. Lechan RM, Toni R, Clark BD, et al. Immunoreactive interleukin-1beta localization in the rat forebrain. Brain Res 1990; 514:135–140.

933. Spangelo BL, Login IS, Judd AM, et al. Release of interleukin-6 from rat hypothalamus (abstract). Soc Neurosci 1989; 8.

934. Tatro JB, Romero LI, Beasley D, et al. Borrelia burgdorferi and Escherichia coli lipopolysaccharides induce nitric oxide and interleukin-6 production in cultured rat brain cells. J Infect Dis 1994; 169:1014–1022.

935. Munck A, Guyre PM, Holbrook NJ. Physiological functions of glucocorticoids in stress and their relation to pharmacological actions. Endocr Rev 1984; 5:25–44.

936. Reichlin S. Neuroendocrine consequences of systemic inflammation. In: Mazzaferri EL, Bar RS, Kreisberg RA, eds. Advances in Endocrinology and Metabolism. Vol 5. St. Louis: CV Mosby, 1994: 83–96.

937. Chikanza IC, Petrou P, Kingsley G, et al. Defective hypothalamic response to immune and inflammatory stimuli in patients with rheumatoid arthritis. Arthritis Rheum 1992; 35:1281–1288.

938. Dreyfuss D, Leviel F, Paillard M, et al. Acute infectious pneumonia is accompanied by a latent vasopressin-dependent impairment of renal water excretion. Am Rev Respir Dis 1988; 138:583–589.

939. Reichlin S, Glaser RJ. Thyroid function in experimental streptococcal pneumonia in the rat. J Exp Med 1958; 107:219–236.

940. Rivest S, Rivier C. The role of corticotropin-releasing factor and interleukin-1 in the regulation of neurons controlling reproductive functions. Endocr Rev 1995; 16:177–199.

941. Shalts E, Feng YJ, Ferin M. Vasopressin mediates the interleukin-1 alpha–induced decrease in luteinizing hormone secretion in the ovariectomized rhesus monkey. Endocrinology 1992; 131:153–158.

942. MacLean D, Reichlin S. Neuroendocrinology and the immune process. In: Ader R, ed. Psychoneuroimmunology. New York: Academic, 1981: 475–520.

943. Romero LI, Kakucska I, Lechan RM, et al. Interleukin-6 (IL-6) is secreted from the brain after intracerebroventricular injection of IL-1β in rats. Am J Physiol, Reg Integr Comp Physiol 1996; 270:R518–R524.

944. Ahlqvist J. Hormonal influences on immunologic and related phenomena. In: Ader R, ed. Psychoneuroimmunology. New York: Academic, 1981: 355–403.

945. Goff BL, Roth JA, Arp LH, et al. Growth hormone treatment stimulates thymulin production in aged dogs. Clin Exp Immunol 1987; 68:580–587.

946. Hartman DP, Holaday JW, Bernton EW. Inhibition of lymphocyte proliferation by antibodies to prolactin. FASEB J 1989; 3:2194–2202.

947. Cross RJ, Roszman TL. Neuroendocrine modulation of immune function: the role of prolactin. Prog Neuroendocr Immunol 1989; 2:17–20.

948. Bernton EW. Prolactin and immune host defenses. Prog Neuroendocr Immunol 1989; 2:21–29.

949. Dardenne M, Savino W, Gagnerault MC, et al. Neuroendocrine control of thymic hormonal production. I: Prolactin stimulates in vivo and in vitro the production of thymulin by human and murine thymic epithelial cells. Endocrinology 1989; 125:3–12.

950. Reber PM. Prolactin and immunomodulation. Am J Med 1993; 95:637–644.

951. Hiestand PC, Mekler P, Nordmann R, et al. Prolactin as a modulator of lymphocyte responsiveness provides a possible mechanism of action for cyclosporine. Proc Natl Acad Sci USA 1986; 83:2599–2603.

952. Schwartz RS, Datta SK. Autoimmunity and autoimmune disease. In: Paul WE, ed. Fundamental Immunology. New York: Raven, 1989: 819–866.

953. Kalman B, Olsson O, Link H, et al. Estradiol potentiates poke-weed mitogen-induced B cell stimulation in multiple sclerosis and healthy subjects. Acta Neurol Scand 1989; 79:340–346.

954. Lipton JM, Glyn JR, Zimmer JA. ACTH and α-melanotropin in central temperature control. Fed Proc 1981; 40:2760–2764.

955. Tatro JB, Entwhistle ML. Heterogeneity of brain melanocortin receptors suggested by differential ligand binding in situ. Brain Res 1994; 635:148–158.

956. Cannon JG, Tatro JB, Reichlin S, et al. α-Melanocyte stimulating hormone inhibits immunostimulatory and inflammatory actions of interleukin 1. J Immunol 1986; 137:2232–2236.

957. Daynes RA, Robertson BA, Cho BH, et al. α-Melanocyte-stimulating hormone exhibits target cell selectivity in its capacity to affect interleukin 1-inducible responses in vivo and in vitro. J Immunol 1987; 139:103–109.

958. Mason MJ, Van Epps D. Modulation of IL-1, tumor necrosis factor, and CSa-mediated murine neutrophil migration by α-melanocyte-stimulating hormone. J Immunol 1989; 1142:1646–1651.

959. Kidd BL, Mapp PI, Gibson SJ, et al. A neurogenic mechanism for symmetrical arthritis. Lancet 1989; 2:1128–1130.

960. Lotz M, Vaugn JH, Carson DA. Effect of neuropeptides on production of inflammatory cytokines by human monocytes. Science 1988; 241:1218–1221.

961. Sreedharan SP, Kodama KT, Peterson KE, et al. Distinct subsets of somatostatin receptors on cultured human lymphocytes. J Biol Chem 1989; 264:949–952.

962. Ottaway CA. Vasoactive intestinal peptide as a modulator of lymphocyte and immune function. Ann NY Acad Sci 1988; 527:486–500.

963. Smith EM, Meyer WJ, Blalock JE. Virus-induced corticosterone in hypophysectomized mice: a possible lymphoid adrenal axis. Science 1982; 218:1311–1312.

964. Dunn AJ, Powell ML, Moreshead WV, et al. Effects of Newcastle disease virus administration to mice on the metabolism of cerebral biogenic amines, plasma corticosterone and lymphocyte proliferation. Brain Behav Immun 1987; 1:216–230.

965. Dupont AGG, Somers AC, Van Steviteghem AC, et al. Ectopic adrenocorticotropin production: disappearance after removal of inflammatory tissue. J Clin Endocrinol Metab 1984; 58:654–658.

966. Smith EM, Brosnan P, Meyer WJ, et al. An ACTH receptor on human mononuclear leukocytes. Relation to adrenal ACTH-receptor activity. N Engl J Med 1987; 317:1266–1269.

967. Moore PS, Couch RM, Perry YS, et al. Allgrove syndrome: an autosomal recessive syndrome of ACTH insensitivity, azchalasia and alacrima. Clin Endocrinol 1991; 34:107–114.

968. Lysle DT, Cunnick JE, Fowler H, et al. Pavlovian conditioning of shock-induced suppression of lymphocyte reactivity: acquisition, extinction, and preexposure effects. Life Sci 1988; 42:2185–2194.

969. Stein M, Schleifer SJ, Keller SE. Hypothalamic influences on immune responses. In: Ader R, ed. Psychoneuroimmunology. New York: Academic, 1981: 429–447.

970. Felten DL, Felten SY, Carlson SL, et al. Noradrenergic and peptidergic innervation of lymphoid tissue. J Immunol 1985; 135:755s–765s.

971. Reichlin S. Neuroendocrine–immune interactions. N Engl J Med 1993; 329:1246–1253.

9

THE ANTERIOR PITUITARY

Michael O. Thorner, Mary Lee Vance, Edward R. Laws, Jr.,
Eva Horvath, and Kalman Kovacs

INTRODUCTION

The anterior pituitary gland regulates various endocrine organs by integrating the signals from the brain and the feedback effects of peripheral hormones to stimulate intermittent hormone release by a particular gland. The pituitary synthesizes at least six hormones, which regulate growth, development, and function of the thyroid gland, adrenal cortex, gonads, and breasts. Peripheral nonendocrine tissues are also the target for some pituitary hormones. Thus disorders of pituitary function may produce selective overstimulation of one target gland, such as the adrenal gland in Cushing's disease, or cause pituitary hormone deficiency, which may or may not be selective. By virtue of the anatomic location of the pituitary in the sella turcica, expanding lesions of the gland may cause visual disturbances, cavernous sinus syndromes, and headache.

The function and importance of the pituitary were recognized in the second half of the 19th century. The name *pituitary* originates from the Greek *ptuo* (to spit) and the Latin *pituita* (mucus). It was thought that mucus, produced by the brain, was excreted through the nose by the pituitary. The term *hypophysis* is also derived from the Greek (*hypo*, under; *physis*, growth).

The beginning of pituitary physiology is often dated to 1886, when Pierre Marie, a French neurologist, described pituitary enlargement in acromegaly and postulated that the pituitary plays an important role in the pathogenesis of this disease. Marie's contribution focused attention on the pituitary and stimulated research to gain insight into the structure and function of the gland in health and disease.

During this century the hormones of the hypothalamus and pituitary have been purified, characterized, and sequenced, and their physiological roles have been defined. The importance of hypothalamic control of the anterior pituitary via secretion of regulatory hormones into the hypothalamic-hypophyseal portal circulation has been established. The consequences of excessive or deficient secretion of the various anterior pituitary hormones have been characterized. The study of these conditions and the evaluation of patients with pituitary disease were revolutionized by the development of sensitive, specific, and reliable radioimmunoassays (RIAs) for the pituitary hormones and for the hormones secreted by the target glands. A similar revolution in noninvasive imaging techniques, such as magnetic resonance imaging (MRI) and computed tomography (CT), allows precise anatomic evaluation of the hypothalamus, pituitary, and surrounding structures. Finally, the application of modern histochemical techniques—including immunocytochemistry, electron microscopy, and in situ hybridization—makes it possible to identify pituitary cell types and provides a logical framework for the classification of pituitary tumors.

Similar advances have been made in the treatment of hypothalamic and pituitary disease with the development of effective replacement therapy for hormone deficiency states. The advent of transsphenoidal pituitary microsurgery and the development of medical therapies to control certain types of hormone excess have improved the treatment of many patients.

PITUITARY MORPHOLOGY

Embryology

The pituitary is derived from two sources.[1–4] The epithelial portion includes the pars distalis, intermediate lobe, and pars tuberalis and originates from evagination of the stomodeal ectoderm, *Rathke's pouch*, named after its discoverer. The neural portion, which includes the infundibulum, the neural stalk, and the posterior lobe, arises in the saccus infundibuli in the diencephalon. Rathke's pouch is apparent in the 3-mm embryo during the third week of gestation. Initially it is composed of a small, thin-walled vesicle in the roof of the primitive buccal cavity, termed the *stomodeum*, and it subsequently expands in the direction of the saccus infundibuli and adheres to it. After the fusion of the epithelial and neural components, the distal end narrows and forms the craniopharyngeal canal, a hollow stalk that usually is obliterated in the 17-mm embryo. In some embryos, however, the canal remains patent until the end of intrauterine life and may persist after birth. Nests of adenohypophyseal tissue may be deposited along the route of the craniopharyngeal canal. A resulting pharyngeal hypophysis[5, 6] may be capable of hormone synthesis and may give rise to ectopic adenomas. The cells at the distal end of Rathke's pouch gradually disappear, whereas those at the proximal end begin to proliferate at about the third month of gestation. Cell proliferation occurs at the attachment site of the ectoderm and the neural tube; cell accumulation is more rapid and extensive at the anterior wall than at the posterior wall. The anterior wall gives rise to the pars distalis of the adenohypophysis, and the posterior wall develops into the intermediate lobe. In the human adult the latter is rudimentary, constituting only a small part of the anterior lobe. At approximately the fifth week of gestation the anterolateral portion of Rathke's pouch extends upward bilaterally, fuses in front of the infundibulum, and forms the pars tuberalis.

By the end of the third month of gestation the characteristic features of the adult pituitary are recognizable. The infundibulum elongates, and the pituitary becomes embedded deeper in the sella turcica that is formed by the sphenoid bone. Thus the close proximity of the pituitary and the infundibulum is lost. The neurohypophysis differentiates proximally into the median eminence and distally into the posterior lobe, connected to the median eminence by the pituitary stalk.

The timing of the onset of synthesis and release of pituitary hormones by the embryo has been investigated in considerable detail.[1, 2, 4, 7, 8] Acidophilic cells are detectable in the anterior lobe of the human embryo about the third month of gestation; basophilic cells become detectable somewhat later. Cells that produce growth hormone (GH) and corticotropin (also called adrenocorticotropic hormone [ACTH], adrenocorticotropin) are identifiable at about the ninth week of gestation; the synthesis of these hormones is followed by the production of the α subunit and subsequently the β subunits of the glycoprotein hormones. At about the eighth week of gestation connective tissue and blood vessels grow into the anterior lobe and establish a direct neurohormonal link between the anterior lobe and the hypothalamus. Neurosecretory material is demonstrable in the posterior lobe at about the fifth month of gestation. The last cell type to develop in the anterior lobe is the lactotrope at about the fifth month of gestation. The functional activity of the pituitary in embryonic life is not understood in every regard (also see Chapter 28).

Hormone-producing cells can differentiate in the absence of hypothalamic stimulation, and hormone synthesis in the absence of hypothalamic stimulation has been documented in the embryonic pituitary in several in vitro studies. In addition in anencephaly all cell types of the anterior pituitary except corticotropes develop and are capable of some degree of hormone synthesis and release.

Anatomy

The pituitary is located under the brain in the sella turcica or hypophyseal fossa of the skull.[3, 4] It is protected by the sphenoid bone, which surrounds it laterally and inferiorly and is covered by the dura, a dense layer of connective tissue that lines the sella turcica. Superiorly the pituitary is covered by the diaphragma sellae, or sellar diaphragm, a dural sheath that forms the roof of the sella. The diaphragma sellae has a 5-mm-wide central opening that is penetrated by the hypophyseal stalk. In some individuals this opening is wider and is thought to allow transmission of pulsations of cerebrospinal fluid (CSF) pressure and lead to the development of the empty sella syndrome or cisternal herniation.

The pituitary is an oval, bean-shaped, symmetrical, brownish red organ. It averages 13 mm transversely, 9 mm anteroposteriorly, and 6 mm vertically. At birth the pituitary weighs approximately 100 mg. The weight of the pituitary in adults averages 0.6 g (range 0.4 to 0.9 g) and is somewhat larger in women than in men. During pregnancy the gland enlarges and may weigh 0.9 to 1.0 g.[9] The pituitary is usually heavier in multiparous than in nulliparous women and decreases in size with advancing age. In senescence connective tissue accumulates in the anterior lobe, but pituitary hormone production is preserved.

The anterior lobe constitutes 80% of the gland. The two lobes are clearly demarcated and are distinguishable with the naked eye; the cut surface of the anterior lobe is brownish red, whereas the posterior lobe is grayish brown.

Space-occupying lesions of the pituitary can compress neighboring structures. The lateral walls of the sella are close to the cavernous sinuses, which contain the internal carotid arteries, the oculomotor (III), trochlear (IV), and abducens (VI) nerves, and the V_1 and V_2 divisions of the trigeminal (V) nerve. The sphenoid sinus is anterior and inferior to the pituitary and is separated from it by the inferior portion of the sella, a thin layer of bone. When a pituitary tumor enlarges, this bone may be resorbed and eroded, allowing tumor extension into the sphenoid sinus. The optic chiasm lies directly above the diaphragma sellae in front of the hypophyseal stalk; suprasellar growth of a pituitary tumor may compress the chiasm and impair vision. The tuber cinereum of the hypothalamus and the third ventricle of the brain lie above the roof of the sella. Space-occupying lesions in or above the pituitary may compress and compromise the tuber cinereum and cause hypothalamic-hypophyseal dysfunction, usually manifested as hypopituitarism associated with mild hyperprolactinemia.

Minor anatomic variations in the shape and size of the pituitary and in the size of the opening of the diaphragma sellae are common.[10, 11] These differences do not affect pituitary function but may cause confusion in the interpretation of imaging studies.

The anterior lobe of the pituitary is composed of three divisions: pars distalis, pars intermedia, and pars tuberalis.[3, 4] The pars distalis is the largest division and is the site of the hormone-producing cells. The pars intermedia is poorly developed in the human and consists of a few dilated cavities lined by a single layer of cuboidal or columnar epithelium and filled with an amorphous proteinaceous material often containing cell debris. The pars tuberalis is the upward extension of the anterior lobe and is attached to the pituitary stalk. It contains small groups of cells that mainly produce glycoprotein hormones and may contain squamous cell nests.

The neurohypophysis or posterior pituitary consists of the median eminence of the tuber cinereum, the infundibular stem or hypophyseal stalk, and the infundibular process or posterior or neural lobe.[10, 12]

The hypophyseal circulation plays an important role in the regulation of the anterior pituitary.[13–16] The pituitary receives blood from the superior and the inferior hypophyseal arteries, which are branches of the internal carotid arteries. Some branches of the superior hypophyseal arteries terminate in the infundibulum where they form gomitoli or adjacent capillaries. The gomitoli—central arteries with a well-developed muscular layer surrounded by many capillaries—are approximately 1 to 2 mm long and 50 to 100 μm wide and are present in large numbers in the infundibulum and proximal part of the hypophyseal stalk. Their function has not been established, but they may control blood flow to adjacent capillaries and the adenohypophysis and thereby regulate the transport of hypothalamic hormones, neuropeptides, and neurotransmitters to the anterior pituitary. The hypothalamic hormones are produced in neurons that originate in various parts of the hypothalamus and terminate at the infundibulum, where they permeate fenestrations in the perigomitolar capillaries to enter the portal circulation. The large parallel veins, the portal veins or long portal vessels, contain a high density of capillaries. Levels of hypothalamic hormones are high in the portal blood, which transports the hormones to the capillaries in the anterior pituitary. The long portal vessels arise in the infundibulum and proximal part of the pituitary stalk, and the short portal vessels originate in the posterior lobe and distal portion of the pituitary stalk to provide a direct vascular connection between the posterior and anterior lobes of the pituitary.

The portal circulation provides approximately 80 to 90% of the blood supply to the anterior lobe. The adenohypophysis also receives blood from other sources. The capsular arteries carry blood to superficial cell layers of the adenohypophysis. In addition, arteries bypass the infundibulum to carry arterial blood directly from the superior hypophyseal arteries, providing 10 to 20% of the blood supply to the pituitary. The superior hypophyseal arteries arise from the carotid circulation, and the blood is relatively devoid of hypothalamic hormones. The capsular arteries arise from the inferior hypophyseal arteries, provide blood to the hypophyseal fibrous capsule, and penetrate the superficial layers of the anterior lobe to supply these layers with arterial blood.

The posterior pituitary receives its blood supply from the inferior hypophyseal arteries, which do not supply blood to the anterior lobe, except through the capsular arteries. Venous blood leaves the pituitary through dural channels into the cavernous sinuses, which drain to the inferior petrosal sinus and the internal jugular veins. The venous pathway from the cavernous sinus to the jugular vein may contain many anastomoses from one petrosal sinus to another or be otherwise anomalous, which can cause confusing findings with petrosal sinus sampling.[17]

Most blood flow is from the hypothalamus to the anterior pituitary, but under some circumstances reversal of blood flow might affect the function of neural centers, producing ultrashort-loop feedback.

The adenohypophyseal capillaries are lined by a single layer of fenestrated endothelial cells with a well-defined subendothelial space and basement membrane. Hormones secreted by the adenohypophyseal cells pass through the cell membrane, the basement membrane of the capillary, the subendothelial layer, and the endothelium before they enter the blood. The hormone-containing secretory granules become undetect-

able by current morphologic techniques after they are discharged from the cells.

Despite its proximity to the brain, the anterior lobe is innervated by only a few sympathetic nerve fibers that reach the tissue along the blood vessels. These nerve fibers are not believed to have major importance in the control of hormone synthesis or release. Hypothalamic regulation is exerted via the hypothalamic regulatory peptides that reach the pituitary via the portal vessels.

The posterior lobe possesses a rich nerve supply (see Chapter 10). Unmyelinated nerve fibers originate in the supraoptic and paraventricular nuclei and other areas of the hypothalamus and enter the posterior lobe via the pituitary stalk. They affect the posterior lobe by neural influences and also contain vasopressin (arginine vasopressin [AVP], also called antidiuretic hormone [ADH]) and oxytocin and their respective neurophysins or carrier proteins. These neurohypophyseal hormones are synthesized in the hypothalamus, transported and stored in the posterior lobe, and released into the peripheral circulation. When the pituitary stalk is sectioned, the posterior lobe atrophies and diabetes insipidus develops.

Histology of the Normal Anterior Pituitary Gland

The "normal" human pituitary is one of the least studied organs. Compounding the inaccessibility of the tissue, the pituitary contains several types of hormone-producing cells whose number, endocrine activity, and morphologic features are affected by changes in the endocrine milieu. The morphologic responses to stimulatory and inhibitory influences differ among cell types, further complicating studies of pituitary cytologic characteristics. The following summary is based chiefly on the study of more than 1000 autopsied pituitaries and of pituitaries removed surgically either for therapeutic hypophysectomy or in conjunction with adenomectomy.[18] Changes in the human pituitary gland also occur with pregnancy.[9, 19]

The five cell types of the human anterior pituitary gland have different regional distributions. In horizontal cross-section the adenohypophysis is composed of two lateral wings and a central mucoid (median) wedge. The cytologic features and distribution of each cell type will be considered in the discussion of the principal hormone it secretes.

PITUITARY HORMONES

Hypothalamic-Pituitary Regulation

Each pituitary hormone is regulated by hypothalamic regulatory hormones synthesized in the hypothalamus and transported from the median eminence to the anterior pituitary via the hypothalamic-pituitary portal circulation. Hypothalamic hormones bind to specific high-affinity cell membrane receptors in individual pituitary cells to regulate hormone secretion from that cell. With the possible exception of prolactin, anterior pituitary hormones are under feedback regulation via the hormones secreted by the target glands on which the pituitary hormones act. Thus signals from the brain and the periphery interact to regulate pituitary hormone secretion and maintain a normal endocrine state. If a target gland fails, reduction in negative feedback leads to augmented secretion of the tropic hypothalamic hormone (and reduced secretion of any tonic hypothalamic inhibiting hormone). This results in enhancement of pituitary responsiveness to the hypothalamic tropic stimulus. Thus negative feedback occurs at both the pituitary

TABLE 9–1. Relationships Among Hypothalamic, Pituitary, and Target Gland Secretion

Hypothalamic Hormone	Pituitary Hormone	Target Gland	Feedback Hormone
TRH	Thyrotropin	Thyroid	T_4 and T_3
LHRH	LH	Gonad	E_2 (women), T (men)
	FSH	Gonad	Inhibin and (?) E_2 and T
SS	GH	Multiple	IGF 1
GHRH	GH	Multiple	IGF 1
DA	Prolactin	Breast	?
CRH	Corticotropin	Adrenal	Cortisol
AVP	Corticotropin	Adrenal	Cortisol

AVP, arginine vasopressin; CRH, corticotropin-releasing hormone; DA, dopamine; E_2, estradiol; FSH, follicle-stimulating hormone; GH, growth hormone; GHRH, growth hormone–releasing hormone; IGF-1, insulin-like growth factor 1; LH, luteinizing hormone; LHRH, luteinizing hormone–releasing hormone; SS, somatostatin; T, testosterone; T_3, triiodothyronine; T_4, thyroxine; TRH, thyrotropin-releasing hormone.

and hypothalamic levels (Table 9–1). In addition pituitary hormones are probably transported directly to the hypothalamus, the short-loop feedback, to inhibit secretion of the pituitary hormone by reducing hypothalamic stimulation (Fig. 9–1).

All anterior pituitary hormones are secreted in a pulsatile fashion. Thus measurement of a single random sample may not provide adequate assessment of hormone secretion, and more frequent measurements may be necessary. The development of computer algorithms to identify hormone pulses and

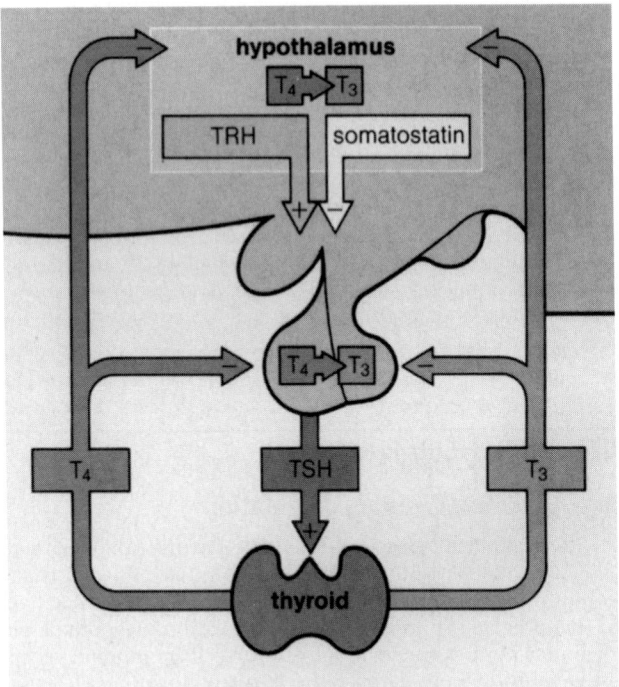

Figure 9–1. Schematic representation of the hypothalamic-pituitary-target gland axis. Hypothalamic hormones regulate secretion of pituitary hormones, which in turn stimulate target gland hormone production. Peripheral hormones feed back on the hypothalamus and pituitary to modulate secretion in a classic negative fashion. For example hypothalamic thyrotropin-releasing hormone (TRH) stimulates pituitary release of thyrotropin (TSH), which stimulates thyroid hormone release. Thyroid hormones inhibit TRH and thyrotropin in the hypothalamus and pituitary, respectively. In addition there is a "short loop" by which the pituitary hormone feeds back at the hypothalamic level to inhibit hypothalamic stimulation of pituitary hormone secretion. T_3, triiodothyronine; T_4, thyroxine. (From Reichlin S. Neuroendocrine control of pituitary function. In: Besser GM, Cudworth AG, eds. Clinical Endocrinology: An Illustrated Text. London: Gower Medical, 1987: 1.1–1.14.)

calculate the quantitative characteristics has facilitated such studies. Two such programs are Cluster[20] and Ultra.[21] The pulsatile pattern of pituitary hormone release is important for efficient and effective signaling of target tissues so that the effects of intermittently generated endocrine signals are enhanced and prolonged despite ongoing metabolic clearance of the hormone. Some pituitary hormone production and clearance rates are illustrated in Table 9–2. The study of pituitary hormone secretion has been facilitated by the development of deconvolution techniques that mathematically neutralize the effects of metabolic clearance and calculate the underlying hormone secretory rates.[22–24] This methodology has revealed that about 95% of luteinizing hormone (LH) secretion occurs during approximately one fourth of the day even though serum LH concentrations are consistently detectable because of the slow metabolic clearance.[22] In contrast although 95% of GH secretion occurs during 37% of the day, serum GH concentrations are undetectable in conventional assays during approximately half of the day because of rapid clearance of GH from the plasma.[25] The pulsatile pattern of pituitary hormone release is altered in Cushing's disease, in which the circadian pattern of pulsatile corticotropin release is altered,[26] and in acromegaly, in which serum GH concentrations remain detectable throughout the day.[27]

Corticotropin

Corticotropin stimulates the adrenal cortex to secrete cortisol, adrenal androgens, and mineralocorticoids. Pituitary corticotropin secretion is regulated by hypothalamic corticotropin-releasing hormone (CRH) and AVP, which stimulate corticotropin secretion. The feedback loop is closed by the negative feedback of cortisol on AVP, CRH, and corticotropin secretion. In addition corticotropin acts via a short-loop feedback to suppress CRH secretion.[28] (For a detailed discussion of the hypothalamic-pituitary-adrenal axis see Chapter 12.)

STRUCTURE OF CORTICOTROPIN, RELATED PEPTIDES, AND PRO-OPIOMELANOCORTIN. Corticotropin, a 39-amino-acid peptide, is synthesized as part of a large, 241-amino-acid precursor molecule, pro-opiomelanocortin (POMC). The human *POMC* gene is located on chromosome 2 and has three exons; exon 2 codes for the signal sequence and 18 amino acids of the NH_2 terminus of the molecule, and exon 3 codes for the remaining translated portion of the molecule.[29] POMC undergoes extensive post-translational processing, including glycosylation, enzymatic cleavage and phosphorylation, NH_2-terminal acetylation, and COOH-terminal amidation of certain cleaved peptides. This processing is species and tissue specific. In the human anterior pituitary gland POMC is cleaved at dibasic amino acids into β-lipotropin (β-LPH), corticotropin, joining peptide, and an NH_2-terminal peptide. In the human intermediate lobe, which is vestigial except during fetal life and at the end of pregnancy, corticotropin is cleaved into α-melanocyte-stimulating hormone [corticotropin (1–13)] and corticotropin-like peptide [corticotropin (18–39)], and β-LPH is split into LPH and β-endorphin.

The first 18 amino acids of corticotropin have full biologic activity, and the first 24 amino acids are identical across species. Synthetic corticotropin (1–24) has a longer half-life than native corticotropin (1–18) and is useful in clinical evaluations.

Because the peptides produced by the corticotrope are derived from the same precursor molecule, they are secreted in equimolar amounts. However the circulating levels of the peptides do not vary in tandem because the half-lives are different. The half-life of β-LPH is longer than that of corticotropin, and hence the β-LPH/corticotropin ratio increases after administration of hydrocortisone, which inhibits secretion of both corticotropin and β-LPH. Similarly β-LPH levels

TABLE 9–2. Anterior Pituitary Hormones: Pituitary Content and Metabolic Characteristics in Normal Adult Men

Hormone	Pituitary Content (mg)	Production (μg/24 h)	Metabolic Clearance Rate (mL/min/m²)	Half-Life (min)* Mono	Half-Life (min)* Alpha	Half-Life (min)* Beta
Corticotropin	0.25	25–50		8		
GH	5–10	1000–2000	100–150	20	3.5	21
Prolactin	0.1	200	45	20		
Thyrotropin	0.1–0.15	50–200	50			
LH	700 IU	1000 IU	34	47	18	90
FSH	200 IU	200 IU	4–12	220	100	500

*Mono, monoexponential decay; alpha, first component of biexponential decay; beta, second component of biexponential decay.

increase in renal failure because of slower metabolic clearance. The hyperpigmentation in corticotropin hypersecretory states and in uremia is not a result of secretion of intermediate-lobe peptides but is due to the stimulation of melanocytes by β-LPH and corticotropin.

CORTICOTROPES. The human pituitary contains approximately 250 μg of corticotropin. Corticotropes are located primarily in the median wedge where they make up about 10% of the cells. The corticotrope may represent only one subtype of the POMC-producing cell line. Other POMC-producing cell populations, the putative sources of silent "corticotrope" adenoma subtypes 1 and 2, may have morphologic features similar to those of corticotrope cells. The typical corticotrope is ovoid or angular and displays basophilia, bright periodic acid–Schiff (PAS) positivity, and immunoreactivity for corticotropin and other POMC-derived peptides such as endorphins, β-LPH, and the NH₂-terminal fragment. When seen by electron microscopy the cells are ovoid or angular and contain relatively electron-dense cytoplasm with numerous secretory granules in the size range of 150 to 450 nm. The granules are morphologically characteristic, being spherical, dented, heart shaped, and drop shaped, often with variable electron density. The specific markers of the human corticotrope cell are type 1 filaments[30] composed of cytokeratin.[30, 31] Crooke's hyalinization occurs when there is functional suppression of corticotrope cells, as in the nontumorous (and sometimes tumorous) areas of pituitaries harboring corticotrope adenomas, in individuals with ectopic corticotropin production or adrenal adenoma, or with chronic administration of large doses of glucocorticoid. The hyalinization is due to the accumulation of keratin-positive type 1 filaments associated with loss of rough endoplasmic reticulum (RER) and Golgi membranes, a finding unique to the human corticotrope cell. These changes are reversible with correction of glucocorticoid excess.

REGULATION OF CORTICOTROPIN SECRETION. CRH stimulates corticotropin secretion by binding to high-affinity CRH receptors on the corticotrope and by stimulating the accumulation of cAMP, which activates protein kinase A. CRH rapidly releases corticotropin and related peptides and increases *POMC* gene transcription and POMC synthesis. Administration of exogenous CRH stimulates the secretion of both corticotropin and cortisol; the magnitude of the response is dependent on the time of day and the level of circulating glucocorticoids. The cortisol response is greater in the afternoon than in the morning.[32] Exogenous glucocorticoids inhibit both the corticotropin and cortisol responses to CRH. Conversely lowering endogenous cortisol levels with metyrapone enhances the corticotropin and cortisol responses to CRH.[33] AVP alone is a weak secretagogue of corticotropin but acts synergistically with CRH to regulate corticotropin release.[34] Additional peptides and neurotransmitters have been implicated in the control of CRH, AVP, and corticotropin secretion.

CORTICOTROPIN SECRETION. Corticotropin is secreted in bursts that cause similar sharp peaks in plasma cortisol levels. The corticotropin secretory bursts increase in frequency after 3 to 5 h of sleep and are maximal prior to awakening and the hour thereafter. Corticotropin secretion is also under circadian control that is regulated by a number of factors including light. Blind persons have a free-running corticotropin rhythm of about 25 h.[35, 36] In normal individuals corticotropin levels decline over the morning and reach a nadir in the evening. The rhythm is established after the first year of life; the timing of the peak level (acrophase) shifts to 3 h earlier in the elderly. The circadian rhythm is resilient and is unaffected by short-term sleep deprivation, continuous feeding, prolonged bed rest, or even working on a night shift if a normal sleep pattern is preserved on weekends. The rhythm can be disrupted by a major time shift as occurs with transmeridian jet travel. In that circumstance it usually takes several days for the rhythm to be restored to normal.[37]

Psychological and physical stress can activate the hypothalamic-pituitary-adrenal axis with an increase in both corticotropin and cortisol secretion. Such stresses include trauma, major surgery, fever, hypoglycemia, and burn injury. Hypoglycemia activates the hypothalamic-pituitary axis by direct action at the basomedial hypothalamus,[38] and fever activates it indirectly through the release of the cytokines interleukin-1, interleukin-2, and interleukin-6, which in turn enhance CRH release from the hypothalamus.[39] Plasma cortisol levels are activated by psychological stress, which can vary from anticipation of physical injury to intense mental activity. Elevation of plasma cortisol levels also occurs in patients with anorexia nervosa and depression but is not a feature of schizophrenia or chronic anxiety.

Glucocorticoids inhibit corticotropin secretion at multiple sites within the corticotrope, including the inhibition of the corticotropin response to CRH and the inhibition of corticotropin synthesis via blockade of *POMC* gene transcription and POMC synthesis. Glucocorticoids also inhibit CRH and AVP synthesis and release from the hypothalamus.

CORTICOTROPIN ACTIONS. Corticotropin binds to specific high-affinity cell membrane receptors with a dissociation constant (K_d) of approximately 1.6 nmol/L. Extracellular calcium is required for the binding of corticotropin to its receptor. The actions of corticotropin are mediated by activation of adenylate cyclase, which leads to accumulation of intracellular cAMP, increased protein kinase A activity, and phosphorylation of proteins. Corticotropin stimulates cortisol synthesis and secretion; only small amounts of cortisol are stored in the adrenal.[40] The acute effects of corticotropin occur within minutes and involve an increase in adrenal blood flow and stimulation of the initial, rate-limiting step of cholesterol conversion to pregnenolone. In addition there is an increase in the supply of free cholesterol ester. The prolonged effects of corticotropin promote maintenance (and growth) of the adrenal by increasing protein synthesis, including the synthesis of the enzymes involved in steroid hormone biosynthesis. Although corticotropin has actions in other tissues, the physiological significance of most of these actions is uncertain. However in Nelson's syndrome and Addison's disease, circulating corticotropin concentrations are extremely high, and both corticotropin and β-LPH act on melanocytes to increase skin pigmentation.

Prolactin–Growth Hormone Family

Human GH, prolactin, and human placental lactogen (hPL, also called human chorionic somatomammotropin [hCS]) share amino acid sequence homologies and are thought to be derived from a common ancestral gene.[41] The genes for these three hormones also have a common structural organization, and the nucleotide homologies are greater than the amino acid sequence homologies of the encoded proteins.[42, 43] Each gene has four introns separating five coding exons.[44, 45] The introns occur at homologous sites in the coding regions despite differences in the gene sizes. The prolactin gene is greater than 10 kb in length and is located on chromosome 6[46]; the *GH* gene is less than 2.5 kb in length and is located on chromosome 17.[47]

The prolactin-GH family can be divided into prolactin and GH subfamilies based on homologies and chromosomal segregation. In the human a single prolactin gene is present, whereas in rodent species several prolactin genes are expressed at different times during gestation, and cDNAs have been cloned that code for placental lactogens, prolactin-like proteins, proliferin, and prolactin-related proteins.[48] These various peptides are also likely to exist in the human but await identification. Primate GH and its receptor have relatively little homology with those in other mammalian species and the GHs of other species are biologically inactive in humans. The human GH (hGH) subfamily consists of five members, all of which are located on a 78-kb section of chromosome 17. They include the normal *GH* gene, a GH variant gene, two expressed hPL genes, and an incompletely characterized hPL-like gene, which is thought not to be expressed, i.e., a pseudogene.[49] The GH variant protein differs from GH by 13 amino acids and has two additional different amino acids in the leader sequence. The genes in the GH subfamily share more amino acid and nucleotide homology than they do with prolactin.

PROLACTIN STRUCTURE. Prolactin was identified in animal species as a distinct anterior pituitary hormone in 1928[50] and was purified and named in 1932,[51–53] but human prolactin was not purified until 1971.[54, 55] Human prolactin consists of 199 amino acids and has three intramolecular disulfide bonds, one more than hGH. Only 16% of the amino acids of prolactin are homologous with those of GH. Prolactin circulates in blood predominantly in a monomeric form ("little prolactin," 23 kd) but also exists in dimeric ("big" prolactin, 48 to 56 kd) and polymeric (>100 kd) forms.[56–61] Glycosylated forms of prolactin also exist.[62] The biologic significance of these different forms is unclear, although the larger forms may have reduced receptor-binding affinity and biologic activity.[58, 60, 62, 63] Monomeric prolactin may be cleaved to liberate 8- and 16-kd forms.[64] The biologic significance of the cleaved forms is also unknown, but they may be mitogenic for mammary cells.[65]

LACTOTROPE CELLS AND PITUITARY PROLACTIN CONTENT. Lactotrope cells have a wide distribution throughout the pars distalis; they account for most of the cells in the posterolateral rim of the pars distalis in the vicinity of the posterior lobe. The number of lactotrope cells in this region varies from 10 to 30%, being lowest in men and highest in multiparous women.[66] Lactotrope cells in the normal pituitary gland are small, polyhedral, and sparsely granulated with fine multiple cytoplasmic processes and a well-developed RER and Golgi complex. Densely granulated lactotrope cells that exhibit strong, diffuse cytoplasmic immunopositivity are rare,

particularly in the pituitaries of older individuals. Knowledge about these densely granulated lactotrope cells is sketchy because of their rarity and the inadequate amount of material for study. In contrast to the apparently stable somatotrope, the fine structure of the lactotrope depends on secretory activity.[18] Pleomorphic secretory granules within Golgi sacculi and secretory granule extrusions at the vascular surface of the cells are useful markers of lactotrope cells. Lactotrope hyperplasia during pregnancy and during estrogen treatment and in some cases of Cushing's disease and primary hypothyroidism is associated with progressive cellular enlargement, accumulation of highly organized RER, formation of concentric whorls (nebenkern), and accumulation of immature granules within the Golgi complex. Because of enhanced exocytic discharge of secretory material, stimulated lactotropes contain few cytoplasmic storage granules. Suppressed lactotrope cells adjacent to a tumorous prolactinoma are small and have a decreased quantity of RER and Golgi membranes. Suppressed lactotrope cells can be distinguished from null cells (cells that contain scant secretory granules and no morphologic markers indicating their derivation) only by the presence of occasional granule extrusions.

REGULATION OF PROLACTIN SECRETION. Prolactin, like all anterior pituitary hormones, is secreted in an episodic manner. Its secretion is inhibited by dopamine and enhanced by various prolactin-releasing factors. Prolactin is unique among the anterior pituitary hormones in that it is under tonic hypothalamic inhibition via dopamine produced by tuberoinfundibular neurons. Dopamine acts by stimulating the lactotrope D_2 receptor to inhibit adenylate cyclase and consequently to inhibit both prolactin synthesis and prolactin release. The putative prolactin-releasing factors include thyrotropin-releasing hormone (TRH), vasoactive intestinal peptide, PHM-27 (a peptide with structural homology to vasoactive intestinal peptide), pituitary adenylate cyclase activating polypeptide (PACAP),[67] and yet unidentified posterior pituitary hormones[68–70] (see Chapter 8). The physiological significance of prolactin-releasing factors in humans is unknown, and it is not known which prolactin-releasing factor is predominant. Vasoactive intestinal peptide is produced in the anterior pituitary and may act as the autocrine or paracrine hormone to regulate prolactin secretion.[71–73]

Normal baseline serum prolactin levels are less than 20 μg/L in adults and usually less than 10 μg/L in men. Prolactin is secreted in an episodic manner with a distinct 24-h pattern.[74, 75] Circulating prolactin levels are lowest at midday, and a modest increase occurs during the afternoon. Prolactin levels increase shortly after onset of sleep, although peak levels occur during the middle to end of the night.[76–79] Studies involving either sleep deprivation or jet lag have demonstrated that there is also an important circadian component.[80] In normal men there are approximately 14 pulses of prolactin secretion per day with an average interpulse interval of 95 min.[79] Prolactin release in young men appears to have a close temporal coupling with LH release.[81] Enhanced prolactin secretion during the night is due to increased pulse amplitude rather than to increased pulse frequency.[81]

Prolactin synthesis is also regulated by effects of estrogen on prolactin gene expression so that serum prolactin levels are higher in normal premenopausal women than in men. Similarly prolactin levels rise during menarche[82] and during pregnancy in both the mother and the fetus (Fig. 9–2).[83] After delivery serum prolactin levels in the mother decline to the normal range over the course of the first 3 mo if the mother does not breast-feed the infant. With suckling maternal prolactin levels rise; this response is greatest early after delivery. If breast-feeding is intermittently supplemented with bottle-feeding, the suckling-induced increase in the mother's serum prolactin level wanes. However normal mean prolactin levels

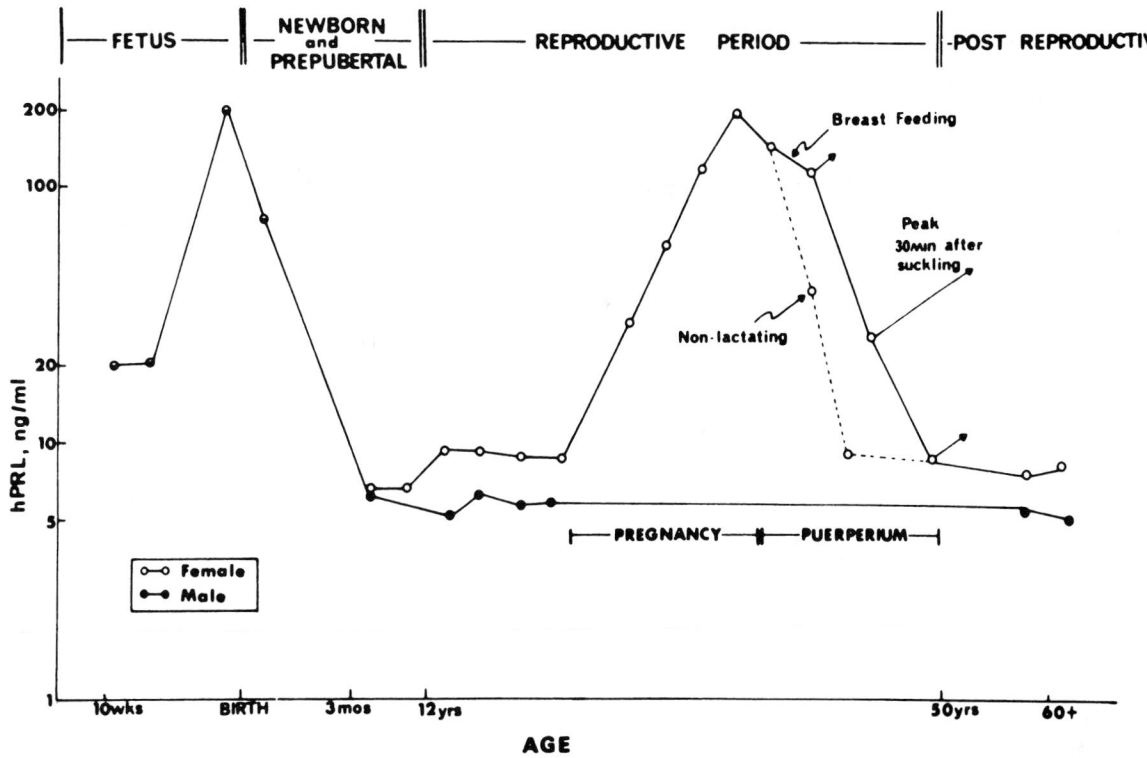

Figure 9–2. Average serum prolactin levels during various periods of life in men and women. The length of the arrows for nursing women indicates the magnitude of increase in serum prolactin level after each episode of suckling. To convert prolactin (hPRL) values to micrograms per liter, multiply by 1.0. (From Friesen HG. Human prolactin. Ann R Coll Phys Surg Can 1978; 11:275–281.)

in such women are high enough to sustain established lactation. Prolactin levels increase in women during stimulation of the nipple and during orgasm. In both men and women prolactin levels rise in response to stress.

Disruption of the hypothalamus or of the hypothalamic-hypophyseal stalk or administration of drugs that interfere with dopamine synthesis or action can cause hyperprolactinemia. In some patients with primary hypothyroidism, increased hypothalamic TRH levels may cause mild hyperprolactinemia. In such patients thyroid hormone replacement lowers thyrotropin (also called thyroid-stimulating hormone, TSH) concentrations, although it may require months for prolactin levels to reach normal.

PROLACTIN SECRETION. Prolactin is synthesized by the fetal anterior pituitary from the fifth week of gestation,[84] although lactotrope cells are not distinguishable histologically until the fifth month. From the 10th week of gestation until term there are progressive increases in the weight of the pituitary and in the prolactin content so that at term the pituitary contains approximately 2 μg of prolactin.[85] Serum prolactin levels in the fetus remain low until approximately week 26 and rise to levels in excess of 150 μg/L at term. The adult human pituitary contains about 100 μg of prolactin, compared with 5 to 10 mg of GH.

Circulating prolactin in the fetus presumably originates from the fetal pituitary. In contrast amniotic fluid prolactin is 50% glycosylated and originates from decidual cells. Maximal amniotic fluid prolactin levels are 100-fold higher than those of fetal or maternal blood and occur at midtrimester, whereas maximal serum levels in both the fetus and the mother occur at term.[86] Decidual prolactin, which is also produced by endometrial cells of the uterus from day 22 to day 28 of the menstrual cycle, is not under tonic dopaminergic inhibition but is instead stimulated by progesterone.[87, 88] mRNA for prolactin is present in chorion and decidua, and a prolactin

cDNA cloned from human term decidua is identical with that for pituitary prolactin except for four silent nucleotide changes.[89, 90]

PROLACTIN ACTIONS. Prolactin acts through prolactin receptors in multiple tissues, including breast, liver, ovary, testis, and prostate (also see Chapter 5). In the human these receptors are stimulated by GH and prolactin with equal potency. The prolactin and GH receptors and a number of cytokine receptors share sequence homology.[91] The receptors are not linked to G proteins nor do they have tyrosine kinase activity. Different forms of the prolactin receptor differ in the length of the cytoplasmic domains.

The main site of prolactin action is the mammary gland. Prolactin initiates and maintains lactation. During pregnancy the breast undergoes considerable development of the secretory apparatus through an interaction of several hormones (see Chapter 17). Insulin, cortisol, and thyroid hormone are all involved in breast development, but the major stimuli are estrogen, progesterone, prolactin, and placental mammotropic hormones, probably including GH (or its placental variant). Lactation is inhibited during pregnancy by the high levels of estrogen and progesterone. After delivery the rapid fall in estrogen and progesterone concentrations enables prolactin to initiate lactation. If prolactin secretion is inhibited after delivery with a dopamine agonist, lactation is prevented.

Prolactin acts at sites other than the breast, but the physiological function of these actions is poorly understood. Prolactin acts in the hypothalamus to regulate dopamine turnover and influence gonadotropin secretion. Physiological hyperprolactinemia during pregnancy and lactation and pathologic hyperprolactinemia are associated with suppression of the hypothalamic-pituitary-gonadal axis. This probably results from prolactin-mediated inhibition of pulsatile secretion of luteinizing hormone–releasing hormone (LHRH, also called gonadotropin-releasing hormone, GnRH), which results in impaired gonadotropin secretion and inhibition of gonadal function. Prolactin directly inhibits LHRH release and possibly *LHRH* gene expression in GT1 neuronal cell lines.[92]

GROWTH HORMONE STRUCTURE. Approximately 75% of pituitary GH is a nonglycosylated, single chain, 191-amino-acid, 22-kd protein with two intramolecular disulfide bonds, and 5 to 10% is a 20-kd form produced by alternate splicing of the second coding exon that deletes the codons for amino acids 32 to 46 from the RNA.[93, 94] GH is present in several different forms in the anterior pituitary, but some of the reported forms are due to analytic artifacts (Table 9–3).[95]

The hGH variant secreted by the placenta during pregnancy is a 22-kd protein that is not produced by the anterior pituitary.[96–99] hPL, like hGH and the hGH variant, contains 191 amino acids, 161 of which are identical with those of hGH, and has two S—S bonds located in the same position as in hGH. hPL has only about 0.001 of the growth-promoting activity of GH.

SOMATOTROPE CELL AND PITUITARY GROWTH HORMONE CONTENT. The somatotrope cells that secrete GH make up about 50% of the hormone-producing cells of the anterior pituitary and occupy the lateral wings; a minority of somatotropes are scattered throughout the median section. The ovoid, middle-sized somatotropes exhibit strong immunoreactivity for GH,[18, 100] and some GH-producing cells may contain prolactin or α subunit as well, suggesting the existence of subsets of somatotropes. Electron microscopy demonstrates abundant, large (500 nm or greater) secretory granules and rare small granules (150 to 200 nm). Sparsely granulated variants of the GH-secreting cell are also present.[18] The derivation and function of the latter subpopulation are unknown.

Somatotropes are remarkably stable, and the number, morphologic features, and immunoreactivity are unchanged by age or disease. There is one report of a decline of somatotrope cell number in senescence.[101] No significant changes are observed in somatotropes in normal areas of pituitaries that harbor somatotrope adenomas that cause acromegaly. In somatotrope hyperplasia, which occurs in response to chronic stimulation by ectopically produced growth hormone–releasing hormone (GHRH), the most characteristic alteration is hypertrophy of the Golgi complex.[102] The consistent appearance of somatotropes, determined chiefly by the abundance of large secretory granules, may mask wide fluctuations in secretory activity.

The human adenohypophysis contains 5 to 10 mg of GH that is synthesized and stored in somatotropes; GH in the secretory granules accounts for as much as 30% of the protein in the cells.

GROWTH HORMONE VARIANTS, GROWTH HORMONE RECEPTOR, AND BINDING PROTEIN. hGH circulates in several forms, including a 22-kd form, a 20-kd form, and at

TABLE 9–3. Human Growth Hormone Variants and Their Abundance in the Pituitary

Variant	Abundance (%)*
MONOMERIC	
22-kd form	75
20-kd form	5–10
Desamido–hGH (Gln-137 and Asn-152)	5
N-acylated hGH	5
DIMERIC	
Dimers (noncovalent and disulfide dimers)	5–10
Oligomers	5

*Values represent an average.
From Baumann G. Molecular variants of human growth hormone in serum and circulating growth hormone binding proteins. In: Frisch H, Thorner MO, eds. Hormonal Regulation of Growth. Serono Symposia Publications. Vol 58. New York: Raven, 1989: 175–184.

TABLE 9–4. Human Growth Hormone Variants in the Circulation*

Variant	Percent
22 kd	76
20 kd	16
Acidic GH (desamido, *N*-acyl-)	8
Monomeric	55
Dimeric	27
Tri-, tetra-, and pentameric	18
Complexed 22 kd	45
Complexed 20 kd	25

*During the second and third trimesters of pregnancy the variant form becomes the predominant form of GH in the maternal circulation and the pituitary forms decrease.[97]
From Baumann G. Molecular variants of human growth hormone in serum and circulating growth hormone binding proteins. In: Frisch H, Thorner MO, eds. Hormonal Regulation of Growth. Serono Symposia Publications. Vol. 58. New York: Raven, 1989: 175–184.

least one acidic form (Table 9–4). A mixture of GH oligomers (up to a pentamer) is also detectable in peripheral blood. Two thirds of the oligomers are noncovalently bound, and one third are linked by intermolecular disulfide bonds; it is likely that they are secreted in these forms.[103, 104] The nature of the secretory stimulus (i.e., its magnitude, duration, and mechanism) does not affect the relative proportions of the mixture of circulating GH forms, nor does sex, age, or pathologic state.[105–107] Fragments of 16 and 12 kd are detectable during periods of low secretory activity[108]; it is not known whether these are secreted or are produced in the periphery by degradation, and their biologic function is unknown.

The proportions of the GH variants in the circulation are similar to those in the pituitary except that the 20-kd form and oligomeric forms are more prominent in the circulation because of their slower metabolic clearance (see Table 9–4).

Growth Hormone Receptor. The rabbit GH receptor was purified from liver, and the binding protein was purified from serum. The structures of the binding protein and the extracellular domain of the GH receptor are identical. cDNA clones were of the rabbit GH receptor[110] used to screen a human cDNA library to obtain cDNA clones encompassing the hGH receptor. A 30 base pair enhancer element 3.4 kb upstream of the transcription start site may play a part in developmental expression of the GH receptor gene.[111] The rabbit and human receptor cDNAs contain a single long open reading frame encoding 638 amino acids (Fig. 9–3). A stretch of 24 hydrophobic amino acids in the middle of the protein constitutes the transmembrane domain and divides the molecule into extracellular and intracytoplasmic domains of similar size. The rabbit and human receptors have 620 amino acids and share considerable sequence homology (84% amino acid identity). The newly synthesized receptor is 70 kd, which is smaller than the purified receptor (130 kd), a difference partly accounted for by glycosylation. The prolactin receptor shares sequence homology with the GH receptor.[112] Each GH molecule has two binding sites for the GH receptor and forms a complex containing 1 GH:2 GH receptors.[113, 114] The prolactin and GH receptors are part of the cytokine receptor superfamily. These receptors signal through activation of the JAK family of intracellular tyrosine kinases and the STAT family of transcription factors.[115] GH activates JAK2 (to a lesser extent JAK1 and JAK3) and STAT 1, STAT 3, and STAT 5.[116] The specifics of the activation of the JAK-STAT pathway depend on the cell type.[117, 118]

Of the GH receptor mutations responsible for the resistance to GH in Laron syndrome, the majority involve the extracellular domain and affect either GH binding[119] or dimerization of the GH receptor or cause deletion of a portion of molecule.[120] There has been one report of a patient with two mutations in the intracellular domain (exon 10) of the receptor, although this patient responded to GH treatment.[121] A

Figure 9–3. Schematic representation of the GH receptor mRNA and protein. Scales of nucleotides and amino acids, the locations of the exon boundaries, and the major features of the protein and mRNA are illustrated. (Modified from Gowdowski PJ, Leung DW, Meacham LR, et al. Characterization of the human growth hormone receptor gene and demonstration of a partial gene deletion in two patients with Laron-type dwarfism. Proc Natl Acad Sci USA 1989; 86:8083–8087.)

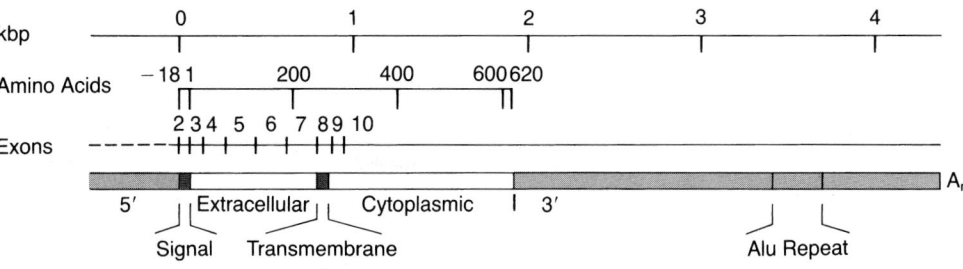

splice mutation in exon 8 that results in a receptor lacking the transmembrane and intracellular domains has been described in a patient with Laron syndrome and elevated GH-binding protein.[122] The potential exists, therefore, that additional mutations in the transmembrane or intracellular domains of the receptor can cause Laron syndrome. Mutations might also arise in other genes that encode proteins required for expression of the receptor or for transduction of the GH signal, causing a phenotype similar to that of Laron dwarfism.

Growth Hormone–Binding Protein. A GH-binding protein in human plasma is identical in amino acid sequence to the extracellular domain of the hGH receptor.[94, 109, 110] Absence of the binding protein in the plasma of patients with Laron dwarfism, in whom there is a resistance to GH action, supports the relationship between the GH-binding protein and receptor.[123, 124] The principal binding protein binds 22-kd GH with high affinity (association constant K_a of 50 nmol/L) and limited binding capacity, i.e., a limited number of binding sites per molecule. Its affinity for 20-kd GH is somewhat lower. The binding protein is a 61-kd glycoprotein and has an apparent molecular mass of 80 to 85 kd when complexed with GH. The complex coelutes on cross-linked dextran beads (Sephadex) columns with "big" and "big, big" GH. Thus "big" GH forms consist of both GH oligomers and GH-binding protein complexes. GH-binding protein, 100 kd, in human plasma has saturable, specific binding for GH, although the binding affinity is less than that of the 61-kd binding protein. The 100-kd binding protein is present in patients deficient in the GH receptor, suggesting that it is not related to the GH receptor.

Forty-five percent of 22-kd GH and 25% of 20-kd GH are complexed with the binding proteins, and the high-affinity binding protein accounts for 85% of this binding.[108] When circulating GH concentrations rise to greater than 10 to 20 μg/L, a progressively smaller proportion is bound to the binding protein.

The association rate of GH and its binding protein is such that the complex forms in the circulation.[104] Administration of monomeric, recombinant-derived, 22-kd GH to normal young men with suppressed endogenous GH secretion results in binding similar to that observed in vitro when radiolabeled GH is added to normal human plasma.[104] Thirty-eight percent of the GH is bound to binding protein at plasma GH levels of 32 to 59 μg/L, and 46% is bound at a serum GH concentration of 7 μg/L. The proportions bound to the high-affinity and low-affinity binding proteins are also similar in vivo and in vitro. No oligomeric GH forms appear to develop in vitro, suggesting that the pituitary is the source of these forms.

The biologic significance of the binding proteins is unclear. Protein-bound GH is metabolized differently than is monomeric GH and persists 10 times longer in plasma. The volume of distribution of protein-bound GH is twice the intravascular compartment, whereas monomeric GH is distributed throughout the extracellular space.[125, 126] These two effects of protein binding may enhance the biologic activity of GH. Alternatively the high-affinity binding protein may compete

with receptor for the binding of GH and thus impair GH action.[127]

The plasma concentrations of the binding proteins appear to remain fairly constant in an individual but vary widely among individuals. Levels of binding proteins are low prenatally and at birth and increase throughout childhood.[108, 128] Levels of the low-affinity (but not the high-affinity) binding protein increase during pregnancy. Binding is decreased in Laron dwarfism and in pygmies, during prolonged fasting, and with uremia.[108, 123, 124]

REGULATION OF GROWTH HORMONE SECRETION.

The pulsatile secretion of GH is regulated by two hypothalamic regulatory hormones, GHRH and somatostatin (also called somatotropin release-inhibiting factor, SRIF). GHRH controls GH synthesis by regulating transcription of GH mRNA via control of cAMP levels.[129] Somatostatin appears to determine the timing and amplitude of GH pulses but has no effect on GH synthesis. The neuroendocrine regulation of GHRH and somatostatin secretion is discussed in Chapter 8.

The mechanisms of action of GHRH and somatostatin have been studied in cultured rat anterior pituitary cells, clonal cell lines and, occasionally, human pituitary cells. The rat somatotrope has spontaneous intracellular calcium oscillations (Fig. 9–4). Binding of somatostatin to its receptor on the somatotrope inhibits GH release by decreasing intracellular calcium concentrations and inhibiting adenylate cyclase.[130] These effects are mediated by a G protein that is sensitive to pertussis toxin, although the exact molecular mechanisms have not been established.[131–133] GHRH interacts with a cell membrane receptor to stimulate adenylate cyclase and increase intracellular cAMP levels[134–137] and to increase intracel-

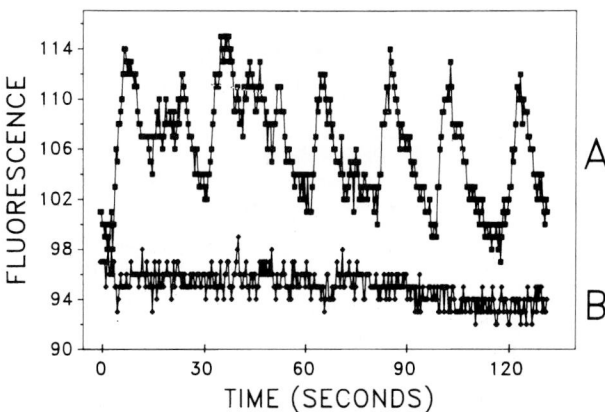

Figure 9–4. Pattern of calcium oscillations in a rat somatotrope (A) and nonsomatotrope pituitary cell (B) in the same field. Fluorescence intensity (arbitrary units) was measured every 300 ms from a continuous recording (excitation at 340 nm) that allows high temporal resolution and qualitative changes in cytosolic calcium concentrations. (From Holl RW, Thorner MO, Mandell GL, et al. Spontaneous oscillations of intracellular calcium and growth hormone secretion. J Biol Chem 1988; 263:9682–9685.)

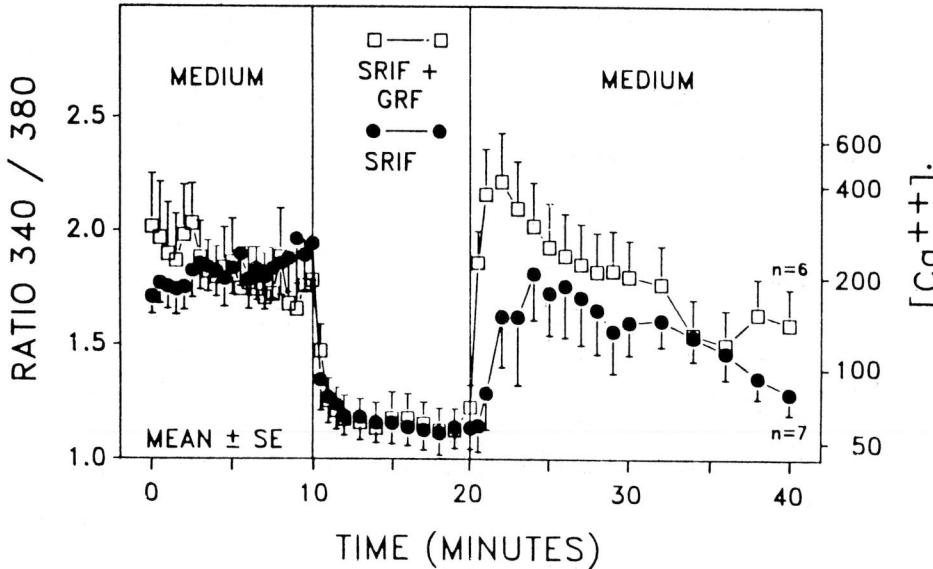

Figure 9–5. Identical reduction of intracellular calcium concentration ($[Ca^{2+}]_i$) in normal rat somatotropes treated with somatostatin (SRIF) plus GHRH (GRF) and cells exposed to somatostatin alone. Recordings of $[Ca^{2+}]_i$ were made every 30 s. Basal recordings were made for 10 min, followed by the addition of either 10 nmol/L GHRH or 1 nmol/L somatostatin. After an additional 10 min, the regulatory peptides were replaced by medium alone. Data points represent the mean ± SE of a group of six or seven somatotropes, respectively, as identified by reverse hemolytic plaque assay. The ratio of fluorescence with excitation at 340 and 380 nm is given on the left axis; the corresponding free cytosolic calcium concentration is shown on the right axis. (From RW Holl, MO Thorner, DA Leong. Intracellular calcium concentration and growth hormone secretion in individual somatotropes: effects of growth hormone–releasing factor and somatostatin, Endocrinology 122:2927–2932, 1988, © by The Endocrine Society.)

lular calcium concentrations.[131] When cells are exposed to both somatostatin and GHRH, somatostatin exerts the dominant effect; intracellular calcium concentration decreases and GH release is inhibited (Fig. 9–5). There is significant interaction among the various intracellular second messenger pathways, and it is likely that the phospholipase C–diacylglycerol–protein kinase C pathway is also involved in regulation of GH secretion both by modulating intracellular calcium concentrations and by activating protein kinase C.[138]

An overview of the regulation of GH secretion is shown in schematic form in Figure 9–6. In addition to the hypothalamic influences the somatotrope is regulated by negative feedback by circulating somatomedins such as insulin-like growth factor

I (IGF-I, also called somatomedin-C) at the pituitary and hypothalamic levels and by short-loop feedback by GH itself on the hypothalamus (also see Chapter 8).

GH is detectable in fetal serum at the end of the first trimester, and its concentration increases rapidly thereafter to reach a peak of 100 to 150 µg/L at about the 20th week of gestation.[84] GH is not thought to be essential for normal intrauterine development and growth. Premature infants have higher serum GH levels than do full-term infants. Mean levels decrease to about 30 µg/L in cord serum and continue to fall during the early postnatal months. The amount of GH secreted is greatest during adolescence and decreases with age (Fig. 9–7). Premenopausal women have higher GH production rates than do young men.[139]

The pattern of GH secretion depends on a number of factors, including stage of development, nutritional state, sleep stage, stress, and exercise. Metabolic clearance may also vary. Characteristic profiles of GH concentrations in normal men and women are shown in Figure 9–8.

The mean half-life of exogenously administered GH in normal individuals ranges from 9 to 27 min.[140–143] The monoexponential half-life of endogenous GH has been estimated by deconvolution analysis (17 ± 1.7 min) and by sequential

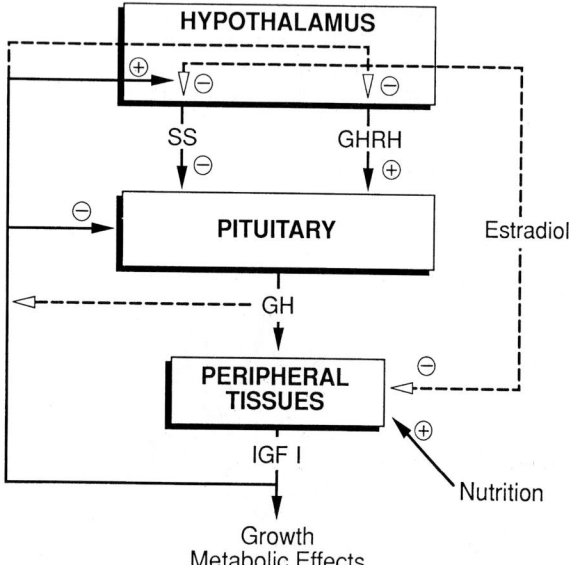

Figure 9–6. Schematic illustration of regulation of serum GH secretion. GH is secreted in a pulsatile fashion under coordinate regulation by hypothalamic somatostatin (SS) and GHRH. GH acts on multiple tissues to regulate metabolic functions and growth. Peripheral tissues produce IGF-I, which is secreted into the circulation and acts as a paracrine factor. Circulating and hypothalamic- or pituitary-derived IGF-I may also inhibit GH secretion at the pituitary or hypothalamic levels or both. GH also regulates its own secretion by short-loop feedback. Estrogen stimulates GH secretion in humans; the mechanism of action is unclear but the effect may be either to inhibit the action of GH peripherally or stimulate GH secretion at the hypothalamic level.

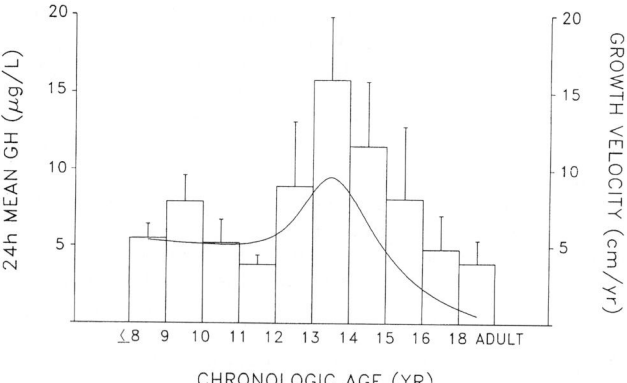

Figure 9–7. Histogram of the 24-h mean (± SE) concentration of growth hormone (GH) (left axis) from 60 24-h GH profiles by chronologic age. An idealized growth velocity curve (50th percentile values) for North American boys[1052] is superimposed (right axis). From Martha PM Jr, Rogol AD, Veldhuis JD, et al. Alterations in the pulsatile properties of circulating growth hormone concentrations during puberty in boys. J Clin Endocrinol Metab 1989; 69:563–570.

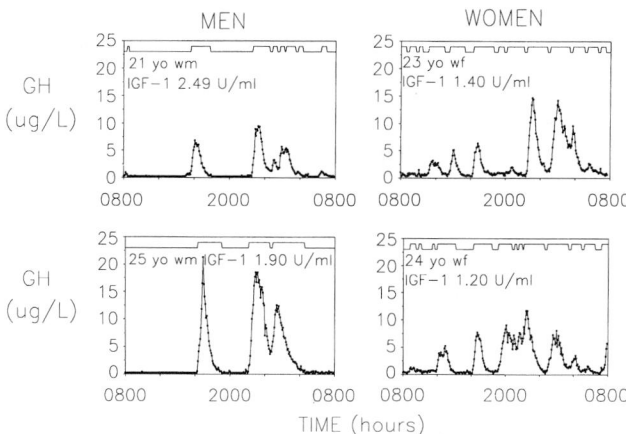

Figure 9–8. Representative 24-h serum GH concentration profiles of two normal men and two normal women. Blood sampling was performed every 5 min for 24 h. The continuous schematized line in the upper portion of each panel identifies individually significant GH pulses detected by cluster analysis. (From ML Hartman, JD Veldhuis, ML Vance, et al., Somatotropin pulse frequency and basal concentrations are increased in acromegaly and are reduced by successful therapy, J Clin Endocrinol Metab 70:1375–1384, 1990, © by The Endocrine Society.)

administration of intravenous boluses of GHRH and somatostatin, followed by a somatostatin infusion (18 ± 0.8 min).[25, 144] The latter technique made possible the delineation of two components of GH disappearance: a distribution alpha phase of 3.5 ± 0.7 min and a metabolic clearance beta phase of 20.7 ± 0.7 min.[144] Twenty-four–hour GH production rates for adult men range from 0.25 to 0.52 mg/m² surface area.[25, 145, 146]

The effects of age and sex on GH release have been studied by measuring GH concentrations in samples drawn every 20 min for 24 h from young men, young women, older men, and older women. Levels of serum estradiol but not testosterone correlated with the 24-h integrated GH concentration,[139] and when the effects of estradiol were excluded, neither age nor sex influenced the integrated GH concentration. This study and studies of GH secretion during puberty[147] suggest that gonadal steroids, particularly estradiol, are important in the regulation of GH secretion. The site of estrogen action may be in the periphery or at the pituitary or hypothalamic level. In rats gonadal steroids affect GHRH and somatostatin gene expression,[148, 149] and estrogens may also influence the synthesis of IGF-I or IGF-I binding proteins and GH-binding proteins, or both.

Between bursts of GH release, serum GH concentrations are undetectable in conventional assays (<0.2 µg/L). GH is secreted in volleys of multiple secretory bursts that probably arise from multiple GHRH secretory bursts into the hypophyseal-portal blood during periods of reduced somatostatin secretion.[25] Regardless of nutritional state, the amplitude of GH secretory bursts is maximal during the night. The most consistent period of GH secretion in children and young adults (and possibly other age groups) coincides with the onset of the first slow-wave sleep (stages III and IV), usually within the first hour of sleep. Delay in the onset of deep sleep usually delays the onset of the major GH peak. GH levels are highest during slow-wave sleep and lowest during rapid eye movement sleep. Plasma levels of glucose, fatty acids, and insulin do not change with the burst of GH secretion, although resistance to exogenous insulin and decreased glucose tolerance develop after the peak of GH secretion. Rapid eye movement sleep may be responsible for the termination of sleep-related GH secretion. Studies involving GHRH administration during different stages of sleep, at different times during the night, and with sleep deprivation[150] support the hypothesis that decreased hypothalamic somatostatin secretion

initiates GH secretory bursts. There is a circadian rhythm for GH secretion in humans, and variations of somatostatin secretion may account for differences in sensitivity to GHRH during different phases of sleep. Thus slow-wave sleep may be associated with low levels of hypothalamic somatostatin secretion, and rapid eye movement sleep may be associated with high levels.

Although fasting increases both the number and amplitude of GH secretory bursts,[151] the predominant effect is an increase in the amplitude of the secretory bursts (Fig. 9–9). Fasting may cause decreased hypothalamic somatostatin secretion. In contrast GH secretion is decreased in obese subjects; again the predominant effect appears to be a reduction in the amplitude of the GH secretory bursts (Fig. 9–10).[153] The metabolic clearance rate of GH is accelerated in obesity.[152] The diminished GH secretion in obesity may be due to high levels of somatostatin. The decline in GH secretion in hypothyroidism and in normal aging are also associated primarily with decreased GH burst amplitudes. Attributes of GH secretion in humans as determined by deconvolution analysis are shown in Table 9–5.

Studies of patients with GHRH-secreting tumors and of normal adults given intravenous GHRH infusions support the concept that somatostatin is the zeitgeber (time giver) for pulses of GH secretion. The significance of pulsatile GH secretion is not established but, as discussed earlier, the pattern of secretion may influence tissue responses. Pulsatile GH secretion may be particularly important for growth and for the effects of the hormone on metabolism.[154]

GH secretion is also influenced acutely by neurogenic, metabolic, and hormonal factors (Table 9–6). For example hyperglycemia in normal individuals acutely suppresses GH secretion,[155] whereas in individuals with poorly controlled diabetes mellitus GH levels are increased.[156] Similarly although acute increases in free fatty acid concentrations inhibit GH release, fatty acid levels are increased during starvation when GH secretion is augmented. GH secretion appears to be inversely related to insulin concentrations. For example GH secretion is augmented in fasting, anorexia nervosa, insulin-dependent diabetes mellitus, and cirrhosis of the liver when circulating insulin levels are low. In contrast in obesity, hyperinsulinemia is present and GH secretion is suppressed. Amino acids such as arginine and leucine stimulate GH secretion (Fig. 9–11).

Although exercise, stress, and some neurogenic factors stimulate GH secretion, emotional deprivation can inhibit its

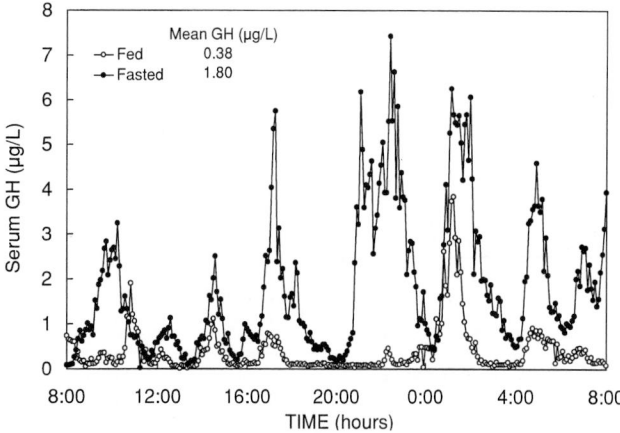

Figure 9–9. Profiles of serum GH concentrations measured in a sensitive chemiluminescence assay in blood collected at 5-min intervals over 24 h from an 81-year-old woman. Serial GH concentrations and mean 24-h GH results from a control day *(fed, open circles)* and the second day of a fast *(fasted, closed circles)* are shown.

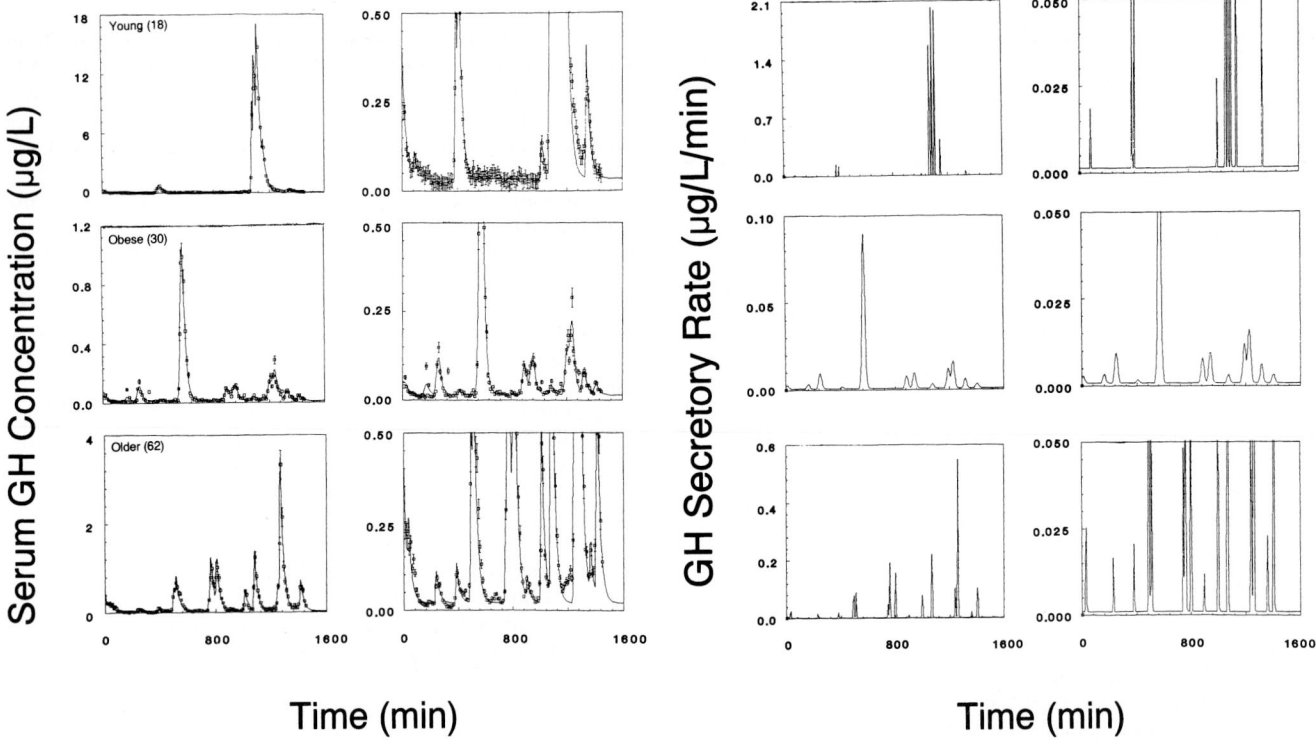

Figure 9–10. Illustrative individual profiles of serum GH concentrations determined in blood collected at 10-min intervals over 24 h in male volunteers. Ages are given in parentheses. Data are shown for the GH chemiluminescence (CL) assay and are plotted on two different scales (note different axes). The right hand scales are expanded to show the low values. Note that in the IRMA less than 0.10 μg/L of the serum GH concentration would be undetectable. In contrast all measurements exceeded the CL assay sensitivity of 0.005 μg/L. The measured serum GH concentrations (two left panels) and the calculated GH secretory rates (two right panels) using multiparameter deconvolution analysis are shown for each profile. Again both nominal *(left)* and expanded *(right)* scales are given. (From Iranmanesh A, Grisso B, Veldhuis JD. Low basal and persistent pulsatile growth hormone secretion are revealed in normal and hyposomatotropic men studied with a new ultrasensitive chemiluminescence assay. J Clin Endocrinol Metab 1994; 78:526–535.)

release in children and impair linear growth.[157, 158] Central α-adrenergic agonists (norepinephrine and clonidine) stimulate GH secretion.[159] β-Adrenergic antagonists augment the efficacy of various stimuli for GH secretion, and dopamine agonists stimulate GH secretion in normal individuals by stimulating dopamine receptors. Acetylcholine agonists stimulate GH release[160, 161] and agents that lower acetylcholine tone suppress it. Stimulation of GH release by dopamine agonists, α-adrener-gic agonists, glucagon, and amino acids is inhibited by pirenzepine, a cholinergic muscarinic blocking drug.[162–165] In addition sleep-induced GH secretion is blocked by the cholinergic blocking agent methscopolamine. These agents are thought to act at the level of the hypothalamus or the median eminence. GH secretory responses to a number of stimuli are augmented by treatment with estrogens (e.g., diethylstilbestrol 3 mg/d for 3 d). The role of serotonin in GH secretion is unclear,[142] and histamine does not appear to play a role. Endogenous opiates probably do not directly influence GH secretion because spontaneous GH secretion is not modified by naloxone. Morphine and β-endorphin do not affect GH secretion, but nalorphine and an enkephalin analogue (DAMME, FK33824) stimulate GH secretion through naloxone-sensitive mechanisms.[166] The pharmacologic agent GH-releasing peptide (GHRP-6)[167] is a potent stimulator of GH release; this hexapeptide was developed from an enkephalin series of peptides, but it does not act through characterized GHRH, somatostatin, or enkephalin receptors.

The cloning of the GH secretagogue receptor[168, 169] is of major importance because GHRP-6, GHRP-2, L-692,429 and MK-677 all act through this receptor to stimulate GH secretion. MK-677 is orally active and enhances GH secretion in normal[170] and elderly individuals[171] and increases serum IGF-I levels. Whether these compounds can enhance GH secretion in GH-deficient individuals or in pathologic states in which GH is suppressed remains to be determined.[172, 173]

GROWTH HORMONE ACTIONS. There are two theories regarding the actions of GH: the GH hypothesis and the somatomedin hypothesis (see Chapter 30).[174, 175] Figure 9–12 illustrates the various direct actions of GH. The existence of somatomedins was invoked as the result of the finding that

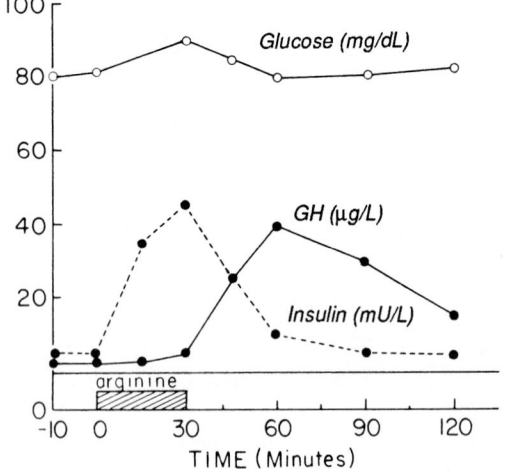

Figure 9–11. Effects of intravenous arginine (0.5 g/kg body weight) on plasma glucose, GH, and insulin concentrations. To convert plasma glucose values to millimoles per liter, multiply by 0.0555. To convert insulin values to picomoles per liter, multiply by 7.175.

TABLE 9–5. Deconvolution Analysis–Derived Features of Growth Hormone Secretion

	Growth Hormone Secreted (µg/24 h)*	No. Secretory Bursts	Mass of Growth Hormone Secreted per Burst (µg)*	Half-Life (mins)
IMMUNORADIOMETRIC ASSAY				
Normal young men[25]†	540 ± 44	12 ± 1.2	45 ± 3.7	17 ± 1.7
Fasted men[995]†	2171 ± 333	32 ± 2.4	64 ± 9.4	18 ± 2.2
Obese men[152]‡	77 ± 20	3.2 ± 0.5	24 ± 4.6	12 ± 1.6
Normal middle-aged men[152]‡	196 ± 65	9.7 ± 0.7	20 ± 6.3	16 ± 0.8
IMMUNOFLUOROMETRIC ASSAY§ (Van den Berghe,[1000] sensitivity 0.0125 µg/L)				
Middle-aged women (n = 10)	187 ± 24	19 ± 1.1	9.7 ± 1.4	18 ± 1.6
Middle-aged men (n = 7)	108 ± 22	20 ± 1.7	5.1 ± 0.83	16 ± 1.6
CHEMILUMINESCENCE ASSAY‖ (Veldhuis et al,[153, 1001] sensitivity 0.002 µg/L)				
Young men (n = 2, range)	176–223**	8–16	3–22	13–17
Middle-aged (n = 2, range)	149–165	9–14	2–4	10–16
Hypothyroid men (n = 2, range)	19–28	12–14	0.2–0.6	11–17
Older men (n = 3, range)	36–138	7–15	0.4–3.0	14–16
Obese (n = 2, range)	23–41	12–19	0.2–0.4	13–17

*Assuming mean GH volume of distribution of 7.9% body weight.
†Samples obtained at 5-min intervals; age of individuals = 22 to 28 y; BMI = 21 to 29 kg/m².
‡Samples obtained at 10-min intervals; mean age of obese individuals = 40 ± 3.1 y; normal individuals = 48 ± 4.7 y; mean BMI obese = 46 ± 1.6 kg/m²; mean BMI normal individuals = 28 ± 1.3 kg/m².
§Women   Age: 48 ± 5 y   BMI (kg/m²) 23 ± 0.9
 Men   Age: 47 ± 3.5 y   23 ± 0.6
‖Young (ages 18 and 19, 12% body fat)
 Middle-aged (ages 43 and 54)
 Obese (ages 30 and 46, BMI 38 and 43 kg/m²)
 Older (ages 62 and 63)
 Hypothyroid (ages 34 and 43)
**Range

growth and mitotic activity of cartilage are dependent on GH in vivo but that the direct addition of GH in vitro is ineffective in promoting either action. Likewise proliferation of cartilage from hypophysectomized rats is stimulated by serum from normal rats but not by serum from GH-deficient rats, and treatment of GH-deficient individuals with GH restores the stimulatory effect of the serum within 24 to 48 h. The active components of the serum are two closely related peptides, IGF-I and IGF-II, single chain peptides that exhibit sequence homology with human proinsulin. Serum IGF-I concentrations are elevated in acromegaly and low in GH deficiency; IGF-II levels are unchanged in acromegaly and modestly reduced in GH deficiency. These observations suggest that IGF-I is the

important mediator of GH action, and the fact that IGF-I inhibits GH secretion lends support to this hypothesis.[176–179] Whether IGF-I acts locally or as a circulating hormone has been difficult to establish. Insight into this issue came from an experiment in which tissue concentrations of IGF-I were measured in normal and hypophysectomized rats; a striking reduction in IGF-I occurred after hypophysectomy in all tissues except the brain. After GH administration tissue IGF-I concentrations increased many hours before the increase in circulating levels, providing an explanation for the lack of a clear relationship between IGF-I levels and growth response during GH treatment (Table 9–7).

Based on studies of GH action in a preadipocyte cell line, a dual-effector model of GH action has been proposed (Fig.

TABLE 9–6. Factors Influencing Normal Growth Hormone Secretion

Factor	Growth Hormone Secretion	
	Augmented	Inhibited
Neurogenic	Stages III and IV sleep	REM sleep
	Stress (traumatic, surgical, inflammatory, psychogenic)	Emotional deprivation
	α-Adrenergic agonist	α-Adrenergic antagonist
	β-Adrenergic antagonist	β-Adrenergic agonist
	Dopamine agonist	
	Acetylcholine agonist	Acetylcholine antagonist
Metabolic	Hypoglycemia	Hyperglycemia
	Fasting	
	Falling fatty acid level	Rising fatty acid level
	Amino acids	
	Uncontrolled diabetes mellitus	Obesity
	Uremia	
	Hepatic cirrhosis	
Hormonal	GHRH	Somatostatin
	Low IGF-I level	High IGF-I level
	Estrogens	Hypothyroidism
	Glucagon	High glucocorticoid levels
	AVP	

REM, rapid eye movement; GHRH, growth hormone–releasing hormone; IGF-I, insulin-like growth factor I; AVP, arginine vasopressin.

TABLE 9–7. Extractable Tissue Insulin-Like Growth Factor I Concentrations in Normal and Hypophysectomized Male Rats

	Insulin-Like Growth Factor I (µg/g)		
Tissue	Normal Rats*	Hypophysectomized Rats*	% of Normal
Serum	28.7 ± 0.98	0.74 ± 0.12	2.6
Liver	1.91 ± 0.23	0.23 ± 0.08	12.0
Lung	2.04 ± 0.86	0.57 ± 0.13	27.9
Kidney	2.59 ± 0.80	0.77 ± 0.29	29.7
Heart	0.92 ± 0.43	0.48 ± 0.14	52.2
Muscle (iliopsoas)	0.42 ± 0.05	<0.08	<19.1
Brain	0.26 ± 0.09	0.28 ± 0.04	107.7
Testes	1.88 ± 0.42	0.52 ± 0.32	27.7
Prostate	1.06	0.40	37.7
Thymus	0.33	0.10	30.3
Lymph nodes	0.48	0.08	16.7
Cartilage (sternum)	0.67	0.53	79.1
Fat pad (perirenal)	0.67 ± 0.19	0.25 ± 0.10	37.3
Submaxillary gland	1.73	0.78	45.1

*Values are mean ± SD.
From D'Ercole AJ, Stiles AD, Underwood LE. Tissue concentrations of somatomedin C: further evidence for multiple sites of synthesis and paracrine or autocrine mechanisms of action. Proc Natl Acad Sci USA 1984; 81:935–939.

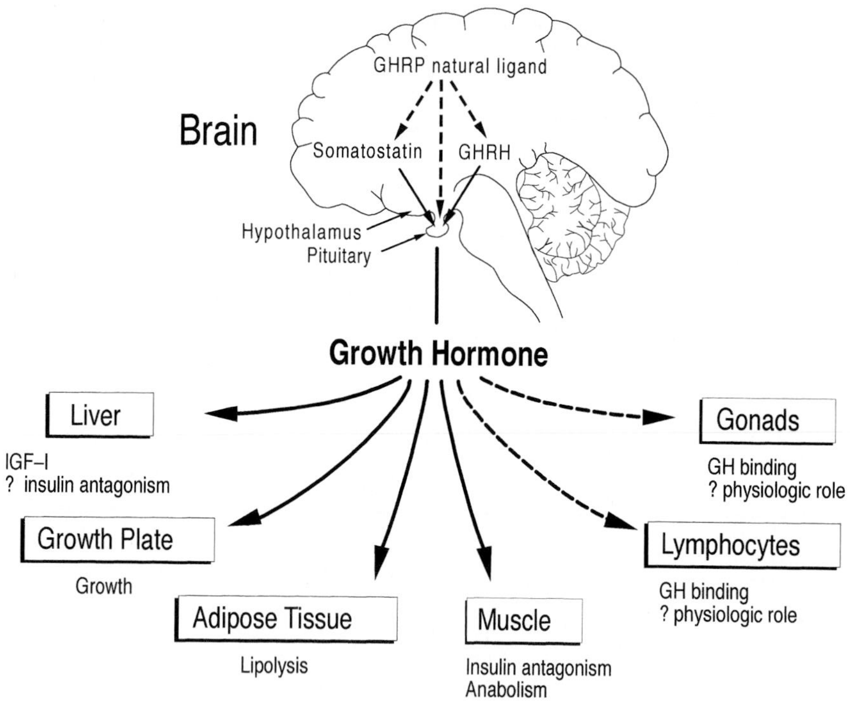

Brain

GHRP natural ligand

Somatostatin | GHRH

Hypothalamus
Pituitary

Growth Hormone

Liver

IGF–I
? insulin antagonism

Growth Plate

Growth

Adipose Tissue

Lipolysis

Muscle

Insulin antagonism
Anabolism

Gonads

GH binding
? physiologic role

Lymphocytes

GH binding
? physiologic role

Figure 9–12. Schematic representation of multiple sites of growth hormone (GH) action.

9–13) in which GH first stimulates precursor cells to undergo differentiation, and somatomedins then act as mitogens to stimulate clonal growth of the differentiated cells.[180] Evidence supporting this hypothesis comes from experiments in which the injection of GH into the epiphyseal plate of hypophysectomized rats stimulated growth only in the injected limb,[98, 181, 182] and the effect was prevented by passive immunization with IGF-I antibodies.[183] IGF-I is present in the proliferative chondrocytes of rat epiphyseal growth plates[184] and in skeletal muscle.[185] In addition IGF-I levels increase in response to GH administration in many of these tissues.[184, 185] Thus locally produced IGF-I, under GH regulation, contributes to the stimulatory effects of GH, particularly the enhancement of longitudinal growth.[186, 187] Administration of IGF-I to hypophysecto

mized rats does not promote growth equivalent to that achieved with GH.[188, 189]

Metabolic Actions of Growth Hormone. Many GH actions described in isolated tissues and organs (Table 9–8) must be interpreted with the knowledge that such studies are subject to all the limitations inherent in in vitro studies. The effect of GH on metabolism in vivo is the subject of intensive study in humans and animals because of the potential for promoting protein synthesis and either lipolysis or reduced fat deposition. The availability of biosynthetic GH produced by recombinant DNA technology and the development of methods for assessing subtle metabolic changes make it possible to define the role of this hormone in human metabolism. GH is described as anabolic, lipolytic, and diabetogenic, concepts de

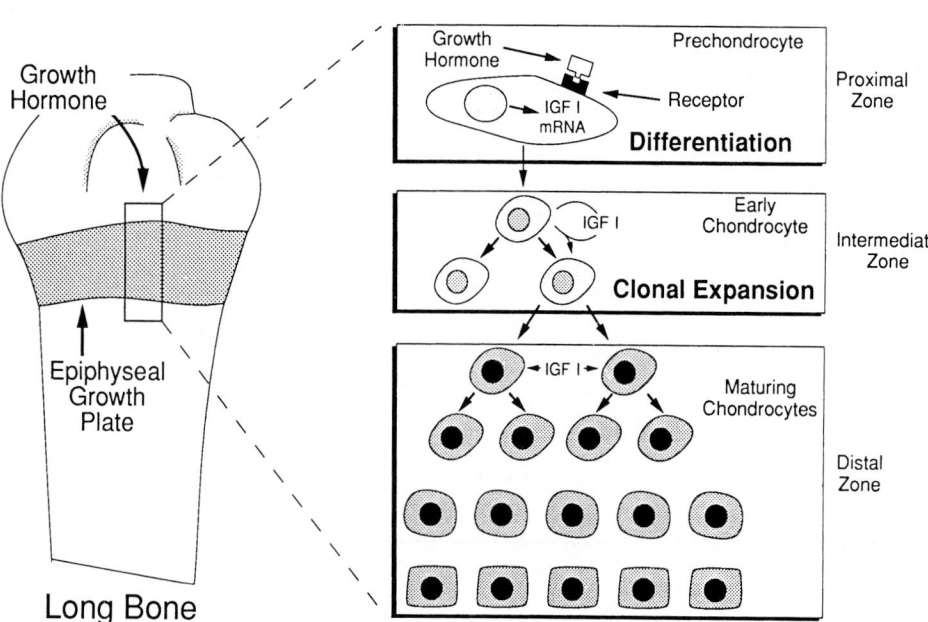

Growth
Hormone

Epiphyseal
Growth
Plate

Long Bone

Growth
Hormone → Receptor

Prechondrocyte

IGF I
mRNA

Differentiation

Proximal
Zone

IGF I

Early
Chondrocyte

Clonal Expansion

Intermediate
Zone

IGF I

Maturing
Chondrocytes

Distal
Zone

Figure 9–13. Schematic representation of the dual-effector hypothesis proposed by Green and colleagues.[180] GH acts directly at the epiphyseal plate to stimulate linear growth. GH stimulates differentiation of prechondrocytes into early chondrocytes, which then secrete IGF-I. In turn IGF-I stimulates clonal expansion and maturation of chondrocytes. (Modified from Isaksson OGP, Isgaard J, Nilsson A, et al. Direct action of growth hormone. In: Bercu BB, ed. Basic and Clinical Aspects of Growth Hormone. New York: Plenum, 1988: 199–211.)

TABLE 9–8. Direct Actions of Growth Hormone on Isolated Tissues and Organs

Tissue or Organ	Action
Liver	
Perfusion	RNA synthesis[1002]
	Plasma protein synthesis[1003]
	Somatomedin release[1004]
Cell culture	Replication[1005]
Muscle	
Isolated rat diaphragm incubation	Amino acid transport and incorporation[1006]
Rat heart perfusion	Amino acid transport and incorporation[1007]
Human vascular smooth muscle cell culture	Outgrowth[1008]
Rat adipocyte incubations	Amino acid incorporation[1009]
	Lipolysis[1010]
Human fibroblast culture	Somatomedin production[1011]
Rabbit and rat chondrocytes	DNA synthesis[1012]
	Sulfate incorporation[1012]
Hematopoietic cell culture	
Rat thymic lymphocyte culture	Mitosis[1013]
Human leukemic lymphoblast culture	[³H]Thymidine, [³H]uridine, and [³H]leucine incorporation[1014]
Human erythrogenic precursors	[³H]Thymidine uptake[1015]
Isolated rat hypothalamus	Somatostatin secretion[177]

rived primarily from in vitro studies of isolated tissues deprived of the normal hormonal milieu and from in vivo studies involving administration of pharmacologic amounts of GH either acutely or in a nonphysiological manner.

Effects of Growth Hormone in Animals. Administration of GH to growing animals improves nutrient "partitioning" and utilization. Administration of pharmacologic GH doses to growing pigs and cattle increases nitrogen retention, improves feed efficiency, and alters carcass composition (reduced fat and increased protein content).[190–192] For example treatment of castrated male pigs with porcine GH for 35 d increased feed efficiency, caused a 25% decrease in carcass lipid, and increased carcass muscle 16% when compared with controls.[193] GH effects cannot be extrapolated from one species to another or from one age group to another, but studies in animals provide a rationale for studies in humans.

Effects of Growth Hormone in Humans. The metabolic effects of GH administration on various aspects of metabolism have been studied in normal, diabetic, and GH-deficient individuals. Most studies either involved intermittent (once daily) pharmacologic administration or were of limited duration and designed to study only the acute effects of GH on a specific aspect of metabolism.

The effects of GH on serum glucose, insulin, and fatty acid levels vary among individuals and among different study protocols. Continuous intravenous infusion of GH that produces serum concentrations of 6 to 10 μg/L causes lipolysis and ketosis in individuals with diabetes mellitus but not in normal individuals.[194] Continuous intravenous GH infusion in normal individuals, producing serum GH concentrations of 10 to 50 μg/L, causes insulin resistance without hyperglycemia, ketonemia, or consistent changes in lipid concentrations. More prolonged GH infusion produces fasting hyperglycemia, hyperinsulinemia, and increased nonesterified fatty acid concentrations without ketonemia or change in serum glycerol concentrations.[195] Eight hours of continuous GH infusion in normal men (serum GH concentrations 30 to 35 μg/L) increases serum nonesterified fatty acid, ketone, and insulin concentrations and causes glucose intolerance but no change in fasting glucose level.[196] GH induction of insulin resistance at a postreceptor site may be the mechanism for these effects, as suggested by studies involving pharmacologic amounts of GH[197] and by studies employing euglycemic insulin and hyper-

glycemic clamp techniques.[198] Hyperglycemic clamp studies with a continuous 14-h GH infusion suggest that the site of insulin resistance is the liver.[199] In summary despite minor differences in study designs, both continuous GH exposure and pharmacologic GH doses produce alterations in carbohydrate and lipid utilization.

Administration of GH in physiological amounts to GH-deficient children enhances positive nitrogen balance, decreases urea production, redistributes body fat, and reduces carbohydrate utilization but does not increase the incidence of diabetes mellitus. A single dose of GH decreases levels of free fatty acid, blood glucose, and amino acids for only a few hours. Similar effects occur in normal individuals, albeit to a lesser extent.[200]

Increased nitrogen retention occurs during short-term (1 to 3 wk) daily or alternate-day GH administration to normal and obese individuals during caloric restriction and to older adults during surfeit nutrition;[201–203] this effect does not persist during more prolonged treatment (5 wk) in obese individuals.[204]

Growth Hormone and Aging. Both integrated and pulsatile GH secretion declines in men and women with age,[139, 205–208] accompanied by a decrease in serum IGF-I concentration. Other changes in metabolism with age include loss of muscle mass and increased body fat despite maintenance of normal weight.[209, 210] The administration of GH for 6 mo to older adults with diminished GH secretion caused an increase in serum IGF-I concentrations, and changes in body composition included a 10% increase in lean body mass, a 15% decrease in adipose tissue, and a 2% increase in vertebral bone density. These changes were associated with increased fasting serum glucose and insulin concentrations.[211, 212] It is not known whether improvements in exercise capacity or changes in carbohydrate, lipid, and protein metabolism occur with chronic GH treatment of the elderly.

Growth Hormone in Catabolic Illness. Burn injury and surgery are associated with a catabolic state despite nutritional support and treatment of associated complications such as infection and anemia. Serum GH concentrations are inappropriately low. In seven postoperative patients receiving a hypocaloric diet of 400 kcal/d as 5% dextrose, the median serum GH level was 3 μg/L (range 3 to 22 μg/L) and did not change when oral nutrition was introduced.[213]

Studies involving administration of large doses of GH to burn patients have focused primarily on the nitrogen-sparing effect. In several studies of burn patients the administration of GH over a 4- to 12-d period decreased urinary nitrogen excretion, suggesting that GH exerts an "anabolic" effect,[214–217] although this methodology does not distinguish between an increase in protein synthesis and a decrease in catabolism. Treatment of burn patients with GH also increases basal plasma insulin levels without causing glucose intolerance.[217] Effects of GH on glucose and lipid turnover are less well defined, but indirect calorimetry studies suggest that lipid utilization is increased by GH.[216]

Administration of pharmacologic doses of glucocorticoids produces a catabolic state by promoting protein degradation. Treatment with GH for 7 d prevents glucocorticoid-induced protein catabolism in normal volunteers.[218] These findings have wide-ranging implications for potential applications of GH treatment in a variety of patients with catabolic illnesses.

Glycoprotein Hormone Family[227, 228]

The three anterior pituitary glycoprotein hormones are thyrotropin, LH (lutropin), and follicle-stimulating hormone (FSH, follitropin). Each consists of two noncovalently linked subunits, αβ. The α subunit is common to all three hormones, but the β subunit is unique for each and confers biologic specificity.[219] The subunits are synthesized as separate peptides from distinct mRNAs.[220-222] Microheterogeneity of the carbohydrate constituents of the individual hormones causes differences in receptor affinity, biologic potency, and metabolic clearance.

The α subunit is more abundant than the unique β subunit. Free serum α subunits are secreted and are present in serum in concentrations equivalent to the combined levels of thyrotropin, LH, and FSH. Free levels of serum β subunit are usually lower than the level of detectability in conventional assays.[223-225] The overabundance of α subunit suggests that regulation of β subunit synthesis is the rate-limiting step in modulating the levels of thyrotropin, LH, and FSH. The glycosylation step is probably also regulated.[226]

α Subunit

The α subunits are approximately 20 to 22 kd, have 92 amino acid residues in the human and 96 amino acid residues in other species, and contain two N-linked carbohydrate groups. The human, cow, mouse, and rat α subunit genes are similar. The human gene is located on chromosome 6q21.1-q23,[229] is 13.5 kb in size, and consists of four exons and three introns. The 5'-untranslated region is encoded by exon 1 and by 14 base pairs of exon 2. A large first intron, approximately 6.4 kb (in humans), interrupts this 5'-untranslated region. The coding portion of the gene is present in exons 2, 3, and 4, and the 3'-untranslated region is within exon 4. The α subunit has a single transcriptional start site. All species have a single mRNA that is between 730 and 800 bases long and that encodes the precursor of the α subunit and a leader sequence of an average of 24 amino acids. In all species except the human, intron 2 interrupts the coding sequence after the first nucleotide of codon $+10$; in the human it interrupts the codon $+6$ after its first nucleotide. In the human a four-codon deletion at the beginning of exon 3[230-236] results in an apoprotein of 92 amino acids, compared with 96 in other species.

Thyrotropin β Subunit

The thyrotropin β subunit is approximately 18 kd, consists of 110 amino acids, and contains one N-linked complex carbohydrate.[219] The human thyrotropin β subunit gene is located on chromosome 1p22[237] and consists of three exons separated by two introns.[238] The genes for the β subunit of thyrotropin of mouse,[239, 240] rat,[233, 241] and cow[242] and portions of the human thyrotropin β gene[238, 243, 244] have been cloned. The thyrotropin beta mRNA encodes the precursor thyrotropin β subunit with a 20-amino-acid leader sequence and a 117- or 118-amino-acid coding region. There is at least 80 to 89% homology at the amino acid level among the sequences of rat, mouse, and bovine species, and at the nucleotide level there is 91% homology between rat and mouse.

Unlike the rat and mouse genes, the human gene may have only one transcriptional start site. Two transcriptional start sites, a major one and a minor one, were present in a human thyrotropin-secreting tumor, similar to the thyrotropin β genes of other species.[245] A point mutation in the thyrotropin β subunit gene that causes a glycine-to-arginine substitution caused a congenital isolated thyrotropin deficiency in two siblings.[246, 247]

Although both the α and β subunits of thyrotropin are negatively regulated by thyroid hormone, there is no consensus sequence in the 5'-flanking regions of each gene that would suggest a common thyroid hormone response element. Thyroid hormone receptors do bind to the 5'-flanking regions of the α and β subunit genes, and these binding sites confer negative regulation for thyrotropin β. The human alpha gene

is regulated by a more complex mechanism.[248, 249] It is unclear which thyroid hormone receptor is responsible and whether it acts directly or by interacting with other transcription regulatory factors.

THYROTROPES AND THYROTROPIN CONTENT. Thyrotropes account for only about 5% of anterior pituitary cells and are located in the anteromedial portion of the gland. These fairly large cells display angular outlines and cytoplasmic processes in immunohistochemical studies. By electron microscopy normal thyrotropes have a spherical nucleus, well-developed and somewhat dilated RER, and a global Golgi network with numerous vesicles. The secretory granules range from 50 to 300 nm but are usually 200 to 300 nm in diameter. Large lysosomes are common. Less typical sparsely granulated cells may be identified by immunoelectron microscopy. Sustained stimulation of the thyrotrope cell, as occurs in primary hypothyroidism, causes development of "thyroid deficiency" cells and thyrotrope hyperplasia.[250] The thyroid deficiency cells are massively enlarged with extensive well-developed, dilated RER. In thyrotoxicosis the thyrotropes are small, and thyrotropin immunoreactivity may not be detectable.[251] The human pituitary contains approximately 100 to 150 μg of thyrotropin.

REGULATION OF THYROTROPIN SECRETION.[227] mRNAs that encode α and thyrotropin β subunits both are regulated by thyroid hormone; the degree of suppression of thyrotropin β by thyroid hormone is greater than suppression of the α subunit.[240] The response to triiodothyronine (T_3) is rapid (1 h). In the hypothyroid rat the amount of thyrotropin β mRNA increases up to 10-fold, but the ratios of mRNAs for α and β are relatively constant. In euthyroid, hypothyroid, and T_3-treated animals, the ratios were 1.1:1.7, 0.4:1.3, and 2:3, respectively. These studies demonstrate that T_3 feedback occurs at the level of the thyrotrope.[240, 252, 253] The reduction in steady-state mRNA levels in response to thyroid hormone is due to a reduction in gene transcription that is demonstrable within 30 min.[254] The mRNAs that encode the subunits appear to have a short half-life in hyperthyroid animals, but it is not known whether the half-life is altered during hypothyroidism. The degree of T_3 receptor occupancy, time course of binding of the T_3 receptor, and suppression of thyrotropin gene transcription are correlated.[253, 255, 256]

TRH increases thyrotropin α and β mRNA levels within 30 min, and levels decline thereafter.[257, 258] The extent of stimulation is similar for both α and β, in contrast to the more profound reduction of thyrotropin β mRNA levels after thyroid hormone administration. TRH stimulates transcription of thyrotropin β via the pituitary specific transcription factor (pituitary factor 1, Pit-1); both cAMP response element-binding protein and Pit-1 are important in human alpha gene transcription.[249, 259-261] Dopamine inhibits thyrotropin secretion, reducing both basal and TRH-stimulated thyrotropin secretion by more than 50%. In vitro dopamine decreases mRNA levels for both subunits and suppresses transcription by 60 to 75%. Effects are demonstrable within 15 min and are maximal after 30 min.[257] The mode of action of dopamine is unknown.

After injection radiolabeled thyrotropin is distributed in a space slightly larger than the plasma volume. The plasma half-life is approximately 50 min, the relatively slow clearance being due to glycosylation of the hormone. The secretion rate of thyrotropin in euthyroid individuals is 50 to 200 μg/d and increases up to fivefold during hypothyroidism.

THYROTROPIN SECRETION. Secretion of thyrotropin is regulated by both hypothalamic hormones and circulating thyroid hormones. The hypothalamic tripeptide TRH stimulates thyrotropin release.[262] If the hypothalamic-pituitary stalk is interrupted, secondary hypothyroidism develops and thyrotropin secretion is reduced but not absent. Somatostatin and dopamine inhibit thyrotropin secretion, but it is not clear

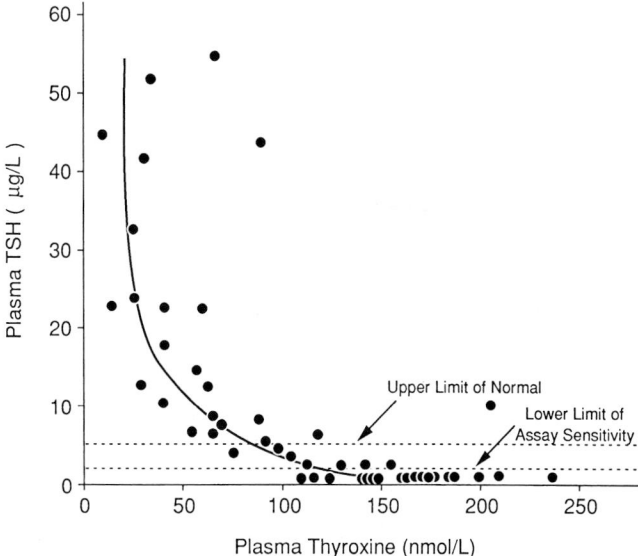

Figure 9–14. Relationship between plasma T$_4$ and plasma thyrotropin levels. When the plasma T$_4$ value decreases to less than 7.77 µg/dL (100 nmol/L) plasma thyrotropin concentration increases to greater than normal. (Modified from S Reichlin, RD Utiger. Regulation of the pituitary-thyroid axis in man: relationship of TSH concentration to concentration of free and total thyroxine in plasma. J Clin Endocrinol Metab 27:251–255, 1967, © by The Endocrine Society.)

whether these actions are important in the physiological regulation of thyrotropin. The circadian rhythm of thyrotropin secretion is preserved during constant TRH infusions in humans.

The principal regulator of thyrotropin secretion is feedback by thyroid hormones. Thyroid hormone acts at the hypothalamic level to inhibit TRH synthesis[263, 264] and at the pituitary to inhibit thyrotropin secretion. Intracellular T$_3$ in the thyrotrope regulates thyrotropin secretion, although plasma thyroxine (T$_4$) levels correlate better with thyrotropin levels than do T$_3$ levels in normal individuals and in hypothyroid patients. When T$_4$ levels decline to the lower range of normal, thyrotropin levels rise exponentially, as shown in Figure 9–14. This is because the thyrotrope has a potent intracellular 5'-deiodinase that converts T$_4$ to T$_3$.[265] Approximately three quarters of intracellular T$_3$ in the pituitary is derived from local conversion of T$_4$ and the remainder is derived from the circulation. In contrast in hypothyroid patients receiving hormone

replacement with levothyroxine, the serum T$_3$ level correlates better with suppression of thyrotropin levels than does the serum T$_4$ level.[266]

Thyrotropin is measured by either RIA or immunoradiometric assay (IRMA). The IRMAs for thyrotropin are more sensitive, have fewer cross-reacting substances, and are better able to distinguish between normal and low thyrotropin levels, which often is not possible with RIAs.

Thyrotropin is secreted in a pulsatile fashion with low-amplitude peaks[267] and in a circadian fashion. Thyrotropin levels are low during the day and increase at approximately 8 PM; higher levels are present during the night and decrease in the early hours of the morning. During sleep deprivation the nighttime increase in thyrotropin secretion is enhanced.[267] Although pharmacologic doses of glucocorticoids inhibit thyrotropin secretion,[268] the normal circadian change in plasma cortisol level is probably not an important regulator of thyrotropin secretion.[269] During the night circulating T$_4$ and T$_3$ levels decline as a consequence of the posture-related fall in plasma protein levels.[269]

The IRMAs have resulted in improved sensitivity so that it is now possible to distinguish between a normal serum thyrotropin value and a suppressed value in hyperthyroidism (Fig. 9–15).[270] In thyroid failure serum thyrotropin levels may rise before the serum thyroid hormone levels decline to less than the normal range; this rise is often considered to be a harbinger of incipient hypothyroidism, as occurs in Hashimoto's thyroiditis. Both serum thyrotropin and T$_4$ levels should be measured simultaneously to exclude hypothyroidism, because in hypothalamic-pituitary disease the thyrotropin level may be in the "normal" range for euthyroid individuals but inappropriately low for the measured thyroid hormone level.

As a diagnostic test for thyrotropin reserve, TRH can be administered to amplify the thyrotropin signal in order to distinguish among low, normal, and high thyrotropin levels and to assess feedback inhibition by peripheral thyroid hormones. Figure 9–16 shows the thyrotropin responses to TRH in normal individuals, in patients with primary hypothyroidism, and in pituitary and hypothalamic hypothyroidism. Patients with thyrotoxicosis do not respond to TRH because of negative feedback by thyroid hormone. The need for this test to exclude hyperthyroidism has largely been eliminated with the development of the sensitive IRMA for thyrotropin. However the TRH test is still helpful in two situations. In the patient with elevated thyroid hormone levels and "normal" thyrotropin levels, the absence of a thyrotropin response to

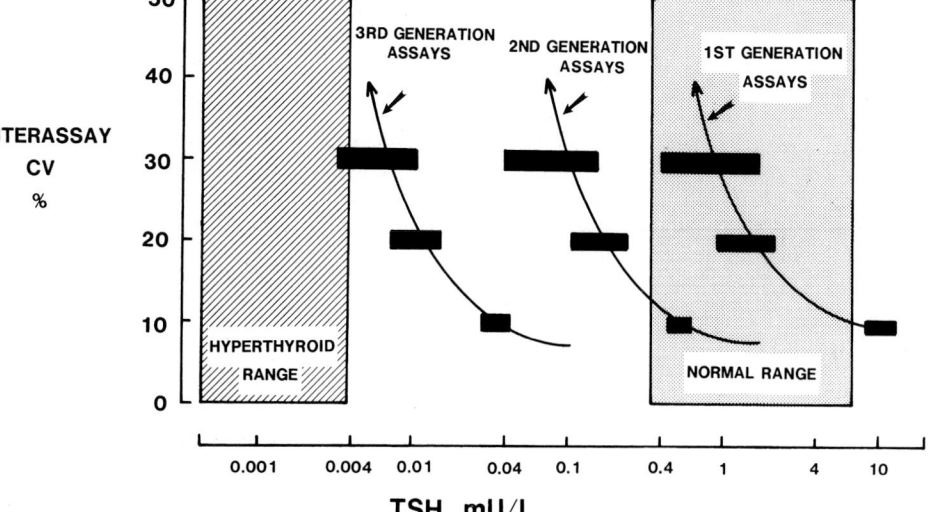

Figure 9–15. With the development of modern thyrotropin assays with greater sensitivity, it is possible to distinguish between normal thyrotropin concentrations and the suppressed values of hyperthyroidism.[1053] Each generation of assays represents a 10-fold improvement in functional sensitivity (20% interassay coefficient of variation value). The black bars denote the 95% confidence limits of measurement at different thyrotropin concentrations. (From Nicoloff JT, Spencer CA. Clinical Review 12: the use and misuse of the sensitive thyrotropin assays. J Clin Endocrinol Metab 1990; 71:553–558.)

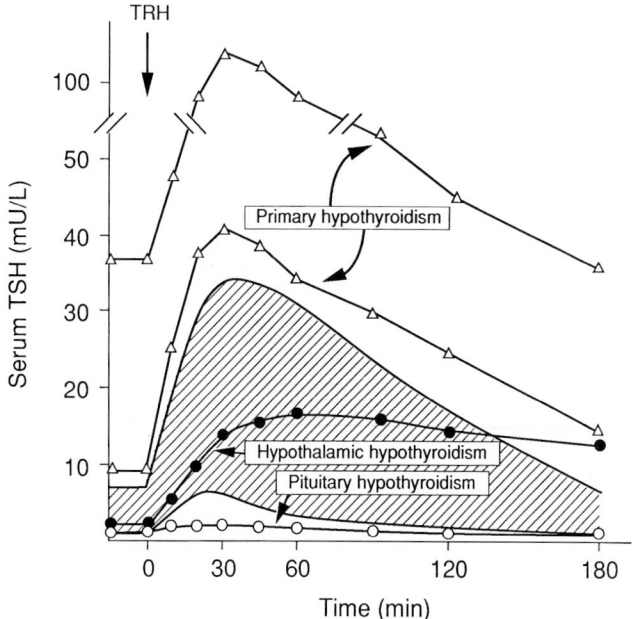

Figure 9–16. Serum thyrotropin (TSH) changes after TRH administration in normal subjects *(shaded area)* and in patients with primary hypothyroidism, hypothalamic disease, and pituitary hypothyroidism. Patients with hypothalamic disease may have a delayed thyrotropin response to TRH. (Modified from Utiger RD. Tests of the hypothalamic-pituitary-thyroid axis. In: Ingbar SH, Braverman LE, eds. The Thyroid. 5th ed. Philadelphia: JB Lippincott, 1986: 515.)

TRH is compatible with either hyperthyroidism or a thyrotrope adenoma (see later), and the presence of a response to TRH may suggest pituitary resistance to thyroid hormone. TRH is also administered to distinguish between pituitary and hypothalamic hypothyroidism in which the peripheral thyroid hormone level is low and the thyrotropin level is normal or low. If the thyrotropin response to TRH is adequate, the abnormality is most likely hypothalamic in origin; in this case the 60-min thyrotropin level is often higher than the 20-min level. No thyrotropin response to TRH is more likely to reflect pituitary failure, often associated with other pituitary hormone deficiencies.

THYROTROPIN ACTIONS. Thyrotropin binds to receptors in the thyroid cell plasma membrane. Specific thyrotropin binding also occurs in other cells, including adipocytes, but the physiological role of the extrathyroidal binding sites is unknown. The thyrotropin receptor also binds human thyroid-stimulating immunoglobulins (see Chapter 11). The binding of thyrotropin to its receptor activates adenylate cyclase, increases intracellular cAMP levels, and activates protein kinase A, leading to phosphorylation of proteins that regulate the thyroid cells.

Thyrotropin regulates both synthesis and secretion of thyroid hormones by increasing the size and the vascularity of the gland. Thyrotropin increases the height of the follicular epithelium and decreases the amount of colloid. The consequences are increased iodide transport, thyroglobulin synthesis, iodotyrosine and iodothyronine formation, thyroglobulin proteolysis, and T_4 and T_3 release.

Gonadotropins

β SUBUNITS OF LUTEINIZING HORMONE, FOLLICLE-STIMULATING HORMONE, AND HUMAN CHORIONIC GONADOTROPIN. The β subunits of both LH and FSH are composed of 115 amino acids and have two carbohydrate side chains. The structure of the β subunit of LH is similar to that of human chorionic gonadotropin (hCG) except that the hCG

β subunit has an additional 32 amino acids and additional carbohydrate residues on the COOH end. A terminal sialic acid is frequently present on the carbohydrate side chains of the β subunit of hCG and FSH. Sialic acid is not necessary for receptor binding but does decrease the metabolic clearance of these hormones, compared with the clearance of thyrotropin and LH (which do not have sialic acid side chains).

The human LH β subunit gene is located on chromosome 19q13.32 and is close to the hCG β genes.[229] Each of the glycoprotein β subunits is coded for by a single gene except hCG β. There are at least seven hCG β genes and pseudogenes, and only primates and horses are known to have these genes. The LH and hCG β genes are approximately 1.5 kb in size and consist of three exons and two introns. The LH β gene encodes a prohormone with a 24-amino-acid leader sequence and a mature peptide of 121 amino acids. The hCG β protein differs from the other β subunits in having a 24-amino-acid COOH-terminal extension, and a longer 5′-untranslated portion. The 5′-flanking region of the LH β gene contains a putative estrogen response element.

The human FSH β gene is located on chromosome 11p13[271] and contains three exons and two introns. The nucleotide and amino acid sequences of the coding regions of the rat and human FSH β subunits show 79 and 80% homology, respectively. In contrast to a single mRNA in rat and cow, the human FSH β subunit gene is transcribed into four mRNA species as the result of alternate splicing of exon 1 and two polyadenylation sites.[272]

GONADOTROPES AND PITUITARY LUTEINIZING HORMONE AND FOLLICLE-STIMULATING HORMONE CONTENT. Gonadotropes are ovoid, medium-sized or smaller, and widely distributed throughout the pars distalis of the pituitary[18, 273]; their prevalence in the human gland is about 20%. The morphologic features and immunoreactivity of gonadotropes vary with different hormonal states. The gonadotrope elaborates both FSH and LH; during the menstrual cycle the secretion of these hormones varies and their concentrations in the gonadotrope change. The cells have a large interface with capillary basement membranes[18] and are often close to lactotropes, raising the possibility of a paracrine interaction between the two.[274] Gonadotropes have a spherical, conspicuously euchromatic nucleus and low-density cytoplasm that contains well-developed, mildly dilated RER and a prominent Golgi apparatus. In women the secretory granules tend to be larger (200 to 600 nm), but no specific histologic changes occur with physiological hormonal variations. In men the small (<200 nm) secretory granules are usually more numerous. In nontumorous human gonadotropes "light bodies,"[275] thought to be markers for gonadotropes in the rat pituitary, are rare. Chronic sustained stimulation of gonadotrope cells, such as after castration, results in the development of "castration cells" that are massively enlarged with abundant, markedly dilated RER, a prominent Golgi complex, and few granules.[276] Little or minimal FSH and LH is present in inactive gonadotropes,[277] such as the gonadotropes in hypogonadotropic hypogonadism or nontumorous parts of pituitaries that harbor gonadotrope cell adenomas.[277] Inactive gonadotropes are small and ovoid and have heterochromatic nuclei, scant membranous organelles and secretory granules, and large compartmentalized lysosomes.

The content of gonadotropins is low in the pituitaries of prepubertal children. In men and in menstruating women, the pituitary contains approximately 700 IU of LH and 200 IU of FSH. After menopause the content of pituitary LH rises to approximately 1700 IU, but there is no change in FSH content. hCG was previously thought to originate only from the placenta and from trophoblastic tumors but is now known to be present in small amounts in the pituitary, testis, and other nonplacental tissues.[278–280]

REGULATION OF LUTEINIZING HORMONE AND FOL-LICLE-STIMULATING HORMONE SECRETION.

Secretion from the gonadotrope is regulated by integration of the LHRH signal and feedback effects of gonadal steroids and peptides (e.g., inhibin). LHRH interacts with a membrane receptor to regulate both LH and FSH release and synthesis and is necessary for gonadotrope function; gonadal steroids and peptides are ineffective alone in regulating release. However once LHRH is present, the effects of gonadal steroids and inhibin are demonstrable. There is uncertainty regarding the mechanism of LHRH action.[281] Interaction of LHRH with the gonadotrope membrane receptor leads to receptor microaggregation, which in turn influences the number of receptors and the cellular response. Gonadotropin secretion is initiated by mobilization of intracellular calcium followed by mobilization of extracellular calcium. Synergism between the calcium-calmodulin system and the inositol trisphosphate–diacylglycerol–protein kinase C cascade allows optimal gonadotropin secretion. cAMP is also likely to have a role in the regulation of gonadotropins, although it is not the primary second messenger for the action of the hormone. Gonadal steroids act by binding to gonadotrope nuclear receptors that affect transcription of various genes by binding to appropriate response elements on DNA.[282, 283] In addition gonadal peptides affect gonadotropin synthesis by binding to cell-surface receptors and indirectly regulating hormone synthesis (see later).

Regulation of gonadotropin synthesis can be assessed by measuring incorporation of labeled amino acids in the glycoproteins or by measuring gonadotropin subunit mRNA synthesis.

Estradiol. Transcription of α and LH β and FSH β subunit mRNAs from ovariectomized rats is increased 2.5-, 10-, and 3.5-fold over that in intact rats, and estradiol treatment causes a decline in the synthesis of the three subunit mRNAs (α, 70%; LH β, 88%; and FSH β, 74%).[284] The estrogen effects appear to be mediated indirectly through the hypothalamus. For example hypothalamic estradiol implants have selective effects in gonadectomized rats to prevent the development of castration cells. In addition in ovariectomized monkeys the LHRH pulse generator is slowed by injection of estradiol.[285] These studies do not exclude additional effects of estradiol at the pituitary level, and pituitary actions have been demonstrated in animals.[286] The negative effects of estradiol on pituitary gonadotropin secretion appear to be mediated by modulation of LHRH action at the pituitary rather than by a direct effect on transcription of subunit mRNAs.[227] The inhibition by estradiol of LH secretion may be a membrane effect. Although a membrane receptor for estrogen has not been described, a membrane receptor for progesterone is present in *Xenopus laevis* oocytes.[287, 288] At high levels estradiol can enhance LH secretion, probably as a result of effects at the pituitary level[286] to increase transcription of LH β subunit mRNA,[283] and at the level of the hypothalamus to enhance LHRH secretion.[289, 290] LHRH receptor levels are positively regulated by estradiol and by LHRH.[291]

Progesterone regulates gonadotropin secretion by slowing the LHRH pulse generator in the hypothalamus. Thus LH pulse frequency is decreased during the luteal phase of the menstrual cycle.[292–294]

Androgens decrease levels of α and LH β mRNAs by suppressing LHRH secretion[295] but have no effect on FSH β mRNA.[296] Testosterone inhibits human alpha gene expression through binding of the androgen–androgen receptor complex to the gene.[297] In vitro, androgens increase levels of FSH β mRNA by a direct effect on the pituitary.[228, 296] Androgen feedback is best exemplified by the study of patients with androgen resistance because of a defect in the androgen receptor. In these individuals the mean LH levels are elevated, and there is an increase in the number of LH secretory

episodes per day.[298] LH levels in these patients are not suppressed by elevated endogenous testosterone levels or by administration of nonaromatizable androgens.

LHRH is essential for gonadotropin secretion, and the timing of LHRH pulses is crucial in the regulation of LH and FSH secretion. In ovariectomized sheep each LH pulse is preceded by a pulse of LHRH release into the hypothalamic-pituitary portal blood. Gonadotropin secretion can be restored in monkeys with hypothalamic lesions and in humans with isolated LHRH deficiency by pulsatile LHRH administration.[299–301] The frequency and amplitude of LHRH pulses are important in regulating LH and FSH secretion differentially. The pulsatile secretion of both LH and FSH is maintained with one LHRH pulse per hour; more frequent LHRH pulses initially increase the frequency of LH pulses and mean LH concentrations.[302, 303] In contrast when the LHRH pulse frequency is decreased to once every 3 h, FSH secretion is preferentially stimulated.[302, 304] In gonadectomized sheep and rats either surgical separation of the hypothalamus from the pituitary or suppression of the hypothalamus by administration of testosterone[295] causes a progressive decline in mRNA levels for α, LH β, and FSH β subunits,[305–308] and LHRH administration to rats increased levels of alpha and LH β mRNA.[308–310] One pulse per 8 min increased only alpha mRNA levels; one pulse per 30 min increased alpha, LH β, and FSH β subunit mRNA levels; and one pulse every 2 h produced an increase in only FSH β mRNA levels. These frequency-dependent effects are mediated through changes in transcription[311] and are consistent with the clinical effects of administration of LHRH on gonadotropin secretion in humans.

In vitro studies have confirmed that the administration of LHRH in a pulsatile fashion increases transcription of α subunit and LH β by rat anterior pituitary fragments.[312] Continuous LHRH exposure stimulated α subunit mRNA synthesis threefold, whereas pulsatile LHRH administration increased the transcription of LH β mRNA and FSH β mRNA, and α subunit mRNA.

Gonadal Peptides. Gonadal peptides have important effects on the secretion of gonadotropins and possibly other pituitary hormones. Inhibin plays an important role in the regulation of FSH secretion, and gonadal secretion of inhibin is regulated by gonadotropins, growth factors, and gonadal steroids. Gonadectomy is followed by increased FSH secretion, indicating that the gonad produces factors that inhibit FSH secretion. Although gonadal steroids (in physiological concentrations) lower LH levels of castrated animals to normal, FSH levels remain elevated.[313, 314]

Inhibin is a member of a larger family of glycoprotein hormones and growth factors that includes antimüllerian hormone (also known as müllerian-inhibiting factor), transforming growth factor β, an erythroid differentiation factor, and an insect protein that plays an important role in cellular differentiation. The two forms of inhibin[315–317] are heterodimers that have a common α subunit and one of two distinct β subunits, type A or type B. Both forms of inhibin, types αβ_A and αβ_B, inhibit FSH secretion. However the two β subunit heterodimers or homodimers (β_Aβ_A, β_Bβ_B, or β_Aβ_B) stimulate FSH secretion in vitro (activin or FSH-releasing protein).[318, 319] It remains to be determined whether this phenomenon is of physiological significance.

Inhibin is synthesized by Sertoli cells of the testis, granulosa cells of the ovary, the placenta,[320] pituitary gonadotropes,[321] and the brain.[322, 323] Thus inhibin may regulate LHRH and gonadotropin secretion not only as a hormone but also by local production as an autocrine or paracrine factor. In the juvenile monkey *(Macaca mulatta)* puberty is accelerated by administering pulsatile LHRH at 3-h intervals (selective for FSH). The administration of a similar regimen to 2-d postorchiectomized monkeys causes a two- to threefold

ALPHA AND LH-BETA mRNA DURING THE RAT ESTROUS CYCLE

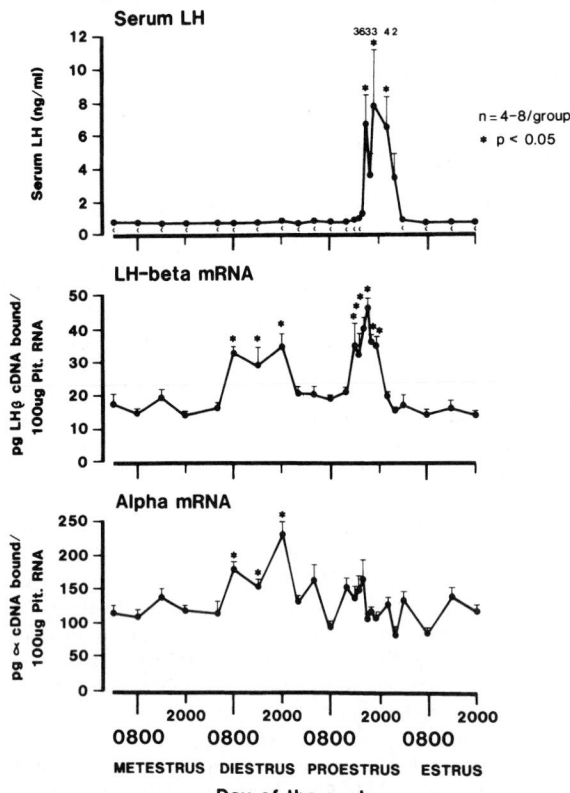

Figure 9–17. Changes in serum LH concentrations and subunit mRNA levels during the rat estrous cycle. Serum LH and pituitary alpha and LH β mRNA levels from individual pituitaries were measured at various times during the rat estrous cycle. Mean (±SEM) serum LH, LH β and alpha mRNA levels are shown in the upper, middle, and lower panels, respectively. < denotes undetectable LH levels. Asterisks denote significant increases over values observed at metestrus. (Modified from SM Zmeili, SS Papavasiliou, et al. Alpha and luteinizing hormone beta subunit messenger ribonucleic acids during the rat estrous cycle. Endocrinology 1986; 119:1867–1869, © by The Endocrine Society.)

increase in FSH levels. Passive immunization of intact monkeys with an antibody directed at the α subunit of inhibin produces an additional two- to threefold increase in FSH levels after LHRH administration.[324] Passive immunization to endogenous inhibin in the diestrous female rat also increases FSH release. In addition the frequency and amplitude of LH pulsatile secretion are enhanced, and responsiveness to exogenous LHRH is increased. Inhibin selectively reduces and activin selectively increases levels of FSH β subunit mRNA.[325–327]

Follistatin, a single chain glycosylated ovarian polypeptide that is not a member of the inhibin family,[328, 329] selectively decreases levels of FSH β mRNA and inhibits FSH secretion in vitro, as does inhibin.[326]

Estrous Cycles. During estrous cycles regulation of LH and FSH secretion is dissociated. Steady-state mRNA levels and transcription of RNA encoding the α, LH β, and FSH β subunits have not been measured in primate pituitaries during the menstrual cycle, but changes in both the steady-state levels[330, 331] and transcription rates occur during the rat estrous cycle.[283] The proestrous LH surge at 7 PM is preceded by an increase in LH β mRNA levels at 6 PM (Fig. 9–17). A rapid increase in the FSH β mRNA level occurs at 8 PM immediately after the LH surge, and α subunit mRNA levels do not change at the time of the preovulatory LH surge. A modest increase occurs in both α and LH β levels at 8 PM in diestrus. In addition FSH β mRNA levels increase from 11 PM in estrus

until 5 PM in diestrus. Similarly transcription rates for LH β mRNA are twofold higher on the afternoon of proestrus when compared with metestrus, and FSH β mRNA transcription is increased at proestrus and continues to increase until the morning of metestrus.

LUTEINIZING HORMONE AND FOLLICLE-STIMULATING HORMONE SECRETION. Circulating levels of gonadotropins as measured by immunologic and bioassay techniques are not always closely correlated.[332] After a single injection of LH in men, the half-time of the first phase of biexponential kinetics was 18 ± 5 min, and that of the second phase was 90 ± 15 min for immunoreactive LH. Corresponding values for bioactive LH were 32 ± 8 min and 85 ± 7 min.[333] In a monoexponential model immunoreactive and bioactive LH half-times were 47 ± 7 min and 65 ± 5 min, respectively. The prolonged bioactive half-lives of LH and FSH are due to the oligosaccharide content. Asialoglycoproteins (i.e., proteins stripped of sialic acid) are cleared rapidly by the liver.[334] The volume of distribution of LH is approximately 3 L in a 70-kg man. The metabolic clearance rate for bioactive LH is 26 ± 3 mL/min/m² and for immunoreactive LH it is 34 ± 3 mL/min/m².[333] The half-time of immunoreactive FSH is greater than that of LH. With a monoexponential model the half-time of FSH was 3.7 h, and with a two-compartment model it was 1.7 h for the first component and 8.3 h for the second component. Similarly metabolic clearance of FSH is less than that of LH, being 6 to 14 mL/min in women and 4 to 12 mL/min in men.[335] Gonadal function does not affect the metabolic clearance rate.[332, 336, 337] Circulating LH and FSH are degraded by the liver and kidneys; small amounts of intact LH and FSH are excreted in the urine (e.g., 3 to 5% for FSH).

Table 9–9 shows estimates of production of immunoreactive LH and FSH in normal men. The production rates of LH and FSH increase 3- to 15-fold in women after menopause.

The two principal functions of the gonads, to produce gonadal steroids and gametes, are regulated precisely by coordinated secretion of LH and FSH, which in turn is regulated by hypothalamic LHRH secretion and feedback effects of gonadal steroids and peptides. These hormones are also responsible for the timing and control of pubertal development and sexual maturation. With aging some reduction in gonadal function may occur in men; this reduction may be centrally mediated (a reduction of bioactive LH levels) and is different from the primary ovarian failure of menopause. The pulsatile patterns of gonadotropin and LHRH secretion are necessary for normal gonadal stimulation. Destruction of the arcuate nucleus in the monkey results in a reduction of gonadotropin secretion.[338] The cells responsible for pulsatile LHRH secretion (the LHRH pulse generator) reside in the mediobasal hypothalamus, but in the female rhesus monkey disconnection of the mediobasal hypothalamus from the rest of the brain does not interfere with the menstrual cycle. In gonadecto-

TABLE 9–9. Production Rates of Immunoradiometric Luteinizing Hormone and Follicle-Stimulating Hormone Determined by Deconvolution Analysis

Subjects	Luteinizing Hormone (IU/24 h)*	Follicle-Stimulating Hormone (IU/24 h)*
Men	230[1016]†	53 ± 12.8[1017]
Ovulating women	200[294]‡	NA§
Postmenopausal women	3500[1018]†	NA

*Assuming mean volume of distribution of 2.5 L.
†The bioactive LH production rate is considerably higher at 2400 IU/24 h[1019] in men and 10,000 IU/24 h in postmenopausal women.[1018]
‡Immunoreactive LH production rates do not vary significantly with various stages of the menstrual cycle.[294]
§NA, not available.

mized monkeys electrolytic destruction of the mediobasal hypothalamus showed that the mode of LHRH administration (continuous or intermittent) is critical. Continuous LHRH infusion initially stimulates LH and FSH secretion; after 7 to 10 d the response diminishes, and LH and FSH concentrations return to baseline, essentially undetectable levels. In contrast intermittent pulsatile administration of LHRH every hour stimulates gonadotropin secretion indefinitely in ovariectomized animals; in animals with ovaries and mesiobasal hypothalamic lesions, pulsatile administration of LHRH sustains the menstrual cycle. Variation in the frequency of LHRH administration to gonadectomized animals alters the ratio of LH to FSH; increasing the interval between LHRH pulses from 1 to 3 h preferentially increases FSH secretion. These findings have been the basis for many human studies, particularly in individuals with isolated gonadotropin deficiency (Kallmann's syndrome). Kallmann's syndrome involves either disordered LHRH secretion or deficiency of LHRH neuronal development or migration. In one fetus with this condition, migration of LHRH neurons from the fetal olfactory pit was impaired.[339]

Pulsatile administration of LHRH reverses human hypothalamic hypogonadism of either a congenital or an acquired cause.[340] Long-acting LHRH agonist analogues are administered to control gonadotropin-dependent precocious puberty; to inhibit ovarian function, for example, in endometriosis; and to treat metastatic prostate cancer ("medical gonadectomy"). LHRH antagonists may replace the LHRH agonists because they have the advantage of immediately suppressing, rather than initially stimulating, gonadotropin secretion and because receptor down-regulation is not required to suppress gonadotropin secretion.

The secretory profile of LHRH in the portal circulation of humans is unknown, but in other species LHRH pulses have brief duration and high amplitude.[341–344] A number of neurotransmitters influence LHRH secretion and mediate the effects of gonadal steroids on LHRH secretion (Table 9–10). For example the suppressive effects of estradiol and dihydrotestosterone on LH secretion are blocked by opiate antagonists. Androgens exert negative feedback by suppressing the frequency of LHRH pulsatile secretion and may also reduce the release of bioactive LH. Estrogen administration to men reduces the amplitude, but not the frequency, of LH pulsations and may also reduce the ratio of bioactivity to immunologic activity. Positive feedback by estradiol is responsible for the midcycle LH surge in women, and positive feedback by estradiol is not normally operative in men. The ontogeny of gonadotropin secretion in humans has been reviewed by Grumbach and Kaplan.[345] A schematic representation of the components and interactions of the hypothalamic-pituitary-gonadal axis and their respective characteristics are shown in Figure 9–18.

Gonadal maturation is regulated by gonadotropin. Before puberty the release of FSH is greater than that of LH; this relationship is reversed at puberty.[346] The prepubertal pattern can be overridden in primates by pulsatile chemical stimulation of the hypothalamus to activate LHRH neurons[315] or by pulsatile LHRH administration to stimulate the pituitary[347]; induction of an adult pattern of gonadotropin secretion is followed by puberty. However if exogenous LHRH is discontinued, gonadotropin secretion regresses to the prepubertal pattern, and puberty will commence at the appropriate time. Thus the pubertal response to LHRH likely reflects the hormonal input rather than the stage of development. The differential release of LH or FSH is not well understood but may reflect effects of inhibin. The major restraint on prepubertal LHRH secretion originates in the central nervous system (CNS). Grumbach and Kaplan[345] analyzed the ontogeny of development of the human hypothalamic–pituitary gonadotropin–gonadal axis and divided the process into five stages: fetus, early infancy, late infancy and childhood, late prepubertal period, and puberty (also see Chapter 31.)

Fetus. By day 80 of gestation the mediobasal hypothalamic LHRH neurons (pulse generator) are operative and stimulate pulsatile LH and FSH secretion, and from days 100 to 150 of gestation LHRH secretion is unrestrained. Negative feedback control by gonadal steroids develops by day 150 of gestation. After day 150 suppression of LHRH appears to be greater in the male fetus, a phenomenon attributed to the effect of testosterone.

Early Infancy. At term the secretion of LHRH is low, and after delivery levels of plasma hCG, α subunit, and placental steroids decline in both sexes, and testosterone levels decline in the male. Hypothalamic LHRH pulsatile secretion is active by 12 d of age, and prominent FSH and LH episodic discharges occur until approximately 6 mo of age in boys and 12 mo of age in girls. Transient increases in plasma testosterone and estradiol occur in boys and girls, respectively.

Late Infancy and Childhood. The CNS intrinsically inhibits hypothalamic LHRH secretion, and by 4 y of age inhibition of LHRH is maximal. The negative feedback of LH and FSH secretion is exquisitely sensitive to gonadal steroids (low set point). Both the amplitude and frequency of LHRH discharges are low so that secretion of FSH, LH, and gonadal steroids is minimal.

Late Prepubertal Period. The intrinsic CNS inhibitory influences and the sensitivity of the hypothalamus and pituitary to gonadal steroids decrease concomitantly, resulting in an increased set point and an increased amplitude and frequency of LHRH pulses. Initially these pulses are most prominent during sleep. Gonadotrope sensitivity to LHRH increases, secretion of FSH and LH rises, gonadal responsiveness to FSH and LH increases, and gonadal hormone secretion increases.

Puberty. Both the CNS restraint of the hypothalamic "LHRH pulse generator" and the sensitivity to negative feedback by gonadal steroids decrease further. The sleep-associated increase in episodic secretion of LHRH gradually changes to the adult pattern of one pulse approximately every 90 min

TABLE 9–10. Effects of Various Factors on Secretion of Luteinizing Hormone and Follicle-Stimulating Hormone in Men

Factor	Luteinizing Hormone		Follicle-Stimulating Hormone	
	Frequency	Amplitude	Frequency	Amplitude
Androgen (nonaromatized)	↓	None	None	↓
Estrogen	↓ *	↓ *	None (decreases half-life)	
Opiate antagonist†	↑ *	↑ *	NT‡	
Alpha-adrenergic antagonist	None in men		NT	

* Demonstrated in women also, in whom stage of the menstrual cycle influences the exact nature of the response.
† Effect dependent on adequate negative feedback by gonadal steroids.
‡ NT, not tested.

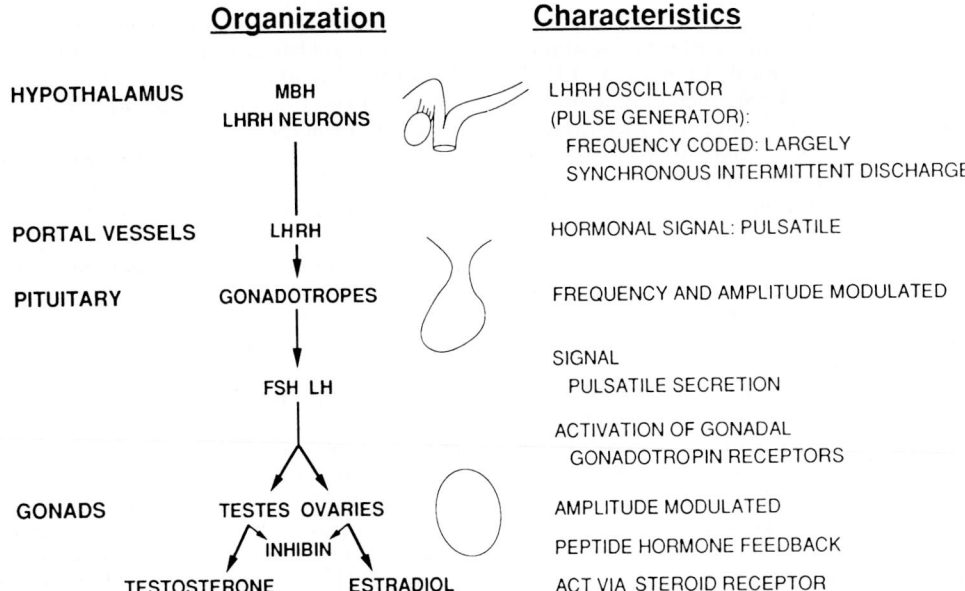

Figure 9–18. Organization and characteristics of the hypothalamic-pituitary-gonadal axis. The medial basal hypothalamus (MBH) contains the LHRH neurons, which translate neural signals into a periodic, oscillatory chemical signal, LHRH. This MBH complex functions as an oscillator (LHRH pulse generator), which is frequency coded and releases LHRH from its axon terminals at the median eminence into the hypothalamic-hypophyseal portal circulation with synchronous intermittent discharge. The LHRH pulse generator is influenced by neurotransmitters, peptidergic neuromodulators, neuroexcitatory amino acids, and neural pathways. During the follicular phase in adult women and men, an LHRH pulse occurs approximately every 90 to 120 min throughout the day. Changes in the frequency and amplitude of the LHRH-secretory episodes modulate the pattern of LH and FSH secretion. Circulating inhibin and gonadal steroids influence the secretion of gonadotropins by acting on both the hypothalamus and the pituitary. LH, luteinizing hormone, LHRH, luteinizing hormone–releasing hormone, FSH, follicle-stimulating hormone. (Modified from Grumbach MM, Kaplan SL. The neuroendocrinology of human puberty: an ontogenetic perspective. In: Grumbach MM, Sizonenko PC, Aubert ML, eds. Control of the Onset of Puberty. Baltimore: Williams & Wilkins, 1990: 1–68. © 1990, the Williams & Wilkins Co., Baltimore.)

throughout the day; the pulsatile pattern of LH follows this LHRH pattern. Secondary sexual development occurs, and spermatogenesis is initiated in boys. In girls during middle to late puberty, the capacity for estrogen positive feedback develops, culminating in a midcycle LH surge and ovulation.

This schema provides a logical explanation for the changes in gonadotropin levels during normal puberty and in agonadal children. The latter have relatively low levels of LH and FSH at birth, but LH and FSH levels rise during the first 2 y of life to levels similar to those observed in castrated adults. From 2 to 4 y of age both LH and FSH levels decline progressively, reflecting the maturation of intrinsic CNS inhibition. This decrease persists until the normal age of the late prepubertal period, when the intrinsic CNS inhibition declines and LH and FSH levels again rise to those of castrated adults. Central precocious puberty results either from premature cessation or inadequate development of the intrinsic CNS inhibition of pulsatile LHRH secretion.

Menstrual Cycle. The complicated changes in gonadotropin secretion during the menstrual cycle can be reproduced in women given invariant pulsatile LHRH stimulation (e.g., LHRH pump therapy at one fixed dose administered hourly for the full cycle of 28 d). This finding suggests that the feedback effects of gonadal steroids and peptides occur predominantly at the pituitary level. However additional levels of regulation probably involve the hypothalamus because during the normal menstrual cycle the frequency and amplitude of LHRH bursts secreted into the portal circulation change.

Figure 9–19 shows changes in gonadotropins, 17-hydroxy-progesterone, progesterone, and basal body temperature during a normal menstrual cycle synchronized around the day of the midcycle preovulatory peak. LH levels rise slightly during the follicular phase, peak at the time of the midcycle surge, and decrease during the luteal phase. The serum FSH level rises during the late luteal phase, increases more during the early follicular phase of the next cycle, and decreases just before a midcycle FSH surge that is smaller than that of LH.

FSH levels then decrease during the luteal phase and increase again before the next menses. In sampling studies every 10 or 20 min at different stages of the menstrual cycle the frequency of LH peaks varies with the phase of the cycle.[348–350] Estimates of LH secretion using deconvolution analysis indicate that the number (mean ± SEM) of LH secretory bursts per 24 h is maximal in the late follicular phase (27 ± 1.6), minimal in the midluteal phase (10 ± 1), and intermediate in the early follicular phase (18 ± 1.4).[294] There is no evidence of tonic (i.e., secretion between bursts) LH secretion during any phase of the menstrual cycle, and no differences have been documented in the LH half-life or in the total daily secretion of LH during the cycle. These studies suggest that the mode of pulsatile LH secretion is the distinct signal for the ovary because the total amount of LH secreted over 24 h is the same in early follicular, late follicular, and luteal phases of the menstrual cycle. If the LH pulses reflect hypothalamic LHRH pulsatility, variations in the frequency of LHRH secretion probably also occur during the menstrual cycle. In sheep, for example, there is concordance between peripheral LH peaks and peaks of LHRH in the hypothalamic-pituitary portal blood.[341]

LUTEINIZING HORMONE AND FOLLICLE-STIMULATING HORMONE ACTIONS. LH regulates gonadal steroid production by Leydig cells of the testis and by the ovarian follicles. The preovulatory LH surge in women produces rupture and luteinization of the follicle. FSH stimulates gametogenesis. FSH stimulates Sertoli cells, which have an important role in spermatogenesis, and is critical for the development of ovarian follicles. FSH also controls the number of LH receptors on the Leydig cell.

hCG is produced primarily by the placenta, but small amounts are synthesized by the pituitary and other tissues. hCG has a longer half-life than LH, but the two have similar actions. hCG is involved in maintaining the corpus luteum during pregnancy and is used as replacement therapy for LH

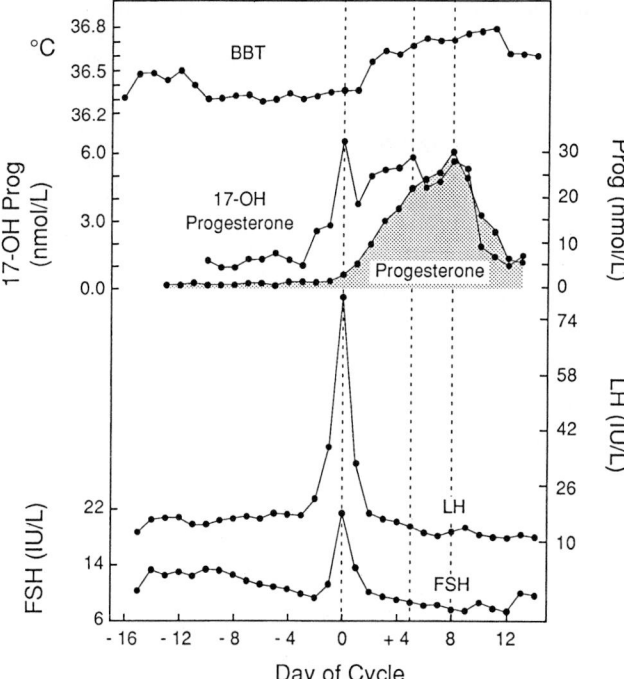

Figure 9–19. Mean daily plasma follicle-stimulating hormone (FSH) luteinizing hormone (LH), progesterone, and 17-hydroxyprogesterone concentrations and basal body temperature (BBT) during 16 presumptive ovulatory cycles in 15 young women. (Modified from Ross GT, Cargille CM, Lipsett MB, et al. Pituitary and gonadal hormones in women during spontaneous and induced ovulatory cycles. Recent Prog Horm Res 1970; 26:1–62.)

to treat delayed puberty or infertility. (For more detail see Chapters 15 and 16.)

UNSOLVED PROBLEMS IN PITUITARY FUNCTION

The identification of tumor cells that secrete several classes of hormones, e.g., GH, prolactin, and thyrotropin, is difficult to reconcile with our understanding of the lineage of different pituitary cell types, but characterization of the molecular biology of the pituitary may provide new insights into this ontogeny. For example demonstration that defects in the gene encoding the GH receptor are associated clinically with GH resistance (i.e., Laron dwarfism) provided insight into the pathogenesis of the disorder and into the function of the normal receptor.[119, 351, 352] Other defined factors of the anterior pituitary include elucidation of the structures of inhibin and the receptors for dopamine (D_2), GH, prolactin, LH, insulin and IGF-I, TRH,[353] LHRH,[354, 355] CRH,[356, 357] and GHRH.[358, 359] A man with a homozygous point mutation in the estrogen receptor that caused a premature stop codon progressed through puberty, but was eunuchoid, had failure of closure of the epiphyses, and had reduced bone mineral density.[360] The serum testosterone level was that of an adult man; serum estradiol, LH, and FSH levels were high; and serum prolactin levels were low. This experiment of nature documents the role of estrogen receptor function in negative feedback on LH and FSH, for fusion of the epiphyses, and in the maintenance of bone mineral density.

Anterior Pituitary Ontogeny

Five phenotypically distinct cell types appear during anterior pituitary ontogeny in a characteristic order. The expression of the α-glycoprotein subunit before the formation of Rathke's pouch heralds the onset of pituitary organogenesis.[361] The order of appearance of distinct cell types is corticotropes, somatotropes, thyrotropes, gonadotropes, and lactotropes. The coexpression of GH and prolactin in precursor cells and in some mature anterior pituitary cells suggests that prolactin and GH genes are regulated similarly. In mice that express a transgene in which 181 base pairs of the rat GH promoter are linked to the hGH gene, the hGH gene is expressed in somatotrope cells and in a subset of cells that produce thyrotropin and prolactin, suggesting a functional relationship in the expression of the GH, prolactin, and thyrotropin genes.[362]

The ontogeny of somatotropes and lactotropes has been analyzed by gene knockout experiments in transgenic mice.[363, 364] Data from such animals demonstrate that most lactotropes are derived from the presomatotrope (or mammosomatotrope) line. Prolactin expression and lactotrope differentiation appear to be postmitotic events, and postmitotic somatotropes cannot progress toward lactotrope cells. Replicating and potentially self-renewing GH-expressing cells (the presomatotropes) are the common precursors of terminally differentiated somatotropes and lactotropes, supporting a model of direct descent.[363] The existence of presomatotropes is well established, and there is evidence for somatotrope-lactotrope transformation[365–367] and reversible somatotrope-thyrotrope transdifferentiation in the rat.[368] Homozygous female mice carrying null mutation of the prolactin receptor gene are infertile because of a failure of embryonic implantation.[369] In addition they have irregular cycles, reduced fertilization rates, defective preimplantation embryonic development, and lack of pseudopregnancy. Half the homozygous males carrying this null mutation were infertile or showed reduced fertility. Thus the prolactin receptor plays a key role in reproduction in the mouse.

Transcription Factors and the Anterior Pituitary

The Pit-1 protein is a 33-kd protein that binds cell-specific DNA elements in the rat prolactin and GH genes.[370–372] The Pit-1 gene transcript is initially detected in most cells of the anterior pituitary of the rat during embryonic day 15. Although all pituitary cell types express the Pit-1 gene transcript, the Pit-1 protein is detected in the nuclei only in thyrotropes, lactotropes, and somatotropes. The binding of Pit-1 to specific regions of the 5'-flanking promoter regions of the GH and prolactin genes permits full basal and hormonally regulated tissue expression of the genes. When transfected into nonpituitary cells, Pit-1 permits expression of GH or prolactin reporter genes. Pit-1 and other (to be identified) transcription factors are believed to be responsible for tissue-specific expression and possibly for pituitary cell differentiation. Pit-1 is found in thyrotropes, as well as in somatotropes and lactotropes, and its expression in thyrotrope cells may explain why GH, prolactin, and thyrotropin can be produced by the same cell. This hypothesis also provides a conceptual framework for explaining the occurrence of multiple pituitary hormones in a single pituitary tumor cell. In some forms of dwarf mice—including the Jackson, Snell, and Ames strains—thyrotropes, lactotropes, and somatotropes do not develop. The Jackson mouse has a major deletion in the Pit-1 gene and the Snell has a point mutation in the Pit-1 gene, whereas the coding sequence of the Pit-1 gene appears to be normal in the Ames mouse[364] (personal communication, MG Rosenfeld). Mutations of Pit-1 in the human cause deficiencies of GH, prolactin, and thyrotropin.[373–376]

The expression in the rat pituitary of Pit-1 on embryonic day 15 precedes the onset of prolactin and GH synthesis, indicating that additional transcription factors are required to achieve full expression. The estrogen receptor appears to act in concert with Pit-1 to regulate prolactin transcription.[361, 377] Because lactotropes arise from presomatotropes, secondary mechanisms must restrict GH expression. Additional mechanisms must also prevent the expression of GH and prolactin in thyrotropes[361, 377] and of prolactin and thyrotropin in somatatropes. Post-transcriptional factors also influence the physiological patterns of gene expression in pituitary cells.[378] Some cell-specific transcription factors are likely involved, such as thyrotrope embryonic factor[379] and thyrotrope-specific splice variant of Pit-1,[260, 380] which are involved in thyrotropin beta gene expression.

Molecular Defects and Tumorigenesis
(see Chapter 6)

Landis and colleagues[381] described G protein mutations in four of eight GH-secreting human pituitary tumors. The point mutations cause constitutive activation of $G_{\alpha S}$, the GTP-binding subunit of the G_s protein.[381] This mutation was present only in the pituitary tumor cells and not in leukocytes from the same patients.

Besides $G_{\alpha s}$ few mutations have been detected in benign pituitary adenomas. Mutations of the *ras* oncogene are common in benign and malignant thyroid tumors[382] and occur rarely in pituitary neoplasia, such as a mutation in the H-*ras* gene at codon 12 in a highly invasive prolactinoma but not in a large series of typical micro- and macroprolactinomas.[383, 384] Three *ras* mutations have also been observed in metastatic deposits of pituitary carcinomas despite the presence of intact *ras* genes in the primary pituitary tumor.[385]

In human cancers gene alterations, including point mutations, deletions, or rearrangements, are common in the *p53* gene, but were not detected in 52 pituitary adenomas.[386] Likewise abnormalities of the retinoblastoma tumor suppressor gene *(RB)* are important in the pathogenesis of many human tumors but do not appear to be involved in pituitary adenomas.[387, 388] Furthermore no evidence of amplification or rearrangement of 10 recognized cellular oncogenes—namely N-*ras*, *myc*L1, *myc*N, *myc*, H-*ras*, *bcl*1, H-*stf*1, *sea*, *kra*S2, and *fos*—was found in a study of 88 pituitary adenomas.[389]

In contrast growth factors and their receptors have been implicated in the tumorigenesis of pituitary tumors. Interleukin-6 is a cytokine that plays a role in the stimulation, inhibition, differentiation, and regulation of cell growth. Interleukin-6 is expressed in normal pituitary tissue, and nonfunctioning GH-secreting and prolactin-secreting adenomas express increased levels of interleukin-6, and the interleukin-6 receptor gene is expressed in nonfunctioning adenomas.[390] The epidermal growth factor receptor is also overexpressed in most nonfunctioning tumors,[391] suggesting a role for epidermal growth factor and its receptor in the development or progression, or both, of such tumors.

Hereditary pituitary tumor formation occurs in multiple endocrine neoplasia type I (MEN1) (also see Chapter 32), and experience with colon and breast cancer suggests that the inherited forms of cancer may point to mutated genes involved in the sporadic development of these tumors. For example although germline *BRCA*1 mutations account for less than 5% of all breast cancers, somatic mutations in *BRCA*1 may account for 30 to 60% of sporadic breast cancers.[392, 393] Thus an uncommon inherited trait may be an acquired defect in sporadic cases. MEN1 is characterized by the combined occurrence of tumors of the parathyroid glands, the pancreatic islet cells, and the anterior pituitary gland. In addition tumors of the adrenal cortex, carcinoids, and lipomas also occur.[394] The *MEN1* gene has been mapped to a 900-kb region on the long arm of chromosome 11,[395, 396, 398] and approximately 20% of adenomas of all types, including prolactinomas,

somatotropinomas, and nonfunctioning pituitary tumors, have a deletion in chromosome 11.[386, 397, 399] Parathyroid adenomas have been extensively studied; chromosome 11 deletions are present in 67% of MEN1-associated tumors and 27% of sporadically occurring parathyroid adenomas.[400–402a] The *MEN1* gene has been cloned.[402b]

The *MEN1* gene may normally function as a tumor suppressor gene. Tumor tissues from patients with MEN1 have loss of heterozygosity at the putative *MEN1* location, indicating that allele losses in MEN1-associated tumors eliminate the normal allele at 11q13 derived from the unaffected parent.[400] In this situation somatic loss of the normal *MEN1* gene represents a "second hit" at the suppressor gene locus, thereby leading to tumorigenesis. One of the candidate *MEN1* genes encodes for phospholipase C-β3; the gene was expressed in all normal tissues tested but not in several endocrine tumors.[403]

In contrast loss of heterozygosity (LOH) at the *Rb* locus is not common in benign sporadic human pituitary adenomas,[404] but LOH at the *Rb* locus has been described in rare human pituitary carcinomas and in a subset of aggressive benign tumors.[405, 406] Thus primary *Rb* inactivation is not common in human pituitary tumors.

Clonality of Human Pituitary Tumors

It is possible to determine whether tumors result from polyclonal proliferation or monoclonal expansion of a single aberrant cell by assessing restriction fragment length polymorphisms in X-linked genes for two enzymes, phosphoglycerate kinase and hypoxanthine phosphoribosyltransferase. In normal tissues in females the two X chromosomes are randomly inactivated, whereas in monoclonal tumors only one of the two is inactivated, and this pattern persists through each cell cycle. By using such an approach several pituitary tumors have been demonstrated to be monoclonal in origin, including "nonfunctioning" tumors, somatotrope adenomas, prolactinomas, and corticotrope adenomas.[407, 408] Whether all pituitary tumors are monoclonal is not known.

Chromosomal Location of Human Genes Related to Anterior Pituitary Function

Although cDNAs that code for several hypothalamic and pituitary hormones and their receptors have been cloned, few hypothalamic-pituitary diseases appear to be caused by single gene defects. Inherited thyrotropin deficiency results from a point mutation in thyrotropin β subunit, and some cases of Laron dwarfism are a result of either a point mutation or partial deletion of the gene coding for the hGH receptor. Table 9–11 shows the known chromosomal locations of some of the relevant genes.

APPROACH TO PITUITARY DISEASE

Pituitary tumors account for 10 to 15% of intracranial tumors at surgery and 6 to 23% of intracranial tumors at autopsy.[409] Pituitary tumors are usually classified as microadenomas (diameter <10 mm) and macroadenomas (diameter >10 mm). Patients with a pituitary tumor can present with symptoms of a mass lesion or endocrine dysfunction, or both. The endocrine abnormality can be hyperfunction or hypofunction, or a combination of the two.

Clinical Manifestations

PITUITARY MASS. The manifestations of a sellar mass (Fig. 9–20) include headache and symptoms secondary to

TABLE 9–11. Chromosomal Location of Human Genes Related to Anterior Pituitary

Hormone	Chromosome	MIM No.*	Clinical Disorder†
HYPOTHALAMIC			
CRH	8q13	122560	Isolated corticotropin deficiency
GHRH	20	139190	GH deficiency
LHRH	8p21 − q11.2	152760	Kallmann's syndrome
Oxytocin	20	167050	Absent milk let-down reflex
PACAP	18p11	102980	
Somatostatin	3q28	182450	
TRH	3p	275120	
VP	20	192340	Diabetes insipidus
PITUITARY			
α Subunit	6q21.1 − q23	118850	Glycoprotein hormone deficiency
CG β	19q13.32	118860	Infertility
FSH β	11p13	136530	Isolated FSH deficiency
GH/prolactin	17q22 − q24	139250	GH and prolactin deficiency
LH β	19q13.32	152780	Isolated LH deficiency
POMC	2p25	176830	Corticotropin deficiency
Prolactin	6p22.2 − q21.3	176760	Prolactin deficiency
TSH β	1p22	188540	Thyrotropin[246, 247]
Vasoactive intestinal peptide	6q26 − q27	192320	
HYPOTHALAMIC HORMONE RECEPTORS			
CRH-R	17q12 − q22	122561	Adrenal insufficiency
Dopamine D₂-R	11q23	126450	Hyperprolactinemia
GHRH-R	7p15 − p14	139191	GH deficiency[1020]
LHRH-R	4q21.2	138850	Hypogonadism
SST-R2	17q24	182452	
TRH-R	8q23	188545	Hypothyroidism
PACAP-R1	7p14	102981	
OTHER RELEVANT GENES			
GH receptor	5p13.1 − p12	600946	Laron dwarfism[352]
LH receptor	2p21	152790	Resistant gonad syndrome Delayed puberty
Prolactin receptor	5p13 − p12	176761	? Lethal ? Reproductive and immune dysfunction
Thyrotropin receptor	22q11 − 13	275200	Hypothyroidism and hyperthyroidism

*MIM No. is the entry number in Mendelian Inheritance in Man and its on-line version (OMIM).
†Only referenced clinical disorders have been proved to give rise to these clinical disorders.
CRH, corticotropin-releasing hormone; GHRH, growth hormone–releasing hormone; GH, growth hormone; LHRH, luteinizing hormone–releasing hormone; PACAP, pituitary adenylate cyclase activating peptide; TRH, thyrotropin-releasing hormone; VP, vasopressin; CG, chorionic gonadotropin; GH, growth hormone; LH β, luteinizing hormone beta; POMC, pro-opiomelanocortin; TSH β, thyrotropin-stimulating hormone beta; CRH-R, corticotropin-releasing hormone receptor; D₂-R, dopamine D₂ receptor; GHRH-R, growth hormone–releasing hormone receptor; LHRH-R, luteinizing hormone–releasing hormone receptor; SST-R2, somatostatin receptor type 2; TRH-R, thyrotropin-releasing hormone receptor; PACAP-R1, pituitary adenylate cyclase activating peptide receptor 1.

compression of adjacent tissues or intracranial nerves, i.e., visual field disturbances, ophthalmoplegia and, occasionally, facial pain from compression of the first or second branch of the trigeminal nerve. The extent of abnormality depends on the size of the tumor and its anatomic position. Microadenomas and macroadenomas can both cause headache, and any sized tumor can produce endocrine dysfunction. The extent of visual field defects varies with the size and location of macroadenomas. The classic finding with suprasellar extension is bitemporal hemianopsia, but any visual disturbance can occur, depending on the extent of suprasellar extension and the location of the optic chiasm, i.e., whether it is prefixed or postfixed (see Fig. 9–28). Pituitary tumors can also cause diminished visual acuity, scotomata, quadrantic defects, and blindness of one or both eyes.[410] The course of the fibers of the optic nerve depends on the site of origin in the retina. Thus fibers from the temporal halves of the retina (for nasal vision) do not cross but course posteriorly along the ipsilateral optic tract. The fibers from the nasal half of the retina (for temporal vision) cross in the chiasm and course posteriorly along the contralateral optic tract, and the chiasm is particularly susceptible to encroachment from pituitary masses. Bitemporal hemianopsia, when present, may be asymmetrical.

Headache from pituitary tumor can be variable and is nonspecific. It may be occipital, retro-orbital, or bitemporal; some are worse on awakening and may improve over the course of the day. The headache is often ameliorated by aspirin or other analgesics. It may result from stretching of the dura mater (i.e., diaphragma sellae) above the pituitary fossa. Large pituitary tumors or suprasellar hypothalamic tumors, e.g., craniopharyngioma, may extend sufficiently superiorly or posteriorly to compress either the foramen of Monro or the aqueduct of Sylvius. The former leads to obstruction of the lateral ventricles, and the latter obstructs CSF flow from the third ventricle to the fourth ventricle, causing hydrocephalus of the third ventricle or lateral and third ventricles, respectively. The relationship of the pituitary gland to the cavernous sinus is shown in Figure 9–21. Extensive lateral extension of a pituitary tumor may produce dysfunction of cranial nerves III, IV, V₁, V₂, and VI.

The incidence of headache and visual disturbance in patients with pituitary tumors is not clear. Patients with macroadenomas usually have symptoms from the mass lesion, although large tumors may be discovered incidentally during evaluation for other complaints. In a series of 1000 patients with a pituitary tumor described by Hollenhorst and Younge,[411] visual disturbance occurred in 61%. Loss of vision was the presenting complaint in 42%, and diplopia occurred in less than 1%. If the tumor extends inferiorly, the patient may have no symptoms and sphenoid sinusitis may not develop. Rare complications include CSF rhinorrhea and recurrent meningitis from erosion of the sella turcica and loss of the barrier between the CSF and the exterior. Giant tumors may extend into the temporal lobes and cause temporal lobe epilepsy and occasionally extend to the cerebral peduncles to cause motor or sensory disturbances, or both.

Headaches

(a) stretching of dura by tumor

(b) hydrocephalus (rare)

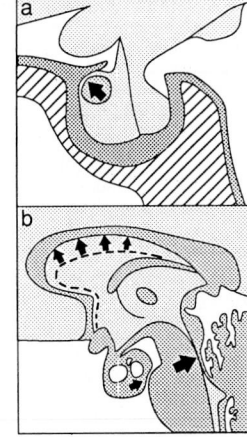

Visual Field Defects

nasal retinal fibers compressed by tumor

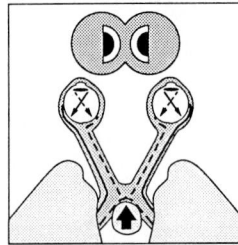

Cranial Nerve Palsies and Temporal Lobe Epilepsy

lateral extension of tumor

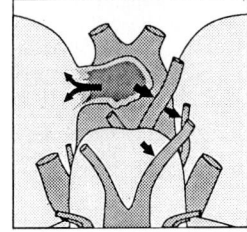

Cerebrospinal Fluid Rhinorrhea

downward extension of tumor

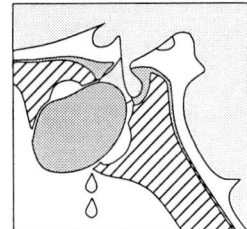

Figure 9–20. Various symptoms of a pituitary tumor. Headaches are rarely caused by hydrocephalus. Visual field defects caused by extension of the tumor are plotted by using the Goldmann perimeter. (From Wass JAH. Hypopituitarism. In: Besser GM, Cudworth AG, eds. Clinical Endocrinology: An Illustrated Text. London: Gower Medical, 1987: 2.1–2.14.)

MANIFESTATIONS OF ANTERIOR PITUITARY HORMONE DEFICIENCY. Total or partial hypopituitarism may occur in patients with pituitary adenomas, with parasellar diseases (see later), following pituitary surgery or radiation (including head and neck radiation for malignancy), or after head injury. Deficiency of any or all of the six major hormones (LH, FSH, GH, thyrotropin, corticotropin, and prolactin) can occur. The most common symptom in both men and women is secondary hypogonadism because of LH and FSH deficiency or secondary to hyperprolactinemia. The classic sequence is loss of pituitary hormones in the following order: gonadotropin (LH, FSH), GH, thyrotropin, corticotropin. However some patients have corticotropin or thyrotropin deficiency, or both, as the presenting feature. Prolactin deficiency is uncommon except with pituitary infarction. In children cessation of growth and delayed puberty are common.

GROWTH HORMONE DEFICIENCY. GH deficiency in adults is now recognized as a disorder, and GH replacement

is approved in most European countries and in the United States. GH deficiency in adults may be a factor in increased mortality in patients with hypopituitarism who receive replacement of hormones other than GH. The predominant cause of excess mortality in such patients is cardiovascular disease.[412] Symptoms of GH deficiency in adults include decreased muscle strength and exercise tolerance and reduced sense of physical and psychological well-being (e.g., less energetic, emotional lability, sense of social isolation, and diminished libido).[413–416] GH deficiency in adults also causes an increase in total body fat and abnormal distribution of fat. Body fat is approximately 6 to 8 kg higher in GH-deficient adults than in matched control subjects,[417, 418] and the fat is primarily subcutaneous and intra-abdominal and is more pronounced in men than in women.[419] Excessive intra-abdominal (visceral) fat is associated with an increased risk of cardiovascular disease.[420, 421] Lean body mass is 8 to 11% lower than in normal adults[417, 422] and is associated with a reduction in muscle strength and exercise capacity.[423] Bone density, particularly in the lumbar spine, is reduced in some patients with adult-onset GH deficiency.[424–427] Serum low-density lipoprotein cholesterol may be increased, whereas high-density lipoprotein cholesterol is in the normal range.[423] The effects of GH deficiency in adults are not surprising, given the effects of GH on all aspects of metabolism; GH replacement partially reverses the abnormalities. Specifically GH replacement increases lean body mass, decreases fat mass (particularly abdominal fat), increases bone density, and increases serum high-density lipoprotein levels. Improvement in exercise tolerance, muscle strength,

TABLE 9–12. Causes of Growth Hormone Deficiency and Their Relative Incidence in 369 Cases (1970–1981), Hôpital des Enfants Malades, Paris, France

Growth Hormone Deficiency	Relative Incidence
IDIOPATHIC, N = 82 (22%)	
Sporadic (isolated or part of multiple anterior pituitary deficiencies)	64
Familial (only two associated with absence of GH because of GH gene deletion)	10
Associated with idiopathic diabetes insipidus	8
ORGANIC, N = 287 (78%)	
Secondary to cranial radiation[1054–1056] (n = 191)	
Acute lymphocytic leukemia	77
Retinoblastoma	18
Medulloblastoma	35
Other head and neck tumors	21
Optic glioma	40
Secondary tumors (before or after surgery) (n = 49)	
Craniopharyngioma	35
Other tumors in hypothalamic-pituitary area	14
Associated with cranial malformations (n = 25)	
Suprasellar arachnoid cyst	6
Hydrocephalus	2
Cleft lip and palate or single incisor and other midline defects	17
Associated with cranial trauma	1
Associated with various diseases (n = 21)	
Diabetes insipidus with histiocytosis X	6
Thalassemia major	1
Diabetes mellitus, insulin dependent	3
Athyroidism	1
Gonadal dysgenesis	1
Nephroblastoma	1
Renal hypoplasia	1
Constitutional bone dysplasia	1
Gastrointestinal tract, facial malformations with omphalocele	2
William-Beuren syndrome	1
Blackfan-Diamond syndrome	1
Mitochondrial defect	1
Dandy-Walker syndrome	1

Personal communication, R. Rappaport.
GH, growth hormone.

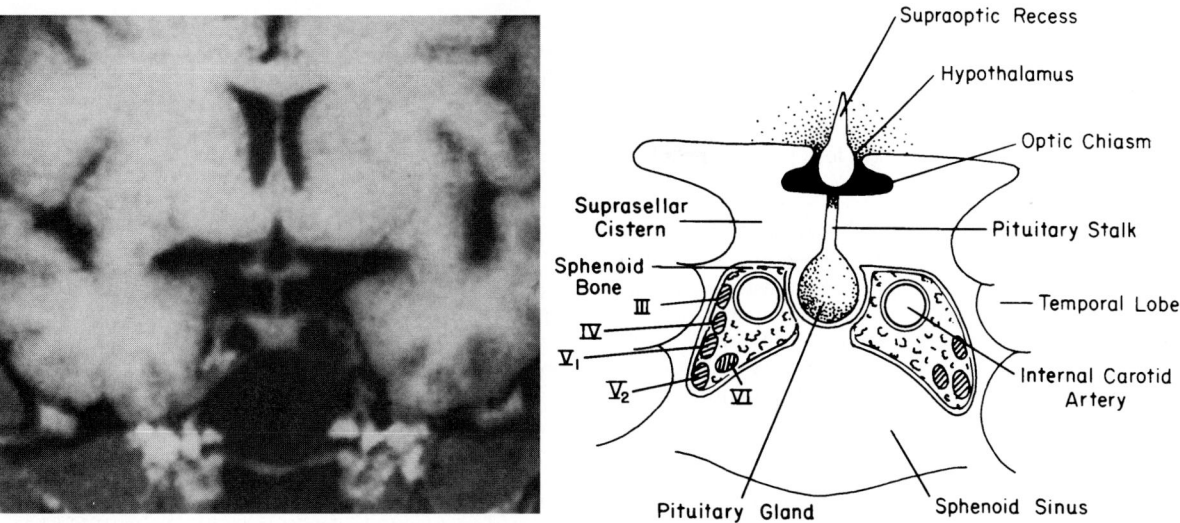

Figure 9–21. MRI scan *(left)* and schematic diagram *(right)* of the normal pituitary fossa. The pituitary is bordered laterally by the cavernous sinus, which contains the internal carotid artery and cranial nerves III, IV, V_1, V_2, and VI. The optic chiasm lies immediately above the pituitary gland and is separated from it by a CSF-filled cistern. Note the location of the sphenoid sinus and temporal lobes. CSF, cerebrospinal fluid. (From Lechan RM. Neuroendocrinology of pituitary hormone regulation. Endocrinol Metab Clin North Am 1987; 16:475–502.)

and psychosocial assessments has also been reported.[212, 428–439] It is not known if GH replacement in adults will improve the cardiovascular mortality observed in adults with hypopituitarism. The most common side effects of GH include fluid retention, carpal tunnel syndrome, and arthralgia; these side effects are usually dose related and may disappear with dose reduction.[212, 428]

The manifestations of GH deficiency in children depend on the age of onset and include short stature and reduced growth velocity. Neonatal GH deficiency is characterized by hypoglycemia that is particularly severe when associated with other anterior pituitary failure but can occur with isolated GH deficiency. GH is not required for normal intrauterine growth so that GH-deficient children are usually of normal weight and length at birth; during the first 2 y growth velocity decreases with a decline in the height and growth velocity percentiles. Weight is normal for length or height, and bone age is delayed. It is important to measure the growth velocity as well as the height and weight percentiles because height reflects only the cumulative growth. For example a child starting off in the 70th percentile would have had a prolonged reduction in growth velocity before being observed to be in the third percentile for height (also see Chapter 30).

GH deficiency in children can be either congenital or acquired (for a detailed discussion see Chapter 30). Idiopathic GH deficiency is usually due to deficiency of hypothalamic GHRH, and mutations of the *GH* gene itself are rare. Other causes of GH deficiency are associated with developmental abnormalities such as aplasia or hypoplasia of the pituitary and midline brain abnormalities. Acquired causes include tumors of the hypothalamus or pituitary, other intracranial tumors such as optic nerve glioma, hypopituitarism secondary to cranial radiation, head injury (including injury at birth), and infection or inflammation. GH deficiency may also occur in the setting of severe psychosocial deprivation. The incidence of different causes of GH deficiency depends on the population studied. Table 9–12 shows the incidence of the various causes of GH deficiency in a large clinic in France. In contrast to experience in the United States, the majority of the French children had radiation-induced GH deficiency.

GONADOTROPIN DEFICIENCY. Gonadotropin deficiency results from either a pituitary defect or deficiency of hypothalamic LHRH stimulation of the gonadotrope. Gonado-

tropin deficiency may be due to hypothalamic disease, disease of the pituitary stalk, or a functional abnormality such as occurs with hyperprolactinemia, anorexia nervosa, secondary adrenal insufficiency, or secondary hypothyroidism.

Gonadotropin deficiency often occurs early in the course of hypopituitarism. In adolescents it causes delayed or arrested puberty. In women it causes infertility, menstrual disorders, or amenorrhea. The resulting low serum estradiol levels are in the range of those of the follicular phase of the menstrual cycle. Hypoestrogenemia is often associated with lack of libido and dyspareunia, and long-standing estrogen deficiency produces breast atrophy. However in women who are hypogonadal from hyperprolactinemia, breast atrophy does not occur. Long-standing estrogen deficiency of any cause results in osteopenia. In men the hypogonadism may be undiagnosed because the syndrome develops slowly and because the diminished libido and impotence may be discounted as a function of "age." Hypogonadism is often diagnosed retrospectively when the patient presents with the symptoms of a mass lesion. Even if the man is unaware of deficiencies, the sexual partner may provide an objective assessment of sexual dysfunction. As in women gonadotropin deficiency in men may result from hyperprolactinemia (see later). Low gonadotropin concentrations cause serum testosterone levels in the prepubertal range; testicular size may decrease and the testes may be soft. Acquired gonadotropin deficiency is a rare cause of male infertility. Spermatogenesis is preserved, and the principal abnormality of the semen analysis is a reduced ejaculate volume. Beard growth and muscle mass may be reduced; osteopenia also develops with long-standing hypogonadism. Hypogonadal men and women experience fine wrinkling of the skin of the face, particularly around the mouth and eyes.

THYROTROPIN DEFICIENCY. Secondary hypothyroidism usually occurs relatively late in the course of hypopituitarism and is characterized by malaise, weight gain, lack of energy, cold intolerance, and constipation. The degree of hypothyroidism depends on the duration of thyrotropin deficiency.

CORTICOTROPIN DEFICIENCY. Secondary adrenal failure may occur as an isolated deficiency or in the course of the development of panhypopituitarism. The symptoms are essentially the same as those of primary adrenal insufficiency (see Chapter 12) but differ in two important respects. Secondary adrenal insufficiency results from lack of corticotropin stimulation of the adrenal and therefore affects only adrenal steroids under predominant corticotropin regulation, namely cortisol and adrenal androgens. Mineralocorticoid secretion, primarily regulated by renin and angiotensin, is preserved, although it may not be optimal. The usual symptoms are malaise, loss of energy, anorexia, weight loss, postural hypotension, orthostatic dizziness, and sometimes headache. Such patients may be misdiagnosed as malingerers. Women tend to lose pubic and axillary hair and have decreased libido, but beard and body hair are preserved in men unless there is coexistent gonadotropin deficiency. In contrast to patients with primary adrenal insufficiency, these patients have a pale and sometimes slightly sallow complexion; corticotropin levels are low, and there is no hyperpigmentation. Severe cortisol deficiency may result in hypoglycemia and hyponatremia; hyperkalemia usually occurs only with coexisting aldosterone deficiency. These patients, particularly those with panhypopituitarism, may deteriorate gradually, and a relatively trivial illness may precipitate vascular collapse, coma, or hypoglycemia. Adrenal insufficiency, regardless of the cause, is a medical emergency.

Morphologic Classification of Pituitary Adenomas

The old tinctorial classification of pituitary adenomas, originating at the beginning of this century, has survived into the era of electron microscopy and immunohistochemistry despite the fact that not all acidophilic adenomas produce GH and more than half of chromophobe adenomas are endocrinologically active. Before 1970 there were few ultrastructural studies of adenomas associated with acromegaly or Cushing's disease.[440–442] Introduction of modern imaging techniques, development of improved hormone assays, and renewed interest in transsphenoidal pituitary surgery created an increasing volume of material for electron microscopy, immunohistochemistry,[443] and in situ hybridization for measurement of mRNA (Fig. 9–22). Assessment of cell proliferation markers such as MIB-1 by light microscopy in fixed sections may be useful in predicting biologic behavior and aggressiveness of the tumor.[444]

The mutated form of *p53*, a tumor suppressor gene, can also be examined histologically. Although the presence of immunoreactivity does not prove mutation of the gene, *p53* immunopositivity is an indication of a rapid pace of growth and aggressive behavior. In one study *p53* was demonstrated in some invasive pituitary adenomas and carcinomas but not in slowly growing, noninvasive adenomas.[445]

The functional classification of pituitary adenomas required histologic, immunohistochemical, and electron microscopic investigation of surgical pituitary specimens and an attempt to characterize every normal and adenomatous cell type. Morphologic findings are correlated with the clinical and laboratory information. This approach has resulted in the delineation of several previously unknown entities. For example three types of ultrastructurally distinct and, as judged by their features, hormonally active adenomas are now recognized that are not related to the known cell types.[446–448] These findings indicate that the cytologic study of the pituitary is not yet complete and that additional cell types are likely to be discovered. Table 9–13 shows the functional morphologic classification of pituitary adenomas and their prevalence in unselected surgical specimens.

This classification,[449] which has gained wide acceptance, is useful for predicting the biologic behavior, natural history, growth pattern, and age-related occurrence of various adenoma types. Electron microscopy is particularly useful for investigating the effect of drugs, such as dopamine agonists and

TABLE 9–13. Prevalence of Pituitary Adenoma Types in Unselected Surgical Material

Adenoma Type	Prevalence (%)
GH-producing adenoma	13.3
Prolactin-producing adenoma	27.3
GH- and prolactin-producing adenoma	7.5
Corticotrope adenoma	10.1
Silent corticotrope adenoma, subtypes 1, 2, 3	5.1
Thyrotrope adenoma	1.0
Gonadotrope adenoma	9.0
Null cell adenoma, including oncocytoma	25.6
Plurihormonal adenoma	1.1

E. Horvath and K. Kovacs, personal communication.
GH, growth hormone.

somatostatin analogues, on the structure of adenomas and for correlating morphologic characteristics with clinical results.

Application of immunohistochemistry demonstrated that more than one hormone can be produced by the same tumor and by the same cells within a tumor[449–452]; this was first demonstrated in an acidophil stem cell adenoma[452] and later in monomorphous-bihormonal mammosomatotrope adenomas.[453] In addition many (densely granulated) GH cell adenomas express α subunit, thyrotropin, and sometimes even FSH and LH.[454] Glycoprotein hormone–producing adenomas often display minor immunoreactivity for GH and, rarely, for prolactin.[450] Thus immunohistochemistry, instead of sharply defining entities, created ambiguity in the classification of some tumors. Until its nature and significance are clarified, plurihormonality should be accommodated within the existing, well-characterized categories. The diagnosis of a plurihormonal adenoma is warranted only if clinical findings or multiple morphologic phenotypes, or both, are compatible with overproduction of more than one hormone.

The most important issue is whether the presence of multiple hormones in adenomas represents abnormal gene expression or is due to amplification of genes normally expressed at a low level. It is not possible to provide an unequivocal solution to this problem, but GH and prolactin and GH and α subunit co-localize in normal human pituitary cells.[18] Furthermore in lactotrope hyperplasia during pregnancy and lactation many cells express both prolactin and GH.[19] In rats estrogen-induced lactotrope hyperplasia is also often bihormonal.[455] In addition a subset of somatotropes in the rat pituitary are capable of transforming into bihormonal thyroidectomy cells.[368] Thus a new perception of the pituitary gland is emerging; the seemingly homogeneous population of five (or more) cell types is not uniform but consists of subsets of cells with one primary function and the potential of producing other hormones. Thus plurihormonality in adenomas may not be due to abnormal gene expression but to deregulation and amplification of genes expressed in the stem cell that gave rise to the tumor.

In some instances a discrepancy exists between clinical presentation, serum hormone levels, and the immunoreactivity of the tumor cells. Some clinically silent tumors are immunoreactive for a hormone, e.g., corticotropin and glycoprotein hormones, without producing clinical or biochemical signs of hormone excess. This discrepancy may be due to incomplete processing or release of the hormone, premature intracellular degradation, or some other discrepancy between the immunoreactivity and biologic activity of FSH-LH or α subunit, or both.

The growth rate, biologic behavior, prognosis, and treatment of null cell adenomas and gonadotrope adenomas are similar and may represent the same tumor type; some patholo-

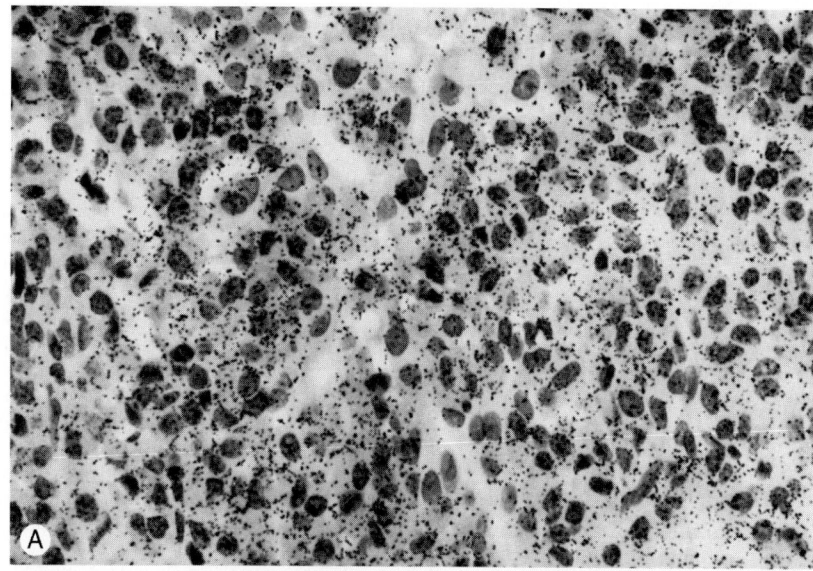

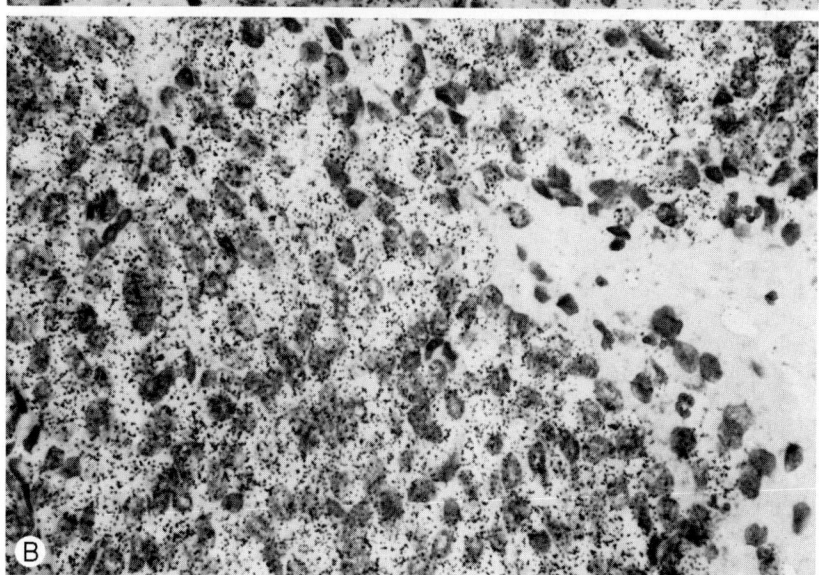

Figure 9–22. *A,* In situ hybridization using autoradiography. The small granules are silver grains corresponding to POMC mRNA in a corticotroph adenoma removed surgically from a 34-year-old female patient with Nelson's syndrome. Original magnification × 400. *B,* In situ hybridization combined with autoradiography demonstrates the presence of estrogen receptor mRNA in a silent subtype 3 pituitary adenoma removed surgically from a 31-year-old man. Original magnification × 400.

gists accept that null cell adenomas may show focal immunoreactivity, whereas others classify tumors with focal immunoreactivity as gonadotrope adenomas. By electron microscopy, however, null cell adenomas do not resemble mature nontumorous gonadotropes. These tumors can express FSH-LH–α subunit, prolactin, GH, or corticotropin mRNA. We believe that null cell adenomas originate in precursor cells that undergo multidirectional differentiation, most frequently to FSH-LH–α subunit–producing cells and less frequently to other hormone-producing cells.

Evaluation of Suspected Pituitary Disease

Therapy for pituitary tumors is dictated by the tumor type and tumor size. The evaluation of the patient with a pituitary tumor should determine (1) the presence and type of hormone hypersecretion, (2) any hormonal deficiencies and need for replacement therapy, (3) the presence of any visual abnormalities, and (4) pituitary anatomy, including the presence of extrasellar extension. Each of these areas needs to be evaluated before therapeutic intervention.

Assessment of Hypothalamic Pituitary Function

Specific tests are performed to confirm the suspicion of a hyperfunctioning pituitary adenoma. In assessment of

pituitary function several factors must be considered: (1) interpretation of the level of the pituitary hormone in relation to the level of the target hormone, (2) pulsatile secretion of anterior pituitary hormones, and (3) specific factors that affect the concentration of each of the pituitary hormones, e.g., time of day, stress, nutritional status (fed or fasting), whether the patient is asleep or awake, and age or stage of development. In general, screening for hyperfunction and hypofunction can usually be achieved by taking a history, performing a physical examination, and assessing pituitary and target organ hormone levels in urine or blood, or both. More subtle abnormalities require functional studies of hormone dynamics.

Table 9–14 shows the pituitary hormones and the target gland hormones. Normal ranges are not listed because they vary from assay to assay. Each laboratory should provide a normal range of values for each test.

Interpretation of hormone concentrations requires consideration of several issues. Currently hormone concentrations are measured by RIA or by IRMA. IRMAs are usually more rapid, more specific, and more sensitive and have a wider working range of levels than do RIAs. However IRMAs are subject to matrix effects and may give artifactual results, as do RIAs, when heterophile antibodies are present.[456–458] Binding proteins, precursors, and metabolites may interfere with both assays and produce spuriously low values.

TABLE 9–14. Pituitary and Target Hormones

Pituitary Hormone	Target Gland	Feedback Hormone
Corticotropin	Adrenal	Cortisol
Thyroid-stimulating hormone	Thyroid	T_4, T_3
Luteinizing hormone	Gonad	Testosterone (men) Estradiol (women)
Follicle-stimulating hormone	Gonad	Testosterone (men) Estradiol (women) Inhibin
Growth hormone	Liver, bone, adipocytes, and other tissues	IGF-I
Prolactin	Breast	Unknown

IGF-I, insulin-like growth factor-I.

Plasma Corticotropin

Measurement of corticotropin is probably required only in the evaluation of adrenal failure or Cushing's syndrome (see Chapter 12). The short plasma half-life of corticotropin requires that samples be collected in a cold syringe, placed in an ethylenediaminetetra-acetic acid (EDTA) tube, centrifuged quickly at 4°C, and stored immediately in a freezer. If these precautions are not followed the peptide is degraded, and the results are not interpretable. Corticotropin is secreted in a pulsatile fashion with a circadian rhythm and increased levels during stress. Therefore corticotropin results must be interpreted with a knowledge of time of sample collection, whether the sample was drawn from an indwelling cannula (in place for at least 2 h), whether the patient was stressed, and whether exogenous synthetic glucocorticoids were administered. A simultaneously obtained plasma cortisol sample is necessary to interpret the appropriateness of the plasma corticotropin level. Furthermore since corticotropin is the prime regulator of cortisol secretion, the plasma cortisol level and 24-h urine free cortisol are useful measures of hypothalamic-pituitary-adrenal function. An 8 AM cortisol value between 10 and 20 µg/dL effectively excludes adrenal insufficiency, although it does not assess corticotropin reserve.

Serum Thyrotropin

Ultrasensitive IRMAs make it possible to distinguish among low, normal, and high levels of thyrotropin. Older RIAs could distinguish between normal and high levels only. The ultrasensitive thyrotropin assay has decreased the need for dynamic function tests, particularly the TRH test. If the thyrotropin concentration is in the normal range in association with normal serum thyroid hormone levels, the patient is euthyroid and requires no further testing. If the serum thyroid hormone levels are low and the thyrotropin level is normal (but inappropriately low for the prevailing thyroid hormone levels) or low, the patient has secondary thyroid failure. Distinction between pituitary and hypothalamic failure can be attempted by administering TRH, but in long-standing thyrotropin deficiency of hypothalamic cause a single dose of TRH may not stimulate intrinsically normal but quiescent thyrotropes. As a practical consideration the serum T_4 level should also be measured, and the value should be interpreted in conjunction with the serum thyrotropin concentration.

Serum Growth Hormone

GH is secreted in a pulsatile fashion, and values in a normal individual may vary from undetectable (during an interpulse interval) to more than 40 µg/L. GH secretion is affected by food ingestion; it is suppressed by hyperglycemia and stimulated by amino acids and hypoglycemia. Sleep stages III and IV (slow-wave sleep) are associated with increased GH secretion, particularly in young adults and children. For these reasons a random serum GH measurement is of limited value. If GH deficiency is suspected, a stimulation test is required (Table 9–15). If GH hypersecretion is suspected, a suppression test (i.e., the oral glucose tolerance test) is employed. Because the bursts of spontaneous GH secretion may occur at any time of day, the timing of the sample is not helpful. The secretion of GH, like corticotropin and prolactin, increases in response to psychological or physical stress or pain. Therefore evaluation of spontaneous GH secretion requires measurement of multiple samples over time via an indwelling venous cannula.[459] GH secretion can also be estimated by measuring urinary excretion. However less than 1% of circulating GH is excreted, and urinary measurement requires a sensitive assay.[460, 461] In addition urinary GH assays are subject to interfering substances and are affected by renal disease. Consequently measurement of urinary GH is not used in clinical practice. The serum IGF-I level provides an overall index of GH secretion and is particularly useful as a screening test for acromegaly. GH secretion is influenced by age and nutritional status and is increased by fasting for 24 h.[462] GH secretion is also increased in type I diabetes mellitus,[156] anorexia nervosa,[463] and hepatic failure and is reduced in obesity.[152] GH secretion increases during puberty, is greater in girls than in boys, and is accompanied by an increase in the serum IGF-I concentration. Thus at puberty the diagnosis of acromegaly may be difficult. GH secretion is suppressed during pregnancy by the hGH variant secreted by the placenta, which presumably feeds back on the maternal hypothalamus and pituitary to inhibit GH secretion. However serum IGF-I levels are increased, indicating that the placental GH has a biologic effect.

Serum Luteinizing Hormone and Follicle-Stimulating Hormone

Serum LH and FSH are also secreted in a pulsatile fashion. In men the levels of these hormones, despite pulsatile secretion, are within a fairly narrow range; therefore marked abnormalities of secretion are easily diagnosed from a pool of three blood samples drawn at 20-min intervals, particularly when interpreted with the clinical findings, simultaneous testosterone level, and possibly semen analysis.

In women marked changes in gonadotropin secretion occur during different phases of the menstrual cycle, and measurement of serum LH and FSH in a woman who is not taking an oral contraceptive and who has regular menstrual cycles is usually not useful. Documentation of a normal menstrual cycle and normal luteal phase serum progesterone level excludes significant gonadotropin dysfunction.

In amenorrheic women measurement of serum LH and FSH, estradiol, prolactin, and hCG concentrations can provide insight into the following diagnoses: (1) primary ovarian fail-

TABLE 9–15. Provocative Tests of Growth Hormone Secretion

1. Insulin 0.15 U/kg body weight causes a peak GH response in 45–60 min. A physician should be in attendance. Severe hypoglycemic symptoms should be reversed with intravenous glucose.
2. Arginine hydrochloride, 0.5 g/kg body weight in normal saline, is administered intravenously over 30 min. GH peak occurs at 45–60 min.
3. Levodopa (>30 kg body weight, 500 mg; 15–30 kg, 250 mg; <15 kg, 125 mg) is given by mouth. Transient nausea is common and vomiting may occur. Side effects are minimized if patient is kept in a supine position in a quiet room. Peak GH response usually occurs between 45 and 90 min.
4. Glucagon, 1 mg, is given intramuscularly. Peak GH response usually occurs 2–3 h later. Nausea and vomiting may result.

GH, growth hormone.

ure with resulting increases in LH and FSH levels (FSH is greater than LH) and usually normal or low serum prolactin levels; (2) hyperprolactinemia with normal or follicular phase LH, FSH, and estradiol levels; and (3) pregnancy with a positive hCG test result, normal or high serum prolactin level, high serum LH level (if hCG cross-reacts in the assay), and high serum estradiol level.

Serum Prolactin

Prolactin is also secreted in a pulsatile fashion, and the pulses increase in the early hours of the morning, particularly just before awakening. Levels of prolactin rise in response to psychological and physical stress, including pain; rise in response to nipple stimulation; and may increase during sexual intercourse. Prolactin secretion is increased in response to estrogens. During pregnancy serum levels may reach 200 to 500 μg/L.

Clinically measurement of a random serum prolactin level is useful if the level is normal or markedly elevated. If the serum prolactin concentration is greater than 200 to 250 μg/L it is almost certain that the patient harbors a prolactinoma, and further prolactin measurements are unnecessary. However mild elevation of serum prolactin levels, e.g., 25 μg/L, likely reflects the stress of venipuncture or physical examination, including the examination of the breasts. In this situation it is necessary to repeat the measurement once or twice. Alternatively samples can be obtained from an indwelling venous cannula after a rest period of 2 h; samples should be obtained at 20-min intervals over the ensuing 2 h.[464] If the prior elevation was a result of stress, samples obtained with this procedure are usually normal. Although prolactin concentrations vary during the day, being lower in the afternoon, the time of sampling is usually not critical. Similarly although changes in prolactin secretion can occur with eating, the magnitude of the change is so small that for clinical purposes fasting is not necessary.

Interpretation of Hormone Levels During Pregnancy

Pregnancy is associated with several alterations in hormonal balance, primarily because the placenta is a pleiotropic endocrine gland (also see Chapter 27). During pregnancy estrogen levels rise many hundredfold. In response prolactin secretion increases and gonadotrope function is suppressed. The high estrogen concentration stimulates the production by the liver of binding proteins for thyroid hormone, cortisol, and androgens (and estrogens) so that total serum T_4, T_3, and cortisol concentrations are elevated, although the free (unbound) levels are normal.

During the first 2 wk of pregnancy hCG levels increase progressively, reach a peak at about 10 wk, and then decline to a nadir at about 120 d. Many LH assays do not cross-react with hCG, but if cross-reactivity occurs, serum LH levels are spuriously elevated, whereas FSH levels are low (in contrast to changes at midcycle, when both are high).

The placenta produces a number of prolactin- and GH-like hormones, two different hPLs, and an hGH variant (also see Chapter 27). The hGH variant suppresses maternal pituitary GH secretion and is thought to be responsible for the high levels of IGF-I during normal pregnancy.

Posterior Pituitary Failure

Diabetes insipidus is discussed in detail in Chapter 10. AVP is synthesized in the magnicellular neurons in the supraoptic and paraventricular nuclei that terminate in the posterior pituitary for storage and direct secretion of AVP into the peripheral circulation. AVP acts on the renal distal tubule to stimulate reabsorption of free water. Diabetes insipidus occurs in patients with hypothalamic tumors or a history of trauma to the pituitary stalk or in those who have undergone pituitary surgery. However when the nuclei are not involved or an adequate amount of the pituitary stalk is preserved, the condition is usually temporary. Diabetes insipidus is unusual in primary anterior pituitary disease.

Diabetes insipidus is characterized by polyuria and polydipsia that persist throughout 24 h. Patients may have a craving for iced water and typically drink large amounts of water at night. Patients with combined corticotropin (or cortisol) deficiency and AVP deficiency may not manifest diabetes insipidus until after cortisol is replaced because renal free water excretion is decreased in the absence of cortisol. Thus before patients are tested for diabetes insipidus it is essential to document normal adrenal function or adequate glucocorticoid replacement. A diagnosis of diabetes insipidus is confirmed by simultaneous measurement of plasma and urine osmolality and, if necessary, a water deprivation test (see Chapter 10). Typically patients with diabetes insipidus have a plasma osmolality greater than 287 mOsm/L and a simultaneous urine osmolality less than 200 mOsm/L. The hallmark of diabetes insipidus is inappropriately dilute urine for plasma osmolality.

Dynamic Tests of Pituitary Function

COMBINED ANTERIOR PITUITARY TEST. Simultaneous administration of four hypothalamic releasing hormones and measurement of the response of target pituitary hormone concentrations permits assessment of pituitary reserve in an ambulatory care setting.

Rationale. The previous exposure of pituitary cells to endogenous hypothalamic hormones "primes" the cells and enables them to respond to the exogenous hypothalamic hormone and to the feedback effects of target cell hormones on the hypothalamus and pituitary.

Indication. The combined anterior pituitary test is a screening tool in suspected pituitary dysfunction. It is particularly useful in assessing pituitary function after pituitary surgery or radiation. If there is a clinical indication of a deficiency, definitive testing is performed, e.g., insulin hypoglycemia or metyrapone administration for suspected corticotropin deficiency.

Test Procedure. The four hypothalamic hormones, GHRH, CRH, LHRH, and TRH, are administered intravenously (sequentially) over 20 s. The doses are LHRH, 100 μg; TRH, 200 μg; CRH, 1 μg/kg body weight; and GHRH, 1 μg/kg body weight.[465] Samples are drawn at −30, 0, 15, 30, 60, 90, and 120 min for measurement of corticotropin, cortisol, thyrotropin, LH, FSH, GH, and prolactin. Results must be interpreted in the light of the baseline levels of the target gland hormones. Baseline samples are obtained at 8 AM for cortisol, T_4, T_3 resin uptake, estradiol (amenorrheic women), testosterone (men), and IGF-I.

Interpretation. Results of administration of the hypothalamic hormones may be of limited utility, but pituitary reserve is likely to be normal if the pituitary hormone response is normal in the setting of an appropriate peripheral target hormone level. The combined anterior pituitary test is useful for amplifying subtle abnormalities; thus if the thyrotropin level and peripheral T_4 levels are both low, the probability of secondary hypothyroidism is high; a lack of thyrotropin response to TRH confirms the suspicion. Deficient response to a hypothalamic hormone may be due to absent or dysfunctional pituitary cells or to increased negative feedback by the peripheral hormone. An example of the latter situation is a lack of a thyrotropin response to TRH in thyrotoxicosis. An absent or a diminished pituitary response may also be due to insufficient priming because of insufficient exposure to the hypothalamic hormone, as in isolated gonadotropin deficiency, usually the result of LHRH deficiency. Administration of CRH may also be useful in distinguishing between ectopic corticotropin production and Cushing's disease; differentiating between these two conditions remains difficult (see Chapter 12). The administration of GHRH to GH-deficient children causes an increase in the serum GH level of greater than 7 μg/L in more than 70% of GH-deficient children; in those with an initial subnormal response the GH response may become normal after repeated GHRH injections. Thus a single injection of GHRH is not useful in identifying the cause of GH deficiency, which is usually a result of a hypothalamic GHRH deficiency. However a deficient GH response to GHRH makes a diagnosis of GH deficiency likely.

The combined anterior pituitary test is useful in documenting the presence of a specific type of functional cells in the anterior pituitary. It cannot be used for diagnosis of hypopituitarism or hyperpituitarism but may aid in defining pituitary function, for example, after pituitary surgery, pituitary or cranial radiation, or pituitary infarction before administering chronic replacement therapy. Patients receiving chronic hormone replacement therapy may also be reassessed after hormone withdrawal to determine the extent of hypopituitarism.

INSULIN TOLERANCE TEST. The insulin tolerance test is most widely used to determine corticotropin and GH reserve.[466, 467]

Rationale. Insulin-induced hypoglycemia activates hypothalamic neurons to stimulate pituitary secretion of corticotropin, GH, and prolactin.

Indication. This test is used to determine corticotropin and GH reserve in a patient suspected of having hypothalamic-pituitary dysfunction.

Test Procedure. If performed by experienced personnel in a properly equipped facility, the test is effective and safe. Contraindications to the insulin tolerance test include an 8 AM plasma cortisol level less than 140 nmol/L (<5 μg/dL) or a history of a seizure disorder, altered mental status, or ischemic heart disease. If the 8 AM plasma cortisol level is less than 140 nmol/L (<5 μg/dL) the patient has adrenal failure and requires a test to distinguish primary from secondary adrenal failure, i.e., simultaneous measurement of plasma corticotropin and plasma cortisol and a short corticotropin (cosyntropin) test followed by a 48-h corticotropin (cosyntropin) infusion (see Chapter 12). Hypoglycemia can precipitate seizures in patients with seizure disorders; it can also cause myocardial infarction in patients with ischemic heart disease. In patients with seizure disorders or ischemic heart disease, an alternative test such as metyrapone administration should be performed (see Chapter 12).

The insulin tolerance test must be performed only when a physician is present. Before insulin is administered a history should be obtained, a physical examination and electrocardiogram should be performed and interpreted, and the 8 AM plasma cortisol level must be documented to be greater than 140 nmol/L (>5 μg/dL). The insulin tolerance test and symptoms of hypoglycemia must be explained in detail to the patient, who must fast from midnight but may take water as desired. A heparin-lock venous cannula is placed about 1 h before beginning the test in the morning. Blood is drawn for plasma glucose, cortisol (and, if indicated, corticotropin), prolactin, and GH determination at −30, 0, 30, 45, 60, and 90 min after the administration of 0.15 U/kg of insulin injection intravenously. Pulse rate and blood pressure are measured, and patients are examined at the times of blood sampling. Symptoms of hypoglycemia usually do not develop during the first 30 min after insulin administration, but between 30 and 45 min, sweating, tachycardia, drowsiness, and hunger usually

occur. If there are no signs of hypoglycemia and the plasma glucose level does not fall to less than 2.2 mmol/L (40 mg/dL), a second dose of insulin, 0.3 U/kg, is administered. In the event of adverse effects, such as seizure, the hypoglycemia is corrected with intravenous glucose, and 1 mg dexamethasone is administered intravenously. Sampling should continue until the end of the test because a subnormal response during this stress indicates a compromised hypothalamic-pituitary-adrenal axis. In patients with insulin resistance (e.g., those with acromegaly) a dose of 0.3 U/kg body weight may be used initially. However if doubt exists, it is safer to start with the standard dose and then double it. There is no point repeating the same dose because it is unlikely to induce hypoglycemia if initially unsuccessful.

Interpretation. Clinical manifestations of hypoglycemia and a plasma glucose level less than 2.2 mmol/L (40 mg/dL) are required for the interpretation of corticotropin and GH levels (Fig. 9–23). If these two criteria are fulfilled, the plasma cortisol level should rise to more than 580 nmol/L (20 μg/dL), and the GH level should increase to more than 10 μg/L.[466, 467] If these levels are not achieved, corticotropin or GH deficiency, or both, are present.

GLUCOSE TOLERANCE TEST
Rationale. GH secretion is inhibited by acute hyperglycemia. The glucose tolerance test is performed to diagnose or exclude acromegaly.

Indication. The test is performed if acromegaly is suspected.

Test Procedure. The patient fasts from midnight and is allowed to take water as desired. A heparin-lock cannula is placed in a forearm vein 1 h before beginning the test. Blood samples for plasma glucose (serum insulin) and serum GH are obtained at −30, 0, 30, 60, 90, and 120 min after ingestion of glucose (75 or 100 g) dissolved in iced orange- or lemon-flavored water immediately after the 0-min blood sample is obtained.

Interpretation. Serum GH level, as assayed by a sensitive IRMA, should decrease to less than 1 μg/L (<2 mU/L) after ingestion of oral glucose.[155] When GH is measured with an ultrasensitive assay (chemiluminescence) that detects levels as low as 0.002 μg/L, GH decreases to less than 0.71 μg/L in women and to less than 0.06 μg/L in men.[468] In older, less sensitive assays for GH, the levels fall to less than 2 μg/L after ingestion of glucose. In acromegalic patients serum GH concentrations remain unchanged, are partially lowered, or increase paradoxically.

Pituitary Imaging

Skull x-ray, hypocycloidal sellar tomography, cerebral arteriography, and pneumoencephalography provide limited visualization of the gland, and arteriography and pneumoencephalography are associated with risk and discomfort. CT and MRI techniques allow noninvasive imaging of the pituitary gland directly. With MRI the structures surrounding the pituitary gland can also be seen. Consequently the evaluation of suspected pituitary or hypothalamic disease is best done with MRI or CT. X-ray, sellar tomography, cerebral arteriography, and pneumoencephalography are rarely indicated. For example a normal skull x-ray film or sellar tomogram does not exclude a pituitary mass, and a skull x-ray or sellar tomogram is of little value in the evaluation of pituitary anatomy. Cerebral angiography may be required before surgical intervention but has no place in the initial evaluation. The best visualization of hypothalamic-pituitary anatomy is usually obtained by MRI and the second best method is high-resolution coronal CT with 1.5-mm sections through the pituitary. MRI is superior because the optic chiasm can be distinguished from the diaphragma sellae, vascular structures can be defined, and tumor

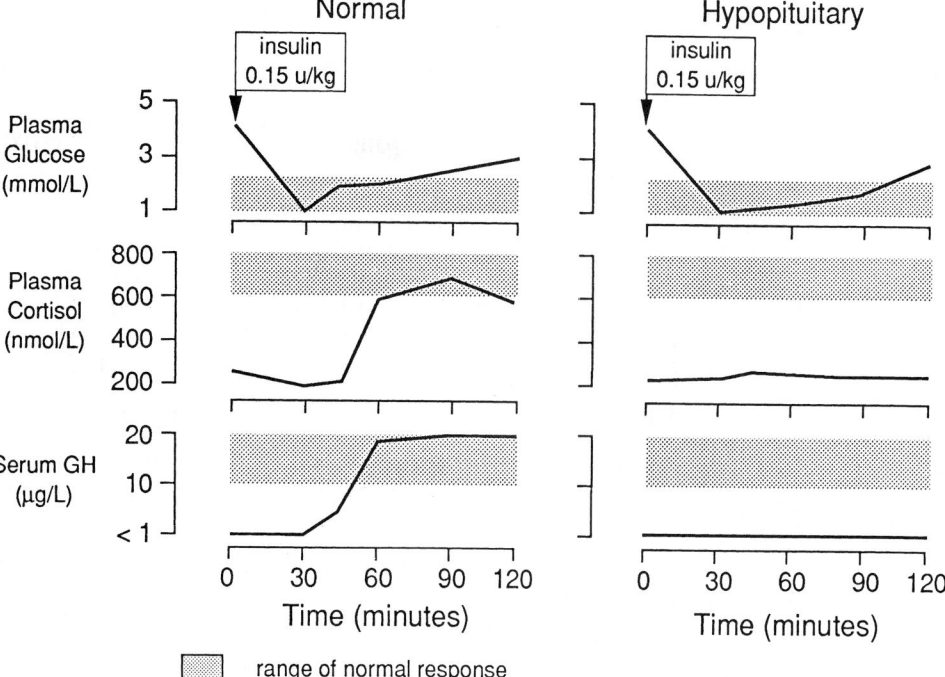

Figure 9–23. The insulin hypoglycemia test in the diagnosis of hypopituitarism. Plasma glucose, cortisol, and serum GH concentrations in a normal subject *(left)* and a subject with hypopituitarism *(right)* are shown. GH levels should rise to a minimum of 10 μg/L, and cortisol levels should increase to 580 nmol/L (21 μg/dL) with achievement of adequate hypoglycemia, namely a blood glucose concentration less than or equal to 2.2 mmol/L (40 mg/dL). (Modified from Wass JAH. Hypopituitarism. In: Besser GM, Cudworth AG, eds. Clinical Endocrinology: An Illustrated Text. London: Gower Medical, 1987: 2.1–2.14.)

extension into the cavernous sinus and sphenoid sinus can be delineated.

NORMAL PITUITARY ANATOMY. High-resolution CT provides insight into pituitary anatomy, particularly into gland size and the presence of focal hypodense or hyperdense lesions in normal glands. Routine axial images of 5-mm thickness do not provide adequate visualization of the pituitary unless a large lesion is present. Direct coronal 1.5-mm images of the pituitary fossa after intravenous contrast administration is optimal (Fig. 9–24). If the neck cannot be hyperextended for a coronal study, sagittal and coronal reconstructions of 1.5-mm images are usually adequate.

The normal pituitary gland ranges from 3 to 9 mm in height, with the average being 6 to 7 mm.[469, 470] Larger glands in women of reproductive age do not correlate with the serum prolactin level. The superior margins of the gland are also more convex in younger (18 to 36 y) than in older (37 to 70 y) women,[469] and gland density is heterogeneous, described as "mottled," in most women. Focal hypodense areas occur in 13 to 36% of normal women,[469, 470] and hyperdense focal areas are present in 9% of normal women. An empty or partially empty sella may be present in up to 18% of normal women.[469] The pituitary gland normally enlarges during the second and third trimesters of pregnancy.

Hypothalamic and pituitary anatomy is best visualized with MRI after administration of gadolinium diethylenetriaminepenta-acetic acid (Gd-DTPA) to enhance lesions such as adenomas. Gland size on MRI correlates with both CT and autopsy findings. Approximately 75% of the pituitary is the anterior lobe, which is usually isointense with brain white matter on most pulse sequences, although heterogeneity may be present. The posterior pituitary has a high signal intensity due to lipid within the AVP-containing neurons; this high signal may be absent in patients with diabetes insipidus. The optic chiasm is directly above the pituitary fossa in 80% of individuals and is usually well visualized; the hypothalamic infundibulum is posterior to the optic chiasm. The cavernous sinus is isointense with and lateral to the pituitary and contains cranial nerves III, IV, and VI and the V_1 and V_2 divisions of cranial nerve V; the nerves are lower in signal intensity than

the pituitary. The low signal intensity (signal void) in the cavernous sinus reflects blood flow in the internal carotid artery. Incidental hemorrhage in the pituitary gland is occasionally present. A partially empty sella may be present in normal individuals.[471]

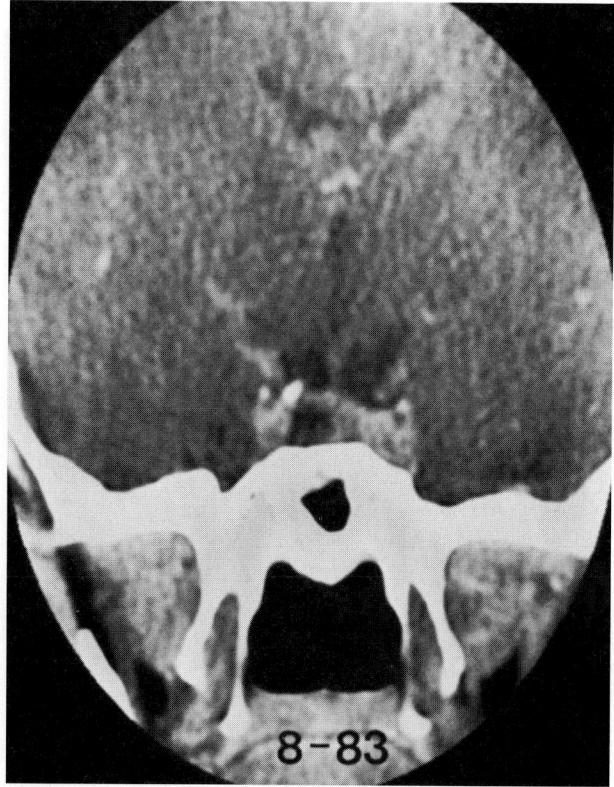

Figure 9–24. Coronal computed tomographic scan with intravenous contrast enhancement demonstrating a 1-cm adenoma of low density. Note the elevation of the diaphragma sellae and deviation of the pituitary stalk.

Hemorrhage into the brain, and presumably into a pituitary tumor, has a characteristic appearance, depending on the age of the hemorrhage and the degree of disruption of the blood-brain barrier. An acute hemorrhage less than 1 wk old, consisting of deoxyhemoglobin, is isointense with the gland on T1-weighted images and has low signal intensity on T2-weighted images. A subacute hemorrhage, 1 to 4 wk old, contains methemoglobin that forms from the periphery to the central region and is of high signal intensity on both T1- and T2-weighted images. A hemorrhage of more than 4 wk duration produces a homogeneously high signal on both T1- and T2-weighted images; hemosiderin appears as a ring around the hemorrhage and is of low signal intensity on T1- and T2-weighted images.[472]

PITUITARY MASS. Although CT and MRI are equally effective in identifying large pituitary tumors, MRI is superior in defining the full extent and relationship to surrounding structures (Fig. 9–25) and is more accurate in identifying small lesions. In patients with surgically proven microadenomas, all the lesions were visualized by MRI; whereas only half of the lesions were visualized with CT scan.[473] A pituitary microadenoma on an MRI scan is round and hypointense to the normal gland on T1-weighted images; lesions exhibit higher signals on T2-weighted scans. The infundibulum may deviate away from the tumor. Macroadenomas tend to have signal characteristics similar to those of the normal gland but may contain cystic or hemorrhagic areas (Fig. 9–26).[471] Intravenous administration of Gd-DTPA enhances the MRI of the normal pituitary maximally after approximately 30 min; adenomas enhance more slowly and the enhancement persists for a longer period. Gd-DTPA and coronal images increase the probability of identifying small lesions and should be used when a pituitary tumor is suspected.[474] MRI may also identify nonpituitary intrasellar masses such as meningioma or internal carotid artery aneurysm (Fig. 9–27). Although MRI is the most sensitive method for identifying microadenomas, small tumors may not be detectable. For example only 83% of the tumors in patients with Cushing's disease were detectable by MRI.[474]

Neuro-ophthalmologic Evaluation

Every patient with a suspected or documented pituitary macroadenoma should undergo a complete ophthalmologic examination before therapeutic intervention as well as careful follow-up during and after treatment. Use of MRI has aided the assessment of the anatomic relationship between the pituitary and the optic chiasm. A distinct separation between the mass and the optic chiasm and absence of tumor invasion into the cavernous sinus suggest that the ophthalmologic examination will be normal. CT cannot provide this information.

Visual acuity and visual fields should be assessed grossly at the initial examination either with the use of a Snellen chart or estimation of visual fields by confrontation. Confrontational screening is performed by finger counting or comparison of two targets. The patient is asked to identify the number of fingers or the appearance of paired objects in each quadrant of one field. Confrontational testing with a red object (e.g., tip of a pen) may detect color desaturation even when the object can be identified, thus revealing subtle visual field loss.

A normal confrontational examination does not exclude subtle abnormalities detectable only with perimetry. Manual perimetry requires a skilled technician; automated perimetry does not require as much technical expertise, and a standardized strategy is used for each field. All types of visual field measurements require cooperation by the patient. An adequate instrument should test both central and peripheral fields, automatically retest missed points, monitor the patient's fixation, and calibrate the background and target luminance.[475]

In approximately 80% of persons the chiasm lies directly

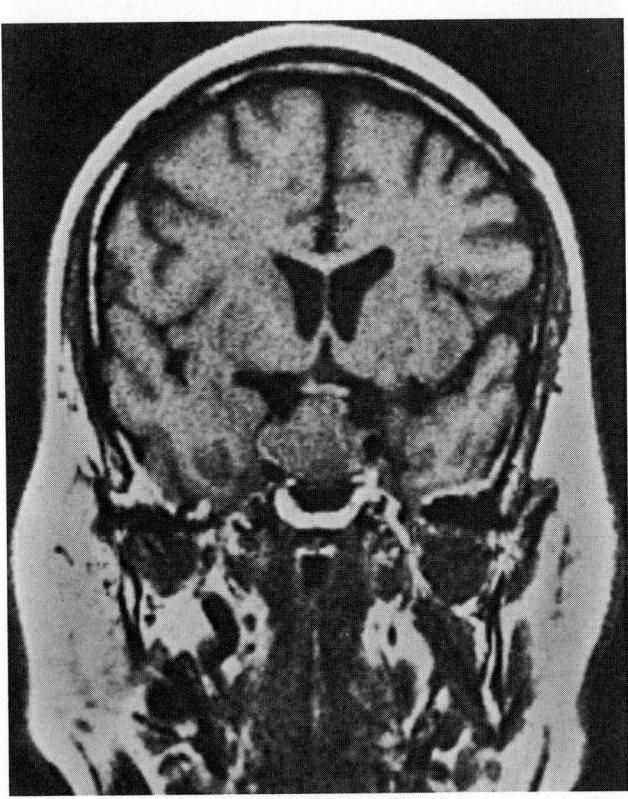
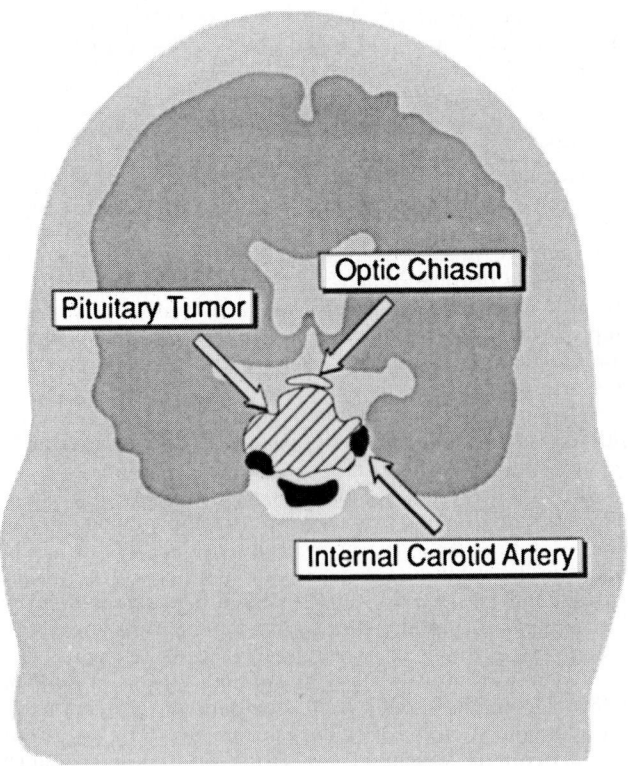

Figure 9–25. Coronal MRI scan and schematic drawing demonstrating a large pituitary tumor extending laterally into both cavernous sinuses and superiorly abutting the optic chiasm. MRI, magnetic resonance imaging.

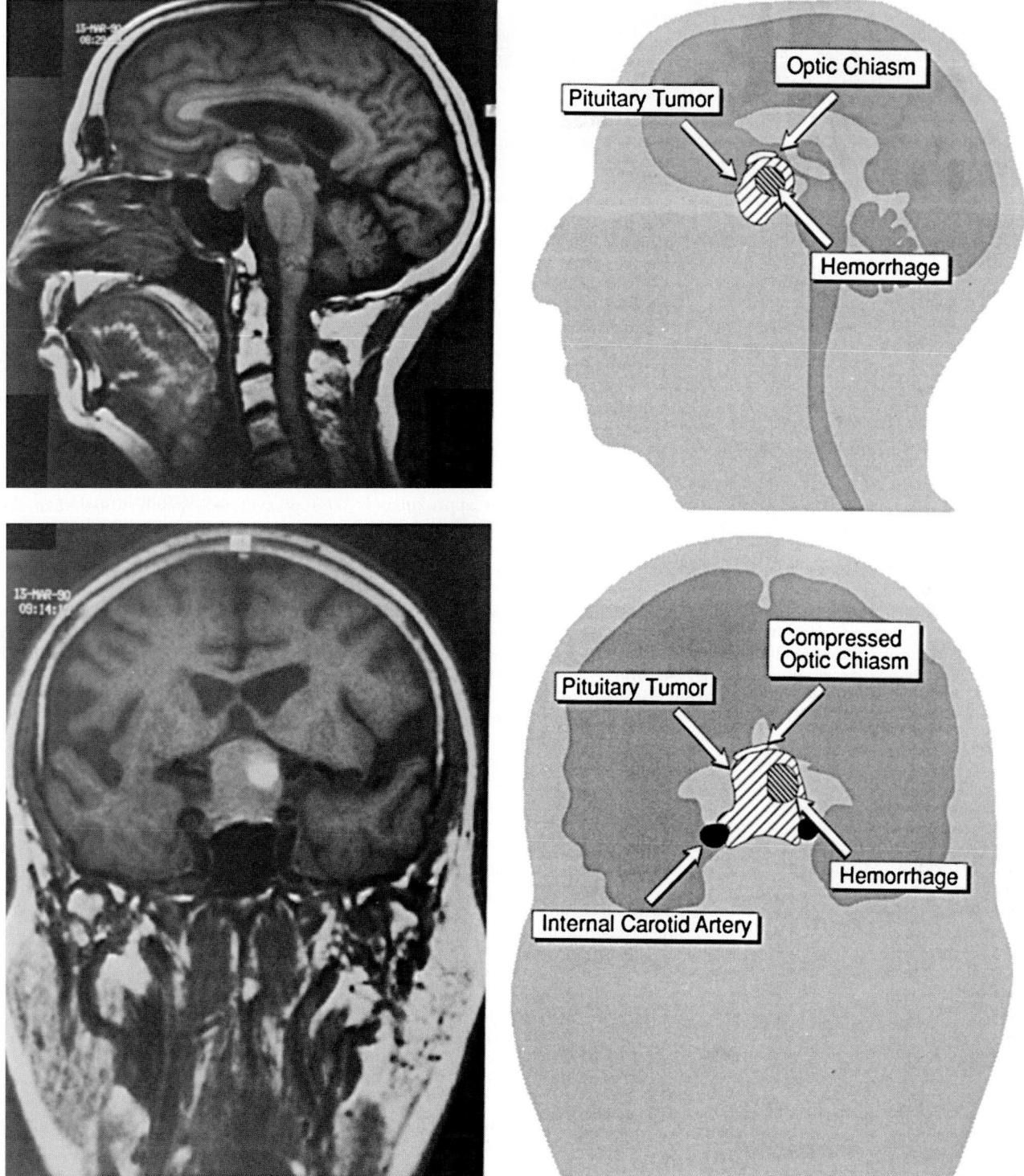

Figure 9–26. Sagittal *(top left)* and coronal *(bottom left)* MRI scans and corresponding schematic drawings of a patient with a macroadenoma with superior extension compressing the optic chiasm and inferior extension into the sphenoid sinus. Note area of high signal intensity suggestive of hemorrhage. (Unpublished observations, courtesy of MO Thorner.)

over the pituitary gland, in 15% the chiasm is anterior to the pituitary and lies above the tuberculum sellae (prefixed chiasm), and in the remaining 5% the chiasm is posterior to the pituitary or the dorsum sellae (postfixed chiasm) (Fig. 9–28).[410] The optic chiasm is separated from the tuberculum sellae, diaphragma sellae, and dorsum sellae by the basal cistern of the subarachnoid space, the height of the cistern ranging between 0 and 10 mm. The infundibulum and hypothalamus are posterior and superior to the optic chiasm.

The pattern of visual field loss caused by a pituitary tumor depends on the location of the chiasm, the course of the optic nerves, and the degree of nerve compression. Permanent loss of vision and permanent visual field defects are usually the consequence of long-standing nerve compression; however the exact relation between duration of compression and permanent damage is not known. If one eye is normal, the patient may fail to notice an abnormality or may describe the vision as dim or foggy. Vision is usually lost gradually, except when

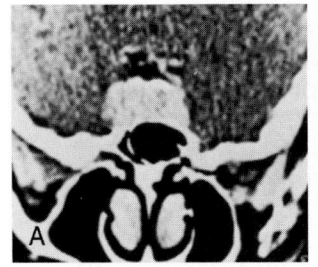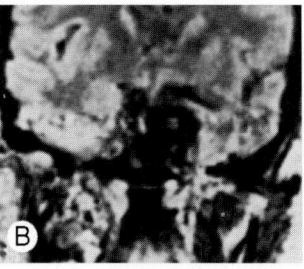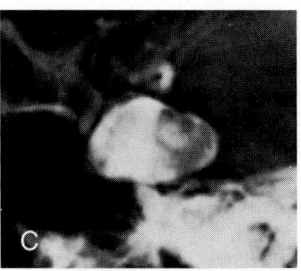

Figure 9–27. *A,* Coronal computed tomographic scan with contrast enhancement of a large pituitary mass. *B,* Coronal MRI scan of the pituitary mass with a signal void from free-flowing blood. *C,* Lateral cerebral arteriogram demonstrating an internal carotid artery aneurysm mimicking a pituitary tumor on CT. (Unpublished observations, courtesy of ML Vance.)

there is significant hemorrhage into the tumor (pituitary apoplexy). Visual impairment may be sudden in pituitary apoplexy, with loss of central vision and development of bitemporal field defects, ophthalmoplegia, and changes in mental function. Visual acuity may range from normal to near or complete blindness. Loss of perception of color, particularly red, and a decreased pupillary light reaction may accompany decreased visual acuity. If the optic nerve is compromised for at least 6 wk, as occurs in 33 to 70% of patients with large tumors, the optic discs may be pale.[411, 476–478]

Although less common, ophthalmoplegia may occur if the tumor extends laterally. Tumors extend into the cavernous sinus in up to 15% of patients but are usually not clinically apparent. Symptoms include diplopia or ptosis, or both, or altered facial sensation. Depending on the degree of cavernous sinus invasion, cranial nerves III, IV, and VI and the V_1 and V_2 divisions of cranial nerve V may be impaired, the most common being third nerve involvement.

Pituitary tumors cause five characteristic patterns of visual field loss and changes in visual acuity (Fig. 9–29).[479, 480] Compression of an optic nerve by anterior and superior extension of tumors produces decreased central acuity and a normal contralateral visual field, findings characteristic and suggestive of optic neuritis. A junctional syndrome—contralateral superotemporal field loss and ipsilateral decreased acuity—results from compression of inferonasal fibers from the contralateral eye that form a loop into the proximal optic nerve (Wilbrand's knee) at its junction with the chiasm. Superior bitemporal field loss with normal acuity occurs when compression of the chiasm below impairs the crossing inferior nasal retinal fibers. This may progress to complete bitemporal loss. Compression of the posterior portion of the chiasm produces central bitemporal scotomatous defects with normal acuity. A homonymous hemianopia with normal acuity results from compression of an optic tract in the setting of a prefixed chiasm or tumor extension superiorly and posteriorly. The last two patterns of visual field loss also occur with hypothalamic tumors such as craniopharyngioma, hypothalamic glioma, and germinoma.

Successful decompression of the optic nerves and chiasm by either resection or medical therapy (e.g., in prolactinoma

or acromegaly) is often followed by improvement in visual function. Surgical removal causes improvement in visual abnormalities in 62 to 80% of patients.[411, 477, 481] The improvement is usually evident within hours or days of surgery and may continue for months. In 4 to 10% of patients visual abnormalities worsen after surgical decompression.[411, 481] Risk of visual deterioration appears to be less with the transsphenoidal approach. Prognostic factors for visual improvement include absence of optic atrophy and short duration of visual impairment. Improvement in visual acuity occurs in most eyes with a preoperative visual acuity of 20/100 or better and in approximately 60% of eyes with acuity worse than 20/100.[410, 477]

Careful ophthalmologic examination and imaging studies must be performed after surgery and after institution of medical therapy to assess the efficacy of treatment and to allow early detection of tumor recurrence. An ophthalmologic examination should be performed shortly after the operation or institution of medical therapy and at least at 6-mo intervals for the first year. Objective assessment of visual fields requires that the patient be alert and cooperative. The frequency of follow-up examinations is determined by the individual abnormalities, type of treatment, and presence of residual tumor on imaging studies. Changes in visual acuity and fields may indicate tumor recurrence even when imaging studies are unchanged, emphasizing the need for regular ophthalmologic examination.

Hormone Replacement Therapy

Hormone replacement is possible for all the target organ hormones (cortisol, thyroid hormone, estrogen, testosterone) and some of the pituitary hormones (gonadotropins, GH, AVP). Replacement must be tailored to the individual hormone deficiency and if possible should not be instituted until the hypothalamic-pituitary-target organ axis has been assessed. For example thyroid hormone replacement before institution of glucocorticoid therapy in an individual with cortisol deficiency may precipitate adrenal crisis.

MEDICAL ALERT (MEDIC ALERT) BRACELET. Every patient receiving adrenal or posterior pituitary (or thyroid hor-

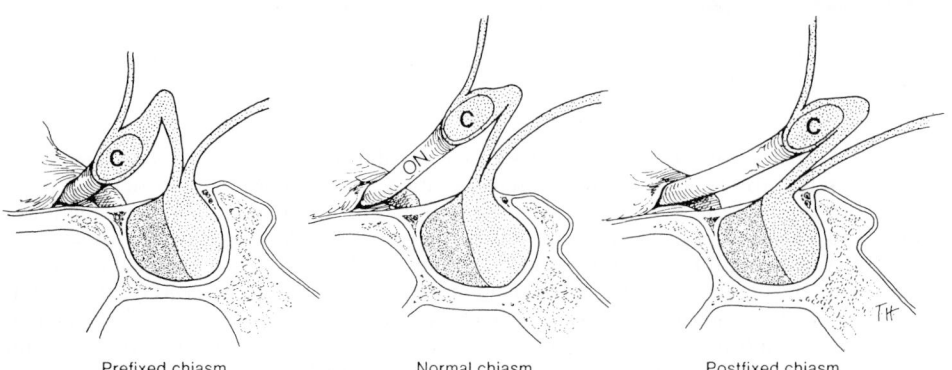

Prefixed chiasm   Normal chiasm   Postfixed chiasm

Figure 9–28. Three different positions of the chiasm in relation to the pituitary gland. C, chiasm; ON, optic nerve. (From Miller NR. Anatomy and physiology of the optic chiasm. In: Miller NR, ed. Walsh and Hoyt's Clinical Neuroophthalmology. Baltimore: Williams & Wilkins, 1982: 60–69. © 1982, the Williams & Wilkins Co., Baltimore.)

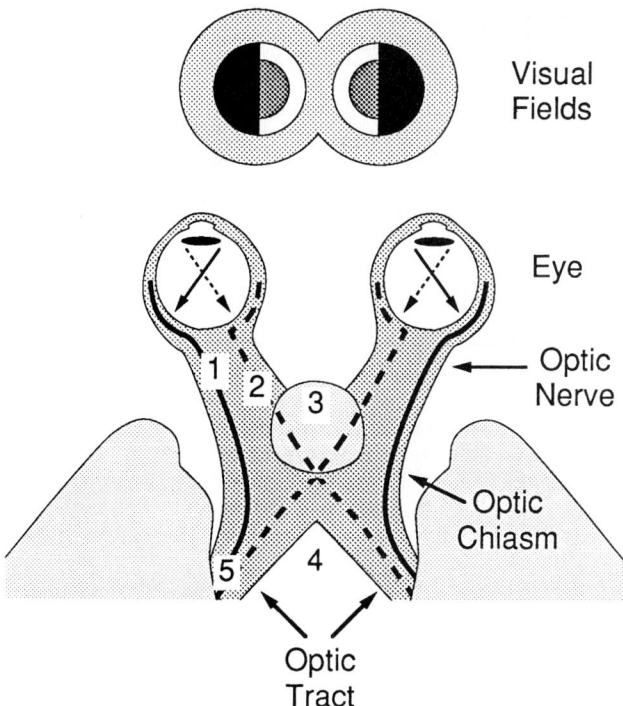

Figure 9–29. The most common visual field defect, bitemporal hemianopia (black areas of visual fields) is caused by compression of the posterior aspect of the chiasm (4) from below. Visual disturbances resulting from compression of the optic nerves, chiasm, and tracts are listed below. The site of lesion is indicated by number.

Pattern	Visual Field/Acuity	Anatomic Correlate
1. Optic neuropathy	Normal contralateral field; decreased central acuity	Postfixed chiasm–anterior extension
2. Junctional syndrome	Contralateral superotemporal field cut; decreased acuity	Junction of Wilbrand's knee
3. Bitemporal	Superior bitemporal desaturation; normal acuity	Inferior fibers cross first
4. Bitemporal scotoma	Relative central bitemporal defect; normal acuity	Relative macular involvement related to posterior compression
5. Tract	Homonymous hemianopia: normal acuity	Prefixed chiasm–posterior extension

(Figure modified from Wass JAH. Hypopituitarism. In: Besser GM, Cudworth AG, eds. Clinical Endocrinology: An Illustrated Text. London: Gower Medical, 1987: 2.1–2.14. Table from Newman SA. Advances in diagnosis and treatment of pituitary tumors. Reprinted with permission from International Ophthalmology Clinics, vol 26, pages 285–300, 1986.)

mone) replacement therapy should have and wear an identifying necklace or bracelet in the event of an emergency.

CORTISOL DEFICIENCY. Cortisol deficiency is usually treated by oral administration of 15 mg hydrocortisone on awakening and 5 mg at 6 PM. This is the simplest way to simulate the circadian rhythm of cortisol secretion. Some patients require an additional 5 mg at midday or early afternoon, and others, particularly very small patients, may require a lower dose. Alternatively synthetic glucocorticoids may be used—either a prednisone dose of 5 mg on awakening and 2.5 mg at 6 PM (some patients do well with only 5 mg on awakening) or 0.5 mg dexamethasone on awakening. The choice of the appropriate replacement dose usually is determined clinically; in patients receiving hydrocortisone, measurement of plasma cortisol through the day may be helpful, but assessment of urinary free cortisol is not helpful. Dose adjustment is made on the basis of symptoms. Overreplace-

ment causes Cushing's syndrome and accelerates bone loss. During stress (whether psychological or physical), fever, and illness, the dose is usually increased to an equivalent of 20 mg hydrocortisone every 6 to 8 h during the intercurrent illness. If parenteral administration is required, 100 mg hydrocortisone is given intravenously every 6 h or intramuscularly every 8 h. Alternatively dexamethasone is given intravenously or intramuscularly at a dose of 1 mg every 12 h; this regimen is frequently used in patients undergoing surgery. The patient should be instructed to increase the oral dose during times of illness, and if vomiting occurs a prepared syringe of dexamethasone, 4 mg, should be available for intramuscular injection.

THYROID HORMONE DEFICIENCY. This deficiency is treated with levothyroxine; the oral dose usually ranges from 0.075 to 0.15 mg once daily. The dose is adjusted according to the clinical response, and the serum thyroid hormone levels (free T_4, T_3) should be in the middle to upper part of the normal range. Measurement of serum thyrotropin is of no value in assessing a response to levothyroxine in patients with hypothalamic-pituitary disease.

GONADAL STEROIDS. Testosterone enanthate for hypogonadal men is usually administered intramuscularly, 200 mg every 2 wk or 300 mg every 3 wk.[482] Testosterone replacement via the transdermal route is also available. One type of patch is placed on the scrotum daily; shaving the scrotum may be necessary for adequate adhesion. The other type of patch usually requires application of two patches each day, these can be placed on the back, chest, abdomen, thighs, and upper arms. Transdermal testosterone provides continuous absorption of the amount of testosterone normally secreted by the testes (approximately 6 mg/d) and is more physiological than the intramuscular injections.[482–485] With the scrotal patch some men have an increase in serum dihydrotestosterone concentrations to greater than normal, presumably because of scrotal skin 5α-reductase activity. Advantages of transdermal testosterone administration include avoidance of wide fluctuations in serum testosterone concentrations and avoidance of intramuscular injection. When initiating testosterone therapy it is our practice to begin with a low dose and gradually increase it, particularly if the plasma testosterone is undetectable. An initial dose of 50 mg testosterone enanthate is given and the dose is doubled every 2 wk until the final dose is reached. Adequacy of therapy is assessed by measuring serum testosterone concentration just before the scheduled injection or at a fixed time of the day in men treated by the transdermal route. Men older than 40 years should have the prostate-specific antigen level measured and a prostate examination before beginning testosterone replacement and periodically thereafter (see also Chapter 16).

Estrogen replacement therapy is given to hypogonadal women to reduce the risk of osteoporosis, to improve the woman's sense of well-being, and to maintain or promote feminization. Estrogen replacement also reduces the risk of premature cardiovascular disease. Calcium supplementation is usually necessary to provide the recommended amount of elemental calcium (1.5 to 2.0 g/d). If the uterus has not been removed, estrogens are administered cyclically or continuously with appropriate progestogens (see Chapter 15). One such regimen consists of conjugated estrogens at 0.625 mg/d for 3 wk together with medroxyprogesterone acetate at 5 or 10 mg/ d for the last 7 or 10 d. Withdrawal menses should occur within a few days of stopping the medications during the fourth week of the cycle. If avoidance of withdrawal bleeding is desired, conjugated estrogens with medroxyprogesterone acetate can be given daily throughout the month. A combined conjugated estrogen and medroxyprogesterone preparation is now available. Regular pelvic examination, Papanicolaou's smear, and mammography are necessary for adequate follow-up.

GONADOTROPINS AND LUTEINIZING HORMONE–RELEASING HORMONE. Gonadotropins and LHRH are administered to initiate puberty and to restore fertility. (Regimens are discussed in detail in Chapters 15 and 16.)

GROWTH HORMONE. GH is available for treatment of GH-deficient children and is approved in the United States and several European countries for replacement in adults. GH is most often given as a daily subcutaneous injection (often administered at bedtime). The recommended beginning dose for children is 0.18 mg/kg/wk (0.025 mg/kg/d) with a maximal dose of 0.3 mg/kg/wk (0.04 mg/kg/d). The recommended starting dose for adults is 0.006 μg/kg/d with a maximal dose of 0.0125 mg/kg/d. Dose adjustment is based on the clinical response, e.g., linear growth in children, and achievement of an appropriate serum IGF-I level for age- and sex-matched normal individuals. GH treatment of GH-deficient children (given three times weekly or daily) results in similar increases in linear growth during the first 6 to 12 mo, and the daily regimen minimizes the decline in growth velocity during the second and third years of treatment (see Chapter 30).

GROWTH HORMONE–RELEASING HORMONE. GHRH has been administered to GH-deficient children by once- or twice-daily injections and by pulsatile subcutaneous administration.[486, 487] Additional experience is needed to determine whether chronic GHRH administration is equivalent to or has advantages over GH treatment.

VASOPRESSIN. Treatment of central diabetes insipidus is discussed in detail in Chapter 10. The major drug for this purpose is desmopressin, an analogue of AVP that is more potent in increasing distal tubular water reabsorption and has less vasopressor activity. Desmopressin has improved the therapy of central diabetes insipidus and can be given by three routes: nasal spray, 10 μg once or twice daily; oral tablets, 0.1 to 0.2 mg once or twice daily; or subcutaneous injection, usually 1 or 2 μg once or twice daily.

Pituitary Surgery

Modern pituitary surgery offers the possibility of selective resection of pituitary adenomas, leaving the normal pituitary intact. Harvey Cushing pioneered the transsphenoidal technique but abandoned it in favor of the transcranial approach. Modern transsphenoidal pituitary surgery was developed by Gerard Guiot and Jules Hardy.[488, 489] Use of intraoperative fluoroscopy to confirm entry into the sella turcica and avoid the risk of being misdirected superiorly or inferiorly (which could lead to catastrophic consequences) and use of the operating microscope to visualize the sellar contents make it possible to identify and selectively remove the tumor and leave the normal gland intact and functional.[489] By decompressing the pituitary fossa from below, a defect results in the sellar floor that usually allows any recurrent tumor growth to extend inferiorly instead of laterally or superiorly. Other advantages include minimal disturbance of the brain, absence of external scars, and no requirement to shave the head. The operation is often well tolerated by elderly or frail patients for whom the risks of a craniotomy might be prohibitive. Blood loss is minimal and transfusion is usually not required. However transsphenoidal surgery requires great skill and experience. Published studies indicate that the better outcomes, in terms of cure and limitation of complications, usually occur when the surgeon performs the operation frequently and has performed several hundred such operations (Table 9–16).[490–492]

It is beyond the scope of this chapter to provide a detailed analysis of transcranial versus transsphenoidal surgery. The guiding principle is that unless contraindicated, the favored approach to the pituitary is transsphenoidal. Contraindications to transsphenoidal surgery include (1) anatomic features

TABLE 9–16. Pituitary Adenomas Treated by Transsphenoidal Microsurgery by ER Laws, Jr, M.D. 1972–1995

Type of Tumor	Number Treated	Recurrences Treated
Clinically nonfunctioning adenomas	741	57
Prolactinoma	803	15
Somatotrope adenoma	425	29
Corticotrope adenomas		
Cushing's disease	319	29
Nelson's syndrome	59	8
Other	26	0
TOTALS	2373	138

that prevent the approach, such as lack of pneumatization of the sphenoid sinus or hyperostosis; (2) suprasellar extension that precludes removal from below; and (3) ambiguity regarding the type of lesion, such as aneurysm or meningioma that cannot be adequately treated transsphenoidally.

Goals of Contemporary Pituitary Surgery

The goals of contemporary pituitary surgery are summarized in Table 9–17. In many cases the primary goal is correction of hormonal hypersecretion, as in patients with acromegaly-gigantism, prolactinoma, Cushing's disease, Nelson's syndrome, and rare thyrotropin-secreting adenomas with associated hyperthyroidism. Ideally excess levels of pituitary hormones are reduced to the normal range, and the hypothalamic-pituitary-target organ responses, both stimulatory and inhibitory, are restored.

Patients with large pituitary adenomas (usually clinically nonfunctioning) usually have symptoms of mass effect. These include headache, visual loss, hypopituitarism from compression of normal pituitary gland, and occasionally involvement of the brain and the paranasal sinuses and other structures at the anterior skull base. Relief of headaches, reversal of visual loss, recovery of lost pituitary function, and reconstruction of the skull base may all be the goals of successful surgery. Occasionally pituitary tumors extend into the cavernous sinus and cause diplopia (from involvement of cranial nerves III, IV, and VI) or facial numbness or pain (from involvement of cranial nerve V). Successful surgery may also reverse these symptoms related to mass effect. Additional goals of pituitary surgery include the avoidance of iatrogenic hypopituitarism and diabetes insipidus, CSF leaks, meningitis, carotid injury, and visual loss. The preservation of normal pituitary function has been aided by the use of the microsurgical approach.[493]

Prevention of recurrence is perhaps the most difficult of the goals of pituitary tumor surgery. Slowly growing indolent lesions often are locally invasive, and tumor cells may infiltrate or invade unresectable structures such as the wall of the cavernous sinus so that radical surgical resection is difficult, hazardous to the patient, or impossible to accomplish.[494, 495] Extensive tumor debulking and decompression of the floor of the sella help decrease the incidence of recurrence and may prevent recurrent tumor from extending rostrally to involve the

TABLE 9–17. Goals of Surgical Management of Pituitary Adenomas

Relief of mass effect causing visual loss, headache, hypopituitarism, or secondary hyperprolactinemia
Correction of endocrine hyperfunction
Avoidance of iatrogenic hypopituitarism and diabetes insipidus
Prevention of recurrence
Definitive histopathologic and immunocytochemical characterization of the lesion

optic chiasm and the brain, permitting a recurrent lesion to follow a less dangerous path of least resistance toward the sphenoid sinus.

Finally surgery provides the opportunity for a complete histopathologic characterization of the lesion. Because the differential diagnosis of sellar masses is so wide (Table 9–18) and because so many lesions can present as "pseudoprolactinomas" with hyperprolactinemia secondary to interference with dopaminergic inhibition of prolactin secretion, a tissue diagnosis is desirable, if not mandatory. In patients with pituitary adenomas immunocytochemical characterization of the tumor helps guide therapy and allow accurate prognosis. Electron microscopy, application of the techniques of molecular biology such as in situ hybridization, and research into the molecular pathologic features of these lesions are possible when surgery provides adequate amounts of tissue to examine.[444, 445, 496–500]

Indications for Pituitary Surgery

PITUITARY APOPLEXY. Minor pituitary hemorrhage into a pituitary tumor probably occurs frequently and may be clinically insignificant; most such cases are probably not diagnosed. A severe hemorrhage leading to prostration, visual disturbance, profound headache, and coma is a neurosurgical emergency. If visual compromise is sudden, neurosurgical intervention is mandatory. The usual approach is by the transsphenoidal route.[501, 502]

PITUITARY TUMOR. If pituitary tumors hypersecrete active pituitary hormones or if they are large enough to produce mass effects, therapy is indicated. With the exception of prolactin-secreting pituitary adenomas, transsphenoidal surgery is usually the treatment of choice. Extirpation of the tumor theoretically, and often practically, cures the hypersecretion of the pituitary hormone or hormones and leads to decompression of any involved structures such as the optic chiasm and cavernous sinus. In most cases lateral extension of the tumor into the cavernous sinus can also be treated with transsphenoidal surgery.

FAILURE OF OTHER THERAPIES. Patients in whom previous therapy has failed are candidates for surgery. For example children with Cushing's disease and adults with acromegaly who have not been cured by pituitary irradiation are candidates for surgery. Patients with prolactinomas whose prolactin levels have been restored to normal but whose "tumor" continues to grow are also candidates for surgery. Uncommonly two lesions may occur simultaneously; e.g., in a patient with a prolactinoma and a sellar meningioma, the growth of the prolactinoma was controlled by bromocriptine and the growth of the tumor was due to the growth of the meningioma.[503] Intolerance of bromocriptine or other dopamine agonist drugs may also be an indication for surgical removal of the tumor. Prolactinomas are not always fully responsive to dopamine agonist therapy, so the prolactin does not return to normal, gonadal function is not restored, and the tumor does not adequately decrease in size. In such cases surgery may reduce the bulk of the tumor and allow better control with medical therapy.

Results of Pituitary Surgery

Because most pituitary tumors are benign, the results of surgery are usually gratifying, particularly in patients with suprasellar extension and visual abnormalities. Improvement in visual field abnormalities occurs in 80% of such patients, progression of visual disturbance is arrested in 16%, and visual deterioration occurs in 4%.[481, 504]

The results of pituitary surgery for hyperfunctioning tumors are discussed in the relevant sections of this chapter. However many of the same issues determine the results for all tumors: (1) the experience and expertise of the surgeon, (2) the size of the tumor, (3) tumor invasion of bone or dura, and (4) previous therapy.

The complications of pituitary surgery in large series are few, but every operation carries a risk. Mortality rates of 0.86, 0.27, and 2.5% have been reported in patients with macroadenomas, microadenomas, and macroadenomas previously treated by other modalities, respectively.[505] For patients with previous treatment or macroadenomas, respectively, visual loss occurred in 2.5 and 0.1%, CSF leak in 5.7 and 1.3%, stroke or vascular injury in 1.3 and 0.2%, meningitis or abscess in 1.3 and 0.1%, and oculomotor palsy in 0.6 and 0.1%.[505] The incidence of postoperative hypopituitarism is about 3% in patients with microadenomas and increases slightly with invasiveness of the tumor.

Pituitary Radiation

Before the improvement in microsurgical techniques and the development of medical therapies, pituitary radiation was the only treatment for many patients with pituitary tumors. Radiation therapy to a pituitary tumor usually prevents further tumor growth and eventually results in a reduction in hormone hypersecretion. However prompt reduction in either tumor size or hormone hypersecretion is rare. In addition hypopituitarism, either total or partial, is a risk. Currently pituitary radiation is most often recommended for patients with residual disease after surgery and patients who cannot undergo surgical resection.

The different types of radiotherapy include conventional supervoltage teletherapy, implantation of radioactive isotopes (rarely used at present), stereotactic radiosurgery using a linear accelerator, alpha particles or proton beam therapy, and single, high-dose, focused stereotactic radiation from the gamma knife. The type of radiation treatment administered must be individualized according to the tumor size and location (proximity to the optic chiasm and cavernous sinus) and the availability of the radiation source. The most commonly used radiation is conventional supervoltage therapy administered in daily fractions 5 d/wk over 4 or 5 wk to provide a total dose of 45 to 50 Gy. This type of treatment may be used in patients with large or small pituitary tumors. Alpha particle or proton beam radiotherapy can be used to treat small tumors only and requires a cyclotron for the energy source, thus limiting availability. Focused radiation from a gamma knife (radiosurgery) decreases the risks of damage to the hypothalamus and other brain structures and can be given effectively as a single dose.

Each method of radiation has advantages and limitations. The results of these treatments are, in general, similar; however information for gamma knife therapy is inadequate to

TABLE 9–18. Differential Diagnosis of Pituitary Adenoma

Pituitary hyperplasia	Teratoma
Lymphocytic hypophysitis	Hamartoma
Granulomatous hypophysitis	Astrocytoma
Sarcoidosis	Schwannoma
Pituitary abscess	Meningioma
Craniopharyngioma	Hemangiopericytoma
Rathke's cleft cyst	Granular cell myoblastoma
Pars intermedia cyst	Choristoma
Colloid cyst	Plasmacytoma
Arachnoid cyst	Lymphoma
Empty sella	Leukemia
Aneurysm	Histiocytosis X
Germinoma	Chordoma
Dermoid tumor	Melanoma
Epidermoid tumor	Metastatic carcinoma

compare it with other techniques. In most studies relatively few patients have progression of disease after radiotherapy, but the recurrence rate despite radiation therapy was 10% in one series.[506] Reduction in hormone hypersecretion may occur within 3 to 6 mo of therapy, but attainment of normal values usually requires at least 5 y and often 10 y.[507–509]

Hypopituitarism, a common consequence of radiotherapy, may be partial or complete and may occur at any time after treatment. In one study half of the patients treated with conventional supervoltage radiation acquired hypopituitarism within 26 mo of therapy,[510] and in other series at least a third of patients had pituitary deficiencies within 2 to 3 y. The incidence of hypopituitarism increases with length of follow-up and consequently all patients treated with pituitary radiation should be monitored lifelong with appropriate hormone measurements and dynamic studies as indicated for early detection of pituitary gland failure.

Other complications of radiotherapy include damage to the optic chiasm or optic nerves, or both, and cranial nerves with consequent visual loss or ophthalmoplegia; vascular damage causing cerebral ischemia; seizures; and development of a pituitary or brain malignancy.[506, 511–514] The loss of cognition is a further concern but is less well documented. The incidence of these complications varies among centers and with the type of radiation administered. Complications of radiotherapy occur more frequently in patients who have received prior surgery.[515] As with surgical excision of tumors radiotherapy should be performed in centers with expertise in these techniques.

Patterns of care for patients with pituitary tumors other than prolactinomas in the United States usually involve transsphenoidal surgery as initial management. Operative removal of the tumor is followed by a recommendation for radiation therapy in patients with endocrine active tumors when the hormonal hypersecretion persists following surgery (acromegaly, Cushing's disease, Nelson's syndrome). In patients with clinically nonfunctioning macroadenomas, radiation therapy is generally recommended when the likelihood of recurrence is high,[516] as in incompletely resected tumors, grossly invasive tumors, and some histologic subtypes (e.g., "silent" corticotropin adenomas) in which recurrence is common. Although conventional methods of radiation therapy (teletherapy) are effective, many patients have recurrence despite this treatment. This fact, along with the convenience for patients of single-dose, stereotactically delivered radiotherapy, has rekindled interest in this modality. The results are being followed carefully and appear to be satisfactory in properly selected patients. Adjunctive postoperative medical therapy is used when possible to control persistent hormonal hypersecretion in anticipation of the radiation effect that may occur in delayed, graded fashion.

PITUITARY DISORDERS

Prolactinoma

Hyperprolactinemia is the most common disorder of the anterior pituitary. A cause of increased prolactin production is prolactin-secreting pituitary adenomas (prolactinoma), the most common secretory pituitary tumor.

NATURAL HISTORY. The natural history of prolactinoma is not known precisely, but most of these tumors grow slowly over years. Autopsy studies demonstrate that 23 to 27% of individuals have pituitary microadenomas[11, 517]; the vast majority of such individuals have no antemortem evidence of endocrine dysfunction, but 40% of the tumors are positive for prolactin by immunocytochemical staining.[11] Serial observations of untreated patients with microadenoma indicate that serum prolactin concentration or tumor size, or both, increase in a minority and that serum prolactin levels in others decrease over time. Table 9–19 summarizes the course in untreated patients. The factors responsible for tumor enlargement and further rises in prolactin levels in a subset of individuals are not known.

ETIOLOGY. Several theories of the genesis of prolactinomas have been proposed. Administration of estrogen in the form of an oral contraceptive has been suggested as a cause of prolactinoma formation,[518, 519] but studies of large numbers of women who used oral contraceptives document no association between use of oral contraceptives, particularly those with lower estrogen doses, and development of prolactinoma.[520–525] Abnormalities of hypothalamic regulation have also been based primarily on abnormal prolactin responses to stimulatory (e.g., TRH, dopamine antagonists) and inhibitory agents (e.g., dopamine agonists). Responses to these agents are inconsistent, both before and after "curative" resection, so a unitary hypothesis as to the pathogenesis cannot be devised. In all likelihood prolactinomas arise de novo and are not a result of hypothalamic dysfunction.[526] Clonal analysis of tumor DNA indicates that prolactinomas are monoclonal in origin.[408]

CLINICAL FEATURES. The clinical presentation of hyperprolactinemia varies with age and sex, the duration of hyperprolactinemia, and the size of the tumor. Men and postmenopausal women usually come to medical attention because of symptoms of a pituitary mass such as headache and visual abnormalities, e.g., decreased visual acuity, visual field deficits, or ophthalmoplegia, or a combination. The most common visual abnormality is bitemporal hemianopsia secondary to compression of the optic chiasm.

Hypogonadism is an almost invariable consequence of hyperprolactinemia. Women of reproductive age commonly seek medical attention because of delayed menarche or disturbance of menstrual function, including amenorrhea, oligomenorrhea, menorrhagia, or regular menses with infertility. Galactorrhea is present in 30 to 80% of these women, and the incidence may be related to the duration of gonadal dysfunction; women with long-standing amenorrhea are less likely to have galactorrhea, probably the consequence of prolonged estrogen deficiency. Other features of estrogen deficiency may include decreased libido, vaginal dryness, and dyspareunia. The majority of premenopausal, hyperprolactinemic women have microadenoma.

In men hypogonadism may be complete or partial, producing decreased libido, complete or partial impotence, or infertility, or a combination. Many hyperprolactinemic men

TABLE 9–19. Natural History of Untreated Prolactin-Secreting Microadenomas

Author, Year	Number of Patients	Mean Duration of Observation (y)	Serum Prolactin Level		
			Unchanged	Decreased	Increased
March et al, 1981[1021]	43	4	38	3	2
von Werder et al, 1983[1022]	30	3–6	26	2	2
Koppelman et al, 1984[1023]	20	5.3	2	14	4
Martin et al, 1985[1024]	41	5.5	11	23	7
Sisam et al, 1987[1025]	38	4.2	5	21	12

report "normal" sexual function and realize that there is a problem only after successful treatment of the hyperprolactinemia. With long-standing hypogonadism, beard and body hair may be decreased and the testes are usually soft but of normal size (>12 mL in volume). Galactorrhea has been reported in 14 to 33% of men with marked hyperprolactinemia but in practice is less common[527, 528]; demonstration may require vigorous breast manipulation. True gynecomastia is uncommon, but the breasts may appear enlarged because of fatty tissue. In arrested puberty body habitus may be immature, and the testes are small (<12 mL in volume) and soft. Symptoms in men with prolactinomas include decreased libido (83%), adiposity (69%), apathy (63%), and headache (63%).[529] As many as 8% of such men in some series are hyperprolactinemic, emphasizing the importance of measuring the serum prolactin level.[530]

In addition a pituitary tumor may be incidentally imaged when a CT or MRI scan is obtained because of head trauma or for evaluation of headaches. A less common presentation is that of severe headache or prostration secondary to hemorrhage into a previously undiagnosed pituitary tumor. This may cause hypopituitarism, including secondary adrenal insufficiency and hypothyroidism, requiring immediate evaluation and treatment.

COMPLICATIONS. The effects of prolactin-secreting pituitary tumors can be due to mass effects of the tumor or to hyperprolactinemia itself. Because microadenomas are intrasellar, visual abnormalities do not occur, but headache occurs more often (50%) than in normal individuals (27%).[531] A larger tumor that extends beyond the confines of the sella turcica can cause headache and visual abnormalities. The classic presentation is bitemporal hemianopsia from compression of the optic chiasm by a tumor that extends superiorly. If the chiasm is prefixed or if the tumor extends posteriorly, compression of a single optic tract produces a homonymous visual field defect. Lateral extension into the cavernous sinus can cause impaired oculomotor function involving cranial nerves III, IV, and VI and the V_1 and V_2 divisions of cranial nerve V, either singly or in combination. Occasionally large tumors may extend into the temporal lobe and cause seizures.

Patients with large tumors are at risk for compromise of other anterior pituitary function due to compression of normal pituitary tissue, causing GH, corticotropin, LH, FSH, or thyrotropin deficiency, singly or in combination. GH deficiency is probably the most common, but this has not been studied systematically. Hyperprolactinemia is associated with impaired pulsatile gonadotropin (LH, FSH) release, most likely via alteration in hypothalamic LHRH secretion. The diminished pulsatile LH and FSH release is restored toward normal by the opiate antagonist naloxone, suggesting that increased endogenous opiate tone plays a role in the impairment of gonadotropin secretion.[532-534] Gonadal insufficiency is secondary to impaired LH and FSH release and is reversed with reduction of prolactin levels.

Chronic hyperprolactinemia causes decreased bone density in both men and women.[535-538] In men suppression of hyperprolactinemia and restoration of gonadal function cause an increase in radial shaft bone density but little change in vertebral bone density; suppression of hyperprolactinemia without restoration of gonadal function does not increase bone density.[537] In hyperprolactinemic, amenorrheic women bone mineral content is decreased when compared with that in amenorrheic women with normal serum prolactin and in eugonadal women, suggesting that prolactin itself has a direct effect on bone.[536]

BIOCHEMICAL EVALUATION. Before embarking on extensive, and frequently expensive, testing in patients with suspected or documented pituitary tumor, a thorough history of drug ingestion should be obtained because some medications

may produce hyperprolactinemia. Common causes of pathologic hyperprolactinemia are listed in Table 9–20.

Evaluation of patients with a suspected or documented pituitary tumor should be focused on the clinical findings, such as evidence of Cushing's syndrome, acromegaly, or hyperthyroidism. Studies should include measurement of serum prolactin, α subunit, LH, FSH, IGF-I (to exclude coexistent excessive GH secretion), hCG β (in women, to exclude pregnancy), T_4, and thyrotropin (to exclude primary hypothyroidism). A single prolactin measurement may be sufficient to diagnose a prolactinoma if the value is greater than 200 μg/L. Because prolactin is secreted in a pulsatile fashion and in response to breast manipulation, a mildly increased concentration of 20 to 60 μg/L may be difficult to interpret; in this situation several measurements should be made before diagnosing hyperprolactinemia. A morning cortisol level is measured to assess adrenal function, but a normal morning cortisol concentration does not assess hypothalamic-pituitary reserve; a stimulatory test such as insulin-induced hypoglycemia or metyrapone administration is necessary to determine whether the hypothalamic-pituitary-adrenal reserve is functionally intact. Induction of hypoglycemia can also be used to determine GH reserve. Additional helpful studies include measurement of plasma testosterone (men) and a careful menstrual history (women).

An increased serum prolactin level must be interpreted in conjunction with the anatomic findings (MRI and CT) to determine whether the hyperprolactinemia is due to a prolactinoma or is secondary to some other process. A serum prolactin concentration of 200 μg/L or greater in the presence of a macroadenoma (>10 mm) is most likely a prolactinoma. Conversely serum prolactin levels of less than 200 μg/L in the setting of a large pituitary tumor are usually elevated because of the mechanical effects of non–prolactin-secreting tumors that cause pituitary stalk compression or interfere with dopamine transport from the hypothalamus to the anterior pituitary. This distinction is particularly important in selecting appropriate therapy; dopamine agonist drugs reduce serum prolactin levels in both instances, but shrinkage of the tumor

TABLE 9–20. Causes of Hyperprolactinemia

Hypothalamic disease
    Tumor, e.g., metastases, craniopharyngioma, germinoma, cyst, glioma, hamartoma
    Infiltrative disease, e.g., sarcoidosis, tuberculosis, histiocytosis X, granuloma
    Pseudotumor cerebri
    Cranial radiation
Pituitary disease
    Prolactinoma
    Acromegaly
    Cushing's disease
    Pituitary stalk section
    Empty sella syndrome
    Other tumors, e.g., metastases, nonsecretory, gonadotrope adenoma, meningioma
    Intrasellar germinoma
    Infiltrative disease, e.g., sarcoidosis, giant cell granuloma, tuberculosis
Drugs
    Dopamine receptor antagonists, e.g., chlorpromazine, fluphenazine, haloperidol, perphenazine, promazine, domperidone, metoclopramide, sulpiride
    Other drugs
        Antihypertensives, e.g., methyldopa, reserpine, verapamil
        Estrogens
        Opiates
        Cimetidine
Primary hypothyroidism
Chronic renal failure
Cirrhosis
Neurogenic, e.g., breast manipulation, chest wall lesions, spinal cord lesions
Stress, e.g., physical, psychological
Idiopathic

is unlikely with secondary hyperprolactinemia.[539] Patients with a prolactin-secreting microadenoma usually have serum prolactin levels less than 200 μg/L. Hyperprolactinemia can also be caused by nonpituitary intracranial lesions; serum prolactin concentrations may be increased, usually to less than 100 μg/ L, with craniopharyngioma, meningioma, ectopic pinealoma, metastatic tumor, or third ventricle tumor.[540]

Stimulatory tests devised to determine whether an elevated prolactin concentration is a result of a prolactinoma include administration of TRH, dopamine antagonists (e.g., sulpiride, chlorpromazine), and drugs that act through diverse mechanisms (e.g., cimetidine and dextroamphetamine). For example patients with prolactinomas have a diminished prolactin response to TRH, but the response is not consistent and cannot be used to diagnose or exclude a tumor or distinguish between hypothalamic and pituitary disease.[541] These tests are nonspecific and are not useful in evaluating a patient with a suspected prolactinoma.

PATHOLOGIC FEATURES. As assessed on surgical material the lactotrope adenoma is the most common pituitary adenoma in women, but there is no gender difference in the incidence of prolactinomas in unselected adult autopsy material.[449] The frequency was approximately 31% before the introduction of dopamine agonist therapy and now approximates 20%. With the exception of rare acidophilic tumors, lactotrope adenomas are chromophobes or acidophiles with a diffuse histologic pattern. Small tumors may rarely be papillary. Prolactin production can be substantiated by immunohistochemistry in the form of the Golgi region of adenoma cells. Cytoplasmic immunostaining is diffuse in the rare, densely granulated variant. Accumulation of spherical calcified bodies (calcospherites) in these tumors[542–544] is important because with the exception of craniopharyngioma and meningioma, calcification is uncommon in sellar tumors. A form of endocrine amyloid may be present intra- and extracellularly.[449, 545]

The ultrastructural appearance of the sparsely granulated lactotrope adenoma is highly characteristic.[449, 546, 547] The middle-sized, polyhedral adenoma cells have nuclei with large, dense nucleoli. The ample cytoplasm contains abundant, highly organized RER and a prominent Golgi apparatus with pleomorphic, immature secretory granules (Fig. 9–30). The cytoplasmic storage granules are sparse, are between 120 and 300 nm in size, and are involved in exocytosis. The number of granule extrusions varies among tumors. The electron microscopic features of the rare, densely granulated variant are similar to those of densely granulated somatotrope adenomas, including a similar size of the secretory granules (400 to 700 nm). A distinguishing feature is the presence of granule extrusions in the lactotrope. The different biologic behavior of different lactotrope adenomas is not reflected in the light microscopic or electron microscopic features.

The variable response[548–550] of lactotrope adenomas to dopaminergic agonists is reflected in the histologic features of these tumors.[546, 551] Optimally dopaminergic agonists produce significant decreases or a return of serum prolactin levels to normal and reduction in tumor volume. The lactotrope tumor that is suppressed by dopamine agonists is cellular and contains little, sometimes barely detectable, prolactin immunoreactivity. When examined by electron microscopy, the tumor tissue is seen to consist of small cells with heterochromatic, multiply indented nuclei and a small rim of cytoplasm containing involuted RER and Golgi membranes (Fig. 9–31). Secretory granules and granule extrusions vary in number (Fig. 9–32).[552–554] In addition some tumors contain a mixed population of suppressed cells and cells displaying varying degrees of synthetic activity,[546, 551] and cell necrosis may occur. In a minority of tumors dopaminergic agonists do not cause a decrease in the serum prolactin concentration or morphologic evidence of suppression.[551]

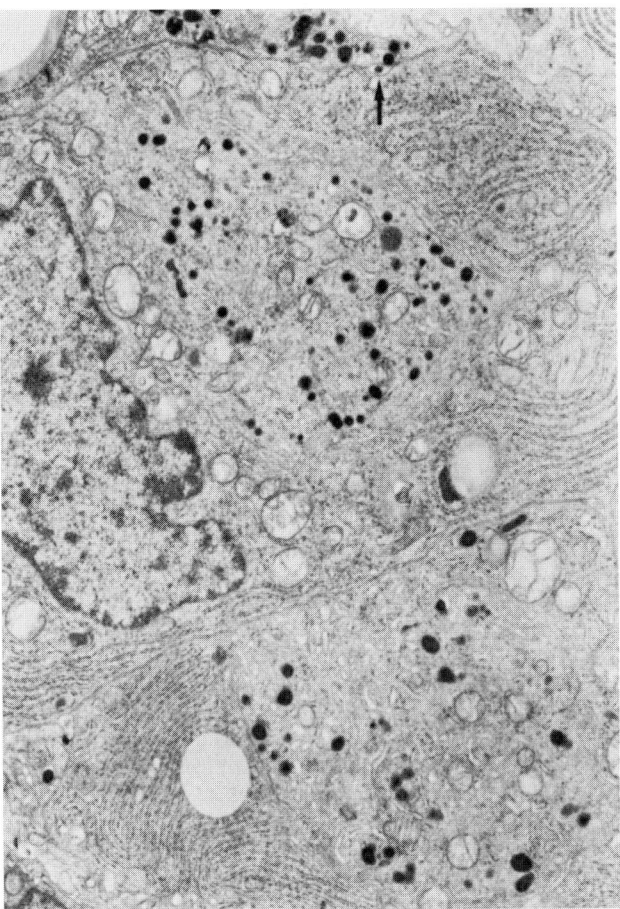

Figure 9–30. Typical sparsely granulated prolactin cell adenoma with abundant RER, prominent Golgi apparatus with numerous immature secretory granules, and granule extrusion (arrow). Magnification × 11,800. RER, rough endoplasmic reticulum.

Estrogen receptor mRNA is expressed in untreated prolactinomas and decreases after bromocriptine treatment.[555] Dopamine receptor D_2 mRNA is present in prolactinomas, and bromocriptine causes a significant increase in dopamine receptor D_2 mRNA in responsive tumors. In bromocriptine-resistant tumors, D_2 receptor mRNA is present, and loss of D_2 receptor mRNA does not explain resistance to bromocriptine.[556]

The variability of responsiveness to dopaminergic agonists is also evident after withdrawal of drug treatment.[551] Under such conditions the original structure of cells may be restored within 2 wk, but in some lactotrope adenomas groups of cells are still suppressed 1 mo or more after cessation of treatment. This phenomenon may partly explain why serum prolactin concentrations do not always return to pretreatment values.[557]

Individual prolactin-producing adenomas respond in different ways to dopaminergic drugs.[558] Significant reductions of the serum prolactin level and of tumor volume are due to decreases in prolactin gene expression and thus in hormone synthesis.[558] Mild or moderate decreases in serum prolactin concentration without morphologic signs of suppression are probably due to tissue insensitivity to dopamine.

Protracted medical treatment of prolactinomas may lead to marked calcification, deposition of endocrine amyloid, and perivascular and interstitial fibrosis.[559–562] The latter, if extensive, may decrease the chance for successful surgery.[560, 563] Only rare cases of prolactin cell carcinoma have been reported.[564–566]

Lactotrope hyperplasia is rare in surgical material as the

sole demonstrable pathologic lesion responsible for hyperprolactinemia, but the number of lactotropes may be increased in the nontumorous pituitary adjacent to the prolactinoma.[449, 567] Hyperplasia of lactotropes may also occur in association with thyrotrope hyperplasia of primary hypothyroidism,[568] and lactotropes may be hyperplastic in glands harboring corticotrope adenomas.[569] Because of limited availability of tissue, lactotrope hyperplasia is probably underreported in surgical specimens; even when observed the extent has not been established, and the cause is unknown.

GOALS OF TREATMENT. Treatment should return hormonal hypersecretion to normal, reduce tumor size, and correct visual or cranial nerve abnormalities, or both; restore any abnormal pituitary function; and, if possible, preclude the need for chronic hormone replacement therapy. These objectives are the ideal, but in the case of large tumors, these goals may be only partially achieved.

Successful treatment of prolactinoma is most often accomplished with administration of a dopamine agonist. In addition to medical and surgical therapy pituitary radiation may be employed, usually as adjunctive therapy. Some patients require more than one type of treatment to correct prolactin levels and decrease tumor size.

MEDICAL THERAPY. The semisynthetic ergot alkaloid bromocriptine, an orally active dopamine agonist, was introduced in 1971 for the treatment of hyperprolactinemia and prolactinomas. During the ensuing years numerous studies have documented the effectiveness of dopamine agonists in lowering serum prolactin levels, reducing tumor size, improv-

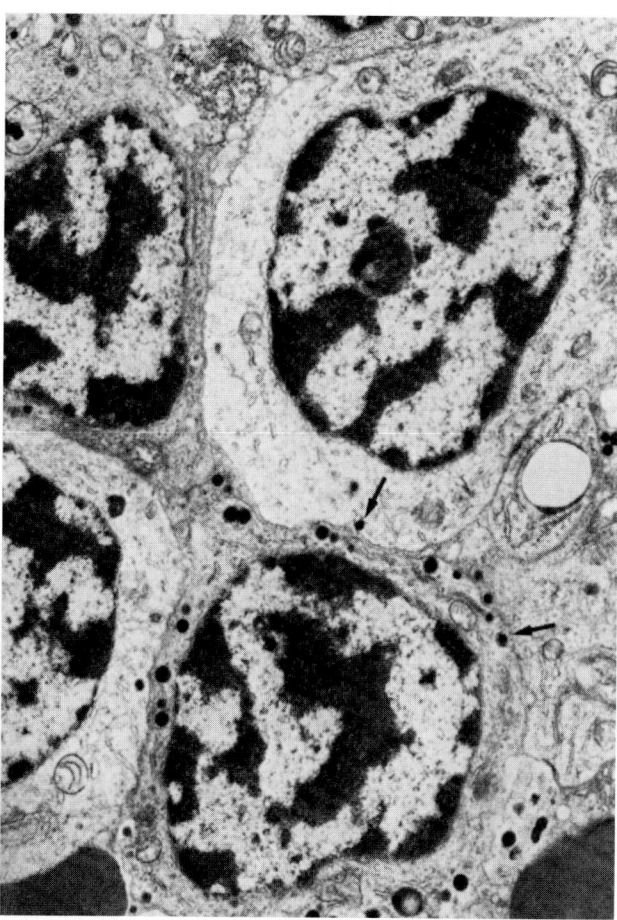

Figure 9–32. Same prolactin cell adenoma as depicted in Figure 9–31. Despite bromocriptine-induced involution of cytoplasmic organelles, granules are still being extruded *(arrows)*. Magnification × 13,200.

ing visual field and cranial nerve abnormalities, and restoring gonadal function.

Dopamine agonists lower serum prolactin concentrations in most patients, but the degree of prolactin suppression varies (Fig. 9–33). In 13 series involving 286 hyperprolactinemic women, bromocriptine lowered serum prolactin levels to normal in 64 to 100%, galactorrhea was improved in 57 to 100%, and menses and ovulation returned in 57 to 100%.[570] Suppression of prolactin secretion depends on the number and affin-

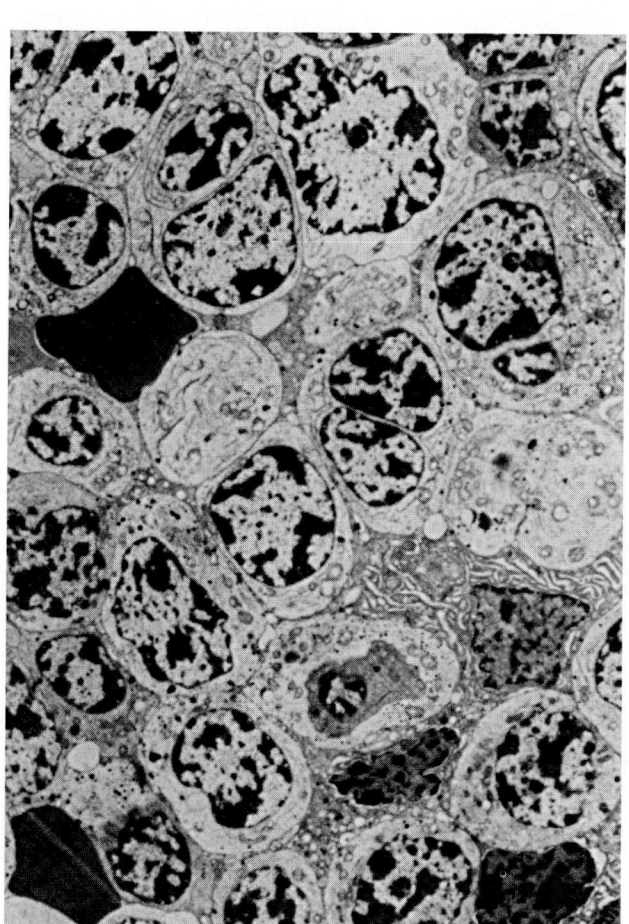

Figure 9–31. Marked bromocriptine effect in a sparsely granulated prolactin cell adenoma. Note the irregular, heterochromatic nuclei and the tiny rim of cytoplasm containing few membranous organelles and secretory granules. Magnification × 4450.

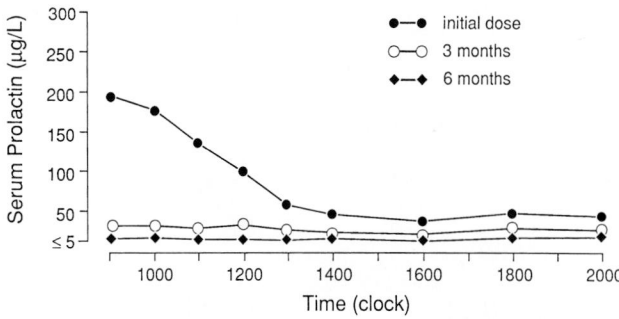

Figure 9–33. Effects of bromocriptine in vivo. After a single 2.5-mg dose of bromocriptine administered at 9 AM, prolactin secretion was inhibited within 2 h and reached a nadir at 7 h. With chronic treatment (2.5 mg three times daily) of 3 and 6 mo, prolactin levels were maintained within the normal range throughout a 24-h period. (Modified from Thorner MO. Hyperprolactinaemia. In: Besser GM, Cudworth AG, eds. Clinical Endocrinology: An Illustrated Text. London: Gower Medical, 1987: 4.1–4.12.)

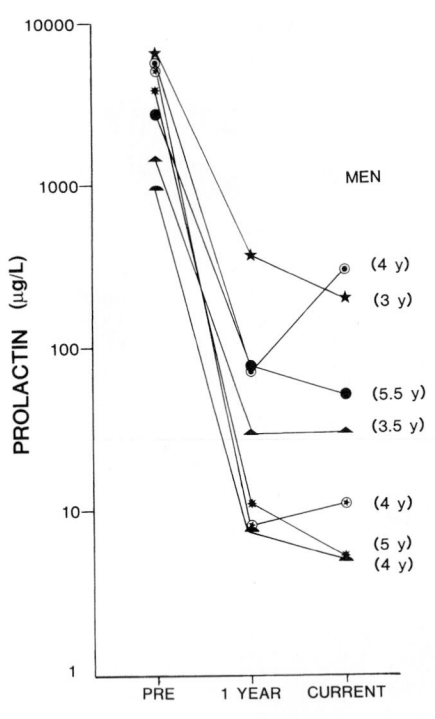

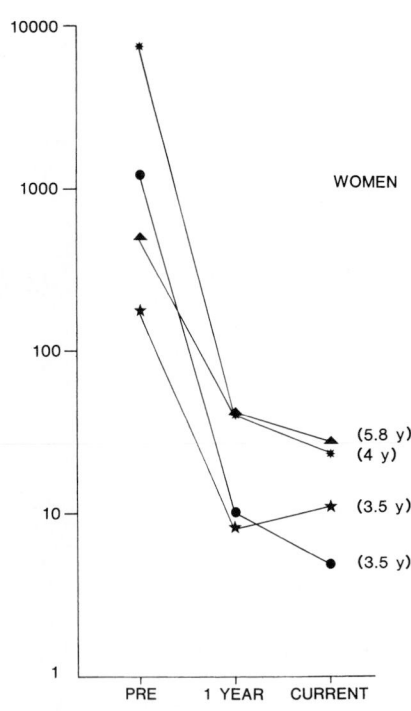

Figure 9–34. Serum prolactin concentrations in patients with prolactin-secreting macroadenomas before and after long-term treatment with bromocriptine, 2.5 mg three times a day. Note continued suppression of prolactin over time. Values are plotted on a semi-logarithmic scale. (Unpublished observations, courtesy of ML Vance.)

ity of tumor dopamine receptors as demonstrated by studies of surgically resected adenomas. Adenomas from patients with the greatest suppression of serum prolactin by bromocriptine contain the largest number of dopamine receptors, and receptor binding activity is greater in these adenomas than in those from patients less responsive to bromocriptine.[571] As an example of the variable response, either partial or almost complete

suppression of serum prolactin can occur after a single dose of 2.5 mg bromocriptine. Serum prolactin is suppressed for 9 h by 47 to 97%; chronic treatment produces a further decrease in serum prolactin level.[550, 572] In addition although patients with markedly increased serum prolactin concentrations, such as 1000 μg/L, have reductions in prolactin with dopamine agonist administration, prolactin levels may not return to nor-

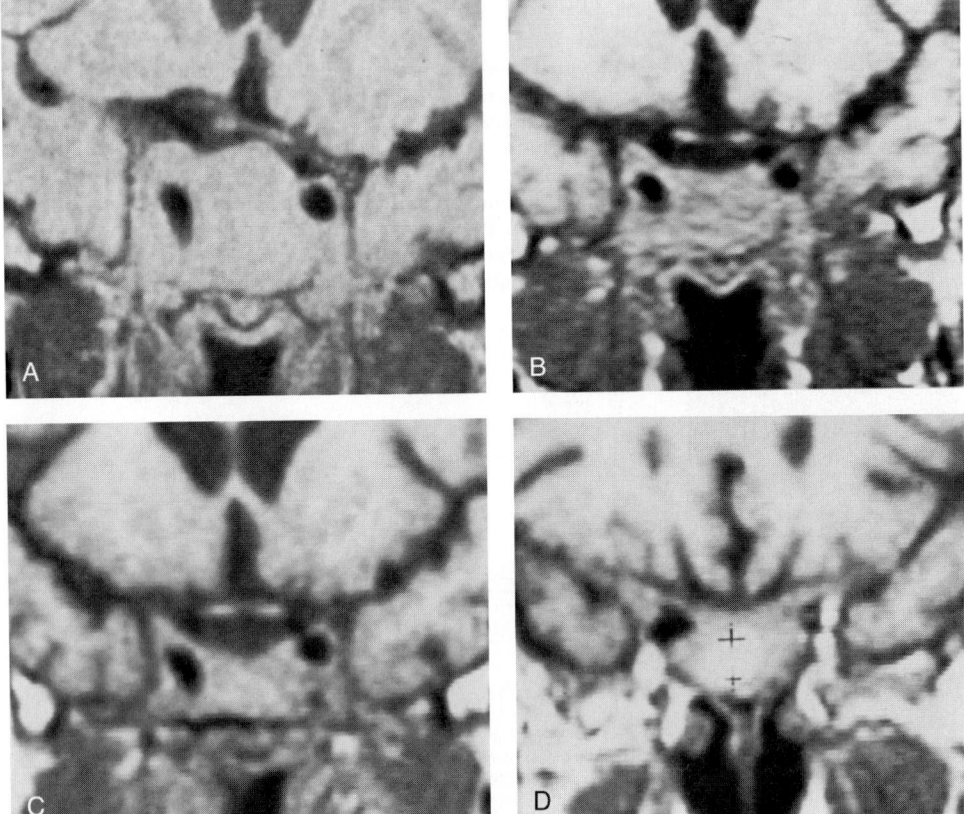

Figure 9–35. T1-weighted coronal MRI scan of a 67-year-old man treated with the dopamine agonist CV 205-502. *A,* Homogeneous tumor extending to the optic chiasm and into the cavernous sinus bilaterally, serum prolactin level 15,000 μg/L. *B,* After 8 wk of treatment the height of the tumor decreased by 20 mm. *C,* After 24 wk of treatment gland height decreased by 30 mm from baseline, serum prolactin level was 11 μg/L. *D,* After 24 wk of treatment—more anterior image demonstrating an area of high signal consistent with hemorrhage that was not present on previous scans. (From Vance ML, Lipper M, Klibanski A, et al. Treatment of prolactin-secreting pituitary macroadenomas with the long-acting nonergot dopamine agonist CV 205–502. Ann Intern Med 1990; 112:668–673.)

mal as rapidly as in patients with lesser degrees of elevation; this variability may be related to the number of adenoma cells.

The results of dopamine agonist treatment in patients with macroadenomas are similar to those in patients with microadenomas (Fig. 9–34). Reduction in tumor size, improvement in visual abnormalities, and partial suppression of serum prolactin are usually evident before the serum prolactin level reaches the normal range. In a prospective study of bromocriptine therapy in 27 patients with macroadenomas 67% had return of prolactin concentration to normal during 15 mo of treatment, all had a reduction in tumor size, and 9 of 10 had improvement in visual field defects.[550] In 38 patients treated with either lisuride or bromocriptine for 30 to 88 mo, 79% had reduction of prolactin level to normal and 76% had a decrease in tumor size.[573] Even when serum prolactin levels do not return to normal, there is usually a substantial reduction in the level. Visual field defects may improve before a demonstrable decrease in tumor size is seen by CT or MRI, emphasizing the fact that careful monitoring of vision and visual fields is a more sensitive indicator of tumor response than are imaging studies.

Available dopamine agonists include bromocriptine, lisuride, pergolide, metergoline, quinagolide, and cabergoline. Figure 9–35 shows the results of treatment of a macroprolactinoma with quinagolide. All of these drugs act by direct stimulation of neuronal and pituitary dopamine receptors (D_2).[574–576] A single dose of 2.5 mg bromocriptine can suppress serum prolactin levels for up to 14 h,[548, 577] and the biologic effect may persist up to 24 h in some patients.[548, 578] The most common side effects are nausea and orthostatic hypotension, which occur on initiation of treatment and can be minimized by beginning with a small dose (1/4 tablet) administered with food at bedtime and by increasing the dose gradually (every 3 d) over 1 to 2 wk. Less common side effects include headache, fatigue, nasal stuffiness, abdominal cramping, and constipation.[570] Despite taking the medication with food, some patients have gastrointestinal intolerance. Administration of bromocriptine intravaginally to women suppresses prolactin levels with fewer side effects.[579] Hallucinations and psychosis have also been observed. The incidence of psychosis was 1.3% in one study of 600 patients treated with bromocriptine; the symptoms included auditory hallucinations, delusions, and mood changes that abated when the drug was discontinued.[580] Concomitant alcohol ingestion may exacerbate nausea and abdominal discomfort.[581] Patients usually acquire a tolerance to the side effects, but there is no loss of effectiveness in suppressing prolactin secretion.

The usual dose of bromocriptine is 2.5 mg three times daily. It is uncommon for a patient to require a higher dose; the size of the tumor and the serum prolactin level have no bearing on the dose required. In patients who achieve a normal serum prolactin level, the dose may be reduced to 2.5 mg twice daily; suppression may continue with the reduced dose. Some patients have been given larger doses of bromocriptine (e.g., 20 to 30 mg/d) in an attempt to suppress prolactin concentration to normal, but there is no conclusive evidence that a larger dose is more effective than the standard regimen. The standard dose of lisuride is 0.2 mg three times daily. In 30 patients treated with either bromocriptine or lisuride, 21 had continued suppression of prolactin level to normal and no increase in tumor size after reduction of the dose.[573] Pergolide is usually administered in a starting dose of 0.05 mg once or twice daily and may be increased to 0.2 mg twice daily as indicated. This drug lowers serum prolactin levels and has also been used to treat patients with acromegaly.[582] Quinagolide is administered once daily, usually at bedtime with food, to minimize side effects; doses range from 0.075 to 0.5 mg/d.[583, 584] Cabergoline is given once or twice weekly in doses ranging from 0.5 to 2.0 mg/dose.[585–588]

A dopamine agonist is usually taken chronically and thus functions as a hormone "replacement" because, for whatever reason, these patients have a functional pituitary dopamine deficiency. Withdrawal of treatment usually results in an increase in serum prolactin concentrations (Fig. 9–36) and re-expansion of the tumor.[549, 570, 576, 589] Occasionally a patient with a microadenoma or no demonstrable tumor has no increase in prolactin concentration after discontinuing dopamine agonist therapy. Whether spontaneous infarction of the tumor occurred is not known. If medication is discontinued, the patient should be followed closely with frequent measurement of the serum prolactin concentration; if the level increases, medical therapy should be restarted.

Resumption of ovulatory menses occurs in 80 to 90% of hyperprolactinemic women during bromocriptine therapy.[570, 590] The fertility rate of these patients should be the same as that of other women of the same age. A standard recommendation for women attempting to become pregnant is that barrier contraception should be used until there has been two or three regular cycles so that cycle length can be determined. After discontinuation of mechanical contraception, a serum hCG β measurement is made to confirm pregnancy as soon as there is a delay in expected menses. This regimen makes possible early diagnosis of pregnancy and early discontinuation of dopamine agonist therapy. Surveillance of more than 2000 pregnancies indicates that bromocriptine use is not associated with an increased risk of multiple pregnancies, spontaneous abortions, ectopic pregnancy, trophoblastic disease, or congenital malformations.[591–595] Tumor expansion may occur during pregnancy, particularly in women with macroadenomas. The incidence of significant tumor enlargement

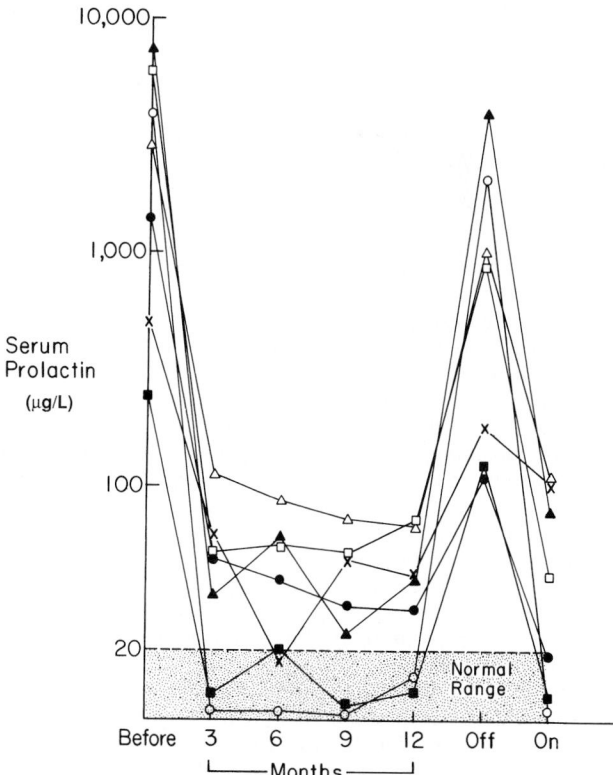

Figure 9–36. Serum prolactin concentrations in seven patients with prolactin-secreting macroadenomas before and during treatment with bromocriptine, 2.5 mg three times a day, and after discontinuation and reinstitution of treatment. Bromocriptine reduces serum prolactin concentrations; withdrawal of treatment results in an increase toward pretreatment values. Serum concentrations decrease with reinstitution of therapy. Values are plotted on a semilogarithmic scale. (From Vance ML, Evans WS, Thorner MO. Drugs five years later. Bromocriptine. Ann Intern Med 1984; 100:78–91.)

during pregnancy is about 1.4% in women with microadenomas and 16% in women with macroadenomas.[590] Both of these percentages may be overestimates resulting from observer bias. In our experience the incidence in microadenomas and macroadenomas is less than 1%. Therapies in the event of significant tumor enlargement include surgical resection, high-dose glucocorticoid therapy, and reinstitution of bromocriptine. Bromocriptine is effective and is the most benign therapy. Patients with macroadenomas treated with bromocriptine continuously during pregnancy do not have tumor-related complications. Similarly those given bromocriptine because of tumor expansion had improvement or resolution of headaches and visual field defects.[596–600] Because of the risk of tumor expansion in women with macroadenomas, a thorough ophthalmologic examination, including visual field testing, is recommended before conception is attempted so that baseline values can be documented.

After cyclic menses have been restored, the need for contraception for those not desiring pregnancy should be addressed. Because estrogens stimulate prolactin synthesis and lactotrope mitotic activity, there is a theoretical risk of promoting enlargement of a prolactinoma with oral contraceptive use. However in hyperprolactinemic women who have had a suppression of prolactin concentration to normal levels with bromocriptine, addition of an oral contraceptive is not associated with an increase in serum prolactin level.[601]

The treatment of men with a dopamine agonist enhances libido and potency as the serum testosterone level increases. Some men note improvement in function before the testosterone concentration becomes normal. The semen analysis (sperm count and semen volume) improves with lowering of the prolactin level to normal and restoration of pulsatile secretion of LH and FSH.[596]

The nonergot long-acting dopamine agonist quinogalide is given once daily and may be useful in patients intolerant of bromocriptine and other ergot derivatives. The suppression of serum prolactin, restoration of gonadal function, and decrease in tumor size with this drug are comparable to other dopamine agonists.[583, 584, 602]

Cabergoline is a long-acting ergot derivative that is administered once or twice weekly and is also better tolerated than bromocriptine by some patients. This drug lowers prolactin concentrations, restores gonadal function, and reduces tumor size.[585–588]

Although most patients have a good response to dopamine agonists, some respond partially or not at all. The clinical response to medical therapy and the number and affinity of tumor dopamine receptors are correlated. Surgically resected adenomas from bromocriptine-responsive patients have twice as many dopamine receptors and higher binding affinity for dopamine than do adenomas from bromocriptine-resistant patients.[571] These observations probably explain occasional tumor growth during bromocriptine therapy, loss of responsiveness, and occasional metastasis of tumors.[564, 603–605] Resistance to bromocriptine is uncommon, but all patients should be closely monitored during medical therapy, and surgical resection should be considered if a patient fails to respond to medical treatment.

SURGICAL THERAPY. Before the development of medical therapy, surgery was the most effective treatment for a prolactinoma. Transsphenoidal microsurgical resection of the adenoma is associated with better results and less morbidity than are other surgical approaches.[606, 607] Although surgical resection offers the potential for cure, in fact cure is effected in a minority of patients with large tumors and is associated with a risk of recurrence in all patients. The results depend on the skill and experience of the surgeon. Resection of microadenomas (<10 mm) at centers where the procedure is performed frequently results in a return of serum prolactin levels to

normal 60 to 87% of the time, whereas serum prolactin levels become normal in only 0 to 40% of patients with macroadenomas (>10 mm).[608–613] The most important factors predictive of successful surgery are the preoperative serum prolactin concentration and the tumor size and stage (degree of invasion of parasellar structures). Of 266 women with prolactinoma, a normal postoperative serum prolactin level was achieved in 86% when the preoperative prolactin concentration was 20 to 250 μg/L, in 48% when the preoperative concentration was 250 to 500 μg/L, and in 6% when the preoperative concentration was greater than 1000 μg/L; similar results have been reported in hyperprolactinemic men.[613] A summary of surgical series is shown in Table 9–21.

Although surgery is effective in debulking large tumors and may be curative for microadenomas, recurrence rates over 5 y of follow-up range from 10 to 50% in patients with microadenomas and from 0 to 91% in those with macroadenomas.[614–619] Risk of mortality with transsphenoidal surgery is less than 1%[620]; complications include CSF rhinorrhea, diabetes insipidus, infection, damage to the visual system (less common with transsphenoidal surgery than with craniotomy), and anterior pituitary insufficiency. The cumulative risk for these complications is on the order of 2% for patients with microadenomas and 14% for patients with macroadenomas.[620] The risk of morbidity is increased with a second surgical procedure.[621] Thus surgical resection of a microadenoma offers the greatest potential for cure, but the usual outcome for patients with large tumors is persistent hyperprolactinemia requiring additional therapy.[622]

RADIATION THERAPY. Primary treatment of prolactinoma by pituitary radiation prevents further growth of the tumor but is less effective in promoting a prompt reduction of the serum prolactin concentration, although a progressive reduction in serum prolactin concentration may occur over time. Of 28 patients treated with conventional radiation therapy, only 2 had a normal serum prolactin level 2 to 10 y (mean, 4.2 y) after treatment[623]; similar results have been reported by others.[507, 624, 625] Combined therapy with a dopamine agonist and radiotherapy produces somewhat better results in regard to plasma prolactin levels and restoration of fertility.[626] The restoration of fertility was probably due to dopamine agonist treatment because 92% of those who conceived did so within 4 mo of combined dopamine agonist and radiation therapy. None had a significant increase in tumor size during pregnancy.[626]

The recommended radiation dose is a total of 45 Gy administered as 1.8 Gy/d over 25 d. A high-energy linear accelerator, rather than a cobalt 60 teletherapy apparatus, combined with a rotational arc technique provides maximal limitation of the high-dose region and usually produces little or no hair loss.[627] A total radiation dose of less than 40 Gy results in poor tumor control, and total doses greater than 50 Gy or daily doses greater than 2 Gy are associated with higher complication rates and no demonstrable improvement in the overall results.[506] Complications of pituitary radiation include hypothalamic insufficiency;[628] hypopituitarism; optic chiasm or optic nerve injury, or both; vascular damage with stroke; brain necrosis; and development of malignant tumors (fibrosarcoma, osteosarcoma). Radiation-induced hypopituitarism has been best documented in acromegalic patients treated with radiotherapy, and the incidence increases with time; gonadotropin deficiency is most common, occurring in 47 to 70% of patients treated with either radiation alone or surgery and radiation. Second most common is corticotropin deficiency (15 to 67%), followed by thyrotropin deficiency (15 to 55%).[515, 629, 630] There have been no adequate studies of GH secretion after radiotherapy, but plasma GH is frequently undetectable in random measurements in these patients. It is possible that stereotactic radiosurgery with the gamma knife

TABLE 9–21. Surgical Results in Patients with Prolactinomas

Author, Year	No. of Patients*	% Normal Postoperative Prolactin	% Recurrence (Time, y)
Aubourg, 1980[1026]	90		NR
	23 micro	57	
	67 macro	39	
Chang et al, 1977[609]	33		NR
	17 micro	59	
	6 macro	0	
Charpentier, 1985[1027]	347		17 (1.5±0.4)
	PRL <100	89	
	PRL <200	72	
	PRL >200	21	
Ciric, 1983[1028]	41		NR
	41 macro	27	
Faria, 1982[1029]	100		
	72 PRL <200	76	13 (0.6–7)
	28 PRL >200	46	36 (0.6–7)
Grisoli, 1980[1030]	20		NR
	PRL <100	100	
	PRL >100	25	
Hardy et al, 1978[610]	80		NR
	PRL <200	87	
	PRL >200	19	
Hubbard et al, 1987[622]	31 micro	68	NR
	24 macro	17	
Keye, 1979[1031]	43	85	NR
Landolt, 1981[1032]	70		NR
	PRL <200	88	
	PRL >200	18	
Laws, 1985[1033]	68 micro	50	24 (5.5, mean)
	32 macro	25	27
Nelson et al, 1983[614]	40	63	36 (1.3±0.2)
Parl et al, 1986[619]	24		
	13 micro	100	31 (5.2, mean)
	11 macro	100	91 (5.2, mean)
Post et al, 1979[612]	30		NR
	17 micro	82	
	13 macro	46	
Randall et al, 1983[607]	100		NR
	54 micro	69	
	36 macro	34	
Rawe, 1980[1034]	30		NR
	21 micro	81	
	9 macro	33	
Rodman et al, 1984[617]	65		
	42 micro	88	17 (4.2±0.3)
	23 macro	39	20 (4.2±0.3)
Schlechte, 1981[1035]	67	43	NR
Soule, 1996[1036]	11 micro	45.5	NR
	23 macro	17.4	
Thomson et al, 1985[618]	69		
	61 micro	75	10 (5)
Thomson, 1994[1037]	45 micro	86.5	13 (10)
	8 macro	50	50 (5)
Tindall et al, 1978[611]	37		NR
	26 PRL <200	73	
	11 PRL >200	27	
Tucker et al, 1981[615]	45		12 (3.2)
	27 micro	74	
	15 macro	53	
van't Verlaat, 1993[1038]	11 micro	100	9 (3.9, mean)
Woosley et al, 1982[616]	36		
	22 micro	72	5 (0.3–3)
	14 macro	29	0 (0.3–3)

*Characterization of patients is reported: micro = tumor less than 10-mm diameter; macro = tumor greater than 10 mm diameter. PRL < or > indicates preoperative prolactin level, in micrograms per liter. NR = not reported.

or focused linear accelerator may produce less hypopituitarism because of the sparing of the hypothalamus with these methods.

Acromegaly

In 1886 Pierre Marie used the term *acromegaly* to describe two patients and reviewed eight previously published papers describing patients with presumed acromegaly.[631] Minkowski, in 1887, deduced a relationship between a pituitary tumor and the development of acromegaly.[632] Four years later the New Sydenham Society published a translation of Marie's original paper and a review of 48 patients.[633]

The prevalence of acromegaly in the United States is unknown. In Newcastle-upon-Tyne in England the estimated prevalence of acromegaly was 38 per million with an annual incidence of 3 per million.[634] In Göteborg, Sweden the prevalence and annual incidence were estimated to be 69 per million and 3.3 per million, respectively.[635] The percentage of acromegalic patients in two large surgery series, each involving more than 1000 pituitary tumors, were 13.7 and 17.1%, respectively.[636, 637] Acromegaly occurs with equal frequency in men and women, may occur at any age, and is most frequent in the fourth and fifth decades. When it occurs before puberty, gigantism results—a syndrome that accounts for less than 5% of acromegalic patients.[636] Acromegaly may occur as a part of the MEN1 syndrome; the prevalence of MEN1 in the Mayo Clinic surgical series was 15 of 254 (5.9%) acromegalic patients.[636] The MEN1 syndrome most commonly includes parathyroid adenoma (hyperparathyroidism), pancreatic islet cell tumor (insulinoma), and pituitary adenomas, of which prolactinoma is the most common type.

ETIOLOGY. Table 9–22 lists the various causes of acromegaly. More than 99% of cases result from a primary pituitary adenoma.[638] Excessive production of GHRH accounts for less than 1% of cases and can arise from gangliocytomas of the hypothalamic or pituitary (eutopic) or peripheral tumors (ectopic).[639] Ectopic GH secretion by a pancreatic islet cell tumor has been described.[640]

Most evidence suggests that somatotrope adenomas originate in the pituitary. Somatotrope adenomas are circumscribed tumors; the remaining pituitary is normal without evidence of somatotrope hyperplasia. With successful tumor removal and reduction of GH concentration to normal, recurrence is rare. If acromegaly were a hypothalamic disease, recurrence would be expected to be common. Reichlin wrote in 1986, "In my view, the etiology of most cases [of acromegaly] will more likely be found in the genetic analysis of clonal tumors that encode chromosomal growth factors, an insight we have gained from the study of oncogene pathogenesis of cancer."[641] This prediction has been fulfilled in part by the description of a point mutation in α_S, the guanosine triphosphate–binding subunit of the stimulatory regulator of adenylate cyclase (G_S), in several somatotrope tumors that causes adenylate cyclase to be activated constitutively.[381] Somatotrope tumors appear to be monoclonal in origin.[408]

Ectopic GHRH production is probably more common than suggested by most series. Approximately 20% of neuroendocrine tumors, including carcinoid, pancreatic endocrine tumors, medullary carcinoma of the thyroid, small cell carcinoma of the lung, and pheochromocytoma, contain GHRH when examined by immunocytochemistry,[642, 643] and approximately 60% are positive for GHRH when tissue is analyzed by RIA.[644, 645] The elaboration of GHRH by these tumors may be more common than the clinical expression for three reasons:

TABLE 9–22. Etiology of Acromegaly

Gangliocytoma—hypothalamic or pituitary[639]
Pituitary adenoma—pure somatotrope, mammosomatotrope, mixed
Ectopic GHRH-secreting tumors[1039]
    59% carcinoid: bronchus (55%), gastrointestinal/pancreas (25%), undetermined (20%)
    21% pancreatic islet tumor
    7% small cell carcinoma
    3% adrenal adenoma
Ectopic GH secretion (one case)[640]

GHRH, growth hormone–releasing hormone; GH, growth hormone.

(1) somatostatin is often also present in these tumors and is presumably cosecreted, minimizing stimulation of the somatotrope[646-648]; (2) the tumor mass and the efficiency of GHRH synthesis may be inadequate to produce circulating GHRH levels that stimulate pituitary GH secretion; and (3) symptoms of acromegaly may be mild, and the patient's life span may be too short for the condition to be detected clinically. With highly malignant tumors, death can occur before the condition is evident.

CLINICAL FEATURES (Table 9–23). Patients with acromegaly have a gradual progression of symptoms and signs so that the diagnosis is often delayed for as many as 15 to 20 y. The symptoms usually begin insidiously, and the changes occur so gradually as to go unnoticed until complications develop (Figs. 9–37 and 9–38). Manifestations may be caused by the pituitary tumor itself, hypopituitarism, or excessive GH secretion, or a combination.

The tumor mass may produce headaches or visual disturbances, including visual field defects or diplopia from ophthalmoplegia. Hypopituitarism can occur if the tumor is large; gonadal dysfunction is more common than hypothyroidism or adrenal insufficiency.

The most common manifestations are due to excessive secretion of GH. If the condition occurs before puberty, excessive linear growth results in gigantism, which causes a multitude of physical, medical, social, and personal problems (see also Chapter 30).

More commonly the condition occurs after puberty, resulting in acromegaly. Thickening and oiliness of the skin, particularly of the face, occur. Facial changes include thick lips, exaggerated nasolabial folds, and thickening and folding of the scalp (cutis verticis gyrata) that are visible on skull x-ray film or CT. Acanthosis nigricans may occur. The vocal cords thicken, which, in conjunction with sinus enlargement, results in a characteristically deep and resonant voice. The overall appearance and deep voice give acromegalic women a rather masculinized appearance, and mild hirsutism may be present. The hands and feet enlarge. Rings become tight, cannot be removed, and may have to be cut off. The increased hand and finger size may cause difficulty with performing fine tasks such as picking up pins; glove size also increases. The foot increases in both length and width. Head size increases because of increases in both soft tissue and skull mass. The calvarium of the skull thickens; hyperostosis frontalis and

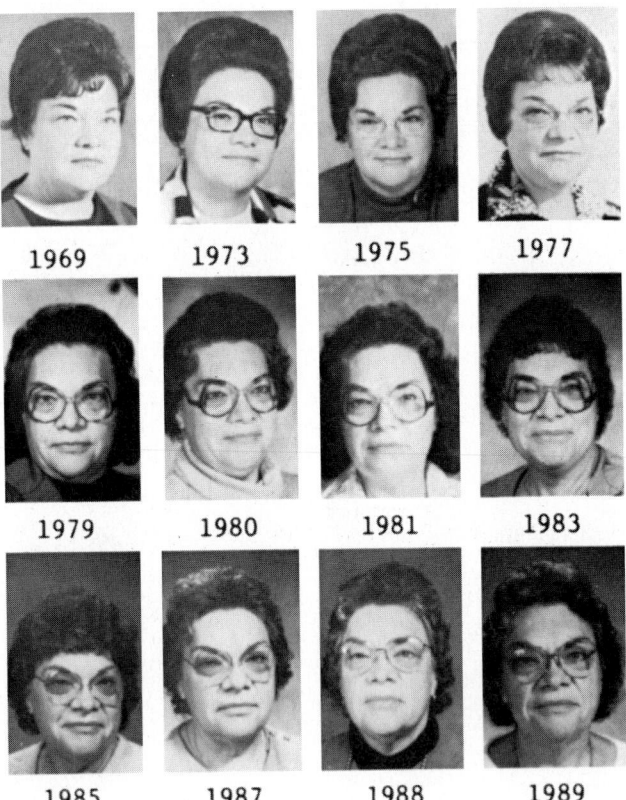

Figure 9–37. Photographs taken over 20 y of a woman with acromegaly from 1969 (age 41) through 1989 (age 61). Note progressive coarsening of facial features. Other characteristics of acromegaly included bilateral carpal tunnel syndrome (1973), hypertension (1975), arthralgias (1979), colonic polyps (1987), and diabetes mellitus (1988). (Unpublished observations, courtesy of ML Vance.)

expansion of the frontal sinuses cause protrusion of the brows (frontal bossing). The zygomatic arch enlarges to produce prominence of the cheek bones and relative hollowness of the temporal fossae. This feature is particularly evident after successful treatment when the soft tissues regress. Growth of the mandible in length and breadth leads to protrusion of the lower jaw, malocclusion, and development of temporomandibular arthritis. The changes in the lower jaw and the temporomandibular arthritis are sometimes the initial features leading to the diagnosis.

Joint pain from accelerated osteoarthrosis may be misdiagnosed as degenerative arthritis. The shafts of the metacarpals, metatarsals, and phalanges and of the articular cartilages thicken. Tufting of the terminal phalanges develops, and exostoses occur in the bones of the hands and feet. Arthralgias occur in 62 to 75% of acromegalic patients, and arthropathy is present in 16 to 62%. Between 10 and 40% of patients have joint symptoms severe enough to limit daily activities. The knees, hips (main weight-bearing joints), and shoulders are frequently affected; elbows and ankles are usually spared. The lumbosacral spine may be affected. The initial symptom is joint stiffness, particularly in the hands, which may reflect the increase of subcutaneous tissue that is reversible with reduction of circulating GH levels.

Early in the course of the disease joint spaces are increased secondary to cartilage proliferation. The synovial and periarticular swelling produces joint swelling without effusion. Weight bearing on proliferating cartilage in joints leads to ulceration, development of osteoarthritis, and irreversible cartilage degeneration[649, 650] that may be so disabling as to require artificial joint replacement. The arthropathy is often severe at the time of diagnosis, but if acromegaly is treated before the

TABLE 9–23. Clinical and Laboratory Findings in 57 Patients with Acromegaly

Finding	Present/Total
Recent acral growth	57/57
Arthralgias	41/57
Excessive sweating	52/57
Weakness	50/57
Malocclusion	39/57
New skin tags	33/57
Hypertension (blood pressure >150/95)	21/57
Carpal tunnel syndrome	25/57
Fasting blood glucose >6 mmol/L	17/57
Abnormal glucose tolerance test (blood glucose >6.1 mmol/L [>110 mg/dL])	39/57
Heel pad thickness >22 mm	48/53
Serum prolactin >25 µg/L	8/51
Serum phosphorus >1.5 mmol/L (>4.5 mg/dL)	26/54
Sella volume >1300 mm³	55/57
Serum T₄ <53 nmol/L (<4.1 µg/dL)	0/57*
Serum testosterone (men) <10 nmol/L (<3 ng/mL)	7/30
8 AM serum cortisol <200 nmol/L (<8 µg/dL)	2/57

*Eleven patients were receiving T₄ replacement at the time of the study.
From Clemmons DR, Van Wyk JJ, Ridgway EC, et al. Evaluation of acromegaly by radioimmunoassay of somatomedin-C. Reprinted, by permission of The New England Journal of Medicine, 301; 1138–1142, 1979.

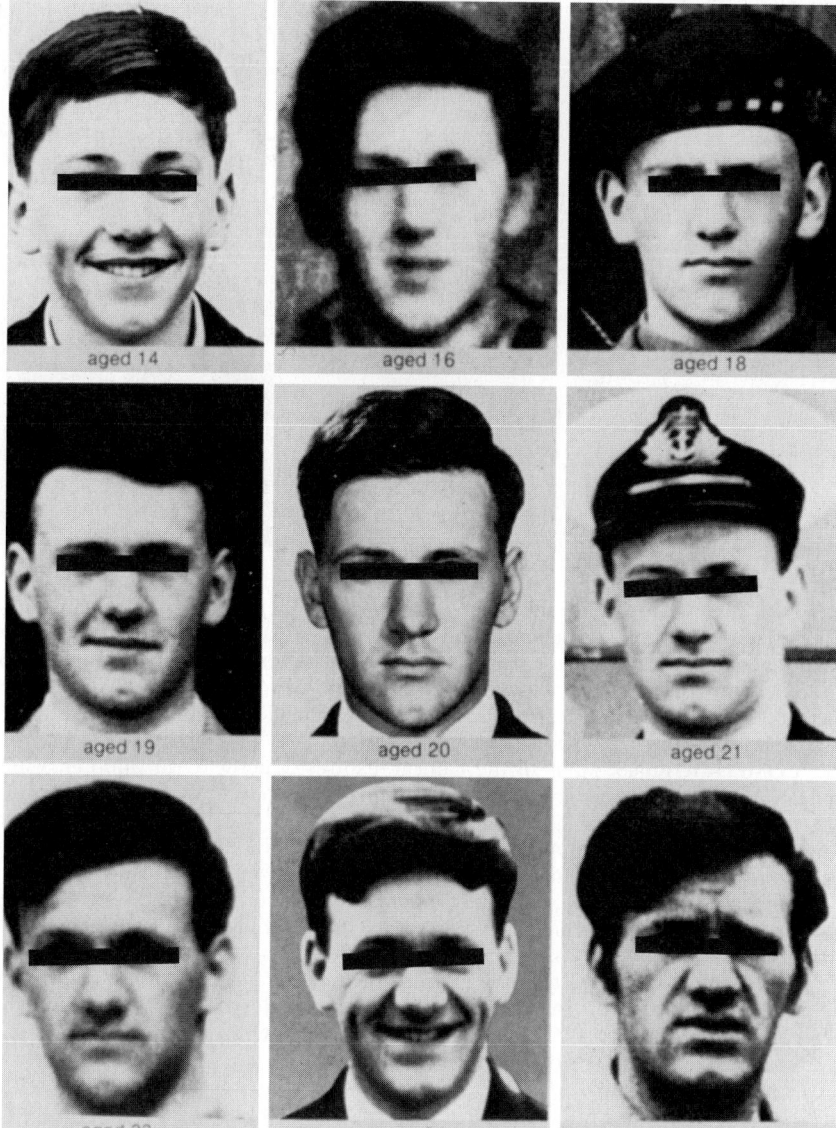

Figure 9–38. Change in facial appearance of a patient with acromegaly over a 13-y period. The development of an acromegalic appearance is seen with enlargement of the supraorbital ridges and nose, thickening of the lips, and generalized coarsening of the features. (From Wass JAH. Acromegaly. In: Besser GM, Cudworth AG, eds. Clinical Endocrinology: An Illustrated Text. London: Gower Medical, 1987: 3.1–3.12.)

articular cartilage is destroyed, joint symptoms are reversible.[651, 652]

Backache is associated with dorsal kyphosis. Disc spaces are increased, and anterior osteophytes are common. Spinal mobility is normal or increased because the discs are resilient, and paraspinal ligaments become hypertrophied and lax.[649, 650]

Patients with acromegaly often acquire a characteristic barrel chest caused by changes in the vertebrae and the ribs. The vertebral bodies become elongated and widened by periosteal apposition of bone along the anterior and lateral surfaces. The intervertebral discs in the cervical and lumbar region thicken, and discs in the thoracic area become thin, resulting in development of kyphosis.[653] Because the epiphyses of the osteochondral junctions fail to close, the ribs elongate to cause an increase in the anteroposterior diameter of the chest.[654] Thus rib elongation and the thoracic kyphosis contribute to the development of a barrel chest.

Excessive GH secretion is associated with excessive sweating, particularly of the face, head, hands, and feet; sweating may be a presenting symptom. The increase in soft tissue mass can compress median nerves and cause carpal tunnel syndrome, and this possibility should be considered in patients with newly diagnosed carpal tunnel syndrome.

Galactorrhea is common in acromegalic women but is rare in men. Hyperprolactinemia may be present in up to 40% of acromegalic patients, but galactorrhea can occur in the absence of hyperprolactinemia, possibly as a result of the lactogenic effects of GH.[655] Between 32 and 87% of acromegalic women younger than age 45 have menstrual abnormalities, and decreased libido and impotence occur in 27 to 46% of men.[656] Gonadal dysfunction can be due to hyperprolactinemia or to the lactogenic effects of GH. Hyperprolactinemic women should also undergo serum IGF-I measurement to exclude cosecretion of GH because early acromegaly may not be clinically evident.

Physical examination demonstrates the typical facial appearance with soft tissue thickening, greasiness of the skin, coarse features, increased breadth of the nose, thickening of the lips, macroglossia, and prognathism. The growth of the lower jaw may produce widened spaces between the teeth. In women mild hirsutism may be present. The hands are usually spade-like with sausage-shaped fingers (Fig. 9–39), thenar wasting, weakness of thumb abduction, and loss of pinprick sensation in the distribution of the median nerve. The chest may be kyphotic. Organomegaly may include thyroid gland enlargement and palpable thyroid nodules. The skinfold thickness is increased and the skin, particularly the palms of the hands and soles of the feet, is moist. Multiple skin tags corre-

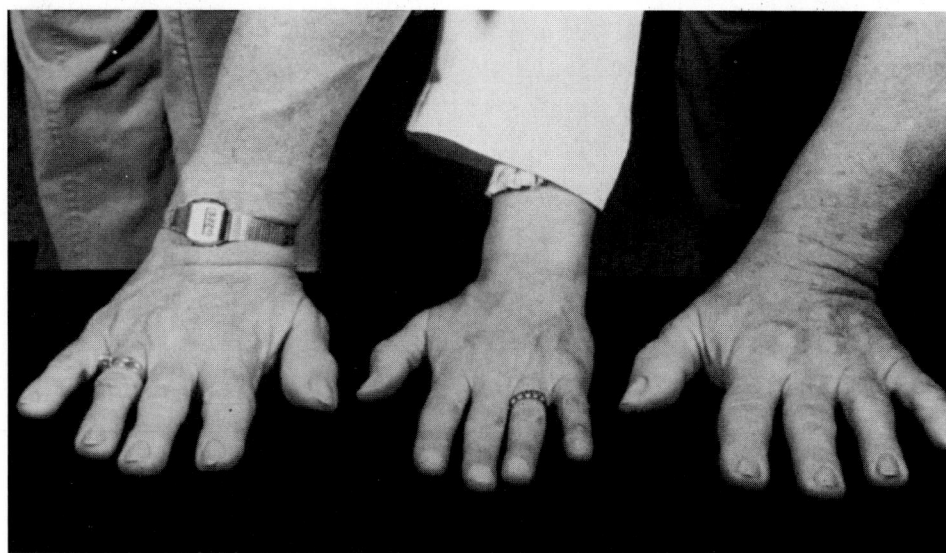

Figure 9–39. Hands of a 49-year-old acromegalic woman *(right* and *left)* compared with the hand of a normal woman *(middle).* (Unpublished observations, courtesy of ML Vance.)

late with the occurrence of colonic polyps. The testes may be enlarged. There are often signs of arthritis, particularly in the knees and hips. The feet have soft tissue thickening and an increase in the heel pad thickness. The relative frequencies of these clinical findings are shown in Table 9–23.

COMPLICATIONS. Many of the clinical features of acromegaly are a result of the effects of long-standing overproduction of GH.

Metabolic and Endocrine. Hypersecretion of GH induces insulin resistance and glucose intolerance in 29 to 45% of acromegalic patients and overt diabetes mellitus in 10 to 20%.[656] In nondiabetic acromegalic patients excessive GH secretion is associated with an exaggerated insulin response to intravenous glucose. In those with impaired glucose tolerance or diabetes mellitus, the insulin response is inadequate to overcome the insulin resistance. The human leukocyte antigen (HLA) phenotype, family history of diabetes mellitus, and duration of acromegaly do not appear to be major risks for the development of overt diabetes mellitus in these patients.[657]

Hypertriglyceridemia occurs in 19 to 44% of acromegalic patients.[658, 659] There is a positive correlation between the serum insulin response to glucose and increased serum triglyceride concentrations. Hepatic triglyceride lipase and lipoprotein lipase activities are decreased in acromegaly. After successful lowering of GH levels, the activities of these enzymes rise. No consistent abnormalities of cholesterol have been observed.

Respiratory. Pulmonary complications account for some of the increased mortality. A threefold increase in respiratory deaths occurred in the study reported by Wright and colleagues.[660] Pulmonary function tests are abnormal in both men and women; total lung capacity is increased in 81% of men and 56% of women, 36% have small airway narrowing, and 26% have upper airway narrowing.[661, 662] It is likely that airway narrowing and possibly sleep apnea account for the increased morbidity and mortality of the disease. Airway obstruction caused by exacerbation of upper airway narrowing during upper respiratory tract infections may cause acute dyspnea and stridor. Intubation may be difficult during induction of anesthesia, and the airway may be obstructed by an enlarged tongue after extubation. The risks of anesthesia can be minimized by proper preparation, use of fiberoptic laryngoscopy, and careful monitoring.

Many acromegalic patients have the obstructive sleep apnea syndrome. Symptoms include excessive daytime sleepiness, habitual snoring, and apneic episodes during sleep; the syndrome is diagnosed by polysomnography studies during sleep because pulmonary function tests when the person is awake are not helpful. Sleep apnea is said to be present if more than 5 apneic episodes occur per hour of sleep or more than 30 apneic episodes occur during the night. The prevalence of obstructive sleep apnea was 38% in one study and was 81% in another, with men being more commonly affected than women.[663–666] Both the prolapse of an enlarged tongue and the inspiratory collapse of the hypopharynx have been implicated in the pathogenesis of this disorder.[667, 668] Cure of acromegaly does not necessarily correct the sleep apnea.[665, 668] In short-term studies of somatostatin analogue therapy (6 d) or bromocriptine therapy (3 mo), 41 and 75% fewer apneic episodes occurred, respectively.[669, 670]

Cardiovascular. The cardiovascular complications of acromegaly include hypertension and cardiomyopathy. The precise nature of acromegalic heart disease is not clear, but cardiovascular disease is the most common cause of death in acromegalic patients.[635, 660] The coexistence of hypertension and diabetes mellitus makes it difficult to determine whether the cardiac disease is secondary to these disorders or directly related to GH excess; indeed there is controversy whether a specific acromegalic cardiomyopathy exists. The problem is exemplified by the results of a prospective study; 9 of 57 patients had heart disease, but in 7 of the 9 individuals hypertension, coronary heart disease, or hypothyroidism was also present.[671] Of 256 patients studied retrospectively, 10 had heart disease without evidence of hypertension, diabetes mellitus, thyroid disease, or coronary or valvular heart disease.[672] No specific pathologic findings have been demonstrated at autopsy.[673] Myocardial hypertrophy occurred in 93%, interstitial fibrosis in 85%, and lymphomononuclear myocarditis in 59% of 27 cases. However in approximately 80% of acromegalic patients, cardiac enlargement, usually an increase of left ventricular mass, can be detected by echocardiography and is independent of hypertension or ischemic heart disease.[674–678] Left ventricular function is impaired in some patients. Although the severity of these abnormalities does not consistently correlate with GH levels, the duration of the disease may be an important determinant.[676–678] Increases in left ventricular mass, end-systolic wall stress (afterload), and fractional shortening and decreased cardiac index were present in 12 acromegalic patients (39 ± 5 y of age) with a relatively short duration of disease (6 ± 3 y). These patients did not have hypertension or overt cardiac disease.

Expanded blood volume and increased peripheral blood flow may lead to left ventricular hypertrophy and a hyperkinetic left ventricle. With prolonged disease hypertension develops, and left ventricular function declines. Cardiac abnormalities may persist in some patients after restoration of normal GH levels; in others restoration of normal GH levels is associated with significant improvement. A specific acromegalic cardiomyopathy is unproved.

Hypertension of the low renin type occurs in 18 to 41% of acromegalic patients.[656, 671, 673, 679–682] Sodium retention, extracellular fluid volume expansion, and suppression of renin-angiotensin-aldosterone secretion occur in both hypertensive and normotensive acromegalic patients. Overactivity of the sympathetic nervous system may be involved.[683] Hypertension is associated with higher mean GH concentrations and longer duration of acromegaly; it is usually mild and uncomplicated and responds to conventional antihypertensive medications. Rarely hypertension may result from other endocrine causes, such as pheochromocytoma,[684] primary hyperparathyroidism, or an aldosterone-secreting adenoma.[685]

Calcium and Bone Metabolism. Serum 1,25-dihydroxycholecalciferol (1,25-$(OH)_2$D) levels are increased in acromegaly, 25-hydroxycholecalciferol (25-OHD) levels are low, and serum parathyroid hormone and calcitonin levels are normal. The increase in 1,25-$(OH)_2$D concentrations is a result of GH stimulation of renal 1α-hydroxylase activity. The consequence is an increase in intestinal calcium absorption and hypercalciuria; serum calcium levels are normal unless coincidental hyperparathyroidism is present. GH increases tubular phosphate reabsorption and causes hyperphosphatemia in approximately half of patients. The metabolic consequences are reversed with lowering of serum GH levels to normal. Urolithiasis occurs in 6 to 12.5% of patients. Acromegaly is associated with increased bone turnover and increased bone density; osteoporosis does not occur unless hypogonadism is also present.[686–688]

Neuromuscular. Although acromegalic patients have a muscular appearance, they are usually weak, possibly because of myopathy.[689–691] The bony changes of the vertebral column may cause nerve root compression at the vertebral foramina and lumbar radiculopathy. Spinal stenosis and a syndrome resembling amyotrophic lateral sclerosis may occur.[692, 693] Carpal tunnel syndrome was present in 35% of one series[694] and 43% of another.[695]

Colonic Polyps and Malignancies. The increased prevalence of colonic polyps in acromegalic patients raised the concern that these patients may be at increased risk for the development of colon cancer, and 4 of 44 acromegalic patients developed colon cancer in one study.[696] Two other studies also suggest an increased incidence of gastrointestinal malignancies in acromegaly. In one series 3 of 12 patients had colon cancer[697] and in another study 2 of 48 acromegalic patients had carcinoma of the stomach and 3 had colon cancer.[698] The increased prevalence of colon polyps has been confirmed in large studies as ranging from 22 to 65%.[699, 700] It is of note that acromegalic patients appear to develop polyps at a younger age than does the control population (50 vs. 59 y, respectively)[699] and have a higher risk of colon cancer if there is a family history of colon cancer.[701] In a prospective study by a single endoscopist, 129 patients with biochemically proven acromegaly were evaluated to determine the prevalence of colorectal carcinoma, premalignant tubulovillous adenomas, and hyperplastic colonic polyps.[702] At least one lesion was visualized in 63 patients and adenocarcinoma was present in 6 patients (5%). Compared with a normal group the odds ratio of colorectal cancer is increased at 13.5 (95% confidence interval, 3.1 to 75). One or more tubulovillous adenomas were found in 34 patients (26%), occurring in 39% of patients 70 y or older. Acromegalic patients with a tubulovillous adenoma were older than unaffected patients (61.9 y vs. 54.1 y, *P* <0.001). However a survey of mortality in acromegaly (194

patients) did not reveal an increased mortality from malignant neoplasms[660]; similar mortality rates have been reported in other studies of malignant disease in acromegalic patients.[703, 704]

PROGNOSIS. In retrospective reviews, acromegalic patients have a risk of premature mortality, usually from cardiovascular and pulmonary causes. In one study of 151 patients treated with various regimens, survival was reduced an average of 10 y compared with the general population.[705] However lowering the serum GH concentrations appears to reduce the risk of premature mortality. In a retrospective study of 79 acromegalic patients treated with various regimens, patients who achieved an average daytime GH level (mean of five values over the day) of less than 2.5 μg/L had a survival equal to that of the general population.[706] Reversal of the adverse metabolic effects of excessive GH secretion prevents progression of the manifestations and leads to some regression, as indicated by reduced soft tissue swelling, diminished sweating, and restoration of normal glucose tolerance. Increased awareness of the early symptoms and signs of acromegaly, ease of diagnosis, ability to determine the correct cause, results of modern transsphenoidal pituitary microsurgery (which demonstrate that the smaller the tumor at the time of operation, the better the outcome), and results of radiotherapy and medical therapy all suggest that patients with acromegaly are more likely to be cured today than in the past.

BIOCHEMICAL EVALUATION. The clinical diagnosis of acromegaly is confirmed by biochemical tests that should be performed before imaging studies are undertaken.

Growth Hormone Secretion in Acromegaly. Serum GH concentrations are elevated but fluctuate widely in acromegaly.[707, 708] Frequent venous sampling over 24 h (every 5 or 20 min) and use of objective pulse detection algorithms make it possible to characterize GH release (Fig. 9–40).[27, 709] Acromegalic patients may have a 10- to 15-fold increase in 24-h integrated GH concentrations. The number of discrete GH pulses over 24 h is 2- to 3-fold higher than in normal individuals, and basal GH concentrations are increased 16- to 20-fold

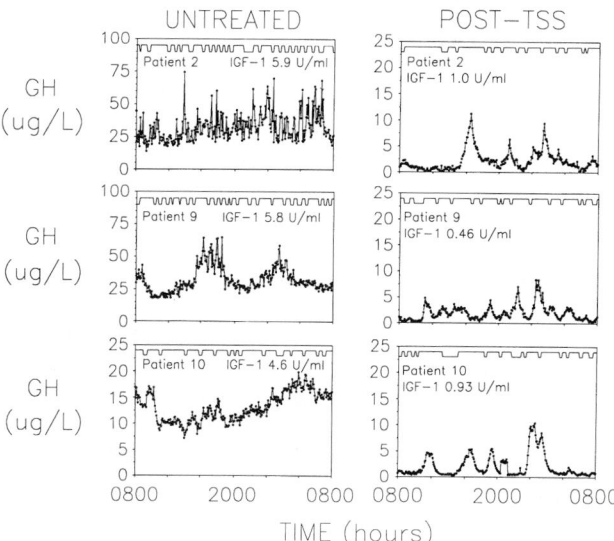

Figure 9–40. Serum GH concentration profiles (24 h) of three acromegalic patients before and after transsphenoidal surgery that induced biochemical and clinical remission. Samples were measured every 5 min over 24 h. The continuous schematized line in the upper portion of each panel defines the individually significant GH pulses detected by cluster analysis. Different scales are used for the vertical axes because of the wide range of serum GH concentrations. After surgery the serum GH concentrations were reduced, and the pattern of GH release closely resembled that of normal young individuals. (From ML Hartman, JD Veldhuis, ML Vance, et al., Somatotropin pulse frequency and basal concentrations are increased in acromegaly and are reduced by successful therapy. J Clin Endocrinol Metab, 70, 1375–1384, 1990, © by The Endocrine Society.)

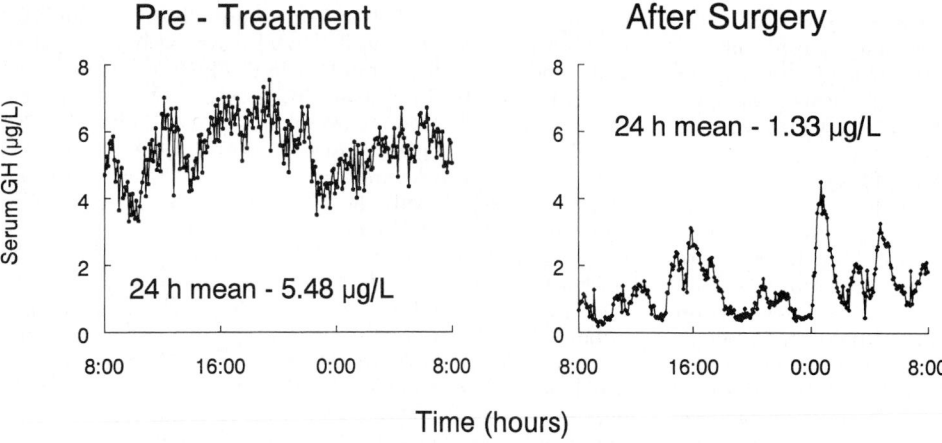

Figure 9–41. Profiles of serum GH concentrations in a 62-year-old acromegalic woman, measured in samples collected at 5-min intervals over 24 h before *(left panel)* and after *(right panel)* transsphenoidal tumor resection. Serum GH was measured by IRMA, with an assay sensitivity of 0.2 μg/L. Although the mean 24-h GH level before surgery of 5.48 μg/L is observed in normal young women (<30 y), in the patient all GH values are detectable and there is loss of intermittent GH pulses. After surgery the mean GH concentration is normal for age and the pulsatile GH pattern is near normal. IRMA, immunoradiometric assay.

above normal. There is an associated attenuation of the underlying 24-h rhythm, which may be secondary to the intrinsic pathologic characteristics of adenomatous somatotropes or effects of altered hypothalamic regulation, or both. With biochemical remission after therapy, acromegalic patients have resumption of normal GH profiles. A less common pattern is the patient with clinical acromegaly in whom measurement of GH (every 5 min for 24 h) demonstrates that although the 24-h mean GH level is similar to that observed in normal young adults, the GH pattern is abnormal. In contrast to normal individuals who have many undetectable values, acromegalic patients have detectable GH levels throughout 24 h using a sensitive IRMA. Figure 9–41 demonstrates this; before treatment GH is secreted continuously; after surgery, the 24-h GH secretory pattern approximates normal (serum IGF-I was normal after surgery). When GH is measured by an ultrasensitive assay with a sensitivity of 0.002 μg/L, all values are detectable, but again the pattern is abnormal. Figure 9–42 shows the 24-h GH profile in a 63-year-old acromegalic woman and a 68-year-old normal woman.

A single random serum GH measurement may not be helpful for diagnosing or excluding acromegaly because a "normal" value may be a nadir level in an acromegalic patient; conversely a "high" value may be a peak value in a normal individual. Measurement of GH levels every 5 or 10 min over 24 h is possible only in a research setting. However the diagnosis of acromegaly can be made readily in an outpatient setting with two biochemical tests and reliable assays.

Serum Insulin-Like Growth Factor I Concentration. The serum IGF-I level is the best screening test for acromegaly; an elevated value suggests excessive GH secretion except during pregnancy or puberty, when IGF-I levels are normally increased. Serum IGF-I levels reflect overall GH secretion during the previous 24 h, vary minimally during the day, and provide a reliable indicator of GH secretion. In studies correlating the serum IGF-I concentration with the clinical activity of acromegaly and fasting GH level, some investigators report excellent correlation,[695, 710, 711] whereas others do not.[712, 713] The circulating IGF-I level does, however, correlate with the 24-h integrated serum GH level when GH is measured at frequent intervals (every 5 or 20 min).[27, 709] IGF-I assays are variable in reliability because of problems related to IGF-I binding to serum IGF-I–binding proteins. Proper interpretation of the values requires knowledge of details of the assay, such as whether the serum is pretreated to remove the binding proteins. The predominant IGF-I binding protein is positively regulated by GH (see Chapter 30). The normal range for serum IGF-I varies with age and sex and declines with age (as does GH). Thus it is important to know normal ranges for age and sex for the laboratory. Serum IGF-I concentration should be assessed as an initial screen, as an index of disease activity, and to indicate efficacy of therapy.

Oral Glucose Tolerance Test. The definitive test result for the diagnosis of acromegaly is a failure of serum GH level to decrease to less than 1 μg/L, using the IRMA method, after ingestion of glucose.[155] With the ultrasensitive GH assay (sensitivity 0.002 μg/L), GH declines to less than 0.71 μg/L in normal women and to less than 0.06 μg/L in normal men.[468] The older criterion for a normal GH response to oral glucose, using the RIA method, of a GH level less than 2 μg/L[707, 708, 714–716] has been supplanted by the use of more precise assays.

In acromegaly the serum GH level may decrease partially, remain unchanged, or increase paradoxically after glucose ingestion. The dose of oral glucose ranges from 50 to 100 g; in normal individuals the serum GH level, measured by the old RIA method, decreases to less than 2 μg/L with as little as 50 g.[707, 708, 714–716] The oral glucose test should be performed after an overnight fast. In the morning a heparin-lock cannula is placed in a forearm vein for blood sampling; 1 h later a −30-min sample is obtained, followed 30 min later by a 0-min sample, at which time the patient drinks a flavored iced drink containing 75 or 100 g of glucose. Blood samples are obtained through the cannula 30, 60, 90, and 120 min after glucose ingestion, and serum GH, plasma glucose and, if indicated,

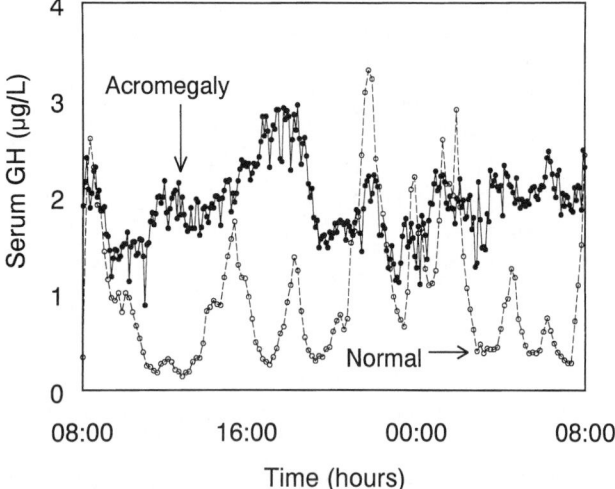

Figure 9–42. Profiles of serum GH concentrations in a 63-year-old woman with acromegaly *(closed circles)* and a 68-year-old normal woman *(open circles),* measured in samples collected at 5-min intervals over 24 h. Serum GH was measured in a chemiluminescence assay, with a sensitivity of 0.002 μg/L. GH was detectable in all samples in both individuals. Note the high basal GH concentrations and the loss of a pulsatile GH pattern in the acromegalic patient.

serum insulin levels are measured.[708] In patients with acromegaly the serum GH level does not decrease to normal levels.

Other tests have been proposed for the diagnosis of acromegaly, including administration of TRH, LHRH, levodopa, and other dopamine agonists.[717-721] These compounds produce different (paradoxical) effects in acromegalic patients than in normal individuals. In the latter, GH concentrations are unaffected by TRH or LHRH, whereas GH secretion in many acromegalic patients is stimulated by these agents. These responses are not as uniform as is the blunted response to oral glucose and therefore are not routinely used. Levodopa and dopamine agonists stimulate GH secretion in normal individuals; GH secretion is acutely inhibited by these agents in 50 to 70% of acromegalic patients.[721, 722]

Administration of the two physiological hypothalamic regulators of GH secretion, somatostatin and GHRH, does not discriminate between normal and excessive GH secretion. Both normal individuals and patients with acromegaly have an increase in GH concentrations after GHRH administration and a decrease in GH release during somatostatin infusion.[716, 723]

Insulin-induced hypoglycemia is used in acromegalic patients to evaluate the hypothalamic-pituitary-adrenal axis.[466, 467] Patients with acromegaly exhibit insulin resistance and frequently require higher doses of insulin injection to decrease the blood glucose level to less than 2.2 mmol/L (40 mg/dL). Until the degree of insulin resistance is known, however, the usual intravenous dose of regular insulin, 0.15 U/kg body weight, is administered. If there is insufficient reduction in serum glucose or absence of hypoglycemic symptoms within 45 min, a second dose of insulin, 0.3 U/kg body weight, is administered. If after another 45 min the response is inadequate, the dose is again increased, to 0.6 U/kg body weight. Results are interpretable when the blood glucose level has decreased to less than 2.2 mmol/L (40 mg/dL), which is associated with hypoglycemic symptoms such as tachycardia, palpitations, diaphoresis, somnolence, or hunger. The plasma cortisol level should increase to greater than 580 nmol/L (20 μg/dL); serum GH levels also increase, even in acromegalic patients, to greater than 10 μg/L.

The differential diagnosis of acromegaly includes a primary pituitary adenoma, either a microadenoma or a macroadenoma, and GH hypersecretion from a hyperplastic pituitary gland that is hyperstimulated by eutopic (hypothalamic tumor) or ectopic (peripheral tumor) GHRH.[102, 639, 724, 725] There is one documented case of acromegaly associated with ectopic GH secretion from a pancreatic tumor.[640] More than 99% of acromegalic patients have a primary pituitary tumor, but it is important to make the correct diagnosis because initial therapy should be directed to the primary lesion. Unfortunately imaging studies cannot distinguish between an enlarged pituitary with an adenoma and an enlarged hyperplastic gland.[102, 726] To date no patient with hypothalamic acromegaly associated with a GHRH-secreting hypothalamic tumor has been diagnosed prior to surgery or postmortem examination, but patients with presumed pituitary adenomas have been retrospectively recognized as having extension into the pituitary of hypothalamic gangliocytoma neurons that produce surrounding somatotrope hyperplasia.[639] A mass lesion in the hypothalamus in association with acromegaly presumptively suggests eutopic GHRH secretion by a hypothalamic tumor as indicated by pathologic studies.[639] A "hypothalamic hamartoma" secondarily producing acromegaly can exist as an intrasellar lesion primarily involving the region of the neurohypophysis. Ectopic GHRH secretion is more common than eutopic secretion, but few cases of ectopic GHRH production have been diagnosed prospectively.[727] Ectopic GHRH secretion should be suspected in a patient with acromegaly and elevated circulating GHRH levels.[638, 727, 728] Plasma GHRH

levels in normal individuals are less than 100 ng/L; in contrast patients with acromegaly from ectopic GHRH secretion have plasma GHRH levels of micrograms per liter. If a patient has an elevated GHRH level, a peripheral or hypothalamic tumor should be sought; however since GHRH can be secreted even by tumors in a pulsatile fashion, a modestly elevated GHRH level may not exclude ectopic GHRH secretion. The most likely peripheral sites are the pancreas, lung, thymus, adrenal (in association with pheochromocytoma), or gastrointestinal tract. A whole body CT or MRI scan should be obtained, and single-photon emission computed tomography (SPECT) octreotide scanning should be considered. Occasionally no ectopic source is found.[728]

PATHOLOGIC FEATURES. Histologic, immunocytochemical, and ultrastructural investigations have revealed a variety of findings in patients with acromegaly or gigantism:[449, 725, 729, 730] (1) densely granulated somatotrope adenoma; (2) sparsely granulated somatotrope adenoma; (3) mixed somatotrope-lactotrope adenoma; (4) acidophilic stem cell adenoma; (5) mammosomatotrope adenoma; (6) plurihormonal adenoma producing GH and one or more glycoprotein hormones, principally α subunit; (7) somatotrope carcinoma; (8) somatotrope hyperplasia; and (9) no distinct morphologic change. Densely granulated somatotrope adenomas and sparsely granulated somatotrope adenomas are the most common tumors in patients with acromegaly; bihormonal somatotrope-lactotrope adenomas and mammosomatotrope adenomas usually occur in younger individuals with acromegaly or gigantism.

Densely granulated somatotrope adenomas are acidophilic, PAS-negative tumors that contain immunoreactive GH. Sparsely granulated somatotrope adenomas are chromophobic on hematoxylin and eosin staining, exhibit no PAS positivity, and are GH immunopositive. Densely granulated somatotrope adenomas are composed of well-differentiated cells that resemble normal somatotropes and contain numerous spherical or ovoid, homogeneous, electron-dense secretory granules 150 to 600 nm in diameter (Fig. 9–43).[449, 725, 729-733]

Cells of sparsely granulated somatotrope adenomas are different from normal somatotropes and contain a few randomly distributed secretory granules up to 250 nm in diameter.[449, 730-732, 734, 735] Sparsely granulated somatotrope adenomas often contain fibrous bodies or cytoplasmic filamentous aggregates (Fig. 9–44) consisting of keratin-positive intermediate filaments, mitochondria, centrioles, and secretory granules. The genesis and functional significance of these fibrous bodies, most often located adjacent to the concave nucleus, are unclear.

Densely granulated somatotrope adenomas and sparsely granulated somatotrope adenomas produce similar clinical and biochemical alterations. Endocrine amyloid may occur in both variants.[545, 736, 737] However the tumors differ in biologic behavior, emphasizing the importance of precise pathologic identification. The sparsely granulated tumors occur in somewhat younger individuals, grow faster, are usually larger and more difficult to remove, and recur more often.

Mixed somatotrope-lactotrope adenomas[738] are bihormonal tumors that produce both GH and prolactin[738, 739] and contain two separate cell types that resemble somatotropes and lactotropes, respectively. Hematoxylin and eosin–stained sections are either acidophilic or chromophobic or contain an admixture of acidophilic and chromophobic cells. Electron microscopy reveals densely granulated or sparsely granulated somatotropes and lactotropes (Fig. 9–45).[738, 739] Although these tumors contain two principal cell types, bihormonal cells that contain both GH and prolactin may also be present.[740-743]

Acidophilic stem cell adenomas are chromophobic or slightly acidophilic tumors with no PAS positivity.[452] Patients rarely exhibit features of acromegaly. The usual finding is

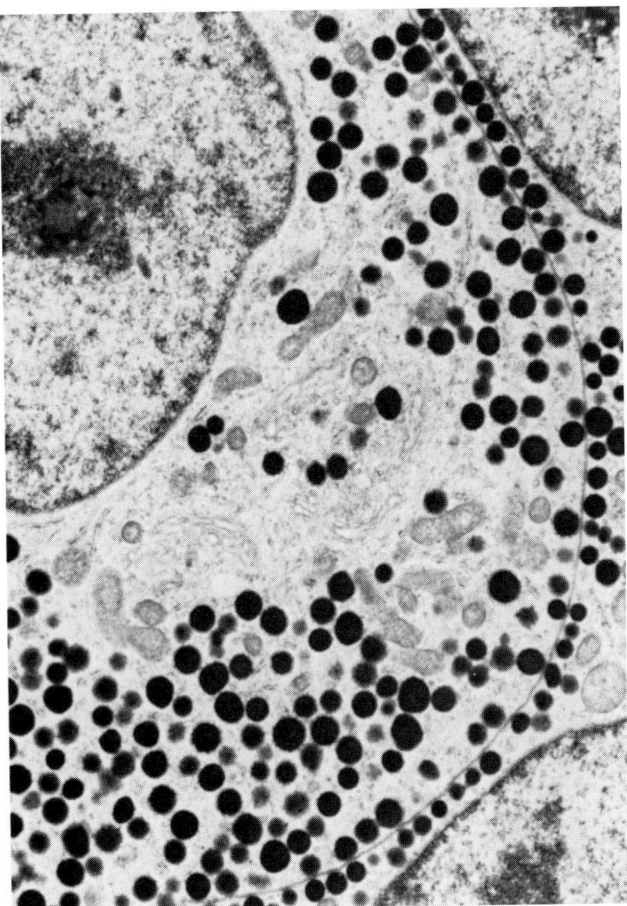

Figure 9–43. Densely granulated GH cell adenoma with well-developed membranous organelles and numerous large secretory granules. Magnification × 12,700.

results obtained by light microscopic immunocytochemistry, electron microscopy, and immunoelectron microscopy are not always in agreement. The origin of these tumors is not clear. They may arise from a precursor cell that undergoes multidirectional differentiation so that it is capable of producing several hormones or from plurihormonal clones that are normally present in the pituitary.

Only a few cases of somatotrope carcinomas have been documented,[749, 750] but some somatotrope adenomas are pleomorphic, contain multiple mitotic figures, are invasive, and have a high growth rate. These tumors are pleomorphic or invasive adenomas and not carcinomas and do not metastasize. The rare somatotrope carcinomas may be acidophilic or chromophobic, and the cells are pleomorphic and contain GH seen by immunocytochemistry. Somatotrope carcinomas usually have a high index of cell proliferation and are immunopositive for the tumor antigen p53. Sites of distant metastases include lymph nodes, liver, brain, heart, and bones.

Somatotrope hyperplasia is rare.[102, 638, 751] The number of somatotropes is normally constant in the pituitary, and somatotrope hyperplasia results from excessive GHRH secretion by extrapituitary tumors, including pancreatic endocrine (islet cell) tumor; pheochromocytoma; bronchial, thymic, and intestinal carcinoids; medullary carcinoma of the thyroid; small cell carcinoma of the lung; and hypothalamic gangliocytoma. In some cases GHRH immunopositivity of the peripheral tumor cells is not associated with increased serum levels of GHRH, GH, and IGF-I, but when large quantities of GHRH are released from the tumors, stimulation of pituitary somato-

hyperprolactinemia of various degrees; serum GH levels may be elevated or within the normal range. This tumor consists of one cell type that produces both GH and prolactin and is assumed to originate in the common precursor cell of somatotropes and lactotropes. The tumors usually occur in younger individuals and grow faster than other tumors of this lineage. By electron microscopy the tumor cells have features of both somatotropes and lactotropes, including fibrous bodies and misplaced exocytosis of secretory granules (Fig. 9–46).

Mammosomatotrope adenomas[453] cause acromegaly and varying degrees of hyperprolactinemia. The tumors are acidophilic, PAS-negative tumors in which the same cells are immunoreactive for both GH and prolactin.[744] By electron microscopy the densely granulated tumor cells are well differentiated and contain numerous large secretory granules, some of which are engaged in misplaced exocytosis (Fig. 9–47). The tumors grow slowly and occur more commonly than was previously thought.

Plurihormonal adenomas produce GH and one or more glycoprotein hormones, primarily α subunit.[450, 454, 745–748] Patients have acromegaly, and serum α subunit levels may also be elevated. Hyperthyroidism occurs rarely in association with increased levels of serum thyroid hormone and inappropriately elevated serum thyrotropin levels. Histologically the tumors usually contain one acidophilic cell type, but on occasion more than one cell type may be present. Immunocytochemistry demonstrates the presence of cells producing GH and α subunit, thyrotropin, prolactin, and rarely FSH or LH, or both. Bimorphous tumors contain densely granulated somatotropes and cells that produce glycoprotein hormone. The

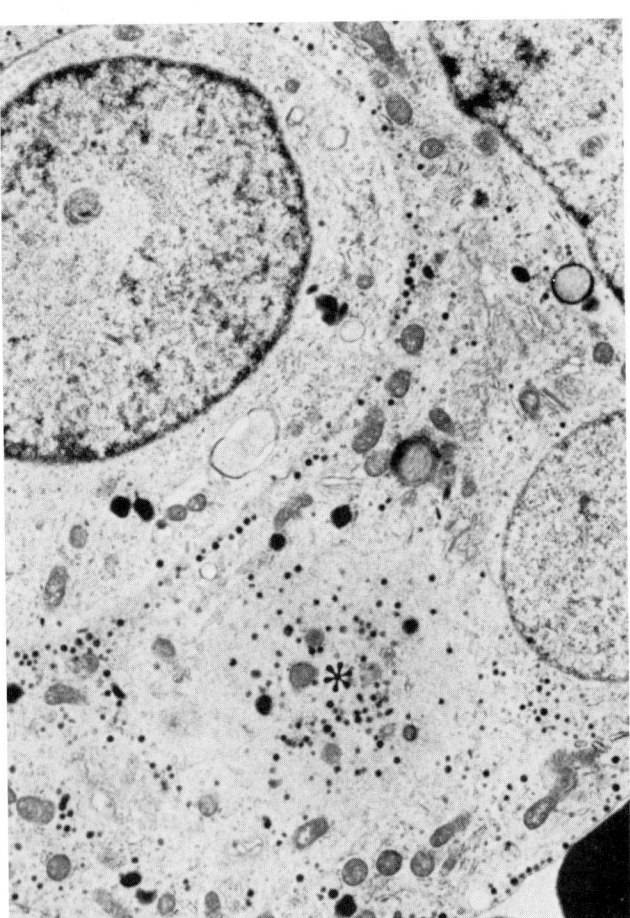

Figure 9–44. Typical features of a sparsely granulated GH cell adenoma. Note the small (< 200 nm), scant secretory granules and the fibrous body (asterisk) trapping secretory granules, mitochondria, and a few lysosomes. Magnification × 12,150.

tropes causes GH hypersecretion and acromegaly or gigantism. Somatotrope hyperplasia can cause pituitary enlargement as assessed by various imaging techniques. Whether hyperplasia can transform into adenoma is not known. Although theoretically adenoma is distinguishable from hyperplasia, practically there are often difficulties in making the distinction because the pathologist receives only small fragments of surgically removed tissue. Furthermore the pathologist is often not informed as to the location of the biopsy site in relation to the tumor and the normal gland. However in some cases hyperplasia is indistinguishable from adenoma. It is not clear whether there is a histologic continuum or whether protracted chronic stimulation results in neoplastic growth. According to the multistep theory of tumorigenesis, protracted GHRH stimulation promotes but does not initiate tumor growth. Alternatively hyperplastic somatotropes are more prone to undergo neoplastic transformation.

In a few patients with acromegaly no morphologic changes were identified in the pituitary,[752] but immunohistochemistry and electron microscopy were not performed. The diagnosis of a normal pituitary is acceptable only if the entire pituitary is studied by serial section. More cases must be studied by modern morphologic methods before definite conclusions can be drawn.

Tumor recurrence after surgery depends on whether tumor tissue was left behind during surgery. Somatotrope adenomas are practically never associated with somatotrope hyperplasia (except in cases of GHRH-producing extrapituitary tumors), and the theory that new tumors develop from proliferating hyperplastic cells after surgery is not tenable.

Morphologic changes after radiotherapy include vascular

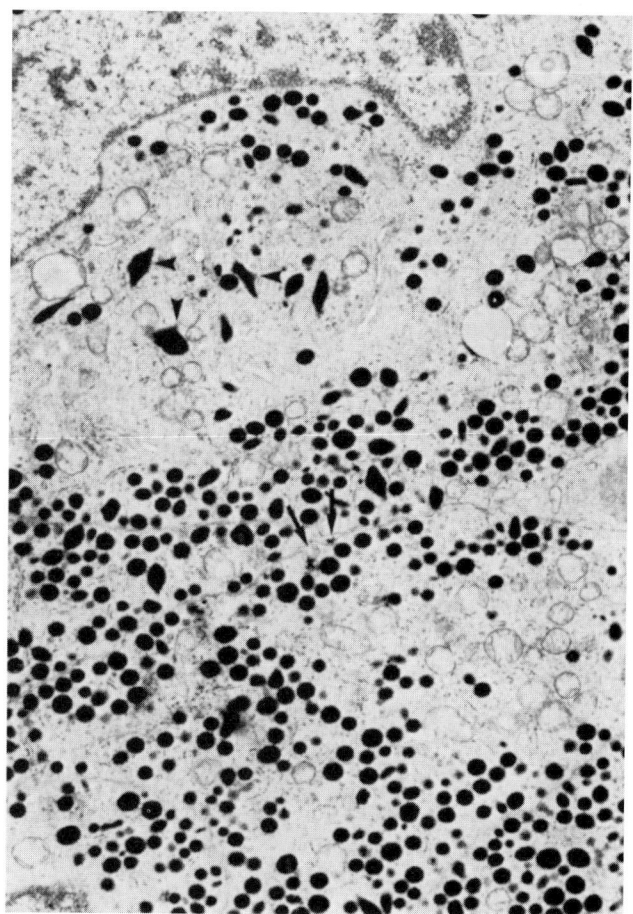

Figure 9–46. The appearance of this mammosomatotrope adenoma is similar to that of densely granulated GH cell adenomas with the added feature of granule extrusions *(arrows)*. Note the geometrically shaped secretory granules seen chiefly in the Golgi area *(arrowhead)*, which sometimes occur in GH-producing adenomas. Magnification × 11,550.

changes, interstitial fibrosis, cell loss, and degenerative features such as oncocytic change and nuclear pleomorphism. Bizarre nuclei may be present in multinucleated cells.

Demonstration that somatotrope adenoma cells have dopamine or somatostatin receptors, or both, raised the possibility that these tumors could be treated effectively with dopamine agonists or long-acting somatostatin analogues. However somatotrope adenomas are not affected morphologically by dopamine agonists even when large doses of the drug are administered for long periods (months to years). The only change is accumulation of mitochondria in a few adenoma cells, but the significance of mitochondrial accumulation in somatotrope adenomas during dopamine agonist treatment is uncertain.

Treatment with somatostatin analogues also produces no consistent morphologic changes.[753–755] In some tumors the cells and the cytoplasm are somewhat smaller than in untreated tumors.[755, 756] Mitochondrial accumulation, amyloid formation, lysosomal accumulation, crinophagy, perivascular and interstitial fibrosis, and increases in the size and number of secretory granules have also been reported. In some cases in which clinical and biochemical responses have occurred, no morphologic changes are observed even with electron microscopic examination.

GOALS OF TREATMENT. The goals of treatment are to return GH secretion to normal, correct clinical symptoms and signs, reverse mass effects of the tumor such as headache and visual abnormalities, and preserve other anterior pituitary

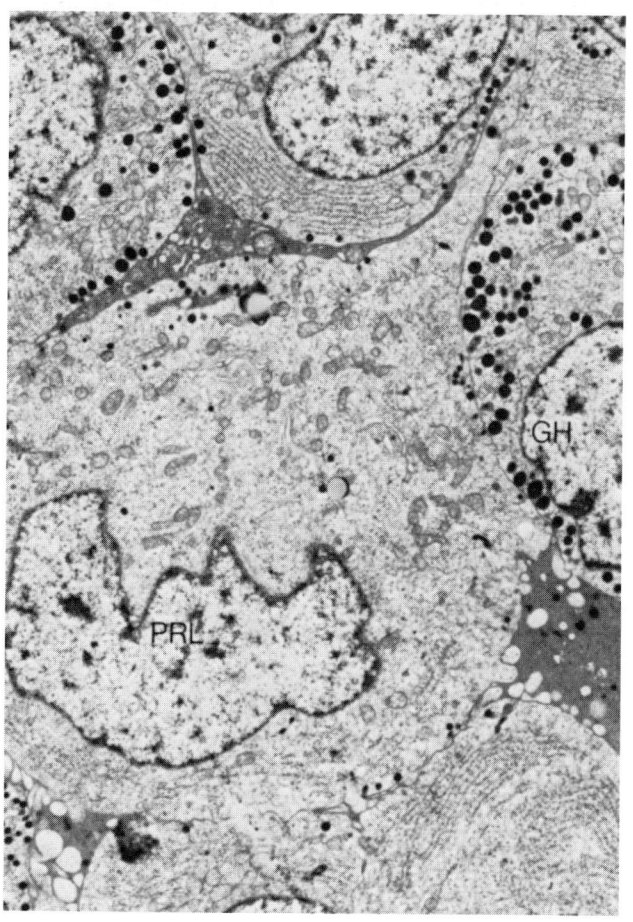

Figure 9–45. Mixed adenoma consisting of sparsely granulated prolactin cells (PRL) and densely granulated GH cells (GH). Magnification × 6500.

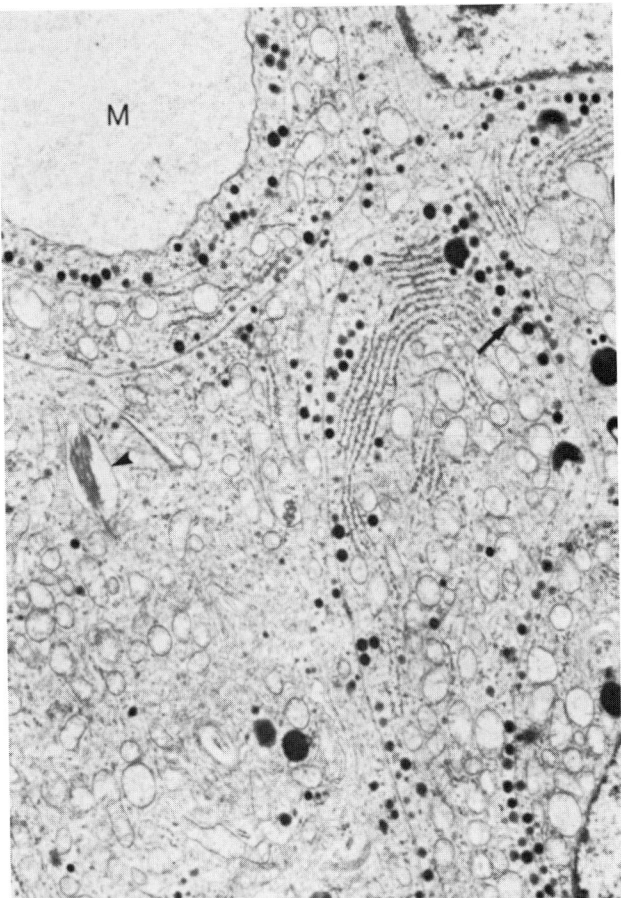

Figure 9–47. Acidophilic stem cell adenoma displaying the characteristic oncocytic change with development of giant mitochondria (M) and occurrence of intramitochondrial electron-dense tubular structures *(arrowhead)*. Note granule extrusion site *(arrow)*. Magnification × 11,550.

TABLE 9–24. Results of Transsphenoidal Surgery for Acromegaly: Patients with Postoperative Serum Growth Hormone Less Than 5 μg/L and Normal Oral Glucose Tolerance Test*

Author, Year	Number of Patients	Basal Growth Hormone <5 μg/L	Oral Glucose Tolerance Test Growth Hormone <2 μg/L†
Arafah et al, 1980[764]	28	20 (78%)	13 (46%)
Tucker et al, 1980[765]	32	24 (75%)	22 (71%)
Quabbe, 1982[766]	152		
114 micro‡		68 (60%)	39 (39%)
38 macro		13 (40%)	9 (26%)
Grisoli et al, 1985[1040]	100	60 (60%)	43 (43%)
Serri et al, 1985[1041]	25		
8 micro		8 (100%)	8 (100%)
17 macro		14 (82%)	13 (76%)
Davis et al, 1993[758]	174	90 (52%)*§	—
	54	—	28 (52%)

*Growth hormone <2 μg/L after glucose ingestion.
†Percentage based on number of patients tested.
‡When possible results are presented according to preoperative tumor size; micro, intrasellar tumor; macro, extrasellar extension or invasion of dura or bone.
§Basal growth hormone <2 μg/L.

function. The definition of cure is a reduction of the serum IGF-I level to normal for age and sex and the return of a normal GH response to oral glucose, i.e., reduction of the GH level to less than 1 μg/L (as measured by IRMA) after ingestion of 75 or 100 g of glucose. In many series a single postoperative GH concentration of less than 10 μg/L or less than 5 μg/L was considered indicative of "cure." A serum GH level less than 10 μg/L is not normal and is not a valid indication of successful surgery. Frequent GH measurements over 24 h indicate that even when postoperative IGF-I levels and GH response to oral glucose are normal, the pattern of pulsatile GH release may not be completely normal so that some acromegalic patients have persistent elevation of basal GH concentrations.[27] This observation is of unknown significance and requires long-term follow-up.

Treatments for GH-secreting pituitary adenomas include surgical resection, pituitary radiation, and medical therapies with dopamine agonists or somatostatin analogues. Many patients, particularly those with large tumors, require more than one type of treatment to produce clinical improvement and reduction in serum GH levels.

SURGICAL THERAPY. The preferred surgical approach is the transsphenoidal route because it permits visualization of the tumor, usually avoids contact with the optic chiasm and nerves, potentially allows complete resection, and causes less morbidity than do transcranial procedures.[757] As with all pituitary tumors the surgical outcome depends on the size of the tumor and the expertise of the surgeon. An intrasellar microadenoma (<10 mm in diameter) offers the greatest

possibility for a surgical cure. The presence of a macroadenoma (>10 mm in diameter), particularly with suprasellar extension or extension into the cavernous sinus, decreases the probability of a surgical cure. Nevertheless surgery may reduce tumor mass and cause immediate improvement in visual abnormalities, headaches, and symptoms of excessive GH and is the preferred initial therapy.

As shown in Tables 9–24 and 9–25 the results of transsphenoidal surgery, although variable, are fairly consistent in that a basal postoperative GH concentration of less than 5 μg/L is achieved in approximately 60% of patients, the best outcomes occurring with small tumors.[758] These results are representative of medical centers in which transsphenoidal surgery is performed frequently. Although a basal serum GH concentration of less than 5 μg/L may be indicative of successful surgery, dynamic studies, particularly the oral glucose tolerance test, are more accurate for evaluating postoperative GH secretion. As shown in Table 9–24, when suppression of GH to less than 2 μg/L after oral glucose ingestion is used as the criterion, some patients with a postoperative serum GH level of less than 5 μg/L are not cured. Furthermore in patients with a preoperative paradoxical GH response to TRH or LHRH, or both, the basal GH concentration may be less than 5 μg/L postoperatively despite a persistently abnormal GH response to TRH or LHRH, or both.

The serum IGF-I level should be measured before and

TABLE 9–25. Results of Transsphenoidal Surgery for Acromegaly: Patients with Postoperative Serum Growth Hormone Less Than 5 μg/L

Author, Year	Number of Patients	Basal Growth Hormone <5 μg/L (%)
Williams et al, 1975[761]	59	39 (66%)
Richards and Thomas, 1980[767]	34	27 (80%)
Balagura et al, 1981[1042]	132	76 (58%)
Laws et al, 1985[724]	75	40 (53%)
Roelfsema et al, 1985[768]	60	37 (62%)
Fahlbusch and Buchfelder, 1988[1043]	38	21 (55%)
Ross and Wilson, 1988[630]	214	117 (54%)
van't Verlaat et al, 1988[762]	25	14 (56%)
Davis et al, 1993[758]	174	90 (52%)*

*Basal growth hormone <2 μg/L.

after surgery, but it does not decrease as rapidly as GH concentrations with tumor removal[759] because it is complexed with a serum binding protein. A potentially useful method of assessing somatotrope function after surgery is measurement of serum GH concentration after the administration of GHRH. A lack of a GH response to GHRH may be indicative of a cure; an increase is difficult to interpret because nonadenomatous somatotropes release GH in response to GHRH. Even if all tests of GH secretion are normal postoperatively, late recurrence of acromegaly can occur, emphasizing the need for careful follow-up and monitoring. The incidence of recurrence is not known, but after an average follow-up of 2 to 3.5 y recurrence rates ranged from 0 to 13%.[630, 758, 760–762] IGF-I levels are useful in monitoring the effects of therapy, as is the documentation of recurrent or residual disease. Even with successfully treated patients, however, IGF-I levels may not fall for a period of months, so they are not useful in the immediate postoperative assessment.

Surgical mortality is low. Particular care must be taken with intubation and extubation because an enlarged tongue can cause airway obstruction, and many patients have sleep apnea and relative upper airway obstruction. Surgical complications include transient diabetes insipidus and CSF rhinorrhea in less than 5% of patients, and meningitis, sinusitis, hematoma, and cranial nerve palsy in less than 1%.[630, 763] The incidence of postsurgical anterior pituitary dysfunction depends on the amount of tissue removed, reported incidences ranging from 2 to 67% for corticotropin, 5 to 61% for thyrotropin, and 3 to 58% for gonadotropins.[630, 761, 762, 764–768] Diabetes insipidus is permanent in 1 to 9% of patients.[630, 763, 767–769]

RADIATION THERAPY. Before the widespread use of transsphenoidal surgery, radiation was the primary treatment for pituitary tumors. Currently pituitary radiation is usually reserved for patients with persistent disease after surgery to prevent tumor growth and reduce hormone hypersecretion. Limitations of radiotherapy include an inability to effect a prompt reduction in tumor size and hormone hypersecretion, a limitation that is particularly important for patients with visual abnormalities and severe acromegaly. Available radiotherapies include conventional high-dose therapy, radioisotope implantation, stereotactic radiosurgery with alpha particles or proton beam therapy, and focused radiation using the Gamma Knife or Lineac (radiosurgery).

Conventional supervoltage pituitary radiation involves administration of a total dose of 45 to 50 Gy in daily fractions 5 d/wk over 4 or 5 wk. Lower or higher radiation doses are associated with suboptimal control of the disease and increased risk of complications, respectively. Of 43 acromegalic patients treated with pituitary radiation only, 16 (37%) had a reduction in serum GH concentrations to less than 5 μg/L; this reduction required 2 y in 4 patients, 5 y in 8 patients, and 10 y in 4 patients. None had evidence of tumor enlargement; 5 of 39 (13%) developed secondary hypothyroidism, and 11 of 40 (28%) required glucocorticoid replacement.[508] In another study of the effects of conventional radiation as primary treatment, 19% of patients required glucocorticoid replacement and 26% required thyroid hormone replacement; the recurrence rate was 10%, and radiation-induced visual abnormalities occurred in 13%.[506] In a third study radiation-induced hypopituitaritism occurred in 50% of patients at a mean follow-up of 26 mo, emphasizing the need for close monitoring of any patient who undergoes radiotherapy.[510] Impairment of endocrine function after conventional radiation therapy is due to both effects on the pituitary and hypothalamic damage. Other complications include visual loss secondary to optic nerve damage, cerebral ischemia, and development of a pituitary or brain malignancy. Of 139 patients given 40 to 60 Gy, 3 acquired radiation necrosis of the brain, 10 developed cerebral ischemia, and 1 had a glioblastoma of the temporal lobe.[512] Radiation-induced hypopituitarism occurs more frequently in patients previously treated with pituitary surgery.[515]

Alpha particle pituitary radiotherapy, using a cyclotron as the energy source, delivers a maximal tumor dose of 90 Gy. This treatment is usually given on one occasion. Serum GH concentrations are reduced to less than 5 μg/L 5 y after therapy in patients with macroadenomas and 3 y after treatment in those with microadenomas. Anterior pituitary deficiency occurs in approximately one third of patients, 34% requiring glucocorticoid replacement, 33% requiring thyroid hormone replacement, and 25% requiring gonadal steroid replacement. Other complications of alpha particle therapy include the development of visual field abnormalities (29%), cranial nerve palsy (43%), and temporal lobe epilepsy (29%), but these complications occur only in patients who have received prior conventional therapy. The incidence of CNS complications in patients treated solely with alpha particle radiation is less than 1%.[511] Because of the current lack of suitable nuclear reactors, alpha particle therapy is not an option for management.

Proton beam radiation, generated by a cyclotron, delivers up to 120 Gy to the tumor mass and is administered as a single treatment. Of 435 acromegalic patients given proton beam therapy, 30% had a serum GH concentration less than 5 μg/L 2 y after treatment, 50% achieved this result after 5 y, 78% after 10 y, and 88% after 20 y. The median time for the development of hypopituitarism was 2.8 y after treatment, with 10% requiring thyroid replacement, 9% requiring glucocorticoid replacement, and 7% requiring gonadal steroids. Other complications of proton beam therapy included temporal lobe seizures in three patients, an arachnoid cyst in one patient, pituitary carcinoma in two patients, and a CNS sarcoma in one patient.[509] Newer methods of stereotactic proton beam therapy are under development.

Surgical implantation of radioactive yttrium 90 seeds into the pituitary is no longer in general use for treating acromegaly. Of 22 patients given these implants, 11 had a reduction in serum GH level to less than 5 μg/L 3 to 11 mo after treatment.[770] Complications included transient cranial nerve palsy in two patients and fever in two patients. Seven of 22 patients required hormone replacement therapy, including glucocorticoid therapy in 6 patients, gonadal steroid replacement in 4 patients, levothyroxine in 2 patients, and AVP in 1 patient.

Stereotactic radiotherapy using the Gamma Knife employs a heavily shielded central body containing 202 sources of ^{60}Co. The radiation sources are radially distributed over a segment of a sphere, and the beams are individually collimated toward the center of the lesion.[771] This method of radiation delivery has been applied to brain tumors, arteriovenous malformations, aneurysms, craniopharyngiomas, and pituitary tumors. It has modest efficacy for the treatment of acromegaly.[772] The procedure is usually limited to patients with small, clearly delineated lesions so that the optic chiasm, optic nerves, and structures in the cavernous sinus can be protected from damage.

MEDICAL THERAPY

Bromocriptine. Bromocriptine, the orally active dopamine agonist used to treat hyperprolactinemia, also reduces serum GH concentrations in acromegalic patients and has been used to treat acromegaly since 1974.[721] Most patients have improvement in clinical symptoms (70 to 90%) and a reduction in serum GH concentrations during chronic bromocriptine therapy (approximately 70% of patients). However, as shown in Table 9–26, reduction of serum GH concentration to less than 5 μg/L occurs rarely. Other effects include reduction in urinary hydroxyproline excretion, improvement of diabetes mellitus control, resolution of hyperprolactinemia (if present), and improvement in visual field abnormalities. A larger bro-

TABLE 9–26. Results of Bromocriptine Therapy for Acromegaly

Author, Year	Number of Patients (%)					
	Total	Suppression of Growth Hormone	Normal Growth Hormone*	↓ Sweating	↓ Ring Size	Dose (mg/d)
Thorner et al, 1975[722]	11	9/11 (82)	0/11	11/11	6/11 (55)	20
Thorner and Besser, 1976[1044]	25	10/15 (67)	Not reported	24/25 (96)	17/18 (94)	15–60
Wass et al, 1977[1045]	73	58/73 (79)	15/73 (21)	60/63 (95)	30/34 (88)	10–60
Belforte et al, 1977[1046]	30	17/30 (57)	6/30 (21)	"Most"	5/14 (36)†	10–20
Halse et al, 1977[1047]	8	7/8 (88)	0/8	7/7	7/7	10–20
Eskildsen et al, 1978[1048]	14	10/14 (71)‡	10/14 (71)§	7/9 (78)	7/11 (64)	30–55
Lundin et al, 1978[1049]	11	9/11 (82)	1/11 (9)	7/11 (64)	10/11 (91)	15–40
Besser et al, 1980[1050]	101	78/101 (77)	NR‖	59/63 (94)	17/19 (89)	20–60
Lindholm et al, 1981[1051]	18	6/18 (33)	0/18	NR	NR	20
Moses et al, 1981[713]	7	6/7 (86)	2/7 (29)	NR	6/7 (86)¶	10–40

*Normal growth hormone level <5 μg/L.
†Reduction in hand volume.
‡24-h urinary levels.
§Urinary excretion <100 μg/24 h.
‖NR, not reported.
¶Decrease in shoe size.
From Vance ML, Evans WS, Thorner MD. Drugs five years later. Bromocriptine. Ann Intern Med 1984; 100:78–91.

mocriptine dose (10 to 20 mg/d or more in divided doses) is required to treat acromegaly than to treat hyperprolactinemia. As noted in the discussion of the treatment of hyperprolactinemia, to minimize side effects bromocriptine therapy should be initiated with a small dose followed by a gradual increase.

Although suppression of GH secretion may be incomplete during bromocriptine therapy, this drug is useful for symptomatic treatment of patients with residual postoperative disease or until radiation therapy is effective.

Somatostatin Analogues. Somatostatin is a 14-amino-acid cyclic peptide in the brain, hypothalamus, pancreas, and gastrointestinal tract[773] that functions as the GH release–inhibiting hormone and, in conjunction with GHRH, negates episodic GH release. Intravenous administration of somatostatin produces a prompt reduction in serum GH levels in normal individuals and in patients with acromegaly. After cessation of the infusion, serum GH levels rebound rapidly.[716] Somatostatin must be administered by continuous intravenous infusion because its half-life is less than 3 min, making it impractical for clinical use. Octreotide is an 8-amino-acid cyclic peptide analogue of somatostatin that has a serum half-life of approximately 90 min and that suppresses GH release for up to 8 h in normal and acromegalic individuals.[774, 775] This peptide is administered subcutaneously and suppresses GH release 20 times more effectively than does the native peptide and is 22 times more suppressive of GH release than of insulin release. Despite its greater selectivity for GH, insulin release is decreased for approximately 3 h after octreotide administration, and postprandial hyperglycemia may occur.[774, 775]

Octreotide has been used to treat acromegaly and other secretory endocrine tumors since 1984. About 90% of patients have improvement in disease manifestations and reduction in serum GH and IGF-I concentrations. Relief of headache can occur without a substantial reduction in tumor size.[756, 776–802] Additionally administration of octreotide to acromegalic patients with sleep apnea causes a 40% decrease in the number of apneic episodes and a 50% decrease in the respiratory disturbance index; improvement is variable among patients.[803] A minority of patients have a 30% reduction or less in pituitary tumor size.[756, 798, 801, 802] Serum GH levels are reduced within an hour of administration and remain reduced for 6 to 8 h in most patients; insulin release is inhibited for less than 3 h after administration.[776] Although serum IGF-I levels are reduced to normal in 40 to 50% of patients, other patients have only a partial suppression of GH release. The heterogeneity of response is likely a function of the density of somatostatin receptors in the adenoma and variable binding affinities for octreotide. In patients who underwent surgical resection of the adenoma after receiving octreotide, those with the greatest degree of GH suppression had a higher density of somatostatin receptors on the tumors than did patients with a poor response.[801]

The recommended octreotide dose is 100 μg every 8 h; some patients have adequate GH suppression with a dose of 50 μg three times a day, and others require as much as 1500 μg/d in divided doses.[796] Some patients respond better to continuous subcutaneous octreotide infusion than to intermittent injections.[782, 783, 787, 804] Occasional patients have better GH suppression with the combination of octreotide and bromocriptine.[779, 781, 801] The precise dose and frequency of administration should be adjusted according to the clinical response and serum IGF-I concentration.

Octreotide inhibits gallbladder contractility and facilitates formation of gallstones;[805] approximately 18% of patients treated chronically develop either gallbladder sludge or stones. A minority become symptomatic and require cholecystectomy. Because postprandial gallbladder motility is decreased by octreotide, a potential method of decreasing the risk of gallstone formation is administration of the drug 2 to 3 h after meals.

In addition to treating patients not cured by or unresponsive to other therapy, octreotide may be useful for reducing pituitary tumor size before surgical resection. In 10 patients studied by Barkan and colleagues, pituitary tumor size decreased by 20 to 54% when octreotide was administered for 3 to 30 wk before surgery.[756] Presurgical octreotide treatment has also been reported to result in a higher surgical remission rate of 76% compared with a remission rate of 30% in patients who did not receive octreotide before surgery.[806]

A slow-release somatostatin analogue, lanreotide, is given every 10 to 14 d and is also effective in suppressing serum GH and IGF-I concentrations. Preliminary studies suggest that this preparation is as effective as octreotide.[807]

Treatment of acromegaly frequently requires more than one approach, including surgery, radiation, and medical treatment. Because uncontrolled acromegaly is associated with enhanced mortality and morbidity, all therapies should be considered in an attempt to reduce GH secretion to normal.

Ectopic Growth Hormone–Releasing Hormone Secretion. Somatotrope stimulation by a GHRH-secreting tumor causes less than 1% of cases of acromegaly.[638] If an ectopic GHRH-secreting tumor is identified, surgical resection is curative in the absence of metastases. Patients with metastatic disease respond to octreotide therapy, which lowers circulating GHRH and GH concentrations.[808, 809] Differential sensitivity to octreotide is observed, with greater suppression of GH than of GHRH.[804]

Cushing's Disease

Cushing's disease is most commonly caused by a pituitary corticotrope adenoma, but excess adrenal cortical function (Cushing's syndrome) can be due to multiple causes. A rare condition of corticotrope hyperplasia from excessive CRH secretion is also referred to as Cushing's disease.[810] The disease has a female to male preponderance of 3:1 to 8:1; it commonly occurs in women of childbearing age but may occur at any age. It accounts for approximately 70% of all cases of spontaneous (endogenous) Cushing's syndrome. The other corticotropin-dependent Cushing's syndrome is ectopic corticotropin syndrome from a malignant peripheral tumor and is frequently associated with weight loss, hypokalemic alkalosis, and hyperglycemia. Causes include oat cell carcinoma, bronchial and foregut (including thymus) carcinoid tumors, pancreatic islet cell tumors, pheochromocytoma, medullary carcinoma of the thyroid and, occasionally, ovarian tumors (<1%). Rarely ectopic CRH production may cause Cushing's syndrome. Non–corticotropin-dependent causes include adrenal adenomas and carcinomas.

In this section Cushing's disease is discussed in outline form because a detailed discussion is included in Chapter 12.

ETIOLOGY. The diagnosis of Cushing's syndrome is usually straightforward when a patient has the classic features. However patients in the early stages of the disease may have only a few features. Weight gain is usually present and is often attributed to overeating and depression. Once the diagnosis of Cushing's syndrome has been made, the cause must be ascertained to determine appropriate therapy. Cushing's syndrome is either corticotropin dependent or corticotropin independent. In this section we consider only the corticotropin-dependent causes, including Cushing's disease, ectopic corticotropin secretion, and the rare disorder of ectopic or eutopic production of CRH. Identifying the source of excessive corticotropin production (pituitary or ectopic tumor) often requires several diagnostic tests and is the most problematic aspect of evaluating these patients. Perhaps the most difficult distinction is between chronic ectopic corticotropin secretion by a relatively benign tumor (e.g., bronchial carcinoid) and a pituitary adenoma, since patients with ectopic corticotropin production may have responses to suppression tests that are similar to those of patients with pituitary adenoma.

Whether Cushing's disease is primarily a pituitary or a hypothalamic disease is unclear (see Chapter 12); a pituitary cause is likely. Thus selective removal of the adenoma returns hypothalamic-pituitary-adrenal function to normal and is associated with a low rate of recurrence. The often prolonged delay in recovery of the hypothalamic-pituitary-adrenal axis (months) is also incompatible with a hypothalamic cause. Furthermore if the cause were hypothalamic, corticotrope hyperplasia would be common, whereas this is rare.

CLINICAL FEATURES. The clinical features of Cushing's syndrome are a result of chronically elevated cortisol concentrations and include weight gain, centripetal obesity, moon facies, violaceous striae, easy bruisability, proximal myopathy, and psychiatric disturbances, most commonly depression.

Although the florid case of Cushing's syndrome is easy to diagnose, the more subtle case presents a diagnostic challenge. In children and prepubertal adolescents the presentation is usually one of obesity and growth retardation. Adult women may have weight gain, menstrual irregularities, and depres-

sion. Occasionally patients have skin manifestations only, particularly thinning, bruising, and poor wound healing. Similarly the diagnosis may be made incidentally by x-ray findings of healed fractures (e.g., rib) with no known history of fracture. Because of the severe pain normally associated with a rib fracture, a painless rib fracture should always raise the possibility of Cushing's syndrome.

Manifestations involve almost every system in the body but may be obvious only after the diagnosis is made. In patients who diet or exercise regularly, it is possible to have Cushing's syndrome without obesity. Hypertension is present in many.

Skin changes include thinning of the epidermis and purple striae that are often more than 1 cm wide. This contrasts with the striae of rapid weight gain or pregnancy, which are narrower and either very pale or pink. In severe Cushing's syndrome the skin of the back of the hand is paper thin and easily peeled off or torn (e.g., by removing adhesive tape). Women with Cushing's disease typically have fine, downy, facial lanugo hair and may have acne, hirsutism, and temporal scalp hair loss secondary to increased adrenal androgen secretion. Superficial fungal infections, particularly tinea versicolor, are common. The shins often show signs of lacerations that have healed poorly and may be hyperpigmented. Patients with Cushing's disease often have had the disease for 3 to 6 y before diagnosis, and it may be possible to date the onset of the condition by determining which scars are pigmented. Such scars develop after the onset of the condition (an effect of excessive secretion of corticotropin and other melanotropins).

Virtually all patients with Cushing's disease have some psychiatric manifestations. The most common is depression, but psychotic and manic behavior may also occur. Depression may be so severe that the patient is suicidal.

Women with Cushing's disease have disturbed menstruation because of several abnormalities. Adrenal androgen secretion is increased as a result of the increased corticotropin secretion and may adversely affect the development of the ovarian follicles. Both the increased androgens and cortisol exert a negative effect on gonadotropin secretion. Men often have decreased libido, which may be a result of decreased gonadotropin secretion or depression, or both.

Because the diagnosis of Cushing's disease is often delayed, significant osteopenia or vertebral collapse, or both, or other fractures may be present. The osteopenia is unlike other forms of osteoporosis in that it is reversible with cure of the Cushing's disease. Although only about half of patients complain of muscle weakness, proximal myopathy is demonstrable in most; such patients are unable to rise from a deep knee bend or unassisted from a seated position.

Excessive glucocorticoid levels cause insulin resistance and glucose intolerance in 75% of patients and overt diabetes mellitus in 8 to 10%. Hypercalciuria results in an increased incidence of renal calculi.

Patients with small cell carcinoma of the lung and ectopic corticotropin production usually have a fulminate form of Cushing's syndrome. Corticotropin levels are high and cortisol production rates may be increased more than 10-fold. Because the condition is acute in onset and progresses rapidly, weight is lost instead of gained and proximal myopathy is severe. Common features include pigmentation (from the high levels of plasma corticotropin and other melanotropin hormones), electrolyte disturbances (especially hypokalemia), and hyperglycemia with insulin resistance that may lead to overt diabetes mellitus. Hypokalemic alkalosis results from the mineralocorticoid effects of high cortisol levels. The hypokalemic alkalosis may be a medical emergency. This syndrome is different from that of typical Cushing's syndrome because of chronic ectopic corticotropin production by a relatively benign tumor such as a carcinoid.

BIOCHEMICAL EVALUATION. The evaluation of patients with Cushing's syndrome is designed to establish the diagnosis and determine the cause of the excessive cortisol production and is discussed in detail in Chapter 12. It cannot be stressed too strongly that the differential diagnosis is primarily addressed by functional studies. Radiologic imaging of the adrenal glands or the pituitary, or both, does not have a role at this stage of the evaluation because imaging provides information on anatomy, not function, and "nonfunctioning" adenomas ("incidentaloma") are common in the pituitary and adrenal glands. Thus without the biochemical tests the results of imaging studies may be misleading.

Establishing the Diagnosis of Cushing's Syndrome. The evaluation of Cushing's syndrome can usually be performed on an outpatient basis. The disorder is most commonly a result of iatrogenic administration of excessive quantities of synthetic glucocorticoids for treatment of other disorders. Therefore the first step is to determine whether the patient is receiving such medications, including prior intramuscular or intra-articular injections of dexamethasone or other synthetic glucocorticoids that can have effects lasting over many months.[811, 812] This condition is suspected if the patient has clinical evidence of Cushing's syndrome but has undetectable or low urinary or plasma cortisol levels. Having excluded iatrogenic Cushing's syndrome, the next step is to determine if the 24-h glucocorticoid secretion is increased. This can be achieved most easily by performing a 24-h urine collection for measurement of urinary free cortisol.[813] Usually two baseline collections are obtained, with measurement of total volume and creatinine to assess the adequacy of the collections and to correct for body mass. Some assay methods for urinary free cortisol are more precise than others; the normal range in the older RIA method is higher than in the high-pressure liquid chromatography method, probably reflecting detection of interfering substances by the RIA. When interpreting the results of tests, urine cortisol levels cannot be compared if the assay used is different from that used for the published reference data. It is also necessary to make sure the patient is not using any hemorrhoid medications that contain hydrocortisone because this may be detected as cortisol in the assay. Prior to the development of urinary free cortisol assays, 17-hydroxysteroid excretion was measured and may still be useful in selected patients, but this assay may also detect interfering substances. If the 24-h urinary free cortisol excretion is increased, the next step is to assess the response to dexamethasone, a synthetic steroid that is not detected appreciably in assays of urine free cortisol and serum cortisol. The initial screening test is often the 1-mg dexamethasone overnight suppression test. Dexamethasone, 1 mg, is given orally at 11 PM, and serum cortisol is measured at 8 AM; the normal response is a plasma cortisol concentration less than 138 nmol/L (<5 μg/dL). This test is associated with significant false-positive and false-negative results.[813, 814] False-positive results (lack of suppression) occur most frequently in hospitalized patients, so the test is most useful as an outpatient *screening* test. The standard low-dose dexamethasone test (0.5 mg every 6 h for 48 h) is used to confirm the diagnosis of Cushing's syndrome. This dexamethasone dose is equivalent to approximately four times normal cortisol production. In normal individuals this amount of dexamethasone exerts a negative feedback on the hypothalamus and pituitary to suppress corticotropin secretion. Thus adrenal cortisol secretion ceases. The standard low-dose dexamethasone suppression test is performed by administering 0.5 mg orally at 8 AM, 2 PM, 8 PM, and 2 AM for 2 d. Doses for children are corrected on the basis of weight.[815] Urine collections are made from 8 AM through 8 AM for each of the two baseline days and two dexamethasone test days. The criteria for normal suppression for the low-dose test is a plasma cortisol level 6 h after the last dose of dexamethasone of less than 138 nmol/L (<5 μg/dL) or a urinary cortisol level of less than 55 nmol/d (<20 μg/24 h) as measured by competitive protein-binding analysis and high-pressure liquid chromatography (see Chapter 12).[816] In another study normal suppression was defined as a urinary free cortisol level of less than 99 nmol/d (<36 μg/24h) and a serum cortisol level of less than 39 nmol/L (<1.4 μg/dL).[817] The administration of CRH at the end of the test appears to increase the sensitivity of the low-dose dexamethasone test to diagnose Cushing's syndrome.[817] Table 9–27 shows the sensitivity and specificity of the low-dose dexamethasone test with and without the addition of CRH in the diagnosis of Cushing's syndrome. In patients with Cushing's syndrome, regardless of cause, neither plasma cortisol nor urinary cortisol excretion is suppressed in response to 2 d of dexamethasone administration. Patients who metabolize dexamethasone rapidly may not have suppressed excretion; this can be determined by measuring a plasma dexamethasone level at 0800 h after the last dose of dexamethasone (0200 h). Six hours after the last 0.5-mg dose in the low-dose test, the plasma dexamethasone level should be 5.1 to 15 nmol/L (200 to 600 ng/dL), with a mean of 9.4 nmol/L (370 ng/dL). Six hours after the last 2-mg dose in the high-dose test, the plasma dexamethasone level should be 18 to 51 nmol/L (700 to 2000 ng/dL), with a mean of 35 nmol/L (1350 ng/dL).[818, 819] This assessment is particularly important in patients receiving drugs such as carbamazepine, phenobarbital, or other drugs that stimulate the cytochrome P450 system of the liver. This measurement also helps document patient compliance with the regimen.

Distinction of Corticotropin-Dependent and Corticotropin-Independent Causes. The cornerstone for determining whether the syndrome is corticotropin dependent or corticotropin independent is measurement of the plasma corticotropin concentration. Corticotropin levels are suppressed in patients with adrenal adenoma or adrenal carcinoma, whereas levels are easily detectable but may overlap with the normal range in patients with ectopic corticotropin syndrome, Cushing's disease, or ectopic CRH syndrome (Fig. 9–48). It is vital that the sample be collected properly—on ice, spun immediately in a cold centrifuge, separated, and frozen until assay. Failure to collect and process the sample correctly leads to erroneous results.

Distinction of Pituitary from Nonpituitary Sources of Corticotropin. Once the syndrome is determined to be corticotro-

TABLE 9–27. Cushing's Syndrome: Comparison of 2-D Low-Dose Dexamethasone (0.5 mg Every 6 h for 48 h) and 2-D Low-Dose Dexamethasone + Corticotropin-Releasing Hormone Tests

Test	Measurements	Sensitivity (%)	Specificity (%)
Dex, 0.5 mg q 6 h × 48 h	Day 2 UFC >99 nmol/d (>36 μg/24h)	56	100
Dex, 0.5 mg q 6 h × 48 h	Day 2, serum cortisol >39 nmol/L (>1.4 μg/dL)	90	100
Dex, 0.5 mg q 6 h × 48 h + CRH	15″ post CRH: serum cortisol >39 nmol/L (>1.4 μg/dL)	100	100

Patients: Cushing's syndrome, n = 39; Pseudo-Cushing's, n = 19.

Dex, dexamethasone; CRH, corticotropin-releasing hormone; UFC, 24-h urine free cortisol.

From Yanovski JA, Cutler GB Jr, Chrousos GP, et al. Corticotropin-releasing hormone stimulation following low-dose dexamethasone administration: a new test to distinguish Cushing's syndrome from pseudo-Cushing's states. JAMA 1993; 269:2232–2238. Copyright 1993, American Medical Association.

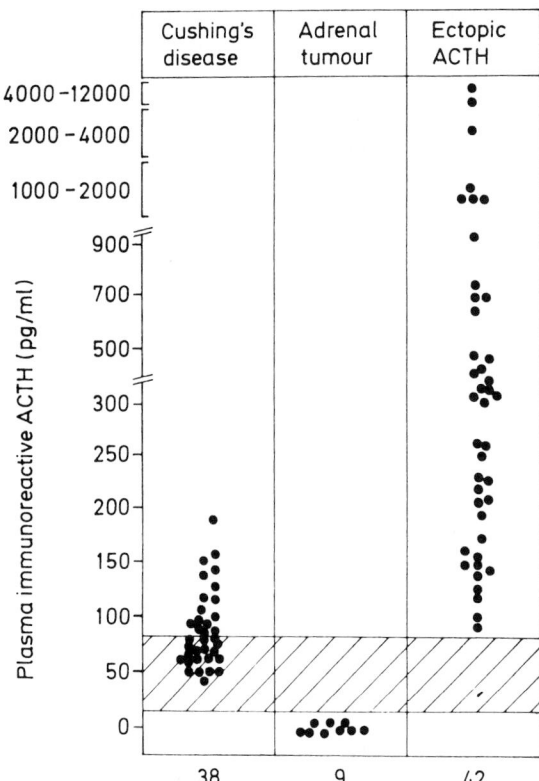

Figure 9–48. Plasma corticotropin concentrations in patients with excessive cortisol production of different causes. To convert corticotropin values to picomoles per liter, multiply by 0.2202. (Modified from Rees LH, Holdaway IM, Phenekos C, et al. ACTH secretion and clinical investigations. In: Some Aspects of Hypothalamic Regulation of Endocrine Functions. Symposium Vienna, June 3–6, 1973. Stuttgart: Schattauer Verlag, 1974.)

pin dependent, it is necessary to determine the origin of the corticotropin: the pituitary gland or an ectopic source. Hypokalemic alkalosis is rare in Cushing's disease, and the occurrence of hypokalemic alkalosis in the absence of diuretic ingestion is suggestive of ectopic corticotropin secretion. The rationale for tests to distinguish between pituitary and ectopic corticotropin production is that in pituitary-dependent disease, the pituitary gland is responsive to high levels of glucocorticoid and to marked reductions in circulating glucocorticoid concentrations. The negative feedback control of corticotropin secretion is present but is relatively insensitive. Thus administration of a high dose of dexamethasone usually suppresses corticotropin production by a pituitary adenoma and decreases adrenal cortisol secretion. Extrapituitary tumors that produce corticotropin are generally unresponsive to high doses of dexamethasone. The standard high-dose dexamethasone suppression test of 2 mg every 6 h for 48 h (8 mg/d) is

TABLE 9–29. Cushing's Disease: Comparison of Overnight 8-mg Dexamethasone and 2-D 8-mg Dexamethasone Tests

Test	% Suppression vs. Baseline	Sensitivity (%)	Specificity (%)
Overnight dex: 8 mg	Serum cortisol: >50%	88	57
Overnight dex: 8 mg	Serum cortisol: >80%	57	100
2-D dex: 2 mg q 6 h × 48 h	17 OH: >50%	88	71
2-D dex: 2 mg q 6 h × 48 h	17 OH: >69%	65	100
2-D dex: 2 mg q 6 h × 48 h	UFC: >90%	65	100

Patients: Cushing's disease, n = 34; ectopic corticotropin syndrome, n = 7.
Dex, dexamethasone; UFC, 24-h urine free cortisol; 17 OH, 24-h urine 17 hydroxysteroids.
From Dichek HL, Nieman LK, Oldfield EH, et al. A comparison of the standard high dose dexamethasone suppression test and the overnight 8-mg dexamethasone suppression test for the differential diagnosis of adrenocorticotropin-dependent Cushing's syndrome. J Clin Endocrinol Metab 1994; 78:418–422. Copyright © The Endocrine Society.

used to distinguish between a pituitary and an ectopic source of corticotropin. Urinary excretion of 17-hydroxysteroid concentrations is usually reduced to 50% or more of the baseline value in patients with pituitary-dependent disease.[820] This 50% suppression has been adopted as a required value by some investigators, but this criterion is probably incorrect (see Chapter 12). Measurement of urinary free cortisol excretion is helpful because any reproducible suppression of cortisol is indicative of pituitary-dependent disease. If a pituitary cause is suspected and adequate suppression of urinary steroids does not occur with usual high-dose dexamethasone administration, it is prudent to retest the patient using a total dexamethasone dose of 16, 32, or 64 mg/d, because a few patients with pituitary adenomas respond to these higher doses. The same criteria for suppression of urinary steroid excretion are used for the 8 mg/d test. If there is no suppression of adrenal cortisol production, even with the highest dexamethasone doses, it can be assumed that a peripheral tumor is the source of corticotropin. Administration of a single dose of 8 mg of dexamethasone with measurement of serum cortisol the following morning has also been used to diagnose pituitary-dependent Cushing's disease. As shown in Tables 9–28 and 9–29 the utility of this test approaches that of the traditional 2-d high-dose dexamethasone test, depending on the criteria for suppression. Table 9–30 shows a comparison of urinary free cortisol and 17-hydroxysteroid excretion with the traditional 2-d high dose test.

The metyrapone test is also used to distinguish between a pituitary and an ectopic corticotropin source and is comple-

TABLE 9–28. Cushing's Disease: Comparison of Overnight 8-mg Dexamethasone and 2-D 8-mg Dexamethasone Tests

Test	% Suppression vs. Baseline	Sensitivity (%)	Specificity (%)
Overnight dex: 8 mg	Serum cortisol: >50%	88	100
2-D dex: 2 mg q 6 h × 48 h	Urine 17 OH: >50%	92	94

Patients: Cushing's disease, n = 73; ectopic corticotropin syndrome, n = 12.
Dex, dexamethasone; 17 OH, 24-h urine 17 hydroxysteroids.
From Kaye TB and Crapo L. The Cushing syndrome: an update on diagnostic tests (see comments) (review). Ann Intern Med 1990; 112:434–444.

TABLE 9–30. Cushing's Disease: 2-D High-Dose Dexamethasone Test (2 mg Every 6 h for 48 h): Comparison of Urine Free Cortisol and Urine 17 Hydroxysteroids

Criterion for Suppression (% Suppression from Baseline)	Sensitivity (%)	Specificity (%)	Misclassification of Patients with Ectopic Corticotropin (%)
UFC >50%	90	79	40
UFC >90%	69	100	0
17 OH >50%	78	92	20
17 OH >64%	69	100	0

Patients: Cushing's disease, n = 94; ectopic corticotropin syndrome, n = 10; primary adrenal disease, n = 14.
UFC, 24-h urine free cortisol; 17 OH, 24-h urine 17 hydroxysteroids.
From Flack MR, Oldfield EH, Cutler GB Jr, et al. Urine free cortisol in the high-dose dexamethasone suppression test for the differential diagnosis of the Cushing syndrome. Ann Intern Med 1992; 116:211–217.

mentary to the high-dose dexamethasone test. The normal pituitary and corticotropin-producing pituitary adenomas respond to the inhibition of cortisol synthesis by metyrapone by increasing corticotropin secretion; this increase does not occur with ectopic corticotropin-producing tumors. Metyrapone inhibits cortisol synthesis at several steps, the most prominent being inhibition of the conversion of 11-deoxycortisol to cortisol. The commencement of the test should be delayed at least 48 h after the high-dose dexamethasone suppression test, preferably longer, for two reasons: (1) dexamethasone must be metabolized and its biologic effects must be eliminated so that reduction of endogenous cortisol synthesis during metyrapone administration is detected by the pituitary and (2) 48 h of high-dose dexamethasone may suppress corticotropin sufficiently that the adrenals are transiently unresponsive to corticotropin stimulation during metyrapone administration (because of reduction of steroidogenic enzymes) (personal communication, David Orth). With ectopic corticotropin secretion hypothalamic-pituitary function is chronically suppressed and cannot be reactivated by a short-term (24-h) reduction in plasma cortisol concentrations such as occurs with metyrapone. Conversely patients with pituitary-dependent disease remain responsive to a sudden reduction in circulating cortisol levels, corticotropin secretion increases, and the additional corticotropin stimulation of the adrenal glands produces an increase in levels of circulating cortisol precursors, with plasma 11-deoxycortisol being the most frequently measured. The metyrapone test involves the oral administration of 750 mg every 4 h (with food to minimize the development of nausea) for 24 h (six doses) and measurement of the plasma 11-deoxycortisol concentration before and 4 h after the last metyrapone dose. Plasma cortisol is also measured 4 h after the last metyrapone dose to assess the adequacy of 11β-hydroxylase blockade.[821] Patients with pituitary-dependent disease have an increase in plasma 11-deoxycortisol levels to more than 144 nmol/L (>5 μg/dL) in the setting of an undetectable or very low plasma cortisol level. Urinary 17-hydroxysteroid excretion may also be measured to distinguish between a pituitary and an ectopic corticotropin cause. Twenty-four–hour urine collections must be obtained on the day before, during, and on the day after metyrapone administration. Because the cortisol precursors are metabolized and excreted as urinary 17-hydroxysteroids, a two- to threefold increase in 17-hydroxysteroid excretion occurs in pituitary-dependent disease. Table 9–31 shows a comparison of the sensitivity and specificity of the metyrapone test and the 2-d high-dose dexamethasone test. If the ectopic corticotropin syndrome is of recent onset, the hypothalamic-pituitary-adrenal axis may not be completely suppressed, resulting in either an attenuated or a normal response to metyrapone.

TABLE 9–31. Cushing's Disease: Comparison of 2-D 8-mg Dexamethasone and 1-D Metyrapone Tests

Test	Measurements	Sensitivity (%)	Specificity (%)
2-D Dex: 2 mg q 6 h × 48 h	UFC: ↓ >90% of baseline	59	73
Metyrapone: 750 mg q 4 h × 24 h	17 OH: ↑ >70% over baseline	60	77
Metyrapone: 750 mg q 4 h × 24 h	Serum 11-deoxycortisol: ↑ >400 over baseline	38	73

Patients: Cushing's disease, n = 170; ectopic corticotropin syndrome, n = 15; adrenal adenoma, n = 1.
Dex, dexamethasone; UFC, 24-h urine free cortisol; 17 OH, 24-h urine 17 hydroxysteroids.
From Avgerinos PC, Yanovski JA, Oldfield EH, et al. The metyrapone and dexamethasone suppression tests for the differential diagnosis of the adrenocorticotropin-dependent Cushing syndrome: a comparison. Ann Intern Med 1994; 121:318–327.

CRH administration was initially believed to be useful in distinguishing between pituitary-dependent disease and ectopic corticotropin syndrome in that CRH administration appeared to stimulate corticotropin release in patients with pituitary adenomas but not in those with the ectopic corticotropin syndrome.[822] However some patients with ectopic corticotropin syndrome have an increase in corticotropin release in response to CRH.[823] CRH has also been administered during petrosal sinus catheterization with simultaneous measurement of petrosal sinus and peripheral corticotropin concentrations.[824] This technique allows definitive identification of a pituitary source of corticotropin but is less accurate (range 50 to 80%) in identifying which side of the pituitary contains the adenoma. Some investigators recommend that this procedure be performed in every corticotropin-dependent patient to confirm the diagnosis of Cushing's disease.[825–828] Petrosal sinus sampling with CRH administration is useful *only* in determining the central or peripheral (ectopic) source of corticotropin; the test cannot distinguish among normal individuals, patients with pseudo-Cushing's and patients with Cushing's syndrome.[829] Furthermore in patients with recent onset of ectopic corticotropin syndrome, the pituitary may still respond to CRH. In patients in whom the diagnosis is clear from the noninvasive studies, this procedure is usually not necessary. The test should be performed if there is doubt about the source of corticotropin but should be performed only by an experienced interventional radiologist who is skilled in this technique.

Summary of Evaluation. A logical strategy for evaluating a patient with Cushing's syndrome has been outlined (Table 9–32). Because a small number of patients with Cushing's syndrome of all causes have cyclic disease, it is possible to be misled by the results of either the dexamethasone or the metyrapone test when the results are due to spontaneous cyclic variation. However both tests should be performed, and if the results are consonant with each other greater certainty in the diagnosis is achieved.

Based on our knowledge of feedback mechanisms, Cushing's syndrome due to ectopic CRH would be expected to respond as in Cushing's disease. In the few cases described, however, the response is similar to that in ectopic corticotropin syndrome, possibly because these ectopic tumors often secrete both corticotropin and CRH. The best-studied case of ectopic CRH production causing Cushing's syndrome was in a patient with prostatic carcinoma metastatic to the median eminence.[830]

Hypothalamic CRH-producing gangliocytoma causing Cushing's syndrome has been diagnosed only retrospectively at pathologic examination; the responses to dynamic function tests are unknown. Again this is an extremely rare cause of Cushing's syndrome, but it is likely that these patients would respond with a pattern similar to that of patients with Cushing's disease.

RADIOLOGIC EVALUATION. Once the diagnosis of Cushing's disease is established, the therapeutic strategy must be defined. In most instances, unless there is a contraindication, transsphenoidal surgery will be performed, and the surgeon will be aided if the location and size of the pituitary tumor are defined by either a high-resolution CT scan or an MRI scan. MRI scanning does not show the bony structures but is useful for defining vascular structures, the optic chiasm, the optic nerves, and the cavernous sinuses. Only about half of adenomas that cause Cushing's disease are detectable by CT or MRI because they may be very small.[831, 832] The findings vary from upward bulging of the diaphragma sellae to a low-density or enhancing area that represents the microadenoma. Macroadenomas are a rare cause of Cushing's disease and are usually invasive and difficult to cure. It should be remembered that patients with ectopic corticotropin syndrome may have

TABLE 9–32. Test Results in Patients with Cushing's Syndrome of Various Causes

Cause	Low-Dose Dexamethasone*	Plasma Corticotropin	High-Dose Dexamethasone†	Metyrapone‡
Pituitary	No or partial suppression	Normal or elevated	Suppression	Increase in serum 11-deoxycortisol More than doubling urinary 17-hydroxycorticosteroid
Ectopic corticotropin	No suppression	Normal or elevated	No suppression§	No change
Adrenal	No suppression	Low	No suppression	Fall

*Normal response: plasma cortisol <138 nmol/L (<5 μg/dL) at 48 h; urinary free cortisol <55 nmol/d (<20 μg/24 h).
†24-h urinary 17-hydroxycorticosteroid decreases reliably.
‡24-h urinary 17-hydroxycorticosteroid and plasma deoxycortisol.
§5% suppressed: approximately 50% of bronchial carcinoid tumors suppressed.

incidental pituitary adenomas, such as nonfunctioning adenomas or prolactinomas; this emphasizes the importance of making the correct diagnosis based on the biochemical tests.[833]

Because corticotropin levels in a few patients with ectopic corticotropin secretion from bronchial or thymic carcinoids are suppressed by dexamethasone, it is advisable that patients thought to have Cushing's disease have a CT or MRI scan of the chest to exclude a bronchial or thymic tumor. If the results are normal, it is probably worthwhile to obtain an abdominal CT scan to search for pancreatic islet tumor or pheochromocytoma. These studies identify approximately 90% of tumors that cause chronic ectopic corticotropin secretion, but some lesions are too small to be detected and may take as long as 18 y to become manifested.[834]

In contrast occasional patients with biochemical evidence suggesting ectopic corticotropin syndrome may in fact have an aggressive pituitary adenoma. Aggressive corticotropin-secreting pituitary adenomas or carcinomas may not be under negative feedback control by glucocorticoids. In all patients with Cushing's disease a CT or MRI scan of the pituitary should be obtained to exclude this unlikely possibility.

PATHOLOGIC FEATURES. In Cushing's disease the most frequent anatomic finding is a corticotropin-producing microadenoma, measuring less than 1 cm in diameter, in the anterior lobe. It is not surprising that some of these adenomas are difficult or impossible to localize preoperatively even using sensitive and sophisticated methods such as MRI and petrosal sinus catheterization with CRH stimulation and measurement of corticotropin concentrations. In some cases the adenoma is not visible on gross examination of the resected tissue. In these cases serial histologic sections of the removed tissue must be examined to identify an adenoma.

The tumor cells are basophilic and stain positive with the PAS method.[449, 835] Immunocytochemistry demonstrates the presence of corticotropin and other POMC-related peptides such as endorphins and lipotropin in the cytoplasm of adenoma cells.[449, 835–837] Corticotrope adenomas are usually monomorphous and monohormonal. In some cases they exhibit immunoreactivity for α subunit, LH,[838] or prolactin.[839]

The findings on electron microscopy of corticotrope adenomas are characteristic and diagnostic.[449, 835–837] The adenoma cells are elongate or angular with ovoid nuclei that manifest some indentation. The cytoplasm is abundant and has prominent RER, free ribosomes and polysomes, a prominent Golgi complex, a few bundles of keratin that are immunopositive intermediary filaments or type 1 microfilaments, and many secretory granules in the size range of 150 to 450 nm. The granules are spherical, indented, and heart shaped and vary in electron density (Fig. 9–49). Corticotrope adenomas that are large and invade adjacent structures may contain cells with varying degrees of pleomorphism and mitotic figures. The immunocytochemical features of these tumor cells do not differ and in many cases are indistinguishable from those of corticotrope microadenomas.

Another variant is the chromophobe pituitary adenoma

with mild or no PAS positivity and scant immunoreactivity for corticotropin and other POMC-related peptides.[449] By electron microscopy chromophobe tumors contain fewer and smaller secretory granules and contain more free ribosomes and mitochondria and few type 1 filaments.[449] The small basophilic tumors usually grow slowly but are hormonally active. The chromophobic tumors are larger, often invasive, hormonally less active despite larger size, and grow rapidly. It is not clear whether these two types of tumors that differ in morphologic characteristics and biologic behavior arise from the same cell type and differentiate or dedifferentiate after neoplastic transformation, originate from two different clones, or undergo mutation. In brief it is not clear if the morphologic and functional differences are due to heterogeneity or variability of tumor cells. Aggressive, large corticotrope adenomas and

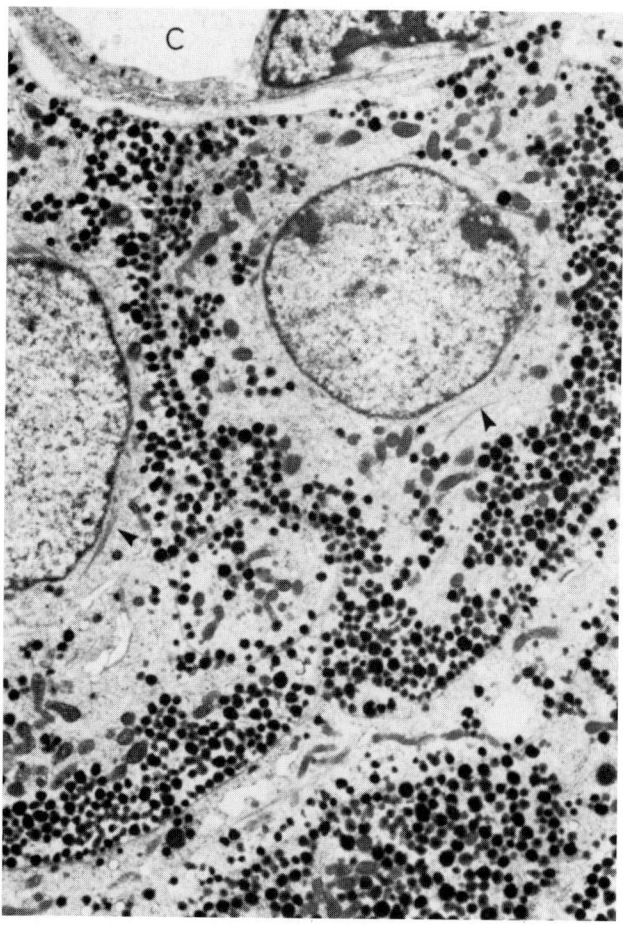

Figure 9–49. Corticotrope cell adenoma with numerous irregular, dented, and heart-shaped secretory granules. Note bundles of type 1 filaments (arrowheads). C, capillary. Magnification × 8150.

carcinomas are often MIB-1 and *p53* immunoreactive. These two immunocytochemical techniques are useful markers to indicate aggressiveness.

Another rare morphologic variant is the so-called Crooke's cell adenoma.[840, 841] It was once thought that Crooke's hyalinization, the morphologic indicator of functional suppression of corticotropes, occurred only in nontumorous corticotropes and not in adenomas. However various degrees of Crooke's hyaline change may occur in some adenomas, suggesting that such tumors are not fully autonomous. The hyaline change is due to accumulation of keratin-positive intermediate filaments and is easily identified[31, 842] on electron microscopy because it consists of bundles of 7-nm-wide type 1 filaments that have no periodicity, are not membrane bound, and are located in the perinuclear areas.[449, 835–837] In advanced forms the filaments almost completely occupy the cytoplasm, and only a few secretory granules are located under the plasmalemma and the Golgi area (Fig. 9–50). Crooke's cell adenomas cause heterogeneous manifestations. Some produce severe Cushing's disease, and others produce mild disease.[841] The reason for these differences is not understood.

Nelson's syndrome develops after bilateral adrenalectomy in patients with Cushing's disease. Nelson's syndrome is now uncommon because patients with Cushing's disease are usually treated with pituitary surgery instead of bilateral adrenalectomy. The adenomas of Nelson's syndrome are rapidly growing, often invasive, basophilic, and PAS-positive.[449, 835] The tumor cells are immunoreactive for corticotropin and other POMC-related peptides, and the electron microscopic features are indistinguishable from those of patients with Cushing's

disease and intact adrenal glands. The only ultrastructural difference is the scarcity or absence of type 1 filaments in the adenoma of Nelson's syndrome, further evidence that glucocorticoid hormones are probably essential for the formation of cytoplasmic type 1 filaments. Another difference between Nelson's syndrome and Cushing's disease is that in Nelson's syndrome the tumors are usually larger, grow more rapidly, are frequently invasive, and have nuclear and cellular pleomorphism; mitotic figures are more frequent. These differences are consistent with the concept that corticotrope adenomas are not completely autonomous but are responsive tumors whose secretory activity and growth rate can be suppressed or modulated by glucocorticoid hormones.

Another tumor type that should be mentioned is the silent "corticotrope" adenoma, subtype 1.[446, 447, 449, 835–837, 843] These tumors are not associated with clinical or biochemical evidence of corticotropin hypersecretion and are classified as nonfunctioning or nonsecretory. However these tumors are morphologically indistinguishable from those of Cushing's disease, and the tumor cells are immunoreactive for corticotropin and other POMC-related peptides. On electron microscopy there is no difference between subtype 1 silent corticotrope adenomas and functional corticotropin-secreting tumors. The silent corticotrope adenoma contains large amounts of POMC mRNA, implying that the gene product is probably processed differently[844] and does not lead to hypercortisolism.

Corticotrope hyperplasia may be found in pituitaries of elderly patients who die of unrelated causes. The hyperplasia is discovered incidentally at autopsy in patients who had no endocrine symptoms. Hormone levels are usually not measured. This idiopathic corticotrope hyperplasia with no obvious functional consequences is not understood.

Corticotrope hyperplasia is a controversial issue, although there is no doubt that non-neoplastic accumulation of corticotropes may be responsible for pituitary Cushing's disease.[449, 835–837, 845–853] However the pathologic diagnosis of corticotrope hyperplasia in the usually fragmented surgical biopsy specimens is difficult and in some cases impossible. Because corticotrope hyperplasia and adenoma may rarely coexist, serial sectioning of all available tissue is required in suspected cases of hyperplasia. Corticotrope hyperplasia may be diffuse but is usually present in a combination of diffuse and nodular forms.[851] The light microscopic and electron microscopic features of corticotropes with diffuse hyperplasia resemble those of Crooke's cells, whereas the smaller, angular corticotropes in nodules are similar to those of adenomatous corticotropes. Corticotrope hyperplasia has been observed in CRH-producing gangliocytoma,[853] CRH-producing extrapituitary tumors,[830, 854–856] and pituitaries of patients with adrenal insufficiency.[857]

Corticotrope carcinomas are rare.[31, 858, 859] The diagnosis is made only when invasion and distant metastases are present. The carcinomas may cause Cushing's disease and exhibit considerable nuclear and cytoplasmic pleomorphism and many mitotic figures. The tumor cells are often chromophobic and either PAS-negative or slightly PAS-positive. However basophilic, PAS-positive tumors may also behave as carcinomas; the tumor cells are immunoreactive for corticotropin and other POMC-related peptides. Electron microscopy shows rather poorly differentiated pleomorphic corticotropes that are usually sparsely granulated. In corticotrope carcinoma, MIB-1 and *p53* immunopositivity is present.

In some cases the pituitary appears normal in patients with biochemical evidence of Cushing's disease, except that Crooke's hyaline change is present. These cases are difficult to interpret. An adenoma may have been present, but either it was not removed or, if removed, it was not identified in the available sections. Alternatively corticotropes may have been hyperactive without an increase in the cell mass.

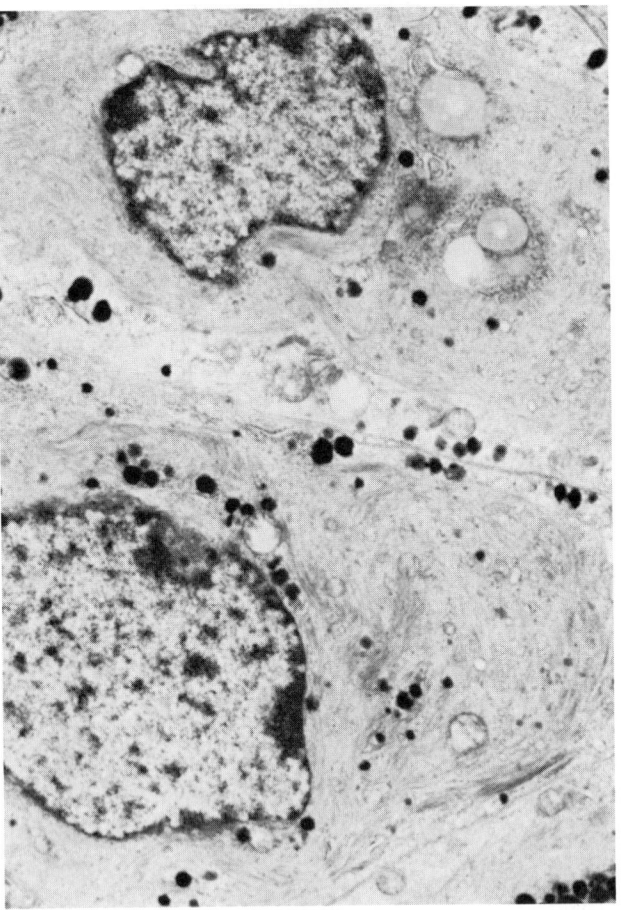

Figure 9–50. Corticotrope cell adenoma displaying advanced Crooke's hyalinization. Most of the cytoplasm is occupied by a thick ring of type 1 filaments displacing secretory granules to the cell periphery. Magnification × 12,550.

Cushing's syndrome includes all patients with hypercortisolism who have no primary pituitary abnormalities. In patients with a nonpituitary cause of Cushing's syndrome, the pituitary shows various degrees of Crooke's hyaline change; no adenoma or corticotrope hyperplasia is present. However the Crooke's hyaline change is a valuable morphologic indicator of glucocorticoid excess. There is substantial individual variation, and the degree of Crooke's hyaline change does not indicate the severity or duration of glucocorticoid excess. The Crooke's hyaline change is reversible; after correction of glucocorticoid excess the corticotropes regain normal morphologic features.

In some cases the morphologic characteristics of corticotropes do not permit distinction between Cushing's disease and Cushing's syndrome. In CRH excess caused by a CRH-producing extrahypothalamic tumor, Crooke's hyaline change and corticotrope hyperplasia are both present. In the ectopic corticotropin syndrome Crooke's hyaline change may be marked, but the number of corticotropes is normal and no corticotrope adenoma is found. In Nelson's syndrome and adrenal insufficiency, Crooke's hyaline change is not present. Some extrapituitary tumors (bronchial carcinoids) may produce both corticotropin and CRH.[856]

It appears that some corticotrope adenomas may arise in the pars intermedia corticotropes.[860] This concept is controversial and has not been confirmed.[861] Corticotropin immunoreactivity is rarely present in plurihormonal adenomas, which are not associated with Cushing's disease.

TREATMENT. In this section the therapeutic strategy for Cushing's disease is discussed; the strategy for other types of Cushing's syndrome is discussed in Chapter 12.

The diagnosis of Cushing's disease should be made after a thorough evaluation, and there should be little doubt that the patient has a corticotropin-secreting pituitary adenoma. The therapeutic objective is to effect a cure without causing permanent pituitary insufficiency. The ideal approach is to remove the pituitary adenoma selectively, whereas in the past the treatment was total bilateral adrenalectomy. The advantages of pituitary surgery are that it restores normal physiology, obviates the risk of Nelson's syndrome, and avoids bilateral adrenalectomy, which is associated with greater morbidity and mortality and requires chronic glucocorticoid and mineralocorticoid replacement.

Surgical Therapy. Selective removal of a pituitary adenoma can be achieved by transsphenoidal surgery. Other than standard contraindications to surgery, such as cardiac or severe pulmonary disease, the specific contraindications to transsphenoidal surgery include a pituitary gland that is inaccessible because of abnormal bony or vascular structures at the skull base. In patients with microadenomas operated on by a surgeon experienced with transsphenoidal microadenectomy, the cure rate is approximately 80%.[862–868] If a tumor is not visible after careful and methodical exploration of the gland, either a total hypophysectomy (in a patient without the capacity or desire for reproduction) or a hemihypophysectomy is usually performed. If a tumor is not visualized on imaging studies, petrosal sampling[17, 829] that suggests lateralization of the side of corticotropin production makes hemihypophysectomy more rational. In all cases the median wedge is carefully explored and usually resected, as the concentration of corticotropin cells is highest there. The operative results are less successful if dural invasion is present resulting from an inability to remove the tumor totally because of invasion of bone or dura, or both.

The patient with Cushing's disease is treated like any other patient with a pituitary tumor, including evaluation of all anterior pituitary function and assessment of visual function before surgery. If the effects of excessive cortisol production are marked and if there is concern about operative morbidity, medical therapy to inhibit cortisol synthesis (ketoconazole or metyrapone) should be initiated before surgery. Glucocorticoids are not usually administered before or during surgery so that the effect of surgery can be determined during the immediate postoperative period. If surgery is successful, glucocorticoid therapy may need to be continued for several months until the hypothalamus and residual corticotrope cells resume function. Successfully treated patients are initially given hydrocortisone, 20 mg on waking and 10 mg at 6 PM or 15 mg on waking and 5 mg at 6 PM. Hydrocortisone has the advantage of being short-acting and thus encourages recovery of the hypothalamic-pituitary axis. Patients may have symptoms of steroid withdrawal after successful surgery, even with adequate replacement. The longer the delay in recovery of the hypothalamic-pituitary-adrenal axis, the better the prognosis for sustained cure; total recovery may take as long as 18 mo. Replacement principles in children treated for Cushing's disease are similar, but the recurrence rate in children is higher than in adults.

Radiation Therapy. Another treatment of Cushing's disease is pituitary radiation. Usually 45 to 50 Gy is given by conventional fractionated teletherapy with a linear accelerator over a 5-wk period. This is successful in about 80% of cases of childhood Cushing's disease[869] but is successful in only 15 to 20% of adults.[870] Similar pituitary radiation (for acromegaly) carries a risk of anterior pituitary dysfunction that may develop 10 y or more after treatment.[508] It is unlikely that patients with Cushing's disease are immune to this effect. Less common complications of radiotherapy include damage to the optic nerves or chiasm, damage to the vascular system, and development of secondary brain tumors. Other forms of radiation therapy, including alpha particle and proton beam therapy, are contraindicated in tumors with extrasellar extension (suprasellar or lateral extension). They also carry a significant risk of hypopituitarism and cranial nerve injury. Focused stereotactic radiotherapy and "radiosurgery" using the Gamma Knife, stereotactic linear accelerator, or a stereotactic proton beam has been applied to the treatment of Cushing's disease and other pituitary adenomas. Most of these treatments are single dose. The short-term outcome with regard to disease control, incidence of iatrogenic hypothalamic dysfunction and hypopituitarism, and complications such as damage to visual pathways is at least as good as with conventional radiation therapy, and these methods may offer advantages for some patients.

Radiation therapy is recommended routinely for patients who undergo bilateral adrenalectomy for Cushing's disease to avoid the risk of Nelson's syndrome, the aggressive growth of the pituitary adenoma after bilateral adrenalectomy, and loss of negative feedback effects of adrenal steroids.[870]

Because radiation therapy and transsphenoidal surgery produce similar results in children, it is difficult to be dogmatic about the best approach. In a center with excellent transsphenoidal surgery, however, this procedure is recommended with the hope of effecting a cure and avoiding hypopituitarism. The surgeon will be more conservative in a child than in an adult and if no tumor is found, a hemihypophysectomy may be considered. If the patient is not cured, postoperative radiation therapy remains an option.

Medical Therapy. Medical therapy for Cushing's disease is adjunctive only. It is used to reduce cortisol production in preparing an extremely ill patient for surgery and to maintain normal plasma cortisol levels while awaiting the full effects of radiation. The goal is to inhibit the enzymes responsible for cortisol synthesis with drugs such as metyrapone, aminoglutethimide, and ketoconazole. Metyrapone and aminoglutethimide have been the standard therapy, and when the two agents are used in combination, side effects may be decreased. Steroid synthesis may be inhibited completely so that replacement glucocorticoid therapy is required. Because aminoglutethimide stimulates hepatic enzymes that degrade dexamethasone, hydrocortisone should be used for replacement therapy. Ketoconazole, a broad-spectrum antimycotic drug, inhibits adrenal steroid biosynthesis at several sites, including side chain cleavage and 11β-hydroxylation.[871, 872] It is administered 800 to 1200 mg/d until normal plasma cortisol levels are achieved, after which the dose may be adjusted to maintain that state. All these drugs are expensive and have significant side effects.[872, 873]

Other medical therapies, such as the use of cyproheptadine and bromocriptine to reduce pituitary corticotropin secretion, are effective in few patients. Those who respond to bromocriptine may have intermediate lobe tumors,[860] but this concept is unconfirmed.[861]

Nelson's Syndrome

Nelson's syndrome results from the development of an aggressive corticotropin-secreting pituitary adenoma in patients who have undergone bilateral adrenalectomy for Cushing's disease.[874] These patients experience symptoms of a mass, including headaches, visual field defects, and external ophthalmoplegia. The high corticotropin levels cause hyperpigmentation similar to that seen in adrenal insufficiency. Because a pituitary tumor that secreted corticotropin was present prior to surgery, this syndrome presumably represents enhancement of the tumor growth by removal of the negative feedback of excessive cortisol from the adrenal glands. The incidence of Nelson's syndrome may be 10 to 50%. This syndrome has been shown to be preventable by external pituitary radiation in some[869, 870] but not all studies.[875, 876]

The diagnosis is suspected from the characteristic history and physical findings. Plasma corticotropin levels are high, often ranging from 220 pmol/L (1000 pg/mL) to 2200 pmol/L (10,000 pg/mL) or higher. However the level of corticotropin does not accurately reflect the size or aggressiveness of the tumor. The presence of the tumor is confirmed by CT or MRI scan. In contrast to the tumors of Cushing's disease, these tumors are usually macroadenomas.

Nelson's syndrome is preventable. Because pituitary microsurgery is the preferred initial treatment of Cushing's disease, this condition is likely to become of historical interest. Once the diagnosis of Nelson's syndrome is made, the treatment should be aggressive, as these tumors are locally invasive and grow rapidly. Pituitary surgery is the preferred treatment. Most neurosurgeons approach the tumor by the transsphenoidal route and resect as much tumor as possible. If residual tumor is known to be present, the patient should undergo pituitary radiation, particularly if the tumor was not previously radiated.[790] The secretion of corticotropin by the tumor is responsive to endogenous CRH and AVP. Thus by optimizing negative feedback to the hypothalamus through a long-acting glucocorticoid and judiciously timing its administration to reverse the normal glucocorticoid rhythm, hypothalamic stimulation of the tumor can be minimized; a suggested regimen is 0.25 to 0.5 mg dexamethasone on retiring. This approach has not been demonstrated to be superior but is logical and is used by several groups.

Glycoprotein-Producing Adenomas

Glycoprotein adenomas produce LH, FSH, thyrotropin, or the α subunit, either alone or in combination, and may or may not result in increased serum hormone levels. When the serum hormone concentrations are normal, glycoprotein hormone production may be detectable by in vitro studies such as RIA of medium from pituitary tumor cell cultures, detection of specific mRNAs in tumor extracts, in situ hybrid-ization, or immunocytochemical staining of surgical specimens. Identification of hormone production by serum measurements and by in vitro techniques indicates that glycoprotein production may occur in as many as 24% of surgical specimens.[877] These tumors may arise spontaneously without an identifiable cause,[878] although one hypothesis about the origin of FSH-secreting tumors is that gonadotrope hyperplasia can develop into an adenoma in the setting of primary gonadal failure. However gonadal failure rarely precedes tumor development, and there is no gonadotrope hyperplasia in the nontumorous pituitary. In addition the gonadal failure of menopause is not associated with an increase in the incidence of this tumor. Another theory is that increased FSH production results from a nonsecretory adenoma that impairs LH but not FSH secretion.[879]

Patients with glycoprotein-producing adenomas usually come to medical attention because of manifestations of a mass lesion or, in the case of a thyrotropin-secreting tumor, because of hyperthyroidism. Glycoprotein tumors are usually diagnosed in middle-aged men (mean age 55 y) because of symptoms of headache, visual disturbance, and acquired hypogonadism. The tumors are uncommon in women of reproductive age, and the prevalence in postmenopausal women is unknown because serum LH and FSH concentrations may be appropriately increased. However in some patients the gonadotropin concentrations are depressed. Mild hyperprolactinemia (<200 μg/L) may result from stalk compression. Men commonly have a subnormal serum testosterone level associated with low, normal, or increased LH and FSH concentrations. The reasons for hypogonadism are unclear, and it has been attributed to depressed bioactive LH secretion, secretion of abnormally glycosylated gonadotropins, or abnormal gonadotropin pulsations.[878]

THYROTROPE ADENOMA. The thyrotropin adenoma is the least common type of pituitary tumor, representing less than 1% of the total, and is the only glycoprotein tumor that produces a syndrome of hormone excess.[880] Common features include symptoms due to the pituitary mass lesion and hyperthyroidism with goiter. The most important biochemical feature is elevation of serum thyroid hormone levels (T_4 and T_3) with an inappropriately "normal" or increased serum thyrotropin level. Because the use of a sensitive thyrotropin assay distinguishes between normal and suppressed values, the diagnosis of a thyrotropin-secreting adenoma is easy. Although this tumor is uncommon, it should be excluded by measurement of the serum thyrotropin concentration in patients with hyperthyroidism. Serum thyrotropin levels may be markedly increased, but about one third of patients with a thyrotropin-secreting adenoma have values less than 10 mU/L.[878, 881] The tumor also frequently secretes free α subunit, which is elevated in more than 80% of patients.[882, 883] The molar ratio of α subunit to thyrotropin may be helpful in distinguishing a thyrotropin-secreting adenoma from other forms of hyperthyroidism; a ratio of serum α subunit to thyrotropin greater than 1 is common in thyrotropin tumors. Other secretory products of thyrotrope adenomas include GH and prolactin. The diagnosis of acromegaly or hyperprolactinemia may be evident only when the patient seeks medical care for symptoms of hyperthyroidism. As noted measurement of the serum α subunit concentration is helpful for the diagnosis of a thyrotropin-secreting adenoma and aids in excluding the syndrome of pituitary resistance to thyroid hormone, in which serum thyrotropin concentrations are inappropriately increased in the setting of hyperthyroxinemia (see Chapter 11). Serum α subunit concentrations are not increased in the syndrome of pituitary resistance to thyroid hormone. In addition administration of TRH to patients with thyrotropin-secreting tumors does not produce an increase in serum thyrotropin, but patients with pituitary resistance to thyroid hormone may have an exaggerated increase in serum thyrotropin level.[882]

The initial treatment of a thyrotropin-secreting adenoma is surgical. As with all large pituitary tumors, however, complete resection may not be possible. Medical treatment with octreotide lowers serum thyrotropin concentrations, results in a euthyroid state, and promotes tumor shrinkage.[884] Postoperative pituitary radiation may be employed for residual tumor. If hyperthyroidism persists, treatment with antithyroid drugs may be necessary.

Pathologic Features of Thyrotrope Tumors. Morphologically indistinguishable thyrotrope tumors may be associated with hyperthyroidism,[885–888] hypothyroidism,[889–891] or euthyroidism. Thus the morphologic features of these tumors do not reflect the endocrine function and no conclusions can be drawn regarding hormone secretion from morphologic studies.

Thyrotrope adenomas are chromophobic tumors that may contain a few PAS-positive granules or larger globules, especially in patients with prolonged primary hypothyroidism.[449] Densely granulated tumors with cytoplasmic basophilia are rare. By immunocytochemistry the adenoma cells immunostain for the βα subunits of thyrotropin. The tumor cells are polyhedral, elongated, and sometimes tall and columnar, forming pseudorosettes around vessels. The adenomas have a distinct border, and the cells show no major pleomorphism. By electron microscopy[449, 890, 892, 893] the tumor cells are elongated and polar and have long cytoplasmic processes, a spherical or ovoid nucleus, and prominent nucleoli. The RER and Golgi complexes are moderately or well developed, and cytoplasmic microtubules often form a rich network. The secretory granules are small and spherical, vary slightly in electron density, most commonly measure between 50 and 200 nm, and are frequently arranged under the plasmalemma in a single row. Exocytosis is not observed (Fig. 9–51).

In autopsy studies the various other cell types in the nontumorous area of the hypophysis harboring a thyrotropin-producing adenoma are normal.[894] In hyperthyroidism thyrotropes are normal or small, suggesting functional inhibition. In patients with prolonged primary hypothyroidism the thyrotropes are numerous and large with abundant cytoplasm ("thyroidectomy cells"), and increased mass of the pituitary may simulate a pituitary adenoma. In the thyrotrope tumor large hypothyroid-associated (thyroidectomy) cells are rare.

Some plurihormonal tumors produce several hormones, including thyrotropin.[449, 450] Synthesis of thyrotropin is not uncommon in plurihormonal adenomas, and densely granulated somatotrope adenomas often contain thyrotropin-positive cells and other α subunit immunoreactive cells.[454] Few of these plurihormonal tumors cause hyperthyroidism; instead the thyrotropin-producing component is usually clinically silent. Thus structural features and functional activity are not always correlated.

Thyrotrope hyperplasia is a well-defined pathologic entity and is easily recognizable in patients with long-standing primary hypothyroidism.[895, 896] Morphologically thyrotrope hyperplasia consists of enlarged, stimulated thyrotropes or thyroid deficiency cells.[250, 568] In some cases overactivity of lactotropes or frank lactotrope hyperplasia is also present.[568] Whether hyperplastic thyrotropes can undergo neoplastic transformation, are the predecessors of a thyrotrope adenoma, and are more susceptible to neoplastic transformation than are normal thyrotropes has not been clarified. One thyrotrope carcinoma has been described, which responded to octreotide and chemotherapy.[897]

GONADOTROPE ADENOMA. Gonadotrope adenomas are identified by increased serum LH, FSH, or α subunit levels or by immunocytochemistry, electron microscopy, or tumor cell culture studies.

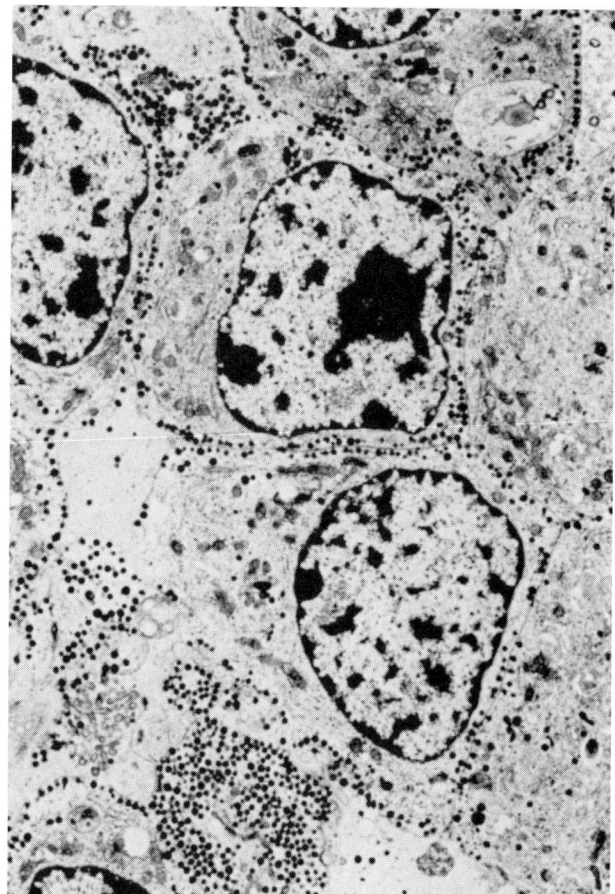

Figure 9–51. Thyrotrope cell adenoma. The angular shape of cells is accentuated by the peripheral localization of small secretory granules. Magnification × 6650.

The prevalence of gonadotrope adenomas is unknown. In one series of 139 men with untreated macroadenomas, 24% had gonadotrope tumors; 17% had hypersecretion of FSH, either alone or in combination with αβ, and FSH β subunits; and 7% had hypersecretion of only the α subunit.[877] Most of these men (87%) had visual impairment indicative of a large tumor. In two studies of surgical specimens, gonadotrope adenomas were present in 3.5 and 4.1% of cases, respectively.[898, 899]

The most commonly observed glycoprotein hormone secreted is FSH, which appears by gel filtration chromatography to be intact FSH.[900] This may be accompanied by an increase in circulating α subunit concentrations, as also occurs in association with LH-secreting tumors. Hypersecretion of intact LH is less common than secretion of intact FSH or free FSH βα subunits. Furthermore the serum LH level may be raised as a result of assay cross-reactivity with free α subunit or LH β subunit; gel filtration chromatography is necessary for precise identification of the secretory product. In most men the serum testosterone concentration is either normal or low because intact LH is not produced. Thus serum LH concentrations are inappropriately normal in the setting of reduced testosterone production. When intact LH is produced, the serum testosterone concentration is greater than normal. Administration of TRH may cause an increase in LH or FSH level after TRH stimulation in about half of patients with gonadatropin adenoma.[877] The FSH and LH responses to exogenous LHRH are variable; approximately 50% of patients with an FSH-secreting tumor have an increase in serum FSH concentration, and serum LH concentration increases less frequently.[901–910]

Gonadotrope adenomas are most commonly diagnosed in middle-aged or older men (mean age 45) who seek medical attention because of visual abnormality or headaches.[877] On testing, they may have biochemical secondary hypogonadism. These tumors are more common in men than in women. The distinction between a nonsecretory adenoma and a gonadotrope adenoma may not be possible clinically or biochemically and may require electron microscopic or immunocytochemical study of the excised tumor. Pre-existing hypogonadism is common.

A history of normal pubertal development, sexual function, and fertility in men with hypersecretion of FSH suggests that the gonadotrope tumor developed spontaneously and did not result from primary hypogonadism. Most tumors do not hypersecrete intact LH, and the serum testosterone level in men may be normal or subnormal. Diagnostic difficulty arises when the serum testosterone level is less than normal and the serum immunoreactive LH level is increased because of increased free α subunit or LH β subunit secretion with assay cross-reactivity; an increased immunoreactive serum LH concentration may erroneously suggest the diagnosis of primary gonadal failure. In this circumstance it is prudent to consider the possibility of a gonadotrope tumor, particularly if there is a history of headache or change in vision. In a man with a subnormal serum testosterone level and an inappropriately normal serum LH concentration, the diagnosis of secondary hypogonadism is evident. A pituitary tumor, gonadotrope or other type, cannot be excluded without an appropriate imaging study.

The initial treatment of a gonadotrope tumor is surgical resection, particularly if visual function is abnormal. Transsphenoidal surgery improves vision in most patients and may correct hormonal hypersecretion, hypogonadism, and the abnormal gonadotropin response to TRH.[911] Persistent hormonal hypersecretion and the presence of residual tumor may require postoperative pituitary radiation treatment.

Medical treatment of gonadotrope adenomas is generally unsatisfactory but a few patients have responded to the dopamine agonist bromocriptine and the somatostatin analogue octreotide. Long-acting LHRH agonists and antagonists may lower serum gonadatropin concentrations but are ineffective in reducing tumor size. Dopamine and its agonists may decrease basal and LHRH-stimulated secretion of gonadotropins and free α subunit.[878] In some patients treatment with bromocriptine has reduced hormone hypersecretion, improved visual abnormalities, and decreased tumor size.[907, 912] However these effects are not consistent; most patients have no response to bromocriptine.[561, 913, 914]

Somatostatin inhibits gonadotropin secretion in vitro and in vivo. The infusion of somatostatin decreases serum levels of α subunit, LH, and FSH by 40 to 60% in patients with gonadotrope tumors,[878] and administration of octreotide decreased serum LH levels in a patient with a gonadatrope adenoma that secreted LH- and α subunit.[915] In another patient octreotide treatment had variable effects on residual tumor mass and serum α subunit concentrations.[916] Studies of the effects of octreotide therapy are necessary before the efficacy can be determined.

Another experimental treatment for gonadotrope adenomas is administration of long-acting LHRH agonists and antagonists to inhibit gonadotropin secretion. LHRH agonists are not consistently successful in reducing hormone hypersecretion or tumor size and may increase serum α subunit levels.[917–920] The LHRH antagonist Nal-Glu LHRH decreased serum FSH levels in several patients with FSH-secreting adenomas but had no effect on tumor size.[921]

In summary the efficacy of the medical treatment of gonadotrope adenomas is not established but is used in an attempt to reduce hormone hypersecretion and tumor size after unsuccessful surgery, while awaiting the effects of pituitary radiation, or in patients who cannot undergo or refuse surgery. Careful monitoring and medical evaluations are necessary.

Pathologic Features of Gonadotrope Adenomas. The frequency of gonadotrope adenomas in surgical specimens ranged from less than 1% to 10% between 1979 and 1989.[903, 922] Gonadotrope adenomas are not as well characterized as other types of pituitary tumors but exhibit clear-cut sex-related ultrastructural dichotomy.[899]

Preoperative diagnosis of gonadotrope adenoma in men is based on the finding of inappropriately high gonadotropin levels.[877, 923–927] The tumors may also cause local mass effects such as visual disturbances, nausea, headaches, and cranial nerve palsies. Gonadotrope adenomas in men[899, 903] are chromophobic or acidophilic. The histologic pattern is usually sinusoidal with pseudorosette formation around vessels. Strong immunoreactivity for FSH or LH, or both, are consistent features and the best diagnostic marker in men. Some adenomas, however, exhibit modest immunoreactivity for FSH or LH (or both) that does not exceed that of many null cell adenomas. The α subunit, which is a fairly consistent clinical marker in gonadotrope adenomas,[904, 928] is not a reliable morphologic indicator. The electron microscopic appearance, which is useful in diagnosing other adenoma types, is variable in gonadotrope adenomas in men.[898, 899, 929] One histologic pattern is that of a well-differentiated tumor consisting of elongate, polar cells with uniform nuclei; well-developed, slightly dilated RER; and a prominent Golgi complex (Fig. 9–52) with sparse secretory granules, 200 nm in diameter, unevenly distributed and more numerous in the basal part of the cytoplasm. Another type of adenoma has the appearance of null cell adenomas.[899, 903] Intermediate forms with cells displaying features of varying degrees of functional differentiation are common. There is no correlation between serum FSH or LH levels and immunoreactivity or ultrastructure. Because of these uncertainties, one method may not be sufficient for diagnosis.

In women with gonadotrope adenomas gonadotropin levels are usually within normal limits and are rarely elevated.[899] The morphologic features of gonadotrope adenoma in women are enigmatic. The well-differentiated chromophobe adenomas display little, if any, immunoreactivity for gonadotropins; strong generalized immunostaining is rare. However by electron microscopy these sparsely granulated tumors are characterized by a unique morphologic marker, the "honeycomb Golgi complex" (Fig. 9–53). The sacculi of Golgi apparatus is transformed into clusters of spheres containing low-density proteinaceous substance. Few if any immature secretory granules are present in these membrane systems, probably indicating impaired packaging of secretory material, which in turn may be the cause of sparse immunoreactivity in these tumors.

No gonadotropin-producing carcinoma has been reported.

Hyperplasia of gonadotrope cells is poorly studied. One case of diffuse, massive gonadotrope hyperplasia at autopsy was associated with Klinefelter's syndrome. In contrast to what might have been expected, gonadatrope hyperplasia does not occur after menopause.

Nonsecretory Adenoma

A nonsecretory or nonfunctioning pituitary tumor, sometimes called a chromophobe adenoma, is characterized by the absence of a distinct clinical syndrome and the presence of normal serum hormone levels. About 25 to 30% of tumors are classified as nonsecretory. However on morphologic examination, these tumors always contain secretory granules suggesting hormone synthesis and storage.[930] Many of these tumors are gonadotrope, α subunit, or corticotrope tumors. In addition a tumor may be immunopositive for more than one hormone, with combinations including α subunit, LH β, FSH β, hCG β, thyrotropin β, and corticotropin.[931] In vitro studies of cultured cells and techniques using in situ hybridization have confirmed that these tumors may produce α subunit, LH β subunit, and hCG β subunit.[932] Normal serum hormone levels are believed to be due to defective post-translational processing. With increased availability of specific glycoprotein subunit assays, more presumptive nonfunctioning tumors will probably be recognized as glycoprotein-producing tumors.

The majority of nonsecretory adenomas are diagnosed because of mass effects (headache, visual disturbance) or symptoms of hypopituitarism such as adrenal insufficiency, hypothyroidism or, more commonly, hypogonadism. These tumors are more common in men and postmenopausal women. A mild or moderate elevation of serum prolactin level (<200 µg/L) is common and is thought to reflect stalk compression. Despite an increase in serum prolactin level, large tumors with a mild hyperprolactinemia are not prolactinomas.

Pretreatment evaluation includes investigation of pituitary function, including measurement of serum levels of prolactin, IGF-I (as a measure of GH secretion), LH, FSH, thyrotropin, and α subunit. If assays are available, LH β, and thyrotropin β subunit should also be measured. The need for hormone replacement, particularly cortisol and levothyroxine, should be assessed by measuring basal levels of T_4, cortisol, and testosterone (men). If these values are abnormal, replacement is necessary. A normal morning cortisol level is not sufficient to

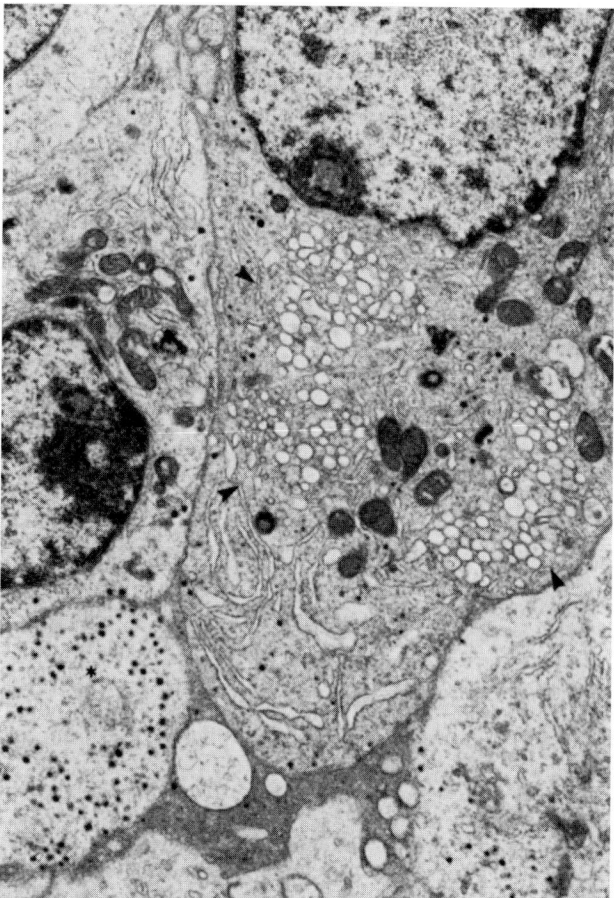

Figure 9–53. Gonadotrope adenoma, female type, containing "honeycomb Golgi complex," the diagnostic marker of the tumor type *(arrowheads)*. Most of the small (150 nm) secretory granules collect in cytoplasmic processes *(asterisk)*. Magnification × 12,750.

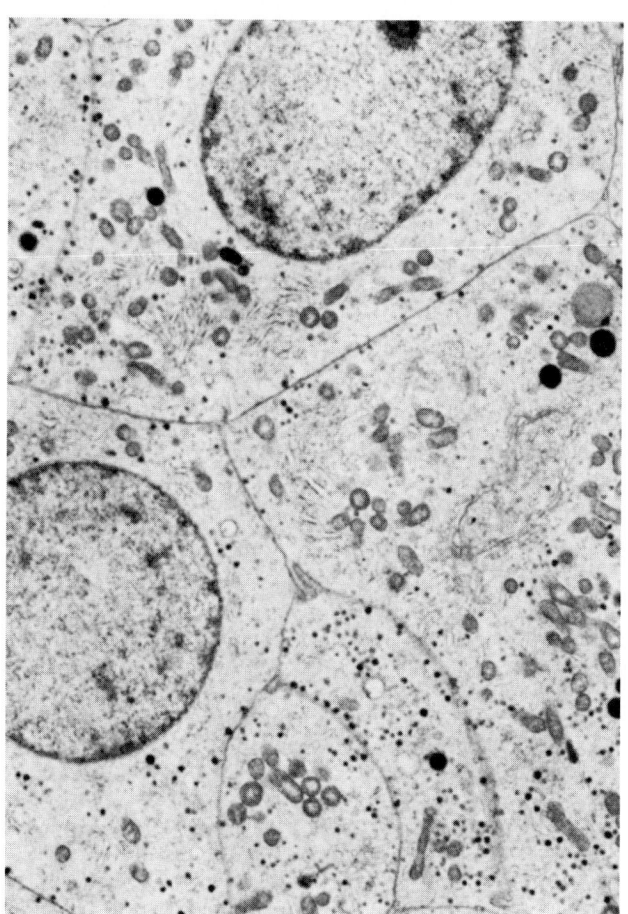

Figure 9–52. Gonadotrope adenoma, male type, featuring uniform euchromatic nuclei, slightly dilated RER, a prominent Golgi complex with regular appearance, and small, unevenly distributed secretory granules. Magnification × 10,000. RER, rough endoplasmic reticulum.

exclude impairment of the hypothalamic-pituitary-adrenal axis; a stimulatory test, such as insulin-induced hypoglycemia or the metyrapone test, is required for assessment. The ophthalmologic examination includes funduscopy, ocular motility determination, assessment of visual acuity, and quantitative assessment of visual fields. A gadolinium-enhanced MRI or coronal CT scan with contrast should be obtained.

The recommended treatment for a nonsecretory tumor is surgical excision, usually via the transsphenoidal approach. A large tumor with extrasellar extension may not be completely resectable, but debulking of the tumor may improve visual abnormalities or minimize the potential for future loss. The transfrontal approach is rarely used because of the higher rates of morbidity and mortality unless most of the tumor is suprasellar, producing signs of brain compression. Transsphenoidal resection usually results in improvement in visual abnormalities and amelioration of headaches. In one study significant residual tumor or recurrence of tumor was present in 20% of patients after 1 y. Tumor recurred in 18% of patients who received postoperative radiotherapy and in 12% who did not. However because radiotherapy was administered to those with known or suspected residual disease, the two groups are not comparable.[516]

Residual tumor is usually treated with postoperative conventional or focused (e.g., Gamma Knife) radiotherapy. If the patient is unable to undergo surgery or if the tumor is asymptomatic and intrasellar (uncommon) and vision is normal, pituitary radiation with monitoring of pituitary function, tumor size, and vision is an alternative primary therapy. The response to pituitary radiation is similar to that of other pituitary tumors; prompt reduction in tumor size is rare but additional tumor growth may be inhibited.

Medical treatment of nonsecretory tumors with dopamine agonists has been used in a small number of patients. Nonsecretory tumors have fewer high-affinity membrane-bound dopamine receptors than are found in prolactin-secreting tumors,[933] and despite isolated reports of reduction in tumor size, dopamine agonist treatment is unsuccessful in most patients.[563, 914, 933–935] However because occasional patients respond to dopamine agonist treatment, a trial of bromocriptine may be warranted if a patient is unwilling or unable to undergo surgery.

The postoperative management is identical to that of any patient undergoing pituitary surgery and should include assessment of the visual system and the endocrine system. Anatomic assessment should include MRI or CT within 4 to 6 wk after surgery and yearly thereafter. If there is evidence of residual tumor, pituitary radiation is usually given to prevent an increase in tumor size. If no tumor is visible on the postoperative or the 6- and 12-mo scans, radiologic evaluation can be performed at yearly intervals.

PATHOLOGIC FEATURES OF NONFUNCTIONING PITUITARY ADENOMAS. These adenomas represent approximately 25% of pituitary tumors in surgical material.[449] The histologic appearance was confusing for many years, and several names were used for these tumors,[449] including chromophobic, nonfunctioning, undifferentiated, precursor cell, fetal, and embryonic adenomas. None of these names satisfactorily expresses their real nature. Nonfunctioning pituitary adenomas can be divided into two groups: null cell adenomas (including oncocytomas) and silent adenomas. The term *null cell adenoma*[936, 937] reflects the main characteristic of these tumors, the lack of morphologic, immunocytochemical, or ultrastructural markers that reveal their cellular origin. Null cell adenomas are histologically chromophobic or slightly acidophilic PAS-negative tumors.[449, 451, 936–938] Either immunocytochemistry yields negative results for anterior pituitary hormones or groups of adenoma cells may be immunoreactive for one or more pituitary hormones—most frequently FSH or the α subunit, or both, less frequently thyrotropin, LH, GH, prolactin, or corticotropin. Null cell adenomas do not secrete hormones, as shown by in vitro studies in which hormones were measured in the culture media by RIA and by the reverse hemolytic plaque assay.[939, 940] mRNA for glycoprotein hormones can be demonstrated in many of these tumors,[932] and corticotropin and prolactin mRNAs may also be present.[941] Electron microscopy shows that null cell adenomas contain secretory granules characteristic of endocrine differentiation,[449, 936, 937] but the hormone-producing machinery of the cells is poorly developed (Fig. 9–54). The secretory granules are sparse and small, 50 to 200 nm in diameter, and no exocytosis is observed. Some null cell adenomas have immunoreactivity for neuron-specific enolase, chromogranin, or synaptophysin, or a combination.[937]

Null cell adenomas can be divided into nononcocytic and oncocytic tumors;[449, 936, 937] oncocytomas contain large numbers of mitochondria[942–945] that cause the cytoplasm to be granular and take up acidic dyes. Oncocytomas also show focal immunostaining for one or more anterior pituitary hormones, mainly FSH and the α subunit.[937] They produce hormones in vitro, release mainly FSH and α subunit[939] as shown by the reverse hemolytic plaque assay, and express mRNA primarily for glycoprotein hormones.[932] The cause of mitochondrial accumulation is not known. Oncocytomas are characteristic on electron microscopy because of the numerous mitochondria (Fig. 9–55),[945] which may account for 40 to 45% of cytoplasmic volume. Despite mitochondrial abundance, RER membranes, Golgi complexes, and secretory granules can be recognized.

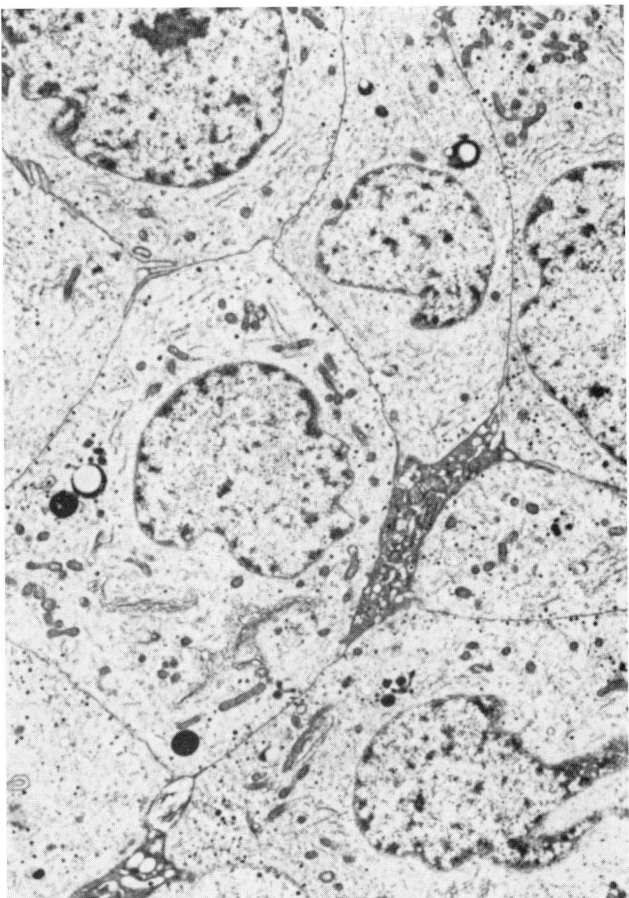

Figure 9–54. Null cell adenoma with poorly developed RER and Golgi complex and scant secretory granules. Magnification × 6850. RER, rough endoplasmic reticulum.

Null cell adenomas contain various receptors, including those for dopamine[933] and somatostatin.[946]

Null cell adenomas resemble gonadotrope adenomas.[899, 937, 939, 947] The histologic and ultrastructural features are indistinguishable in some tumors in men,[899] and the immunocytochemical profile may also be similar. Both null cell adenomas and gonadotrope adenomas may be immunoreactive for FSH and the α subunit,[939, 945, 947] and the FSH, LH, and α subunit genes are expressed in both tumor types.[932] Thus the question arises whether one should distinguish between null cell adenomas and gonadotrope adenomas or consider null cell adenomas as a variant of gonadotrope adenomas. However some null cell adenomas are not immunoreactive for glycoprotein hormones and do not express their genes, whereas others are immunoreactive and express genes for additional hormones such as prolactin or corticotropin,[941] clearly indicating that the null cell adenoma–oncocytoma category is heterogeneous. With refinement of diagnostic techniques, some null cell adenomas will be categorized as functioning tumors. Derivation of others may remain obscure because of the absence of endocrine activity; these are usually slowly growing large tumors that cause local symptoms such as visual defects.

Silent adenomas encompass three morphologic subtypes of well-differentiated tumors with characteristic ultrastructural appearances, distinct in two of the subtypes from those of other adenomas.[446–448, 843] These adenomas are apparently functionless and, apart from occasional hyperprolactinemia,[843] are not associated with elevated serum levels of known pituitary hormones. Although the cause of the lack of function is not established, it is assumed that silent adenomas are derived from pituitary cell types not yet characterized and elaborate hormones that do not cause conspicuous clinical syndromes.

Silent "corticotrope" adenoma subtype 1 is morphologicly indistinguishable from corticotrope adenomas that cause Cushing's disease.[446, 447, 843, 844] The tumors are macroadenomas at the time of diagnosis, and approximately 40% are associated with symptoms of recent hemorrhage.[449] The type is somewhat more common in women. Electron microscopy may reveal accumulation of lysosomes and follicle formation.[446] These structural features are common in the pars intermedia and in the posterior lobe basophils that may be the precursor cell of the tumor. In all cases examined, in situ hybridization reveals strong expression of the *POMC* gene.[844] The post-translational processing of the gene product has not been characterized.

Silent "corticotrope" adenoma subtype 2 is clinically similar to a nonfunctional macroadenoma.[447, 449] This tumor type displays a marked (4:1) male preponderance. Histologically these tumors are chromophobes or show mild basophilia and PAS positivity. Varying degrees of immunoreactivity for corticotropin and other POMC-derived peptides are present. Ultrastructurally the adenomas are well differentiated and consist of polyhedral cells without polarity (Fig. 9–56). The secretory granules are similar morphologically to corticotrope granules, including numerous drop-shaped forms, but are smaller (less than 400 nm, chiefly 200 to 300 nm). Unlike subtype 1, subtype 2 tumors contain no type 1 filaments. Morphologic studies suggest that the tumor also produces POMC and a hormone as yet uncharacterized. The cell of derivation is unknown. Cells morphologically similar to cells of silent corticotrope adenoma subtype 2 are present in normal, nontumorous pituitary gland.

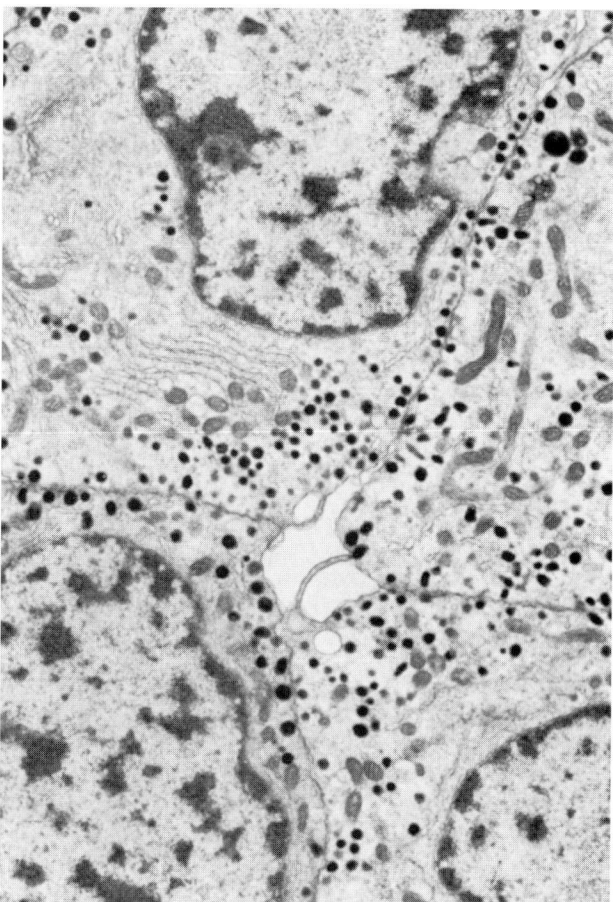

Figure 9–56. Silent "corticotrope" adenoma, subtype 2. The rather small, polyhedral cells contain irregular nuclei, moderately developed RER and Golgi complex, and numerous, often drop-shaped, rod-shaped, or dented secretory granules. Magnification × 11,900.

Subtype 3 silent adenomas[447, 449] were originally thought to consist of POMC-producing cells because several tumors showed variable immunoreactivity for corticotropin and other POMC-related peptides. However some such tumors are immunonegative for corticotropin. Scattered adenoma cells are immunoreactive for GH, prolactin, or one or more glycoprotein hormones.[448] By electron microscopy the tumor cells resemble well-differentiated gonadatropes (Fig. 9–57) and are composed of large, irregular polar cells with abundant cytoplasm containing well-developed rough (and often smooth) endoplasmic reticulum membranes and prominent Golgi complexes. The secretory granules are sparse, more numerous in cell processes, and measure about 200 nm. Ultrastructural studies suggest that these cells are in a hyperactive state, but the hormonal product is unknown. There is no sex predilection for this tumor type. In young women the tumors may be mistaken for prolactin-producing adenomas because of the associated hyperprolactinemia. Treatment with a dopamine agonist reduces serum prolactin levels but does not affect tumor size, and the excess prolactin appears to be secreted by nontumorous lactotropes. Because hyperprolactinemia is present when the tumor is still small, stalk compression is not likely to play a role. One possibility is that the tumor produces a factor that stimulates prolactin release from nontumorous lactotropes.

Silent tumors also occur in adenomas with known cell derivation. Several gonadotrope adenomas and a few thyrotrope tumors are not associated with clinical evidence of hormone overproduction. Some sparsely granulated GH cell ade-

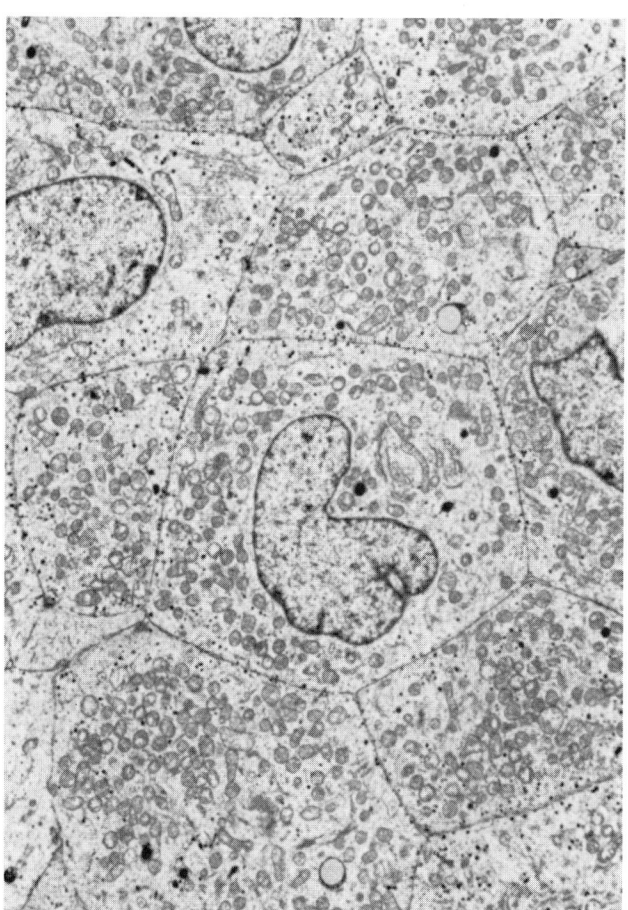

Figure 9–55. Pituitary oncocytoma showing abundance of mitochondria. Magnification × 5050.

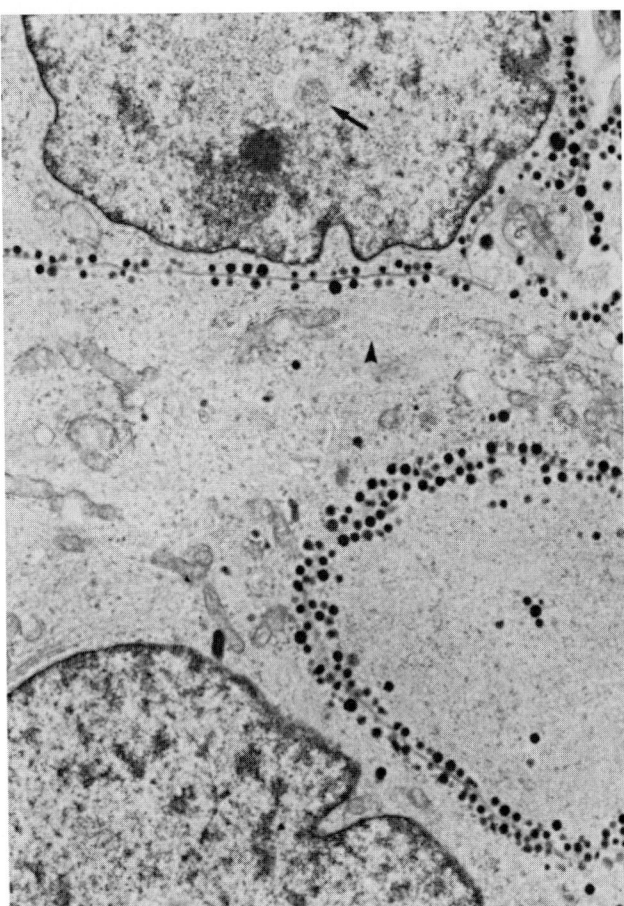

Figure 9–57. Silent adenoma subtype 3. The large cytoplasm is filled with arrays of delicate, partly rough and partly smooth endoplasmic reticulum *(arrowhead)* and Golgi membranes. The small secretory granules are often located at the cell periphery. Note prominent nuclear inclusion (spheridium) *(arrow)*. Magnification × 12,550.

nomas may also be clinically silent.[948] Such tumors have a typical ultrastructure, but GH immunoreactivity is sparse or almost absent. However in situ hybridization shows expression of the GH gene in some tumor cells. This finding indicates that the GH gene is transcribed, but either the message is not translated or the gene product is not processed into a biologically active hormone in sufficient amounts to be clinically detectable.

Plurihormonal adenomas also have silent areas.[449, 450] With the exception of mixed GH cell–prolactin cell adenomas, one morphologic cell type is predominant in plurihormonal adenomas, and the corresponding hormone is oversecreted and causes clinical manifestations, whereas other hormones are detectable in trace quantities only.

The discrepancy between morphologic features and endocrine activity in silent adenomas is difficult to explain. In reality many silent adenomas are pseudosilent. As judged by their ultrastructure, all three subtypes of silent adenomas are believed to produce and release unknown hormones that cause no obvious manifestations. The silence of some GH adenomas may be explained by the lack of bioactivity of the product, by subtlety of the clinical features, or by abnormal processing of GH. The silent products of plurihormonal adenomas are probably produced and released in small quantities that do not produce elevated hormone levels. The same circumstance may also explain the lack of function in cases of null cell adenomas.

Nonpituitary Sellar Mass

Lesions that can occur in the region of the hypothalamus and pituitary but are not pituitary tumors include craniopharyngioma, hypophysitis, germinoma, Rathke's cleft cyst, arachnoid cyst,[949] chordoma, optic nerve glioma, meningioma, Langerhans cell histiocytosis (histiocytosis X), leukemias, lymphomas, and metastatic cancers.[950] Only the first four are discussed, as the management of the others follows standard medical lines. It is important to make the correct diagnosis because treatment is often different. For example the transsphenoidal approach can be disastrous for an internal carotid artery aneurysm. Modern imaging techniques have facilitated diagnosis of aneurysm before therapeutic intervention.

CRANIOPHARYNGIOMA. A craniopharyngioma or Rathke's pouch tumor arises from embryonic squamous cell rests that persist after the upward migration of stomodeal epithelium to form the anterior pituitary. Because a tumor may arise from any position along the craniopharyngeal canal, it may be intrasellar or extrasellar. The tumor is usually well encapsulated and composed of cystic and solid components.[951–953] The cysts may be multiloculated and contain dark brown, oily fluid. The tumor cells are keratin immunoreactive, do not contain secretory granules on electron microscopy, and have characteristic bundles of tonofilaments and desmosomes. Tumor cells contain estrogen receptor mRNA.[954] Calcification is common but may also occur in prolactinomas and meningiomas. These tumors may occur at any age but are most common in children, accounting for 5 to 10% of primary brain tumors in childhood. Approximately one quarter are diagnosed after age 40.[951, 955]

Clinical Presentation. Children are usually diagnosed because of growth failure or manifestations of increased intracranial pressure (headache, vomiting, somnolence). Sixty percent of children have visual disturbances, and growth and sexual retardation are usual.[953] Eighty percent of adults have symptomatic visual disturbance and on examination more than 90% have visual abnormalities.[956] Disturbance of intellectual function in approximately 30% of adults may include dementia.[955, 957]

A prospective study of endocrine function in 20 patients with craniopharyngioma (6 adults and 14 children and adolescents) revealed a variable degree of hypopituitarism.[958] GH and gonadotropin deficiencies were present in 19 of 20. Sixty-five percent had secondary hypothyroidism, and half had corticotropin deficiency; none had diabetes insipidus, but diabetes insipidus is common after surgical resection of the tumor, particularly after surgery involving craniotomy.

Assessments of hypothalamic-pituitary function and vision and anatomic evaluation are identical to those of all patients with pituitary or suprasellar masses. Craniopharyngiomas are characteristically suprasellar lesions but may extend inferiorly into the sella turcica and destroy the bony margins of the sella and dorsum sellae. They may also extend superiorly into the third ventricle and obstruct the foramen of Monro to cause hydrocephalus.[951] The CT scan may be helpful in suggesting the diagnosis preoperatively. The tumor is calcified in 70 to 90% of children and in 40 to 60% of adults; calcification is detectable on CT but not on MRI. The solid portion of the tumor may appear enhanced on CT after administration of intravenous contrast agent. The high cholesterol content of cyst fluid produces a characteristic MRI signal that may also aid in the diagnosis.[959, 960]

Therapy. The primary treatment of craniopharyngioma, surgical resection,[951, 961–964] is associated with considerable morbidity and mortality, usually from the standard surgical approach (craniotomy) and from diabetes insipidus and other hypothalamic-pituitary dysfunction.[965] Transsphenoidal surgery is often successful in obtaining an accurate diagnosis, debulking the tumor mass, and setting the stage for subsequent radiotherapy. Tumor recurrence is a definite risk. Because these tumors are relatively radioresistant and grow slowly, it is difficult to assess the efficacy of radiotherapy.[966]

With the use of CT and MRI to evaluate patients with complaints referable to the cranium, more asymptomatic patients are being diagnosed with craniopharyngioma. These patients are a therapeutic dilemma. Craniotomy is associated with greater risk, and if the patient is asymptomatic an argument can be made for an anticipatory approach with careful follow-up, including a repeat imaging study at 6 mo or 1 y. The interval between scans may be doubled if there has been no increase in tumor size or tumor symptoms.

LYMPHOCYTIC HYPOPHYSITIS. Lymphocytic infiltration of the pituitary gland is associated with complete or partial hypopituitarism and a pituitary mass and occurs typically in women, often during pregnancy or in the postpartum period; a few cases have been described in men. Occasional maternal deaths with this entity are likely due to unrecognized adrenal failure, emphasizing the need for consideration of the diagnosis in a pregnant or post partum woman with symptoms of headache, visual disturbance, weakness, and fatigue.

Lymphocytic hypophysitis was first described in an autopsy specimen in 1962; more than 30 cases have been reported subsequently.[967-979] Seventy percent of women were either pregnant or post partum; in 30% there was no relationship to pregnancy. The clinical manifestations are due to hypopituitarism, frequently adrenal insufficiency, and to a pituitary mass. Pituitary deficiencies include corticotropin, thyrotropin, LH, FSH, and AVP, either alone or in combination; serum prolactin concentration is elevated in half of patients. The most common mass effects are headache in most and visual field loss in 32%. Evidence of suprasellar extension of the mass was present in 64% of patients.[971] Although most women had permanent destruction of all or part of the pituitary and required chronic hormone replacement therapy, one patient had transient hypopituitarism of 12 mo duration, suggesting that pituitary regeneration may have occurred.[973] Patients should probably be evaluated at regular intervals to determine the necessity for continued hormone replacement. The cause is unknown, but animal studies have implicated an autoimmune cause. Antipituitary antibodies were present in the sera of some women, and autoimmune endocrine disorders, including thyroiditis and adrenalitis, have been seen in others. Another proposed cause is virus-induced autoimmune destruction of the gland. The common association with pregnancy has been attributed to increased exposure to pituitary antigens or changes in maternal immunologic status.

Although the diagnosis may be suspected in a pregnant or post partum woman with the typical clinical features, confirmation requires surgical biopsy and histologic examination of the tissue. Diffuse infiltration with lymphocytes and plasma cells, lymphoid follicles with germinal centers, and destruction of normal pituitary cells are characteristic morphologic features on light and electron microscopy. Immunoperoxidase staining is positive for all pituitary cell types that remain intact.[970] The differential diagnosis based on light microscopic findings includes sarcoidosis, Langerhans histiocytosis, syphilis, tuberculosis, granulomatous hypophysitis, and postpartum hemorrhagic infarction. Examination of the specimen with electron microscopy is helpful in demonstrating characteristic interdigitation of lymphocytes and pituitary cells, fusion of lysosomes and secretory granules, and swollen mitochondria indicative of oncocytic transformation. Vascular injury or immune complex deposition was not evident in the cases examined with electron microscopy.[970, 971]

SUPRASELLAR GERMINOMAS. Germ cell tumors in the brain usually arise in the midline structures. The most common location is the pineal region, where germinomas, em-

bryonal cell carcinomas, yolk sac tumors, and teratomas occur. Germinomas, the most common pineal tumors, may also occur in the suprasellar region (usually related to the infundibulum) or along the floor of the third ventricle. The germinomas resemble germ cell tumors of the gonads and of other extragonadal sites such as the mediastinum and may be typical seminomas or nonseminoma germinomas with elements of teratoma, choriocarcinoma, or embryonal cell carcinoma. The tumors are more common in males, appear to be more frequent in Japan, and are usually diagnosed before age 30. The embryologic origin and derivation of these tumors is unsettled.[980] The characteristic histologic feature is the finding of tumor cells surrounded by a granulomatous infiltrate with multifocal accumulation of lymphocytes; the lymphocytic infiltration may make the histologic diagnosis difficult.[981] Large suprasellar germinomas often compress the optic nerves and chiasm and may extend inferiorly into the pituitary; extension into the third ventricle can cause hydrocephalus, and posterior third ventricle germinomas can cause Parinaud's syndrome.

Clinical Presentation.[982, 983] Untreated germinomas may behave in a malignant fashion. They often are multifocal and may metastasize within or outside the CNS. The clinical manifestations depend on the size and location of the tumor mass (or masses) within the CNS. The most common presenting abnormality is diabetes insipidus, which occurs in more than 80% of patients and may be the sole disturbance at the time of diagnosis. Less common manifestations include visual disturbance, symptoms of increased intracranial pressure (headache, nausea, vomiting), obesity (presumably due to hypothalamic damage), anterior pituitary deficits (including growth retardation and hypogonadism), and evidence of increased intracranial pressure.

The radiologic features are not distinctive.[984] In one MRI study 5 of 14 suprasellar lesions had extension into the sella, and the tumors enhanced consistently with gadolinium. Tumors that present with diabetes insipidus can be small, may involve only the pituitary stalk, and may be detectable only with contrast-enhanced MRI. The diagnosis should be considered in all individuals with diabetes insipidus and a suprasellar mass.

In addition to the tests that would be performed for patients with suspected pituitary disease, potential tumor markers for germ cell tumors should be measured, including hCG β, α-fetoprotein, and lactate dehydrogenase. These markers are elevated in only about 5% of individuals with typical germinoma but may be positive in 30% or more of patients with germinomas that contain other (usually malignant) germ cell components. When levels of these markers are normal in plasma, the CSF should be examined cytologically and for measurement of the three tumor markers. Elevation of either hCG β or α-fetoprotein is sufficient to make the diagnosis of malignant germ cell tumor. In the absence of diagnostic levels of tumor markers, the establishment of a tissue diagnosis is desirable because of the potential curability of some germinomas. In many cases the diagnosis can be made on cytologic smear preparations at the time of surgery.[985]

The first step in treatment is to correct any pituitary hormone deficiencies. Diabetes insipidus should be treated with desmopressin (see Chapter 10). Because of the location of this tumor and because it is frequently multifocal, surgery is not likely to effect a cure but may be useful to relieve hydrocephalus or decrease the size of tumors that do not respond to chemotherapy or radiation, or both.

CNS germinomas have a good response to both radiotherapy and cisplatin-based chemotherapy, but each of these treatments has undesirable side effects and is associated with a recurrence rate of 20% or more after apparent complete remission.[986, 987] One strategy that appears promising, particularly in children, is to treat initially with chemotherapy and then to administer a reduced dose of radiotherapy to those that express a complete response; if less than a complete response is obtained additional chemotherapy and radiotherapy are given as indicated.[988] This approach minimizes the chance of radiation injury to the brain in adolescents and young adults, and cure is possible in most patients (75 to 80%).

Because most germinomas are exquisitely sensitive to conventional radiotherapy, some investigators recommend a therapeutic trial of 1500 cGy of fractionated radiotherapy. If posttreatment imaging studies showed marked reduction in the size of the lesion, a presumptive diagnosis of germinoma is made, and radiation therapy can be completed.

EMPTY SELLA. An empty sella is usually an incidental anatomic finding that results in abnormal pituitary function in occasional patients. Pituitary fossa enlargement is a result of a communicating extension of the subarachnoid space into the pituitary fossa, which promotes remodeling and enlargement of the bony sella and flattening of the pituitary gland against the sella floor. An empty sella may occur as a result of a congenital diaphragmatic defect (primary empty sella) or as a result of damage to the diaphragm by surgery, radiotherapy, or pituitary tumor infarction (secondary empty sella). A primary empty sella is a fairly common incidental finding and is usually associated with only minor disturbances of pituitary function.

If the empty sella is associated with destruction of the pituitary gland, hypopituitarism is the outcome. Pituitary destruction occurs when a large pituitary adenoma undergoes infarction (usually a hemorrhage) or as a consequence of surgical resection. Hypopituitarism may be partial or complete, and measurement of serum pituitary and target organ hormones is necessary to establish the diagnosis of hormone deficiency and to determine the central (hypothalamic or pituitary) cause of the dysfunction (e.g., serum thyrotropin and T_4; corticotropin, cortisol; LH and testosterone). In the case of primary empty sella (congenital diaphragmatic incompetence), mild hyperprolactinemia (usually <100 μg/L, with or without galactorrhea) occurs in approximately 15% of patients. Since even a mild elevation of prolactin may interfere with normal gonadal function, this may require treatment, but the patient should be reassured that this problem does not usually result in additional pituitary dysfunction.

Children with an empty sella most commonly have GH deficiency, although other pituitary hormone dysfunction may occur. In children with isolated GH deficiency or multiple pituitary deficiencies, empty sella was observed in 48% but was present in only 2% of children with normal pituitary function.[989]

PITUITARY APOPLEXY. This condition is an acute, life-threatening infarction of the pituitary gland. Hemorrhagic infarction usually occurs in the presence of a pituitary tumor; ischemic infarction may occur spontaneously in a normal gland, after obstetric hemorrhage (Sheehan's syndrome), or in the setting of increased intracranial pressure or systemic anticoagulation therapy. Other predisposing states include diabetes mellitus, bleeding disorders, pituitary radiation, pneumoencephalography, carotid angiography, mechanical ventilation, trauma, and upper respiratory tract infection.[990-994] Pituitary infarction usually results in anterior pituitary hypofunction that may be permanent or transient, the degree of impairment being dependent on the amount of tissue destruction. Hormone deficiencies include GH (88%), gonadotropins (58 to 76%), and corticotropin (66%). Secondary hypothyroidism occurs in 42 to 53% of patients, and prolactin secretion is deficient in 67 to 100% of patients. Diabetes insipidus occurs in 2 to 3% of patients.[995] The precise incidence of pituitary infarction and hemorrhage is unknown. In unse-

lected autopsy studies, infarction of more than 25% of the gland was present in 1 to 3% of specimens. The frequency of apoplexy in patients with a known pituitary tumor was 17% in one series of 560 patients undergoing pituitary surgery; 8% had no clinical symptoms of hemorrhage.[994] Apoplexy may decrease hormone excess by pituitary tumors and result in spontaneous "cure" of the tumor. CT and MRI studies of patients with known pituitary tumors indicate that hemorrhage into tumors can occur without clinical evidence of apoplexy.[584] Of 12 patients with radiographically proven hemorrhage in one study, only 3 had clinical evidence of apoplexy.[996] Apoplexy may occur in a nontumorous pituitary gland in post partum women who had excessive blood loss during delivery. After a period of complete ischemia, revascularization and vascular congestion with thrombosis of the anterior lobe are observed.[990]

The pattern of tumor growth, the size of the tumor, and the extent of hemorrhage and necrosis and edema in the gland determine the symptoms. Infarction with hemorrhage and edema may cause rapid expansion of the lesion, compression of surrounding structures, and neurologic manifestations. In conscious patients the initial symptom is usually a severe retro-orbital headache, frequently accompanied by nausea and vomiting. Extravasation of blood or necrotic tissue into the subarachnoid space may cause meningeal irritation, fever, clouding of consciousness, or coma. Superior expansion produces compression of the optic chiasm or optic nerve, or both, with acute visual field loss or decreased visual acuity, or both. Lateral expansion into the cavernous sinus may impair the function of cranial nerves III, IV, and VI and the first division of cranial nerve V. The most common abnormality is unilateral involvement of cranial nerve III with ophthalmoplegia (impaired medial and downward gaze), diplopia, ptosis, and mydriasis. Expansion that causes mechanical compression of the carotid siphon against the anterior clinoid process can cause hemispheric dysfunction, seizures, and hemiplegia. Hemispheric dysfunction can also be due to vasospasm secondary to irritation by subarachnoid hemorrhage.

Clinical evaluation of the patient with a sudden change in sensorium, headache, ophthalmoplegia, visual loss, or prostration should include an immediate imaging study of the pituitary area and orbits, either non–contrast-enhanced CT or an MRI scan. If CT is performed, thin (1.5 mm) sections should be obtained through the pituitary in the coronal plane to identify the lesion; an unenhanced scan is necessary to identify hemorrhage, and contrast agent may be administered intravenously after initial images are obtained. Increased intensity, signifying hemorrhage, is also seen on a T1-weighted MRI scan. CT may be superior for visualizing intratumoral hemorrhage within the first few days of the event, but the MRI scan is more sensitive in following the hemorrhage in the subacute stage.[996]

If pituitary apoplexy is suspected, the patient should be presumed to have anterior pituitary insufficiency and must be treated accordingly. Blood should be obtained for measurement of serum cortisol and T_4 levels, and glucocorticoid should be administered immediately. The glucocorticoid dose must be adequate for the stress of the illness and for presumptive cerebral edema (e.g., dexamethasone 2 mg every 6 h). Ophthalmologic examination is performed to determine the nature and extent of deficits. If visual deficits or altered sensorium is present, emergent neurosurgical intervention is required. Immediate surgical decompression of the hemorrhage and tumor can result in recovery of visual deficits and alleviation of increased intracranial pressure. After recovery from surgery the patient should undergo a complete endocrinologic evaluation to determine the nature and degree of hormone deficits. Because hormone deficits may be transient, function should be re-evaluated several months after the event.[997, 998] Evidence for hormone hypersecretion should also be sought. Surgical decompression may not be necessary in the setting of normal sensorium and visual function. The patient should be hospitalized and treated with glucocorticoid replacement, and serial ophthalmologic and imaging examinations should take place. Complete endocrine evaluation may be performed after recovery to assess the need for chronic hormone replacement. With modern imaging techniques objective assessment of the visual system, prompt hormone replacement, and surgical decompression as indicated, pituitary gland apoplexy is rarely lethal.

REFERENCES

Pituitary Morphology

1. Asa SL, Kovacs K. Functional morphology of the human fetal pituitary (review). Pathol Annu 1984; 19(Pt 1):275–315.
2. Asa SL, Kovacs K, Laszlo FA, et al. Human fetal adenohypophysis. Histologic and immunocytochemical analysis. Neuroendocrinology 1986; 43:308–316.
3. Ikeda H, Suzuki J, Sasano N, et al. The development and morphogenesis of the human pituitary gland. Anat Embryol 1988; 178:327–336.
4. Goodyer CG. Ontogeny of pituitary hormone secretion. In: Collu R, Ducharme JR, Guyda HJ, eds. Pediatric Endocrinology. New York: Raven Press, 1989: 125–169.
5. Boyd JD. Observations on human pharyngeal hypophysis. J Endocrinol 1956; 14:66–77.
6. McGrath P. Volume and histology of the human pharyngeal hypophysis. Aust NZ J Surg 1967; 37:16–27.
7. Frawley LS, Miller HA. Ontogeny of prolactin secretion in the neonatal rat is regulated posttranscriptionally. Endocrinology 1989; 124:3–6.
8. Lugo DI, Roberts JL, Pintar JE. Analysis of proopiomelanocortin gene expression during prenatal development of the rat pituitary gland. Mol Endocrinol 1989; 3:1313–1324.
9. Scheithauer BW, Sano T, Kovacs K, et al. The pituitary gland in pregnancy: a clinicopathologic and immunohistochemical study of 69 cases. Mayo Clin Proc 1990; 65:461–474.
10. Sheehan HL, Kovacs K. Neurohypophysis and hypothalamus. In: Bloodworth JMB, Jr, ed. Endocrine Pathology. Baltimore: Williams & Wilkins, 1982: 45–99.
11. Burrow GN, Wortzman G, Rewcastle NB, et al. Microadenomas of the pituitary and abnormal sellar tomograms in an unselected autopsy series. N Engl J Med 1981; 304:156–158.
12. Scheithauer BW. The hypothalamus and neurohypophysis. In: Kovacs K, Asa SL, eds. Functional Endocrine Pathology. Boston: Blackwell Scientific, 1991: 170–244.
13. Stanfield JP. The blood supply of the human pituitary gland. J Anat 1960; 94:257–273.
14. Sheehan HL, Stanfield JP. The pathogenesis of post-partum necrosis of the anterior lobe of the pituitary gland. Acta Endocrinol 1961; 37:479–510.
15. Bergland RM, Page RB. Pituitary-brain vascular relations: a new paradigm (review). Science 1979; 204:18–24.
16. Gorczyca W, Hardy J. Arterial supply of the human anterior pituitary gland. Neurosurgery 1987; 20:369–378.
17. Landolt AM, Schubiger O, Maurer R, et al. The value of inferior petrosal sinus sampling in diagnosis and treatment of Cushing's disease. Clin Endocrinol (Oxf) 1994; 40:485–492.
18. Horvath E, Kovacs K. Fine structural cytology of the adenohypophysis in rat and man (review). J Electron Microsc Tech 1988; 8:401–432.
19. Stefaneanu L, Kovacs K, Lloyd RV, et al. The pituitary in pregnancy. A morphologic study including immunocytochemistry and in situ hybridization (abstract). FASEB J 1991; 5(5 Part II):A1391–A5290.

Pituitary Hormones

Hypothalamic-Pituitary Regulation

20. Veldhuis JD, Johnson ML. Cluster analysis: a simple, versatile, and robust algorithm for endocrine pulse detection. Am J Physiol 1986; 250:E486–E493.
21. Van Cauter E. Estimating false-positive and false-negative errors in analyses of hormonal pulsatility. Am J Physiol 1988; 254:E786–E794.
22. Veldhuis JD, Carlson ML, Johnson ML. The pituitary gland secretes in bursts: appraising the nature of glandular secretory impulses by simultaneous multiple-parameter deconvolution of plasma hormone concentrations. Proc Natl Acad Sci USA 1987; 84:7686–7690.
23. Polonsky KS, Licinio Paixao J, Given BD, et al. Use of biosynthetic human C-peptide in the measurement of insulin secretion rates in normal volunteers and type I diabetic patients. J Clin Invest 1986; 77:98–105.
24. Polonsky KS, Given BD, Van Cauter E. Twenty-four-hour profiles and pulsatile patterns of insulin secretion in normal and obese subjects. J Clin Invest 1988; 81:442–448.

25. Hartman ML, Faria ACS, Vance ML, et al. Temporal structure of in vivo growth hormone secretory events in man. Am J Physiol 1991; 260:E101–E110.
26. Van Cauter E, Refetoff S. Evidence for two subtypes of Cushing's disease based on the analysis of episodic cortisol secretion. N Engl J Med 1985; 312:1343–1349.
27. Hartman ML, Veldhuis JD, Vance ML, et al. Somatotropin pulse frequency and basal concentrations are increased in acromegaly and are reduced by successful therapy. J Clin Endocrinol Metab 1990; 70(5):1375–1384.
28. Jones MT, Gillham B. Factors involved in the regulation of adrenocorticotropic hormone/beta-lipotropic hormone (review). Physiol Rev 1988; 68:743–818.
29. Lundblad JR, Roberts JL. Regulation of proopiomelanocortin gene expression in pituitary (review). Endocr Rev 1988; 9:135–158.
30. Kovacs K, Horvath E, Stratmann IE, et al. Cytoplasmic microfilaments in the anterior lobe of the human pituitary gland. Acta Anat 1974; 87:414–426.
31. Neumann PE, Horoupian DS, Goldman JE, et al. Cytoplasmic filaments of Crooke's hyaline change belong to the cytokeratin class. An immunocytochemical and ultrastructural study. Am J Pathol 1984; 116:214–222.
32. DeCherney GS, DeBold CR, Jackson RV, et al. Diurnal variation in the response of plasma adrenocorticotropin and cortisol to intravenous ovine corticotropin-releasing hormone. J Clin Endocrinol Metab 1985; 61:273–279.
33. DeBold CR, Jackson RV, Kamilaris TC, et al. Effects of ovine corticotropin-releasing hormone on adrenocorticotropin secretion in the absence of glucocorticoid feedback inhibition in man. J Clin Endocrinol Metab 1989; 68:431–437.
34. DeBold CR, Sheldon WR, DeCherney GS, et al. Arginine vasopressin potentiates adrenocorticotropin release induced by ovine corticotropin-releasing factor. J Clin Invest 1984; 73:533–538.
35. Moore-Ede MC, Czeisler CA, Richardson GS. Circadian timekeeping in health and disease. Part 1: Basic properties of circadian pacemakers (review). N Engl J Med 1983; 309:469–476.
36. Orth DN, Besser GM, King PH, et al. Free-running circadian plasma cortisol rhythm in a blind human subject. Clin Endocrinol (Oxf) 1979; 10:603–617.
37. Desir D, Van Cauter E, Fang VS, et al. Effects of "jet lag" on hormonal patterns. I: Procedures, variations in total plasma proteins, and disruption of adrenocorticotropin-cortisol periodicity. J Clin Endocrinol Metab 1981; 52:628–641.
38. Widmaier EP, Plotsky PM, Sutton SW, et al. Regulation of corticotropin-releasing factor secretion in vitro by glucose. Am J Physiol 1988; 255:E287–E292.
39. Bateman A, Singh A, Kral T, et al. The immune-hypothalamic-pituitary-adrenal axis (review). Endocr Rev 1989; 10:92–112.
40. Simpson ER, Waterman MR. Regulation of the synthesis of steroidogenic enzymes in adrenal cortical cells by ACTH (review). Annu Rev Physiol 1988; 50:427–440.

Prolactin–Growth Hormone Family

41. Niall HD, Hogan ML, Sauer R, et al. Sequences of pituitary and placental lactogenic and growth hormones: evolution from a primordial peptide by gene reduplication. Proc Natl Acad Sci USA 1971; 68:866–870.
42. Cooke NE, Coit D, Weiner RI, et al. Structure of cloned DNA complementary to rat prolactin messenger RNA. J Biol Chem 1980; 255:6502–6510.
43. Cooke NE, Baxter JD. Structural analysis of the prolactin gene suggests a separate origin for its 5′ end. Nature 1982; 297:603–606.
44. Cooke NE, Coit D, Shine J, et al. Human prolactin. cDNA structural analysis and evolutionary comparisons. J Biol Chem 1981; 256:4007–4016.
45. Truong AT, Duez C, Belayew A, et al. Isolation and characterization of the human prolactin gene. Embo J 1984; 3:429–437.
46. Owerbach D, Rutter WJ, Cooke NE, et al. The prolactin gene is located on chromosome 6 in humans. Science 1981; 212:815–816.
47. Owerbach D, Rutter WJ, Martial JA, et al. Genes for growth hormone, chorionic somatomammotropin, and growth hormone-like gene on chromosome 17 in humans. Science 1980; 209:289–292.
48. Cooke NE. Prolactin: normal synthesis, regulation, and actions. In: DeGroot LJ, Besser GM, Cahill GF Jr, et al, eds. Endocrinology. Philadelphia: WB Saunders, 1989: 384–407.
49. Barsh GS, Seeburg PH, Gelinas RE. The human growth hormone gene family: structure and evolution of the chromosomal locus. Nucleic Acids Res 1983; 11:3939–3958.
50. Stricker S, Grueter F. Action du lobe anterieur de l'hypophyse sur la montee laiteuse. Compt Rend Soc Biol 1928; 99:1978–1980.
51. Riddle O, Braucher PF. Studies on the physiology of reproduction in birds. XXX: Control of the special secretion of the crop-gland in pigeons by anterior pituitary hormones. Am J Physiol 1931; 97:617–627.
52. Riddle O, Bates RW, Dykshorn SW. The preparation, identification and assay of prolactin—a hormone of the anterior pituitary. Am J Physiol 1933; 105:191–216.
53. Riddle O, Bates RW, Dykshorn SW. A new hormone of the anterior pituitary. Proc Soc Exp Biol Med 1932; 29:1211–1215.
54. Lewis UJ, Singh RN, Seavey BK. Human prolactin: isolation and some properties. Biochem Biophys Res Commun 1971; 44:1169–1176.

55. Hwang P, Guyda H, Friesen H. Purification of human prolactin. J Biol Chem 1972; 247:1955–1958.
56. Sinha YN, Gilligan TA, Lee DW. Detection of a high molecular weight variant of prolactin in human plasma by a combination of electrophoretic and immunologic techniques. J Clin Endocrinol Metab 1984; 58:752–754.
57. Suh HK, Frantz AG. Size heterogeneity of human prolactin in plasma and pituitary extracts. J Clin Endocrinol Metab 1974; 39:928–935.
58. Farkouh NH, Packer MG, Frantz AG. Large molecular size prolactin with reduced receptor activity in human serum: high proportion in basal state and reduction after thyrotropin-releasing hormone. J Clin Endocrinol Metab 1979; 48:1026–1032.
59. Benveniste R, Helman JD, Orth DN, et al. Circulating big human prolactin: conversion to small human prolactin by reduction of disulfide bonds. J Clin Endocrinol Metab 1979; 48:883–886.
60. Whittaker PG, Wilcox T, Lind T. Maintained fertility in a patient with hyperprolactinemia due to big, big prolactin. J Clin Endocrinol Metab 1981; 53:863–866.
61. Soong YK, Ferguson KM, McGarrick G, et al. Size heterogeneity of immunoreactive prolactin in hyperprolactinaemic serum. Clin Endocrinol (Oxf) 1982; 16:259–265.
62. Lewis UJ, Singh RN, Sinha YN, et al. Glycosylated human prolactin. Endocrinology 1985; 116:359–363.
63. Andersen AN, Pedersen H, Djursing H, et al. Bioactivity of prolactin in a woman with an excess of large molecular size prolactin, persistent hyperprolactinemia and spontaneous conception. Fertil Steril 1982; 38:625–628.
64. Sinha YN, Gilligan TA, Lee DW, et al. Cleaved prolactin: evidence for its occurrence in human pituitary gland and plasma. J Clin Endocrinol Metab 1985; 60:239–243.
65. Mittra I. A novel "cleaved prolactin" in the rat pituitary. Part II: In vivo mammary mitogenic activity of its N-terminal 16K moiety. Biochem Biophys Res Commun 1980; 95:1760–1767.
66. Asa SL, Penz G, Kovacs K, et al. Prolactin cells in the human pituitary. A quantitative immunocytochemical analysis. Arch Pathol Lab Med 1982; 106:360–363.
67. Coleman DT, Bancroft C. Pituitary adenylate cyclase–activating polypeptide stimulates prolactin gene expression in a rat pituitary cell line. Endocrinology 1993; 133:2736–2742.
68. Steinmetz R, Gutierrez-Hartmann A, Bigsby RM, et al. Activation of the prolactin promoter in transfected GH3 cells by posterior pituitary cells. Endocrinology 1994; 135:2737–2741.
69. Liu JW, Ben-Jonathan N. Prolactin-releasing activity of neurohypophysial hormones: structure-function relationship. Endocrinology 1994; 134:114–118.
70. Corcia A, Steinmetz R, Liu JW, et al. Coculturing posterior pituitary and GH3 cells: dramatic stimulation of prolactin gene expression. Endocrinology 1993; 132:80–85.
71. Lam KS, Lechan RM, Minamitani N, et al. Vasoactive intestinal peptide in the anterior pituitary is increased in hypothyroidism. Endocrinology 1989; 124:1077–1084.
72. Nagy G, Mulchahey JJ, Neill JD. Autocrine control of prolactin secretion by vasoactive intestinal peptide. Endocrinology 1988; 122:364–366.
73. Hagen TC, Arnaout MA, Scherzer WJ, et al. Antisera to vasoactive intestinal polypeptide inhibit basal prolactin release from dispersed anterior pituitary cells. Neuroendocrinology 1986; 43:641–645.
74. Nokin J, Vekemans M, L'Hermite M, et al. Circadian periodicity of serum prolactin concentration in man. Br Med J 1972; 3:561–562.
75. Parker DC, Rossman LG, Vander Laan EF. Sleep-related, nychthermeral and briefly episodic variation in human plasma prolactin concentrations. J Clin Endocrinol Metab 1973; 36:1119–1124.
76. Sassin JF, Frantz AG, Weitzman ED, et al. Human prolactin: 24-hour pattern with increased release during sleep. Science 1972; 177:1205–1207.
77. Sassin JF, Frantz AG, Kapen S, et al. The nocturnal rise of human prolactin is dependent on sleep. J Clin Endocrinol Metab 1973; 37:436–440.
78. Parker DC, Rossman LG, Vanderlaan EF. Relation of sleep-entrained human prolactin release to REM-nonREM cycles. J Clin Endocrinol Metab 1974; 38:646–651.
79. Van Cauter E, L'Hermite M, Copinschi G, et al. Quantitative analysis of spontaneous variations of plasma prolactin in normal man. Am J Physiol 1981; 241:E355–E363.
80. Desir D, Van Cauter E, L'Hermite M, et al. Effects of "jet lag" on hormonal patterns. III: Demonstration of an intrinsic circadian rhythmicity in plasma prolactin. J Clin Endocrinol Metab 1982; 55:849–857.
81. Veldhuis JD, Johnson ML. Operating characteristics of the hypothalamo-pituitary-gonadal axis in men: circadian, ultradian, and pulsatile release of prolactin and its temporal coupling with luteinizing hormone. J Clin Endocrinol Metab 1988; 67:116–123.
82. Thorner MO, Round J, Jones A, et al. Serum prolactin and oestradiol levels at different stages of puberty. Clin Endocrinol (Oxf) 1977; 7:463–468.
83. Friesen HG. Human prolactin. Ann R Coll Phys Surg Can 1978; 11:275–281.
84. Gluckman PD, Grumbach MM, Kaplan SL. The neuroendocrine regulation and function of growth hormone and prolactin in the mammalian fetus (review). Endocr Rev 1981; 2:363–395.
85. Suganuma N, Seo H, Yamamoto N, et al. Ontogenesis of pituitary prolactin in the human fetus. J Clin Endocrinol Metab 1986; 63:156–161.
86. Tyson JE, Hwang P, Guyda H, et al. Studies of prolactin secretion in human pregnancy. Am J Obstet Gynecol 1972; 113:14–20.
87. Maslar IA, Riddick DH. Prolactin production by human endometrium during the normal menstrual cycle. Am J Obstet Gynecol 1979; 135:751–754.
88. Riddick DH, Daly DC. Decidual prolactin production in human gestation (review). Semin Perinatol 1982; 6:229–237.
89. Clements J, Whitfeld P, Cooke N, et al. Expression of the prolactin gene in human decidua-chorion. Endocrinology 1983; 112:1133–1134.
90. Takahashi H, Nabeshima Y, Ogata K, et al. Molecular cloning and nucleotide sequence of DNA complementary to human decidual prolactin mRNA. J Biochem 1984; 95:1491–1499.
91. Goodwin RG, Friend D, Ziegler SF, et al. Cloning of the human and murine interleukin-7 receptors: demonstration of a soluble form and homology to a new receptor superfamily. Cell 1990; 60:941–951.
92. Milenkovic L, D'Angelo G, Kelly PA, et al. Inhibition of gonadotropin hormone–releasing hormone release by prolactin from GT1 neuronal cell lines through prolactin receptors. Proc Natl Acad Sci USA 1994; 91:1244–1247.
93. Cooke NE, Ray J, Watson MA, et al. Human growth hormone gene and the highly homologous growth hormone variant gene display different splicing patterns. J Clin Invest 1988; 82:270–275.
94. DeNoto FM, Moore DD, Goodman HM. Human growth hormone DNA sequence and mRNA structure: possible alternative splicing. Nucleic Acids Res 1981; 9:3719–3730.
95. Baumann G. Molecular variants of human growth hormone in serum and circulating growth hormone binding proteins. In: Frisch H, Thorner MO, eds. Hormonal Regulation of Growth. Serono Symposia Publications. Vol 58. New York: Raven Press, 1989: 175–184.
96. Frankenne F, Rentier Delrue F, Scippo ML, et al. Expression of the growth hormone variant gene in human placenta. J Clin Endocrinol Metab 1987; 64:635–637.
97. Frankenne F, Closset J, Gomez F, et al. The physiology of growth hormones (GHs) in pregnant women and partial characterization of the placental GH variant. J Clin Endocrinol Metab 1988; 66:1171–1180.
98. Isgaard J, Nilsson A, Lindahl A, et al. Effects of local administration of GH and IGF-1 on longitudinal bone growth in rats. Am J Physiol 1986; 250:E367–E372.
99. Igout A, Scippo ML, Frankenne F, et al. hGH V gene: specific placental expression, isolation and structure of the related cDNA. Proceedings of the 70th meeting of the Endocrine Society, New Orleans, LA, 1988: 303 (abstract).
100. Pelletier G, Robert F, Hardy J. Identification of human anterior pituitary cells by immunoelectron microscopy. J Clin Endocrinol Metab 1978; 46:534–542.
101. Sano T, Kovacs KT, Scheithauer BW, et al. Aging and the human pituitary gland. Mayo Clin Proc 1993; 68:971–977.
102. Thorner MO, Perryman RL, Cronin MJ, et al. Somatotroph hyperplasia. Successful treatment of acromegaly by removal of a pancreatic islet tumor secreting a growth hormone–releasing factor. J Clin Invest 1982; 70:965–977.
103. Stolar MW, Baumann G. Big growth hormone forms in human plasma: immunochemical evidence for their pituitary origin. Metabolism 1986; 35:75–77.
104. Baumann G, Vance ML, Shaw MA, et al. Plasma transport of human growth hormone in vivo. J Clin Endocrinol Metab 1990; 71:470–473.
105. Stolar MW, Baumann G, Vance ML, et al. Circulating growth hormone forms after stimulation of pituitary secretion with growth hormone–releasing factor in man. J Clin Endocrinol Metab 1984; 59:235–239.
106. Baumann G, Stolar MW. Molecular forms of human growth hormone secreted in vivo: nonspecificity of secretory stimuli. J Clin Endocrinol Metab 1986; 62:789–790.
107. Baumann G, Winter RJ, Shaw M. Circulating molecular variants of growth hormone in childhood. Pediatr Res 1987; 22:21–22.
108. Baumann G, Shaw MA, Merimee TJ. Decreased growth hormone–binding protein in pygmy plasma (abstract). Clin Res 1988; 36:551A.
109. Leung DW, Spencer SA, Cachianes G, et al. Growth hormone receptor and serum binding protein: purification, cloning and expression. Nature 1987; 330:537–543.
110. Spencer SA, Hammonds RG, Henzel WJ, et al. Rabbit liver growth hormone receptor and serum binding protein. Purification, characterization, and sequence. J Biol Chem 1988; 263:7862–7867.
111. Menon RK, Stephan DA, Singh M, et al. Cloning of the promoter-regulatory region of the murine growth hormone receptor gene. Identification of a developmentally regulated enhancer element. J Biol Chem 1995; 270:8851–8859.
112. Boutin JM, Jolicoeur C, Okamura H, et al. Cloning and expression of the rat prolactin receptor, a member of the growth hormone/prolactin receptor gene family. Cell 1988; 53:69–77.
113. Cunningham BC, Ultsch M, de Vos AM, et al. Dimerization of the extracellular domain of the human growth hormone receptor by a single hormone molecule. Science 1991; 254:821–825.
114. de Vos AM, Ultsch M, Kossiakoff AA. Human growth hormone and extracellular domain of its receptor: crystal structure of the complex. Science 1992; 255:306–312.
115. Ihle JN, Kerr IM. Jaks and Stats in signaling by the cytokine receptor superfamily (review). Trends Genet 1995; 11:69–74.
116. Carter-Su C, Schwartz J, Smit LS. Molecular mechanism of growth hormone action. Annu Rev Physiol 1996; 58:187–207.

117. Silva CM, Lu H, Day RN. Characterization and cloning of STAT 5 from IM-9 cells and its activation by growth hormone. Mol Endocrinol 1996; 10:508–518.

118. Silva CM, Lu H, Weber MJ, et al. Differential tyrosine phosphorylation of JAK1, JAK2, and STAT1 by growth hormone and interferon-gamma in IM-9 cells. J Biol Chem 1994; 269:27532–27539.

119. Bass S, Wells J. Growth hormone–receptor gene in Laron dwarfism. N Engl J Med 1990; 332(12):854–855.

120. Rosenfeld RG, Rosenbloom AL, Guevara-Aguirre J. Growth hormone (GH) insensitivity due to primary GH receptor deficiency (review). Endocr Rev 1994; 15:369–390.

121. Kou K, Lajara R, Rotwein P. Amino acid substitutions in the intracellular part of the growth hormone receptor in a patient with the Laron syndrome. J Clin Endocrinol Metab 1993; 76:54–59.

122. Woods KA, Fraser NC, Postel-Vinay MC, et al. A homozygous splice site mutation affecting the intracellular domain of the growth hormone (GH) receptor resulting in Laron syndrome with elevated GH-binding protein (see comments). J Clin Endocrinol Metab 1996; 81:1686–1690.

123. Baumann G, Shaw MA, Winter RJ. Absence of the plasma growth hormone–binding protein in Laron-type dwarfism. J Clin Endocrinol Metab 1987; 65:814–816.

124. Daughaday WH, Trivedi B. Absence of serum growth hormone binding protein in patients with growth hormone receptor deficiency (Laron dwarfism). Proc Natl Acad Sci USA 1987; 84:4636–4640.

125. Baumann G, Amburn KD, Buchanan TA. The effect of circulating growth hormone–binding protein on metabolic clearance, distribution, and degradation of human growth hormone. J Clin Endocrinol Metab 1987; 64:657–660.

126. Baumann G, Shaw MA, Buchanan TA. In vivo kinetics of a covalent growth hormone–binding protein complex. Metabolism 1989; 38:330–333.

127. Herington AC, Ymer S, Stevenson J. Identification and characterization of specific binding proteins for growth hormone in normal human sera. J Clin Invest 1986; 77:1817–1823.

128. Daughaday WH, Trivedi B, Andrews BA. The ontogeny of serum GH binding protein in man: a possible indicator of hepatic GH receptor development. J Clin Endocrinol Metab 1987; 65:1072–1074.

129. Barinaga M, Yamonoto G, Rivier C, et al. Transcriptional regulation of growth hormone gene expression by growth hormone–releasing factor. Nature 1983; 306:84–85.

130. Holl RW, Thorner MO, Mandell GL, et al. Spontaneous oscillations of intracellular calcium and growth hormone secretion. J Biol Chem 1988; 263:9682–9685.

131. Holl RW, Thorner MO, Leong DA. Intracellular calcium concentration and growth hormone secretion in individual somatotropes: effects of growth hormone–releasing factor and somatostatin. Endocrinology 1988; 122:2927–2932.

132. Dorflinger LJ, Schonbrunn A. Somatostatin inhibits vasoactive intestinal peptide–stimulated cyclic adenosine monophosphate accumulation in GH pituitary cells. Endocrinology 1983; 113:1541–1550.

133. Koch BD, Blalock JB, Schonbrunn A. Characterization of the cyclic AMP-independent actions of somatostatin in GH cells. I: An increase in potassium conductance is responsible for both the hyperpolarization and the decrease in intracellular free calcium produced by somatostatin. J Biol Chem 1988; 263:216–225.

134. Cronin MJ, Rogol AD, Dabney LG, et al. Selective growth hormone and cyclic AMP stimulating activity is present in human pancreatic islet cell tumor. J Clin Endocrinol Metab 1982; 55:381–383.

135. Cronin MJ, Hewlett EL, Evans WS, et al. Human pancreatic tumor growth hormone (GH)–releasing factor and cyclic adenosine 3′,5′-monophosphate evoke GH release from anterior pituitary cells: the effects of pertussis toxin, cholera toxin, forskolin, and cycloheximide. Endocrinology 1984; 114:904–913.

136. Schettini G, Cronin MJ, Hewlett EL, et al. Human pancreatic tumor growth hormone–releasing factor stimulates anterior pituitary adenylate cyclase activity, adenosine 3′,5′-monophosphate accumulation, and growth hormone release in a calmodulin-dependent manner. Endocrinology 1984; 115:1308–1314.

137. Holl RW, Thorner MO, Leong DA. Cytosolic free calcium in normal somatotropes: effects of forskolin and phorbol ester. Am J Physiol 1989; 256:E375–E379.

138. Borges JL, Schran HF, Evans WS, et al. Mesulergine, a new dopamine agonist: effects on anterior pituitary function and kinetics. Clin Pharmacol Ther 1984; 36:696–703.

139. Ho KY, Evans WS, Blizzard RM, et al. Effects of sex and age on the 24-hour profile of growth hormone secretion in man: importance of endogenous estradiol concentrations. J Clin Endocrinol Metab 1987; 64:51–58.

140. Hendricks CM, Eastman RC, Takeda S, et al. Plasma clearance of intravenously administered pituitary human growth hormone: gel filtration studies of heterogeneous components. J Clin Endocrinol Metab 1985; 60:864–867.

141. Hindmarsh PC, Matthews DR, Brain CE, et al. The half-life of exogenous growth hormone after suppression of endogenous growth hormone secretion with somatostatin. Clin Endocrinol (Oxf) 1989; 30:443–450.

142. Owens D, Srivastava MC, Tompkins CV, et al. Studies on the metabolic clearance rate, apparent distribution space and plasma half-disappearance time of unlabelled human growth hormone in normal subjects and in patients with liver disease, renal disease, thyroid disease and diabetes mellitus. Eur J Clin Invest 1973; 3:284–294.

143. Parker ML, Utiger RD, Daughaday WH. Studies on human growth hormone. II: The physiological disposition and metabolic rate of human growth hormone in man. J Clin Invest 1962; 41:262–268.

144. Faria AC, Veldhuis JD, Thorner MO, et al. Half-time of endogenous growth hormone (GH) disappearance in normal man after stimulation of GH secretion by GH-releasing hormone and suppression with somatostatin. J Clin Endocrinol Metab 1989; 68:535–541.

145. MacGillivray MH, Frohman LA, Doe J. Metabolic clearance and production rates of human growth hormone in subjects with normal and abnormal growth. J Clin Endocrinol Metab 1970; 30:632–638.

146. Thompson RG, Rodriguez A, Kowarski A, et al. Growth hormone: metabolic clearance rates, integrated concentrations, and production rates in normal adults and the effect of prednisone. J Clin Invest 1972; 51:3193–3199.

147. Martha PM Jr, Rogol AD, Veldhuis JD, et al. Alterations in the pulsatile properties of circulating growth hormone concentrations during puberty in boys. J Clin Endocrinol Metab 1989; 69:563–570.

148. Zeitler P, Argente J, Chowen-Breede JA, et al. Growth hormone releasing hormone messenger ribonucleic acid in the hypothalamus of the adult male rat is increased by testosterone. Endocrinology 1990; 127:362–368.

149. Werner H, Koch Y, Baldino F, et al. Steroid regulation of somatostatin mRNA in the rat hypothalamus. J Biol Chem 1988; 263:7666–7671.

150. Van Cauter E, Kerkhofs M, Van Onderbergen A, et al. Modulation of spontaneous and GHRH-stimulated GH secretion by sleep. Proceedings of the 71st meeting of the Endocrine Society, Seattle, WA, 1989: 220 (abstract).

151. Fiddes JC, Goodman HM. The gene encoding the common alpha subunit of the four human glycoprotein hormones. J Molec Appl Genet 1981; 1:3–18.

152. Veldhuis JD, Iranmanesh A, Ho KK, et al. Dual defects in pulsatile growth hormone secretion and clearance subserve the hyposomatotropism of obesity in man. J Clin Endocrinol Metab 1991; 72(1):51–59.

153. Veldhuis JD, Liem AY, South S, et al. Differential impact of age, sex steroid hormones, and obesity on basal versus pulsatile growth hormone secretion in men as assessed in an ultrasensitive chemiluminescence assay. J Clin Endocrinol Metab 1995; 80:3209–3222.

154. Jansson JO, Isaksson OG, Eden S, et al. Effects of plasma GH pattern on growth factors and body growth. In: Frisch H, Thorner MO, eds. Hormonal regulation of growth. Serono Symposia, Vol 58. New York: Raven Press, 1989: 185–199.

155. Stewart PM, Smith S, Seth J, et al. Normal growth hormone response to the 75 g oral glucose tolerance test measured by immunoradiometric assay. Ann Clin Biochem 1989; 26:205–206.

156. Asplin CM, Faria AC, Carlsen EC, et al. Alterations in the pulsatile mode of growth hormone release in men and women with insulin-dependent diabetes mellitus. J Clin Endocrinol Metab 1989; 69:239–245.

157. Silver HK, Finkelstein M. Deprivation dwarfism. J Pediatr 1967; 70:317–324.

158. Powell GF, Brasel JA, Blizzard RM. Emotional deprivation and growth retardation simulating idiopathic hypopituitarism. I: Clinical evaluation of the syndrome. N Engl J Med 1967; 276:1271–1278.

159. Delitala G. Clinical neuropharmacology in the management of disorders of the pituitary and hypothalamus. In: Endocrinology. DeGroot LJ, Besser GM, Cahill GF Jr, et al, eds. Philadelphia: WB Saunders, 1989: 454–473.

160. Soulairac A, Schaub C, Franchimont P, et al. A study of the pharmacological activation of the central pole of the hypothalamo-hypophyseal axis. Ann Endocrinol (Paris) 1968; 29(1):45–54.

161. Salvadorini F, Galeone F, Nicotere M. Clinical evaluation of CDP-choline: efficacy as antidepressant treatment. Curr Ther Res Clin Exp 1968; 18:513–520.

162. Mendelson WB, Sitaram N, Wyatt RJ, et al. Methoscopolamine inhibition of sleep-related growth hormone secretion. Evidence for a cholinergic secretory mechanism. J Clin Invest 1978; 61:1683–1690.

163. Delitala G, Frulio T, Pacifico A, et al. Participation of cholinergic muscarinic receptors in glucagon- and arginine-mediated growth hormone secretion in man. J Clin Endocrinol Metab 1982; 55:1231–1233.

164. Delitala G, Grossman A, Besser GM. Opiate peptides control growth hormone through a cholinergic mechanism in man. Clin Endocrinol (Oxf) 1983; 18:401–405.

165. Delitala G, Maioli M, Pacifico A, et al. Cholinergic receptor control mechanisms for L-dopa, apomorphine, and clonidine-induced growth hormone secretion in man. J Clin Endocrinol Metab 1983; 57:1145–1149.

166. Stubbs WA, Delitala G, Jones A, et al. Hormonal and metabolic responses to an enkephalin analogue in normal man. Lancet 1978; 2:1225–1227.

167. Bowers CY, Reynolds GA, Durham D, et al. Growth hormone (GH)–releasing peptide stimulates GH release in normal men and acts synergistically with GH-releasing hormone. J Clin Endocrinol Metab 1990; 70:975–982.

168. Pong SS, Chaung LYP, Dean DC, et al. Identification of a new G-protein-linked receptor for growth hormone secretagogues. Mol Endocrinol 1996; 10:57–61.

169. Howard AD, Feighner SD, Cully DF, et al. A receptor in pituitary and hypothalamus that functions in growth hormone release (see comments). Science 1996; 273:974–977.

170. Copinschi G, Vanonderbergen A, Lhermitebaleriaux M, et al. Effects of a

7-day treatment with a novel, orally active, growth hormone (GH) secretagogue, MK-677, on 24-hour GH profiles, insulin-like growth factor I, and adrenocortical function in normal young men. J Clin Endocrinol Metab 1996; 81:2776–2782.

171. Chapman IM, Bach MA, Van Cauter E, et al. Stimulation of the growth hormone (GH)–insulin-like growth factor I axis by daily oral administration of a GH secretagogue (MK-677) in healthy elderly subjects. J Clin Endocrinol Metab 1996; 81:4249–4257.

172. Conn PM, Bowers CY. A new receptor for growth hormone-release peptide (comment; review). Science 1996; 273:923.

173. Chapman IM, Bach MA, Van Cauter E, et al. Stimulation of the growth hormone (GH)–insulin-like growth factor I axis by daily oral administration of a GH secretagogue (MK-677) in healthy elderly subjects. J Clin Endocrinol Metab 1996; 81:4249–4257.

174. Salmon WD Jr, Daughaday WH. A hormonally controlled serum factor which stimulates sulfate incorporation by cartilage in vitro. J Lab Clin Med 1957; 49:825.

175. Daughaday WH, Reeder C. Synchronous activation of DNA synthesis in hypophysectomized rat cartilage by growth hormone. J Lab Clin Med 1966; 68:357–368.

176. Abe H, Molitch ME, Van W, et al. Human growth hormone and somatomedin C suppress the spontaneous release of growth hormone in unanesthetized rats. Endocrinology 1983; 113:1319–1324.

177. Berelowitz M, Szabo M, Frohman LA, et al. Somatomedin-C mediates growth hormone negative feedback by effects on both the hypothalamus and the pituitary. Science 1981; 212:1279–1281.

178. Brazeau P, Guillemin R, Ling N, et al. Inhibition par les somatomedines de la secretion de l'hormone de croissace stimulee par le facteur hypothalamique somatocrinine (GRF) ou le peptide de synthese hpGRF. C R Acad Sci 1982; 295:651–654.

179. Melmed S, Yamashita S. Insulin-like growth factor-I action on hypothyroid rat pituitary cells: suppression of triiodothyronine-induced growth hormone secretion and messenger ribonucleic acid levels. Endocrinology 1986; 118:1483–1490.

180. Green H, Morikawa M, Nixon T. A dual effector theory of growth-hormone action (review). Differentiation 1985; 29:195–198.

181. Isaksson OG, Jansson JO, Gause IA. Growth hormone stimulates longitudinal bone growth directly. Science 1982; 216:1237–1239.

182. Russell SM, Spencer EM. Local injections of human or rat growth hormone or of purified human somatomedin-C stimulate unilateral tibial epiphyseal growth in hypophysectomized rats. Endocrinology 1985; 116:2563–2567.

183. Schlechter NL, Russell SM, Spencer EM, et al. Evidence suggesting that the direct growth-promoting effect of growth hormone on cartilage in vivo is mediated by local production of somatomedin. Proc Natl Acad Sci USA 1986; 83:7932–7934.

184. Nilsson A, Isgaard J, Lindahl A, et al. Regulation by growth hormone of number of chondrocytes containing IGF-I in rat growth plate. Science 1986; 233:571–574.

185. D'Ercole AJ, Stiles AD, Underwood LE. Tissue concentrations of somatomedin C: further evidence for multiple sites of synthesis and paracrine or autocrine mechanisms of action. Proc Natl Acad Sci USA 1984; 81:935–939.

186. Isaksson OG, Eden S, Jansson JO. Mode of action of pituitary growth hormone on target cells (review). Annu Rev Physiol 1985; 47:483–499.

187. Isaksson OG, Lindahl A, Nilsson A, et al. Mechanism of the stimulatory effect of growth hormone on longitudinal bone growth (review). Endocr Rev 1987; 8:426–438.

188. Skottner A, Clark RG, Robinson IC, et al. Recombinant human insulin-like growth factor: testing the somatomedin hypothesis in hypophysectomized rats. J Endocrinol 1987; 112:123–132.

189. Guler HP, Zapf J, Scheiwiller E, et al. Recombinant human insulin-like growth factor I stimulates growth and has distinct effects on organ size in hypophysectomized rats. Proc Natl Acad Sci USA 1988; 85:4889–4893.

190. Bauman DE, Eisemann JH, Currie WB. Hormonal effects on partitioning of nutrients for tissue growth: role of growth hormone and prolactin. Fed Proc 1982; 41:2538–2544.

191. Muir LA, Wien S, Duquette PF, et al. Effects of exogenous growth hormone and diethylstilbestrol on growth and carcass composition of growing lambs. J Anim Sci 1983; 56:1315–1323.

192. Evock CM, Etherton TD, Chung CS, et al. Pituitary porcine growth hormone (pGH) and a recombinant pGH analog stimulate pig growth performance in a similar manner. J Anim Sci 1988; 66:1928–1941.

193. Etherton TD, Wiggins JP, Evock CM, et al. Stimulation of pig growth performance by porcine growth hormone: determination of the dose-response relationship. J Anim Sci 1987; 64:433–443.

194. Gerich JE, Lorenzi M, Bier DM, et al. Effects of physiologic levels of glucagon and growth hormone on human carbohydrate and lipid metabolism. Studies involving administration of exogenous hormone during suppression of endogenous hormone secretion with somatostatin. J Clin Invest 1976; 57:875–884.

195. Metcalfe P, Johnston DG, Nosadini R, et al. Metabolic effects of acute and prolonged growth hormone excess in normal and insulin-deficient man. Diabetologia 1981; 20:123–128.

196. Sherwin RS, Schulman GA, Hendler R, et al. Effect of growth hormone on oral glucose tolerance and circulating metabolic fuels in man. Diabetologia 1983; 24:155–161.

197. Rosenfeld RG, Wilson DM, Dollar LA, et al. Both human pituitary growth hormone and recombinant DNA–derived human growth hormone cause insulin resistance at a postreceptor site. J Clin Endocrinol Metab 1982; 54:1033–1038.

198. Bratusch-Marrain PR, Smith D, DeFronzo RA. The effect of growth hormone on glucose metabolism and insulin secretion in man. J Clin Endocrinol Metab 1982; 55:973–982.

199. Orskov L, Schmitz O, Jorgensen JO, et al. Influence of growth hormone on glucose-induced glucose uptake in normal men as assessed by the hyperglycemic clamp technique. J Clin Endocrinol Metab 1989; 68:276–282.

200. Frohman LA. Diseases of the anterior pituitary. In: Felig P, Baxter JD, Broadus AE, et al, eds. Endocrinology and Metabolism. New York: McGraw-Hill, 1981: 151–231.

201. Manson JM, Wilmore DW. Positive nitrogen balance with human growth hormone and hypocaloric intravenous feeding. Surgery 1986; 100:188–197.

202. Clemmons DR, Snyder DK, Williams R, et al. Growth hormone administration conserves lean body mass during dietary restriction in obese subjects. J Clin Endocrinol Metab 1987; 64:878–883.

203. Binnerts A, Wilson JH, Lamberts SW. The effects of human growth hormone administration in elderly adults with recent weight loss. J Clin Endocrinol Metab 1988; 67:1312–1316.

204. Snyder DK, Clemmons DR, Underwood LE. Treatment of obese, diet-restricted subjects with growth hormone for 11 weeks: effects on anabolism, lipolysis, and body composition. J Clin Endocrinol Metab 1988; 67:54–61.

205. Carlson HE, Gillin JC, Gorden P, et al. Absence of sleep-related growth hormone peaks in aged normal subjects and in acromegaly. J Clin Endocrinol Metab 1972; 34:1102–1105.

206. Finkelstein JW, Boyar RM, Roffwarg HP, et al. Age-related change in the twenty-four-hour spontaneous secretion of growth hormone. J Clin Endocrinol Metab 1972; 35:665–670.

207. Dudl RJ, Ensinck JW, Palmer HE, et al. Effect of age on growth hormone secretion in man. J Clin Endocrinol Metab 1973; 37:11–16.

208. Rudman D, Kutner MH, Rogers CM, et al. Impaired growth hormone secretion in the adult population: relation to age and adiposity. J Clin Invest 1981; 67:1361–1369.

209. Young VR, Uauy R, Winterer JC. Protein metabolism and needs in elderly people. In: Rockstein M, Sussman ML, eds. Nutrition, Longevity and Aging. New York: Academic Press, 1976: 67–102.

210. Forbes GB, Reina JC. Adult lean body mass declines with age: some longitudinal observations. Metabolism 1970; 19:653–663.

211. Rudman D, Feller AG, Nagraj HS, et al. Effects of human growth hormone in men over 60 years old. N Engl J Med 1990; 323:1–6.

212. Salomon F, Cuneo RC, Hesp R, et al. The effects of treatment with recombinant human growth hormone on body composition and metabolism in adults with growth hormone deficiency. N Engl J Med 1989; 321:1797–1803.

213. Ward HC, Halliday D, Sim AJ. Protein and energy metabolism with biosynthetic human growth hormone after gastrointestinal surgery. Ann Surg 1987; 206:56–61.

214. Soroff HS, Pearson E, Green NL, et al. The effect of growth hormone on nitrogen balance at various levels of intake in burned patients. Surg Gynecol Obstet 1960; 111:259–273.

215. Liljedahl SO, Gemzell CA, Plantin LO, et al. Effect of human growth hormone in patients with severe burns. Acta Chir Scand 1961; 122:1–14.

216. Soroff HS, Rozin RR, Mooty J, et al. Role of human growth hormone in the response to trauma. I: Metabolic effects following burns. Ann Surg 1967; 166:739–752.

217. Wilmore DW, Moylan JA Jr, Bristow BF, et al. Anabolic effects of human growth hormone and high caloric feedings following thermal injury. Surg Gynecol Obstet 1974; 138:875–884.

218. Horber FF, Haymond MV. Human growth hormone prevents the protein catabolic side effects of prednisone in humans. J Clin Invest 1990; 86:265–272.

Glycoprotein Hormone Family

219. Pierce JG, Parsons TF. Glycoprotein hormones: structure and function (review). Annu Rev Biochem 1981; 50:465–495.

220. Vamvakopoulos NC, Kourides IA. Identification of separate mRNAs coding for the alpha and beta subunits of thyrotropin. Proc Natl Acad Sci USA 1979; 76:3809–3813.

221. Giudice LC, Weintraub BD. Evidence for conformational differences between precursor and processed forms of thyroid-stimulating hormone beta subunit. J Biol Chem 1979; 254:12679–12683.

222. Godine JE, Chin WW, Habener JF. Luteinizing and follicle-stimulating hormones. Cell-free translations of messenger RNAs coding for subunit precursors. J Biol Chem 1980; 255:8780–8783.

223. Blackman MR, Gershengorn MC, Weintraub BD. Excess production of free alpha subunits by mouse pituitary thyrotropic tumor cells in vitro. Endocrinology 1978; 102:499–508.

224. Kourides IA, Landon MB, Hoffman BJ, et al. Excess free alpha relative to beta subunits of the glycoprotein hormones in normal and abnormal human pituitary glands. Clin Endocrinol (Oxf) 1980; 12:407–416.

225. Ross DS, Downing MF, Chin WW, et al. Changes in tissue concentrations of thyrotropin, free thyrotropin beta, and alpha-subunits after thyroxine

administration: comparison of mouse hypothyroid pituitary and thyrotropic tumors. Endocrinology 1983; 112:2050–2053.

226. Weintraub BD, Stannard BS, Magner JA, et al. Glycosylation and posttranslational processing of thyroid-stimulating hormone: clinical implications (review). Recent Prog Horm Res 1985; 41:577–606.

227. Shupnik MA, Ridgway EC, Chin WW. Molecular biology of thyrotropin (review). Endocr Rev 1989; 10:459–475.

228. Gharib SD, Wierman ME, Shupnik MA, et al. Molecular biology of the pituitary gonadotropins (review). Endocr Rev 1990; 11:177–199.

229. Fiddes JC, Talmadge K. Structure, expression, and evolution of the genes for the human glycoprotein hormones (review). Recent Prog Horm Res 1984; 40:43–78.

230. Chin WW, Kronenberg HM, Dee PC, et al. Nucleotide sequence of the mRNA encoding the pre-alpha-subunit of mouse thyrotropin. Proc Natl Acad Sci USA 1981; 78:5329–5333.

231. Schorr Toshav NL, Gurr JA, Catterall JF, et al. Thyrotropin and alpha-subunit in the brain: evidence for biosynthesis within the pituitary. Endocrinology 1983; 112:1434–1440.

232. Godine JE, Chin WW, Habener JF. Alpha subunit of rat pituitary glycoprotein hormones. Primary structure of the precursor determined from the nucleotide sequence of cloned cDNAs. J Biol Chem 1982; 257:8368–8371.

233. Croyle ML, Maurer RA. Thyroid hormone decreases thyrotropin subunit mRNA levels in rat anterior pituitary. DNA 1984; 3:231–236.

234. Nilson JH, Thomason AR, Cserbak MT, et al. Nucleotide sequence of a cDNA for the common alpha subunit of the bovine pituitary glycoprotein hormones. Conservation of nucleotides in the 3'-untranslated region of bovine and human pre–alpha subunit mRNAs. J Biol Chem 1983; 258:4679–4682.

235. Erwin CR, Croyle ML, Donelson JE, et al. Nucleotide sequence of cloned complementary deoxyribonucleic acid for the alpha subunit of bovine pituitary glycoprotein hormones. Biochemistry 1983; 22:4856–4860.

236. Fiddes JC, Goodman HM. Isolation, cloning and sequence analysis of the cDNA for the alpha-subunit of human chorionic gonadotropin. Nature 1979; 281:351–356.

237. Dracopoli NC, Rettig WJ, Whitfield GK, et al. Assignment of the gene for the beta subunit of thyroid-stimulating hormone to the short arm of human chromosome 1. Proc Natl Acad Sci USA 1986; 83:1822–1826.

238. Wondisford FE, Radovick S, Moates JM, et al. Isolation and characterization of the human thyrotropin beta-subunit gene. Differences in gene structure and promoter function from murine species. J Biol Chem 1988; 263:12538–12542.

239. Gurr JA, Catterall JF, Kourides IA. Cloning of cDNA encoding the pre-beta subunit of mouse thyrotropin. Proc Natl Acad Sci USA 1983; 80:2122–2126.

240. Chin WW, Shupnik MA, Ross DS, et al. Regulation of the alpha and thyrotropin beta-subunit messenger ribonucleic acids by thyroid hormones. Endocrinology 1985; 116:873–878.

241. Chin WW, Muccini JA Jr, Shin L. Evidence for a single rat thyrotropin-beta-subunit gene: thyroidectomy increases its mRNA. Biochem Biophys Res Commun 1985; 128:1152–1158.

242. Maurer RA, Croyle ML, Donelson JE. The sequence of a cloned cDNA for the beta subunit of bovine thyrotropin predicts a protein containing both NH_2- and COOH-terminal extensions. J Biol Chem 1984; 259:5024–5027.

243. Hayashizaki Y, Miyai K, Kato K, et al. Molecular cloning of the human thyrotropin-beta subunit gene. Febs Lett 1985; 188:394–400.

244. Whitfiled GK, Powers RE, Gurr JA, et al. Isolation of a gene encoding human thyrotropin beta subunit. In: Medeiros-Neto G, Gaitan E, eds. Frontiers in Thyroidology. New York: Plenum Medical, 1986: 173–176.

245. Samuels MH, Wood WM, Gordon DF, et al. Clinical and molecular studies of a thyrotropin-secreting pituitary adenoma. J Clin Endocrinol Metab 1989; 68:1211–1215.

246. Miyai K, Hayashizaki Y, Matsubara K. Familial hypothyroidism due to thyrotropin gene abnormality. Int Congr Endocrinol (Jpn) 1988; 1:545–550.

247. Hayashizaki Y, Hiroaka Y, Endo Y, et al. Thyroid-stimulating hormone (TSH) deficiency caused by a single base substitution in the CAGYC region of the beta subunit. Embo J 1989; 8:2291.

248. Bodenner DL, Mroczynski MA, Weintraub BD, et al. A detailed functional and structural analysis of a major thyroid hormone inhibitory element in the human thyrotropin beta-subunit gene. J Biol Chem 1991; 266:21666–21673.

249. Pennathur S, Madison LD, Kay TW, et al. Localization of promoter sequences required for thyrotropin-releasing hormone and thyroid hormone responsiveness of the glycoprotein hormone alpha-gene in primary cultures of rat pituitary cells. Mol Endocrinol 1993; 7:797–805.

250. Khalil A, Kovacs K, Sima AA, et al. Pituitary thyrotroph hyperplasia mimicking prolactin-secreting adenoma. J Endocrinol Invest 1984; 7:399–404.

251. Scheithauer BW, Kovacs KT, Young WF Jr, et al. The pituitary gland in hyperthyroidism. Mayo Clin Proc 1992; 67:22–26.

252. Gurr JA, Kourides IA. Ratios of alpha to beta TSH mRNA in normal and hypothyroid pituitaries and TSH-secreting tumors. Endocrinology 1984; 115:830–832.

253. Shupnik MA, Ridgway EC. Thyroid hormone control of thyrotropin gene expression in rat anterior pituitary cells. Endocrinology 1987; 121:619–624.

254. Shupnik MA, Chin WW, Habener JF, et al. Transcriptional regulation of the thyrotropin subunit genes by thyroid hormone. J Biol Chem 1985; 260:2900–2903.

255. Shupnik MA, Ardisson LJ, Meskell MJ, et al. Triiodothyronine (T_3) regulation of thyrotropin subunit gene transcription is proportional to T_3 nuclear receptor occupancy. Endocrinology 1986; 118:367–371.

256. Gershengorn MC. Thyroid hormone regulation of thyrotropin production and interaction with thyrotropin-releasing hormone in thyrotropic cells in culture. In: Oppenheimer JH, Samuels HH, eds. Molecular Basis of Thyroid Hormone Action. New York: Academic Press, 1983: 387–411.

257. Shupnik MA, Greenspan SL, Ridgway EC. Transcriptional regulation of thyrotropin subunit genes by thyrotropin-releasing hormone and dopamine in pituitary cell culture. J Biol Chem 1986; 261:12675–12679.

258. Lippman SS, Amr S, Weintraub BD. Discordant effects of thyrotropin (TSH)-releasing hormone on pre- and posttranslational regulation of TSH biosynthesis in rat pituitary. Endocrinology 1986; 119:343–348.

259. Steinfelder HJ, Hauser P, Nakayama Y, et al. Thyrotropin-releasing hormone regulation of human TSHB expression: role of a pituitary-specific transcription factor (Pit-1/GHF-1) and potential interaction with a thyroid hormone–inhibitory element. Proc Natl Acad Sci USA 1991; 88:3130–3134.

260. Mason ME, Friend KE, Copper J, et al. Pit-1/GHF-1 binds to TRH-sensitive regions of the rat thyrotropin beta gene. Biochemistry 1993; 32:8932–8938.

261. Kim DS, Ahn SK, Yoon JH, et al. Involvement of a cAMP-responsive DNA element in mediating TRH responsiveness of the human thyrotropin alpha-subunit gene. Mol Endocrinol 1994; 8:528–536.

262. Reichlin S. TRH: historical aspects (review). Ann NY Acad Sci 1989; 553:1–6.

263. Dyess EM, Segerson TP, Liposits Z, et al. Triiodothyronine exerts direct cell-specific regulation of thyrotropin-releasing hormone gene expression in the hypothalamic paraventricular nucleus. Endocrinology 1988; 123:2291–2297.

264. Lechan RM. Neuroendocrinology of pituitary hormone regulation. Endocrinol Metab Clin North Am 1987; 16:475–502.

265. Larsen PR. Thyroid-pituitary interaction: feedback regulation of thyrotropin secretion by thyroid hormones (review). N Engl J Med 1982; 306:23–32.

266. Fish LH, Schwartz HL, Cavanaugh J, et al. Replacement dose, metabolism, and bioavailability of levothyroxine in the treatment of hypothyroidism. Role of triiodothyronine in pituitary feedback in humans. N Engl J Med 1987; 316:764–770.

267. Parker DC, Rossman LG, Pekary AE, et al. Effect of 64-hour sleep deprivation on the circadian waveform of thyrotropin (TSH): further evidence of sleep-related inhibition of TSH release. J Clin Endocrinol Metab 1987; 64:157–161.

268. Brabant G, Brabant A, Ranft U, et al. Circadian and pulsatile thyrotropin secretion in euthyroid man under the influence of thyroid hormone and glucocorticoid administration. J Clin Endocrinol Metab 1987; 65:83–88.

269. Chan V, Jones A, Liendo-Ch P, et al. The relationship between circadian variations in circulating thyrotrophin, thyroid hormones and prolactin. Clin Endocrinol (Oxf) 1978; 9:337–349.

270. Nicoloff JT, Spencer CA. Clinical Review 12: The use and misuse of the sensitive thyrotropin assays. J Clin Endocrinol Metab 1990; 71(3):553–558.

271. Watkins PC, Eddy R, Beck AK, et al. DNA sequence and regional assignment of the human follicle-stimulating hormone beta-subunit gene to the short arm of human chromosome 11. DNA 1987; 6:205–212.

272. Jameson JL, Becker CB, Lindell CM, et al. Human follicle-stimulating hormone beta-subunit gene encodes multiple messenger ribonucleic acids. Mol Endocrinol 1988; 2:806–815.

273. Pelletier G, Leclerc R, Labrie F. Identification of gonadotropic cells in the human pituitary by immunoperoxidase technique. Mol Cell Endocrinol 1976; 6:123–128.

274. Denef C. Paracrine interactions in the anterior pituitary (review). Clin Endocrinol Metab 1986; 15:1–32.

275. Holck S, Albrechtsen R, Wewer UM. Laminin in the anterior pituitary gland of the rat. Laminin in the gonadotrophic cells correlates with their functional state. Lab Invest 1987; 56:481–488.

276. Kovacs K, Horvath E. Gonadotrophs following removal of the ovaries: a fine structural study of human pituitary glands. Endokrinologie 1975; 66:1–8.

277. Kovacs K, Sheehan HL. Pituitary changes in Kallmann's syndrome: a histologic, immunocytologic, ultrastructural, and immunoelectron microscopic study. Fertil Steril 1982; 37:83–89.

278. Braunstein GD, Rasor J, Wade ME. Presence in normal human testes of a chorionic-gonadotropin-like substance distinct from human luteinizing hormone. N Engl J Med 1975; 293:1339–1343.

279. Chen HC, Hodgen GD, Matsuura S, et al. Evidence for a gonadotropin from nonpregnant subjects that has physical, immunological, and biological similarities to human chorionic gonadotropin. Proc Natl Acad Sci USA 1976; 73:2885–2889.

280. Odell WD, Griffin J. Pulsatile secretion of human chorionic gonadotropin in normal adults. N Engl J Med 1987; 317:1688–1691.

281. Conn PM. GnRH regulation of gonadotropin release and target cell responsiveness. In: DeGroot LJ, ed. Endocrinology. Vol 1. Philadelphia: WB Saunders, 1989: 284–295.

282. Shupnik MA, Weinmann CM, Notides AC, et al. An upstream region of the rat luteinizing hormone beta gene binds estrogen receptor and confers estrogen responsiveness. J Biol Chem 1989; 264:80–86.

283. Shupnik MA, Gharib SD, Chin WW. Divergent effects of estradiol on gonadotropin gene transcription in pituitary fragments. Mol Endocrinol 1989; 3:474–480.

284. Shupnik MA, Gharib SD, Chin WW. Estrogen suppresses rat gonadotropin gene transcription in vivo. Endocrinology 1988; 122:1842–1846.

285. Yamaji T, Dierschke DJ, Bhattacharya AN, et al. The negative feedback control by estradiol and progesterone of LH secretion in the ovariectomized rhesus monkey. Endocrinology 1972; 90:771–777.

286. Knobil E. The neuroendocrine control of the menstrual cycle (review). Recent Prog Horm Res 1980; 36:53–88.

287. Blondeau JP, Baulieu EE. Progesterone receptor characterized by photoaffinity labelling in the plasma membrane of *Xenopus laevis* oocytes. Biochem J 1984; 219:785–792.

288. Baulieu EE, Godeau F, Schorderet M, et al. Steroid-induced meiotic division in *Xenopus laevis* oocytes: surface and calcium (review). Nature 1978; 275:593–598.

289. Clarke IJ, Cummins JT. Increased gonadotropin-releasing hormone pulse frequency associated with estrogen-induced luteinizing hormone surges in ovariectomized ewes. Endocrinology 1985; 116:2376–2383.

290. Neill JD, Patton JM, Dailey RA, et al. Luteinizing hormone releasing hormone (LHRH) in pituitary stalk blood of rhesus monkeys: relationship to level of LH release. Endocrinology 1977; 101:430–434.

291. Kaiser UB, Jakubowiak A, Steinberger A, et al. Regulation of rat pituitary gonadotropin-releasing hormone receptor mRNA levels in vivo and in vitro. Endocrinology 1993; 133:931–934.

292. Marshall JC, Kelch RP. Gonadotropin-releasing hormone: role of pulsatile secretion in the regulation of reproduction (review). N Engl J Med 1986; 315:1459–1468.

293. Soules MR, Steiner RA, Clifton DK, et al. Progesterone modulation of pulsatile luteinizing hormone secretion in normal women. J Clin Endocrinol Metab 1984; 58:378–383.

294. Sollenberger MJ, Carlsen EC, Johnson ML, et al. Specific physiological regulation of LH secretory events throughout the human menstrual cycle: new insights into the pulsatile mode of gonadotropin release. J Neuroendocrinol 1990; 2(6):845–852.

295. Steiner RA, Bremner WJ, Clifton DK. Regulation of luteinizing hormone pulse frequency and amplitude by testosterone in the adult male rat. Endocrinology 1982; 111:2055–2061.

296. Wierman ME, Gharib SD, LaRovere JM, et al. Selective failure of androgens to regulate follicle stimulating hormone beta messenger ribonucleic acid levels in the male rat. Mol Endocrinol 1988; 2:492–498.

297. Clay CM, Keri RA, Finicle AB, et al. Transcriptional repression of the glycoprotein hormone alpha subunit gene by androgen may involve direct binding of androgen receptor to the proximal promoter. J Biol Chem 1993; 268:13556–13564.

298. Boyar RM, Moore RJ, Rosner W, et al. Studies of gonadotropin-gonadal dynamics in patients with androgen insensitivity. J Clin Endocrinol Metab 1978; 47:1116–1122.

299. Belchetz PE, Plant TM, Nakai Y, et al. Hypophysial responses to continuous and intermittent delivery of hypothalamic gonadotropin-releasing hormone. Science 1978; 202:631–633.

300. Valk TW, Corley KP, Kelch RP, et al. Hypogonadotropic hypogonadism: hormonal responses to low dose pulsatile administration of gonadotropin-releasing hormone. J Clin Endocrinol Metab 1980; 51:730–738.

301. Hoffman AR, Crowley WF Jr. Induction of puberty in men by long-term pulsatile administration of low-dose gonadotropin-releasing hormone. N Engl J Med 1982; 307:1237–1241.

302. Pohl CR, Richardson DW, Hutchison JS, et al. Hypophysiotropic signal frequency and the functioning of the pituitary-ovarian system in the rhesus monkey. Endocrinology 1983; 112:2076–2080.

303. Clarke IJ, Cummins JT, Findlay JK, et al. Effects on plasma luteinizing hormone and follicle-stimulating hormone of varying the frequency and amplitude of gonadotropin-releasing hormone pulses in ovariectomized ewes with hypothalamo-pituitary disconnection. Neuroendocrinology 1984; 39:214–221.

304. Wildt L, Hausler A, Marshall G, et al. Frequency and amplitude of gonadotropin-releasing hormone stimulation and gonadotropin secretion in the rhesus monkey. Endocrinology 1981; 109:376–385.

305. Mercer JE, Clements JA, Funder JW, et al. Luteinizing hormone–beta mRNA levels are regulated primarily by gonadotropin-releasing hormone and not by negative estrogen feedback on the pituitary. Neuroendocrinology 1988; 47:563–566.

306. Hamernik DL, Crowder ME, Nilson JH, et al. Measurement of messenger ribonucleic acid for luteinizing hormone beta-subunit, alpha-subunit, growth hormone, and prolactin after hypothalamic pituitary disconnection in ovariectomized ewes. Endocrinology 1986; 119:2704–2710.

307. Hamernik DL, Nett TM. Gonadotropin-releasing hormone increases the amount of messenger ribonucleic acid for gonadotropins in ovariectomized ewes after hypothalamic-pituitary disconnection. Endocrinology 1988; 122:959–966.

308. Papavasiliou SS, Zmeili S, Khoury S, et al. Gonadotropin-releasing hormone differentially regulates expression of the genes for luteinizing hormone alpha and beta subunits in male rats. Proc Natl Acad Sci USA 1986; 83:4026–4029.

309. Haisenleder DJ, Katt JA, Ortolano GA, et al. Influence of gonadotropin-releasing hormone pulse amplitude, frequency, and treatment duration on the regulation of luteinizing hormone (LH) subunit messenger ribonucleic acids and LH secretion. Mol Endocrinol 1988; 2:338–343.

310. Dalkin AC, Haisenleder DJ, Ortolano GA, et al. The frequency of gonado-

tropin-releasing-hormone stimulation differentially regulates gonadotropin subunit messenger ribonucleic acid expression. Endocrinology 1989; 125:917–924.

311. Haisenleder DJ, Dalkin AC, Ortolano GA, et al. A pulsatile gonadotropin-releasing hormone stimulus is required to increase transcription of the gonadotropin subunit genes: evidence for differential regulation of transcription by pulse frequency in vivo. Endocrinology 1991; 128:509–517.

312. Shupnik MA. Effects of gonadotropin-releasing hormone on rat gonadotropin gene transcription in vitro: requirement for pulsatile administration for luteinizing hormone–beta gene stimulation. Mol Endocrinol 1990; 4:1444–1450.

313. Abeyawardene SA, Plant TM. Bilateral orchidectomy and concomitant testosterone replacement in the juvenile male rhesus monkey (*Macaca mulatta*) receiving an invariant intravenous gonadotropin-releasing hormone (GnRH) infusion results, as in the hypothalamus lesioned GnRH-driven adult male, in a selective hypersecretion of follicle-stimulating hormone. Endocrinology 1989; 125:257–259.

314. Dubey AK, Zeleznik AJ, Plant TM. In the rhesus monkey (*Macaca mulatta*), the negative feedback regulation of follicle-stimulating hormone secretion by an action of testicular hormone directly at the level of the anterior pituitary gland cannot be accounted for by either testosterone or estradiol. Endocrinology 1987; 121:2229–2237.

315. Plant TM, Gay VL, Marshall GR, et al. Puberty in monkeys is triggered by chemical stimulation of the hypothalamus. Proc Natl Acad Sci USA 1989; 86:2506–2510.

316. Ying SY. Inhibins and activins: chemical properties and biological activity (review). Proc Soc Exp Biol Med 1987; 186:253–264.

317. de Jong FH. Inhibin (review). Physiol Rev 1988; 68:555–607.

318. Vale W, Rivier J, Vaughan J, et al. Purification and characterization of an FSH releasing protein from porcine ovarian follicular fluid. Nature 1986; 321:776–779.

319. Ling N, Ying SY, Ueno N, et al. Pituitary FSH is released by a heterodimer of the beta-subunits from the two forms of inhibin. Nature 1986; 321:779–782.

320. Petraglia F, Sawchenko P, Lim AT, et al. Localization, secretion, and action of inhibin in human placenta. Science 1987; 237:187–189.

321. Roberts V, Meunier H, Vaughan J, et al. Production and regulation of inhibin subunits in pituitary gonadotropes. Endocrinology 1989; 124:552–554.

322. Ramasharma K, Li CH. Human seminal alpha-inhibins: detection in human pituitary, hypothalamus, and serum by immunoreactivity. Proc Natl Acad Sci USA 1986; 83:3484–3486.

323. Sawchenko PE, Plotsky PM, Pfeiffer SW, et al. Inhibin beta in central neural pathways involved in the control of oxytocin secretion. Nature 1988; 334:615–617.

324. Medhamurthy R, Abeyawardene SA, Culler MD, et al. Immunoneutralization of circulating inhibin in the hypophysiotropically clamped male rhesus monkey (*Macaca mulatta*) results in a selective hypersecretion of follicle-stimulating hormone. Endocrinology 1990; 126:2116–2124.

325. Mercer JE, Clements JA, Funder JW, et al. Rapid and specific lowering of pituitary FSH beta mRNA levels by inhibin. Mol Cell Endocrinol 1987; 53:251–254.

326. Carroll RS, Corrigan AZ, Gharib SD, et al. Inhibin, activin, and follistatin: regulation of follicle-stimulating hormone messenger ribonucleic acid levels. Mol Endocrinol 1989; 3:1969–1976.

327. Attardi B, Keeping HS, Winters SJ, et al. Rapid and profound suppression of messenger ribonucleic acid encoding follicle-stimulating hormone beta by inhibin from primate Sertoli cells. Mol Endocrinol 1989; 3:280–287.

328. Ueno N, Ling N, Ying SY, et al. Isolation and partial characterization of follistatin: a single-chain Mr 35,000 monomeric protein that inhibits the release of follicle-stimulating hormone. Proc Natl Acad Sci USA 1987; 84:8282–8286.

329. Ying SY, Becker A, Swanson G, et al. Follistatin specifically inhibits pituitary follicle stimulating hormone release in vitro. Biochem Biophys Res Commun 1987; 149:133–139.

330. Zmeili SM, Papavasiliou SS, Thorner MO, et al. Alpha and luteinizing hormone beta subunit messenger ribonucleic acids during the rat estrous cycle. Endocrinology 1986; 119:1867–1869.

331. Ortolano GA, Haisenleder DJ, Dalkin AC, et al. Follicle-stimulating hormone beta subunit messenger ribonucleic acid concentrations during the rat estrous cycle. Endocrinology 1988; 123:2149–2151.(Erratum Endocrinology 1988; 123(6):2942.)

332. Veldhuis JD. Male hypothalamic–pituitary–gonadal axis. In: Yen SSC, Jaffe RB, eds. Reproductive Endocrinology. Philadelphia: WB Saunders (in press).

333. Veldhuis JD, Fraioli F, Rogol AD, et al. Metabolic clearance of biologically active luteinizing hormone in man. J Clin Invest 1986; 77:1122–1128.

334. Van Hall EV, Vaitukaitis JL, Ross GT, et al. Effects of progressive desialylation on the rate of disappearance of immunoreactive HCG from plasma in rats. Endocrinology 1971; 89:11–15.

335. Urban RJ, Veldhuis JD. Kinetics of distribution and metabolic clearance of human FSH in men. Tenth annual NIH Testis Workshop, Baltimore, MD, 1988: 34 (abstract).

336. Coble YD, Kohler PO, Cargille CM, et al. Production rates and metabolic clearance rates of human follicle-stimulating hormone in premenopausal and postmenopausal women. J Clin Invest 1969; 48:359–363.

337. Amin HK, Hunter WM. Human pituitary follicle-stimulating hormone: distribution, plasma clearance and urinary excretion as determined by radioimmunoassay. J Endocrinol 1970; 48:307–317.

338. Plant TM, Krey LC, Moossy J, et al. The arcuate nucleus and the control of gonadotropin and prolactin secretion in the female rhesus monkey (Macaca mulatta). Endocrinology 1978; 102:52–62.

339. Schwanzel-Fukuda M, Bick D, Pfaff DW. Luteinizing hormone–releasing hormone (LHRH)–expressing cells do not migrate normally in an inherited hypogonadal (Kallmann) syndrome. Brain Res Mol Brain Res 1989; 6:311–326.

340. Crowley WF Jr, Filicori M, Spratt DI, et al. The physiology of gonadotropin-releasing hormone (GnRH) secretion in men and women (review). Recent Prog Horm Res 1985; 41:473–531.

341. Clarke IJ, Cummins JT. The temporal relationship between gonadotropin releasing hormone (GnRH) and luteinizing hormone (LH) secretion in ovariectomized ewes. Endocrinology 1982; 111:1737–1739.

342. Clarke IJ, Thomas GB, Yao B, et al. GnRH secretion throughout the ovine estrous cycle. Neuroendocrinology 1987; 46:82–88.

343. Levine JE, Pau KY, Ramirez VD, et al. Simultaneous measurement of luteinizing hormone–releasing hormone and luteinizing hormone release in unanesthetized, ovariectomized sheep. Endocrinology 1982; 111:1449–1455.

344. Levine JE, Ramirez VD. Luteinizing hormone–releasing hormone release during the rat estrous cycle and after ovariectomy, as estimated with push-pull cannulae. Endocrinology 1982; 111:1439–1448.

345. Grumbach MM, Kaplan SL. The neuroendocrinology of human puberty: an ontogenetic perspective. In: Grumbach MM, Sizonenko PC, Aubert ML, eds. Control of the Onset of Puberty. Baltimore: Williams & Wilkins, 1990: 1–68.

346. Germak JA, Knobil E. Control of puberty in the rhesus monkey. In: Grumbach MM, Sizonenko PC, Aubert ML, eds. Control of the Onset of Puberty. Baltimore: Williams & Wilkins, 1990: 69–81.

347. Wildt L, Marshall G, Knobil E. Experimental induction of puberty in the infantile female rhesus monkey. Science 1980; 207:1373–1375.

348. Santen RJ, Bardin CW. Episodic luteinizing hormone secretion in man. Pulse analysis, clinical interpretation, physiologic mechanisms. J Clin Invest 1973; 52:2617–2628.

349. Reame N, Sauder SE, Kelch RP, et al. Pulsatile gonadotropin secretion during the human menstrual cycle: evidence for altered frequency of gonadotropin-releasing hormone secretion. J Clin Endocrinol Metab 1984; 59:328–337.

Unsolved Problems in Pituitary Function

350. Filicori M, Santoro N, Merriam GR, et al. Characterization of the physiological pattern of episodic gonadotropin secretion throughout the human menstrual cycle. J Clin Endocrinol Metab 1986; 62:1136–1144.

351. Amselem S, Duquesnoy P, Attree O, et al. Laron dwarfism and mutations of the growth hormone–receptor gene. N Engl J Med 1989; 321:989–995.

352. Godowski PJ, Leung DW, Meacham LR, et al. Characterization of the human growth hormone receptor gene and demonstration of a partial gene deletion in two patients with Laron-type dwarfism. Proc Natl Acad Sci USA 1989; 86:8083–8087.

353. Straub RE, Frech GC, Joho RH, et al. Expression cloning of a cDNA encoding the mouse pituitary thyrotropin-releasing hormone receptor. Proc Natl Acad Sci USA 1990; 87(24):9514–9518.

354. Tsutsumi M, Zhou W, Millar RP, et al. Cloning and functional expression of a mouse gonadotropin-releasing hormone receptor. Mol Endocrinol 1992; 6:1163–1169.

355. Reinhart J, Mertz LM, Catt KJ. Molecular cloning and expression of cDNA encoding the murine gonadotropin-releasing hormone receptor. J Biol Chem 1992; 267:21281–21284.

356. Chen R, Lewis KA, Perrin MH, et al. Expression cloning of a human corticotropin-releasing-factor receptor. Proc Natl Acad Sci USA 1993; 90:8967–8971.

357. Vita N, Laurent P, Lefort S, et al. Primary structure and functional expression of mouse pituitary and human brain corticotrophin releasing factor receptors. Febs Lett 1993; 335:1–5.

358. Gaylinn BD, Harrison JK, Zysk JR, et al. Molecular cloning and expression of a human anterior pituitary receptor for growth hormone–releasing hormone. Mol Endocrinol 1993; 7:77–84.

359. Mayo KE. Molecular cloning and expression of a pituitary-specific receptor for growth hormone–releasing hormone. Mol Endocrinol 1992; 6:1734–1744.

360. Smith EP, Boyd J, Frank GR, et al. Estrogen resistance caused by a mutation in the estrogen-receptor gene in a man (see comments). N Engl J Med 1994; 331:1056–1061. (Erratum N Engl J Med 1995; 332(2):131.)

361. Simmons DM, Voss JW, Ingraham HA, et al. Pituitary cell type phenotypes involve cell-specific Pit-1 mRNA translation and synergistic interactions with other classes of transcription factors. Genes Dev 1990; 4:696–711.

362. Lira SA, Crenshaw EB, Glass CK, et al. Identification of rat growth hormone genomic sequences targeting pituitary expression in transgenic mice. Proc Natl Acad Sci USA 1988; 85:4755–4759.

363. Borrelli E, Heyman RA, Arias C, et al. Transgenic mice with inducible dwarfism. Nature 1989; 339:538–541.

364. Behringer RR, Mathews LS, Palmiter RD, et al. Dwarf mice produced by genetic ablation of growth hormone–expressing cells. Genes Dev 1988; 2:453–461.

365. Frawley LS, Boockfor FR, Hoeffler JP. Identification by plaque assays of a pituitary cell type that secretes both growth hormone and prolactin. Endocrinology 1985; 116:734–737.

366. Frawley LS, Boockfor FR. Mammosomatotropes: presence and functions in normal and neoplastic pituitary tissue. Endocr Rev 1991; 12(4):337–355.

367. Goth MI, Lyons CE, Ellwood MR, et al. Chronic estrogen treatment in male rats reveals mammosomatotropes and allows inhibition of prolactin secretion by somatostatin. Endocrinology 1996; 137:274–280.

368. Horvath E, Lloyd RV, Kovacs K. Propylthiouracil-induced hypothyroidism results in reversible trans-differentiation of somatotrophs into thyroidectomy cells. A morphologic study of the rat pituitary including immunoelectron microscopy. Lab Invest 1990; 63(4):511–520.

369. Ormandy CJ, Camus A, Barra J, et al. Null mutation of the prolactin receptor gene produces multiple reproductive defects in the mouse. Genes Dev 1997; 11:167–178.

370. Ingraham HA, Chen RP, Mangalam HJ, et al. A tissue-specific transcription factor containing a homeodomain specifies a pituitary phenotype. Cell 1988; 55:519–529.

371. Castrillo JL, Bodner M, Karin M. Purification of growth hormone–specific transcription factor GHF-1 containing homeobox. Science 1989; 243:814–817.

372. Mangalam HJ, Albert VR, Ingraham HA, et al. A pituitary POU domain protein, Pit-1, activates both growth hormone and prolactin promoters transcriptionally. Genes Dev 1989; 3:946–958.

373. Pfaffle RW, DiMattia GE, Parks JS, et al. Mutation of the POU-specific domain of Pit-1 and hypopituitarism without pituitary hypoplasia. Science 1992; 257:1118–1121.

374. Radovick S, Nations M, Du Y, et al. A mutation in the POU-homeodomain of Pit-1 responsible for combined pituitary hormone deficiency. Science 1992; 257:1115–1118.

375. Cohen LE, Wondisford FE, Salvatoni A, et al. A "hot spot" in the Pit-1 gene responsible for combined pituitary hormone deficiency: clinical and molecular correlates. J Clin Endocrinol Metab 1995; 80:679–684.

376. Haugen BR, Ridgway CE. Transcription factor Pit-1 and its clinical implications: from bench to bedside. Endocrinologist 1995; 5:132–139.

377. Crenshaw EB, Kalla K, Simmons DM, et al. Cell-specific expression of the prolactin gene in transgenic mice is controlled by synergistic interactions between promoter and enhancer elements. Genes Dev 1989; 3:959–972.

378. Crenshaw EB III, Li S, Simmons DM, et al. The role of Pit-1 in phenotypic development in the anterior pituitary. Proceedings of the 72nd meeting of the Endocrine Society, Atlanta, GA, 1990: p 17 (abstract).

379. Drolet DW, Scully KM, Simmons DM, et al. TEF, a transcription factor expressed specifically in the anterior pituitary during embryogenesis, defines a new class of leucine zipper proteins. Genes Dev 1991; 5:1739–1753.

380. Haugen BR, Wood WM, Gordon DF, et al. A thyrotrope-specific variant of Pit-1 transactivates the thyrotropin beta promoter. J Biol Chem 1993; 268:20818–20824.

381. Landis CA, Masters SB, Spada A, et al. GTPase inhibiting mutations activate the alpha chain of Gs and stimulate adenylyl cyclase in human pituitary tumours. Nature 1989; 340:692–696.

382. Fagin JA. Genetic basis of endocrine disease. 3: Molecular defects in thyroid gland neoplasia (review). J Clin Endocrinol Metab 1992; 75:1398–1400.

383. Cai WY, Alexander JM, Hedley-Whyte ET, et al. Ras mutations in human prolactinomas and pituitary carcinomas. J Clin Endocrinol Metab 1994; 78:89–93.

384. Karga HJ, Alexander JM, Hedley-Whyte ET, et al. Ras mutations in human pituitary tumors. J Clin Endocrinol Metab 1992; 74:914–919.

385. Pei L, Melmed S, Scheithauer B, et al. H-ras mutations in human pituitary carcinoma metastases. J Clin Endocrinol Metab 1994; 78:842–846.

386. Herman V, Drazin NZ, Gonsky R, et al. Molecular screening of pituitary adenomas for gene mutations and rearrangements. J Clin Endocrinol Metab 1993; 77:50–55.

387. Cryns VL, Alexander JM, Klibanski A, et al. The retinoblastoma gene in human pituitary tumors. J Clin Endocrinol Metab 1993; 77:644–646.

388. Zhu J, Leon SP, Beggs AH, et al. Human pituitary adenomas show no loss of heterozygosity at the retinoblastoma gene locus. J Clin Endocrinol Metab 1994; 78:922–927.

389. Boggild MD, Jenkinson S, Pistorello M, et al. Molecular genetic studies of sporadic pituitary tumors. J Clin Endocrinol Metab 1994; 78:387–392.

390. Rezai AR, Rezai A, Martinez-Maza O, et al. Interleukin-6 and interleukin-6 receptor gene expression in pituitary tumors. J Neurooncol 1994; 19:131–135.

391. Chaidarun SS, Eggo MC, Sheppard MC, et al. Expression of epidermal growth factor (EGF), its receptor, and related oncoprotein (erbB-2) in human pituitary tumors and response to EGF in vitro. Endocrinology 1994; 135:2012–2021.

392. Leone A, McBride OW, Weston A, et al. Somatic allelic deletion of nm23 in human cancer. Cancer Res 1991; 51:2490–2493.

393. Sato T, Akiyama F, Sakamoto G, et al. Accumulation of genetic alterations and progression of primary breast cancer. Cancer Res 1991; 51:5794–5799.

394. Thakker RV. The role of molecular genetics in screening for multiple endocrine neoplasia type 1 (review). Endocrinol Metab Clin North Am 1994; 23:117–135.

395. Larsson C, Skogseid B, Oberg K, et al. Multiple endocrine neoplasia type 1 gene maps to chromosome 11 and is lost in insulinoma. Nature 1988; 332:85–87.
396. Teh BT, Cardinal J, Shepherd J, et al. Genetic mapping of the multiple endocrine neoplasia type 1 locus at 11q13. J Intern Med 1995; 238:249–253.
397. Thakker RV, Pook MA, Wooding C, et al. Association of somatotrophinomas with loss of alleles on chromosome 11 and with gsp mutations. J Clin Invest 1993; 91:2815–2821.
398. Bystrom C, Larsson C, Blomberg C, et al. Localization of the MEN1 gene to a small region within chromosome 11q13 by deletion mapping in tumors. Proc Natl Acad Sci USA 1990; 87:1968–1972.
399. Friedman E, De Marco L, Gejman PV, et al. Allelic loss from chromosome 11 in parathyroid tumors. Cancer Res 1992; 52:6804–6809.
400. Thakker RV, Bouloux P, Wooding C, et al. Association of parathyroid tumors in multiple endocrine neoplasia type 1 with loss of alleles on chromosome 11. N Engl J Med 1989; 321:218–224.
401. Bale AE, Norton JA, Wong EL, et al. Allelic loss on chromosome 11 in hereditary and sporadic tumors related to familial multiple endocrine neoplasia type 1. Cancer Res 1991; 51:1154–1157.
402a. Friedman E, Sakaguchi K, Bale AE, et al. Clonality of parathyroid tumors in familial multiple endocrine neoplasia type 1. N Engl J Med 1989; 321:213–218. (Erratum, N Engl J Med 1989; 321(15):1057.)
402b. Chandrasekharappa SC, Guru SC, Manickam P, et al. Positional cloning of the gene for multiple endocrine neoplasia-1. Science 1997; 276:404–407.
403. Lagercrantz J, Larsson C, Grimmond S, et al. Candidate genes for multiple endocrine neoplasia type 1. J Intern Med 1995; 238:245–248.
404. Woloschak M, Roberts JL, Post KD. Loss of heterozygosity at the retinoblastoma locus in human pituitary tumors. Cancer 1994; 74:693–696.
405. Pei L, Melmed S, Scheithauer B, et al. Frequent loss of heterozygosity at the retinoblastoma susceptibility gene (RB) locus in aggressive pituitary tumors: evidence for a chromosome 13 tumor suppressor gene other than RB. Cancer Res 1995; 55:1613–1616.
406. Woloschak M, Yu A, Xiao J, et al. Abundance and state of phosphorylation of the retinoblastoma gene product in human pituitary tumors. Int J Cancer 1996; 67:16–19.
407. Alexander JM, Biller BMK, Bikkal H, et al. Clinically nonfunctioning pituitary tumors are monoclonal in origin. J Clin Invest 1990; 86:336–340.
408. Herman I, Gonsky R, Fagin J, et al. Clonal origin of secretory and nonsecretory pituitary tumors. Clin Res 1990; 38:296A (abstract).

Approach to Pituitary Disease

409. Kovacs K, Horvath E. Pathology of pituitary tumors (review). Endocrinol Metab Clin North Am 1987; 16:529–551.
410. Melen O. Neuro-ophthalmologic features of pituitary tumors (review). Endocrinol Metab Clin North Am 1987; 16:585–608.
411. Hollenhorst RW, Younge BR. Ocular manifestations produced by adenomas of the pituitary gland: analysis of 1000 cases. In: Kohler PO, Ross GT, eds. Diagnosis and Treatment of Pituitary Tumors. New York: American Elsevier, 1973: 53–64.
412. Rosen T, Bengtsson BA. Premature mortality due to cardiovascular disease in hypopituitarism. Lancet 1990; 336:285–288.
413. McGauley GA. Quality of life assessment before and after growth hormone treatment in adults with growth hormone deficiency. Acta Paediatr Scand 1989; 356(Suppl):70–72 (discussion).
414. Bjork S, Jonsson B, Westphal O, et al. Quality of life of adults with growth hormone deficiency: a controlled study. Acta Paediatr Scand 1989; 356(Suppl):55–59 (discussion).
415. Rosen T, Wiren L, Wilhelmsen L, et al. Decreased psychological well-being in adult patients with growth hormone deficiency. Clin Endocrinol (Oxf) 1994; 40:111–116.
416. Stabler B, Turner JR, Girdler SS, et al. Reactivity to stress and psychological adjustment in adults with pituitary insufficiency. Clin Endocrinol (Oxf) 1992; 36:467–473.
417. Binnerts A, Deurenberg P, Swart GR, et al. Body composition in growth hormone–deficient adults. Am J Clin Nutr 1992; 55:918–923.
418. Rosen T, Bosaeus I, Tolli J, et al. Increased body fat mass and decreased extracellular fluid volume in adults with growth hormone deficiency. Clin Endocrinol (Oxf) 1993; 38:63–71.
419. de Boer H, Blok GJ, Voerman HJ, et al. Body composition in adult growth hormone–deficient men, assessed by anthropometry and bioimpedance analysis. J Clin Endocrinol Metab 1992; 75:833–837.
420. Larsson B, Svardsudd K, Welin L, et al. Abdominal adipose tissue distribution, obesity, and risk of cardiovascular disease and death: 13 year follow up of participants in the study of men born in 1913. Br Med J 1984; 288:1401–1404.
421. Peiris AN, Sothmann MS, Hoffmann RG, et al. Adiposity, fat distribution, and cardiovascular risk. Ann Intern Med 1989; 110:867–872.
422. Adler S, Waterman ML, He X, et al. Steroid receptor–mediated inhibition of rat prolactin gene expression does not require the receptor DNA-binding domain. Cell 1988; 52:685–695.
423. de Boer H, Blok GJ, Van der Veen EA. Clinical aspects of growth hormone deficiency in adults (review). Endocr Rev 1995; 16:63–86.
424. Wuster C, Slenczka E, Ziegler R. Increased prevalence of osteoporosis and arteriosclerosis in conventionally substituted anterior pituitary insufficiency: need for additional growth hormone substitution? (German). Klin Wochenschr 1991; 69:769–773.
425. Rosen T, Hansson T, Granhed H, et al. Reduced bone mineral content in adult patients with growth hormone deficiency (see comments). Acta Endocrinol 1993; 129:201–206.
426. Holmes SJ, Economou G, Whitehouse RW, et al. Reduced bone mineral density in adult onset growth hormone deficiency. J Clin Endocrinol Metab 1994; 78:669–674.
427. Hyer SL, Rodin DA, Tobias JH, et al. Growth hormone deficiency during puberty reduces adult bone mineral density. Arch Dis Child 1992; 67:1472–1474.
428. Jorgensen JOL, Pedersen SA, Thuesen L, et al. Beneficial effects of growth hormone treatment in GH-deficient adults. Lancet 1989; 1:1221–1225.
429. Whitehead HM, Boreham C, McIlrath EM, et al. Growth hormone treatment of adults with growth hormone deficiency: results of a 13-month placebo controlled cross-over study. Clin Endocrinol (Oxf) 1992; 36:45–52.
430. Binnerts A, Swart GR, Wilson JH, et al. The effect of growth hormone administration in growth hormone deficient adults on bone, protein, carbohydrate and lipid homeostasis, as well as on body composition. Clin Endocrinol (Oxf) 1992; 37:79–87.
431. Degerblad M, Elgindy N, Hall K, et al. Potent effect of recombinant growth hormone on bone mineral density and body composition in adults with panhypopituitarism. Acta Endocrinol 1992; 126:387–393.
432. Bengtsson BA, Eden S, Lonn L, et al. Treatment of adults with growth hormone (GH) deficiency with recombinant human GH. J Clin Endocrinol Metab 1993; 76:309–317.
433. O'Halloran DJ, Tsatsoulis A, Whitehouse RW, et al. Increased bone density after recombinant human growth hormone (GH) therapy in adults with isolated GH deficiency. J Clin Endocrinol Metab 1993; 76:1344–1348.
434. Cuneo RC, Salomon F, Wiles CM, et al. Skeletal muscle performance in adults with growth hormone deficiency. Horm Res 1990; 33(Suppl 4):55–60.
435. Cuneo RC, Salomon F, Wiles CM, et al. Growth hormone treatment in growth hormone-deficient adults. I: Effects on muscle mass and strength. J Appl Physiol 1991; 70:688–694.
436. Cuneo RC, Salomon F, Wiles CM, et al. Growth hormone treatment in growth hormone-deficient adults. II: Effects on exercise performance. J Appl Physiol 1991; 70:695–700.
437. Cuneo RC, Salomon F, Watts GF, et al. Growth hormone treatment improves serum lipids and lipoproteins in adults with growth hormone deficiency. Metabolism 1993; 42:1519–1523.
438. Jorgensen JO, Thuesen L, Muller J, et al. Three years of growth hormone treatment in growth hormone–deficient adults: near normalization of body composition and physical performance. Eur J Endocrinol 1994; 130:224–228.
439. Almqvist O, Thoren M, Saaf M, et al. Effects of growth hormone substitution on mental performance in adults with growth hormone deficiency: a pilot study. Psychoneuroendocrinology 1986; 11:347–352.

Morphologic Classification of Pituitary Adenomas

440. Foncin JF, LeBeau J. Light and electron microscope study of a pituitary tumor with adrenocorticotopic function. C R Soc Biol 1963; 157:249–252.
441. Cardell RR Jr, Knighton RS. The cytology of a human pituitary tumor: an electron microscopic study. Trans Am Microsc Soc 1966; 85:58–78.
442. Peake GT, McKeel DW, Jarett L, et al. Ultrastructural, histologic and hormonal characterization of a prolactin-rich human pituitary tumor. J Clin Endocrinol Metab 1969; 29:1383–1393.
443. Nakane PK. Classifications of anterior pituitary cell types with immunoenzyme histochemistry. J Histochem Cytochem 1970; 18:9–20.
444. Thapar K, Kovacs K, Scheithauer BW, et al. Proliferative activity and invasiveness among pituitary adenomas and carcinomas: an analysis using the MIB-1 antibody. Neurosurgery 1996; 38:99–107.
445. Thapar K, Scheithauer BW, Kovacs K, et al. p53 expression in pituitary adenomas and carcinomas: correlation with invasiveness and tumor growth fractions. Neurosurgery 1996; 38:763–770.
446. Kovacs K, Horvath E, Bayley TA, et al. Silent corticotroph cell adenoma with lysosomal accumulation and crinophagy. A distinct clinicopathologic entity. Am J Med 1978; 64:492–499.
447. Horvath E, Kovacs K, Killinger DW, et al. Silent corticotropic adenomas of the human pituitary gland: a histologic, immunocytologic, and ultrastructural study. Am J Pathol 1980; 98:617–638.
448. Horvath E, Kovacs K, Smyth HS, et al. A novel type of pituitary adenoma: morphological features and clinical correlations. J Clin Endocrinol Metab 1988; 66:1111–1118.
449. Kovacs K, Horvath E. Tumors of the pituitary gland. In: Hartmann WH, ed. Atlas of Tumor Pathology, Fascicle 21, 2nd series. Washington, DC: Armed Forces Institute of Pathology, 1986: 1–264.
450. Scheithauer BW, Horvath E, Kovacs K, et al. Plurihormonal pituitary adenomas. Semin Diagn Pathol 1986; 3:69–82.
451. Heitz PU, Landolt AM, Zenklusen HR, et al. Immunocytochemistry of pituitary tumors. J Histochem Cytochem 1987; 35:1005–1011.
452. Horvath E, Kovacs K, Singer W, et al. Acidophil stem cell adenoma of the human pituitary: clinicopathologic analysis of 15 cases. Cancer 1981; 47:761–771.
453. Horvath E, Kovacs K, Killinger DW, et al. Mammosomatotroph cell ade-

noma of the human pituitary: a morphologic entity. Virchows Arch [A] 1983; 398:277–289.

454. Horvath E, Kovacs K, Scheithauer BW, et al. Pituitary adenomas producing growth hormone, prolactin, and one or more glycoprotein hormones: a histologic, immunohistochemical, and ultrastructural study of four surgically removed tumors. Ultrastruct Pathol 1983; 5:171–183.

455. Stratmann IE, Ezrin C, Sellers EA. Estrogen-induced transformation of somatotrophs into mammotrophs in the rat. Cell Tissue Res 1974; 152:229–238.

Evaluation of Suspected Pituitary Disease

456. Felder RA, Holl RW, Martha P Jr, et al. Influence of matrix on concentrations of somatotropin measured in serum with commercial immunoradiometric assays. Clin Chem 1989; 35:1423–1426.

457. Boscato LM, Stuart MC. Heterophilic antibodies: a problem for all immunoassays. Clin Chem 1988; 34:27–33.

458. Boscato LM, Stuart MC. Incidence and specificity of interference in two-site immunoassays. Clin Chem 1986; 32:1491–1495.

459. Evans WS, Faria AC, Christiansen E, et al. Impact of intensive venous sampling on characterization of pulsatile GH release. Am J Physiol 1987; 252:E549–E556.

460. Winer LM, Shaw MA, Baumann G. Urinary growth hormone excretion rates in normal and acromegalic man: a critical appraisal of its potential clinical utility. J Endocrinol Invest 1989; 12:461–467.

461. Hattori N, Kato Y, Murakami Y, et al. Urinary growth hormone levels measured by ultrasensitive enzyme immunoassay in patients with renal insufficiency. J Clin Endocrinol Metab 1988; 66:727–732.

462. Ho KY, Veldhuis JD, Johnson ML, et al. Fasting enhances growth hormone secretion and amplifies the complex rhythms of growth hormone secretion in man. J Clin Invest 1988; 81:968–975.

463. Hurd HP, Palumbo PJ, Gharib H. Hypothalamic-endocrine dysfunction in anorexia nervosa. Mayo Clin Proc 1977; 52:711–716.

464. Jeffcoate SL. Diagnosis of hyperprolactinaemia. Lancet 1978; 2:1245–1247.

465. Sheldon WR Jr, DeBold CR, Evans WS, et al. Rapid sequential intravenous administration of four hypothalamic releasing hormones as a combined anterior pituitary function test in normal subjects. J Clin Endocrinol Metab 1985; 60:623–630.

466. Landon J, Greenwood FC, Stamp TC, et al. The plasma sugar, free fatty acid, cortisol, and growth hormone response to insulin, and the comparison of this procedure with other tests of pituitary and adrenal function. II: In patients with hypothalamic or pituitary dysfunction or anorexia nervosa. J Clin Invest 1966; 45:437–449.

467. Greenwood FC, Landon J, Stamp TCB. The plasma sugar, free fatty acid, cortisol, and growth hormone response to insulin. I: In control subjects. J Clin Invest 1966; 45:429–436.

468. Chapman IM, Hartman ML, Straume M, et al. Enhanced sensitivity growth hormone (GH) chemiluminescence assay reveals lower postglucose nadir GH concentrations in men than women. J Clin Endocrinol Metab 1994; 78:1312–1319.

469. Wolpert SM, Molitch ME, Goldman JA, et al. Size, shape, and appearance of the normal female pituitary gland. Am J Roentgenol 1984; 143:377–381.

470. Swartz JD, Russell KB, Basile BA, et al. High-resolution computed tomographic appearance of the intrasellar contents in women of childbearing age. Radiology 1983; 147:115–117.

471. Chakeres DW, Curtin A, Ford G. Magnetic resonance imaging of pituitary and parasellar abnormalities (review). Radiol Clin North Am 1989; 27:265–281.

472. Gomori JM, Grossman RI, Zimmerman RA, et al. Intracranial hematomas: imaging by high-field MRI. Radiology 1985; 157(1):87–93.

473. Kulkarni MV, Lee KF, McArdle CB, et al. 1.5-T MR imaging of pituitary microadenomas: technical considerations and CT correlation. Am J Neuroradiol 1988; 9:5–11.

474. Dwyer AJ, Frank JA, Doppman JL, et al. Pituitary adenomas in patients with Cushing disease: initial experience with Gd-DTPA–enhanced MR imaging. Radiology 1987; 163:421–426.

475. Beck RW. Automated perimetry: principles and practice. Int Ophthalmol Clin 1986; 26(4):163–174.

476. Chamlin F, Davidoff LM, Feiring EH. Ophthalmologic changes produced by pituitary tumors. Am J Ophthalmol 1955; 40:353–368.

477. Cohen AR, Cooper PR, Kupersmith MJ, et al. Visual recovery after transsphenoidal removal of pituitary adenomas. Neurosurgery 1985; 17:446–452.

478. Wilson P, Falconer MA. Patterns of visual failure with pituitary tumors: clinical and radiological correlations. Br J Ophthalmol 1968; 52:94–110.

479. Wass JAH. Hypopituitarism. In: Besser GM, Cudworth AG, eds. Clinical Endocrinology: An Illustrated Text. Philadelphia: JB Lippincott, 1987: 2.1–2.14.

480. Newman SA. Advances in diagnosis and treatment of pituitary tumors. Int Ophthalmol Clin 1986; 26(4):285–300.

481. Trautmann JC, Laws ER Jr. Visual status after transsphenoidal surgery at the Mayo Clinic, 1971–1982. Am J Ophthalmol 1983; 96:200–208.

Hormone Replacement Therapy

482. Snyder PJ, Lawrence DA. Treatment of male hypogonadism with testosterone enanthate. J Clin Endocrinol Metab 1980; 51(6):1335–1339.

483. Carey PO, Howards SS, Vance ML. Transdermal testosterone treatment of hypogonadal men. J Urol 1988; 140:76–79.

484. Arver S, Dobs AS, Meikle AW, et al. Improvement of sexual function in testosterone deficient men treated for 1 year with a permeation enhanced testosterone transdermal system. J Urol 1996; 155:1604–1608.

485. Meikle AW, Mazer NA, Moellmer JF, et al. Enhanced transdermal delivery of testosterone across nonscrotal skin produces physiological concentrations of testosterone and its metabolites in hypogonadal men. J Clin Endocrinol Metab 1992; 74:623–628.

486. Thorner MO, Rogol AD, Blizzard RM, et al. Acceleration of growth rate in growth hormone–deficient children treated with human growth hormone–releasing hormone. Pediatr Res 1988; 24:145–151.

487. Thorner MO, Rochiccioli P, Colle M, et al. Once daily subcutaneous growth hormone–releasing hormone therapy accelerates growth in growth hormone–deficient children during first year of therapy. J Clin Endocrinol Metab 1996; 81:1189–1196.

Pituitary Surgery

488. Guiot G. Transsphenoidal approach in surgical treatment of pituitary adenomas: general principles and indications in nonfunctioning adenomas. In: Kohler PO, Ross GT, eds. Diagnosis and Treatment of Pituitary Tumors. New York: American Elsevier, 1973: 159–178.

489. Hardy J. Transsphenoidal microsurgery of the normal and pathological pituitary. Clin Neurosurg 1969; 16:185–217.

490. Laws ER Jr. Surgical management of pituitary tumors. In: Mazzaferri EL, Samaan N, eds. Endocrine Tumors. Boston: Blackwell, 1993: 215–222.

491. Thapar K, Laws ER Jr. Tumors of the central nervous system. In: Murphy GP, Lawrence W Jr, Lenhard RE Jr, eds. American Cancer Society Textbook of Clinical Oncology. Atlanta: American Cancer Society, 1995: 378–410.

492. Thapar K, Laws ER Jr. Pituitary tumors. In: Kaye AH, Laws ER Jr, eds. Brain Tumors. London: Churchill Livingstone, 1995: 759–777.

493. Laws ER Jr, Fode NC, Randall RV, et al. Pregnancy following transsphenoidal resection of prolactin-secreting pituitary tumors. J Neurosurg 1983; 58:685–688.

494. Scheithauer BW, Kovacs KT, Laws ER Jr, et al. Pathology of invasive pituitary tumors with special reference to functional classification. J Neurosurg 1986; 65:733–744.

495. Selman WR, Laws ER Jr, Scheithauer BW, et al. The occurrence of dural invasion in pituitary adenomas. J Neurosurg 1986; 64:402–407.

496. Jacoby LB, Hedley-Whyte ET, Pulaski K, et al. Clonal origin of pituitary adenomas. J Neurosurg 1990; 73:731–735.

497. Alexander JM, Biller BM, Bikkal H, et al. Clinically nonfunctioning pituitary tumors are monoclonal in origin. J Clin Invest 1990; 86:336–340.

498. Friend KE, Chiou YK, Laws ER Jr, et al. Pit-1 messenger ribonucleic acid is differentially expressed in human pituitary adenomas. J Clin Endocrinol Metab 1993; 77:1281–1286.

499. Friend KE, Chiou YK, Lopes MB, et al. Estrogen receptor expression in human pituitary: correlation with immunohistochemistry in normal tissue, and immunohistochemistry and morphology in macroadenomas. J Clin Endocrinol Metab 1994; 78:1497–1504.

500. Alexander JM, Bikkal HA, Zervas NT, et al. Tumor-specific expression and alternate splicing of messenger ribonucleic acid encoding activin/transforming growth factor-beta receptors in human pituitary adenomas. J Clin Endocrinol Metab 1996; 81:783–790.

501. Ebersold MJ, Laws ER Jr, Scheithauer BW, et al. Pituitary apoplexy treated by transsphenoidal surgery. A clinicopathological and immunocytochemical study. J Neurosurg 1983; 58:315–320.

502. Bills DC, Meyer FB, Laws ER Jr, et al. A retrospective analysis of pituitary apoplexy (discussion). Neurosurgery 1993; 33:602–608.

503. Zentner J, Gilsbach J. Pituitary adenoma and meningioma in the same patient. Report of three cases. Eur Arch Psychiatry Neurol Sci 1989; 238:144–148.

504. Laws ER Jr, Trautmann JC, Hollenhorst RW Jr. Transsphenoidal decompression of the optic nerve and chiasm. Visual results in 62 patients. J Neurosurg 1977; 46:717–722.

505. Laws ER Jr. Pituitary surgery (review). Endocrinol Metab Clin North Am 1987; 16:647–665.

506. Bloom B, Kramer S. Conventional radiation therapy in the management of acromegaly. In: Black PMcL, Zervas NT, Ridgway EC, et al, eds. Secretory Tumors of the Pituitary Gland. Progress in Endocrine Research and Therapy. Vol 1. New York: Raven Press, 1984: 179–190.

Pituitary Radiation

507. Frantz AG, Cogon PH, Chang CH, et al. Long-term evaluation of the results of transsphenoidal surgery and radiotherapy in patients with prolactinoma. In: Crosignan PG, Rubin BL, eds. Endocrinology of Human Infertility: New Aspects. New York: Grune & Stratton, 1981: 161–170.

508. Eastman RC, Gorden P, Roth J. Conventional supervoltage irradiation is an effective treatment for acromegaly. J Clin Endocrinol Metab 1979; 48:931–940.

509. Kliman B, Kjellberg RN, Swisher B, et al. Proton beam therapy of acromegaly: a 20-year experience. In: Black PMcL, Zervas NT, Ridgway EC, et al, eds. Secretory Tumors of the Pituitary Gland. Progress in Endocrine Research and Therapy. Vol 1. New York: Raven Press, 1984: 191–211.

510. Nelson PB, Goodman ML, Flickenger JC, et al. Endocrine function in patients with large pituitary tumors treated with operative decompression and radiation therapy. Neurosurgery 1989; 24:398–400.

511. Linfoot JA. Alpha particle pituitary irradiation in the primary and post-surgical management of pituitary microadenomas. In: Faglia G, Giovanelli MA, McLeod RM, eds. Pituitary Microadenomas. London: Academic Press, 1978: 515–529.

512. Hashimoto N, Handa H, Yamashita J, et al. Long-term follow-up of large or invasive pituitary adenomas. Surg Neurol 1986; 25:49–54.

513. Brada M, Ford D, Ashley S, et al. Risk of second brain tumour after conservative surgery and radiotherapy for pituitary adenoma. BMJ 1992; 304:1343–1346.

514. Al-Mefty O, Kersh JE, Routh A, et al. The long-term side effects of radiation therapy for benign brain tumors in adults (see comments) (review). J Neurosurg 1990; 73:502–512.

515. Snyder PJ, Fowble BF, Schatz NJ, et al. Hypopituitarism following radiation therapy of pituitary adenomas. Am J Med 1986; 81:457–462.

516. Ebersold MJ, Quast LM, Laws ER Jr, et al. Long-term results in transsphenoidal removal of nonfunctioning pituitary adenomas. J Neurosurg 1986; 64:713–719.

Pituitary Disorders

Prolactinoma

517. Costello RT. Subclinical adenoma of the pituitary gland. Am J Pathol 1936; 12:205–215.

518. Abu Fadil S, DeVane G, Siler TM, et al. Effects of oral contraceptive steroids on pituitary prolactin secretion. Contraception 1976; 13:79–85.

519. Dericks Tan JS, Taubert HD. Elevation of serum prolactin during application of oral contraceptives. Contraception 1976; 14:1–8.

520. Jacobs HS, Knuth UA, Hull MG, et al. Post-"pill" amenorrhoea—cause or coincidence? Br Med J 1977; 2:940–942.

521. Coulam CB, Annegers JF, Abboud CF, et al. Pituitary adenoma and oral contraceptives: a case-control study. Fertil Steril 1979; 31:25–28.

522. Wingrave SJ, Kay CR, Vessey MP. Oral contraceptives and pituitary adenomas. Br Med J 1980; 280:685–686.

523. Franks S. Regulation of prolactin secretion by oestrogens: physiological and pathological significance (review). Clin Sci 1983; 65:457–462.

524. Franks S, Jacobs HS, Hull MGR. The oral contraceptive and hyperprolactinemic amenorrhea. In: Molinatti GM, Crosignani PG, Muller EE, eds. Pituitary Hyperfunction: Physiopathology and Clinical Aspects. New York: Raven Press, 1984: 175–178.

525. Davis JR, Selby C, Jeffcoate WJ. Oral contraceptive agents do not affect serum prolactin in normal women. Clin Endocrinol (Oxf) 1984; 20:427–434.

526. Molitch ME. Pathogenesis of pituitary tumors. Endocrinol Metab Clin North Am 1987; 16:503–527.

527. Thorner MO, Edwards CRW, Hanker JP, et al. Prolactin and gonadotropin interaction in the male. In: Troen P, Nankin H, eds. The Testis in Normal and Infertile Men. New York: Raven Press, 1977: 351–366.

528. Carter JN, Tyson JE, Tolis G, et al. Prolactin-screening tumors and hypogonadism in 22 men. N Engl J Med 1978; 299:847–852.

529. Cohen LM, Greenberg DB, Murray GB. Neuropsychiatric presentation of man with pituitary tumors (the 'four A's'). Psychosomatics 1984; 25:925–928.

530. Schwartz MF, Bauman JE, Masters WH. Hyperprolactinemia and sexual disorders in men. Biol Psychiatry 1982; 17:861–876.

531. Kemmann E, Jones JR. Hyperprolactinemia and headaches. Am J Obstet Gynecol 1983; 145:668–671.

532. Quigley ME, Sheehan KL, Casper RF, et al. Evidence for an increased opioid inhibition of luteinizing hormone secretion in hyperprolactinemic patients with pituitary microadenoma. J Clin Endocrinol Metab 1980; 50:427–430.

533. Lightman SL, Jacobs HS, Maguire AK, et al. Constancy of opioid control of luteinizing hormone in different pathophysiological states. J Clin Endocrinol Metab 1981; 52:1260–1263.

534. Grossman A, Moult PJ, McIntyre H, et al. Opiate mediation of amenorrhoea in hyperprolactinaemia and in weight-loss related amenorrhoea. Clin Endocrinol (Oxf) 1982; 17:379–388.

535. Klibanski A, Neer RM, Beitins IZ, et al. Decreased bone density in hyperprolactinemic women. N Engl J Med 1980; 303:1511–1514.

536. Schlechte JA, Sherman B, Martin R. Bone density in amenorrheic women with and without hyperprolactinemia. J Clin Endocrinol Metab 1983; 56:1120–1123.

537. Greenspan SL, Neer RM, Ridgway EC, et al. Osteoporosis in men with hyperprolactinemic hypogonadism. Ann Intern Med 1986; 104:777–782.

538. Jackson JA, Kleerekoper M, Parfitt AM. Symptomatic osteoporosis in a man with hyperprolactinemic hypogonadism. Ann Intern Med 1986; 105:543–545.

539. Boulanger CM, Mashchak CA, Chang RJ. Lack of tumor reduction in hyperprolactinemic women with extrasellar macroadenomas treated with bromocriptine. Fertil Steril 1985; 44:532–535.

540. Balagura S, Frantz AG, Housepian EM, et al. The specificity of serum prolactin as a diagnostic indicator of pituitary adenoma. J Neurosurg 1979; 51:42–46.

541. Klijn JG, Lamberts SWJ, de Jong FH, et al. The value of the thyrotropin-releasing hormone test in patients with prolactin-secreting pituitary tumors and suprasellar non-pituitary tumors. Fertil Steril 1981; 35:155–161.

542. Landolt AM, Rothenbuhler V. Pituitary adenoma calcification. Arch Pathol Lab Med 1977; 101:22–27.

543. Rilliet B, Mohr G, Robert F, et al. Calcifications in pituitary adenomas. Surg Neurol 1981; 15:249–255.

544. Mukada K, Ohta M, Uozumi T, et al. Ossified prolactinoma: case report. Neurosurgery 1987; 20:473–475.

545. Landolt AM, Kleihues P, Heitz PU. Amyloid deposits in pituitary adenomas. Differentiation of two types. Arch Pathol Lab Med 1987; 111:453–458.

546. Horvath E, Kovacs K. Pathology of prolactin cell adenomas of the human pituitary. Semin Diagn Pathol 1986; 3:4–17.

547. Saeger W, Mohr K, Caselitz J, et al. Light and electron microscopical morphometry of pituitary adenomas in hyperprolactinemia. Pathol Res Pract 1986; 181:544–550.

548. Thorner MO, Schran HF, Evans WS, et al. A broad spectrum of prolactin suppression by bromocriptine in hyperprolactinemic women: a study of serum prolactin and bromocriptine levels after acute and chronic administration of bromocriptine. J Clin Endocrinol Metab 1980; 50:1026–1033.

549. Thorner MO, Perryman RL, Rogol AD, et al. Rapid changes of prolactinoma volume after withdrawal and reinstitution of bromocriptine. J Clin Endocrinol Metab 1981; 53:480–483.

550. Molitch ME, Elton RL, Blackwell RE, et al. Bromocriptine as primary therapy for prolactin-secreting macroadenomas: results of a prospective multicenter study. J Clin Endocrinol Metab 1985; 60:698–705.

551. Horvath E, Kovacs K, Killinger DW, et al. Diverse ultrastructural response to dopamine agonist's medication in human pituitary prolactin cell adenomas. In: Hoshino K, ed. Prolactin Gene Family and Its Receptors. Amsterdam: Elsevier Science, 1988: 307–311.

552. Tindall GT, Kovacs K, Horvath E, et al. Human prolactin-producing adenomas and bromocriptine: a histological, immunocytochemical, ultrastructural, and morphometric study. J Clin Endocrinol Metab 1982; 55:1178–1183.

553. Bassetti M, Spada A, Pezzo G, et al. Bromocriptine treatment reduces the cell size in human macroprolactinomas: a morphometric study. J Clin Endocrinol Metab 1984; 58:268–273.

554. Saitoh Y, Mori S, Arita N, et al. Cytosuppressive effect of bromocriptine on human prolactinomas: stereological analysis of ultrastructural alterations with special reference to secretory granules. Cancer Res 1986; 46:1507–1512.

555. Stefaneanu L, Kovacs K, Horvath E, et al. In situ hybridization study of estrogen receptor messenger ribonucleic acid in human adenohypophysial cells and pituitary adenomas. J Clin Endocrinol Metab 1994; 78:83–88.

556. Kovacs K, Stefaneanu L, Horvath E, et al. Prolactin-producing pituitary tumor: resistance to dopamine agonist therapy. Case report. J Neurosurg 1995; 82:886–890.

557. Arita K, Uozumi T, Ohta M. A case of large prolactinoma supposed to be cured by bromocriptine therapy. Endocrinol Jpn 1988; 35:503–509.

558. Maurer RA. Transcriptional regulation of the prolactin gene by ergocryptine and cyclic AMP. Nature 1981; 294:94–97.

559. Gen M, Uozumi T, Ohta M, et al. Necrotic changes in prolactinomas after long term administration of bromocriptine. J Clin Endocrinol Metab 1984; 59:463–470.

560. Landolt AM, Osterwalder V. Perivascular fibrosis in prolactinomas: is it increased by bromocriptine? J Clin Endocrinol Metab 1984; 58:1179–1183.

561. Esiri MM, Bevan JS, Burke CW, et al. Effect of bromocriptine treatment on the fibrous tissue content of prolactin-secreting and nonfunctioning macroadenomas of the pituitary gland. J Clin Endocrinol Metab 1986; 63:383–388.

562. Hallenga B, Saeger W, Ludecke DK. Necroses of prolactin-secreting pituitary adenomas under treatment with dopamine agonists: light microscopical and morphometric studies. Exp Clin Endocrinol 1988; 92:59–68.

563. Bevan JS, Adams CB, Burke CW, et al. Factors in the outcome of transsphenoidal surgery for prolactinoma and non-functioning pituitary tumour, including pre-operative bromocriptine therapy. Clin Endocrinol (Oxf) 1987; 26:541–556.

564. Martin NA, Hales M, Wilson CB. Cerebellar metastasis from a prolactinoma during treatment with bromocriptine. J Neurosurg 1981; 55:615–619.

565. U HS, Johnson C. Metastatic prolactin-secreting pituitary adenoma. Hum Pathol 1984; 15:94–96.

566. Scheithauer BW, Randall RV, Kramer S, et al. Prolactin cell carcinoma of the pituitary: clinicopathologic, immunohistochemical and ultrastructural study of a case with cranial and extracranial metastases. Cancer 1985; 55:598–604.

567. Landolt AM, Minder H. Immunohistochemical examination of the paraadenomatous "normal" pituitary. An evaluation of prolactin cell hyperplasia. Virchows Arch [A] 1984; 403:181–193.

568. Pioro EP, Scheithauer BW, Kramer S, et al. Combined thyrotroph and lactotroph cell hyperplasia simulating prolactin-secreting pituitary adenoma in long-standing primary hypothyroidism. Surg Neurol 1988; 29:218–226.

569. Wowra B, Peiffer J. An immunoperoxidase study of a human pituitary adenoma associated with Cushing's syndrome. Pathol Res Pract 1984; 178:349–354.

570. Vance ML, Evans WS, Thorner MO. Drugs five years later. Bromocriptine (review). Ann Intern Med 1984; 100:78–91.

571. Pellegrini I, Rasolonjanahary R, Gunz G, et al. Resistance to bromocriptine in prolactinomas. J Clin Endocrinol Metab 1989; 69:500–509.

572. Thorner MO, McNeilly AS, Hagan C, et al. Long-term treatment of galactorrhoea and hypogonadism with bromocriptine. Br Med J 1974; 2:419–422.

573. Liuzzi A, Dallabonzana D, Oppizzi G, et al. Low doses of dopamine agonists in the long-term treatment of macroprolactinomas. N Engl J Med 1985; 313:656–659.

574. Hokfelt T, Fuxe K. On the morphology and the neuroendocrine role of the hypothalamic catecholamine neuron. In: Knigge KM, Jacobs HS, Weindl A, eds. Brain-Endocrine Interaction. Median Eminence: Structure and Function. Basel: Karger, 1972: 181–223.

575. Corrodi H, Fuxe K, Hokfelt T, et al. Effect of ergot drugs on central catecholamine neurons: evidence for a stimulation of central dopamine neurons. J Pharm Pharmacol 1973; 25:409–412.

576. Calabro MA, MacLeod RM. Binding of dopamine to bovine anterior pituitary gland membranes. Neuroendocrinology 1978; 25:32–46.

577. Muller EE, Panerai AE, Cocchi D, et al. Endocrine profile of ergot alkaloids (review). Life Sci 1977; 21:1545–1558.

578. Schran HF, Bhuta SI, Schwarz HJ, et al. The pharmacokinetics of bromocriptine in man. Adv Biochem Psychopharmacol 1980; 23:125–139.

579. Kletzky OA, Vermesh M. Effectiveness of vaginal bromocriptine in treating women with hyperprolactinemia. Fertil Steril 1989; 51:269–272.

580. Turner TH, Cookson JC, Wass JA, et al. Psychotic reactions during treatment of pituitary tumours with dopamine agonists. Br Med J 1984; 289:1101–1103.

581. Ayres J, Maisey MN. Alcohol increases bromocriptine's side effects (letter). N Engl J Med 1980; 302:806, 1980.

582. Kleinberg DL, Boyd AE, Wardlaw S, et al. Pergolide for the treatment of pituitary tumors secreting prolactin or growth hormone. N Engl J Med 1983; 309:704–709.

583. Vance ML, Cragun JR, Reimnitz C, et al. CV 205–502 treatment of hyperprolactinemia. J Clin Endocrinol Metab 1989; 68:336–339.

584. Vance ML, Lipper M, Klibanski A, et al. Treatment of prolactin-secreting pituitary macroadenomas with the long-acting non-ergot dopamine agonist CV 205–502. Ann Intern Med 1990; 112:668–673.

585. Ciccarelli E, Giusti M, Miola C, et al. Effectiveness and tolerability of long term treatment with cabergoline, a new long-lasting ergoline derivative, in hyperprolactinemic patients. J Clin Endocrinol Metab 1989; 69:725–728.

586. Webster J, Piscitelli G, Polli A, et al. Dose-dependent suppression of serum prolactin by cabergoline in hyperprolactinaemia: a placebo controlled, double blind, multicentre study. European Multicentre Cabergoline Dose-finding Study Group. Clin Endocrinol (Oxf) 1992; 37:534–541.

587. Webster J, Piscitelli G, Polli A, et al. A comparison of cabergoline and bromocriptine in the treatment of hyperprolactinemic amenorrhea. Cabergoline Comparative Study Group (see comments). N Engl J Med 1994; 331:904–909.

588. Biller BMK, Molitch ME, Vance ML, et al. Treatment of prolactin-secreting macroadenomas with the once-weekly dopamine agonist cabergoline. J Clin Endocrinol Metab 1996; 81:2338–2343.

589. Werder K, Fahlbusch R, Landgraf R, et al. Treatment of patients with prolactinomas. J Endocrinol Invest 1978; 1:47–58.

590. Molitch ME. Pregnancy and the hyperprolactinemic woman (review). N Engl J Med 1985; 312:1364–1370.

591. Mornex R, Orgiazzi J, Hugues B, et al. Normal pregnancies after treatment of hyperprolactinemia with bromoergocryptine, despite suspected pituitary tumors. J Clin Endocrinol Metab 1978; 47:290–295.

592. Lamberts SWJ, Klijn JG, de Lange SA, et al. The incidence of complications during pregnancy after treatment of hyperprolactinemia with bromocriptine in patients with radiologically evident pituitary tumors. Fertil Steril 1979; 31:614–619.

593. Turkalj I, Braun P, Krupp P. Surveillance of bromocriptine in pregnancy. JAMA 1982; 247:1589–1591.

594. Krupp P, Turkalj I. Surveillance of Parlodel (bromocriptine) in pregnancy and offspring. In: Jacobs HS, Harrison RF, Bonnar J, et al, eds. Prolactinomas and Pregnancy. Lancaster: MTP Press, 1983: 45–50.

595. Raymond JP, Goldstein E, Konopka P, et al. Follow-up of children born of bromocriptine-treated mothers. Horm Res 1985; 22:239–246.

596. Thorner MO, Martin WH, Rogol AD, et al. Rapid regression of pituitary prolactinomas during bromocriptine treatment. J Clin Endocrinol Metab 1980; 51:438–445.

597. Canales ES, Garcia IC, Ruiz JE, et al. Bromocriptine as prophylactic therapy in prolactinoma during pregnancy. Fertil Steril 1981; 36:524–526.

598. van Roon E, van der Vijver JCM, Gerretsen G, et al. Rapid regression of a suprasellar extending prolactinoma after bromocriptine treatment during pregnancy. Fertil Steril 1981; 36:173–177.

599. Konopka P, Raymond JP, Merceron RE, et al. Continuous administration of bromocriptine in the prevention of neurological complications in pregnant women with prolactinomas. Am J Obstet Gynecol 1983; 146:935–938.

600. Maeda T, Ushiroyama T, Okuda K, et al. Effective bromocriptine treatment of a pituitary macroadenoma during pregnancy. Obstet Gynecol 1983; 61:117–121.

601. Moult PJ, Dacie JE, Rees LH, et al. Oral contraception in patients with hyperprolactinaemia. Br Med J 1982; 284(6319):868.

602. Newman CB, Hurley AM, Kleinberg DL. Effect of CV 205–502 in hyperprolactinaemic patients intolerant of bromocriptine. Clin Endocrinol (Oxf) 1989; 31:391–400.

603. Breidahl HD, Topliss DJ, Pike JW. Failure of bromocriptine to maintain reduction in size of a macroprolactinoma. Br Med J 1983; 287:451–452.

604. Gasser RW, Finkenstedt G, Skrabal F, et al. Multiple intracranial metastases from a prolactin secreting pituitary tumour. Clin Endocrinol (Oxf) 1985; 22:17–27.

605. Plangger CA, Twerdy K, Grunert V, et al. Subarachnoid metastases from a prolactinoma. Neurochirurgia 1985; 28:235–237.

606. Randall RV, Scheithauer BW, Laws ER Jr, et al. Pituitary adenomas associated with hyperprolactinemia: a clinical and immunohistochemical study of 97 patients operated on transsphenoidally. Mayo Clin Proc 1985; 60:753–762.

607. Randall RV, Kramer S, Abboud CF, et al. Transsphenoidal microsurgical treatment of prolactin-producing pituitary adenomas. Results in 100 patients. Mayo Clin Proc 1983; 58:108–121.

608. Antunes JL, Housepian EM, Frantz AG, et al. Prolactin-secreting pituitary tumors. Ann Neurol 1977; 2:148–153.

609. Chang RJ, Keye WR Jr, Young JR, et al. Detection, evaluation, and treatment of pituitary microadenomas in patients with galactorrhea and amenorrhea. Am J Obstet Gynecol 1977; 128:356–363.

610. Hardy J, Beauregard H, Robert F. Prolactin-secreting pituitary adenomas: transsphenoidal microsurgical treatment. In: Robyn C, Harter M, eds. Progress in Prolactin Physiology and Pathology. Developments in Endocrinology. Vol 2. Amsterdam: Elsevier/North Holland Biomedical, 1978: 361–370.

611. Tindall GT, McLanahan CS, Christy JH. Transsphenoidal microsurgery for pituitary tumors associated with hyperprolactinemia. J Neurosurg 1978; 48:849–860.

612. Post KD, Biller BJ, Adelman LS, et al. Selective transsphenoidal adenomectomy in women with galactorrhea-amenorrhea. JAMA 1979; 242:158–162.

613. Hardy J. Transsphenoidal microsurgery of prolactinomas. In: Black PMcL, Zervas NT, Ridgway EC, et al, eds. Secretory Tumors of the Pituitary Gland. Progress in Endocrine Research and Therapy. Vol 1. New York: Raven Press, 1984: 73–81.

614. Nelson PB, Goodman M, Maroon JC, et al. Factors in predicting outcome from operation in patients with prolactin-secreting pituitary adenomas. Neurosurgery 1983; 13:634–641.

615. Tucker HS, Grubb SR, Wigand JP, et al. Galactorrhea-amenorrhea syndrome: follow-up of forty-five patients after pituitary tumor removal. Ann Intern Med 1981; 94:302–307.

616. Woosley RE, King JS, Talbert L. Prolactin-secreting pituitary adenomas: neurosurgical management of 37 patients. Fertil Steril 1982; 37:54–60.

617. Rodman EF, Molitch ME, Post KD, et al. Long-term follow-up of transsphenoidal selective adenomectomy for prolactinoma. JAMA 1984; 252:921–924.

618. Thomson JA, Teasdale GM, Gordon D, et al. Treatment of presumed prolactinoma by transsphenoidal operation: early and late results. Br Med J 1985; 291:1550–1553.

619. Parl FF, Cruz VE, Cobb CA, et al. Late recurrence of surgically removed prolactinomas. Cancer 1986; 57:2422–2426.

620. Zervas NT. Surgical results for pituitary adenomas: results of an international survey. In: Black PMcL, Zervas NT, Ridgway EC, et al, eds. Secretory Tumors of the Pituitary Gland. Progress in Endocrine Research and Therapy. Vol 1. New York: Raven Press, 1984: 377–385.

621. Laws ER Jr, Fode NC, Redmond MJ. Transsphenoidal surgery following unsuccessful prior therapy. An assessment of benefits and risks in 158 patients. J Neurosurg 1985; 63:823–829.

622. Hubbard JL, Scheithauer BW, Abboud CF, et al. Prolactin-secreting adenomas: the preoperative response to bromocriptine treatment and surgical outcome. J Neurosurg 1987; 67:816–821.

623. Sheline GE, Grossman A, Jones AE, et al. Radiation therapy for prolactinomas. In: Black PMcL, Zervas NT, Ridgway EC, et al, eds. Secretory Tumors of the Pituitary Gland. Progress in Endocrine Research and Therapy. Vol 1. New York: Raven Press, 1984: 93–108.

624. Krieg RJ Jr, Thorner MO, Evans WS. Sex differences in beta-adrenergic stimulation of growth hormone secretion in vitro. Endocrinology 1986; 119:1339–1342.

625. Nabarro JD. Pituitary prolactinomas (review). Clin Endocrinol (Oxf) 1982; 17:129–155.

626. Grossman A, Cohen BL, Charlesworth M, et al. Treatment of prolactinomas with megavoltage radiotherapy. Br Med J 1984; 288:1105–1109.

627. Halberg FE, Sheline GE. Radiotherapy of pituitary tumors. Endocrinol Metab Clin North Am 1987; 16:667–684.

628. Constine LS, Woolf PD, Cann D, et al. Hypothalamic-pituitary dysfunction after radiation for brain tumors. N Engl J Med 1993; 328:87–94.(Erratum 1993; 328(16):1208) (see comments).

629. Feek CM, McLelland J, Seth J, et al. How effective is external pituitary irradiation for growth hormone–secreting pituitary tumors? Clin Endocrinol (Oxf) 1984; 20:401–408.

630. Ross DA, Wilson CB. Results of transsphenoidal microsurgery for growth hormone–secreting pituitary adenoma in a series of 214 patients. J Neurosurg 1988; 68:854–867.

Acromegaly

631. Marie P. Sur deux cas d'acromegalie. Hypertrophie singuliere non congenitale des extremites superieures, inferieures et cephaliques. Rev Med 1886; 6:297–333.

632. Minkowski O. Uber einen Fall von Akromegalie. Berl Klin Wochenschr 1887; 24:371–374.

633. Marie P, de Souza-Leite JD. Essays on Acromegaly. London: New Sydenham Society, 1891.

634. Alexander L, Appleton D, Hall R, et al. Epidemiology of acromegaly in the Newcastle region. Clin Endocrinol (Oxf) 1980; 12:71–79.

635. Bengtsson BA, Eden S, Ernest I, et al. Epidemiology and long-term survival in acromegaly. A study of 166 cases diagnosed between 1955 and 1984. Acta Med Scand 1988; 223:327–335.

636. Randall RV. Acromegaly and gigantism. In: DeGroot LJ, ed. Endocrinology. Vol 1. Philadelphia: WB Saunders, 1989: 330–350.

637. Wilson CB. A decade of pituitary microsurgery. The Herbert Olivecrona lecture. J Neurosurg 1984; 61:814–833.

638. Thorner MO, Frohman LA, Leong DA, et al. Extrahypothalamic growth hormone–releasing factor (GRF) secretion is a rare cause of acromegaly: plasma GRF levels in 177 acromegalic patients. J Clin Endocrinol Metab 1984; 59:846–849.

639. Asa SL, Scheithauer BW, Bilbao JM, et al. A case for hypothalamic acromegaly: a clinicopathological study of six patients with hypothalamic gangliocytomas producing growth hormone–releasing factor. J Clin Endocrinol Metab 1984; 58:796–803.

640. Melmed S, Ezrin C, Kovacs K, et al. Acromegaly due to secretion of growth hormone by an ectopic pancreatic islet-cell tumor. N Engl J Med 1985; 312:9–17.

641. Reichlin S. Etiology of acromegaly from the neuroendocrine point of view: a historical perspective. In: Robbins RJ, Melmed S, eds. Acromegaly. A Century of Scientific and Clinical Progress. New York: Plenum, 1987: 7–15.

642. Asa SL, Kovacs K, Thorner MO, et al. Immunohistological localization of growth hormone–releasing hormone in human tumors. J Clin Endocrinol Metab 1985; 60:423–427.

643. Dayal Y, Lin HD, Tallberg K, et al. Immunocytochemical demonstration of growth hormone–releasing factor in gastrointestinal and pancreatic endocrine tumors. Am J Clin Pathol 1986; 85:13–20.

644. Frohman LA. Growth hormone–releasing factor: a neuroendocrine perspective. J Lab Clin Med 1984; 103:819–832.

645. Christofides ND, Stephanou A, Suzuki H, et al. Distribution of immunoreactive growth hormone–releasing hormone in the human brain and intestine and its production by tumors. J Clin Endocrinol Metab 1984; 59:747–751.

646. Frohman LA, Thominet JL, Szabo M. Ectopic growth hormone releasing factor syndromes. In: Raiti S, Tolman R, eds. Human Growth Hormone. New York: Plenum, 1986: 347–360.

647. Frohman LA, Szabo M, Berelowitz M, et al. Partial purification and characterization of a peptide with growth hormone-releasing activity from extrapituitary tumors in patients with acromegaly. J Clin Invest 1980; 65:43–54.

648. Guillemin R, Brazeau P, Bohlen P, et al. Growth hormone–releasing factor from a human pancreatic tumor that caused acromegaly. Science 1982; 218:585–587.

649. Bluestone R, Bywaters EG, Hartog M, et al. Acromegalic arthropathy. Ann Rheum Dis 1971; 30:243–258.

650. Detenbeck LC, Tressler HA, O'Duffy JD, et al. Peripheral joint manifestations of acromegaly. Clin Orthop 1973; 91:119–127.

651. Dons RF, Rosselet P, Pastakia B, et al. Arthropathy in acromegalic patients before and after treatment: a long-term follow-up study. Clin Endocrinol (Oxf) 1988; 28:515–524.

652. Layton MW, Fudman EJ, Barkan A, et al. Acromegalic arthropathy. Characteristics and response to therapy. Arthritis Rheum 1988; 31:1022–1027.

653. Steinbach HL, Feldman R, Goldberg MB. Acromegaly. Radiology 1959; 72:535–549.

654. Jones DR, Bahn RC, Randall RV, et al. The human costochondral junction. II: Patients with acromegaly. Mayo Clin Proc 1969; 44:330–334.

655. Fradkin JE, Eastman RC, Lesniak MA, et al. Specificity spillover at the hormone receptor—exploring its role in human disease (review). N Engl J Med 1989; 320:640–645.

656. Jadresic A, Banks LM, Child DF, et al. The acromegaly syndrome. Relation between clinical features, growth hormone values and radiological characteristics of the pituitary tumours. Q J Med 1982; 51:189–204.

657. Wass JA, Cudworth AG, Bottazzo GF, et al. An assessment of glucose intolerance in acromegaly and its response to medical treatment. Clin Endocrinol (Oxf) 1980; 12:53–59.

658. Nikkila EA, Pelkonen R. Serum lipids in acromegaly. Metabolism 1975; 24:829–838.

659. Takeda R, Tatami R, Ueda K, et al. The incidence and pathogenesis of hyperlipidaemia in 16 consecutive acromegalic patients. Acta Endocrinol 1982; 100:358–362.

660. Wright AD, Hill DM, Lowy C, et al. Mortality in acromegaly. Q J Med 1970; 39:1–16.

661. Evans CC, Hipkin LJ, Murray GM. Pulmonary function in acromegaly. Thorax 1977; 32:322–327.

662. Harrison BD, Millhouse KA, Harrington M, et al. Lung function in acromegaly. Q J Med 1978; 47:517–532.

663. Perks WH, Horrocks PM, Cooper RA, et al. Sleep apnoea in acromegaly. Br Med J 1980; 280:894–897.

664. Hart TB, Radow SK, Blackard WG, et al. Sleep apnea in active acromegaly. Arch Intern Med 1985; 145:865–866.

665. Pekkarinen T, Partinen M, Pelkonen R, et al. Sleep apnoea and daytime sleepiness in acromegaly: relationship to endocrinological factors. Clin Endocrinol (Oxf) 1987; 27:649–654.

666. Grunstein RR, Ho KY, Sullivan CE. Sleep apnea in acromegaly. Ann Intern Med 1991; 115:527–532.

667. Mezon BJ, West P, MacLean JP, et al. Sleep apnea in acromegaly. Am J Med 1980; 69:615–618.

668. Cadieux RJ, Kales A, Santen RJ, et al. Endoscopic findings in sleep apnea associated with acromegaly. J Clin Endocrinol Metab 1982; 55:18–22.

669. Chanson P, Timsit J, Benoit O, et al. Rapid improvement in sleep apnoea of acromegaly after short-term treatment with somatostatin analogue SMS 201–995 (letter). Lancet 1986; 1:1270–1271.

670. Ziemer DC, Dunlap DB. Relief of sleep apnea in acromegaly by bromocriptine. Am J Med Sci 1988; 295:49–51.

671. McGuffin WL Jr, Sherman BM, Roth F, et al. Acromegaly and cardiovascular disorders. A prospective study. Ann Intern Med 1974; 81:11–18.

672. Hayward RP, Emanuel RW, Nabarro JD. Acromegalic heart disease: influence of treatment of the acromegaly on the heart. Q J Med 1987; 62:41–58.

673. Lie JT. Pathology of the heart in acromegaly: anatomic findings in 27 autopsied patients. Am Heart J 1980; 100:41–52.

674. Jonas EA, Aloia JF, Lane FJ. Evidence of subclinical heart muscle dysfunction in acromegaly. Chest 1975; 67:190–194.

675. Savage DD, Henry WL, Eastman RC, et al. Echocardiographic assessment of cardiac anatomy and function in acromegalic patients. Am J Med 1979; 67:823–829.

676. Luboshitzki R, Hammerman H, Barzilai D, et al. The heart in acromegaly: correlation of echocardiographic and clinical findings. Isr J Med Sci 1980; 16:378–383.

677. O'Keefe JC, Grant SJ, Wiseman JC, et al. Acromegaly and the heart—echocardiographic and nuclear imaging studies. Aust NZ J Med 1982; 12:603–607.

678. Csanady M, Gaspar L, Hogye M, et al. The heart in acromegaly: an echocardiographic study. Int J Cardiol 1983; 2:349–361.

679. Gordon DA, Hill FM, Ezrin C. Acromegaly: A review of 100 cases. Can Med Assoc J 1962; 87:1106–1109.

680. Hejtmancik MR, Bradfield JY Jr, Herrmann GR. Acromegaly and the heart: a clinical and pathologic study. Ann Intern Med 1951; 34:1445–1456.

681. Balzer R, McCullagh EP. Hypertension in acromegaly. Am J Med Sci 1959; 237:449–452.

682. Hamwi GJ, Skillman TG, Tufts KC. Acromegaly. Am J Med 1960; 29:690–699.

683. Sowers JR, Tuck ML. Hypertension associated with diabetes mellitus, hypercalcaemic disorders, acromegaly and thyroid disease (review). Clin Endocrinol Metab 1981; 10:631–656.

684. Anderson RJ, Lufkin EG, Sizemore GW, et al. Acromegaly and pituitary adenoma with phaeochromocytoma: a variant of multiple endocrine neoplasia. Clin Endocrinol (Oxf) 1981; 14:605–612.

685. Rioperez E, Botella JM, Valdivieso L, et al. Conn's syndrome in a patient with acromegaly. Horm Metab Res 1981; 13:186–187.

686. Riggs BL, Randall RV, Wahner HW, et al. The nature of the metabolic bone disorder in acromegaly. J Clin Endocrinol Metab 1972; 34:911–918.

687. Seeman E, Wahner HW, Offord KP, et al. Differential effects of endocrine dysfunction on the axial and the appendicular skeleton. J Clin Invest 1982; 69:1302–1309.

688. Diamond T, Nery L, Posen S. Spinal and peripheral bone mineral densities in acromegaly: the effects of excess growth hormone and hypogonadism. Ann Intern Med 1989; 111:567–573.

689. Mastaglia FL, Barwich DD, Hall R. Myopathy in acromegaly. Lancet 1970; 2:907–909.

690. Mastaglia FL. Pathological changes in skeletal muscle in acromegaly. Acta Neuropathol 1973; 24:273–286.

691. Pickett JB, Layzer RB, Levin SR, et al. Neuromuscular complications of acromegaly. Neurology 1975; 25:638–645.

692. Epstein N, Whelan M, Benjamin V. Acromegaly and spinal stenosis. Case report. J Neurosurg 1982; 56:145–147.

693. McCullagh EP, Hewlett JS. Acromegaly with amyotrophic lateral sclerosis of the amyotrophic type. J Clin Endocrinol 1947; 7:636–643.

694. O'Duffy JD, Randall RV, MacCarty CS. Median neuropathy (carpal-tunnel syndrome) in acromegaly. Ann Intern Med 1973; 78:379–383.

695. Clemmons DR, Van Wyk JJ, Ridgway EC, et al. Evaluation of acromegaly by radioimmunoassay of somatomedin-C. N Engl J Med 1979; 301:1138–1142.

696. Klein I, Parveen G, Gavaler JS, et al. Colonic polyps in patients with acromegaly. Ann Intern Med 1982; 97:27–30.

697. Ituarte EM, Petrini J, Hershman JM. Acromegaly and colon cancer. Ann Intern Med 1984; 101:627–628.

698. Pines A, Rozen P, Ron E, et al. Gastrointestinal tumors in acromegalic patients. Am J Gastroenterol 1985; 80:266–269.

699. Terzolo M, Tappero G, Borretta G, et al. High prevalence of colonic polyps in patients with acromegaly. Influence of sex and age (see comments). Arch Intern Med 1994; 154:1272–1276.

700. Vasen HF, van Erpecum KJ, Roelfsema F, et al. Increased prevalence of colonic adenomas in patients with acromegaly. Eur J Endocrinol 1994; 131:235–237.

701. Brunner JE, Johnson CC, Zafar S, et al. Colon cancer and polyps in acromegaly: increased risk associated with family history of colon cancer. Clin Endocrinol (Oxf) 1990; 32:65–71.

702. Jenkins PJ, Fairclough PD, Richards T, et al. Acromegaly, colonic polyps and carcinoma. Clin Endocrinol (Oxf) 1997; 47:17–22.

703. Evans HM, Briggs JH, Dixon JS. The physiology and chemistry of growth hormone. In: Harris GW, Donovan BT, eds. The Pituitary Gland. Vol 1. Berkeley: University of California Press, 1966: 439–491.

704. Mustacchi P, Shimkin MB. Occurrence of cancer in acromegaly and hypopituitarism. Cancer 1957; 10:100–104.

705. Rajasoorya C, Holdaway IM, Wrightson P, et al. Determinants of clinical outcome and survival in acromegaly. Clin Endocrinol (Oxf) 1994; 41:95–102.

706. Bates AS, Van't Hoff W, Jones JM, et al. An audit of outcome of treatment in acromegaly. Q J Med 1993; 86:293–299.

707. Cryer PE, Daughaday WH. Regulation of growth hormone secretion in acromegaly. J Clin Endocrinol Metab 1969; 29:386–393.

708. Jaquet P, Guibout M, Jaquet C, et al. Circadian regulation of growth hormone secretion after treatment in acromegaly. J Clin Endocrinol Metab 1980; 50:322–328.

709. Barkan AL, Stred SE, Reno K, et al. Increased growth hormone pulse frequency in acromegaly. J Clin Endocrinol Metab 1989; 69:1225–1233.

710. Wass JA, Clemmons DR, Underwood LE, et al. Changes in circulating somatomedin-C levels in bromocriptine-treated acromegaly. Clin Endocrinol (Oxf) 1982; 17:369–377.

711. Rieu M, Girard F, Bricaire H, et al. The importance of insulin-like growth factor (somatomedin) measurements in the diagnosis and surveillance of acromegaly. J Clin Endocrinol Metab 1982; 55:147–153.

712. Stonesifer LD, Jordan RM, Kohler PO. Somatomedin C in treated acromegaly: poor correlation with growth hormone and clinical response. J Clin Endocrinol Metab 1981; 53:931–934.

713. Moses AC, Molitch ME, Sawin CT, et al. Bromocriptine therapy in acromegaly: use in patients resistant to conventional therapy and effect on serum levels of somatomedin. J Clin Endocrinol Metab 1981; 53:752–758.

714. Beck P, Parker ML, Daughaday WH. Paradoxical hypersecretion of growth hormone in response to glucose. J Clin Endocrinol Metab 1966; 26:463–469.

715. Earll JM, Sparks LL, Forsham PH. Glucose suppression of serum growth hormone in the diagnosis of acromegaly. JAMA 1967; 201:628–630.

716. Besser GM, Mortimer CH, McNeilly AS, et al. Long-term infusion of growth hormone release inhibiting hormone in acromegaly: effects on pituitary and pancreatic hormones. Br Med J 1974; 4:622–627.

717. Lawrence AM, Goldfine ID, Kirsteins L. Growth hormone dynamics in acromegaly. J Clin Endocrinol Metab 1970; 31:239–247.

718. Irie M, Tsushima T. Increase of serum growth hormone concentration following thyrotropin-releasing hormone injection in patients with acromegaly or gigantism. J Clin Endocrinol Metab 1972; 35:97–100.

719. Hanew K, Kokubun M, Sasaki A, et al. The spectrum of pituitary growth hormone responses to pharmacological stimuli in acromegaly. J Clin Endocrinol Metab 1980; 51:292–297.

720. Liuzzi A, Chiodini PG, Botalla L, et al. Inhibitory effect of L-dopa on GH release in acromegalic patients. J Clin Endocrinol Metab 1972; 35:941–943.

721. Liuzzi A, Chiodini PG, Botalla L, et al. Decreased plasma growth hormone (GH) levels in acromegalics following CB 154(2-Br-alpha ergocryptine) administration. J Clin Endocrinol Metab 1974; 38:910–912.

722. Thorner MO, Chait A, Aitken M, et al. Bromocriptine treatment of acromegaly. Br Med J 1975; 1:299–303.

723. Gelato MC, Merriam GR, Vance ML, et al. Effects of growth hormone–releasing factor on growth hormone secretion in acromegaly. J Clin Endocrinol Metab 1985; 60:251–257.

724. Laws ER Jr, Scheithauer BW, Carpenter S, et al. The pathogenesis of acromegaly. Clinical and immunocytochemical analysis in 75 patients. J Neurosurg 1985; 63:35–38.

725. Scheithauer BW, Kovacs K, Randall RV, et al. Pathology of excessive production of growth hormone (review). Clin Endocrinol Metab 1986; 15:655–681.

726. Ramsay JA, Kovacs K, Asa SL, et al. Reversible sellar enlargement due to growth hormone–releasing hormone production by pancreatic endocrine tumors in a acromegalic patient with multiple endocrine neoplasia type I syndrome. Cancer 1988; 62:445–450.

727. Barth RJ, Constant RB, Parker MW, et al. Preoperative diagnosis of acromegaly by growth hormone–releasing factor radioimmunoassay. Mil Med 1991; 156(7):375–378.

728. Penny ES, Penman E, Price J, et al. Circulating growth hormone releasing factor concentrations in normal subjects and patients with acromegaly. Br Med J 1984; 289:453–455.

729. Melmed S, Braunstein GD, Horvath E, et al. Pathophysiology of acromegaly (review). Endocr Rev 1983; 4:271–290.

730. Kovacs K, Horvath E. Pathology of growth hormone-producing tumors of the human pituitary. Semin Diagn Pathol 1986; 3:18–33.

731. Trouillas J, Girod C, Lheritier M, et al. Morphological and biochemical relationships in 31 human pituitary adenomas with acromegaly. Virchows Arch [A] 1980; 389:127–142.

732. Kanie N, Kageyama N, Kuwayama A, et al. Pituitary adenomas in acromegalic patients: an immunohistochemical and endocrinological study with special reference to prolactin-secreting adenoma. J Clin Endocrinol Metab 1983; 57:1093–1101.

733. Saeger W, Rubenach Gerz K, Caselitz J, et al. Electron microscopical morphometry of GH producing pituitary adenomas in comparison with normal GH cells. Virchows Arch [A] 1987; 411:467–472.

734. Horvath E, Kovacs K. Morphogenesis and significance of fibrous bodies in human pituitary adenomas. Virchows Arch [B] 1978; 27:69–78.

735. Neumann PE, Goldman JE, Horoupian DS, et al. Fibrous bodies in growth hormone–secreting adenomas contain cytokeratin filaments. Arch Pathol Lab Med 1985; 109:505–508.

736. Mori H, Mori S, Saitoh Y, et al. Growth hormone–producing pituitary adenoma with crystal-like amyloid immunohistochemically positive for growth hormone. Cancer 1985; 55:96–102.

737. Saitoh Y, Mori H, Matsumoto K, et al. Accumulation of amyloid in pituitary adenomas. Acta Neuropathol 1985; 68:87–92.

738. Corenblum B, Sirek AM, Horvath E, et al. Human mixed somatotrophic and lactotrophic pituitary adenomas. J Clin Endocrinol Metab 1976; 42:857–863.

739. Bassetti M, Spada A, Arosio M, et al. Morphological studies on mixed growth hormone (GH)- and prolactin (PRL)-secreting human pituitary adenomas. Coexistence of GH and PRL in the same secretory granule. J Clin Endocrinol Metab 1986; 62:1093–1100.

740. Halmi NS. Occurrence of both growth hormone- and prolactin-immunoreactive material in the cells of human somatotropic pituitary adenomas containing mammotropic elements. Virchows Arch [A] 1983; 398:19–31.

741. Zurschmiede C, Landolt AM. Distribution of growth hormone and prolactin in secretory granules of the normal and neoplastic human adenohypophysis. Virchows Arch [B] 1987; 53:308–315.

742. Bassetti M, Arosio M, Spada A, et al. Growth hormone and prolactin secretion in acromegaly: correlations between hormonal dynamics and immunocytochemical findings. J Clin Endocrinol Metab 1988; 67:1195–1204.

743. Beckers A, Courtoy R, Stevenaert A, et al. Mammosomatotropes in human pituitary adenomas as revealed by electron microscopic double gold immunostaining method. Acta Endocrinol 1988; 118:503–512.

744. Felix IA, Horvath E, Kovacs K, et al. Mammosomatotroph adenoma of the pituitary associated with gigantism and hyperprolactinemia. A morphological study including immunoelectron microscopy. Acta Neuropathol 1986; 71:76–82.

745. Kovacs K, Horvath E, Ezrin C, et al. Adenoma of the human pituitary producing growth hormone and thyrotropin. A histologic, immunocytologic and fine-structural study. Virchows Arch [A] 1982; 395:59–68.

746. Carlson HE, Linfoot JA, Braunstein GD, et al. Hyperthyroidism and acromegaly due to a thyrotropin- and growth hormone–secreting pituitary tumor. Lack of hormonal response to bromocriptine. Am J Med 1983; 74:915–923.

747. Beck-Peccoz P, Bassetti M, Spada A, et al. Glycoprotein hormone alpha-subunit response to growth hormone (GH)-releasing hormone in patients with active acromegaly. Evidence for alpha-subunit and GH coexistence in the same tumoral cell. J Clin Endocrinol Metab 1985; 61:541–546.

748. Beck-Peccoz P, Piscitelli G, Amr S, et al. Endocrine, biochemical, and morphological studies of a pituitary adenoma secreting growth hormone, thyrotropin (TSH), and alpha-subunit: evidence for secretion of TSH with increased bioactivity. J Clin Endocrinol Metab 1986; 62:704–711.

749. Asai A, Matsutani M, Funada N, et al. Malignant growth hormone-secreting pituitary adenoma with hematogenous dural metastasis: case report (review). Neurosurgery 1988; 22:1091–1094.

750. Mountcastle RB, Roof BS, Mayfield RK, et al. Pituitary adenocarcinoma in an acromegalic patient: response to bromocriptine and pituitary testing: a review of the literature on 36 cases of pituitary carcinoma (review). Am J Med Sci 1989; 298:109–118.

751. Horvath E, Scheithauer BW, Kovacs K. Morphologic aspects of growth hormone–producing pituitary adenomas with emphasis on novel concepts. In: Ludecke DK, Tolis G, eds. Growth Hormone, Growth Factors, and Acromegaly. New York: Raven, 1987: 107–114.

752. Kovacs K. The relation of the endocrine system to tumors of non-endocrine organs (German) (review). Deutsch Gesundh 1966; 21:1105–1108.

753. Landolt AM, Osterwalder V, Stackmann G. Preoperative treatment of acromegaly with SMS 201–995: surgical and pathological observations. In: Ludecke DK, Tolis G, eds. Growth Hormone, Growth Factors, and Acromegaly. New York: Raven, 1987: 229–244.

754. George SR, Kovacs K, Asa SL, et al. Effect of SMS 201–995, a long-acting somatostatin analogue, on the secretion and morphology of a pituitary growth hormone cell adenoma. Clin Endocrinol (Oxf) 1987; 26:395–405.

755. Beckers A, Stevenaert A, Kovacs K, et al. The treatment of acromegaly with SMS 201–995. Adv Biosci 1988; 69:227–228.

756. Barkan AL, Lloyd RV, Chandler WF, et al. Preoperative treatment of acromegaly with long-acting somatostatin analog SMS 201–995: shrinkage of invasive pituitary macroadenomas and improved surgical remission rate. J Clin Endocrinol Metab 1988; 67:1040–1048.

757. Wass JA, Kramer R, Randall RV, et al. The treatment of acromegaly (review). Clin Endocrinol Metab 1986; 15:683–707.

758. Davis DH, Laws ER Jr, Ilstrup DM, et al. Results of surgical treatment for growth hormone-secreting pituitary adenomas. J Neurosurg 1993; 79:70–75.

759. Kao PC, Laws ER Jr, Zimmerman D. Somatomedin C/insulin-like growth factor I levels after treatment of acromegaly. Ann Clin Lab Sci 1992; 22:95–99.

760. Laws ER Jr, Piepgras DG, Randall RV, et al. Neurosurgical management of acromegaly. Results in 82 patients treated between 1972 and 1977. J Neurosurg 1979; 50:454–461.

761. Williams RA, Jacobs HS, Kurtz AB, et al. The treatment of acromegaly with special reference to trans-sphenoidal hypophysectomy. Q J Med 1975; 44:79–98.

secreting pituitary tumors. Endocrinol Metab Clin North Am 1989; 18(2):339–358.

879. Snyder PJ. Gonadotroph cell pituitary adenomas (review). Endocrinol Metab Clin North Am 1987; 16:755–764.

880. Weintraub BD, Gershengorn MC, Kourides IA, et al. Inappropriate secretion of thyroid-stimulating hormone. Ann Intern Med 1981; 95:339–351.

881. Smallridge RC. Thyrotropin-secreting pituitary tumors (review). Endocrinol Metab Clin North Am 1987; 16:765–792.

882. Kourides IA, Weintraub BD, Rosen SW, et al. Secretion of alpha subunit of glycoprotein hormones by pituitary adenomas. J Clin Endocrinol Metab 1976; 43:97–106.

883. Ridgway EC. Glycoprotein hormone production by pituitary tumors. Prog Endocr Res Ther 1984; 1:343.

884. Comi RJ, Gesundheit N, Murray L, et al. Response of thyrotropin-secreting pituitary adenomas to a long-acting somatostatin analogue. N Engl J Med 1987; 317:12–17.

885. Afrasiabi A, Valenta L, Gwinup G. A TSH secreting pituitary tumour causing hyperthyroidism: presentation of a case and review of the literature. Acta Endocrinol 1979; 92:448–454.

886. Hill SA, Falko JM, Wilson CB, et al. Thyrotrophin-producing pituitary adenomas. J Neurosurg 1982; 57:515–519.

887. Cravioto H, Fukaya T, Zimmerman EA, et al. Immunohistochemical and electron-microscopic studies of functional and non-functional pituitary adenomas including one TSH secreting tumor in a thyrotoxic patient. Acta Neuropathol 1981; 53:281–292.

888. Grisoli F, Leclercq T, Winteler JP, et al. Thyroid-stimulating hormone pituitary adenomas and hyperthyroidism. Surg Neurol 1986; 25:361–368.

889. Samaan NA, Osborne BM, Mackay B, et al. Endocrine and morphologic studies of pituitary adenomas secondary to primary hypothyroidism. J Clin Endocrinol Metab 1977; 45:903–911.

890. Katz MS, Gregerman RI, Horvath E, et al. Thyrotroph cell adenoma of the human pituitary gland associated with primary hypothyroidism: clinical and morphological features. Acta Endocrinol 1980; 95:41–48.

891. Wajchenberg BL, Tsanaclis AM, Marino J. TSH-containing pituitary adenoma associated with primary hypothyroidism manifested by amenorrhoea and galactorrhoea. Acta Endocrinol 1984; 106:61–66.

892. Saeger W, Ludecke DK. Pituitary adenomas with hyperfunction of TSH. Frequency, histological classification, immunocytochemistry and ultrastructure. Virchows Arch [A] 1982; 394:255–267.

893. Girod C, Trouillas J, Claustrat B. The human thyrotropic adenoma: pathologic diagnosis in five cases and critical review of the literature. Semin Diagn Pathol 1986; 3:58–68.

894. Scheithauer BW, Kovacs K, Randall RV, et al. Pituitary gland in hypothyroidism. Histologic and immunocytologic study. Arch Pathol Lab Med 1985; 109:499–504.

895. Vagenakis AG, Dole K, Braverman LE. Pituitary enlargement, pituitary failure, and primary hypothyroidism. Ann Intern Med 1976; 85:195–198.

896. Farley JD, Toth EL, Ryan EA. Primary hypothyroidism presenting as growth delay and pituitary enlargement. Can J Neurol Sci 1988; 15:35–37.

897. Mixson AJ, Friedman TC, Katz DA, et al. Thyrotropin-secreting pituitary carcinoma. J Clin Endocrinol Metab 1993; 76:529–533.

898. Trouillas J, Girod C, Sassolas G, et al. Human pituitary gonadotropic adenoma; histological, immunocytochemical, and ultrastructural and hormonal studies in eight cases. J Pathol 1981; 135:315–336.

899. Horvath E, Kovacs K. Gonadotroph adenomas of the human pituitary: sex-related fine-structural dichotomy. A histologic, immunocytochemical, and electron-microscopic study of 30 tumors. Am J Pathol 1984; 117:429–440.

900. Snyder PJ, Johnson J, Muzyka R. Abnormal secretion of glycoprotein alpha-subunit and follicle-stimulating hormone (FSH) beta-subunit in men with pituitary adenomas and FSH hypersecretion. J Clin Endocrinol Metab 1980; 51:579–584.

901. Snyder PJ, Sterling FH. Hypersecretion of LH and FSH by a pituitary adenoma. J Clin Endocrinol Metab 1976; 42:544–550.

902. Koide Y, Kugai N, Kimura S, et al. A case of pituitary adenoma with possible simultaneous secretion of thyrotropin and follicle-stimulating hormone. J Clin Endocrinol Metab 1982; 54:397–403.

903. Kovacs K, Horvath E, Van Loon GR, et al. Pituitary adenomas associated with elevated blood follicle-stimulating hormone levels: a histologic, immunocytologic, and electron microscopic study of two cases. Fertil Steril 1978; 29:622–628.

904. Borges JL, Ridgway EC, Kovacs K, et al. Follicle-stimulating hormone–secreting pituitary tumor with concomitant elevation of serum alpha-subunit levels. J Clin Endocrinol Metab 1984; 58:937–941.

905. Wide L, Lundberg PO. Hypersecretion of an abnormal form of follicle-stimulating hormone associated with suppressed luteinizing hormone secretion in a woman with a pituitary adenoma. J Clin Endocrinol Metab 1981; 53:923–930.

906. Berezin M, Olchovsky D, Pines A, et al. Reduction of follicle-stimulating hormone (FSH) secretion in FSH-producing pituitary adenoma by bromocriptine. J Clin Endocrinol Metab 1984; 59:1220–1223.

907. Vance ML, Ridgway EC, Thorner MO. Follicle-stimulating hormone– and alpha-subunit-secreting pituitary tumor treated with bromocriptine. J Clin Endocrinol Metab 1985; 61:580–584.

908. Friend JN, Judge DM, Sherman BM, et al. FSH-secreting pituitary adenomas: stimulation and suppression studies in two patients. J Clin Endocrinol Metab 1976; 43:650–657.

909. Cunningham GR, Huckins C. An FSH and prolactin-secreting pituitary tumor: pituitary dynamics and testicular histology. J Clin Endocrinol Metab 1977; 44:248–253.

910. Demura R, Kubo O, Demura H, et al. FSH and LH secreting pituitary adenoma. J Clin Endocrinol Metab 1977; 45:653–657.

911. Harris RI, Schatz NJ, Gennarelli T, et al. Follicle-stimulating hormone secreting pituitary adenomas: correlation of reduction of adenoma size with reduction of hormonal hypersecretion after transsphenoidal surgery. J Clin Endocrinol Metab 1983; 56:1288–1293.

912. Klibanski A, Deutsch PJ, Jameson JL, et al. Luteinizing hormone–secreting pituitary tumor: biosynthetic characterization and clinical studies. J Clin Endocrinol Metab 1987; 64:536–542.

913. Barrow DL, Tindall GT, Kovacs K, et al. Clinical and pathological effects of bromocriptine on prolactin-secreting and other pituitary tumors. J Neurosurg 1984; 60:1–7.

914. Grossman A, Ross R, Charlesworth M, et al. The effect of dopamine agonist therapy on large functionless pituitary tumours. Clin Endocrinol (Oxf) 1985; 22:679–686.

915. Vos P, Croughs RJ, Thijssen JH, et al. Response of luteinizing hormone secreting pituitary adenoma to a long-acting somatostatin analogue. Acta Endocrinol (Copenh) 1988; 118:587–590.

916. Sassolas G, Serusclat P, Claustrat B, et al. Plasma alpha-subunit levels during the treatment of pituitary adenomas with the somatostatin analog (SMS 201-995). Horm Res 1988; 29:124–128.

917. Chapman AJ, MacFarlane IA, Shalet SM, et al. Discordant serum alpha-subunit and FSH concentrations in a woman with a pituitary tumour. Clin Endocrinol (Oxf) 1984; 21:123–129.

918. Roman SH, Goldstein M, Kourides IA, et al. The luteinizing hormone–releasing hormone (LHRH) agonist [D-Trp⁶-Pro⁹-NEt]LHRH increased rather than lowered LH and alpha-subunit levels in a patient with an LH-secreting pituitary tumor. J Clin Endocrinol Metab 1984; 58:313–319.

919. Sassolas G, Lejeune H, Trouillas J, et al. Gonadotropin-releasing hormone agonists are unsuccessful in reducing tumoral gonadotropin secretion in two patients with gonadotropin-secreting pituitary adenomas. J Clin Endocrinol Metab 1988; 67:180–185.

920. Zarate A, Fonseca ME, Mason M, et al. Gonadotropin-secreting pituitary adenoma with concomitant hypersecretion of testosterone and elevated sperm count. Treatment with LRH agonist. Acta Endocrinol 1986; 113:29–34.

921. Daneshdoost L, Molitch ME, Synder PJ. Inhibition of follicle stimulating hormone secretion from gonadotroph adenomas by repetitive administration of a GnRH antagonist. Proceedings of the 72nd Meeting of the Endocrine Society, Atlanta, GA, 1990; p 366 (abstract).

922. Kovacs K, Horvath E, Rewcastle NB, et al. Gonadotroph cell adenoma of the pituitary in a women with long-standing hypogonadism. Arch Gynecol 1980; 229:57–65.

923. Nicolis GL, Modhi G, Gabrilove JL. Gonadotropin producing pituitary adenomas. A case report and review of the literature. Mt Sinai J Med 1982; 49:297–304.

924. Beckers A, Stevenaert A, Mashiter K, et al. Follicle-stimulating hormone–secreting pituitary adenomas. J Clin Endocrinol Metab 1985; 61:525–528.

925. Miura M, Matsukado Y, Kodama T, et al. Clinical and histopathological characteristics of gonadotropin-producing pituitary adenomas. J Neurosurg 1985; 62:376–382.

926. Snyder PJ. Gonadotroph cell pituitary adenomas. Endocrinol Metab Clin North Am 1987; 16(3):755–764.

927. Nicolis G, Shimshi M, Allen C, et al. Gonadotropin-producing pituitary adenoma in a man with long-standing primary hypogonadism. J Clin Endocrinol Metab 1988; 66:237–241.

928. Demura R, Jibiki K, Kubo O, et al. The significance of alpha-subunit as a tumor marker for gonadotropin-producing pituitary adenomas. J Clin Endocrinol Metab 1986; 63:564–569.

929. Trouillas J, Girod C, Sassolas G, et al. The human gonadotropic adenoma: pathologic diagnosis and hormonal correlations in 26 tumors. Semin Diagn Pathol 1986; 3:42–57.

Nonsecretory Adenoma

930. Klibanski A. Non-secretory pituitary tumors. Endocrinol Metab Clin North Am 1987; 16:793–804.

931. Heshmati HM, Turpin G, Kujas M, et al. The immunocytochemical heterogeneity of silent pituitary adenomas. Acta Endocrinol 1988; 118:533–537.

932. Jameson JL, Klibanski A, Black PM, et al. Glycoprotein hormone genes are expressed in clinically nonfunctioning pituitary adenomas. J Clin Invest 1987; 80:1472–1478.

933. Bevan JS, Burke CW. Non-functioning pituitary adenomas do not regress during bromocriptine therapy but possess membrane-bound dopamine receptors which bind bromocriptine. Clin Endocrinol (Oxf) 1986; 25:561–572.

934. D'Emden MC, Harrison LC. Rapid improvement in visual field defects following bromocriptine treatment of patients with non-functioning pituitary adenomas. Clin Endocrinol (Oxf) 1986; 25:697–702.

935. Johnston DG, Hall K, McGregor A, et al. Bromocriptine therapy for "nonfunctioning" pituitary tumors. Am J Med 1981; 71:1059–1061.

936. Kovacs K, Horvath E, Ryan N, et al. Null cell adenoma of the human pituitary. Virchows Arch [A] 1980; 387:165–174.

937. Kovacs K, Asa SL, Horvath E, et al. Null cell adenomas of the pituitary: attempts to resolve their cytogenesis. In: Lechago J, Kameya T, eds. Endocrine Pathology Update. Philadelphia: Field and Wood, 1990: 17–31.

938. Martinez AJ. The pathology of nonfunctional pituitary adenomas. Semin Diagn Pathol 1986; 3:83–94.

939. Asa SL, Gerrie BM, Singer W, et al. Gonadotropin secretion in vitro by human pituitary null cell adenomas and oncocytomas. J Clin Endocrinol Metab 1986; 62:1011–1019.

940. Yamada S, Asa SL, Kovacs K, et al. Analysis of hormone secretion by clinically nonfunctioning human pituitary adenomas using the reverse hemolytic plaque assay. J Clin Endocrinol Metab 1989; 68:73–80.

941. Sakurai T, Seo H, Yamamoto N, et al. Detection of mRNA of prolactin and ACTH in clinically nonfunctioning pituitary adenomas. J Neurosurg 1988; 69:653–659.

942. Kovacs K, Horvath E. Pituitary "chromophobe" adenoma composed of oncocytes. A light and electron microscopic study. Arch Pathol 1973; 95:235–239.

943. Landolt AM, Oswald UW. Histology and ultrastructure of an oncocytic adenoma of the human pituitary. Cancer 1973; 31:1099–1105.

944. Gunzl HJ, Saeger W, Diehl S, et al. Immunohistochemical analyses of oncocytic and chromophobe pituitary adenomas. Exp Clin Endocrinol 1988; 92:51–58.

945. Yamada S, Asa SL, Kovacs K. Oncocytomas and null cell adenomas of the human pituitary: morphometric and in vitro functional comparison. Virchows Arch [A] 1988; 413:333–339.

946. Peillon F, Le D, Garnier P, et al. Receptors and neurohormones in human pituitary adenomas. Horm Res 1989; 31:13–18.

947. Asa SL, Gerrie BM, Kovacs K, et al. Structure-function correlations of human pituitary gonadotroph adenomas in vitro. Lab Invest 1988; 58:403–410.

948. Kovacs K, Lloyd R, Horvath E, et al. Silent somatotroph adenomas of the human pituitary. A morphologic study of three cases including immunocytochemistry, electron microscopy, in vitro examination, and in situ hybridization. Am J Pathol 1989; 134:345–353.

Nonpituitary Sellar Mass

949. Meyer FB, Carpenter SM, Laws ER Jr. Intrasellar arachnoid cysts. Surg Neurol 1987; 28:105–110.

950. Branch CL Jr, Laws ER Jr. Metastatic tumors of the sella turcica masquerading as primary pituitary tumors. J Clin Endocrinol Metab 1987; 65:469–474.

951. Carmel PW. Craniopharyngiomas. In: Wilkins RH, Rengachary SS, eds. Neurosurgery. Vol 1. New York: McGraw-Hill, 1985: 905–916.

952. Hunt WE, Sayers MP, Yashon D. Tumor of the sellar and parasellar area. In: Youmans JR, ed. Neurological Surgery. III: Philadelphia: WB Saunders, 1973: 1412–1431.

953. Matson DD. Neurosurgery of Infancy and Childhood. Springfield, IL: Charles C Thomas, 1969.

954. Thapar K, Stefaneanu L, Kovacs K, et al. Estrogen receptor gene expression in craniopharyngiomas: an in situ hybridization study. Neurosurgery 1994; 35:1012–1017.

955. Ross-Russell RW, Pennybaker JB. Craniopharyngioma in the elderly. J Neurol Neurosurg Psychiatry 1961; 24:1–13.

956. Baskin DS, Wilson CB. Surgical management of craniopharyngiomas. J Neurosurg 1986; 65:22–27.

957. Bartlett JR. Craniopharyngiomas—a summary of 85 cases. J Neurol Neurosurg Psychiatry 1971; 34:37–41.

958. Jenkins JS, Gilbert CJ, Ang V. Hypothalamic-pituitary function in patients with craniopharyngiomas. J Clin Endocrinol Metab 1976; 43:394–399.

959. Daniels DL, Williams AL, Thornton RS, et al. Differential diagnosis of intrasellar tumors by computed tomography. Radiology 1981; 141:697–701.

960. Naidich TP, Pinto RS, Kushner MJ, et al. Evaluation of sellar and parasellar masses by computed tomography. Radiology 1976; 120:91–99.

961. Streja D, Teichner F, Marliss EB. Fifty-year survival after surgery for craniopharyngioma. JAMA 1975; 234:510–512.

962. Laws ER Jr, Thapar K. Treatment of craniopharyngioma. Growth Genet Horm 1994; 10:6–10.

963. Laws ER Jr. Transsphenoidal removal of craniopharyngioma. Pediatr Neurosurg 1994; 21(Suppl) 1:57–63.

964. Laws ER Jr. Diagnosis and management of craniopharyngioma in children and adolescents. Curr Opin Endocrinol Diabetes 1996; 3:110–114.

965. Lyen KR, Grant DB. Endocrine function, morbidity, and mortality after surgery for craniopharyngioma. Arch Dis Child 1982; 57:837–841.

966. Lichter AS, Wara WM, Sheline GE, et al. The treatment of craniopharyngiomas. Int J Radiat Oncol Biol Phys 1977; 2:675–683.

967. Miyamoto M, Sugawa H, Mori T, et al. A case of hypopituitarism due to granulomatous and lymphocytic adenohypophysitis with minimal pituitary enlargement: a possible variant of lymphocytic adenohypophysitis. Endocrinol Jpn 1988; 35:607–616.

968. Mayfield RK, Levine JH, Gordon L, et al. Lymphoid adenohypophysitis presenting as a pituitary tumor. Am J Med 1980; 69:619–623.

969. Hassoun P, Anayssi E, Salti I. A case of granulomatous hypophysitis with hypopituitarism and minimal pituitary enlargement. J Neurol Neurosurg Psychiatry 1985; 48:949–951.

970. Asa SL, Bilbao JM, Kovacs K, et al. Lymphocytic hypophysitis of pregnancy resulting in hypopituitarism: a distinct clinicopathologic entity. Ann Intern Med 1981; 95:166–171.

971. McDermott MW, Griesdale DE, Berry K, et al. Lymphocytic adenohypophysitis (review). Can J Neurol Sci 1988; 15:38–43.

972. Jensen MD, Handwerger BS, Scheithauer BW, et al. Lymphocytic hypophysitis with isolated corticotropin deficiency. Ann Intern Med 1986; 105:200–203.

973. McGrail KM, Beyerl BD, Black PM, et al. Lymphocytic adenohypophysitis of pregnancy with complete recovery. Neurosurgery 1987; 20:791–793.

974. Meichner RH, Riggio S, Manz HJ, et al. Lymphocytic adenohypophysitis causing pituitary mass. Neurology 1987; 37:158–161.

975. Vanneste JA, Kamphorst W. Lymphocytic hypophysitis. Surg Neurol 1987; 28:145–149.

976. Gal R, Schwartz A, Gukovsky Oren S, et al. Lymphoid hypophysitis associated with sudden maternal death: report of a case review of the literature. Obstet Gynecol Surv 1986; 41:619–621.

977. Wild RA, Kepley M. Lymphocytic hypophysitis in a patient with amenorrhea and hyperprolactinemia. A case report. J Reprod Med 1986; 31:211–216.

978. Okamoto T, Moriyama E, Mizukawa N. Lymphoid adenohypophysitis. Acta Pathol Jpn 1986; 36:751–756.

979. Lee JH, Laws ER Jr, Guthrie BL, et al. Lymphocytic hypophysitis: occurrence in two men (discussion). Neurosurgery 1994; 34:159–62.

980. Sano K. So-called intracranial germ cell tumors: are they really of germ cell origin? Br J Neurosurg 1995; 9:391–401.

981. Newelt EA, Frenkel EP, Smith RG. Suprasellar germinomas (ectopic pinealomas): aspects of immunological characterization and successful chemotherapeutic responses in recurrent disease. Neurosurgery 1980; 7:65–70.

982. Abboud CF, Randall RV, Laws ER Jr. Clinical manifestations of suprasellar germinomas. In: Givens JR, ed. The Hypothalamus. Chicago: Year Book Medical, 1984: 355–359.

983. Shivdasani RA, Kantoff PW. Extragonadal germ cell tumors. In: Raghavan D, Scher HI, Leibel SA, et al, eds. Principles and Practice of Genitourinary Oncology. Philadelphia: Lippincott-Raven, 1997: 751–764.

984. Sumida M, Uozumi T, Kiya K, et al. MRI of intracranial germ cell tumors. Radiology 1995; 37:32–37.

985. Ng HK. Cytological diagnosis of intracranial germinomas in smear preparations. Acta Cytol 1995; 39:693–697.

986. Allen JC, DaRosso RC, Donahue B, et al. A phase II trial of preirradiation carboplatin in newly diagnosed germinoma of the central nervous system. Cancer 1994; 74:940–944.

987. Vijayaraghavan S, Brock C, Monson JP, et al. Does the rapid response to cisplatin-based chemotherapy justify its use as primary treatment for intracranial germ-cell tumors? Q J Med 1993; 86:801–812.

988. Patel SR, Buckner JC, Smithson WA, et al. Cisplatin-based chemotherapy in primary central nervous system germ cell tumors. J Neurooncol 1992; 12:47–52.

989. Pocecco M, De Campo C, Marinoni S, et al. High frequency of empty sella syndrome in children with growth hormone deficiency. Helv Paediatr Acta 1989; 43:295–301.

990. Reid RL, Quigley ME, Yen SSC. Pituitary apoplexy. Arch Neurol 1985; 42:712–719.

991. Cardoso ER, Peterson EW. Pituitary apoplexy: a review. Neurosurgery 1984; 14(3):363–373.

992. Jacobi JD, Fishman LM, Daroff RB. Pituitary apoplexy in acromegaly followed by partial pituitary insufficiency. Arch Intern Med 1974; 134:559–561.

993. Markowitz S, Sherman L, Kolodny HD, et al. Acute pituitary vascular accident (pituitary apoplexy). Med Clin North Am 1981; 65(1):105–116.

994. Wakai S, Fukushima T, Teramoto A, et al. Pituitary apoplexy: its incidence and clinical significance. J Neurosurg 1981; 55:187–193.

995. Veldhuis JD, Hammond JM. Endocrine function after spontaneous infarction of the human pituitary: report, review, and reappraisal (review). Endocr Rev 1980; 1:100–107.

996. Ostrov SG, Quencer RM, Hoffman JC, et al. Hemorrhage within pituitary adenomas: how often associated with pituitary apoplexy syndrome? Am J Roentgenol 1989; 153:153–160.

997. Pelkonen R, Kuusisto A, Salmi J, et al. Pituitary function after pituitary apoplexy. Am J Med 1978; 65:773–778.

998. Wright RL, Ojemann RG, Drew JH. Hemorrhage into pituitary adenomata. Arch Neurol 1965; 12:326–331.

Miscellaneous References

999. Hartman ML, Veldhuis JD, Thorner MO. Augmented growth hormone (GH) secretory burst frequency and amplitude mediate enhanced GH secretion during a two-day fast in normal men. Second International Pituitary Congress, Palm Desert, CA, 1989; p. 13 (abstract).

1000. Van den Berghe G, Frolich M, Veldhuis JD, et al. Growth hormone secretion in recently operated acromegalic patients. J Clin Endocrinol Metab 1994; 79:1706–1715.

1001. Iranmanesh A, Grisso B, Veldhuis JD. Low basal and persistent pulsatile growth hormone secretion are revealed in normal and hyposomatotropic men studied with a new ultrasensitive chemiluminescence assay. J Clin Endocrinol Metab 1994; 78:526–535.

1002. Jefferson LS, Korner A. A direct effect of growth hormone on the incorporation of precursors into proteins and nucleic acids of perfused rat liver. Biochem J 1967; 104:826–832.

1003. Griffin EE, Miller LL. Effects of hypophysectomy of liver donor on net synthesis of specific plasma proteins by the isolated perfused rat liver: modulation of synthesis of albumin, fibrinogen, alpha₁-acid glycoprotein, alpha₂-(acute phase)-globulin, and haptoglobin by insulin, cortisol, triiodothyronine, and growth hormone. J Biol Chem 1974; 249:5062–5069.

1004. McConaghey P, Sledge CB. Production of "sulphation factor" by the perfused liver. Nature (Lond) 1970; 225:1249–1250.

1005. Moon HD, Jentoft VL, Li CH. Effect of human growth hormone on growth of cells in tissue culture. Endocrinology 1962; 70:31–38.

1006. Kostyo JL, Hotchkiss J, Knobil E. Stimulation of amino acid transport in isolated diaphragm by growth hormone added in vitro. Science 1959; 130:1653–1654.

1007. Hjalmarson A, Isaksson O, Ahrén K. Effects of growth hormone and insulin on amino acid transport in perfused rat heart. Am J Physiol 1969; 217:1795–1802.

1008. Ledet T. Growth hormone stimulating the growth of arterial medial cells in vitro: absence of effect of insulin. Diabetes 1976; 25:1011–1017.

1009. Goodman HM. Multiple effects of growth hormone on lipolysis. Endocrinology 1968; 83:300–308.

1010. Fain JN, Kovacev VP, Scow RO. Effect of growth hormone and dexamethasone on lipolysis and metabolism in isolated fat cells of the rat. J Biol Chem 1965; 240:3522–3529.

1011. Atkison PR, Weidman ER, Bhaumick B, et al. Release of somatomedin-like activity by cultured WI-38 human fibroblasts. Endocrinology 1980; 106:2006–2012.

1012. Madsen K, Makower AM, Friberg U, et al. Effect of human growth hormone on proteoglycan synthesis in cultured rat chondrocytes. Acta Endocrinol (Copenh) 1985; 108:338–342.

1013. Whitfield JF, MacManus JP, Rixon RH. Stimulation by growth hormone of deoxyribonucleic acid synthesis and proliferation of rat thymic lymphocytes. Horm Metab Res 1971; 3:28–33.

1014. Desai LS, Lazarus H, Li CH, et al. Human leukemic cells: effect of human growth hormone. Exp Cell Res 1973; 81:330–332.

1015. Golde DW, Bersch N, Li CH. Growth hormone: species-specific stimulation of erythropoiesis in vitro. Science 1977; 196:1112–1113.

1016. Veldhuis JD, Johnson ML. In vivo dynamics of luteinizing hormone secretion and clearance in man: assessment by deconvolution mechanics. J Clin Endocrinol Metab 1988; 66:1291–1300.

1017. Urban RJ, Dahl KD, Padmanabhan V, et al. Specific regulatory actions of dihydrotestosterone and estradiol on the dynamics of FSH secretion and clearance in man. J Androl 1991; 12:27–35.

1018. Urban RJ, Veldhuis JD, Dafau ML. Estrogen regulates the gonadotropin-releasing hormone–stimulated secretion of biologically active luteinizing hormone. J Clin Endocrinol Metab 1991; 72:660–668.

1019. Veldhuis JD, Johnson ML, Dafau ML. Physiological attributes of endogenous bioactive luteinizing hormone secretory bursts in man. Am J Physiol 1989; 256:E199–E207.

1020. Wajnrajch MP, Gertner JM, Harbison MD, et al. Nonsense mutation in the human growth hormone–releasing hormone receptor causes growth failure analogous to the little (lit) mouse. Nat Genet 1996; 12:88–90.

1021. March CM, Kletzky OA, Davajan V, et al. Longitudinal evaluation of patients with untreated prolactin-secreting pituitary adenomas. Am J Obstet Gynecol 1981; 139:835–844.

1022. von Werder K, Fahlbusch R, Rjosk H-K. Macroprolactinomas: clinical and therapeutic aspects. In: Tolis G, Stefanis C, Mountokalakis T, et al, eds. Prolactin and Prolactinomas. New York: Raven Press, 1983: 415–429.

1023. Koppelman MC, Jaffe MJ, Rieth KG, et al. Hyperprolactinemia, amenorrhea, and galactorrhea: a retrospective assessment of twenty-five cases. Ann Intern Med 1984; 100:115–121.

1024. Martin TL, Kim M, Malarkey WB. The natural history of idiopathic hyperprolactinemia. J Clin Endocrinol Metab 1985; 60:855–858.

1025. Sisam DA, Sheehan JP, Sheeler LR. The natural history of untreated microprolactinomas. Fertil Steril 1987; 48:67–71.

1026. Aubourg PR, Derome PJ, Peillon F, et al. Endocrine outcome after transsphenoidal adenomectomy for prolactinoma: prolactin levels and tumor size as predicting factors. Surg Neurol 1980; 14:141–143.

1027. Charpentier G, de Plunkett T, Jedynak P, et al. Surgical treatment of prolactinomas. Short- and long-term results, prognostic factors. Horm Res 1985; 22:222–227.

1028. Ciric I, Mikhael M, Stafford T, et al. Transsphenoidal microsurgery of pituitary macroadenomas with long-term follow-up results. J Neurosurg 1983; 59:395–401.

1029. Faria MA Jr, Tindall GT. Transsphenoidal microsurgery for prolactin-secreting pituitary adenomas. J Neurosurg 1982; 56:33–43.

1030. Grisoli F, Vincentelli F, Jaquet P, et al. Prolactin-secreting adenoma in 22 men. Surg Neurol 1980; 13:241–247.

1031. Keye WR Jr, Chang RJ, Monroe SE, et al. Prolactin-secreting pituitary adenomas in women. II. Menstrual function, pituitary reserves, and prolactin production following microsurgical removal. Am J Obstet Gynecol 1979; 134:360–365.

1032. Landolt AM. Surgical treatment of pituitary prolactinomas: postoperative prolactin and fertility in seventy patients. Fertil Steril 1981; 35:620–625.

1033. Laws ER Jr, Ebersold MJ, Piepgras DG, et al. The role of surgery in the management of prolactinomas. In: MacLeod RM, Thorner MO, Scapagnini U, eds. Prolactin, Basic and Clinical Correlates. New York: Springer-Verlag, 1985; 849–853.

1034. Rawe SE, Williamson HO, Levine JH, et al. Prolactinomas: surgical therapy, indications and results. Surg Neurol 1980; 14:161–167.

1035. Schlechte JA, Sherman BM. Abnormal regulation of prolactin secretion after successful surgery for prolactin-secreting pituitary tumours. Clin Endocrinol (Oxf) 1981; 15:165–174.

1036. Soule SG, Farhi J, Conway GS, et al. The outcome of hypophysectomy for prolactinomas in the era of dopamine agonist therapy. Clin Endocrinol (Oxf) 1996; 44:711–716.

1037. Thomson JA, Davies DL, McLaren EH, et al. Ten-year follow-up of microprolactinoma treated by transsphenoidal surgery. Br Med J 1994; 309:1409–1410.

1038. van't Verlaat JW. The use of surgery for the treatment of prolactinomas. Acta Endocrinol (Copenh) 1993; 129(Suppl 1):34–37 (review).

1039. Frohman LA, Downs TR. Ectopic GRH syndromes. In: Robbins RJ, Melmed S, eds. Acromegaly: A Century of Scientific and Clinical Progress. New York: Plenum Press, 1987: 115–125.

1040. Grisoli F, Leclercq T, Jaquet P, et al. Transsphenoidal surgery for acromegaly: long-term results in 100 patients. Surg Neurol 1985; 23:513–519.

1041. Serri O, Somma M, Comtois R, et al. Acromegaly: biochemical assessment of cure after long-term follow-up of transsphenoidal selective adenomectomy. J Clin Endocrinol Metab 1985; 61:1185–1189.

1042. Balagura S, Derome P, Guiot G. Acromegaly: analysis of 132 cases treated surgically. Neurosurgery 1981; 8:413–416.

1043. Fahlbusch R, Buchfelder M. Transsphenoidal surgery of parasellar pituitary adenomas. Acta Neurochir 1988; 92:93–99.

1044. Thorner MO, Besser GM. Successful treatment of acromegaly with bromocriptine. Postgrad Med J 1976; 52:71–74.

1045. Wass JA, Thorner MO, Morris DV, et al. Long-term treatment of acromegaly with bromocriptine. Br Med J 1977; 1:875–878.

1046. Belforte L, Camanni F, Chiodini PG, et al. Long-term treatment with 2-Br-alpha-ergocryptine in acromegaly. Acta Endocrinol (Copenh) 1977; 85:235–248.

1047. Halse J, Haugen HN, Bohmer T. Bromocriptine treatment in acromegaly: clinical and biochemical effects. Acta Endocrinol 1977; 86:464–472.

1048. Eskildsen PG, Svendsen PA, Vang L, et al. Long-term treatment of acromegaly with bromocriptine. Acta Endocrinol 1978; 87:687–700.

1049. Lundin L, Ljunghall S, Wide L, et al. Bromocriptine therapy in eleven patients with acromegaly. Acta Endocrinol Suppl 1978; 216:207–216.

1050. Besser GM, Wass JAH, Thorner MO. Bromocriptine in the medical management of acromegaly. In: Goldstein M, Calne DB, Lieberman A, et al, eds. Ergot Compounds and Brain Function: Neuroendocrine and Neuropsychiatric Aspects. New York: Raven Press, 1980: 191–198.

1051. Lindholm J, Riishede J, Vestergaard S, et al. No effect of bromocriptine in acromegaly: a controlled trial. N Engl J Med 1981; 304:1450–1454.

1052. Tanner JM, Davies PS. Clinical longitudinal standards for height and height velocity for North American children. J Pediatr 1985; 107:317–329.

1053. Spencer CA. Thyroid profiling for the 1990's: free T₄ estimate or sensitive TSH measurement. J Clin Immunol 1989; 12:82–89.

1054. Brauner R, Malandry F, Rappaport R, et al. Growth and endocrine disorders in optic glioma. Eur J Pediatr 1990; 149:825–828.

1055. Rappaport R, Brauner R. Growth and endocrine disorders secondary to cranial irradiation. Pediatr Res 1989; 25:561–567.

1056. Sulmont V, Brauner R, Fontoura M, et al. Response to growth hormone treatment and final height after cranial or craniospinal irradiation. Acta Paediatr Scand 1990; 79:542–549.

10

POSTERIOR PITUITARY AND WATER METABOLISM

W. Brian Reeves, Daniel G. Bichet, and Thomas E. Andreoli

INTRODUCTION

This chapter considers the anatomy, function, and pathophysiology of the posterior pituitary neurohypophyseal system. Dysfunction of the neurohypophysis causes failure of regulation of the osmolality of body fluid. Alterations in osmolality may cause death from abrupt changes in the volume of the central nervous system (CNS): brain shrinkage in the hypertonic syndromes and brain swelling in the hypotonic syndromes. The coordinated responses involving vasopressin (arginine vasopressin [AVP], also called antidiuretic hormone [ADH]), thirst, and the kidney that maintain osmotic homeostasis are described here.

A convenient way of introducing osmoregulatory disorders is to consider briefly two of the cardinal physiological processes in osmotic homeostasis: the water repletion reaction and the cell volume regulatory response. The former provides a reference for understanding the pathogenesis of these disorders, and the latter makes it possible to understand changes in brain volume with osmoregulatory disorders.

Water Repletion Reaction

In normal individuals the serum osmolality is virtually constant from day to day and the serum sodium concentration is an accurate index of body water osmolality. The normal ranges for serum sodium levels and osmolality values in healthy individuals depend on small differences among individuals rather than on variations in a given individual.

Figure 10–1 presents a brief analysis of the key elements in water homeostasis. The solid lines on the figure indicate mechanisms that are activated by changes in effective extracellular fluid (ECF) osmolality and consequently by changes in cell volume; the dashed lines indicate mechanisms activated by changes in effective circulating volume; and the dotted lines indicate negative feedback limbs. Osmoreceptors, both for AVP release and for thirst, respond to small changes in effective ECF osmolality, whereas baroreceptors respond to changes in effective circulating volume. As little as a 2% increase in ECF osmolality causes shrinkage of osmoreceptor cells and stimulation of both thirst and AVP release from the posterior pituitary. Volume-dependent mechanisms operate independently of changes in plasma osmolality so that AVP release and thirst are stimulated when the effective circulating volume is reduced by approximately 10%. Suppression of thirst and of AVP release depends on two factors: the oropharyngeal reflex and the release of atrial natriuretic peptide (ANP), the latter occurring in all likelihood both systemically and in the CNS. These issues are discussed later.

When considered in these terms certain features of the water repletion reaction are particularly noteworthy. First,

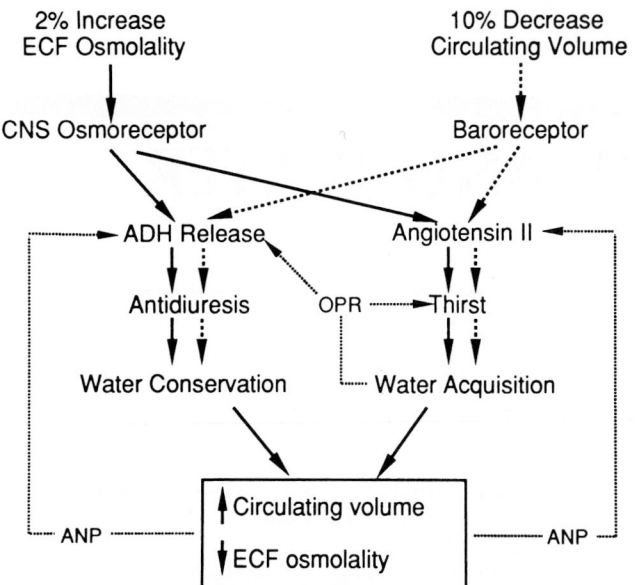

Figure 10–1. A schematic illustration of the water repletion reaction. Solid lines indicate osmotically stimulated pathways and dashed lines indicate volume-stimulated pathways. The dotted lines indicate negative feedback pathways. ANP, atrial natriuretic peptide; AVP, vasopressin; CNS, central nervous system; ECF, extracellular fluid; OPR, oropharyngeal reflex.

redundant mechanisms—namely thirst and AVP release—protect osmotic homeostasis. Second, release of AVP and stimulation of thirst require rather small changes in effective ECF osmolality, whereas nonosmotic stimuli of thirst and AVP release operate only in association with rather large decreases (approximately 10%) in effective circulating volume.

Cell Volume Regulation

Fluid transport between extracellular and intracellular compartments is designed to maintain constancy of cell volume and a negligible hydrostatic pressure gradient between the cells and the ECF. Because cell membranes are freely permeable to water, the two goals are achieved when the ECF osmolality is normal and when intracellular and extracellular osmolality values are identical. The water repletion reaction (see Fig. 10–1) functions to maintain a normal ECF osmolality and involves the balance between the tendency for dissipative processes (i.e., ionic "leak" processes) to reach equilibrium and the action of Na^+,K^+-ATPase to extrude Na^+ from cells while pumping K^+ into cells.

More specifically, sodium leakage from the ECF into cells and potassium leakage out of cells into the ECF are counterbalanced exactly by active outward sodium transport and inward potassium transport, both mediated by Na^+,K^+-ATPase. These active transport events maintain the intracellular cation (and therefore osmolar) content equal to that of ECF. Thus in normal individuals Na^+,K^+-ATPase maintains the equality of intracellular cation concentrations, whereas the water repletion reaction (see Fig. 10–1) determines the solute/water ratio in body fluids.

Finally when the effective ECF osmolality is increased or decreased, additional processes maintain the constancy of cell volume. When cells are exposed to an elevated extracellular osmolality the initial response is the loss of cell water and an increase in the *concentration* of solutes within the cell.[1] Conversely extracellular hypotonicity causes water movement into cells and a dilution of the cell contents. Thus, acutely, cells establish osmotic equilibrium with their surroundings at the expense of cell volume.

Many cells also possess osmoregulatory mechanisms that enable them to gain solute, as is the case in hypertonicity, or to lose solute, as is the case in hypotonicity, and thereby to return cell volume toward normal (Fig. 10–2). The transport processes responsible for gain or loss of solute vary from tissue to tissue. In the kidney medulla, in which large changes in extracellular osmolality are common, cells adjust to hypertonicity in two phases. Initially cell volume is increased as a result of NaCl transport into cells[2] and NaCl is subsequently replaced by organic solutes, or osmolytes, such as betaine, sorbitol, and glycerophosphocholine, which are less perturbing to cell function.[1, 3]

Clinical Syndromes: Definitions

Derangements in osmotic homeostasis are the consequences of derangements in the water repletion reaction. The manifestations of these disorders are due to alterations in cell volume, particularly in the CNS; changes in effective circulating volume; and local disturbances produced, e.g., by an intracranial neoplasm.

The *hypertonic syndromes* develop when the ratio of solutes to water in body fluids is increased. These disorders occur when water intake is less than the sum of renal plus extrarenal water losses; in the steady state the net water balance may be zero.

The *hypotonic syndromes* occur when the ratio of solutes to water in body fluids is reduced. The hypotonic syndromes develop when water intake exceeds the sum of renal plus extrarenal water losses, but in chronic hyponatremia water intake and water output may be equal.

THE NEUROHYPOPHYSIS

Structure of the Neurohypophysis

The neurohypophysis consists of a set of hypothalamic nuclei that house the perikarya of the magnicellular neurons responsible for synthesis of oxytocin and AVP; the axons of

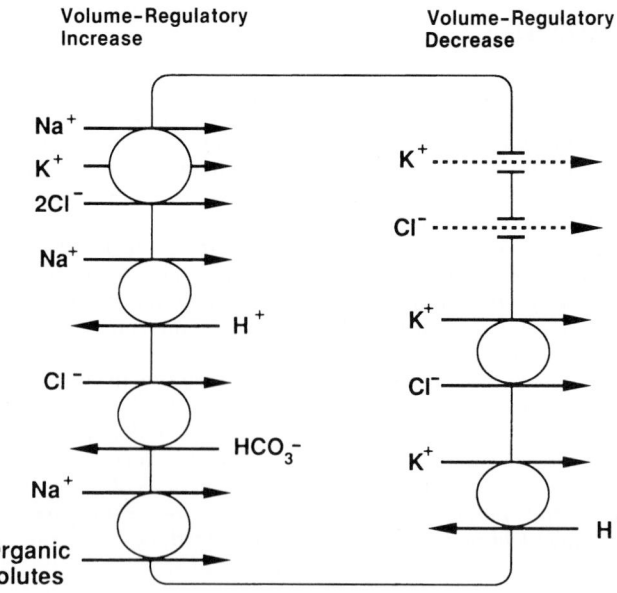

Figure 10–2. A schematic representation of some of the cell membrane transport systems that help to regulate cell volume. Cell shrinkage stimulates solute uptake pathways (*left*) and results in an increase in cell volume. Cell swelling activates solute loss primarily via conductive pathways for K^+ and Cl^-.

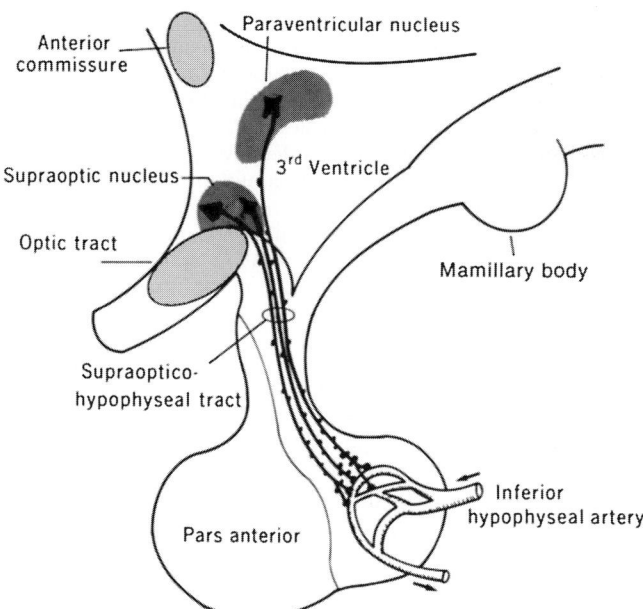

Figure 10–3. A schematic illustration of the neurohypophysis showing hypothalamic magnicellular nuclei, the supraopticohypophyseal tract with Herring bodies, and nerve endings forming on capillaries of the posterior pituitary.

these neurons, which form the supraopticohypophyseal tract; and the termini of these neurons in the posterior lobe of the pituitary. The posterior pituitary also contains pituicytes, small glial cells apparently unrelated to the neuroendocrine function of the gland.

The locations of the neurohypophyseal nuclei are shown schematically in Figure 10–3. The supraoptic nucleus (SON) is situated along the proximal half of the optic tract, whereas the paraventricular nucleus (PVN) lies vertically within the wall of the third ventricle; scattered neurons bridge the two principal nuclei in some species, forming the internuclear group. The SON consists almost entirely of magnicellular neurons that project to the posterior pituitary[4]; the PVN contains magnicellular neurons that project to the posterior pituitary and parvicellular neurons that project to the median eminence or to autonomic centers in the brain stem.[5] Immunocytochemical studies have demonstrated cells containing AVP and oxytocin in both nuclei.[6, 7] However the hormones are located in different cells.[7, 8] In humans AVP-containing magnicellular neurons occupy the more ventral aspects of the SON and are located more centrally in the PVN, whereas oxytocin-containing magnicellular neurons tend to be in the dorsal portion of the SON and in the periphery of the PVN.[9] AVP is also found in certain parvicellular neurons in the PVN and in some magnicellular neurons near the organum vasculosum of the lamina terminalis (OVLT).[10] AVP secretion by parvicellular neurons, which terminate in the hypophyseal-portal capillary bed, accounts for the high AVP levels in portal blood.[11, 12] These cells also secrete corticotropin-releasing hormone (CRH) and after adrenalectomy the number of neurons that stain for both CRH and AVP increases.[13, 14] AVP secretion into the portal blood may potentiate the effect of CRH on corticotropin (also called adrenocorticotropic hormone [ACTH] or adrenocorticotropin) secretion[11] through the action of AVP on V_3 receptors.[15, 16] The physiological role of AVP release at the OVLT is unknown.

The unmyelinated axons of the magnicellular neurons average less than 1 μm in diameter but they include numerous varicosities (Herring bodies), approximately 20 μm in diameter, that contain clusters of granules.[17] Microtubules can be traced down the length of the axons but do not appear to radiate into the granule-filled dilations. The axons terminate in the posterior lobe (pars nervosa) of the pituitary gland where they make up about 40% of the bulk of the gland.

The axonal nerve endings are distinctive in two respects.[17] First, terminal sacculations contain electron-lucent vesicles and preterminal dilations contain granules. Second, the terminal sacculations abut directly onto basement membranes that are separated from basement membranes of capillaries of the inferior hypophyseal artery by a perivascular space, whereas the preterminal dilations do not have direct capillary contact.

The secretion of AVP or oxytocin requires that the neurosecretory cells in the PVN and SON receive information from various sensor elements. Information from low-pressure baroreceptors is carried to the brain stem by afferents from cranial nerves IX and X, which relay in the nucleus tractus solitarius and a noradrenergic nucleus (A_1) and project to the magnicellular regions of the PVN and SON.[18] Additional noradrenergic afferents from the locus coeruleus (A_6) and solitary tract project to the AVP and CRH parvicellular neurons of the medial PVN.[19] Cholinergic innervation of the SON is provided by cholinergic neurons situated adjacent to the SON.[20, 21] Nicotinic and muscarinic receptors are present in the SON and PVN, respectively, and stimulation of these receptors increases AVP secretion.[22]

Two circumventricular organs, the subfornical organ (SFO) and the OVLT, also provide input to the AVP neurons of the SON and PVN. These organs lie outside the blood-brain barrier and therefore may be important for osmoreception and interaction with blood-borne hormones such as angiotensin II (AII).[23] Both the anatomy and the physiology of the afferent pathways to the PVN and the SON are poorly defined.

Hormone Biosynthesis, Transport, and Metabolism

The hormones that are elaborated by most mammalian neurohypophyses are oxytocin and AVP.[24–26] As shown in Figure 10–4 both oxytocin and AVP are nonapeptides with a molecular mass of approximately 1.1 kd. In both molecules a sulfhydryl bond between the cysteine residues at positions 1 and 6 forms a single cystine moiety, yielding a ring structure. AVP is the antidiuretic hormone in all mammals except hogs and other members of the suborder Suina, in which lysine vasopressin (containing lysine rather than arginine in position 8) occurs. The antidiuretic hormone among lower vertebrates is arginine vasotocin, which contains the same three COOH-terminal acyclic amino acids as AVP but the "tocin" ring structure of oxytocin.

Neurophysins

The neurophysins are sulfur-rich proteins with molecular masses of 9 to 10 kd; they are soluble in 10% NaCl solutions at acid pH (3.9) and form insoluble ionic complexes with neurohypophyseal hormones.[27–29] Neurophysins contain 92 to 95 amino acid residues with conservation of the central domain in all species[28]; a high content of cysteine residues causes extensive disulfide binding within the molecule. The high cysteine content of neurophysin also accounts for the Gomori staining of neurosecretory granules (NSGs). Neurophysins are believed to be transported as polymeric aggregates within NSGs, thereby reducing the osmotic activity of the intravesicular protein.[28, 30]

Separate hormone-specific neurophysins exist for vasopressin and oxytocin.[31] The AVP-associated neurophysin is designated NpII and the oxytocin-associated neurophysin is called NpI. Neurophysin plays an important role in the processing

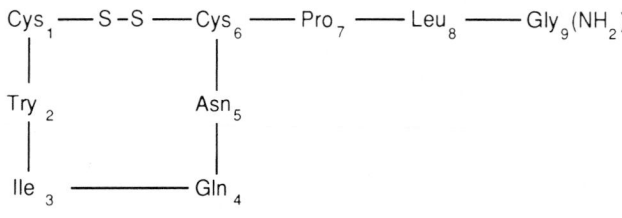

Arginine Vasopressin (AVP)

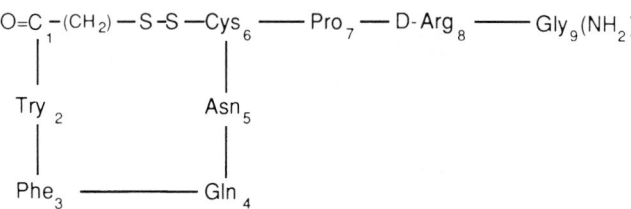

Oxytocin

1-Desamino-8-D-Arginine Vasopressin (Desmopressin)

Figure 10–4. Chemical structures of the major posterior pituitary hormones and desmopressin, a commonly used synthetic vasopressin analogue.

and secretion of AVP, and mutations in the pre-proneurophysin II gene have been identified in familial central diabetes insipidus, a condition in which AVP secretion is impaired.

Hormone Biosynthesis

The cardinal steps[32–36] in hormone biosynthesis are summarized in Figure 10–5. AVP and neurophysin are derived from a common precursor[37, 38] and the organization of the

AVP precursor peptide and the AVP gene of the rat are illustrated in Figure 10–6. The hormone precursor contains three peptide regions: a signal peptide and AVP at the NH_2 terminus, a neurophysin II region, and a COOH-terminal glycoprotein region of unknown significance.[39] Each of these regions of the precursor protein is encoded by one of three exons of the AVP precursor gene. The human AVP gene is on chromosome 20.[40]

Thus the steps in AVP biosynthesis are as follows: transcription of the AVP precursor mRNA; translation of the mRNA to a pre-prohormone of 166 amino acids; removal of the signal peptide sequence while the peptide is still attached to the ribosome to yield the prohormone; and conversion of the prohormone peptide into AVP and neurophysin II. This final step occurs within the NSG during its transport to the neurohypophysis.[32–36, 41]

These types of studies have yielded insight into the pathogenesis of hereditary central diabetes insipidus. In the Brattleboro rat, which lacks the ability to produce hypothalamic AVP, the defect is due to a single base deletion in the exon encoding neurophysin II.[42] Although the AVP-containing region of the precursor is translated normally, the frameshift that results from the nucleotide deletion causes misreading of the COOH-terminal codons, including the normal stop codon, so that translation proceeds to the extreme 3′ end of the poly(A) tail of the mRNA. The resulting protein is not processed normally into AVP and neurophysin II, so no hormone is detectable in the pituitary even though AVP mRNA is present in hypothalamic nuclei.[42] Mutations in neurophysin II have also been identified in humans with familial central diabetes insipidus.

Neurosecretory Cells

NSGs that appear to be identical with those in cell bodies of the SON and PVN are present along the length of the supraopticohypophyseal tract leading to the posterior pituitary[9] and in nerve endings in the posterior pituitary. The neurosecretory material is depleted in proportion to the reduction in AVP content of the posterior pituitary gland after dehydration, and repletion of NSGs in the posterior pituitary occurs with hydration.[43] Thus the posterior pituitary is a storage depot for AVP that is produced in hypothalamic cells and transported via the axons in NSGs.[43] NSG is transported at rates of about 200 mm/d, in contrast to approximately 4 mm/d for axonal protoplasmic flow, indicating that axonal transport of NSGs is facilitated.[17] The fact that NSG transport is inhibited by the microtubule disrupter colchicine[17] suggests that microtubules participate in NSG movement. NSGs are packets of hormone and binding protein.[44, 45]

Form	Molecular Weight	Synthetic Step
Pre-prohormone	≃ 21,000	Protein synthesis; magnicellular neuron ribosomes
↓		
Prohormone	≃ 23,000	Glycosylation and membrane packaging; magnicellular neuron Golgi apparatus
↓		
Neurosecretory granule (NSG)	$(23,000)_n$	Transport down supraopticohypophyseal tract as osmotically inactive granules
↓		
Neurophysin	≃ 10,000	Storage in posterior pituitary; cleavage within NSG
+		
Hormone	≃ 1,100	

Figure 10–5. Flow diagram for the pathway of posterior pituitary hormone biosynthesis.

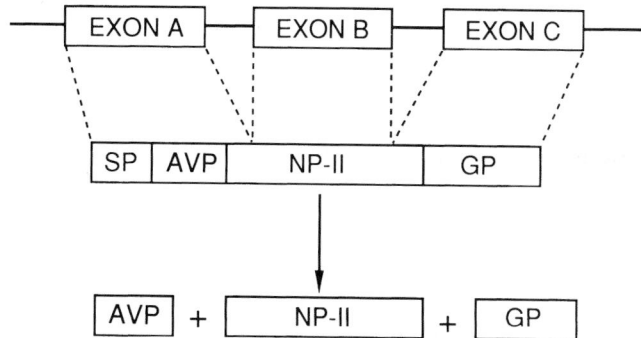

Figure 10–6. A schematic representation of the organization of the AVP gene and its relation to the pre-prohormone and final peptide products. GP, glycoprotein; NP-II, neurophysin II; SP, signal peptide.

Neuropeptide Release

Electrical stimulation of the neurohypophysis causes inhibition of urine flow.[46] Magnicellular neurons that secrete AVP respond to osmotic stimulation by firing in a characteristic phasic pattern, with bursts of 5 to 15 Hz separated by silent periods. Stimulation of AVP secretion by dehydration causes a progressive recruitment of neurons into phasic activity,[47] titrating hormone release to the magnitude of osmolar derangement.

Although cells of the SON generate action potentials after application of hyperosmotic solutions in vitro,[48] the magnicellular neurons are believed to be at least one synapse removed from the osmoreceptors.[49] Cholinergic stimuli, such as nicotine, release AVP directly.[50, 51] The microiontophoretic application of acetylcholine in the presence of selective nicotinic or muscarinic receptor blockers indicates that excitatory nicotinic receptors and inhibitory muscarinic receptors modulate activity in the SON.[50] Acetylcholine may be the synaptic transmitter between osmoreceptor and magnicellular neurons.

Neurohypophyseal secretion occurs by exocytosis,[50] which involves fusion of membranes from NSGs with plasma membranes; opening of the granules at the site of fusion; and release of granule material, including AVP and neurophysin II, into the extracellular space. Because not all AVP-neurophysin complexes within the posterior pituitary gland are readily available for release, the complexes may be segregated into two pools: a readily released pool and a storage pool.[52] The readily released pool is composed of NSGs located adjacent to plasma membranes, whereas the storage pool NSGs are remote from plasma membranes.

Exocytosis of the NSGs is triggered by neurotransmitter-induced depolarization of the hypothalamic magnicellular neurons. The control of AVP-producing neuron electrical activity is discussed later, but partial depolarization by these neurotransmitters results in the generation and propagation of a sodium-dependent, tetrodotoxin-sensitive[53] action potential. Voltage-sensitive calcium channels, which are opened by the membrane depolarization, allow calcium to flow into the nerve endings.[50, 54, 55] The calcium entry in turn activates exocytosis of NSGs and release of AVP and neurophysin II into the circulation. The rate of AVP secretion depends on both the rate and the pattern of neuron firing. For example stimulation of AVP-producing neurons in rapid intermittent bursts results in more AVP secretion than does the same degree of stimulation delivered at regular intervals.[56]

Distribution and Metabolism

Lysine vasopressin or AVP is distributed in a volume approximately equal to the extracellular space[57] and nearly all the hormone in plasma is in an unbound form,[57] which, because of its relatively low molecular weight, permeates peripheral and glomerular capillaries readily. In humans the clearance time of AVP, which represents both metabolic degradation and renal excretion, is in the range of 30 to 40 min.[58, 59] Consequently suppression of endogenous AVP release results in a change from the antidiuretic to the water diuretic state after approximately 30 min.[57, 59, 60]

Metabolic degradation of AVP follows binding of biologically active AVP to hormone receptors.[58–61] At least four sites of proteolytic cleavage for the hormone have been identified. AVP (see Fig. 10–4) may undergo cleavage: within the liver by rupture of the 1,6-disulfide bond[62, 63]; within the brain by cleavage at position 6,7 and subsequent hydrolysis of 9-glycinamide from the tripeptide[64]; within a variety of tissues by hydrolysis of the peptide bond between the hemicystine residue in position 1 and tyrosine in position 2[64, 65]; and within the kidney by proteolysis of the peptide bond between residues 8 and 9, resulting in glycinamide release.[66] A peptidase of 442 kd, which cleaves glycinamide and results in biologic inactivation, is present in kidney plasma membranes.[67] Renal excretion accounts for about one fourth of metabolic clearance.[57, 68]

The metabolic clearance rate of AVP is increased three- to fourfold during middle and late pregnancy.[69, 70] This increased clearance, which occasionally results in diabetes insipidus, is due to the production of an AVP-degrading enzyme, or vasopressinase, by the placenta.[70–72] Circulating vasopressinase activity declines rapidly after delivery and does not contribute to AVP metabolism in the nongravid state.

Chemistry

The hormones that are elaborated by most mammalian neurohypophyses include oxytocin and AVP. Figure 10–4 shows the structure of AVP and that of a synthetic analogue, 1-desamino-8-D-arginine vasopressin (desmopressin, DDAVP; see later). Most analogues possess antidiuretic, vasopressor, and uterotonic activities. Other analogues function as competitive antagonists of the vasopressor and antidiuretic actions.

AVP acts via V_1 receptors in smooth muscle and V_2 receptors in renal epithelia; only the latter receptors activate adenylate cyclase.[73] Antidiuretic activity depends on the ability of a peptide to bind to the V_2 receptor, to stimulate adenylate cyclase, and to resist metabolic degradation. Synthetic analogues of AVP with reduced receptor affinity and reduced ability to activate adenylate cyclase in vitro may exhibit potent and specific antidiuretic activity in the intact animal,[74–78] indicating that metabolic stability plays an important role in determining in vivo activity.

Deamination at position 1 reduces receptor affinity and renders the compound more resistant to metabolic degradation. As a result 1-desamino-arginine vasopressin (dAVP) possesses antidiuretic activity fourfold higher than that of AVP. Substitution of D-arginine for L-arginine at position 8 decreases the pressor activity so that the product DAVP has an antidiuretic/pressor activity a factor of 28.[78] Deamination at position 1 combined with substitution of D-arginine for L-arginine at position 8 yields desmopressin, which has a long duration of action and an antidiuretic/pressor factor of approximately 3000.[78] Desmopressin is the most widely used synthetic AVP analogue. Substitution of the hydrophobic amino acid valine for glutamine at position 4 (dDVAVP) prolongs the duration of action and abolishes the pressor effects, thus making the compound the most specific antidiuretic agonist reported.[78]

The first selective antagonist to AVP contains a pentamethylene ring at position 1, an *O*-ethyltyrosine substitution at position 2, and a valine substitution for glutamine at position 4.[79] This compound, d(CH$_2$)$_5$ Tyr (ET)VAVP, is a potent

AVP antagonist for both V_1 and V_2 receptors. Selective modification of d(CH$_2$)$_5$ Tyr (ET)VAVP can yield compounds with enhanced antidiuretic antagonist activity and increased selectivity for antidiuretic over antivasopressor activity.[80] The substitution of the L-Tyr (ET) at position 2 of d(CH$_2$)$_5$ Tyr (ET)VAVP by aliphatic D-amino acids, such as D-isoleucine, D-leucine, or D-valine, results in increased antidiuretic-antivasopressor selectivity.[81] Further substitution at position 4 with aminobutyric acid, isoleucine, or alanine leads to even greater antidiuretic-antivasopressor selectivity.[82] Finally the COOH-terminal glycine–NH$_2$ may be deleted or substituted by amino acid amides with full retention of antagonist activity.[83] These analogues competitively inhibit the antidiuretic response to exogenous and endogenous vasopressin and cause a water diuresis in normally hydrated rats that is equal to that seen in AVP-deficient Brattleboro rats.[79] These antagonists also inhibit lysine vasopressin binding and adenylate cyclase activation in renal medullary membrane preparations.[84–86]

In isolated segments of collecting ducts and medullary thick ascending limbs these antagonists inhibit the AVP-induced increase in adenylate cyclase activity but do not affect the response of adenylate cyclase to other agonists such as glucagon or parathyroid hormone.[87] In isolated perfused collecting duct segments[87] and in toad urinary bladder[88] d(CH$_2$)$_5$ Tyr (ET)VAVP prevents the AVP-induced increase in water permeability but has no effect on the response to forskolin, an agent that directly activates adenylate cyclase. In other words, these agents antagonize the effect of AVP by preventing the binding of AVP to its receptor.[85] Such antagonists are useful for physiological studies and may be useful clinically in the management of acute water intoxication associated with the syndrome of inappropriate vasopressin secretion (syndrome of inappropriate antidiuretic hormone secretion [SIADH]) (see later).

CONTROL OF VASOPRESSIN RELEASE

To maintain plasma osmolality at a constant level, AVP secretion must vary in response to small changes in plasma osmolality. AVP can also be released when the plasma osmolality is less than normal if the effective circulating volume is reduced.

Osmotic Regulation of Vasopressin Release

Injections of hypertonic NaCl or sucrose, but not urea solutions, cause prompt antidiuresis, indicating the presence of osmoreceptors that stimulate AVP release when osmolality is raised by solutes to which osmoreceptors are impermeable.[89] The osmoreceptors are located in an area of the brain that lacks an effective blood-brain barrier.[90] The precise location of the osmoreceptors is unresolved.

Leng[91] showed that the neurons of the SON are themselves osmosensitive in that microinjections of hypertonic saline into the SON produce a depolarization of the membrane potential and increased frequency of action potentials, suggesting that the SON itself is the site of osmoreception.[92] Other evidence, however, suggests that the osmoreceptor is separate from the SON and probably involves afferent fibers from the OVLT.[93–96]

Because individuals are not normally in a state of water diuresis, maintenance of plasma osmolality is believed to require tonic secretion of AVP. It is instructive in this regard to consider the relationship between serum osmolality and plasma AVP levels.[97] As shown in Figure 10–7, with plasma

osmolalities less than 280 mmol/L, plasma AVP levels are in the range of 0.45 to 1.4 pmol/L (0.5 to 1.5 ng/L); for osmolality greater than 280 mmol/L, plasma AVP levels rise with plasma osmolality according to the following relation: plasma AVP = 0.38 (plasma osmolality − 280).[98–100] Thus a plasma osmolality of 280 mmol/L is the osmotic threshold for AVP release, a view that coincides well with the concept that maintenance of normal plasma osmolality depends on the tonic secretion of AVP. In practical terms a 0.9 pmol/L (1 ng/L) rise in the level of plasma AVP translates into an increase in urine osmolality of about 200 mmol/kg. As a consequence maximal urine concentrations are produced at a plasma osmolality of about 290 to 292 mmol/kg and a plasma AVP level of 4.6 to 5.5 pmol/L (5 to 6 ng/L).

Nonosmotic Regulation of Vasopressin Release

Volume-mediated release of AVP can occur as a consequence of stimuli arising from "volume receptors," or baroreceptors.[101] Loci in the venous bed of the systemic circulation, the right side of the heart, and the left atrium are termed *low-pressure baroreceptors* and loci within the systemic arterial system of the carotid sinus and aortic arch are *high-pressure baroreceptors*.[102] The electrical activity of the baroreceptor is related to the degree of stretch in the vessel wall. Increases in pressure and wall tension cause an increase in the rate of firing of the receptor, and decreases in blood pressure or blood volume decrease the electrical activity of the baroreceptor.[103]

The afferent pathways for the atrial and carotid bifurcation baroreceptors appear to be the vagus and the glossopharyngeal nerves, respectively. Following synapses in the nucleus tractus solitarius, noradrenergic projections relay baroreceptor input to the PVN and SON.[49, 103] Baroreceptors inhibit AVP secretion under resting conditions and severing of all baroreceptor afferents increases plasma AVP levels. In addition stimulation of baroreceptors by balloon distention of either the left atrium or the carotid bifurcation inhibits electrical activity in the SON,[49] an inhibition prevented by section of the vagus nerve or local anesthesia of the carotid bifurcation.

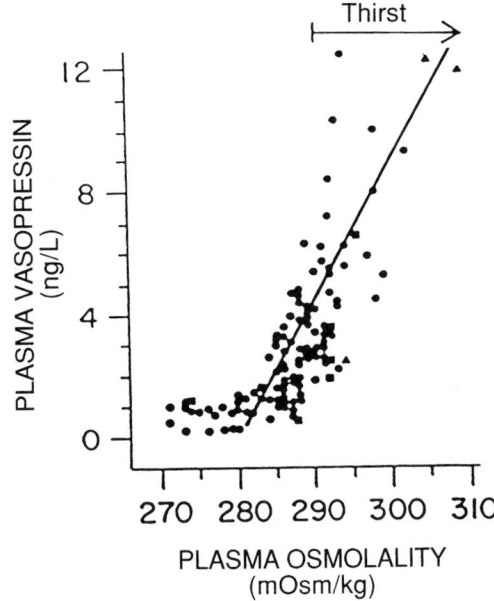

Figure 10–7. The relationship between plasma osmolality and plasma AVP level. To convert AVP values to picomoles per liter, divide by 1.1. (Adapted from Robertson GL, Berl T. Water metabolism. In: Brenner BM, Rector FC Jr, eds. The Kidney. 3rd ed. Philadelphia: WB Saunders, 1986: 385–432, with permission.)

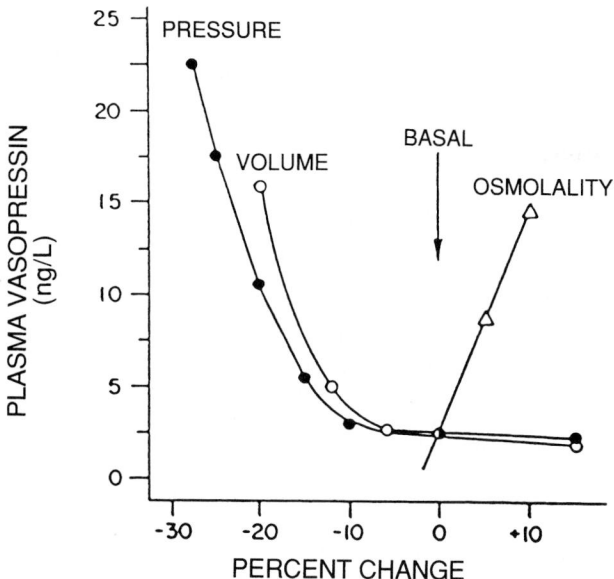

Figure 10–8. The relationship between plasma AVP and changes in plasma osmolality, blood volume, and mean arterial pressure in humans. To convert AVP values to picomoles per liter, divide by 1.1. (Adapted from Robertson GL, Berl T. Water metabolism. In: Brenner BM, Rector FC Jr, eds. The Kidney. 3rd ed. Philadelphia: WB Saunders, 1986: 385–432, with permission.)

TABLE 10–1. Agents That Alter Vasopressin Release

Agents That Enhance Release	Agents That Suppress Release
Prostaglandin E_2	Phenytoin
Morphine and narcotic analogues	Alcohol
Nicotine	α-Adrenergic agents
β-Adrenergic agents	Atrial natriuretic peptide
Angiotensin II	
Anesthetic agents	
Hypoxia	
Hypercapnia	
Vincristine	
Cyclophosphamide	
Clofibrate	
Carbamazepine	
Barbiturates	
Acetylcholine	
Histamine	
Metoclopramide	

Although each of the baroreceptors can influence AVP secretion, the left atrial baroreceptor is most important.[103] Atrial baroreceptors respond to smaller changes in blood volume than do arterial receptors[104, 105]; balloon distention of the left atrium inhibits AVP secretion more effectively than does distention of the right atrium; and cardiac denervation attenuates the secretion of AVP in response to hemorrhage.[106]

The sensitivity of the baroreceptor mechanism is illustrated in Figure 10–8. Acute reductions in arterial blood pressure exceeding 5 to 10% cause an exponential rise in AVP secretion.[100] Volume depletion in humans[107] and in animals[108–110] produces little elevation in plasma AVP levels until blood volume decreases by more than 8 to 10%. Further volume depletion results in exponential increases in plasma AVP levels.

In conscious dogs whose left atrial pressure was manipulated, decreases in left atrial pressure reduced the osmotic threshold and increased the sensitivity for osmotic AVP release, whereas increases in left atrial pressure raised the threshold and dampened the sensitivity for osmotic AVP release (Fig. 10–9).[109] This change in set point was confirmed by demonstrating that adequate water loading can suppress AVP secretion further even in the presence of hyponatremia.[108, 111] The resetting of the osmotic threshold in response to nonosmotic stimuli can be abolished by opioid antagonists.[111]

Chemical Mediators of Vasopressin Release

AVP release can also be modulated by agents that have either systemic hemodynamic effects or CNS actions. Table 10–1 lists some drugs, neurotransmitters, and other agents that modulate AVP release via either the peripheral nervous system or CNS effects.

Catecholamines

Evidence for a hemodynamic role of α- and β-adrenergic agents in mediating AVP release as the primary means of affecting renal water excretion has been summarized by Schrier and colleagues.[112] The β-agonist isoproterenol causes antidiuresis in normal rats, whereas the α-agonist norepinephrine reduces urine osmolality. Neither agent has an effect on Brattleboro rats that lack AVP. Thus the effects on water excretion are secondary to stimulation (β-agonists) or suppression (α-agonists) of endogenous AVP release.[113]

Adrenergic agents may also act as neurotransmitters to stimulate central release of AVP. Nerve terminals containing norepinephrine are abundant in both the SON and the PVN, as indicated by histochemical and immunocytochemical studies.[51, 114] Central norepinephrine fibers stimulate AVP secretion via α_1-receptors on AVP-producing neurons.[115–117]

Angiotensin II

The renin-angiotensin system participates in the regulation of AVP release. Nerve cells and fibers that contain AII are present in the SFO and in the magnicellular division of the PVN and SON.[118] Likewise AII stimulates the electrical activity of many neurons in the SFO, PVN, and SON.[119] The SFO lies outside the blood-brain barrier and may convey blood-borne signals to the hypothalamic nuclei. The administration of AII peripherally or centrally increases AVP secretion in the rat,[120, 121] a response that can be abolished by lesions of the SFO[120] or by transection of the SFO efferents.[122]

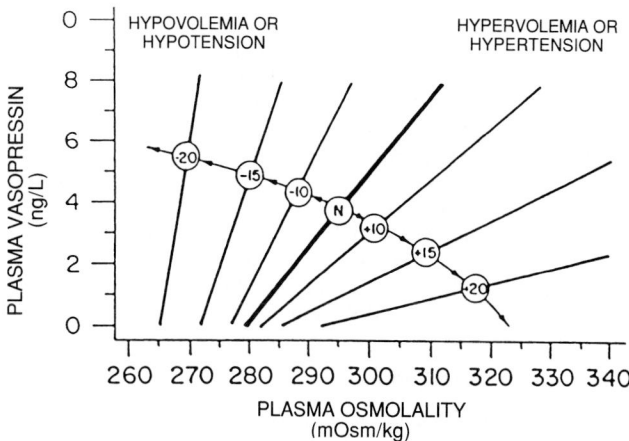

Figure 10–9. The effect of changes in blood volume or arterial pressure on the relation between plasma osmolality and plasma AVP activity. To convert AVP values to picomoles per liter, divide by 1.1. (Modified from Robertson GL, Berl T. Water metabolism. In: Brenner BM, Rector FC Jr, eds. The Kidney. 3rd ed. Philadelphia: WB Saunders, 1986: 385–432, with permission.)

Electrophysiological evidence also suggests that AII modulates AVP release. Neurons in the SFO with efferent projections to the PVN, identified by antidromic stimulation, are stimulated by intravenously administered AII.[122] In addition, in rat brain slices AII stimulates AVP-producing cells in the SON.[119] Thus AII may stimulate AVP release through a direct action on AVP-producing neurons and by stimulating afferent pathways from other regions of the brain. In humans the intravenous infusion of AII stimulates AVP release,[123] and reduction of AII by the converting enzyme inhibitor captopril inhibits AVP release.[124] However in one study in which plasma AII levels were increased fivefold by sodium depletion, no change in plasma AVP levels was detected.[125]

Opiates

Morphine induces antidiuresis, and the demonstration of endogenous opiates within the neurohypophysis and of the association of leu-enkephalin (see Chapter 8) with AVP-containing nerve terminals[126] led to a reinvestigation of the relation between opiates and AVP release. In isolated rat neurohypophyses[116, 127] and in conscious dogs[128] and rats[129, 130] opioids act through κ-receptors[107, 130] to inhibit rather than stimulate AVP secretion. In addition opioids suppress AVP secretion by inhibiting the release of norepinephrine from neurohypophyseal nerve terminals.[116] As mentioned earlier, norepinephrine stimulates AVP secretion.

Prostaglandins

Endogenous CNS prostaglandins may modulate AVP release in response to osmotic stimulation. Intraventricular infusions of E prostaglandins[51] raise plasma AVP levels in the absence of changes in systemic hemodynamics, and inhibition of intraventricular prostaglandin synthesis by indomethacin attenuates AVP release to an osmotic stimulus, although release can be effected by exogenous prostaglandin E_2 (PGE_2) even with indomethacin present.[131]

Anesthetics

Although surgical procedures commonly cause antidiuresis Forsling and Ullmann[132] found that only halothane anesthesia leads to a persistent antidiuretic state. These results coincide with studies in humans undergoing anesthesia for surgery in whom plasma AVP levels rise only after the initiation of the surgical procedure.[131]

Chemoreceptors

A fall in arterial oxygen tension (PaO_2) to less than 60 mm Hg causes a rise in mean arterial pressure and a rise in plasma AVP concentrations; the catecholamine-depleting agent guanethidine prevents the rise in plasma AVP levels,[132] a finding that is consistent with an adrenergic role in the stimulation of AVP release. Electrophysiological activity of SON neurons increases when the PCO_2 of arterial blood is elevated[49]; local anesthesia of the carotid bodies eliminates this response, indicating that arterial chemoreceptors also influence the secretion of AVP from the neurohypophysis.

Atrial Natriuretic Peptide

As indicated in Figure 10–1, ANP may provide negative feedback for the release of AVP. The latter, principally through its vasopressor action, may stimulate the release of ANP[133] and ANP in turn inhibits the release of AVP and the effect of AVP on the permeability of the renal collecting duct to water.[134] ANP-containing nerve cell bodies are present in the AV3V

region of the brain,[135] a region that surrounds the third ventricle, includes the OVLT and connections to the SFO, and plays an important role in body fluid homeostasis. Injection of ANP into the cerebral ventricles of rats[136, 137] or superfusion of hypothalamus-pituitary explants with ANP[136, 138, 139] inhibits the secretion of AVP.

Oropharyngeal Stimulation

A second level of feedback control of AVP release involves the oropharyngeal reflex, which is responsible for prompt suppression of AVP secretion after the ingestion of water (see Fig. 10–1). In both animals and humans[140–143] suppression occurs prior to the absorption of the ingested water and before any fall in the plasma osmolality; i.e., AVP secretion is inhibited in anticipation of the subsequent absorption of water and fall in plasma osmolality. AVP secretion is suppressed even if the ingested water is diverted from the stomach through a fistula.[140] Moreover the ingested fluid need not be hypotonic. Ingestion of isotonic[140] and even hypertonic[144] solutions (but not solid foods[142]) also suppresses AVP release, at least transiently, and cold liquids elicit a stronger oropharyngeal reflex than do warm liquids.[143] This finding may explain the clear-cut preference of patients with diabetes insipidus for ice water. The rapidity with which AVP secretion and hypothalamic electrical activity are suppressed[145] and the lack of a requirement for the gastric absorption of fluid suggest that neural mechanisms mediate the response. The similarities between the oropharyngeal suppression of AVP release and the anticipatory control of drinking are striking and may indicate a common mediator, such as intracerebral ANP.

THIRST

The ingestion of water to preserve body fluid tonicity is governed by the sense of thirst, which in turn is regulated by many of the same factors that determine AVP release. The response of thirst to osmotic (hypertonic) stimuli is sufficiently powerful that significant hypertonicity does not develop even in the absence of AVP in conscious individuals who have free access to water. The osmotic threshold for thirst in humans and other primates occurs with a 2 to 3% increase in plasma osmolality, a value about 10 mmol/L higher than the value that stimulates AVP release.[141, 146, 147] Thirst-mediated water intake also occurs with falls in effective ECF volume and may continue, as with severe loss of gastrointestinal fluids, decompensated cirrhosis with ascites, and congestive heart failure, despite a decrease in body fluid osmolality.

Osmotic Regulation of Thirst

The concept of a thirst center in the CNS[148] was substantiated by the demonstration that injections of hypertonic NaCl into the medial hypothalamus elicit drinking in water-replete goats.[149] Ablation of tissue surrounding the OVLT of sheep reduces water intake subsequent to intracarotid infusion of hypertonic NaCl,[150] suggesting that an osmoreceptor for thirst stimulation is located in or close to the OVLT, just as osmoregulation of AVP is controlled from this region.[94–96] Osmoregulation of thirst and of AVP release are similar: hypertonic NaCl stimulates both thirst and AVP release, whereas hypertonic urea or glucose stimulates neither. Nevertheless electrophysiological studies indicate that thirst and AVP are mediated by distinct but adjacent osmoreceptors. Immediate drinking can be induced in animals by electrical stimulation of the anterior wall of the third ventricle, whereas stimulation at the SON or PVN does not elicit drinking but causes antidiuresis.[151]

AII is a potent inducer of thirst when injected directly into the third ventricle[152] and may mediate osmotically stimulated thirst. Intraventricular infusion of the AII inhibitor saralasin slowed the onset of drinking in one study of dehydrated animals but had no effect on water consumption in another study.[152, 153] However the addition of the cholinergic inhibitor atropine to saralasin suppressed drinking in the latter group.[153] Thus there may be parallel pathways for thirst regulation, with AII being more important in the response to a nonosmotic stimulus. A further association between AII and osmotic thirst stimulation has been shown by documenting the presence of AII receptors on the OVLT and by the ablation of the enhancement of thirst by intraventricular AII when the OVLT is destroyed.[152]

Volume-Mediated Thirst

Alterations in baroreceptor function, such as with underfilling of the low-pressure thoracic circulation, elicit drinking,[149] and crushing of the left atrial appendage in sheep abolishes the drinking response to hypovolemia but leaves intact the response to hyperosmolality.[154] This response is mediated by the vagus nerve. Conversely although hypovolemia stimulates the renin-angiotensin system, it is not clear whether blood-borne AII has access to the thirst centers or if peripherally generated AII participates in the hypovolemic thirst response. Stimulation of thirst by AII may be mediated via a renin-angiotensin system within the brain.[149]

Satiation of Thirst

There appear to be two major patterns of water repletion in response to hypertonic dehydration.[155] When given access to water, dogs, sheep, goats, and camels drink an amount that approximates the amount lost during dehydration.[156] Passage of water through the pharynx and out an esophageal fistula or distention of the stomach by a balloon temporarily suppresses drinking, yet drinking in these species normally halts before any water can have been absorbed into the bloodstream.[157] The second pattern—exhibited by rats, rabbits, and humans—involves replenishment of about half the water lost in 10 to 12 min, which is about the time required for ingested water to arrive at body tissues[156]; further water intake takes place over another 20 to 30 min.

In animals with hypertonic volume depletion intracarotid infusions of water that are sufficient to restore the osmolality of the carotid circulation to normal, but not to affect peripheral osmolality, cause a 70% decrease in drinking.[157] Restoration of the ECF volume deficit in these animals with isotonic NaCl, which does not ameliorate the plasma hypertonicity, reduces drinking by about 30%. In contrast, thirst in primates depends almost totally on osmolality, with minimal dependence on ECF volume.[147] These findings are in accord with observations that left atrial stretch receptors do little to regulate AVP release in primates[158] and have led to the suggestion that decreased dependence of thirst on volume stimuli is an adaptive correlate to the upright posture of primates.[147, 158] In humans the ingestion of water is even more complex, influenced by pharyngeal, gastrointestinal, thermal, chemical, and social factors, but "permanent" satisfaction of thirst occurs only when the volume of water ingested returns body fluid osmolality to normal.[149]

OXYTOCIN

General

Oxytocin is the second cyclic octapeptide hormone produced in magnicellular nuclei and is stored in the posterior pituitary. Oxytocin, like AVP, is synthesized as a single 20-kd peptide molecule termed *prooxyphysin*, which consists of the 1-kd peptide hormone and its nonglycosylated 10-kd carrier protein type I neurophysin.[28] Neurons that synthesize oxytocin are present in both the SON and the PVN, oxytocin-containing cells tending to cluster in more rostral aspects of these nuclei. Like AVP, oxytocin is packaged in secretory granules, stored in the posterior pituitary, and enters the portal system of the neurohypophysis by calcium-dependent exocytosis of the membrane-bound granules. However, oxytocin secretion is characterized by distinct bursts of electrical activity superimposed on a background of continuous firing activity,[49] a pattern that is distinct from the phasic electrical discharge and progressive recruitment of AVP-secreting neurons.[49]

Oxytocin Release

The primary stimuli for oxytocin release are mechanical distention of the reproductive tract (vagina) and suckling of the nipples; both stimuli effect this release through neural pathways. Like AVP release, oxytocin release is stimulated by plasma hypertonicity. In conscious dogs and rats the rise in the plasma level of oxytocin is comparable to that of AVP at any given rise in plasma osmolality.[159, 160] Likewise isotonic volume contraction causes an increase in plasma oxytocin levels, although of a lesser magnitude than that of AVP.[159]

As noted earlier, magnicellular neurons of the hypothalamus receive input from the AV3V region. Electrical stimulation of the AV3V region increases the firing rate of oxytocin-secreting neurons and causes oxytocin release, and lesions in the AV3V region abolish oxytocin release in response to hyperosmolality but not in response to suckling or parturition.[161] The electrical activity of oxytocin-secreting neurons, and hormone secretion, depends on the physiological stimulus: suckling causes firing in brief synchronized bursts; parturition causes bursts of activity superimposed on a background of increased activity; and hyperosmolality causes a gradual increase in the rate of firing.[161]

Like AVP secretion the secretion of oxytocin is modulated by several chemical mediators (Table 10–2). Endogenous opioids inhibit the secretion of oxytocin,[116, 162-164] an inhibition mediated both at the cell body to reduce electrical activity and at the neurosecretory terminals to reduce the amount of hormone secretion.[116] In addition, opioids may modulate oxytocin secretion indirectly by inhibiting norepinephrine release from neurohypophyseal terminals.[117, 163, 164]

Intraventricular injection of AII stimulates oxytocin secretion in the rat[130] and perfusion of rat brain slices with AII evokes excitatory responses in oxytocin-secreting neurons in the SON and in cells of the AV3V and SFO.[119] These pathways may convey blood-borne signals to the hypothalamic nuclei.[165]

Nausea, satiety, and cholecystokinin, each acting through vagal afferents, stimulate oxytocin secretion[166] but oxytocin is not believed to play a role in regulating food intake.

TABLE 10–2. Factors That Influence Oxytocin Secretion

Physiological	Chemical
Parturition	***Stimulatory***
Suckling, breast stimulation	
ECF hypertonicity	Angiotensin II
Nausea	Cholecystokinin
Volume contraction	Vasoactive intestinal peptide
Satiety	Norepinephrine
	Inhibitory
	Opioids
	Relaxin
	ANP

ECF, extracellular fluid; ANP, atrial natriuretic peptide.

TABLE 10–3. Localization of Oxytocin in Peripheral Tissues

Tissue	Immunoreactive Oxytocin	Oxytocin mRNA	Possible Function
Ovary	+	+	Modulation of uterine prostaglandin release
Uterus	+	−	?
Placenta	+	−	Uterine contraction
Testis	+	+	Modulation of seminiferous tubule contraction
Adrenal	+	+	Modulation of steroidogenesis or cathecolamine secretion, or both
Thymus	+	+	Lymphokine production
Anterior pituitary	+	+	Regulation of corticotropin and prolactin secretion

Modified from Clements JA, Funder JW. Arginine vasopressin and oxytocin in organs outside the nervous system. In: Martini L, Ganong WF, eds. Frontiers in Neuroendocrinology. Vol 10. New York: Raven, 1988: 117–152.

Relaxin, an ovarian peptide hormone that suppresses uterine contraction and relaxes pelvic connective tissue during parturition,[167] may also affect oxytocin secretion. Intravenous or intraventricular injection of relaxin suppresses reflex milk ejection in lactating rats,[168] and in isolated neural lobes and neurosecretory terminals relaxin inhibits the basal release of oxytocin and AVP but potentiates their release in response to electrical stimulation.[169] It is not known if the effects on oxytocin release are due to locally produced or circulating relaxin.

Actions of Oxytocin

Oxytocin stimulates uterine contractions at parturition and smooth muscle contraction in the mammary gland during suckling. It also promotes maternal behavior.[170] Oxytocin may have other functions in other tissues; e.g., oxytocin or oxytocin mRNA, or both, are present in ovary, uterus, placenta, testis, renal medulla, thymus, and anterior pituitary.[171] The physiological role of oxytocin in these tissues is not defined (Table 10–3).

Finally oxytocin and AVP have similar effects on water homeostasis. In anuran epithelia[172] oxytocin binds to high-affinity receptors, stimulates cellular accumulation of cAMP, and increases the natriferic and hydro-osmotic responses of the tissue, actions analogous to the action of AVP on anuran epithelia and mammalian renal tubules. Whether oxytocin secretion affects water homeostasis in normal individuals is unknown but pharmacologic doses of oxytocin, such as those used for pregnancy termination and occasionally for induction of labor, alter the metabolism of water by the kidney.[174] One unit of oxytocin, as defined by uterotonic activity, has about 0.01 IU of antidiuretic activity. Severe water intoxication can occur in women who receive infusions of oxytocin at high rates, usually greater than 20 mIU/min, and who are simultaneously given hypotonic fluids, usually in excess of 3.5 L.[173–175] Antidiuresis is notable at infusion rates of 15 mIU/min and is near maximal at 30 mIU/min, the antidiuretic effect becoming apparent 10 to 15 min after the onset of infusion and continuing 10 to 15 min after its cessation.

RENAL CONTRIBUTION TO OSMOTIC HOMEOSTASIS

Renal Countercurrent Mechanisms

From the evolutionary standpoint the ability to concentrate urine coincides with the appearance of the loop of Henle. This structure consists of three anatomically and functionally distinct regions interposed between proximal and distal tubules: the thin descending limb, the thin ascending limb, and the thick ascending limb. Although all mammalian kidneys possess a loop of Henle, the maximal level to which the urine can be concentrated depends on the fraction of nephrons whose loops of Henle dip deep into the papilla, the so-called long loops of Henle. The average human kidney contains about 1 million nephrons, about 15% of which are long-looped.

The descending and ascending loops of Henle are parallel tubes that are joined by a hairpin turn; oppositely directed flows in the two tubes permit small differences in osmolality between fluid in the descending and ascending limbs at any level of the renal medulla (the so-called single effect) to be amplified many times along the length of the loop of Henle.[176] Urine in the loop of Henle at the papillary tip is as concentrated as that in the collecting duct during antidiuresis; fluid entering the early distal convolution is hypotonic to plasma both in the absence and in the presence of AVP[177]; and approximately 20% of the glomerular filtrate is absorbed in the loop of Henle.[178] Because proximal tubular fluid absorption is an isotonic process, more solute than water is removed from tubular fluid during transit through the loop and therefore the factor driving the countercurrent multiplier is solute abstraction from the ascending limbs.[178]

The thick ascending limb of the loop of Henle (TALH) is impermeable to water and transports solute actively, thus providing both for dilution of the urine leaving the loop of Henle and for the active step (single effect) in countercurrent multiplication.[179, 180] Because the cortical and the outer medullary collecting ducts are relatively impermeable to water in the absence of AVP and permeable to water in the presence of AVP, the fate of the dilute tubular fluid leaving the loop of Henle—and therefore final urine osmolality—depends on the presence or absence of AVP.

These findings have been integrated[181] into a model that provides two sites for countercurrent amplification: an active step in the outer medulla and a passive step in the inner medulla (Fig. 10–10). The first amplification depends on NaCl efflux from water-impermeable thick ascending limbs; thus fluid entering the distal tubule is both hypotonic and salt poor. During antidiuresis AVP-enhanced water abstraction from urea-impermeable cortical and outer medullary collecting ducts results in accumulation of urea in fluid entering the papillary collecting ducts. Because these ducts are permeable to urea, passive urea transport down a chemical gradient from tubular fluid to medullary interstitium contributes to medullary hypertonicity, thereby providing a second, passive amplification. Simultaneously, osmotic equilibration of papillary collecting duct fluid with the medullary interstitium results in the formation of hypertonic urine.

The progressive concentration and dilution of tubular fluid in descending and ascending thin limbs can be rationalized in terms of passive flow. Consider, e.g., a medulla whose osmolality ranges from 300 mmol/L at the corticomedullary junction to 1400 mmol/L at the papillary tip (see Fig. 10–10). About half of medullary hypertonicity is due to NaCl and the remainder is due to urea.[182] Isotonic fluid containing 280

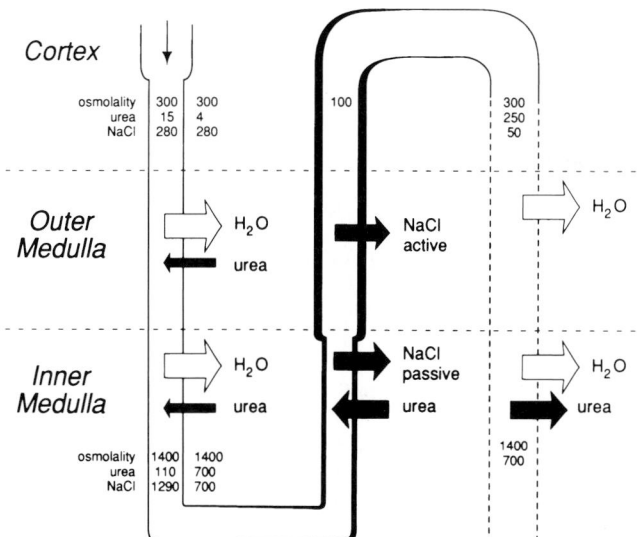

Figure 10–10. Schematic illustration of the model of Kokko and Rector for the renal concentrating mechanism. (From Reeves WB, Andreoli TE. Nephrogenic diabetes insipidus. In: Scriver CR, Beaudet AL, Sly WS, et al, eds. The Metabolic Basis of Inherited Disease. 6th ed. New York: McGraw-Hill, 1989: 1985–2011. Copyright © 1989 by McGraw-Hill, Inc. Used by permission of McGraw-Hill Book Co.)

mmol/L of NaCl enters the water-permeable, but urea- and Na$^+$-impermeable, thin descending limb and is concentrated almost entirely by water abstraction so that fluid entering the thin ascending limb has a higher NaCl concentration and a lower urea concentration than does the medullary interstitium. These passive driving forces between lumen and interstitium, coupled with the fact that the thin ascending limb is more permeable to NaCl than to urea, poise the system for fluid dilution. As fluid moves up the water-impermeable thin ascending limb, passive NaCl efflux from lumen to interstitium exceeds passive urea influx from interstitium to tubular fluid and concomitantly the rate of urea recycling from papillary collecting ducts through the interstitium to thin ascending limbs. Finally the process begins again by active NaCl transport from the thick ascending limb.

Vascular Countercurrent Exchange

Maintenance of a hypertonic medullary interstitium requires that the rate of solute removal by medullary blood flow be slow enough to prevent equilibration of medullary interstitial fluid with isotonic plasma. These requirements are satisfied by countercurrent exchange processes within medullary capillary loops.

The medullary vasa recta form a counterflow system. In descending vasa recta, water leaves the blood and solute enters, so that the osmolality at the bend of the vasa recta is the same as that at the tip of the loop of Henle and presumably also the same as that of the medullary interstitium at the same point.[183] As blood flows from the tip of the vasa recta to venules in the inner cortex it gains water and loses NaCl to the progressively less hypertonic medullary interstitium. The net effect of this countercurrent exchange in the vasa recta is to reduce the rate of solute loss from the medulla with respect to a linear blood flow system.

Effects of Filtration Rate and Solute Excretion

Factors in addition to AVP and counterflow processes also affect concentration and dilution of urine. For example the permeability of the collecting duct to water, even in the ab-

sence of AVP, is finite and by varying the rate of fluid delivery to collecting ducts, and hence the time available for water efflux from these ducts, the glomerular filtration rate (GFR) can influence urine osmolality, even in animals lacking circulating AVP.[184, 185] Presumably with low urine flow rates in the collecting duct, osmotic equilibration of urine with the medullary interstitium is at least partial. Conversely increased GFRs produced by expansion of the ECF volume can cause a hypoosmotic urine, even in the presence of high levels of AVP.

In clinical terms solute excretion has more influence on urine osmolality than does GFR. The effect of osmotic diuresis on urine composition may be viewed by considering solute excretion in terms of the osmolar clearance (C$_{osm}$, in milliliters per minute), which is the urine flow rate required to produce a urine that is isotonic to plasma. In antidiuresis solute-free water, termed *negative free water clearance*, is removed from urine and the urine flow rate is less than the C$_{osm}$. In water diuresis the urine flow rate exceeds the C$_{osm}$; the difference between the urine flow rate and the C$_{osm}$, termed *positive free water clearance*, is the amount of solute-free water that is excreted. During progressive osmotic diuresis an increasingly greater volume of isotonic fluid containing nonabsorbed solute escapes proximal tubular absorption and is delivered to the loop of Henle. As a consequence the C$_{osm}$ becomes sufficiently large that even if the magnitude of either positive (during water diuresis) or negative (during antidiuresis) free water clearance stays unchanged urine osmolality approaches isotonicity (Fig. 10–11).

At relatively low rates of solute excretion the urine may be either concentrated maximally or diluted maximally, but as urine solute excretion increases, i.e., as C$_{osm}$ increases, the osmolality of urine approaches isotonicity.[186] Stated in another way, during a massive solute diuresis the ability of the renal concentrating or diluting mechanisms to modify the osmolality of proximal tubular fluid is progressively blunted (see Fig. 10–11A). Even though the urine osmolality may approach isotonicity during progressive solute diuresis, the absolute free water clearance continues to rise. Thus for C$_{osm}$ values as high as 20 mL/min, the formation of free water—i.e., salt absorption in the thick ascending limb—is not saturable.[187, 188] In addition the urine osmolality in a solute diuresis does not approach isotonicity until solute excretion exceeds 8000 mmol/d. By comparison a healthy individual eating a normal diet excretes 600 to 800 mmol/d of solute.

Collecting Tubule

The major antidiuretic contribution of AVP is to increase the water permeability of terminal nephron segments, specifically the cortical collecting duct, the outer medullary collecting duct, and the papillary collecting duct. The increase in the water permeability in these segments augments osmotic water flow from tubular lumen into a hypertonic medullary interstitium, thus providing for maximal urine concentration during antidiuresis.

Water and Solute Permeability

AVP increases the water permeability of apical plasma membranes in hormone-responsive epithelia.[189, 190] The standard method for the study of the action of AVP uses in vitro microperfusion of isolated tubule segments. In freshly dissected rabbit cortical collecting duct segments, the initial water permeability declines, and when AVP is introduced into the bathing solution the water permeability rises to its initial high value.[191–193] The stability of the AVP-dependent hydro-osmotic effect depends on the experimental conditions.[194, 195]

In spite of the increase in the osmotic water permeability with AVP, the cortical collecting duct remains impermeable to

A

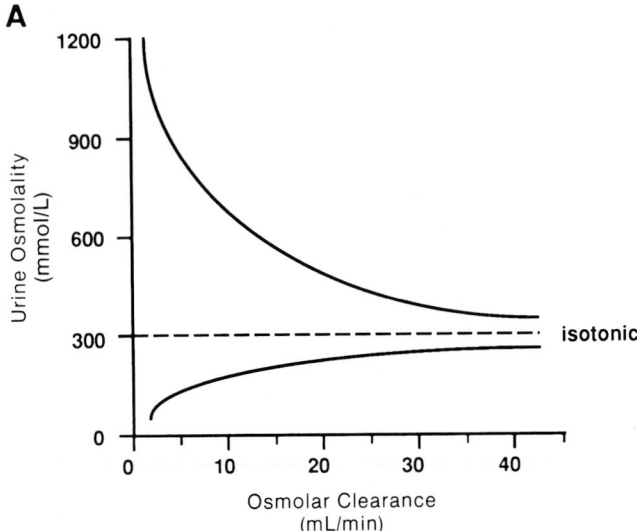

B

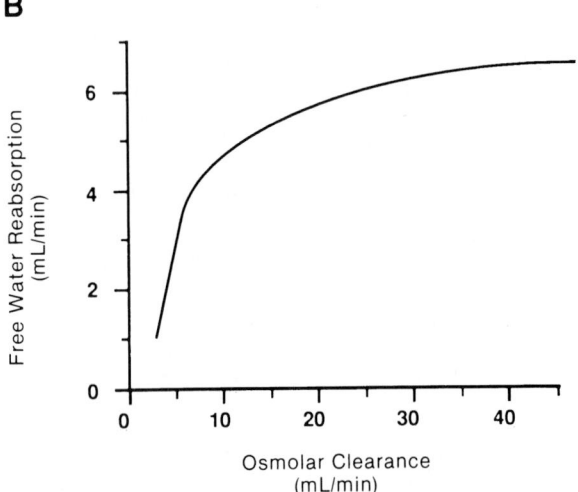

Figure 10–11. The effect of varying rates of urine osmolar clearance (C_{osm}) on urine osmolality (A) and free water reabsorption (B). As C_{osm} increases hypertonic urine becomes progressively diluted and approaches isotonicity; hypotonic urine becomes less dilute and also approaches isotonicity. In spite of the approach to isotonicity free water reabsorption continues to increase as C_{osm} increases (B). (From data in Rapoport S, Brodsky WA, West CD, et al. Urinary flow and excretion of solutes during osmotic diuresis in hydropenic man. Am J Physiol 1949; 156:433–442; and Goldberg M, McCurdy DK, Foltz EL, et al. Effects of ethacrynic acid (a new saluretic agent) on renal diluting and concentrating mechanisms: evidence for site of action in the loop of Henle. J Clin Invest 1964; 43:201–216, with permission.)

even the smallest hydrophilic nonelectrolytes.[191, 196, 197] Thus the antidiuretic response involves a profound increase in the water permeability of an epithelium that can discriminate more than 1000-fold between water and hydrophilic solutes, such as urea, that have effective radii less than twice as large as that of a water molecule. These findings suggest that water moves through narrow (radius of 0.2 nm [2 Å]) pores.[198]

Morphologic Studies of the Vasopressin Response

AVP acts on water permeability at the apical epithelial surface. The bulk of water flow across the collecting tubule proceeds through epithelial cells rather than through the junctional complexes, and AVP changes water permeability in the apical membranes of the collecting duct cells.[199]

A number of ultrastructural changes occur in the apical membranes of granular cells of urinary bladders of frogs and toads after the application of serosal AVP, including aggregation of apical membrane intramembranous particles.[200–202] These aggregates represent AVP-induced water channels. The appearance of aggregates is induced by serosal but not mucosal application of AVP and by cAMP or forskolin[201, 203, 204] and can be inhibited by drugs that inhibit the AVP-induced increase in water flow.[205] The number of membrane aggregates is proportional to the AVP-induced increase in water permeability.[201, 202, 206]

In the absence of AVP aggregates are present in the walls of small vacuoles beneath the apical membranes of granular cells in both toad and frog urinary bladders.[207] These vacuoles, or aggrephores, have a tubular shape and measure 1 to 2 μm long and 0.1 μm in diameter. The aggrephores have a high permeability to water that is inhibited by mercurial agents[208–211] and contain the AVP-sensitive water channel.[208] The walls of the aggrephores are densely packed with particles arranged in a helical array. At one or both ends of the aggrephore is a spherical head that appears to be coated with clathrin.[212] The significance of this clathrin coat is unknown. In the presence of AVP the number of aggrephores decreases and the number of aggregates in the apical membrane increases. Occasionally aggrephores can be seen fusing with the apical membrane. The fact that frequency of fusion events correlates with the accumulation of aggregates in the apical membrane[205] suggests that water permeation sites are "shuttled" from the membranes of these aggrephores to the apical membrane under the influence of AVP (Fig. 10–12).[207, 213, 214]

On removal of AVP from the basolateral solution the water permeability of the toad bladder decreases and aggregates and aggrephore fusion sites disappear from the apical membrane.[215, 216] Enzymatic, electron-dense, or fluorescent markers from the mucosal solution are taken up into tubular vesicles during retrieval of fused aggrephores from apical membrane. Early after AVP is removed, fluid-phase markers such as horseradish peroxidase or fluorescent dextran become localized in cytoplasmic tubular vacuoles that resemble aggrephores.[215, 217] It is not clear whether aggrephores cycle into and out of the apical membrane without some intervening step.[208]

The general scheme of AVP action in the anuran bladder, namely insertion of water channels into the apical membrane and their subsequent retrieval, also occurs in mammalian col-

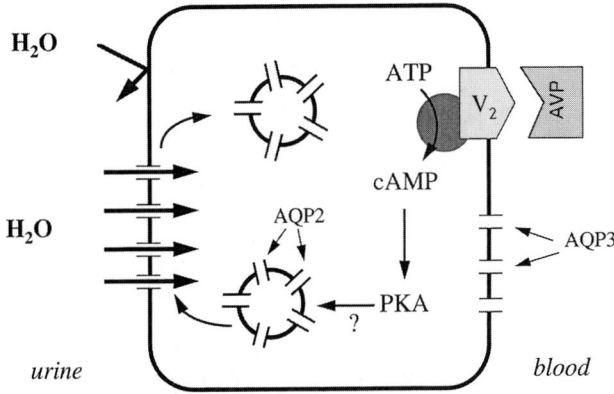

Figure 10–12. A schematic model of the shuttle mechanism for the action of AVP in the collecting tubule. In the absence of AVP, AQP2 water channels are located in vesicles beneath the apical membrane and the apical membrane is impermeable to water. On stimulation by AVP these vesicles fuse with the apical membrane delivering water channels to the cell surface. Water channels are retrieved from the cell surface by endocytosis of clathrin-coated vesicles. AQP3 water channels are present in the basolateral membrane and facilitate the efflux of water from the cell.

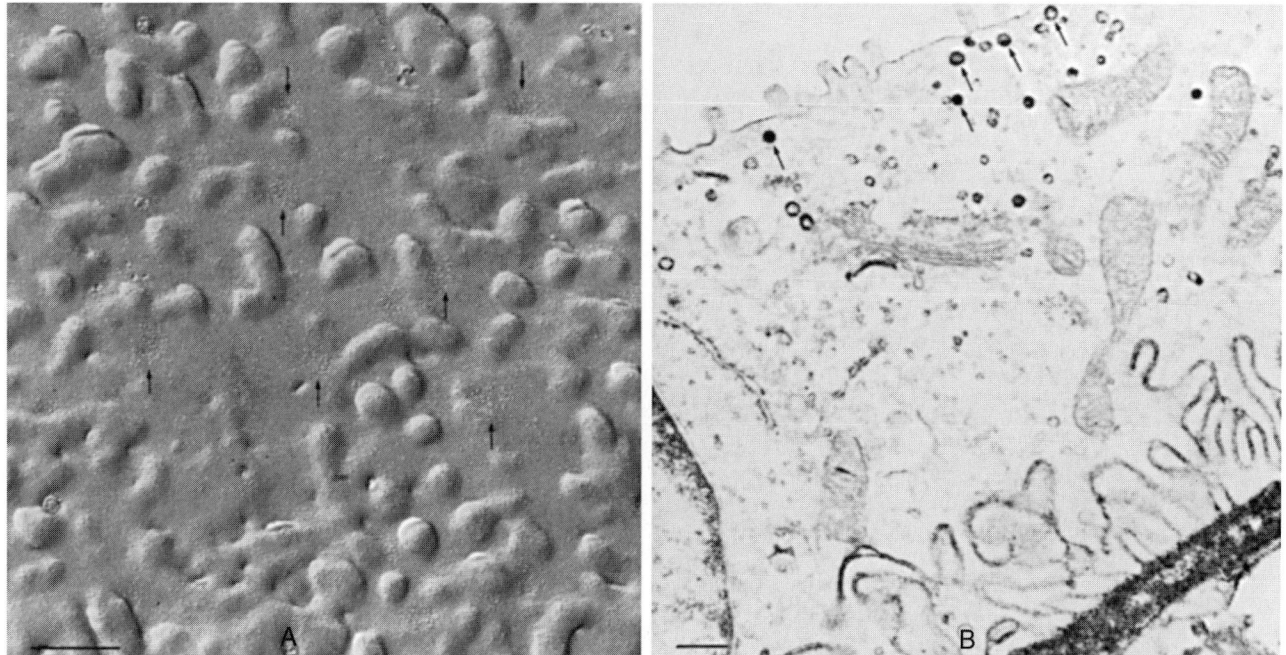

Figure 10–13. Electron micrographs of collecting duct principal cells. *A,* Freeze-fracture electron micrograph of the apical plasma membrane P face of a principal cell from a normal mouse. Numerous clusters of intramembranous particles *(arrows)* are visible on this membrane. The clusters of intramembranous particles are the hallmark of the AVP-induced water permeability response in these apical plasma membranes. The rounded projections that are also visible on this membrane are stubby microvilli that characterize these cells. Bar = 0.5 μm. *B,* Thin section of a principal cell from a normal Long-Evans rat that was injected with 6 mg/mL horseradish peroxidase 15 min before fixation. Many vesicles loaded with horseradish peroxidase–diaminobenzidine reaction product are present in the cytoplasm, where they are concentrated below the apical plasma membrane *(arrows).* Most of the peroxidase-labeled endocytotic vesicles are smooth (noncoated), which is consistent with the known rapid decoating of clathrin-coated vesicles after they detach from the plasma membrane. *(A* from Brown D, Shields GI, Valtin H, et al. Lack of intramembranous particle clusters in collecting ducts of mice with nephrogenic diabetes insipidus. Am J Physiol 1985; 249:F582–F589, with permission. *B* from Brown D, Weyer P, Orci L. Vasopressin stimulates endocytosis in kidney collecting duct principal cells. Eur J Cell Biol 1988; 46:336–341, with permission.)

lecting ducts.[214] Thus apical intramembranous particle aggregates are present in rat medullary collecting ducts (Fig. 10–13)[218–220] and in the apical membranes of the outer medullary and cortical collecting ducts of rabbits.[221] The particle aggregates in mammalian tubules are similar to, but not identical with, those of anuran epithelia. Furthermore cytoplasmic aggrephores that are typical of the anuran bladder have not been found in mammalian collecting ducts. Instead movement of water channels into and out of the apical membrane of collecting duct cells may be mediated by the exocytosis and endocytosis of clathrin-coated vesicles.[210, 211, 218, 222, 223]

As will be discussed later in the section on intracellular mediators of AVP action, the cDNA for the water channel of the apical membrane of the collecting duct has been cloned.[224, 225] The protein, AQP2, also known as AQP-CD, is a member of the aquaporin family of water channels.[226] AQP2 is expressed exclusively in the collecting duct—more specifically in the apical membrane and subapical region of the principal cell.[224, 226, 228] Moreover the intracellular distribution of AQP2 is regulated by AVP. In Brattleboro rats, which lack endogenous AVP, AQP2 is localized primarily within cytoplasmic vesicles in collecting duct principal cells and after vasopressin stimulation, AQP2 is found mainly in the apical membrane.[229, 230] Likewise, apical membrane AQP2 levels were greater in dehydrated antidiuretic rats than in well-hydrated rats[228, 231, 232] and were decreased after treatment with a vasopressin receptor antagonist.[232] Additional support of the shuttle hypothesis comes from microperfusion studies.[233] Acute exposure to AVP increased water permeability of the collecting ducts, increased apical membrane AQP2 levels, and increased the ratio of apical membrane to intracellular vesicle AQP2 levels. Following AVP removal water permeability fell in parallel with a decrease in apical membrane AQP2 and a decrease in the apical membrane–to–intracellular AQP2 ratio.[233] Thus

AVP increases the water permeability of collecting duct cells through a translocation of AQP2 water channels from cytoplasmic vesicles into the apical membrane. AVP may also affect water permeability through other pathways. For example AVP may also increase the activity of individual water channels, possibly via phosphorylation of AQP2 by cAMP-dependent protein kinase.[234]

Intracellular Mediators of Vasopressin Action

Understanding the cellular actions of AVP has been enhanced by the characterization of the vasopressin V_2 receptor[235, 236] and the discovery of a family of water channel proteins, the aquaporins.[226] These elements mediate the initial and final events in AVP action in the collecting duct cell, i.e., the binding of the hormone to its receptor at the basolateral membrane and the movement of water across the apical membrane through water channels. The effects of AVP are mediated primarily by the intracellular second messenger cAMP.[237] AVP binds to specific receptors, the V_2 receptors, on basolateral membrane surfaces of hormone-responsive epithelial cells and activates membrane-associated adenylate cyclase to catalyze cAMP generation from ATP (see also Chapter 5). V_2 receptors are expressed at high levels throughout the collecting duct and at lower levels in the thick ascending limb of Henle's loop.[238, 239] This receptor belongs to the growing family of G protein–coupled seven-transmembrane domain receptors.[235, 236] As will be discussed later, mutations in the V_2 receptor have been identified in a large number of families with X-linked nephrogenic diabetes insipidus.[240]

Adenylate cyclase is a multicomponent enzyme system (Fig. 10–14) in which the catalytic subunit is under regulation by two guanosine triphosphate–binding proteins, G_s and G_i.[241] G_s and G_i require guanosine triphosphate binding for activity

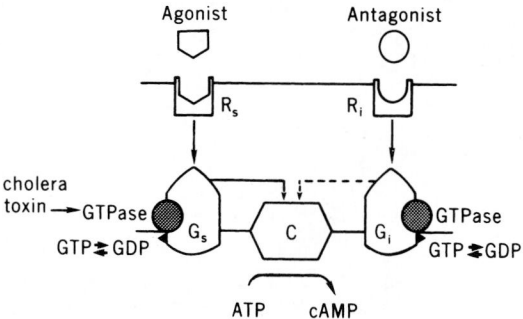

Figure 10–14. A schematic model for the regulation of adenylate cyclase activity by G_s and G_i guanine nucleotide regulatory subunits.

and when activated stimulate or inhibit the activity of the catalytic subunit, respectively.[241] Consequently these proteins, the guanine nucleotide–binding proteins or G proteins, are responsible for the transduction of hormone-receptor interactions into changes in cAMP formation.[243] When hormone action is mediated by cAMP, the hormone-receptor complex activates the G_s subunit of the adenylate cyclase enzyme; G_s may also be activated by cholera toxin.[242] The activated guanosine triphosphate–bound G_s stimulates the catalytic subunit (C) of adenylate cyclase to produce more cAMP. Hormones that antagonize the tissue effects of cAMP bind to receptors that are coupled to the G_i subunit. Activation of G_i inhibits the activity of the catalytic subunit of adenylate cyclase; the G_i subunit is also inactivated by pertussis toxin.[242] Because the effects of AVP on epithelia are mediated by cAMP, the V_2 receptor is believed to be associated with the G_s regulatory subunit.

Vasopressin-stimulated adenylate cyclase is present in the medullary TALH (mTALH) and along the entire collecting duct.[243] The intimate relation between hormone binding and adenylate cyclase activation was firmly established by demonstrating close correlation between binding of analogues of lysine vasopressin and adenylate cyclase activation.[244]

The role of G_s and G_i in AVP-responsive renal epithelia has been demonstrated in the mouse mTALH[245, 246] and in the rabbit cortical collecting tubule[247] and the presence of G_s and G_i proteins has also been demonstrated in mouse and rabbit TALH,[248] in the cortical collecting tubule,[249] and in medullary collecting tubules.[248] Enzymatic cleavage of cAMP to 5'-AMP by cytosolic phosphodiesterase terminates hormone action.

cAMP-dependent protein phosphorylation is believed to be the next step in AVP action on renal epithelial transport.[250] The activation of protein kinase in intact renal medullary tissue is proportional to the concentration of AVP bathing the tissue and the concentration of cAMP within the tissue.[251]

After the addition of AVP to isolated collecting duct segments there is a time lag of approximately 23 s (Fig. 10–15) before water permeability begins to rise.[252] With the addition of a cAMP analogue, the time lag is reduced to 11 s. Thus approximately 12 s is required for AVP to bind to its receptor and to generate sufficient intracellular cAMP, and 11 s is required for the more distal steps in the cascade (e.g., activation of protein kinase A, phosphorylation of cytoskeletal elements, and insertion of water channels).

AVP and oxytocin also produce a spike-like increase in the intracellular calcium level in the rabbit cortical collecting tubule[253] and in the rat medullary collecting tubule.[254, 255] The ability of AVP and oxytocin to mobilize intracellular calcium in the medullary collecting duct is mediated by oxytocin receptors and perhaps the V_{1b} receptor.[253] However the concentration of AVP required to increase intracellular calcium concentration exceeds the physiological range, and it is unlikely

that changes in intracellular calcium mediate the hydro-osmotic effects of AVP.[253, 254]

The biophysical characteristics of water flow in renal proximal tubules and collecting ducts and in red blood cells suggested that transmembrane water movement in these cells occurs through pores, or channels, rather than by diffusion across the lipid bilayer. The first membrane protein demonstrated to be a water channel was a protein purified from red blood cells and now termed AQP1.[256] AQP1 is expressed in the renal proximal tubule and descending thin limb,[257] nephron segments that are highly permeable to water. However, AQP1 is not present in the collecting duct. A second water channel, AQP2, shares 42% amino acid identity with AQP1 and is the AVP-regulated water channel of the collecting duct.[224] AQP2 is expressed in the cortical and inner medullary collecting ducts[224] and is present primarily in the apical membrane and subapical vesicles of collecting duct principal cells (Fig. 10–16A).[224, 228, 230, 231] As discussed earlier, vasopressin induces the movement of AQP2 from the subapical vesicles into the apical membrane,[233] and mutations in the AQP2 gene that inactivate the protein have been found in certain individuals with congenital nephrogenic diabetes insipidus.[258, 259] The expression of AQP2 is increased by dehydration and by AVP.[230, 231] Thus vasopressin regulates collecting duct water permeability acutely through the translocation, and perhaps phosphorylation (see earlier) of AQP2 channels, and chronically by increasing the number of AQP2 channels.

The basolateral membrane of the collecting duct principal cell has a high constitutive water permeability such that the apical membrane is always limiting to flow, even in the presence of AVP.[260] A third member of the aquaporin family of water channels, termed *AQP3*, is located in the basolateral membrane of the collecting duct (see Fig. 10–16B) and in stomach and intestines, lung, urinary bladder, and spleen.[227, 261]

The AQP1 channel is a homotetramer of 28-kd subunits

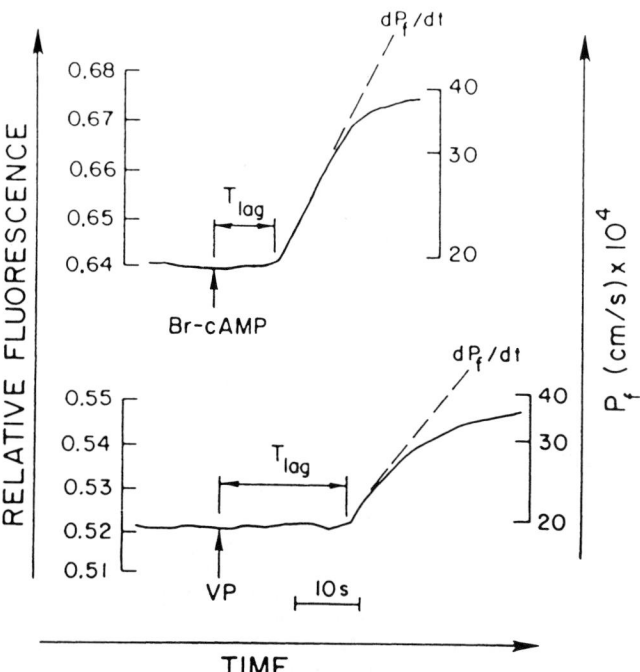

Figure 10–15. The early time course of the AVP response in cortical collecting tubules measured by using a fluorescent technique capable of providing rapid time resolution. P_f began to increase 23 ± 3 s after the addition of AVP (VP on figure) and only 11 ± 2 s after the addition of Br-cAMP. (From Kuwahara M, Verkman AS. Pre–steady state analysis of the turn-on and turn-off of water permeability in the kidney collecting tubule. J Membr Biol 1989; 110:57–65, with permission.)

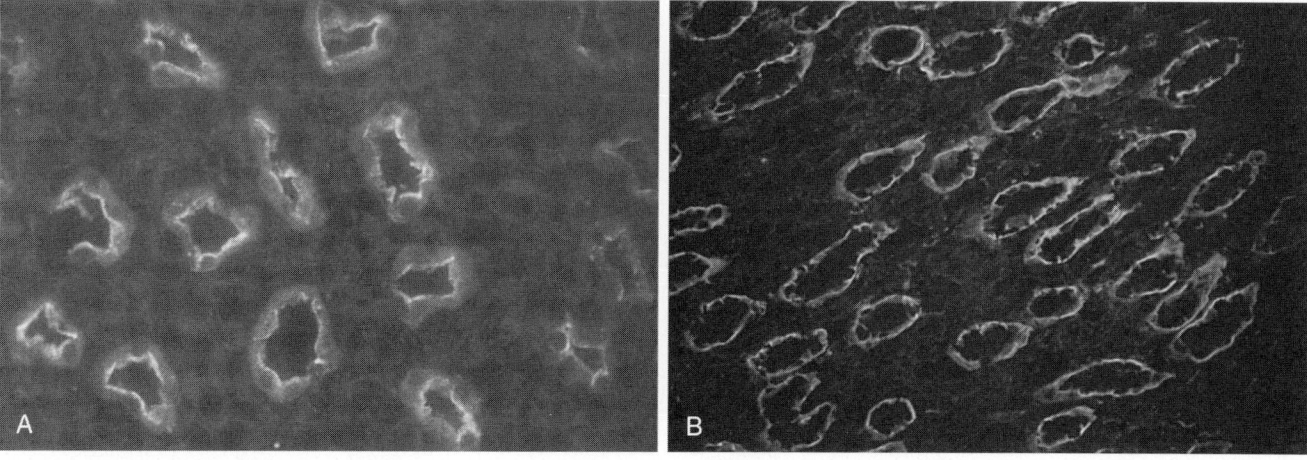

Figure 10–16. *A,* Immunolocalization of AQP2 in the rat kidney medulla. Staining is limited to collecting duct cells and is more intense in the apical region. *B,* Immunolocalization of AQP3 in the rat kidney outer medulla. Staining is limited to the basolateral membrane of collecting duct cells. (From Sasaki S, Fushimi K, Ishibashi K, et al. Water channels in the kidney collecting duct. Kidney Int 1995; 48:1082–1087, with permission.)

and each subunit contains six-transmembrane spanning domains. Although the proteins form tetramers, each subunit is believed to function independently as a channel.[262–264] Presumably the other AQP channels have similar structures.

As noted earlier, stimulation of amphibian urinary bladder or mammalian collecting ducts with AVP leads to the insertion of patches of membrane that contain AQP2 water channels into the apical membrane,[214, 233, 265] a process that depends on the integrity of the cytoskeleton.[266] Treatment of amphibian bladders with agents that disrupt microtubules and microfilaments impairs the fusion of aggrephores and the apical membrane, decreases the number of aggregates on the cell surface, and impairs the hydro-osmotic response to AVP.[266, 267] Likewise, treatment of rats with the microtubule inhibitor colchicine causes AQP2 water channels to move from apical and subapical locations and become diffusely distributed.[229]

A number of proteins appear to be involved in the docking and fusion of synaptic vesicles with neuronal membranes. A vesicle-associated membrane protein is thought to bind a soluble *N*-ethylmaleimide–sensitive attachment protein receptor on the target membrane, and vesicle-associated membrane proteins (vesicle-associated membrane protein 2 or cellulobrevin, or both) are present on AQP2-containing intracellular vesicles in principal cells of the collecting duct.[268–270]

In summary AVP, working via cAMP and protein kinase, alters water transport in hormone-responsive epithelia by causing the microtubule-dependent insertion of specialized membrane units into the apical plasma membranes of these cells. In other tissues, such as the mTALH, AVP may act by different mechanisms to increase the functional number of Na⁺,K⁺,2Cl⁻ cotransport units and K⁺ channels in apical membranes.

Modulation of Vasopressin Action

A number of physiological and pharmacologic agents influence the effects of AVP on the water permeability in the collecting duct (Table 10–4).

α-ADRENERGIC AGENTS. In addition to their effects on AVP secretion, α-adrenergic agents acting at the level of the collecting duct may decrease water permeability.[271] Moreover the inhibitory effects of the α-adrenergic agonists clonidine and epinephrine are attenuated by preincubation of collecting ducts with pertussis toxin,[248, 249] an agent that inactivates the inhibitory guanine regulatory protein G_i. Thus α-adrenergic agonists inhibit AVP action in the collecting duct by activating

the G_i subunit and by decreasing cAMP formation. These effects however may be species specific. For example α₂-adrenergic agonists inhibit AVP-stimulated cAMP production in rat cortical and medullary collecting ducts but have no effect on cAMP accumulation in dog or human collecting ducts.[272]

ATRIAL NATRIURETIC PEPTIDE. This agent inhibits the hydro-osmotic effect of AVP in isolated rabbit cortical collecting tubules at a site proximal to the catalytic subunit of adenylate cyclase because ANP has no effect on cAMP- and forskolin-stimulated water flow.[134]

PROSTAGLANDINS. In the mammalian cortical collecting tubule, the medullary interstitial cell, and the toad urinary bladder AVP stimulates the production of PGE_2,[273, 274] and inhibition of prostaglandin production increases the rate of Na⁺ transport and the rate of osmotic water permeation.[274] In both the rabbit cortical collecting tubule and the toad urinary bladder prostaglandins inhibit AVP-stimulated accumulation of cAMP within the cell and exert little or no inhibitory action on transport events beyond the accumulation of cAMP within the cell.[192, 247, 275]

PGE_2 does not inhibit the hydro-osmotic effect of the nonhormonal catalytic subunit activator forskolin but does inhibit the stimulation of water flow by cholera toxin, which activates adenylate cyclase by irreversible binding to G_s, the stimulatory guanine nucleotide–binding subunit of adenylate cyclase. Thus PGE_2 probably inhibits AVP-stimulated generation of cAMP in the cortical collecting tubule by interacting with G_i.[247] The same mechanism has been reported for prostaglandin-mediated inhibition of NaCl transport in isolated

TABLE 10–4. Agents That Alter Collecting Duct Responsiveness to Vasopressin

Increase AVP action
Chlorpropamide
Carbamazepine
Chronic dehydration
Nonsteroidal anti-inflammatory agents
Decrease AVP action
α-Adrenergic agents
Atrial natriuretic peptide
PGE_2
Hypokalemia
Hypercalcemia
Protein kinase C
Lithium
Demeclocycline

AVP, arginine vasopressin; PGE_2, prostaglandin E_2.

mTALH.[246, 248] It is noteworthy in this connection that AVP appears to stimulate PGE$_2$ synthesis in medullary interstitial cells[273, 276] and in medullary collecting duct cells,[277] although some studies have failed to show this effect.[278–280]

CALCIUM. Hypercalcemia causes an AVP-resistant decrease in maximal urine osmolality. In the toad urinary bladder[281, 282] the hydro-osmotic effect of AVP is inhibited by high concentrations of calcium in serosal solutions but calcium has no effect on the cAMP-induced hydro-osmotic effect, suggesting that the high serosal calcium concentration interferes with the generation of cAMP. In contrast, in the rabbit collecting duct an increase in the peritubular calcium concentration enhances the hydro-osmotic effect of AVP but not cAMP.[283] Furthermore increasing the peritubular calcium concentration from 1 to 5 mmol/L (4.8 to 24 mg/dL) does not inhibit AVP-dependent cAMP production in the mouse collecting duct.[248] In the mTALH, however, high peritubular calcium levels inhibit AVP-induced cAMP generation.[248, 284] Preincubation of tubule segments with pertussis toxin abolishes this inhibition, indicating that inhibition of cAMP generation by high calcium levels is mediated through activation of G$_i$.[248] Although high extracellular calcium concentrations have little effect on cAMP generation, increases in intracellular calcium levels produced by the calcium ionophore A23187[285] or by permeabilization of the cell membrane inhibit AVP-induced cAMP accumulation in the collecting duct.

PROTEIN KINASE C. AVP acts in the collecting duct via intracellular cAMP but in hepatocytes and vascular smooth muscle cells AVP activates a V$_1$ receptor leading to phosphoinositide turnover, and the phosphoinositide–protein kinase C pathway may down-regulate the activation by AVP of the water transport pathway through protein kinase A. In toad urinary bladder,[286] frog skin,[287] and rabbit cortical collecting tubules,[285, 288] phorbol esters, which activate protein kinase C, inhibit the hydro-osmotic effect of AVP. Studies with the toad[286] and the frog[287] suggest that phorbol esters act on the generation of cAMP, because they do not inhibit the response to exogenous cAMP, whereas in the rabbit collecting duct a "post-cAMP" effect has been proposed.[285]

Medullary Thick Ascending Limb of Henle

The concept that AVP might regulate renal concentrating power by modulating the rate of NaCl absorption in the mTALH was set forth by Wirz and co-workers[289] and has been discussed generally by others.[290] Figure 10–17 presents a general model for net NaCl absorption in the mTALH. Net transepithelial Cl$^-$ absorption in the TALH involves a transport process in which luminal Cl$^-$ entry into cells is mediated by an electroneutral Na$^+$,K$^+$,2Cl$^-$ cotransport mechanism.[291, 292] The cDNA for protein responsible for this transport, which is the target of the loop-acting diuretics, has been cloned[293] and the protein is localized in the apical membrane of the thick ascending limb.[294]

Apical membranes of diluting segments, either mammalian[291, 295] or amphibian,[296] also contain barium (Ba^{2+})-sensitive K$^+$ conductances that account almost entirely for the electrical conductance of apical membranes. These channels constitute the route for active K$^+$ secretion in renal tubular diluting segments[297, 298] but most K$^+$ that is secreted from cells to lumen is recycled into cells via the Na$^+$,K$^+$,2Cl$^-$ cotransport process. Thus the rate of net K$^+$ secretion constitutes less than 10% of the rate of net Cl$^-$ absorption, whereas the calculated K$^+$ current across apical membranes is approximately 60% of the rate of net Cl$^-$ absorption.[297]

The apical membrane K$^+$ channel is a member of the family of ATP-sensitive K$^+$ channels. Increases in intracellular ATP or decreases in intracellular pH inhibit the activity of the

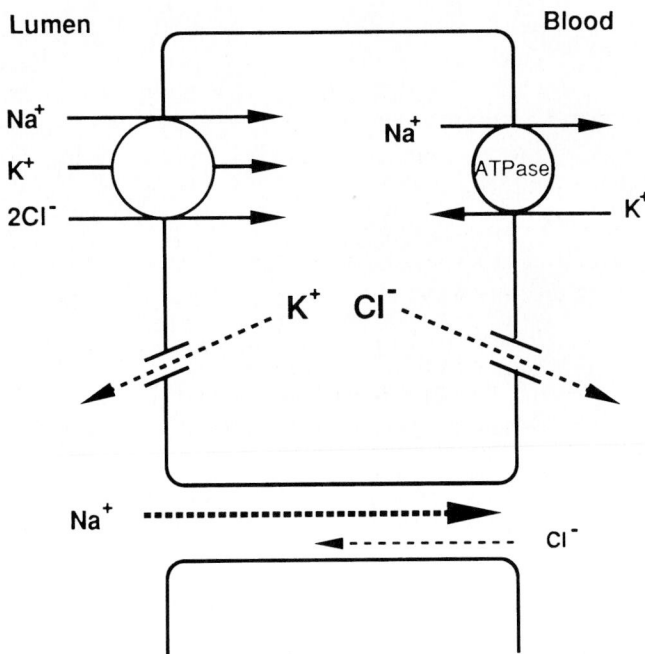

Figure 10–17. A model for salt absorption in mouse mTALH. The solid lines denote conservative (primary or secondary) processes and the dashed lines denote dissipative processes.

channel.[299] The cDNA that encodes the K$^+$ channel has been cloned from the rat outer medulla[300] and the primary product ROMK1, and its alternative splice products ROMK2 and ROMK3, are expressed in the apical membranes of the thick ascending limb and cortical collecting duct.[301, 302]

Cl$^-$ exit from the cell across the basolateral membrane of the TALH appears to be primarily conductive.[303] The large intracellular negative voltage of -40 to -70 mV (cell with respect to bath) provides a portion of the driving force for transport of Cl$^-$ across the basolateral membrane in these segments.[297, 304] A large fraction of Cl$^-$ uptake into basolaterally enriched renal medullary vesicles proceeds through conductive pathways.[305] These pathways have been identified as Cl$^-$ channels by incorporating vesicles into planar lipid bilayers.[306] The channel activity increases as the intracellular Cl$^-$ is increased from 2 to 50 mmol/L[307] and although phosphorylation of the channel by cAMP-dependent protein kinase increases channel activity at low (2 mmol/L) Cl$^-$ levels, phosphorylation has no added effect when the cytosolic Cl$^-$ is high (50 mmol/L).[308] As discussed later these characteristics may account for the rise in basolateral membrane Cl$^-$ conductance in AVP-stimulated TALH segments. RbClC-Ka, which belongs to the ClC[308b] family of Cl$^-$ channels, is expressed in the thick ascending limb, and treatment of cultured TALH cells with an rbClC-Ka antisense oligonucleotide eliminates Cl$^-$ channel activity.[308c] These findings suggest that rbClC-Ka is the basolateral membrane Cl$^-$ channel of the TALH.

The model for NaCl absorption in the TALH shown in Figure 10–17 has at least two general implications. First, about half of the total net Na$^+$ absorption occurs through the paracellular route. In other words the combination of a lumen-positive transepithelial voltage and a high shunt conductance reduces—with respect to exclusively transcellular active Na$^+$ absorption—the metabolic energy expenditure for net Na$^+$ absorption. Second, the regulatory mechanisms in epithelial cells promote the rapid adjustment of the rate of Na$^+$ entry to equal the rate of Na$^+$ exit, thus preventing changes in cell volume ("flush-through" effect) when net Na$^+$ absorption is varied.[309] The flush-through effect is also minimized in diluting segments in which half the net Na$^+$ absorption proceeds through the paracellular route.

Effect of Vasopressin on Net Salt Absorption

AVP increases both the net rate of salt absorption and the spontaneous transepithelial voltage in isolated mouse mTALH segments.[292, 310] This stimulating effect on net salt absorption occurs at peritubular hormone concentrations found in the plasma of mammalian species during ordinary antidiuresis, and cAMP analogues produce the same effect on mouse mTALH segments.[310] Moreover AVP also increases the rate of salt absorption from the mTALH of homozygous Brattleboro rats with central diabetes insipidus.[311]

MECHANISM OF THE VASOPRESSIN EFFECT. AVP simultaneously increases the net rate of salt absorption and transepithelial voltage in the mouse mTALH, the transepithelial electrical conductance, and the rate of net K$^+$ secretion in that nephron segment.[297, 303] Moreover these effects are probably linked; a synopsis of the argument in favor of this suggestion is as follows.

A primary effect of AVP in increasing salt absorption in the mTALH appears to depend on a hormone-mediated increase in the number of conductive K$^+$ channels and Na$^+$,K$^+$,2Cl$^-$ cotransporters in apical plasma membranes. For example in membrane vesicles from outer renal medulla, exposure to cAMP-dependent protein kinase in vitro increases barium-sensitive K$^+$ uptake,[312] an increase that may account for AVP- or cAMP-mediated increases in net K$^+$ secretion.[295]

AVP also increases transepithelial conductance and the Cl$^-$ conductance of basolateral membranes,[313, 314] an effect that is abolished when net salt absorption is inhibited by furosemide.[314] The latter observation has been rationalized by assuming that the increase in cell Cl$^-$ activity is responsible for the AVP-dependent increase in basolateral conductance.[295, 314] In this regard the activity of Cl$^-$ channels in basolateral medullary membrane vesicles is increased by increasing intracellular Cl$^-$ activity.[306] AVP may also activate basolateral Cl$^-$ channels directly.[313, 314]

AVP also increases the functional number of Na$^+$,K$^+$,2Cl$^-$ cotransport units in apical membranes.[295] Because AVP increases net Cl$^-$ absorption in the mouse mTALH, the rate of Cl$^-$ flux across apical membranes is greater with hormone than without hormone but, as noted earlier, it is likely that cell Cl$^-$ concentrations rise in the presence of AVP. Consequently the chemical driving force for electroneutral Na$^+$,K$^+$,Cl$^-$ cotransport (see Fig. 10–17) from lumen to cell may be less in the presence of AVP than in its absence. According to this view AVP increases the functional number of Na$^+$,K$^+$,2Cl$^-$ cotransport units as well as K$^+$ conductance units in apical plasma membranes.[295, 314]

Modulation of Function of Thick Ascending Limb of Henle

In isolated mouse mTALH segments, increases in peritubular osmolality, produced either with permeant solutes such as urea or with impermeant solutes such as mannitol, inhibit the AVP-stimulated rate of net Cl$^-$ absorption.[315, 316] This inhibition of transcellular NaCl absorption occurs at a locus beyond the generation of cAMP because supramaximal concentrations of either AVP or cAMP are unable to reverse the effect. Thus increasing interstitial osmolality provides a negative feedback signal, which can reduce AVP-dependent NaCl absorption by the mTALH.

PGE$_2$ also participates in a negative feedback system that modulates the rate of net NaCl absorption by the mTALH.[317–319] In the in vitro mouse mTALH,[246, 320] PGE$_2$ has no effect on NaCl absorption when AVP is absent, but in the presence of

AVP, PGE$_2$ reduces the AVP-dependent values for transepithelial voltage and net NaCl absorption to AVP-independent values. Likewise, PGE$_2$ has no effect on cellular cAMP concentrations in the absence of AVP, and PGE$_2$ inhibits the AVP-dependent stimulation of cytosolic cAMP concentrations.[321] PGE$_2$ probably inhibits AVP-stimulated generation of cAMP in the mTALH by activating G$_i$.[246]

The significance of these interactions of prostaglandins and AVP on concentrating ability has been affirmed by in vivo studies. Inhibition of renal prostaglandin synthesis, either with indomethacin or with meclofenamate, causes antinatriuresis and an enhanced urine concentration in response to administration of vasopressin.[322, 323] In addition an increase in medullary NaCl content follows inhibition of prostaglandin synthesis even in the absence of a change in papillary blood flow.[324]

PGE$_2$ is synthesized in the medullary collecting duct and in interstitial cells. AVP and increases in osmolality produced with urea or NaCl appear to influence PGE$_2$ synthesis by affecting the calcium-dependent acyl hydrolase activity that regulates the availability of arachidonic acid in these cells.[276] Increases in local osmolality in the renal medulla produced by AVP-mediated increases in NaCl absorption from the mTALH and the consequent enhancement in countercurrent multiplication may play a role in PGE$_2$ synthesis in vivo. For example hypertonic NaCl stimulates PGE$_2$ release from medullary cells and hypertonic urea suppresses this effect and the PGE$_2$ release that is mediated by pharmacologic levels of AVP.

Integration of Vasopressin Action on Concentration of Urine

The in vivo and in vitro data summarized in this section can be integrated into a model for the modulation of renal concentrating mechanisms (Fig. 10–18). AVP-stimulated NaCl absorption by the mTALH is regulated by two negative feedback loops (the dashed lines in Fig. 10–18), each of which

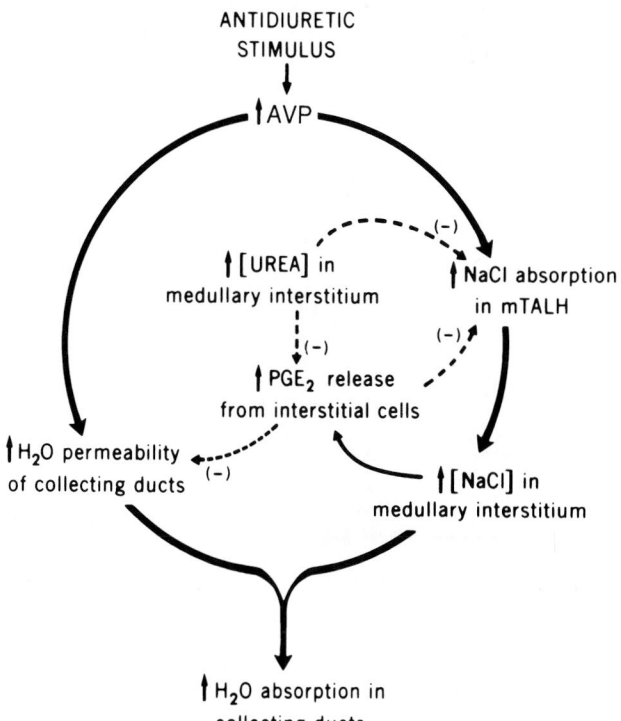

Figure 10–18. Model for the feedback regulation of renal concentrating mechanisms. (From Hebert SC, Andreoli TE. Control of NaCl transport in the thick ascending limb. Am J Physiol 1984; 246:F745–F756, with permission.)

depends on increases in interstitial osmolality due to enhancement of countercurrent multiplication. During the early stages of antidiuresis an AVP-mediated increase in NaCl absorption by the mTALH increases the interstitial NaCl concentration and stimulates the release of PGE_2 from interstitial cells, which in turn decreases the rate of AVP-stimulated NaCl absorption. Later, during antidiuresis, a rise in medullary interstitial urea concentration inhibits PGE_2 release from interstitial cells and the AVP-mediated increase in NaCl absorption from the mTALH.[283]

Thus the inhibition by interstitial hyperosmolality of AVP-dependent NaCl absorption by the mTALH is coupled to PGE_2 production, which modulates AVP action through the second messenger cAMP; the net effect is a negative feedback loop on AVP-dependent NaCl addition to the medullary interstitium. A similar negative feedback loop operates at the level of the collecting duct, where endogenous PGE_2 production, stimulated by AVP, decreases the AVP-induced increase in water permeability at the level of cellular cAMP.

CLINICAL DERANGEMENTS OF WATER BALANCE

The control of plasma osmolality and its primary determinant, the plasma sodium concentration, is achieved through AVP-mediated water conservation and thirst-induced water acquisition (see Fig. 10–1). The integrated actions of the two effector limbs of the water repletion reaction are required: water conservation and water intake. Likewise, abnormal plasma osmolality, i.e., hyponatremia or hypernatremia, is usually due to a derangement in water balance rather than salt balance.

As illustrated in Figure 10–7, the principal physiological stimulus for AVP secretion is plasma osmolality.[325] At low plasma osmolalities AVP secretion is suppressed but when plasma osmolality exceeds the threshold value, usually about 280 mmol/L, AVP secretion increases in a linear fashion. AVP in turn concentrates urine. Figure 10–19 depicts the relation,

at a given solute excretion rate, between the plasma AVP level and urine osmolality. A comparison of Figures 10–7 and 10–19 indicates that at a plasma osmolality of 290 mmol/L, 10 mmol/L above the AVP threshold, a plasma AVP level of 4 to 5 pmol/L (4 to 5 ng/L) is sufficient to concentrate urine maximally. Conversely, at a plasma osmolality of 280 mmol/L, plasma AVP is completely suppressed and urine is maximally dilute. In other words a 3% increase in plasma osmolality causes a change in a normal individual from a state of maximal diuresis to one of maximal antidiuresis.

Urine flow varies inversely with the urine osmolality. Thus when plasma AVP is suppressed to allow maximal urine dilution, the rate of water excretion increases dramatically. At solute excretion rates of 800 to 900 mmol/d, e.g., the free water clearance can approach 20 L/d; i.e., a normal individual can ingest up to 20 L of water daily and not risk water intoxication.

The osmotic threshold for thirst is roughly 290 mmol/kg water, 10 mmol/kg water above the AVP threshold. Small increases in plasma osmolality past this threshold cause intense thirst and increased water intake. Thus the thresholds for AVP secretion and thirst form the lower and upper boundaries, respectively, for plasma osmolality. A fall in plasma osmolality toward the AVP threshold causes water diuresis and increased plasma osmolality. An increase in plasma osmolality past the thirst threshold, in contrast, increases water intake to cause a fall in plasma osmolality. Within the range defined by these thresholds plasma osmolality is determined primarily by AVP-mediated changes in urine concentration.

HYPERTONIC SYNDROMES

As discussed earlier, increases in ECF osmolality are caused by substances to which cells are impermeable (NaCl, mannitol and, in the case of insulin deficiency, glucose). The hypertonic syndromes cause cellular dehydration and shrinkage. Because body fluids are in osmotic equilibrium, the plasma osmolality is determined by the ratio of total body solutes to total body water. The major extracellular and intracellular solutes are salts of sodium and potassium, respectively. Accordingly hypertonicity can result from an increase in total body sodium or potassium, or both, or from a decrease in total body water.

Hypertonicity due to increased total body sodium most often results from the administration of hypertonic sodium bicarbonate during cardiopulmonary resuscitation. Hyperkalemia is lethal before increases in total body potassium cause hypertonicity. Hypertonicity can also result from increases in the concentration of other solutes such as mannitol or glycerol. In these cases the serum sodium concentration can be normal or depressed. However as the solute is excreted with its obligate water load the serum sodium concentration may become elevated.

Hypertonic syndromes usually result from decreases in total body water resulting from losses of renal or extrarenal water in the face of inadequate water replacement.

Classification

Failure of water homeostasis can result from inadequacy of either AVP-dependent water conservation or thirst-mediated water acquisition (see Fig. 10–1) and the clinical circumstances that lead to hypernatremia can be grouped into several categories (Table 10–5).

Deficiency of renal concentrating mechanisms does not lead to hypertonicity if free access to water is ensured, and hypertonic volume depletion usually occurs in the very young

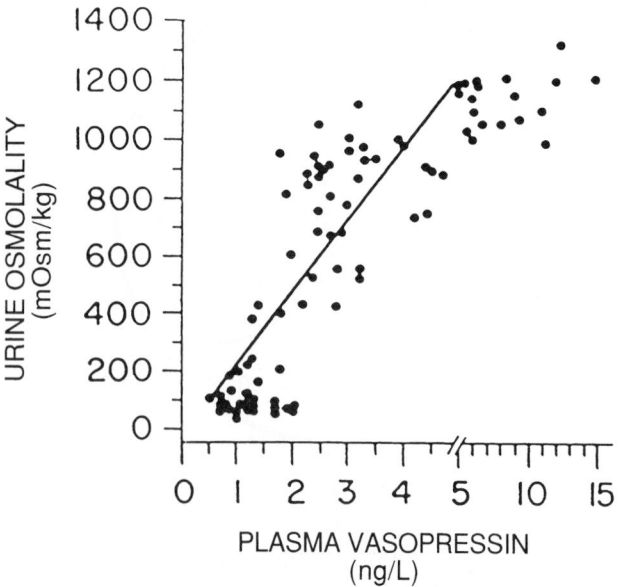

Figure 10–19. The relation between plasma AVP concentrations and urine osmolality. (Adapted from Robertson GL, Berl T. Water metabolism. In: Brenner BM, Rector FC Jr, eds. The Kidney. 3rd ed. Philadelphia: WB Saunders, 1986: 385–432, with permission.)

TABLE 10–5. Major Causes of Hypernatremia

Impaired Thirst	Solute Diuresis
Coma	Glucose
Essential hypernatremia	Diabetic ketoacidosis
	Nonketotic hyperosmolar coma
Excessive Water Losses	Other
	Mannitol administration
Renal	Glycerol administration
Central diabetes insipidus	
Nephrogenic diabetes insipidus	**Sodium Excess**
Impaired medullary	
Hypertonicity	Administration of hypertonic NaCl
Extrarenal	Administration of hypertonic
Sweating	NaHCO₃
Osmotic diarrhea	
Burns	

or the very old, in whom either immaturity or debility prevents the translation of thirst into water-acquiring behavior, or in individuals such as comatose patients who are unable to communicate thirst. In a subset of patients with essential hypernatremia the osmoregulatory centers malfunction so that osmotic stimulation of both AVP release and thirst is impaired.

Central diabetes insipidus is characterized by the failure of appropriate osmotic, volume, or chemical stimuli to evoke antidiuresis and by a normal response to exogenous vasopressin. Congenital nephrogenic diabetes insipidus is identified by polyuria that has been present since birth, generally in males, and persistent unresponsiveness to exogenous vasopressin. Acquired nephrogenic diabetes insipidus is characterized by unresponsiveness to AVP in a person with a history of exposure to agents (e.g., lithium, demeclocycline, or methoxyflurane anesthesia) that antagonize the action of AVP on collecting ducts. The history and laboratory data are adequate to identify disorders such as sickle cell disease or interstitial nephritis, both of which impair the ability to generate a hypertonic medullary interstitium. Finally hypercalcemia or hypokalemia can be identified on routine laboratory screening.

Diabetes mellitus, which produces a solute diuresis, is characterized by an isotonic urine and glycosuria. Therapeutic administration of mannitol or glycerol is likewise associated with large volumes of relatively isotonic urine. In other words, hypertonic disorders that are associated with solute diuresis are characterized by high rates of solute excretion (i.e., by a high C_{osm}; see Fig. 10–11), whereas the central or nephrogenic diabetes insipidus syndromes are characterized by defects in water conservation with normal rates of solute excretion. Rarely hypernatremia is due to the administration of hypertonic NaCl.

Clinical Syndromes

Essential Hypernatremia

Essential hypernatremia[326, 327] is characterized by chronic hypernatremia with euvolemia, normal renal function, decreased thirst perception, and a normal renal response to exogenous vasopressin. Despite elevations of serum sodium levels and ECF osmolalities these patients exhibit hypodipsia and an inappropriately dilute urine.[326, 327] The disorder may be due to a resetting of the threshold sensitivity of osmoreceptors in the CNS.[326, 327] However, the osmotic threshold for AVP release is normal but the amount of AVP release at any level of plasma osmolality is attenuated.[328, 329] This syndrome has been reported in association with CNS histiocytosis, pineal tumors, surgery for craniopharyngioma, and head trauma.[326, 327]

A common finding is normal AVP release (measured either as a rise in urine osmolality[326, 327] or as an increase in plasma AVP levels determined by radioimmunoassay[328, 329]) to baroreceptor stimulation. This finding has been interpreted

to indicate adequate AVP production and storage but a dissociation between the neurohypophysis and the osmoreceptors.

Given the combination of diminished thirst sensation and decreased release of AVP in response to osmotic stimulation, the disorder is probably the consequence of ablation of hypothalamic osmoreceptor function. Forced hydration does not consistently correct the hypernatremia but chlorpropamide, a drug that augments the antidiuretic effect of low levels of circulating AVP,[330] is useful in restoring osmotic homeostasis.[326, 327]

Central Diabetes Insipidus

Central diabetes insipidus is a polyuric syndrome due to a level of AVP that is insufficient to concentrate the urine. The disease is identified by three features: persistence of an inappropriately dilute urine in the presence of strong osmotic or nonosmotic stimuli for AVP secretion, absence of intrinsic renal disease, and a rise in urine osmolality after the administration of vasopressin.

ETIOLOGY. The factors that cause central diabetes insipidus (Table 10–6) have changed over time. In early series more than half of cases were due to tumors of the basilar surface of the brain, one tenth of cases were caused by head trauma, and one fourth of cases involved inflammation of the basal meninges.[331] In contrast, in a series published in 1980[332] 30% of cases were idiopathic, 25% were related to malignant or benign tumors of the brain or pituitary, 16% were secondary to head trauma, and 20% followed cranial surgery. A retrospective study of central diabetes insipidus in children found brain tumors (60%) and cerebral malformations (25%) to be the most common causes.[333]

Primary intracranial tumors that cause diabetes insipidus are often craniopharyngiomas or pineal tumors,[334] and metastatic tumors are most often from lung or breast.[335–338] The appearance of other hypothalamic manifestations may be delayed up to 10 y after the onset of diabetes insipidus.[339, 340] Periodic follow-up of patients diagnosed as having idiopathic central diabetes insipidus is necessary to detect slowly growing

TABLE 10–6. Causes of Central Diabetes Insipidus

Congenital central diabetes insipidus
  Familial (autosomal dominant)
  Septo-optic dysplasia
  Familial hypopituitarism
  Congenital cytomegalovirus infection
Acquired central diabetes insipidus
  Idiopathic
  Trauma
  Postsurgical
  Neoplastic
    Craniopharyngioma
    Pineal tumors
    Pituitary tumors
    Lymphoma
    Meningioma
    Metastatic tumors
  Ischemic
    Sheehan's syndrome
    Brain death
  Granulomatous
    Sarcoidosis
    Histiocytosis
    Wegener's granulomatosis
    Bronchocentric granulomatosis
  Infections
    Tuberculosis
    Blastomycosis
    Syphilis
    Viral encephalitis
    Bacterial meningitis
  Autoimmune

intracranial lesions. Finally histiocytosis (either eosinophilic granuloma or Hand-Schüller-Christian disease), encephalitis or meningitis, granulomatous diseases such as sarcoidosis or Wegener's granulomatosis, lymphocytic hypophysitis, and intraventricular hemorrhage can cause central diabetes insipidus.[332, 341-346]

A rare hereditary form of the disorder is transmitted as an autosomal dominant trait.[347, 348] These patients may maintain a persistently hypotonic urine even when hyperosmolality is induced by dehydration or infusion of hypertonic saline or when hypotension is induced pharmacologically. Nevertheless all patients respond to exogenous vasopressin with reduction in urine volume and elevation of urine osmolality. This disorder is clearly different from familial nephrogenic diabetes insipidus in which vasopressin is ineffective.[349] Some patients with familial central diabetes insipidus experience increased plasma AVP levels in response to strong osmotic or nonosmotic stimuli of AVP release.[348, 350] This finding suggests that the disorder is due to a progressive degenerative process of magnicellular neurons.[347, 350] Genetic studies have uncovered several mutations involving the AVP-neurophysin gene (Table 10–7).[351-354] As noted earlier AVP and neurophysin II are encoded by a single gene, with post-translational cleavage of AVP and neurophysin II. None of the mutations studied to date involve the coding region for vasopressin itself but affect either the signal peptide region or, more commonly, neurophysin II. The mechanism by which the mutations impair AVP release is not understood. Neurophysin II consists of two beta sheets that form a pocket in which AVP binds.[355] Disruption of the secondary structure of neurophysin II by mutations could impair proteolytic cleavage of the precursor protein, binding of AVP to neurophysin II, or the intracellular transport of the AVP-neurophysin II complexes.[352] Moreover the accumulation of abnormal AVP-neurophysin II precursor might be cytotoxic to magnicellular neurons and lead to loss of AVP-producing cells in the hypothalamus.

TABLE 10–7. *Prepro-AVP-NPII* Mutations Causing Autosomal Dominant Neurogenic Diabetes Insipidus

Name*	Type of Mutation	Nucleotide Change	Predicted Amino Acid Change	Restriction-Enzyme Analysis	Comments and Putative Functional Consequences	References†
S17F	Missense	C→T at 274	Ser→Phe at codon 17	*Mbo* II site created		Rittig et al, 1996
A19T	Missense	G→A at 279	Ala→Thr at codon 19	*Bst* UI site abolished, *Pml* I site created	CG CA; alteration of the cleavage of the leader peptide	Ito et al, 1993; Krishnamani et al, 1993; McLeod et al, 1993; Rittig et al, 1996; (total of five families)
A19V	Missense	C→T at 280	Ala→Val at codon 19	*Bst* UI site abolished		Rittig et al, 1996
G45R	Missense	G→C at 1730	Gly→Arg at codon 45 (NP$_{14}$)	*Bsl* I site created		Rittig et al, 1996
G48V	Missense	G→T at 1740	Gly→Val at codon 48 (NP$_{17}$)	*Bgl* I site abolished	Disruption of a beta turn in AVP-NPII precursor	Bahnsen et al, 1992
R51C	Missense	C→T at 1748	Arg→Cys at codon 51 (NP$_{20}$)			Rittig et al, 1996
P55L	Missense	C→T at 1761	Pro→Leu at codon 55 (NP$_{24}$)	*Dde* I site created	De novo mutation, amino acid substitution in NPII	Repaske and Browning, 1994
E77	Inframe deletion	Deletion of three nucleotides in region 1824–1829	Deletion of Glu (glutamic acid) at codon 77 (NP$_{46}$)	*Mnl* I site abolished	Two sets of staggered 3-base pair tandem repeats; unable to form a salt bridge between AVP and NPII	Yuasa et al, 1993; Rittig et al, 1996
E78G	Missense	A→G at 1830	Glu→Gly at codon 78 (NP$_{47}$)			Rittig et al, 1996
L81P	Missense	T→C at 1839	Leu→Pro at codon 81 (NP$_{50}$)			Rittig et al, 1996
G88R	Missense	G→C at 1859	Gly→Arg at codon 88 (NP$_{57}$)	*Msp* I and *Bgl* I sites abolished		Rittig et al, 1996
G88S	Missense	G→A at 1859	Gly→Ser at codon 88 (NP$_{57}$)	*Msp* I and *Bgl* I sites abolished	Failure of dimerization of NPII, alteration of axonal transport, or posttranslational processing	Ito et al, 1991; Rittig et al, 1996 (two families)
C92S	Missense	G→C at 1872	Cys→Ser at codon 92 (NP$_{61}$)	*Hga* I site created		Rittig et al, 1996
C92X	Nonsense	C→A at 1873	Cys→stop at codon 92 (NP$_{61}$)	*Mnl* I site created		Rittig et al, 1996
G93W	Missense	G→T at 1874	Gly→Trp at codon 93 (NP$_{62}$)	*Bpm* I site created	—	Nagasaki et al, 1995
G96C	Missense	G→T at 1883	Gly→Cys at codon 96 (NP$_{65}$)			Rittig et al, 1996
C98X	Nonsense	C→A at 1891	Cys→stop at codon 99 (NP$_{68}$)	*Dde* I site created	—	Nagasaki et al, 1995
C110X	Nonsense	C→A at 2094	Cys→stop at codon 110 (NP$_{79}$)	*Bbv* I site abolished		Rittig et al, 1996
2106 CG GT	Nonsense	C→G at 2106	Pro→Pro at 114 (NP$_{83}$)			Rittig et al, 1996
		G→T at 2107	Glu→stop at 115 (NP$_{84}$)			
E118X	Nonsense	G→T at 2116	Glu→stop at 118 (NP$_{87}$)	*Mae* I site created		Rittig et al, 1996

*The names were assigned following the suggested nomenclature for mutations (Beaudet AL, Tsui LC. A suggested nomenclature for designating mutations. Hum Mutat 1993; 2:245–248).
†References are found in Rittig R, Robertson GL, Siggaard C, et al. Identification of 13 new mutations in the vasopressin-neurophysin II gene in 17 kindreds with familial autosomal dominant neurohypophyseal diabetes insipidus. Am J Hum Genet 1996; 58:107–117.
The nucleotides and amino acids are numbered according to the *prepro-AVP-NPII* gene sequence published by Sausville et al. The human vasopressin gene is linked to the oxytocin gene and is selectively expressed in a cultured lung cancer cell line. J Biol Chem 1985; 260:10236–10241 and GenBank accession number M11166. The codons corresponding to the moieties are 1 to 19—signal peptide, 20 to 28—AVP, 29 to 31—cleavage site, 32 to 124—NPII, and 126 to 164—glycopeptide. NP$_{14}$ is the 14th amino acid of the protein neurophysin; likewise NP$_{17}$ is the 17th amino acid of the protein neurophysin, and so on.
AVP-NPII, arginine vasoporessin–neurophysin II.

Central diabetes insipidus occurs in about one third of patients with the DIDMOAD syndrome (diabetes insipidus, diabetes mellitus, optic atrophy, and deafness; [Wolfram syndrome][356, 357]) and in about one third of patients with congenital septo-optic dysplasia.[358] Both congenital and acquired central diabetes insipidus may include anterior pituitary dysfunction.[358, 359]

PATHOPHYSIOLOGY. Two features are noteworthy regarding the development of diabetes insipidus after injury to the neurohypophyseal system: the first relates to the site and degree of injury necessary to reduce AVP levels sufficiently to impair normal water homeostasis and the second is the characteristic triphasic response of neurohypophyseal function to injury.

Removal of the posterior pituitary gland does not necessarily lead to diabetes insipidus.[360] Rather persistent polyuria develops only when injury is sufficiently high in the supraopticohypophyseal tract to cause bilateral neuron degeneration in the SON and the PVN.[361] Approximately 90% of the magnicellular neurons in the SON and PVN have to be lost before diabetes insipidus develops.[362, 363] Consequently anterior pituitary tumors commonly compress the posterior pituitary but rarely cause diabetes insipidus[341, 364] and diabetes insipidus is uncommon in patients with hemorrhagic infarction of the anterior pituitary gland (Sheehan's syndrome).[365, 366] In short, although transient diabetes insipidus may follow any injury to the neurohypophysis, permanent diabetes insipidus occurs only when neurohypophyseal damage is high in the pituitary stalk.

Diabetes insipidus after surgery or trauma to the pituitary or hypothalamus may exhibit one of three patterns: transient, permanent, or triphasic. Transient diabetes insipidus usually has an abrupt onset within the first postoperative day and resolves within several days. This is the most common pattern (50 to 60%) of postsurgical diabetes insipidus and may occur after limited transsphenoidal resections of microadenomas. Permanent or prolonged diabetes insipidus also has an abrupt and early onset but persists for weeks or is permanent. This form of diabetes insipidus follows damage to the neurohypophyseal stalk or hypothalamus or wide resection of the pituitary for large masses with extrasellar extension.[367] In the triphasic pattern, shown in Figure 10–20, there is an immediate increase in urine volume after injury and a concomitant fall in urine osmolality, lasting 4 to 5 d; an intervening period of 5 to 7 d (the interphase) during which urine flow falls abruptly and urine osmolality rises; and a final phase consisting of permanent diabetes insipidus. This triphasic pattern also occurs after destruction of the supraopticohypophyseal tract in cats.[361]

The initial diuresis of the triphasic response is assumed to be due to an injury-related neuronal shock, during which time no hormone release occurs,[341, 364] or to the release of biologically inactive precursors from the damaged neurohypophysis.[368] The interphase appears to be due to the leak of hormone from degenerating neurons because the urinary excretion of water cannot be altered either by water loading or by hypotonic saline infusions[369] and because complete removal of the posterior pituitary together with hypothalamic nuclei of the neurohypophyseal system prevents the appearance of an interphase.[341]

Patients in whom central diabetes insipidus develops postoperatively can osmoregulate effectively despite these extreme fluctuations in AVP levels as long as they control water intake through thirst. However, severe water intoxication can develop during the phase of autonomous AVP release if infusion of hypotonic fluids is continued. Urine and serum osmolalities should be monitored carefully in patients undergoing surgery in the area of the neurohypophysis. Moreover if hormone replacement is needed in the early postoperative period, short-

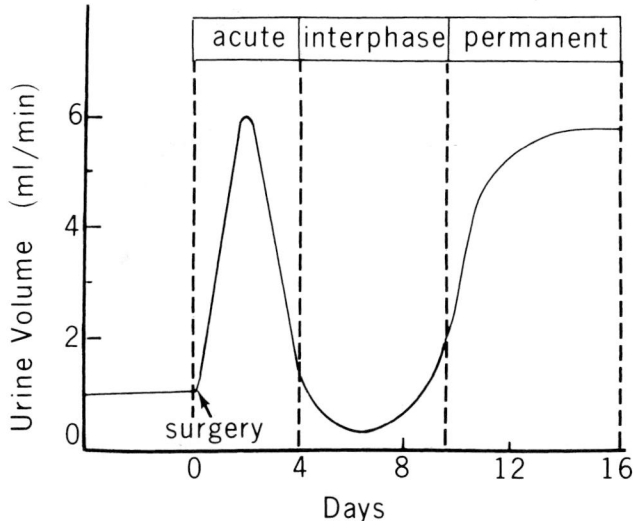

Figure 10–20. Triphasic response of urine volume after injury to the supraopticohypophyseal tract. (From C Fisher, WR Ingram. The effect of interruption of the supraopticohypophyseal tracts on the antidiuretic, pressor and oxytocic activity of the posterior lobe of the hypophysis. Endocrinology 20, 762–768, 1936, © by The Endocrine Society.)

acting agents (i.e., aqueous vasopressin) should be used to minimize the risk of subsequent hyponatremia if a phase of autonomous AVP release develops.

CLINICAL MANIFESTATIONS. The primary symptoms of diabetes insipidus are persistent polyuria and its companions, thirst and polydipsia.[370, 371]

The volume of urine may vary from only a few liters per day in the case of a partial hormone deficiency to a maximum of about 18 L/d, the average volume of glomerular filtrate delivered to collecting ducts in the total absence of AVP. Thus patients with partial central diabetes insipidus may be inconvenienced so little as to ignore their symptoms, the disorder being noticed only when they are deprived of water. Nocturia is almost invariably present in these patients as opposed to patients with primary polydipsia in whom nocturia is uncommon.

Most patients with central diabetes insipidus have abrupt onset of polyuria and polydipsia in contrast to the slow onset of polyuria due to impaired renal handling of water. The central diabetes insipidus that follows intracranial surgery usually shows a triphasic pattern (see earlier) with permanent polyuria commencing 10 to 14 d after surgery.

Patients with central diabetes insipidus usually show a particular predilection for cold or iced drinks to quench thirst. The most striking manifestations ensue if access to water is interrupted and hypertonic volume depletion develops. This condition, described later, is characterized by CNS manifestations beginning with irritability, followed by mental dullness, and progressing to coma with secondary signs of ataxia, hyperthermia, and hypotension. Finally in patients with diabetes insipidus due to intracranial lesions, neurologic manifestations of the primary lesion may be prominent.

LABORATORY MANIFESTATIONS. Persistent hyposthenuria, with a urine specific gravity of 1.005 or less and a urine osmolality less than 200 mmol/L, is the hallmark of diabetes insipidus.[332, 341] Partial deficiency of AVP may be recognized only as an inappropriately dilute urine in the face of elevated serum osmolality.[372] In euvolemic patients the GFR is normal.[332, 341] Because water is ingested in response to plasma hypertonicity, random plasma osmolality determinations are, on average, greater than 287 mmol/L.[373] Serum sodium levels are also elevated and account for the increases in plasma

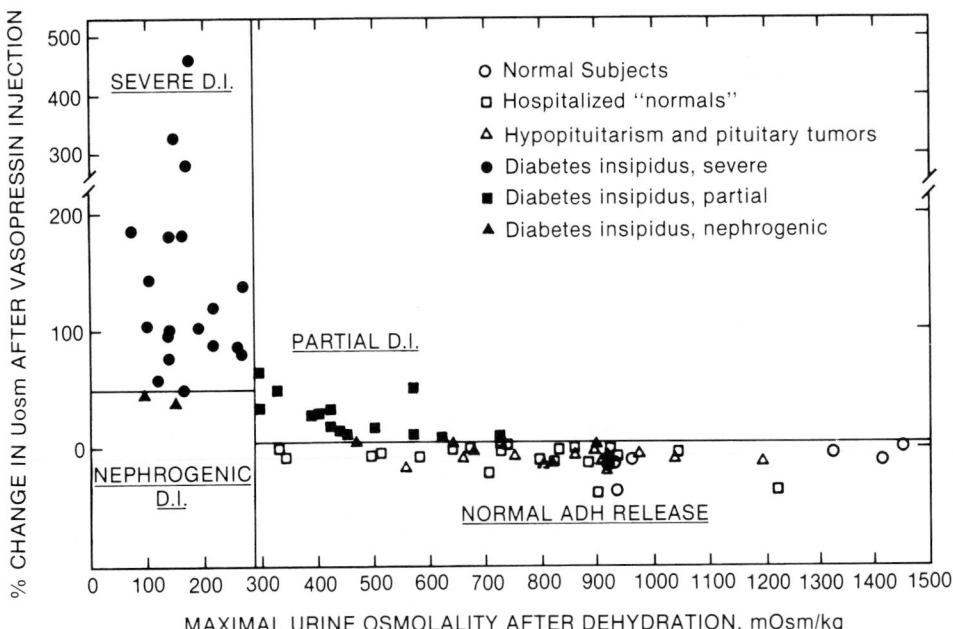

Figure 10–21. Response of urine osmolality to water deprivation and vasopressin injection in normal subjects, in patients with central or nephrogenic diabetes insipidus, and in patients with hypopituitarism. (Reproduced with permission, from Miller M, Dalakos T, Moses AM, et al. Recognition of partial defects in antidiuretic hormone secretion. Ann Intern Med 1970; 73:721–729.)

osmolality. In contrast individuals with primary polydipsia have an aberrant thirst mechanism and ingest water independent of physiological stimuli and often have mild dilutional hyponatremia.[373] When diabetes insipidus, either central or nephrogenic, begins in childhood, dilation of the urinary bladder, ureters, and renal pelvis may impair renal function.[374, 375]

DIAGNOSIS. Central diabetes insipidus must be separated from other polyuria states such as solute diuresis, impaired renal concentrating ability, or nephrogenic diabetes insipidus (see Table 10–5). Measurement of serum and urine solute levels should disclose osmotic diuretics (glucose, mannitol, urea) and measurements of serum creatinine and serum electrolyte levels identify GFR reductions, hypokalemia, and hypercalcemia. A history of recent head trauma, intracranial surgery, or neurologic deficits (bitemporal hemianopsia) that suggest midline tumors obviously points to central diabetes insipidus as the cause of polyuria.

Separation of patients with partial or complete deficiency of AVP from those with primary polydipsia is more difficult.[372, 373, 376] A 24-h urine volume greater than 18 L, a random plasma osmolality determination lower than 285 mmol/L, and a history of episodic polyuria suggest compulsive water drinking. A history of head trauma or neoplasm, the sudden onset of unrelenting polyuria, and a random plasma osmolality determination greater than 290 mmol/L suggest central diabetes insipidus. These distinguishing features depend on the fact that patients with central diabetes insipidus ingest water only in response to physiological stimuli and do not ingest water to the point of becoming hyponatremic.

Functional tests for central diabetes insipidus depend on the ability of the kidney to excrete a hypertonic urine after an osmotic stimulus. The simplest maneuver is to produce hypertonicity of body fluids by water deprivation, but the absolute level of urine concentration with water deprivation is nondiagnostic because maximal concentrating ability depends on the degree of medullary hypertonicity and on the presence of adequate amounts of AVP. For example Miller and co-workers[372] found the maximal urine osmolality produced by water deprivation in a group of randomly selected hospitalized patients to be 764 mmol/L compared with 1067 mmol/L in healthy volunteers. Presumably the lower value for maximal concentrating ability in hospitalized patients reflects a reduction in medullary interstitial hypertonicity. However even in patients with reduced medullary interstitial tonicity, the maximal urine osmolality with water deprivation depends on the amount of endogenous AVP release in response to dehydration. Therefore in individuals with intact AVP production and release, the administration of exogenous vasopressin does not produce an increase in the maximal urine osmolality beyond that achieved via water deprivation. This rationale forms the framework for a test scheme,[332, 372] which is illustrated in Figure 10–21, that distinguishes central diabetes insipidus (complete or partial) from other polyuria syndromes.

With mild polyuria water deprivation may begin the night preceding the test; patients with severe polyuria should have water restricted during the day to allow close observation. The test begins with paired measurements of osmolality of urine and plasma. All water intake is then withheld and hourly measurements of urine osmolality and body weight are made. When two sequential urine osmolality values vary by less than 30 mmol/L or when 3 to 5% of body weight is lost, 5 U of aqueous vasopressin is injected subcutaneously. A final urine osmolality measurement is taken 60 min later. This test must be carried out under supervision to avoid water intoxication in patients with primary polydipsia who may continue to ingest water secretly and then are given vasopressin.

The time required to achieve maximal urine concentration varies from 4 to 18 h.[332] In normal individuals water deprivation results in a urine osmolality two to four times greater than that of plasma osmolality. More important, the subsequent administration of exogenous vasopressin results in less than 9% further increase in urine osmolality. Patients with primary polydipsia, who have a reduced medullary interstitial tonicity as a result of prolonged water diuresis, may concentrate urine only slightly after water deprivation but they also have maximal endogenous AVP release and exhibit a less than 9% rise in urine osmolality with supplemental vasopressin.

Patients with complete central diabetes insipidus do not have an increase in urine osmolality to greater than plasma osmolality in response to water deprivation but have a greater than 50% increase in urine osmolality after vasopressin administration.[332, 372] Patients with partial central diabetes insipidus may concentrate the urine to some degree in response to water deprivation but also increase urine osmolality by at least 10% after vasopressin injection.[332, 372] Patients with partial central diabetes insipidus often show a peak urine osmolality that decreases with further water restriction, suggesting a limited reserve of neurohypophyseal hormone that becomes depleted after an initial secretory burst. Finally deprivation of water in patients with nephrogenic diabetes insipidus fails to increase urine osmolality to greater than plasma osmolality even when exogenous vasopressin is given.

When a diagnosis of central diabetes insipidus is made a careful evaluation for neoplasms involving the hypothalamus or the neurohypophyseal tract is mandatory. Magnetic resonance imaging is the preferred imaging technique. A curious observation in this regard is that T1-weighted images of the normal posterior pituitary yield a hyperintense signal, which is presumed to be due to some constituent of the AVP-containing NSGs. In patients with central diabetes insipidus the hyperintense signal in the posterior pituitary is usually absent[377, 378] but may persist in the rare patient with familial central diabetes insipidus. Patients with primary polydipsia and nephrogenic diabetes insipidus have normal posterior pituitary hyperintensity.[378] In addition to the loss of the hyperintense signal, magnetic resonance imaging in patients with central diabetes insipidus may reveal thickening of the pituitary stalk or masses caused by primary or metastatic tumors.[377] Thus magnetic resonance imaging is a useful adjunct, particularly in differentiating patients with primary polydipsia from those with central diabetes insipidus.[378]

Levels of circulating AVP can be measured by radioimmunoassay. Zerbe and Robertson[376] compared the diagnostic accuracy of the indirect test for AVP release described earlier with actual measurements of plasma AVP levels by radioimmunoassay. The diagnosis of severe central diabetes insipidus or nephrogenic diabetes insipidus that was made by the indirect test was confirmed in every case by direct measurements of plasma AVP levels. In contrast two patients who were diagnosed as having partial diabetes insipidus by the indirect test had normal plasma AVP levels when subjected to dehydration; one proved to have primary polydipsia and the other nephrogenic diabetes insipidus. Finally 3 of 10 patients who were classified as having primary polydipsia by the indirect test had plasma AVP levels that were consistent with partial central diabetes insipidus. These authors concluded that direct measurement of plasma AVP levels can improve the diagnostic accuracy of indirect tests for diagnosing the polyuria syndromes but care must be taken in interpreting results from available radioimmunoassay procedures.[376, 379]

Hypertonic saline infusion has also been used to test for release of AVP.[332] In this procedure hypertonic saline is briefly infused to raise the serum sodium concentration to between 145 and 150 mmol/L and one or more blood samples are obtained for measurement of serum osmolality and AVP level. Patients with primary polydipsia or nephrogenic diabetes insipidus have normal AVP release in response to the hypertonicity, whereas patients with central diabetes insipidus have little or no rise in plasma AVP levels. This procedure may be hazardous in patients with limited cardiac reserve in whom volume expansion may cause cardiac decompensation.

Finally measurement of the urinary excretion of the AQP2 water channel may provide an index of collecting duct function. As AQP2 channels are shuttled to and from the apical membrane of the collecting duct in response to AVP (see earlier), some AQP2 protein is shed into the urine. In normal individuals the amount of AQP2 in the urine is increased by water deprivation, vasopressin infusion, or hypertonic saline administration and is decreased by water loading.[380, 381] Kanno and colleagues[380] examined the urinary excretion of AQP2 in a small group of patients with diabetes insipidus. Patients with either central or nephrogenic diabetes insipidus excreted low amounts of AQP2 at baseline and the values did not increase after fluid deprivation. After an infusion of desmopressin, however, the urinary AQP2 excretion

increased promptly in the patients with central diabetes insipidus but remained low in patients with nephrogenic diabetes insipidus.[380] All the patients with nephrogenic diabetes insipidus in that study had familial forms of the disease (see later). Further studies will be required to determine if urinary AQP2 excretion is abnormal in acquired forms of nephrogenic diabetes insipidus as well. In any case, measurement of urinary AQP2 excretion does not provide any advantage over the measurement of urine osmolality following vasopressin administration in separating patients with central and nephrogenic diabetes insipidus.

THERAPY

Estimation of Free Water Deficit. Patients with diabetes insipidus, either central pituitary or nephrogenic, may require emergency treatment for hypertonic encephalopathy consequent to polyuria and inadequate water intake. The goal in treating hypertonic encephalopathy is to replenish body water thereby restoring osmotic homeostasis and repleting cell volume at a rate that avoids significant complications. Because the brain adjusts to hypertonicity (at least in part) by increasing the intracellular solute content via the accumulation of "idiogenic osmoles"[382, 383] (see later), the rapid repletion of body water with ECF dilution causes translocation of water into cells and can cause cerebral edema. Accordingly seizures occur in up to 40% of patients treated for severe hypernatremia by rapid infusion of hypotonic solutions.[384] If slower water repletion is undertaken brain cells lose the accumulated intracellular solutes and osmotic equilibration can occur without cell swelling. A good rule of thumb is to administer fluids at a rate that reduces the serum sodium concentration by about 1 mmol/L every 2 h.

The magnitude of acute water loss when hypernatremia is due to water loss exclusively can be estimated by using the assumption that the total ECF sodium content has remained nearly constant. This concept can be formulated as follows:

$$\text{Body water}_N \times [\text{Na}^+]_N = \text{body water}_H \times [\text{Na}^+]_H$$

where the subscript N denotes total body water and serum sodium concentration in the normal state and the subscript H denotes the same values in the hypertonic state. Because body water is approximately 60% of body weight in kilograms this equation can be rearranged to obtain

$$\text{Water deficit} = 0.6 \times \text{BW} \times ([\text{Na}^+] - 140)/140$$

As stressed earlier, this formulation is most applicable when there is no deficit in total ECF sodium content. In hypernatremic states with net sodium deficits the formulation underestimates the total water deficit.

The choice of fluid to be administered in diabetes insipidus depends on three factors: whether circulatory collapse is present, the rate at which hypernatremia developed, and the magnitude of the hypernatremia. Hypotonic NaCl solutions or oral fluids are appropriate as initial therapy in patients with modest volume contraction and mild elevations of serum sodium levels, i.e., Na$^+$ less than 160 mmol/L. Five percent glucose solutions may be used to replenish body water in acute hypernatremia in the absence of significant circulatory collapse but the infusion rate must be less than the rate of glucose metabolism to avoid glycosuria; otherwise the resulting osmotic diuresis will thwart attempts to replenish body free water. However with more severe hypernatremia, particularly if it has developed gradually over more than 24 h and is accompanied by circulatory collapse, it is appropriate to administer normal saline solutions for two reasons: (1) normal saline is dilute relative to body fluid osmolality and thus will dilute the latter while minimizing the risk of iatrogenic cerebral swelling and (2) at the same time normal saline provides an effective means of volume expansion.

TABLE 10–8. Therapy of Central Diabetes Insipidus

Type of Therapy	Dose	Route	Duration of Action (h)	Usage/Comments
AVP replacement				
Aqueous vasopressin	5–10 U	SC, IM	4–6	Useful for diagnostic testing; acute management after trauma or surgery
Vasopressin tannate in oil	1.5–5 U	IM	24–72	Long-term management failures can be due to improper mixing of emulsion Side effects includes smooth muscle contraction, angina, abdominal cramps
Lysine vasopressin	5–10 U	Nasal spray	4–6	Short-acting, relatively nonirritating
Desmopressin	5–20 μg	Nasal drops	12–24	Preferred drug
	10–40 μg	Nasal spray	12–24	Side effects are few
	1–4 μg	SC	12–24	
	0.1–0.8 mg	PO	12	
Adjunctive therapy				
Thiazide diuretics, e.g., hydrochlorothiazide	50–100 mg/d	PO	12–24	Also useful in nephrogenic diabetes insipidus Na$^+$ loading diminishes effectiveness
Chlorpropamide	250–750 mg/d	PO	24–36	Useful only in partial central diabetes insipidus Hypoglycemia is not uncommon
Clofibrate	250–500 mg every 6–8 h	PO	6–8	Useful only in partial central diabetes insipidus Side effects are frequent

AVP, arginine vasopressin; SC, subcutaneous; IM, intramuscularly; PO, orally.

Chronic Therapy. Because the most troublesome manifestations of central diabetes insipidus are persistent polyuria, inevitable nocturia, and constant thirst, the goal of treatment is to reduce the daily volume of urine excretion. Patients with partial hormonal deficiency and urine volumes of 2 to 6 L daily may require no treatment as long as they have access to water. For most patients, however, the therapy for central diabetes insipidus is some form of AVP replacement. Hormone preparations differ in the mode of administration and the duration of biologic effect (Table 10–8).

Aqueous vasopressin is active for only a few hours and is not practical for long-term therapies, although nasal sprays of aqueous lysine vasopressin may be used for intermittent relief of polyuria.[332, 341] Neither of these preparations prevents nocturia.

A widely used preparation in the past was vasopressin tannate in oil given intramuscularly. As little as 1.5 U (0.3 mL) daily may provide adequate hormone levels for 24 to 48 h.[332, 341] Great care must be exercised in preparing the injection by careful warming and mixing of the ampule to suspend the hormone uniformly in the oil. Failure to do so may result in injection of the oil vehicle alone and thus in apparent vasopressin resistance. Pain at injection sites and sterile abscesses are frequent and recurrent abdominal pain may result from the effect of vasopressin on intestinal motility.

A synthetic analogue of vasopressin, desmopressin (DDAVP, see earlier), provides antidiuretic activity for 8 to 20 h with negligible pressor effect, can be taken as nasal drops or as a nasal spray, and is the drug of choice for both adults and children.[332, 341, 385] The drug is best started at night to find the lowest dose that prevents nocturia. This dose, usually 5 to 10 μg intranasally, can be given twice daily or can be doubled as a single morning dose. A nasal catheter is calibrated for convenient dosing in the 5- to 20-μg range. Headache and flushing may be troublesome side effects with large doses but usually disappear with a reduction of dosage.[386] A parenteral formulation is available for patients who are unable to take the drug by nasal insufflation. The parenteral route is also effective when desmopressin is used for its hemostatic effects in patients with uremia or von Willebrand's disease. Desmopressin can also be given by mouth[387, 388] but the bioavailability of oral desmopressin is low. Accordingly the doses required for oral administration are higher than those for the nasal

route,[388] the recommended starting dose being 0.05 mg twice a day with subsequent dose adjustment to provide optimal water balance.

For patients having some residual AVP production the oral hypoglycemic agent chlorpropamide may provide adequate amelioration of symptoms. Chlorpropamide was originally thought to stimulate AVP release[389] but there is now general agreement[332, 341, 385, 389, 390] that it enhances the action of AVP on renal tubules to augment urine-concentrating ability.

The mechanism of the potentiating effect is unclear. Chlorpropamide may enhance AVP stimulation of renal medullary cAMP by augmenting adenylate cyclase sensitivity to AVP or by inhibiting phosphodiesterase.[341] Inhibition of PGE$_2$ synthesis, thereby removing an antagonist of AVP, may also be involved in chlorpropamide potentiation.[341] Finally in microdissected tubules from normal and AVP-deficient Brattleboro rats, AVP-stimulated cAMP accumulation is enhanced in mTALH of chlorpropamide-treated animals,[391] and chlorpropamide treatment might augment AVP-dependent NaCl absorption in mTALH, thereby increasing the driving force for water absorption in collecting ducts.

Doses of 250 to 750 mg chlorpropamide daily reduce polyuria in between 50 and 80% of patients with partial central diabetes insipidus.[341] Hypoglycemia, which is common in children and in patients taking more than 500 mg daily of the drug, limits its usefulness.

The hypolipidemic agent clofibrate[392] and the anticonvulsant carbamazepine[393] may also curtail polyuria in patients with partial central diabetes insipidus. Both drugs seem to work by stimulating the release of AVP from the hypothalamus and carbamazepine may also increase the sensitivity of the kidney to AVP.[394] The combination of clofibrate and chlorpropamide is useful on some patients.[341]

Finally thiazide diuretics may reduce urine volume in patients with all forms of diabetes insipidus, i.e., either central or nephrogenic, by causing mild salt depletion. This depletion causes a secondary increase in isotonic proximal tubular fluid absorption and a decrease in the volume of fluid delivered to the collecting duct. The effect is produced by 50 to 100 mg of hydrochlorothiazide daily, is sustained by salt restriction, and can be abolished by salt loading even with continued diuretic administration.[395]

Patients with diabetes insipidus, either central or nephrogenic, should carry some form of identification, such as a Medic-Alert bracelet, to warn physicians and emergency workers of their condition in the event of an accident or hypertonic encephalopathy (see later).

Nephrogenic Diabetes Insipidus

Nephrogenic diabetes insipidus is a polyuric disorder characterized by normal rates of renal filtration and solute excretion, a persistently hypotonic urine, normal or high levels of plasma AVP, and a failure of exogenous vasopressin to raise urine osmolality or reduce urine volume. Some of the conditions associated with a failure of the renal tubule to respond to AVP are noted in Table 10–9.

A review of hereditary diabetes insipidus[396, 397] was published in 1945 by Forssman who added new data on five kindreds involving 32 male patients:[398] male-to-male transmission does not occur; descendants of phenotypically normal males are healthy; polyuria invariably has its onset in infancy; daily urine volumes in adults exceed 4 L; urine specific gravity values after water deprivation are in the range of 1.003 to 1.008; and female carriers frequently have unusual thirst, nocturnal water consumption, and impaired urine-concentrating ability after water deprivation. In three affected men from one kindred, water deprivation and injections of posterior pituitary extracts failed to reduce urine volume or increase urine specific gravity. In 1947 Williams and Henry[399] applied the term *nephrogenic diabetes insipidus* to the disease and concluded that renal tubular insensitivity to AVP is the primary pathophysiological disturbance.

CLINICAL MANIFESTATIONS. The picture in dehydrated patients with nephrogenic diabetes insipidus is one of volume contraction, hypernatremia, and hyperthermia attended by potentially lethal effects, particularly on the CNS.[400] Because of the nonspecific nature of symptoms in early stages, the disorder may be difficult to identify in the first few months of life. Mental and physical retardation may occur or children with the disorder may have normal intelligence and normal physical maturation. Inadequate caloric ingestion associated with incessant water intake accounts for growth retardation, and repeated bouts of hypernatremia may lead to mental impairment.[349]

RENAL FUNCTION. The cardinal abnormality is the failure of collecting ducts to increase water permeability in response to AVP, causing excretion of urine that is hypotonic to plasma. The concentrating defect is due to end organ refractoriness to AVP because doses of vasopressin sufficient

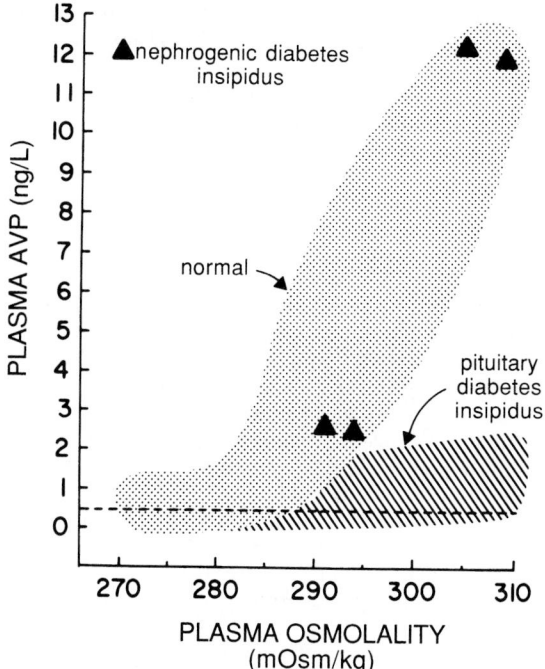

Figure 10–22. Relation between plasma AVP levels and serum osmolality in normal subjects, in patients with central diabetes insipidus, and in patients with nephrogenic diabetes insipidus. (Adapted from Robertson GL, Mahr EA, Athar S, et al. Development and clinical application of a new method for the radioimmunoassay of arginine vasopressin in human plasma. Adapted from the Journal of Clinical Investigation, 1973, vol. 52, pp. 2340–2352 by copyright permission of the American Society of Clinical Investigation; and Robertson GL. Vasopressin in osmotic regulation in man. Adapted, with permission, from the Annual Review of Medicine, Vol. 25, © 1974 by Annual Reviews Inc.)

to cause abdominal cramps and cutaneous blanching have no effect on urine volume and concentration.[399]

As in some patients with central diabetes insipidus[374] the dilation of the urinary tract may progress to hydroureter, hydronephrosis, and a urinary bladder capacity of more than 1 L.

SERUM VASOPRESSIN LEVELS. In normal subjects and in patients with nephrogenic diabetes insipidus, serum osmolality values higher than 280 mmol/L cause near-linear increases in serum AVP concentrations, whereas in patients with central diabetes insipidus, plasma AVP concentrations change negligibly or not at all in response to an osmotic challenge (Fig. 10–22).[97, 98] Normal subjects and patients with central diabetes insipidus also exhibit a near-linear relationship between urine osmolality and plasma AVP concentrations, whereas patients with nephrogenic diabetes excrete a consistently hypotonic urine despite 15-fold variations in plasma AVP levels. These observations confirm that familial nephrogenic diabetes insipidus is due to end organ unresponsiveness to AVP.

PATHOPHYSIOLOGY. In normal individuals or in patients with central diabetes insipidus, administration of exogenous vasopressin increases the rate of urinary cAMP excretion. In the majority of patients with familial nephrogenic diabetes insipidus, however, vasopressin and desmopressin have little or no effect on cAMP excretion,[401–403] whereas epinephrine stimulates cAMP excretion normally in these individuals.[403] Thus the defect is specific to AVP responses and appears to reside at a pre-cAMP locus.

The lack of response to vasopressin is restricted to the responses mediated by the V_2 receptor. V_1 receptor–mediated effects, such as vasoconstriction and enhancement of corticotropin release and renal prostaglandin production, are preserved in familial nephrogenic diabetes insipidus.[404, 405] Extra-

TABLE 10–9. Causes of Nephrogenic Diabetes Insipidus

Familial
X-linked
Autosomal recessive (rare)

Acquired
Tubulointerstitial renal disease
  Sickle cell disease or trait
  Amyloidosis
  Polycystic kidney disease
  Obstructive uropathy
  Medullary sponge kidney
Electrolyte Disorders
  Hypokalemia
  Hypercalcemia
Drugs
  Lithium
  Demeclocycline
  Methoxyflurane
  Amphotericin B
  Vincristine
Pregnancy

renal vasopressin effects mediated by V_2 receptors include an increase in levels of von Willebrand's factor and factor VIII, a fall in diastolic blood pressure, and stimulation of renin release. In most patients with familial nephrogenic diabetes insipidus these extrarenal V_2 receptor–mediated responses are absent, indicating a generalized defect in the V_2 receptor signal transduction pathway.[403, 406] Obligate carriers of the disorder, e.g., mothers of affected individuals, have intermediate extrarenal responses to the administration of the selective V_2 agonist desmopressin. In occasional families extrarenal V_2 receptor–mediated responses are preserved.[407, 408]

MOLECULAR BASES OF FAMILIAL NEPHROGENIC DIABETES INSIPIDUS

Two Genes* (AVPR2 and AQP2), *One Disease: Familial or Congenital Nephrogenic Diabetes Insipidus. Since polyuric manifestations are usually present during the first week of life, familial nephrogenic diabetes insipidus is also known as congenital nephrogenic diabetes insipidus. This rare entity is secondary either to mutations in the *AVPR2* gene that codes for the AVP antidiuretic (V_2) receptor or to mutations in the *AQP2* gene[240, 409, 410] that codes for the AVP-dependent water channel.[258, 411] Of 75 families with congenital nephrogenic diabetes insipidus referred to our laboratory in Montreal, 71 families have *AVPR2* mutations and 4 have *AQP2* mutations.

The Human V_2 Receptor Gene, AVPR2, Is Located in Chromosome Region Xq28. The human V_2 receptor[235, 236] is encoded by a 2-kb gene that contains the entire coding sequence on three exons separated by two small introns, 100 base pairs of 5' untranslated sequence with a putative TATA (Goldberg-Hogness) box and 460 base pairs of 3' untranslated sequence terminating at the polyadenylation signal (Fig. 10–23).[412, 413] The gene is located in the telomeric region of the long arm of the X chromosome (Xq28),[235, 413–415] the same region as the nephrogenic diabetes insipidus locus deduced from restriction fragment length polymorphism analysis.[416]

The first mutation identified in individuals with nephrogenic diabetes insipidus was a single base deletion causing a shift in the open reading frame in a North American family.[417] Since then approximately 72 different *AVPR2* mutations have been reported in 102 unrelated families with the disorder.[240, 418–426]

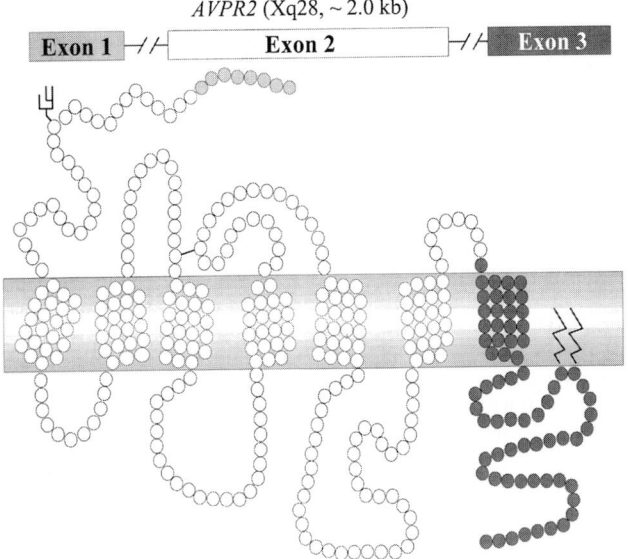

AVPR2 (Xq28, ~ 2.0 kb)

Figure 10–23. Exon/intron organization of the *AVPR2* gene and secondary structure model of the human V_2 receptor. The depicted membrane topology is consistent with the hydropathy profile of the polypeptide chain of the V_2 receptor and assumed to be analogous to that of bacteriorhodopsin, a bacterial light-driven pump. Similar models have been proposed for the V_1, V_3, and oxytocin receptors.

Incidence, Population Genetics, Ancestral Mutations and De Novo Mutations, and Mechanisms of AVPR2 Mutations. X-linked nephrogenic diabetes insipidus[427] is a rare recessive X-linked disease.[428, 429] In Quebec the incidence of this disease among males is approximately 4 in 1 million.[430] A founder effect for a particular *AVPR2* mutation in Ulster Scot immigrants increased the prevalence of X-linked nephrogenic diabetes insipidus in Nova Scotia, where it affects 24 in 1000 males in some communities. The W71X mutation is the cause of nephrogenic diabetes insipidus in the extended "Hopewell" kindred[431] and in families in the Canadian Maritime provinces[432, 433] and is also thought to result from a founder effect although a common ancestor has not been identified in all cases. Among X-linked nephrogenic diabetes insipidus patients in North America the W71X mutation is the common mutation.

The diversity of *AVPR2* mutations (described in Fig. 10–24) in different ethnic groups (whites, Japanese, blacks, Africans) and the rareness of the disease is consistent with an X-linked recessive disease that was lethal in the past for male patients and was balanced by new mutations in the gene. Loss of mutant alleles from the population occurs because of the higher mortality of affected males compared with normal males, whereas gain of mutant alleles occurs by mutation. If affected males with a rare X-linked recessive disease do not reproduce at a normal rate and if mutation rates are equal in mothers and fathers, at equilibrium as many as one third of new cases of affected males will be due to new mutations.[434] The origins of new mutations could be identified or inferred in 18 families and included five maternal gametes, nine grandpaternal gametes, two grandmaternal gametes, one great-grandmaternal gamete, and one gamete of grandpaternal or grandmaternal origin.[412, 418, 419, 421] Figure 10–25 illustrates the identification of a new mutation.

Eleven different *AVPR2* mutations are present in more than one family that does not appear to share a common ancestor, suggesting that there are hot spots for mutations. For example mutations at serine 167 have been described in at least eight unrelated families.[418, 419, 421, 422] These data are reminiscent of those obtained from patients with late-onset autosomal dominant retinitis pigmentosa in which many different mutations (>100) are spread throughout the coding region of the rhodopsin gene.[435, 436] Seven of nine mutations at the CpG nucleotide in the *AVPR2* gene (V88M, R113W, R137H, S167L, R181C, R202C, and R337X) are recurrent mutations, i.e., they have arisen de novo in unrelated families. The hypermutability of methylated CpG dinucleotides[439] is a frequent cause of single base pair substitution. Thirteen of 18 small deletion or insertion mutations (1 to 35 base pairs) involved direct or complementary repeats (2 to 9 base pairs) or strings of four to six guanines. This finding suggests that these deletions, like many others that have been described in other genes, resulted from DNA strand slippage and mispairing during replication.[439] Examples of mutations generated by the slipped mispairing model are presented in Figure 10–26.

Expression of* AVPR2 *Mutants. The cause of impairment of function of 28 different V_2 mutations has been studied in cells transiently or stably transfected with plasmids encoding the mutant receptors.[420, 438–441] A classification of these mutation analogues to the classification of low-density lipoprotein receptor mutations[442] has been proposed by Tsukaguchi and co-workers[420] to explain the molecular pathophysiology of the disease. Type 1 mutations reach the cell surface but have impaired binding; type 2 mutations are not transported normally to the cell surface; and type 3 mutations are ineffectively translated or rapidly degraded, or both.

A defect in protein processing has been found in the mutants L44P and W164S and in mutations with substitutions at codon 167 (S167L, S167T).[441] These mutant proteins lack

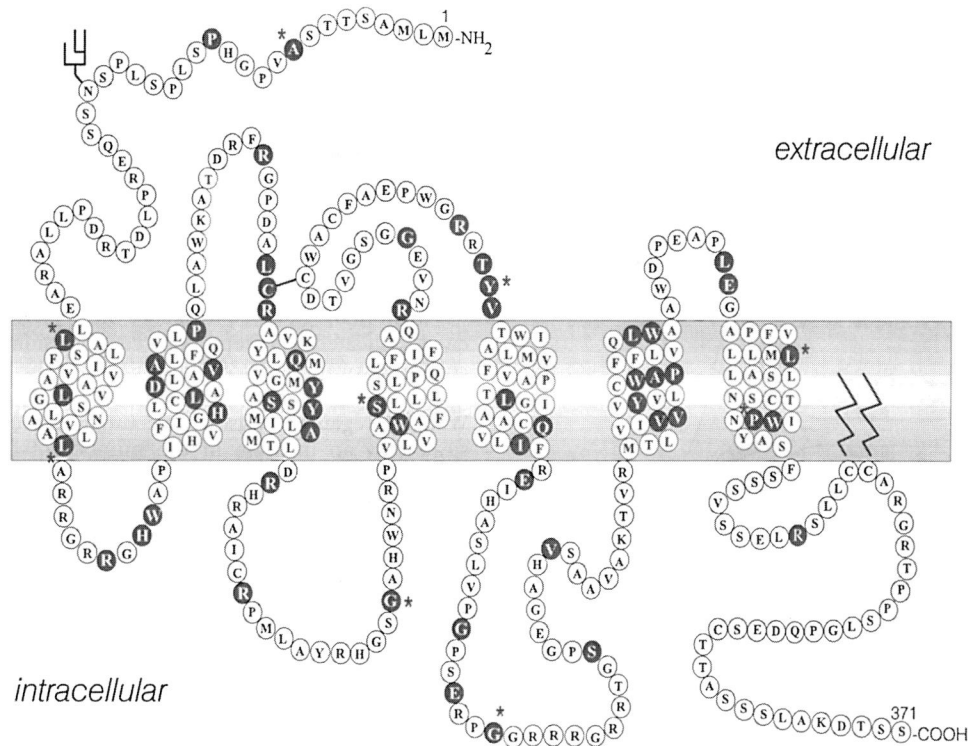

Figure 10–24. Schematic representation of the V_2 receptor and identification of 72 *AVPR2* mutations, which include 36 missense, 10 nonsense, 18 frameshift, 2 inframe deletion, 1 splice-site, and 5 large deletion mutations. The five large deletions are incompletely characterized and are not included in the figure. Predicted amino acids are given as the one-letter code. Solid symbols indicate the predicted location of the mutations; an asterisk indicates two different mutations in the same codon. The names of the mutations were assigned according to the conventional nomenclature. The extracellular (E_I to E_{IV}), cytoplasmic (C_I to C_{IV}), and transmembrane domains (TM_I to TM_{VII}) are labeled from the N terminus to the C terminus according to Sharif and Hanley (Nature 357:279–280, 1992). E_I: 98del28, 98ins28, 113delCT. TM_I: L44F, L44P, L53R, L62P. TM_I and C_I: 253del35, 255del9. C_I: 274insG, W71X. TM_{II}: H80R, L83P, D85N, V88M, 337delCT, P95L. E_{II}: R106C, 402delCT, C112R, R113W. TM_{III}: Q119X, Y124X, S126F, Y128S, A132D. C_{II}: R137H, R143P, 528del7, 528delG. TM_{IV}: W164S, S167L, S167T. E_{III}: R181C, G185C, R202C, T204N, 684delTA, Y205C, V206D. TM_V: L219R, Q225X, 753insC. C_{III}: E231X, 763delA, 786delG, E242X, 804insG, 804delG, 834delA, 855delG. TM_{VI}: V277A, V278, Y280C, W284X, A285P, P286L, P286R, L292P, W293X. E_{IV}: 977delG, 982–2A→G. TM_{VII}: L312X, P322H, P322S, W323R. C_{IV}: R337X.

complex glycosylation and are expressed at low levels, probably due to misfolding, retention in the endoplasmic reticulum, and subsequent degradation. However, most mutations impair the transport of the V_2 receptor to the cell surface.

Missense mutations in the first (R113W)[439] and second extracellular loops (R181C and R202C)[420, 440] have a lowered or nondetectable binding affinity for AVP, supporting the assumption that these loops are the binding site for AVP.[443, 444] In addition the missense mutations Y128S,[440, 445] in the second transmembrane domain, and P286R,[440] in the sixth transmembrane domain, cause a complete loss of AVP-binding activity

although the mutant receptors are expressed at the cell surface. A decrease or loss of binding activity may also be the primary defect of the L44F mutation at the junction of the extracellular N terminus and the first transmembrane domain.[441] This would explain why this mutant, although normally processed and therefore most likely expressed on the cell surface, is not capable of stimulating adenylate cyclase in response to AVP. The missense mutation R137H,[438] in the second intracellular loop close to the third transmembrane domain, does not affect binding affinity for AVP but abolishes stimulation of adenylate cyclase, indicating that residues of

Figure 10–25. Parental origin of a de novo mutation. The mother of the affected male (solid symbol) is a carrier of the S167L mutation. None of her three sisters carries this mutation although all the daughters received the same haplotype from their father. These data are consistent with a new mutation arising during spermatogenesis in the maternal grandfather of the patient. The distance spanned by the markers is sufficiently large that recombination between the markers has been observed.[419] In this pedigree the affected male inherited a recombinant chromosome; recombination occurred between *AVPR2* and *G6PD*. (From Fujiwara TM, Morgan K. Molecular biology of diabetes insipidus. Annu Rev Med 1995; 46:331–343, with permission. © 1995 Annual Reviews Inc.)

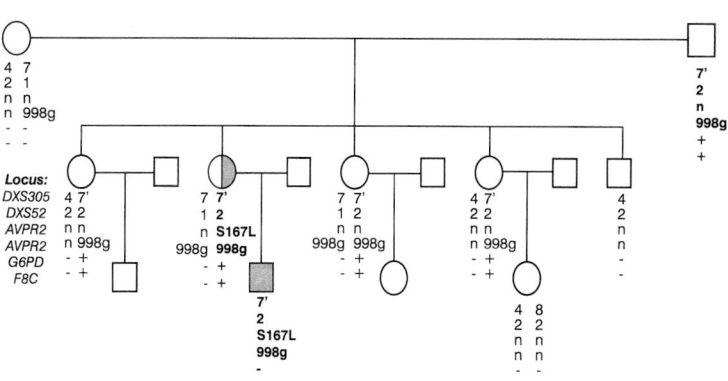

cation of mutations in *AVPR2* and *AQP2* allows the early diagnosis and management of at-risk members of families with identified mutations. We encourage physicians who follow families with X-linked nephrogenic diabetes insipidus to recommend mutation analysis before the birth of a male infant because early diagnosis and treatment can avert the physical and mental retardation associated with episodic dehydration. Diagnosis of X-linked nephrogenic diabetes insipidus within 48 hours of birth was made by testing of cord blood DNA[419] in three patients. These neonatal diabetes insipidus patients were treated with abundant water intake, a low-sodium diet, and hydrochlorothiazide; they have had no episodes of dehydration and their physical and mental development is normal. Early diagnosis of autosomal recessive nephrogenic diabetes insipidus is equally important to avoid repeated episodes of dehydration.

DRUG-INDUCED NEPHROGENIC DIABETES INSIPIDUS.
AVP-unresponsive hyposthenuria can occur in patients receiving demeclocycline; both the concentrating defect and the unresponsiveness to AVP are reversible and disappear after discontinuing the drug.[453] In toad urinary bladder serosal demeclocycline inhibits the increase in water permeability produced by either AVP or cAMP.[453] In human renal medulla demeclocycline noncompetitively inhibits basal adenylate cyclase activity, AVP-stimulated adenylate cyclase activity, and cAMP-dependent protein kinase activity but does not affect cyclic nucleotide phosphodiesterase activity.[454] These in vitro observations suggest that demeclocycline-induced nephrogenic diabetes insipidus may be due to inhibition of both cAMP accumulation and the action of cAMP on urinary membranes.[453]

Methoxyflurane anesthesia can also cause vasopressin-resistant polyuria and hyposthenuria. Both fluoride and oxalic acid, which are metabolic products of methoxyflurane, contribute to the nephrotoxicity but the polyuric state is due to the inorganic fluoride alone,[453] which causes vasopressin-resistant polyuria in dogs[455] and reduces collecting duct water permeability in rats without affecting salt transport in the ascending limb.[456]

Finally serum lithium concentrations of 0.5 to 1.5 mmol/L, the therapeutic range for affective disorders, can produce AVP-resistant diabetes insipidus in 12 to 30% of patients; the disorder is usually reversible when lithium is discontinued although several months may be required for full restoration of concentrating ability.[453]

Lithium induces nephrogenic diabetes insipidus by impairment of cAMP production in the collecting duct[457] although the precise mechanism is unclear. Acute exposure of rabbit collecting ducts to lithium inhibits the action of G_s[458] and chronic exposure of rats to lithium inhibits adenylate cyclase through stimulation of G_i.[459] Chronic treatment with lithium may also blunt urine concentrating capacity by reducing the expression of AQP2 water channels in the renal medulla.[460] This reduction in water channel expression is partially reversed 1 wk after discontinuing lithium. The latter finding may explain why lithium-induced polyuria may persist for weeks or months after stopping the drug.[461]

DIAGNOSIS. Familial nephrogenic diabetes insipidus is characterized by onset during infancy; a positive family history; persistent thirst, polyuria, and hyposthenuria that is unresponsive to the administration of vasopressin; and serum AVP levels that vary appropriately with changes in serum osmolality (see Fig. 10–22). In the absence of dehydration renal function is normal. Likewise acquired drug-induced nephrogenic diabetes insipidus is characterized by vasopressin-resistant polyuria. In the water deprivation test described earlier (see Fig. 10–21) urine osmolality achieved at maximal dehydration in patients with nephrogenic diabetes insipidus increases by less than 10% after administration of vasopressin.

TREATMENT. There is no specific therapy. Adequate hydration is easily achieved by oral intake in children and adults but sometimes requires parenteral supplementation in infants. Hydration is essential to prevent the damaging effects of hypernatremia and circulatory collapse, particularly in children. Although polyuria can be minimized by reducing solute intake this measure is rarely necessary except in children. Neither vasopressin nor its analogues lysine vasopressin and desmopressin have any effect on the disease. Likewise drugs that stimulate endogenous AVP release, such as clofibrate,[392] or that enhance AVP action, such as chlorpropamide,[391] are also ineffective.

Nonsteroidal anti-inflammatory drugs reduce the urine volume and free water clearance in children with nephrogenic diabetes insipidus.[462–465] Indomethacin is used most frequently. An agent such as sulindac, which does not inhibit renal prostaglandin synthesis, would not be expected to be effective. In one comparison ibuprofen was not as effective as indomethacin in reducing urine volume.[465] The effect of nonsteroidal anti-inflammatory drugs appears to be secondary to a reduction in the delivery of solute to the distal tubule rather than to an alleviation of prostaglandin antagonism to the tubular action of AVP.

An effective therapy for nephrogenic diabetes insipidus is to produce mild volume depletion, thereby reducing urine volume, nocturia, and dilation of the urinary bladder and ureters. The most widely used approach is the combination of thiazide diuretics and mild salt depletion.[395] With volume depletion the fractional absorption of fluid in the proximal tubule is increased, resulting in less solute and fluid delivery to the distal nephron and therefore less urine output. Thiazide diuretics may lead to hypokalemia, which may further aggravate the renal concentrating defect. The combination of amiloride, a potassium-sparing diuretic, and thiazides is less likely to produce hypokalemia and may have an additive effect in decreasing urine volume.[466, 467] Amiloride is particularly effective in limiting the polyuria in lithium-induced diabetes insipidus.[468, 469]

Mineralocorticoid Excess

Mild hypernatremia (serum sodium concentration >145 mmol/L) often occurs in syndromes of primary mineralocorticoid excess. The hypernatremia is due to an increase in the osmotic threshold for AVP release as a result of chronic hypervolemia (see Fig. 10–9). Reduction of the effective circulating volume with diuretics corrects the hypernatremia. Hypokalemia related to mineralocorticoid excess can impair renal concentrating ability, as discussed later, and can contribute to hypernatremia.

Electrolyte Disorders

Both potassium depletion and hypercalcemia can cause concentrating defects manifested primarily as a limitation in maximal renal concentrating ability rather than as persistent hyposthenuria. In hypokalemia the defect in concentrating ability usually occurs when both GFR and urine-diluting ability are near normal.

Several factors may contribute to the genesis of hypokalemic polyuria. The Na^+ concentrations and osmolalities of the renal medulla and papilla are both decreased.[470] The polyuria is also associated with an increased excretion of PGE_2, and the administration of indomethacin, which inhibits prostaglandin synthesis, can partially correct the concentrating defect.[471] In addition Berl and co-workers[472] suggested that potassium depletion results in polydipsia, thus accentuating polyuria independently of the concentrating defect.

In hypercalcemic states the concentrating defect is accompanied by a reduction in GFR. Additional factors may include the reduction in medullary solute content[173] and inhibition by calcium of adenylate cyclase activation by AVP in hormone-sensitive epithelia.[474] As mentioned previously, increases in extracellular calcium level inhibit AVP-sensitive adenylate cyclase activity in the mTALH.[248] Increases in the intracellular calcium level also inhibit the AVP-induced cAMP accumulation in the collecting duct.[248, 288]

Pregnancy

Diabetes insipidus is a rare complication of pregnancy.[71, 475–477] This disorder has features of both central and nephrogenic diabetes insipidus and is thought to be caused by the degradation of circulating AVP by the enzyme vasopressinase.[69, 71, 72, 475, 476] The polyuria usually begins in the third trimester and resolves spontaneously after delivery. Plasma AVP levels are low but polyuria may not respond to exogenous vasopressin. In contrast, desmopressin promptly controls the polyuria.[71, 476] The serum contains high levels of vasopressinase,[71] a cysteine aminopeptidase that degrades AVP but not desmopressin. Serum vasopressinase activity falls after delivery. In pregnant women the turnover rate of AVP normally increases during the later stages of pregnancy, presumably because of the high activity of vasopressinase in the placenta,[70] and women with subclinical forms of central diabetes insipidus may be the ones who experience symptomatic polyuria during pregnancy caused by the increased rate of AVP catabolism.[69]

Nephrogenic diabetes insipidus has also been reported during pregnancy. This condition, which is characterized by high plasma AVP levels and no response to either exogenous vasopressin or desmopressin, also remits after delivery. The pathogenesis is not known.[478]

Women with pre-existing diabetes insipidus are generally managed with desmopressin. Because this drug is not metabolized by placental vasopressinase the dosage does not need to be adjusted during pregnancy. Use of desmopressin during pregnancy does not appear to cause fetal morbidity or mortality.[479]

Osmotic Diuresis

A type of vasopressin-resistant polyuria that can be confused with nephrogenic diabetes insipidus is osmotic diuresis. This syndrome is commonly iatrogenic and is typically seen in intensive care or postoperative patients who receive infusions of large volumes of colloid or saline and in patients with uncontrolled diabetes mellitus. Analysis of the fluid therapy and measurement of the urine solute excretion rate generally are sufficient to diagnose this problem.

In diabetes insipidus, either nephrogenic or central, the polyuria represents a true water diuresis and the solute excretion rate is normal. In contrast, the urine during an osmotic diuresis is nearly isotonic and the solute excretion rate is elevated. Thus the finding of isotonic or hypertonic urine in a polyuric patient usually indicates osmotic diuresis. The reason for this is that the excretion of a normal solute load (800 mmol/d) in isotonic urine (300 mmol/d) obligates only 2.7 L of urine daily. Urine volumes greater than 3 L/d therefore require either an increased solute excretion rate or hypotonic urine. Treatment is achieved by reducing the rate of solute administration.

Osmotic diuresis also affects the plasma sodium concentration. The accumulation of either exogenous solutes, e.g., glycerol or mannitol, which are given to reduce intracranial pressure, or endogenous solutes, e.g., glucose in uncontrolled diabetes mellitus, can cause plasma hypertonicity. The serum sodium concentration, however, may be normal or even reduced in the face of an elevated measured serum osmolality.

Comparison of the measured osmolality and the calculated osmolality provides a clue to the diagnosis of these disorders.

Osmotic diuresis may also cause true hypernatremia (see Table 10–5). In the initial phases of an osmotic diuresis, patients are hypertonic because of accumulation of nonsodium solutes but are not hypernatremic. As the nonsodium solutes are excreted the plasma osmolality falls slightly because of a positive free water balance (see Fig. 10–11B), whereas sodium is left to represent an increasing fraction of the plasma osmolality; i.e., as the nonsodium osmolality decreases the sodium osmolality increases. Thus osmotic diuresis per se does not cause hypertonicity but results in the conversion of a normonatremic hypertonic state to a hypernatremic hypertonic state.

Hypertonic Encephalopathy

The consequences of the hypertonic syndromes—more specifically, disorders in which ECF osmolality is increased with solutes that are excluded from cells—include hypertonic encephalopathy and volume contraction. Virtually all cells, including those of the CNS, are permeable to water. Accordingly an increase in ECF osmolality inevitably causes osmotic equilibration between cells and ECF and consequently an increase in intracellular osmolality. This equilibration may occur in one of three ways: (1) in acute hypertonic states water is lost from cells and the acute shrinkage in brain volume results in hypertonic encephalopathy; (2) in chronic hypertonic states CNS cells accumulate solutes and brain shrinkage is minimized so that CNS symptoms are also minimized; or (3) a combination of these two processes may occur.[382] In other words, the relations among increases in effective ECF osmolality, changes in brain volume, and the occurrence of hypertonic encephalopathy depend on the magnitude of the ECF osmolality increase, the duration of the increase, and the solute responsible for the osmolality increase.

Hypernatremia may cause irreversible damage to the CNS, particularly in infants. An example of this phenomenon occurred in 1962 when a group of infants was inadvertently given a nursery formula containing salt rather than sugar and hypernatremic encephalopathy developed, with more than a 50% fatality rate.[480] In rabbits neurologic symptoms commence when the serum osmolality reaches 350 to 375 mmol/L; nystagmus and ataxia occur at a serum osmolality value of 375 to 400 mmol/L; and coma, stupor, and death occur when the serum osmolality value is in the range of 400 to 435 mmol/L.[481]

Because hypernatremic encephalopathy and death can occur in the absence of pathologic changes in the CNS other than brain shrinkage and an increase in brain NaCl content[482] the combination of hyperosmolality and cellular shrinkage is probably the major factor responsible for the encephalopathy.[382]

Cell Volume Adjustments to Extracellular Fluid Hypertonicity

The adjustments in brain cell volume and in the cellular content of osmotically active solutes during acute (1 to 2 h) and chronic (2 h to 2 wk) increases in osmolality produced by endogenous and exogenous solutes are shown in Table 10–10. Although these data derive from experiments involving animals,[382, 483] similar changes are believed to occur during the development of hypertonic states in humans. The term *idiogenic osmoles* refers to osmotically active solutes measured as the difference between total cell osmolality and the sum of the osmolalities of Na^+, K^+, and Cl^-.[484]

During acute increases in osmolality caused by endogenous or exogenous solutes, osmotic equilibrium between intracellular and extracellular water is achieved almost completely

TABLE 10–10. Brain Volume Adjustment During Hyperosmolality

Variable	Adjustment for Endogenous Solutes			Adjustment for Exogenous Solutes
	Na+	Glucose	Urea	Mannitol, Glycerol, Sucrose
Acute (1–2 h) hyperosmolality				
Brain water	↓↓	↓↓	↓↓	↓↓
Electrolyte content	Normal	Normal	Normal	Normal
Idiogenic osmoles	Absent	Absent	Absent	Absent
Chronic (2 h–2 wk) hyperosmolality				
Brain water	Normal	Normal	Normal	↓↓
Electrolyte content	↑	↑	Normal	Normal
Idiogenic osmoles	↑↑↑	↑↑	↑	Absent

Data from Arieff AI, Guisado R, Lazarowitz VC. The pathophysiology of hyperosmolar states. In: Andreoli TE, Grantham JJ, Rector FC, eds. Disturbances in Body Fluid Osmolality. Bethesda: American Physiological Society, 1977: 227–250; and Chan PH, Fishman RA. Elevation of rat brain amino acids and idiogenic osmoles induced by hyperosmolality. Brain Res 1979; 161:293–301.

by cell water loss (see Table 10–10). In this case increases in intracellular Na+, K+, and Cl− concentrations account for the increase in cell osmolality, and idiogenic osmoles are absent. The rapid changes in brain cell volume appear to account for the CNS symptoms and the high mortality from acute increases in ECF osmolality (see earlier).

In chronic hypertonic states brain cell volume returns toward normal (volume regulatory increase) when the increase in osmolality is produced by endogenous solutes such as Na+, glucose, and urea but not with exogenous solutes such as glycerol, mannitol, or sucrose (see Table 10–10).[382] Why the exogenous solutes do not produce a brain cell volume regulatory increase is not understood but this result provides a rationale for the use of these solutes to reduce brain volume during episodes of cerebral edema.

The extent to which brain cell volume is regulated by solute or electrolyte uptake or by accumulation of organic idiogenic osmoles differs for different endogenous solutes. About 50 to 60% of the brain osmoles responsible for brain cell volume regulation during chronic hypernatremia are amino acids[382, 383] and the remaining 40 to 50% of cell volume regulation results from the cellular accumulation of Na+, K+, and Cl−. The transport mechanism that mediates intracellular accumulation of these ions has not been defined but may be similar to the coupled Na+,K+,2Cl− cotransport process (see Fig. 10–2) that is responsible for hypertonic volume regulation in other cells.[485] Dissipation of the hypernatremia-induced organic osmoles after returning to the isotonic state is not rapid but takes hours to a day.

During hyperglycemia brain volume regulation is by insulin-independent cellular uptake of glucose (20%), electrolyte uptake, and accumulation of idiogenic osmoles. These osmoles are not amino acids, however, and their nature is unknown. In contrast to the hypernatremia-induced amino acids, the idiogenic osmoles that accumulate during hyperglycemia dissipate rapidly with decreasing plasma glucose levels.[382] This difference may account for the clinical axiom that rapid reduction in serum sodium concentrations in diabetes insipidus patients with chronic hypernatremia is more dangerous than are reductions in plasma glucose concentrations during a 6- to 8-h period in patients with nonketotic hyperglycemic coma.

HYPOTONIC SYNDROMES

The hypotonic syndromes are derangements of the water repletion reaction (see Fig. 10–1) so that free water is not excreted at a rate sufficient to maintain the serum sodium concentration and the body fluid osmolality at normal values. Such a circumstance can occur for any of several reasons: (1) ingestion of a quantity of water that exceeds the capacity of the kidney to excrete it (primary polydipsia), (2) diminished

capacity to excrete a water load because of inadequate solute delivery to the diluting segment, and (3) diminished capacity to excrete a water load because of sustained nonosmotic release of AVP.

Classification

In principle, hyponatremia can develop if the rate of water intake exceeds the normal ability of the kidney to excrete free water, but the hyponatremia that occurs in primary polydipsia is generally slight, with serum sodium concentrations generally in the range of 135 mmol/L.[373] The usual reason for the mild hyponatremia in primary polydipsia may be inferred from Figure 10–10. In normal individuals salt abstraction in the TALH results in the formation of a dilute distal tubular fluid with an osmolality of approximately 50 mmol/kg and a volume of about 18 L, or approximately 10% of the GFR.[177] Thus, because patients with primary polydipsia generally ingest less than 18 L of water daily, they are protected from profound hyponatremia.

The most common reason for severe hyponatremia is a disturbance in the rate of water excretion due to an inability of the kidney to excrete a maximally dilute urine. Such inability can occur because of (1) a reduction in the rate of salt delivery to the diluting segment, (2) sustained nonosmotic AVP release, or (3) a combination of these factors. Table 10–11 presents a summary of the commonly encountered hyponatremic states based on this classification. Although the primary derangement in these disorders is a defect in the rate of renal free water excretion, the development of hyponatremia also requires that free water intake exceed the rate of free water excretion. In other words, the development of hyponatremia in the disorders listed in Table 10–11 also re-

TABLE 10–11. The Hypotonic Syndrome

Excessive water ingestion
Decreased water excretion
  Decreased solute delivery to diluting segments
    Starvation
    Beer potomania
  AVP excess
    Syndrome of inappropriate antidiuretic hormone
    Drug-induced AVP secretion
  AVP excess with decreased distal solute delivery
    Congestive heart failure
    Cirrhosis of the liver
    Nephrotic syndrome
    Cortisol deficiency
    Hypothyroidism
    Diuretic use
    Renal failure

AVP, arginine vasopressin.

quires that factors other than cellular shrinkage stimulate thirst.

Clinical Syndromes

Increased Water Ingestion

As noted, primary polydipsia alone rarely causes significant hyponatremia because of the large capacity of the kidney to excrete free water. However, polydipsia may cause severe hyponatremia in individuals with some underlying psychiatric illness.[486-488] Episodic polydipsia and hyponatremia occur in 3 to 5% of institutionalized patients with mental illness and polyuria occurs in more than 60% of institutionalized patients.[487] The cause of the polydipsia and hyponatremia is uncertain. Most patients have, in addition to polydipsia, some abnormality in water excretion such as excessive AVP secretion.[488-490] Carbamazepine, which is sometimes used to control agitation in psychotic patients, may also cause hyponatremia.[491, 492]

Reduced Salt Delivery to the Diluting Segment

A reduced rate of salt delivery to the TALH and, consequently, a reduction in the volume of dilute urine formed may be responsible for hyponatremia in patients with euvolemic disorders such as beer potomania[493, 494] and in the hyponatremia associated with volume contraction, such as adrenal insufficiency, and with edematous disorders, such as congestive heart failure or cirrhosis. An analysis of hyponatremia in association with sodium depletion was provided by McCance[495] who showed that salt depletion induced by sweating (involving 150 to 200 mmol of sodium) regularly led to hyponatremia. Harrington[496] evaluated the contribution of AVP to this derangement by comparing the hyponatremic response to sodium depletion in control rats and rats with hypothalamic diabetes insipidus (Fig. 10-29). The hyponatremic response to sodium depletion is similar in the two groups of animals, implying that water retention during sodium depletion can occur without AVP and that water ingestion in hyponatremia is driven by nonosmotic, volume-mediated factors.

Berliner and Davidson[497] subsequently showed that a diminished rate of sodium delivery to the diluting segment could result in concentrated urine in the absence of AVP and

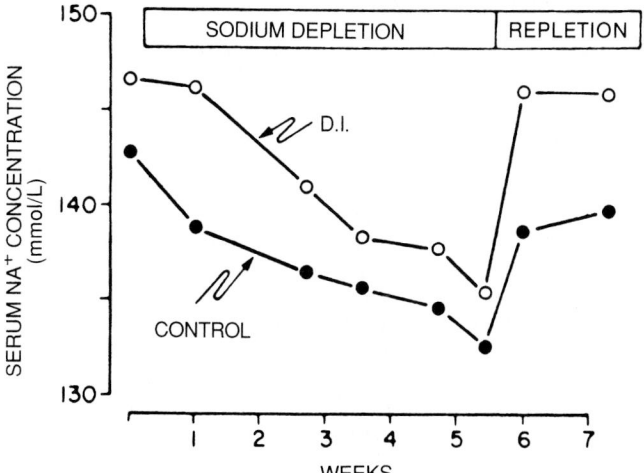

Figure 10–29. Hyponatremic response of normal and Brattleboro rats with diabetes insipidus to salt depletion. (Adapted from Harrington AR. Hyponatremia due to sodium depletion in the absence of vasopressin. Am J Physiol 1972; 222:768–774, with permission.)

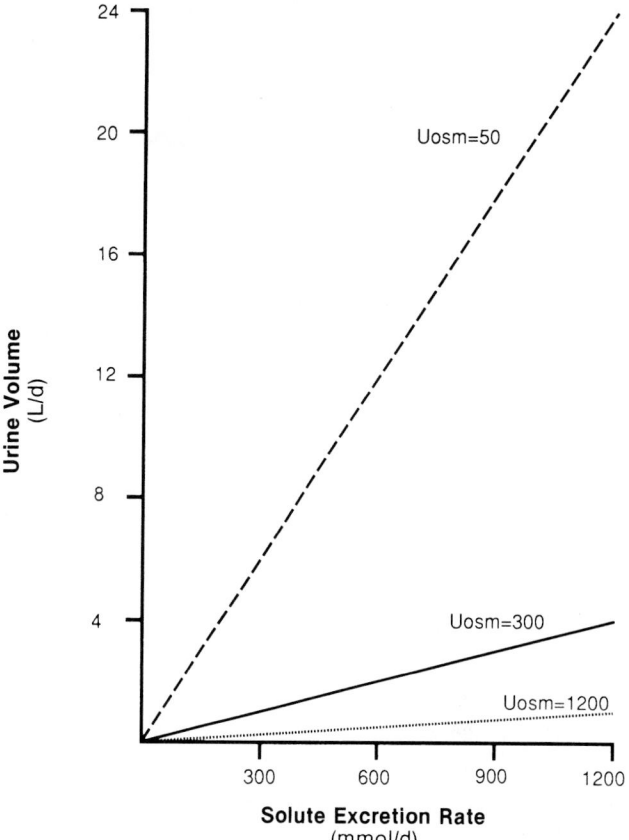

Figure 10–30. The relationship among daily solute excretion rate, urine osmolality (U_{osm}), and urine volume.

Edwards and co-workers[185] showed that this effect occurred with relatively small changes in the GFR. Because renal sodium retention is provoked[498] by an ECF volume loss as small as 200 mL (which corresponds to a sodium loss of approximately 28 mmol), even small sodium losses may compromise the renal excretion of free water.

Beer potomania is the prototype of hyponatremia resulting from a reduction in distal solute delivery. Individuals with beer potomania can acquire profound hyponatremia with urine osmolality in the range of 70 mmol/L and no weight loss.[493, 494] Thus the defect in free water excretion need not be in the degree to which urine is diluted maximally but in the amount of maximally dilute urine that is formed. Patients with beer potomania derive a large part of their caloric intake from beer, which contains little salt or protein. Because sodium and urea are the major solutes in normal urine, dietary sodium restriction increases the fractional rate of proximal sodium absorption, diminishes the rate of salt delivery to diluting segments, and limits the formation of dilute urine. The relationship between daily solute excretion and the formation of dilute urine is depicted in Figure 10–30. As the daily urine solute excretion falls, the maximal rate of urine formation is reduced. Moreover partial equilibration of reduced volumes of collecting duct fluid with the renal medullary interstitium further impairs the excretion of dilute urine. Hyponatremia related to reduced solute intake can also occur with starvation, particularly in the elderly, when solute intake may be dramatically reduced without parallel reductions in water intake.

Thus reduced solute intake may predispose subjects with primary polydipsia to the development of hyponatremia. With regard to Figure 10–30 consider, e.g., a polydipsic patient who excretes 800 mmol/d of solute. This patient could excrete up to 16 L of dilute (50 mmol/kg) urine daily. If the solute excretion rate were reduced to 300 mmol/d this same patient could excrete only 6 L of dilute urine. If more than this volume of water were ingested the excess would be retained and hyponatremia would ensue.

Mixed Derangements: Nonosmotic Vasopressin Release and Reduced Distal Solute Delivery

Hyponatremia occurs commonly in states of volume contraction and in edematous states such as congestive heart failure and cirrhosis. The former disorders include those in which both the ECF volume and total body water are reduced; the latter group includes states with deranged Starling forces such as local or systemic increases in venous pressure that result in inadequate filling of the arterial tree. In both types of disorders two factors may contribute, individually or in unison, to a renal defect in water excretion: (1) nonosmotic volume-mediated AVP release and (2) reductions in sodium delivery to the diluting segment.

As indicated in Figure 10–8 there is a linear relation between increases in plasma osmolality and increases in plasma AVP levels but a nonlinear relation between blood volume depletion and plasma AVP levels. Moreover with volume depletion the threshold for the osmotic release of AVP is reduced. Thus when blood volume is depleted more than 7 to 10%, plasma AVP levels rise and can produce an antidiuretic effect even when the plasma osmolality is less than normal.[97, 98] In other words, volume-mediated nonosmotic AVP release occurs when circulatory dynamics are moderately to severely advanced; in that circumstance volume-mediated stimuli mediate AVP release so that hyponatremia ensues. Accordingly low urine osmolality does not exclude the possibility of volume-mediated AVP release in a hyponatremic patient. However, as shown in Figure 10–9, severe plasma hypotonicity suppresses AVP release even in the presence of volume depletion.

A second cause of hyponatremia in volume-contracted states is the inability to dilute urine because the rate of sodium delivery to diluting segments in the TALH is reduced.[185, 493–499] The significance of volume contraction in this type of hyponatremia can be gauged, as indicated earlier, by noting that hyponatremia occurs during volume contraction in Brattleboro rats with hypothalamic diabetes insipidus.[496, 499] Finally the hyponatremia in volume-contracted states requires that water ingestion continue in the face of hypotonicity. Presumably, volume-mediated mechanisms drive thirst in such circumstances.

VOLUME-EXPANDED STATES. Hyponatremia occurs in advanced stages of disorders characterized by edema formation and a reduced effective circulating volume, particularly in intractable heart failure and hepatic cirrhosis with ascites. As noted earlier, reduced rates of salt delivery to diluting segments in these disorders contribute to the impairment in water excretion. Plasma AVP levels in patients with heart failure or severe ascites are inappropriately high with respect to the plasma osmolality.[500] Furthermore because nonosmotic AVP release occurs only with significant reductions in blood volume (see Fig. 10–8), hyponatremia in congestive failure or cirrhosis indicates profound arterial underfilling, a concept that fits with the ominous prognosis of hyponatremia in these disorders.

VOLUME-CONTRACTED STATES. The hyponatremia in volume-contracted states may be rationalized most readily, as indicated earlier, in terms of a reduction in sodium delivery rates to the loop of Henle and consequently a reduction in the rate of renal free water formation. Thus hyponatremia commonly accompanies prolonged administration of diuretics.[493, 501] In this regard two factors warrant particular consideration.

First, the most commonly used diuretics include loop diuretics such as furosemide, bumetanide, and ethacrynic acid and terminal nephron diuretics such as the thiazides, triamterene, spironolactone, and amiloride. Because loop diuretics inhibit salt absorption in the mTALH[179, 180] they inhibit both renal concentrating and diluting power[502] (see Fig. 10–10). In contrast, thiazide diuretics inhibit salt absorption in cortical rather than medullary diluting segments and consequently inhibit renal dilution but not renal concentration.[502] Accordingly, the risk of diuretic-induced hyponatremia is greater with thiazides than with furosemide.

Second, Fichman and colleagues[503] have described a group of patients in whom diuretic-associated hyponatremia referable to thiazide diuretics persisted even after correction of sodium depletion but was corrected with potassium repletion. These authors postulated that potassium depletion may cause sustained AVP release because approximately half the patients had relatively hypertonic urine. Alternatively a portion of the hyponatremia may have been due to the polydipsia that accompanies potassium depletion[472] or to a dipsogenic effect of thiazide diuretics.[504]

It is often impossible to distinguish between volume contraction and normovolemia on the basis of physical examination and history. In these cases the most reliable indicators of volume contraction are a low urine sodium concentration (<30 mmol/L) and the response to saline administration.[505] Thus patients with either volume expansion or volume contraction tend to have mixed disorders, whereas normovolemic patients usually have excess AVP as the primary pathogenic factor. Volume-expanded states can usually be detected on the basis of the history and physical examination.

ADRENAL INSUFFICIENCY. Hyponatremia may complicate untreated adrenal insufficiency. In mineralocorticoid deficiency the combination of ECF volume contraction, reduced GFR, enhanced proximal tubular salt absorption, and volume-mediated, nonosmotic AVP release is responsible for an inability to handle water loads.[493, 501, 506] In Brattleboro rats with hypothalamic diabetes insipidus, bilateral adrenalectomy causes hyponatremia that is partially reversed by the concomitant administration of glucocorticoids and salt[501]; thus in adrenal insufficiency volume depletion can cause hyponatremia even in the absence of AVP. Glucocorticoids are required for the complete correction of the defect in water excretion in adrenal insufficiency[493, 501] and glucocorticoid-mediated impairment of cardiac function may contribute to the reduction in effective circulating volume in adrenal insufficiency.[493]

Finally nonosmotic AVP release contributes to water retention.[507] Glucocorticoid-deficient rats have inappropriately high plasma AVP levels and an inability to excrete a water load[507, 508] and AVP antagonists largely correct the deficit in water excretion.[509] As noted earlier, AVP and CRH are coproduced by certain parvicellular neurons in the PVN[10] and both hormones are under negative feedback control by cortisol. After adrenalectomy the number of AVP-containing cells in this region increases[13] and AVP synthesis is increased in the absence of glucocorticoids.[14]

HYPOTHYROIDISM. The cause for the hyponatremia in hypothyroid patients is not clear. Hyponatremia might occur because of sustained AVP release[510] or because of a "reset osmostat,"[493] i.e., normal modes for regulating plasma osmolality but at reduced plasma osmolality levels. Alternatively, DeRubertis and co-workers[511] inferred that reduced salt delivery to the loop of Henle in hypothyroidism accounted for the defect in free water excretion. Regardless of the mechanism involved, restoration of the euthyroid state restores renal concentrating and diluting capacities.[512]

Vasopressin Excess

In the third group of disorders associated with hyponatremia, release of AVP is sustained in the absence of either osmotic or nonosmotic stimuli. By definition, therefore, the diagnosis requires that salt depletion is absent so that salt delivery to diluting segments is normal, effective circulating volume is not reduced, and there are no volume-mediated nonosmotic stimuli for AVP release. In general a primary excess of AVP occurs in two settings: in the syndrome of inappropriate vasopressin release (syndrome of inappropriate antidiuretic hormone [SIADH]) or as a consequence of drugs that enhance AVP release or action. Measurements of AVP levels indicate that SIADH is the most common cause of hyponatremia,[513–515] accounting for more than 95% of hyponatremia in hospitalized patients.[513, 514, 516]

SYNDROME OF INAPPROPRIATE ANTIDIURETIC HORMONE. Studies by Leaf and co-workers[517] in 1953 provided convincing evidence that the increments in urine salt excretion that accompany exogenous vasopressin administration are the result of hormone-induced volume expansion related to water retention rather than to a direct effect of AVP on renal tubular salt absorption (Fig. 10–31).

The administration of vasopressin, coupled with unrestricted fluid intake, initially results in hyponatremia, urine concentration and antidiuresis, and a weight gain of approximately 3 kg. After 3 d, body weight and serum sodium concentration approach a steady state and a natriuresis occurs; this natriuresis is termed *sodium escape*. Moreover when fluid is restricted, hyponatremia is corrected, body weight declines, and urine sodium excretion falls even in the face of continued vasopressin administration. Thus the natriuresis after 3 d of vasopressin administration is the consequence of volume expansion. The natriuresis with volume expansion, either hypotonic or isotonic, is in part due to a reduction in the fractional rate of proximal tubular salt absorption, i.e., to a resetting of glomerulotubular balance.[518] After prolonged vasopressin administration there may also be a partial escape from vasopressin action.[519]

In 1957 Schwartz and co-workers[520] provided the first clear account of SIADH in a patient with bronchogenic carcinoma, and the disorder has subsequently been observed in a variety of disorders, particularly pulmonary diseases such as bronchogenic carcinoma and cranial disorders.

In most patients with SIADH there is persistent production of AVP or an AVP-like peptide despite body fluid hypotonicity and an expanded effective circulating volume.[501, 521, 522] There are four patterns of serum AVP response to osmotic and nonosmotic stimuli in patients with SIADH:

1. The most common derangement (40%) is wide fluctuations of AVP levels independent of osmotic or nonosmotic control.

2. About a third of patients have a low osmotic threshold for AVP release but at higher osmolalities the correlation between plasma AVP levels and plasma osmolality is normal. These patients can maximally dilute urine if they are sufficiently hyponatremic.

3. In a fifth of patients, AVP release is sustained ("AVP leak") below serum osmolality values of 278 mmol/L and AVP release is normal in response to osmotic stimuli.

4. Approximately a sixth of patients have no detectable abnormality of AVP levels but fail to dilute urine maximally. The pathogenesis of this type of SIADH is poorly understood.

The fluid and electrolyte abnormalities in SIADH are illustrated in Figure 10–31. Specifically, as a result of the sustained release of AVP or AVP-like substances, retention of ingested water causes hyponatremia, modest volume expansion, and increased body weight of 5 to 10%. The volume expansion causes reduced rates of proximal tubular sodium absorption and a natriuresis, albeit at a total expansion of total body weight. Increased levels of ANP also contribute to the natriuresis. Aldosterone secretion is stimulated by hyponatremia and may contribute to reducing renal sodium losses in volume-expanded hyponatremic patients. There are also increased urinary losses of substances like uric acid, whose excretion rates vary directly with effective circulating volume and rates of sodium excretion. Consequently hypouricemia is common in SIADH. The GFR is normal as are adrenal and thyroid function.

PHARMACOLOGIC STIMULI. Hyponatremia can also result from drug therapy. As indicated earlier, diuretics can cause hyponatremia because of volume contraction or less commonly because of potassium depletion.[503] Certain agents (see Table 10–1) can stimulate AVP release or, as in the case of chlorpropamide, potentiate the effects of AVP on renal tubules. Thus either class of agents can result in an SIADH-like syndrome, namely sustained hyponatremia in the absence of a reduction in effective circulating volume.

Finally, as indicated earlier (see Fig. 10–18), renal medullary prostaglandins, particularly of the E series, inhibit salt absorption in the mTALH and antagonize the effects of AVP on collecting tubules. Prostaglandins also aid in the maintenance of glomerular blood flow during volume contraction.[523] Accordingly aspirin or other nonsteroidal anti-inflammatory drugs can, by interfering with prostaglandin synthesis, cause hyponatremia, particularly in patients with volume contraction.[524–526]

Pseudohyponatremia

In the disorders just discussed plasma hyponatremia is accompanied by parallel decreases in plasma osmolality, i.e., they are true hypotonic syndromes. In some patients, however, plasma hyponatremia may be associated with a normal or even an increased plasma osmolality, a situation referred to as *pseudohyponatremia* (Table 10–12). The importance of detecting pseudohyponatremia lies in the fact that attempts to increase the plasma sodium concentrations are contraindicated. In severe hyperlipidemia or hyperproteinemia the fractional volume of plasma that is composed of water may fall

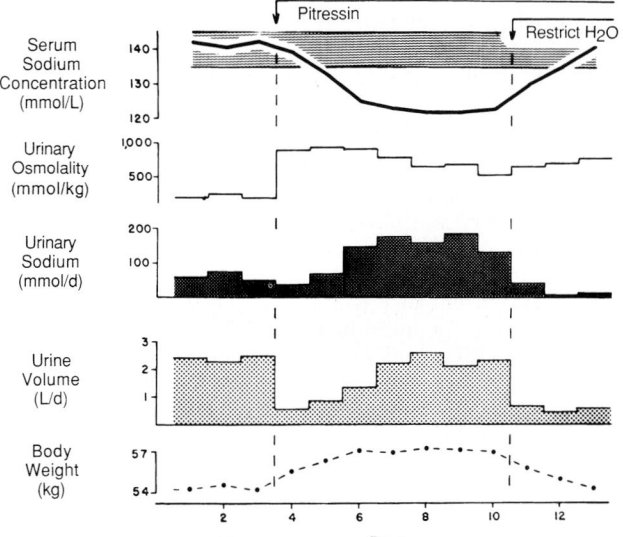

Figure 10–31. The role of volume expansion in vasopressin (Pitressin)-induced natriuresis. (Adapted from Goldberg M. Abnormalities in renal excretion of water. Med Clin North Am 1963; 47:915–933, with permission.)

TABLE 10–12. Causes of Pseudohyponatremia

Normal plasma osmolality
  Hyperproteinemia
  Hyperlipidemia
  Prostate surgery, with use of irrigant fluid containing glycine or sorbitol
Elevated plasma osmolality
  Hyperglycemia
  Mannitol
  Glycerol

from a normal range of 93 to 95% to 70 to 75%. Because sodium is confined to the aqueous phase, the sodium content of whole plasma, in millimoles per liter, falls in parallel with the fall in plasma water content. The plasma osmolality and the sodium concentration of the plasma water remain normal. Another reason for a falsely depressed sodium concentration in hyperproteinemia relates to hyperviscosity, as in multiple myeloma, in which resistance to flow may limit the delivery of plasma to automated flame photometers.

Pseudohyponatremia related to hyperlipidemia or hyperproteinemia is becoming less common because of advances in laboratory medicine.[527] The measurement of plasma sodium concentration by using sodium-selective electrodes assesses directly the activity of sodium dissolved in the aqueous phase of plasma and is not susceptible to the errors introduced by hyperlipidemia and hyperproteinemia.

Pseudohyponatremia may also occur after urologic procedures, typically transurethral prostatectomy,[528, 529] in which large amounts of isotonic irrigant fluid containing glycine or sorbitol can be absorbed and lower the plasma sodium concentration but not the plasma osmolality. Hence a comparison of the measured plasma osmolality and the calculated osmolality reveals an elevated osmolar gap (see later).[529]

As discussed in the section on osmotic diuresis, nonsodium solutes such as glucose or mannitol may create hypertonicity with a normal or low plasma sodium concentration. When these poorly permeable solutes are added to the ECF, an osmotic gradient is created that draws water out of cells and into the extracellular space and results in a dilutional hyponatremia. Indeed this effect is responsible for the efficacy of mannitol and glycerol in the treatment of increased intracranial pressure. Again measurement of plasma osmolality discloses these conditions. Except in hyperglycemia the measured plasma osmolality exceeds the calculated osmolality to produce an osmolar gap. The other common causes of an increased osmolar gap—e.g., ethanol, methanol, isopropanol, and ethylene glycol—are solutes that are freely permeable through cell membranes and do not cause shifts of water and hyponatremia.

Water Intoxication

The syndrome of water intoxication[530] varies in severity, depending on the degree and duration of hyponatremia. In acute hyponatremia with serum sodium concentrations of less than 120 mmol/L, the disorder is characterized by somnolence, seizures, coma, and mortality rates as high as 50%[531, 532] and the autopsy findings are those of cerebral edema.[532] In animals made acutely hyponatremic there is a reduction in brain electrolyte concentrations and in brain osmolality and a mortality rate of approximately 85%.[532]

Chronic hyponatremia differs from the acute form in two respects: (1) approximately half of patients with chronic hyponatremia are asymptomatic, even with serum sodium concentrations less than 125 mmol/L and (2) the fatality rate is nil in asymptomatic patients and is approximately 10 to 15% in symptomatic patients.[531] In animals chronic hyponatremia causes a greater decrease in brain sodium, potassium, and

chloride levels and organic osmolyte concentrations for a given reduction in serum sodium concentration than does acute hyponatremia.[531, 533] Consequently in chronic hyponatremia there is less of an increase in brain water content for a given reduction in serum Na[+] level than in acute hyponatremia and a correspondingly lower mortality rate.[531, 532]

Several factors are responsible for the differences between acute and chronic hyponatremia. First, water permeability of the blood-brain barrier and brain cells is so high that osmotic equilibrium between brain and plasma occurs quickly. Second, in acute hyponatremia the approach to osmotic equilibrium between brain cells and the ECF involves primarily water gain that causes both the cerebral edema and the high fatality rates. Finally for a given reduction in serum Na[+] level, brain electrolyte concentrations and brain water content are lower in chronic than in acute hyponatremia. In other words, when hyponatremia occurs slowly solutes are extruded from cells so that osmotic equilibration between the brain and the ECF occurs with smaller increases in brain volume.

A wide variety of cell types exhibit a volume regulatory decrease (VRD) in response to a hypotonic ECF, i.e., an initial period of cellular swelling, in which the cell acts as an osmometer, and a subsequent period of cellular shrinkage accompanied by solute loss. The initial VRD response (<24 h) involves principally the loss of intracellular electrolytes through the activation of membrane transport processes other than Na[+],K[+]-ATPase, whose role in the VRD response is largely permissive. The nature of the solute efflux processes differs among various cell types.[534] In brain the initial VRD response involves principally a loss of intracellular KCl and NaCl,[532, 534, 535] and a subsequent brain VRD response over a period of days involves the loss of organic solutes.[536] In chronic hyponatremia the brain levels of taurine, *myo*-inositol, glycerophosphocholine, and creatine are reduced.[536–538]

The VRD response in chronic hyponatremia has major therapeutic implications. The rapid correction of chronic hyponatremia to normal leads to CNS disturbances, particularly in children. The reason for such an occurrence is that when the brain electrolyte content is adaptively reduced in chronic hyponatremia the rapid correction of serum sodium concentrations to normal levels will cause an acute hypertonic encephalopathy. Indeed central pontine myelinolysis can follow the rapid correction of hyponatremia both in animals[539] and in humans.[540–542]

Diagnosis and Treatment

The diagnosis of hyponatremia is most commonly made from routine laboratory findings. Hyponatremia should also be considered whenever there is a sudden deterioration in CNS function, particularly with intractable heart failure, hepatic cirrhosis and ascites, or the administration of large volumes of intravenous fluids.

The history and physical examination are generally adequate for recognizing disorders such as beer potomania, compulsive water ingestion, and the use of drugs that stimulate AVP release or enhance AVP action. The presence of edema is characteristic of individuals with hyponatremia due to a reduced effective circulating volume and ECF volume expansion. In hypothyroidism and adrenal insufficiency typical clinical and laboratory findings are generally present.

The most difficult differential diagnosis among hyponatremic disorders involves the distinction between patients with modest volume contraction and those who have SIADH. In both circumstances the serum sodium level and the serum osmolality are reduced and the urine osmolality is inappropriately high with respect to the reduced serum osmolality. Nonosmotic water conservation in SIADH and in volume contraction is recognized by the presence of a urine osmolality value higher than 120 to 150 mmol/L in association with reduced serum osmolality.

Patients with volume contraction may provide a history of volume losses or of diuretic ingestion and exhibit signs of ECF volume contraction. When the volume losses are due to extrarenal causes the urine sodium concentration is less than 10 to 15 mmol/L, and the fractional excretion of sodium is generally less than 1%. Hyperuricemia and azotemia are useful indices of volume contraction. In contrast, patients with SIADH are generally normovolemic or have slight volume expansion and therefore have no signs of volume contraction. The blood urea nitrogen and creatinine values are normal and the serum uric acid level is generally reduced. The urine sodium concentration usually exceeds 30 mmol/L and the fractional excretion of sodium is greater than 1%. Tests of adrenal function are normal.

The previously mentioned studies usually discriminate between SIADH and extrarenal volume contraction but when ECF volume contraction is due to renal salt wasting, urine sodium losses generally persist unless volume contraction is profound. A useful diagnostic and therapeutic maneuver in this situation is to observe the results of water restriction. When water intake is restricted to 600 to 800 mL daily patients with SIADH exhibit a highly characteristic response: a 2- to 3-kg weight loss accompanied by correction of hyponatremia and cessation of salt wasting usually over a period of 2 to 3 d. If weight loss fails to correct both hyponatremia and urine sodium wasting simultaneously the diagnosis of SIADH is doubtful. Rather renal sodium wasting with ECF volume contraction, related to adrenal insufficiency or the other renal salt-losing disorders listed in Table 10–11, is the more probable diagnosis.

Therapy

The goal of treatment is to correct body water osmolality and to restore cell volume to normal by raising the ratio of sodium to water in the ECF. The increase in ECF osmolality draws water from cells and therefore reduces their volume. The therapeutic approach, as well as whether net sodium and water balance is adjusted to be positive or negative during therapy, depends on the serum sodium concentration, the rate at which hyponatremia has developed, the clinical state, and the underlying disorder.

SYMPTOMATIC HYPONATREMIA. Severe hyponatremia with a serum sodium concentration less than 120 to 125 mmol/L and CNS manifestations requires immediate treatment. In states of volume contraction the treatment of choice is to raise the serum sodium level to 125 mmol/L by administering hypertonic (3 to 5%) saline. Because the desired effect is to correct osmolality, the amount of sodium that is administered must be sufficient to raise total body water osmolality to approximately 250 mmol/L, i.e., to approximately twice the desired serum sodium level. A convenient formula for calculating this sodium requirement is

$$[125 - \text{measured serum Na}] \times 0.6 \text{ body weight} = \text{required mmol of Na}$$

The serum sodium concentration is in millimoles per liter and the body weight is in kilograms. Because 60% of body weight is water, the formula allows an estimate of the amount of sodium required to raise body water osmolality to 250 mmol/L.

The administration of hypertonic saline is hazardous in volume-expanded, salt-retaining states such as congestive heart failure. Furthermore in SIADH associated with volume expansion and sodium wasting, hypertonic saline may be ineffective in correcting hyponatremia because the administered salt is excreted promptly in a relatively concentrated urine. In such

circumstances normal saline or hypertonic saline solutions may be used in combination with furosemide (Fig. 10–32).[543] The diuretic induces urine salt loss and therefore reduces the risk of ECF volume expansion. Moreover, as illustrated in Figure 10–32, the diuresis induced by furosemide is characterized by the excretion of dilute urine. Consequently the combination of intravenously administered normal or hypertonic saline and a furosemide-induced diuresis of urine that is dilute with respect to plasma provides an effective way of raising the serum sodium level in SIADH or other volume-expanded states. By adjusting the rates of salt administration to be less than urine salt losses, the ECF volume can be reduced simultaneously.

As indicated in the preceding section, the rapid elevation of serum sodium concentrations to levels greater than 125 mmol/L is potentially hazardous. Because loss of brain solute represents one of the compensatory mechanisms for preserving brain cell volume in dilutional states,[532–535] a serum sodium level of 140 mmol/L is relatively hypertonic to brain cells that are partially depleted of solute as a result of hyponatremia. Consequently, raising the serum sodium level rapidly to greater than 120 to 125 mmol/L can cause CNS damage such as central pontine myelinolysis.[534–536, 539–542, 544] Moreover, raising the serum sodium concentration to greater than 120 mmol/L is both hazardous and unnecessary.

The major, and still unresolved, controversy surrounding the treatment of hyponatremia concerns the rate at which hyponatremia should be corrected.[545, 546]

Mortality rates for severe hyponatremia of 33 to 86% have been cited in support of its prompt correction. These estimates, however, derive largely from single case reports and small series of patients and may overestimate the mortality from hyponatremia. In a prospective study of 33 patients with symptomatic hyponatremia there were no deaths.[547] Likewise in studies of patients with severe hyponatremia (serum sodium level less than 110 mmol/L) the mortality rate was 8%, with most deaths attributed to underlying diseases.[544, 548] Slow or delayed correction of hyponatremia was not associated with higher mortality or with neurologic complications. Indeed the risk of neurologic complications was greatest when serum sodium levels were corrected at a rate greater than 0.6 mmol/L/h (14 mmol/d).[544, 548] In part the discrepant mortality rates may relate to differences in the patient populations under study. Arieff and others[545, 547, 549–551] have described more than 80 healthy young women in whom symptomatic hyponatremia

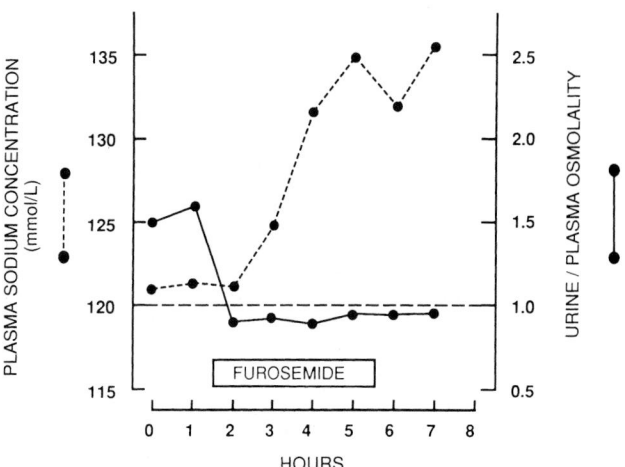

Figure 10–32. Effect of furosemide plus saline in treatment of hyponatremia in SIADH. (Modified from Hartman D, Rossier B, Fohlman R, et al. Rapid correction of hyponatremia in the syndrome of inappropriate secretion of antidiuretic hormone. Ann Intern Med 1973; 78:870–875, with permission.)

developed after elective surgery and who subsequently died or suffered permanent brain damage. Although women do not appear to be any more prone to the development of postoperative hyponatremia than are men, they have a 25-fold increased risk of death or permanent neurologic damage as a result of the hyponatremia.[551] Children also seem to be at increased risk of death or permanent neurologic damage from hyponatremia.[552] The gender and age differences are also seen in animal models of hyponatremia.[553–556] In rats the mortality from acute hyponatremia decreases steadily with increasing age and the mortality rate from chronic hyponatremia in adult male rats was 13% compared with 62% in adult females. The mortality rate in males was increased by estrogens, whereas the mortality rate in female rats was decreased by testosterone.[555] Finally the imposition of a hypoxic cerebral insult in the setting of hyponatremia increases the mortality rate dramatically.[557] Hypoxia or ischemia impairs the adaptive mechanisms to hyponatremia and results in worse cerebral edema than in uncomplicated hyponatremia.[557] This may have clinical relevance because many of the women described by Arieff and others[550, 551] had respiratory arrests in the course of the hyponatremia. In contrast the patients reported in the prospective studies tend to be older men who have underlying illnesses or are receiving diuretics. In these patients the hyponatremia does not carry as grave a prognosis.

As just noted, rapid correction of hyponatremia may lead to central pontine myelinolysis, a demyelinating lesion of the pons with destruction of myelin sheaths but sparing of the axis cylinders and nerve cells. The majority of patients have suffered from debilitating disease, malnutrition, or alcoholism and, occasionally, hyponatremia. The manifestations include flaccid quadriplegia or paraplegia, facial weakness, dysphagia, dysarthria, and coma. The role of the rate of correction of hyponatremia in its development remains uncertain.[543] For example the incidence of this disorder in hyponatremia is low and the rate of correction in patients who experience the complication is no faster than in those who do not.[545] Patients who have central pontine myelinolysis generally have additional risk factors, such as alcoholism or malnutrition, which could be responsible for the lesion. Finally the neurologic lesion that develops in hyponatremic patients often is not myelinolysis but rather a diffuse lesion that may be caused by anoxia.[547] In rats rapid correction of severe hyponatremia to normonatremic levels results in diffuse necrotic brain lesions, whereas rapid correction to mildly hyponatremic levels (serum sodium concentration of 139 mmol/L) does not.[558] Thus the extent of correction, as well as the rate of correction, may be important in the development of neurologic complications.

On the basis of available data it seems prudent to correct the sodium concentration at a rate of 0.5 mmol/L/h until the serum sodium concentration reaches 120 to 125 mmol/L. However, young women with acute symptomatic hyponatremia are at risk for respiratory arrest, severe neurologic sequelae, and death. It is reasonable to treat these patients with hypertonic saline to raise the serum sodium concentration to 125 mmol/L at a rate of 1 to 2 mmol/L/h.[544, 559] At this point the patient should be asymptomatic and the serum sodium concentration can be returned to normal gradually over several days with water restriction. Overcorrection of the serum sodium concentration (to greater than 130 mmol/L) is unnecessary and potentially harmful. Even in acute hyponatremia, symptoms and CNS signs are uncommon until the serum sodium concentration falls to less than 120 mmol/L. Patients with chronic hyponatremia may tolerate much greater degrees of hyponatremia.[542, 546]

ASYMPTOMATIC HYPONATREMIA. Mild asymptomatic chronic hyponatremia is generally managed by correction of the underlying disorder when the hyponatremia occurs in volume contraction or in salt-regaining states such as conges-

tive heart failure or hepatic cirrhosis with ascites. Chronic hyponatremia in SIADH may be easily corrected by restricting water intake to 800 to 1000 mL daily provided that patients can adhere to water restriction.

An alternative approach involves the use of lithium or demeclocycline, which interferes with the renal tubular effects of AVP. However, the response to lithium is variable and lithium itself causes multiple side effects, including renal tubular acidosis, cardiotoxicity, and thyroid dysfunction.[453, 457, 465, 468, 560] In contrast, demeclocycline reproducibly inhibits renal concentrating ability in SIADH patients.[560, 561] However, demeclocycline should be used cautiously in patients with liver disease because of the risk of toxic nephropathy produced by accumulation of the drug.[562] As another alternative some workers[563] have recommended reducing renal concentrating ability by administering oral urea loads that are sufficient to produce osmotic diuresis. A maneuver that is effective in patients who are not edematous, hypertensive, or in congestive heart failure is to administer oral furosemide (see Fig. 10–32) in association with a high-salt diet. Finally the competitive antagonists of AVP binding to renal tubular receptors[84] may be useful in the treatment of acute and chronic water intoxication. A nonpeptide AVP antagonist, OPC-31260, can be administered orally and was effective in increasing free water excretion in rats with either cirrhosis[564] or SIADH.[565] The short-term use of this agent in humans appears to be safe[566] but its therapeutic efficacy in the treatment of hyponatremia in humans is not established.

REFERENCES

1. Burg MB, Kador PF. Sorbitol, osmoregulation, and the complications of diabetes. J Clin Invest 1988; 81:635–640.
2. Blumenfeld JD, Grossman EB, Sun AM, et al. Sodium-coupled ion cotransport and the volume regulatory increase response. Kidney Int 1989; 36:434–440.
3. Bagnasco SM, Uchida S, Balaban RS, et al. Induction of aldose reductase and sorbitol in renal inner medullary cells by elevated extracellular NaCl. Proc Natl Acad Sci USA 1987; 84:1718–1720.
4. Morris JF. Organization of neural inputs to the supraoptic and paraventricular nuclei: anatomical aspects. Prog Brain Res 1983; 60:3–18.
5. Sawchenko PE, Swanson LW. The organization and biochemical specificity of afferent projections to the paraventricular and supraoptic nuclei. Prog Brain Res 1983; 60:19–29.
6. Vandesande F, Dierickx K. Identification of the vasopressin producing and of the oxytocin producing neurons in the hypothalamic magnocellular neurosecretory system of the rat. Cell Tissue Res 1975; 164:153–162.
7. Zimmerman EA, Robinson AG. Hypothalamic neurons secreting vasopressin and neurophysin. Kidney Int 1976; 10:12–24.
8. Morris JF, Sokol HW, Valtin H. One neuron—one hormone? In: Moses AM, Share L, eds. Neurohypophysis. Basel: S Karger, 1977: 58–66.
9. Zimmerman EA, Defendi R. Hypothalamic pathways containing oxytocin, vasopressin and associated neurophysins. In: Moses AM, Share L, eds. Neurohypophysis. Basel: S Karger, 1977: 22–29.
10. Sawchenko PE, Swanson LW, Vale WW. Co-expression of corticotropin-releasing factor and vasopressin immunoreactivity in parvocellular neurosecretory neurons of the adrenalectomized rat. Proc Natl Acad Sci USA 1984; 81:1883–1887.
11. Zimmerman EA, Silverman AJ. Vasopressin and adrenal cortical interactions. Prog Brain Res 1983; 60:493–504.
12. Whitnall MH, Mezey E, Gainer H. Co-localization of corticotropin-releasing factor and vasopressin in median eminence neurosecretory vesicles. Nature 1985; 317:248–252.
13. Kiss JZ, Mezey E, Skirboll L. Corticotropin-releasing factor—immunoreactive neurons of the paraventricular nucleus become vasopressin-positive after adrenalectomy. Proc Natl Acad Sci USA 1984; 81:1854–1858.
14. Davis LG, Arentzen R, Reid JM, et al. Glucocorticoid sensitivity of vasopressin mRNA levels in the paraventricular nucleus of the rat. Proc Natl Acad Sci USA 1986; 83:1145–1149.
15. Sugimoto T, Saito M, Mochizuki S, et al. Molecular cloning and functional expression of a cDNA encoding the human V_{1b} vasopressin receptor. J Biol Chem 1994; 269:27088–27092.
16. deKeyzer Y, Auzan C, Lenne F, et al. Cloning and characterization of the human V3 pituitary vasopressin receptor. FEBS Lett 1994; 356:215–220.
17. Cross BA, Dyball REJ, Dyer RG, et al. Endocrine neurons. Recent Prog Horm Res 1975; 31:243–294.
18. Carter DA, Lightman SL. Neuroendocrine control of vasopressin secretion. In: Baylis PH, Padfield PL, eds. The Posterior Pituitary. Hormone Secretion in Health and Disease. New York: Marcel Dekker, 1985: 53–118.

19. Sawchenco PE, Swanson LW. Central noradrenergic pathways for the integration of hypothalamic neuroendocrine and autonomic responses. Science 1981; 214:685–687.

20. Saper CB, Standaert DG, Currie MG, et al. Atriopeptin-immunoreactive neurons in the brain: presence in cardiovascular regulatory areas. Science 1985; 227:1047–1049.

21. Johnson AK, Cunningham JT. Brain mechanisms and drinking: the role of lamina terminalis–associated systems in extracellular thirst. Kidney Int 1987; 32:S35–S42.

22. Iitake K, Share L, Ouchi Y, et al. Central cholinergic control of vasopressin release in conscious rats. Am J Physiol 1986; 251:E146–E150.

23. Russell JA, Blackburn RE, Leng G. The role of the AV3V region in the control of magnocellular oxytocin neurons. Brain Res Bull 1988; 20:803–810.

24. Kamm O, Aldrich TB, Grote IW, et al. The active principles of the posterior lobe of the pituitary gland. J Am Chem Soc 1928; 50:573–601.

25. du Vigneaud V. Hormones of the mammalian posterior pituitary gland and their naturally occurring analogues. Johns Hopkins Med J 1969; 124:53–65.

26. du Vigneaud V. Experiences in the polypeptide field: insulin to oxytocin. Ann NY Acad Sci 1960; 88:537–548.

27. van Dyke HB, Chow BF, Greep RO, et al. The isolation of a protein from the pars neuralis of the ox pituitary with constant oxytocic, pressor and diuresis-inhibiting activities. J Pharmacol Exp Ther 1942; 74:190–209.

28. Pickering BT, Jones CW. Neurophysins. In: Li CH, ed. Hormonal Proteins and Peptides. Vol 5. New York: Academic, 1978: 103–158.

29. Archer R, Manoussos G, Olivry G. Sur les relations entre l'oxytocine et la vasopressine d'une part et la protéine de van Dyke d'autre part. Biochim Biophys Acta 1955; 16:155–156.

30. Robinson AG. Radioimmunoassay of neurophysin proteins: utilization of specific neurophysin assays to demonstrate independent secretion of different neurophysins in vivo. Ann NY Acad Sci 1975; 248:246–256.

31. Robinson AG. The neurophysins. In: Reichlin S, ed. The Neurohypophysis: Physiological and Clinical Aspects. New York: Plenum, 1984: 65–93.

32. Sachs H, Fawcett P, Takabatake Y, et al. Biosynthesis and release of vasopressin and neurophysin. Recent Prog Horm Res 1969; 25:447–484.

33. Sachs H, Takabatake Y. Evidence for a precursor in vasopressin biosynthesis. Endocrinology 1964; 75:943–948.

34. Takabatake Y, Sachs H. Vasopressin biosynthesis. III. In vitro studies. Endocrinology 1964; 75:934–942.

35. Brownstein MJ, Russell JT, Gainer H. Synthesis, transport and release of posterior pituitary hormones. Science 1980; 207:373–378.

36. Russell JT, Brownstein MJ, Gainer H. Time course of appearance and release of [^{35}S]cysteine labelled neurophysins and peptides in the neurohypophysis. Brain Res 1981; 205:299–311.

37. Land H, Schuetz G, Schmale H, et al. Nucleotide sequence of cloned cDNA encoding bovine arginine vasopressin–neurophysin II precursor. Nature 1982; 295:299–303.

38. Schmale H, Heinsohn S, Richter D. Structural organization of the rat gene for the arginine vasopressin–neurophysin II precursor. EMBO J 1983; 2:763–767.

39. Schmale H, Fehr S, Richter D. Vasopressin biosynthesis: from gene to peptide hormone. Kidney Int 1987; 32:S8–S13.

40. Riddell DC, Mallonee R, Phillips JA, et al. Chromosomal assignment of human sequences encoding arginine vasopressin–neurophysin II and growth hormone releasing factor. Somat Cell Mol Genet 1985; 11:189–195.

41. Gainer H, Sarne Y, Brownstein MJ. Neurophysin biosynthesis: conversion of a putative precursor during axonal transport. Science 1977; 195:1354–1356.

42. Schmale H, Richter D. Single base deletion in the vasopressin gene is the cause of diabetes insipidus in Brattleboro rats. Nature 1984; 308:705–709.

43. Scharrer E, Scharrer B. Hormones produced by neurosecretory cells. Recent Prog Horm Res 1954; 10:183–240.

44. Weinstein H, Malamed S, Sachs H. Isolation of vasopressin-containing granules from the neurohypophysis of the dog. Biochim Biophys Acta 1961; 50:386–389.

45. Russell JT, Brownstein MJ, Gainer H. Biosynthesis of vasopressin, oxytocin and neurophysins: isolation and characterization of two common precursors (propressophysin and prooxyphysin). Endocrinology 1980; 107:1880–1891.

46. Harris GW. The innervation and actions of the neurohypophysis: an investigation using the method of remote-control stimulation. Philos Trans Soc Lond (Biol) 1947; 232:425–439.

47. Wakerly JB, Poulain DA, Brown D. Comparison of firing patterns in oxytocin- and vasopressin-releasing neurones during progressive dehydration. Brain Res 1978; 148:425–440.

48. Hatton GI, Armstrong WE, Gregory WA. Spontaneous and osmotically-stimulated activity in slices of rat hypothalamus. Brain Res Bull 1978; 3:497–508.

49. Poulain DA, Wakerley JB. Electrophysiology of hypothalamic magnocellular neurones secreting oxytocin and vasopressin. Neuroscience 1982; 7:773–808.

50. Dreifuss JJ. A review on neurosecretory granules: their contents and mechanisms of release. Ann NY Acad Sci 1975; 248:184–201.

51. Sklar AH, Schrier RW. Central nervous system mediators of vasopressin release. Physiol Rev 1983; 63:1243–1280.

52. Sachs H, Haller EW. Further studies on the capacity of the neurohypophysis to release vasopressin. Endocrinology 1968; 83:251–262.

53. Dreifuss JJ, Kalnins I, Kelly JS, et al. Action potentials and release of neurohypophyseal hormones in vitro. J Physiol (Lond) 1971; 215:805–817.

54. Nordmann JJ. Stimulus-secretion coupling. Prog Brain Res 1983; 60:281–304.

55. Nordmann JJ, Dyball REJ. Effects of veratridine on Ca fluxes and the release of oxytocin and vasopressin from the isolated rat neurohypophysis. J Gen Physiol 1978; 72:297–304.

56. Nordmann JJ, Diayanithi G, Cazalis M. Coupling between the bioelectrical activity of a neurosecretory cell and the release at its terminals of neuropeptides. In: Schrier RW, ed. Vasopressin. New York: Raven, 1985: 375–383.

57. Bauman G, Dingman JF. Distribution, blood transport, and degradation of antidiuretic hormone in man. J Clin Invest 1976; 57:1109–1116.

58. Weitzman RE, Fisher DA. Arginine vasopressin metabolism in dogs. I: Evidence for a receptor-mediated mechanism. Am J Physiol 1978; 235:E591–E597.

59. Czaczkes JW, Kleeman CR, Koenig M. Physiologic studies of antidiuretic hormone by its direct measurement in human plasma. J Clin Invest 1964; 43:1625–1640.

60. Nitschke U, Balzar H. Die Inaktivierung von infundiertem Vasopressin bei Diabetes insipidus-Probanden. Acta Endocrinol 1969; 62:270–282.

61. Wilson KC, Weitzman RE, Fisher DA. Arginine vasopressin metabolism in dogs. II: Modeling and systems analysis. Am J Physiol 1978; 235:E598–E605.

62. Barth T, Krejci I, Kupkova B, et al. Pharmacology of cyclic analogues of deamino-oxytocin not containing a disulphide bond (carba analogues). Eur J Pharmacol 1973; 24:183–188.

63. Koida M, Glass JD, Schwartz IL, et al. Mechanism of inactivation of oxytocin by rat kidney enzymes. Endocrinology 1971; 88:633–643.

64. Marks N, Abrash L, Walter R. Degradation of neurohypophyseal hormones by brain extracts and purified brain enzymes. Proc Soc Exp Biol Med 1973; 142:455–460.

65. Cort JH, Schück O, Stribrna J, et al. Role of the disulfide bridge and the C-terminal tripeptide in the antidiuretic action of vasopressin in man and the rat. Kidney Int 1975; 8:292–302.

66. Walter R, Bowman RH. Mechanism of inactivation of vasopressin and oxytocin by the isolated perfused rat kidney. Endocrinology 1973; 92:189–193.

67. Nardacci NJ, Mukhopadhyay S, Campbell BJ. Partial purification and characterization of the antidiuretic hormone–inactivating enzyme from renal plasma membranes. Biochim Biophys Acta 1975; 377:146–157.

68. Shade RE, Share L. Renal vasopressin clearance with reductions in renal blood flow in the dog. Am J Physiol 1977; 232:F341–F347.

69. Lindheimer MD, Davison JM. Osmoregulation, the secretion of arginine vasopressin and its metabolism during pregnancy. Eur J Endocrinol 1995; 132:133–143.

70. Davison JM, Sheills EA, Barron WM, et al. Changes in the metabolic clearance of vasopressin and in plasma vasopressinase throughout human pregnancy. J Clin Invest 1989; 83:1313–1318.

71. Durr JA, Hoggard JG, Hunt JM, et al. Diabetes insipidus in pregnancy associated with abnormally high circulating vasopressinase activity. N Engl J Med 1987; 316:1070–1074.

72. Gordge MP, Williams DJ, Huggett NJ, et al. Loss of biological activity of arginine vasopressin during its degradation by vasopressinase from pregnancy serum. Clin Endocrinol 1995; 42:51–58.

73. Sawyer WH. Evolution of neurohypophyseal hormones and their receptors. Fed Proc 1977; 36:1842–1847.

74. Butlen D, Guillon G, Rajerison RM, et al. Structural requirements for activation of vasopressin-sensitive adenylate cyclase, hormone binding, and antidiuretic actions: effects of highly potent analogues and competitive inhibitors. Mol Pharmacol 1978; 14:1006–1017.

75. Barth T, Rajerison MR, Roy C, et al. Activation of rat kidney adenylate cyclase by vasopressin analogues: lack of correlation with antidiuretic activity. Mol Cell Endocrinol 1975; 2:69–80.

76. Hechter O, Terada S, Nakahara T, et al. Neurohypophyseal hormone-responsive adenylate cyclase. II: Relationship between hormonal occupancy of neurohypophyseal hormone receptor sites and adenylate cyclase activation. J Biol Chem 1978; 253:3219–3229.

77. Roy C, Barth T, Jard S. Vasopressin-sensitive kidney adenylate cyclase. Structural requirements for attachment to the receptor and enzyme activation: studies with vasopressin analogues. J Biol Chem 1975; 250:3144–3156.

78. Sawyer WH, Acosta M, Balaspiri L, et al. Structural changes in the arginine vasopressin molecule that enhance antidiuretic activity and specificity. Endocrinology 1974; 94:1106–1115.

79. Sawyer WH, Pang PKT, Seto J, et al. Vasopressin analogs that antagonize antidiuretic responses by rats to the antidiuretic hormone. Science 1981; 212:49–51.

80. Manning M, Sawyer WH. Synthesis and receptor specificities of vasopressin antagonists. J Cardiovasc Pharmacol 1986; 8:S29–S32.

81. Manning M, Klis WA, Olma A, et al. Design of more potent and selective antagonists of the antidiuretic responses to arginine vasopressin. J Med Chem 1982; 25:414–419.

82. Manning M, Nawrocka E, Misicka A, et al. Potent and selective antagonists of the antidiuretic responses to arginine vasopressin based on modification of [1-(β-mercapto-β,β-cyclopentamethylenepropionic acid) 2-D-isoleucine, 4-valine] arginine vasopressin at position 4. J Med Chem 1984; 27:423–429.

83. Manning M, Sawyer WA. Development of selective agonists and antagonists of vasopressin and oxytocin. In: Schrier RW, ed. Vasopressin. New York: Raven, 1985: 131–144.

84. Stassen FL, Heckman GD, Schmidt DB, et al. Actions of vasopressin antagonists: molecular mechanisms. In: Schrier RW, ed. Vasopressin. New York: Raven, 1985: 145–154.

85. Kinter LB, Huffman WF, Stassen FL. Antagonists of the antidiuretic activity of vasopressin. Am J Physiol 1988; 254:F165–F177.

86. Stassen FL, Erickson RW, Huffman WF, et al. Molecular mechanisms of novel antidiuretic antagonists: analysis of the effects on vasopressin binding and adenylate cyclase activation in animal and human kidney. J Pharmacol Exp Ther 1982; 223:50–54.

87. Kim JK, Schrier RW. Cellular effect of arginine vasopressin antagonist on the isolated renal tubule. In: Schrier RW, ed. Vasopressin. New York: Raven, 1985: 155–158.

88. Mann WA, Kinter LB, Stassen F, et al. Mechanism of action and structural requirements of vasopressin analog inhibition of transepithelial water flow in toad urinary bladder. J Pharmacol Exp Ther 1986; 238:401–406.

89. Verney EB. The antidiuretic hormone and the factors which determine its release. Proc Soc Lond (Biol) 1947; 135:25–105.

90. McKinley MJ, Denton DA, Weisinger RS. Sensors for antidiuresis and thirst—osmoreceptors or CSF sodium detectors? Brain Res 1978; 141:89–103.

91. Leng G. Rat supraoptic neurones: the effects of locally applied hypertonic saline. J Physiol (Lond) 1980; 304:405–414.

92. Leng G, Dyball REJ, Mason WT. Electrophysiology of osmoreceptors. In: Schrier RW, ed. Vasopressin. New York: Raven, 1985: 333–342.

93. Thrasher TN, Brown CJ, Keil LC, et al. Thirst and vasopressin release in the dog: an osmoreceptor or sodium receptor mechanism? Am J Physiol 1980; 238:R333–R339.

94. Thrasher TN, Keil LC, Ramsay DJ. Lesions of the organum vasculosum of the lamina terminalis (OVLT) attenuate osmotically-induced drinking and vasopressin secretion in the dog. Endocrinology 1982; 110:1837–1839.

95. Bealer SL, Crofton JT, Share L. Hypothalamic knife cuts alter fluid regulation, vasopressin secretion and natriuresis during water deprivation. Neuroendocrinology 1983; 36:364–370.

96. Honda K, Negoro H, Higuchi T, et al. Activation of neurosecretory cells by osmotic stimulation of anteroventral third ventricle. Am J Physiol 1987; 252:R1039–R1045.

97. Robertson GL, Mahr EA, Athar S, et al. Development and clinical application of a new method for the radioimmunoassay of arginine vasopressin in human plasma. J Clin Invest 1973; 52:2340–2352.

98. Dunn FL, Brennan JT, Nelson AE, et al. The role of blood osmolality and volume in regulating vasopressin secretion in the rat. J Clin Invest 1973; 52:3212–3219.

99. Robertson GL. Vasopressin in osmotic regulation in man. Annu Rev Med 1974; 25:315–322.

100. Robertson GL, Berl T. Water metabolism. In: Brenner BM, Rector FC Jr, eds. The Kidney. 3rd ed. Philadelphia: WB Saunders, 1986: 385–432.

101. Peters JP. Body Water. The Exchange of Fluids in Man. Springfield, IL: Charles C Thomas, 1935: 274–313.

102. Gauer OH, Henry JP. Circulatory basis of fluid volume control. Physiol Rev 1963; 43:423–481.

103. Sved AF. Central neural pathways in baroreceptor control of vasopressin secretion. In: Schrier RW, ed. Vasopressin. New York: Raven, 1985: 443–453.

104. Share L. Vasopressin, its bioassay and the physiological control of its release. Am J Med 1967; 42:701–712.

105. Gupta PD, Henry JP, Sinclair R, et al. Responses of atrial and aortic baroreceptors to nonhypotensive hemorrhage and to transfusion. Am J Physiol 1966; 211:1429–1437.

106. Wang BC, Sundet WD, Hakumäki MOK, et al. Vasopressin and renin responses to hemorrhage in conscious, cardiac-denervated dogs. Am J Physiol 1983; 245:H399–H405.

107. Caillens H, Pruszczynski W, Meyrier A, et al. Relationship between change in volemia at constant osmolality and plasma antidiuretic hormone. Miner Electrolyte Metab 1980; 4:161–171.

108. Stricker EM, Verbalis JG. Interaction of osmotic and volume stimuli in regulation of neurohypophyseal secretion in rats. Am J Physiol 1986; 250:R267–R275.

109. Quillen EW, Cowley AW. Influence of volume changes on osmolality-vasopressin relationships in conscious dogs. Am J Physiol 1983; 244:H73–H79.

110. Ross MG, Ervin MG, Leake RD, et al. Continuous ovine fetal hemorrhage: sensitivity of plasma and urine arginine vasopressin response. Am J Physiol 1986; 251:E464–E469.

111. Robertson GL. Physiology of ADH secretion. Kidney Int 1987; 32:S20–S26.

112. Schrier RW, Berl T, Anderson RJ, et al. Non-osmotic regulation of renal water excretion. Trans Am Clin Climatol Assoc 1976; 87:161–169.

113. McDonald KM, Kuruvila KC, Aisenbrey GA, et al. Effect of alpha and beta adrenergic stimulation on renal water excretion and medullary cyclic AMP in intact and diabetes insipidus rats. Kidney Int 1977; 12:96–103.

114. Sladek JR, McNeill TH. Simultaneous monoamine histofluorescence and neuropeptide immunocytochemistry. IV. Verification of catecholamine-neurophysin interactions through single section analysis. Cell Tissue Res 1980; 210:181–190.

115. Willoughby JO, Jervois PM, Menadue MF, et al. Noradrenaline, by activation of alpha-1-adrenoceptors in the region of the supraoptic nucleus, causes secretion of vasopressin in the unanesthetized rat. Neuroendocrinology 1987; 45:219–226.

116. Zhao BG, Chapman C, Brown D, et al. Opioid-noradrenergic interactions in the neurohypophysis. II: Does noradrenaline mediate the actions of endogenous opioids on oxytocin and vasopressin release? Neuroendocrinology 1988; 48:25–31.

117. Zhao BG, Chapman C, Bicknell RJ. Opioid-noradrenergic interactions in the neurohypophysis. I: Differential opioid receptor regulation of oxytocin, vasopressin and noradrenaline release. Neuroendocrinology 1988; 48:16–24.

118. Lind RW, Swanson LW, Ganten D. Organization of angiotensin II immunoreactive cells and fibers in the rat central nervous system. Neuroendocrinology 1985; 40:2–24.

119. Okuya S, Inenaga K, Kaneko T, et al. Antiotensin II sensitive neurons in the supraoptic nucleus, subfornical organ and anteroventral third ventricle of rats in vitro. Brain Res 1987; 402:58–67.

120. Iovino M, Steardo L. Vasopressin release to central and peripheral angiotensin II in rats with lesion of the subfornical organ. Brain Res 1984; 322:365–368.

121. Knepel W, Nutto D, Meyer DK. Effects of transection of subfornical organ efferent projections on vasopressin release induced by angiotensin or isoprenaline in the rat. Brain Res 1982; 248:180–184.

122. Tanaka J, Kaba H, Saito H, et al. Electrophysiological evidence that circulating angiotensin II sensitive neurons on the subfornical organ alter the activity of hypothalamic paraventricular neurohypophyseal neurons in the rat. Brain Res 1985; 342:361–365.

123. Usberti M, Federico S, Cianciaruso B, et al. Effects of angiotensin II on plasma ADH, PGE₂ synthesis and water excretion in normal man. Am J Physiol 1985; 248:F254–F259.

124. Usberti M, DiMinno G, Ungaro B, et al. Angiotensin II inhibition with captopril on plasma ADH, PG synthesis, and renal function in humans. Am J Physiol 1985; 250:F986–F990.

125. Morton JJ, Connell JM, Hughes MJ, et al. The role of plasma osmolality, angiotensin II and dopamine in vasopressin release in man. Clin Endocrinol 1985; 23:129–138.

126. Martin R, Voigt KH. Enkephalins co-exist with oxytocin and vasopressin in nerve terminals of rat neurohypophysis. Nature 1981; 289:502–504.

127. Iversen LL, Iversen SD, Bloom FE. Opiate receptors influence vasopressin release from nerve terminals in rat neurohypophysis. Nature 1980; 284:350–351.

128. Matsui K, Kimura T, Ota K, et al. Attenuation of the osmotic release of vasopressin by enkephalins in dogs. Am J Physiol 1989; 256:E270–E276.

129. Yamada T, Nakao K, Itoh H, et al. Inhibitory action of leumorphin on vasopressin secretion in conscious rats. Endocrinology 1988; 122:985–990.

130. Oiso Y, Iwasaki Y, Kondo K, et al. Effect of the opioid kappa-receptor agonist U50488H on the secretion of arginine vasopressin. Study on the mechanism of U50488H-induced diuresis. Neuroendocrinology 1988; 48:658–662.

131. Hoffman PK, Share L, Crofton JT, et al. The effect of intracerebroventricular indomethacin on osmotically stimulated vasopressin release. Neuroendocrinology 1982; 34:132–139.

132. Forsling ML, Ullmann EA. Non-osmotic stimulation of vasopressin release. In: Moses AM, Share L, eds. Neurohypophysis. Basel: S Karger, 1977: 128–135.

133. Manning PT, Schwartz D, Katsube NC, et al. Vasopressin-stimulated release of atriopeptin: endocrine antagonists in fluid homeostasis. Science 1985; 229:395–397.

134. Dillingham MA, Anderson RJ. Inhibition of vasopressin action by atrial natriuretic factor. Science 1986; 231:1572–1573.

135. Zimmerman EA, Ma L-Y, Nilaver G. Anatomical basis of thirst and vasopressin secretion. Kidney Int 1987; 32:S14–S19.

136. Poole CJM, Carter DA, Vallejo M, et al. Atrial natriuretic factor inhibits the stimulated in vivo and in vitro release of vasopressin and oxytocin in the rat. J Endocrinol 1987; 112:97–102.

137. Iitake K, Share L, Crofton JT, et al. Central atrial natriuretic factor reduces vasopressin secretion in the rat. Endocrinology 1986; 119:438–440.

138. Obana K, Natuse M, Inagami T, et al. Atrial natriuretic factor inhibits vasopressin secretion from rat posterior pituitary. Biochem Biophys Res Commun 1985; 132:1088–1094.

139. Crandall ME, Gregg CM. In vitro evidence for an inhibitory effect of atrial natriuretic peptide on vasopressin release. Neuroendocrinology 1986; 44:439–445.

140. Thrasher TN, Nistal-Herrera JF, Keil LC, et al. Satiety and inhibition of vasopressin secretion after drinking in dehydrated dogs. Am J Physiol 1981; 240:E394–E401.

141. Geelen G, Keil LC, Kravik SE, et al. Inhibition of plasma vasopressin after drinking in dehydrated humans. Am J Physiol 1984; 247:R968–R971.

142. Thrasher TN, Keil LC, Ramsay DJ. Drinking, oropharyngeal signals, and inhibition of vasopressin secretion in dogs. Am J Physiol 1987; 253:R509–R515.

143. Salata RA, Verbalis JG, Robinson AG. Cold water stimulation of oropharyngeal receptors in man inhibits release of vasopressin. J Clin Endocrinol Metab 1987; 65:561–567.

144. Seckl JR, Williams TDM, Lightman SL. Oral hypertonic saline causes transient fall of vasopressin in humans. Am J Physiol 1986; 251:R214–R217.

145. Arnauld E, duPont J. Vasopressin release and firing of supraoptic neurosecretory neurones during drinking in the dehydrated monkey. Pflugers Arch 1982; 394:195–201.

146. Robertson GL, Shelton RL, Athar S. The osmoregulation of vasopressin. Kidney Int 1976; 10:25–37.
147. Wood RJ, Rolls ET, Rolls BJ. Physiological mechanisms for thirst in the nonhuman primate. Am J Physiol 1982; R423–R428.
148. Nothnagel H. Durst und Polydipsie. Virchows Arch Pathol Anat Physiol 1881; 86:435–447.
149. Andersson B, Rundgren M. Thirst and its disorders. Annu Rev Med 1982; 33:231–239.
150. McKinley MJ, Denton DA, Leksell LG, et al. Osmoregulatory thirst in sheep is disrupted by ablation of the anterior wall of the optic recess. Brain Res 1982; 236:210–215.
151. Andersson B, McCann SM. Drinking, antidiuresis and milk ejection from electrical stimulation within the hypothalamus of the goat. Acta Physiol Scand 1956; 35:191–201.
152. Phillips MI, Hoffman WE, Bealer SL. Dehydration and fluid balance: central effects of angiotensin. Fed Proc 1982; 41:2520–2527.
153. Hoffman WE, Ganten U, Phillips MI, et al. Inhibition of drinking in water-deprived rats by combined central angiotensin II and cholinergic receptor blockade. Am J Physiol 1978; 234:F41–F47.
154. Zimmerman MB, Blaine EH, Stricker EM. Water intake in hypovolemic sheep: effects of crushing the left atrial appendage. Science 1981; 211:489–491.
155. Dill DB. Life, Heat and Altitude. Cambridge: Harvard University Press, 1938.
156. Adolph, EF. Termination of drinking: satiation. Fed Proc 1982; 41:2533–2535.
157. Ramsay DJ, Rolls BJ, Wood RJ. Thirst following water deprivation in dogs. Am J Physiol 1977; 232:R93–R100.
158. Gilmore JP, Zucker IH. Failure of left atrial distension to alter renal function in the nonhuman primate. Circ Res 1978; 42:267–270.
159. Weitzman RE, Glatz TH, Fisher DA. The effect of hemorrhage and hypertonic saline upon plasma oxytocin and arginine vasopressin in conscious dogs. Endocrinology 1978; 103:2154–2160.
160. Landgraf R, Neumann I, Schwarzberg H. Central and peripheral release of vasopressin and oxytocin in the conscious rat after osmotic stimulation. Brain Res 1988; 457:219–225.
161. Russell JA, Blackburn RE, Leng G. The role of the AV3V region in the control of magnocellular oxytocin neurons. Brain Res Bull 1988; 20:803–810.
162. Hartman RD, Rosella-Dampman LM, Emmert SE, et al. Inhibition of release of neurohypophyseal hormones by endogenous opioid peptides in pregnant and parturient rats. Brain Res 1986; 382:352–359.
163. Bicknell RJ, Zhao BG, Chapman C, et al. Opioid inhibition of secretion from oxytocin and vasopressin nerve terminals following selective depletion of neurohypophyseal catecholamines. Neurosci Lett 1988; 93:281–286.
164. Carter DA, Lightman SL. Opioid control of oxytocin secretion: evidence of distinct regulatory actions of two opiate receptor types. Life Sci 1987; 40:2289–2296.
165. Johnson AK. The periventricular anteroventral third ventricle (AV3V): its relationship with the subfornical organ and neural systems involved in maintaining body fluid homeostasis. Brain Res Bull 1985; 15:595–601.
166. Verbalis JG, McCann MJ, McHale CM, et al. Oxytocin secretion in response to cholecystokinin and food: differentiation of nausea from satiety. Science 1986; 232:1417–1419.
167. Bradshaw JMC, Downing SJ, Moffatt A, et al. Demonstration of some of the physiological properties of rat relaxin. J Reprod Fertil 1981; 63:145–153.
168. Summerlee AJS, O'Byrne KT, Paisley AC, et al. Relaxin affects the central control of oxytocin release. Nature 1984; 309:372–374.
169. Dayanithi G, Cazalis M, Nordmann JJ. Relaxin affects the release of oxytocin and vasopressin from the neurohypophysis. Nature 1987; 325:813–816.
170. Rosenblatt JS, Mayer AD, Giodano AL. Hormonal basis during pregnancy for the onset of maternal behavior in the rat. Psychoneuroendocrinology 1988; 13:29–46.
171. Clements JA, Funder JW. Arginine vasopressin and oxytocin in organs outside the nervous system. In: Martini L, Ganong WF, eds. Frontiers in Neuroendocrinology. Vol 10. New York: Raven, 1988: 117–152.
172. Rajerison RM, Montegut M, Jard S, et al. The isolated frog skin epithelium: permeability characteristics and responsiveness to oxytocin, cyclic AMP and theophylline. Pflugers Arch 1972; 332:302–312.
173. Balment RJ, Brimble MJ, Forsling ML. Oxytocin release and renal actions in normal and Brattleboro rats. Ann NY Acad Sci 1982; 394:241–253.
174. Ahmad AJ, Clark EH, Jacobs HS. Water intoxication associated with oxytocin infusion. Postgrad Med J 1975; 51:249–252.
175. Feeney JG. Water intoxication and oxytocin. Br Med J 1982; 285:243.
176. Kuhn W, Ryffel K. Herstellung konzentrierter Lösungen aus verdünnten durch blosse Membranwirkung. Ein Modellversuch zur Funcktion der Niere. Z Physiol Chemie 1942; 276:145–178.
177. Gottschalk CW, Mylle M. Micropuncture study of the mammalian urinary concentrating mechanism: evidence for the countercurrent hypothesis. Am J Physiol 1959; 196:927–936.
178. Gottschalk CW. Osmotic concentration and dilution of the urine. Am J Med 1964; 36:670–685.
179. Burg MB, Green N. Function of the thick ascending limb of Henle's loop. Am J Physiol 1973; 224:659–668.
180. Rocha AS, Kokko JP. Sodium chloride and water transport in the medullary thick ascending limb of Henle. Evidence for active chloride transport. J Clin Invest 1973; 52:612–623.
181. Kokko JP, Rector FC Jr. Countercurrent multiplication system without active transport in inner medulla. Kidney Int 1972; 2:214–223.
182. Valtin H. Sequestration of urea and nonurea solutes in renal tissues of rats with hereditary hypothalamic diabetes insipidus: effect of vasopressin and dehydration on the countercurrent mechanism. J Clin Invest 1966; 45:337–345.
183. Stephenson JL. Concentration of urine in a central core model of the renal counterflow system. Kidney Int 1972; 2:85–94.
184. Gellai M, Edwards BR, Valtin H. Urinary concentrating ability during dehydration in the absence of vasopressin. Am J Physiol 1979; 237:F100–F104.
185. Edwards BR, Gallai M, Valtin H. Concentration of urine in the absence of ADH with minimal or no decrease in GFR. Am J Physiol 1980; 239:F84–F91.
186. Rapoport S, Brodsky WA, West CD, et al. Urinary flow and excretion of solutes during osmotic diuresis in hydropenic man. Am J Physiol 1949; 156:433–442.
187. Goldberg M, McCurdy DK, Foltz EL, et al. Effects of ethacrynic acid (a new saluretic agent) on renal diluting and concentrating mechanisms: evidence for site of action in the loop of Henle. J Clin Invest 1964; 43:201–216.
188. DeWardener HE, Del Greco F. The influence of solute excretion rate on the production of a hypotonic urine in man. Clin Sci 1955; 14:715–723.
189. Hebert SC, Schafer JA, Andreoli TE. The effects of antidiuretic hormone (ADH) on solute and water transport in the mammalian nephron. J Membr Biol 1981; 58:1–19.
190. Hebert SC, Andreoli TE. Water permeability of biological membranes. Lessons from antidiuretic hormone–responsive epithelia. Biochim Biophys Acta 1982; 650:267–280.
191. Grantham JJ, Burg MB. Effect of vasopressin and cyclic AMP on permeability of isolated collecting tubules. Am J Physiol 1966; 211:255–259.
192. Grantham JJ, Orloff J. Effect of prostaglandin E_1 on the permeability response of the isolated collecting tubule to vasopressin, adenosine 3',5'-monophosphate and theophylline. J Clin Invest 1968; 47:1154–1161.
193. Schafer JA, Andreoli TE. Cellular constraints to diffusion: the effect of antidiuretic hormone on water flows in isolated mammalian collecting tubules. J Clin Invest 1972; 51:1264–1278.
194. Hall DA, Grantham JJ. Temperature effect on ADH response of isolated perfused rabbit collecting tubules. Am J Physiol 1980; 239:F595–F601.
195. Reif MC, Troutman SL, Schafer JA. Sustained response to vasopressin in isolated rat cortical collecting tubules. Kidney Int 1984; 26:725–732.
196. Burg MB, Helman S, Grantham JJ, et al. Effect of vasopressin on the permeability of isolated rabbit cortical collecting tubules to urea, acetamide, and thiourea. In: Schmidt-Nielsen B, ed. Urea and the Kidney. Amsterdam: Excerpta Medica, 1970: 193–208.
197. Schafer JA, Andreoli TE. The effect of antidiuretic hormone on solute flows in mammalian collecting tubules. J Clin Invest 1972; 51:1279–1286.
198. Hebert SC, Andreoli TE. Interactions of temperature and ADH on transport processes in cortical collecting tubules: evidence for ADH-induced narrow aqueous channels in apical membranes. Am J Physiol 1980; 238:F470–F480.
199. Verkman AS. Mechanisms and regulation of water permeability in renal epithelia. Am J Physiol 1989; 257:C837–C850.
200. Chevalier J, Bourguet J, Hugon JJ. Membrane-associated particles: distribution in frog urinary bladder epithelium at rest and after oxytocin treatment. Cell Tissue Res 1974; 152:129–140.
201. Kachadorian WA, Wade JB, DiScala VA. Vasopressin: induced structural change in toad bladder luminal membranes. Science 1975; 190:67–69.
202. Kachadorian WA, Wade JB, Uiterwyk CC, et al. Membrane structural and functional responses to vasopressin in toad urinary bladder. J Membr Biol 1977; 30:381–401.
203. Kachadorian WA, Levine SD, Wade JB, et al. Relationship of aggregated intramembranous particles to water permeability in vasopressin-treated toad urinary bladder. J Clin Invest 1977; 59:576–581.
204. Kachadorian WA, Coleman RA, Wade JB. Water permeability and particle aggregates in ADH-, cAMP-, and forskolin-treated toad bladder. Am J Physiol 1987; 253:F14–F20.
205. Muller J, Kachadorian WA, DiScala VA. Evidence that ADH-stimulated intramembrane particle aggregates are transferred from cytoplasmic to luminal membranes in toad bladder epithelial cells. J Cell Biol 1980; 85:83–95.
206. Levine SD, Kachadorian WA. Barriers to water flow in vasopressin-treated toad urinary bladder. J Membr Biol 1981; 61:135–139.
207. Wade JB, Stetson DL, Lewis SA. ADH action: evidence for a membrane shuttle mechanism. Ann NY Acad Sci 1981; 372:106–117.
208. Zeidel ML, Hammond TG, Wade JB, et al. Fate of antidiuretic hormone water channel proteins after retrieval from apical membrane. Am J Physiol 1993; 265:C822–C833.
209. Harris HW Jr, Zeidel ML, Jo I, et al. Characterization of purified endosomes containing the antidiuretic hormone–sensitive water channel from rat renal papilla. J Biol Chem 1994; 269:11993–12000.
210. Verkman AS, Lencer WI, Brown D, et al. Endosomes from kidney collecting tubule cells contain the vasopressin-sensitive water channel. Nature 1988; 333:268–269.
211. Verkman AS, Weyer P, Brown D, et al. Functional water channels are present in clathrin-coated vesicles from bovine kidney but not from brain. J Biol Chem 1989; 264:20608–20613.

212. Franki N, Ding G, Quintana N, et al. Evidence that heads of ADH-sensitive aggrephores are clathrin-coated vesicles: implications for aggrephore structure and function. Tissue Cell 1986; 18:803–807.

213. Wade JB. Membrane structural studies of the action of vasopressin. Fed Proc 1985; 44:2687–2692.

214. Brown D. Membrane recycling and epithelial cell function. Am J Physiol 1989; 256:F1–F12.

215. Harris HW, Wade JB, Handler JS. Fluorescent markers to study membrane retrieval in ADH treated toad urinary bladder. Am J Physiol 1986; 251:C274–C284.

216. Harris HW, Wade JB, Handler JS. Transepithelial water flow regulates apical membrane and retrieval on ADH-stimulated toad urinary bladder. J Clin Invest 1986; 78:703–712.

217. Muller J, Kachadorian WA. Aggregate-carrying membranes during ADH stimulation and washout in toad bladder. Am J Physiol 1984; 247:C90–C98.

218. Brown D, Orci L. Vasopressin stimulates formation of coated pits in rat kidney collecting ducts. Nature 1983; 302:253–255.

219. Harmanci MC, Kachadorian WA, Valtin H, et al. Antidiuretic hormone–induced intramembranous alteration in mammalian collecting ducts. Am J Physiol 1978; 235:F440–F443.

220. Harmanci MC, Stern P, Kachadorian WA, et al. Vasopressin and collecting duct intramembranous particle clusters: a dose-response relationship. Am J Physiol 1980; 239:F560–F564.

221. Harmanci MC, Lorenzen M, Kachadorian WA. Vasopressin-induced intramembranous particle aggregates in isolated rabbit collecting duct. Kidney Int 1982; 21:275A.

222. Strange K, Willingham MC, Handler JS, et al. Apical membrane retrieval via clathrin-coated pits is stimulated by removal of ADH from isolated perfused rabbit cortical tubule. J Membr Biol 1988; 103:17–28.

223. Brown D, Weyer P, Orci L. Vasopressin stimulates endocytosis in kidney collecting duct principal cells. Eur J Cell Biol 1988; 46:336–341.

224. Fushimi K, Uchida S, Hara Y, et al. Cloning and expression of apical membrane water channel of rat kidney collecting tubule. Nature 1993; 361:549–552.

225. Sasaki S, Fushimi K, Saito H, et al. Cloning, characterization, and chromosomal mapping of human aquaporin of collecting duct. J Clin Invest 1994; 93:1250–1256.

226. Nielsen S, Agre P. The aquaporin family of water channels in kidney. Kidney Int 1995; 48:1057–1068.

227. Sasaki S, Fushimi K, Ishibashi K, et al. Water channels in the kidney collecting duct. Kidney Int 1995; 48:1082–1087.

228. Nielsen S, Digiovanni SR, Christensen EI, et al. Cellular and subcellular immunolocalization of vasopressin-regulated water channel in rat kidney. Proc Natl Acad Sci USA 1993; 90:11663–11667.

229. Sabolic I, Katsura T, Verbavatz JM, et al. The AQP2 water channel: effect of vasopressin treatment, microtubule disruption, and distribution in neonatal rats. J Membr Biol 1995; 143:165–175.

230. Digiovanni SR, Nielsen S, Christensen EI, et al. Regulation of collecting duct water channel expression by vasopressin in Brattleboro rat. Proc Natl Acad Sci USA 1994; 91:8984–8988.

231. Yamamoto T, Sasaki S, Fushimi K, et al. Localization and expression of a collecting duct water channel, aquaporin, in hydrated and dehydrated rats. Exp Nephrol 1995; 3:193–201.

232. Hayashi M, Sasaki S, Tsuganezawa H, et al. Expression and distribution of aquaporin of collecting duct are regulated by vasopressin V_2 receptor in rat kidney. J Clin Invest 1994; 94:1778–1883.

233. Nielsen S, Chou C-L, Marples D, et al. Vasopressin increases water permeability of kidney collecting duct by inducing translocation of aquaporin-CD water channels to plasma membrane. Proc Natl Acad Sci USA 1995; 92:1013–1017.

234. Kuwahara M, Fushimi K, Terada Y, et al. cAMP-dependent phosphorylation stimulates water permeability of aquaporin-collecting duct water channel protein expressed in Xenopus oocytes. J Biol Chem 1995; 270:10384–10387.

235. Lolait SJ, O'Carroll AM, McBride OW, et al. Cloning and characterization of a vasopressin V_2 receptor and possible link to nephrogenic diabetes insipidus. Nature 1992; 357:336–339.

236. Birnbaumer M, Seibold A, Gilbert S, et al. Molecular cloning of the receptor for human antidiuretic hormone. Nature 1992; 357:333–335.

237. Dousa TP. Cyclic nucleotides in the cellular action of neurohypophyseal hormones. Fed Proc 1977; 36:1867–1871.

238. Fahrenholz F, Jurzak M, Gerstberger R, et al. Renal and central vasopressin receptors: immunocytochemical localization. Ann NY Acad Sci 1993; 689:194–206.

239. Firsov D, Mandon B, Morel A, et al. Molecular analysis of vasopressin receptors in the rat nephron: evidence for alternative splicing of the V_2 receptor. Pflugers Arch 1994; 429:79–89.

240. Fujiwara TM, Morgan K, Bichet DG. Molecular biology of diabetes insipidus. Annu Rev Med 1995; 46:331–343.

241. Hildebrandt J, Sekura R, Codina J, et al. Stimulation and inhibition of adenyl cyclases mediated by distinct regulatory proteins. Nature 1983; 302:706–709.

242. Gilman AG. Guanine nucleotide–binding regulatory proteins and dual control of adenylate cyclase. J Clin Invest 1984; 73:1–4.

243. Rodbell M. The role of hormone receptors and GTP-regulatory proteins in membrane transduction. Nature 1980; 284:17–22.

244. Jard S, Roy C, Barth T, et al. Antidiuretic hormone–sensitive kidney adenylate cyclase. Adv Cyclic Nucleotide Res 1975; 5:31–52.

245. Seamon KB, Daly JW. Forskolin, cyclic AMP and cellular physiology. Trends Pharmacol Sci 1983; 4:120–123.

246. Culpepper RM, Andreoli TE. PGE_2, forskolin, and cholera toxin interactions in modulating NaCl transport in mouse mTALH. Am J Physiol 1984; 247:F784–F792.

247. Nadler SP, Hebert SC, Brenner BM. PGE_2, forskolin, and cholera toxin interaction in rabbit cortical collecting tubule. Am J Physiol 1986; 250:F127–F135.

248. Takaichi K, Kurokawa K. Inhibitory guanosine triphosphate–binding protein-mediated regulation of vasopressin action in isolated single medullary tubules of mouse kidney. J Clin Invest 1988; 82:1437–1444.

249. Ribeiro CP, Ribeiro-Neto F, Field JB, et al. Prevention of α_2-adrenergic inhibition on ADH action by pertussis toxin in rabbit CCT. Am J Physiol 1987; 253:C105–C112.

250. Dousa TP, Valtin H. Cellular actions of vasopressin in the mammalian kidney. Kidney Int 1976; 10:46–63.

251. Dousa TP, Barnes LD, Kim JK. The role of cyclic AMP–dependent protein phosphorylations and microtubules in the cellular action of vasopressin in mammalian kidney. In: Moses AM, Share L, eds. Neurohypophysis. Basel: S Karger, 1977: 220–235.

252. Kuwahara M, Verkman AS. Pre–steady state analysis of the turn-on and turn-off of water permeability in the kidney collecting tubule. J Membr Biol 1989; 110:57–65.

253. Yasuhiro A, Breyer MD, Jacobson HR. Dose-dependent heterogenous actions of vasopressin in rabbit cortical collecting ducts. Am J Physiol 1989; 256:F556–F562.

254. Star RA, Nonoguchi H, Balaban R, et al. Calcium and cyclic adenosine monophosphate as second messengers for vasopressin in the rat inner medullary collecting duct. J Clin Invest 1988; 81:1879–1888.

255. Maeda Y, Han JS, Gibson CC, et al. Vasopressin and oxytocin receptors coupled to Ca^{2+} mobilization in rat inner medullary collecting duct. Am J Physiol 1993; 265:F15–F25.

256. Preston BM, Carroll TP, Guggino WB, et al. Appearance of water channels in Xenopus oocytes expressing red cell CHIP28 protein. Science 1992; 256:385–387.

257. Nielsen S, Smith B, Christensen EI, et al. CHIP28 water channels are localized in constitutively water-permeable segments of the nephron. J Cell Biol 1993; 120:371–383.

258. Deen PMT, Verdijk MA, Knoers NVAM, et al. Requirement of human renal water channel aquaporin-2 for vasopressin-dependent concentration of urine. Science 1994; 264:92–95.

259. Deen PMT, Croes H, vanAubel RAMH, et al. Water channels encoded by mutant aquaporin-2 genes in nephrogenic diabetes insipidus are impaired in their cellular routing. J Clin Invest 1995; 95:2291–2296.

260. Strange K, Spring KR. Cell membrane water permeability of rabbit cortical collecting duct. J Membr Biol 1987; 96:27–43.

261. Ishibashi K, Sasaki S, Fushimi K, et al. Molecular cloning and expression of a member of the aquaporin family with permeability to glycerol and urea in addition to water expressed at the basolateral membrane of kidney collecting duct cells. Proc Natl Acad Sci USA 1994; 91:6269–6273.

262. Jung JS, Preston GM, Smith BL, et al. Molecular structure of the water channel through aquaporin CHIP. J Biol Chem 1994; 269:14648–14654.

263. Walz T, Smith BL, Zeidel ML, et al. Biologically active two-dimensional crystals of aquaporin CHIP. J Biol Chem 1994; 269:1583–1586.

264. Verkman AS, Shi L-B, Frigeri A, et al. Structure and function of kidney water channels. Kidney Int 1995; 48:1069–1081.

265. Wade JB. Dynamics of apical membrane responses to ADH in amphibian bladder. Am J Physiol 1989; 257:R998–R1003.

266. Valenti G, Hugon JS, Bourguet J. To what extent is microtubular network involved in antidiuretic response? Am J Physiol 1988; 255:F1098–F1106.

267. Kachadorian WA, Muller J, Rudich S, et al. Temperature dependence of ADH-induced water flow and intramembranous particle aggregates in toad bladder. Science 1979; 205:910–913.

268. Nielsen S, Marples D, Birn H, et al. Expression of VAMP2-like protein in kidney collecting duct intracellular vesicles. J Clin Invest 1995; 96:1834–1844.

269. Franki N, Macaluso F, Schubert W, et al. Water channel–carrying vesicles in the rat IMCD contain cellubrevin. Am J Physiol 1995; 269:C797–C801.

270. Jo I, Harris HW, Amendt-Raduege AM, et al. Rat kidney papilla contains abundant synaptobrevin protein that participates in the fusion of antidiuretic hormone–regulated water channel–containing endosomes in vitro. Proc Natl Acad Sci USA 1995; 92:1876–1880.

271. Krothapalli RK, Duffy WB, Senekjian HO, et al. Modulation of the hydro-osmotic effect of vasopressin on the rabbit cortical collecting tubule by adrenergic agents. J Clin Invest 1983; 72:287–294.

272. Edwards RM, Stack EJ, Gellai M, et al. Inhibition of vasopressin-sensitive cAMP accumulation by alpha 2-adrenoceptor agonists in collecting tubules is species dependent. Pharmacology 1992; 44:26–32.

273. Beck TR, Dunn MJ. The relationship of antidiuretic hormone and renal prostaglandins. Miner Electrolyte Metab 1981; 6:46–59.

274. Handler JS. Vasopressin-prostaglandin interactions in the regulation of epithelial cell permeability to water. Kidney Int 1981; 19:831–838.

275. Orloff J, Handler JS, Bergstrom S. Effect of prostaglandin (PGE-1) on the permeability response of toad bladder to vasopressin, theophylline and adenosine 3',5'-monophosphate. Nature 1965; 205:397–398.

276. Craven PA, DeRubertis FR. Effects of vasopressin and urea on Ca^{2+}-calmodulin–dependent renal prostaglandin E. Am J Physiol 1981; 241:F649–F658.

277. Wuthrich RP, Loup R, Favre L, et al. Dynamic response of PG synthesis to peptide hormones and osmolality in renal tubular cells. Am J Physiol 1986; 250:F790–F797.

278. Sato M, Dunn MJ. Interaction of vasopressin, prostaglandins and cAMP in rat papillary collecting tubule cells in culture. Am J Physiol 1984; 247:F423–F433.

279. Schlondorff D, Satriano JA, Schwartz GJ. Synthesis of prostaglandin E₂ in different segments of isolated collecting tubules from adult and neonatal rabbits. Am J Physiol 1985; 248:F134–F144.

280. Portilla D, Shayman JA, Morrison AR. Vasopressin does not hydrolyze polyphosphoinositides in rabbit collecting tubule cells. Biochim Biophys Acta 1987; 928:305–311.

281. Argy WP, Handler JS, Orloff J. Ca⁺⁺ and Mg⁺⁺ effects on toad bladder response to cyclic AMP, theophylline and ADH analogues. Am J Physiol 1967; 213:803–808.

282. Peterson MJ, Edelman IS. Calcium inhibition of the action of vasopressin on the urinary bladder of toad. J Clin Invest 1964; 43:583–594.

283. Goldfarb S. Effects of calcium on ADH action in the cortical collecting tubule perfused in vitro. Am J Physiol 1982; 243:F481–F486.

284. Takaichi K, Uchida S, Kurokawa K. High Ca²⁺ inhibits AVP-dependent cAMP production in thick ascending limbs of Henle. Am J Physiol 1986; 250:F770–F776.

285. Ando Y, Jacobson HR, Breyer MD. Phorbol ester and A23187 have additive but mechanistically separate effects on vasopressin action in rabbit collecting tubule. J Clin Invest 1988; 81:1578–1584.

286. Schlondorff D, Levine SD. Inhibition of vasopressin-stimulated water flow in toad bladder by phorbol myristate acetate, dioctanoylglycerol and RHC-80267. J Clin Invest 1985; 76:1071–1078.

287. Casavola V, Iacovelli L, Svelto M. Phorbol ester effect on the hydro-osmotic response to vasopressin in frog skin. Pflugers Arch 1987; 408:318–320.

288. Ando Y, Jacobson HR, Bryer MD. Phorbol myristate acetate, dioctanoylglycerol and phosphatidic acid inhibit the hydro-osmotic effect of vasopressin on rabbit cortical collecting tubule. J Clin Invest 1987; 80:590–593.

289. Wirz H, Hargitay B, Kuhn W. Lokalisation des Konzentrierungsprozesses in der Niere durch direkte Kryoskopie. Helv Physiol Acta 1951; 9:196–207.

290. Morel F. Regulation of kidney functions by hormones: a new approach. Recent Prog Horm Res 1983; 39:271–304.

291. Greger R, Schlatter E. Properties of the lumen membrane of the cortical thick ascending limb of Henle's loop of rabbit kidney. Pflugers Arch 1983; 396:315–324.

292. Molony DA, Reeves WB, Andreoli TE. Na⁺:K⁺:2Cl⁻ cotransport and the thick ascending limb. Kidney Int 1989; 36:418–426.

293. Gamba G, Miyanoshita A, Lombardi M, et al. Molecular cloning, primary structure, and characterization of two members of the mammalian electro-neutral sodium-(potassium)-chloride cotransporter family expressed in kidney. J Biol Chem 1994; 269:17713–17122.

294. Kaplan MR, Plotkin MD, Lee W-S, et al. Apical localization of the Na-K-Cl cotransporter, rBSCl, on rat thick ascending limbs. Kidney Int 1996; 49:40–47.

295. Hebert SC, Andreoli TE. Effects of antidiuretic hormone on cellular conductive pathways in mouse medullary thick ascending limbs of Henle. II: Determinants of the ADH-mediated increases in transepithelial voltage and in net Cl⁻ absorption. J Membr Biol 1984; 80:221–233.

296. Oberleithner H, Guggino W, Giebisch G. Mechanism of distal tubular chloride transport in Amphiuma kidney. Am J Physiol 1982; 242:F331–F339.

297. Hebert SC, Friedman PA, Andreoli TE. The effects of antidiuretic hormone on cellular conductive pathways in mouse medullary thick ascending limbs of Henle. I: ADH increases transcellular conductance pathways. J Membr Biol 1984; 80:201–219.

298. Stokes JB. Consequences of potassium recycling in the renal medulla. Effects on ion transport by the medullary thick ascending limb of Henle's loop. J Clin Invest 1982; 70:219–229.

299. Wang W, White S, Giebel J, et al. A potassium channel in the thick ascending limb of Henle's loop of rabbit kidney. Am J Physiol 1990; 258:F244–F253.

300. Ho K, Nichols CG, Lederer WJ, et al. Cloning and expression of an inwardly rectifying ATP-regulated potassium channel. Nature 1993; 362:31–37.

301. Lee W-S, Hebert SC. ROMK inwardly rectifying ATP-sensitive K⁺ channel. I: Expression in rat distal nephron segments. Am J Physiol 1995; 268:F1124–F1131.

302. Boim MA, Ho K, Shuck ME, et al. ROMK inwardly rectifying ATP-sensitive K⁺ channel II. Cloning and distribution of alternative forms. Am J Physiol 1995; 268:F1132–F1140.

303. Hebert SC, Andreoli TE. Control of NaCl transport in the thick ascending limb. Am J Physiol 1984; 15:F745–F756.

304. Greger R, Schlatter E. Properties of the basolateral membrane of the cortical thick ascending limb of Henle's loop of rabbit kidney: a model for secondary active chloride transport. Pflugers Arch 1983; 396:325–334.

305. Bayliss JM, Reeves WB, Andreoli TE. Cl⁻ transport in basolateral renal medullary vesicles. I: Cl⁻ transport in intact vesicles. J Membr Biol 1990; 113:49–56.

306. Reeves WB, Andreoli TE. Cl⁻ transport in basolateral renal medullary vesicles. II: Cl⁻ channels in planar lipid bilayers. J Membr Biol 1990; 113:57–65.

307. Winters CJ, Reeves WB, Andreoli TE. Cl⁻ channels in basolateral renal medullary membranes. III: Determinants of single channel activity. J Membr Biol 1991; 118:269–278.

308. Winters CJ, Reeves WB, Andreoli TE. Cl⁻ channels in basolateral renal medullary membrane vesicles. IV: Analogous channel activation by Cl⁻ or cAMP-dependent protein kinase. J Membr Biol 1991; 122:89–95.

308a. Zimniak L, Winters CJ, Reeves WB, et al. Cl⁻ channels in basolateral renal medullary vesicles. X: Cloning of a basolateral mTAL Cl⁻ channel. Kidney Int 1995; 48:1828–1836.

308b. Jentsch TJ, Gunther W, Pusch M, et al. Properties of voltage-gated chloride channels of the ClC gene family. J Physiol 1995; 482:19S–25S.

308c. Zimniak L, Winters CJ, Reeves WB, et al. Cl⁻ channels in basolateral renal medullary vesicles. XI: RbClC-Ka encoded basolateral mTAL Cl⁻ channels. Am J Physiol (in press).

309. Schultz SG. Homocellular regulatory mechanisms in sodium-transporting epithelia: avoidance of extinction by "flush-through." Am J Physiol 1981; 241:F579–F590.

310. Hebert SC, Culpepper RM, Andreoli TE. NaCl transport in mouse medullary thick ascending limbs. I: Functional nephron heterogeneity and ADH-stimulated NaCl cotransport. Am J Physiol 1981; 241:F412–F431.

311. Work J, Galla JH, Booker BB, et al. Effect of ADH on chloride reabsorption in the loop of Henle of the Brattleboro rat. Am J Physiol 1985; 249:F698–F703.

312. Reeves WB, McDonald GA, Mehta P, et al. Activation of K⁺ channels in renal medullary vesicles by cAMP-dependent protein kinase. J Membr Biol 1989; 109:65–72.

313. Schlatter E, Greger R. cAMP increases the basolateral Cl⁻-conductance in the isolated perfused medullary thick ascending limb of Henle's loop of the mouse. Pflugers Arch 1985; 405:367–376.

314. Molony DA, Reeves WB, Hebert SC, et al. ADH increases apical Na⁺,K⁺,2Cl⁻ entry in mouse medullary thick ascending limbs of Henle. Am J Physiol 1987; 252:F177–F187.

315. Hebert SC, Culpepper RM, Andreoli TE. NaCl transport in mouse medullary thick ascending limbs. III: Modulation of the ADH effect by peritubular osmolality. Am J Physiol 1981; 241:F443–F451.

316. Molony DA, Andreoli TE. Diluting power of thick ascending limbs of Henle. I: Peritubular hypertonicity blocks basolateral Cl⁻ channels. Am J Physiol 1988; 255:F1128–F1137.

317. Higashihara E, Stokes JB, Kokko JP, et al. Cortical and papillary micropuncture examination of chloride transport in segments of the rat kidney during inhibition of prostaglandin production. J Clin Invest 1979; 64:1277–1287.

318. Kauker ML. Prostaglandin E₂ effect from the luminal side on renal tubular ²²Na efflux: tracer microinjection studies. Proc Soc Exp Biol Med 1977; 154:274–277.

319. Stokes JB. Effect of prostaglandin E₂ on chloride transport across the rabbit thick ascending limb of Henle. J Clin Invest 1979; 64:495–502.

320. Culpepper RM, Andreoli TE. Interactions among prostaglandin E₂, antidiuretic hormone, and cyclic adenosine monophosphate in modulating Cl⁻ absorption in single mouse medullary thick ascending limbs of Henle. J Clin Invest 1983; 71:1588–1601.

321. Torikai S, Kurokawa K. Effect of PGE₂ on vasopressin-dependent cell cAMP in isolated single segments. Am J Physiol 1983; 245:F58–F66.

322. Fejes-Tóth G, Magyar A, Walter J. Renal response to vasopressin after inhibition of prostaglandin synthesis. Am J Physiol 1977; 232:F416–F423.

323. Berl T, Raz A, Wald H, et al. Prostaglandin synthesis inhibition and the action of vasopressin: studies in man and rat. Am J Physiol 1977; 232:F529–F537.

324. Ganguli M, Tobian L, Azar S, et al. Evidence that prostaglandin synthesis inhibitors increase the concentration of sodium and chloride in rat renal medulla. Circ Res 1977; 40(Suppl 1):I135–I139.

325. Robertson GL, Athar S, Shelton RL. Osmotic control of vasopressin function. In: Andreoli TE, Grantham JJ, Rector FC, eds. Disturbances in Body Fluid Osmolality. Bethesda: American Physiological Society, 1977: 125–148.

326. Mahoney JH, Goodman AD. Hypernatremia due to hypodipsia and elevated threshold for vasopressin release. N Engl J Med 1968; 279:1191–1196.

327. DeRubertis FR, Michelis MF, Beck N, et al. "Essential" hypernatremia due to ineffective osmotic and intact volume regulation of vasopressin secretion. J Clin Invest 1971; 50:97–111.

328. Halter JB, Goldbert AP, Robertson GL, et al. Selective osmoreceptor dysfunction in the syndrome of chronic hypernatremia. J Clin Endocrinol Metab 1977; 44:609–616.

329. Fernandez CM, Vendrell SJM, Ricard W, et al. Arginine-vasopressin in essential hypernatremia. J Endocrinol Invest 1986; 9:331–335.

330. Miller M, Moses AM. Potentiation of vasopressin action by chlorpropamide in vivo. Endocrinology 1970; 86:1024–1027.

331. Fink EB. Diabetes insipidus. Arch Pathol Lab Med 1928; 6:102–120.

332. Moses AM, Notman DD. Diabetes insipidus and syndrome of inappropriate antidiuretic hormone secretion (SIADH). Adv Intern Med 1973; 27:73–100.

333. Wang LC, Cohen ME, Duffner PK. Etiologies of central diabetes insipidus in children. Pediatr Neurol 1994; 11:276–277.

334. Tarng DC, Huang TP. Diabetes insipidus as an early sign of pineal tumor. Am J Nephrol 1995; 15:161–164.

335. Genka S, Soeda H, Takahashi M, et al. Acromegaly, diabetes insipidus, and visual loss caused by metastatic growth hormone–releasing hormone–producing malignant pancreatic endocrine tumor in the pituitary gland. J Neurosurg 1995; 83:719–723.

336. Kawamura J, Tsukamoto K, Yamakawa K, et al. Diabetes insipidus due to pituitary metastasis from bladder cancer. Urol Int 1991; 46:217–220.

337. Tham LC, Millward MJ, Lind MJ, et al. Metastatic breast cancer presenting with diabetes insipidus. Acta Oncol 1992; 31:679–680.

338. Koshiuyama H, Ohgaki K, Hida S, et al. Metastatic renal cell carcinoma to the pituitary gland presenting with hypopituitarism. J Endocrinol Invest 1992; 15:677–681.

339. Sherwood MC, Stanhope R, Preece MA, et al. Diabetes insipidus and occult intracranial tumours. Arch Dis Child 1986; 61:1222–1224.

340. Randall RV, Clark EC, Bahn RC. Classification of the causes of diabetes insipidus. Mayo Clin Proc 1959; 34:299–302.

341. Weitzman RE, Kleeman CR. The clinical physiology of water metabolism. Part II: renal mechanisms for urinary concentration; diabetes insipidus. West J Med 1979; 131:486–515.

342. Imura H, Nakao K, Shimatsu A, et al. Lymphocytic infundibuloneurohypophysitis as a cause of central diabetes insipidus. N Engl J Med 1993; 329:683–689.

343. Ashmed SR, Aiello DP, Page R, et al. Necrotizing infundibulo-hypophysitis: a unique syndrome of diabetes insipidus and hypopituitarism. J Clin Endocrinol Metab 1993; 76:1499–1504.

344. Czarnechi EJ, Spickler EM. MR demonstration of Wegener granulomatosis of the infundibulum, a cause of diabetes insipidus. Am J Neuroradiol 1995; 16:968–970.

345. Rossi GP, Pavan E, Chiesura-Corona M, et al. Bronchocentric granulomatosis and central diabetes insipidus successfully treated with corticosteroids. Eur Respir J 1994; 7:1893–1898.

346. Matsumot AT, Sanno K, Osamura Y. Lymphocytic hypophysitis: case report. Neurosurgery 1995; 36:1016–1019.

347. Martin MR. Familial diabetes insipidus. Q J Med 1959; 28:573–582.

348. Baylis PH, Robertson GL. Vasopressin function in familial cranial diabetes insipidus. Postgrad Med J 1981; 57:36–40.

349. Reeves WB, Andreoli TE. Nephrogenic diabetes insipidus. In: Schriver CR, Beaudet AL, Sly WS, et al, eds. Metabolic and Molecular Bases of Inherited Disease. New York: McGraw-Hill, 1995: 3045–3071.

350. Kaplowitz PB, D'Ercole AJ, Robertson GL. Radioimmunoassay of vasopressin in familial central diabetes insipidus. J Pediatr 1982; 100:76–81.

351. Repaske D, Browning D. A de novo mutation in the coding sequence for neurophysin-II (Pro24–Leu) is associated with onset and transmission of autosomal dominant neurohypophyseal diabetes insipidus. J Clin Endocrinol Metab 1994; 79:421–427.

352. Bahnsen U, Oosting P, Swaab DF, et al. A missense mutation in the vasopressin-neurophysin precursor gene cosegregates with human autosomal dominant neurohypophyseal diabetes insipidus. EMBO 1992; 11:19–23.

353. Nagasaki H, Ito M, Yuasa H, et al. Two novel mutations in the coding region for neurophysin-II associated with familial central diabetes insipidus. J Clin Endocrinol Metab 1995; 80:1352–1356.

354. Rittig R, Robertson GL, Siggaard C, et al. Identification of 13 new mutations in the vasopressin-neurophysin II gene in 17 kindreds with familial autosomal dominant neurohypophyseal diabetes insipidus. Am J Hum Genet 1996; 58:107–117.

355. Chen LQ, Rose JP, Breslow E, et al. Crystal structure of a bovine neurophysin II dipeptide complex at 2.8 Å determined from the single-wavelength anomalous scattering signal of an incorporated iodine atom. Proc Natl Acad Sci USA 1991; 88:4240–4245.

356. Dreyer M, Rüdiger HW, Bujara K, et al. The syndrome of diabetes insipidus, diabetes mellitus, optic atrophy, deafness, and other abnormalities. Klin Wochenschr 1982; 60:471–475.

357. Blasi C, Pierelli F, Rispoli E, et al. Wolfram's syndrome: a clinical, diagnostic, and interpretative contribution. Diabetes Care 1986; 9:521–528.

358. Masera N, Grant DB, Stanhope R, et al. Diabetes insipidus with impaired osmotic regulation in septo-optic dysplasia and agenesis of the corpus callosum. Arch Dis Child 1994; 70:51–53.

359. Yagi H, Nagashima K, Miyake H, et al. Familial congenital hypopituitarism with central diabetes insipidus. J Clin Endocrinol Metab 1994; 78:884–889.

360. Camus J, Roussy G. Experimental researches on the pituitary body. Endocrinology 1920; 4:507–522.

361. Fisher C, Ingram WR. The effect of interruption of the supraopticohypophyseal tracts on the antidiuretic, pressor and oxytocic activity of the posterior lobe of the hypophysis. Endocrinology 1936; 20:762–768.

362. Heinbecker P, White HL. Hypothalamico-hypophysial system and its relation to water balance in the dog. Am J Physiol 1944; 133:582–593.

363. Rasmussen AT, Gardner WJ. Effects of hypophysial stalk resection on the hypophysis and hypothalamus of man. Endocrinology 1940; 27:219–226.

364. Lipsett MB, MacLean JP, West CD, et al. An analysis of the polyuria induced by hypophysectomy in man. J Clin Endocrinol Metab 1956; 16:183–195.

365. Velhuis JD, Hammond JM. Endocrine function after spontaneous infarction of the human pituitary: report, review, and reappraisal. Endocr Rev 1980; 1:100–107.

366. Jialal E, Desai RK, Rajput MC. An assessment of posterior pituitary function in patients with Sheehan's syndrome. Clin Endocrinol 1987; 27:91–95.

367. Bononi PL, Robinson AG. Central diabetes insipidus: management in the postoperative period. Endocrinologist 1996; 1:180–185.

368. Seckl JR, Dunger DB, Lightman SL. Neurohypophyseal peptide function during early postoperative diabetes insipidus. Brain 1987; 110:737–746.

369. Mudd RH, Dodge HW, Clark EC, et al. Experimental diabetes insipidus: a study of the normal interphase. Proc Staff Meet Mayo Clin 1957; 32:94–108.

370. Quain R. Polyuria. In: Quain R, ed. A Dictionary of Medicine. New York: D Appleton, 1883: 1239–1241.

371. Osler W. The Principles and Practice of Medicine. New York: D Appleton, 1893.

372. Miller M, Dalakos T, Moses AM, et al. Recognition of partial defects in antidiuretic hormone secretion. Ann Intern Med 1970; 73:721–729.

373. Barlow E, deWardener HE. Compulsive water drinking. Q J Med 1959; 28:235–258.

374. Manson AD, Yalowitz PA, Randall RV, et al. Dilatation of the urinary tract associated with pituitary and nephrogenic diabetes insipidus. J Urol 1970; 103:327–331.

375. Streitz JM Jr, Streitz JM. Polyuric urinary tract dilatation with renal damage. J Urol 1988; 139:784–785.

376. Zerbe RL, Robertson GL. A comparison of plasma vasopressin measurements with a standard indirect test in the differential diagnosis of polyuria. N Engl J Med 1981; 305:1539–1546.

377. Tien R, Kucharczyk J, Kucharczyk W. MR imaging of the brain in patients with diabetes insipidus. Am J Neuroradiol 1991; 12:533–542.

378. Moses AM, Clayton B, Hochhauser L. Use of T1-weighted MR imaging to differentiate between primary polydipsia and central diabetes insipidus. Am J Neuroradiol 1992; 13:1273–1277.

379. Robertson GL. The use of vasopressin assays in physiology and pathophysiology. Semin Nephrol 1994; 14:368–383.

380. Kanno K, Sasaki S, Hirata Y, et al. Urinary excretion of aquaporin-2 in patients with diabetes insipidus. N Engl J Med 1995; 332:1540–1545.

381. Elliot S, Goldsmith P, Knepper M, et al. Urinary excretion of aquaporin-2 in humans: a potential marker of collecting duct responsiveness to vasopressin. J Am Soc Nephrol 1996; 7:403–409.

382. Arieff AI, Guisado R, Lazarowitz VC. The pathophysiology of hyperosmolar states. In: Andreoli TE, Grantham JJ, Rector FC, eds. Disturbances in Body Fluid Osmolality. Bethesda: American Physiological Society, 1977: 227–250.

383. Chan PH, Fishman RA. Elevation of rat brain amino acids and idiogenic osmoles induced by hyperosmolality. Brain Res 1979; 161:293–301.

384. Morris-Jones PH, Houston IB, Evans RC. Prognosis of the neurological complications of acute hyponatremia. Lancet 1967; 2:1385–1389.

385. Robertson GL, Harris A. Clinical use of vasopressin analogues. Hosp Pract 1989; 24:114–139.

386. Cobb WE, Spare S, Reichlin S. Neurogenic diabetes insipidus: management with dDAVP (1-desamino-8-D-arginine vasopressin). Ann Intern Med 1978; 88:183–188.

387. Cunnah D, Ross G, Besser GM: Management of cranial diabetes insipidus with oral desmopressin (dDAVP). Clin Endocrinol 1986; 24:253–257.

388. Fjellestad-Paulson A, Paulsen O, D'Agay-Abensour L, et al. Central diabetes insipidus: oral treatment with dDAVP. Regul Pept 1993; 45:303–307.

389. Moses AM, Numann P, Miller M. Mechanism of chlorpropamide-induced antidiuresis in man: evidence for release of ADH and enhancement of peripheral action. Metab Clin Exp 1973; 22:59–66.

390. Pokracki FJ, Robinson AG, Seif SM. Chlorpropamide effect: measurement of neurophysin and vasopressin in humans and rats. Metabolism 1981; 30:72–78.

391. Kusano E, Braun-Werness JL, Vick DJ, et al. Chlorpropamide action on renal concentrating mechanism in rats with hypothalamic diabetes insipidus. J Clin Invest 1983; 72:1298–1313.

392. Moses AM, Howanitz J, van Gemert M, et al. Clofibrate-induced antidiuresis. J Clin Invest 1973; 52:535–542.

393. Kimura T, Matsui K, Sato T, et al. Mechanism of carbamazepine (Tegretol)–induced antidiuresis: evidence for release of antidiuretic hormone and impaired excretion of a water load. J Clin Endocrinol Metab 1974; 38:356–362.

394. Gold PW, Robertson GL, Ballenger JC, et al. Carbamazepine diminishes the sensitivity of the plasma arginine vasopressin response to osmotic stimulation. J Clin Endocrinol Metab 1983; 57:952–957.

395. Crawford JD, Kennedy GC. Clinical results of treatment of diabetes insipidus with drugs of the chlorthiazide series. N Engl J Med 1960; 262:737–742.

396. McIlraith CH. Notes on some cases of diabetes insipidus with marked family and hereditary tendencies. Lancet 1892; 2:767.

397. deLange C. Über erblichen Diabetes insipidus. Jahrb Kinderheilk 1935; 145:1.

398. Forssman H. On hereditary diabetes insipidus. Acta Med Scand 1945; 121(Suppl 159):3–196.

399. Williams RH, Henry C. Nephrogenic diabetes insipidus: transmitted by females and appearing during infancy in males. Ann Intern Med 1947; 27:84–95.

400. Waring AJ, Kajdi L, Tappan V. A congenital defect of water metabolism. Am J Dis Child 1945; 69:323–324.

401. Fichman MP, Brokker G. Deficient renal cyclic adenosine 3′,5′-monophosphate production in nephrogenic diabetes insipidus. J Clin Endocrinol Metab 1972; 35:35–47.

402. Bell NH, Clark CM Jr, Avery S, et al. Demonstration of a defect in the formation of adenosine 3′,5′-monophosphate in vasopressin-resistant diabetes insipidus. Pediatr Res 1974; 8:223–230.

403. Bichet DG, Razi M, Arthus M-F, et al. Epinephrine and dDAVP administration in patients with congenital nephrogenic diabetes insipidus. Evidence

for a pre–cyclic AMP V_2 receptor defective mechanism. Kidney Int 1989; 36:859–866.

404. Orr FR, Filipich RL. Studies with angiotensin in nephrogenic diabetes insipidus. Can Med Assoc J 1967; 97:841–845.

405. Moses AM, Scheinman SJ, Schroeder ET. Antidiuretic and PGE_2 responses to AVP and dDAVP in subjects with central and nephrogenic diabetes insipidus. Am J Physiol 1985; 248:F354–F359.

406. Bichet DG, Razi M, Lonergan M, et al. Hemodynamic and coagulation responses to 1-desamino/8-D-arginine vasopressin in patients with congenital nephrogenic diabetes insipidus. N Engl J Med 1988; 318:881–887.

407. Brenner B, Seligsohn U, Hochberg Z. Normal response of factor VIII and von Willebrand factor to 1-desamino-8-D-arginine vasopressin in nephrogenic diabetes insipidus. J Clin Endocrinol Metab 1988; 67:191–193.

408. Moses AM, Miller JL, Levine MA. Two distinct pathophysiological mechanisms in congenital nephrogenic diabetes insipidus. J Clin Endocrinol Metab 1988; 66:1259–1264.

409. Knoers N, Monnens LAH. Invited review: nephrogenic diabetes insipidus: clinical symptoms, pathogenesis, genetics and treatment. Pediatr Nephrol 1992; 6:476–482.

410. Holtzman EJ, Kolakowski LF, Ausiello DA. The molecular biology of congenital nephrogenic diabetes insipidus. In: Bonventre J, ed. Molecular Nephrology. New York: Marcel Dekker, 1994: 887–912.

411. van Lieburg AF, Verdijk MAJ, Knoers NVAM, et al. Patients with autosomal nephrogenic diabetes insipidus homozygous for mutations in the aquaporin 2 water-channel gene. Am J Hum Genet 1994; 55:648–652.

412. Pan Y, Metzenberg A, Das S, et al. Mutations in the V_2 vasopressin receptor gene are associated with X-linked nephrogenic diabetes insipidus. Nature Genet 1992; 2:103–106.

413. Seibold A, Brabet P, Rosenthal W, et al. Structure and chromosomal localization of the human antidiuretic hormone receptor gene. Am J Hum Genet 1992; 51:1078–1083.

414. Jans DA, van der Oost BA, Ropers HH, et al. Derivatives of somatic cell hybrids which carry the human gene locus for nephrogenic diabetes insipidus (NDI) express functional vasopressin renal V_2-type receptors. J Biol Chem 1992; 265:15379–15382.

415. van den Ouweland AMW, Dreesen JCFM, Verdijk M, et al. Mutations in the vasopressin type 2 receptor gene (AVPR2) associated with nephrogenic diabetes insipidus. Nature Genet 1992; 2:99–102.

416. Knoers N, van der Heyden H, van der Oost BA, et al. Nephrogenic diabetes insipidus: close linkage with markers from the distal long arm of the human X chromosome. Hum Genet 1988; 30:31–38.

417. Rosenthal W, Seibold A, Antaramian A, et al. Molecular identification of the gene responsible for congenital nephrogenic diabetes insipidus. Nature 1992; 359:233–235.

418. Knoers NVAM, van den Ouweland AMW, Verdijk M, et al. Inheritance of mutations in the V_2 receptor gene in thirteen families with nephrogenic diabetes insipidus. Kidney Int 1994; 46:170–176.

419. Bichet DG, Birnbaumer M, Lonergan M, et al. Nature and recurrence of AVPR2 mutations in X-linked nephrogenic diabetes insipidus. Am J Hum Genet 1994; 55:278–286.

420. Tsukaguchi H, Matsubara H, Taketani S, et al. Binding-, intracellular transport-, and biosynthesis-defective mutants of vasopressin type 2 receptor in patients with X-linked nephrogenic diabetes insipidus. J Clin Invest 1995; 96:2043–2050.

421. Wildin RS, Antush MJ, Bennett RL, et al. Heterogeneous AVPR2 gene mutations in congenital nephrogenic diabetes insipidus. Am J Hum Genet 1994; 55:266–277.

422. Oksche A, Dickson J, Schülein R, et al. Two novel mutations in the vasopressin V_2 receptor gene in patients with congenital nephrogenic diabetes insipidus. Biochem Biophys Res Commun 1994; 205:552–557.

423. Yuasa H, Ito M, Kurokawa K, et al. Novel mutations in the V_2 vasopressin receptor gene in two pedigrees with congenital nephrogenic diabetes insipidus. J Clin Endocrinol Metab 1994; 79:361–365.

424. Tajima T, Nakae J, Takekoshi Y, et al. Three novel AVPR2 mutations in three Japanese families with X-linked nephrogenic diabetes insipidus. Pediatr Res 1996; 39:522–526.

425. Yokoyama K, Yamauchi A, Izumi M, et al. A low-affinity vasopressin V_2-receptor gene in a kindred with X-linked nephrogenic diabetes insipidus. J Am Soc Nephrol 1996; 7:410–414.

426. Jinnouchi H, Araki E, Miyamura N, et al. Analysis of vasopressin receptor type II (V2R) gene in three Japanese pedigrees with congenital nephrogenic diabetes insipidus: identification of a family with complete deletion of the V2R gene. Eur J Endocrinol 1996; 134:689–698.

427. Online Mendelian Inheritance in Man, OMIM (TM). Johns Hopkins University, Baltimore, MD. MIM Numbers: 304800 diabetes insipidus nephrogenic; 222000 diabetes insipidus, renal type, autosomal recessive. World Wide Web URL: http://www3.ncbi.nlm.nih.gov/omim/.

428. Bichet DG. Nephrogenic diabetes insipidus. In: Cameron JS, Davison AM, Grünfeld JP, et al, eds. Oxford Textbook of Clinical Nephrology. 2nd ed. New York: Oxford University Press (in press).

429. van Lieburg AF, Verdijk MAJ, Schoute F, et al. Clinical phenotype of nephrogenic diabetes insipidus in females heterozygous for a vasopressin type 2 receptor mutation. Hum Genet 1995; 96:70–78.

430. Bichet DG, Hendy GN, Lonergan M, et al. X-linked nephrogenic diabetes insipidus: from the ship Hopewell to restriction fragment length polymorphism studies. Am J Hum Genet 1992; 51:1089–1102.

431. Bode HH, Crawford JD. Nephrogenic diabetes insipidus in North America—the Hopewell hypothesis. N Engl J Med 1969; 280:750–754.

432. Bichet DG, Arthus MF, Lonergan M, et al. X-linked nephrogenic diabetes insipidus mutations in North America and the Hopewell hypothesis. J Clin Invest 1993; 92:1262–1268.

433. Holtzman EJ, Kolakowski LF Jr, O'Brien D, et al. A null mutation in the vasopressin V_2 receptor gene (AVPR2) associated with nephrogenic diabetes insipidus in the Hopewell kindred. Hum Mol Genet 1993; 2:1201–1204.

434. Vogel F, Motulsky AG. Human Genetics: Problems and Approaches. 2nd ed. Berlin: Springer, 1986: 347–349.

435. Souied E, Gerber S, Rozet J-M, et al. Five novel missense mutations of the rhodopsin gene in autosomal dominant retinitis pigmentosa. Hum Mol Genet 1994; 3:1433–1434.

436. Vaithinathan R, Berson EL, Dryja TP. Further screening of the rhodopsin gene in patients with autosomal dominant retinitis pigmentosa. Genomics 1994; 21:461–463.

437. Cooper DN, Krawczak M, Antaonarakis SE. The nature and mechanisms of human gene mutation. In: Scriver CR, Beaudet AL, Sly WS, et al, eds. The Metabolic and Molecular Bases of Inherited Disease. 7th ed, Vol I. New York: McGraw-Hill, 1995: 259–291.

438. Rosenthal W, Antaramian A, Gilbert S, et al. Nephrogenic diabetes insipidus. J Biol Chem 1993; 268:13030–13033.

439. Birnbaumer M, Gilbert S, Rosenthal W. An extracellular congenital nephrogenic diabetes insipidus mutation of the vasopressin receptor reduces cell surface expression, affinity for ligand, and coupling to the G_s/adenylyl cyclase system. Mol Endocrinol 1994; 8:886–894.

440. Pan Y, Wilson P, Gitschier J. The effect of eight V_2 vasopressin receptor mutations on stimulation of adenyl cyclase and binding to vasopressin. J Biol Chem 1994; 269:31933–31937.

441. Oksche A, Schülein R, Rutz C, et al. Vasopressin V_2 receptor mutants causing X-linked nephrogenic diabetes insipidus: analysis of expression, processing and function. Mol Pharmacol 1996 (in revision).

442. Hobbs HH, Russell DW, Brown MS, et al. The LDL receptor locus in familial hypercholesterolemia: mutations analysis of a membrane protein. Annu Rev Genet 1990; 24:133–170.

443. Kojro E, Eich P, Gimpl G, et al. Direct identification of an extracellular agonist binding site in the renal V_2 vasopressin receptor. Biochemistry 1993; 32:13537–13544.

444. Chini B, Mouillac B, Ala Y, et al. Tyr115 is the key residue for determining agonist selectivity in the V_{1a} vasopressin receptor. EMBO J 1995; 14:2176–2182.

445. Schöneberg T, Yun J, Wenkert D, et al. Functional rescue of mutant V_2 vasopressin receptors causing nephrogenic diabetes insipidus by a coexpressed receptor polypeptide. EMBO J 1996; 15:1283–1291.

446. Schülein R, Rutz C, Rosenthal W. Membrane targeting and determination of transmembrane topology of the human vasopressin V_2 receptor. J Biol Chem (in revision).

447. Uchida S, Sasaki S, Fushimi K, et al. Isolation of human aquaporin-CD gene. J Biol Chem 1994; 269:23451–23455.

448. Deen PMT, Weghuis DO, Sinke RJ, et al. Assignment of the human gene for the water channel of renal collecting duct aquaporin 2 (AQP2) to chromosome 12 region q12 q13. Cytogenet Cell Genet 1994; 66:260–262.

449. Knoers N, Monnens AH. A variant of nephrogenic diabetes insipidus: V_2 receptor abnormality restricted to the kidney. Eur J Pediatr 1991; 150:370-373.

450. Langley JM, Balfe JW, Selander T, et al. Autosomal recessive inheritance of vasopressin-resistant diabetes insipidus. Am J Med Genet 1991; 38:90-94.

451. Lonergan M, Birnbaumer M, Arthus MF, et al. Non–X-linked nephrogenic diabetes insipidus: phenotype and genotype features. J Am Soc Nephrol 1993; 4:264 (abstract).

452. Bichet DG, Arthus MF, Lonergan M, et al. Autosomal dominant and autosomal recessive nephrogenic diabetes insipidus: novel mutations in the AQP2 gene. J Am Soc Nephrol 1995; 6:717 (abstract).

453. Singer I, Forrest JN. Drug-induced states of nephrogenic diabetes insipidus. Kidney Int 1976; 10:82–95.

454. Dousa TP, Wilson DM. Effects of demethylchlortetracycline on cellular action of antidiuretic hormone in vitro. Kidney Int 1974; 5:279–284.

455. Frascino JA, O'Flaherty J, Olmo C, et al. Effect of inorganic fluoride on the renal concentrating mechanism. Possible nephrotoxicity in man. J Lab Clin Med 1972; 79:192–203.

456. Wallin JD, Kaplan RA. Effect of sodium fluoride on concentrating and diluting ability in the rat. Am J Physiol 1977; 232:F335–F340.

457. Jackson BA, Edwards RM, Dousa TP. Lithium-induced polyuria: effect of lithium on adenylate cyclase and adenosine $3',5'$-monophosphate phosphodiesterase in medullary ascending limb of Henle's loop and in medullary collecting tubules. Endocrinology 1980; 107:1693–1698.

458. Goldberg H, Clayman P, Skorecki K. Mechanism of Li inhibition of vasopressin-sensitive adenylate cyclase in cultured renal epithelial cells. Am J Physiol 1988; 255:F995–F1002.

459. Yamake M, Kusano E, Toshifumi T, et al. Cellular mechanism of lithium-induced nephrogenic diabetes insipidus in rats. Am J Physiol 1991; 261:F505–F511.

460. Marples D, Christensen S, Christensen EI, et al. Lithium-induced downregulation of aquaporin-2 water channel expression in rat kidney medulla. J Clin Invest 1995; 95:1838–1845.

461. Boton R, Gaviria M, Batlle DC. Prevalence, pathogenesis, and treatment of

renal dysfunction associated with chronic lithium therapy. Am J Physiol 1987; 10:329–345.

462. Usberti M, Decaux M, Guillot M, et al. Renal prostaglandin E₂ in nephrogenic diabetes insipidus: effects of inhibition of prostaglandin synthesis in indomethacin. J Pediatr 1980; 97:476–478.

463. Delaney V, de Pertuz Y, Nixon D, et al. Indomethacin in streptozocin-induced nephrogenic diabetes insipidus. Am J Kidney Dis 1987; 9:79–83.

464. Allen HM, Jackson RL, Winchester MD, et al. Indomethacin in the treatment of lithium-induced nephrogenic diabetes insipidus. Arch Intern Med 1989; 149:1123–1126.

465. Libber S, Harrison H, Spector D. Treatment of nephrogenic diabetes insipidus with prostaglandin synthesis inhibitors. J Pediatr 1986; 108:305–311.

466. Alon U, Chan JCM. Hydrochlorothiazide-amiloride in the treatment of congenital nephrogenic diabetes insipidus. Am J Nephrol 1985; 5:9–13.

467. Knoers N, Monnens LAH. Amiloride-hydrochlorothiazide versus indomethacin-hydrochlorothiazide in the treatment of nephrogenic diabetes insipidus. J Pediatr 1990; 117:499–502.

468. Kosten TR, Forrest JN. Treatment of severe lithium-induced polyuria with amiloride. Am J Psychiatry 1986; 143:1563–1568.

469. Batlle DC, von Riotte AB, Gaviria M, et al. Amelioration of polyuria by amiloride in patients receiving long-term lithium therapy. N Engl J Med 1985; 312:408–414.

470. Manitius A, Levitin H, Beck D, et al. On the mechanisms of impairment of renal concentrating ability in potassium deficiency. J Clin Invest 1960; 39:684–692.

471. Galvez OG, Roberts BW, Bay WH, et al. Studies on the mechanism of polyuria with hypokalemia. Kidney Int 1976; 10:583A.

472. Berl T, Linas SL, Aisenbery GA, et al. On the mechanism of polyuria in potassium depletion. J Clin Invest 1977; 60:620–625.

473. Manitius A, Levitin H, Beck D, et al. On the mechanism of impairment of renal concentrating ability in hypercalcemia. J Clin Invest 1960; 39:693–697.

474. Campbell BJ, Woodward G, Broberg V. Calcium-mediated interactions between the antidiuretic hormone and renal plasma membranes. J Biol Chem 1972; 247:6167–6175.

475. Barron WM, Cohen LH, Ulland LA, et al. Transient vasopressin-resistant diabetes insipidus of pregnancy. N Engl J Med 1984; 310:442–444.

476. Hughes JM, Barron WM, Vance ML. Recurrent diabetes insipidus associated with pregnancy: pathophysiology and therapy. Obstet Gynecol 1989; 73:462–464.

477. Shah SV, Thakur V. Vasopressinase and diabetes insipidus of pregnancy. Ann Intern Med 1988; 109:435–436.

478. Ford SM Jr. Transient vasopressin-resistant diabetes insipidus of pregnancy. Obstet Gynecol 1986; 68:288–289.

479. Kallen BA, Carlsson SS, Bengtsson BK. Diabetes insipidus and use of desmopressin (Minirin) during pregnancy. Eur J Endocrinol 1995; 132:144–146.

480. Finberg L, Kiley S, Lettrell CN. Mass accidental salt poisoning in infancy. JAMA 1963; 184:187–190.

481. Dodge PR, Sotos JF, Gamstorp I, et al. Neurophysiologic disturbances in hypertonic dehydration. Trans Am Neurol Assoc 1962; 87:33–36.

482. Sotos JF, Dodge PR, Meara P, et al. Studies in experimental hypertonicity: pathogenesis of the clinical syndrome, biochemical abnormalities and cause of death. Pediatrics 1960; 26:925–937.

483. Holliday MA, Kalayci MN, Harrah J. Factors that limit brain volume changes in response to acute and sustained hyper- and hyponatremia. J Clin Invest 1968; 47:1916–1928.

484. Arieff AI, Guisado R. Effects on the central nervous system of hypernatremic and hyponatremic states. Kidney Int 1976; 10:104–116.

485. Cala PM. Volume regulation by red blood cells: mechanisms of ion transport. Mol Physiol 1983; 4:33–52.

486. Cronin RE. Psychogenic polydipsia with hyponatremia: report of eleven cases. Am J Kidney Dis 1987; 4:410–416.

487. Victor W, Vieweg R, Godleski LS, et al. Failure of antipsychotic drug dose to explain abnormal diurnal weight gain among 129 chronically psychotic inpatients. Prog Neuropsychopharmacol Biol Psychiatry 1989; 13:709–723.

488. Kramer DS, Drake ME. Acute psychosis, polydipsia, and inappropriate secretion of antidiuretic hormone. Am J Med 1983; 75:712–714.

489. Levine S, McManus BM, Blackbourne BD, et al. Fatal water intoxication, schizophrenia, and diuretic therapy for systemic hypertension. Am J Med 1987; 82:153–155.

490. Goldman MB, Luchins DJ, Robertson GL. Mechanisms of altered water metabolism in psychotic patients with polydipsia and hyponatremia. N Engl J Med 1988; 318:397–403.

491. Vieweg V, Glick JL, Herring S, et al. Absence of carbamazepine-induced hyponatremia among patients also given lithium. Am J Psychiatry 1987; 144:943–947.

492. Yassa R, Iskandar H, Nastase C, et al. Carbamazepine and hyponatremia in patients with affective disorder. Am J Psychiatry 1988; 145:339–342.

493. Fanestil DA. Hyposmolar syndromes. In: Andreoli TE, Grantham JJ, Rector FC, eds. Disturbances in Body Fluid Osmolality. Bethesda: American Physiological Society, 1977: 267–284.

494. Hilden T, Svendsen TL. Electrolyte disturbances in beer drinkers: a specific "hypo-osmolality syndrome." Lancet 1975; 2:245–246.

495. McCance RA. Experimental sodium chloride deficiency in man. Proc R Soc Lond (Biol) 1936; 119:245–268.

496. Harrington AR. Hyponatremia due to sodium depletion in the absence of vasopressin. Am J Physiol 1972; 222:768–774.

497. Berliner RW, Davidson DG. Production of hypertonic urine in the absence of pituitary antidiuretic hormone. J Clin Invest 1957; 36:1416–1427.

498. Kassirer JP, Berkman PM, Lawrenz DR, et al. The critical role of chloride in the correction of hypokalemic alkalosis in man. Am J Med 1965; 38:172–189.

499. Valtin H, Sokol HW, Sunde D. Genetic approaches to the study of the regulation and actions of vasopressin. Recent Prog Horm Res 1975; 31:447–486.

500. Szatalowicz VL, Arnold PE, Chaimovitz C, et al. Radioimmunoassay of plasma arginine vasopressin in hyponatremic patients with congestive heart failure. N Engl J Med 1981; 305:263–266.

501. Weitzman RE, Kleeman CR. The clinical physiology of water metabolism. III: The water depletion (hyperosmolar) and water excess (hypoosmolar) syndromes. West J Med 1980; 132:16–38.

502. Seldin DW, Eknoyan G, Suki WN, et al. Localization of diuretic action from the pattern of water and electrolyte excretion. Ann NY Acad Sci 1966; 139:328–343.

503. Fichman MP, Vorherr H, Kleeman CR, et al. Diuretic-induced hyponatremia. Ann Intern Med 1971; 75:853–863.

504. Friedman E, Shadel M, Halkin H, et al. Thiazide-induced hyponatremia: reproducibility by single-dose rechallenge and an analysis of pathogenesis. Ann Intern Med 1989; 110:24–30.

505. Chung H-M, Kluge R, Schrier RW, et al. Clinical assessment of extracellular fluid volume in hyponatremia. Am J Med 1987; 83:905–908.

506. Schrier RW, Linas SL. Mechanisms of the defect in water excretion in adrenal insufficiency. Miner Electrolyte Metab 1980; 4:1–7.

507. Raff H. Glucocorticoid inhibition of neurohypophysial vasopressin secretion. Am J Physiol 1987; 252:R635–R644.

508. Linas SL, Berl T, Robertson GL, et al. Role of vasopressin in the impaired water excretion of glucocorticoid deficiency. Kidney Int 1980; 18:58–67.

509. Ishikawa S-E, Kim JK, Schrier RW. Effects of arginine vasopressin antidiuretic and vasopressor antagonists in glucocorticoid and mineralocorticoid deficient rats. In: Schrier RW, ed. Vasopressin. New York: Raven, 1985: 171–180.

510. Chinitz A, Turner FL: The association of primary hypothyroidism and inappropriate secretion of the antidiuretic hormone. Arch Intern Med 1965; 116:871–874.

511. DeRubertis FR, Mechelis MF, Bloom ME, et al. Impaired water excretion in myxedema. Am J Med 1971; 51:41–53.

512. DiScala VA, Kinney MJ. Effects of myxedema on the renal diluting and concentrating mechanism. Am J Med 1971; 50:325–335.

513. Anderson RJ, Chung H-M, Kluge R, et al. Hyponatremia: a prospective analysis of its epidemiology and the pathogenetic role of vasopressin. Ann Intern Med 1985; 102:164–168.

514. Chung H-M, Kluge R, Schrier RW, et al. Postoperative hyponatremia: a prospective study. Arch Intern Med 1986; 146:333–336.

515. Gross PA, Pehrisch H, Rascher W, et al. Pathogenesis of clinical hyponatremia: observations of vasopressin and fluid intake in 100 hyponatremic medical patients. Eur J Clin Invest 1987; 17:123–129.

516. Gross P, Pehrisch H, Rascher W, et al. Vasopressin in hyponatremia: what stimuli? J Cardiovasc Pharmacol 1986; 8:S92–S95.

517. Leaf A, Bartter FC, Santos RF, et al. Evidence in man that urinary electrolyte loss induced by polydipsia is a function of water retention. J Clin Invest 1953; 32:868–871.

518. Gertz KH, Boylan J. Glomerulotubular balance. In: Orloff J, Berliner RW, eds. Handbook of Physiology. Sect 8: Renal Physiology. Bethesda: American Physiological Society, 1973: 763–790.

519. Chan WY. A study on the mechanism of vasopressin escape: effects of chronic vasopressin and overhydration on renal tissue osmolality and electrolytes in dogs. J Pharmacol Exp Ther 1973; 184:244–252.

520. Schwartz WB, Bennett W, Curelop S, et al. A syndrome of renal sodium loss and hyponatremia probably resulting from inappropriate secretion of antidiuretic hormone. Am J Med 1957; 23:529–542.

521. Zerbe R, Stropes L, Robertson G. Vasopressin function in the syndrome of inappropriate diuresis. Annu Rev Med 1980; 31:315–327.

522. Goldberg M. Abnormalities in the renal excretion of water. Med Clin North Am 1963; 47:915–933.

523. Clive DM, Stoff JS. Renal syndromes associated with nonsteroidal antiinflammatory drugs. N Engl J Med 1984; 310:563–572.

524. Blum M, Aviram A. Ibuprofen induced hyponatremia. Rheumatol Rehabil 1980; 19:258–259.

525. Reeves WB, Foley RJ, Weinman EJ. Nephrotoxicity from non-steroidal anti-inflammatory drugs. South Med J 1985; 78:318–321.

526. Petersson I, Nilsson G, Hansson BG, et al. Water intoxication associated with non-steroidal anti-inflammatory drug therapy. Acta Med Scand 1987; 221:221–223.

527. Weisberg LS. Pseudohyponatremia: a reappraisal. Am J Med 1989; 86:315–318.

528. Rao PN. Fluid absorption during urological endoscopy. Br J Urol 1987; 60:93–99.

529. Campbell HT, Fincher ME, Sklar AH. Severe hyponatremia without severe hypo-osmolality following transurethral resection of the prostate (TURP) in end-stage renal disease. Am J Kidney Dis 1988; 12:152–155.

530. Weir JF, Larson EE, Rowntree LG. Studies in diabetes insipidus, water balance and water intoxication. Arch Intern Med 1922; 29:321–330.

531. Arieff AI, Llach F, Massry SG. Neurological manifestations and morbidity of hyponatremia: correlation with brain water and electrolytes. Medicine 1976; 55:121–129.

532. Pollock AS, Arieff AI. Abnormalities of cell volume regulation and the functional consequences. Am J Physiol 1980; 239:F195–F205.

533. Sterns RH, Baer J, Ebersol S, et al. Organic osmolytes in acute hyponatremia. Am J Physiol 1993; 264:F833–F836.

534. Grantham J, Linshaw M. The effect of hyponatremia on the regulation of intracellular volume and solute composition. Circ Res 1984; 54:483–491.

535. Sterns RH, Thomas DJ, Herndon RM. Brain dehydration and neurologic deterioration after rapid correction of hyponatremia. Kidney Int 1989; 35:69–75.

536. Kurtz I. Measuring intracerebral osmolytes in hyponatremic disorders. J Clin Invest 1995; 95:441–442.

537. Lien Y-HH, Shapiro JI, Chan L. Study of brain electrolytes and organic osmolytes during correction of chronic hyponatremia. J Clin Invest 1991; 88:303–309.

538. Videen JS, Michaelis T, Pinto P. Human cerebral osmolytes during chronic hyponatremia. J Clin Invest 1995; 95:788–793.

539. Kleinschmidt-DeMasters BK, Norenberg MD. Rapid correction of hyponatremia causes demyelination: relation to central pontine myelinolysis. Science 1981; 211:1068–1070.

540. Telfer AB, Miller EM. Central pontine myelinolysis following hyponatremia, demonstrated by computerized tomography. Ann Neurol 1979; 6:455–456.

541. Norenberg MD, Leslie KO. Correction of hyponatremia and central pontine myelinolysis. Am J Med 1982; 73:882.

542. Sterns RH. Neurological deterioration following treatment for hyponatremia. Am J Kidney Dis 1989; 13:434–437.

543. Hantman D, Rossier B, Zohlman R, et al. Rapid correction of hyponatremia in the syndrome of inappropriate secretion of antidiuretic hormone. Ann Intern Med 1973; 78:870–875.

544. Sterns RH, Cappucio JD, Silver SM, et al. Neurologic sequelae after treatment of severe hyponatremia: a multicenter perspective. J Am Soc Nephrol 1994; 4:1522–1530.

545. Arieff AI. Hyponatremia associated with permanent brain damage. Adv Intern Med 1987; 32:325–344.

546. Berl T. Treating hyponatremia: damned if we do and damned if we don't. Kidney Int 1990; 37:1006–1018.

547. Ayus JC, Krothapalli RK, Arieff AI. Treatment of symptomatic hyponatremia and its relation to brain damage: a prospective study. N Engl J Med 1987; 317:1190–1195.

548. Sterns RH. Severe symptomatic hyponatremia: treatment and outcome. Ann Intern Med 1987; 107:656–664.

549. Fraser CL, Arieff AI. Fatal central diabetes mellitus and insipidus resulting from untreated hyponatremia: a new syndrome. Ann Intern Med 1990; 112:113–119.

550. Arieff AI. Hyponatremia, convulsions, respiratory arrest, and permanent brain damage after elective surgery in healthy women. N Engl J Med 1986; 314:1529–1535.

551. Ayus JC, Wheeler JM, Arieff AI. Postoperative hyponatremic encephalopathy in menstruant women. Ann Intern Med 1992; 117:891–897.

552. Arieff AI, Ayus JC, Fraser CL. Hyponatraemia and death or permanent brain damage in healthy children. Br Med J 1992; 304:1218–1222.

553. Ayus JC, Krothapalli RK, Arieff AI. Sexual difference in survival with severe symptomatic hyponatremia. Kidney Int 1988; 33:180.

554. Fraser CL, Kucharczyk J, Arieff AI, et al. Sex differences result in increased morbidity from hyponatremia in female rats. Am J Physiol 1989; 256:R880–R885.

555. Arieff AI, Kozniewska E, Roberts TP, et al. Age, gender, and vasopressin affect survival and brain adaptation in rats with metabolic encephalopathy. Am J Physiol 1995; 268:R1143–R1152.

556. Kozniewska E, Roberts TP, Vexler ZS, et al. Hormonal dependence of the effects of metabolic encephalopathy on cerebral perfusion and oxygen utilization in the rat. Circ Res 1995; 76:551–558.

557. Vexler ZS, Ayus JC, Roberts TP, et al. Hypoxic and ischemic hypoxia exacerbate brain injury associated with metabolic encephalopathy in laboratory animals. J Clin Invest 1994; 93:256–264.

558. Ayus JC, Krothapalli RK, Armstrong DL. Rapid correction of severe hyponatremia in the rat: histopathological changes in the brain. Am J Physiol 1985; 248:F711–F719.

559. Sterns RH. The management of hyponatremic emergencies. Crit Care Clin 1991; 7:127–142.

560. Forrest JN Jr, Cox M, Hong C, et al. Superiority of demeclocycline over lithium in the treatment of chronic syndrome of inappropriate secretion of antidiuretic hormone. N Engl J Med 1978; 298:173–177.

561. Dias N, Hocken AG. Oliguric renal failure complicating lithium carbonate therapy. Nephron 1972; 10:246–249.

562. Schrier RW. New treatments for hyponatremia. N Engl J Med 1978; 298:214–215.

563. Decaux G, Brimioulle S, Genette F, et al. Treatment of the syndrome of inappropriate secretion of antidiuretic hormone by urea. Am J Med 1980; 69:99–106.

564. Tsuboi Y, Ishikawa S, Fujisawa G, et al. Therapeutic efficacy of the non-peptide AVP antagonist OPC-31260 in cirrhotic rats. Kidney Int 1994; 46:237–244.

565. Fujisawa G, Ishikawa S, Tsuboi Y, et al. Therapeutic efficacy of non-peptide ADH antagonist OPC-31260 in SIADH rats. Kidney Int 1993; 44:19–23.

566. Ohnishi A, Orita Y, Okahara R, et al. Potent aquaretic agent: a novel nonpeptide selective vasopressin 2 antagonist (OPC-31260) in men. J Clin Invest 1993; 92:2653–2659.

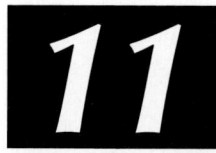

THE THYROID GLAND

P. Reed Larsen, Terry F. Davies, and Ian D. Hay

INTRODUCTION

Dysfunction and anatomic abnormalities of the thyroid are among the most common diseases of the endocrine glands. This chapter is designed to provide an up-to-date physiological and biochemical background, describe the various tests for evaluating patients with suspected disease of the thyroid gland, and discuss the pathophysiology and treatment of thyroid diseases.

PHYLOGENY

The phylogeny, embryogenesis, and certain aspects of thyroid function are closely interlinked with the gastrointestinal tract. The capacity of the thyroid to metabolize iodine and incorporate it into a variety of organic compounds occurs widely throughout the animal and plant kingdoms. Monoiodotyrosine (3-monoiodo-L-tyrosine [MIT]) and diiodotyrosine (3,5-diiodo-L-tyrosine [DIT]) are present in a variety of invertebrate species, including mollusks, crustaceans, coelenterates, annelids, insects, and certain marine algae. In these lower forms, however, no recognizable thyroid tissue is present. Thyroid tissue is confined to and is present in all vertebrates. A close link to the thyroid of higher vertebrates is evident in the ammocoete, the larval form of the lamprey.[1] Here the endostyle is capable of carrying out iodinations, but prior to metamorphosis a protease is expressed in the endostyle that can hydrolyze the iodoprotein formed. Presumably this permits the endostyle to lose its connection with the pharynx during metamorphosis and to assume its adult function as an endocrine organ that secretes iodothyronines, including 3,5,3',5'-tetraiodo-L-thyronine (thyroxine [T_4]) and 3,5,3'-triiodo-L-thyronine (T_3). Figure 11–1 shows the structural formulas of the thyroid hormones, their precursors, and certain of their metabolites.

Except perhaps in some lower vertebrates, control of thyroid function is mediated by pituitary thyrotropin (thyroid-stimulating hormone [TSH]). In higher vertebrates, control of TSH secretion is, in turn, influenced by a thyrotropin-releasing hormone (TRH) of hypothalamic origin. In many lower vertebrates the pituitary-thyroid axis does not respond to TRH, although TRH is present within the brain.

The phylogenetic association of the thyroid gland and the gastrointestinal tract is evident in several functions. Thus the salivary and gastric glands, like the thyroid, are capable of concentrating iodide in their secretions, although iodide transport in these sites is not responsive to stimulation by TSH. The salivary gland contains enzymes that are capable of iodinating tyrosine in the presence of hydrogen peroxide, although it forms insignificant quantities of iodoproteins under normal circumstances.

ANATOMIC AND FUNCTIONAL EMBRYOLOGY

The human thyroid anlage is first recognizable about 1 mo after conception, when the embryo is approximately 3.5 to 4.0 mm in length. The primordium begins as a thickening of epithelium in the pharyngeal floor, which later forms a diverticulum. With continuing development, the median diverticulum is displaced caudally, and the primitive stalk connecting the primordium with the pharyngeal floor elongates (thyroglossal duct). During its caudal displacement, the primordium assumes a bilobate shape, coming into contact and fusing with the ventral aspect of the fourth pharyngeal pouch. Normally the thyroglossal duct undergoes dissolution and fragmentation by about the second month after conception, leaving at its point of origin a small dimple at the junction of the middle and posterior thirds of the tongue, the foramen caecum. Cells of the lower portion of the duct differentiate into thyroid tissue, forming the pyramidal lobe of the gland. Concomitantly, histologic alterations occur throughout the gland. Complex interconnecting cord-like arrangements of cells interspersed with vascular connective tissue replace the solid epithelial mass and become tubule-like structures at

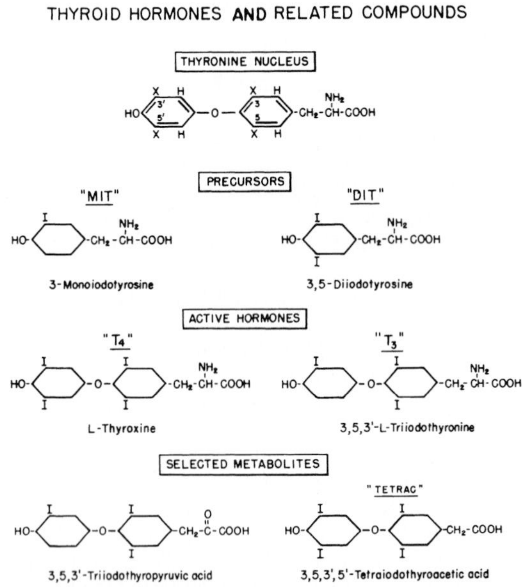

THYROID HORMONES **AND** RELATED COMPOUNDS

Figure 11–1. Structure of thyroid hormones and related compounds. The thyronine nucleus of the hormonally active iodinated amino acids, T_4 and T_3, is shown above. Iodinated thyronines are formed by the oxidative coupling of the precursor iodotyrosines MIT and DIT in varying combination. 3,5,3'-Triiodothyropyruvic acid is derived by oxidative deamination from T_3. TETRAC is derived from T_4 by oxidative deamination and decarboxylation.

about the third month of fetal life; shortly thereafter, follicular arrangements devoid of colloid appear, and eventually the follicles fill with colloid.

The ontogeny of thyroid function and its regulation in the human fetus are fairly well defined.[2, 3] Future follicular cells acquire the capacity to form thyroglobulin (Tg) as early as the 29th day of gestation, whereas the capacities to concentrate iodide and synthesize T_4 are delayed until about the 11th week. Radioactive iodine given to the mother is accumulated by the fetal thyroid soon thereafter. Early growth and development of the thyroid do not seem to be TSH dependent, because the capacity of the pituitary to synthesize and secrete TSH is not apparent until the 10th to 12th weeks. Subsequently, rapid changes in pituitary and thyroid function take place. Probably as a consequence of hypothalamic maturation and increasing secretion of TRH, the serum TSH concentration increases from about 18 to 26 wk, after which levels remain higher than those in the mother.[3, 4] The higher levels may reflect a higher set point of the negative-feedback control of TSH secretion during fetal life than at maturity. In the fetal rat and lamb T_3 has little ability to inhibit the response to TRH,[5] and in the human fetus the response to TRH is greater than that in the adult.[6] Thyroxine-binding globulin (TBG), the major thyroid hormone–binding protein in plasma, is detectable in the serum by the 10th gestational week and increases in concentration progressively to term. This increase in TBG concentration accounts in part for the progressive increase in the serum T_4 concentration in the second and third trimesters, but increased secretion of T_4 must also play a role because the concentration of unbound, or free, T_4 also rises.

The peripheral metabolism of T_4 in the human fetus differs markedly from that in the adult both quantitatively and qualitatively. Overall, rates of production and degradation of T_4 in unit per body mass exceed those in the adult. In addition, the enzymatic pathways by which T_4 is metabolized differ from those in the adult, favoring the formation of 3,3′,5′-triiodo-L-thyronine (reverse T_3 [rT_3]) at the expense of T_3.

Several aspects of fetal thyroid development are of note from the clinical standpoint.[7] Rarely, thyroid tissue may develop from remnants of the thyroglossal duct near the base of the tongue. Such lingual thyroid tissue may be the sole functioning thyroid present; its surgical removal will lead to hypothyroidism. More commonly, elements of the thyroglossal duct may persist and later give rise to thyroglossal duct cysts, or thyroid tissue progenitors may migrate to occupy a place within the mediastinum.

The fetal pituitary-thyroid axis functions as a unit that is essentially independent of the mother.[4, 8] Transplacental passage of TSH from mother to fetus is negligible or nearly so, but the same is not true of maternal T_4. In infants with congenital hypothyroidism caused by either thyroid peroxidase deficiency or athyrosis, serum concentrations of T_4 in cord blood can be one third to one half of normal.[9] Thus, at least when the maternal-fetal concentration gradient is high, there can be significant transfer of T_4 to the fetal circulation. This transfer may be significant, given the capacity of the fetal brain to increase the efficiency of T_4-to-T_3 conversion.[3, 10, 11] Thyroid hormones almost certainly condition skeletal maturation, influence prenatal maturation of the lung, and are required for normal development of the brain and intellectual function, either before birth or soon thereafter, making the diagnosis of neonatal hypothyroidism urgent.[12]

ANATOMY AND HISTOLOGY

The thyroid is one of the largest of the endocrine organs, weighing approximately 15 to 20 g in North American adults.

Moreover, the potential of the thyroid for growth is tremendous. Goiters can weigh many hundreds of grams. The normal thyroid is made up of two lobes joined by a thin band of tissue, the isthmus. The latter is approximately 0.5 cm thick, 2 cm wide, and 2 cm high. The individual lobes normally have a pointed superior pole and a poorly defined, blunt inferior pole that merges medially with the isthmus. Each lobe is approximately 2.0 to 2.5 cm in thickness and width at its largest diameter and is approximately 4.0 cm in length. Occasionally, especially when the remainder of the gland is goitrous, a pyramidal lobe is discernible as a finger-like projection directed upward from the isthmus, generally just lateral to the midline, usually on the left. The right lobe is normally more vascular than the left, is often the larger of the two, and tends to enlarge more in disorders associated with a diffuse increase in size.

Two pairs of vessels constitute the major arterial blood supply, namely the superior thyroid artery, arising from the external carotid artery, and the inferior thyroid artery, arising from the subclavian artery. Estimates of thyroid blood flow range from 4 to 6 mL/min/g, well in excess of the blood flow to the kidney (3 mL/min/g). In diffuse toxic goiter, blood flow rates may exceed 1 L/min. Increased flow is evidenced by the presence of a thrill or an audible bruit over the gland or in its immediate vicinity. The rich lymphatic drainage is of uncertain function relative to the endocrine activity of the gland, but the lymph contains a higher concentration of newly released radioiodine than does thyroid venous blood, probably in the form of iodoprotein.

The thyroid is innervated by both adrenergic and cholinergic nervous systems via fibers arising from the cervical ganglia and the vagus nerve, respectively. Afferent fibers pass through the laryngeal nerves and regulate an active vasomotor system. One function of neurogenic stimuli is to regulate blood flow to the thyroid. Although acute changes in blood flow do not appear to alter the rate of hormonal release, the rate of perfusion influences the delivery of TSH, iodide, and metabolic substrates and may eventually influence glandular function and growth.

In addition to vasomotor innervation, there is a network of adrenergic fibers that terminates near the basement membrane of the follicular wall. Moreover, adrenergic receptors are present in thyroid plasma membranes. These findings, together with the capacity of adrenergic (and other) amines to affect metabolism of the thyroid, indicate that the adrenergic nervous system can influence thyroid function by direct effects on the follicle cell as well as by changing blood flow.

The gland is composed of closely packed sacs, called acini or follicles, which are invested with a rich capillary network. The interior of the follicle is filled with the clear proteinaceous colloid that normally is the major constituent of the total thyroid mass. The diameter of the follicles varies considerably even within a single gland but averages about 200 μm. The iodine-accumulating function of the individual follicle varies with its surface area. The wall of the follicle is lined by a single layer of closely packed cuboidal cells, approximately 15 μm high. The cells of the acinar epithelium vary in height with the degree of glandular stimulation, becoming columnar when active and cuboidal when inactive. The epithelium rests on a basement membrane that is rich with mucopolysaccharides and that separates the follicular cells from the surrounding capillaries. From 20 to 40 follicles are demarcated by connective tissue septa to form a lobule supplied by a single artery. The function of a given lobule may vary from that of its neighbors.

With electron microscopy the thyroid epithelium has many features in common with other secretory cells and some peculiar to the thyroid. From the apex of the follicular cell, numerous microvilli extend into the colloid. It is at or near this surface of the cell that iodination, exocytosis, and the initial phase of hormone secretion, namely colloid resorption, occur.[10] The nucleus of the follicular cell has no distinctive features. The cytoplasm contains an extensive endoplasmic reticulum laden with microsomes. The endoplasmic reticulum is composed of a network of wide irregular tubules that contain the precursor of Tg. The carbohydrate component of Tg is probably added to this precursor in the Golgi apparatus, which is located apically.[13] Lysosomes and mitochondria are scattered throughout the cytoplasm. Stimulation by TSH results in enlargement of the Golgi apparatus, formation of pseudopodia at the apical surface, and appearance in the apical portion of the cell of many droplets that contain colloid taken up from the follicular lumen.

The thyroid also contains parafollicular, or C, cells that are the source of the calcium-lowering hormone calcitonin. These cells arise during embryonic development from the last pair of pharyngeal pouches but ultimately come to rest either among the cells of the follicular epithelium or in the thyroid interstitium.[14] They differ from the cells of the follicular epithelium in never bordering on the follicular lumen and in being rich in both mitochondria and α-glycerophosphate dehydrogenase. C cells undergo hyperplasia early in the syndrome of familial medullary carcinoma of the thyroid and give rise to this tumor in both its familial and its sporadic forms (see Chapter 32).

FORMATION AND SECRETION OF THYROID HORMONES

The function of the thyroid is to secrete such quantities of hormone as are necessary to meet the demands of the peripheral tissues. This requires the daily thyroidal uptake of sufficient iodide to allow the synthesis of approximately 100 μg of T_4, which is 65% iodine by weight.

Iodine Metabolism

Formation of normal quantities of thyroid hormone requires the availability of adequate quantities of exogenous iodine. The mechanisms for conserving iodine in the presence of iodine deficiency do not entirely succeed in preventing depletion of iodine stores, which ultimately may lead to insufficient hormone production. Given the fact that at least 1 billion individuals live in iodine-deficient areas of the world, it is not surprising that iodine-deficiency disorders (IDD), including endemic goiter and cretinism, are the most common thyroid-related human illnesses, indeed the most common endocrine disorders worldwide. Normally iodine balance is maintained from dietary sources, i.e., food and water, but iodine may enter the body via medications, diagnostic agents, dietary supplements, and food additives. Increases in available iodine modify both the metabolism of iodine and the clinical tests by which it is assessed.

The daily dietary intake of iodine varies widely throughout the world, depending on the iodine content of soil and water and on dietary practice (Table 11–1). Even in a single area, iodine intake varies among different individuals and in the same individual from day to day. A minimum of 60 μg of elemental iodine/d is required for thyroid hormone synthesis, and at least 100 μg is required to eliminate all signs of iodine deficiency from the population. In North America the dietary iodine intake is in the range of 500 μg daily, largely owing to the iodination of salt, and in Japan, where large quantities of foods rich in iodine are consumed, intakes may be as high as several milligrams per day. In most of western Europe, iodine

TABLE 11–1. Typical Values for Iodine Content of Diet and of Various Medications

Typical Iodine Intakes	μg I/Day
North America (1970)	240–740
Chile (1981)	<50–150
Belgium (1993)	50–60
Germany (1993)	20–70
Switzerland (1993)	130–160
Recommended Daily Intake	**μg I/Day**
Adults	150
During pregnancy	200
Children	90–120
Quantity Required to Suppress RAIU to <2%	>15 mg I/day
Iodine Content of Various Iodinated Pharmaceuticals	
Saturated solution of potassium iodide (SSKI)	38 mg/drop
Lugol's solution	6 mg/drop
Iodized salt (1 pt KI/10,000 pt NaCl)	760 μg/10 g
Amiodarone	75 mg/200 mg tablet
Iopanoate, ipodate	350 mg/tablet
Angiographic and CT dyes	400–4000 mg/dose
Povidone-iodine	10 mg/mL
Kelp tablets	150 μg/tablet
Prenatal vitamins	150 μg/tablet
Iodinated glycerol	25 mg/mL

intakes of approximately 50 to 100 μg/d are tolerated without symptomatic thyroid dysfunction except during pregnancy.[15–17] The resulting marginal iodine deficiency, however, predisposes to the development of hyperthyroidism on exposure to large quantities of additional iodine in individuals with underlying Graves' disease or multinodular goiter (see later).

Variations in dietary iodine intake, when sustained, cause differences in the kinetics of iodine metabolism and hence must be taken into account in assigning normal limits to tests designed to evaluate thyroid function. Figure 11–2 is a schema of the major pathways of overall iodine metabolism, summarizing the movement of iodide into, out of, and among the various compartments of body iodine. The numeric values presented are approximations of the normal means in the United States. Iodine used in the synthesis of thyroid hormone is drawn from the inorganic iodide (I^-) of the extracellular fluid. Iodide refers to the biologic form of the free element (inorganic), while iodine includes both I^- and iodine cova-

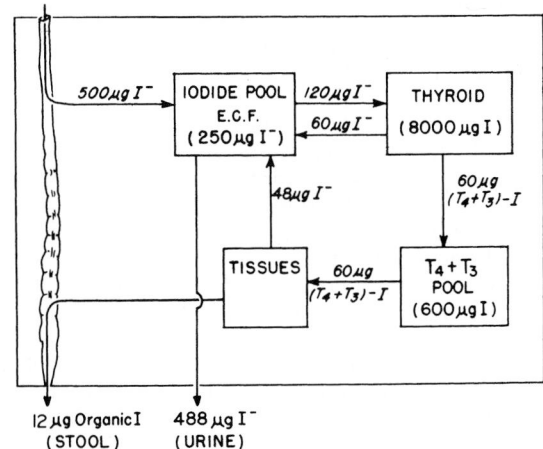

Figure 11–2. Iodine metabolism in a state of iodine balance. Most (approximately 90%) of body iodine is present in the thyroid (chiefly in the organic form), and approximately 10% is iodide. Arrows indicate daily flux of iodine from one compartment to another. In this example, one fifth of the iodide entering the iodide space (120/608) is accumulated by the thyroid. Peak thyroid uptake of I* should be approximately 20%, and the rate of turnover of thyronine-iodine is approximately 10%/d.

lently bound to tyrosine. The iodide thereby cleared is partly replenished both by iodide lost from the thyroid into the blood (iodide leak) and by iodide liberated through deiodination of thyroid hormones in peripheral tissues. Ultimately, however, the diet is the most important source of iodide. Iodine is ingested in both inorganic and organically bound forms. The rapidity of absorption of organically bound iodine and the form in which it is absorbed are uncertain, but eventually it is made available as inorganic iodide. Iodide per se (NaI) is rapidly (within 30 min) and efficiently absorbed from the gastrointestinal tract, and little is lost in the stool.

In the body iodide is confined largely to the extracellular fluid. It is also found, however, in the red blood cell and is concentrated in the intraluminal fluids of the gastrointestinal tract, notably the saliva and gastric juice, from which it is reabsorbed, and reenters the extracellular fluid. Until oxidized and bound to tyrosyl residues in Tg, iodide brought into the thyroid by active transport is, in essence, a portion of the extracellular iodide, because it is in rapid equilibrium with the main compartment. The concentration of iodide in the extracellular fluid is normally approximately 10 to 15 µg/L, and the content of the peripheral pool is approximately 250 µg. Thus only a very small percentage of total body iodine is present in the extracellular iodide compartment, and this is turned over several times daily.

There are two main avenues for the removal of iodide from the extracellular fluid. Small quantities are lost in expired air and through the skin, but most iodine is cleared via the thyroid and the kidneys. Renal removal of iodide determines the availability of iodide to the thyroid (and vice versa). Although iodide is almost completely filterable at the glomerulus, the renal clearance rate in adults approximates only 30 to 40 mL/min. Thus filtered iodide is largely reabsorbed by a passive process. In humans, unlike other animals, the renal iodide clearance rate is unaffected by the excretion of chloride or other anions and is apparently independent of the plasma iodide concentration and hence of the filtered load. Iodide clearance is minimally affected by the rate of urine flow per se and is uninfluenced by TSH or by drugs that alter thyroidal iodide transport. As with other urinary components that are passively reabsorbed, the renal clearance of iodide varies with changes in glomerular filtration rate, the iodide clearance increasing or decreasing disproportionately when the glomerular filtration rate is suddenly increased or decreased, respectively. Thus the kidneys are passive participants in iodide metabolism and do not make physiological adjustments to maintain iodine homeostasis.

About 500 µg of iodine are cleared into the urine daily in individuals living in North America, almost entirely in the inorganic form. About 12 µg of iodine are lost in the stool daily, mainly in the organic form. Fecal loss of organic iodine may be excessive when gastrointestinal absorption is impaired, as in chronic diarrheal states or under the influence of certain dietary constituents, such as soybean products, or of anionic resins, such as cholestyramine, that bind iodothyronines. Finally, iodine may be lost through lactation.

The second major site of removal of iodide from the extracellular fluid is the thyroid. The thyroid contains the largest pool of body iodine, under normal circumstances approximately 8000 µg, most of which is in the form of iodinated amino acids. Normally this pool of iodine turns over slowly (about 1%/d).

IODIDE TRANSPORT. Except when the plasma concentration of inorganic iodide is very high, synthesis of normal quantities of hormone requires that iodide enter the thyroid more rapidly than would be possible by simple diffusion from the extracellular fluid. The thyroid contains a transport mechanism (the iodide-concentrating, transporting, or trapping mechanism) that provides sufficient iodide substrate for hormone formation. The DNA for iodide carrier has been cloned and encodes a typical transporter protein with eight membrane-spanning domains.[18] Iodide transported into the gland is either oxidized and organified or diffuses back into the extracellular fluid. Under normal circumstances the rate of inward clearance of iodide exceeds the combined rates of organic binding* and backdiffusion, with the result that intrathyroid concentration gradients are about 50 to 100. Such gradients are referred to as the thyroid/plasma ratio. Although most of the inorganic iodide within the thyroid is located within the follicular lumen, the iodide-concentrating mechanism is located within the acinar cell itself. The interior of the cell maintains a negative electrical potential with respect to both the interstitium and the follicular lumen. Iodide is thus actively transported into the cell against this negative potential and then diffuses along the electrochemical gradient into the luminal area.

Like other active transport mechanisms, thyroid iodide transport is energy-requiring, dependent on continued generation of ATP. In addition, active iodide transport is closely related to the function of the Na^+, K^+-ATPase system, and a mechanism for the cotransport of sodium and iodide has been proposed. Although TSH increases the activity of both the iodide transport and the ATPase systems, the two do not respond in parallel in other circumstances. Hence the precise nature of their relationship remains uncertain.

The activity of the iodide transport mechanism is influenced by physiological factors, the most important being the level of TSH. Iodide transport is enhanced by TSH and decreased by hypophysectomy. TSH may enhance the expression of the iodide transporter protein, possibly reflecting the capacity of TSH to increase cyclic AMP (cAMP) concentration within the follicular cell; dibutyryl cAMP reproduces the effects of TSH on iodide transport in isolated thyroid cells. There is also an internal autoregulatory system through which the activity of the iodide transport mechanism and its responsiveness to TSH vary inversely with the glandular content of organic iodine. This reflects an autoregulatory effect on the cotransport of iodide and sodium. As a result of these influences, thyroid/plasma ratios rise when the thyroid is depleted of organic iodine or is stimulated by TSH. Under such conditions, ratios of several hundred have been observed, and high ratios are also common in patients with thyroid hyperfunction, regardless of its cause. The capacity of the thyroid to transport iodide and maintain iodide concentration gradients against the extracellular fluid is not unlimited, however. Thus increases in the concentration of iodide in the extracellular fluid are associated with decreasing values of the thyroid/plasma ratio, and the concentration of iodide that is actively transported into the gland decreases progressively, ultimately reaching a maximum. Absolute values of both the thyroid/plasma ratio and the iodide transport maximum vary with the functional state of the gland.

The thyroid mechanism for concentrating iodide is shared by other monovalent anions, including pertechnetate (TcO_4^-) perchlorate (ClO_4^-), and thiocyanate (SCN^-). These anions act as competitive inhibitors of iodide transport, a property that is likely related to the similarity of their partial specific molar volumes and negative charge. The capacity of perchlorate and thiocyanate to inhibit iodide transport is the basis of their use in the perchlorate- or thiocyanate-discharge test for defects in the thyroid organic-binding mechanism.[19] Concentration of the radioactive anion $^{99m}TcO_4^-$ makes it a useful agent for thyroid imaging, since it is concentrated by

---

*For brevity, *organic binding*, *organic iodine*, *organified*, and similar terms are often used. These expressions signify that iodide is bound to organic compounds, chiefly as iodotyrosine.[19]

the thyroid cell without a requirement for further metabolism (see the section on laboratory tests).

The capacity of the thyroid to concentrate iodide is shared by certain other tissues of endodermal origin, including the salivary and mammary glands, gastric mucosa, and choroid plexus. The effect of metabolic inhibitors and inhibitory anions on iodide transport in these other tissues is similar to that on iodide transport in the thyroid, and presumably those tissues express the iodide transporter protein. A rare cause of congenital goitrous hypothyroidism is the absence of an effective thyroid iodide transport mechanism.[20] In patients with this disorder, the salivary and gastric iodide concentration mechanisms are also lacking, suggesting that expression or structure of the transporter protein itself is impaired. Whether the result of a genetic defect or of the action of competitive inhibitors such as $NaClO_4$, inadequate iodide transport results in goiter and hypothyroidism, both of which can be overcome by administering sufficient iodine to increase plasma iodide concentration and permit sufficient iodine for hormone synthesis to enter the gland by simple diffusion.[20]

In addition to iodide brought into the thyroid by active transport from the extracellular fluid, iodide is generated in the thyroid by the deiodination of iodotyrosines liberated during the hydrolysis of Tg. A portion of this iodide is reorganified, and the remainder is lost from the gland as the so-called iodide leak (see Fig. 11–2). This conservation process is interrupted when antithyroid drugs, such as methimazole (MMI) or propylthiouracil (PTU), are given, thus further enhancing the effectiveness of these agents in blocking thyroid hormone synthesis.

Synthesis and Secretion of Thyroid Hormones

The structures of the thyroid hormones and several related compounds are shown in Figure 11–1, and the major steps in their synthesis and secretion are shown in Figure 11–3. The biosynthesis of thyroid hormone involves oxidation of iodide by H_2O_2 and thyroid peroxidase (TPO), the iodination of tyrosyl residues within Tg to yield the hormonally inactive iodotyrosines, and the coupling of iodotyrosines in Tg

to form the hormonally active iodothyronines T_4 and T_3. The hormones thus formed are held in peptide linkage within Tg, the major component of the intrafollicular colloid. Release of hormones involves reuptake of colloid at the apical thyroid cell membrane, proteolysis of Tg to liberate free iodinated amino acids, and release of the iodothyronines into the blood. The iodotyrosines released during Tg hydrolysis undergo intrathyroidal deiodination with salvage of most of the resulting free iodide for reutilization (see Fig. 11–3). The synthesis of thyroid hormones requires the expression of a number of thyroid cell–specific proteins. In addition to Tg and TPO, the TSH receptor is also required to transduce the effects of extracellular TSH for efficient hormone synthesis. Several thyroid cell–specific proteins, thyroid transcription factors 1 and 2 (TTF 1 and 2) and PAX8, stimulate transcription of the Tg and TPO genes.[21–24] One or more of these proteins may also influence expression of the TSH receptor.

OXIDATION OF IODIDE AND ORGANIC IODINATIONS. Within the thyroid, iodide participates in a series of reactions that lead to the synthesis of the active thyroid hormones. The first of these reactions involves oxidation of iodide and incorporation of the resulting intermediate into the hormonally inactive iodotyrosines MIT and DIT. Iodide is normally oxidized rapidly, immediately appearing in organic combination, mainly in Tg. The iodinations that lead to formation of iodotyrosines occur within Tg, rather than in free amino acids that are then incorporated into protein. Oxidation of thyroidal iodide is mediated by a heme-containing protein, TPO. The cDNA for human thyroid peroxidase has been cloned, and the deduced sequence contains 933 amino acids and has a molecular size of 103 kd, 10% of which is due to carbohydrate. The protein contains a putative membrane-spanning region near the COOH terminus, and it is oriented in the apical membrane of the thyroid cell to face the follicular lumen.[25–28] TPO is the major thyroid microsomal antigen, and recombinant human TPO is used for the assay of antithyroid "microsomal" antibodies (see the section on laboratory tests).

Since peroxidase is a heme protein, organic iodinations require molecular oxygen and are inhibited by cyanide and azide. In vitro, TPO, in the presence of hydrogen peroxide, iodinates Tg as well as other proteins. The reaction catalyzed by peroxidase in vitro has many properties of the iodination reaction in vivo, including inhibition by antithyroid agents and by high concentrations of iodide (Wolff-Chaikoff effect). The evanescent product of the peroxidation of iodide, i.e., the active iodinating form, may be free hypoiodous acid.[29] The hydrogen peroxide that serves as the oxidant of iodide is generated through the auto-oxidation of flavin enzymes acting as NADH and particularly NADPH oxidases. In this way, generation of hydrogen peroxide is linked to electron transfers due to substrate oxidations within the thyroid.

Radioautographic and histochemical evidence suggests that the iodination reactions occur at the cell-colloid interface.[29] Thus mitochondrial systems provide a source of hydrogen peroxide and cell membranes possess the iodide peroxidase, and the cytoplasmic fraction may contain regulatory inhibitors of organic iodinations.

Organic iodinations are conditioned by the extent of thyroid stimulation by TSH. Iodinations are susceptible to inhibition by a number of pharmacologic agents, including the usual antithyroid drugs, most of which are inhibitors of peroxidase and have intrinsic reducing activity. Defects in the organic-binding mechanism in humans lead to the development of goitrous hypothyroidism or, if less severe, to goiter without hypothyroidism. In some instances the thyroid is lacking in peroxidase.[9] In others, the defect may reside in inadequate production of hydrogen peroxide or abnormalities in Tg that render it less readily iodinated.

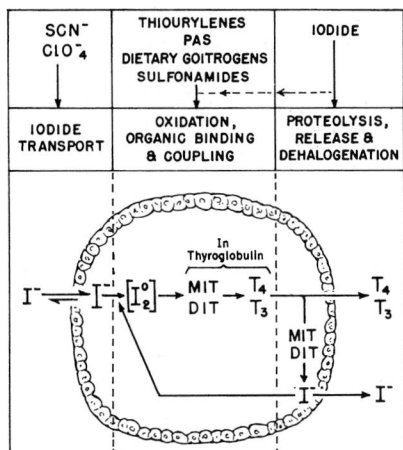

Figure 11–3. The major steps in thyroid hormone biosynthesis; the outline is intended to differentiate the intrathyroid from the interstitial compartment and does not imply that the reactions necessarily occur in the follicular lumen. Note that the concentration of intrathyroid iodide is greater than that in the extracellular fluid. Iodide oxidation, organic binding, and coupling of iodotyrosines appear to be closely related reactions. An uncertain fraction of iodide liberated from iodotyrosines by dehalogenation is reused or released into the extracellular fluid. Large quantities of iodide inhibit organic binding and coupling *(dashed lines)* transiently. Although not shown, the lithium ion, like iodide, inhibits proteolysis and release.

FORMATION OF IODOTHYRONINES OCCURS IN THY-ROGLOBULIN. Formation of MIT and DIT via oxidation and organic binding of iodide is followed by synthesis of the hormonally active iodothyronines T_4 and T_3. Because noniodinated thyronine cannot be demonstrated in Tg, T_4 and T_3 must arise from iodinated precursors. Synthesis of T_4 from DIT requires the fusion of two DIT molecules to yield a structure with two diiodinated rings linked by an ether bridge. Concomitantly a residual dehydroalanine is formed at the site of the DIT residue, contributing the phenolic hydroxyl group (beta or outer ring). This process is termed the *coupling reaction*.

Efficient synthesis of T_4 and T_3 in the thyroid requires Tg. The Tg gene has been cloned and is large (greater than 260 kb).[30] The human gene is localized on chromosome 8 close to the oncogene *MYC*. The Tg messenger RNA (mRNA) is 8 to 8.5 kb in length and encodes a 330 kd (12s) subunit that is 10% carbohydrate by weight. There are 134 tyrosyl residues in the homodimer of molecular size 660 kd (19s). Only about 25 to 30 of these are iodinated, and only 6 to 8 form iodothyronines. Specific portions of the molecule are involved in the formation of thyroid hormones. The primary T_4 acceptor tyrosine is residue 5 and constitutes about 50% of the T_4 in Tg.[31] Two other acceptor tyrosine residues are near the COOH terminus. Interestingly, the third tyrosyl residue from the COOH terminus is the major T_3-forming site and accounts for more than 50% of this hormone. The T_4-forming acceptor residues of Tg from different species are in a Glu/Asp-Tyr sequence, whereas T_3-forming Tyr residues are in the Thr/Ser-Tyr-Ser sequence.

There are approximately three to four T_4 molecules per mole of human Tg under conditions of normal iodination (25 atoms/molecule, approximately 0.5% iodine by weight), but only about one in five molecules of human Tg contains a T_3 residue.[32] In Tg from patients with untreated Graves' disease, however, the content of T_4 residues remains approximately the same, but the number of T_3 residues is doubled to an average of 0.4 per molecule.[32] This difference is independent of the iodination state of the Tg and presumably is a consequence of thyroidal stimulation.

Synthesis of iodothyronines requires oxidative conditions. It is thought that the coupling reaction is mediated by TPO, the same enzyme that mediates the initial oxidation of iodide. Virtually all agents that inhibit organic binding also inhibit coupling. Moreover, synthesis of labeled iodothyronines from prelabeled iodotyrosines is demonstrable when prelabeled Tg is incubated with TPO and a source of hydrogen peroxide in the absence of free iodide.

STORAGE AND RELEASE OF HORMONES. The thyroid is unique among the endocrine glands by virtue of the large store of hormone it contains and the low rate at which the hormone normally turns over (1%/d). This aspect of thyroid hormone economy has homeostatic value in that the reservoir provides prolonged protection against depletion of circulating hormone should synthesis cease. In normal humans the administration of blocking doses of antithyroid agents for as long as 2 wk results in little lowering of the serum T_4 concentration. Thus the storage function is an important aspect of thyroid hormone economy. As noted earlier, the normal thyroid contains about 8000 μg of iodine, of which at least 90% is organic. There are approximately 250 μg T_4/g wet weight in normal human thyroid or about 5000 μg T_4 in a 20-g gland.[33] This would be sufficient T_4 for approximately 50 d.

Tg is present in the plasma of normal individuals at concentrations up to 50 ng/mL, having escaped from the thyroid through the lymphatics. It is very unlikely, however, that peripheral hydrolysis of Tg contributes significantly to the T_4 and T_3 in the circulation.

HYDROLYSIS OF THYROGLOBULIN AND RELEASE OF T_3 AND T_4. The first step in thyroid hormone release is the endocytosis of colloid from the follicular lumen by two processes: macropinocytosis by pseudopods formed at the apical membranes or face, and micropinocytosis by small coated vesicles at the apical surface. Both processes are stimulated by TSH, but the relative importance of the two pathways varies among species, with micropinocytosis thought to predominate in humans. Following endocytosis, endocytotic vesicles fuse with lysosomes, and proteolysis is catalyzed by cathepsin L– and D–like thiol proteases, all of which are active at the acidic pH of the lysosome. The iodotyrosines released from Tg are rapidly deiodinated by an NADPH-dependent iodotyrosine deiodinase, and the released iodine is recycled (see Fig. 11–3). The T_4 is released into the thyroid cells, but it is not clear how its transfer into the plasma is regulated. Release is acutely stimulated by TSH, as may be the 5′-monodeiodination of T_4 to T_3 by the types 1 and 2 iodothyronine deiodinases (D1 and D2).[34-37]

While basal and TSH-stimulated conversion of T_4 to T_3 is easily demonstrated in the perfused dog thyroid, the contribution of thyroidal T_4 deiodination to T_3 secretion in humans under physiological conditions is not known. The ratio of T_4 to T_3 in normal fully iodinated human Tg is about 15:1, and the T_4/T_3 ratio of the secreted hormones is about 10:1. This modest difference may be due to T_4 monodeiodination. In the rat FRTL5 cell, both TSH and T_3 increase D1 activity, and in Graves' disease thyroidal D1 and D2 activities are markedly stimulated by thyroid-stimulating immunoglobulins.[35, 37-40] Therefore, thyroidal D1 and D2 may play a role in the enhanced T_3 production in patients with hyperthyroidism due to Graves' disease.[41]

The thyroid does not function as a single homogeneous unit. Radioautographic studies reveal variations among different areas of the gland and in different follicles. In truth, there may be many iodine pools in the thyroid that turn over at different rates, just as there are subtle differences in the Tg molecules within a single thyroid. The storage function of the thyroid is not perfectly maintained, even under normal conditions. As already noted, Tg can be detected by radioimmunoassay in the blood of normal individuals, and increased concentrations are present in the serum of patients with nontoxic goiter, Graves' disease, and thyroid neoplasia. Large quantities of Tg are released into the blood during surgical manipulation of the thyroid, with radiation thyroiditis, and in patients with subacute thyroiditis.[42]

Tg proteolysis and T_4 (and T_3) release are inhibited by several agents, the most important of which is iodide. Inhibition of hormone release is responsible for the rapid improvement that iodide induces in hyperthyroid patients. The complete mechanism by which this effect is mediated is uncertain, but iodine inhibits the stimulation of thyroid adenylate cyclase by TSH and by the stimulatory immunoglobulins of Graves' disease. Increasing iodination of Tg also increases its resistance to hydrolysis by acid proteases in the lysosomes. Lithium inhibits thyroid hormone release, although its mechanism of action is poorly understood and may differ from that of iodine.[43-45]

Role and Mechanism of Action of Thyrotropin (TSH) and Other Factors Regulating Thyroid Cell Function

All steps in the formation and release of thyroid hormones are stimulated by TSH from the pituitary thyrotropes (see Chapters 5 and 9). The regulation of TSH secretion by thyroid hormones is discussed further later, and its effects on thyroid cell function are reviewed in this section. Thyroid cells express the TSH receptor, a member of the G protein–coupled receptor family. The deduced amino acid sequence of this receptor predicts a large extracellular domain, seven mem-

TABLE 11–2. TSH-Responsive Events in Human Thyroid Cells

Cyclic AMP–Mediated	Phospholipase C–Mediated
Iodide transport	H_2O_2 generation (human)
Tg synthesis	I^- efflux
TPO synthesis	
Hormone secretion	
Type 1 deiodinase	
Growth	

brane-spanning domains, and an intracellular domain that transduces the signal to the Gs and Gp proteins.[46–49] This receptor also interacts with thyroid-stimulating (TSAb) and blocking antibodies (TBAb), and these aspects of the TSH receptor are discussed under the section on laboratory tests and the section on Graves' disease.

Studies of the effects of TSH are complicated by the fact that the same pathway is stimulated by protein kinase A–related mechanisms in one species or cell model and by protein kinase C–directed pathways in another.[50, 51] The effects of activation by TSH of each of the individual pathways in human thyroid cells are summarized in Table 11–2.

The effects on iodide kinetics include both an early stimulation of iodide efflux into the follicular lumen and a later increase in the V_{max} for iodide transport. The latter is likely due to enhanced expression of the iodide carrier.[18] H_2O_2 generation in human thyrocytes is activated by Ca^{2+} and diacylglycerol, although 10-fold higher concentrations of TSH are required for activation of this limb of the TSH receptor pathways than for activation of adenylate cyclase. TSH increases the levels of both TPO protein and mRNA, even though no CREB binding sequences have been identified in the promoter of this gene.[52] The effect on TPO may be secondary to cAMP stimulation of thyroid cell–specific proteins, such as TTF 1 or 2 or PAX8 (see earlier), but this remains to be shown. Similarly, transcription of the Tg gene is also stimulated by cAMP through indirect pathways, perhaps involving the same mechanism.[52, 53] Interestingly, TSH can increase TSH receptor mRNA in human thyroid cells, although at high TSH receptor concentrations there may be a modest decrease in receptor expression. Nonetheless, the persistence of functional TSH receptor that is not down-regulated by autophosphorylation can explain the hyperthyroidism of Graves' disease and that associated with TSH-producing thyrotrope tumors. TSH or cAMP also stimulates the ingestion and hydrolysis of colloid and the release of Tg and T_4 from the thyroid.

Thyroid cell proliferation is stimulated by cAMP, phorbol esters, and epidermal growth factor (EGF) through tyrosine kinase.[52] However, cAMP causes proliferation while maintaining differentiated function, while EGF and phorbol esters lead to dedifferentiation. Similarly insulin-like growth factor I (IGF-I) and fibroblast growth factor (FGF) stimulate cell division and dedifferentiation, although there are species differences in the effects of these agents.[46, 52] In human thyrocytes the events stimulated by the adenylate cyclase pathway are probably the most critical for thyroid growth and explain the goitrous changes associated with prolonged TSH stimulation such as occurs with iodine deficiency.

Drugs That Inhibit Thyroid Hormone Synthesis

A wide variety of chemical agents can inhibit the synthesis of thyroid hormones. When these agents reduce thyroid hormones to subnormal levels, secretion of TSH is increased, and goiter ensues. Hence such agents are termed goitrogens. In practice, goitrogenic agents are encountered as drugs used in the treatment of hyperthyroidism, as pharmacologic agents used for other purposes, and as agents occurring naturally in foodstuffs.

Antithyroid agents can be grouped into two classes: agents that inhibit thyroid iodide transport and those that inhibit the organic binding and coupling processes. Inhibitors of iodide transport are monovalent anions. Of these, thiocyanate and perchlorate have been used clinically, but neither is now used in the routine treatment of hyperthyroidism because of their toxicity. However, perchlorate has been advocated as a supplement to methimazole in the treatment of hyperthyroidism due to amiodarone-induced hyperthyroidism.[54] These competitive inhibitors of iodide transport are effective when the plasma iodide concentration is normal or low. However, if iodine intake is increased, hormone overproduction will resume. Thus control is unpredictable, and such agents cannot be used with iodine in preparing patients for subtotal thyroidectomy.

The second class of antithyroid agents inhibits the thyroid organic binding and coupling reactions. Compounds that exert this effect can be classified into three main groups: thionamides, aminoheterocyclic compounds, and substituted phenols (Fig. 11–4). The thionamide agents, of which methimazole, carbimazole, and propylthiouracil are members, exert their antithyroid action primarily by inhibiting the oxidation and binding of iodide in the thyroid.

As a class, the thionamide compounds are the most potent inhibitors of thyroid hormone formation and are characterized by the following substituent grouping:

$$S = C \begin{matrix} N— \\ \diagup \\ \diagdown \\ R— \end{matrix}$$

in which R may be a sulfur, an oxygen, or a nitrogen atom. In contrast to the agents that inhibit thyroid iodide transport, the action of the thionamides is not completely prevented by large doses of iodide, although it is attenuated.

The aminoheterocyclic compounds and substituted phenols are less potent than the thionamides and are not used in the treatment of hyperthyroidism. Their effects on the thyroid are sometimes manifested, however, during their use in the treatment of other disease. A number of other agents of

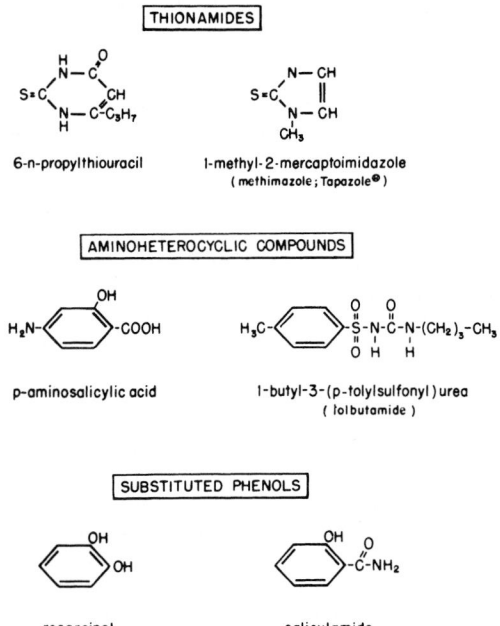

Figure 11–4. Structural formulas of several representative antithyroid compounds.

diverse chemical nature also have antithyroid activity. Phenylbutazone decreases the thyroid uptake of I* and can cause goitrous hypothyroidism in humans. Antithyroid activity has also been ascribed to ethionamide and 6-mercaptopurine, both of which contain the thionamide grouping.[55, 56*]

Goiter with or without hypothyroidism can occur in patients treated with lithium, usually for bipolar manic-depressive psychosis.[43–45, 57] Like iodide, lithium inhibits thyroid hormone release, and, in high concentrations, can inhibit organic binding reactions.[43–45, 58] At least acutely, iodide and lithium act synergistically in the latter respect. The mechanisms underlying the several effects of lithium are uncertain. Also uncertain is what differentiates patients who develop goiter during lithium therapy from those who do not. Underlying autoimmune thyroiditis may be at least one factor.[58]

Antithyroid agents also occur naturally in foods. These are widely distributed in the family Cruciferae or Brassicaceae, particularly in the genus *Brassica*, including cabbages, turnips, kale, kohlrabi, rutabaga, mustard, and a number of plants that are not eaten by humans but serve as animal fodder. It is likely that some thiocyanate is present in such plants (particularly cabbage).[59] Cassava meal, a dietary staple in many regions of the world, contains linamarin, a cyanogenic glycoside whose metabolism leads to the formation of thiocyanate. Ingestion of cassava can accentuate goiter formation in some areas of endemic iodine deficiency. Except for thiocyanate, dietary goitrogens influence thyroid iodine metabolism in the same manner as do the thionamides, which they resemble chemically; their role in the induction of disease in humans is uncertain. Water-borne, sulfur-containing goitrogens of mineral origin are believed to contribute to the development of endemic goiter in certain areas of Colombia.[59, 60]

THYROID HORMONES IN PERIPHERAL TISSUES

The metabolic transformations of thyroid hormones in peripheral tissues determine their biologic potency and regulate their biologic effects. Consequently, an understanding of thyroid physiopathology requires a knowledge of the pathways of thyroid hormone metabolism.

A wide variety of iodothyronines and their metabolic derivatives exist in plasma. Of these, T_4 is highest in concentration and the only one that arises solely from direct secretion by the thyroid gland. In normal humans T_3 is also released from the thyroid, but most plasma T_3 is derived from the peripheral tissues by the enzymatic removal of a single iodine atom (monodeiodination) from T_4 (Fig. 11–5). The remaining iodothyronines and their derivatives are almost entirely generated in the peripheral tissues from T_4 and T_3. Principal among them are $3,3',5'$-triiodothyronine (rT$_3$) and $3,3'$-diiodo-L-thyronine ($3,3'$-T$_2$). Trace concentrations of other diiodothyronines, monoiodothyronines, and conjugates thereof with glucuronic or sulfuric acid are also present.[61] Deaminated derivatives of T_4 and T_3 that bear an acetic acid rather than an alanine side chain are also present in low concentrations (see Figs. 11–1 and 11–5).

Plasma Transport

The major secretory products of the normal thyroid gland, T_4 and T_3, are bound in a firm but reversible bond to

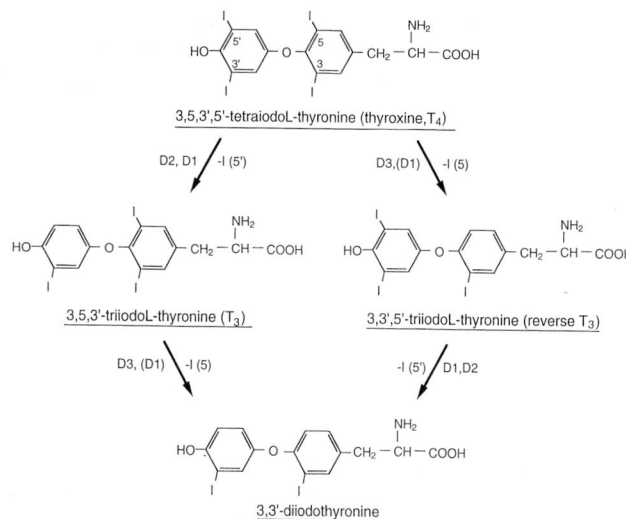

Figure 11–5. Pathways of thyroid hormone activation and inactivation catalyzed by human iodothyronine deiodinases. Numbers refer to the iodine positions in the iodothyronine nucleus. The iodothyronine deiodinases are abbreviated D1, D2, and D3 for types 1, 2, and 3 deiodinases, respectively. Arrows refer to nonodeiodination of the outer or inner ring of the iodothyronine nucleus, which is termed 5' or 5 by convention. A parenthesis reflects the fact that D3 is very likely the major enzyme catalyzing inner-ring deiodination of T_4 and T_3 (see also Table 11–4 for a comparison of the properties of these deiodinases).

several proteins, all of which are synthesized in the liver.[62–64] The two plasma proteins with which T_4 is mainly associated are TBG and transthyretin (TTR), formerly termed T_4-binding prealbumin (TBPA) (Table 11–3). About 75 to 80% of T_3 is bound by TBG, and the remainder by TTR and albumin (Fig. 11–6).

THYROXINE-BINDING GLOBULIN (TBG). TBG is a glycoprotein with a molecular mass of about 54 kd, about 20% of which is carbohydrate.[65] The gene that encodes the protein is on the X chromosome. The nucleotide sequence of TBG resembles that of the serine antiproteases α_1-antichymotrypsin and α_1-antitrypsin.[65] Because there is one iodothyronine binding site per TBG molecule, the binding capacity of TBG in normal human serum is equivalent to its concentration, which is approximately 270 nmol/L (15 μg/mL) (see Table 11–3). The half-time of the protein in plasma is about 5 d, and the metabolic clearance rate is approximately 800 mL/d.

The glycosylation of TBG influences its clearance from the plasma and its behavior during isoelectric focusing.[66, 67] Four to six bands are present after isoelectric focusing, but

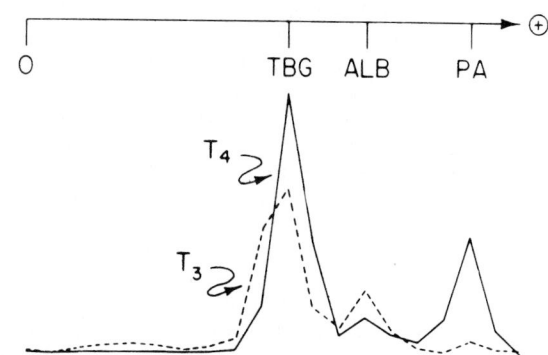

Figure 11–6. Diagram depicting the electrophoretic migration of radioiodine-labeled T_4 and T_3 in normal human serum. T_4 is bound predominantly by thyroxine-binding globulin (TBG), to a lesser extent by transthyretin (TTR), and to a slight extent by albumin. T_3 is bound by TBG and by albumin, but little binds to transthyretin.

The abbreviation I is employed to denote any of the radioactive isotopes of iodine that cannot be distinguished from one another physiologically or biochemically. When a specific isotope of iodine is referred to, it will be appropriately designated.

TABLE 11–3. Comparison of the Major Human Thyroid Hormone–Binding Proteins

	Thyroxine-Binding Globulin	Transthyretin	Albumin
Mol wt of holoprotein (kd)	54,000	54,000 (4 subunits)	66,000
Plasma concentrations (μmol/L)	0.27	4.6	640
T_4 binding capacity as μg T_4/dL	21	350	50,000
Association constants of the major binding site (L/M)			
T_4	1×10^{10}	7×10^7	7×10^5
T_3	5×10^8	1.4×10^7	1×10^5
Fraction of sites occupied by T_4 in euthyroid plasma	0.31	0.02	<0.001
Distribution volume (L)	7	5.7	7.8
Turnover rate (%/d)	13	59	5
Distribution of iodothyronines (%/protein)			
T_4	68	11	20
T_3	80	9	11

after exposure to neuraminidase these differences are lost, indicating that they are due to variations in the numbers of sialic acid residues. In estrogen-treated patients there is an increase in the prevalence of the more acidic bands of TBG.[66] The more highly sialylated TBG is cleared more slowly from plasma than is the more positively charged TBG, because increased sialylation inhibits the hepatic uptake of glycoproteins. Sera from pregnant patients, women receiving oral contraceptives, and patients with acute hepatitis have increased fractions of acidic TBG (see Table 11–7).[67] Patients with inherited TBG excess have normal amounts of highly sialylated TBG, as do nonpregnant women and men.

Other abnormalities of TBG can alter the susceptibility to heat denaturation and the capacity to bind thyroid hormone. One such variant has been described in the Australian aborigines, and a TBG with increased heat lability occurs in blacks.[68] All of these abnormalities are inherited in an X-linked fashion. L-Asparaginase blocks the synthesis of TBG in HEP G2 cells, which explains the low TBG concentrations in patients receiving this agent.[69, 70, 71] The overall frequency of TBG deficiency is about 1 in 5000 newborns.[62–64]

TRANSTHYRETIN (TTR). TTR exists in part as a complex with retinol (vitamin A)-binding protein, hence its name. It consists of four identical polypeptide chains whose total molecular mass is approximately 55 kd.[63, 64, 72] Its concentration in plasma is approximately 4 mmol/L (250 μg/mL). Each mole of TTR can bind 1 mole of T_4 with high affinity, and a second T_4 molecule is bound with lower affinity at high concentrations of T_4.[63] Binding of T_4 by TTR is independent of the association with retinol-binding protein. TTR is devoid of carbohydrate but rich in tryptophan. Its half-time in plasma is normally about 2 d but decreases during illness.[73] TTR is expressed in the choroid plexus and thus in the cerebrospinal fluid, where it is the major thyroid hormone–binding protein.[74] The choroid plexus may be an important site for T_4 concentration in the brain.[75–77] Targeted TTR gene-disruption studies in mice show that, aside from the predictable decrease in total plasma T_4 concentration and reciprocal increase in the free T_4 fraction (since TTR is a major T_4-binding protein in mice), absence of the gene causes no developmental abnormality,[78] a finding that argues against a requirement for TTR in the transport of T_4 into the central nervous system in this species.

Variant forms of TTR are associated with familial amyloidotic polyneuropathy.[63, 64, 79] In affected families the TTR monomer has one of several different point mutations, and TTR accumulates in the amyloid tissue deposits. Neither thyroid dysfunction nor altered vitamin A metabolism has been reported, although there is altered affinity of some of the mutant proteins for T_4. Two types of abnormalities have been reported in the total T_4 concentrations associated with rare abnormalities in TTR:[64] occasional families with a TTR of high affinity[80, 81] and a few families with increased TTR levels.[82]

COMPARISON OF T_4 BINDING BY TBG AND TTR. The TBG binding site has an affinity for T_3 that is about 20-fold less than that for T_4 (see Table 11–3). TBG binds both the dextroisomer of T_4 and the naturally occurring levoisomer. Deamination of the iodothyronine molecule reduces binding to TBG and increases the affinity for TTR; the acetic and propionic acid analogues of T_4 and T_3 bind poorly, if at all, to this protein. Binding of T_4 by TBG is inhibited by phenytoin,[83] salicylate,[84, 85] barbital,[84] furosemide,[86] fenclofenac,[87] and mitotane. The affinity of these compounds for TBG binding is weaker than that of T_4 or T_3, but the concentration in plasma may be sufficient to interfere with T_4 and T_3 binding and lower total hormone levels. Inhibitors of the T_4-TTR interaction include barbital, salicylate, and some of its congeners, 2,4-dinitrophenol, penicillin, and plant flavonoids.[57, 63, 64]

ALBUMIN. The affinity of albumin for T_4 and T_3 binding is much lower than that of either TBG or TTR, but the high concentration of this protein results in the binding of 10% of the plasma thyroid hormones (see Table 11–3). Changes in albumin concentration per se have little influence on the total hormone levels, unless accompanied by alterations in TBG and TTR, all three of which are synthesized in the liver. Therefore hepatic failure or nephrotic syndrome leads to decreases in the plasma concentration of all three, and measurement of the albumin concentration serves as an index of the severity of the problem. The role of albumin in thyroid economy becomes chemically important in patients with familial dysalbuminemic hyperthyroxinemia (FDH).[88–91] In this autosomal dominant disorder, the plasma contains high amounts of a usually minor albumin variant that binds T_3—but not T_3—with increased avidity. This leads to the presence of an increased total T_4 but normal free T_4 and normal total T_3 in an otherwise euthyroid patient with a normal TSH level. Such patients may have a confusing pattern of test results, which are discussed further in the section on laboratory tests.

OTHER PLASMA THYROID HORMONE–BINDING PROTEINS. Between 3 and 6% of plasma T_4 and T_3 are bound to lipoproteins.[92] The T_4-binding lipoprotein is 27 kd in size on gel electrophoresis and is present in serum as a dimer.[92] The affinity of T_4 for this protein is lower than that for TBG. This binding is of uncertain physiological significance but could play a role in targeting T_4 delivery to specific tissues.

Free Thyroid Hormones

TBG is normally responsible for the transport of most of the T_4 (about 77%) and is the major determinant of the free or unbound fraction of T_4. Interaction of the thyroid hormones with the transport proteins alters their metabolism.

The negligible urinary excretion of T_3 and T_4 is due to the limited filterability of the hormone-binding protein complexes at the glomerulus. The volume of distribution and rate of turnover of the hormones are also affected by their protein associations, so that they resemble more closely those of the plasma proteins rather than those of unbound amino acids. In vitro, the interaction between the thyroid hormones and their binding proteins conforms to a reversible binding equilibrium that can be expressed by conventional equilibrium equations. For the formulations that follow, T_4 is used as the prototype, with the understanding that similar interactions apply in the case of T_3. The interaction between T_4 and TBG can be expressed as follows:

$$T_4 + TBG \overset{k}{\rightleftharpoons} T_4 \cdot TBG$$

Here TBG represents the unoccupied binding sites of the protein, k the equilibrium association constant for the interaction; T_4 refers to the concentration of free T_4; $T_4 \cdot TBG$ represents the T_4 bound to TBG. This interaction can also be expressed by the mass action relationship, wherein

$$\frac{T_4 \cdot TBG}{(T_4)\,(TBG)} = k$$

Rearranging

$$\frac{T_4}{T_4 \cdot TBG} = \frac{1}{(TBG)k}$$

and

$$T_4 = \frac{T_4 \cdot TBG}{(TBG)k}$$

These expressions illustrate that T_4 exists in the plasma in both the bound and the free forms, and that the free fraction of T_4 is inversely proportional to the concentration of unoccupied TBG binding sites. The free T_4 concentration can be quantitated in serum by indirect radioimmunoassay[93, 94] or by the dialysis technique. With the aid of I*-labeled T_4, the proportion that is unbound by protein is determined, and the concentration of free T_4 can then be calculated as the product of the total hormone concentration and the fraction that is free. In normal serum, the free T_4 is approximately 0.02% of the total (about 20 pmol/L) (see Table 11–5). The approximately 10-fold lower affinity of TBG for T_3 results in a proportion of free T_3 (0.30%) that is about 15 times that of T_4.

The free hormone is available to the tissues, induces the metabolic effects, and undergoes degradation. The bound hormone acts merely as a reservoir. It follows that the concentration of the free hormone is an important determinant of the metabolic state and is defended by homeostatic mechanisms. In the presence of an increase in the overall net binding affinity for T_4, a normal free T_4 concentration can be maintained only if the bound T_4 level increases. This is true whether the causative factor is an increase in the concentration of TBG or the appearance of abnormal T_4-binding proteins.

Two factors influence the plasma concentration of T_4: its rate of entry into the plasma and the efficiency of its removal from plasma. The metabolic clearance rate relates the quantity of T_4 removed from the plasma per unit time to the quantity available for removal, i.e., its plasma concentration. Thus

$$MCR = D/[P]$$

where MCR is the metabolic clearance rate (volume/time), D is the absolute disposal or removal rate (amount/time), and [P] is the plasma concentration (amount/volume). Transposing,

$$[P] = D/MCR$$

However, under steady-state conditions, the production rate of T_4 (PR) and the disposal rate (D) are equal. Hence,

$$[P] = PR/MCR$$

Thus, for any level of T_4 production, be it increased, normal, or decreased, the total plasma T_4 level varies inversely with its MCR. However, if only the free T_4 is readily able to leave the plasma and enter the cells, while the bound T_4 is confined largely to the intravascular space, then changing the fraction of total T_4 that is free, by changing the fraction that is available to the tissues, changes the MCR in a parallel manner. This would explain why a primary increase in hormone binding, as occurs when TBG concentrations are increased during pregnancy, without any change in thyroid function, increases the plasma total T_4 concentration and why a decrease in hormone binding has the converse effect (Fig. 11–7).

This formulation is termed the *free thyroid hormone hypothesis*.[95] If it is free hormone that diffuses into the tissue, what is the role, if any, of the hormone-binding proteins? If a protein-free solution containing tracer T_3 is perfused through rat liver via the portal vein, there is a steep concentration gradient with a decreasing quantity of T_3 in cells as the distance from the center of the portal lobule increases.[96–99] Virtually all of the T_3 is taken up by the first cells to be contacted by the bolus. In contrast, if 4% serum albumin is added to the perfusate, the distribution of tracer is uniform throughout the lobule, with only 46% of the tracer removed from the bolus. Thus, plasma-binding proteins function to ensure uniform distribution of hydrophobic ligands such as T_4 and T_3 throughout the circulatory system and within various organs. Efflux from the same tissues is also rapid. Thus, intracellular T_3 and T_4 are in equilibrium with the free hormone pool in plasma, consistent with the free hormone hypothesis. In the steady state, the rate of T_3 and T_4 metabolism, not the dissociation rate from plasma proteins, determines the rate of removal of these hormones from the plasma.

Cellular Uptake and Intracellular Binding

Carrier-mediated transport of thyroid hormone has been demonstrated into hepatocytes, human fibroblasts, rat skeletal

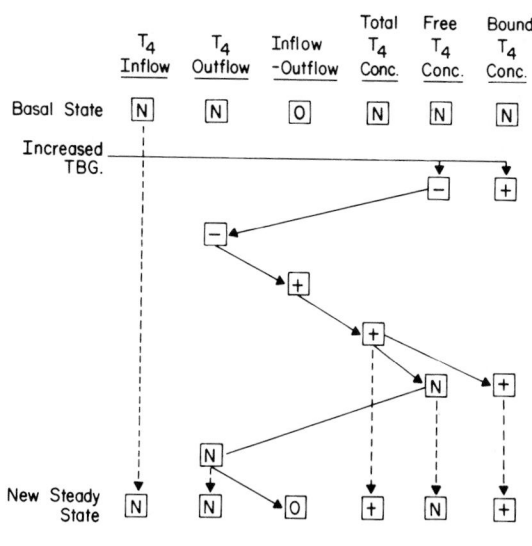

Figure 11–7. The sequence of events after an increase in TBG: effects on the turnover of T_4 and on the serum total and free T_4 levels. Converse consequences follow a decrease in TBG.

muscle cells, and neuroblastoma cells.[100–102] The carrier transport system for T_3 and T_4 is saturable, is stereospecific, and requires ATP, but the two iodothyronines do not compete for uptake.[100, 103] Extracellular sodium is required, and sodium ionophore increases the uptake of thyroid hormone by rat skeletal muscle.[102] Iopanoic acid, monodansylcadaverine, phenytoin, phloretin, ATP-depleting compounds, and nonsteroidal anti-inflammatory agents interfere with the uptake.[104, 105] In addition, certain compounds in the sera of patients with renal failure, such as indoxyl sulfate and furan fatty acid, also inhibit T_4 transport.[106] In patients on a low-calorie diet for 1 wk, T_3 and T_4 uptake into both rapidly equilibrating (liver and kidney) and slowly equilibrating pools (muscle) is decreased.[107] Thus inhibition of T_4 and rT_3 transport into these organs may well explain the low production of T_3 and the elevation of rT_3 concentrations in the serum of sick or fasting individuals.

CELLULAR BINDING PROTEINS. The characterization of the sites on the cell surface with which T_4 and T_3 bind is incomplete. Proteins that bind T_4 and T_3 have been identified in the cytosol of many tissues, and some studies suggest that the cytosol binding proteins for T_4 and T_3 are distinct from one another.

The intracellular free T_3 concentration can be estimated by evaluating the binding affinity of intracellular and nuclear binding proteins and by measuring the T_3 concentration in cytosol.[108] Such analyses suggest that there is a free hormone gradient of twofold to threefold across the cell membrane. These concentration gradients, however, are not as high as those calculated for the nuclear/cytosolic ratios in liver, kidney, heart, and brain, which are 50:1 to 250:1.

Thyroid Hormone Activation and Inactivation by the Selenodeiodinases

MOLECULAR BIOLOGY, BIOCHEMISTRY, AND PHYSIOLOGY OF IODOTHYRONINE DEIODINATION. The most important pathway for metabolism of T_4 is the monodeiodination of its outer ring to form the active thyroid hormone T_3.[109, 110] Inner-ring deiodination of T_4 and T_3 and further deiodination reactions deactivate the hormones (see Table 11–8 and Fig. 11–5).[61, 111–113] Three deiodinases have been identified in mammalian tissues (Table 11–4). The structures of the enzymes as deduced from the cDNAs are similar from tadpoles to humans.[114–119] Deiodinases 1 and 2 (abbreviated D1 and D2) catalyze outer-ring monodeiodination, thereby producing T_3. D1 also catalyzes removal of an inner-ring iodine from T_3 and T_4 but prefers the sulfated derivatives as substrates.[61, 120, 121] The type 3 deiodinase (D3) is an obligate

inner-ring monodeiodinase with a preference for T_3 as substrate.

All three enzymes contain selenocysteine in the active center, which is the region of highest homology among them (Fig. 11–8). This rare amino acid has properties that make it ideal for catalysis of oxidoreductive reactions such as iodothyronine deiodination and the reduction of H_2O_2[113, 122–124] by the glutathione peroxidases. The reaction catalyzed by D1 is schematized in Figure 11–9.[124] Mutagenesis of selenocysteine in D1 to cysteine, e.g., replacing Se with S, reduces the enzyme velocity by 100-fold and renders it less sensitive to inhibition by PTU and by gold.[124–126] A low substrate turnover number can explain the insensitivity of the D2 and D3 enzymes to PTU even though they contain selenocysteine.[114, 116–118, 127]

SELENOPROTEIN SYNTHESIS. Selenocysteine is encoded by the "stop" codon UGA.[128, 129] Thus the translational machinery must distinguish between the "stop" message and the "selenocysteine insertion function" of UGA. While the details of the process are still being worked out in eukaryotes, in prokaryotes at least four gene products, termed SEL A, B, C, and D, and a stem-loop structure in the coding region of the mRNA are required.[130] In eukaryotes the process appears quite similar with the important exception that the stem-loop sequence is found in the 3′-untranslated region of the mRNA.[131–135] This structure, termed a "*selenocysteine insertion sequence*," or SECIS element, is present in virtually all eukaryotic mRNAs encoding selenoproteins.[136]

SELENIUM AND IODOTHYRONINE METABOLISM. Given the important role of selenocysteine in deiodination, the supply of this trace element can have an important bearing on thyroid physiology (reviewed in reference 123). Selenium deficiency reduces D1 activity in liver and kidney of rats.[137, 138] Furthermore, selenium supplementation of the diets of people with deficiency of iodine and selenium in Zaire resulted in significant decreases in serum T_4 levels. This suggests that when T_4 synthesis is impaired (as in iodine deficiency), deiodination by D1 regulates the level of T_4 in the circulation.[139, 140] Since T_4 is required for the generation of much of the T_3 in the central nervous system via the action of D2, selenium deficiency protects the brain from T_3 deficiency (see later).[110, 141] Therefore indiscriminate supplementation of selenium in iodine-deficient populations has adverse effects on the overall thyroid economy.[140] However, effects of selenium deficiency are mitigated by the fact that the thyroid, brain, and testis conserve selenium, so the synthesis of D2 and D3 in these tissues is not impaired by selenium deficiency.[142, 143]

TYPE 1 DEIODINASE (D1). In the rat and probably in humans the D1 enzyme provides T_3 to the plasma and deiodinates 3,3′, 5′-triiodothyronine (rT_3) to produce 3,3′-diiodo-

TABLE 11–4. Human Iodothyronine Selenodeiodinases

Parameter	Type 1 (5′ and 5)	Type 2 (5′)	Type 3 (5)
Physiological role	Provide T_3 to plasma Inactivate T_3 and T_4 Degrade rT_3	Provide intracellular T_3 in specific tissues, provide plasma T_3	Inactivate T_3 and T_4
Tissue location	Liver, kidney, thyroid, central nervous system, pituitary (?)	Central nervous system, pituitary, brown fat, placenta, thyroid, skeletal muscle, heart	Central nervous system, placenta, skin
Substrate preference	$rT_3 \gg T_4 > T_3$	$T_4 \geq rT_3$	$T_3 > T_4$
Molecular weight of human protein (? monomer)	29,000	30,500	31,500
K_m (apparent)	$\sim 10^{-7}$ M (reverse T_3) $\sim 10^{-6}$ M (T_4)	$\sim 10^{-9}$ M (T_4) $\sim 10^{-8}$ M (rT_3)	$\sim 10^{-9}$ M (T_3) $\sim 10^{-8}$ M (T_4)
Deiodination site	Outer and inner ring	Outer ring	Inner ring
Active site	Selenocysteine	Selenocysteine	Selenocysteine
Apparent K_i for Propylthiouracil Gold	2×10^{-7} M (sensitive) $\sim 5 \times 10^{-9}$ M (sensitive)	4×10^{-3} M (resistant) $\sim 2 \times 10^{-6}$ M (resistant)	10^{-3} M (resistant) 5×10^{-6} M (resistant)
Response to T_3	Increase	Decrease	Increase

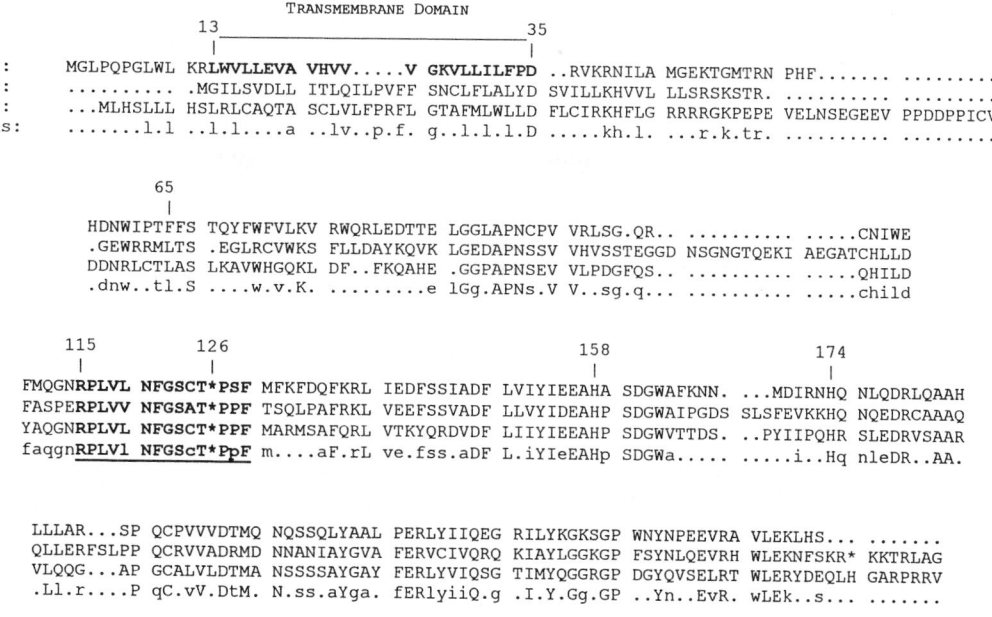

TRANSMEMBRANE DOMAIN

```
                                13                              35
                                |                               |
HD1:    MGLPQPGLWL KRLWVLLEVA VHVV.....V GKVLLILFPD ..RVKRNILA MGEKTGMTRN PHF...... .........S
HD2:    .......... .MGILSVDLL ITLQILPVFF SNCLFLALYD SVILLKHVVL LLSRSKSTR. .......... ..........
HD3:    ...MLHSLLL HSLRLCAQTA SCLVLFPRFL GTAFMLWLLD FLCIRKHFLG RRRRGKPEPE VELNSEGEEV PPDDPPICVS
Cons:   ......l.l ..l.l....a ..lv..p.f. g..l.l.l.D .....kh.l. ..r.k.tr. .......... .........s


                   65
                   |
        HDNWIPTFFS TQYFWFVLKV RWQRLEDTTE LGGGLAPNCPV VRLSG.QR.. .......... .....CNIWE
        .GEWRRMLTS .EGLRCVWKS FLLDAYKQVK LGEDAPNSSV VHVSSTEGGD NSGNGTQEKI AEGATCHLLD
        DDNRLCTLAS LKAVWHGQKL DF..FKQAHE .GGPAPNSEV VLPDGFQS.. .......... ....QHILD
        .dnw..tl.S ....w.v.K. .........e lGg.APNs.V V..sg.q... .......... ....child


        115          126                          158                  174
        |            |                            |                    |
        FMQGNRPLVL NFGSCT*PSF MFKFDQFKRL IEDFSSIADF LVIYIEEAHA SDGWAFKNN. ...MDIRNHQ NLQDRLQAAH
        FASPERPLVV NFGSAT*PPF TSQLPAFRKL VEEFSSVADF LLVYIDEAHP SDGWAIPGDS SLSFEVKKHQ NQEDRCAAAQ
        YAQGNRPLVL NFGSCT*PPF MARMSAFQRL VTKYQRDVDF LIIYIEEAHA SDGWVTTDS. ..PYIIPQHR SLEDRVSAAR
        faqgnRPLVl NFGScT*PpF m....aF.rL ve.fss.aDF L.iYIeEAHp SDGWa..... .....i..Hq nleDR..AA.


        LLLAR...SP QCPVVVDTMQ NQSSQLYAAL PERLYIIQEG RILYKGKSGP WNYNPEEVRA VLEKLHS... .......
        QLLERFSLPP QCRVVADRMD NNANAIAYGVA FERVCIVQRQ KIAYLGGKGP FSYNLQEVRH WLEKNFSKR* KKTRLAG
        VLQQG...AP GCALVLDTMA NSSSSAYGAY FERLYVIQSG TIMYQGGRGP DGYQVSELRT WLERYDEQLH GARPRRV
        .Ll.r....P qC.vV.DtM. N.ss.aYga. fERlyiiQ.g .I.Y.Gg.GP ..Yn..EvR. wLEk..s... .......
```

* = Selenocysteine

Figure 11–8. Amino acid sequences of the three human selenodeiodinases. The proteins have in common a hydrophobic amino terminus and a conserved sequence of amino acids around the selenocysteine in the active center of each enzyme. Selenocysteine is denoted by an asterisk.

thyronine ($3,3'$-T_2). Since PTU, a D1 specific inhibitor (see Table 11–4), causes only a 20% inhibition of conversion of T_4 to T_3 in euthyroid humans,[144–146] the PTU-insensitive D2 pathway may be more important in serum T_3 production in humans (see Fig. 11–9). Fasting reduces hepatic T_4 uptake, thereby reducing the access of T_4 and rT_3 to D1 action.[100, 147] A patient has been described with impaired uptake of T_4 into T_3 producing tissues,[148] and a similar effect in muscle could block access of T_4 to D2.[118, 119]

The high K_m of D1 for T_4 ($\sim 10^{-6}$ M) indicates that at normal or elevated free T_4 concentrations this enzyme will not be saturated. D1 activity is increased in hyperthyroidism and decreased in hypothyroidism (reviewed in reference 123). Two thyroid hormone response elements (TRE) are in the human *dio1* gene promoter.[149]

D1 also catalyzes monodeiodination of the inner ring of T_4 and T_3.[150] Sulfation of the phenolic hydroxyl of T_4 or T_3 reduces the K_m for inner-ring deiodination and increases the V_{max} for the reaction.[120, 151–153] Sulfate conjugates are present in cord sera and in amniotic fluid,[3, 154–158] and sulfated conjugates accumulate in fetal serum owing to the low levels of D1 in fetal tissues.[3, 159] While T_3-SO_4 has little biologic activity, it

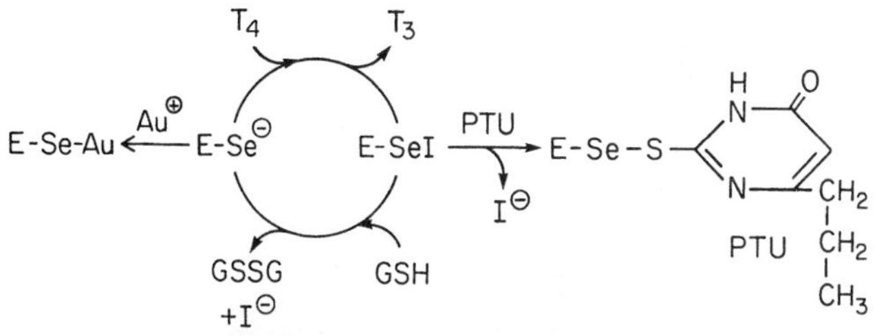

could serve as a local source of T_3 in tissues that express sulfatase, such as the liver and brain of fetal rats.[3] T_3-SO_4 is not a substrate for inner-ring deiodination by D3,[160] and in adult humans T_3-SO_4 is not deconjugated.[161]

A sulfhydryl-containing cytosolic cofactor, which is required for all deiodination reactions, maybe glutathione, requires NADPH for regeneration. Fasting could reduce both T_4 and rT_3 5'-deiodination by reducing the levels of NADPH, and glucose can reverse the fasting-induced decrease in circulating T_3. PTU acts by competing with the cytosolic cofactor for reactivation of D1 (see Fig. 11–9). For example, PTU administration causes a marked inhibition of rT_3 deiodination in humans, but only a modest decrease in total T_3 production.[144–146] As mentioned, in hyperthyroidism propylthiouracil causes a 50% fall in serum T_3 and a decrease in the ratio of T_3 to T_4.[41, 162] The activity of D1 in the thyroid is increased by TSH in the rat and is higher in the thyroids of patients with Graves' disease.[34, 35] However, thyroidal D2 activity is also enhanced in Graves' disease.[37] The enhanced D1 activity in the liver and kidneys may explain the greater sensitivity of T_3 production to inhibition by PTU in the hyperthyroid patient.[41]

TYPE 2 DEIODINASE. Type 2 deiodinase (D2) is present in the pituitary gland, central nervous system, brown fat, and placenta of rats and humans (see Table 11–4) and also in human skeletal, cardiac, and thyroid tissue.[37, 118, 119] The apparent K_m is three orders of magnitude lower than for the D1 enzyme, and D2 catalyzes only the outer ring of deiodination of T_4 and rT_3. Catalysis by D2 is resistant to inhibition by propylthiouracil or gold.[113, 118, 122, 123] The D2 enzyme is thought to act primarily to maintain intracellular T_3 concentrations in tissues, but the widespread expression of D2 in human tissues suggests a role for D2 in the generation of circulating T_3.[37, 118, 119] A reduction in serum T_4 concentration leads to an increase in the activity of D2, and vice versa.[163, 164] This regulation of D2 is not dependent on the metabolic potency of the iodothyronine involved.[163, 165] The mechanism of the regulation of D2 by iodothyronine substrates is not well understood but is both pretranslational and post-translational.[119, 165, 166]

D2 also provides the mechanism by which the thyrotropic

Figure 11–9. Schematic diagram of T_4 5'-deiodination by type 1 iodothyronine deiodinase (D1). The reaction assumes the formation of a selenolyl-iodide intermediate that must be regenerated by a cystolic cofactor that is probably an -SH compound such as reduced glutathione (GSH). Heavy metals with a single positive charge such as gold (Au) inhibit deiodination by interaction with the negatively charged selenium atom. Propylthiouracil (PTU) forms a stable Se-S complex and blocks regeneration of the active enzyme.

cells of the pituitary monitor the serum T_4 concentration.[167] As shown in Figure 11-10, D2 activity is necessary for the physiological suppression of TSH release by T_4.[168] If T_4 level falls, the consequent increase in serum TSH maintains serum T_3 concentrations by increasing the ratio of T_3 to T_4 in thyroid hormone secretion. This sequence occurs in subjects living in endemic goiter areas, in animal models of iodine deficiency (see later), and in early hypothyroidism.[169-172]

TYPE 3 DEIODINASE. The role of D3 is to inactivate T_3 and T_4. It increases in response to T_3 (see Table 11-4), suggesting that it is part of a homeostatic mechanism for maintaining the T_3 concentration constant in the central nervous system and for protecting the fetus from maternal T_4 and T_3.[3, 114, 173, 174] A decrease in D3 activity in the hypothyroid or iodine-deficient state blocks T_3 and T_4 inactivation and facilitates the adaptation to these situations. Inner-ring deiodination of T_4 by D3 is thought to be the most important source of circulating rT_3 in humans.

QUANTITATIVE ASPECTS OF DEIODINATIVE PATHWAYS. About 80% of T_4 is deiodinated, and the remainder is eliminated principally as the glucuronide by fecal excretion, probably as a mixture of T_4, T_3, and their various conjugated and unconjugated derivatives. Deamination and decarboxylation reactions that produce tetraiodothyroacetic acid (TETRAC) and triiodothyroacetic acid (TRIAC) account for 5% or less of daily T_4 disposal.

About 35 to 40% of secreted T_4 is monodeiodinated in the 5' position to yield T_3, and a similar fraction is deiodinated in the 5 position to yield rT_3 (see Fig. 11-5). Hence, with the normal T_4 production rate of 100 nmol (78 µg)/d, 40 nmol (26 µg) of T_3 and rT_3 are produced by peripheral deiodination. In brief, most (at least 80%) of T_3 and all of rT_3 production can be accounted for by peripheral deiodination of T_4 (Table 11-5), findings consonant with the high ratio of T_4 to T_3 (15:1) and rT_3 (>100:1) in the normal thyroid gland. Although much of the T_3 and rT_3 produced from T_4 in peripheral tissues exits those tissues and enters the blood, an uncertain fraction of T_3 and rT_3 is degraded locally prior to exit. As discussed later, in some tissues the T_3 in the cell nuclei is derived to a large extent from local T_3 generation, rather than from the blood (Fig. 11-11).[110] Thus, estimates of the rate of conversion of T_4 to T_3 and rT_3, based solely on measurements in plasma, are minimal values.

T_3 is metabolized mainly by 5-monodeiodination, and rT_3 is metabolized by 5'-monodeiodination; both processes yield $3,3'-T_2$ (see Fig. 11-5), which is rapidly degraded to monoiodothyronine and thyronine.[175] Thyronine and the iodide that escapes uptake by the thyroid are excreted in the urine.

TABLE 11-5. Comparison of T_3 and T_4 in Humans

	T_3	T_4
Production rate (nmol/d)	50	100
Fraction from thyroid	0.2	1.0
Relative metabolic potency	1.0	0.3
Serum concentration		
Total (nmol/L)	1.8	100
Free (pmol/L)	5	20
Fraction of total hormone in free form ($\times 10^{-2}$)	0.3	0.02
Distribution volume (L)	40	10
Fraction intracellular	0.64	0.15
Half-life (d)	0.75	7.0

To convert T_4 from nmol/L to µg/dL (total) or pmol/L to ng/dL (free), divide by 12.87. To convert T_3 from nmol/L to ng/dL (total) or pmol/L to pg/dL (free), multiply by 65.1.

TETRAC and TRIAC are metabolized by deiodination or by conjugation and are excreted into the bile (see Fig. 11-1).

PHYSIOLOGICAL IMPLICATIONS. In view of the tissue distribution of the various deiodinases, their different K_m values, and the characteristics of iodothyronine tissue uptake systems, it is not surprising that various tissues obtain the active thyroid hormone T_3 from different sources.[100] Because the T_3 regulates gene expression, it is especially relevant to compare the quantity and source of this nuclear T_3 in various tissues of the rat (Fig. 11-11). In the rat kidney and liver, most of the nuclear T_3 is derived directly from the plasma T_3. In the rat cerebral cortex, pituitary, and brown fat, all of which contain D2, half or more of intracellular T_3 is generated locally from T_4 within the tissue. The tissues that depend on D2 for nuclear T_3 are those in which a constant supply of thyroid hormone is critical for either normal development (cerebral cortex), function (pituitary), or survival during cold stress (brown adipose tissue). These tissues are also characterized by a high degree of saturation of the nuclear T_3 receptors. In rat liver, kidney, and heart, on the other hand, nuclear receptor sites are only about 50% occupied at normal serum T_3 concentrations. This arrangement allows multiple levels of regulation of thyroid hormone action. The supply of T_3 to tissues such as kidney, liver, and perhaps heart can be decreased by reducing the conversion of T_4 to the plasma T_3. For example, in the rat, starvation, surgical stress, glucocorticoid therapy, and diabetes mellitus all decrease D1 activity (Table 11-6).[123] As mentioned earlier, in humans serum T_3 decreases to about a third of its normal value after overnight fasting, possibly acting to conserve protein and reduce metabolic rate,[176] and the inverse relation between D2 and serum T_4 allows nuclear receptor-bound T_3 in the brain to remain at

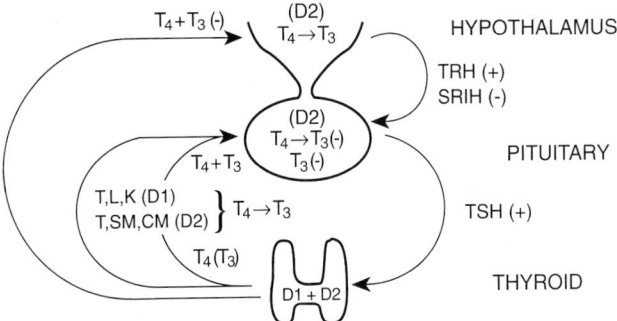

Figure 11-10. Schematic diagram of the role of T_4 and T_3 in the regulation of TRH and TSH secretion. Thyroidal T_4 must be converted to T_3 to produce its effects. This conversion may take place in the liver (L), kidney (K), and thyroid (T) catalyzed by either the propylthiouracil-sensitive iodothyronine 5'-deiodinase (D1) or the propylthiouracil-insensitive 5'-deiodinase (D2). D2 is present in the human pituitary, central nervous system, thyroid, skeletal muscle (SM), and possibly cardiac muscle (CM).

QUANTITY AND SOURCE OF NUCLEAR T_3 IN VARIOUS TISSUES

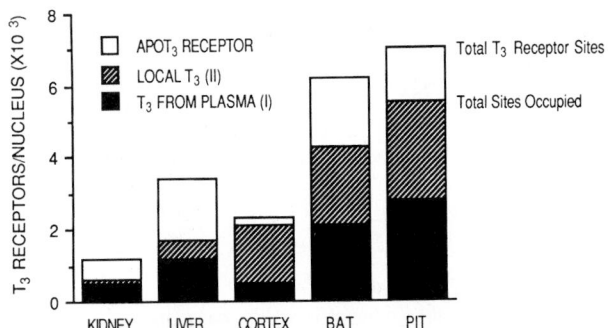

Figure 11-11. Origin of nuclear T_3 in various tissues of the rat. Data are derived from studies in which specifically bound nuclear T_3 was estimated with double-isotope labeling techniques. In tissues in which the receptor saturation is above 50%, the additional T_3 is provided by D2. T_3 in rat plasma is derived from D1-catalyzed conversion of T_4 to T_3 in liver and kidney and by the thyroid.

TABLE 11–6. Factors That Impair Peripheral Conversion of T₄ to T₃

Physiological
Fetal and early neonatal life
Old age?

Pathologic
Fasting, malnutrition
Hepatic or renal dysfunction
Systemic illness
Trauma, postoperative state

Pharmacologic
Drugs (propylthiouracil, glucocorticoids, propranolol, amiodarone)
Oral cholecystographic agents

nearly normal levels despite a fall in serum T_4 levels. This, plus some transplacental passage of maternal T_4,[9] may account for normal brain development in athyreotic infants if they are identified and treated soon after birth.[3, 177] Thus only in certain tissues is it possible to predict the nuclear T_3 concentration from its level in plasma. T_3 is three to four times more active than T_4, and because one third of T_4 is converted to T_3, it is likely that all the metabolic activity of T_4 can be ascribed to the T_3 that it gives rise to, i.e., T_4 is a prohormone. Indeed there is considerable evidence that T_4 has no independent physiological effects as long as conversion of T_4 to T_3 can occur. The fact that rT_3 has no known metabolic effect, together with the fact that outer- or inner-ring T_4 deiodination can vary independently, has given rise to the concept that these two pathways cause either hormone activation or hormone inactivation.

Thyroid Hormone Turnover

In the normal adult, T_4 has a volume of distribution of approximately 10 L (see Table 11–5). Because the concentration of T_4 in plasma is approximately 100 nmol/L (8 µg/dL), the extrathyroidal pool of T_4 is approximately 1 µmol (about 800 µg). In the young or middle-aged adult, the fractional rate of turnover of T_4 in the periphery is normally about 10%/d (half-time, 6.7 d). Thus about 1.1 L of the peripheral T_4 distribution space is cleared of hormone daily, a volume that contains approximately 110 nmol (85 µg) of T_4. The fact that the fractional rate of turnover and rate of clearance of total T_4 are smaller than those of most hormones is a reflection of the extent to which T_4 is bound to plasma proteins. The clearance rate of free T_4 is at least 5500 L/d.

The kinetics of T_3 metabolism differ greatly from those of T_4, partly because of differences in the intensity of its binding to TBG. A single bolus of T_3 disappears from the plasma over several hours as a result of its distribution and consequent rapid cellular metabolism. The volume of distribution of T_3 in the normal adult is about 40 L, and its fractional turnover rate is about 60%/d. Hence, the MCR of total T_3 is about 24 L/d. At a mean normal serum T_3 concentration of 1.8 nmol/L (120 ng/dL), the daily production rate of T_3 is approximately 50 nmol (36 µg) or about 40% that of T_4.

The rapid metabolic clearance rate of rT_3 and a low concentration in plasma (0.25 nmol/L, 15 ng/dL) combine to yield daily production rates for rT_3 of about 45 nmol. The turnover and metabolism of $3,3'-T_2$ are even faster than those of rT_3.

Alterations in Transport, Turnover, and Metabolism of Thyroid Hormones

The level of free hormones is the major determinant of the amount available to the cells, the rate of hormone turnover, and the metabolic state of the individual.

EXTRACELLULAR ABNORMALITIES. Perturbations in the interaction between thyroid hormones and the binding proteins can result from a change in the number or affinity of available binding sites or from a change in the concentration of the hormone. The consequences of these two types of changes differ. Consider first the consequences of an increase in the level of TBG in plasma (Table 11–7; see Fig. 11–7). Initially, the number of unoccupied binding sites increases, causing a shift of hormone from the free to the bound state, a decrease in the MCR and in the quantity of hormone removed from the plasma, and an increase in TSH. With the same or increased T_4 secretion, the total hormone level would increase progressively until the concentration of free hormone is restored to normal, so that both the absolute concentration of free T_4 and its dependent variable, the rate of hormone disposal to the tissues, are normal. The patient remains euthyroid. This sequence occurs for both T_4 and T_3 with an increase in TBG levels in plasma. The opposite sequence occurs with decreased levels of TBG (see Table 11–7).

Thus, although primary alterations in TBG alter the total concentrations of hormone in plasma and the kinetics of T_4 metabolism, they do not ultimately influence the quantity of hormone that enters the cell, acts, and is degraded per unit time. Therefore they do not influence the total turnover of hormone or the metabolic state in the steady state.

Different consequences occur with a primary alteration in the rate of hormone supply. For example in hyperthyroid states, hypersecretion of hormone leads to an increase in total hormone concentration. As a result, the concentration of unoccupied binding sites on TBG decreases, and the concentrations of bound and free hormone rise. In vivo these changes are reflected in an increase in the MCR of T_4, an increase in the rate of hormone delivery to the tissues, and a hypermetabolic state. The opposite consequences occur when the supply of hormone is decreased, as in hypothyroidism. In the final analysis, the metabolic state over any prolonged period is determined by the rate of hormone production.

CELLULAR ABNORMALITIES. Phenobarbital, phenytoin, and carbamazepine can accelerate the peripheral metabolism of T_4.[83, 178–182] There is no uniformity of data concerning the effect of phenytoin on serum T_3 and TSH concentrations. Some data suggest, however, that phenytoin accelerates the peripheral conversion of T_4 to T_3, thereby maintaining the serum T_3 concentration and obviating the need for increased TSH secretion, despite the subnormal serum concentrations of total and free T_4.[181] Phenytoin may also have thyromimetic activity at least at the level of the pituitary.[57] Any such effects, however, are minor, and there is no indication for administering supplemental levothyroxine to otherwise normal patients receiving this drug, although therapy with these agents may increase levothyroxine requirements in hypothyroidism.[180, 181]

In patients with thyrotoxicosis, the metabolic clearance

TABLE 11–7. Circumstances Associated with Altered Binding of T₄ by TBG

Increased Binding	Decreased Binding
Pregnancy	Androgens
Neonatal state	Large doses of glucocorticoids
Estrogens and hyperestrogenemic states	Active acromegaly
Tamoxifen	Nephrotic syndrome
Oral contraceptives	Major systemic illness
Acute intermittent porphyria	Genetic factors
Infectious and chronic active hepatitis	Asparaginase
Biliary cirrhosis	
Genetic factors	
Perphenazine	
HIV infection	

HIV, human immunodeficiency virus.

rates of T_4 and T_3 are increased, and the converse is true in patients with hypothyroidism. These changes are partly due to alterations in extracellular binding of the hormones and partly due to cellular factors. In experimental thyrotoxicosis and hypothyroidism, overall degradation of T_4 in liver and brain preparations in vitro is accelerated or retarded, respectively, both D1 and D3 activities varying in parallel with the metabolic state. In the pituitary, in contrast, D2 activity varies inversely with the metabolic state (see Table 11–4).

IMPAIRMENT OF THYROXINE ACTIVATION. The conversion of T_4 to T_3 is impaired in conditions that have come to be known as the *low-T_3 syndrome*, the *euthyroid sick syndrome*, or *nonthyroidal illness*.[183] Circumstances that can lead to the syndrome are listed in Table 11–6. Serum T_3 concentration and T_3 production rate fall, and the serum rT_3 level rises because of impairment of outer-ring deiodination of this compound. An example of this phenomenon occurs in individuals given the antiarrhythmic agent amiodarone, which partially blocks T_4-to-T_3 conversion.[184, 185] The response to the administration of this agent is to increase TSH secretion and, consequently, serum T_4 until a new equilibrium is established, at which point the TSH level returns to normal. At this time all tests of thyroid hormone economy indicate a euthyroid state despite the reduced T_3/T_4 ratio and elevated serum T_4 concentration. It is not known whether amiodarone inhibits both D1 and D2 or how much of its effect is due to inhibition of pituitary T_4-to-T_3 conversion in the thyrotrope. Whatever the cause, if amiodarone is given to an individual who is hypothyroid, the requirement for levothyroxine increases.[186] Similar effects have been demonstrated with the oral cholecystographic agent iopanoic acid.[57]

Another cause of impaired T_4-to-T_3 conversion is illness or trauma (see Table 11–7).[183, 187] Whether ill patients with serum T_3 concentrations less than one third of normal are hypothyroid is unclear because of a paucity of tests for assessing thyroid hormone action in vivo. The problem is further compounded by the dual feedback of TSH by serum T_3 and intrapituitary T_4-to-T_3 conversion (see Fig. 11–10). Thus serum TSH is not always a valid reflection of the thyroid state. Because of these complexities, it cannot be certain whether hypothyroidism is, in fact, present when the serum T_3 level is reduced. Administration of levothyroxine or liothyroxine does not change the outcome in seriously ill patients.[188, 189]

Peripheral iodothyronine metabolism in the fetus differs from that in adults. 5′-Monodeiodination of T_4 is retarded[3, 8, 190] and 5-monodeiodination is accelerated, so that rT_3 formation and the degradation of any T_3 formed are increased. At about the time of delivery, iodothyronine metabolism switches to a more mature pattern.[2–4, 8]

REGULATION OF THYROID FUNCTION

The thyroid participates with the hypothalamus and pituitary in a classic type of feedback control (see Fig. 11–10). In addition, there is an inverse relationship between the glandular organic iodine level and the rate of hormone formation. Such autoregulatory mechanisms serve to stabilize the rate of hormone synthesis despite fluctuations in the availability of a substrate such as iodine. Stability in hormone production is achieved in part because the large intraglandular store of hormone buffers the effect of acute increases or decreases in hormone synthesis. Autoregulatory mechanisms within the gland, in turn, tend to maintain the constancy of the thyroid hormone pool. Finally, the hypothalamic-pituitary feedback mechanism senses variations in the availability of thyroid hormones and serves to correct abnormalities in the concentration of free thyroid hormones in the blood, however small, once they occur.

The Hypothalamic-Pituitary-Thyroid Complex

There is a close relationship between the hypothalamus, the anterior pituitary, the thyroid gland, and still higher centers in the brain, the function of the entire complex being modified in a typical negative-feedback manner by the availability of the thyroid hormones.

THYROTROPIN-RELEASING HORMONE (TRH) SYNTHESIS AND SECRETION. TRH, a modified tripeptide (pyroglutamyl-histidyl-proline-amide; Fig. 11–12), is derived from a large prepro-TRH molecule that contains five progenitor sequences.[191–194] The TRH peptides are released from the prepro molecule by a peptidase that acts at flanking lysine-arginine residues.[195] TRH is expressed in the hypothalamus, the brain, the C cells of the thyroid gland, the beta cells of the pancreas, the myocardium, the reproductive organs including prostate and testis, and the spinal cord.[196, 197] The parvocellular region of the paraventricular nuclei of the hypothalamus is the source of the hypothalamic portal TRH that regulates TSH secretion. The 5′-flanking region of the gene encoding TRH has sequences for mediating responses to glucocorticoids and cAMP. In addition, at least two elements in this region of the gene can confer negative regulation of thyroid hormone receptor complexes.[193, 198] TRH travels in the axons of the peptidergic neurons through the median eminence and is released close to the hypothalamic-pituitary portal plexus. The neuron bodies producing TRH are innervated by catecholamine-, neuropeptide Y–, and somatostatin-containing axons, all of which potentially influence the rate of synthesis of the prepro-TRH molecule.

T_3 suppresses the levels of prepro-TRH mRNA by T_3 in the hypothalamus,[199, 200] but normal feedback regulation of prepro-TRH mRNA synthesis by thyroid hormone requires a combination of T_3 and T_4 in the circulation, the latter giving rise to T_3 via direct local synthesis in the central nervous system.[201]

TRH binds to a receptor in the thyrotrope membrane,[202, 203] and calcium and cGMP are the second messengers for induction of the thyrotrope response.[204, 205] The calcium is derived from endoplasmic reticulum, owing to increases in inositol triphosphate secondary to G protein activation of phospholipase C. Both phorbol esters and calcium ionophores can stimulate TSH gene transcription.[206, 207] In addition to inhibiting the synthesis of prepro-TRH mRNA, thyroid hormone also blocks the capacity of TRH to stimulate TSH release from the pituitary thyrotrope. The mechanism for this is unknown, but the stimulating effects of both phorbol esters and calcium ionophores are blocked by prior incubation with thyroid hormone.[208–210]

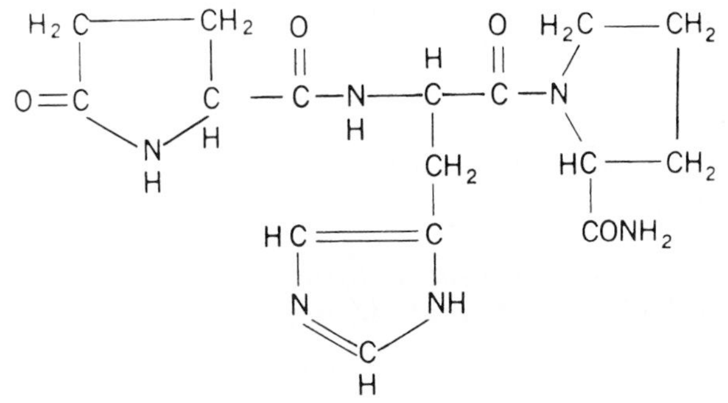

Figure 11–12. Formula of TRH (pyroglutamyl-histidyl-proline amide).

Exogenous TRH elicits the secretion of prolactin at threshold doses that are the same as those for stimulation of TSH secretion. As with TSH, the prolactin response to TRH is modified by the prevailing levels of thyroid hormones, although not to as marked an extent. The role of TRH as a physiological modulator of prolactin secretion is uncertain, however. Nursing increases the serum prolactin concentration, but the serum TSH concentration is unchanged. TRH may also act as a neurotransmitter. Exogenous TRH elicits the secretion of growth hormone in some patients with renal failure and acromegaly. The basis for these anomalous responses is also unknown.

THYROTROPIN (THYROID-STIMULATING HORMONE) SYNTHESIS AND SECRETION. TSH is the major regulator of the morphologic and functional states of the thyroid, but not all adjustments in thyroid function are mediated by TSH. Intrinsic autoregulatory mechanisms (e.g., those induced when the supply of iodide is altered) also operate to alter thyroid cell sensitivity to TSH.

TSH is a glycoprotein secreted by the thyrotropes in the anteromedial portion of the adenohypophysis. TSH is composed of an α subunit of about 14 kd that is common to luteinizing hormone (LH), follicle-stimulating hormone (FSH), and human chorionic gonadotropin (hCG) and a specific β subunit that, in the case of TSH, is a 112-amino-acid protein.[211, 212] The peptide sequence cysteine-alanine-glycine-tyrosine-cysteine (CAGYC) is highly conserved in the β subunits of TSH, FSH, LH, and hCG and is required for heterodimerization with the α subunit.[213] An autosomal recessive form of hypothyroidism is associated with a G (glycine)–to–R (arginine) mutation in this sequence of the TSH β subunit which blocks its capacity to heterodimerize and renders it nonfunctional.[214] Transcription of both the α and β subunits are suppressed by thyroid hormone, although the effect on the β subunit is greater.[212, 215] Even in thyrotrope tumors, synthesis of α subunit is in excess, indicating that the quantity of β subunit is rate-limiting for TSH secretion. TRH increases and dopamine suppresses the transcription of both subunits.[207, 212]

The glycosylation of TSH involves addition of preformed asparagine-linked oligosaccharides in rough endoplasmic reticulum, modifications in proximal and distal Golgi apparatus, and the appearance of the intact folded hormone in the secretory granules.[216] The glycosylation of the subunits protects them from intracellular degradation and permits normal folding of the protein chains so that internal disulfide linkages are correctly formed. Glycosylation is also required for full biologic activity, and sialylation protects circulating TSH from interaction with hepatic galactose receptors, thus increasing its half-life.[217, 218]

The biologic activity of TSH in the serum of patients with pituitary tumors or hypothalamic disorders is inappropriately low compared with immunologic activity, suggesting the formation of an abnormal product.[219, 220] Long-term administration of TRH can enhance the biologic activity of TSH in patients with hypothalamic hypothyroidism and lead to increased thyroid hormone levels.[217] Thus TRH not only regulates both α and β TSH subunit synthesis but also post-translational processing.

Levels of α subunit in serum range from 0.5 to 2 μg/L but are increased in postmenopausal women. In normal serum, TSH is present at concentrations between 0.5 and 5 μU/L. The level is increased in hypothyroidism and reduced in hyperthyroidism (see later). The plasma half-life of TSH is about 30 min, and production rates in humans are 40 to 150 mU/d.[221]

Circulating TSH displays both pulsatile and circadian variations. The former is characterized by fluctuations at 1- to 2-h intervals. The magnitude of TSH pulsations is decreased during fasting, illness, or after surgery.[222–224] The circadian variation is characterized by a nocturnal surge that precedes the onset of sleep and appears to be independent of the cortisol rhythm and fluctuations in the serum and T_4 and T_3 concentrations.[225] When the onset of sleep is delayed, the nocturnal TSH surge is enhanced and prolonged, and the early onset of sleep results in a surge of lesser magnitude and shorter duration.

TRH acts in the thyrotrope to stimulate the release and later the synthesis of TSH, while thyroid hormones inhibit these functions. The inhibitory effects can be observed when the hypothalamic source of TRH is destroyed or the pituitary gland is separated from the hypothalamus. Moreover, the degree of thyroid hypofunction after destruction of the hypothalamus is less severe than that which follows hypophysectomy, and residual thyroid function in the former circumstance can be altered by raising or lowering the concentration of thyroid hormones in the blood. Thus thyroid hormones mediate the feedback regulation of TSH secretion, and TRH determines its set point.

The relationship between serum T_4 and T_3 levels and pituitary TSH release is demonstrated in Figure 11–10. The acute inhibition of TSH release by physiological quantities of T_4 is mediated by the T_3 produced in the pituitary gland.[167] If pituitary deiodinase is blocked by an inhibitor such as iopanoic acid, the effect of T_4 is reduced or eliminated.[168] The mechanism by which the nuclear binding of T_3 leads within minutes to inhibition of TSH release is not known.

In rats a decrease in either plasma T_3 or T_4 causes an increase in TSH release because both T_3 directly, and T_4 via intrapituitary and intracerebral T_4-to-T_3 conversion, contribute to T_3 (see Fig. 11–11).[110] However, the plasma T_3 concentration must be increased to about twice normal levels to replace intracellular T_4-to-T_3 conversion as a source of pituitary nuclear T_3. It follows that exogenous T_4 is an effective suppressor of TSH secretion both because it is converted to plasma T_3 and because it serves as the prohormone for T_3 in the central nervous system and pituitary. Since nuclear T_3 in most tissues is exclusively from plasma T_3 (see Fig. 11–11), the degree of TSH suppression for a given dose of T_4 is likely to be greater than, for example, hepatic enzyme induction. This may offer a therapeutic advantage when TSH suppression is desired for treatment of thyroid carcinoma.

Small doses of thyroid hormone, sufficient to produce only minimal increases in plasma concentration, greatly diminish the basal TSH and/or the response to exogenous TRH.[226–228] By contrast, in euthyroid subjects large doses of iodide can transiently inhibit T_3 and T_4 release and produce very slight decreases in serum T_4 and T_3 concentrations. Even though these levels remain within the normal range, such changes are uniformly accompanied by increases in the basal and TRH-stimulated TSH concentrations (Fig. 11–13).

Somatostatin (somatotropin release-inhibiting factor [SRIF]), acting through inhibitory G protein (G_i), decreases the response to TRH in vitro and in vivo,[229, 230] but prolonged treatment with a somatostatin analogue does not cause hypothyroidism.[231, 232] Prolonged administration of levodopa decreases the basal serum TSH concentration in hypothyroid patients and decreases the response to TRH. Similar effects follow dopamine infusion and the administration of bromocriptine, a dopamine agonist.[232, 233] Both of these agents inhibit adenylate cyclase. Conversely, blockade of the dopamine receptor by metoclopramide increases the basal serum TSH concentration in both euthyroid and hypothyroid patients and increases the response to TRH.[234] These findings indicate that dopamine is a regulator of TSH secretion, but chronic administration of dopamine agonists for the treatment of prolactinoma does not cause central hypothyroidism, indicating that compensatory mechanisms negate these acute effects. Pharma-

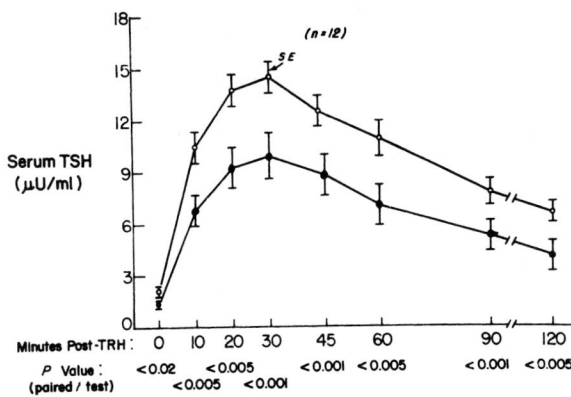

Figure 11–13. Iodide (190 mg twice daily for 10 d) increases response of the serum TSH level to administration of TRH in euthyroid volunteers. During iodide administration, mean serum T_4 concentration decreased from 8.0 to 6.6 μg/dL, and mean serum T_3 concentration decreased from 128 to 110 ng/dL. (From Vagenakis AG, Rappoport B, Azizi F, et al. Accelerated response to TRH accompanying small decreases in serum thyroid hormone concentrations. Reproduced from the Journal of Clinical Investigation 1974; 54:913–918. By permission of the American Society of Clinical Investigation.)

cologic doses of glucocorticoids transiently inhibit the release of TSH in response to TRH and may decrease secretion of TRH as well[235] but, when given chronically, do not suppress the hypothalamic-pituitary-thyroid axis. The cytokines interleukin-1β (IL-1β), IL-6, and tumor necrosis factor α (TNF α), or cachectin, inhibit TSH release.[236–239] Since IL-1β is produced in thyrotropes and is increased by bacterial lipopolysaccharide, it, together with TNF α, could act to decrease TSH secretion during illness.[240]

TSH enhances essentially all processes leading to the synthesis and secretion of hormone (see earlier). Abolition of TSH secretion by hypophysectomy or suppression is followed by decreased thyroid iodide transport and inhibition of organic binding.

The Influence of Iodine Availability

In contrast to the feedback control effected via TSH, which maintains the plasma or tissue concentrations of the thyroid hormones, intrinsic autoregulatory mechanisms maintain the constancy of thyroid hormone stores and play a role in the capacity of the thyroid to overcome factors that impair hormone synthesis.

Iodine Excess

EFFECTS ON THYROID HORMONE SYNTHESIS. The quantity of iodine that undergoes organification displays a biphasic response to increasing doses of iodide, at first increasing and then decreasing as a result of a relative blockade of organic binding. This decreasing yield of organic iodine from increasing doses of iodide, termed the Wolff-Chaikoff effect,[241–243] depends on the establishment within the thyroid of a sufficient concentration of inorganic iodide.

Susceptibility to the Wolff-Chaikoff effect can be increased either by stimulation of the iodide-trapping mechanism, as occurs in patients with Graves' disease or after TSH administration, or by impairment of organic iodine formation, as may occur after radioiodine therapy, during propylthiouracil treatment, or in patients with Hashimoto's disease. In such situations goiter or hypothyroidism can develop if iodide is given for long periods.

When moderate or large doses of iodide are administered repeatedly, the relative inhibition of organic binding and inhibition of iodothyronine formation are partly relieved. This

"escape" or "adaptation" phenomenon occurs because iodide transport activity decreases and the thyroid iodide concentration is insufficient to maintain a full Wolff-Chaikoff effect. This response is a manifestation of the thyroid autoregulatory inhibition of iodide transport discussed earlier and prevents development of goitrous hypothyroidism in normal people. In unusual circumstances, adaptation does not occur, and chronic inhibition of hormone synthesis leads to the development of goiter and hypothyroidism (iodide myxedema). This disorder is discussed more fully in the section on hypothyroidism.

EFFECTS ON THYROID HORMONE RELEASE. The most important clinical effect of pharmacologic doses of iodine is the prompt inhibition of hormone release. Iodine decreases not only the fractional turnover of thyroidal iodine but also the actual T_4 secretion rate. This effect is the mechanism by which iodine rapidly lowers the serum T_4 concentration in the patient with diffuse toxic goiter (see the section on Graves' disease). The mechanism by which iodine inhibits secretion of T_4 is unknown, but the effect is mediated at the thyroid level, rather than through an action on TSH. For example, the effect is demonstrable in the autonomously hyperfunctioning thyroid nodule and in Graves' disease in which secretion of TSH is suppressed.

INVOLUTION OF THYROID HYPERPLASIA. Iodine diminishes the hypervascularity and hyperplasia that characterize the diffuse toxic goiter of Graves' disease.[244] This effect facilitates surgical therapy for the disorder.

Iodine Deficiency

The responses of vertebrates to iodine deficiency are designed to conserve this limited resource and involves adjustments at the hypothalamic-pituitary, thyroid, and peripheral levels (Fig. 11–14).[245–247] Removal of iodine from the diet causes a rapid decrease in serum T_4 concentrations and a simultaneous increase in serum TSH. Circulating T_3 concentrations are maintained despite the marked fall in T_4, but eventually T_3 levels fall if restriction is continued.[248, 249] Thyroidal T_4 is progressively depleted, while T_3 synthesis is maintained in the enlarging thyroid.[247] The increase in TSH and decrease in iodine availability cause changes in Tg, namely an increase in the ratio of MIT to DIT and in the ratio of T_3 to T_4 owing to a decrease in T_4 synthesis. In addition, iodine uptake and organification are enhanced owing to the increased TSH stimulation, a decrease in the autoregulatory suppression of thyroid function by iodine (reviewed earlier), and an increase in the efficiency of intrathyroidal conservation of iodine. TSH stimulates the rate of thyroid cell division, leading to goiter. In humans thyroidal T_4-to-T_3 conversion by D2 may also be stimulated. All of these changes have been well documented in humans in areas of iodine deficiency[250–252] and in rare patients with absence of the iodide trapping mechanism.[20, 253] Thus the bulk of T_3 in the iodine-deficient vertebrate is derived not from peripheral T_4 monodeiodination, but directly from the thyroid. In humans the presence of D2 in skeletal and cardiac muscle provides another mechanism by which serum T_3 concentration can be maintained when serum T_4 falls.

The changes in circulating T_4, T_3, and TSH in iodine deficiency are similar to those that occur during the development of primary hypothyroidism in humans.[170] The pathophysiology of iodine deficiency is also reproduced when the efficiency of iodide trapping and organification is reduced in Hashimoto's disease or in the patient with Graves' disease receiving thiourea drugs.[33] The physiological rationale for this series of events is clear. T_3 has approximately three times the potency of the prohormone T_4 and contains only three iodine atoms. In terms of metabolic potency, this represents a four-

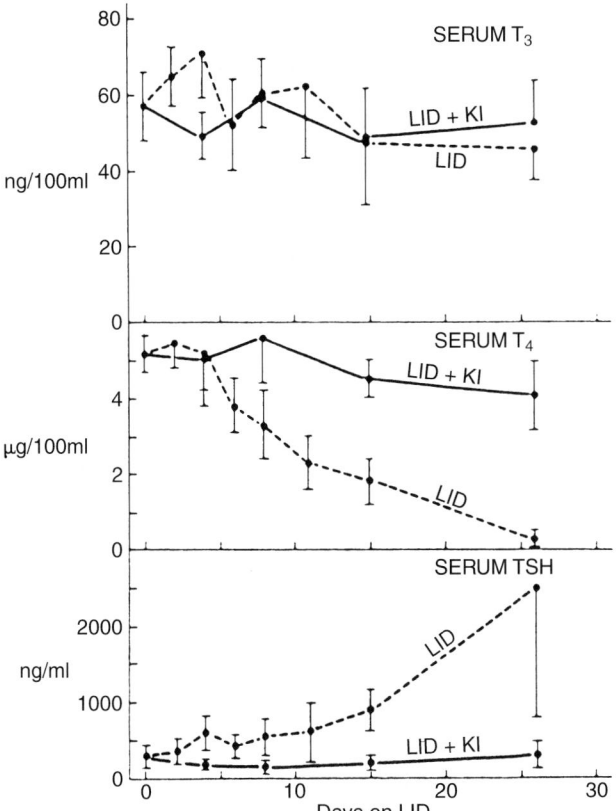

Figure 11–14. Effect of acute depletion of dietary iodine on serum T_3, T_4, and TSH in rats. Animals received a low-iodine diet (LID) without or with supplementation of potassium iodide (KI) in drinking water. (From Riesco G, Taurog A, Larsen PR, et al. Acute and chronic responses to iodine deficiency in rats. Endocrinology 1977; 100:303–313. © The Endocrine Society.)

fold more efficient use of an iodine atom. Since T_3 is the active hormone, maintenance of normal circulating levels provides T_3 for tissues in which nuclear T_3 is completely derived from the plasma (see Fig. 11–11).

How is this remarkable adaptation effected? While the changes in iodine availability clearly affect the thyroid, the central role is played by the hypothalamic-pituitary axis. The increase in TSH occurs *pari passu* with a decrease in serum T_4 (see Fig. 11–14). Since T_4 is an obligate source of intracellular T_3 to the pituitary and central nervous system (see earlier and Fig. 11–11) via deiodination by D2, the feedback suppression of TSH secretion is reduced. The compensatory increase in D2 when T_4 falls would be expected to partially or completely negate this effect. It clearly does not, possibly because D2 levels in the thyrotrope are less sensitive to the effects of a reduced T_4 than are those in other pituitary cells.[254] The consequence is that when T_4 falls, peripheral euthyroidism is maintained by the increased TSH consequent to the effects of hypothyroidism in the pituitary. In humans, these compensatory alterations in thyroid function come into operation when total iodine intake falls below 75 to 80 μg/d (see Table 11–1), the situation in many countries in Europe and South America and for hundreds of millions of individuals in areas of iodine-deficiency in China, India, Indonesia, and Africa.[251, 252]

Adrenergic Nervous System and Bioactive Amines or Peptides

Despite the adrenergic innervation of the human thyroid (see earlier), the role of the sympathetic nervous system in normal thyroid function is unclear. Depending on the magni-

tude and timing of the dose, the administration of epinephrine may either increase or decrease the radioactive iodine uptake (RAIU), and thyroid function is normal in most patients with pheochromocytoma. Thyroid function or serum T_4 concentrations are normal in patients given pharmacologic doses of adrenergic blocking agents.

OTHER EXOGENOUS AND ENDOGENOUS FACTORS THAT INFLUENCE THYROID HORMONE ECONOMY

PREGNANCY AND MATERNAL-FETAL INTERACTIONS.
Pregnancy affects virtually all aspects of thyroid hormone economy (Fig. 11–15).[3, 255, 256] The total serum T_4 and T_3 concentrations rise to levels twice those of nonpregnant women[257] owing to the increase in TBG concentration in the first trimester.[66, 67] Free T_4 and T_3 levels also increase slightly during the first trimester,[3, 257, 258] but return to normal by about 20 wk of gestation and remain so until delivery. This pattern coincides with that of hCG levels, which is the probable cause of the increase in free hormone levels in the first trimester.[259–263] A slight decrease in serum TSH during the first trimester indicates that the free T_4 and T_3 changes are not dependent on the hypothalamic-pituitary axis.[15, 259, 261, 262, 264] Owing to the increase in the glomerular filtration rate (GFR), iodide clearance increases during gestation, leading to increased dietary requirements. If these are not met, serum T_4 falls, TSH increases, and goiter ensues. There is no clinically significant change in the size of the thyroid during pregnancy in normal women receiving adequate quantities of iodide.

Human chorionic gonadotropin stimulates thyroid function in patients with hydatidiform mole or choriocarcinoma, in whom increases in serum free T_4 and T_3 may cause clinical thyrotoxicosis.[265–267] Serum TSH is suppressed, in keeping with the nonpituitary source of the thyroid stimulation. The hyper-

Mother

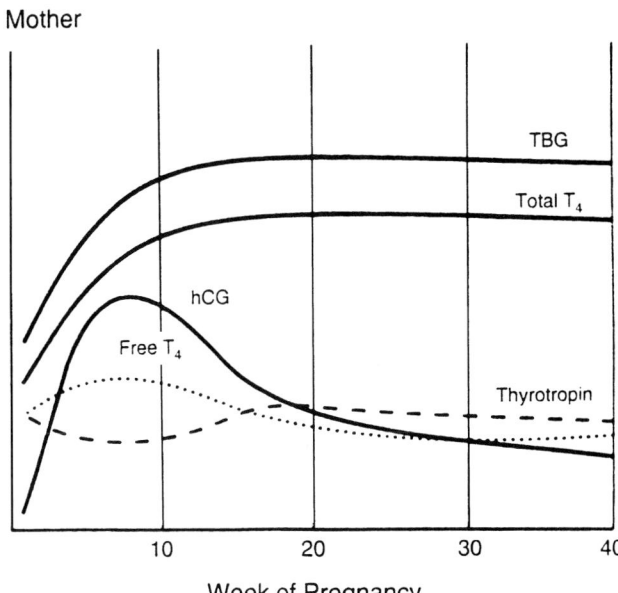

Figure 11–15. Schematic diagram of changes in the thyroid-pituitary axis during pregnancy. Note the early increase in free T_4 probably due to stimulation of the thyroid by hCG, which causes a reciprocal modest suppression of serum TSH during the late first trimester. (From Burrow GN, Fisher DA, Larsen PR. Mechanisms of disease: maternal and fetal thyroid function. New England Journal of Medicine 1994; 331:1072–1078. © 1994, Massachusetts Medical Society.)

concentration may persist until circulating free T_4 and T_3 levels return to normal. This pattern can be confusing in occasional patients in whom the elevated TSH concentration is associated with the still-reduced concentrations of free T_4 and T_3. Such patients meet all diagnostic criteria for primary hypothyroidism with the exception that the manifestations are not usually convincing. Except when the findings are strongly suggestive, it is appropriate to follow such patients for 1 or 2 wk or more without instituting therapy to ascertain the course of thyroid axis recovery.

A fourth category of patients is thought to be intrinsically euthyroid with systemic illness; their serum T_3 concentrations are subnormal, and serum T_4 levels are increased but return to normal after recovery.[326–328] This pattern may also occur during normal pregnancy, in patients with hyperemesis gravidarum,[329] and patients with acute psychosis.[330–333] In the latter group, the serum T_3 level may also be increased. The serum TSH concentration and/or its response to TRH infusion is also generally reduced. In the authors' experience, such patients may have underlying subtle evidence of autonomous thyroid function that causes persistent T_4 secretion despite impairment of T_4 metabolic clearance by illness. The latter group may be difficult to separate from those with T_4 thyrotoxicosis or Graves' disease complicated by serious illness. In those without intrinsic hyperthyroidism, serum T_3 levels tend to be reduced to less than 1 nmol/L (60 ng/dL), whereas patients with hyperthyroidism have higher levels.[326]

By contrast, the levels of TBG and T_4 in plasma may be elevated in patients with acute hepatitis, human immunodeficiency virus (HIV) infection, chronic active hepatitis, or biliary cirrhosis.

LABORATORY TESTS OF THYROID HORMONE ECONOMY

In considering the patient with known or suspected thyroid disease, the physician should seek to arrive at both etiologic or anatomic and functional diagnoses. The one encompasses an appreciation of the underlying cause or nature and the associated pathology in the gland. The other involves a decision about whether there is an excess, a normal, or an insufficient supply of thyroid hormone.

Laboratory evaluation can be divided into five major categories: (1) direct tests of thyroid function that provide information about the handling of iodine, (2) tests that assess the state of the hypothalamic-pituitary-thyroid axis, (3) tests that assess the concentration and binding of the thyroid hormones in the blood, (4) tests that assess the impact of thyroid hormone on tissues, and (5) miscellaneous tests.

Radioiodine Uptake: A Direct Test of Thyroid Function

The only direct test of thyroid function employs a radioactive isotope of iodine as a tag for the body's stable form of iodine, ^{127}I. The most common test is the measurement of the fractional uptake by the thyroid of a tracer (chemically inconsequential) dose of radioiodine, the thyroid RAIU, but several factors make this test less frequently used than in the past. The first is the improvement in indirect methods for assessing thyroid status. The second is the decrease in normal values for thyroid RAIU consequent to the widespread increase in daily dietary iodine intake,[334] reducing the usefulness of the test in the diagnosis of hypothyroidism.

^{131}I (half-life 8.1 d) and ^{123}I (half-life 0.55 d) both emit gamma radiation, which permits their external detection and quantitation at sites of accumulation, such as the thyroid. These isotopes are physiologically indistinguishable, not only from one another but also from the naturally occurring ^{127}I, which permits their use as valid tracers. The shorter half-life of ^{123}I is preferable because the radiation delivered to the thyroid per amount of administered ^{123}I is only about one hundredth of that delivered by ^{131}I.

Measurements of Thyroid Iodine Accumulation

PHYSIOLOGICAL BASIS. When tracer quantities of inorganic radioiodine are administered either orally or intravenously, the isotope quickly mixes with the endogenous stable iodide in the extracellular fluid and begins to be removed by the two major sites of clearance, the thyroid and the kidneys. As this process continues, the plasma level of I* decreases exponentially. Normally, low values are reached by 24 h, and inorganic I* is virtually undetectable in the plasma by 72 h after its administration. The thyroid content of I* increases rapidly during the early hours, then at a decreasing rate until a plateau is approached. The proportion of administered I* ultimately accumulated by the thyroid is a function of the clearance of iodide by the thyroid and kidneys. The relation is simply expressed as follows:

$$\text{RAIU at plateau} = \frac{C_T}{C_T + C_K}$$

where C_T represents the thyroid iodide clearance rate, and C_K the renal iodide clearance rate. The normal thyroid iodide clearance rate is approximately 0.4 L/h, and the renal iodide clearance rate is 2.0 L/h, so the uptake of I* normally approximates 0.05 to 0.25 of the administered dose.

Measurements of RAIU are generally made at 24 h, both as a matter of convenience and because the value at 24 h is usually near the plateau. The RAIU usually indicates the rate of thyroid hormone synthesis and, by inference, the rate of thyroid hormone release into the blood.

RADIOACTIVE IODINE UPTAKE (RAIU). Little difference will be noted if the uptake is measured at any time during the day following the day on which the isotope was administered, and for the calculation of therapeutic radioiodine doses in treating thyrotoxic Graves' disease an early uptake at 3 to 6 h may produce results comparable to those found at 20 to 28 h.[335] With the use of this modified early RAIU measurement, diagnosis and treatment of thyrotoxic Graves' disease can be done on the same day.

In general, the range of normal values in North America is approximately 5 to 25%. Higher values indicate thyroid hyperfunction, but as with other procedures, patients with mild hyperthyroidism may display values at or just above the upper limit of the normal range (Table 11–8).

States Associated with Increased RAIU

HYPERTHYROIDISM. Hyperthyroidism causes increased RAIU unless body iodide stores are increased. Such increases in uptake are always evident except in patients with severe thyrotoxicosis, in whom release of hormone can be so rapid that the thyroid content of I* has decreased to the normal range by the time the measurement is made. This condition is rare and is usually associated with obvious thyrotoxicosis.

ABERRANT HORMONE SYNTHESIS. RAIU can be increased in the absence of hyperthyroidism in disorders in which iodine accumulation is normal but the secretion of hormone is impaired, such as in patients with abnormal thyroglobulin synthesis.[335a] The magnitude of the increase in uptake and the time at which the plateau is achieved vary with the

TABLE 11–8. Factors That Influence 24-h Thyroid Iodide Uptake

Factors That Increase Uptake

Increased hormone synthesis
  Hyperthyroidism
  Response to glandular hormone depletion
    Recovery from thyroid suppression
    Recovery from subacute thyroiditis
    Antithyroid agents
  Excessive hormone losses
    Nephrotic syndrome
    Chronic diarrheal states
    Soybean ingestion
Normal hormone synthesis
  Iodine deficiency
    Dietary insufficiency
    Excessive loss (dehalogenase defect, pregnancy)
  Hormone biosynthetic defects

Factors That Decrease Uptake

Decreased hormone synthesis
  Primary hypofunction
    Primary hypothyroidism
    Antithyroid agents
    Hormone biosynthetic defects
    Hashimoto's disease
    Subacute thyroiditis
  Secondary hypofunction
  Exogenous thyroid hormones
Not reflecting decreased hormone synthesis
  Increased availability of iodine
    Diet or drugs
    Cardiac or renal insufficiency
  Increased hormone release
    Very severe hyperthyroidism (rare)

nature and severity of the disorder. Differentiation of the foregoing states from hyperthyroidism is generally not difficult, because in the former, clinical findings and laboratory evidence of hyperthyroidism are lacking, and indeed hypothyroidism may be present.

IODINE DEFICIENCY. RAIU is increased in acute or chronic iodine deficiency, as demonstrated by measurement of urinary iodine excretion, with values lower than 100 μg/d indicating deficiency. Chronic iodine deficiency is usually the result of an inadequate content of iodine in the food and water (endemic iodine deficiency). Patients with cardiac, renal, or hepatic disease may develop iodine deficiency if given diets severely restricted in salt, especially if diuretic agents are administered.

RESPONSE TO THYROID HORMONE DEPLETION. Rebound increases in RAIU are seen after withdrawal of antithyroid therapy, after subsidence of transient or subacute thyroiditis, and after recovery from prolonged suppression of thyroid function by exogenous hormone. A striking increase in uptake occurs in patients with iodide-induced myxedema after cessation of iodide administration. The duration of the rebound depends on the time required to replenish thyroid hormone stores.

EXCESSIVE HORMONE LOSSES. In *nephrotic syndrome* excessive losses of hormone in the urine occurring in association with urinary loss of binding protein cause a compensatory increase in hormone synthesis and RAIU. A similar sequence may occur when losses of hormone via the gastrointestinal tract are abnormal, as in chronic diarrheal states or during ingestion of agents, such as soybean protein and cholestyramine, that bind T_4 in the gut.

States Associated with Decreased RAIU

A general increase in iodine intake has made values of the RAIU in hypothyroidism indistinguishable from those at the lower end of the normal range. Therefore the major

indication for measuring the RAIU is to establish the causes of thyrotoxicosis associated with decreased values of the RAIU.

HYPOTHYROIDISM. The problems involved in utilizing the RAIU as an aid to the diagnosis of hypothyroidism have been discussed.

EXOGENOUS THYROID HORMONE: THYROTOXICOSIS FACTITIA. Except in disorders in which homeostatic control is disrupted or overridden (e.g., Graves' disease or autonomously functioning thyroid nodules), administration of exogenous thyroid hormone suppresses TSH secretion and reduces the RAIU, usually to values below 5%. Failure of the RAIU to suppress when doses of exogenous hormone adequate to suppress TSH to subnormal levels are given to patients with nontoxic goiter suggests the presence of autonomous function. This can be confirmed by thyroid scintiscan while exogenous hormone therapy is continued (T_4 suppression scan).

Low values of the RAIU in a patient who is clinically thyrotoxic may indicate the presence of thyrotoxicosis factitia, the syndrome produced by the ingestion of excess thyroid hormone. The subnormal serum TSH concentration and unmeasurably low level of Tg in serum differentiate thyrotoxicosis factitia from other causes of thyrotoxicosis with decreased RAIU.[336]

DISORDERS OF HORMONE STORAGE. The RAIU is usually low in the early phase of subacute thyroiditis and in chronic thyroiditis with transient hyperthyroidism. Here inflammatory follicular disruption leads to loss of the normal storage function of the gland and leakage of hormone into the blood. In the early stage of subacute thyroiditis, leakage of hormone is usually sufficient to suppress TSH secretion and the RAIU. Transient hypothyroidism often occurs late in both diseases, when stores of preformed hormone are depleted; the RAIU may return to normal or increased values at that time.

EXPOSURE TO EXCESSIVE IODINE. Exposure to excessive iodine is the most common cause of a subnormal RAIU. Such decreases are spurious in the clinical sense because they do not indicate decreased absolute iodine uptake or decreased hormone production but can be produced by the introduction of excessive iodine in any form—inorganic, organic, or elemental (see Table 11–1). Special offenders are organic iodinated dyes used as x-ray contrast media and amiodarone. The duration of suppression of the uptake varies among individuals and with the compound administered. In general, dyes used for pyelography are cleared relatively rapidly, whereas some used for cholecystography may influence the uptake for months. A single large dose of inorganic iodide can decrease uptake for several days, and chronic ingestion of iodide may depress the uptake for many weeks. Lugol's solution or saturated solution of potassium iodide (SSKI) in the dosage usually given (two to five drops three times/d) delivers up to about 500 mg of iodine daily, as opposed to the customary intake of 500 μg/d in the United States. Excessive quantities of iodine may be present in vitamin and mineral preparations, vaginal or rectal suppositories, and iodinated antiseptics such as povidone. Because of its storage in fat, the iodinated antiarrhythmic agent amiodarone may serve as a source of excess iodine for many months. Some preparations of barium sulfate used in x-ray diagnosis also contain iodine, and large quantities of iodine are ingested in the form of kelp by dietary faddists. Inhibition of uptake by excess stable iodine is of shorter duration in hyperthyroid than in normal individuals.

The measurement of urinary iodine excretion is an invaluable means of establishing or excluding the existence of excessive body iodide stores; a random urine sample can be obtained, and the 24-h iodine excretion extrapolated from the iodine/creatinine ratio. Values in excess of several mg/d can explain a low RAIU value, whereas values less than 1 mg/

d suggest that a low RAIU value is due to one of the other disorders discussed in this section.

Tests That Assess the State of the Hypothalamic-Pituitary-Thyroid Axis

Tests that assess the state of the hypothalamic-pituitary TSH-secretory mechanism play a critical role in the diagnosis of thyroid disease. With few exceptions, all varieties of thyrotoxicosis or hypothyroidism are associated with changes in thyroregulatory function that represent either the primary cause of or the response to thyroid hormone excess or insufficiency.

SERUM TSH CONCENTRATION. Measurements of the serum TSH concentration are valuable in the diagnosis and management of hypothyroidism and thyrotoxicosis. Immunometric assay technology now makes it possible to define the upper and the lower limits of serum TSH and hence to ascertain both when thyroid function is inadequate and when the hormone supply is excessive. There is a close relationship between basal and TRH-stimulated TSH values.[318, 319, 337]

The immunometric TSH assay uses the TSH molecule as a link between one TSH-antibody bound to an inert surface and a second antibody directed against a different TSH epitope that is labeled with a detectable marker (^{125}I or an enzyme or chemiluminescent reagent). Thus, the signal generated is proportional to the concentration of TSH in the serum. This technique is more specific, sensitive, and rapid than radioimmunoassay.[338] The normal range of the serum TSH concentration varies in different laboratories, being most commonly 0.5 to 5 mU/L or 0.3 to 3.5 mU/L, depending on the reference preparation and assay used. Patients with primary thyroid failure have serum TSH concentrations greater than 3.5 to 5 mU/L (Fig. 11–17), often markedly so. Individuals with clinical thyrotoxicosis have concentrations less than 0.1 mU/L. The zone between 0.1 and 0.5 mU/L indicates intermediate degrees of suppression of the normal hypothalamic-pituitary axis. Patients with such values usually have variable degrees of autonomous function or are receiving slightly excessive quantities of exogenous hormone.[337] Not all available commercial "sensitive" assays perform equally well,[318, 339, 340] but a more useful functional categorization is in terms of the minimal detectable TSH that can be quantified with a less than 20% coefficient of variation.[318, 338, 339, 341] Each generation offers a 10-fold improvement over that of the earlier one. Most currently available clinical assays fall into the second or third-generation classification. The first generation (TSH radioimmunoassay) had lower limits of detectability of approximately 1 mU/L, whereas the fourth-generation assay has minimal detectable limits of 0.004 mU/L (see Chapter 3). A suitable "sensitive" TSH assay should be able to quantitate concentrations of TSH of 0.1 mU/L with a coefficient of variation of less than 20%.

An artifactually elevated result may be obtained with the immunometric technique with serum containing heterologous antibodies against mouse immunoglobulin G (IgG).[189] Such antibodies may substitute for TSH and cause falsely high values. Most manufacturers add mouse IgG to the assay matrix to obviate this problem, but the quantity added may be insufficient for the rare individual with a high concentration of heterophilic antibodies. In general, results for such patients are elevated out of proportion to the clinical state or to the levels of the serum T_4 and are readily recognized as artifactual (see later, Table 11–9).

The free α subunit common to TSH, FSH, LH, and hCG is generally detectable in serum with a normal range of 1 to 5 μg/L,[342, 343] but the TSH β subunit is not. When FSH and LH production are increased, as in postmenopausal women, or when TSH production is increased, as in primary hypothy-

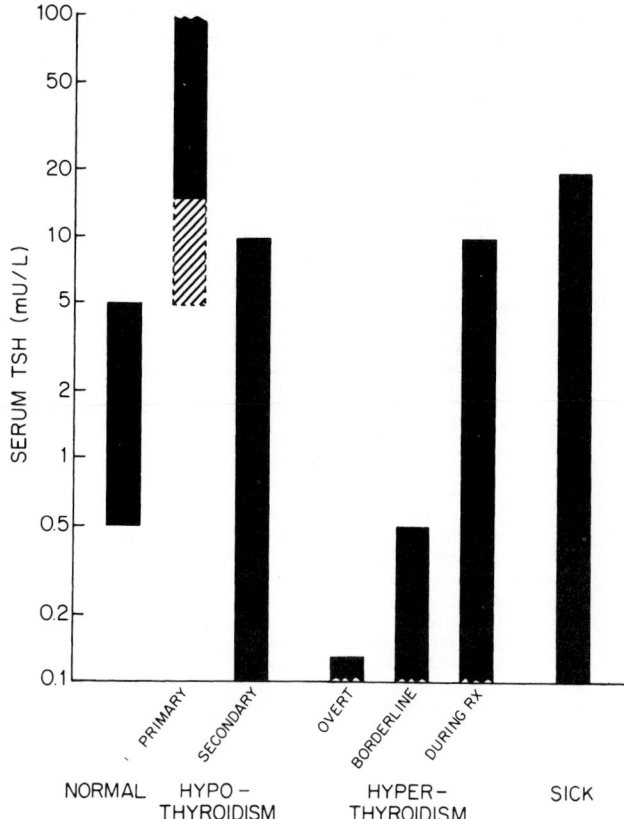

Figure 11–17. Typical serum TSH levels in individuals with various disorders measured with the use of immunometric assay technology. In primary hypothyroidism, serum TSH concentrations can exceed 100 mU/L, but TSH values between 5 and 15 mU/L are not generally associated with symptoms of thyroid hormone deficiency. In secondary hypothyroidism serum TSH levels range from undetectable to slightly elevated. The presence of overt hyperthyroidism causes a reduction in the TSH concentration below the lower limit of normal of 0.1 mU/L, and euthyroid persons with autonomous thyroid function may have values between 0.1 and 0.5 mU/L. During therapy, hyperthyroid patients may continue to have undetectable serum TSH concentrations, depending on the duration of therapy and the degree of suppression of thyroid function by antithyroid drugs. In illness TSH can range from undetectable to modestly elevated levels.

roidism, the free α subunit level is also increased. The α subunit level can also be increased with tumors of the anterior pituitary (see Chapter 9). Its measurement may be useful in the rare patient with hyperthyroidism and a detectable or elevated TSH to differentiate between tumorous and nontumorous causes of TSH excess.[166, 342–349]

TSH IN PATIENTS WITH THYROID DYSFUNCTION. Patients with primary hypothyroidism have serum TSH levels that range from minimally elevated to 1000 mU/L (Table 11–9; see Fig. 11–17). In general, the degree of TSH elevation correlates with the clinical severity. Patients with serum TSH values in the range of 6 to 15 mU/L have few if any symptoms,[350] and the serum free T_4 index (FT_4I) may be low-normal or even slightly reduced, but serum T_3 concentrations are typically normal.[170] Such findings characterize early thyroidal decompensation with a compensatory increase in TSH secretion.

Patients with subnormal TSH values fall into two general categories: values between the lower limit of normal and 0.1 mU/L, and those with values less than 0.1 mU/L. Individuals in the latter category almost invariably have hyperthyroidism and elevations in the FT_4I. Patients with hypothalamic or pituitary hypothyroidism generally have normal values for serum TSH, although rarely the TSH level may be slightly elevated.[347, 348] In some of these patients the circulating TSH is not biologically active by cytochemical bioassay.[217, 219, 351]

TABLE 11–9. Thyroid Status and Free Thyroid Hormone Levels in Clinical States Associated with Abnormal Serum TSH Concentrations

	Expected TSH (mU/L)	Clinical Thyroid Status	Free T₄ Index	Free T₃ Index
Thyrotropin Reduced				
1. Hyperthyroidism of any cause	<0.1	↑	↑	↑
2. "Euthyroid" Graves' disease	0.2–0.5	N, (↑)	N	N, (↑)
3. Autonomous nodule or multinodular goiter	0.2–0.5	N, (↑)	N	↑
4. Exogenous thyroid hormone excess	0.1–0.5	N, ↑	N, ↑	↑
5. Thyroiditis (subacute or painless)	0.1–0.5	N, ↑	N, ↑	↑, (N)
6. Recent thyrotoxicosis due to any cause	<0.1–0.5	↑, N, ↓	N, ↓	N, ↓
7. Illness with or without dopamine infusion	0.1–5.0	N	↑, N, ↓	↓
8. First trimester of pregnancy	0.2–0.5	N, (↑)	N, (↑)	↑
9. Hyperemesis gravidarum	0.2–0.5	N, (↑)	↑, (N)	↑
10. Hydatidiform mole	0.1–0.4	↑	↑	↑
11. Acute psychosis or depression (rare)	0.4–10	N	N, (↑)	N, (↓ or ↑)
12. Elderly (small fraction)	0.2–0.5	N	N	N
13. Glucocorticoids (acute, high dose)	0.1–0.5	N	N	↓
14. Congenital TSH deficiency				
a. PIT1 deficiency	0	↓	↓	↓
b. CAGYC mutant	0	↓	↓	↓
Thyrotropin Elevated				
1. Primary hypothyroidism	6–500	↓	↓	N, ↓
2. Recovery from severe illness	5–30	N, (?)	N, ↓	N, ↓
3. Iodine deficiency	6–150	N, ↓	↓	N
4. Thyroid hormone resistance	1–20	↑, N, ↓	↑	↑
5. Thyrotrope tumor of pituitary	0.5–50	↑	↑	↑
6. Hypothalamic-pituitary disease	1–20	↓	↓	N, ↓
7. Psychiatric illnesses	0.4–10	N	N	N, ↓
8. Adrenal insufficiency	5–30	N	N	N, ↓
9. Artifact (endogenous anti-mouse γ globulin antibodies)	10–500	N	N	N

Arrows indicate the nature of the abnormality in the T₄ or T₃ index. Parentheses indicate that such a result is unusual but may occur.

Although TSH excess may be involved in the pathogenesis of simple or nontoxic goiter, TSH is not usually elevated in these patients unless the pathogenetic factors that led to goiter produce hypothyroidism (goitrous hypothyroidism). In endemic goiter due to iodine deficiency, serum TSH levels are usually elevated and in part responsible for the elevated T₃. In areas of less severe iodine deficiency, endemic goiter is associated with normal serum TSH concentrations, much as it is in sporadic nontoxic goiter (already discussed).

The proposal has been made that the *immunometric TSH assay* could be used to screen for suspected thyroid disease. This strategy is proving to be successful for outpatients[341, 352] but has some limitations in hospitalized individuals.[318, 338, 353] First, some ill individuals have elevated serum TSH concentrations but do not have primary hypothyroidism.[315, 317, 324] Second, illness or the administration of dopamine or high doses of glucocorticoids can suppress serum TSH in the absence of hyperthyroidism.[318, 338, 341, 353–355] However, this overlap is less significant with a third-generation assay. Because normal serum TSH does not eliminate the possibility of hypothalamic or pituitary hypothyroidism, an FT₄I must also be measured if this is a diagnostic consideration.

TRH STIMULATION TEST. When a reliable immunometric TSH assay is not available, TRH testing may be needed. The extent of increase in the serum TSH concentration after TRH administration correlates with the basal serum TSH concentration.[130, 318] Hence in most circumstances exogenous TRH acts as an amplifier to exaggerate any underlying abnormality in TSH secretion and, hence, in the plasma TSH concentration.

A dose of 400 μg, which produces a maximal response, is administered as a single intravenous bolus (Fig. 11–18). In normal individuals, the serum TSH concentration rises rapidly, reaches a peak in 20 to 30 min, and returns to basal values in 2 or 3 h. In practice, specimens for TSH analysis need be drawn only just before and 30 min after TRH administration. Normal increments usually range between 5 and 30

mU/L and average about 15 mU/L. Responses to TRH are decreased by pharmacologic doses of glucocorticoids and by somatostatin. Diminished responses also occur in patients receiving levodopa, dopamine, and bromocriptine, and responses are augmented by the dopaminergic antagonists metoclopramide and domperidone.

The negative-feedback inhibition of TSH secretion and of TRH responsiveness is so exquisitely sensitive that doses of exogenous hormone insufficient to increase the serum T₄ and T₃ concentrations above the normal range can decrease the response to TRH. Conversely, small decreases in serum T₄ and T₃ levels cause increased basal serum TSH concentrations and an increased response to TRH (see Fig. 11–13). Differentiation between hypothalamic and pituitary causes with TRH testing is not reliable, and other diagnostic technologies such

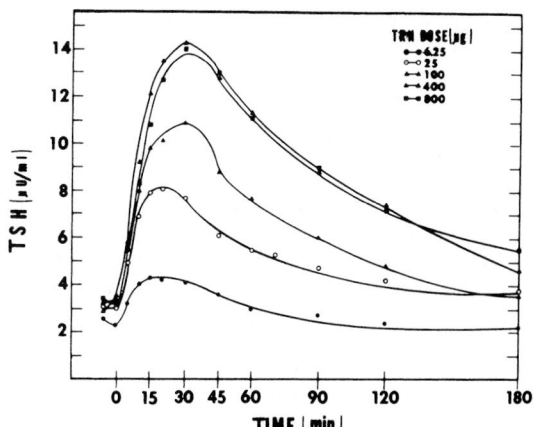

Figure 11–18. Response of serum TSH level to intravenous TRH in normal subjects. (From Snyder PJ, Utiger RD. Response to thyrotropin-releasing hormone [TRH] in normal man. J Clin Endocrinol Metab 1972; 34:380–385. With permission of The Endocrine Society.)

as magnetic resonance imaging (MRI) are required for a final differentiation (see Chapter 9).[319]

As mentioned earlier, the TRH test may be useful in the evaluation of hyperthyroidism accompanied by a detectable TSH to separate artifactual results due to circulating endogenous TSH antibodies, thyroid hormone resistance in which TSH responsiveness to TRH is normal, and a TSH-secreting pituitary tumor in which TSH production may be high but relatively fixed.[348, 349]

Tests Related to Concentration and Binding of Thyroid Hormones in Blood

Quantitation of circulating hormone levels is essential for determining the functional thyroid state, but these tests must be interpreted in the context of the serum TSH and the clinical picture (see Table 11–9). In many situations serum hormone concentrations are used to confirm the presence and/or determine the severity of thyroid dysfunction suspected from an abnormal TSH result. When thyroid dysfunction is obvious on clinical grounds, the serum TSH and FT_4I are ordered simultaneously to provide an immediate assessment of the severity and cause of the abnormality.

GENERAL CONSIDERATIONS. Sensitive, specific radioimmunoassays are available for measuring the total concentrations of serum thyroid hormones. Since the metabolic state correlates more closely with the free hormone than with the total hormone concentration, the physician must obtain some estimate of the free hormone concentration either by measurement of the free hormone concentration itself, an estimate as in a free hormone index, or by measurement of the concentration of TBG.

The degree of abnormality in free hormone level generally correlates with the severity of the disturbance, so the serum TSH measurement is an indication of the impact of this level of thyroid hormone for that patient. Many factors other than the supply or production of T_4 and T_3 and the concentration of TBG in plasma can influence the concentration of the two hormones. Because of the diverse combinations of changes that can be seen and the many factors that produce them, no comprehensive and consistent classification can be devised. Table 11–10 provides a summary of the most commonly encountered patterns of abnormalities in the concentrations of serum free T_4 and T_3, and Table 11–9 describes these test results in the context of the TSH measurement.

MEASUREMENTS OF HORMONE CONCENTRATIONS. Total concentrations of T_4 and T_3 are measured in whole serum by immunoassays. Errors peculiar to tests for the thyroid hormones result from competition for the labeled antigen between the specific antibody and other binding proteins if binding of the hormone-antigen to plasma proteins is not adequately inhibited by the agents used for this purpose or if the serum contains an endogenous antibody to the hormone that is being measured.

SERUM T_4 AND T_3 CONCENTRATIONS. The normal range for total T_4 in healthy, euthyroid adults with normal circulating binding protein levels is between 64 and 142 nmol/L (5 and 11 μg/dL). A serum T_3 is not usually ordered in the initial evaluation, and, in this respect, serum T_3 measurements are tertiary tests of thyroid status that supplement serum TSH and FT_4I assays only in specific situations. Measurements of the serum T_3 concentration are most useful in the patient with clinical features of hyperthyroidism, a suppressed TSH, and a normal FT_4I. Normal serum T_3 concentrations are 1.1 to 2.9 nmol/L (70 to 190 ng/dL).[356] At birth (cord serum) T_3 concentrations are below those in normal adults,[3] but within a few hours the level rises abruptly, peaking at about 24 h at values in the low thyrotoxic range for adults.[3, 4, 8] The T_3 concentration gradually decreases during the next few weeks but remains about 25% higher than values in adults through early adolescence. Serum T_3 values do not decrease with age in healthy individuals.[280]

OTHER CIRCULATING IODOTHYRONINES AND THE PRODUCTS OF T_4 AND T_3 CATABOLISM. Radioimmunoassays for rT_3, T_3SO_4, TRIAC, TETRAC, and the diiodothyronines are of primary interest in the research setting because all these iodothyronines are derived from the circulating T_4 or T_3, both of which can be easily quantitated. An exception to this may be "compound W," thought to be a product of T_4 metabolism in the fetal circulation that appears in maternal sera.[156, 357] If this is indeed the case, measurements of compound W could serve as a much needed index of the state of fetal thyroid function when one monitors the effects of maternal antithyroid drug therapy on fetal thyroid function.

MEASUREMENTS OF HORMONE BINDING. Tests that reflect hormone binding in serum are the most convenient means of estimating free thyroid hormone levels.

PROPORTION AND CONCENTRATION OF FREE T_4 AND T_3. Measurements of the concentrations of free T_4 and free T_3 in serum are most accurate when performed by dialysis or ultracentrifugation techniques.[358–360] In one method, serum is enriched with tracer amounts of the labeled hormone, and the fraction of hormone that dialyzes through a semipermeable membrane is then measured. The absolute concentration of free hormone can then be calculated as the product of the total hormone concentration and the fraction that is dialyzable, or the concentration of T_3 or T_4 can be measured directly in the dialysate.[316, 358–360] The normal value for the proportion of free T_4 is about 2×10^{-4} (0.02%). Because of the lower affinity of T_3 for TBG, the proportion of T_3 that is free is about 15 times that of T_4, i.e., 3×10^{-3} (0.3%) (see Table 11–5).

The free T_4 concentration can be measured indirectly. In one approach, serum is allowed to interact briefly with anti-T_4 antibodies coated on an inert matrix, often the inner surface of a plastic tube. The free T_4 in the serum is bound by the immobilized antibody, and a solution containing labeled T_4 is added. The quantity of labeled T_4 bound to the antibody during the second incubation is inversely related to the number of occupied T_4-binding sites on the tube surface and hence to the free T_4 level of the test specimen.

In the other approach to the direct measurement of free T_4, serum and a labeled analogue of T_4 are incubated in tubes coated with anti-T_4 antibody. Free, unlabeled T_4 in the serum is bound by the antibody, decreasing the availability of antibody-binding sites; so the quantity of labeled hormone bound is inversely related to the amount of free T_4 in the test specimen. Spurious results may occur, possibly because the tracer analogue can bind to serum albumin and perhaps other proteins.[361] As a consequence, values may be low in nonthyroidal illness or hypoalbuminemic states including pregnancy, and values may be high in patients with FDH or endogenous anti-T_4 antibodies.[361]

Both two-step and single-step methods provide falsely low free T_4 estimates owing to nonspecific absorption of free T_4 to antibodies or reagents in the matrix or the tube itself.[358, 360] Thus since the "free T_4" measurements do not provide much additional information, an FT_4I estimate is considered satisfactory by many thyroidologists. Nevertheless if the "free T_4" result deviates from the expectation based on clinical examination and/or the TSH level, it is not possible to ascertain whether this is due to an altered total T_4 concentration or an unusual value for the free fraction.

IN VITRO UPTAKE TESTS: THE THYROID HORMONE BINDING RATIO (THBR). The traditional means of circumventing the technical difficulties inherent in direct estimates of the free concentration has been the in vitro T_3 or T_4 uptake test. Such tests are performed by enriching the patient's serum with a tracer quantity of labeled T_4 or T_3, incubating the serum with a solid-phase matrix coated with T_3 or T_4 antibody, and quantitating the proportion of labeled T_4 or T_3 bound by the solid phase. This value, like the free T_4 measured directly by dialysis, varies inversely with the concentration of unoccupied high-affinity (usually TBG) binding sites in the serum and is proportional to the free fraction of T_3 and T_4 in the original serum. Because of its lower fractional binding to serum proteins, which leads to higher uptake values and thereby reduces both counting time and error, T_3 was more commonly used than was T_4 in the performance of the earlier generations of in vitro uptake tests. Because of this, such determinations are called "T_3 uptake" or "T_3 resin uptake" tests, which can be confused with the T_3 radioimmunoassay result. However, this nomenclature remains entrenched in clinical parlance.[340] Even when tracer T_3 is used in such tests, distribution among the proteins is determined by the ratio of T_4, not T_3, to TBG in the test sample, because T_4 is present in 50- to 60-fold higher levels than T_3 and has a higher affinity for these proteins. Tracer T_4 is now used in many of these tests.

The results of such tests are compared with those simultaneously obtained for standard control sera with normal thyroid hormone–binding proteins and serum T_4 levels.[340] This comparison is generally done by dividing the result for the unknown sample by that obtained for the control serum in the same assay. The quotient is termed the thyroid hormone binding ratio (THBR) and typically has a value of 0.85 to 1.10.[340] A value of 1.0 indicates that the two values are identical. Because the THBR is proportional to the free fraction of the endogenous thyroid hormone in the serum, it can be multiplied by the total hormone concentration to obtain an estimate of the free thyroid hormone concentration, termed the *free T_4* or *free T_3 index* (FT$_4$I or FT$_3$I). A schematic demonstration of the relationships between total and free T_4, occupied and unoccupied TBG binding sites, and the THBR is shown in Figure 11–19 for normal individuals and those with alterations in TBG, and in Figure 11–20 for subjects with alterations in thyroid function.

Figure 11–19 illustrates the utility of the FT$_4$I calculation. Estrogen, pregnancy, and severe illness are more common causes of changes in T_4 levels than are hyperthyroidism and hypothyroidism (see Table 11–7). Under normal circumstances, only about one third of the available binding sites on TBG are occupied by T_4, and the free fraction for T_4 is 2×10^{-4}. During pregnancy the TBG binding capacity, the serum T_4, and the number of unoccupied binding sites double, lead-

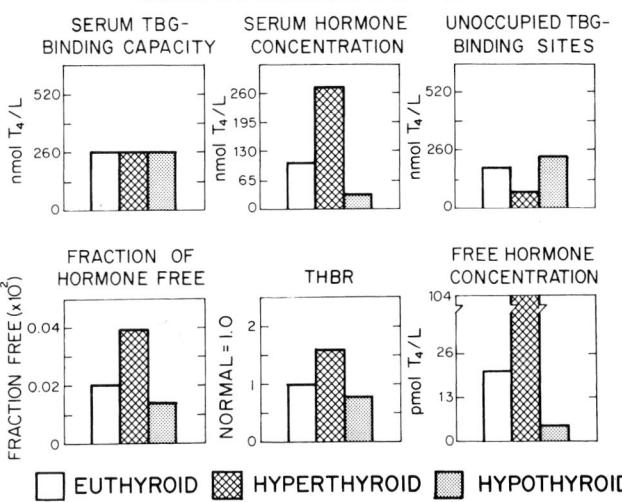

Figure 11–20. Change in total serum T_4 concentration and thyroid hormone binding ratio (THBR) in patients with hyperthyroidism or hypothyroidism and normal serum TBG concentration.

ing to a reduction of about the same degree in the free fraction, which is reflected in the THBR. If the reduced THBR or free fraction is multiplied by the increased serum hormone concentration, an accurate reflection of the free hormone concentration is obtained. When the serum T_4 concentration is reduced owing to decreased TBG in a euthyroid patient, the concentration of unoccupied binding sites is reduced to an even greater extent. This reduction leads to an increase in the free T_4 and T_3 fractions or THBR, so free hormone levels and the FT$_4$I remain in the normal range.

The THBR is linearly related to the free fraction of thyroid hormones except at the extremes of the range. Therefore it is important to examine both the calculated FT$_4$I and the pattern of the deviations of total hormone measurements and THBR from normal to derive the maximum information when levels of binding proteins are altered; the deviation of the total T_4 measurements from normal is in the direction opposite to that of the THBR (see Fig. 11–19). In this circumstance one should be suspicious that an alteration in binding protein concentration is responsible for the abnormality in the total thyroid hormone level, rather than an alteration in thyroid hormone production.

On the other hand, when the T_4 level is elevated, the concentration of unoccupied TBG binding sites is reduced, and both the free fraction and the THBR are increased. Therefore the free hormone concentration and the index are increased more than would be suspected from the change in the total hormone level.

The changes in hypothyroidism are in the opposite direction, but of lower magnitude. The concentration of unoccupied TBG binding sites does not increase greatly when the serum T_4 decreases from a normal mean of 100 nmol/L to 30 nmol/L, and the decreases in the free fraction of T_4 and the THBR are not large. Thus the reduced FT$_4$I is due predominantly to the decrease in T_4, rather than to a decrease in the free fraction. The two central panels in Figure 11–20 show the parallel alterations in total hormone and THBR when thyroid hormone production is altered.

Simultaneous abnormalities in both TBG and thyroid hormone production may also occur. One should suspect hyperthyroidism during pregnancy when the T_4 concentration is high and the THBR is not *subnormal*. Likewise, a serum T_4 level in the normal range for a nonpregnant individual accom-

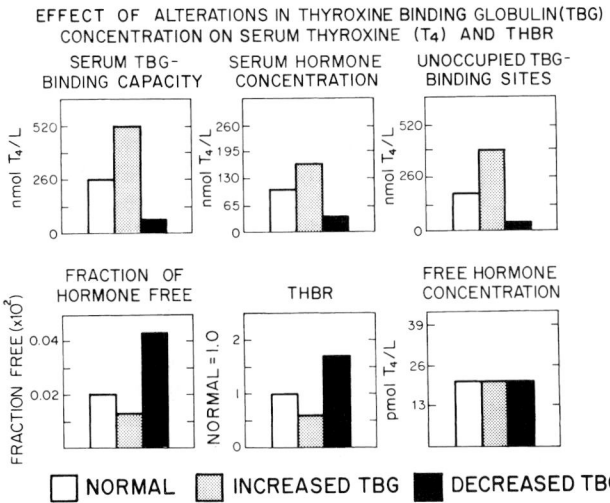

Figure 11–19. Change in total serum T_4 concentrations and the thyroid hormone binding ratio (THBR) in euthyroid patients with alterations in the circulating concentrations of TBG.

decreased and the free T_4, free T_3, and TSH values return to normal.[84] Marked lowering of the serum T_4 concentration and moderate decreases in the serum T_3 level may also occur in patients receiving the nonsteroidal anti-inflammatory agent fenclofenac. The patients are clinically euthyroid, and serum TSH levels are normal.

Both acute and chronic alterations in nutritional state and systemic illness influence the pathways of peripheral iodothyronine metabolism and the concentrations of the metabolites of T_4, T_3, and rT_3 (see the previous section on factors that influence hormone economy).

Tests That Assess the Metabolic Impact of Thyroid Hormones

Abnormalities in the supply of hormone to the peripheral tissues are associated with alterations in a number of metabolic processes, some of which provide a means of assessing whether hormone action is normal. Such tests, often referred to as *metabolic indices*, are the sole means of evaluating the metabolic impact of thyroid hormones in the peripheral tissues but now have no diagnostic usefulness.

BASAL METABOLIC RATE. Thyroid hormones increase energy expenditure and heat production, as manifested by weight loss, increased caloric requirement, and heat intolerance. Because it is impractical to measure heat production directly, the BMR test measures oxygen consumption under specified conditions of fasting, rest, and tranquil surroundings. Under these conditions, the energy equivalent of 1 L of oxygen is equivalent to 4.83 kcal.

Under basal conditions, approximately 25% of oxygen consumption is due to energy expenditure in visceral organs, including the liver, kidneys, and heart; 10% in the brain; 10% in respiratory activity; and the remainder in skeletal muscles. Because energy expenditure is related to functioning tissue mass, oxygen consumption is related to some index thereof, most often body surface area. Calculated in this way, basal oxygen consumption is higher in men than in women and declines rapidly from infancy to the third decade, and more slowly thereafter. Values in patients, calculated as a percentage of established normal means for sex and age, normally range from -15 to $+5\%$. In severely hypothyroid patients, values may be as low as -40%, and in thyrotoxic patients deviations in excess of the norm can be greater. Abnormal, usually elevated values are seen in burn patients and in systemic disorders, such as febrile illnesses, pheochromocytoma, myeloproliferative disorders, anxiety, and disorders associated with involuntary muscular activity.

ACHILLES REFLEX TIME. The duration of the deep tendon reflexes is prolonged in hypothyroidism and shortened in thyrotoxicosis. These differences are due to differences in the speed of both muscular contraction and relaxation, particularly the latter. In about 90% of patients with hypothyroidism, the delay is clinically apparent. A delay in reflex relaxation also occurs in diabetes mellitus, pernicious anemia, anorexia nervosa, edematous states, peripheral vascular disease, and hypothermia from any cause. Morphine, propranolol, quinidine, and procainamide also prolong the relaxation time.

ENZYMES AND METABOLITES IN BLOOD. The concentrations in serum of several muscle enzymes are usually elevated in hypothyroidism. The principal enzymes are the MM variant of creatine phosphokinase, lactate dehydrogenase, and serum aspartate aminotransferase.[387, 388] Levels of these enzymes may be low in patients with thyrotoxicosis and elevated in hypothyroidism. Such alterations are of no value in the diagnosis of thyroid dysfunction.

The serum cholesterol concentration is frequently elevated in patients with hypothyroidism and is low in patients with thyrotoxicosis. In hypothyroidism there is both increased production and decreased degradation of low-density lipoprotein (LDL).[389–393] Cholesterol measurements are of no diagnostic value but may have some value in following the response to therapy in hypothyroidism.

DETERMINING THE EFFECTS OF THYROID HORMONE ON THE HEART. The interval between the initiation of the QRS complex and the arrival of the pulse wave at the brachial artery at diastolic pressure (QKd) is normally in the range of 200 ms and is shortened in thyrotoxicosis and lengthened in hypothyroidism.[394, 395] The degree of abnormality correlates with the extent of thyroid dysfunction. However, values are also decreased in high-output states, in conditions with increased adrenergic tone, and with age-related decreases in arterial elasticity. Prolongation of the interval occurs in aortic stenosis, with β-adrenergic blockade, and in the presence of ventricular conduction defects. If extrathyroidal factors such as these can be excluded, the QKd interval can be utilized to assess the impact of thyroid hormone on the heart.

A related index of myocardial contractility, the pre-ejection period (PEP), is shortened in patients with thyrotoxicosis, owing mainly to a decrease in the period of isovolumetric systole; the PEP may lengthen in hypothyroidism. The PEP is shortened in patients with aortic stenosis and insufficiency or by the administration of epinephrine. Measurements of systolic time intervals, as determined from these indices, have been used in evaluating the time course and magnitude of responses to thyroid hormone replacement in hypothyroidism.[396]

Miscellaneous Tests of Thyroid Function

ASSESSMENT OF ORGANIC BINDING OF IODIDE. In normal or hyperfunctioning thyroids, oxidation of iodide and organic binding are rapid, so little free iodide is present in the thyroid at any time. Consequently little loss of iodide from the normal thyroid can be demonstrated after the administration of agents, such as perchlorate, that inhibit iodide transport and thereby discharge accumulated iodide. When organic binding is incomplete, however, accumulation of iodide occurs, and significant discharge follows inhibition of iodide transport. Two tests of the integrity of the organic binding mechanism are the standard perchlorate discharge test and the iodide-perchlorate discharge test. In the former, radioiodine (^{123}I) is allowed to accumulate in the thyroid, and after measurement of the thyroid I* content with an external Geiger counter, a blocking dose of perchlorate (1 g) is administered orally. A significant decrease (greater than 20%) in epithyroid radioactivity within 1 h constitutes a positive response and indicates a defect in organic binding. Administration of iodide (0.5 mg) as KI with the radioiodine enhances the sensitivity of the test. A positive response to the standard test occurs in patients with inherited defects in organic binding, in some patients with Hashimoto's disease, and in patients with diffuse toxic goiter after treatment with radioiodine. A positive response to the iodide-perchlorate discharge test is seen in all the foregoing disorders, in some patients with untreated hyperthyroidism, in some patients receiving amiodarone,[19] and in previous hyperthyroid patients treated surgically or with radioiodine or antithyroid drugs. A positive response to the iodide-perchlorate discharge test is thought to be a forerunner of thyroid failure and a likely indication that the patient is prone to the development of hypothyroidism if iodides are given for a prolonged period.

THYROGLOBULIN. Thyroglobulin (Tg) is normally present in the serum, the concentration ranging up to 30 pmol/L (20 ng/mL); mean normal values vary with the assay used but are on the order of 15 pmol/L (10 ng/mL). Concentrations are somewhat higher in women than in men and are

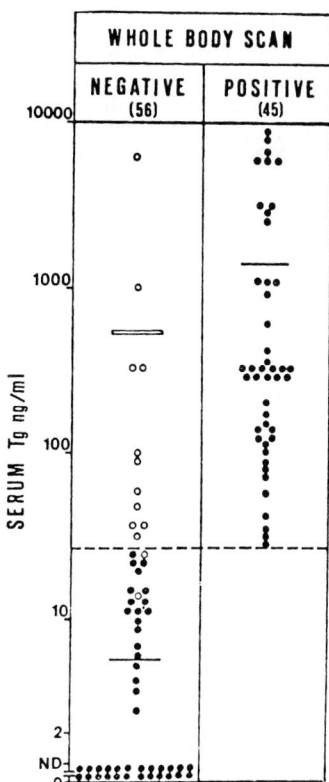

Figure 11–22. Serum thyroglobulin levels in patients with differentiated thyroid carcinoma after surgical and ^{131}I ablation of residual thyroid tissue; results classified according to the findings on whole-body scan. Note the log scale. In the left column, solid circles indicate values in patients with no detectable metastatic tissue; open circles indicate those with detectable but nonfunctioning metastases. The right column depicts the findings in patients with metastases that are detectable with radioiodine. Dashed line, upper limit of normal bar; horizontal bar, mean for each group. (From Baschieri L, Giani C, Taddei P, et al. Serum thyroglobulin as a marker of thyroid carcinoma. In: Andreoli M, Monaco F, Robbins J, eds. Advances in Thyroid Neoplasia 1981. Rome: Field Education Italia, 1981; 187–199, with permission.)

several-fold elevated in pregnant women and in the newborn. Levels are elevated in three types of thyroid disorders: goiter and thyroid hyperfunction, inflammatory or physical injury to the thyroid, and differentiated thyroid tumors. Values are elevated in both endemic and sporadic nontoxic goiter, and the degree of elevation correlates with the thyroid size. Transient elevations occur in patients with subacute thyroiditis and as a result of trauma to the gland during thyroid surgery or after ^{131}I therapy.[42] Subnormal or undetectable concentrations are found in patients with thyrotoxicosis factitia and aid in differentiating this disorder from other causes of thyrotoxicosis with a low RAIU.[336] Antithyroglobulin antibodies interfere with measurements of the serum Tg concentration, and there are few data concerning the concentration of Tg in the serum of patients with Hashimoto's disease.

A major clinical value of measurements of serum Tg level is in the management—but not in the diagnosis—of differentiated thyroid carcinoma. Serum Tg concentrations are increased in patients with both benign and differentiated malignant tumors of the thyroid and do not serve to distinguish between the two. After removal of thyroid malignancies, values decrease into the normal range and remain normal if metastatic disease is not present. Secretion of Tg is often TSH-dependent, so the serum Tg level may rise when suppressive therapy is withdrawn.[397] Thus serum Tg is a sensitive marker of persistent or recurrent thyroid carcinoma, assuming that normal thyroid tissue has been removed by surgery and/or radioiodine. Indeed elevation of the serum Tg concentration can indicate the presence of metastatic disease, even when ^{131}I scans are negative (see later section on thyroid malignancies; Fig. 11–22).[397]

Tests for Thyroid Autoantibodies

Graves' and Hashimoto's diseases are interrelated autoimmune thyroid disorders (AITD). Thus, circulating antibodies against one or another thyroid antigen are often present. Three varieties of thyroid autoantibodies are useful for diagnostic testing (Table 11–11).

METHODS FOR MEASURING AUTOANTIBODIES TO THYROID PEROXIDASE AND THYROGLOBULIN. Table 11–12 summarizes some advantages and disadvantages of available techniques for measuring thyroid autoantibodies. Hemagglutination is not IgG-specific, has low sensitivity, and is operator dependent. The enzyme immunoassays tend to be imprecise. However, radioassay techniques have better precision than other methods because other techniques depend on the indirect measurement of the interaction between autoantibody and autoantigen. In contrast, the radioassay technique is based on the interaction between radiolabeled thyroid antigen and the patient's serum. In general, the more sensitive an assay, the more it tends to be specific and precise. Since many normal individuals exhibit low levels of autoantibodies, the specificity of the more sensitive tests is reduced.

STANDARDIZATION. To compare levels of thyroid antibodies from one office visit to the next and to compare results between patients and among laboratories, it is important that assays for thyroid autoantibodies be standardized; e.g., results should be expressed in relation to a widely available standard preparation, as for immunoassays. Although there are no formal "International Standards" for human thyroid autoantibodies, TgAb and TPOAb standard sera are available from the National Institute for Biological Standards in the United Kingdom and are an essential component of many thyroid autoantibody assays. Such results can then be expressed in units per milliliter.

PATHOGENIC ROLE OF TgAb AND TPOAb. Thyroid autoantibodies are a secondary response to thyroid injury. Both types of antibodies are polyclonal and, although of the IgG class, are not restricted to one particular IgG subclass. Polyclonality mitigates against a primary role in disease, but the antibodies may be determinants of chronicity. While both TPOAb and TgAb levels correlate with lymphocytic infiltration of the thyroid, they do not transfer disease from mother to fetus or between animals. These observations again confirm

TABLE 11–11. Common Thyroid Autoantibodies

Antigen	Molecular Size	Abbreviation	Notes
TSH receptor	100 kd	TSHRAb	Antibody that causes Graves' disease
		TSHR-blocking Ab	Present in some thyroiditis patients
Thyroglobulin	330 kd	TgAb	Often undetectable using older techniques
Thyroid peroxidase	107 kd	TPOAb	Useful diagnostic marker

TABLE 11–12. Advantages and Disadvantages of Different Methods for Measurement of Autoantibodies to TPO and Tg

Technique	Precision	Sensitivity	Specificity	Cost
Immunofluorescence	Low	Low	High	High
Hemagglutination	Low	Low	Variable	High
ELISA	Variable	High	High	Low
Radioassay	High	High	High	Low

ELISA, enzyme-linked immunosorbent assay.

that thyroid autoantibodies to Tg and TPO do not initiate disease. However, both antibodies have complement-fixing cytotoxic activity, and TPOAb autoantibodies correlate with thyroidal damage and lymphocytic infiltration. Patients with AITD have autoantibody "fingerprints," a characteristic spectrum of Tg and TPO autoantibodies belonging to IgG1, IgG2, IgG3, and IgG4 subclasses.[398] Since IgG1 antibodies fix complement while, for example, IgG4 antibodies do not, this pattern of distribution may affect thyroidal pathology.

THYROID AUTOANTIBODIES IN HASHIMOTO'S DISEASE. The disease most associated with TgAb and TPOAb is *autoimmune thyroiditis*, a term that embraces both goitrous (Hashimoto's disease) and atrophic thyroid failure. The titers of these antibodies correlate with the degree of thyroidal lymphocytic infiltration. The conventional assay for TPOAb is more sensitive in the diagnosis of autoimmune thyroiditis than TgAb, but with immunoassays both autoantibodies are found in almost 100% of such patients, TPOAb being of higher affinity and in higher concentrations. In an unclear clinical situation therefore, strongly positive Tg-Ab and TPO-Ab levels are diagnostic of primary autoimmune thyroid disease. Antibody measurements may also be useful prognostically in subclinically hypothyroid patients (those with an elevated TSH and normal T$_4$), since patients with a mildly increased TSH level and positive thyroid autoantibodies develop overt hypothyroidism at a rate of approximately 5% per year.[399]

THYROID AUTOANTIBODIES IN GRAVES' DISEASE. Antibodies to Tg and TPO are also commonly detectable in 50 to 90% of patients with Graves' disease, indicative of the associated thyroiditis that is evident histologically. While the presence of such autoantibodies favors autoimmune hyperthyroidism over other etiologies, the tests are neither sensitive nor specific in this setting and are interpretable only as part of the clinical scenario. Limited data suggest that higher titers of TgAb and TPOAb in hyperthyroid Graves' disease are predictive of future hypothyroidism after treatment with antithyroid drugs.[400] The prevalence of thyroid autoantibodies in different disorders is shown in Table 11–13.

THYROID AUTOANTIBODIES IN NON-AITD. Antibodies to Tg and TPO are more common in patients with sporadic goiter, multinodular goiter, and isolated thyroid nodules and cancer than in the general population. This finding usually represents an associated thyroiditis on histology. Thyroid cancer patients with thyroid autoantibodies may have a better prognosis than those without,[401] but significant levels of TgAb in a patient may limit the utility of serum Tg radioimmunoassay measurements in tracking the status of patients with thyroid cancer. Low levels of thyroid autoantibodies may occur transiently in patients with subacute (de Quervain's) thyroiditis, but they correlate poorly with disease course and are probably a nonspecific response to thyroid injury. There is also a higher prevalence of thyroid autoantibodies in other autoimmune diseases, such as insulin-dependent diabetes mellitus (IDDM).

THE "NORMAL" POPULATION. The prevalence of thyroid autoantibodies is dependent on the technique used for detection, but autoantibodies to Tg and TPO are common in the general population (Table 11–13), and at all ages are up to five times more common in women than in men. The tendency to secrete thyroid autoantibodies is inherited in a mendelian dominant manner,[402] and selected at-risk groups, such as younger women and relatives of patients with AITD, have higher incidences. Low levels of autoantibodies to TPO and Tg are of uncertain significance in the presence of normal thyroid function.

SUMMARY OF CLINICAL UTILITY OF TgAb AND TPOAb ASSAY

Establishment of Disease Etiology. Thyroid failure has a variety of causes, and autoimmune thyroid disease can be inferred by the presence of a family history of Graves' or Hashimoto's disease. However, the presence of significant levels of thyroid autoantibodies is the only simple way of confirming the autoimmune diathesis. The measurement of thyroid autoantibodies also allows the generation of data on the prevalence of AITD within the patient's family.

Prediction of Disease Onset. Patients with an increased TSH level and normal T$_4$ will progress to overt thyroid failure at a rate of about 5% per year if levels of thyroid autoantibodies are elevated.[399] Hence patients with subclinical hypothyroidism (increased TSH levels but apparently normal free T$_4$ values) and thyroid autoantibodies are at risk for developing thyroid failure.

Thyroid Nodule and Unnecessary Surgery. A nodular gland or a particularly hard, prominent nodule may be mistakenly diagnosed as thyroid cancer. The presence of high titers of thyroid autoantibodies and lymphocytes on aspiration biopsy establishes the diagnosis of autoimmune thyroiditis.

Risk Analysis for Postpartum Thyroid Disease (PPTD). In the United States the prevalence of PPTD is about 8 to 10% in the first 4 to 8 mo after delivery. More than 33% of women who are anti-TPO positive early in pregnancy develop some form of PPTD, particularly those patients with high levels of thyroid autoantibodies.[403] Hence the measurement of anti-TPO and TSH levels is helpful in pregnancy screening.

Risk Analysis for Early Pregnancy Loss. Thyroid autoantibodies may be useful markers of at-risk pregnancy[404] but do not imply that thyroid dysfunction causes the increased risk. Rather, the generation of autoantibodies appears to be a signal that all is not well with the developing fetus.

Thyroid Disease Screening in Associated Autoimmune Conditions. AITD occur commonly with other forms of autoimmune disease. For example, patients with IDDM are at particular risk, and the presence of thyroid autoantibodies is helpful in selecting patients for monitoring of thyroid function.

Tests for Antibodies Most Often Related to Graves' Disease

TSH RECEPTOR. The TSH receptor (TSHR) is G protein–linked and employs cAMP and the phosphoinositol pathways for signal transduction.[405] The human TSHR (hTSHR) is the primary autoantigen of Graves' disease. Putative extrathyroidal

TABLE 11–13. Prevalence of Thyroid Autoantibodies

Group	TSHRAb (%)	hTgAb (%)	hTPOAb (%)
General population	0	5–20	8–27
Graves' disease	80–95	50–70	50–80
Autoimmune thyroiditis	10–20	80–90	90–100
Relatives of patients	0	40–50	40–50
Patients with IDDM	0	40	40
Pregnant women	0	14	14

IDDM, insulin-dependent diabetes mellitus.

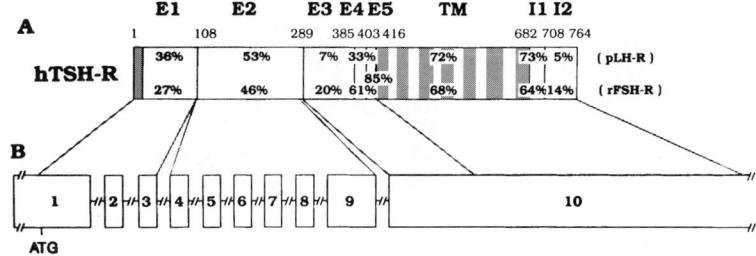

Figure 11–23. TSHR exon structure. Outline structure of the TSHR (A) in comparison with the LH and FSH receptor genes and (B) the exon/intron organization of the TSHR gene. A, The similarity (%) between the human TSHR and the porcine LH and rat FSH receptors, respectively. (From Gross B, Misrahi M, Sar S, et al. Composite structure of the human TSH receptor gene. Biochem Biophys Res Comm 1991; 177:679–687, with permission.)

TSHR and mRNA has been reported in other tissues, but the physiological role of TSH receptors in these sites is not known.[406, 407]

MOLECULAR BIOLOGY OF THE hTSHR. Cloning of TSHR cDNAs of animals and humans[408–411] made it possible to define the structure of the hTSHR gene and its chromosomal location (14q31).[412, 413] The hTSHR gene spans more than 60 kb and is split into 10 exons (Fig. 11–23). Seven hydrophobic transmembrane spanning regions in the hTSHR indicate that it is a member of the G protein–coupled receptor gene superfamily, and those receptors with large extracellular domains have been designated subgroup B. The hTSHR-specific mRNA of human thyroid consists of a major 4.3-kb transcript and additional smaller species, indicating that the mRNA undergoes alternate splicing.[414]

PROTEIN STRUCTURE OF THE hTSHR. The hTSHR consists of a 100-kd, glycosylated, 744-amino-acid sequence and a 20-amino-acid signal peptide. Pro-TSHR is cleaved to two subunits, A (or α) and B (or β), which are linked by disulfide bonds to form the physiological receptor (Fig. 11–24).[405, 415] The 50-kd A subunit is water-soluble and may contain the TSH-binding site, previously referred to as long-acting thyroid stimulator (LATS)–absorbing activity (LAA).[416] The 30-kd B subunit is water-insoluble, contains the membrane-spanning domain[405] with its three extracellular loops and three cytoplasmic loops, and is 70 to 75% homologous with the LH/hCG receptor.

AUTOANTIBODIES TO THE TSH RECEPTOR. In Graves' disease TSH receptor autoantibodies (TSHRAb) bind to the TSH receptor, activate adenylate cyclase, induce thyroid growth, increase vascularity, and cause an increased rate of thyroid hormone production and secretion (Fig. 11–25).[405] The TSHRAb in patients with Graves' disease is referred to as the stimulating or agonist type of TSHRAb, as first described by Adams and Purves.[417, 418] However, other varieties of TSHRAb may also be present, namely a receptor antibody that acts as a TSH antagonist and is referred to as a blocking TSHRAb. Blocking TSHRAb may be coincident with stimulating antibodies, and they may also be found to predominate in certain patients after treatment with radioiodine, antithyroid drugs, or surgery. They can also be found in 15% of patients with autoimmune thyroiditis, particularly those without a goiter (the atrophic variety).[419] TSHRAb are not detectable in the normal population with the use of currently available methods.

MEASURING TSHRAb. Two types of tests are most often employed for the detection of TSHRAb. The first assesses the capacity of patient serum or IgG to inhibit the binding of ^{125}I-labeled TSH to TSH receptors from thyroid membrane preparations (available commercially) or to Chinese hamster ovary (CHO) cells expressing recombinant human TSHR. This protein-binding inhibition assay is of low cost and good precision, and the frequency of positive results in patients with active and untreated disease is on the order of 80 to 90%. The second type of test assesses the capacity of patient serum or IgG to stimulate adenylate cyclase or to enhance thyroid hormone or Tg secretion or iodine uptake in isolated thyroid epithelial cells or CHO-TSHR cells.[420] Tests of this type are more expensive, have relatively poor precision, and are positive in 80% or more of the patients with active untreated Graves' disease. Because of the proliferation of acronyms describing these antibodies, the authors encourage the designation of the specific assay used.[340] Both types of tests are now available commercially.

STANDARDIZATION. As with all autoantibody tests, it is best to use an internationally accepted standard to allow comparison of results from different laboratories. A TSHRAb standard from the Medical Research Council (MRC) in Britain

The hTSHR: primary antigen in Graves' disease

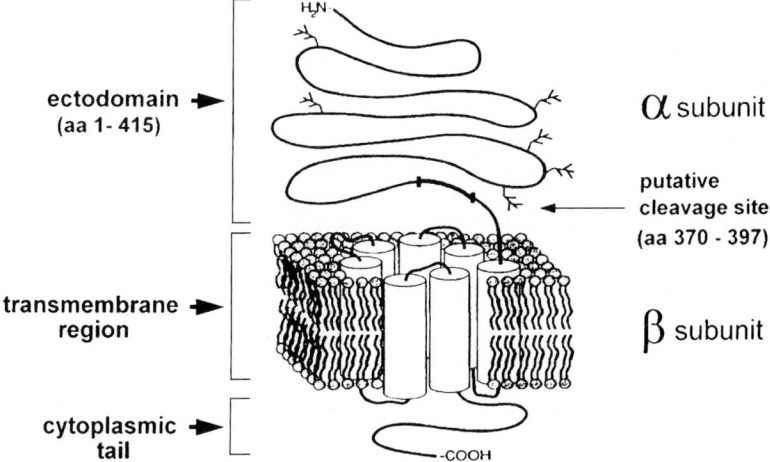

Figure 11–24. A current model of the hTSHR structure. The TSHR has seven transmembrane domains, a large extracellular domain, and a small intracellular domain. The receptor is cleaved, probably after activation, into A (or α) and B (or β) subunits. The A subunit is shed from the cell.

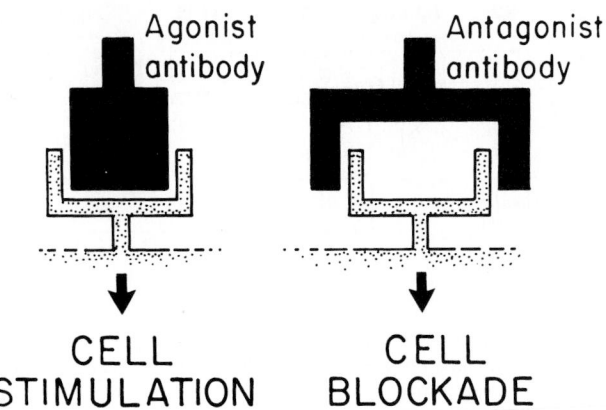

Figure 11–25. Schematic diagram of thyroid cell stimulation and blockade by antibodies to the TSHR. Such autoantibodies may act as agonists or antagonists, depending on how they interact within the extracellular domain.

is sometimes employed. Results may be reported in MRC Units. Alternatively, results have often been reported in terms of equivalent TSH Units. However, the hTSHRAbs from different patients may not give parallel results with the MRC standards or TSH standards when measured in different dilutions. This means that the conversion of hTSHRAb data into MRC Units or TSH can be erroneous.

INDICATIONS FOR MEASURING TSHRAb. The level of TSHRAb may be a useful indicator of the degree of disease activity in an individual patient and confirm the clinical diagnosis. Demonstration of TSHRAb may be of diagnostic value in the euthyroid patient with exophthalmos, especially when it is unilateral. High TSHRAb titers in the pregnant woman with Graves' disease indicate the possibility that neonatal thyrotoxicosis will be present in her offspring, and in this situation a bioassay is preferred to a radioassay. Another use of TSHRAb testing is in the prognosis of patients with Graves' disease who are treated with antithyroid agents. A persisting high titer of TSHRAb is an excellent predictor of relapse on stopping the drug. Unfortunately, in patients with low or negative titers, the test is much less helpful.[421]

IMAGING TECHNIQUES

External Scintiscanning

Localization of functioning or nonfunctioning thyroid tissue in the area of the thyroid gland or elsewhere is made possible by techniques of external scintiscanning. The underlying principle is that isotopes that are differentially accumulated by thyroid tissue can be detected and quantified in situ and the data transformed into a visual display. Two types of apparatus are available.

The rectilinear scanner is a device that moves a highly collimated (focused) scintillation detector back and forth across the area of study in a series of parallel tracks. A printing device that moves in concert with the detector records a mark whenever a predetermined number of counts have been received to provide a visual representation of the localization of radioactivity, areas of greater radioactivity corresponding to areas of greater density in the scan. Other modifications make use of a light source whose intensity is proportional to the counting rate. The light exposes a sheet of x-ray film, and the degree of darkening of the image corresponds to the counting rate at different sites in the thyroid photographic scan.

The second type of apparatus is a stationary scintillation camera equipped with a pinhole collimator that views the

entire field of interest and translates the counting rates from specific areas of the field into photographic or visual images. Electronic and recording instruments permit the quantification of radioactivity in specific areas and the subtraction of extrathyroid radioactivity. The information can be recorded on tape for later study. These cameras provide better resolution than rectilinear scanners, but careful attention must be given to patient positioning to prevent problems caused by magnification and distortion.[422]

Several radioisotopes are employed in thyroid imaging. ^{99m}Tc-pertechnetate (TcO$_4^-$) is a monovalent anion that, like iodide, is actively concentrated by the thyroid gland, undergoes negligible organic binding, and diffuses out of the thyroid as its concentration in the plasma decreases. The short physical half-life of ^{99m}Tc (6 h) and its transient stay within the thyroid make the radiation delivered to the thyroid by a standard dose very low. Consequently, the administration of large doses (> 37 MBq [1 mCi]) permits high counting rates and adequate imaging of the thyroid when the fractional uptake is too low to permit scintiscanning with radioiodine. Pertechnetate is usually given as a single intravenous bolus, and imaging is performed about 30 min later. Serial imaging makes possible studies of the dynamics of thyroid blood flow and isotope accumulation.

Three radioactive isotopes of iodine have been used in thyroid imaging. ^{131}I was commonly used in the past, and it is still useful when functioning metastases of thyroid carcinoma are being sought. The physical half-life of ^{125}I (60 d) is longer than that of ^{131}I (8 d), but its lower radiation energy results in the delivery of a radiation dose to the thyroid per unit of radioactivity administered that is only about two thirds that delivered by ^{131}I. The third isotope, ^{123}I, is in many respects ideal. Its short half-life and the absence of beta radiation result in a radiation dose to the thyroid that is about 1% of that delivered by a comparable dose of ^{131}I. All three isotopes of iodine provide satisfactory images of the thyroid in its normal location. Because of the low radiation dose to the thyroid, ^{123}I is the isotope of choice for thyroid scintigraphy in pediatric practice.[423, 424]

Imaging of thyroid tissue can be used to provide some evidence of overall thyroid size, but its most important use is to define areas of increased or decreased function ("hot" or "cold" areas, respectively) relative to function of the remainder of the gland, provided that they are 1 cm in diameter or larger. Small, cold nodules may be obscured by overlying functioning tissue, but superior discrimination can be achieved if the gland is scanned in the lateral or oblique and anteroposterior projections. Although most nonfunctioning nodules are not malignant, lack of function increases the likelihood of malignant disease, particularly if only one nodule is present. Conversely, functioning nodules, particularly if they are either more active than surrounding tissue or the sole functioning tissue ("hot nodules"), are virtually never malignant. Occasionally, scintiscans may be normal in the absence of palpable abnormalities. Scintiscanning of the thyroid is most useful when the palpable findings are correlated with the areas of increased or decreased function.

After administration of exogenous TSH, scintiscans may demonstrate the presence of hemiagenesis of the thyroid and document the functional capability of suppressed thyroid tissue. Conversely, scans performed after a period of exogenous thyroid hormone administration (suppression scans) can reveal areas of autonomous function that may not be detectable in baseline studies. Scintiscanning can also be used to demonstrate that substernal or intrathoracic masses represent thyroid tissue, to detect ectopic thyroid tissue in the tongue or ovary, and to detect functioning metastases of thyroid carcinoma.

Choice of the scanning agent depends on many factors. Pertechnetate delivers a small dose of radiation to the thyroid and is readily available, and because imaging is performed soon after administration of the scanning agent, the entire procedure requires only a single visit to the laboratory. However, pertechnetate provides information only about iodide transport—and not about organic binding or retention. Therefore pertechnetate may be used in patients receiving propylthiouracil or methimazole, but some tumors of the thyroid appear to be functioning when examined with pertechnetate—but not with radioiodine. Because pertechnetate imaging is done early, radiation from intravascular sources or from salivary tissue may obscure or confuse the findings. For the same reason, pertechnetate is inappropriate for scans of substernal or intrathoracic goiter.

All three isotopes of iodine provide satisfactory thyroid scans, but many researchers believe that superior scans are obtained with ^{123}I. The short half-life, which limits the radiation dose delivered to the thyroid, precludes its use in the search for functioning thyroid metastases. The low-energy emissions of ^{125}I preclude scanning from deep sources, such as substernal goiter and distant metastases, so either ^{123}I or ^{131}I should be used in the former, and ^{131}I should be used in the latter.

Fluorescent Scans

Fluorescent scanning provides information concerning the content of stable iodine within the gland.[425] In this technique, discrete zones of the thyroid are subjected to gamma radiation from radioactive americium (^{241}Am). When ^{241}Am encounters ^{127}I, a fluorescent x-ray is emitted, which is appreciated by a suitable detector. Thus whereas gamma scintillation imaging localizes and quantifies the continuing accumulation of iodine, the fluorescent scan localizes and quantifies iodine stored within the gland. The technique has limited clinical utility. Nonfunctioning nodules generally have a low iodine content and are therefore "cold" on fluorescent scan. The technique may be useful when isotopic scanning is either unsuccessful or contraindicated, as in iodine overload or during pregnancy.[426]

Ultrasonography

Sonography is noninvasive, less expensive than computed tomography (CT) or magnetic resonance imaging (MRI), and produces no known tissue damage. The technique may be performed while the patient is taking thyroid hormone therapy. No contrast material is administered. No special patient preparation is necessary, and the technique requires only portable equipment and can be performed in the office.

Sonography uses high-frequency sound waves that are emitted by a transmitter and reflected as they pass through the body, whereupon the returning echoes are received by the transmitter, which also acts as a receiver. The amplitude of the reflections of the sound waves is influenced by differences in the acoustic impedance of the tissues encountered by the sound; for example, fluid-filled structures reflect few echoes and therefore have no or few internal echoes and well-defined margins. Solid structures reflect varying amounts of sound and therefore have varying degrees of internal echoes and less well-defined margins. Calcified structures reflect virtually all incoming sound and yield pronounced echoes with an acoustic "shadow" posteriorly. High-frequency sound waves, such as are used in current thyroid sonography, are attenuated rapidly in the body tissues. Therefore they cannot be used to image structures deeper than about 5 cm from the skin. Fortunately, the thyroid gland is usually well within this limit and can be completely imaged.[427]

Since the middle 1980s, high-frequency (7.5 to 10.0 MHz), "small-parts" instruments have become widely available

and provide good spatial resolution and image quality.[428] The theoretical axial resolution of these systems is about 1 mm; no other thyroid imaging method can achieve this degree of resolution.[427] Intrathyroidal nodules as small as 3 mm in diameter and cystic nodules as small as 2 mm can be readily detected with transducers with frequencies between 7.5 and 10.0 MHz.[429]

Thyroid sonography is typically performed with the patient in a supine position. The patient's neck is hyperextended by a pad centered under the scapulae to provide optimal exposure. The examiner usually sits at the head of the examining table and can steady the transducer by resting an elbow or a forearm on the table next to the patient's head. The thyroid gland must be examined thoroughly in transverse and longitudinal planes. Imaging of the lower poles can be enhanced by swallowing, which momentarily raises the thyroid gland in the neck. The examination should cover the entire gland, including the isthmus. Imaging should also include the region of the carotid artery and jugular vein to identify enlarged cervical lymph nodes.[427]

The normal thyroid parenchyma has a characteristic homogeneous medium-level echogenicity, with little identifiable internal architecture (Fig. 11–26). The surrounding muscles have the appearance of hypoechoic structures. The air-filled trachea in the midline gives a characteristic curvilinear reflecting surface, with an associated reverberation artifact. The esophagus is usually hidden from sonographic visualization by the tracheal air shadow. A portion of the esophagus, however, may swing laterally, usually toward the left, where it may lie adjacent to the posteromedial surface of the thyroid.

Neck ultrasound is an ideal technique for establishing whether a palpable cervical mass is within or adjacent to the thyroid and for differentiating thyroid nodules from other neck masses such as cystic hygromas, thyroglossal duct cysts, and enlarged lymph nodes. In addition, sonography may confirm the presence of a thyroid nodule when the findings on physical examination are equivocal. A diagrammatic representation of the neck showing the location or locations of any abnormal findings is a useful supplement to the routine film images recorded during an ultrasound examination.[427] Such a cervical "map" (Fig. 11–27) can help communicate the anatomic relationships of the pathology more clearly to the referring clinician and serve as a reference for the radiologist and sonographer on follow-up examinations.

In patients with known thyroid cancer, sonography can be useful in evaluating the extent of disease, both preoperatively and postoperatively. In most instances sonography is not performed routinely prior to thyroidectomy, but it can be useful in patients with large cervical masses to evaluate nearby structures, such as the carotid artery and internal jugular vein, for direct invasion or encasement by the tumor. Alternatively, in patients who present with cervical lymphadenopathy caused by papillary thyroid cancer but in whom the gland is palpably normal, sonography may be used preoperatively to detect an occult, primary intrathyroid focus.

After surgery for thyroid cancer, sonography is the preferred method for detecting residual, recurrent, or metastatic disease in the neck.[430] In patients who have had subtotal thyroidectomy, the sonographic appearances of the remaining thyroid tissue may serve as an important factor in deciding whether completion thyroidectomy is recommended. If a mass is identified, its nature can be determined by sonographic-guided fine-needle aspiration (FNA) biopsy.[431] If no masses are seen, the clinician may choose to follow the patient with periodic sonographic studies. After total or near-total thyroidectomy, sonography is more sensitive than neck palpation in detecting recurrent disease within the thyroid bed and metastatic disease in cervical lymph nodes.[431, 432]

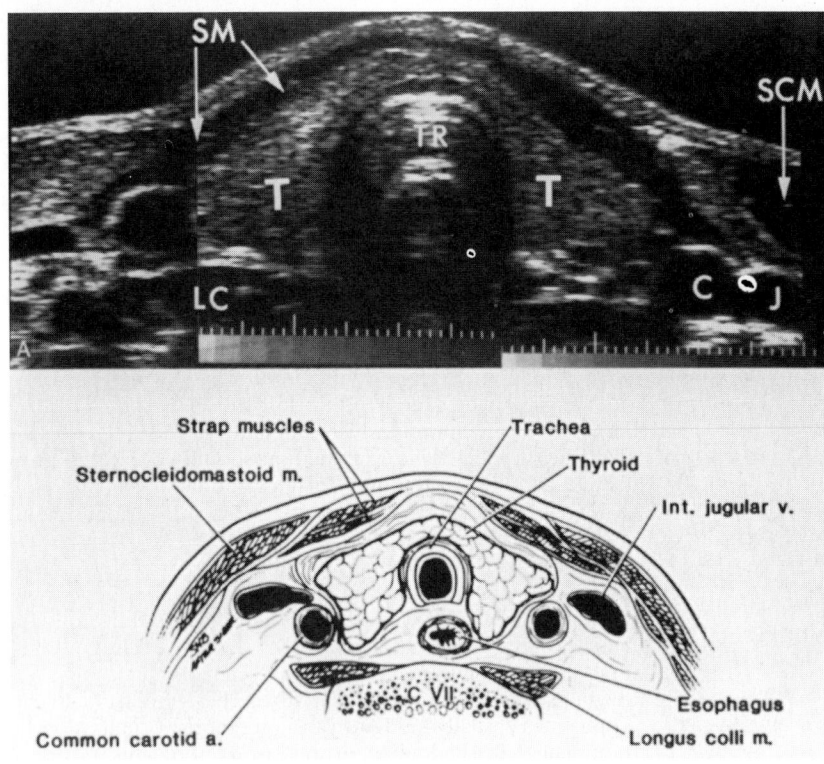

Figure 11–26. Transverse composite sonogram of the normal thyroid gland. T, thyroid; TR, trachea; C, common carotid artery; LC, longus colli muscle; SM, strap muscles; SCM, sternocleidomastoid muscle; CVII, seventh cervical vertebra. (From Rifkin MD, Charboneau JW, Laing FC. Special course: Ultrasound 1991. In: Reading CC, ed. Syllabus: Thyroid, Parathyroid, and Cervical Lymph Nodes. Oak Brook, IL: Radiological Society of North America, 1991: 363–377, with permission.)

Computed Tomography

The appearance of the anatomic structures in the CT image depends on the tissue. The thyroid gland, because of its high concentration of iodine, has a higher attenuation than the surrounding soft tissues.[433]

The usefulness of CT in the evaluation of nodular thyroid disease is limited because thyroid masses, whether benign or malignant, may be hypodense, hyperdense, or isodense, compared to adjacent normal thyroid tissue.[434] Malignant tumors may be inhomogeneous, with irregular margins, or homogeneous, with cystic components. In aggressive pathologic processes, such as anaplastic thyroid carcinoma, CT can define the relationship of the mass to surrounding structures such as

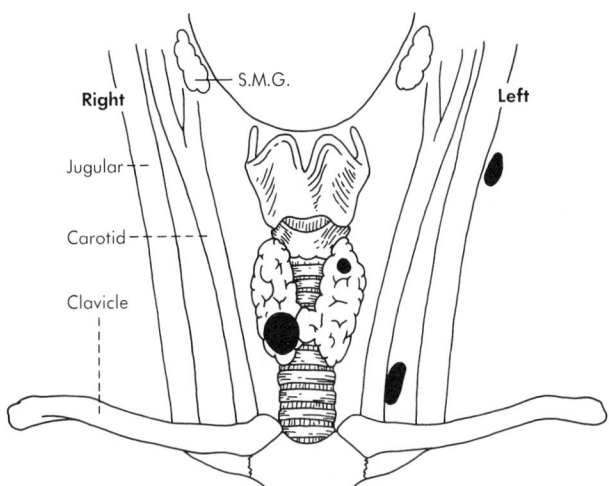

Figure 11–27. Cervical "map" derived from sonographic images helps communicate anatomic relationships of pathology to clinicians and serves as a reference for follow-up examinations. SMG, submandibular gland. (From James EM, Charboneau JW, Hay ID. The Thyroid. In: Rumack CM, Wilson SR, Charboneau JW, eds. Diagnostic Ultrasound. Vol 1. St. Louis: Mosby–YearBook, 1991: 507–528.)

the carotid artery, jugular vein, and trachea before attempted surgical excision. In patients with known thyroid cancer, CT is used most frequently to search for distant metastases in the chest and abdomen. It is less useful in evaluating recurrence in the neck because of the difficulty in detecting small masses in the indistinct tissue planes in the postoperative neck.[435] There is a considerable overlap in the appearance of malignant and inflammatory nodes, and CT lacks the ability to guide the needle biopsy of minimally enlarged nodes.[428]

CT can provide useful information regarding the presence and extent of intrathoracic (substernal) goiters. The CT findings of an intrathoracic mass in continuity with the thyroid gland that contains punctate, coarse, or ring-like calcifications and has high attenuation on non–contrast-enhanced images and marked enhancement following intravenous contrast material injection all suggest intrathoracic goiter.[436] Radionuclide scanning can also be performed in this clinical setting, but false-negative results can occur when little or no functional tissue is present in the intrathoracic goiter. The necessity of infusing iodine-containing contrast agents may limit the application of CT in patients being considered for radioiodine therapy.[435]

Magnetic Resonance Imaging

Because the hydrogen atoms of different tissues have different relaxation times (termed T1 and T2), a computer-assisted analysis of T1-weighted and T2-weighted signals is used to differentiate the thyroid gland from skeletal muscle, blood vessels, or regional lymph nodes. The normal thyroid tissue tends to be slightly more intense than muscle on a T1-weighted image, and tumors frequently appear more intense than normal thyroid.

Unfortunately, MRI is an uncomfortable procedure for patients. Claustrophobic reactions occur, and the technique is noisy. The images obtained have superior tissue contrast resolution but poorer spatial resolution than comparable CT images. Because of its relatively high cost and limitations due to spatial resolution and motion artifact, MRI is used less frequently than other thyroid imaging methods.[428]

As with CT, MRI does not distinguish benign from malignant nodules and does not assess functional status.[437] MRI, however, can define the anatomic extent of large goiters with great clarity.[438] Coronal and sagittal images provide a simultaneous view of the cervical and thoracic components of substernal goiters. The relation of the goiter to surrounding vessels in the mediastinum is also well visualized.[439]

Recurrent neoplasm in the thyroid bed or regional lymph nodes can be detected with MRI. Recurrence is characterized by a mass with low-to-medium intensity on T1-weighted images and medium-to-high signal intensity on T2-weighted images. Conversely, scar tissue or fibrous tissue is of low signal intensity on both T1- and T2-weighted images. Tumor invasion of adjacent skeletal muscle will be of high signal intensity on T2-weighted images.[437] Edema or inflammation in the muscle can cause a similar appearance and can be difficult to differentiate from recurrent tumor.[437]

THYROID BIOPSY AND FINE-NEEDLE ASPIRATION

Biopsy of the thyroid, usually closed percutaneous needle biopsy, is employed to obtain an anatomic diagnosis in certain situations. Although biopsy can be applied to the diagnosis of a variety of thyroid disorders, the major rationale is to differentiate between benign and malignant thyroid nodules. Initially, open biopsy, a surgical procedure performed with the patient under general or local anesthesia, was the sole type of biopsy performed. In diseases involving the thyroid diffusely, a specimen was taken for histologic examination, but nodular lesions were usually removed in toto. Hence the procedure was often therapeutic as well as diagnostic.

Subsequently, closed percutaneous biopsies were developed to obtain a core of tissue for histologic diagnosis. In these office procedures, a large Vim-Silverman or Tru-Cut needle (about 15-gauge) is introduced through a small nick in the skin, and one or more specimens are obtained for histologic examination. In experienced hands, cutting needle biopsies are safe, and a diagnostic accuracy of about 90% is obtained.[440] In less experienced hands, complications such as hemorrhage, tracheal puncture, laryngoparalysis, and transient injury to the recurrent laryngeal nerve are more common, and specimens may be insufficient for histologic diagnosis.[441]

Use of thyroid biopsy has become even more widespread as the result of a lessening fear of disseminating malignant cells[442] and the introduction of FNA biopsy.[443] In this technique, which is simple, safe, and rarely requires local anesthesia, the patient is placed in a supine position with the neck extended. The nodule is penetrated with a fine (25-gauge) needle attached to a 10-mL disposable plastic syringe in a mechanical syringe holder, and suction is applied manually. The contents of the needle are spread on a glass slide, dried or fixed, and stained.[444]

Both large- and fine-needle biopsies have limitations. In both techniques, the amount of tissue obtained is limited and may not be representative of the entire lesion. Neither technique is reliable in the diagnosis of differentiated follicular carcinoma, in which evidence of capsular or blood vessel invasion is required for diagnosis, and neither allows separation of Hashimoto's disease and lymphoma of the thyroid on pure cytologic grounds. In the case of fine-needle biopsy, the strongest caveat, however, is that slides must be read by an experienced thyroid cytologist. In general, 20 to 30% of patients are referred for surgery on the basis of the biopsy's

cytologic features.[445] About one third (17 to 51%) of those operated on have a malignancy. False-negative rates[446] range from 1% to more than 11% (mean 5%).

Thyroid biopsy of any type should not be performed as an isolated diagnostic procedure, but rather as part of a systematic approach to the management of the thyroid nodule that includes careful clinical evaluation and, when indicated, scintiscanning or ultrasonography.[447–449]

APPROACH TO THE CLINICAL DIAGNOSIS OF THYROID DISEASE AND INITIAL LABORATORY TESTING

Manifestations of thyroid disease are usually due to excessive or insufficient production of thyroid hormone, local symptoms in the neck (principally goiter but occasionally pain or compression of adjacent structures), or in the case of Graves' disease ophthalmopathy or dermopathy. Although attention is directed initially at the major features, it is critical to define the metabolic state and ascertain the nature of the underlying disorder.

A functional diagnosis of thyroid disease is based on a carefully taken history, a thorough search for the physical signs of hypothyroidism or thyrotoxicosis, and an appraisal of the results of laboratory tests. Although conditioned by the functional diagnosis, the anatomic diagnosis depends largely on the examination of the thyroid gland itself (Fig. 11–28).

Local examination of the neck is best accomplished with the patient seated in a good light with the neck moderately extended. The patient should be provided with a glass of water to facilitate swallowing. The physician should first inspect the neck from the front and on the sides. The presence of old surgical scars, distended veins, and redness or fixation of the overlying skin should be noted. If a mass is present, attention should be directed to its location and to whether it moves when the patient swallows. The position of the trachea should be noted. Movement on swallowing is a characteristic of the thyroid gland because it is ensheathed by the pretracheal fascia; this feature distinguishes a goiter from most other neck masses. However, if a goiter is so large that it occupies all the available space in the neck or if the thyroid gland is the seat of an invasive carcinoma or Riedel's thyroiditis that has caused fixation to adjacent structures, movement on swallowing may be lost. The physician should also inspect the dorsum of the tongue, which is the origin of the thyroglossal duct and occasionally the seat of a lingual goiter.

The neck may be examined with the physician standing behind the seated patient and palpating with the fingertips of both hands. The position of the cricoid cartilage is first determined because the superior border of the isthmus lies just below it. The isthmus is a band of tissue crossing the front of the trachea and joining the two lateral lobes. The examiner then attempts to outline the thyroid gland and to determine the limits of the lower borders of the lateral lobes, while the patient swallows sips of water at appropriate intervals. A normal thyroid gland can usually be palpated.

An alternative approach is for the physician to stand facing the patient using the thumb to locate the thyroid isthmus. The right thumb is then moved laterally to compress the right lobe of the thyroid against the trachea as the patient swallows. A similar strategy with the left thumb is used for the left lobe. This technique may be especially useful for evaluating small nodules that might not be easily appreciated with the posterior approach.

The examiner should note the shape of the gland, its size in relation to normal, and its consistency, which is usually

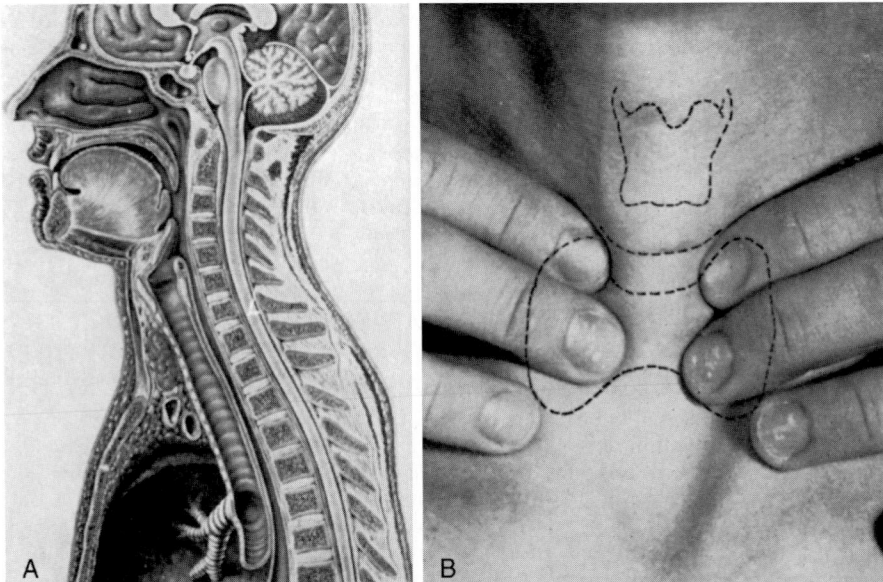

Figure 11–28. *A,* Sagittal section demonstrating the relation of the isthmus of the normal thyroid gland. The superior border is inferior to the cricoid cartilage. The inferior thyroid border is essentially at the level of the superior surface of the manubrium. The inferior portions of the lateral lobes (not shown) extend more inferiorly than the isthmus. *B,* The cricoid cartilage is an important landmark. Especially when the thyroid gland is thought to be essentially normal or subnormal in size, the cricoid should be located. The index fingers are then inserted so that their superior portion rests against the inferior portion of the cricoid, while the inferior portion of these fingers is over the superior portion of the thyroid. The second and third fingers are rotated over other portions of the gland, evaluating its size, contour, consistency, possible adherence to surrounding structures, and other features. Because there is marked variation among different subjects in the length and thickness of the neck and in the length of the trachea superior to the level of the manubrium, the relative position of the thyroid also varies. In some cases, essentially all of the thyroid rests posterior to the sternum. In most instances, however, by having the patient extend the neck maximally (short of markedly tightening the neck muscles) and swallow repeatedly, it is possible to palpate most or all of the gland. Despite variations in neck-chest relations, thyroid tissue, when present, is found within 1 cm of the cricoid. By concentrating the palpation in the area where the thyroid is normally found, with rare exceptions it is possible to outline small as well as enlarged glands.

rubbery. The normal thyroid lobe has approximately the same size in frontal projection as the terminal phalanx of the thumb. Whereas the diffuse colloid goiter and the hyperplastic gland of Graves' disease tend to be softer than normal, the gland of Hashimoto's disease tends to be firm, and the gland that is the seat of carcinoma or Riedel's thyroiditis may be "stony" hard. Irregularities of the surface, variations in consistency, and tender areas should be noted. If nodules are palpated, their shape, size, position, opacity, and consistency in relation to the surrounding tissue should be determined. A search should be made for the pyramidal lobe; this is a band of tissue extending upward from the isthmus to the right or left of the midline. The pyramidal lobe may be mistaken for the pretracheal or "delphian" lymph node that sometimes accompanies thyroid carcinoma or thyroiditis. Thyroglossal cysts are midline masses that remain attached to the base of the tongue by the obliterated thyroglossal duct and move upward when the tongue is protruded. During palpation a vascular thrill may be felt that, in the absence of cardiac disease, is suggestive of hyperthyroidism. Finally, palpation should always include examination of the regional lymph nodes.

Auscultation of the neck provides some indication of the vascularity of the gland. A systolic or continuous bruit is commonly heard over a hyperplastic gland. Care should be taken to distinguish a thyroid bruit from a murmur transmitted from the base of the heart or from a venous hum that can be obliterated by compression of the external jugular vein or by turning the head.

An arm-raising test is useful when a retrosternal goiter is suspected. The basis for this maneuver is that if the size of the thoracic inlet is already reduced by a retrosternal goiter, raising both arms until they touch the sides of the head further narrows the thoracic inlet and causes congestion and venous engorgement of the face and respiratory distress (Pemberton's sign) or even (rarely) syncope.

In addition to examination of the thyroid gland and regional lymph nodes, evidence of compression or displacement of adjacent structures should be sought. Hoarseness may indicate compression of the recurrent laryngeal nerve, usually by a malignant thyroid neoplasm, and this should be confirmed by laryngoscopy. Displacement of the trachea may be evident, and inspiratory stridor may indicate compression of the trachea. Radiologic examination may reveal retrosternal extension of a goiter, displacement or narrowing of the trachea, and, during a barium swallow, displacement of the esophagus. Calcification in the thyroid gland may also be seen and, by its nature, aid in distinguishing between benign and malignant lesions.

THYROTOXICOSIS

The term *thyrotoxicosis* refers to the biochemical and physiological manifestations of excessive quantities of the thyroid hormones. The authors prefer the term *thyrotoxicosis* rather than *hyperthyroidism* to describe this disorder, because it need not originate in the thyroid gland. The term *hyperthyroidism* is reserved for disorders that result from overproduction of hormone by the thyroid itself, Graves' disease being the most common. The manifestations depend on the severity of the disease, the age of the patient, the presence or absence of extrathyroidal manifestations, and the specific disorder producing the thyrotoxicosis.

Peripheral Clinical Manifestations of Thyrotoxicosis
Skin and Hair

The most characteristic change is the warm, moist feel of the skin that results from cutaneous vasodilation and excessive sweating. While the hands are usually warm and moist, the texture of the hands may be altered by occupational or environmental factors; hence, texture is best assessed on the inner aspect of the arm or thigh or over the chest. The elbows are smooth and pink; the complexion is rosy; and the patient blushes readily. Palmar erythema may resemble "liver palms," and telangiectasia may be present. Increased diffuse pigmentation resembles that in adrenal insufficiency, but buccal pigmentation does not occur. The hair is fine and friable, and hair loss may be excessive. A history of early graying in the patient or in relatives is said to be common in Graves' disease. The nails are often soft and friable. A characteristic finding is Plummer's nails, a term applied to separation of the distal margin of the nail from the nail bed, with irregular recession of the junction (onycholysis).

Eyes

Retraction of the upper eyelid, evident as the presence of a rim of sclera between the lid and the limbus, is frequent in all forms of thyrotoxicosis, regardless of the underlying cause, and is responsible for the bright-eyed "stare" or "fish eyes" of the patient with thyrotoxicosis. Lid lag is the phenomenon in which the upper lid lags behind the globe when the patient is asked to gaze slowly downward, and globe lag occurs when the globe lags behind the upper lid when the patient gazes slowly upward. The movements of the lids may be jerky and spasmodic, and a fine tremor of the lightly closed lids can often be observed in severe cases. These ocular manifestations appear to be the result of increased adrenergic activity. *It is important to differentiate these ocular manifestations, which occur in all forms of thyrotoxicosis, from those of infiltrative orbitopathy, which are characteristic of Graves' disease and are described below.*

Cardiovascular System

Alterations in cardiovascular function are due to increased circulatory demands that result from the hypermetabolism and the need to dissipate the excess heat produced.[450] At rest, peripheral vascular resistance is decreased, and cardiac output is increased as a result of an increase in stroke volume and heart rate. Thyroid hormones in excess have a direct ionotropic effect mediated by alterations of contractile proteins. Tachycardia is almost always present, and tachycardia during sleep (pulse rate greater than 90 beats/min) serves to distinguish tachycardia of thyrotoxic origin from that of psychogenic cause. Widening of the pulse pressure is due to an increase in systolic pressure and a decrease in diastolic pressure. The increased force of cardiac contraction is often felt by the patient as palpitation and may be evident on inspection or palpation of the precordium. Because of the diffuse and forceful nature of the apex beat, the heart may seem enlarged, but echocardiography is usually normal. Heart sounds are loud and ringing, and a systolic or even a late diastolic or presystolic murmur (Means-Lerman scratch) may be present at the apex. A scratchy systolic sound along the left sternal border, resembling a pleuropericardial friction rub, may also be heard. These manifestations usually abate when a normal metabolic state is restored. Mitral valve prolapse occurs more frequently than in the normal population and may persist indefinitely.[451]

Cardiac arrhythmias are almost invariably supraventricular. Approximately 10% of patients with thyrotoxicosis have atrial fibrillation, and a similar percentage of patients with otherwise unexplained atrial fibrillation are thyrotoxic. In a study of more than 2000 individuals of 60 years of age or older, 28% of those with a suppressed TSH developed atrial fibrillation.[452] Paroxysmal supraventricular tachycardia may be demonstrable or may be suggested by the history. Systolic

time intervals are altered in thyrotoxicosis; the pulse wave propagation is accelerated; the pre-ejection period is shortened; and the ratio of pre-ejection period–to–left ventricular ejection time is decreased.

The adequacy of the circulation is a question of importance in the patient with thyrotoxicosis. The increased cardiovascular cost of a standard workload or metabolic challenge is adequately met if the patient is not or has not previously been in heart failure. Thus, *in most patients without underlying heart disease, cardiac competence is maintained.* Mild edema may occur in the absence of heart failure. Thyrotoxicosis may lead to congestive heart failure, but, even so, the circulation time may remain short. Heart failure usually occurs in patients with pre-existing heart disease, but it may not be possible to determine whether underlying heart disease is present until after thyrotoxicosis is relieved. Atrial fibrillation decreases the efficiency of the cardiac response to any increased circulatory demand and may play a role in causing cardiac failure. Attempts to convert atrial fibrillation to sinus rhythm are usually of no avail while thyrotoxicosis is present. Regardless of the type of rhythm, the response to digitalis is decreased, possibly because of accelerated metabolism of the drug, and large quantities may be required to produce a clinical effect. Resistance to digitalis and failure of cardiac decompensation to respond to a usually adequate regimen should suggest the possibility of thyrotoxicosis. It is obviously important to deal definitively with thyrotoxicosis in a patient with concomitant heart disease.

Sympathetic Nervous System

Many of the manifestations of thyrotoxicosis and of sympathetic nervous system activation are similar. As judged from the plasma concentrations of epinephrine and norepinephrine, as well as their urinary excretion and that of their metabolites, the activity of the sympathetic nervous system is not increased in patients or animals with thyrotoxicosis, and thyroid hormones may exert effects separate from, but similar and additive to, those of the catecholamines. Consideration of the relationship between catecholamines and thyroid hormone excess and deficiency reveals the futility of attempting a generalization in this area.[453] The reduction in heart rate and in some clinical manifestations of hyperthyroidism induced by β-blockade in patients with this condition has led to the concept that there is increased sympathetic tone or increased cardiac sensitivity to the sympathetic nervous system. Careful studies have shown that this is clearly not the case in terms of the heart.[454, 455] Adequate β-adrenergic blockade reduces the basal level of cardiac output, but the slope of the epinephrine dose-response curve is not altered in hyperthyroidism. In other tissues the situation may be even more complex, and species differences may exist.

In hyperthyroid humans there are no alterations in β-adrenergic receptor number on lymphocytes and no changes in lymphocyte β-adrenergic responsiveness. In normal subjects receiving 100 μg of liothyronine for 10 d, the β-adrenergic receptor number in fat and skeletal muscle increased 60 and 30%, respectively, but metabolic and hemodynamic sensitivity to infused epinephrine in vivo was not altered.[456] There was no evidence of increased glycemic, lipolytic, glycogenolytic, or ketogenic sensitivity to catecholamines, possibly because of a concomitant increase in endogenous insulin secretion that compensated for these changes.

In another study, the accelerated basal energy expenditure and body protein catabolism caused by 150 μg of liothyronine/d were unaffected by doses of propranolol that completely blocked the stimulatory effect of epinephrine infusion on these parameters. These results indicate that the calorigenic stimulation by thyroid hormone is independent of catecholamines. However, because basal energy expenditure was increased by liothyronine, the absolute increment in energy expenditure during epinephrine infusion was also greater. Thus propranolol blockade of epinephrine-induced increases in energy expenditure had a greater effect in the thyrotoxic subjects than in normal individuals. This would justify the use of β-adrenergic blockade in thyrotoxic subjects, particularly in states of marked sympathetic activation such as thyroid storm or during emergency surgery.

Respiratory System

Dyspnea is common in severe thyrotoxicosis, and several factors may contribute to this condition. Vital capacity is commonly reduced; this reduction appears to result mainly from weakness of the respiratory muscles, but decreased pulmonary compliance may also play a role. During exercise, ventilation is increased out of proportion to the increase in oxygen uptake; the diffusing capacity of the lung is normal, however. Pulmonary function returns to normal when a normal metabolic state is restored.

Alimentary System

An increase in appetite is common but is usually not seen in patients with mild disease. In severe disease the increased intake of food is usually inadequate to meet the increased caloric requirements, and weight is lost at a variable rate. However, in the occasional, usually younger, patient with mild disease, weight gain may occur when caloric intake exceeds the metabolic demand. Anorexia, rather than hyperphagia, occurs in about one third of elderly thyrotoxic patients and contributes to the picture of "apathetic" thyrotoxicosis.

Stools are frequently soft, and the frequency of bowel movements is increased, but diarrhea is rare. When constipation has anteceded the development of thyrotoxicosis, bowel function may become normal. Anorexia, nausea, and vomiting are uncommon but may occur with severe disease. These symptoms, as well as abdominal pain, may be forerunners of accelerated thyrotoxicosis. The increased gastric emptying and intestinal motility in thyrotoxicosis appear to be responsible for slight malabsorption of fat, and these functions return to normal when a normal metabolic state has been restored. Celiac disease and Graves' disease may coexist more frequently than can be accounted for by chance. A high proportion of patients have gastric achlorhydria. In most, acid secretion returns after relief of the thyrotoxicosis. Autoantibodies against gastric parietal cells are detectable in about one third of patients with Graves' disease, and approximately 3% have pernicious anemia. In the oral glucose tolerance test the glycemic peak is frequently delayed.

Hepatic dysfunction occurs, particularly when thyrotoxicosis is severe; hypoproteinemia and increases in serum alanine aminotransferase (ALT) and alkaline phosphatase levels may be present. Hepatomegaly and jaundice occasionally develop. Splanchnic oxygen consumption is increased, while splanchnic blood flow is essentially unchanged. As a result, the arteriovenous oxygen difference across the splanchnic bed is increased; hence hypoxia may contribute to hepatic dysfunction.[457] Hypoxia and the relative caloric deprivation may partly account for the depletion of hepatic glycogen that is evident both in the response to glycogenolytic agents and on direct analysis. In the absence of severe thyrotoxicosis or congestive heart failure, the liver usually appears normal on light microscopic examination. In severe cases centrilobular fatty infiltration, patchy portal fibrosis, lymphocytic infiltration, and proliferation of bile ducts can occur. Ultramicroscopic examination of the liver reveals enlarged mitochondria and hypertrophic smooth endoplasmic reticulum. Graves' disease and autoimmune hepatitis coexist more often than can be explained by chance.

Nervous System

Alterations in the function of the nervous system in thyrotoxicosis are manifested by nervousness, emotional lability, and hyperkinesia. The nervousness is not typical of the patient who is chronically anxious, but rather is characterized by restlessness, shortness of attention span, and a compulsion to be moving around, sometimes referred to as almost "levitating." Unlike the patient with neurocirculatory asthenia, the thyrotoxic patient wishes to be active but is hampered by fatigue and is tired from the neck down, rather than from the top of the head down. Fatigue may be due both to muscle weakness and to the insomnia that is commonly present. In some patients, severe wasting and fatigue impair overall activity. Emotional lability causes patients to lose their tempers easily and to have episodes of crying with only slight provocation. In rare cases mental disturbance may be severe; manic-depressive, schizoid, or paranoid reactions may emerge.

The hyperkinesia of the thyrotoxic patient is characteristic. During the interview the patient cannot sit still, drums on the table, taps a foot, or shifts positions frequently. Movements are quick, jerky, exaggerated, and often purposeless. In children, in whom such manifestations tend to be more severe, Sydenham's chorea may be suggested. Examination also reveals a fine rhythmic tremor of the hands, tongue, or lightly closed eyelids. With the aid of a magnifying glass, a tremor of the eyeballs may be seen. The tremor may sometimes mimic that of parkinsonism, and a pre-existing parkinsonian tremor can be accentuated. The electroencephalogram reveals an increase in fast-wave activity, and in patients with convulsive disorders, the frequency of seizures is increased.

The physiological basis of the nervous system findings is not well understood. They may reflect increased adrenergic activity because some improvement occurs during treatment with adrenergic antagonists. The widespread distribution of thyroid hormone receptors in the brain makes it likely that alterations in cerebral metabolism are induced by thyroid hormone excess. Nevertheless oxygen consumption by the brain is not altered.

Muscle

Weakness and fatigability are usually not accompanied by objective evidence of muscle disease save for the generalized wasting associated with loss of weight. Often the weakness is most prominent in the proximal muscles of the limbs, causing difficulty in climbing stairs or in maintaining the leg in an extended position. The latter maneuver can be employed to assess the degree of muscle weakness. Occasionally, in severe untreated cases, muscle wasting that again tends to be proximal develops out of proportion to the overall loss of weight (*thyrotoxic myopathy*). In the extreme form, the patient may be unable to rise from a sitting or lying position and may be virtually unable to walk. This disorder may resemble progressive muscular atrophy or polymyositis; however, fasciculation is absent, and little if any inflammatory change is evident on biopsy. Instead the muscle is atrophic and infiltrated with fat cells and lymphocytes. Electron microscopy reveals abnormal mitochondria and dilations of the myotubular system. Electromyograms reveal a decreased duration of action potentials and an increased number of polyphasic potentials. The biochemical basis of the muscle weakness is uncertain but may be related to the impaired ability to phosphorylate creatine.

Myopathy affects men with thyrotoxicosis more commonly than women and may overshadow the other manifestations of the syndrome. In the most severe forms, the myopathy may involve the more distal muscles of the extremities and the muscles of the trunk and face. Although myopathy of ocular muscles is unusual, the disorder may mimic myasthenia gravis. In uncomplicated thyrotoxic myopathy, some improvement of muscular strength may follow the administration of edrophonium, but, unlike that in myasthenia, the response is incomplete. Muscular strength returns to normal when a normal metabolic state is restored, but muscle mass takes longer to recover.

Graves' disease occurs in about 3 to 5% of the patients with myasthenia gravis, and about 1% of the patients with Graves' disease develop myasthenia gravis. These associations are of interest in view of the frequent association of thymic enlargement with Graves' disease.[458] Furthermore antibodies and T cells specific for receptors (i.e., the TSH receptor and the acetylcholine receptor) are involved in the pathogenesis of the two diseases. Unlike thyrotoxic myopathy, the association of myasthenia gravis with Graves' disease has a distinct female sex preponderance. The effect of both thyrotoxicosis and its alleviation on the course of myasthenia gravis is variable, but in the majority of instances, myasthenia is accentuated during the thyrotoxic state and improves when a normal metabolic state is restored.

Periodic paralysis of the hypokalemic type may occur together with thyrotoxicosis, and its severity is accentuated by the latter disorder. The coincidence of the two disorders is particularly common in Asian and Latino males.[459]

Skeletal System: Calcium and Phosphorus Metabolism

Thyrotoxicosis is generally associated with increased excretion of calcium and phosphorus in urine and stool; with demineralization of bone, as demonstrated by densitometry; and occasionally with pathologic fractures, especially in elderly women. In such instances the pathologic changes are variable and may include osteitis fibrosa, osteomalacia, or osteoporosis. Urinary excretion of collagen breakdown products is increased in thyrotoxicosis, indicating increased turnover of collagen. Kinetic studies indicate an increase in the exchangeable calcium pool and acceleration of both bone resorption and accretion, particularly the former. The changes lead to decreased bone density and a propensity to hip fractures in later years.[460] As the thyrotoxicosis is treated, bone density may return to almost predisease levels in premenopausal patients.[461] Postmenopausal women, however, may have a permanent reduction in bone density that may require treatment with agents that increase bone density (see Chapter 25).

Hypercalcemia can occur in patients with thyrotoxicosis. The total serum calcium concentration is increased in as many as 27% of patients, and the ionized serum calcium level is elevated in 47%.[462] The concentrations of heat-labile serum alkaline phosphatase and osteocalcin are also frequently elevated.[463–465] These findings resemble those of primary hyperparathyroidism, but the concentration of immunoreactive parathyroid hormone in serum is decreased in most thyrotoxic patients with hypercalcemia. True primary hyperparathyroidism and thyrotoxicosis may sometimes coexist. Hypercalcemia may be severe enough to induce anorexia, nausea, vomiting, polyuria, and occasionally impairment of renal function. The alterations in calcium metabolism in thyrotoxicosis may be due to a direct effect of thyroid hormones in stimulating bone resorption and are reversed when the eumetabolic state is restored. Plasma 25-hydroxycholecalciferol levels are decreased in thyrotoxic patients, and this alteration could contribute to the decreased intestinal absorption of calcium and osteomalacia noted in some patients.

Renal Function: Water and Electrolyte Metabolism

Thyrotoxicosis produces no symptoms referable to the urinary tract save for mild polyuria. Nevertheless renal blood flow, glomerular filtration, and tubular reabsorptive and secretory maxima are increased. Total amounts of body water and exchangeable potassium are decreased, possibly because of a decrease in lean body mass, but the amount of exchangeable sodium tends to be increased. Serum sodium, potassium, and chloride concentrations are normal, however. In thyrotoxicosis the level of exchangeable magnesium is normal, the serum magnesium concentration is often decreased, and urinary magnesium excretion is increased.

Hematopoietic System

The red blood cells are usually normal, as judged by the usual indices, but the red blood cell mass is increased. The increase in erythropoiesis appears to be due both to the direct effect of thyroid hormones on the erythroid marrow and to increased production of erythropoietin. A parallel increase in plasma volume also occurs, with the result that the hematocrit is normal. Other abnormalities in thyrotoxicosis include a reduced content of zinc and carbonic anhydrase 1 and an increased content of sodium in red blood cells, probably because the activity of Na^+,K^+-ATPase is impaired (in contrast to the increased Na^+,K^+-ATPase activity that may be seen in other tissues).

Approximately 3% of patients with Graves' disease have pernicious anemia, and a further 3% have antibodies to intrinsic factor but normal absorption of vitamin B_{12}. Autoantibodies against gastric parietal cells are present in about one third of the patients with Graves' disease, and the requirements for vitamin B_{12} and folic acid appear to be increased. Rarely thyrotoxicosis is associated with a mild hypochromic anemia characterized by adequate stores of iron in the marrow and responsive to large doses of pyridoxine.

The total white blood cell count is often low because of a decrease in the number of neutrophils. The absolute lymphocyte count is normal or increased, leading to a relative lymphocytosis. The numbers of monocytes and eosinophils may also be increased. Splenic enlargement occurs in about 10% of the patients, and thymic and lymph node enlargement is common.[458] It is assumed that these abnormalities are a reflection of the autoimmune aspects of Graves' disease, since it does not occur in thyrotoxicosis due to other causes.

Platelet levels and the intrinsic clotting mechanism are normal, but the concentration of factor VIII is often increased and returns to normal when the thyrotoxicosis is treated.[466] Despite this increase, there is an enhanced sensitivity to anticoagulants of the coumarin series because of accelerated clearance of the vitamin K–dependent clotting factors. Somewhat paradoxically then, the dosage of such anticoagulants may have to be reduced in thyrotoxic patients and is increased in hypothyroid patients.[467]

Pituitary and Adrenocortical Function

The thyrotoxic state imposes several challenges on pituitary and adrenocortical function. The inactivation of cortisol is accelerated, including reduction of the A ring, which is rapidly followed by conjugation, and oxidation of the 11-hydroxy group to a keto group as a result of an increase in 11β-hydroxysteroid dehydrogenase activity. As a result of these changes the disposal of cortisol is accelerated, but its rate of secretion is also increased, so the plasma cortisol concentration remains normal. The concentration of corticosteroid-binding globulin in plasma is normal. The urinary excretion of free cortisol and 17-hydroxycorticosteroids (17-OHCS) is normal or slightly increased, whereas the urinary excretion of 17-ketosteroids (17-KS) may be reduced.[468]

Basal pituitary-adrenal function is adequate, as indicated by normal plasma cortisol concentrations, and the response to an acute challenge, such as that imposed by insulin-induced hypoglycemia, is adequate. The rate of turnover of aldosterone is increased, but the plasma level is normal. Plasma renin activity is increased, and sensitivity to angiotensin II is reduced.

The response of plasma growth hormone concentration to insulin-induced hypoglycemia is subnormal, particularly with severe disease. This observation may not indicate deficient growth hormone production but rather reflect depletion of pituitary stores from caloric inadequacy or accelerated removal of growth hormone from plasma. Incomplete suppression of plasma growth hormone concentration by induced hyperglycemia may also reflect prolonged caloric deprivation.

Reproductive Function

Thyrotoxicosis in early life may cause delayed sexual maturation, although physical development is normal and skeletal growth may be accelerated. Thyrotoxicosis after puberty influences reproductive function, especially in women. An increase in libido sometimes occurs in both sexes. The intermenstrual interval may be prolonged or shortened, and menstrual flow is initially diminished and ultimately ceases. Fertility may be reduced, and if conception takes place, there is an increased risk of miscarriage. The association of thyroid autoantibodies and increased pregnancy loss is not related to changes in thyroid function[404]; the thyroid autoantibodies are thought to represent a marker of immune instability predisposing to pregnancy interruption.

In some patients, menstrual cycles are predominantly anovulatory with oligomenorrhea, but in most, ovulation occurs, as indicated by a secretory endometrium. In the former, a subnormal midcycle surge of LH may be responsible. In premenopausal women with thyrotoxicosis, basal plasma concentrations of LH and FSH are reportedly normal but may display enhanced responsiveness to luteinizing hormone–releasing hormone (LHRH).

Thyrotoxicosis, whether spontaneous or induced by T_3, is accompanied by an increase in the concentration of testosterone-binding globulin (TeBG) in plasma. As a result the plasma concentrations of total testosterone, dihydrotestosterone, and estradiol are increased, but their unbound fractions are normal or transiently decreased. The increased binding in plasma is responsible for the decreased metabolic clearance rate of testosterone and dihydrotestosterone. In the case of estradiol, however, the metabolic clearance rate is normal, suggesting that tissue metabolism of the hormone is increased. Conversion rates of androstenedione to testosterone, estrone, and estradiol, and of testosterone to dihydrotestosterone are increased. The increased rate of conversion of androgens to estrogens may be the mechanism for gynecomastia in some 10% of thyrotoxic men and one mechanism for menstrual irregularities in women.

Catecholamines and Serotonin

Many effects induced by thyroid hormones are reminiscent of those induced by epinephrine, including tachycardia, increased cardiac output, and enhanced glycogenolysis, lipolysis, and calorigenesis (see earlier). Moreover, the fact that some of the manifestations of thyrotoxicosis, among them eyelid retraction, tremor, excessive sweating, and tachycardia, are at least partly alleviated by adrenergic antagonists has been interpreted as indicating that a state of increased adrenergic activity exists in the thyrotoxic organism. However, as discussed earlier, this apparent adrenergic hyperactivity appears to be a consequence of a direct effect of thyroid hormones on these tissues because there is no evidence for increased cardiac sensitivity to catecholamines in hyperthyroid subjects.[453–455, 469] The secretion rates and plasma levels of epinephrine and norepinephrine are normal.[470, 471]

Some manifestations of thyrotoxicosis, such as flushing, sweating, tachycardia, and gastrointestinal hypermotility, are also reminiscent of those of carcinoid syndrome. However, plasma serotonin levels, urinary 5-hydroxy-indoleacetic acid excretion, and platelet monoamine oxidase activity are normal.

Energy Metabolism: Protein, Carbohydrate, and Lipid Metabolism

The stimulation of energy metabolism and heat production is reflected in the increased BMR, increased appetite, and heat intolerance and in the sometimes slightly elevated basal body temperature. Despite the increased food intake, a state of chronic caloric and nutritional inadequacy often ensues, depending on the degree of increased metabolism.

Both synthesis and degradation of protein are increased, the latter to a greater extent than the former, with the result that there is a net decrease in tissue protein, as indicated by negative nitrogen balance, loss of weight, muscle wasting, weakness, and mild hypoalbuminemia.

The oral glucose tolerance curve is often abnormal and varies from one in which the peak glycemia is increased and somewhat delayed to one that is frankly diabetic. Plasma insulin concentrations, however, are increased, suggesting insulin resistance. The pathogenesis of these alterations remains to be defined. Pre-existing diabetes mellitus is aggravated by thyrotoxicosis, one cause being increased degradation of insulin.

Both synthesis and degradation of triglycerides and of cholesterol are increased, but the net effect is one of lipid degradation, as reflected by an increase in the plasma concentration of free fatty acids and glycerol and a decrease in the serum cholesterol level; serum triglyceride levels are usually slightly decreased. Postheparin lipolytic activity is reported to be decreased in some studies and increased in others. The enhanced mobilization and oxidation of free fatty acids in response to fasting, catecholamines, and growth hormone are probably due to activation of adenylate cyclase and result in a tendency to ketosis and to fatty infiltration of the liver, depending on the degree of caloric deprivation.

Composite Clinical Picture and Laboratory Tests in Thyrotoxic States

The effects of thyrotoxicosis on the major organ systems are the same regardless of the underlying etiology. Their frequency and intensity and other findings with which they are associated are influenced by the nature of the underlying disorder. To a large extent, the same is true of laboratory test results. Consequently the clinical picture, laboratory features, and differential diagnosis will be considered in relation to the specific etiologies (Table 11–14).

GRAVES' DISEASE

Background

OVERVIEW. The disorder known as Graves' disease in the English-speaking world and as von Basedow's disease on the

TABLE 11–14. Varieties of Thyrotoxicosis

Sustained Hormone Overproduction (Hyperthyroidism)*

Graves' disease
Toxic multinodular goiter
Toxic adenoma
Iodine-induced (jodbasedow)
Trophoblastic tumor
Increased TSH secretion

No Associated Hyperthyroidism†

Thyrotoxicosis factitia
Subacute thyroiditis
Chronic thyroiditis with transient thyrotoxicosis (painless thyroiditis, silent thyroiditis, post-partum thyroiditis)
Ectopic thyroid tissue (struma ovarii, functioning metastatic thyroid cancer)

*Except for iodine-induced hyperthyroidism, associated with increased values of RAIU.
†Associated with decreased values of RAIU.

continent of Europe is the most enigmatic and, in areas of iodine abundance, the most common of thyroid diseases.[471a]

PRESENTATION. Graves' disease is characterized by diffuse goiter, thyrotoxicosis, infiltrative orbitopathy, and occasionally infiltrative dermopathy. In the individual patient the thyroid disease and the infiltrative phenomena may occur singly or together but run courses that are largely independent. The thyroid component is closely related to autoimmune thyroiditis (Hashimoto's disease) in its pathogenesis and clinical course. In Grave's disease, hyperthyroidism occurs in the presence of some degree of chronic thyroiditis and may ultimately be replaced, in the long term, by thyroid hypofunction. Conversely hyperthyroidism may occasionally supervene in patients with pre-existing Hashimoto's disease.[204, 472]

AUTOIMMUNE CHARACTERISTICS. Autoimmune thyroid disease is characterized by the occurrence in the serum of antibodies against thyroid peroxidase (the "microsomal" antigen), Tg, and the TSH receptor.[473] T cell–mediated autoimmunity can be demonstrated against the three primary thyroid antigens, as judged by a variety of criteria, including the ability of the T cells to elaborate various lymphokines and to exhibit a mitogenic response when exposed to thyroid antigens or to peptide sequences from the antigens. Autoimmune thyroid disease is also characterized by lymphocytic infiltration of the thyroid gland or remnant thyroid bed. In patients and their relatives there is an increased frequency of other disorders of autoimmune origin, such as insulin-dependent diabetes mellitus (IDDM), pernicious anemia, myasthenia gravis, adrenal atrophy, Sjögren's syndrome, lupus erythematosus, rheumatoid arthritis, and idiopathic thrombocytopenic purpura (see Chapter 33). Circulating autoantibodies specific to hyperthyroid Graves' disease are against the TSH receptor (TSHRAb) and behave as thyroid-stimulating antibodies.[405] These antibodies can compete for the binding of TSH to its specific receptor site in the cell membrane (Fig. 11–29) and are able to activate adenylate cyclase, as TSH agonists (Fig. 11–30). Similar but distinct autoantibodies in the sera of some patients with autoimmune thyroiditis do not stimulate the thyroid cell and therefore block the ligand-binding site and act as TSH antagonists[474] (see Fig. 11–25). The thyroid gland itself is a site of thyroid autoantibody secretion in autoimmune thyroid disease. Transplantation of Graves' thyroid tissue into the T cell– and B cell–deficient mice with severe combined immunodeficiency (*scid* mice) results in the appearance of

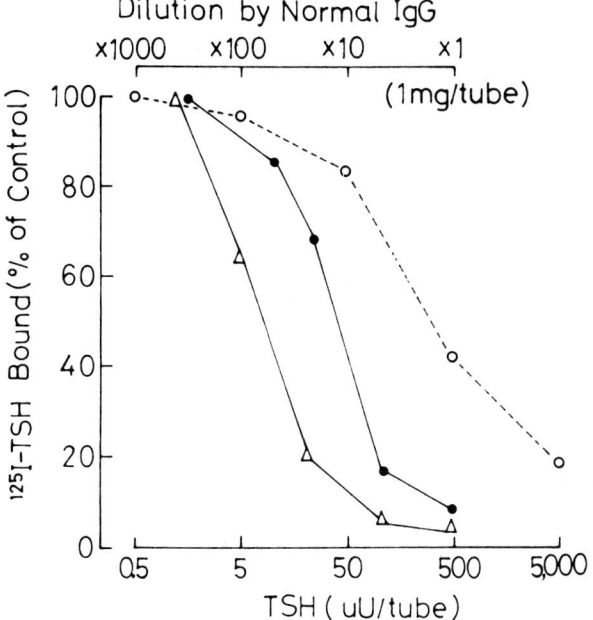

Figure 11–29. Inhibition of the binding of ¹²⁵I-labeled TSH to human thyroid TSH receptors by increasing concentrations of bovine TSH (O---O) and by increasing concentrations of IgG containing TSH-binding inhibitory immunoglobulin (TBII) activity (●---● and △---△). (From Endo K, Kashagi K, Konishi J, et al. Detection and properties of TSH-binding inhibitor immunoglobulins in patients with Graves' disease and Hashimoto's thyroiditis. J Clin Endocrinol Metab 1978; 46:734–739. © 1978, The Endocrine Society.)

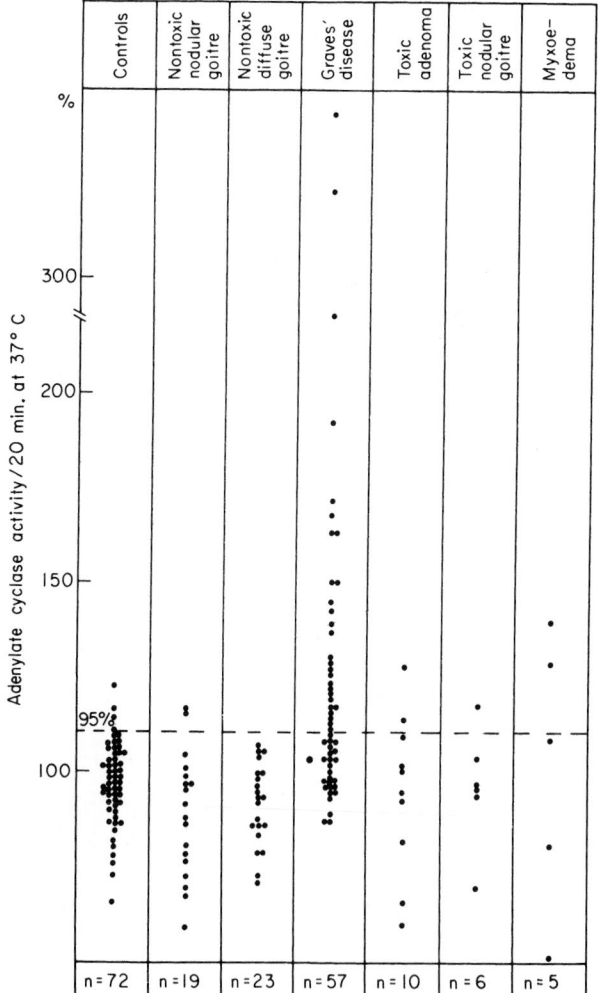

Figure 11–30. Stimulation of adenylate cyclase activity in human thyroid membranes by serum IgG in normal control subjects and patients with thyroid disease. (From Bech K, Nistrup Madsen SN. Thyroid adenylate cyclase stimulating immunoglobulins in thyroid disease. Clin Endocrinol 1979; 11:47–58.)

human thyroid autoantibodies, including TSHRAb, in the serum.[475] Additional evidence for a role of the thyroid itself in antibody production comes from animal models of thyroiditis and from the decline in thyroid autoantibody levels after antithyroid drug treatment,[476, 477] thyroidectomy, or radioiodine ablation.[478] However, a few post-thyroidectomy patients and post-radioiodine treatment patients have no decline in autoantibody secretion, implying extrathyroidal sources of continued production.

PATHOLOGY. The thyroid in Graves' disease is characterized by a nonhomogeneous lymphocytic infiltration with an absence of follicular destruction[479] (Fig. 11–31). Antithyroid drug treatment may reduce the degree of infiltration.[480] Although the intrathyroidal lymphocyte population is mixed, the majority are T lymphocytes; B-cell germinal centers are less common than in autoimmune thyroiditis.[481] However, both intraepithelial T cells and plasma cells can be seen in peripolesis within the thyroid follicles.[481–483] Follicular epithelial cell size correlates with the intensity of the local infiltrate, suggesting local thyroid cell stimulation by TSHRAb.[484] Memory T cells may predominate within the T-cell population, but this finding can vary from patient to patient. Activated B-cell and T-cell markers are more frequent in intrathyroidal lymphocyte cultures than in peripheral blood cultures.

PREVALENCE. In the United States, the prevalence of Graves' disease is uncertain. A well-designed epidemiologic survey in Wickham, in the northeast of England (population about 2800), an area thought to be representative of the United Kingdom, indicated a prevalence of 2.7%, past and present, in women and a prevalence about one tenth as frequent in men. Overall, the incidence was estimated, in women, to be 1 case per 1000 per year over a 20-year follow-up.[485] Graves' disease is the most common cause of spontaneous hyperthyroidism in patients younger than age 40, and the hazard rate does not change with age. The overall prevalence of autoimmune thyroid disease, comprising Graves' disease and autoimmune thyroiditis, approaches or exceeds that of diabetes mellitus.

Pathogenesis

PRINCIPLES OF ANTIGENIC RECOGNITION (see Chapter 7). Antibodies interact with either linear or nonlinear (conformationally dependent) areas of a target molecule called the epitope. The strength of the binding of antibodies to target antigen (the affinity of the antibody) is dependent largely on the number of binding sites the antibody has with the antigen. These sites contribute to the binding energy, which is therefore likely to be greater for large nonlinear epitopes than for small linear peptides.[486] High-affinity antibodies are therefore most likely to interact with nonlinear epitopes and to be dependent on the natural conformation of the target molecule. The T-cell receptor is also a member of the immunoglobulin receptor superfamily[487] but interacts only with a complex of antigen and HLA molecule. The CD8+ T cells recognize target antigen complexed with HLA class I molecules (A, B, and C), and CD4+ T cells recognize antigen complexed with HLA class II molecules (D, P, and Q). The antigen that interacts with T cells when complexed with autologous HLA molecules is a 15-amino-acid linear peptide derived from the whole antigen molecule.[488] Thyroid antigens are endocytosed by antigen-presenting cells (APCs), such as

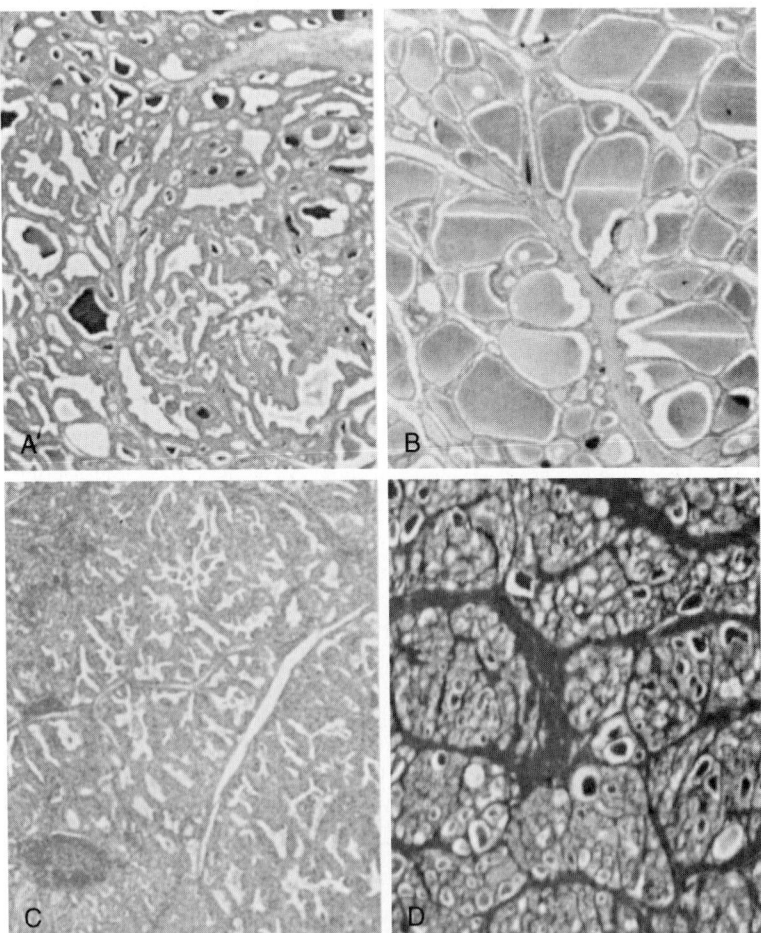

Figure 11–31. Section of thyroid gland of four patients with Graves' disease. *A*, Untreated. *B*, After therapy with potassium iodide for 3 wk. *C*, After treatment with thiouracil for 5 wk. *D*, Three months after three treatments with radioiodine. Note the marked hypertrophy and hyperplasia of the acinar cells and scant amount of colloid in sections *A*, *C*, and *D*. A lymph follicle is present in *C*. Note the broad bands of scar tissue in *D*. Section *B* is almost normal in appearance. Each patient, except the first one, was euthyroid at the time of thyroidectomy.

macrophages or dendritic cells; peptide breakdown products are then bound to HLA molecules, and the entire complex is transported to the cell surface where the peptide lies within a clearly defined binding groove within the HLA molecule.[489] In addition to the recognition of antigen (the first immune cell signal), immune cells, both T and B, also respond to secondary signals to enter an active proliferative and secretory state.[490] Cytokines originating from T cells serve as secondary B-cell signals. The most important second signals for the T cells themselves are the B7 family of cell surface molecules found on APCs such as macrophages and dendritic cells.

B cells and T cells that interact with specific antigen in the absence of the appropriate second signal are *deleted* by apoptosis, but immune cells in similar circumstances may survive in a state of *anergy* (i.e., desensitized). Hence deletion and anergy combine to help define the repertoire of immune responses in an individual.

THE AUTOIMMUNE RESPONSE. It is helpful to know whether autoimmune reactions are multireactive (representative of a secondary polyclonal immune response) or more focused, involving a restricted number of B cells and T cells.[491] In autoimmune disease a restricted immune response has been observed at the onset of the disease, and the authors discuss below some of the evidence for this in Graves' disease.

TSHR AUTOANTIBODIES. Long-acting thyroid stimulator (LATS) was discovered by Adams and Purves[492] in 1956 during a search for the thyroid-stimulating activity of Graves' disease. Patient sera stimulated radioiodine release from prelabeled guinea pig thyroid for a much longer time period than a pituitary TSH preparation. LATS was present in the IgG fraction of serum and could compete with TSH for receptor occupancy[493] and was postulated to be a TSHRAb acting as a TSH agonist. Hence in patients with Graves' disease the thyroid gland is no longer under the control of pituitary TSH but is continuously stimulated by a circulating antibody or antibodies with TSH-like activity (Fig. 11–32). As a consequence, T_3 suppression of RAIU is ineffective, and the TSH levels are suppressed and poorly responsive to TRH.

BIOACTIVITY OF TSHR ANTIBODIES. Demonstration that the self-infusion of sera from patients with Graves' disease

caused thyroid stimulation was the first demonstration of the role of TSHRAb in the induction of human hyperthyroidism.[494] Another demonstration of the in vivo effects of TSHRAb came from studies in neonates demonstrating the transplacental stimulation of the fetal thyroid in mothers with high titers of TSHRAb.[495] The TSHR antibodies demonstrate light chain restriction in many patients with Graves' disease, and those that exhibit TSH agonist bioactivity are in the IgG1 subclass, both suggesting oligoclonality.[496, 497] Autoantibodies that bind to the TSH receptor may or may not activate adenylate cyclase and may therefore be either TSHR-stimulating or TSHR-blocking[474] (see Fig. 11–24). Further complicating this issue is the fact that many patients have both TSHR-stimulating and TSHR-blocking antibodies, the degree of thyroid stimulation depending on the relative concentration and bioactivities of the different autoantibodies.[498]

PREVALENCE OF TSHRAb IN GRAVES' DISEASE. The fact that TSHR autoantibodies are detectable only in patients with autoimmune thyroid disease indicates that the autoantibodies are disease specific, in contrast to the high prevalence of TgAb and TPOAb in the normal population. Furthermore, TSHR autoantibodies are unique human autoantibodies; there are no known animal models of TSHRAb or Graves' disease. A total of 80 to 100% of untreated hyperthyroid patients with Graves' disease have detectable TSHRAb with thyroid-stimulating activity. The titers of TSHRAb are decreased by treatment of the disease[480] and, when they persist, are predictive of failure of response to antithyroid drug treatment.[499, 500] With time, TSHR-blocking autoantibodies may become the prevalent autoantibody after treatment of Graves' disease.

TSHRAb EPITOPES. The extracellular domain (ecd) of the TSHR is the major site of TSHRAb binding (see Fig. 11–24). The difference in functional activity of different TSHR autoantibodies is dependent on receptor conformation and affinity. The use of recombinant chimeric TSH/LH receptors has suggested two major regions of TSHRAb binding that may convey thyroid-stimulating activity (the NH_2-terminal end) and thyroid-blocking activity (the COOH-terminal end).[500a, 500b] Prokaryotic TSHR-ecd has also been used to identify immunogenic regions in the hTSHR-ecd, using antibodies from immunized mice and from patients with Graves' disease.[501] These data suggest that some TSHR autoantibodies also recognize linear epitopes.

CONTROL OF TSHR FUNCTION IN GRAVES' DISEASE. Like TSH, TSHR autoantibodies cause cAMP-mediated generation of thyroid hormone and Tg, uptake and release of iodine, stimulation of protein synthesis, and cell growth. Desensitization of the thyroidal cAMP response by prolonged exposure to TSHRAb can be observed in vitro but cannot be complete in vivo, or patients would not remain hyperthyroid.[502, 503] At lower levels of stimulation, the TSH receptor is positively regulated by TSH both in vivo and in vitro,[504, 505] and such resistance to desensitization by TSH may allow the hyperthyroid state to persist.

INTRATHYROIDAL T CELLS. As described earlier, T cells in patients with autoimmune thyroid disease are reactive to thyroid antigens and to peptides derived from these antigens (Fig. 11–33).[506–510] Such memory T cells enhance thyroid autoantibody secretion and may have both helper and cytotoxic T-cell activity. About 10% of activated T cells infiltrating the thyroid gland in patients with autoimmune thyroid disease proliferate in response to thyroid cell antigens.[511] Attempts to characterize intrathyroidal T cells from patients with Graves' disease as helper T subset 1 (Th1) (which secrete IL-2 and interferon γ) or Th2 helper T cells (which secrete IL-4) have been difficult.[512] However, these T cells secrete considerable amounts of interferon γ, suggesting that most CD4+ T cells may be Th1 cells.[513, 514]

T-CELL RECEPTOR V GENE REPERTOIRE. T-cell receptors

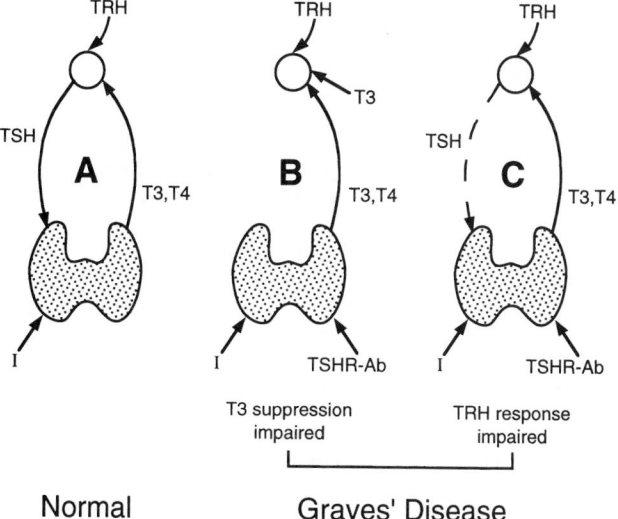

Figure 11–32. Schematic diagram of the pathophysiology of Graves' disease. *A,* TSH is normally inhibited by thyroid hormone, resulting in feedback control of thyroid hormone secretion. *B,* In the presence of stimulating TSH receptor antibodies (TSHRAb), TSH release is no longer regulated by thyroid hormone. *C,* Similarly, in the presence of stimulating TSHRAb, TRH is unable to release normal amounts of TSH. (Adapted from Hall R, Rees Smith B, Mukhtar ED. Thyroid stimulators in health and disease. Clinic Endocrinol 1975; 4:213–230.)

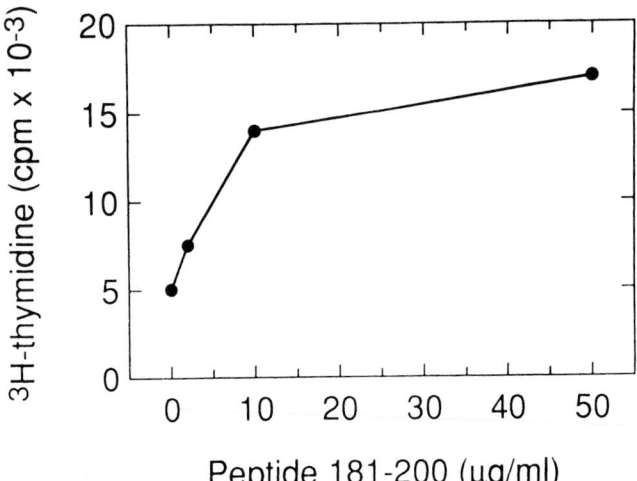

Figure 11–33. T cells from a patient with Graves' disease demonstrate a dose-related proliferative response to a TSH receptor peptide (aa 181–200). Data shown as ³H-thymidine uptake at 18 h.

(TCR) consist of two noncovalently linked chains (α and β or less commonly γ and δ), each with variable (V), diversity (D; mainly β), and junctional (J) regions (Fig. 11–34). The V, D, and J genes code for the antigen-HLA recognition site on the TCR that determines antigen specificity. In addition to the many V (more than 100) and J (more than 50) genes, random nucleotide (N) additions and deletions to the D region (the CDR3 region or N-D-N region) provide additional complexity to the TCR repertoire.[487, 515] Studies of the V_α and V_β families expressed by intrathyroidal T cells from patients with Graves' disease[516, 517] demonstrate that hTCR V gene expression by T cells from within the thyroid is different from hTCR V gene expression found in peripheral blood from the same individuals. Additional evidence has been obtained for the presence in the thyroid of clonally expanded T cells based on the presence of multiple identical sequences within the generated fragments.[518, 519] Such information further documents that Graves' disease is an antigen-driven disorder that causes oligoclonal T-cell expansion. Similar data have been obtained in rheumatoid arthritis, multiple sclerosis, and other autoimmune diseases.[520, 521]

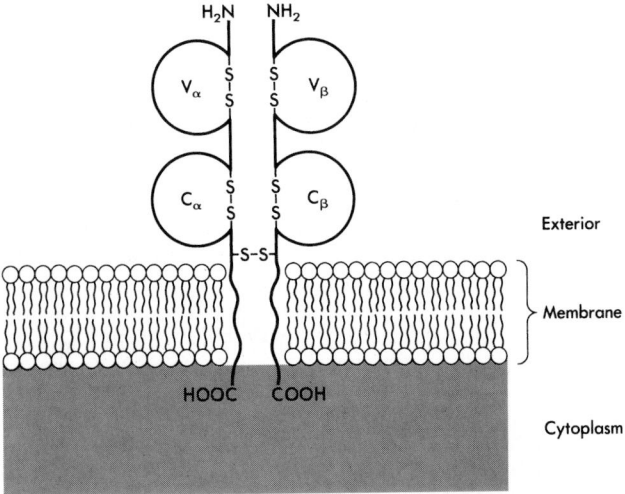

Figure 11–34. Schematic diagram of a T-cell receptor dimer showing the alpha and beta chains retained by transmembrane regions. V, variable region; C, constant region. (From Davis MM, Chien YH, Gascoigne NR, et al. A murine T cell receptor gene complex. Immunol Rev 1984; 81:235–258.)

REGULATORY T CELLS. The presence of reduced levels of circulating CD8 + (suppressor/cytotoxic) T cells in patients with Graves' disease suggested that a lack of suppressor/cytotoxic T cells might be responsible for the breakdown of tolerance in Graves' disease.[522] Whether true thyroid antigen-specific human suppressor T cells exist has been questioned,[523] but the immune system does exert some of its overall control via "regulatory" cells, including the secretion of T-cell cytokines and the suppressive influence of "anergized" T cells. In addition to regulatory cells, both positive and negative selection of T cells and B cells occurs in the thymus, and deletion of immature immune cells via antigen-initiated apoptosis takes place in the peripheral immune system.[524, 525] Deletion probably occurs when T cells and B cells see antigen in the absence of second signals, as discussed earlier. When a mature immune cell sees antigen in the absence of second signal, it may become desensitized rather than deleted, a phenomenon known as "anergy." Together, deletion and anergy account for immune suppression, but certain HLA-DR haplotypes are associated with reduced suppressor T-cell function. For example normal individuals with HLA-DR3[526, 527] have reduced suppressor activity compared with non-DR3 individuals.

Susceptibility Mechanisms

THE CONCEPT OF CRYPTIC ANTIGENIC EPITOPES. T-cell tolerance depends on self-antigens being seen in sufficient amounts to initiate continuous T-cell deletion and anergy induction. However, many self-antigens are not seen in sufficient concentrations to cause the removal of T cells that may react to them. These antigens contain what are called cryptic epitopes. Hence, T cells specific for these cryptic epitopes may be present in normal immune repertoires and become autoaggressive only if such an epitope is uncovered or increased in concentration. The question therefore is what mechanisms can cause cryptic thyroid antigens to increase.

GENETIC SUSCEPTIBILITY AND CANDIDATE GENES. Whatever the etiology, both the development and the subsequent course of Graves' disease are influenced by heredity. The role of hereditary factors is evidenced by the increased incidence in patients with Graves' disease and in members of their families of other autoimmune disorders, such as Hashimoto's disease or pernicious anemia, and of autoantibodies against endocrine tissues, gastric parietal cells, and intrinsic factor. Indeed, the propensity to develop thyroid autoantibodies appears to be an autosomal dominant trait.[528] In addition, monozygotic twins have a higher concordance rate of Graves' disease than do dizygotic twins. However, Graves' disease appears to be a polygenic disorder with a number of candidate polymorphic genetic loci that may contribute to disease susceptibility. These can be divided into thyroid-specific and non–thyroid-specific genes. The thyroid specific-group includes the TSHR and hTPO genes, and the thyroid nonspecific group includes HLA genes, the TAP (protein transporter) genes, the cytokine genes, the TCR cell receptor genes, and loci with linkage to IDDM.[529] There is an increased frequency of haplotype HLA-B8/DR3 in whites with Graves' disease, although this HLA region is unlikely to be the site of the major susceptibility genes.[530–532]

NONIMMUNE CELL EXPRESSION OF MHC ANTIGENS. The human major histocompatibility (MHC) genes are referred to as the HLA genes. Normal thyroid epithelial cells do not express HLA class II antigens, but they are expressed in thyroids from patients with autoimmune thyroid disease (Fig. 11–35; see color section between pages 875 and 877).[533] As proposed by Bottazzo and colleagues,[533] a local viral infection of the thyroid gland could cause production of interferon γ or other cytokines in the thyroid, which in turn would induce HLA class II expression. This first-time expression would lead

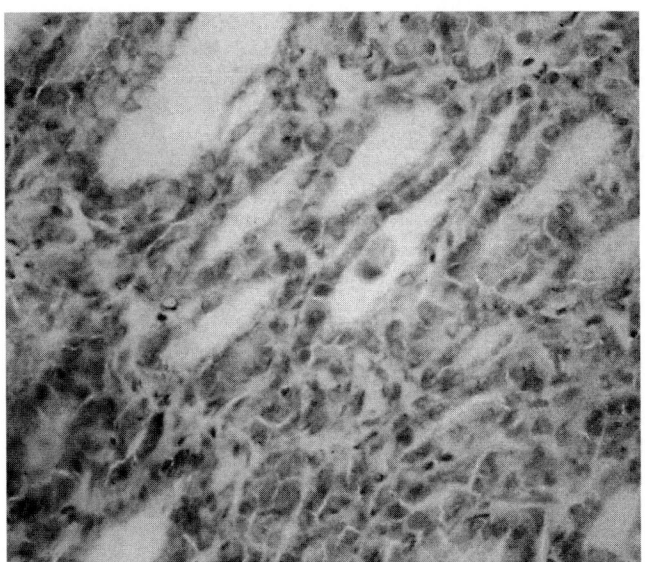

Figure 11–35. This photomicrograph of Graves' thyroid tissue is stained for HLA class II (DR) antigen expression using the immunoperoxidase technique. Note the brown thyroid epithelial cells indicating the presence of DR antigen. Note also the relative lack of lymphocytic infiltration in this region (see color section between pages 875 and 877).

to enhanced presentation of thyroid autoantigens and activation of autoreactive T cells in a susceptible individual. Support for this concept comes from the in vivo induction of MHC class II molecules on mouse thyrocytes by interferon γ that also induced autoimmune thyroiditis.[534] A number of viruses can induce MHC class II expression independent of cytokine secretion,[535] including reovirus types 1 and 3[536] and cytomegalovirus (CMV).[537]

SPECIFICITY CROSSOVER. In addition to enhanced presentation of normally cryptic thyroid antigens within the thyroid gland, T cells may become activated in other ways. Structural similarity between different antigens can lead to specificity crossover (often called molecular mimicry). Antigenic similarity between bacteria and viruses and human proteins is common, and in one study 4% of monoclonal antibodies raised against a variety of viruses cross-reacted with antigens in tissues.[538] Furthermore, mice infected with reovirus type 1 developed an autoimmune polyendocrinopathy with autoantibodies directed against normal pancreas, pituitary, thyroid, and gastric mucosa, suggesting molecular mimicry between a reoviral antigen and a common tissue antigen.[539] Molecular mimicry has also been reported between *Yersinia enterocolitica* and the TSHR based on the observed cross-reaction between sera from patients with Yersinia infection and sera from patients with Graves' diseise and between retroviral sequences and the TSH receptor.[540]

INFECTION. If infection were the cause of Graves' disease, an identifiable agent should be present in most patients, and transfer of the agent to susceptible recipients should transfer the disease. Indeed it has been suggested that Graves' disease is "associated" with infectious agents (e.g., *Y. enterocolitica*,[541, 542] but no studies meet the necessary criteria. Infections of the thyroid gland itself (e.g., subacute thyroiditis, congenital rubella) are associated with thyroid autoimmune phenomena.[543] Nevertheless a causative role for infectious agents has not been definitively demonstrated in Graves' disease, although autoimmune thyroid disease can be induced in experimental animals by certain viral infections.[543, 544] Reports of retroviral sequences in the thyroid glands of patients with Graves' disease[545–547] have not been confirmed.[545, 548, 549]

STRESS. Graves' disease frequently appears to become evident either after severe emotional stress, such as the actual or threatened separation from a loved one, or after an acute fright, such as an automobile accident. There are in fact many clinical experiences and reports associating major stress with the onset of Graves' disease, including data on the high incidence of thyrotoxicosis among refugees from Nazi prison camps.[550] Some data suggest that stress induces an overall state of immune suppression by non–antigen-specific mechanisms,[551] perhaps secondary to the effects of cortisol and corticotropin-releasing hormone (CRH) action at the level of the immune cell. Furthermore more patients with Graves' disease are said to give a history of major stresses than are control groups.[552–554] Following the acute immune suppression by stress, there is presumably an overcompensation by the immune system when suppression is released. This would precipitate autoimmune thyroid disease, as in the postpartum period during which Graves' disease may occur 3 to 9 mo after delivery.[555, 556] The rebound phenomenon would result in greater immune activity than normal and initiate disease if the individual were genetically susceptible.

GENDER AND GONADAL STEROIDS. Graves' disease is more common in women than in men (7 to 10:1) and has a tendency to become manifest during puberty, pregnancy, and the menopause. In men the disease tends to occur at a later age, to be more severe, and to be accompanied more often by ophthalmopathy. The female preponderance and the fact that the disorder is uncommon before puberty suggest that gonadal steroids may be responsible for this difference. In addition, estrogen influences the immune system, particularly the B-cell repertoire.[557, 558] During pregnancy, both T-cell and B-cell functions are diminished, and the rebound from this immunosuppression may contribute to the development of postpartum thyroid disease.[555, 556]

Pathogenesis of Graves' Orbitopathy and Dermopathy

The pathogenesis of the orbitopathy and dermopathy is unknown. The extraocular muscle tissue is swollen by the accumulation in the extracellular matrix of glycosaminoglycans that are secreted by fibroblasts under the influence of cytokines such as interferon γ from local lymphocytes (Fig. 11–36; see color section between pages 875 and 877).[559, 560] This accumulation disrupts and impairs the function of muscle. As the disease runs its course and inflammation decreases, the damaged muscles become fibrosed. Hence histologic examination shows a patchy muscle infiltrate predominantly of T cells, and some muscle cells exhibit HLA class II antigen as seen within the thyroid gland. Such T cells react in vitro with retro-orbital tissue.[561] Hence the working hypothesis is that the immune system recognizes an antigen(s) common to the thyroid and retro-orbital tissues (and skin). Such antigens may be the same molecule or a molecule similar enough to be mistaken as the same antigen by the phenomenon of "specificity crossover." Retro-orbital and dermal fibroblasts appear to be the primary site of this antigen, which has not been fully characterized.[562] Expression of TSHR mRNA by retro-orbital fibroblasts has provoked speculation that TSHR may also be involved in the pathogenesis of orbitopathy,[559] a concept that would fit with data demonstrating that patients with severe orbitopathy have the highest titers of TSHRAb. However, TSHR mRNA is found in many fibroblasts and a wide variety of cells, including lymphocytes. There is currently no convincing evidence that specific antibodies against orbital tissue contents play a primary pathogenic role.[563] More likely, antigen-specific T cells have the major role in initiating the disorder.

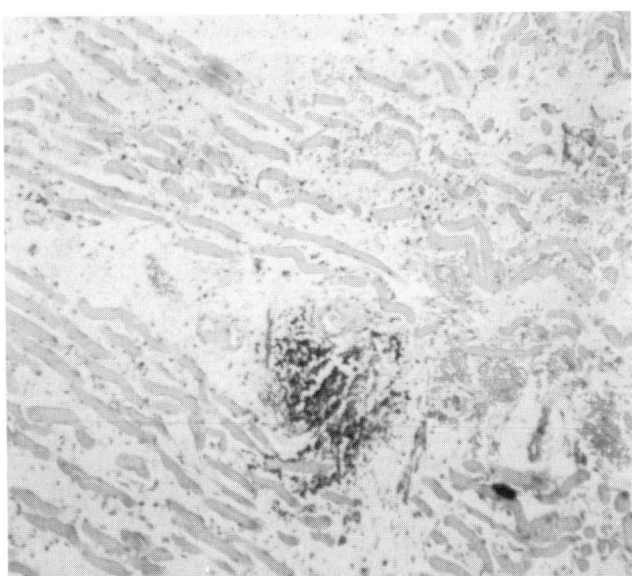

Figure 11–36. A section of extraocular muscle from a biopsy taken from a patient with severe Graves' orbitopathy. Note that within the muscle fibers is a patch of lymphocytic infiltration (see color section between pages 875 and 877). (Provided by Dr. D. Kendler, University of British Columbia, Vancouver, Canada.)

Natural History and Course of Graves' Disease

The course of the thyrotoxic component of Graves' disease is variable and often erratic. In some patients thyrotoxicosis persists, although it may vary in severity. In others, the course may be cyclic, exhibiting remissions of varying frequency, intensity, and duration. This cyclic feature has an important bearing on treatment. With the passage of months or years thyrotoxicosis tends to give way to euthyroidism. Approximately one third of patients become hypothyroid within 20 y of treatment with antithyroid agents.[564]

The orbitopathy may or may not commence together with the thyrotoxic component. Thus thyrotoxic patients may initially be free from eye disease but develop this manifestation months or years later, or not at all. Conversely the disease may begin with orbitopathy and only later, if at all, be associated with thyrotoxicosis. In euthyroid patients with orbitopathy, so-called "euthyroid Graves' disease," some show no evidence of a thyroid abnormality, as judged from tests for TSHRAb, thyroid suppressibility, or response to exogenous TRH. Others have suppressed TSH levels and thyroid nonsuppressibility. Some patients become hypothyroid within a few years, some become hyperthyroid, and others remain euthyroid. Many have evidence of chronic thyroiditis.[565] Importantly, most patients with euthyroid Graves' disease have defective thyroregulatory control and evidence of thyroid autoimmunity. In brief, the course of thyroid function in these patients is unpredictable. These considerations are important in establishing the diagnosis of thyroid-related eye disease.

Histopathology

THYROID. The designation *diffuse toxic goiter* denotes that the gland is both enlarged and uniformly affected. These glands vary in consistency from softer than normal to firm and rubbery. The outer surface is usually smooth but may be somewhat lobular; rarely, the gland is grossly nodular prior to treatment. The cut surface is red and glistening. Microscopically, the follicles are small and lined with hyperplastic columnar epithelium and contain scant colloid that displays much marginal scalloping and vacuolization (see Fig. 11–31). The nuclei are vesicular and basally located and exhibit occasional mitoses. Papillary projections of the hyperplastic epithelium extend into the lumina of the follicles. Vascularity is increased, and there is a varying infiltration by lymphocytes and plasma cells that collect in aggregates and may form germinal centers. In such regions the thyroid epithelial cells express HLA class II antigens not seen in normal thyroid and are large, perhaps due to local stimulation by TSHR autoantibodies (see Fig. 11–33) When the patient is treated with iodine, the thyroid undergoes *involution*, in which the hyperplasia and vascularity regress, the papillary projections recede, and the follicles enlarge and become filled with colloid.

EYES. In patients with infiltrative orbitopathy, the volume of orbital contents is increased because of both an increase in retrobulbar connective tissue and an increase in mass of the extraocular muscles (Fig. 11–37). Some of the increase in connective tissue is due to edema resulting from accumulation in the ground substance of hyaluronic acid and chondroitin sulfates, which are hydrophilic.[559] The extraocular muscles are swollen, and some fibers have loss of striation, fragmentation, and lymphocytic infiltration. The lacrimal glands may also be involved. Ultimately, the tissues fibrose.

SKIN. Dermopathy (Fig. 11–38; see color section between pages 875 and 877) is usually a late manifestation, and 99%

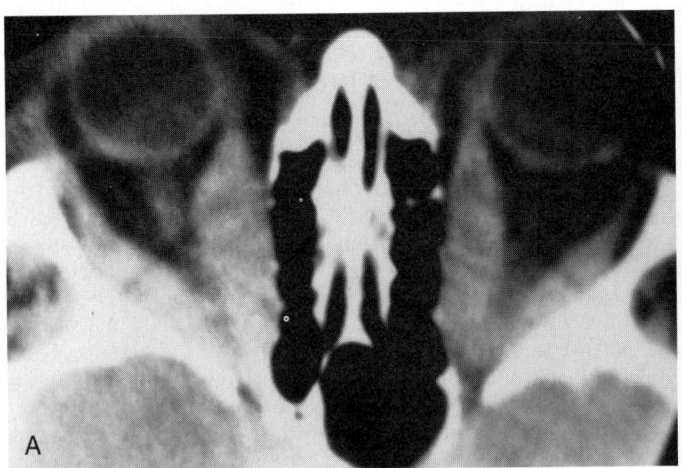
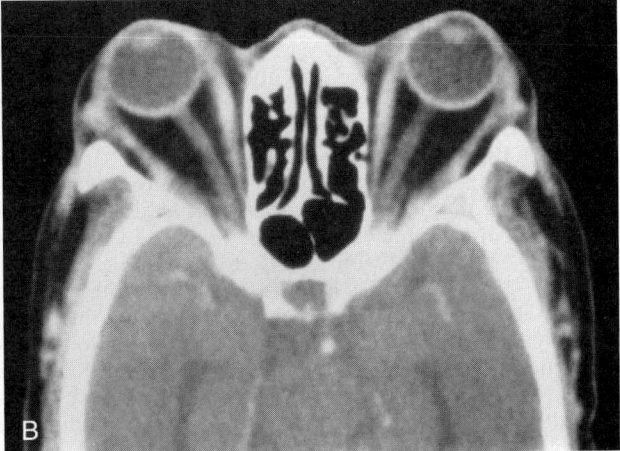

Figure 11–37. CT scans of orbits in two patients with Graves' orbitopathy. *A,* Note the obviously grossly swollen medial rectus extraocular muscles in both orbits and the resulting proptosis. *B,* The patient shows considerable proptosis with only minimal muscle enlargement, suggesting the presence of a large amount of retro-orbital fat. (Kindly provided by Dr. Peter Som, New York, NY.)

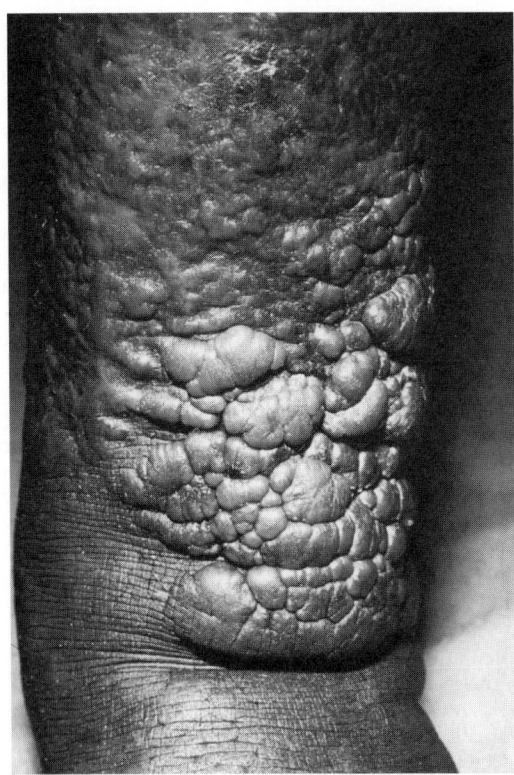

Figure 11–38. Chronic pretibial myxedema in a patient with Graves' disease and orbitopathy. The lesions are firm and nonpitting with a clear edge to feel (see color section between pages 875 and 877). (Kindly provided by Dr. Andrew Werner, New York, NY.)

of patients with infiltrative dermopathy have Graves' orbitopathy.[566] The content of hyaluronic acid and chondroitin sulfates in the dermis is increased, presumably by lymphokine activation of fibroblasts, causing compression of the dermal lymphatics and nonpitting edema[567]; the collagen fibers are separated and fragmented, and early lesions contain lymphocytic infiltrate. Nodular and plaque formation may occur in chronic lesions. The cause of the characteristic location of the dermopathy is unclear but presumably is dependent on inadequate lymphatic drainage.

Pathophysiology

All aspects of thyroid hormone economy are abnormal in patients with diffuse toxic goiter, including disruption of the regulatory control of thyroid function; alterations in thyroid function itself; changes in the concentration, binding, and metabolism of thyroid hormones; and manifestations of thyroid hormone excess in the peripheral tissues. Abnormalities in these parameters also occur in other forms of thyrotoxicosis but may differ in kind or amount.

An abnormality or override of normal regulatory control is inherent in all forms of thyrotoxicosis, as illustrated by the re-emergence of TSH secretion when thyrotoxicosis is relieved. In Graves' disease, regulatory mechanisms are overridden by the action of TSHR autoantibodies of the stimulating variety. The resulting hyperfunction of the thyroid leads to suppression of TSH secretion that is reflected in a suppressed or an undetectable serum TSH level. The basal TSH level may also be suppressed in patients with euthyroid Graves' disease (indicating the presence of mild excess of thyroid hormone) and in patients in apparent remission, indicating that thyroid hormone excess is not necessarily associated with clinical thyrotoxicosis.

In this context, the term *functional autonomy* is often misused when the intent is to imply that thyroid function is independent of TSH stimulation. True functional autonomy occurs when the thyroid is capable of functioning at a normal or an increased pace in the absence of both TSH and any other circulating thyroid stimulator. Defined in this way, functional autonomy occurs with toxic multinodular goiter and toxic adenoma but not in Graves' disease. In Graves' disease, the thyroid is controlled by an abnormal stimulator (as in molar pregnancy). When that stimulator is withdrawn—i.e., when the disease enters remission—hyperfunction subsides, and the nonautonomous nature of thyroid function becomes evident in the re-emergence of normal TSH secretion and control of thyroid function.

The disturbance of thyroid function in Graves' disease leads to hypersecretion of thyroid hormones. Thyroid avidity for iodine is enhanced, so thyroid iodide clearance is increased from its normal rate of 6 to 7 mL/min to 2 L/min in the most severe cases. The increase in iodide clearance rate reflects in past enhanced thyroid blood flow, even if extraction of iodine is assumed to be complete, and hypervascularity most likely mediated by local angiogenic factors secreted by the thyroid cells.[568] The enhanced thyroid iodide clearance rate is also due to an increase in the overall glandular mass and its unit functional activity so that iodide transport and probably organic binding are enhanced. The increase in iodide transport is partly responsible for the enhanced susceptibility of the hyperthyroid gland to the inhibitory effects of iodide on organic binding reactions. As judged from the normal ratio of iodotyrosines to iodothyronines, the rate of the coupling reaction must also be increased. The molar ratio of T_3 to T_4 in Tg is about twice normal and this increase in T_3 production cannot be ascribed to intrathyroidal iodine deficiency because the iodine content of Tg and the number of T_4 residues per molecule are normal. It may simply reflect chronic hyperstimulation of the gland.[32] The rates of turnover and release of the glandular iodine pool are increased, often greatly so. The major product of glandular secretion is T_4, but the ratio of T_3 to T_4 in the thyroid secretion is increased in proportion to the overproduction of T_3. In some instances, T_3 appears to be the major secretory product, so that the serum T_3 level is increased while serum T_4 concentration is within the normal range (T_3 toxicosis). Direct secretion of rT_3 may augment the increase in serum rT_3 concentration due to enhanced generation from T_4 in peripheral tissue.

The proportion of total plasma T_4 and T_3 in the free or unbound state is increased (see Fig. 11–20) both because of a slight decrease in concentration of TBG and because of the increase in the concentration of T_4. The fractional turnover rates of T_4 and T_3 are increased, leading to increased amounts of hormone in the peripheral pool and to an increase in total daily turnover of T_4 and T_3. In severe cases, this rate may increase from the normal of about 100 nmol T_4 and 50 nmol T_3/d to more than 600 nmol/d for both hormones. The total daily disposal of T_3 is disproportionately increased relative to that of T_4, indicating that the production rate of T_3 is disproportionately increased, probably owing to both a preferential increase in thyroid secretion of T_3 and increased peripheral conversion of T_4 to T_3.

Clinical Picture

Graves' disease is most common in the third and fourth decades of life, is rare before the age of 10 years, and occurs in the elderly, sometimes in an "apathetic" form. Like other thyroid diseases, it is more common in women, approximately 7 to 10:1. The features include diffuse goiter, thyrotoxicosis, infiltrative orbitopathy, and occasionally infiltrative dermopathy. Because the orbitopathy and dermopathy may be independent of other manifestations, they will be discussed separately.

Hyperthyroidism of Graves' Disease

Thyroid enlargement is the most common manifestation of Graves' disease but on occasion may be absent. The signs and symptoms usually begin gradually and include nervousness, irritability, palpitation, fatigue, heat intolerance, weight loss, and change in menstrual pattern. A single symptom or sign may predominate (Table 11–15). Enlargement of the thyroid may cause only a sense of fullness in the neck or obstructive symptoms. In about one third of cases, ocular manifestations begin coincidentally with thyrotoxicosis. Symptoms may remain mild or moderate or progress to a florid state characterized by aggravation of the foregoing symptoms, together with weakness, insomnia, voracious appetite, and excessive sweating, so-called *accelerated thyrotoxicosis.*

Nervousness, the most common symptom, may be manifested as a feeling of apprehension and inability to concentrate. Emotional lability and irritability can lead to difficulty in interpersonal relationships and to crying. Fatigue limits the desire of the patient to be continuously active. On the patient's climbing stairs weakness is striking, and all activities can produce breathlessness. Heat intolerance and sweating may be a cause of family discord. The patient prefers a cool environment and may lower the thermostat, open the windows, sleep with fewer blankets, or kick off the covers while asleep. The patient usually prefers winter to summer and finds hot weather intolerable. Oligomenorrhea with a variable intermenstrual period can occasionally progress to amenorrhea. Diarrhea is uncommon, but increased frequency of bowel movements and softening of the stools are common. Palpitations may be continuous or episodic, suggesting paroxysmal arrhythmia. Mitral valve prolapse is more common than in the normal population and may be one reason for frequent palpitations.[451, 569] Although weight loss is common despite an increase in appetite, the occasional patient gains weight, and the appetite may be decreased. Women may note excessive fineness of the hair and inability to hold a wave. The skin may become more pigmented. Itching may be present, and urticaria can develop, sometimes on exposure to the sun. Development of urticarial rash on exposure to the sun may occur only when patients are taking propylthiouracil. The ocular manifestations of thyrotoxicosis per se, and not Graves'

orbitopathy, are due to spasm and retraction of the eyelids and are noted as a bright-eyed (or fish-eyed) staring appearance.

This symptom complex may develop over a period of months or even years before the patient is first seen or may be fulminant in its emergence, the full picture developing within a few weeks or less. In such patients emotional stress may be a forerunner. In patients with pre-existing heart disease, mild or moderate thyrotoxicosis may precipitate heart failure, which dominates the clinical picture. In others severe weakness and wasting of muscles are the major manifestations, often designated "masked" or "apathetic" hyperthyroidism. This term implies that the typical features of thyrotoxicosis are absent, but a careful history and examination usually reveal that this is not the case.

The physical findings are manifold. Apart from the goiter and eye signs, which in themselves may establish the diagnosis, the appearance and behavior may be virtually pathognomonic; namely exaggerated alertness, fidgeting, quick response to questions or commands, and flushed appearance.

The thyroid is enlarged in most patients; thyrotoxicosis in Graves' disease occurs in a gland of normal size in about 3% of patients, and in the elderly goiter may be absent in 20%. The thyroid is most commonly two to three times normal and may be massively enlarged. The consistency varies from soft to firm and rubbery. The enlargement is usually symmetrical, but the right lateral lobe may be larger than the left. The surface is generally smooth but may feel lobular. In severe cases a thrill may be felt, usually over the upper poles, and a thrill is always accompanied by an audible bruit. The thrills and bruits are due to increased blood flow and are usually continuous but sometimes are present only in systole. The bruit is most easily detected at the upper or lower poles and should not be confused with a venous hum or murmur arising from the base of the heart. A thrill or bruit is suggestive, but not pathognomonic, of hyperthyroidism.

Spasm and retraction of the eyelids lead to widening of the palpebral fissure so that the sclera are exposed above the superior margin of the limbus. Lid retraction may be asymmetrical. When the patient looks downward the upper lid lags behind the globe, exposing more sclera, and when the patient gazes upward the globe lags behind the lid (lid lag and globe lag). The movements of the lids are jerky and spasmodic, and the lightly closed lids may have a tremor.

The remaining peripheral manifestations of thyrotoxicosis are described in a previous section; they include warm, smooth, moist texture of the skin; Plummer's nails; signs of a hyperdynamic circulation; tremor of the hands and tongue; muscular wasting; and a rapid reflex response.

In general, men tend to develop the disease at a somewhat older age than women, and although the degree of thyroid hyperfunction is often more severe in men, symptoms may be less severe. Men are prone to developing myopathy and severe orbitopathy. In older patients the circulatory manifestations may predominate, while the nervous manifestations are lacking or minimal. Orbitopathy is less common in elderly patients, who are more likely to develop muscular weakness, prostration, and anorexia (apathetic hyperthyroidism).

Manifestations of Infiltrative Orbitopathy and Dermopathy

DIFFERENTIAL DIAGNOSIS. Eye changes are major and usually a specific manifestation of Graves' disease. As noted, the ocular changes that are more proximately related to the disease process pose serious problems in treatment and prognosis and must be separated from ocular changes that result from thyrotoxicosis per se. The former is called *infiltrative orbitopathy* or *ophthalmyopathy.* The thyrotoxic ocular manifestations have already been described; if present alone these mani-

TABLE 11–15. Manifestations of Thyrotoxicosis

Symptom	%	Symptom	%
Nervousness	99	Increased appetite	65
Increased sweating	91	Eye complaints	54
Hypersensitivity to heat	89	Swelling of legs	35
Palpitation	89	Hyperdefecation (without diarrhea)	33
Fatigue	88	Diarrhea	23
Weight loss	85	Anorexia	9
Tachycardia	82	Constipation	4
Dyspnea	75	Weight gain	2
Weakness	70		

Sign	%	Sign	%
Tachycardia*	100	Eye signs	71
Goiter†	100	Atrial fibrillation	10
Skin changes	97	Splenomegaly	10
Tremor	97	Gynecomastia	10
Bruit over thyroid	77	Liver palms	8

*In other studies, thyrotoxic patients with normal pulse rate have been observed.
†Data in this table from Williams RH. Thiouracil treatment of thyrotoxicosis. J Clin Endocrinol 1946; 6:1–22. In the experience of the present authors, enlargement of the thyroid is lacking in approximately 3% of patients with thyrotoxicosis.

festations abate when the thyrotoxicosis is relieved. Infiltrative orbitopathy, on the other hand, may follow an independent course from the thyrotoxic manifestations and is often uninfluenced by their treatment (Figs. 11–39 to 11–41). Infiltrative orbitopathy is evident in about 50% of patients, but ultrasonographic, CT, or MRI examination of the orbits reveals changes, such as swelling of extraocular muscles and increased retroorbital fat, in virtually all patients with Graves' disease, including those in whom the clinical changes are minimal or absent (see Fig. 11–37).[570, 571] Occasionally, infiltrative ophthalmopathy occurs in the absence of diffuse toxic goiter (euthyroid Graves' disease).

SIGNS AND SYMPTOMS. The disease symptoms and signs of infiltrative ophthalmopathy may appear in varying combinations. Early symptoms and signs include a sense of irritation in the eyes, resembling that caused by a foreign body, and excessive tearing that is often made worse by exposure to air or wind, especially if exophthalmos is present. The conjunctivae may be injected. Exophthalmos is frequently asymmetrical and may cause a feeling of pressure behind the globes. When exophthalmos is pronounced, the eyes may not close during sleep, a condition termed *lagophthalmos*. Exophthalmos may be masked by periorbital edema, which is a common accompaniment and source of complaint. Patients frequently describe blurred vision and easy tiring of the eyes. Double vision may occur in combination with the foregoing symptoms or alone. In severe cases visual acuity may be decreased or lost, and the corneas may ulcerate or become infected.

PHYSICAL EXAMINATION. The ocular findings are variable (see Fig. 11–40). Exophthalmos is usually bilateral and is often asymmetrical. True unilateral exophthalmos is uncommon but can occur in the absence of thyrotoxicosis; the other eye usually becomes affected eventually. In following the course of the disease, the degree of exophthalmos must be measured objectively with the Hertel or Luedde exophthalmometer. These instruments permit measurement of the distance between the lateral angle of the bony orbit and an imaginary perpendicular tangent to the most anterior part of the cornea. Generally the upper limit of normal is 20 mm, although in African Americans 22 mm is normal. In severe exophthalmos

readings may be as high as 30 mm. To obtain an estimate of the degree of exophthalmos, the physician stands behind the seated patient and looks downward from above to ascertain the extent to which the eyes protrude beyond the plane of the forehead. The lids are often reddened, and enlarged lacrimal glands may cause a bulging of the surface of the eyelids. The extent to which the upper and lower lids can be completely apposed should be determined, because failure of apposition promotes drying and ulceration of the cornea. Injection of the bulbar conjunctiva may be accompanied by edema or frank chemosis, in which the edematous conjunctiva bulges from under the lids and around the corneal limbus. Weakness of the extraocular muscles is evident in the patient's inability to achieve or maintain convergence. Upward gaze and especially superolateral gaze may be limited. Occasionally upward gaze is paralyzed; in such cases, that neck is extended and the head is tilted backward to make possible a field of vision above the horizontal. Rarely, downward or inward gaze is impaired. Ophthalmoplegia usually occurs in association with other signs of infiltrative ophthalmopathy but may occur alone. In some cases only a single muscle is affected (see Fig. 11–41).

Some indication of the severity of the ophthalmopathy is provided by an assessment of intraorbital tension, which can be assessed with a specially devised instrument (orbitonometer) or by clinical assessment by having the patient close the eyes lightly and determining the ease with which the globe can be displaced posteriorly by pressure from the thumb. The manifestations of extreme orbitopathy can be catastrophic and include subluxation of the globe. Blindness may result from ulceration or infection of the cornea secondary to incomplete apposition of the lids or to optic nerve ischemia due to reduced blood flow caused by increased intraorbital pressure. Ophthalmoscopic examination may reveal venous congestion and papilledema; these may be accompanied by visual field defects.

CLASSIFICATION AND OBJECTIVE ASSESSMENT OF GRAVES' ORBITOPATHY. The eye changes of Graves' disease have been classified by the American Thyroid Association using a mnemonic system in which the first letters of each category constitute the term *NOSPECS* (Table 11–16). NO

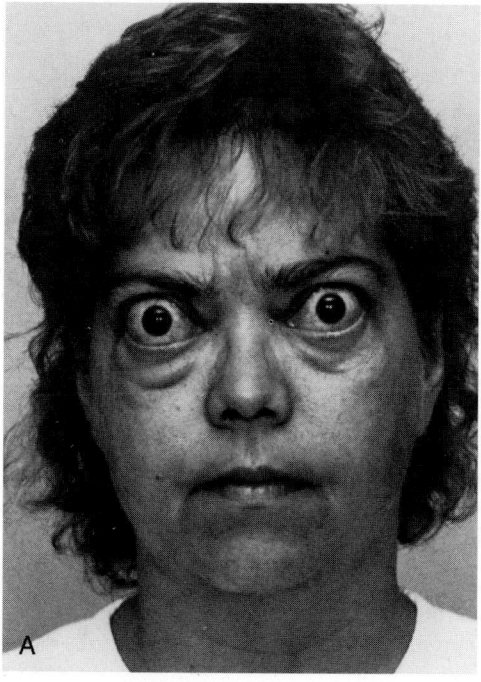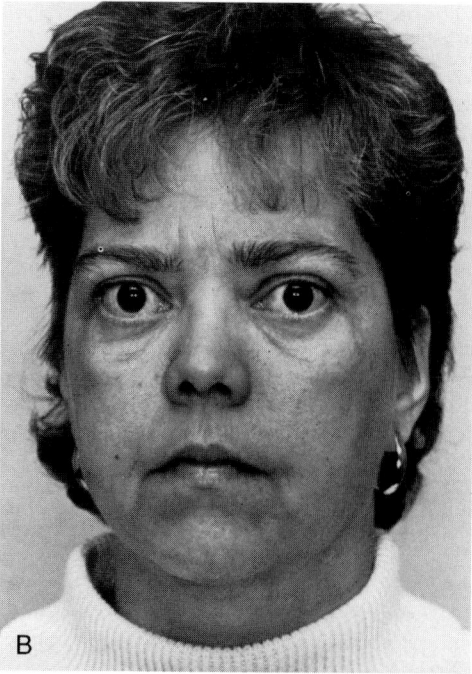

Figure 11–39. Characteristic signs of Graves' orbitopathy *(A)* subsequently corrected by orbital decompression surgery *(B)*. Note the thyroid stare, the asymmetry, the proptosis, and the periorbital edema prior to correction. (Kindly provided by Dr. Jack Rootman, University of British Colombia, Vancouver, Canada.)

A

B

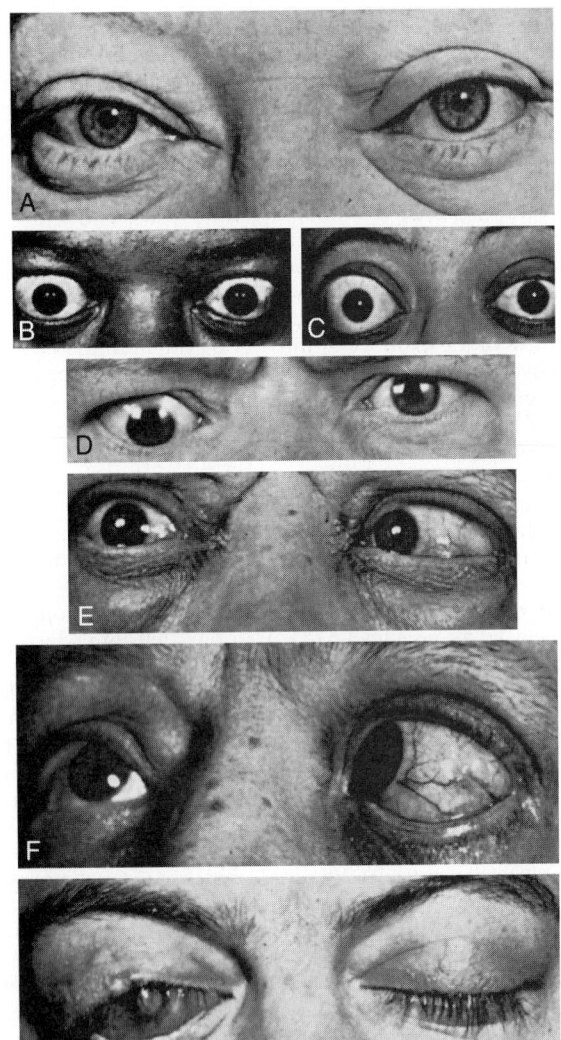

Figure 11–40. Graves' orbitopathy. *A,* Palpebral edema. This patient's eyes protruded anteriorly 1 cm more than normal, but there is no "pop-eye" appearance, owing to edema of the surrounding structures. *B,* Marked widening of palpebral fissures; slight palpebral swelling. *C,* Unequal degrees of ophthalmopathy. *D,* Unilateral lid retraction. *E,* Palpebral swelling, presumably because of fat pads and edema; paralysis of right external rectus muscle. *F,* Marked conjunctival injection and chemosis, together with ophthalmoplegia. *G,* Failure to close lids on right because of marked exophthalmos, corneal scarring, and panophthalmitis; the eye had to be enucleated.

connotes the absence or a mild degree of involvement. SPECS represents the more serious degrees of involvement. NO-SPECS and the numerical indices derived from it are useful as a memory tool for physical examination. The system is less satisfactory for objective assessment of orbital changes.[572] Objective measurements for each eye separately should include documentation of maximum lid fissure width, assessment of exposure keratitis with rose bengal or fluorescein, quantitation of extraocular muscle function (with the use of the Hess chart or Maddox rod test), measurement of intraocular pressure, and measurements of visual acuity, fields and color vision. An overall ACTIVITY SCORE is helpful in the follow-up of such patients and can be determined by assigning 1 point for the presence of spontaneous retrobulbar pain, pain on eye movement, eyelid erythema, conjunctival injection, chemosis, swelling of the caruncle, or eyelid edema or fullness. The range is, therefore, 0 to 7. More sophisticated orbitopathy indices require careful assessment for their reproducibility (Table 11–17).[573]

TABLE 11–16. American Thyroid Association Classification of Eye Changes of Graves' Disease

Class	Definition
0	*No physical signs or symptoms*
1	*Only signs, no symptoms (signs limited to upper lid retraction, stare, lid lag, and proptosis to 22 mm)*
2	*Soft tissue involvement (symptoms and signs)*
3	*Proptosis > 22 mm*
4	*Extraocular muscle involvement*
5	*Corneal involvement*
6	*Sight loss (optic nerve involvement)*

INFILTRATIVE DERMOPATHY. Dermopathy occurs in 5 to 10% of Graves' patients and is almost always accompanied by infiltrative orbitopathy, usually of severe degree. These lesions cause hyperpigmented, nonpitting induration of the skin of the legs, commonly over the pretibial area (pretibial myxedema) and the dorsa of the feet, usually in the form of individual nodules and plaques but occasionally becoming confluent with a smooth characteristic edge or shoulder (see Fig. 11–38). Rarely, lesions develop on the face, elbows, or dorsa of the hands. Clubbing of the digits is occasionally associated with long-standing thyrotoxicosis (thyroid acropachy; Fig. 11–42; see color section between pages 875 and 877).

Laboratory Tests

In moderate or severe Graves' disease, laboratory findings are consonant with the pathophysiology. The serum TSH level is almost totally suppressed and serum T_4 and T_3 levels are increased. The free T_4 and free T_3 indices are increased more than are the T_4 and T_3 levels (see Fig. 11–20). The serum T_3 concentration is typically more elevated than the serum T_4 level. The increase in thyroid iodide clearance rate is reflected

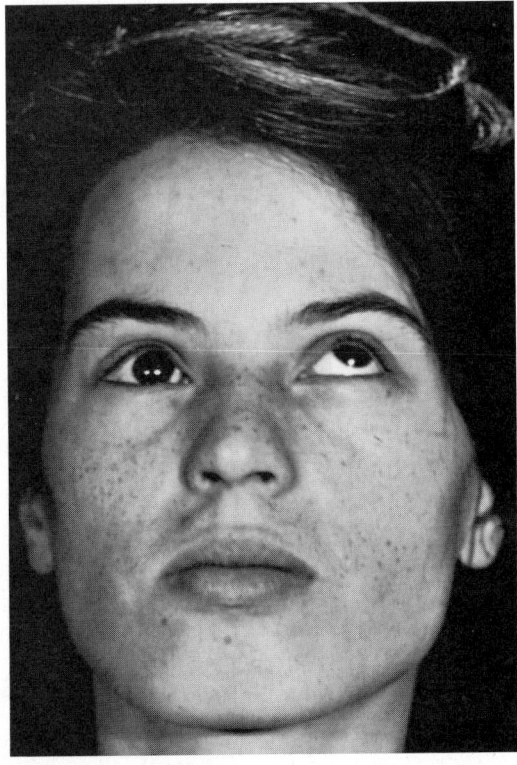

Figure 11–41. Ophthalmoplegia in Graves' disease. Other than slight conjunctival injection, the only ocular abnormality was paralysis of upward gaze on the right in this woman with severe Graves' disease.

TABLE 11–17. Assessment of Severity of Eye Disease by Orbitopathy Activity Score

Degree of Involvement	Score
Soft tissue inflammation	
slight	1
moderate	2
severe	3
Exophthalmos (mm)	
16	0.2
17	0.4
18	0.6
19	0.8
20	1
21	2
22	3
≥23	4
Palpebral aperture (mm)	
8	0.15
9	0.45
10	0.75
11	1.05
12	1.35
13	1.65
14	1.95
15	2.25
16	2.55
17	2.85
18	3
Differential IOP (mm Hg)	
1	0.1
2	0.2
3	0.3
4	0.4
5	0.5
6	0.6
7	0.7
8	0.8
9	0.9
10	1.0
Diplopia	
intermittent	1
inconstant	2
constant	3
Cornea	
initial lesions	1
ulcers	2
clouding/perforation	3
Optic neuropathy	
abnormal VEP	3
VA = 0.5–0.9	5
VA = 0.1–0.4	7
VA < 0.1	9

IOP, intraocular pressure; VEP, visual evoked potentials; VA, visual acuity.
From Perros P, Crombie AL, Matthews JNS, et al. Age and gender influence the severity of thyroid-associated ophthalmopathy: a study of 101 patients attending a combined thyroid-eye clinic. Clin Endocrinol 1993; 38:367–372, with permission.

in the increased RAIU. In patients with severe accompanying illness, conversion of T_4 to T_3 may be impaired, permitting the return to normal of the serum T_3 concentration but usually not the free T_4 (T_4 toxicosis); a similar effect on the relation between serum T_4 and T_3 levels can be seen in patients with diffuse toxic goiter who have been exposed to iodine. Occasionally, the discrepancy between T_4 and T_3 levels is exaggerated, the serum T_4 concentration being normal and the serum T_3 concentration alone being elevated (T_3 toxicosis). In this circumstance, the RAIU may be within the normal range.

The physiological basis of these tests and the manner in which they are affected by factors other than thyroid disease have been discussed earlier. Some practical aspects of the use of the tests in the diagnosis of Graves' disease deserve emphasis. It is neither desirable nor feasible that all the major laboratory tests be used to make the diagnosis. Documentation that TSH is suppressed by an appropriate assay establishes or excludes the diagnosis of hyperthyroidism in most cases and excludes the possibility of TSH-induced hyperthyroidism (see later). However, since there are other causes of suppressed TSH, such as depression and hypothalamic-pituitary disease (see Table 11–9), and to exclude the possibility that an increase in serum T_4 concentration is the result of an increase in hormone binding in the blood, measurement of either the free T_4 concentration or the FT_4I should be made. When values for serum total or free T_4 concentrations are not increased, serum T_3 or FT_3I should be measured to exclude T_3 thyrotoxicosis.

The diagnostic accuracy of the RAIU in hyperthyroidism does not approach that of measuring the TSH plus FT_4I (FT_3I) levels. Therefore measurement of RAIU is not useful in straightforward Graves' disease but is useful for excluding thyrotoxicosis not due to hyperthyroidism. Very low values of the RAIU in association with thyrotoxicosis signal the presence of *thyrotoxicosis factitia*, ectopic thyroid tissue, subacute thyroiditis, or the thyrotoxic phase of autoimmune (silent) thyroiditis. A low value may also alert one to unsuspected iodine-induced hyperthyroidism, in which, of course, production of hormone by the thyroid gland is indeed increased.

In subtle or mild cases of thyrotoxicosis, laboratory tests are most important, particularly when values are only slightly abnormal. With the improved sensitivity of the immunometric TSH assay, there is now no indication for the TRH stimulation test. In the appropriate clinical setting, a TSH concentration of less than 0.2 mU/L is virtually pathognomonic of an excessive thyroid hormone supply. A value between 0.2 and 0.4 mU/L suggests a supranormal exposure to thyroid hormones but not a condition likely to be associated with significant clinical manifestations.

The presence of TSHRAb of the stimulating variety in the serum is diagnostic of Graves' disease but does not always correlate with the clinical state. Measurement of TSHRAb is particularly useful in two situations. In pregnant patients very high levels of TSHRAb raise the likelihood of neonatal thyrotoxicosis in the offspring; in patients on long-term antithyroid drug therapy, the continued presence of TSHRAb augurs badly for a long-term remission after withdrawal of therapy.

Differential Diagnosis

The patient with major manifestations of Graves' disease, namely thyrotoxicosis, goiter, and infiltrative orbitopathy, does not pose a diagnostic problem. In some patients, however, one of the major manifestations either dominates the clinical picture or is present alone, and the disorder may mimic other disease. Because the major manifestations differ, the conditions from which they require differentiation will be considered separately.

The Thyroid Disease

The disorder that most frequently simulates thyrotoxicosis is an anxiety state with fatigue, palpitations, nervous irritability, and insomnia. Fatigue differs from that in thyrotoxicosis in that it is not accompanied by a desire to be active. The patient is listless and often feels tired on awakening. Tachycardia is common during examination of the anxiety patient, but the sleeping pulse rate is normal. The palms are cool and clammy, rather than warm and moist. Hyperreflexia is present in both disorders. *Chronic obstructive pulmonary disease* may require differentiation from thyrotoxicosis when retention of carbon dioxide may lead to a warm, flushed skin, tremulousness, and a bounding pulse. Mild exophthalmos may also be present.

Pheochromocytoma may mimic thyrotoxicosis by causing tachycardia and hypermetabolism (see Chapter 13). Other similarities include nervous irritability, eyelid retraction, trem-

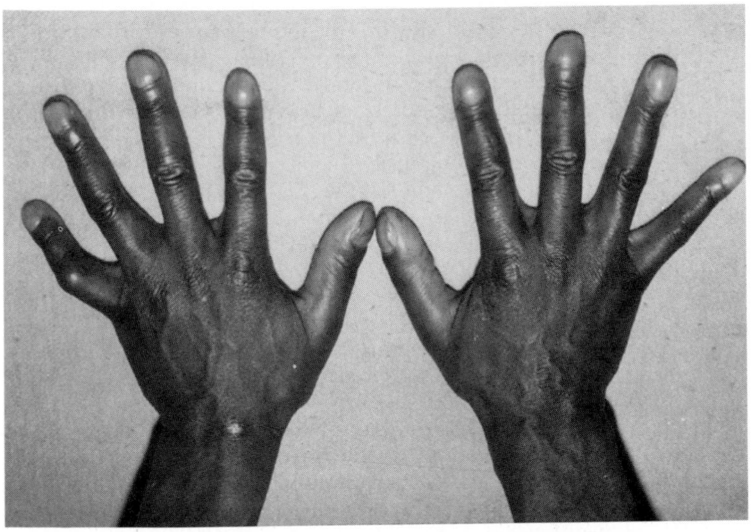

Figure 11–42. Rare thyroid acropachy in a patient with Graves' disease. The hypermetabolic state leads to axial bone destruction, presumably secondary to enhanced osteoclast activity. Not to be confused with clubbing, which is usually painless (see color section between pages 875 and 877). (Kindly provided by Dr. Andrew Werner, New York, NY.)

ulousness, and excessive sweating. Weight loss may occur despite a good appetite, and hyperglycemia can cause glucosuria. However, diastolic hypertension is often present in the patient with pheochromocytoma (as opposed to reduced diastolic pressure in thyrotoxicosis), and urinary excretion of vanillylmandelic acid, metanephrine, and catecholamines is increased. In the patient with pheochromocytoma, goiter is absent, and the laboratory indices of thyroid function are almost always normal.

In *diabetes mellitus*, weight loss despite a good appetite, muscle wasting, and occasionally diarrhea may suggest thyrotoxicosis, but other features of thyrotoxicosis are absent. However, the incidence of thyroid disease in patients with diabetes mellitus is higher than in the general population.

Myeloproliferative disorders may be accompanied by signs of hypermetabolism, such as sweating, weight loss, and tachycardia, especially if anemia is present. Goiter is absent, and laboratory indices of thyroid function are normal.

Cirrhosis of the liver may require differentiation from thyrotoxicosis because patients with cirrhosis often display weight loss, excessive sweating, a bounding pulse, and occasionally mild exophthalmos. Furthermore the RAIU may be increased in cirrhosis as a result of iodine deficiency secondary to inadequate intake. However, serum TSH and T_4 concentrations are normal, serum T_3 concentration is often low, and goiter is generally absent.

Thyrotoxic myopathy may resemble progressive muscular atrophy or polymyositis. In *progressive muscular atrophy*, fasciculation is present and the deep tendon jerks are diminished or absent, and in *polymyositis* muscle biopsy discloses inflammatory and degenerative changes. In both progressive muscular atrophy and polymyositis, other features of thyrotoxicosis are lacking, and laboratory indices of thyroid function are normal.

The diffuse goiter of Graves' disease may rarely be confused with that of other thyroid diseases if thyrotoxicosis is present. In subacute thyroiditis, particularly the painless variant, asymmetry of the gland, tenderness, and systemic evidence of inflammation assist in the diagnosis. The subnormal RAIU distinguishes this disease from Graves' disease. When Graves' disease is in a latent or inactive phase and thyrotoxicosis is absent, the goiter may require exclusion of Hashimoto's thyroiditis or simple nontoxic goiter as possible diagnoses. The goiter of Hashimoto's disease is somewhat lobulated and firmer and rubbery compared with that of Graves' disease. Serum titers of thyroid antibodies are generally higher in Hashimoto's disease but may not be helpful in distinguishing individual patients. In the absence of thyrotoxicosis the diffuse goiter of Graves' disease cannot be distinguished from nontoxic, or simple, goiter. An abnormal serum TSH concentration and the presence of TSHRAb indicate underlying Graves' disease, but their absence does not exclude the diagnosis.

The Eye Disease

The orbitopathy of Graves' disease, if bilateral and associated with thyrotoxicosis past or present, does not require differentiation from exophthalmos of other origin. However, unilateral exophthalmos, even when associated with thyrotoxicosis, should alert the physician to the possibility of a local cause. Other diseases that may produce either unilateral or bilateral exophthalmos include orbital neoplasms, carotid-cavernous sinus fistulae, cavernous sinus thrombosis, infiltrative disorders affecting the orbit, and pseudotumor of the orbit. Mild bilateral exophthalmos, generally without infiltrative signs, is occasionally present on a familial basis and also sometimes occurs in patients with Cushing's syndrome, cirrhosis, uremia, chronic obstructive pulmonary disease, and the superior vena cava syndrome. Ophthalmoplegia as the sole manifestation of the orbitopathy of Graves' disease requires exclusion of diabetes mellitus and other disorders affecting the brain stem and its connections. The demonstration of swelling of the extraocular muscles by orbital ultrasonography or CT[570, 571] is diagnostic of Graves' orbitopathy, as is the detection of TSHRAb in serum or the demonstration of a suppressed TSH.

Treatment of Hyperthyroidism

It is not yet possible to treat the basic pathogenetic factors in Graves' disease. Existing therapies for both the thyrotoxic and the ophthalmopathic manifestations are palliative in that they may relieve but do not cure the disease.

The lack of general agreement as to which therapy is the best is due to the fact that none is ideal, as reflected in the treatment guidelines of the American Thyroid Association.[574] Because the therapeutic problems posed by thyrotoxicosis and orbitopathy differ and because they run independent courses, their treatments will be discussed separately. Treatment of thyrotoxicosis is designed to impose restraint on hormone secretion either by means of chemical agents that inhibit hormone synthesis or release or by reducing the quantity of thyroid tissue.

Antithyroid Agents

The mechanisms of action of the various antithyroid drugs are discussed in the section on formation and secretion of thyroid hormones.

IODIDE TRANSPORT INHIBITORS. Both thiocyanate and perchlorate inhibit thyroid iodide transport, but as discussed earlier, theoretical and practical disadvantages attend their use except in special circumstances.

THIONAMIDES. The major agents for treating thyrotoxicosis are drugs of the thionamide class (see Fig. 11–4), most commonly propylthiouracil, methimazole, and carbimazole.[575] These agents inhibit the oxidation and organic binding of thyroid iodide and therefore produce intrathyroidal iodine deficiency that further increases the ratio of T_3 to T_4 in the thyroid secretion, as reflected in the high T_3/T_4 ratio in the serum. In addition propylthiouracil, but not methimazole, impairs the conversion of T_4 to T_3 by D1 in the peripheral tissues (see Fig. 11–9). Because of this additional action, propylthiouracil may provide rapid alleviation of severe thyrotoxicosis (Fig. 11–43).[41, 575–577]

The half-life in plasma of methimazole is about 6 h, whereas that of propylthiouracil is about 1 1/2 hours. However, both drugs are accumulated by the thyroid, and a single 30-mg dose of methimazole may exert an antithyroid effect for longer than 24 h. This provides a rational basis for the single-daily-dose regimen of methimazole for mild or moderate thyrotoxicosis.[578] The propylthiouracil concentration in serum correlates with the extent of blockade of organic binding of iodine within the thyroid.[575] These drugs cross the placenta and can inhibit thyroid function in the fetus. Methimazole may cross the placenta more readily than propylthiouracil (see later section on hyperthyroidism and thyrotoxicosis in pregnancy).

Immunosuppressive Action of Thionamides. Thionamide drugs may also directly influence the immune response in patients with autoimmune thyroid disease.[477] This action occurs within the thyroid where the drugs are concentrated and involves immunosuppresive mechanisms. First, the action on the thyroid cells themselves decreases thyroid antigen expression, and decreases prostaglandin and cytokine release from thyroid cells with a subsequent impairment of the autoimmune response.[480, 579, 580] Second, thionamides inhibit the generation of oxygen radicals in T cells, B cells, and particularly the antigen-presenting cells and hence may cause a decline in thyroid autoantibody titers.[581] The clinical importance of immunosuppression compared with inhibition of thyroid hormone formation is unclear.

Use of Thionamides. The initial dose of propylthiouracil most commonly employed is 200 mg given orally every 8 h. An equivalent dose of methimazole is 20 mg every 12 h. Carbimazole, which is converted to methimazole in vivo and is equivalent in potency, is not used in the United States. These doses are effective in most patients, but in some no therapeutic response is seen, and in some patients doses of up to 1200 mg propylthiouracil or an equivalent amount of methimazole daily may be required. It is unlikely that a true state of complete resistance to these agents ever occurs. The higher doses are required in patients with severe thyrotoxicosis and large thyroid glands, possibly because of more rapid degradation of the drug within the gland or extrathyroidally. When large amounts are required, doses should be administered at 4- to 6-h intervals.

The therapeutic response to effective antithyroid therapy invariably occurs after a latent period because the agents inhibit the synthesis but not the release of hormone; hence reduction in the supply of hormone to the tissues does not occur until glandular hormone stores are depleted (see Figs. 11–31 and 11–43). Although propylthiouracil differs from methimazole in having the additional effect of inhibiting the peripheral conversion of T_4 to T_3, there appears to be little difference in the duration of the latent period when either of these agents is employed alone in the usual dosage because the extrathyroidal effect of propylthiouracil on conversion of T_4 to T_3 is more apparent at dosages greater than 600 mg/d. This effect may be an advantage in the acute treatment of severe hyperthyroidism.[41] Factors that influence the duration of the latent period include the quantity of hormone initially stored in the thyroid, its inherent rate of release, and the effectiveness of blockade of new hormone synthesis achieved. In the thyroid rich in iodine, as when the patient has received medications containing iodine, the clinical response to antithyroid agents may be delayed for months. As would be expected, the latent period is shortened by administration of large doses (more than 600 mg daily of propylthiouracil), and such doses should be given when a more rapid therapeutic response is required. Generally, improvement within the first 2 wk includes decreased nervousness and palpitations, increased strength, and weight gain. Usually, the metabolic state becomes normal within about 6 wk. At this time, the dosage can often be reduced substantially to maintain a normal metabolic state.

During treatment the size of the thyroid decreases in one third to one half of the patients. In the remainder it may remain unchanged or enlarge. The latter change signals either an intensification of the disease process, which often requires that the dosage of drug be increased, or the production of hypothyroidism and increased TSH secretion as a result of excessive dosage. It is important to differentiate between these causes. Clinical criteria are the main guidelines by which the adequacy of treatment is judged, but confirmation may be sought in the serum T_4 and T_3 levels. Mild thyrotoxicosis may persist despite a serum T_4 concentration in the normal range, because the serum T_3 concentration may still be elevated. The latter phenomenon may also account for maintenance of a normal metabolic state in the setting of a subnormal serum T_4 level. The serum TSH concentration may remain subnormal for many months, presumably secondary to accelerated conversion of T_4 to T_3.

Antithyroid agents can cause hypothyroidism if given in excessive amounts over long periods. When this occurs, the patient often complains of gain in weight, sluggishness, and

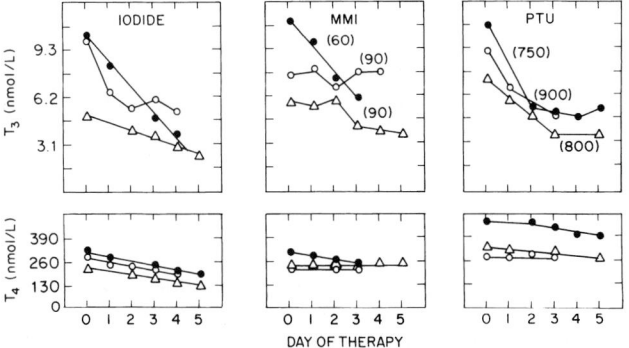

Figure 11–43. Effects of antithyroid agents on the serum levels of T_3 and T_4 in patients with Graves' disease. The first panel shows the effects of potassium iodide (SSKI, 5 drops every 8 h). A rapid reduction in T_3 concentration occurs in all patients over the first 5 d of therapy. Methimazole (MMI) at the indicated doses has a variable effect on serum T_3 concentrations. In one patient the serum T_3 level falls rapidly over the first 3 d, whereas in the other two individuals, despite an even larger dosage, there is no change. Serum T_4 concentration does not change significantly over this time interval. Administration of high-dose propylthiouracil (PTU) causes a marked decrease in serum T_3 concentrations to one third to one half of initial levels. This decrease is due to the propylthiouracil-induced inhibition of type 1 iodothyronine 5′-deiodinase. (Data from Abuid J, Larsen PR. Triiodothyronine and thyroxine in thyrotoxicosis: acute response to therapy with anti-thyroid agents. J Clin Invest 1974; 39:263–268.)

fatigue, and signs of mild hypothyroidism may be present, especially a delay in the relaxation phase of the deep tendon reflexes. Signs of incipient hypothyroidism are enlargement of the thyroid gland and the appearance or accentuation of a bruit, both consequences of the hypersecretion of TSH. The hypothyroidism can be reversed by reducing the dosage of the antithyroid drug or by administering supplemental thyroid hormone. To forestall this development, which may have adverse effects on pre-existing orbitopathy, some physicians employ supplemental thyroid hormone routinely, the "block-and-replace" approach.

"Block-and-Replace" Regimens. The logic behind prescribing a full dose of a thionamide drug and adding thyroxine supplements to prevent the patient from becoming hypothyroid is twofold. First, a few patients are very difficult to keep euthyroid on thionamides alone, and a block-and-replace regimen can be helpful and requires fewer office visits. Second, the immunosuppressive action of the thionamides may be helpful in attenuating the natural history of the autoimmune thyroid diseases directly. However, some investigators found the relapse rate after the block-and-replace approach to be much reduced,[582] whereas others have found no difference.[583, 584] One group has reported that continuing levothyroxine replacement after withdrawal of antithyroid drugs also increases the remission rate,[585] possibly because suppression of pituitary TSH inhibits expression of thyroid antigens and reduces immune stimulation (an effect influenced by the level of TSHRAb). Such studies have not been reproduced,[586] and this approach is not recommended.

Predicting the Response to Drug Withdrawal. Thus, a central question in the treatment of Graves' disease to which there is no simple answer is the appropriate duration of antithyroid drug treatment. As discussed earlier, antithyroid therapy may alter the course of the underlying autoimmune process, but remission after withdrawal of treatment will persist only if the disorder has entered a latent or inactive phase. This latter transition and natural decline in the titers of TSHRAb are more likely to occur the longer the course of treatment. This reasoning is the basis for the traditional practice of continuing antithyroid treatment for 6 to 12 mo or longer.

However, persistence of high levels of circulating TSHRAb during treatment of Graves' disease portends recurrence after withdrawal of antithyroid drugs.[499, 587, 588] Factors preventing a recurrence include a change from stimulating antibody to blocking antibody, which occurs rarely, or the progression of concomitant thyroiditis. These factors may explain why a few authors failed to confirm the predictive value of TSHRAb measurement.[589] The use of poorly validated assays for TSHRAb may compound this problem. However, most patients do not have persisting high levels of TSHRAb, and the prediction of their outcome is more difficult.[499]

Additional features associated with the likelihood of long-term remission after withdrawal of therapy (Table 11–18) include the initial presence of T_3 toxicosis, a small thyroid (less than twice normal), decrease in size of the thyroid, and, in particular, return of the TSH concentration to normal during treatment. HLA typing is not helpful in such predictions.[590] Hence treatment should generally be continued for about 6 to 12 mos and then withdrawn if the titer for TSHRAb is negative. About three quarters of relapses occur in the first 3

TABLE 11–19. Incidence of Toxic Reactions with Antithyroid Drugs

Drug	All Reactions (%)	Agranulocytosis (%)
Methimazole	7.1	0.1
Carbimazole	1.9	0.8
Propylthiouracil	3.3	0.4
Methylthiouracil	13.8	0.5

mo after withdrawal of therapy, and most of the remainder occurs during the subsequent 6 mo. Suppression of TSH and elevation of serum T_3 concentration first signal a return of the disease even in the presence of a normal serum T_4 level.

Long-Term Remission. The frequency with which long-term remission occurs after withdrawal of antithyroid therapy has decreased over the past 30 y,[591, 592] in part because of the increase in dietary iodine intake but also occurring in geographic regions where iodine intake has remained constant and low. Nevertheless about one third of patients experience a lasting remission. *This fact alone indicates that antithyroid agents have a significant role as sole therapy in the first treatment of thyrotoxicosis.*

Adverse Reactions. Adverse reactions occur in a small number of patients taking thionamide drugs (Table 11–19). Agranulocytosis occurs in less than 1% of the patients, generally within the first few weeks or months of treatment. It is accompanied by fever and sore throat, and when therapy is begun the patient should be instructed to discontinue the drug and notify the physician immediately should these symptoms develop. This precaution is more important than the frequent measurement of leukocyte counts, because agranulocytosis may develop within a day or two. If agranulocytosis occurs the drug should be discontinued immediately, and the patient treated with antibiotics as appropriate. Granulocyte colony-stimulating factor (G-CSF) has been used to speed the recovery that invariably takes place. Lymphocytes of patients who have developed agranulocytosis while taking propylthiouracil undergo blast transformation when exposed in vitro to propylthiouracil or methimazole,[593] and consequently they should not be given a thionamide drug again. Granulocytopenia occurs during antithyroid therapy and is sometimes a forerunner of agranulocytosis, but it can also be a manifestation of thyrotoxicosis itself. For this reason, a total white blood cell count and differential is useful prior to the initiation of treatment with thionamide drugs. Granulocytopenia that develops during the first few weeks of therapy may be difficult to interpret; namely whether or not treatment should be continued. In this circumstance, serial measurements of the leukocyte count should be made, and if they display a downward trend the antithyroid drugs should be discontinued. When serial measurements of the white blood cell count remain constant or return to normal, treatment need not be interrupted. A rash that can take many forms, including hives, occurs in as many as 10% of patients. Less frequent reactions include arthralgia, myalgia, neuritis, hepatitis (with PTU) or cholestasis (with methimazole) and rare liver necrosis necessitating transplantation, thrombocytopenia, loss of or abnormal pigmentation of the hair, loss of taste sensation, enlargement of lymph nodes or salivary glands, edema, a lupus-like syndrome, and toxic psychoses. The mechanisms underlying these reactions are not known, although some disappear with continuance of treatment. It is obviously helpful to have a baseline complete blood count (CBC) and liver function studies before the initiation of antithyroid drugs to help interpret the presence of some of these side effects. It is the authors' view that the appearance of any serious manifestation may be an indication for abandonment of antithyroid therapy and recourse to surgery or [131]I.

TABLE 11–18. Factors Favoring Long-Term Remission After Antithyroid Therapy for Graves' Disease

T_3 toxicosis	Normal thyroid function tests
Small goiter	Normal serum TSH
Decrease in goiter size during therapy	Negative tests for TSHRAb

Iodine and Iodine-Containing Agents

Iodine is now rarely used as sole therapy. The mechanism of action of iodine in relieving thyrotoxicosis differs from that of the thionamides. Although quantities of iodine in excess of several milligrams can acutely inhibit organic binding (acute Wolff-Chaikoff effect), this transient phenomenon probably does not contribute to the therapeutic effect.

Instead the major action of iodine is to inhibit hormone release. First, administration of iodine increases glandular stores of organic iodine. Second, the beneficial effect of iodine is evident more quickly than the effects of even large doses of agents that inhibit hormone synthesis. Third, in patients with diffuse toxic goiter, iodine acutely retards the rate of secretion of T_4, an effect that is rapidly lost when iodine is withdrawn. These features of iodine action provide both disadvantages and advantages. The enrichment of glandular organic iodine stores that occurs when this agent is given alone may retard the clinical response to subsequently administered thionamide, and the decrease in RAIU produced by iodine prevents the use of radioiodine as treatment for weeks or more. Furthermore if iodine is withdrawn resumption of accelerated release of hormone from an enriched glandular hormone pool may exacerbate the disorder. Another reason for not using iodine alone is that the therapeutic response on occasion is either incomplete or absent, and even if initially effective iodine may lose its effect with time. (This phenomenon, which has been termed *iodine escape*, should not be confused with the escape from the acute Wolff-Chaikoff effect; see earlier section on thyroid autoregulation.) Nevertheless the rapid slowing of hormone release by iodine makes it more effective than the thionamide drugs when prompt relief of thyrotoxicosis is mandatory (see Fig. 11–43). Therefore, aside from its use in preparation for subtotal thyroidectomy, iodine is useful mainly in patients with actual or impending thyrotoxic crisis, severe thyrocardiac disease, or acute surgical emergencies.

If iodine is used in these circumstances, it should be administered with large doses of a thionamide, as the severity of the thyrotoxicosis itself indicates. The dose of iodine required for control of thyrotoxicosis is approximately 6 mg daily, a quantity less than that usually given. Six milligrams of iodine is present in one eighth of a drop of saturated solution of potassium iodide (SSKI) or eight tenths of a drop of Lugol's solution; many physicians, however, prescribe 5 to 10 drops of one of these agents three times daily. Although it is advisable to administer amounts larger than the suggested minimal effective dose, huge quantities of iodine are more likely to produce adverse reactions, including iodide myxedema. The authors recommend the use of three drops of SSKI three times daily. In patients who are so ill that medications cannot be taken by mouth, antithyroid agents can be triturated and administered by stomach tube; iodine can be given by the same route. When use of a stomach tube is contraindicated, thionamide drugs cannot be administered because no parenteral preparations are available. Here, the disadvantages attendant on administration of iodine may be accepted if the clinical situation is sufficiently serious, and some physicians use intravenous sodium iodide at the same dosage as that for oral use (0.5 to 1.0 mg every 12 h). Iodine appears to be particularly effective after administration of a therapeutic dose of ^{131}I for the rapid alleviation of thyrotoxicosis.

REACTIONS TO IODINE. Adverse reactions to iodine are unusual and are generally not serious[594, 595] but include rash, which may be acneiform; drug fever; sialadenitis; conjunctivitis and rhinitis; vasculitis; and a leukemoid eosinophilic granulocytosis. Sialadenitis may respond to reduction of dosage; in the case of the other reactions, iodine should be stopped.

IPODATE. In doses of 1 g daily, the iodine-containing cholecystographic contrast agent sodium ipodate (or iopanoate) causes a prompt decrease in serum T_4 and serum T_3 concentrations in patients with hyperthyroidism.[596] These effects are the result of both the release of iodine and the ability of the agent to inhibit peripheral T_3 neogenesis, a combination that can be useful in the seriously ill patient. However, as with iodine itself, withdrawal of the drug carries the risk of an exacerbation. Hence if the patient is sufficiently ill to warrant treatment with ipodate, large doses of antithyroid agents should be administered concomitantly.

Other Antithyroid Agents

LITHIUM. Lithium carbonate also inhibits thyroid hormone secretion, but unlike iodine it does not interfere with the accumulation of radioiodine. Lithium at a dose of 300 to 450 mg every 8 h is employed only to provide temporary control of thyrotoxicosis in patients who are allergic to both thionamide and iodide.[596] The goal is to maintain a serum concentration of 1 mEq/L.

DEXAMETHASONE. Dexamethasone in a dosage of 2 mg every 6 h inhibits the glandular secretion of hormone, inhibits the peripheral conversion of T_4 to T_3, and has immunosuppressive effect.[284] The inhibitory effect of dexamethasone on the conversion of T_4 to T_3 is additive to that of propylthiouracil, suggesting a different mechanism of action. Concurrent administration of propylthiouracil, SSKI, and dexamethasone to the patient with severe thyrotoxicosis effects a rapid reduction in serum T_3 concentration, often to within the normal range in 24 to 48 h.[597] Addition of ipodate to this regimen, or substitution of ipodate for SSKI, may be even more effective.

BETA-BLOCKING AGENTS. Agents that block the response to catecholamines at the receptor site (e.g., propranolol) ameliorate some of the manifestations of thyrotoxicosis and are often used as adjuncts in management. Tremulousness, palpitations, excessive sweating, eyelid retraction, and heart rate decrease; effects are rapidly manifested and appear to be mediated largely through the adrenergic nervous system, although propranolol may also impair the conversion of T_4 to T_3. Adrenergic antagonists are most useful in the interval when a response to thionamide or radioiodine therapy is being awaited. They are of limited usefulness in patients with mild to moderate disease but are useful in patients with severe thyrotoxicosis, such as those with impending or actual thyrotoxic crisis (see later section on special aspects of thyrotoxicosis). Adrenergic antagonists are especially useful when tachycardia is contributing to cardiac insufficiency. However, the fact that β-adrenergic blockers can reduce cardiac output without altering oxygen consumption can have adverse effects in some organs, such as the liver, where the arteriovenous oxygen difference is already elevated in the hyperthyroid state.[458] Moreover, since thyroid hormone has a direct effect on the myocardium independent of the adrenergic nervous system, adrenergic antagonists reduce the heart rate by an independent mechanism (see earlier discussion of catecholamine-thyroid interrelationships).

Propranolol is the most widely used agent, as it is relatively free from adverse effects and can be given orally in a dose of 20 to 80 mg every 6 or 8 h. For intravenous use, a shorter-acting agent may be preferable (see section on treatment of thyroid crisis). Propranolol is contraindicated in patients with asthma or chronic obstructive pulmonary disease because it aggravates bronchospasm. Because of its myocardial depressant action, it is also contraindicated in patients with heart block and in patients with congestive failure, unless severe tachycardia is a contributory factor. Whether propranolol should be given chronically to pregnant women with hyperthyroidism is unclear, although these authors avoid it. Some studies indicate that its use causes no significant complications,[598, 599] whereas others report an association with small size of the fetus, low Apgar scores, and postnatal bradycardia and hypoglycemia. Other β-blocking agents include metoprolol, a longer acting drug that allows a once-a-day regimen. Calcium channel blockers such as diltiazem may be used when β-blocking agents are contraindicated.[600]

Surgery

Both types of ablative therapy, i.e., surgery and radioiodine, ameliorate thyrotoxicosis by permanent removal or destruction of thyroid tissue, impairing the capacity of the gland to synthesize hormone. Antithyroid therapy, aimed at preserving the thyroid gland, and ablative therapy are different, and their opposite properties may be advantageous or disadvantageous, depending on one's point of view. The impermanence of antithyroid therapy leads to a relatively frequent recurrence, whereas recurrence is uncommon with ablative therapy. However, antithyroid therapy probably does not cause permanent hypothyroidism, whereas the frequency of permanent hypothyroidism is very high with ablative therapy.

The surgical procedure of choice for the treatment of Graves' disease is a bilateral subtotal thyroidectomy that avoids the dangers of hypoparathyroidism and laryngeal nerve injury. Surgery is effective in relieving hyperthyroidism, the frequency of recurrent hyperthyroidism after subtotal thyroidectomy in adults being less than 5% when the procedure is performed by experienced surgeons. Nevertheless the high prevalence of postoperative hypothyroidism makes surgery an imperfect treatment.

Table 11–20 is taken from a summary of the results of surgery in eight series.[601] The incidence of permanent hypothyroidism ranged in frequency from 4% to approximately 30% and was highest in clinics in which internists did the follow-ups on the patients. In a study conducted by internists, a mean frequency of postoperative hypothyroidism of 28% was found in patients followed for 1 to 16 y, and the frequency in patients followed for 10 y was 43%. Although it was previously assumed that hypothyroidism usually develops within 1 y after operation, long-term studies indicate a progressive increase in the cumulative incidence with time, similar to that produced by radioiodine but of lesser magnitude. It is likely that the frequency of partial impairment of thyroid function is even higher than that of hypothyroidism because the aim of subtotal thyroidectomy is to decrease thyroid reserve. The increasing frequency with time of hypothyroidism may result from progressive restriction of blood supply or from autoimmune destruction of the thyroid remnant. If eventual thyroid failure is a frequent consequence of the Graves' disease process itself, the increase in the cumulative frequency with time of hypothyroidism after either surgery or radioiodine therapy is to be expected and is unavoidable. Treatment that destroys thyroid tissue would accelerate the emergence of hypothyroidism resulting from the disease process itself.

There is an inverse relationship between the frequency of recurrence and that of hypothyroidism, and both partly depend on the amount of thyroid tissue left in place. When one considers that thyroid glands vary in size and degree of

hyperfunction and that the techniques of surgeons vary to a considerable extent, it is remarkable that a normal metabolic state is restored for long periods in most patients. The reason for this favorable outcome may be that the amount of tissue remaining after operation is insufficient to sustain a normal metabolic state and hence becomes stimulated by endogenous TSH. In this way, the patient's homeostatic mechanism provides the adjustment in thyroid function that surgery alone could not. This hypothesis is supported by the return of serum TSH to normal in patients restored to a normal metabolic state by surgery. However, this explanation would suffice only in the absence of TSHRAb, which rapidly decreases and disappears in many patients after surgery. How the autoimmune disease is suppressed following surgery is unclear.

COMPLICATIONS OF SURGERY. The hazards of subtotal thyroidectomy are inversely related to the experience and skill of the surgical team, so it is impossible to generalize about the frequency of complications. Furthermore data from the era in which surgery was common are probably no longer applicable (see Table 11–20). Unless circumstances are otherwise compelling, thyroidectomy should not be performed by surgeons who do the operation only occasionally. Bleeding into the operative site, the most serious postoperative complication, can rapidly produce death by asphyxia and requires immediate evacuation of the blood and ligation of the bleeding vessel. The recurrent laryngeal nerve can be damaged even with subtotal surgery. If unilateral, such damage causes dysphonia that usually improves in a few weeks but may leave the patient slightly hoarse. If laryngeal nerve damage is bilateral, obstruction of the airway can cause stridor within hours; tracheostomy is then required, at which time the nature of the damage to the nerves should be explored. Hypoparathyroidism can be either transient or permanent. Transient hypoparathyroidism results from inadvertent removal of some parathyroids and impairment of blood supply to those that remain. Depending on the severity of these insults, symptoms and signs of hypocalcemia appear, usually within 1 to 7 d after surgery. The earliest evidence of hypoparathyroidism may be anxiety and mental depression, followed by paresthesias and heightened neuromuscular excitability, such as Chvostek's and Trousseau's signs and carpopedal spasm. The serum calcium level is subnormal, and the serum inorganic phosphate level is increased. Severe hypoparathyroidism should be treated with intravenous calcium gluconate. Milder cases can be treated with oral calcium carbonate in a dose of 1 g three times daily. It is impossible at the onset to predict whether hypoparathyroidism will be permanent or regress within a few weeks, as usually occurs.

The hypocalcemia that occurs immediately after surgery for thyrotoxicosis may not be due to transient hypoparathyroidism, because it occurs more frequently here than after surgery for other thyroid disorders. Instead, it may be due to retention of calcium by bone,[602] because the demineralization of bone that occurs in hyperthyroidism[464–466] is rapidly reversed after cure of the hyperthyroid state and may contribute to the modest elevation in alkaline phosphatase during recovery. The frequency of permanent hypoparathyroidism correlates with the proportion of the thyroid removed and with the frequency of postoperative hypothyroidism. The incidence of mild hypoparathyroidism (or diminished parathyroid reserve) detectable years after surgery is probably greater than is generally supposed. The treatment of hypoparathyroidism is discussed in Chapter 24.

PREPARATION FOR SURGERY. Preoperative use of antithyroid agents has greatly decreased the morbidity and mortality rates of surgery for Graves' disease because these drugs deplete glandular hormone stores and restore the metabolic state to normal surgery. However, these agents do not improve the hyperplasia and hypervascularity of the gland. Iodine

TABLE 11–20. Effects of Surgery for Hyperthyroidism in Eight Clinics

Result	%
Mortality	0.0–3.1
Recurrent hyperthyroidism	0.6–17.9
Vocal cord paralysis	0.0–4.4
Permanent hypoparathyroidism	0.0–3.6
Permanent hypothyroidism	4.0–29.7

From Hershman, JM. The treatment of hyperthyroidism. Ann Intern Med 1966; 64:1306–1314.

causes a decrease in height of the follicular cells, enlargement of follicles with retention of colloid, and reduction of hypervascularity. Hence the aim of preoperative management is to restore the metabolic state to normal with antithyroid agents and then to induce involution of the gland with iodine. Patients who are to undergo subtotal thyroidectomy are first given antithyroid therapy in the manner described earlier. Often, relatively large doses are given, both to hasten the clinical response and because surgical candidates are frequently patients with severe disease and/or large goiters. After the metabolic state is restored to normal, SSKI is added (three drops three times daily) for a further 7 to 10 d. During this period, a pre-existing bruit or thrill may decrease in intensity or disappear entirely, and the gland usually becomes firm.

Several cautions should be observed. First, no date for surgery should be set until a normal metabolic state has been restored. Much too often the operation is planned well in advance, and the patient is given a standardized regimen independent of the clinical progress. Second, therapy with iodine should not be started until a normal metabolic state has been restored; iodine should not be relied on to complete an as yet incomplete response to antithyroid therapy because iodine will enrich glandular hormone stores if the antithyroid drug is not entirely effective. Finally, antithyroid agents should not be withdrawn when iodine therapy is begun.

THYROID SURGERY IN THE HYPERTHYROID PATIENT. Propranolol may be a useful adjunct in controlling signs and symptoms (see earlier) while the patient is being prepared for surgery. Propranolol has been used alone in preoperative preparation of the patient in whom surgery is to be undertaken,[603] and although this mode of therapy is probably safe and effective in many patients with mild disease, thyroid crises can occur in patients receiving propranolol. Therefore the authors believe that unless there is some compelling indication for the use of propranolol alone, restoration of the patient to a eumetabolic state, as outlined earlier, is appropriate before subjecting the patient to the stress of general anesthesia and surgery.

Radioiodine

Radioiodine produces the ablative effects but not the complications of surgery. The principal disadvantage of radioiodine is the high frequency of late hypothyroidism. Previously there was concern that this form of therapy might also produce thyroid carcinoma, leukemia, or an increase in mutation rates. However, during the half century in which radioiodine has been in use, no increased prevalence of thyroid carcinoma in treated patients has been noted. Indeed the prevalence may be lower than that in the general population, presumably because the effective dose interferes with cell replication. This phenomenon is to be contrasted with the increased prevalence of thyroid carcinoma in patients treated with lower amounts of radiation in childhood or adolescence. The prevalence of leukemia is also no greater in adults treated with radioiodine, and the frequency of genetic damage in the offspring of patients treated earlier with radioiodine does not appear to be increased. Indeed the conventional dose of radioiodine employed in the treatment of thyrotoxicosis delivers to the gonads a radiation dose about equivalent to that delivered by a barium enema examination or intravenous urogram. In view of the lack of evidence of serious toxicity from radioiodine in doses generally employed for treating hyperthyroidism, the age limit for the use of radioiodine has been lowered progressively from the initial limit of 40—in some clinics it is employed in children and adolescents. Experience from the Chernobyl nuclear accident, which caused a large increase in the number of childhood thyroid cancers, may alter this trend, particularly for adolescents,[604–607] and many physicians think

that the use of any radioactivity in children should be avoided if possible. Hence there is regional and international variation in the use of radioiodine therapy.

Attempts have been made to standardize the radiation delivered to the thyroid gland by varying the dose of radioiodine according to the size of the gland, the uptake of ^{131}I, and its subsequent rate of release. However, such calculations do not provide uniform results, probably because of variations in individual sensitivity. Hence many clinics have settled on an arbitrary dose calculated to result in the delivery of 185 to 222 MBq (5 to 7 mCi) of ^{131}I to the thyroid gland 24 h after administration. Others aim to deliver 50 to 100 Gy (5 to 10,000 rad/g) to the gland.

HYPOTHYROIDISM AFTER RADIOIODINE. In 1961, however, there appeared the first of many reports documenting that the incidence of hypothyroidism is significant during the first year or two after treatment and continues to increase at a rate of approximately 5%/y thereafter. The incidence of postradioiodine hypothyroidism at 5 y is approximately 30% and at 10 y is approximately 40%, although values as high as 70% have been reported (Fig. 11–44).

The beneficial effect of radioiodine and the early induction of hypothyroidism are both the consequence of radiation-induced destruction of thyroid parenchyma. Radiation thyroiditis develops within the first few weeks of treatment, as evidenced by epithelial swelling and necrosis, disruption of follicular architecture, edema, and infiltration with leukocytes. Resolution of the acute phase is followed by fibrosis, vascular narrowing, and lymphocytic infiltration. These changes account for the early response to radioiodine, be it favorable or excessive, but do not appear sufficient to account for the continuing development of hypothyroidism with time. In some studies, the likelihood of hypothyroidism is increased by the presence of high titers of thyroid antibodies and presumably of thyroid-specific T cells, at the time of treatment and with increasing age of the patient. The two predisposing factors may be related to one another. If this is true, it is unlikely that the early ablative effects can be obtained free from subsequent late effects, and doses of radioiodine sufficient to exert an early therapeutic action will inevitably be associated with a high frequency of delayed hypothyroidism.

This therapeutic dilemma with respect to radioiodine therapy is handled differently in different clinics. Some continue to administer the conventional dose because of its effectiveness and because hypothyroidism, when it eventually occurs, can be treated. A disadvantage of such an approach is

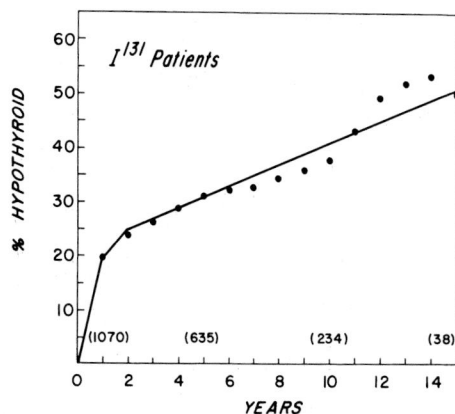

Figure 11–44. Incidence of postradioiodine hypothyroidism in relation to the duration of follow-up. The total number of patients followed for each of the indicated time periods is shown in parentheses. (From Dunn JT, Chapman EM. Rising incidence of hypothyroidism after radioactive-iodine therapy in thyrotoxicosis. Reprinted by permission of The New England Journal of Medicine, 1964; 271:1037–1042.)

that the onset and progression of hypothyroidism may be insidious, that prolonged follow-up of patients may not be possible, and that patients may not associate symptoms arising long after therapy with a complication. The advantage of this approach is that it minimizes the dangers of persistent or recurrent thyrotoxicosis, which may be hazardous, especially in the elderly.

One approach to minimizing the frequency of hypothyroidism is to administer a dose per gram of estimated weight that is larger the greater the gland size. In this way, many large thyroids are treated with large doses, and the converse is true for thyroids that are small. However, regimens of this type do not appear to improve the treatment of hyperthyroidism in the short run, and it is too early to know their success in the late development of hypothyroidism. A second approach involved the use of ^{125}I, rather than ^{131}I, with the rationale being that the lower energy and shorter path length of the beta emission might localize radiation to the apical portion of the thyroid cell and impair hormone biosynthesis, while sparing the nucleus and its replicative machinery. However, the frequency of hypothyroidism in patients treated with ^{125}I is similar to that following ^{131}I. Consequently, ^{125}I offers no advantages.

Another approach employs smaller than usual doses of radioiodine, the rationale being that the small dose may be sufficient to prevent both delayed hypothyroidism and the recurrence of thyrotoxicosis. Although such doses are usually insufficient to control thyrotoxicosis acutely, control can be achieved by administration of antithyroid drugs or stable iodine after radioiodine has been given. The efficacy of this last approach is unclear. In a controlled prospective study, the effects of a single conventional dose of approximately 5.2 MBq/g (140 μCi/g) of estimated glandular weight were compared with the effects of half the dose.[608] Although the therapeutic effect of radioiodine developed more slowly in patients receiving the half-dose and although a greater proportion required antithyroid drug therapy until this effect became apparent, the frequency of remission after 2 y was the same as that in patients receiving the conventional dose, and recurrence of thyrotoxicosis was no more common. Importantly, in the full-dose group the incidence of hypothyroidism was 8% at 1 y and 29% at 5 y, whereas in the half-dose group the corresponding values were 4 and 7%. However, thereafter the cumulative frequency with time with the low dose is similar to that observed with conventional doses.[609] For these reasons, some physicians advocate the ablative approach to treatment.[610]

ORBITOPATHY AND RADIOIODINE. As discussed earlier, Graves' orbitopathy is most likely the result of a crossover specificity between retro-orbital and thyroid antigens. Any worsening of the autoimmune thyroid response, might therefore worsen the orbital immune response. Following radioiodine therapy, the levels of circulating TSHR autoantibodies increase strikingly,[478] perhaps secondary to impairment of immune restraint caused by the intrathyroidal irradiation. This change is in keeping with exacerbation of pretibial myxedema after radioiodine administration.[611] Likewise, carefully conducted studies indicate that eye disease worsens in patients with Graves' orbitopathy who are treated with radioiodine[612, 613] (Fig. 11–45). Such changes are usually mild and temporary but on occasion can involve dramatic deterioration. Some physicians advocate the use of glucocorticoids at the time of radiodine treatment to prevent such effects.[614] One regimen involves prednisone, 0.4 to 0.5 mg/kg 1 mo prior to ^{131}I treatment, with a gradual taper over 3 to 4 mo. Others suggest that radioiodine may not be the treatment of choice in patients with significant orbitopathy. However, maneuvers such as careful control of thyroid function before and after therapy

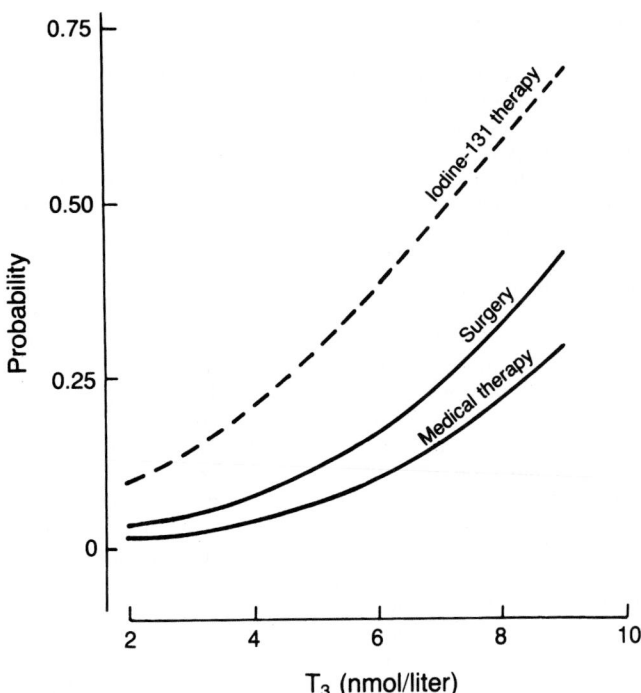

Figure 11–45. Probability of the development of worsening of orbitopathy in patients with Graves' disease. The serum T_3 levels are shown before treatment, and the type of therapy is shown as a variable. (From Tallestedt L, Lundell G, Torring O, et al. Occurrence of ophthalmopathy after treatment for Graves' disease. N Engl J Med 1992; 326:1733–1738. Copyright © 1992, Massachusetts Medical Society. All rights reserved.)

and cessation of smoking by the patient may minimize the eye changes.

OTHER SIDE EFFECTS OF RADIOIODINE. Additional hazards may attend the use of radioiodine, particularly large doses. The parathyroids are exposed to radiation in patients treated with radioiodine, but although parathyroid reserve may be diminished in some patients, development of overt hypoparathyroidism is rare. The effect of radioiodine on other tissues that concentrate iodide, such as the salivary and gastric glands, has received little attention. The radiation thyroiditis itself may lead to an exacerbation of thyrotoxicosis 10 to 14 d after the radioiodine is administered that has occasionally had serious consequences, including precipitation of thyrotoxic crisis and aggravation of patients with severe thyrotoxicosis or cardiac insufficiency. In thyrocardiac disease, therefore, antithyroid drugs should be given for several weeks before radioiodine is given to deplete glandular hormone stores. This prevents an outpouring of hormone if severe radiation thyroiditis occurs. The antithyroid agent is withdrawn about 3 to 5 d before administration of the radioiodine and, if the clinical condition warrants, can be begun again 7 d later.

Because ^{131}I administration is contraindicated during pregnancy, a pregnancy test should be carried out in women of childbearing age before ^{131}I therapy if there is any possibility of pregnancy.

GENERAL MEASURES. Several general measures may contribute to the well-being of the thyrotoxic patient. Bed rest is an excellent treatment. Help with family responsibilities and avoidance of physical exertion are also important. In addition, a diet rich in protein, calories, and vitamins may repair the nutritional deficiencies that are common in thyrotoxic patients.

CHOICE OF THERAPY. The choice of therapy for thyrotoxicosis is influenced by emotional attitudes, economic considerations, and family and personal issues. The authors' choice of therapy takes into account the natural history of the disease, the advantages and disadvantages of the available therapies, and the features of the population group in which the patient falls. Apart from patients directly requesting surgery, surgery is recommended only when shortcomings of other modes of therapy are of particular importance; for example, patients with antithyroid drug allergy and those with very large goiters and/or the need for a rapid return to normal. Occasionally, in young adults, it is necessary to remove a diffuse toxic goiter because of obstructive symptoms or cosmetic disfigurement. Nevertheless only a small percentage of patients with Graves' disease are recommended for surgery. The remainder of this section is confined to the choice of therapy in adults. One approach to the therapy in adults is to initiate treatment with antithyroid drugs in all patients to produce a euthyroid state before reaching a final decision regarding a definitive therapeutic strategy. This allows the patient to return to a euthyroid status as rapidly as possible and provides an estimate of the antithyroid drug dose requirement. The magnitude of the drug requirement and the size of the thyroid gland are factors considered in the evaluation of the patient with regard to the likelihood of a remission. The three options for treatment are explained to the patient during these first months of contact, and individual recommendations are then formulated. This approach allows the establishment of a workable physician-patient relationship, which is especially important in addressing anxieties about the use of radioiodine. Such concerns lead many patients, especially those younger than age 50, to elect a trial of antithyroid drugs before definitive therapy with ^{131}I. Individuals with large thyroid glands, maintenance thionamide dose requirement of more than 400 mg propythiouracil/d, and high titers of TSHRAb require prolonged antithyroid drug treatment and are advised that the chance of spontaneous remission is less than 30%. A therapeutic trial is generally pursued for 6 to 12 mo if long-term thionamide therapy is selected. One can, in theory, treat forever unless side effects become a problem. When a decision in favor of radioiodine is made, ^{131}I is prescribed at a dose designed to result in the retention of 186 to 222 MBq (5 to 6 mCi) ^{131}I in the thyroid gland at 24 h. This estimate is based on a ^{123}I uptake test performed immediately before treatment and at least 5 d after stopping thionamides. Because ^{131}I is given when the patient is euthyroid and this is a relatively large dose, no additional therapy is required immediately after treatment except for patients in whom a recurrence of hyperthyroidism poses a medical risk; for example, patients with coronary artery disease or congestive heart failure. Patients are seen at 4-wk intervals after ^{131}I administration, and hypothyroidism is treated when it appears, generally within 3 mo. Women planning to become pregnant are advised to wait for an arbitrary period of 6 mo after ^{131}I therapy to allow for resolution of any transient effects of gonadal radiation. If, after a period of 6 to 8 mo, hyperthyroidism is still present and the patient is symptomatic, the treatment is repeated, generally using about 1.5 times the initial dose of ^{131}I.

Although the foregoing reflects the authors' approach to therapy, it is important to be aware that the opinions of thyroidologists differ widely.[615] In view of the several approaches to treatment available, each with its advantages and disadvantages, it is incumbent on the physician to explain these factors thoroughly to patients, to indicate a preference and the reasons for it, and to allow the final choice to rest with the patient.

HYPOTHYROIDISM IN THE RECENTLY HYPERTHYROID PATIENT. The early onset of hypothyroidism may cause distinct symptoms in the previously thyrotoxic patient after ^{131}I or surgical treatment or even with high doses of thionamide drugs. Such patients may develop severe muscle cramps, often in large muscle groups such as the trapezius or latissimus dorsi or the proximal muscles of the extremities. Such symptoms can develop even when the serum hormone levels are only low-normal or slightly decreased and before the TSH level has risen. It is possible to mistake symptoms such as back pain for an unrelated illness unless the patient is warned in advance. It is also not unusual for patients to complain of hypothyroid symptoms when thyroid function tests return to within the normal range. Such patients appear to have trouble adjusting to the normal thyroid hormone levels after being exposed to excessive amounts for long periods.

Treatment of Infiltrative Orbitopathy or Infiltrative Dermopathy

Infiltrative orbitopathy varies in severity from the common mild form to a severe form that threatens the vision. Fortunately the latter is rare, because it is difficult to treat. Indeed the most effective therapies are merely palliative. The natural course of the disorder, which is variable and characterized by exacerbations and remissions, makes conclusions about the efficacy of any treatment difficult. A further source of confusion is the variable terminology for describing the manifestations of orbitopathy and the lack of rigid criteria for defining their severity. Use of the American Thyroid Association classification and its expanded indices, described earlier, is strongly recommended (see Tables 11–16 and 11–17).

INFLUENCE OF TREATING THE THYROID. The first question that arises is whether different treatments for thyrotoxicosis affect the course of the orbitopathy differently. Subtotal thyroidectomy and thionamide drug therapy do not influence ophthalmopathy except if they lead to the development of hypothyroidism.[616] Hypothyroidism has an adverse effect on the disorder and should be treated fully when it occurs. However, exogenous thyroid hormone in the absence of hypothyroidism does not improve the ophthalmopathy. As discussed earlier, controlled studies suggest that radioiodine treatment may lead to a slight but significant worsening of orbitopathy,[614] and it may be best to avoid radioiodine in patients with severe orbitopathy. Alternatively, as mentioned earlier, coincidental glucocorticoid therapy may prevent deterioration of orbitopathy after radioiodine but may, itself, cause significant side effects.[613] Controlled, prospective studies of the influence of antithyroid drug treatment prior to radioiodine on the eye changes are needed.

SYMPTOMATIC TREATMENT. Treatment modalities can be divided into those that are largely symptomatic (useful mainly in the mild form) and those that attempt to arrest or reverse the progression of the disorder. In milder forms little treatment is required.[617] The patient who experiences photophobia and sensitivity to wind or cold air is benefited by wearing dark glasses, which also afford protection from foreign bodies. Elevation of the head of the bed at night and instillation of lubricants, such as 1% methylcellulose, may help when the lids do not appose completely during sleep. Artificial tears can be used during the day. Since the ophthalmic manifestations tend to be self-limited and the progression to a more severe form is uncommon, such measures usually suffice to tide the patient over until the disorder regresses spontaneously.

GLUCOCORTICOIDS. The appearance of increasing proptosis with inability to appose the lids or of severe infiltrative manifestations such as chemosis warrants the use of more vigorous therapeutic measures. Such changes, even when severe, may respond favorably and rapidly to glucocorticoids. Some physicians use massive doses of prednisone (120 to 140 mg/d), and if improvement occurs, the dose is decreased to the lowest level at which improvement is maintained. The latter dose is still likely to be large, but it is hoped that a halt to the progression or actual regression of the disease will occur before untoward effects make withdrawal of the drug necessary. Other physicians find that much smaller doses of prednisone (20 to 30 mg/d) can be highly effective with rapid reduction to a longer-term maintenance dose (10 to 15 mg/d). Intravenous hydrocortisone pulse therapy is said to have the advantage of fewer side effects than high doses of prednisone.[560, 618] To circumvent the inevitable side effects of large doses of glucocorticoids, periodic injection of depot preparations of glucocorticoids subconjunctivally or into the retro-orbital space has been tried but is not recommended. Such treatment may have a dramatic effect on irritative symptoms as well as on diplopia, but the efficacy varies, and systemic effects of the glucocorticoids are sometimes seen. Moreover, this treatment entails the risk of puncture of the globe or a retro-orbital hematoma.

EXTERNAL IRRADIATION. The value of external radiation to the orbits is established now by controlled trials[618] but is in fact a steroid-sparing rather than steroid-replacing therapy. Whether it is more effective than prednisone therapy is unclear, and combined therapy has long been advocated.[619] The safe administration of highly collimated supervoltage radiation to the retro-orbital space requires experienced personnel, but it does provide seemingly rapid and beneficial effects on infiltrative and inflammatory manifestations; exophthalmos and ophthalmoparesis are usually little affected.[620] There is a clear need for a reliable disease marker to monitor the effects of such treatment.

ORBITAL DECOMPRESSION. If glucocorticoid therapy and/or external radiation fail to halt progression of the disease and if loss of vision is threatened either by ulceration or infection of the cornea or by changes in the retina or optic nerve, orbital decompression can be performed.[621] In some patients a desire for a nearly complete cosmetic correction may be such that decompression surgery is the only therapy. This procedure usually involves removal of either the lateral wall or the roof of the orbit or resection of the lateral wall of the ethmoid sinus and the roof of the maxillary sinus.[622] This surgery usually causes diplopia, and even in the best of hands corrective muscle surgery may be necessary later.

AN APPROACH TO THE TREATMENT OF ORBITOPATHY. There is no merit to the suggestion that infiltrative ophthalmopathy is benefited or that its progression is retarded by total ablation of the thyroid, whether performed surgically, by radioiodine, or by a combination of the two. Hence the authors recommend a trial of oral glucocorticoid therapy for patients with severe or progressive ophthalmopathy. If effective doses cannot be tolerated, a course of external radiation may be attempted if edema predominates. Local measures should be employed, along with these major forms of treatment. Ulceration and infection of the cornea should be treated with antibiotics, lubricants, and protective shields. An attempt to appose the lids by means of sutures (tarsorrhaphy) should be performed only by an experienced ophthalmologist, as the sutures may tear out and cause scarring. The management of severe ophthalmopathy should never be undertaken by the endocrinologist or by the ophthalmologist acting alone. Close and coordinated observation of the effects of medical therapy and the progress of the disease is necessary to determine whether and when surgery is appropriate. Surgery almost invariably halts the progress of the disease and preserves vision if performed in time. This decision is influenced by the ability of the available surgical team because the degree of success of such procedures is proportional to experience.

INFILTRATIVE DERMOPATHY. Treatment of infiltrative dermopathy is necessary as soon as it is recognized. The application of a topical, high-potency glucocorticoid preparation with an occlusive dressing may cause regression or disappearance of the lesion. Long-standing untreated dermopathy is more resistant to treatment.

Hyperthyroidism and Thyrotoxicosis in Pregnancy

As discussed earlier, postpartum thyroiditis with transient thyrotoxicosis may occur with some frequency (approximately 5 to 10%) during the postpartum period. However, when thyrotoxicosis is present during pregnancy, it is usually more severe and is usually due to Graves' disease. Difficulty in conception and fetal wastage are increased in women with Graves' disease, but occasional patients become pregnant despite antecedent untreated hyperthyroidism. More commonly, a woman under treatment for hyperthyroidism becomes pregnant, or hyperthyroidism develops after pregnancy is under way. Whatever the sequence, pregnancy complicates the diagnosis and treatment of hyperthyroidism in Graves' disease and influences its severity and course.[623]

DIAGNOSIS. Pregnancy and hyperthyroidism are both accompanied by thyroid enlargement, a hyperdynamic circulation, and hypermetabolism. Amenorrhea may occur in thyrotoxicosis not associated with pregnancy. In both conditions, the total serum T_4 and T_3 levels are increased. The most useful laboratory test in this differentiation is measurement of the serum TSH level. TSH is suppressed in hyperthyroidism during pregnancy, just as it is in nonpregnant individuals. However, there is sometimes a modest suppression of TSH (between 0.1 and 0.5 mU/L) during the 8th to 14th weeks of normal pregnancy because of stimulation of the thyroid by hCG during this interval.[257, 259, 260, 264] A TSH level of 0.1 mU/L and an elevated FT_4 and/or FT_3 strongly suggest coexistent hyperthyroidism.

TREATMENT. The management of hyperthyroidism during pregnancy is an even greater problem. Surgery during the last trimester, and probably during the first trimester as well, is not desirable because of the possible induction of premature labor. Although surgery may be successful during the middle trimester, it is best to avoid major surgery during pregnancy if possible. Because antithyroid drug treatment poses no greater risk to the mother or fetus than does surgery and possibly involves less risk, medical therapy is the method of choice. Furthermore pregnancy has an attenuating influence on the hyperthyroid state because of the immunosuppression associated with pregnancy, manifested here by a decrease in the level of thyroid autoantibodies.[624] Although levels of TSHR autoantibodies decrease during pregnancy, the levels may not correlate with the clinical disease under these conditions.[625–627] The consequence is that the dosage of antithyroid drug required to control the disease in the latter phases of pregnancy is generally much less than that required in the same patient when she is not pregnant.

Certain aspects of placental physiology are relevant to the use of antithyroid drugs. First, propylthiouracil and methimazole readily cross the placenta,[628] are concentrated in the fetal thyroid, and in sufficient quantity can cause goitrous hypothyroidism in the fetus. The administration of as little as 100 to 300 mg propylthiouracil/d to the mother causes a slight decrease in serum T_4 concentration and an elevated TSH level in neonates.[629, 630] The long-term complication of this mild hypothyroidism is unknown but should be kept in mind. Although maternal T_4 crosses the placenta (as evidenced by infants with congenital hypothyroidism), placental transfer is not efficient and varies from patient to patient.[9] For these reasons the flux of antithyroid agent to the fetus should be limited by giving the mother the smallest dosage of antithyroid agent that induces a physiological state consistent with normal pregnancy. The serum free T_4 level should be maintained in the upper normal range. However, the concentration of hormone is not as critical as the clinical status of the patient. A modest tachycardia is a physiological response to the increased metabolic demands of pregnancy; and pulse rates of 90 to 100/min are well tolerated without evidence of myocardial decompensation during delivery. The daily maintenance dose of propylthiouracil should in most cases be 200 mg or less, although doses up to 450 mg may occasionally be required. Propylthiouracil is preferred to methimazole because of the greater transplacental passage of the latter drug.[628] In a compliant patient, a dose requirement in excess of 400 mg propylthiouracil/d is a reasonable threshold for considering subtotal thyroidectomy, preferably in the second trimester. All pregnant patients with significant Graves' disease should be managed in close cooperation with obstetricians experienced with modern techniques for monitoring the fetus for intrauterine thyroid dysfunction. These techniques normally include fetal heart rate monitoring and ultrasound assessment of fetal growth rate. With advanced ultrasound it may be possible to examine the fetus for the presence of goiter. Convincing evidence of fetal hyperthyroidism would be a strong indication to switch the mother to methimazole (60 to 120 mg/d) to attempt in utero treatment of the fetus.[625] Levothyroxine supplementation of the mother would be required in these rare situations. The concern regarding a congenital defect, *aplasia cutis*, in infants of mothers receiving methimazole or carbimazole have been allayed to some extent but cannot be dismissed.[631]

Iodine should not be used as therapy for any length of time in the pregnant woman, because it readily crosses the placenta and can induce in the fetus a very large goiter that may cause airway obstruction and even death. Whether propranolol should be used in the pregnant woman with hyperthyroidism is a matter of debate. In the experience of some, it can cause intrauterine growth retardation and neonatal hypoglycemia or depression, but other studies suggest that it can be employed with safety.[598, 599]

Assays for TSHRAb in the serum of pregnant women with Graves' disease may be of value in selected cases.[625] Because maternal immunoglobulins cross the placenta, there is a rough correlation between the maternal level of stimulatory TSHRAb, as measured by bioassay, and the development of fetal thyrotoxicosis. Although thyrotoxicosis occurs in only 1% of infants of mothers with Graves' disease, it is helpful to know the level of maternal TSHRAb by radioassay, and in those women in whom the titer remains high in the third trimester a formal bioassay should be obtained to estimate the stimulatory capacity of the TSHRAb. Pregnant women at risk include those with more severe hyperthyroidism and those with significant Graves' orbitopathy or infiltrative dermopathy. In addition, the prior ablative treatment of the mother with either surgery or radioiodine may not be accompanied by a reduction in TSHRAb. Thus the fetus of a treated patient with Graves' disease is still at risk for developing neonatal thyrotoxicosis and might require in utero treatment, as described earlier.

Pregnancy and the postpartum state apparently influence the course of hyperthyroidism in Graves' disease. Patients in clinical remission during pregnancy are prone to postpartum relapse.[626, 627] In 41 pregnancies in 35 patients in remission, 78% were followed by development of thyrotoxicosis during the postpartum period. The patients with Graves' disease and postpartum thyrotoxicosis could be classified into three categories. Some had persistent recurrent hyperthyroidism with an elevated RAIU; this outcome was associated with an increase in the FT_4 early in pregnancy. Others had a transient disorder associated with a normal or an elevated RAIU, and still others, those with the highest titers of TPOAb, developed a transient thyrotoxicosis with a decreased RAIU, similar to that in the postpartum thyroiditis syndrome.

A special problem related to hyperthyroidism and pregnancy is presented by the patient who is in early remission after a course of antithyroid treatment or is being treated with antithyroid agents and wants to become pregnant in the near future. Management with antithyroid agents can be continued through pregnancy or reinstituted should hyperthyroidism recur, but in such instances definitive therapy (radioiodine or surgery) should be considered to forestall the complexities of managing hyperthyroidism during pregnancy. As with the therapy of Graves' disease in general, such decisions must involve education of the patient so that the risks and benefits of the various alternatives are clearly appreciated.

Relatively more methimazole than propylthiouracil appears in breast milk of women receiving these drugs.[632] Women who take antithyroid drugs are best advised not to nurse their infants. However, no untoward effects in the infants have been found, although periodic thyroid function tests are appropriate.

Graves' Disease in Children and Adolescents

Thyrotoxicosis in childhood and adolescence is almost always the result of Graves' disease. Thyrotoxicosis in this age group is worthy of special consideration because treatment is less satisfactory than in adults. Hence there is more uncertainty concerning its management,[633] probably because the disease tends to be more severe in children. In addition several factors weigh against the use of radioiodine in children. First, the enhanced carcinogenic potential of radiation in the thyroid gland of the infant or child is evidenced by the correlation between childhood thyroid carcinoma and a history of x-ray therapy to the head, neck, or chest in childhood.[634] Second, among patients with thyrotoxicosis, those treated in childhood or adolescence are feared to be at greatest risk for transmitting genetic damage, although available data suggest that this may not be likely.[635] Finally, postradioiodine hypothyroidism is a particularly undesirable complication in young children because inadequate or interrupted therapy can impair growth, development, and scholastic performance. For these reasons the authors do not often use radioiodine in the treatment of childhood thyrotoxicosis.

The choice between surgical and antithyroid therapy is a difficult one. The data indicate that children have a lower incidence of long-term remission after antithyroid therapy than adults, although some believe that thyrotoxicosis often undergoes remission after adolescence. On the other hand, most surgical series reveal a relatively high frequency of postoperative hypothyroidism in children. Recurrences are also more frequent, presumably as a result of attempts to avoid hypothyroidism. Complications such as hypoparathyroidism and recurrent laryngeal nerve damage must be borne over a longer life span. On the basis of these considerations, a course of 1 to 2 y of antithyroid therapy seems most reasonable. A second course of antithyroid therapy is regularly employed if recrudescence or relapse occurs after the first course. If sustained remission does not follow a second course of therapy and, particularly if the patient has passed through adolescence during this period, radioiodine therapy or surgery may be considered.

OTHER CAUSES OF THYROTOXICOSIS

Toxic Multinodular Goiter

Toxic multinodular goiter is a disorder in which hyperthyroidism arises in a multinodular goiter, usually of long standing, and is the result of one of several pathogenetic factors. It is important to avoid the term *toxic nodular goiter* because this encompasses both toxic multinodular goiter, as here described, and toxic adenoma of the thyroid gland, which will be discussed in a succeeding section.

PATHOGENESIS. The pathogenesis of toxic multinodular goiter cannot be considered apart from that of its invariable forerunner, nontoxic multinodular goiter, from which it emerges slowly and surreptitiously. Two hallmarks of the disorder, structural and functional heterogeneity and functional autonomy, evolve over time; the increase in the extent of autonomous function causes the disease to move from the nontoxic to the toxic phase, but the mechanisms of this change are uncertain. The somatic mutations in the TSHR gene demonstrated in toxic adenomas have not been demonstrated in toxic multinodular goiter. Sometimes, hyperthyroidism develops abruptly, usually after exposure to increased quantities of iodine, which permits autonomous foci to increase hormone secretion to excessive levels and which may simply exacerbate already established mild hyperthyroidism (iodine-induced hyperthyroidism, jodbasedow). In addition Graves' disease may develop in a multinodular gland.

Radioiodine becomes localized in one or more discrete nodules, while iodine accumulation in the remainder of the gland is usually suppressed in toxic multinodular goiter. No further suppression is produced by exogenous thyroid hormone, but TSH stimulates iodine uptake in the previously inactive areas, indicating that the suppression is due to the lack of TSH. Histopathologically, the functioning areas resemble adenomas in being reasonably well demarcated from surrounding tissue. They generally consist of large follicles, sometimes with hyperplastic epithelium, but here, too, architecture correlates poorly with functional state. The remaining tissue appears inactive, and zones of degeneration are present in both functioning and nonfunctioning areas. These findings suggest that the functioning areas are independent of TSH and can therefore be termed *areas of adenomatous hyperfunction.* The remaining areas, in contrast, retain TSH dependence, their function being suppressed as a consequence of hyperfunction in the autonomous zones. Hence from the pathophysiological standpoint, this thyroid harbors multiple solitary hyperfunctioning and hypofunctioning adenomas. Whether the hyperfunctioning areas represent adenomas, with their now well-defined somatic mutations in the TSHR gene, is still unclear.

PRESENTATION. The overproduction of thyroid hormone in toxic multinodular goiter is usually less than that in Graves' disease. First, the clinical manifestations of thyrotoxicosis are rarely flagrant. Second, the serum T_4 and T_3 concentrations may be only marginally increased, and a suppressed TSH may be the only abnormality.[367] Finally, the RAIU is slightly increased or within the normal range. The mildness of the hyperthyroidism is consistent with either of its presumed pathogenetic origins. The effectiveness of any stimulus to hyperfunction may be blunted in a thyroid that is the seat of a pre-existing nontoxic multinodular goiter, because of the associated impairment in the efficiency of hormone synthesis. Toxic multinodular goiter is a common complication of nontoxic multinodular goiter, but its precise incidence is unknown. Toxic multinodular goiter usually occurs after the age of 50 in patients who have had nontoxic multinodular goiter for many years. Like its forerunner, toxic multinodular goiter is many times more common in women than in men. Toxic multinodular goiter is almost never accompanied by infiltrative ophthalmopathy, and when the two coexist, it represents the emergence of Graves' disease. Indeed Graves' disease in the presence of multinodular goiter is a well-defined variant.

The clinical manifestations differ from those in Graves' disease. Cardiovascular manifestations tend to predominate,

possibly because of the age of the patient, and include atrial fibrillation or tachycardia, with or without heart failure. A large survey indicated that TSH was suppressed in 28% of elderly patients with atrial fibrillation (see Table 11–15).[367] A decreased response to digitalis may alert the physician to the presence of thyrotoxicosis. Weakness and wasting of muscles are common. The nervous manifestations are less prominent than in younger patients with thyrotoxicosis, but emotional lability may be pronounced. Because of the physical characteristics of the thyroid gland and its frequent retrosternal extension, obstructive symptoms are more common than in Graves' disease. On palpation, the characteristics of the goiter are the same as those of the more common nontoxic multinodular goiter, discussed later. In as many as 20% of elderly patients with thyrotoxicosis, the thyroid gland is firm and irregular but not distinctly enlarged. Ultrasound examination confirms the diagnosis as toxic multinodular goiter rather than toxic adenoma or Graves' disease.

LABORATORY TESTS AND DIFFERENTIAL DIAGNOSIS. The challenge to determine whether the patient with a multinodular goiter is thyrotoxic can be resolved only with laboratory tests. If the FT_4I or FT_3I is elevated and the TSH level is suppressed, the diagnosis of hyperthyroidism is established. TSH levels intermediate between 0.1 and the 0.2 mU/L lower limit of normal are not usually associated with significant symptoms. Such patients have thyroid autonomy but are not thyrotoxic. The pituitary-hypothalamic axis provides the most sensitive indicator of the level of thyroid hormone that is specifically relevant to the individual patient. Monitoring the concentration of serum TSH takes advantage of this sensitivity and is one of the most useful ways of establishing the existence of autonomous thyroid function. The RAIU is of little help because thyrotoxicosis may exist in association with values that are normal or only slightly increased.

TREATMENT. Radioiodine is the treatment of choice for most patients with toxic-multinodular goiter, despite disagreement about the size and number of doses required to achieve a therapeutic response. Along the eastern seaboard of the United States the responsiveness of toxic multinodular goiter to radioiodine differs little from that of the diffuse toxic goiter of Graves' disease. However, in areas where goiter was formerly endemic, such as the Great Lakes area of the United States, toxic multinodular goiter is said to be more resistant to radioiodine. Although no studies to support this hypothesis have been reported, the type of toxic multinodular goiter that readily responds to radioiodine may resemble diffuse toxic goiter in displaying a relatively diffuse accumulation of iodine. The more resistant variety of toxic multinodular goiter, on the other hand, may be associated with adenomatous hyperfunction in which focal accumulation of radioiodine occurs; here tissue previously suppressed may regain function and ultimately achieve autonomy after the hyperactive tissue has been destroyed.

Because of the age of the patient and variations in sensitivity to radioiodine, conventional doses should be administered. In any event, these are likely to be larger than those used in diffuse toxic goiter, because the uptake of ^{131}I tends to be lower and the gland larger. Many patients with this disorder have underlying heart disease. Therefore the administration of radioiodine should be preceded by a course of antithyroid therapy until a eumetabolic state is achieved. Medication is then discontinued for 3 d before radioiodine is administered. Seven days thereafter the antithyroid drug is reinstituted so that the thyrotoxicosis is controlled until radioiodine takes effect. After 6 to 8 wk the antithyroid drug is gradually withdrawn, and if thyrotoxicosis recurs a second course of therapy is given. This entire treatment sequence should be accompanied by adequate β-blockade if the cardiac status permits. Surgical therapy is often recommended after adequate preoperative preparation in patients with obstructive manifestations or when it is feared that such manifestations may result from the temporary thyroid enlargement that radioiodine sometimes produces, particularly in patients with retrosternal extensions of the goiter. In these patients, MRI is recommended to define the extent of the goiter and the adequacy of the tracheal walls. Respiratory function studies may also be helpful in assessing the need for surgery. When surgery is contraindicated, even significant obstructive symptoms can be relieved by adequate radioiodine therapy.[636]

Toxic Adenoma (Plummer's Disease)

A third, less common form of hyperthyroidism is caused by one or more autonomous adenomas of the thyroid gland. As herein employed, the term *toxic adenoma* refers to tumors in a thyroid that is intrinsically normal, differentiating this lesion from areas of adenomatous hyperfunction within a toxic multinodular goiter. The disorder is usually caused by a single adenoma that is palpable as a solitary nodule and hence is sometimes referred to as *hyperfunctioning solitary nodule* or *toxic nodule*. Occasionally, two or three adenomas of similar character are present.

PATHOGENESIS. Toxic adenomas are true follicular adenomas (for histopathologic characteristics, see section on thyroid neoplasms). The basic pathogenesis of a large fraction of them is one of several somatic point mutations in the TSHR gene, commonly in the third transmembrane loop. These amino acid changes lead to constitutive activation of the TSH receptor in the absence of TSH (Fig. 11–46).[637] It appears therefore that the TSHR is "tripped" from an "off state" to an "on state." Similarly, loss-of-function rather than gain-of-function mutations may also occur in the TSHR gene (see later). A small number of autonomous adenoma have mutations in the G protein genes that lead to a similar state of constitutive activation.[638]

The course is one of progressive growth and increasing function over many years. At first the adenoma may be present as a small nodule or may be impalpable, but in either case it can be detected in the scintiscan as a localized area of increased radioiodine accumulation. On administration of exogenous thyroid hormone the function of the remainder of the gland is suppressed, but function in the adenoma persists. Later, with further growth, a progressively increasing share of glandular function is assumed by the adenoma, with the result that the remaining tissue is increasingly suppressed. Ultimately the remainder of the gland is completely suppressed and atrophic, and the scintiscan reveals function only in the adenoma (hot nodule). Although continued growth of the adenoma causes secretion of excessive quantities of hormone, some time may pass before thyrotoxicosis becomes overt. The extranodular tissue usually retains its capacity to function if TSH is provided, either by exogenous administration or as a result of ablation of the nodule. Some adenomas secrete T_3 predominantly.

CLINICAL PICTURE. Toxic adenoma occurs in a younger age group than does toxic multinodular goiter, often in patients in their 30s or 40s. Frequently there is a history of a long-standing, slowly growing lump in the neck. It is unusual for adenomas to produce thyrotoxicosis until they have achieved a diameter of 2.5 to 3 cm. The adenoma can undergo central necrosis and hemorrhage; as a result, the thyrotoxicosis may be relieved, the remainder of the thyroid may resume its function, and the adenoma may appear on the scintiscan as a cold area, suggesting a thyroid carcinoma. Calcification in the area of hemorrhage may take place and may be evident on x-ray examination. Such calcification is usually gross and irregular and does not resemble the finely stippled calcification of the psammoma bodies seen in papillary cancers.

The peripheral manifestations of toxic adenoma are generally milder than those of Graves' disease and are notable for the absence of infiltrative orbitopathy and myopathy; cardio-

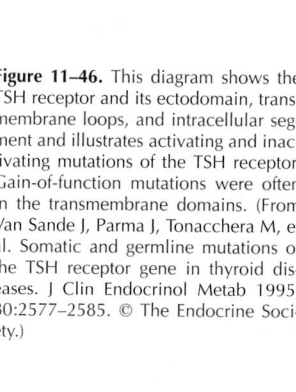

Figure 11–46. This diagram shows the TSH receptor and its ectodomain, transmembrane loops, and intracellular segment and illustrates activating and inactivating mutations of the TSH receptor. Gain-of-function mutations were often in the transmembrane domains. (From Van Sande J, Parma J, Tonacchera M, et al. Somatic and germline mutations of the TSH receptor gene in thyroid diseases. J Clin Endocrinol Metab 1995; 80:2577–2585. © The Endocrine Society.)

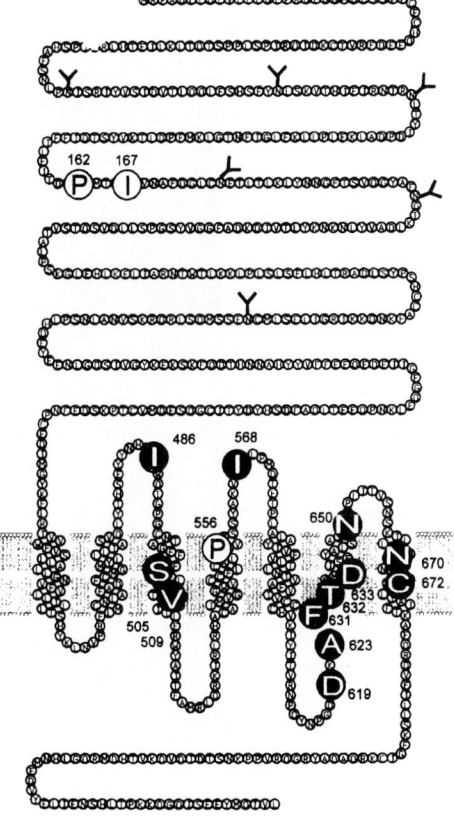

Loss of function:

Pro	162	Ala
Ile	167	Asn
Pro	556	Leu (mouse)

Gain of function:

Ile	486	Phe/Met
Ser	505	Arg
Val	509	Ala
Ile	568	Thr
Asp	619	Gly
Ala	623	Ile/Val
Phe	631	Leu/Cys
Thr	632	Ile
Asp	633	Glu/Tyr
Asn	650	Tyr
Asn	670	Ser
Cys	672	Tyr

vascular manifestations may be prominent. The nodule is usually felt as a smooth, well-defined, round or ovoid mass that is firm and moves freely on swallowing. Often the remainder of the gland is not palpable. A bruit is never present.

LABORATORY TESTS. The results of laboratory tests depend on the stage of the disorder. At first, serum thyroid hormone concentrations may be normal except for borderline suppression of the serum TSH. This, together with ultrasound examination to exclude multiple nodules, confirms the diagnosis. Later a thyroid scintiscan may show localization of radioisotope in the palpated nodule, but this does not occur until TSH secretion is suppressed. If the nodule continues to grow, frank hyperthyroidism is accompanied by elevation of serum thyroid hormone levels and metabolic indices. When the nodule is small, the RAIU is normal but cannot be suppressed completely by exogenous thyroid hormone. However, TSH and therefore function in the extranodular tissue will be suppressed by exogenous hormone, allowing identification of the autonomous nature of the nodular lesion by scanning even before the lesion has become sufficiently large to suppress serum TSH. Occasionally, values for serum T_4 concentration are normal, and only the serum T_3 level is increased (T_3 toxicosis). Relative to its overall rate of occurrence, toxic adenoma is the most frequent cause of T_3 toxicosis. If there is any question about the presence of the suppressed lobe, exogenous TSH may be administered before scintiscanning to demonstrate uptake in this tissue. Incidental thyroid carcinoma may rarely coexist within a gland exhibiting a hyperfunctioning adenoma, although malignant nodules that cause functional hyperthyroidism are rare.

TREATMENT. Although many hyperfunctioning adenomas eventually cause hyperthyroidism, some do so slowly, and others not at all. Therefore treatment of asymptomatic patients with functional adenomas is decided on an individual basis. The degree of TSH suppression is an index of the progression of thyroid hormone production by the adenoma. Suppression below the lower limits of normal indicates that hyperthyroidism is present and that therapy should be given except in unusual situations. Two therapies are available: radioiodine and surgery. Large nodules with concomitant physical symptoms are most readily treated with surgical excision. Surgical excision is also used in patients younger than age 20, in whom radiation from ^{131}I to the perinodular normal thyroid tissue could theoretically predispose to the development of radiation-related thyroid neoplasia.[639]

In terms of the specificity of treatment, functioning thyroid nodules are ideal candidates for radioiodine therapy. The radiation is directed almost exclusively to the diseased tissue; because TSH is suppressed, the normal thyroid tissue surrounding the nodule does not take up radioiodine, although many patients develop thyroid failure. For the patient older than age 20 with a nodule 5 cm in diameter or smaller, ^{131}I is an appropriate treatment if the risk of eventual hypothyroidism is acceptable. In general, higher doses of radioiodine are required than in Graves' disease, namely 185 to 370 MBq (5 to 10 mCi) deposited at 24 h.[640] Because of the potential for hypothyroidism with higher ^{131}I doses, prolonged follow-up is mandatory.[641] Suppression of TSH by exogenous liothyronine (T_3), 25 μg/d for 7 d, may be used in appropriate patients to reduce ^{131}I uptake by the normal thyroid tissue during therapy.

The toxic adenoma is not diffusely hypervascular, and consequently preoperative preparation with iodine is not required. In the patient with overt thyrotoxicosis, however, a normal metabolic state should be restored with an antithyroid drug before surgery.

Inherited Nonautoimmune Autosomal Dominant Hyperthyroidism

Toxic thyroid hyperplasia without the pathologic characteristics of autoimmune disease has been reported in a few families and appears to be inherited as an autosomal dominant.[642] Polymorphic genomic mutations in the TSHR gene have been reported to cause constitutively activated TSHRs differing from family to family. These gain-of-function mutations in the transmembrane regions of the TSHR are similar to those seen in toxic adenomas (see Fig. 11–16).[637] Treatment is by radioiodine ablation or thyroidectomy, depending on the age of the patient.

Transient Hyperthyroidism

Subacute Thyroiditis

Subacute thyroiditis has been termed granulomatous giant cell or de Quervains' thyroiditis. It is thought to be caused by a viral infection of the thyroid gland and often follows an upper respiratory illness. A tendency to a seasonal and geographic aggregation of cases has been noted. The mumps virus has been implicated in some cases, and coxsackievirus, influenza virus, echoviruses, and adenoviruses may also be etiologic agents.[643] Evidence of thyroid autoimmunity is often present during the active phase of the disease.[644] This autoimmunity is usually transitory, although some patients may retain evidence of thyroid autoimmunity for many years.[645] A small number of patients eventually develop autoimmune thyroid disease.

Subacute thyroiditis is uncommon, but mild cases may be mistakenly diagnosed as pharyngitis. Women are more frequently affected than men, and the peak incidence is in the fourth and fifth decades.

HISTOPATHOLOGY. The histopathologic changes (Fig. 11–47) are different from those in Hashimoto's disease. The lesions are patchy in distribution and vary in their stage of development from area to area. Affected follicles are infiltrated predominantly with mononuclear cells and show disruption of epithelium, partial or complete loss of colloid, and fragmentation and duplication of the basement membrane.

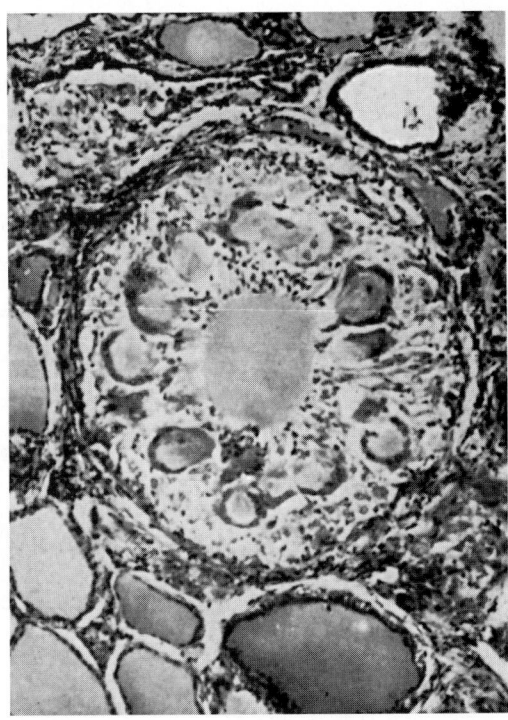

Figure 11–47. Subacute thyroiditis. Intrafollicular giant cell surrounding a central core of colloid. (From Meachim G, Young MH. De Quervain's subacute granulomatous thyroiditis: histological identification and incidence. J Clin Pathol 1963; 16:189–199.)

To this extent, the histopathologic appearance may resemble that in Hashimoto's disease. A characteristic feature is the well-developed follicular lesion that consists of a central core of colloid surrounded by the multinucleate giant cells, from which stems the designation "giant cell" thyroiditis. Colloid may be found in the interstitium or within the giant cells (colloidophagy). The follicular changes progress to form granulomas. Interfollicular fibrosis and an interstitial inflammatory reaction are present to varying degrees. When the disease subsides, an essentially normal histologic appearance is restored.

PATHOPHYSIOLOGY. Destruction of follicular epithelium and loss of follicular integrity are the primary events in the pathophysiology. Tg, preformed hormone, and abnormal iodinated materials are released, often in quantities sufficient to elevate not just the serum Tg level but also the serum T_4 and T_3 concentrations, produce clinical thyrotoxicosis, and suppress TSH secretion. As a result of the latter, thyroid function is suppressed, the RAIU decreases to low levels, and hormone synthesis ceases. Destruction of the follicular epithelium contributes to lowering of the RAIU and disruption of hormone synthesis, because TSH may fail to increase the RAIU normally. Later in the disease, when stores of preformed hormone are depleted, serum T_4 and T_3 concentrations decline, sometimes into the hypothyroid range, and the serum TSH level rises, often to elevated values (Fig. 11–48). As the disease becomes inactive, the RAIU may be greater than normal for a time as hormone stores are repleted. Ultimately, when hormone secretion resumes, serum T_4 and T_3 concentrations rise, and serum TSH concentration decreases to normal values.

CLINICAL PICTURE. The characteristic feature is the gradual or sudden appearance of pain in the region of the thyroid gland with or without fever. The pain, which is aggravated by turning the head or swallowing, characteristically radiates to the ear, jaw, or occiput and may mimic disorders arising in these areas. The absence of pain does not exclude the diagnosis, because biopsy-proven painless subacute thyroiditis occurs, but it must be distinguished from autoimmune thyroiditis.[646] Hoarseness and dysphagia may be present; patients may complain of palpitation, nervousness, and lassitude; lassitude can be extreme, considering the local nature of the disease, and indicating a systemic component. Although acute manifestations are present in severe cases, in milder disease, which is often wrongly diagnosed, symptoms may be present

for months. On palpation at least part of the thyroid is slightly to moderately enlarged, firm, often nodular, and usually exquisitely tender, one lobe frequently being more severely affected than the other. Indeed the symptoms may be truly unilateral. The overlying skin may be warm and red. Occasionally the locus of maximal involvement migrates over the course of a few weeks to other parts of the gland. The disease usually subsides within a few months, leaving no residual deficiency of thyroid function, but often passes through a transient phase of hypothyroidism, resembling the syndrome of transient silent autoimmune thyroiditis with transient thyrotoxicosis (see Fig. 11–48). In rare cases the disease may smolder, with repeated exacerbations over many months, hypothyroidism sometimes being the final result.

LABORATORY TESTS. The laboratory findings vary with the phase of the disease. During the active phase, the erythrocyte sedimentation rate can be increased, to a remarkable extent. Indeed a diagnosis of active subacute thyroiditis is hardly tenable when the sedimentation rate is normal. The leukocyte count is normal or, at most, moderately increased. The serum Tg level is characteristically high, in keeping with the degree of thyroid destruction.

Subacute thyroiditis is one of several causes of "low-uptake thyrotoxicosis," the others being so-called silent thyroiditis (see earlier), thyrotoxicosis factitia, and iodine-induced hyperthyroidism. For reasons described earlier, the RAIU is subnormal, despite the presence of normal, or often elevated, values of serum T_4 and T_3 concentrations. At this point in the course, basal serum TSH is suppressed. In the typical patient, TPO and Tg autoantibodies are either not detectable or present in low levels. In milder cases some uptake of radioiodine may persist in unaffected portions of the gland, as revealed by scintiscan, but this is unusual, and a diagnosis of active subacute thyroiditis should be viewed with suspicion if the RAIU is normal.

In the hypothyroid phase, serum T_4 and T_3 concentrations are low, and the serum TSH concentration is appropriately elevated (see Fig. 11–48). With recovery, the RAIU returns to normal or high levels and values for serum T_4 and T_3 concentrations are restored to normal.

DIFFERENTIAL DIAGNOSIS. Subacute thyroiditis must be differentiated from acute hemorrhagic degeneration in a pre-existing thyroid nodule, Hashimoto's disease of acute onset, silent thyroiditis, and acute pyogenic thyroiditis. Differentiation from hemorrhage into a nodule presents no difficulty

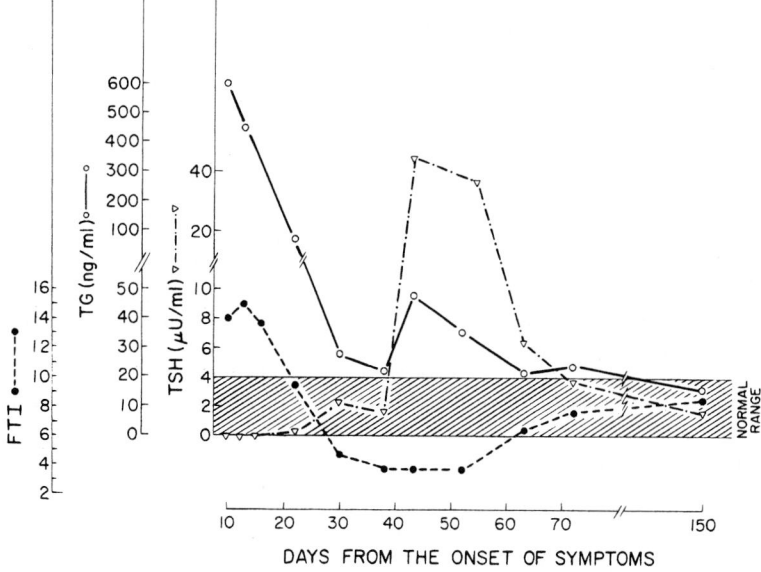

Figure 11–48. Thyroid function in a patient in the course of de Quervain's (subacute) thyroiditis. During the thyrotoxic phase (days 10 to 20) the serum Tg concentration was elevated, the FTI was high, and TSH was suppressed. The erythrocyte sedimentation rate was 86 mm/h, and the thyroidal RAIU was 2%. The Tg level and FTI declined in parallel. During the phase of hypothyroidism (days 30 to 63), when the FTI was below normal, the serum Tg level transiently increased in parallel with the increase in serum TSH. All parameters of thyroid function were normal by day 150, 5 mo after the onset of symptoms. (From DeGroot LJ, Larsen PR, Hennemann G, eds. Acute and subacute thyroiditis. In: The Thyroid And Its Diseases. 6th ed. New York: Churchill Livingstone, 1996: 705.)

DAYS FROM THE ONSET OF SYMPTOMS

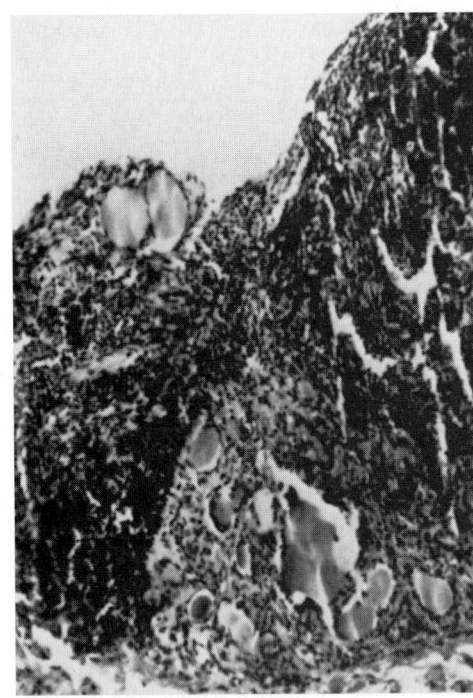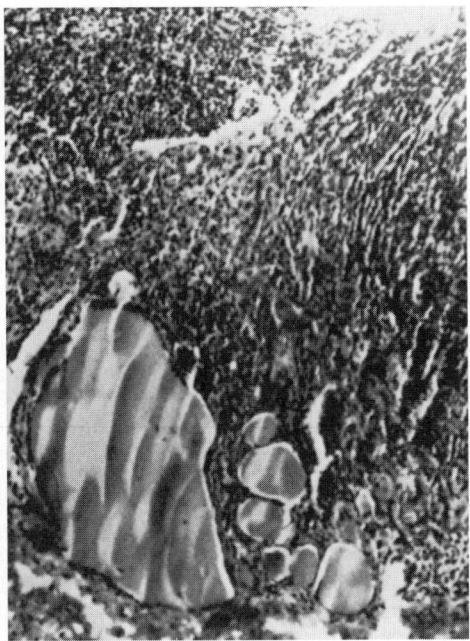

Figure 11–49. High- and low-power magnification of a thyroid gland biopsy during the hypothyroid phase of "silent thyroiditis." Note the extensive lymphocytic infiltration and patchy distribution of poorly preserved follicles. (From Woolf PD. Transient painless thyroiditis with hyperthyroidism: a variant of lymphocytic thyroiditis? Endocr Rev 1980; 1:411–420. © 1980, The Endocrine Society.)

when this occurs in a multinodular goiter, because other non-tender nodules will be felt. Detection is more difficult when there is hemorrhage into a solitary nodule, but this should be easily seen on ultrasound. In both varieties of hemorrhage, function in the remainder of the gland persists, and the sedimentation rate is rarely elevated. Hashimoto's disease of acute onset may be accompanied by pain and tenderness in the thyroid gland, but the gland usually is diffusely affected. Painless thyroiditis with thyrotoxicosis and a decreased RAIU but with a histologic picture of autoimmune thyroiditis and no giant cells, often termed *hashitoxicosis*, may be difficult to distinguish from painless subacute thyroiditis. Lack of elevation of the erythrocyte sedimentation rate and high titers of thyroid autoantibodies strongly suggest the former. Acute pyogenic thyroiditis is distinguished by the presence of a septic focus elsewhere, by a greater inflammatory reaction in the tissues adjacent to the thyroid, and by much greater leukocytic and febrile responses. The RAIU is usually preserved in acute pyogenic thyroiditis. Rarely, widespread infiltrating cancer of the thyroid can present with a clinical and laboratory picture almost indistinguishable from that of subacute thyroiditis.[647]

TREATMENT. In mild cases, aspirin or nonsteroidal anti-inflammatory drugs generally control the symptoms. In more severe cases, glucocorticoids (e.g., prednisone up to 40 mg/d) alleviate the manifestations but do not influence the underlying disease process. Hence the symptoms may be exacerbated if treatment is withdrawn too early but will again respond if treatment is reinstituted. The chance of relapse may be minimized if glucocorticoid therapy is continued at a dose that maintains the patient in an asymptomatic state until the RAIU has returned to normal.[648] Thyroid hormone replacement therapy may decrease the size of the gland by suppressing TSH and relieving the pressure on the thyroid capsule. However, TSH is needed for thyroid cell regeneration, so such therapy should be decreased as the symptoms subside.

Silent or Painless Thyroiditis

Thyrotoxicosis is associated with the early phase of subacute thyroiditis, in both painful and painless variants. Thyrotoxicosis can also occur without pain in early autoimmune thyroiditis, in which biopsy of the thyroid reveals the histopathologic changes of Hashimoto's disease rather than those of subacute thyroiditis (Fig. 11–49).[649] This syndrome has variously been alluded to as silent or painless thyroiditis with thyrotoxicosis, "hyperthyroidism," or "hashitoxicosis."

The cardinal features are thyrotoxicosis associated with depressed values of the RAIU in the absence of excess body iodide stores, lack of pain or tenderness in the thyroid area, and spontaneous resolution of the thyrotoxic phase of the disease. There is a tendency to pass through a transient euthyroid and then a hypothyroid phase before a long-term return to euthyroidism and a tendency for the syndrome to recur (Fig. 11–50). The thyroid gland is enlarged in only about 50% of cases, and enlargement is usually mild and unaccompanied by nodularity. Thyrotoxicosis is usually mild, and this is reflected in the extent of elevation of serum T_4 and T_3 levels. Although TPO autoantibodies can be detected in most patients by sensitive assays, agglutination assays reveal antithyroid antibodies in only about one half of the patients. Systemic manifestations of inflammation are lacking, and the erythrocyte sedimentation rate is normal or nearly normal.

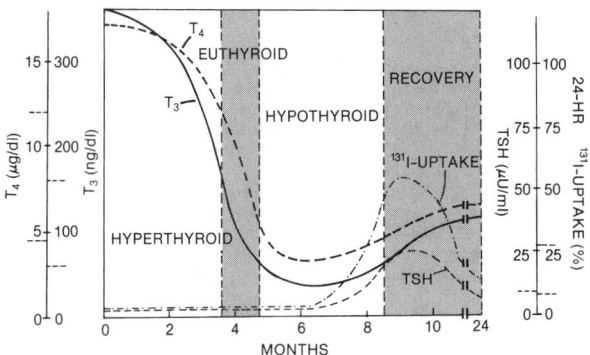

Figure 11–50. Schematic of the typical course in chronic thyroiditis with transient thyrotoxicosis. The duration of each phase may vary, and some patients do not experience a discernible hyperthyroid or hypothyroid phase. (From Woolf PD. Transient painless thyroiditis with hyperthyroidism: a variant of lymphocytic thyroiditis? Endocr Rev 1980; 1:411–420. © 1980, The Endocrine Society.)

Several aspects of the pathophysiology of this disorder are instructive. Reduction in the RAIU cannot be explained by iodine excess, as it is in the jodbasedow phenomenon. Thus, as in subacute thyroiditis, the rate of ongoing synthesis of thyroid hormones is negligible, justifying the classification of this disorder among those that lead to thyrotoxicosis without hyperthyroidism. Decreased values of the RAIU are due partly to suppression of TSH secretion by the excess of circulating hormones, because the serum TSH level is suppressed. But function of the thyroid follicular cell is also impaired because the RAIU does not increase after administration of TSH, presumably secondary to T cell– and antibody-mediated thyroid cell lysis. Although not grossly excessive, urinary iodine excretion is at the upper limit or slightly above normal because of the subnormal RAIU. Finally the tendency of the disorder to pass through a hypothyroid phase is not surprising in view of the extensive depletion of glandular hormone stores that occur while hormone is leaking from the gland and new hormone synthesis is impaired.

The duration of the thyrotoxic phase averages about 2 mo. About one half of the patients return to a euthyroid phase and remain well, at least for some time. In the remaining half, a hypothyroid phase may follow and last from 2 to 9 mo. In most, there is eventual restoration of euthyroidism, but some develop permanent hypothyroidism years later.[650] About one third retain a goiter, usually with persistence of thyroid autoantibodies in the serum. The opposite sequela, recurrence of thyrotoxicosis, may also occur months or years after restoration of a euthyroid state, and some patients have multiple recurrences.

Treatment of the thyrotoxic phase consists of alleviation of the peripheral manifestations through the use of propranolol or sedatives. Reportedly, prednisone (30 to 50 mg/d) decreases the duration of the thyrotoxic phase without the risk of relapse on its withdrawal, but is not needed.[651] If mild and brief, the hypothyroid phase may not require treatment. When treatment is required, it should be undertaken with the understanding that it will be withdrawn approximately 6 mo later, because the hypothyroidism is unlikely to be permanent.

The underlying nature of this disorder is an autoimmune dysregulation. Extensive lymphocytic infiltration and the presence of plasma cells within the thyroid are reminiscent of, although not identical to, those in Hashimoto's thyroiditis, as are the circulating thyroid autoantibodies. The latter, however, may merely reflect a response to the inflammatory release of antigens. The occurrence of the syndrome in patients known to have Graves' disease, which the authors and others have observed, and the later emergence of hypothyroidism or Hashimoto's disease are also consonant with an autoimmune etiology. On the other hand, the absence of high titers of circulating antithyroid antibodies and the permanent resolution indicate that the immune system regains its equilibrium in an unknown manner.

Postpartum Thyroiditis

The postpartum thyroiditis syndrome is similar in presentation, course, and pathophysiology to silent thyroiditis (Fig. 11–51).[652] Transient thyrotoxicosis with low RAIU may develop within 3 to 12 mo after delivery and is often followed by a period of hypothyroidism of several months' duration and an eventual return to a euthyroid state. In some patients, only a hypothyroid phase is evident. Postpartum hypothyroidism may occur in as many as 10% of women and in more than 30% of those with positive TPO autoantibodies.[653, 654] This argues for prenatal assessment for the presence of TPOAb and postpartum assessment in women with TPOAb of thyroid function at 2, 4, 6, and 12 mo. As in the similar syndrome not temporally related to pregnancy, recurrences are common after subsequent pregnancies. Most patients have a small goiter and positive tests for TPOAb, although titers may be low. The syndrome has also been observed post partum in patients known to have Graves' disease. There is a strong association with the HLA-DR3 and HLA-DR5 haplotypes,[654] which are also associated with Hashimoto's disease. The occurrence of the disorder post partum is probably due to a rebound of immune activity after its suppression during pregnancy.[624]

Reports from Japan indicated that approximately 5% of women developed postpartum thyroiditis syndrome; of these, about 50% had transient thyrotoxicosis alone, 25% had transient hypothyroidism alone, and the remainder had both phases of the disease.[655] This, and even higher frequencies, have been reported in other centers and appear to average nearer 10% in the United States. Thyroid function should be surveyed with measurements of serum T_4, T_3, and TSH levels, if not in all women in the postpartum period, at least in those who have serum TPOAb and in all women with symptoms suggestive of thyroid dysfunction, some of which were ascribed

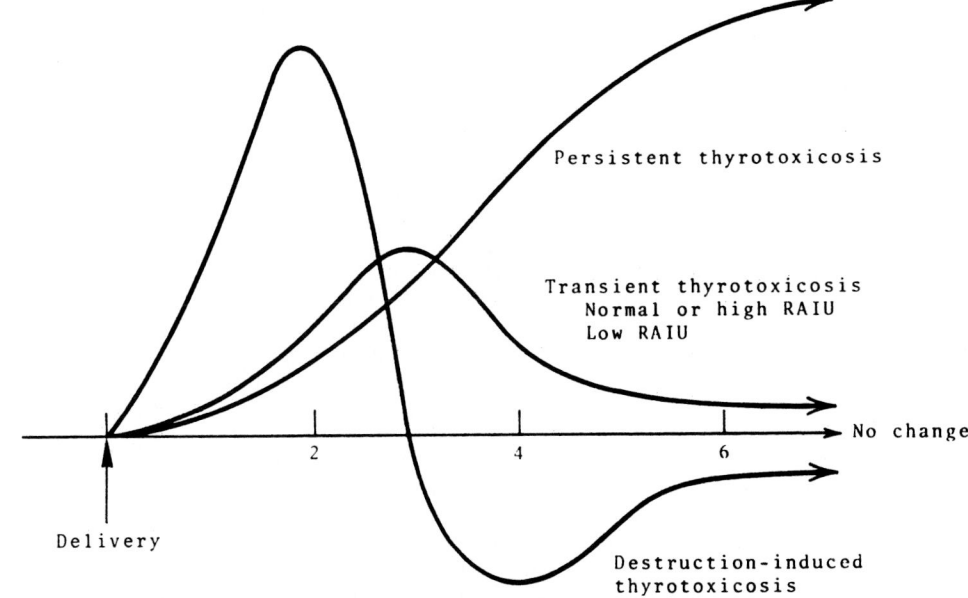

Figure 11–51. Changes in free thyroxine in various types of postpartum thyroid disease. The numbers indicate months postpartum. (From Amino N, Miyai H. In: Davies TF, ed. Autoimmune Endocrine Disease. New York: Wiley, 1983: 255.)

to psychological factors or other disease in the past. Furthermore patients who have experienced one episode of the postpartum thyroiditis syndrome should be considered at risk for recurrence of the syndrome both after and between pregnancies. By the same token, women of childbearing age who have had thyrotoxicosis unrelated to pregnancy should be considered at risk for development of the postpartum syndrome after pregnancy.

Hyperthyroidism Due to TSH or TSHR Agonists

Rarely hyperthyroidism results from hypersecretion of TSH or TSH-like activity because of three causative factors: (1) a TSH-secreting pituitary adenoma, (2) inappropriate hypersecretion of TSH secondary to localized pituitary resistance to thyroid hormones or increased secretion of TRH, and (3) excessive secretion of hCG from trophoblastic tumors. All varieties are associated with a diffuse hyperfunctioning goiter. Features of autoimmune thyroid disease are absent in patients and in the families of patients. When TSH is the cause, the serum TSH concentrations are not suppressed at a time when serum free T_4 and/or T_3 concentrations are elevated.[349]

TSH-SECRETING PITUITARY TUMORS. In the adenomatous variety, a mass lesion is present in the pituitary (see Chapter 9). The concentration of free α subunits of TSH in serum is elevated, and serum TSH concentrations may fail to increase after TRH administration. In patients with nonadenomatous TSH hypersecretion, in contrast, α subunits are not present in the blood in high concentrations, and the response to TRH is usually normal.[342, 348, 349] Patients with thyroid hormone resistance may respond to oral T_3 rather than T_4. Patients with excess TSH in the absence of resistance present a difficult therapeutic problem. In some cases, TSH secretion can be suppressed if very large doses of thyroid hormone are administered, but this results in worsening of the thyrotoxicosis. Hyperthyroidism can be controlled, of course, by thyroid ablation, but the serum TSH level then increases still further, raising the question as to whether a TSH-producing adenoma may ultimately develop. Bromocriptine, a dopamine agonist, may suppress TSH secretion and alleviate the hyperthyroidism in this disorder.[656] Somatostatin analogues have also been used. However, TSH-producing tumors usually require surgical resection.[657, 658] Treatment with 3,5,3′-triiodothyroacetic acid has also been successful.[659]

The occurrence of TSH-induced hyperthyroidism is further support for the argument that a serum TSH concentration should be measured as part of the initial work-up of every patient who is hyperthyroid and has a diffuse goiter. The remote possibility that a patient with Graves' disease might have an artifactual elevation of TSH concentration because of a heterophilic antibody cross-reacting with mouse immunoglobulin (see discussion of TSH assay) must be kept in mind.[189] For some sera, the use of a different assay kit may confirm the elevated level. Alternatively, mouse serum may be added to the assay tube to absorb the heterophile antibody.

PITUITARY RESISTANCE TO THYROID HORMONE. In some patients with inherited thyroid hormone resistance due to mutations in the β thyroid hormone receptor, the hypothalamic pituitary feedback mechanism may be more resistant to the effects of thyroid hormone than are peripheral tissues such as the heart.[373, 660, 661] These patients may have a hyperthyroid appearance with tachycardia, nervousness, and goiter associated with an elevated FT_4I. However, since the thyroid hormone hyperproduction is TSH-driven, serum TSH concentrations are detectable (>0.1 mU/L) or even elevated inappropriately for the circulating thyroid hormone levels. In general, the manifestations are due not to excessive but rather to inadequate thyroid hormone action, and these individuals may

require treatment with thyroid hormone or thyroid hormone analogues and/or β-adrenergic receptor–blocking agents rather than antithyroid drugs.[372, 660, 661] This argues again for the appropriateness of at least one serum TSH measurement in every hyperthyroid patient, since this is the only way that an accurate diagnosis can be achieved (see also the discussion of thyroid hormone resistance in the section on hypothyroidism). Rarely, families with pituitary resistance to thyroid hormone (PRTH), possibly due to a deficiency of type 2 deiodinase (D2), may respond to treatment with liothyronine.[662]

HYPERTHYROIDISM IN TROPHOBLASTIC DISEASE. Thyroid hyperfunction often accompanies hydatidiform mole, choriocarcinoma, or metastatic embryonal carcinoma of the testis. Such neoplasms, particularly hydatidiform mole, elaborate differentially glycosylated hCG molecules that exhibit crossover specificity for binding to the TSH receptor and can induce thyroid overactivity.[259, 260, 264] Some patients have clinically overt thyrotoxicosis; however, clinical manifestations are usually not prominent, and goiter is absent or minimal despite laboratory evidence of a hyperthyroid state. Free T_4 and/or free T_3 levels are increased, and TSH values are suppressed. The reason for this discordance between the clinical and the laboratory indices is not known but may be due to the relatively short duration of thyroid hormone excess. The possibility of a molar pregnancy should always be considered in a young woman with thyrotoxicosis, because appropriate therapy is evacuation of the uterus.

Iodine-Induced Hyperthyroidism

Administration of supplemental iodine to subjects with endemic iodine-deficiency goiter can result in iodine-induced Graves' disease. This response, termed *iodine-induced hyperthyroidism* or the *jodbasedow* effect, occurs in only a small fraction of individuals at risk. The best studied experience has been in Tasmania, where a temporary increase in thyrotoxicosis occurred shortly after the addition of small quantities of iodine to bread as a means of correcting iodine deficiency. Studies revealed two major patterns of underlying thyroid disorder. In the first, especially common in older individuals, nodular goiter with areas of autonomous function were present, and TSHR autoantibodies of the type found in Graves' disease were not detectable in the blood. The second pattern occurred in younger individuals with diffuse goiter, and here stimulating TSHR autoantibodies were often present. These findings suggest that jodbasedow occurs only in thyroid glands in which function is independent of TSH stimulation. The occurrence of jodbasedow should not be construed as a reason for failing to treat endemic iodine deficiency. Apart from the many other benefits that accrue from iodine treatment and prophylaxis, over the long run the frequency of spontaneous hyperthyroidism associated with the development of autonomous nodules is diminished.

Iodine-induced hyperthyroidism is an important disorder in areas of the world in which dietary iodine intake is high.[595] In regions in which iodine intake is marginal but overt iodine deficiency is absent, moderate increments in iodine intake may induce hyperthyroidism in patients with autonomous thyroid nodules, and large pharmacologic doses of iodine, such as those employed in the treatment of pulmonary disease, can do so in geographic areas in which the iodine intake is more than adequate. Consequently the physician must be alert to the possibility of inducing hyperthyroidism when administering large quantities of iodine in expectorants, x-ray contrast media, medications containing iodine, or any other form to patients with nodular goiter. Because nodular goiter is generally a disease of older people, induction of the jodbasedow phenomenon can have serious consequences, particularly because enrichment of the thyroid with iodine forestalls administration of ^{131}I and delays the response to antithyroid agents.

In these patients, serum T_3 concentration is sometimes normal, although total and free T_4 concentrations are increased and TSH is suppressed. Confirmation that the patient has been exposed to large quantities of iodine can be obtained by demonstrating that the RAIU is low and urinary iodine excretion increased (more than several milligrams per day).

Although the jodbasedow phenomenon can occur only when the thyroid is free from normal regulatory control, patients with iodine-induced hyperthyroidism have been reported in whom thyroid function was normal and normally suppressible after iodine was withdrawn and a euthyroid state restored. The mechanism by which iodine induces thyrotoxicosis in such instances is unknown. The treatment of these individuals may be difficult. Even after discontinuation of exogenous iodide, the uptake of ^{131}I by the thyroid gland may remain low, not adequate for conventional doses of radioiodine. The elevated thyroid hormone content also makes thionamide drugs less effective. In some cases it may be necessary to treat such individuals for prolonged periods (6 to 9 mo) before administering radioiodine therapy. On the other hand, if uptake is detectable, larger doses of radioiodine may be given to destroy thyroid tissue.

Thyrotoxicosis Due to Nonthyroid Sources of Thyroid Hormone

THYROTOXICOSIS FACTITIA. Thyrotoxicosis that arises from the ingestion, usually chronic, of excessive quantities of thyroid hormone usually occurs in individuals with a background of underlying psychiatric disease, especially in paramedical personnel who have access to thyroid hormone or in patients for whom thyroid hormone medication has been prescribed in the past.[663] Generally the patient is aware of taking thyroid hormone but may adamantly deny it. In other instances large doses of thyroid hormone or other thyroactive material, such as iodocasein, may be given without the knowledge of the patient, usually as part of a regimen for weight reduction. Symptoms are typical of thyrotoxicosis and may be severe. In the absence of pre-existing disease of the thyroid, diagnosis is made from the combination of typical thyrotoxic manifestations, together with thyroid atrophy and hypofunction. Infiltrative ophthalmopathy never occurs, but lid lag, stare, and other "thyrotoxic" eye signs may be present. Hypofunction of the thyroid gland is evidenced by suppressed serum Tg levels and subnormal values of the RAIU, which can be increased by administration of TSH. Serum T_4 concentrations are increased unless the patient is taking T_3, in which case they will be subnormal. Serum T_3 concentrations are increased in either case. TSH levels are suppressed. The presence of low, rather than elevated, values of serum Tg concentration is a clear indication that the thyrotoxicosis results from exogenous hormone, rather than thyroid hyperfunction.[336] This disorder may be confused with other varieties of thyrotoxicosis associated with a subnormal RAIU and absence of goiter, including the syndrome of chronic thyroiditis with transient thyrotoxicosis; ectopic thyroid tissue; and hyperfunctioning metastatic follicular carcinoma. Evidence for the two latter disorders can be obtained by demonstration of the ectopic focus or foci by external scintiscanning. Differentiation from painless thyroiditis may be difficult. The presence of circulating TPOAb and TgAb points to painless chronic autoimmune thyroiditis, whereas a firm thyroid and brief history suggest the painless variant of subacute thyroiditis. Treatment of thyrotoxicosis factitia consists of withdrawing the offending medication. Psychiatric help may be necessary.

HAMBURGER THYROTOXICOSIS. An unusual form of exogenous thyrotoxicosis occurred in the midwestern portion

of the United States in 1984 and 1985. The source was the inclusion of large quantities of bovine thyroid in ground beef preparations.[664] When the slaughtering practices were changed, this condition disappeared. Such a possibility, however remote, should be considered, especially if one is confronted with epidemic exogenous thyrotoxicosis.

ECTOPIC THYROID TISSUE. Thyroid tissue may be present in teratomas, especially in the ovary (struma ovarii), and such foci may produce thyrotoxicosis.[664a] Rarely, hyperfunctioning metastases of follicular carcinoma can produce thyrotoxicosis. The distinguishing features of such lesions were discussed earlier.

Special Aspects of Thyrotoxicosis

T_3 TOXICOSIS. Concurrent measurements of T_4 and T_3 production rates have revealed a disproportionate increase in T_3 production in most patients with hyperthyroidism.[184] Whether this phenomenon results solely from the preferential increase in thyroid synthesis of T_3, preferential intrathyroidal T_4-to-T_3 conversion, or a disproportionate increase in peripheral conversion of T_4 to T_3 is uncertain, but the preferential synthesis is likely responsible in the majority.[32] In the extreme case, the production rate of T_3 alone is increased; the thyrotoxic state resulting therefrom has been designated T_3 toxicosis. In some patients T_3 toxicosis may be the forerunner of the usual form of thyrotoxicosis in which production of both T_3 and T_4 is increased, and in other patients it persists as such. T_3 toxicosis may occur with Graves' disease, toxic multinodular goiter, or toxic adenoma. Its prevalence is not known, but it appears to be more common than the conventional types of hyperthyroidism in areas of iodine deficiency. In the authors' experience, it tends to be more frequent in the elderly; consequently in the elderly, reliance should not be placed solely on measurement of the serum T_4 concentration to diagnose hyperthyroidism.

The diagnosis of T_3 toxicosis should be suspected in a patient with clinical manifestations of thyrotoxicosis in whom the serum T_4 level and free T_4 concentration or index are normal or decreased while the serum TSH concentration is suppressed, and documentation of an elevated free T_3 level confirms the diagnosis. The presence of a palpable goiter and normal or increased RAIU exclude the diagnosis of thyrotoxicosis factitia induced by ingestion of T_3. Experience suggests that patients with T_3 toxicosis are more likely to have a long-term remission after withdrawal of antithyroid drug therapy than patients with the usual form of thyrotoxicosis.

T_4 TOXICOSIS. T_4 toxicosis refers to thyrotoxicosis with an increased serum T_4 concentration and free T_4 concentration or index but a normal or decreased serum T_3 concentration. This phenomenon occurs in two circumstances. One is iodine-induced thyrotoxicosis,[595] in which about one third of the patients have a normal serum T_3 concentration and the remainder display proportionate elevations of serum T_3 and T_4 concentrations.[665] The second is thyrotoxicosis accompanied by severe intercurrent illness.[326, 327] Here, that component of the serum T_3 usually contributed by peripheral T_4 5'-monodeiodination is decreased or lacking, so the serum T_3 concentration, sustained mainly or entirely by direct thyroid secretion, is normal or low although the serum T_4 concentration is high. Concomitantly the serum rT_3 concentration is increased, often markedly, owing to inhibition of its 5'-monodeiodination. With recovery from the intercurrent illness, serum rT_3 concentration declines, and serum T_3 concentration increases into the thyrotoxic range.[666] T_4 toxicosis of this type is to be differentiated from the low serum T_3 level and elevated serum T_4 concentration that are occasionally found in the euthyroid sick syndrome.[328] A reduced serum TSH level may not distinguish patients who are mildly hyperthyroid from those who are not.

Thyrotoxic Crisis

Thyrotoxic crisis or accelerated hyperthyroidism or thyroid storm is an extreme accentuation of thyrotoxicosis. The crisis, however, may be exaggerated by an inexperienced physician. It is an uncommon but serious complication, usually occurring in association with Graves' disease but sometimes with toxic multinodular goiter. Before the availability of adequate means for achieving full preoperative control, crisis frequently followed subtotal thyroidectomy ("surgical crisis"); "medical crisis" is now the more common term. Thyrotoxic crisis is usually of abrupt onset and occurs in patients in whom pre-existing thyrotoxicosis has been treated incompletely or has not been treated at all. Crisis is usually precipitated by infection, trauma, surgical emergencies, or operations and less commonly by radiation thyroiditis, diabetic ketoacidosis, toxemia of pregnancy, or parturition. The mechanism by which such factors worsen thyrotoxicosis may be related to cytokine release and acute immunologic disturbance caused by the precipitating condition. The serum thyroid hormone levels in crisis are not appreciably greater than those in uncomplicated thyrotoxicosis. The clinical picture is one of severe hypermetabolism. Fever is almost invariable and may be severe; sweating is profuse. Marked tachycardia of sinus or ectopic origin and arrhythmias may be accompanied by pulmonary edema or congestive heart failure. Early, tremulousness and restlessness are present; delirium or frank psychosis may supervene. Nausea, vomiting, and abdominal pain occur early in the course. As the disorder progresses, apathy, stupor, and coma may supervene, and hypotension can develop. If unrecognized, the condition is invariably fatal. This clinical picture in a patient with a history of pre-existing thyrotoxicosis or with goiter or exophthalmos or both is sufficient to establish the diagnosis, and emergency treatment should not await laboratory confirmation.

There are no foolproof criteria by which severe thyrotoxicosis complicated by some other serious disease can be distinguished from thyrotoxic crisis induced by that disease. In any event, the differentiation between these alternatives is of no great significance because treatment of the two is the same. Treatment of thyrotoxic crisis aims to correct both the severe thyrotoxicosis and the precipitating illness and to provide general support. The patient suspected of having thyroid crisis should be monitored in a medical intensive care unit during the initial phases of therapy. The therapy of crisis per se is designed to inhibit hormone synthesis and release and to antagonize the adrenergically mediated aspects of peripheral thyroid hormone action. Large doses of an antithyroid agent (300 to 400 mg of propylthiouracil every 4 h) are given by mouth, by stomach tube, or, if necessary, per rectum. Propylthiouracil is preferable to methimazole, since it has the additional action of inhibiting the peripheral generation of T_3 from T_4.[41, 577] Administration of propylthiouracil initiates therapy for the postcrisis period and prevents enrichment of glandular hormone stores by the iodine, whose administration is of more immediate importance. The latter agent, administered either as SSKI (five drops every 6 h), ipodate (0.5g bid) or, if available, sodium iodide intravenously (0.250 g/6 h), retards acutely the release of hormone from the thyroid. Propylthiouracil should be administered before iodine to inhibit the synthesis of additional thyroid hormones therefrom. Nonetheless, because iodine blocks release of preformed thyroid hormones from the thyroid gland, its administration *should not be delayed or omitted* in the severely toxic patient if propylthiouracil (or methimazole) is not immediately available. The latter agents may be given by intragastric infusion if necessary. Large

doses of dexamethasone (2 mg orally every 6 h) are given to inhibit both the release of hormone from the gland and the peripheral generation of T_3 from T_4, synergizing with iodide and propylthiouracil, respectively, in these actions. Indeed the combined use of propylthiouracil, iodide, and dexamethasone restores serum T_3 concentration to within the normal range in 24 to 48 h,[597] and the substitution of sodium ipodate or iopanoate for iodide may be even more effective.[596] In the absence of cardiac insufficiency a β-adrenergic blocking agent should be given to ameliorate the manifestations. Most experience has been with propranolol given at a dose of 40 to 80 mg orally every 6 h or 2 mg intravenously, but a short-acting β-adrenergic blocker such as labetalol may be safer than propranolol in this situation. Patients with severe thyrotoxicosis can develop high-output congestive heart failure, and a β-adrenergic antagonist may further reduce cardiac output.

Supportive measures include correction of dehydration and hypernatremia, if present, and administration of glucose. Hyperpyrexia should be treated vigorously. In mild cases, acetaminophen may suffice, but wet packs, fans, or ice packs may be required. Salicylates should be avoided because they compete with T_3 and T_4 for binding to TBG and TTR and therefore increase the free hormone levels.[84] In addition, in large doses, salicylates increase the metabolic rate. If heart failure or pulmonary congestion is present, digitalis and diuretics are indicated. Digitalis derivatives or possibly calcium channel blockers should be used in patients with atrial fibrillation with a rapid ventricular response to block atrioventricular node conduction.

The foregoing regimens have reduced the mortality in this disorder to about 20%, a figure that is still disturbingly high. When treatment is successful, improvement is usually manifested within 1 or 2 d, and recovery occurs within a week. At this time, iodide and dexamethasone are gradually withdrawn, and plans for long-term management are made.

THYROID HORMONE DEFICIENCY

Many structural or functional abnormalities can impair production of thyroid hormones (Table 11–21) and cause the clinical state termed hypothyroidism. The causes can be divided into three main categories: (1) permanent loss or atrophy of thyroid tissue (primary hypothyroidism), (2) hypothyroidism with compensatory thyroid enlargement due to transient or progressive impairment of hormone biosynthesis (goitrous hypothyroidism), and (3) insufficient stimulation of a normal gland as a result of hypothalamic or pituitary disease or defects in the TSH molecule itself (control hypothyroidism). Primary and goitrous hypothyroidism together account for approximately 95% of cases, only 5% or less being due to TSH deficiency.

PREVALENCE. Neonatal screening programs for congenital hypothyroidism in many areas of the world show that hypothyroidism is present in 1 of every 4000 newborns.[11] Acquired impairment of thyroid function affects about 2% of adult women and about 0.1 to 0.2% of adult men in North America.

Peripheral Manifestations of Thyroid Hormone Deficiency

Hypothyroidism can be manifested in all organ systems, and these manifestations are largely independent of the underlying disorder but are a function of the degree of hormone deficiency (Table 11–22).

SKIN AND APPENDAGES. Accumulation of hyaluronic

TABLE 11–21. Causes of Hypothyroidism

Primary Atrophic Hypothyroidism

Primary idiopathic hypothyroidism (probably end-stage Hashimoto's disease)
Postablative (iatrogenic) ^{131}I or surgery or therapeutic radiation for nonthyroidal malignancy
Sporadic athyreotic hypothyroidism (agenesis or dysplasia)
Endemic cretinism (less common, agoitrous form)
Unresponsiveness to TSH

Goitrous Hypothyroidism

Hashimoto's (chronic lymphocytic) thyroiditis
Riedel's struma
Endemic iodine deficiency
Iodine-induced hypothyroidism
Antithyroid agents (thionamides, thiourylenes, thiocyanate, perchlorate, lithium, resorcinol, p-aminosalicylic acid, cyanogenic glucosides, plants from the genus Brassica, etc.)
Inherited defects of hormone synthesis
Amyloidosis, cystinosis, sarcoidosis, hemochromatosis, scleroderma

Transient

Withdrawal of thyroid hormone treatment in patients with an intact thyroid
Removal of toxic adenoma or subtotal thyroidectomy for Graves' disease
Following de Quervain's (subacute or postviral) thyroiditis
Following postpartum lymphocytic thyroiditis
Following ^{131}I treatment for Graves' disease

Central Hypothyroidism

Secondary (pituitary) hypothyroidism
Panhypopituitarism (Sheehan's syndrome, tumors, infiltrative disorders)
Isolated TSH deficiency
TSH synthesis defect
Defect in TSH receptor
Tertiary (hypothalamic) hypothyroidism (idiopathic, traumatic, tumors, infiltrative disorders)

Resistance to Thyroid Hormone Action

---

acid alters the composition of the ground substance in the dermis and other tissues. This material binds water, producing the mucinous edema that is responsible for the thickened features and puffy appearance (termed *myxedema*) with full-blown hypothyroidism (Fig. 11–52). Myxedema is characteristically boggy and nonpitting and is apparent around the eyes, on the dorsa of the hands and feet, and in the supraclavicular fossae. It causes enlargement of the tongue and thickening of the pharyngeal and laryngeal mucous membranes. A histologically similar deposit may occur in patients with Graves' disease, usually over the pretibial area (infiltrative dermopathy or pretibial myxedema). In addition to having a puffy appearance,

TABLE 11–22. Symptoms of Hypothyroidism

Symptom	% of Cases	Symptom	% of Cases
Weakness	99	Constipation	61
Dry skin	97	Gain in weight	59
Coarse skin	97	Loss of hair	57
Lethargy	91	Pallor of lips	57
Slow speech	91	Dyspnea	55
Edema of eyelids	90	Peripheral edema	55
Sensation of cold	89	Hoarseness or aphonia	52
Decreased sweating	89	Anorexia	45
Cold skin	83	Nervousness	35
Thick tongue	82	Menorrhagia	32
Edema of face	79	Palpitation	31
Coarseness of hair	76	Deafness	30
Pallor of skin	67	Precordial pain	25
Memory impairment	66		

Data from Means JH. The Thyroid and Its Diseases. 2nd ed. Philadelphia: JB Lippincott, 1948:233.

the skin is pale and cool as a result of cutaneous vasoconstriction. Anemia may contribute to the pallor; hypercarotenemia gives the skin a yellow tint but does not cause scleral icterus. The secretions of the sweat glands and sebaceous glands are reduced, leading to dryness and coarseness of the skin, which in extreme cases may resemble ichthyosis. Wounds of the skin tend to heal slowly. Easy bruising is due to an increase in capillary fragility. Head and body hair is dry and brittle, lacks luster, and tends to fall out. Hair may be lost from the temporal aspects of the eyebrows. Growth of hair is retarded so that haircuts and shaves are required less often. The nails are brittle and grow slowly.

In secondary hypothyroidism, the changes in the skin and its appendages may be less striking than in primary hypothyroidism. The skin is pale and cool and tends to be thinner and finely wrinkled, and infiltration of the tissues is less prominent. Depigmentation of areas that are normally pigmented, such as the areolae, occurs in pituitary but not primary hypothyroidism.

Histopathologic examination of the skin reveals hyperkeratosis with plugging of hair follicles and sweat glands. The dermis is edematous, and the connective tissue fibers are separated by an increased amount of metachromatically staining, periodic acid–Schiff (PAS)-positive mucinous material. This material consists of protein complexed with two mucopolysaccharides, hyaluronic acid and chondroitin sulfate B. The glycosaminoglycans are mobilized early during treatment with thyroid hormone, leading to an increase in urinary excretion of nitrogen and hexosamines.[667]

CARDIOVASCULAR SYSTEM. The cardiac output at rest is decreased because of reduction in both stroke volume and heart rate, reflecting loss of the inotropic and chronotropic effects of thyroid hormones. Peripheral vascular resistance at rest is increased, and blood volume is reduced. These hemodynamic alterations cause narrowing of pulse pressure, prolongation of circulation time, and decrease in blood flow to the tissues.[394, 668, 669] The decrease in cutaneous circulation is responsible for the coolness and pallor of the skin and the sensitivity to cold. In most tissues the decrease in blood flow is proportional to the decrease in oxygen consumption, so the arteriovenous oxygen difference remains normal. The hemodynamic alterations at rest resemble those of congestive heart failure, but cardiac output increases and peripheral vascular resistance decreases normally in response to exercise unless the hypothyroid state is severe and of long standing.

In severe primary hypothyroidism the heart is enlarged (Fig. 11–53), and the heart sounds are diminished in intensity. These findings are due largely to effusion into the pericardial sac of fluid rich in protein and glycosaminoglycans, but the "flabby" myocardium may also be dilated.[394, 670] Pericardial effusion is rarely of sufficient magnitude to cause tamponade. In pituitary hypothyroidism, the heart is frequently small.

Angina pectoris is uncommon, but it may appear or worsen during treatment of the hypothyroid state with thyroid hormone.[671, 672] There has been much discussion as to whether the hypercholesterolemia that accompanies primary hypothyroidism accelerates the development of coronary atherosclerosis.[389] Necropsy data suggest that the hypercholesterolemia of hypothyroidism predisposes to coronary atherosclerosis only in the presence of hypertension; in normotensive hypothyroid patients the degree of coronary atherosclerosis appears to be similar to that in age- and sex-matched normotensive control subjects.[673] Hypertension is present in 10 to 20% of patients with hypothyroidism.[390]

Electrocardiographic changes include sinus bradycardia, prolongation of the PR interval, low amplitude of the P wave and QRS complex, alterations of the ST segment, and flattened or inverted T waves. Pericardial effusion is probably responsible for the low amplitude. Rarely, complete heart

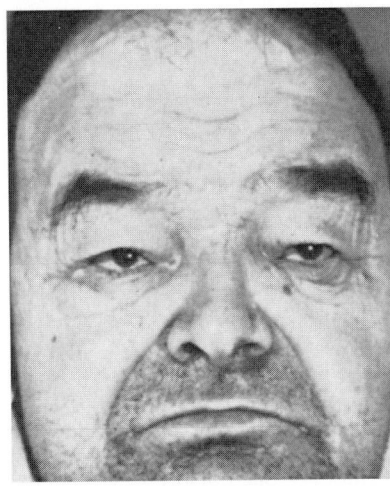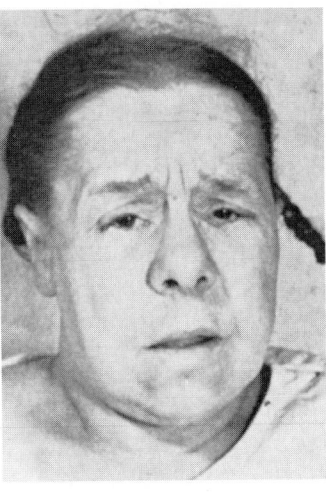

Figure 11–52. Typical facial appearance of severely hypothyroid (myxedematous) patients.

block may be present, but this disappears when hypothyroidism is treated.[674] Systolic time intervals are altered; the pre-ejection period is prolonged, and the ratio of pre-ejection period to left ventricular ejection time is increased. Echocardiographic studies have revealed a high frequency of asymmetrical septal hypertrophy and apparent obstruction of the left ventricular outflow tract, suggesting idiopathic hypertrophic subaortic stenosis. These findings disappear when myxedema is treated, and their hemodynamic significance is uncertain.

The serum levels of creatine kinase, aspartate aminotransferase, and lactate dehydrogenase may be increased.[387, 388] Furthermore the isoenzyme patterns sometimes suggest that the source of the increased creatine kinase and lactate dehydrogenase is cardiac muscle.

The combination of large heart, hemodynamic and electrocardiographic alterations, and the serum enzyme changes has been termed *myxedema heart.* If myxedema heart is ever the sole cause of heart failure,[668, 669] this must be quite rare because the usual hemodynamic response to exercise in hypothyroidism is normal.[396] Furthermore in the patient with hypothyroidism, as in the normal individual, the Valsalva maneuver leads to a decrease in pulse pressure, whereas in the patient with heart failure the pulse pressure does not decrease but displays the so-called square-wave response. In the absence

of coexisting organic heart disease, treatment with thyroid hormone corrects the hemodynamic, electrocardiographic, and serum enzyme alterations of myxedema heart and restores heart size to normal (see Fig. 11–53).

On pathologic examination, the pericardial space contains fluid rich in glycoproteins. The heart is dilated, and the myocardium is pale and flabby. Coronary atherosclerosis is not unusual. Histopathologic examination of the myocardium reveals interstitial edema and swelling of the muscle fibers with loss of striations.

RESPIRATORY SYSTEM. Pleural effusions usually are evident only on radiologic examination but rarely may cause dyspnea. Lung volumes are usually normal, but maximal breathing capacity and diffusing capacity are reduced. In severe hypothyroidism myxedematous involvement of respiratory muscles and depression of both the hypoxic and the hypercapnic ventilatory drives may cause alveolar hypoventilation and carbon dioxide retention, which in turn can contribute to the development of myxedema coma.[675] Obstructive sleep apnea is common but is reversible with restoration of a euthyroid state.[676]

ALIMENTARY SYSTEM. Although most patients have a modest gain in weight, the appetite is usually reduced, and true obesity is not a feature of hypothyroidism per se. The

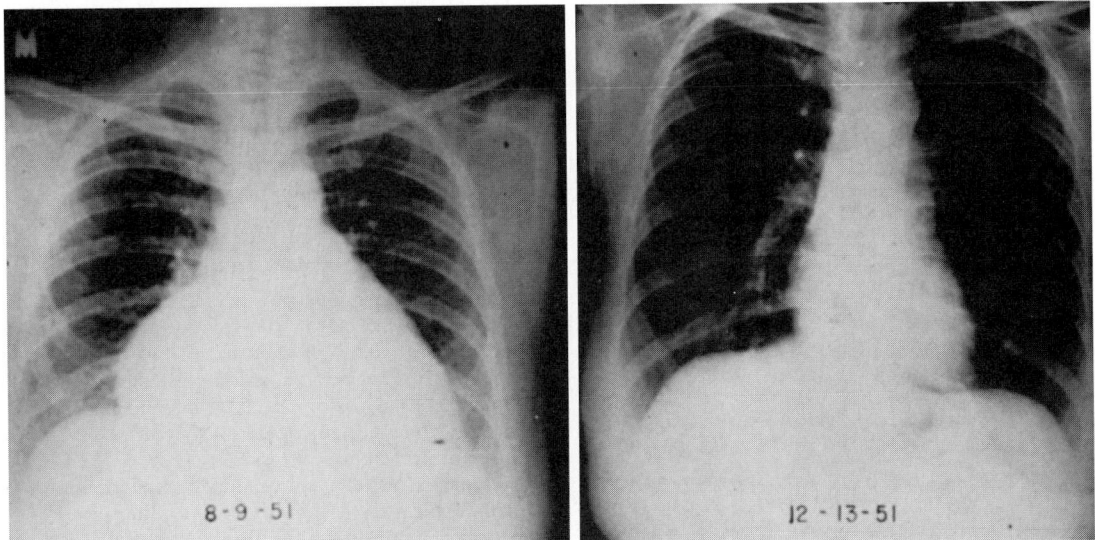

Figure 11–53. Chest roentgenograms in a patient with myxedema heart disease. The patient had signs suggestive of severe congestive heart failure and was treated with thyroid hormone alone. Within 4 mo, the heart had returned to normal size, and there was no evidence of underlying heart disease.

weight gain that occurs is due largely to retention of fluid by the hydrophilic glycoprotein deposits in the tissues. Peristaltic activity is decreased and, together with the decreased food intake, is responsible for the frequent complaint of constipation. The latter may lead to fecal impaction (myxedema megacolon). Gaseous distention of the abdomen (myxedema ileus), if accompanied by colicky pain and vomiting, may mimic mechanical ileus. Elevations in the serum levels of carcinoembryonic antigen, which may occur on the basis of hypothyroidism alone,[677] add to the impression that an organic obstruction is present. Ascites in the absence of another cause is unusual in hypothyroidism, but it can occur, usually in association with pleural and pericardial effusions. Like pericardial and pleural effusions, the ascitic fluid is rich in protein and glycosaminoglycans.

Achlorhydria after maximal histamine stimulation may be present in patients with primary hypothyroidism. Circulating antibodies against gastric parietal cells have been found in about one third of patients with primary hypothyroidism and may be secondary to atrophy of the gastric mucosa. Overt pernicious anemia is reported in about 12% of patients with primary hypothyroidism. The coexistence of pernicious anemia and other autoimmune diseases with primary hypothyroidism supports the view that autoimmunity plays the central role in the pathogenesis of primary hypothyroidism (see Chapter 33).

Hypothyroidism has complex effects on intestinal absorption. Although the rates of absorption for many substances are decreased, the total amount absorbed may be normal or even increased because the decreased bowel motility may allow more time for absorption. Malabsorption is occasionally overt.

Liver function tests are usually normal, but levels of aminotransaminases may be elevated, probably because of impaired clearance. Cholecystography often reveals a distended gallbladder that contracts sluggishly, but whether these changes predipose to the development of gallstones is unknown.

Atrophy of the gastric and intestinal mucosa and myxedematous infiltration of the bowel wall may be demonstrated histologically. The colon may be greatly distended (myxedema megacolon), and the volume of fluid in the peritoneal cavity is usually increased. The liver and pancreas are normal.

NERVOUS SYSTEM. Thyroid hormone is essential for the development of the central nervous system. Deficiency in fetal life or at birth caused retention of the infantile characteristics of the brain, hypoplasia of cortical neurons with poor development of cellular processes, retarded myelination, and reduced vascularity[678] (see Chapter 28). If the deficiency is not corrected in early postnatal life, the damage is irreversible. Deficiency of thyroid hormone beginning in adult life causes less severe manifestations that usually respond to treatment with thyroid hormone. Cerebral blood flow is reduced, but cerebral oxygen consumption is usually normal; this finding is in accord with the finding that the oxygen consumption of isolated brain tissue in vitro, unlike that of most other tissues, is not stimulated by administration of thyroid hormones. In severe cases, decreased cerebral blood flow may lead to cerebral hypoxia.

All intellectual functions, including speech, are slowed. There is loss of initiative; slow-wittedness and memory defects are common; lethargy and somnolence are prominent; dementia in the elderly patient may be mistaken for senile dementia. Psychiatric disorders are common and are usually of the paranoid or depressive type and may induce agitation (myxedema madness).[679] Headaches are frequent. Cerebral hypoxia due to circulatory alterations may predispose to confusional attacks and syncope. Syncope may be prolonged and lead to stupor or coma. Other factors predisposing to coma in hypothyroidism include exposure to severe cold, infection, trauma, hypoventilation with carbon dioxide retention, and depressant drugs. Epileptic seizures have been reported and are prone to occurring in myxedema coma. Night blindness is due to deficient synthesis of the pigment required for dark adaptation. Hearing loss of the perceptive type is frequent. Perceptive deafness may also occur in association with a defect in the organic binding of thyroidal iodide (Pendred's syndrome) or with endemic cretinism, but in these instances it is not due to hypothyroidism per se. Thick, slurred speech and hoarseness are due to myxedematous infiltration of the tongue and larynx, respectively. Body movements are slow and clumsy, and cerebellar ataxia may occur. Numbness and tingling of the extremities are frequent; in the fingers these symptoms may be due to compression by glycosaminoglycan deposits in and around the median nerve in the carpal tunnel (carpal tunnel syndrome).[680, 681] The tendon reflexes are slow, especially during the relaxation phase, producing the characteristic "hung-up reflexes"; this phenomenon is due to a decrease in the rate of muscle contraction and relaxation rather than a delay in nerve conduction. The presence of extensor plantar responses or diminished vibration sense should alert the physician to the possibility of coexisting pernicious anemia with combined system disease. Electroencephalographic changes include slow alpha wave activity and general loss of amplitude. The concentration of protein in the cerebrospinal fluid is often increased, but cerebrospinal pressure is normal.

On histopathologic examination of untreated hypothyroidism, the nervous system is edematous with mucinous deposits in and around nerve fibers. In patients with cerebellar ataxia, neural myxedematous infiltrates of glycogen and mucinous material are present in the cerebellum. There may be foci of degeneration and an increase in glial tissue. The cerebral vessels may show atherosclerosis, but this is much more common if the patient has had coexistent hypertension.[682]

MUSCULAR SYSTEM. Stiffness and aching of muscles are common and are aggravated by cold temperatures.[680, 681] Delayed muscle contraction and relaxation cause the slowness of movement and delayed tendon jerks. Muscle strength is usually normal. Muscle mass may be slightly increased, and the muscles tend to be firm. Rarely, a profound increase in muscle mass with slowness of muscular activity may be the predominant manifestation (the Kocher-Debré-Sémélaigne, or Hoffmann syndrome). Myoclonus may be present. The electromyogram may be normal or may exhibit disordered discharge, hyperirritability, and polyphasic action potentials.

On histopathologic examination, the muscles appear pale and swollen. The muscle fibers may show swelling, loss of normal striations, and separation by mucinous deposits. Type I muscle fibers tend to predominate.[683]

SKELETAL SYSTEM: CALCIUM AND PHOSPHORUS METABOLISM. Thyroid hormone is essential for normal growth and maturation of the skeleton, and growth failure is due both to impaired protein synthesis and to reduction in IGF-I levels[684–686] (see Chapter 30). The human growth hormone gene, unlike that of the rat, does not contain a thyroid hormone response element and does not respond directly to thyroid hormone.[687, 688] Before puberty, thyroid hormone plays a major role in the maturation of bone. Deficiency of thyroid hormone in early life leads to both a delay in the development of and an abnormal, stippled appearance of the epiphyseal centers of ossification (epiphyseal dysgenesis). Impairment of linear growth leads to dwarfism in which the limbs are disproportionately short in relation to the trunk.[684] Bone age is retarded in relation to chronologic age.

Urinary excretion of calcium is decreased as is the GFR, whereas fecal excretion of calcium and both urinary and fecal excretion of phosphorus are variable. Calcium balance is also variable, and any changes are slight. The exchangeable pool of calcium and its rate of turnover are reduced, changes that reflect decreased bone formation and resorption.[465, 689] Because levels of parathyroid hormone are often slightly increased, some degree of resistance to its action may be present; levels of 1,25-dihydroxycholecalciferol are also increased.

Levels of calcium and phosphorus in serum are usually normal, but calcium may be slightly elevated. The alkaline phosphatase level is usually below normal in infantile and juvenile hypothyroidism. Bone density may be increased. The radiologic appearances of the skeleton in cretinism and juvenile hypothyroidism are discussed subsequently.

RENAL FUNCTION: WATER AND ELECTROLYTE METABOLISM. Renal blood flow, glomerular filtration rate, and tubular reabsorptive and secretory maxima are reduced. Blood urea nitrogen and serum creatinine levels are normal, but uric acid levels may be increased. Urine flow is reduced, and delay in the excretion of a water load may result in reversal of the normal diurnal pattern of urine excretion. The delay in water excretion appears to be due to decreased volume delivery to the distal diluting segment of the nephron as a result of the diminished renal perfusion as well as to inappropriate secretion of vasopressin (syndrome of inappropriate antidiuretic hormone [SIADH]).[690, 691] These changes are reversed by treatment with thyroid hormone. The ability to concentrate urine may be slightly impaired. Mild proteinuria may occur.

The impaired renal excretion of water and the retention of water by the hydrophilic deposits in the tissues result in an increase in total body water, even though plasma volume is reduced. This increase accounts for the hyponatremia commonly noted, because the level of exchangeable sodium is increased. The amount of exchangeable potassium is usually normal in relation to lean body mass. Serum magnesium concentration may be increased, but exchangeable magnesium level and urinary magnesium excretion are decreased.

HEMATOPOIETIC SYSTEM. In response to the diminished oxygen requirements and decreased production of erythropoietin, the red blood cell mass is decreased; this is evident in the mild normocytic, normochromic anemia that often occurs. Less commonly, the anemia is macrocytic, sometimes from deficiency of vitamin B_{12}. Reference has already been made to the high incidence of pernicious anemia (and of achlorhydria and vitamin B_{12} deficiency without overt anemia) in primary hypothyroidism. Conversely, overt and subclinical hypothyroidism is present in 12 and 15% of patients, respectively, with pernicious anemia. Hyperthyroidism was present in 9%, and TSH was suppressed in an additional 6%. Folate deficiency from malabsorption or dietary inadequacy may also cause macrocytic anemia. The frequent menorrhagia and the defective absorption of iron resulting from achlorhydria may contribute to a microcytic, hypochromic anemia.

The total and differential white blood cell counts are usually normal, and platelets are adequate, although platelet adhesiveness may be impaired. If pernicious anemia or significant folate deficiency is present, the characteristic changes in peripheral blood and bone marrow will be found. The intrinsic clotting mechanism may be defective because of decreased concentrations in plasma of factors VIII and IX, and this, together with an increase in capillary fragility and the decrease in platelet adhesiveness, may account for the bleeding tendency that sometimes occurs.[467, 692–694]

PITUITARY AND ADRENOCORTICAL FUNCTION. In long-standing hypothyroidism of thyroid origin, hyperplasia of the thyrotropes may cause the pituitary gland to be enlarged, and this can be detected radiologically as an increase in the volume of the pituitary fossa.[695–697] Rarely, the pituitary enlargement compromises the function of other pituitary cells and causes pituitary insufficiency or visual field defects.[698] Patients with severe hypothyroidism may have an increase in serum prolactin level that correlates with the level of serum TSH, and some patients develop galactorrhea.[699] Treatment

with thyroid hormone corrects serum prolactin and TSH levels and causes disappearance of galactorrhea, if present. The cause of hyperprolactinemia in hypothyroidism is uncertain but may result from enhanced sensitivity of the lactotropes to TRH. In severe primary hypothyroidism, the response of growth hormone to provocative stimuli, such as insulin-induced hypoglycemia or growth hormone–releasing hormone may be subnormal.[170, 684]

As a result of the decreased rate of turnover of cortisol, the 24-h urinary excretion of cortisol and 17-hydroxycorticosteroids is decreased, but the plasma cortisol level is usually normal (see Chapter 12). The responses of urinary 17-hydroxycorticosteroid to exogenous vasopressin and metyrapone are usually normal but may be decreased. The response of plasma cortisol to insulin-induced hypoglycemia may be impaired.[170, 700, 701] In severe, long-standing primary hypothyroidism pituitary and adrenal function may be secondarily decreased, and adrenal insufficiency may be precipitated by stress or by rapid replacement therapy with thyroid hormone.[702] The rate of turnover of aldosterone is decreased, but the plasma level is normal. Plasma renin activity is decreased, and sensitivity to angiotensin II is increased[702] (see Chapter 14). In primary hypothyroidism, pituitary histology shows an increase in the number of thyrotropes. The adrenals are usually normal but may show cortical atrophy.[469]

REPRODUCTIVE FUNCTION. In both sexes thyroid hormones influence sexual development and reproductive function. Infantile hypothyroidism, if untreated, leads to sexual immaturity, and juvenile hypothyroidism causes a delay in the onset of puberty followed by anovulatory cycles. Paradoxically, primary hypothyroidism may also cause precocious sexual development and galactorrhea.

In adult women severe hypothyroidism may be associated with diminished libido and failure of ovulation. Secretion of progesterone is inadequate, and endometrial proliferation persists, resulting in excessive and irregular breakthrough menstrual bleeding. These changes may be due to deficient secretion of LH. Rarely, in primary hypothyroidism, secondary depression of pituitary function may lead to ovarian atrophy and amenorrhea. Fertility is reduced, and spontaneous abortion may result, although many pregnancies are successful.[703, 704] Hypothyroidism in men may cause diminished libido, impotence, and oligospermia.

Values for plasma gonadotropins are usually in the normal range in primary hypothyroidism; in postmenopausal women the levels are usually somewhat lower than in euthyroid women of the same age but are nevertheless within the menopausal range. This provides a valuable means of differentiating primary from secondary hypothyroidism.

The metabolism of both androgens and estrogens is altered in hypothyroidism. Secretion of androgens is decreased, and the metabolism of testosterone is shifted toward etiocholanolone rather than androsterone. With respect to estradiol and estrone, hypothyroidism favors metabolism of these steroids via 16α-hydroxylation over that via 2-oxygenation, with the result that formation of estriol is increased and that of 2-hydroxyestrone and its derivative, 2-methoxyestrone, is decreased. The binding activity of TeBG in plasma is decreased, with the result that the plasma concentrations of both testosterone and estradiol are decreased, but the unbound fractions are increased. The alterations in steroid metabolism are corrected by restoration of the euthyroid state.[469]

CATECHOLAMINES AND SEROTONIN. The plasma cAMP response to epinephrine is decreased, suggesting a state of decreased adrenergic activity. The fact that the responses of plasma cAMP to glucagon and parathyroid hormone are also decreased suggests that thyroid hormones have a general modulating influence on cAMP action. The mechanism underlying the decreased adrenergic responsiveness is uncertain.

The secretion rate and plasma concentration of epinephrine are normal, but the corresponding norepinephrine functions are increased.[470, 471]

ENERGY METABOLISM: PROTEIN, CARBOHYDRATE, AND LIPID METABOLISM. The decrease in energy metabolism and heat production is reflected in the low BMR, decreased appetite, cold intolerance, and slightly low basal body temperature. Both the synthesis and the degradation of protein are decreased, the latter especially so, with the result that nitrogen balance is usually slightly positive. The decrease in protein synthesis is reflected in retardation of both skeletal and soft tissue growth. In addition, thyroid hormone deficiency impairs both the secretion and effectiveness of growth hormone, the latter perhaps related to impaired formation of IGF-I.[684–686, 705, 706]

Permeability of capillaries to protein is increased, accounting for the high levels of protein in effusions and in cerebrospinal fluid. In addition, the albumin pool is increased because of the greater decrease in albumin degradation than in albumin synthesis. A greater than normal fraction of exchangeable albumin is in the extravascular space. The total concentration of serum proteins may be increased.

The oral glucose tolerance curve is characteristically flat, and the insulin response to glucose is delayed.[707] These alterations may be due to a decreased rate of absorption of glucose from the gut. The disappearance from plasma of an intravenous load of glucose is delayed because of the slow rate of glucose uptake by tissues. Degradation of insulin is slow, so the sensitivity to exogenous insulin may be increased.[708, 709] Increased insulin sensitivity and the decrease in appetite presumably account for the decrease in insulin requirement when hypothyroidism develops in a patient with pre-existing diabetes mellitus.[701]

Both the synthesis and the degradation of lipid are depressed, the latter especially so, the net effect being one of lipid accumulation, especially of LDL and triglycerides.[391, 392, 710–712] The decrease in the lipid degradation rate may reflect the decrease in postheparin lipolytic activity, as well as reduced LDL receptors.[393, 713] High-density lipoprotein (HDL) concentrations are reduced.[714] The increase in serum cholesterol in primary (but not central) hypothyroidism is accompanied by increased levels of serum phospholipids, serum triglycerides, and LDL.[715, 716] Plasma free fatty acid levels are decreased, and the mobilization of free fatty acids in response to fasting, catecholamines, and growth hormone is impaired.

Composite Clinical Picture of Hypothyroidism

ADULT HYPOTHYROIDISM. The onset of hypothyroidism is usually so insidious that the typical manifestations may take months or years to appear and may go unnoticed by family and friends. The gradual development of the hypothyroid state is due to slow progression both of thyroid hypofunction and of the clinical manifestations after thyroid failure is complete. This course is in contrast with the more rapid development of the hypothyroid state when replacement therapy is discontinued in a patient with treated primary hypothyroidism or when the thyroid gland of a normal subject is surgically removed. In such patients manifestations of frank hypothyroidism are present by 6 wk; by 3 mo myxedema is usually full-blown.

The early symptoms are variable and nonspecific (see Table 11–22). Tiredness and lethargy are common and lead to difficulty in performing a full day's work. Constipation may develop or become worse. The presence of sensitivity to cold is often suggested by the use of more blankets on the bed or a preference for warm weather. Drowsiness and slowing of intellectual and motor activity appear. The patient becomes

apathetic and listless and loses interest in work and environment. Women frequently complain of hair loss, brittle nails, and dry skin. Despite a reduction in appetite, modest weight gain often occurs owing to accompanying fluid retention. The voice becomes husky, which may be attributed to laryngitis, but is due to myxedema of the vocal cords and oropharyngeal structures. Periorbital puffiness may be present (see Fig. 11–52). Stiffness and aching of muscles may be attributed to "rheumatism." Numbness and tingling of the fingers may occur. Progressive deafness may lead the patient to seek medical advice. Eventually, the picture of full-blown myxedema results, with thickened features, enlarged tongue, hoarseness, nonpitting edema, and extreme mental and physical lethargy.

The unusual syndrome of acute hypothyroidism in the previously hyperthyroid patient and characterized by cramping of large muscle has been discussed in the section on radioiodine treatment of Graves' disease.

INFANTILE HYPOTHYROIDISM AND CRETINISM. Severe hypothyroidism is seldom apparent at birth.[717, 718] The age at which symptoms appear depends on the degree of impairment of thyroid function. Severe hypothyroidism in infancy is termed *cretinism*. As the age at onset increases, the clinical picture of cretinism merges imperceptibly with that of juvenile hypothyroidism (see Chapter 31). Retardation of mental development and growth, the hallmarks of cretinism, become manifest only in later infancy and are largely irreversible. Consequently, early recognition is crucial and can be achieved by measuring serum T_4 or TSH concentrations routinely in neonates. During the first few months of life, symptoms of hypothyroidism include feeding problems, failure to thrive, constipation, a hoarse cry, and somnolence. In succeeding months, especially in severe cases, protuberance of the abdomen, dry skin, poor growth of hair and nails, and delayed eruption of the deciduous teeth become evident. Retardation of mental and physical development is manifested by delay in reaching the normal milestones of development, such as holding up the head, sitting, walking, and talking.

Impairment of linear growth results in dwarfism, with the limbs disproportionately short in relation to the trunk. Delayed closure of the fontanelles causes the head to be large in relation to the body. The naso-orbital configuration remains infantile. Maldevelopment of the femoral epiphyses results in a waddling gait. The teeth are malformed and susceptible to caries. The characteristic appearance includes a broad, flat nose, widely set eyes, periorbital puffiness, large protruding tongue, sparse hair, rough skin, short neck, and protuberant abdomen with an umbilical hernia. Mental deficiency is usually severe.

Radiologic examination of the skeleton is diagnostic. The skull shows a poorly developed base, delayed closure of the fontanelles, widely set orbits, and a short, flat nasal bone. The pituitary fossa may be enlarged. Shedding of deciduous teeth and eruption of permanent teeth are delayed. The radiologic picture of epiphyseal dysgenesis is virtually pathognomonic of hypothyroidism in infancy and childhood and may involve any center of endochondral ossification, depending on the age at onset of the hypothyroid state; it is usually best seen in the femoral and humeral heads and the navicular bone of the foot. The centers of ossification appear late, so bone age is retarded in relation to chronologic age, and when they eventually appear, instead of a single center, multiple small centers are scattered through a misshapen epiphysis. These small centers of ossification eventually coalesce and form a single center with an irregular outline and a stippled appearance (*stippled epiphysis*). Epiphyseal dysgenesis is evident only in centers that normally ossify at a time after the onset of the hypothyroidism. After a normal metabolic state is restored by treatment, centers destined to ossify at a later age develop normally.

Hypothyroidism beginning in childhood is termed *juvenile*

hypothyroidism. The clinical manifestations are intermediate between those of infantile and those of adult hypothyroidism, in that the developmental retardation is not as severe as that of cretinism and the manifestations of full-blown adult myxedema are rarely seen. Growth and sexual development are affected predominantly. Linear growth is severely retarded, and the rate of linear growth is usually less than that of weight gain. Maturation of the facial bones is impaired, so that the naso-orbital configuration of the infant or young child is retained. Eruption of permanent teeth is delayed. Sexual maturation and the onset of puberty are delayed. The result is a child who appears much younger than the chronologic age. Rarely, precocious puberty and galactorrhea occur (see Chapter 31). Intellectual performance is poor, but the mental deficiency is not as severe as that in cretinism. The manifestations of adult hypothyroidism are present to a varying, but usually milder, degree. On radiologic examination, epiphyseal dysgenesis may be present, and epiphyseal union is always delayed, resulting in a bone age that is retarded in relation to chronologic age.

LABORATORY TESTS. A decrease in secretion of the thyroid hormones is common to all varieties of hypothyroidism, irrespective of underlying etiology. In patients with primary thyroid disease, the decrease in feedback inhibition of TSH secretion and increase in basal serum TSH concentration (see Fig. 11–17) are the earliest laboratory abnormalities (Table 11–23). With time serum T_4 and T_3 concentrations become subnormal, the former more rapidly than the latter. This is due to preferential synthesis and secretion of T_3 by residual functioning thyroid tissue under the influence of increased plasma TSH levels. In addition the efficiency of conversion of T_4 to T_3 by D2 is increased in the thyroid and skeletal muscle as the serum T_4 level falls.[719] Consequently the serum T_3 concentration may be within the normal range. Since the serum T_3 concentration is frequently decreased in euthyroid patients with severe systemic illness, the serum T_3 concentration is a less specific reflection of thyroid function and is not as useful in confirming the diagnosis as is serum T_4. The decrease in circulating hormone concentrations and the slight increase in the concentration of TBG result in low-normal values for the THBR or the free fractions of T_4 and T_3 (see Fig. 11–20). Calculated values for the FT_4I are also low.

Serum cholesterol concentration may be increased to values in excess of 8 mmol/L (300 mg/dL), whereas in secondary hypothyroidism the levels may be normal or low. Other manifestations of the hypothyroid state include increased serum concentrations of creatine kinase, serum aspartate aminotransferase, lactate dehydrogenase, and carcinoembryonic antigen. In infantile and juvenile hypothyroidism the serum alkaline phosphatase concentration does not display the usual increase characteristic of active growth.

Tests that employ radioiodine and assess the function of the thyroid gland per se display a variable pattern, depending on the underlying thyroid disorder. When the amount of thyroid tissue is reduced (primary hypothyroidism), the RAIU is subnormal. However, the diagnostic value of this finding in North America is minimized by the decrease in the range of normal values that resulted from the increase in dietary iodine

TABLE 11–23. Laboratory Evaluation* of Patients with Suspected Hypothyroidism or Thyroid Enlargement

TSH, Free T_4 Estimate	TPO or TgAb	Diagnosis
TSH > 10 mU/L		
FREE T_4 ESTIMATE:		
Low	+	Primary hypothyroidism due to autoimmune thyroid disease
Low-normal	+	Primary "subclinical" hypothyroidism (autoimmune)
Low or low-normal	−	Recovery from systemic illness
		External irradiation, drug-induced, congenital hypothyroidism
		Iodine deficiency
		Seronegative autoimmune thyroid disease
		Rare thyroid disorders (amyloidosis, sarcoidosis, etc.)
		Recovery from subacute granulomatous thyroiditis
Normal	+, −	Consider TSH or T_4 assay artifacts
Elevated	−	Thyroid hormone resistance
		Blockade of T_4-to-T_3 conversion (amiodarone) or a congenital 5'-deiodinase deficiency
		Consider assay artifacts
TSH 5–10 mU/L		
FREE T_4 ESTIMATE:		
Low, low-normal	+	Early primary autoimmune hypothyroidism
Low, low-normal	−	Milder forms of nonautoimmune hypothyroidism (see above)
		Central hypothyroidism with impaired TSH bioactivity
Elevated	−(+)	Consider thyroid hormone resistance
		T_4-to-T_3 conversion blockade (e.g., amiodarone)
TSH 0.5–5 mU/L		
FREE T_4 ESTIMATE:		
Low, low-normal	−(+)	Central hypothyroidism
		Salicylate or phenytoin therapy
		Desiccated thyroid or T_3 replacement
TSH <0.5 mU/L		
FREE T_4 ESTIMATE:		
Low, low-normal	−(+)	"Posthyperthyroid" hypothyroidism (^{131}I or surgery), central hypothyroidism
		T_3 or desiccated thyroid excess
		Post–excess levothyroxine withdrawal

Initial Tests: Serum TSH, serum free T_4 index, antibodies to TPO or Tg.

intake. On the other hand, when hypothyroidism results primarily from biochemical rather than anatomic failure and when compensatory goitrogenesis occurs, the RAIU may be normal or increased. Specific functional patterns are discussed later in relation to the specific causes of hypothyroidism. Measurement of the RAIU is almost never required for the diagnosis of primary hypothyroidism.

The differentiation of hypothyroidism due to intrinsic thyroid failure (primary and goitrous hypothyroidism) from hypothyroidism due to diminished TSH secretion from hypothalamic or pituitary disease (central or secondary hypothyroidism) is important, because failure to recognize the latter may have serious consequences when thyroid replacement is instituted. The measurement of the serum TSH concentration is the most discriminating, because it is increased in intrinsic thyroid failure regardless of underlying etiology but is normal, decreased, or only slightly increased in central hypothyroidism (see Table 11–23). In some patients with pituitary tumors the basal serum TSH concentration and the response to TRH may be elevated, but the TSH has reduced biologic potency even though it is immunologically reactive.[217, 218] On occasion patients with the euthyroid sick syndrome have modest elevations in serum TSH levels, particularly during recovery,[317, 324] but the elevated serum TSH concentrations in such patients are rarely in excess of 20 mU/L and usually return to normal as the serum thyroid hormone concentrations rise to normal.

In summary, laboratory confirmation of hypothyroidism and discrimination between the two general causes of reduced thyroid function are readily achieved through measurement of the TSH and FT$_4$I concentrations.

DIFFERENTIAL DIAGNOSIS. The clinical picture of fully developed myxedema is usually characteristic enough to leave the diagnosis in little doubt, but milder forms of hypothyroidism may require differentiation from several other states. The fact that these disorders tend to occur in elderly patients is partly responsible for diagnostic uncertainty. In some elderly patients, slowing of mental and physical activity, dry skin, and loss of hair, especially from the lateral third of the eyebrows, may mimic similar findings in hypothyroidism. Furthermore the elderly often become hypothermic on exposure to cold. In patients with chronic renal insufficiency, anorexia, torpor, periorbital puffiness, sallow complexion, and anemia may suggest hypothyroidism and require specific testing. The differentiation of nephrotic states from hypothyroidism on clinical examination alone may be even more difficult. Here, waxy pallor, edema, hypercholesterolemia, and hypometabolism may suggest hypothyroidism. In addition serum T$_4$ concentration may be decreased if significant TBG is lost in the urine, but the FT$_4$I and TSH will be normal. In pernicious anemia psychiatric abnormalities, sallow skin, and numbness and tingling of the extremities may mimic similar findings in hypothyroidism. Although there is a clinical and immunologic overlap between primary hypothyroidism and pernicious anemia, this association is not invariable.

The presence of hypothyroidism is often suspected in patients who are severely ill, especially the elderly.[280] In ill patients, the serum T$_4$ concentration may be decreased, often markedly so, but the FT$_4$I is generally normal.[94, 314, 315] These features, together with the absence of an elevation of serum TSH, usually serve to differentiate the ill euthyroid patient from one with primary hypothyroidism.

Primary Hypothyroidism Without Goiter

Disorders characterized by loss or atrophy of thyroid tissue result in decreased production of thyroid hormone despite stimulation of the thyroid remnant by TSH (see Table 11–21).

PRIMARY HYPOTHYROIDISM. Primary hypothyroidism (also termed *idiopathic hypothyroidism* or *myxedema*) is more common in women than in men and occurs most often between the ages of 40 and 60. The presence of circulating thyroid autoantibodies in as many as 80% of the patients and the clinical and immunologic overlap with autoimmune diseases indicate that it usually represents the end stage of an autoimmune thyroiditis in which goiter either did not develop or went unnoticed (see the section on thyroiditis, later). Although most are due to autoimmune destruction of the thyroid parenchyma, some cases of nongoitrous hypothyroidism are caused by antibodies that block the response of thyroid cells to endogenous TSH (see Fig. 11–25).[405, 419, 720] In others thyroid atrophy may reflect the action of antibodies that specifically inhibit thyroid growth. Primary hypothyroidism can also occur as part of the polyglandular autoimmune syndromes in association with one or more of the following: adrenal atrophy, hypoparathyroidism, hypogonadism, IDDM, and pernicious anemia (see Chapter 33). Primary thyroid failure may also develop in patients with Hodgkin's disease after treatment with mantle irradiation[721] or after high-dose neck radiation for other forms of lymphoma or carcinoma.[722]

The clinical manifestations have been discussed. The thyroid is not usually palpable but may be normal in size or even somewhat enlarged and of firm consistency. Laboratory indices include the expected low serum FT$_4$I and elevated TSH levels. Circulating autoantibodies to thyroid peroxidase (TPOAb) or Tg (TgAb) are detectable in as many as 80% of patients but may be absent in long-standing disease.

POSTABLATIVE HYPOTHYROIDISM. Postablative hypothyroidism is a common cause of thyroid failure in the adult. One type follows total thyroidectomy usually performed for thyroid carcinoma. Although functioning remnants may be present, as indicated by foci of radioiodine accumulation, hypothyroidism invariably develops. The most common cause of postoperative hypothyroidism is subtotal resection of the diffuse goiter of Graves' disease or multinodular goiter. Its frequency depends on the amount of tissue remaining, but continued autoimmune destruction of the thyroid remnant in patients with Graves' disease may be a factor, because some studies suggest a correlation between the presence of circulating thyroid autoantibodies in thyrotoxicosis and the development of hypothyroidism after surgery. Hypothyroidism can become manifest during the first year after surgery, but, as with postradioiodine hypothyroidism, the incidence increases with time to approach a frequency of 50% or more.[602] In some patients mild hypothyroidism appears during the early postoperative period and then remits, as also occurs after radioiodine treatment.[723] In adults with mild postoperative hypothyroidism it may be appropriate to withhold replacement therapy for 1 or 2 mo to determine whether the hypothyroidism is permanent, provided that close observation is maintained. Alternatively, replacement therapy can be administered and withdrawn later to determine whether thyroid function has recovered. In children treatment should be instituted whenever hypothyroidism supervenes.

Hypothyroidism after destruction of thyroid tissue with radioiodine is common and is the only established disadvantage of this form of treatment for hyperthyroidism in adults. Its frequency is determined in large part by the dose of radioiodine but is also influenced by variations in individual susceptibility, including autoimmune factors.[564] The incidence of postradioiodine hypothyroidism increases with time. At 10 y the incidence is approximately 40%, although values as high as 70% have been reported.

While FT$_4$I is low in patients with postablative hypothyroidism, the serum TSH may be anomalously low for several months after either surgical or ^{131}I-induced hypothyroidism if the patient's TSH had been suppressed for a long period prior to treatment.[366, 723, 724]

Either surgical or radioiodine therapy may lead to a state of *subclinical hypothyroidism*, which usually represents an interim phase in the evolution of thyroid failure. During this phase, the patient is eumetabolic but has a modest increase in the serum TSH level (5 to 15 mU/L), a normal serum T_3 concentration, and low-normal or slightly decreased serum FT_4I levels (see Table 11–23).

SPORADIC CRETINISM. Developmental defects of the thyroid are responsible for most hypothyroidism in 1 in every 4000 newborns.[717, 725–727] These defects may take the form of complete absence of thyroid tissue or failure of the thyroid to descend properly during embryologic development. Thyroid tissue may then be found anywhere along its normal route of descent from the foramen caecum at the junction of the anterior two thirds and posterior third of the tongue (lingual thyroid) to the normal site or below. Absence of thyroid tissue or its ectopic location can be ascertained by scintiscanning. In a small number of patients, neonatal hypothyroidism results from biosynthetic defects in the thyroid or from pituitary or hypothalamic failure (see later). Hypothyroidism has also been described in one family with a mutation in the gene coding for the TSH β subunit.[213, 214]

Goitrous Hypothyroidism

Patients may develop hypothyroidism either because of some extrinsic factor or because of an intrinsic, usually heritable, defect in hormone biosynthesis. Inadequate synthesis of hormone leads to hypersecretion of TSH, which in turn produces both goiter and stimulation of all steps in hormone biosynthesis capable of response. If the compensatory response is inadequate, goitrous hypothyroidism results. In some instances, however, the compensatory response overcomes the impairment in hormone biosynthesis, and the patient has euthyroid goiter. The latter condition will be discussed later in the section on simple or nontoxic goiter. Hashimoto's disease is the most common cause of goitrous hypothyroidism in areas where dietary iodine is sufficient. It is discussed separately in the section on thyroiditis.

ENDEMIC GOITER. The term *endemic goiter* denotes any goiter occurring in a region where goiter is prevalent.[251, 252, 728, 729] Endemic goiter usually occurs in areas of environmental iodine deficiency (see earlier) and is due to the deficiency although other factors may also contribute. While this disease is estimated to affect more than 200 million people throughout the world and is of major public health significance, it does not occur in North America and is very mild in western Europe. It is most common in mountainous areas, such as the Alps, Himalayas, and Andes, owing to the persistence of glacial runoff in these areas. The causative role of iodine deficiency in the genesis of endemic goiter is supported by the inverse correlation between the iodine content of soil and water and the incidence of goiter, the kinetics of iodine metabolism in patients with the disorder, and a decrease in incidence after iodine prophylaxis. The occurrence of endemic goiter can be spotty, even within an area of known iodine deficiency; the role of dietary minerals or naturally occurring goitrogens and of pollution of water supplies has been suggested in instances of this type. For example, in the Cauca Valley of Colombia, water-borne goitrogens have been implicated, and in many areas of endemic iodine deficiency, consumption of cassava meal, which gives rise to thiocyanate, aggravates the iodine-deficient state by inhibiting thyroid iodide transport.

Most abnormalities in iodine metabolism in patients with endemic goiter are consistent with the expected effects of iodine deficiency, as mentioned earlier under the discussion of iodine. Thyroid iodide clearance rates and RAIU are increased in proportion to the decrease in the urinary excretion of stable iodine. The absolute iodine uptake is normal or low. In areas of moderate iodine deficiency, the serum T_4 concentration is usually in the lower range of normal; in areas of severe deficiency, however, values may be decreased. Nevertheless, most patients in these areas do not appear to be hypothyroid because of an increase in the synthesis of the calorigenically more efficient T_3 at the expense of T_4 and because of an increase in the activity of thyroidal deiodinases 1 and 2 (see Fig. 11–14).

The incidence and severity of endemic goiter and the metabolic state of the goitrous patient depend mainly on the degree of iodine deficiency. In the absence of hypothyroidism the effects of the goiter are mainly cosmetic. When the goiter becomes nodular, however, hemorrhage into a nodule may cause acute pain and swelling, mimicking subacute thyroiditis or neoplasia. Occasionally, a goiter may compress adjacent structures, such as the trachea, esophagus, and recurrent laryngeal nerves. The borderline nature of the iodine supply in many countries of western Europe is exemplified by the development in Belgium of compensatory goiter during pregnancy,[15, 16, 288, 728, 730–732] due to the increased requirement for thyroid hormone during gestation.[271, 733]

The incidence of endemic goiter has been greatly reduced in many areas by the introduction of iodized salt. In the United States, table salt is enriched with potassium iodide to a concentration of 0.01%, which, if the intake of salt is average, would provide an iodine intake of approximately 500 μg/d, the desired amount in an adult (see Table 11–1). An annual injection of iodized oil is another effective means of administering iodine, and endemic goiter can be treated by the addition of iodine to communal drinking water.

Administration of iodine has little, if any, effect on a long-standing endemic goiter, but it causes the early endemic hyperplastic goiter of iodine deficiency to regress. Similarly, thyroid hormone usually has no effect on goiters of long standing or on established mental or skeletal changes, but it should be given in full replacement doses if there is evidence of hypothyroidism; this is of paramount importance in pregnant women. Surgical treatment is indicated if the adjacent structures are compressed or if the goiter is either very large or enlarging rapidly.

ENDEMIC CRETINISM. Endemic cretinism is a developmental disorder that occurs in regions of severe endemic goiter.[251, 727, 728, 734] Both parents of an endemic cretin are usually goitrous, and in addition to the features of sporadic cretinism described earlier, endemic cretins often have deaf-mutism, spasticity, motor dysfunction, and abnormalities in the basal ganglia demonstrable by MRI.[734, 735] Thus one can distinguish three types of cretins: hypothyroid cretins, neurologic cretins, and those with combined features of the two. The pathogenesis of neurologic cretinism is obscure, but it may be due to severe thyroid hormone deficiency during a critical early phase of central nervous system development.[727] Some cretins are goitrous, but the thyroid may be atrophic, possibly as a consequence of exhaustion atrophy from continuous overstimulation, or a requirement for iodine in normal thyroid growth. Neither explanation seems wholly satisfactory, however.[251, 252, 728]

Goiter and Hypothyroidism Due to Agents That Inhibit Thyroid Hormone Synthesis

The ingestion of compounds that block thyroid hormone synthesis is an occasional cause of goiter with or without hypothyroidism. Apart from the agents used in the treatment of thyrotoxicosis, antithyroid agents may be encountered either as drugs for the treatment of disorders unrelated to the thyroid gland or as natural agents in foodstuffs.[57]

Of the drugs with potential goitrogenic action, lithium is

the most important.[44, 58, 178, 736, 737] Lithium, like iodide, decreases thyroid hormone synthesis and inhibits release of preformed hormone.[43] Lithium-induced hypothyroidism appears to occur principally in women, particularly women older than 40, many of whom have evidence of thyroid autoimmunity. This finding suggests that autoimmune thyroid disease may be a predisposing factor.

Other drugs that occasionally produce goitrous hypothyroidism include para-aminosalicylic acid, phenylbutazone, topically applied resorcinol, and ethionamide (see Fig. 11–4).[55] Like the thionamides, these drugs interfere with both the organic binding of iodine and the later steps in hormone biosynthesis (see Fig. 11–3).

Although soybean is not an antithyroid agent, soybean products in feeding formulas formerly resulted in goiter in infants by enhancing fecal loss of hormone, which, together with the low iodine content of soybean products, produced a state of iodine deficiency. Feeding formulas containing soybean products are now enriched with iodine.

Both the goiter and the hypothyroidism usually subside after the antithyroid agent is withdrawn, but if continued administration of pharmacologic goitrogens is required replacement therapy with thyroid hormone will cause the goiter to regress.

IODIDE GOITER AND HYPOTHYROIDISM. Goiter and hypothyroidism, either alone or in combination, are sometimes induced by chronic administration of large doses of iodine in either organic or inorganic form.[172, 241, 242, 738] However, iodide goiter develops in only a small proportion of adults given iodine. Iodine goiter was formerly seen in patients with chronic respiratory disease, who were given potassium iodide as an expectorant. The development of iodide goiter has also been reported after a single administration of radiographic contrast medium from which iodide is released slowly over a long period and may occur during amiodarone administration.[57, 739] Iodide goiter without hypothyroidism may occur endemically, such as on the island of Hokkaido, Japan, where seaweed is consumed in large quantity.

From an analysis of reported cases and from the fact that only a small percentage of patients who receive iodides chronically develop goiter, it appears that the disorder develops on a background of underlying thyroid dysfunction. Categories of susceptible individuals include those with Hashimoto's disease; patients with Graves' disease, especially after treatment of the latter with radioiodine; and those with cystic fibrosis. Among these groups, many but not all individuals display a positive iodide-perchlorate discharge test, indicating a defect in the thyroid organic binding mechanism (see section on diagnostic tests). However, intrinsic thyroid disease need not be present, because a propensity to develop iodide goiter and hypothyroidism has also been demonstrated in patients who have undergone hemithyroidectomy for a solitary thyroid nodule and in whom the remaining lobe was histologically normal. In these patients, as in those with Hashimoto's disease or Graves' disease studied prospectively, individuals with the highest basal serum TSH concentrations, even within the normal range, were the ones who developed iodide goiter.

Goiter and hypothyroidism commonly occur in newborn infants born to women given large quantities of iodine during pregnancy, and death from neonatal asphyxia has been reported. In such cases, the mother is usually free from goiter. Pregnant women should not receive large doses of iodine (>1 mg/d) over prolonged periods (more than 10 d) especially near term. It is not known whether iodide goiter in newborns results from an inherent hypersensitivity of the fetal thyroid or from the fact that the placenta concentrates iodide severalfold or both.[241, 242]

As discussed earlier, large doses of iodine cause an acute inhibition of organic binding that abates in the normal indi-

vidual, despite continued iodine administration (acute Wolff-Chaikoff effect and escape).[243] Iodide goiter appears to result from a more pronounced inhibition of organic binding and a failure of escape. As a consequence of decreased hormone synthesis, iodide transport is enhanced. Because inhibition of organic binding is a function of the intrathyroidal concentration of iodide, a cycle, augmented by an increase in serum TSH, is set in motion. The disorder usually appears as a goiter with or without hypothyroidism; rarely, iodine may produce hypothyroidism unaccompanied by goiter. Usually the thyroid is firm and diffusely enlarged, often greatly so. Histopathologic examination reveals hyperplasia that is often intense.

The FT_4I level is low, TSH concentration is increased, and the 24-h urinary iodine excretion and the serum inorganic iodide concentration are increased. The disorder regresses after iodine is withdrawn. Thyroid hormone may also be given to relieve severe symptoms.

Inherited Defects in Thyroid Hormone or TSH Biosynthesis

Inherited defects in hormone biosynthesis are rare causes of goitrous hypothyroidism.[2, 52, 729] In most instances, the defect appears to be transmitted as an autosomal recessive trait. Individuals with goitrous hypothyroidism are believed to be homozygous for the abnormal gene, whereas euthyroid relatives with slightly enlarged thyroids are presumably heterozygous. In the latter, appropriate functional testing may disclose a mild abnormality of the same biosynthetic step that is defective in the homozygous individual. In contrast to nontoxic goiter, which is more common in females than in males, these defects, as a group, affect females only slightly more commonly than males.

Although goiter may be present at birth, it usually does not appear until several years later. Therefore, the absence of goiter in a child with functioning thyroid tissue does not exclude the presence of hypothyroidism. The goiter is initially diffusely hyperplastic, often intensely so, suggesting papillary carcinoma, but eventually becomes nodular. In general the more severe the biosynthetic defect, the earlier the goiter appears, the larger it is, and the greater the likelihood of early development of hypothyroidism, or even cretinism. Five specific defects in the pathways of hormone synthesis have been identified.

IODIDE TRANSPORT DEFECT. This defect, which is rare, is characterized by impaired iodide transport mechanism and is reflected in a low RAIU.[253] Defective iodide transport is also demonstrable in other tissues, such as salivary gland and gastric mucosa, that share a similar embryologic origin with the thyroid and normally also transport iodide actively. Administration of iodine, by raising the plasma concentration, increases the intrathyroidal concentration of iodide sufficiently to permit the synthesis of normal quantities of hormone and thereby causes regression of both goiter and hypothyroidism.[20]

ORGANIFICATION DEFECT. This is a heterogeneous group of disorders that impair organic iodination in the thyroid. The enzymatic defects have been defined in only a few patients and include quantitative and/or qualitative abnormalities of thyroid peroxidase, abnormality of hydrogen peroxide generation, and alterations of the amino acid sequences in Tg that serve as the iodine acceptors. The most common presentation in such patients is a mild defect in organification accompanied by sensory nerve deafness (Pendred's syndrome). The common features of these conditions is a goiter associated with an enhancement of iodide transport, as manifested by a high uptake of ^{123}I or TcO_4^-. The ^{123}I can be discharged almost completely by subsequent administration of 500 mg of perchlorate, which competes with the circulating iodide for reuptake by the thyroidal trapping mechanism. The deafness associated with Pendred's syndrome may be present at birth or may develop during early childhood, but it is not due to hypothyroidism per se because most patients with this syndrome, although goitrous, are euthyroid.[740]

IODOTYROSINE-COUPLING DEFECT. This defect appears to cause an inability to couple iodotyrosines to form iodothyronines. The thyroid accumulation of I* is rapid, approaching 100% of the administered dose within the first 2 h. Kinetic analysis reveals very rapid turnover and recycling of thyroid iodine. Analysis of thyroid tissue in this disorder reveals little or no T_4 and T_3, most of the organic iodine being in the form of MIT and DIT. Of the several defects in hormone biosynthesis, this is the least well characterized.

IODOTYROSINE DEHALOGENASE DEFECT. The pathogenesis of goiter and hypothyroidism in this defect is complex. The major abnormality is an impairment of both intrathyroidal and peripheral deiodination of iodotyrosines, presumably because of absence of iodotyrosine dehalogenase in these tissues. As a consequence both of intense thyroid stimulation and of lack of intrathyroidal recycling of iodide derived from dehalogenation, I* is rapidly accumulated by the thyroid gland and rapidly released; labeled MIT and DIT are present in the blood and, together with their deaminated derivatives, in the urine. Hypothyroidism is presumed to result from an intense stimulation of the thyroid release mechanism, leading to the loss of large quantities of MIT and DIT in the urine and to secondary iodine deficiency. The goiter and hypothyroidism are relieved by administration of large doses of iodine. The most specific diagnostic test for the presence of this defect is the appearance in the urine of a large proportion of unchanged MIT or DIT after their systemic administration. A milder defect occurs in some patients with nontoxic goiter and in nongoitrous relatives of patients with the severe defect.

ABNORMAL SECRETION OF IODOPROTEINS. Release of abnormal iodinated proteins or polypeptides occurs in a variety of thyroid diseases, including Hashimoto's disease, benign adenomas, diffuse toxic goiter, thyroid carcinoma, and endemic goiter. Rarely release of similar compounds appears to be the sole or major abnormality leading to goiter with or without hypothyroidism. Goiter presumably develops because these calorigenically inactive compounds make up a major proportion of the products of hormone biosynthesis. These proteins collectively are measured as protein-bound iodine (PBI), but not as T_4, resulting in an abnormally large difference between the value for the PBI and the calculated value of the T_4 iodine. In years past, this discrepancy was the laboratory hallmark of the disorder. Increase in the RAIU reflects the diversion of iodine into hormonally inactive iodoproteins and the elevation of TSH. A small quantity of similar iodoproteins is present in the serum of normal individuals. Hence the abnormality in the goitrous group appears to be quantitative rather than qualitative. In their physical properties these compounds usually resemble serum albumin, but an iodoprotein resembling TTR is present in some. A more extensive discussion of the nature of these iodoproteins and their relation to intrathyroidal proteins other than Tg appears in the earlier section dealing with thyroid hormone synthesis. The severity of the defect ranges from cretinism to nontoxic goiter in the adult. The frequency with which the disorder is familial has not been established.

CONGENITAL HYPOTHYROIDISM NOT ASSOCIATED WITH GOITER. In addition to thyroid gland aplasia or dysgenesis, several individuals have been described with what appears to be either a mutation in the TSH molecule that causes it to be ineffective as a thyroid stimulator[213, 214] or a defect in the TSH receptor that impairs the ability of the thyroid cell to respond to TSH.[741] Such patients have congenital hypothyroidism of a moderate or severe degree, depending on the nature of the biochemical abnormality and may respond to exogenous TSH (in the case of a defect in TSH synthesis) or not (if the defect is in the TSH receptor). Decreased responsiveness to TSH also occurs in pseudohypoparathyroidism type I (see Chapter 24).[742] Transplacental passage of thyrotropin receptor–blocking antibodies may cause transient neonatal hypothyroidism without goiter.[743]

Thyroid Hormone Resistance

Patients with resistance to thyroid hormone (RTH) may have features of hypothyroidism if the resistance affects all tissues or symptoms suggesting hyperthyroidism if the resistance is more severe in the pituitary than in the rest of the tissues (see earlier section on hyperthyroidism). In clinical terms the patients in the former group are said to have *generalized resistance to thyroid hormone* (GRTH), while the latter syndrome is referred to as *pituitary resistance to thyroid hormone* (PRTH).[373, 660, 744] Virtually all patients with RTH have mutations in one allele of the TR beta gene that interferes with the capacity of that TR beta receptor to respond normally to T_3, usually by reducing its binding affinity for T_3 (Fig. 11–54). Furthermore the mutant receptor inhibits the function of the remaining normal receptors, both TR alpha and TR beta, which are products of the three normal alleles. This phenomenon, termed *dominant negative inhibition* (see Chapter 4), accounts for the autosomal dominant pattern of inheritance. About 300 families have been identified with this condition; however, systematic population screening has not been performed, and its true prevalence is unknown. The study of the function of the mutant receptors in this disorder has provided major insight into the mechanism of action of thyroid hormone (see Chapter 4).[745, 746]

Patients with any form of inherited resistance to thyroid hormone have growth retardation and goiter but may be relatively euthyroid. The serum total and free T_4 and T_3 concentrations are increased, but the presence of a detectable or an elevated serum TSH indicates that the thyrotropes are not under normal feedback regulation and are the cause of the elevated T_4 and T_3. Closer examination may reveal attention-deficit hyperactivity disorder, hypercholesterolemia or hearing disorders, and tachycardia. Paradoxically, these findings may suggest hyperthyroidism and occur because the heart is more responsive to elevated thyroid hormones than are other tissues, perhaps owing to the greater role played by TR alpha in this tissue than in tissues in which TR beta is dominant. In some circumstances, the mutation affects the feedback effects of thyroid hormone on TSH more than that in any other organ (PRTH). Such patients appear to have TSH-induced hyperthyroidism (see earlier section on TSH-induced hyperthyroidism). The family history often allows recognition of the inherited nature of the problem. Unfortunately, a satisfactory treatment has not yet been developed.[372, 373]

Central Hypothyroidism

Central hypothyroidism is due to TSH deficiency caused by either hypothalamic or pituitary disease (see Chapters 8 and 9). One may subdivide causes of TSH deficiency into pituitary (secondary hypothyroidism) and hypothalamic (tertiary hypothyroidism) causes, but this distinction is not necessary in the initial separation of primary from central hypothyroidism. When the intrinsically normal thyroid gland is deprived of TSH stimulation as a result of hypothalamic or pituitary disease, the thyroid undergoes partial atrophy, and the production of thyroid hormones is decreased. In most cases hyposecretion of TSH is accompanied by decreased secretion of other pituitary hormones, with the result that evidence of gonadal and adrenocortical insufficiency is also present. Hyposecretion of TSH as the sole demonstrable ab-

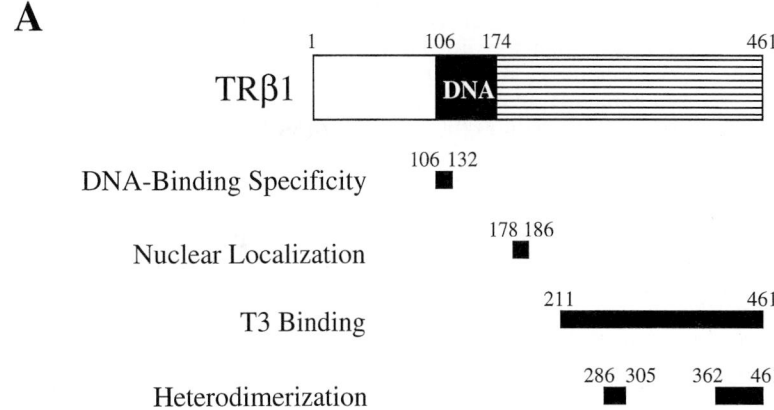

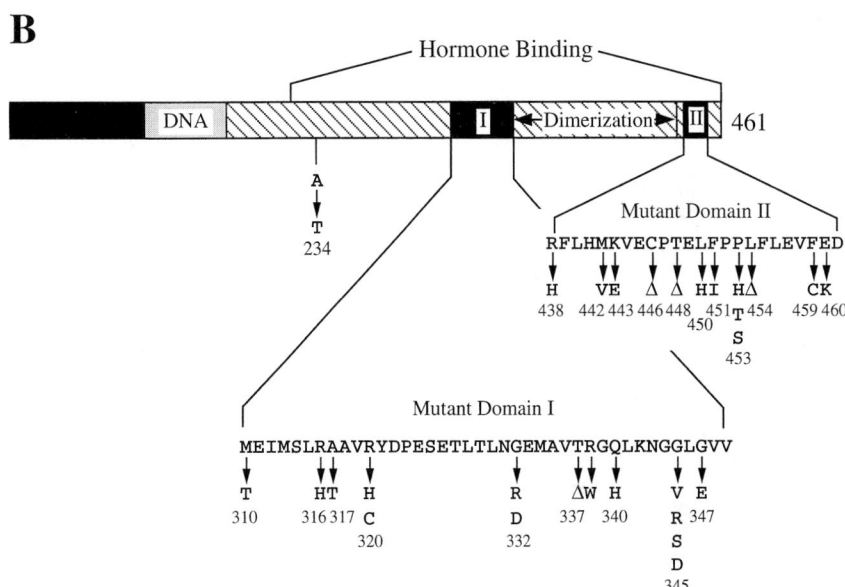

Figure 11–54. The cause of familial resistance to thyroid hormone. *A*, Schematic diagram of the thyroid hormone receptor (TR) and its functional domains correlated with (*B*) the locations of common mutations in families with resistance to thyroid hormone (RTH). The amino acid substitutions typically affect the T_3-binding domain (residues 211–461), reducing the T_3 affinity of the receptor encoded by the mutant allele, but not affecting its capacity to heterodimerize with other DNA-binding nuclear receptors such as those of the retinoid-X-receptor class. The presence of the mutant TRβ1 interferes with the function of the normal TRα1 and TRβ1, leading to a pattern of dominant inheritance of the resistance phenotype in almost all families. (*A* from Lazar MA. Thyroid hormone receptors: multiple forms, multiple possibilities. Endocr Rev 1993; 14:270–278. © The Endocrine Society; *B* from Jameson JL. Mechanisms by which thyroid hormone receptor mutations cause clinical syndromes of resistance to thyroid hormones. Thyroid 1994; 4:485–492.)

normality (monotropic deficiency) is less common. Hypothyroidism due to pituitary insufficiency varies in severity from instances in which it is mild and overshadowed by features of gonadal and adrenocortical failure to those in which the features of the hypothyroid state are predominant.

The differentiation of secondary from primary hypothyroidism is important because, in the former, treatment with thyroid hormone alone fails to correct the associated endocrine abnormalities and indeed, by precipitating acute adrenocortical insufficiency, may be dangerous. Three major aspects serve to differentiate pituitary from hypothalamic hypothyroidism: (1) features arising from the cause of the pituitary insufficiency itself, (2) differences in clinical manifestations, and (3) the laboratory results. Secondary and tertiary hypothyroidism are discussed in Chapters 8 and 9.

Conclusive differentiation of secondary from primary hypothyroidism depends on the results of laboratory tests. In pituitary insufficiency serum FT_4I is usually not as low as in primary hypothyroidism, values at or near the lower limit of the normal range being common. Measurement of serum TSH is the most direct means of differentiating between secondary and primary hypothyroidism; in secondary hypothyroidism serum TSH is usually normal or mildly elevated, whereas in primary hypothyroidism the serum TSH concentration is invariably increased. Measurements of the response of serum TSH to exogenous TRH are rarely required to confirm

the diagnosis of secondary hypothyroidism but may provide useful information in separating pituitary from hypothalamic disease. Subnormal responses would be expected in the former, and normal, but perhaps delayed, responses would be expected in the latter. Frequently, however, the pattern is not as predicted, and the TRH test has not been particularly helpful in differentiating between the two. Sometimes in patients with pituitary or hypothalamic disease, basal serum TSH concentrations are increased, and responses to TRH are augmented. These unexpected findings have been ascribed to secretion of a form of TSH that is immunoreactive but has little or no bioactivity.[217, 218, 747, 748] In pituitary insufficiency the increases in plasma growth hormone and cortisol concentrations that normally occur in response to insulin-induced hypoglycemia either are blunted or fail to occur (see Chapter 9). However, subnormal responses can also occur in severe primary hypothyroidism, so this test does not provide a useful means of differentiating between these two varieties of hypothyroidism.[170]

Treatment of Hypothyroidism

Hypothyroidism, either primary or central, is one of the most gratifying diseases to treat because of the ease and completeness with which it responds to thyroid hormone. Treatment is nearly always with the prohormone, *levothyroxine*, and the proper use of this preparation has been reviewed extensively.[733, 749, 750] A primary advantage of levothyroxine therapy is that the peripheral deiodination mechanisms can continue to produce the amount of T_3 required. If one accepts the principle that replicating the natural state is the goal of hormone replacement, it is logical to provide the prohormone and allow the peripheral tissues to activate it by physiologically regulated mechanisms.

PHARMACOLOGIC CONSIDERATIONS. Levothyroxine has a 7-d half-life, is absorbed relatively slowly, and equilibrates rapidly in its distribution volume, therefore avoiding significant postabsorptive perturbations in FT_4I levels.[751] With its long half-life, omission of a single day's tablet has no significant effect, and the patient may safely take an additional tablet the following day. In fact, levothyroxine dosage can be calculated almost as satisfactorily on a weekly as on a daily basis.

According to the U.S. Pharmacopeia (USP) the levothyroxine content of replacement tablets must be between 90 and 110% of the stated amount. The availability of a multiplicity of tablet strengths with contents ranging from 25 to 300 µg allows precise titration of the daily levothyroxine dosage for most patients with a single tablet, improving compliance significantly. The typical dose of levothyroxine of approximately 1.4 to 1.6 µg/kg ideal body weight per day will generally result in the prescription of between 75 and 112 µg/d for women and 125 to 200 µg/d in men. In patients with primary hypothyroidism, such doses usually result in serum TSH concentrations that are within the normal range. Because of the 7-d half-life, approximately 6 wk is required before there is complete equilibration of the FT_4I and the biologic effects of levothyroxine. Accordingly assessments should not be made of the adequacy of a given dose or the effects of a change in dosage until this interval has passed.

A number of effective levothyroxine products in North America are clinically equivalent. However, the variation permitted by the USP in tablet content can result in slight variations in serum TSH (in patients with primary hypothyroidism) even when they are using the same brand. While serum TSH is an *indirect reflection* of levothyroxine effect, it is superior to any other method of assessing the adequacy of therapy. Return of serum TSH level to normal is therefore the goal of levothyroxine therapy in the patient with primary hypothyroidism. Some patients may require slightly higher or lower doses than the 0.6 to 0.7 µg/lb ideal body weight generally used, owing to individual variations in absorption, and a number of conditions or associated medications may change levothyroxine requirements in patients with established hypothyroidism (see later).

In decades past, desiccated thyroid was successfully employed for the treatment of hypothyroidism and still accounts for 10 to 20% of the prescriptions written for thyroid replacement in the United States.[752] While this approach was successful, desiccated thyroid preparations contain thyroid hormone derived from animal thyroids, which, in general, have higher ratios of T_3 to T_4 than does normal human thyroid.[383, 384] Accordingly, the quantity of *liothyronine* (T_3) in such preparations can lead to supraphysiological levels of T_3 in the immediate postabsorptive period owing to the rapid release of T_3 from Tg, its immediate absorption, and the relatively long period (1 d) required for T_3 to equilibrate with its 40-L volume of distribution (see Table 11–5).[382] Mixtures of liothyronine and levothyroxine (generic term, *liotrix*) contain in a 1-grain (64-mg) equivalent tablet the amounts of T_3 (approximately 12.5 µg) and T_4 (approximately 50 µg) present in the most popular desiccated thyroid tablet used in the United States (Thyrolar).[383, 384, 753] The levothyroxine equivalency of a 1-grain desiccated thyroid tablet or its liotrix equivalent can be estimated as follows. The 12.5 µg of liothyronine (T_3) is rapidly

and completely absorbed from desiccated thyroid or from liotrix (T_3 + T_4) tablets.[382] Levothyroxine is approximately 80% absorbed,[754, 755] and about 40% of the 40 µg of levothyroxine absorbed is converted to T_3, and the molecular weight of T_3 (651) is 84% that of T_4(777). Accordingly, a 1-grain tablet should provide approximately 26 µg of T_3 (12.5 + 13.4), which would be approximately equivalent to that obtained from 97 µg of T_4. This equivalency ratio can be used as an initial guide in converting patients from desiccated thyroid or liotrix to levothyroxine.

Liothyronine is also available for use but is used only when there is a need for rapid reinstitution of a euthyroid state or for special purposes during levothyroxine withdrawal for patients with thyroid carcinoma. The daily T_3 production rate in a 70-kg individual is approximately 35 µg, and this provides a guide for estimating the quantity of liothyronine required (see Table 11–5). Because of the rapid absorption of T_3, however, serum FT_3I concentrations will be supraphysiological 2 to 6 h after ingestion.[382] Thus the effect of a given dose of liothyronine is also best assessed by serum TSH measurements.

INSTITUTION OF REPLACEMENT THERAPY. When initially diagnosed, primary hypothyroidism is usually of long duration and seldom requires immediate reversal. Thus, the restoration of a normal metabolic state can be undertaken gradually. The initial dose of levothyroxine depends on the degree of hypothyroidism and the age and general health of the patient. At one extreme, the young, otherwise healthy individual with no associated cardiovascular or other abnormalities and mild to moderate hypothyroidism can be given a complete replacement dose of ~1.3 µg/kg (0.6 µg/lb) ideal body weight. The increase in serum T_4 concentration during such treatment is sufficiently gradual and the biologic effects of T_3 are so delayed that these individuals do not experience adverse effects. At the other extreme, the elderly patient with heart disease, particularly angina pectoris, should be given small initial doses of thyroid hormone (12.5 to 25 µg levothyroxine/d), and the dosage should be increased in 12.5-µg increments at 2- to 3-mo intervals after careful clinical and laboratory evaluation.[756] The therapeutic goal is to return the serum FT_4I and FT_3I to normal, as reflected in the return of serum TSH concentrations to normal in the patient with primary hypothyroidism. In the patient with central hypothyroidism, serum TSH is not a reliable index of adequate replacement, and the serum FT_4I should be restored to the upper half of the normal range. Such patients should be evaluated and treated when appropriate for glucocorticoid deficiency prior to institution of thyroid replacement (see Chapter 9).

While adverse effects of rapid institution of therapy are unusual, pseudotumor cerebri has been reported in profoundly hypothyroid juveniles between the ages of 8 and 12 who were given even modest initial levothyroxine replacement.[757] This complication appears 1 to 10 mo after initiation of treatment and responds to acetazolamide and dexamethasone.

The interval between initiation of treatment and the first evidence of improvement depends on the size of dose given. An early clinical response in moderate to severe hypothyroidism is a diuresis of 2 to 4 kg. The serum Na^+ level will increase even sooner if hyponatremia was present initially. Thereafter, pulse rate and pulse pressure increase, appetite improves, and constipation may disappear. Later, psychomotor activity increases, and the delay in the deep tendon reflex disappears. Hoarseness abates slowly, and changes in skin and hair do not disappear for several months. In individuals started on a complete replacement dose, the serum FT_4I level should return to normal after 6 wk, but serum TSH may require a somewhat longer period, perhaps up to 3 mo.

In addition to myxedema coma, which is discussed later,

it is appropriate to alleviate hypothyroidism rapidly on occasion. For example, patients with severe hypothyroidism withstand acute infections or other serious illnesses poorly and may develop myxedema coma as a complication. In such circumstances, rapid repletion of the peripheral hormone pool can be accomplished by a single intravenous dose of 500 μg of levothyroxine in the average adult. Alternatively, by virtue of its rapid onset of action, liothyronine (25 μg orally every 12 h) can be administered if the patient is able to take medication by mouth. With both approaches, the initial effect is achieved within 24 h. Parenteral therapy with levothyroxine is continued using a dose that is 80% of the oral dose. Because of the possibility that acute increases in metabolic rate will overtax the existing pituitary-adrenocortical reserve, supplemental glucocorticoid (5 mg hydrocortisone/h intravenously) should also be given to patients receiving high initial doses of thyroid hormones. Finally, in view of the tendency of hypothyroid patients to retain free water, intravenous fluids should be given judiciously.

When hypothyroidism results from administration of iodine-containing or antithyroid drugs, withdrawal of the offending agent usually relieves both the hypothyroidism and the accompanying goiter. An exception is amiodarone, which may remain in tissues for many months.

INFANTS AND CHILDREN. In the infant with congenital hypothyroidism, the determining factor for eventual intellectual attainment is the age at which *adequate treatment* with thyroid hormone is begun. The treatment for infants with congenital hypothyroidism should consist of initially raising the serum T_4 level to more than 130 nmol/L (10 μg/dL) as rapidly as possible and maintaining at that level for the first 3 to 4 y of life. This is usually accomplished by administering an initial levothyroxine dose of 50 μg/d,[758] which is higher than the adult dose on a weight basis and in keeping with the higher metabolic clearance of the hormone in the infant.[3] The serum TSH concentration may not return to normal on this high dose because of an apparent residual reset of the pituitary feedback mechanism,[759] but after age 2, a TSH level in the normal range is an index of optimal therapy, as it is in adults.

MONITORING REPLACEMENT THERAPY. Monitoring the adequacy of and compliance with thyroid hormone therapy in the patient with primary hypothyroidism is easily done by measurement of serum TSH. This measure should be within the normal range for an assay sufficiently sensitive to measure, *with confidence*, the lower limit of the normal range. The normal serum TSH varies between 0.5 and 5.0 mU/L in most second- and third-generation assays, and results within this range are associated with the elimination of all clinical and biochemical manifestations of primary hypothyroidism, except in the patient with thyroid hormone resistance. After the first 6 mo of therapy, the dose should be reassessed because restoration of euthyroidism increases the metabolic clearance of T_4. A dose that was adequate during the early phases of therapy may not be adequate when the same patient is euthyroid. Under normal circumstances the finding of a normal serum TSH level on an annual basis is adequate to ensure that the proper dose is prescribed and is being taken by the patient. If serum TSH is outside the normal range and noncompliance is not the explanation, then small adjustments, usually in 12-μg increments, can be made with reassessment of TSH concentrations after full equilibration with the new dose (at 6 wk) to confirm that such adjustments are appropriate.[756] In North America, this strategy is simplified by the availability of many tablet strengths, many of which differ by only 12 μg. Most patients can receive the same dose until they reach the seventh or eighth decade, at which point a downward adjustment of 20 to 30% may be indicated owing

to the fact that thyroid hormone clearance decreases in the elderly.[280, 760, 761]

Thyroid hormone requirements may be altered in several situations (Table 11–24). A reduction in replacement dosage may be required in the female patient who receives androgen therapy for adjuvant treatment of breast carcinoma.[762] Most other conditions or medications increase the levothyroxine requirement in the patient on maintenance therapy. During pregnancy there is usually a 50 to 100% increase in levothyroxine requirement.[271, 272] Hypothyroid patients who are planning pregnancy should be advised to increase the dose by 50% as soon as the diagnosis is confirmed because the change in requirement appears very early after implantation. The reason for the increased requirement is probably due to a combination of factors, including increases in TBG and the volume of distribution of T_4, increase in body mass, and increases in inner-ring deiodination due to the expression of D3 in the placenta.[3, 173] The increase in requirement persists throughout pregnancy but returns to normal within a few weeks of delivery. Therefore the dose should be reduced to the original prepregnancy level at the time of delivery. Maternal T_4 is critically important to the athyreotic fetus, and pregnant patients should be monitored carefully.[3, 9, 12]

Other conditions in which levothyroxine requirements are increased are shown in Table 11–24.[57] They include malabsorption due to either bowel disease or adsorption of levothyroxine to coadministered medications such as sucralfate,[763] aluminum hydroxide,[294] ferrous sulfate,[764] lovastatin,[765] or various resins.[766, 767] Certain medications, including rifampin,[386] carbamazepine,[385] and phenytoin,[181] will increase the metabolic clearance of levothyroxine by inducing cytochrome p450 enzymes. Amiodarone will increase levothyroxine requirements by blocking conversion of T_4 to T_3 and perhaps by interfering with T_3-thyroid-hormone receptor binding.[186] Selenium deficiency is rare, but since it is rate-limiting in the synthesis of D1 (see Figs. 11–8 and 11–9), a deficiency could require an increase in levothyroxine dosage.[122, 139, 768]

Occasionally, in patients who have been treated with radioactive iodine for Graves' disease or toxic nodular goiter, some degree of thyroid hormone secretion persists and, while inadequate, is autonomous. Such patients usually have suppressed TSH values on what otherwise would be considered a

---

TABLE 11–24. Conditions That Alter Levothyroxine Requirements

Increased Levothyroxine Requirements

Gastrointestinal Disorders

Mucosal diseases of the small bowel (e.g., sprue)
After jejunoileal bypass and small bowel resection
Diabetic diarrhea

Pregnancy

Therapy with Certain Pharmacologic Agents

Drugs that interfere with levothyroxine absorption
   Cholestyramine
   Sucralfate
   Aluminum hydroxide
   Ferrous sulfate
   Possibly lovastatin or similar agents
Drugs that increase nondeiodinative T_4 clearance
   Rifampin
   Carbamazepine
   Possibly phenytoin
Drugs that block T_4 conversion to T_3
   Amiodarone
Conditions that may block deiodinase synthesis
   Selenium deficiency
   Cirrhosis

Decreased Levothyroxine Requirements

Aging (65 years and older)

Androgen therapy in women

replacement dose of levothyroxine. The levothyroxine dose in these individuals should be reduced until TSH rises to normal, keeping in mind that some time may be required before TSH secretion recovers after prolonged suppression. Because of either the delayed effects of radioiodine or the natural history of Graves' disease per se, this autonomous T_4 secretion may decrease with time, causing an increase in levothyroxine requirements in subsequent years.

Rarely, the opposite occurs; that is, a patient treated with radioiodine develops an increased TSH, but after several months of therapy the requirement for such replacement is either reduced or eliminated. This may reflect transient impairment of thyroid function by a combination of preirradiation antithyroid drug therapy and immediate effects of radiation on the thyroid. In such patients, frequent monitoring of levothyroxine replacement is required to avoid overreplacement.

In North America, clinical experience with the most commonly used levothyroxine preparations suggests that these products are equally effective; although rigorously controlled, crossover studies in the same patients have not been published.[769, 770, 771] Again, clinical experience suggests that interchange between the various preparations in patients being treated for primary hypothyroidism does not result in significant differences in serum TSH in the majority. Nonetheless the possibility of a difference in tablet content should be kept in mind if a change in preparation leads to a change in dose requirement.

ADVERSE EFFECTS OF LEVOTHYROXINE THERAPY. While the administration of excessive doses of levothyroxine causes osteoporosis in the postmenopausal patient,[772] most authorities believe that returning thyroid status to normal does not have adverse effects on bone density.[773–776] Administration of excessive doses also increases cardiac wall thickness and contractility and, in elderly patients, increases the risk of atrial fibrillation.[777, 778]

In some patients TSH will remain elevated despite the prescription of adequate replacement doses. This is most often a consequence of poor compliance. The combination of normal or even elevated serum T_4 values and elevated TSH levels can occur if the patient does not take levothyroxine regularly but attempts to remedy this by taking a bolus of the drug before visiting the physician. The integrated dose of levothyroxine over prior weeks is best reflected in the serum TSH, and noncompliant patients require careful education as to the rationale for treatment. Subtle changes in dietary habits, such as increasing the ingestion of bran, may decrease levothyroxine absorption. Recognition of such changes requires a careful history.

Special Aspects of Hypothyroidism

SUBCLINICAL HYPOTHYROIDISM. The term *subclinical hypothyroidism* designates a situation in which an asymptomatic patient has low-normal FT_4I indices but a slightly elevated serum TSH. Other terms for this condition are *mild hypothyroidism, preclinical hypothyroidism, biochemical hypothyroidism,* and *decreased thyroid reserve* (see Table 11–23). The elevation of the TSH in such patients is modest, between 5.5 and 15 mU/L. This syndrome is most often seen in patients with Hashimoto's disease or with Graves' disease after treatment with surgery or radioactive iodine. Patients with type I diabetes mellitus, primary biliary cirrhosis, and vitiligo[779] are prone to developing subclinical or frank hypothyroidism, as are patients with pernicious anemia and progressive systemic sclerosis.[780]

A number of studies on the effects of thyroid hormone treatment in such patients have utilized physiological endpoints such as measurements of various serum enzymes, systolic time intervals, and serum lipids and psychometric testing,

and the results have been variable. In the most carefully controlled studies, one or another of the parameters has returned to normal in about 25% of such patients.[346, 350, 781–784] In one study that employed a double-blind crossover approach, the 4 of 17 women who improved could be differentiated from the remainder only by a somewhat lower serum free T_3 concentration at the start of the study.[350] In other studies LDL has decreased,[784] and HDL has increased.[783] Modest improvements in cardiac indices have been noted in some[781, 785] but not all reports.[346] Thus when one is confronted with this clinical situation, there is no clearly correct approach. With respect to the issue of the relative roles of T_4 and T_3 in the regulation of TSH in humans, it is of interest that in virtually all such studies, levothyroxine treatment causes an increase in the FT_4I, the serum TSH returns to normal, but the FT_3I does not change. This is consistent with studies in animals that showed that T_4, via its conversion to T_3 in the central nervous system and pituitary, has an independent effect to suppress TSH (see Fig. 11–11).[110, 171]

One factor favoring a decision to recommend levothyroxine therapy is the presence of antibodies to TPO or Tg or the presence of a goiter. There is a risk of progression of thyroid dysfunction in patients with Hashimoto's disease, and this premonitory sign of thyroid failure may be justification for initiation of therapy. To be weighed against this are the expense and bother of daily medication, not acceptable to some patients, and the possibility that overdosage with levothyroxine may aggravate osteoporosis. If a therapeutic trial is performed, the TSH concentration should be monitored carefully and should not be reduced below normal. If no therapy is given, such patients should be monitored at intervals of 6 to 12 mo both clinically and with measurements of serum TSH.

METABOLIC INSUFFICIENCY. Nonspecific symptoms of true hypothyroidism (see Table 11–22) include mild lassitude, fatigue, slight anemia, constipation, apathy, cold intolerance, menstrual irregularities, loss of hair, and weight gain. For this reason, some patients with such complaints but with normal laboratory results have been considered for levothyroxine therapy. The response to thyroid hormone therapy is sometimes gratifying, at least initially, but symptomatic improvement usually disappears after a time unless the dose is increased. Eventually, even larger doses fail to alleviate the symptoms, suggesting that the symptoms do not arise from deficiency of thyroid hormone. Thus thyroid hormone therapy should be avoided in patients for whom there is no biochemical documentation of impaired thyroid function. Furthermore even in patients with preclinical or subclinical hypothyroidism shown by biochemical tests, symptoms may be out of proportion to these abnormalities. It is unwise to raise the patient's expectations regarding the relief of symptoms by treatment of mild biochemical abnormalities.

WITHDRAWAL OF THYROID HORMONE THERAPY. Physicians are frequently confronted with patients in whom the diagnosis of hypothyroidism, often mild, has been made and to whom replacement therapy has been given. In this circumstance it may be impossible to determine from retrospective clinical or laboratory findings that thyroid hormone replacement is truly required. An indication that the patient is not truly hypothyroid can be obtained from the nature of the initial complaints or from peculiarities in the response to treatment, as already described. If TSH is in the normal range in such patients and primary hypothyroidism is suspected, a simple way of assessing whether levothyroxine therapy is appropriate is to reduce the levothyroxine therapy to every other day and to re-evaluate TSH and FT_4I after 4 wk. If there has been no significant increase in TSH concentration and FT_4I remains constant during that period, levothyroxine is completely withdrawn, and blood tests are repeated 4 and 8 wk later. If the initial TSH is suppressed, indicating chronic overreplacement, the dose should be reduced until TSH becomes detectable prior to instituting this trial. If secondary hypothyroidism is suspected, the FT_4I must be followed during this test.

EMERGENT SURGERY IN THE HYPOTHYROID PATIENT. The perioperative course of patients with untreated hypothyroidism has been evaluated in several studies. In general, such patients were not recognized to be hypothyroid or did not require surgery despite the presence of significant hypothyroidism. Most of these patients had few complications. In one series[786] perioperative hypotension, ileus, and central nervous system disturbances were more common in hypothyroid patients, and hypothyroid patients with major infections had fewer episodes of fever than euthyroid control subjects.[389] Other complications were delayed recovery from anesthesia and abnormal hemostasis, possibly owing to an acquired form of von Willebrand's disease.[692] One may conclude from these studies that emergent surgery should not be postponed in hypothyroid patients but that such patients should be rigorously monitored for evidence of carbon dioxide retention, bleeding, infection, and hyponatremia. These findings are also relevant to the treatment of hypothyroid individuals with symptomatic coronary artery disease. Considering the lack of significant increase in perioperative complications in the hypothyroid patient, the option of surgery for remediable coronary artery lesions is open to hypothyroid individuals without the risk of a myocardial infarction in association with restitution of the euthyroid state (see later).

TREATMENT OF THE PATIENT WITH COEXISTING CORONARY ARTERY DISEASE AND HYPOTHYROIDISM. In many patients with coronary artery disease and primary hypothyroidism, cardiac function improves during institution of levothyroxine therapy because of a decrease in peripheral vascular resistance and improvement in myocardial function.[787–793] However, patients with pre-existing angina pectoris should be evaluated for correctable lesions of the coronary arteries and treated appropriately prior to the institution of levothyroxine treatment. Retrospective studies indicate that this approach is safer than the institution of replacement therapy prior to angiography and angioplasty or even coronary artery bypass grafting.[786, 794–796] In a few patients lesions are not remediable, or small vessel disease is severe even after bypass grafting so that complete replacement cannot be instituted. Such patients must be treated with optimal antianginal therapy, and thyroid hormone replacement must be compromised.[672]

PATIENTS WHO CONTINUE TO HAVE HYPOTHYROID SYMPTOMS DESPITE RESTITUTION OF NORMAL THYROID FUNCTION BY BIOCHEMICAL TESTS. In rare patients symptoms consistent with hypothyroidism persist despite appropriate treatment of the hypothyroid state. Such patients should be educated as to the relationship between symptoms of hypothyroidism and the role of thyroid hormone in relieving these, and other causes should be sought for the symptomatology. In very rare patients hypothyroid symptoms are associated with hypometabolism despite normal levels of serum thyroid hormones and TSH.[797] Such patients could have resistance to thyroid hormone in peripheral but not central tissues, a situation that has been documented only rarely.[373]

Myxedema Coma

Myxedema coma is the ultimate stage of severe longstanding hypothyroidism. This state, which almost invariably affects the elderly patient, occurs most commonly during the winter months and is associated with a high mortality. It is usually, but not always, accompanied by a subnormal temperature, values as low as 23.3°C having been recorded. The external manifestations of severe myxedema, bradycardia, and severe hypotension are invariably present. The characteristic

delay in deep tendon reflexes may be lacking if the patient is areflexic. Seizures may accompany the comatose state.

Although the pathogenesis of myxedema coma is not clear, factors that predispose to its development include exposure to cold, infection, trauma, and central nervous system depressants or anesthetics. Alveolar hypoventilation, leading to carbon dioxide retention and narcosis, and dilutional hyponatremia resembling that seen with inappropriate secretion of vasopressin may also contribute to the clinical state.

From the foregoing, it appears that the diagnosis of myxedema coma is easy, but this is not the case. After a brain stem infarction, elderly patients with features suggestive of hypothyroidism may be both comatose and hypothermic. In addition, hypothermia of any cause, due for example to exposure to cold, may cause changes suggestive of myxedema, including delayed relaxation of deep tendon reflexes. The importance of the difficulty in diagnosing myxedema coma is that a delay in therapy worsens the prognosis. Consequently the diagnosis should be made on clinical grounds, and therapy should be initiated without awaiting the results of confirmatory tests because mortality may be 20% or higher.[798]

Treatment consists of administration of thyroid hormone and correction of the associated physiological disturbances.[798, 799] Because of the sluggish circulation and severe hypometabolism, absorption of therapeutic agents from the gut or from subcutaneous or intramuscular sites is unpredictable, and medications should be administered intravenously if possible. Administration of levothyroxine as a single intravenous dose of 500 to 800 μg serves to replete the peripheral hormone pool and may cause improvement within hours. Daily doses of 100 μg intravenously are given thereafter. Hydrocortisone (5 to 10 mg/h) should also be administered because of the possibility of associated adrenocortical insufficiency as the metabolic rate increases.

Alternatively, liothyronine[801, 802] is given at a dose of 25 μg intravenously every 12 h. Others have used a combination of 200 to 300 μg T_4 and 25 μg T_3 intravenously as a single dose[803] followed by 25 μg T_4 and 100 μg T_4 24 h later and then by 50 μg T_4 daily until the patient regains consciousness. Hypotonic fluids should not be given because of the danger of water intoxication owing to SIADH and because of the reduced renal perfusion. Hypertonic saline and glucose may be required to alleviate severe dilutional hyponatremia and the occasional hypoglycemia. A critical element in therapy is support of respiratory function by means of assisted ventilation and controlled oxygen administration. Internal warming by gastric perfusion may be useful, but external warming should be avoided because it may lead to vascular collapse. Further heat losses can be prevented with blankets. An increase in temperature may be seen within 24 h in response to levothyroxine. General measures applicable to the comatose patient should be undertaken, such as frequent turning, prevention of aspiration, and attention to fecal impaction and urinary retention. Finally, the physician should be alert to the presence of coexisting disease, such as infection and cardiac or cerebrovascular disease. As soon as the patient is able to take medication by mouth, treatment with oral levothyroxine should be instituted.

AUTOIMMUNE AND INFECTIOUS THYROIDITIS

Definition of Autoimmune Thyroiditis

Autoimmune thyroid disease has been redefined in recent years. Many use the term *autoimmune thyroiditis* to cover both primary myxedema (nongoitrous) and Hashimoto's disease (goitrous).[804] These are differing clinical manifestations of a disorder that is closely related to Graves' disease. Autoantibodies to the TSH receptor that act as TSH antagonists may be the cause of some cases of the thyroid atrophy seen in primary myxedema and are seen less often in goitrous Hashimoto's disease.[805, 806] However, both Graves' and Hashimoto's diseases may occur within the same families and may share HLA susceptibility haplotypes.[531, 807] Furthermore some patients with Graves' disease later develop thyroid failure,[564] and some patients with Hashimoto's disease develop hyperthyroidism[808] and even orbitopathy.[809] Both types of patients may have autoantibodies to Tg, TPO, and the TSH receptor. Hence the diseases must be closely related, and autoimmune thyroid disease can be viewed as a spectrum from hyperthyroidism to hypothyroidism.

To bring some clarity to this situation, it is also necessary to redefine the term *thyroiditis*.[810] In pathological terms, thyroiditis implies the presence of both a lymphocytic infiltrate and destruction of thyroid follicles. However, these are arbitrary criteria. The term *thyroiditis* is more appropriately defined simply as evidence of "intrathyroidal lymphocytic infiltration" without the necessity for follicular damage. Since by this definition patients with both Graves' disease and Hashimoto's disease have thyroiditis, replacement of the term *autoimmune thyroid disease* with the more correct term *autoimmune thyroiditis* allows a new classification for autoimmune thyroid disease (Table 11–25).

Hashimoto's Disease (Autoimmune Thyroiditis Type 2A)

Until the demonstration of circulating thyroid antigen-specific T cells and thyroid autoantibodies, Hashimoto's dis-

---

TABLE 11–25. Classification of Autoimmune Thyroiditis

Type 1 Autoimmune Thyroiditis (Hashimoto's Disease Type 1)

1A Goitrous
1B Nongoitrous
Status
Euthyroid with normal TSH level. Autoantibodies to Tg and TPO usually present.

Type 2 Autoimmune Thyroiditis (Hashimoto's Disease Type 2)

2A Goitrous (classic Hashimoto's disease)
2B Nongoitrous (primary myxedema, atrophic thyroiditis)
Status
Persistent hypothyroidism with increased TSH levels. Autoantibodies to Tg and TPO usually present. Some type 2B is associated with blocking-type TSH receptor autoantibodies.
2C Transient aggravation of thyroiditis
Status
May start as transient thyrotoxicosis (increased serum thyroid hormones with low thyroidal radioactive iodine uptake). Often followed by transient hypothyroidism. However, patients may show transient hypothyroidism without the preceding thyrotoxicosis. Autoantibodies to Tg and TPO present. Example: postpartum thyroiditis.

Type 3 Autoimmune Thyroiditis (Graves' Disease)

3A Hyperthyroid Graves' disease
3B Euthyroid Graves' disease
Status
Hyperthyroid or euthyroid with suppressed TSH. Stimulatory autoantibodies to the TSH receptor are present. Autoantibodies to Tg and TPO are also usually present.
3C Hypothyroid Graves' disease
Status
Orbitopathy with hypothyroidism. Diagnostic levels of autoantibodies to the TSH receptor of the blocking or stimulating variety may be detected. Autoantibodies to Tg and TPO are usually present.

From Davies TF, Amino N. A new classification for human autoimmune thyroid disease. Thyroid 1993; 3:332, with permission.

---

ease could be diagnosed with certainty only by biopsy of the thyroid. The ease with which we can now demonstrate high titers of circulating antibodies and cell-mediated immunity to thyroid antigens in most patients with Hashimoto's disease has led to the use of the term *autoimmune thyroiditis* to describe this disorder. Although its true prevalence is uncertain, Hashimoto's disease is common and may be increasing in frequency. The mean incidence in women is in the order of 3.5 cases per 1000 people per year and in men is 0.8 cases per 1000 people per year.[811] No age is exempt, although the prevalence increases with age. Hashimoto's disease is the most common cause of goitrous hypothyroidism in areas of iodine sufficiency. There is often a family history of Hashimoto's disease, goiter, hypothyroidism, or Graves' disease, and circulating thyroid autoantibodies may be detected in relatives without overt thyroid disease. Other diseases with autoimmune components, such as pernicious anemia, diabetes mellitus, adrenal insufficiency, rheumatoid arthritis, chronic active hepatitis, vitiligo, early graying of the hair, biliary cirrhosis, and Sjögren's syndrome, may occur in patients with Hashimoto's disease and in their relatives more often than can be accounted for by chance (see Chapter 33).

PATHOGENESIS. The presence of lymphocytic infiltration of the thyroid (hence the older term *lymphocytic thyroiditis*), circulating thyroid autoantibodies, and clinical or immunologic overlap with other diseases with autoimmune components indicates that Hashimoto's disease is an autoimmune thyroid disorder. The current understanding of autoimmune mechanisms has been discussed in the section on Graves' disease. However, autoimmune thyroiditis is characterized by thyroid destruction rather than thyroid stimulation. Although both TPOAb and TgAb may be cytotoxic, the thyroid is infiltrated predominantly by T cells that elaborate a variety of lymphokines and undergo blast transformation when exposed to thyroid antigens (TSHR, TPO and Tg) in vitro, suggesting that cell-mediated autoimmune mechanisms are pathogenetically involved. Indeed a T-cell clone specifically cytotoxic for autologous thyroid cells in a patient with Hashimoto's disease (Fig. 11–55) is reminiscent of animal models of cytotoxic T cells associated with experimental autoimmune thyroiditis.[812] These manifestations of autoimmunity in Hashimoto's disease and other autoimmune thyroid disorders reflect a hereditary susceptibility to thyroid disease that allows the survival and persistence of B cells and T cells directed against thyroid antigens.[491] The fact that infusion of IL-2 and lymphokine-activated killer cells causes progression or development of hypothyroidism in patients with detectable TPOAb is additional evidence of the autoimmune nature of this disease.[813]

GENETIC SUSCEPTIBILITY. Reference has already been made to the familial predisposition to autoimmune disease in patients with Hashimoto's disease. As with Graves' disease, there is a significant but weak association between Hashimoto's disease and HLA-DR3, perhaps also HLA-DR5,[814] and certain DQ alleles.[815] Unlike in diabetes mellitus, formal linkage of specific histocompatibility antigens with autoimune thyroid disease has been difficult to demonstrate. Hashimoto's disease occurs with increased frequency in Down's syndrome and (probably) gonadal dysgenesis.[816] The fact that thyroid cells can express HLA-DR antigens, at least as a secondary phenomenon, indicates the potential role of these cells in perpetuating the immune response and may be related to the propensity of autoimmune disease for certain HLA-DR subgroups.[817] Hashimoto's disease almost certainly is associated with a polygenetic susceptibility, HLA being one gene involved. Efforts are under way to identify non-HLA susceptibility genes in families with autoimmune thyroid disease.

HISTOPATHOLOGY. The thyroid is pale and firm. The histopathologic changes vary in type and extent but usually consist of diffuse lymphocytic infiltration with germinal center

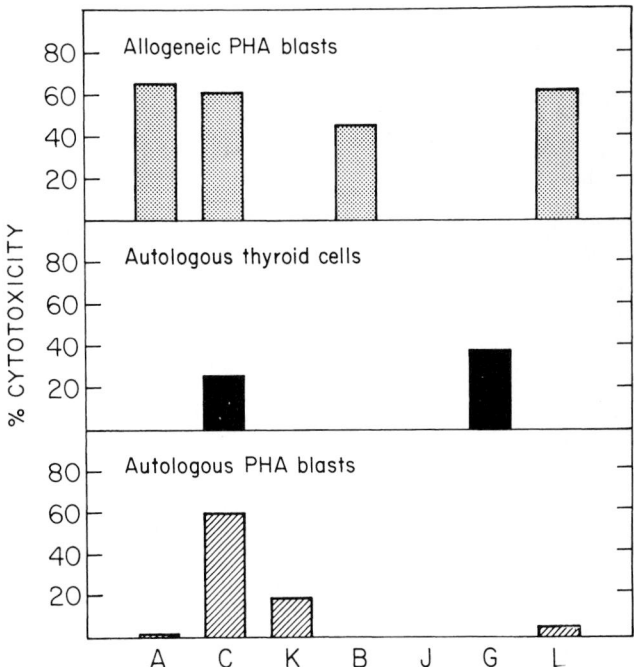

Figure 11–55. A T-cell clone (G) from a patient with Hashimoto's disease was able to lyse autologous thyroid cells. Data are shown as % cytotoxicity from a radioactive chromium release assay. Note that clone C was able to lyse all cell targets and was therefore not thyroid cell specific. (From McKenzie WA, Davies TF. An intrathyroidal T cell clone specifically cytotoxic for human thyroid cells. Immunology 1987; 61:101–103.)

formation, obliteration of thyroid follicles, and fibrosis (Fig. 11–56). In most cases there is destruction of epithelial cells and degeneration and fragmentation of the follicular basement membrane. The remaining epithelial cells may be larger and show oxyphilic changes in the cytoplasm; these so-called Askanazy cells are virtually pathognomonic. In some cases epithelial hyperplasia may be prominent. Colloid is sparse. The interstitial tissue is infiltrated with lymphocytes that may form typical lymphoid follicles with germinal centers. Plasma cells may be prominent. Fibrosis is generally present in the older lesions but not to the extent seen in Riedel's thyroiditis. Histologically, two variants can be distinguished. The oxyphilic variant displays more oxyphilic change, less fibrosis, and striking infiltration with lymphocytes forming germinal centers. The fibrous variant is infiltrated mainly with plasma cells and displays more fibrosis. Clinical differences between the two are described below, but there is no evidence that the etiologies are different.

Lymphocytic infiltration of a focal or diffuse nature may be found in the thyroid gland in Graves' disease, in thyroid neoplasms including multinodular goiter, and in simple or nontoxic goiter. In the past the diagnosis of Hashimoto's disease required the presence of Askanazy cells or lymphoid follicles. Because the lymphocytic infiltrations are usually associated with circulating thyroid autoantibodies, the pathogenetic mechanisms leading to lymphocytic infiltration in these disorders may be similar. In Graves' disease, lymphocytic infiltration and associated antibodies may favor the development of hypothyroidism in the long term, accelerated by partial thyroidectomy or radioiodine therapy.

PATHOPHYSIOLOGY. Impairment of hormone synthesis is due to the autoimmune destruction of the thyroid cells and involves a defect in organic binding of thyroid iodide, as evidenced by a positive perchlorate discharge test, and accelerated turnover of a depleted organic iodine pool. In addition, release of iodoproteins, mostly Tg, is enhanced. The foregoing

abnormalities in hormone biosynthesis may occur in relatives of patients with Hashimoto's disease who are normal or have only circulating thyroid autoantibodies as evidence of ongoing thyroiditis. Approximately 90% of the thyroid gland must be destroyed before hypothyroidism develops, but many patients with mild Hashimoto's disease, but decreased thyroid reserve, develop iodide-induced myxedema if iodide is taken chronically.

Because of the faulty synthesis of hormone, hypersecretion of TSH causes thyroid hyperactivity without thyrotoxicosis. Stimulation by endogenous TSH may be maximal, so exogenous TSH causes no further stimulation (decreased thyroid reserve).

CLINICAL PICTURE. Goiter, the hallmark of Hashimoto's disease, usually develops gradually and may be found during routine examination. On occasion, the thyroid enlarges rapidly and, when accompanied by pain and tenderness, may mimic de Quervain's or subacute thyroiditis. Some patients, particularly those with the fibrous variant, are hypothyroid when first seen. The goiter is generally moderate in size and firm in consistency and moves freely on swallowing. The surface is either smooth or scalloped, but well-defined nodules are unusual. Both lobes are enlarged, but the gland may be asymmetrical. The pyramidal lobe may be enlarged, and adjacent structures, such as the trachea, esophagus, and recurrent laryngeal nerves, may be compressed. Enlargement of regional lymph nodes is unusual.

Although atrophic hypothyroidism (see later) is thought to be the end result of autoimmune destruction of the thyroid, the progression of goitrous Hashimoto's disease to the atrophied state is not often seen in the individual patient. Indeed the histopathologic picture tends to remain rather static, except for some increase in fibrous tissue. Clinically, the untreated goiter remains unchanged or enlarges gradually over many years. The manifestations of hypothyroidism may develop over several years in patients who are initially euthyroid. Some but not all studies suggest an increased prevalence of thyroid carcinoma in Hashimoto's disease.[818] As mentioned earlier, the presence of coexistent Hashimoto's disease may be a favorable prognostic factor in patients with papillary carcinoma.

Occasional patients with Hashimoto's disease develop hyperthyroidism. Other patients with early autoimmune thyroiditis develop transitory thyrotoxicosis (painless or silent thyroiditis with thyrotoxicosis) as the result of thyroid cell destruction. Here evidence of ongoing thyroid hyperfunction is lacking because the thyroid RAIU is depressed. As described earlier, a phase of transient hypothyroidism begins 3 to 6 mo post partum in 30% of women with autoimmune thyroiditis, as evidenced by the presence of TPOAb.[624, 652–655] There may be a history suggesting earlier mild thyrotoxicosis (see earlier discussion of syndromes associated with transient hyperthyroidism).

LABORATORY TESTS. The results of the common tests of thyroid function depend on the stage of the disease. At first, the tests may suggest thyroid hyperfunction with a suppressed TSH but without overproduction of hormone. The RAIU may be increased, but serum T_4 and T_3 levels may remain normal. At this stage, the patient may be eumetabolic. As the TSH rises, the glandular response at first compensates for the impairment of hormone biosynthesis. With time, the ability of the thyroid to respond to TSH diminishes, and the RAIU and serum T_4 level decline to subnormal values. The serum T_3 concentration, however, may be slightly increased, probably reflecting maximal stimulation of the failing thyroid by the increased serum TSH level. The foregoing sequence with still normal T_4 and T_3 and an increased TSH reflects the development of *subclinical hypothyroidism* (see Table 11–23). Ultimately,

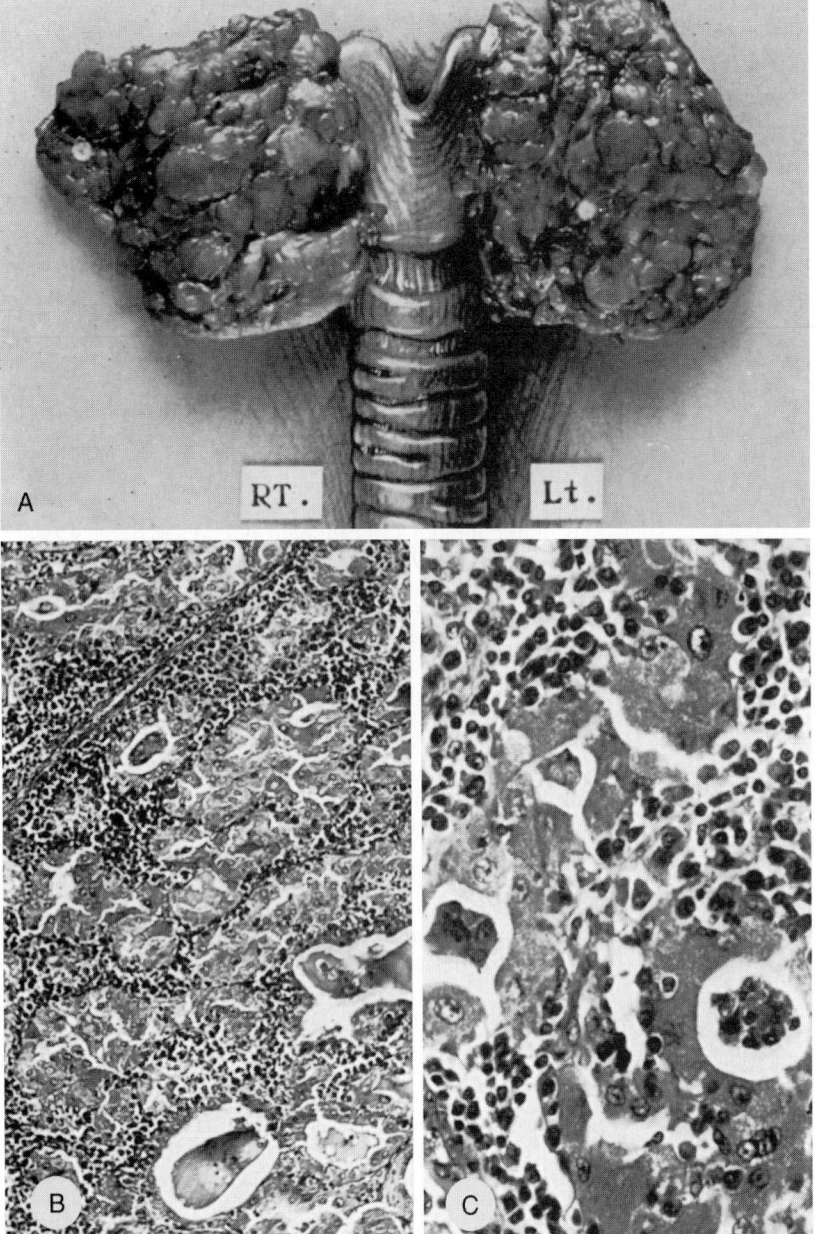

Figure 11–56. Hashimoto's disease. *A,* Note the exaggeration of the normal lobular pattern. *B,* Interfollicular infiltration by lymphocytes and plasma cells. *C,* Granular, oxyphilic changes in the cytoplasm of the follicular epithelium (Askanazy cells). (From Woolner LB, McConahey WM, Beahrs OH. Struma lymphomatosa [Hashimoto's thyroiditis] and related thyroidal disorders. J Clin Endocrinol Metab 1959; 19:53–83. © 1959, The Endocrine Society.)

the serum T_4 and sometimes the T_3 levels also decrease and cause frank hypothyroidism.

The diagnosis of Hashimoto's disease is confirmed by the finding of thyroid autoantibodies, usually of high titer, in the serum. TPO autoantibodies are more common and higher in titer than Tg autoantibodies. Sometimes, part of a gland with autoimmune thyroiditis may look and feel like a hard thyroid nodule. When neoplasia is suspected, fine-needle aspiration biopsy should be undertaken.

DIFFERENTIAL DIAGNOSIS. Differentiation of Hashimoto's disease from other uncomplicated disorders of the thyroid is facilitated by the demonstration that high levels of thyroid autoantibodies occur more commonly in Hashimoto's disease than in other thyroid disorders. The frequent coexistence of hypothyroidism and Hashimoto's disease serves to distinguish this disease from nontoxic goiter and thyroid neoplasms. Differentiation of euthyroid Hashimoto's disease from diffuse nontoxic goiter is often difficult, although diffuse nontoxic goiter tends to be softer than that of Hashimoto's disease. In adolescents differentiation of Hashimoto's disease from diffuse nontoxic goiter is even more difficult because in this age group Hashimoto's disease may not be accompanied by the high levels of thyroid autoantibodies. The presence of well-defined nodules usually distinguishes nontoxic multinodular goiter from Hashimoto's disease. Differentiation between Hashimoto's disease and thyroid carcinoma can sometimes be made on clinical grounds. Thyroid carcinoma is usually nodular and firm or hard and may be fixed to adjacent structures. Compression of the recurrent laryngeal nerve with hoarseness is virtually pathognomonic of thyroid carcinoma but occurs late in the disease progression. A history of a recent enlargement of the goiter is more common in thyroid carcinoma than in Hashimoto's disease. Enlargement of regional lymph nodes also suggests thyroid carcinoma. In thyroid carcinoma ultrasound examination or scintiscanning of the thyroid may reveal only the isolated lesion, whereas in Hashimoto's disease activity is usually heterogeneous.

TREATMENT. In many patients no treatment is required because the goiter is small and the disease is asymptomatic, with the TSH remaining in the normal range (type 1). In others, treatment with thyroid hormone is directed at alleviating goiter, hypothyroidism, or both (type 2). Levothyroxine treatment is indicated in patients when the goiter presses on adjacent structures or is unsightly and is most effective in goiters of recent onset. In long-standing goiter, treatment with thyroid hormone is usually ineffective, possibly because of fibrosis. Glucocorticoids may cause regression of the goiter and decrease autoantibody levels, but these agents are not recommended in the usual case because of untoward side effects and the return of activity after treatment is withdrawn. Full replacement doses of thyroid hormone should be given when hypothyroidism or when subclinical hypothyroidism supervenes (see earlier section on hypothyroidism). Surgery is justified only if pressure symptoms or unsightly enlargement persists after a trial of suppressive therapy. Administration of levothyroxine should be continued after surgery, because hypothyroidism is inevitable. The importance of maintaining the serum TSH within the normal range is dealt with elsewhere in this chapter.

Atrophic Autoimmune Thyroiditis (Autoimmune Thyroiditis Type 2B, or Primary Myxedema)

Atrophic autoimmune thyroiditis (primary myxedema) is, after postablative hypothyroidism, the most common cause of thyroid failure in the adult. It is more common in women than in men and usually occurs between the ages of 40 and 60. The presence of circulating thyroid autoantibodies in as many as 80% of the patients and overlap of the clinical and immunologic features with the autoimmune diseases indicate that what was once thought to be a separate disease in fact represents the end stage of an autoimmune thyroiditis in which goiter either was absent or had gone unnoticed prior to atrophy. Although most cases probably reflect autoimmune destruction of the thyroid parenchyma, some cases of nongoitrous hypothyroidism are due to antibodies that block the response to endogenous TSH, so-called blocking TSHR autoantibodies.[720] Primary hypothyroidism may also occur as part of an autoimmune syndrome of polyglandular failure in association with one or more of the following: adrenal insufficiency, hypoparathyroidism, hypogonadism, IDDM, and pernicious anemia (see Chapter 33).

On histopathologic examination the thyroid remnant consists largely of fibrous tissue with an occasional thyroid follicle and foci of lymphocytic infiltration. The thyroid is usually impalpable or normal in size. Typical laboratory findings include low serum T_4 and high serum TSH levels. Autoantibodies to TPO and to Tg are detectable in the serum in as many as 80% of patients but may be absent in long-standing disease.

Riedel's Thyroiditis

Riedel's chronic sclerosing thyroiditis is rare and occurs chiefly in middle-aged women.[819, 820] The etiology is unknown. Some cases are considered to be an advanced state of Hashimoto's disease,[821] but there is also evidence that it is a separate disease entity. It is characterized by fibrosis of the thyroid gland and adjacent structures and may be associated with fibrosis elsewhere, especially in the retroperitoneal area.[819] The presence of eosinophils has recently been demonstrated histologically, suggesting a unique autoimmune response to fibrous tissue.[822]

Symptoms develop insidiously and are related chiefly to compression of adjacent structures, including the trachea, esophagus, and recurrent laryngeal nerves. Constitutional evidence of inflammation is uncommon. The thyroid gland is moderately enlarged, stony hard, and usually asymmetrical. The consistency of the gland and the invasion of adjacent structures suggest carcinoma, but there is no enlargement of regional lymph nodes. Temperature, pulse, and leukocyte count are normal. Hypothyroidism is unusual. The RAIU may be normal or low. Circulating thyroid autoantibodies are less frequent and are found in lower titers than in Hashimoto's disease.

Surgery may be required to preserve tracheal and esophageal function. If extensive involvement of perithyroid tissues is present, resection of the isthmus may relieve some symptoms. Treatment with thyroid hormone relieves the hypothyroidism but has no effect on the primary process.

MISCELLANEOUS TYPES OF THYROIDITIS. Acute pyogenic thyroiditis is a rare disorder that is due to an infection of the thyroid by pyogenic organisms, usually as a result of dissemination from a septic focus elsewhere or a piriform sinus fistula.[823] It is characterized by pain and tenderness in the thyroid, dysphagia, fever, and malaise. There are signs of acute inflammation in the gland and in the surrounding tissues. Needle biopsy of the thyroid should be performed so that the infecting organism can be identified and treated with the appropriate antibiotic. Surgical drainage is indicated when pus is present. Rarely, the thyroid gland is the seat of tuberculosis, coccidioidomycosis, or other fungal infection disseminated from another focus. Patients with acquired immunodeficiency syndrome (AIDS) should be suspected of such complications.

SIMPLE OR NONTOXIC GOITER: DIFFUSE AND MULTINODULAR

Simple or nontoxic goiter may be defined as any thyroid enlargement that is not associated with hyperthyroidism or hypothyroidism and that does not result from inflammation or neoplasia. The term is usually restricted to the form that occurs sporadically, i.e., in regions that are not the locus of endemic goiter. Although useful in indicating the presence of the characteristics just noted, the term *simple goiter* can be a result of different underlying abnormalities.[824]

Pathogenesis and Pathophysiology

Any comprehensive theory of the pathogenesis of simple goiter must take into account the fact that the cause may differ from one patient to another and must explain the natural history. Diffuse symmetrical goiters tend to increase in size but may regress when TSH is suppressed. Multinodular goiters are structurally and functionally heterogeneous and tend to develop areas of functional autonomy.

The traditional theory about the pathogenesis suggests that it is a response to any of several factors that impair hormone synthesis. When such factors are operative, hypersecretion of TSH stimulates thyroid growth and increases the aspects of hormone biosynthesis that are capable of response. As a consequence of the increase in thyroid mass and functional activity, a normal rate of hormone secretion is restored, and the patient is goitrous but eumetabolic. Thus the disorder differs from goitrous hypothyroidism only in degree and is presumed to result from the same etiologies, discussed in the previous section. This sequence is evident in some patients with iodine deficiency and in others who develop goiter in response to specific agents. For example, lithium administration can cause goiter with or without hypothyroidism. Goiter (if early) regresses when iodine is administered (if iodine deficiency is the cause), when lithium or another offending agent is withdrawn, or if suppressive doses of exogenous thyroid hormone are administered. In most patients with nontoxic goiter, however, no extrinsic goitrogenic factor can be identified. As a consequence, the cause may be some intrinsic, probably inborn, abnormality in thyroid hormone synthesis akin to those that produce goitrous hypothyroidism. In some cases defects of this type can be detected, as by the perchlorate discharge test, but more often no abnormality can be demonstrated.[825] In such instances the abnormality is believed to be too mild to be detected by the relatively insensitive available in vivo techniques.

This concept of the pathogenesis of nontoxic goiter is inconsistent with the fact that the serum TSH concentration is normal in most patients with nontoxic goiter.[826, 827] Nonetheless a participatory role of TSH in the maintenance of goiter is indicated by the regression of goiter that sometimes follows administration of suppressive doses of thyroid hormone. Several possible mechanisms may accommodate these seemingly divergent findings. The mechanism with experimental support is that iodine depletion in rats enhances the promotion of thyroid growth by TSH.[827] Hence any factor that impairs intrathyroidal iodine levels might lead to gradual development of goiter in response to normal concentrations of TSH. A second possibility is that the increase in serum TSH concentration is significant but too small to be detected by the immunoassay methods now available. Finally, a goitrogenic stimulus may have been present in the past but may no longer be detectable at the time of study, so the residual normal TSH concentration can maintain but not initiate the goiter.

An alternative concept to explain thyroid growth in nontoxic goiter[828] is that a class of "thyroid growth immunoglobulins" (TGIs) stimulate growth but do not stimulate thyroid adenylate cyclase activity, as do TSH and autoantibodies, thus explaining why the thyroid is not hyperfunctioning.[743] These observations, however, remain controversial because of the difficult relationships involved. TGIs and their inhibitory counterparts have been detected with extremely sensitive cytochemical bioassays[829] or by measurements of thymidine incorporation by reconstituted thyroid follicles[830] or rat thyroid cells in culture.[831] Patients in whom "autoimmune nontoxic goiter" is likely have a high incidence of other autoimmune phenomena in themselves or their families or have recurrence of goiter after subtotal thyroidectomy. More study of this phenomenon is needed.[743, 832]

Neither TSH nor TGI would explain why long-standing nontoxic goiter becomes nodular and develops anatomic and functional heterogeneity and functional autonomy. These characteristics have been assumed to result from either prolonged hyperstimulation by TSH or repeated cycles of hyperstimulation and involution.[833] Hyperstimulation or cycles of hyperstimulation and involution could lead to the emergence of areas of hyperplasia, possibly associated with functional autonomy, coupled with areas of involution (exhaustion atrophy), the whole made more heterogeneous by localized hemorrhage, fibrosis, and sometimes calcification.

Another pathogenetic concept is based on autoradiographic and clinical studies of normal, nontoxic, and toxic multinodular goiters.[834] Early in the course, areas of microheterogeneity of structure and function are intermixed and include areas of functional autonomy and small areas of focal hemorrhage. Indeed, as judged from the presence of scattered foci of persistent radioiodine uptake in the thyroids of patients given suppressive doses of thyroid hormone before surgery,

some cells with functional autonomy are present in the normal thyroid gland. Thus in addition to variability in the thyroid microcirculation, heterogeneity may result from clonal differences among the cells that give rise to thyroid follicles, some being more and some less responsive to external stimulation by TSH and some being autonomous at the outset. Individual responses to TSH might also vary from clone to clone in respect to iodine accumulation, exocytosis of Tg, and resorption of colloid. This concept implies that the anatomic and functional heterogeneity within the thyroid at the outset of the disease is exaggerated by prolonged stimulation.

Further insights into the pathogenesis of sporadic multinodular goiter have been gained by assessment of the clonality of individual thyroid nodules. Polyclonality implies multicellular origin due to the proliferation of a group of cells, whereas a monoclonal tumor is thought to be formed by an expansion of a single cell.[835] Studies involving X-chromosome inactivation analysis have produced variable results in multinodular goiters. Some dominant nodules are monoclonal, especially if they showed evidence of recent rapid growth.[836] Other researchers have found a monoclonal pattern in only a minority of large nodules.[837] Two groups reported that in multinodular glands more than one nodule could be monoclonal and that both monoclonal and polyclonal nodules can coexist within the same gland.[838, 839] Analysis of hyperplastic nodules by rigid criteria[840] also indicates that morphologically indistinguishable hyperplastic thyroid nodules may be either monoclonal or polyclonal. "Monoclonal adenomas within hyperplastic thyroid glands may reflect a stage in progression along the hyperplasia-neoplasia spectrum; accumulation of multiple somatic mutations may subsequently confer a selective growth advantage to this single cell clone."[840] Cytogenetic[841] and in situ hybridization[842] studies also support the idea of a biologic continuum and karyotypic evolution between hyperplastic nodules and follicular adenomas.

Eventually the amount of functionally autonomous tissue in a multinodular goiter may be sufficient to suppress TSH secretion. Formerly, this was recognized by a subnormal response to TRH or a lack of thyroid suppression during administration of exogenous hormone.[826] Such abnormalities are now identified on the basis of suppression of the basal TSH level.[843] Ultimately, autonomous hyperfunction may be sufficient to produce thyrotoxicosis, or thyrotoxicosis may supervene when the patient is exposed to an iodine load. For this reason, patients with nontoxic multinodular goiter should not be given medications that contain iodine and should be observed after radiologic procedures that involve administration of iodinated contrast media. Some investigators administer antithyroid agents to patients with nodular goiter who are to receive agents containing iodine; this is a reasonable suggestion especially in areas of iodine deficiency where jodbasedow is prone to occur.

The role of heredity in the genesis of nontoxic goiter is evident in twin studies[844] and in rare families.[845] Nontoxic goiter has a female preponderance (7 to 9:1) and seems to occur more commonly during adolescence or pregnancy. There appears to be no physiological increase in thyroid volume during normal adolescence, and development of a goiter during adolescence is a pathologic rather than a physiological process.[846] However, as evidenced by sonography to measure thyroid volume in patients living in an area of moderate iodine intake, normal pregnancy, especially in women with pre-existing thyroid disorders, is goitrogenic.[16] The increased thyroid volume during pregnancy is associated with biochemical features of thyroid stimulation (i.e., an increased T_3/T_4 ratio), owing to slightly elevated serum TSH levels at delivery or a high hCG concentration during the first trimester. Repeated pregnancies may play a role in the development of later thyroid disorders, a relation that might explain the high prevalence of thyroid disorders in women.[847]

Pathology

Simple goiter is a noninflammatory, non-neoplastic, diffuse or nodular enlargement of the thyroid gland without hyperthyroidism.[848] The gland is usually large or very large, weighing from 60 g to more than 1000 g and may have a distorted shape (Fig. 11–57). The cut surface shows areas of nodularity, fibrosis, hemorrhage, and calcification. The nodules vary in size, number, and appearance, the latter according to their colloid or cellular content. Single or multiple cystic areas may contain colloid or brown fluid, representing previous hemorrhage.

Histologically, nodules contain irregularly enlarged, involuted follicles distended with colloid or clusters of smaller follicles lined by taller epithelium and containing small colloid droplets. These microfollicles may be surrounded by an edematous or a fibrous stroma. Large nodules tend to compress the surrounding parenchyma and may have a partially developed fibrous capsule. Markedly distended follicles may coalesce to form colloid cysts measuring several millimeters in diameter. The nodules tend to be incompletely encapsulated and are poorly demarcated from and merge with the internodular tissue, which also has an altered architecture. However, the nodules in some glands appear to be localized, with areas of apparently normal architecture elsewhere. Here the distinction from a follicular adenoma may be difficult, and some pathologists apply terms such as *colloid* or *adenomatous nodules* to such lesions. Studies of clonality may be helpful in distinguishing between focal or nodular hyperplasia and true adenomas.[849, 850] While nodular goiters are polyclonal in origin,

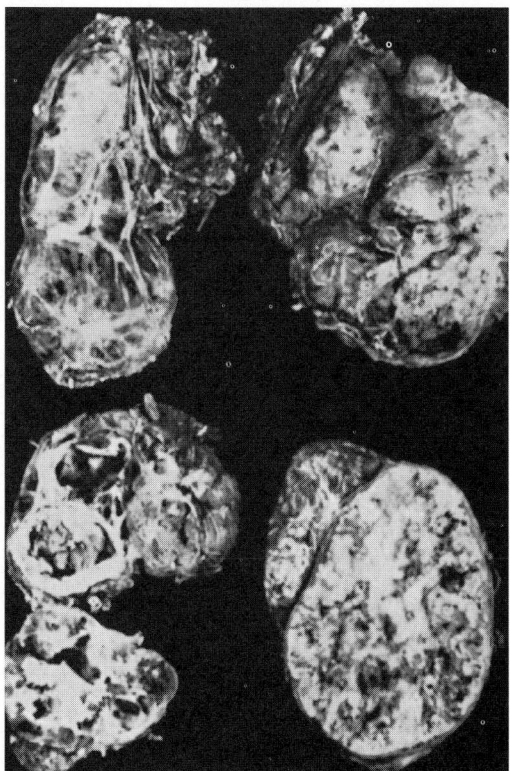

Figure 11–57. Outer and cut surfaces of a nontoxic nodular goiter of 15 y duration. Note variations in size and structure of the nodules; there are thick areas of fibrous tissue, flecks of calcium, scattered areas of thyroid tissue, cysts, and small hemorrhages.

solitary thyroid nodules are monoclonal and therefore true benign neoplasms.[837]

Clinical Picture

The clinical features of nontoxic goiter are those of thyroid enlargement. Most commonly, the effect either is merely disfiguring or is felt as a tightening of garments worn about the neck. Nearly 70% of patients with sporadic nontoxic goiter complain of neck discomfort; the remainder have cosmetic concerns or a fear of possible malignancy.[851] Large goiters may displace or compress the esophagus or trachea, leading to dysphagia, a choking sensation, and inspiratory stridor. Narrowing of the thoracic inlet may compromise the venous return from the head, neck, and upper limbs sufficiently to produce venous engorgement. This obstruction is accentuated when the patient's arms are raised (Pemberton's sign); dizziness and even syncope may result. Compression of the recurrent laryngeal nerve, with hoarseness, suggests carcinoma rather than nontoxic goiter, but vocal cord paralysis can occasionally result from benign nodular goiter.[852] Hemorrhage into a nodule or cyst produces acute, painful enlargement locally and may enhance or induce obstructive symptoms.

Laboratory Tests

Serum T_4 and T_3 concentrations, by definition, are within the normal range. However, the T_3/T_4 ratio may be increased, perhaps reflecting defective iodination of Tg.[853] Serum Tg concentrations are elevated in most.[854] The RAIU is usually normal but may be increased, either because of mild iodine deficiency or because of a biosynthetic defect. Patients with sporadic nontoxic goiter tend to have high free T_4 and T_3 concentrations and low TSH levels.[851] The prevalence of subclinical hyperthyroidism is higher when patients with nodular goiter have clear-cut autonomous areas on scintigraphy.[853]

In a cross-sectional study of 102 patients with sporadic nontoxic goiter, the plasma TSH level correlated negatively with the thyroid volume, which in turn correlated positively with both the age of the patient and the duration of the goiter.[851] In a prospective study of 242 patients with nodular goiter, no correlation was found between thyroid volume and any thyroid biochemical parameters, but there were significant negative correlations between the number of nodules identified by ultrasonography and the levels of free T_4 and T_3, basal TSH, and the TSH response to TRH stimulation.[853]

Differential Diagnosis

The differential diagnosis of nontoxic goiter can be considered in functional and anatomic terms. As indicated, the same factors that lead to goitrous hypothyroidism can, if less severe, cause nontoxic goiter. Consequently, some patients with putative nontoxic goiter are slightly hypothyroid. On the other hand, foci of autonomous function may develop in multinodular goiters in which the spectrum of function can range from clinical euthyroidism with intact regulatory control to euthyroidism with some degree of functional autonomy to thyrotoxicosis (toxic multinodular goiter).[855]

Anatomically, the diffuse stage of nontoxic goiter can resemble the thyroid of either Graves' or Hashimoto's disease. If Graves' disease is not in an actively thyrotoxic phase and if the ocular manifestations are lacking, there is no way of differentiating the two except to demonstrate the presence of TSHRAb in the serum. In one study of 108 patients with diffuse nontoxic goiter followed for more than 5 y, 33% had a family history of autoimmune thyroid disease, and 5 developed Graves' disease during follow-up.[856] Diffuse nontoxic goiter is sometimes also difficult to differentiate from Hashimoto's disease, although the thyroid of Hashimoto's disease is usually firmer and more irregular. Demonstration of high titers of antithyroid antibodies indicate Hashimoto's disease.

In its multinodular stage, nontoxic goiter may suggest thyroid carcinoma. The approach to differentiating between the two is discussed in the section on thyroid neoplasms.

Treatment

For more than a century "thyroid feeding" has been employed to reduce the size of nontoxic goiters.[857] The 1953 report of Greer and Astwood, in which in two thirds of patients' goiters regressed with thyroid therapy,[858] led to widespread acceptance of suppressive therapy,[858] despite some doubts about the value of such therapy.[859, 860] In a prospective placebo-controlled double-blind randomized clinical trial, 58% of the thyroxine-treated group had a significant response at 9 mo, as measured by ultrasonography, in contrast with 5% after placebo.[861] However, after treatment was discontinued, thyroid volume returned to baseline within 9 mo. An overview of studies performed from 1960 to 1992 suggests that 60% or more of sporadic nontoxic goiters respond to suppressive therapy.[859] However, maintenance of the reduction may require continuous long-term treatment. Ultrasonographic measurement of goiter size has demonstrated a return to pretherapy values within 3 mo of discontinuation.[862] Nodular goiters appear to be less responsive than diffuse goiters, and efficacy is increased in younger patients and in those with small or recently diagnosed goiters.[859]

It has been proposed that a basal serum TSH greater than 1 mU/L in a patient with sporadic nontoxic goiter is an indication to administer levothyroxine to lower the serum TSH level to the low-normal range (0.5 to 1.0 mU/L). If the goiter size decreases or remains stable, treatment should be continued indefinitely, with periodic monitoring of serum TSH levels to detect possible development of functional autonomy.[733] Others[863] have suggested that TSH levels on treatment should be subnormal but not profoundly suppressed (0.1 to 0.3 mU/L). The validity of this approach remains to be ascertained.

A major concern in relation to long-term thyroxine suppressive therapy is the possibility of detrimental effects to the skeleton and heart.[864] It has been reported that thyroxine suppression therapy is associated with variable degrees of bone loss, particularly in postmenopausal women.[865] However, other studies failed to demonstrate significant change in bone mass after long-term thyroxine therapy.[866, 867] Furthermore, although marginal cardiac changes may occur with thyroxine therapy, there is no evidence that levothyroxine per se is detrimental to the heart.[864] It is now generally accepted that TSH should be suppresed with the lowest effective dose of levothyroxine,[733, 859, 864, 866] usually between 1.5 and 2.0 µg/kg body weight/d; the risk of deleterious effects can be minimized by monitoring serum TSH and free T_3 concentrations.[864]

Surgery for simple nontoxic goiter is physiologically unsound because it further restricts the ability of the thyroid to meet hormone requirements. Nevertheless surgery may become necessary because of persistence of obstructive manifestations despite a trial of levothyroxine. Surgery rapidly and effectively removes the goiter, but recurrence is seen in about 10 to 20% within 10 y.[868] Surgical complications are seen in 7 to 10% of cases and are more common with large goiters and with reoperation.[869] Postoperative hypothyroidism rates depend largely on the extent of surgical resection; prophylactic treatment with levothyroxine after goiter resection probably does not prevent recurrence of goiter.[870, 871]

Traditionally the role of ^{131}I therapy in nontoxic goiter was to reduce the size of massive goiter in elderly patients who

were poor candidates for surgery[872, 873] or to treat goiter that recurs after resection.[874] However, several studies have demonstrated that primary treatment of multinodular goiter with ^{131}I is followed by a reduction in thyroid volume and is associated with a low incidence of hypothyroidism[875, 876] (Fig. 11–58). In one study thyroid volume (assessed by ultrasonography) was reduced by 40% after 1 y and 55% after 2 y, with no further reduction thereafter[875]; most of the patients were given one dose of ^{131}I, and 60% of the total reduction occurred within the first 3 mo. It was formerly argued that treatment of large goiters or goiters with substernal extension with ^{131}I should be avoided because of the risks of acute swelling of the gland and consequent tracheal compression.[729] Ultrasonographic studies of thyroid volume after ^{131}I have failed to demonstrate significant early volume increase.[877] Moreover decreased tracheal deviation and increased tracheal lumen size were demonstrable by MRI in patients who had compression from nontoxic goiters with substernal extension.[873]

Therefore it appears that ^{131}I treatment of nontoxic multinodular goiter is effective and safe,[860] but hypothyroidism may occur in 22 to 40% within 5 y after ^{131}I therapy.[875, 876] If young patients with goiter are treated with ^{131}I, the incidence of hypothyroidism will obviously increase with time, and regular follow-up, preferably by a systematic annual recall scheme, is necessary.[878] Although reassuring data are available on the long-term cancer risk after ^{131}I treatment in hyperthyroidism,[879] follow-up of ^{131}I-treated nontoxic goitrous patients is short term and involves small numbers of patients. No data are available on the long-term risk of high-dose ^{131}I treatment for this condition, and long-term randomized studies comparing the effects, side-effects, and cost-benefits of surgery and ^{131}I treatment should be performed.[860]

THYROID NEOPLASIA

In an era when patients are advised on self-examination to detect cancer at an early stage, the finding of a palpable mass in such a superficial location as the thyroid gland can be disconcerting. The affected patient will likely seek medical evaluation. At the end of an appropriate investigation, the clinician can usually reassure the patient that the nodule is

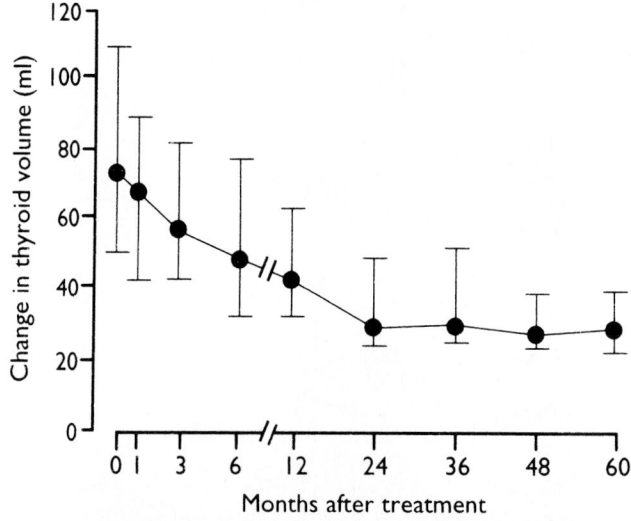

Figure 11–58. Median changes in thyroid volume alterations after iodine-131 treatment in 39 patients with nontoxic multinodular goiter who remained euthyroid after a single dose. Bars are quartiles. (From Nygaard B, Hegedus L, Gervil M, et al. Radioiodine treatment of multinodular nontoxic goiter. BMJ 1993; 307:828–832.)

benign. Alternatively if the discovered lesion proves to be suspicious for malignancy, the patient can be advised that the management of typical thyroid cancer is effective[880] and usually consists of surgical resection,[881] followed by medical therapy[882] and regular surveillance.[883] The major challenge in this circumstance is to define whether the discovered thyroid nodule represents a true neoplasm and to determine whether the biologic behavior will be malignant.

Some degree of consensus has been achieved with regard to both the initial evaluation of nodular thyroid disease[884-886] and the management of differentiated thyroid cancer,[887-889] but important clinical and biologic questions remain unanswered.[890, 891] In the following sections a clinical approach to nodular thyroid disease will be described, and a widely used scheme for classifying and staging tumors of the thyroid gland will be presented. The features of the principal types of benign and malignant thyroid neoplasms will be discussed, and controversies in the management of differentiated thyroid carcinoma will be reviewed.

Nodular Thyroid Disease

Thyroid tumors are the most common endocrine neoplasms. They usually present as anterior neck nodules that in most cases can be localized to the thyroid gland by palpation. The majority of these nodules are benign hyperplastic (or colloid) nodules, but between 5 and 20% of nodules coming to medical attention are true neoplasms, either benign follicular adenoma or carcinomas of follicular or parafollicular (C) cells. Differentiating true neoplasms from hyperplastic nodules and distinguishing benign from malignant tumors are major challenges. Moreover with the widespread practice of medical "check-ups" in healthy individuals and the common use of sophisticated imaging technology, this problem is likely to become more common. High-resolution ultrasound studies in large groups of normal volunteers suggest that the prevalence of nodular thyroid disease (NTD) in healthy adults is over 60%.[892] However, in the United States during 1996 only about 15,600 new cases of thyroid cancer were diagnosed.[893] Given that the prevalence of clinical thyroid cancer in most populations is much less than 1%, the majority of these thyroid incidentalomas are obviously benign.[894]

In identifying those nodules that are likely to be malignant, a thorough history and a careful physical examination should be supplemented with laboratory testing, imaging procedures, and, most important, fine-needle aspiration biopsy of the nodule in question. With the use of this approach, it is possible in the majority of patients to assess the likelihood of malignancy and to advise appropriate treatment.

HISTORY AND PHYSICAL EXAMINATION. Historical features that favor benign disease include (1) a family history of Hashimoto's thyroiditis, benign thyroid nodule, or goiter; (2) symptoms of hypothyroidism or hyperthyroidism; and (3) pain or tenderness associated with the nodule. Historical features that suggest malignancy include (1) young (<20 years old) or old (>70 years old) patient age; (2) male sex; (3) history of external neck radiation during childhood or adolescence; (4) previous history of thyroid cancer; (5) recent changes in speaking, breathing, or swallowing; and (6) a family history of thyroid cancer or multiple endocrine neoplasia type 2. On physical examination, manifestations of thyroid malignancy should be sought, including firm consistency of the nodule, irregular shape, and fixation to underlying or overlying tissues. Evidence of suspicious regional lymphadenopathy may be present in up to a third of patients with papillary or medullary carcinoma but is absent in most patients with hyperplastic nodules or follicular neoplasms (benign or malignant).

In both prospective[895] and retrospective[896, 897] studies, the sensitivity and specificity rates for detecting thyroid malignancy by history and physical examination were around 60 and 80%, respectively. Only about 20% of patients with later confirmed malignancy had, when initially seen, neither suspicious historical features nor evidence of potential malignancy on neck examination. If the likelihood of malignancy is felt to be very low on clinical grounds, observation may initially be justified. However, if cancer is thought to be likely, even negative results on further testing should be interpreted with extreme caution. Further testing may include assessment of thyroid function, measurement of tumor markers, genetic screening, thyroid imaging, and tissue sampling, usually via fine-needle aspiration biopsy.

LABORATORY EVALUATION. Measurement of a serum TSH level in a sensitive immunometric assay should be performed to exclude thyroid dysfunction. If the screening TSH proves to be abnormal, free T_4 and T_3 should be measured. Patients with thyroid cancer rarely have abnormalities in serum TSH levels, and an abnormal TSH concentration decreases but does not eliminate the likelihood of malignancy in a thyroid nodule. Measurement of serum antithyroid peroxidase (anti-TPO) antibody and anti-Tg antibody levels may be helpful for diagnosing chronic autoimmune thyroiditis, especially if the serum TSH level is increased. In chronic autoimmune thyroiditis the thyroid may have a size and consistency that simulates either a solitary nodule or bilateral nodules. Evidence for autoimmune thyroiditis, however, does not preclude the presence of cancer within the gland.

Follicular cell–derived thyroid cancers (FCTCs) may produce excessive amounts of Tg or release stored Tg in increased amounts into the bloodstream. Unfortunately, there is overlap in serum levels in FCTC and in a number of benign conditions. Although a serum Tg level of greater than 10 times the normal upper limit is suspicious for thyroid malignancy in the absence of thyrotoxicosis,[898] measurement of the baseline serum Tg level is not a useful or cost-effective test in the initial work-up of nodular thyroid disease.[886] Similarly, some investigators[899] routinely measure calcitonin (Ct) levels in all patients with nodular thyroid disease to identify cases of medullary thyroid carcinoma (MTC). In the absence of clinical suspicion for MTC or multiple endocrine neoplasia type 2 (MEN 2) syndrome, it is neither cost-effective nor necessary to measure Ct levels in patients with nodular thyroid disease.

In patients who have a family history of MTC (either familial MTC or associated with MEN 2), measurements of basal and pentagastrin-stimulated Ct levels have now been largely replaced by more specific genetic screening tests (see Chapter 32). The molecular abnormality in more than 90% of these familial cases is a mutation of the *RET* proto-oncogene that is located on the short arm of chromosome 10.[900] Once the mutation in the *RET* gene is sequenced in an affected individual, asymptomatic members of the family can be tested for the presence of the mutation in this locus. Such tests are now commercially available and are highly accurate, reproducible, and reliable.[901] A negative test obviates the need for any further testing, and individuals who harbor such mutations should undergo prophylactic total thyroidectomy to prevent later development of the multicentric MTC that occurs in this disorder.[901] Some investigators advocate RET mutation testing in all patients with MTC, including sporadic cases without a family history; 4 to 6% of such patients have mutations of the gene.[902] If such a mutation is found, family members at risk are then tested to identify affected individuals. This approach may be justifiable in apparently sporadic MTC patients younger than age 50, but in older MTC patients the incidence of undetected familial disease is so low that genetic testing is probably appropriate only in unusual circumstances, such as previous or present history of pheochromocytoma or patients with bilateral multicentric MTC.

THYROID IMAGING. The traditional imaging procedure

is thyroid scintigraphy using ^{131}I, ^{123}I, or ^{99m}Tc. Most thyroid carcinomas are inefficient in trapping and organifying iodine and appear on scanning as areas of diminished isotope uptake, so-called "cool" or "cold" nodules. Unfortunately, most benign nodules also do not concentrate iodine and therefore are "cold" nodules. In fact, 80% of thyroid nodules scanned for possible cancer may be scintigraphically cold. Furthermore not all nodules with normal or slightly increased uptake are benign because there is little difference in cancer rate between cold and warm nodules.[903] The only situation where an iodine scan can exclude malignancy with reasonable certainty is in the case of a toxic adenoma, which is characterized by significantly increased uptake within the nodule and markedly suppressed or absent uptake in the remainder of the gland. These lesions are almost invariably benign.[898] When isotopic scanning with iodine and related compounds is compared with history and physical examination, most authors have found scanning to be of negligible or no value.[903, 904]

In an attempt to improve the performance of isotopic scanning, a number of radioisotopes other than iodine-related compounds have been tried. Thallium-201(^{201}Tl) scanning is used in conjunction with radioiodine scanning. The absence of ^{201}Tl uptake in a nodule that has decreased uptake on radioiodine or technetium scanning may have a negative predictive value (i.e., excludes malignancy) as high as 97%.[905] A positive thallium scan under the same circumstances may have a positive predictive value of about 90%.[905] However, not all investigators have obtained such excellent results, and ^{201}Tl scanning has a false-negative rate of about 40% when used without prior radioiodine imaging.[906] The situation is similar with other nonradioiodine isotopic scanning, such as ^{99m}Tc-labeled methoxyisobutyl isonitrile (MIBI).[907] In the hands of dedicated experts these techniques may be valuable, but widespread use will have to await more extensive evaluation.

Ultrasonography is capable of detecting even minute thyroid nodules and increases the sensitivity of carcinoma detection but does little to enhance specificity. In fact, in 1000 normal control subjects, 65% had detectable nodularity on high-resolution scanning.[892] Attempts have been made to develop criteria for distinguishing benign and malignant nodules. Echo-free (cystic) and homogeneously hyperechoic lesions are reputed to carry a low risk of malignancy,[908, 909] but positive predictive criteria of malignancy are less well defined, with only 64% of malignant nodules displaying patterns typical for malignancy in one study.[910] In addition, nodules that can be clearly identified as benign by sonography are uncommon, limiting the usefulness of ultrasound scanning. Despite these limitations, ultrasonography is capable of identifying up to 80% of thyroid malignancies and may have a specificity as high as 90% in experienced hands.[897]

The experience with CT scanning and MRI in the initial diagnosis of thyroid malignancy is limited, and no judgment about their ultimate usefulness is possible. It appears, however, that these techniques do not provide better quality images of the thyroid and cervical nodes than those of sonography. Computed tomographic examination of the lower central neck is preferable to sonography when tracheal invasion is suspected, as this technique can delineate the presence of intraluminal tumor; air in the trachea produces an acoustic shadow on ultrasound that impairs the quality of the image in the paratracheal area.

FINE-NEEDLE ASPIRATION BIOPSY. Fine-needle aspiration biopsy (FNAB) of thyroid nodules has eclipsed all other techniques for diagnosing thyroid cancer, with reported overall rates of sensitivity and specificity exceeding 90% in iodine-sufficient areas.[911, 912] The technique is easy to perform and safe, with only a handful of complications having been reported in the literature,[913–915] and causes little discomfort. However, care must be taken to obtain an adequate specimen,

with most authors recommending between 3 and 6 aspirations.[911, 912] A satisfactory specimen contains at least five or six groups of 10 to 15 of well-preserved cells. The cells are categorized by their cytologic appearances into benign, indeterminate or suspicious, and malignant. The diagnosis of papillary thyroid carcinoma (PTC) by FNAB is particularly reliable and accurate; few cancers are missed, and most malignant specimens are readily identified as such, with sensitivity and specificity both approaching 100%. However, for follicular neoplasms the technique performs much less well. If strict criteria for malignancy are used, sensitivity may be as low as 8%.[897] If any follicular neoplasm that is not clearly benign on cytologic examination is classified as cancerous, sensitivity rises to around 90% or more. Unfortunately, this is associated with a considerable drop in specificity to less than 50% (i.e., a large number of false-positives). This seriously limits the usefulness of this technique in iodine-deficient regions, where the incidence of follicular thyroid carcinoma (FTC) approaches that of PTC and where both follicular adenomas and hyperplastic adenomatous nodules are very prevalent.

Thyroid peroxidase (TPO) immunochemistry with a monoclonal antibody (MoAb 47) shows promise in improving the accuracy of FNAB in follicular lesions.[916] For 100% sensitivity a specificity of almost 70% has been achieved with this technique. Pending independent confirmation of these results, TPO immunocytochemistry may be a valuable adjunct to the standard cytologic techniques for the elevation of thyroid FNAB. The use of large-needle biopsy in addition to standard FNAB has improved diagnostic accuracy in difficult FNA cases,[917, 918] but the technique is more exacting than FNAB alone and is associated with increased morbidity and possibly increased complication rates.

Particularly for cystic thyroid nodules, sampling from the margin of the nodule, rather than from the cystic fluid and debris in the center, increases accuracy.[912] Ultrasonographically guided FNA can be used for this purpose (Fig. 11–59). Although such guided biopsies may sometimes be helpful, routine use of ultrasound-guided biopsy in clinically palpable nodules is not any better than "free-hand" aspiration.[919]

Preoperative FNAB and intraoperative frozen section are combined in some European centers with high rates of follicular tumors.[920] In the hands of experienced surgeon-pathologist teams, this approach results in less than 5% misdiagnoses, as evidenced by subsequent review of paraffin-embedded specimens, and thereby avoids unnecessarily extensive surgery in patients with benign tumors, achieves resection of nearly all malignant tumors, and rarely necessitates a second operation for completion thyroidectomy.[920] This approach is employed at the Mayo Clinic, where intraoperative frozen section is routine.

Apart from its limited utility in the evaluation of follicular neoplasms, the only other limitation of FNAB is "nondiagnostic" specimens, which may be obtained in up to 20% of cases.[911] Although repeated aspiration increases both the accuracy and the rate of diagnostic aspirations, even repeated attempts may sometimes fail. Many persistently nondiagnostic FNABs may be neoplastic, possibly 50%.[921] Hence either close observation or surgical removal of the nodule is probably the best option. Some authorities recommend a trial of TSH suppression, which can sometimes shrink benign nodules.[912] However, a significant proportion of benign nodules will fail to shrink, and some carcinomas shrink; consequently, the value of TSH suppression is doubtful. Whether ultrasound-guided FNAB will help overcome this problem is not known but may be possible.[919] Figure 11–60 shows an algorithmic scheme[911] for the management of nodular thyroid disease where FNAB is the first diagnostic test and subsequent management is based on cytologic results.

CONCLUSION. The most expeditious way of diagnosing

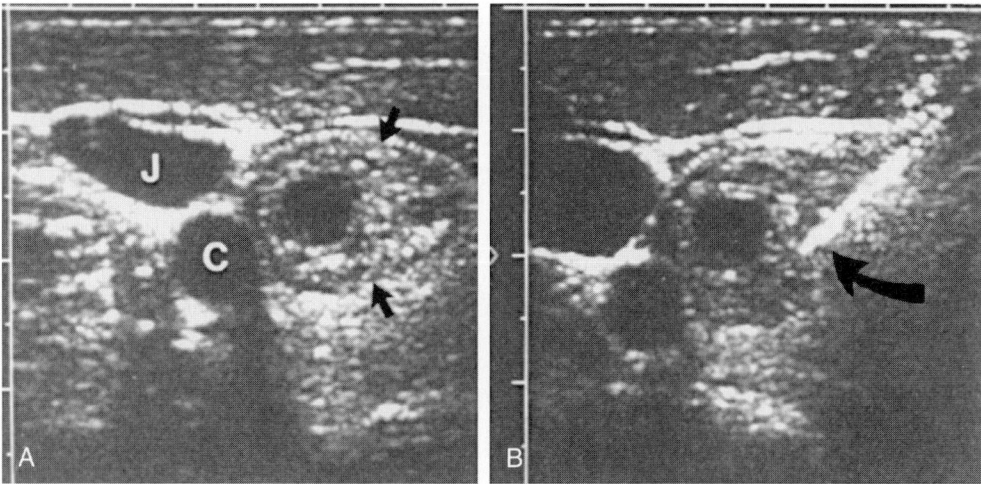

Figure 11–59. *A,* Sonographically guided thyroid nodule FNA. Transverse sonogram of the right thyroid lobe shows a 1.5-cm solid thyroid nodule *(arrows)* containing a central cystic component. J, jugular vein; C, common carotid artery. *B,* Palpation-guided aspiration biopsy obtained nondiagnostic fluid only. Sonographically guided needle aspiration/biopsy *(curved arrow)* of the solid portion of the nodule proved that this was a benign adenomatous nodule. (From Rifkin MD, Charboneau JW, Laing FC. Special course: Ultrasound 1991. In: Reading CC, ed. Syllabus: Thyroid, Parathyroid, and Cervical Lymph Nodes. Oak Brook, IL: Radiological Society of North America, 1991: 363–377, with permission.)

thyroid malignancy is to obtain a thorough history and physical examination, followed by FNAB and evaluation of the sample by an experienced cytologist. In some cases a guided biopsy should be done under ultrasound scanning. Imaging procedures, in addition to ultrasound, and other tests may occasionally be helpful, but diagnostic radioactive iodine scanning, as traditionally practiced, is of little or no value and should be abandoned. In iodine-sufficient areas with a high relative prevalence of PTC, the combination of history and physical examination, FNAB, and ultrasound is usually sufficient to confirm malignancy. Conversely, if history and physical examination, FNAB, and ultrasound do not suggest malignancy, the chances of missing PTC are probably less than 1%.[897] In areas where the prevalence of follicular tumors is higher, more patients may require neck exploration, and in experienced hands intraoperative frozen sections can limit the number of unnecessarily extensive, bilateral procedures. MTC differs from PTC and FTC in that it is often familial and may be diagnosed at the presymptomatic stage by genetic testing.

Classification of Thyroid Tumors

Two monographs have had a major impact on the histologic classification of thyroid tumors. The first is from the World Health Organization (WHO) Collaborating Centre for the Histological Classification of Thyroid Tumours,[922] and the second is from the Armed Forces Institute of Pathology (AFIP).[923] The classification described in Table 11–26 is modified from the guidelines described by both the WHO[922] and the AFIP.[923]

Primary thyroid epithelial tumors can be divided into three major categories, depending on the cell type involved, and subdivided further into benign and malignant tumors. Lesions with follicular cell differentiation constitute more than 95% of the cases, and the remainder are largely made up of tumors exhibiting C-cell differentiation.[924] Mixed medullary and follicular carcinomas, made up of cells with both C-cell and follicular differentiation, are rare and of uncertain histogenesis.[922] Nonepithelial thyroid tumors include sarcomas, malignant hemangioendotheliomas, and malignant lymphomas, which may involve the thyroid as the only manifestation of the disease or as part of systemic disease. Blood-borne metastases to the thyroid are not uncommon at autopsy in patients with widespread malignancy but rarely cause clinically detectable thyroid enlargement.

Staging of Thyroid Carcinoma

While the WHO and AFIP groups developed a histologic classification of thyroid tumors, the International Union Against Cancer (UICC) and the American Joint Committee on Cancer (AJCC) agreed on a staging system in thyroid cancer.[925] The AJCC system was developed after the analysis of

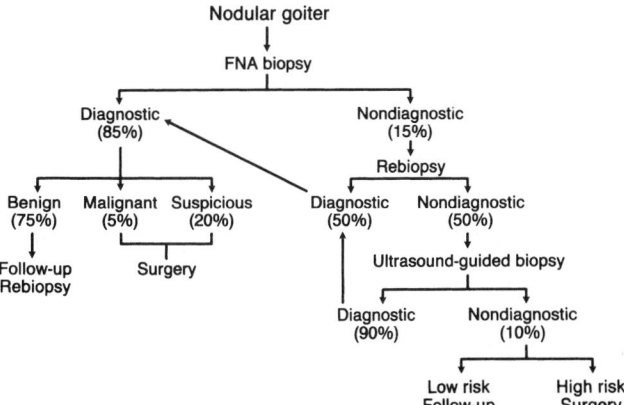

Figure 11–60. Management of nodular goiter based on FNA biopsy as the first diagnostic test. Subsequent management is based on cytologic results. Percentages in parentheses indicate satisfactory or unsatisfactory biopsy results. (From Gharib H. Fine-needle aspiration biopsy of thyroid nodules: advantages, limitations, and effect. Mayo Clinic Proc 1994; 69:44–49, with permission.)

TABLE 11–26. Classification of Thyroid Neoplasms

Primary Epithelial Tumors	**Tumors of C Cells**
Tumors of Follicular Cells	Medullary carcinoma
Benign: follicular adenoma	***Tumors of Follicular and C Cells***
Malignant: carcinoma	Mixed medullary-follicular
Differentiated	carcinoma
Papillary	
Follicular	**Primary Nonepithelial Tumors**
Poorly differentiated	***Malignant Lymphomas***
Insular	
Others	***Sarcomas***
Undifferentiated (anaplastic)	***Others***
	Secondary Tumors

more than 1000 case protocols. As stated by the AJCC, "the principal purpose served by international agreement on the classification of cancer cases by extent of disease was to provide a method of conveying clinical experience to others without ambiguity."[925] The AJCC based their system of classification on the TNM system, which relies on assessing three components: the extent of the primary tumor (T), the absence or presence of regional lymph node metastases (N), and the absence or presence of distant metastases (M). The addition of numbers to these three components indicates the extent of the malignant disease, thus showing progressive increase in tumor size or involvement. In effect, the TNM system is a "shorthand notation for describing the clinical extent" of the malignancy.[925]

The TNM system allows a reasonably precise description and recording of the anatomic extent of disease. The classification may be either clinical (cTNM), based on evidence (including biopsy) acquired before treatment, or pathologic (pTNM), where intraoperative and surgical pathology data are available. Obviously, pTNM classification is preferable, since a precise size can be assigned to the primary tumor, the histotype is identified, and extrathyroid invasion is demonstrated unequivocally. Typically the primary thyroid tumor (T) status is defined according to the size of the primary lesion: T1, greatest diameter 1 cm or smaller; T2, larger than 1 cm but not larger than 4 cm; T3, larger than 4 cm; and T4, direct (extrathyroid) extension/invasion through the thyroid capsule. A thyroid tumor with four degrees of T, two degrees of N, and two degrees of M could have 16 different TNM categories. For purposes of tabulation and analysis, these categories have been condensed into a convenient number of TNM stage-groupings (Table 11–27). Although head and neck cancer is usually staged entirely on the basis of anatomic extent, thyroid cancer staging differs in that both the histologic diagnosis and the age of the patient are included because of their importance in predicting the behavior and prognosis of thyroid cancer.[926]

According to this staging scheme, all patients younger than age 45 with papillary or follicular cancer are stage I, unless they have distant metastases, in which circumstance they would be stage II. Older patients (age 45 or older) with node-negative papillary or follicular microcarcinoma (T1N0M0) are stage I. Tumors between 1.1 and 4.0 cm are stage II, and either nodal spread or extrathyroid invasion in older papillary/follicular patients is stage III. For MTC, the scheme is similar in that microcarcinoma is stage I, and node-positive is stage III. However, there is no age distinction for MTC, and local (extrathyroid) invasion is defined as stage II. For both MTC and older patients with papillary or follicular cancer, stage IV denotes the presence of distant metastases. Independent of age or tumor extent, all patients with undifferentiated (anaplastic) cancer are considered stage IV.

Follicular Adenoma

Follicular adenoma is a benign encapsulated tumor with evidence of follicular cell differentiation.[922, 923] It is the most common thyroid neoplasm and may be found in 4 to 20% of glands examined at autopsy.[927, 928] The tumor is usually solitary and has a well-defined fibrous capsule that is grossly and microscopically complete. There is sharp demarcation and distinct structural difference from and compression of the surrounding parenchyma. The size of follicular adenomas is variable, but most have a diameter of 1 to 3 cm at the time of excision. Occasionally, lesions may weigh several hundred grams. Secondary degenerative changes are common in the larger tumors but are less frequent than in hyperplastic nodules. Degenerative changes include hemorrhage, edema, fibrosis, calcification, ossification, and cystic degeneration.

Follicular adenomas can be classified into subtypes (Table 11–28), according to the size or presence of follicles and degree of cellularity, each adenoma tending to have a consistent architectural pattern. Trabecular adenomas are very cellular and consist of columns of cells arranged in compact cords. They show little follicle formation and rarely contain colloid. A variant, the hyalinizing trabecular adenoma, has a prominent hyaline appearance, both in the cytoplasm and in the extracellular space.[929] It may resemble either medullary or papillary carcinoma, but it is benign.

Microfollicular, normofollicular, and macrofollicular adenomas owe their names to the size of their follicles compared with follicles in the neighboring, non-neoplastic areas of the gland. The histologic differences between these subtypes are striking but of no clinical importance. The only practical value of the classification is that the more cellular a follicular nodule is, the more one should search for evidence of malignancy in the form of invasion of blood vessels and capsule, either singly or in combination.[923]

The most important cytologic variant is the oxyphilic or oncocytic (Hürthle cell) adenoma, which is composed predominantly (at least 75%) or entirely of large cells with granular, eosinophilic cytoplasm.[930] Ultrastructurally the cells are rich in mitochondria and may exhibit nuclear pleomorphism with distinct nucleoli. Although all such neoplasms are thought by some to be potentially malignant,[931] the biologic behavior and clinical course of oncocytic tumors correlate closely with the histology of the initial lesion, and the absence of invasion predicts a benign outcome.[932–935]

Some normofollicular adenomas may contain pseudopapillary structures that can be confused with the papillae of papillary carcinoma. These structures are probably an expression of localized hyperactivity and are most common in adenomas that show autonomous function. These rare tumors produce excessive amounts of thyroid hormone independent of TSH and on scintiscans exhibit preferential uptake of isotope, in contrast to the suppression of uptake in the remaining gland, including the contralateral lobe. When such a tumor is accompanied by clinical hyperthyroidism, the lesion is termed a hyperfunctioning or "toxic" adenoma. Such adenomas are usually microfollicular or normofollicular; the cells lining the pseudopapillae tend to be tall and cuboidal and have the

---

TABLE 11–28. Subtypes of Follicular Adenoma

Conventional

Trabecular/solid (embryonal) adenoma
Microfollicular (fetal) adenoma
Normofollicular (simple) adenoma
Macrofollicular (colloid) adenoma

Variants

Hyalinizing trabecular adenoma
Oncocytic (oxyphilic or Hürthle cell) tumor
Adenomas with papillary hyperplasia
Hyperfunctioning ("toxic") adenoma
Atypical (hypercellular) adenoma

TABLE 11–27. AJCC Stage Groupings for Thyroid Carcinoma

Stage	Papillary or Follicular (age <45 y)	Papillary or Follicular (age ≥45 y)	Medullary (any age)	Anaplastic (any age)
I	M0	T1	T1	—
II	M1	T2–T3	T2–T4	—
III	—	T4 or N1	N1	—
IV	—	M1	M1	Any

T, size of primary thyroid tumor (T1, ≤1 cm; T2 >1≤4 cm; T3 >4 cm; T4, extrathyroid invasion); N, regional nodal metastases (0, absent; 1, present); M, distant metastases (0, absent; 1, present).

features of secreting follicular cells, comparable to those in Graves' disease.[936] Point mutations in the TSH receptor in some hyperfunctioning follicular adenomas[937, 938] cause constitutive activation of the receptor in the absence of TSH and are associated with high cAMP production.[939] In other hyperfunctioning adenomas, point mutations have been identified[940, 941] in the α subunit of the stimulatory guanyl nucleotide protein (G_s); these mutations impair GTPase activity, trapping the G protein in a state of constitutive activation and enhancing cAMP production.[942] Activating point mutations of the RAS oncogenes have also been identified in toxic adenomas but at a lesser frequency than in macrofollicular adenomas or thyroid carcinomas.[943]

Atypical adenomas are hypercellular tumors with gross and histologic appearances that suggest the possibility of malignancy but do not invade. They account for fewer than 3% of all follicular adenomas.[944] Follow-up indicates that this lesion behaves in a benign fashion, although some would designate the entity as preinvasive adenocarcinoma or follicular carcinoma in situ.[945, 946] The fact that the tumor does not recur or produce metastases after removal does not prove that it is actually benign; removal may have interrupted a natural history that would have culminated in invasion and metastases.[848]

Papillary Thyroid Carcinoma

Papillary thyroid carcinoma has been defined as "a malignant epithelial tumor showing evidence of follicular cell differentiation, and characterized by the formation of papillae and/or a set of distinctive nuclear changes."[947] The most common thyroid malignancy, PTC constitutes 50 to 90% of differentiated FCTCs worldwide.[948] Papillary thyroid microcarcinoma (PTM) is defined by the WHO as a PTC 1.0 cm in diameter or smaller.[949] The incidence rates for clinically diagnosed PTC in the United States approximate 5 per 100,000 for tumors larger than 1 cm in diameter and 1 per 100,000 for PTM. By contrast, the incidence of PTM in autopsy material from various continents ranges from 4 to 36%.[947]

The nuclei of PTC cells have a distinctive appearance, which has a diagnostic significance comparable to that of the papillae. Indeed the preoperative diagnosis of PTC can often be made on the basis of the characteristic nuclear changes seen in FNA material. Typically, PTC shows a predominance of papillary structures, but the papillae are usually admixed with neoplastic follicles having similar nuclear features. When the lining cells of the neoplastic follicles have the same nuclear features as those seen in typical PTC and the follicular predominance over the papillae is complete, the tumor is designated a "follicular variant" of PTC.[947]

Another subtype of PTC is the diffuse sclerosing variant, which is characterized by widespread lymphatic permeation, prominent fibrosis, and diffuse involvement of one or both thyroid lobes. The tall cell variant is characterized by well-formed papillae that are covered by cells twice as tall as they are wide. The columnar cell variant differs from other forms of PTC because of the presence of prominent nuclear stratification. The tall and columnar cell variants are considered more aggressive,[947] but controversy exists regarding outcome in the diffuse sclerosing variant.

MOLECULAR PATHOGENESIS. The thyroid follicular cell may give rise to both benign and malignant tumors, and the malignancy can be of either papillary or follicular histotype. Whether hyperplastic nodules or follicular adenomas can be transformed into follicular cancers has been the subject of much speculation, but there is no evidence that benign tumors ever undergo malignant transformation into classic PTC. DNA aneuploidy as determined by flow cytometry occurs in fewer than 20% of PTCs and may in fact occur less commonly than in follicular adenoma.[950] By contrast, structural abnormalities

of the chromosomes may occur in about 50% of PTCs, frequently involving the long arm of chromosome 10.[951]

The structural defect in chromosome 10 frequently involves an intrachromosomal inversion of the RET proto-oncogene, a member of the receptor tyrosine kinase family. This commonly results in the formation of a chimeric fusion gene with the H4 (D10S170) gene, resulting in an oncogene, designated RET/PTC 1.[952, 953] The H4 gene is not homologous to any known gene but contains an open reading frame that encodes a 585-amino-acid sequence with putative alpha-helical domains.[954] The chimeric RET/PTC 1 gene encodes a fusion protein containing the NH₂-terminus of H4 upstream of the RET tyrosine kinase domain, such that RET/PTC 1 expression is driven by the H4 gene promoter.[955] In other PTCs, translocation of the RET locus to chromosome 17q23 results in formation of the RET/PTC 2 oncogene by fusion with part of the gene coding for the regulatory subunit RIα of protein kinase A. Still another intrachromosomal rearrangement involving the RET locus leads to a fusion with the ele 1 gene and formation of the RET/PTC 3 chimeric gene, which functions as an oncogene as a consequence of RET overexpression under the control of the strong ele 1 promoter.[953, 956] Together, the three RET/PTC chromosomal rearrangements are present is about 30% of PTCs.[953] RET/PTC was expressed in 11 of 26 occult PTCs, suggesting that activation represents an early, possible crucial, event in the process of thyroid oncogenesis.[957] Furthermore RET activation is specific for PTC,[958] again suggesting that it represents a critical event in the transition of a normal follicular thyroid cell into a PTC cell. RET/PTC expression might serve as an indicator of aggressive behavior[959] and correlate with "biologically aggressive histologic features." However, no such rearrangements were found in either 15 patients with tall cell PTC or three tumors with focal or anaplastic dedifferentiation.[960]

Several additional oncogenes may be occasionally involved in PTC, including NTR K1 (also named TRKA), which, like RET, codes for a receptor tyrosine kinase and which is activated in 10 to 20% of PTCs.[961] Theoretically, any event leading to an increased frequency of chromosomal breakage and subsequent rearrangement could be responsible for the RET and NTR K1 gene rearrangements. That radiation may be one mechanism for generating such RET/PTC oncogenes is suggested by the fact that 4 of 7 PTC tumors that developed after the Chernobyl disaster had an RET gene rearrangement.[962]

PRESENTING FEATURES. Although PTC can occur at any age, most occur in patients between 30 and 50 years of age (mean age 45). Women are affected more frequently (female predominance 60 to 80%). Most primary tumors are 1 to 4 cm in size, the average about 2 to 3 cm in greatest diameter.[948, 963] Ninety-five percent of PTC tumors are classified on the basis of degree of differentiation as histologic grade 1[948, 963]; 80% of primary tumors are diploid by flow cytometry.[948] Extrathyroid invasion of adjacent soft tissues is present in about 15% (range 5 to 34%) at primary surgery, and about one third of PTC patients have clinically evident lymphadenopathy at presentation.[963] About 35 to 50% of excised neck nodes have histologic evidence of involvement, and in patients 17 years of age or younger nodal involvement may be present in up to 90%.[964] The primary disease is confined to the neck in 93 to 99% of PTC patients at diagnosis.[948, 964] Spread to superior mediastinal nodes is usually associated with extensive neck nodal involvement. Only 1 to 7% of PTC patients have distant metastases diagnosed before or within 30 d of primary treatment.[948]

The TNM classification is a widely used system for tumor staging.[965] Postoperative stage assessment in PTC is dependent not only on TNM categories but also on whether the patient is younger than age 45 or older.[948, 965] Most PTC patients

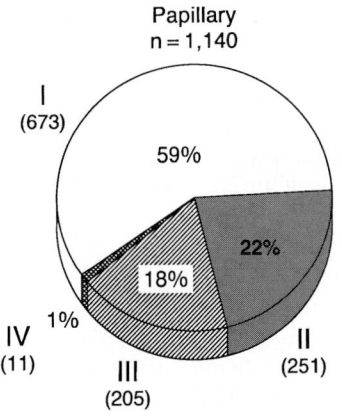
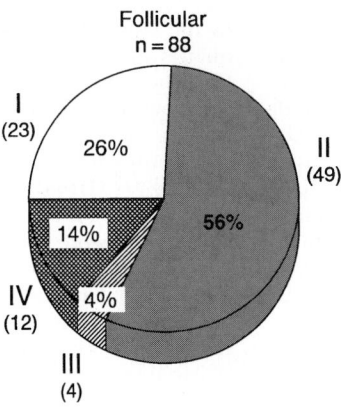

Figure 11–61. Distribution of pathologic-Tumor-Node-Metastases (pTNM) stages in 1140 patients with papillary thyroid carcinoma (PTC) and 88 patients with follicular thyroid carcinoma (FTC) undergoing primary surgical treatment at the Mayo Clinic from 1940 to 1990. Oxyphilic (Hürthle cell) variant tumors were excluded from this comparison of pTNM stages.

present as either stage I (60%) or stage II (22%). Patients aged 45 years or older with either nodal metastases or extrathyroid extension (stage III) account for fewer than 20% of cases.[948] Only about 1 to 3% of PTC patients present with distant metastases and have stage IV disease (age 45 years or older with any T, any N, M1). Figure 11–61 illustrates distribution of TNM stages in 1140 PTC cases seen at the Mayo Clinic, and Figure 11–62 demonstrates survival by TNM stage in 1851 PTC patients treated from 1940 through 1990.

RECURRENCE AND MORTALITY. Three types of tumor recurrence may occur with PTC: (1) postoperative nodal metastases (NM), (2) local recurrences (LR), and (3) postoperative distant metastases (DM). Local recurrence may be defined as "histologically confirmed tumor occurring in the resected thyroid bed, thyroid remnant, or other adjacent tissues of the neck (excluding lymph nodes)" after complete surgical removal of the primary tumor.[966] Nodal or distant spread is considered postoperative if the metastases are discovered within 180 d or 30 d, respectively.[948] Ideally tumor recurrence should be considered only as it occurs in patients without initial DM who had complete surgical resection of the primary tumors. Figures 11–63 and 11–64 illustrate rates of PTC recurrence at local, nodal, and distant sites and compare these rates with those of nonpapillary thyroid cancers treated at one institution during 5 decades. After 25 y of follow-up, postoperative NM had been discovered in 9%, while LR and DM occurred in 6% and 5%, respectively. Both LR and DM are less common in PTC than in FTC. However, postoperative cases of NM were more frequent in PTC.

Survival rates for differentiated thyroid cancer are shown in Figure 11–64. Survival rates for PTC were 98% at 5 y, 96%

at 10 y, and 95% at 20 y. Of those with lethal PTC, 20% of deaths occurred in the first year after diagnosis, and 80% of the deaths occurred within 10 y. The 25-y cause-specific survival rate of 94% for PTC was higher than the 79% rate with MTC and the 71% rates with FTC and Hürthle cell cancer.

OUTCOME PREDICTION. Only a fraction (about 15%) of patients with PTC are liable to relapse of disease, and even fewer (around 5%) have a lethal outcome. Exceptional patients, who have an aggressive course, tend to relapse early (Fig. 11–65), and the rare fatalities usually occur within 5 to 10 y of diagnosis.[948, 949, 963, 964] Multivariate analyses have been utilized to identify variables predictive of cause-specific mortality.[967–970] Increasing patient age and presence of extrathyroid invasion are independent prognostic factors in all studies.[967–970] The presence of initial DM and large size of the primary tumor are also significant variables in most studies,[967, 969, 970] and some groups[948, 967, 968] have reported that histopathologic grade (degree of differentiation) is an independent variable. The completeness of initial tumor resection (postoperative status) is also a predictor of mortality.[948, 969, 971] The presence of initial neck NM, although relevant to future nodal recurrence, did not influence cause-specific mortality (Fig. 11–66).[948, 963, 971]

A scoring index devised to assign PTC patients to prognostic risk groups[967] was named the AGES score after the five independent variables of patient's *a*ge, tumor *g*rade, tumor *e*xtent (local invasion, distant metastasis) and tumor *s*ize. With the use of such a scoring system, 86% of patients were in the "minimal risk" group (AGES score <4), and they experienced a 20-y cause-specific mortality rate of only 1%.[948] By contrast, patients with AGES scores of 4+ (high-risk; 14% of the total)

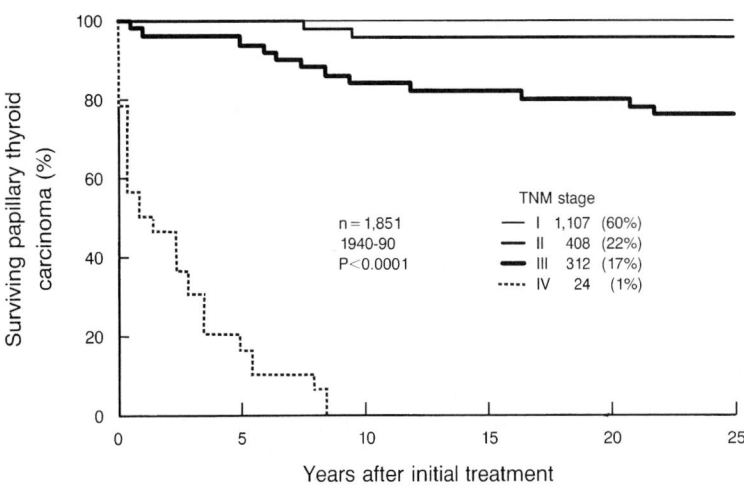

Figure 11–62. Cause-specific survival according to pathologic-Tumor-Node-Metastases (pTNM) stage in a cohort of 1851 patients with papillary thyroid carcinoma (PTC) treated at the Mayo Clinic from 1940 to 1990. The numbers in parentheses represent the percentages of patients in each pTNM stage grouping.

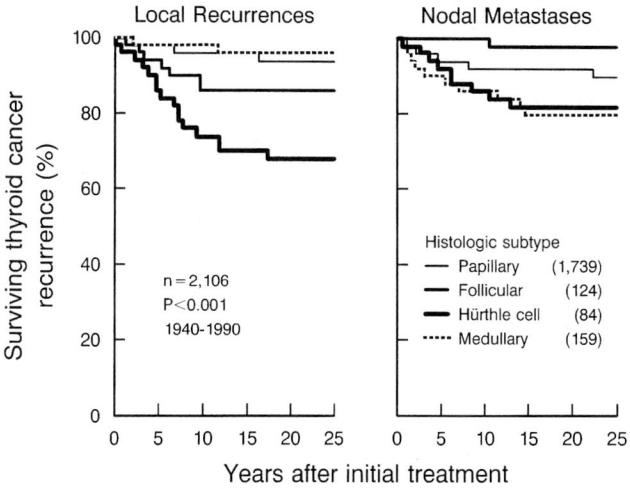

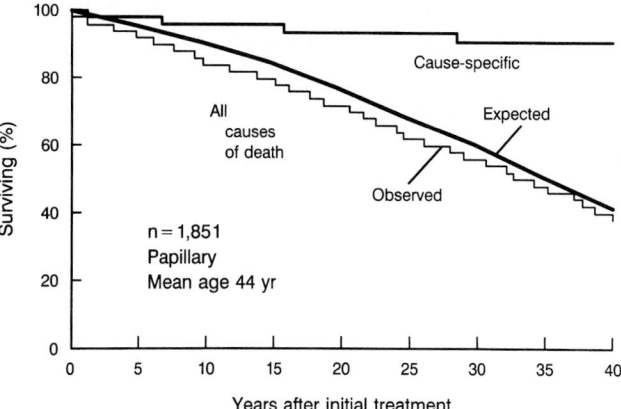

Figure 11–63. Development of local recurrences *(left panel)* and neck nodal metastases *(right panel)* in the first 25 y after definitive surgery for differentiated thyroid carcinoma (DTC) at the Mayo Clinic from 1940 to 1990. Based on 2106 consecutive patients (1739 papillary thyroid carcinoma [PTC], 124 nonoxyphilic follicular thyroid carcinoma [FTC], 84 Hürthle cell carcinoma [HCC], and 159 medullary thyroid carcinoma [MTC]) who had complete surgical resection (i.e., had no gross residual disease), and were without distant metastases on initial examination.

Figure 11–65. Survival to all causes of death and to death from thyroid cancer (cause-specific mortality) in 1851 consecutive patients with papillary thyroid carcinoma (PTC) undergoing initial management at the Mayo Clinic from 1940 to 1990. Also plotted is the expected survival (all causes) of persons of same age and sex and with the same date of treatment and living under mortality conditions of the northwest central United States.

had a 20-y cause-specific mortality of 40%. Figure 11–67 compares the AGES (1987) scores with TNM stage and with two other schemes designed to stratify PTC patients into groups at either minimal risk or high risk of cancer-related death. The prognostic scoring system makes it possible to counsel patients and to aid in the planning of individualized postoperative management programs in PTC.[967, 971]

Although the AGES scheme had the potential for universal application, some academic centers could not include the differentiation (G) variable because their surgical pathologists did not recognize higher grade PTC tumors.[972] Accordingly a prognostic scoring system for predicting PTC mortality rates was devised with the use of candidate variables that included completeness of primary tumor resection but excluded histologic grade.[971] Cox model analysis and stepwise variable selection led to a final prognostic model that included five variables abbreviated by *m*etastasis, *a*ge, *c*ompleteness of resection, *inva*-sion, and *s*ize (MACIS). The final score was defined as MACIS = 3.1 (if age is 39 years or less) or 0.08 × age (if age is 40 years or more), + 0.3 × tumor size (in centimeters), +1 (if tumor not completely resected), +1 (if locally invasive), +3 (if distant metastases present). As illustrated by Figure 11–68 the MACIS scoring system permits identification of patient groups with a broad range of risk of death from PTC. Twenty-year cause-specific survival rates for patients with MACIS scores of less than 6, 6 to 6.99, 7 to 7.99, and 8+ were 99%, 89%, 56%, and 24%, respectively (*P* < .0001). When cumulative mortality from all causes of death was considered, approximately 85% of PTC patients who had scores of AGES < 4 or MACIS < 6 had no excess mortality over rates predicted for control subjects.[967, 971]

It should be emphasized that the five variables in MACIS scoring are easy to define after primary operation, and consequently the system can be applied in any clinical setting with access to chest and skeletal radiographs and good surgical pathology. The MACIS system can also be used for counseling individual PTC patients and can help guide decision-making as to the intensity of the postoperative tumor surveillance and the appropriateness of adjunctive radioiodine therapy. Since the CIS variables require information obtained at surgery, the system cannot be used to decide the extent of primary surgery.[972]

Follicular Thyroid Carcinoma

Follicular thyroid carcinoma (FTC) is "a malignant epithelial tumor showing evidence of follicular cell differentiation but lacking the diagnostic features of papillary carcinoma."[947] Such a definition excludes the follicular variant of PTC,[973] and it is customary also to exclude both the poorly differentiated insular carcinoma[974] and the rare mixed medullary and follicular carcinoma.[975] The correct classification of tumors with predominant oncocytic features (Hürthle cell carcinomas) is controversial.[930] The WHO committee has taken the stance that this tumor is an oxyphilic variant of FTC.[947] The AFIP, by contrast, believes that "the tumors made up of this cell type have gross, microscopic, behavioral, cytogenetic (and conceivably etiopathogenic) features that set them apart from all others and justify discussing them in a separate section."[923] Thus categorized, FTC is a relatively rare neoplasm whose identification requires invasion of the capsule, blood vessel, or adjacent thyroid. In epidemiologic surveys FTC constitutes from 5 to 50% of differentiated thyroid cancers and tends to

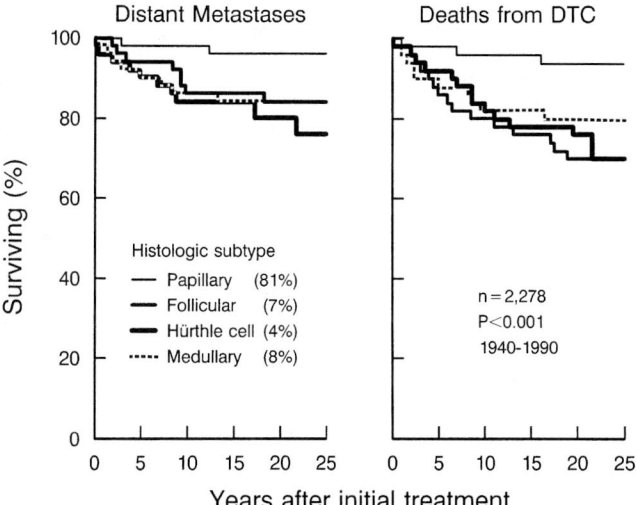

Figure 11–64. Survival to development of distant metastases *(left panel)* in 2106 differentiated thyroid carcinoma (DTC) patients, as described for Figure 11–65. Cause-specific survival *(right panel)* in 2278 DTC patients presenting to the Mayo Clinic for initial management from 1940 to 1990.

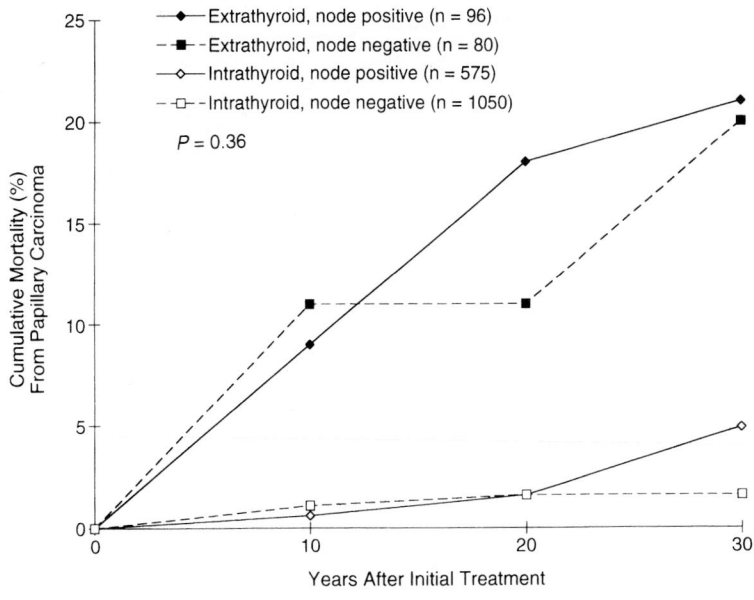

Figure 11–66. Lack of influence of nodal metastases at initial operation on cumulative mortality from papillary thyroid carcinoma (PTC) in 1625 patients with intrathyroid tumors (completely confined to the thyroid) and 176 patients with extrathyroid (locally invasive) tumors. All patients had initial surgical treatment at the Mayo Clinic from 1940 to 1991. (From Grebe SKG, Hay ID. Thyroid cancer nodal metastases: biologic significance and therapeutic considerations. Surg Oncol Clin North Am 1996; 5:43–63, with permission.)

be more common in areas with iodine deficiency.[976] Owing to a combination of changing diagnostic criteria and an increase in the incidence of PTC associated with dietary iodine supplementation, the diagnosis of FTC has decreased in frequency; in one North American experience minimally invasive nonoxyphilic FTC made up fewer than 2% of thyroid malignancies.[977]

The microscopic appearance of FTC varies from well-formed follicles to a predominantly solid growth pattern.[924] Poorly formed follicles and atypical patterns (e.g., cribriform) may occur, and multiple architectural types may coexist.[923] Mitotic activity is not a useful indicator of malignancy. Focal or extensive clear cell changes can occur. A rare clear cell variant of FTC has been described in which glycogen accumulation or dilatation of the granular endoplasmic reticulum is responsible for the clear cells.[978] When more than 75% of cells in an FTC exhibit Hürthle cell or oncocytic features, the tumor is classified as a Hürthle cell carcinoma,[979] oncocytic carcinoma,[923] or oxyphilic variant FTC.[848] Such oncocytes are characterized by abundant granular acidophilic cytoplasm due to numerous mitochondria, large nuclei with prominent

nucleoli, and occasional, bizarre, hyperchromatic forms.[848, 924] Independent of the predominant cellular type, FTC is best divided into two categories on the basis of degree of invasiveness: (1) minimally invasive or encapsulated, and (2) widely invasive. There is little overlap between these two widely disparate types of FTC.

Minimally invasive FTC is an encapsulated tumor whose growth pattern resembles that of a trabecular/solid, microfollicular, or atypical adenoma. The diagnosis of malignancy depends on the demonstration of blood vessel and/or capsular invasion. The criteria for invasion must therefore be strict.[924] Blood vessel invasion is almost never seen grossly. Microscopically the vessels "should be of venous caliber, be located in or immediately outside of the capsule and contain one or more clusters of tumor cells attached to the wall and protruding into the lumen."[924] Interruption of the capsule must involve the full thickness to qualify as capsular invasion. Penetration of only the inner half or the presence of tumor cells embedded in the capsule does not qualify for the diagnosis of FTC. Foci of capsular invasion must be distinguished from the capsular rupture that can result from FNA. The acronym WHAFFT (*w*orrisome *h*istologic *a*lterations *f*ollowing *F*NA of the *t*hyroid) is applied to such changes.[980] In contrast to the minimally invasive (encapsulated) FTC, the rare "widely invasive" FTC can be distinguished easily from benign lesions. While it may be partially encapsulated, the margins are infiltrative even on gross examination, and vascular invasion is often extensive. The structural features are variable with solid and trabecular areas, but a follicular element is always present. When follicular differentiation is poor or absent, the tumor may be classified as a poorly differentiated (insular) carcinoma.[848, 924]

MOLECULAR PATHOGENESIS. There is still no accepted paradigm for the pathogenesis of follicular thyroid cancer, but some evidence suggests a multistep adenoma-to-carcinoma pathogenesis, similar to that for colon cancer and other adenocarcinomas.[981, 982] This concept is not universally accepted, since pathologists do not recognize follicular carcinoma in situ, and documentation of the evolution of adenoma to carcinoma is rare. Nevertheless several facts about the evolution of FTC are firmly established:

First, most follicular adenomas and all FTCs are probably of monoclonal origin.[837, 849, 850] Second, oncogene activation, particularly by mutation or translocation of the *RAS* oncogene, is common both in follicular adenomas and in FTC (around

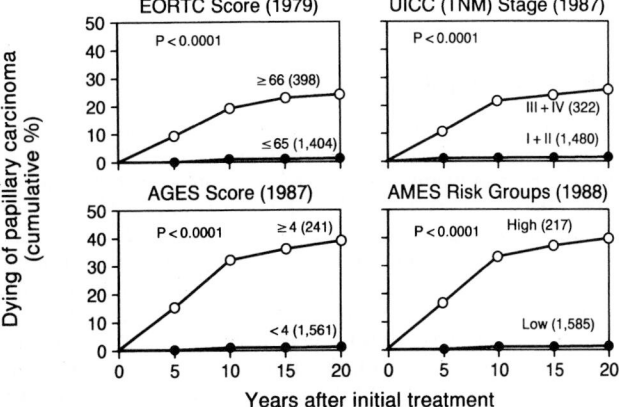

Figure 11–67. Cumulative mortality from papillary thyroid carcinoma (PTC) in patients at either minimal risk or higher risk for cancer-related death as defined by EORTC (European Organization for Research and Treatment of Cancer) score *(upper left)*, pathologic Tumor-Node-Metastases (pTNM) stage *(upper right)*, AGES (age, tumor grade, tumor extent, and tumor size) score *(lower left)*, and AMES risk groups *(lower right)*. The minimal risk group constitutes 82% of the 1802 patients when defined by pTNM stages I and II, and 87% of the total when defined by an AGES score <4.

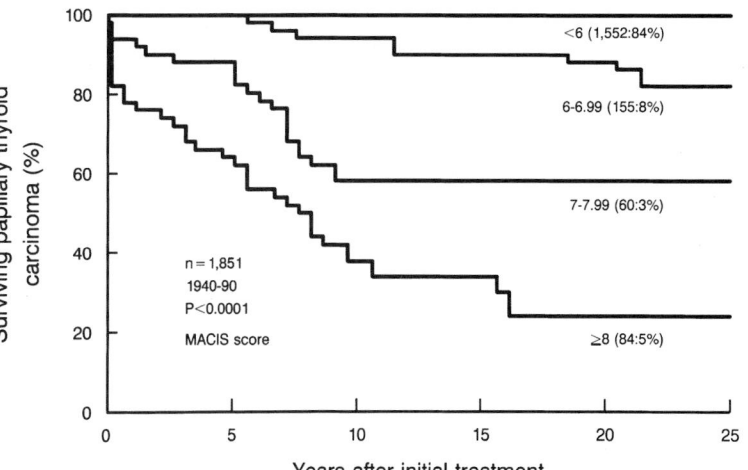

Figure 11–68. Cause-specific survival according to MACIS (metastasis, age, completeness of resection, invasion, and size) scores of <6, 6–6.99, 7–7.99, and 8+ in a cohort of 1851 consecutive papillary thyroid carcinoma (PTC) patients undergoing initial treatment at the Mayo Clinic from 1940 to 1990. The numbers in parentheses represent the number and percentages of PTC patients in each of the four risk groups.

40%), supporting a role in early tumorigenesis.[943, 981] Such *RAS* mutations are not specific for follicular tumors and occur in PTC.[943] The *RET* oncogene seems to be specific for PTC and does not appear to be significant in follicular tumors.[958] Third, cytogenetic abnormalities and evidence of genetic loss are more common in FTC than in PTC and also occur in follicular adenomas,[950, 983–985] suggesting that cell cycle control, mitotic spindle formation, DNA repair, or more than one of these mechanisms may be impaired in these neoplasms, possibly at an early stage. These changes may be associated with loss of function of one or more tumor suppressor genes. Potential candidate genes may be localized by analyzing the pattern of genetic loss; losses in FTC are particularly associated with chromosomes 3, 10, 11, and 17.[983–986]

Of the cytogenetic abnormalities described in FTC,[987] the most common are deletions, partial deletions, and deletion/rearrangements involving the p arm of chromosome 3.[985, 988] Loss of heterozygosity (LOH) studies corroborate the cytogenetic studies, particularly with regard to a 3p locus.[983] Since LOH at 3p can occur in both a primary tumor and its metastasis, loss of genetic material on the p arm of chromosome 3 may be a nonrandom, inherited property of certain FTCs and of possible etiologic and prognostic significance.[985] Small cell lung cancer and renal cell carcinoma also exhibit frequent LOH on 3p, suggesting that one or more tumor suppressor genes are located on the short arm of chromosome 3.[989, 990] LOH on chromosome 3p appears to be limited to FTC, since no evidence for 3p LOH has been found with follicular adenomas or PTC.[983, 984] In summary, loss of a tumor suppressor on 3p could be specific for FTC and may be involved in an adenoma-to-carcinoma progression. However, because loss of function of one of the tumor suppressor alleles usually involves a major genetic deletion, it is possible that these losses occur only when the genomic stability of the tumor cell population is already compromised by an initiating event.

PRESENTING FEATURES. FTC tends to occur in older persons, with the mean age in most studies being more than 50 years, about 10 years older than for typical PTC.[976, 991] The median age of patients with oxyphilic FTC (Hürthle cell cancer [HCC]) averages around 60 years.[976, 979] As in most thyroid malignancies, women outnumber men by more than 2 to 1. Most patients with FTC present with a painless thyroid nodule, with or without background thyroid nodularity. In contrast to PTC where almost 40% have palpable lymph nodes, patients with FTC rarely (4 to 6%) have clinically evident lymphadenopathy at presentation.[976] Lymph node metastases to the neck in FTC are so exceptional that "wherever they are observed, the alternative possibilities of follicular variant papil-

lary carcinoma, oncocytic carcinoma, and poorly differentiated (insular) carcinoma should be considered."[923]

In most series where tumor sizes are reported, the average tumor in FTC (oxyphilic or nonoxyphilic) is larger than those seen with PTC.[976, 979, 991] When tumor histopathologic grading is performed, higher grade tumors, indicating less differentiation, are more common than with PTC.[979, 991] Nuclear aneuploidy is present in about 60% of FTC tumors and in up to 90% of patients with HCC.[932, 950, 992] Direct extrathyroid extension, by definition, does not occur with minimally invasive FTC but is not uncommon in the rare patient with invasive FTC. Nonspecific systematic signs of malignancy are more common in FTC than PTC, because between 5 and 20% of patients may have distant metastases at presentation.[976, 991] It is unusual for patients with FTC to have thyrotoxicosis, but this occurs, owing to either massive tumor burden or functioning metastatic disease.[993] The most common sites for distant metastases in FTC are lung and bone.[923, 991] Bone metastases (which are usually osteolytic) may be the first manifestations of the disease. Pathologic fracture of a long bone may be due to metastasis of previously occult FTC. The bones most often involved are long bones (e.g., femur) and flat bones (particularly the pelvis, sternum, and skull). Occasionally, patients present because of persistent neck or lumbar pain due to involvement of vertebrae by metastatic FTC.

Most patients (54 to 70%) with FTC or HCC have pTNM stage II disease. Patients aged 45 years or older with nodal metastases or extrathyroid extension (stage III) account for only 4% of FTC and 8% of HCC (Fig. 11–69). In contrast to PTC, in which only 1 to 3% present with stage IV cases, about 5% of HCC and 15% or more of nonoxyphilic FTC have distant metastases at the time of diagnosis.

RECURRENCE AND MORTALITY. Nodal metastases are rare in typical FTC, and nodal recurrence rates at 10 and 20 postoperative years are the lowest in differentiated thyroid carcinoma, 1 and 2% respectively (see Fig. 11–61). About 6% of HCC patients have node involvement at presentation,[994] but within 20 to 30 y after primary surgery 18 and 24% of HCC patients have nodal recurrence.[976] When recurrences at either neck or distant sites are taken into consideration, patients with HCC (Fig. 11–70) have the highest numbers of tumor recurrences after 10 to 20 y. As illustrated by Figures 11–63 and 11–64, local recurrences account for most postoperative events, since the numbers of distant metastases in HCC patients are comparable with FTC or MTC, i.e., about 20% after 20 postoperative years.

Cause-specific mortality rates vary with the presenting TNM stage in both FTC (Fig. 11–69) and HCC. The death

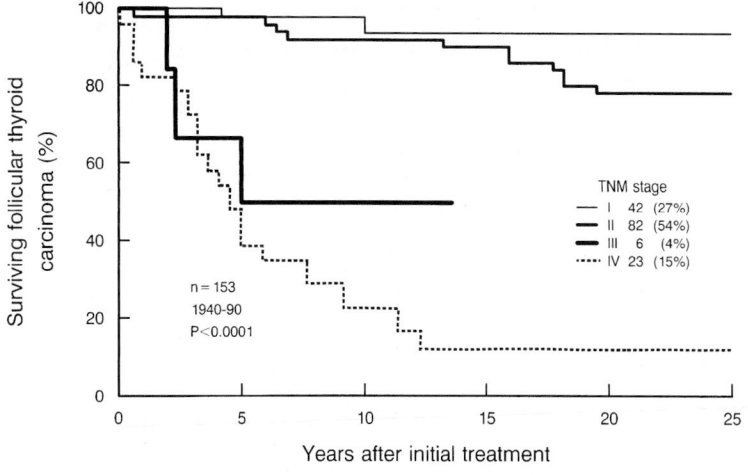

Figure 11–69. Cause-specific survival according to pathologic-Tumor-Node-Metastases (pTNM) stages in a cohort of 153 patients with nonoxyphilic follicular thyroid carcinoma (FTC) treated at the Mayo Clinic from 1940 to 1990. The numbers in parentheses represent the percentages of patients in each pTNM stage grouping.

rates (Figs. 11–63 and 11–64) tend to parallel the curves for development of distant metastases. Clearly the cause-specific mortality from PTC is less than with other forms of differentiated thyroid carcinoma (FTC, HCC, or MTC). In 5 decades of experience at the Mayo Clinic, the mortality rate for FTC initially exceeds that of HCC, but by 20 to 30 postoperative years there are no significant differences in cause-specific survival rates between FTC and HCC (Fig. 11–71), both being around 80% at 20 and 70% at 30 postoperative years.[976] All-causes mortality curves differ in FTC and HCC. FTC patients are younger, tend to die within the first 10 postoperative years, and have high all-causes mortality for 10 to 30 postoperative years (Fig. 11–72). Deaths due to HCC occur gradually over the first 15 y, but by 15 to 20 y the average survivor from HCC is 73 to 78 years old, and by that time almost 50% of the treated cohort would be predicted by the actuarial curve to have died from other causes.

OUTCOME PREDICTION. The risk factors that predict outcome are largely the same in FTC and PTC[976]: distant metastases at presentation, increasing patient age, large tumor size, and the presence of local (extrathyroidal) invasion. To a lesser degree, increased mortality is associated with male sex and higher grade (less well-differentiated) tumors. In addition, vascular invasiveness, lymphatic involvement at presentation, DNA aneuploidy, and oxyphilic histology are potential prognostic variables unique to FTC.[976] The importance of vascular invasion is underscored by a study showing that FTC patients with minimal capsular invasion and no evidence of vascular invasion had 0% cause-specific mortality at 5- and 10-y follow-up.[995]

In all types of thyroid cancer the importance of regional lymph node involvement is debated.[976] One review concluded that nodal metastases are irrelevant to mortality in PTC but may play a minor role in FTC.[994] The importance of DNA aneuploidy is also controversial. In typical FTC, some investigators find it to be predictive of an adverse outcome, and others demonstrate no effect on prognosis.[950, 976] By contrast, in HCC, DNA ploidy measurements are of prognostic significance.[932, 950]

Prognostic scoring systems for FTC[991, 996] allow stratification of patients into high- and low-risk categories. A multivariate analysis at the Mayo Clinic found that distant metastases at presentation, patient age greater than 50 years, and marked vascular invasion predict a poor outcome.[991] As illustrated by Figure 11–73, if two or more of these factors are present, the 5-y survival rate is only 47%, and 20-y survival is 8%. By contrast, if only one of these factors is present, 5-y survival is 99%, and 20-y survival is 86%.[991]

Systems developed to predict outcome in either PTC or FTC have been applied to FTC patients. Specifically, the AMES risk-group categorization (*age, metastasis, extent, size*) is useful in FTC.[997] From a multivariate analyses of 228 FTC patients treated at Sloan-Kettering, the independent adverse prognostic factors were identified as age older than 45 years, Hürthle cell histotype, extrathyroidal extension, tumor size exceeding 4 cm, and the presence of distant metastasis.[998] The prognostic importance in FTC of histologic grade was also confirmed,[998, 999] and this factor is included in assignment of risk-groups to low, intermediate, or high categories (Fig. 11–74). The AGES scheme, originally developed for PTC, has also been successfully applied to FTC.[1000, 1001] It therefore appears

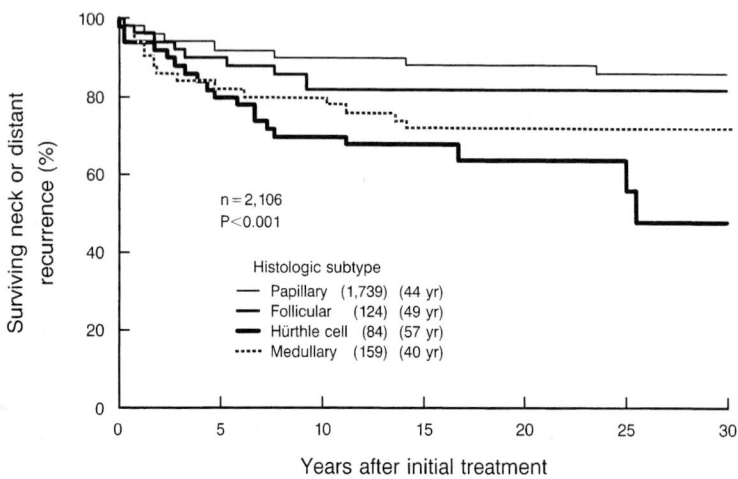

Figure 11–70. Postoperative recurrence (any site) in the first 25 y after definitive surgery for differentiated thyroid carcinoma (DTC) at the Mayo Clinic from 1940 to 1990. Based on 2106 consecutive patients (1739 papillary thyroid carcinoma [PTC], 124 nonoxyphilic follicular thyroid carcinoma [FTC], 84 Hürthle cell carcinoma [HCC], and 159 medullary thyroid carcinoma [MTC]) who had complete tumor resection and had no distant metastases at presentation. The numbers of years in parentheses represent the mean ages of the patients according to the four histologic subtypes.

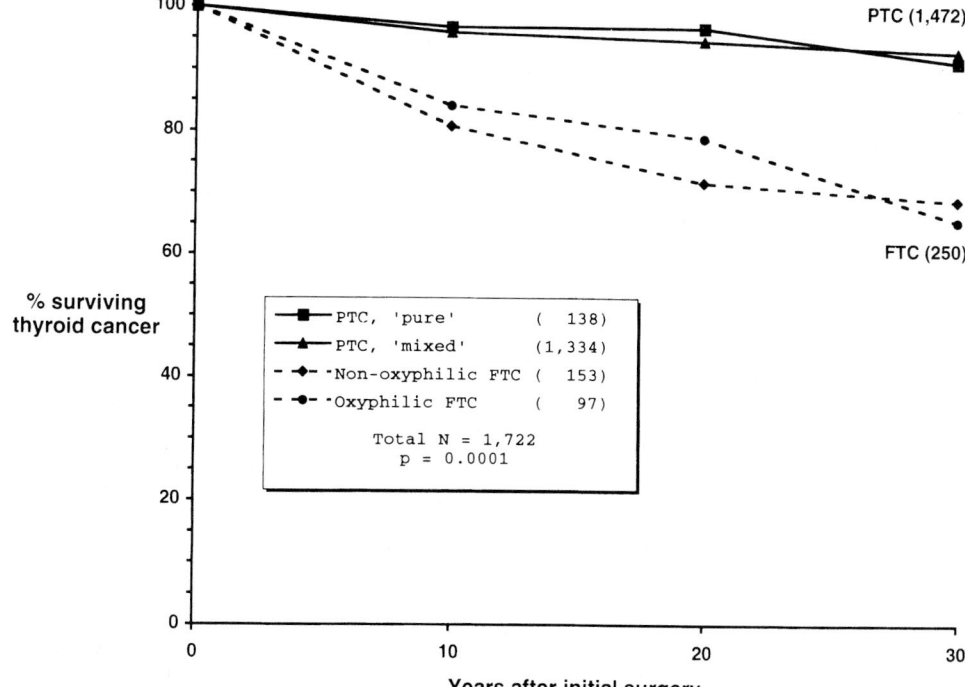

Figure 11–71. Comparison of cause-specific survival in 1472 papillary thyroid carcinoma (PTC) and 250 follicular thyroid carcinoma (FTC) patients treated at the Mayo Clinic from 1940 to 1991. A total of 128 of the papillary thyroid carcinoma (PTC) patients were "pure" papillary in histotype (no follicular elements). A total of 97 of the FTC patients had predominantly oxyphilic tumors. There is a significant difference ($P = .0001$) between the PTC and the FTC survival curves. However, within either the PTC and the FTC groups, the two survival curves are insignificantly different. (From Grebe SKG, Hay ID. Follicular thyroid cancer. Endocrinol Metab Clin North Am 1995; 24:761–801, with permission.)

that scoring systems used in PTC may be cautiously applied in FTC, as long as some of the unique features of this tumor, such as vascular invasiveness and the remarkable significance of DNA aneuploidy in HCC, are kept in mind.[976]

Poorly Differentiated (Insular) Carcinoma

This cancer has been defined as "a tumor of follicular cell origin with morphological and biologic attributes intermediate between differentiated and anaplastic carcinomas of the thyroid."[848] The most distinctive histologic feature is the presence of round or oval nests (insulae) composed of small cells with round nuclei and scant cytoplasm. The predominant pattern of growth is solid, but microfollicles are also seen, some of which contain dense colloid. Growth is infiltrative, and blood vessel invasion is common. Most such tumors exhibit foci of necrosis, are larger than 5 cm in diameter at

diagnosis, and have an invasive margin on gross examination, often with extrathyroid extension.

The mean age at diagnosis is around 55 years, and the female-to-male ratio is about 2:1.[848] Insular carcinoma is aggressive and often lethal. Metastases are common in regional nodes and distant sites (lung, bone, brain). In one series 56% of patients died from their tumor within 8 y of initial therapy.[974] The tumor is viewed by the WHO committee[922] as a morphologic variant of FTC, but others[848, 924] view it as a poorly differentiated variant of either PTC or FTC. It has developed after a typical PTC of either the conventional or the follicular-

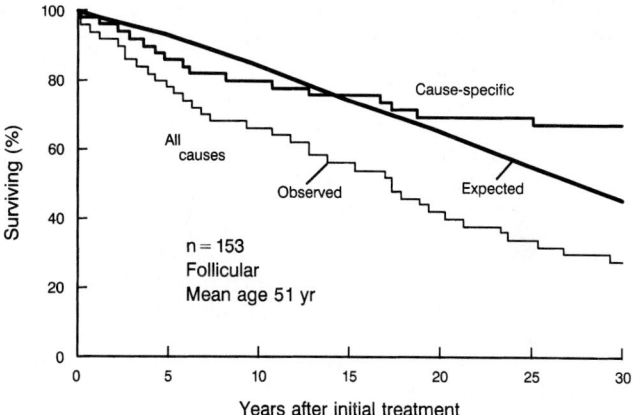

Figure 11–72. Survival to all causes of death and to death from thyroid cancer (cause-specific mortality) in 153 consecutive patients with nonoxyphilic follicular thyroid carcinoma (FTC) undergoing initial management at the Mayo Clinic from 1940 to 1990. Also plotted is the expected survival (all causes) of persons of the same age and sex and with the same date of treatment and living under mortality conditions of the northwest central United States.

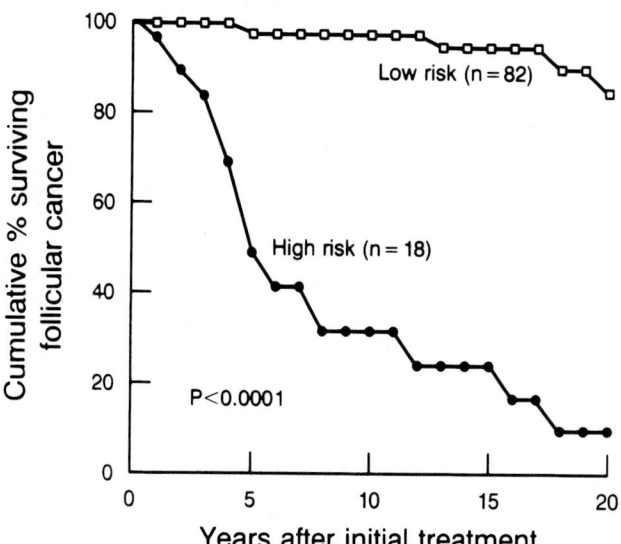

Figure 11–73. Cumulative cause-specific survival among 100 patients with non-oxyphilic follicular thyroid carcinoma (FTC) treated at the Mayo Clinic from 1946 to 1970 and plotted by high-risk and low-risk categories. High-risk = two or more of the following factors present: age greater than 50 years, marked vascular invasion, and metastatic disease at time of initial diagnosis. (From Brennan MD, Bergstralh EJ, van Heerden JA, et al. Follicular thyroid cancer treated at the Mayo Clinic, 1946 through 1970: initial manifestations, pathologic findings, therapy, and outcome. Mayo Clinic Proc 1991; 66:11–22, with permission.)

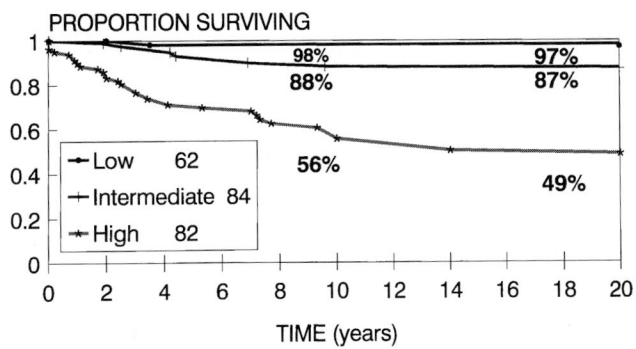

Figure 11–74. Survival differences with low/intermediate/high risk groups for 228 consecutive patients with follicular thyroid carcinoma (FTC) who were seen and treated at Memorial Sloan-Kettering Cancer Center during a period of 55 years from 1930 to 1985. (From Shaha AR, Loree TR, Shah JP. Prognostic factors and risk group analyses in follicular carcinoma of the thyroid. Surgery 1995; 118:1131–1138, with permission.)

variant type.[923] In other circumstances progression from a typical papillary to an insular pattern is accompanied by a gradual change in the ground-glass appearance of PTC nuclei to the smaller hyperchromatic forms characteristic of insular tumors.[923] Some tumors formerly classified as the compact form of undifferentiated small cell carcinoma probably belonged to this category.[848] The AFIP group also believe that a large proportion of "low-risk" young patients with aggressive PTC or FTC belong to this category of high-grade poorly differentiated follicular cell–derived thyroid carcinomas.[923]

Undifferentiated (Anaplastic) Carcinoma

Anaplastic carcinoma constitutes about 5 to 10% of all thyroid carcinomas,[1002] usually occurs after the age of 60, and is slightly more common in women (1.3 to 1.5:1). It is highly malignant, rapidly invading adjacent structures and metastasizing throughout the body.

Anaplastic carcinoma is nonencapsulated and extends widely, distorting the shape of the thyroid. It is stony hard in some areas and soft or friable in others. Evidence of invasion of adjacent structures, such as the skin, muscle, nerve, blood vessels, larynx, and esophagus, is common. On histopathologic examination, the lesion is composed of atypical cells that exhibit numerous mitoses and form a variety of patterns. Spindle-shaped cells and multinucleate giant cells usually predominate, and a third histologic pattern is described as squamoid, in which cells are undifferentiated but retain an epithelial appearance.[923, 924] Areas of necrosis and polymorphonuclear infiltration are common, and the presence of PTC or FTC suggests that they may be the precursors of anaplastic carcinoma. Thorough sampling may be necessary to detect the residual well-differentiated thyroid. Mutations of the p53 gene are present in many undifferentiated carcinomas but may not be found in the residual well-differentiated component,[1003, 1004] suggesting that these mutations occurred after the development of the original tumor and may have played a key role in tumor progression.

The usual clinical complaint is of a rapid, often painful enlargement of a mass that may have been present in the thyroid gland for many years. The tumor invades adjacent structures, causing hoarseness, inspiratory stridor, and difficulty in swallowing. On examination, the overlying skin is often warm and discolored. The mass is tender and is often fixed to adjacent structures, with the result that it moves poorly on swallowing. It is stony hard in consistency, but some areas may be soft or fluctuant. The regional lymph nodes are enlarged, and there may be evidence of distant metastases. The patient usually succumbs within months after diagnosis.

In general, anaplastic carcinomas do not accumulate iodine. Rarely, extensive replacement of the thyroid parenchyma may produce hypothyroidism.

Medullary Thyroid Carcinoma

Medullary thyroid carcinoma (see Chapter 32) accounts for as many as 10% of thyroid malignancies, usually occurs after the age of 40, and is slightly more common in women. This carcinoma readily invades the intraglandular lymphatics and spreads to other parts of the gland and to the pericapsular and regional lymph nodes.[1005, 1006] In this respect it resembles PTC, but it also regularly spreads via the bloodstream to the lungs, bone, and liver.[1005]

Medullary thyroid carcinoma is firm and usually unencapsulated. On histopathologic examination, the tumor is composed of cells that vary in morphologic features and arrangement. Round, polyhedral, and spindle-shaped cells form a variety of patterns but do not form papillary folds or follicles. The cells may appear undifferentiated and exhibit mitoses, but unlike the findings in anaplastic carcinoma, necrosis and polymorphonuclear infiltration are absent. There is an abundant hyaline connective tissue stroma that stains positively with Congo red for amyloid.[1007] Gross or microscopic foci of carcinoma may be present in other parts of the gland, and blood vessels may be invaded. The histopathologic appearance of the metastases resembles that of the primary lesion.

Medullary thyroid carcinoma first appears either as a hard nodule or mass in the thyroid gland or as an enlargement of the regional lymph nodes. Occasionally a metastatic lesion in a distant site is found first. Lesions are sometimes bilateral but are usually localized to the upper two thirds of the gland, which is the anatomic location of the parafollicular cells.

Medullary thyroid carcinoma arises from the C cells of the thyroid rather than the follicular epithelium; secretes a characteristic hormone, calcitonin; is frequently associated with one or more paraendocrine manifestations; may be familial; and provides an early biochemical signal (hypersecretion of calcitonin) that permits its early detection, treatment, and cure.[1008] The tumor occurs in both sporadic and familial forms, the latter making up about 20% of the total. The familial variety usually appears at a younger age, is more often bilateral, is less likely to have associated cervical metastases when diagnosed, and has a better prognosis.[1009] Most important, the familial variety is preceded by a premalignant C-cell hyperplasia (CCH) that can be cured by total thyroidectomy.[1010, 1011]

The entity of MTC was described in 1959, and early series of MTC mainly described sporadic cases, in which 80% of patients presented with TNM stages II or III.[1007] As more patients with familial MTC[1012] or MEN 2A have been diagnosed, more patients have curable (stage I) disease, and the survival has improved, a trend that should continue with widespread application of *RET* proto-oncogene testing in MTC.[1013] MTC patients now have similar or better outcomes than patients with nonpapillary follicular cell–derived cancers (see Fig. 11–64). The cause-specific survival curves for 181 consecutive MTC cases treated from 1940 to 1990 at the Mayo Clinic, according to TNM stage, are presented in Figure 11–75. Unlike PTC, nodal metastases at presentation (stage III) influence mortality.

Other prognostic factors relevant to outcome in MTC include age at diagnosis, male gender, vascular invasion, calcitonin immunoreactivity and amyloid staining in tumor tissue, presence or absence of postoperative gross residual disease, and abnormal postoperative plasma calcitonin levels.[1005–1007] In a multivariate analysis, only the presence of extrathyroid invasion and postoperative gross residual disease were significant in the prediction of cause-specific survival.[1006] Another study

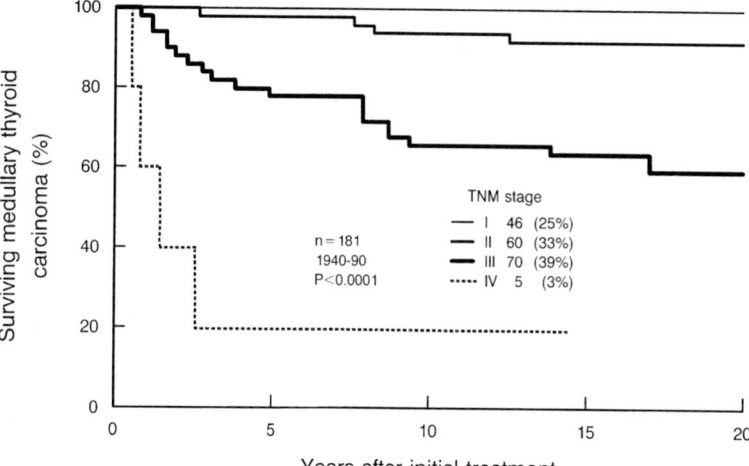

Figure 11–75. Cause-specific survival according to pathologic-Tumor-Node-Metastases (pTNM) stage in a cohort of 181 patients with medullary thyroid carcinoma (MTC) treated at the Mayo Clinic from 1940 to 1990. The numbers in parentheses represent the percentages of patients in each pTNM stage grouping.

concluded that the only factors remaining in the final Cox model were: TNM stages III or IV disease, negative Congo red staining for amyloid, and postoperative gross residual disease.[1007] Based on these three independent prognostic variables, a scoring system was devised to define four risk-groups (Fig. 11–76). Patients with stages I or II disease, complete tumor resection, and positive amyloid staining were at "minimal" risk for death from MTC (5% at 10 y), whereas patients with all three adverse features died within 1 of primary surgery. The presence of only one or two (of the three) features imparted either a low risk (10-y rate of 22%) or a high risk (10-y rate of 74%) of death from MTC.

In patients with MTC the carcinoid syndrome and Cushing's syndrome may occur, owing to secretion of serotonin and corticotropin, respectively, by the tumors. Prostaglandins, kinins, and vasoactive intestinal peptide may also be secreted and are variously responsible for the attacks of watery diarrhea that about one third of patients experience. In the familial disorder, there is often clinical or laboratory evidence of hyperparathyroidism and pheochromocytoma (Sipple's syndrome; multiple endocrine neoplasia type 2A [MEN 2A]; see Chapter 32). Hyperparathyroidism is usually due to parathyroid hyperplasia rather than adenoma. Pheochromocytomas are often bilateral and are prone to secreting epinephrine, so urinary total catecholamine and vanillylmandelic acid excre-

tions may be normal. Specific measurements of urinary epinephrine excretion often reveal some elevation, however. In MEN 2B MTC, pheochromocytoma are associated with ganglioneuromas, multiple mucosal neuromas ("bumpy lip" syndrome), a marfanoid habitus, and typical facies but usually not hyperparathyroidism.[1011] Differentiation of patients with sporadic MTC from other types of thyroid nodule on clinical grounds alone may be difficult. In patients with a family history of thyroid cancer, hypertension, hyperparathyroidism, or nephrolithiasis, the MEN 2A syndrome should be suspected. Basal plasma calcitonin levels are elevated in about one third to two thirds of patients with MTC. Infusions of pentagastrin or calcium elicit secretion of calcitonin, and the response is exaggerated in patients with either MTC or the antecedent C-cell hyperplasia (see Chapter 32). Patients are usually normocalcemic, but those suspected of having MEN should be evaluated for hyperparathyroidism and for pheochromocytoma.

When the diagnosis of MTC is made from calcitonin measurements or FNAB, total thyroidectomy with removal of regional nodes should be performed.[1008] In patients with MEN, pheochromocytomas should be operated on before operation on MTC. First-degree relatives of patients with MEN, including small children, should undergo DNA testing for the presence of the mutant gene or be screened regularly for the emergence of one or more manifestations of the syndrome[1010] (see Chapter 32). Patients diagnosed with familial MTC or MEN by DNA testing or serum calcitonin elevations should undergo a prophylactic total thyroidectomy.[1014] The current practice is to perform a total thyroidectomy on children with positive *RET* mutations between 5 and 7 years of age.[1009, 1010]

Primary Malignant Lymphoma

Thyroid lymphoma is responsible for only 1 to 2% of thyroid malignancies. It may cause manifestations that suggest anaplastic carcinoma. Differentiation of the two is important because the prognoses and the therapeutic approaches are different. The most common form of thyroid lymphoma is the diffuse large cell type, and immunoblastic lymphoma is the second most common.[924] Most low-grade lymphomas of the thyroid may belong to the MALT (mucosa-associated lymphoid tissue) category, and nearly all thyroid lymphomas are of B-cell derivation.[1015] Hashimoto's thyroiditis is usually present in the surrounding thyroid, and the risk of thyroid lymphoma is more than 60-fold higher in Hashimoto's thyroiditis than in nodular goiter. Nonetheless the disease is a rare complication of Hashimoto's thyroiditis, in one series occurring in only 4 of 829 patients.[1016] The clinical picture is that of a rapidly enlarging thyroid mass in a patient with a history of Hashi-

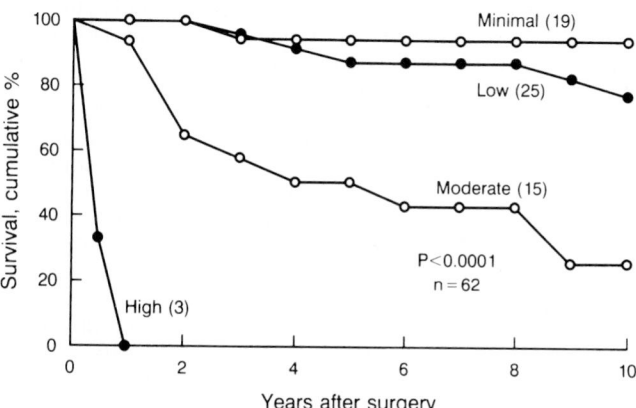

Figure 11–76. Survival until death from medullary thyroid carcinoma (MTC) according to four risk groups, based on the presence or absence of adverse independent prognostic factors, that is, pathologic-Tumor-Node-Metastases (pTNM) stages III or IV, negative amyloid stain, and incomplete tumor resection. (From Pyke CM, Hay ID, Goellner JR, et al. Prognostic significance of calcitonin immunoreactivity, amyloid staining, and flow cytometric DNA measurements in medullary thyroid carcinoma. Surgery 1991; 110:964–971, with permission.)

moto's thyroiditis or of hypothyroidism. The lesion is nonfunctional on thyroid scintiscan, and the tumor may compress adjacent tissues. Surgical decompression can often be avoided by the use of radiation therapy once an appropriate diagnosis is made. The diagnosis is made with either FNA or Vim-Silverman needle biopsy with appropriate immunohistochemical staining.[1015, 1017] It is especially important to make a pathologic distinction between the lesion formerly referred to as small cell carcinoma of the thyroid and lymphoma; lymphoma is a curable lesion, whereas undifferentiated thyroid carcinoma is rapidly fatal. The best success rates are obtained with combined therapy involving systemic chemotherapy and external radiation to the neck and mediastinum.[1017]

Treatment of Thyroid Carcinoma

There is controversy as to the extent of surgery appropriate for thyroid malignancy.[966, 967] Factors that influence this decision include the histologic diagnosis, the size of the original lesion, the presence of distant metastasis, the age of the patient, and the risk-group category.[997, 999] Obviously the surgeon must be skilled in thyroid surgery. General guidelines are as follows: papillary microcancers (tumor size not more than 1.0 cm in diameter) and possibly small (less than 2 cm) FTC without invasion of blood vessels can usually be treated with ipsilateral total lobectomy and isthmectomy with exploration of the ipsilateral lymph nodes.[949, 995] However, for larger PTC lesions and especially for those that have extended through the thyroid capsule into periglandular tissues, a total lobectomy on the involved side and a subtotal or nearly total thyroidectomy on the contralateral side are recommended.[948, 963] Such patients are likely candidates for postoperative ^{131}I remnant ablation. All patients with PTC should have exploration for, and resection of, involved lymph nodes. Preoperative ultrasound may be of assistance to the surgeon in planning such a procedure.[427]

For larger follicular lesions and Hürthle cell tumors that invade the capsule or vessels, a total resection on the ipsilateral side and at least subtotal resection of the contralateral side are indicated, because of the more aggressive nature of this lesion and the probable need for radioactive iodine ablation.[991] Medullary thyroid carcinoma is usually treated with total thyroidectomy with removal of involved soft tissue and nodes in the central portion of the neck and upper mediastinum.[1008] Systematic nodal dissection may be required for MTC affecting lateral neck nodes.[1018] Patients with anaplastic carcinoma generally have lesions that are too extensive for any procedure but palliative surgery.[1002] Individuals with primary thyroid lymphoma should be evaluated in collaboration with an oncologist, and appropriate therapy for the lymphoma should be initiated. In some patients with lymphoma, the thyroid gland is the only organ involved, and resection may be appropriate[1015]; in most cases radiation and chemotherapy will be employed.[1017] For the very rare individual with malignant epithelial lesions in whom immediate surgery cannot be performed, institution of TSH suppression with levothyroxine is indicated when the basal serum TSH concentrations are normal or elevated. This can usually be accomplished by administering levothyroxine at approximately 1.8 to 2.0 µg/kg body weight.

In recommending surgery the endocrinologist should discuss the potential complications with the patient. Unilateral lobectomy virtually never causes permanent hypocalcemia but can cause vocal cord paralysis in as many as 3% of patients. Near-total thyroidectomy causes temporary hypocalcemia in 7 to 10% of patients and permanent hypocalcemia in 0.5 to 1%; temporary vocal cord paralysis occurs in about 1 to 2%. A total extracapsular thyroidectomy may lead to hypoparathyroidism in as many as 30% of individuals, an unacceptable complication rate for patients with indolent malignancy. In addition, vocal cord paralysis is more common after such a procedure. The experience of the surgeon is important in terms of the finer technical points of thyroidectomy, including preservation of the external branch of the recurrent laryngeal nerve, which is important in the fine regulation of voice pitch. This is especially pertinent for individuals who depend on the voice for a livelihood.

APPROACH TO IRRADIATED PATIENTS. A history of radiation in childhood increases the risk of both benign and malignant thyroid nodules in later life.[1019] The risk varies with the type of radiation, the size of the radiation port, and the dose. Several issues are relevant for the thyroidologist. First, given that surgical exploration may be required for patients with a history of thyroid radiation and suspicious thyroid nodules, what should be the extent of initial surgery and how should such patients be treated subsequently? With respect to the extent of surgery, opinions vary from near-total thyroidectomy at the time of the initial procedure to an individual assessment, the extent of surgery depending on the degree of thyroid involvement. Individuals with bilateral nodular disease should have a near-total or total thyroidectomy, and residual thyroid tissue should be considered for remnant ablation. If there is no involvement of the opposite lobe at the time of surgery, one must weigh the relative risk of complications associated with a more extensive surgical procedure against the possibility of recurrence of thyroid nodules in the residual thyroid tissue. In one irradiated population, both benign and malignant nodules recurred after previous subtotal thyroidectomy.[1020] The risk of recurrence overall in this study was approximately 20% and was lower in those who had more thyroid tissue removed than in those who had less extensive procedures. In those patients, suppression of TSH by thyroid hormone led to a reduction in recurrence from 35% to approximately 8%, but TSH suppression had no influence on the prevalence of malignant nodules. Thus the recommendations for such patients must take into account the nature of the radiation exposure and the experience of the operating surgeon, and no general rule can be given. All irradiated patients who have had thyroid nodules removed should receive TSH-suppressive doses of levothyroxine regardless of the extent of surgery. The appearance of new thyroid nodules is common, and such patients should be monitored indefinitely for this possibility. It is not clear whether this experience should be extrapolated to prescribe routine TSH suppression therapy for all irradiated patients, even if nodularity is not present. This approach cannot be recommended at present because patients who do not have thyroid nodules may not have received sufficient exposure to have a propensity for thyroid neoplasia and because the risks of long-term TSH suppression in women, especially vis-a-vis osteoporosis, have not been clearly defined and may be significant.[866, 867, 1021]

POSTOPERATIVE MANAGEMENT. In view of the foregoing uncertainties and the different needs of individual patients, postoperative treatment of thyroid carcinoma cannot always accord with a rigid algorithm.[1014] One must consider the extent of disease at surgery, the histotype and differentiation of the tumor, the age of the patient, and the risk-group category.[902, 999]

In a large group of patients with differentiated carcinoma (PTC, FTC, and HCC), only 9% developed distant metastasis.[1022] Most of the patients had PTC, and of these 7% developed distant metastasis, as opposed to 19% of patients with FTC and 34% of patients with HCC. Mortality rates at 5 and 10 y after diagnosis of metastasis were 65 and 75% for all patients with distant metastasis, and nearly 80% of the deaths were due to thyroid cancer. Thus distant metastases are an ominous development. Younger patients have a better prognosis, and the prognosis is better for individuals whose metastases concentrate radioiodine. Micronodular (diffuse) pulmonary metastases tend to concentrate radioiodine better and have a better prognosis than do macronodular lesions. As expected, patients with multiple-organ involvement (usually bone and lung) have a worse outcome than those with single-site involvement. In the total group only a small number of patients could be evaluated for the efficacy of ^{131}I therapy, and this therapy did not have a positive influence on survival. In contrast, other studies have reported that radioiodine prolonged life.[1023, 1024]

The treatment of individuals with well-differentiated carcinoma depends to a great extent on the risk-group. Papillary microcarcinomas (<1.0 cm) can be followed postoperatively by physical examination and serum Tg estimations. Levothyroxine should be given in quantities adequate to suppress TSH to just below the euthyroid range. Patients younger than 10 years of age with PTC or FTC are usually candidates for postoperative radioiodine studies and therapy, because pulmonary metastases are more common in this age group and may not be detectable with standard radiographs.[1025, 1026] Attempts are usually made to ablate these lesions, although it is difficult to prove that this prolongs survival. Adults with PTC larger than 1 cm in diameter, especially if it extends through the thyroid capsule into the surrounding tissues, and patients with widely invasive FTC or with unresectable or metastatic disease, are also candidates for radioiodine therapy. Men older than age 40 and women older than age 50 with PTC should also be considered for ablative radioiodine therapy.[997] Alternatively, radioiodine treatment may be considered for PTC patients at high-risk by AGES[948] or MACIS[971] criteria and for those FTC patients at high-risk by Mayo,[991] Lahey,[997] or Sloan-Kettering criteria.[998]

RADIOIODINE TREATMENT. The use of radioiodine in the treatment of thyroid carcinoma has a sound theoretical basis.[1027] Iodine organification is a thyroid-specific function, and ^{131}I is an effective agent for delivering radiation to the thyroid tissue with low spillover to other portions of the body. To be useful, however, ^{131}I must be concentrated by the tissue,[1028] which is usually not the case in euthyroid patients because most tumors are cold. For either primary or metastatic thyroid tumors to concentrate ^{131}I, function usually must be stimulated by TSH administration. However, since TSH is a less effective stimulator of neoplastic than of normal thyroid tissue, not all thyroid tumors can be treated with this modality. In practice, the patient is rendered hypothyroid to stimulate endogenous TSH secretion either by performing a near-total thyroidectomy at the initial operation or by the subsequent administration of radioiodine to patients with residual thyroid tissue. When sufficient normal thyroid tissue has been destroyed to cause hypothyroidism, the patient may receive a "tracer" dose of ^{131}I, usually 110 MBq (3 mCi) while hypothyroid, and dosimetric studies may be performed with the help of computerized data collection systems.[1029]

Despite the theoretical suitability of thyroid carcinoma for radioiodine treatment, it is not clear whether such therapy prolongs life. Various series report either no effect[1022, 1030] or an effect only in a subset of patients.[1023, 1031] However, the modality is commonly employed because of the paucity of long-term complications and acute adverse effects at least in the adult. This consideration does not apply when the accumulated ^{131}I dose exceeds 19 GBq (0.5 Ci), at which point the incidence of leukemia increases.

It is essential to establish that significant quantities of the administered dose will accumulate in the residual tumor lesions before employing this treatment.[1028, 1029] The effectiveness of radioiodine in the ablation of thyroid tissue can be appreciated from the fact that the deposition of 186 MBq (5 mCi) of ^{131}I in a typical 50-g Graves' disease thyroid (resulting in an average radioiodine content of approximately 3.7 MBq/g [100 μCi/g]) causes hypothyroidism in most patients and could theoretically provide the same radiation dose in a 1-g metastasis. Such an amount of ^{131}I is accumulated in a nodule with only 0.1% uptake after administration of 3.7 GBq (100 mCi) [131]I. This oversimplifies the situation because the hyperthyroid gland is more homogeneous than tumor metastases and because the mean residence time of ^{131}I may differ between the hyperthyroid and the carcinomatous follicular cell. Nonetheless the detection system for evaluating radioiodine uptake and the dose given should be sensitive enough to quantitate radioiodine uptakes in this range.

The full details of administering radioiodine therapy are beyond the scope of this chapter,[1027–1029] but several general guidelines should be followed.[1014] First, several months should elapse between surgery and radioiodine therapy if patients are exposed to povidone-iodine during the procedure. No contrast agents should be administered in the 6 wk before scanning, and, if required, myelography should be performed only with water-soluble dyes because residual iodine will be present for many years after administration of lipid-soluble agents such as Lipiodol (iodized oil). Patients should be given a low-iodine diet at least 1 wk before administration of radioiodine and should avoid all iodine-containing foods (especially seafoods), medicines, and antiseptics. After surgery, the patient can be given replacement doses of levothyroxine, but the drug should be discontinued about 4 wk before the planned uptake study, and liothyronine should be given at 25 μg bid or qd (depending on lean body mass) for 2 wk. Ten days to 2 weeks after stopping liothyronine and after documenting that the TSH level is elevated (preferably above 30 mU/L), the patient is given about 110 MBq (3 mCi) [131]I. This hormonal withdrawal approach allows controlled timing of the onset of hypothyroidism. In the future it is likely to be superseded by the administration of recombinant human TSH.[1032]

The mean residence time of radioiodine in metastases does not always increase with increasing TSH concentration because TSH may accelerate both iodine uptake and hormone turnover in the lesion.[1033] In general, total-body scans are performed 3 to 4 d after administration of radioiodine. Complete absence of uptake in the neck should lead to a determination of a urinary iodine-to-creatinine ratio to determine whether unsuspected iodine in the body is saturating iodine uptake in tumor tissue. Doses of radioiodine greater than 7.4 GBq (200 mCi) are rarely given outside specialized centers, and the calculated uptake in a metastasis should be sufficient to allow accumulation of a significant amount of radioiodine in the tumor tissue after administration of this amount or less. Furthermore, the upper limits of radioiodine deposition should not be exceeded; because of the possibility of radiation fibrosis and pneumonitis, less than 3 GBq (80 mCi) should be retained in the lungs at 48 h when diffuse metastases are present. The total-body retention should be less than 4.5 GBq (120 mCi) at 48 h, and less than 2 Gy (200 rad) should be delivered to whole blood by the radioiodine dose given.[1034] In adults such limitations are rarely an issue, but in children appropriate adjustments in the administered dosage should be made.

In general, radioiodine is more useful in the treatment of soft tissue metastases than of bone metastases, which are generally treated by at least 20 Gy (2000 rad) of external radiation. Anaplastic carcinoma rarely concentrates ^{131}I, and this modality is also not useful for patients with MTC or lymphoma. After ablation of the thyroid gland and radioiodine therapy, patients should be followed with assessments of serum Tg and serum TSH levels. The appearance of Tg in the serum of the patient without residual normal thyroid tissue (i.e., after radioiodine ablation) indicates the development of metastases and should lead to further evaluation for additional therapy.[1035] On the other hand, an undetectable serum Tg level during TSH suppression therapy does not indicate that tumor tissue is absent. The most sensitive use of the serum Tg determination is when the patient is no longer receiving thyroid hormone and the TSH level is elevated.[1036] Under these circumstances, the absence of serum Tg indicates that little functioning tumor tissue is present, although poorly differentiated thyroid carcinoma may not synthesize this protein.

Should ^{131}I treatments of asymptomatic patients with residual thyroid metastases be repeated? There is no conclusive evidence that such an approach prolongs life. An initial treatment with ^{131}I can be justified as an attempt to destroy small residual deposits of tumor, but it is difficult to demonstrate that additional radioiodine therapy is either effective or, when the total dose accumulates beyond 19 GBq (500 mCi), safe. Because TSH may stimulate thyroid tumor cells, repeated exposure of the tumor to TSH is undesirable. However, radioiodine therapy may be beneficial when unresectable lesions are symptomatic. When symptomatic lesions (e.g., bone and soft tissue) do not concentrate ^{131}I, palliative external radiation should be considered.[1037]

LONG-TERM FOLLOW-UP. Patients with PTC and FTC on TSH suppression are followed at 3-mo and then 6-mo intervals for the first 2 y after initial surgical or radioiodine treatment. If no abnormality appears, they are then followed on an annual basis. In the absence of specific indications, chest radiographs are performed each year, and the serum FT$_4$, TSH, and Tg levels are measured. Solitary recurrences in lymph nodes or in the neck can be detected by palpation and/or sonography, confirmed by FNA, and resected.[1038] Depending on the situation, such a recurrence may be an indication for re-evaluation for radioiodine treatment after resection of the lesion.[1039, 1040] Development of pulmonary nodules, particularly in a military pattern, should lead to an evaluation for ^{131}I treatment.[1025, 1026, 1041] Without such indications, it is probably not necessary to obtain regular ^{131}I scans or bone radiographs, especially if the serum Tg level is acceptably low (<0.5 μg/L) on suppressive therapy. Because more than 80% of recurrences of PTC appear in the first 10 y after treatment, this is the earliest time at which one may begin to feel secure about the success of the initial surgery.[948, 963] One may consider a reduction in levothyroxine at that time, particularly in women at risk for osteoporosis. The death rate from PTC in one large series was 5.5% at 20 y, and more than 70% of those who died did so within 10 y of the diagnosis.[948, 963] Only 1% of the patients with positive lymph nodes but no other metastatic lesion at the time of initial presentation died of PTC, again emphasizing the lack of correlation of lymph node metastases with prognosis.[948, 963, 994] The presence of a distant metastasis is an alarming sign and is an indication for more aggressive therapy with radioiodine, but only 30 to 60% of such tumors concentrate sufficient ^{131}I to allow this.[1022, 1030]

For patients with MTC the tumor marker for diagnosis and follow-up is the calcitonin level, both basal and stimulated. In young patients with an *RET* oncogene mutation, whose disease is treated at a very early premetastatic stage, the postoperative calcitonin level may return to normal, and peak levels after stimulation with either pentagastrin or combined pentagastrin-calcium may also be normal.[1010] In adults with sporadic MTC, who most often present with TNM stage III (node-positive) disease, postoperative calcitonin levels are rarely normal, and normal responsiveness to pentagastrin stimulation is very unusual.[1042] In general, basal and stimulated calcitonin levels correlate with MTC tumor mass,[1008, 1010] but many MTC patients who have surgery with curative intent and have no gross residual disease after initial surgery still have postoperative elevation in calcitonin levels without clinical or imaging evidence of persistent disease.[1008, 1042] Such a situation may in fact exist for several postoperative years, and slowly rising calcitonin levels may not necessarily imply a worsening prognosis, beyond that predicted by the presenting stage of disease.[1042]

A second major tumor marker for MTC is carcinoembryonic antigen (CEA). In general, CEA levels are higher in more malignant MTC, whereas the calcitonin level is higher in those with better differentiated tumors, leading some authorities to suggest that a rising CEA level postoperatively correlates better with the emergence of a potentially aggressive tumor recurrence.[1043, 1044]

REFERENCES

1. Ericson LE, Frederickson G. Phylogeny and ontogeny of the thyroid gland. In: Greer MA, ed. The Thyroid Gland: Comprehensive Endocrinology. New York: Raven, 1990: 1–35.
2. Fisher DA, Klein AH. Thyroid development and disorders of thyroid function in the newborn. N Engl J Med 1981; 304:702–712.
3. Burrow GN, Fisher DA, Larsen PR. Mechanisms of disease: maternal and fetal thyroid function. N Engl J Med 1994; 331:1072–1078.
4. Thorpe-Beeston JG, Nicolaides KH, Felton CV, et al. Maturation of the secretion of thyroid hormone and thyroid-stimulating hormone in the fetus. N Engl J Med 1991; 324:532–536.
5. Fisher DA. Thyroid system ontogeny in the sheep: a model for precocial mammalian species. N Engl J Med 1991; 324:532–536.
6. Roti E, Gnudi A, Braverman LE, et al. Human cord blood concentrations of thyrotropin, thyroglobulin, and iodothyronines after maternal administration of thyrotropin-releasing hormone. J Clin Endocrinol Metab 1981; 53:813–817.
7. Mansberger AR, Wei JP. Surgical embryology and anatomy of the thyroid and parathyroid glands. Surg Clin North Am 1993; 73:727–746.
8. Thorpe-Beeston JG, Nicolaides KH, McGregor AM. Fetal thyroid function. Thyroid 1992; 2:207–217.
9. Vulsma T, Gons MH, DeVijlder JMM. Maternal fetal transfer of thyroxine in congenital hypothyroidism due to a total organification defect of thyroid dysgenesis. N Engl J Med 1989; 321:13–16.
10. Ericson LE. Exocytosis and endocytosis in the thyroid follicle cell. Mol Cell Endocrinol 1981; 22:1–24.
11. Larsen PR. Ontogenesis of thyroid function, thyroid hormone and brain development, diagnosis and treatment of congenital hypothyroidism. In: DeGroot LJ, Larsen PR, Hennemann G, eds. The thyroid and Its Diseases. 6th ed. New York: Churchill Livingstone, 1996: 541–567.
12. deZegher F, Pernasetti F, Vanhole C, et al. The prenatal role of thyroid hormone evidenced by fetomaternal pit-1 deficiency. J Clin Endocrinol Metab 1995; 80:3127–3130.
13. Ekholm R, Bjorkman U. Structural and functional integration of the thyroid gland. In: Greer MA, ed. The Thyroid Gland: Comprehensive Endocrinology. New York: Raven, 1990: 37–81.
14. Pearse AGE. Genesis of the neuroendocrine system. In: Friesen SR, Thompson NW, eds. Surgical Endocrinology Clinical Syndromes. 2nd ed. New York: Lippincott-Raven, 1990: 15–21.
15. Glinoer D, De Nayer P, Bourdoux P, et al. Regulation of maternal thyroid during pregnancy. J Clin Endocrinol Metab 1990; 71:276–287.
16. Glinoer D, Leome M. Goiter and pregnancy: a new insight into an old problem. Thyroid 1992; 2:65–69.
17. Glinoer D, Delange F, Laboureur I, et al. Maternal and neonatal thyroid function at birth in an area of marginally low iodine intake. J Clin Endocrinol Metab 1992; 75:800–805.
18. Dai G, Carrasco L, Carrasco N. Cloning and characterization of the thyroid iodide transporter. Nature 1996; 379:458–460.
19. Roti E, Minelli R, Gardini E, et al. Impaired intrathyroidal iodine organification and iodine-induced hypothyroidism in euthyroid women with a previous episode of postpartum thyroiditis. J Clin Endocrinol Metab 1991; 73:958–963.
20. Gershengorn MC, Wolff J, Larsen PR. Thyroid-pituitary feedback during iodine repletion. J Clin Endocrinol 1976; 43:601–605.
21. Sinclair AJ, Lonigro R, Civitareale D, et al. The tissue-specific expression of the thyroglobulin gene requires interaction between thyroid-specific and ubiquitous factors. Eur J Biochem 1990; 193:311–318.
22. Civitareale D, Lonigro R, Sinclair AJ, et al. A thyroid-specific nuclear protein essential for tissue-specific expression of the thyroglobulin promoter. EMBO J 1989; 8:2537–2542.
23. Zannini M, Francis Lang H, Plachov D, et al. Pax-8, a paired domain-containing protein, binds to a sequence overlapping the recognition site of a homeodomain and activates transcription from two thyroid-specific promoters. Mol Cell Biol 1992; 12:4230–4241.
24. Javaux F, Bertaux F, Donda A, et al. Functional role of TTF-1 binding sites in bovine thyroglobulin promoter. FEBS Lett 1992; 300:222–226.
25. Magnusson B, Chazenbalk GD, Gestautas J, et al. Molecular cloning of the complementary deoxyribonucleic acid for human thyroid peroxidase. Mol Endocrinol 1987; 1:856–861.
26. Portmann L, Fitch FW, Havran E, et al. Characterization of the thyroid microsomal antigen, and its relationship to thyroid peroxidase, using monoclonal antibodies. J Clin Invest 1988; 81:1217–1224.

27. Libert F, Ruel J, Ludgate M, et al. Complete nucleotide sequence of the human thyroperoxidase-microsomal antigen cDNA. Nucleic Acids Res 1987; 15:6735.

28. Kimura S, Kotani T, McBride OW, et al. Human thyroid peroxidase: complete cDNA and protein sequence, chromosome mapping, and identification of two alternately spliced mRNAs. Proc Natl Acad Sci USA 1987; 84:5555–5559.

29. Bjorkman U, Ekholm R, Denef JF. Cytochemical localization of hydrogen peroxide in isolated thyroid follicles. J Ultrastruc Res 1981; 74:105–115.

30. Di Lauro R, Obici S, Condliffe D, et al. The sequence of 967 amino acids at the carboxyl-end of rat thyroglobulin: location and surroundings of two thyroxine-forming sites. Eur J Biochem 1985; 148:7–11.

31. Dunn JT, Anderson PC, Fox JW, et al. The sites of thyroid hormone formation in rabbit thyroglobulin. J Biol Chem 1987; 262:16948–16952.

32. Izumi M, Larsen PR. Triiodothyronine, thyroxine and iodine in purified thyroglobulin from patients with Graves' disease. J Clin Invest 1977; 59:1105–1112.

33. Larsen PR. Thyroidal triiodothyronine and thyroxine in Graves' disease: correlation with presurgical treatment, thyroid status and iodine content. J Clin Endocrinol Metab 1975; 41:1098–1104.

34. Erickson VJ, Cavalieri RR, Rosenberg LL. Thyroxine-5'-deiodinase of rat thyroid, but not that of liver, is dependent on thyrotropin. Endocrinology 1982; 111:434–440.

35. Ishii H, Inada M, Tanaka K, et al. Induction of outer and inner ring monodeiodinases in human thyroid gland by thyrotropin. J Clin Endocrinol Metab 1983; 57:500–505.

36. Laurberg P. Mechanisms governing the relative proportions of thyroxine and 3,5,3'-triiodothyronine in thyroid secretion. Metabolism 1984; 33:379–392.

37. Salvatore D, Tu H, Harney JW, et al. Type 2 iodothyronine deiodinase is highly expressed in human thyroid. J Clin Invest 1996; 98:962–968.

38. Toyoda N, Nishikawa M, Mori Y, et al. Thyrotropin and triiodothyronine regulate iodothyronine 5'-deiodinase messenger ribonucleic acid levels in FRTL-5 rat thyroid cells. Endocrinology 1992; 131:389–394.

39. Toyoda N, Nishikawa M, Horimoto M, et al. Graves' immunoglobulin G stimulates iodothyronine 5'-deiodinating activity in FRTL-5 rat thyroid cells. J Clin Endocrinol Metab 1990; 70:1506–1511.

40. Borges M, Ingbar SH, Silva JE. Iodothyronine deiodinase activities in FRTL5 cells: predominance of type I 5'-deiodinase. Endocrinology 1990; 126:3059–3068.

41. Abuid J, Larsen PR. Triiodothyronine and thyroxine in hyperthyroidism. J Clin Invest 1974; 54:201–208.

42. Izumi M, Larsen PR. Correlation of sequential changes in serum thyroglobulin, triiodothyronine, and thyroxine in patients with Graves' disease and subacute thyroiditis. Metabolism 1978; 27:449–460.

43. Spaulding SW, Burrow GN, Bermudez F, et al. The inhibitory effect of lithium on thyroid hormone release in both euthyroid and thyrotoxic patients. J Clin Endocrinol Metab 1972; 35:905–911.

44. Perrild H, Hegedus L, Baastrup PC, et al. Thyroid function and ultrasonically determined thyroid size in patients receiving long-term lithium treatment. Am J Psychiatry 1990; 147:1518–1521.

45. Bocchetta A, Bernardi A, Pedditzi M, et al. Thyroid abnormalities during lithium treatment. Acta Psychiatr Scand 1991; 83:193–198.

46. Vassart G, Dumont JE. The thyrotropin receptor and the regulation of thyrocyte function and growth. Endocr Rev 1992; 13:596–611.

47. Parmentier M, Libert F, Maenhaut C, et al. Molecular cloning of the thyrotropin receptor. Science 1989; 246:1620–1622.

48. Nagayama Y, Kaufman KD, Seto P, et al. Molecular cloning, sequence and functional expression of the cDNA for the human thyrotropin receptor. Biochem Biophys Res Commun 1989; 165:1184–1190.

49. Nagayama Y, Rapoport B. The thyrotropin receptor 25 years after its discovery: new insight after its molecular cloning. Mol Endocrinol 1992; 6:145–156.

50. Van Sande J, Lejeune C, Ludgate M, et al. Thyroid-stimulating immunoglobulins, like thyrotropin, activate both the cyclic AMP and PIP2 cascades in CHO cells expressing the TSH receptor. Mol Cell Endocrinol 1992; 88:R1–R5.

51. Brabant G, Bergmann P, Kirsch CM, et al. Early adaptation of thyrotropin and thyroglobulin secretion to experimentally decreased iodine supply in man. Metabolism 1992; 41:1093–1096.

52. Dumont JE, Lamy F, Roger P, et al. Physiological and pathological regulation of thyroid cell proliferation and differentiation by thyrotropin and other factors. Physiol Rev 1992; 72:667–697.

53. Christophe D, Gerard C, Juvenal G, et al. Identification of a cAMP-responsive region in thyroglobulin gene promoter. Mol Cell Endocrinol 1989; 64:5–18.

54. Martino E, Aghini-Lombardi F, Mariotti S, et al. Treatment of amiodarone-associated thyrotoxicosis by simultaneous administration of potassium perchlorate and methimazole. J Endocrinol Invest 1986; 9:201–207.

55. Drucker D, Eggo MD, Salit IE, et al. Ethionamide-induced goitrous hypothyroidism. Ann Intern Med 1984; 100:837–839.

56. Jubiz W, Nolan G. The effects of 6-mercaptopurine (6-MP) on the thyroid gland. Endocrinology 1974; 94:1583–1586.

57. Surks MI, Sievert R. Drugs and thyroid function. N Engl J Med 1995; 333:1688–1694.

58. Transbol I, Christiansen C, Bastrup PC, et al. Endocrine effects of lithium. I. Hypothyroidism, its prevalence in long-term patients. Acta Endocrinol 1978; 87:759–767.

59. Ermans AM. Goitrogens of vegetable origin as possible aetiological factors in endemic goiter. Ann Endocrinol 1981; 42:435–438.

60. Meyer JD, Gaitan E, Merino H, et al. Geologic implications in the distribution of endemic goiter in Colombia, South America. Int J Epidemiol 1978; 7:25–30.

61. Hennemann G, ed. Thyroid Hormone Metabolism. New York: Marcel Dekker, 1986.

62. Refetoff S. Inherited thyroxine-binding globulin abnormalities in man. Endocr Rev 1989; 10:275–293.

63. Bartalena L. Recent achievements in studies on thyroid hormone–binding proteins. Endocr Rev 1990; 11:47–64.

64. Bartalena L. Thyroid hormone–binding proteins: update 1994. Endocr Rev 1994; 13:140–142.

65. Flink IL, Bailey TJ, Gustafson TA, et al. Complete amino acid sequence of human thyroxine-binding globulin deduced from cloned DNA: close homology to the serine antiproteases. Proc Natl Acad Sci USA 1986; 83:7708–7712.

66. Ain KB, Mori Y, Refetoff S. Reduced clearance rate of thyroxine-binding globulin (TBG) with increased sialylation: a mechanism for estrogen-induced elevation of serum TBG concentration. J Clin Endocrinol Metab 1987; 65:689–696.

67. Ain KB, Refetoff S. Relationship of oligosaccharide modification to the cause of serum thyroxine-binding globulin excess. J Clin Endocrinol Metab 1988; 66:1037–1043.

68. Murata Y, Takamatsu J, Refetoff S. Inherited abnormality of thyroxine-binding globulin with no demonstratable thyroxine-binding activity and high serum levels of denatured thyroxine-binding globulin. N Engl J Med 1986; 314:694–699.

69. Garnick MB, Larsen PR. Acute deficiency of thyroxine-binding globulin during L-asparaginase therapy. N Engl J Med 1979; 301:252–253.

70. Bartalena L, Martino E, Antonelli A, et al. Effect of the antileukemic agent L-asparaginase on thyroxine-binding globulin and albumin synthesis in cultured human hepatoma (HEP G2) cells. Endocrinology 1985; 119:1185–1188.

71. Heidemann PH, Stubbe P, Beck W. Transient secondary hypothyroidism and thyroxine-binding globulin deficiency in leukemic children during polychemotherapy: an effect of L-asparaginase. Eur J Pediatr 1981; 136:291–295.

72. Blake CCF, Geisow MJ, Oatley SJ, et al. Structure of prealbumin: secondary, tertiary and quaternary interactions determined by Fourier refinement at 1.8 A. J Mol Biol 1978; 121:339.

73. Surks MI, Oppenheimer JH. Postoperative changes in the concentration of thyroxine-binding prealbumin and serum free thyroxine. J Clin Endocrinol 1964; 24:794–801.

74. Dickson PW, Aldred AR, Marley PD, et al. Rat choroid plexus specializes in the synthesis and secretion of transthyretin (prealbumin). J Biol Chem 1985; 261:3475.

75. MacDonald PN, Bok D, Ong DE. Localization of cellular retinol-binding protein and retinol-binding protein in cells comprising the blood-brain barrier of rat and human. Proc Natl Acad Sci USA 1990; 87:4265–4269.

76. Schreiber G, Aldred AR, Jaworowski A, et al. Thyroxine transport from blood to brain via transthyretin synthesis in choroid plexus. Am J Physiol 1990; 258:R338–R345.

77. Chanoine JP, Alex S, Fang SL, et al. Role of transthyretin in the transport of thyroxine from the blood to the choroid plexus, the cerebrospinal fluid and the brain. Endocrinology 1992; 130:933–938.

78. Episkopou V, Maeda S, Nishiguchi S, et al. Disruption of the transthyretin gene results in mice with depressed levels of plasma retinol and thyroid hormone. Proc Natl Acad Sci USA 1993; 90:2375–2379.

79. Refetoff S, Dwulet FE, Benson MD. Reduced affinity for thyroxine in two of three structural thyroxine-binding prealbumin variants associated with familial amyloidotic polyneuropathy. J Clin Endocrinol Metab 1986; 63:1432–1437.

80. Rosen HN, Moses AC, Murrell JR, et al. Thyroxine interactions with transthyretin: a comparison of 10 different naturally occurring human transthyretin variants. J Clin Endocrinol Metab 1993; 77:370–374.

81. Curtis AJ, Scrimshaw BJ, Topless DJ, et al. Thyroxine binding by human transthyretin variants: mutations at position 119, but not positions 54, increase thyroxine binding affinity. J Clin Endocrinol Metab 1994; 78:459–462.

82. Skiest D, Braverman LE, Emerson CH. Concentration of free thyroxine in serum of a patient with euthyroid hyperthyroxinemia secondary to increased thyroxin-binding prealbumin: results by various methods compared. Clin Chem 1986; 32:687–689.

83. Larsen PR, Atkinson AJ, Jr, Wellman HN, et al. The effect of diphenylhydantoin on thyroxine metabolism in man. J Clin Invest 1970; 49:1266–1279.

84. Larsen PR. Salicylate-induced increases in free triiodothyronine in human serum: evidence of inhibition of triiodothyronine binding to thyroxine-binding globulin and thyroxine-binding prealbumin. J Clin Invest 1972; 51:1125–1134.

85. McConnel RJ. Abnormal thyroid function test results in patients taking salsalate. JAMA 1992; 267:1242–1243.

86. Stockigt JR, Lim C-F, Barlow JW, et al. High concentrations of furosemide

inhibit serum binding of thyroxine. J Clin Endocrinol Metab 1984; 59:62–66.

87. Kurtz AB, Capper SJ, Clifford J, et al. The effect of fenclofenac on thyroid function. Clin Endocrinol 1981; 15:117–124.

88. Doctor R, Bos G, Krenning EP, et al. Inherited thyroxine excess: a serum abnormality due to an increased affinity for modified albumin. Clin Endocrinol 1981; 15:363–371.

89. Ruiz M, Rajatanavin R, Young RA, et al. Familial dysalbuminemic hyperthyroxinemia: a syndrome that can be confused with thyrotoxicosis. N Engl J Med 1981; 306:635–639.

90. Mendel CM, Cavalieri RR. Thyroxine distribution and metabolism in familial dysalbuminemic hyperthyroxinemia. J Clin Endocrinol Metab 1984; 59:499–504.

91. Sarne DH, Refetoff S. Normal cellular uptake of thyroxine from serum of patients with familial dysalbuminemic hyperthyroxinemia or elevated thyroxine-binding globulin. J Clin Endocrinol Metab 1988; 67:1166–1170.

92. Benvenga S. The 27-kilodalton thyroxine (T_4)-binding protein is human apolipoprotein A-I: identification of a 68-kilodalton high-density lipoprotein that binds T_4. Endocrinology 1989; 124:1265–1269.

93. Faber J, Waetjen I, Siersbaek-Nielson K. Free thyroxine measured in undiluted serum by dialysis and ultrafiltration: effects of non-thyroidal illness, and an acute load of salicylate or heparin. Clin Chim Acta 1993; 223:159–167.

94. Surks MI, Hupart KH, Pan C, et al. Normal free thyroxine in critical nonthyroidal illnesses measured by ultrafiltration of undilated serum and equilibrium dialysis. J Clin Endocrinol Metab 1988; 67:1031–1039.

95. Mendel CM. The free hormone hypothesis: a physiologically based mathematical model. Endocr Rev 1989; 10:232–274.

96. Pardridge WM. Plasma protein-mediated transport of steroid and thyroid hormones. Am J Physiol 1987; 252:E158–E164.

97. Mendel CM, Cavalieri RR, Gavin LA, et al. Thyroxine transport and distribution in Nagase analbuminemic rats. J Clin Invest 1989; 83:143–148.

98. Mendel CM, Weisiger RA, Cavalieri RR. Uptake of 3,5,3'-triiodothyronine by the perfused rat liver: return to the free hormone hypothesis. Endocrinology 1988; 123:1817–1824.

99. Mendel CM, Weisiger RA, Jones AL, et al. Thyroid hormone–binding proteins in plasma facilitate uniform distribution of thyroxine within tissues: a perfused rat liver study. Endocrinology 1987; 120:1742–1749.

100. Docter R, Krenning EP. Role of cellular transport systems in the regulation of thyroid hormone bioactivity. In: Greer MA, ed. The Thyroid Gland. New York: Raven, 1990: 233–254.

101. Docter R, Krenning EP, Bernard HF, et al. Active transport of iodothyronines into human cultured fibroblasts. J Clin Endocrinol Metab 1987; 65:624–628.

102. Cetanni M, Robbins J. Role of sodium in thyroid hormone uptake by rat skeletal muscle. J Clin Invest 1987; 80:1068–1072.

103. Hennemann G, Docter R. Plasma transport proteins and their role in tissue delivery of thyroid hormone. In: Greer MA, ed. The Thyroid Gland. New York: Raven, 1990: 221–231.

104. Topliss DJ, Kolliniatis E, Barlow JW, et al. Uptake of 3,5,3'-triiodothyronine by cultured rat hepatoma cells is inhibitable by nonbile acid cholephils, diphenylhydantoin, and nonsteroidal antiinflammatory drugs. Endocrinology 1989; 124:980–986.

105. Movius EG, Phyillaier MM, Robbins J. Phloretin inhibits cellular uptake and nuclear receptor binding of triiodothyronine in human hep G2 hepatocarcinoma cells. Endocrinology 1989; 124:1988–1997.

106. Lim C-F, Bernard BF, De Jong M, et al. A furan fatty acid and indoxyl sulfate are the putative inhibitors of thyroxine hepatocyte transport in uremia. J Clin Endocrinol Metab 1993; 76:318–324.

107. van der Heyden JTM, Docter R, van Toor H, et al. Effects of caloric deprivation on thyroid hormone tissue uptake and generation of low-T_3 syndrome. Am J Physiol 1986; 251:E156–E163..

108. Oppenheimer JH, Schwartz HL. Stereospecific transport to triiodothyronine from plasma to cytosol and from cytosol to nucleus in rat liver, kidney, brain and heart. J Clin Invest 1985; 75:147–154.

109. Braverman LE, Ingbar SH, Sterling K. Conversion of thyroxine (T_4) to triiodothyronine (T_3) in athyreotic subjects. J Clin Invest 1970; 49:855–864.

110. Larsen PR, Silva JE, Kaplan MM. Relationships between circulating and intracellular thyroid hormones: physiological and clinical implications. Endocr Rev 1981; 2:87–102.

111. Larsen PR, Berry MJ. Nutritional and hormonal regulation of thyroid hormone deiodinases. Annu Rev Nutr 1995; 15:323–352.

112. Berry MJ, Larsen PR. The molecular cloning of Type I iodothyronine deiodinase: new insights into thyroid hormone action. Thyroid Today 1991; 14:1–9.

113. Berry MJ, Larsen PR. Selenocysteine and the structure, function, and regulation of iodothyronine deiodination: update 1994. Endocr Rev 1994; 3:265–269.

114. Salvatore D, Low SC, Berry MJ, et al. Type 3 iodothyronine deiodinase: cloning, in vitro expression, and functional analysis of the placental selenoenzyme. J Clin Invest 1995; 95:2421–2430.

115. Mandel SJ, Berry MJ, Kieffer JD, et al. Cloning and in vitro expression of the human selenoprotein, type I iodothyronine deiodinase. J Clin Endocrinol Metab 1992; 75:1133–1139.

116. St. Germain DL, Schwartzman RA, Croteau W, et al. A thyroid hormone–regulated gene in Xenopus laevis encodes a type III iodothyronine 5-deiodinase. Proc Natl Acad Sci USA 1994; 91:7767–7771.

117. Davey JC, Becker KB, Schneider MJ, et al. Cloning of a cDNA for the type II iodothyronine deiodinase. J Biol Chem 1995; 270:26786–26789.

118. Salvatore D, Bartha T, Harney JW, et al. Molecular biological and biochemical characterization of the human Type 2 selenodeiodinase. Endocrinology 1996; 137:3308–3315.

119. Croteau W, Davey JC, Galton VA, et al. Cloning of the mammalian Type II iodothyronine deiodinase: a selenoprotein differentially expressed and regulated in human and rat brain and other tissues. J Clin Invest 1996; 98:405–417.

120. Otten MH, Mol JA, Visser TJ. Sulfation preceding deiodination of iodothyronines in rat hepatocytes. Science 1983; 221:81–83.

121. Visser TJ, Kaptein E, Terpstra OT, et al. Deiodination of thyroid hormone by human liver. J Clin Endocrinol Metab 1988; 67: 17–24.

122. Berry MJ, Larsen PR. The role of selenium in thyroid hormone action. Endocr Rev 1992; 13:207–219.

123. Larsen PR, Berry MJ. Nutritional and hormonal regulation of thyroid hormone deiodinases. Annu Rev Nutr 1995; 15:323–352.

124. Berry MJ, Kieffer JD, Harney JW, et al. Selenocysteine confers the biochemical properties of the type I iodothyronine deiodinase. J Biol Chem 1991; 266:14155–14158.

125. Berry MJ, Kieffer JD, Larsen PR. Evidence that cysteine, not selenocysteine, is in the catalytic site of type II iodothyronine deiodinase. Endocrinology 1991; 129: 550–552.

126. Berry MJ, Maia AL, Kieffer JD, et al. Substitution of cysteine for selenocysteine in type I iodothyronine deiodinase reduces the catalytic efficiency of the protein but enhances its translation. Endocrinology 1992; 131:1848–1852.

127. Croteau W, Whittemore SL, Schneider MJ, et al. Cloning and expression of a cDNA for a mammalian Type III iodothyronine deiodinase. J Biol Chem 1995; 270:16569–16575.

128. Böck A, Forchhammer K, Heider J, et al. C. Selenoprotein synthesis: an expansion of the genetic code. Trends Biochem Sci 1991; 16:463–467.

129. Böck A, Forchhammer K, Heider J, et al. Selenocysteine: the 21st amino acid. Mol Microbiol 1991; 5:515–520.

130. Heider J, Baron C, Böck A. Coding from a distance: dissection of the mRNA determinants required for the incorporation of selenocysteine into protein. EMBO J 1992; 11:3759–3766.

131. Berry MJ, Banu L, Chen Y, et al. Recognition of UGA as a selenocysteine codon in type I deiodinase requires sequences in the 3' untranslated region. Nature 1991; 353:273–276.

132. Berry MJ, Banu L, Harney JW, et al. Functional characterization of the eukaryotic SECIS elements which direct selenocysteine insertion at UGA codons. EMBO J 1993; 12:3315–3322.

133. Berry MJ, Harney JW, Ohama T, et al. Selenocysteine insertion or termination: factors affecting UGA codon fate and complementary anticodon:codon mutations. Nucleic Acids Res 1994; 22:3753–3759.

134. Low SC, Berry MJ. Knowing when not to stop: selenocysteine incorporation in eukaryotes. Trends Biochem Sci 1996; 21:203–208.

135. Berry MJ, Larsen PR. Recognition of UGA as a selenocysteine codon in eukaryotes: a review of recent progress. Biochem Soc Trans 1993; 21:827–832.

136. Low SC, Berry MJ. Knowing when not to stop: selenocysteine incorporation in eukaryotes. Trends Biochem Sci 1996; 21:203–208.

137. Beckett GJ, Beddows SE, Morrice PC, et al. Inhibition of hepatic deiodination of thyroxine is caused by selenium deficiency in rats. Biochem J 1987; 248:443–447.

138. Arthur JR, Nicol F, Beckett GJ. Hepatic iodothyronine 5'-deiodinase: the role of selenium. Biochem J 1990; 272:537–540.

139. Contempre B, Dumont JE, Bebe N, et al. Effect of selenium supplementation in hypothyroid subjects of an iodine and selenium deficient area: the possible danger of indiscriminate supplementation of iodine-deficient subjects with selenium. J Clin Endocrinol Metab 1991; 73:213–215.

140. Vanderpas JB, Contempre B, Duale NL, et al. Iodine and selenium deficiency associated with cretinism in northern Zaire. Am J Clin Nutr 1990; 52:1087–1093.

141. Crantz FR, Silva JE, Larsen PR. Analysis of the sources and quantity of 3,5,3'-triiodothyronine specifically bound to nuclear receptors in rat cerebral cortex and cerebellum. Endocrinology 1982; 110:367–375.

142. Meinhold H, Campos-Barros A, Walzog B, et al. Effects of selenium and iodine deficiency on Type I, Type II and Type III iodothyronine deiodinases and circulating thyroid hormones in the rat. Exp Clin Endocrinol 1993; 101:87–93.

143. Behne D, Hilmert H, Scheid S, et al. Evidence for specific selenium target tissues and new biologically important selenoproteins. Biochim Biophys Acta 1988; 966:12–21.

144. Geffner DL, Azukizawa M, Hershman JM. Propylthiouracil blocks extrathyroidal conversion of thyroxine to triiodothyronine and augments thyrotropin secretion in man. J Clin Invest 1975; 55:224–229.

145. Saberi M, Sterling FH, Utiger RD. Reduction in extrathyroidal triiodothyronine production by propylthiouracil in man. J Clin Invest 1975; 55:218–223.

146. LoPresti JS, Eigen A, Kaptein E, et al. Alterations in 3,3',5'-triiodothyronine metabolism in response to propylthiouracil, dexamethasone, and thyroxine administration in man. J Clin Invest 1989; 84:1650–1656.

147. van der Heijden JTM, Krenning EP, van Toor H, et al. Three-compartmental analysis of effects of D-propranolol on thyroid hormone kinetics. Am J Physiol 1988; 255:E80–E86.

148. Hennemann G, Vos RA, de Johng M, et al. Decreased peripheral 3,5,3'-triiodothyronine (T₃) production from thyroxine (T₄): a syndrome of impaired thyroid hormone activation due to transport inhibition of T₄ into T₃-producing tissues. J Clin Endocrinol Metab 1993; 77:1431–1435.

149. Toyoda N, Zavacki AM, Maia AL, et al. A novel retinoid X receptor-independent thyroid hormone response element is present in the human Type I deiodinase gene. Mol Cell Biol 1995; 15:5100–5112.

150. Moreno M, Berry MJ, Horst C, et al. Activation and inactivation of thyroid hormone by type I iodothyronine deiodinase. FEBS Lett 1994; 344:143–146.

151. Mol JA, Visser TJ. Rapid and selective inner ring deiodination of thyronine sulfate by rat liver deiodinase. Endocrinology 1985; 117:8–12.

152. Rooda SJE, Kaptein E, Rutgers M, et al. Increased plasma 3,5,3'-triiodothyronine sulfate in rats with inhibited Type I iodothyronine deiodinase activity, as measured by radioimmunoassay. Endocrinology 1989; 124:740–745.

153. Rooda SJE, Kaptein E, Visser TJ. Serum triiodothyronine sulfate in man measured by radioimmunoassay. J Clin Endocrinol Metab 1989; 69:552–556.

154. Behr M, Loos U. A point mutation (Ala²²⁹ to Thr) in the hinge domain of the c-erbAβ thyroid hormone receptor gene in a family with generalized thyroid hormone resistance. Mol Endocrinol 1992; 6:1119–1126.

155. Chopra IJ, Wu SY, Chua Teco GN, et al. A radioimmunoassay for measurement of 3,5,3'-triiodothyronine sulfate: studies in thyroidal and nonthyroidal disease, pregnancy and neonatal life. J Clin Endocrinol Metab 1992; 75:189–194.

156. Wu S-Y, Huang W-S, Polk D, et al. The development of a radioimmunoassay for reverse triiodothyronine sulfate in human serum and amniotic fluid. J Clin Endocrinol Metab 1993; 76:1625–1630.

157. Takeda K, Sakurai A, DeGroot LJ, et al. Recessive inheritance of thyroid hormone resistance caused by complete deletion of the protein-coding region of the thyroid hormone receptor-β gene. J Clin Endocrinol Metab 1992; 74:49–55.

158. Koenig RJ, Warne RL, Brent GA, et al. Isolation of a cDNA clone encoding a biologically active thyroid hormone receptor. Proc Natl Acad Sci 1988; 85:5031–5035.

159. Rutgers M, Bonthuis F, deHerder WW, et al. Accumulation of plasma triiodothyronine sulfate in rats treated with propylthiouracil. J Clin Invest 1987; 80:758–762.

160. Santini F, Hurd RE, Chopra IJ. A study of metabolism of deaminated and sulfoconjugated iodothyronines by rat placental iodothyronine 5-monodeiodinase. Endocrinology 1992; 131:1689–1694.

161. LoPresti JS, Mizuno L, Nimalysuria A, et al. Characteristics of 3,5,3'-triiodothyronine sulfate metabolism in euthyroid man. J Clin Endocrinol Metab 1991; 73:703–709.

162. Laurberg P, Boye N. Propylthiouracil, ipodate, dexamethasone and periods of fasting induce different variations in serum rT₃ in dogs. Metabolism 1984; 33:323–325.

163. Leonard JL, Kaplan MM, Visser TJ, et al. Cerebral cortex responds rapidly to thyroid hormones. Science 1981; 214:571–573.

164. Visser TJ, Kaplan MM, Leonard JL, et al. Evidence for two pathways of iodothyronine 5'-deiodination in rat pituitary that differ in kinetics, propylthiouracil sensitivity, and response to hypothyroidism. J Clin Invest 1983; 71:992–1002.

165. Leonard JL, Silva JE, Kaplan MM, et al. Acute post-transcriptional regulation of cerebrocortical and pituitary iodothyroinine 5'-deiodinase by thyroid hormone. Endocrinology 1984; 114:998–1004.

166. Leonard JL, Visser TJ. Biochemistry of deiodination. In: Hennemann, G, ed. Thyroid Hormone Metabolism. New York: Marcel Dekker, 1986: 189–229.

167. Silva JE, Larsen PR. Pituitary nuclear 3,5,3'-triiodothyronine and thyrotropin secretion: an explanation for the effect of thyroxine. Science 1977; 198:617.

168. Larsen PR, Dick TE, Markovitz MM, et al. Inhibition of intrapituitary thyroxine to 3,5,3'-triiodothyronine conversion prevents the acute suppression of thyrotropin release by thyroxine in hypothyroid rats. J Clin Invest 1979; 64:117–128.

169. Riesco G, Taurog A, Larsen PR, et al. Acute and chronic responses to iodine deficiency in rats. In: Robbins J, Braverman LE, eds. Proceedings of the Seventh International Thyroid Conference. New York: American Elsevier, 1976: 490–492.

170. Bigos ST, Ridgway EC, Kourides IA, et al. Spectrum of pituitary alterations with mild and severe thyroid impairment. J Clin Endocrinol Metab 1978; 46:317.

171. Larsen PR. Thyroid-pituitary interactions: feedback regulation of thyrotropin secretion by thyroid hormones. N Engl J Med 1982; 306:23.

172. Silva JE. Effects of iodine and iodine-containing compounds on thyroid function. Med Clin North Am 1985; 69:881–898.

173. Koopdonk-Kool JM, deVijlder JJM, Veenboer GJM, et al. Type II and Type III deiodinase activity in human placenta as a function of gestational age. J Clin Endocrinol Metab 1996; 81:2154–2158.

174. Campos-Barros A, Hoell T, Musa A, et al. Phenolic and tyrosyl ring iodothyronine deiodination and thyroid hormone concentrations in the human central nervous system. J Clin Endocrinol Metab 1996; 81:2179–2185.

175. Engler D, Burger AG. The deiodination of the iodothyronines and of their derivatives in man. Endocr Rev 1984; 5:151–184.

176. Gardner DF, Kaplan MM, Stanley CA, et al. Effect of triiodothyronine replacement on the metabolic and pituitary responses to starvation. N Engl J Med 1979; 3000:579–584.

177. New England Congenital Hypothyroid Collaborative. Correlation of cognitive test scores and adequacy of treatment in adolescents with congenital hypothyroidism. J Pediatr 1994; 124:383–387.

178. Smith PJ, Surks MI. Multiple effects of 5,5'-diphenylhydantoin on the thyroid hormone system. Endocr Rev 1984; 5:514–524.

179. Liewendahl K, Tikanoja S, Helenius T, et al. Free thyroxin and free triiodothyronine as measured by equilibrium dialysis and analog radioimmunoassay in serum of patients taking phenytoin and carbamazepine. Clin Chem 1985; 31:1993–1996.

180. Isojarvi JI, Pakarinen AJ, Myllyla VV. Thyroid function with antiepileptic drugs. Epilepsia 1992; 33:142–148.

181. Faber J, Lumholtz IB, Kirkegaard C, et al. The effects of phenytoin on the extrathyroidal turnover of thyroxine, 3,5,3'-triiodothyronine, 3,3',5'-triiodothyronine, and 3',5'-diiodothyronine in man. J Clin Endocrinol Metab 1985; 61:1093–1099.

182. Chin W, Schussler GC. Decreased serum free thyroxine concentration in patients treated with diphenylhydantoin. J Clin Endocrinol 1968; 28:181–186.

183. Wartofsky L, Burman KD. Alterations in thyroid function in patients with systemic illness: the "euthyroid sick syndrome." Endocr Rev 1982; 3:164.

184. Wiersinga WM, Trip MD. Amiodarone and thyroid hormone metabolism. Postgrad Med J 1986; 62:909–914.

185. Phillips DI, Lazarus JH, Butland BK. The influence of pregnancy and reproductive span on the occurrence of autoimmune thyroiditis. Clin Endocrinol 1990; 32:301–306.

186. Figge J, Dluhy RG. Amiodarone-induced elevation of thyroid-stimulating hormone in patients receiving levothyroxine for primary hypothyroidism. Ann Intern Med 1990; 113:553–555.

187. Wartofsky L. The low T₃ or "sick euthyroid syndrome": update 1994. Endocr Rev 1994; 3:248–251.

188. Brent GA, Hershman JM. Thyroxine therapy in patients with severe nonthyroidal illness and low serum thyroxine concentrations. J Clin Endocrinol Metab 1986; 63:1.

189. Kahn BB, Weintraub BD, Csako G, et al. Factitious elevation of thyrotropin in a new ultrasensitive assay: implications for the use of monoclonal antibodies in "sandwich" immunoassay. J Clin Endocrinol Metab 1988; 66:526–533.

190. Eng SJ, LoPresti JS, Liang H, et al. Dynamics of T₄ and T₃ deiodination in man: dominant role of extrahepatic metabolism. Thyroid 1994; 4(Suppl 1):S-47.

191. Lechan RM, Wu P, Jackson IMD, et al. Thyrotropin-releasing hormone precursor: characterization in rat brain. Science 1986; 231:159–161.

192. Yamada M, Wondisford FE, Radovick S, et al. Assignment of human preprothyrotropin-releasing hormone (TRH) gene to chromosome 3. Somat Cell Mol Genet 1991; 17:97–100.

193. Lee SL, Stewart K, Goodman RH. Structure of the gene encoding rat thyrothropin-releasing hormone. J Biol Chem 1988; 263:16604–16609.

194. Yamada M, Radovick S, Wondisford FE, et al. Cloning and structure of human genomic DNA and hypothalamic cDNA encoding human preprothyrotropin-releasing hormone. Mol Endocrinol 1990; 4:551–556.

195. Bulant M, Roussel JP, Astier H, et al. Processing of thyrotropin-releasing hormone prohormone (pro-TRH) generates a biologically active peptide, prepro-TRH-(160–169), which regulates TRH-induced thyrotropin secretion. Proc Natl Acad Sci 1990; 87:4439–4443.

196. Engler D, Scanlon M, Jackson IMD. Thyrotropin-releasing hormone in the systemic circulation of the neonatal rat is derived from the pancreas and other extraneural tissues. J Clin Invest 1981; 67:800–808.

197. Gkonos PJ, Tavianini MA, Liu CC, et al. Thyrotropin-releasing hormone gene expression in normal thyroid parafollicular cells. Mol Endocrinol 1989; 3:2101–2109.

198. Hollenberg AN, Monden T, Flynn TR, et al. The human thyrotropin-releasing hormone gene is regulated by thyroid hormone through two distinct classes of negative thyroid hormone response elements. Mol Endocrinol 1995; 9:540–550.

199. Segerson TP, Kauer J, Wolfe H, et al. Thyroid hormone regulates TRH biosynthesis in the paraventricular nucleus of the rat hypothalamus. Science 1987; 238:78–80.

200. Dyess EM, Segerson TP, Liposits Z, et al. Triiodothyronine exerts direct cell-specific regulation of thyrotropin-releasing hormone gene expression in the hypothalamic paraventricular nucleus. Endocrinology 1988; 123:2291–2297.

201. Kakucska I, Rand W, Lechan RM. Thyrotropin-releasing hormone (TRH) gene expression in the hypothalamic paraventricular nucleus is dependent upon feedback regulation by both triiodothyronine and thyroxine. Endocrinology 1992; 130:2845–2850.

202. Straub RE, Frech GC, Joho RH, et al. Expression cloning of a cDNA encoding the mouse pituitary thyrotropin-releasing hormone receptor. Proc Natl Acad Sci 1990; 87:9514–9518.

203. Zhao D, Yang J, Jones KE, et al. Molecular cloning of a complementary

deoxyribonucleic acid encoding the thyrotropin-releasing receptor and regulation of its messenger ribonucleic acid in rat GH cells. Endocrinology 1992; 130:3529–3536.

204. Brenner-Gati L, Gershengorn MC. Effects of thyrotropin-releasing hormone on phosphoinositides and cytoplasmic free calcium in thyrotropic pituitary cells. Endocrinology 1986; 118:163–169.

205. Kolesnick RN, Gershengorn MC. Thyrotropin-releasing hormone and the pituitary. Am J Med 1985; 79:729–739.

206. Carr FE, Shupnik MA, Burnside J, et al. Thyrotropin-releasing hormone stimulates the activity of the rat thyrotropin β-subunit gene promoter transfected into pituitary cells. Mol Endocrinol 1989; 3:717.

207. Carr FE, Galloway RJ, Reid AH, et al. Thyrotropin-releasing hormone regulation of thyrotropin β-subunit gene expression involves intracellular calcium and protein kinase C. Biochemistry 1991; 30:3721–3728.

208. Gard TG, Bernstein B, Larsen PR. Studies on the mechanism of 3,5,3′-triiodothyronine-induced suppression of secretagogue-induced thyrotropin release *in vitro*. Endocrinology 1981; 1:44.

209. Koenig RJ, Senator D, Larsen PR. Phorbol esters as probes of the regulation of thyrotropin secretion. Biochem Biophys Res Commun 1984; 125:353–359.

210. Schrey MP, Larsen PR. Evidence for a possible role of Ca^{++} in the 3,3,3′-triiodothyronine inhibition of thyrotropin-releasing hormone-induced secretion of thyrotropin by rat anterior pituitary *in vitro*. Endocrinology 1981; 108:1690.

211. Chin WW, Carr FE, Burnside J, et al. Thyroid hormone regulation of thyrotropin gene expression. Recent Prog Horm Res 1993; 48:393–414.

212. Shupnik MA, Ridgway EC, Chin WW. Molecular biology of thyrotropin. Endocr Rev 1989; 10:459–475.

213. Hayashizaki Y, Hiraoka Y, Endo Y, et al. Thyroid-stimulating hormone (TSH) deficiency caused by a single base substitution in the CAGYC region of the β-subunit. EMBO J 1989; 8:2291–2296.

214. Hayashizaki Y, Hiraoka Y, Tatsumi K. Deoxyribonucleic acid analyses of five families with familial inherited thyroid stimulating hormone deficiency. Clin Endocrinol Metab 1990; 71:792.

215. Shupnik MA, Ardisson LJ, Meskell MJ, et al. Triiodothyronine (T_3) regulation of thyrotropin subunit gene transcription is proportional to T_3 nuclear receptor occupancy. Endocrinology 1986; 118:367.

216. Magner JA. Thyroid-stimulating hormone: biosynthesis, cell biology and bioactivity. Endocr Rev 1990; 11:354.

217. Beck-Peccoz P, Amir S, Menezes-Ferreira MM, et al. Decreased receptor binding of biologically inactive thyrotropin in central hypothyroidism: effect of treatment with thyrotropin-releasing hormone. N Engl J Med 1985; 312:1085.

218. Menezes-Ferreira MM, Petrick PA, Weintraub BD. Regulation of thyrotropin (TSH) bioactivity by TSH-releasing hormone and thyroid hormone. Endocrinology 1986; 118:2125.

219. Faglia G, Bitensky L, Pinchera A, et al. Thyrotropin secretion in patients with central hypothyroidism: evidence for reduced biological activity of immunoreactive thyrotropin. J Clin Endocrinol Metab 1979; 48:989.

220. Taylor R, Weintraub BD. Altered thyrotropin (TSH) carbohydrate structures in hypothalamic hypothyroidism created by paraventricular nuclear lesions are corrected by *in vivo* TSH-releasing hormone administration. Endocrinology 1989; 125:2198–2203.

221. Kourides IA, Re RN, Weintraub BD, et al. Metabolic clearance and secretion rates of subunits of human thyrotropin. J Clin Invest 1977; 59:508.

222. Brabant G, Frank K, Ranft U. Physiological regulation of circadian and pulsatile thyrotropin secretion in normal man and woman. J Clin Endocrinol Metab 1990; 70:403.

223. Romijn JA, Wiersinga WM. Decreased nocturnal surge of of thyrotropin in non-thyroidal illness. J Clin Endocrinol Metab 1990; 70:35.

224. Romijn JA, Adriaanse R, Brabant G, et al. Pulsatile secretion of thyrotropin during fasting: a decrease of thyrotropin pulse amplitude. J Clin Endocrinol Metab 1990; 70:1631–1636.

225. Bartalena L, Placidi GF, Martino E, et al. Nocturnal serum thyrotropin (TSH) surge and the TSH response to TSH-releasing hormone: dissociated behavior in untreated depression. J Clin Endocrinol Metab 1990; 71:650–655.

226. Seth J, Kellett HA, Caldwell G, et al. A sensitive immunoradiometric assay for serum thyroid-stimulating hormone: a replacement for the thyrotropin-releasing hormone test? Br J Med 1984; 289:1334–1336.

227. Burmeister LA, Goumaaz MO, Mariash CN, et al. Levothyroxine dose requirements for thyrotropin suppression in the treatment of differentiated thyroid cancer. J Clin Endocrinol Metab 1992; 75:344–350.

228. Sawin CT, Hershman JM, Chopra IJ. The comparative effect of T_4 to T_3 on the TSH response to TRH in young adult men. J Clin Endocrinol Metab 1977; 44:273–278.

229. Weeke J, Hansen AAP, Lundbaek K. Inhibition by somatostatin of basal levels of serum thyrotropin (TSH) in normal men. J Clin Endocrinol Metab 1975; 41:168.

230. Weeke J, Christensen SE, Hansen AP, et al. Somatostatin and the 24th levels of serum TSH, T_3, T_4 and reverse T_3 in normals, diabetics and patients treated for myxedema. Acta Endocrinol 1980; 94:30.

231. Comi RJ, Gesundheit N, Murray L. Response of thyrotropin-secreting pituitary adenomas to a long-acting somatostatin analogue. N Engl J Med 1987; 317:12–17.

232. Beck-Peccoz P, Mariotti S, Guillausseau PJ. Treatment of hyperthyroidism due to inappropriate secretion of thyrotropin with somatostatin analogue SMS 201-995. J Clin Endocrinol Metab 1989; 68:208–214.

233. Yaoita Y, Shi YB, Brown DD. *Xenopus laevis* α and β thyroid hormone receptors. Proc Natl Acad Sci 1990; 87:7090–7094.

234. Pourmand M, Rodriguez-Arnao MD, Weightman DR, et al. A novel agent for the investigation of anterior pituitary function and control in man. Clin Endocrinol 1980; 12:211.

235. Brabant G, Brabant A, Ranft U. Circadian and pulsatile thyrotropin secretion in euthyroid man under the influence of thyroid hormone and glucocorticoid administration. J Clin Endocrinol Metab 1987; 65:83.

236. Rogers EB, Hosler BA, Gudas LJ. Specific expression of a retinoic acid–regulated, zinc-finger gene, Rex-1, in preimplantation embryos, trophoblast and spermatocyte. Development 1991; 113:815–824.

237. Dubuis JM, Dayer JM, Siegrist-Kaiser CA, et al. Human recombinant interleukin-1β decreases plasma thyroid hormone and thyroid-stimulating hormone levels in rats. Endocrinology 1988; 123:2175–2181.

238. Van der Poll T, Romijn JA, Wiersinga WM, et al. Tumor necrosis factor: a putative mediator of the sick euthyroid syndrome in man. J Clin Endocrinol Metab 1990; 71:1567–1572.

239. van Haasteren GA, van der Meer MJ, Hermus AR, et al. Different effects of continuous infusion of interleukin-1 and interleukin-6 on the hypothalamic-hypophysial-thyroid axis. Endocrinology 1994; 135:1336–1345.

240. Koenig JI, Snow K, Clark BD, et al. Intrinsic pituitary interleukin-1 beta is induced by bacterial lipopolysaccharide. Endocrinology 1990; 126:3053.

241. Wolff J. Physiological aspects of iodide excess in relation to radiation protection. J Mol Med 1980; 4:151–165.

242. Wolff I. Iodide goiter and the pharmacologic effects of excess iodide. Am J Med 1969; 47:101–124.

243. Wolff J, Chaikoff IL. Plasma inorganic iodide as a homeostatic regulator of thyroid function. J Biol Chem 1948; 174:555.

244. Michalkiewicz M, Huffman JM. Alterations in thyroid blood flow induced by varying levles of iodine intake in the rat. Endocrinology 1989; 125:54–60.

245. Abrams GM, Larsen PR. Triiodothyronine and thyroxine in the serum and thyroid glands of iodine-deficient rats. J Clin Invest 1973; 52:2522.

246. Fukuda H, Yasuda N, Greer MA, et al. Changes in plasma thyroxine, triiodothyronine, and TSH during adaptation toiodine deficiency in the rat. Endocrinology 1975; 97:307.

247. Riesco G, Taurog A, Larsen PR, et al. Acute and chronic responses to iodine deficiency in rats. Endocrinology 1977; 100:303–313.

248. Okamura K, Taurog A, Krulich L. Hypothyroidism in severely iodine-deficient rats. Endocrinology 1981; 109:464–468.

249. Pazos-Moura CC, Moura EG, Egberto GM, et al. Effect of iodine deficiency and cold exposure on thyroxine 5′-deiodinase activity in various rat tissues. Am J Physiol 1991; 260:E175–E182.

250. Chopra IJ, Hershman JM, Hornabrook RW. Serum thyroid hormone and thyrotropin levels in subjects from endemic goiter regions of New Guinea. J Clin Endocrinol Metab 1975; 40:326.

251. Boyages SC. Clinical review 49: iodine deficiency disorders. J Clin Endocrinol Metab 1993; 77:587–591.

252. Boyages SC, Halpern JP. Endemic cretinism: toward a unifying hypothesis. Thyroid 1993; 3:59–69.

253. Wolff J. Congenital goiter with defective iodide transport. Endocrinol Rev 1983; 4:240.

254. Koenig RJ, Leonard JL, Senator D, et al. Regulation of thyroxine 5′-deiodinase activity by T_3 in cultured rat anterior pituitary cells. Endocrinology 1984; 115:324–329.

255. Burrow GN. Thyroid function and hyperfunction during gestation. Endocr Rev 1993; 14:194–202.

256. Burrow GN. Thyroid status in normal pregnancy. J Clin Endocrinol Metab 1990; 71:274–275.

257. Guillaume J, Schussler GC, Goldman J. Components of the total serum thyroid hormone concentrations during pregnancy: high free thyroxine and blunted thyrotropin (TSH) response to TSH-releasing hormone in the first trimester. J Clin Endocrinol Metab 1985; 60:678–684.

258. Weeke J, Dybkjaer L, Granlie K, et al. A longitudinal study of serum TSH, and total and free iodothyronines during normal pregnancy. Acta Endocrinol 1982; 101:531–537.

259. Pekonen F, Alfthan H, Stenman UH, et al. Human chorionic gonadotropin (hCG) and thyroid function in early human pregnancy: circadian variation and evidence for intrinsic thyrotropic activity of hCG. J Clin Endocrinol Metab 1988; 66:853–856.

260. Hershman JM, Lee HY, Sugawara M, et al. Human chorionic gonadotropin stimulates iodide uptake, adenylate cyclase, and deoxribonucleic acid synthesis in cultured rat thyroid cells. J Clin Endocrinol Metab 1988; 67:74–79.

261. Kimura M, Amino N, Tamaki H, et al. Physiologic thyroid activation in normal early pregnancy is induced by circulating hCG. Obstet Gynecol 1990; 75:775–778.

262. Ballabio M, Poshyachinda M, Ekins RP. Pregnancy-induced changes in thyroid function: role of human chorionic gonadotropin as putative regulator of maternal thyroid. J Clin Endocrinol Metab 1991; 73:824–831.

263. Glinoer D, De Nayer P, Robyn C, et al. Serum levels of intact human chorionic gonadotropin (HCG) and its free alpha and beta subunits, in relation to maternal thyroid stimulation during normal pregnancy. J Endocrinol Invest 1993; 16:881–888.

264. Yoshikawa N, Nishikawa M, Horimoto M, et al. Thyroid-stimulating activity in sera of normal pregnant women. J Clin Endocrinol Metab 1989; 69:891–895.

265. Norman RJ, Green-Thompson RW, Jialal I, et al. Hyperthyroidism in gestational trophoblastic neoplasia. Clin Endocrinol 1981; 15:395–401.

266. Berghout A, Endert E, Wiersinga WM, et al. The application of an immunoradiometric assay of plasma thyrotropin (TSH-IRMA) in molar pregnancy. J Endocrinol Investi 1988; 11:15–19.

267. Nagataki S, Mizuno M, Sakamoto S, et al. Thyroid function in molar pregnancy. J Clin Endocrinol Metab 1977; 44:254–263.

268. Goodwin TM, Montoro M, Mestman JH. Transient hyperthyroidism and hyperemesis gravidarum: clinical aspects. Am J Obstet Gynecol 1992; 167:648–652.

269. Lao TT, Chin KH, Chang AMZ. The outcome of hyperemetic pregnancies complicated by transient hyperthyroidism. Aust NZ J Obstet Gynaecol 1987; 27:99–101.

270. Wilson R, McKillop JH, MacLean M, et al. Thyroid function tests are rarely abnormal in patients with severe hyperemesis gravidarum. Clin Endocrinol 1992; 37:331–334.

271. Mandel SJ, Larsen PR, Seely EW. Increased need for thyroxine during pregnancy in women with primary hypothyroidism. N Engl J Med 1990; 323:91–95.

272. Kaplan MM. Monitoring thyroxine treatment during pregnancy. Thyroid 1992; 2:147–152.

273. Roti E, Fang SL, Green K, et al. Human placenta is an active site of thyroxine and 3,3′,5-triiodothyronine tyrosyl ring deiodination. J Clin Endocrinol Metab 1981; 53:498–501.

274. Roti E, Gnudi A, Braverman LE. The placental transport, synthesis and metabolism of hormones and drugs which affect thyroid function. Endocr Rev 1983; 4:131–149.

275. El-Zaheri MM, Vagenakis AG, Hinerfeld L, et al. Maternal thyroid function is the major determinant of amniotic fluid 3,3′,5′-triiodothyronine in the rat. J Clin Invest 1981; 67:1126–1133.

276. Dowling JT, Appleton WG, Nicoloff JT. Thyroxine turnover during human pregnancy. J Clin Endocrinol Metab 1964; 27:1749–1750.

277. Burman KD, Read J, Dimond RC, et al. Measurements of 3,3′,5′-triiodo-thyronine (reverse T_3), 3,3′-L-diiodothyronine, T_3, and T_4 in human amniotic fluid and in cord and maternal serum. J Clin Endocrinol Metab 1976; 43:1351–1359.

278. Thorpe-Beeston JG, Nicolaides KH, Snijders RJ, et al. Thyroid function in small-for-gestational-age fetuses. Obstet Gynecol 1991; 77:701–706.

279. Houstek J, Vizek K, Stanislav P, et al. Type II iodothyronine 5′-deiodinase and uncoupling protein in brown adipose tissue of human newborns. J Clin Endocrinol Metab 1993; 77:382–387.

280. Mariotti S, Franceschi C, Cossarizza A, et al. The aging thyroid. Endocr Rev 1995; 16:686–715.

281. Robuschi G, Safran M, Braverman LE, et al. Hypothyroidism in the elderly. Endocr Rev 1987; 8:142–153.

282. Duick DS, Wahner HW. Thyroid axis in patients with Cushing's syndrome. Arch Intern Med 1979; 139:767.

283. Nicoloff JT, Fisher DA, Appleman MD, Jr. The role of glucocorticoids in the regulation of thyroid function in man. J Clin Invest 1970; 49:1922.

284. Williams DE, Chopra IJ, Orgiazzi J, et al. Acute effects of corticosteroids on thyroid activity in Graves' disease. J Clin Endocrinol Metab 1975; 41:354–361.

285. Duick DS, Warren DW, Nicoloff JT, et al. Effect of single-dose dexamethasone on the concentration of serum triiodothyronine in man. J Clin Endocrinol Metab 1974; 39:1151.

286. Farah DA, Boag D, Moran F, et al. High concentrations of thyroid-stimulating hormone in untreated glucocorticoid deficiency: indications of primary hypothyroidism? Br Med J 1982; 172:285.

287. Topliss DJ, White EL, Stockigt JR. Significance of thyrotropin excess in untreated primary adrenal insufficiency. J Clin Endocrinol Metab 1980; 50:52–56.

288. Glinoer D, Soto MF, Bourdoux P, et al. Pregnancy in patients with mild thyroid abnormalities: maternal and neonatal repercussions. J Clin Endocrinol Metab 1991; 73:421–427.

289. Faglia G, Beck-Peccoz P, Ferrari C, et al. Enhanced plasma thyrotropin response to thyrotrophin-releasing hormone following oestradiol administration in man. Clin Endocrinol 1974; 2:207.

290. Gershengorn MC, Marcus-Samuels BE, Geras E. Estrogens increase the number of thyrotropin-releasing hormone receptors on mammotropic cells in culture. Endocrinology 1979; 105:171.

291. Arafah BM. Decreased levothyroxine requirement in women with hypothyroidism during androgen therapy for breast cancer. Ann Intern Med 1994; 121:247–251.

292. Porter BA, Refetoff S, Rosenfeld RL, et al. Abnormal thyroxine metabolism in hyposomatotrophic dwarfism and inhibition of responsiveness to TRH during GH therapy. Pediatrics 1975; 51:668.

293. Lippe BM, Van Herle AJ, LaFranchi SH, et al. Reversible hypothyroidism in growth-hormone deficient children treated with growth hormone. J Clin Endocrinol Metab 1975; 40:143.

294. Laurberg P, Jakobsen PE, Hoeck HC, et al. Growth hormone and thyroid function: is secondary thyroid failure underdiagnosed in growth hormone–deficient patients? Thyroidology 1994; 6:73–79.

295. Jorgensen JOL, Pedersen SA, Laurberg P, et al. Effects of growth hormone therapy on thyroid function of growth hormone–deficient adults with and without concomitant thyroxine-substituted central hypothyroidism. J Clin Endocrinol Metab 1989; 69:1127–1132.

296. Radovick S, Nations M, Du Y, et al. A mutation in the POU-homeodomain of Pit-1 responsible for combined pituitary hormone deficiency. Science 1992; 257:1115–1118.

297. Pfaffle RW, DiMattia GE, Parks JS, et al. Mutation of the POU-specific domain of Pit-1 and hypopituitarism without pituitary hypoplasia. Science 1992; 257:1118–1121.

298. Tatsumi K, Miyai K, Notomi T, et al. Cretinism with combined hormone deficiency caused by a mutation in the PIT1 gene. Nat Genet 1992; 1:56–58.

299. Smals AG, Ross HA, Kloppenborg PWC. Seasonal variation in serum T_3 and T_4 levels in man. J Clin Endocrinol Metab 1977; 44:998–1001.

300. Balsam A, Ingbar SH. The influence of fasting, diabetes and several pharmacological agents on the pathways of thyroxine metabolism in rat liver. J Clin Invest 1978; 62:415–424.

301. Portnay GI, O'Brien JT, Bush J, et al. The effect of starvation on the concentration and binding of thyroxine and triiodothyronine in serum and on the response to TRH. J Clin Endocrinol Metab 1974; 39:191.

302. Chopra IJ, Smith SR. Circulating thyroid hormones and thyrotropin in adult patients with protein-calorie malnutrition. J Clin Endocrinol Metab 1975; 40:221.

303. Spaulding SW, Chopra IJ, Sherwin RS, et al. Effects of caloric restriction and dietary composition on serum T_3 and rT_3 in man. J Clin Endocrinol Metab 1976; 42:197–200.

304. Hugues J, Burger AG, Pekary AE, et al. Rapid adaptations of serum thyrotropin, triiodothyronine and reverse triiodothyronine levels to short-term starvation and refeeding. Acta Endocrinol 1984; 105:194.

305. Borst GC, Osburne RC, O'Brian JT, et al. Fasting decreases thyrotropin responsiveness to thyrotropin-releasing hormone: a potential cause of misinterpretation of thyroid function tests in the critically ill. J Clin Endocrinol Metab 1983; 57:380.

306. Carlson HE, Drenick EJ, Chopra IJ, et al. Alterations in basal and TRH-stimulated serum levels in thyrotropin, prolactin, and thyroid hormones in starved obese men. J Clin Endocrinol Metab 1977; 45:707–713.

307. Chopra IJ, Solomon DH, Chopra U, et al. Pathways of metabolism of thyroid hormones. Recent Prog Horm Res 1978; 34:521–657.

308. Danforth E, Jr, Horton ES, O'Connell M, et al. Dietary-induced alterations in thyroid hormone metabolism during overnutrition. J Clin Invest 1979; 64:1336–1347.

309. Berry MJ, Grieco D, Taylor BA, et al. Physiological and genetic analyses of inbred mouse strains with a type I iodothyronine 5′ deiodinase deficiency. J Clin Invest 1993; 92:1517–1528.

310. Maia AL, Kieffer JD, Harney JW, et al. Effect of 3,5,3′-triiodothyronine (T_3) administration on Dio1 gene expression and T_3 metabolism in normal and Type 1 deiodinase-deficient mice. Endocrinology 1995; 136:4842–4849.

311. Kaplan MM, Tatro JB, Breibart R, et al. Comparison of thyroxine and 3,3′,5′-triiodothyronine metabolism in rat kidney and liver homogenates. Metabolism 1979; 28:1139–1146.

312. Balsam A, Ingbar SH. Observations on the factors that control the generation of triiodothyronine from thyroxine in rat liver and the nature of the effect induced by fasting. J Clin Invest 1979; 63:1145.

313. Harris ARC, Fang SL, Hinerfeld L, et al. The role of sulfhydryl groups on the impaired hepatic 3′,3,5-triiodothyronine generation from thyroxine in the hypothyroid, starved, fetal and neonatal rodent. J Clin Invest 1979; 63:516–524.

314. Kaplan MM, Larsen PR, Crantz FR, et al. Prevalence of abnormal thyroid function test results in patients with acute medical illnesses. Am J Med 1982; 72:9–16.

315. Faber J, Kirkegaard C, Rasmussen B, et al. Pituitary-thyroid axis in critical illness. J Clin Endocrinol Metab 1987; 65:315.

316. Nelson JC, Weiss RM. The effect of serum dilution on free thyroxine (T_4) concentrations in the low T_4 syndrome of nonthyroidal illness. J Clin Endocrinol Metab 1985; 61:239–246.

317. Brent GA, Hershman JM, Braunstein GD. Patients with severe nonthyroidal illness and serum thyrotropin concentrations in the hypothyroid range. Am J Med 1986; 81:463–466.

318. Spencer CA, LoPresti JS, Patel A, et al. Applications of a new chemiluminometric thyrotroin assay to subnormal measurement. J Clin Endocrinol Metab 1990; 70:453–460.

319. Spencer CA, Schwarzbein D, Guttler RB, et al. Thyrotropin (TSH)-releasing hormone stimulation test responses employing third- and fourth-generation TSH assays. J Clin Endocrinol Metab 1993; 76:494–498.

320. Ramos-Gabatin A, Jacobson JM, Young RL. In vivo comparison of levothyroxine preparations. JAMA 1982; 247:203–205.

321. Bartalena L, Martino E, Brandi LS. Lack of nocturnal serum thyrotropin surge after surgery. J Clin Endocrinol Metab 1990; 70:293.

322. Custro N, Scafidi V, Gallo S, et al. Deficient pulsatile thyrotropin secretion in the low-thyroid-hormone state of severe non-thyroidal illness. Eur J Endocrinol 1994; 130:132–136.

323. Becker RA, Vaughan GM, Ziegler MD, et al. Hypermetabolic low triiodothyronine syndrome of burn injury. Crit Care Med 1982; 10:870–875.

324. Bacci V, Schussler GC, Kaplan TB. The relationship between serum triiodothyronine and thyrotropin during systemic illness. J Clin Endocrinol Metab 1982; 54:1229.

325. Hamblin PS, Dyer SA, Mohr VS, et al. Relationship between thyrotropin and thyroxine changes during the recovery from severe hypothyroxinemia of critical illness. J Clin Endocrinol Metab 1986; 62:717–722.

326. Gavin LA, Rosenthal M, Cavalieri RR. The diagnostic dilemma of isolated hyperthyroxinemia in acute illness. JAMA 1979; 242:251–253.

327. Birkhauser M, Burer T, Busset R, et al. Diagnosis of hyperthyroidism when serum thyroxine alone is raised. Lancet 1977; 2:53–56.

328. Burman KD, Borst GC, Eil C. Euthyroid hyperthyroxinemia. Ann Intern Med 1983; 98:366–378.

329. Bouillon R, Naesens M, Van Assche FA, et al. Thyroid function in patients with hyperemesis gravidarum. Am J Obstet Gynecol 1982; 143:922–926.

330. Spratt DI, Pont A, Miller MB, et al. Hyperthyroxinemia in patients with acute psychiatric disorders. Am J Med 1982; 73:41–48.

331. Morley JE, Shafer RB. Thyroid function screening in new psychiatric admissions. Arch Intern Med 1982; 142:592–593.

332. Chopra IJ, Solomon DH, Huang TS. Serum thyrotropin in hospitalized psychiatric patients: evidence for hyperthyrotropinemia as measured by an ultrasensitive thyrotropin assay. Metabolism 1990; 39:538–543.

333. O'Shanick GD, Ellinwood EH, Jr. Persistent elevation of thyroid-stimulating hormone in women with bipolar affective disorder. Am J Psychiatry 1982; 139:513–514.

334. Pittman JA, Jr, Dailey GE, III, Beschi RJ. Changing normal values for thyroidal radioiodine uptake. N Eng J Med 1969; 280:1431–1441.

335. Hayes AA, Akre CM, Gorman CA. Iodine-131 treatment of Graves' disease using modified early iodine-131 uptake measurements in therapy dose calculations. J Nucl Med 1990; 31:519–522.

335a. Medeiros-Neto G, Kim PS, Vono J, et al. Congenital hypothyroid goiter with deficient thyroglobulin. J Clin Invest 1996; 98:2838–2844.

336. Mariotti S, Martino E, Cupini C, et al. Low serum thyroblobulin as a clue to the diagnosis of thyrotoxicosis factitia. N Engl J Med 1982; 307:410–412.

337. Spencer CA, Lai-Rosenfeld AO, Guttler RB, et al. Thyrotropin secretion in thyrotoxic and thyroxine-treated patient: assessment by a sensitive immunoenzymometric assay. J Clin Endocrinol Metab 1986; 63:349–355.

338. Spencer C, Eigen A, Shen D, et al. Specificity of sensitive assays of thyrotropin (TSH) used to screen for thyroid disease in hospitalized patients. Clin Chem 1987; 33:1391–1396.

339. Laurberg P. Persistent problems with the specificity of immunometric TSH assays. Thyroid 1993; 3:279–283.

340. Larsen PR, Alexander NM, Chopra IJ, et al. Revised nomenclature for tests of thyroid hormones and thyroid-related proteins in serum. J Clin Endocrinol Metab 1987; 64:1089–1092.

341. Nicoloff JT, Spencer CA. Clinical review 12: the use and misuse of the sensitive thyrotropin assays. J Clin Endocrinol Metab 1990; 71:553–558.

342. Kourides IA, Ridgway EC, Weintraub BD, et al. Thyrotropin-induced hyperthyroidism: use of alpha and beta subunit levels to identify patients with pituitary tumors. J Clin Endocrinol Metab 1977; 45:534.

343. Kuzuya N, Kinji I, Ishibashi M. Endocrine and immunohistochemical studies on thyrotropin (TSH)-secreting pituitary adenomas: responses of TSH, α-subunit, and growth hormone to hypothalamic releasing hormones and their distribution in adenoma cells. J Clin Endocrinol Metab 1990; 71:1103–1111.

344. Gesundheit N, Petrick PA, Nissim M, et al. Thyrotropin-secreting pituitary adenomas: clinical and biochemical heterogeneity. Ann Intern Med 1989; 11:827–835.

345. Weintraub BD, Gershengorn MC, Kourides IA, et al. Inappropriate secretion of thyroid-stimulating hormone. Ann Intern Med 1981; 95:339.

346. Cooper DS, Halpern R, Wood LC, et al. L-Thyroxine therapy in subclinical hypothyroidism: a double-blind, placebo-controlled trial. Ann Intern Med 1984; 101:18–24.

347. Blunt S, Woods CA, Joplin GF, et al. The role of a highly sensitive amplified enzyme immunoassay for thyrotrophin in the evaluation of thyrotroph function in hypopituitary patients. Clin Endocrinol 1988; 29:387–393.

348. Faglia G, Beck-Peccoz P, Piscitelli G, et al. Inappropriate secretion of thyrotropin by the pituitary. Horm Res 1987; 26:79–99.

349. Smallridge RC. Thyrotropin-secreting pituitary tumors. Endocrinol Metab Clin North Am 1987; 16:765–792.

350. Nystrom E, Caidahl K, Fager G, et al. A double-blind cross-over 12-month study of L-thyroxine treatment of women with "subclinical" hypothyroidism. Clin Endocrinol 1988; 29:63–76.

351. Petersen VB, McGregor AM, Belchetz PE, et al. The secretion of thyrotrophin with impaired biological activity in patients with hypothalamic-pituitary disease. Clin Endocrinol 1978; 8:397.

352. Ross DS, Daniels GH, Goveia D. The use and limitations of a chemiluminescent thyrotropin assay as a single thyroid function test in an outpatient endocrine clinic. J Clin Endocrinol Metab 1990; 71:764–769.

353. Franklyn JA, Black EG, Betteridge J, et al. Comparison of second- and third-generation methods for measurement of serum thyrotopin in patients with overt hyperthyroidism, patients receiving thyroxine therapy, and those with nonthyroidal illness. J Clin Endocrinol Metab 1994; 78:1368–1371.

354. Kaptein EM, Spencer CA, Kamiel MB, et al. Prolonged dopamine administration and thyroid hormone economy in normal and critically ill subjects. J Clin Endocrinol Metab 1980; 51:387.

355. Ross DS, Ardisson LJ, Meskell MJ. Measurement of thyrotropin in clinical and subclinical hyperthyroidism using a new chemiluminescent assay. J Clin Endorcinol Metab 1989; 64:684–688.

356. Larsen PR. Triiodothyronine: a review of recent studies of the physiology and pathophysiology of this hormone in man. Metabolism 1972; 21:1073–1091.

357. Wu SY, Huang WS, Polk D, et al. Identification of thyroxine sulfate (T_4S) in human serum and amniotic fluid by a novel T_4S radioimmunoassay. Thyroid 1992; 2:101–105.

358. Nelson JC, Weiss RM, Wilcox RB. Underestimates of serum free thyroxine (T_4) concentrations by free T_4 immunoassays. J Clin Endocrinol Metab 1994; 79:76–79.

359. Nelson JC, Wilcox RB, Pandian MR. Dependence of free thyroxine estimates obtained with equilibrium tracer dialysis on the concentration of thyroxine-binding globulin. Clin Chem 1992; 38:1294–1300.

360. Nelson JC, Nayak SS, Wilcox RB. Variable underestimates by serum free thyroxine (T_4) immunoassays of free T_4 concentrations in simple solutions. J Clin Endocrinol Metab 1994; 79:1373–1375.

361. Faix JD, Rosen HN, Velazquez FR. Indirect estimation of thyroid hormone–binding proteins to calculate free thyroxine index: comparison of nonisotopic methods that use labeled thyroxine ("T-uptake"). Clin Chem 1995; 41:41–47.

362. Nagaya T, Madison LD, Jameson JL. Thyroid hormone receptor mutants that cause resistance to thyroid hormone: evidence for receptor competition for DNA sequences in target genes. J Biol Chem 1992; 267:13014–13019.

363. Glass CK, Holloway JM, Devary OV, et al. The thyroid hormone receptor binds with opposite transcriptional effects to a common sequence motif in thyroid hormone and estrogen response elements. Cell 1988; 54:313–323.

364. Mendel CM, Frost PH, Kunitake ST, et al. Mechanism of the heparin-induced increase in the concentration of free thyroxine in plasma. J Clin Endocrinol Metab 1987; 65:1259–1264.

365. Davies P, Franklyn JA, Daykin J, et al. The significance of TSH values measured in a sensitive assay in the follow-up of hyperthyroid patients treated with radioiodine. J Clin Endocrinol Metab 1992; 74:1189–1194.

366. Toft AD, Irvine WJ, Hunter WM, et al. Anomalous plasma TSH levels in patients developing hypothyroidism in the early months after ^{131}I therapy for thyrotoxicosis. J Clin Endocrinol Metab 1974; 39:607.

367. Sawin CT, Geller A, Wolf PA, et al. Low serum thyrotropin concentrations as a risk factor for atrial fibrillation in older persons. N Engl J Med 1994; 331:1249–1252.

368. Sawin CT, Geller A, Hershman JM, et al. The aging thyroid. JAMA 1989; 261:2653–2655.

369. Ree RN, Kourides AA, Ridgway EC, et al. The effect of glucocorticoid administration on human pituitary secretion of thyrotropin and prolactin. J Clin Endocrinol Metab 1976; 43:338.

370. Kaptein EM. Thyroid hormone metabolism and thyroid diseases in chronic renal failure. Endocr Rev 1996; 17:45–63.

371. Weiss RE, Refetoff S. Thyroid hormone resistance. Annu Rev Med 1992; 43:363–375.

372. Refetoff S. Resistance to thyroid hormone: an historical overview. Thyroid 1994; 4:345–349.

373. Refetoff S, Weiss RE, Usala SJ. The syndromes of resistance to thyroid hormone. Endocr Rev 1993; 14:348–399.

374. Refetoff S, Weiss RE, Wing JR, et al. Resistance to thyroid hormone in subjects from two unrelated families is associated with a point mutation in the thyroid hormone receptor β gene resulting in the replacment of the normal proline 453 with serine. Thyroid 1994; 4:249–253.

375. Jameson JL. Mechanisms by which thyroid hormone receptor mutations cause clinical syndromes of resistance to thyroid hormone. Thyroid 1994; 4:485–491.

376. Wiersinga WM, Endert E, Trip MD, et al. Immunoradiometric assay of thyrotropin in plasma: its value in predicting response to thyroliberin stimulation and assessing thyroid function in amiodarone-treated patients. Clin Chem 1986; 32:433–436.

377. Trip MD, Wiersinga W, Plomp TA. Incidence, predictability, and pathogenesis of amiodarone-induced thyrotoxicosis and hypothyroidism. Am J Med 1991; 91:507–511.

378. Borowski GD, Garofano CD, Rose LI, et al. Effect of long-term amiodarone therapy on thyroid hormone levels and thyroid function. Am J Med 1985; 78:443–450.

379. Norman MF, Lavin TN. Antagonism of thyroid hormone action by amiodarone in rat pituitary tumor cells. J Clin Invest 1989; 83:306–313.

380. Cooper DS, Daniels GH, Ladenson PW, et al. Hyperthyroxinemia in patients treated with high-dose propranolol. Am J Med 1982; 73:867–871.

381. Perrild H, Molhom Hansen J, Skovsted L, et al. Different effects of propranolol, alprenolol, sotalol, atenolol, and metoprolol on serum T_3 and serum rT_3 in hyperthyroidism. Clin Endocrinol 1983; 18:139–142.

382. LeBoff MS, Kaplan MM, Silva JE, et al. Bioavailability of thyroid hormones from oral replacement preparations. Metabolism 1982; 31:900–905.

383. Rees-Jones RW, Larsen PR. Triiodothyronine and thyroxine content of desiccated thyroid tablets. Metabolism 1977; 26:1213–1218.

384. Rees-Jones RW, Rolla AR, Larsen PR. Hormone content of thyroid replacement preparations. JAMA 1980; 243:549–550.

385. DeLuca F, Arrigo T, Pandullo E, et al. Changes in thyroid function tests induced by 2-month carbamazepine treatment in L-thyroxine-substituted hypothyroid children. Euro J Pediatr 1986; 145:77–79.

386. Isley WL. Effect of rifampin therapy on thyroid function tests in a hypothyroid patient on replacement L-thyroxine. Ann Intern Med 1987; 107:517–518.

387. Klein I, Mantell P, Parker M, et al. Resolution of abnormal muscle enzyme studies in hypothyroidism. Am J Med Sci 1980; 279:159.

388. Hickman PE, Silvester W, McLellan GH, et al. Cardiac enzyme changes in myxedema coma. Clin Chem 1987; 33:622.

389. Becker C. Hypothyroidism and atherosclerotic heart disease: pathogenesis, medical management, and the role of coronary artery bypass surgery. Endocr Rev 1985; 6:432–440.

390. Tunbridge WMG, Evered DC, Hall R, et al. Lipid profiles and cardiovascular disease in the Whickham area with particular reference to thyroid failure. Clin Endocrinol 1977; 7:495–508.

391. Abrams JJ, Grundy SM, Ginsberg H. Metabolism of plasma triglycerides in hypothyroidism and hyperthyroidism in man. J Lipid Res 1981; 22:307–353.

392. Abrams JJ, Grundy SM. Cholesterol metabolism in hypothyroidism and hyperthyroidism in man. J Lipid Res 1981; 22:323–338.

393. Thompson GR, Soutar AK, Spengel FA, et al. Defects of receptor-mediated low-density lipoprotein catabolism in homozygous familial hypercholesterolemia and hypothyroidism *in vivo*. Proc Natl Acad Sci 1981; 78:2591–2595.

394. Polikar R, Burger AG, Scherrer U, et al. The thyroid and heart. Circulation 1993; 87:1435–1441.

395. Crowley WF, Jr, Ridgeway EC, Bough EW, et al. Noninvasive evaluation of cardiac function in hypothyroidism. N Engl J Med 1977; 296:1–6.

396. Landenson PW, Goldenheim PD, Ridgway EC. Rapid pituitary and peripheral tissue responses to intravenous L-triiodothyronine in hypothyroidism. J Clin Endocrinol Metab 1983; 56:1252–1259.

397. Schneider AB, Ikekubo K. Sequential serum thyroglobulin determinations, ^{131}I scans, and ^{131}I uptakes after triiodothyronine withdrawal in patients with thyroid cancer. J Clin Endocrinol Metab 1981; 53:1199–1206.

398. McLachlan SM, Feldt-Rasmussen U, Young ET, et al. IgG subclass distribution of thyroid autoantibodies: a "fingerprint" of an individual's response to thyroglobulin and thyroid microsomal antigen. Clin Endocrinol 1987; 26:335–346.

399. Vanderpump MPJ, Tunbridge WMG, French JM, et al. The incidence of thyroid disorders in the community: a twenty-year follow-up of the Whickham survey. Clin Endocrinol 1995; 43:55–68.

400. Wood LC, Ingbar SH. Hypothyroidism as a late sequela in patients with Graves' disease treated with antithyroid agents. J Clin Invest 1979; 64:1429–1436.

401. Baker J, Fosso CK. Immunological aspects of cancers arising from thyroid follicular cells. Endocr Rev 1993; 14:729–746.

402. Phillips D, Prentice L, Upadhyaya M, et al. Autosomal dominant inheritance of autoantibodies to thyroid peroxidase and thyroglobulin: studies in families not selected for autoimmune thyroid disease. J Clin Endocrinol Metab 1991; 72:973–975.

403. Stagnaro-Green A, Roman SH, Cobin RH, et al. A prospective study of lymphocyte-initiated immunosuppression in normal pregnancy: evidence of a T-cell etiology for postpartum thyroid dysfunction. J Clin Endocrinol Metabolism 1992; 74:645–653.

404. Stagnaro-Green A, Roman SH, Cobin RH, et al. Detection of at-risk pregnancy by means of highly sensitive assays for thyroid autoantibodies. JAMA 1990; 264:1422–1426.

405. Rees Smith B, McLachlan SM, Furmaniak J. Autoantibodies to the thyrotropin receptor. Endocr Rev 1988; 9:106–121.

406. Janson A, Karlsson FA, Micha-Johansson G, et al. Effects of stimulatory and inhibitory thyrotropin receptor antibodies on lipolysis in infant adipocytes. J Clin Endocrinol Metab 1995; 80:1712–1716.

407. Kruger T, Smith LR, Harbour DV, et al. Thyrotropin: an endogenous regulator of the in vitro immune response. J Immunol 1989; 142:744–747.

408. Parmentier M, Libert F, Maenhaut C, et al. Molecular cloning of the TSH receptor. Science 1989; 246:1620–1622.

409. Misrahi M, Loosfelt H, Atger M, et al. Cloning, sequencing, and expression of human TSH receptor. Biochem Biophys Res Commun 1990; 166:394–403.

410. Nagayama Y, Kaufman KD, Seto P, et al. Molecular cloning, sequence and functional expression of the cDNA for the human thyrotropin receptor. Biochem Biophys Res Commun 1989; 165:1184–1190.

411. Libert F, Lefort A, Gerard C, et al. Cloning, sequencing and expression of the human TSH receptor: evidence for binding of autoantibodies. Biochem Biophys Res Commun 1989; 165:1250–1255.

412. Gross B, Misrahi M, Sar S, et al. Composite structure of the human thyrotropin receptor gene. Biochem Biophys Res Commun 1991; 177:679–687.

413. Libert F, Passage E, Lefort A, et al. Localization of human thyrotropin receptor gene to chromosome 14q31 by in situ hybridization. Cytogenet Cell Genet 1991; 54:82–83.

414. Graves PN, Tomer Y, Davies TF. Cloning and sequencing of a 1.3 kb variant of human thyrotropin receptor mRNA lacking the transmembrane domain. Biochem Biophys Res Commun 1992; 187:1135–1143.

415. Loosfelt H, Pichon C, Jolivet A, et al. Two-subunit structure of the human thyrotropin receptor. Proc Natl Acad Sci USA 1992; 89:3765–3769.

416. Rees Smith B. Characterisation of long-acting thyroid stimulator gamma globulin binding protein. Biochem Biophys Acta 1971; 229:649–662.

417. Adams DD. The presence of an abnormal thyroid-stimulating hormone in the serum of some thyrotoxic patients. J Clin Endocrinol Metab 1958; 18:699–712.

418. Adams DD, Purves HD. Abnormal responses in the assay of thyrotropin. Proc Univ Otago Med Sch 1956; 34:11–12.

419. Kraiem Z, Lahat N, Glaser B, et al. Thyrotropin receptor blocking antibodies: incidence, characterization and in-vitro synthesis. Clin Endocrinol 1987; 27:409–421.

420. Davies TF, Platzer M, Schwartz A, et al. Functionality of thyroid-stimulating antibodies assessed by cryopreserved human thyroid cell bioassay. J Clin Endocrinol Metab 1983; 57:1021–1027.

421. Zakarija M, McKenzie JM, Banovac K. Clinical significance of assay of thyroid-stimulating antibody in Graves' disease. Ann Intern Med 1980; 93:28–32.

422. Nishiyama H, Sodd VJ, Berke RA, et al. Evaluation of clinical value of ^{123}I and ^{131}I in thyroid disease. J Nucl Med 1974; 15:261–265.

423. Paltiel HJ, Summerville DA, Treves ST. Iodine-123 scintigraphy in the evaluation of pediatric thyroid disorders: a ten-year experience. Pediatr Radiol 1992; 22:251–256.

424. Price DC. Radioisotopic evaluation of the thyroid and the parathyroids. Radiol Clin North Am 1993; 31:991–1015.

425. Hoffer PB, Goltschalk A, Refetoff S. Thyroid scanning technics: the old and the new. Curr Probl Radiol 1972; 2:1–26.

426. Rapoport B, Block MB, Hofer PB, et al. Depletion of thyroid iodine during subacute thyroiditis. J Clin Endocrinol Metab 1973; 36:610–611.

427. James EM, Charboneau JW, Hay ID. The thyroid, In: Rumack CM, Wilson SR, Charboneau JW, eds. Diagnostic Ultrasound. St. Louis: Mosby, Year-Book, 1991: 507–523.

428. Reading CC, Gorman CA. Thyroid imaging techniques. Clin Lab Med 1993; 13:711–724.

429. James EM, Charboneau JW. High-frequency (10MHz) thyroid ultrasonography. Semin Ultrasound CT MR 1985; 6:294–309.

430. Simeone JF, Daniels GH, Hall DA, et al. Sonography in the follow-up of 100 patients with thyroid carcinoma. Am J Radiol 1987; 148:45–49.

431. Sutton RT, Reading CC, Charboneau JW, et al. US-guided biopsy of neck masses in postoperative management of patients with thyroid cancer. Radiology 1988; 168:769–772.

432. Boland GW, Lee MJ, Mueller PR, et al. Efficacy of sonographically-guided biopsy of thyroid masses and cervical lymph nodes. Am J Radiol 1993; 161:1053–1056.

433. Reede DL, Berceron RT. The CT evaluation of the normal and diseased neck. Semin Ultrasound CT MR 1986; 22:239–250.

434. Silverman PM, Newman GE, Korobkin M. Computed tomography in the evaluation of thyroid disease. Am J Radiol 1984; 141:897–902.

435. Blum M, Reede DL, Seltzer TF, et al. Computerized tomography in the diagnosis of thyroid and parathyroid disorders. Am J Med Sci 1984; 287:34–39.

436. Bashist B, Ellis K, Gold RP. Computed tomography of intrathoracic goiters. Am J Radiol 1983; 140:455–460.

437. Higgins CB, Aufferman W. MR imaging of thyroid and parathyroid glands: a review of current status. Am J Radiol 1988; 151:1095–1106.

438. Mountz JM, Glazer GM, Dmuchowski C, et al. MR imaging of the thyroid: comparison with scintigraphy in the normal and diseased gland. J Comput Tomogr 1987; 11:612–621.

439. Brown LR, Aughenbaugh GL. Masses of the anterior mediastinum: CT and MR imaging. Am J Radiol 1991; 157:1171–1180.

440. Wang C, Vickery AI, Jr, Maloof F. Needle biopsy of the thyroid. Surg Gynecol Obstet 1976; 143:365–368.

441. Broughan TA, Esselstyn CB, Jr. Large-needle thyroid biopsy: still necessary. Surgery 1986; 100:1138–1141.

442. Smith EH. The hazards of fine-needle aspiration biopsy. Ultrasound Med Biol 1984; 10:629–634.

443. Solomon D. Fine-needle aspiration of the thyroid: an update. Thyroid Today 1993; 16:1–9.

444. Gharib H, Goellner JR. Fine-needle aspiration of thyroid nodules. Endocr Pract 1995; 1:410–417.

445. Gharib H, Goellner JR. Fine-needle aspiration biopsy of the thyroid: an appraisal. Ann Intern Med 1993; 118:282–289.

446. Gharib H. Fine-needle aspiration biopsy of thyroid nodules: advantages, limitations, and effect. Mayo Clin Proc 1994; 69:44–49.

447. Ridgway EC. Clinician's evaluation of a solitary thyroid nodule. J Clin Endocrinol Metab 1992; 74:231–235.

448. Mazzaferri EL. Management of a solitary thyroid nodule. N Engl J Med 1993; 329:553–559.

449. Gharib H. Current evaluation of thyroid nodules. Trends Endocrinol Metab 1994; 5:365–369.

450. Woeber KA. Thyrotoxicosis and the heart. N Engl J Med 1992; 327:94–98.

451. Channick BJ, Adlin EV, Marks AD. Hyperthyroidism and mitral valve prolapse. N Engl J Med 1981; 305:497–500.

452. Sawin CT, Geller A, Wolf PA, et al. Low serum thyrotropin concentrations as a risk factor for atrial fibrillation in older persons. N Engl J Med 1994; 331:1249–1252.

453. Bilezekian JP, Loeb JN. The influence of hyperthyroidism and hypothyroidism on the α- and β-adrenergic receptor system and adrenergic responsiveness. Endocr Rev 1983; 4:378–388.

454. Aoki VS, Wilson WR, Theilen EO, et al. The effects of triiodothyronine

on hemodynamic responses to epinephrine and norepinephrine in man. J Pharmacol Exp Ther 1967; 157:62–68.

455. Landsberg L. Catecholamines and hyperthyroidism. Clin Endocrinol Metab 1977; 6:697–718.

456. Liggett SB, Shah SD, Cryer PE. Increased fat and skeletal muscle β-adrenergic receptors but unaltered metabolic and hemodynamic sensitivity to epinephrine *in vivo* in experimental human thyrotoxicosis. J Clin Invest 1989; 83:803–809.

457. Gelfand RA, Hutchinson-Williams KA, Bonde AA, et al. Catabolic effects of thyroid hormone excess: the contribution of adrenergic activity to hypermetabolism and protein breakdown. Metabolism 1987; 36:562–569.

458. Myers JD, Brannon ES, Holland BC. A correlative study of the cardiac output and the hepatic circulation in hyperthyroidism. J Clin Invest 1950; 29:1069–1077.

459. Bergman TA, Mariash CN, Oppenheimer JH. Anterior mediastinal mass in a patient with Graves' disease. J Clin Endocrinol Metab 1982; 55:587–588.

460. Engel AG. Neuromuscular manifestations of Graves' disease. Mayo Clin Proc 1972; 47:919–925.

461. Wejda B, Hintze G, Katschinski B, et al. Hip fractures and the thyroid: a case-control study. J Intern Med 1995; 237:241–247.

462. Diamond T, Vine J, Smart R, et al. Thyrotoxic bone disease in women: a potentially reversible disorder. Ann Intern Med 1994; 120:8–11.

463. Burman RD, Monchik JM, Earll JM, et al. Ionized and total serum calcium and parathyroid hormone in hyperthyroidism. Ann Intern Med 1976; 84:668–671.

464. Garrel DR, Delmas PD, Malaval L, et al. Serum bone Gla protein: a marker of bone turnover in hyperthyroidism. J Clin Endocrinol Metab 1986; 62:1052–1055.

465. Eriksen EF, Mosekilde L, Melsen F. Trabecular bone remodeling and bone balance in hyperthyroidism. Bone 1985; 6:421–428.

466. Rhone DP, Berlinger FG, White FM. Tissue sources of elevated serum alkaline phosphatase activity in hyperthyroid patients. Am J Clin Pathol 1980; 74:381–386.

467. Rogers JS, Shane SR, Jencks FS. Factor VIII activity and thyroid function. Ann Intern Med 1982; 97:713.

468. Self TH, Straughn AB, Weisburst MR. Effect of hyperthyroidism on hypoprothrombinemic response to warfarin. Am J Hosp Pharm 1976; 33:387–389.

469. Gordon GG, Southren AL. Thyroid-hormone effects on steroid-hormone metabolism. Bull NY Acad Med 1977; 53:241–259.

470. Coulombe P, Dussault JH, Walker P. Plasma catecholamine concentrations in hyperthyroidism and hypothyroidism. Metabolism 1976; 25:973–979.

471. Coulombe P, Dussault JH, Walker P. Catecholamine metabolism in thyroid disease II. Norepinephrine secretion rate in hyperthyroidism and hypothyroidism. J Clin Endocrinol Metab 1977; 44:1185–1189.

471a. Taylor S. Robert Graves: The Golden Years of Irish Medicine. London: Royal Society of Medicine, 1989.

472. Kohut WD, Gharib H, Anderson MW. Triiodothyronine thyrotoxicosis complicating primary hypothyroidism in a patient with autoimmune thyroiditis. Am J Med 1982; 72:843–846.

473. Salvi M, Fukazawa H, Bernard N, et al. Role of autoantibodies in the pathogenesis and association of endocrine autoimmune disorders. Endocr Rev 1988; 9:450.

474. Kraiem Z, Lahat N, Glaser B, et al. Thyrotropin receptor blocking antibodies: incidence, characterization and in-vitro synthesis. Clin Endocrinol 1987; 27:409–421.

475. Martin A, Valentine M, Unger P, et al. Engraftment of human lymphocytes and thyroid tissue into Scid and Rag2-deficient mice: absent progression of lymphocytic infiltration. J Clin Endocrinol Metab 1994; 79:716–723.

476. McGregor AM, Petersen MM, McLachlan SM, et al. Carbimazole and the autoimmune response in Graves' disease. N Engl J Med 1980; 303:302–307.

477. Weetman AP. The immunomodulatory effects of antithyroid drugs. Thyroid 1994; 4:145–146.

478. McGregor AM, Petersen MM, Capifferi R, et al. Effects of radioiodine on thyrotrophin binding inhibiting immunoglobulins in Graves' disease. Clin Endocrinol 1979; 11:437–444.

479. Livolsi VA. Surgical Pathology of the Thyroid. Philadelphia: WB Saunders, 1990:68–97.

480. Weetman AP, McGregor AM, Hall R. Evidence for an effect of antithyroid drugs on the natural history of Graves' disease. Clin Endocrinol 1984; 21:163–172.

481. Martin A, Goldsmith NK, Friedman EW, et al. Intrathyroidal accumulation of T cell phenotypes in autoimmune thyroid disease. Autoimmunity 1990; 6:269–281.

482. Paschke R, Bruckner N, Schmeidl R, et al. Predominant intraepithelial localization of primed T cells and immunoglobulin-producing lymphocytes in Graves' disease. Acta Endocrinol 1991; 124:630–636.

483. Roman SH, Goldsmith NK, Leiderman IZ, et al. Induction of microsomal antigen and comparison with histologic localization of HLA-DR in Graves thyroid tissue. Autoimmunity 1989; 2:253–263.

484. Paschke R, Bruckner N, Eck T, et al. Regional stimulation of thyroid epithelial cells in Graves' disease by lymphocytic aggregates and plasma cells. Acta Endocrinol 1991; 125:459–465.

485. Tunbridge WMG, Evered DE, Hall R, et al. The spectrum of thyroid disease in a community: the Wickham Survey. Clin Endocrinol 1977; 7:481–493.

486. Tainer JA, Deal CD, Geysen HM, et al. Defining antibody-antigen recognition: towards engineered antibodies and epitopes. Int Rev Immunol 1991; 7:165–188.

487. Weiss A. Structure and function of the T cell antigen receptor. J Clin Invest 1990; 86:1015–1022.

488. Brown JH, Jardetzky S, Gorga JC, et al. Three-dimensional structure of the human class II histocompatibility antigen HLA-DR1. Nature 1993; 364:33–39.

489. Bjorkman PJ, Saper MA, Samraoui B, et al. Structure of the human class I histocompatibility antigen, HLA-A2. Nature 1987; 329:506–512.

490. Schwartz RH. T cell anergy. Sci Am 1993; 269:66–71.

491. Martin A, Davies TF. T cells and human autoimmune thyroid disease: emerging data show lack of need to invoke suppressor T-cell problems. Thyroid 1992; 2:247–261.

492. Adams DD, Purves HD. Abnormal responses in the assay of thyrotropin. Proc Univ Otago Med School 1956; 34:11–12.

493. Rees Smith B, McLachlan SM, Furmaniak J. Autoantibodies to the thyrotropin receptor. Endocr Rev 1988; 9:106–121.

494. Adams DD, Fastier FN, Howie JB, et al. Stimulation of the human thyroid by infusions of plasma containing LATS protector. J Clin Endocrinol Metab 1974; 39:826–832.

495. Zakarija M, McKenzie JM. Pregnancy-associated changes in thyroid-stimulating antibody of Graves' disease and the relationship to neonatal hyperthyroidism. J Clin Endocrinol Metab 1983; 57:1036–1040.

496. Zakarija MJ. Immunochemical characterization of the thyroid-stimulating antibody (TSab) of Graves' disease: evidence for restricted heterogeneity. J Clin Lab Immunol 1983; 10:77–85.

497. Weetman AP, Yateman ME, Ealey PA, et al. Thyroid-stimulating antibody activity between different immunoglobulin G subclasses. J Clin Invest 1990; 86:723–727.

498. Zakarija M, McKenzie JM, Eidson MS. Transient neonatal hypothyroidism: characterization of maternal antibodies to the thyrotropin receptor. J Clin Endocrinol Metab 1990; 70:1239–1246.

499. Davies TF, Yeo PP, Evered DC, et al. Value of thyroid-stimulating-antibody determinations in predicting short-term thyrotoxic relapse in Graves' disease. Lancet 1977; 1:1181–1182.

500. Wilson R, McKillop JH, Henderson N, et al. The ability of the serum TSH receptor antibody index and HLA status to predict long-term remission of thyrotoxicosis following medical therapy for Graves' disease. Clin Endocrinol 1986; 25:151–156.

500a. Nagayama Y, Izumi M, Ashizawa K, et al. Inhibitory effect of interferon-gamma on the response of human thyrocytes to thyrotropin (TSH) stimulation: relationship between the response to TSH and the expression of DR antigen. J Clin Endocrinol Metab 1987; 64:949–953.

500b. Kosugi S, Ban T, Akamizu T, et al. Site-directed mutagenesis of a portion of the extracellular domain of the rat thyrotopin receptor important in autoimmune thyroid disease and nonhomologous with gonadotropin receptors—relationship of functional and immunogenic domains. J Biol Chem 1991; 266:19413–19418.

501. Vlase H, Graves PN, Magnusson R, et al. Human autoantibodies to the TSH receptor: recognition of linear, folded and glycosylated recombinant extracellular domain. J Clin Endocrinol Metab 1995; 80:46–53.

502. Damante G, Foti D, Catalfamo R, et al. Desensitization of thyroid cyclic AMP response to thyroid-stimulating immunoglobulin: comparison with TSH. Metabolism 1987; 36:768–773.

503. Kraiem Z, Alkobi R, Sadeh O. Sensitization and desensitization of human thyroid cells in culture: effects of thyrotropin and thyroid-stimulating immunoglobulin. J Endocrinol 1988; 119:341–349.

504. Davies TF. Positive regulation of the guinea pig thyrotropin receptor. Endocrinology 1985; 117:201–207.

505. Huber G, Concepcion LE, Graves P, et al. Positive regulation of the human TSH receptor mRNA by recombinant human TSH is at the nuclear level. Endocrinology 1992; 130:2858–2864.

506. Male DK, Champion BR, Pryce G, et al. Antigenic determinants of human thyroglobulin differentiated using antigen fragments. Immunology 1985; 54:419–427.

507. Dayan CM, Londei M, Corcoran AE, et al. Autoantigen recognition by thyroid-infiltrating T cells in Graves disease. Proc Natl Acad Sci USA 1991; 88:7415–7419.

508. Acuto O, Reinhertz EL. The human T cell receptor: structure and function. N Engl J Med 1985; 312:1100–1111.

509. Benacerraf B. Role of the MHC gene products in immune regulation. Science 1981; 212:1229–1238.

510. Tandon N, Freeman MA, Weetman AP. T cell response to synthetic TSH receptor peptides in Graves' disease. Clin Exp Immunol 1992; 89:468–473.

511. Mackenzie WA, Schwartz AE, Friedman EW, et al. Intrathyroidal T cell clones from patients with autoimmune thyroid disease. J Clin Endocrinol Metab 1987; 64:818–824.

512. Grubeck-Loebenstein B, Turner M, Pirich K, et al. CD4+ T-cell clones from autoimmune thyroid tissue cannot be classified according to their lymphokine production. Scand J Immunol 1990; 32:433–440.

513. Del Prete GF, Tiri A, Mariotti S, et al. Enhanced production of gamma-interferon by thyroid-derived T cell clones from patients with Hashimoto's thyroiditis. Clin Exp Immunol 1987; 69:323–331.

514. Watson PF, Pickerill AP, Davies R, et al. Analysis of cytokine gene expression in Graves' disease and multinodular goiter. J Clin Endocrinol Metab 1994; 79:355–360.

515. Davis MM, Bjorkman PJ. T-cell antigen receptor genes and T-cell recognition. Nature 1988; 334:395–402.

516. Davies TF, Martin A, Concepcion ES, et al. Evidence of limited variability of antigen receptors on intrathyroidal T cells in autoimmune thyroid disease. N Engl J Med 1991; 325:238–244.

517. Davies T, Concepcion E, Ben-Nun A, et al. T-cell receptor V gene usage in autoimmune thyroid disease: direct assessment by thyroid aspiration. J Clin Endocrinol Metab 1993; 76:660–666.

518. Matsuoka N, Martin A, Concepcion ES, et al. Preservation of functioning human thyroid organoids in the scid mouse. II. Biased use of intrathyroidal T cell receptor V genes. J Clin Endocrinol Metab 1993; 77:311–315.

519. De Riu S, Martin A, Valentine M, et al. Graves' disease thyroid transplants in Scid mice: persistent selectivity in hTcR V alpha gene family use. Autoimmunity 1994; 19:271–277.

520. Oksenberg JR, Stuart S, Begovich AB, et al. Limited heterogeneity of rearranged T cell receptor V alpha transcripts in brains of multiple sclerosis patients. Nature 1990; 345:344–346.

521. Ben-Nun A, Liblau RS, Cohen L, et al. Restricted T cell receptor V beta usage by myelin basic protein-specific T cell clones in multiple sclerosis: predominant genes vary in individuals. Proc Natl Acad Sci USA 1991; 88:2466–2470.

522. Sridama V, Pacini V, DeGroot LJ. Decreased suppressor T lymphocytes in autoimmune thyroid diseases detected by monoclonal antibodies. J Clin Endocrinol Metab 1982; 54:316–329.

523. Moller G. Do suppressor T cells exist Scand J Immunol 1988; 27:247–250.

524. Jenkins M. The role of cell division in the induction of clonal anergy. Immunology Today 1992; 13:69–73.

525. Morahan G, Hoffmann M, Miller J. A. nondeletional mechanism of peripheral tolerance in T-cell receptor transgenic mice. Proc Natl Acad Sci 1992; 88:11421–11425.

526. Ambinder JM, Chiorazzi N, Gibofsky A, et al. Special characteristics of cellular immune function in normal individuals of the HLA-DR3 type. Clin Immunol Immunopathol 1982; 23:269–274.

527. Kallenberg CGM, Klaassen RJL, Beelen JM, et al. HLA-B8/DR3 phenotype and the primary immune response. Clin Immunol Immunopathol 1985; 34:135–140.

528. Phillips D, Prentice L, Upadhyaya M, et al. Autosomal dominant inheritance of autoantibodies to thyroid peroxidase and thyroglobulin: studies in families not selected for autoimmune thyroid disease. J Clin Endocrinol Metab 1991; 72:973–975.

529. Davies JL, Kawauchi Y, Bennet ST, et al. A genome-wide search for human type 1 diabetes susceptibility genes. Nature 1994; 371:130–136.

530. Dahlberg PA, Holmlund G, Karlsson FA, et al. HLA-A, -B, -C and -DR antigens in patients with Graves' disease and their correlation with signs and clinical course. Acta Endocrinol 1981; 97:42–47.

531. Roman SH, Greenberg D, Rubinstein P, et al. Genetics of autoimmune thyroid disease: lack of evidence for linkage to HLA within families. J Clin Endocrinol Metab 1992; 74:496–503.

532. O'Connor G, Neufeld DS, Greenberg DA, et al. Lack of disease-associated HLA-DQ restriction fragment length polymorphisms in families with autoimmune thyroid disease. Autoimmunity 1993; 14:237–241.

533. Bottazzo GF, Pujol Borrell R, Hanafusa T, et al. Role of aberrant HLA-DR expression and antigen presentation in induction of endocrine autoimmunity. Lancet 1983; 2:1115–1119.

534. Kawakami Y, Kuzuya N, Watanabe T, et al. Induction of experimental thyroiditis in mice by recombinant interferon gamma administration. Acta Endocrinol (Copen) 1990; 122:41–48.

535. Massa PT, Dorries R, Meulen V. Viral particles induce Ia antigen expression on astrocytes. Nature 1986; 320:543–546.

536. Neufeld DS, Platzer M, Davies TF. Reovirus induction of MHC class II antigen in rat thyroid cells. Endocrinology 1989; 124:543–545.

537. Khoury EL, Pereira L, Greenspan FS. Induction of HLA-DR expression on thyroid follicular cells by cytomegalovirus infection in vitro: evidence for a dual mechanism of induction. Am J Pathol 1991; 138:1209–1223.

538. Srinivasappa J, Saegusa J, Prabhakar BS, et al. Molecular mimicry: frequency of reactivity of monoclonal antiviral antibodies with normal tissues. J Virol 1986; 57:397–401.

539. Haspel MV, Onodera T, Prabhakar BS, et al. Virus-induced autoimmunity: monoclonal antibodies that react with endocrine tissues. Science 1983; 220:304–306.

540. Burch HB, Nagy EV, Lukes YG, et al. Nucleotide and amino acid homology between the human thyrotropin receptor and HIV-1 nef protein: identification and functional analysis. Biochem Biophys Res Commun 1991; 181:498–505.

541. Lidman K, Eriksson U, Norberg R, et al. Indirect immunofluorescence staining of human thyroid by antibodies occurring in Yersinia enterocolitiea infections. Clin Exp Immunol 1976; 23:429–435.

542. Wenzel BE, Heeseman J, Wenzel KW, et al. Antibodies to plasmid-encoded proteins of enteropathogenic Yersinia in patients with autoimmune thyroid disease. Lancet 1988; 1:56–59.

543. Tomer Y, Davies TF. Infection, thyroid disease and autoimmunity. Endocr Rev 1993; 14:107–120.

544. Carter JK, Smith RE. Rapid induction of hypothyroidism by an avian leukosis virus. Infect Immun 1983; 40:795–805.

545. Ciampolillo A, Mirakian R, Schulz T, et al. Retrovirus-like sequences in Graves' disease: implications for human autoimmunity. Lancet 1989; 1:1096–1099.

546. Wick G, Trieb K, Aguzzi A, et al. Possible role of human foamy virus in Graves' disease. Intervirology 1993; 35:101–107.

547. Lagaye S, Vexiau P, Morozov V, et al. Human spumaretrovirus-related sequences in the DNA of leukocytes from patients with Graves' disease. Proc Natl Acad Sci 1992; 89:10070–10074.

548. Humphrey M, Baker JR Jr, Carr FE, et al. Absence of retroviral sequences in Graves' disease. Lancet 1991; 337:17–18.

549. Neumann-Haefelin D, Fleps U, Renne R, et al. Foamy viruses. Intervirology 1993; 35:196–207.

550. Weisman SA. Incidence of thyrotoxicosis among refugees from Nazi prison camps. J Clin Endocrinol Metab 1958; 48:747–752.

551. Locke S, Ader R, Besedovsky H, et al. Foundations of Psychoneuroimmunology. New York: Aldine, 1985.

552. Leclere J, Weryha S. Stress and autoimmune endocrine diseases. Horm Res 1989; 31:90–93.

553. Winsa B, Adami H, Bergstrom R, et al. Stressful life events and Graves' disease. Lancet 1991; 338:1475–1479.

554. Sonino N, Girelli ME, Boscaro M, et al. Life events in the pathogenesis of Graves' disease: a controlled study. Acta Endocrinol 1993; 128:293–296.

555. Amino N, Miyai K. Postpartum Autoimmune Endocrine Syndromes. New York: Wiley, 1983; 247–272.

556. Stagnaro-Green A, Roman SH, Cobin RH, et al. A prospective study of lymphocyte-initiated immunosuppression in normal pregnancy: evidence of a T-cell etiology for postpartum thyroid dysfunction. J Clin Endocrinol Metab 1992; 74:645–653.

557. Paavonen T. Hormonal regulation of immune responses. Ann Med 1994; 26:255–258.

558. Da Silva JAP. Sex hormones, glucocorticoids, and autoimmunity: facts and hypotheses. Ann Rheum Dis 1995; 54:6–16.

559. Bahn RS, Heufelder AE. Pathogenesis of Graves' ophthalmopathy. N Engl J Med 1993; 329:1468–1475.

560. Burch HB, Wartofsky L. Graves' ophthalmopathy: current concepts regarding pathogenesis and management. Endocr Rev 1993; 14:747–793.

561. Grubeck-Loebenstein B, Trieb K, Holter W, et al. Retrobulbar T cells from patients with Graves' ophthalmopathy are CD8+ and specifically autologous fibroblasts. J Clin Invest 1993; 93:2738–2743.

562. Wall JR, Bernard N, Boucher A, et al. Pathogenesis of thyroid-associated ophthalmopathy: an autoimmune disorder of the eye muscle associated with Graves' hyperthyroidism and Hashimoto's thyroiditis. Clin Immunol Immunopathol 1993; 68:1–8.

563. Wall JR, Henderson J, Strakosch CR, et al. Graves' ophthalmopathy. Can Med Assoc J 1981; 124:855–866.

564. Wood LC, Ingbar SH. Hypothyroidism as a late sequela in patients with Graves' disease treated with antithyroid agents. J Clin Invest 1979; 64:1429–1436.

565. Solomon DH, Chopra IJ, Chopra U, et al. Identification of subgroups of euthyroid Graves' ophthalmopathy. N Engl J Med. 1977; 296:181–186.

566. Fatourechi V, Fransway AF. Dermopathy of Graves' disease (pretibial myxedema). Medicine 1994; 73:1–7.

567. Bull RH, Coburn PR, Mortimer PS. Pretibial myxedema: a manifestation of lymphoedema? Lancet 1993; 341:403–404.

568. Sato K, Yamazaki K, Shizume K, et al. Stimulation by TSH and Graves' immunoglobulin G of vascular endothelial growth factor mRNA expression in human thyroid follicles in vitro flt mRNA expression in the rat thyroid in vivo. J Clin Invest 1995; 96:1295–1302.

569. Marks AD, Bertram BJ, Channick J, et al. Chronic thyroiditis and mitral valve prolapse. Ann Intern Med 1995; 102:479–483.

570. Forrester JV, Sutherland GR, McDougall IR. Dysthyroid ophthalmopathy: orbital evaluation with beta-scan ultrasonography. J Clin Endocrinol Metab 1977; 45:221–224.

571. Dallow RH, Mormose KJ, Weber AL, et al. Comparison of ultrasonography, computerized tomography (EMI scan) and radiographic techniques in evaluation of exophthalmos. Trans Am Acad Ophthalmol Otolaryngol 1976; 81:305–322.

572. Wartofsky L. Classification of eye changes of Graves' disease. Thyroid 1992; 3:235–236.

573. Perros P, Crombie AL, Matthews JNS, et al. Age and gender influence the severity of thyroid-associated ophthalmopathy: a study of 101 patients attending a combined thyroid-eye clinic. Clin Endocrinol 1993; 38:367–372.

574. Singer PA, Cooper DS, Levy E, et al. Treatment guidelines for patients with hyperthyroidism and hypothyroidism. JAMA 1995; 273:808–812.

575. Cooper DS. Antithyroid drugs. N Engl J Med 1984; 311:1353–1362.

576. Geffner DL, Azukizawa M, Herhsman JM. Propylthiouracil blocks extrathyroidal conversion of thyroxine to triiodothyronine and augments thyrotropin secretion in man. J Clin Invest 1975; 55:218–223.

577. Laurberg P, Weeke J. Dynamics of inhibition of iodothyronine deiodination during propylthiouracil treatment of thyrotoxicosis. Horm Metab Res 1981; 13:289–292.

578. Jansson R, Dahlberg PA, Johansson H, et al. Intrathyroid concentrations of methimazole in patients with Graves' disease. J Clin Endocrinol Metab 1983; 57:129–132.

579. Weetman AP, McGregor AP, Hall R, Methimazole inhibits thyroid autoan-

tibody production by an action on accessory cells. Clin Immunol Immunopathol 1983; 28:39–45.

580. Volpe R. Evidence that the immunosuppressive effects of antithyroid drugs are mediated through actions on the thyroid cell, modulating thyrocyte-immunocyte signaling: a review. Thyroid 1994; 4:217–223.

581. McGregor AM, Ibbertson HK, Rees Smith B, et al. Carbimazole and autoantibody synthesis in Hashimoto's thyroiditis. BMJ 1995; 281:968–969.

582. Romaldini JH, Bromberg N, werner RS, et al. Comparison of effects of high and low dosage regimens of antithyroid drugs in the management of Graves' hyperthyroidism. J Clin Endocrinol Metab 1983; 57:563–570.

583. Tamai H, Hayaki I, Kawai K, et al. Lack of effect of thyroxine administration on elevated thyroid-stimulating hormone receptor antibody levels in treated Graves' disease patients. J Clin Endocrinol Metab 1995; 80:1481–1484 (see comments).

584. McIver B, Rae P, Beckett G, et al. Lack of effect of thyroxine in patients with Graves' hyperthyroidism who are treated with an antithyroid drug. N Engl J Med 1996; 334:220–224 (see comments).

585. Hashizume K, Ichikawa K, Sakurai A, et al. Administration of thyroxine in treated Graves' disease: effects on the level of antibodies to thyroid-stimulating hormone receptors and on the risk of recurrence of hyperthyroidism. N Engl J Med 1991; 324:947–953.

586. Tamai H, Hayaki I, Kawai K, et al. Lack of effect of thyroxine administration on elevated thyroid-stimulating hormone receptor antibody levels in treated Graves' disease. J Clin Endocrinol Metab 1995; 80:1481–1484.

587. O'Donnell J, Trokoudes K, Silverberg J, et al. Thyrotrophin displacement activity of serum immunoglobulins from patients with Graves' disease. J Clin Endocrinol Metab 1978; 46:770–777.

588. Bliddal H, Kirkegaard C, Siersback-Nielsen K, et al. Prognostic value of thyrotropin binding inhibiting immunoglobulins (TBII) in long-term antithyroid treatment, ^{131}I therapy given in combination with carbimazole and in euthyroid ophthalmopathy. Acta Endocrinol 1981; 98:364–369.

589. Feldt-Rasmussen U, Schleusner H, Carayon P. Meta-analysis evaluation of the impact of thyrotropin receptor antibodies on long-term remission after medical therapy of Graves' disease. J Clin Endocrinol Metab 1994; 78:98–102.

590. Weetman A, Ratanchaiyavong S, Middleton GW, et al. Prediction of outcome in Graves' disease after carbimazole treatment. Q J Med 1986; 59:409–419.

591. Greer MA, Kammer H, Bouma DJ. Short-term antithyroid drug therapy for the thyrotoxicosis of Graves' disease. N Engl J Med 1977; 297:173–176.

592. Solomon BL, Evaul JE, Burman KD, et al. Remission rates with antithyroid drug therapy: continuing influence of iodine intake? Ann Intern Med 1987; 107:510–512.

593. Wall JR, Fang SL, Kuroki T, et al. In vitro immunoreactivity to propylthiouracil, methimazole, and carbimazole in patients with Graves' disease: a possible cause of antithyroid drug-induced agranulocytosis. Clin Endocrinol Metab 1984; 58:868–872.

594. Becker DV, Braverman LE, Dunn JT, et al. The use of iodine as a thyroidal blocking agent in the event of a reactor accident. JAMA 1984; 252:659–661.

595. Fradkin JE, Wolff J. Iodide-induced thyrotoxicosis. Medicine 1983; 62:1–20.

596. Wu SY, Shyh TP, Chopra I, et al. Comparison of sodium ipodate (Orografin) and propylthiouracil in early treatment of hyperthyroidism. J Clin Endocrinol Metab 1982; 54:630–634.

596a. Lazarus JH, Richards AR, Addison GM, et al. Treatment of thyrotoxicosis with lithium carbonate. Lancet 1974; 2:1160–1163.

597. Croxson MS, Hall TD, Nicoloff JT. Combination drug therapy for treatment of hyperthyroid Graves' disease. J Clin Endocrinol Metab 1977; 45:623–630.

598. Rubin PC. Beta-blockers in pregnancy. N Engl J Med 1981; 305:1323–1326.

599. Gladstone R, Hordf A, Gersony WM. Propranolol administration during pregnancy: effects on the fetus. J Pediatr 1975; 86:962–964.

600. Milner MR, Gelman KM, Phillips RA, et al. Double-blind cross-over trial of diltiazem versus propranolol in the management of thyrotoxic symptoms. Pharmacotherapy 1990; 10:100–106.

601. Hershman JM. The treatment of hyperthyroidism. Ann Intern Med 1966; 64:1306–1314.

602. Michie W, Stowers JM, Duncan T, et al. Mechanism of hypocalcemia after thyroidectomy for thyrotoxicosis. Lancet 1971; 1:508–514.

603. Toft AD, Irvine WJ, McIntosh D, et al. Propranolol in the treatment of thyrotoxicosis by subtotal thyroidectomy. J Clin Endocrinol Metab 1976; 43:1312–1316.

604. Kazakov VS, Demidchik EP, Astakhova LN. Thyroid cancer after Chernobyl. Nature 1992; 359:21 (letter; see comments).

605. Nikiforov Y, Gnepp DR. Pediatric thyroid cancer after the Chernobyl disaster: pathomorphologic study of 84 cases (1991–1992) from the Republic of Belarus. Cancer 1994; 74:748–766.

606. Baverstock KF. Thyroid cancer in children in Belarus after Chernobyl. World Health Stat Q 1993; 46:204–208.

607. Williams ED. Fallout from Chernobyl: thyroid cancer in children increased dramatically in Belarus. BMJ 1994; 309:1298 (letter).

608. Smith RN, Wilson GM. Clinical trial of different doses of ^{131}I in treatment of thyrotoxicosis. BMJ 1967; 1:129–132.

609. Malone JF, Cutten MJ. Hypothyroidism after ^{125}I therapy. Ann Intern Med 1977; 86:823–824.

610. Wise PH, Ahmad A, Burnet RB, et al. Intentional radioiodine ablation for Graves' disease. Lancet 1975; 2:1231–1233.

611. Harvey RD, Metclafe RA, Morteo C, et al. Acute pretibial myxedema following radioiodine therapy for thyrotoxic Graves' disease. Clin Endocrinol 1995; 42:657–660.

612. Tallestedt L, Lundell G, Torring O, et al. Occurrence of ophthalmopathy after treatment for Graves' disease. N Engl J Med 1992; 326:1733–1738.

613. Bartalena L, Marcocci C, Bogazzi F, et al. Use of corticosteroids to prevent progression of Graves' ophthalmopathy after radioiodine therapy for hyperthyroidism. N Engl J Med 1989; 321:1349–1352.

614. Wartofsky L. Therapeutic controversies, summation, commentary, and overview: concerns over aggravation of Graves' ophthalmopathy by radioactive iodine treatment and the use of retrobulbar radiation therapy. J Clin Endocrinol Metab 1995; 80:347–349.

615. Dunn JT. Choice of therapy in young adults with hyperthyroidism of Graves' disease. Ann Intern Med 1984; 100:891–893.

616. Sridama V, DeGroot LJ. Treatment of Graves' disease and the course of ophthalmopathy. Am J Med 1989; 87:70–73.

617. Jacobson DH, Gorman CA. Endocrine ophthalmopathy: current ideas concerning etiology, pathogenesis, and treatment. Endocr Rev 1984; 5:200–220.

618. Prummel MF, Wiersinga WM. Medical management of Graves' ophthalmopathy. Thyroid 1995; 5:231–234.

619. Bartalena L, Marcocci C, Chiovato L, et al. Orbital cobalt irradiation combined with systemic corticosteroids for Graves' ophthalmopathy: comparison with systemic corticosteroids alone. J Clin Endocrinol Metab 1983; 56:1139–1144.

620. Teng CS, Crombie AL, Hall R, et al. An evaluation of supervoltage orbital irradiation for Graves' disease. Clin Endocrinol 1980; 13:545–551.

621. Lyons CJ, Rootman J. Orbital decompression for disfiguring exophthalmos in thyroid orbitopathy. Ophthalmopathy 1994; 101:223–230.

622. Ogura J, Wessler S, Avioli LV, et al. Surgical approach to the ophthalmopathy of Graves' disease. JAMA 1971; 216:1627–1631.

623. Davis LE, Lucas MJ, Hankins GDV, et al. Thyrotoxicosis complicating pregnancy. Am J Obstet Gynecol 1989; 160:63–70.

624. Amino N, Kuro R, Tanizawa O, et al. Changes of serum antithyroid antibodies during and after pregnancy in autoimmune thyroid diseases. Clin Exp Immunol 1978; 31:30–37.

625. Zakarija M, McKenzie JM, Hoffman WH. Prediction and therapy of intrauterine and late-onset neonatal hyperthyroidism. J Clin Endocrinol Metab 1986; 62:368–371.

626. Yabu Y, Amino N, Mori H, et al. Postpartum recurrence of hyperthyroidism and changes of thyroid-stimulating immunoglobulins in Grave's disease. J Clin Endocrinol Metab 1980; 51:1454–1458.

627. Amino N, Tanizawa O, Mori H, et al. Aggravation of thyrotoxicosis in early pregnancy and after in delivery in Graves' disease. J Clin Endocrinol Metab 1982; 55:108–112.

628. Marchant B, Brownlie BEW, Hart DM, et al. The placental transfer of propylthiouracil, methimazole and carbamizole. J Clin Endocrinol Metab 1977; 45:1187–1193.

629. Cheron RG, Kaplan MM, Larsen PR, et al. Neonatal thyroid function after propylthiouracil therapy for maternal Graves' disease. N Engl J Med 1981; 304:525–528.

630. Momotani N, Noh J, Oyanagi H, et al. Antithyroid drug therapy for Graves' disease during pregnancy: optimal regimen for fetal thyroid status. N Engl J Med 1986; 315:24–28.

631. van Dijke CP, Heydendael RJ, de Kleine MJ. Methimazole, carbimazole, and congenital skin defects. Ann Intern Med 1987; 106:60–61.

632. Low LCK, Lang J, Alexander WD. Excretion of carbimazole and propylthiouracil in breast milk. Lancet 1979; 2:1011.

633. Hayles AB. Problem of childhood Graves' disease. Mayo Clin Proc 1972; 47:850–853.

634. Favus MJ, Schneider AB, Stachura ME, et al. Thyroid cancer occurring as a late consequence of head-and-neck irradiation. N Engl J Med 1976; 294:1019–1025.

635. Safa AM, Schneider AB, Stachura ME, et al. Long-term follow-up results in children and adolescents treated with radioactive iodine (^{131}I) for hyperthyroidism. N Engl J Med 1975; 292:167–171.

636. Huysmans DAKC, Hermus RMM, Corstens FHM, et al. Large, compressive, goiters treated with radioiodine. Ann Intern Med 1994; 121:757–762.

637. Van Sande J, Parma J, Tonacchera M, et al. Somatic and germline mutations of the TSH receptor gene in thyroid diseases. J Clin Endocrinol Metab 1995; 80:2577–2585.

638. Clapham DE. Mutations in G protein–linked receptors: novel insights on disease. Cell 1993; 75:1237–1239.

639. Gorman CA, Robertson JS. Radiation dose in the selection of ^{131}I or surgical treatment for toxic thyroid adenoma. Ann Intern Med 1978; 89:85–90.

640. Ross DS, Ridgway EC, Daniels GH. Successful treatment of solitary toxic thyroid nodules with relatively low-dose iodine-131, with low prevalence of hypothyroidism. Ann Intern Med 1984; 101:488–490.

641. Goldstein R, Hart IA. Follow-up of solitary autonomous thyroid nodules treated with ^{131}I. N Engl J Med 1983; 309:1473–1476.

642. Duprez L, Parma J, Van Sande J, et al. Germline mutations in the thyrotropin receptor gene cause non-autoimmune autosomal dominant hyperthyroidism. Nat Genet 1994; 7:396–401.

643. Stancek D, Stancekova-Gressnerova M, Janotka M, et al. Isolation and some serological and epidemiological data on the viruses recovered from patients with subacute thyroiditis de Quervain. Med Microbiol Immunol 1975; 161:133–144.

644. Wall JR, Fang SL, Ingbar SH, et al. Lymphocytic transformation in response to human thyroid extract in patients with subacute thyroiditis. J Clin Endocrinol Metab 1976; 43:587–590.

645. Weetman AP, Smallridge RC, Nutman TB, et al. Persistent thyroid autoimmunity after subacute thyroiditis. J Clin Lab Immunol 1987; 23:1–6.

646. Papapetrou PD, Jackson IMD. Thyrotoxicosis due to "silent" thyroiditis. Lancet 1975; 361:363.

647. Rosen IB, Strawbridge HG, Walfish PG, et al. Malignant pseudothyroiditis: a new clinical entity. Am J Surg 1978; 136:445–449.

648. Vagenakis AG, Abreau CM, Braverman LE. Prevention of recurrence in acute thyroiditis following corticosteroid withdrawal. J Clin Endocrinol Metab 1970; 31:705–708.

649. Woolf PD. Transient painless thyroiditis with hyperthyroidism: a variant of lymphocytic thyroiditis? Endocr Rev 1980; 1:411–420.

650. Nikolai TF, Coombs GJ, McKenzie AK. Lymphocytic thyroiditis with spontaneously resolving hyperthyroidism and subacute thyroiditis. Arch Intern Med 1981; 141:1455–1458.

651. Nikolai TF, Brosseau J, Kettrick MA, et al. Lymphocytic thyroiditis with spontaneously resolving hyperthyroidism (silent thyroiditis). Arch Intern Med 1980; 140:478–482.

652. Jansson R, Bernander S, Karlsson A. et al. Autoimmune thyroid dysfunction in the postpartum period. J Clin Endocrinol Metab 1984; 58:681–687.

653. Freeman R, Rosen H, Thysen B. Incidence of thyroid dysfunction in an unselected postpartum population. Arch Intern Med 1986; 146:1361–1364.

654. Tachi J, Amino N, Tamaki H, et al. Long-term follow-up and HLA association in patients with postpartum hypothyroidism. J Clin Endocrinol Metab 1986; 66:480–484.

655. Amino N, Mori H, Iwatani Y, et al. High prevalence of transient postpartum thyrotoxicosis and hypothyroidism. N Engl J Med 1982; 306:849–852.

656. Kourides IA. A patient with thyroid-stimulating hormone (TSH) hypersecretion. Med Grand Rounds 1983; 2:222–228.

657. Wemeau JL, Dewailly D, Leroy R, et al. Long-term treatment with the somatostatin analog SMS 201–995 in a patient with a thyrotropin- and growth hormone-secreting pituitary adenoma. J Clin Endocrinol Metab 1988; 66:636–639.

658. Oppenheim DS, Klibanski A. Medical therapy of glycoprotein hormone-secreting pituitary tumors. Endocrinol Metab Clin North Am 1989; 18:339–358.

659. Beck-Peccoz P, Piscitelli G, Cattaneo MG, et al. Successful treatment of hyperthyroidism due to nonneoplastic pituitary TSH secretion with 3,5,3′-triiodothyroacetic acid (TRIAC). J Endocrinol Invest 1983; 6:217–223.

660. Refetoff S, Weiss RE, Usala SJ, et al. The syndromes of resistance to thyroid hormone: update 1994. Endocr Rev 1994; 3:336–342.

661. Beck-Peccoz P, Chatterjee VKK. The variable clinical phenotype in thyroid hormone resistance syndrome. Thyroid 1994; 4:225–231.

662. Rosler A, Litvin Y, Hage C, et al. Familial hyperthyroidism due to inappropriate thyrotropin secretion successfully treated with triiodothyronine. J Clin Endocrinol Metab 1982; 54:76–82.

663. Cohen JH, Ingbar SH, Braverman LE. Thyrotoxicosis due to ingestion of excess thyroid hormone. Endocr Rev 1989; 10:113–124.

664. Hedberg CW, Fishbein DB, Janssen RS, et al. An outbreak of thyrotoxicosis caused by the consumption of bovine thyroid gland in ground beef. N Engl J Med 1987; 316:993–998.

664a. Brown WW, Shetty KR, Rosenfeld PS. Hyperthyroidism due to struma ovarii: demonstration by radioiodine scan. Acta Endocrinol (Copenh) 1973; 73:266–272.

665. Sobrinho LG, Limbert ES, Santos MA. Thyroxine toxicosis in patients with iodine-induced thyrotoxicosis. J Clin Endocrinol Metab 1977; 45:25–29.

666. Engler D, Donaldson EB, Stockigt JR, et al. Hyperthyroidism without triiodothyronine excess: an effect of severe non-thyroidal illness. J Clin Endocrinol Metab 1978; 46:77–82.

667. Smith TJ, Horwitz AL, Refetoff S. The effect of thyroid hormone on glycosaminoglycan accumulation in human skin fibroblasts. Endocrinology 1981; 108:2397–2399.

668. Ladenson PW. Recognition and management of cardiovascular disease related to thyroid dysfunction. Am J Med 1990; 88:638–641.

669. Ladenson PW, Sherman SI, Baughman KL, et al. Reversible alterations in myocardial gene expression in a young man with dilated cardiomyopathy and hypothyroidism. Proc Natl Acad Sci 1992; 89:5251–5255.

670. Hardisty CA, Naik DR, Munro DS. Pericardial effusion in hypothyroidism. Clin Endocrinol 1980; 13:349–354.

671. Keating FR Jr, Parkin TW, Selby JB, et al. Treatment of heart disease associated with myxedema. Prog Cardiovasc Dis 1961; 3:364–381.

672. Levine HD. Compromise therapy in the patient with angina pectoris and hypothyroidism: a clinical assessment. Am J Med 1980; 69:411–418.

673. Steinberg AD. Myxedema and coronary artery disease: a comparative autopsy study. Ann Intern Med 1968; 68:338–344.

674. Lee JK, Lewis JA. Myxedema with complete A-V block and Adams-Stokes disease abolished with thyroid medication. Br Heart J 1962; 24:253–256.

675. Zwillich CW, Pierson DJ, Hofeldt FD, et al. Ventilatory control in myxedema and hypothyroidism. N Engl J Med 1975; 292:662–665.

676. Orr WC, Males JL, Imes NK. Myxedema and obstructive sleep apnea. Am J Med 1981; 70:1061–1066.

677. Amino N, Kuro R, Yabu Y, et al. Elevated levels of circulating carcinoembryonic antigen in hypothyroidism. J Clin Endocrinol Metab 1981; 52:457–462.

678. Rosman NP. Neurological and muscular aspects of thyroid dysfunction in childhood. Pediatr Clin North Am 1976; 23:575–594.

679. Hall RCW. Psychiatric effects of thyroid hormone disturbance. Psychosomatics 1983; 24:7.

680. Bland JH, Frymoyer JW. Rheumatic syndromes of myxedema. N Engl J Med 1970; 282:1171–1174.

681. Frymoyer JW, Bland JH. Carpal-tunnel syndrome in patients with myxedematous arthropathy. J Bone Joint Surg 1973; 55-A:78–82.

682. Sanders V. Neurologic manifestations of myxedema. N Engl J Med 1962; 266:547–552, 599–603.

683. Khaleeli AA, Griffith DG, Edwards RHT. The clinical presentation of hypothyroid myopathy. Clin Endocrinol 1983; 19:365–376.

684. Chernausek SD, Underwood LE, Utiger RD, et al. Growth hormone secretion and plasma somatomedin-C in primary hypothyroidism. Clin Endocrinol 1983; 19:337–344.

685. Valcavi R, Jordon V, Kieguez C, et al. Growth hormone responses to GRF 1-29 in patients with primary hypothyroidism before and during replacement therapy with thyroxine. Clin Endocrinol 1986; 24:693–696.

686. Cavaliere H, Knobel M, Medeiros-Neto G. Effect of thyroid hormone therapy on plasma insulin-like growth factor I levels in normal subjects, hypothyroid patients and endemic cretins. Horm Res 1987; 25:132–139.

687. Brent GA, Harney JW, Moore DD, et al. Multihormonal regulation of the human, rat, and bovine growth hormone promoters: differential effects of 3′,5′-cyclic adenosine monophosphate, thyroid hormone, and glucocorticoids. Mol Endocrinol 1988; 2:792–798.

688. Koenig RJ, Brent GA, Warne RL, et al. Thyroid hormone receptor binds to a site in the rat growth promoter required for induction by thyroid hormone. Proc Natl Acad Sci 1987; 84:5670–5674.

689. Eriksen EF. Normal and pathological remodeling of human trabecular bone: three-dimensional reconstruction of the remodeling sequence in normals and in metabolic bone disease. Endocr Rev 1986; 7:379–408.

690. Skowsky WR, Kikuchi TA. The role of vasopressin in the impaired water excretion of myxedema. Am J Med 1978; 64:613–621.

691. Iwasaki Y, Oiso Y, Yamauchi K, et al. Osmoregulation of plasma vasopressin in myxedema. J Clin Endocrinol Metab 1990; 70:534–539.

692. Dalton RG, Dewar MS, Savidge GF, et al. Hypothyroidism as a cause of acquired von Willebrand's disease. Lancet 1987; 1:1007–1009.

693. Tachman ML, Guthrie GP Jr. Hypothyroidism: diversity of presentation. Endocr Rev 1984; 5:456–465.

694. Edson JR, Fecher DR, Doe RP. Low platelet adhesiveness and other hemostatic abnormalities in hypothyroidism. Ann Intern Med 1975; 82:342.

695. Yamada T, Tsukui T, Ikejiri K, et al. Volume of sella turcica in normal subjects and in patients with primary hypothyroidism and hyperthyroidism. J Clin Endocrinol Metab 1976; 421:817–822.

696. Lecky BR, Williams TD, Lightman SL, et al. Myxoedema presenting with chiasmal compression: resolution after thyroxine replacement. Lancet 1987; 1:1347–1350.

697. Vagenakis AG, Dole K, Braverman LE. Pituitary enlargement, pituitary failure, and primary hypothyroidism. Ann Intern Med 1976; 85:195–198.

698. Yamamoto K, Saito K, Takai T, et al. Visual field defects and pituitary enlargement in primary hypothyroidism. J Clin Endocrinol Metab 1983; 57:283–287.

699. Onishi T, Miyai K, Aono T, et al. Primary hypothyroidism and galactorrhea. Am J Med 1977; 63:373–378.

700. Reichlin S, Utiger RD. Regulation of the pituitary-thyroid axis in man: relationship of TSH concentration to concentration of free and total thyroxine in plasma. J Clin Endocrinol Metab 1967; 27:251.

701. Clausen N, Lins PE, Adamson U, et al. Counterregulation of insulin-induced hypoglycaemia in primary hypothyroidism. Acta Endocrinol 1986; 111:516–521.

702. Kamilaris TC, DeBold CR, Pavlou SN, et al. Effect of altered thyroid hormone levels on hypothalamic-pituitary-adrenal function. J Clin Endocrinol Metab 1987; 65:994–999.

703. Montoro M, Collea JV, Frasier SD, et al. Successful outcome of pregnancy in women with hypothyroidism. Ann Intern Med 1981; 94:31–34.

704. Davis LE, Leveno KJ, Cunningham FG. Hypothyroidism complicating pregnancy. Obstet Gynecol 1988; 72:108.

705. Katz HP, Youlton SL, Kaplan SL, et al. Growth and growth hormone. III. Growth hormone release in children with primary hypothyroidism and thyrotoxicosis. J Clin Endocrinol Metab 1969; 29:346–351.

706. Chernausek SD, Turner R. Attenuation of spontaneous nocturnal growth hormone secretion in children with hypothyroidism and its correlation with plasma insulin-like growth factor I concentrations. J Pediatr 1989; 114:968–972.

707. Sterman BM, Ganguli S, Devaskar SU, et al. Hypothyroidism and glucocorticoids modulate the development of hepatic insulin receptors. Pediatr Res 1983; 17:111–116.

708. Shah JH, Motto GS, Papagiannes E, et al. Insulin metabolism in hypothyroidism. Diabetes 1975; 24:922–925.

709. Pederson O, Richelsen B, Bak J, et al. Characterization of the insulin

841. Roque L, Gomes P, Correia C, et al. Thyroid nodular hyperplasia: chromosomal studies in 14 cases. Cancer Genet Cytogenet 1993; 69:31–34.

842. Criado B, Barros A, Suijkerbuijk RF, et al. Detection of numerical alterations for chromosomes 7 and 12 in benign thyroid lesions by in situ hybridization. Am J Pathol 1995; 147:136–144.

843. Bartalena L, Martino E, Vellozzi F, et al. The lack of nocturnal serum TSH surge in patients with nontoxic nodular goiter may predict the subsequent occurrence of hyperthyroidism. J Clin Endocrinol Metab 1991; 72:604–609.

844. Greig WR, Boyle JA, Duncan A, et al. Genetic and non-genetic factors in simple goiter formation: evidence from a twin study. Q J Med 1967; 36:175–185.

845. Murray IPC, Thomson JA, McGirr EM. Unusual familial goiter associated with intrathyroidal calcification. J Clin Endocrinol 1966; 26:1039–1049.

846. Foley TP. Goiter in adolescents. Endocrinol Metab Clin North Am 1993; 22:593–606.

847. Hennemann G. Goiter and pregnancy: a new insight into an old problem—comment. Thyroid 1992; 2:71–72.

848. Murray D. The thyroid gland. In: Kovacs K, Asa SL, eds. Functional Endocrine Pathology. Boston: Blackwell Scientific Publications, 1991: 293–374.

849. Hicks DG, Livolsi VA, Neidich JA, et al. Clonal analysis of solitary follicular nodules in the thyroid. Am J Pathol 1990; 137:553–562.

850. Namba H, Matsuo K, Fagin JA. Clonal composition of benign and malignant human thyroid tumors. J Clin Invest 1990; 86:120–125.

851. Berghout A, Wiersinga WM, Smits NJ, et al. Interrelationships between age, thyroid volume, thyroid nodularity, and thyroid function in patients with sporadic nontoxic goiter. Am J Med 1990; 89:602–608.

852. Collazo-Clavell ML, Gharib H, Maragos NE. Relationship between vocal cord paralysis and benign thyroid disease. Head Neck 1995; 17:24–30.

853. Rieu M, Bekka S, Sambor B, et al. Prevalence of subclinical hyperthyroidism and relationship between thyroid hormonal states and thyroid ultrasonographic parameters in patients with nontoxic nodular goiter. Clin Endocrinol 1993; 39:67–71.

854. Pezzino V, Vigneri R, Squatrito S. Increased serum thyroglobulin levels in patients with nontoxic goiter. J Clin Endocrinol Metab 1978; 46:653–657.

855. Kristensen HL, Vadstrup S, Knudsen N, et al. Development of hyperthyroidism in nodular goiter and thyroid malignancies in an area of relatively low iodine intake. J Endocrinol Invest 1995; 18:41–43.

856. Hara T, Tamai H, Mukata T, Fukata S, Kuma K, Nakayama T. A long-term follow-up study of patients with nontoxic diffuse goiter in Japan. Clin Endocrinol 1993; 39:541–546.

857. Bruns P. Ueber die Kropfbehandlung mit Schilddrusenfutterung. Beitr Klin Chirurg 1894; 12:847–853.

858. Greer MA, Astwood EB. Treatment of simple goiter with thyroid. J Clin Endocrinol 1953; 13:1312–1331.

859. Ross DS. Thyroid hormone suppressive therapy of sporadic nontoxic goiter. Thyroid 1992; 2:263–269.

860. Nygaard B, Faber J, Hegedus L, et al. 131I treatment of nodular nontoxic goitre. Eur J Endocrinol 1996; 134:15–20.

861. Berghout A, Wiersinga WM, Drexhage HA, et al. Comparison of placebo with L-thyroxine alone or with carbimazole for treatment of sporadic nontoxic goitre. Lancet 1990; 336:193–197.

862. Perrild H, Hansen JM, Hegedus L. Triiodothyronine and thyroxine treatment of diffuse nontoxic goitre evaluated by ultrasound scanning. Acta Endocrinol 1982; 100:382–387.

863. Baran DT, Braverman LE. Thyroid hormone and bone mass. J Clin Endocrinol Metab 1991; 72:1182–1184.

864. Bartalena L, Pinchera A. Levothyroxine suppressive therapy: harmful and useless or harmless and useful? J Endocrinol Invest 1994; 17:675–677.

865. Faber J, Galloe AM. Changes in bone mass during prolonged subclinical hyperthyroidism due to L-thyroxine treatment: a meta-analysis. Eur J Endocrinol 1994; 13:350–356.

866. Marcocci C, Golia F, Bruno-Bosoro G, et al. Carefully monitored levothyroxine suppressive therapy is not associated with bone loss in premenopausal women. J Clin Endocrinol Metab 1994; 78:818–823.

867. Muller CG, Baylel TA, Harrison JE, et al. Possible limited bone loss with suppressive thyroxine therapy is unlikely to have clinical relevance. Thyroid 1995; 5:81–87.

868. Berghout A, Wiersinga WM, Drexhage HA, et al. The long-term outcome of thyroidectomy for sporadic nontoxic goitre. Clin Endocrinol 1989; 31:193–199.

869. Agerback H, Pilegaard HK, Watt-Boolsen S, et al. Complications of 2,028 operations for benign thyroid disease. Ugeskr Laeger 1988; 150:533–536.

870. Berglund J, Bondesson L, Christensen SB, et al. Indications for thyroxine therapy after surgery for nontoxic benign goitre. Acta Chirurg Scand 1990; 156:433–438.

871. Bistrup C, Nielsen JD, Gregersen G, et al. Preventive effect of levothyroxine in patients operated for nontoxic goitre: a randomized trial of one hundred patients with nine years follow-up. Clin Endocrinol 1994; 40:323–327.

872. Verelst J, Bonnyns M, Glinoer D. Radioiodine therapy in voluminous multinodular nontoxic goiter. Acta Endocrinol 1990; 122:417–421.

873. Huysmans DAKC, Hermus ARMM, Corstens FHM, et al. Large compressive goiters treated with radioiodine. Ann Intern Med 1994; 121:757–762.

874. Kay TW, d'Emden MC, Andrews JT, et al. Treatment of nontoxic multinodular goiter with radioactive iodine. Am J Med 1988; 84:19–22.

875. Nygaard B, Hegedus L, Gervil M, et al. Radioiodine treatment of multinodular nontoxic goiter. BMJ 1993; 307:828–832.

876. Wesche MF, Tiel-V-Buul MM, Smits NJ, et al. Reduction in goiter size by 131I therapy in patients with nontoxic multinodular goiter. Eur J Endocrinol 1995; 132:86–87.

877. Nygaard B, Faber J, Hegedus L. Acute changes in thyroid volume and function following 131I therapy of multinodular goiter. Clin Endocrinol 1994; 41:715–718.

878. Glinoer D. Radioiodine therapy of nontoxic multinodular goiter. Clin Endocrinol 1994; 41:713–714.

879. Hall P, Berg G, Bjelkengren G, et al. Cancer mortality after iodine-131 therapy for hyperthyroidism. Int J Cancer 1992; 50:886–890.

880. Mazzaferri EL. Impact of initial tumor features and treatment selected on the long-term course of differentiated thyroid cancer. Thyroid Today 1995; 18:1–13.

881. Tezelman S, Clark OH. Current management of thyroid cancer. Adv Surg 1995; 28:191–221.

882. Dulgeroff AJ, Hershman JM. Medical therapy for differentiated thyroid carcinoma. Endocr Rev 1994; 15:500–515.

883. Pacini F, Elisei R, Fugazzola L, et al. Post-surgical follow-up of differentiated thyroid cancer. J Endocrinol Invest 1995; 18:165–166.

884. Mazzaferri EL. Management of a solitary thyroid nodule. N Engl J Med 1993; 328:553–559.

885. Woeber KA. Cost-effective evaluation of the patient with a thyroid nodule. Surg Clin North Am 1995; 75:357–363.

886. Feld S, Garcia M, Baskin HJ, et al. AACE clinical practice guidelines for the diagnosis and management of thyroid nodules. Endocr Pract 1996; 2:78–84.

887. Van De Velde CJH, Hamming JF, Goslings BM, et al. Report of the consensus development conference on the management of differentiated thyroid cancer in the Netherlands. Eur J Cancer Clin Oncol 1988; 24:287–292.

888. Baldet L, Manderscheid JC, Glinoer D, et al. The management of differentiated thyroid cancer in Europe in 1988: results of an international survey. Acta Endocrinol 1989; 120:547–558.

889. Pasieka JL, Rotstein LE. Consensus conference on well-differentiated thyroid cancer: a summary. Can J Surg 1993; 36:298–301.

890. DeGroot LJ. Long-term impact of initial and surgical therapy on papillary and follicular thyroid cancer. Am J Med 1994; 97:499–500.

891. Solomon BL, Wartofsky L, Burman KD. Current trends in the management of well-differentiated papillary thyroid carcinoma. J Clin Endocrinol Metab 1996; 81:333–339.

892. Bruneton JN, Balu-Maestro C, Marcy PY, et. Very high frequency (13 Mhz) ultrasonographic examination of the normal neck: detection of normal lymph nodes and thyroid nodules. J Ultrasound Med 1994; 13:87–90.

893. Parker SL, Tong T, Bolden S, et al. Cancer statistics. CA Cancer J Clin 1996; 65:5–27.

894. Tan GH, Gharib H. Thyroid incidentalomas: management approaches to nonpalpable nodules discovered incidentally on thyroid imaging. Ann Intern Med 1997; 126:226–231.

895. Blum M, Rothschild M. Improved nonoperative diagnosis of the solitary 'cold' thyroid nodule: surgical selection based on risk factors and three months of suppression. JAMA 1980; 243:242–245.

896. Piromalli D, Martelli G, DelPrato I, et al. The role of fine-needle aspiration in the diagnosis of thyroid nodules: analysis of 795 consecutive cases. J Surg Oncol 1992; 50:247–250.

897. Okamato T, Yamashita T, Harasawa A, et al. Test performances of three diagnostic procedures in evaluating thyroid nodules: physical examination, ultrasonography and fine-needle aspiration cytology. Endocr J 1994; 41:243–247.

898. Christensen SB, Bondeson L. Ericsson UB, et al. Prediction of malignancy in the solitary thyroid nodule by physical examination, thyroid scan, fine-needle biopsy and serum thyroglobulin: a prospective study of 100 surgically treated patients. Acta Chir Scand 1984; 150:433–439.

899. Pacini F, Fontanelli M, Fugazzola L, et al. Routine measurement of serum calcitonin in nodular thyroid diseases allows the preoperative diagnosis of unsuspected sporadic medullary thyroid carcinoma. J Clin Endocrinol Metab 1994; 78:826–829.

900. Ledger GA, Khosla S, Lindor NM, et al. Genetic testing in the diagnosis and management of multiple endocrine neoplasia type II. Ann Intern Med 1995; 122:118–124.

901. Wells SA, Chi DD, Toshima K, et al. Predictive DNA testing and prophylactic thyroidectomy in patients at risk for multiple endocrine neoplasia type 2A. Ann Surg 1994; 220:237–250.

902. Gagel RF, Geopfert H, Callender DL. Changing concepts in the pathogenesis and management of thyroid carcinoma. CA Cancer J Clin 1996; 46:261–283.

903. Nelson RL, Wahner HW, Gorman CA. Rectilinear thyroid scanning as a predictor of malignancy. Ann Intern Med 1978; 88:41–44.

904. Hughes FC, Baudet M, Laccourreye H. Le nodule thyroidien: une etude retrospective de 200 observations. Ann Otolaryngol Chir Cervicofac 1989; 106:77–70.

905. Hermans J, Schmitz A, Merlo P, et al. Le thallium 201, permet-il de differencier le nodule thyroidien benin du nodule malin? Ann Endocrinol 1993; 54:248–240.

906. Kumar A, Ahuja MM, Chattopadhyay TK, et al. Fine-needle aspiration cytology, sonography and radionuclide scanning in solitary thyroid nodule. J Assoc Physicians India 1992; 40:302–306.

907. Synbinski Z, Huszno B, Golkowski F, et al. Technetium 99m–methoxyisobutylisonitrile in early diagnosis of thyroid cancer. Endokrynol Polska 1993; 44:427–433.

908. Leisner B. Ultrasound evaluation of thyroid diseases. Horm Res 1987; 26:33–41.

909. Solbiati L, Volterrani L, Rizzatto G, et al. The thyroid gland with low uptake lesions: evaluation by ultrasound. Radiology 1985; 155:187–191.

910. Seya A, Oeda T, Terano T, et al. Comparative studies on fine-needle aspiration cytology with ultrasound scanning in the assessment of thyroid nodule. Jpn J Med 1990; 29:478–480.

911. Gharib H. Management of thyroid nodules: another look. Thyroid Today 1997; 20:1–11.

912. Hamburger JI. Diagnosis of thyroid nodules by fine-needle biopsy: use and abuse. J Clin Endocrinol Metab 1994; 79:335–339.

913. Hales MS, Hsu FS. Needle tract implantation of papillary carcinoma of the thyroid following aspiration biopsy. Acta Cytol 1990; 34:801–804.

914. Jones JD, Pittman DL, Sanders LR. Necrosis of thyroid nodules after fine-needle aspiration. Acta Cytol 1985; 29:29–32.

915. Keyhani-Rofagha S, Kooner DS, Keyhani M, et al. Necrosis of Hürthle cell tumor of the thyroid following fine-needle aspiration: case report and literature review. Acta Cytol 1990; 34:805–808.

916. DeMicco C, Vasko V, Garcia S, et al. Fine-needle aspiration of thyroid follicular neoplasm: diagnostic use of thyroid peroxidase immunochemistry with monoclonal antibody 47. Surgery 1994; 116:1031–1035.

917. Carpi A, Ferrari E, DeGaudio C, et al. The value of aspiration needle biopsy in evaluating thyroid nodules. Thyroidology 1994; 6:5–9.

918. Liu Q, Castelli M, Gattuso P, et al. Simultaneous fine-needle aspiration and core-needle biopsy of thyroid nodules. Am Surgeon 1995; 61:628–632.

919. Takashima S, Fukuda H, Kobayashi T. Thyroid nodules: clinical effect of ultrasound-guided fine-needle aspiration biopsy. J Clin Ultrasound 1994; 22:535–542.

920. Schmid KW, Ladurner D, Zechmann W, et al. Clinicopathologic management of tumors of the thyroid gland in an endemic goiter area: combined use of preoperative fine-needle aspiration biopsy and intraoperative frozen section. Acta Cytol 1989; 33:27–30.

921. McHenry CR, Walfish PG, Rosen IB. Non-diagnostic fine-needle aspiration biopsy: a dilemma in management of nodular thyroid disease. Am Surgeon 1993; 59:415–419.

922. Hedinger C, Williams ED, Sobin LH. Histological typing of thyroid tumours. In: International Histological Classification of Tumours. 2nd ed, No. 11. World Health Organization. New York: Springer-Verlag, 1988: 1–20.

923. Rosai J, Carganio ML, Delellis RA. Tumors of the Thyroid Gland. Washington, DC: Armed Forces Institute of Pathology, 1992: 1–343.

924. Rosai J. Thyroid gland. In: Rosai J, ed. Ackerman's Surgical Pathology. 8th ed. St. Louis: Mosby-YearBook 1996: 493–567.

925. Beahrs OH, Henson DE, Hutter RVP, et al. Manual for Staging of Cancer. 4th ed. American Joint Committee on Cancer. Philadelphia: JB Lippincott, 1992: 53–56.

926. Robbins J. Prognostic factors in the management of thyroid cancer. J Endocrinol Invest 1995; 18:159–160.

927. Doniach I. The thyroid gland. In: Symmers W St C, ed. Systemic Pathology. 2nd ed, Vol 14. Edinburgh: Churchill Livingstone, 1978: 1976–2037.

928. Bisi H, Fernandes VS, Asato de Camargo RY, et al. The prevalence of unsuspected thyroid pathology in 300 sequential autopsies, with special reference to the incidental carcinoma. Cancer 1989; 64:1888–1893.

929. Carney JA, Ryan J, Goellner JR. Hyalinizing trabecular adenoma of the thyroid gland. Am J Surg Pathol 1987; 11:583–592.

930. Tallini G, Carcangiu ML, Rosai J. Oncocytic neoplasms of the thyroid gland. Acta Pathol Jpn 1992; 42:305–315.

931. Gundry SR, Burney RE, Thompson NW, et al. Total thyroidectomy for Hurthle cell neoplasm of the thyroid. Arch Surg 1983; 118:529–532.

932. Ryan JJ, Hay ID, Grant CS, et al. Flow cytometric DNA measurements in benign and malignant Hurthle cell tumors of the thyroid. World J Surg 1988; 12:482–487.

933. Grant CS, Barr D, Goellner JR, et al. Benign Hürthle cell tumors of the thyroid: a diagnosis to be trusted? World J Surg 1988; 12:488–494.

934. Flint A, Lloyd RV. Hurthle-cell neoplasms of the thyroid gland. Pathol Annu 1990; 25:37–52.

935. Carcangiu ML, Bianchi S, Savino D, et al. Follicular Hürthle cell neoplasms of the thyroid gland: a study of 153 cases. Cancer 1991; 68:1944–1953.

936. Pauke TW, Croxson MS, Parker JW, et al. Triiodothyronine-secreting (toxic) adenoma of the thyroid gland: light and electron microscopic characteristics. Cancer 1978; 41:528–537.

937. Parma J, Duprez L, Van Sande J, et al. Somatic mutations of the thyrotropin receptor gene cause hyperfunctioning thyroid adenomas. Nature 1993; 365:649–651.

938. Porcellini A, Ciullo I, Laviola L, et al. Novel mutations of thyrotropin receptor gene in thyroid hyperfunctioning adenomas. J Clin Endocrinol Metab 1994; 76:657.

939. Parma J, Van Sande J, Swillens S, et al. Somatic mutations causing constitutive activity of the thyrotropin receptor are the major cause of hyperfunctioning thyroid adenomas: identification of additional mutations activating both the cyclic adenosine 3'5'-monophosphate and inositol phosphate–Ca^{++} cascades. Mol Endocrinol 1995; 9:725–733.

940. O'Sullivan CO, Barton CM, Staddon SL, et al. Activating point mutations of the gsp oncogene in human thyroid adenomas. Mol Carcinog 1991; 4:345–349.

941. Suarez HG, Du Villard JA, Caillou B, et al. Gsp mutations in human thyroid tumors. Oncogene 1991; 6:677–679.

942. Duh Q-Y, Grossman RF. Thyroid growth factors, signal transduction pathways, and oncogenes. Surg Clin North Am 1995; 75:421–437.

943. Du Villard JA, Schlumberger M, Wicker R, et al. Role of ras and gsp oncogenes in human epithelial thyroid tumorigenesis. J Endocrinol Invest 1995; 18:124–126.

944. Hazard JB, Kenyon R. Atypical adenoma of the thyroid. Arch Pathol 1954; 58:554–563.

945. Lang W, Georgii A, Stauch G, et al. The differentiation of atypical adenomas and encapsulated follicular carcinomas in the thyroid gland. Virch Arch [A] 1980; 385:125–141.

946. Greenebaum E, Koss LG, Elequin F, et al. The diagnostic value of flow cytometric DNA measurements in follicular tumors of the thyroid gland. Cancer 1985; 56:2011–2018.

947. Rosai J. Papillary carcinoma. Monogr Pathol 1993; 35:138–165.

948. Hay ID. Papillary thyroid carcinoma. Endocrinol Metab Clin North Am 1990; 19:545–576.

949. Hay ID, Grant CS, vanHeerden JA, et al. Papillary thyroid microcarcinoma: a study of 535 cases observed in a 50-year period. Surgery 1992; 112:1139–1147.

950. Hay ID. Cytometric DNA ploidy analysis in thyroid cancer. Diagn Oncol 1991; 1:181–185.

951. Teyssier JR, Liautaud-Roger F, Ferre D, et al. Chromosomal changes in thyroid tumors: relation with DNA content, karyotypic features, and clinical data. Cancer Genet Cytogenet 1990; 50:249–263.

952. Pierotti MA, Santoro M, Jenkins RB, et al. Characterization of an inversion on the long arm of chromosome 10 juxtaposing D10S170 and ret and creating the oncogenic sequence ret/ptc. Proc Natl Acad Sci 1992; 89:1616–1620.

953. Bongarzone I, Butti MG, Coronelli S, et al. Frequent activation of ret protooncogene by fusion with a new activating gene in papillary thyroid carcinomas. Cancer Res 1994; 54:2979–2985.

954. Grieco M, Cerrato A, Santoro M, et al. Cloning and characterization of H4 (D10S170), a gene involved in RET rearrangements in vivo. Oncogene 1994; 9:2531–2535.

955. Tong Q, Li YS, Smanik PA, et al. Characterization of the promoter region and oligomerization domain of h4 (d10s170), a gene frequently rearranged with the ret protooncogene. Oncogene 1995; 10:1781–1787.

956. Sozzi G, Bongarzone I, Miozzo M, et al. A t(10;17) translocation creates the RET/PTC2 chimeric transforming sequence in papillary thyroid carcinoma. Genes Chromosomes Cancer 1994; 9:244–250.

957. Viglietto G, Chiappetta G, Martinez-Tello FJ, et al. RET/PTC oncogene activation is an early event in thyroid carcinogenesis. Oncogene 1995; 11:1207–1210.

958. Santoro M, Carlomagno F, Hay ID, et al. Ret oncogene activation in human thyroid neoplasms is restricted to the papillary cancer subtype. J Clin Invest 1992; 89:1517–1522.

959. Jhiang SM, Mazzaferri EL. The RET/PTC oncogene in papillary thyroid carcinoma. J Lab Clin Med 1994; 123:331–337.

960. Sugg SL, Zheng L, Rosen IB, et al. RET/PTC-1, -2, and -3 oncogene rearrangements in human thyroid carcinomas: implications for metastatic potential. J Clin Endocrinol Metab 1996; 81:3360–3365.

961. Bongarzone I, Pierotti MA, Monzini N, et al. High frequency of activation of tyrosine kinase oncogenes in human papillary thyroid carcinoma. Oncogene 1989; 4:1457–1462.

962. Klugbauer S, Lengfelder E, Demidchik EP, et al. High prevalence of RET rearrangement in thyroid tumors of children from Belarus after the Chernobyl reactor accident. Oncogene 1995; 11:2459–2467.

963. McConahey WM, Hay ID, Woolner LB, et al. Papillary thyroid cancer treated at the Mayo Clinic, 1946 through 1970: initial manifestations, pathologic findings, therapy and outcome. Mayo Clin Proc 1986; 61:978–996.

964. Zimmerman D, Hay ID, Gough IR, et al. Papillary thyroid carcinoma in children and adults: long-term follow-up of 1,039 patients conservatively treated at one institution during three decades. Surgery 1988; 104:1157–1166.

965. Kukkonen ST, Haapiainen RK, Fransila KO, et al. Papillary thyroid carcinoma: the new, age-related TNM classification system in a retrospective analysis of 199 patients. World J Surg 1990; 14:837–842.

966. Grant CS, Hay ID, Gough IR, et al. Local recurrence in papillary thyroid carcinoma: is extent of surgical resection important? Surgery 1988; 104:954–962.

967. Hay ID, Grant CS, Taylor WF, et al. Ipsilateral lobectomy versus bilateral lobar resection in papillary thyroid carcioma: a retrospective analysis of surgical outcome using a novel prognostic scoring system. Surgery 1987; 102:1088–1095.

968. Simpson WJ, McKinney SE, Carruthers JS, et al. Papillary and follicular thyroid cancer: prognostic factors in 1,578 patients. Am J Med 1987; 83:479–488.

969. DeGroot LJ, Kaplan EL, McCormick M, et al. Natural history, treatment and course of papillary thyroid carcinoma. J Clin Endocrinol Metab 1990; 71:414–424.

970. Shah JP, Loree TR, Dharker D, et al. Prognostic factors in differentiated carcinoma of the thyroid gland. Am J Surg 1992; 164:658–661.

971. Hay ID, Bergstralh EJ, Goellner JR, et al. Predicting outcome in papillary thyroid carcinoma: development of a reliable prognostic scoring system in a cohort of 1,779 patients surgically treated at one institution during 1940 through 1989. Surgery 1993; 114:1050–1058.

972. DeGroot LJ, Kaplan EL, Straus FH, et al. Does the method of management of papillary thyroid carcinoma make a difference in outcome? World J Surg 1994; 18:123–130.

973. Tielens ET, Sherman SI, Hruban RH, et al. Follicular variant of papillary thyroid carcinoma: a clinicopathologic study. Cancer 1994; 73:424–431.

974. Carcangiu MC, Zempi G, Rosai J. Poorly differentiated ("insular") thyroid carcinoma: a reinterpretation of Langhens "wuchernde Struma." Am J Surg Pathol 1984; 8:655–668.

975. Sobrinho-Simoes M. Mixed medullary and follicular carcinoma of the thyroid. Histopathology 1993; 23:187–189.

976. Grebe SKG, Hay ID. Follicular thyroid cancer. Endocrinol Metab Clin North Am 1996; 24:761–801.

977. Livolsi VA, Asa SL. The demise of follicular carcinoma of the thyroid gland. Thyroid 1994; 4:233–236.

978. Ishimaru Y, Fukuda S, Kurano R, et al. Follicular thyroid carcinoma with clear cell change showing unusual ultrastructural features. Am J Surg Pathol 1988; 12:240–246.

979. Watson RG, Brennan MD, Goellner JR, et al. Invasive Hürthle cell carcinoma of the thyroid: natural history and management. Mayo Clin Proc 1984; 59:851–855.

980. Livolsi VA, Merino MJ. Worrisome histologic alterations following fine-needle aspiration of the thyroid. Pathol Annu 1994; 29:99–120.

981. Farid NR, Zou M, Shi Y. Genetics of follicular thyroid cancer. Endocrinol Metab Clin North Am 1995; 24:865–883.

982. Santoro M, Grieco M, Melillo R, et al. Molecular defects in thyroid carcinomas: role of the RET oncogene in thyroid neoplastic transformation. Eur J Endocrinol 1995; 133:513–522.

983. Herrmann MA, Hay ID, Bartlet DH, et al. Cytogenetic and molecular genetic studies of follicular and papillary thyroid cancers. J Clin Invest 1991; 88:1596–1603.

984. Matsuo K, Tang SH, Fagin JA. Allelotype of human thyroid tumors: loss of chromosome 11q13 sequences in follicular neoplasms. Mol Endocrinol 1991; 5:1873–1879.

985. Roque L, Cestedo S, Clode A, et al. Deletion of 3p 25-pter in a primary thyroid follicular carcinoma and its metastasis. Genes Chromosomes Cancer 1993; 8:199–206.

986. Zedenius J, Wallin G, Svensson A, et al. Deletions of the long arm of chromosome 10 in progression of follicular thyroid tumors. Hum Genet 1996; 97:299–303.

987. Soares P, Sobrinhoe-Simoes M. Recent advances in cytometry, cytogenetics and molecular genetics of thyroid tumors and tumor-like lesions. Pathol Res Pract 1995; 191:304–317.

988. Jenkins RB, Hay ID, Herath JF, et al. Frequent occurrence of cytogenetic abnormalities in sporadic nonmedullary thyroid carcinoma. Cancer 1990; 66:1213–1220.

989. Gazdav AF. The molecular and cellular basis of human lung cancer. Anticancer Res 1994; 14:261–267.

990. Kovacs G. Molecular differential pathology of renal cell tumors. Histopathology 1993; 22:1–8.

991. Brennan MD, Bergstralh EJ, vanHeerden JA, et al. Follicular thyroid cancer treated at the Mayo Clinic, 1946 through 1970: initial manifestations, pathologic findings, therapy and outcome. Mayo Clinic Proc 1991; 66:11–19.

992. Grant CS, Hay ID, Ryan JJ, et al. Diagnostic and prognostic utility of flow cytometric DNA measurements in follicular thyroid tumors. World J Surg 1990; 14:183–190.

993. Paul SJ, Sisson JC. Thyrotoxicosis caused by thyroid cancer. Endocrinol Metab Clin North Am 1990; 19:593–612.

994. Grebe SKG, Hay ID. Thyroid cancer nodal metastases: biologic significance and therapeutic considerations. Surg Oncol Clin North Am 1996; 5:43–63.

995. van Heerden JA, Hay ID, Goellner JR, et al. Follicular thyroid carcinoma with capsular invasion alone: a non-threatening malignancy. Surgery 1992; 112:1130–1136.

996. Mueller-Gaertner HW, Brzac HT, Rehpenning W. Prognostic indices for tumor relapse and tumor mortality in follicular thyroid carcinoma. Cancer 1991; 67:1903–1908.

997. Cady R, Rossi R. An expanded view of risk-group definition in differentiated thyroid carcinoma. Surgery 1985; 98:1171–1176.

998. Shaha AR, Loree TR, Shah JP. Prognostic factors and risk group analysis in follicular carcinoma of the thyroid. Surgery 1995; 118:1131–1138.

999. Loree TR. Therapeutic implications of prognostic factors in differentiated carcinoma of the thyroid gland. Semin Surg Oncol 1995; 11:246–255.

1000. Emerick GT, Duh QY, Siperstein AE, et al. Diagnosis, treatment, and outcome of follicular thyroid carcinoma. Cancer 1993; 72:3287–3294.

1001. Davis NL, Bugis SD, McGregor GI, et al. An evaluation of prognostic scoring systems in patients with follicular thyroid cancer. Am J Surg 1995; 170:476–480.

1002. Nel CJ, van Heerden JA, Goellner JR, et al. Anaplastic carcinoma of the thyroid: a clinicopathologic study of 82 cases. Mayo Clinic Proc 1985; 60:51–58.

1003. Fagin JA, Matsuo K, Karmakar A, et al. High prevalence of mutation of the p53 gene in poorly differentiated human thyroid carcinomas. J Clin Ivest 1993; 91:179–184.

1004. Ito T, Segama T, Mizuno T, et al. Unique associations of p53 mutations with undifferentiated, but not with differentiated, carcinoma of the thyroid gland. Cancer Res 1992; 52:1369–1371.

1005. Gharib H, McConahey WM, Tiegs RD, et al. Medullary thyroid carcinoma: clinicopathologic features and long-term follow-up of 65 patients treated during 1946 through 1970. Mayo Clin Proc 1992; 67:934–940.

1006. Brierley J, Tsang R, Simpson WJ, et al. Medullary thyroid cancer: analyses of survival and prognostic factors and the role of radiation therapy in local control. Thyroid 1996; 6:305–310.

1007. Pyke CM, Hay ID, Goellner JR, et al. Prognostic significance of calcitonin immunoreactivity, amyloid staining, and flow cytometric DNA measurements in medullary thyroid carcinoma. Surgery 1991; 110:964–970.

1008. Moley JF. Medullary thyroid cancer. Surg Clin North Am 1995; 75:405–420.

1009. Wohlik N, Cote GJ, Evans DB, et al. Applications of genetic screening information to the management of medullary thyroid carcinoma and multiple neoplasia type 2. Endocrinol Metab Clin North Am 1996; 25:1–25.

1010. Lips CJM, Landsvater RM, Hoppener JWM, et al. Clinical screening as compared with DNA analysis in families with multiple endocrine neoplasia type 2A. N Engl J Med 1994; 331:828–835.

1011. Chong GC, Beahrs OH, Sizemore GW. Medullary carcinoma of the thyroid gland. Cancer 1975; 35:695–704.

1012. Farndon JR, Leight GS, Dilley WG, et al. Familial medullary thyroid carcinoma without associated endocrinopathies: a distinct clinical entity. Br J Surg 1986; 42:287–296.

1013. Wohlik N, Cote GJ, Bugalho MMJ, et al. Relevance of RET proto-oncogene mutations in sporadic medullary thyroid carcinoma. J Clin Endocrinol Metab 1996; 81:3740–3745.

1014. Singer PA, Cooper DS, Daniels GH, et al. Treatment guidelines for patients with thyroid nodules and well-differentiated thyroid cancer. Arch Intern Med 1996; 156:2165–2172.

1015. Pyke CM, Grant CS, Habermann TM, et al. Non-Hodgkin's lymphoma of the thyroid: is more than biopsy necessary? World J Surg 1992; 16:604–609.

1016. Holm LE, Blomgren H, Lowhagen T. Cancer risks in patients with chronic lymphocytic thyroiditis. N Engl J Med 1985; 312:601–604.

1017. Matsuzuka F, Migauchi A, Katayama S, et al. Clinical aspects of primary thyroid lymphoma: diagnosis and treatment based on our experience of 119 cases. Thyroid 1993; 3:93–98.

1018. Buhr HJ, Kallinowski F, Raue F, et al. Microsurgical neck dissection for metastasizing medullary thyroid carcinoma. Eur J Surg Oncol 1995; 21:195–197.

1019. Sarne D, Schneider AB. External radiation and thyroid neoplasia. Endocrinol Metab Clin North Am 1996; 25:181–195.

1020. Fogelfeld L, Wiviott MBT, Shore-Freedman P, et al. Recurrence of thyroid nodules after surgical removal in patients irradiated in childhood for benign conditions. N Engl J Med 1989; 320:835–840.

1021. Hawkins F, Rigopoulou D, Papapretro K, et al. Spinal bones mass after long-term treatment with L-thyroxine in postmenopausal women with thyroid cancer and chronic lymphocytic thyroiditis. Calcif Tissue Int 1994; 54:16–19.

1022. Ruegemer JJ, Hay ID, Bergstralh EJ, et al. Distant metastases in differentiated thyroid carcinoma: a multivariate analysis of prognostic variables. J Clin Endocrinol Metab 1988; 63:960–967.

1023. Schlumberger M, Tubiana M, De Vathaire F, et al. Long-term results of treatment of 283 patients with lung and bone metastases from differentiated thyroid carcinoma. J Clin Endocrinol Metab 1986; 63:960–967.

1024. Samaan NA, Schultz PN, Hickey RC, et al. The results of various modalities of treatment of well-differentiated thyroid carcinomas: a retrospective review of 1,599 patients. J Clin Endocrinol Metab 1992; 75:714–720.

1025. Schlumberger M, Arcangioli O, Piekarski JD, et al. Detection and treatment of lung metastases of differentiated thyroid carcinoma in patients with normal chest x-rays. J Nucl Med 1988; 29:1790–1794.

1026. Vassilopoulou-Sellin R, Klein MJ, Smith TH, et al. Pulmonary metastases in children and young adults with differentiated thyroid cancer. Cancer 1993; 71:1348–1352.

1027. Sweeney DC, Johnston GS. Radioiodine therapy for thyroid cancer. Endocrinol Metab Clin North Am 1995; 24:803–839.

1028. Maxon HR, Thomas SR, Hertzberg VS, et al. Relation between effective radiation dose and outcome of radioiodine therapy for thyroid cancer. N Engl J Med 1983; 309:937–941.

1029. Maxon HR, Englaro EE, Thomas SR, et al. Radioiodine-131 therapy for well-differentiated thyroid cancer: a quantitative radiation dosimetric approach—outcome and validation in 85 patients. J Nucl Med 1992; 33:1132–1140.

1030. Dinneen SF, Valimaki MJ, Bergstralh EJ, et al. Distant metastases in papillary thyroid carcinoma: 100 cases observed at one institution during 5 decades. J Clin Endocrinol Metab 1995; 80:2041–2045.

1031. Mazzaferri EL, Jhiang SM. Long-term impact of initial surgical and medical therapy on papillary and follicular thyroid cancer. Am J Med 1994; 97:418–428.

1032. Meier CA, Braverman LE, Ebner SA, et al. Diagnostic use of recombinant human thyrotropin in patients with thyroid carcinoma (phase I/II study). J Clin Endocrinol Metab 1994; 78:188–196.

1033. Goldman JM, Line BR, Aamodt RL, et al. Influence of triiodothyronine withdrawal time on ^{131}I uptake post-thyroidectomy for thyroid cancer. J Clin Endocrinol Metab 1980; 50:734–739.

1034. Leeper RD. Thyroid cancer. Med Clin North Am 1985; 69:1079–1096.

1035. Spencer CA, Wang CC. Thyroglobulin measurement: techniques, clinical benefits, and pitfalls. Endocrinol Metab Clin North Am 1995; 24:841–863.

1036. Ozata M, Suzuki S, Miyamoto T, et al. Serum thyroglobulin in the follow-up of patients with treated differentiated thyroid cancer. J Clin Endocrinol Metab 1994; 79:98–105.

1037. Brierley JD, Tsang RW. External radiation therapy in the treatment of thyroid malignancy. Endocrinol Metab Clin North Am 1996; 25:141–157.

1038. Soh EY, Clark OH. Surgical considerations and approach to thyroid cancer. Endocrinol Metab Clin North Am 1996; 25:115–140.

1039. Pacini F, Cetani F, Miccoli P, et al. Outcome of 309 patients with metastatic differentiated thyroid carcinoma treated with radioiodine. World J Surg 1994; 18:600–604.

1040. Coburn M, Teates D, Wanebo HJ. Recurrent thyroid cancer: role of surgery versus radioactive iodine (I-131). Ann Surg 1994; 219:587–593.

1041. Samaan NA, Schultz PN, Haynie TP, et al. Pulmonary metastasis of differentiated thyroid carcinoma: treatment results in 101 patients. J Clin Endocrinol Metab 1985; 65:376–380.

1042. van Heerden JA, Grant CS, Gharib H, et al. Long-term course of patients with persistent hypercalcitoninemia after apparent curative primary surgery for medullary thyroid carcinoma. Ann Surg 1990; 212:395–400.

1043. Saad MF, Fritsche HA, Samaan NA. Diagnostic and prognostic values of carcinoembryonic antigen in medullary carcinoma of the thyroid. J Clin Endocrinol Metab 1984; 58:889–894.

1044. Mendelsohn G, Wells SA, Baylin SB. Relationship of tissue carcinoembryonic antigen and calcitonin to tumor virulence in medullary thyroid carcinoma. Cancer 1984; 54:657–664.

12

THE ADRENAL CORTEX

David N. Orth and William J. Kovacs

THE NORMAL ADRENAL CORTEX

History

The anatomy of the adrenal glands appears to have been described first in 1563 by Bartholomeo Eustachius as the "glandulae renis incumbentes" in his *Tabulae Anatomicae,* edited and published in 1714 by Lancisius.[1-4] Emil Huschke first differentiated the cortex from the medulla anatomically.[5] Edme F. A. Vulpian[6] demonstrated the differential staining of the two regions, and Rudolph Albert von Kölliker[7] described the formation of the fetal adrenal cortex and its subsequent invasion by the neural precursors of the medulla, which were called "chromaffin" cells because they stained selectively with potassium dichromate.[8] The three concentric zones of the cortex were subsequently given their current designations: zonae glomerulosa, fasciculata, and reticularis.[9]

Ideas about the function of the adrenal glands lagged behind. Thomas Bartholin[10] proposed that these "capsulae atrabilariae" purified black bile that subsequently drained into the renal veins. In 1716 the Academie des Sciences de Bordeaux offered a prize for the answer to the question, "What is the purpose of the suprarenal glands?" Charles de Montesquieu, judging the responses, found the essays so unsatisfactory that he was unable to award the prize, concluding that "Perhaps some day chance will reveal what all of this work was unable to do."[2] As early as 1639 Walter Charleton distinguished glands with ducts from those without them. John Ranby showed in 1725 that the adrenal "ducts" are arteries,

and Théophile de Bordeu[11] espoused the theory of internal secretion by such glands. William B. Carpenter[12] wrote in 1852 that the "vascular glands," including the adrenals, produced substances that, "instead of being carried out of the body, are destined to be restored to the circulating current, apparently in a state of more complete adaptiveness to the wants of the nutritive function." Claude Bernard[13] popularized the concept and introduced the term "sécrétion interne"—by which he meant glucose, however, not the hormones, which were yet to be discovered. Some 40 y later the physiologist Edward A. Schäfer[14] elevated Bernard's concept about internal secretions to the status of full-fledged theory.

Evidence for a central physiological role for adrenal glands came from clinical observation. On March 15, 1849, Thomas Addison[15] presented a paper to the South London Medical Society entitled, "On anaemia: disease of the suprarenal capsules," a result of his interest in idiopathic, or pernicious, anemia. Three of the patients he described had adrenal disease at autopsy, and it was the only abnormality that was identified in two of them. However, 6 y passed before he was persuaded to publish his classic monograph, *On the Constitutional and Local Effects of Disease of the Supra-renal Capsules,*[16] describing the "anaemia, general languor and debility, remarkable feebleness of the heart's action, irritability of the stomach, and a peculiar change of colour of the skin" he observed in 11 patients with the disease that has since borne his name.[17] The following year, Charles E. Brown-Séquard[18] provided experimental confirmation of the theory that the adrenal glands are essential to life by performing adrenalectomies in several species of animals, although his operative technique and conclusions were challenged. Neither Brown-Séquard's nor Addison's conclusions were quickly or universally accepted.

The importance of the adrenal cortex relative to the medulla was a matter of debate well into the 20th century. Oliver and Schäfer described their discovery of a vasopressor agent in extracts of the medulla in 1894, and epinephrine was subsequently characterized[19, 20] and purified.[21] The issue was settled for most scientists by the demonstration that removal of one adrenal and half of the other and cauterization of the medulla in the remaining half-adrenal was compatible with healthy survival in dogs,[22] a result corroborated by Bernardo A. Houssay and Juan T. Lewis.[23] Nonetheless, some persisted in considering epinephrine the vital adrenal principle on into the 1920s.

Early studies on the physiological role of adrenal steroids were complicated because their actions appeared almost ubiquitous, adrenocortical extracts were usually contaminated with catecholamines, and the chemical nature of what was assumed to be a single active cortical principle was unknown. The turning point came in 1930, when it was found that lipid extracts of adrenal cortex had high potency for maintaining normal health and growth of adrenalectomized cats.[24–26] The extracts were immediately but unsuccessfully applied to treating human adrenal insufficiency by Sir William Osler[3] and later successfuly by others.[27] The isolation, identification, and synthesis of the adrenal steroids then began in earnest. Deoxycorticosterone (DOC), synthesized by M. von Steiger and Tadeus Reichstein[28] in 1937, had weak mineralocorticoid and negligible glucocorticoid activity, but it established the steroidal nature of the adrenocortical hormones. Cortisone was identified at about the same time, but it was not until 1949 that cortisone acetate was synthesized in quantities sufficient for therapeutic use. The possible existence of a salt-retaining principle had been suggested in 1916 by evidence of decreased plasma volume in adrenalectomized cats[29] and by the observation that adrenalectomized dogs developed hyponatremia, hypomagnesemia, and hyperkalemia and that their lives were prolonged by administration of sodium salts.[30] However, aldosterone was the most elusive of the steroids to isolate and characterize and by far the most difficult to synthesize, a feat not accomplished until 1955.[31, 32]

The mechanisms by which adrenocortical function is regulated were elucidated in the 20th century. Philip E. Smith[33] documented the existence of a functional pituitary-adrenal axis, and D.J. Ingle and Edward C. Kendall[34] showed in 1937 that adrenocortical extracts inhibited the adrenocorticotropic effect of the pituitary, establishing the presence of a homeostatic negative feedback mechanism characteristic of most endocrine regulatory systems. They also observed the existence of other control mechanisms, such as the one mediating the response to stressful stimuli. The development of bioassays of adrenocortical stimulation—reduction in circulating eosinophils, depletion of adrenal cholesterol, and depletion of adrenal ascorbic acid—facilitated the identification of corticotropin (ACTH, adrenocorticotropic hormone, adrenocorticotropin), the structure of which was determined in the decade beginning in 1956.[35] Geoffrey W. Harris[36] predicted the existence of a hypothalamic factor that is secreted into the hypothalamic-hypophyseal portal blood and stimulates ACTH release from the anterior pituitary. This factor, corticotropin-releasing hormone (CRH), was characterized and synthesized by Wylie W. Vale and his coworkers in 1981.[37]

Until the late 1940s, the only clinical use of steroids was as replacement therapy in patients with adrenal insufficiency. However, it had been observed that the inflammation of rheumatoid arthritis is often mitigated in patients who are jaundiced or pregnant. Philip S. Hench, reasoning that the effect must be mediated by an endogenous factor that was unusually abundant in those conditions, eliminated a number of other possible factors before deciding to test glucocorticoids in 1941. In 1949, sufficient cortisone was available for Hench and his co-workers[38] to demonstrate that both it and ACTH are effective in improving "certain clinical and biochemical features of rheumatoid arthritis" and that, when "use of them was discontinued, symptoms and signs of rheumatoid arthritis usually, but not always, returned or increased promptly." The effect was entirely unexpected. Glucocorticoids have since been used with enormous benefit as antiinflammatory agents, but their adverse side effects and inappropriate use have also resulted in enormous harm.

Knowledge of the function of the adrenal gland and its products has increased rapidly since 1949. Advances include the synthesis of potent steroids such as prednisone, prednisolone, dexamethasone, triamcinolone, and fludrocortisone; elucidation of the relations between steroid structure and function; and diagnostic, therapeutic, and experimental application of these insights. Development of inhibitors of steroid biosynthesis such as metyrapone, aminoglutethimide, and ketoconazole; inhibitors of steroid action such as cyproterone and mifepristone (RU486); and the cytotoxic drug for the adrenal cortex, mitotane, has provided important diagnostic and therapeutic agents and investigative tools. There have been advances in knowledge of the structure and physiology of the hypothalamic factors such as CRH and arginine vasopressin (AVP, also called antidiuretic hormone, ADH) that regulate pituitary ACTH secretion and of the precursor of ACTH, pro-opiomelanocortin (POMC), and the enzymes that process it into ACTH and the other POMC peptides. The messenger RNAs (mRNAs) and genes that encode these peptides and their membrane-spanning G-protein–coupled receptors have all been described. The normal levels and metabolic fate of ACTH and other POMC peptides in plasma have been characterized. The pulsatile nature and circadian pattern of release of these peptides and their intracellular mechanisms of action are now understood in considerable detail. Many aspects of steroid biosynthesis, including the intracellular location and structure of the steroidogenic CYP (cytochrome P450) enzymes, the genes that encode these enzymes, and the mutations of these genes that cause various hereditary human diseases have been revealed. The discovery of cytoplasmic receptors for steroids and the elucidation of the structures of the genes that encode them have provided insights into how the steroid-receptor complex interacts with specific DNA response elements, in concert with other *trans*-acting factors, to regulate the transcription of target genes. Proteins such as the heat shock proteins and the lipocortins, which may be involved in steroid hormone action, have been identified. Finally, nontranscriptional actions of steroids, some of which involve activation of the complex of their plasma-binding protein and its cell surface receptor, have been described. Despite these advances, one need not probe deeply to discover the limits of present knowledge.

Anatomy

Embryology

Each adrenal consists of two functionally distinct endocrine glands within a single capsule. The cortex derives from mesenchymal cells attached to the coelomic cavity lining adjacent to the urogenital ridge. The fetal adrenal is recognizable by 2 mo of gestation, when it is invaded by neuroectodermal cells that will form the medulla. It becomes quite vascular and increases rapidly in size to become larger than the kidney at midgestation.[39] By the second trimester, the thin, outer *definitive* zone that will form the adult cortex is distinct; the inner *fetal* zone comprises most of the adrenal mass and still represents three quarters of the cortex at birth. The fetal zone degenerates rapidly after birth, accounting for only one quarter of the cortical mass at 2 mo and vanishing by 1 y. The definitive zone, which has distinct zonae glomerulosa and fasciculata at birth, proliferates, but total adrenal weight declines until age 2 to 3 mo. Adrenal growth thereafter parallels somatic growth. The zona reticularis develops during the first year of life.[40] Steroidogenic factor-1 (SF-1), an orphan nuclear receptor, is essential for the development of the adrenal cortex and the gonads and for the regulation of steroidogenesis.[41, 42]

Gross Structure

Each adult adrenal is a roughly pyramidal structure, 2 to 3 cm wide, 4 to 6 cm long, and about 1 cm thick, lies above or posteromedial to and occasionally attached to the upper pole of the kidney and is usually surrounded by perirenal fat. Each gland is encased in a thin layer of loose areolar connective tissue and a thick fibrous capsule. The right adrenal usually lies lower and slightly more lateral than the left. Each weighs about 4 g, regardless of age, weight, or sex, but may weigh as much as 22 g at autopsy, apparently as a result of the stress of terminal illness.[43] About 10% of adrenal weight is medulla.[4] Up to 3% of normal adults may have macroscopic nodules in the adrenal gland,[44] and micronodular changes are seen in two thirds of normal adults.[45] Most of these nodules are variants of normal structure, but on occasion they must be differentiated from those that arise under conditions of abnormal stimulation or that secrete steroids autonomously (see later discussion).

Ectopic Adrenal Tissue

Adrenal tissue can develop in ectopic sites. Except when situated medial to the gland's normal location, it consists only of cortical cells. Ectopic adrenal tissue can be located in the retroperitoneal celiac plexus, in the hilum of the spleen, adjacent to or within the ovaries, in the broad ligaments, in the scrotum, in the liver, in the wall of the gallbladder, or adjacent to the brain.[4]

Vascular Supply

The adrenals are supplied with blood by an average of 11 or 12 small arteries that branch from the aorta and the inferior phrenic, renal, often intercostal, and occasionally left ovarian or left internal spermatic arteries.[46] Sixty or more small branches form a subcapsular arteriolar plexus that drains into a rich array of radial capillaries, some of which anastomose as they penetrate the deeper zona fasciculata. These vessels then create a dense sinusoidal plexus around the cells of the zona reticularis and coalesce to form veins that traverse the medulla to empty into the central vein (Fig. 12–1). There is no direct arterial blood supply to the zonae fasciculata and reticularis.[47] A separate medullary capillary sinusoidal network, supplied by medullary arteries that penetrate the cortex, also drains into the central vein.[48] Therefore, only a minority of chromaffin cells (those that lie adjacent to the smaller radicles of the central vein) are exposed to cortical venous blood. The central vein has two to four conspicuous longitudinal smooth muscle bundles, the function of which is unknown but which presumably constrict outflow from the gland and thereby increase the exposure of cortical cells to systemic factors such as ACTH and of medullary cells to cortisol.[49] In humans the central vein and its main branches are surrounded by a cuff of cortical tissue that invaginates at the head and fuses with the cortex in the tail.[50] The right adrenal vein is short and drains into the inferior vena cava, and the

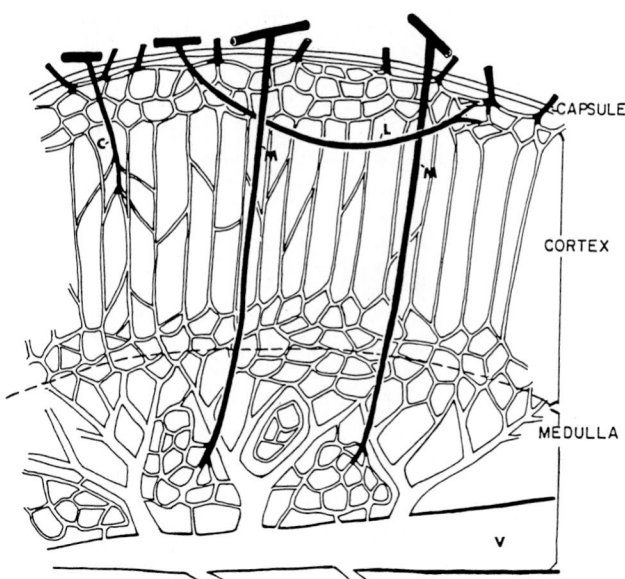

Figure 12–1. Vasculature of the mammalian adrenal gland. Arterial supply is indicated in black, venous drainage in white. C, cortical artery; L, looped artery; M, medullary arteries; V, central vein. (From Coupland RE. Blood supply of the adrenal gland. In: Greep RO, Astwood EB, eds. Handbook of Physiology. Sect 7: Endocrinology. Vol VI: Adrenal Gland. Washington, DC: American Physiological Society, 1975: 283–294.)

longer left adrenal vein usually drains into the left renal vein, either directly or after being joined by the left inferior phrenic vein. Smaller emissary veins may drain into the inferior phrenic, the renal, or, rarely, the hepatic portal veins.[51, 52]

Nerve Supply

Efferent sympathetic axons from lower thoracic and upper lumbar plexus preganglionic neurons and efferent parasympathetic axons from the celiac branch of the posterior vagal trunk form a plexus medial to the adrenal, enter the gland with the arterioles, and traverse the cortex to terminate in the medulla. Sympathetic axons also innervate the subcapsular arteriolar plexus and regulate adrenal blood flow.[53] Nerves that enter the adrenal also have endings on glomerulosa cells; they contain catecholamines and neuropeptide Y. Zona glomerulosa cells and the subcapsular plexus are also innervated by axons containing vasoactive intestinal peptide (VIP), but most of these axons arise and radiate outward from adrenomedullary cells that are under splanchnic regulation.[54] In addition, chromaffin cells may be scattered throughout all three zones of the cortex.[55] The function of these nerves is unknown, but β-adrenergic agonists and VIP may influence secretion of aldosterone and cortisol.[55, 56] An afferent pathway that is postulated to exist between the adrenal and the hypothalamus may modulate stress-induced secretion of ACTH.[57]

Light Microscopic Structure

Arnold's division of the cortex into three concentric zones[9] was based primarily on differences in vascular and connective tissue structure that are most evident in species (e.g., humans) whose adrenocortical cells contain abundant cytoplasmic lipid inclusions (Fig. 12–2). The outer zona glomerulosa constitutes about 15% of the cortex and consists of a poorly demarcated layer of U-shaped or spherical nests, several cells in diameter, lying just under the capsule. The middle zona glomerulosa is penetrated by extensions of the zona fasciculata that may reach the capsule. The glomerulosa

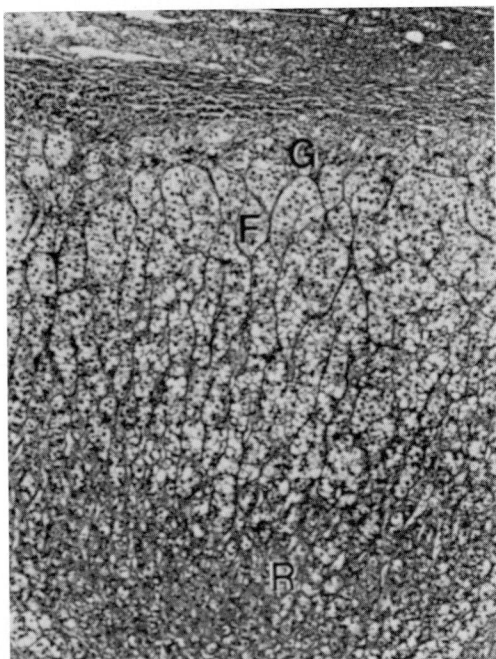

Figure 12–2. Light microscopic section of the human adrenal cortex from an unstressed individual who died of a gunshot wound. The narrow zona glomerulosa (G) lies just within the capsule, shown at the top. The broad lipid-filled zona fasciculata (F) lies between the zona glomerulosa and the dense compact cells of the zona reticularis (R). The medulla, which lies below the zona reticularis at the bottom, is not shown. (From Page DL, DeLellis RA, Hough AJ Jr. Tumors of the adrenal. In: Hartmann WH, Sobin LE, eds. Atlas of Tumor Pathology. 2nd Ser. Fasc 23. Washington, DC: Armed Forces Institute of Pathology, 1986.)

cells are small and have a lower cytoplasmic/nuclear ratio, an intermediate number of lipid inclusions, and smaller nuclei containing more condensed chromatin than the other two layers. The zona fasciculata constitutes about 75% of the cortex, is not sharply demarcated from the glomerulosa, and consists of radial cords of cells lying between delicate fibrovascular trabeculae. Its large cells have a high cytoplasmic/nuclear ratio and a foamy, vacuolated, "clear" cytoplasm because of the many lipid inclusions. The innermost zona reticularis is sharply demarcated from both the fasciculata and the medulla and consists of irregular anastomosing cords of cells separated by thin-walled sinusoids. The cytoplasmic/nuclear ratio is intermediate, and the "compact" cytoplasm is lipid poor and, in the adult, contains numerous lipofuscin granules. The cortical cuff around the central vein resembles zona glomerulosa centrally and fasciculata peripherally.[4]

As discussed later, the zona glomerulosa cells produce the mineralocorticoid aldosterone, whereas the zonae fasciculata and reticularis secrete cortisol and dehydroepiandrosterone (DHEA), which is sulfated in the zona reticularis. However, these functional differences do not explain the different arrangement and morphology of the cells in the three cortical zones.

Ultrastructure

The ultrastructure of adrenocortical cells is similar to that of other steroid-secreting cells (Fig. 12–3). Zona glomerulosa cells have small, elongated mitochondria with lamelliform cristae; scanty, finely vesiculated smooth endoplasmic reticulum; occasional lipid inclusions; and few lysosomes, lipofuscin granules, or microvilli. These cells gradually blend into typical fasciculata cells that contain small, spherical to ovoid mitochondria with vesicular cristae, abundant smooth and occasional rough endoplasmic reticulum arrayed as large vesicles

in a honeycomb pattern, abundant lipid inclusions, increased numbers of lipofuscin granules, and prominent microvilli. Cells of the zona reticularis possess small, mostly ovoid mitochondria with tubulovesicular cristae, densely packed smooth endoplasmic reticulum, rare lipid inclusions, abundant lipofuscin granules in the adult, and numerous microvilli.[4, 47]

Growth, Regeneration, and Hypertrophy

The factors that regulate adrenal growth in the fetus and maintenance of adrenal size in the adult are only partially understood. Because the adrenal gland of the anencephalic fetus develops normally for about 15 wk,[58] its early growth is presumed to be independent of fetal pituitary ACTH stimulation. From midterm until term, ACTH is essential for adrenal growth and maturation; its actions may be mediated by enhanced synthesis of insulin-like growth factor II (IGF-II) and IGF receptor by adrenocortical cells.[59] The role of placental ACTH,[60] if any, is unknown, and there is no evidence that chorionic gonadotropin or other placental factors are involved in growth of the fetal adrenal (see Chapter 28). Activin inhibits fetal zone proliferation and potentiates the ACTH-stimulated shift of steroid production from dehydroepiandrosterone sulfate (DHEAS) to cortisol by the fetal adrenal.[61] Estradiol and IGF-II also influence the pattern of fetal ACTH-stimulated steroidogenesis.[62] Inhibin appears to act as a tumor suppressor in steroidogenic tissues.[63] Factors that may regulate adrenal weight in the adult[64] include the NH_2-terminal fragment of POMC,[65, 66] epidermal growth factor, fibroblast growth factor, and IGF-I (also known as somatomedin-C).[67]

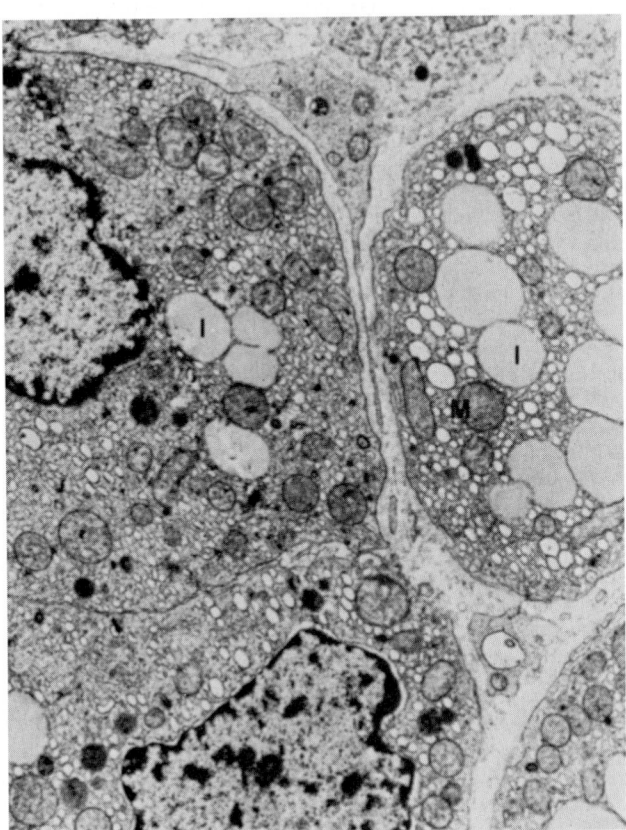

Figure 12–3. Ultrastructure of the human adrenal cortex. Cells from the inner zona fasciculata containing prominent lipid droplets (I), numerous ovoid mitochondria (M), and abundant smooth endoplasmic reticulum, which fills the cytoplasm. Uranyl acetate–lead citrate. (From Page DL, DeLellis RA, Hough AJ Jr. Tumors of the adrenal. In: Hartmann WH, Sobin LE, eds. Atlas of Tumor Pathology. 2nd Ser. Fasc 23. Washington, DC: Armed Forces Institute of Pathology, 1986.)

Maintenance of normal adrenal size and function may involve cell division in the zona glomerulosa, subsequent centripetal cell migration and differentiation in the fasciculata, and eventual senescence and death in the reticularis. Although the zonae fasciculata and reticularis of the adult adrenal can regenerate from subcapsular remnants,[68] even in ectopic locations,[69] it is less clear whether this capability is utilized in the maintenance of normal adrenal anatomy.[70] The thin layer between the zonae glomerulosa and fasciculata, termed the transitional or intermediate zone, is composed of cells that contain neither CYP11B1 or CYP11B2 and therefore cannot synthesize either cortisol or aldosterone.[71] These cells may be progenitors of glomerulosa cells and/or fasciculata cells. Studies with [³H]thymidine labeling provided evidence for centripetal cell movement.[72] Furthermore, chronic ACTH stimulation and the consequent exposure to increased ambient glucocorticoid concentrations change the phenotype of glomerulosa cells to that of fasciculata cells in regard to structure, response to stimuli, and the steroids they produce.[47, 73, 74] Chronic ACTH stimulation also converts the innermost fasciculata cells to the reticularis phenotype, a process that extends outward until the reticularis may completely replace the zona fasciculata, initially causing cell hypertrophy and then hyperplasia that is reversible when ACTH is withdrawn.[75]

Cells divide mainly within the zona glomerulosa, but the mechanisms that regulate the rate of their division and the differentiation of some glomerulosa-type cells into the fasciculata phenotype are poorly understood. The glomerulosa phenotype of some cells persists. Chronic administration of angiotensin II[76] or its physiological equivalent, dietary salt restriction, causes hypertrophy of the zona glomerulosa and increased aldosterone secretion without increasing fasciculata size or function. Furthermore, adequate basal secretion of aldosterone can persist despite years of ACTH and cortisol deficiency.[77] Finally, some patients who are "medically adrenalectomized" with mitotane, a cytotoxic drug that preferentially destroys zona fasciculata cells, maintain normal aldosterone secretion without recovery of normal cortisol secretion.[78] On the basis of these observations it appears either that the glomerulosa and fasciculata/reticularis cells arise from different stem cells or that unknown (presumably local) factors stimulate the differentiation of a common stem cell into the two major types of adrenocortical cells.

After the loss of one adrenal gland, the remaining gland can undergo compensatory hypertrophy. Such hypertrophy does not occur in the absence of the pituitary gland. ACTH appears to be the most important pituitary factor, but other hormones, such as growth hormone (hGH) and the NH₂-terminal fragment of POMC, which may be processed locally to a bioactive product,[65, 66] may also be involved. Release from chronic β-adrenergic inhibition[54, 56] and, possibly, other neurally mediated factors may also play a role.[79]

Steroid Biochemistry

The steroid hormones produced by the adrenal cortex are members of a large family of compounds derived from the cyclopentanoperhydrophenanthrene ring structure that comprises three cyclohexane rings and one cyclopentane ring (Fig. 12–4). Steroids are widely distributed in the plant and animal kingdoms. They exert a remarkable diversity of biologic effects, depending on the nature of the chemical modifications of the basic steroid nucleus, such as unsaturation of the carbon-carbon bonds in the rings and the attachment of hydroxyl, ketone, or other groups to specific carbon atoms.

Nomenclature

Steroid nomenclature follows either the chemical system established by the International Union of Pure and Applied

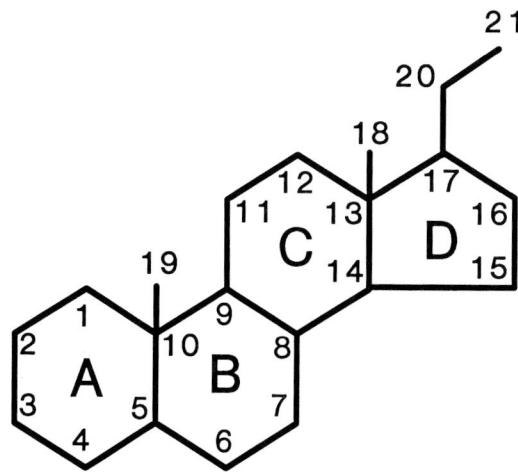

Figure 12–4. Basic steroid ring structure. The four rings are identified by letters. Individual carbon atoms comprising the steroid ring are numbered as shown. Substituent groups in derivative steroid molecules are designated by the number of the carbon atom to which they are attached. Double bonds in the ring structure are identified by the lower-numbered of the two carbon atoms they bind.

Chemistry (IUPAC) or trivial names based in part on biologic properties (Table 12–1).

IUPAC NOMENCLATURE. Begun in the early 1950s, the rules for nomenclature have subsequently been refined.[80, 81] The rings are referred to by letter and the individual carbon atoms by number (see Fig. 12–4). Parent structures have unique names. The unsaturated 17-carbon ring structure is termed *gonane*. Steroids with 18 carbons (C₁₈-steroids) derived from this molecule by addition of a methyl group at C₁₃ are *estranes*. A C₁₉-steroid formed by the addition of an another methyl at C₁₀ is an *androstane*. Further addition of an ethyl group at C₁₇ produces a *pregnane* (a C₂₁-steroid). A double bond is indicated by adding *-ene* to the name of the parent compound, its position designated by the lower-numbered carbon to which it is attached. The position of a group is indicated by the number of the carbon to which it is attached. The stereochemistry of modifying groups is designated by the letter α for those projecting behind the plane of the steroid ring and β for those in front. In structural formulas the α-configuration is denoted by a dotted line, the β-configuration by a solid line.

TRIVIAL NOMENCLATURE. The IUPAC system is too cumbersome for clinical applications, and trivial names are generally used for most steroid hormones. Table 12–1 lists both systematic and trivial names for some commonly encountered steroid hormones. Estrogens are C₁₈-steroids with an aromatized (fully unsaturated) A ring, androgens are C₁₉-steroids, and progestagens and glucocorticoids are C₂₁-derivatives. The symbol Δ indicates an unsaturated bond; its superscript number indicates the lower-numbered carbon to which it is attached.

Steroid Biosynthesis

SOURCES OF CHOLESTEROL FOR ADRENAL STEROIDOGENESIS. All human steroid hormones are derived from cholesterol. The cells of steroidogenic tissues can synthesize cholesterol de novo from acetate, mobilize intracellular cholesteryl ester pools, or import lipoprotein cholesterol from plasma. About 80% of the cholesterol precursor for steroid hormone formation in the adrenal is provided by circulating plasma lipoproteins.[82–84] Adrenal tissue in vitro utilizes low-density lipoprotein (LDL) cholesterol by a specific receptor-mediated pathway.[85–87] Such receptors are present in mouse

by virtue of the subcellular localization of the enzyme involved. The rate-limiting process in steroidogenesis is the transport of free cholesterol through the cytosol to the inner mitochondrial membrane, the site of the enzyme (CYP11A1) that catalyzes the first step in steroidogenesis. A number of factors appear to play a role in this transport,[106] including a 13.5-kd sterol carrier protein-2 (SCP-2),[107, 108] a 3.2-kd "steroidogenesis activator peptide,"[109, 110] an 8.2-kd protein,[111] and the peripheral benzodiazepine receptor.[112–114] All these proteins are believed to enhance cholesterol transfer to the inner membrane of mitochondria and to stimulate the first step in steroidogenesis, but their precise physiological roles are poorly understood at present.[106, 115] A 30-kd protein designated StAR (steroidogenic acute regulatory protein) is rapidly induced by cyclic AMP and also functions to enhance cholesterol delivery to the inner mitochondrial membrane.[116–120] Clear evidence for the role of StAR in regulation of adrenal steroidogenesis has been adduced from the study of human mutations.[116]

Within the mitochondrion, the removal of the side chain at C_{20} that converts cholesterol to pregnenolone was thought to proceed through the generation of several intermediates: 20-hydroxycholesterol, 22-hydroxycholesterol, and 20,22-dihydroxycholesterol.[121–125] Three distinct enzymes were thought be involved: 20- and 22-hydroxylases and a 20,22-lyase. However, a single protein catalyzes the complete reaction,[126–129] and a single mRNA species encodes the enzyme in steroidogenic tissues.[130, 131] The *CYP11A1* gene is present on the long arm of human chromosome 15 (q24-q25).[131]

The electrons transferred by CYP11A1 during the side-chain cleavage reaction are provided through an electron transport system comprised of adrenodoxin, a non-heme iron-binding protein that exists in soluble form in the mitochondrial matrix, and adrenodoxin reductase, a mitochondrial membrane–bound flavoprotein. Adrenodoxin reductase accepts electrons from NADPH and transfers them to adrenodoxin, which serves as a shuttle to deliver reducing equivalents to various CYPs (Fig. 12–6).[132] Humans have a single expressed gene for adrenodoxin on chromosome 11 (q13-qter), two adrenodoxin pseudogenes on chromosome 20, and a single gene for adrenodoxin reductase on chromosome 17 (q24-q25).[133, 134] Alternative splicing produces two forms of adrenodoxin reductase mRNA,[135] the functional significance of the resulting two forms being unknown.[136]

Conversion of Pregnenolone to Progesterone by 3β-HSD/Δ⁴,⁵-Isomerase. Newly synthesized pregnenolone is returned to the cytosolic compartment, where a series of microsomal enzymes convert it to 11-deoxycortisol. First, it is converted to progesterone by dehydrogenation of the 3-hydroxyl group of pregnenolone and isomerization of the double bond at C_5. These enzymatic processes are carried out by a 3β-HSD enzyme that is expressed in the adrenal and gonads.[137] This

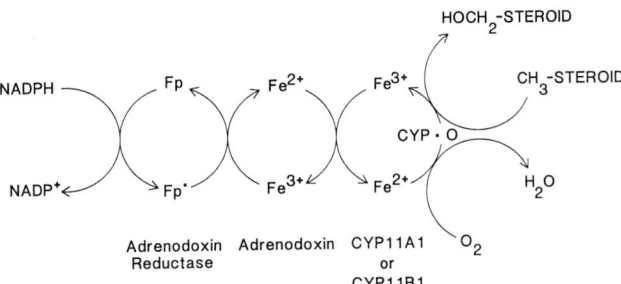

Figure 12–6. Electron shuttle system for the mitochondrial enzymes, CYP11A1 and CYP11B1. Adrenodoxin reductase receives electrons from NADPH and reduces adrenodoxin, which transfers reducing equivalents to the CYP enzyme. The enzyme then transfers electrons, by way of oxygen, to the steroid. Fp, flavoprotein; Fp•, reduced form of flavoprotein.

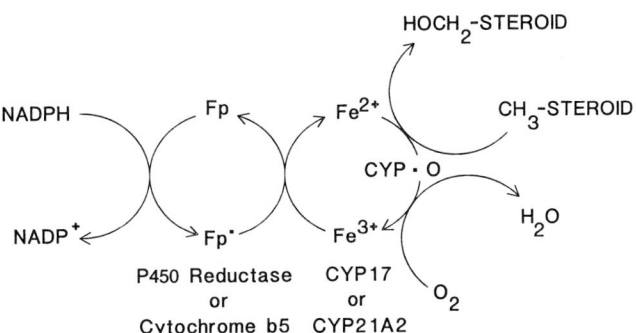

Figure 12–7. Electron shuttle system for the microsomal enzymes, CYP17 and CYP21A2. P450 reductase, a flavoprotein, accepts electrons from NADPH and transfers them to the NADPH-P450 enzyme. The enzyme then transfers electrons, by way of oxygen, to the steroid. A second reducing equivalent may be supplied to CYP17 by NADPH-P450 reductase or cytochrome b_5.

enzyme, human 3β-HSD type II, is encoded by a gene, *HSD3B2*, distinct from that for the placental form of the enzyme (type I).

Conversion of Progesterone to 17α-Hydroxyprogesterone by CYP17. CYP17 is a microsomal enzyme that catalyzes both the hydroxylation of the C_{17} of progesterone or pregnenolone (17α-hydroxylase activity) and the cleavage of the residual two-carbon side chain at C_{17} (17,20-lysase activity).[138, 139] Human CYP17 is encoded by a gene on chromosome 10 (q24.3).[140, 141] The dual function of this enzyme allows direction of the steroid precursors along several different pathways: 17α-hydroxylated substrates with the side chain intact are glucocorticoid precursors, whereas generation of C_{19} steroids by both 17α-hydroxylase and 17,20-lyase activities directs substrate toward androgen and estrogen synthesis. In the zona glomerulosa, which lacks either CYP17 activity, pregnenolone is converted into mineralocorticoids. Whether a given steroid molecule undergoes both 17α-hydroxylation and lysis of the 17,20 bond appears to depend on the supply of electrons to CYP17 from a flavoprotein distinct from mitochondrial adrenodoxin. This protein, NADPH-P450 reductase, also supplies electrons to CYP21A2, the other microsomal CYP enzyme.[142] NADPH-P450 reductase transfers two electrons sequentially from NADPH to CYP17. Cytochrome b_5 may also donate the second electron (Fig. 12–7). Since CYP17, with both its 17α-hydroxylase and 17,20-lyase activities, and CYP21A2 are present in large molar excess compared with the reductase, they compete for the same pool of electrons.[105, 143–145] With a sufficient flux of electrons from NADPH-P450 reductase or cytochrome b_5 (or both), both 17α-hydroxylation and C_{21} side-chain cleavage occur.

Conversion of 17α-Hydroxyprogesterone to 11-Deoxycortisol by CYP21A2. Both progesterone and its 17α-hydroxylated derivative undergo 21-hydroxylation by the CYP21A2 enzyme located in the smooth endoplasmic reticulum.[142] Two genes encoding 21-hydroxylase enzymes are located on the short arm of chromosome 6,[146–150] but only *CYP21A2* is active in humans; the other, *CYP21A1P*, is a pseudogene.[151]

Conversion of 11-Deoxycortisol to Cortisol by CYP11B1. The last step in cortisol biosynthesis is the 11β-hydroxylation of 11-deoxycortisol, catalyzed by the mitochondrial enzyme CYP11B1. Like CYP11A1, the other P450 enzyme of the inner mitochondrial membrane, CYP11B1 receives electrons from NADPH via adrenodoxin reductase and adrenodoxin.[152, 153] CYP11B1 is encoded by a gene on the long arm of chromosome 8.[154] The enzyme is a 479-amino-acid protein of molecular weight 51 kd that is almost identical to the P450 enzyme responsible for the terminal steps of aldosterone synthesis (see later discussion), but it lacks the ability to convert corticosterone into aldosterone. CYP11B1 is more closely related to CYP11A1 than to the microsomal CYPs.[154-156]

Mineralocorticoid Biosynthesis. Progesterone is also the substrate for mineralocorticoid synthesis (see Fig. 12-5). In the zona glomerulosa progesterone is hydroxylated at C_{21} by CYP21A2 to yield DOC. All three terminal steps in the conversion of this intermediate to aldosterone (11β-hydroxylation, 18-hydroxylation, and 18-methyl oxidation) are catalyzed by a single mitochondrial P450 enzyme.[157] The human CYP11B2 (aldosterone synthase) is encoded by a gene on the long arm of chromosome 8 that shares more than 90% sequence homology with CYP11B1 at the protein level.[158] On denaturing polyacrylamide gel electrophoresis the CYP11B2 appears to have a molecular weight of 49 kd.[157, 159]

Adrenal Androgen Biosynthesis. Adrenal steroids with 19 carbon atoms include DHEA and its sulfate, DHEAS, the most abundant products of the adrenal glands (see Fig. 12-5). They are formed from 17α-hydroxypregnenolone by the 17,20-lyase activity of CYP17. Androstenedione, another 19-carbon steroid (Table 12-3), is produced by side-chain cleavage of 17α-hydroxyprogesterone by CYP17. DHEA and androstenedione can serve as substrate for the formation of testosterone in peripheral tissues; synthesis of testosterone in the adrenal is minimal.

Adrenal Estrogen Biosynthesis. Estrogens are produced from 19-carbon androgens by the microsomal CYP enzyme, aromatase,[105, 160] whose net effect is removal of carbon 19 and creation of a conjugated double bond system (aromatization) in the A ring with a hydroxyl group in the 3 position. Only small amounts of estrogen are synthesized by the normal adrenal,[161] but DHEA, DHEAS, and androstenedione are substrates for estrogen production by peripheral tissues such as adipose tissue, which contain considerable aromatase activity (see Chapters 15 through 17).[162]

Fetal Adrenal Steroid Biosynthesis. A morphologically and functionally distinct "fetal zone" exists in the human fetal adrenal gland until birth, after which it rapidly involutes.[163] Under ACTH stimulation, the fetal zone both imports LDL cholesterol[164-166] and synthesizes cholesterol de novo[167] to serve as substrate for the formation of pregnenolone sulfate and DHEAS,[168-170] which are detectable at about 25 wk of gestation.[171] Predominant secretion of Δ^5 steroids such as DHEAS apparently results from the low 3β-HSD/$\Delta^{4,5}$-isomerase activity required to convert 17α-hydroxypregnenolone to 17α-hydroxyprogesterone.[172] DHEAS is converted in peripheral fetal tissues to 16α-hydroxy-DHEAS,[173] which serves as substrate for the synthesis of estriol in the placenta. Estrogen, in turn, inhibits 3β-HSD activity in the fetal adrenal, thus enhancing production of DHEAS.[174]

FUNCTIONAL ANATOMY. The structural zones of the adrenal cortex roughly correlate with the biosynthesis of different steroids. As already noted, the fetal zone of the fetal adrenal is deficient in 3β-HSD and therefore produces little cortisol but prodigious amounts of DHEAS. The definitive zone of the fetal adrenal produces mainly cortisol, the major glucocorticoid in humans. In the mature gland, the zona glomerulosa and the outermost portion of the fasciculata synthesize the major mineralocorticoid, aldosterone. The fascicu-

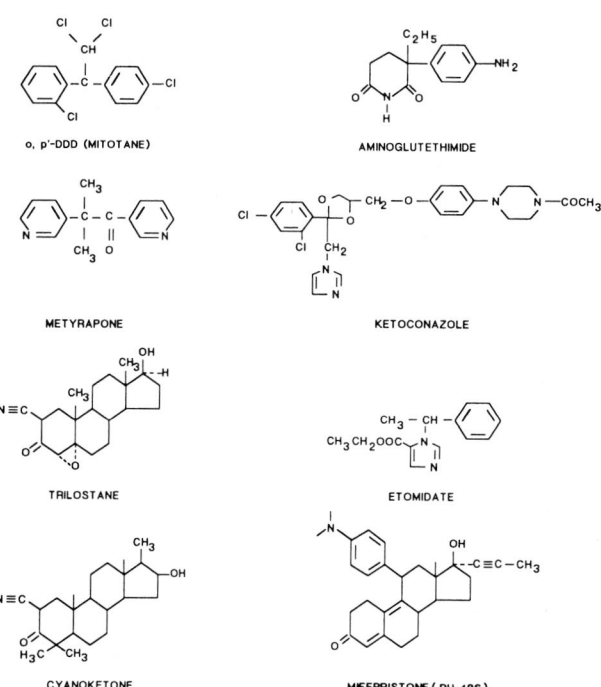

Figure 12-8. Structures of inhibitors of steroid synthesis or action. Mitotane is an adrenocorticolytic drug. Aminoglutethimide, metyrapone, cyanoketone, ketoconazole, trilostane, and etomidate are inhibitors of steroidogenesis. Mifepristone (RU486) is a competitive antagonist of glucocorticoid that binds to its receptor in target cells and is an even more potent antagonist of progesterone, binding to its receptor.

lata and, less importantly, the reticularis synthesize cortisol. In addition to DOC and 18-hydroxy-DOC, which are mainly products of the zona glomerulosa, DHEA and other adrenal androgens and estrogens are also synthesized by the fasciculata and reticularis,[175-178] sulfation occurring exclusively in the reticularis.[179] DHEAS is the major steroid product of the mature adrenal in terms of amount, but it is not the most important one physiologically.

INHIBITORS OF STEROIDOGENESIS. A number of compounds (Fig. 12-8) can inhibit adrenal steroidogenesis by interfering with one or more of the enzymatic processes described earlier. These compounds have been useful not only for characterization of the enzymes involved in steroid synthesis but also in the therapy of conditions of glucocorticoid excess (see later discussion).

Adrenocorticolytic: Mitotane. In 1949 the insecticide DDT was recognized to produce adrenal deficiency in dogs.[180] The active component is 2,2-bis(2-chlorophenyl-4-chlorophenyl)-1,1-dichloroethane, or o,p'-DDD, termed *mitotane*.[181] Administration of mitotane to dogs causes necrosis and hemorrhage in the zonae fasciculata and reticularis, with relative sparing of the zona glomerulosa.[182] There is considerable intraspecies variation in sensitivity to the drug, but normal and neoplastic human adrenal glands are sensitive to the cytotoxic effect, and the agent is used to produce a medical adrenalectomy under certain circumstances (see later discussion).[183-185] Mitotane also alters the peripheral metabolism of cortisol.[186] Ordinarily, cortisol is metabolized to compounds measurable in urine as 17-hydroxycorticosteroids (17-OHCS; see later discussion). Mitotane causes a 50 to 80% reduction in these metabolites by diverting metabolism toward formation of a more polar compound, 6β-hydroxycortisol, that is not measured in the assay.[186]

CYP11A1 Inhibition: Aminoglutethimide. Aminoglutethimide was developed for clinical use as an anticonvulsant be-

TABLE 12-3. Relative Androgenic Activity of Adrenal Androgens

Steroid	Activity
Dihydrotestosterone	300
Testosterone	100
Androstenedione	10
DHEA, DHEAS	5

Adapted from Nelson DH. The Adrenal Cortex: Physiological Function and Disease. Philadelphia, WB Saunders, 1980: 1122.

fore discovery of its antisteroidogenic activity.[187] The compound inhibits CYP11A1, which converts cholesterol to Δ^5-pregnenolone,[188] resulting in decreased cortisol levels and a compensatory increase in pituitary ACTH secretion,[189] which tends to override the drug-induced blockade. Because an early step in steroidogenesis is inhibited, mineralocorticoid biosynthesis is also decreased. The compensatory increase in plasma renin activity cannot completely overcome the blockade, and persons treated with the compound have decreased aldosterone secretion.[189] Aminoglutethimide is useful for controlling hypercortisolism in patients with Cushing's syndrome caused by autonomous secretion of cortisol or ACTH (see later discussion).

CYP11B1 Inhibition: Metyrapone. Metyrapone is mainly an inhibitor of CYP11B1, which catalyzes the final step in cortisol biosynthesis, conversion of 11-deoxycortisol to cortisol.[190-192] Metyrapone also inhibits aldosterone secretion[193] (presumably by inhibition of CYP11B2), but its effect on electrolyte metabolism is mitigated by increased production of DOC. Production of adrenal androgen precursors is also increased. Metyrapone is useful for diagnostic testing of hypothalamic-pituitary-adrenal axis function and for controlling hypercortisolism in patients with Cushing's syndrome caused by autonomous secretion of cortisol or ACTH (see later discussion).

3β-HSD Inhibition: Cyanoketone. Cyanoketone (2α-cyano-4,4,17α-trimethylandrost-5-ene-17β-ol-3-one) is a 19-carbon steroid analogue that inhibits 3β-HSD activity in rats.[194] It inhibits the enzyme in all steroidogenic tissues and thereby reduces production of both gonadal and adrenal steroids. It has not been used clinically.

Multiple Enzyme Inhibition: Ketoconazole and Etomidate. Several imidazole-derived antifungal drugs have antisteroidogenic actions in humans. These compounds inhibit a fungal CYP enzyme system.[195] Effects on human testosterone production were first recognized[196] after men taking the drug developed gynecomastia.[197] Ketoconazole acts in the adrenal primarily by inhibiting CYP11B1, but it also inhibits CYP11A1.[198, 199] Like aminoglutethimide and metyrapone, it is useful in treating some patients with Cushing's syndrome (see later discussion). Etomidate, another imidazole derivative, is a parenteral anesthetic that is used to sedate patients on mechanical ventilators in intensive care units. As with ketoconazole, the major effect of etomidate is inhibition of CYP11B1,[200-204] but higher doses also inhibit CYP11A1.[200, 205] Etomidate can also be used to control cortisol secretion in hospitalized patients with Cushing's syndrome (see later discussion).[206]

Blockade of Cortisol Action: Mifepristone. Mifepristone does not inhibit steroidogenesis, but it antagonizes the peripheral actions of glucocorticoids and progestagens because it is a competitive inhibitor for binding to their cytosolic receptor proteins.[207, 208] It is an effective abortifacient and has been used in patients with Cushing's syndrome (see later discussion).

Regulation of Glucocorticoid Secretion

The Hypothalamic-Pituitary-Adrenal Axis

Glucocorticoid secretion is regulated by hormonal interactions among the hypothalamus, pituitary, and adrenal glands and by neural and other stimuli (Fig. 12–9).[209-211] Neural stimuli from the brain, as in the response to stress, cause the release of CRH, AVP, and other agents from hypothalamic neurons into the hypothalamic-hypophyseal portal blood. They are carried to the pituitary, where they stimulate ACTH secretion into the systemic blood. ACTH acts on the adrenal cortex to cause secretion of cortisol and other steroids. The negative feedback loop is completed by the inhibitory effect

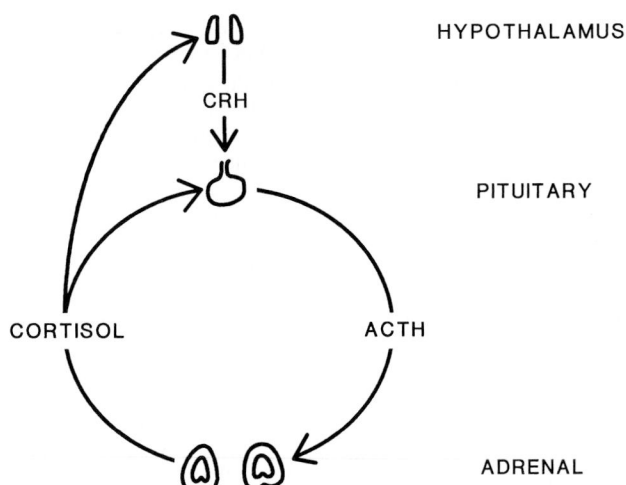

Figure 12–9. Normal regulation of adrenal glucocorticoid secretion. CRH and other hypothalamic releasing factors, such as AVP, are regulated by central nervous system afferents mediating the circadian rhythm and responses to stress. ACTH and other POMC peptides are released from anterior pituitary corticotropes. ACTH stimulates the cells of the inner two zones of the adrenal cortex to produce cortisol, which inhibits the synthesis and release of CRH and the action of CRH, AVP, and other secretagogues on the pituitary corticotrope.

of glucocorticoids on synthesis and secretion of CRH, AVP, and ACTH.

Pro-opiomelanocortin

STRUCTURE, SYNTHESIS, AND PROCESSING

The POMC Gene. ACTH is synthesized as part of a 241-amino-acid precursor, POMC, which also contains the sequences for the lipotropins (LPHs), melanocyte-stimulating hormones (MSHs), and β-endorphin (β-END) (Fig. 12–10).[212-214] The human POMC gene is located on chromosome 2.[212, 213, 215] The gene structure is the same among different species, and there is considerable sequence homology. Exon 3 codes for most of the translated sequence, whereas exon 2 codes for the signal peptide and the 18 NH$_2$-terminal amino acids of POMC.

Post-Translational Processing. POMC undergoes extensive post-translational processing, including cleavage, glycosylation, phosphorylation, sulfation, and NH$_2$-terminal acetylation and COOH-terminal amidation of certain cleaved peptides (see Fig. 12–10).[216-218] Multiple peptides are produced from the POMC precursor by tissue-specific enzymatic cleavage. In the anterior pituitary the principal peptide products are the NH$_2$-terminal (NT) peptide, the joining peptide (JP), ACTH, and β-LPH. In the intermediate lobe, which is fully developed in most subprimates but is active in humans only during fetal life and pregnancy, ACTH is cleaved into ACTH(1–14), the precursor of α-MSH, and ACTH(18–39), the corticotropin-like intermediate lobe peptide (CLIP); β-LPH is completely processed into γ-LPH and β-END; and the NT peptide is cleaved to yield γ$_3$-MSH. Glycosylation can occur at Thr^{45} and Asn^{65} of the NT peptide.[219] ACTH is glycosylated in rodents but not in humans. The JP and ACTH(1–14) are further modified by cleavage of the COOH-terminal glycine and amidation of the adjacent amino acid.[220] β-END and ACTH(1–13) amide (desacetyl-α-MSH) can be modified by the addition of one or two acetyl groups to the NH$_2$-termini, yielding acetyl-β-END and α-MSH [acetyl-ACTH(1–13) amide] or diacetyl-α-MSH.[221] In the anterior lobe, less than 1% of ACTH and β-LPH undergoes similar cleavage, and the products are not acetylated[222] because the necessary enzyme is not present. In the testis and other nonpituitary tissues, four or five amino

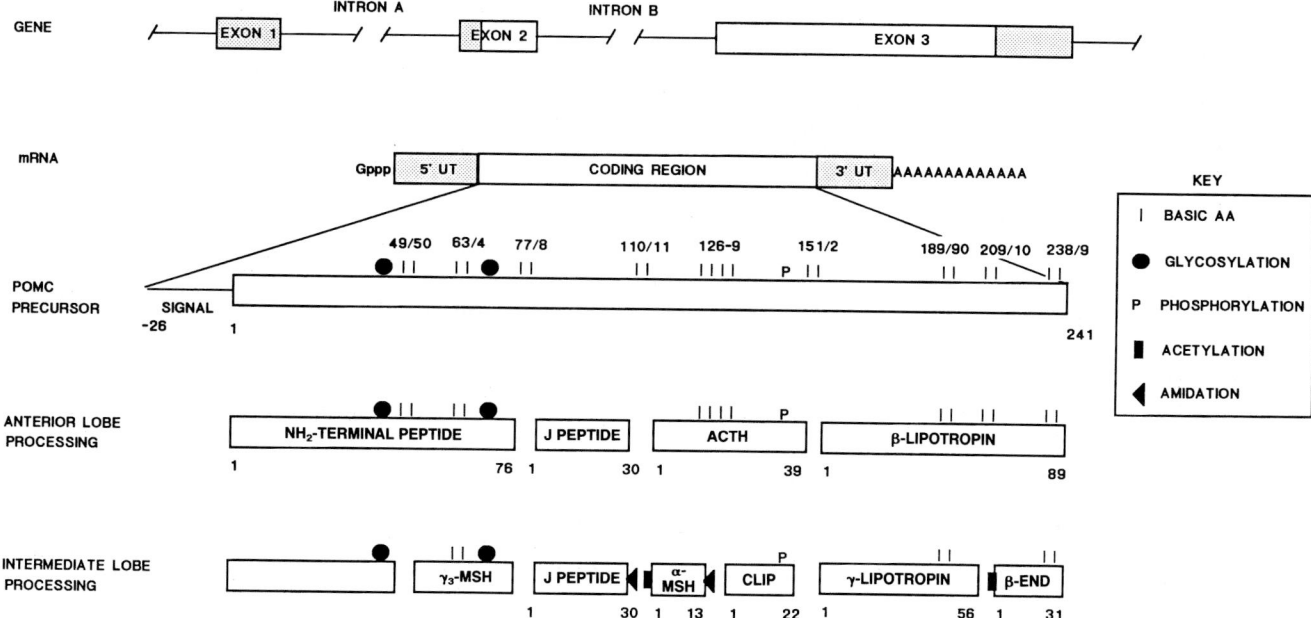

Figure 12–10. Structures of the human POMC gene, its mRNA, precursor POMC with its 26-amino-acid signal sequence, and the mature peptides produced from POMC by cleavage at basic dipeptides in the anterior lobe and, in the fetus and pregnant woman, the intermediate lobe-like corticotropes. UT, flanking untranslated region; J PEPTIDE, joining peptide; and CLIP, corticotropin-like intermediate lobe peptide.

acids can be cleaved from the COOH-terminal end of β-END to produce γ-END [β-END(1–27)], or α-END [β-END(1–26)].[223] About one third of ACTH in the human pituitary is phosphorylated at Ser-31,[224] and the carbohydrate side chains of POMC peptides may be sulfated[225]; the significance of these modifications is unknown. Although the sequence for met-enkephalin is present in the NH₂ terminus of β-END, this peptide arises from a different precursor protein.

PLASMA POMC-DERIVED PEPTIDES AND THEIR ACTIONS

Anterior Lobe Peptides. POMC and intermediate precursor forms have no steroidogenic activity; in fact, POMC may be a competitive antagonist of ACTH in the fetal adrenal.[226] ACTH is a 39-amino-acid peptide that stimulates secretion of glucocorticoids, androgenic steroids, and, to a lesser extent, mineralocorticoids from the adrenal cortex (Fig. 12–11). The first 24 NH₂-terminal amino acids of ACTH are the same in all species studied, but there are minor species differences in the COOH-terminal portion of the molecule. The half-life of circulating ACTH depends on how it is measured. Bioactivity disappears from the circulating blood with a half-life of 4 to 8 min, whereas immunoreactivity may disappear more or less rapidly, depending on which part of the ACTH amino acid sequence the antibody recognizes.[227–229] The biologically active portion of ACTH is the first 18 NH₂-terminal amino acids. Because of rapid metabolic degradation of this molecule, synthetic ACTH(1–24) or, in some countries, synthetic ACTH(1–18) amide is used for clinical purposes.

ACTH, β-LPH, JP, and the NT peptide arise from the same precursor protein, so they are secreted in approximately equimolar amounts, resulting in similar plasma levels basally and after stimulation by hypocortisolemia (e.g., during metyrapone administration), hypoglycemia, or the administration of CRH or AVP.[230–233] However, the longer half-life of circulating

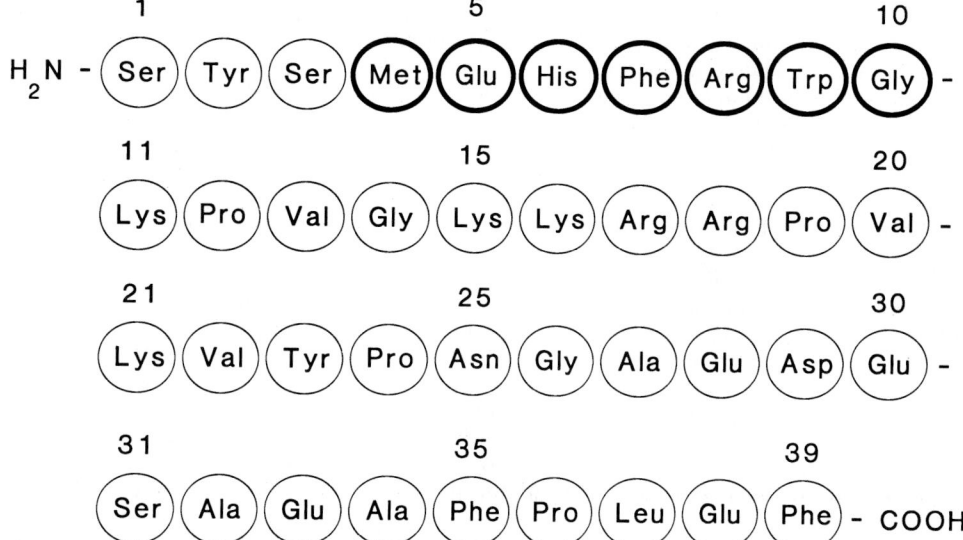

Figure 12–11. Amino acid sequence of ACTH. The heptapeptide core sequence common to ACTH, α-MSH, β-MSH, and, with slight modification, γ-MSH is indicated by the heavy circles.

β-LPH compared with ACTH results in a slower decline in the plasma level of β-LPH and an elevated plasma β-LPH/ACTH ratio after a secretory episode or during prolonged hypersecretion. The ratio is also elevated in patients undergoing chronic hemodialysis.[234] These observations imply that β-LPH has no direct or indirect feedback effect on POMC synthesis or secretion. The physiological function of β-LPH, an 89-amino-acid peptide in humans, is unknown, although it has weak steroidogenic and lipolytic activities.[235, 236] It was thought to have potent melanotropic activity,[237] but β-MSH and presumably β-LPH bind relatively weakly to the human melanocortin-1 (i.e., MSH) receptor.[238] The NT peptide and its NH$_2$-terminal fragments may be adrenal growth factors,[65, 66, 239] and the NT peptide and β-LPH may modulate the action of ACTH on steroidogenesis and have weak steroidogenic activity of their own.[236]

The three MSH regions in the POMC precursor, α, β, and γ, consist of identical six-amino-acid core sequences and similar flanking regions. MSH darkens skin by binding to melanocortin-1 receptors on melanocytes, activating adenylyl cyclase and thus tyrosinase, and thereby stimulating melanin synthesis. Although they are flanked by basic dipeptides that are the sites of post-translational cleavage, the MSHs are not produced in appreciable amounts by the human pituitary gland. Therefore, the hyperpigmentation that occurs in primary adrenal insufficiency and in Nelson's syndrome is presumably caused by the melanotropic activity of the elevated plasma level of ACTH, which binds avidly to the human melanocortin-1 (i.e., MSH) receptor.[238, 240, 241] Other reported effects of α-MSH include stimulation of aldosterone secretion in hypophysectomized rats,[242] enhancement of growth of the adrenal zona glomerulosa,[243] gonadotropin-releasing activity,[244] potentiation of the acute stimulatory effect of ACTH on aldosterone secretion, and reduction of inflammation.[245, 246] However, plasma α-MSH levels are too low to exert any of these effects in humans.

Intermediate Lobe Peptides. The intermediate lobe peptides are not present in significant amounts in normal human plasma but may be secreted by some pituitary and nonpituitary tumors. α-MSH and diacetyl-α-MSH are potent melanotropins,[245] β-MSH has intermediate melanotropic activity, and CLIP is a weak insulin secretagogue[247] and may stimulate pancreatic exocrine function.[248] β-END has potent opioid activity in the central nervous system, but its function in peripheral plasma is unknown. Acetyl-β-END is devoid of opioid activity.

Nonpituitary Production of ACTH and POMC-Related Peptides. It was originally thought that the POMC gene is expressed only in the pituitary, but in fact the gene is widely expressed in nonpituitary tissues,[218, 249–253] including brain, hypothalamus, liver, kidney, gastrointestinal tract, reproductive tissues, placenta, lymphocytes, and monocytes. Except perhaps in the placenta, the peptide levels are so low that it is unlikely they contribute significantly to circulating levels. The POMC-like mRNA in all tissues except the hypothalamus is shorter than in the pituitary and lacks exons 1 and 2 and part of exon 3.[254] Consequently, it may not be translated efficiently[252] and, because the product lacks a signal peptide, may not be secreted.[255] The POMC peptide levels in nonpituitary tissues are not altered by dexamethasone treatment,[250] but gonadal POMC peptide and POMC-like mRNA levels are increased by gonadotropins and lowered by androgen treatment.[256, 257] The function of these peptides in nonpituitary tissues is uncertain, but they may have paracrine or autocrine actions. Melanocortin receptors are widely distributed in the brain and peripheral tissues.[258, 259]

ACTIONS OF ACTH ON THE ADRENAL CORTEX

Steroidogenesis. The primary action of ACTH on the adrenal cortex is to increase cortisol synthesis and secretion.

Intra-adrenal cortisol storage is minimal.[260, 261] ACTH depletes adrenal cholesterol content,[262] which correlates with steroid synthesis.[263]

ACTH acts by binding to a cell-surface receptor on adrenal cells, the melanocortin-2 receptor,[264, 265] which has an apparent dissociation constant (K$_d$) of about 1 nM.[266] About 3560 receptor molecules are present on each adrenocortical cell, and ACTH up-regulates expression of the receptor, thereby enhancing the steroidogenic response to ACTH stimulation.[267, 268] ACTH binding activates adenylate cyclase activation and increases cAMP concentration, which in turn activates cAMP-dependent protein kinase (protein kinase A) and phosphorylation of a number of proteins.[269] Extracellular calcium is required for optimal ACTH binding[270] and ACTH-induced steroidogenesis.[271] Extracellular calcium enters through T-type calcium (Ca^{2+}) channels, independent of adenylyl cyclase activation; low-voltage A-type potassium (K$^+$) channels may also be important.[272] Release of intracellular calcium may also play a role in steps subsequent to ACTH binding.[261, 273] Most actions of ACTH, except T-type Ca^{2+} channel activation, appear to be mediated through cAMP.[274–276] Optimal adrenal responses may require cell-cell communication through gap junctions[277] that facilitate the passage of Ca^{2+} or other cytoplasmic mediators of ACTH action. ACTH-stimulated increases in expression of proto-oncogenes such as *fos-B*, *jun B*, *c-fos*, and *c-jun* may be involved both in steroidogenesis and in cell proliferation[278, 279] via the cAMP-dependent protein kinase pathway.[280] ACTH, the major cortisol secretagogue, may interact with a number of other factors in regulating adrenal steroidogenesis, especially in the fetus. These include angiotensin II,[281] transforming growth factor (TGF),[281–283] pancreatic polypeptide,[284] CRH,[285] IGF-II,[286] prolactin,[287] estradiol,[62] and epinephrine.[288] Some of these and other factors, such as tumor necrosis factor α (TNF-α),[289] are produced in the adrenal gland, and some, such as inhibin, are regulated by ACTH.[290] Activin selectively inhibits fetal zone proliferation and potentiates the ACTH-stimulated shift from DHEAS to cortisol production by the fetal adrenal[61]; estradiol and IGF-II also modulate the pattern of fetal ACTH-stimulated steroidogenesis.[62] Inhibin appears to act as a tumor suppressor in steroidogenic tissues; mice in which the inhibin gene has been inactivated by homologous recombination develop adrenal and gonadal tumors.[63]

The effects of ACTH on steroidogenesis can be divided into acute effects, which occur within minutes, and chronic effects, which require hours or days.[291, 292] The acute effect of ACTH is to increase conversion of cholesterol to Δ^5-pregnenolone, the initial step in cortisol biosynthesis.[261, 291, 292] As discussed earlier, this effect is mediated by activation of cholesterol delivery to the inner mitochondrial membrane, where CYP11A1 is located.[116] In contrast, the chronic effects of ACTH involve increased synthesis of most of the enzymes of the steroidogenic pathway and more general actions on the synthesis of RNA and DNA and growth of adrenocortical cells.[261, 291, 292] When ACTH levels are low, such as after hypophysectomy or during glucocorticoid administration, steroid biosynthesis declines, and the levels of all steroidogenic CYP enzymes[291] and of protein and RNA synthesis decline.[269, 292] With prolonged ACTH deficiency the adrenal glands become small and atrophic. These changes are reversed by ACTH administration, although steroidogenesis may take several days to return to normal, and return of adrenal size takes even longer. ACTH is essential for normal steroidogenesis and is required but is not sufficient, by itself, to maintain normal adrenal size.[64, 293]

In bovine adrenocortical cells, ACTH increases the rate of synthesis of all steroidogenic CYP enzymes, including CYP11A1,[294] CYP17,[295] CYP21A2,[296] and CYP11B1,[297] as well as adrenodoxin[298] and adrenodoxin reductase.[292] Protein synthesis is maximal 24 to 36 h after ACTH stimulation.[292] The levels of mRNAs coding for all of these enzymes increase, some within 4 h of exposure to ACTH.[292] The increased mRNA levels are the result of increased rates of gene transcription.[292, 299] These effects, like the acute effects of ACTH, are reproduced by cAMP analogues, indicating that they are mediated by cAMP.[292, 300] The exact mechanism by which cAMP increases adrenocortical CYP enzyme gene transcription is not fully understood, but it involves cAMP-dependent protein kinase[301] and may involve a cAMP response element (CRE), as in bovine granulosa cells,[302] but through a non–CRE-binding, non–SF-1 protein that binds to an SF-1–like regulatory sequence.[303] Cycloheximide, which inhibits protein synthesis at the level of translation, blocks the ACTH-induced increase in CYP mRNA levels, suggesting that the mechanism involves a *trans*-acting nuclear protein that turns over rapidly.[299]

ACTH also increases the synthesis of other proteins required for steroidogenesis, such as the LDL receptor, apolipoprotein AI, and the HDL receptor,[101] which are involved in the uptake of circulating cholesterol; adrenodoxin,[298] which is needed for transfer of reducing equivalents; SCP-2,[163, 304] which is required for transportation of cholesterol from intracellular lipid stores to mitochondria; and, in fetal but not adult adrenals, HMG-CoA reductase,[305] which catalyzes the rate-limiting step in cholesterol biosynthesis. The increase in HMG-CoA reductase and part of the increase in LDL receptors are thought to occur secondary to cholesterol depletion, rather than as direct actions of ACTH or cAMP.[163, 305] It was thought that the major source of cholesterol for steroid synthesis is circulating LDL,[85, 163, 292] but HDL cholesterol, taken up through HDL receptors present on adrenal cells,[100] is required for cholesteryl ester formation and normal adrenal steroid production in mice.[101] It is not known whether HDL receptor expression is regulated by ACTH or whether HDL is an important source of cholesterol in the human adrenal.

Maintenance of Adrenal Weight. ACTH stimulates adrenal growth as well as steroidogenesis. Supraphysiological plasma ACTH concentrations stimulate adrenocortical hypertrophy and hyperplasia, and ACTH deficiency results in adrenal atrophy.[306] An early effect of ACTH is increased adrenal blood flow.[307] Longer exposure to ACTH increases total RNA and protein synthesis and, later, DNA content and adrenal weight.[306] Removal of one adrenal gland in rats causes compensatory growth of the remaining adrenal that occurs mainly by cell proliferation. The role of ACTH in this process is in some doubt, because administration of ACTH antibodies, which decrease steroidogenesis, does not alter adrenal growth[308] and because physiological concentrations of ACTH inhibit compensatory hypertrophy of the remaining adrenal[309] and inhibit proliferation of cultured adrenal cells.[310, 311] Therefore, it is likely that other factors participate in maintaining normal adrenal weight. One candidate, a peptide consisting of the 28 NH$_2$-terminal amino acids of POMC, has mitogenic effects on adrenal cells in vivo and in vitro and partially prevents adrenal atrophy after hypophysectomy.[65, 66] Other studies suggest that neural stimuli originate from the site of the removed adrenal gland, ascend through the spinal cord to the medial basal hypothalamus, and descend to the remaining adrenal gland, stimulating compensatory hypertrophy.[312, 313]

EXTRA-ADRENAL ACTIONS OF ACTH. Large doses of ACTH increase glucose and amino acid transport into muscle cells,[314] increase hepatic protein synthesis,[315] and increase cAMP and stimulate lipolysis in adipocytes,[316] which have both melanocortin-2 receptors and the much more widely distributed melanocortin-5 receptors, which respond to α-MSH.[317] Physiological levels of ACTH do not cause these effects, but elevated plasma ACTH concentrations, as in patients with Nelson's syndrome or untreated primary adrenal insufficiency, may be sufficient. As already mentioned, ACTH binds avidly to the human melanocortin-1 (or MSH) receptor[240, 241, 318] and

is the cause of melanocyte proliferation and hyperpigmentation when plasma POMC peptide levels are elevated.[241]

Corticotropin-Releasing Hormone

STRUCTURE AND SYNTHESIS. In 1955 two groups demonstrated independently that a hypothalamic factor increases ACTH release from pituitary cells.[319, 320] More than 25 y later, ovine CRH was finally isolated and sequenced.[37, 321] Subsequently, the CRHs of other species were characterized.[322–324] CRH is a 41-amino-acid peptide that appears to be the major physiological ACTH secretagogue (Fig. 12–12).[325–327] There is considerable sequence homology among species, particularly in the NH$_2$-terminal region, which is required for biologic activity. Rat and human CRHs are identical. CRH belongs to a family of peptides that includes sauvagine from frog skin and urotensin I from teleost fish, both of which have ACTH-releasing and hypotensive activities like those of CRH.[321, 328, 329] Analyses of ovine[330] and rat[331] CRH cDNAs and human[332] and rat[333] genomic DNAs indicate that CRH is synthesized as a larger precursor (191 amino acids in humans), from which it is cleaved at flanking basic amino acid pairs. The single human CRH gene is located on chromosome 8.[334]

BIOSYNTHESIS. CRH is synthesized by neurons of the parvicellular division of the hypothalamic paraventricular nucleus.[335–337] Their axons project to the median eminence, where CRH is secreted into the hypophyseal portal blood. These neurons, particularly after adrenalectomy, may also contain other ACTH secretagogues, such as AVP[338, 339] and cholecystokinin[340]; opioid peptides, such as met-enkephalin[341] and dynorphin(1–8)[342]; and the 27-amino-acid peptide (P) having NH$_2$-terminal histidine (H) and COOH-terminal isoleucine (I) amide residues (PHI-27), a prolactin secretagogue.[341] In addition, CRH is present in a subpopulation of oxytocin-containing neurons in the magnocellular division of the paraventricular nucleus that project to the posterior pituitary.[343] CRH is also widely distributed throughout the brain and spinal cord[335, 336] and in peripheral tissues, such as the adrenal medulla,[344] testis,[345] gastrointestinal tract,[346, 347] pancreas,[347, 348] and placenta.[349, 350] The presence of CRH and its two receptor types[351–355] in the brain suggests that CRH functions as a neurotransmitter (see Chapter 8). In other tissues, CRH may exert local regulatory effects. For instance, CRH inhibits human chorionic gonadotropin–stimulated androgen production by the testis.[356]

MECHANISM OF ACTION. CRH acts on the anterior pituitary corticotrope by binding to type 1 CRH cell-surface receptors[352, 357, 358] and activating adenylate cyclase, thereby increasing intracellular cAMP levels and activating cAMP-dependent protein kinase A,[359] increasing the influx of extracellular calcium through L-type Ca^{2+} channels,[360, 361] increasing the production of lipoxygenase metabolites of arachidonic acid,[362] and other as yet unknown events. This results within a few seconds in secretion of ACTH and other POMC-related peptides[363] and subsequently in increased POMC mRNA synthesis.[214, 364, 365] Chronic CRH stimulation causes corticotrope hyperplasia.[366] Corticotrope CRH receptor number may modulate the ACTH response, because receptors are reduced in the anterior pituitary but not in brain by immobilization stress, adrenalectomy, and administration of CRH, AVP, or glucocorticoid.[357, 367–370] The effects of adrenalectomy and glucocorticoids appear to be mediated, at least in part, by AVP and CRH levels and may be exerted at translational or post-translational levels.[368, 371] Stress increases CRH receptors in the paraventricular nucleus.[372] The effects of CRH and AVP on CRH receptor expression are additive.[368, 373] CRH also stimulates intermediate-lobe melanotropes to synthesize POMC mRNA[365] and secrete α-MSH.[374] Intermediate-lobe CRH receptors are increased by dopamine.[375]

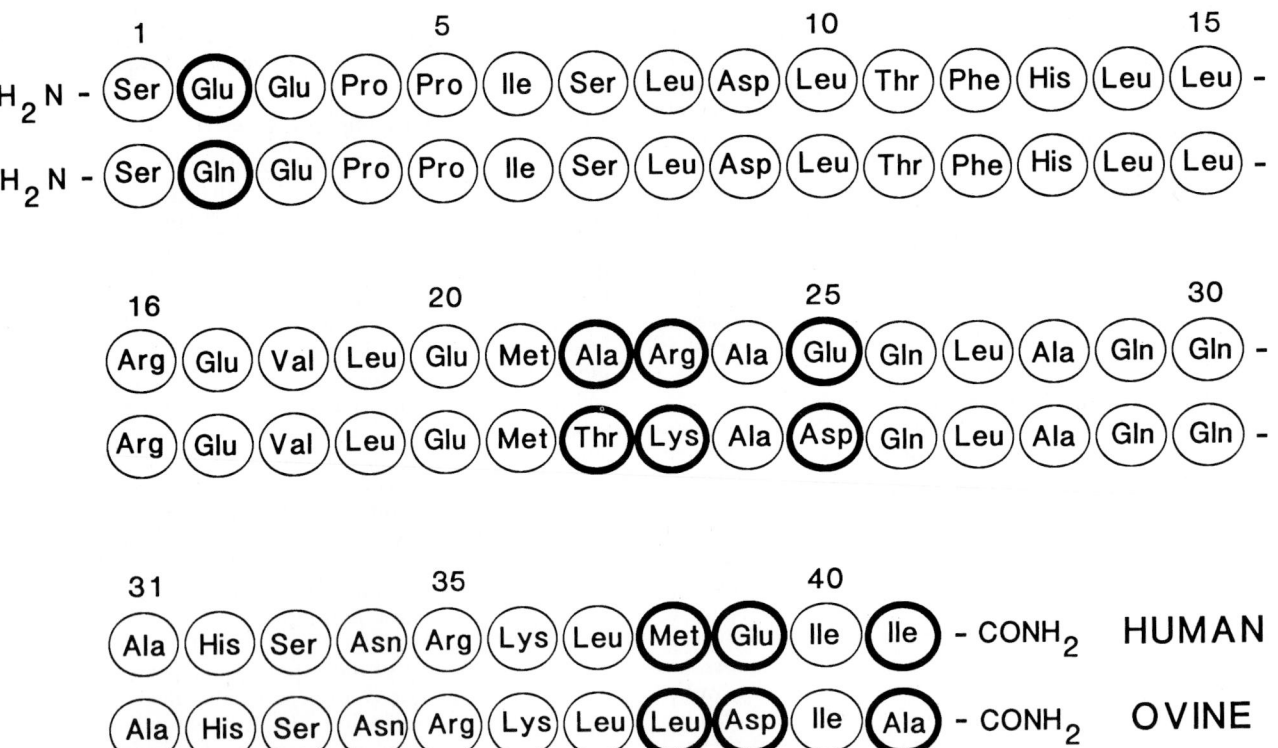

Figure 12–12. Amino acid sequences of human and ovine CRH. The latter is used in most diagnostic testing and is equipotent and longer-acting than human CRH. Differences between the two sequences are indicated by the heavy circles.

PLASMA LEVELS. There is disagreement as to whether peripheral plasma CRH levels reflect hypothalamic secretion.[376] This disagreement may be caused by methodologic differences, but it more likely indicates that peripheral plasma CRH levels reflect nonhypothalamic secretion of CRH.[377–380] Under certain circumstances, such as insulin-induced hypoglycemia, small increments in plasma CRH level may reflect hypothalamic CRH release.[381] Plasma CRH levels increase in third-trimester pregnancy because the placenta secretes CRH (see Chapters 27 and 28).[350, 382] CRH circulates in human plasma bound to a high-affinity binding protein,[383] in which state its bioactivity is reduced,[384] probably explaining why the high levels of CRH in pregnancy do not cause increased ACTH secretion. In complicated pregnancy, however, CRH-binding protein levels may be decreased[385] at the same time that plasma CRH levels are increased.[386, 387] A similar binding protein has not been found in other species.[383, 388, 389] Despite binding to this protein, the circulating half-life of human CRH is only 4 min.[390] Ovine CRH is used for most clinical studies because despite the fact that it does not bind to the binding protein[383] it has a half-life of 55 min and, consequently, a prolonged duration of action.[391, 392]

EFFECTS ON PITUITARY ACTH SECRETION. Human and ovine CRH cause a rapid, dose-dependent increase in plasma ACTH without affecting the plasma levels of other anterior pituitary hormones, vasopressin, or catecholamines.[390, 393, 394] Human CRH is equipotent to ovine CRH, but because of its shorter circulating half-life the duration of plasma ACTH elevation is shorter and less total ACTH is secreted,[390, 395] although the plasma cortisol response is similar.[395] The specific binding of human CRH to the CRH-binding protein found in human plasma[383, 396] may facilitate its removal from circulating blood.[397] The ACTH released by CRH stimulates secretion of cortisol and other adrenal steroids, such as aldosterone and DHEA.[394, 398] There is no sex or age difference in the plasma ACTH or cortisol response to CRH[398–400]; however, the DHEA response is reduced in elderly men, and the cortisol response is blunted in obese subjects.[398, 401] African-American subjects have greater plasma immunoreactive ACTH responses but similar plasma cortisol responses to those of whites, apparently because they release a larger fraction of bioactive ACTH.[402] Time of day has little effect on the plasma ACTH response to CRH, but the increment in plasma cortisol is greater in late afternoon or evening than in the morning.[403] A major factor influencing the magnitude of the plasma ACTH response to CRH is the circulating glucocorticoid concentration. For example, the plasma response to CRH varies inversely with the basal plasma cortisol concentration.[403] Therefore, the ACTH response is enhanced during metyrapone-induced hypocortisolemia[404] and reduced by glucocorticoid administration.[404, 405]

EXTRAPITUITARY EFFECTS. The peripheral and central effects of CRH may be mediated by binding of CRH to type 1 and type 2 CRH receptors and to CRH-binding protein.[355, 406–408] Systemic administration causes mesenteric vasodilation, which at high doses can result in hypotension and tachycardia,[393, 409] and stimulation of respiration through a central effect.[410] Intracerebroventricular injection activates the autonomic nervous system[411]; increases plasma concentrations of catecholamine, glucagon, and glucose; elevates blood pressure and heart rate; decreases gastric acid secretion[412]; and induces behavioral changes in animals.[413] CRH may modulate reproductive function, since it reduces female rat sexual receptivity,[414] lowers luteinizing hormone (LH) levels by inhibiting secretion of LH-releasing hormone (LHRH),[415] and inhibits human chorionic gonadotropin–stimulated testosterone production by cultured Leydig cells.[416]

Multihormonal Control of ACTH Secretion

CRH and AVP are physiologically the most important regulators of ACTH secretion, but other agents, such as catecholamines, angiotensin II, serotonin, oxytocin, atrial natriuretic peptide (ANP), cholecystokinin, VIP, PHI-27, and gastrin-releasing peptide have been implicated.[209–211] Some agents, such as interleukin-1 (IL-1) and IL-6, act by regulating hypothalamic CRH secretion.[417, 418]

CRH is the most important ACTH secretagogue.[37] AVP is a weak stimulator of ACTH secretion, but it potentiates the action of CRH in vivo and in vitro.[419, 420] AVP alone does not increase cAMP levels, but it augments CRH-induced cAMP levels. AVP exerts its effect by binding to a novel vasopressin receptor (the V_3 receptor, also known as the V_{1B} receptor),[421, 422] thereby activating phospholipase C–mediated hydrolysis of phosphatidylinositol 4,5-bisphosphate (PIP_2) to produce inositol 1,4,5-trisphosphate (IP_3), which mobilizes intracellular calcium, and diacylglycerol, which activates phospholipid- and calcium-dependent protein kinase C.[423–425] Unlike CRH, AVP does not by itself stimulate POMC gene transcription.[426] Oxytocin probably acts through the AVP receptor and postreceptor pathway.[427] Angiotensin II presumably binds to type 1 angiotensin receptors[428] to activate the phosphatidylinositol pathway.[429] Cholecystokinin binds to type A receptors,[430] but its postreceptor signaling pathway is not fully understood. Angiotensin II and cholecystokinin may act mainly by central mechanisms to stimulate CRH release.[431] The role of oxytocin is controversial because in vivo studies in humans have shown either no effect or an inhibitory effect on ACTH secretion.[432] It is not entirely clear how VIP and PHI-27, both gastrointestinal and hypothalamic peptides, stimulate ACTH secretion; they presumably bind to VIP type 2 receptors[433] but may activate different postreceptor mechanisms.[434] VIP may be involved in the plasma ACTH response to food ingestion.[435] ANP(1–28) has been detected in hypothalamic neurons, and it inhibits CRH-induced ACTH release from anterior pituitary cells in vitro[436] and in humans,[437] apparently by binding to type B ANP receptors and activating guanylyl cyclase.[438] ANP may modulate the ACTH response to stress.[439, 440] Opioid peptides inhibit ACTH secretion in humans,[441, 442] perhaps by binding to δ- or κ-receptors. In contrast, opioid agonists stimulate ACTH secretion in rats by means of central μ- or κ-receptors.[443] Tonic inhibition by opioids can be blocked by naloxone, resulting in release of ACTH.[444, 445] The role of catecholamines is unclear.[446] Circulating plasma catecholamines have no role in humans, but activation of central α_1-adrenergic receptors may be an important stimulus for CRH and therefore ACTH secretion; central β-adrenergic receptor activation has minimal effect. The inhibitory effect of opioids may be exerted on central α_1-adrenergic neurons that stimulate CRH-containing neurons in the hypothalamus.[447]

Interactions with the Immune System

Many interactions occur between the immune system and the hypothalamic-pituitary-adrenal axis (see Chapters 7 and 8).[448] IL-1 and IL-6 are secreted by monocytes in response to an antigenic challenge. They increase ACTH secretion by stimulating hypothalamic CRH release.[417, 418] IL-2, secreted by T lymphocytes, also stimulates ACTH secretion by indirect and possibly direct pituitary actions. TNF, released by macrophages in response to infection, directly stimulates pituitary ACTH secretion.[449] Lymphocytes, like many other tissues, have low levels of POMC mRNA and may or may not release small amounts of ACTH and other POMC peptides.[450–453] However, immune cells probably do not secrete sufficient ACTH or other POMC peptides to influence the hypothalamic-pituitary-adrenal axis.[454]

Regulation of Intermediate-Lobe POMC Peptide Secretion

Regulation of secretion of α-MSH, β-END, and other POMC peptides from the pituitary intermediate lobe differs from that in the anterior lobe. Secretion is mainly under tonic inhibitory control by hypothalamic dopamine,[455] and glucocorticoids do not inhibit secretion. CRH and β-adrenergic agonists stimulate α-MSH secretion through a cAMP-mediated mechanism, which is inhibited by dopamine. However, dopamine actually increases expression of intermediate-lobe CRH receptors.[375] γ-Aminobutyric acid, a neurotransmitter, also inhibits secretion of POMC peptides.[456] As already noted, a functional intermediate lobe exists in humans only during fetal life and in late pregnancy.

Normal Patterns of ACTH and Cortisol Secretion

PULSATILE SECRETION. ACTH is secreted in brief episodic bursts, which cause sharp rises in plasma concentrations of ACTH and cortisol followed by slower declines in cortisol levels, as a result of the slower clearance of cortisol from plasma (Fig. 12–13). The normal diurnal rhythm is caused by ACTH secretory episodes of varying amplitude at different times of the day.[457–460] The secretory episodes increase in amplitude (Fig. 12–14) but not in frequency after 3 to 5 h of sleep, reach a maximum in the hours before and the hour after awakening, decline throughout the morning, and are minimal in the evening.[459] Consequently, plasma ACTH and cortisol levels are highest at about the time of waking in the morning, are low in the late afternoon and evening, and reach their nadir an hour or two after beginning sleep. Additional secretory episodes frequently occur during lunch and sometimes with dinner, depending on the protein content of the meal.[461, 462]

CIRCADIAN RHYTHM. An endogenous pacemaker, presumably located in the suprachiasmatic nucleus of the hypothalamus, generates a circadian (literally, "about a day") rhythm in a variety of physiological processes, including the activity of the hypothalamic-pituitary-adrenal axis. The timing of the circadian rhythm is synchronized to the solar day by dark-light shifts, which normally are a reflection of the habitual sleep-wake pattern.[463–466] As long as it is thus synchronized, it is a diurnal rhythm. In blind subjects (i.e., persons without a dark-light synchronizer), the diurnal rhythm reverts to a

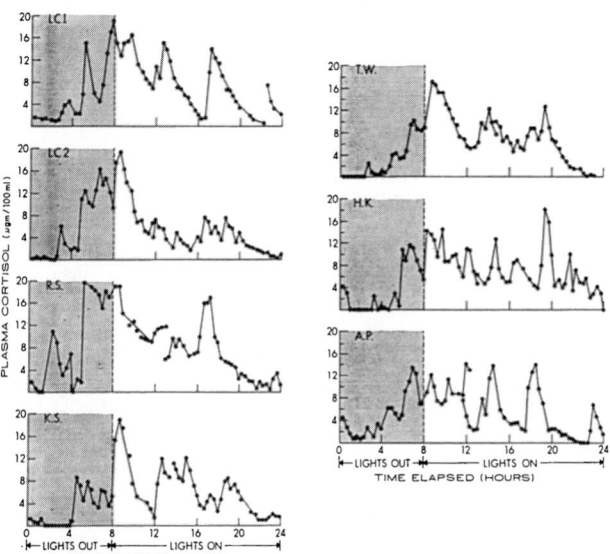

Figure 12–13. Circadian rhythm in plasma cortisol concentration in seven normal subjects. Samples were drawn every 20 to 30 minutes. (From Weitzman ED, Fukushima DK, Nogeire C, et al. Twenty-four hour pattern of the episodic secretion of cortisol in normal subjects. J Clin Endocrinol Metab 1971; 33:14–22. Copyright © 1971, by The Endocrine Society.)

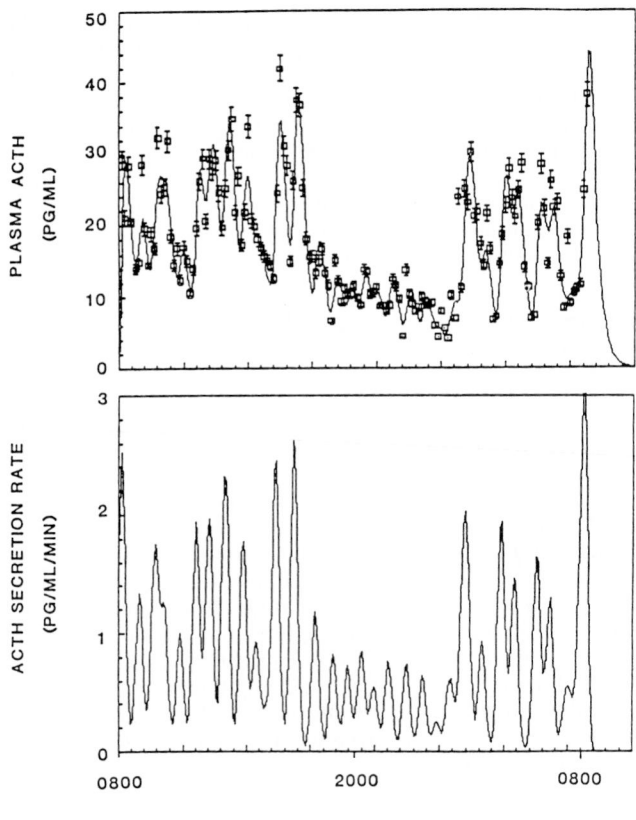

Figure 12–14. Pulse analysis of plasma ACTH sampled at 10-minute intervals for 24 hours. The upper panel shows the measured serial plasma ACTH concentrations *(boxes)*, the concentration-dependent standard deviation of the assay *(brackets)*, and the ACTH concentrations predicted by the deconvolution program *(solid line)*. The lower panel shows the computer-calculated ACTH secretion rate plotted as a function of time. To convert pg/mL to pmol/L, multiply by 0.22. Variation in the amplitude, not the frequency, of the pulses is responsible for the circadian rhythmicity of plasma ACTH concentration. (From Veldhuis JD, Iranmanesh A, Johnson ML, et al. Amplitude, but not frequency, modulation of adrenocorticotropin secretory bursts gives rise to the nyctohemeral rhythm of the corticotropic axis in man. J Clin Endocrinol Metab 1990; 71:452–463. Copyright © 1990, by The Endocrine Society.)

free-running circadian rhythm with a periodicity of 24.5 to 25 h.[464] In the chronic absence of external time cues, both the plasma cortisol and the sleep-wake cycles gradually revert to a similar, synchronized circadian rhythm.[465]

The normal diurnal rhythm becomes apparent only after 1 y of age and is well established only after 3 y.[467, 468] The rhythm probably establishes itself at different ages in different individuals, possibly related to establishment of adult sleep-wake patterns.[469] In the elderly, the rhythm shifts about 3 h earlier[470] but it is not clear whether this shift is caused by the earlier time of awakening in elderly persons, whether earlier awakening is dictated by the shift in cortisol rhythm, or whether both result from some other factor.[471] The cortisol secretory pattern is resistant to acute change. Prolonged bed rest, continuous feeding, 5 d of fasting,[472] or 2 to 3 d of sleep deprivation do not alter the rhythm.[473] After a major time shift, for example after long-distance jet travel, it takes 1 to 2 weeks for the rhythm to return to normal.[474] Exposure to bright light after such a change can speed the readjustment and perhaps lessen the symptoms of jet lag.[475, 476] The mechanisms responsible for the circadian rhythm are poorly understood, except that neurons in or fibers passing through the suprachiasmatic nucleus of the ventral hypothalamus are essential.[477] Molecular models of the suprachiasmat-

ic oscillator have been proposed from studies of invertebrates.[478, 479] CRH is the most potent ACTH secretagogue, but its role in the ACTH circadian rhythm is unclear. In the rat, either a peak[480] or a nadir[481] in hypothalamic CRH immunoreactivity has been observed before peak ACTH secretion. A diurnal rhythm in plasma CRH in humans, with the highest levels at 6:00 AM, has been reported by some investigators[482] but not by others.[380, 483] When CRH is infused continuously in humans, the plasma ACTH circadian rhythm persists,[484] suggesting that factors other than CRH must be involved in generation of the circadian ACTH rhythm.

Factors independent of ACTH release regulate adrenal responsiveness to ACTH in some animals, but they have not been confirmed under basal conditions in humans.[480, 485–487] In rats the plasma corticosterone rhythm persists even though endogenous ACTH secretion is suppressed with dexamethasone, and in hypophysectomized rats plasma corticosterone levels show a diurnal pattern during continuous administration of exogenous ACTH.[485] Adrenal innervation may be responsible for these changes in adrenal sensitivity, because the rhythm is lost with spinal cord transection at T7 but not at L1.[488] Cutting of the splanchnic nerves reduced sensitivity to ACTH in lambs.[489] Adrenal autotransplantation abolished the rhythm in some[490] but not all studies.[491] This neural influence on adrenal sensitivity may be caused by changes in adrenal blood flow.[492, 493]

EFFECT OF STRESS. Acute physical or psychological stress activates the hypothalamic-pituitary-adrenal axis and increases plasma levels of ACTH and cortisol. Stress is a poorly defined term. It usually cannot be quantified, nor are the mechanisms by which it elicits a response completely understood. Physical stresses include severe trauma, burns or illness, major surgery, hypoglycemia, fever, hypotension, exercise, cold exposure, and cigarette smoking.[494–498] Surgery is one of the most potent activators of the hypothalamic-pituitary-adrenal axis. Plasma ACTH levels may increase at the time of incision and during the surgery, but the greatest ACTH secretion occurs during reversal of anesthesia, extubation, and the immediate postoperative recovery period.[497, 499] This response can be reduced by use of morphine-like analgesics,[499, 500] which blunt the pituitary ACTH response to CRH and may also act centrally to inhibit secretion of ACTH secretagogues.[499, 501] The ACTH and cortisol response to surgery can be abolished by interrupting the neural connections from the operative site, such as by sectioning of the spinal cord[502] or epidural anesthesia,[503] indicating that afferent nerve impulses mediate the response. Pretreatment with glucocorticoids blocks the pituitary-adrenal response to minor stress but may not alter the response to major stress.[499, 504, 505] The pituitary-adrenal response is proportional to the extent of a burn[494] or intensity of exercise.[498]

Acute psychological stress also enhances ACTH and cortisol secretion. Its degree may appear to be relatively mild, as with anticipation of athletic competition,[506] surgery,[507] or mental tasks.[508] Chronic anxiety and schizophrenia are not usually associated with increased adrenal activity, but hypercortisolemia is a common feature of severe endogenous depression, in which the nocturnal quiescent period is shortened, the morning rise occurs early,[509] and the overall cortisol level is increased.[509–511] The abnormality disappears after spontaneous recovery from or successful treatment of the depression. The abnormality is less common in mild or atypical depression.

Stress exerts its effects through unknown central pathways that stimulate the hypothalamus to release multiple ACTH secretagogues, CRH and AVP being the most important.[211, 512] Hypoglycemia exerts a direct effect on the medial basal hypothalamus[513] and stimulates CRH release from isolated rat hypothalami[514] but has no direct effect on pituitary ACTH secretion. Hypoglycemia also increases plasma levels of CRH, AVP, epinephrine, and norepinephrine.[482] AVP probably plays a role in the pituitary response to hypoglycemia, but peripheral catecholamines are not involved.[446, 515] Fever, caused either by infection or by pyrogen administration, stimulates ACTH and cortisol secretion.[516] Infection or exposure of mononuclear leukocytes to bacterial endotoxin causes release of IL-1 and IL-6, which stimulate hypothalamic CRH secretion; IL-2, which causes ACTH secretion by indirect[517, 518] and possibly direct[519, 520] actions on the pituitary; and TNF, which directly stimulates pituitary ACTH release.[449, 521]

GLUCOCORTICOID NEGATIVE FEEDBACK. This feedback occurs at the pituitary and hypothalamic levels and perhaps at higher centers. In the anterior pituitary, glucocorticoids inhibit both ACTH secretion and POMC gene transcription, resulting in reduced POMC mRNA levels and reduced POMC synthesis.[214] To a lesser extent, glucocorticoids also decrease CRH and AVP mRNA and peptide levels in the hypothalamic paraventricular nuclei.[522–524] In addition, glucocorticoids block the stimulatory effect of CRH on POMC gene transcription[525] and ACTH release.[361] As already mentioned, they also inhibit anterior pituitary CRH receptor expression.[368, 371] As a consequence of these actions of glucocorticoids, plasma ACTH levels are markedly elevated in untreated primary adrenal insufficiency and are suppressed in patients with Cushing's syndrome caused by a cortisol-secreting adrenal tumor or exogenous steroid administration.

Glucocorticoid feedback inhibition of ACTH secretion in rats appears to consist of at least two phases.[526] Fast feedback occurs in seconds to minutes and is proportional to the rate of increase in glucocorticoid concentration rather than its absolute level. It is believed to represent a membrane-stabilizing effect. Delayed feedback occurs in hours to days; it is proportional to the glucocorticoid dose, potency, duration of administration,[526] and, therefore, plasma levels. It presumably is mediated through the glucocorticoid receptor. Initially, secretion but not synthesis of ACTH and CRH is inhibited. Later, decreased POMC and CRH gene transcription leads to decreased hormone synthesis.[525]

Data on the mechanisms of glucocorticoid negative feedback in humans are limited. Any glucocorticoid can suppress ACTH secretion, but the degree of suppression depends on the dose, potency, and duration of action of the steroid and the duration and time of its administration. The shorter the interval before the normal early morning peak of ACTH secretion, the greater the suppressive effect of the steroid. The longer its duration of action and the larger the dose administered, the greater the duration of suppression. After withdrawal of chronic administration of pharmacologic doses of glucocorticoid, the hypothalamic-pituitary-adrenal axis may remain suppressed for weeks to months (see later discussion).

The possibility of short-loop glucocorticoid negative feedback has been suggested by evidence of a direct inhibitory effect on adrenal steroidogenesis in cultured adrenal cells.[527] This effect must be minimal in vivo, however, because dexamethasone administration does not inhibit ACTH-stimulated cortisol production.[528, 529]

Regulation of Mineralocorticoid Secretion

The major circulating mineralocorticoid is aldosterone, which is synthesized exclusively in the zona glomerulosa. Its precursors, 18-hydroxycorticosterone, corticosterone, and DOC, also have some mineralocorticoid activity. The three precursors are synthesized in all three adrenocortical zones, but 18-hydroxycorticosterone is produced predominantly in the zona glomerulosa, so its secretion correlates with that of aldosterone. Much more corticosterone and DOC are produced in the zona fasciculata than in the zona glomerulosa. Their secretion correlates with that of cortisol and is ACTH-depen-

dent.[530, 531] Cortisol also has modest mineralocorticoid activity, which becomes significant in Cushing's syndrome. Secretion of 18-oxygenated cortisol derivatives, which have weak mineralocorticoid activity and have been implicated in the hypertension of glucocorticoid-suppressible aldosteronism, is also ACTH-dependent.[532] 19-Nor-DOC is a potent mineralocorticoid that is produced by nonadrenal conversion of 19-oxygenated DOC precursors and may be a cause of hypertension.[533] The factors regulating its secretion are not clear, although ACTH administration acutely increases its plasma concentration.[533]

Aldosterone secretion is governed by multiple factors that exert complex regulatory interactions (Fig. 12–15).[534, 535] The renin-angiotensin system and potassium ion are the major regulators, whereas ACTH and other POMC peptides, sodium ion, vasopressin, dopamine, ANP, β-adrenergic agents, serotonin, and somatostatin are minor modulators. These various factors regulate aldosterone secretion by modulating one or both of two biosynthetic steps. The early step is the conversion of cholesterol to Δ^5-pregnenolone, and the late step is the conversion of corticosterone to aldosterone,[534] which is catalyzed by a single mitochondrial enzyme, CYP11B2 (aldosterone synthase); this was previously referred to as the corticosterone 18-hydroxylase/18-methyloxidase (CMO I/CMO II) or 18-hydroxylase/isomerase reaction.[536]

The Renin-Angiotensin System

Renin is an enzyme that cleaves renin substrate, angiotensinogen, an α_2-globulin (approximately 60 kd) that is synthesized by the liver, to produce the decapeptide, angiotensin I (Fig. 12–16).[537] Angiotensin I is rapidly cleaved by angiotensin-converting enzyme in the lungs and other tissues to form the octapeptide, angiotensin II. Cleavage of the NH_2-terminal Asp residue from angiotensin II produces the heptapeptide, angiotensin III, whose circulating levels are only 20% of those of angiotensin II. Angiotensin I has no known biologic action. Angiotensin II and III are equipotent in stimulating aldosterone secretion, but angiotensin II is a more potent vasopressor agent.[537, 538] Neither stimulates cortisol production. The angiotensins are inactivated within minutes by tissue and plasma peptidases.

The level of circulating renin is the rate-limiting factor in this process. Renin is synthesized by the juxtaglomerular cells in the renal cortex, and its secretion is controlled by renal arteriolar blood pressure, by the sodium concentration of

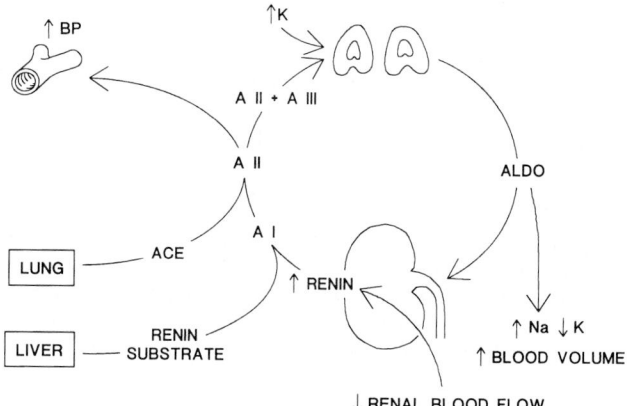

Figure 12–15. The normal renin-angiotensin-aldosterone regulatory system. Renin, secreted by the kidney, cleaves angiotensin I from renin substrate (angiotensinogen), an α_2-globulin produced by the liver. Angiotensin I is converted into biologically active angiotensin II by angiotensin-converting enzyme (ACE), mainly in the lung. Angiotensin II increases peripheral vascular resistance, and it and angiotensin III stimulate aldosterone secretion, which results in sodium retention and increased plasma volume.

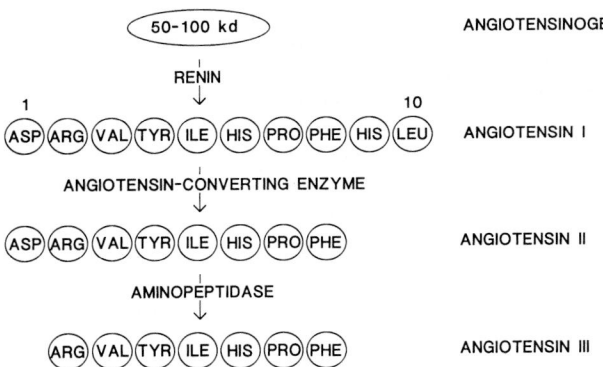

Figure 12–16. Amino acid sequences of angiotensins I, II, and III and the sequence of their production from angiotensinogen (renin substrate).

tubular fluid sensed by the macula densa, and by renal sympathetic nerve activity.[537] Factors that decrease renal blood flow, such as hemorrhage, dehydration, salt restriction, upright posture, or renal artery narrowing, increase plasma renin levels. Factors that increase blood pressure, such as high salt intake, peripheral vasoconstrictors, or supine posture, decrease renin secretion. Acute infusions of norepinephrine stimulate renin release. β-Adrenergic blockers and central α_1-blockers, such as clonidine, inhibit renin release, whereas peripheral α-blockers are without effect. In addition, angiotensin II inhibits renin secretion by direct short-loop feedback.[535] Aldosterone administration reduces renin by an indirect pathway through increased sodium reabsorption and plasma volume expansion. Hypokalemia increases and hyperkalemia decreases renin release.[535] Prostaglandins may play a role in renin release, because prostaglandin A_1 infusion increases and inhibition of prostaglandin biosynthesis by indomethacin reduces basal and stimulated renin release.[539] An additional complexity of uncertain physiological importance is the ability of the adrenal zona glomerulosa, itself, to synthesize both angiotensinogen and renin and to generate angiotensin II.[540]

The effect of angiotensins II and III on the adrenal glomerulosa is initiated by binding to high-affinity cell-surface receptors, which may be coupled to one or more guanosine triphosphate–binding proteins.[534] The primary intracellular signal transduction mechanism is activation of phospholipase C. Phospholipase C hydrolyzes PIP_2 to IP_3, which releases intracellular calcium ions, and 1,2-diacylglycerol, which activates protein kinase C and thereby causes influx of extracellular calcium.[534] These events lead to stimulation of the conversion of cholesterol to Δ^5-pregnenolone and corticosterone to aldosterone.[541–543] Angiotensin II does not stimulate adenylate cyclase activity.[544] The mechanism of the increased conversion of cholesterol to Δ^5-pregnenolone is similar to that mediating the acute effect of ACTH on cortisol biosynthesis in the zona fasciculata.[292] A series of steps are initiated that transfer cholesterol to the inner mitochondrial membrane for CYP11A1 action.[543] However, in contrast to cortisol biosynthesis, there is no effect on cholesterol ester synthesis or hydrolysis, and protein synthesis apparently is not required. Protein synthesis is required to activate 18-hydroxylation by CYP11B1.[543] There is little evidence that prostaglandins regulate aldosterone secretion, but lipoxygenase pathway metabolites of arachidonic acid, such as 12-hydroxyeicosatetraenoic acid, may play an important role in angiotensin II–mediated aldosterone production.[545] Sodium and potassium intake affect the response to angiotensin II (see later discussion).

Potassium

There is a reciprocal relation between serum potassium and aldosterone concentrations. Potassium directly increases aldosterone secretion by the adrenal cortex, and aldosterone lowers serum potassium by stimulating its excretion by the kidney. Small changes in serum potassium concentration within the physiological range affect aldosterone secretion. For instance, an increase in serum potassium of as little as 0.1 mmol/L increases aldosterone by 35%, and a decrease of only 0.3 mmol/L reduces aldosterone by 46%.[546] High dietary potassium intake increases plasma aldosterone and enhances the aldosterone response to a subsequent potassium or angiotensin II infusion, whereas reduced potassium intake results in decreased responsiveness.[534, 547, 548]

The initial signal transduction mechanism by which potassium stimulates aldosterone secretion is different from that of the other aldosterone secretagogues. The primary action of potassium is to depolarize the plasma membrane, which activates voltage-dependent calcium channels, permitting influx of extracellular calcium.[534, 549] Potassium may also cause some release of calcium from intracellular stores. In addition, there is a small increase in cAMP levels after exposure to potassium.[534, 549] The increased cytosolic calcium stimulates the same two steps in aldosterone biosynthesis as angiotensin II does.[541, 542] Cortisol production is not influenced by serum potassium concentrations.

Pituitary Factors

POMC PEPTIDES. ACTH, other POMC-derived peptides, and possibly other pituitary factors influence aldosterone secretion. CRH administration or stresses that cause ACTH secretion increase circulating aldosterone levels,[394, 535] an effect that is blocked by hypophysectomy.[535] However, the role of ACTH in aldosterone secretion is minor. Aldosterone secretion usually remains normal after hypophysectomy because the renin-angiotensin system and potassium are the major regulators. ACTH acutely increases aldosterone secretion in humans, but, in contrast to the effect of angiotensin II, this effect lasts less than 24 h despite continued ACTH administration.[550] The lack of a prolonged response to ACTH appears to result from a direct effect on the glomerulosa cells, such as down-regulation of ACTH receptors or the postreceptor signal transduction mechanism, rather than from an indirect effect, such as suppression of renin or lowering of serum potassium caused by the mineralocorticoid action of cortisol.[551] Other POMC peptides, such as NT peptide, α-MSH, β-MSH, β-LPH, and β-END, have been shown to stimulate aldosterone secretion,[242, 552–556] and γ-MSH potentiates ACTH-induced aldosterone secretion.[556] However, pharmacologic peptide concentrations were often used in these studies. The weak effect of β-LPH is probably caused by contamination with ACTH,[557] and β-END has no effect on rat glomerulosa cells in vitro.[553] POMC peptides are produced by the adrenal medulla, but because of centripetal blood flow they presumably do not reach the cortex.

ACTH increases aldosterone secretion by binding to glomerulosa cell-surface melanocortin-2 receptors, activating adenylate cyclase, and increasing intracellular cAMP,[264, 265, 545, 558] just as it increases cortisol production by fasciculata cells. The response depends on extracellular calcium influx[534] and can be partially blocked by calmodulin inhibitors.[559] Like other agents, ACTH stimulates the same two early and late steps of aldosterone biosynthesis.[542]

VASOPRESSIN. AVP has a modest, transient stimulatory effect on aldosterone secretion from zona granulosa cells in vitro.[560] This effect is probably mediated through binding to V_2-type vasopressin receptors and activation of phospholipase C to generate IP_3 and diacylglycerol.[534, 560]

Sodium

Sodium intake influences aldosterone secretion by indirect effects through changes in renin secretion and to a minor extent by direct effects on zona glomerulosa responsiveness to angiotensin II. High sodium intake increases vascular volume, which suppresses renin secretion and angiotensin II generation, whereas sodium deprivation leads to increased renin secretion. A low-sodium diet increases and a high-sodium diet decreases the sensitivity and magnitude of the aldosterone response to angiotensin II in vivo and in vitro.[561, 562]

Other Stimulatory Agents

Administration of ammonium chloride induces a metabolic acidosis that stimulates aldosterone secretion without changes in serum potassium, renin, angiotensin II, or cortisol concentrations, which suggests a direct effect of hydrogen ion concentration.[563] β-Adrenergic agonists,[564] neuropeptide Y,[74] VIP,[565] leu-enkephalin,[566] calcitonin gene-related product,[567] and serotonin[534] have been reported to affect aldosterone secretion, but their physiological importance is not clear.

Inhibitory Agents

DOPAMINE. Dopamine inhibits aldosterone secretion in humans by a mechanism that is independent of effects on prolactin, ACTH, electrolytes, and the renin-angiotensin system.[568, 569] The adrenals must be under maximal tonic dopaminergic inhibition because dopamine infusion does not lower basal, angiotensin II–stimulated, or ACTH-stimulated aldosterone levels, but dopaminergic blockade with metoclopramide increases aldosterone secretion.[569] The mechanism of the inhibitory dopamine effect may involve binding to D_2 receptors on glomerulosa cells.[570] There are conflicting reports on the effect of dopamine on cAMP levels.[570]

ATRIAL NATRIURETIC PEPTIDE. ANP directly inhibits aldosterone secretion and blocks the stimulatory effects of angiotensin II, potassium, and ACTH, partly by interfering with extracellular calcium influx.[571, 572] ANP may inhibit zona glomerulosa growth, because chronic infusion in the setting of constant ACTH and renin stimulation can induce glomerulosa atrophy.[572]

SOMATOSTATIN. Somatostatin inhibits angiotensin II–stimulated aldosterone production in vitro. The mechanism is not clear, but high-affinity binding sites have been found on glomerulosa cells.[534]

Regulation of Adrenal Androgen and Estrogen Secretion

Adrenal Androgens

The major 19-carbon steroids secreted by the adrenal cortex are DHEA, DHEAS, and androstenedione.[573, 574] They are probably not effective androgens themselves (see Table 12–2) but can be converted to the potent androgens, testosterone and 5α-dihydrotestosterone (DHT), in peripheral tissues. Peripheral conversion contributes significantly to circulating testosterone levels in women (Fig. 12–17), but not in men, in whom testosterone is largely produced by the testis. Peripheral tissues also interconvert DHEA and DHEAS. During the follicular phase of the menstrual cycle, the adrenal glands of women secrete 3 to 4 mg of DHEA, 7 to 14 mg of DHEAS, 1 to 1.5 mg of androstenedione, and 50 μg of testosterone per day.[573] This accounts for about 50%, more than 90%, and about 50% of their circulating levels of DHEA, DHEAS, and androstenedione, respectively. An additional 30% of circulating DHEA arises from peripheral conversion of DHEAS. In women, about 67% of the plasma testosterone and 50% of the dihydrotestosterone comes from androstenedione (see Fig. 12–17).[573, 575] The ovaries produce the remainder. Androstenedione and testosterone levels rise at midcycle because of in-

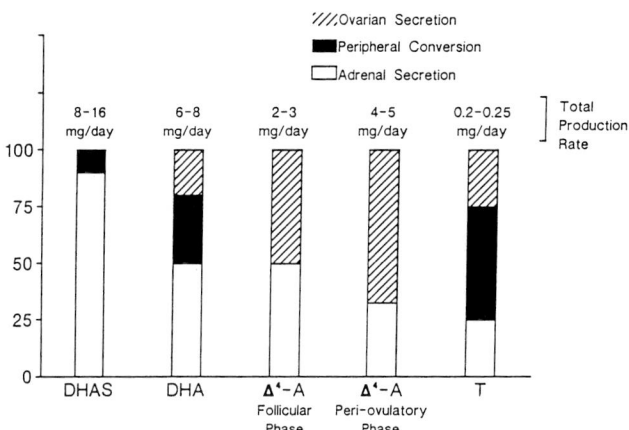

Figure 12–17. Percent contributions to total androgen production in women of adrenal secretion, conversion in peripheral tissues, and ovarian secretion. DHA, dehydroepiandrosterone (DHEA); DHAS, DHEA-S; Δ⁴-A, Δ⁴-androstenedione; T, testosterone. Total daily production is shown at the top. To convert values to moles per day, multiply DHAS by 2.721, DHA by 3.467, Δ⁴-A by 3.491, and T by 3.467. (From Longcope C. Adrenal and gonadal androgen secretion in normal females. Clin Endocrinol Metab 1986; 15:213–228 © 1986, The Endocrine Society.)

creased ovarian secretion. Adrenal secretion of androgens in men is about the same as in women during the follicular phase.

POSSIBLE STIMULATORS OF ADRENAL ANDROGEN SECRETION

ACTH. Control of adrenal androgen secretion is less well understood than that of glucocorticoids and mineralocorticoids. ACTH clearly plays a role. Plasma DHEA, androstenedione, and testosterone concentrations closely parallel the circadian rhythm in plasma cortisol (Fig. 12–18).[576, 577] Plasma DHEAS does not exhibit a circadian rhythm because of its much longer circulating half-life.[574] Similarly, ACTH acutely increases circulating DHEA and androstenedione levels, but 1 or 2 d of treatment are needed before an increase in DHEAS can be detected.[573, 578] Dexamethasone administration lowers plasma adrenal androgen levels.[573, 578]

Cortical Androgen-Stimulating Hormone. Factors other than ACTH also appear to be involved, because the ACTH-induced increase in androgens is relatively small compared with the cortisol response. Furthermore, chronic dexamethasone administration, which completely suppresses cortisol production, fails to reduce androgen levels below 20% of baseline in castrate subjects.[578] Most importantly, adrenal androgen secretion diverges from that of ACTH and cortisol in a number of circumstances. For example, plasma adrenal androgen concentrations begin to increase during adrenarche at age 6 to 8 y, reaching adult levels during puberty,[578] and they decrease during fasting[578] and aging[579] and in anorexia nervosa[580, 581] and severe illness,[578, 582] without concomitant changes in ACTH and cortisol levels. In addition, adrenal androgen secretion suppresses more readily than cortisol with low doses of dexamethasone[583] and recovers more slowly after glucocorticoid withdrawal,[578] despite the incomplete suppression with high-dose dexamethasone, mentioned previously.

Evidence for a non-ACTH pituitary factor that stimulates adrenal androgen secretion was provided by a study of hypophysectomized chimpanzees in which ACTH replacement produced normal secretion of cortisol but not of DHEA and DHEAS.[584] A 60-kd glycopeptide[585] and an 18-amino-acid peptide corresponding to the NH₂-terminal region of the JP of POMC[586] have been proposed as possible cortical androgen-stimulating hormones. Other studies have not confirmed an androgen-stimulating activity of the POMC derivative.[587, 588]

Other hormones and cytokines, such as triiodothyronine, pituitary adenylyl cyclase–activating polypeptide, vitamin D, retinoic acid, and IL-6, influence CBG synthesis by hepatocytes in vitro,[625–627] possibly acting through *cis*-regulatory elements that have been identified in the CBG promoter.[628] Decreased CBG concentrations can be seen with polycystic ovary syndrome, cirrhosis, hyperthyroidism, nephrosis, and other protein-losing conditions.[616, 622, 629] Increased CBG levels can occur during chronic active hepatitis[630] and during treatment with anticonvulsant drugs.[622] Inherited abnormalities of CBG are less common than those of TBG. Three families have been described with partial CBG deficiency, one with total CBG deficiency, two with variant CBGs that had decreased cortisol-binding affinity, and one with high CBG concentrations.[608, 631–633] In states of altered plasma CBG concentration, free plasma cortisol concentrations remain within the normal range despite changes in total cortisol. The exception is during third-trimester pregnancy, when serum free cortisol is slightly increased.[616, 622] There is no effect of short-term administration of pharmacologic doses of glucocorticoids or ACTH on CBG levels, although decreased levels have been reported in Cushing's syndrome.[616, 622] CBG levels are normal in adrenal insufficiency.[616, 622]

OTHER STEROID-BINDING PROTEINS

Albumin. Albumin has a greater binding capacity for cortisol than does CBG, because its circulating level of about 550 μmol/L (38 g/L) is almost 800 times greater than that of CBG. However, the binding affinity is weaker, with an association constant of 1 mmol/L, about 1300-fold lower than that of CBG. Synthetic steroids bind to albumin with an affinity similar to or slightly greater than that of cortisol.

Testosterone-Binding Globulin. TeBG is produced mainly by the liver and binds testosterone, dihydrotestosterone, and estradiol (see Table 12–4). It is a 90-kd glycoprotein homodimer composed of two 373-amino-acid subunits.[634, 635] The 18–177 sequence is required for full steroid binding and is probably sufficient for dimerization.[636] It is structurally related to cytoplasmic androgen-binding protein, which is synthesized in Sertoli cells.[637] In fact, these two proteins may arise from the same gene by alternate splicing of exons.[595] Two major alleles of the TeBG gene have equal steroid-binding characteristics.[638] CBG mRNA is found in fetal mouse liver and exocrine pancreas and in human placenta.[620, 639] Plasma TeBG levels are increased by estrogens and pregnancy and decreased by administration of testosterone, suggesting that estrogens and androgens regulate hepatic TeBG production.[596, 640, 641] However, these may represent pharmacologic effects on liver metabolism, since physiological changes in gonadal steroid levels do not always correlate with changes in TeBG levels.[641] For instance, TeBG levels do not vary during the menstrual cycle, are only slightly greater in women than in men, are greater in children than in adults, and fall in both boys and girls before and during puberty.[641, 642] Increased TeBG levels are also associated with thyrotoxicosis, cirrhosis, end-stage nonalcoholic liver disease, hypogonadism, and fasting, and levels are decreased in hypothyroidism, acromegaly, and obesity.[596, 640, 641, 643] Levels are not altered in patients with euthyroid sick syndrome and low thyroxine or triiodothyronine levels[644] and are unaltered or increased in men with human immunodeficiency virus (HIV) infection.[645] Estrogens and thyroxine stimulate TeBG mRNA levels and TeBG production by cultured hepatoma cells, whereas insulin, epidermal growth factor, prolactin, and perhaps hGH decrease them.[596, 646–649] Insulin decreases plasma TeBG levels in men[650, 651] and low levels of TeBG predict development of type 2 diabetes mellitus in men[652]; the TeBG levels reflect hepatic portal insulin levels, not insulin sensitivity.[653] IGF-I does not appear to affect plasma TeBG levels.[647] Androgens decrease circulating TeBG levels in vivo but increase its synthesis and secretion in vitro.[596] There is no diur-

nal rhythm in plasma TeBG levels.[654] TeBG slows testosterone clearance from circulating plasma and its transport from plasma into cerebrospinal fluid.[655]

Like CBG, TeBG has specific high-affinity (about 0.6 nM) receptors on estrogen and androgen target cells, including epididymus, testis, prostate, skeletal muscle, and liver.[656–658] The dynamics of non–ligand-bound TeBG binding to the receptors and activation of adenylyl cyclase are similar to those of CBG.[659] Estradiol binds TeBG and the TeBG-receptor complex and increases cAMP levels in human prostate, an effect that is not mimicked by dihydrotestosterone or blocked by antiestrogens.[660] 5α-Androstan-3α,17β-diol, a metabolite of dihydrotestosterone, also increases cAMP levels in human prostate by binding to the TeBG-receptor complex, but dihydrotestosterone itself does not do so.[661] The estradiol–TeBG-receptor complex inhibits estradiol-stimulated proliferation of the human mammary carcinoma cell line MCF-7.[662]

Orosomucoid. Orosomucoid, or α₁-acid glycoprotein, is a 41-kd plasma protein that plays a minor role in the plasma binding of progesterone and other steroids. It has an association constant for cortisol of only 0.2 mmol/L.[663] It is an acute-phase reactant that is involved in the binding of many drugs.[664]

Hucolin. Hucolin is a 200-kd disulfide-linked heterotetrameric plasma protein related to β-ficolin, a TGF β₁–binding protein purified from uterus, that binds cortisol.[665]

Role of Steroid-Binding Plasma Proteins

FREE HORMONE HYPOTHESIS. According to this widely held hypothesis, the intracellular concentration of a hormone and therefore its biologic activity are proportional to the concentration of free hormone in plasma, not to the plasma protein-bound hormone concentration.[666] This hypothesis is not valid for every hormone (e.g., progesterone) in every tissue because other factors, such as blood flow and rate of dissociation from plasma binding proteins, influx into cells, and intracellular degradation, may play a rate-limiting role in net hormone uptake. Evidence supporting the free hormone hypothesis for cortisol is the following: (1) addition of CBG inactivates the suppressive effect of cortisol on mononuclear cell DNA synthesis in vitro,[667] (2) CBG-bound cortisol[668] or prednisolone[669] is partially or completely protected from metabolic degradation, (3) mechanisms that regulate cortisol production correlate with free plasma cortisol rather than with total cortisol level, and (4) plasma free cortisol concentration and urinary free cortisol excretion are usually normal in subjects with abnormal CBG levels.[666]

FREE HORMONE TRANSPORT HYPOTHESIS. This hypothesis, as distinguished from the free hormone hypothesis just described, postulates that a hormone enters tissues exclusively from the pool of free hormone after dissociation from its binding protein in the circulating blood during its passage through a tissue.[666] Protein binding presumably inhibits diffusion of the hormone into a tissue. However, hepatic uptake of cortisol is several times greater than the amount of free cortisol in plasma. It is possible that albumin-bound or even CBG-bound cortisol can be transported into some tissues,[594, 670] but the apparent paradox can probably be explained by the fact that the dissociation half-time of cortisol from CBG (<1 s) is brief compared with its transit time in blood through the hepatic capillary/sinusoidal system (9 s).[670] Thus, protein-bound hormone may be available for intracellular transport in tissues, such as liver, in which the circulation time exceeds the dissociation rate. In fact, the rate of uptake of cortisol and other steroids from protein-free solutions by perfused rat liver is rapid enough to account for the observed hepatic uptake of the steroids from serum.[671] Therefore, all of the cortisol taken up from plasma can be accounted for by the pool of free cortisol, which is rapidly replenished by the dissociation of cortisol from binding proteins. Dissociation may be enhanced by a transient conformational change of the binding protein or by receptor-mediated uptake.[672]

PHYSIOLOGICAL ROLE. The physiological role of plasma protein binding of steroid hormones is not fully understood. Binding is not necessary for the transport of all steroid hormones because many are sufficiently water soluble at physiological concentrations. The traditional explanation is that hormone-binding proteins serve as reservoirs to lessen the rapid swings in free steroid hormone levels such as would occur with cortisol, for example, because of episodic ACTH secretion.[592, 616, 666] It is noteworthy in this regard that the upper limit of normal plasma cortisol concentration corresponds approximately to the binding capacity of CBG (i.e., about 690 nmol/L, or 25 μg/dL). When radiolabeled thyroxine is perfused through the portal vein in a solution containing TBG, it is uniformly distributed, but in the absence of TBG virtually all of the hormone is taken up by the first cells it contacts.[673] Therefore, the principal function of hormone-binding proteins may be to assure uniform hormone distribution among the cells of target tissues.[672]

Steroid Metabolism

The processes that terminate the physiological actions of steroids in their target tissues are not completely known. However, catabolism of the biologically active hormone to inactive forms is one mechanism by which this could be achieved. The complex processes by which adrenal steroids are inactivated and prepared for excretion are understood in some detail. The relative abundance of various urinary metabolites is shown in Table 12–6.

Hepatic Metabolism of Glucocorticoids
(Fig. 12–20)

REDUCTION. The Δ^4 double bond, usually in conjugation with a 3-ketone, is a structural feature of many steroid hormones, including cortisol and its precursors. Most of these steroids are inactivated by reduction of this unsaturated ketone system. Reduction of the double bond results in an asymmetric carbon at position 5, with two possible isomers. The liver, principal site of this modification, expresses stereospecific enzymes that catalyze the process.[674] 5α-Reductase produces the isomer with the hydrogen atom below, and 5β-reductase produces the isomer with the hydrogen above the plane of the steroid ring. In rat liver, 5α-reductase activity occurs in the endoplasmic reticulum, whereas 5β-reductase is a cytosolic enzyme.[675]

Reduction of the Δ^4 double bond is the rate-limiting step in cortisol metabolism.[674] Human liver expresses 5α-reductase type 1, encoded by a gene on the end of the short arm of chromosome 5.[676, 677] A second form of the enzyme (5α-reduc-

tase type 2) is expressed in reproductive tract tissues, where it functions as an amplifier of androgen action rather than as a catabolic enzyme.[678] Similarly, several substrate-specific 5β-reductases are thought to exist, but an electrophoretically pure preparation of rat liver 5β-reductase is capable of reducing a variety of steroids.[679] The 5β-reduction of cortisol predominates in humans,[680] so that 5β-dihydrocortisol is produced in considerable excess over the 5α-isomer.[675]

The 3-keto group of 5α- and 5β-dihydrocortisol can be reduced by 3α-HSD to yield tetrahydrocortisols. Only trace amounts of 3β-hydroxytetrahydrocortisols are formed,[680] and the major tetrahydrocortisol excreted in urine is 3α,5β-tetrahydrocortisol (THF).

Cortisol, cortisone, and their tetrahydro derivatives may also be reduced by 20α- and 20β-HSDs to yield cortols and cortolones.

OXIDATION. Three types of oxidative reactions involving cortisol and its metabolites occur in the liver. Oxidative removal of the side chain yields a 19-carbon steroid with a 17-ketone group.[681] These compounds mostly have the 5β-configuration. A second reaction is conversion of the 11β-hydroxyl group to a ketone, as in the reversible conversion of cortisol to cortisone.[682] This reaction is catalyzed by 11β-HSD type I, an NADP+-dependent enzyme with both dehydrogenase and oxoreductase activities. The enzyme therefore has the capacity to inactivate cortisol, but the reverse reaction (cortisone conversion into cortisol) is believed to predominate in vivo.[683] The third hepatic oxidative process is conversion of the C_{21}-hydroxyl to a carboxylic acid. The products are called cortolic acids if they are cortisol derivatives (11β-hydroxyl) or cortolonic acids if they are derived from cortisone (11-ketone).

HYDROXYLATION. 6β-Hydroxylation of cortisol occurs in the liver, normally only to a minor extent. The resultant product is highly soluble in water. When plasma cortisol levels are elevated, as in Cushing's syndrome, the normal pathways apparently become saturated, and disproportionately large amounts of 6β-hydroxycortisol are produced and excreted in the urine.[684]

CONJUGATION. The metabolites of cortisol are rendered more water soluble by conjugation with glucuronic acid or sulfate. Glucuronidation predominates and is catalyzed by one of the family of uridine diphosphoglucuronyl transferases. These enzymes catalyze the glucuronidation of xenobiotics, bilirubin, and steroids in the hepatic endoplasmic reticulum.[685] Distinct isoenzymes catalyze the glucuronidation of different substrates, even among the steroid hormones.[686, 687] Glucuronide may be conjugated to any hydroxyl group, but the 3α-hydroxyl is preferred. Most 3α,5β-tetrahydro derivatives of cortisol are excreted as glucuronides. Sulfation, catalyzed by cytosolic sulfotransferases, accounts for only a minor fraction of conjugates of the 3α-hydroxysteroids but for most of the 3β-hydroxysteroids (both 19- and 21-carbon metabolites).[688]

ALTERATIONS IN HEPATIC METABOLISM OF CORTISOL. Factors that can alter the hepatic metabolism of cortisol include hormones, age, intercurrent disease states, obesity, and drugs.

Hormonal Factors. In hyperthyroid states, the turnover rate of cortisol is accelerated but plasma cortisol levels remain normal.[689] In hypothyroid states, the turnover of cortisol is slowed; plasma cortisol levels remain normal, but urinary excretion of cortisol metabolites is decreased. The effect of thyroxine results primarily from regulation of hepatic 5α- and 5β-reductase activity.[690] There are few data in humans, but hepatic steroid-metabolizing hormones are sexually dimorphic in the rat.[691] 5β-Reductase is apparently androgen-induced, since its concentration is twofold to threefold greater in males than in females,[691] whereas hepatic 5β-reductase activity is

TABLE 12–6. Relative Amounts of Various Metabolites of Cortisol in Urine

Steroid	Approximate % of Total
Tetrahydrocortisols	20
Tetrahydrocortisones	20
Cortolones	20
Cortols	10
Cortolic and cortolonic acids	10
11-Hydroxyetiocholanolone	5
6β-Hydroxycortisol	1
11-Hydroxyandrostenedione	1
Cortisol	1

Data from reviews of cortisol metabolism by Peterson[674] and Monder and Bradlow.[2193]

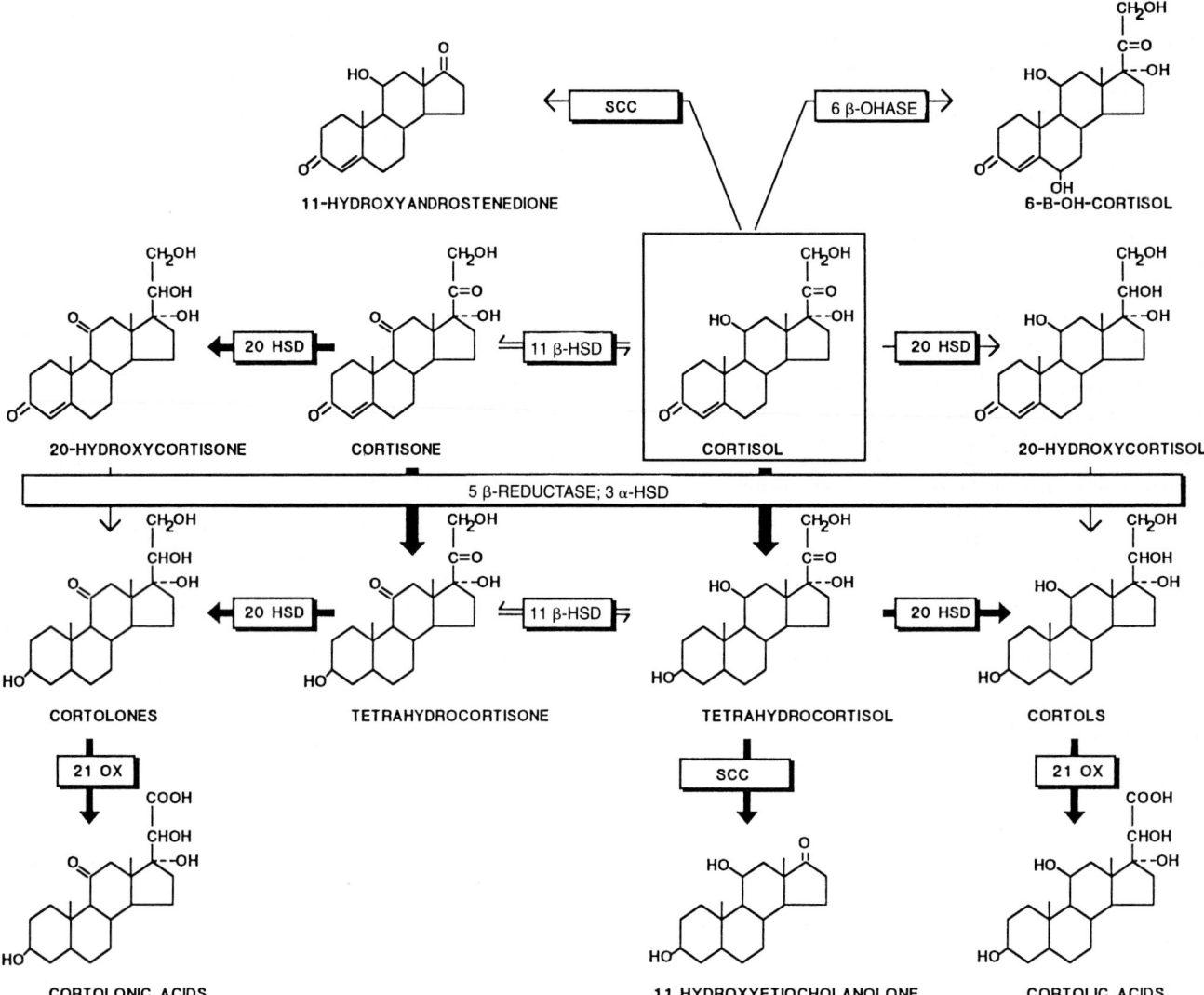

Figure 12–20. Cortisol metabolism in vivo. The relative importance of the pathways under normal conditions is indicated by the width of the arrows. Both 5α- and 5β-reduction occur, but the 5β-pathway predominates. Enzymes are indicated by the boxes. SCC, side-chain cleavage activity; 6 β-OHASE, 6β-hydroxylase; 20 HSD, 20α-hydroxysteroid dehydrogenase; 11 β-HSD, 11β-hydroxysteroid dehydrogenase; 3 α-HSD, 3α-hydroxysteroid dehydrogenase; and 21 OX, 21-oxidase.

higher in female rats. Glucocorticoids in high concentrations (as in exogenous steroid therapy or from endogenous production in Cushing's syndrome) also affect cortisol metabolism.[684] Proportional excretion of cortols and cortolones, tetrahydrocortisone, and 5α-tetrahydrocortisol is decreased in states of glucocorticoid excess.[674] Glucocorticoids stimulate and insulin and IGF-I inhibit hepatic 11β-HSD activity.[683]

Age and Disease. Urinary excretion of 17-hydroxycorticosteroids (tetrahydrocortisols, tetrahydrocortisone) diminishes with age,[692] but plasma cortisol levels remain normal. Enzymatic metabolism of cortisol usually is unaffected by renal impairment, but clearance of glucuronides is diminished and these inactive compounds may accumulate in plasma.[674] In patients with cirrhosis of the liver, 5α- and 5β-reductase activities are selectively decreased but 3α-HSD and glucuronyl transferase activities are normal.[693]

Obesity. Obese persons excrete greater amounts of cortisol metabolites than do lean individuals, a difference that persists even when the data are normalized for body surface area.[694] The cortisol production rate is accelerated in obese subjects, however, so that plasma cortisol levels are normal.[694]

Drugs. Hepatic metabolism of cortisol is altered by a number of drugs. As discussed earlier, the adrenolytic drug

mitotane alters the flux of cortisol metabolites from the usual pathway (tetrahydro metabolites) to the pathway of direct 6β-hydroxylation. Phenytoin and phenobarbital have similar effects.[695, 696] The antituberculosis drug, rifampin, appears to accelerate the metabolism of synthetic steroids (including 9α-fluorohydrocortisone) and of cortisol.[697–699] The enzymatic mechanism is not known. However, increased quantities of 6β-hydroxycortisol are found in the urine of rifampin-treated patients,[700] and induction of 6β-hydroxylase may be the underlying mechanism. The effect may be quantitatively more significant in the case of synthetic steroids. Although cimetidine inhibits hepatic CYP enzymes, it does not affect prednisolone metabolism.[701]

Extrahepatic Metabolism of Cortisol

The kidney is the major site of extrahepatic inactivation of cortisol in humans, where it is converted to the bioinactive metabolite, cortisone.[702] The kidney expresses a high-affinity, NAD-dependent form of 11β-HSD that is encoded by a gene on the long arm of chromosome 16.[703, 704] In the kidney 11β-HSD type II serves to limit cortisol access to the mineralocorticoid receptor,[705, 706] which binds cortisol and aldosterone with equal affinity.[707] Inactivation of cortisol in mineralocorticoid target tissues allows aldosterone to exert physiological effects by means of these receptors. Genetic or pharmacologic impairment of 11β-HSD type II results in cortisol-mediated mineralocorticoid effects (see Chapter 14).

Hepatic Metabolism of Aldosterone
(Fig. 12–21)

REDUCTION. Like cortisol, aldosterone is reduced predominantly by a 5β-reductase and 3α-HSD, so that the product is 3α,5β-tetrahydroaldosterone, which accounts for 35 to 40% of the metabolites of aldosterone in urine.[708] A 21-deoxy form of tetrahydroaldosterone[709] is further reduced to the 20α-hydroxy form. The 20α-hydroxyl group can then condense with the hydroxyl of the C_{18} hemiacetal to form a unique aldosterone metabolite with bicyclic acetal rings.[710]

CONJUGATION. Tetrahydroaldosterone is conjugated in the liver to glucuronide at the 3-keto position. Tetrahydroaldosterone glucuronide is the major urinary metabolite of aldosterone.[711] Another conjugate, aldosterone-18-glucuronide, is produced by direct conjugation of unreduced aldosterone. Therefore, unaltered aldosterone can be recovered from urine by acid hydrolysis of the glucuronides followed by nonpolar solvent extraction[712]; it accounts for approximately 10% of the aldosterone metabolites excreted in urine.

ALTERATIONS IN THE METABOLISM OF ALDOSTERONE. In patients with cirrhosis of the liver and ascites, the production rate and plasma levels of aldosterone are frequently elevated.[693] The liver apparently has reduced ability to metabolize the aldosterone in plasma, so greater amounts are metabolized extrahepatically.[713, 714] Patients with severe congestive heart failure and resultant hypoperfusion of the liver also have decreased aldosterone clearance.[715]

Metabolism of Adrenal Androgens (Fig. 12–22)

The steroid produced in greatest quantity by the adrenal, and its major 19-carbon androgenic steroid, is DHEA and its sulfate ester (DHEAS). Most of the unconjugated steroid is converted to androstenedione by oxidation of the 3β-hydroxyl group and isomerization of the Δ^5 double bond to the Δ^4 position. Androstenedione is metabolized to yield androsterone and etiocholanolone, which are 17β-reduced to yield the respective diol derivatives, conjugated, and excreted.[674] DHEAS can be excreted directly in the urine; the sulfate group can be hydrolyzed to yield free DHEA, which is metabolized as described earlier; or the intact ester can be metabolized by 16- or 7-hydroxylation (or both) or by reversible 17β-reduction to yield androstenediol sulfate.[716] DHEAS and its metabolites are cleared more slowly from plasma by the kidney than are their nonsulfated analogues.[716] Fecal excretion of DHEA and its metabolites is quantitatively more significant than for other adrenal steroids. Thirty to 45% of the radiolabeled metabolites of an intravenous dose of radioactive DHEAS may appear in the feces.[674] Biliary excretion of DHEA and DHEAS metabolites accounts for several percent of the metabolites of these steroids.[674]

Molecular Mechanisms of Adrenal Steroid Action*

Glucocorticoids

Glucocorticoids exert their effects on every system of the body, although their name derives from their effects on carbohydrate metabolism. Because so many physiological processes are affected, it is difficult to formulate a unifying definition of glucocorticoid action.[717] Since most physiological actions of glucocorticoids are mediated by binding to a specific intracellular protein receptor molecule, this receptor mediation could serve as a functional definition of a "glucocorticoid effect." Glucocorticoids may also exert nontranscriptional effects by binding to CBG that has bound to specific cell-surface CBG receptors in target tissues.[612, 614]

The naturally occurring glucocorticoids are 21-carbon steroids with a Δ^4 configuration and 11β- and 21-hydroxyl and 3- and 20-ketone groups (Fig. 12–23). These structural features are necessary for high-affinity binding of the steroids to the glucocorticoid receptor.

MOLECULAR AND CELLULAR MECHANISMS OF ACTION
The Glucocorticoid Receptor
Biochemistry and Physiology. Glucocorticoids, like other steroid hormones, exert their effects on target cells by interacting with soluble intracellular receptor proteins (Fig. 12–24; also see Chapter 4).[718] The steroid is thought to enter the cell by passive diffusion, although possible transport systems have been described.[719–721] Once inside the cell, the steroid binds to the glucocorticoid receptor. Receptor purification[722, 723] and affinity labeling[724–727] studies have shown that the receptor is a single-chain polypeptide with a molecular weight of about 94 kd that binds glucocorticoids with high affinity and in a saturable and specific manner. The glucocorticoid receptor exists in cells complexed with a number of other proteins, including the heat shock protein hsp90,[728–733] the immunophilins hsp56[734, 735] or CyP40,[736] and a 23-kd acidic protein.[737] The

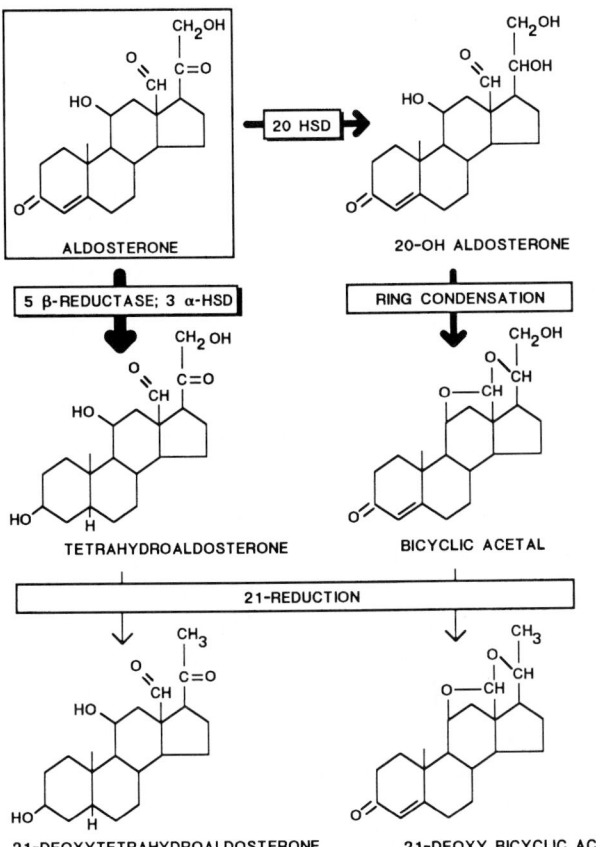

Figure 12–21. Aldosterone metabolism in vivo. The relative importance of the pathways under normal conditions is indicated by the width of the arrows. Enzymes are indicated by the boxes. 20 HSD, 20α-hydroxysteroid dehydrogenase; 3 α-HSD, 3α-hydroxysteroid dehydrogenase. Ring condensation proceeds after reduction at C_{20}.

*See Chapter 4.

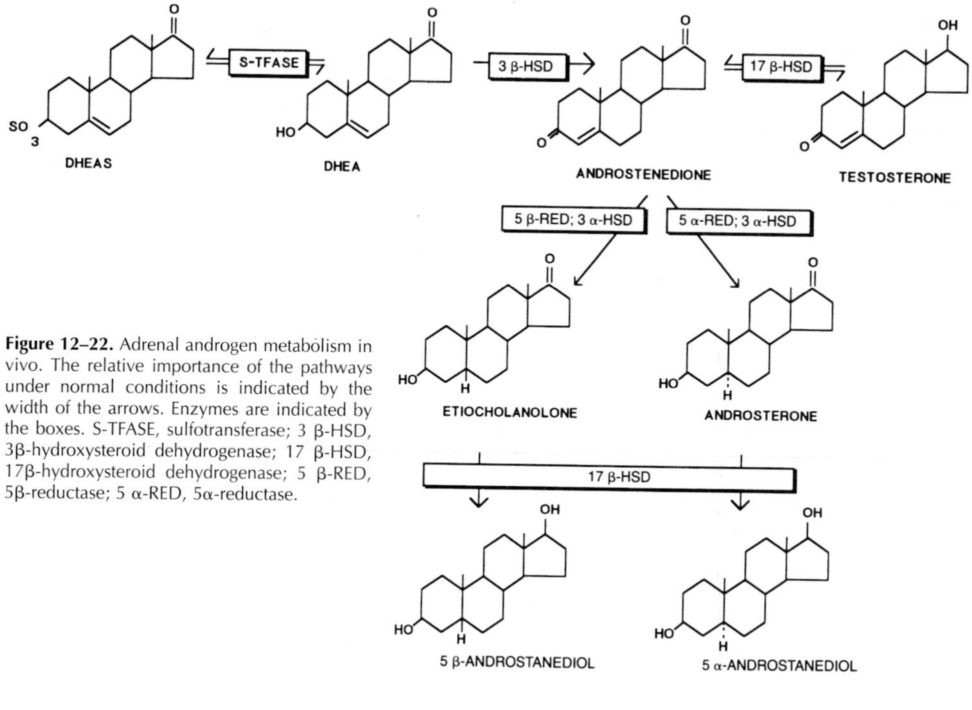

Figure 12–22. Adrenal androgen metabolism in vivo. The relative importance of the pathways under normal conditions is indicated by the width of the arrows. Enzymes are indicated by the boxes. S-TFASE, sulfotransferase; 3 β-HSD, 3β-hydroxysteroid dehydrogenase; 17 β-HSD, 17β-hydroxysteroid dehydrogenase; 5 β-RED, 5β-reductase; 5 α-RED, 5α-reductase.

functions of these proteins are not completely understood, but hsp90 and the 23-kd acidic protein are required for proper folding and assembly of the glucocorticoid receptor-protein complex and its maintenance in a state capable of binding glucocorticoid.[738, 739] The immunophilin component may be involved in trafficking from the cytoplasm to the nucleus.[734]

Once the steroid is bound, the hormone-receptor complex acquires the capacity to bind to DNA.[740] The nature of this activation process is uncertain, but involves dissociation of the hsp90 moiety from the steroid-binding domain of the receptor.[726, 741] Transformation of the complex to a DNA-binding form can be achieved in vitro by increasing temperature or the ionic strength. Cell fractionation experiments,[742] immunocytochemical studies,[743-745] and confocal microscopic examination of the intracellular localization of a green fluorescent protein–glucocorticoid receptor fusion protein[746] all indicate that the unliganded receptor resides in the cell cytoplasm

and, after binding the steroid, translocates to the nuclear compartment.

Domain Structure. Specific domains of the glucocorticoid receptor molecule are associated with its steroid- and DNA-binding functions. The steroid-binding site is at the COOH-terminal region of the protein.[747] Studies with covalently bound ligands suggest that specific residues are involved in steroid binding. The DNA-binding region is located in mid-molecule.[748] Most antibodies prepared against purified receptor protein react with the NH₂-terminal "immunogenic" domain.[749-753]

The structural features of the glucocorticoid receptor have been more precisely defined by molecular cloning methods.[754-757] Human glucocorticoid receptor cDNA sequence predicts two forms of the receptor protein, a more abundant 777-residue α isoform and a 742-amino-acid β isoform. Their sequences are identical up to residue 727 but diverge thereafter.[756] The glucocorticoid receptor is a member of a family of DNA-binding proteins that act as regulators of gene transcription, including receptors for all classes of steroid hormones, the thyroid hormone receptor (c-*erbA* or *THRA1* oncogene),

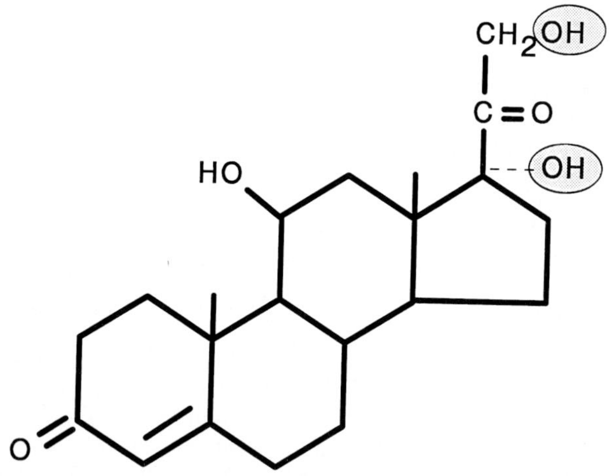

Figure 12–23. Basic structure of a glucocorticoid. The features that are not essential for basic glucocorticoid activity but enhance glucocorticoid potency are shown in the shaded areas. (Adapted from Liddle GW. The adrenals. In: Williams RW, ed. Textbook of Endocrinology. 6th ed. Philadelphia: WB Saunders, 1981: 242–292.)

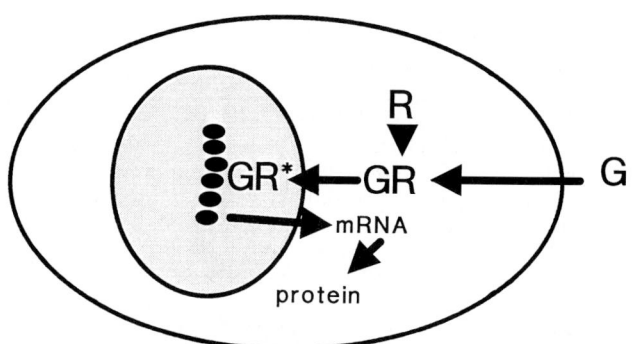

Figure 12–24. Glucocorticoid (G) action in target cells. Like other steroids, glucocorticoids are thought to enter cells by a passive process. They bind to a cytoplasmic glucocorticoid receptor protein (R) to form a glucocorticoid-receptor complex (GR) capable of activating transcription of target genes. The mRNA is translated into new proteins that express the biologic activity of the glucocorticoid.

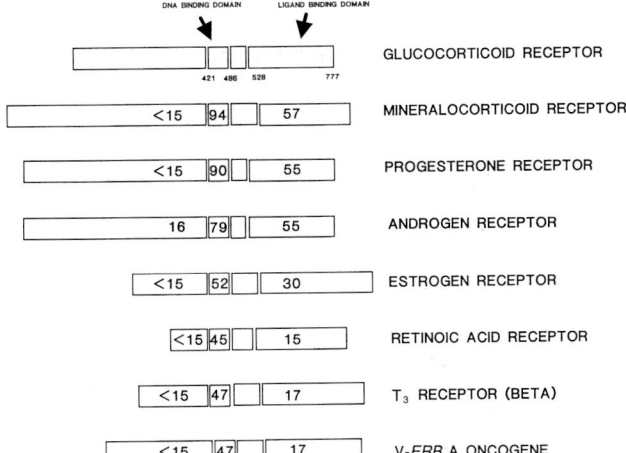

Figure 12–25. Domain structure of the glucocorticoid receptor protein and its homology with other steroid receptors, the retinoic acid receptor, the thyroid hormone receptor, and the v-*erb-A* oncogene. The 777–amino acid α form of the receptor contains DNA-binding (residues 421–486) and ligand-binding (residues 528–777) domains. The DNA-binding region is highly conserved among the various receptors (figures indicate the percent homology in each domain).

and the retinoic acid receptor (Fig. 12–25; see Chapter 4).[758] The hormone-binding domain of these proteins is relatively conserved, but the most distinctive feature is the highly conserved zinc finger domain (Fig. 12–26).[758] This cysteine-rich region is in the central DNA-binding domain. A similar structure in the DNA-binding protein, *Xenopus* transcription factor IIIA (TFIIIA), forms a finger-like loop structure of 12 amino acids anchored at the base by a zinc ion chelated between two pairs of cysteine and histidine residues.[759] Similar finger-like structures are assumed to exist in the glucocorticoid and other steroid hormone receptors and to interact with the coils of the DNA double helix.

The steroid-binding domain of the glucocorticoid receptor is at the COOH terminus.[760–762] Mutant human receptors lose dexamethasone-binding ability when small three- to four-codon segments are inserted into their genomic DNA past the codon for amino acid number 527, whereas insertions before the codon for amino acid 500 have no effect.[760] Deletional mutations in the same region also impair steroid binding, whereas deletions in other parts of the coding sequence do not.[761] The DNA-binding zinc finger domain of the human glucocorticoid receptor lies between amino acids 421 and 486.[763] Mutant human receptors with deletions in this region do not bind to DNA.[761] Studies of naturally occurring mutations of the glucocorticoid receptor in murine S49 lymphoma cells yield similar conclusions.[757] Other regions of the glucocorticoid receptor control nuclear translocation[764] and gene transcription (see later discussion).

MECHANISMS OF GENE REGULATION BY GLUCOCORTICOIDS

Induction of Transcription. Glucocorticoid receptor complexes regulate gene expression by interacting with specific regulatory DNA sequences or glucocorticoid response elements (GREs), which are usually located near the promoter region of target genes.[765, 766] A consensus sequence has been deduced for one such GRE,[765, 767–770] although not all functional GREs share this sequence.[771] The GRE is a partially palindromic structure with the sequence GGTACAnnnTGTTCT. Dimerization of the steroid-receptor complex appears to be necessary for it to bind to the GRE and exert its regulatory effect. Other steroid hormone–receptor complexes can bind to this GRE, although some (e.g., the estrogen–estrogen receptor complex) apparently cannot induce transcription of the target

gene.[772] Some specificity for induction appears to be conferred by the first zinc finger, since a chimeric estrogen receptor whose first zinc finger is replaced with the first finger of the glucocorticoid receptor is capable of inducing transcription from a GRE.[773]

Exactly how binding of the hormone-receptor complex to the hormone response element affects gene transcription is the subject of intense investigation. Sequences in the NH₂-terminal region of the receptor, the DNA-binding domain, and the COOH-terminal half of the molecule all appear to be required for full transcriptional activation,[760, 774–776] but the quantitative contributions of these domains to the total *trans*-activation effect is not clear.[765] The unoccupied steroid-binding domain of the glucocorticoid receptor appears to exert tonic inhibitory influence over the transcriptional activation function of the receptor. Mutant receptors missing the steroid-binding domain are constitutive activators (i.e., no longer hormone dependent) of target gene transcription.[763, 774, 777] The glucocorticoid receptor β isoform is widely expressed, and although it cannot function as an activator of synthetic target gene expression, it exerts dominant negative effects on the function of the α isoform.[778]

Transcriptional activation not only depends on interaction of the DNA-binding and activation domains of the receptor with the GRE but also requires the interaction of other transcription factors, including general transcription factors such as transcription factor IIB (TFIIB)[779] and co-activator molecules such as glucocorticoid receptor interacting protein (GRIP) 170, hRPF I,[780] and GRIP 1,[781] among others.[782] These co-activators are believed to function in the linking of the hormone receptor to the general transcription factors and in the remodeling of the chromatin during assembly of the transcription complex.[779]

Inhibition of Transcription. Glucocorticoids increase the transcriptional activity of many genes and suppress the transcription of others, such as the genes that encode POMC, prolactin, and glycoprotein hormone α-subunit.[783] No clear consensus sequence for a negative response element has emerged from studies of these genes.[765] Mechanisms that have been proposed to explain the inhibitory effects of glucocorticoids in these systems include interference with other transcription factors by direct protein-protein interaction,[784–786] interference with binding of another transcription factor to its own response element near the negative GRE,[787, 788] or direct action by binding of the receptor to negative response elements that prevent transcriptional activation.[789]

Nontranscriptional Effects. CBG that is not liganded with glucocorticoid can bind to specific cell-surface CBG receptors

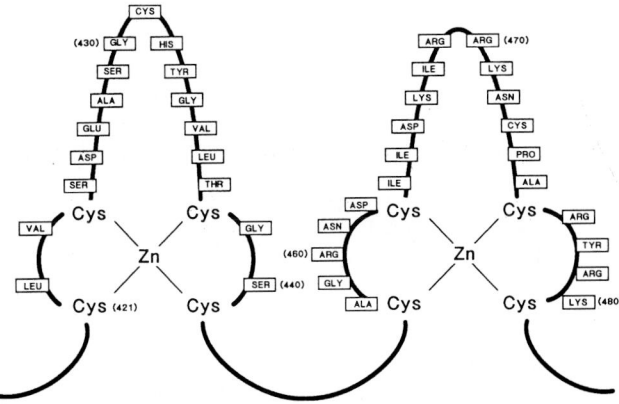

Figure 12–26. Putative zinc finger structures in the DNA-binding domain of the glucocorticoid receptor. The eight highly conserved cysteine residues are believed to chelate Zn²⁺ ions to form the "finger" structure observed in other *trans*-acting transcriptional regulatory factors.

in target tissues such as the liver; liganded CBG does not bind. Glucocorticoid can bind to the CBG-receptor complex[612] and activate adenylyl cyclase[614] and, presumably, the cAMP-dependent protein kinase A signal transduction pathway. This mechanism provides a rapid, nontranscriptional mode of action for glucocorticoids that may function when glucocorticoid levels initially are low, so that CBG can bind to its receptor, and then rise, activating the CBG-receptor–adenylyl cyclase complex.

Mineralocorticoids

Mineralocorticoids are named for their ability to regulate electrolyte transport across epithelial surfaces. The principal physiological mineralocorticoid is aldosterone. The main target tissues of its action are the kidney, colon, and salivary glands[790, 791]; all have high-affinity type I glucocorticoid (i.e., mineralocorticoid) receptors that bind aldosterone.[792–794] Type I receptors are also found in liver, brain (particularly hippocampus), pituitary, and peripheral blood mononuclear cells.[795–798] Aldosterone promotes active sodium transport and excretion of potassium in its major target tissues. These effects are presumably mediated by transcriptional activation mechanisms similar to those of other members of the steroid/thyroid hormone/retinoic acid receptor family,[765] although rapid, nongenomic mechanisms may be responsible for some effects.[799]

MOLECULAR AND CELLULAR MECHANISMS OF ACTION

The Mineralocorticoid Receptor

Structure. Aldosterone binds to at least two different proteins in kidney, at high-affinity type I binding sites and at the more abundant low-affinity type II binding sites.[800, 801] The type I site is thought to be the receptor that mediates the action of aldosterone. The type II site is the glucocorticoid receptor. The type I receptor displays a curious lack of specificity.[802] Radiolabeled aldosterone can be displaced from the receptor by approximately equimolar concentrations of glucocorticoids such as corticosterone, provided that steroid-binding contaminants such as CBG are excluded from the extracts. Therefore it was not clear at first how the type I receptor specifically recognizes mineralocorticoids in the presence of physiological concentrations of glucocorticoids.

The predicted 984-amino-acid protein (107 kd) of the type I receptor is similar to but distinct from the human glucocorticoid receptor.[707] Their NH$_2$ termini are unrelated. The DNA-binding zinc finger domain has 94% homology with the corresponding portion of the glucocorticoid receptor.[759] The COOH-terminal, steroid-binding domain is about 50% homologous with that of the glucocorticoid and progesterone receptors.[707] When expressed in mammalian cells, the recombinant receptor, like the native receptor, cannot distinguish between mineralocorticoids and glucocorticoids.[707]

Basis of Specificity of Response. The nature of the specificity of mineralocorticoid receptor–mediated response was unclear for several years.[803, 804] Specificity is conferred by the 11β-HSD enzyme that is present in the microsomes of mineralocorticoid target tissues and that converts cortisol into cortisone, which has low affinity for the type I (mineralocorticoid) receptor.[702, 706] Aldosterone-responsive tissues express 11β-HSD activity at higher levels than nonresponsive tissues.[705, 706] In some tissues in which the 11β-HSD system is lacking, such as hippocampus and heart, glucocorticoids express their biologic effects by type I receptor binding. In fetal lung, the activity appears to require two independent enzymes, an 11β-HSD and an 11β-oxosteroid reductase.[805] There are both inherited and acquired states of 11β-HSD deficiency (see later discussion).

Effects of Glucocorticoids

Effects on Metabolism

GLYCOGEN METABOLISM. It was known by the mid-19th century that the adrenal glands are essential for life. Their role in intermediary metabolism was recognized when it was noted that adrenalectomized animals cannot maintain hepatic glycogen stores[806] and that replacement of adrenocortical steroids reverses both glycogen depletion and hypoglycemia in fasting adrenalectomized animals.[807] Glucocorticoids activate glycogen synthase[808, 809] and inactivate the glycogen-mobilizing enzyme, glycogen phosphorylase.[809] The total amount of glycogen synthase remains unchanged, but it is activated by dephosphorylation. It is not known whether glucocorticoids exert their effects on glycogen synthase by activating a hepatic phosphatase or indirectly, by inactivating glycogen phosphorylase, a phosphatase inhibitor.

GLUCONEOGENESIS. Glucocorticoids increase hepatic glucose production in part by increasing substrate availability as the result of stimulating release of glucogenic amino acids from peripheral tissues, such as skeletal muscle (Fig. 12–27).[810] Their effect is most apparent when a physiological replacement dose is administered to adrenalectomized animals.[807] Glucocorticoids also directly activate key hepatic gluconeogenic enzymes, such as glucose-6-phosphatase and phosphoenolpyruvate carboxykinase (PEPCK).[810] The increased PEPCK activity results from glucocorticoid-induced activation of PEPCK gene transcription,[811, 812] which is mediated by interaction of the glucocorticoid receptor complex with a specific GRE located in the 5′ flanking region of the gene.[771, 812]

Other gluconeogenic hormones, such as glucagon and epinephrine, are ineffective without the permissive effect of glucocorticoids.[810, 813] Glucocorticoids enhance the sensitivity of lipolysis to catecholamines in target tissues.[810] The glycerol released during lipolysis provides substrate for glucose production, and released fatty acids provide an energy source for the

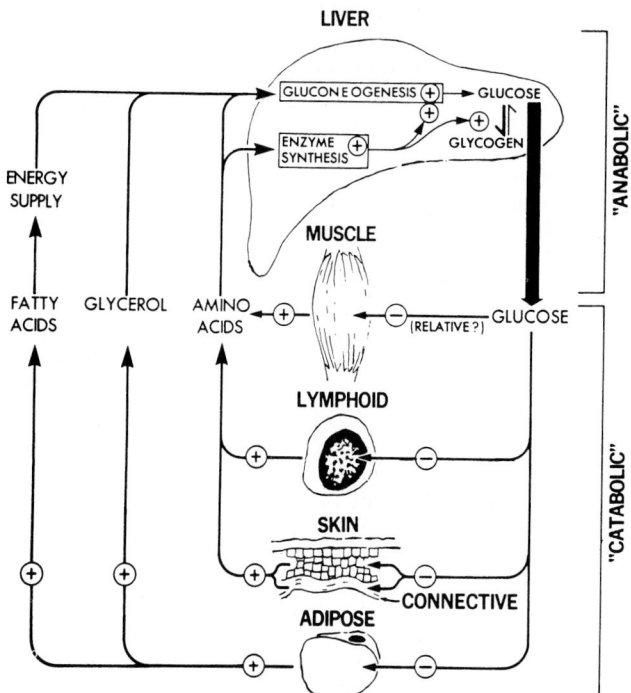

Figure 12–27. Glucocorticoid effects on hepatic glucose metabolism and peripheral tissue metabolism of protein and fat. Stimulation is indicated by plus signs, inhibition by minus signs. (From Baxter JD, Rousseau GG. Glucocorticoid hormone action: an overview. In: Baxter JD, Rousseau GG, eds. Glucocorticoid Hormone Action. New York: Springer-Verlag, 1979: 25–48.)

process. Glucocorticoids also enhance the sensitivity of lactate production to catecholamine stimulation in muscle. Increased sensitivity also underlies the permissive effect of glucocorticoids on glucagon action, but the mechanism is unknown.[810]

PERIPHERAL GLUCOSE UTILIZATION. In addition to mobilizing substrate for hepatic gluconeogenesis, glucocorticoids inhibit glucose uptake and utilization by peripheral tissues,[814–817] in part through inhibition of glucose transport into the cells (see Fig. 12–27).[818, 819] The number of glucose transporters in adipocytes is decreased by glucocorticoids, apparently because transporter mRNA levels are decreased.[820]

LIPID METABOLISM. Glucocorticoids acutely activate lipolysis in adipose tissue (see Fig. 12–27).[817] Lipolytic activity and, consequently, plasma free fatty acid levels are reduced in adrenalectomized animals and return to normal within 2 h after glucocorticoid administration.[821, 822] This permissive effect may be mediated by altered sensitivity to other lipolytic hormones, such as catecholamines and hGH,[821–823] but the molecular mechanisms are not known.

Glucocorticoids also exert chronic effects on lipid metabolism. One of the most striking in humans is the redistribution of body fat observed after chronic glucocorticoid excess. There is relative sparing of the extremities, whereas the dorsocervical and supraclavicular regions in particular, the trunk, and the anterior mediastinum and mesentery are sites of marked fat deposition. Animals exposed to excess glucocorticoids generally do not exhibit similar fat redistribution and may actually lose total body weight, although protein loss exceeds that of fat.[824] Hyperinsulinemia resulting from glucocorticoid effects on glucose metabolism may underlie the lipogenic effect,[825] but the mechanism underlying the central predisposition is unknown.

Effects on Immunologic Function and Inflammatory Processes

Endogenous glucocorticoid excess suppresses immunologic responses,[826] and latent infections (e.g., tuberculosis) may be reactivated by administration of pharmacologic doses of glucocorticoids. The immunosuppressive properties of glucocorticoids are exploited in the treatment of autoimmune diseases and inflammatory states and in the field of organ transplantation. A variety of effects on components of the immunologic and inflammatory responses have been described in vitro and in animal models, but which phenomena are most relevant to the physiological role of glucocorticoids in immunomodulation remains to be demonstrated (see Chapter 7).

TRAFFIC OF CELLS OF THE IMMUNE SYSTEM. Glucocorticoids alter the traffic of immune cells to and from the peripheral circulation. Glucocorticoids produce a marked decrease in human peripheral lymphocyte numbers within about 4 h, with greater depletion of thymus-derived lymphocytes (T cells) than marrow-derived lymphocytes (B cells). The effect is caused by temporary redistribution of lymphocytes from the intravascular compartment to the spleen, lymph nodes, thoracic duct, and bone marrow.[827, 828] Glucocorticoids cause a similar redistribution of monocytes but have the opposite effect on granulocytes, causing them to leave the bone marrow and enter the circulating blood. At the same time, glucocorticoids inhibit the accumulation of neutrophils at sites of inflammation.[829] These effects are manifested by increased numbers of circulating neutrophils and suppression of local inflammatory responses.

LYMPHOCYTE APOPTOSIS. Glucocorticoids promote the process of apoptosis or programmed cell death in lymphoid cells. Apoptosis is characterized by cytoplasmic changes, such as water loss and protein degradation, and by nuclear changes including chromatin condensation and internucleosomal

DNA fragmentation.[830] Since the apoptotic pathway is the mechanism for negative selection of thymocytes, the process is of central importance in the development of the immune repertoire. Glucocorticoid-induced apoptosis is mediated by the glucocorticoid receptor, but transcriptional activation is apparently not required, because mutant glucocorticoid receptors lacking transcriptional activation function can mediate induction of apoptosis.[831, 832]

T-CELL FUNCTION. Lymphocytes have long been recognized as targets for glucocorticoid action.[833] The effects of glucocorticoids on glucose uptake and amino acid incorporation were first defined in these cells.[834, 835] Inhibition of the synthesis of a wide variety of cytokines by glucocorticoids is believed to underlie their immunosuppressive properties and appears to be mediated by a common mechanism. Glucocorticoids inhibit the activation of nuclear factor kappa B (NF-κB), a transcription factor with a central role in induction of cytokine gene expression,[836, 837] through induction of a cytoplasmic inhibitor of NF-κB (IκB) that binds NF-κB, sequestering it in the cytoplasm and preventing its nuclear translocation.[836, 837]

B-CELL FUNCTION. Glucocorticoids modulate B-cell function directly and indirectly by effects on monocytes and T-cell subpopulations. Resting B cells presumably are activated and then proliferate in response to T cell–derived growth factors (e.g., IL-4) and terminally differentiate to produce immunoglobulins.[838] Glucocorticoids appear to modulate the steps in this process differently. Early events, such as B-cell activation and proliferation, are inhibited.[839] Terminal B-cell differentiation is less sensitive to glucocorticoid inhibition,[839] and glucocorticoids may actually enhance immunoglobulin production in certain situations.[838, 840–842] In some lymphoid organs, glucocorticoids may induce apoptosis of immature B cells.[843]

MONOCYTE AND MACROPHAGE FUNCTION. Glucocorticoids inhibit the proliferative response of monocytes to colony-stimulating factor[844] and their differentiation into macrophages.[845] They also inhibit the phagocytic and cytotoxic functions of macrophages.[846]

MEDIATORS OF INFLAMMATION. Glucocorticoids inhibit the movement of cells and fluid from the intravascular compartment that characterizes the local inflammatory response.[847] They inhibit the action of histamine, a potent vasoactive agent,[848] by an unknown mechanism. Prostaglandins are probable mediators of the inflammatory response,[849] and glucocorticoids inhibit prostaglandin synthesis,[850–853] possibly by inducing increased levels of one of the lipocortins, a family of Ca^{2+}/phospholipid-dependent proteins that inhibit phospholipase A_2 activation and therefore synthesis of prostaglandins and other arachidonic acid derivatives.[854–856] Lipocortin I, also called annexin I, is a 35-kd substrate of epidermal growth factor receptor tyrosine kinase activity[857] and is a potential inhibitor of phospholipase A_2,[858, 859] but its role in mediating glucocorticoid effects on phospholipase A_2 activity in inflammatory cells is unclear.[857, 860–863] Another possible mechanism of anti-inflammatory glucocorticoid action is inhibition of plasminogen activators (PAs),[864–866] serine proteases that convert plasminogen into active plasmin. Plasmin cleaves the plasma globulin, kininogen, into potent kinins that cause the vasodilatation and increased capillary permeability characteristic of inflammation. It is not known whether glucocorticoids regulate PA biosynthesis, PA inhibitor synthesis, or both. In vitro studies suggest that, although glucocorticoids may actually increase transcription of some PA genes, the increase is offset by induction of PA inhibitor gene expression.[867]

Effects on Musculoskeletal and Connective Tissues

BONE AND MINERAL METABOLISM. Chronic glucocorticoid excess causes osteopenia. Glucocorticoids inhibit osteoblast function and decrease new bone formation.[868–870] Synthesis of IGF-I, which promotes osteoblast proliferation and differentiation, is down-regulated in osteoblasts by glucocorticoids.[871] Bone histology in steroid-induced osteopenia reveals increased osteoclast numbers,[870] and glucocorticoids enhance the ability of osteoclasts to bind to bone surfaces as a consequence of altered expression of N-acetylglucosamine and N-acetylgalactosamine on the cell surface.[872] Whether osteoclast-mediated bone resorption is stimulated or suppressed is unclear.[873, 874]

Glucocorticoids also exert indirect effects on bone by decreasing intestinal calcium absorption,[870, 875–877] which does not appear to be caused by decreased levels of serum 25-hydroxycholecalciferol or 1,25-dihydroxycholecalciferol[870, 878, 879] or to decreased sensitivity of intestinal epithelial cells to vitamin D.[880]

A secondary effect of glucocorticoids is increased serum parathyroid hormone (PTH) levels,[870, 881] presumably caused by impaired intestinal calcium absorption. The increase is reversed by administration of vitamin D and calcium. Glucocorticoids may also have a direct effect on the parathyroid glands. Serum PTH rapidly increases without a measurable change in intestinal calcium absorption in hyperparathyroid patients given glucocorticoids,[882] and glucocorticoids stimulate PTH release from rat parathyroid glands in vitro.[883]

Glucocorticoids increase renal calcium excretion by decreasing reabsorption.[884, 885] In hyperparathyroidism, the combination of an increased filtered load of calcium and decreased calcium reabsorption produces marked hypercalciuria.[882]

SKELETAL MUSCLE. Glucocorticoid effects on intermediary metabolism (see previous discussion) involve skeletal muscle, a major source of amino acid substrate for gluconeogenesis. The catabolic effect on muscle protein is the basis for the profound myopathy that can result from glucocorticoid excess.

CONNECTIVE TISSUE. Glucocorticoids modulate proliferation of fibroblasts and a number of their differentiated functions. Most effects are inhibitory, such as suppression of fibroblast DNA, RNA, and protein synthesis.[886] Glucocorticoids also suppress synthesis of the extracellular matrix components, collagen[887–891] and hyaluronidate.[892, 893] The clinical result of chronic glucocorticoid excess is impaired wound healing and friable connective tissues.[894] Another deleterious effect on wound healing is defective macrophage recruitment to the wound site.[894] TGF-β may reverse these defects.[895]

Glucocorticoids stimulate production of some fibroblast products, such as fibronectin, an extracellular matrix glycoprotein.[896–898] TGF-β also induces fibronectin biosynthesis and acts synergistically with glucocorticoids. Glucocorticoids appear to stabilize fibronectin mRNA, whereas TGF-β stimulates fibronectin mRNA transcription.[898] Elastin, a product of fibroblasts that have differentiated into ligament cells, is also increased by glucocorticoids.[899] This effect may also result from mRNA stabilization, rather than transcriptional regulation.

Effects on Fluid and Electrolyte Homeostasis

MINERALOCORTICOID ACTIVITY. Patients with glucocorticoid excess usually have hypertension, which may occur in the absence of elevated plasma mineralocorticoid concentrations or evidence of functional mineralocorticoid excess such as hypokalemia or suppressed plasma renin activity.[900, 901] The principal endogenous glucocorticoids in humans and rodents, cortisol and corticosterone, respectively, have weak intrinsic mineralocorticoid activity. However, in a rat model of glucocorticoid-induced hypertension the elevated blood pressure is not caused by supraphysiological concentrations of glucocorticoids acting on type I mineralocorticoid receptors.[902] Therefore, although it is generally assumed that exces-

sive concentrations of glucocorticoids exert a direct mineralocorticoid effect on target tissues, in the presence of normally functioning 11β-HSD this may not be the case (see Chapter 14). Other glucocorticoid-mediated phenomena have been implicated. Glucocorticoids induce hepatic production of angiotensinogen, but it is unclear whether its increased circulating levels result in increased generation of angiotensin II. There is little evidence for an angiotensin II–induced increase in aldosterone secretion. Enhanced vascular sensitivity to the pressor effects of infused angiotensin II and norepinephrine occurs in patients with Cushing's syndrome,[901] but its mechanism also is unknown. Finally, levels of the vasodilators prostaglandin E₂ and kallikrein are decreased in the urine of animals and humans with glucocorticoid excess.[901, 903] The actual basis for the hypertension in patients with glucocorticoid excess is not fully understood.

Patients with glucocorticoid deficiency may be hypotensive and refractory to the effects of pressor agents, in part because of the associated deficiency in renin substrate.[904] Decreased inhibition by glucocorticoids of production of prostaglandin I₂, a potent vasodilator, may decrease peripheral vascular tone.[904]

VASOPRESSIN. Free water clearance is decreased in patients with glucocorticoid deficiency[905, 906] in association with increased plasma AVP concentrations.[907] Glucocorticoid deficiency increases vasopressin mRNA levels in the paraventricular nucleus but not in the supraoptic or suprachiasmatic nuclei of the rat.[522] It is not known whether this increase and the increased plasma AVP concentrations are direct effects of loss of glucocorticoid negative feedback on vasopressin gene expression or are secondary to changes in intravascular volume and plasma osmolality. However, glucocorticoid receptors are present in AVP-producing cells of the parvicellular division of the paraventricular nucleus.[908] Increased circulating levels of vasopressin may play a role in maintaining normal blood pressure in adrenal insufficiency.[909]

ATRIAL NATRIURETIC PEPTIDE. Animals subjected to adrenal enucleation (removal of the adrenals, with the capsules and adherent zona glomerulosa cells left intact) are unable to excrete a salt load.[910, 911] Glucocorticoid replacement results in a natriuresis that was at first thought to be caused by a glucocorticoid-induced increase in glomerular filtration rate[912] but now appears to involve ANP. Both human and rat ANP genes contain putative GREs,[913–915] and glucocorticoids induce increased plasma ANP levels in intact[916] and adrenalectomized animals.[917] Glucocorticoids stimulate increased ANP mRNA content,[917] ANP synthesis and secretion, and processing of the ANP(1–126) precursor into mature ANP(99–126) by cardiac myocytes in vitro.[918–920] Glucocorticoids also potentiate ANP action on the kidney by both cyclic guanosine monophosphate (cGMP)–dependent and cGMP–independent mechanisms.[921]

Neuropsychiatric and Behavioral Effects

MOOD. Glucocorticoids influence diverse aspects of human behavior, including sleep patterns, mood, cognition, and reception of sensory input.[922] The duration of rapid eye movement sleep is decreased in patients with Cushing's syndrome[923] and in normal subjects given pharmacologic doses of glucocorticoid[924] or ACTH.[925] Evidence for steroid-induced alterations of mood and cognitive function comes largely from clinical observation. About half of patients with either spontaneous or iatrogenic Cushing's syndrome have psychological disturbances, depression being the most common.[926–930] Patients with exogenous Cushing's syndrome have been thought to have euphoria more often than those with spontaneous Cushing's, but there is little evidence for this. Varying degrees of manic behavior and even overt psychosis can occur. Patients with adrenal insufficiency also may suffer from psychiatric disturbances, mainly depression, apathy, and lethargy. The mechanisms that mediate the behavioral effects of glucocorticoids are unknown.

CENTRAL NERVOUS SYSTEM. Cells in several parts of the central nervous system contain glucocorticoid receptors, but some neuronal responses seem too rapid to be mediated by transcriptional activation of target genes by glucocorticoid-receptor complexes. These responses include changes in electrical activity, such as hyperpolarization of the cell membrane[931] or suppression of spontaneous electrical activity.[932, 933] They occur so rapidly (i.e., within 2 min of exposure to the hormone) that a direct membrane effect is likely. Hyperpolarization is blocked by antiglucocorticoids, suggesting involvement of a receptor-like molecule.[932] Chronic exposure causes inhibition of the regenerative axon sprouting that follows deafferentation of hippocampal neurons[934, 935] and reduction in their number.[936] Central nervous system glial cells such as astrocytes[937–939] and oligodendrocytes[940, 941] also appear to be targets for glucocorticoids. The effects appear to be exerted at the transcriptional level.[942]

Gastrointestinal Effects

ION TRANSPORT. Glucocorticoids have direct effects on ion transport in the colon.[943] Although the colon also contains mineralocorticoid receptors that may mediate such effects (see later discussion), two lines of evidence suggest that glucocorticoid-induced sodium transport is mediated by glucocorticoid (type II) receptors. First, the use of steroid analogues specific for glucocorticoid receptors shows a saturable effect on sodium transport.[944] Second, blockade of mineralocorticoid receptors with spironolactone does not diminish the response of sodium transport to low doses of dexamethasone.[945]

ULCER FORMATION. Chronic administration of pharmacologic doses of glucocorticoids is believed to increase the risk of peptic ulcer in the upper gastrointestinal tract.[946] The mechanism by which ulcers may be induced is not known but may involve inhibition of healing of ulceration caused by other factors. Acute administration of even pharmacologic doses of glucocorticoids is not associated with increased ulcer formation.

Developmental Effects

LINEAR GROWTH. Supraphysiological levels of endogenous glucocorticoids or pharmacologic doses of exogenous glucocorticoids inhibit linear skeletal growth in children.[947, 948] The mechanism is unknown. hGH may be suppressed,[949] but usually not markedly so in children, and serum IGF-I levels are not decreased.[950] Furthermore, hGH gene transcription is activated by glucocorticoids in vitro.[951] Therefore, growth arrest is presumably caused by direct inhibitory effects of glucocorticoids on bone and connective tissue (see earlier discussion). In addition, circulating inhibitors of IGF-I action are induced by glucocorticoids,[952] but their nature is unknown.

LUNG. Glucocorticoids stimulate differentiation of many cell types.[953] In the developing lung, for example, endogenous glucocorticoid induces surfactant production by type II pneumocytes, a normal developmental process that is accelerated by pharmacologic amounts of exogenous glucocorticoid.[954] Glucocorticoids induce morphologic changes in type II cells,[955, 956] apparently induce enzymes involved in phospholipid biosynthesis, and regulate transcription of the genes for the surfactant proteins (SP-A, SP-B, and SP-C).[956–960] Mice in whom the glucocorticoid receptor genes have been disrupted by homologous recombination have atelectatic lungs and die shortly after birth from respiratory failure.[961]

NERVOUS SYSTEM AND ADRENAL MEDULLA. In the nervous system, glucocorticoids regulate the differentiation of neural crest epithelial cells into chromaffin cells. Neural crest cells are precursors for a variety of more differentiated cell types, including autonomic ganglion cells and adrenomedullary cells, and their hormonal environment plays a major role in determining their developmental fate.[962] Under the influence of nerve growth factor, for example, sympathetic ganglion cells enlarge, develop neuronal processes and synaptic vesicles, and produce a variety of neuron-specific proteins, such as SCG-10 (cloned from a superior cervical ganglion cDNA library), guanosine triphosphatase–activating protein or GAP-43 (a growth associated protein believed to be involved in neuronal growth and plasticity), and NF-68 (a neurofilament component).[963–967] Under the influence of glucocorticoids, neural crest precursor cells that invade the embryonic adrenal gland acquire the characteristic morphology of adrenomedullary chromaffin cells.[967] They also lose their neural processes and begin to produce catecholamine-synthesizing enzymes, such as phenylethanolamine N-methyltransferase (PNMT). The exact mechanism by which glucocorticoids induce this differentiation is not known. Mice in which the glucocorticoid receptor gene is disrupted by homologous recombination lack an organized adrenal medulla.[961]

Dissociation of Biologic Effects

There is an obvious attraction to finding synthetic glucocorticoids that exert desirable therapeutic effects and lack undesirable side effects. The synthesis of fludrocortisone, which has salt-retaining activity out of proportion to its glucocorticoid activity, was such an accomplishment. However, the search for synthetic glucocorticoids that exert anti-inflammatory effects but are devoid of effects on intermediary metabolism or calcium metabolism has been generally unsuccessful. One such synthetic glucocorticoid is deflazacort, an oxaziline derivative of prednisolone. Deflazacort in some studies is an effective anti-inflammatory agent but has less propensity to exert adverse effects on carbohydrate and bone mineral metabolism.[968, 969] This sparing of side effects has not been observed in all studies of the drug, and, since all glucocorticoid effects are believed to be mediated by the same type II glucocorticoid receptor, the mechanism by which such a dissociation might occur is unexplained.

DISEASES OF THE ADRENAL CORTEX

Hypofunction

Adrenal insufficiency may be caused by destruction of the adrenal cortex (primary adrenal insufficiency, Addison's disease), deficient pituitary ACTH secretion (secondary adrenal insufficiency), or deficient hypothalamic secretion of CRH or other ACTH secretagogues (tertiary adrenal insufficiency) (see Fig. 12–28; see Chapter 9.) Although the prevalence of primary adrenal insufficiency is only about 40 to 110 cases per 1 million adults and the incidence is only about 6 cases per 1 million adults per year,[970–972] it causes considerable morbidity and frequent mortality. The disorder can be reliably diagnosed and easily treated. The symptoms of weakness, fatigue, weight loss, and gastrointestinal complaints are common to many other disorders, so adrenal insufficiency must be considered in their differential diagnosis. Secondary adrenal insufficiency from natural causes is also uncommon, but iatrogenic tertiary adrenal insufficiency caused by suppression of hypothalamic-pituitary-adrenal function secondary to glucocorticoid administration is common.

Pathophysiology

Primary adrenal insufficiency results from adrenal gland destruction or dysfunction caused by a local lesion or disease process. Secondary adrenal insufficiency is caused by inadequate pituitary ACTH secretion and consequent insufficient adrenal cortisol secretion. Tertiary adrenal insufficiency results from inadequate secretion of CRH or other hypothalamic ACTH secretagogues and secondary hyposecretion of pituitary ACTH.

PRIMARY ADRENAL INSUFFICIENCY. In primary adrenal insufficiency all three zones of the adrenal cortex are usually involved by a disease process. The process can be local or, more commonly, a manifestation of systemic disorders; these include autoimmune diseases (either isolated or as part of the polyglandular autoimmune [PGA] syndromes), granulomatous diseases such as tuberculosis and histoplasmosis, metastatic malignancies such as lung and breast carcinoma, hemorrhage associated with anticoagulant therapy or meningococcemia, and rare hereditary diseases. The result is inadequate secretion of glucocorticoids, mineralocorticoids, and androgens (Fig. 12–28). Clinical signs and symptoms do not become manifest until at least 90% of the adrenal cortex is destroyed.[973, 974] Therefore, the onset of clinical manifestations is usually gradual, going first through a phase of partial glucocorticoid deficiency that results only in an inadequate cortisol increase in response to stress and, rarely, because of deficiencies of both glucocorticoid and epinephrine, mild postprandial hypoglycemia. The initial mineralocorticoid deficiency may be manifested only as mild transient postural hypotension.[975, 976] Manifestations of complete glucocorticoid deficiency include a decreased sense of well-being, gastrointestinal disturbances, and abnormal glucose metabolism. Mineralocorticoid deficiency results in decreased renal potassium and hydrogen ion excretion and reduced sodium retention, the latter leading to contraction of intravascular volume, hypotension, and dehydration. Volume depletion is compounded by reduced peripheral vascular adrenergic tone caused by glucocorticoid deficiency and can lead to vascular collapse and shock. Potassium retention leads to high serum potassium levels that can cause cardiac arrhythmias and death. A mild

acidosis contributes to the hyperkalemia by permitting potassium to shift from the intracellular to the extracellular space. Adrenal androgen deficiency is evident only in women, as decreased pubic and axillary hair and decreased libido; men derive most of their androgens from the testes. Decreased adrenal epinephrine secretion[977] may contribute to postprandial hypoglycemia.

The lack of cortisol negative feedback increases hypothalamic CRH and AVP synthesis and secretion, leading to increased synthesis and secretion of pituitary ACTH and other POMC-related peptides (see Fig. 12–28). However, peripheral plasma CRH and AVP concentrations are not elevated.[978] The increased plasma ACTH levels reflect increased amplitude of the secretory pulses; pulse frequency is normal.[978] ACTH causes hyperpigmentation of the skin and mucous membranes.[240, 318] CRH and possibly other growth factors cause corticotrope hyperplasia, which, especially in the absence of adequate glucocorticoid replacement therapy, can become evident on computerized tomography (CT) scan of the pituitary[979–981] and rarely can lead to an autonomous corticotrope adenoma.[982] However, ACTH secretion, though increased, usually retains a normal circadian rhythm[983] and is normally suppressed by glucocorticoid administration.[978]

SECONDARY AND TERTIARY ADRENAL INSUFFICIENCY. In secondary adrenal insufficiency, cortisol production is inadequate due to insufficient pituitary ACTH secretion (see Fig. 12–28). As a result of decreased negative feedback inhibition by cortisol, the synthesis and secretion of hypothalamic CRH (and possibly of AVP) presumably are increased. In tertiary adrenal insufficiency, the defect is a lack of normal CRH secretion (see Fig. 12–28). The intrinsically normal pituitary gland can secrete ACTH in response to exogenous CRH.[984–986] In secondary and tertiary adrenal insufficiency, the clinical presentation is one of pure glucocorticoid deficiency and, in women, loss of adrenal androgen secretion. In isolated ACTH deficiency, hypoglycemia may be the initial manifestation.[987, 988] Because ACTH secretion is decreased rather than increased, patients are not hyperpigmented. Mineralocorticoid secretion usually is normal because it is regulated by the renin-angiotensin system. Therefore, hypotension, dehydration, and shock are unusual, and adrenal crisis is rare. As with

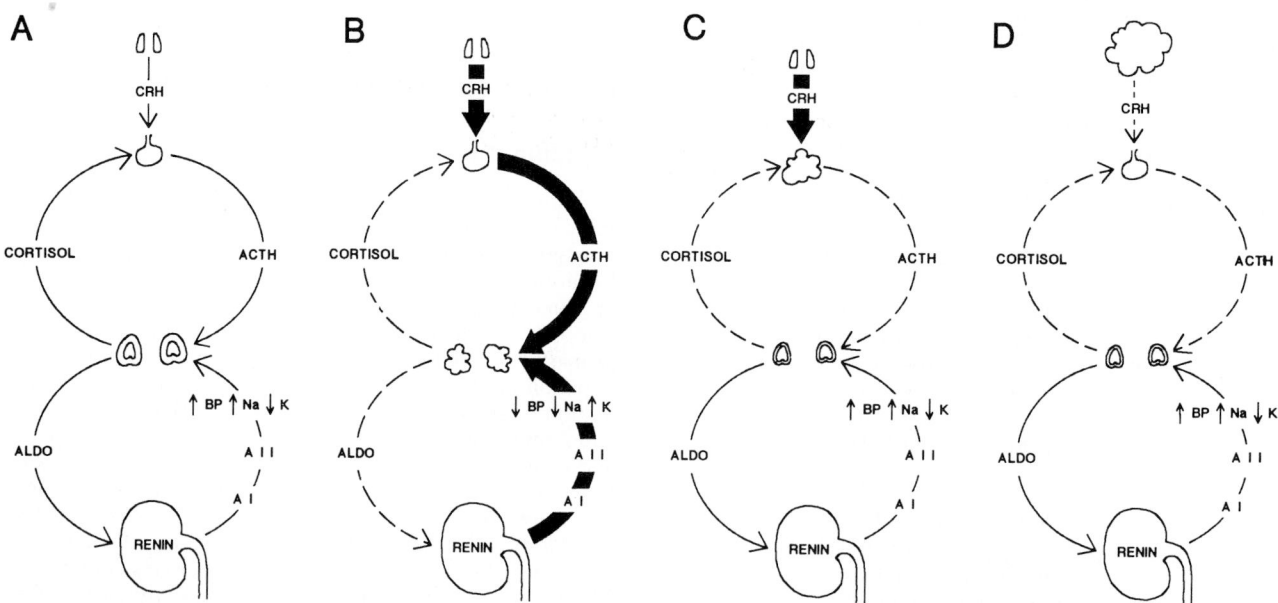

Figure 12–28. Hypothalamic-pituitary-adrenal and renin-angiotensin-aldosterone regulatory system function in normal individuals *(A)* and in patients with primary *(B),* secondary *(C),* and tertiary *(D)* hypoadrenocorticism.

primary adrenal insufficiency, the process is usually gradual, going first through a stage of partial ACTH deficiency that is evident only in inadequate ACTH and cortisol responses to stress. With prolonged and more profound ACTH deficiency, the adrenal fasciculata and reticularis atrophy and lose the ability to respond acutely to ACTH. However, the adrenal cortex can recover its ability to produce cortisol in response to continuous maximal ACTH stimulation over a period of a few days to a week. In chronic untreated secondary or tertiary adrenal insufficiency, mineralocorticoid deficiency may develop. It is usually responsive to glucocorticoid replacement.

Clinical Presentation

The signs and symptoms depend on the rate and degree of loss of adrenal function, on whether mineralocorticoid production is preserved (as is usually the case in secondary and tertiary adrenal insufficiency), and on the degree of physiological stress. Adrenal insufficiency is often insidious in onset and may go undetected until an intercurrent illness or stress precipitates a crisis.

ADRENAL CRISIS: ACUTE ADRENAL INSUFFICIENCY

Primary Adrenal Insufficiency. Acute adrenal insufficiency, or adrenal crisis, usually manifests as shock in a previously undiagnosed patient with primary adrenal insufficiency who has been subjected to a major physiological stress or in a patient with established adrenal insufficiency who does not increase glucocorticoid replacement during a bacterial infection or other major illness or cannot retain medication because of persistent vomiting due to viral gastroenteritis or other causes. In addition to shock, patients often have other nonspecific symptoms, such as anorexia, nausea, vomiting, abdominal pain, weakness, fatigue, lethargy, confusion, or coma (Table 12–7). Abdominal tenderness on deep palpation without localizing signs is common but of unknown cause. Fever is often present, usually caused by a precipitating infection, and may be exaggerated because of the hypocortisolemia. The abdominal pain and fever may lead to incorrect diagnosis of an acute surgical abdomen and potentially catastrophic surgical exploration without steroid replacement. Hypoglycemia rarely may be the presenting manifestation; it is more common in secondary adrenal insufficiency caused by isolated ACTH deficiency.[987, 988] Patients with long-standing adrenal insufficiency who present in crisis may be hyperpigmented and have weight loss and other evidence of chronic adrenal insufficiency (see Table 12–7).[987]

It is important to recognize that a major pathophysiological factor in the precipitation of adrenal crisis is mineralocorticoid deficiency. In fact, adrenal crisis can occur in patients who are receiving physiological or even pharmacologic dosages of synthetic glucocorticoids if their mineralocorticoid requirements are not met.[989, 990] However, glucocorticoid deficiency contributes to the hypotension, perhaps as a result of decreased vascular sensitivity to angiotensin II and norepinephrine,[901] decreased synthesis of renin substrate,[991] and increased prostaglandin I_2 production.[992]

Adrenal crisis may also occur as a result of sudden, bilateral adrenal infarction caused by hemorrhage, embolus, or sepsis or, very rarely, by adrenal vein thrombosis after a back injury.[993, 994] Such patients do not have evidence of pre-existing adrenal insufficiency. Until the development of the CT scan, the diagnosis of adrenal hemorrhage usually was made at autopsy.[994] Manifestations include hypotension or shock (>90%); abdominal, flank, back, or lower chest pain (86%); fever (66%); anorexia, nausea, or vomiting (47%); neuropsychiatric manifestations, such as confusion or disorientation (42%); and abdominal rigidity or rebound tenderness (22%).[993] Hypotension occurs in only about half of the patients before shock develops. Evidence of occult hemorrhage, such as a sudden fall in hemoglobin and hematocrit, and progressive hyperkalemia, hyponatremia, and volume contraction should suggest the diagnosis. Major risk factors include anticoagulant therapy or coagulopathy, thromboembolic disease such as recurrent intravascular thrombosis, and the postoperative state. In patients treated with anticoagulants, clotting indices usually are within the therapeutic range, and spontaneous bleeding elsewhere is not evident.[993] Adrenal hemorrhage is difficult to recognize clinically and must be considered whenever these symptoms develop in a patient with one or more risk factors. Without appropriate therapy, shock can progress to coma and death. Adrenal hemorrhage and death have been associated with meningococcemia (Waterhouse-Friderichsen syndrome),[995] but *Pseudomonas aeruginosa* was the most common pathogen in 51 children dying of sepsis and bilateral adrenal hemorrhage.[996]

Chronic Secondary/Tertiary Adrenal Insufficiency. Adrenal crisis is uncommon in patients with secondary or tertiary adrenal insufficiency because normal renin-angiotensin-aldosterone physiology is usually maintained and hypovolemia is rare.[987, 988, 997, 998] These patients often also have deficiency of other anterior pituitary hormones. Patients with pituitary apoplexy resulting from infarction of a large tumor usually complain of severe headache and may have acute visual loss or reduction in visual fields (see Chapter 9). Because glucocorticoids have a role in maintaining peripheral vascular adrenergic tone, sudden loss of ACTH secretion, particularly in conjunction with other serious illness, can cause hypotension and shock.

CHRONIC ADRENAL INSUFFICIENCY.

Patients with chronic primary adrenal insufficiency have signs and symptoms of glucocorticoid, mineralocorticoid, and androgen deficiency. Patients with secondary or tertiary adrenal insufficiency usually maintain adequate mineralocorticoid function. The diagnosis is usually obvious in patients with the full-blown syndrome of adrenal insufficiency. However, its onset is often insidious, with gradual development of signs and symptoms, each of which alone is nonspecific. In its early stage, therefore, the disease presents a difficult problem of differential diagnosis.

Primary Adrenal Insufficiency. The most common clinical features of chronic primary adrenal insufficiency are listed in Table 12–8.[971, 987, 999–1001] Regardless of the immediate complaint, patients with adrenal insufficiency consistently have chronic malaise, lassitude, fatigability, weakness, weight loss, and anorexia. The weakness is generalized, rather than being limited to particular muscle groups. The fatigue is worsened by exertion and improved with bed rest. Weight loss, which results mostly from anorexia but partly from dehydration, may vary from 2 to as much as 15 kg but may not become evident until adrenal failure is advanced.[999] Patients may exhibit extreme sensitivity to drugs, such as narcotics or anesthetics, or

---

TABLE 12–7. Clinical and Laboratory Features Suggesting Adrenal Crisis in a Patient with Chronic Primary Adrenal Insufficiency

Dehydration, hypotension, or shock out of proportion to severity of current illness
Nausea and vomiting with a history of weight loss and anorexia
Abdominal pain, so-called acute abdomen
Unexplained hypoglycemia
Unexplained fever
Hyponatremia, hyperkalemia, azotemia, hypercalcemia, or eosinophilia
Hyperpigmentation or vitiligo
Other autoimmune endocrine deficiencies, such as hypothyroidism or gonadal failure

Adapted from Burke CW. Adrenocortical insufficiency. Clin Endocrinol Metab 1985; 14:947–976. Copyright 1985, The Endocrine Society.

TABLE 12–8. Major Manifestations in Patients with Primary Adrenal Insufficiency

Symptom, Sign, or Laboratory Finding	Frequency (%)
Symptom	
Weakness, tiredness, fatigue	100
Anorexia	100
Gastrointestinal symptoms	92
Nausea	86
Vomiting	75
Constipation	33
Abdominal pain	31
Diarrhea	16
Salt craving	16
Postural dizziness	12
Muscle or joint pains	6–13
Sign	
Weight loss	100
Hyperpigmentation	94
Hypotension (<110 mm Hg systolic)	88–94
Vitiligo	10–20
Auricular calcification	5
Laboratory Finding	
Electrolyte disturbances	92
Hyponatremia	88
Hyperkalemia	64
Hypercalcemia	6
Azotemia	55
Anemia	40
Eosinophilia	17

Data from Thorn,[1001] Irving and Barnes,[1000] Nerup,[971] Jarvis et al.,[1002] Dunlop,[999] and Burke.[987]

they may recover very slowly from illnesses or operations that do not precipitate an adrenal crisis.

Gastrointestinal complaints, usually nausea and occasionally vomiting, abdominal pain, or diarrhea that may alternate with constipation, are common and correlate with the severity of adrenal insufficiency. Vomiting and abdominal pain often herald an adrenal crisis (see previous discussion). The mechanism of these gastrointestinal disorders has not been systematically investigated. Esophagogastroduodenoscopy and gastrointestinal radiography findings are usually normal,[1002] but gastric emptying time may be delayed.[1003] Peptic ulcer disease is rare.[1004] Steatorrhea, responsive to glucocorticoid replacement, has occasionally been reported and occurs in adrenalectomized rats, in which it may be caused by decreased activity of intestinal mucosal enzymes.[1004, 1005]

Cardiovascular symptoms include postural dizziness or syncope. In most patients the blood pressure is low, but initially only postural hypotension may be evident. Blood pressure control improves in patients with pre-existing hypertension. Therefore, the presence of systolic hypertension is strong evidence against a diagnosis of adrenal insufficiency.[999–1001] Salt craving, sometimes with massive salt ingestion, is a distinctive feature in some patients.[1001] Salt is often "chased" with lemon juice. Increased thirst for iced liquids is often reported.

The loss of the gluconeogenic effects of cortisol may cause hypoglycemia after prolonged fasting or, rarely, several hours after a high-carbohydrate meal.[999–1001, 1006] It is infrequent in adults in the absence of infection, fever, or alcohol ingestion. In contrast, hypoglycemia is more common in infants and children with primary adrenal insufficiency[1007] (see later discussion) and in patients with secondary adrenal insufficiency caused by isolated ACTH deficiency.[987, 988] Hypoglycemia is thought to be the result of increased peripheral glucose utilization associated with increased sensitivity to insulin[1008] and impairment of gluconeogenesis, hepatic glucose production, and glycogen synthesis.[987] Patients with adrenal insufficiency may tolerate hypoglycemia without developing symptoms.[1006] Presumably, other symptoms usually develop in

patients with primary adrenal insufficiency or panhypopituitarism before symptomatic hypoglycemia occurs.

Hyperpigmentation, which is evident in most but not all[1009] patients with primary adrenal insufficiency (see Table 12–8), is one of the characteristic physical findings (Fig. 12–29; see color section between pages 875 and 877). Patients often are aware of the darkening of the skin. It is caused by increased content of melanin in the skin, which results from the melanocyte-stimulating activity of the increased circulating ACTH levels.[240, 318] α-MSH, the most potent melanotropin in frogs and lizards and equipotent in human melanocytes,[240, 318] may be synthesized in the human pituitary gland[1010, 1011] in addition to desacetyl-α-MSH,[222, 1012] which is about one tenth as potent but is absent from the peripheral plasma of patients with primary adrenal insufficiency.[1013] Skin darkening in frogs and lizards reflects acute dispersion of intracellular melanin granules within stellate cells called *melanophores*. In humans, chronic darkening of the skin involves synthesis of melanin by epidermal melanocytes subjacent to the basal cells. The melanin is packaged in secretory granules, called *melanosomes*, which are phagocytosed by the basal cells of the epidermis.[1014] The resulting brown pigmentation is generalized but is most conspicuous in areas exposed to light, such as the face, neck, and backs of hands, and areas exposed to chronic mild trauma, friction, or pressure, such as the elbows, knees, spine, knuckles, waist (belt), midriff (girdle), and shoulders (brassiere straps). Patchy buccal pigmentation occurs on the inner surface of lips and on the buccal mucosa along the line of dental occlusion, sites of repeated trauma (see Fig. 12–29). It may also occur under the tongue, along the gingival border in patients with chronic periodontal disease, and on the hard palate. Generalized buccal, vaginal, and anal mucosal membrane hyperpigmentation usually is seen only in patients whose skin is normally pigmented, such as African-Americans and Native Americans. Pigmentation is also prominent in the palmar creases, where it escapes being worn away by friction, and in areas that are normally pigmented, such as the areola, axillae, perineum, and umbilicus (see Fig. 12–29).[999–1001] Existing freckles (lentigines) become darker, and numerous new brown or black freckles may appear. Hyperpigmentation in African-Americans may cause generalized darkening of the skin but it is usually less noticeable than in light-skinned persons. Scars acquired during untreated primary adrenal insufficiency are permanently pigmented; those acquired before the onset of adrenal failure remain unpigmented, and those acquired after treatment do not become pigmented (see Fig. 12–29). The hair and nails may become darker, the nails showing longitudinal bands of darkening. The cutaneous hyperpigmentation begins to fade within several days and disappears after weeks to months of adequate adrenal hormone replacement; fading of hair and nails takes longer, and scars never fade.

Patchy, often bilaterally symmetrical areas of depigmented skin (vitiligo) occur on the trunk or extremities in 10 to 20% of patients with autoimmune types but not in those with other varieties of adrenal insufficiency (see Fig. 12–29).[1000, 1001, 1015]

Decreased axillary and pubic hair and loss of libido are common in women but not in men,[1000] because most androgen in women is produced by the adrenal glands. Amenorrhea occurs in about 25% of women and may result from the effects of chronic illness, weight loss, or autoimmune-mediated primary ovarian failure.[1000] About 7% of women experience premature menopause because of autoimmune-mediated gonadal failure.[1015]

Diffuse myalgias and arthralgias often are present (see Table 12–8). Occasionally musculoskeletal complaints and rarely flexion contractures of the lower extremities predominate.[1016, 1017] Muscle enzyme analyses, muscle histology, and electromyography results usually are normal. Relief often oc-

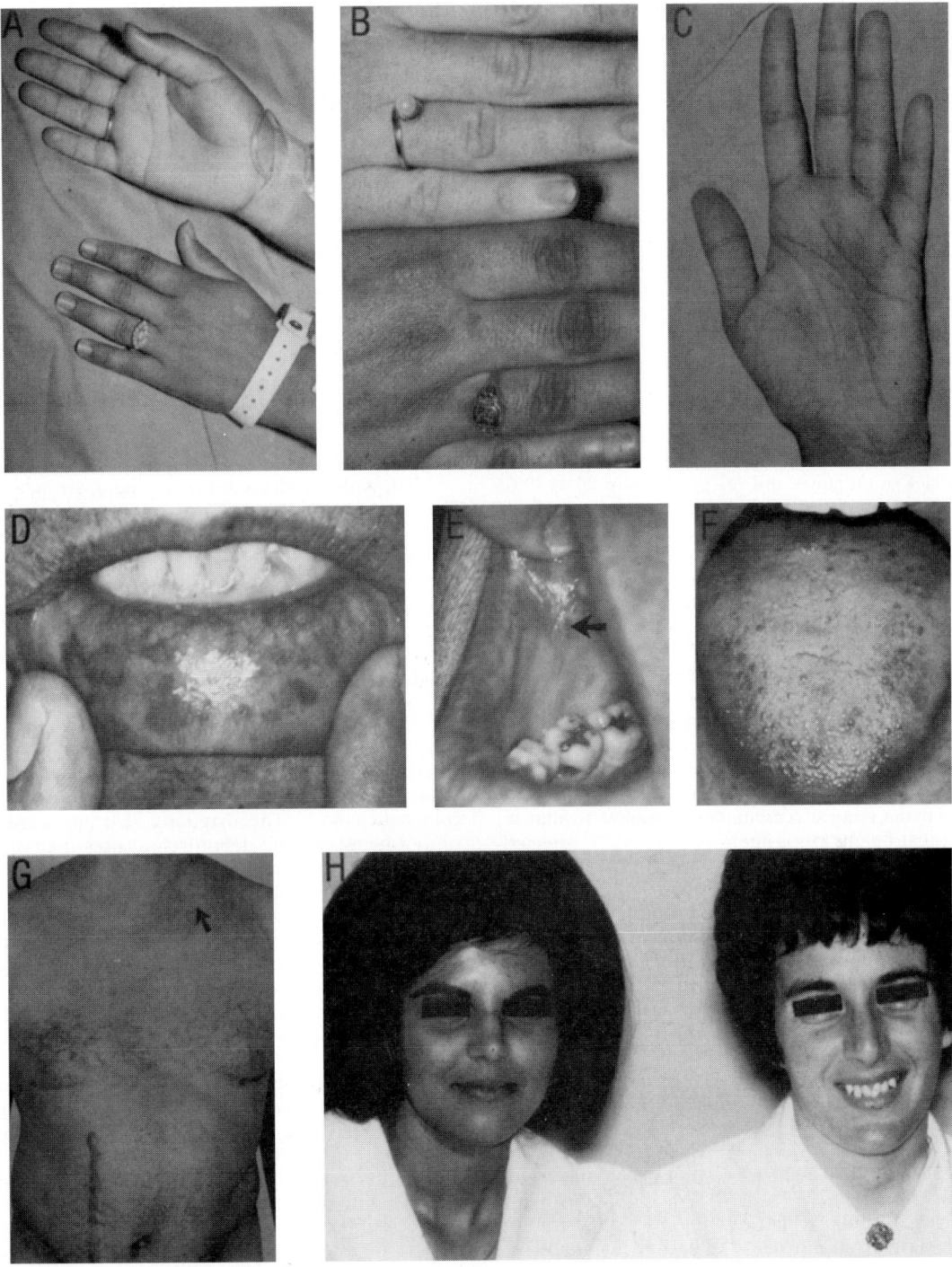

Figure 12–29. Cutaneous hyperpigmentation related to POMC-derived peptide hypersecretion (see color section between pages 875 and 877). *A,* Hands of an 18-year-old woman with polyglandular autoimmune syndrome and Addison's disease. Note vitiligo above the left thumb. *B,* Hand of a 16-year-old girl with Nelson's syndrome 2 y after bilateral adrenalectomy for Cushing's disease, compared with a normal girl's hand. Note deep pigmentation of the knuckles. *C,* Hand of the same young woman as in *B* at the age of 24 years. Note deep pigmentation of the palmar creases. *D,* Buccal pigmentation in a 32-year-old man with tuberculous Addison's disease. Note clustering along the line of dental occlusion on the lower lip and inflammatory periodontal disease on the gums. *E,* Same man as in *D.* Note pigmentation in the cheek mucosa along the line of dental occlusion *(arrow). F,* Pigmentation of the tongue in a 20-year-old girl with Nelson's syndrome 1 y after bilateral adrenalectomy for Cushing's disease. *G,* Pigmented scar from a right adrenalectomy in a 47-year-old man with Cushing's disease. The linear traumatic scar above the left medial clavicle *(arrow),* which was formed before the onset of Cushing's disease, is nonpigmented. *H,* Generalized deep pigmentation in a 19-year-old white woman with Nelson's syndrome 5 y after bilateral adrenalectomy for Cushing's disease *(left),* compared with a normally pigmented woman *(right). (B, C, F,* and *H* courtesy of Dr. H. Patrick Higgins.)

curs rapidly with glucocorticoid and mineralocorticoid replacement, but reversal of the contractures may take months and may require orthopedic measures. Hyperkalemic neuromyopathy with symmetrical, ascending flaccid quadriplegia has been reported in a few patients.[1018]

Calcification of the auricular cartilages may occur in longstanding primary or secondary adrenal insufficiency.[1002, 1019, 1020] Adrenal insufficiency is the most common associated systemic disorder.[1019] It occurs exclusively in men, is postulated to result from chronic cortisol deficiency, and does not improve with glucocorticoid replacement.[1019] The incidence of multiple dental caries may be high.[1002]

Splenomegaly and lymphoid tissue hyperplasia, particularly of the tonsils, may occur.[987, 1001] Patients with PGA syndrome type I (PGA I) often have chronic moniliasis of the vagina and mouth, and sometimes of the nails, that does not respond to replacement hormone therapy; antifungal agents afford only temporary relief.

Psychiatric symptoms in patients with severe or longstanding adrenal insufficiency[1021] can include (1) mild to moderate organic brain syndrome in 5 to 20%, usually impairment of memory that can progress to confusion, delirium, and stupor; (2) depression in 20 to 40%, manifested by apathy, poverty of thought, and lack of initiative; and (3) psychosis in 20 to 40%, manifested by social withdrawal, irritability, negativism, poor judgment, agitation, hallucinations, paranoid delusions, and bizarre or catatonic posturing. Perceptual disturbances can include enhanced sensitivity to, but impaired recognition and interpretation of, auditory, tactile, gustatory, and olfactory stimuli. These psychiatric manifestations occur early in the disease and may predate other physical findings, making diagnosis of the cause difficult. Most symptoms disappear within a few days after adequate glucocorticoid therapy is begun, but the psychosis may persist for several months. Improvement does not correlate with correction of electrolyte imbalance except, on occasion, in patients with severe hyponatremia and organic brain syndrome.

In children the clinical presentation is similar to that in adults, except that weight loss is not as prominent.[1022] Affected children usually are short, between the 3rd and 25th percentile for their ages. Those with PGA I often have antecedent moniliasis of the mouth and nails and hypocalcemia caused by hypoparathyroidism,[1023] whereas those with adrenoleukodystrophy or adrenomyeloneuropathy may initially have neurologic symptoms.[1024, 1025] Neonates with primary adrenal insufficiency (usually caused by congenital adrenal hypoplasia or adrenoleukodystrophy) are particularly susceptible to hypoglycemia.[1007]

Secondary Adrenal Insufficiency. The clinical features of secondary adrenal insufficiency are similar to those of primary adrenal insufficiency with two major exceptions. First, hyperpigmentation is not present because plasma ACTH levels are not elevated. Second, dehydration does not occur, and hypotension is less prominent.[987, 988, 997, 998] Weakness, fatigability, myalgias, arthralgias, and psychiatric symptoms are as common as in primary adrenal insufficiency, indicating that most of these symptoms are caused by glucocorticoid rather than mineralocorticoid deficiency. However, gastrointestinal symptoms are less common,[987] suggesting that electrolyte disturbances may be involved in their genesis. Hypoglycemia is more common in secondary than in primary adrenal insufficiency.[987] The increased incidence of hypoglycemia is not simply a result of concomitant loss of hGH secretion, because it is the presenting feature in more than one third of the patients with isolated ACTH deficiency.[987, 988] Perhaps hypoglycemia occurs frequently because, in the absence of dehydration and severe hypotension, these patients tolerate their illness longer and present with symptoms of chronic glucocorticoid deficiency rather than those of mineralocorticoid deficiency. These patients may show evidence of a pituitary or hypothalamic tumor, such as signs and symptoms of other hormone deficiencies or excess, headaches, or visual field defects (see Chapter 9).

Laboratory Findings

PRIMARY ADRENAL INSUFFICIENCY

Hormonal Findings. Cortisol secretion is low and does not increase normally with acute or chronic ACTH stimulation. Plasma ACTH and other POMC peptides, such as β-LPH and β-END,[1026] are elevated but exhibit a normal diurnal rhythm.[983] Secretion of aldosterone, DHEA, DHEAS, and androstenedione is low.[1027, 1028] Serum testosterone level is normal in men but low in women, in whom it is derived in large part from peripheral conversion of adrenal androgens.

Increase in the basal plasma AVP level is caused partly by a decreased circulating volume and partly by a lower osmotic threshold for AVP secretion.[1029] The increased AVP level impairs free water clearance, which is one of the causes of the hyponatremia. It also plays an important role in maintaining the blood pressure of these patients, as demonstrated by the acute hypotensive effect of an AVP antagonist in adrenalectomized dogs.[909] Plasma ANP is appropriately low.[1030]

The volume depletion resulting from aldosterone deficiency causes increased plasma renin concentration and activity.[904] Glucocorticoid deficiency reduces angiotensinogen (renin substrate) levels,[904] but plasma concentrations of angiotensin II are increased,[1031] and, because of a direct peripheral vasoconstrictor effect, they play an important role in maintaining blood pressure in primary adrenal insufficiency.[1032] Serum angiotensin-converting enzyme levels are also elevated.[1033]

Serum thyroxine levels are normal or low, and thyrotropin (TSH) concentration is often elevated. The levels of both usually return to normal after several months of steroid replacement.[1034] These changes may reflect associated autoimmune thyroiditis, or they may be a direct effect of glucocorticoid deficiency.[987] The diagnosis of primary hypothyroidism cannot be established definitively at presentation, so the decision to begin thyroid hormone replacement must be based on clinical findings and the serum thyroxine level. Thyroid function must be re-evaluated after the adrenal insufficiency has been corrected. Modest hyperprolactinemia (up to 50 ng/L), with hyperresponsiveness to thyrotropin-releasing hormone, may be observed[987] and usually returns to normal after steroid replacement.

Other Findings. Electrolyte abnormalities are the rule (see Table 12–8).[971, 987, 1000] Hyponatremia and hyperkalemia are present at diagnosis in 88% and 64% of patients, respectively.[971] The hyperkalemia is caused by aldosterone deficiency. The hyponatremia, which occurs mostly with glucocorticoid deficiency, is caused by elevated AVP levels and resulting increased free water retention,[1029] decreased sodium pump activity and shift of extracellular sodium into cells,[1035] and decreased delivery of filtrate to diluting segments of the nephron as a result of decreased glomerular filtration rate.[1036] Mild hyperchloremic acidosis and increased ratio of blood urea nitrogen to creatinine are the results of prerenal azotemia from dehydration and decreased cardiac output.[987, 1000] Mild to moderate hypercalcemia occurs in up to 6% of patients.[1037] Elevated calcium-binding proteins caused by hemoconcentration are a factor, but volume repletion with saline does not restore calcium concentration to normal, for which glucocorticoid replacement therapy is required.[1038]

Serum levels of hepatic aspartate transaminase may be elevated, but they fall to normal after a few days of glucocorticoid replacement.[987] Fasting blood glucose is usually in the low-normal range, but occasionally fasting or, rarely, postprandial hypoglycemia may occur.

Mild to moderate eosinophilia, relative lymphocytosis, and anemia are common. The normocytic, normochromic anemia, which may initially be masked by hemoconcentration, is probably a direct effect of glucocorticoid deficiency.[987] A macrocytic anemia may occur in patients with PGA syndrome and associated pernicious anemia. Some patients also have a neutropenia, which presumably is caused by increased sequestration of neutrophils in the marginal pool.[987]

Electrocardiographic abnormalities are frequently seen in adrenal insufficiency. Hyperkalemia is responsible for peaked T waves, low P waves, and wide QRS complexes and, in the extreme case, atrial asystole, intraventricular block, and, ultimately, ventricular asystole.[1018] Flattened or inverted T waves, prolonged QT_c interval, and low QRS voltage are caused by glucocorticoid deficiency, because they are seen when the electrolytes are normal and are reversed by glucocorticoid replacement.[987, 1039]

SECONDARY ADRENAL INSUFFICIENCY. The laboratory findings in secondary adrenal insufficiency are the same as those in primary adrenal insufficiency, except that (1) plasma ACTH levels are not elevated, (2) hyperkalemia does not occur and azotemia is less common in the unstressed patient because of continued mineralocorticoid secretion, (3) hypoglycemia is more common,[987, 988] and (4) hypercalcemia is less common.[987] Hyponatremia can occur in secondary adrenal insufficiency, largely because of increased AVP levels.[987] In contrast to primary adrenal insufficiency, plasma renin levels are usually normal, but in chronic secondary adrenal insufficiency both plasma renin activity and aldosterone concentrations may be low.[997, 998]

Radiologic Findings

PRIMARY ADRENAL INSUFFICIENCY. Adrenal enlargement associated with tuberculosis or other granulomatous diseases, metastatic cancer, or hemorrhage may be seen on abdominal CT scans.[993, 1040] Adrenal enlargement is not seen in patients with autoimmune adrenal destruction (Fig. 12–30).[1002] Tuberculous glands are enlarged initially but atrophy and become calcified over months to years.[1041, 1042] Chest radiographs frequently reveal a small heart.[971, 999, 1002] In chronic untreated or inadequately treated primary adrenal insufficiency, the sella turcica may be enlarged on skull radiographs,[1002, 1043] and CT scan may reveal pituitary enlargement that is reversible with steroid treatment.[979] This is usually caused by corticotrope hyperplasia,[980, 981] but in rare cases an ACTH-secreting adenoma can develop.[982]

SECONDARY AND TERTIARY ADRENAL INSUFFICIENCY. Adrenal atrophy cannot reliably be demonstrated by CT or magnetic resonance imaging (MRI) scan. Primary or metastatic mass lesions in the hypothalamus, median eminence, or pituitary fossa can usually be detected by CT or MRI scan (see Chapter 9).

Pathogenesis

PRIMARY ADRENAL INSUFFICIENCY. When Addison first described primary adrenal insufficiency,[16] bilateral adrenal destruction by tuberculosis was the most common cause, and it remained so until the advent of effective treatment for tuberculosis. Today, tuberculosis causes 7 to 20% of cases,

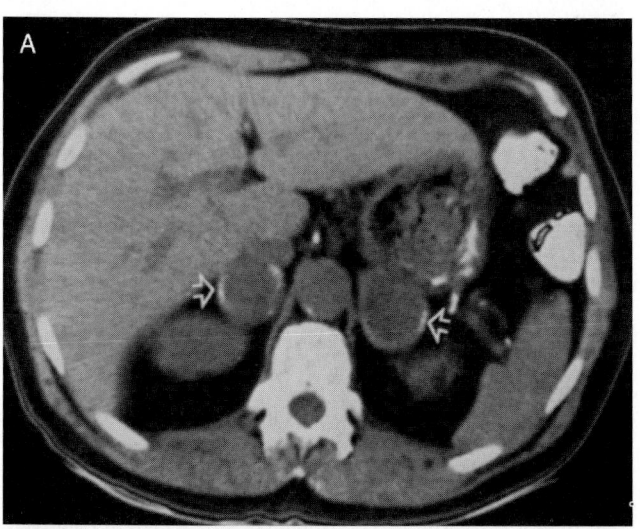
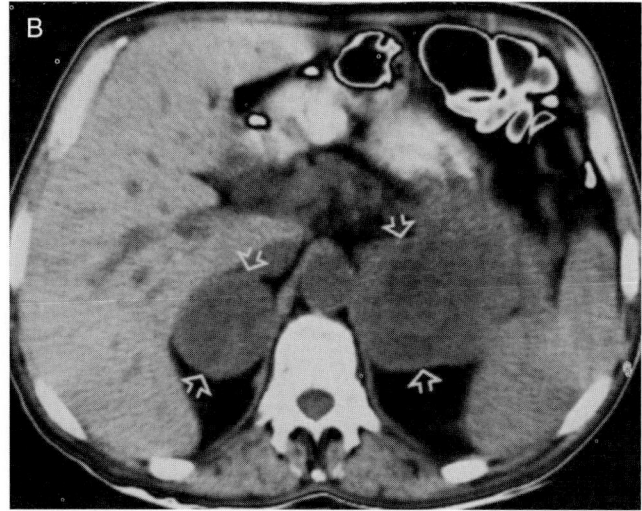
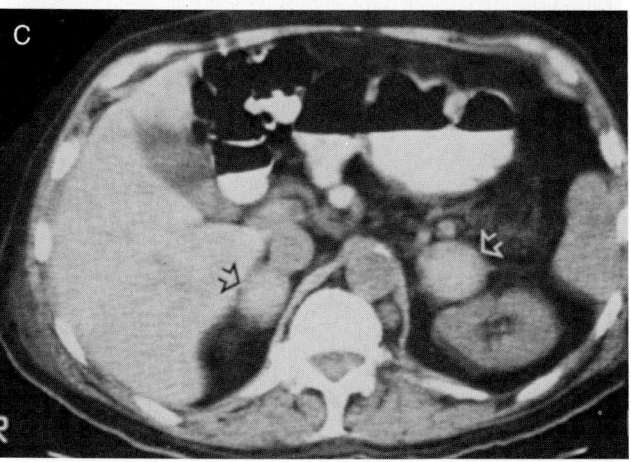

Figure 12–30. CT scans of patients with primary adrenal insufficiency. The affected adrenal glands are indicated by arrows. *A,* CT scan of a 59-year-old man with histoplasmosis. Note the subcapsular calcium in both glands. *B,* CT scan of a 59-year-old man with metastatic melanoma. *C,* CT scan of an 80-year-old man with bilateral adrenal hemorrhage resulting from anticoagulation for pulmonary emboli. (*A* and *B* courtesy of Dr. William D. Salmon, Jr.; *C* courtesy of Dr. Craig R. Sussman.)

TABLE 12–9. Incidence of Antiadrenal Antibodies in Patients with Nonadrenal Autoimmune Endocrine Diseases

Autoimmune Endocrine Disease	Incidence of Antiadrenal Antibodies (%)
Hypoparathyroidism	16
Hashimoto's thyroiditis	1.9
Diabetes mellitus	1.2
Thyrotoxicosis	1.9
Atrophic hypothyroidism	1.7
Pernicious anemia	<1

Compiled from Irvine and Barnes,[1000] Ketchum et al.,[1075] Blizzard et al.,[1073] Scherbaum and Berg,[1076] Betterle et al.,[975] and Nerup.[971]

autoimmune destruction accounts for 70 to 90%, and the remainder are caused by other granulomatous or fungal diseases or by replacement by lymphoma, metastatic cancer, or adrenal hemorrhage.[999, 1000, 1015, 1044–1047] However, disseminated tuberculosis or fungal infection is still a major cause of adrenal insufficiency in those populations with a high prevalence of these infectious diseases,[1048, 1049] and as tuberculosis is controlled, the overall incidence of adrenal insufficiency decreases.[1050] Bilateral metastatic small cell lung carcinoma, breast carcinoma, and melanoma are probably the most common causes on oncology services.

Autoimmune Adrenalitis. What previously was known as idiopathic primary adrenal insufficiency appears to be the result of an autoimmune process that destroys the adrenal cortex. Evidence of both humoral and cell-mediated immune mechanisms directed at the adrenal cortex, including lymphocytic infiltration of the adrenal glands, is found in association with autoimmune destruction of other endocrine glands and a genetic predisposition manifested by familial aggregation and increased prevalence of certain human leukocyte antigen (HLA) subtypes (see Chapter 33).

Patients with autoimmune adrenal insufficiency and PGA syndrome are predominantly female (70%). In contrast, patients with isolated autoimmune adrenal insufficiency are predominantly male (71%) in the first two decades of life, equally male and female in the third decade, and predominantly female (81%) thereafter.[1051] The explanation for these sex differences is unknown.

Humoral Immunity. Antibodies that react with all three zones of the adrenal cortex have been identified by complement fixation, immunofluorescent, or radiolabeled antibody—binding techniques. They are found in the serum of 60 to 75% of patients with autoimmune primary adrenal insufficiency but rarely in serum from patients with other causes of adrenal insufficiency, from first-degree relatives of patients with idiopathic primary adrenal insufficiency who themselves have no autoimmune endocrine disease, or from normal subjects.[1000, 1037, 1052–1056] Antibodies are more common in women, particularly those with PGA syndrome. After onset of overt adrenal insufficiency, the titers decrease and sometimes disappear completely. Some patients with other autoimmune endocrine diseases but without adrenal insufficiency also have antiadrenal antibodies (Table 12–9). The presence of antiadrenal antibodies seems to precede the development of adrenal insufficiency by several years.[975, 1057, 1058] Although all patients who have antiadrenal antibodies do not have adrenal insufficiency, as a group they develop adrenal insufficiency at a rate of up to 19% per year.[975] The first sign of adrenal insufficiency is an increase in plasma renin activity in association with a normal or low serum aldosterone level, which suggests that the zona glomerulosa is affected initially.[975, 976] After months to years, zona fasciculata dysfunction becomes evident, first by a decreasing plasma cortisol response to ACTH, later by increasing

basal plasma ACTH, and, finally, by decreasing basal plasma cortisol and overt symptoms.[975, 1057]

The main antigens with which the antiadrenal antibodies react are the steroidogenic enzymes CYP11A1, CYP17, and CYP21A2.[1055, 1059, 1060] Patients who have primary adrenal insufficiency associated with PGA I have autoantibodies to CYP11A1 and CYP17, whereas those with isolated primary adrenal insufficiency or primary adrenal insufficiency associated with PGA II have autoantibodies to CYP21A2 and CYP17.[1061, 1062] Some antibodies may react with two related epitopes in the COOH-terminal halves of CYP17 and CYP21A2.[1060, 1063] Antibodies to other CYP enzymes may also be present.

Immunoglobulins from most patients with autoimmune adrenal insufficiency block the stimulatory effect of ACTH on adrenal cortisol production and DNA synthesis in vitro.[1064] Preliminary results indicate that antibodies to the ACTH receptor are not present in patients with adrenal insufficiency.[1065] Antibodies to CYP21A2 block the activity of recombinant CYP21A2 in vitro,[1066] but it is uncertain whether the antibodies gain access to CYP21A2 in vivo.

Cell-Mediated Immunity. Cell-mediated immune processes may also be important in the development of adrenal insufficiency.[1067] Decreased suppressor T-cell function[1068] and increased circulating Ia-positive T lymphocytes[1069] have been described in patients with idiopathic adrenal insufficiency. Human adrenal homogenate inhibited the in vitro migration of leukocytes from 14 of 30 patients with idiopathic adrenal insufficiency but from only 1 of 7 patients with tuberculous adrenal insufficiency,[1070] and activated mouse macrophages blocked ACTH-induced steroidogenesis in cultured rabbit adrenocortical cells.[1071] The presence of lymphocytic infiltration in the adrenal glands further supports this concept.[1072]

Associated Endocrine Autoimmunity. Antibodies against other endocrine glands are common in patients with autoimmune adrenal insufficiency but rare in control populations (Table 12–10).[1000, 1015, 1052, 1054, 1073, 1074] Thyroid microsomal antibodies are present in about 60% of the patients.[1015] Of this group, almost half have overt hypothyroidism, and many of the others have subclinical hypothyroidism (i.e., increased serum TSH, normal serum thyroxine, and exaggerated responses to thyrotropin-releasing hormone) and are at risk for development of overt hypothyroidism.[1052, 1054, 1074] The increased incidence of gastric parietal cell and intrinsic factor antibodies correlates with atrophic gastritis and pernicious anemia, respectively. The presence of antigonadal antibodies correlates with premature ovarian failure in women. Antigonadal antibodies are less common in men, as is the incidence of testicular failure.

In contrast, the incidence of antiadrenal antibodies in serum from patients with other autoimmune endocrine diseases, but not adrenal insufficiency, is low (<2%), except in hypoparathyroidism (16%) (see Table 12–9).[971, 975, 1000, 1073, 1075, 1076]

TABLE 12–10. Incidence of Autoantibodies in Patients with Autoimmune Adrenal Insufficiency

Tissue	Incidence of Antibodies (%)
Adrenal	60–70
Thyroid Microsomal	50
Parathyroid	26
Islet Cell	8
Gonad	
Ovary	22
Testis	5
Stomach	
Parietal cell	30
Intrinsic factor	9

Data from Irvine et al.,[1054] Blizzard et al.,[1052] McHardy-Young et al.,[1074] Irving and Barnes,[1000] Blizzard et al.,[1073] and Zelissen et al.[1015]

Associated Disorders—Polyglandular Autoimmune Syndromes. About 50% of patients with autoimmune adrenal insufficiency have one or more other autoimmune endocrine disorders (Table 12–11).[971, 1000, 1015, 1052] On the other hand, patients with the more common autoimmune endocrine disorders, such as insulin-dependent diabetes mellitus or thyroid diseases, rarely develop adrenal insufficiency. The disorders associated with autoimmune adrenal insufficiency are referred to as PGA I and II and by many other names.[1023, 1077–1079] Other types of PGA syndrome not associated with adrenal insufficiency are not discussed further here (see Chapters 7 and 33).

PGA I, also referred to as the autoimmune polyendocrinopathy-candidiasis-ectodermal dysplasia (APECED) syndrome, is a rare familial syndrome inherited in an autosomal recessive pattern in which females are affected 0.8 to 1.7 times more frequently than males.[1023, 1051, 1077–1079] Hypoparathyroidism or mucocutaneous candidiasis is usually the first manifestation and characteristically appears during childhood or early adolescence, always by the early 20s (Table 12–12).[1023, 1051, 1077–1079] The candidiasis is chronic or recurrent, relatively resistant to conventional therapy, and usually involves the mouth,[1077] but it may involve just the nail beds or be more extensive. Adrenal insufficiency usually develops later, at a mean age of 12 to 13 years. About half of patients are found to develop all three of these features, if observed carefully.[1077] Diabetes mellitus is relatively infrequent, and autoimmune thyroid disease is uncommon. Atrophic thyroiditis and Hashimoto's thyroiditis are seen with equal frequency, and Graves' disease does not occur with this syndrome. Other endocrine and nonendocrine autoimmune disorders are even less common (see Table 12–12). In a large series of 68 Finnish patients,[1077] the incidence of various manifestations was different from that reported in other series and reviews of the literature, diabetes mellitus being 12 times more prevalent, for example. Furthermore, manifestations of ectodermal dysplasia, including dental enamel hypoplasia, pitted dystrophy of the nails, keratopathy, and calcified plaques on the tympanic membranes, were present in one third to two thirds of the patients. These differences may reflect a peculiar variant of the disorder or a more complete description of the several components of the syndrome.

In the more common PGA II, primary adrenal insufficiency is the principal manifestation.[1023, 1078–1080] Primary hypothyroidism, nontoxic goiter, and Graves' disease occur in 20 to 25% of patients with autoimmune adrenal insufficiency, and diabetes mellitus, hypoparathyroidism, pernicious anemia, Sjögren's syndrome, and celiac disease occur in 1 to 11% (see Table 12–12).[971, 1000, 1015, 1023, 1052, 1078] Patients with autoimmune thyroid disease or diabetes mellitus who have adrenal autoantibodies but do not yet have adrenal insufficiency, and relatives

TABLE 12–12. Clinical Manifestations of Polyglandular Autoimmune Syndromes Associated with Adrenal Insufficiency

Disorder	Prevalence (%)
Type I	
Endocrine	
Hypoparathyroidism	89
Chronic mucocutaneous candidiasis	75
Adrenal insufficiency	60
Gonadal failure	45
Hypothyroidism	12
Insulin-dependent diabetes mellitus	1
Hypopituitarism	<1
Diabetes insipidus	<1
Nonendocrine	
Malabsorption syndromes	25
Alopecia totalis or areata	20
Pernicious anemia	16
Chronic active hepatitis	9
Vitiligo	4
Type II	
Endocrine	
Adrenal insufficiency	100
Autoimmune thyroid disease	70
Insulin-dependent diabetes mellitus	50
Gonadal failure	5–50
Diabetes insipidus	<1
Nonendocrine	
Vitiligo	4
Alopecia, pernicious anemia, myasthenia gravis, immune thrombocytopenia purpura, Sjögren's syndrome, rheumatoid arthritis	<1

Compiled from Leshin M. Polyglandular autoimmune syndromes. Am J Med Sci 1985; 290:77–88 and Neufeld M, Maclaren NK, Blizzard RM. Two types of autoimmune Addison's disease associated with different polyglandular autoimmune (PGA) syndromes. Medicine 1981; 60:355–362.

with one or more components of the syndrome, should also be included. About half of the cases are familial, but various modes of inheritance have been reported.[1023, 1051, 1078] Women are affected 1.8 times more frequently than men.[1023, 1078] Onset ranges from childhood to late adulthood, most cases occurring between ages 20 and 40 years.[971, 1023, 1051] Adrenal insufficiency is the initial manifestation in about 50% of patients, occurs simultaneously with thyroiditis or diabetes mellitus in about 20%, and follows their development in about 30%.[971, 1051, 1078] Hypogonadism may occur first, and, as in PGA I, ovarian failure is more frequent than testicular failure.[971, 1023, 1078] Hypoparathyroidism does not occur in this syndrome, and alopecia and pernicious anemia are less frequent than in PGA I. Other nonendocrine autoimmune disorders, such as vitiligo, myasthenia gravis, thrombocytopenic purpura, Sjögren's syndrome, rheumatoid arthritis, and primary antiphospholipid syndrome (recurrent deep vein thrombosis with antibodies to cardiolipin) are occasionally associated.[1023, 1078, 1080–1082] Serositis with pericardial or pleural involvement, or both, has been reported.[1083]

Genetics. Autoimmune adrenal insufficiency may be familial or nonfamilial. It is somewhat less likely to be familial when it occurs alone: about one third of such patients have affected family members, whereas about one half of patients with adrenal insufficiency as part of PGA I or PGA II have positive family histories.[971, 1023, 1051, 1078] PGA I is inherited as an autosomal recessive trait, whereas pedigrees with autosomal recessive, autosomal dominant, or polygenic inheritance have been reported for PGA II.[1023, 1051, 1078, 1084]

Genetic susceptibility to autoimmune adrenal insufficiency is strongly linked with HLA-B8, -DR3, and -DR4 alleles, except when it occurs as part of PGA I, in which no HLA association has been found.[1023, 1085, 1086] The gene responsible for PGA I has been located on the long arm of human chromosome 21 (21q22.3).[1087] A number of specific HLA antigens,

TABLE 12–11. Incidence of Other Endocrine and Autoimmune Diseases in Patients with Autoimmune Adrenal Insufficiency (N = 448)

Disease	Incidence (%)
Thyroid disease	
Hypothyroidism	8
Nontoxic goiter	7
Thyrotoxicosis	7
Gonadal failure	
Ovarian	20
Testicular	2
Insulin-dependent diabetes mellitus	11
Hypoparathyroidism	10
Pernicious anemia	5
None	53

Compiled from Irvine and Barnes,[1000] Blizzard et al.,[1052] Nerup,[971] and Zelissen et al.[1015]

including DPB1*0101, DQA1*0501, DQB1*0201, and DRB1*0301, are associated with sporadic autoimmune adrenal insufficiency and PGA II.[1088, 1089] DQA1*0501 is associated with adrenal insufficiency, diabetes mellitus, and Graves' disease, and an Arg[52] substitution in either DQA1*0501 or DQA1*0301 also links strongly with adrenal insufficiency.[1089] These associations appear to result from the location of the CYP21A2 and CYP21B genes in the class III major histocompatibility (MHC) region between the class I and class II MHC loci on the short arm of human chromosome 6,[105] and a strong association has been noted with the C4A-plus-CYP21A2 gene deletion and with the TNFB*1 allele, located about 450 kilobases upstream from CYP21A2.[1088] However, some families with PGA II do not have an HLA linkage,[1084, 1085] and similar markers are found in controls.[1088] Furthermore, Hashimoto's thyroiditis, pernicious anemia, and premature primary gonadal failure, all components of PGA II, do not have strong HLA linkage.[1085, 1086] These observations suggest that a gene or genes linked to certain HLA antigens convey susceptibility to autoimmune adrenal insufficiency and diabetes mellitus and that different, non–HLA-associated genes are involved in Hashimoto's thyroiditis and gastric autoimmune disease and in PGA I. The CYP11A1 and CYP17 genes lie on long arms of human chromosomes 15 (15q23-q24) and 10 (10q24-q25), respectively,[134] and therefore are not linked to HLA antigens. Because normal adrenocortical cells express MHC class II antigens, inappropriate expression of these proteins does not appear to be involved in the pathogenesis of autoimmune adrenal insufficiency.[1090]

Pathology. In the initial stage of autoimmune adrenal insufficiency, the glands may be enlarged, with extensive lymphocytic infiltration.[1053, 1072, 1091] In long-standing disease, the adrenal glands are small and sometimes difficult to locate. The capsule is thickened and fibrotic. The cortex is completely destroyed, although there may be a few small clusters of adrenocortical cells surrounded by lymphocytes. The medulla is relatively spared. Adrenal insufficiency becomes clinically manifest only after at least 90% of the cortex is destroyed.[973, 974] Patients with other associated autoimmune endocrine diseases have lymphocytic infiltration and varying degrees of destruction and fibrosis of the involved glands.[1053] The expression of MHC class II antigens is increased.[1090] In untreated adrenal insufficiency there is pituitary corticotrope hyperplasia with the corticotropes forming micronodules.[1092]

Infectious Adrenalitis. The incidence of tuberculous primary adrenal insufficiency has declined in the last few decades from about 80 to 20% because of effective prevention and drug treatment of tuberculosis.[999, 1000, 1044, 1050] Tuberculous adrenalitis results from hematogenous spread from infection elsewhere in the body.[1091] Extra-adrenal tuberculosis usually is evident but may be clinically latent.[1040, 1091] Adrenal destruction is gradual. The medulla is more frequently destroyed than the cortex, for unknown reasons.[1091] The adrenal glands usually are enlarged in the early stage of the disease, often enough to be seen on CT or MRI scan[1040–1042, 1093]; they become completely replaced by caseous nodules and fibrosis.[1040] After about 2 y of adrenal insufficiency, the adrenals become normal or small in size.[1040–1042, 1093] Calcifications can be seen radiographically in 50% of cases.[1002, 1040, 1093] However, absence of enlarged or calcified adrenal glands does not rule out tuberculosis as the cause of adrenal insufficiency. Recovery of adrenal function can occur after effective anti-tuberculous therapy.[1094]

Disseminated fungal infections can involve the adrenal glands and cause adrenal insufficiency. Histoplasmosis[1095] and paracoccidioidomycosis (South American blastomycosis)[1046, 1096] have a predilection for invading and destroying the adrenal glands and are important causes of adrenal insufficiency in endemic areas. In contrast, cryptococcosis,[1097] coccidioidomycosis,[1098] and North American blastomycosis[1099] are rare causes. The adrenal glands are enlarged and may become calcified. Recovery of adrenal function after prolonged antifungal treatment has been reported.[1100, 1101] Syphilis causes adrenal insufficiency but rarely. The adrenals are sclerotic, with gumma formation and demonstrable spirochetes.[1091] African trypanosomiasis is also reported to cause adrenal insufficiency unrelated to its treatment with suramin, a drug that can impair adrenal function when given in high doses.[1102]

Metastatic Replacement. Infiltration of the adrenal glands by metastatic cancer is common, probably because of the ample sinusoidal blood supply. Most autopsy series report adrenal metastases in 40 to 60% of patients with disseminated lung or breast cancer, 30% of those with melanoma, and 14 to 20% of those with stomach or colon cancer, but clinically recognized adrenal insufficiency is uncommon.[974, 1103–1105] Primary or systemic lymphoma often involves the adrenals but rarely causes adrenal insufficiency.[1045, 1106] The apparently low incidence of clinical adrenal insufficiency may occur in part because most of the adrenal cortex must be destroyed before hypofunction becomes evident[973, 974] and in part because symptoms are mistakenly attributed to cancer. Two small studies have suggested that one fifth to one third of patients with bilateral adrenal metastases have partial adrenal insufficiency and benefit from glucocorticoid treatment.[1104, 1105]

Miscellaneous Causes

Acquired Immunodeficiency Syndrome. Endocrine abnormalities are common in asymptomatic patients who are HIV positive and in those with acquired immunodeficiency syndrome (AIDS), but the adrenocortical abnormalities are the most clinically significant.[1107] The adrenal glands often show a necrotizing adrenalitis caused by cytomegalovirus infection, but infection with Mycobacterium avium-intracellulare or Cryptococcus and involvement with metastatic Kaposi's sarcoma also occur.[1108] Adrenal insufficiency has been reported in patients with AIDS[1109]; cortisol responses to the short-term high-dose (250-μg) cosyntropin stimulation test is decreased in 8 to 14% of AIDS patients, and most AIDS patients have decreased adrenal reserve as measured by the cortisol response to prolonged (3-d) ACTH stimulation.[1110, 1111] In addition, there is a defect in 17-deoxysteroid production by the zona fasciculata.[1111] Even patients with AIDS-related complex may have a subnormal cortisol response to ACTH administration.[1111] Therefore, all HIV-infected patients should be considered at risk for development of adrenal insufficiency.

Some AIDS patients have symptoms of adrenal insufficiency but high plasma cortisol levels. These patients may have peripheral resistance to glucocorticoid action because of decreased affinity of type II receptors for glucocorticoids; receptor density is increased.[1112, 1113] The mechanism of the abnormality is unknown. Plasma ACTH concentrations are normal or slightly elevated but lack a diurnal rhythm and are resistant to low-dose dexamethasone suppression.[1112] The response to the short-term high-dose cosyntropin test is usually normal, but the response to CRH may be blunted.[1114] The intense cutaneous hyperpigmentation that is observed cannot be attributed to ACTH, but interferon-α, which is increased in AIDS patients with peripheral glucocorticoid resistance, may stimulate melanocortin-1 receptor expression and melanin synthesis.[1115, 1116]

Some drugs used to treat opportunistic infections in AIDS, such as ketoconazole, which inhibits cortisol synthesis,[1117] and rifampicin, which increases cortisol metabolism,[699, 1118] may precipitate adrenal crisis in patients with unrecognized partial adrenal insufficiency[1119]

Adrenoleukodystrophy and Adrenomyeloneuropathy. The two phenotypes of this X-linked recessive disorder affect 1 in 20,000 males and are characterized by progressive neurologic dysfunction and primary adrenal insufficiency. Adrenoleukodystrophy (ALD) begins in childhood and progresses rapidly to dementia, blindness, and quadraplegia. Adrenomyeloneuropathy (AMN) begins in adolescence and early adulthood with weakness, spasticity, and distal polyneuropathy as the initial neurologic complaints. It is milder and more slowly progressive.[1024, 1025] It was thought that the neurologic symptoms of both disorders appeared before adrenal insufficiency, but up to 60% of males with idiopathic adrenal insufficiency have the biochemical defect of ALD/AMN, the likelihood being greatest when the adrenal insufficiency occurs before the age of 15 years.[1120, 1121] Therefore, ALD/AMN should be considered in any boy presenting with adrenal insufficiency. The disorders are caused by defective fatty acid beta oxidation in peroxisomes, which leads to elevated plasma concentration of very-long-chain saturated fatty acids and accumulation of their cholesterol esters and gangliosides in the membranes of cells in the brain, adrenal cortex, and other organs.[1122] Response of bovine adrenocortical cells to ACTH in vitro is inhibited by very-long-chain saturated fatty acids, perhaps because they induce changes in cell membrane viscosity.[1123] The responsible gene is located on Xq28[1124] and encodes a peroxisomal membrane protein[1125] that belongs to the ATP-binding cassette superfamily of transporter proteins.[1126] A variety of point mutations cause ALD/AMN, with single amino acid substitutions concentrated in the ATP-binding domain.[1127–1129] A large deletion of the unrelated acyl-CoA oxidase gene is found in isolated peroxisomal acyl-CoA oxidase deficiency (pseudoneonatal ALD).[1130] Dietary therapy, such as Lorenzo's oil, may prevent or delay the neurologic manifestations of ALD/AMN, but it does not improve symptoms once they occur.[1129, 1131] There are no data on the effects of dietary therapy on adrenal function.

Congenital Adrenal Hypoplasia. Congenital adrenal hypoplasia is a rare familial condition in which the adult adrenal cortex does not develop normally. The disorder is evident at birth with any of four forms of primary adrenal insufficiency: (1) a sporadic form associated with pituitary hypoplasia, (2) an autosomal recessive form, (3) an X-linked cytomegalic form associated with hypogonadotropic hypogonadism, and (4) an X-linked form associated with glycerol kinase deficiency, psychomotor retardation, and, in most cases, muscular dystrophy and characteristic facies.[1132–1134] Maternal estriol secretion is reported to be decreased in late pregnancy.[1135] Congenital adrenal hypoplasia occurs in about 1 of 12,500 births.[1136] The X-linked forms are caused by mutations of a gene that is located on the short arm of the X chromosome (Xp21) and encodes DAX1, a member of the nuclear hormone receptor gene superfamily, or by deletions involving the DAX1 gene and the contiguous centromeric glycerol kinase gene.[1133, 1137–1139] DAX1 is expressed in the affected endocrine tissues: adrenal cortex, gonads, hypothalamus, and pituitary gland.[1140] Patients with congenital adrenal hypoplasia also may have a variety of point mutations that alter or truncate the COOH-terminal 11-amino-acid residues of the DAX1 protein.[1141] SF-1 is a transcription factor that regulates gene expression of the CYP steroid hydroxylases and is essential for development of the adrenal cortex.[41] A potential SF-1 response element has been identified in the 5' flanking region of the DAX1 gene.[1140] The SF-1 gene is found on chromosome 9q33.[1142] The Duchenne's muscular dystrophy locus is centromeric to the glycerol kinase gene in the Xp21 locus.[1143]

Familial Glucocorticoid Deficiency. Familial glucocorticoid deficiency is a rare autosomal recessive disorder in which glucocorticoid and androgen secretion is deficient and unresponsive to ACTH stimulation. Plasma cortisol concentrations are low or undetectable and plasma ACTH levels are elevated. Mineralocorticoid secretion is normal or only partially deficient and responds to postural stimuli and volume depletion.[1144] The disorder usually presents in childhood with hyperpigmentation, muscle weakness, hypoglycemia, and seizures and may be associated with achalasia and alacrima (Allgrove's

syndrome, triple-A syndrome).[1144, 1145] Patients with isolated familial glucocorticoid deficiency have defective melanocortin-2 receptors[1146] and are homozygotes or compound heterozygotes for point mutations that alter a critical amino acid, alter the reading frame, or truncate the receptor.[1146, 1147] Patients with Allgrove's syndrome and some patients with isolated familial glucocorticoid deficiency do not have ACTH receptor mutations[1147, 1148] but may have postreceptor defects.[1149]

Defective Cholesterol Metabolism. In humans, the majority of cortisol is thought to be synthesized from cholesterol provided to the adrenals from circulating LDL.[87] Therefore, patients with no LDL, such as those with abetalipoproteinemia,[97] or with no LDL receptors, such as those with homozygous familial hypercholesterolemia,[99] have a moderate impairment of cortisol response to ACTH, although they maintain normal basal cortisol production and do not have clinically significant adrenal insufficiency. Hypocholesterolemic drugs (e.g., lovastatin) that inhibit cholesterol biosynthesis at the HMG-CoA reductase step do not further impair adrenal function in patients with familial hypercholesterolemia.[1150] It has long been known that cattle and rodents are more dependent than humans on circulating HDL cholesterol for cortisol and corticosterone biosynthesis, respectively. Evidence indicates that HDL is taken up by scavenger receptors,[100] and apolipoprotein AI knockout mice, in which HDL particles cannot form, have severe adrenal insufficiency.[101] Adrenal function studies in patients with the rare syndrome of apolipoprotein AI deficiency have not been reported, however, and most of the data on LDL involvement were obtained from in vitro cell culture studies. Therefore, the relative importance of HDL and LDL in human steroidogenesis remains uncertain.

Drugs. A number of drugs may cause adrenal insufficiency by inhibiting cortisol biosynthesis, including aminoglutethimide,[189, 1151] etomidate,[200] ketoconazole,[1117] metyrapone[190] and suramin.[1152, 1153] These agents usually do not produce clinical adrenal insufficiency in subjects with normal hypothalamic-pituitary-adrenal function because enzyme inhibition is incomplete and increased ACTH secretion overrides the blockade. However, patients with limited pituitary or adrenal reserve may develop symptomatic adrenal insufficiency. Other drugs accelerate the metabolism of cortisol and most synthetic steroids by inducing hepatic mixed-function oxygenase enzymes. They include phenytoin,[118, 1154] barbiturates,[118] and rifampicin.[699, 1118] These agents can also provoke adrenal insufficiency in patients with limited pituitary or adrenal reserve and in those with adrenal insufficiency who are receiving replacement steroids. The adrenocorticolytic agent mitotane accelerates the metabolism of halogenated synthetic steroids such as dexamethasone[1155] and fludrocortisone but has little or no effect on cortisol or prednisolone metabolism (D. Gaitan, W.E. Nicholson, and D.N. Orth, unpublished observations). Mitotane can provoke adrenal insufficiency in patients with adrenal insufficiency who are receiving replacement halogenated steroids.

SECONDARY ADRENAL INSUFFICIENCY

Panhypopituitarism. Any process that involves the pituitary and interferes with its ability to secrete ACTH will cause secondary adrenal insufficiency. Large pituitary tumors or craniopharyngiomas, infectious processes (e.g., tuberculosis, histoplasmosis), infiltrative diseases, lymphocytic hypophysitis, head trauma, and large intracranial artery aneurysms can destroy the normal pituitary tissue. Pituitary metastases are common (about 5%) in patients with disseminated cancer at autopsy but rarely disrupt hormone secretion.[1156] Pituitary infarction may occur in pregnant women at the time of delivery if excessive blood is lost and hypotension occurs (Sheehan's syndrome) or with hemorrhage into a pituitary tumor (pituitary apoplexy). These patients usually have evidence of other pituitary hormone deficiencies.

Isolated ACTH Deficiency. Isolated ACTH deficiency is rare.[988] The defect probably is at the pituitary level because ACTH secretion does not increase in response to CRH or vasopressin, as usually occurs in hypothalamic disorders.[1157–1159] Occasionally a patient has hypothyroxinemia and hyperprolactinemia that are corrected with glucocorticoid replacement.[1160, 1161] This disorder can have multiple causes, but its frequent association with other autoimmune endocrine disorders,[1161] the lymphocytic hypophysitis and selective corticotrope absence observed in several patients,[1162] the antipituitary antibodies in the serum of half of 21 patients in another study,[1163] and the anticorticotrope antibodies in the serum of at least one patient[1164] suggest that most cases are caused by an autoimmune process. Some cases may be caused by deficient post-translational processing of POMC.[1165]

TERTIARY ADRENAL INSUFFICIENCY

Chronic Pharmacologic Administration of Glucocorticoids. Suppression of hypothalamic-pituitary-adrenal function by chronic administration of pharmacologic dosages of glucocorticoids is the most common cause of adrenal insufficiency. Such regimens decrease CRH synthesis and secretion by the hypothalamus, block its trophic and secretagogue actions on the pituitary corticotropes, and secondarily decrease synthesis and secretion of ACTH by the anterior pituitary corticotropes, which decrease in size and in the amount of stored ACTH. Eventually, the number of identifiable corticotropes decreases.[1166] In the absence of ACTH stimulation, the adrenal zonae fasciculata and reticularis atrophy and can no longer secrete cortisol. However, cortisol production can be restored after prolonged ACTH administration, a feature that also distinguishes primary from secondary adrenal insufficiency. In tertiary adrenal insufficiency the adrenals retain almost normal mineralocorticoid secretion, because this function depends mostly on the renin-angiotensin system rather than on ACTH. This condition is treated in greater detail later in this chapter.

After Cure of Cushing's Syndrome. Tertiary adrenal insufficiency also occurs in patients who are cured of Cushing's syndrome by removal of a pituitary or nonpituitary ACTH-secreting or adrenal cortisol-secreting tumor. The chronic endogenous hypercortisolemia suppresses the hypothalamic-pituitary-adrenal axis in the same manner as exogenous glucocorticoids.

Other Causes. Any process that involves the hypothalamus and interferes with CRH secretion will result in tertiary adrenal insufficiency. Such processes include tumors, infiltrative diseases (e.g., sarcoidosis), and cranial radiation. The CRH test can be used to differentiate secondary from tertiary adrenal insufficiency. In patients with pituitary disease, the ACTH secretory response to CRH is inappropriately low or absent, whereas in those with a hypothalamic defect, the ACTH response usually is exaggerated and prolonged.[209, 1167]

Diagnosis

DIFFERENTIAL DIAGNOSIS. When classic signs and symptoms of advanced disease are present, the diagnosis of adrenal insufficiency is obvious. However, early symptoms, such as fatigue and lassitude, are nonspecific. Consequently, the diagnosis is sometimes overlooked while other possibilities are pursued. The weight loss and gastrointestinal complaints often raise suspicion of gastric carcinoma. Even the hyperpigmentation is not always reliable, because primary adrenal insufficiency can occur without hyperpigmentation[1009] and because hyperpigmentation can be caused by antineoplastic and antimalarial drugs, and by tetracyclines, phenothiazines, zidovudine,[1168] and heavy metals.[1169] The pigmentation of hemochromatosis is similar except that it seldom involves the mucous membranes. Nail pigment abnormalities may occur in Peutz-Jeghers syndrome and with pregnancy or radiotherapy.[1170] Secondary and tertiary adrenal insufficiency are not associated with hyperpigmentation. Even when the diagnosis appears obvious, endocrine evaluation must be undertaken to confirm the diagnosis and determine the type of adrenal insufficiency and its cause before initiating lifelong therapy.

LABORATORY DIAGNOSIS

Adrenal Insufficiency

Basal Cortisol Secretion. A scheme for establishing the diagnosis of adrenal insufficiency and determining its cause is shown in Figure 12–31. The diagnosis depends on demonstration of inadequate cortisol production. Plasma cortisol concentration is normally high in the early morning (i.e., before 8:00 AM) and increases with stress. Therefore, a low plasma cortisol level (i.e., <140 nmol/L [5 μg/dL]) in these situations provides presumptive evidence of adrenal insufficiency, and a value of less than 275 nmol/L (10 μg/dL) strongly suggests the diagnosis. Conversely, a level of 550 nmol/L (20 μg/dL) or greater precludes the diagnosis. An intermediate plasma cortisol level is not diagnostic. Plasma cortisol is normally low in the late afternoon and evening, so its determination in a sample drawn at these times is of no diagnostic value. Although a basal morning plasma cortisol of more than 275 nmol/dL (10 μg/dL) predicts a normal cortisol response to insulin-induced hypoglycemia or the short ACTH test in most patients,[1171, 1172] patients with partial adrenal insufficiency may have normal basal cortisol levels but an inadequate adrenal response to stress. As with basal serum cortisol levels, basal urinary free cortisol and 17-OHCS levels are low in patients with severe adrenal insufficiency, but they may be low normal in patients with partial adrenal insufficiency.

Response to Acute ACTH Stimulation. A short ACTH stimulation test should be performed for virtually all patients in whom the diagnosis is being considered. The details of the test are discussed later in this chapter. The low-dose (1 μg, or 0.5 μg/1.73 m² surface area) ACTH stimulation test[1173, 1174] reveals partial adrenal insufficiency that may be missed by the standard (250 μg) test.[1175] A normal response is a rise in plasma cortisol concentration after 30 or 60 min to a peak of 550 nmol/L (20 μg/dL) or more.[1173, 1174, 1176] An impaired

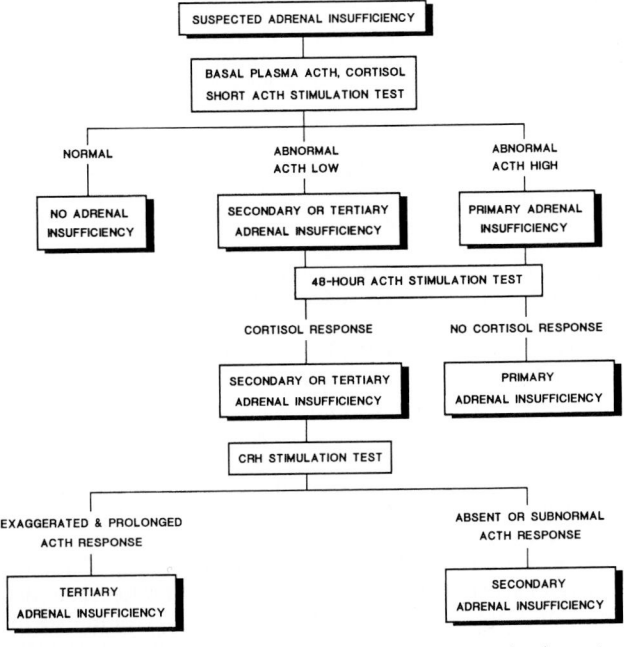

Figure 12–31. A diagnostic laboratory approach to confirming the diagnosis of adrenocortical insufficiency and determining whether it is primary, secondary, or tertiary.

response confirms adrenal insufficiency, but additional studies are necessary to establish its type and cause. A normal response in the short ACTH stimulation test excludes primary adrenal insufficiency[1177] but does not eliminate secondary adrenal insufficiency of recent onset (e.g., within 1 or 2 wk after pituitary surgery); in the latter setting, only an insulin-induced hypoglycemia or metyrapone test is reliable.[1178, 1179] The overnight metyrapone test is quicker than and as reliable as the standard 3-d metyrapone test.[1180] Neither should be performed in an outpatient in whom adrenal insufficiency is considered a possibility.

Treatment of patients who present in possible adrenal crisis should not be delayed while diagnostic tests are performed. Blood for plasma cortisol and electrolytes should be drawn, and therapy should be initiated immediately with intravenous saline and dexamethasone, as discussed later in this chapter. The short ACTH stimulation test can be performed after initiation of glucocorticoid treatment provided that (1) glucocorticoid therapy has not been given for more than a few days, after which it could suppress the hypothalamic-pituitary-adrenal axis and compromise the adrenal response,[1175] and (2) neither hydrocortisone (cortisol) nor cortisone (which is converted to cortisol) is used for glucocorticoid therapy, because both are measured in cortisol radioimmunoassays. Dexamethasone is the drug of choice in this circumstance.

Primary Versus Secondary or Tertiary Adrenal Insufficiency

Basal Plasma ACTH. In primary adrenal insufficiency, basal 8:00 AM plasma ACTH concentrations are elevated, sometimes as high as 880 pmol/L (4000 pg/mL) and occasionally even higher (see Fig. 12–28). In secondary or tertiary adrenal insufficiency, plasma ACTH levels are low or low normal. The ACTH level must be drawn before the initiation of glucocorticoid therapy, or at least 24 h after the last dose of a short-acting glucocorticoid, such as hydrocortisone. Otherwise, the ACTH level may be suppressed by glucocorticoid negative feedback. If the patient has been on replacement glucocorticoids, the steroid must be replaced with hydrocortisone for several days before morning plasma ACTH is measured. If the sample is drawn in the proper setting and the ACTH assay is reliable, this measurement by itself is sufficient to establish whether the adrenal insufficiency is primary.[1177]

Response to Prolonged ACTH Stimulation. Prolonged ACTH stimulation also differentiates primary from secondary or tertiary adrenal insufficiency, because the atrophic adrenal glands in secondary or tertiary adrenal insufficiency recover cortisol secretory capacity if chronically exposed to ACTH, whereas the adrenal glands in primary adrenal insufficiency are partially or completely destroyed, are already exposed to maximally stimulating levels of endogenous ACTH, and do not respond to further ACTH stimulation (Fig. 12–32A). This test is performed by administering ACTH as a continuous infusion for 48 h[1181] or as daily 8-h infusions or twice-daily intramuscular injections for 4 to 5 d, while measuring daily urinary 17-OHCS or free cortisol excretion and plasma cortisol concentrations (discussed in the section on testing). Glucocorticoid replacement should be given as dexamethasone, 0.5 to 1 mg daily for at least 24 h before and during the test, because it does not affect adrenal response to ACTH or significantly interfere at this dosage with either plasma or urinary steroid measurements. Cortisol secretion increases progressively in secondary or tertiary adrenal insufficiency but changes little or not at all in primary adrenal insufficiency. The 48-h ACTH infusion is preferred because it reliably separates primary from secondary or tertiary adrenal insufficiency in the shortest time.

Secondary Versus Tertiary Adrenal Insufficiency

ACTH Response to Corticotropin-Releasing Hormone. The differentiation between secondary and tertiary adrenal insufficiency can be made with a CRH test (Fig. 12–33), although from a therapeutic standpoint this distinction is rarely important. There is little or no ACTH response in patients with secondary adrenal insufficiency, whereas patients with tertiary adrenal insufficiency usually have an exaggerated and prolonged ACTH response.[209, 1167]

Cause of Adrenal Insufficiency. It is important to determine the cause of adrenal insufficiency, because the underlying disease may have other clinical ramifications, such as tuberculosis in primary adrenal insufficiency or a pituitary tumor in secondary adrenal insufficiency.

Primary Adrenal Insufficiency. The age of the patient, the

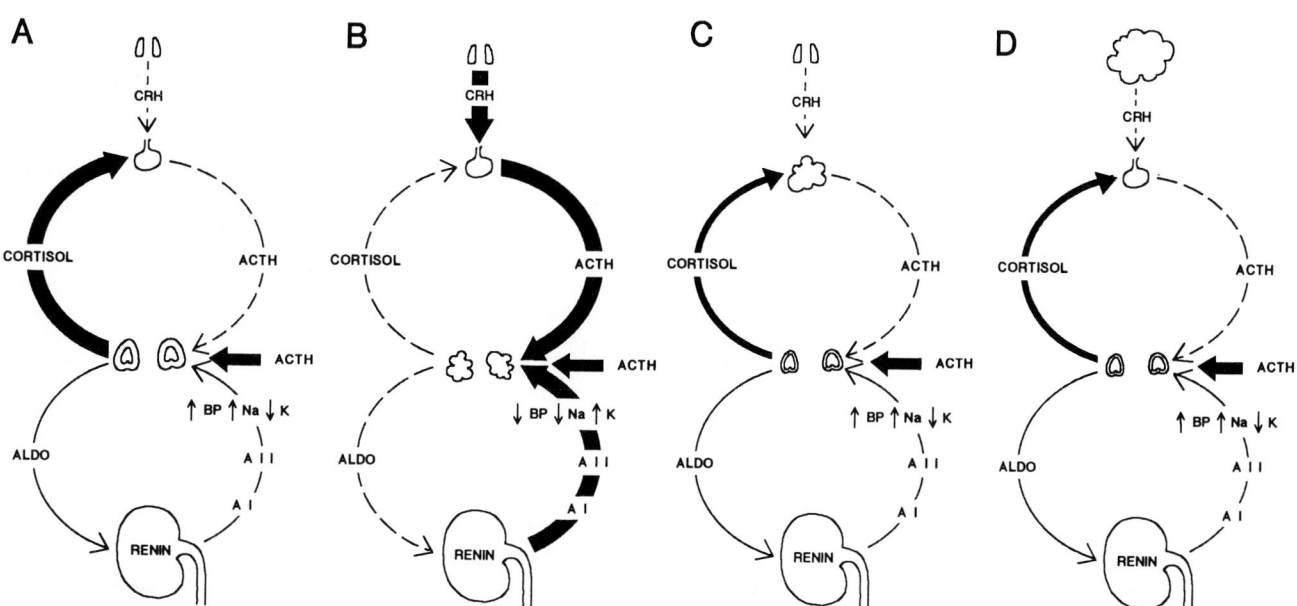

Figure 12–32. The response of a normal individual (A) and those of patients with primary (B), secondary (C), and tertiary (D) adrenal insufficiency to prolonged (i.e., 48-h) stimulation with maximal dosages of ACTH.

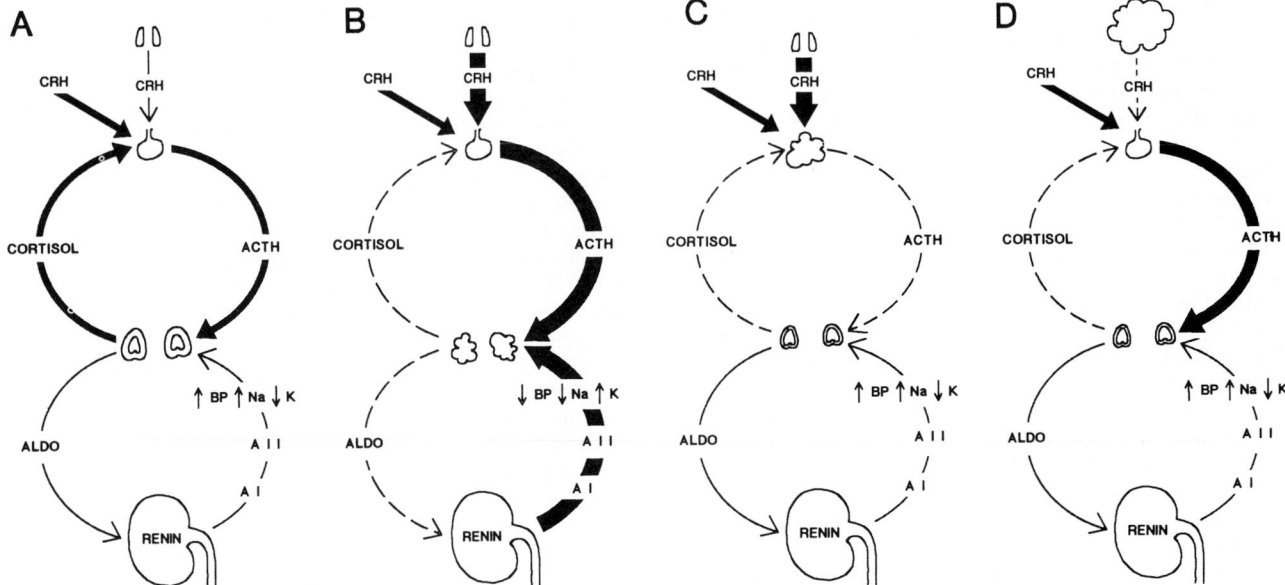

Figure 12–33. The response of a normal individual *(A)* and those of patients with primary *(B)*, secondary *(C)*, and tertiary *(D)* adrenal insufficiency to CRH stimulation.

clinical setting (e.g., anticoagulation), and the presence of other autoimmune-mediated endocrine disorders are important. An abdominal CT scan provides useful information, because enlarged adrenal glands or the presence of adrenal calcium deposits eliminates an autoimmune process and suggests an infectious, hemorrhagic, metastatic, or, rarely, primary lymphomatous cause.[1040, 1093, 1182, 1183] However, absence of enlarged or calcified adrenal glands does not exclude tuberculosis as the cause. Patients presenting initially with tuberculous adrenal insufficiency usually have obvious active tuberculosis elsewhere.[1040, 1091] Chest radiography, urine culture for *Mycobacterium tuberculosis*, and tuberculin skin testing should be done if the diagnosis is not clear. Complement fixation titers for histoplasmosis should be obtained. The diagnosis of autoimmune adrenal insufficiency is based on the presence of associated autoimmune disorders and exclusion of other causes, at least until assays for antiadrenal antibodies become widely available. In patients thought to have autoimmune primary adrenal insufficiency, the presence of other endocrine gland dysfunction should be sought by measuring serum levels of calcium, phosphorus, glucose, free thyroxine, TSH, and thyroid antibodies. If the serum calcium concentration is low, serum PTH should be assayed. If there is oligomenorrhea or amenorrhea, the possibility of hypogonadism should be investigated by measuring serum levels of follicle-stimulating hormone and LH. CT-directed percutaneous fine-needle aspiration of enlarged adrenal glands can establish the cause.[1097, 1184] The treatable causes of primary adrenal insufficiency can almost always be identified by other, noninvasive means. However, this procedure may establish the presence of metastases from a previously unsuspected malignancy, especially small cell lung carcinoma or breast carcinoma. ALD/AMN should be excluded by measuring serum levels of very-long-chain fatty acids in young men, certainly in boys younger than 15 years old, who have idiopathic adrenal insufficiency without accompanying neurologic symptoms.[1120, 1121, 1185]

Secondary or Tertiary Adrenal Insufficiency. A pituitary CT or MRI scan should be performed to exclude a tumor as the cause. A variety of other disorders, some of which are treatable, can cause secondary or tertiary adrenal insufficiency (see Chapter 9).

Treatment

The introduction of synthetic cortisone for therapeutic use in 1948[38, 1186] first made it possible to treat adrenal insufficiency easily and successfully.[999]

ACUTE ADRENAL INSUFFICIENCY: ADRENAL CRISIS. Adrenal crisis is a life-threatening emergency that requires immediate and appropriate treatment (Table 12–13). When there is strong clinical suspicion of the diagnosis, therapy should not be delayed to perform diagnostic studies or await laboratory results. If there is not strong evidence of adrenal insufficiency, consideration should be given to other possible causes of shock. The initial goal of therapy is reversal of the hypotension and electrolyte abnormalities. Large volumes (i.e., 2 to 3 L) of 0.9% saline solution or 5% dextrose in saline should be infused intravenously as quickly as possible. Hypotonic saline solution should not be used because of the risk of worsening hyponatremia. Dexamethasone sodium phosphate (4 mg) or a soluble form of injectable cortisol (e.g., hydrocortisone sodium succinate, 100 mg) should be injected intravenously immediately. Dexamethasone is preferred, because its effect lasts 12 to 24 h and it does not interfere with measurement of plasma or urinary steroids during subsequent ACTH stimulation tests. If hydrocortisone is used, 100 mg should be given every 6 to 8 h for the first 24 h. Mineralocorticoid is not useful acutely because it takes several days for its sodium-retaining effects to become manifest and because adequate sodium replacement can be achieved by intravenous saline administration. After initial treatment, the precipitating cause of the adrenal crisis (e.g., bacterial infection, viral gastroenteritis) should be sought and appropriately treated. After the patient's condition is stable, the diagnosis can be confirmed in patients not known to have adrenal insufficiency with a short ACTH stimulation test (see section on testing), and studies can be performed to determine the type and cause of the adrenal insufficiency (see earlier discussion). Unless there is a major precipitating or complicating illness, glucocorticoid therapy can be tapered over 1 to 3 d to an oral maintenance dose. Most patients who present with adrenal crisis have primary adrenal insufficiency and therefore require lifelong mineralocorticoid replacement as well. Fludrocortisone can be started when the saline infusion is

TABLE 12–13. Treatment of Suspected Acute Adrenal Insufficiency (Adrenal Crisis)

Emergency Measures
1. Establish intravenous access with a large-gauge needle.
2. Draw blood for stat serum electrolytes and glucose and routine measurement of plasma cortisol and ACTH. Do not wait for laboratory results.
3. Infuse 2 to 3 L of 154 mmol/L NaCl (0.9% saline) solution or 50 g/L (5%) dextrose in 154 mmol/L NaCl (0.9% saline) solution as quickly as possible. Monitor for signs of fluid overload by measuring central or peripheral venous pressure and listening for pulmonary rales. Reduce infusion rate if indicated.
4. Inject 4 mg of dexamethasone phosphate intravenously. Intravenous hydrocortisone (100 mg immediately and every 6 h thereafter) may also be used but will interfere with measurement of plasma cortisol during the short ACTH stimulation test. Mineralocorticoids are unnecessary at this time.
5. Use supportive measures as needed.

Subacute Measures After Stabilization of the Patient
1. Continue intravenous 154 mmol/L NaCl (0.9% saline) solution at a slower rate for next 24 to 48 h.
2. Search for and treat possible infectious precipitating causes of the adrenal crisis.
3. Perform a short ACTH stimulation test to confirm the diagnosis of adrenal insufficiency, if patient does not have known adrenal insufficiency.
4. Determine the type of adrenal insufficiency and its cause if not already known.
5. Taper glucocorticoids to maintenance dosage over 1 to 3 d, if precipitating or complicating illness permits.
6. Begin mineralocorticoid replacement with fludrocortisone (0.1 mg by mouth daily) when saline infusion is stopped.

stopped and the patient is taking food and fluids by mouth; 0.1 mg/d is the traditional dosage, but many patients require 0.2 mg/d or more to maintain a normal plasma renin activity level.[1031, 1187]

CHRONIC PRIMARY ADRENAL INSUFFICIENCY

Education of the Patient and Emergency Precautions. Education of the patient is the key to successful treatment of this disease. The patient must be taught that an active and vigorous life of normal length can be led as long as the prescribed medication regimen is followed and a few commonsense precautions are observed. The patient and responsible family members should be instructed about (1) the nature of the hormonal deficit and the rationale for replacement therapy, (2) maintenance medications, (3) changes in medications during minor illnesses, (4) when to consult a physician, and (5) when and how to inject dexamethasone for emergencies.

Every patient should at all times wear a medical alert (MedicAlert) bracelet or necklace and carry the Emergency Medical Information Card that is supplied with it. Both should indicate the diagnosis and daily medications. Every patient should have at least three 1-mL syringes prefilled with dexamethasone sodium phosphate (4 mg/mL in 154 mmol/L

NaCl solution): one at home, one at work or school, and one in the car. In addition, it is wise for the patient to carry such a syringe at all times, particularly while away from home, work, or car. The 1-mL prefilled syringes (Organon Inc., West Orange, NJ) can be obtained from some large pharmacies, or the pharmacist can prepare regular 1-mL syringes from a multidose vial. Larger 2.5-mL syringes prefilled with the same strength dexamethasone solution are also available (Merck Sharp & Dohme), but the patient should be instructed that only 1 mL of the contents is needed.

Maintenance Therapy (Table 12–14). Traditionally, cortisone acetate (25 to 37.5 mg/d) or cortisol (hydrocortisone) (20 to 30 mg/d) tablets were given for glucocorticoid replacement orally in two or three divided doses, often with two thirds taken upon arising in the morning and one third in the early afternoon, to simulate the normal circadian rhythm in plasma cortisol concentrations. There is no reason to give late afternoon or evening doses of these agents, because normal individuals secrete almost no cortisol from about 6:00 PM to 3:00 AM. There is also no rationale for using cortisone acetate under any circumstances. It is not biologically active but must first undergo hepatic metabolism to cortisol, over

TABLE 12–14. Treatment of Chronic Primary Adrenal Insufficiency

Maintenance Therapy
Glucocorticoid Replacement
• Dexamethasone 0.5 (0.25–0.75) mg or prednisone 5 (2.5–7.5) mg orally at bedtime. Supplement with hydrocortisone 5–10 mg orally in mid-afternoon if indicated.
• Alternative therapy is with hydrocortisone 15–20 mg on awakening and 5–10 mg in early afternoon.
• Monitor clinical symptoms and morning plasma ACTH.

Mineralocorticoid Replacement
• Fludrocortisone 0.1 (0.05–0.2) mg orally.
• Liberal salt intake.
• Monitor lying and standing blood pressure and pulse, edema, serum potassium, and plasma renin activity.
• Educate patient about the disease, how to manage minor illnesses and major stresses, and how to inject dexamethasone intramuscularly.
• Obtain MedicAlert bracelet/necklace, Emergency Medical Information Card, and prefilled syringes containing dexamethasone 4 mg in 1 mL saline.

Treatment of Minor Febrile Illness or Stress
• Increase glucocorticoid dose twofold to threefold for the few days of illness; do not change mineralocorticoid dose.
• Contact physician if illness worsens or persists for more than 3 d.
• No extra supplementation is needed for most uncomplicated, outpatient dental procedures under local anesthesia. General anesthesia or intravenous sedation should not be used in the office.

Emergency Treatment of Severe Stress or Trauma
• Inject contents of prefilled dexamethasone (4-mg) syringe intramuscularly.
• Get to physician as quickly as possible.

Steroid Coverage for Illness or Surgery in Hospital
• For moderate illness give hydrocortisone 50 mg twice a day orally or intravenously. Taper rapidly to maintenance dose as patient recovers.
• For severe illness give hydrocortisone 100 mg intravenously every 8 h. Taper dose to maintenance level by decreasing by half every day. Adjust dose according to course of illness.
• For minor procedures under local anesthesia and most radiologic studies, no extra supplementation is needed.
• For moderately stressful procedures, such as barium enema, endoscopy, or arteriography, give a single 100 mg intravenous dose of hydrocortisone just before the procedure.
• For major surgery, give hydrocortisone 100 mg intravenously just before induction of anesthesia and continue every 8 h for first 24 h. Taper dose rapidly, decreasing by half per day, to maintenance level.

which it holds no advantage. Furthermore, when given intramuscularly, it is either largely unabsorbed or not metabolized.[1188] Unfortunately, the administration of cortisone acetate or hydrocortisone does not achieve the desired goal of mimicking the normal daily rhythm, because the plasma cortisol concentration increases rapidly in the 30 min or so after ingestion, quickly exceeds the CBG binding capacity of about 690 nmol/L (25 μg/dL), reaches much higher than normal levels, and then very rapidly declines to 690 nmol/L (25 μg/dL) before slowing to a disappearance half-time of about 80 min. This results in transient very high cortisol concentrations followed by low levels until the next dose.[1189] In addition, by the time the patient takes the morning cortisol dose, plasma cortisol levels would normally already be at or near the circadian peak. This transient adrenal insufficiency probably accounts for the symptoms of fatigue, lassitude, mild nausea, or headache of which many patients complain on awakening and that are relieved within 30 to 60 min of taking the morning dose of glucocorticoid. Furthermore, plasma ACTH levels are much higher than normal for several hours in the early morning and for about 3 h after the cortisol is taken.[1189, 1190] The elevated plasma ACTH concentrations account for the persistent hyperpigmentation frequently seen in patients treated with this regimen. Moreover, because ACTH secretion is chronically inadequately inhibited by glucocorticoid negative feedback, ACTH secretion may eventually become relatively nonsuppressible,[979, 980, 1191, 1192] and pituitary hyperplasia[979, 981,1092] or, rarely, corticotrope adenomas may develop.[982, 1043, 1191, 1192]

Therefore, replacement therapy with a long-acting synthetic glucocorticoid, dexamethasone or prednisone, is preferred to replacement with short-acting cortisol or cortisone acetate, because the longer duration of action provides a smoother physiological effect and avoids the extremes of plasma glucocorticoid level that occur even when multiple daily doses of shorter-acting steroids are given. The usual oral daily replacement dosages are 0.5 mg and 5 mg for dexamethasone and prednisone, respectively. Occasionally patients require dosage adjustments ranging from 0.25 to 0.75 mg for dexamethasone or from 2.5 to 7.5 mg for prednisone. A larger dosage may be required for very large patients or those who metabolize the steroid more rapidly than normal, and a smaller dosage for children or small adults and for those who metabolize the steroid less rapidly. The dosage must be increased in patients taking drugs that accelerate hepatic steroid metabolism, such as phenytoin,[1118] barbiturates,[1118] rifampin,[699, 1118] mitotane,[1155] and aminoglutethimide.[1193] The dosage can be adjusted based on relief of clinical symptoms of adrenal insufficiency, decreased hyperpigmentation, and return of morning plasma ACTH concentration to less than 18 pmol/L (80 pg/mL). Excessive weight gain, facial plethora, or other signs and symptoms of Cushing's syndrome, and a suppressed morning plasma ACTH concentration (i.e., <4 pmol/L [20 pg/mL]) suggest excessive glucocorticoid replacement.

The ideal time to administer the glucocorticoid would be at 3:00 or 4:00 AM, just as circadian ACTH secretion normally begins to increase. Because a timed-release preparation is not available, the next best option is to give the dexamethasone or prednisone at bedtime. This lowers morning plasma ACTH levels into the normal range and provides adequate circulating glucocorticoid activity when the patient awakens. It can be given on awakening for the rare patient in whom the bedtime dose causes insomnia. A 5- to 10-mg dose of hydrocortisone may be given in early to middle afternoon for the occasional patient who seems to require more glucocorticoid in the late afternoon. Steroid is virtually never required later in the day. Occasionally patients experience gastrointestinal symptoms

from steroids that can be minimized by taking the drug with food or milk.

Mineralocorticoid replacement is required for all patients with primary adrenal insufficiency to prevent sodium loss, intravascular volume depletion, and hyperkalemia. The natural mineralocorticoids, aldosterone and DOC, are not used because of rapid hepatic degradation after oral ingestion and the high cost of synthesizing aldosterone. DOC, which is available in a long-acting, oil-based preparation for intramuscular injection, was used extensively when it was introduced in the 1940s but is little used at present. Fludrocortisone (9α-fluorohydrocortisone), a potent synthetic mineralocorticoid, is given orally in a usual dose of 0.1 mg daily; many patients require up to 0.2 mg daily to lower plasma renin activity to the upper-normal range.[1031, 1187] Patients receiving hydrocortisone, which in doses large enough to overcome renal 11-HSD inactivation has some mineralocorticoid activity, may require a lower dose, such as 0.05 mg daily. Adequacy of mineralocorticoid replacement can be monitored by inquiring for symptoms of postural hypotension and measuring supine and upright blood pressure and pulse, serum potassium concentration, and plasma renin activity. The dose may have to be doubled during the summer, when salt loss in perspiration increases, especially if the patient is routinely exposed to temperatures above about 29°C (85°F). Salt intake should be liberal, especially when exercising. Hypertension, edema, and hypokalemia are signs of excessive mineralocorticoid replacement, and some investigators caution against too vigorous attempts to lower plasma renin activity to normal.[1194]

Essential hypertension in patients with adrenal insufficiency should be treated with restriction of dietary sodium and reduced mineralocorticoid replacement, rather than sodium-wasting diuretics.[1194, 1195] Antihypertensive agents other than sodium-wasting diuretics or spironolactone should be used. Mineralocorticoid therapy usually cannot be discontinued without risking sodium depletion.

Treatment During Illness or Surgery. Cortisol secretion normally increases with the stress of illness and surgery. Recommendations for increased glucocorticoid treatment during minor or major illnesses, minor procedures, and major surgery are given in Table 12–14. Despite evidence from studies in monkeys that supraphysiological glucocorticoid doses may not be required for successful survival of major surgery,[1196] the prudent approach is to provide high doses of glucocorticoid to all patients with proven or suspected adrenal insufficiency, starting before induction of anesthesia.

Pregnancy in Adrenal Insufficiency. Before glucocorticoid replacement therapy became available, pregnancy in patients with adrenal insufficiency was associated with a maternal mortality rate as high as 35 to 45%.[1197] Now most patients with adrenal insufficiency go through pregnancy, labor, and delivery without difficulty. The usual glucocorticoid and mineralocorticoid replacement dosages are continued.[1000, 1198] Some patients may require slightly more glucocorticoid in the third trimester. During labor, adequate saline hydration and 25 mg of intravenous cortisol (hydrocortisone sodium succinate) every 6 h should be administered. At the time of delivery or if labor is prolonged, high-dosage parenteral hydrocortisone should be administered as 100 mg every 6 h or as a continuous infusion. After delivery, the dosage can be tapered rapidly to maintenance within 3 d.[1198] The occasional patient with severe nausea and vomiting in the first trimester may require intramuscular dexamethasone at a slightly increased dosage (i.e., 1 mg daily). If the patient cannot take medicines by mouth, 1 to 2 mg/d of desoxycorticosterone acetate in sesame oil may be administered intramuscularly as mineralocorticoid replacement.

CHRONIC SECONDARY AND TERTIARY ADRENAL INSUFFICIENCY. Treatment of chronic secondary or tertiary adrenal insufficiency is identical to that of chronic primary adrenal insufficiency (see Table 12–14), except that mineralocorticoid replacement is rarely required and replacement for other pituitary hormones may be necessary. In most patients with hypoaldosteronism, plasma renin activity is low[997, 998] because of the lack of cortisol's stimulatory effect on angiotensinogen production.[904] Plasma renin activity and aldosterone levels return to normal with glucocorticoid replacement alone.[997] Treatment of adrenal insufficiency caused by pharmacologic administration of glucocorticoids and withdrawal of the steroids is discussed later in this chapter.

Prognosis and Survival

The prognosis for patients with adrenal insufficiency was grim before the availability of glucocorticoids in 1950s; more than 80% of patients died within 2 y after diagnosis.[999] Today, a patient with autoimmune adrenal insufficiency should have a normal life span and can lead a fully active life, including vigorous exercise.[999, 1000] The prognosis for patients with other causes of adrenal insufficiency depends mostly on the underlying disease. However, heart failure was reported in 7 of 22 patients with long-standing primary adrenal insufficiency receiving conventional treatment after a mean of 26 years[1195]; the causal relation, if any, is unclear. Essential hypertension occasionally occurs[1195] and must be treated. Linear growth and pubertal development proceed normally in correctly treated children with adrenal insufficiency (i.e., those adequately but not overly treated).[1022, 1028] Increased osteopenia in women but not men treated chronically for adrenal insufficiency was reported in one study,[1199] and in men but not women in another.[1200] A third study found no increase in bone loss after chronic replacement with hydrocortisone 30 mg/d or prednisone 7.5 mg/d.[1201]

Isolated Mineralocorticoid Deficiency

Aldosterone is deficient in conditions other than adrenal insufficency. Isolated mineralocorticoid deficiency states include acquired secondary aldosterone deficiency (hyporeninemic hypoaldosteronism), acquired primary aldosterone deficiency, and inherited enzymatic defects in aldosterone biosynthesis.

HYPORENINEMIC HYPOALDOSTERONISM. The most common form of isolated hypoaldosteronism is caused by impaired renin release from the kidney. The syndrome was first described in 1957,[1202] and the hyporeninemia was first recognized in 1972.[1203, 1204] The typical patient is 50 to 70 years old and has unexplained, chronic, asymptomatic hyperkalemia and mild to moderate renal insufficiency (creatinine clearance >15 mL/min).[1205] A minority of patients present with muscle weakness or cardiac arrhythmias. About half have diabetes mellitus.[1205] Other associated disease states include systemic lupus erythematosus, multiple myeloma, renal amyloidosis, cirrhosis, sickle cell anemia, AIDS, POEMS syndrome (polyneuropathy, organomegaly, endocrinopathy, M protein, and skin changes), and primary autonomic insufficiency.[1206–1215] Hyporeninemic hypoaldosteronism may occur transiently in association with use of nonsteroidal anti-inflammatory drugs,[1216] cyclosporin A,[1217] mitomycin C,[1218] cosyntropin,[1219] and other agents in susceptible individuals.

Pathophysiology

Aldosterone Deficiency. Urinary aldosterone excretion, an index of aldosterone production, is low under basal conditions and fails to increase after sodium restriction.[1203] Plasma renin activity is also low and does not increase appropriately during sodium restriction, periods of prolonged upright posture, or diuretic administration.[1203] It was postulated that interstitial renal disease and damage to the juxtaglomerular apparatus result in a primary defect in renin generation or release and secondary deficiency of aldosterone secretion.[1203] However, no specific anatomic lesion has been identified to explain the deficient renin production. Aldosterone secretory capacity appears to respond to administration of angiotensin II in some patients,[1220–1222] but the response is absent[1223] or blunted[1205] in others. Failure to respond could indicate a coexisting primary defect in aldosterone secretion or reflect atrophy of the zona glomerulosa caused by chronic renin deficiency. Instances of frankly elevated[1224] or inappropriately high basal levels and normal responsiveness of plasma 18-hydroxycorticosterone to angiotensin II infusion[1225] suggest a defect in a terminal enzymatic step in aldosterone biosynthesis. However, it is not known whether this defect is primary or is a consequence of chronic renin deficiency.

Renin Deficiency. Various mechanisms have been invoked to explain the hyporeninemia. One explanation is physiological suppression of renin secretion by hypervolemia. In hypertensive patients (up to 50% of patients with hyporeninemic hypoaldosteronism have elevated blood pressure), expanded extracellular fluid volume may suppress renin. Prolonged sodium restriction and diuretic administration increase plasma renin activity in these patients,[1226] but the increments in plasma renin activity and aldosterone concentration are less than those in normal subjects. A second possible mechanism is insufficiency of the autonomic nervous system, particularly in patients with diabetic neuropathy, in whom impairment of the norepinephrine response to postural change is thought to contribute to deficient renin release. Furthermore, these patients exhibit decreased sensitivity to administered β-adrenergic agonists, suggesting defects in both catecholamine production and action.[1227] A third proposed mechanism is secretion of abnormal forms of renin, such as a defect in the conversion of prorenin to renin.[1224, 1228, 1229] Kallikrein, a neutral serine protease produced in the macula densa, activates prorenin, and some patients with hyporeninemic hypoaldosteronism have low kallikrein levels.[1229] However, the suppression of kallikrein can be a secondary phenomenon, since mineralocorticoid replacement may restore kallikrein levels to normal.[1230] A fourth possibility is prostaglandin deficiency, because vasodilatory prostaglandins, particularly prostaglandin I_2, mediate renin release.[1231] Furthermore, cyclooxygenase inhibitors, such as indomethacin, produce a reversible defect in renin production.[1232] The finding of low prostaglandin E_2 levels in hyporeninemic hypoaldosteronism[1232] has not been confirmed,[1233, 1234] but prostaglandin I_2 (prostacyclin) production, as assessed by measurement of the stable urinary metabolite 6-keto-prostaglandin $F_{1\alpha}$, apparently is diminished in these patients.[1235] Furthermore, the prostaglandin I_2 in these patients was unresponsive to the potent stimulators, norepinephrine and calcium. Prostaglandin I_2 deficiency may cause hyporeninemic hypoaldosteronism from resulting defects in the conversion of prorenin to renin[1236, 1237] and in renin release. TGF-β, which may be elevated in patients with diabetes mellitus, inhibits renin release.[1238] Conversion of inactive to active renin may also be impaired in diabetes mellitus.[1239]

Hyperkalemia. The pathogenesis of hyperkalemia is probably multifactorial. Factors that interact to regulate ion transport processes in the distal nephron include rates of tubular flow and sodium reabsorption, transepithelial voltage gradients, dietary potassium intake, systemic pH, and mineralocorticoid action. Aldosterone has an acute effect on epithelial potassium transport in isolated renal tubules in vitro,[1240, 1241] and chronic exposure to mineralocorticoids increases the potassium-secretory capacity of the tubule, presumably by indirect means. An additional factor operative in diabetes mellitus is loss of insulin effect on internal potassium balance.[1242]

Acidosis. Patients with hyporeninemic hypoaldosteronism have a unique form of renal tubular acidosis, termed type

IV.[1243] The acidosis is a consequence of decreased renal ammoniagenesis, reduced hydrogen ion–secretory capacity in the distal nephron, and mild reduction in the proximal tubular threshold for bicarbonate reabsorption. The impaired ammoniagenesis is not directly attributable to aldosterone deficiency but is the consequence of hyperkalemia. Correction of hyperkalemia by means other than mineralocorticoid replacement improves urinary ammonium excretion and sometimes corrects the urinary acidification defect.[1244] Mineralocorticoid replacement also corrects the hyperkalemia and thereby increases urinary ammonium excretion, but net acid excretion also rises, implying that mineralocorticoid has an additional effect on hydrogen ion–secretory capacity.[1243] Aldosterone acutely increases sodium-independent hydrogen ion secretion in the medullary collecting duct in vitro.[1245]

Clinical Diagnosis. The diagnosis of hypoaldosteronism must be considered in any patient with unexplained chronic hyperkalemia. Spurious serum potassium values associated with in vitro hemolysis, thrombocytosis, or leukocytosis must be excluded. Dietary or medicinal sources of excess potassium should be sought but usually do not cause sustained hyperkalemia if renal function is normal. Renal function should be evaluated, and drugs that impair renal tubular potassium excretion should be withdrawn.

The clinical diagnosis is confirmed by finding low plasma renin activity and low plasma or urinary aldosterone concentration under conditions that ordinarily activate the renin-angiotensin-aldosterone axis. The standard methods for achieving this are maintenance of an upright posture for 3 or 4 h and administration of furosemide (see Chapter 14). A low random plasma aldosterone level associated with a normal ratio of aldosterone to plasma renin activity is also diagnostic.[1246–1248]

Treatment. The therapeutic approach must take into consideration the age of the patient and the other associated disorders. If the hyperkalemia is moderate and if no electrocardiographic changes are evident, periodic measurement of serum potassium concentration should suffice. Drugs that tend to promote hyperkalemia, such as β-adrenergic antagonists, cyclooxygenase inhibitors, angiotensin-converting enzyme inhibitors, heparin, and potassium-sparing diuretics, should be avoided. Dietary potassium intake should be reduced, if possible. Diuretic therapy should be the initial treatment for patients who have coexisting diseases associated with sodium retention, such as hypertension and congestive heart failure. Mineralocorticoid replacement with fludrocortisone is reserved for patients who have more severe hyperkalemia and no hypertension or congestive heart failure. The usual starting dose is 0.1 mg of fludrocortisone per day, but some patients require higher doses.

PRIMARY HYPOALDOSTERONISM

CYP11B2 (Aldosterone Synthase) Deficiency. Congenital hypoaldosteronism is a rare inherited disorder transmitted as an autosomal recessive trait. The clinical presentation is typical of aldosterone deficiency and in infants is characterized by recurrent dehydration, salt wasting, and failure to thrive.[1249] The deficiency is in the activity of the terminal enzyme in the aldosterone biosynthetic pathway, CYP11B2. Corticosterone 18-methyloxidase I (CMO I) refers to the enzymatic activity of CYP11B2 responsible for hydroxylation of corticosterone at C_{18}; the isomerase (CMO II) activity of CYP11B2 converts the 18-hydroxyl group to an aldehyde.[1250] CYP11B2 type I deficiency would be expected to produce low plasma levels of products derived from corticosterone (18-hydroxycorticosterone and aldosterone) and low urinary excretion of their metabolites,[1251] whereas CYP11B2 type II deficiency should be associated with high plasma 18-hydroxycorticosterone and low plasma aldosterone.[1252] Urinary excretion of tetrahydro-18-hydroxy,11-dehydrocorticosterone, the major metabolite of 18-

hydroxycorticosterone, is increased, but urinary excretion of tetrahydroaldosterone is decreased.[1251] Reanalysis of the original two reports of CMO I defects[1253, 1254] indicates that the patients actually had CMO II deficiency,[1251] but 20 to 30 cases of type I deficiency have subsequently been reported,[1255] accounting for about half of all reported cases of CYP11B2 deficiency.

Mitochondrial CYP11B2, the product of a single gene, *CYP11B2*, catalyzes both 11β-hydroxylation and 18-hydroxylation to convert DOC to aldosterone.[536] The *CYP11B2* gene is located on chromosome 8q21-22 and is the site of mutations causing both type I and type II deficiency. *CYP11B2* is located near *CYP11B1*, which encodes CYP11B1, the enzyme that converts deoxycortisol to cortisol.

Some patients with CYP11B2 type I deficiency have a 5-nucleotide deletion in exon 1 which leads to a frameshift and premature stop codon[1256, 1257]; they produce no functional CYP11B2. Other type I patients have a point mutation causing a R384P substitution; the arginine is highly conserved and presumably important for enzyme activity.[1255] Patients with CYP11B2 type II deficiency have either of two point mutations resulting in R181W and V386A substitutions that do not affect 11β-hydroxylase activity but reduce 18-hydroxylase activity and abolish 18-oxidase activity.[1257, 1258] A mutation that greatly reduces the activity of the enzyme in vitro is associated with normal aldosterone secretion,[1258] so only the most severe enzyme deficiencies must be manifested clinically. The diagnosis can be established by assay of 11-DOC, corticosterone, 18-hydroxycorticosterone, 18-hydroxy-DOC, and aldosterone levels in plasma.[1249] The ratio of plasma 18-hydroxycorticosterone to plasma aldosterone differentiates the two disorders: it is less than 10 in type I and more than 100 in type II deficiency.[1249] Patients with type II deficiency tend to have increased plasma cortisol levels that may result from increased adrenal sensitivity to ACTH induced by the increased plasma angiotensin II levels in response to sodium depletion.[1259] Both forms of the syndrome are treated by replacement of mineralocorticoid with the usual dosage of fludrocortisone.

Acquired Forms of Primary Hypoaldosteronism. Several conditions may be associated with aldosterone biosynthetic defects. Heparin therapy causes natriuresis, with or without frank hyperkalemia in certain patients,[1260–1262] some of whom may have diabetes mellitus. Heparin suppresses aldosterone synthesis, leading to a compensatory rise in plasma renin activity, which in most subjects is sufficient to prevent aldosterone deficiency.[1262] The compensatory mechanism apparently is insufficient in some persons because of an impaired renin-angiotensin system, as may exist in diabetes mellitus.[1262] Persistently hypotensive, critically ill patients also have inappropriately low plasma aldosterone concentrations in relation to the activity of the renin-angiotensin system. The defect is at the level of the adrenal but has not been associated with any particular disease state or therapy[1263]; the mechanism is unknown. Isolated primary hypoaldosteronism is occasionally associated with carcinoma metastatic to the adrenal glands.[1264]

PSEUDOHYPOALDOSTERONISM.

This rare salt-wasting syndrome of infancy was described in 1958[1265] and postulated to be caused by renal tubular insensitivity to mineralocorticoids. It may be inherited as an autosomal dominant or recessive disorder,[1266–1268] may occur sporadically, or may be associated with other conditions, such as prematurity and hydramnios,[1269, 1270] obstructive uropathy,[1271] acute pyelonephritis,[1272] or renal transplantation.[1273] The autosomal dominant form exhibits resistance to aldosterone action that is confined to the renal tubule, whereas the recessive form is more severe and also affects the sweat glands, salivary glands, and colon.[1274] Some patients and relatives of patients may be asymptomatic but have elevated plasma aldosterone and renin levels.[1275] The clinical hallmarks of pseudohypoaldosteronism are those of aldosterone deficiency: hyponatremia, hyperkalemia, hyper-reninemia, and renal salt wasting. However, plasma aldosterone levels and urinary excretion are markedly elevated,[1266] and the ratio of plasma 18-hydroxycorticosterone to aldosterone is normal. Hypothalamic-pituitary-adrenal function is normal. Neither the clinical nor the biochemical abnormalities respond to mineralocorticoid treatment; sodium chloride supplementation (2 to 8 g/d) and potassium-binding resins usually are successful. One study documented spontaneous improvement in electrolyte balance with increasing age, although plasma renin activity and aldosterone concentrations remained elevated.[1276] Salt supplements can be discontinued after a few years in some patients. Carbenoxolone, an 11β-HSD inhibitor, may be beneficial; it presumably acts by allowing cortisol, which circulates in much higher concentrations than aldosterone in plasma, access to the renal tubular type I (mineralocorticoid) receptor.[1277]

In five of seven kindreds studied, type 1 familial pseudohypoaldosteronism resulted from homozygous mutations of the amiloride-sensitive epithelial sodium channel. One is a G37S substitution in the β-subunit, which reduces the channel's activity by 60%.[1278] The β-subunit gene is located on the short arm of chromosome 16 and is the same gene in which mutations causing COOH-terminal truncation result in Liddle syndrome (pseudohyperaldosteronism).[1279] The other mutations are frameshift or point mutations that introduce a premature termination codon and truncate the α-subunit of the sodium channel, the gene for which is on chromosome 12.[1278] α-Subunit knockout mice die of respiratory failure because of inability to clear alveolar fluid[1280]; patients with type 1 pseudohypoaldosteronism also have respiratory problems.[1281] Type I (mineralocorticoid) receptors, which are normally expressed in circulating blood mononuclear cells,[1282] were found to be absent or reduced in number in a kindred with the autosomal recessive form of the disorder,[1283] and aldosterone had no effect on transmembrane sodium-potassium flux.[1284] Immunofluorescence studies have demonstrated type I receptor protein in the peripheral mononuclear cells of patients with both the sporadic and the autosomal dominant forms of the disorder, but none in patients with the autosomal recessive form.[1285] However, there is no linkage between the locus for the type I receptor gene, which is located on chromosome 4q31.1, and the gene for autosomal recessive type 1 pseudohypoaldosteronism.[1286] No type I receptor mutation has been found in patients with familial or sporadic pseudohypoaldosteronism,[1277, 1287–1289] although polymorphisms have been described,[1277] and mRNA levels appear to be normal.[1287] The low type I receptor levels may result from down-regulation by the chronic high plasma aldosterone levels. Low erythrocyte Na+,K+-ATPase activity was found in twins with pseudohypoaldosteronism, whereas a child with hypoaldosteronism had a normal level.[1290] Enzyme activity increased to normal by 6 to 8 mo of age, and salt supplementation requirement decreased concomitantly.[1290]

Hyperfunction

Glucocorticoids: Hypercortisolism (Cushing's Syndrome)

HISTORY

Cushing's syndrome, the constellation of clinical signs and symptoms resulting from chronic glucocorticoid excess, was probably first described by Sir William Osler in 1899.[1291] In 1912 Osler's colleague and friend, Harvey Cushing, reported on a 23-year-old woman with "painful obesity, hypertrichosis and amenorrhea"[1292] and postulated 20 y later that the "polyglandular syndrome" was caused by primary pituitary dysfunction ("pituitary basophilism") (Fig. 12–34).[1293] By then

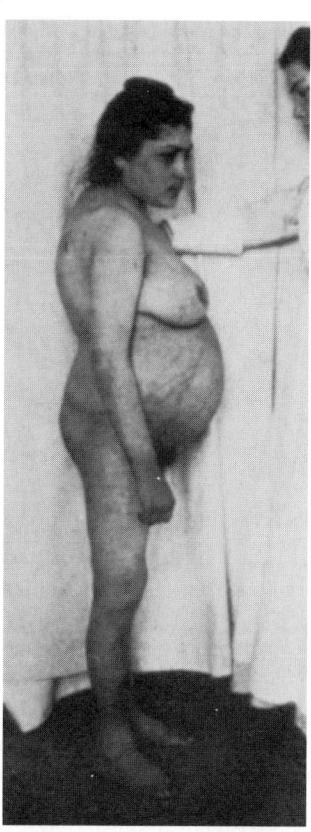

Figure 12–34. Minnie G., Cushing's index patient, at age 23 years. (From Cushing H. The basophil adenomas of the pituitary body and their clinical manifestations [pituitary basophilism]. Bull Johns Hopkins Hosp 1932; 50:137–195.)

a pituitary factor was thought to regulate the adrenal cortex,[33, 34] but neither ACTH nor adrenal steroids had yet been discovered. Adrenal tumors were known to cause the syndrome in some patients.[1294] A patient with Cushing's syndrome and a nonendocrine tumor was described in 1928,[1295] but ectopic ACTH production was not demonstrated until 1962.[1296]

CLINICAL PRESENTATION

The more common features of Cushing's syndrome are listed in Table 12–15. None is pathognomonic, but initial development or increasing severity of several of these features should arouse suspicion. The manifestations depend on the degree and duration of hypercortisolism, the presence or absence of androgen excess (pure hypercortisolism does not cause hirsutism or seborrhea), and the additional tumor-related effects in the case of adrenal carcinoma or ectopic ACTH syndrome. These clinical manifestations are now usually less severe than in Cushing's day[1293] because of earlier diagnosis.

Progressive obesity is the most common sign. It is usually central (centripetal), involving the face, neck, trunk, and abdomen, with the extremities spared or even wasted (Fig. 12–35A; see color section between pages 875 and 877). Some authors report generalized obesity in most patients,[1297] but in our experience a minority of adults develop generalized obesity. The amount of intra-abdominal fat is greater and the amount of fat on the arms is less than in patients with exogenous obesity.[1298] In contrast, generalized obesity is almost the rule in children, in whom linear growth is slowed or arrested; often it is the first indication of glucocorticoid excess. A child whose weight begins to rise across the percentiles as height begins to fall across the percentiles (Fig. 12–36) should be

TABLE 12–15. Signs and Symptoms of Cushing's Syndrome

Sign or Symptom	Reported Incidence (%)
Centripetal obesity	79–97
Facial plethora	50–94
Glucose intolerance	39–90
Weakness, proximal myopathy	29–90
Hypertension	74–87
Psychological changes	31–86
Easy bruisability	23–84
Hirsutism	64–81
Oligomenorrhea or amenorrhea	55–80
Impotence	55–80
Acne, oily skin	26–80
Abdominal striae	51–71
Ankle edema	28–60
Backache, vertebral collapse, fracture	40–50
Polydipsia, polyuria	25–44
Renal calculi	15–19
Hyperpigmentation	4–16
Headache	0–47
Exophthalmos	0–33
Tinea versicolor infection	0–30
Abdominal pain	0–21

Adapted from a table in Howlett TA, Rees LH, Besser GM. Cushing's syndrome. Clin Endocrinol Metab 1985; 14:911–945. Copyright 1985, The Endocrine Society. Data summarized from Cushing,[1293] Plotz et al.,[1299] Ross et al.,[1301] Gold,[2194] Jeffcoate et al.,[926] Cohen,[927] Liddle,[1512] Urbanic and George,[1306] and Ross and Linch.[1297]

considered to have Cushing's syndrome until proven otherwise. Facial fat accumulation can produce a moon face, often accompanied by plethora over the cheeks, anterior neck, and sun-exposed chest (see Fig. 12–35C). The neck is thick and appears shortened. There is usually a dorsocervical fat pad, or buffalo hump, consistent with the degree of obesity. Enlarged fat pads that fill the supraclavicular fossae are more characteristic of Cushing's syndrome (see Fig. 12–35C) and are much less common in exogenous obesity. Patients who diet and exercise rigorously may have little or no weight gain, facial rounding, or central weight redistribution (see Fig. 12–35L to O). Exophthalmos is present in about 6% of patients,[1299] probably as a result of increased retro-orbital fat deposition.[1300] There is no inflammatory component.

Weakness is common, and it is usually associated with proximal muscle wasting, including wasting of the gluteus maximus; reduction in the arm muscle mass is most striking.[1298] Many patients cannot rise from a squatting position without assistance, and those with more severe disease may be unable to climb stairs, get up from a deep chair, or raise their arms long enough to comb their hair. In patients with extreme hypercortisolemia and those receiving thiazide diuretics, hypokalemia may aggravate weakness.

Cardiovascular complications are a major cause of morbidity and death in untreated Cushing's syndrome.[1299] Moderate hypertension (diastolic blood pressure >100 mm Hg) is common.[1301] Dependent edema is another sign of mineralocorticoid excess, one of several causes of hypertension in Cushing's syndrome.[901, 1302] Congestive heart failure was present in almost half of patients older than 40 years of age in one series[1301] but is much less frequent in our experience. Like other features, it presumably reflects both the chronicity and the severity of the disease. The mineralocorticoid excess results at least in part from increased accessibility of cortisol to the type I (mineralocorticoid) receptor because of defective 11β-HSD activity, reflected by an increased ratio of cortisol to cortisone metabolites in urine.[1303] This phenomenon is most pronounced in the ectopic ACTH syndrome.

The skin is atrophic, the stratum corneum is thinned, and there is loss of subcutaneous fat,[1304] allowing subcutaneous blood vessels to be seen. The skin becomes fragile and, in extreme cases, peels off with adhesive tape like damp tissue

paper (Liddle's sign). Minor wounds heal slowly, and surgical wounds may dehisce. Loss of connective tissue results in easy bruising on the forearms and shins after minimal, unremembered trauma; patients are sometimes initially thought to have senile purpura[1305] or a bleeding diathesis. Extensive ecchymoses at venipuncture sites are common, and it is often difficult to maintain intravenous lines without infiltrating fluid. The fragile skin is stretched by the rapidly enlarging trunk and abdomen, producing striae (see Fig. 12–35). Unlike the striae of pregnant women, they appear purplish or reddish because the thin, transparent skin reveals the color of venous blood in the dermis. They are also more numerous and often more than 1 cm wide. Such striae are most frequent on the lower flanks and abdomen, but can occur on the breasts, hips, buttocks, upper abdomen, shoulders, and upper thighs and in the axillae. They occur more frequently in younger patients (see Fig. 12–35).[1306] Cutaneous fungal infections, especially tinea versicolor, are often found on the chest. Oral candidiasis is encountered only in severe hypercortisolism. Fungal infections of the nails are occasionally observed. Hyperpigmentation is not caused by hypercortisolism but by increased plasma ACTH.[240] Hyperpigmentation may occur with Cushing's disease and, more frequently, with the ectopic ACTH syndrome, but not with adrenocortical tumors. The distribution of the melanin deposits resembles that seen in adrenal insufficiency but is less pronounced. Acanthosis nigricans may occur in the axillae and around the neck.

Androgen excess is manifested by oily facial skin, acne, and mild hirsutism in women. Hirsutism is usually limited to the face (see Fig. 12–35) but can be generalized. Thinning scalp hair is common, but temporal balding is rare. Oligomenorrhea in women, impotence in men, and decreased libido in both sexes are common, presumably because of hypercortisolemia in men and the combination of cortisol and androgen excess in women.

Low back pain is common. Back pain, vertebral compression fractures, pathologic rib fractures, and, less commonly, long bone fractures result from osteoporosis, which can usually be demonstrated even in young patients with dual-energy X-ray absorptiometry or CT scan densitometry of the lumbosacral vertebrae. Up to 22% of patients develop radiologically demonstrable vertebral compression fractures.[1301, 1307] We have encountered several patients with aseptic necrosis of the femoral heads, and in one instance of the humeral heads (Fig. 12–37), a condition known to be associated with chronic administration of exogenous glucocorticoids. Because of increased bone reabsorption, hypercalciuria and renal calculi may be present. Hypercalcemia is unusual and, when it is encountered, suggests primary hyperparathyroidism.

Polydipsia and polyuria are seen most frequently in patients with hypercalciuria or glycosuria. Glucose intolerance and hyperinsulinemia are common because of the effect of cortisol on gluconeogenesis, but true diabetes mellitus occurs in only 10 to 15% of patients, usually those with a family history of the disease. Ketoacidosis is rare and indicates unsuspected insulin-dependent diabetes mellitus that has been exacerbated by the hypercortisolism.

Psychiatric complications occur in more than half of patients with Cushing's syndrome of all causes[926, 930, 1299, 1308] and are, therefore, presumably a result of hypercortisolemia. Emotional lability, agitated depression, loss of energy and libido, irritability, anxiety, panic attacks, and mild paranoia are most common.[930] Most patients have increased appetite and weight gain, but anorexia may rarely predominate.[1309] Some patients are suicidal[1299]; the physician must be alert to this possibility and take precautions to protect the patient. Some patients appear euphoric or manic, particularly during the early course of the disease. Children tend to be tireless overachievers, often ranking near the top of their class in school. Some patients

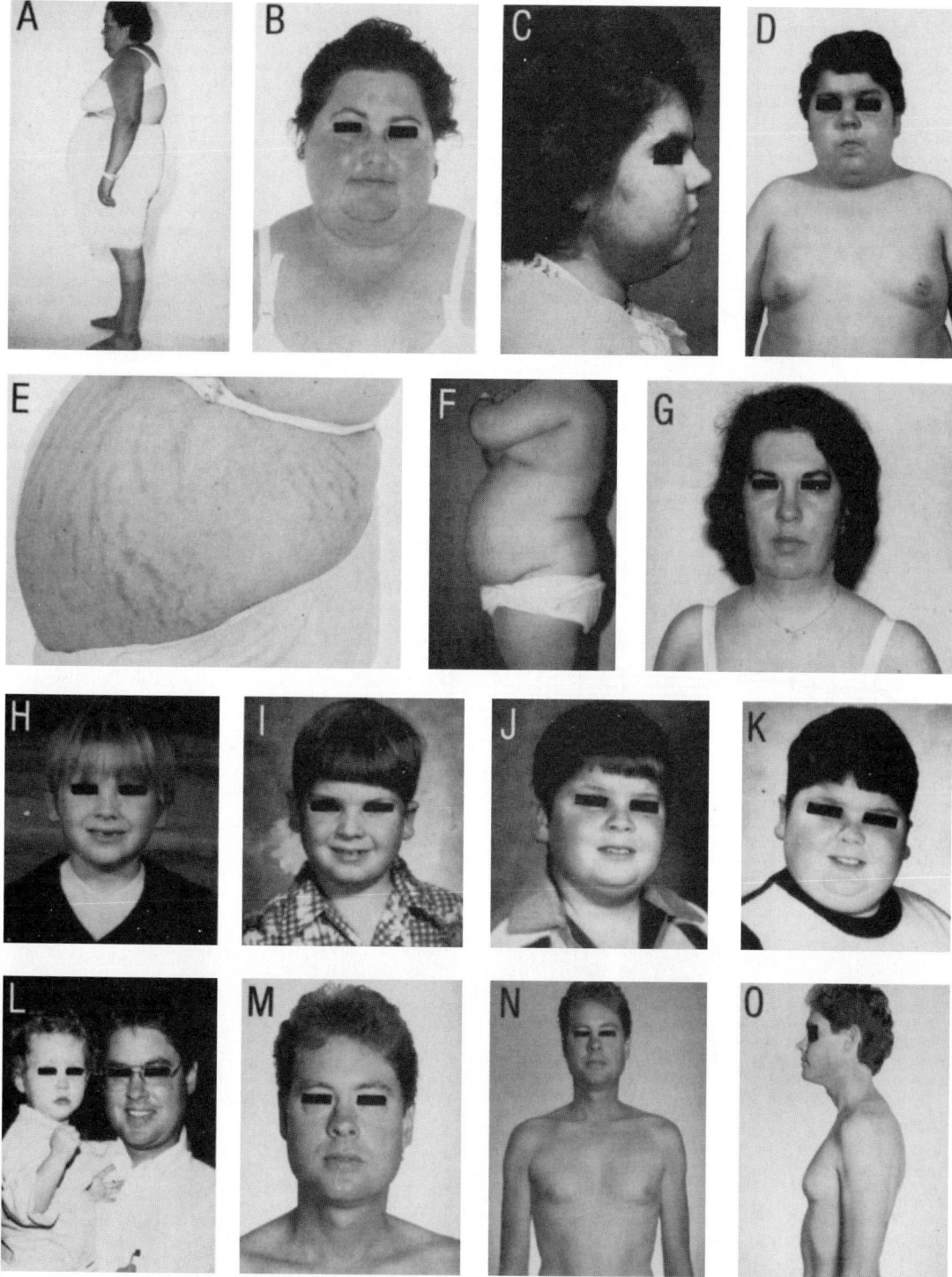

Figure 12–35. Physical appearance of patients with Cushing's syndrome (see color section between pages 875 and 877). *A,* Centripetal and some generalized obesity and dorsal kyphosis in a 30-year-old woman with Cushing's disease. *B,* Same woman as in *A,* showing moon facies, plethora, hirsutism, and enlarged supraclavicular fat pads. *C,* Facial rounding, hirsutism, and acne in a 14-year-old girl with Cushing's disease. *D,* Central and generalized obesity and moon facies in a 14-year-old boy with Cushing's disease. *E,* Abdominal striae in the 30-year-old patient shown in *A. F,* Striae on the breast, abdomen, and thigh of a 9-year-old girl with generalized obesity and Cushing's disease. *G,* Facial plethora, mild hirsutism, and increased supraclavicular fat pads in a 42-year-old woman with a centripetal shift in weight distribution without weight gain. *H* through *K,* Development of childhood Cushing's disease from normal at age 7 years and early Cushing's disease at age 8 years to progressive Cushing's disease at ages 9 and 11 years. *L* through *O,* Effects of diet and exercise on Cushing's syndrome. The patient at age 37 years with a 2-y history of Cushing's disease before and after 8 mo of self-imposed diet and rigorous exercise; minimal central fat distribution and mild residual loss of proximal muscle mass are seen. *(C* courtesy of Dr. H. Patrick Higgins.)

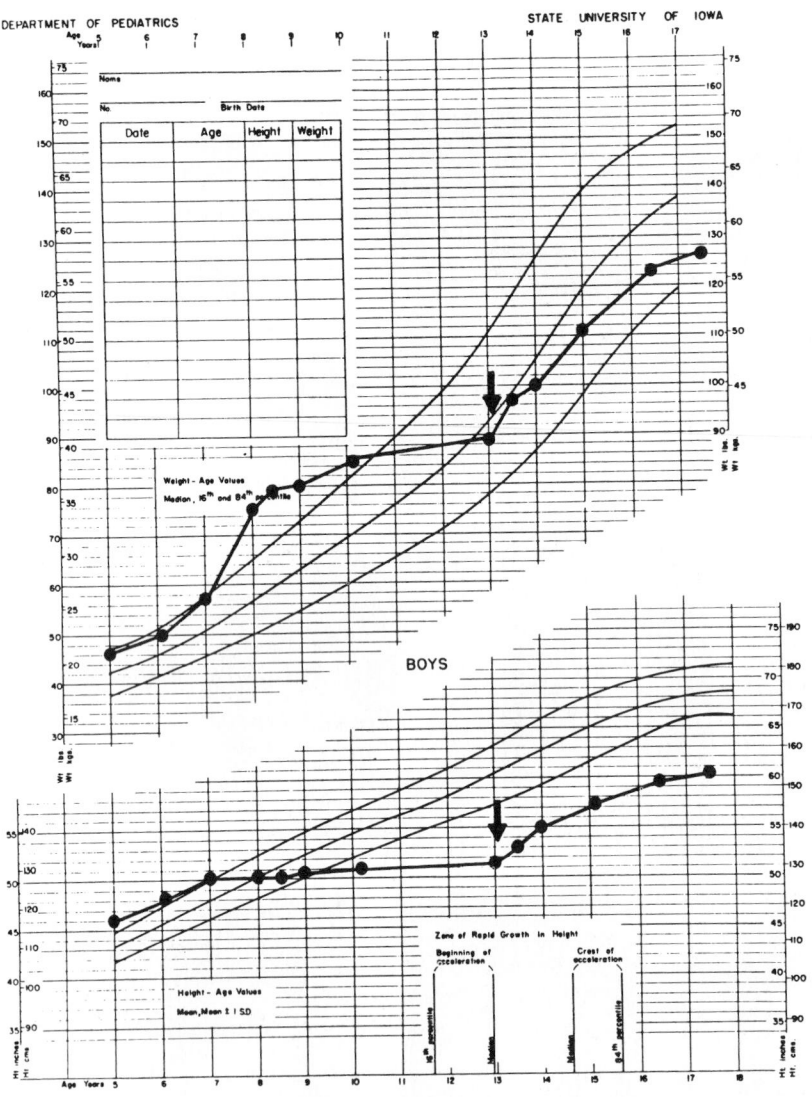

Figure 12–36. Growth chart of a boy with childhood Cushing's syndrome beginning at about 7 years of age. Weight gain was minimized from the age of 8½ to 13 years by rigorous diet and exercise. He received 40 Gy (4000 rad) of megavoltage pituitary radiation at age 13 years (*arrows*). Note the lack of catch-up linear growth. At age 25 years, the height was unchanged, the weight was 70 kg, and pituitary function was normal.

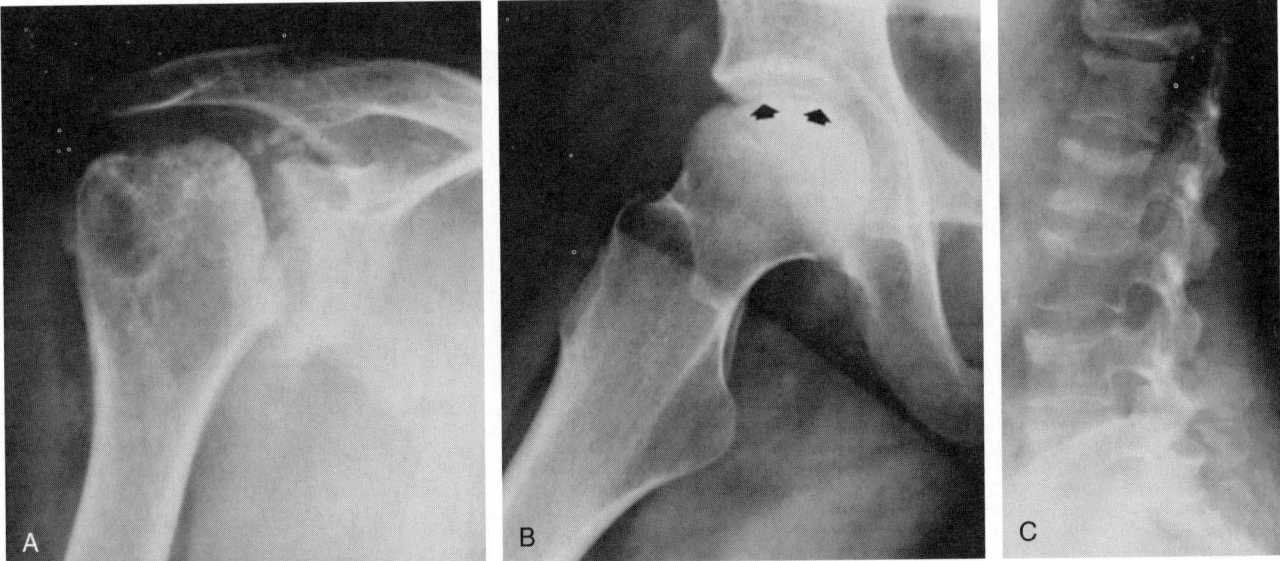

Figure 12–37. Aseptic necrosis of bone in Cushing's disease. *A,* Aseptic necrosis of the right humeral head of a 43-year-old woman with Cushing's disease of about 8 mo duration. *B,* Aseptic necrosis of the right femoral head in a 24-year-old woman with Cushing's disease of about 4½ y duration. The arrows indicate the crescent subchondral radiolucency, best seen in this lateral view. *C,* Diffuse osteoporosis, vertebral collapse, and subchondral sclerosis in the patient whose shoulder is shown in *A.* (From Phillips KA, Nance EP Jr, Rodriguez RM, et al. Avascular necrosis of bone: a manifestation of Cushing's disease. Reprinted by permission from the Southern Medical Journal 1986; 79:825–829.)

with psychiatric complications have underlying personality disorders that were present before the hypercortisolism occurred[1310] and persist after it is cured. Insomnia is common, often an early symptom, and is presumably caused by high cortisol levels at night.[930, 1311, 1312] Both rapid eye movement sleep[1313] and delta-wave sleep[1314] are reduced; plasma delta-sleep–inducing peptide levels are decreased,[1314] but a causal relation is unproved. Patients with Cushing's disease report incidences of depression in female relatives and of alcoholism in male relatives that are similar to those of families of patients with major depressive disorder.[930]

Phlebothrombosis and thromboembolic events are said to be increased in frequency,[1297, 1315] presumably related to increased levels of plasma clotting factors and prothrombin,[1316] but others dispute this claim.[1317]

Glucocorticoids suppress immune function, but infection with organisms of low pathogenicity occurs only with severe hypercortisolemia.[826] Inflammatory and febrile responses to bacterial infection are suppressed, masking its presence. Asymptomatic urinary tract infection is common and may become symptomatic only after cure of hypercortisolism.

Intraocular pressure is reversibly increased in about one quarter of patients[1318] and aggravates pre-existing glaucoma. Chronic hypercortisolism results in several nonspecific abnormalities in laboratory screening tests. Packed red blood cell volume and hemoglobin concentration tend to be high normal, but a real increase in red blood cell mass is unusual.[1301] The total leukocyte count is usually normal but may be elevated. There is relative or absolute lymphopenia in half of all patients.[1301] Total eosinophils are usually low ($<10/mm^3$ in one third of patients). Hypercalciuria occurs in almost half of patients,[1301] but serum calcium and phosphorus are normal. Electrolyte levels are normal except in extreme hypercortisolism; mild fasting hyperglycemia occurs in about 15% of patients; and serum cholesterol and triglyceride concentrations are often elevated, owing to increased levels of very-low-density lipoprotein (VLDL), LDL, and HDL.[1319] Clotting factors V and VIII and prothrombin may be elevated.[1316]

Cushing's syndrome occurs only rarely in pregnant women[1320] because of the ovulatory disturbances and relative infertility caused by the hypercortisolism. When it does occur during prenancy it may be difficult to detect clinically because of the central weight gain, abdominal striae, dependent edema, increased blood pressure, and glucose intolerance associated with normal pregnancy.[1321]

PATHOPHYSIOLOGY

Cushing's syndrome may be either ACTH-dependent or ACTH-independent. The ACTH-dependent varieties are: Cushing's disease (primary pituitary ACTH hypersecretion), the ectopic ACTH syndrome (secretion of ACTH by nonpituitary tumors),and the ectopic CRH syndrome (pituitary hypersecretion of ACTH caused by secretion of CRH by nonhypothalamic tumors). Iatrogenic or factitious Cushing's syndrome caused by administration of exogenous ACTH is rare. These conditions all cause bilateral adrenocortical hyperplasia and cortisol hypersecretion. The ACTH-independent varieties of Cushing's syndrome are primary adrenocortical adenoma or carcinoma, the more rare bilateral micronodular dysplasia,[1322–1326] and the even more rare bilateral ACTH-independent macronodular hyperplasia.[1327–1330] Iatrogenic or factitious Cushing's syndrome is usually ACTH-independent and is caused by administration of potent synthetic glucocorticoids, usually for their anti-inflammatory effects.

Normal hypothalamic-pituitary-adrenal relationships and the aberrations observed in different types of Cushing's syndrome are diagrammed in Figure 12–38.

NORMAL RELATIONSHIPS. CRH and other hypothalamic factors are released into hypophyseal portal blood in the median eminence and carried to the anterior pituitary, where they stimulate synthesis and release of ACTH and other POMC peptides (see Fig. 12–38A). The increased plasma ACTH concentrations stimulate increased adrenocortical cortisol secretion. Increased plasma cortisol inhibits hypothalamic CRH synthesis and secretion, blocks the action of CRH and other secretagogues on pituitary corticotropes, and inhibits synthesis of POMC and release of ACTH and other POMC peptides. Falling plasma ACTH levels reduce the stimulus for cortisol production, and the system returns to the basal state. The circadian rhythm in ACTH secretion results in maximal secretion rates at about the time of awakening and minimal rates about an hour after beginning sleep. Plasma ACTH and cortisol concentrations reflect this changing rate. Finally, various stressful stimuli increase ACTH and, consequently, increase cortisol secretion. Plasma free cortisol is filtered into saliva and urine, its metabolites are excreted in the urine as 17-OHCS or 17-ketogenic steroids (17-KGS), and some of its precursors are excreted in the form of 17-ketosteroids (17-KS).

ACTH-DEPENDENT CUSHING'S SYNDROME

Cushing's Disease. In Cushing's disease, the amplitude and length but not the frequency of ACTH secretory episodes are increased,[1331–1336] and the normal ACTH circadian rhythm is lost in most patients (Fig. 12–39). The increased plasma level of ACTH, alone or with other growth factors,[64, 65, 67, 1337] stimulates the development of bilateral adrenocortical hyperplasia and the hypersecretion of cortisol (see Fig. 12–38B). The normal circadian rhythm in cortisol secretion is also lost. Morning plasma ACTH and cortisol levels may be normal, but late evening concentrations are elevated (Fig. 12–40; see Fig. 12–39). Increased cortisol secretion is reflected by increased urinary free cortisol and 17-OHCS excretion. ACTH secretion is increased more than that of cortisol (19-fold versus 7-fold), suggesting that the adrenal cortex is relatively unresponsive to the increased plasma ACTH levels.[1336] Since the cortisol biosynthetic enzymes are normal, production and excretion of cortisol precursors are increased proportionately. The chronic hypercortisolemia suppresses hypothalamic CRH secretion and inhibits ACTH secretion by the normal, nonadenomatous pituitary corticotropes, which atrophy. CRH levels in the cerebrospinal fluid are low.[1338] The adenomatous cells respond to decreased plasma cortisol by increasing ACTH secretion and to increased plasma glucocorticoid concentration by decreased ACTH secretion, but the hallmark of the disorder is the relative resistance of ACTH secretion to glucocorticoid negative feedback inhibition. In effect, the adenoma functions at a higher than normal set point for cortisol feedback.[1339] As the adrenals become increasingly hyperplastic, they secrete proportionately more cortisol in response to a given increment in plasma ACTH, levels of which fall as the result of "autosuppression." This phenomenon is especially pronounced in patients with severe bilateral macronodular hyperplasia,[4, 47, 987, 1340–1344] in whom plasma ACTH may not exceed 3 pmol/L (15 pg/mL) (D.N. Orth, unpublished observations). Such cases may be interpreted erroneously as being ACTH-independent.[1345] No case of Cushing's disease has been documented to progress to ACTH-independent adrenocortical Cushing's syndrome.

Ectopic ACTH Syndrome. In the ectopic ACTH syndrome[1346] the nonpituitary tumor secretes ACTH, which stimulates bilateral adrenal hyperplasia and hyperfunction (see Fig. 12–38D). Increased plasma cortisol concentration suppresses hypothalamic CRH synthesis and secretion and blocks CRH action on the normal pituitary corticotropes, suppressing pituitary ACTH secretion. Except in some bronchial carcinoid tumors,[1347–1349] tumor ACTH secretion is not regulated by plasma glucocorticoid concentrations. As in Cushing's disease,

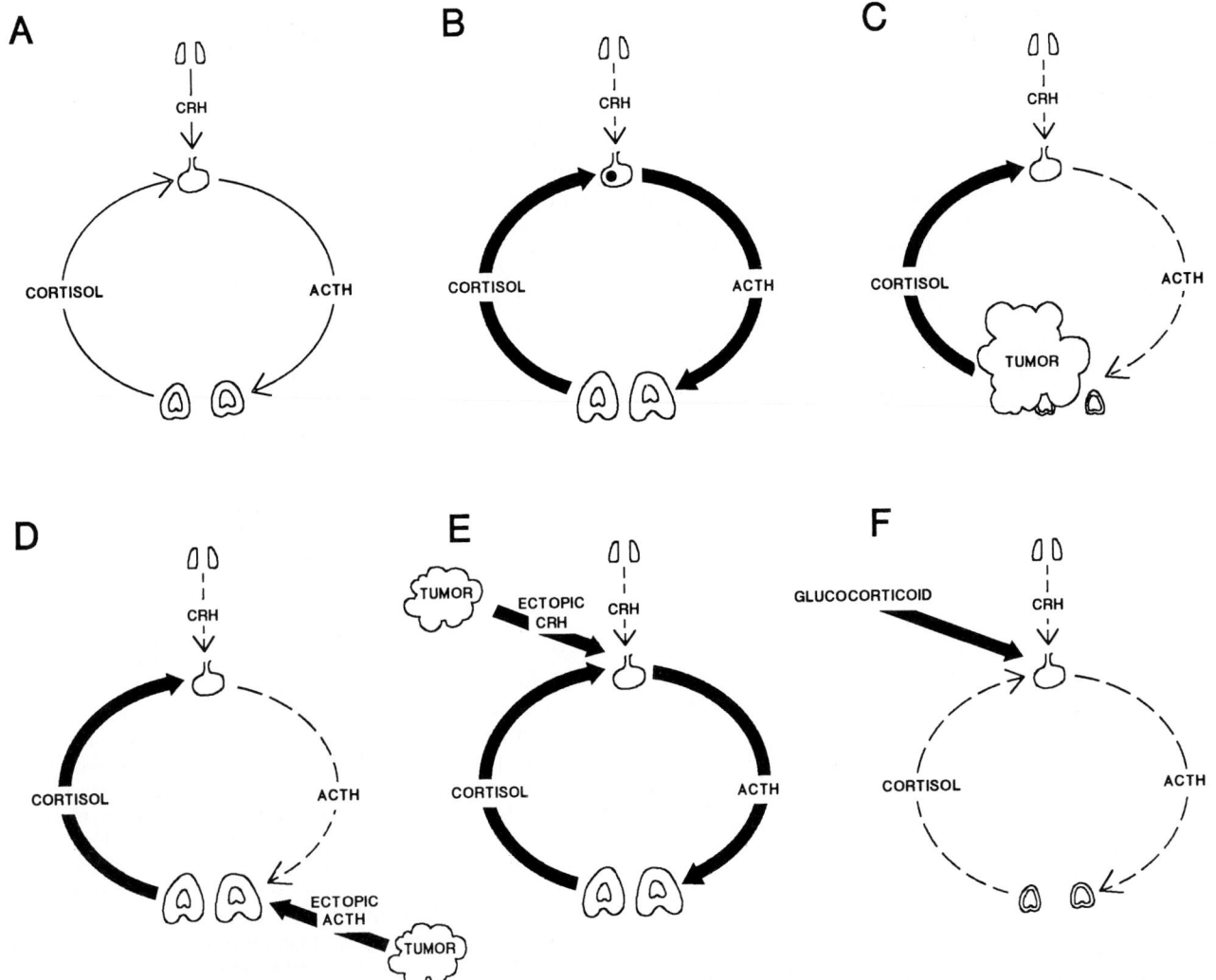

Figure 12–38. Hypothalamic-pituitary-adrenal function in normal individuals *(A)* and the pathophysiologic aberrations in pituitary ACTH-dependent Cushing's disease *(B),* primary adrenocortical disease (i.e., cortisol-secreting adrenal tumor, bilateral micronodular dysplasia, and bilateral ACTH-independent macronodular hyperplasia) *(C),* ectopic ACTH syndrome *(D),* ectopic CRH syndrome *(E),* and iatrogenic Cushing's syndrome caused by pharmacologic dosage of glucocorticoids *(F).*

urinary excretion of cortisol and its precursors is increased proportionately.

Ectopic CRH Syndrome. The ectopic CRH syndrome[1350] is similar to the ectopic ACTH syndrome, except that secretion of CRH by the nonhypothalamic tumor stimulates hyperplasia of anterior pituitary corticotropes[1350] and hypersecretion of ACTH (see Fig. 12–38E). The ACTH stimulates bilateral adrenocortical hyperplasia and hypersecretion of cortisol,[1350] which presumably suppresses hypothalamic CRH secretion. Somewhat surprisingly, ACTH secretion is often not suppressed by high glucocorticoid concentrations.[1350, 1351] This may be because the majority of these tumors also produce ACTH[376, 1352–1356] and because in those cases the hypercortisolism is actually caused by ectopic ACTH, not CRH. When CRH alone is produced, dosages of dexamethasone higher than 8 mg/d may be required to suppress ACTH secretion.[1357]

An interesting variant of this syndrome was produced by a CRH-secreting gangliocytoma composed of hypothalamic-like neurons within the sella turcica and adjacent to the pituitary gland.[1358] There was partial (i.e., 40%) suppression with low-dose dexamethasone; the high-dose test was not performed. There was also a fourfold increase in urinary 17-OHCS excretion in response to metyrapone, further indicating that ACTH secretion was responsive to glucocorticoid

negative feedback. The corticotropes were hyperplastic, and the patient recovered normal hypothalamic-pituitary-adrenal function after the tumor was removed.[1358] One CRH-producing prostatic carcinoma metastasized to the median eminence and pituitary stalk.[1350] ACTH secretion was not suppressed by high-dose dexamethasone, presumably because of very high local concentrations of CRH.

ACTH-INDEPENDENT CUSHING'S SYNDROME

Primary Adrenocortical Hyperfunction. In Cushing's syndrome caused by primary adrenocortical disease (i.e., adrenocortical tumor, micronodular dysplasia, or ACTH-independent macronodular hyperplasia), increased cortisol secretion suppresses CRH synthesis, release, and action, thereby suppressing POMC synthesis and ACTH secretion (see Fig. 12–38C). Pituitary corticotropes atrophy, as does the normal adrenal cortex. Adrenal carcinomas produce excessive adrenal steroids only because of their size; they are usually inefficient per unit weight in converting cholesterol to cortisol, and production of cortisol precursors is disproportionately high. In contrast, adrenal adenomas can exhibit very efficient steroidogenesis, and urinary excretion of DHEAS and 17-KS is often low in relation to that of 17-OHCS or free cortisol and may even be normal. The occasional adenoma may produce relatively large amounts of androgen due to increased expression

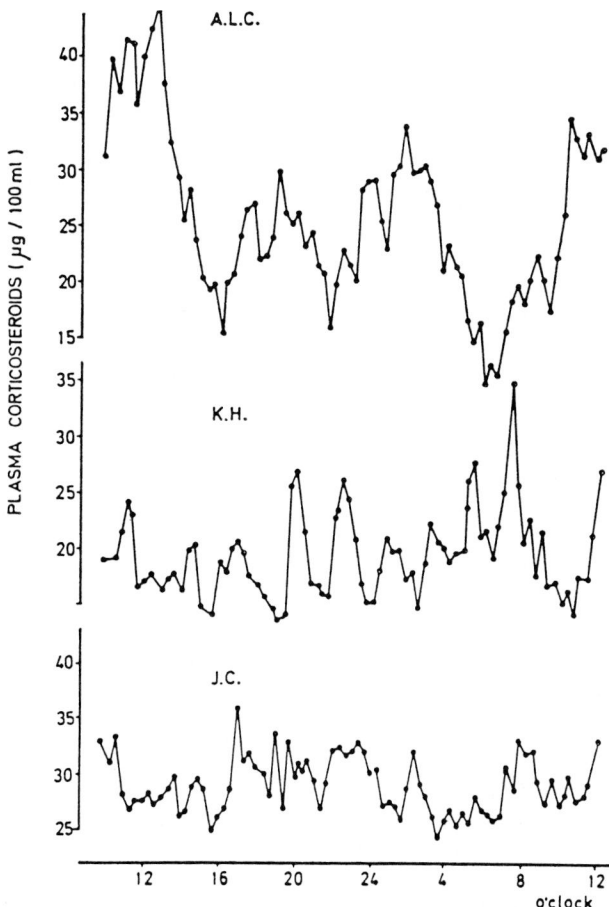

Figure 12–39. Abnormal circadian rhythm in plasma cortisol in Cushing's disease. Samples were drawn every 20 min. To convert values to nmol/L, multiply by 27.59. Note that the ordinate scales do not extend to zero, and compare with Fig. 12–14. (From Sederberg-Olsen P, Binder C, Kehlet H, et al., Episodic variation in plasma corticosteroids in subjects with Cushing's syndrome of differing etiology. J Clin Endocrinology Metab 1973; 36:906–910. Copyright © 1973, by The Endocrine Society.)

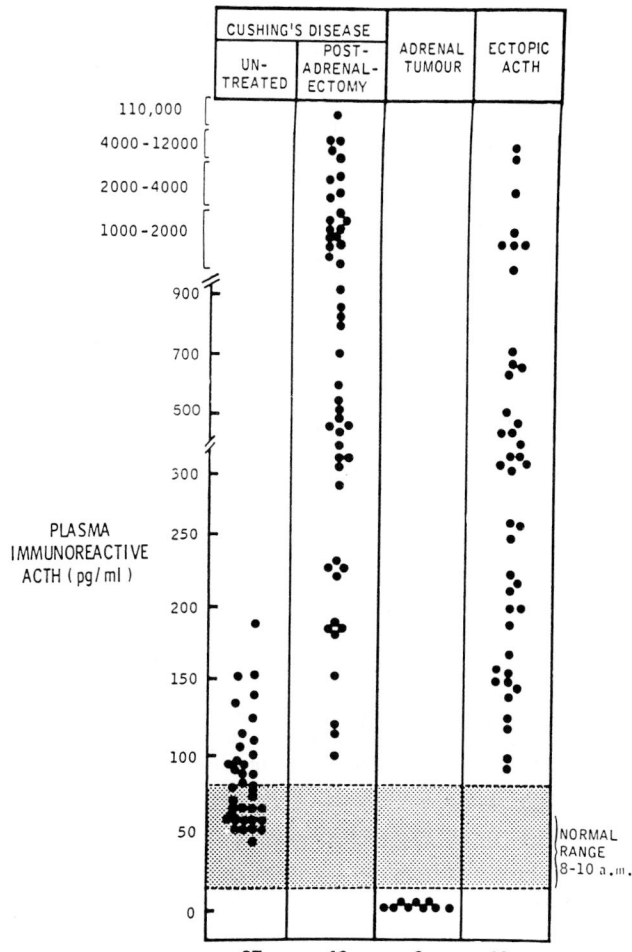

Figure 12–40. Plasma ACTH concentrations in patients with Cushing's disease and Cushing's syndrome associated with adrenocortical tumors and ectopic ACTH syndrome. To convert values to pmol/L, multiply by 0.2202. (From Besser GM, Edwards CRW. Cushing's syndrome. Clin Endocrinol Metab 1972; 1:451–490.)

of cytochrome b_5 with consequent increased 17,20-lyase activity of CYP17.[1359] Low serum aldosterone levels and normal or increased plasma concentrations of aldosterone precursors (i.e., DOC, 18-hydroxy-DOC, corticosterone, and 18-hydroxycorticosterone) are found in most adrenal carcinomas but not in adenomas.[1360]

On rare occasions Cushing's syndrome may become evident or more pronounced during pregnancy and may improve or remit spontaneously postpartum.[1320, 1361, 1362] Most of these patients have adrenal adenomas.[1363] The role of placental ACTH and CRH in these cases is unclear. One patient had apparent estrogen-dependent bilateral nodular adrenal hyperplasia.[1364]

Iatrogenic Cushing's Syndrome. Iatrogenic Cushing's syndrome is usually caused by administration of excessive amounts of potent synthetic glucocorticoids, rarely by ACTH administration. The exogenous steroid inhibits hypothalamic synthesis and secretion of CRH, suppresses pituitary ACTH synthesis and secretion (see Fig. 12–38*F*), and results in bilateral adrenocortical atrophy. Levels of plasma ACTH and cortisol (unless cortisol is the steroid administered) are suppressed.

ENDOCRINE LABORATORY FINDINGS

The laboratory findings in endogenous Cushing's syndrome of all causes (Table 12–16) reflect increased synthesis

and secretion of cortisol. The early morning plasma cortisol level may be normal, but the normal circadian rhythm is lost, the late evening plasma cortisol level is elevated, and the mean plasma cortisol concentration is increased. This leads to increased excretion of free cortisol in saliva[1365] and of free cortisol and 17-OHCS in urine. Urinary and salivary free cortisol reflect plasma free cortisol concentration and are more sensitive indicators of increased cortisol secretion than urinary 17-OHCS excretion because they increase more rapidly after plasma cortisol exceeds the binding capacity of CBG at about 690 nmol/L (25 μg/dL). Similarly, the normal hepatic metabolic pathway becomes saturated at high plasma cortisol concentrations, shunting metabolism toward 6β-hydroxycortisol, which is disproportionately increased in the urine.[684] 5α-Re-

TABLE 12–16. Endocrine Laboratory Abnormalities in Cushing's Syndrome of Any Cause

Increased cortisol secretory rate
Increased 24-h urinary excretion of free cortisol and its metabolites (17-OHCS or 17-KGS)
Loss of normal diurnal rhythm in plasma cortisol concentration with increased late evening and mean daily plasma cortisol concentrations
Relative or absolute resistance to glucocorticoid negative feedback suppression of cortisol secretion

ductase is also deficient, resulting in greater excretion of 5β metabolites.[1366] Cortisol precursor production also increases, and plasma levels of DHEA and DHEAS and urinary excretion of 17-KS and DHEAS increase. Plasma concentrations of DOC, 18-hydroxy-DOC and corticosterone, all 17-deoxysteroids, are elevated, but levels of 18-hydroxycorticosterone and aldosterone are normal or decreased.[531] Plasma renin substrate levels are increased[901, 1367] as a result of the action of cortisol on the liver[1367]; plasma renin activity[900, 901, 1367] and aldosterone[1368] are usually normal; but urinary excretion of the depressor substances kallikrein and prostaglandin E₂ is decreased.[901] Plasma ANP concentrations are elevated,[1369] presumably owing to the direct stimulatory effect of cortisol on ANP synthesis and secretion[919] and the indirect effect of increased plasma volume caused by cortisol and other weak mineralocorticoids.

Serum TSH concentration is often decreased[1370] as a result of glucocorticoid effects at both hypothalamic and pituitary levels.[1371–1373] Serum triiodothyronine concentration is decreased because glucocorticoids inhibit peripheral conversion of thyroxine[1374]; reverse triiodothyronine is normal, total thyroxine level is low because of decreased TSH and TBG, but free thyroxine concentration is normal.[1370] Clinically, thyroid function is normal.

Serum concentrations of PTH, 25-hydroxycholecalciferol, and 1,25-dihydroxycholecalciferol are normal, but tubular reabsorption of phosphate increases, serum phosphorus concentration rises, and serum 1,25-dihydroxycholecalciferol concentration falls after cure.[879] The causes of the decreased intestinal absorption and renal reabsorption of calcium and the severe loss of calcium from bone may be multifactorial.[1375]

Serum testosterone concentrations are low in men,[1376] in part because of direct glucocorticoid action on the Leydig cell.[1377] However, serum LH concentration is low normal,[1376, 1378] and LH and follicle-stimulating hormone responses to LHRH are inhibited, indicating a reversible hypogonadotropic hypogonadism,[1378] which is mild in adults but may be profound in children.

Serum insulin and glucagon levels are higher than can be accounted for by obesity alone.[1379–1381] The hyperinsulinemia may modulate the hypertriglyceridemia by affecting substrate availability, triglyceride clearance, and hepatic synthesis.[1381] Serum hGH concentrations tend to be low[1382] and respond subnormally to a variety of stimuli,[1382, 1383] perhaps because the hypercortisolism increases somatostatin secretion.[1384, 1385] Priming with growth hormone–releasing hormone for a week increases the response,[1386] suggesting that the defect is at the pituitary level and may reflect a decrease in releasable hGH. Serum IGF-I, IGF-I–binding protein, and hGH-binding protein levels tend to be normal.[1382] Low hGH levels may contribute to the growth arrest observed in children with Cushing's syndrome.[1384, 1385]

INCIDENCE

Estimates of the incidence of Cushing's syndrome are imprecise. All series grossly underestimate the incidence of iatrogenic Cushing's and the ectopic ACTH syndrome.[1387] With perhaps 10 million Americans receiving pharmacologic doses of glucocorticoids each year, iatrogenic Cushing's must be more common than any other cause, but it is seldom reported. Ectopic ACTH syndrome is probably the second most common cause of Cushing's syndrome but it is not often diagnosed. Because (1) about 1% of patients with small cell lung cancer have ectopic ACTH syndrome, (2) small cell lung carcinoma causes half of all cases,[1346] and (3) the incidence of small cell lung carcinoma is about 33,000 per 1 million population per year,[1388] the incidence of ectopic ACTH syndrome can be estimated to be about 660 per 1 million per year.

Adrenal masses discovered incidentally at autopsy or by radiographic studies range from 1.3 to 8.7%, and more than 99% of these do not cause clinical disease.[1389] Adrenal carcinoma is somewhat more common than adenoma, but each causes a similar proportion of cases of Cushing's syndrome in most series. However, a large preponderance of Cushing's syndrome caused by adrenal adenoma has been described in the population of Hokkaido, Japan.[1389] The incidence of adrenal carcinoma is unknown[1390] but is estimated by the National Cancer Institute to be 2 per 1 million population per year.[1391] Cushing's disease is five to six times more common than Cushing's syndrome caused by benign and malignant adrenal tumors combined.[1387] Therefore, the incidence of Cushing's disease may be 5 to 25 per 1 million population per year. All other causes of Cushing's syndrome are rare.

The distribution of Cushing's syndrome between the sexes varies with the cause. Men had a three times greater incidence of ectopic ACTH syndrome 25 y ago, but the increasing incidence of lung cancer in cigarette-smoking women has narrowed that margin. Women are three to eight times more likely than men to develop Cushing's disease,[1387] about three times more likely to have either benign or malignant adrenal tumors, and four to five times more likely to have Cushing's syndrome associated with an adrenal tumor.[1387, 1392–1395] The reasons for this female preponderance are unknown. About 70 cases of Cushing's syndrome occurring during pregnancy have been reported.[1321, 1363] Approximately half of these patients had ACTH-independent Cushing's syndrome (42% adenoma and 10% carcinoma); most of the rest had bilateral adrenal hyperplasia, and in about one third a diagnosis of pituitary Cushing's disease was established. Three pregnant woman with the ectopic ACTH syndrome have been reported.[1321, 1396, 1397]

The age at which ectopic ACTH syndrome develops parallels the development of lung carcinoma, increasing rapidly after age 50 years. Ectopic ACTH secretion caused by carcinoid tumors can occur at earlier ages but is uncommon in children. Cushing's disease occurs mainly in women aged 25 to 45 years. It is unusual in children but still accounts for about one third of childhood Cushing's syndrome, occurring mostly after puberty. Boys and girls are about equally affected. Adrenal tumors have a bimodal age distribution, with small peaks in the first decade of life for both adenomas and carcinomas and major peaks at about 52 years for adenomas and 39 years for carcinomas.[1393, 1394] About one quarter of adrenal tumors occur in children. Adrenal carcinoma is the cause of one half of all cases of childhood Cushing's syndrome, and adenoma accounts for another one sixth.[1398] Girls are affected slightly more frequently than boys.

COMMON CAUSES OF CUSHING'S SYNDROME

ACTH-Dependent Cushing's Syndrome

CUSHING'S DISEASE
Distinctive Clinical Features. Cushing's disease is usually characterized by chronic, moderate hypersecretion of ACTH and other POMC peptides. Consequently, its clinical features are usually those of chronic, moderate cortisol excess of gradual onset. Central obesity, moon facies, striae, muscle wasting, easy bruising, menstrual abnormalities, low back pain, depression, decreased libido, and impotence are the predominant features. Hirsutism is usually mild because, although secretion of DHEA, a weak adrenal androgen, is increased, testosterone secretion is normal or low.[1378] Virilization is rare. Hyperpigmentation is uncommon and mild because the plasma levels of ACTH usually are not very high. Patients frequently are moderately hypertensive and have mild to moderate glucose intolerance. Most have symptoms for 3 to 6 y before diagnosis.

Pathogenesis. Most patients have ACTH-secreting anterior pituitary corticotrope microadenomas, but a small number have diffuse corticotrope hyperplasia.[1399–1401] Some patients are reported to have "intermediate lobe-like" microadenomas that tend to be multifocal, suppress poorly with dexamethasone, and respond to the dopaminergic agonist bromocriptine.[1402] We have not encountered these tumors, nor have others, and their distinctive pathology has been challenged.[1403, 1404] If they occur, they are very uncommon. Rarely, a corticotrope adenocarcinoma causes Cushing's disease.[1405, 1406] Cushing's disease has twice been reported to arise from a previously nonfunctioning pituitary tumor.[1407, 1408]

The nature of the basic defect in Cushing's disease is unclear. The hypothalamic hypothesis proposes that hypersecretion of CRH (or other hypothalamic factors) causes corticotrope hyperplasia and that the hyperplastic corticotropes subsequently undergo adenomatous change, proliferating and secreting ACTH independent of stimulation by CRH,[1409] secretion of which is suppressed by the resulting hypercortisolemia (Fig. 12–41).[1410] The pituitary hypothesis proposes that the corticotrope adenoma develops as the result of loss of normal restraints on cell growth and secretes excessive amounts of ACTH and that the resulting chronic hypercortisolemia suppresses CRH secretion (see Fig. 12–41). Neither hypothesis explains the cause of CRH hypersecretion on the one hand or of the autonomous growth of the corticotropes on the other.

Several types of evidence suggest that Cushing's disease is a primary pituitary abnormality. Pituitary stalk section does not cure Cushing's disease.[1411] The prolonged period of ACTH and cortisol deficiency[1412, 1413] and subsequent recovery of normal plasma ACTH circadian rhythm, the dexamethasone suppressibility, and the response to CRH that is seen after successful microadenomectomy[1333, 1413–1417] support the pituitary hypothesis. Chronic CRH hypersecretion in animal models sometimes causes corticotrope hyperplasia but not adenomas,[366, 1418, 1419] as does ectopic CRH secretion in humans.[1350, 1358, 1420, 1421] A patient with an intrasellar CRH-secreting gangliocytoma and a coincident ACTH-secreting corticotrope microadenoma has been described,[1422] but a causal relation was not established. Peripheral plasma CRH levels are not a reliable index of hypothalamic-hypophyseal portal blood, and plasma and cerebrospinal fluid CRH levels tend to be suppressed.[1338, 1423] Abnormalities in the secretion of hGH,[1424–1426] prolactin,[1427–1430] TSH,[1431] and gonadotropin,[1376, 1378] invoked as evidence of a hypothalamic disorder,[1409] resolve after cure.[1333, 1412, 1413, 1416, 1432] Responses to neurotransmitter drugs are probably mediated by their direct actions on the pituitary.[1433–1438] CRH physiology has not been carefully studied after cure, but there is no evidence of CRH hypersecretion. Soon after cure, patients respond suboptimally to exogenous CRH.[1417] If a hypothalamic abnormality were present, one might expect to see recurrent disease after successful microadenomectomy. Cushing's disease recurs in about 20% of patients as long as

8 y after documented cure,[1439–1445] probably because of growth of residual tumor cells.[1446] Furthermore, corticotrope adenomas are monoclonal,[1447, 1448] whereas hyperplastic corticotropes are polyclonal,[1448] arguing against (although not disproving) a role for hypothalamic hyperstimulation. Somatic mutation of the gene encoding the subunit of the G_s protein that regulates adenylate cyclase activity, rendering adenylate cyclase constitutively active, has been reported to be the cause of some tumors causing acromegaly,[1449] but this mutation was not found in any of seven corticotrope tumors.[1450]

The pathogenesis of some cases of Cushing's disease may involve a two-hit phenomenon. Ten to 20% of clinically silent pituitary microadenomas synthesize ACTH but do not cause hypercortisolism.[1451] There is a high incidence of major depressive disorder and chronic alcoholism in the families of patients with Cushing's disease.[930] Perhaps chronic hyperactivation of the hypothalamic-pituitary-adrenal axis in members of such kindreds, a result of dysregulation of their response to stress, coupled with a somatic mutation in a pituitary corticotrope that results in abnormal growth like that of silent microadenomas, can cause development of corticotrope microadenomas that secrete supernormal amounts of ACTH independent of continued CRH stimulation.

Finally, there may be more than one kind of Cushing's disease, one of which may have a primary hypothalamic origin.[1452, 1453] Patients with corticotrope hyperplasia would seem to be the most likely candidates for this form of the disorder.

Laboratory Findings. Early morning plasma ACTH and cortisol concentrations may be normal, but late evening levels are elevated (see Figs. 12–39 and 12–40). Levels of other POMC peptides parallel those of ACTH.[1454] Plasma concentration and urinary excretion of cortisol precursors (e.g., DHEA, DHEAS, 17-KS) are usually increased in proportion to those of cortisol. Mild hyperprolactinemia is present in perhaps 25% of patients with Cushing's disease but not in those with adrenocortical tumors.[1429] Prolactin responses to thyrotropin-releasing hormone and hypoglycemia are normal or only slightly blunted.[1428, 1429] The tumors themselves contain prolactin-secreting cells.[1429] Hypokalemia occurs in fewer than 2% of patients who are not receiving diuretics.[1387]

Radiographic/Nuclear Medicine Findings. The tumors are usually microadenomas (<10 mm in diameter), most of which are not visible in conventional x-ray views of the sella turcica. Even high-resolution, contrast-enhanced, thin-section CT scans detect only about one third of adenomas,[1387, 1455–1458] which appear hypodense with contrast medium or reveal themselves only by displacement of the diaphragm of the sella upward or by local bone resorption (Fig. 12–42). CT scans define bony structures, however, and are useful to the neurosurgeon. Coronal projections of high-resolution MRI scans at 1.5 T with gadolinium-diethylenetriaminepentaacetic acid enhancement localize microadenomas in about two thirds of patients (Fig. 12–43).[1458–1460] False-positive CT or MRI scans can be obtained in 10% of individuals without endocrine disorders,[1461] who may or may not have "nonfunctioning" microadenomas,[1462] and false-negative scans can be reported when an adenoma is present in an empty sella.[1463] Interpretation of MRI scans can be particularly challenging in children with Cushing's disease.[1464]

The adrenal glands may appear normal in size on high-resolution thin-section CT or MRI scans, or bilateral diffuse enlargement or unilateral or bilateral macronodular enlargement may be seen (Fig. 12–44A and B).[1465] Nodules smaller than 1 cm in diameter may be detected on occasion.[1466] Scintiscans with ^{131}I-labeled cholesterol and adrenal arteriograms, venograms, or venous cortisol sampling are rarely indicated, and ultrasonography is not useful.

Osteopenia may be observed on plain films and can be documented by dual-energy photon or x-ray absorptiometry

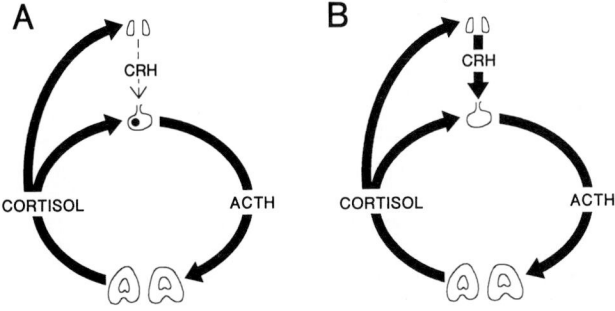

Figure 12–41. Hypothalamic-pituitary-adrenal relationships in the pituitary *(A)* and the hypothalamic hypothesis about the pathogenesis of Cushing's disease *(B)*.

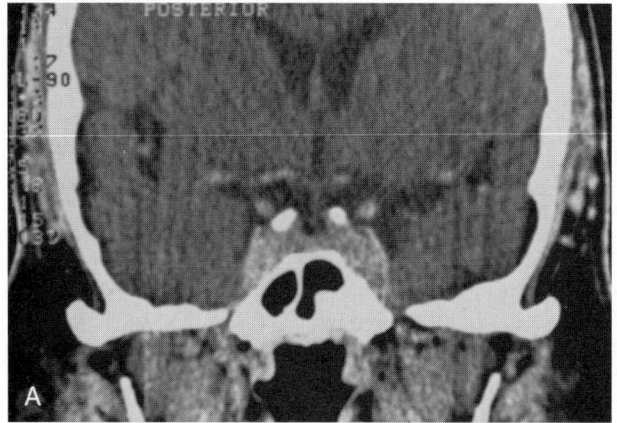

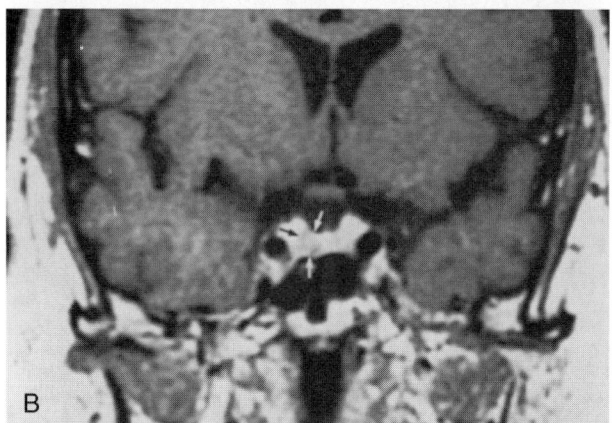

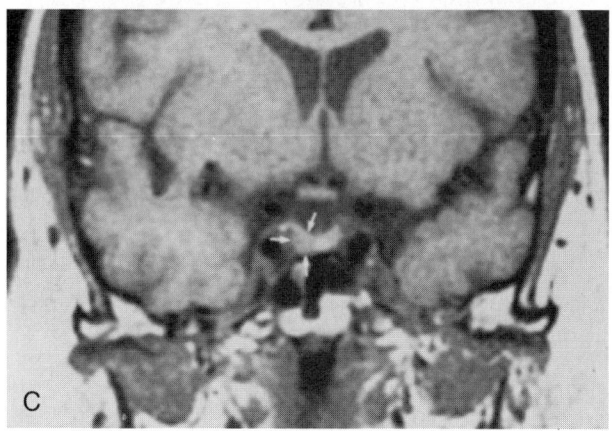

Figure 12–42. Coronal sections of CT and T1-weighted MRI scans of the sella turcica of a 59-year-old man with Cushing's disease of about 2 y duration. *A,* The CT scan is normal. *B,* The gadolinium-enhanced MRI scan reveals a 5- to 6-mm microadenoma *(arrows)* in the right side of the pituitary gland that is visible as an area of decreased signal in the nonenhanced scan *(C).* *(B and C courtesy of Dr. Jorge Pino.)*

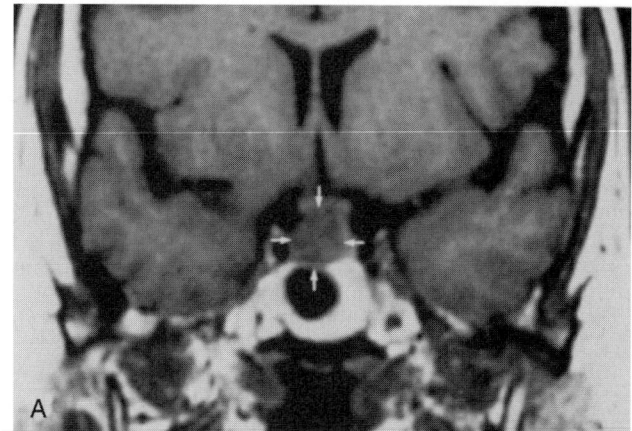

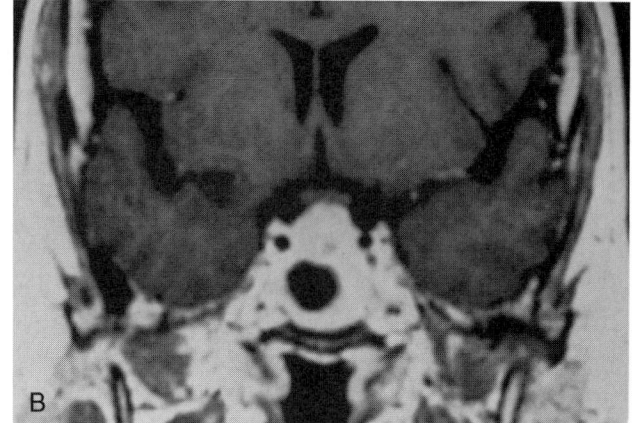

Figure 12–43. Coronal sections of T1-weighted MRI scan of the sella turcica of a 37-year-old woman with Cushing's disease of 10 y duration caused by a 14 × 11 × 9 mm pituitary microadenoma *(arrows),* before *(A)* and after *(B)* gadolinium enhancement.

to confirm the clinical diagnosis of Cushing's syndrome and define its cause. The scheme we follow is shown in Figure 12–45.[1470] The diagnosis of Cushing's disease involves demonstrating (1) increased basal cortisol production, (2) depen-

TABLE 12–17. Relative Prevalence of Various Endogenous Causes of Cushing's Syndrome

Diagnosis	Percent of Patients
ACTH-dependent Cushing's syndrome	
Cushing's disease	68
Ectopic ACTH syndrome	12
Ectopic CRH syndrome	<<1
ACTH-independent Cushing's syndrome	
Adrenocortical adenoma	10
Adrenocortical carcinoma	8
Bilateral micronodular hyperplasia	1
Macronodular hyperplasia	<<1
Pseudo-Cushing's syndrome	
Melancholic depressive psychosis	1
Chronic alcoholism	<<1

Summary of 630 patients referred to four major medical centers: 146 consecutive patients seen at Vanderbilt University Medical Center before 1993 and published reports describing 484 patients (Oldfield et al.,[2181] Findling et al.,[1546] and Trainer and Besser[2195]). Patients with unusual causes of Cushing's syndrome may be over-represented. The prevalence of pseudo-Cushing's syndrome depends on the individual physician's threshold of clinical suspicion. The relative prevalence of various causes of Cushing's syndrome among children and adolescents may differ somewhat from that in adults; for example, the ectopic ACTH syndrome is less common in children.[2196]

Modified from Orth DN. Medical progress: Cushing's syndrome. Reproduced by permission of The New England Journal of Medicine, 1995;332:791–803. Copyright 1995, Massachusetts Medical Society. All rights reserved.

or CT bone densitometry in most patients.[1467] Cerebral cortical atrophy, without an apparent functional deficit, is an incidental finding.[1468] The hippocampus is also often decreased in size.[1469] The anterior mediastinal fat pad is often enlarged and can be confused with a pulmonary or thymic tumor.

Laboratory Diagnosis. The prevalence of the various causes of Cushing's syndrome (Table 12–17) defines the diagnostic aim as (1) differentiating ACTH-independent (i.e., primary adrenal) hypercortisolism from ACTH-dependent hypercortisolism (i.e., Cushing's disease and ectopic ACTH syndrome) and (2) identifying the few patients with ectopic ACTH syndrome. There is no current consensus on how best

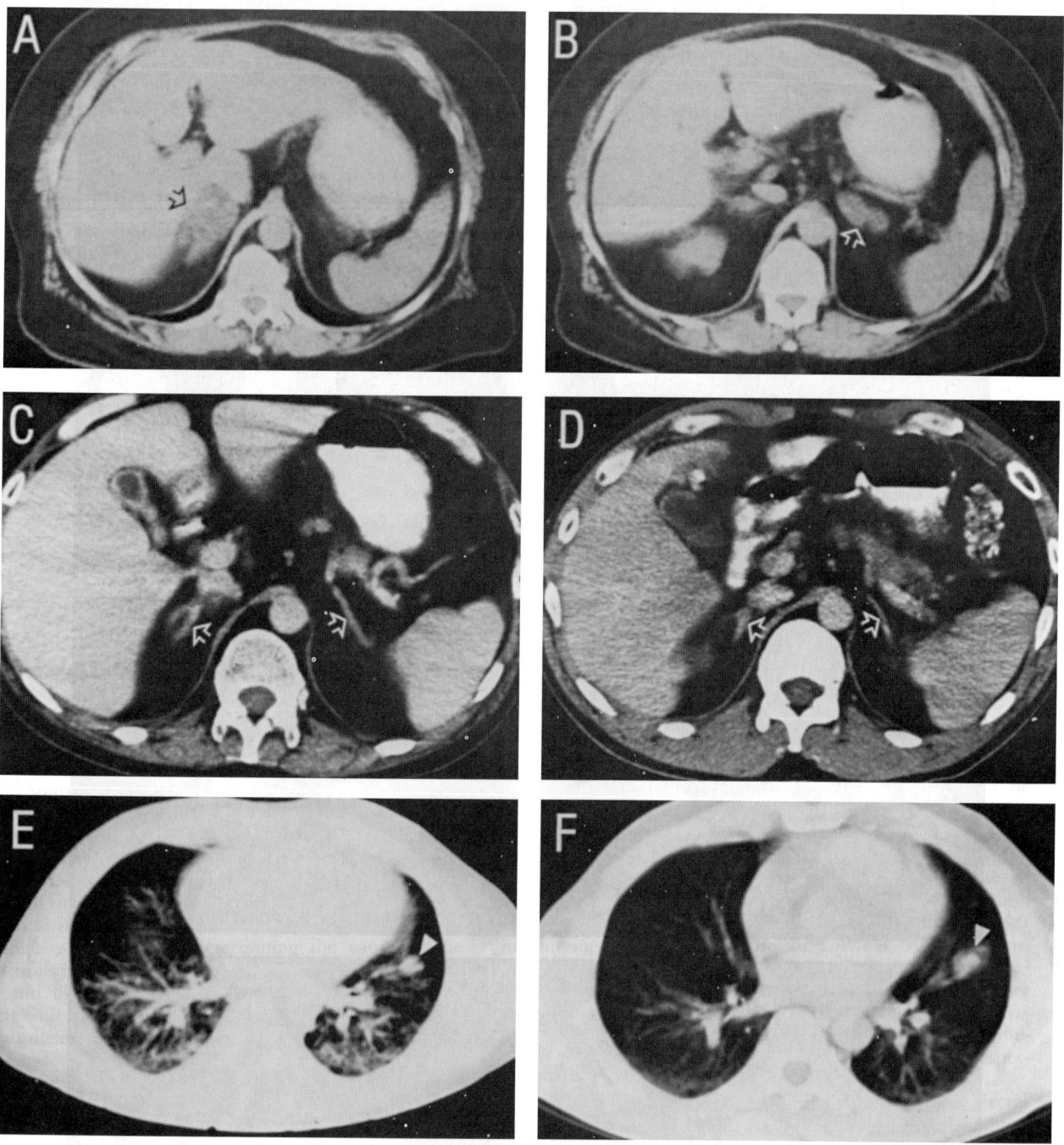

Figure 12–44. CT and MRI scans of the adrenal glands in Cushing's syndrome. The adrenals and other objects of interest are shown by the arrows. *A* and *B*, CT scans of a 57-year-old woman with a 2-y history of Cushing's syndrome demonstrating bilateral macronodular hyperplasia. CT scans of the adrenal glands *(C)* and the chest *(E)* of a 32-year-old man with a 2-y history of Cushing's syndrome. He has diffuse bilateral adrenal hyperplasia and a left lung lesion thought to represent old granulomatous disease. *D* and *F*, The same patient as in *C*, 3 y later, during which time hypercortisolism was controlled with the use of adrenal enzyme inhibitors, showing no change in the adrenal glands but an increase in the size of the lung lesion, an ACTH-secreting bronchial carcinoid tumor.

Illustration continued on following page

tions of these drugs, additive or synergistic therapeutic effects can be achieved at lower individual dosages and therefore with fewer side effects. Aminoglutethimide increases the metabolism of dexamethasone but not of cortisol.[1634] Therefore, cortisol or cortisone acetate may be the glucocorticoid therapy of choice with this drug. Aminoglutethimide therapy, which may cause aldosterone deficiency without a compensatory increase in DOC level, may occasionally necessitate fludrocortisone replacement. In addition to their other limitations as long-term treatment, the enzyme inhibitors are expensive drugs. A therapeutic dosage of aminoglutethimide is by far the least expensive of the four currently clinically available. Metyrapone and aminoglutethimide have been used in pregnant women with Cushing's syndrome, but their efficacy is unclear.[1321, 1363] Ketoconazole is teratogenic and toxic to animal embryos but has been used successfully and without harm to the fetus in the late stages of pregnancy.[1635]

Mifepristone (see Fig. 12–8) is an antiprogestational drug that at higher dosages also competes with glucocorticoids for binding to the receptor and thus blocks their action. This drug has been used acutely in Cushing's disease.[1636] Plasma cortisol levels increase about twofold. The agent appears to be effective, but it also blocks exogenous glucocorticoids. Therefore it is difficult to assess and treat the systemic functional glucocorticoid deficiency induced by mifepristone. At present, it is an investigational drug.

The long-acting somatostatin analogue, octreotide, appears to have little role in treating Cushing's disease.[1637, 1638] It may act at the level of the adrenal gland, not the pituitary.[1637]

Prognosis. Cushing's syndrome is often fatal, owing to cardiovascular, thromboembolic, or hypertensive complications or increased susceptibility to bacterial infection. There was once a 50% mortality rate by 5 y after development of symptoms,[1299] but the prognosis is now much improved. Cushing's disease is virtually always curable, although patients may in rare instances die of perioperative or other complications. In addition, patients with large, locally invasive or metastatic tumors can succumb to effects of the tumor itself. No patient should die from persistent hypercortisolism, since it can always be controlled by adrenal enzyme inhibitors, mitotane, or surgical adrenalectomy.

Signs and symptoms of Cushing's syndrome disappear gradually over a period of 2 to 12 mo. Hypertension and glucose intolerance improve but may not be cured. Unlike other forms of osteoporosis, the osteopenia of Cushing's syndrome improves rapidly during the first 2 y after hypercortisolemia is cured, more gradually thereafter.[1467, 1639] However, vertebral compression fractures and aseptic necrosis of proximal long bones[1640] cause permanent deformity and are a major reason for the importance of early cure of Cushing's syndrome.

Patients have low plasma cortisol levels for up to 12 mo after microadenomectomy and require glucocorticoid replacement therapy, which must be supplemented during stress. The rationale and methods for ensuring rapid, safe recovery are discussed later in this chapter.

The incidence of recurrence after cure by transsphenoidal microadenomectomy is not known, but one center at which more than 200 operations were performed reported recurrences in about 2%, occurring as long as 8 to 10 y after operation.[1439, 1587] The rate is higher in children, with 42% recurrence at 10 y.[1445] Patients with recurrent Cushing's syndrome should be evaluated and treated as if they had developed the disorder for the first time.

Patients who have been adrenalectomized, particularly those who have not undergone pituitary radiation, may develop Nelson's syndrome, in which an enlarging pituitary tumor is associated with progressive hyperpigmentation. Plasma ACTH levels range from as low as 175 pmol/L (800 pg/mL) to as high as 5500 pmol/L (25,000 pg/mL) or higher. The syndrome appears several months to many years after adrenalectomy, but the average is about 3 y. The pathogenesis of these tumors is uncertain. Presumably they represent the growth of pre-existing microadenomas, but it is not clear why some but not all of these tumors continue to grow in size. In some, a somatic mutation reduces glucocorticoid receptor expression or function,[1641] and therefore glucocorticoid resistance may play a role. There are no certain predictive clinical or laboratory indices. Younger age may[1642] or may not[1587, 1602] be a risk factor. The plasma ACTH level in those who subsequently develop tumors increases more during prolonged preadrenalectomy treatment with mitotane (but not during acute suppression of cortisol biosynthesis with metyrapone) and during the first year after adrenalectomy during equivalent steroid replacement therapy (500 pmol/L [2300 pg/mL], versus 77 pmol/L [350 pg/mL] in those who do not develop tumors) (J.-P. Luton, H. Escourelle, X.Y. Bertagna, B. Guilhaume, personal communications).[1611] Because the development of Nelson's syndrome appears to be a chronic rather than an acute response to decreased glucocorticoid negative feedback, it presumably reflects the tendency of these tumors to grow and produce more ACTH-secreting cells when the effect of glucocorticoids is reduced. Alternatively, the development may simply reflect the growing mass of corticotrope adenoma cells, which, because of reduced glucocorticoid inhibition, produce more POMC-derived peptides per cell. Detectable tumors may appear soon thereafter.[1611] Once the tumors become large enough to expand the sella, they become locally invasive and are difficult to cure. Therefore, adrenalectomized patients should be monitored with periodic CT or MRI scans of the pituitary and measurements of basal and dexamethasone-suppressed plasma ACTH levels.[1613, 1643] Transsphenoidal surgery or radiation therapy should be performed before the tumors become macroadenomas. Proton beam radiation is more successful than conventional radiation, although satisfactory results can be achieved with the latter in most patients.[1589] Stereotactic ^{60}Co gamma knife[1594] or linear accelerator photon knife[1595] radiation may prove useful.[1644] Sustained remission after a course of cyproheptadine therapy has been reported,[1645] but this is an isolated instance and may represent spontaneous infarction of the tumor.[1646, 1647]

Cushing's syndrome in pregnancy, if untreated, is associated with spontaneous abortion, premature delivery, and, rarely, neonatal adrenal insufficiency.[1321] Maternal complications include hypertension, gestational diabetes mellitus, and congestive heart failure. Maternal death occurs in about 4% of patients.[1321]

ECTOPIC ACTH SYNDROME

Distinctive Clinical Features. The majority of patients with ectopic ACTH syndrome have malignant tumors, half of them small cell lung carcinoma (see Chapter 36).[1346] Plasma ACTH concentrations can be very high and cause hyperpigmentation. The metabolic manifestations, which appear suddenly and progress rapidly, are caused by the acute salt-retaining and gluconeogenic effects of extreme hypercortisolemia: hypertension, edema, hypokalemia, weakness, and glucose intolerance.[1296, 1346] The typical Cushing's habitus is often absent. Hirsutism is unusual. The findings may be complicated by secretion of other ectopic hormones, such as AVP.[1346] Anorexia, weight loss, and anemia are frequent, unrelated manifestations of the malignancy causing the hypercortisolism. About 20% of patients have more indolent tumors, such as bronchial, thymic, and pancreatic carcinoid tumors or medullary carcinoma of the thyroid. The manifestations in patients with more indolent tumors may be indistinguishable from those of patients with Cushing's disease, and the tumors, in contrast to those in the typical patient with ectopic ACTH syndrome, may not be apparent without careful investigation.

Pathogenesis. A wide variety of tumors, most of them carcinomas, have been reported to secrete ACTH and other POMC peptides.[1346] Very low concentrations of POMC-like mRNA and peptides can be found in many normal tissues and tumors not associated with ectopic ACTH syndrome.[253] As discussed previously, POMC mRNA in most normal tissues is smaller than in the pituitary,[1648] whereas the mRNA in ACTH-secreting tumors tends to be the same size or larger, suggesting that alternative initiation sites are responsible for the transcription of the gene in normal and neoplastic nonpituitary tissues.[1648–1650] Transcription factors different from those in pituitary corticotropes may regulate expression of the POMC gene in ectopic ACTH-secreting tumors,[1651] but it is not known whether these factors regulate POMC expression in normal nonpituitary cells. Therefore it is not clear whether ectopic hormone secretion is merely inappropriate secretion of a normal product[1652] or is truly ectopic.[1346] Examples of both phenomena may exist. With only rare exceptions,[1347] ACTH production by these tumors is not regulated by glucocorticoid negative feedback, either because of absent or defective glucocorticoid receptors[1653, 1654] or because of a more distal defect in steroid action.[1655] POMC gene expression occurs in all types of lung tumors,[253, 1650] but the ectopic ACTH syndrome occurs only with the occasional tumor that expresses large amounts of the pituitary-sized mRNA.[1650]

Laboratory Findings. Hypokalemic, hypernatremic alkalosis is often observed, presumably because of mineralocorticoid effects of the high steroid levels in these patients. Plasma ACTH levels usually exceed the normal range (i.e., about 20 pmol/L [90 pg/mL]) and may be 175 pmol/L (800 pg/mL) or higher, but they overlap with the levels seen in Cushing's disease and may occasionally be only 9 pmol/L (40 pg/mL) (see Fig. 12–40). Other POMC peptides are similarly elevated. Plasma cortisol reflects the increased ACTH and ranges from 550 to more than 5500 nmol/L (20 to >200 μg/dL). Typically, ACTH and cortisol concentrations are two to four times normal morning values. The NH_2-terminal 22-kd intermediate of POMC (31 kd) processing is found in plasma of some of these patients but not plasma of most patients with pituitary tumors.[1516, 1656] Similarly, more 18-amino-acid β-MSH, CLIP, and γ-LPH are made by POMC-producing nonpituitary tumors than by pituitary tumors,[1657–1660] suggesting altered posttranslational processing by these tumors.[1656] There is no circadian rhythm in plasma ACTH or cortisol levels. Urinary steroid excretion is increased in proportion to the increase in plasma steroids. The enzymatic machinery for cortisol biosynthesis is normal, and levels of androgenic precursors (DHEA, DHEAS, 17-KS) are increased in proportion to those of cortisol and 17-OHCS. Serum aldosterone levels usually are normal, and plasma renin activity usually is normal or slightly increased[901]; sodium retention and hypertension are caused by the action of high levels of cortisol, which saturate the renal tubular 11β-HSD[703] and thus gain access to the type I (mineralocorticoid) receptor.[1303, 1661] The renal 11β-HSD isoform has a high affinity for cortisol,[1662] which is consistent with overload saturation in ectopic ACTH syndrome. However, 11β-HSD activity is also decreased in the ectopic ACTH syndrome[1303, 1663] as a result of inhibition by its product, cortisone,[1664] by ACTH,[1663] or by other factors.

Radiographic/Nuclear Medicine Findings. The tumors are often obvious, and about half of them are found on routine x-ray films or CT scans of the chest. Usually, both adrenal glands are diffusely enlarged. Macronodular hyperplasia is uncommon, presumably because the duration of ACTH hypersecretion is usually brief. Bronchial carcinoid tumors are typically small (see Fig. 12–41A), and some cannot be identified even with high-resolution thin-section CT scans.[1508] MR imaging may be more successful in identifying carcinoids in the middle third of the lung.[1665] Hyperplasia of the anterior mediastinal fat (see Fig. 12–41B) may be mistaken for a bronchial or thymic tumor. Pituitary CT and MRI are normal.

Laboratory Diagnosis. Diagnosis of ectopic ACTH syndrome (see Fig. 12–45) is based on demonstration of (1) increased basal cortisol production, (2) dependence of cortisol secretion on ACTH stimulation, and (3) resistance to glucocorticoid negative feedback. Characteristics useful in differentiating some patients from those with Cushing's disease include a reduced ACTH response to falling plasma cortisol levels and lack of response to CRH and/or AVP. Details for performing these tests are provided at the end of this chapter.

Increased Basal Cortisol Production: Basal Plasma Concentrations and Urinary Excretion of Cortisol and/or Its Metabolites (see Fig. 12–49A). The means for demonstrating increased basal cortisol production by measurement of urinary excretion of cortisol and plasma cortisol concentration are discussed in the section on Cushing's disease. There is more likely to be day-to-day variation in hormone secretion in patients with ectopic ACTH syndrome than in those with Cushing's disease, and some patients have cyclic or episodic secretion,[1480, 1666, 1667] making interpretation of results more difficult.

Dependence of Cortisol Secretion on ACTH Stimulation: Basal Plasma ACTH Concentrations (Fig. 12–49A). Plasma ACTH and cortisol levels are measured in the same blood specimens. Plasma ACTH concentrations tend to be higher in ectopic ACTH syndrome, but there is overlap with levels in patients with Cushing's disease. Although the processing of POMC is abnormal,[1516, 1656–1660, 1668] there are no specific peptides in plasma that distinguish these tumors from pituitary tumors.

Abnormal Resistance to Glucocorticoid Negative Feedback: The High-Dose Dexamethasone Suppression Test (see Fig. 12–49B and C). Unless basal steroid production is unequivocally increased, the patient should first have measurements of plasma cortisol taken between 11:00 PM and midnight or a low-dose dexamethasone suppression test to confirm the diagnosis of Cushing's syndrome. Among patients with ACTH-dependent hypercortisolism, the high-dose test differentiates most of those who have Cushing's disease, who are only relatively resistant to glucocorticoid negative feedback inhibition, from those with ectopic ACTH syndrome, almost all of whom demonstrate absolute resistance. Suppression is reported in about half of the 5% of patients with ectopic ACTH syndrome associated with bronchial carcinoid tumors[1347–1349, 1669] as well as in the occasional patient with thymic carcinoid.[1346] No more than about 3% of all patients with ectopic ACTH syndrome fall into this category. In one study,[1349] 69% of 94 patients with Cushing's disease but none of 10 patients with ectopic ACTH syndrome and none of 14 patients with primary adrenal Cushing's syndrome had more than 90% suppression of their basal urinary cortisol excretion (Fig. 12–50). This criterion provides 69% sensitivity and 100% specificity for Cushing's disease. In a subsequent report from the same investigators, 59% of 170 patients with Cushing's disease, many of whom were included in the earlier study,[1349] met the cutoff criterion.[1475] If either suppression of urinary free cortisol by more than 90% or suppression of urinary 17-OHCS by more than 64% is used as the criterion, the sensitivity is increased to 72%[1475] to 83%.[1349] As discussed previously, an ^{111}In-octreotide scintiscan should be obtained in patients in whom suppression does not meet this criterion. A scintiscan identifies most of the patients who have the ectopic ACTH syndrome. Patients who have a negative scintiscan should be subjected to inferior petrosal sinus sampling for ACTH before and after CRH administration.

There are three other tests that may occasionally be useful in the differential diagnosis: the metyrapone, CRH or CRH-plus-AVP, and ACTH stimulation tests.

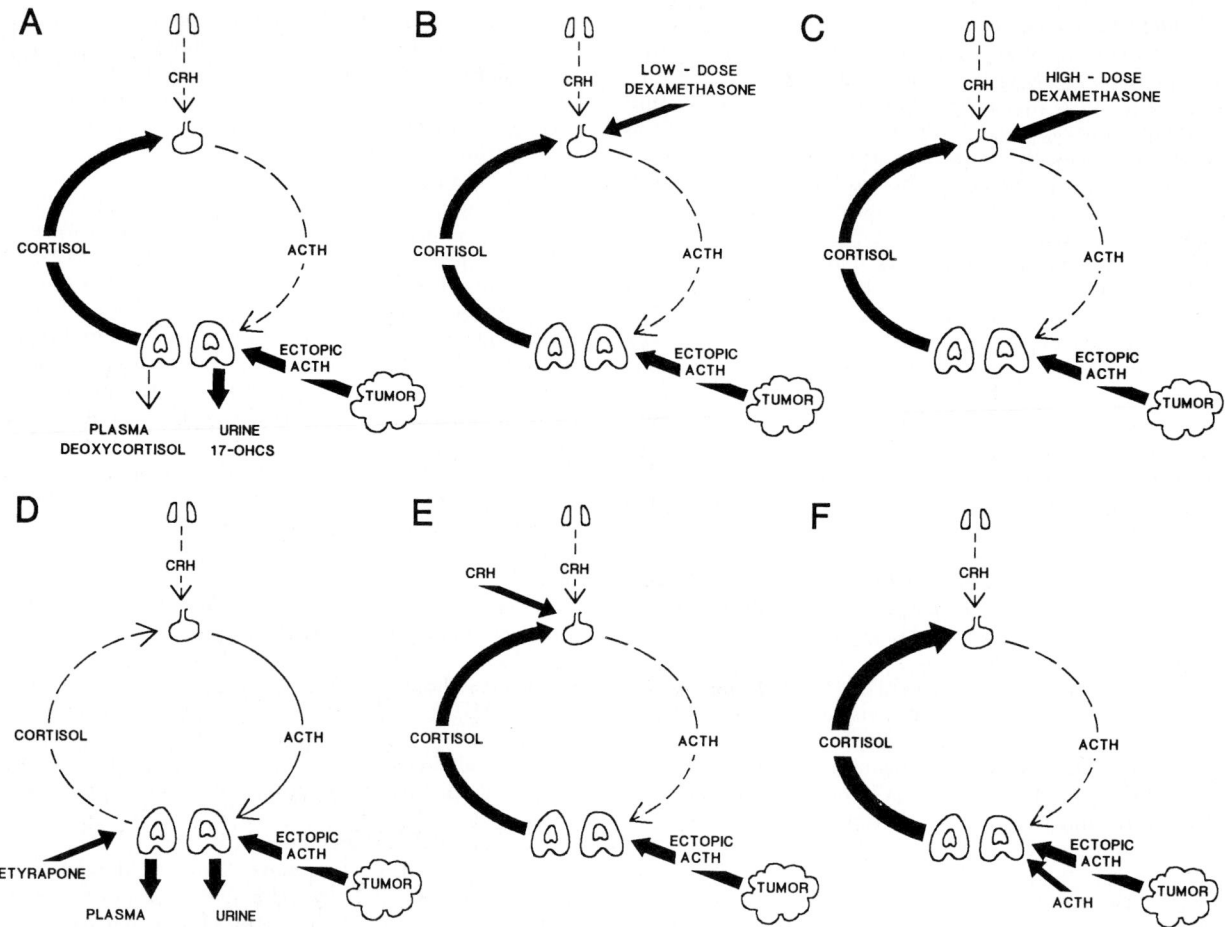

Figure 12–49. Responses of a patient with ectopic ACTH syndrome *(A)* to the low-dose *(B)* and high-dose *(C)* dexamethasone suppression, metyrapone *(D)*, CRH *(E)*, and ACTH *(F)* stimulation tests.

Reduced ACTH Response to Falling Plasma Cortisol Levels: The Metyrapone Test (see Fig. 12–49*D*). ACTH-secreting nonpituitary tumors do not respond to falling plasma cortisol by increasing ACTH secretion. However, patients with acute ectopic ACTH syndrome, usually caused by small cell lung carcinoma, may not have prolonged or profound suppression of pituitary ACTH secretion. Moreover, the hyperplastic adrenal glands in these patients may be capable of responding to increased ACTH stimulation. Urinary 17-OHCS levels rise in response to metyrapone in about half of these patients, albeit subnormally,[1659] and they remain constant in almost all of the others rather than increasing normally (as in almost all patients with Cushing's disease) or falling (as in patients with benign or malignant adrenal tumors).[1393] Therefore, the metyrapone test is an adjunctive means of distinguishing among

the causes of Cushing's syndrome in patients whose cortisol secretion is not suppressible with dexamethasone. Documentation of suppressed plasma ACTH should identify patients with primary adrenal disease.

Lack of Tumor Response to CRH and/or AVP: The CRH and AVP Tests (see Fig. 12–49*E*). In general, these patients do not respond to CRH nor, presumably, to other normal ACTH secretagogues.[1524] However, some patients respond normally, and at least some responders are those with bronchial carcinoid tumors, who are difficult to differentiate from patients with Cushing's disease.[1669] It has not been determined whether the tumor or the pituitary responds in these patients, but it is probably the pituitary in at least some cases. The incidence of such false-positive CRH tests is probably about 5 to 8%. It is surprising that more tumors do not respond to AVP, because the AVP V_3 receptor[421] appears to be expressed by pituitary corticotropes and by most POMC peptide-secreting nonpituitary tumors.[1670] Two patients with occult bronchial carcinoid tumors that secreted ACTH apparently responded to vasopressin,[1670] as have some other patients.[1671] The AVP stimulation test has not routinely been administered to patients with ectopic ACTH syndrome, however, so the frequency of positive responses is not known.

Cortisol Response to Exogenous ACTH Stimulation: The Short ACTH Test (see Fig. 12–49*F*). As in Cushing's disease, patients with ectopic ACTH syndrome have adrenocortical hyperplasia and respond to intravenous injection of ACTH (cosyntropin) with normal or exaggerated increases in plasma cortisol concentration and in urinary excretion of free cortisol

```
        ┌─────────────────────────────────┐
        │  SURGICAL RESECTION OF TUMOR    │
        └─────────────────────────────────┘
         │                              │
BENIGN (<10%) CURED        MALIGNANT (>90%) NOT CURED
                             ┌──────────────────────────┐
                             │ ADRENAL ENZYME INHIBITORS │
                             └──────────────────────────┘
              │                              │
CUSHING'S CONTROLLED              INDOLENT TUMOR
                        ┌──────────────────────────────────┐
                        │ MEDICAL/SURGICAL ADRENALECTOMY    │
                        └──────────────────────────────────┘
                                      │
                              CUSHING'S CURED
```

Figure 12–50. Treatment of patients with ectopic ACTH syndrome.

and 17-OHCS. Rare exceptions may occur when endogenous plasma ACTH levels are already maximally stimulating. This test is seldom clinically useful, although it further distinguishes these patients from those with adrenal carcinoma or ACTH-unresponsive adrenal adenoma.

Other Procedures: Demonstrating the Source of ACTH Secretion: Venous ACTH Sampling and Percutaneous Biopsy. Occasionally it is possible to localize the tumor by measuring plasma ACTH levels in simultaneous central and peripheral samples obtained by venous catheterization.[1668, 1672] However, most of these tumors are located in the pulmonary or splanchnic vascular beds, where the veins directly draining the tumor are inaccessible by procedures other than trans–left ventricular pulmonary vein or transhepatic portal vein catheterization. Consequently, the yield from venous sampling is very low. Percutaneous aspiration biopsy of bronchial or thymic carcinoid tumors under CT or ultrasound guidance may provide sufficient tissue in which to measure ACTH and thereby confirm the source of ACTH.[1673] Measurement of ACTH in lavage fluid obtained during bronchoscopy is not helpful.[1674]

Pathology. The nonpituitary tumors are distinguished from others of the same histologic type only by the fact that they contain ACTH and ACTH precursors, which can be measured in tumor extracts or demonstrated by immunocytochemical techniques.[1656, 1657, 1675, 1676] Secretory granules can usually be found by electron microscopy; they tend to be relatively numerous in tumors such as bronchial carcinoids and scarce in small cell carcinomas but their number does not correspond closely to the concentration of ACTH in the tumor.[1677] These tumors also contain neuroendocrine cell markers, such as neuron-specific enolase and carcinoembryonic antigen.[1678, 1679]

The adrenal glands are diffusely enlarged, weighing 12 to 30 g each. The cut surface reveals a thickened, regular, uniformly brown cortex without nodules. The cortex consists almost exclusively of straight columns of compact cells. There are few clear cells, and compact cells often penetrate the zona glomerulosa to reach the capsule.[4] The typical appearance is distinct from that in Cushing's disease and reflects relatively acute stimulation by very high concentrations of ACTH.

Treatment. The therapy for ectopic ACTH syndrome is outlined diagrammatically in Figure 12–50. When possible, the tumor should be surgically excised, removing the source of ectopic ACTH and thereby curing the metabolic disorder. In most patients, however, the tumor is nonresectable at the time of diagnosis. Chemotherapy or radiation therapy, or both, may be helpful. In any case, hypercortisolism, which may pose a more immediate threat than the tumor, should quickly be controlled by pharmacologic means.

Adrenal enzyme inhibitors are ideal agents in this situation. Tumor ACTH secretion does not respond to falling plasma cortisol, so there is no tendency to override the pharmacological blockade. Aminoglutethimide, ketoconazole, and metyrapone should be administered, alone or in combination. Etomidate may be useful in hospitalized patients.[1680] Hypercortisolism usually is easily controlled within a few days with one or two of these agents (e.g., 200 to 400 mg ketoconazole and/or 250 to 750 mg metyrapone three times a day) (Fig. 12–51), and acute adrenal insufficiency may develop. Because it is difficult to adjust the dose of inhibitor to achieve normal adrenal function, a replacement dosage of glucocorticoid (e.g., 0.5 mg dexamethasone) should be started at the same time as the enzyme inhibitor. Aminoglutethimide induces increased hepatic clearance of steroids, so higher than normal glucocorticoid dosage may be required.

Patients can escape suddenly from enzymatic blockade, even though their peripheral venous ACTH concentration remains constant. Metastases to the adrenal are common, particularly with small cell carcinoma,[4] and can produce ex-

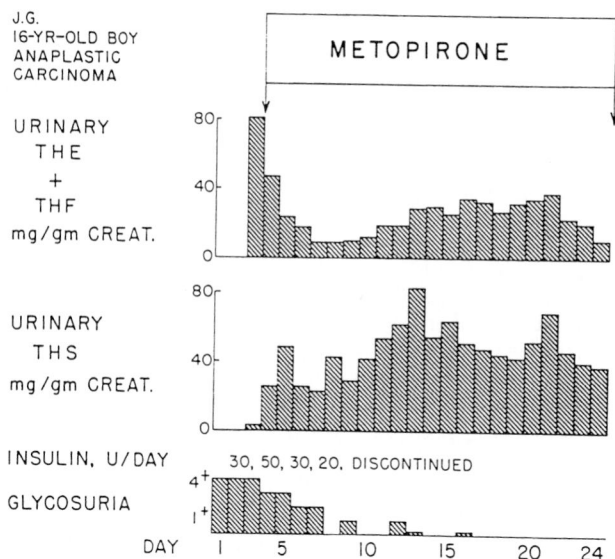

Figure 12–51. Changes in urinary steroid excretion, serum K$^+$ concentration, and insulin requirements in an adolescent patient with severe hypercortisolemia caused by ectopic ACTH secretion after treatment with metyrapone (metopirone). Metabolites of cortisol (tetrahydrocortisol, THF, its major renal metabolite), and cortisone (tetrahydrocortisone, THE) rapidly fall and are replaced with the tetrahydro-metabolite of 11-deoxycortisol (THS), the biologically inactive immediate precursor of cortisol. This is reflected by the normalization of serum K$^+$ concentration (not shown) and reduction in and elimination of the patient's insulin requirement. The patient, who was moribund on arrival at hospital, returned to a fully active life before dying suddenly from intracranial metastatic disease. (From Liddle GW, Nicholson WE, Island DP, et al. Clinical and laboratory studies of ectopic hormone syndromes. Recent Prog Horm Res 1969; 25:283–314.)

tremely high local concentrations of ACTH, resulting in increased steroidogenesis. When escape is not overcome by increasing the dosage of the drug or drugs, addition of small daily doses (1 to 3 g) of the adrenocorticolytic drug mitotane usually induces adrenal insufficiency within a few days.

When a tumor cannot be identified, enzyme inhibitors can be administered and the patient re-examined periodically with ^{111}In-octreotide, CT, or MRI scans for several years, if necessary, until the tumor can be located and treated. In patients with indolent tumors and a long life expectancy who cannot be cured surgically, mitotane can be used, as already described for the treatment of Cushing's disease, to achieve a medical adrenalectomy; pituitary radiation is unnecessary, of course. In appropriate patients, bilateral surgical adrenalectomy may be an alternative to mitotane.

The glucocorticoid antagonist mifepristone was used successfully for 9 wk in one patient.[1681] Its limitations have already been discussed. Octreotide, a long-acting analogue of somatostatin, can rapidly reduce ectopic ACTH secretion by some nonpituitary tumors[1637, 1682, 1683] but usually does not reduce tumor size. Uptake of ^{111}In-octreotide predicts a positive response to the drug.[1684] Octreotide must be injected twice daily and is expensive. It has limited value in treating ectopic ACTH syndrome.

Patients whose hypercortisolism is controlled by any means occasionally develop rebound thymic hyperplasia that may be confused radiologically with tumor recurrence or metastases in the anterior mediastinum.[1685, 1686]

Prognosis. The prognosis is dictated by the nature of the tumor and is usually poor. Most patients succumb to the malignant disease within 1 year, whereas patients with indolent tumors may survive for more than a decade. No patient should suffer from the effects of persistent hypercortisolism, which can be controlled.

ACTH-Independent Cushing's Syndrome

ADRENOCORTICAL TUMORS

Distinctive Clinical Features. Patients with adrenal adenoma usually have gradual onset of signs of hypercortisolism. In contrast, patients with adrenocortical carcinoma tend to have a more acute and progressive course, and virilizing effects may predominate.[1393] The carcinoma may be palpable, or the left kidney may be displaced downward, making its lower pole readily palpable. Abdominal, back, and flank pain and other tumor-related symptoms may be present. Nonfunctioning adrenal masses, most of which are benign, usually cause no symptoms[1389] and are discovered incidentally.[1687]

Although most adrenal tumors cause Cushing's syndrome, with or without accompanying hypertension or virilization, adrenal adenomas may cause only virilization,[1688, 1689] and adrenal carcinomas may cause only hypertension, virilization, or feminization, or they may produce no endocrine syndrome.[1393, 1394, 1690] In tumors that do not secrete cortisol, levels of DOC, testosterone, estradiol, estrone, or no steroid may be elevated, basal plasma ACTH and cortisol concentrations may be normal, and basal cortisol production by the normal adrenal cortex may be normal and suppressible with low-dose dexamethasone. The reported incidence of nonfunctional carcinomas varies considerably, depending in part on how rigorously autonomous steroid secretion was excluded. The true incidence probably does not exceed 20%.[1393, 1394]

Pathogenesis. The cause of these tumors is not known. There are isolated instances in which adenomas[1691] or carcinomas[1692] occur in a setting of chronic ACTH excess and nodular hyperplasia, but there is no compelling evidence that either excessive stimulation by or increased sensitivity to ACTH plays a role in their development. They are monoclonal neoplasms.[1693] Some of them may result from the expression of inappropriate or promiscuous G protein–coupled receptors[1694] that activate adenylate cyclase[1695] in response to factors (e.g., β-adrenergic agonists[1696]) that are not regulated by glucocorticoid negative feedback. Other tumors may result from the overexpression of receptors that are found on normal adrenocortical cells, such as the vasopressin V_3 receptor.[1697, 1698] They do not appear to result from activation of mutations of the ACTH receptor[1699] and may[1450] or may not[1700] have mutations of the $G_{\alpha i2}$ adenylate cyclase–inhibitory G protein. Some adenomas may have G_s α-subunit mutations,[1701] and some carcinomas have mutations of the p53 tumor suppressor gene.[1702, 1703] Mice in which the inhibin gene has been knocked out have an almost 100% incidence of adrenal tumors, which secrete estradiol but not cortisol.[63] Inhibin is expressed in normal human adrenal cells,[290, 1704] is stimulated by both protein kinase A and protein kinase C signal transduction pathways,[1704] binds to adrenal cells,[1705] and is also expressed in adrenal adenomas associated with Cushing's syndrome.[1706] Inhibin may be an extracellular tumor suppressor, so that loss of inhibin secretion or action may be involved in adrenal tumorigenesis.[61, 1707]

Laboratory Findings. Plasma cortisol concentration may be normal in the morning but inappropriately high in late evening. Plasma ACTH is suppressed and may be undetectable (<1 pmol/L [<5 pg/mL]). Urinary 17-OHCS and free cortisol levels are elevated to a similar degree in patients with benign or malignant tumors causing Cushing's syndrome. In patients with adenoma, plasma DHEAS and urinary DHEAS and 17-KS levels may be normal or increased in proportion to cortisol and 17-OHCS levels; urinary 17-KS are usually less than 20 mg/d. In carcinoma the precursors tend to be disproportionately elevated, and urinary 17-KS are usually greater than 20 mg/d and sometimes very high.[1393] In some "nonfunctioning" carcinomas, measurement of steroid precursors such as pregnenolone[1708] or determination of the ratio of aldosterone to its precursor, 18-hydroxydeoxycorticosterone,[1709] may provide the diagnosis.

Radiographic/Nuclear Medicine Findings. Both adenomas and carcinomas are usually visible on high-resolution, thin-section CT or MRI scan (see Fig. 12–44G to N). Adrenal arteriograms may be of value to the surgeon but are usually unnecessary for diagnosis. Intravenous pyelograms are seldom indicated except to define renal involvement; sonography can define large adrenal cysts but provides little additional useful information. Venacaval contrast studies are useful in patients with carcinoma to define external compression, invasion, or thrombus formation by the tumor. CT or MRI scans are superior to and less time-consuming and less expensive than ^{131}I-labeled cholesterol scans,[1710–1712] which may miss relatively large adenomas causing Cushing's syndrome (D.N. Orth, unpublished observations). Most carcinomas do not take up the labeled cholesterol efficiently, although even some allegedly nonfunctioning tumors may take up the agent.[1713] Furthermore, T2-weighted MR images differentiate adrenal adenomas from carcinomas.[1714] However, imaging techniques cannot differentiate between a nonfunctioning adenoma or "incidentaloma" (see later discussion) and one causing hypercortisolism. When the results of endocrine function studies disagree with the radiographic results, the latter should always be questioned first.

Laboratory Diagnosis. Establishing the diagnosis of Cushing's syndrome caused by adrenal tumor (see Fig. 12–46) involves demonstrating increased basal cortisol production and independence of cortisol secretion from ACTH stimulation.

Increased Basal Cortisol Production: Basal Plasma Cortisol Concentrations and Urinary Excretion of Cortisol and/or Its Metabolites. The procedure for establishing the presence of hypercortisolism was described in the section on Cushing's disease. As with other causes of Cushing's syndrome, day-to-day hormone secretion by adrenal tumors, especially carcinomas, may be variable. This renders interpretation of results more difficult. As already noted, secretion of steroids in addition to, or instead of, cortisol may be observed.

Independence of Cortisol Secretion from ACTH Stimulation: Basal Plasma ACTH Concentration (Fig. 12–52). In these patients and others with primary adrenocortical hyperfunction, basal plasma ACTH levels are low or undetectable at all times of the day. The ACTH concentration must be demonstrated to be suppressed at a time when cortisol is actively being secreted (i.e., when plasma cortisol concentration is 414 nmol/L [15 μg/dL] or greater).

Absolute Resistance to Glucocorticoid Negative Feedback: The High-Dose Dexamethasone Suppression Test. The existence of Cushing's syndrome must be demonstrated before the high-dose dexamethasone suppression test is performed. Because the hypercortisolemia has suppressed pituitary ACTH secretion in these patients and because dexamethasone has no direct effect on adrenal steroidogenesis, even high-dose dexamethasone has no effect on steroid production (see Fig. 12–52).

The following three tests may be useful adjunctive tests in patients with suspected adrenal tumors.

Unresponsiveness to Falling Plasma Cortisol Concentration: The Metyrapone Test (see Fig. 12–52). In these patients pituitary ACTH secretion is suppressed, all adrenocortical carcinomas and about half of the adenomas are nonresponsive to ACTH, and the remaining normal adrenal cortex is atrophic. Furthermore, metyrapone blocks not only conversion of deoxycortisol to cortisol but also conversion of cholesterol to pregnenolone. Therefore, even though plasma ACTH may rise in some patients whose pituitary function is not profoundly suppressed, serum 11-deoxycortisol does not rise normally, and urinary 17-OHCS excretion uniformly falls.[1393]

Unresponsiveness to CRH: The CRH Test (see Fig. 12–52). Because pituitary ACTH secretion is suppressed and the high

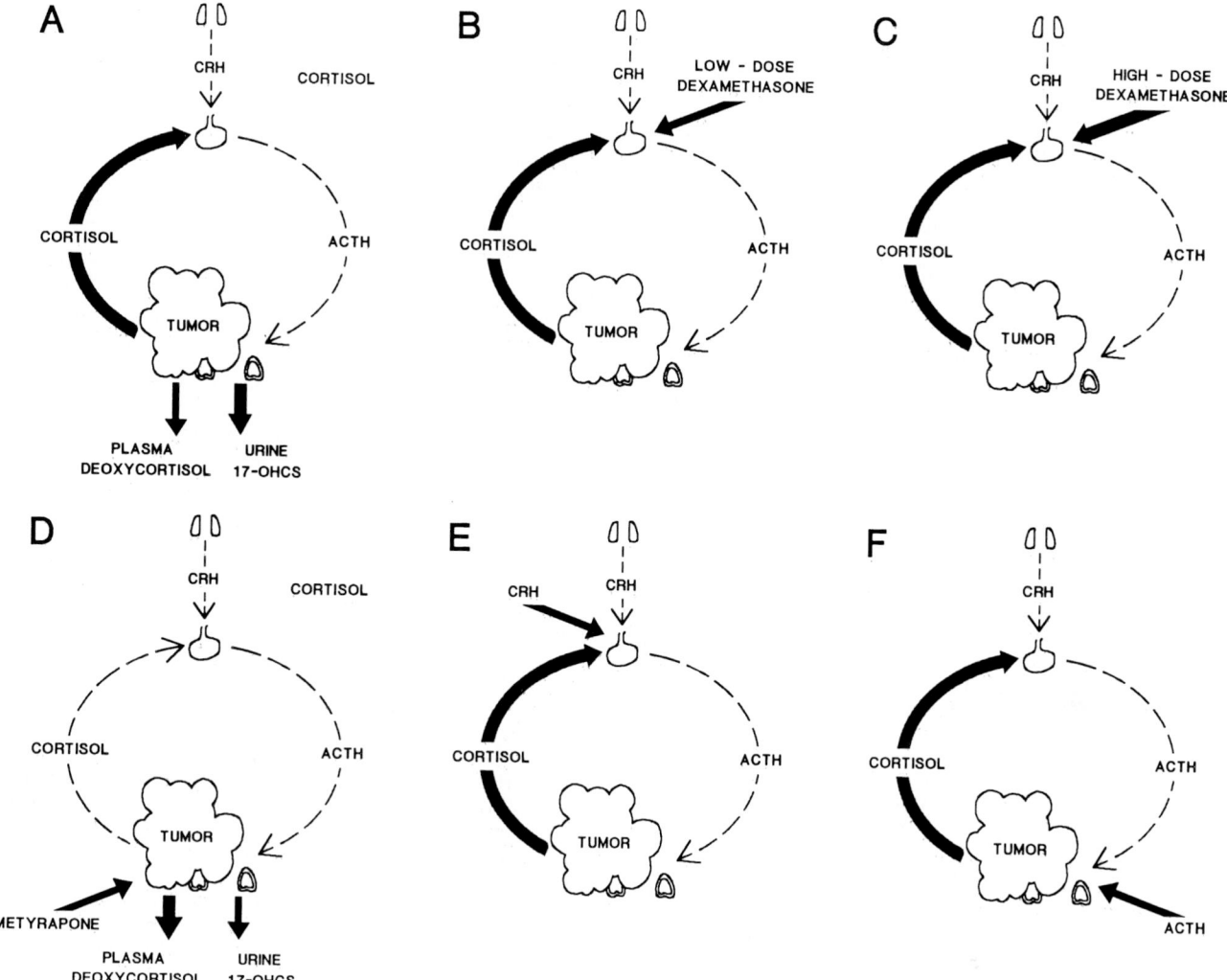

Figure 12–52. Responses of a patient with Cushing's syndrome caused by an adrenocortical tumor *(A)* to the low-dose *(B)* and high-dose *(C)* dexamethasone suppression, metyrapone *(D),* CRH *(E),* and ACTH *(F)* stimulation tests.

plasma cortisol level blocks the actions of CRH and AVP, most patients with adrenal tumors do not respond to CRH.[1524] However, some patients whose cortisol is not markedly elevated at the time of the test and whose disease is presumably of short duration, so that the pituitary is not profoundly suppressed, do respond (D.N. Orth, C.R. DeBold, unpublished observations). The AVP and CRH-plus-AVP tests are not reliable, because normal human adrenocortical cells have AVP type V_{1a} receptors,[1697, 1698] adrenal tumors may respond to AVP,[1715] and tumors and ACTH-independent macronodular adrenal glands may respond to lysine vasopressin.[1716] Some adrenal tumors fail to respond to desmopressin,[1526] but it is not clear whether this is a general phenomenon.

Responsiveness, or Lack Thereof, to ACTH Stimulation: The ACTH Stimulation Test (see Fig. 12–52). Although by definition no adrenocortical tumor that causes Cushing's syndrome is dependent on ACTH secretion, about 60% of adenomas are responsive to pharmacologic ACTH stimulation and, because of their large size, may sometimes produce exaggerated steroid responses.[1393] The remaining adenomas and virtually all carcinomas are unresponsive.[1393] Some of these adenomas may also have small responses to vasopressin.[1716]

Pathology. True adenomas of the adrenal are rare, if incidental adrenocortical nodules are discounted.[4] The left and right adrenal glands are about equally affected. True bilateral adenomas and familial adenomas are rare.[1717] On occasion, ectopic adenomas are found in the scrotum, broad ligaments, ovary, perirenal area, or body of the pancreas or liver.[1718] The cut surface of the adenoma is usually yellow and mottled with brown, but rarely they are filled with lipofuscin pigment and are black. They average 4 cm in diameter and are encapsulated, and the remaining cortex is atrophied because pituitary ACTH secretion is suppressed. Characteristically, the adenoma is composed of mixtures of compact, zona reticularis–type cells and clear, zona fasciculata–type cells. Clear cells predominate in the adenomas that respond to ACTH. Necrosis and nuclear pleomorphism are unusual, but myelolipomatous foci are common.[4] Atrophic normal cortex shows decreased or absent reticularis cells or thinning of both inner zones. The zona glomerulosa is intact, and the capsule appears thickened.[4] The ultrastructure resembles that of normal cortex, with some variation in mitochondrial morphology.[4]

Adrenocortical carcinoma affects the left and right adrenal glands with equal frequency. Bilateral tumors and ectopic sites are uncommon. Tumors can weigh more than 5 kg; carcinomas weighing less than 100 g (5.5 cm in diameter) are rare. Carcinomas are usually encapsulated, soft masses, colored pink, gray, brown, or yellow, with areas of hemorrhage and necrosis. Larger tumors may be cystic and quite vascular. Local tissue invasion is common. It is often difficult to find the normal adrenal remnant. The histologic appearance of carcinomas varies markedly among tumors and from one area to another within a tumor. Clear and compact cell types are mixed. Nuclear pleomorphism is usually prominent, even when the cells look uniform under low power. Mitotic figures and vascular invasion are uncommon but are indicative of malignancy, as are large areas of necrosis and broad fibrous connective tissue bands traversing the tumor.[4] There is not a perfect correlation between histology and biologic behavior,[1719] but, when combined with certain clinical criteria, histologic features can be highly predictive of metastatic potential.[1720] The ultrastructure is more abnormal than that of adenomas in terms of mitochondrial number and morphology, increased numbers of microvilli, and loss of integrity of the basement membrane surrounding alveolar groups of cells.[4] The normal cortex is atrophic. Rarely, carcinomas arise in ectopic adrenocortical tissue in the kidney, liver, para-aortic region, and gonads. Needle aspiration biopsy has been used for the diagnosis of adrenal tumors.[1721, 1722]

Treatment. The treatment of adrenal tumors is outlined in Figure 12–53. When possible, the tumor should be removed surgically; this not only corrects the steroid excess and cures the syndrome but removes a neoplasm that may threaten the health of the patient. Small adenomas can be removed by laparascopy[1607]; larger adenomas and carcinomas require an open flank or transabdominal approach. The cure with surgical removal of adrenal adenoma is virtually 100%.[1393, 1569, 1723] These patients usually have profound suppression of the hypothalamic-pituitary-adrenal axis and require glucocorticoid replacement for months after resection of the tumor. The principles of management are identical to those for patients cured of Cushing's disease by microadenomectomy (see earlier discussion).

Results in adrenal carcinoma, in contrast, are dismal and are unrelated to the size of the tumor or the duration of symptoms but do relate to tumor stage.[1394] It is almost always impossible to resect malignant adrenocortical tumors completely.[1393, 1394, 1724] Even when the surgeon believes that the entire tumor has been resected and there is no radiologic or hormonal evidence of residual tumor, one must assume that micrometastases are present in the liver, lungs, or other sites (see Fig. 12–45*M* and *N*) and will become clinically apparent within months. In adults, median survival time after diagnosis is 14.5 mo[1394] to 3 y[1393]; without treatment, survival averages 3 mo.[1724] Children may have somewhat less aggressive tumors,[1725] and patients younger than 40 years of age survive longer than older patients.[1394] Reoperation to resect abdominal recurrences or distant metastases may prolong survival.[1726–1728]

Mitotane has been used for nonresectable or recurrent disease.[1392, 1393, 1729, 1730] It is usually given to tolerance (10 to 20 g/d) to produce serum levels of at least 44 to 78 μmol/L (14 to 25 μg/mL).[1731] It has been reported to return hormonal findings to normal in up to 75% of patients and to reduce

tumor size in up to 30%,[1392, 1732, 1733] but these results have not been confirmed by others.[1393, 1729, 1730] Treatment is never curative, and tumor regression is transient.[1394] In the most optimistic series, median survival time was only 6.5 mo after beginning the drug,[1392, 1732] and there is no evidence that mitotane prolonged life.[1394, 1734, 1735] Even those who have an objective response are often incapacitated by the side effects of large dosages of mitotane,[1736] although a preparation available outside the United States is better tolerated.[1394, 1724]

Administration of mitotane in the absence of metastatic disease may delay or prevent recurrent disease in some patients.[1734, 1737] Mitotane is begun immediately after removal of the primary tumor and is continued indefinitely. Two of four patients in one series remained free of metastases, and mean survival time (75 ± 33 mo) was longer than in those who received no mitotane (10 ± 8.7 mo).[1726] Four of another 11 treated patients survived for 4 to 15.5 years without recurrent tumor.[1737] However, patients may develop recurrent local or metastatic disease despite taking mitotane, and in one report adjuvant mitotane treatment was associated with a worse outcome.[1733] The optimal dosage and duration of treatment are not established. Nevertheless, this disease is so uniformly fatal that it is rational to treat every patient, beginning immediately after tumor resection, with 4 g of mitotane per day, or the maximum lesser dose the patient can tolerate, half of it at bedtime to minimize nausea, and to maintain treatment indefinitely. Efficacy can be assessed periodically by CT or MRI scan of the chest and upper abdomen and by measuring 24-h urinary free cortisol excretion. As mentioned previously, mitotane increases the rate of metabolism of dexamethasone[1155] and of fludrocortisone, but not of prednisone or hydrocortisone (D. Gaitan, W.E. Nicholson, D.N. Orth, unpublished observations). Therefore, prednisone, which is less expensive and has a longer effective half-life than hydrocortisone, is the best choice for glucocorticoid replacement. Some symptoms ascribed to mitotane may be caused by adrenal insufficiency, and regimens of up to seven times the usual maintenance dosages of dexamethasone and fludrocortisone may be required to cure the symptoms and maintain normal serum electrolytes and blood pressure.

Other chemotherapeutic drugs that have been tested in adrenal carcinoma, alone and in combination with mitotane, do not have greater efficacy than mitotane.[1738, 1739] Oral gossypol, a spermatotoxin extracted from crude cottonseed oil, in doses of 40 to 50 mg/d produced partial responses in 3 of 17 patients with metastatic disease that had progressed despite mitotane treatment; responses lasted 6 to 12 months.[1740]

It is generally agreed that radiotherapy is not useful in this disease, but one study reported a 10-y survival time for three of nine patients.[1741] However, two of the three died of other malignancies.

Excess steroid production can usually be controlled by use of adrenal enzyme inhibitors in these patients, and none should suffer from persistent Cushing's syndrome. The adrenal enzyme inhibitors already mentioned, administered alone or in combination, should be used to render the patient hypoadrenal, because it is too difficult to achieve and maintain normal serum cortisol levels. Replacement steroid therapy should be given. There is no advantage to using antiglucocorticoids such as mifepristone, because enzyme inhibitors are less expensive, readily available, and less difficult to manage.

Prognosis. As already noted, the prognosis with adrenal adenoma is excellent because surgery is usually curative. The prognosis with adrenal carcinoma is poor because most patients have distant metastases at diagnosis and because there is no effective therapy for metastatic or recurrent disease. The symptoms of steroid excess, however, can be controlled.

IATROGENIC, FACTITIOUS, OR EXOGENOUS CUSHING'S SYNDROME

Distinctive Clinical Features. These patients usually have signs of pure glucocorticoid excess, because most have re-

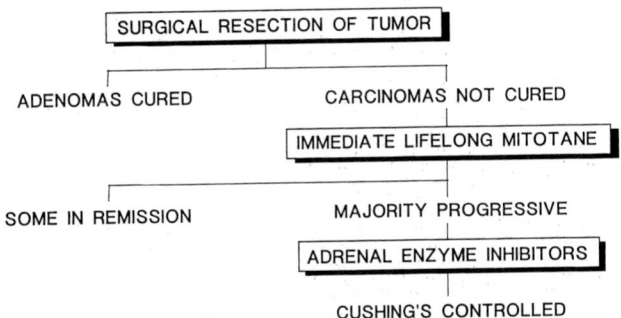

Figure 12–53. Treatment of patients with adrenocortical tumors causing Cushing's syndrome.

ceived potent synthetic steroids, such as dexamethasone or prednisone, which have little or no mineralocorticoid activity and no androgenic activity. Hirsutism is absent, and hypertension is observed only if the patient has incidental hypertension or is taking hydrocortisone or cortisone. A careful medical history is necessary because some patients take medications that, unbeknownst to them, contain glucocorticoids, or have received depot injections of glucocorticoids weeks or longer before seeking assistance. Most cases are caused by use of synthetic glucocorticoids, but one case was caused by prolonged (7-y) administration of high dosages (400 mg/d) of medroxyprogesterone acetate.[1742]

Laboratory Findings. Laboratory results are characteristic of suppressed hypothalamic-pituitary-adrenal function: low or undetectable morning plasma ACTH and cortisol levels; suppressed excretion of urinary steroids; and failure to respond to metyrapone, cosyntropin, or CRH. Patients taking hydrocortisone or cortisone may have residual cortisol in plasma and have variable amounts of 17-OHCS and free cortisol but suppressed 17-KS in urine. Even in malingering patients, it is usually not difficult to establish the diagnosis. Such patients may, for example, add cortisol to their urine collections; however, urinary steroid levels do not correlate with plasma cortisol concentrations, and levels of urinary 17-OHCS, corticosterone, and cortisone are normal.[1743]

Treatment. The treatment is to stop the steroid. Most patients who have taken enough steroid long enough to cause Cushing's syndrome have a period of hypothalamic-pituitary-adrenal insufficiency when steroids are discontinued, so gradual steroid withdrawal is necessary.

UNCOMMON CAUSES OF CUSHING'S SYNDROME

ACTH-Dependent Cushing's Syndrome

PSEUDO-CUSHING'S SYNDROMES

Depression. Patients with depression, especially older women with typical melancholic symptoms severe enough to warrant hospitalization, can have all of the hormonal abnormalities of patients with Cushing's disease, including characteristic responses to most of the standard pituitary-adrenal function tests.[1744] Circadian rhythmicity of ACTH and cortisol secretion is maintained, but ACTH pulse frequency may be increased, and the resultant cortisol pulses are of greater amplitude and duration.[1745] In general, depressed patients do not have the physical signs of Cushing's syndrome and are thus not difficult to distinguish. However, depression is common in Cushing's syndrome, and depressed patients can be obese, hypertensive, and diabetic. There are several ways to differentiate this disorder from Cushing's disease. The most efficient way is to measure late evening (11:00 PM to 1:00 AM) plasma cortisol concentrations. Depressed patients have levels lower than 140 nmol/L (5 μg/dL), whereas patients with Cushing's disease have levels greater than 207 nmol/L (7.5 μg/dL).[1487] In another study in which plasma cortisol was drawn at midnight, when the patient appeared to be asleep (an indication of lack of stress), normal subjects had cortisol concentrations lower than 50 nmol/L (2 μg/dL), whereas 150 patients with Cushing's syndrome had levels ranging from 70 to 2000 nmol/L (2.5 to 72 μg/dL).[1488] Depressed patients have greater sensitivity to dexamethasone suppression, and patients with Cushing's disease have greater plasma cortisol responses to exogenous CRH. Therefore, plasma cortisol concentration is lower after the standard 2-d dexamethasone suppression test and remains lower after CRH is administered 8 h after the last 0.5-mg dexamethasone dose.[1746] The third method is based on the ability of naloxone to release endogenous CRH secretion from tonic opioid inhibition.[447] Endogenous CRH secretion is presumably suppressed in Cushing's

disease but normal or increased in depression, so the response to naloxone is decreased in Cushing's disease. However, the responses of depressed patients and patients with Cushing's disease overlap somewhat,[1747] so this is not a specific test. A fourth method relies on the fact that hypercortisolism in depression is usually mild and transient, so suppression of hypothalamic-pituitary-adrenal function is incomplete and can be overcome by hypoglycemic stress. Plasma cortisol concentrations increase in response to insulin-induced hypoglycemia in depressed patients but not in patients with chronic Cushing's syndrome.[1748] Finally, patients with severe, typical, melancholic depression may have blunted responses to CRH[1749] because their hypercortisolemia, as in acutely stressed patients,[393] blocks the effect of CRH on the intrinsically normal corticotropes. The hormonal abnormalities disappear as soon as the depression is corrected, whether spontaneously, by psychotherapy, or by antidepressant drug therapy. The pathogenesis of the hormonal disorder and its role in the manifestations of depression are unknown. Therapy is directed solely at the psychiatric disorder. Transient hypothalamic-pituitary-adrenal insufficiency does not occur after cure.

Alcoholism. A few cases of alcoholic pseudo-Cushing's syndromes have been reported,[1750, 1751] but the disorder is rare.[1752] These patients may have round, plethoric faces, centripetal obesity, thin extremities, and other features of Cushing's syndrome, but whether these features result from hypercortisolism or other causes is uncertain. A careful history and laboratory evidence of abnormal liver function are the keys to diagnosis. These patients have significant alcoholic liver disease, with elevated hepatic enzymes in the serum. The pathogenesis is unknown, but altered hepatic metabolism of cortisol alone cannot explain the abnormality. An alcohol-induced central nervous system disorder may be a major factor. The treatment is abstinence from alcohol.

ECTOPIC CORTICOTROPIN-RELEASING HORMONE SYNDROME

Distinctive Clinical Features. Ectopic CRH secretion is rare.[376, 1422, 1753, 1754] No clinical features distinguish this disorder from the ectopic ACTH syndrome. The patients have had a variety of tumors, mostly carcinoids.

Laboratory Findings. Material that appears immunologically, biologically, and physicochemically identical to human CRH has been extracted from normal and neoplastic nonhypothalamic tissues.[344] Plasma ACTH and cortisol levels and urinary steroid excretion are increased, as in ectopic ACTH syndrome. Plasma CRH levels, when measured, are increased.[1350, 1352, 1354] Responses to pituitary-adrenal function tests are identical to those in ectopic ACTH syndrome.

As noted earlier, steroid production in about half of these patients is resistant to high-dose dexamethasone suppression, although one would assume that the action of endogenous ectopic CRH, like that of exogenous CRH, could be blocked by glucocorticoids.[404] Steroid hypersecretion caused by one intrasellar gangliocytoma that produced CRH was partially suppressed by low-dose dexamethasone,[1358] but in another it was not suppressed by high-dose dexamethasone.[1422] However, most[1352-1354, 1356] but not all[1350, 1351, 1420] CRH-producing tumors also contain ACTH, suggesting that the adrenal glands in at least some of these patients are stimulated by ectopic ACTH, secretion of which is not dexamethasone-suppressible. It is unlikely that the co-secreted ectopic CRH stimulates pituitary ACTH secretion in the face of the resulting ACTH-induced hypercortisolemia. Therefore, whereas tumors may synthesize and secrete CRH, patients whose tumors also secrete ACTH and display resistance to dexamethasone suppression should be considered to be examples of the ectopic ACTH syndrome until proved otherwise. The proof should include inferior petrosal sinus sampling for ACTH before and after stimulation with exogenous CRH. There should be a central-to-peripheral

ACTH gradient if ectopic CRH is involved. Furthermore, intraoperative sampling of CRH in the tumor venous drainage and in a peripheral vein should reveal a tumor-to-peripheral CRH gradient.

Pathology. The pituitary corticotropes may be hyperplastic,[1350] but CT scan of the pituitary is normal, the adrenal glands are both enlarged, and the tumor may or may not be detected by CT or MRI scan. The histopathology of the tumors is unremarkable, except that they stain for CRH and, in most cases, for ACTH. The two hormones may be contained in the same or different populations of cells. Two instances have been reported of intrasellar, extrapituitary, CRH-secreting gangliocytomas consisting of hypothalamic-like neurons.[1358, 1422] The corticotropes were hyperplastic in one case,[1358] and an ACTH-secreting microadenoma was present in the other.[1422]

Treatment. Therapy is the same as for the ectopic ACTH syndrome. The prognosis is also similar: the Cushing's syndrome can easily be controlled, but the ultimate prognosis depends on the malignancy of the tumor and whether it can be completely resected.

ECTOPIC GASTRIN-RELEASING PEPTIDE SECRETION.
One medullary carcinoma of the thyroid secreted gastrin-releasing peptide, the mammalian homologue of bombesin, which acted together with hypothalamic CRH to cause Cushing's syndrome.[1755] However, there is disagreement whether gastrin-releasing peptide has an independent effect on ACTH secretion.[1756, 1757]

FACTITIOUS CUSHING'S SYNDROME CAUSED BY ACTH ADMINISTRATION.
These rare patients can resemble those with endogenous ACTH hypersecretion, and if a careful history and a search for injection sites do not reveal the cause and the patient wishes to deceive, diagnosis can be difficult. No pituitary or ectopic source of ACTH can be identified, of course, but neither is one found in some patients with endogenous Cushing's syndrome. Commercial ACTH prepared from animal sources is contaminated with α-MSH derived from the intermediate lobe. Because α-MSH is minimally increased in endogenous Cushing's syndrome, if it is increased at all[1012] (D.N. Orth, unpublished observations), plasma α-MSH measurement may be helpful. Many patients receiving ACTH develop anti-ACTH antibodies,[1758] which also can be measured. If the patient can be isolated from the source of ACTH, hypothalamic-pituitary-adrenal insufficiency will develop in a matter of days, just as in the patient with Cushing's disease after microadenomectomy.

ACTH-Independent Cushing's Syndrome

BILATERAL MICRONODULAR DYSPLASIA
Distinctive Clinical Features. About half of the patients with this disorder have no distinctive clinical presentation other than being young—always younger than 30 years of age, half younger than 15 years, and some infants.[1322, 1759] Median duration of symptoms before diagnosis is 1 y, although intervals of up to 18 y have been reported.[1326] The other half of patients have a familial form of the disorder (Carney's syndrome) that is inherited as an autosomal dominant trait and is accompanied by pigmented lentigines and blue nevi on the face, neck, and trunk, including the lips, conjunctiva, or sclera. These patients may also have cutaneous, mammary, and atrial myxomas, psammomatous melanotic schwannomas, Sertoli cell tumors of the testis, and other benign and malignant tumors.[1325, 1326, 1759–1761] Only about 20 to 30% of the patients with Carney's syndrome have Cushing's syndrome, and none has all the features of Carney's syndrome. Conversely, more than 80% of patients with bilateral micronodular dysplasia have Cushing's syndrome.[1759] Two siblings presented in infancy with hypertelorism, profuse dark hair, heavy eyebrows, large fontanelles, and marked hypotonia; the girl had clitoral enlargement and the boy had severe hypertension.[1324] Acromegaly occurs in about 10% of the patients, and precocious puberty is present in about 25% of male patients.[1759]

Pathogenesis. The pathogenesis is unknown. Linkage analysis has placed the gene on chromosome 2p16.[1761] The *POMC* gene, which is located about 15 cM telomeric to the Carney locus, is not responsible.[1761] The gene may encode a tumor suppressor that affects multiple cell types,[1272] but a gene that functions as an oncogene, growth factor, or constitutively activated growth factor receptor or postreceptor effector seems likely.[1760] A circulating immunoglobulin that stimulates steroidogenesis[1762] and adrenal cell growth[1763] has been reported. However, it is unclear why the cells that form the nodules, but not the intervening cells, should be susceptible to stimulation by these autoantibodies.[1764] Other autoimmune disorders are not common in these patients or in their families, and no evidence of an immune disorder or adrenal-stimulating immunoglobulins has been found by others.[1761]

Laboratory Findings. Plasma cortisol is usually moderately elevated and exhibits no diurnal rhythm. Cortisol precursors have not often been measured but appear to be proportionately elevated.[1324] Plasma ACTH concentration is low or undetectable. Steroid production may be irregular[1564] or cyclic.[1565]

Radiographic/Nuclear Medicine Findings. The adrenal glands are normal or slightly enlarged and may or may not have discernible nodules on CT or MRI scan.[1765] Scans with ^{131}I-labeled cholesterol reveal bilateral symmetrical uptake. The pituitary appears normal. A high percentage of patients have marked osteopenia that is out of proportion to other manifestations of hypercortisolism and that presumably occurs in both the sporadic[1322, 1564] and familial[1325, 1565] forms of the disease.

Laboratory Diagnosis. As with adrenal tumor, another example of primary adrenal hypercortisolism, ACTH secretion is suppressed, so steroid production is not suppressed by either low- or high-dose dexamethasone. Urinary 17-OHCS levels fall, and plasma 11-deoxycortisol does not rise normally during metyrapone administration.[1322, 1564, 1759] The cells forming the dysplastic nodules do not respond to ACTH[1564, 1759]; the occasional responses are subnormal and are probably caused by variable daily steroid production or by the response of the atrophic adrenocortical cells. There is no ACTH response to CRH (D.N. Orth, unpublished observations) or, presumably, to vasopressin.

Pathology. The adrenals are either of normal size or slightly enlarged. Both glands contain many nodules, ranging from microscopic to 5 mm in diameter and from yellow-brown to bluish-black in color, most often brown or black. The nodules consist of large cells with eosinophilic cytoplasm containing brown lipofuscin pigment. Nuclei are enlarged and somewhat pleomorphic. The ultrastructure of the cells resembles that of fasciculata cells. The intervening non-nodular cortex consists of small cells with clear cytoplasm characteristic of adrenal atrophy.[1759]

Treatment. Surgical bilateral adrenalectomy, either by the open flank or laparoscopic approach, is the treatment of choice. The pituitary is intrinsically normal, so pituitary surgery or radiation is not helpful, nor is subtotal adrenalectomy.[1326]

Prognosis. Results of treatment are excellent. The surgery produces permanent adrenal insufficiency. Nelson's syndrome has not been described in patients adrenalectomized for this disorder. One infant died of refractory hypertension and heart failure a month after subtotal adrenalectomy.[1324]

BILATERAL ACTH-INDEPENDENT MACRONODULAR HYPERPLASIA.
This syndrome[1327–1329, 1568, 1716, 1766–1769] has been reported in an infant[1768] and in men and women patients of all ages, as has familial incidence.[1767] Plasma and urinary steroids are increased; plasma ACTH is undetectable in the basal

state and after metyrapone or CRH. Steroid production is suppressed minimally, if at all, during high-dose dexamethasone administration. The response to metyrapone is usually minimal,[1327] but in one patient it was normal despite failure to suppress with high-dose dexamethasone.[1568] Plasma cortisol may increase after administration of cosyntropin, and in one case[1327] estrone was reported to increase. Pituitary CT and MRI scans are normal. The adrenal glands weigh from 24 to 500 g or more and contain multiple macroscopic nonpigmented nodules larger than 5 mm in diameter. The nodules appear to be typical benign adrenal nodules, but the internodular cortex may be hypertrophic rather than atrophic. Bilateral adrenalectomy cures the hypercortisolemia. The pathogenesis is unknown, but there is no evidence that ACTH hypersecretion is involved. In one instance, an activating somatic mutation of the α-subunit of G_s was associated with the syndrome in an infant.[1768] In two patients, early morning plasma cortisol levels were low but increased in response to eating.[1328, 1329] ACTH secretion was induced by gastric inhibitory polypeptide (also known as glucose-dependent insulinotropic peptide), but not by ACTH. This presumably represents another example of the promiscuous receptor concept.[1770] Two other patients had a doubling of plasma cortisol in response to vasopressin, but not to CRH administration.[1716] Vasopressin V_{1a} receptors are expressed on normal adrenocortical cells.[1697, 1698]

CORTISOL HYPERREACTIVE SYNDROME. One 54-year-old man has been described with centripetal obesity, moon facies, and non–insulin-dependent diabetes mellitus but normal blood pressure and no striae.[1771] He had low cortisol production; undetectable plasma ACTH (i.e., <2 pmol/L [<9 pg/mL]); normal CBG concentration; markedly decreased responses to cosyntropin, insulin-induced hypoglycemia, and repeated CRH-plus-lysine vasopressin administration; and an absent response to metyrapone. However, the plasma cortisol concentration increased to about 660 nmol/L (24 μg/dL), urinary 17-OHCS excretion increased to 64 μmol/d (23 mg/d), and urinary free cortisol excretion rose to 1800 nmol/d (650 μg/d) after 2 d of intramuscular depot cosyntropin administration. CT scans of the pituitary and adrenal glands were normal. Prolonged observation in hospital and low glucocorticoid radioreceptor activity of the patient's serum excluded surreptitious self-medication with glucocorticoids. Aromatase activity in cultured skin fibroblasts was 1.5- to 1.8-fold greater than normal, and [³H]thymidine incorporation was inhibited 33 to 44% more than normal. In vitro studies of his receptors did not fully explain the greater glucocorticoid sensitivity. The authors concluded that the patient's Cushing's syndrome was caused by hyper-reactivity to cortisol. It is unclear, however, why the patient developed Cushing's syndrome, given the very low basal cortisol production and suppressed ACTH secretion, or why he developed it only in his sixth decade. This cause of Cushing's syndrome, if it exists, requires further explanation.

Mineralocorticoid: Hyperaldosteronism

PRIMARY ALDOSTERONISM. Inappropriate hypersecretion of aldosterone is an uncommon cause of hypertension, accounting for fewer than 1% of cases. The initial patient in whom this disorder was described had asymptomatic hypertension, hypokalemia, and a single adrenal adenoma.[1772]

Clinical Presentation. The diagnosis should be considered in patients with hypertension and spontaneous hypokalemia. Early reports described a higher incidence of physical symptoms than has subsequently been observed.[1773] Some patients may have frontal headaches, muscular weakness or flaccid paralysis caused by hypokalemia,[1774] or polyuria. The peak incidence occurs between 30 and 50 years of age, and most

patients are women. The hypertension may be severe. Malignant hypertension is a rare complication.[1775, 1776]

Pathophysiology. Primary aldosteronism is usually caused by solitary unilateral adrenal adenomas, which were thought to account for 70 to 80% of all cases of hyperaldosteronism.[1777] Most of the remaining cases were caused by bilateral adrenal hyperplasia, so-called idiopathic hyperaldosteronism. However, bilateral adrenal hyperplasia now accounts for almost 50% of cases in some referral centers.[1778] The apparent shift in frequency is probably a result of more careful evaluation of hypertensive patients. A heritable form of hyperaldosteronism that can be suppressed by glucocorticoid therapy accounts for a small percentage of cases.[1779, 1780] Adrenal carcinoma is a rare cause of primary hyperaldosteronism.[1781] Unilateral adrenal hyperplasia is even more unusual.[1782]

Adrenal Adenoma. The pathogenesis of aldosterone-secreting adrenocortical adenomas is unknown. The manifestations of primary hyperaldosteronism of all causes result from excess aldosterone secretion. Increased renal distal tubular sodium reabsorption causes an increase in total body sodium content. Water is also retained, so serum sodium concentration remains normal. Continued exposure to excess mineralocorticoid results in an "escape" phenomenon, possibly mediated by a compensatory increase in ANP secretion.[1783–1786] For this and other reasons, the hypertension in hyperaldosteronism may not result solely from volume expansion; peripheral vascular resistance may also be elevated.[1787–1789] In animal models of mineralocorticoid-induced hypertension, increased intracellular vascular smooth muscle cell sodium content is believed to cause vasoconstriction and increased peripheral vascular resistance.[1790, 1791]

Aldosterone also causes potassium loss in the distal renal tubule, resulting in hypokalemia. The electrochemical gradient generated by avid sodium retention also causes hydrogen ion loss in the distal tubule. Ammonia synthesis by the kidney increases in parallel with hypokalemia, contributing to the alkalosis. Hypokalemia impairs renal concentrating capacity, causing polyuria. Inappropriate urinary potassium excretion continues despite hypokalemia. Plasma renin activity is suppressed and remains unresponsive to maneuvers that deplete intravascular volume.[1792–1794]

Bilateral Adrenocortical Hyperplasia. The pathogenesis of zona glomerulosa hyperplasia is unknown. Possible causes include the action of normal intermediate-lobe POMC products, such as β-MSH,[553, 1795] γ-MSH,[1796, 1797] and β-END.[554, 1798] Additional putative aldosterone-stimulating pituitary factors unrelated to POMC have been reported but not structurally characterized.[1799, 1800] Indirect evidence for possible intermediate lobe involvement is the serotoninergic control of aldosterone secretion observed in these patients.[1801, 1802] However, the intermediate lobe normally is functional only in the fetus and during pregnancy in humans, and there is no evidence that any of its POMC products circulates in sufficient concentration to stimulate glomerulosa cell function.

The manifestations of idiopathic hyperaldosteronism are usually less severe than with adenomas: aldosterone levels are not as high, and the hypokalemia and suppression of renin are not as profound. Consequently, some authorities believe that this syndrome is not clinically distinct from "low-renin" essential hypertension.[1803]

Glucocorticoid-Remediable Hyperaldosteronism. This form of dexamethasone-suppressible hyperaldosteronism is transmitted as an autosomal dominant disorder.[1779, 1780, 1804, 1805] Aldosterone levels fall after glucocorticoid administration and remain suppressed during chronic therapy, indicating the dependence of aldosterone secretion on ACTH stimulation. In one patient, however, exogenous glucocorticoids lost the capacity to suppress aldosterone secretion after 7 y.[1806] Individuals with the syndrome have a distinctive biochemical phenotype characterized by excretion of large amounts of the novel urinary metabolites 18-hydroxycortisol and 18-oxotetrahydrocortisol.[532, 1807] The underlying molecular defect is now recognized. Unequal recombination events between the ACTH-regulated *CYP11B1* gene that encodes the 11β-hydroxylase enzyme in the zona fasciculata and the homologous *CYP11B2* gene that encodes aldosterone synthetase in the zona glomerulosa create a chimeric gene with ACTH-responsive regulatory elements from the *CYP11B1* gene located upstream of the promoter for the coding region of the *CYP11B2* gene. The result is ACTH-regulated aldosterone production in the zona fasciculata.[1808, 1809]

Rare Forms of Adrenocortical Hyperplasia. One type of bilateral adrenal hyperplasia has been described as primary hyperplasia, because subtotal (75%) adrenalectomy apparently results in permanent cure.[1810] The pathogenesis is unknown. In rare instances unilateral adrenal hyperplasia causes hyperaldosteronism,[1782, 1811] and mineralocorticoid excess may be cured by resecting the affected adrenal. The pathogenesis of this disorder is also unknown.

Laboratory Diagnosis. The diagnostic approach consists of two phases. It is first necessary to differentiate primary hyperaldosteronism from other causes of hypertension by documenting hyperaldosteronemia and suppressed plasma renin activity. Second, dynamic tests and imaging procedures are used to distinguish between surgically remediable forms of hyperaldosteronism and those that respond to medical management.

The criterion for deciding which hypertensive patients to evaluate is the presence of unprovoked hypokalemia.[1812] Diuretics should be discontinued 2 to 4 weeks before evaluation, and dietary sodium intake should be at least 100 mmol/d. As many as 12% of patients with adrenal adenoma and 50% of those with bilateral hyperplasia have serum potassium levels higher than 3.5 mmol/L.[1794] A level of less than 4.0 mmol/L increases the sensitivity to 100%, but the specificity falls to 64%.[1813, 1814] Urinary potassium excretion is inappropriately high in aldosteronism. A rate of less than 30 mmol/24 h is very unusual.[1814] Adequate dietary sodium (i.e., urinary excretion of at least 100 mmol/d) is required to allow normal renal sodium-potassium exchange and demonstrate the kaliuresis.

Increased Basal Aldosterone Secretion, Suppressed Plasma Renin Activity. Screening aldosterone measurements can be made on plasma or 24-h urine collections. Plasma aldosterone is usually measured after 4 h of upright posture. Plasma renin activity should be measured in the same sample. Increased plasma aldosterone in the face of suppressed plasma renin activity is highly suggestive of the diagnosis. The ratio of plasma aldosterone concentration (in nanograms per deciliter) to plasma renin activity (in nanograms per milliliter per hour) best discriminates between patients with essential hypertension and those with primary hyperaldosteronism. A ratio of plasma aldosterone to plasma renin activity greater than 20 to 25 indicates the need for further study.[1778, 1815]

Failure of Aldosterone Secretion to be Suppressed Normally. In the hypertensive patient with hypokalemia and/or kaliuresis or with an elevated plasma aldosterone–renin ratio, the diagnosis of hyperaldosteronism is confirmed by demonstrating failure of normal suppression of plasma aldosterone. Medications that affect the renin-angiotensin-aldosterone system must be discontinued, preferably for several weeks before testing, and potassium deficits must be corrected.[1778] Urine aldosterone excretion of more than 39 nmol (14 µg)/d after oral sodium loading over 3 d establishes the diagnosis.[1816] The intravenous saline suppression test[1817] is also widely used. Isotonic saline is infused intravenously at a rate of 300 to 500 mL/h for 4 h, after which plasma aldosterone and renin activity are measured. Aldosterone levels normally fall to less than 0.28 nmol/L (10 ng/dL), and renin activity is sup-

pressed. Failure to suppress normally identifies patients with aldosterone-producing adenomas[1812]; most patients with secondary forms of hyperaldosteronism suppress normally. False-negative results (i.e., suppressibility) are most often seen in patients with bilateral hyperplasia.[1818–1820]

An alternative test uses the angiotensin-converting enzyme inhibitor, captopril, to inhibit the generation of angiotensin II. This has the same net effect on plasma angiotensin II concentration and, consequently, on plasma aldosterone concentration as suppression of renin secretion with saline infusion. The captopril test is recommended in patients in whom the risks from volume overload preclude performance of the saline infusion test. Plasma aldosterone is measured 2 h after oral administration of 25 mg of captopril. Plasma aldosterone normally suppresses to less than 0.42 nmol/L (15 ng/dL).[1821–1823] The test may not always be diagnostic, but it is a useful alternative when saline suppression cannot be performed.[1824, 1825]

Adenoma Versus Bilateral Hyperplasia. Once the diagnosis of primary hyperaldosteronism is established, one must distinguish between aldosterone-producing adrenal adenoma and bilateral adrenal hyperplasia. The hypertension caused by adenomas can be cured by surgical therapy, whereas the hypertension associated with bilateral hyperplasia is often not cured even by total bilateral adrenalectomy and should be treated medically. Adenomas tend to produce more severe hyperaldosteronism, and consequently more severe hypertension, more profound hypokalemia, and more complete renin suppression,[1792] but these findings do not reliably differentiate them from hyperplasia. However, one widely used test is based on the less complete suppression of renin activity in hyperaldosteronism caused by bilateral hyperplasia. Plasma renin activity rises slightly and aldosterone concentration increases significantly after the stimulation of 2 to 4 h of upright posture in these patients, presumably because the hyperplastic glands are sensitive to small increments in plasma renin activity. In contrast, renin remains suppressed and aldosterone does not rise in patients with adenomas,[1826] in whom plasma aldosterone level may fall paradoxically.[1827] A diagnostic accuracy of 85% was reported in a review of 246 cases,[1828] although others have not found it as reliable.[1829] The plasma concentration of 18-hydroxycorticosterone, a late precursor in the aldosterone biosynthetic pathway, is elevated in most patients with aldosterone-producing adenomas but not in those with bilateral adrenal hyperplasia.[1812, 1830]

Patients with glucocorticoid-suppressible hyperaldosteronism, like those with adenomas, may have an anomalous postural decrease in plasma aldosterone concentration.[1831] If the patient has no evidence of an adenoma on CT or MRI, particularly if there is a family history of hypertension and hypokalemia, the diagnosis should be excluded by administering dexamethasone at a dosage of 2 mg every day for 3 to 4 weeks. Plasma concentration and urinary excretion of aldosterone should remain suppressed; transient suppression can occur in patients with adenomas or the common form of bilateral adrenal hyperplasia.[1831] Primary adrenal hyperplasia causes abnormalities in dynamic tests similar to those seen in patients with adrenal adenoma but does not lateralize by CT, MRI, [6β-131I]-iodomethyl-19-norcholesterol (NP-59) imaging, or adrenal venous sampling.[1810, 1812] Adrenal carcinomas usually are remarkable for the severity of hypertension and hypokalemia they produce but may be similar to adenomas in respect to all dynamic tests. However, a large adrenal mass is usually found by imaging procedures, whereas adenomas are typically quite small.[1781, 1832–1835]

Lateralization of Aldosterone Secretion. Adrenal venous sampling can be useful when all else fails,[1836] but it is reliable only in experienced hands. Catheterization of the right adrenal vein is technically difficult and is unsuccessful about 25%

of the time.[1778] However, adenomas reportedly can be localized despite failure of catheterization.[1837] Cosyntropin (5 IU/h) is administered continuously during the test to minimize episodic adrenocortical steroid secretion caused by stress-induced release of endogenous ACTH.[1794] Ideally, both adrenal veins should be catheterized, and aldosterone and cortisol should be measured in plasma obtained simultaneously from both veins and a peripheral site. Well-validated criteria for lateralization are lacking, but adrenal vein aldosterone concentration on the side of the tumor is usually at least 10 times higher than in the nontumorous, presumably suppressed adrenal gland.[1823] The minimal amount of contrast material necessary to document proper catheter placement is used, because of the risk of adrenal hemorrhage.

Radiographic/Nuclear Medicine Findings. Imaging procedures can assist in differentiating causes of hyperaldosteronism and in lateralizing adenomas. CT scanning of the adrenals is usually done first. Several percent of upper abdominal CT scans performed for other reasons reveal incidental adrenal masses, most of which are not associated with abnormal hormone secretion.[1838] The clinical significance of such nonfunctioning "incidentalomas" is unclear (see later discussion and Chapters 13 and 14). The current highest-resolution CT scanners can detect adrenal tumors as small as 7 to 8 mm in diameter.[1812, 1839, 1840] The diagnostic accuracy is only about 70% for aldosterone-producing adenomas, largely because of the occurence of nonfunctioning adrenal adenomas.[1778, 1838] Aldosterone-producing adenomas usually have attenuation values lower than those of cortisol-secreting adenomas or pheochromocytomas but similar to some incidental adenomas.[1841] MRI is no better than CT in differentiating aldosterone-secreting tumors from other adrenal tumors.[1842] Scintigraphic imaging with ^{131}I-labeled cholesterol derivatives during dexamethasone suppression provides an image based on functional properties of the adrenal; NP-59 is currently used.[1713, 1843] Dexamethasone and stable iodide treatment are necessary to suppress ACTH secretion and prevent uptake of the tracer by the thyroid. Asymmetric uptake after 48 h indicates an adenoma, whereas symmetric uptake after 72 h indicates bilateral hyperplasia. Diagnostic accuracy in 308 reported cases was 72%.[1778] However, if the adrenal CT scan is normal, iodocholesterol scanning is unlikely to be helpful.[1710] This procedure is generally used only when other data are contradictory. Adrenal venography is associated with greater risk of adrenal hemorrhage and has been abandoned as a diagnostic technique, but, as noted previously, it may be used in a final attempt to lateralize the source of proven aldosterone hypersecretion.

Treatment. Total unilateral surgical adrenalectomy is the treatment of choice for adrenal adenoma, if the patient does not face unacceptable operative risk. Cure rates as high as 90% are reported, but the long-term cure rate in a review of 694 cases was 69%.[1778] Laparoscopic adrenalectomy has been used with good success and allows faster recovery and less pain for patients.[1844, 1845] The patient should be prepared for surgery with spironolactone (200 to 400 mg/d) for several weeks to control blood pressure and restore normal potassium balance. The dosage may be reduced after control is achieved. Electrolyte imbalances disappear promptly after successful surgery, but blood pressure may not return to normal for months. Some patients with primary bilateral hyperplasia may be cured by subtotal adrenalectomy,[1810, 1812] but there is no reliable method for identifying these patients preoperatively. Ease of control of blood pressure and of serum potassium with spironolactone before surgery may be a favorable prognostic sign.[1810]

Medical therapy is indicated for patients with bilateral adrenal hyperplasia and for those with adenomas who are not surgical candidates. Spironolactone (200 to 400 mg/d) usually controls the hypokalemia, but additional antihypertensive therapy may be needed, especially in patients with hyperplasia. Side effects of spironolactone include menstrual disturbances in women and gynecomastia, impotence, and decreased libido in men and result mainly from inhibition of steroid biosynthesis. Amiloride, an inhibitor of distal tubular sodium transport, has been used in hyperaldosteronism[1846] but rarely controls blood pressure in subjects with hyperplasia. Some authorities consider it the drug of choice for men with hyperaldosteronism who are not cured by surgery.[1778] Calcium channel blockers have also been used, because increased cytoplasmic free calcium stimulates aldosterone synthesis. They also inhibit vascular smooth muscle contraction and lower peripheral vascular resistance. Although they initially appeared to decrease plasma aldosterone and blood pressure,[1847, 1848] subsequent studies demonstrated no effect on aldosterone levels and incomplete blood pressure control.[1849, 1850]

11β-HYDROXYSTEROID DEHYDROGENASE DEFICIENCY. Both inherited and acquired states of 11β-HSD deficiency cause syndromes of apparent mineralocorticoid excess.

Hereditary 11β-HSD Deficiency. The inherited disorder causes low-renin hypertension and hypokalemia not accompanied by increased plasma aldosterone levels but responds to spironolactone therapy.[1851] These individuals excrete tetrahydro metabolites of cortisol but not of cortisone, whereas normal humans excrete more metabolites of cortisone than of cortisol.[1852] Furthermore, the sodium retention, potassium wastage, and renin suppression are corrected by suppressing endogenous cortisol production with dexamethasone administration, whereas the administration of exogenous hydrocortisone with the dexamethasone re-creates the syndrome.[1851] Therefore, cortisol acts as a mineralocorticoid in the kidney if the 11β-HSD system fails to "protect" the relatively nonspecific type I (mineralocorticoid) receptor from exposure to it. The 11β-HSD type II, which is present in the distal convoluted tubule and collecting duct,[1853] is the product of a gene on chromosome 16q22.[1854] A number of point mutations have been reported in affected families,[1855] of which the R337C mutation has a 10-fold higher K_m (Michaelis constant) for cortisol, compromising its ability to convert it to cortisone.[1856]

Acquired 11β-HSD Deficiency. Additional evidence for the protection hypothesis comes from studies of patients with licorice-induced pseudohyperaldosteronism. Chronic excessive ingestion of glycyrrhizic acid, the active principle in licorice, suppresses the renin-aldosterone system and causes kaliuresis.[1857-1859] The adrenal glands must be present for licorice to have a mineralocorticoid effect in animals,[1860] and licorice is an effective mineralocorticoid replacement in human primary adrenal insufficiency only if given with hydrocortisone.[1861, 1862] The explanation for these observations is that glycyrrhizic acid inhibits 11β-HSD deficiency[1863] and allows glucocorticoids to exert effects through the mineralocorticoid receptor. The 3β-D-monoglucuronyl-glycyrrhetinic acid metabolite, which is increased in the blood of patients with licorice-induced pseudohyperaldosteronism, may be the active agent.[1864]

BARTTER'S SYNDROME AND GITELMAN'S SYNDROME. Bartter's syndrome is a rare disorder of hyperreninemia, hyperaldosteronism, hypokalemia, and alkalosis without hypertension or edema.[1865] Renal juxtaglomerular cell hyperplasia and increased urinary prostaglandin E_2 excretion are present.[1866] The disorder usually begins in childhood, and patients present with muscle weakness, cramps, urinary frequency, and, in many cases, growth delay and impaired intellectual development. The more severe variant (Bartter's syndrome) is associated with polyhydramnios, premature delivery, and hypercalciuria and volume depletion in infancy.[1867, 1868] Affected offspring of one consanguineous kindred also had sensorineural deafness.[1869] The diagnosis can be established prepartum by finding increased aldosterone in the amniotic fluid.[1870] Early onset of nephrocalcinosis and nephrolithiasis is common[1867, 1868] and

nal tumor may not produce excessive amounts of cortisol each day, yet most or all of the daily cortisol production may be autonomous, the hypothalamic-pituitary axis may be partially suppressed, and the remaining normal adrenal cortex may be atrophic. The purpose of dynamic tests of hypothalamic-pituitary-adrenal function is to define abnormalities in the functional relations between the elements of the axis that may not be reflected in altered basal secretion.

Tests For Evaluating Primary and Secondary Adrenal Insufficiency

Hypocortisolism can result from (1) a primary adrenal disorder resulting in failure to produce cortisol (primary adrenal insufficiency), (2) a primary pituitary disorder resulting in lack of ACTH secretion (secondary adrenal insufficiency), or (3) a primary hypothalamic disorder resulting in lack of CRH secretion and secondarily in lack of ACTH secretion (tertiary adrenal insufficiency). Measurement of basal plasma ACTH and cortisol concentrations, urinary steroid excretion, and the responses of the anterior pituitary gland and adrenal cortex to a variety of stimuli define the site of the defect.

A major problem with relying on observations of unstimulated plasma hormone levels as the basis for diagnosis is that hormone secretion is episodic. A single plasma level, if it falls within the range of normal, is inconclusive. Furthermore, the normal ranges are broad, and an individual can have pituitary or adrenal insufficiency but maintain secretion of ACTH or cortisol, or both, within the range of the normal population. For these reasons, dynamic function tests should be performed when there is reasonable doubt about the hypothalamic-pituitary-adrenal status.

Nevertheless, a basal early morning plasma cortisol value can be very helpful in excluding adrenal hypofunction. If the value is greater than 300 nmol/L (11 μg/dL) it is unlikely that the patient has clinically important hypothalamic-pituitary-adrenal insufficiency, whereas if it is less than about 80 nmol/L (3 μg/dL) the probability of adrenal insufficiency is high.[1171, 2149] Conversely, a patient whose plasma cortisol level 1 h after sleep is less than 140 nmol/L (5 μg/dL) has virtually no probability of having Cushing's syndrome. Similarly, patients whose salivary cortisol level at 8:00 AM is greater than 16 nmol/L (5.8 ng/mL) are highly unlikely to have adrenal insufficiency, whereas if the level is less than about 5 nmol/L (1.8 ng/mL) the probability of adrenal insufficiency is high. A patient whose late evening salivary cortisol level is less than 4 nmol/L (1.4 ng/mL) is unlikely to have Cushing's syndrome, but if the level is greater than 16 nmol/L (5.8 ng/mL) the probability is high. Patients whose basal plasma or salivary cortisol concentrations do not meet these criteria are the major candidates for dynamic function testing.

ACTH TEST: THE ADRENOCORTICAL RESPONSE TO EXOGENOUS ACTH

Rationale. If the primary disorder is hypopituitarism with deficient ACTH secretion and secondary adrenal insufficiency, then the intrinsically normal adrenal gland should respond to maximally stimulating concentrations of exogenous ACTH (see Fig. 12–32C and D). Conversely, in primary adrenal insufficiency, endogenous ACTH levels are already elevated, and there should be no adrenal response to exogenous ACTH (see Fig. 12–32B).

Procedure

One-Hour Low-Dose ACTH Stimulation Test. It has been argued that a test involving more physiological plasma concentrations of ACTH provides a more sensitive index of adrenocortical responsiveness. The low-dose ACTH test is performed by measuring plasma cortisol concentration immediately before and 30 min after intravenous injection of cosyntropin [synthetic ACTH(1–24)], 1 μg (350 pmol, or 160 mIU)[1173] or

0.5 μg (175 pmol, 80 mIU)/1.73 m².[2150] The latter dose has the advantage of compensating for plasma volume, but it is half the former dose and may not result in the same peak plasma cortisol concentrations at 30 min because the peak tends to be reached earlier.[1175, 2150] Therefore, a cosyntropin dose of 1 μg (350 pmol, 160 mIU)/1.73 m² is recommended. Plasma ACTH can also be measured in the basal sample, as in all ACTH stimulation tests. The test can be performed on an outpatient basis. There are no untoward side effects. Allergic reactions, which were rare with purified animal ACTH, are almost unheard of with cosyntropin.

One-Hour Standard ACTH Stimulation Test. Plasma cortisol measurements are made immediately before and 30 and 60 min after intravenous injection of 250 μg (85 nmol, 40 IU) of cosyntropin. This dose of cosyntropin produces pharmacologic concentrations of plasma ACTH for the 60-min duration of the test. The test can be performed on an outpatient basis. There are no untoward side effects.

Eight-Hour ACTH Stimulation Test. This test is performed by infusing 250 μg (85 nmol, 40 IU) cosyntropin or 40 IU purified bovine ACTH continuously over 8 h in 500 mL of normal saline. A 24-h urine specimen is collected the day before and the day of the infusion for 17-OHCS and creatinine determination, and plasma cortisol concentration is measured at the end of the infusion. Plasma ACTH levels are maintained at supraphysiological levels for the duration of the infusion. The infusion solution must contain isotonic saline (154 mmol/L [9 g/L] NaCl), because patients with adrenal insufficiency, who may already be hyponatremic and lack salt-retaining aldosterone, can become severely hyponatremic if infused with hypotonic solutions. This is a particular problem with purified bovine ACTH, which is contaminated with variable amounts of AVP; the AVP promotes renal free water retention, aggravating hyponatremia. Cosyntropin is also preferable to bovine ACTH because of rare instances of allergic reactions to contaminating proteins in purified ACTH preparations. In countries where it is available, 1 mg (444 nmol) of a long-acting cosyntropin preparation [ACTH(1–18)-NH₂] can be injected intramuscularly. The 8-h ACTH infusion test is rarely performed.

Two-Day ACTH Infusion Test. The 2-d ACTH infusion test[1181] is similar to the 8-h infusion test, except that the same dose of ACTH is infused every 8 h for 48 h. Alternatively, 40 IU of a depot formulation of purified bovine ACTH in gelatin is injected intramuscularly every 12 h for 48 h. Daily 444-nmol (1-mg) intramuscular injections of long-acting ACTH(1–18)-NH₂ can be used outside the United States. The same precautions should be observed as during the 8-h test. This test is the most widely used prolonged ACTH stimulation test.

Three- to Five-Day ACTH Infusion Tests. The 3- to 5-d ACTH stimulation tests are generally conducted in the same way as the 2-d test, but are prolonged an additional 1 to 3 d.

Normal Values

One-Hour Low-Dose ACTH Stimulation Test. Using radioimmunoassay to determine plasma cortisol, an increment of 200 nmol/L (7.2 μg/dL) and/or a level of 500 nmol/L (18 μg/dL) or more at any time during the test, including before injection, is indicative of normal adrenal function.[1173, 2150] Criteria that require a minimum increment in plasma cortisol[1173] are invalid,[51] because patients who have a high basal plasma cortisol, because of either normal circadian rhythmicity or acute stress, may be almost maximally stimulated and unable to increase cortisol secretion further.

One-Hour ACTH Stimulation Test. Using radioimmunoassay to determine plasma cortisol, a value of 550 nmol/L (20 μg/dL) or more at any time during the test, including before injection, is indicative of normal adrenal function.[1176] Earlier criteria that required a minimum increment in plasma cortisol are invalid for the reasons already mentioned.[2151] Salivary cortisol increases to 52 ± 2.2 nmol/L (19 ± 0.8 ng/mL) (range, 24 to 99 nmol/L [8.7 to 36 ng/mL]) 1 h after injection.[1491]

Eight-Hour ACTH Stimulation Test. The 24-h urinary excretion of 17-OHCS should increase threefold to fivefold over baseline on the day of ACTH infusion. Plasma cortisol should reach 550 nmol/L (20 μg/dL) 30 to 60 min after and exceed 690 nmol/L (25 μg/mL) 6 to 8 h after the infusion is begun.

Two-Day ACTH Stimulation Test. Urinary excretion of 17-OHCS should exceed 74 nmol (27 mg) during the first 24 h of infusion and 130 nmol (47 mg) during the second 48 h. If measured, plasma cortisol should reach 550 nmol/L (20 μg/dL) 30 to 60 min after and exceed 690 nmol/L (25 μg/dL) 6 to 8 h after the infusion is begun. Both plasma and urinary steroids increase progressively thereafter, but ranges of normal for plasma cortisol are not standardized.

Three- to Five-Day ACTH Stimulation Test. Urinary 17-OHCS should increase threefold to fivefold fold over baseline on the first day of ACTH infusion. If measured, plasma cortisol should reach 550 nmol/L (20 μg/dL) 30 to 60 min after and exceed 690 nmol/L (25 μg/dL) 6 to 8 h after the infusion is begun. Both plasma and urinary steroids increase progressively thereafter, but ranges of normal are not standardized.

Interpretation. A subnormal response to the 1-h ACTH stimulation test is diagnostic of primary, secondary, or tertiary adrenal insufficiency, whereas a normal response excludes these disorders.[2152] The low-dose ACTH stimulation test is more sensitive in detecting adrenal insufficiency than the standard test.[1175, 2153] The tests do not distinguish between the primary and secondary or tertiary forms of adrenal insufficiency. However, if the response is inadequate, one can measure the plasma ACTH concentration in the basal sample. If it is higher than normal the patient has primary adrenal insufficiency, and if it is low the diagnosis is secondary or tertiary adrenal insufficiency. In primary adrenal insufficiency, prolonged stimulation with exogenous ACTH for 1 to 5 d results in little, if any, increase in cortisol production. In secondary or tertiary adrenal insufficiency, the adrenal gland is intrinsically normal but is atrophic because of chronic ACTH deficiency; in most of these patients, stimulation for 1 d (8 h) is too brief to exert a major effect. Continuous infusion of ACTH for 2 d increases 24-h urinary 17-OHCS excretion to 25 nmol (9 mg) or more during the second day of infusion in most patients with hypopituitarism. Some patients may require 3 to 5 d of stimulation. However, even after 5 d, plasma cortisol levels may not attain those observed after 1 to 8 h of ACTH stimulation in normal individuals,[2154] and 24-h urinary 17-OHCS may increase only threefold over baseline.[2155] In practice the prolonged ACTH stimulation tests are seldom used because sensitive assays of plasma ACTH, used in conjunction with the 1-h tests, have supplanted them.

An area in which there continues to be controversy is whether the standard 1-h ACTH test accurately predicts the ability to respond adequately to stress (e.g., major surgery). Some patients have normal responses to cosyntropin but subnormal responses to insulin-induced hypoglycemia,[1179, 2156] although the hypoglycemia has not always been adequate.[2151] Rarely, patients who respond normally to the 1-h ACTH test have a subnormal cortisol response to surgery,[2151] but these patients tolerate surgery normally.[2157] Furthermore, the plasma cortisol responses of most persons to the 1-h ACTH test and to insulin-induced hypoglycemia, a standard stress, are virtually identical.[2156] Presumably, the reason is that the endogenous plasma ACTH levels elicited in response to insulin-induced hypoglycemia are maximally stimulating during the hour or less that the test lasts, as are the plasma levels of exogenous ACTH achieved during the standard 1-h ACTH stimulation test; plasma cortisol responses indicate that such maximally stimulating ACTH levels are not achieved during the low-dose 1-h ACTH test.[1175, 2153] In all three tests a normal response is

predicated on the fact that the adrenal gland has been stimulated daily with sufficient endogenous ACTH to prevent adrenal atrophy and maintain the required basal activity of the steroidogenic CYP enzymes. The reason why patients do well during major surgery even though their cortisol levels do not rise normally may be that no more than basal daily cortisol secretion is required to survive surgery.[1196]

With one exception, anyone who responds normally to the 1-h ACTH test does not require glucocorticoid supplementation for stress, surgical or otherwise. The exception is the patient who is acutely ACTH-deficient, such as the patient who has just had a hypophysectomy.[2156] During the several days after cessation of ACTH secretion, the adrenocortical zonae fasciculata and reticularis undergo functional and anatomic atrophy. During part of that interval the adrenals may respond normally to pharmacologic doses of exogenous ACTH, but the pituitary gland is unable to release ACTH in response to stress. These patients respond normally to the 1-h ACTH test but fail to respond to insulin-induced hypoglycemia and require steroid supplementation during surgical or other stresses.

Because the results of the standard 1-h ACTH test are identical to those of the insulin-induced hypoglycemia test, because the standard test can be performed in an outpatient setting without a physician's being present and without risk, and because it is less expensive to perform, the 1-h ACTH test has supplanted the insulin-induced hypoglycemia test in practice except in patients with suspected recent loss of ACTH secretory capacity. The low-dose 1-h ACTH stimulation test is intermediate in sensitivity between the metyrapone and insulin-induced hypoglycemia tests and may detect more subtle deficiency than the insulin-induced hypoglycemia test,[2153] but the clinical relevance of this finding is uncertain.

INSULIN-INDUCED HYPOGLYCEMIA TEST: THE HYPOTHALAMIC-PITUITARY RESPONSE TO HYPOGLYCEMIC STRESS

Rationale. Stress is difficult to define, let alone to reproduce. However, hypoglycemia produces a major stress response, with increases in plasma ACTH, cortisol, hGH, and prolactin and activation of the adrenergic system.[2158] Furthermore, (1) the degree of hypoglycemia can easily be quantified; (2) the test is safe, if a physician is present, in patients without a history of seizures or cardiovascular or cerebrovascular disease; and (3) the hypoglycemia can be corrected within seconds by intravenous infusion of hypertonic glucose solution. The magnitude of the response depends on the degree of hypoglycemia. Criteria that are adequate to elicit a maximal hGH response (i.e., rate and degree of fall in plasma glucose) are inadequate to ensure a maximal ACTH response. Because the purpose of the test is to define the magnitude of a maximal stress response, stringent criteria of adequate hypoglycemia must be applied. In a patient with a morning plasma cortisol of less than 140 nmol/L (5 μg/dL) and 24-h urinary free cortisol excretion of less than 55 nmol (20 μg), there is rarely any indication for this test.

Procedure. The patient must fast for at least 8 h before and remain supine during the procedure. A physician must be present during the entire procedure. A 30-mL syringe containing 50% glucose solution should be at bedside. An intravenous line is established, and insulin (0.15 U/kg body weight) is injected intravenously. The insulin dose is decreased to 0.1 U/kg for patients thought to have hypopituitarism or primary adrenal insufficiency; it is increased because of insulin resistance to 0.25 U/kg for obese patients, as well as for patients with diabetes mellitus or suspected acromegaly or Cushing's syndrome. Blood is obtained for plasma glucose and cortisol assays immediately before insulin is injected and at 30 and 45 min thereafter. All patients in whom adequate hypoglycemia is achieved (1.9 mmol/L [35 mg/dL] or less) develop a profuse cold sweat. In fact, if the patient does not have a sweat, irrespective of plasma glucose level, the adequacy of stress stimulus is suspect. Most patients have a hyperactive precordium (but not tachycardia or hypotension, because they are supine) and feelings of hunger, drowsiness, detachment, or anxiety. The last is common and sometimes severe, and many patients find this an unpleasant experience. Hypoglycemia is usually achieved 30 to 45 min after insulin injection. If adequate hypoglycemia is not achieved, a second identical dose of regular insulin should be injected intravenously. Adequate hypoglycemia should be achieved within 30 to 45 min. Ideally, an automated glucose oxidase analyzer should be available at the bedside; most glucose oxidase strips are inaccurate at low plasma glucose levels and tend to underestimate the plasma glucose concentration, leading to premature termination of the test. The final, definitive blood sample should be obtained 5 to 10 min after the patient develops a profuse sweat or, if it can reliably be measured, when plasma glucose falls below 1.9 mmol/L (35 mg/dL). Patients with primary or secondary adrenal insufficiency or long-standing diabetes mellitus have an impaired compensatory response to hypoglycemia. Therefore, it is prudent to terminate the test, after achieving a plasma glucose concentration of 1.9 mmol/L, by infusing 10% glucose solution in addition to giving sweetened orange juice or cola by mouth. If seizure, chest pain, confusion, disorientation, or other potentially serious complications occur, a 50% glucose solution should be infused over a period of 1 min or so (because of its hypertonicity); this produces hyperglycemia within 30 s.

Normal Values. Plasma cortisol concentration is measured by radioimmunoassay and should reach 550 nmol/L (20 μg/dL) at some point during the test. If this level is achieved, it is unimportant whether hypoglycemia was adequate. However, failure to reach this level indicates an inadequate response only if plasma glucose fell to 1.9 mmol/L (35 mg/dL) or less. Otherwise, the stimulus was inadequate and the test must be repeated. The increment in plasma cortisol is irrelevant, as discussed in the section on the 1-h ACTH stimulation test. Plasma ACTH concentration can also be measured. The response has not been carefully standardized, but the level should exceed 33 pmol/L (150 pg/mL).[232, 2159-2162] Finally, as discussed in greater detail in Chapter 9, plasma hGH levels should also increase; measurement of ACTH and hGH provides another index of anterior pituitary function.

Interpretation. An inadequate response can result from hypopituitarism of any cause, including hypothalamic CRH deficiency, isolated ACTH deficiency, partial or panhypopituitarism, and acute or chronic ingestion of synthetic glucocorticoids. Because adrenocortical secretion of cortisol is used as a bioassay of ACTH secretion, both primary and secondary adrenal insufficiency can cause an abnormal cortisol response. Hypoglycemia is a much stronger stimulus for secretion of ACTH than is hypocortisolemia. Consequently, patients may have a normal response to hypoglycemia but an inadequate response to metyrapone administration. The reverse is almost never true. As already mentioned, the low-dose 1-h ACTH stimulation test does not produce maximally stimulating plasma ACTH levels, so patients may have a normal response to hypoglycemia but an inadequate response to low-dose cosyntropin.

Although the insulin-induced hypoglycemia test is valid and perhaps the most rational test of hypothalamic-pituitary-adrenal response to stress, the 1-h ACTH test provides the same information, is less difficult and less expensive to perform, and can be performed without risk in any patient. Consequently, there is little, if any, reason for performing the insulin-induced hypoglycemia test in clinical practice, except in patients with suspected recent ACTH deficiency.[2156] The test is discussed further in Chapter 9.

METYRAPONE TEST: THE PITUITARY RESPONSE TO HYPOCORTISOLEMIA

Rationale. The metyrapone test (see Fig. 12–46D) is based on the fact that ACTH secretion is inhibited by plasma cortisol. Metyrapone blocks the conversion of 11β-deoxycortisol to cortisol by CYP11B1, the last step in the biosynthetic pathway from cholesterol to cortisol (see Fig. 12–5). 11-Deoxycortisol is essentially devoid of glucocorticoid bioactivity and does not inhibit ACTH secretion. As plasma cortisol concentration falls, therefore, ACTH secretion increases, adrenal steroidogenesis is stimulated, and the secretion of cortisol precursors, especially 11-deoxycortisol, increases rapidly (see Fig. 12–45D). The 11-deoxycortisol can be measured either in blood, by protein-binding radioassay,[2163, 2164] radioimmunoassay, or high-performance liquid chromatography, or in urine as a 17-OHCS,[1520] providing an index of the increase in ACTH secretion.

Procedure. Metyrapone administration can result in hypotension, nausea, and vomiting in patients with primary or secondary adrenal insufficiency; testing with this compound should be performed with great caution. If symptoms of adrenal insufficiency occur, the patient should be infused with physiological saline solution and the test should be continued. Saline can usually be stopped a few hours after the last dose of metyrapone.

Standard Three-Day Metyrapone Test. This test[1520] is performed by obtaining a baseline (8:00 AM to 8:00 AM) 24-h urine collection. Immediately after completing this collection, the patient begins taking metyrapone (750 mg every 4 h for six doses) by mouth with a glass of milk or a small snack to minimize gastrointestinal symptoms. The 24-h urine specimens are collected the day of and the day after metyrapone administration for measurement of urinary 17-OHCS and creatinine excretion. Plasma 11-deoxycortisol, cortisol, and ACTH can also be measured 4 h after the last dose of metyrapone.[2163, 2164] The metyrapone test cannot be performed in a patient who is taking any glucocorticoid.

Two-Day Metyrapone Test. This test[1475] is a slight variation on the standard 3-d test: 24-h urine and 8:00 AM blood specimens are collected during a baseline day and the day the patient takes 750 mg of metyrapone by mouth every 4 h. Urinary 17-OHCS and plasma 11-deoxycortisol are measured.

Overnight Single-Dose Metyrapone Test. This test[2164] is performed by oral administration of metyrapone (30 mg/kg body weight, or 2 g for <70 kg, 2.5 g for 70 to 90 kg, and 3 g for >90 kg body weight) at midnight with a glass of milk or a small snack. Plasma 11-deoxycortisol and cortisol are measured by radioimmunoassay in an 8:00 AM blood sample.[2165] Plasma ACTH concentration can also be measured.[2166-2168]

Normal Values. A normal response to the standard 3-d test is a twofold to threefold increase above the baseline 24-h urinary 17-OHCS excretion on either the day of metyrapone administration or, more often, the day after.[1520] A normal response to the 2-d test, which has been used to differentiate patients with Cushing's disease from those with the ectopic ACTH syndrome,[1475] has not been defined. An increase in urinary 17-OHCS excretion greater than 70% or an increase in plasma 11-deoxycortisol greater than 400-fold is required to establish the diagnosis of Cushing's disease; if either was observed, the sensitivity was 71%. A normal response to the overnight single-dose test is an 8:00 AM plasma 11-deoxycortisol concentration of 210 to 660 nmol/L (7 to 22 μg/dL) or more.[2163, 2164] Plasma ACTH concentrations should exceed 17 pmol/L (75 pg/mL), with a mean of about 44 pmol/L (200 pg/mL) at 8:00 AM after the overnight dose[2167, 2168] and, presumably, 4 h after the last dose in the 3-d test.

Interpretation. The metyrapone test is the most sensitive test of pituitary ACTH secretory reserve. It depends on the release of pituitary ACTH secretion from negative feedback inhibition by cortisol, which is a much less powerful stimulus to increased ACTH secretion than hypoglycemia or other stresses. Therefore, a patient with partial hypopituitarism may maintain normal daily ACTH and cortisol secretion and respond to insulin-induced hypoglycemia or other stresses with a normal increase in ACTH and cortisol secretion, yet be unable to increase ACTH secretion normally when cortisol biosynthesis is blocked by metyrapone. Conversely, a patient who responds normally to metyrapone usually responds normally to hypoglycemia or other stresses.

An individual who responds normally to any of the metyrapone tests has an intact hypothalamic-pituitary-adrenal axis and requires no further investigation. An abnormal test can result from several causes. Because adrenal steroid secretion is used as the assay of ACTH activity, primary adrenal insufficiency can be the cause. This can be determined by finding a high ACTH concentration in the basal plasma specimen[2167] and can be confirmed, if necessary, by lack of a normal plasma cortisol response to cosyntropin. Acute or chronic ingestion of synthetic glucocorticoids can also result in a subnormal response. Any of the drugs that interfere in the assay of 17-OHCS can interfere with interpretation of the standard 3-d or the 2-d test results.

In the differential diagnosis of Cushing's syndrome, a positive response indicates that the ACTH-secreting tumor responds to falling plasma cortisol levels. Most ectopic ACTH-secreting tumors, such as small cell lung carcinomas, do not respond, just as they do not respond to the increased plasma glucocorticoid levels produced by the high-dose dexamethasone suppression test. Some bronchial carcinoid tumors may respond, although most respond minimally.[1475, 1669]

One of the more common causes of a factitious abnormal result is unusually rapid clearance of metyrapone from plasma, resulting in inadequate blockade of cortisol biosynthesis. This is manifested by a plasma cortisol level greater than 210 nmol/L (7.5 μg/dL) in the sample drawn at 8:00 AM in the overnight test, by a plasma cortisol greater than 140 nmol/L (5 μg/dL) 4 h after the last dose of metyrapone, or by urinary free cortisol excretion greater than 55 nmol (20 μg)/24 h on the day metyrapone was administered in the standard 2-d test. Rapid clearance occurs in about 4% of the normal population.[2165, 2168] Metyrapone is metabolized by hepatic CYP enzymes that are induced by many of the same agents that increase steroid metabolism (e.g., phenobarbital, phenytoin, rifampicin, mitotane, glucocorticoids), so these drugs should be stopped before the metyrapone test is performed. An alternative is to perform the 3-d test with twice the dosage of metyrapone (750 mg every 2 h for 12 doses; presumably, 1.5 g every 4 h for six doses would be equally effective). A normal response is said to be indicated by a plasma 11-deoxycortisol level greater than 300 nmol/L (10 μg/dL) 2 h after the last dose or by urinary 17-OHCS excretion of more than 17 nmol (6 mg)/24 h on the day of metyrapone administration.[2169] However, because the double dosage of metyrapone is given to overcome the increased metabolic clearance, it is not apparent why the criterion for a normal response should be different than for the standard 3-d test. Consequently, a twofold to threefold increase above the baseline 24-h 17-OHCS excretion during the day of or the day after metyrapone administration can reasonably be assumed to be indicative of normal ACTH secretory reserve. Furthermore, if baseline 17-OHCS excretion is 17 nmol (6 mg)/24 h, a similar value on the day of metyrapone administration indicates a lack of response.

CORTICOTROPIN-RELEASING HORMONE TEST: THE PITUITARY RESPONSE TO CRH

Rationale.
The conceptual basis of the CRH test is the use of a maximally stimulating dose of exogenous CRH to stimulate ACTH secretion by anterior pituitary corticotropes. If the defect in hypothalamic-pituitary-adrenal function lies at the hypothalamic level, CRH administration should cause release of ACTH, whereas if the primary defect is in the pituitary, ACTH secretion should be subnormal or absent even after maximal CRH stimulation. Synthetic ovine CRH is equipotent to human CRH and has a more prolonged duration of action than human CRH,[390–392] which makes it useful for clinical testing.[1473]

Procedure.
The patient usually fasts for 4 h or longer, after which an intravenous access line is established and synthetic ovine CRH (1 μg [200 nmol]/kg body weight) is injected as a bolus. Blood samples for plasma ACTH and cortisol assays are drawn 15 and 0 min before and 5, 10, 15, 30, 45, 60, 90, and 120 min after CRH injection. However, if one measures only the plasma ACTH response, the samples at 0, 15 and 30 min are sufficient,[399, 2170] and if one measures only the cortisol response, the samples at 15 min before and 0, 45, and 60 min after injection are sufficient.[399] Some patients experience mild, brief facial flushing immediately after injection, but there are no other side effects at this dose level.[393] Allergic reactions have not been reported.

Normal Values.
The normal range of the ACTH response to ovine CRH has not been standardized. Absolute increments in plasma ACTH are quite variable among individuals and from one time to another in the same person[2171] (D.R. Davis, M.T. McDermott, T.F. Culclasure, M.E. Dorogy, W.E. Nicholson, D.N. Orth, unpublished observations). The cause of this variability is unknown, but it cannot be accounted for simply by inhibition by variable basal plasma cortisol concentrations (D.R. Davis, M.T. McDermott, T.F. Culclasure, M.E. Dorogy, W.E. Nicholson, D.N. Orth, unpublished observations). However, in our experience basal ACTH increases twofold to fourfold in 95% of normal subjects and reaches a peak of 4.4 to 22 pmol/L (20 to 100 pg/mL) 10 to 30 min after CRH injection; plasma cortisol usually increases to 550 to 690 nmol/L (20 to 25 μg/dL), reaching a peak 30 to 60 min after CRH injection.[392, 393, 399, 1524] Others have proposed that an increase in plasma cortisol of 20% or more is a normal response.[1474, 1525, 2170] Whereas the increment in ACTH is the same in the morning and evening, the peak ACTH value is higher in the morning, when basal ACTH is higher. In contrast, the peak cortisol value is similar at both times of day, but the increment is smaller in the morning, when the basal cortisol level is higher.[403] In patients with Cushing's syndrome, an increase of 35% or more above basal plasma ACTH concentration distinguishes those with Cushing's disease from those with ectopic ACTH syndrome.[2170] In patients with Cushing's syndrome, in whom the normal circadian rhythm in ACTH secretion is absent, the CRH test can be performed at any time of day with similar results.

Interpretation.
Patients with primary pituitary ACTH deficiency (secondary adrenal insufficiency) have decreased primary plasma ACTH and cortisol responses to CRH. In general, patients with hypothalamic CRH deficiency (tertiary adrenal insufficiency) have exaggerated and prolonged plasma ACTH responses; plasma cortisol responses are subnormal. Patients with primary adrenal insufficiency have high basal plasma ACTH concentrations and exaggerated responses to CRH, and plasma cortisol concentrations are low before and after CRH injection. The CRH test is not recommended for differentiating primary from secondary adrenal insufficiency but may be useful for differentiating secondary from tertiary adrenal insufficiency.

This test can be performed as part of a combined anterior pituitary function test, in which CRH, hGH-releasing hormone, LHRH, and thyrotropin-releasing hormone are administered simultaneously and plasma concentrations of all of the anterior pituitary hormones are measured.[399] This test is useful in evaluating the site (i.e., hypothalamic versus pituitary) and extent (i.e., partial versus panhypopituitarism) of deficiency in patients with suspected pituitary dysfunction and in evaluating residual pituitary function after pituitary surgery and radiation. This test is discussed further in Chapter 9.

UPRIGHT PLASMA RENIN ACTIVITY/ALDOSTERONE TEST: THE RENAL-ADRENAL RESPONSE TO UPRIGHT POSTURE

Rationale. Renin secretion is regulated by effective renal perfusion, so anything that decreases renal blood flow will increase plasma renin levels. If the adrenal is intact, increased plasma renin concentration stimulates increased aldosterone secretion. Patients with primary adrenal insufficiency also lack aldosterone secretion, whereas those with secondary adrenal insufficiency usually have normal aldosterone response (see Fig 12–29). Although it is not necessary to document this fact to establish the diagnosis, it is sometimes important to assess the status of the renin-angiotensin-aldosterone system in a patient with primary adrenal insufficiency in whom electrolyte disturbances are mild or absent.

Procedure. Salt should not be restricted without careful monitoring in a patient with primary adrenal insufficiency, and diuretics are dangerous. On the other hand, the patient should not be overly hydrated with saline solution. In these patients upright posture alone suffices to stimulate increased renin secretion. The patient maintains an upright posture, preferably standing, sitting when necessary, but never lying down, for 3 h. Blood pressure should be monitored. If the patient becomes hypotensive, the test can be terminated after a blood sample is obtained. Otherwise, blood is obtained before and at the end of the 3-h period for assay of plasma renin activity and aldosterone concentration.

Normal Values. Normal upright plasma renin activity is 0.5 to 2.6 nmol/L/h (0.7 to 3.3 ng/mL/h). Normal upright plasma aldosterone concentrations range from 140 to 560 pmol/L (5 to 20 ng/dL).

Interpretation. Patients with primary adrenal insufficiency have low plasma aldosterone and increased plasma renin activity in response to upright posture. Patients with secondary adrenal insufficiency (hypopituitarism) usually have a normal response, although some patients with chronic ACTH deficiency may develop aldosterone deficiency.[997, 998] Tests of renin-angiotensin-aldosterone axis function are discussed in Chapter 14.

OTHER TESTS. The blood eosinophil response[1001] and water-loading tests[2172] no longer have a role in the evaluation of pituitary insufficiency.

Tests for Evaluating Adrenocortical Hypersecretion: Cushing's Syndrome

DEXAMETHASONE SUPPRESSION TESTS: PITUITARY RESPONSE TO GLUCOCORTICOID NEGATIVE FEEDBACK INHIBITION OF ACTH SECRETION. Dexamethasone (see Fig. 12–62) is a potent glucocorticoid, about 40 times more potent than cortisol (see Table 12–19). The average daily maintenance dosage of dexamethasone for an Addison's patient is 0.5 mg, whereas the average daily dosage of cortisol is 20 mg. Dexamethasone and its tetrahydro metabolite both form Porter-Silber chromogens and are measured as 17-OHCS. As in the case of cortisol, only about one third of the urinary metabolites of dexamethasone are detected as 17-OHCS. Because so little dexamethasone is required to suppress pituitary ACTH secretion, its contribution to total urinary 17-OHCS is relatively small, about 0.7 mg/d in the standard two-d low-dose dexamethasone suppression test, and about 2.4 mg/d in the 2-d high-dose test. Furthermore, current antibodies used in cortisol radioimmunoassay are directed toward the D ring of the molecule and react very poorly with dexamethasone, which has a 16α-methyl modification of the D ring. Therefore measurements of plasma cortisol and urinary free cortisol are unaffected by the presence of dexamethasone. The low-dose and high-dose dexamethasone suppression tests are considered separately.

LOW-DOSE DEXAMETHASONE SUPPRESSION TESTS

Rationale. The purpose of the low-dose dexamethasone suppression test is to differentiate patients with Cushing's syndrome of any cause (see Figs. 12–47B, 12–49B, and 12–53B) from patients with normal hypothalamic-pituitary-adrenal function (see Fig. 12–47B). Type II glucocorticoid receptors in the adrenal cortex bind dexamethasone, and dexamethasone may directly inhibit steroidogenesis to a degree in rat adrenals.[2173] However, dexamethasone has no inhibitory effect on steroid production when exogenous ACTH is infused in humans; if anything, it augments its effect.[2174] Therefore, for the purpose of this test, one can assume that the only action of dexamethasone is to suppress pituitary ACTH secretion (see Fig. 12–46B). If the hypothalamic-pituitary axis is intrinsically normal, the excess dosage of dexamethasone is sufficient to suppress most of pituitary ACTH secretion. Consequently, adrenal cortisol secretion falls, and the plasma concentration and urinary excretion of cortisol and cortisol metabolites also decrease.

Procedure. No special precautions are required for the dexamethasone suppression tests; untoward side effects are virtually absent; and either test can be conducted on an outpatient basis by an intelligent and compliant patient. Obviously, these tests cannot be conducted with a patient who is receiving exogenous ACTH or glucocorticoids.

Standard Two-Day Test. At least one basal 24-h urine specimen is collected, usually beginning at 8:00 AM, for 17-OHCS, free cortisol, and creatinine assays. Immediately after the basal urine collection is completed, the patient begins taking 0.5 mg dexamethasone orally every 6 h for a total of eight doses while urine collection is continued. The dose can be modified in children who weigh less than about 45 kg (100 pounds).[2136] Six hours after the last dose of dexamethasone, the last urine collection is completed and blood can be drawn for assay of cortisol, ACTH, and dexamethasone.

Overnight Screening Test. Dexamethasone (1 mg) is taken orally between 11:00 PM and midnight, and a single blood sample is drawn at 8:00 AM the next morning for assay of cortisol and, if desired, ACTH and dexamethasone. A dose of 0.3 mg/m^2 surface area can be used in children.[2175]

Normal Values

Standard Two-Day Test. Urinary 17-OHCS excretion should fall to 6.9 mol (2.5 mg) or less per 24 h, irrespective of creatinine excretion (i.e., lean body weight), and urinary free cortisol should fall to less than 27 nmol (10 μg)/24 h on the second day of dexamethasone administration. Although the test does not require it, confirmatory data are provided by a plasma cortisol value of less than 140 nmol/L (5 μg/dL), a plasma ACTH concentration of less than 2.2 pmol/L (10 pg/mL), and a plasma dexamethasone level of about 5 to 17 nmol/L (2 to 6.5 ng/mL).[1496]

Overnight Test. The 8:00 AM plasma cortisol concentration should be less than 140 nmol/L (5 μg/dL), plasma ACTH level should always be less than 2.2 pmol/L (10 pg/mL) and usually less than 1.1 pmol/L (5 pg/mL), and plasma dexamethasone should range from about 5 to 17 nmol/L (2 to 6.5 ng/mL).[1496] Salivary cortisol concentration at 8:00 AM should be 2.1 ± 1.1 nmol/L (0.8 ± 0.4 ng/mL), with a range of 1.7 to 3 nmol/L (0.6 to 1.1 ng/mL).[1491]

Interpretation. The overnight test is a quick screening test for Cushing's syndrome but has a 12 to 15% rate of false-positive results.[2176, 2177] If the criterion is increased to 200 nmol/L (7.2 μg/dL), however, this rate falls to 7.3%.[2177] If the morning plasma cortisol is less than 140 nmol/L (5 μg/dL), the syndrome is essentially excluded. With plasma levels between 140 and 275 nmol/L (5 and 10 μg/dL), the test is equivocal, and the standard 2-d test should be performed. If the 8:00 AM plasma cortisol level is greater than 275 nmol/L (10 µg/mL), the patient has a high probability of having Cushing's syndrome, and further diagnostic tests must be performed to confirm the diagnosis and determine the cause.

Measurement of plasma cortisol at the end of the standard 2-d test provides reassurance that the urinary steroid values are correct. Measurement of plasma ACTH, if either of the tests is positive, gives an indication of the cause of the hypercortisolism: plasma ACTH usually is high normal or elevated in ectopic ACTH syndrome, within the normal range in Cushing's disease, and undetectable in adrenal tumor.

Measurement of plasma dexamethasone concentration for all dexamethasone suppression tests provides verification that the drug was taken and indicates whether the plasma concentration is within the limits expected in an person who metabolizes the drug normally. Nomograms are available that relate plasma dexamethasone levels to plasma cortisol concentrations in normal subjects and in some patients with Cushing's disease,[1496, 1497] but these are not widely applied. However, a finding of an abnormally high or low dexamethasone level allows one to interpret the cause of an unusual cortisol response and to repeat the test, if necessary, with the same or another dexamethasone dosage. In two forms of pseudo-Cushing's syndrome (severe bipolar depression and severe alcoholism), results of the low-dose dexamethasone suppression tests may be abnormal. These disorders are considered elsewhere in this chapter.

HIGH-DOSE DEXAMETHASONE SUPPRESSION TESTS

Rationale. The basis for the high-dose suppression tests is the fact that ACTH secretion in Cushing's disease is not completely, but only relatively, resistant to glucocorticoid negative feedback inhibition.[1339, 1512] Therefore, by increasing the dosage of dexamethasone fourfold to eightfold (i.e., 16 times the usual daily maintenance dosage), ACTH secretion can almost always be suppressed (see Fig. 12–47C). In contrast, most nonpituitary tumors that produce ectopic ACTH are not responsive to glucocorticoid negative feedback, and adrenal tumors that cause Cushing's syndrome are not dependent on ACTH secretion. In both of these varieties of Cushing's syndrome, pituitary ACTH secretion is already suppressed (see Figs. 12–49A and 12–53A). Therefore, dexamethasone cannot suppress ACTH secretion further and has no effect on cortisol secretion at any dosage (see Figs. 12–49C and 12–53C).

Procedure

Standard Two-Day Test. The patient collects at least one baseline 24-h urine specimen, usually beginning at 8:00 AM. After the baseline collection is completed, the patient begins taking 2 mg dexamethasone orally every 6 h for a total of eight doses, and the urine collections are continued. In practice, this test is often performed immediately after completing the low-dose dexamethasone suppression test, and no intervening baseline urine collection is obtained. The urine collections are assayed for 17-OHCS, free cortisol, and creatinine. In addition, a blood specimen can be collected 6 h after the last dose of dexamethasone for cortisol, dexamethasone, and ACTH radioimmunoassays.

Overnight Test. Dexamethasone (8 mg) is taken orally between 11:00 PM and midnight, and a single blood sample is drawn at 8:00 AM the next morning for assay of plasma cortisol and, if desired, ACTH and dexamethasone.

Normal Values

Standard Two-Day Test. Urinary 17-OHCS are suppressed to less than 6.9 µmol (2.5 mg)/24 h, most of which consist of dexamethasone metabolites. Urinary free cortisol excretion is less than 14 nmol (5 µg)/d, and plasma cortisol and ACTH concentrations are low and usually undetectable. Plasma dexamethasone concentrations range from about 20 to 51 nmol/L (8 to 20 ng/mL).[1496]

Overnight Test. The 8:00 AM plasma cortisol level is less than 140 nmol/L (5 µg/dL) and is usually undetectable. Plasma ACTH is also low and usually undetectable. Plasma dexamethasone concentrations have not been published.

Interpretation. Most patients with Cushing's disease demonstrate a significant decrease (i.e., greater than day-to-day baseline variation) in urinary free cortisol and 17-OHCS excretion,[1339] and about 70% suppress urinary free cortisol excretion by more than 90% or urinary 17-OHCS excretion by more than 64%.[1349] As in the low-dose tests, plasma cortisol levels respond similarly and reinforce the urinary steroid results. Plasma ACTH levels are also significantly suppressed in Cushing's disease, and plasma dexamethasone concentrations provide information about compliance and steroid metabolism. Excretion of free cortisol and 17-OHCS in patients with Cushing's syndrome caused by primary adrenal disease is not suppressed, but this test should not be used to distinguish these two causes of hypercortisolism. Most patients with ectopic ACTH syndrome also fail to suppress with high-dose dexamethasone, but about half of patients with ACTH-secreting bronchial carcinoid tumors and occasionally those with other tumors (e.g., thymic carcinoid tumors, hepatomas, pheochromocytomas) respond with decreased tumor secretion of ACTH and reduced urinary steroid excretion.[1346, 1347, 1349] Taken together, these patients represent fewer than 5% of all patients with ectopic ACTH syndrome, but they pose a difficult diagnostic problem because they may have chronic cortisol excess and typical Cushing's features. Patients who fail to meet the current criteria[1349] must undergo additional differential diagnostic procedures.[1470]

There are five common sources of error in the dexamethasone suppression tests: (1) improper urine collection, (2) day-to-day variation in hormone secretion by tumors, particularly by malignant pituitary and nonpituitary ACTH-secreting and cortisol-secreting adrenocortical tumors, (3) failure of the patient to take the dexamethasone, (4) abnormal metabolism of the dexamethasone, and (5) application of improper criteria for normal suppression. The first of these errors can be detected by measuring creatinine excretion; the second can be detected only by serial baseline 24-h urine steroid[1480, 1481, 2178] or salivary cortisol[1486] determinations; the third and fourth can be detected by measuring dexamethasone levels in blood a few hours after the last dose. The drugs that influence the metabolism of dexamethasone have already been discussed. Because cortisol may be less affected than fluorinated steroids such as dexamethasone, it has been suggested that a cortisol suppression test be substituted; in this case the index of suppression would be plasma corticosterone levels measured by radioimmunoassay, because exogenous cortisol cannot be distinguished from endogenous cortisol in the urinary 17-OHCS and free cortisol assays or in the plasma cortisol assay.[2179] Like most other variations on the original dexamethasone suppression tests, this suggestion has not been widely applied.

The urinary steroid excretion of most patients with Cushing's disease is suppressed by high-dose dexamethasone, but in general the higher the baseline ACTH and cortisol secretion the greater the resistance to suppression. In fewer than 5% of patients with Cushing's disease, higher dosages of dexamethasone (16 to 100 mg/d) are required to produce significant suppression. These patients tend to have large tumors. There are also rare reports of "paradoxical" responses to dexamethasone (i.e., cortisol secretion that increases in response to dexamethasone administration),[2180] but most of these are poorly documented in terms of reproducibility of the response. In only one well-documented case has the cause (spontaneous variation in tumor ACTH secretion) been defined.[1481] As in the other three cases with which we have been acquainted (D.N. Orth, unpublished observations), this patient had a malignant pituitary tumor.

1434. Ishibashi M, Yamaji T. Direct effects of thyrotropin-releasing hormone, cyproheptadine, and dopamine on adrenocorticotropin secretion from human corticotroph adenoma cells in vitro. J Clin Invest 1981; 68:1018–1027.

1435. Shibasaki T, Masui H. Effects of various neuropeptides on the secretion of proopiomelanocortin-derived peptides by a cultured pituitary adenoma causing Nelson's syndrome. Clin Endocrinol Metab 1982; 55:872–876.

1436. Lamberts SWJ, Verleun T, Bons EG, et al. Effect of cyproheptadine, desmethylcyproheptadine, gamma-amino-butyric acid and sodium valproate on adrenocorticotrophin secretion by cultured pituitary tumour cells from three patients with Nelson's syndrome. J Endocrinol 1983; 96:401–406.

1437. Tucci JR, Nowakowski KJ, Jackson IM. Cyproheptadine may act at the pituitary in Cushing's disease: evidence from CRF stimulation. J Endocrinol Invest 1989; 12:197–200.

1438. Whitehead HM, Beacom R, Sheridan B, et al. The effect of cyproheptadine and/or bromocriptine on plasma ACTH levels in patients cured of Cushing's disease by bilateral adrenalectomy. Clin Endocrinol (Oxf) 1990; 32:193–201.

1439. Carpenter PC. Cushing's syndrome: update of diagnosis and management. Mayo Clin Proc 1986; 61:49–58.

1440. Tagliaferri M, Berselli ME, Loli P. Transsphenoidal microsurgery for Cushing's disease. Acta Endocrinol 1986; 113:5–11.

1441. Guilhaume B, Bertagna X, Thomsen M, et al. Transsphenoidal pituitary surgery for the treatment of Cushing's disease: results in 64 patients and long term follow-up studies. J Clin Endocrinol Metab 1988; 66:1056–1064.

1442. Friedman RB, Oldfield EH, Nieman LK, et al. Repeat transsphenoidal surgery for Cushing's disease. J Neurosurg 1989; 71:520–527.

1443. Arnott RD, Pestell RG, McKelvie PA, et al. A critical evaluation of transsphenoidal pituitary surgery in the treatment of Cushing's disease: prediction of outcome. Acta Endocrinol 1990; 123:423–430.

1444. Bochicchio D, Losa M, Buchfelder M, et al. Factors influencing the immediate and late outcome of Cushing's disease treated by transsphenoidal surgery: a retrospective study by the European Cushing's Disease Survey Group. J Clin Endocrinol Metab 1995; 80:3114–3120.

1445. Leinung MC, Kane LA, Scheithauer BW, et al. Long term follow-up of transsphenoidal surgery for the treatment of Cushing's disease in childhood. J Clin Endocrinol Metab 1995; 80:2475–2479.

1446. Mindermann T, Kovacs K, Wilson CB. Changes in the immunophenotype of recurrent pituitary adenomas. Neurosurgery 1994; 35:39–44.

1447. Gicquel C, Le Bouc Y, Luton J-P, et al. Monoclonality of corticotroph macroadenomas in Cushing's disease. J Clin Endocrinol Metab 1992; 75:472–475.

1448. Biller BMK, Alexander JM, Zervas NT, et al. Clonal origins of adrenocorticotropin-secreting pituitary tissue in Cushing's disease. J Clin Endocrinol Metab 1992; 75:1303–1309.

1449. Landis CA, Masters SB, Spada A, et al. GTPase inhibiting mutations activate the α chain of Gs and stimulate adenylyl cyclase in human pituitary tumours. Nature 1989; 340:692–696.

1450. Lyons J, Landis CA, Harsh G, et al. Two G protein oncogenes in human endocrine tumors. Science 1990; 249:655–659.

1451. Yamada S, Kovacs K, Horvath E, et al. Morphological study of clinically nonsecreting pituitary adenomas in patients under 40 years of age. J Neurosurg 1991; 75:902–905.

1452. Pieters GFFM, Smals AGH, Goverde HJM, et al. Adrenocorticotropin and cortisol responsiveness to thyrotropin-releasing hormone and luteinizing hormone-releasing hormone discloses two subsets of patients with Cushing's disease. J Clin Endocrinol Metab 1982; 55:1188–1197.

1453. Van Cauter E, Refetoff S. Evidence for two subtypes of Cushing's disease based on the analysis of episodic cortisol secretion. N Engl J Med 1985; 312:1343–1349.

1454. Suda T, Demura H, Demura R, et al. Anterior pituitary hormones in plasma and pituitaries from patients with Cushing's disease. J Clin Endocrinol Metab 1980; 51:1048–1053.

1455. Aron DC, Findling JW, Tyrrell JB. Cushing's disease. Endocrinol Metab Clin North Am 1987; 16:705–730.

1456. Marcovitz S, Wee R, Chan J, et al. The diagnostic accuracy of preoperative CT scanning in the evaluation of pituitary ACTH-secreting adenomas. AJR Am J Roentgenol 1987; 149:803–806.

1457. Saris SC, Patronas NJ, Doppman JL, et al. Cushing syndrome: pituitary CT scanning. Radiology 1987; 162:775–777.

1458. Escourolle H, Abecassis JP, Bertagna X, et al. Comparison of computerized tomography and magnetic resonance imaging for the examination of the pituitary gland in patients with Cushing's disease. Clin Endocrinol (Oxf) 1993; 39:307–313.

1459. Dwyer AJ, Frank JA, Doppman JL, et al. Pituitary adenomas in patients with Cushing disease: initial experience with Gd-DTPA-enhanced MR imaging. Radiology 1987; 163:421–426.

1460. Peck WW, Dillon WP, Norman D, et al. High-resolution MR imaging of pituitary microadenomas at 1.5 T: experience with Cushing disease. AJR Am J Roentgenol 1989; 152:145–151.

1461. Hall WA, Luciano MG, Doppman JL, et al. Pituitary magnetic resonance imaging in normal human volunteers: occult adenomas in the general population. Ann Intern Med 1994; 120:817–820.

1462. Parent AD, Bebin J, Smith RR. Incidental pituitary adenomas. J Neurosurg 1981; 54:228–231.

1463. Lipkin EW, Fujimoto WY. Cushing's syndrome in a patient with suppressible hypercortisolism and an empty sella. West J Med 1984; 140:613–615.

1464. Kalifa G, Adamsbaum C, Carel JC, et al. Diagnosis of Cushing's disease in children: a challenge for the radiologist. Pediatr Radiol 1994; 24:547–549.

1465. Doppman JL, Miller DL, Dwyer AJ, et al. Macronodular adrenal hyperplasia in Cushing disease. Radiology 1988; 166:347–352.

1466. White FE, White MC, Drury PL, et al. Value of computed tomography of the abdomen and chest in investigation of Cushing's syndrome. BMJ 1982; 284:9–12.

1467. Hermus AR, Smals AG, Swinkels LM, et al. Bone mineral density and bone turnover before and after surgical cure of Cushing's syndrome. J Clin Endocrinol Metab 1995; 80:2859–2865.

1468. Momose KJ, Kjellberg RN, Kliman B. High incidence of cortical atrophy of the cerebral and cerebellar hemispheres in Cushing's disease. Radiology 1971; 99:341–348.

1469. Starkman MN, Gebarski SS, Berent S, et al. Hippocampal formation volume, memory dysfunction, and cortisol levels in patients with Cushing's syndrome. Biol Psychiatry 1992; 32:756–765.

1470. Orth DN. Medical Progress: Cushing's syndrome. N Engl J Med 1995; 332:791–803.

1471. Yanovski JA, Cutler GB Jr, Doppman JL, et al. The limited ability of inferior petrosal sinus sampling with corticotropin-releasing hormone to distinguish Cushing's disease from pseudo-Cushing states or normal physiology. J Clin Endocrinol Metab 1993; 77:503–509.

1472. Grossman AB, Howlett TA, Perry L, et al. CRF in the differential diagnosis of Cushing's syndrome: a comparison with the dexamethasone suppression test. Clin Endocrinol (Oxf) 1988; 29:167–178.

1473. Nieman LK, Cutler GB Jr, Oldfield EH, et al. The ovine corticotropin-releasing hormone (CRH) stimulation test is superior to the human CRH stimulation test for the diagnosis of Cushing's disease. J Clin Endocrinol Metab 1989; 69:165–169.

1474. Kaye TB, Crapo L. The Cushing syndrome: an update on diagnostic tests. Ann Intern Med 1990; 112:434–444.

1475. Avgerinos PC, Yanovski JA, Oldfield EH, et al. The metyrapone and dexamethasone suppression tests for the differential diagnosis of the adrenocorticotropin-dependent Cushing syndrome: a comparison. Ann Intern Med 1994; 121:318–327.

1476. Dichek HL, Nieman LK, Oldfield EH, et al. A comparison of the standard high dose dexamethasone suppression test and the overnight 8-mg dexamethasone suppression test for the differential diagnosis of adrenocorticotropin-dependent Cushing's syndrome. J Clin Endocrinol Metab 1994; 78:418–422.

1477. Orth DN. The old and the new in Cushing's syndrome. N Engl J Med 1984; 310:649–651.

1478. Liddle GW. Cushing's syndrome. Ann N Y Acad Sci 1977; 297:594–602.

1479. Murphy BEP. Clinical evaluation of urinary cortisol determinations by competitive protein-binding radioassay. J Clin Endocrinol Metab 1968; 28:343–348.

1480. Bailey RE. Periodic hormonogenesis—a new phenomenon. Periodicity in function of a hormone-producing tumor in man. J Clin Endocrinol Metab 1971; 32:317–327.

1481. Brown RD, Van Loon GR, Orth DN, et al. Cushing's disease with periodic hormonogenesis: one explanation for paradoxical response to dexamethasone. J Clin Endocrinol Metab 1973; 36:445–451.

1482. Jordan RM, Ramos-Gabatin A, Kendall JW, et al. Dynamics of adrenocorticotropin (ACTH) secretion in cyclic Cushing's syndrome: evidence for more than one abnormal ACTH biorhythm. J Clin Endocrinol Metab 1982; 55:531–537.

1483. Atkinson AB, Kennedy AL, Carson DJ, et al. Five cases of cyclical Cushing's syndrome. Br Med J Clin Res Ed 1985; 291:1453–1457.

1484. Kuchel O, Bolté E, Chrétien M, et al. Cyclical edema and hypokalemia due to occult episodic hypercorticism. J Clin Endocrinol Metab 1987; 64:170–174.

1485. Atkinson AB, McCance DR, Kennedy L, et al. Cyclical Cushing's syndrome first diagnosed after pituitary surgery: a trap for the unwary. Clin Endocrinol (Oxf) 1992; 36:297–299.

1486. Hermus AR, Pieters GF, Borm GF, et al. Unpredictable hypersecretion of cortisol in Cushing's disease: detection by daily salivary cortisol measurements. Acta Endocrinol 1993; 128:428–432.

1487. Papanicolaou DA, Yanovski JA, Cutler GB, et al. A single midnight cortisol measurement discriminates Cushing syndrome from pseudo-Cushing states. Program of 76th Annual Meeting Endocr Soc, Anaheim CA, June 15–18 1994: 518 (abstract #1270).

1488. Newell-Price J, Trainer P, Perry L, et al. A single sleeping midnight cortisol has 100% sensitivity for the diagnosis of Cushing's syndrome. Clin Endocrinol (Oxf) 1995; 43:545–550.

1489. Vining RF, McGinley RA, Maksvytis JJ, et al. Salivary cortisol: a better measure of adrenal cortical function than serum cortisol. Ann Clin Biochem 1983; 20:329–335.

1490. Lo MS, Ng ML, Azmy BS, et al. Clinical applications of salivary cortisol measurements. Singapore Med J 1992; 33:170–173.

1491. Laudat MH, Cerdas S, Fournier C, et al. Salivary cortisol measurement: a practical approach to assess pituitary-adrenal function. J Clin Endocrinol Metab 1988; 66:343–348.

1492. Allolio B, Hoffmann J, Linton EA, et al. Diurnal salivary cortisol patterns during pregnancy and after delivery: relationship to plasma corticotrophin-releasing-hormone. Clin Endocrinol (Oxf) 1990; 33:279–289.

1493. Reincke M, Nieke J, Krestin GP, et al. Preclinical Cushing's syndrome in adrenal "incidentalomas": comparison with adrenal Cushing's syndrome. J Clin Endocrinol Metab 1992; 75:826–832.

1494. Nugent CA, Nichols T, Tyler FH. Diagnosis of Cushing's syndrome: single dose dexamethasone test. Arch Intern Med 1965; 116:172–176.

1495. Lindholm J. Endocrine function in patients with Cushing's disease before and after treatment. Clin Endocrinol (Oxf) 1992; 36:151–159.

1496. Meikle AW, Lagerquist LG, Tyler FH. Apparently normal pituitary-adrenal suppressibility in Cushing's syndrome: dexamethasone metabolism and plasma levels. J Lab Clin Med 1975; 86:472–478.

1497. Meikle AW. Dexamethasone suppression tests: usefulness of simultaneous measurement of plasma cortisol and dexamethasone. Clin Endocrinol (Oxf) 1982; 16:401–408.

1498. Meikle AW, Clarke DH, Tyler FH. Cushing syndrome from low doses of dexamethasone: a result of slow plasma clearance. JAMA 1976; 235:1592–1593.

1499. Haigh SE, Tevaarwerk GJM. A rise in the glomerular filtration rate as the cause of a "paradoxical" increase in urinary free cortisol during dexamethasone suppression in a patient with an adrenal adenoma: a case report. Clin Endocrinol (Oxf) 1981; 15:53–56.

1500. Arana GW, Reichlin S, Workman R, et al. The dexamethasone suppression index: enhancement of DST diagnostic utility for depression by expressing serum cortisol as a function of serum dexamethasone. Am J Psychiatry 1988; 145:707–411.

1501. Ramirez G, Gomez-Sanchez C, Meikle AW, et al. Evaluation of the hypothalamic hypophyseal adrenal axis in patients receiving long-term hemodialysis. Arch Intern Med 1982; 142:1448–1452.

1502. Workman RJ, Vaughn WK, Stone WJ. Dexamethasone suppression testing in chronic renal failure: pharmacokinetics of dexamethasone and demonstration of a normal hypothalamic-pituitary-adrenal axis. J Clin Endocrinol Metab 1986; 63:741–746.

1503. Vierhapper H, Derfler K, Nowotny P, et al. Impaired conversion of cortisol to cortisone in chronic renal insufficiency—a cause of hypertension or an epiphenomenon? Acta Endocrinol 1991; 125:160–154.

1504. Carroll BJ, Feinberg M, Greden JF, et al. A specific laboratory test for the diagnosis of melancholia: standardization, validation, and clinical utility. Arch Gen Psychiatry 1981; 38:15–22.

1505. Noth RH, Walter RMJ. The effects of alcohol on the endocrine system. Med Clin North Am 1984; 68:133–146.

1506. Phlipponneau M, Lenne F, Proeschel MF, et al. Plasma immunoreactive joining peptide in man: a new marker of proopiomelanocortin processing and corticotroph function. J Clin Endocrinol Metab 1993; 76:325–329.

1507. Tyrrell JB, Findling JW, Aron DC, et al. An overnight high-dose dexamethasone suppression test for rapid differential diagnosis of Cushing's syndrome. Ann Intern Med 1986; 104:180–186.

1508. Leinung MC, Young WF Jr, Whitaker MD, et al. Diagnosis of corticotropin-producing bronchial carcinoid tumors causing Cushing's syndrome. Mayo Clin Proc 1990; 65:1314–1321.

1509. Howlett TA, Rees LH. Is it possible to diagnose pituitary-dependent Cushing's disease? Ann Clin Biochem 1985; 22:550–558.

1510. Nieman LK, Chrousos GP, Oldfield EH, et al. The ovine corticotropin-releasing hormone stimulation test and the dexamethasone suppression test in the differential diagnosis of Cushing's syndrome. Ann Intern Med 1986; 105:862–867.

1511. Hermus ARMM, Pieters GFFM, Pesman GJ, et al. The corticotropin-releasing-hormone test versus the high-dose dexamethasone test in the differential diagnosis of Cushing's syndrome. Lancet 1986; 2:540–544.

1512. Liddle GW. The adrenals. In: Williams RW, ed. Textbook of Endocrinology. 6th ed. Philadelphia: WB Saunders, 1981: 242–292.

1513. Miller J, Crapo L. The biochemical analysis of hypercortisolism. Endocrinologist 1994; 4:7–16.

1514. Biemond P, de Jong FH, Lambers SWJ. Continuous dexamethasone infusion for seven hours in patients with the Cushing syndrome: a superior differential diagnostic test. Ann Intern Med 1990; 112:738–742.

1515. Linn JE Jr, Bowdoin B, Farmer TA, et al. Observations and comments on failure of dexamethasone suppression. N Engl J Med 1967; 277:403–405.

1516. Hale AC, Millar JBG, Ratter SJ, et al. A case of pituitary dependent Cushing's disease with clinical and biochemical features of the ectopic ACTH syndrome. Clin Endocrinol (Oxf) 1985; 22:479–488.

1517. Carey RM. Suppression of ACTH by cortisol in dexamethasone-nonsuppressible Cushing's disease. N Engl J Med 1980; 302:275–279.

1518. Komor J, Laeng RH, Heitz PU, et al. Cushing-syndrom bei Bronchuskarzinoid: supprimierbare ektopische ACTH-Sekretion. Schweiz Med Wochschr 1982; 112:1507–1514.

1519. Ward PS, Mott MG, Smith J, et al. Cushing's syndrome and bronchial carcinoid tumour. Arch Dis Child 1984; 59:375–377.

1520. Liddle GW, Estep HL, Kendall JW Jr, et al. Clinical application of a new test of pituitary reserve. J Clin Endocrinol Metab 1959; 19:875–894.

1521. Orth DN, DeBold CR, DeCherney GS, et al. Pituitary microadenomas causing Cushing's disease respond to corticotropin-releasing factor. J Clin Endocrinol Metab 1982; 55:1017–1019.

1522. Müller OA, Stalla GK, Von Werder K. Corticotropin releasing factor: a new tool for the differential diagnosis of Cushing's syndrome. J Clin Endocrinol Metab 1983; 57:227–229.

1523. Pieters GFFM, Hermus ARMM, Smals AGH, et al. Responsiveness of the hypophyseal-adrenocortical axis to corticotropin-releasing factor in pituitary-dependent Cushing's disease. J Clin Endocrinol Metab 1983; 57:513–516.

1524. Chrousos GP, Schulte HM, Oldfield EH, et al. The corticotropin-releasing factor stimulation test: an aid in the evaluation of patients with Cushing's syndrome. N Engl J Med 1984; 310:622–626.

1525. Dickstein G, DeBold CR, Gaitan D, et al. Plasma corticotropin and cortisol responses to ovine corticotropin-releasing hormone (CRH), arginine vasopressin (AVP), CRH plus AVP, and CRH plus metyrapone in patients with Cushing's disease. J Clin Endocrinol Metab 1996; 81:2934–2941.

1526. Malerbi DA, Mendonca BB, Liberman B, et al. The desmopressin stimulation test in the differential diagnosis of Cushing's syndrome. Clin Endocrinol (Oxf) 1993; 38:463–472.

1527. de Herder WW, Krenning EP, Malchoff CD, et al. Somatostatin receptor scintigraphy: its value in tumor localization in patients with Cushing's syndrome caused by ectopic corticotropin or corticotropin-releasing hormone secretion. Am J Med 1994; 96:305–312.

1528. Hoefnagel CA. Metaiodobenzylguanidine and somatostatin in oncology: role in the management of neural crest tumours. Eur J Nucl Med 1994; 21:561–581.

1529. Phlipponneau M, Nocaudie M, Epelbaum J, et al. Somatostatin analogs for the localization and preoperative treatment of an adrenocorticotropin-secreting bronchial carcinoid tumor. J Clin Endocrinol Metab 1994; 78:20–24.

1530. Findling JW, Aron DC, Tyrrell JB, et al. Selective venous sampling for ACTH in Cushing's syndrome: differentiation between Cushing disease and the ectopic ACTH syndrome. Ann Intern Med 1981; 94:647–652.

1531. Manni A, Latshaw RF, Page R, et al. Simultaneous bilateral venous sampling for adrenocorticotropin in pituitary-dependent Cushing's disease: evidence for lateralization of pituitary venous drainage. J Clin Endocrinol Metab 1983; 57:1070–1073.

1532. Oldfield EH, Chrousos GP, Schulte HM, et al. Preoperative lateralization of ACTH-secreting pituitary microadenomas by bilateral and simultaneous inferior petrosal venous sinus sampling. N Engl J Med 1985; 312:100–103.

1533. Calzolari F, Ambrosio MR, Trasforini G. Diagnosis of Cushing's disease in children: the role of inferior petrosal sinus sampling. Pediatr Radiol 1995; 25:575 (letter).

1534. Schulte HM, Allolio B, Günther RW, et al. Selective bilateral and simultaneous catheterization of the inferior petrosal sinus: CRF stimulates prolactin secretion from ACTH-producing microadenomas in Cushing's disease. Clin Endocrinol (Oxf) 1988; 28:289–295.

1535. Doppman JL, Nieman LK, Chang R, et al. Selective venous sampling from the cavernous sinuses is not a more reliable technique than sampling from the inferior petrosal sinuses in Cushing's syndrome. J Clin Endocrinol Metab 1995; 80:2485–2489.

1536. Doppman JL, Oldfield E, Krudy AG, et al. Petrosal sinus sampling for Cushing syndrome: anatomical and technical considerations. Radiology 1984; 150:99–103.

1537. Oldfield EH, Girton ME, Doppman JL. Absence of intercavernous venous mixing: evidence supporting lateralization of pituitary microadenomas by venous sampling. J Clin Endocrinol Metab 1985; 61:644–647.

1538. Doppman JL, Krudy AG, Girton ME, et al. Basilar venous plexus of the posterior fossa: a potential source of error in petrosal sinus sampling. Radiology 1985; 155:375–378.

1539. Zovickian J, Oldfield EH, Doppman JL, et al. Usefulness of inferior petrosal sinus venous endocrine markers in Cushing's disease. J Neurosurg 1988; 68:205–210.

1540. McCance DR, McIlrath E, McNeill A, et al. Bilateral inferior petrosal sinus sampling as a routine procedure in ACTH-dependent Cushing's syndrome. Clin Endocrinol (Oxf) 1989; 30:157–166.

1541. Mamelak AN, Dowd CF, Tyrrell JB, et al. Venous angiography is needed to interpret inferior petrosal sinus and cavernous sinus sampling data for lateralizing adrenocorticotropin-secreting adenomas. J Clin Endocrinol Metab 1996; 81:475–481.

1542. Miller DL, Doppman JL, Peterman SB, et al. Neurologic complications of petrosal sinus sampling. Radiology 1992; 185:143–147.

1543. Seyer H, Honegger J, Schott W, et al. Raymond's syndrome following petrosal sinus sampling. Acta Neurochir (Wien) 1994; 131:157–159.

1544. Midgette AS, Aron DC. High-dose dexamethasone suppression testing versus inferior petrosal sinus sampling in the differential diagnosis of adrenocorticotropin-dependent Cushing's syndrome: a decision analysis. Am J Med Sci 1995; 309:162–170.

1545. Yamamoto Y, Davis DH, Nippoldt TB, et al. False-positive inferior petrosal sinus sampling in the diagnosis of Cushing's disease: report of two cases. J Neurosurg 1995; 83:1087–1091.

1546. Findling JW, Kehoe ME, Shaker JL, et al. Routine inferior petrosal sinus sampling in the differential diagnosis of adrenocorticotropin (ACTH)-dependent Cushing's syndrome: early recognition of the occult ectopic ACTH syndrome. J Clin Endocrinol Metab 1991; 73:408–413.

1547. Lüdecke DK. Intraoperative measurement of adrenocorticotropic hormone in peripituitary blood in Cushing's disease. Neurosurgery 1989; 24:201–205.

1548. de Herder WW, Uitterlinden P, Pieterman H, et al. Pituitary tumour localization in patients with Cushing's disease by magnetic resonance imaging: is there a place for petrosal sinus sampling? Clin Endocrinol (Oxf) 1994; 40:87–92.

1549. Hardy J. Cushing's disease: 50 years later. Can J Neurol Sci 1982; 9:375–380.

1550. Fahlbusch R, Buchfelder M, Müller OA. Transsphenoidal surgery for Cushing's disease. J R Soc Med 1986; 79:262–269.

1551. Chandler WF, Schteingart DE, Lloyd RV, et al. Surgical treatment of Cushing's disease. J Neurosurg 1987; 66:204–212.

1552. Mampalam TJ, Tyrrell JB, Wilson CB. Transsphenoidal microsurgery for Cushing disease: a report of 216 cases. Ann Intern Med 1988; 109:487–493.

1553. Rovitt RL, Duane TD. Cushing's syndrome and pituitary tumors: pathophysiology and ocular manifestations of ACTH-secreting pituitary adenomas. Am J Med 1969; 46:416–427.

1554. Gabrilove JL, Anderson PJ, Halmi NS. Pituitary pro-opiomelanocortin-cell carcinoma occurring in conjunction with a glioblastoma in a patient with Cushing's disease and subsequent Nelson's syndrome. Clin Endocrinol (Oxf) 1986; 25:117–126.

1555. Lenhard L, Deftos LJ. Adenohypophyseal hormones in the CSF. Neuroendocrinology 1982; 34:303–308.

1556. Nakao N, Oki S, Tanaka I, et al. Immunoreactive β-endorphin and adrenocorticotropin in human cerebrospinal fluid. J Clin Invest 1980; 66:1383–1390.

1557. Robert F, Pelletier G, Hardy J. Pituitary adenomas in Cushing's disease: a histologic, ultrastructural, and immunocytochemical study. Arch Pathol Lab Med 1978; 102:448–455.

1558. Olivier L, Vila-Porcile E, Dubois MP. Localisations cellulaires des peptides dérivés de la pro-opiocortine dans l'adenohypophyse humaine normale et dans les tumeurs de la maladie de Cushing. Horm Res 1980; 13:211–329.

1559. Sherry SH, Guay AT, Lee AK, et al. Concurrent production of adrenocorticotropin and prolactin from two distinct cell lines in a single pituitary adenoma: a detailed immunohistochemical analysis. J Clin Endocrinol Metab 1982; 55:947–955.

1560. Burke CW, Adams CB, Esiri MM, et al. Transsphenoidal surgery for Cushing's disease: does what is removed determine the endocrine outcome? Clin Endocrinol (Oxf) 1990; 33:525–537.

1561. Taylor HC, Velasco ME, Brodkey JS. Remission of pituitary-dependent Cushing's disease after removal of nonneoplastic pituitary gland. Arch Intern Med 1980; 140:1366–1368.

1562. Kruse A, Klinken L, Holck S, et al. Pituitary histology in Cushing's disease. Clin Endocrinol (Oxf) 1992; 37:254–259.

1563. Schteingart DE, Tsao HS. Coexistence of pituitary adrenocorticotropin-dependent Cushing's syndrome with a solitary adrenal adenoma. J Clin Endocrinol Metab 1980; 50:961–966.

1564. Ruder HJ, Loriaux DL, Lipsett MB. Severe osteopenia in young adults associated with Cushing's syndrome due to micronodular adrenal disease. J Clin Endocrinol Metab 1974; 39:1138–1147.

1565. Carson DJ, Sloan JM, Cleland J, et al. Cyclical Cushing's syndrome presenting as short stature in a boy with recurrent atrial myxomas and freckled skin pigmentation. Clin Endocrinol (Oxf) 1988; 28:173–180.

1566. Hashimoto K, Kawada Y, Murakami K, et al. Cortisol responsiveness to insulin-induced hypoglycemia in Cushing's syndrome with huge nodular adrenocortical hyperplasia. Endocrinol Jpn 1986; 33:479–487.

1567. Makino S, Hashimoto K, Sugiyama M, et al. Cushing's syndrome due to huge nodular adrenocortical hyperplasia with fluctuation of urinary 17-OHCS excretion. Endocrinol Jpn 1989; 36:655–663.

1568. Cheitlin RA, Westphal M, Cabrera CM, et al. Cushing's syndrome due to bilateral adrenal macronodular hyperplasia with undetectable ACTH: cell culture of adenoma cells on extracellular matrix. Horm Res 1988; 29:162–167.

1569. Orth DN, Liddle GW. Results of treatment in 108 patients with Cushing's syndrome. N Engl J Med 1971; 285:243–247.

1570. Casson IF, Davis JC, Jeffreys RV, et al. Successful management of Cushing's disease during pregnancy by transsphenoidal adenectomy. Clin Endocrinol (Oxf) 1987; 27:423–428.

1571. Laws ER, Ebersold MJ, Peipgras DG, et al. The results of transsphenoidal surgery in specific clinical entities. In: Laws ER, ed. Management of Pituitary Adenomas and Related Lesions with Emphasis on Transsphenoidal Microsurgery. New York: Appleton-Century-Crofts, 1982: 277–305.

1572. Styne DM, Grumbach MM, Kaplan SL, et al. Treatment of Cushing's disease in childhood and adolescence by transsphenoidal microadenomectomy. N Engl J Med 1984; 310:889–893.

1573. Aron DC, Findling JW, Fitzgerald PA, et al. Cushing's syndrome: problems in management. Endocr Rev 1982; 3:229–244.

1574. Burch W. A survey of results with transsphenoidal surgery in Cushing's disease. N Engl J Med 1983; 308:103–104.

1575. Kammer H, George R. Cushing's disease in a patient with an ectopic pituitary adenoma. JAMA 1981; 246:2722–2724.

1576. Wilson CB, Mindermann T, Tyrrell JB. Extrasellar, intracavernous sinus adrenocorticotropin-releasing adenoma causing Cushing's disease. J Clin Endocrinol Metab 1995; 80:1774–1777.

1577. Rasmussen P, Lindholm J. Ectopic pituitary adenomas. Clin Endocrinol (Oxf) 1979; 11:69–74.

1578. Trainer PJ, Lawrie HS, Verhelst J, et al. Transsphenoidal resection in Cushing's disease: undetectable serum cortisol as the definition of successful treatment. Clin Endocrinol (Oxf) 1993; 38:73–78.

1579. Hotta MN, Shibasaki T, Suda T, et al. The use of the corticotropin-releasing hormone test to monitor the recovery of patients with Cushing's disease or Cushing's syndrome due to an adrenal adenoma after adenomectomy. Endocrinol Jpn 1985; 32:113–125.

1580. Ram Z, Nieman LK, Cutler GB Jr, et al. Early repeat surgery for persistent Cushing's disease. J Neurosurg 1994; 80:37–45.

1581. Favia G, Boscaro M, Lumachi F, et al. Role of bilateral adrenalectomy in Cushing's disease. World J Surg 1994; 18:462–466.

1582. Tahir AH, Sheeler LR. Recurrent Cushing's disease after transsphenoidal surgery. Arch Intern Med 1992; 152:977–981.

1583. Jennings AS, Liddle GW, Orth DN. Results of treating childhood Cushing's disease with pituitary irradiation. N Engl J Med 1977; 297:957–962.

1584. Salassa RM, Kearns TP, Kernohan JW, et al. Pituitary tumors in patients with Cushing's syndrome. J Clin Endocrinol Metab 1959; 19:1523–1539.

1585. Nelson DH, Meakin JW, Thorn GW. ACTH-producing pituitary tumors following adrenalectomy for Cushing's syndrome. Ann Intern Med 1960; 52:560–569.

1586. Lamberts SWJ, de Jong FH, Birkenhäger JC. Evaluation of a therapeutic regimen in Cushing's disease. Acta Endocrinol 1977; 86:146–155.

1587. Sonino N, Zielezny M, Fava GA, et al. Risk factors and long-term outcome in pituitary-dependent Cushing's disease. J Clin Endocrinol Metab 1996; 81:2647–2652.

1588. Sharpe GF, Kendall-Taylor P, Prescott RWG, et al. Pituitary function following megavoltage therapy for Cushing's disease: long term follow up. Clin Endocrinol (Oxf) 1985; 22:169–177.

1589. Howlett TA, Plowman PN, Wass JAH, et al. Megavoltage pituitary irradiation in the management of Cushing's disease and Nelson's syndrome: long-term follow-up. Clin Endocrinol (Oxf) 1989; 31:309–323.

1590. Linfoot JA. Heavy ion therapy: alpha particle therapy of pituitary tumors. In: Linfoot JA, ed. Recent Advances in Diagnosis and Treatment of Pituitary Tumors. New York: Raven Press, 1979: 245–267.

1591. Kjellberg RN, Kliman B, Swisher B, et al. Proton beam therapy of Cushing's disease and Nelson's syndrome. In: Black PML, et al, eds. Secretory Tumors of the Pituitary Gland. New York: Raven Press, 1984: 295–307.

1592. Burke CW, Doyle FH, Joplin GF, et al. Cushing's disease: treatment by pituitary implantation of radioactive gold or yttrium seeds. Q J Med 1973; 168:693–714.

1593. Cassar J, Doyle FH, Mashiter K, et al. Treatment of Cushing's disease in juveniles with interstitial pituitary irradiation. Clin Endocrinol (Oxf) 1979; 11:313–321.

1594. Lunsford LD, Flickinger J, Lindner G, et al. Stereotactic radiosurgery of the brain using the first United States 201 cobalt-60 source gamma knife. Neurosurgery 1989; 24:151–159.

1595. Friedman WA, Bova FJ. The University of Florida radiosurgery system. Surg Neurol 1989; 32:334–342.

1596. Constine LS, Woolf PD, Cann D, et al. Hypothalamic-pituitary dysfunction after radiation for brain tumors. N Engl J Med 1993; 328:87–94.

1597. Luton J-P, Mahoudeau JA, Bouchard P, et al. Treatment of Cushing's disease by o,p'-DDD: survey of 62 cases. N Engl J Med 1979; 300:459–464.

1598. Schteingart DE, Tsao HS, Taylor CI, et al. Sustained remission of Cushing's disease with mitotane and pituitary irradiation. Ann Intern Med 1980; 92:613–619.

1599. Leiba S, Weinstein R, Shindel B, et al. The protracted effect of o,p'-DDD in Cushing's disease and its impact on adrenal morphogenesis of young human embryo. Ann Endocrinol (Paris) 1989; 50:49–53.

1600. Takamatsu J, Kitazawa A, Nakata K, et al. Does mitotane reduce endogenous ACTH secretion? N Engl J Med 1981; 305:957 (letter).

1601. Hogan TF, Citrin DL, Johnson BM, et al. O,p'-DDD (mitotane) therapy of adrenal cortical carcinoma: observations on drug dosage, toxicity, and steroid replacement. Cancer 1978; 42:2177–2181.

1602. Kelly WF, MacFarlane IA, Longson D, et al. Cushing's disease treated by total adrenalectomy: long-term observations of 43 patients. Q J Med 1983; 52:224–231.

1603. Landau B, Leiba S, Kaufman H, et al. Unilateral adrenalectomy and pituitary irradiation in the treatment of ACTH-dependent Cushing's disease in children and adolescents. Clin Endocrinol (Oxf) 1978; 9:221–226.

1604. Grabner P, Hauer-Jensen M, Jervell J, et al. Long-term results of treatment of Cushing's disease by adrenalectomy. Eur J Surg 1991; 157:461–464.

1605. Hardy JD. Surgical management of Cushing's syndrome with emphasis on adrenal autotransplantation. Ann Surg 1978; 188:290–307.

1606. Scott HW Jr, Orth DN. Hypercortisolism (Cushing's syndrome). In: Scott HW Jr, ed. Surgery of the Adrenal Glands. Philadelphia: JB Lippincott, 1990: 115–151.

1607. Gagner M, Lacroix A, Prinz RA, et al. Early experience with laparoscopic approach for adrenalectomy. Surgery 1993; 114:1120–1124; discussion 1124–1125.

1608. Chalmers RA, Mashiter K, Joplin GF. Residual adrenocortical function after bilateral "total" adrenalectomy for Cushing's disease. Lancet 1981; 2:1196–1199.

1609. Herwig KR, Schteingart DE. Successful removal of an adrenal remnant localized by ¹³¹I-19-iodocholesterol. J Urol 1974; 111:713–714.

1610. Barnett AH, Livesey JH, Friday K, et al. Comparison of preoperative and postoperative ACTH concentrations after bilateral adrenalectomy in Cushing's disease. Clin Endocrinol (Oxf) 1983; 18:301–305.

1611. Moreira AC, Castro M, Machado HR. Longitudinal evaluation of adrenocorticotrophin and β-lipotrophin plasma levels following bilateral adrenalectomy in patients with Cushing's disease. Clin Endocrinol (Oxf) 1993; 39:91–96.

1612. Ray DW, Gibson S, Crosby SR, et al. Elevated levels of adrenocorticotropin (ACTH) precursors in post-adrenalectomy Cushing's disease and their regulation by glucocorticoids. J Clin Endocrinol Metab 1995; 80:2430–2436.

1613. Hopwood NJ, Kenny FM. Incidence of Nelson's syndrome after adrenalectomy for Cushing's disease in children. results of a nationwide survey. Am J Dis Child 1977; 131:1353–1356.

1614. Cohen KL, Noth RH, Pechinski T. Incidence of pituitary tumors following adrenalectomy: a long-term follow-up study of patients treated for Cushing's disease. Arch Intern Med 1978; 138:575–579.

1615. McArthur RG, Hayles AB, Salassa RM. Childhood Cushing disease: results of bilateral adrenalectomy. J Pediatr 1979; 95:214–219.

1616. Wilson CB, Tyrrell JB, Fitzgerald PA, et al. Cushing's disease and Nelson's syndrome. Clin Neurosurg 1980; 27:19–30.

1617. Jenkins PJ, Trainer PJ, Plowman PN, et al. The long term outcome after adrenalectomy and prophylactic pituitary radiotherapy in adrenocorticotropin-dependent Cushing's syndrome. J Clin Endocrinol Metab 1995; 80:165–171.

1618. Moore TJ, Dluhy RG, Williams GH, et al. Nelson's syndrome: frequency, prognosis, and effect of prior pituitary irradiation. Ann Intern Med 1976; 85:731–734.

1619. Wild W, Nicolis GL, Gabrilove JL. Appearance of Nelson's syndrome despite pituitary irradiation prior to bilateral adrenalectomy for Cushing's syndrome. Mt Sinai J Med 1973; 40:68–71.

1620. Krieger DT, Amorosa L, Linick F. Cyproheptadine-induced remission of Cushing's disease. N Engl J Med 1975; 293:893–896.

1621. Lamberts SWJ, Birkenhäger JC. Effect of bromocriptine in pituitary-dependent Cushing's syndrome. J Endocrinol 1976; 70:315–316.

1622. Dornhorst A, Jenkins JS, Lamberts SWJ, et al. The evaluation of sodium valproate in the treatment of Nelson's syndrome. J Clin Endocrinol Metab 1983; 56:985–991.

1623. Koppeschaar HPF, Croughs RJM, Thijssen JHH, et al. Response to neurotransmitter modulating drugs in patients with Cushing's disease. Clin Endocrinol (Oxf) 1986; 25:661–667.

1624. Child DF, Burke CW, Burley DM, et al. Drug control of Cushing's syndrome: combined aminoglutethimide and metyrapone therapy. Acta Endocrinol 1976; 82:330–341.

1625. Komanicky P, Spark RF, Melby JC. Treatment of Cushing's syndrome with trilostane (WIN 24,540), an inhibitor of adrenal steroid biosynthesis. J Clin Endocrinol Metab 1978; 47:1042–1051.

1626. Loli P, Berselli ME, Tagliaferri M. Use of ketoconazole in the treatment of Cushing's syndrome. J Clin Endocrinol Metab 1986; 63:1365–1371.

1627. Verhelst JA, Trainer PJ, Howlett TA, et al. Short and long-term responses to metyrapone in the medical management of 91 patients with Cushing's syndrome. Clin Endocrinol (Oxf) 1991; 35:169–178.

1628. Schöneshöfer M, Fenner A, Claus M. Suppressive effect of metyrapone on plasma corticotrophin immunoreactivity in normal man. Clin Endocrinol (Oxf) 1983; 18:363–370.

1629. Jeffcoate WJ, Rees LH, Tomlin S, et al. Metyrapone in long-term management of Cushing's disease. BMJ 1977; 2:215–217.

1630. Orth DN. Metyrapone is useful only as adjunctive therapy in Cushing's disease. Ann Intern Med 1978; 89:128–130.

1631. Stalla GK, Stalla J, Huber M, et al. Ketoconazole inhibits corticotropic cell function in vitro. Endocrinology 1988; 122:618–623.

1632. McCance DR, Hadden DR, Kennedy L, et al. Clinical experience with ketoconazole as a therapy for patients with Cushing's syndrome. Clin Endocrinol (Oxf) 1987; 27:593–599.

1633. Semple CG, Beastall GH, Gray CE, et al. Trilostane in the management of Cushing's syndrome. Acta Endocrinol 1983; 102:107–110.

1634. Santen RJ, Wells SA, Runic S, et al. Adrenal suppression with aminoglutethimide. I. Differential effects of aminoglutethimide on glucocorticoid metabolism as a rationale for use of hydrocortisone. J Clin Endocrinol Metab 1977; 45:469–479.

1635. Amado JA, Pesquera C, Gonzalez EM, et al. Successful treatment with ketoconazole of Cushing's syndrome in pregnancy. Postgrad Med J 1990; 66:221–223.

1636. Bertagna X, Bertagna C, Laudat MH, et al. Pituitary-adrenal response to the antiglucocorticoid action of RU 486 in Cushing's syndrome. J Clin Endocrinol Metab 1986; 63:639–643.

1637. Invitti C, de Martin M, Brunani A, et al. Treatment of Cushing's syndrome with the long-acting somatostatin analogue SMS 201-995 (sandostatin). Clin Endocrinol (Oxf) 1990; 32:275–281.

1638. Stalla GK, Brockmeier SJ, Renner U, et al. Octreotide exerts different effects in vivo and in vitro in Cushing's disease. Eur J Endocrinol 1994; 130:125–131.

1639. Lufkin EG, Wahner HW, Bergstralh EJ. Reversibility of steroid-induced osteoporosis. Am J Med 1988; 85:887–888.

1640. Wicks IP, Calligeros D, Kidson W, et al. Cushing's disease presenting with avascular necrosis of the femoral heads and complicated by pituitary apoplexy. Ann Rheum Dis 1987; 46:783–786.

1641. Karl M, Von Wichert G, Kempter E, et al. Nelson's syndrome associated with a somatic frame shift mutation in the glucocorticoid receptor gene. J Clin Endocrinol Metab 1996; 81:124–129.

1642. Kemink L, Pieters G, Hermus A, et al. Patient's age is a simple predictive

factor for the development of Nelson's syndrome after total adrenalectomy for Cushing's disease. J Clin Endocrinol Metab 1994; 79:887–889.

1643. Kasperlik-Zaluska AA, Nielubowicz J, Wisawski J, et al. Nelson's syndrome: incidence and prognosis. Clin Endocrinol (Oxf) 1983; 19:693–698.

1644. Rahn T, Thoren M, Hall K, et al. Stereotactic radiosurgery in the treatment of MB Cushing. In: Szikla G, ed. Sterotactic Cerebral Irradiation. INSERM Symp No. 12. Amsterdam: Elsevier/North Holland Biomedical Press, 1979: 207–212.

1645. Aronin N, Krieger DT. Sustained remission of Nelson's syndrome after stopping cyproheptadine treatment. N Engl J Med 1980; 302:453–455.

1646. Dickstein G, Spindel A, Shechner C, et al. Spontaneous remission in Cushing's disease. Arch Intern Med 1991; 151:185–189.

1647. Ishibashi M, Shimada K, Abe K, et al. Spontaneous remission in Cushing's disease. Arch Intern Med 1993; 153:251–255.

1648. DeBold CR, Mufson EE, Menefee JK, et al. Proopiomelanocortin gene expression in a pheochromocytoma using upstream transcription initiation sites. Biochem Biophys Res Commun 1988; 155:895–900.

1649. de Keyzer Y, Bertagna X, Lenne F, et al. Altered proopiomelanocortin gene expression in adrenocorticotropin-producing nonpituitary tumors. J Clin Invest 1985; 76:1892–1898.

1650. Texier P-L, de Keyzer Y, Lacave R, et al. Proopiomelanocortin gene expression in normal and tumoral human lung. J Clin Endocrinol Metab 1991; 73:414–420.

1651. Picon A, Leblond-Francillard M, Raffin-Sanson ML, et al. Functional analysis of the human pro-opiomelanocortin promoter in the small cell lung carcinoma cell line DMS-79. J Mol Endocrinol 1995; 15:187–194.

1652. Odell WD. Ectopic ACTH secretion: a misnomer. Endocrinol Metab Clin North Am 1991; 20:371–379.

1653. Garroway NW, Orth DN, Harrison RW. Binding of cytosol receptor–glucocorticoid complexes by isolated nuclei of glucocorticoid-responsive and nonresponsive cultured cells. Endocrinology 1976; 98:1100–1100.

1654. Gaitan D, DeBold CR, Turney MK, et al. Glucocorticoid receptor structure and function in an adrenocorticotropin-secreting small cell lung cancer. Mol Endocrinol 1995; 9:1193–1201.

1655. Clark AJL, Stewart MF, Lavender PM, et al. Defective glucocorticoid regulation of proopiomelanocortin gene expression and peptide secretion in a small cell lung cancer cell line. J Clin Endocrinol Metab 1990; 70:485–490.

1656. Stewart PM, Gibson S, Crosby SR, et al. ACTH precursors characterize the ectopic ACTH syndrome. Clin Endocrinol (Oxf) 1994; 40:199–204.

1657. Orth DN, Nicholson WE, Mitchell WM, et al. Biologic and immunologic characterization and physical separation of ACTH and ACTH fragments in the ectopic ACTH syndrome. J Clin Invest 1973; 52:1756–1769.

1658. Bertagna X, Lenne F, Comar D, et al. Human β-melanocyte stimulating hormone revisited. Proc Natl Acad Sci U S A 1986; 83:9719–9723.

1659. Howlett TA, Drury PL, Perry L, et al. Diagnosis and management of ACTH-dependent Cushing's syndrome: comparison of the features in ectopic and pituitary ACTH production. Clin Endocrinol (Oxf) 1986; 24:699–713.

1660. Vieau D, Massias JF, Girard F, et al. Corticotrophin-like intermediary lobe peptide as a marker of alternate pro-opiomelanocortin processing in ACTH-producing non-pituitary tumours. Clin Endocrinol (Oxf) 1989; 31:691–700.

1661. Ulick S, Wang JZ, Blumenfeld JD, et al. Cortisol inactivation overload: a mechanism of mineralocorticoid hypertension in the ectopic adrenocorticotropin syndrome. J Clin Endocrinol Metab 1992; 74:963–967.

1662. Stewart PM, Murry BA, Mason JI. Human kidney 11β-hydroxysteroid dehydrogenase is a high affinity nicotinamide adenine dinucleotide-dependent enzyme and differs from the cloned type I isoform. J Clin Endocrinol Metab 1994; 79:480–484.

1663. Walker BR, Campbell JC, Fraser R, et al. Mineralocorticoid excess and inhibition of 11β-hydroxysteroid dehydrogenase in patients with ectopic ACTH syndrome. Clin Endocrinol (Oxf) 1992; 37:483–492.

1664. Rusvai E, Naray-Fejes-Toth A. A new isoform of 11β-hydroxysteroid dehydrogenase in aldosterone target cells. J Biol Chem 1993; 268:10717–10720.

1665. Doppman JL, Pass HI, Nieman LK, et al. Detection of ACTH-producing bronchial carcinoid tumors: MR imaging vs CT. AJR Am J Roentgenol 1991; 156:39–43.

1666. Estopinan V, Varela C, Riobo P, et al. Ectopic Cushing's syndrome with periodic hormonogenesis: a case suggesting a pathogenetic mechanism. Postgrad Med J 1987; 63:887–889.

1667. Stewart PM, Venn P, Heath DA, et al. Cyclical Cushing's syndrome. Br J Hosp Med 1992; 48:186–187.

1668. Howlett TA, Rees LH, Besser GM. Cushing's syndrome. Clin Endocrinol Metab 1985; 14:911–945.

1669. Malchoff CD, Orth DN, Abboud C, et al. Ectopic ACTH syndrome caused by a bronchial carcinoid tumor responsive to dexamethasone, metyrapone, and corticotropin-releasing factor. Am J Med 1988; 84:760–764.

1670. de Keyzer Y, Lenne F, Auzan C, et al. The pituitary V3 vasopressin receptor and the corticotroph phenotype in ectopic ACTH syndrome. J Clin Invest 1996; 97:1311–1318.

1671. Tabarin A, San Galli F, Dezou S, et al. The corticotropin-releasing factor test in the differential diagnosis of Cushing's syndrome: a comparison with the lysine-vasopressin test. Acta Endocrinol 1990; 123:331–338.

1672. Schteingart DE, Conn JW, Orth DN, et al. Secretion of ACTH and β-

changes in neuropeptide expression.[14] Neither the sequence of developmental events nor the identification of all neurotrophic factors leading to the development of mature chromaffin cells and sympathetic neurons is precisely defined (see Fig. 13–4).

NEUROTROPHINS

Like nerve cells within the CNS, protoadrenergic neurons are produced in abundance, but only a minority eventually become terminally differentiated sympathetic neurons. The others undergo apoptosis, the process of programmed cell death.[15] The elaboration of specific neuron survival factors by peripheral target tissues prevents apoptosis from occurring in all precursor cells. Neurotrophins, the best known of these survival factors, are a family of homologous proteins produced by the innervated tissue that act in a paracrine manner to prevent apoptosis in adrenergic neurons.[16] Members of this family include NGF, brain-derived neurotrophic factor (BDNF), neurotrophin-3 (NT-3) and neurotrophin-4/5 (NT-4/5), among others, although only NGF and NT-3 are specifically linked to the preservation of sympathetic innervation in vivo.[17–19]

Neurotrophins exert other effects in addition to suppression of apoptosis. During fetal development these factors, along with other growth factors like bFGF, insulin, and insulin-like growth factor I (IGF-I), promote proliferation of adrenergic neurons,[11, 20] although preservation of neuronal cell populations in sympathetic ganglia during postnatal life results more from a reduction in cell loss than from an increase in neuronal division.[21] In mature neurons the neurotrophins induce sprouting of dendrites and increased arborization of the network of sympathetic fibers in innervated tissues.[20, 22] Consequently, the density of sympathetic innervation, reflected in tissue NE levels, correlates with NGF protein expression in peripheral tissues.[23, 24]

In addition to production by target tissues in some species, NGF is synthesized and released from salivary glands.[25] Although NGF is secreted principally into saliva,[26] it is absorbed by intestinal transport[27] and exerts systemic effects after oral administration in neonatal animals.[28] In adult animals, salivary glands are an important source of NGF in the circulation.[29]

Sympathetic Nervous System

The peripheral sympathetic nerves originate from neurons in the paravertebral and preaortic ganglia (see Fig. 13–3). Small, nonmyelinated postganglionic fibers arising from these ganglia are distributed widely to the viscera and blood vessels. In sympathetically innervated tissues, the sympathetic nerve endings ramify extensively and form a plexus of terminal fibers rather than discrete nerve endings. Each sympathetic nerve fiber appears to control many effector cells, and each effector cell is in turn innervated by many nerve fibers. Neurotransmitters are not distributed homogeneously in the nerve endings but rather show numerous discrete areas of high NE concentration (Fig. 13–5). These dense collections of neurotransmitter are called varicosities. In some mammalian species the length of the terminal fiber of a single sympathetic neuron is about 10 cm, and each neuron contains approximately 25,000 varicosities. The membrane-bound vesicles of the sympathetic nerve endings are about 50 nm in diameter, and many contain NE. The NE-containing granules, which have an electron-dense core, are concentrated in varicosities (Fig. 13–6). Each varicosity contains about 1000 granules, and each granule contains about 15,000 molecules of NE.

The peripheral sympathetic nerve endings synthesize and store NE and release it in response to sympathetic nerve

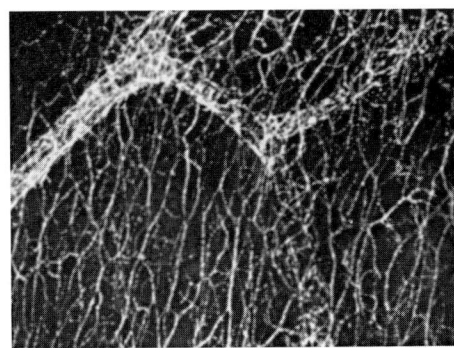

Figure 13–5. Peripheral adrenergic nerve endings demonstrated by fluorescence histochemical technique. The ground plexus of terminal sympathetic fibers is shown in a normal rat iris. The plexus is particularly dense around a heavily innervated arteriole that courses through the field. Numerous discrete areas of high norepinephrine concentration (varicosities) are visible. Magnification × 160. (From Malmfors T. Studies on adrenergic nerves. Acta Physiol Scand 1965; 64[Suppl 248]:7–93.)

impulses. The nerve endings also take up catecholamines from the extracellular fluid. These processes are described later.

COTRANSMITTERS AND NEUROMODULATORS

Central and peripheral adrenergic nerves contain additional chemical mediators that are stored and released along with NE,[30] including peptides (neuropeptide Y, somatostatin, substance P, galanin, and enkephalins), purines (ATP, adenosine), and amines (serotonin). These substances, when released with NE from adrenergic nerves, may act as neuromodulators or cotransmitters. The term *neuromodulation* refers to effects on transmitter release (prejunctional) or modification of the response of the effector tissue (postjunctional). The term *cotransmission* implies direct stimulation of the effector tissue by interaction with a specific (nonadrenergic) receptor.

Adrenal Medulla

The human adrenal medulla is enveloped within the adrenal cortex. The combined weight of the medullae from both

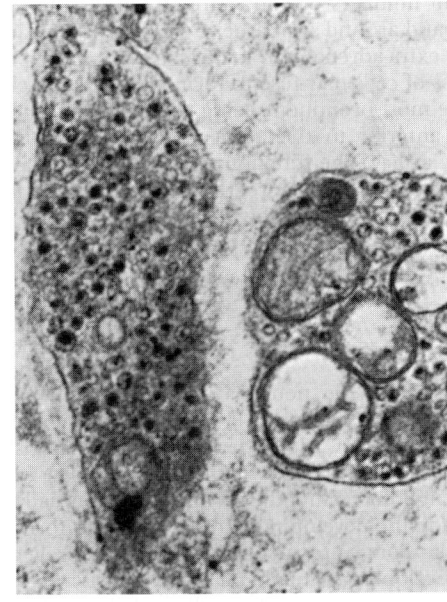

Figure 13–6. Electron photomicrograph of a sympathetic nerve ending in rat pineal gland. Note vesicles with electron-dense cores containing norepinephrine. Magnification × 45,000. (Courtesy of Dr. Floyd Bloom.)

glands is about 1.0 g, or 10% of the total adrenal mass. The adrenal medulla is composed almost entirely of chromaffin cells arranged in irregularly shaped polyhedrons that are organized into cords or small clumps and surrounded by nerves, connective tissue, and blood vessels. They contain numerous chromaffin granules, which are electron-dense vesicles 100 to 300 nm in diameter that resemble the granules of the sympathetic nerve endings (Fig. 13–7). These granules are important in the storage and secretion of catecholamines. Individual chromaffin cells contain large amounts of either NE or epinephrine; in humans 85% of the adrenomedullary catecholamine store is epinephrine. As with the sympathetic nerve endings, a variety of potential noncatecholamine mediators are also present in adrenomedullary chromaffin cells.

The blood supply of the adrenal gland is derived from three adrenal arteries: the superior artery is a branch of the inferior phrenic artery; the middle artery arises directly from the aorta; and the inferior artery arises from the renal artery. Cortical arteries supply the cortex from the subcapsular plexus, which drains centripetally toward the medulla; medullary arteries traverse the cortex and supply the medulla directly. In the zona reticularis the capillaries coalesce to form progressively larger venous sinuses that drain centrally.[31] Medullary capillaries arise from medullary arteries and join these venous channels,[32] which eventually form a single adrenal vein that usually drains into the vena cava on the right and into the renal vein on the left. Careful anatomic studies have failed to substantiate the thesis that a portal venous system exists in which steroid-rich cortical venous blood percolates around chromaffin cells of the medulla.[31, 32] The distribution of epinephrine- and NE-containing chromaffin cells also appears to be unrelated to the vascular anatomy, decreasing the likelihood that the phenotype of a chromaffin cell is determined by its spatial proximity to cortical venous blood.[33]

The adrenal medulla is innervated by typical cholinergic preganglionic sympathetic neurons in the splanchnic nerves that originate in the intermediolateral cell column between T-3 and L-3. The major portion of the innervation is from the ipsilateral greater splanchnic nerve (T5 through T9). In addition, postganglionic sympathetic fibers, either from ganglia in the sympathetic chain or from the suprarenal ganglion, innervate cortical blood vessels and possibly secretory tissue as well.[34] Spinal cord transections above T-3 are usually associated with deficient epinephrine secretion, whereas transections at a lower level may not influence epinephrine output.

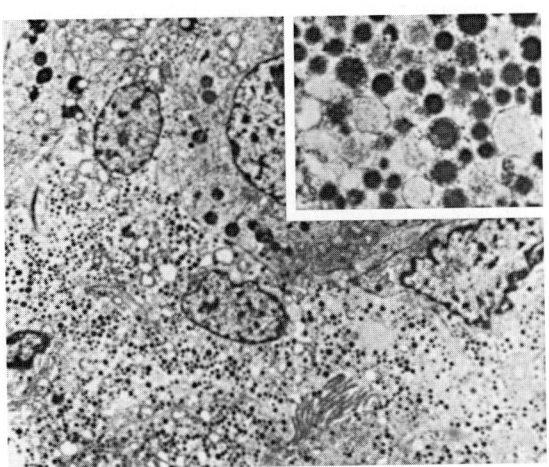

Figure 13–7. Electron photomicrograph of human adrenal medulla. Cells at the lower left containing small, electron-dense particles are adrenomedullary chromaffin cells with chromaffin granules; those above are adrenocortical cells. Magnification × 7250. Inset *(upper right)* shows chromaffin granules with clearly defined limiting membranes under higher magnification (× 50,000). (Courtesy of Dr. James Connolly.)

CATECHOLAMINES

Catecholamines in Mammalian Tissues

Catecholamines have a wide distribution in the plant and animal kingdoms.[35, 36] In higher vertebrates catecholamines are localized predominantly in the sympathetic neurons, the adrenal medulla, and the CNS. The level of catecholamines in mammalian adrenal is of the order of several millimoles per kilogram (several milligrams per gram) of tissue. The amounts of epinephrine in brain and sympathetic ganglia are small. NE, on the other hand, is widely distributed; it is found in the peripheral sympathetic nerves, in the CNS, and (in very small amounts) in the extra-adrenal chromaffin cells, in addition to the adrenal medulla. Because virtually all NE outside the CNS and the adrenal gland is located in the sympathetic nerve endings, the NE content of a particular tissue reflects the extent of its sympathetic innervation. Heavily innervated organs such as heart have NE concentrations in the range of 5 to 10 μmol/kg (1 to 2 μg/g) of tissue. The concentration in the nerve ending itself is much greater and has been estimated to be in the range of 5 to 50 mmol/kg (1 to 10 mg/g) of nerve cytoplasm. In the brain the concentration of NE is greatest in the hypothalamus, with somewhat lower levels in the brain stem and other regions.

DA is also present in high concentrations in the brain, particularly in the basal ganglia and the median eminence. DA outside the CNS is present in specialized interneurons in the sympathetic ganglia (in SIF cells, discussed previously), in the carotid body, and in some enterochromaffin cells. Lower levels of DA are found in peripheral nerves. The extent to which this represents DA stored in typical sympathetic nerve endings or in distinct dopaminergic neurons is uncertain.

The regulation of physiological processes by catecholamines is mediated by both sympathetic nerves and the adrenal medulla. The concentration of catecholamines in the sympathoadrenal system remains relatively constant despite marked changes in the level of sympathetic activity. This steady state is the result of a careful balance among catecholamine biosynthesis, storage, release, and reuptake.

Catecholamine Biosynthesis

Biosynthetic Pathway

The major pathway for the biosynthesis of catecholamines is shown in Figure 13–8.[37] The precursor tyrosine can be derived from dietary sources or synthesized from phenylalanine in the liver. It is uncertain whether specific uptake processes for tyrosine exist in adrenergic structures, but there is no evidence that tyrosine uptake is rate-limiting.

TYROSINE HYDROXYLASE. TH (EC 1.14.16.2) catalyzes the conversion of tyrosine to 3,4-dihydroxyphenylalanine (dopa) and requires iron (Fe^{+2}), molecular oxygen, and a reduced pteridine cofactor (tetrahydrobiopterin) for activity.[38] The cofactor is oxidized in the reaction and is subsequently regenerated by the enzyme dihydropteridine reductase. TH exists in both cytoplasmic and membrane-bound forms and is expressed only in tissues that synthesize catecholamines.[39] At physiological tyrosine levels, TH is probably saturated with regard to tyrosine but not with regard to the pteridine cofactor. The hydroxylation of tyrosine is the rate-limiting step in the biosynthetic pathway; regulation of catecholamine biosynthesis involves changes in either the activity of TH or its rate of synthesis. TH is inhibited by catechols (dopa, NE, DA), which act as competitive antagonists for activation by the reduced pteridine cofactor.

TH exists as a homotetramer and therefore is structurally and functionally related to the hydroxylases for phenylalanine

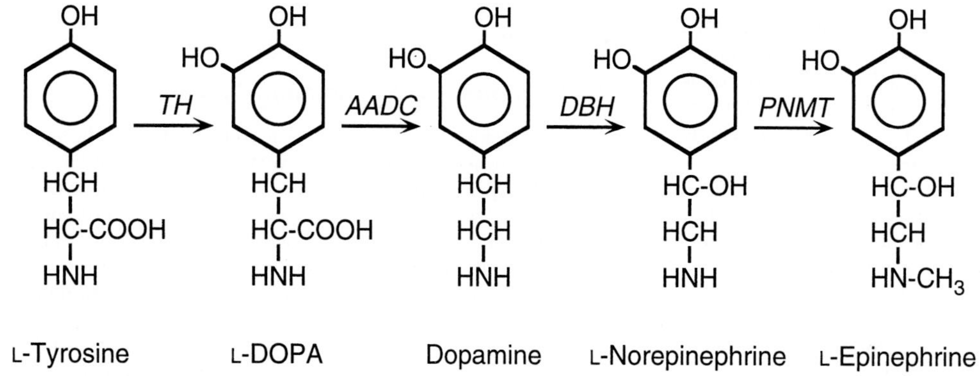

Figure 13–8. Biosynthetic pathway for catecholamines. Tyrosine hydroxylase (TH), aromatic-L-amino acid decarboxylase (AADC), and dopamine β-hydroxylase (DBH) catalyze formation of NE from tyrosine. Subsequent formation of epinephrine, catalyzed by phenylethanolamine-N-methyltransferase (PNMT), takes place in the adrenal medulla and in neurons of the CNS and peripheral ganglia that use epinephrine as a neurotransmitter.

and tryptophan, which also require Fe^{+2} and the tetrahydrobiopterin cofactor for activity. Each subunit of about 60 kd is assumed to contain a catalytic center at the COOH-terminal end that binds substrates and cofactor and a regulatory site in the NH$_2$-terminal region.[38] Mutational analysis suggests that the subunits are held together through interactions among leucine zipper motifs in the COOH-terminal ends.[40] In human brain and adrenal medulla, four isoforms of TH arise from alternative splicing of a single primary transcript.[38] Nonhuman primates exhibit only two of these isoforms, and lower animals have only one.[41] The significance of multiple isoforms is unclear. The human TH gene is located on the short arm of chromosome 11.[42]

AROMATIC-L-AMINO ACID DECARBOXYLASE. AADC (EC 4.1.1.28) catalyzes the decarboxylation of dopa to DA. The enzyme exists as a dimer of identical subunits approximately 50 kd in size.[38] It requires pyridoxal phosphate as a cofactor, is located in the cytosol, and is expressed in nonneuronal as well as neuronal tissues. AADC decarboxylates a variety of aromatic amino acids in addition to dopa, including 5-hydroxytryptophan (to serotonin). Unlike the other reactions in catecholamine biosynthesis, which are limited to the sympathetic nerve endings and the adrenal medulla, the decarboxylation of circulating dopa occurs in non-neuronal tissues, with the local production of DA. Much of the DA in urine, for example, originates from the decarboxylation of circulating dopa in renal tubules. The human AADC gene is located on the short arm of chromosome 7.[43]

DOPAMINE β-HYDROXYLASE. DBH (EC 1.14.17.1) catalyzes the beta hydroxylation of the DA side chain to form NE. The enzyme is a glycoprotein composed of four identical 75-kd subunits with two copper ions each.[38] DBH requires molecular oxygen, uses ascorbate as a hydrogen donor, and is structurally related to TH. Like TH, DBH is expressed only in tissues that synthesize and store catecholamines. DBH and TH genes contain common regulatory elements and respond in parallel to NGF, glucocorticoids, and cAMP.[44] The enzyme is not specific for DA and beta hydroxylates a variety of phenylethylamines. DBH is located in the granulated vesicles of sympathetic nerve endings and the chromaffin granules of the adrenomedullary chromaffin cells, where it is both a structural component in the granule wall and a soluble component inside the vesicle. Both forms are encoded by the same mRNA,[45] and the post-translational events giving rise to these two forms have not been defined. The soluble DBH fraction is released along with catecholamines during the neurosecretory process. DA or alternative substrates must be taken up into these storage particles before beta hydroxylation can occur. The human DBH gene is located on the long arm of chromosome 9 in close proximity to the ABO blood group locus.[46] This co-localization may account for genetic linkage between serum levels of DBH and the ABO blood group.[47]

PHENYLETHANOLAMINE N-METHYLTRANSFERASE.

PNMT (EC 2.1.1.28) catalyzes the N-methylation of NE to epinephrine. PNMT is a 30-kd monomeric cytosolic enzyme that is expressed only in epinephrine-containing cells of the adrenal medulla and in some neurons in the CNS and retina that use epinephrine as a neurotransmitter. S-Adenosylmethionine is the methyl donor. PNMT is not substrate specific for NE; it N-methylates a variety of phenylethanolamine derivatives. Adrenomedullary PNMT is inducible by glucocorticoids, by cholinergic stimulation through both nicotinic and muscarinic mechanisms,[48] and by angiotensin II. Corticotropin (ACTH) also increases PNMT activity by preventing PNMT degradation, possibly through an indirect action involving alterations in cofactor metabolism.[49] The human PNMT gene is located on the long arm of chromosome 17.[50]

REGULATION OF CATECHOLAMINE BIOSYNTHESIS

COUPLING OF CATECHOLAMINE RELEASE AND BIOSYNTHESIS. Stimulation of the adrenal medulla or of adrenergic nerves results in release of catecholamines without much change in the catecholamine content within the tissue. This stability of catecholamine levels in the face of enhanced release is the result of simultaneous increase in catecholamine biosynthesis. (In the peripheral sympathetic nerve ending, recapture of released NE also contributes to the constancy of NE stores, as described later.) Changes in catecholamine biosynthesis are coupled to nerve activity in two ways. In the short run, changes in the activity of TH adjust the rate of biosynthesis in parallel with that of catecholamine release. In the long run, a variety of factors induce TH synthesis, creating a greater reserve of enzyme for enhanced catecholamine biosynthesis.

ACTIVATION OF TYROSINE HYDROXYLASE. The rapid increase in tyrosine hydroxylation after neurally-mediated stimulation of catecholamine release does not require de novo protein synthesis. This change in enzyme activity is caused by alterations in the interactions among TH, catecholamines, and the pteridine cofactor.[39] Catecholamines normally are tightly bound to TH through coordination to FE^{+3}, limiting access of the cofactor to the active site.[51] TH, in turn, is a substrate for protein phosphorylation by any of a number of protein kinases and undergoes phosphorylation at multiple sites.[39] Phosphorylation, specifically at serine-40, reduces TH affinity for catecholamines, increases binding of cofactor, and enhances enzyme activity.[52, 53]

This model of regulation of TH activity by acute alterations in catecholamine and cofactor binding helps explain discordant changes in enzyme activity with alterations in catecholamine release. In some circumstances TH activity does not increase appreciably despite catecholamine depletion, and in others TH activity increases in the absence of nerve stimulation. Furthermore, phosphorylation of serine-40 is common to many intracellular signaling pathways, possibly accounting for

for the diversity of physiological and pharmacological stimuli that increase TH activity.[39]

INDUCTION OF TYROSINE HYDROXYLASE. Prolonged stimulation of the sympathoadrenal system increases the amount of TH in the adrenal medulla and sympathetic nerves by a process termed *trans-synaptic induction*. Induction of TH is presumably secondary to preganglionic release of acetylcholine, because it can be abolished by denervation of the adrenal, decentralization of sympathetic ganglia, or pharmacologic ganglionic blockade.[54] Stimulation of postganglionic sympathetic neurons, however, does not induce long-term changes in TH, although it increases TH activity acutely.[55, 56] Factors other than acetylcholine also stimulate TH synthesis, including NGF, glucocorticoids, angiotensin II, androgens, and neuropeptide Y. The importance of these factors for regulation of TH synthesis is unclear, although the effects of NGF and angiotensin II are additive to those of nerve activity.[57] The synthesis of TH presumably reflects interactions with regulatory elements in the promoter region of the TH gene, including a cAMP response element and an AP-1 site; the former is implicated in TH induction by nicotine,[58] and the latter is involved in induction by cold exposure.[59] Increase in TH increases the capacity of sympathetic neurons or chromaffin cells to synthesize catecholamines in response to physiological demand.

ALTERATIONS IN TETRAHYDROBIOPTERIN. Because tetrahydrobiopterin is present in subsaturating amounts, TH activity depends on the availability of cofactor under conditions of heightened demand. In vitro, induction of the biosynthetic enzymes for tetrahydrobiopterin occurs in parallel with that of TH,[60] and cofactor levels within the adrenal medulla increase in response to neural stimulation.[61]

CATECHOLAMINE UPTAKE INTO SUBCELLULAR STORAGE PARTICLES. The location of DBH within the catecholamine storage particles in adrenergic neurons and adrenal medulla means that DA must be taken up into these particles before beta hydroxylation to NE can occur. Uptake into these particles is stereospecific, energy-requiring, saturable, and competitive with regard to substrate. ATP and magnesium are required. This particle uptake process is unrelated to the axonal membrane uptake process; both of these processes are described later. Nerve stimulation leads to trans-synaptic induction of both DBH and the amine carrier but not of all granule constituents.[62]

In adrenergic neurons and NE-containing chromaffin cells the NE formed from DA is stored in the granule. In epinephrine-containing adrenomedullary chromaffin cells the situation is more complex. Because PNMT is localized in the cytosol, the NE that is formed in the chromaffin granule must leave the granule for *N*-methylation to epinephrine, which in turn must re-enter the granule for storage. Granular uptake may protect DA from oxidative deamination by monoamine oxidase (MAO), because DA is a better substrate for MAO than either NE or epinephrine and therefore is more liable to enzymatic destruction.

ROLE OF ADRENAL CORTEX IN BIOSYNTHESIS OF EPINEPHRINE

Activity of rat adrenal PNMT, the epinephrine-forming enzyme, is reduced by hypophysectomy and restored by pharmacologic but not by physiological doses of glucocorticoids.[63] Because transcription of PNMT is also induced by glucocorticoids, the view is widely held that high levels of glucocorticoids in cortical venous blood percolating through the adrenal medulla are required both for initial induction of PNMT and for subsequent maintenance of adrenal epinephrine synthesis. Moreover, epinephrine-containing, PNMT-positive chromaffin cells contain glucocorticoid receptors, but NE-containing,

PNMT-negative cells do not.[64] Although the role of fetal glucocorticoids in the expression of the PNMT-positive phenotype is unclear,[65–67] the spatial distribution of epinephrine- and NE-containing medullary cells does not reflect proximity to venous channels.[31, 33] Furthermore, changes in PNMT activity in response to glucocorticoids or during postnatal development do not always correspond to alterations in PNMT mRNA,[67–69] suggesting that the role of glucocorticoids in the maintenance of epinephrine synthesis may involve both post-transcriptional and transcriptional controls. One potential mechanism is stabilization of PNMT itself through alterations in metabolism of the co-substrate *S*-adenosylmethionine.[49] Nonetheless, PNMT activity is not known to be rate-limiting in epinephrine biosynthesis, and a direct regulatory role for glucocorticoids in epinephrine synthesis or secretion cannot be inferred.

Catecholamine Storage and Release

The processes of catecholamine storage and release are similar in the sympathetic nerve endings and in the adrenal medulla and also share common features with mechanisms of hormone secretion in other neural and endocrine cells. The sympathetic nerve ending, by virtue of its relation to the adrenergic synapse and the effector tissue, is subject to local regulatory influences that affect the adrenal medulla to a lesser degree.

ADRENAL MEDULLA

A pair of normal human adrenals contains about 33 μmol (6 mg) of catecholamine in the chromaffin granules. Approximately 10,000 to 30,000 chromaffin granules are present in each chromaffin cell.

CHROMAFFIN GRANULES. It was established in 1953 that catecholamines are localized predominantly in a particulate fraction.[70] The chromaffin granules are electron-dense, membrane-bound vesicles between 50 and 350 nm in diameter (see Fig. 13–7) that are analogous to the secretory vesicles of neural and endocrine cells (Table 13–1).[70] Chromaffin cells also contain synaptic-like microvesicles, although their role is currently undefined.[71] The chromaffin granules contain both small molecules and proteins, but in molar terms catecholamines are the most abundant species in the granules, followed by ATP, ascorbic acid, and calcium.[72] The ascorbic acid present is predominantly (>90%) in the reduced form, functioning as an antioxidant to preserve the catecholamine store and as a source of electrons for DBH in the synthesis of NE from DA.

The protein in the granules consists of soluble and insoluble components, the soluble fraction being released during exocytosis or on hypotonic lysis of the granules. About 80% of the protein is soluble; the remainder is associated with the limiting membrane of the chromaffin granule. DBH is present in both soluble and insoluble fractions and is the major protein of the granule membrane.[73] Proteins involved in granular transport functions and in exocytosis are also present in chromaffin granule membranes, and most of the soluble proteins belong to the enkephalin or chromogranin protein families. Post-translational processing of both enkephalins and chromogranins occurs during storage within the granule.[74] Neuropeptide Y, neurotensin, substance P, and galanin have been identified as well.

Chromogranins was the name given to the soluble proteins isolated from chromaffin granules more than 25 years ago.[70] This family of acidic glycoproteins is a component of large dense-core vesicles (LDVs), which are widely distributed in endocrine as well as nervous tissue.[75] The most abundant of these proteins in bovine chromaffin granules is chromogranin-A. Chromogranin-B and chromogranin-C (secretogranins I and II, respectively[76]) are present in lower concentrations. In

TABLE 13–1. Secretory Vesicles in Chromaffin Cells, Adrenergic Neurons, and Endocrine Secretory Cells

	Small Synaptic Vesicles (SSV)	Small Dense-Core Vesicles (SDV)	Large Dense-Core Vesicles (LDV)
Size (diameter)	50 nm	50 nm	70–200 nm
Appearance on electron microscopy	Translucent core	Electron-dense core	Electron-dense core
Soluble contents	Nonpeptide neurotransmitters, including biogenic amines	Norepinephrine, nucleotides, dopamine β-hydroxylase*	Biogenic amines, chromogranins, neuropeptides, nucleotides, peptide-processing enzymes, secretogranins, dopamine β-hydroxylase*
Vesicle membrane proteins	ATPase proton pumps, neurotransmitter transporters, vesicle proteins for exocytosis	ATPase proton pumps, neurotransmitter transporters, cytochrome b-561, vesicle proteins for exocytosis, dopamine β-hydroxylase*	ATPase proton pumps, neurotransmitter transporters, cytochrome b-561, glycoproteins, vesicle proteins for exocytosis, dopamine β-hydroxylase*
Location:			
Adrenal medulla	Neurotransmitter storage and secretion?	—	Chromaffin granules
Adrenergic nerves	—	Neurotransmitter release at active zones	LDV of sympathetic nerves
Endocrine secretory cells	Synaptic-like microvesicles	—	Secretory granules

*Present only in granules of adrenergic neurons and chromaffin cells.

the human chromogranin-B predominates.[77] Chromogranins are present in the parathyroids, anterior pituitary, thyroid (parafollicular or C cells), and pancreatic islets, but the adrenal medulla contains the largest store of chromogranin-A.[75] The precise function of chromogranin-A remains unknown; it possibly plays a role in stabilization of catecholamines within the granule.[78] Several of its proteolytic products exert inhibitory effects on hormone secretion; chromostatin, a 20-amino-acid peptide, inhibits adrenal medullary responses to cholinergic stimulation.[79]

After DBH, cytochrome b-561 is the second most common membrane protein; it is involved in transmembrane electron transport linking the ascorbic acid cycle with DBH and other mono-oxygenases.[70] The membrane proteins include two distinct ATPases, one of which (ATPase I) translocates protons from the cytoplasm to the interior matrix.[62] In addition to protein carriers for amines and nucleotides, chromaffin granule membranes also contain several glycoproteins and other vesicular proteins that may be involved in the intracellular transport of organelles or in exocytosis.[70]

UPTAKE AND STORAGE IN CHROMAFFIN GRANULES. The catecholamine store within the chromaffin granule is maintained by synthesis, active uptake from the cytosol, and storage in a poorly characterized intragranular complex. Several aspects of these processes are summarized in Figure 13–9. A critical feature is the inwardly directed H^+-ATPase, which maintains a steep electrochemical proton gradient because the granule membrane has a low ionic permeability.[80] The energy is derived from ATP, which translocates two protons per ATP molecule hydrolyzed. The acidic internal pH (approximately 5.5) tends to trap intragranular catecholamines in a protonated form.

The proton gradient alone is not sufficient to explain amine uptake into the granules, a process that is stereospecific, saturable, and inhibited by reserpine and related compounds. Amine uptake depends on specific carrier proteins.[81, 82] Two distinct vesicle monoamine transporters have been identified in rats, one in chromaffin granules and the other in brain (VMAT1 and VMAT2, respectively). Although both transporters map to separate chromosomes in humans, at present only transporters similar to VMAT2 have been identified in humans.[83] The vesicle monoamine transporters share sequence homology with transport proteins that are found in microorganisms and confer multidrug resistance.[81, 83] These vesicular transporters, like neurotransmitter transport proteins in the plasma membrane, contain 12 membrane-spanning domains.[84] The energy for vesicular uptake is provided by the proton gradient established by the H^+ transporter and the impermeable granule membrane (see Fig. 13–9). This is in contrast to transport of neurotransmitter across the plasma membrane,

which is sodium dependent. In chromaffin granules the egress of H^+ along its concentration gradient is coupled to amine uptake against a huge concentration gradient.[83]

Osmotic requirements necessitate an intragranular storage mechanism, because the concentration of catecholamines within the granule (0.55 mol/L) would cause osmotic rupture if they existed free in solution.[80] Although the nature of the storage complex is not known, ATP may be involved for the following reasons: (1) ATP in the chromaffin granules is metabolically inert; (2) the molar ratio of catecholamine to ATP is approximately 4:1; and (3) ATP forms complexes with catecholamines in vitro in the presence of calcium. These findings suggest that catecholamines interact with ATP in some rapidly reversible way involving positively charged catecholamine mol-

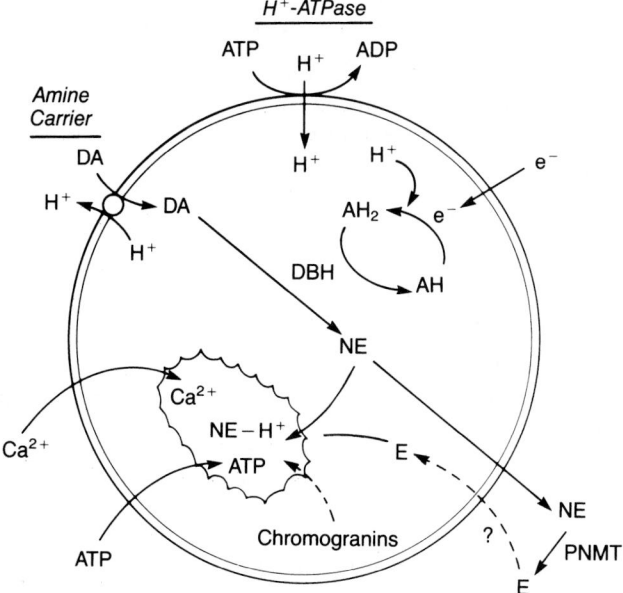

Figure 13–9. Schematic representation of a chromaffin granule. The amine carrier for dopamine (DA) and other catecholamines, H^+-ATPase, electron shuttle (e^-), and uptake processes for calcium and ATP are shown in the granule membrane, along with a putative process for epinephrine (E) uptake linked to norepinephrine (NE) egress. Stoichiometric relations are not shown. AH_2 refers to reduced ascorbate, which is an essential cofactor for dopamine β-hydroxylase (DBH), which is regenerated by the electron shuttle. Calcium, ATP, catecholamines in protonated form, and chromogranins participate in a poorly understood storage complex. Synthesis of E occurs in the cytoplasm and therefore requires translocation of NE and uptake of E for storage within the granule. Although the energetics of a linkage between NE egress (down a huge concentration gradient) and E uptake appear to be quite favorable, conclusive evidence for such a process has not appeared.

ecules with negatively charged sites on ATP. However, ATP-catecholamine–divalent cation complexes can account for only a portion of the catecholamine store; chromogranins and other as yet undefined factors may be involved in intragranular macromolecular binding.[78]

The chromaffin granule membrane also plays an important role in the synthesis of NE from DA. Optimum synthetic rates depend on the local concentration of reduced ascorbate, which is an essential cofactor for DBH; reduced ascorbate is oxidized to semidehydroascorbate during the synthesis of NE. Activity of soluble DBH within the granule depends on the intragranular concentration of reduced ascorbate, whereas the activity of vesicle membrane-bound DBH depends more on the cytoplasmic concentration.[85] Regeneration of reduced ascorbate within the granule occurs by means of a transmembrane electron shuttle because transport of ascorbate itself across the granule membrane is inefficient.[86] Cytochrome b-561 may be involved in this transfer.[80]

ATP and calcium levels are maintained within chromaffin granules against high concentration gradients.[80] The transport of ATP and calcium into the granule is poorly understood.

As noted previously, the synthesis of epinephrine requires transport of NE from the chromaffin granule into the cytosol, where PNMT is localized, and subsequent reuptake of epinephrine. The cytoplasmic synthesis of epinephrine suggests the possibility of an exchange mechanism coupling NE efflux down its concentration gradient with epinephrine uptake, although supportive evidence is inconclusive.[80]

RELEASE BY EXOCYTOSIS. The principal physiological stimulus for catecholamine release from the adrenomedullary chromaffin cell is acetylcholine that originates in the preganglionic sympathetic nerve endings. Acetylcholine acts on nicotinic receptors to induce depolarization of the chromaffin cell; this in turn increases its permeability to calcium.[87] The increase in intracellular calcium is sufficient to trigger catecholamine secretion, which involves extrusion of the soluble contents of the chromaffin granule into the extracellular space (exocytosis; Fig. 13–10). The following evidence has been marshaled in support of this mechanism: (1) the major soluble macromolecular constituents of the chromaffin granule—ATP, chromogranins, DBH, and the opioid peptides (enkephalins)—are released along with catecholamines in proportion to their concentration in the soluble fraction of the chromaffin granule; (2) cytoplasmic macromolecules are not simulta-neously released; (3) the major insoluble (membrane) components of the chromaffin granules are retained in the chromaffin cell; and (4) in certain species extrusion of granule contents has been demonstrated by electron microscopy. These observations demonstrate that the soluble contents of the granule are extruded through a temporary defect in the cell membrane, with retention of the structural granule components. Secretion of catecholamines from single chromaffin cells is quantal, which is consistent with all-or-none release of the contents of individual chromaffin granules.[88, 89]

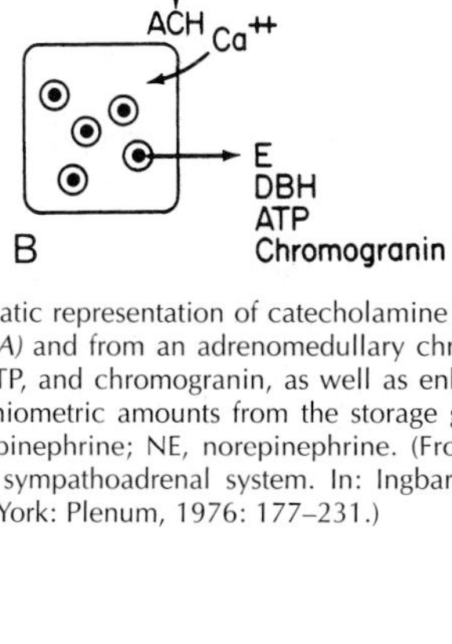

Several components of the cellular mechanisms involved in the triggering of exocytosis have been identified. Chromaffin cells contain a network of actin filaments beneath the plasma membrane. Although a few granules normally are present in this region, most are excluded. In response to stimulation the actin network is disassembled to permit access of granules to the plasma membrane and subsequent exocytotic fusion of granule and plasma membranes.[90] Actin reorganization is activated by calcium entry, which may transiently achieve concentrations of 100 μmol/L within the immediate vicinity of the plasma membrane, or by protein kinase C.[87] Actin disassembly is necessary but not sufficient for exocytosis; interactions among membrane proteins on the chromaffin granule and those on the inner surface of the cell membrane promote the docking of granules and subsequent exocytosis. Members of the annexin family of calcium-binding proteins (e.g., synexin, annexin II) and other vesicular or nucleotide-binding proteins may be participants in these processes.[90, 91] The chromaffin granule membranes are retrieved from the plasma membrane after exocytosis and recycled into newly formed chromaffin granules.

Chromaffin cells also possess receptors for hormones, neurotransmitters, and metabolic substances.[87] These factors affect catecholamine secretion in vitro primarily through alterations in calcium availability, but their importance in vivo is as yet undefined.

NEUROPEPTIDES OF THE ADRENAL MEDULLA. A large number of peptides have been identified in the mammalian adrenal medulla (Table 13–2). These peptides are stored both in the chromaffin granules of chromaffin cells and in the neurons innervating the adrenal medulla. Substantial variation in peptide expression exists among species, although the patterns do not differ demonstrably between epinephrine- and NE-containing chromaffin cells. Neuropeptides play at least three roles in adrenal medullary function. First, some peptides, vasoactive intestinal peptide (VIP) in particular, stimulate catecholamine secretion from chromaffin cells.[92] Second, other peptides, although not acting directly, modulate responses to acetylcholine. For example, chromostatin, neuropeptide Y, and the enkephalins reduce and substance P increases catecholamine responses to nicotinic receptor stimulation.[93–96] Third, in a few circumstances peptides released from the adrenal medulla exert systemic effects. Adrenal opioid peptides may mediate stress-associated analgesia and contribute to the regulation of cerebral blood flow and oxygen consumption.[97, 98] Neuropeptide Y from the adrenal medulla may provide blood pressure support during endotoxemia.[99]

SYMPATHETIC NERVES. NE in tissues that do not contain chromaffin cells is localized in the sympathetic nerve terminals. The concentration of NE within a particular tissue is a measure of the density of sympathetic innervation. Heavily innervated tissues such as myocardium contain about 6 μmol/kg (1 μg/g) of NE, whereas less well innervated tissues such as liver or skeletal muscle contain less than 10% of that amount.

STORAGE GRANULES. NE in sympathetic nerves is localized predominantly in small synaptic vesicles (approximately 50 nm in diameter) that are called small dense-core vesicles (SDVs) because they develop an electron-opaque core after tissue fixation (see Table 13–1). These vesicles are similar to

Figure 13–10. Schematic representation of catecholamine release from a sympathetic nerve ending *(A)* and from an adrenomedullary chromaffin cell *(B)*. Catecholamines, DBH, ATP, and chromogranin, as well as enkephalins (not shown), are released in stoichiometric amounts from the storage granule in response to nerve impulses. E, epinephrine; NE, norepinephrine. (From Landsberg L. Catecholamines and the sympathoadrenal system. In: Ingbar SH, ed. The Year in Endocrinology. New York: Plenum, 1976: 177–231.)

TABLE 13–2. Neuropeptides in Adrenal Medulla and Sympathetic Nerves

	Adrenal Medulla		Sympathetic Nerves	
Neuropeptide	Chromaffin Cells	Adrenal Nerves	Adrenergic Fibers	Cholinergic Fibers
Adrenomedullin	X	—	—	—
Calcitonin gene-related peptide	X	X	—	X
Chromogranins/secretogranins				
Chromogranin A	X	—	—	—
Chromostatin	X	—	—	—
Secretoneurin	X	—	—	—
Dynorphin	Adrenal medulla		X	—
Endothelins	Adrenal medulla		—	—
Enkephalins	X	X	X	—
Erythropoietin	Pheochromocytoma only		—	—
Galanin	X	X	X	—
Natriuretic peptides (A-, B-, and C-types)	X	—	—	—
Neuropeptide Y	X	X	X	—
Neurotensin	X	X	—	X
Parathyroid hormone-related protein	Adrenal medulla		—	—
Peptide histidine isoleucine or histidine methionine	—	—	—	X
Pituitary adenylate cyclase–activating peptide	—	X	—	X
Pro-opiomelanocortin–related peptides				
Corticotropin	Pheochromocytoma only		—	—
Corticotropin-releasing hormone	X	—	—	—
Endorphins	X	—	—	—
Somatostatin	X	X	X	—
Somatotropin-releasing hormone	Pheochromocytoma only		—	—
Substance P	X	X	—	X
Vasoactive intestinal peptide	X	X	—	X

other small synaptic vesicles (SSV) that take up and release neurotransmitters such as acetylcholine and glutamate. Because of their small size both SDVs and SSVs contain little protein other than those peptides required to concentrate the neurotransmitters and to regulate exocytosis, though SDVs appear also to contain DBH.[100] (Although NE storage vesicles have also been referred to as SSVs, the hybrid nature of NE-containing vesicles suggests that SDV may be a more accurate and less confusing term). Distinct from these small vesicles are the LDVs, 70 to 100 nm in diameter, that contain neuropeptides and monoamines and that are the neuronal counterpart to the chromaffin granule. LDVs are also found in nerve endings, although in less abundance.[101]

On the basis of different contents of membrane proteins, SSVs and LDVs appear to represent two distinct organelles, rather than one being a derivative of the other.[101] LDV membranes are made in the trans-Golgi network of the cell body and transported down the axon to the nerve terminal.[102, 103] SSVs may also originate in the trans-Golgi network or in the endosomes located near the nerve terminal.[102, 104] SDVs that contain DBH and cytochrome b-561, which are not normally present in SSVs, may be formed in the nerve terminal from components derived from both SSVs and LDVs.[62, 105] Although LDVs (or their constituent parts) must be returned to the cell body for recycling, the SDVs appear to be capable of refilling with NE many times. The refilling of SDVs may reflect local recycling of vesicle membrane rather than recycling of the intact vesicle, although the mechanism is not fully understood.

UPTAKE AND STORAGE IN SYNAPTIC VESICLES. Synaptic vesicles of the sympathetic nerve endings accumulate amines by a carrier-mediated process similar to that in adrenomedullary chromaffin granules. LDVs and SDVs also appear to possess the capacity to take up monoamines.[103] Energy for this amine transport process derives from the proton gradient established by a vesicular H^+-ATPase. The exchange of two H^+ ions for every cationic monoamine transported means that a pH gradient of 1.5 units and a vesicular membrane potential of 50 mV generates a monoamine gradient from inside to outside the vesicle of about 10,000:1.[83] Although the plasma membrane transport proteins are specific for DA, NE, or

serotonin (see later discussion), the synaptic vesicle amine transporter does not distinguish among cationic monoamines. Consequently, many hydroxylated phenylethylamines may be stored in the granules. Reserpine, guanethidine, and some sympathomimetic amines block vesicular uptake.

Unlike chromaffin granules, in which catecholamines are stored in complex form to limit the osmotic effects of high intravesicular concentrations, catecholamines in synaptic vesicles are stored in osmotic equilibrium with the cytoplasm.[106] In addition to catecholamines, synaptic vesicles and LDVs contain ATP. Under ordinary circumstances the storage granules are not filled to capacity; NE stores rise with reduction in impulse traffic.

RELEASE BY EXOCYTOSIS. The release of NE at the sympathetic nerve ending is triggered by depolarization of the axonal membrane by an action potential (see Fig. 13–10). Depolarization is followed by the influx of calcium. Although the molecular events consequent to calcium entry are not clearly established, they appear to involve phosphorylation of proteins on the cytoplasmic surface of the synaptic vesicle, including the synapsins, synaptophysin, and synaptotagmin.[107] NE release is presumed to occur by exocytosis for the following reasons: (1) electrophysiological properties of effector cells are consistent with quantal release of NE; (2) cytoplasmic NE, the level of which can be increased by pretreatment with an MAO inhibitor and reserpine, is not released by nerve impulses; (3) phenylethylamine derivatives that are stored in the granules (false transmitters) are released by nerve stimulation, and the proportion of false transmitter released reflects the proportion in the granule store; and (4) exocytotic structures have been identified in electron photomicrographs of bovine splenic nerve. Quantitative measures of NE release from a single site on a nerve ending support the hypothesis of quantal release of the entire contents of a single vesicle but indicate that the probability of releasing even a single vesicle in response to a nerve impulse is low. As impulse frequency increases, the probability of vesicular release rises, leading to facilitation in NE release.[108]

Because the interval between membrane depolarization and NE release by sympathetic nerves is short (less than 1 ms) compared with a lag time on the order of 50 ms for chromaffin cells,[89] the mechanisms of exocytosis in the two cell types must differ. First, NE release from sympathetic nerves occurs only at specialized sites on the presynaptic membrane, the so-called action zones. Second, the rapid, initial release of NE represents NE contained in vesicles already docked at release sites in the action zone.[107] Third, further release of NE after continued stimulation appears to reflect the movement of reserve vesicles to the plasma membrane and subsequent exocytosis.[107] The proportion of reserve vesicles within the nerve terminal in proximity to the action zones may be influenced by the phosphorylation state of the synaptic vesicle protein, synapsin I.[107]

This model of synaptic regulation explains several aspects of neuronal function. First, the storage pool of NE in sympathetic nerve endings is heterogeneous. Newly synthesized NE, for example, is released in preference to stored NE during stimulation of the sympathetic nerves.[109] Although the anatomic basis for this nonhomogeneity has not been established, proximity to the axonal membrane may be an important factor in differential release. Second, facilitation of transmitter release occurs in response to increased frequency of nerve impulses or activation of presynaptic receptors, both of which increase phosphorylation of synapsin I.[107]

FALSE NEUROTRANSMITTERS. Under certain circumstances, compounds other than NE can be stored in the sympathetic nerve endings. The lack of absolute specificity of the enzymes involved in catecholamine biosynthesis and in the mechanisms for granular uptake and storage permits the introduction of other compounds into the neurotransmitter pool. Storage of alternative transmitters may occur if MAO is inhibited or after administration of compounds that can be stored but are not substrates for MAO (e.g., metaraminol) or that are metabolized to such compounds (e.g., α-methyldopa, which forms α-methyldopamine and α-methylnorepinephrine). These compounds are released in response to nerve stimulation. Because almost all the false transmitters are less potent adrenergic agonists than NE, a sympatholytic effect is the usual result of false neurotransmitter accumulation. Under certain circumstances, epinephrine derived from the adrenal medulla may be stored in sympathetic nerve endings and released by sympathetic stimulation.

NOREPINEPHRINE RELEASE BY SYMPATHOMIMETIC AMINES. Indirect-acting sympathomimetic amines, such as tyramine and metaraminol, release NE from sympathetic nerve endings. To function as sympathomimetics, amines must be substrates for the axonal membrane transport process (see later discussion) and must mobilize NE from the granule store by competing with cytoplasmic NE for vesicular uptake.[110] The release of stored NE and the inhibition of NE reuptake by competition for the axonal membrane transport system are responsible for a major portion of the sympathomimetic effects of these agents. This mechanism of release is, however, different from NE release in response to nerve impulses. NE release by sympathomimetic amines does not require calcium, occurs from the cytoplasmic pool as well as from the storage granules, and is not associated with a concomitant release of DBH. Therefore, sympathomimetic amines do not release NE by exocytosis but appear to displace NE from storage sites and to promote its outward diffusion by facilitated exchange.

NEUROPEPTIDES OF THE SYMPATHETIC NERVOUS SYSTEM. The peptides stored in sympathetic nerve terminals (see Table 13–2) are found exclusively in LDVs and are released in response to nerve impulses. These neuropeptides may function as modulators that influence the prejunctional release or synthesis of NE or the postjunctional effector response to NE.[111] They may serve as cotransmitters by influencing the responses of effector tissues through interaction with specific nonadrenergic receptors. The peptides co-localized with NE

have specific distributions within the sympathetic nervous system.[30] Neuropeptide Y, for example, is distributed principally in sympathetic fibers innervating vascular structures. Although the distribution of other neuropeptides differs among mammalian species, the correspondence in the distribution of neuropeptides within populations of autonomic nerves has led to the concept of chemical coding of autonomic neurons—the idea that particular combinations of neurotransmitters and peptides subserve specific functions.[30]

Co-localized peptides and other mediators may play an important physiological role. The situation is complicated by the fact that these compounds have both prejunctional and postjunctional effects that may differ in their impact on a given adrenergic response. Neuropeptide Y decreases NE release prejunctionally, potentiates the effect of NE postjunctionally, and exerts a direct stimulatory effect on vascular smooth muscle.[111] Potential competition by different co-released modulators from the same nerve ending complicate the attempts to define the physiological role of these compounds. Also, because neuropeptides are not present in the synaptic vesicles that contain the preponderance of NE in sympathetic neurons, variations in impulse traffic (frequency and pattern) affect the release of neuropeptides and NE differently under different physiological circumstances.[112, 113] In addition, postsynaptic events may have different effects, depending on the transmitter mediating the response. For example, vasoconstrictor responses to sympathetic nerve stimulation are triphasic, possibly reflecting sequential effects of ATP, NE, and neuropeptide Y.[30]

NEUROPEPTIDE Y. This 36-amino-acid peptide is structurally related to pancreatic polypeptide and is stored and released with NE from sympathetic nerve endings that innervate the cardiovascular system.[114, 115] It is also stored in central neurons involved in the regulation of autonomic function and in the adrenal medulla. In peripheral sympathetic nerve endings it is found in the LDVs of perivascular sympathetic fibers and in the heart but not in fibers innervating exocrine glands and other structures. It is also present in nonadrenergic neurons innervating nonvascular structures. When infused exogenously, it exerts a potent pressor response that is not antagonized by adrenergic blockade.[114] It is released in response to sympathetic nerve stimulation, particularly when the stimulation frequency rate is high, and plasma levels are increased during sympathoadrenal stimulation in humans.[115] Compared with NE, the vasoconstrictor response to neuropeptide Y develops more slowly and is more prolonged. At the adrenergic synapse neuropeptide Y acts postjunctionally as a direct agonist and as a modulator that potentiates the effects of NE. The cerebral and coronary circulations may be particularly sensitive to the direct effects. Neuropeptide Y acts prejunctionally to decrease NE release.[114] These paradoxical prejunctional and postjunctional effects may conserve NE during periods of intense sympathetic stimulation.[114] In summary, neuropeptide Y appears to participate in cardiovascular responses mediated by the sympathetic nervous system.

GALANIN. This is a 29-amino-acid peptide that is amidated at its COOH terminus. Galanin originally was isolated from porcine intestine, and it shares little homology with other known peptides.[116] The peptide is found in the central nervous system, the adrenal medulla, the respiratory tract, the enteric nervous system, and the vascular adrenergic nerves.[30] Galanin causes contraction of intestinal smooth muscle and inhibits ion transport stimulated by electrical activation of submucosal neurons.[116, 117] Galanin is present in pancreatic sympathetic nerves and is released in response to electrical stimulation.[118, 119] Administration of the peptide induces mild hyperglycemia as a result of inhibition of insulin and stimulation of glucagon secretion.[116, 120] In the central nervous system

bind to the transporter. If the substrate also competes with NE for vesicular uptake, levels of NE in the cytoplasm rise, further increasing the binding of NE to the transporter on the inside of the plasma membrane. For any substrate for uptake-1 to elicit a sympathomimetic effect, the compound must also compete successfully with NE for vesicular uptake.[110]

EXTRANEURONAL UPTAKE. Although catecholamines induce physiological effects by interacting with specific receptors on the plasma membrane of effector cells (see later discussion), the formation of catecholamine metabolites in liver, kidney, lung, and gut implies catecholamine uptake into a wide variety of cells. The uptake-2 process is probably carrier-mediated because it exhibits stereospecificity for some substrates.[153] Uptake-2 differs from uptake-1 in having a preference for isoproterenol (a poor substrate for uptake-1) as substrate, in being highly sensitive to inhibition by glucocorticoids, and in being independent of extracellular levels of sodium and chloride.[153] Outward transport of catecholamines by uptake-2 occurs commonly, not under the special conditions required for uptake-1.[153] The carrier has not been iso-

lated, but it shares many features with organic cation transport in the renal tubule.[154]

METABOLIC PATHWAYS

The metabolic transformations of NE and epinephrine are shown in Figure 13-12, and the metabolites of dopa and DA are shown in Figure 13–13. The major changes include 3-O-methylation, oxidative deamination, and conjugation with sulfate and glucuronide. The combinations of uptake-1 with MAO and uptake-2 with COMT and MAO (COMT > MAO) form two separate metabolizing systems for the inactivation of neurally released and circulating catecholamines.[110]

MONOAMINE OXIDASE. MAO (EC 1.4.3.4) catalyzes the oxidative deamination of a variety of amines with production of the corresponding aldehydes, which are metabolized to their related carboxylic acids or alcohols by aldehyde dehydrogenase or alcohol dehydrogenase, respectively.

MAO is present in most tissues; the activity is low in skeletal muscle and blood and high in liver, kidney, intestine,

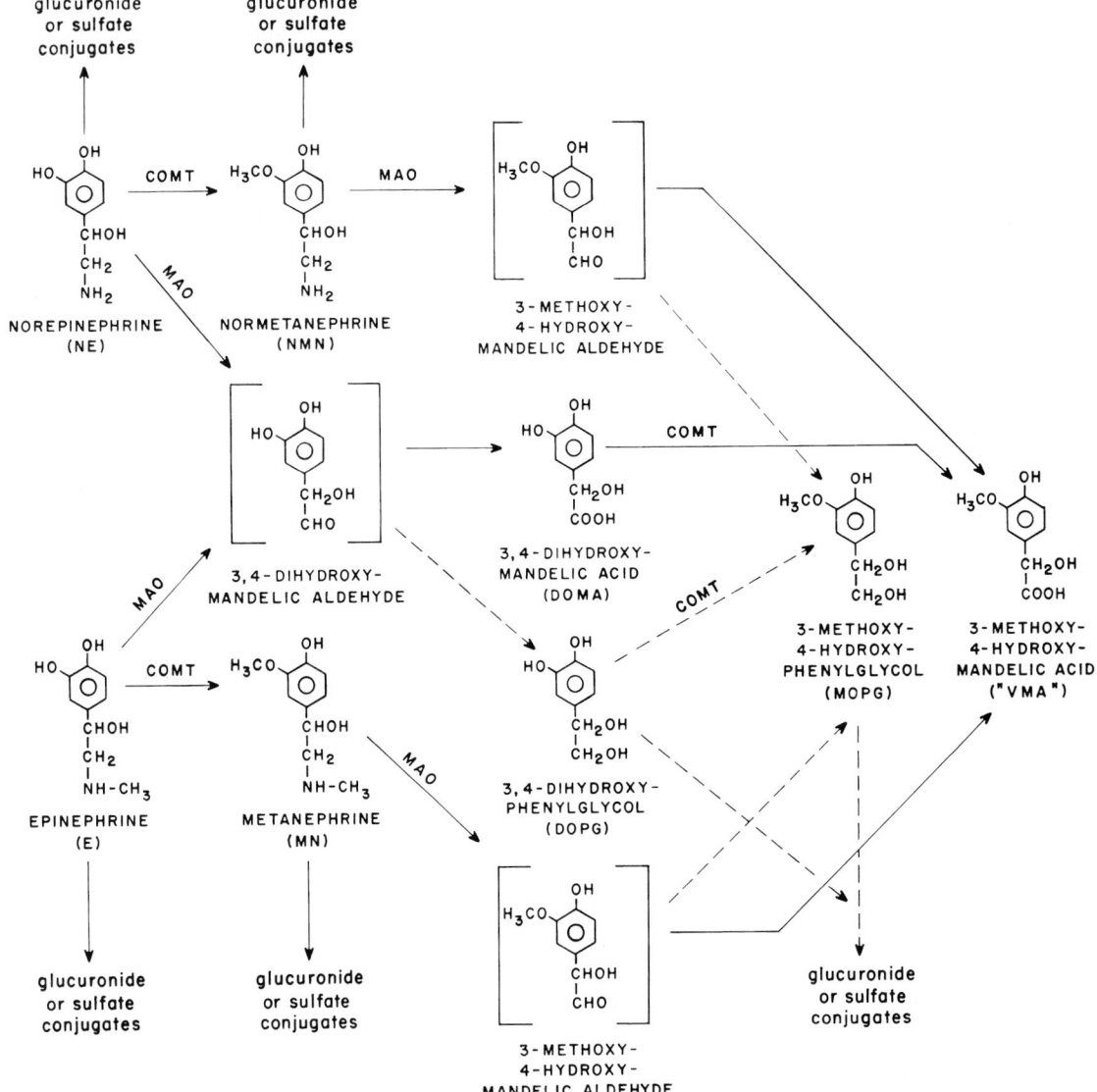

Figure 13–12. Metabolism of norepinephrine (NE) and epinephrine (E) by catechol O-methyltransferase (COMT) and monoamine oxidase (MAO). The dashed lines represent the glycol pathway. Aldehyde intermediates (in brackets) exist only transiently; they are rapidly metabolized to corresponding acids and glycols by aldehyde and alcohol dehydrogenases. Conjugation of the phenolic hydroxyl group with sulfate or glucuronide also occurs. (From Landsberg L, Young JB. Catecholamines and the adrenal medulla. In: Bondy PK, Rosenberg LE, eds. Metabolic Control and Disease. 8th ed. Philadelphia: WB Saunders, 1980: 1621–1693.)

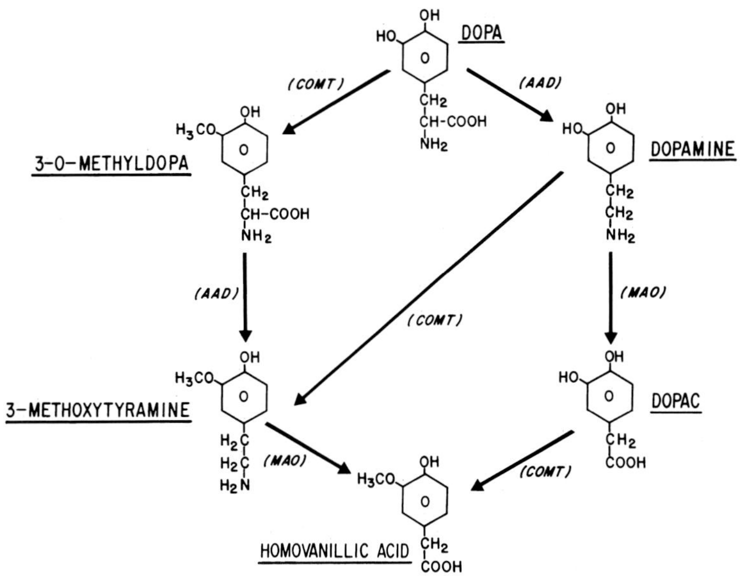

Figure 13–13. Metabolism of dopa and DA. Dopa is converted into DA by aromatic-L-amino acid decarboxylase (AAD) or into 3-O-methyldopa by catechol O-methyltransferase (COMT). The deaminated product of DA is 3,4-dihydroxyphenylacetic acid (DOPAC); the O-methylated deaminated metabolite is 3-methoxy-4-hydroxyphenyl-acetic acid (homovanillic acid, HVA). (From Landsberg L, Berardino MB, Silva R. Metabolism of ^{3}H-L-dopa by the rat gut in vivo: evidence for glucuronide conjugation. Reprinted with permission from Biochemical Pharmacology 1975; 24:1167–1174. Copyright © 1975, by Pergamon Press, Ltd.)

and stomach.[155] MAO is a mitochondrial flavoprotein located in the outer mitochondrial membrane. MAO oxidizes primary, secondary, and tertiary amines but requires an unsubstituted methylene group attached to the amine; alpha substituents on congeners of NE prevent metabolism by MAO. Partial substrate specificity favors the naturally occurring levo isomer of NE. More than one form of the enzyme has been identified on the basis of substrate specificity, sensitivity to different inhibitors, genetic analysis, and monoclonal antibodies. The MAO-A subtype has a higher affinity for NE and is localized in central catecholamine-containing neurons. Both MAO-A and MAO-B are present in liver.

The action of MAO on NE or epinephrine produces the alcohol 3,4-dihydroxyphenylglycol or the acid 3,4-dihydroxymandelic acid (see Fig. 13–12). The O-methylated metabolites of epinephrine and NE (the metanephrines) are better substrates; oxidative deamination of the metanephrines produces 3-methoxy-4-hydroxymandelic acid (vanillylmandelic acid, VMA) or the corresponding alcohol 3-methoxy-4-hydroxy-phenylglycol (MOPG). The relative proportions of the glycol and the acid metabolites vary with species and tissues. In humans free plasma MOPG is converted into VMA. The action of MAO on DA produces 3,4-dihydroxyphenylacetic acid; the O-methylated metabolite of DA (3-methoxytyramine) is converted to 3-methoxy-4-hydroxyphenylacetic acid (homovanillic acid, HVA; see Fig. 13–13).

MAO plays an important role in the regulation of intraneuronal metabolism of DA and NE. NE in vesicular storage sites is protected from metabolism by MAO, whereas cytoplasmic NE and DA are substrates for oxidative deamination by MAO. MAO therefore participates in regulating storage of NE in the nerve ending. When MAO is inhibited, NE stores in the cytosol and in the granules increase. In addition, MAO is responsible for metabolism of ingested dietary amines and metabolism of circulating catechols and their O-methylated metabolites.

CATECHOL O-METHYLTRANSFERASE. COMT (EC 2.1.1.6) catalyzes the meta-O-methylation of epinephrine, NE, and their deaminated metabolites 3,4-dihydroxyphenylglycol and 3,4-dihydroxymandelic acid (see Figs. 13–12 and 13–13). COMT was isolated originally from the soluble fraction of cells; liver and kidney have the highest levels. A similar but distinct membrane-bound form of COMT has a higher affinity for catecholamines. The enzyme utilizes S-adenosylmethionine as the methyl donor, requires a divalent cation, and is specific for the catechol group. COMT is primarily extraneuronal, but some of the enzyme may be intraneuronal.

COMT metabolizes circulating catechols in the liver and kidney and locally released NE in the effector tissue. O-Methylation is more important than deamination in the metabolism of circulating and locally released catechols. The relative importance at the adrenergic synapse of local metabolism by COMT, reuptake, and diffusion into the circulation depends on local factors in the innervated tissue, the density of the adrenergic innervation, and blood flow. As described previously, neuronal recapture is of prime importance in transmitter inactivation.

The action of COMT produces normetanephrine from NE, metanephrine from epinephrine, VMA or MOPG from 3,4-dihydroxymandelic acid or 3,4-dihydroxyphenylglycol (see Fig. 13–12), 3-methoxytyramine from DA, and HVA from 3,4-dihydroxyphenylacetic acid (see Fig. 13–13).

CONJUGATION WITH SULFATE OR GLUCURONIDE. The phenolic hydroxyl group of catecholamines can be conjugated with sulfate or glucuronide. In the rat glucuronide is the principal conjugate; in humans the sulfate predominates; but both conjugates occur in both species. The liver and gut are important sites of conjugation. Ingested catechols are conjugated to an important degree, and catechols in the diet appear in plasma and urine principally as conjugates. The enzyme that catalyzes sulfation of catechols is phenol sulfotransferase (EC 2.8.2.1). It occurs in two forms and is important in the inactivation of many phenolic compounds. The enzyme is present at high concentrations in platelets, brain, liver, and gut.

EXCRETION OF CATECHOLAMINES AND CATECHOLAMINE METABOLITES

Mammalian kidney contains COMT and MAO, metabolizes circulating catecholamines, and excretes both catecholamines and the metabolites in urine. Renal tubules also secrete unconjugated epinephrine and NE. The liver is capable of excreting catechols and catechol metabolites in bile, but the quantitative significance of this route is unknown.

Most of the catecholamines are excreted as deaminated metabolites (VMA, MOPG, HVA); a small fraction is excreted unchanged or as metanephrines (Table 13–3). Excretion of nonmetabolized catecholamines provides a better index of physiological activity of the sympathoadrenal system than ex-

TABLE 13–3. Excretion of Catecholamines and Metabolites in Urine of Normal Human Subjects

	Amount Excreted in μmol/d (μg/d)*	% of Total from NE + E	Source†
Epinephrine (E) (free)	0.03 (5)	0.1	Adrenal medulla
Norepinephrine (NE) (free)	0.18 (30)	0.4	Sympathetic nerve endings (Adrenal medulla)
Conjugated NE + E	0.59 (100)	1.6	Dietary catecholamines (Sympathetic nerve endings) (Adrenal medulla)
Metanephrine (total)	0.33 (65)	1.0	Adrenal medulla
Normetanephrine (total)	0.55 (100)	1.6	Sympathetic nerve endings (Adrenal medulla)
Vanillylmandelic acid	20.2 (4000)	63.5	Sympathetic nerve endings Adrenal medulla CNS
3-Methoxy-4-hydroxyphenylglycol	10.9 (2000)	31.8	Sympathetic nerve endings Adrenal medulla CNS
Dopamine (free)	1.5 (225)	—	Kidney
Homovanillic acid	37.9 (6900)	—	CNS Plasma DA

*Average values.
†Secondary sources in parentheses.

cretion of catecholamine metabolites, because the latter also reflects NE that is metabolized within the nerve endings and brain and never released at adrenergic synapses in active form.

Plasma Catecholamines

METHODOLOGIC CONSIDERATIONS

In the most widely used radioenzymatic assay, COMT is used to transfer a labeled methyl group from S-adenosylmethionine to the 3-hydroxyl position of NE, epinephrine, and DA, with the formation of labeled normetanephrine, metanephrine, and 3-methoxytyramine, respectively. The labeled products are extracted, separated chromatographically, oxidized to VMA, extracted, and assayed for radioactivity, and the catecholamine concentration in the plasma is determined from a standard curve or internal standard. An alternative approach employs reverse-phase or cation-exchange high-performance liquid chromatography (HPLC) in conjunction with electrochemical detection. These techniques require an initial purification step followed by separation of NE, epinephrine, and DA on the chromatography column and detection of the catecholamine with an electrochemical detector.

PLASMA CATECHOLAMINES IN HUMANS: SOURCE, BASAL LEVELS, AND PHYSIOLOGICAL VARIATIONS

PROTEIN BINDING AND CONJUGATION. At physiological levels, 50 to 60% of catecholamines in plasma are loosely bound to albumin, globulins, and lipoproteins. A high-affinity, stereospecific, saturable binding site is present in $α_1$-acid glycoprotein.[156] The significance of protein binding is unclear because water-soluble catecholamines do not require protein binding for transport. Most catecholamine assays measure both free and protein-bound catecholamines but do not measure conjugated catecholamines. Conjugated catecholamines can be measured by hydrolysis of the conjugates in the plasma sample before measurement; because conjugates do not reflect acute changes in sympathetic nervous system activity, they are of less interest in most circumstances. When referring to catecholamines, the designation *free* means unconjugated and does not refer to protein binding. Unless specified, reported levels of plasma catecholamines always refer to the free (unconjugated) forms.

SAMPLE COLLECTION. Because catecholamine levels in plasma reflect the activity or functional state of the sympatho-

adrenal system, the physiological state of the subject at the time of sampling is critical to interpretation. Catecholamine levels in plasma samples collected casually, without attention to the technique of phlebotomy or the physiological state of the subject, are uninterpretable. Basal catecholamine levels should be measured in a supine subject in a relaxed environment. Pain and anxiety can transiently activate the sympathoadrenal system, so samples should be taken from an indwelling intravenous line. By convention, after the intravenous line is placed, the patient remains supine for 30 min, at which time blood may be withdrawn. The blood should be collected in chilled tubes with an appropriate reducing agent to prevent oxidation of catecholamines and placed immediately on ice; plasma should be separated promptly and stored at $-70°C$ until analysis. Drugs of diverse types, particularly those that affect the autonomic nervous system, can influence the circulating levels of catecholamines. The α- and β-adrenergic blocking agents and clonidine are of particular concern. Preferably all medications should be discontinued before plasma catecholamines are measured.

NOREPINEPHRINE. Basal plasma NE levels are usually in the range of 0.6 to 2.0 nmol/L (100 to 350 pg/mL). NE that is released from adrenergic synapses is subject to reuptake into sympathetic nerve endings or local metabolism within the effector tissue (see Fig. 13–11); the neurotransmitter that escapes reuptake and local metabolism diffuses into the circulation and constitutes the circulating pool. Under basal conditions, venous levels of NE in the forearm exceed the arterial concentration by approximately 30%. Arteriovenous differences at other sites reflect the relative contributions of metabolism, which extracts NE, and local release, which reflects sympathetic activity in the region being sampled (Fig. 13–14). Under basal conditions the contribution of the adrenal medulla to the circulating pool of NE is small[157]; when the adrenal medulla is stimulated, however, large amounts of NE and epinephrine are released, and under these circumstances the adrenal medulla can contribute substantially to the plasma NE level. Plasma NE turns over rapidly; the half-time of disappearance, calculated from steady-state NE infusions, is between 2.0 and 2.5 min. The metabolic clearance rate of plasma NE approximates 40 mL/min/kg.[158, 159]

NE levels in forearm venous plasma are influenced by the position of the body. Orthostatic activation of the sympathetic nervous system, for example 5 min of quiet standing, results in a doubling of the basal plasma NE concentration.[160, 161] The plasma NE response to upright posture constitutes a

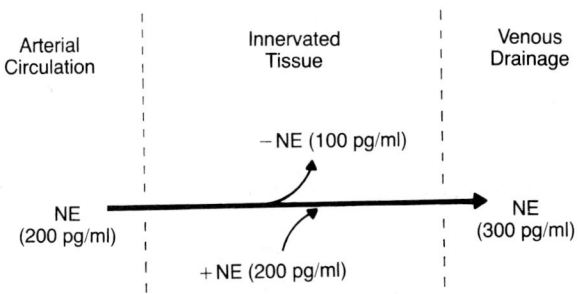

− = NE extracted (uptake in nerve endings and metabolism)
+ = NE added (release from nerve endings)

Figure 13–14. Relation between arterial and venous NE levels. The venous level depends on the amount of NE extracted as the innervated tissue is perfused with arterial blood and on the amount of NE released from nerve endings in response to neuronal impulse traffic in the area served by the venous drainage. Only a fraction of released NE escapes reuptake and local metabolism and diffuses into the venous circulation. Both the extraction process and diffusion from the region of the synapse are influenced by blood flow. To convert NE values to nmol/L, multiply by 0.005911.

convenient test of sympathetic nervous system function, as described later. Basal plasma NE levels are similar in men and women and in whites and African Americans,[162, 163] although the latter two may differ in plasma clearance.[164] Basal NE levels vary throughout the day, with the lowest levels occurring during the night, even in subjects who remain continuously supine.[165] Aging is associated with an increase in supine and upright NE levels, in part as a result of an age-related decrease in NE clearance.[166] More than half of the interindividual variation in plasma NE may be caused by undefined genetic factors.[167]

EPINEPHRINE. Plasma epinephrine is derived from the adrenal medulla. The basal plasma epinephrine level is 100 to 275 pmol/L (20 to 50 pg/mL). The metabolic clearance rate of epinephrine is similar to that of NE, but, in contrast to NE, levels of epinephrine are lower in forearm venous than arterial plasma. This difference reflects substantial extraction and metabolism of epinephrine by tissues, principally by conjugation with sulfate, and the fact that the forearm tissues do not release epinephrine into the circulation. Because plasma epinephrine levels at baseline are near the limit of detection in most assays, the impacts of various factors on adrenal medullary secretion may be underestimated. Epinephrine levels in venous plasma increase minimally in response to upright posture,[160] are lower in women than men,[167] and may be lower in African American than in white men.[168] Circadian variation is present, although its relation to posture and activity is uncertain.[165, 169] The impact of aging on epinephrine levels has not been resolved, because different studies report either a reduction or no difference in older persons. Almost 70% of the interindividual variation in plasma epinephrine may be a result of genetic factors.[167]

DOPAMINE. Basal levels of free DA are in the range of 165 to 330 pmol/L (25 to 50 pg/mL). Levels of conjugated DA are higher, and the sulfate derivative constitutes about 98% of total plasma DA. The source of plasma DA is not known with certainty. Dopa, the immediate precursor of DA, is present at levels of about 7.6 nmol/L (1.5 ng/mL), and dopa may be an important source of circulating DA. The proper interpretation of plasma DA or dopa levels awaits more complete characterization of the peripheral dopaminergic system.

UTILITY OF PLASMA CATECHOLAMINE MEASUREMENTS. There are few clinical indications for the measurement of plasma catecholamines except as a test of sympathetic nervous system function in patients with orthostatic hypoten-

sion (see later discussion). In patients with suspected pheochromocytoma, plasma catecholamine determinations may be helpful in rare circumstances. The major utility of plasma catecholamine measurements is in clinical investigation, especially in evaluation of the role of the sympathoadrenal system in the regulation of physiological processes.

Assessment of Sympathoadrenal Activity

ADRENAL MEDULLA

Assessment of adrenomedullary function is relatively straightforward. Plasma levels of epinephrine accurately reflect medullary activity, although the short half-life in plasma, the extraction by muscle, and the technical difficulty in measuring basal levels limit their usefulness. Urinary epinephrine excretion provides an integrated assessment of adrenomedullary secretion over time, although limited sensitivity of urine epinephrine to changes in adrenal secretion and altered handling of catecholamines with renal disease complicate interpretation of urine data. An increase in epinephrine in plasma or urine is, however, good evidence of adrenomedullary stimulation.

SYMPATHETIC NERVOUS SYSTEM

The assessment of sympathetic nervous system activity is more difficult. Each strategy that has been used to assess the functional state of the sympathetic nerves has strengths and weaknesses, and none is fully satisfactory in terms of sensitivity or specificity. Consequently, it is common to apply more than one approach.

PLASMA AND URINARY NOREPINEPHRINE LEVELS. NE is a neurotransmitter, not a circulating hormone. As described previously, the plasma pool of NE is derived from the small portion of neurotransmitter that escapes reuptake and metabolism at adrenergic synapses throughout the body. As a consequence, plasma levels of NE usually are below the threshold for stimulation of adrenergic receptors. (Epinephrine, in contrast, stimulates adrenergic receptors at physiological levels, as would be expected for a circulating hormone.) The plasma NE level is an insensitive index of sympathetic activity. When NE is infused, the level required to stimulate sympathetically mediated processes exceeds the plasma NE level during physiological stimulation of the same processes. Furthermore, when the sympathetic nervous system is activated, adrenergic processes are stimulated before a rise in circulating NE is seen. Concomitant increases in NE clearance may accompany changes in sympathetic activity, thereby lessening the impact of the change in sympathetic activity on the plasma NE level, and the failure of the NE level to rise in a particular circumstance does not exclude the possibility of significant sympathetic stimulation.

Peripheral plasma NE levels also lack specificity for two reasons. On the one hand, the adrenal medulla secretes NE as well as epinephrine, and increases in plasma NE concentration do not necessarily reflect the activity of sympathetic nerves. On the other hand, as indicated in Figure 13–14, the venous NE concentration is influenced by processes that promote the extraction of NE from arterial plasma or the addition of NE to the venous drainage. Extraction averages 30 to 50% and is highly dependent on blood flow, whereas addition of NE depends on release from the sympathetic nerve endings. Because blood flow and sympathetic nervous system activity vary under different conditions, the venous level depends on these factors, as well as on the arterial level of NE perfusing the innervated tissue. The plasma NE in antecubital venous plasma is derived principally from NE released in the tissues of the forearm (see Fig. 13–14). Because the sympathetic outflow to various tissues or organ systems is not uniform, NE levels in venous plasma from the forearm may not reflect changes in sympathetic activity in other tissues.

Despite these limitations, antecubital venous plasma NE levels can provide a useful estimate of sympathetic activity. Sympathetic nerve impulse traffic and plasma NE concentration correspond under a variety of circumstances, and treatments that diminish sympathetic nerve activity reduce plasma NE concentration in animals and humans. Furthermore, physiological manipulations that increase sympathetic nervous system activity cause increased plasma NE levels, as illustrated by the plasma NE response to upright posture (Fig. 13–15). The magnitude of response is an indication of the functional reserve of the sympathetic nervous system; failure to increase plasma NE in the presence of a fall in blood pressure indicates dysfunction of the sympathetic nervous system.

The same considerations apply to urinary NE excretion. Although a portion of NE in the urine originates from renal sympathetic nerves, the major fraction reflects the NE concentration in arterial blood. Urinary NE excretion is a reasonable estimate of plasma NE concentrations integrated over time and under most circumstances reflects sympathetic nervous system activity.

KINETIC TECHNIQUES. Kinetic studies with infusion of radiolabeled NE may be more sensitive than simple plasma NE measurements in defining the overall level of sympathetic activity.[170] These techniques permit calculation of a rate of appearance of NE in the circulation and correct for alterations in plasma NE clearance that limit changes in plasma NE levels. When coupled with venous catheterization of specific anatomic regions or organ systems, the kinetic method permits calculation of the contribution made by the various regions to the total pool of plasma NE. Under normal circumstances the lungs contribute substantially to the circulating pool of NE, but with hypertension, cirrhosis, or congestive heart failure, the NE release rate in heart and kidney can be increased under circumstances in which the release rate sampled at the forearm is either normal or increased to a lesser degree.[170] Attempts to derive additional information from tracer infusions by application of more complex mathematical models (e.g., compartmental analysis) have not provided in-

formation more useful than that obtained from analyses of the appearance rate and clearance of plasma NE. Despite their power, tracer NE infusions are not practical for clinical use.

In animals plasma catecholamine measurements are often difficult to interpret because activation of the sympathoadrenal system frequently accompanies acquisition of the plasma sample. However, with kinetic techniques measurements of NE turnover within sympathetic nerves in individual tissues are proportional to impulse traffic within the sympathetic nerves and therefore provide tissue-specific information of sympathetic activity in peripheral tissues. Measurement of tissue NE turnover has not been applied to humans.

NERVE RECORDINGS. An alternative approach involves the direct recording of impulse traffic from sympathetic nerves.[171] Recording electrodes are placed transcutaneously, usually into the peroneal nerve in the lower extremity, to assess nerve impulse traffic in sympathetic fibers innervating skeletal muscle. These techniques are invasive, technically demanding, and feasible only for short-term studies but have yielded useful information regarding the regulation of sympathetic activity in this tissue. However, as noted earlier, neurotransmitter release at the sympathetic nerve ending is not linear with incoming nerve impulse traffic. Furthermore, a wide variety of factors act on the presynaptic nerve cell membrane to increase or decrease the likelihood that an incoming impulse will trigger neurotransmitter release. Finally, the density of sympathetic innervation in peripheral tissues is subject to modification during development or with disease. Because efferent impulses are distributed to all terminal branches of the dendritic arbor, changes in the density of sympathetic nerve endings should alter the relation between impulse traffic and neurotransmitter release. This problem is ameliorated, in part, in studies combining measurements of plasma NE with the electrical recordings.

OTHER APPROACHES. Several other methods have been employed in the assessment of sympathetic activity. Heart rate spectral analysis is based on mathematical analysis of spontaneous fluctuations in heart rate.[172, 173] However, heart rate spectral analysis is not a reliable measure of cardiac sympathetic activity.[174]

As described, DBH, chromogranin-A, and catecholamines are released during exocytosis. Although plasma DBH activity and chromogranin-A levels increase in situations that increase sympathetic activity, the changes are small in comparison with changes in plasma NE and the known degree of stimulation of the sympathetic nervous system.[175, 176] These measurements therefore are relatively insensitive indicators of sympathetic activity, and neither DBH nor chromogranin-A is a suitable alternative to plasma NE in the assessment of sympathetic activity in humans.

ADRENERGIC RECEPTORS

General Characteristics and Classification

The interaction between catecholamines and receptors on the surface of effector cells initiates events that begin in the cell membrane, progress to the cell interior, and culminate in a characteristic response. The relation between receptor occupancy and the response of the effector tissue is incompletely understood (see Chapter 5), but the intracellular events within effector cells and the molecular structure and function of the receptor itself are understood in some detail.

Two major categories of physiological response to sympathetic nerve stimulation—inhibitory and excitatory—have been recognized since the early part of the 20th century.[5] On the basis of differential agonist potencies, Ahlquist postulated

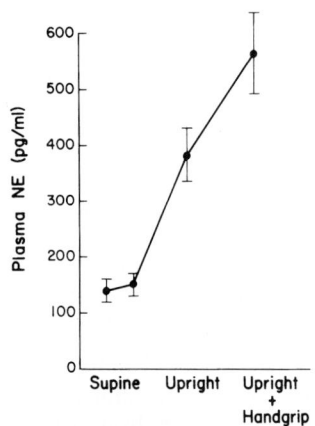

Figure 13–15. Plasma NE responses to upright posture and isometric hand grip. Mean values ± SEM are shown for eight normal male subjects; supine values represent basal plasma NE levels. The increase in the plasma NE concentration after 5 min of quiet upright standing reflects activation of the sympathetic nervous system in response to orthostatic stress. A further increment in plasma NE is demonstrable after 5 min more of standing upright with isometric hand grip exercise at one-third maximal force. These maneuvers permit assessment of sympathetic nervous system reactivity. (From Landsberg L, Young JB. Sympathetic nervous system in hypertension. In: Brenner B, Stein JH, eds. Hypertension: Contemporary Issues in Nephrology. Vol 8. New York: Churchill Livingstone, 1981: 100–141.)

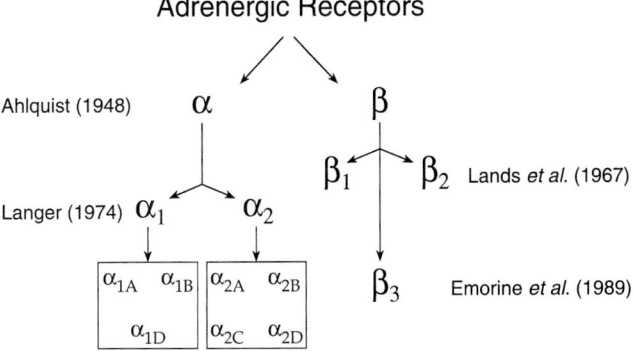

Adrenergic Receptors

Figure 13–16. Historical development of classification for adrenergic receptors.

two distinct adrenergic receptors, which he designated α and β (Fig. 13–16).[177] Ergot derivatives, which were known to block many of the excitatory effects of catecholamines, affect only α-receptor responses; subsequently, antagonists were found that selectively block β-receptor responses.

Almost 20 years later, Lands and co-workers observed that the structural requirements for amine activation of cardioacceleration and lipolysis were distinguishable from those optimal for bronchodilation and vasodilation, leading to the designation of the former as β_1 and the latter as β_2 responses (see Fig. 13–16).[178] In 1974 Langer postulated the existence of an α_2-adrenergic receptor on the membrane of the sympathetic nerve terminal that is involved in presynaptic regulation of NE release (see previous discussion) and is distinct from the postsynaptic α_1-adrenergic receptor.[179]

Continued pharmacologic characterization of adrenergic responses in specific tissues indicated that further subdivision of both α- and β-receptor responses was required. β-Adrenergic responses that did not fit into the β_1- and β_2-categories were referred to as "atypical" β-adrenergic responses. Beginning in the 1980s the discovery by molecular means of a distinct β_3-adrenergic receptor confirmed the strength of this approach.[180] Moreover, cloning of the cDNAs that encode receptor genes made possible the study of recombinant adrenergic receptors expressed in cultured cells. In general, these molecular approaches have reinforced the classification of adrenergic receptors made earlier on pharmacologic grounds. In some cases, however, the subtype assignment of a particular receptor clone has been controversial. The scheme depicted

in Figure 13–16 reflects a consensus for the subdivision of α- and β-adrenoceptors.[181, 182]

Dopaminergic receptors exist in certain peripheral vascular beds, visceral smooth muscle, and the peripheral and central nervous systems and are clearly distinct from α- and β-receptors.

REGULATORY (G) PROTEINS AND SECOND MESSENGERS

The coupling of receptor binding and catecholamine-mediated response depends on membrane-bound regulatory proteins (see Chapter 5) termed *G proteins* because they bind GTP (Fig. 13–17). In the activated state G proteins influence membrane-associated enzymes that control the concentration of intracellular mediators (second messengers), thereby affecting the activity of enzymes and ion channels. G proteins can be stimulatory or inhibitory. The β-adrenergic, dopaminergic, and α_2-adrenergic receptor subtypes interact with the G protein–adenylyl cyclase system.[183] The α_1-adrenergic receptor also interacts with a G protein that regulates the activity of phospholipase C (see Fig. 13–17). These membrane-associated enzymes alter the levels of cAMP, phospholipid metabolites (see later discussion), and intracellular calcium, which act as second messengers that provoke effector responses by stimulating phosphorylation of enzymes and other intracellular proteins.

MOLECULAR STRUCTURE OF ADRENERGIC RECEPTORS

Adrenergic receptors interact with catecholamines on the extracellular side of the plasma membrane and with G proteins within the membrane. cDNAs for various subtypes of the α- and β-adrenergic receptors have been isolated, and the amino acid sequences have been deduced from the cDNAs. These proteins belong to a family of more than 100 membrane proteins that also includes the muscarinic acetylcholine receptors and the visual protein rhodopsin.[184] Regions of the proteins in this family show remarkable sequence homology; particularly well conserved are seven sequences consisting of 20 to 25 hydrophobic amino acids, possibly arranged as alpha-helices, that are believed to form membrane-spanning domains. A schematic representation of this family of proteins is presented in Figure 13–18.

The critical structural features of this model, which appear to be common to many receptors coupled to G proteins,

Figure 13–17. Relations between autonomic agonists and receptors, membrane-bound regulatory proteins and enzymes, and intracellular effector systems. Adrenergic receptors are designated α and β, dopaminergic receptors DA, and muscarinic receptors M. Receptor subtypes are designated with subscripts 1, 2 and 3. G refers to the GTP-associated regulatory protein that stimulates (G_s) or inhibits (G_i) adenylate (adenylyl) cyclase or stimulates phospholipase C (G_q); (+), stimulation; (−), inhibition; PIP_2, phosphatidylinositol 4,5-bisphosphate; DAG, diacylglycerol; IP_3, inositol 1,4,5-trisphosphate. (From Landsberg L, Young JB. Physiology and pharmacology of the autonomic nervous system. In: Wilson JD, Braunwald E, Isselbacher KJ, eds. Harrison's Principles of Internal Medicine. 12th ed. New York: McGraw Hill, 1991: 380–392. Reproduced with permission of McGraw-Hill, Inc.)

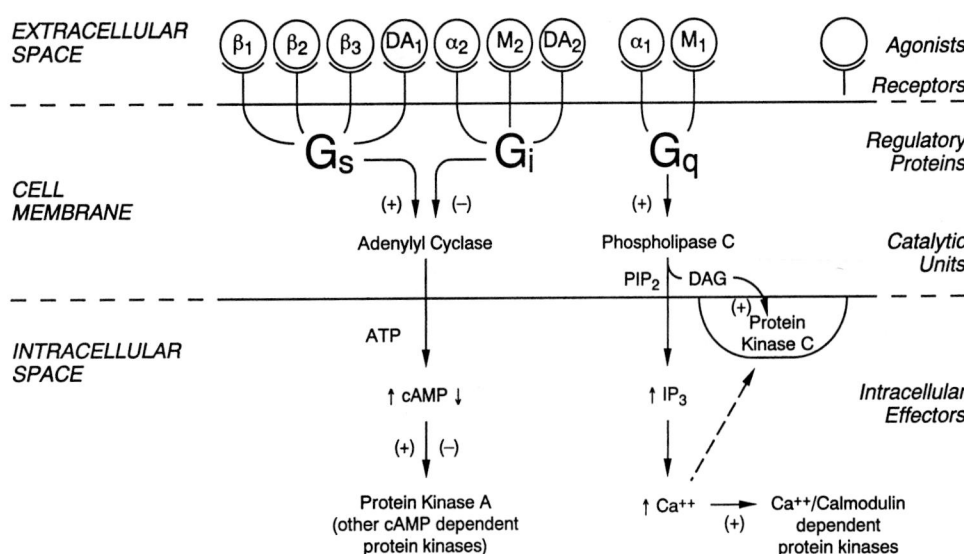

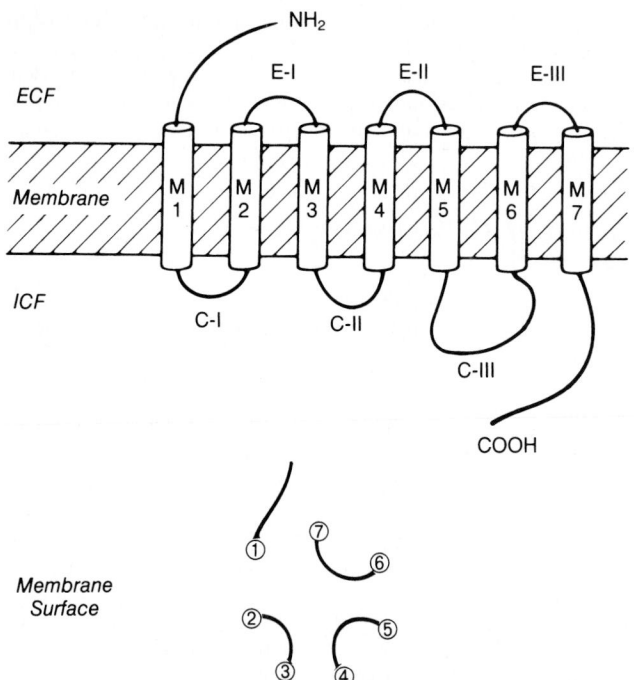

Figure 13–18. Proposed structure of prototypical adrenergic receptor as deduced from primary amino acid sequences. The receptor is composed of a single protein chain with an extracellular (ECF) hydrophilic NH$_2$ terminus, seven hydrophobic membrane-spanning domains (M1 through M7) connected by three extracellular loops (E-I through E-III) and three cytoplasmic loops (C-I through C-III), and an intracellular (ICF) COOH terminus. The α- and β-adrenergic receptors, including subtypes, appear to fit this general model. Variations in structure at the seventh membrane-spanning domain, the third cytoplasmic loop, and the COOH terminus have been shown to be important in agonist binding and in the relation to specific G proteins. The top portion of the figure shows the structure longitudinally; however, the three-dimensional structure within the cell membrane may be more compact. A possible arrangement of the membrane-spanning domains, extracellular loops, and NH$_2$ terminus, as seen from the extracellular membrane surface, is shown in the bottom portion of the figure.

include an extracellular NH$_2$ terminus, an intracellular COOH terminus, and seven hydrophobic membrane-spanning domains connected by three extracellular and three cytoplasmic loops. G protein–linked receptors contain one to three glycosylation sites near the NH$_2$ terminus which may localize the receptor to the cell surface.[185] The membrane-spanning re-

gions appear to be particularly important in determining ligand binding.[184] In one model, the catecholamine agonist forms a three-point attachment within a pocket bounded by the hydrophobic transmembrane domains of the receptor.[184, 185] Interactions between the amino group, the phenolic and β-hydroxyl groups, and the aromatic catechol ring of the agonist with functional groups on the transmembrane domains of the receptor are postulated to account for differences in the binding of different ligands.[185] For α$_2$- and β$_2$-adrenoceptors, specificity of agonist binding apparently resides at the seventh (or the combination of the sixth and the seventh) membrane-spanning domain.[186]

By analogy with rhodopsin, the third cytoplasmic loop and the COOH terminus of the intracellular domain of the adrenergic receptors are responsible for receptor interactions with specific G proteins.[185] Receptors coupling to G$_i$ (see Fig. 13–17) have long third loops and short COOH termini, whereas the β-adrenergic receptors coupled to G$_s$ have relatively short third cytoplasmic loops and long COOH termini.[187] The α$_1$-receptor possesses the longest COOH terminus in the group and is most divergent in this area and in the third cytoplasmic loop. In comparison, cytoplasmic loops 1 and 2 are reasonably well conserved throughout the whole group of related receptors. The members of this family also have potential sites for phosphorylation on the cytoplasmic domains.[187]

α-Adrenergic Receptors

AGONISTS AND ANTAGONISTS

α-Adrenergic receptors mediate a variety of responses, including vasoconstriction (Table 13–4). The α$_1$ subtype mediates a wide variety of effects, most prominently involving smooth muscle. Epinephrine and NE are potent nonselective agonists of the α-receptor; phentolamine and phenoxybenzamine are nonselective α-receptor antagonists. Selective α$_1$-agonists include the synthetic sympathomimetic amines phenylephrine and methoxamine. At low concentrations, phenoxybenzamine is relatively selective for the α$_1$-receptor. Prazosin is a selective α$_1$-antagonist that is useful in the treatment of hypertension. The α$_2$-receptor is located on presynaptic sympathetic neurons, on cholinergic neurons within the gut, on CNS neurons involved in the regulation of cardiovascular function, on platelets, and on blood vessels. The α$_2$-receptor mediates inhibition of NE release from adrenergic neurons, inhibition of acetylcholine release from cholinergic neurons, potentiation of the baroreceptor vasodepressor response medi-

TABLE 13–4. Adrenergic Receptors

| Subtypes | α-Adrenergic Receptors | | β-Adrenergic Receptors | | |
	α$_1$	α$_2$	β$_1$	β$_2$	β$_3$
Agonists	Epi, NE		Isoproterenol, EPi, NE		
Agonist potency	Epi ≥ NE		Iso > NE ≥ Epi	Iso > Epi >> NE	Iso ≥ NE >> Epi
Representative selective agonists	Phenylephrine, methoxamine	Clonidine, α-methyl NE	Denopamine	Terbutaline, clenbuterol	BRL 37344, oxprenolol
Antagonists	Phentolamine, Phenoxybenzamine		Propranolol, nadolol, timolol, oxprenolol		
Representative selective antagonists	Prazosin, terazosin	Yohimbine, rauwolscine	Metoprolol, atenolol	ICI 118551	—
Second messenger	Phosphatidyl inositol turnover, ↑ intracellular Ca^{+2}	↓ Cyclic AMP, ↑ or ↓ Ca^{+2} influx, Na$^+$/H$^+$ exchange	↑ Cyclic AMP	↑ Cyclic AMP	↑ Cyclic AMP
Representative responses	Vasoconstriction, intestinal relaxation, uterine contraction, pupillary dilation	↓ NE (presynaptic), ↑ platelet aggregation, vasoconstriction, ↓ insulin secretion	↑ Heart rate, ↑ contractility, ↑ lipolysis, ↑ renin secretion	Smooth muscle relaxation, ↑ glycogenolysis in skeletal muscle, ↑ NE (presynaptic)	↑ Brown fat thermogenesis, ↑ lipolysis
Desensitization	Yes	Yes	Yes (+)	Yes (+ +)	No

Epi, epinephrine; Iso, isoproterenol; NE, norepinephrine.

ated through central regulatory neurons, platelet aggregation, and vasoconstriction. Differences in selectivity between the agonist and the antagonist for α_1- and α_2-receptors may approach three to four orders of magnitude,[188] a difference greater than the differences in selectivity among the subtypes of the β-receptor. Clonidine and α-methylnorepinephrine (derived in vivo from α-methyldopa) are relatively selective α_2-agonists; central inhibition of sympathetic outflow is the basis for the use of agents in the treatment of hypertension. Some α_2-agonists, such as clonidine and idazoxan, are also agonists for imidazoline receptors, which may confound interpretation of functional studies utilizing these agents.[189] Yohimbine is a specific α_2-antagonist.

α-RECEPTOR SIGNAL TRANSDUCTION

The α_1- and α_2-receptors use different mechanisms to couple receptor occupancy with cellular response.

α_1-RECEPTOR. The induction of α_1-mediated responses in effector tissues involves both calcium mobilization and membrane phospholipids, particularly phosphatidylinositol. α_1-Agonist binding activates phospholipase C, an effect that is mediated through G proteins belonging to the G_q family (see Fig. 13–17).[190] Phospholipase C activation, in turn, catalyzes the hydrolysis of membrane phospholipids such as phosphatidylinositol 4,5-bisphosphate (PIP_2) to form inositol 1,4,5-trisphosphate (IP_3) and 1,2-diacylglycerol (DAG). Both IP_3 and DAG act as second messengers: IP_3 rapidly increases the cytosolic calcium concentration and DAG activates protein kinase C (see Fig. 13–17). The relative contributions of intracellular and extracellular calcium vary among α_1-agonists and by anatomic location and species.[188, 191] The mechanisms by which IP_3 mobilizes calcium appear to involve a specific receptor and to require potassium.

DAG, the other second messenger produced by the action of phospholipase C on membrane phospholipids, remains associated with the plasma membrane and activates cytosolic protein kinase C.[191] Protein kinase C is also stimulated by calcium, so the two second messengers generated by α_1-agonist responses have a synergistic effect on this enzyme.

Other messengers that may mediate α_1-adrenergic effects include phospholipase A_2, phosphatidylcholine, and the phosphodiesterase that degrades cAMP.[192] The importance of these mechanisms is unknown.

α_2-RECEPTOR. Signal transduction of α_2-mediated responses in effector tissues is more complex than that for α_1-adrenergic actions.[192] The common explanation is that α_2-mediated events are related, at least in part, to the inhibition of adenylyl cyclase (see Fig. 13–17). Agonist occupancy of the α_2-receptor activates a G_i protein in the plasma membrane to antagonize the activation of adenylyl cyclase by G_s. Not all α_2-mediated responses, however, involve inhibition of adenylyl cyclase.[191] α_2-Adrenergic–mediated vasoconstriction involves an influx of extracellular calcium,[191] whereas presynaptic suppression of NE release depends on inhibition of calcium entry because of a reduction in N-type calcium channels in the neuronal membrane.[193] An additional mechanism suggested for α_2-mediated responses involves acceleration of sodium-hydrogen exchange leading to an elevation in intracellular pH, release of plasma membrane–bound calcium into the cell, and activation of phospholipase A_2.[191] Subtypes of the α_2-adrenergic receptor are not known to differ substantially in activation of these signaling pathways.[192]

β-Adrenergic Receptors

AGONISTS AND ANTAGONISTS

β-Receptors mediate cardiac stimulation, bronchodilatation, and vasodilatation (see Table 13–4). The subtypes are

designated β_1, β_2, and β_3. cDNAs for all three subtypes have been isolated, and the predicted amino acid sequence homology is only 45 to 50%,[180] although homology increases to 60 to 70% within the membrane-spanning domains.[194] Sequence homologies are considerably higher for the same subtypes among mammalian species than for different subtypes in the same species. All three subtypes are products of separate genes.

Epinephrine, NE, and the synthetic sympathomimetic amine isoproterenol are nonselective β-agonists. Nonselective β-antagonists include propranolol, alprenolol, nadolol, and timolol. NE is a potent agonist of the β_1-receptor (equivalent to or slightly more potent than epinephrine) but is a weak agonist of the β_2-receptor. The β_1-receptor mediates cardiac stimulation and lipolysis; the β_2-receptor mediates bronchodilatation, vasodilatation, and prejunctional stimulation of NE release from sympathetic neurons. Synthetic congeners with selective agonist or antagonist activity for the β_1- and β_2-receptor subtypes are given in Table 13–4. This selectivity is relative and less than that for the corresponding α_1 and α_2 agents. The administration of high doses of these compounds circumvents the relative selectivity and causes effect on both β_1- and β_2-receptors; nonetheless, at less than maximal dosages these agonists and antagonists have selective clinical utility.

NE is a more potent agonist of the β_3-receptor than epinephrine, although the affinity of all β-agonists for the β_3-receptor is lower than that for β_1 or β_2.[195] Furthermore, antagonists of β_1- or β_2-receptors such as oxprenolol may be partial agonists of the β_3-receptor.[196] The difference in receptor affinity for agonists in conjunction with the greater potency of NE suggests that the β_3-receptor is oriented more toward neurally released NE than toward circulating catecholamines. Tissue expression of β_3-adrenergic receptors in humans is limited to adipose tissue (especially brown fat), gallbladder, and colon.[197] Whether "atypical" β-receptor–mediated responses in other tissues are caused by additional β-receptor subtypes is unclear. Finally, across species, the β_3-receptor displays variable responses to pharmacologic agonists and antagonists, a phenomenon that has slowed development of compounds active at these receptors in humans.[198]

PHARMACOLOGIC PROPERTIES OF β-RECEPTOR ANTAGONISTS. The 14 β-blocking agents currently approved for use in the United States have different pharmacologic properties that may be exploited to clinical advantage (Table 13–5). Some of the β-blockers (propranolol, pindolol, acebutolol, betaxolol) possess membrane-stabilizing local anesthetic properties that do not appear to contribute to efficacy or affect safety. Esmolol is rapidly metabolized and is available only for intravenous use. Sotalol is used for the treatment of ventricular arrhythmias; its antiarrhythmic efficacy may arise more from blockade of potassium channels than from antagonism at β-receptors.[199] Labetalol, a combined α- and β-blocking agent approved for the treatment of hypertension, produces selective α_1-blockade and nonselective β-blockade, with relatively greater potency on the β-receptor.

Pharmacologic characteristics that may contribute to clinical utility include β_1 selectivity and partial agonist activity (see Table 13–5). β_1-Selective antagonists theoretically should cause less bronchoconstriction and vasoconstriction and have less impact on hepatic glucose output because bronchodilatation, vasodilatation, glycogenolysis, and gluconeogenesis are mediated principally by the β_2-receptor subtype. However, the advantage of β_1-selective agonists is small and may not apply at clinically relevant dosages.

Some β-blocking agents produce low-level stimulation of the adrenergic receptor but antagonize the effects of endogenous catecholamines.[200] As a consequence, they may have less effect on resting heart rate than agents without agonist activity. The effect of partial agonists on cardiac output and contractil-

TABLE 13–5. Pharmacology and Pharmacokinetics of β-Adrenergic Antagonists

Agent	Selectivity	Partial Agonist	Plasma Half-Life (h)	Dosage Interval*
Acebutolol	β_1	Yes	3–4	bid/qid
Atenolol	β_1	No	6–7	qd
Betaxolol	β_1	No	14–22	qd
Bisoprolol	β_1	No	9–13	qd
Carteolol	Nonselective	Yes	5–6	qd
Esmolol	β_1	No	9 min	prn
Labetalol	Nonselective	No	3–7	bid
Metoprolol	β_1	No	3–7	bid
Nadolol	Nonselective	No	20–24	qd
Penbutolol	Nonselective	Yes	5	qd
Pindolol	Nonselective	Yes	3–4	bid/qid
Propranolol	Nonselective	No	4	bid/qid
Sotalol	Nonselective	No	7–15	bid/tid
Timolol	Nonselective	No	4–5	bid

bid, twice daily; prn, as required; qd, once daily; qid, four times daily; tid, three times daily.
*Depends on indication; some indications may require more frequent dosing.

ity is variable and depends on their potency and on the underlying level of sympathetic stimulation. Partial agonists may also cause a decrease in peripheral resistance because of β-mediated vasodilatation, rather than the increase observed with pure antagonists, and may avoid the rebound increase in sensitivity to catecholamines after withdrawal of β-blockers. β-Adrenergic antagonists with partial agonist activity (particularly at β_2-receptors) may also have less adverse effects on glucose and lipid metabolism.[201, 202]

SELECTIVE AGONISTS. Agonists with selectivity for the β_1-receptor are not in common clinical use. Agonists with selectivity for the β_2-receptor (see Table 13–4) can cause bronchodilatation at low doses with little cardiac stimulation. Other β_2-agonists have been used in the treatment of premature labor. Outside the United States, β_2-agonists (e.g., clenbuterol, cimaterol) are employed in animal husbandry to enhance the efficiency of meat production.[203] β_3-adrenergic agonists are not clinically available. In animal studies, selective β_3-agonists have shown promise in the treatment of obesity and non–insulin-dependent diabetes mellitus.[204]

β-RECEPTOR SIGNAL TRANSDUCTION

Agonists for all three β-receptors stimulate adenylyl cyclase and increase the level of the second messenger, cAMP (see Fig. 13–17). Attachment of the agonist to the receptor induces a conformational change in the receptor; this permits interaction with the membrane-associated regulatory protein G_s, activating the catalytic portion of adenylyl cyclase and enhancing the formation of cAMP. The increase in intracellular cAMP activates protein kinase A (PKA) and other cAMP-dependent protein kinases that phosphorylate a variety of proteins. Alterations in the functional state of these proteins generate the β-receptor response that is characteristic of the effector tissue. β-Receptor antagonists, on the other hand, with the exception of those with partial agonist activity, bind to the receptor but do not induce receptor interaction with the nucleotide regulatory protein and therefore do not activate adenylyl cyclase. As a consequence, agonist-receptor interaction is inhibited and physiological response is blocked. Mechanisms other than G_s-mediated activation of adenylyl cyclase may be involved in mediation of the biologic effects of β_3-adrenergic receptor stimulation.[195]

Alterations in Adrenergic Receptor Number and Function

PHYSIOLOGICAL RESPONSES TO ADRENERGIC STIMULATION

The responsiveness of peripheral effector tissues to adrenergic stimulation can be modified by alterations in tempera-

ture, in the chemical composition of extracellular fluid, and in the levels of various hormones and mediators. Such changes in responsiveness may originate at the adrenergic receptor, by alterations in receptor number or affinity for agonist, or at postreceptor sites. Alterations in receptor response secondary to activation of the receptor by agonists are referred to as *homologous regulation*; those caused by environmental changes or agonist-receptor interactions not involving the affected receptor are designated *heterologous regulation*.

The progressive decline in physiological response despite continued exposure of an effector tissue to an agonist is termed *desensitization* or tachyphylaxis. Among the mechanisms that cause desensitization are a decrease in signal transduction caused by diminished coupling of adrenergic receptors to G proteins (which can occur over minutes) and a reduction in receptor protein on the outer surface of the cell membrane (which can occur in minutes, hours or days). The latter process is referred to as receptor down-regulation, and it can occur secondary to internalization and degradation of membrane receptors or to diminished synthesis of receptor protein. Down-regulation of G proteins or of protein kinase C can also contribute to desensitization.[205, 206] Both desensitization and down-regulation can be homologous or heterologous depending on the role of specific adrenergic agonists in mediating the reduction in end-organ response.

REGULATION OF SHORT-TERM CHANGES IN RECEPTOR FUNCTION

Phosphorylation of receptor protein plays a central role in acute desensitization of adrenergic receptors. Structural analysis of the β-adrenergic receptors reveals multiple potential sites of phosphorylation within the third cytoplasmic loop and COOH terminus.[207] One specific kinase (termed β-adrenergic receptor kinase or β-ARK) recognizes and phosphorylates only the activated conformation of β-adrenergic receptors[207] and also phosphorylates other G-protein–coupled receptors, including α_1- and α_2-adrenergic receptors.[208, 209] β-ARK belongs to a family of serine/threonine protein kinases that recognize and phosphorylate G-protein–coupled receptors in their activated conformation.[208, 209]

After phosphorylation of the β-adrenergic receptor by β-ARK, the affinity of binding of a second protein, β-arrestin, to the cytoplasmic tail of the receptor increases.[207] The β-arrestin–receptor complex sterically blocks coupling of the receptor to the G protein–adenylyl cyclase complex, with rapid loss of responsiveness to further stimulation by agonist. Phosphorylated receptors may then undergo sequestration to an interior compartment of the cell, where the proteins are dephosphorylated and recycled to the cell surface (leading to resensitization) or are degraded and eliminated.[210] The molecular events underlying sequestration are poorly understood, although prior phosphorylation is not required.[211] Desensitization is caused principally by receptor phosphorylation; it occurs too rapidly for sequestration to play a major role.[194] Phosphorylation of agonist-occupied receptors by β-ARK is an example of *homologous desensitization*. Because it is more apparent at high rather than low agonist concentrations, *homologous desensitization* may play an important role in synaptic function.[194]

Adrenergic receptors are also substrates for protein kinase A and protein kinase C, which phosphorylate the receptor protein at sites different from those phosphorylated by β-ARK and related kinases.[210] Consequently, receptor desensitization through phosphorylation mediated by these protein kinases does not involve alterations in binding of β-arrestin to receptor protein.[210] On the other hand, suppression of cAMP production by inhibition of adenylyl cyclase increases β-adrenergic responsiveness.[212] Unlike β-ARK–mediated desensitization, phosphorylation by these kinases does not depend on the conformation of the adrenergic receptors and therefore does not depend on occupancy of the specific receptor by agonist.[194] Because agents such as catecholamines activate kinases capable of phosphorylating adrenergic receptors, these pathways provide a mechanism for acute *heterologous desensitization*, which may be especially important at low agonist concentrations.[207]

Adrenergic receptors differ in their susceptibility to agonist-induced desensitization or sequestration. Of the three subtypes of β-adrenergic receptors, β$_2$ receptors are the most prone and β$_3$-receptors are the least prone to phosphorylation by either β-ARK or protein kinase A; β$_1$-receptors are intermediate in susceptibility.[196] β$_2$-Receptors also undergo agonist-promoted sequestration to a greater extent than either β$_1$- or β$_3$-receptors.[210] As a consequence, short-term desensitization of β$_3$-receptors is not demonstrable in vitro. Differences among α$_2$-receptor subtypes in short-term desensitization are of uncertain functional importance.[213]

REGULATION OF SUBACUTE OR CHRONIC CHANGES IN RECEPTOR NUMBER

Prolonged exposure to adrenergic agonists leads to receptor down-regulation. Although changes in receptor number over minutes to hours primarily reflect sequestration of receptors within the intracellular compartment, changes over a longer interval can reflect decreases in receptor protein synthesis as well.[210] De novo synthesis of receptor protein probably is required for subsequent restoration of receptor number and may be an important determinant of steady-state receptor number during continuous agonist exposure.[211] Adrenergic agonists influence receptor synthesis through effects on gene transcription and on the stability of receptor protein mRNA.[214] The effects of catecholamines on gene transcription are mediated, in part, by changes in intracellular levels of cAMP. Prolonged agonist exposure, however, can lead to a reduction in receptor protein mRNA.[215, 216] For the β$_2$-receptor, the decrease in mRNA is caused by accelerated degradation and occurs coincident with the induction of a specific mRNA-binding protein presumably involved in RNA catabolism.[217] Reduced stability of mRNA also contributes to the agonist-induced decrease in α$_1$-receptor mRNA.[218] As with desensitization, homologous down-regulation has variable effects on the different subtypes of α- and β-adrenergic receptors.[210] The β$_2$ subtype is the most susceptible β-adrenergic receptor to receptor uncoupling, receptor sequestration, and receptor down-regulation.[210]

Glucocorticoids, insulin, thyroid hormone, estrogens, androgens, and mineralocorticoids influence the regulation of adrenergic receptor gene transcription, induce alterations in receptor number and in signal transduction by adrenergic receptor pathways, and ultimately affect adrenergic responsiveness in target tissues. How effects at the nuclear and cellular levels bring about changes in responsiveness at the tissue and system levels is not fully understood. Because the effects of various hormones or mediators on α- and β-adrenergic receptors are tissue- and receptor-subtype specific, it is difficult to predict the net effect of hormone action on adrenergic responsiveness in a particular tissue on the basis of individual cellular events. For example, glucocorticoids induce expression of β-adrenergic receptors in both smooth muscle cells and adipocytes[219, 220]; adrenergic stimulation of cAMP, however, is increased in smooth muscle cells and diminished in adipocytes.[220, 221] The effects of glucocorticoids in smooth muscle cells counter those of β$_2$-adrenergic agonists to down-regulate β$_2$-receptors.[222]

PHYSIOLOGICAL SIGNIFICANCE OF ALTERATIONS IN ADRENERGIC RECEPTOR NUMBER: SPARE RECEPTORS. Because a maximal physiological response can be demonstrated when only a small portion of β-receptors are occupied, the significance of alterations in the number of adrenergic receptors is unclear. Interactions of agonist and receptor, however, follow the law of mass action; increased numbers of adrenergic receptors increase the likelihood of agonist-receptor interaction and shift the dose-response curve to the left, indicating an increase in sensitivity. The presence of "spare" receptors *(receptor reserve)* implies that alterations in receptor number are translated into alterations in sensitivity to agonist. In fact, an alteration in receptor number does correlate with changes in sensitivity to catecholamines in arteries and veins.[223] Furthermore, because of the inactivation of agonist-occupied receptors by homologous desensitization, continued end-organ response to agonist stimulation depends on this receptor reserve. Alteration in receptor number, however, is only one determinant of the sensitivity of effector tissues to catecholamines.

Dopaminergic Receptors

Although DA is a weak agonist of both α- and β-adrenergic receptors, distinct dopaminergic receptors mediate DA responses in several peripheral tissues. The classification of dopaminergic receptors into two categories has been modified with identification of three additional receptors.[224] DA receptors within the CNS are referred to as D$_1$-like and D$_2$-like. D$_{1A}$ and D$_5$/D$_{1B}$ belong to the D$_1$-like family, and D$_{2s}$, D$_{2L}$, D$_3$, and D$_4$ belong to the D$_2$-like family. In peripheral tissues DA receptors are classified as DA$_1$ or DA$_2$ on the basis of synaptic localization, following the work of Goldberg and coworkers.[225, 226] DA$_2$ receptors are located in autonomic ganglia and on presynaptic neuronal membranes, and DA$_1$ receptors are in non-neuronal peripheral tissues. The relation between the central and peripheral dopaminergic receptors has been uncertain because of slight differences in agonist and antagonist potencies, although peripheral DA$_1$ receptors are roughly similar to central D$_{1A}$ and D$_5$/D$_{1B}$ receptors and peripheral DA$_2$ to central D$_2$.[227]

D$_1$-like receptors (both D$_{1A}$ and D$_5$/D$_{1B}$) are coupled to adenylyl cyclase by the G$_s$ regulatory protein.[224] The phosphoprotein DARPP-32 (*d*opamine- and cAMP-*r*egulated *p*hospho*p*rotein, molecular weight 32,000) is present in central and peripheral tissues rich in D$_1$ receptors and may act as a third messenger in the expression of D$_1$ and D$_1$-like effects.[228] Among D$_2$-like receptors most DA$_2$ and D$_2$ responses are caused by inhibition of adenylyl cyclase by interaction with G$_i$ (see Fig. 13–17).[224] In addition, some responses in CNS and peripheral tissues appear to require simultaneous activation of both DA$_1$ and DA$_2$ receptors.[229, 230]

The DA$_1$ receptor mediates vasodilatation in renal, mesenteric, coronary, and cerebral vascular beds. Fenoldopam and the investigational compound SKF 38393 are selective agonists for the DA$_1$ receptor; the investigational compound SCH 23390 is a specific DA$_1$ antagonist. The DA$_2$ receptor inhibits transmission in sympathetic ganglia, reduces NE release from sympathetic nerve endings, inhibits prolactin release from the pituitary and aldosterone secretion from the adrenal cortex, and evokes emesis. Selective agonists for the DA$_2$ receptor include bromocriptine, lergotrile, and apomorphine; selective DA$_2$ antagonists include butyrophenones, such as haloperidol and domperidone, and the benzamide sulpiride. Although DA may affect the lower esophageal sphincter, this dopaminergic response has not been characterized with regard to receptor type.

PHYSIOLOGY AND PATHOPHYSIOLOGY OF SYMPATHOADRENAL SYSTEM

Regulation of Sympathoadrenal Activity

CENTRAL NEURAL CONTROL

Catecholamine release at the sympathetic nerve endings and the adrenal medulla is the result of a downward flow of impulses from sympathetic centers within the CNS (see Fig. 13–2). The functional state of these centers is governed by many factors: (1) the intrinsic activity of the hypothalamic and brain stem nuclei that constitute the sympathetic centers and initiate the downward flow of impulses; (2) other regions in the brain stem, hypothalamus, limbic lobe, and cortex that send projections to the sympathetic centers; (3) visceral and somatic afferents that coordinate the activity of the sympathetic centers with environmental factors; and (4) the composition of the extracellular fluid, including the levels of electrolytes, substrates, and hormones as well as temperature and tonicity, all of which can influence the sympathetic centers and related regions in the CNS. Of the neural afferent pathways involved in regulation of sympathetic activity, only the baroreceptor reflex has been well characterized.[231]

GENERALIZED VERSUS DISCRIMINANT RESPONSES

Generalized or global sympathoadrenal activation results in the fight-or-flight response described by Walter Cannon. The organization of the sympathoadrenal system is consistent with the view that generalized responses are an important aspect of sympathoadrenal function. Amplification of sympathetic outflow occurs at the sympathetic ganglia, where each preganglionic fiber activates several postganglionic neurons, suggesting widespread dispersion of descending nerve impulse traffic. Furthermore, the release of catecholamines from the adrenal medulla into the circulation distributes the neurohumoral signal systematically. However, different components of the sympathoadrenal system are affected differently by physiological stimuli. Not only is sympathetic outflow to peripheral tissues distributed nonhomogeneously, but the activity of postganglionic sympathetic neurons is often dissociated from that of the adrenal medulla. Moreover, release of NE from the adrenal medulla appears to be regulated separately from that of epinephrine.[232]

RELATION BETWEEN SYMPATHETIC NERVOUS SYSTEM AND ADRENAL MEDULLA

The relation between the two limbs of the sympathoadrenal system is complex. The traditional view, implicit in the work of Cannon, envisages the sympathetic nervous system and the adrenal medulla working in tandem, with circulating catecholamines from the adrenal medulla supporting the effects of the sympathetic nerves. This view is consistent with the pattern of sympathoadrenal involvement in conditions such as cold exposure or exercise. In other circumstances (e.g., fasting-associated hypoglycemia, ischemic injury, hemorrhagic hypotension), however, suppression of sympathetic activity occurs in concert with adrenomedullary stimulation.[233, 234] Such divergence between sympathetic and adrenal medullary responses suggests that circulating and locally-released catecholamines (and neuropeptides) serve different functions in cardiovascular and metabolic regulation. Because of difficulties inherent in the assessment of sympathetic and adrenal medullary function, the contributions of the two systems to the regulation of catecholamine-dependent processes are in many cases not well defined.

GENERAL FEATURES OF PHYSIOLOGICAL REGULATION BY SYMPATHOADRENAL SYSTEM

SPEED. Because the sympathoadrenal system is an efferent limb of the nervous system, catecholamine-mediated events take place in seconds compared with the longer time course of action of most hormones. Connections between the cerebral cortex and the sympathetic centers that regulate sympathoadrenal outflow link sympathetic outflow with conscious mental processes.

ANTICIPATION. Anticipation of a particular activity may activate the sympathoadrenal system before the activity begins, thereby stimulating catecholamine-responsive processes in advance.

INTEGRATION. Most catecholamine-mediated responses have both direct and indirect components. Direct effects are mediated by interaction of catecholamines and adrenergic receptors in a particular effector tissue; indirect effects involve alterations in (1) secretion of other hormones that regulate the process under study; (2) delivery of a substrate necessary for the process under observation; or (3) local blood flow. As a general rule, the vascular, metabolic, and hormonal effects of catecholamines reinforce one another. Although the contributions of the sympathoadrenal system to physiological regulation are most often considered in relation to acute responses to stimuli such as hypoglycemia or upright posture, the chronic level of sympathoadrenal activity is also important.

Physiological Effects of Catecholamines

Catecholamines influence virtually all tissues and many functions. In most instances, they participate with other hormonal and neuronal systems in regulation of physiological processes, contributing to a redundancy that ensures both physiological reserve and fine or discriminating control. Involvement of the sympathoadrenal system in multiple processes implies an important integrative role in accordance with the needs of the organism as a whole.

In the following discussion, the effects of catecholamines have arbitrarily been divided into cardiovascular, visceral, and metabolic effects, recognizing that overlap exists. In general terms the cardiovascular effects of catecholamines control cardiac output and apportion blood flow, and the visceral effects regulate vegetative functions in other organs. The metabolic effects involve mobilization of energy reserves from storage depots, regulation of oxygen uptake, and maintenance of the constancy of extracellular fluid.

CARDIOVASCULAR EFFECTS

Sympathetically mediated adjustments in peripheral resistance maintain the integrity of the circulation to provide ade-

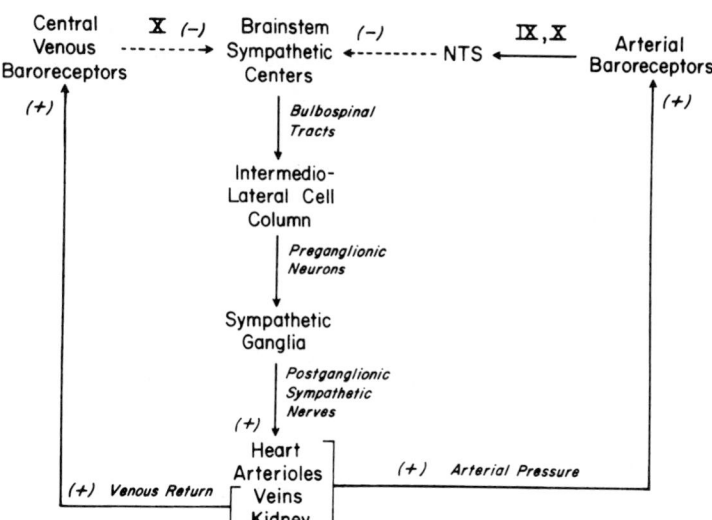

Figure 13–19. Sympathetic regulation of circulation: afferent impulses from resistance and capacitance portions of circulation. Stretch receptors in venous (low-pressure, capacitance) and arterial (high-pressure, resistance) circulations are stimulated by an increase in tension that reflects increased venous filling pressure or increased arterial pressure. Afferent impulses from these receptors are carried to the CNS by the ninth and tenth cranial nerves. The consequence of increased afferent impulse traffic in this system is inhibition of central sympathetic outflow. Although the central connections that are involved in these circulatory reflexes are only partially clarified, the arterial baroreceptor reflex involves a relay in the nucleus tractus solitarius (NTS). If venous filling pressure or arterial blood pressure falls, impulse traffic from stretch receptors diminishes; as a consequence the tonic inhibitory effect of these circulatory afferents is diminished, with a resultant increase in central sympathetic outflow. (+), stimulation; (−), inhibition. (From Landsberg L, Young JB. Physiology and pharmacology of the autonomic nervous system. In: Wilson JD, Braunwald E, Isselbacher K, et al., eds. Harrison's Principles of Internal Medicine. 12th ed. New York: McGraw-Hill, 1991: 380–392. Reproduced with permission of McGraw-Hill, Inc.)

quate perfusion of vital organ systems in the face of changing circumstances. Although the sympathetic nerves to the heart and vasculature are more important in cardiovascular regulation, circulating catecholamines from the adrenal medulla may partially compensate for suppressed or defective sympathetic responses.

AFFERENT PATHWAYS. Stretch receptors in both low-pressure capacitance vessels and high-pressure resistance vessels continuously monitor the status of the circulation; stimulation of these stretch receptors by afferent impulses carried in the ninth and tenth cranial nerves (Fig. 13–19)[231] reduces central sympathetic outflow. The presence of receptors in both capacitance and resistance portions of the circulation permits the sympathetic nervous system to respond to alterations in volume, pressure, or both. Although the high- and low-pressure baroreceptors work in tandem to maintain blood pressure and tissue perfusion, the low-pressure baroreceptors appear to be more sensitive; small decrements in venous return, such as those induced by alterations in position, stimulate the sympathetic nervous system without a fall in arterial pressure.

CENTRAL CONNECTIONS. High-pressure baroreceptor afferents terminate in the nucleus of the tractus solitarius (NTS); increased baroreceptor afferent activity stimulates an inhibitory reflex that originates in the NTS and terminates in

brain stem sympathetic centers. The inhibitory pathway involves an α_2-adrenergic synapse of uncertain location. Centrally acting α-adrenergic agonists that lower blood pressure (clonidine; α-methylnorepinephrine) appear to potentiate this baroreceptor depressor response. The central mechanisms involved in the low-pressure baroreceptor response have not been clarified, although the afferent neural pathway terminates within the NTS and appears to involve the vagus. Excitatory bulbospinal tracts originating in the rostral ventrolateral medulla and inhibitory pathways in the caudal ventrolateral medulla have been identified.[7] The neurotransmitters involved in cardiovascular regulation include epinephrine, NE, and serotonin. Substance P and neuropeptide Y may act as cotransmitters in some pathways.

EFFERENT CARDIOVASCULAR EFFECTS. The efferent limb of the baroreceptor reflex involves sympathetic outflow to the arterioles, heart, kidneys, and veins (Fig. 13–20). Venous return is augmented by α-receptor–mediated venoconstriction and by enhancement of sodium reabsorption (described later). Peripheral resistance is increased by α-receptor–mediated vasoconstriction in the subcutaneous, mucosal, splanchnic, and renal vascular beds. Because sympathetically mediated vasoconstriction is minimal in the coronary and cerebral circulations, flow to these areas is maintained at the

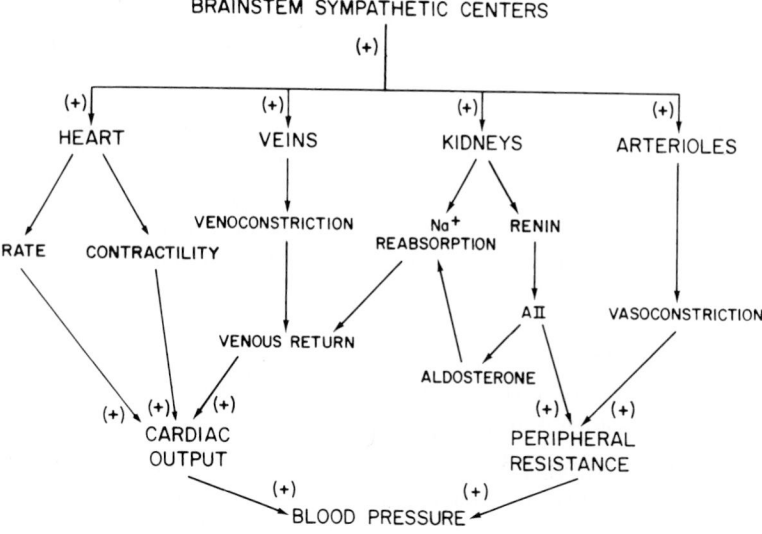

Figure 13–20. Sympathetic regulation of circulation: effects on blood pressure. Sympathetic stimulation (+) increases blood pressure by effects on the heart, veins, kidneys, and arterioles. Both cardiac output and peripheral resistance are increased by direct and indirect effects of the sympathetic nervous system. AII, angiotensin II. (From Young JB, Landsberg L. Obesity and the circulation. In: Sleight P, Jones JV, eds. Scientific Foundations of Cardiology. London: Heinemann, 1983: 201–206.)

expense of that to the other major vascular beds. The distribution of blood flow is regulated by differences in sympathetically mediated arteriolar resistance in different anatomic regions.

VASCULAR RESPONSES. Vasoconstriction throughout the vasculature, including lymphatics, is mediated by α_1- and α_2-receptors. Arterial α-receptors regulate peripheral resistance and tissue perfusion, and venous α-receptors control venous capacitance and hence plasma volume. Arteries and veins in many vascular beds, including the pulmonary, coronary, and renal circulations, are endowed with both α_1- and α_2-receptors,[191] but the distribution of these receptor subtypes is heterogeneous within a single vascular bed. In general, α_1-receptors predominate in large arteries, α_2-receptors predominate in veins, and both receptor types mediate vasoconstriction in resistance vessels.[235] α_2-Receptors also modulate vasomotor tone indirectly through inhibition of NE release from sympathetic nerves. In addition, sympathetic nerves release other mediators and neuropeptides, including ATP, neuropeptide Y, galanin, and opioid peptides, which mediate vasoconstriction.[236] The relative importance of these cotransmitters in vascular regulation is unclear.

Catecholamines and sympathetic nerves also mediate vasodilatation. Low levels of circulating epinephrine cause vasodilatation by stimulation of noninnervated β_2-receptors, particularly in vessels of skeletal muscle.[237] In animals activation of either α- or β-receptors stimulates endothelial production of nitric oxide, resulting in vasodilatation.[238, 239] Impairment in β-mediated vasodilatation in atherosclerotic coronary arteries may be a result of the endothelial dysfunction in this disorder.[240] Cholinergic impulses may also promote vasodilatation by stimulating endothelial production of nitric oxide.[236] The importance of acetylcholine release by sympathetic nerves in vascular regulation is unknown.[241]

Vasoconstrictor responses to sympathetic stimulation are modified by local factors in the innervated vascular bed, such as temperature.[242] α_2-Receptor–mediated vasoconstriction is more susceptible to inhibition by acidosis, hypoxia, and endotoxemia than is that mediated by α_1-receptors.[243, 244] Such differential sensitivity of vasoconstrictor responses in the microcirculation can serve to redirect local blood flow without causing alterations in total peripheral resistance and blood pressure.

CARDIAC EFFECTS. The direct effects of catecholamines on the heart are mediated predominantly by postjunctional β_1-receptors and include increased heart rate, enhanced contractility, and augmented conduction velocity, all of which contribute to the increase in cardiac output. Increased contractility is secondary to an increase in the rate of spontaneous diastolic depolarization in the pacemaker cells and results in enhanced cardiac work in relation to ventricular muscle fiber length at diastole. Increased venous return caused by catecholamine-induced venoconstriction also increases the force of atrial contraction, enhancing ventricular contractility by increasing diastolic fiber length. Finally, an increase in conduction velocity in the junctional tissues causes a more synchronous ventricular contraction, resulting in more useful work per contraction. The biologic cost of catecholamine-induced cardiac stimulation is increased myocardial oxygen consumption.

VISCERAL EFFECTS

The visceral effects of catecholamines are summarized in Table 13–6. The physiological importance in some cases is uncertain.

SMOOTH MUSCLE. As a general rule, catecholamines cause smooth muscle relaxation through β-receptor mechanisms and smooth muscle contraction through α-receptor

TABLE 13–6. Visceral Effects of Catecholamines

Smooth muscle function
 Gastrointestinal motility
 Gallbladder contraction
 Splenic contraction
 Gastrointestinal and genitourinary sphincter
  tone
 Urinary bladder contraction
 Bronchial smooth muscle tone
 Piloerection and activity of ciliated epithelium
 Iris and ciliary muscle function
Fluid and electrolyte transport
 Gastrointestinal tract function
  Salivary secretion
  Gastric acid secretion
  Pancreatic exocrine secretion
  Intestinal absorption
  Gallbladder reabsorption
 Renal tubular function
 Tracheobronchial fluid reabsorption
 Aqueous humor formation
 Corneal epithelium transport
 Choroid plexus secretion
 Sweat gland secretion (apocrine and eccrine)
Protein secretion
 Gastrointestinal tract function
  Salivary secretion
  Gastric secretion of mucus
  Pancreatic exocrine secretion
 Peripheral hormone production
 Bronchial mucin secretion
 Lacrimal secretion
 Factor VIII secretion
Cell growth and division
 Intestinal epithelium
 Erythropoiesis
 Adaptive hypertrophy in heart, vascular
  smooth muscle, and skeletal muscle
 Brown fat hypertrophy
 Prostatic hypertrophy
Hemostasis
 Platelet aggregation
 Vasoconstriction
Immune function
 Cell-mediated immunity
 Humoral immunity
Reproductive function
 Epididymal duct reabsorption
 Prostataic secretion
 Spermatogenesis
 Oviduct and vas deferens contractility
 Uterine contractility
 Ovarian and testicular contractility
 Prostatic smooth muscle tone
 Ejaculation
 Milk duct contractility

stimulation.[245] Sympathetic stimulation decreases tone in intestinal and urinary bladder smooth muscle while constricting the corresponding sphincters. Smooth muscle relaxation traditionally has been attributed to the β_2-receptor subtype, but atypical β-receptors (presumably β_3) may be involved in responses of gastrointestinal and bronchial smooth muscle.[246–248] Dopaminergic receptors also mediate relaxation of gut and vascular smooth muscle.[225] In the intact animal the influence of catecholamines on gut smooth muscle is intimately related to the function of the enteric nervous system. Sympathetic nerve terminals that are close to myenteric ganglion cells and postganglionic sympathetic fibers exert prejunctional inhibitory effects on both cholinergic and nonadrenergic, noncholinergic (possibly nitric oxide) neurotransmission by an α_2 mechanism.[249] The inhibition of intestinal motility by catecholamines therefore may be caused either by β-receptor–mediated relaxation or by α_2-receptor–mediated suppression of acetylcholine (or nitric oxide) release. Normal intestinal motility depends on the balance between sympathetic and parasympathetic effects. Sympathetic dominance can cause paralytic ileus. Neuropeptides co-localized and released with NE, such as neuropeptide Y, may affect gut motility as well.

The bronchial musculature is heavily innervated with parasympathetic nerve endings, and the sympathetic nervous system plays only a minor role in regulation of airway resistance. The effects of catecholamines on diverse pulmonary functions are mediated largely by β₂-adrenergic receptors, which may be a target for circulating epinephrine.[250, 251] A genetic variant of the β₂-receptor that exhibits accelerated agonist-promoted desensitization has been reported in some patients with nocturnal asthma.[252]

Myoepithelial cells that contain contractile elements but are not true smooth muscle cells are present in the breast (in the milk duct) and the ovary (in the wall of the graafian follicle). Catecholamines stimulate contraction of these structures, thereby contributing to milk ejection and ovulation. Contractile cells in the prostate and testicular capsule also respond to NE and to nerve stimulation. Bladder outlet obstruction in men with prostatic enlargement is caused partly by α₁-mediated smooth muscle contraction.[253]

FLUID AND ELECTROLYTE TRANSPORT. Catecholamines influence the movement of water and ions across membrane surfaces, including the intestine, gallbladder, trachea, cornea, and renal epithelium.[254, 255] They likewise alter the secretion of fluid into the aqueous humor, so that both α-adrenergic agonists and β-adrenergic antagonists are useful in the treatment of glaucoma. α-Receptor stimulation promotes and dopaminergic receptor activation antagonizes intestinal absorption of sodium and water,[256, 257] raising the possibility that catecholamine effects on water and electrolyte metabolism in gut may contribute to homeostatic regulation of the extracellular fluid. Apocrine sweating in the axillary and genital areas is stimulated by catecholamines, whereas eccrine sweating in other skin areas involved in temperature regulation is mediated by postganglionic cholinergic sympathetic fibers.

PROTEIN SECRETION. Catecholamines stimulate the secretion of peptides into tears, saliva, pancreatic juice, and prostatic fluid and promote release of mucus from gastric mucosa and bronchial epithelium.

CELL GROWTH AND DIVISION. Catecholamines stimulate cell growth and division in a wide array of tissues, including the parotid glands[258] and continuously replicating cell populations such as intestinal epithelial cells, erythroid precursors in bone marrow, and possibly spermatocytes.[259–261] Catecholamine stimulation contributes to the development of adaptive hypertrophy of cardiac muscle, skeletal muscle, and vascular smooth muscle.[262–264] Sympathetic activation is also associated with hyperplasia of brown adipose tissue and prostate.[265, 266] In general, increased cell proliferation caused by catecholamines or other neurotransmitters results from inhibition of adenylyl cyclase, and reduced cell division results from elevations in cAMP.[267] The role of catecholamines in cancer growth is uncertain.[259, 268]

HEMOSTASIS. Epinephrine increases the platelet count and promotes platelet aggregation through α₂-receptor stimulation.[269] Epinephrine also increases circulating levels of factor VIII, von Willebrand's factor, and tissue plasminogen activator, and it decreases levels of the plasminogen activator inhibitor in plasma.[270, 271] β-Adrenergic blockade attenuates these elevations in factor VIII and von Willebrand's factor.[270] Epinephrine also promotes hepatic synthesis of fibrinogen.[272] Changes in plasma levels of epinephrine frequently correlate with indices of blood coagulation and fibrinolysis, suggesting a role for epinephrine in mediation of these events.

IMMUNE FUNCTION. The spleen and lymph nodes are heavily innervated with sympathetic fibers, and although the role of catecholamines in immunoregulation is uncertain, they may provide a link between the immune system and conditions

that affect sympathoadrenal activity, such as emotional state, nutritional status, and physical activity.[273, 274]

METABOLIC EFFECTS

FUEL METABOLISM. Catecholamines stimulate the breakdown of stored fuels into utilizable substrates for generation of energy (see Chapters 20 and 21). One of the major metabolic functions of catecholamines is the rapid mobilization of substrates from liver, adipose tissue, and skeletal muscle (Fig. 13–21). Substrate mobilization depends on levels of hormones and substrates, on the nerve supply, and on blood flow through storage tissues. The effects of catecholamines, glucagon, and glucocorticoids are generally opposite to those of insulin, and the net activity of a given process reflects the interactions among these regulators.

Liver. Catecholamines promote hepatic glucose output by activating glycogenolysis, accelerating gluconeogenesis, and inhibiting glycogen synthesis. Interaction of catecholamines with the β₂-adrenergic receptor stimulates adenylyl cyclase and leads to generation of cAMP, initiation of the cAMP-dependent enzymatic cascade, and conversion of glycogen phosphorylase from the inactive to the active form.[275] α₁-Receptor stimulation also activates phosphorylase, thereby increasing glycogenolysis, and enhances gluconeogenesis in isolated hepatocytes by mechanisms that are independent of cAMP.[276] Amino acid uptake into liver—and perhaps lactate entry also—is augmented by α-agonists, which increase the availability of substrates for gluconeogenesis. Suppression of insulin and stimulation of glucagon secretion by catecholamines augment their direct effects on hepatic glucose production. The contributions of α- and β-adrenergic receptor mechanisms to hepatic glucose production vary among species and in different conditions within the same species. α-Adrenergic effects predominate in rats, whereas β-adrenergic effects predominate in dogs and humans. α-Adrenergic stimulation also enhances hepatic glucose production in humans.[277]

Epinephrine and NE decrease and dopamine increases hepatic blood flow.[278, 279] In addition, glucagon may decrease catecholamine-induced hepatic arterial vasoconstriction.[278]

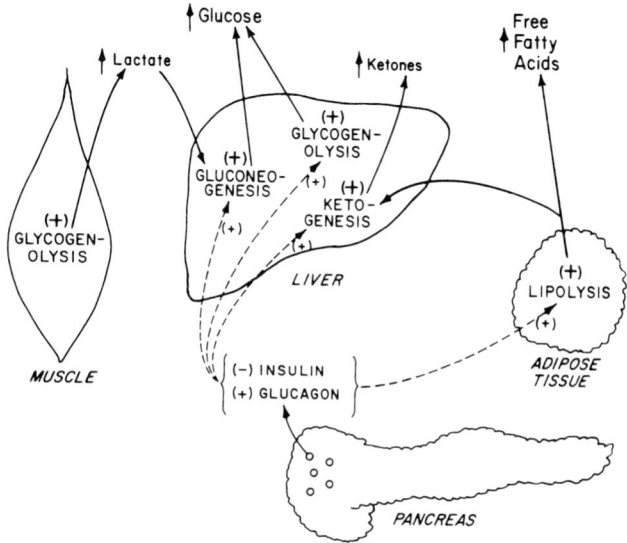

Figure 13–21. Schematic representation of catecholamine effects on fuel mobilization in liver, adipose tissue, and skeletal muscle. Direct effects are reinforced by (but do not require) catecholamine-mediated suppression of insulin and stimulation of glucagon. (+), stimulation; (−), inhibition. (From Landsberg L, Young JB. Catecholamines and the adrenal medulla. In: Bondy PK, Rosenberg LE, eds. Metabolic Control and Disease. 8th ed. Philadelphia: WB Saunders, 1980: 1621–1693.)

otides the free fatty acids stimulate heat production by uncoupling of oxidative phosphorylation in brown adipocyte mitochondria.[333, 334] This physiological uncoupling involves a unique mitochondrial protein named *thermogenin* or *uncoupling protein*, which shares homology with a superfamily of carrier proteins in mitochondria.[335] In the normally coupled state substrate oxidation leads to H^+ transport out of the mitochondria; these protons can re-enter the mitochondria only by means of an ATPase tightly coupled to ATP synthesis. In brown fat mitochondria the proton gradient is dissipated by the uncoupling protein which, in conjunction with purine nucleotides, renders the mitochondrial membrane permeable to protons (or hydroxyl ions) so that ATP is not resynthesized and the energy is released directly as heat.[335] Transcription of the gene that regulates the synthesis of uncoupling protein is also under the direct control of NE through a β_3-receptor mechanism and is amplified by thyroid hormone.[334, 335]

In addition to the β_3-receptor mechanism that regulates heat production in brown adipose tissue, β_1-receptor stimulation enhances differentiation of preadipocytes into mature brown fat cells and proliferation of brown adipocytes both in vivo and in vitro.[334, 336] In addition, an α_1-receptor–mediated process stimulates the deiodination of thyroxine to triiodothyronine (T_3). The brown adipose tissue deiodinase has been designated type 2 and is distinct from the type 1, propylthiouracil-sensitive deiodinase that is present in liver and kidney (see Chapter 11). It provides the high local concentrations of T_3 that are essential for full expression of the thermogenic potential of this tissue and may, under some circumstances, produce T_3 for systemic distribution.[337]

WATER AND ELECTROLYTE METABOLISM. The role of catecholamines in the regulation of the volume and composition of the extracellular fluid involves direct effects, effects on other hormones, and alterations in regional blood flow. In addition, alterations in mineral content of the diet or in the ionic composition of extracellular fluid elicit changes in sympathoadrenal activity and in the response of peripheral tissues to catecholamines.

Water. Catecholamines alter sodium reabsorption in the proximal tubule (discussed later) and water reabsorption in the cortical collecting duct. Infusions of NE increase and those of isoproterenol decrease free water clearance, principally as a result of effects of catecholamines on pituitary secretion of vasopressin. NE inhibits and isoproterenol stimulates vasopressin release through an effect on arterial baroreceptors unrelated to changes in blood pressure.[338] In addition, α_2-adrenergic agonists inhibit vasopressin responses in cortical collecting tubules and renal papillae, though the magnitude of this effect varies among mammalian species.[339] DA may also antagonize the action of vasopressin in cortical collecting tubules,[340] although its principal diuretic effect is secondary to a reduction in proximal tubular sodium reabsorption.

Sodium. In the kidney noradrenergic fibers are found not only in relation to vascular structures but also in proximity to the juxtaglomerular apparatus (where they influence renin secretion) and the renal tubules.[341] Consequently, the effects of sympathetic nerves on renal sodium reabsorption involve vascular, hormonal, and tubular events. Marked sympathoadrenal activation increases sodium reabsorption by reducing glomerular filtration. Lesser degrees of sympathetic stimulation that do not affect glomerular filtration promote sodium reabsorption by redistributing renal blood flow from cortical to juxtamedullary nephrons, by increasing peritubular oncotic pressure, and by reducing intrarenal hydrostatic pressure. Catecholamines also enhance renin release from the juxtaglomerular apparatus (see later discussion). DA, on the other hand, produces renal vasodilatation and inhibits aldosterone secretion, actions that diminish sodium reabsorption.

In addition to the vascular and hormonal effects, catecholamines directly affect renal tubular function throughout the nephron.[342] Renal denervation or suppression of renal sympathetic activity acutely increases sodium excretion. Stimulation of renal nerves does the reverse, and both effects occur in the absence of alterations in glomerular filtration or renal plasma flow. Fluid reabsorption in the proximal tubule is enhanced by NE (α-receptor) and inhibited by DA. The increase in sodium reabsorption with NE may reflect activation of Na^+-H^+ exchange on the luminal cell membrane (α_2) and of Na^+,K^+-ATPase at the basolateral surface (α_1).[343, 344] DA inhibits both transport processes.

Alterations in sodium chloride intake also affect sympathetic and dopaminergic activity. Restriction of salt intake increases renal NE release and increases impulse traffic in sympathetic nerves to skeletal muscle.[345, 346] Urinary excretion of DA, by contrast, is directly related to sodium intake.[340] Impairment of sympathetic function in humans interferes with renal sodium conservation,[347, 348] although adjustments in other systems can compensate for brief periods of sodium restriction.[349] Oral administration of the AADC inhibitor carbidopa decreases renal DA formation and transiently reduces urinary sodium excretion.[340] Therefore, increased sympathetic activity may be a crucial component of renal sodium conservation, and DA may play a role in the regulation of sodium excretion during salt loading.

Potassium. Catecholamines influence the distribution of potassium between the intracellular and the extracellular spaces. α-Receptor stimulation increases potassium efflux and impairs the disposal of an intravenous potassium load,[350, 351] and β_2-receptor activation promotes potassium uptake into liver and skeletal muscle.[350] In part, the β_2-mediated effect represents direct stimulation by catecholamines of membrane-bound Na^+,K^+-ATPase in muscle.[352] DA, on the other hand, antagonizes cellular uptake of potassium and increases potassium excretion in urine.[353, 354]

Despite the effect of adrenergic agents on extrarenal potassium disposal, the physiological role of catecholamines in potassium homeostasis is uncertain. Sympathetic nerves appear to play at least a permissive role in maintenance of potassium homeostasis.[355] Moreover, the reduction in sympathetic activity associated with ingestion of a low potassium diet may limit potassium entry into innervated tissues and thereby help sustain potassium concentrations in extracellular fluid.[356] Although circulating catecholamines are less clearly affected by alterations in potassium concentrations, they may influence potassium disposition when the sympathoadrenal system is stimulated by other factors, such as exercise or respiratory alkalosis.[357, 358] In situations such as these, enhanced catecholamine release, particularly of epinephrine, may act as a buffer against the development of hyperkalemia.

The effects of catecholamines on potassium metabolism have several clinical implications. β-Adrenergic blockade potentiates the increase in potassium concentration during exercise and after cardiopulmonary bypass surgery.[359] This hyperkalemic effect is of therapeutic utility in treatment of hypokalemic periodic paralysis associated with thyrotoxicosis.[360] The hypokalemic effect of β_2-adrenergic agonists is of corresponding benefit in the treatment of patients with hyperkalemic periodic paralysis[361] but can be deleterious in other situations, as when used in the treatment of asthma.[362]

Calcium, Magnesium, and Phosphate. Catecholamines affect calcium, magnesium, and phosphate metabolism both directly, through effects on ion transport mechanisms and possibly on bone metabolism, and indirectly, through effects on the secretion of calcitonin and parathyroid hormone (PTH). Sympathetic fibers are distributed along blood vessels to bone and also within the periosteum, at the growth plate, and among marrow cells.[363, 364] Destruction of sympathetic nerves leads to a reduction in osteoblastic activity and an increase in osteoclastic activity.[365, 366] β-Adrenergic receptors are present on osteoblasts, and NE and various neuropeptides regulate cAMP formation in these cells in vitro.[367, 368] Administration of β₂-agonists also reduces inactivity-induced bone demineralization in animals.[369] The physiological importance of sympathetic innervation to bone is unknown.

Plasma levels of magnesium in humans fall in response to epinephrine infusion.[362, 370] A similar response follows administration of β₂-agonists and occurs in the absence of any changes in insulin or glucose concentration.[362, 370] β₂-Agonists also increase urinary excretion of both calcium and magnesium.[371] Although the hypercalcemia of pheochromocytoma may be caused by tumor secretion of PTH-related protein (PTHrP) rather than by catecholamines (see later discussion), enhanced urinary calcium excretion in these patients may reflect the calciuric effect of catecholamines.

Epinephrine also lowers serum phosphate levels by a β₂-adrenergic receptor mechanism,[372] an effect that probably explains the hypophosphatemia associated with increased sympathoadrenal activity.[373] Stimulation of α₂-adrenergic receptors in the kidney suppresses urinary phosphate excretion, even in response to PTH.[374] DA induces phosphaturia by a direct intrarenal effect involving inhibition of sodium-phosphate cotransport.[375] DA-mediated effects on phosphate excretion may contribute to the phosphaturic responses to PTH and atrial natriuretic peptide.[376, 377] Because renal DA formation is increased in animals fed a high-phosphate diet,[378] the impact of dietary phosphate on phosphaturic responses to PTH may reflect changes in intrarenal DA action.

PURINE METABOLISM. Catecholamines elevate plasma levels of uric acid, in part because of increased urate release, as occurs in isolated, perfused animal tissues in response to NE or nerve stimulation,[379, 380] and in part from reduced renal clearance of urate, as noted in human subjects during NE infusions.[381] Dopamine in the kidney may increase urate excretion, because dopamine blockade with metoclopramide diminishes fractional excretion of uric acid.[382]

Effects of Catecholamines on Hormone Secretion

GENERAL CONSIDERATIONS

NEURAL CONTROL OF HORMONE SECRETION. The sympathetic nerves and adrenal medulla influence the secretion of many peptide and steroid hormones (Table 13–7) in addition to the regulation provided by specific feedback loops. For those feedback loops that do not involve the CNS, the imposition of the sympathoadrenal system introduces advantages inherent in central regulation, including speed of response, anticipation, and integration. Many of the hormones listed in Table 13–7 also are known to affect the activity of the sympathetic nerves or the adrenal medulla, or both. For example, insulin, glucagon, and erythropoietin increase and glucocorticoids reduce sympathetic activity or plasma catecholamine levels. These effects suggest that neural feedback loops involving hormonal modulation of the sympathetic innervation of secretory tissues complement the more well-known feedback regulation of endocrine function by circulating factors.

EFFECTS OF CATECHOLAMINES: AN OVERVIEW. The effects of catecholamines on peripheral hormone secretion have common features. For peptide hormones, β-adrenergic receptor activation causes acute release of preformed hormone through a cAMP-dependent mechanism; this enhancement of hormone secretion is transient despite the continued presence of the agonist. α-Receptor effects are usually inhibitory and antagonize the principal stimulus for hormone secretion (e.g., glucose for insulin release, thyrotropin for thyroid hormone secretion), and they are frequently associated with suppression of cAMP. In addition to influencing secretion, catecholamines also alter hormone synthesis through effects on gene transcription (e.g., stimulation of renin expression by β₁-receptor activation, and suppression of insulin mRNA transcription by a G protein–related mechanism).[383, 384] Steroid hormones are synthesized by members of the cytochrome

TABLE 13–7. Major Effects of Catecholamines on Hormone Secretion

Endocrine Organ	Hormone	Effect	Receptor	Usual Feedback Loop
Kidney				
Juxtaglomerular apparatus	Renin	↑	β	Renal baroreceptor, distal tubular Na
Peritubular cells (?)	Erythropoietin	↑	β	Arterial PO₂
Pancreatic islets				
Alpha cells	Glucagon	↑	α, β	Plasma substrate
Beta cells	Insulin	↑	β	Plasma substrate
		↓	α	
Delta cells	Somatostatin	↑	β	?
		↓	α	
Non-α, β, δ cells	Pancreatic, polypeptide	↑	β	?
		↓	α	
Thyroid				
Follicles	Thyroxine, triiodothyronine	↑	β	Thyrotropin
		↓	α	
C cells	Calcitonin	↑	β	Plasma ionized Ca
		↓	α	
Parathyroid	Parathyroid hormone	↑	Dopamine, β	Plasma ionized Ca
		↓	α	
Gastric antrum and duodenum	Gastrin	↑	β	Gastric luminal pH
Adrenal cortex				
Zona fasciculata	Cortisol	↑	?	Corticotropin
	Androstenedione	↑	β	?
Zona glomerulosa	Aldosterone	↓	Dopamine	Angiotensin II, plasma K, corticotropin
		↑	β	
Ovary and placenta				
Granulosa cells or corpus luteum	Progesterone	↑	β, dopamine	Luteinizing hormone, human chorionic gonadotropin
	Oxytocin	↑	β	?
Theca cells	Androgens	↑	β	?
Testis	Testosterone	↑	β	Luteinizing hormone
Pineal	Melatonin	↑	β	Light-dark cycle
Heart, Atrium	Atrial natriuretic factor	↑	α, β	Atrial distention

P450 (*CYP*) gene superfamily of oxidases. Catecholamines stimulate gene expression of several enzymes of this family in adrenocortical cells, leading to increased synthesis of cortisol, aldosterone, and androstenedione.[385, 386]

EFFECTS OF CATECHOLAMINES ON REGULATION BY FEEDBACK LOOPS. Catecholamines influence the sensitivity of the endocrine cells to feedback regulation by their usual secretogogues. Evidence of these effects is seen in vitro in synergistic hormonal responses to stimulation by a secretogogue in the presence of catecholamines and in vivo in diminished responses to a secretogogue in denervated endocrine tissues. Moreover, the responsiveness to gonadotropin stimulation in the ovary and the neonatal response to corticotropin in the adrenal cortex caused by maternal separation both depend on sympathetic innervation.[387, 388] The mechanisms involved are not fully delineated but may reflect alterations in intracellular calcium or changes in cell surface receptor number or sensitivity for trophic hormone.[389–391] Such effects of catecholamines are of potential clinical importance in the regulation of endocrine function during development, in transplanted tissues, and in patients with autonomic insufficiency.

EFFECTS OF SYMPATHETIC INNERVATION ON COMPENSATING HYPERPLASIA. Sympathetic nerves contribute to the development of compensating hyperplasia. After unilateral adrenalectomy or castration, the contralateral gland increases in size; this hyperplastic response is attenuated by sympathetic denervation of the remaining gland.[392, 393] Such a response in the adrenal gland provides added support for an adrenergic role in glandular function. Sympathetic innervation of the thyroid may also support hypertrophic responses, because the activity of sympathetic nerves is increased in several states of thyroid growth and because hypertrophy is attenuated by preganglionic denervation of the gland.[394] Whether the effects of sympathetic nerves on glandular hypertrophy are caused by NE or by other co-transmitters (or both) is not known.

SYMPATHETIC NERVES VERSUS ADRENAL MEDULLA. As in other areas of metabolism, the relation between the sympathetic nerves and the adrenal medulla in regulation of hormone secretion is unclear. The presence of adrenergic fibers in proximity to the cell of origin of a particular hormone, especially synaptic contact between nerve terminal and secretory cell, provides prima facie evidence of sympathetic neuronal involvement in the secretory regulation of that hormone. In general, simultaneous catecholamine-induced alterations in the secretion of many hormones imply the global effect of adrenomedullary stimulation, whereas a selective change in one or another hormone is probably the result of the local effect of sympathetic nervous system activity.

Renin

Renin is secreted by the juxtaglomerular cells of the kidney in response to changes in perfusion pressure at the afferent arteriole and changes in solute delivery to the distal tubule. Renal nerve stimulation or infusion of catecholamines increases renin secretion independent of changes in renal blood flow or in filtered sodium load. The mammalian juxtaglomerular apparatus is innervated by sympathetic nerve endings in both vascular and tubular components that contain neuropeptide Y as well as norepinephrine.[395, 396] Renin secretion elicited by renal nerve stimulation or administration of adrenergic agonists is mediated in most circumstances by prejunctional β_2-receptors and postjunctional β_1-receptors.[397] The renin response to sympathetic stimulation also depends on macula densa function.[398] A role of the α-receptor independent of prejunctional or vascular effects is less clear.[397] Similarly, an inhibitory effect of neuropeptide Y on renin secretion

may be secondary to vasoconstriction.[396] In addition to the direct effects of catecholamines on renin secretion, renal sympathetic nerves potentiate renin responses to other stimuli.[399]

Catecholamines stimulate renin synthesis in vitro,[400, 401] and stimulation of renal nerves increases renin gene expression in vivo.[383] In vitro evidence supports involvement of both α- and β-adrenergic mechanisms in this process,[400, 401] and induction of renin gene expression in vivo is a result of activation of β_1-receptors.[383] Adrenergic effects on renin gene transcription may be mediated by a cAMP-responsive regulatory element in the renin gene.[402]

Catecholamine stimulation of renin output is an integral part of the physiological response to volume depletion. Renin release is tonically inhibited by a neural arc arising from low-pressure, cardiopulmonary baroreceptors; interruption of these neural afferents increases and distention of the baroreceptors diminishes sympathetically mediated renin secretion.[397] Afferent signals from carotid baroreceptors also participate but are less potent. Deficient or discoordinated renin release in some patients with postural hypotension secondary to autonomic neuropathy demonstrates the importance of sympathetic input for postural renin responses.[403] The rise in plasma renin level that accompanies chronic sodium depletion cannot, however, be attributed entirely to catecholamines. Surgical denervation of the canine or rat kidney lowers but does not abolish the increase in renin synthesis caused by sodium restriction.[404–406] Similarly, plasma renin levels rise in response to a low-sodium diet in patients with autonomic neuropathy.[348]

Epinephrine infusions also increase plasma renin acutely,[407] but the role of the adrenal medulla in renin secretion is unclear. Dopamine may also stimulate renin release by DA_1-receptor activation,[408, 409] although the precise role of DA in the regulation of renin secretion also remains to be established.[402] In most circumstances in which plasma renin activity is elevated, the increase is mediated by renal sympathetic nerves acting through β-adrenergic receptors.

Insulin and Glucagon

Although the endocrine pancreas is regulated predominantly by delivery of substrates, particularly glucose and amino acids, catecholamines influence pancreatic hormone secretion. Sympathetic (and parasympathetic) nerve fibers are close to all islet cell types, and alterations in insulin and glucagon secretion occur in response to pancreatic nerve stimulation or administration of adrenergic agonists. β_2-Receptor activation transiently increases secretion of both insulin and glucagon, whereas α_2-receptor stimulation suppresses insulin secretion and may enhance glucagon secretion.[410, 411] α-Receptor–mediated inhibition of insulin secretion usually predominates over β-receptor–mediated stimulation.[412] In purified alpha and beta cells, epinephrine and NE directly stimulate glucagon secretion from alpha cells and, in the presence of glucagon, inhibit insulin secretion.[413] The effects of catecholamines on islet hormone secretion occur in the context of paracrine regulation of islet function. Adrenergic neural mechanisms influence secretion of somatostatin and pancreatic polypeptide from pancreatic islets,[414, 415] which in turn may also affect insulin and glucagon release.

Neuropeptides in pancreatic sympathetic nerves also influence hormone secretion by islet cells. Galanin and neuropeptide Y are present in adrenergic nerves and are released on electrical stimulation of sympathetic fibers; they diminish pancreatic blood flow, suppress insulin and somatostatin secretion, and increase glucagon release.[416] The effects of these agents are independent of NE, because they are preserved in the presence of specific adrenergic antagonists, and may be responsible for nonadrenergically-mediated alterations in islet hormone secretion after sympathetic activation.[416]

Islet responses to nonadrenergic stimuli are influenced by prior exposure to catecholamines. In vivo treatments that impair sympathetic function limit glucose-induced insulin and calcium-mediated glucagon secretion in vitro,[417, 418] whereas exposure of islets to epinephrine or NE enhances subsequent insulin secretion in response to glucose or acetylcholine in the absence of catecholamine.[389, 419] The synergistic interaction between catecholamines and the nutrient responses of beta and alpha cells may reflect catecholamine-mediated changes in cAMP formation.[420, 421] In addition, the rate of insulin synthesis may be responsive to catecholamines.[384]

The role of the sympathetic innervation of the islets in the physiological regulation of insulin and glucagon release is incompletely understood. The hormonal pattern of impaired insulin (either low insulin levels per se or normal insulin levels despite hyperglycemia) and enhanced glucagon release suggests a role for the sympathoadrenal system in regulation of the endocrine pancreas. For pancreatic beta cells, the improvement in insulin secretion after α-adrenergic blockade or adrenalectomy buttresses the argument favoring active inhibition of insulin secretion by catecholamines. Increased glucagon release often coincides with sympathoadrenal activation and may be mediated by catecholamines in some circumstances.[422] Because both glucose administration and hypoglycemia activate pancreatic sympathetic nerves,[423, 424] islet function is probably under feedback control from the glucoregulatory centers within the CNS through efferent pathways including postganglionic sympathetic fibers. Subtle alterations in regulation of insulin secretion in the denervated pancreas are consistent with neurally mediated feedback suppression of insulin secretion.[425, 426]

THYROID HORMONE

Nerves originating from the cervical ganglia and the vagus nerve terminate within the thyroid gland, innervating blood vessels and nonvascular structures, including the thyroid follicles themselves.[427, 428] Several neuropeptides have been identified within thyroid nerves, including neuropeptide Y in adrenergic fibers.[429]

Catecholamines influence various aspects of thyroid gland metabolism and thyroid hormone biosynthesis and release.[427, 430] Epinephrine, through an α-receptor mechanism, increases uptake of iodine by augmenting organification. Catecholamines also stimulate glucose metabolism and protein synthesis. Both epinephrine and NE inhibit the release of thyroxine (T_4) induced by thyrotropin and thyroid-stimulating immunoglobulin. Stimulation of the superior cervical ganglion in mammals increases and chemical or surgical sympathectomy reduces thyroid hormone release.

Adrenergic nerves also appear to participate in the regulation of thyroid hyperplasia. Sympathetic denervation of the thyroid leads to an enhanced hyperplastic response to goitrogenic stimuli, suggesting growth-inhibiting effects of the sympathetic nerves.[431] Interruption of preganglionic sympathetic nerves, on the other hand, impairs thyroid growth.[394] Because sympathetic activity in the thyroid gland is increased in conditions associated with thyroid growth (e.g., hypothyroidism, pregnancy, iodine deficiency),[394] sympathetic nerves may promote thyroid hyperplasia under physiological conditions. The overall role of sympathetic nerves in the regulation of thyroid function, however, is unclear.

Sympathetic nervous system function is also affected by thyroid state. Despite clinical signs suggestive of adrenergic underactivity in hypothyroidism and overactivity in hyperthyroidism, sympathetic activity is increased in hypothyroid subjects, as evidenced by elevations in plasma NE levels and increased impulse traffic in muscle sympathetic nerves.[432–434] In hyperthyroidism these indices of sympathetic activity are normal or low.[433–436]

PARATHYROID HORMONE AND CALCITONIN

The secretion of PTH and calcitonin is governed primarily by serum calcium, but catecholamines may also play a role.[437, 438] Human parathyroid tissue is innervated by nerve fibers terminating on chief cells.[439] Although sympathetic varicosities occur in interfollicular spaces within the thyroid, synaptic contact with the calcitonin-producing C cells has not been described. β-Receptor stimulation increases and α-receptor stimulation inhibits secretion of both PTH and calcitonin in vitro. Similar results have been obtained in vivo with adrenergic agonists and antagonists in some but not all studies. Stimulation of PTH secretion by catecholamines depends, in part, on the extracellular serum calcium level; hypercalcemia suppresses and hypocalcemia augments the PTH response to catecholamines. PTH secretion is also increased by DA in vitro.[440] PTH responses to DA administration in vivo are variable, but human chief cells contain both the DA-specific phosphoprotein DARPP-32 and dopamine D_1 receptors, implying that they are targets of dopaminergic action.[441]

A role for catecholamines in the regulation of PTH and calcitonin secretion is not defined. After denervation of thyroid and parathyroid glands in rats, the release of PTH and calcitonin in response to hypocalcemia and hypercalcemia, respectively, is transiently reduced.[442, 443] In humans hypoglycemia suppresses PTH and elevates calcitonin[444, 445]; the PTH response is partially attenuated by adrenergic blockade.[445] A postprandial increase in calcitonin in sheep is also blocked by propranolol.[446] Finally, in patients with chronic renal failure, a condition of heightened sympathetic activity,[447] suppression of calcitonin and PTH levels by acute β-blockade suggests increased sympathetic stimulation of hormonal secretion.[448] These data indicate that sympathetic nerves, and to a lesser extent circulating catecholamines, may influence PTH and calcitonin secretion in specific circumstances, although no overall model for catecholamine involvement is available.

ADRENAL STEROID HORMONES

The mammalian adrenal cortex is innervated by adrenergic, cholinergic, and peptidergic fibers that target both nonvascular and vascular structures.[34, 449, 450] In humans cortical cells are found within the adrenal medulla and chromaffin cells are present in the adrenal cortex[451]; this juxtaposition of steroid-producing and chromaffin cells may affect adrenocortical function.

Catecholamines stimulate production of glucocorticoids, aldosterone, and adrenal androgens in animals.[385, 452, 453] The changes in steroid biosynthesis reflect β-receptor–mediated elevation in cAMP and subsequent increase in expression of CYP genes involved in steroid hormone biosynthesis.[385, 454] Denervation of adrenal gland in animals reduces the glucocorticoid response to exogenous corticotropin, whereas electrical stimulation of adrenal nerves potentiates the response.[455] The role of neuropeptides (including corticotropin-releasing hormone) within the adrenal in these neurally-mediated changes in adrenal cortical sensitivity to corticotropin is unknown, although the effects of some neuropeptides on adrenal steroid secretion appear to involve catecholamine-dependent mechanisms.[456, 457]

The physiological importance of adrenergic influence on adrenal cortical function is uncertain. In some experimental conditions the neurally-dependent component of adrenal cortical secretion may mediate as much as 50% of the increase in circulating levels of glucocorticoids.[458] Furthermore, glucocorticoid secretion can increase in the absence of an elevation in circulating corticotropin, as with tooth pulp stimulation, hemorrhage, or acute brain injury.[458] In addition, catecholamines may contribute to the adaptive hyperplasia in the remaining gland after unilateral adrenalectomy.[392]

ROLE OF DOPAMINE IN ALDOSTERONE SECRETION. Although all steroid-secreting cells of the adrenal cortex respond to β-adrenergic stimulation, aldosterone release from the zona glomerulosa may be uniquely susceptible to suppression by DA. Plasma aldosterone levels in human subjects increase after dopaminergic blockade and after peripheral inhibition of DA biosynthesis.[459, 460] Suppression of aldosterone secretion by DA in vivo is demonstrable, but only in the presence of elevated angiotensin II levels.[461, 462] The suppressive effect of DA is more apparent in perfused adrenal glands than in dispersed zona glomerulosa cells,[463] suggesting that the intra-adrenal effect of DA is indirect. Because DA is taken up and converted to NE by sympathetic nerve endings in proximity to zona glomerulosa cells and because ganglionic blockade abolishes the metoclopramide-induced rise in aldosterone,[464–466] efferent autonomic nerves may participate in dopaminergic regulation of aldosterone secretion.

PROGESTERONE

Synthesis and secretion of progesterone in the ovary are influenced by catecholamines and by ovarian sympathetic nerves.[467] The ovary is endowed with an extensive network of sympathetic nerves that innervate interstitial cells and vascular structures.[468] The density of this extrinsic innervation reaches adult levels at about the time of puberty in primates.[469] Peptide-containing nerves also are present in the ovary, including neuropeptide Y in adrenergic fibers.[469]

Addition of catecholamines to granulosa cells increases progesterone production and diminishes progesterone degradation by a β₂-adrenergic mechanism, possibly involving cAMP.[470] Gonadotropins modulate the responsiveness of granulosa cells to catecholamines.[471, 472] α-Adrenergic stimulation can inhibit progesterone responses to gonadotropins.[473] Catecholamine stimulation augments ovarian biosynthesis of androgens as well.[474] Both sympathetic nerves and circulating catecholamines from the adrenal medulla may contribute to the maintenance of steroid secretion by the ovary.[475, 476] Therefore, catecholamines act directly to stimulate progesterone release from ovarian tissue and indirectly through preservation of ovarian responsiveness to gonadotropins. Adrenergic neural mechanisms also may contribute to compensatory ovarian hyperplasia.[468]

The sympathoadrenal influence on progesterone secretion may be important in several circumstances. The temporal association between development of the ovarian sympathetic innervation and onset of puberty suggests a role for peripheral adrenergic mechanisms in the maturation of the female reproductive axis.[387, 477] Sympathetic activation during the luteal phase of the menstrual cycle and in pregnancy raises the possibility of a sympathetic component to progesterone secretion in these situations.[478, 479] Because progesterone administration also stimulates sympathetic nerves,[480] ovarian sympathetic activity may contribute to feedback regulation of progesterone production. Finally, ovarian sympathetic nerves may play a role in the pathophysiology of polycystic ovary syndrome.[481, 482] This syndrome frequently occurs in association with obesity and insulin resistance,[483] conditions in which sympathetic activity may be elevated.

TESTOSTERONE

Adrenergic nerves are present close to the Leydig cells.[484] In vitro catecholamines increase testosterone production, although the cellular mechanisms mediating this response vary among species.[485–487] Denervation of the rat testis reduces the number of testicular leuteinizing hormone (LH) receptors and impairs the enhancement of androgen production by human chorionic gonadotropin (hCG).[391] Although β-adrenergic stimulation raises testosterone synthesis and output from perfused canine testis,[488] catecholamines lower circulating testosterone levels in vivo.[489] The overall role of catecholamines in the regulation of androgen production therefore remains undefined.

GASTRIN

Secretion of gastrin by the G cells of the gastric antrum and proximal duodenum is governed by the interaction of intraluminal, hormonal, and neural factors, including catecholamines.[490] Adrenergic nerve fibers extend into mucosal and submucosal layers of stomach and duodenum.[491, 492] Catecholamines increase gastrin and somatostatin levels acutely by β-adrenergic mechanisms,[493, 494] both effects being potentiated by peptide secretogogues.[494, 495] Both stimulation and inhibition of gastrin and somatostatin release have been linked to activation of adrenergic neural pathways.[496–499] Moreover, gastrin responses to insulin-induced hypoglycemia are abnormal in patients with autonomic insufficiency.[500]

ERYTHROPOIETIN

The release of erythropoietin by the kidney is regulated primarily by arterial PO_2[501] but may also be influenced by catecholamines through β₂-receptor stimulation.[502] Acute splanchnic nerve section or β-adrenergic blockade diminishes the erythropoietin response to hypoxia and hemorrhage,[503, 504] although renal nerves are not required for hypoxic stimulation of erythropoietin synthesis.[505] Anemia associated with diminished erythropoietin levels develops with weightlessness during space flight and in patients with primary autonomic failure.[506] Erythropoietin treatment of anemia leads to an increase in blood pressure, possibly as a result of activation of the sympathetic nervous system.[507–509]

OTHER HORMONES

Catecholamines influence the secretion of melatonin, atrial natriuretic peptide, gastric inhibitory polypeptide,[510] and ovarian oxytocin,[511] among others. The regulation of melatonin secretion is reviewed elsewhere.[512, 513] The function of the pineal gland is coupled to the environmental light-dark cycle by a neuronal pathway originating at the retina and reaching the pineal via adrenergic fibers from the superior cervical ganglion. Release of atrial natriuretic peptide from cardiac atria is stimulated by catecholamines both in vivo and in vitro.[514–516] Activation of α- or β-adrenergic receptors increases atrial natriuretic peptide secretion in vitro[516, 517]; in vivo the atrial natriuretic peptide response to catecholamine infusion appears to be β-mediated.[514] β-Adrenergic mechanisms also increase expression of the atrial natriuretic peptide gene in animal hearts.[518]

Role of Sympathoadrenal System in Various Physiological and Pathophysiological States

COLD EXPOSURE

SYMPATHOADRENAL ACTIVATION DURING COLD EXPOSURE. An intact sympathoadrenal system is essential for defense against cold exposure in mammals. Although the sympathetic nervous system usually plays the dominant role, either the sympathetic nervous system or the adrenal medulla can sustain life when the other is deficient. In mammals cold exposure elicits a prompt rise in sympathetic nervous system activity.[519] The activation does not occur uniformly, but is greatest in brown fat,[520] less in heart, pancreas, and skeletal muscle,[423, 520, 521] and absent in liver and kidney.[423, 522] Adrenomedullary stimulation of a lesser degree results in release of more NE than epinephrine.[523] The adrenal response is exaggerated if sympathetic activation is impaired.[524] With continued exposure to cold the increase in adrenomedullary activity is not sustained.[525]

Sympathetic stimulation during cold exposure is induced by temperature receptors in the skin and by temperature-sensitive neurons in the hypothalamus, lower brain stem, and spinal column.[526, 527] Integration in the hypothalamus of afferent neural input from these areas stimulates sympathetic outflow.[528] Heat conservation is the consequence of diminished subcutaneous blood flow and of piloerection, both of which increase the insulation provided by the skin. Heat production is increased by shivering, which is regulated by the somatic motor system and facilitated by catecholamines, and by the enhancement of nonshivering thermogenesis. The sympathoadrenal system also provides fuel for heat production through mobilization of substrates and regulates the distribution of substrates and oxygen to metabolizing tissues.

REGULATION OF SUBSTRATE SUPPLY. Substrate for heat production during cold exposure is provided by the breakdown of triglyceride from fat tissue and of glycogen from muscle and liver and by the synthesis of glucose and ketone bodies in liver. The mobilization of substrate is regulated by the sympathoadrenal system, because animals that are subjected to adrenalectomy and chemical sympathectomy do not mobilize free fatty acids or increase hepatic glucose output in response to cold.[529] The sympathetic nervous system is more important in mediating lipolysis from adipose tissue, because adrenal demedullation does not prevent the rise in free fatty acids.[530] Sympathetic activation may also foster utilization of intracellular triglyceride stores, because administration of NE or acute cold exposure increases triglyceride lipase activity and decreases triglyceride content in heart.[290, 531] Cold-induced elevations in lipoprotein lipase activity and gene expression in brown fat are mediated by the sympathetic nervous system.[532, 533]

Activation of the adrenal medulla or the sympathetic nervous system during cold exposure accelerates carbohydrate metabolism by promoting glycogenolysis in liver and increased glucose utilization in peripheral tissues.[529, 534–536] Stimulation of glucagon and suppression of insulin release occur during cold exposure, and α-adrenergic blockade antagonizes cold-induced suppression of insulin release.[534, 537] The adrenal medulla mediates suppression of insulin release, whereas the sympathetic nervous system may contribute to stimulation of glucagon secretion.[534, 537]

CARDIOVASCULAR CHANGES DURING COLD EXPOSURE. Cardiovascular changes mediated by the sympathetic nervous system contribute both to heat conservation and to the delivery of oxygen and substrate to metabolizing tissues. Vasoconstriction in subcutaneous vascular beds diminishes heat loss through the skin by an α2-receptor mechanism.[538] The superficial veins are particularly responsive, and venoconstriction shifts blood from the superficial veins to deeper veins. External cooling potentiates α2 responses in superficial veins by enhancing receptor affinity but diminishes α1 responses in the deep venous system by a direct effect on the contractile process.[539] The shunting of cooler blood to the deep system augments the efficiency of countercurrent heat exchange,[540] promoting the transfer of heat from arterial to venous blood.

The importance of α2-receptor mechanisms in the vasoconstrictor response to cold is emphasized by the abrogation of cold-induced vasospasm in patients with Raynaud's disease by α2-antagonists.[541] In addition, ATP released from sympa-

thetic nerves during cold exposure may activate purinergic vascular receptors and increase vasoconstrictor responses to sympathetic nerve stimulation.[542] Release of neuropeptide Y by cold also may contribute to augmented vasomotor tone.[543]

Cold exposure elevates cardiac output coincident with activation of the sympathetic nervous system,[544, 545] and with a rise in oxygen uptake.[544] Acute cold exposure also causes an increase in blood pressure, a response that is greater in older persons.[546]

COLD ACCLIMATION. Chronic exposure to cold, either continuous or intermittent, increases the capacity for heat production on re-exposure to cold and decreases the need to shiver. The hallmark of the cold-acclimated state is enhancement of the thermogenic response to NE (Fig. 13–23).[331] A heightened thermic response to circulating catecholamines is also reflected in the reduction in energy expenditure after adrenal denervation in cold-adapted primates.[547] In small mammals cold acclimation causes hypertrophy and hyperplasia of brown adipose tissue and an increase in the tissue content of the uncoupling protein thermogenin.[548, 549] The sympathetic nervous system is involved in cold acclimation, because chronic administration of NE (or other β-agonists) enhances the thermogenic response to subsequent administration of NE and promotes the development of brown fat, whereas sympathetic denervation of brown adipose tissue retards the thermogenic response.[313, 336, 550] Several of these adaptive responses also depend on thyroid hormone,[551, 552] although the precise relation between sympathetic and thyroid function remains to be determined.

HYPOGLYCEMIA (See Also Chapter 20)

Hypoglycemia elicits a prompt and marked increase in epinephrine output by the adrenal (Fig. 13–24).[553, 554] The effect of hypoglycemia on sympathetic nerves is more variable; small increases in plasma and urinary NE levels occur with acute hypoglycemia, but these increments largely reflect adrenal secretion.[555, 556] Acute hypoglycemia activates sympathetic nerves in muscle, skin and pancreas[424, 556, 557] but not in kid-

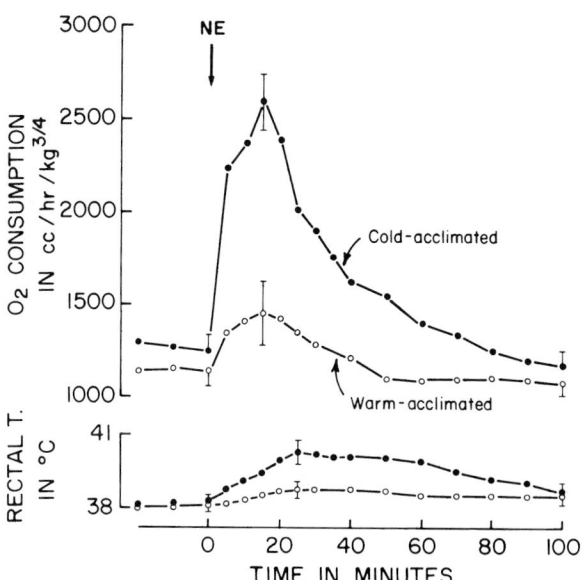

Figure 13–23. NE-stimulated thermogenesis in the rat: effect of cold acclimation. NE increases oxygen consumption (and rectal temperature) in both cold-acclimated (●) and warm-acclimated (○) curarized rats. The effect is markedly enhanced in cold-acclimated animals; it is the hallmark of cold acclimation. (From Hseih ACL, Carlson LD, Gray G. Role of the sympathetic nervous system in the control of chemical regulation of heat production. Am J Physiol 1957; 190:247–251.)

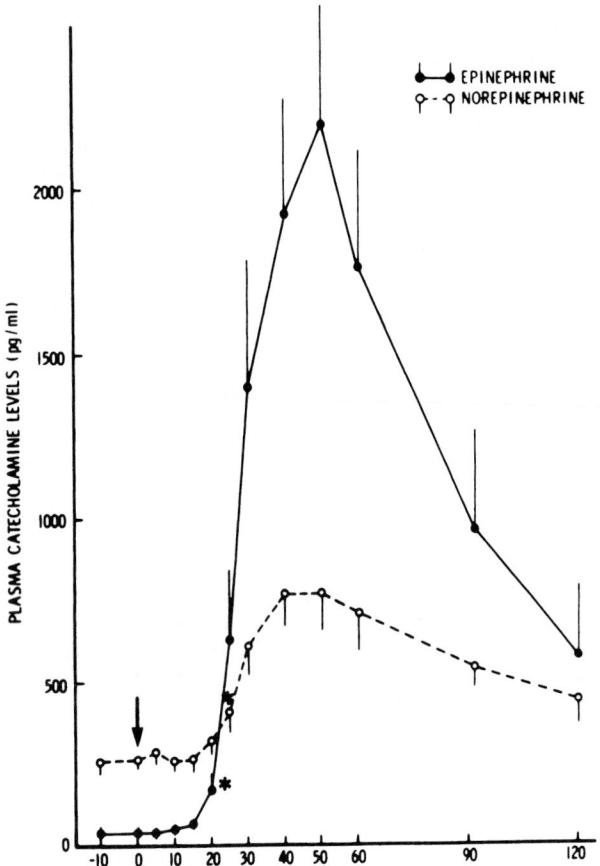

Figure 13–24. Effect of insulin-induced hypoglycemia on plasma epinephrine and norepinephrine levels. After an intravenous injection of 0.15 U/kg of regular insulin at time 0, plasma levels of epinephrine rise 50-fold in normal human subjects. To convert epinephrine values to pmol/L, multiply by 5.45; to convert norepinephrine values to nmol/L, multiply by 0.005911. (From Garber AJ, Cryer PE, Santiago JV, et al. The role of adrenergic mechanisms in the substrate and hormonal response to insulin-induced hypoglycemia in man. Reproduced from The Journal of Clinical Investigation, 1976, vol. 58, pp. 7–15 by copyright permission of The American Society for Clinical Investigation.)

ney.[558] Chronic hypoglycemia, often occurring in the context of fasting, does not stimulate sympathetic nerves.[559] Hypoglycemia also stimulates secretion of neuropeptide Y and enkephalins from the adrenal medulla and of galanin from pancreatic sympathetic nerves.[560, 561]

Adrenal responses are influenced by the circumstances in which hypoglycemia occurs. Because insulin in the absence of hypoglycemia activates sympathetic nerves,[562, 563] some sympathetic responses to hypoglycemia reflect the effect of insulin more than that of blood glucose per se. For example, in animals impulse traffic to the kidney is increased by insulin-induced hypoglycemia but not by 2-deoxyglucose.[564] In humans hyperinsulinemia potentiates catecholamine responses to the same hypoglycemic stimulus,[565] whereas starvation, a low-insulin state, suppresses sympathetic activity despite concurrent stimulation of adrenal medullary secretion.[559] Catecholamine responses to the same glycemic stimulus also are lower in women than in men.[566] Therefore, changes in sympathetic nervous system activity in response to hypoglycemia are more variable than those of the adrenal medulla and may be affected by other factors, such as the prevailing level of insulin.

REGULATION OF ADRENOMEDULLARY RESPONSE: STIMULUS AND CENTRAL RECEPTORS. Plasma epinephrine levels increase as the glucose level falls from 5.3 to 3.3 mmol/ L (95 to 60 mg/dL),[567] indicating that the adrenal medulla is stimulated in response to glucose lowering within the physio-

logical range and at levels above those regarded as hypoglycemic. At glucose levels of about 2.8 mmol/L (50 mg/dL) a further increase in epinephrine secretion occurs, the magnitude depending on both the degree and duration of the hypoglycemia and on the absolute glucose level rather than the rate of glucose fall.[568] The glucose threshold for adrenomedullary stimulation ranges between 2.7 and 4.1 mmol/L (48 to 74 mg/dL) among normal subjects,[568] and appears to decrease with age.[569, 570] In some patients with diabetes mellitus the threshold may lie above 5.5 mmol/L (100 mmol/dL) and may return to normal after months of intensive insulin therapy.[571, 572] Excess insulin, whether resulting from intensive treatment of diabetes mellitus, pancreatic neoplasms, or research protocols in normal subjects,[573, 574] lowers the glucose threshold at which adrenomedullary responses occur.

Sympathoadrenal responses to hypoglycemia are mediated by alterations in the activity of neurons within the CNS. Neither epinephrine secretion by chromaffin cells nor NE release from sympathetic nerves is responsive to local changes in glucose concentration.[424, 575] Several regions of the brain, particularly the ventromedial hypothalamus and brain stem, are capable of triggering an adrenal medullary response to hypoglycemia,[576, 577] and the earliest signals of developing hypoglycemia probably originate from hepatic glucosensors and reach central integrative areas through afferent neuronal pathways.[578, 579] These findings suggest that adrenal medullary secretion and the activity of glucose-sensitive sympathetic efferents (such as those to pancreas) may be regulated by sympathetic impulses in the liver mediated by glucose delivery into the portal veins.

Studies with 2-deoxyglucose in animals and humans indicate that diminished intracellular glucose metabolism rather than glucose concentration per se is the proximate stimulus of the adrenomedullary response. Availability of alternative substrates, such as ketone bodies, blunts the adrenomedullary response to hypoglycemia in humans.[580, 581] This effect within the CNS may contribute to the impaired epinephrine response to insulin-induced hypoglycemia in starvation.[582]

ADRENAL MEDULLA AND COUNTERREGULATORY RESPONSE. Plasma glucose counterregulation after hypoglycemia is considered in Chapter 20. The actions of epinephrine that contribute to the counterregulatory response include (1) enhancement of hepatic glucose output; (2) stimulation of lipolysis in adipose tissue; and (3) inhibition of insulin-mediated glucose uptake in muscle.[583] Epinephrine also contributes to the suppression of insulin and enhancement of glucagon secretion during hypoglycemia, although autonomic outflow to pancreas participates as well.[584, 585] Epinephrine is not required for counterregulation, provided glucagon secretion is normal. Because glucagon response is deficient in most patients with insulin-dependent diabetes mellitus, these patients are especially dependent on the adrenal medullary response. Impairment in this response places individuals at risk for hypoglycemia during insulin therapy.

Of the cardiovascular responses to hypoglycemia, only tachycardia and widened pulse pressure appear to depend on the adrenal medulla.[586] Blood flow increases in the splanchnic circulation, in the upper extremities, and (possibly) in the cerebral circulation and decreases in the kidney.[587] Sweating with hypoglycemia appears to involve sympathetic cholinergic fibers, not apocrine sweating secondary to epinephrine.[588] Sweating increases heat loss and contributes to the lowering of body temperature in hypoglycemia.

FEEDING

SYMPATHETIC NERVOUS SYSTEM. The sympathetic nervous system is activated by food intake in three phases. In the first phase transient elevations in circulating catecholamines occur immediately after ingestion, dissipate within 30 to 40 min, and are caused by oropharyngeal stimulation.[589, 590] The second phase begins about 30 min after ingestion and may be caused by nonspecific factors associated with feeding (e.g., fluid shifts), because it does not depend on the nutritive content of ingested food and may persist for several hours.[591–593] The third phase involves sympathetic nervous system responses to changes in diet and is distinguishable from the second phase by the fact that sympathetic responses to dietary alteration are nutrient specific. Intravenous infusions of glucose and insulin also increase sympathetic activity in humans in the absence of hypoglycemia.[562, 563] The linkage of this response with glucose metabolism suggests that sympathetic activation by euglycemic insulin infusions may be more akin to the sympathetic response to changes in diet than to the immediate postprandial response.

Sympathetic nervous system function is directly related to the level of caloric intake,[594–596] but fat and carbohydrate intake affect sympathetic activity in individual tissues differently, even when caloric intake is constant.[522] Alterations in intake of minerals (sodium, potassium, iron, and iodine) or vitamins (A, E, and perhaps B_{12}) also affect sympathetic activity.

Activation of sympathetic nerves may contribute to the cardiovascular and metabolic changes after feeding, including increased heart rate and cardiac output.[597, 598] The link between postprandial increases in sympathetic activity and changes in energy expenditure is uncertain. However, with long-term dietary modification, alterations in heart rate and blood pressure correspond to alterations in sympathetic activity.[599, 600] β-Blockade diminishes the metabolic rate in human subjects consuming a high- but not a low-energy diet,[601] implying that the difference in energy expenditure caused by different levels of energy intake is, in part, adrenergically mediated. In small animals sympathetic nerves play an important role in dietary regulation of energy expenditure by controlling brown adipose tissue function.[333] Because β-blockade antagonizes a portion of the increase in metabolic rate during insulin and glucose infusions in normal subjects,[602] sympathetically-mediated thermogenesis may be important in humans as well.

ADRENAL MEDULLA. Adrenal catecholamine release is largely unaffected by feeding.[593] However, after an oral glucose load, plasma epinephrine levels fall transiently with hyperglycemia[603] and then rise above baseline as glucose levels decline.[591, 604] Epinephrine secretion thereby helps stabilize the postabsorptive plasma glucose level in a manner analogous to the hypoglycemic response.[605] This postglucose elevation in circulating epinephrine is greater in children than in adults and may contribute to the behavioral effects of sugar ingestion in normal children.[606] In general, the adrenal medulla is not affected by changes in diet, although ingestion of a diet high in animal fat suppresses epinephrine secretion in rats.[294]

FASTING AND STARVATION

SYMPATHETIC NERVOUS SYSTEM. In animals and humans sympathetic nervous system activity is reduced by fasting or caloric restriction.[233, 607] This effect in humans may be difficult to demonstrate because of concomitant sodium restriction,[608] especially early in fasting when sodium excretion is disproportionate to intake, a phenomenon referred to as the natriuresis of fasting.[609] One postulated mechanism linking diet and sympathetic nervous system activity involves insulin-mediated glucose metabolism in glucose-sensitive neurons of the hypothalamus that regulate an inhibitory pathway governing central sympathetic outflow.[610]

ADRENAL MEDULLA. The adrenal medulla, in contrast, is stimulated modestly during fasting.[233] It can be further stimulated in fasting animals by the conditions that stimulate

sympathetic nerves in fed animals, such as cold exposure or exercise,[524, 611] suggesting a compensatory role for the adrenal medulla in the context of sympathetic suppression. With fasting or caloric restriction, epinephrine excretion in urine is less in women than in men.[612]

The fasted or starved state necessitates two major metabolic adaptations: energy expenditure must be reduced to conserve calories, and fuel stores must be mobilized to maintain vital functions. Suppression of sympathetic activity may contribute to a decrease in metabolic rate with caloric restriction, and the increase in epinephrine secretion may foster mobilization of triglyceride from adipose tissue. Lipolysis is sensitive to variations in plasma epinephrine level within the physiological range,[613] and fasting enhances the lipolytic effect of catecholamines.[283] The combination of sympathetic nervous system suppression and adrenomedullary stimulation allows substrate mobilization with a minimal increase in energy expenditure.

EXERCISE

EFFECT OF EXERCISE ON THE SYMPATHOADRENAL SYSTEM. Intense or prolonged exercise activates both parts of the sympathoadrenal system, whereas mild to moderate exercise affects principally the sympathetic nerves. The release of NE from skeletal muscle and the cardiovascular system accounts for much of the increase in plasma NE during exercise.[614–616] The sympathetic response to exercise is mediated by a metabolic reflex arising from the exercising muscle, by baroreflexes, and by activation of other central neural pathways. The metabolic signal from muscle reflects local concentrations of diprotonated phosphate ($H_2PO_4^-$), which is increased by intracellular acidification and phosphate production.[617] Regulation of epinephrine release during exercise is not as well understood but probably does not involve hepatic glucosensing mechanisms.[618] The relation between exercise-induced changes in sympathetic activity and adrenomedullary secretion is influenced by antecedent diet, environmental temperature, and oxygen content of inspired air.

Exercise training lowers resting rates of NE spillover into plasma in young but not in elderly subjects.[619, 620] This effect of training largely reflects reduced renal sympathetic activity without alteration in sympathetic outflow to heart or skeletal muscle.[621, 622] Decreases in peripheral sensitivity to catecholamines may also occur.[623, 624] In contrast, physical training induces adrenal medullary hypertrophy in rats and enhanced epinephrine secretion with various stimuli in human subjects.[625, 626]

EFFECTS OF CATECHOLAMINES DURING EXERCISE. Blood pressure and cerebral blood flow are maintained during exercise by splanchnic and renal vasoconstriction despite vasodilatation in skeletal muscle and cutaneous vascular beds. These cardiovascular adjustments are consistent with the known effects of catecholamines and neuropeptide Y.[627] Adrenergic blockade, surgical denervation, or autonomic neuropathy impairs cardiovascular responses to exercise and diminishes exercise tolerance.

Catecholamines facilitate the mobilization of stored fuel in support of exercising muscle and suppress insulin secretion. Adrenergic blockade but not adrenalectomy abolishes this response, implying mediation by pancreatic sympathetic nerves.[628] The increase in glucagon with exercise is closely related to the ambient glucose concentration.[628] Epinephrine stimulates muscle glycogenolysis in general, although its effect may be more important in resting than in working muscles.[629, 630] Epinephrine also contributes to the increase in hepatic glucose output during exercise,[628] but a role for hepatic sympathetic nerves is controversial.[628, 631] β-Adrenergic blockade attenuates exercise-induced glycerol release from subcutaneous tissue and triglyceride release from red muscle fibers.[632, 633] Catecholamine effects may persist beyond the period of exercise and contribute to heightened glucose turnover and oxygen consumption during recovery from exercise.[634, 635]

Catecholamines contribute to the stabilization of extracellular potassium during exercise. Plasma potassium levels rise during exercise because of release from contracting muscle and fall in the postexercise recovery period.[636] β_2-Receptor activation, which stimulates Na^+, K^+-ATPase in skeletal muscle,[352] increases potassium uptake into nonexercising muscle and other tissues and ameliorates exercise-induced hyperkalemia.[637] Consequently, β-adrenergic blockade impairs redistribution of potassium during exercise and magnifies the hyperkalemia and sensation of fatigue.[637]

TRAUMA, CIRCULATORY FAILURE, AND HYPOXIA

SYMPATHOADRENAL RESPONSES. Sympathoadrenal activity is altered in pathophysiological states that threaten the integrity of the internal environment. Elevations in epinephrine signify enhanced adrenal medullary secretion, a uniform component of the acute response to severe injury or stress. Elevations in NE, on the other hand, do not necessarily imply increased activity of sympathetic nerves, because adrenal medullary release of NE may be substantial. With ischemic injury, hypoxia, and hemorrhage, sympathetic nerve activity may even be suppressed despite concomitant activation of the adrenal medulla.[233, 234] However, with continued stress, sympathetic activation may take place.[233] The mechanisms underlying these responses are not fully understood, although in animals inhibition of renal sympathetic activity during severe hemorrhage involves CNS serotonergic and/or opioid pathways.[638, 639]

PHYSIOLOGICAL CONSEQUENCES OF SYMPATHO-ADRENAL RESPONSE. The sympathoadrenal response to stress has important implications. The increase in mortality in acutely injured animals after sympathoadrenal ablation demonstrates the importance of catecholamines in circulatory support.[640] Catecholamine-mediated vasoconstriction and activation of the renin-angiotensin-aldosterone system are essential components of the defense against injury, but if these responses are prolonged they can cause necrosis of vital organs and potentiate the development of lactic acidosis. Catecholamines also may be involved in the pathogenesis of stress ulceration and paralytic ileus after severe injury or surgery.[641]

In the acute phase, levels of plasma glucose, lactate, glycerol, and free fatty acid are elevated in relation to the severity of injury. Hyperglycemia results largely from the effects of epinephrine, glucagon, and cortisol. Despite elevations in glucose level, insulin secretion is suppressed, primarily by an α-adrenergic effect of adrenal catecholamines. Glucocorticoids stimulate protein degradation and contribute to the negative nitrogen balance in these patients. Epinephrine may act to oppose protein breakdown because activation of β-adrenergic receptors blunts muscle protein catabolism in animals after burn injury.[642] Inhibition of sympathetic nerve activity during stress also may contribute to the reduction in energy expenditure. In the chronic phase after injury, glucose levels are almost normal, glucose cycling is accelerated, and insulin secretion is normal despite increased sympathetic activity. During this phase catecholamines contribute to the increase in energy expenditure.

The effects of catecholamines with injury, hypoxia, or circulatory failure are determined both by changes in sympathoadrenal activity and by alterations in the sensitivity of peripheral tissues to catecholamines. β-Adrenergic receptors and the responses to stimulation are diminished in hypoxic and hypotensive states.[643–645]

REPRODUCTION, MENSES, AND PREGNANCY

Sympathetic nervous system activity increases at the time of ovulation and remains elevated during the luteal phase of the menstrual cycle.[479, 646] In animals the increase in ovarian sympathetic activity follows the surge in LH.[647] Late in pregnancy sympathetic nerve activity is suppressed in kidney, elevated in heart, and unchanged in brown fat, alterations that may be caused by progesterone or its metabolites.[478, 480, 648] Myometrial tone is affected by catecholamines, and the suppression of uterine contractility by β_2-adrenergic agonists inhibits premature labor. Because estrogens and progestogens are capable of altering adrenergic receptors in peripheral tissues, the effects of catecholamines on reproduction reflect changes in tissue responsiveness in addition to changes in sympathoadrenal activity.

Catecholamines and Hypertension

SYMPATHETIC NERVOUS SYSTEM EFFECTS ON BLOOD PRESSURE

VASOCONSTRICTION, VENOCONSTRICTION, AND CARDIAC STIMULATION. Sympathetic stimulation of the vasculature and the heart increases blood pressure (see Fig. 13–20). Peripheral resistance is increased by stimulation of arteriolar vasoconstriction and by activation of the renin-angiotensin system and increased production of angiotensin II. Cardiac output is increased by enhancement of myocardial contractility and by increased venous return, the latter resulting from venoconstriction and enhanced renal sodium reabsorption.

RENAL SYMPATHETIC ACTIVITY. Sympathetic stimulation of the kidney enhances renal sodium reabsorption by both direct and indirect effects. The renal response to an increase in blood pressure is an increase in salt excretion (i.e., pressure natriuresis). Factors that decrease sodium excretion, such as increased renal sympathetic activity, raise the level of blood pressure required to induce the natriuretic response. Intrarenal but not intravenous infusions of NE produce sustained elevations in blood pressure and a positive sodium balance.[649, 650] Likewise, renal denervation increases fractional sodium and water excretion over a wide range of renal perfusion pressures and delays or prevents the rise in blood pressure in animal models of hypertension.[255] Renal sympathetic activity therefore plays a role in the regulation of blood pressure and in the pathogenesis of hypertension.

SYMPATHOADRENAL SYSTEM AND HYPERTENSION

ROLE OF THE SYMPATHETIC NERVOUS SYSTEM. Heightened sympathetic nervous system activity probably plays a role in the pathogenesis of human hypertension. Early reports of plasma catecholamine levels in hypertensive subjects were consistent with the view that sympathetic activity is increased in young hypertensives,[651] and the spillover of NE from kidney and heart is increased in hypertensive patients younger than 40 years of age.[652] Sympathetic activity in skeletal muscle is likewise increased in young subjects with borderline hypertension.[346] Such patients also have increased heart rate and cardiac output, indicative of a so-called hyperkinetic circulation.[653] As these individuals age the hemodynamic pattern in hypertension changes to one characterized by low cardiac output and high peripheral resistance.[654] In older patients with hypertension sympathetic activity is not consistently increased.[651, 655] Nonsuppressed levels of sympathetic activity in older hypertensive subjects, despite the elevations in blood pressure, raise the possibility that the sympathetic nervous system plays a permissive role in the maintenance of hypertension. Decreased cardiac parasympathetic activity or increased adrenal medullary secretion in the hypertensive process may play a role, although evidence in favor of either is limited. Sympathetic activity appears to be increased in patients with renovascular hypertension and reduced in those with primary hyperaldosteronism.[656]

A variety of factors may play a role in the heightened cardiorenal sympathetic activity in young, borderline hypertensives. Because measures of sympathetic activity display intrafamily correlations,[167, 657] genetic or developmental factors may be involved. Weight gain and obesity also are associated with elevated blood pressure. Because sympathetic activity is increased in some obese individuals,[658] body weight or body composition per se may be important. Alternatively, an attribute of the obese state such as insulin resistance, obstructive sleep apnea, or a sedentary lifestyle may contribute to sympathetic stimulation.[652, 659, 660] Dietary constituents that increase both blood pressure and sympathetic activity include macronutrients (elevated fat or carbohydrate and restricted protein), minerals (increased sodium and decreased potassium), and alcohol.[356, 661, 662] Finally, stresses of daily life and the individual reaction to them may also contribute to sympathetic activation in early hypertension.[653]

ROLE OF DOPAMINE. Because stimulation of DA_1 receptors promotes natriuresis and lowers blood pressure in humans,[663] deficient renal DA formation or action may contribute to hypertension.[664] Evidence of diminished DA excretion in hypertensive individuals was first reported more than 30 years ago,[665] and a deficient dopaminergic response to salt loading may play an etiologic role in patients with the salt-sensitive form of hypertension.[666, 667] Because normotensive elderly men have a similar deficit in DA formation,[460] diminished DA production may also contribute to the salt sensitivity that is common among aged individuals. In hypertensive animals the DA_1 receptor function may be defective.[664]

DISORDERS OF SYMPATHETIC NERVOUS SYSTEM

General Considerations

ORTHOSTATIC HYPOTENSION

Under normal circumstances the assumption of erect posture is not associated with a significant decrease in blood pressure. An orthostatic fall in blood pressure is the most prominent sign of a defective sympathetic nervous system. A decrease in systolic pressure of 20 mm Hg or a diastolic fall of 10 mm Hg within 3 min of standing (or within 3 min of passive tilting in the head-up position to an angle of at least 60 degrees) is defined as orthostatic hypotension.[668] Maintenance of arterial pressure during postural stress depends on an adequate circulating blood volume, an unimpaired venous return, and an intact sympathetic nervous system. A postural fall in blood pressure is commonly associated with extracellular fluid volume depletion or with a loss of the sympathetic reflexes that defend arterial pressure by constricting both veins and arterioles. Disruption of the sympathetic reflexes with resultant postural hypotension may occur with a variety of diseases (Table 13–8). It is the most prominent feature of a chronic degenerative disease of the nervous system known as pure autonomic failure (also called idiopathic orthostatic hypotension or progressive autonomic failure) and of other neuropathies of the autonomic nervous system. Drugs that block adrenergic transmission (e.g., guanethidine), ganglionic transmission (e.g., trimethaphan, hexamethonium), or central sympathetic activity (e.g., phenothiazines, tricyclic antidepressants) commonly cause orthostatic hypotension. Postural hypotension also occurs in patients with adrenal insufficiency,

TABLE 13–8. Autonomic Nervous System Disorders That Cause Postural Hypotension

Primary Autonomic Failure
　Pure autonomic failure (also called idiopathic orthostatic hypotension)
　Autonomic failure in multiple system atrophy (also called Shy-Drager syndrome)
　Autonomic failure in Parkinson's disease
Secondary causes of autonomic failure
Lesions of central nervous system and spinal cord
　Tumors of third ventricle, posterior fossa, spinal cord
　Multiple sclerosis
　Syringobulbia and syringomyelia
　Transverse myelitis
Hereditary neuropathies
　Familial dysautonomia (Riley-Day syndrome)
　Familial amyloid polyneuropathy
Inflammatory and autoimmune neuropathies
　Guillain-Barré syndrome
　Acute dysautonomia
　Connective tissue disorders
Infections
　Human immunodeficiency virus infections and AIDS
　Syphilis (tabes dorsalis)
　Chagas' disease
　Leprosy
Metabolic disorders
　Diabetes mellitus
　Primary amyloidosis
　Uremia
　Porphyria
　Vitamin B_{12} deficiency
　Hypokalemia
　Fabry's disease
　Tangier disease
Malignancy, carcinomatous neuropathies
Drugs
Dopamine β-hydroxylase deficiency

Adapted from McLeod JG. Autonomic dysfunction in peripheral nerve disease. J Clin Neurophysiol 1993; 10:51–60; and Mathias CJ. Orthostatic hypotension: causes, mechanisms, and influencing factors. Neurology 1995; 45(Suppl 5):S6–S11. Copyright by Advanstar Communications Inc.

hypopituitarism, primary hypoaldosteronism, and pheochromocytoma.

TESTS OF AUTONOMIC FUNCTION

PHYSIOLOGICAL AND PHARMACOLOGIC TESTS. Autonomic dysfunction can be classified and diagnosed on the basis of clinical, pharmacologic, and biochemical tests. Responsiveness of sympathetic reflexes can be tested by assessing the integrity of cardiovascular responses to the Valsalva maneuver, tilt table, or cold pressor test.[669] An abnormal response to these tests indicates impaired sympathetic function but does not identify the site of dysfunction. The integrity of the peripheral sympathetic nerve endings may be tested with an indirect-acting sympathomimetic amine such as tyramine. A normal pressor response to tyramine indicates that the peripheral sympathetic nerves and NE stores are intact; a poor response is consistent with degeneration of the peripheral sympathetic nerves. Sympathetic denervation is commonly associated with enhanced responsiveness to infusions of NE. Sweating and pupillary responses can be tested pharmacologically.

PLASMA NOREPINEPHRINE LEVELS. Measurements of plasma NE levels are useful in the diagnosis and classification of patients with orthostatic hypotension. The basal supine NE concentration is determined with blood drawn from a previously placed indwelling intravenous line after 30 min of quiet recumbency. The subject is then asked to stand for 3 to 5 min, and blood is resampled. Normally, the basal NE level doubles in the upright position, increasing more than 0.9 nmol/L (150 pg/mL) to an absolute value in excess of 1.5 nmol/L (250 pg/mL). A blood pressure decrease on upright standing coupled with a failure to increase plasma NE indicates a disorder of the sympathetic nervous system. A normal

TABLE 13–9. Frequency of Symptoms in 100 Patients with Pheochromocytoma

Symptom	%	Symptom	%	Symptom	%
Headache	80	Chest pain	19	Tinnitus	3
Excessive perspiration	71	Dyspnea	19	Dysarthria	3
Palpitation (with or without tachycardia)	64	Flushing or warmth	18	Gagging	3
Pallor	42	Numbness or paresthesia	11	Bradycardia	3
Nausea (with or without vomiting)	42	Blurring of vision	11	Back pain	3
Tremor or trembling	31	Tightness of throat	8	Coughing	1
Weakness or exhaustion	28	Dizziness or faintness	8	Yawning	1
Nervousness or anxiety	22	Convulsions	5	Syncope	1
Epigastric pain	22	Neck-shoulder pain	5	Unsteadiness	1
		Extremity pain	4	Hunger	1
		Flank pain	4		

Data from Thomas JE, Rooke ED, Kvale WF. The neurologist's experience with pheochromocytoma: a review of 46 cases. J Urol 1974; 111:715–721.

Clinical Features

The clinical manifestations of pheochromocytomas are largely predictable from the physiological and pharmacologic effects of catecholamines. Presenting manifestations include (1) sustained hypertension that is resistant to conventional treatment; (2) hypertensive crisis with malignant hypertension, hypertensive encephalopathy, or manifestations suggestive of aortic dissection or myocardial infarction; and (3) paroxysmal attacks suggestive of seizure disorder, anxiety attacks, or hyperventilation. Less common manifestations include unexplained hypotension, shock, and severe hypertensive reactions during incidental surgery or in association with trauma.

PAROXYSM

The characteristic paroxysm or crisis of pheochromocytoma is the consequence of catecholamine release from the tumor. The manifestations are variable. Headache occurs in more than 80% of patients (Table 13–9)[686]; it may be severe, frontal, or occipital and throbbing or steady. Excessive sweating and palpitations are also common. In a series of more than 21,000 hypertensive patients, the absence of headache, sweating, and palpitations virtually excluded the diagnosis of pheochromocytoma.[687] Other features include apprehension, often with a sense of impending doom, pain in the chest or abdomen, nausea, vomiting, and occasionally paresthesias. The face can blanch or flush during the paroxysm, with a flushed, warm feeling afterward. Blood pressure is elevated, often to alarming levels. The presence of tachycardia in the face of elevated blood pressure often suggests the diagnosis. The paroxysm may last from minutes to hours; most episodes subside within 40 min. More prolonged episodes are rare.

A paroxysm may be precipitated by any movement that displaces the abdominal contents, such as lifting, straining, or bending, or by strenuous exertion of any kind. In some patients a specific stimulus reproduces an attack in a characteristic manner. In others no precipitating event can be found, and the episodes are random. In contrast to anxiety states, which may be confused with pheochromocytoma, mental stress or psychological tension does not usually provoke a crisis, although anxiety may accompany the attack. A variety of therapeutic or diagnostic maneuvers may provoke a crisis. Vigorous palpation of the abdomen may initiate an episode. In most patients paroxysms occur frequently enough so that over the course of 1 or 2 d it is possible to witness an attack and measure the blood pressure. In some patients the intervals between attacks are weeks or months. As the disease progresses, paroxysms tend to increase in frequency, severity, and duration. Although pheochromocytoma is identified with the characteristic crises, paroxysmal symptoms were present in only 56% of 507 cases in one series.[688]

HYPERTENSION

Although the paroxysm is the most distinctive manifestation, hypertension is the most common feature and occurs in more than 90% of patients. It is usually sustained and may be without definite crises, resembling essential hypertension (Table 13–10).[688] Blood pressure lability is usually present, however, and many patients with sustained hypertension also have distinct paroxysms. In 25 to 40% of patients the hypertension is truly paroxysmal, with an elevated blood pressure demonstrable only intermittently or during symptomatic episodes. The hypertension in patients with pheochromocytoma is often severe and occasionally malignant with retinopathy, severe proteinuria, and secondary aldosteronism. Although it is generally attributed to the direct effects of high circulating levels of catecholamines, the hypertension in patients with pheochromocytoma also may involve the sympathetic nervous system, by mechanisms that remain obscure, and/or release of neuropeptides, with vasoconstrictor activity such as endothelin or neuropeptide Y, by the tumor (see Table 13–2).

Refractoriness of hypertension to conventional antihypertensive treatment may be a clue to the diagnosis. The hypertension in patients with pheochromocytoma, however, responds to α-blocking agents commonly used in the treatment of essential hypertension (e.g., prazosin, terazosin, labetalol), to calcium channel blockers, and to nitroprusside.

OTHER DISTINCTIVE FEATURES

ORTHOSTATIC HYPOTENSION AND SHOCK. Orthostatic hypotension occurs in many patients.[689] In untreated hypertensive patients, a significant postural fall in blood pressure should suggest the diagnosis. Orthostatic hypotension is probably caused by the reduced plasma volume that results from high circulating levels of catecholamines. In addition,

TABLE 13–10. Frequency of Hypertension and Crises in 507 Cases of Pheochromocytoma

Symptom	%	
Sustained hypertension	60.5	
With crises		27.0
Without crises		33.5
Paroxysmal hypertension	26.4	
Hypertension of pregnancy	3.5	
No hypertension	9.5	
Paroxysmal symptoms		2.8
Sustained symptoms		1.2
No symptoms (discovered by chance)		4.3
Local signs		1.2
Paroxysmal symptoms or crises of any kind	56.2	

Data from Hermann H, Mornex R. Human Tumors Secreting Catecholamines. New York: Macmillan, 1964: 1–14.

the postural reflexes that defend upright blood pressure may lose their tone with a prolonged excess of catecholamines. Both factors predispose untreated patients to hypotension or shock when subjected to surgery or trauma. Pheochromocytomas also contain and release a neuropeptide with vasodilatating activity called adrenomedullin (see Table 13–2),[690] but its contribution to hypotension in patients with pheochromocytoma is unknown.

CARDIAC MANIFESTATIONS. The clinical course can be dominated by manifestations of cardiac disease. Chest pain, angina pectoris, and acute myocardial infarction can occur in the absence of coronary artery disease.[691, 692] Catecholamine-induced increase in myocardial oxygen consumption and coronary artery spasm may be the cause. Electrocardiographic changes in the absence of clinical ischemia include nonspecific ST-T wave changes and prominent U waves. Sinus tachycardia, sinus bradycardia, supraventricular tachycardias, and ventricular premature contractions may be associated with palpitations. Conduction disturbances include right and left bundle branch block. Cardiomyopathy of the congestive or hypertrophic type may be associated with congestive heart failure.[693, 694] Noncardiogenic pulmonary edema has also been described, possibly caused by a shift of extracellular fluid volume to the central compartment, increased pulmonary venous tone, and damage to the pulmonary capillary endothelium.[695]

METABOLIC ALTERATIONS. The metabolic rate is increased, excessive sweating and heat intolerance are common, and fever may be present. Activation of brown fat is evident in patients with pheochromocytoma,[696] although its contribution to the increase in energy expenditure is unknown. Weight loss is usual, but obesity does not exclude the diagnosis.

Elevated fasting plasma glucose concentrations or carbohydrate intolerance may be present, most commonly during paroxysms. The elevated plasma glucose level is associated with a low level of plasma insulin, the latter reflecting α-receptor–mediated suppression of insulin release. β-Receptor–mediated stimulation of hepatic glucose output may also contribute. In rare patients hyperglycemia may be caused by Cushing's syndrome or acromegaly secondary to ectopic production of corticotropin, corticotropin-releasing hormone (CRH), or growth-hormone–releasing hormone (GHRH) by the tumor.[697, 698] The carbohydrate intolerance with pheochromocytoma is characteristically mild but may require treatment, and it is reversed by removal of the tumor.

Hypercalcemia, an uncommon complication, may reflect associated hyperparathyroidism, particularly in familial cases (see later discussion), but it can occur in the absence of parathyroid disease, and it resolves after resection of the tumor. PTHrP, the humoral factor associated with the hypercalcemia of malignancy syndrome, is also secreted by some pheochromocytomas, although not all patients with detectable levels of PTHrP are hypercalcemic.[699, 700] Calcium levels fall postoperatively even in patients with undetectable levels of PTHrP before surgery, implying that other factors may contribute to the hypercalcemia.[700] Consequently, hypercalcemia in a patient with pheochromocytoma should be re-evaluated after the pheochromocytoma is resected, because the hypercalcemia may resolve.

Gastrointestinal symptoms can include nausea, vomiting, abdominal pain,[689] and occasionally constipation or diarrhea. The constipation may reflect direct inhibitory effects of catecholamines on gut smooth muscle contraction. The so-called watery diarrhea, hypokalemia, achlorhydria syndrome (WDHA; also known as the Verner-Morrison syndrome) in patients with pheochromocytoma is secondary to the ectopic production of VIP. Either condition resolves after the tumor is removed. Cholelithiasis occurs in as many as 15 to 20% of patients.

HEMATOCRIT. Elevation of the hematocrit in patients with pheochromocytoma usually is associated with a normal red cell mass and therefore reflects the diminished plasma volume. Increased levels of erythropoietin have been demonstrated in plasma and tumor extracts from some patients with pheochromocytoma.[701] Catecholamine-stimulated erythropoietin release from kidney also may occur.

ADVERSE DRUG INTERACTIONS. The course of pheochromocytoma may be adversely affected by drugs or diagnostic studies that affect catecholamine metabolism. Severe and even fatal crises have been induced by opiates, histamine, corticotropin, saralasin, glucagon, metoclopramide, and pancuronium. Of these agents, the effects of opiates have been insufficiently emphasized, and serious paroxysms can be induced by administration of an opiate analgesic in patients with headache or abdominal pain. Glucagon, which is used in a standard provocative test for pheochromocytoma (as described later), may precipitate a crisis if it is administered to relax the bowel during radiologic studies. The opiate agonist fentanyl can precipitate crises during induction of anesthesia in patients with unsuspected pheochromocytoma who are undergoing incidental surgery. The intra-arterial administration of radiographic contrast media also releases catecholamines, and, if pheochromocytoma is suspected, arteriography should be performed only in patients who have received adrenergic blocking agents. Radiopaque contrast media, however, can safely be administered intravenously. Indirect-acting sympathomimetic amines, including intravenously administered methyldopa, may cause an increase in blood pressure by releasing catecholamines from the augmented stores in nerve endings. Proprietary cold medicines and decongestants that contain sympathomimetic amines are common offenders. Drugs that block the neuronal uptake of catecholamines, such as guanethidine or tricyclic antidepressants, may enhance the physiological effects of circulating catecholamines and increase blood pressure. These agents should specifically be avoided in patients with known or suspected pheochromocytoma, and all medications should be administered cautiously.

Pathology

MORPHOLOGY

Pheochromocytomas usually are solitary and are located in or about the adrenal gland.[702] In sporadic cases about 80 to 85% are intra-adrenal (both unilateral and bilateral), and the rest are extra-adrenal (Table 13–11). Sporadic pheochromocytomas usually are unilateral and may be more common on the right side. Familial pheochromocytomas are also intra-adrenal and are often bilateral. Extra-adrenal pheochromocytomas are unusual in familial cases. The incidence of bilateral and extra-adrenal pheochromocytomas is increased in children.

TABLE 13–11. Location of Pheochromocytomas

Location	%	%
Solitary adrenal	70–80	
Bilateral adrenal*	5–10	
Extra-adrenal†	15–20	
Head and neck		3
Thorax		10
Superior para-aortic		46
Inferior para-aortic		29
Bladder		10
Pelvis		2

*In sporadic cases frequency of bilateral pheochromocytomas is <5%; in familial cases it is very common.
†Data on extra-adrenal pheochromocytomas from Whalen RK, Althausen AF, and Daniels GH. Extra-adrenal pheochromocytoma. J Urol 1992; 147:1–10.

ease, or aganglionic megacolon, is also caused by germ-line mutations in the *RET* proto-oncogene.[721, 722] Targeted disruption of the *RET* gene in mice leads to defective enteric neurogenesis, not pheochromocytoma.[723]

About one half of MEN 2B patients show the complete syndrome. Mucosal neuromas occur in all affected subjects. Oral neuromas are most common and occur about the lips, tongue, and buccal mucosa. Although the neuromas and the facial characteristics often are present at an early age, the disease frequently is not recognized until medullary carcinoma or pheochromocytoma is diagnosed later in life. The pathology, clinical behavior, and management of pheochromocytomas are similar in MEN 2A and MEN 2B.

Von Hippel-Lindau Disease (Retinal Cerebellar Hemangioblastomatosis)

Von Hippel-Lindau disease is an autosomal dominant disorder consisting of retinal angioma, hemangioblastoma of the central nervous system, renal carcinoma, renal and pancreatic cysts, and epidermal cystadenoma. Pheochromocytomas occur in 10 to 20% of patients overall.[724, 725] Variations in the disease cluster within affected families causing variability in the prevalence of pheochromocytoma among kindreds. Pheochromocytoma may be present in more than 90% of affected members, or it may be rare.[726] Among patients with pheochromocytoma, about 20% may have von Hippel-Lindau disease,[710] but whether the high prevalence reflects careful screening or the presence of several large kindreds in the geographic area of the study is unknown. Pheochromocytoma in these patients occurs earlier and is more often multifocal than in nonfamilial cases.[710] The gene responsible for this disorder (*VHL*) is located on human chromosome 3 and appears to function as a tumor suppressor gene.[727] Although multiple mutations have been described in the *VHL* gene, most patients with pheochromocytoma have missense mutations, and one mutation carries a 62% risk of tumor development.[728] Genetic abnormalities in the region of chromosome 3 in which the *VHL* gene is located, have been noted in patients with sporadic pheochromocytoma.[729]

Neurofibromatosis

The incidence of pheochromocytomas in kindreds with neurofibromatosis is uncertain, in part because of the presence of two variants of the syndrome (type 1 and type 2). In type 1, neurofibromas arise along peripheral nerves; in the type 2 syndrome, they develop in proximity to the cochlear branch of the eighth cranial nerve. Pheochromocytoma is associated only with type 1 disease. Overall, pheochromocytoma is present in probably 1% of type 1 patients, but among hypertensive patients with neurofibromatosis the prevalence may be higher than 50%.[730] Underlying mutations in this disorder are inactivating mutations in the *NF1* gene, a putative tumor suppressor gene that codes for the protein neurofibromin and is located on chromosome 17.[731] Targeted heterozygous mutations in *NF1* in mice cause a predisposition to develop pheochromocytomas, which otherwise occur rarely in these animals.[732] Although neurofibromatosis type 1 is an autosomal dominant trait, loss of *NF1* gene expression also has been demonstrated in pheochromocytomas removed from patients without neurofibromatosis, raising the possibility that somatic mutation in this gene may contribute to the development of the tumors.[733]

Diagnosis

Urinary Catecholamines and Catecholamine Metabolites

The diagnosis of pheochromocytoma is established by demonstration of increased urinary excretion of catechol-amines or catecholamine metabolites. The problem is to suspect the diagnosis; if the possibility of pheochromocytoma is raised, the diagnosis usually can be made or excluded on the basis of a single 24-h urine collection, provided the patient is symptomatic or hypertensive at the time of collection.

GENERAL CONSIDERATIONS. Assays used in diagnosis of pheochromocytoma include VMA, metanephrines, and unconjugated (free) catecholamines. Of the three determinations, metanephrines and unconjugated catecholamines are probably equivalent and superior to VMA. The combinations of metanephrine and normetanephrine and of NE and epinephrine measured in 24-h urine collections both achieved sensitivities and specificities of almost 100% in detecting pheochromocytoma, substantially higher than that of VMA.[734, 735] The number of 24-h urine collections obtained and the number of different determinations performed on each collection depend on the level of suspicion. Elevated values should be confirmed by at least one repeat determination.

The following general considerations apply to all urinary determinations. (1) Twenty-four-hour urine collections are preferable to random urine samples expressed per unit of creatinine. Creatinine should be measured for each 24-h collection to assess its adequacy. (2) If possible, the collection should be made with the patient at rest, while taking no medication, and without recent exposure to radiographic contrast media. If it is not feasible to discontinue all medications, those known to interfere in the assays should be avoided. Diuretics, some adrenergic blocking agents, vasodilators, calcium channel blockers, and angiotensin-converting enzyme inhibitors do not interfere appreciably. (3) The best assays are reasonably specific, and dietary restrictions are minimal. (4) The urine must be acidified (pH <3.0) and kept cold during and after collection. (5) Although most patients with pheochromocytoma, including those with paroxysmal symptoms, excrete increased amounts of catecholamines and catecholamine metabolites each day, the diagnostic yield is increased in patients with paroxysmal symptoms if a 24-h urine collection is initiated at the onset of a crisis. (6) Interfering substances depend on the specific analysis; specific questions should be referred to the clinical pathologist at the laboratory that performs the assays.

FREE CATECHOLAMINES. The upper limit of normal for total urinary catecholamines is usually between 591 and 890 nmol/d (100 and 150 μg/d). Most patients with pheochromocytoma have values in excess of 1500 nmol/d (250 μg/d). Specific assay of epinephrine often is beneficial because epinephrine excretion in excess of 270 nmol/d (50 μg/d) suggests an adrenal lesion and may be the only abnormality in cases associated with MEN.[708] The major cause of false-positive elevations of catecholamine excretion is administration of exogenous catecholamines such as methyldopa, levodopa, or labetalol, which can elevate urine concentrations for as long as 2 wk. Excessive stimulation of the sympathoadrenal system, as with hypoglycemia, strenuous exertion, increased intracranial pressure, or clonidine withdrawal, may also increase catecholamine excretion sufficiently to confound the diagnosis.

VANILLYLMANDELIC ACID AND TOTAL METANEPHRINES. In most assays the upper limit of normal for VMA excretion is 35 μmol/d (7.0 mg/d); the upper limit of normal for total metanephrines is 7 μmol/d (1.3 mg/d). Patients with pheochromocytoma almost always excrete these metabolites in excess, usually exceeding the normal range by threefold. Total metanephrine (metanephrine and normetanephrine) excretion is modestly increased by exogenous and endogenous catecholamines and can be markedly increased by treatment with MAO inhibitors. A metabolite of propranolol also falsely elevates metanephrine excretion in one of the commonly used assays. VMA excretion is affected less by endogenous and exogenous catecholamines, but a variety of drugs can produce spurious increases. VMA is less sensitive and less specific than either metanephrines or catecholamines in detecting pheochromocytoma.[734, 735]

PLASMA CATECHOLAMINES

Plasma catecholamine determinations are of limited usefulness in the diagnosis. Although many patients with pheochromocytoma have elevations in basal plasma catecholamine levels, considerable care is required in measuring basal catecholamine levels accurately. Casually obtained plasma levels, especially in anxious patients, can overlap levels in persons with pheochromocytoma. Plasma determinations should never be used as a screening test for pheochromocytoma. In an occasional problem patient in whom the clinical suspicion is high and in whom urinary assay results are borderline, plasma catecholamine measurements may be useful. In these circumstances, basal plasma catecholamine levels higher than 12 nmol/L (2 ng/mL) support the diagnosis, whereas values lower than 3 nmol/L (0.5 ng/mL) make the diagnosis unlikely. Assays of catecholamine metabolites in plasma are of limited utility.

SUPPRESSION TESTS. The usefulness of assays of plasma catecholamines may be enhanced by determining the response to agents that diminish sympathetic outflow. Administration of clonidine or the ganglionic-blocking agent pentolinium decreases plasma catecholamine levels in normal people but has a negligible effect in patients with pheochromocytoma.[157, 736] Prompt suppression of plasma catecholamine levels after oral clonidine is, therefore, useful to exclude the diagnosis in patients with suggestive clinical features and elevated plasma catecholamine levels. However, catecholamine levels are not suppressed in all normal individuals, particularly if baseline catecholamine levels are normal or low.[737] Diuretic treatment attenuates clonidine-induced suppression of plasma NE. Clonidine administration also has been used to suppress overnight catecholamine excretion.

PHARMACOLOGIC TESTS

Pharmacologic tests for pheochromocytoma for the most part have been rendered obsolete by measurement of catecholamines and catecholamine metabolites in urine. The pharmacologic tests are of two types: the adrenolytic test was utilized to determine catecholamine dependence in a hypertensive patient by evaluating the fall in blood pressure after administration of the rapidly acting α-receptor antagonist phentolamine; the provocative test was used to precipitate a crisis in normotensive patients with paroxysmal symptoms. The pharmacologic tests lack sensitivity and specificity. Adrenolytic tests have a high incidence of false-positive responses, and provocative tests have a false-negative response rate of 20 to 25%. The pharmacologic tests also are potentially hazardous; fatalities during provocative testing have occurred from cerebral hemorrhage and myocardial infarction. Although in some situations modified pharmacologic tests may be useful, because of the potential hazards these tests must always be carefully supervised and should never be undertaken casually.

ADRENOLYTIC TESTS. In some patients with malignant hypertension the features suggest the possibility of pheochromocytoma; in this setting significant blood pressure reduction by phentolamine not only supports the diagnosis but also indicates that α-adrenergic blockade may be a useful treatment. However, a good response to phentolamine only suggests the diagnosis; it must always be confirmed by documentation of increased urinary catecholamines or catecholamine metabolites.

The phentolamine test is performed with the patient in the supine position and with an intravenous line in place. After a stable baseline blood pressure is established and recorded, an intravenous bolus of phentolamine is administered, and blood pressure is recorded every 30 s for 3 min and then every minute for an additional 7 min or until the original values are regained. It is wise to start with a test dose of 0.5 mg; in the absence of a significant hypotensive response the remainder of a 5-mg ampule may be administered. The test result usually is considered to be positive when the decrease in blood pressure is 35 mm Hg systolic and 25 mm Hg diastolic or greater. The response to phentolamine begins after 2 to 3 min and lasts approximately 10 min; blood pressure decreases during the first 1 to 2 min after injection are nonspecific. An intravenous form of NE or phenylephrine should be available for immediate use in the event of a severe hypotensive reaction. False-positive responses are common in patients with renal failure and in patients treated with vasodilators.

PROVOCATIVE TESTS. Because of the potential hazard associated with induction of a severe paroxysm, provocative tests have limited indication. In the patient with paroxysmal symptoms and normal or borderline catecholamine excretion, it is preferable to document an increase in catecholamine excretion at the time of the crisis by sequential timed urine collections or, if these are not feasible, to initiate a 24-h urine collection after the onset of the paroxysm.

Previously, provocative tests used histamine, glucagon, or tyramine and assessed the blood pressure response to these agents. In addition to the danger of a severe hypertensive crisis, the false-negative rate with these agents was substantial. The sensitivity and specificity of diagnosis may be enhanced by measurement of plasma and urinary catecholamines after administration of glucagon, the safest of these agents.[738] Prior α-adrenergic blockade is an important safety precaution to limit the pressor response.[738, 739]

PLASMA NEUROPEPTIDES

As noted previously, pheochromocytomas release into plasma a variety of peptides; some of these circulate at higher than normal levels in patients with pheochromocytoma, including chromogranin-A, neuropeptide Y, and endothelin-1.[740–742] Plasma chromogranin-A levels are reported to be 83% sensitive and 96% specific in separating patients with pheochromocytoma from normal controls and patients with essential hypertension.[740] Renal dysfunction, however, impairs the diagnostic efficacy of chromogranin-A measurements.[740, 743] Although plasma neuropeptide Y levels are higher on average in patients with pheochromocytoma, the difference appears to be caused solely by elevated levels in patients with intra-adrenal tumors.[744] Measurements of plasma neuropeptides, however, have no proven diagnostic role, because their utility in diagnosing tumors not detectable by conventional methods has not been established.

DIFFERENTIAL DIAGNOSIS

The diagnosis of pheochromocytoma should be considered in patients with suggestive clinical features.

"HYPERADRENERGIC" ESSENTIAL HYPERTENSION. The possibility of pheochromocytoma is often considered in patients with essential hypertension and hyperadrenergic features such as tachycardia, sweating, increased cardiac output, and anxiety. Although increased sympathetic nervous activity may contribute to the hypertension in these subjects, analysis of a 24-h urine collection is usually sufficient to exclude pheochromocytoma. Anxiety attacks resembling pheochromocytoma paroxysms may occur in these patients, and several analyses of urine collected during symptomatic episodes may be necessary before the diagnosis can be excluded with certainty.

MEDICATIONS. Pressor crises in patients who are taking

MAO inhibitors closely resemble pheochromocytoma paroxysms. Clonidine withdrawal also is associated with pressor crises. These crises are caused by increased sympathetic nervous system activity and frequently are associated with increased urinary and plasma catecholamine levels. They can be treated by administration of α-adrenergic blocking agents or by reintroduction of clonidine. Ingestion of crack cocaine also may precipitate adrenergic crisis, and an accurate medication history is critical for identification of the offending agents. Factitious crises can be produced by self-administration of sympathomimetic amines in emotionally disturbed patients, particularly those who work in health care professions. Depending on the medication taken, urinary catecholamine excretion may be normal or abnormal. The direct addition of catecholamines to urine collections can also result in a factitious diagnosis.

INTRACRANIAL LESIONS. Intracranial lesions associated with increased intracranial pressure, particularly posterior fossa tumor or subarachnoid hemorrhage, may be confused with pheochromocytoma. Often it is obvious that these patients have experienced a neurologic catastrophe, and it is usually clear that the neurologic disease is primary. The possibility of subarachnoid or intracranial hemorrhage secondary to pheochromocytoma, however, should not be overlooked.

NEUROPSYCHIATRIC DISEASE. Anxiety attacks, often with hyperventilation, may suggest pheochromocytoma paroxysms. Significant blood pressure elevation during the attacks, especially if associated with tachycardia, supports the diagnosis of pheochromocytoma, because anxiety attacks usually are not associated with hypertension. In some, however, both systolic and diastolic blood pressure may be elevated; in these cases it is difficult to differentiate anxiety attacks from pheochromocytoma paroxysms on clinical grounds. Several 24-h urine catecholamine or metabolite determinations may be required. Seizure disorders, especially the rare autonomic or diencephalic epilepsy, also may be confused with the paroxysms of pheochromocytoma. Modest elevations in plasma catecholamine levels have been reported during autonomic epilepsy, although urinary catecholamine excretion usually is normal. An abnormal electroencephalogram, an aura, and a beneficial response to anticonvulsant therapy usually suffice to exclude pheochromocytoma if urinary catecholamine excretion is normal.

MISCELLANEOUS DISORDERS. The sympathomimetic features of thyrotoxicosis may suggest pheochromocytoma; diastolic hypertension, however, is not a feature of uncomplicated hyperthyroidism, and catecholamine excretion is normal. Some patients with angina pectoris have pressor attacks that resemble the paroxysms of pheochromocytoma, but urinary excretion of catecholamines is normal. Patients with pheochromocytoma may present with chest pain and electrocardiographic abnormalities suggesting myocardial infarction or dissecting aortic aneurysm; the absence of pulse deficits, poor blood pressure response to conventional treatment, and the presence of tachycardia in association with high diastolic blood pressure support the diagnosis of pheochromocytoma. Urinary catecholamine measurements usually distinguish these entities.

SCREENING FOR PHEOCHROMOCYTOMA

It is neither feasible nor necessary to screen all hypertensive patients for pheochromocytoma. Patients with hypertension who have a poor response to conventional antihypertensive medications, signs of sympathetic overactivity, or paroxysms of any kind should undergo a 24-h urine collection while they are symptomatic. Any of the suggestive clinical features in a hypertensive patient (Table 13–12) should raise the suspicion of pheochromocytoma, especially if blood pres-

TABLE 13–12. Findings Suggestive of Pheochromocytoma

Clinical manifestations
  Paroxysmal attacks of any kind
  Signs of excessive adrenergic stimulation
    Tachycardia
    Excessive sweating
  Signs of hypermetabolism
    Fever
    Weight loss
  Orthostatic hypotension
  Anxiety-hyperexcitability
  Signs of cardiomyopathy
  Headaches
  Chest or abdominal pain
  Signs of neurocutaneous disease
    Five or six café au lait spots
    Neuromas or neurofibromas
    Retinal angiomas
    Vertebral abnormalities
  Unusual blood pressure response to surgery, anesthesia, or trauma
  Abdominal mass
Laboratory findings
  Hyperglycemia
  High hematocrit
Associated diseases
  Medullary thyroid carcinoma
  Mucosal neuroma syndrome
  Neurofibromatosis
  Retinocerebellar hemangioblastomatosis
  Hyperparathyroidism
  Islet cell tumors
Family history
  Pheochromocytoma
  Associated diseases

sure control is suboptimal. The personal or familial occurrence of a disorder associated with pheochromocytoma is also an indication for screening. The possibility of pheochromocytoma should be considered in all members at risk in kindreds with MEN 2A, MEN 2B, neurofibromatosis, or von Hippel-Lindau disease. In the MEN kindreds, affected members should be screened yearly for pheochromocytoma. Screening is relatively inexpensive and reasonably effective at establishing the diagnosis.

Management

Surgical removal is the definitive treatment for pheochromocytoma. Before surgery, however, a period of medical management with adrenergic blocking agents is required to reverse the effects of excessive adrenergic stimulation. Nonspecific treatment of hypertension with intravenous sodium nitroprusside or oral calcium-channel antagonists also may control blood pressure acutely.

MEDICAL ASPECTS OF TREATMENT

α-RECEPTOR BLOCKADE. After the diagnosis of pheochromocytoma is established, the patient should immediately be given α-adrenergic blocking agents. Phenoxybenzamine, the agent of choice, produces a stable, noncompetitive α-receptor blockage of long duration and is particularly suitable for preoperative management. Hypertensive crises that occur while the patient is being brought under control with phenoxybenzamine should be treated with intravenous phentolamine in doses of 1 to 5 mg. The usual initial dose of phenoxybenzamine is 10 mg every 12 h; increments of 10 mg may be added every few days until blood pressure is controlled and the paroxysms cease. Because of the long duration of action, the therapeutic effects are cumulative and last for several days. The optimal dose, therefore, must be achieved gradually. Most patients require between 40 and 80 mg/d, although some need 200 mg/d or more. In patients with intermittent hypertension, ascertainment of the appropriate dose of phenoxybenzamine is more difficult. In these individuals the dose should be titrated to the point that paroxysms cease; when postural signs and symptoms develop and persist, the dose should be stabilized. All patients who are being treated with phenoxybenzamine should have blood pressure recorded in the supine and upright positions several times each day. Dosage adjustment is best performed in a hospital setting.

Prazosin, the selective α₁-antagonist, and the longer-acting α₁-selective agents doxazosin and terazosin have been used in preoperative management of patients with pheochromocytoma. The ultimate role of these agents has not been established, but the fact that they are competitive inhibitors may be a disadvantage in comparison with phenoxybenzamine.

α-Adrenergic receptor blockade also increases the blood volume, an important consideration for the success of surgical removal of the tumor. Imposition of a high-salt diet augments restitution of plasma volume. The hematocrit can fall after initiation of α-receptor blockade, presumably a manifestation of volume expansion. α-Adrenergic blockade also improves congestive heart failure and angina pectoris, if these are present, as a consequence of afterload reduction.

Patients with pheochromocytoma should receive full blocking doses of phenoxybenzamine before invasive diagnostic tests or surgery. In normotensive patients preoperative preparation is the same except that it may be more difficult to judge the adequacy of phenoxybenzamine treatment. A 2-wk course of α-adrenergic blockade is the cornerstone of preoperative management.

β-RECEPTOR BLOCKADE. Propranolol (or some other β-adrenergic antagonist) is a useful adjunct in treatment, but it should be administered only after α-adrenergic blockade is effective. If given in the absence of α-adrenergic blockade, propranolol can cause a paradoxical increase in blood pressure by blocking β-receptor–mediated vasodilatation in skeletal muscle. This effect is particularly prominent when the tumor secretes epinephrine. Propranolol may be begun if tachycardia develops during institution of α-adrenergic blockade. Small doses usually are adequate, and a reasonable starting dose is 10 mg three or four times per day, titrated as needed to control the pulse rate. Propranolol is particularly useful in controlling catecholamine-induced arrhythmias that develop during administration of anesthesia. It also decreases sweating by blocking heat production and may improve angina by controlling tachycardia. If an underlying myocarditis is present propranolol may precipitate congestive heart failure.

INHIBITION OF CATECHOLAMINE BIOSYNTHESIS. Metyrosine has been used to inhibit catecholamine biosynthesis by pheochromocytomas. In doses of 0.3 to 4 g/d it inhibits catecholamine biosynthesis by 50 to 80%. This agent has been used both in preoperative preparation and in long-term treatment of inoperable patients. Although usually not required, the agent may be helpful if prolonged medical management is necessary.

LOCALIZATION OF TUMOR

Preoperative localization of the tumor or tumors facilitates surgical removal. Computerized tomography (CT), magnetic resonance imaging (MRI), and radionuclide scanning with iodine 123– or iodine 131–labeled meta-iodobenzylguanidine (^{123}I/^{131}I-MIBG) are all used for tumor localization. Radiolabeled somatostatin analogues and tracers for positron emission tomography (PET) are currently under investigation for use in localization. Previously, arteriography and venography (with or without catecholamine analysis in venous blood) were employed to diagnose and localize lesions, but they have been supplanted by the noninvasive methods.

In general, localization techniques should be used after the diagnosis of pheochromocytoma is confirmed biochemically. Because the incidence of nonfunctioning "incidental" adrenal masses identifiable on CT scan is far from negligible, the finding of a small nodule in the absence of catecholamine hypersecretion is problematic. Judicious use of the CT scan, nonetheless, may be helpful in the unusual difficult case in which the issue cannot be resolved by biochemical determinations. Under these circumstances the demonstration of completely normal adrenals frequently reassures both the patient and the physician that an adrenal pheochromocytoma is not responsible for the clinical picture. The demonstration of an adrenal nodule, on the other hand, may suggest the need for further attempts at biochemical confirmation. It should be emphasized in this context that up to 10% of incidentally discovered adrenal masses may be pheochromocytomas in some series,[745] and appropriate screening is therefore indicated.

ADRENAL TUMORS. Because the normal adrenal gland is surrounded by retroperitoneal fat, CT and MRI are powerful tools to differentiate intra-adrenal lesions from normal glands (Fig. 13–27). Because most of these tumors are at least 2 cm in diameter at the time of diagnosis, the lesions usually fall within the resolving power of these techniques. Adequate visu-

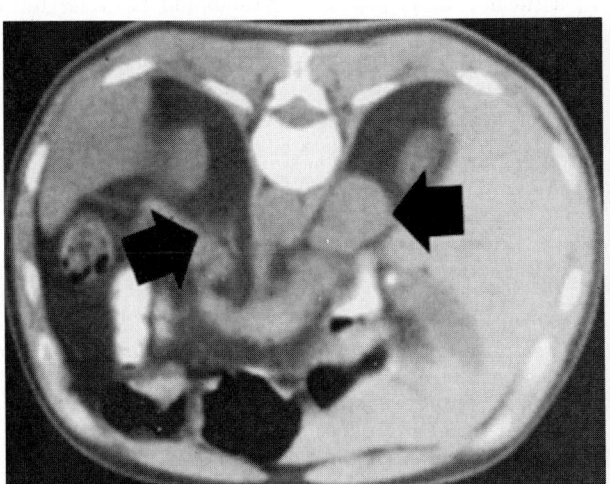
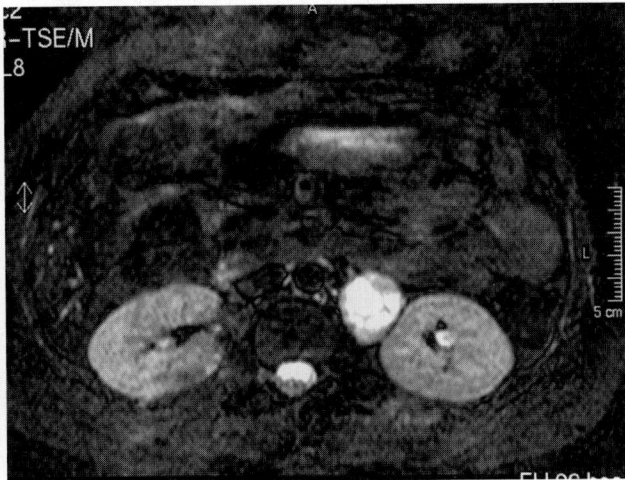

Figure 13–27. Adrenal pheochromocytomas demonstrated by CT and MRI scans. In CT scan *(left)* note the normal adrenal on the left, and the pheochromocytoma on the right *(arrows)*. In the MRI scan *(right)* an extra-adrenal pheochromocytoma is visible in the perihilar region of the left kidney. (CT scan from Landsberg L. Pheochromocytoma. Medical Grand Rounds 1983;2:7–21, with permission.)

alization of a normal-appearing adrenal is ordinarily sufficient to exclude an intra-adrenal pheochromocytoma. CT scanning with contrast enhancement can be performed on unblocked patients, but glucagon should not be used as an antiperistaltic agent because it may induce a severe paroxysm. MRI is as sensitive as CT and may provide additional information regarding the character of the lesion.[746, 747] Pheochromocytomas exhibit high signal intensity on T2-weighted images, although other adrenal lesions may give similar findings. In pregnant women MRI is the preferred approach.

Scintigraphic localization of pheochromocytoma with the radiopharmaceutical ^{131}I-MIBG is also useful. This agent, a substrate for the NE transporter,[748] is concentrated in pheochromocytomas and can provide diagnostic information about an adrenal mass. For identification of intra-adrenal pheochromocytomas before the initial operation, MIBG scintigraphy may be slightly less sensitive than CT or MRI, but it is more specific.[747, 749] In the evaluation of previously operated patients, MIBG scintigraphy appears to be the technique of choice, because it is reportedly as sensitive as MRI, more sensitive than CT, and more specific than either in diagnosing recurrent disease.[747]

Ultrasonography is less sensitive than CT or MRI in detecting adrenal masses, but it may be helpful in children, who usually have less retroperitoneal fat. However, the pressure exerted by the sonogram probe may provoke a paroxysm. Fine-needle biopsy of any adrenal mass should not be undertaken until the diagnosis of pheochromocytoma is excluded, because aspiration of an unsuspected pheochromocytoma can also provoke a serious or fatal paroxysm.

EXTRA-ADRENAL PHEOCHROMOCYTOMAS. The possibility of extra-adrenal pheochromocytoma should be considered in patients with increased catecholamine or catecholamine metabolite excretion in whom the adrenal glands appear normal on CT or MRI scan. One advantage of MIBG scintigraphy in the search for extra-adrenal disease is that it is possible to screen the whole body with high specificity.[750] Most extra-adrenal pheochromocytomas, however, are located within the abdomen between the diaphragm and pelvic floor (see Table 13–11). MRI and MIBG scintigraphy are superior to CT in localizing abdominal extra-adrenal pheochromocytomas. MIBG may be as sensitive as MRI and slightly more specific.[747, 749] For lesions within the thorax CT may be superior to MRI as a complement to MIBG scintigraphy.[751]

Extra-adrenal pheochromocytomas or chemodectomas in the neck may be palpable. Pressure may induce a paroxysm, but a crisis should not be intentionally provoked. If the symptoms are related to micturition, a bladder pheochromocytoma should be sought, as described previously. All diagnostic studies likely to provoke catecholamine release should be performed only after adrenergic blockade.

SURGERY

The extent of surgical exploration depends on the results of preoperative studies that localize the tumor. The exploration can be limited when CT or MRI demonstrates a pheochromocytoma in one adrenal and a normal adrenal on the contralateral side. In patients with familial pheochromocytoma bilateral adrenalectomy is not necessary in every case.[752] If CT or MRI indicates unilateral disease, it is reasonable to leave the normal adrenal and monitor for possible development of pheochromocytoma in the remaining gland, which may occur after a hiatus of many years, or not at all. Even if disease is present on microscopic examination, prophylactic removal of a normal-appearing adrenal subjects the patient to added years of treatment with exogenous steroids and to the potential risks of adrenal crisis.

PREOPERATIVE MANAGEMENT. Successful surgery re-

quires the cooperation of surgeon, anesthesiologist, and endocrinologist. Surgery for pheochromocytoma is technically demanding, should not be undertaken lightly, and is preferably done in centers that have experience with this disease.

The cornerstone of successful surgery is adequate preparation, which entails a 2-wk course of α-adrenergic blockade with phenoxybenzamine. In conjunction with a liberal salt intake, this regimen allows restoration of plasma volume and permits recovery from the untoward effects of excessive adrenergic stimulation. There is no indication for intravenous phenoxybenzamine and the rapid induction of adrenergic blockade that this produces. While adrenergic blockade is being gradually induced, a careful search can be made for a familial diathesis and associated diseases. Features suggesting MEN 2A or MEN 2B greatly increase the likelihood of bilateral tumors. Localization studies also can be performed during this period. There has been some controversy regarding whether phenoxybenzamine should be administered up until the day of surgery. Despite its relatively long duration of action, this agent can be continued until the time of surgery without untoward effects during the operation or in the postoperative period. Intraoperative and postoperative hypotension can be adequately controlled if sufficient time has been allowed for restoration of the extracellular fluid volume before surgery. As noted earlier, β-blockade can be added after α-blockers have been started to control arrhythmias.

ANESTHESIA AND INTRAOPERATIVE MANAGEMENT. Scopolamine and short-acting barbiturates are satisfactory preanesthetic medications. Both pancuronium and succinylcholine have been used as muscle relaxants. The choice of anesthetic agent is controversial. A satisfactory approach utilizes a combination of nitrous oxide, thiopental, narcotics, and enflurane. All halogenated hydrocarbons (including enflurane) sensitize to the arrhythmogenic properties of catecholamines; these arrhythmias are effectively antagonized by β-adrenergic blocking agents. Innovar, which is a combination of droperidol (a butyrophenone) and fentanyl (a narcotic), may provoke paroxysms in patients with unsuspected pheochromocytoma who are undergoing incidental surgery. The safety of this agent in blocked patients is uncertain; prudence dictates the use of other agents. Narcotics, although hazardous in unblocked patients, have been used without ill effects in blocked patients during surgery.

During surgery there should be continuous monitoring of arterial pressure (by intra-arterial catheter), central venous pressure, and electrocardiographic changes. Pulmonary wedge pressure also should be monitored in the presence of known or suspected heart disease. There should be a careful and continuous estimation of blood loss, and particular efforts should be made to keep the rate of fluid replacement (saline, albumin, and blood) equal to the rate of loss. Hypotension usually responds better to volume replacement than to administration of vasoconstrictors. Reduced central venous pressure or pulmonary capillary wedge pressure is a good indication of the need for volume replacement.

Hypertensive reactions and cardiac arrhythmias are most likely to occur during induction of anesthesia, intubation or manipulation of the tumor and are best controlled with intravenous administration of phentolamine or propranolol, respectively (Fig. 13–28). Phentolamine is given as a bolus of 1 to 5 mg intravenously, as needed. Propranolol is administered intravenously in 0.5- to 1-mg doses for tachycardia or ventricular ectopy. Lidocaine and nitroprusside may be required for arrhythmias and hypertension that are poorly responsive to propranolol and phentolamine; these agents are rarely needed in properly prepared patients. If a vasopressor agent is needed, norepinephrine bitartrate or phenylephrine is satisfactory. Indirect-acting sympathomimetic amines that release catecholamines have an unpredictable effect and should be avoided.

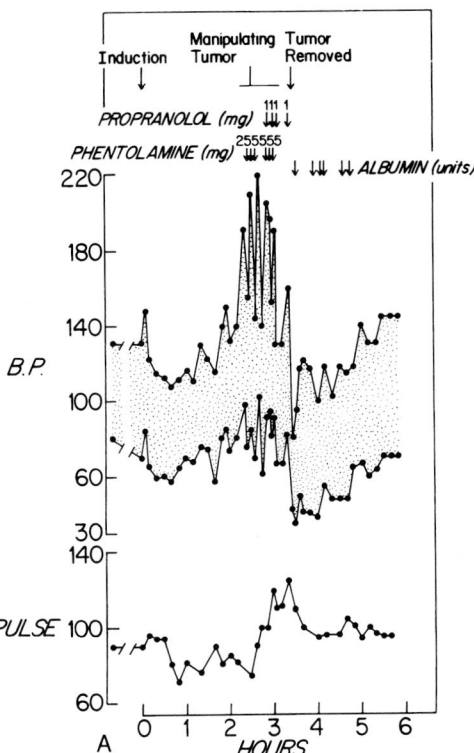

Figure 13–28. Pulse and blood pressure changes during resection of a pheochromocytoma. Note the rise in blood pressure and pulse during induction and during the manipulation of the tumor; blood pressure falls after the tumor is resected. Blood pressure is usually restored by fluid administration. Increased blood pressure and pulse rate respond to intraoperative administration of phentolamine and propranolol. (From Landsberg L, Young JB. Catecholamines and the adrenal medulla. In: Bondy PK, Rosenberg LE, eds. Metabolic Control and Disease. 8th ed. Philadelphia: WB Saunders, 1980: 1621–1693.)

Each pheochromocytoma should be considered potentially malignant and should be removed with the capsule intact. Surrounding connective tissue and fat should also be removed. It is important to remove the entire adrenal gland. Patients with locally recurrent disease commonly have undergone procedures in which an attempt was made to remove the tumor but to spare the normal adrenal tissue. The malignant potential of the pheochromocytoma cannot be predicted with confidence solely on the basis of histologic appearance. Malignancy is suggested by metastatic deposits or microvascular invasion.

Arterial blood pressure usually falls when the pheochromocytoma is removed (see Fig. 13–28); the failure of blood pressure to fall should raise the possibility of an additional tumor.

POSTOPERATIVE MANAGEMENT. A transient episode of hypertension is not uncommon in the immediate postoperative period, usually as a result of fluid shifts and/or autonomic instability. It often responds to administration of diuretics. If there is any doubt about the hypertension being caused by residual pheochromocytoma, phentolamine may be administered. A response to phentolamine suggests that all of the pheochromocytoma may not have been removed. In some patients, vigorous fluid administration is required to support blood pressure in the postoperative period.

For about 1 wk the patient should be regarded as having excessive catecholamine stores in sympathetic nerve endings. Administration of catecholamine-releasing agents should be avoided during this period. Before the patient is discharged from the hospital, preferably 1 wk after removal of the tumor, assays for catecholamines and their metabolites in urine

should be repeated for confirmation that all of the functioning pheochromocytoma has been removed. Levels of catecholamines (or their metabolites) should be measured again if suggestive symptoms reappear or, if the patient remains asymptomatic, at yearly intervals until the likelihood of recurrence is very low (at least 5 y).

MALIGNANT PHEOCHROMOCYTOMA

Malignant pheochromocytoma usually recurs in the retroperitoneum or appears as metastatic deposits in bone, lung, or liver. Recurrence can happen decades after the initial surgery. Radiation therapy is not usually effective but may be of value for controlling symptomatic involvement of bone. Limited success has been reported with combination chemotherapy consisting of cyclophosphamide, vincristine, and dacarbazine. An alternative approach involves the repeated use of ^{131}I-MIBG in higher doses than those employed for diagnostic imaging. Responses to this treatment are incomplete.[753]

LONG-TERM MEDICAL MANAGEMENT

In some patients chronic medical management is necessary because of disseminated malignancy or some other intercurrent illness that makes surgery inappropriate. Most tumors grow slowly, and the major morbidity is caused by excessive catecholamine secretion rather than by local invasion or metastases to other organs. The manifestations may be controlled by adrenergic blocking agents in conjunction with metyrosine, which reduces catecholamine biosynthesis by the tumor.

PREGNANCY

Pheochromocytoma during pregnancy can be difficult to manage. In unprepared patients spontaneous labor with vaginal delivery is usually disastrous for mother and fetus and should be avoided. For tumor localization MRI is the diagnostic option of choice. After the diagnosis is established treatment with adrenergic blocking agents should be initiated. In early or middle pregnancy, the tumor should be removed after the patient is prepared. The pregnancy need not be terminated, but the risk of spontaneous abortion at the time of surgery is considerable. Late in the course, cesarean section followed by excision of the tumor may be undertaken if the fetus is of sufficient size. If the fetus is too immature, the patient may be monitored closely while being given adrenergic blocking drugs, and the operation may be delayed until fetal maturation progresses to the point of viability. If the clinical course deteriorates, however, surgery should not be postponed. Although the safety of adrenergic blocking agents during pregnancy is not established, they have been used in many cases without obvious adverse effect.

Prognosis

In nonmalignant pheochromocytoma the 5-y survival rate is higher than 95%, and the recurrence rate after surgery is less than 10%. In patients with benign pheochromocytoma the survival rate after operation approaches the age-adjusted norm. In experienced hands surgical mortality usually is less than 2 to 3%; casually performed surgery in improperly prepared patients, on the other hand, can be catastrophic. In malignant pheochromocytoma the 5-y survival rate is less than 50%.

Complete resection cures the hypertension in approximately 75% of patients with pheochromocytoma; in the remaining 25%, hypertension recurs but is usually well controlled with a standard antihypertensive regimen. In this group, underlying essential hypertension or irreversible vascular damage induced by catecholamines may cause the persistent elevation of blood pressure.

OTHER TUMORS OF SYMPATHETIC AND ADRENOMEDULLARY ORIGIN

Neuroblastoma

GENERAL FEATURES

Neuroblastoma, ganglioneuroblastoma, and ganglioneuroma, like pheochromocytomas, are derived from the neural crest and are located in the adrenal medulla and sympathetic ganglia (Fig. 13–29). Like pheochromocytomas, they are often associated with excessive production of catecholamines and catecholamine metabolites. The pharmacologic effects of their humoral products are usually minor, but aggressive malignant behavior is common.

Neuroblastomas, the most immature and malignant of these tumors, are derivatives of sympathoadrenal progenitor cells or neuroblasts. Ganglioneuroblastomas are partially differentiated neuroblastomas containing mature ganglion cells and neurofibrils; although these tumors are malignant, the prognosis is better than for neuroblastoma. Ganglioneuroma is a benign tumor derived from the sympathetic ganglion cells. The biology of the three tumors is poorly understood; the immature tumors appear to have a latent capacity to differentiate into more mature tissues, and this feature may account for some of the spontaneous remissions that have occurred.

The excretion of catecholamines and their metabolites is almost always increased in patients with neuroblastomas and is often increased in those with ganglioneuromas. NE (but not epinephrine), VMA, DA, HVA, and dopa may be excreted in increased amounts. Increased excretion of DA and HVA is characteristic of neuroblastomas. Compared with pheochromocytomas, the tumors themselves contain little catecholamine. Metabolism of catecholamines within the tumor may explain the absence of hypertension in most patients. Although catecholamine excretion does not correlate closely with the clinical manifestations in these patients, assays of urinary catecholamine excretion are useful in establishing a diagnosis and in monitoring the results of treatment. Low ratios of VMA to HVA in the urine are correlated with a poor prognosis, perhaps because the more immature tumors have diminished DBH activity.

CLINICAL FEATURES

Neuroblastoma is a common malignant tumor in children. It is characterized by rapid growth and widespread metastasis. The tumors originate either in the sympathetic chain or in the adrenal medulla; the prognosis is poorest for those of adrenomedullary origin. In younger patients the tumor is more aggressive and less likely to undergo spontaneous regression. Neuroblastomas are more likely to undergo spontaneous regression than are any other malignant tumors in humans. The treatment of neuroblastoma is complex and involves surgery (usually partial or palliative resection of the tumor), radiation, and administration of chemotherapeutic agents.

Ganglioneuroma

Ganglioneuromas are benign tumors found in both children and adults. They originate in the sympathetic chain, most commonly in the posterior mediastinum. Some patients exhibit manifestations of excessive catecholamine secretion, particularly hypertension, which is more likely to occur with ganglioneuroma than with neuroblastoma. The clinical features, diagnosis, and management of NE-secreting ganglioneuromas are similar to those of extra-adrenal pheochromocytomas.

A syndrome of chronic diarrhea has been described in children with either ganglioneuroma or ganglioneuroblastoma. The pathogenesis of the diarrhea is obscure; it appears to be mediated by a humoral factor, possibly VIP, and disappears on removal of the tumor.

REFERENCES

1. Oliver G, Schäfer EA. The physiological effects of extracts of the suprarenal capsules. J Physiol (Lond) 1895; 18:230–276.
2. Takamine J. The isolation of the active principle of the suprarenal gland. J Physiol (Lond) 1901; 27:29P–30P.
3. Abel JJ, Taveau RdeM. On the decomposition products of epinephrin hydrate. J Biol Chem 1905; 1:1–32.
4. von Euler US. Identification of the sympathomimetic ergone in adrenergic nerves of cattle (sympathin N) with laevo-noradrenaline. Acta Physiol Scand 1948; 16:63–74.
5. Barger G, Dale HH. Chemical structure and sympathomimetic action of amines. J Physiol (Lond) 1910; 41:19–59.
6. Cabot JB. Sympathetic preganglionic neurons: cytoarchitecture, ultrastructure, and biophysical properties. In: Loewy AD, Spyer KM, eds. Central Regulation of Autonomic Functions. New York: Oxford University Press, 1990: 44–67.
7. Guyenet PG. Role of the ventral medulla oblongata in blood pressure regulation. In: Loewy AD, Spyer KM, eds. Central Regulation of Autonomic Functions. New York: Oxford University Press, 1990: 145–167.
8. Le Douarin NM, Dupin E. Cell lineage analysis in neural crest ontogeny. J Neurobiol 1993; 24:146–161.
9. Anderson DJ. The neural crest cell lineage problem: neuropoiesis? Neuron 1989; 3:1–12.
10. Anderson DJ, Carnahan JF, Michelsohn A, et al. Antibody markers identify a common progenitor to sympathetic neurons and chromaffin cells *in vivo* and reveal the timing of commitment to neuronal differentiation in the sympathoadrenal lineage. J Neurosci 1991; 11:3507–3519.
11. Anderson DJ. Cell fate determination in the peripheral nervous system: the sympathoadrenal progenitor. J Neurobiol 1993; 24:185–198.
12. Cole TJ, Blendy JA, Monaghan AP, et al. Targeted disruption of the glucocorticoid receptor gene blocks adrenergic chromaffin cell development and severely retards lung maturation. Genes Dev 1995; 9:1608–1621.
13. Unsicker K. The chromaffin cell: paradigm in cell, developmental and growth factor biology. J Anat 1993; 183:207–221.
14. Rao MS, Landis SC. Cell interactions that determine sympathetic neuron transmitter phenotype and the neurokines that mediate them. J Neurobiol 1993; 24:215–232.
15. Oppenheim RW. Cell death during development of the nervous system. Annu Rev Neurosci 1991; 14:453–501.
16. Korsching S. The neurotrophic factor concept: a reexamination. J Neurosci 1993; 13:2739–2748.
17. Crowley C, Spencer SD, Nishimura MC, et al. Mice lacking nerve growth factor display perinatal loss of sensory and sympathetic neurons yet develop basal forebrain cholinergic neurons. Cell 1994; 76:1001–1011.
18. Ernfors P, Lee K-F, Kucera J, et al. Lack of neurotrophin-3 leads to deficiencies in the peripheral nervous system and loss of limb proprioceptive afferents. Cell 1994; 77:503–512.
19. Fariñas I, Jones KR, Backus C, et al. Severe sensory and sympathetic deficits in mice lacking neurotrophin-3. Nature 1994; 369:658–661.

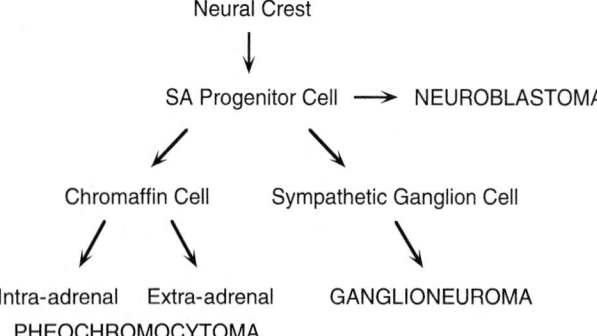

Figure 13–29. Embryologic origin of sympathoadrenal tumors.

20. Black IB, DiCicco-Bloom E, Dreyfus CF. Nerve growth factor and the issue of mitosis in the nervous system. Curr Top Dev Biol 1990; 24:161–192.

21. Hendry IA. Cell division in the developing sympathetic nervous system. J Neurocytol 1977; 6:299–309.

22. Campenot RB. NGF and the local control of nerve terminal growth. J Neurobiol 1994; 25:599–611.

23. Korsching S, Thoenen H. Nerve growth factor in sympathetic ganglia and corresponding target organs of the rat: correlation with density of sympathetic innervation. Proc Natl Acad Sci USA 1983; 80:3513–3516.

24. Shelton DL, Reichardt LF. Expression of the β-nerve growth factor gene correlates with the density of sympathetic innervation in effector organs. Proc Natl Acad Sci USA 1984; 81:7951–7955.

25. Levi-Montalcini R. The nerve growth factor 35 years later. Science 1987; 237:1154–1162.

26. Murphy RA, Saide JD, Blanchard MH, et al. Nerve growth factor in mouse serum and saliva: role of the submandibular gland. Proc Natl Acad Sci USA 1977; 74:2330–2333.

27. Siminoski K, Gonnella P, Bernanke J, et al. Uptake and transepithelial transport of nerve growth factor in suckling rat ileum. J Cell Biol 1986; 103:1979–1990.

28. Aloe L, Calissano P, Levi-Montalcini R. Effects of oral administration of nerve growth factor and of its antiserum on sympathetic ganglia of neonatal mice. Dev Brain Res 1982; 4:31–34.

29. Aloe L, Cozzari C, Levi-Montalcini R. Cyclocytidine-induced release of nerve growth factor from mouse submandibular glands enhances regeneration of sympathetic fibers in adult mice. Brain Res 1985; 332:259–265.

30. Morris JL, Gibbins IL. Co-transmission and neuromodulation. In: Burnstock G, Hoyle CHV, eds. Autonomic Neuroeffector Mechanisms. Chur, Switzerland: Harwood Academic Publishers, 1992: 33–119.

31. Coupland RE, Selby JE. The blood supply of the mammalian adrenal medulla: a comparative study. J Anat 1976; 122:539–551.

32. Kikuta A, Murakami T. Microcirculation of the rat adrenal gland: a scanning electron microscope study of vascular casts. Am J Anat 1982; 164:19–28.

33. Kikuta A, Murakami T. Relationship between chromaffin cells and blood vessels in the rat adrenal medulla: a transmission electron microscopic study combined with blood vessel reconstructions. Am J Anat 1984; 170:73–81.

34. Parker TL, Kesse WK, Mohamed AA, et al. The innervation of the mammalian adrenal gland. J Anat 1993; 183:265–276.

35. Welsh JH. Catecholamines in the invertebrates. In: Blaschko H, Muscholl E, eds. Handbook of Experimental Pharmacology. Vol 33: Catecholamines. Berlin: Springer-Verlag, 1972: 79–109.

36. Holzbauer M, Sharman DF. The distribution of catecholamines in vertebrates. In: Blaschko H, Muscholl E, eds. Handbook of Experimental Pharmacology. Vol 33: Catecholamines. Berlin: Springer-Verlag, 1972: 110–185.

37. Kirshner N. Biosynthesis of the catecholamines. In: Blaschko H, Sayers G, Smith AD, eds. Handbook of Physiology. Section 7: Endocrine. Vol VI: Adrenal Gland. Washington, DC: American Physiological Society, 1975: 341–355.

38. Nagatsu T. Genes for human catecholamine-synthesizing enzymes. Neurosci Res 1991; 12:315–345.

39. Zigmond RE, Schwarzschild MA, Rittenhouse AR. Acute regulation of tyrosine hydroxylase by nerve activity and by neurotransmitters via phosphorylation. Annu Rev Neurosci 1989; 12:415–461.

40. Vrana KE, Walker SJ, Rucker P, et al. A carboxyl terminal leucine zipper is required for tyrosine hydroxylase tetramer formation. J Neurochem 1994; 63:2014–2020.

41. Ichinose H, Ohye T, Fujita K, et al. Increased heterogeneity of tyrosine hydroxylase in humans. Biochem Biophys Res Commun 1993; 195:158–165.

42. Mallet J, Boni C, Darmon M, et al. Molecular biology of rat and human tyrosine hydroxylases. In: Dahlström A, Belmaker RH, Sandler M, eds. Progress in Catecholamine Research. Part A: Basic Aspects and Peripheral Mechanisms. New York: Alan R Liss, 1988: 21–27.

43. Sumi-Ichinose C, Ichinose H, Takahashi E, et al. Molecular cloning of genomic DNA and chromosomal assignment of the gene for human aromatic L-amino acid decarboxylase, the enzyme for catecholamine and serotonin biosynthesis. Biochemistry 1992; 31:2229–2238.

44. Ishiguro H, Kim KT, Joh TH, et al. Neuron-specific expression of the human dopamine β-hydroxylase gene requires both the cAMP-response element and a silencer region. J Biol Chem 1993; 268:17987–17994.

45. Lewis EJ, Asnani LP. Soluble and membrane-bound forms of dopamine β-hydroxylase are encoded by the same mRNA. J Biol Chem 1992; 267:494–500.

46. Craig SP, Buckle VJ, Lamouroux A, et al. Localization of the human dopamine beta hydroxylase (DBH) gene to chromosome 9q34. Cytogenet Cell Genet 1988; 48:48–50.

47. Wilson AF, Elston RC, Siervogel RM, et al. Linkage of a gene regulating dopamine-beta-hydroxylase activity and the ABO blood group locus. Am J Hum Genet 1988; 42:160–166.

48. Evinger MJ, Ernsberger P, Regunathan S, et al. A single transmitter regulates gene expression through two separate mechanisms: cholinergic regulation of phenylethanolamine N-methyltransferase mRNA via nicotinic and muscarinic pathways. J Neurosci 1994; 14:2106–2116.

49. Wong DL, Hayashi RJ, Ciaranello RD. Regulation of biogenic amine meth-
yltransferases by glucocorticoids via S-adenosylmethionine and its metabolizing enzymes, methionine adenosyltransferase and S-adenosylhomocysteine hydrolase. Brain Res 1985; 330:209–216.

50. Kaneda N, Ichinose H, Kobayashi K, et al. Molecular cloning of cDNA and chromosomal assignment of the gene for human phenylethanolamine N-methyltransferase, the enzyme for epinephrine biosynthesis. J Biol Chem 1988; 263:7672–7677.

51. Andersson KK, Cox DD, Que L Jr, et al. Resonance Raman studies on the blue-green–colored bovine adrenal tyrosine 3-monooxygenase (tyrosine hydroxylase): evidence that the feedback inhibitors adrenaline and noradrenaline are coordinated to iron. J Biol Chem 1988; 263:18621–18626.

52. Haavik J, Martinez A, Flatmark T. pH-Dependent release of catecholamines from tyrosine hydroxylase and the effect of phosphorylation of Ser-40. FEBS Lett 1990; 262:363–365.

53. Daubner SC, Lauriano C, Haycock JW, et al. Site-directed mutagenesis of serine 40 of rat tyrosine hydroxylase: effects of dopamine and cAMP-dependent phosphorylation on enzyme activity. J Biol Chem 1992; 267:12639–12646.

54. Stachowiak M, Stricker EM, Zigmond MJ, et al. A cholinergic antagonist blocks cold stress–induced alterations in rat adrenal tyrosine hydroxylase mRNA. Mol Brain Res 1988; 3:193–196.

55. Rittenhouse AR, Schwarzschild MA, Zigmond RE. Both synaptic and antidromic stimulation of neurons in the rat superior cervical ganglion acutely increase tyrosine hydroxylase activity. Neuroscience 1988; 25:207–215.

56. Chalazonitis A, Zigmond RE. Effects of synaptic and antidromic stimulation on tyrosine hydroxylase activity in the rat superior cervical ganglion. J Physiol (Lond) 1980; 300:525–538.

57. Goc A, Stachowiak MK. Bovine tyrosine hydroxylase gene-promoter regions involved in basal and angiotensin II–stimulated expression in nontransformed adrenal medullary cells. J Neurochem 1994; 62:834–843.

58. Hiremagalur B, Nankova B, Nitahara J, et al. Nicotine increases expression of tyrosine hydroxylase gene: involvement of protein kinase A–mediated pathway. J Biol Chem 1993; 268:23704–23711.

59. Miner LL, Pandalai SP, Weisberg EP, et al. Cold-induced alterations in the binding of adrenomedullary nuclear proteins to the promoter region of the tyrosine hydroxylase gene. J Neurosci Res 1992; 33:10–18.

60. Anastasiadis PZ, States JC, Kuhn DM, et al. Co-induction of tetrahydrobiopterin (BH4) levels and tyrosine hydroxylase activity in cultured PC12 cells. Adv Exp Med Biol 1993; 338:227–230.

61. Abou-Donia MM, Viveros OH. Tetrahydrobiopterin increases in adrenal medulla and cortex: a factor in the regulation of tyrosine hydroxylase. Proc Natl Acad Sci USA 1981; 78:2703–2706.

62. Winkler H, Fischer-Colbrie R. Common membrane proteins of chromaffin granules, endocrine and synaptic vesicles: properties, tissue distribution, membrane topography and regulation of synthesis. Neurochem Int 1990; 17:245–262.

63. Wurtman RJ, Axelrod J. Control of enzymatic synthesis of adrenaline in the adrenal medulla by adrenal cortical steroids. J Biol Chem 1966; 241:2301–2305.

64. Ceccatelli S, Dagerlind Å, Schalling M, et al. The glucocorticoid receptor in the adrenal gland is localized in the cytoplasm of adrenaline cells. Acta Physiol Scand 1989; 137:559–560.

65. Seidl K, Unsicker K. The determination of the adrenal medullary cell fate during embryogenesis. Dev Biol 1989; 136:481–490.

66. Ehrlich ME, Evinger MJ, Joh TH, et al. Do glucocorticoids induce adrenergic differentiation in adrenal cells of neural crest origin? Dev Brain Res 1989; 50:129–137.

67. Wong DL, Lesage A, White S, et al. Adrenergic expression in the rat adrenal gland: multiple developmental regulatory mechanisms. Dev Brain Res 1992; 67:229–236.

68. Jiang W, Uht R, Bohn MC. Regulation of phenylethanolamine N-methyltransferase (PNMT) mRNA in the rat adrenal medulla by corticosterone. Int J Dev Neurosci 1989; 7:513–520.

69. Wong DL, Lesage A, Siddall B, et al. Glucocorticoid regulation of phenylethanolamine N-methyltransferase in vivo. FASEB J 1992; 6:3310–3315.

70. Winkler H. The adrenal chromaffin granule: a model for large dense core vesicles of endocrine and nervous tissue. J Anat 1993; 183:237–252.

71. Thomas-Reetz AC, De Camilli P. A role for synaptic vesicles in non-neuronal cells: clues from pancreatic b cells and from chromaffin cells. FASEB J 1994; 8:209–216.

72. Winkler H, Sietzen M, Schober M. The life cycle of catecholamine-storing vesicles. Ann NY Acad Sci 1987; 493:3–19.

73. Winkler H, Westhead E. The molecular organization of adrenal chromaffin granules. Neuroscience 1980; 5:1803–1823.

74. Dillen L, Miserez B, Claeys M, et al. Posttranslational processing of proenkephalins and chromogranins/secretogranins. Neurochem Int 1993; 22:315–352.

75. Winkler H, Fischer-Colbrie R. The chromogranins A and B: the first 25 years and future perspectives. Neuroscience 1992; 49:497–528.

76. Eiden LE, Huttner WB, Mallet J, et al. A nomenclature proposal for the chromogranin/secretogranin proteins. Neuroscience 1987; 21:1019–1021.

77. Fischer-Colbrie R, Hagn C, Schober M. Chromogranins A, B, and C: widespread constituents of secretory vesicles. Ann NY Acad Sci 1987; 493:120–134.

78. Videen JS, Mezger MS, Chang Y-M, et al. Calcium and catecholamine interactions with adrenal chromogranins: comparison of driving forces in binding and aggregation. J Biol Chem 1992; 267:3066–3073.

79. Galindo E, Rill A, Bader M-F, et al. Chromostatin, a 20-amino acid peptide derived from chromogranin A, inhibits chromaffin cell secretion. Proc Natl Acad Sci USA 1991; 88:1426–1430.

80. Johnson RG Jr. Accumulation of biological amines into chromaffin granules: a model for hormone and neurotransmitter transport. Physiol Rev 1988; 68:232–307.

81. Liu Y, Peter D, Roghani A, et al. A cDNA that suppresses MPP+ toxicity encodes a vesicular amine transporter. Cell 1992; 70:539–551.

82. Erickson JD, Eiden LE, Hoffman BJ. Expression cloning of a reserpine-sensitive vesicular monoamine transporter. Proc Natl Acad Sci USA 1992; 89:10993–10997.

83. Schuldiner S, Shirvan A, Linial M. Vesicular neurotransmitter transporters: from bacteria to humans. Physiol Rev 1995; 75:369–392.

84. Nelson N, Lill H. Porters and neurotransmitter transporters. J Exp Biol 1994; 196:213–228.

85. Huyghe BG, Klinman JP. Activity of membranous dopamine β-monooxygenase with chromaffin granule ghosts: interaction with ascorbate. J Biol Chem 1991; 266:11544–11550.

86. Dhariwal KR, Black CDV, Levine M. Semidehydroascorbic acid as an intermediate in norepinephrine biosynthesis in chromaffin granules. J Biol Chem 1991; 266:12908–12914.

87. Burgoyne RD. Control of exocytosis in adrenal chromaffin cells. Biochim Biophys Acta 1991; 1071:174–202.

88. Wightman RM, Jankowski JA, Kennedy RT, et al. Temporally resolved catecholamine spikes correspond to single vesicle release from individual chromaffin cells. Proc Natl Acad Sci USA 1991; 88:10754–10758.

89. Chow RH, von Rüden L, Neher E. Delay in vesicle fusion revealed by electrochemical monitoring of single secretory events in adrenal chromaffin cells. Nature 1992; 356:60–63.

90. Burgoyne RD, Morgan A. Regulated exocytosis. Biochem J 1993; 293:305–316.

91. Schaefer T, Hodel A, Heuss C, et al. The docking protein of chromaffin granules. Ann NY Acad Sci 1994; 733:279–289.

92. Wakade TD, Blank MA, Malhotra RK, et al. The peptide VIP is a neurotransmitter in rat adrenal medulla: physiological role in controlling catecholamine secretion. J Physiol (Lond) 1991; 444:349–362.

93. Galindo E, Zwiller J, Bader M-F, et al. Chromostatin inhibits catecholamine secretion in adrenal chromaffin cells by activating a protein phosphatase. Proc Natl Acad Sci USA 1992; 89:7398–7402.

94. Hexum TD, Zheng J, Zhu J. Neuropeptide Y inhibition of nicotinic receptor–mediated chromaffin cell secretion. J Pharmacol Exp Ther 1994; 271:61–66.

95. Kumakura K, Karoum F, Guidotti A, et al. Modulation of nicotinic receptors by opiate receptor agonists in cultured adrenal chromaffin cells. Nature 1980; 283:489–492.

96. Livett BG, Marley PD, Wan DCC, et al. Peptide regulation of adrenal medullary function. J Neural Transm Suppl 1990; 29:77–89.

97. Lewis JW, Tordoff MG, Sherman JE, et al. Adrenal medullary enkephalin-like peptides may mediate opioid stress analgesia. Science 1982; 217:557–559.

98. Dora E, Hines K, Kunos G, et al. Significance of an opiate mechanism in the adjustment of cerebrocortical oxygen consumption and blood flow during hypercapnic stress. Brain Res 1992; 573:293–298.

99. Evéquoz D, Waeber B, Aubert J-F, et al. Neuropeptide Y prevents the blood pressure fall induced by endotoxin in conscious rats with adrenal medullectomy. Circ Res 1988; 62:25–30.

100. Schwarzenbrunner U, Schmidle T, Obendorf D, et al. Sympathetic axons and nerve terminals: the protein composition of small and large dense-core and of a third type of vesicles. Neuroscience 1990; 37:819–827.

101. De Camilli P, Jahn R. Pathways to regulated exocytosis in neurons. Annu Rev Physiol 1990; 52:625–645.

102. Jahn R, Südhof TC. Synaptic vesicle traffic: rush hour in the nerve terminal. J Neurochem 1993; 61:12–21.

103. Bauerfeind R, Ohashi M, Huttner WB. Biogenesis of secretory granules and synaptic vesicles: facts and hypotheses. Ann NY Acad Sci 1994; 733:233–244.

104. Régnier-Vigouroux A, Huttner WB. Biogenesis of small synaptic vesicles and synaptic-like microvesicles. Neurochem Res 1993; 18:59–64.

105. Bauerfeind R, Jelinek R, Hellwig A, et al. Neurosecretory vesicles can be hybrids of synaptic vesicles and secretory granules. Proc Natl Acad Sci USA 1995; 92:7342–7346.

106. Maycox PR, Hell JW, Jahn R. Amino acid neurotransmission: spotlight on synaptic vesicles. Trends Neurosci 1990; 13:83–87.

107. Greengard P, Valtorta F, Czernik AJ, et al. Synaptic vesicle phosphoproteins and regulation of synaptic function. Science 1993; 259:780–785.

108. Brock JA, Cunnane TC. Neurotransmitter release mechanisms at the sympathetic neuroeffector junction. Exp Physiol 1993; 78:591–614.

109. Kopin IJ, Breese GR, Krauss KR, et al. Selective release of newly synthesized norepinephrine from the cat spleen during sympathetic nerve stimulation. J Pharmacol Exp Ther 1968; 161:271–278.

110. Trendelenburg U. The TiPS Lecture: Functional aspects of the neuronal uptake of noradrenaline. Trends Pharmacol Sci 1991; 12:334–337.

111. Burnstock G. Mechanisms of interaction of peptide and nonpeptide vascular neurotransmitter systems. J Cardiovasc Pharmacol 1987; 10(Suppl 12):S74–S81.

112. Lundberg JM, Rudehill A, Sollevi A, et al. Co-release of neuropeptide Y and noradrenaline from pig spleen in vivo: importance of subcellular storage, nerve impulse frequency and pattern, feedback regulation and resupply by axonal transport. Neuroscience 1989; 28:475–486.

113. Kupfermann I. Functional studies of cotransmission. Physiol Rev 1991; 71:683–732.

114. Potter EK. Neuropeptide Y as an autonomic neurotransmitter. Pharmacol Ther 1988; 37:251–273.

115. Lundberg JM, Franco-Cereceda A, Lacroix J-S, et al. Neuropeptide Y and sympathetic neurotransmission. Ann NY Acad Sci 1990; 611:166–174.

116. Tatemoto K, Rökaeus Å, Jörnvall H, et al. Galanin—a novel biologically active peptide from porcine intestine. FEBS Lett 1983; 164:124–128.

117. Brown DR, Hildebrand KR, Parsons AM, et al. Effects of galanin on smooth muscle and mucosa of porcine jejunum. Peptides 1990; 11:497–500.

118. Dunning BE, Ahrén B, Veith RC, et al. Galanin: a novel pancreatic neuropeptide. Am J Physiol 1986; 251:E127–E133.

119. Dunning BE, Taborsky GJ Jr. Galanin release during pancreatic nerve stimulation is sufficient to influence islet function. Am J Physiol 1989; 256:E191–E198.

120. Ahrén B, Ar'Rajab A, Böttcher G, et al. Presence of galanin in human pancreatic nerves and inhibition of insulin secretion from isolated human islets. Cell Tissue Res 1991; 264:263–267.

121. Leibowitz SF. Specificity of hypothalamic peptides in the control of behavioral and physiological processes. Ann NY Acad Sci 1994; 739:12–35.

122. Cowen T, Haven AJ, Milner P, et al. Increase in neuropeptide Y, but not noradrenaline, in the superior cervical ganglion of rabbits chronically exposed to cold. J Auton Nerv Syst 1988; 24:175–178.

123. Schalling M, Franco-Cereceda A, Hemsén A, et al. Neuropeptide Y and catecholamine synthesizing enzymes and their mRNAs in rat sympathetic neurons and adrenal glands: studies on expression, synthesis and axonal transport after pharmacological and experimental manipulations using hybridization techniques and radioimmunoassay. Neuroscience 1991; 41:753–766.

124. Henion PD, Landis SC. Modulation of the enkephalinergic phenotype of rat sympathetic neurons by hormonal and transsynaptic mechanisms. J Neurobiol 1993; 24:1243–1251.

125. Vanhoutte PM, Verbeuren TJ, Webb RC. Local modulation of adrenergic neuroeffector interaction in the blood vessel well. Physiol Rev 1981; 61:151–247.

126. Langer SZ, Arbilla S. Presynaptic receptors on peripheral noradrenergic neurons. Ann NY Acad Sci 1990; 604:7–16.

127. Göthert M, Molderings GJ, Fink K, et al. α₂-Adrenoceptor-independent inhibition by imidazolines and guanidines of noradrenaline release from peripheral, but not central noradrenergic neurons. Ann NY Acad Sci 1995; 763:405–419.

128. Nedergaard OA, Abrahamsen J. Modulation of noradrenaline release by activation of presynaptic β-adrenoceptors in the cardiovascular system. Ann NY Acad Sci 1990; 604:528–544.

129. Westfall TC. The physiological operation of presynaptic inhibitory autoreceptors. Ann NY Acad Sci 1990; 604:398–413.

130. Kalsner S. The problem with autoreceptors. Ann NY Acad Sci 1990; 604:414–438.

131. Stjärne L, Msghina M, Stjärne E. "Upstream" regulation of the release probability in sympathetic nerve varicosities. Neuroscience 1990; 36:571–587.

132. Westfall TC. Local regulation of adrenergic neurotransmission. Physiol Rev 1977; 57:659–728.

133. Greenberg SS, Diecke FPJ, Curro FA, et al. Presynaptic modulation of sympathetic neurotransmitter release by modulators of cyclic 3′,5′-guanosine monophosphate in canine vascular smooth muscle. Ann NY Acad Sci 1990; 604:305–322.

134. Malik KU, Sehic E. Prostaglandins and the release of the adrenergic neurotransmitter. Ann NY Acad Sci 1990; 604:222–236.

135. Schwieler JH, Kahan T, Nussberger J, et al. Participation of prostaglandins and bradykinin in the effects of angiotensin II and converting enzyme inhibition on sympathetic neurotransmission in vivo. Acta Physiol Scand 1994; 152:83–91.

136. Hurst SM, Collins SM. Mechanism underlying tumor necrosis factor-α suppression of norepinephrine release from rat myenteric plexus. Am J Physiol 1994; 266:G1123–G1129.

137. Cohen RA. Adenine nucleotides and 5-hydroxytryptamine released by aggregating platelets inhibit adrenergic neurotransmission in canine coronary artery. J Clin Invest 1986; 77:369–375.

138. Fuder H, Muth U. ATP and endogenous agonists inhibit evoked [³H]-noradrenaline release in rat iris via A₁ and P₂ₓ-like purinoceptors. Naunyn Schmiedebergs Arch Pharmacol 1993; 348:352–357.

139. Cohen RA. Platelet 5-hydroxytryptamine and vascular adrenergic nerves. News Physiol Sci 1988; 3:185–189.

140. Stjärne L, Msghina M, Stjärne E. Is cyclic AMP the intra-axonal messenger "X" mediating "upstream" control of sympathetic transmitter secretion? Acta Physiol Scand 1989; 136:617–618.

141. Bell C. Peripheral dopaminergic nerves. Pharmacol Ther 1989; 44:157–179.

142. Ordonez LA, Arbrus M, Boyson S, et al. Skeletal muscle: reservoir for exogenous L-dopa. J Pharmacol Exp Ther 1974; 190:187–191.

143. Eldrup E, Richter EA, Christensen NJ. DOPA, norepinephrine, and dopamine in rat tissues: no effect of sympathectomy on muscle DOPA. Am J Physiol 1989; 256:E284–E287.

144. Landsberg L. L-3,4-dihydroxyphenylalanine-induced release of norepinephrine from rat heart. Biochem Pharmacol 1971; 20:3542–3547.
145. Eisenhofer G, Brush JE, Cannon RO III, et al. Plasma dihydroxyphenylalanine and total body and regional noradrenergic activity in humans. J Clin Endocrinol Metab 1989; 68:247–255.
146. Goldstein DS, Udelsman R, Eisenhofer G, et al. Neuronal source of plasma dihydroxyphenylalanine. J Clin Endocrinol Metab 1987; 64:856–861.
147. Peleg D, Munsick RA, Diker D, et al. Distribution of catecholamines between fetal and maternal compartments during human pregnancy with emphasis on L-dopa and dopamine. J Clin Endocrinol Metab 1986; 62:911–914.
148. Ness JC, Morse DE. Regulation of galactokinase gene expression in Tetrahymena thermophila. II: Identification of 3,4-dihydroxyphenylalanine as a primary effector of adrenergic control of galactokinase expression. J Biol Chem 1985; 260:10013–10018.
149. Slominski A, Paus R. Towards defining receptors for L-tyrosine and L-DOPA. Mol Cell Endocrinol 1994; 99:C7–C11.
150. Pacholczyk T, Blakely RD, Amara SG. Expression cloning of a cocaine- and antidepressant-sensitive human noradrenaline transporter. Nature 1991; 350:350–354.
151. Brüss M, Kunz J, Lingen B, et al. Chromosomal mapping of the human gene for the tricyclic antidepressant–sensitive noradrenaline transporter. Hum Genet 1993; 91:278–280.
152. Amara SG, Kuhar MJ. Neurotransmitter transporters: recent progress. Annu Rev Neurosci 1993; 16:73–93.
153. Trendelenburg U. The extraneuronal uptake and metabolism of catecholamines. In: Trendelenburg U, Weiner N, eds. Handbook of Experimental Pharmacology. Vol 90/I: Catecholamines. Berlin: Springer-Verlag, 1988: 279–319.
154. Schömig E, Schönfeld C-L. Extraneuronal noradrenaline transport (uptake2) in a human cell line (Caki-1 cells). Naunyn Schmiedebergs Arch Pharmacol 1990; 341:404–410.
155. Youdim MBH, Finberg JPM, Tipton KF. Monamine oxidase. In: Trendelenburg U, Weiner N, eds. Handbook of Experimental Pharmacology, Vol 90/I: Catecholamines. Berlin: Springer-Verlag, 1988: 119–192.
156. Sager G, Bratlid H, Little C. Binding of catecholamines to alpha-1 acid glycoprotein, albumin and lipoproteins in human serum. Biochem Pharmacol 1987; 36:3607–3612.
157. Brown MJ, Allison DJ, Jenner DA, et al. Increased sensitivity and accuracy of phaeochromocytoma diagnosis achieved by use of plasma-adrenaline estimations and a pentolinium-suppression test. Lancet 1981; 1:174–177.
158. Silverberg AB, Shah SD, Haymond MW, et al. Norepinephrine: hormone and neurotransmitter in man. Am J Physiol 1978; 234:E252–E256.
159. Esler M, Jackman G, Bobik A, et al. Determination of norepinephrine apparent release rate and clearance in humans. Life Sci 1979; 25:1461–1470.
160. Cryer PE, Santiago JV, Shah S. Measurement of norepinephrine and epinephrine in small volumes of human plasma by a single isotope derivative method: response to the upright posture. J Clin Endocrinol Metab 1974; 39:1025–1029.
161. Lake CR, Ziegler MG, Kopin IJ. Use of plasma norepinephrine for evaluation of sympathetic neuronal function in man. Life Sci 1976; 18:1315–1325.
162. Martignoni E, Blandini F, Melzi d'Eril GV, et al. The influence of gender in the evaluation of platelet and plasma catecholamines. Life Sci 1993; 52:1995–2004.
163. Dimsdale JE, Ziegler M, Mills P, et al. Effects of salt, race, and hypertension on reactivity to stressors. Hypertension 1990; 16:573–580.
164. Ziegler MG, Mills PJ, Dimsdale J. The effects of race on norepinephrine clearance. Life Sci 1991; 49:427–433.
165. Cameron OG, Curtis GC, Zelnik T, et al. Circadian fluctuation of plasma epinephrine in supine humans. Psychoneuroendocrinology 1987; 12:41–51.
166. Esler M, Lambert G, Jennings G. The influence of aging on catecholamine metabolism. In: Amery A, Staessen J, eds. Handbook of Hypertension. Vol 12: Hypertension in the Elderly. Amsterdam: Elsevier Science, 1989: 85–98.
167. Williams PD, Puddey IB, Beilin LJ, et al. Genetic influences on plasma catecholamines in human twins. J Clin Endocrinol Metab 1993; 77:794–799.
168. Mills PJ, Dimsdale JE, Ziegler MG, et al. Racial differences in epinephrine and β2-adrenergic receptors. Hypertension 1995; 25:88–91.
169. Linsell CR, Lightman SL, Mullen PE, et al. Circadian rhythms of epinephrine and norepinephrine in man. J Clin Endocrinol Metab 1985; 60:1210–1215.
170. Esler M, Jennings G, Lambert G, et al. Overflow of catecholamine neurotransmitters to the circulation: source, fate, and functions. Physiol Rev 1990; 70:963–985.
171. Vallbo ÅB, Hagbarth K-E, Torebjörk HE, et al. Somatosensory, proprioceptive, and sympathetic activity in human peripheral nerves. Physiol Rev 1979; 59:919–957.
172. Pomeranz B, Macaulay RJB, Caudill MA, et al. Assessment of autonomic function in humans by heart rate spectral analysis. Am J Physiol 1985; 248:H151–H153.
173. Malliani A, Pagani M, Lombardi F, et al. Cardiovascular neural regulation explored in the frequency domain. Circulation 1991; 84:482–492.
174. Kingwell BA, Thompson JM, Kaye DM, et al. Heart rate spectral analysis, cardiac norepinephrine spillover, and muscle sympathetic nerve activity during human sympathetic nervous activation and failure. Circulation 1994; 90:234–240.
175. Kopin IJ. Plasma levels of catecholamines and dopamine-β-hydroxylase. In: Trendelenburg U, Weiner N, eds. Handbook of Experimental Pharmacology, Vol 90/II: Catecholamines. Berlin: Springer-Verlag, 1989: 211–275.
176. Cryer PE, Wortsman J, Shah SD, et al. Plasma chromogranin A as a marker of sympathochromaffin activity in humans. Am J Physiol 1991; 260:E243–E246.
177. Ahlquist RP. A study of the adrenotropic receptors. Am J Physiol 1948; 153:586–600.
178. Lands AM, Arnold A, McAuliff JP, et al. Differentiation of receptor systems activated by sympathomimetic amines. Nature 1967; 214:597–598.
179. Langer SZ. Presynaptic regulation of catecholamine release. Biochem Pharmacol 1974; 23:1793–1800.
180. Emorine LJ, Marullo S, Briend-Sutren M-M, et al. Molecular characterization of the human β3-adrenergic receptor. Science 1989; 245:1118–1121.
181. Bylund DB, Eikenberg DC, Hieble JP, et al. International Union of Pharmacology nomenclature of adrenoceptors. Pharmacol Rev 1994; 46:121–136.
182. Hieble JP, Bylund DB, Clarke DE, et al. International Union of Pharmacology. X. Recommendation for nomenclature of α1-adrenoceptors: consensus update. Pharmacol Rev 1995; 47:267–270.
183. Dohlman HG, Thorner J, Caron MG, et al. Model systems for the study of seven-transmembrane-segment receptors. Annu Rev Biochem 1991; 60:653–688.
184. Strader CD, Fong TM, Tota MR, et al. Structure and function of G protein–coupled receptors. Annu Rev Biochem 1994; 63:101–132.
185. Ostrowski J, Kjelsberg MA, Caron MG, et al. Mutagenesis of the β2-adrenergic receptor: how structure elucidates function. Annu Rev Pharmacol Toxicol 1992; 32:167–183.
186. Kobilka BK, Kobilka TS, Daniel K, et al. Chimeric α2-,β2-adrenergic receptors: delineation of domains involved in effector coupling and ligand binding specificity. Science 1988; 240:1310–1316.
187. Lefkowitz RJ, Caron MG. Adrenergic receptors: Models for the study of receptors coupled to guanine nucleotide regulatory proteins. J Biol Chem 1988; 263:4993–4996.
188. Minneman KP. α1-Adrenergic receptor subtypes, inositol phosphates, and sources of cell Ca2+. Pharmacol Rev 1988; 40:87–119.
189. Hieble JP, Ruffolo RR Jr. Possible structural and functional relationships between imidazoline receptors and α2-adrenoceptors. Ann NY Acad Sci 1995; 763:8–21.
190. Wu D, Katz A, Lee C-H, et al. Activation of phospholipase C by α1-adrenergic receptors is mediated by the a subunits of Gq family. J Biol Chem 1992; 267:25798–25802.
191. Ruffolo RR Jr, Hieble JP. α-Adrenoceptors. Pharmacol Ther 1994; 61:1–64.
192. Milligan G, Svoboda P, Brown CM. Why are there so many adrenoceptor subtypes? Biochem Pharmacol 1994; 48:1059–1071.
193. Lipscombe D, Kongsamut S, Tsien RW. α-Adrenergic inhibition of sympathetic neurotransmitter release mediated by modulation of N-type calcium-channel gating. Nature 1989; 340:639–642.
194. Caron MG, Lefkowitz RJ. Catecholamine receptors: structure, function, and regulation. Recent Prog Horm Res 1993; 48:277–290.
195. Giacobino J-P. β3-Adrenoceptor: an update. Eur J Endocrinol 1995; 132:377–385.
196. Strosberg AD. Structural and functional diversity of β-adrenergic receptors. Ann NY Acad Sci 1995; 757:253–260.
197. Krief S, Lönnqvist F, Raimbault S, et al. Tissue distribution of β3-adrenergic receptor mRNA in man. J Clin Invest 1993; 91:344–349.
198. Pietri-Rouxel F, Strosberg AD. Pharmacological characteristics and species-related variations of β3-adrenergic receptors. Fundam Clin Pharmacol 1995; 9:211–218.
199. Cavusoglu E, Frishman WH. Sotalol: a new β-adrenergic blocker for ventricular arrhythmias. Prog Cardiovasc Dis 1995; 37:423–440.
200. Waller DG. β-Adrenoceptor partial agonists: a renaissance in cardiovascular therapy? Br J Clin Pharmacol 1990; 30:157–171.
201. Frishman WH. Clinical significance of beta1-selectivity and intrinsic sympathomimetic activity in a beta-adrenergic blocking drug. Am J Cardiol 1987; 59:33F–37F.
202. Haenni A, Lithell H. Treatment with a β-blocker with β2-agonism improves glucose and lipid metabolism in essential hypertension. Metabolism 1994; 43:455–461.
203. Yang YT, McElligott MA. Multiple actions of β-adrenergic agonists on skeletal muscle and adipose tissue. Biochem J 1989; 261:1–10.
204. Cawthorne MA, Sennitt MV, Arch JRS, et al. BRL 35135, a potent and selective atypical β-adrenoceptor agonist. Am J Clin Nutr 1992; 55:252S–257S.
205. Gasic S, Green A. Gi down-regulation and heterologous desensitization in adipocytes after treatment with the α2-agonist UK 14304. Biochem Pharmacol 1995; 49:785–790.
206. Hu Z, Azhar S, Hoffman BB. Prolonged activation of α1 adrenoceptors induces down-regulation of protein kinase C in vascular smooth muscle. J Cardiovasc Pharmacol 1992; 20:982–989.
207. Hausdorff WP, Caron MG, Lefkowitz RJ. Turning off the signal: desensitization of β-adrenergic receptor function. FASEB J 1990; 4:2881–2889.
208. Eason MG, Moreira SP, Liggett SB. Four consecutive serines in the third intracellular loop are the sites for β-adrenergic receptor kinase-mediated phosphorylation and desensitization of the α2A-adrenergic receptor. J Biol Chem 1995; 270:4681–4688.

209. Premont RT, Inglese J, Lefkowitz RJ. Protein kinases that phosphorylate activated G protein-coupled receptors. FASEB J 1995; 9:175–182.

210. Lohse MJ. Molecular mechanisms of membrane receptor desensitization. Biochim Biophys Acta 1993; 1179:171–188.

211. Collins S, Lohse MJ, O'Dowd B, et al. Structure and regulation of G protein–coupled receptors: the β_2-adrenergic receptor as a model. Vitam Horm 1991; 46:1–39.

212. Port JD, Hadcock JR, Malbon CC. Cross-regulation between G-protein–mediated pathways: acute activation of the inhibitory pathway of adenylyl-cyclase reduces β_2-adrenergic receptor phosphorylation and increases β-adrenergic responsiveness. J Biol Chem 1992; 267:8468–8472.

213. Eason MG, Liggett SB. Subtype-selective desensitization of α_2-adrenergic receptors: different mechanisms control short and long term agonist-promoted desensitization of α_2C10, α_2C4, and α_2C2. J Biol Chem 1992; 267:25473–25479.

214. Hadcock JR, Malbon CC. Agonist regulation of gene expression of adrenergic receptors and G proteins. J Neurochem 1993; 60:1–9.

215. Izzo NJ Jr, Seidman CE, Collins S, et al. α_1-Adrenergic receptor mRNA level is regulated by norepinephrine in rabbit aortic smooth muscle cells. Proc Natl Acad Sci USA 1990; 87:6268–6271.

216. Hough C, Chuang D-M. Differential down-regulation of β_1- and β_2-adrenergic receptor mRNA in C_6 glioma cells. Biochem Biophys Res Commun 1990; 170:46–52.

217. Tholanikunnel BG, Granneman JG, Malbon CC. The M_r 35,000 β-adrenergic receptor mRNA-binding protein binds transcripts of G-protein–linked receptors which undergo agonist-induced destabilization. J Biol Chem 1995; 270:12787–12793.

218. Izzo NJ Jr, Tulenko TN, Colucci WS. Phorbol esters and norepinephrine destabilize α_{1B}-adrenergic receptor mRNA in vascular smooth muscle cells. J Biol Chem 1994; 269:1705–1710.

219. Collins S, Caron MG, Lefkowitz RJ. β_2-Adrenergic receptors in hamster smooth muscle cells are transcriptionally regulated by glucocorticoids. J Biol Chem 1988; 263:9067–9070.

220. Fève B, Emorine LJ, Briend-Sutren M-M, et al. Differential regulation of β_1- and β_2-adrenergic receptor protein and mRNA levels by glucocorticoids during 3T3-F442A adipose differentiation. J Biol Chem 1990; 265:16343–16349.

221. Norris JS, Brown P, Cohen J, et al. Glucocorticoid induction of β-adrenergic receptors in the DDT1 MF-2 smooth muscle cell line involves synthesis of new receptor. Mol Cell Biochem 1987; 74:21–27.

222. Hadcock JR, Wang H-Y, Malbon CC. Agonist-induced destabilization of β-adrenergic receptor mRNA: attenuation of glucocorticoid-induced up-regulation of β-adrenergic receptors. J Biol Chem 1989; 264:19928–19933.

223. Ruffolo RR Jr. Spare α adrenoceptors in the peripheral circulation: excitation-contraction coupling. Fed Proc 1986; 45:2341–2346.

224. Gingrich JA, Caron MG. Recent advances in the molecular biology of dopamine receptors. Annu Rev Neurosci 1993; 16:299–321.

225. Willems JL, Buylaert WA, Lefebvre RA, et al. Neuronal dopamine receptors on autonomic ganglia and sympathetic nerves and dopamine receptors in the gastrointestinal system. Pharmacol Rev 1985; 37:165–216.

226. Kohli JD, McNay JL, Rajfer SI, et al. Peripheral dopamine receptors in cardiovascular therapy: the legacy of Leon Goldberg (1927–1989). Hypertension 1991; 17:700–706.

227. Jose PA, Raymond JR, Bates MD, et al. The renal dopamine receptors. J Am Soc Nephrol 1992; 2:1265–1278.

228. Meister B, Aperia A. Molecular mechanisms involved in catecholamine regulation of sodium transport. Semin Nephrol 1993; 13:41–49.

229. Walters JR, Bergstrom DA, Carlson JH, et al. D_1 dopamine receptor activation required for postsynaptic expression of D_2 agonist effects. Science 1987; 236:719–722.

230. Bertorello A, Aperia A. Inhibition of proximal tubule Na^+-K^+-ATPase activity requires simultaneous activation of DA_1 and DA_2 receptors. Am J Physiol 1990; 259:F924–F928.

231. Spyer KM. The central nervous organization of reflex circulatory control. In: Loewy AD, Spyer KM, eds. Central Regulation of Autonomic Functions. New York: Oxford University Press, 1990: 168–188.

232. Guo X, Wakade AR. Differential secretion of catecholamines in response to peptidergic and cholinergic transmitters in rat adrenals. J Physiol (Lond) 1994; 475:539–545.

233. Young JB, Rosa RM, Landsberg L. Dissociation of sympathetic nervous system and adrenal medullary responses. Am J Physiol 1984; 247:E35–E40.

234. Victor RG, Thorén P, Morgan DA, et al. Differential control of adrenal and renal sympathetic nerve activity during hemorrhagic hypotension in rats. Circ Res 1989; 64:686–694.

235. Ping P, Faber JE. Characterization of α-adrenoceptor gene expression in arterial and venous smooth muscle. Am J Physiol 1993; 265:H1501–H1509.

236. Morris JL, Gibbins IL, Kadowitz PJ, et al. Roles of peptides and other substances in cotransmission from vascular autonomic and sensory neurons. Can J Physiol Pharmacol 1995; 73:521–532.

237. Russell MP, Moran NC. Evidence for lack of innervation of β-2 adrenoceptors in the blood vessels of the gracilis muscle of the dog. Circ Res 1980; 46:344–352.

238. Vanhoutte PM, Miller VM. Alpha$_2$-adrenoceptors and endothelium-derived relaxing factor. Am J Med 1989; 87(Suppl 3C):1S–5S.

239. Ghaleh B, Béa M-L, Dubois-Randé J-L, et al. Endothelial modulation of β-adrenergic dilation of large coronary arteries in conscious dogs. Circulation 1995; 92:2627–2635.

240. Quyyumi AA, Dakak N, Andrews NP, et al. Nitric oxide activity in the human coronary circulation: impact of risk factors for coronary atherosclerosis. J Clin Invest 1995; 95:1747–1755.

241. Lundberg J, Norgren L, Ribbe E, et al. Direct evidence of active sympathetic vasodilatation in the skin of the human foot. J Physiol (Lond) 1989; 417:437–446.

242. Freedman RR, Sabharwal SC, Moten M, et al. Local temperature modulates α_1- and α_2-adrenergic vasoconstriction in men. Am J Physiol 1992; 263:H1197–H1200.

243. Baker CH, Sutton ET, Price JM, et al. Attenuation of arteriolar α_2-adrenoceptor sensitivity during endotoxemia. Am J Physiol 1994; 267:H2171–H2178.

244. Tateishi J, Faber JE. Inhibition of arteriole α_2- but not α_1-adrenoceptor constriction by acidosis and hypoxia in vitro. Am J Physiol 1995; 268:H2068–H2076.

245. Bülbring E, Tomita T. Catecholamine action on smooth muscle. Pharmacol Rev 1987; 39:49–96.

246. de Boer REP, Brouwer F, Zaagsma J. The β-adrenoceptors mediating relaxation of rat oesophageal muscularis mucosae are predominantly of the β_3-, but also of the β_2-subtype. Br J Pharmacol 1993; 110:442–446.

247. MacDonald A, Forbes IJ, Gallagher D, et al. Adrenoceptors mediating relaxation to catecholamines in rat isolated jejunum. Br J Pharmacol 1994; 112:576–578.

248. Tamaoki J, Yamauchi F, Chiyotani A, et al. Atypical β-adrenoceptor- (β_3-adrenoceptor) mediated relaxation of canine isolated bronchial smooth muscle. J Appl Physiol: Respirat Environ Exercise Physiol 1993; 74:297–302.

249. Boeckxstaens GE, De Man JG, Pelckmans PA, et al. α_2-Adrenoceptor-mediated modulation of the nitrergic innervation of the canine isolated ileocolonic junction. Br J Pharmacol 1993; 109:1079–1084.

250. Barnes PJ. β-Adrenoceptors on smooth muscle, nerves and inflammatory cells. Life Sci 1993; 52:2101–2109.

251. Barnes PJ. Beta-adrenergic receptors and their regulation. Am J Respir Crit Care Med 1995; 152:838–860.

252. Turki J, Pak J, Green SA, et al. Genetic polymorphisms of the β_2-adrenergic receptor in nocturnal and nonnocturnal asthma: evidence that Gly16 correlates with the nocturnal phenotype. J Clin Invest 1995; 95:1635–1641.

253. Lepor H, Gup DI, Baumann M, et al. Comparison of alpha$_1$ adrenoceptors in the prostate capsule of men with symptomatic and asymptomatic benign prostatic hyperplasia. Br J Urol 1991; 67:493–498.

254. Hubel KA. Intestinal nerves and ion transport: stimuli, reflexes, and responses. Am J Physiol 1985; 248:G261–G271.

255. DiBona GF. Role of renal nerves in hypertension. Semin Nephrol 1991; 11:503–511.

256. Barry MK, Maher MM, Gontarek JD, et al. Luminal dopamine modulates canine ileal water and electrolyte transport. Dig Dis Sci 1995; 40:1738–1743.

257. Finkel Y, Eklöf AC, Granquist L, et al. Endogenous dopamine modulates jejunal sodium absorption during high-salt diet in young but not in adult rats. Gastroenterology 1994; 107:675–679.

258. Himms-Hagen J. Effects of catecholamines on metabolism. In: Blaschko H, Muscholl E, eds. Handbook of Experimental Pharmacology, Vol 33: Catecholamines. Berlin: Springer-Verlag, 1972: 363–462.

259. Tutton PJM, Barkla DH. Biogenic amines as regulators of the proliferative activity of normal and neoplastic intestinal epithelial cells (review). Anticancer Res 1987; 7:1–12.

260. Brown JE, Adamson JW. Modulation of in vitro erythropoiesis: the influence of β-adrenergic agonists on erythroid colony formation. J Clin Invest 1977; 60:70–77.

261. Bell C. Autonomic nervous control of reproduction: circulatory and other factors. Pharmacol Rev 1972; 24:657–736.

262. Terzic A, Pucéat M, Vassort G, et al. Cardiac α_1-adrenoceptors: an overview. Pharmacol Rev 1993; 45:147–175.

263. Kim YS, Sainz RD. β-Adrenergic agonists and hypertrophy of skeletal muscles. Life Sci 1992; 50:397–407.

264. Lee RMKW, Owens GK, Scott-Burden T, et al. Pathophysiology of smooth muscle in hypertension. Can J Physiol Pharmacol 1995; 73:574–584.

265. Géloën A, Collet AJ, Bukowiecki LJ. Role of sympathetic innervation in brown adipocyte proliferation. Am J Physiol 1992; 263:R1176–R1181.

266. McVary KT, Razzaq A, Lee C, et al. Growth of the rat prostate gland is facilitated by the autonomic nervous system. Biol Reprod 1994; 51:99–107.

267. Lauder JM. Neurotransmitters as growth regulatory signals: role of receptors and second messengers. Trends Neurosci 1993; 16:233–240.

268. Brenner GJ, Felten SY, Felten DL, et al. Sympathetic nervous system modulation of tumor metastases and host defense mechanisms. J Neuroimmunol 1992; 37:191–201.

269. Kjeldsen SE, Weder AB, Egan B, et al. Effect of circulating epinephrine on platelet function and hematocrit. Hypertension 1995; 25:1096–1105.

270. Larsson PT, Wallén NH, Martinsson A, et al. Significance of platelet β-adrenoceptors for platelet responses in vivo and in vitro. Thromb Haemost 1992; 68:687–693.

271. Larsson PT, Wiman B, Olsson G, et al. Influence of metoprolol treatment on sympatho-adrenal activation of fibrinolysis. Thromb Haemost 1990; 63:482–487.

272. Roy AK, Sarkar J, Bhadra R, et al. Effect of amines on fibrinogen synthesis. Arch Biochem Biophys 1985; 239:364–367.

273. Sanders VM, Munson AE. Norepinephrine and the antibody response. Pharmacol Rev 1985; 37:229–248.

274. Madden KS, Sanders VM, Felten DL. Catecholamine influences and sympathetic neural modulation of immune responsiveness. Annu Rev Pharmacol Toxicol 1995; 35:417–448.

275. Katz MS, Dax EM, Gregerman RI. Beta adrenergic regulation of rat liver glycogenolysis during aging. Exp Gerontol 1993; 28:329–340.

276. Exton JH. Role of phosphoinositides in the regulation of liver function. Hepatology 1988; 8:152–166.

277. Rosen SG, Clutter WE, Shah SD, et al. Direct α-adrenergic stimulation of hepatic glucose production in human subjects. Am J Physiol 1983; 245:E616–E626.

278. Richardson PDI, Withrington PG. Physiological regulation of the hepatic circulation. Annu Rev Physiol 1982; 44:57–69.

279. Gardemann A, Püschel GP, Jungermann K. Nervous control of liver metabolism and hemodynamics. Eur J Biochem 1992; 207:399–411.

280. Kowalyk S, Veith R, Boyle M, et al. Liver releases galanin during sympathetic nerve stimulation. Am J Physiol 1992; 262:E671–E678.

281. Taborsky GJ Jr, Beltramini LM, Brown M, et al. Canine liver releases neuropeptide Y during sympathetic nerve stimulation. Am J Physiol 1994; 266:E804–E812.

282. Ahlborg G, Lundberg JM. Inhibitory effects of neuropeptide Y on splanchnic glycogenolysis and renin release in humans. Clin Physiol 1994; 14:187–196.

283. Lafontan M, Berlan M. Fat cell adrenergic receptors and the control of white and brown fat cell function. J Lipid Res 1993; 34:1057–1091.

284. Lafontan M, Berlan M. Fat cell α₂-adrenoceptors: the regulation of fat cell function and lipolysis. Endocr Rev 1995; 16:716–738.

285. Castan I, Valet P, Quideau N, et al. Antilipolytic effects of α₂-adrenergic agonists, neuropeptide Y, adenosine, and PGE₁ in mammal adipocytes. Am J Physiol 1994; 266:R1141–R1147.

286. Cousin B, Casteilla L, Lafontan M, et al. Local sympathetic denervation of white adipose tissue in rats induces preadipocyte proliferation without noticeable changes in metabolism. Endocrinology 1993; 133:2255–2262.

287. Jones DD, Ramsay TG, Hausman GJ, et al. Norepinephrine inhibits rat pre-adipocyte proliferation. Int J Obes 1992; 16:349–354.

288. Coppack SW, Jensen MD, Miles JM. In vivo regulation of lipolysis in humans. J Lipid Res 1994; 35:177–193.

289. Clark MG, Colquhoun EQ, Rattigan S, et al. Vascular and endocrine control of muscle metabolism. Am J Physiol 1995; 268:E797–E812.

290. Oscai LB, Gorski J, Miller WC, et al. Role of the alkaline TG lipase in regulating intramuscular TG content. Med Sci Sports Exerc 1988; 20:539–544.

291. Garber AJ, Karl IE, Kipnis DM. Alanine and glutamine synthesis and release from skeletal muscle. IV: B-adrenergic inhibition of amino acid release. J Biol Chem 1976; 251:851–857.

292. Kraenzlin ME, Keller U, Keller A, et al. Elevation of plasma epinephrine concentrations inhibits proteolysis and leucine oxidation in man via β-adrenergic mechanisms. J Clin Invest 1989; 84:388–393.

293. Fryburg DA, Gelfand RA, Jahn LA, et al. Effects of epinephrine on human muscle glucose and protein metabolism. Am J Physiol 1995; 268:E55–E59.

294. Uemura K, Young JB. Effects of fat feeding on epinephrine secretion in the rat. Am J Physiol 1994; 267:R1329–R1335.

295. Costelli P, García-Martínez C, Llovera M, et al. Muscle protein waste in tumor-bearing rats is effectively antagonized by a β₂-adrenergic agonist (clenbuterol): role of the ATP-ubiquitin–dependent proteolytic pathway. J Clin Invest 1995; 95:2367–2372.

296. Straumann E, Keller U, Kraenzlin M, et al. Interaction of cortisol and epinephrine in the regulation of leucine kinetics in man. Experientia 1988; 44:176–178.

297. Wirthensohn G, Guder WG. Renal substrate metabolism. Physiol Rev 1986; 66:469–497.

298. McGuinness OP, Fugiwara T, Murrell S, et al. Impact of chronic stress hormone infusion on hepatic carbohydrate metabolism in the conscious dog. Am J Physiol 1993; 265:E314–E322.

299. Stumvoll M, Chintalapudi U, Perriello G, et al. Uptake and release of glucose by the human kidney: postabsorptive rates and responses to epinephrine. J Clin Invest 1995; 96:2528–2533.

300. Deibert DC, DeFronzo RA. Epinephrine-induced insulin resistance in man. J Clin Invest 1980; 65:717–721.

301. Rizza RA, Cryer PE, Haymond MW, et al. Adrenergic mechanisms for the effects of epinephrine on glucose production and clearance in man. J Clin Invest 1980; 65:682–689.

302. Joost HG, Weber TM, Cushman SW, et al. Insulin-stimulated glucose transport in rat adipose cells: modulation of transporter intrinsic activity by isoproterenol and adenosine. J Biol Chem 1987; 261:10033–10036.

303. Challiss RAJ, Lozeman FJ, Leighton B, et al. Effects of the β-adrenoceptor agonist isoprenaline on insulin-sensitivity in soleus muscle of the rat. Biochem J 1986; 233:377–381.

304. Shirakura S, Furugohri T, Tokumitsu Y. Activation of glucose transport by activatory receptor agonists of adenylate cyclase in rat adipocytes. Comp Biochem Physiol A Physiol 1990; 97:81–86.

305. Marette A, Bukowiecki LJ. Stimulation of glucose transport by insulin and norepinephrine in isolated rat brown adipocytes. Am J Physiol 1989; 257:C714–C721.

306. Rattigan S, Appleby GJ, Clark MG. Insulin-like action of catecholamines and Ca²⁺ to stimulate glucose transport and GLUT4 translocation in perfused rat heart. Biochim Biophys Acta 1991; 1094:217–223.

307. Young DA, Wallberg-Henriksson H, Cranshaw J, et al. Effect of catecholamines on glucose uptake and glycogenolysis in rat skeletal muscle. Am J Physiol 1985; 248:C406–C409.

308. van Putten JPM, Krans HMJ. Long-term regulation of hexose uptake by isoproterenol in cultured 3T3 adipocytes. Am J Physiol 1985; 248:E706–E711.

309. Scheidegger K, Robbins DC, Danforth E Jr. Effects of chronic beta receptor stimulation on glucose metabolism. Diabetes 1984; 33:1144–1149.

310. Budohoski L, Challiss RAJ, Dubaniewicz A, et al. Effects of prolonged elevation of plasma adrenaline concentration in vivo on insulin-sensitivity in soleus muscle of the rat. Biochem J 1987; 244:655–660.

311. Widén E, Lehto M, Kanninen T, et al. Association of a polymorphism in the β₃-adrenergic-receptor gene with features of the insulin resistance syndrome in Finns. N Engl J Med 1995; 333:348–351.

312. Torgan CE, Etgen GJ Jr, Kang HY, et al. Fiber type–specific effects of clenbuterol and exercise training on insulin-resistant muscle. J Appl Physiol 1995; 79:163–167.

313. Tsukazaki K, Nikami H, Shimizu Y, et al. Chronic administration of β-adrenergic agonists can mimic the stimulative effect of cold exposure on protein synthesis in rat brown adipose tissue. J Biochem 1995; 117:96–100.

314. Osawa H, Printz RL, Whitesell RR, et al. Regulation of hexokinase II gene transcription and glucose phosphorylation by catecholamines, cyclic AMP, and insulin. Diabetes 1995; 44:1426–1432.

315. Cori CF. The glucose-lactic acid cycle and gluconeogenesis. Curr Top Cell Regul 1981; 18:377–387.

316. Kusaka M, Ui M. Activation of the Cori cycle by epinephrine. Am J Physiol 1977; 232:E145–E155.

317. Forichon J, Jomain MJ, Schellhorn J, et al. Effect of epinephrine upon irreversible disposal and recycling of glucose in dogs. Experientia 1977; 33:1171–1173.

318. Kunihara M, Oshima T. Effects of epinephrine on plasma cholesterol levels in rats. J Lipid Res 1983; 24:639–644.

319. Dimsdale JE, Herd JA, Hartley LH. Epinephrine mediated increases in plasma cholesterol. Psychosom Med 1983; 45:227–232.

320. Edwards PA. The influence of catecholamines and cyclic AMP on 3-hydroxy-3-methylglutaryl coenzyme A reductase activity and lipid biosynthesis in isolated rat hepatocytes. Arch Biochem Biophys 1975; 170:188–203.

321. Deverey R, O'Donnell L, Tomkin GH. Effect of catecholamines on hepatic rate-limiting enzymes of cholesterol metabolism in normally fed and cholesterol-fed rabbits. Biochim Biophys Acta 1986; 887:173–181.

322. Krone W, Naegele H, Behnke B, et al. Opposite effects of insulin and catecholamines on LDL-receptor activity in human mononuclear leukocytes. Diabetes 1988; 37:1386–1391.

323. Smith CCT, Prichard BNC, Betteridge DJ. Plasma and platelet free catecholamine concentrations in patients with familial hypercholesterolaemia. Clin Sci (Colch) 1992; 82:113–116.

324. Brindle NPJ, Ontko JA. α-Adrenergic suppression of very-low-density-lipoprotein triacylglycerol secretion by isolated rat hepatocytes. Biochem J 1988; 250:363–368.

325. O'Donnell L, Owens D, McGee C, et al. Effects of catecholamines on serum lipoproteins of normally fed and cholesterol-fed rabbits. Metabolism 1988; 37:910–915.

326. Miller WC, Gorski J, Oscai LB, et al. Epinephrine activation of heparin-releasable lipoprotein lipase in 3 skeletal muscle fiber types of the rat. Biochem Biophys Res Commun 1989; 164:615–619.

327. Deshaies Y, Géloën A, Paulin A, et al. Tissue-specific alterations in lipoprotein lipase activity in the rat after chronic infusion of isoproterenol. Horm Metab Res 1993; 25:13–16.

328. Miller NE. Effects of adrenoceptor-blocking drugs on plasma lipoprotein concentrations. Am J Cardiol 1987; 60:17E–23E.

329. Materson BJ, Vlachakis ND, Glasser SP, et al. Influence of beta₂ agonism and beta₁ and beta₂ antagonism on adverse effects and plasma lipoproteins: results of a multicenter comparison of dilevalol and metoprolol. Am J Cardiol 1989; 63:581–631.

330. Hooper PL, Woo W, Visconti L, et al. Terbutaline raises high-density-lipoprotein-cholesterol levels. N Engl J Med 1981; 305:1455–1457.

331. Landsberg L, Young JB. Autonomic regulation of thermogenesis. In: Girardier L, Stock MJ, eds. Mammalian Thermogenesis. London: Chapman & Hall, 1983: 99–140.

332. Hsieh ACL, Carlson LD, Gray G. Role of the sympathetic nervous system in the control of chemical regulation of heat production. Am J Physiol 1957; 190:247–251.

333. Himms-Hagen J. Brown adipose tissue thermogenesis and obesity. Prog Lipid Res 1989; 28:67–115.

334. Cannon B. The mammalian prerogative: sympathetically controlled thermogenesis. Verh Dtsch Zool Ges 1995; 88:191–201.

335. Klaus S, Casteilla L, Bouillaud F, et al. The uncoupling protein UCP: a membraneous mitochondrial ion carrier exclusively expressed in brown adipose tissue. Int J Biochem 1991; 23:791–801.

336. Géloën A, Collet AJ, Guay G, et al. β-Adrenergic stimulation of brown adipocyte proliferation. Am J Physiol 1988; 254:C175–C182.

337. Silva JE, Larsen PR. Potential of brown adipose tissue type II thyroxine 5′-deiodinase as a local and systemic source of triiodothyronine in rats. J Clin Invest 1985; 76:2296–2305.

338. Schrier RW, Berl T, Harbottle JA, et al. Catecholamines and renal water excretion. Nephron 1975; 15:186–196.

339. Edwards RM, Stack EJ, Gellai M, et al. Inhibition of vasopressin-sensitive cAMP accumulation by α₂-adrenoceptor agonists in collecting tubules is species dependent. Pharmacology 1992; 44:26–32.

340. Lee MR. Dopamine and the kidney: ten years on. Clin Sci (Colch) 1993; 84:357–375.

341. Moss NG, Colindres RE, Gottschalk CW. Neural control of renal function. In: Windhager EE, ed. Handbook of Physiology. Sect 8: Renal Physiology. Vol 1. New York: Oxford University Press, 1992: 1061–1128.

342. DiBona GF. Neural control of renal tubular solute and water transport. Miner Electrolyte Metab 1989; 15:44–50.

343. Gesek FA, Schoolwerth AC. Hormonal interactions with the proximal Na⁺-H⁺ exchanger. Am J Physiol 1990; 258:F514–F521.

344. Aperia A, Holtbäck U, Syrén ML, et al. Activation/deactivation of renal Na⁺, K⁺-ATPase: a final common pathway for regulation of natriuresis. FASEB J 1994; 8:436–439.

345. Friberg P, Meredith I, Jennings G, et al. Evidence for increased renal norepinephrine overflow during sodium restriction in humans. Hypertension 1990; 16:121–130.

346. Anderson EA, Sinkey CA, Lawton WJ, et al. Elevated sympathetic nerve activity in borderline hypertensive humans: evidence from direct intraneural recordings. Hypertension 1989; 14:177–183.

347. Gill JR, Bartter FC. Adrenergic nervous system in sodium metabolism. II: Effects of guanethidine on the renal response to sodium deprivation in normal man. N Engl J Med 1966; 275:1466–1471.

348. Wilcox CS, Aminoff MJ, Slater JDH. Sodium homeostasis in patients with autonomic failure. Clin Sci Mol Med 1977; 53:321–328.

349. Sutters M, Wakefield C, O'Neil K, et al. The cardiovascular, endocrine and renal response of tetraplegic and paraplegic subjects to dietary sodium restriction. J Physiol (Lond) 1992; 457:515–523.

350. Struthers AD, Reid JL. The role of adrenal medullary catecholamines in potassium homeostasis. Clin Sci (Colch) 1984; 66:377–382.

351. Williams ME, Rosa RM, Silva P, et al. Impairment of extrarenal potassium disposal by α-adrenergic stimulation. N Engl J Med 1984; 311:145–149.

352. Clausen T, Everts ME. Regulation of the Na, K-pump in skeletal muscle. Kidney Int 1989; 35:1–13.

353. Bevilacqua M, Norbiato G, Raggi U, et al. Dopaminergic control of serum potassium. Metabolism 1980; 29:306–310.

354. Finlay GD, Whitsett TL, Cucinell EA, et al. Augmentation of sodium and potassium excretion, glomerular filtration rate and renal plasma flow by levodopa. N Engl J Med 1971; 284:865–870.

355. Silva P, Spokes K. Sympathetic system in potassium homeostasis. Am J Physiol 1981; 241:F151–F155.

356. Lawton WJ, Fitz AE, Anderson EA, et al. Effect of dietary potassium on blood pressure, renal function, muscle sympathetic nerve activity, and forearm vascular resistance and flow in normotensive and borderline hypertensive humans. Circulation 1990; 81:173–184.

357. Williams ME, Gervino EV, Rosa RM, et al. Catecholamine modulation of rapid potassium shifts during exercise. N Engl J Med 1985; 312:823–827.

358. Krapf R, Caduff P, Wagdi P, et al. Plasma potassium response to acute respiratory alkalosis. Kidney Int 1995; 47:217–224.

359. Lundborg P. The effect of adrenergic blockade on potassium concentrations in different conditions. Acta Med Scand Suppl 1983; 672:121–125.

360. Yeung RTT, Tse TF. Thyrotoxic periodic paralysis: effect of propranolol. Am J Med 1974; 57:584–590.

361. Wang P, Clausen T. Treatment of attacks in hyperkalaemic familial periodic paralysis by inhalation of salbutamol. Lancet 1976; 1:221–223.

362. Haffner CA, Kendall MJ. Metabolic effects of β₂-agonists. J Clin Pharm Ther 1992; 17:155–164.

363. Duncan CP, Shim S-S. The autonomic nerve supply of bone: an experimental study of the intraosseous adrenergic nervi vasorum in the rabbit. J Bone Joint Surg Br 1977; 59:323–330.

364. Bjurholm A. Neuroendocrine peptides in bone. Int Orthop 1991; 15:325–329.

365. Herskovits MS, Singh IJ. Effect of guanethidine-induced sympathectomy on osteoblastic activity in the rat femur evaluated by ³H-proline autoradiography. Acta Anat (Basel) 1984; 120:151–155.

366. Sherman BE, Chole RA. A mechanism for sympathectomy-induced bone resorption in the middle ear. Otolaryngol Head Neck Surg 1995; 113:569–581.

367. Moore RE, Smith CK II, Bailey CS, et al. Characterization of beta-adrenergic receptors on rat and human osteoblast-like cells and demonstration that beta-receptor agonists can stimulate bone resorption in organ culture. Bone Miner 1993; 23:301–315.

368. Bjurholm A, Kreicbergs A, Schultzberg M, et al. Neuroendocrine regulation of cyclic AMP formation in osteoblastic cell lines (UMR-106-01, ROS 17/2.8, MC3T3-E1, and Saos-2) and primary bone cells. J Bone Miner Res 1992; 7:1011–1019.

369. Zeman RJ, Hirschman A, Hirschman ML, et al. Clenbuterol, a β₂-receptor agonist, reduces net bone loss in denervated hindlimbs. Am J Physiol 1991; 261:E285–E289.

370. Whyte KF, Addis GJ, Whitesmith R, et al. Adrenergic control of plasma magnesium in man. Clin Sci (Colch) 1987; 72:135–138.

371. Bos WJW, Postma DS, van Doormaal JJ. Magnesiuric and calciuric effects of terbutaline in man. Clin Sci (Colch) 1988; 74:595–597.

372. Hansen O, Johansson BW, Nilsson-Ehle P. Metabolic, electrocardiographic, and hemodynamic responses to increased circulating adrenaline: effects of selective and nonselective beta adrenoceptor blockade. Angiology 1990; 41:175–188.

373. Lovén L, Larsson L, Lindell B, et al. Effect of propranolol on post-traumatic hypophosphataemia and catecholamine secretion. Acta Chir Scand 1985; 151:201–204.

374. Isaac J, Berndt TJ, Knox FG. Stimulation of α₂-adrenoreceptors blunts the phosphaturic response to parathyroid hormone. J Lab Clin Med 1992; 120:305–309.

375. Glahn RP, Onsgard MJ, Tyce GM, et al. Autocrine/paracrine regulation of renal Na⁺-phosphate cotransport by dopamine. Am J Physiol 1993; 264:F618–F622.

376. Isaac J, Berndt TJ, Knox FG. Role of dopamine in the exaggerated phosphaturic response to parathyroid hormone in the remnant kidney. J Lab Clin Med 1995; 126:470–473.

377. Ortola FV, Seri I, Downes S, et al. Dopamine₁-receptor blockade inhibits ANP-induced phosphaturia and calciuria in rats. Am J Physiol 1990; 259:F138–F146.

378. Berndt TJ, Khraibi AA, Thothathri V, et al. Effect of increased dietary phosphate intake on dopamine excretion in the presence and absence of the renal nerves. Miner Electrolyte Metab 1994; 20:158–162.

379. Püschel GP, Nath A, Jungermann K. Increase of urate formation by stimulation of sympathetic hepatic nerves, circulating noradrenaline and glucagon in the perfused rat liver. FEBS Lett 1987; 219:145–150.

380. Clark MG, Richards SM, Hettiarachchi M, et al. Release of purine and pyrimidine nucleosides and their catabolites from the perfused rat hindlimb in response to noradrenaline, vasopressin, angiotensin II and sciatic-nerve stimulation. Biochem J 1990; 266:765–770.

381. Ferris TF, Gorden P. Effect of angiotensin and norepinephrine upon urate clearance in man. Am J Med 1968; 44:359–365.

382. Satoh N, Kikuchi K, Hasegawa T, et al. [The role of the renal dopaminergic and the prostaglandin systems in renal uric acid metabolism in patients with essential hypertension]. Nippon Naibunpi Gakkai Zasshi 1991; 67:1271–1281.

383. Holmer S, Rinne B, Eckardt K-U, et al. Role of renal nerves for the expression of renin in adult rat kidney. Am J Physiol 1994; 266:F738–F745.

384. Zhang H-J, Redmon JB, Andresen JM, et al. Somatostatin and epinephrine decrease insulin messenger ribonucleic acid in HIT cells through a pertussis toxin-sensitive mechanism. Endocrinology 1991; 129:2409–2414.

385. Güse-Behling H, Ehrhart-Bornstein M, Bornstein SR, et al. Regulation of adrenal steroidogenesis by adrenaline: expression of cytochrome P450 genes. J Endocrinol 1992; 135:229–237.

386. Ehrhart-Bornstein M, Bornstein SR, González-Hernández J, et al. Sympathoadrenal regulation of adrenocortical steroidogenesis. Endocr Res 1995; 21:13–24.

387. Lara HE, McDonald JK, Ahmed CE, et al. Guanethidine-mediated destruction of ovarian sympathetic nerves disrupts ovarian development and function in rats. Endocrinology 1990; 127:2199–2209.

388. Walker C-D. Chemical sympathectomy and maternal separation affect neonatal stress responses and adrenal sensitivity to ACTH. Am J Physiol 1995; 268:R1281–R1288.

389. Burr IM, Slonim AE, Burke V, et al. Extracellular calcium and adrenergic and cholinergic effects on islet β-cell function. Am J Physiol 1976; 231:1246–1249.

390. Jena BP, Abramowitz J. Catecholamine-induced heterologous desensitization of rabbit luteal adenylyl cyclase: loss of luteinizing hormone responsiveness is associated with impaired G-protein function. Endocrinology 1989; 124:1942–1948.

391. Campos MB, Chiocchio SR, Calandra RS, et al. Effect of bilateral denervation of the immature rat testis on testicular gonadotropin receptors and in vitro androgen production. Neuroendocrinology 1993; 57:189–194.

392. Kleitman N, Holzwarth MA. Compensatory adrenal cortical growth is inhibited by sympathectomy. Am J Physiol 1985; 248:E261–E263.

393. Gerendai I, Marchetti B, Maugeri S, et al. Prevention of compensatory ovarian hypertrophy by local treatment of the ovary with 6-OHDA. Neuroendocrinology 1978; 27:272–278.

394. Young JB, Saville ME, Burgi U, et al. Sympathetic nervous system (SNS) activity in rat thyroid: evidence for a role in thyroid hypertrophy. Clin Res 1983; 31:280A (abstract).

395. Barajas L, Liu L, Powers K. Anatomy of the renal innervation: intrarenal aspects and ganglia of origin. Can J Physiol Pharmacol 1992; 70:735–749.

396. Persson PB, Gimpl G, Lang RE. Importance of neuropeptide Y in the regulation of kidney function. Ann NY Acad Sci 1990; 611:156–165.

397. Kopp UC, DiBona GF. Neural regulation of renin secretion. Semin Nephrol 1993; 13:543–551.

398. Osborn JL, Thames MD, DiBona GF. Role of macula densa in renal nerve modulation of renin secretion. Am J Physiol 1982; 242:R367–R371.

399. Gibbons GH, Dzau VJ, Farhi ER, et al. Interaction of signals influencing renin release. Annu Rev Physiol 1984; 46:291–308.

400. Johns EJ, Richards HK, Singer B. Effects of adrenaline, noradrenaline, isoprenaline and salbutamol on the production and release of renin by isolated renal cortical cells of the cat. Br J Pharmacol 1975; 53:67–73.

401. Dzau VJ, Carleton JE, Brody T. Sequential changes in renin secretion-synthesis coupling in response to acute β adrenergic stimulation. Clin Res 1987; 35:604A (abstract).

402. Hackenthal E, Paul M, Ganten D, et al. Morphology, physiology, and molecular biology of renin secretion. Physiol Rev 1990; 70:1067–1116.

403. Biaggioni I, Garcia F, Inagami T, et al. Hyporeninemic normoaldosteronism in severe autonomic failure. J Clin Endocrinol Metab 1993; 76:580–586.
404. Mizelle HL, Hall JE, Woods LL, et al. Role of renal nerves in compensatory adaptation to chronic reductions in sodium intake. Am J Physiol 1987; 252:F291–F298.
405. Fernández-Repollet E, Silva-Netto CR, Colindres RE, et al. Role of renal nerves in maintaining sodium balance in unrestrained conscious rats. Am J Physiol 1985; 249:F819–F826.
406. Holmer S, Eckardt K-U, LeHir M, et al. Influence of dietary NaCl intake on renin gene expression in the kidneys and adrenal glands of rats. Pflügers Arch 1993; 425:62–67.
407. Yang HM, Lohmeier TE, Kivlighn SD, et al. Sustained increases in plasma epinephrine concentration do not modulate renin release. Am J Physiol 1989; 257:E57–E64.
408. Girbes ARJ, Smit AJ, Meijer S, et al. Renal and endocrine effects of fenoldopam and metoclopramide in normal man. Nephron 1990; 56:179–185.
409. Antonipillai I, Broers MI, Lang D. Evidence that specific dopamine-1 receptor activation is involved in dopamine-induced renin release. Hypertension 1989; 13:463–468.
410. Oda S, Hagino A, Ohneda A, et al. Adrenergic modulation of pancreatic glucagon and insulin secretion in sheep. Am J Physiol 1988; 254:R518–R523.
411. Hirose H, Maruyama H, Ito K, et al. Effects of α_2- and β-adrenergic agonism on glucagon secretion from perfused pancreata of normal and streptozocin-induced diabetic rats. Metabolism 1993; 42:1072–1076.
412. Lacey RJ, Cable HC, James RFL, et al. Concentration-dependent effects of adrenaline on the profile of insulin secretion from isolated human islets of Langerhans. J Endocrinol 1993; 138:555–563.
413. Schuit FC, Pipeleers DG. Differences in adrenergic recognition by pancreatic A and B cells. Science 1986; 232:875–877.
414. Ahrén B, Veith RC, Paquette TL, et al. Sympathetic nerve stimulation versus pancreatic norepinephrine infusion in the dog. 2: Effects on basal release of somatostatin and pancreatic polypeptide. Endocrinology 1987; 121:332–339.
415. Brunicardi FC, Elahi D, Andersen DK. Splanchnic neural regulation of somatostatin secretion in the isolated perfused human pancreas. Ann Surg 1994; 219:258–266.
416. Dunning BE, Taborsky GJ Jr. Neural control of islet function by norepinephrine and sympathetic neuropeptides. Adv Exp Med Biol 1991; 291:107–127.
417. Burr IM, Jackson A, Culbert S, et al. Glucose intolerance and impaired insulin release following 6-hydroxydopamine administration to intact rats. Endocrinology 1974; 94:1072–1076.
418. Lundquist I, Fanska R, Grodsky GM. Direct calcium-stimulated release of glucagon from the isolation perfused rat pancreas and the effect of chemical sympathectomy. Endocrinology 1976; 98:815–818.
419. Burr IM, Balant L, Stauffacher W, et al. Adrenergic modification of glucose-induced biphasic insulin release from perifused rat pancreas. Eur J Clin Invest 1971; 1:216–224.
420. Pipeleers DG, Schuit FC, Van Schravendijk CFH, et al. Interplay of nutrients and hormones in the regulation of glucagon release. Endocrinology 1985; 117:817–823.
421. Pipeleers DG, Schuit FC, in't Veld PA, et al. Interplay of nutrients and hormones in the regulation of insulin release. Endocrinology 1985; 117:824–833.
422. Havel PJ, Veith RC, Dunning BE, et al. Role for autonomic nervous system to increase pancreatic glucagon secretion during marked insulin-induced hypoglycemia in dogs. Diabetes 1991; 40:1107–1114.
423. Young JB, Landsberg L. Effect of diet and cold exposure on norepinephrine turnover in pancreas and liver. Am J Physiol 1979; 236:E524–E533.
424. Havel PJ, Veith RC, Dunning BE, et al. Pancreatic noradrenergic nerves are activated by neuroglucopenia but not by hypotension or hypoxia in the dog: evidence for stress-specific and regionally selective activation of the sympathetic nervous system. J Clin Invest 1988; 82:1538–1545.
425. Luzi L, Battezzati A, Perseghin G, et al. Lack of feedback inhibition of insulin secretion in denervated human pancreas. Diabetes 1992; 41:1632–1639.
426. Boden G, Chen X, DeSantis R, et al. Evidence that suppression of insulin secretion by insulin itself is neurally mediated. Metabolism 1993; 42:786–789.
427. Ahrén B. Thyroid neuroendocrinology: neural regulation of thyroid hormone secretion. Endocr Rev 1986; 7:149–155.
428. Tice LW, Creveling CR. Electron microscopic identification of adrenergic nerve endings on thyroid epithelial cells. Endocrinology 1975; 97:1123–1129.
429. Grunditz T, Sundler F, Håkanson R, et al. Regulatory peptides in the thyroid gland. Adv Exp Med Biol 1989; 261:121–149.
430. Maayan ML, Volpert EM, Debons AF. Neurotransmitter regulation of thyroid activity. Endocr Res 1987; 13:199–212.
431. Lewinski A, Pawlikowski M, Cardinali DP. Thyroid growth-stimulating and growth-inhibiting factors. Biol Signals 1993; 2:313–351.
432. Polikar R, Kennedy B, Ziegler M, et al. Plasma norepinephrine kinetics, dopamine-β-hydroxylase, and chromogranin-A, in hypothyroid patients before and following replacement therapy. J Clin Endocrinol Metab 1990; 70:277–281.
433. Fagius J, Westermark K, Karlsson A. Baroreflex-governed sympathetic outflow to muscle vasculature is increased in hypothyroidism. Clin Endocrinol (Oxf) 1990; 33:177–185.
434. Matsukawa T, Mano T, Gotoh E, et al. Altered muscle sympathetic nerve activity in hyperthyroidism and hypothyroidism. J Auton Nerv Syst 1993; 42:171–175.
435. Coulombe P, Dussault JH, Walker P. Catecholamine metabolism in thyroid disease. II: Norepinephrine secretion rate in hyperthyroidism and hypothyroidism. J Clin Endocrinol Metab 1977; 44:1185–1189.
436. Esler M. Assessment of sympathetic nervous function in humans from noradrenaline plasma kinetics. Clin Sci (Colch) 1982; 62:247–254.
437. Heath H III. Biogenic amines and the secretion of parathyroid hormone and calcitonin. Endocr Rev 1980; 1:319–338.
438. Fischer JA, Blum JW, Born W, et al. Regulation of parathyroid hormone secretion in vitro and in vivo. Calcif Tissue Int 1982; 34:313–316.
439. Norberg K-A, Persson B, Granberg P-O. Adrenergic innervation of the human parathyroid glands. Acta Chir Scand 1975; 141:319–322.
440. Brown EM. PTH secretion in vivo and in vitro: regulation by calcium and other secretagogues. Miner Electrolyte Metab 1982; 8:130–150.
441. Meister B, Askergren J, Tunevall G, et al. Identification of a dopamine- and 3'5'-cyclic adenosine monophosphate-regulated phosphoprotein of 32 kd (DARPP-32) in parathyroid hormone–producing cells of the human parathyroid gland. J Endocrinol Invest 1991; 14:655–661.
442. Cardinali DP, Ladizesky MG. Changes in parathyroid hormone and calcium levels after superior cervical ganglionectomy of rats. Neuroendocrinology 1985; 40:291–296.
443. Cardinali DP, Sartorio GC, Ladizesky MG, et al. Changes in calcitonin release during sympathetic nerve degeneration after superior cervical ganglionectomy of rats. Neuroendocrinology 1986; 43:498–503.
444. Body J-J, Cryer PE, Offord KP, et al. Epinephrine is a hypophosphatemic hormone in man: physiological effects of circulating epinephrine on plasma calcium, magnesium, phosphorus, parathyroid hormone, and calcitonin. J Clin Invest 1983; 71:572–578.
445. Shearing CH, Ashby JP, Hepburn DA, et al. Suppression of plasma intact parathyroid hormone levels during insulin-induced hypoglycemia in humans. J Clin Endocrinol Metab 1992; 74:1270–1276.
446. Phillippo M, Lawrence CB, Bruce JB, et al. Feeding and calcitonin secretion in sheep. J Endocrinol 1972; 53:419–424.
447. Converse RL Jr, Jacobsen TN, Toto RD, et al. Sympathetic overactivity in patients with chronic renal failure. N Engl J Med 1992; 327:1912–1918.
448. Coevoet B, Desplan C, Sebert JL, et al. Effect of propranolol and metoprolol on parathyroid hormone and calcitonin secretions in uraemic patients. Br Med J 1980; 280:1344–1346.
449. Carlsson S, Jónsdóttir IH, Skarphedinsson JO, et al. Evidence for an adrenergic innervation of the adrenal cortical blood vessels in rats. Acta Physiol Scand 1993; 149:23–30.
450. Gilchrist AB, Leake A, Charlton BG. Innervation of the human adrenal cortex: simultaneous visualisation using acetylcholinesterase histochemistry and dopamine β-hydroxylase immunohistochemistry. Acta Anat 1993; 146:31–35.
451. Bornstein SR, Gonzalez-Hernandez JA, Ehrhart-Bornstein M, et al. Intimate contact of chromaffin and cortical cells within the human adrenal gland forms the cellular basis for important intraadrenal interactions. J Clin Endocrinol Metab 1994; 78:225–232.
452. Pratt JH, Turner DA, McAteer JA, et al. β-Adrenergic stimulation of aldosterone production by rat adrenal capsular explants. Endocrinology 1985; 117:1189–1194.
453. Ehrhart-Bornstein M, Bornstein SR, Güse-Behling H, et al. Sympatho-adrenal regulation of adrenal androstenedione release. Neuroendocrinology 1994; 59:406–412.
454. Lightly ERT, Walker SW, Bird IM, et al. Subclassification of β-adrenoceptors responsible for steroidogenesis in primary cultures of bovine adrenocortical zona fasciculata/reticularis cells. Br J Pharmacol 1990; 99:709–712.
455. Edwards AV, Jones CT. Autonomic control of adrenal function. J Anat 1993; 183:291–307.
456. Bernet F, Bernard J, Laborie C, et al. Neuropeptide Y (NPY)– and vasoactive intestinal peptide (VIP)–induced aldosterone secretion by rat capsule/glomerular zone could be mediated by catecholamines via β_1 adrenergic receptors. Neurosci Lett 1994; 166:109–112.
457. Hinson JP, Kapas S, Orford CD, et al. Vasoactive intestinal peptide stimulation of aldosterone secretion by the rat adrenal cortex may be mediated by the local release of catecholamines. J Endocrinol 1992; 133:253–258.
458. Charlton BG. Adrenal cortical innervation and glucocorticoid secretion. J Endocrinol 1990; 126:5–8.
459. Carey RM, Thorner MO, Ortt EM. Effects of metoclopramide and bromocriptine on the renin-angiotensin-aldosterone system in man. J Clin Invest 1979; 63:727–735.
460. Fukagawa NK, Bandini LG, Lee MA, et al. Effect of age on dopaminergic responses to protein feeding. Am J Physiol 1995; 268:F613–F625.
461. Gordon MB, Moore TJ, Dluhy RG, et al. Dopaminergic modulation of aldosterone responsiveness to angiotensin II with changes in sodium intake. J Clin Endocrinol Metab 1983; 56:340–345.
462. Malchoff CD, Hughes JM, Carey RM. Effect of upright posture on the aldosterone responses to dopamine, metoclopramide, angiotensin II, and adrenocorticotropin. J Clin Endocrinol Metab 1987; 65:203–207.
463. Porter ID, Whitehouse BJ, Price GM, et al. Effects of dopamine, high

588. French EB, Kilpatrick R. The role of adrenaline in hypoglycemic reactions in man. Clin Sci (Colch) 1955; 14:639–651.

589. LeBlanc J, Cabanac M, Samson P. Reduced postprandial heat production with gavage as compared with meal feeding in human subjects. Am J Physiol 1984; 246:E95–E101.

590. LeBlanc J, Brondel L. Role of palatability on meal-induced thermogenesis in human subjects. Am J Physiol 1985; 248:E333–E336.

591. Tse TF, Clutter WE, Shah SD, et al. Neuroendocrine responses to glucose ingestion in man: specificity, temporal relationships, and quantitative aspects. J Clin Invest 1983; 72:270–277.

592. Berne C, Fagius J, Niklasson F. Sympathetic response to oral carbohydrate administration: evidence from microelectrode nerve recordings. J Clin Invest 1989; 84:1403–1409.

593. Cox HS, Kaye DM, Thompson JM, et al. Regional sympathetic nervous activation after a large meal in humans. Clin Sci 1995; 89:145–154.

594. Rappaport EB, Young JB, Landsberg L. Effects of 2-deoxy-D-glucose on the cardiac sympathetic nerves and the adrenal medulla in the rat: further evidence for a dissociation of sympathetic nervous system and adrenal medullary responses. Endocrinology 1982; 110:650–656.

595. O'Dea K, Esler M, Leonard P, et al. Noradrenaline turnover during under- and over-eating in normal weight subjects. Metabolism 1982; 31:896–899.

596. Andersson B, Elam M, Wallin BG, et al. Effect of energy-restricted diet on sympathetic muscle nerve activity in obese women. Hypertension 1991; 18:783–789.

597. Vatner SF, Franklin D, Van Citters RL. Mesenteric vasoactivity associated with eating and digestion in the conscious dog. Am J Physiol 1970; 219:170–174.

598. Bloom SR, Edwards AV, Hardy RN, et al. Cardiovascular and endocrine responses to feeding in the young calf. J Physiol (Lond) 1975; 253:135–155.

599. Kaufman LN, Peterson MM, Smith SM. Hypertension and sympathetic hyperactivity induced in rats by high-fat or glucose diets. Am J Physiol 1991; 260:E95–E100.

600. Rocchini AP, Moorehead CP, DeRemer S, et al. Pathogenesis of weight-related changes in blood pressure in dogs. Hypertension 1989; 13:922–928.

601. Jung RT, Shetty PS, James WPT. The effect of beta-adrenergic blockade on metabolic rate and peripheral thyroid metabolism in obesity. Eur J Clin Invest 1980; 10:179–182.

602. Acheson K, Jéquier E, Wahren J. Influence of β-adrenergic blockade on glucose-induced thermogenesis in man. J Clin Invest 1983; 72:981–986.

603. Trunet P, Lhoste F, Ansquer J-C, et al. Decreased plasma epinephrine concentrations after glucose ingestion in humans. Metabolism 1984; 33:101–103.

604. Astrup A, Bülow J, Christensen NJ, et al. Facultative thermogenesis induced by carbohydrate; a skeletal muscle component mediated by epinephrine. Am J Physiol 1986; 250:E226–E229.

605. Rosen SG, Clutter WE, Berk MA, et al. Epinephrine supports the postabsorptive plasma glucose concentration and prevents hypoglycemia when glucagon secretion is deficient in man. J Clin Invest 1984; 73:405–411.

606. Jones TW, Borg WP, Boulware SD, et al. Enhanced adrenomedullary response and increased susceptibility to neuroglycopenia: mechanisms underlying the adverse effects of sugar ingestion in healthy children. J Pediatr 1995; 126:171–177.

607. Young JB, Landsberg L. Suppression of sympathetic nervous system during fasting. Science 1977; 196:1473–1475.

608. Gougeon R, Mitchell TH, Larivière F, et al. Effects of sodium supplementation during energy restriction on plasma norepinephrine levels in obese women. J Clin Endocrinol Metab 1991; 73:975–981.

609. Boulter PR, Hoffman RS, Arky RA. Pattern of sodium excretion accompanying starvation. Metabolism 1973; 22:675–682.

610. Landsberg L, Young JB. Insulin-mediated glucose metabolism in the relationship between dietary intake and sympathetic nervous system activity. Int J Obes 1985; 9(Suppl 2):63–68.

611. Galbo H, Christensen NJ, Mikines KJ, et al. The effect of fasting on the hormonal response to graded exercise. J Clin Endocrinol Metab 1981; 52:1106–1112.

612. Del Rio G, Carani C, Bonati M, et al. Sexual dimorphism of the autonomic nervous system response to weight loss in obese patients. Int J Obes 1992; 16:897–903.

613. Galster AD, Clutter WE, Cryer PE, et al. Epinephrine plasma thresholds for lipolytic effects in man: measurements of fatty acid transport with [1-¹³C]palmitic acid. J Clin Invest 1981; 67:1729–1738.

614. Savard G, Strange S, Kiens B, et al. Noradrenaline spillover during exercise in active versus resting skeletal muscle in man. Acta Physiol Scand 1987; 131:507–515.

615. Péronnet F, Béliveau L, Boudreau G, et al. Regional plasma catecholamine removal and release at rest and exercise in dogs. Am J Physiol 1988; 254:R663–R672.

616. Wallin BG, Esler M, Dorward P, et al. Simultaneous measurements of cardiac noradrenaline spillover and sympathetic outflow to skeletal muscle in humans. J Physiol (Lond) 1992; 453:45–58.

617. Sinoway LI, Smith MB, Enders B, et al. Role of diprotonated phosphate in evoking muscle reflex responses in cats and humans. Am J Physiol 1994; 267:H770–H778.

618. Latour MG, Cardin S, Hélie R, et al. Effect of hepatic vagotomy on plasma catecholamines during exercise-induced hypoglycemia. J Appl Physiol 1995; 78:1629–1634.

619. Jennings G, Nelson L, Nestel P, et al. The effects of changes in physical activity on major cardiovascular risk factors, hemodynamics, sympathetic function, and glucose utilization in man: a controlled study of four levels of activity. Circulation 1986; 73:30–40.

620. Marker JC, Cryer PE, Clutter WE. Simplified measurement of norepinephrine kinetics: application to studies of aging and exercise training. Am J Physiol 1994; 267:E380–E387.

621. Meredith IT, Friberg P, Jennings GL, et al. Exercise training lowers resting renal but not cardiac sympathetic activity in humans. Hypertension 1991; 18:575–582.

622. Sheldahl LM, Ebert TJ, Cox B, et al. Effect of aerobic training on baroreflex regulation of cardiac and sympathetic function. J Appl Physiol 1994; 76:158–165.

623. Tremblay A, Coveney S, Després J-P, et al. Increased resting metabolic rate and lipid oxidation in exercise-trained individuals: evidence for a role of β-adrenergic stimulation. Can J Physiol Pharmacol 1992; 70:1342–1347.

624. Chen H-I, Li H-T, Chen C-C. Physical conditioning decreases norepinephrine-induced vasoconstriction in rabbits: possible roles of norepinephrine-evoked endothelium-derived relaxing factor. Circulation 1994; 90:970–975.

625. Schmidt KN, Gosselin LE, Stanley WC. Endurance exercise training causes adrenal medullary hypertrophy in young and old Fischer 344 rats. Horm Metab Res 1992; 24:511–515.

626. Kjaer M, Galbo H. Effect of physical training on the capacity to secrete epinephrine. J Appl Physiol 1988; 64:11–16.

627. Ahlborg G, Lundberg JM. Splanchnic release of neuropeptide Y during prolonged exercise with and without β-adrenoceptor blockade in healthy man. Clin Physiol 1991; 11:343–351.

628. Wasserman DH. Regulation of glucose fluxes during exercise in the postabsorptive state. Annu Rev Physiol 1995; 57:191–218.

629. Chesley A, Hultman E, Spriet LL. Effects of epinephrine infusion on muscle glycogenolysis during intense aerobic exercise. Am J Physiol 1995; 268:E127–E134.

630. McDermott JC, Elder GC, Bonen A. Adrenal hormones enhance glycogenolysis in nonexercising muscle during exercise. J Appl Physiol 1987; 63:1275–1283.

631. Miles PDG, Finegood DT, Lickley HLA, et al. Regulation of glucose turnover at the onset of exercise in the dog. J Appl Physiol 1992; 72:2487–2494.

632. Arner P, Kriegholm E, Engfeldt P, et al. Adrenergic regulation of lipolysis in situ at rest and during exercise. J Clin Invest 1990; 85:893–898.

633. Stankiewicz-Choroszucha B, Górski J. Effect of beta-adrenergic blockade on intramuscular triglyceride mobilization during exercise. Experientia 1978; 34:357–358.

634. Marliss EB, Simantirakis E, Miles PDG, et al. Glucoregulatory and hormonal responses to repeated bouts of intense exercise in normal male subjects. J Appl Physiol 1991; 71:924–933.

635. Børsheim E, Bahr R, Hansson P, et al. Effect of β-adrenoceptor blockade on post-exercise oxygen consumption. Metabolism 1994; 43:565–571.

636. Young DB, Srivastava TN, Fitzovich DE, et al. Potassium and catecholamine concentrations in the immediate post exercise period. Am J Med Sci 1992; 304:150–153.

637. Lindinger MI. Potassium regulation during exercise and recovery in humans: implications for skeletal and cardiac muscle. J Mol Cell Cardiol 1995; 27:1011–1022.

638. Morgan DA, Thoren P, Wilczynski EA, et al. Serotonergic mechanisms mediate renal sympathoinhibition during severe hemorrhage in rats. Am J Physiol 1988; 255:H496–H502.

639. Hasser EM, Schadt JC. Sympathoinhibition and its reversal by naloxone during hemorrhage. Am J Physiol 1992; 262:R444–R451.

640. Young JB, Fish S, Landsberg L. Sympathetic nervous system and adrenal medullary responses to ischemic injury in mice. Am J Physiol 1983; 245:E67–E73.

641. Djahanguiri B, Taubin HL, Landsberg L. Increased sympathetic activity in the pathogenesis of restraint ulcer in rats. J Pharmacol Exp Ther 1973; 184:163–168.

642. Chance WT, von Allmen D, Benson D, et al. Clenbuterol decreases catabolism and increases hypermetabolism in burned rats. J Trauma 1991; 31:365–370.

643. Radisavljevic Z. Arterial oxygen consumption after hemorrhagic shock: the effect of β-adrenergic agonist. Am J Med Sci 1991; 302:284–286.

644. Bernstein D, Doshi R, Huang S, et al. Transcriptional regulation of left ventricular β-adrenergic receptors during chronic hypoxia. Circ Res 1992; 71:1465–1471.

645. Tait SM, Wang P, Ba ZF, et al. Downregulation of hepatic β-adrenergic receptors after trauma and hemorrhagic shock. Am J Physiol 1995; 268:G749–G753.

646. Blum I, Nessiel L, David A, et al. Plasma neurotransmitter profile during different phases of the ovulatory cycle. J Clin Endocrinol Metab 1992; 75:924–929.

647. Wolf R, Meier-Fleitmann A, Düker E-M, et al. Intraovarian secretion of catecholamines, oxytocin, beta-endorphin, and gamma-amino-butyric-acid in freely moving rats: development of a push-pull tubing method. Biol Reprod 1986; 35:599–607.

648. Heesch CM, Rogers RC. Effects of pregnancy and progesterone metabolites on regulation of sympathetic outflow. Clin Exp Pharmacol Physiol 1995; 22:136–142.

649. Katholi RE, Carey RM, Ayers CR, et al. Production of sustained hyperten-

sion by chronic intrarenal norepinephrine infusion in conscious dogs. Circ Res 1977; 40(Suppl I):I-118–I-126.

650. Smits JFM, Kleinjans JCS, Janssen BJA, et al. Characterization of hypertension induced by long-term intrarenal norepinephrine infusion in conscious rats. Clin Exp Hypertens [A] 1987; 9(Suppl 1):197–209.

651. Goldstein DS. Plasma catecholamines and essential hypertension: an analytical review. Hypertension 1983; 5:86–99.

652. Esler M, Lambert G, Jennings G. Regional norepinephrine turnover in human hypertension. Clin Exp Hypertens [A] 1989; 11(Suppl 1):75–89.

653. Julius S. Sympathetic hyperactivity and coronary risk in hypertension. Hypertension 1993; 21:886–893.

654. Lund-Johansen P. Twenty-year follow-up of hemodynamics in essential hypertension during rest and exercise. Hypertension 1991; 18(Suppl III):III-54–III-61.

655. Mörlin C, Wallin BG, Eriksson BM. Muscle sympathetic activity and plasma noradrenaline in normotensive and hypertensive man. Acta Physiol Scand 1983; 119:117–121.

656. Miyajima E, Yamada Y, Yoshida Y, et al. Muscle sympathetic nerve activity in renovascular hypertension and primary aldosteronism. Hypertension 1991; 17:1057–1062.

657. Wallin BG, Kunimoto MM, Sellgren J. Possible genetic influence on the strength of human muscle nerve sympathetic activity at rest. Hypertension 1993; 22:282–284.

658. Young JB, Macdonald IA. Sympathoadrenal activity in human obesity: heterogeneity of findings since 1980. Int J Obes 1992; 16:959–967.

659. Landsberg L. Diet, obesity and hypertension: an hypothesis involving insulin, the sympathetic nervous system, and adaptive thermogenesis. Q J Med 1986; 61:1081–1090.

660. Somers VK, Dyken ME, Clary MP, et al. Sympathetic neural mechanisms in obstructive sleep apnea. J Clin Invest 1995; 96:1897–1904.

661. Landsberg L, Young JB. Diet and the sympathetic nervous system. In: Lehnert H, Murison R, Weiner H, Hellhammer D, Beyer J, eds. Endocrine and Nutritional Control of Basic Biological Functions. Seattle: Huber-Hogrefe Publishers, 1993: 3–12.

662. Iwase S, Matsukawa T, Ishihara S, et al. Effect of oral ethanol intake on muscle sympathetic nerve activity and cardiovascular functions in humans. J Auton Nerv Syst 1995; 54:206–214.

663. Carey RM, Stote RM, Dubb JW, et al. Selective peripheral dopamine-1 receptor stimulation with fenoldopam in human essential hypertension. J Clin Invest 1984; 74:2198–2207.

664. Aperia A. Dopamine action and metabolism in the kidney. Curr Opin Nephrol Hypertens 1994; 3:39–45.

665. Serrano PA, Figueroa G, Torres M,Z., et al. Adrenaline, noradrenaline and dopamine excretion in patients with essential hypertension. Am J Cardiol 1964; 13:484–488.

666. Shikuma R, Yoshimura M, Kambara S, et al. Dopaminergic modulation of salt sensitivity in patients with essential hypertension. Life Sci 1986; 38:915–921.

667. Gordon MS, Steunkel CA, Conlin PR, et al. The role of dopamine in nonmodulating hypertension. J Clin Endocrinol Metab 1989; 69:426–432.

668. Consensus statement on the definition of orthostatic hypotension, pure autonomic failure, and multiple system atrophy: the Consensus Committee of the American Autonomic Society and the American Academy of Neurology. Neurology 1996; 46:1470.

669. Low PA. Autonomic nervous system function. J Clin Neurophysiol 1993; 10:14–27.

670. Meredith IT, Eisenfofer G, Lambert GW, et al. Plasma norepinephrine responses to head-up tilt are misleading in autonomic failure. Hypertension 1992; 19:628–633.

671. Benarroch EE, Chang F-LF. Central autonomic disorders. J Clin Neurophysiol 1993; 10:39–50.

672. Low PA, Fealey RD. Structure and function of pre- and postganglionic neurons in pure autonomic failure and multisystem atrophy with autonomic failure. In: Bannister R, ed. Autonomic Failure: A Textbook of Clinical Disorders of the Autonomic Nervous System. Oxford, UK: Oxford University Press, 1988: 544–557.

673. Bannister R. Introduction and classification. In: Bannister R, ed. Autonomic Failure: A Textbook of Clinical Disorders of the Autonomic Nervous System. Oxford, UK: Oxford University Press, 1988: 1–20.

674. Quinn N. Multiple system atrophy: the nature of the beast. J Neurol Neurosurg Psychiatry 1989; 52 Suppl:78–89.

675. Bannister R. Histochemical studies in autonomic failure. A: Sympathetic terminals in autonomic failure. In: Bannister R, ed. Autonomic Failure: A Textbook of Clinical Disorders of the Autonomic Nervous System. Oxford, UK: Oxford University Press, 1988: 558–563.

676. Meredith IT, Esler MD, Cox HS, et al. Biochemical evidence of sympathetic denervation of the heart in pure autonomic failure. Clin Auton Res 1991; 1:187–194.

677. Polinsky RJ, Brown RT, Lee GR, et al. β-endorphin, ACTH, and catecholamine responses in chronic autonomic failure. Ann Neurol 1987; 21:573–577.

678. McLeod JG. Autonomic dysfunction in peripheral nerve disease. J Clin Neurophysiol 1993; 10:51–60.

679. Blumenfeld A, Slaugenhaupt SA, Axelrod FB, et al. Localization of the gene for familial dysautonomia on chromosome 9 and definition of DNA markers for genetic diagnosis. Nat Genet 1993; 4:160–164.

680. Eng CM, Slaughenhaupt SA, Blumenfeld A, et al. Prenatal diagnosis of familial dysautonomia by analysis of linked CA-repeat polymorphisms on chromosome 9q31-q33. Am J Med Genet 1995; 59:349–355.

681. Robertson D, Haile V, Perry SE, et al. Dopamine β-hydroxylase deficiency: a genetic disorder of cardiovascular regulation. Hypertension 1991; 18:1–8.

682. O'Connor DT, Cervenka JH, Stone RA, et al. Dopamine β-hydroxylase immunoreactivity in human cerebrospinal fluid: properties, relationship to central noradrenergic neuronal activity and variation in Parkinson's disease and congenital dopamine β-hydroxylase deficiency. Clin Sci (Colch) 1994; 86:149–158.

683. Robertson D, Davis TL. Recent advances in the treatment of orthostatic hypotension. Neurology 1995; 45(Suppl 5):S26–S32.

684. Jankovic J, Gilden JL, Hiner BC, et al. Neurogenic orthostatic hypotension: a double-blind, placebo-controlled study with midodrine. Am J Med 1993; 95:38–48.

685. Biaggioni I, Robertson RM, Robertson D. Manipulation of norepinephrine metabolism with yohimbine in the treatment of autonomic failure. J Clin Pharmacol 1994; 34:418–423.

686. Thomas JE, Rooke ED, Kvale WF. The neurologist's experience with pheochromocytoma. A review of 100 cases. JAMA 1966; 197:754–758.

687. Plouin PF, Chatellier G, Delahousse M, et al. Recherche, diagnostic et localisation du phéochromocytome. 77 cas dans une population de 21,420 hypertendus. Presse Méd 1987; 16:2211–2215.

688. Hermann H, Mornex R: Human Tumours Secreting Catecholamines: Clinical and Physiopathological Study of the Phaeochromocytomas. New York: Macmillan, 1964: 1–14.

689. Ross EJ, Griffith DNW. The clinical presentation of phaeochromocytoma. Q J Med 1989; 71:485–496.

690. Kitamura K, Kangawa K, Kawamoto M, et al. Adrenomedullin: a novel hypotensive peptide isolated from human pheochromocytoma. Biochem Biophys Res Commun 1993; 192:553–560.

691. Gupta KK. Phaeochromocytoma and myocardial infarction. Lancet 1975; 1:281–282.

692. Radtke WE, Kazmier FJ, Rutherford BD, et al. Cardiovascular complications of pheochromocytoma crisis. Am J Cardiol 1975; 35:701–705.

693. Van Vliet PD, Burchell HB, Titus JL. Focal myocarditis associated with pheochromocytoma. N Engl J Med 1966; 274:1102–1108.

694. Northfield TC. Cardiac complications of phaeochromocytoma. Br Heart J 1967; 29:588–593.

695. de Leeuw PW, Waltman FL, Birkenhäger WH. Noncardiogenic pulmonary edema as the sole manifestation of pheochromocytoma. Hypertension 1986; 8:810–812.

696. Garruti G, Ricquier D. Analysis of uncoupling protein and its mRNA in adipose tissue deposits of adult humans. Int J Obes 1992; 16:383–390.

697. Spark RF, Connolly PB, Gluckin DS, et al. ACTH secretion from a functioning pheochromocytoma. N Engl J Med 1979; 301:416–418.

698. Roth KA, Wilson DM, Eberwine J, et al. Acromegaly and pheochromocytoma: a multiple endocrine syndrome caused by a plurihormonal adrenal medullary tumor. J Clin Endocrinol Metab 1986; 63:1421–1426.

699. Kimura S, Nishimura Y, Yamaguchi K, et al. A case of pheochromocytoma producing parathyroid hormone-related protein and presenting with hypercalcemia. J Clin Endocrinol Metab 1990; 70:1559–1563.

700. Mune T, Katakami H, Kato Y, et al. Production and secretion of parathyroid hormone-related protein in pheochromocytoma: participation of an α-adrenergic mechanism. J Clin Endocrinol Metab 1993; 76:757–762.

701. Shulkin BL, Shapiro B, Sisson JC. Pheochromocytoma, polycythemia, and venous thrombosis. Am J Med 1987; 83:773–776.

702. Manger WM, Gifford RW Jr: Pheochromocytoma. New York: Springer-Verlag, 1977; 1–398.

703. Whalen RK, Althausen AF, Daniels GH. Extra-adrenal pheochromocytoma. J Urol 1992; 147:1–10.

704. Winkler H, Smith AD. Phaeochromocytoma and other catecholamine-producing tumours. In: Blaschko H, Muscholl E, eds. Handbook of Experimental Pharmacology, Vol 33: Catecholamines. Berlin: Springer-Verlag, 1972: 900–933.

705. Johnson RG, Carty SE, Scarpa A. Catecholamine transport and energy-linked function of chromaffin granules isolated from a human pheochromocytoma. Biochim Biophys Acta 1982; 716:366–376.

706. Roizen MP, Isambert MF, Henry JP, et al. Characterization of the monoamine uptake system in catecholamine storage vesicles isolated from a pheochromocytoma taken from a child. Biochem Pharmacol 1984; 33:2245–2252.

707. Grouzmann E, Werffeli-George P, Fathi M, et al. Angiotensin-II mediates norepinephrine and neuropeptide-Y secretion in a human pheochromocytoma. J Clin Endocrinol Metab 1994; 79:1852–1856.

708. Hamilton BP, Landsberg L, Levine RJ. Measurement of urinary epinephrine in screening for pheochromocytoma in multiple endocrine neoplasia Type II. Am J Med 1978; 65:1027–1032.

709. Vistelle R, Grulet H, Gibold C, et al. High permanent plasma adrenaline levels: a marker of adrenal medullary disease in medullary thyroid carcinoma. Clin Endocrinol (Oxf) 1991; 34:133–138.

710. Neumann HPH, Berger DP, Sigmund G, et al. Pheochromocytomas, multiple endocrine neoplasia type 2, and von Hippel-Lindau disease. N Engl J Med 1993; 329:1531–1538.

711. Schimke RN. Multiple endocrine neoplasia: how many syndromes? Am J Med Genet 1990; 37:375–383.

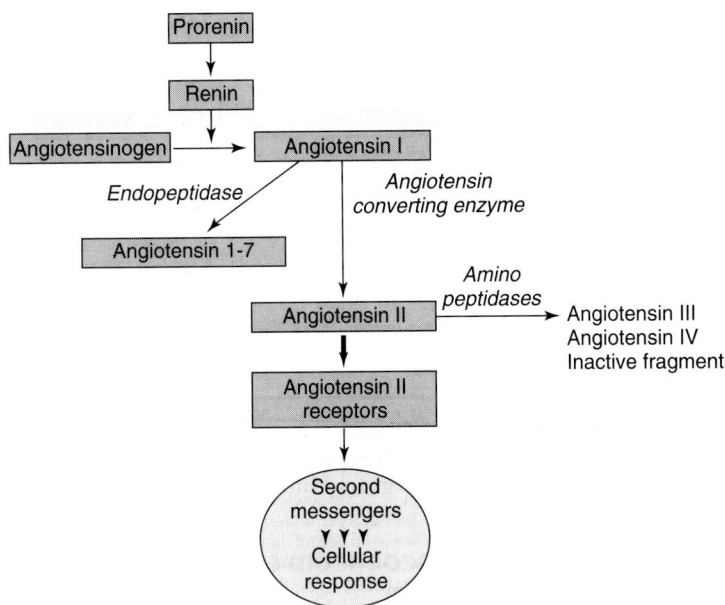

Figure 14–1. Components of the renin-angiotensin system. (Redrawn from Williams GH, Chao J, Chao L. Kidney hormones. In: Conn PM, Melmed S, eds. Endocrinology: Basic and Clinical Principles. Totowa, NJ: Humana Press, 1997, pp 393–404, with permission.)

In tissues that produce renin it is stored in granules and released in response to specific secretagogues. It is a member of the aspartyl proteinase family of enzymes and is synthesized as a pre-proprotein. In humans the gene that encodes renin is located on the short arm of chromosome 1 (1q32–1q42). In the rat the gene is located on chromosome 13, and in the mouse it is located on chromosome 1,[7, 8] (in the mouse, there are two renin genes). In each species the nucleotide sequence is approximately 12 kb, with 10 exons and 9 introns. The transcription product is a 1.5-kb mRNA, and the initial protein consists of 340 amino acids of which the first 43 are a prosegment cleaved to produce the active enzyme.

Renin is termed a "double-domain" enzyme because the N- and the C-terminal halves are very similar.[7] Each domain contains a single aspartic acid residue critical for its catalytic activity. The three-dimensional structure of the enzyme has been characterized. A number of factors can regulate the transcription of the renin gene; consensus elements are present in the 5'-flanking region of the gene, including those for cyclic AMP and a number of steroid receptors (estrogen, progesterone, and glucocorticoids).[7, 8]

Angiotensinogen

Angiotensinogen is the only known substrate for renin and is catabolized to angiotensin peptides. The interaction between enzyme and substrate appears to be species specific, as minor structural variations in the substrate render it relatively inactive in different species.[9] Human angiotensinogen belongs to the serpin superfamily of proteins and is encoded by a gene on chromosome 1q42.3 near the renin gene.[10] The angiotensinogen gene consists of five exons and four introns and is approximately 13 kb long. The transcript encodes a protein of 485 amino acids, 33 of which constitute a presegment that is cleaved following secretion. Angiotensin I is composed of the first 10 amino acid sequence following the presegment. The 5' promoter region has consensus sequences for control by glucocorticoids, estrogens, and cytokines.[11, 12]

Angiotensin-Converting Enzyme

Angiotensin-converting enzyme (ACE), a second enzyme involved in the final production of angiotensin II (see Fig. 14–1), is a dipeptidyl carboxyl zinc metallopeptidase usually found bound to cell membranes.[13] It also is present in intracellular granules in certain tissues that produce angiotensin II. Its molecular weight is considerably larger than renin, and it consists of two homologous domains, suggesting there are two active sites in each molecule. In humans, the ACE gene is located on chromosome 17q23 and consists of 26 exons and 25 introns. Two molecular forms of ACE are products of a single gene but have separate promoter regions. One product is a somatic, or endothelial, ACE that consists of 1306 amino acids, and the second is a germinal ACE with a promoter region upstream from the 13th exon.[14]

Angiotensin Receptors

In humans the two primary forms of the angiotensin receptor are termed "AT$_1$" and "AT$_2$." The AT$_1$ receptor mediates most of the effects of angiotensin II.[15] In humans a single gene on chromosome 3 encodes this receptor, while rats have two genes. The 5'-flanking region contains three putative glucocorticoid response elements. The receptor has seven transmembrane regions, with a disulfide bridge linking the first and fourth extracellular segments. The principal signaling mechanism involved in the AT$_1$ receptor operates through a G$_q$ protein–mediated activation of phospholipase C.[16] However, some data suggest a linkage to protein tyrosine kinase.[17–19] The AT$_2$ receptor gene has three exons and two introns and a seven transmembrane domain structure.[18, 19]

Angiotensin Peptides

At least four angiotensin-like peptides have biologic activity (Table 14–1).[20, 21] The action of renin on angiotensinogen produces angiotensin I, a decapeptide that does not appear to have biologic activity. Angiotensin II is formed by cleavage

TABLE 14–1. Amino Acid Composition of Angiotensin Peptides

AI	Asp-Arg-Val-Tyr-Ile-His-Pro-Phe-His-Leu
AII	Asp-Arg-Val-Tyr-Ile-His-Pro-Phe
A1–7	Asp-Arg-Val-Tyr-Ile-His-Pro
AIII	Arg-Val-Tyr-Ile-His-Pro-Phe
AIV	Val-Tyr-Ile-His-Pro-Phe

A = angiotensin.

of the two carboxyl-terminal peptides by ACE[6] and has full biologic activity. Amino peptidase A can remove the amino-terminal aspartic acid to produce the heptapeptide, angiotensin III. Angiotensin II and III have equivalent efficacy in promoting aldosterone secretion and modifying renal blood flow. However, angiotensin III has less pressor activity. Amino peptidase B can cleave an additional amino acid from angiotensin III to form angiotensin IV (angiotensin 3–8).[21] The function of this peptide is not clear, but it may be involved in the regulation of cerebral circulation and may produce vasodilation rather than vasoconstriction. A fourth biologically active compound is produced from angiotensin I by the action of a propyl endopeptidase to form angiotensin 1–7,[22] the function of which in unclear.

Functions

The effects of the renin-angiotensin system can be mediated by local paracrine effects or through endocrine action.[6, 23] The endocrine system primarily involves renin from the juxtaglomerular apparatus of the kidney and angiotensinogen from the liver. In the circulation the concentrations of each are such that variations in the angiotensinogen levels can modify angiotensin I generation. The half-life in the circulation of angiotensin II is short (probably less than a minute). While circulating levels of angiotensin II are in the picomolar range, its affinity for its receptor is in the nanomolar range, suggesting that some angiotensin II effects may actually be mediated not by the circulating peptide but by its local generation.

Elements of the renin-angiotensin system are present in the adrenal, the kidneys, the heart, and the brain.[23] For example, the adrenal glomerulosa cells contain the proteins needed to produce and secrete angiotensin II.[24] Other tissues contain one or more components of the renin-angiotensin system and require other cells and/or circulating components to generate angiotensin II. For example, fat cells synthesize angiotensinogen, but not renin or ACE, but can generate angiotensin II locally.[25]

Angiotensin II functions to maintain normal extracellular volume and blood pressure in five ways[6]: (1) constriction of vascular smooth muscle, thereby increasing blood pressure and reducing renal blood flow; (2) release of norepinephrine and epinephrine from the adrenal medulla; (3) enhancement of the activity of the sympathetic nervous system by increasing central sympathetic outflow, thereby increasing norepinephrine discharge from sympathetic nerve terminals; (4) promotion of the release of vasopressin; and (5) increasing aldosterone secretion.

Other functions that may possibly contribute to the major function of angiotensin II include (1) central nervous system effects, including modification of thirst or the sense of well-being, or both; (2) modification of the release of corticotropin from the pituitary; (3) possible effects on placental and ovarian function; and (4) modification of growth of the heart, the kidneys, and vascular smooth muscle.[26, 27]

Regulation

Renin

The release of renin into the circulation from the kidneys is controlled by four factors: (1) the macula densa, a specialized group of distal convoluted tubular cells that function as chemoreceptors for monitoring the sodium and chloride loads present in the distal tubule; (2) juxtaglomerular cells acting as miniature pressure transducers that sense renal perfusion pressure; (3) the sympathetic nervous system, which modifies the release of renin, particularly in response to upright posture in humans[6]; and (4) humoral factors including potassium, angiotensin II, and atrial natriuretic peptides. Importantly, the tissue renin-angiotensin systems are not necessarily regulated in the same manner as the circulating renin-angiotensin system.[8, 28, 29] For example, a high potassium intake reduces renal renin release and increases adrenal renin secretion.

Aldosterone

The action of angiotensin II on aldosterone involves a negative-feedback loop that also includes extracellular fluid volume (Fig. 14–2). The major function of this feedback loop is to modify sodium homeostasis and, secondarily, to regulate arterial pressure.[30, 31] Thus, sodium restriction activates the renin-angiotensin-aldosterone axis. The effects of angiotensin II on both the adrenal cortex and the renal vasculature promote renal sodium conservation. Conversely, with suppression of renin release and suppression of the level of circulating angiotensin, aldosterone secretion is reduced, and renal blood flow is increased, thereby promoting sodium loss. In addition to the usual internal regulation of this negative-feedback loop, a secondary fine-tuning component is related to the level of dietary sodium intake.[30, 31] Most endocrine negative-feedback loops are not particularly sensitive to environmental factors. In contrast, the renin-angiotensin-aldosterone loop is exquisitely sensitive to the level of dietary sodium intake. Sodium excess enhances the renal and peripheral vasculature responsiveness and reduces the adrenal responsiveness to angiotensin II (Fig. 14–3). Sodium restriction has the opposite effect. Thus sodium intake modifies, or modulates, target tissue responsiveness to angiotensin II, a fine-tuning that appears to be critical to maintaining normal sodium homeostasis without modifying blood pressure, particularly chronically. The mechanism or mechanisms by which dietary sodium intake induces these changes in the adrenal is unclear, but in the vascular system, the effects are a consequence of angiotensin II's downregulation of the target tissue responsiveness to its agonists.

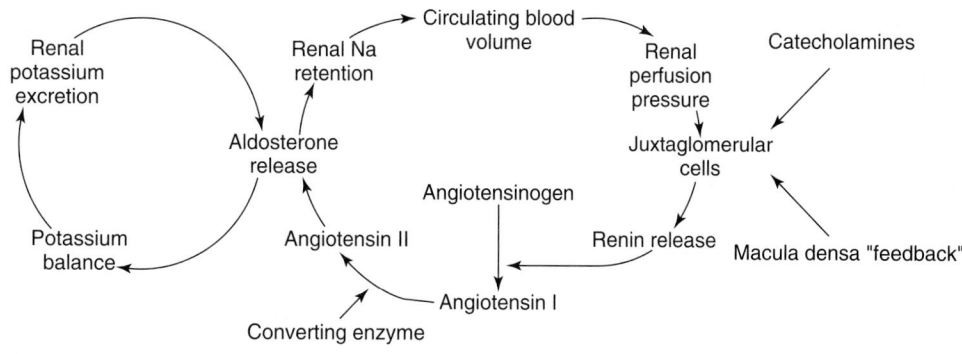

Figure 14–2. Renin-angiotensin-aldosterone and potassium-aldosterone negative-feedback loops. Aldosterone production is determined by input from each loop. (Redrawn from Williams GH, Dluhy RG. Diseases of the adrenal cortex. In: Fauci AD, Braunwald E, Isselbacher KJ, et al, eds. Harrison's Principles of Internal Medicine. 14th ed. New York: McGraw-Hill, 1998, with permission.)

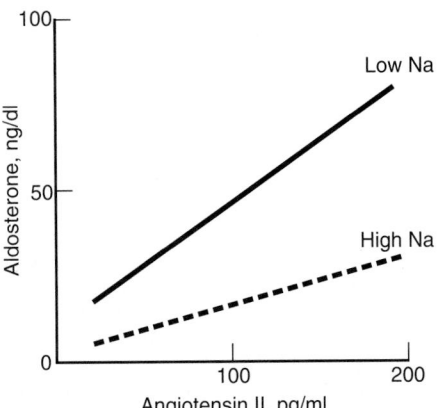
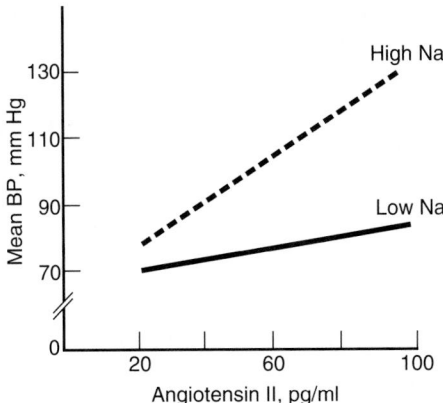

Figure 14–3. Modification of vascular and aldosterone response to angiotensin II by dietary salt intake. Sodium intake has a reciprocal influence on vascular and adrenal responses to angiotensin II. On a high salt intake the vascular response is enhanced while the adrenal response is suppressed. Sodium restriction has the opposite effect. (Redrawn from Williams GH, Hollenberg NK. "Sodium-sensitive" essential hypertension: emerging insights into pathogenesis and therapeutic implications. In: Klahr S, Massry SG, eds. Contemporary Nephrology. Vol 3. New York: Plenum Press, 1985: 303, with permission.)

ESSENTIAL HYPERTENSION

The renin-angiotensin system has a powerful influence on both vasoconstrictor activity and volume regulation. Thus defects in its regulation could lead to a rise in blood pressure by either or both of these mechanisms. Two other hormonal systems are implicated in the pathogenesis of essential hypertension: insulin (either directly or mediated by selective insulin resistance) and the calcium-regulating systems.

Role of the Renin-Angiotensin System in the Pathogenesis of Essential Hypertension

In the late 1960s and early 1970s, Laragh and colleagues developed a classification of hypertension based on the level of circulating renin activity.[32] By controlling dietary sodium and potassium intake, they classified patients into those whose values were low, normal, or high and used this information to define whether an individual case of hypertension was more volume dependent or vasoconstrictor dependent (Fig. 14–4). The model predicted that the individuals with low plasma renin activity (PRA) levels would have a volume-sensitive form of hypertension while those with high plasma levels would have a vasoconstrictor form of hypertension. It was presumed that classifying patients in this manner would lead to a more rational treatment program.

However, several concerns have been raised. First, age modifies the level of renin activity, older subjects having lower renin levels regardless of volume status. Second, race modifies the level of renin activity (whites, in general, have higher levels than blacks). Finally, in individuals who consume a relatively large amount of sodium (greater than 175 mmol/d) low, normal, and high PRA levels are difficult to distinguish from each other. However, the concept of subclassification of hypertensive patients based on the level of renin activity was useful in the development of better approaches to subclassifying patients.

Pathophysiological Mechanisms in Low-Renin Essential Hypertension

Several mechanisms are thought to cause volume expansion and suppress renin activity in some patients with essential hypertension.[33] Adrenal mechanisms may be involved in some subjects with low-renin hypertension because spironolactone (a mineralocorticoid antagonist) and aminoglutethimide (an inhibitor of steroid hormone biosynthesis) substantially reduce blood pressure in them.[34, 35] Wisgerhof and Brown reported that the adrenal response to angiotensin II is enhanced in some low-renin essential hypertensive patients, and that the enhanced responsiveness alters the renin-angiotensin-aldosterone negative-feedback loop, allowing restoration of normal sodium homeostasis with decreased PRA and angiotensin II levels (Fig. 14–5).[36, 37] However, on a normal-to-high sodium intake, this enhanced adrenal response could result in a scenario in which aldosterone secretion would not suppress adequately, thereby promoting sodium retention and an increase in blood pressure. The frequency of this abnormality is unclear, as no population-based studies have been reported.

HIGH RENIN (dry vasoconstriction)		LOW RENIN (wet vasoconstriction)
	PATHOPHYSIOLOGIC DIFFERENCES	
	Arterioles	
Higher	Peripheral resistance	High
High	Aldosterone	Low to High
Low	Plasma volume	High
Low	Cardiac output	High
High	Hematocrit	Low
High	Blood urea	Low
High	Blood viscosity	Low
Low	Tissue perfusion	High
Yes	Postural hypotension	No
	CLINICAL EXAMPLES	
High-renin essential hypertension		Low-renin essential hypertension
Renovascular and malignant hypertension		Primary aldosteronism
	VASCULAR SEQUELAE	
(+)	Stroke	(−)
(+)	Heart attack	(−)
(+)	Renal damage	(−)
(+)	Retinopathy-encephalopathy	(−)
	TREATMENTS	
(+)	Converting enzyme inhibitors	(−)
(+)	β-Blockers	(−)
(−)	Calcium channel blockers	(+)
(−)	Diuretics	(+)
(−)	α-Blockers	(+)

Figure 14–4. Relationship between the activity of the renin-angiotensin system and the mechanisms underlying the hypertension. (Redrawn from Laragh JH, Sealey JE, Niarchos AP, et al. The vasoconstrictor volume spectrum in normotension and in the pathogenesis of hypertension. Fed Proc 41:2415–2423, 1982.)

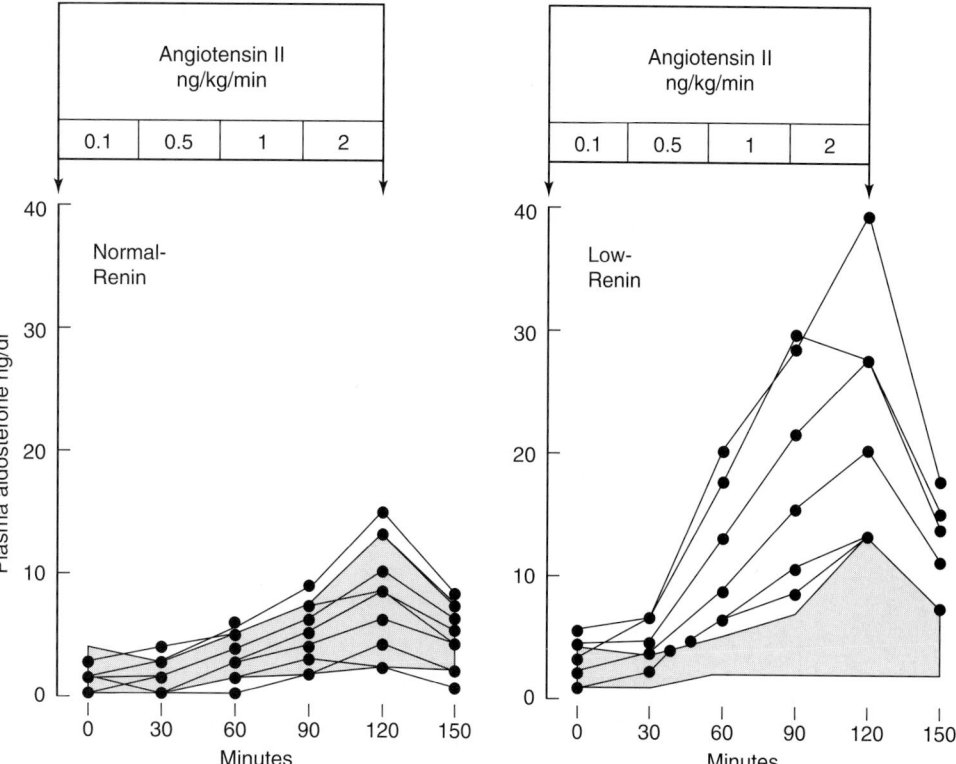

Figure 14–5. Adrenal responses to angiotensin II in normotensive and hypertensive subjects on a normal-to-high sodium intake. The patients with hypertension were divided into low-renin and normal-to-high-renin groups. The responses of normal subjects are shown in the shaded area. Low-renin patients had an enhanced aldosterone response to angiotensin II compared with both normotensive subjects and normal-to-high-renin hypertensive patients. (Redrawn from Wisgerhof M, Brown RD. Increased adrenal sensitivity to angiotensin II in low renin essential hypertension. J Clin Invest 1978; 61:1456–1462, with permission.)

However, even some patients with so-called normal-renin essential hypertension appear to have a similar defect.[38]

Nonmodulating Hypertension: Salt Sensitivity and Normal-to-High Renin Levels

Some patients with normal or high renin levels have a peculiar form of salt-sensitive hypertension in which increased sodium intake failed to change the vascular and the adrenal response to angiotensin II.[39] These patients, termed "nonmodulators," appear to be a subset of the essential hypertensive population, as documented by a bimodal distribution of several of their biochemical features.[40] Patients with these features have been reported from Argentina, Brazil, Japan, the Netherlands, France, Italy, and the United States.[41–43] In whites, the frequency of nonmodulation is between 25 and 30% of hypertensives, and in black hypertensives the frequency is likely to be greater. Nonmodulators share several features in association with low-renin essential hypertensive patients: (1) they both have salt-sensitive hypertension, and (2) they tend to be older than the rest of the hypertensive population. However, nonmodulators have several features that are not similar to low-renin hypertension, including (1) fasting hyperinsulinemia, (2) a positive family history for hypertension and myocardial disease, (3) elevated levels of cholesterol and triglycerides, and (4) a *decreased* adrenal response to angiotensin II as assessed on a sodium-restricted intake. Finally, and perhaps most important, the characteristics associated with nonmodulation distribute in a bimodal fashion in the hypertensive population—suggesting a discrete subgroup.[40, 43–45]

In nonmodulators target tissue responsiveness to angiotensin II does not change when sodium intake is modified. Two functional tests have been used to distinguish them from the rest of the hypertensive population. One measures aldosterone response to a 3 ng/kg/min angiotensin II infusion on a low (10 mEq) salt diet.[39, 40, 46] The other approach is to measure renal blood flow response to the same dose of angio-

tensin II on a high (200 mEq) salt diet.[39, 47] Unless the dietary sodium intake is precisely controlled, a hypertensive subject can be misclassified. The correlation between these two criteria is 70 to 80%.[40, 42] Thus, if feasible, the best approach is to require both criteria to be positive in defining the nonmodulator. Other characteristics of this subset include a failure of renal blood flow to increase when dietary sodium intake is changed from low to high and an enhanced response of atrial natriuretic peptide to infused angiotensin II.[42, 48]

Nonmodulators appear to have an inherited form of hypertension, as evidenced by (1) bimodality of the distribution of the nonmodulating characteristic in the hypertensive population[40]; (2) the presence of the nonmodulating characteristic in normotensive subjects[41]; (3) a strong family history of hypertension in nonmodulators (approximately 80%, compared with about 30% for the rest of the hypertensive population)[45, 48]; (4) familial aggregation of nonmodulating characteristics with hypertension[49]; and (5) the association of the nonmodulating phenotype with individuals who are homozygous for the angiotensinogen 235T genotype (Fig. 14–6).[50]

A defect in the renin-angiotensin system is likely to underlie nonmodulating hypertension, probably a defect in the local renal and adrenal renin-angiotensin systems, as evidenced by the following: (1) a low renal blood flow on a high-sodium diet and a reduced renal vascular response to infused angiotensin II, suggesting inappropriately high local renal angiotensin II levels; (2) correction of the renal blood flow defect by administration of a converting enzyme inhibitor; and (3) correction of the nonmodulating adrenal defect by a converting enzyme inhibitor.[46–48] The effect of sodium intake on blood pressure in nonmodulators has been extensively evaluated. Either short-term (3 d) or chronic (2 wk) salt loading increases blood pressure in nonmodulators, but not in other normal/high renin hypertensive patients.[45, 48] The salt sensitivity of the hypertension is due to the tendency for nonmodulators to retain more of a salt load both acutely and chronically.[48] The abnormality in sodium handling is probably due to the alteration in renal hemodynamics with salt loading described

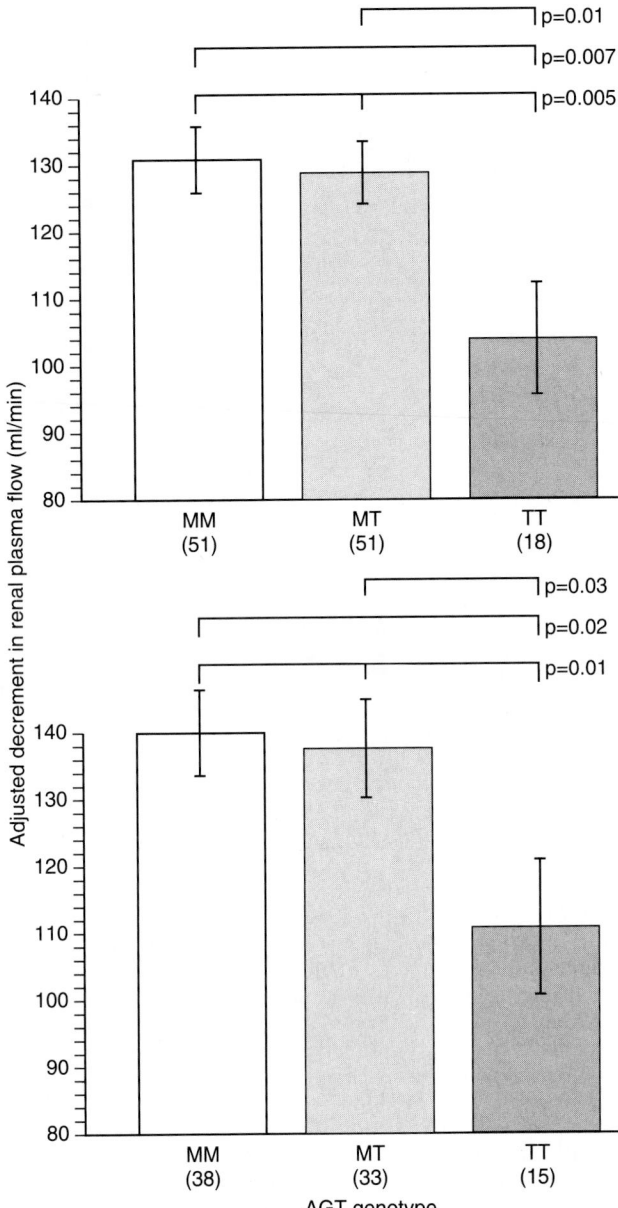

Figure 14–6. Effect of angiotensinogen genotype on renal blood flow responses to angiotensin II infusions. Subjects were classified according to their alleles at the 235 codon of the angiotensinogen gene as to whether they were homozygous for the wild type (MM), heterozygous (MT), or homozygous for the hypertensive-link (TT) alleles. The subjects with the TT235 genotype had a renal blood flow response to angiotensin II similar to that of nonmodulators. (Redrawn from Hopkins P, Lifton RP, Hollenberg NK, et al. Blunted renal vascular response to angiotensin II is associated with a common variant of the angiotensinogen gene and obesity. J Hypertens 1996; 14:199–207, with permission. Copyright 1996, Rapid Science Publishers.)

previously[39, 47] and secondary to an inappropriately high local angiotensin II level. Support for this conclusion comes from correction of salt-sensitive hypertension in nonmodulators by converting enzyme inhibitors.

In summary, nonmodulators are a distinct subgroup of the essential hypertensive population and may constitute as many as 30% of that population. They have a sodium-sensitive form of hypertension, probably owing to a derangement of the local renin-angiotensin system in the kidney and the adrenal (Fig. 14–7). These patients also have insulin resistance, hypercholesterolemia, a family history positive for myocardial infarction, and an association with a specific allelic variant of the angiotensinogen gene. Finally, the defect appears to be correctable by the administration of converting enzyme inhibitors.

Insulin Resistance and Hypertension

Non–insulin-dependent diabetes mellitus (NIDDM), hypertension, and obesity are commonly associated, and the frequency of this association may be greater than their occurrence in the general population (see the review by Hopkins and colleagues[51]), suggesting a common etiology. In support of this possibility is the fact that insulin resistance and hypertension can coexist without obesity or other stigmata of NIDDM.[52–53] There may be a genetic component to this interaction. For example, in whites of European descent there is a strong relation between insulin resistance and blood pressure, while in normotensive blacks or Pima Indians there is no such relationship (Fig. 14–8).[54] However, most hypertensive blacks are insulin resistant.

Causative Role of Insulin in Hypertension

Several mechanisms have been proposed to explain the insulin-resistant state, including abnormalities in insulin binding to its receptor, defects in glucose transport, changes in the signal transduction pathway within insulin-sensitive cells, and metabolic abnormalities in glycolysis, glucose oxidation, and/or glucagon synthesis. Yet little is known concerning the cause of insulin resistance in essential hypertension (reviewed in reference 51)(Fig. 14–9). Several features are relevant. First, insulin resistance is common but not unusual in essential hypertension whether defined by fasting and/or post–glucose load insulin levels or by euglycemic, hyperinsulinemic clamps.[55–57] Second, obesity cannot explain all cases of insulin resistance. Third, insulin directly stimulates the calcium pump in insulin-sensitive tissues and promotes calcium loss from the cell,[58] and raising cytosolic calcium levels in an adipocyte can induce insulin resistance.[59–60] If a cell is resistant to insulin, the insulin-induced calcium loss from cells would be decreased, and in vascular smooth muscle cells the resultant increase in intracellular calcium would enhance responsiveness to vasoconstrictors and increase blood pressure.

Two other mechanisms have been proposed to explain

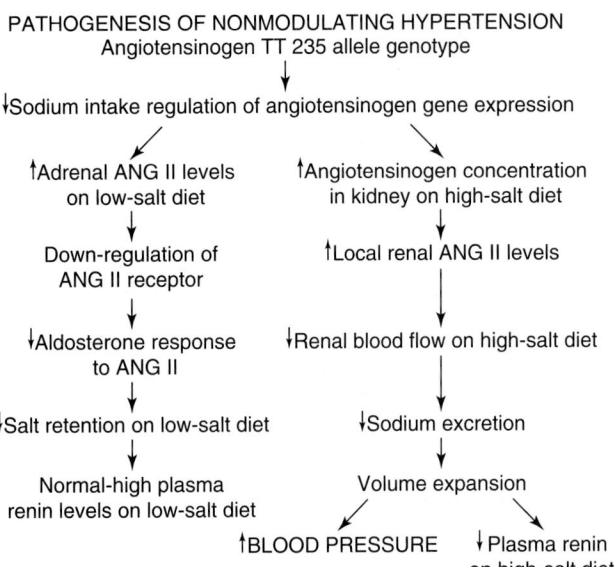

Figure 14–7. Pathogenesis of nonmodulating hypertension.

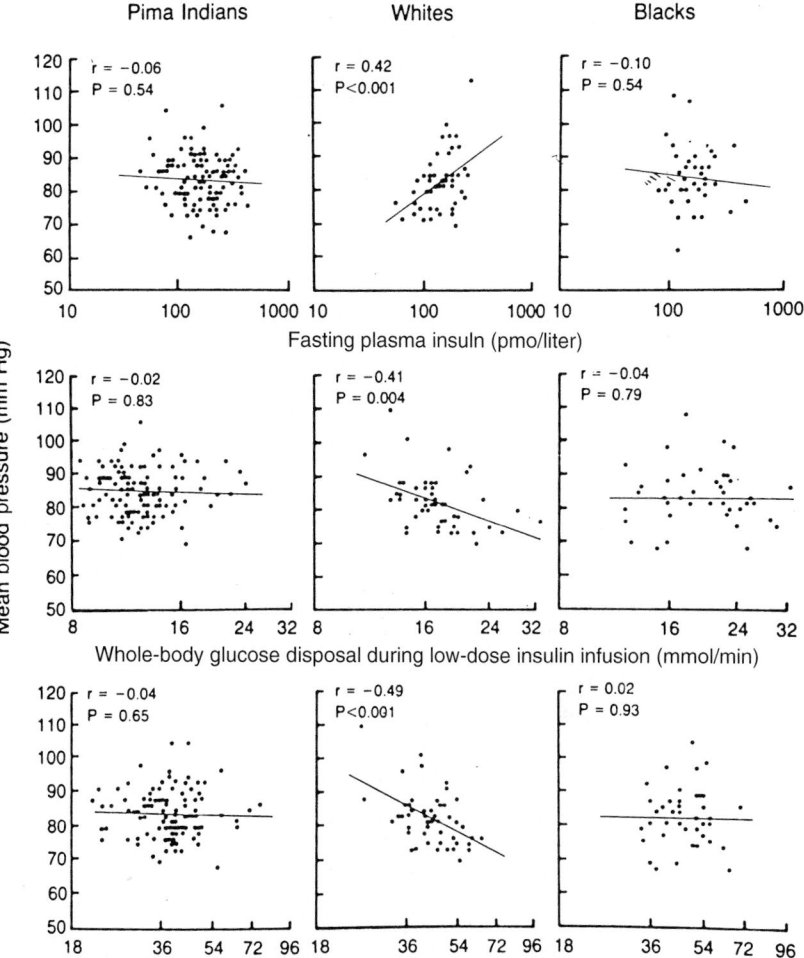

Figure 14–8. Relationship of arterial pressure to insulin resistance in normotensive ethnic subgroups. An index of insulin sensitivity, glucose disposal rate, was determined by an insulin clamp and fasting insulin levels were measured in normotensive blacks, whites, and Pima Indians. There was a significant negative correlation between arterial blood pressure and glucose disposal rates in whites, but not in the other subgroups. (From Saad MF, Lillioja S, Nyomba BL, et al. Racial differences in the relationship between arterial pressure and insulin resistance. N Engl J Med 1991; 324:733–739, with permission. Copyright 1991, Massachusetts Medical Society.)

the linkage between insulin resistance and hypertension: an increased activity of the adrenergic nervous system[61] and increased renal sodium retention.[62] Underlying both these hypotheses is the assumption that insulin resistance in a hypertensive subject may be selective. Accordingly, insulin resistance in the skeletal muscle and/or liver would induce a rise in circulating insulin levels. However, there would be little, if any, resistance at the renal tubule or adrenergic nervous system.

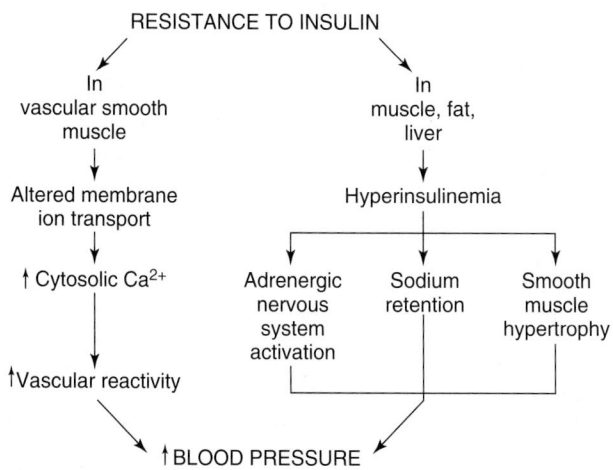

Figure 14–9. Mechanisms by which insulin resistance may produce hypertension.

Finally, for the vasoconstrictor hypothesis to be correct, there would have to be an imbalance between insulin's direct vasodilator effect and the vasoconstriction induced by activation of the adrenergic nervous system.

A hyperinsulinemic response to glucose loading[63] and insulin resistance[64] have been described in salt-sensitive, but not in salt-resistant, normotensives. This salt sensitivity also extends to metabolic abnormalities that are often associated with insulin resistance, such as increased levels of circulating low-density lipoprotein (LDL) cholesterol in salt-sensitive hypertensives, compared with salt-resistant hypertensives.[65] Thus, salt sensitivity of blood pressure is associated with lipid and glucose metabolic abnormalities and increased cardiovascular risk. Impaired insulin sensitivity[66] and hyperlipidemia[67] have been described in healthy volunteers with normal-to-high plasma renin levels, compared with those with low-renin levels. Thus there is an inconsistency in the data derived from these sources. Individuals who are salt sensitive, as noted earlier, are likely to have low PRA. Yet salt-sensitive subjects as a group also have an increased risk of carbohydrate and lipid abnormalities.

In summary, insulin resistance occurs in some patients with essential hypertension who do not have obesity or NIDDM. Several lines of evidence suggest that insulin resistance per se and/or hyperinsulinemia could result in increased sodium reabsorption, enhanced vascular tone, and activation of the adrenergic nervous system. Alternatively, this state could be associated with abnormal regulation of the renin-angiotensin system. Importantly, environmental factors can aggravate this defect. For example, if patients with insulin resistance gain weight and/or receive drugs that increase insulin resistance, e.g., diuretics or β-blockers, the hypertension could be aggravated. However, it is still unclear whether the insulin resistance is a marker for some other abnormality or a primary defect in these patients.

Calcium and Hypertension

In 1982 McCarron and co-workers reported that dietary calcium intake in humans with hypertension was lower than in normotensive controls,[68] and the inverse relation between blood pressure and calcium intake has been confirmed in epidemiologic studies.[69, 70] These studies also suggest an association between the level of calcium intake and the degree of sensitivity of the blood pressure to sodium intake. In part this may not be surprising given the known relationship between the reabsorption of calcium and that of sodium by the proximal tubule of the kidney. Blood pressure, in part, may also correlate with magnesium intake, at least in women.[69] Indeed, the relative risk of developing hypertension was 0.65 when both magnesium (<200 mg/d) and calcium (<400 mg/d) intakes were lower. Importantly, there appears to be a critical threshold for the effect of calcium intake on blood pressure, the effect not being evident unless calcium intake is less than 700 to 800 mg/d.[71] Thus, increasing calcium intake above this threshold may not modify blood pressure.

Clinical trials designed to evaluate the validity of these observational data have provided equivocal results. However, meta-analysis of these trials suggests that high calcium intake causes a minimal reduction of blood pressure in the general population and a modest reduction in individuals who already have hypertension. In one meta-analysis[72] in 2412 subjects, high calcium intake reduced systolic blood pressure 1.33 mm Hg in the general population and 4.3 mm Hg in hypertensive patients. Hypertensive subjects also had a significant reduction in diastolic blood pressure (1.5 mm Hg). A second meta-analysis involving 1231 individuals did not demonstrate as large an effect.[73]

Pathophysiological Mechanisms

Identification of the mechanisms responsible for the impact of calcium intake on blood pressure is uncertain. Some studies have shown that parathyroid hormone (PTH) levels, on average, are higher in hypertensives compared with normal control subjects, suggesting a potential role for PTH in mediating hypertension. However, PTH levels in hypertensive patients are still within the normal range and are not inappropriate for the level of ionized calcium. Thus, it is unclear whether the elevated PTH causes an increase in blood pressure or is simply a reflection of a modest change in calcium homeostasis. Furthermore, when infused, PTH is a vasodilator,[74] and PTH inhibits contraction of vascular smooth muscle, presumably by inhibiting calcium entry.[75]

Pang and colleagues have suggested that there is a specific hypertensive factor from the parathyroid gland, distinct from PTH, that is increased in some patients with essential hypertension.[76] Several studies in experimental hypertension suggest that the plasma level of the factor is elevated and that it can modify vascular smooth muscle function by increasing cytosolic calcium levels.[77] In some patients with hyperparathyroidism and hypertension, parathyroid hypertensive factor is said to be elevated and following parathyroidectomy becomes undetectable as blood pressure decreases.[78] However, only a single group has reported on the presence of such a factor.

PTHrP, a peptide with a structure similar to that of PTH but derived from a different gene, appears to share with PTH an ability to produce vasodilation. It has been suggested that

a deficiency in PTHrP could lead to an elevated blood pressure, as this substance may be produced to counteract the effect of vasoconstrictors.[79]

Finally, the active metabolite of vitamin D (1,25-dihydroxycholecalciferol) increases calcium uptake in cardiac and vascular smooth muscle cells, induces vascular contractions, and exerts a myotrophic effect on vascular smooth muscle.[80] Patients with low-renin or salt-sensitive hypertension tend to have an increase in both PTH and 1,25-dihydroxycholecalciferol levels. With sodium loading, levels of both hormones increase further as the blood pressure increases. However, as with the changes in PTH levels, it is difficult to determine a cause-and-effect relationship. For example, the increase in 1,25-dihydroxycholecalciferol levels in these patients may be secondary to the higher PTH level, since PTH stimulates 1α-hydroxylase activity.

In brief, epidemiologic and experimental evidence suggests that calcium and calcium-regulating hormones play a role in the control of vascular tone. Meta-analyses of clinical trials support a blood pressure–lowering effect of a high calcium intake, particularly in patients with essential hypertension. However, the mechanism or mechanisms involved and the relationship of the effects of calcium intake to the effects of sodium intake on blood pressure are still unclear. Finally, it is uncertain how many of these associations are primary versus secondary events.

Summary

Several lines of evidence suggest that many patients with essential hypertension have an endocrine basis for elevated blood pressure. Increased circulating hormone levels, changes in the responsiveness of target tissues to these hormones, and abnormalities in vascular tone all can contribute to the pathogenesis of the hypertension. Whether these endocrine abnormalities are primary or secondary events is unclear. Intriguingly, most do not fit the classic endocrine pattern for disease, since hormonal overproduction is rare. Rather, there is a change in the response of target tissues to specific hormones, with associated adaptive responses probably the major contributor to the hypertensive process. Finally, a number of the abnormalities appear to have a major genetic component. This fact makes possible a more precise dissection of subgroups or phenotypes of hypertensive patients with the use of genetic markers.

RENIN-ANGIOTENSIN SYSTEM AND SECONDARY HYPERTENSION

In addition to the involvement of the renin-angiotensin system in primary hypertension, it is also a major factor in the most common cause of secondary hypertension: hypertension associated with renal disease. Indeed, many insights into the renin-angiotensin system have come from the study of patients with renal disease.

Renal Vascular Hypertension

Goldblatt and colleagues described the pathologic role of excess renin production in the hypertension associated with constriction of a renal artery,[81] and 4 y after their observations, a nephrectomy in a hypertensive patient with a small kidney led to correction of the hypertension.[82] Thus, renal vascular hypertension is defined as hypertension associated with either unilateral or bilateral ischemia. Unilateral renal vascular disease is likely to be the cause of elevated blood pressure in approximately 1% of the hypertensive population, and bilateral renal parenchymal disease is causative in another 2 to 4%.[83] It is important to distinguish between renal vascular *disease* and renal vascular *hypertension*. Perhaps 50% or more of subjects older than 60 years of age have renal vascular disease, only a minority of whom also have hypertension.[84] This discrepancy is not surprising when one considers Goldblatt's original experiment, which documented that the lumen of the renal artery needs to be reduced to less than 30% of its original size before hypertension develops. Documentation of a *functional abnormality* in association with a radiologically defined renal arterial lesion is a critical diagnostic maneuver prior to therapeutic intervention.

African-Americans and patients with diabetes mellitus seem to have a lower frequency of renal vascular hypertension, even though in both groups the incidence of renal vascular disease is higher than in the nondiabetic white population.[83] Most patients with renal vascular disease have either atherosclerotic plaques or fibromuscular disease, and in 10% of the cases the lesion may not be in the main renal artery, but in a segmental or branch artery (Table 14–2).

Pathophysiology

The initiating event in the hypertension in subjects with renal disease is a reduction in perfusion pressure to the affected kidney, which stimulates the release of renin.[6, 83] The increased production of renin leads to increased angiotensin II levels and increased aldosterone secretion (secondary aldosteronism) (see Fig. 14–2). As a consequence of the hyperaldosteronism, sodium is retained and potassium is lost. The combination of angiotensin II–induced vasoconstriction and sodium retention increases blood pressure and leads to a natriuresis through the contralateral kidney. The increased levels of renin, elevated blood pressure, and sodium retention all act in concert to suppress renin production from the contralateral kidney, an important feature in the diagnostic evaluation of these patients. With bilateral renal arterial disease, the vasculature to both kidneys is compromised, both kidneys are damaged, or both. Thus, the ability of the kidneys to excrete sodium is reduced, a gradual volume expansion occurs, and circulating renin levels are suppressed.

In long-standing unilateral renal artery stenosis, the contralateral kidney may become damaged secondary to the elevated blood pressure.[85] Thus, the affected kidney is protected by the stenotic lesion and may ultimately suffer less damage, except for the ischemia induced by the stenosis. In these cases correction of the renal artery stenosis may not correct the elevated blood pressure, which can be sustained by the diffusely damaged contralateral kidney. Paradoxically, in this circumstance repair of the renal artery stenosis and removal of the contralateral kidney may normalize blood pressure.

While renal vascular hypertension occurs in all age groups, the etiology varies. In individuals younger than 50 years of age, renal vascular hypertension is more common in women and is usually secondary to fibromuscular dysplasia of the renal artery. After the age of 50 it is more likely to be secondary to atherosclerosis and therefore more common in men. In addition to unilateral or bilateral vascular insufficiency, generalized renal ischemia can result from renal compression, such as in hydronephrosis. Initially the kidney is enlarged, but over time cortical atrophy develops.

Diagnosis

Renal vascular hypertension should be suspected in a normotensive individual of any age who has sudden onset of hypertension, in a known hypertensive subject with an acute acceleration of blood pressure, or in an individual younger than 30 years of age who has significant hypertension. Other clinical features are suggestive of this condition (Fig. 14–10). In general, if the hypertension is mild to moderate (diastolic blood pressure ≤ 105 mm Hg) with an onset between ages 30 and 60 years, the probability of renal vascular hypertension is low. In these patients a detailed search for renal vascular hypertension is probably not warranted.

The diagnosis of renal vascular hypertension requires two criteria: (1) the identification of a significant arterial obstruction, and (2) evidence of excess renin secretion by the affected kidney.[86, 87] Previously, the rapid-sequence intravenous pyelogram (IVP) was the standard screening test for renal vascular hypertension; features consistent with chronic renal ischemia include a difference in kidney size greater than 1.5 cm; unilateral early delay in the appearance and excretion of the contrast material in the affected kidney; indentation on the ureter or renal pelvis secondary to dilated collateral ureteral arteries; and hyperconcentration of contrast medium in the smaller kidney in later images. However, in most centers other tests have replaced the IVP:

1. *Captopril renogram.* Captopril, a converting enzyme inhibitor, is administered 30 to 60 min prior to the renogram.[88, 89] This test takes advantage of the dependency of the hemodynamics of the renal vasculature on angiotensin II, since both the efferent and the afferent arterioles are highly sensitive to the vasoconstrictor actions of angiotensin II. Indeed a balanced constriction of these two vessels maintains a normal glomerular filtration rate under a variety of changes in renal blood flow, so-called renal autoregulation. An increase in angiotensin II levels secondary to unilateral stenosis of a renal artery leads to vasoconstriction of the afferent and

---

TABLE 14–2. Causes of Renal Vascular Hypertension

Atherosclerosis (65–75%)
Fibromuscular dysplasia (25–30%)
Miscellaneous (1%)
    Extrinsic, e.g., hematoma, pheochromocytoma, fibrous
      band, retroperitoneal fibrosis
    Intrinsic, e.g., emboli, arteritis, transplant rejection,
      Ask-Upmark kidney

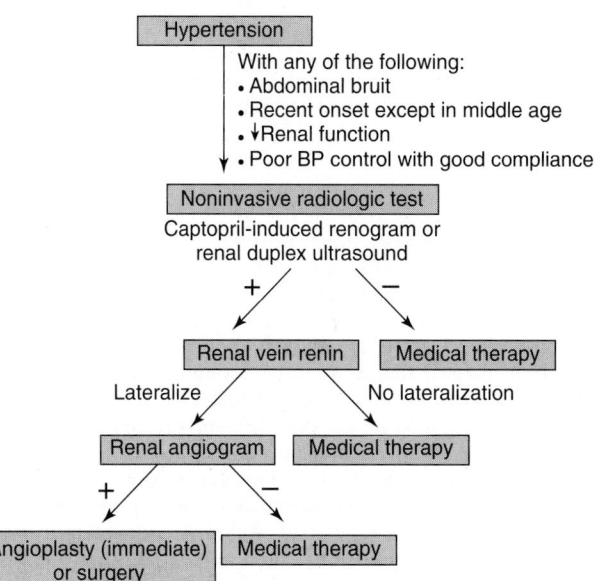

Figure 14–10. Diagnostic and therapeutic flow chart for evaluating patients for renovascular hypertension.

efferent arterioles in both kidneys. Because of the stenotic lesion on the affected side, blood flow to the glomerulus, and therefore glomerular pressure, on this side is determined primarily by the structural lesion. When a converting enzyme inhibitor (which reduces intrarenal angiotensin II levels) is given, angiotensin II–induced afferent arteriolar constriction is reduced in both kidneys. In the unaffected contralateral kidney there is a concomitant reduction in efferent arteriolar tone, an increase in blood flow, and no change in glomerular filtration rate. However in the stenotic kidney, where perfusion of the glomeruli is restricted by the stenosis, a reduction in efferent arteriolar tone results in a fall in glomerular filtration rate and a reduced uptake and delayed excretion of the isotopic tracer as assessed by the renogram.

2. *Digital subtraction angiogram.* This procedure is used in some centers,[86, 90] but because of the cost and the need for arterial rather than venous injection, its role as a screening test is limited.

3. *Renal duplex ultrasound.* This test provides both a functional (from Doppler) and an anatomic (B-mode imaging) evaluation of the renal artery and renal perfusion. While in theory this may be an ideal screening test, in practice its validity is dependent on the skills of the radiologist.[86, 87, 90, 91] Thus it has not been widely utilized.

4. The definitive test for a correctable renal vascular lesion is the combination of *bilateral renal vein renin sampling* and a *selective renal arteriogram.* As noted earlier the renal arteriogram alone defines structural lesions but does not provide insight into their functional significance. Simultaneous bilateral renal vein renin measurement provides a valuable adjunct for predicting whether therapeutic intervention will modify the hypertension. When one kidney is ischemic and the other is normal, nearly all the circulating renin is produced by the affected side. As a result the venous concentration of renin from the ischemic kidney will be at least 1.5 times greater than that from the contralateral kidney. Theoretically, the renin concentration from the contralateral kidney should be the same as that in the peripheral circulation. Unfortunately, in many circumstances there is a varying degree of damage to the contralateral kidney, and therefore total suppression of renin from that kidney does not occur. Some administer captopril before renal vein sampling to exaggerate the renin release from the stenotic side; all agents that suppress renin secretion, such as β-blockers, should be withheld prior to the study. If feasible, the patient also should be placed on a low sodium intake to enhance renin release from the affected kidney. If these procedures are followed, approximately 80% of subjects with unilateral renin elevations that fulfill the aforementioned criteria will have a beneficial response to therapeutic intervention.

Treatment

The treatment of choice in renal artery stenosis is renal angioplasty with or without insertion of a stent.[87, 92, 93] Lesions at the ostium of the renal artery often do not respond well to angioplasty alone, but the addition of a stent may improve outcome. Surgical revascularization, previously the primary approach, is used less frequently in older adults with atherosclerotic lesions because the surgical risk is high in these individuals. Thus surgery is usually reserved for individuals in whom angioplasty has proved unsuccessful.

Medical management may be appropriate in individuals who are not candidates for definitive corrective procedures or in whom those procedures have failed.[94] Converting enzyme inhibitors or an angiotensin II receptor antagonist would be the treatment of choice, given the pathophysiology of the disease. However, for the reasons outlined earlier, these agents may worsen ischemia in the affected kidney. Converting enzyme inhibitors should be used with great caution in individuals who may have bilateral renal artery disease or arterial disease in a solitary kidney, as these agents may reduce glomerular filtration rate, cause renal hypoxia, and precipitate renal failure.

Primary Reninism

Rarely, juxtaglomerular cell tumors of the kidney or ectopic tumors secrete renin.[95] Such individuals have typical features of renal vascular hypertension: hypertension, elevated renin levels, hypokalemia, and hyponatremia. Most, however, are young and have high circulating levels of renin in the blood and also severe hypertension at the time of diagnosis. When a mass lesion is discovered in the kidney, there is unilateral renin secretion but no evidence of renal artery stenosis. Radiologic evaluation with computed tomography scanning is invaluable. Surgical removal of the tumor cures the hypertension and the hyperreninemia.

Renal Parenchymal Disease

A variety of conditions can cause hypertension associated with renal parenchymal disease—the most common of which are hypertension per se, diabetes mellitus, and autoimmune disease (e.g., systemic lupus erythematosus). In these patients there is the potential, depending on the level of sodium intake, of a shift from a vasoconstrictor (angiotensin II) form of hypertension to a volume-sensitive hypertension secondary to decreased capacity for renal sodium excretion. The local (intrarenal) renal renin-angiotensin system is activated to a variable degree in these subjects. This activation results in an elevation of hydraulic pressure in the glomeruli (so-called glomerular hypertension) secondary to the vasoconstrictor effect of angiotensin II on the efferent arteriole as noted earlier.[96] Chronic elevation of glomerular pressure leads to glomerular sclerosis and a progressive loss of functioning nephron units.

The administration of converting enzyme inhibitors can slow the progression of renal damage in both diabetic and nondiabetic renal parenchymal disease.[97, 98] This effect appears to be an added action of converting enzyme inhibitors beyond their ability to lower systemic blood pressure, probably because they also selectively reduce renal glomerular pressure. Thus agents that produce a decrease in systemic blood pressure equivalent to that accomplished by converting enzyme inhibitors do not afford the same degree of protection of renal function. However, caution should be exercised in administering converting enzyme inhibitors to patients who may have an increased risk of bilateral renal artery stenosis. In such circumstances, instead of improvement, converting enzyme inhibitors would cause a sudden deterioration of renal function.[99] Interestingly, the renal-protective actions of converting enzyme inhibitors work in advanced diabetic nephropathy, a condition usually associated with hyporeninemic hypoaldosteronism. Because of the possible further reduction of aldosterone production with converting enzyme inhibitors in such patients, frequent measurement of serum potassium levels is mandatory, with institution of appropriate measures to reduce potassium levels if hyperkalemia occurs (e.g., low-potassium diet, potassium-wasting diuretics). In some instances the converting enzyme inhibitor may have to be discontinued.

Hypertension During Pregnancy

Pregnancy-induced hypertension (PIH), or gestational hypertension, is defined as de novo hypertension arising during the second half of pregnancy. The literature regarding the prevalence and pathophysiological abnormalities in this disorder is clouded by studies that have often included pregnant patients with chronic hypertension. The classification of hypertensive disorders of pregnancy developed by the American College of Obstetricians and Gynecologists has been adopted by the National Institutes of Health[100]:

1. *Chronic hypertension*: blood pressure greater than 140/90 mm Hg before pregnancy or before the 20th wk of pregnancy

2. *Preeclampsia*: a systolic blood pressure increase of at least 30 mm Hg or a diastolic blood pressure increase of at least 15 mm Hg over prepregnancy or early pregnancy values, combined with proteinuria ($\geq$300 mg/24 h) and/or edema

3. *Preeclampsia superimposed on chronic hypertension*: the same criteria as for No. 2, but occurring in women with pre-existing hypertension

4. *Transient hypertension*: a blood pressure increase similar to that in preeclampsia but without proteinuria or edema

Preeclampsia may also progress to eclampsia, defined as the occurrence of convulsions. As viewed by the aforementioned classification, pregnancy-induced hypertension includes preeclampsia and transient hypertension of pregnancy. However, the prognosis of each is different. The preeclampsia form of PIH is self-limited and usually does not occur in subsequent pregnancies, whereas chronic hypertension commonly complicates all pregnancies. Importantly, preeclampsia increases both maternal and fetal morbidity and mortality.

Risk Factors for Pregnancy-Induced Hypertension

Pregnancy-induced hypertension arises in approximately 5% of nulliparous pregnant women, and the prevalence appears to be related to both environmental and genetic factors. For example, the prevalence of PIH is double in indigent, inner-city pregnant women. Other risk factors include nulliparity, low dietary calcium intake, multiple gestations, black race, chronic hypertension, increasing age, and a history of a mother who had this syndrome.[101]

Pathophysiology

Pathophysiological abnormalities in PIH should be divided into those in preeclampsia versus those in transient hypertension of pregnancy. In normal pregnancy, plasma volume increases by 40%,[102] associated with a reduction in peripheral vascular resistance (40 to 80%) and a rise in cardiac output, renal blood flow, and glomerular filtration rate.[103] The renin-angiotensin-aldosterone system is activated despite the increase in plasma volume.[104] This activation is believed to be related to prostanoids, e.g., prostacyclin and prostaglandin E_2 (PGE_2), direct effects of estrogen, and/or an antinatriuretic action of progesterone.

A number of alterations have been reported in subjects with PIH, although many investigations do not clearly distinguish between patients with preeclampsia and those with transient hypertension of pregnancy. Table 14–3 presents the findings in preeclampsia compared with normotensive pregnancy. Plasma volume is reduced in preeclamptics,[105–107] and systemic vascular resistance is increased.[108, 109] Paradoxically, the hormonal markers of volume are consistent with a volume-expanded state: relative suppression of the renin-angiotensin-aldosterone system and increased levels of atrial natriuretic peptide[110–112] and digitalis-like factor (DLF)[113] This apparent paradox is unexplained unless these hormonal changes induce the volume changes or there is a misperception of extracellular fluid volume in this disorder. On the other hand, elevated levels of DLF, an inhibitor of the Na$^+$,K$^+$-ATPase pump, could increase intracellular sodium levels, as has been

TABLE 14–3. Pathophysiological Changes in Preeclampsia Compared with Normal Pregnancy

Cardiovascular Measurements
Reduced circulating plasma volume
Increased systemic vascular resistance
Decreased cardiac index

Hormonal Indicators of Volume
Reduced circulating plasma renin activity (PRA), angiotensin II, and aldosterone
Enhanced angiotensin II pressor responsiveness
Increased levels of atrial natriuretic peptide (ANP)
Increased levels of digitalis-like factor (DLF)

Other Hormonal Alterations
Hyperinsulinemia and insulin resistance
Decreased prostacyclin and/or elevated thromboxane production

reported in red blood cells in patients with PIH.[114] The role of DLF is controversial however, owing to disparate findings between digoxin-like immunoreactivity versus measurement by bioassay, i.e., inhibition of Na$^+$,K$^+$-ATPase.[115]

Enhanced maternal vascular reactivity is also seen in PIH with increased pressor sensitivity to infused angiotensin II even in normotensive phases of pregnancies—before patients progress to PIH. In contrast, in normal pregnancies pressor responsiveness to angiotensin II is blunted. One important hypothesis that could explain these observations includes decreased production of vasodilatory prostaglandins, such as PGE_1 and prostacyclin[116]; in fact, decreased prostacyclin production may precede the appearance of hypertension in PIH.[117] Others propose a relative increase in the vasoconstriction prostaglandin, thromboxane. Reported cation abnormalities include increased intracellular calcium and enhanced responses of intracellular calcium to vasopressin in platelets of patients with PIH.[118] These findings suggest that parallel changes might occur in vascular smooth muscle, where intracellular calcium is a major determinant of peripheral vascular resistance. It is unclear whether the aforementioned abnormalities in PIH reflect initiating events or are secondary alterations that sustain the elevation of blood pressure.

One unifying hypothesis to explain PIH is uteroplacental hypoperfusion. Perhaps secondary to structural abnormalities in the spiral arteries supplying the uterus, uterine blood flow is impaired. Through unknown mechanisms, prostaglandin production is reduced, and there is generalized endothelial damage (endothelin levels are elevated in PIH). Subsequently, platelet aggregation is enhanced, fibrin is deposited in the glomeruli, and proteinuria occurs. Although this is an attractive hypothesis, a number of links need to be established.

Treatment

There is little evidence that sodium restriction improves the outcome of pregnancy in women with PIH or is effective for prophylaxis against PIH.[119] On the other hand, some studies suggest that volume expansion may improve both blood pressure as well as outcome in preeclampsia.[120] It now appears that a moderate-to-liberal sodium diet should be recommended to pregnant women and that the diet should also be adequate in calcium. Bed rest with lateral recumbency is commonly recommended for women with PIH and is believed to cause hemodynamic improvements, including increased renal and uterine blood flow and reduced peripheral vascular resistance with lowering of systemic blood pressure.

Low-dose aspirin (50 to 100 mg/d) may reduce the incidence of PIH, although the results of several large trials remain controversial. The rationale for low-dose aspirin is to restore the balance between vasodilator and vasoconstrictor prostaglandins (primarily by reducing thromboxane A_2 but without affecting prostacyclin levels).[121, 122] Antihypertensive agents are usually given when diastolic blood pressure exceeds 100 mm Hg. Traditional agents include methyldopa and hydralazine. α-Blockers, such as prazosin, and calcium channel blockers, primarily nifedipine, are being used with increased frequency owing to their greater efficacy. These agents also appear to have acceptable safety profiles, although they have not been used as long as have the traditional drugs. Angiotensin-converting enzyme inhibitors and angiotensin receptor antagonists are contraindicated in PIH owing to adverse effects on kidney development in the fetus.

PRIMARY MINERALOCORTICOID-EXCESS STATES

Primary mineralocorticoid-excess states are characterized by suppressed PRA and hypokalemia and include primary aldosteronism, deoxycorticosterone (DOC)-secreting tumors, congenital adrenal hyperplasia, the syndrome of apparent mineralocorticoid excess (AME), including licorice ingestion; and Liddle's syndrome (Table 14–4).

Primary Aldosteronism

Primary aldosteronism, the cause of approximately .05 to 2.2% of all unselected cases of hypertension, was first described in 1955 by Conn in conjunction with an aldosterone-producing adrenal adenoma (APA).[123] Other etiologies include idiopathic bilateral hyperplasia (idiopathic hyperaldosteronism) and glucocorticoid-remediable aldosteronism (GRA).

Clinical Features

The clinical symptoms of primary aldosteronism are nonspecific and result from potassium depletion. Neuromuscular symptoms (weakness, periodic paralysis, cramps, or tetany), fatigue, and paresthesias are not uncommon; polyuria and nocturia probably result from a hypokalemia-induced renal concentrating defect. Hypertensive retinopathy in patients with primary hyperaldosteronism, as in essential hypertension, correlates with the severity and duration of the elevated blood pressure. Despite the continuous high levels of aldosterone, patients rarely exhibit edema presumably owing to "escape," in which the sodium-retaining effects of chronic mineralocorticoid excess are lost. Intracellular potassium depletion can also impair insulin secretion and cause glucose intolerance or overt diabetes mellitus. Resetting of the osmostat can occur in primary aldosteronism, as evidenced by slightly higher than normal serum sodium levels.[124] This is a useful clinical point because there is a tendency toward a reduced serum sodium level in states of secondary aldosteronism.

The hypertension associated with primary aldosteronism is usually moderate to severe with mean blood pressures (±SD) of $184 \pm 28/112 \pm 16$ mm Hg.[125] However, some patients have malignant hypertension, and others have normal or only mildly elevated blood pressure. Individuals with APA tend to have higher blood pressures than those with idiopathic hyperaldosteronism (IHA).[126] Patients with primary aldosteronism may be refractory to conventional antihypertensive agents and may develop severe hypokalemia after institution of potassium-wasting diuretics such as hydrochlorothiazide. Although it would be anticipated that the hypertension is related to volume expansion, measurements of extracellular sodium spaces in APA patients are usually normal, while peripheral resistance is increased.

Mineralocorticoid-excess states are associated with vascular remodeling that results in perivascular fibrosis and vascular wall thickening. Cardiac fibrosis has also been reported in postmortem studies of adrenal adenoma patients with mineralocorticoid hypertension.[127] An excessive number of renal cysts has also been noted in association with hypokalemia and hyperaldosteronism (in as many as 60% of cases).[128] However, other studies report a prevalence of renal cysts similar to that in the normal population.[126, 129]

Etiologies (Table 14–5)

ALDOSTERONE-PRODUCING ADENOMA (APA). The solitary APA is the most common cause of primary aldosteronism and accounts for approximately 65% of cases. These lesions are usually less than 2 cm in diameter, making them difficult to image. They are benign neoplasms and are surrounded by a well-defined capsule; microscopically the most common cell type is a large, clear lipid-filled cell resembling a zona fasciculata cell.[130]

IDIOPATHIC HYPERALDOSTERONISM (IHA). Idiopathic hyperplasia (bilateral adrenal hyperplasia) is the cause of approximately 30% of cases of primary aldosteronism.[131] Microscopically, the glands show hyperplasia of the zona glomerulosa, accompanied by adrenocortical nodules. The aldosterone excess in IHA is usually milder than in APA; as a result, the biochemical abnormalities such as hypokalemia and suppression of PRA are usually less severe than in APA.

Since the plasma aldosterone response to infused angiotensin II is exaggerated compared with that in normal individuals or patients with APA,[132] IHA has been hypothesized to represent a syndrome of enhanced responsiveness to angiotensin II. Others suggest that IHA is a form of essential hypertension representing one end of the distribution of aldosterone production in essential hypertension and is therefore related to the low-renin essential hypertensive in which an enhanced aldosterone response to angiotensin II is seen (see earlier).

ADRENOCORTICAL CARCINOMA. Adrenocortical carcinoma is an extremely rare cause of primary aldosteronism. In contrast with APA these tumors are usually very large at the time of diagnosis (>6 cm).

TABLE 14–5. Causes of Primary Aldosteronism and Their Frequencies

Syndrome	Proportion of Cases
Aldosterone-producing adenoma, including renin-responsive adenoma	65%
Idiopathic hyperaldosteronism, including primary adrenal hyperplasia	30–40%
Glucocorticoid-remediable aldosteronism	1–3%

TABLE 14–4. Mineralocorticoid-Excess States Associated with Low Plasma Renin Levels

Primary aldosteronism
    Aldosterone-producing adenoma (APA)
    Idiopathic hyperplasia (idiopathic hyperaldosteronism)
    Adrenocortical carcinoma
    Glucocorticoid-remediable aldosteronism (GRA)
Congenital adrenal hyperplasia
    11β-hydroxylase deficiency
    17α-hydroxylase deficiency
Apparent mineralocorticoid excess (AME)
    Congenital
    Licorice ingestion
    Ectopic corticotropin production
Liddle's syndrome

GLUCOCORTICOID-REMEDIABLE ALDOSTERONISM
(GRA). This syndrome is inherited in an autosomal dominant fashion and is probably responsible for fewer than 3% of cases of primary aldosteronism. GRA is characterized by hypertension of early onset that is usually severe and refractory to conventional antihypertensive therapies. Prospective screening of GRA pedigrees has revealed that many affected individuals are not hypokalemic.[133]

Regulation of Aldosterone Secretion

The renin-angiotensin system is suppressed in primary aldosteronism and does not contribute to the regulation of aldosterone production.[134] In this sense, aldosterone production is "autonomous." However, studies in patients with APA, for example, demonstrate that the adenomas are regulated by corticotropin (ACTH) and potassium. Thus autonomy is defined by the failure of aldosterone production to respond to maneuvers that normally activate (upright posture) or suppress (sodium loading) the renin-angiotensin system. A variant form of APA has been described in which the adenomas are renin responsive (see later). Moreover in IHA aldosterone production is usually responsive to stimuli that activate the renin-angiotensin system.[134] On the other hand, adrenal carcinomas are truly resistant to all secretagogues.

The sine qua non of GRA is aldosterone production that is solely under the control of corticotropin. As a result, the syndrome can be mitigated by exogenous glucocorticoid therapy. GRA is caused by a chimeric gene duplication that results from unequal crossing over between the highly homologous 11β-hydroxylase (CYP11B) and aldosterone synthase (CYP18) genes.[135] This chimeric gene contains the 3′ corticotropin-responsive portion of the promoter from the 11β-hydroxylase gene fused to the 5′ coding sequence of the aldosterone synthase gene. The result is ectopic expression of aldosterone synthase activity in the cortisol-producing zona fasciculata. Thus, mineralocorticoid production is regulated by corticotropin instead of the normal secretagogue, angiotensin II. This mutation results in the overproduction of aldosterone and also the characteristic hybrid steroids 18-oxocortisol and 18-OH-cortisol, which can be measured in the urine to diagnose affected individuals.

Diagnosis

SCREENING TESTS. Spontaneous hypokalemia is usually present, although some patients may have normal potassium levels, possibly because of self-selected dietary sodium restriction, since aldosterone-induced renal potassium wasting is diminished by decreased sodium delivery to the distal nephron. When potassium-wasting diuretics are given as antihypertensive agents, hypokalemia is more frequent and more severe. Serum potassium measurement is not a good screening test in GRA because many patients have normal potassium levels.[136]

PRA is suppressed in almost all patients ([<0.8 nmol/L/h] <1.0 ng/mL/h) and does not increase appropriately ([>1.6 nmol/L/h] >2 ng/mL/h) after dietary sodium restriction and/or after acute diuretic administration with furosemide followed by 90 to 120 min of upright posture.[137] Although a subset of essential hypertensives (25%) also have low PRA, documentation of a normal or high stimulated PRA excludes primary aldosteronism.

Given the high prevalence of suppressed PRA levels in essential hypertensives, documentation of a concomitant elevation of plasma aldosterone (PA) makes the diagnosis of primary aldosteronism more likely (Fig. 14–11). Thus, a PA/PRA ratio greater than 25 is suggestive, and a ratio of 50 or more is virtually diagnostic of primary aldosteronism (when PRA is expressed as ng/mL/h and PA as ng/dL).[126] Since a number

of drugs (ACE inhibitors, β-blockers, and spironolactone) all alter PRA levels, such antihypertensives should be withdrawn for 2 to 4 wk if possible (6 to 8 wk for spironolactone) before determining the PA/PRA ratio. Since hypokalemia reduces aldosterone levels, diagnostic studies should be performed in a potassium-repleted state. Specimens should be obtained after 2 h of upright posture, since stimulated ratios have been shown to have better diagnostic accuracy than supine values.[138]

The captopril test can also be used to diagnose primary aldosteronism.[139, 140] One protocol is to administer 50 mg orally at 9:00 AM; blood samples are obtained before and 90 min later. In normotensive individuals or essential hypertensives acute inhibition of ACE decreases angiotensin-regulated aldosterone production. However, in primary aldosteronism aldosterone levels fail to decline because the renin-angiotensin system is suppressed and aldosterone production is autonomous. A postcaptopril aldosterone reduction of more than 20%—usually to less than 410 pmol/L (<15 ng/dL)—is considered a normal response. Although the sensitivity of this test ranges from 90 to 100%, the specificity is significantly less (50 to 80%).

DIAGNOSIS OF AUTONOMOUS ALDOSTERONE PRODUCTION. Oral sodium loading for 3 d followed by a 24-h urine collection for determination of aldosterone excretion can discriminate primary aldosteronism from essential hypertension with excellent sensitivity and specificity (96% and 93%, respectively).[141] A 24-h urinary aldosterone excretion rate greater than 28 to 39 nmol/d (10 to 14 μg/d) in the presence of a urinary sodium excretion greater than 250 mmol/d is considered diagnostic of primary aldosteronism.

The diagnosis of autonomous aldosterone production can also be demonstrated by acute intravascular volume expansion with isotonic saline. Isotonic saline is administered intravenously at a rate of 500 mL/h for 4 to 6 h. Post saline plasma aldosterone levels greater than 280 pmol/L (>10 ng/dL)—a more stringent value of greater than 140 to 220 pmol/L (>5 to 8 ng/dL) has also been proposed[142, 143]—confirm the diagnosis of autonomous aldosterone production.

Differential Diagnosis (Table 14–6)

HORMONAL TESTING. Hormonal testing provides supportive data especially if radiography fails to show a solitary tumor. The posture test is the most common study used in the differential diagnosis of primary aldosteronism. Samples are collected for PRA and plasma aldosterone when the subject is recumbent and after 2 to 4 h of standing or walking. The response in normal subjects and in essential hypertensives is an increase in plasma aldosterone levels of at least 50% compared with recumbent levels. Hypokalemia should be corrected before testing with oral potassium supplementation. The accuracy of the test is enhanced by simultaneous measurement of recumbent and upright cortisol levels.[144] In APA patients aldosterone levels generally decline in parallel with the circadian secretion of cortisol, the so-called anomalous postural response.[145] This is because the renin-angiotensin system is suppressed in patients with APA, and therefore changes in posture do not stimulate an increased production of aldosterone. In contrast, in IHA there is usually an increase in renin and aldosterone levels in response to the patient's assuming the upright posture. The predictive value of the posture test in distinguishing between APA and IHA approaches 90%; however, variant forms of APA and IHA reduce the specificity of this test (see later). A postural decline in plasma aldosterone is also seen in GRA because aldosterone secretion is regulated solely by corticotropin in this disorder. Blood levels of 18-OH-corticosterone [18-(OH)-B], an intermediate of the aldosterone biosynthetic pathway, are generally greater

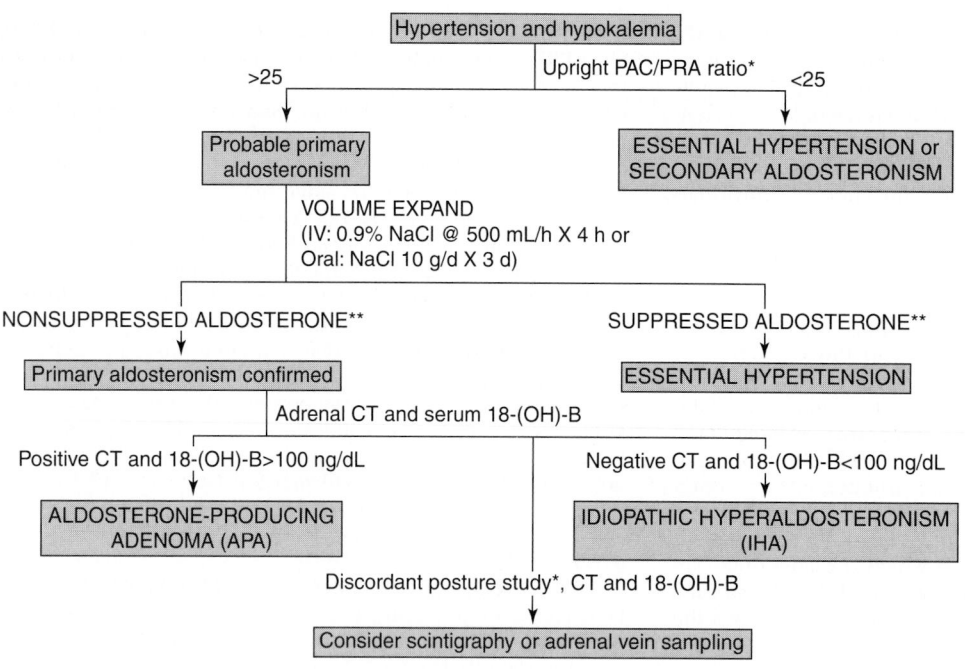

Figure 14-11. Diagnostic flow chart for evaluating the hypokalemic hypertensive patient.

than 2800 nmol/mL (100 ng/dL) in APA subjects, whereas patients with IHA have lower 18-(OH)-B levels.[146]

Documentation of the unique hybrid 18-oxygenated cortisol compounds 18-oxocortisol and 18-OH-cortisol in a 24-h urine collection can successfully diagnose GRA and also differentiate APA from IHA.[147] In contrast with modest elevations in APA[147, 148] and normal levels in IHA levels of these compounds are 10-fold above normal in GRA. A major drawback is the lack of general availability of assays for these compounds.

RADIOLOGIC STUDIES. Tomography using spiral computed tomographic techniques is the imaging modality of first choice. It is critical to make a biochemical diagnosis before imaging the adrenal because of the 2 to 10% incidence of nonfunctioning adrenal masses in computed tomography studies of the abdomen.[149] The use of adrenal scintigraphy with NP-59 ([131]I-6β-iodomethyl-19-norcholesterol) can differentiate APA from IHA because lateralization is seen in the former disorder. However, a lateralizing scan lacks specificity, since it may also be seen in adrenal adenomas that do not produce aldosterone.

Adrenal venous sampling, which should be reserved for cases in which diagnostic imaging and biochemical studies are inconclusive, is the most sensitive means of differentiating APA from IHA. In most cases of APA the ratio of ipsilateral to contralateral aldosterone concentration is greater than 10:1. This procedure is diagnostic in more than 95% of cases when catheterization of the right adrenal vein is successful. However, the incidence of unsuccessful procedures can be as high as 25%.[125] Furthermore, adrenal venous sampling is invasive and is associated with a small but significant risk of venous thrombosis, adrenal hemorrhage, and/or adrenal insufficiency.

Nonclassic Variants of Primary Aldosteronism

The aldosterone-producing renin-responsive adenoma (APRA) and primary adrenal hyperplasia (PAH) are variants of primary aldosteronism[150] that represent important exceptions in terms of both diagnosis and treatment. In contrast with APA, the changes in plasma renin (features characteristically considered diagnostic of IHA) after upright posture in subjects with APRA cause an increase in aldosterone levels. Thus in patients diagnosed with primary aldosteronism the importance of adrenal imaging in documenting a solitary lesion is emphasized by this unusual entity.

Primary unilateral adrenal hyperplasia (PAH) is another

TABLE 14-6. Diagnostic Testing Used to Differentiate Aldosterone-Producing Adenoma from Idiopathic Hyperaldosteronism

	Etiology			
	Adenoma		Hyperplasia	
Diagnostic Test	APA	APRA	IHA	PAH
Posture study (PAC after 2 h of upright posture)	Decreased or no change	Increased	Increased	Decreased or no change
Serum 18-OH-corticosterone	>100 ng/dL	>100 ng/dL	<100 ng/dL	<100 ng/dL
24-h urine 18-OH-cortisol	>60 μg/d	<60 μg/d	<60 μg/d	>60 μg/d
24-h urine tetrahydro-18-(oxo)-cortisol	>15 μg/d	<15 μg/d	<15 μg/d	>15 μg/d
Adrenal computed tomography	Unilateral nodule	Unilateral nodule	Bilateral hyperplasia ± nodularity	Unilateral hyperplasia ± nodularity
Adrenal venous sampling	Lateralization	Lateralization	Nonlateralization	Lateralization

APA = aldosterone-producing adenoma; APRA = aldosterone-producing renin-responsive adenoma; PAH = primary adrenal hyperplasia; IHA = idiopathic (bilateral) hyperaldosteronism; PAC = plasma aldosterone concentration.

"variant" form of primary aldosteronism.[149] The biochemical features resemble those in APA: no increase or a decline in aldosterone levels in response to upright posture and elevated levels of urinary 18-OH-cortisol and 18-oxocortisol. The syndrome can be ameliorated by unilateral adrenalectomy or a reduction in adrenal mass.

Genetic Testing for Glucocorticoid-Remediable Aldosteronism

The diagnosis of GRA was initially based on the family history and the clinical response to dexamethasone suppression. Subsequently GRA was diagnosed by demonstrating markedly elevated levels of 18-oxocortisol and 18-OH-cortisol in a 24-h urine collection. However, the discovery of the genetic basis of GRA by Lifton, Dluhy, and co-workers[135, 151] made it possible to make a genetic diagnosis with the use of Southern blotting techniques from a peripheral blood sample. Genetic testing is both a sensitive and a specific way of diagnosing GRA and obviates the need to measure the urinary levels of 18-oxocortisol and 18-OH-cortisol or to perform dexamethasone suppression testing. Genetic analysis can be arranged by calling the International GRA Registry (1–800–GRA–2262 in North America or 617–732–5761).

Therapy

Surgery is the treatment of choice in patients with APA, APRA, and PAH. Cure rates (defined as blood pressure less than 140/90 off medications 6 to 12 mo after surgery) vary between 35 and 50%. All patients should receive medical treatment prior to surgery to control blood pressure and replete potassium stores (see later). Persistent postoperative hypertension may relate to the chronicity or severity of hypertension, the presence of end-organ changes, or concurrent essential hypertension. On the other hand, the hypertension in IHA responds poorly to bilateral adrenalectomy, although the potassium-wasting state is reversed. Pharmacologic treatment is the therapy of choice in IHA and for preoperative management of APA, or when the patient is not a surgical candidate.[152] A sodium-restricted diet (sodium < 2 g/d) is also prescribed in conjunction with pharmacologic treatment to minimize potassium wasting and lower the blood pressure.

Spironolactone, a competitive antagonist of aldosterone, has traditionally been the drug of first choice, with doses of 100 to 500 mg/d usually being required. Spironolactone also blocks testosterone biosynthesis and action, resulting in erectile dysfunction, decreased libido, and gynecomastia in men; menstrual irregularities are seen in women. Amiloride blocks the apical sodium channel in the distal nephron and is an alternative to spironolactone; it is given in divided doses starting at 5 mg bid, with a maximal dose of 15 mg bid. The sustained-release formulation of the calcium channel blocker nifedipine (dose range 30 to 90 mg/d) also has been used in the medical management of primary aldosteronism[153] because this compound inhibits aldosterone biosynthesis in vitro.[154] However, the antihypertensive response to this agent alone in primary aldosteronism is disappointing,[155] and nifedipine should be viewed as a second-line agent. ACE inhibitors and angiotensin II receptor antagonists also may have a role in the medical management of IHA because the response to angiotensin II may be exaggerated in this disorder.

GRA is unique among the syndromes of primary aldosteronism in that the underlying pathophysiological abnormality is the regulation of aldosterone production solely by corticotropin. As a result glucocorticoid treatment usually reverses the syndrome. Of great importance is an awareness of the potential toxicity (Cushing's syndrome) with excessive doses of glucocorticoids, especially with the use of dexamethasone

in children.[156] When a decision to use glucocorticoids is made, the smallest effective dose of shorter-acting agents such as prednisone or hydrocortisone should be prescribed in relation to body surface area (hydrocortisone, 10 to 12 mg/m²/d). Target blood pressure in children should be guided by age-specific blood pressure percentiles.[157, 158] Children should be followed by pediatricians with expertise in glucocorticoid therapy, with careful attention being paid to preventing retardation of linear growth by overtreatment. Therapeutic alternatives in treating hypertension in GRA are mineralocorticoid antagonists, which also avoid the adverse effects of chronic glucocorticoid therapy. Amiloride or spironolactone are effective as monotherapies in most GRA patients.

Other Low-Renin Mineralocorticoid-Excess States

In the following syndromes the steroids responsible for the mineralocorticoid-excess states include DOC and cortisol. As a result of the suppression of the renin-angiotensin system the aldosterone levels are low—not elevated, as in the previously described syndromes.

Congenital Adrenal Hyperplasia

Deoxycorticosterone excess is seen in several hypertensive forms of congenital adrenal hyperplasia or rarely in neoplasms (adenoma or carcinoma) that overproduce DOC. Congenital adrenal hyperplasia results from a deficiency in cortisol biosynthesis. Deficiencies in both 11β-hydroxylase (CYP11B) and 17α-hydroxylase (CYP17) are associated with hypertension and hypokalemia. In 11β-hydroxylase deficiency the impaired conversion of 11-deoxycorticosterone to corticosterone results in the accumulation of DOC, a potent mineralocorticoid. Virilization in females, usually recognizable in children, results from shunting into the androgen pathway. Blood levels of DOC, 11-deoxycortisol, and adrenal androgens are characteristically elevated. This form of congenital adrenal hyperplasia is more prevalent in Middle Eastern Moslems and Jews.

17α-Hydroxylase deficiency is characterized by hypogonadism, hypokalemia, and hypertension. As in 11β-hydroxylase deficiency this disorder is a result of decreased production of cortisol with shunting into the unblocked mineralocorticoid pathway. Because 17α-hydroxylase is required for the biosynthesis of gonadal testosterone and estrogen, a defect in this enzyme in both sexes is associated with sexual immaturity, high gonadotropin levels, and low urinary 17-ketosteroid excretion. Females have primary amenorrhea and lack of development of secondary sexual characteristics. Males may have ambiguous external genitalia or a female phenotype (male pseudohermaphroditism). Blood levels of 17β-hydroxyprogesterone are low, and corticosterone and DOC levels are elevated.

The elevated blood pressure and hypokalemia in both syndromes result from elevated levels of DOC, a potent mineralocorticoid; excessive sodium retention and hypertension result and lead to suppression of PRA and low levels of aldosterone. The genetic lesions causing 11β-hydroxylase deficiency are in the gene that encodes CYP11B.[159] There are a large number of mutations in the CYP17 gene that can cause 17α-hydroxylase deficiency.[160, 161]

Glucocorticoid suppression with dexamethasone or prednisone restores normal levels of DOC and reverses the mineralocorticoid-excess state in these adrenal hyperplasia syndromes. Caution must be exercised to avoid overdosing and induction of Cushing's syndrome.

Apparent Mineralocorticoid Excess

This syndrome is the result of impaired activity of the enzyme 11β-hydroxysteroid dehydrogenase (11β-HSD), which in the kidney normally inactivates cortisol by converting it to cortisone.[162] As a result of the enzyme deficiency high levels of cortisol accumulate in the kidney. The characteristic abnormal urinary cortisol metabolite profile seen in AME also reflects decreased 11β-HSD activity (ratio of cortisol to cortisone increased 10-fold compared with the normal ratio of approximately 1).[163, 164] As a result of elevated intrarenal levels, cortisol binds to glucocorticoid type I (mineralocorticoid) receptors in the distal tubule, which are normally sites of aldosterone binding.

Underlying the pathogenesis of AME is the nonselectivity of renal mineralocorticoid receptors in that in vitro they bind cortisol with affinity equal to that of aldosterone.[165, 166] Thus 11β-HSD normally excludes physiological glucocorticoids from nonselective mineralocorticoid receptors by converting them to the inactive 11-keto compound, cortisone. 11β-HSD has bidirectional activity in different tissues, acting primarily as a reductase in the liver and a dehydrogenase in the kidney. These different activities are the consequence of two isoenzymes that are expressed in liver and kidney, respectively.[167, 168]

Decreased 11β-HSD activity may be hereditary or secondary to pharmacologic inhibition of enzyme activity by glycyrrhetinic acid, the active principle of licorice root and some chewing tobaccos. The hereditary form contains mutations in the gene coding for isoenzyme 2. The phenotype of patients with AME includes hypertension, low PRA levels, hypokalemia, normal plasma cortisol levels, and low plasma aldosterone levels.

The mineralocorticoid-excess state commonly seen in patients with the ectopic ACTH syndrome is believed to be related to the high rates of cortisol production that cause a relative deficiency of 11β-HSD activity. However, DOC levels are high and could account for the hypokalemia in this disorder.

Liddle's Syndrome

This syndrome is inherited as an autosomal dominant disorder in which affected subjects present with hypertension, suppressed PRA, low aldosterone levels and usually hypokalemia.[169] The hypokalemic state cannot be corrected by the administration of the antimineralocorticoid spironolactone but is ameliorated by triamterene or amiloride, agents that block renal sodium reabsorption and potassium secretion by mineralocorticoid receptor–independent mechanisms. This disorder is caused by mutations in the subunits of the renal sodium epithelial channel.[170, 171] The amiloride-sensitive epithelial channel, considered the rate-limiting step for sodium absorption in the distal nephron, is composed of three subunits (α, β, γ); mutations have been found in two of these subunits.[170, 171] As a result of these mutations, constitutive activity of the epithelial channel leads to increased sodium absorption and volume expansion.

OTHER ENDOCRINE DISORDERS ASSOCIATED WITH HYPERTENSION

Glucocorticoid Excess (Cushing's Syndrome)

Cushing's syndrome, the hypersecretion of cortisol, is associated with elevations in blood pressure in more than 80% of cases. Diastolic blood pressure exceeds 100 mm Hg in more than 50% of patients with endogenous Cushing's syndrome.[172] On the other hand, the incidence of hypertension is less and more variable in patients treated with exogenous glucocorticoids. Nevertheless, hypertension and associated metabolic abnormalities (diabetes mellitus and hyperlipidemia) probably account for the atherosclerotic cardiovascular morbidity and mortality seen in spontaneous Cushing's syndrome.[173]

Mineralocorticoid production is usually normal in endogenous Cushing's syndrome. In Cushing's disease, commonly secondary to corticotropin hypersecretion from a pituitary microadenoma, aldosterone and renin levels are usually normal,[174, 175] and DOC levels are normal or increased modestly.[176] On the other hand, in ectopic corticotropin syndrome increased mineralocorticoid activity and hypokalemia are the rule—as a result of elevated levels of DOC and mineralocorticoid effects of high levels of cortisol. In adrenal carcinomas, DOC and aldosterone may also be elevated. Thus in adrenal carcinomas and in ectopic corticotropin secretion, mineralocorticoid production may contribute to the hypertension; in such situations PRA is usually suppressed.[175, 177]

The elevation of blood pressure by cortisol and synthetic glucocorticoids (which have minimal mineralocorticoid activity) is mediated by multiple mechanisms. Glucocorticoids increase cardiac output[178] and activate the renin-angiotensin system by increasing the hepatic production of angiotensinogen.[175] Other actions of glucocorticoids include reduction in the synthesis of vasodilatory prostaglandins secondary to inhibition of phospholipase A_2, thus blocking the release of arachidonic acid from phospholipids. There is also evidence for reduction in the components of the kallikrein-kinin system[175] as well as enhanced pressor sensitivity to endogenous vasoconstrictors (epinephrine and angiotensin II).[179] Glucocorticoids may also promote sodium influx into vascular smooth muscle cells.[180]

The screening for endogenous cortisol excess is accomplished by measuring the response of plasma cortisol to the 1-mg dexamethasone suppression test or by the measurement of elevated levels of free cortisol in a 24-h urine collection. Further studies to determine the etiology of the cortisol-excess state are outlined in Chapter 12.

Pheochromocytoma

Pheochromocytoma (see Chapter 13) is the cause of high blood pressure in approximately 0.1% of hypertensive individuals. On the other hand, pheochromocytoma is underdiagnosed in that as many as 40% of cases go unsuspected and are diagnosed at autopsy.[181, 182] The majority of pheochromocytomas occur as sporadic cases, but their association with familial syndromes (e.g., multiple endocrine neoplasia ([MEN]), 2A and 2B and von Hippel-Lindau syndrome) in approximately 10% of cases underscores the importance of taking a careful family history in patients in whom this diagnosis is suspected (also see Chapter 32).

Hypertension is one of the most consistent manifestations of pheochromocytoma,[183] the "hallmark" being paroxysmal hypertension. However, paroxysms occur in only a third of patients, and sustained hypertension occurs in about half. Even in the absence of clear paroxysms, lability of blood pressure is common. Orthostatic hypotension is frequent owing to the peripheral vasoconstriction and hypovolemia associated with catecholamine excess. Symptoms suggestive of this disorder include palpitations, sweats, and headache.

When pheochromocytoma is suspected, biochemical screening is indicated. Some recommend the measurement of plasma catecholamines as the initial screening test,[183] but the measurement of metanephrines and urinary catecholamines has the highest sensitivity and that of urine vanillylmandelic acid (VMA) the lowest.[184, 185]

With a positive biochemical screen, computed tomography or magnetic resonance imaging of the abdomen is the best approach to localize a pheochromocytoma. Ninety percent of pheochromocytomas are intra-adrenal; almost all are longer than 1 cm at the time of presentation and thus are easily visualized by either modality.[186] Magnetic resonance imaging may be of additional value in that pheochromocytomas classically appear hyperintense on T2-weighted images with a signal intensity greater than three times that of liver, a characteristic that distinguishes them from "incidentalomas" (see Chapter 12).[187, 188] If adrenal imaging procedures fail to identify a mass when catecholamine levels are elevated, scintigraphy with metaiodobenzylguanidine (MIBG) may be useful in localizing extra-adrenal lesions.[189] Another promising localizing study utilizes somatostatin-receptor imaging with indium—or ^{123}I-labeled [Tyr³]octreotide.[190]

The treatment for pheochromocytoma is surgical unless metastatic disease contraindicates this approach. Preoperative preparation is critical to successful surgery, to prevent hypertensive crises from anesthesia and intraoperative tumor manipulation. Patients should be pretreated for 10 to 14 d preoperatively with an α-receptor antagonist such as phenoxybenzamine (a noncompetitive α-adrenergic blocker)[191] or with α₁-adrenergic receptor antagonists (prazosin, terazosin, doxazosin)[192] (see Chapter 13). Patients who are or have become tachycardic with α-blockade or who experience significant ectopic beats preoperatively are also treated with β-receptor blockers.

Thyroid Disease (See Chapter 11)

Hypothyroidism

Hypothyroidism may account for 1 to 2% of cases of diastolic hypertension in the general population. In a large series of patients screened for the secondary forms of hypertension by age the prevalence of hypothyroidism was 3%.[193] In that study hypothyroidism was thought to be a significant cause of secondary hypertension, especially in female individuals older than 70 years of age. That hypothyroidism can actually cause hypertension was shown by Streeten and colleagues in another study in which 32% of hypertensive hypothyroid patients had a fall in diastolic blood pressure to 90 mm Hg or less following replacement levothyroxine treatment and after withdrawal of all hypertensive drugs.[194] Postulated mechanisms for the elevation of blood pressure include extracellular volume expansion and elevation in systemic vascular resistance.

Hyperthyroidism

In contrast with the diastolic hypertension associated with hypothyroidism, hyperthyroidism usually causes elevated systolic blood pressure. Thyrotoxic patients usually have tachycardia, high cardiac output, increased stroke volume, and decreased peripheral vascular resistance.[195, 196] These hemodynamic alterations are usually ameliorated by β-blocker therapy. In elderly patients atrial fibrillation may be the sole manifestation of thyrotoxicosis.

Acromegaly

Hypertension occurs in one third of patients with acromegaly (see Chapter 9), presumably owing to sodium retention with resultant extracellular volume expansion.[197] This retention of sodium, in the context of an increase in glomerular filtration rate and low PRA, is the consequence of uncharacterized antinatriuretic actions of growth hormone. Sodium retention is also a complication of exogenous administration of growth hormone. The prevalence of primary aldosteronism in acromegaly appears to be increased.[198] As previously discussed, in primary aldosteronism plasma renin levels are suppressed, and aldosterone levels are increased. In acromegaly plasma renin levels also are suppressed owing to volume expansion, but aldosterone levels are not increased.[199]

Hyperparathyroidism (See Chapter 24)

In contrast with the overall incidence of 0.1% of primary hyperparathyroidism in the general population, this disorder occurs in approximately 1% of hypertensive patients. Conversely, approximately, 30 to 40% of individuals with hyperparathyroidism are hypertensive. The mechanisms are unclear because there is no direct correlation with the elevated PTH or calcium levels (see earlier).[200] Hypertension may or may not remit following successful parathyroidectomy.[201-204] Since the blood pressure response to correction of primary hyperparathyroidism is variable and since hypertension is not a clear-cut manifestation of the hyperparathyroid state, hypertension is considered a minor criterion for recommending surgery to patients with mild asymptomatic primary hyperparathyroidism.[205] On the other hand, surgery may cause regression of myocardial hypertrophy in normotensive patients with hyperparathyroidism and may also reverse the increased mortality associated with hyperparathyroidism in subjects younger than 70 years of age.[206, 207] The hypertension associated with hyperparathyroidism also can result as a complication of hypercalcemia-induced renal impairment or when this disorder is part of a multiple endocrine neoplasia syndrome that includes pheochromocytoma or primary aldosteronism.

Exogenous Treatments

Treatment with certain hormones or pharmacologic agents can elevate blood pressure (Table 14–7). Fludrocortisone, a potent mineralocorticoid used in the treatment of patients with primary adrenal insufficiency, can cause hypertension when used in supraphysiological doses, as in the administration to patients with orthostatic hypotension, to cause volume expansion. Licorice and chewing tobacco abuse can result in hypokalemia, sodium and water retention, and blood pressure elevation, as noted earlier. The administration of growth hormone in pharmacologic doses to patients who have received transplants or to severely catabolic hospitalized subjects for its protein-sparing actions can raise blood pressure. The hypertension associated with cyclosporine treatment appears to be related to renal vasospasm and secondary volume expansion. Glucocorticoid treatment in supraphysiological doses for inflammatory and allergic disorders frequently elevates blood pressure, as noted earlier, but less commonly than in endogenous Cushing's syndrome. Oral contraceptive preparations containing higher dose estrogen-progesterone formulations are known to induce hypertension. It is unknown whether current lower dose formulations cause hypertension. However, postmenopausal estrogen replacement therapy does not elevate blood pressure.[208] Androgens in pharmacologic doses can also produce volume expansion and arterial hypertension.[209]

Finally, analogous to the hypertension in pheochromocytoma, ingestion of sympathomimetic amines or substances that potentiate endogenous sympathetic nervous system activity (e.g., cocaine inhibits reuptake of catecholamines at adrenergic nerve endings) produces increased cardiac output, in-

---

TABLE 14–7. Exogenous Causes of Secondary Hypertension

Mineralocorticoids (licorice and licorice-containing chewing tobacco; fludrocortisone)
Growth hormone
Glucocorticoids
Gonadal steroids
    Oral contraceptives
    Androgens
Sympathomimetic amines (amphetamines, cocaine)
Cyclosporine

creased peripheral arteriolar vasoconstriction, and hypertension.

REFERENCES

1. Williams GH. Hypertensive vascular disease. In: Fauci AS, Braunwald E, Isselbacher KJ, et al, eds. Harrison's Principles of Internal Medicine. 4th ed. New York: McGraw-Hill, 1998: 1380–1394.
2. Williams GH, Moore TJ. Hormonal aspects of hypertension. In: DeGroot LJ, Besser M, Burger HG, et al, eds. Endocrinology. 3rd ed. Philadelphia: WB Saunders, 1994: 2917–2934.
3. Williams GH, Hollenberg NK. Pathophysiology of essential hypertension. In: Parmley WW, Chatterjee K, eds. Cardiology. Vol 2. Philadelphia: JB Lippincott, 1990: 1–18.
4. Conlin PR, Dluhy RG, Williams GH. Disorders of the renin-angiotensin-aldosterone system. In: Schrier RW, ed. Renal and Electrolyte Disorders. 5th ed. Boston: Little, Brown, 1997: 349–392.
5. Williams GH, Chao J, Chao L. Kidney hormones: the kallikrein-kinin and renin-angiotensin systems. In: Conn PM, Melmed S, eds. Endocrinology: Basic and Clinical Principles. Totowa, NJ: Humana Press, 1997: 393–404.
6. Williams GH, Dluhy RG. Diseases of the adrenal cortex. In: Fauci AS, Braunwald E, Isselbacher KJ, et al, eds. Harrison's Principles of Internal Medicine. 14th ed. New York: McGraw-Hill, 1998: 1380–1394.
7. Baxter JD, Dunkin K, Chu W, et al. Molecular biology of human renin gene. Recent Prog Horm Res 1991; 47:211–257.
8. Raizada MK, Phillips MI, Sumners C, eds. Cellular and Molecular Biology of the Renin-Angiotensin System. Boca Raton, FL: CRC Press, 1993.
9. Hate T, Takimoto E, Murakami K, et al. Comparative studies on species-specific reactivity between renin and angiotensinogen. Mol Cell Biochem 1994; 131:43–47.
10. Gaillard-Sanchez I, Mattei MG, Clauser E, et al. Assignment by in situ hybridization of angiotensinogen to chromosome band 1q42: the same region as human renin gene. Hum Genet 1990; 84:341–343.
11. Gaillard L, Clauser E, Corvol P. Structure of human angiotensinogen gene. DNA Seq 1989; 8:87–89.
12. Deschepper CF. Angiotensinogen: hormonal regulation and relative importance in the generation of angiotensin II. Kidney Int 1994; 46:1561–1563.
13. Bernstein KE, Shai SY, Howard T, et al. Structure and regulated expression of angiotensin-converting enzyme and the receptor for angiotensin II. Am J Kidney Dis 1993; 21(4S):53–57.
14. Corvol P, Michaud A, Soubrier F, et al. Recent advances in knowledge of the structure and function of the angiotensin I converting enzyme. J Hypertens 1995; 13:S3–S10.
15. Timmermans PB, Wong PC, Chiu AT, et al. Angiotensin II receptors and angiotensin II receptor antagonists. Pharmacol Rev 1993; 45:205–251.
16. Shibata T, Suzuki C, Ohnishi J, et al. Identification of regions in the human angiotensin II receptor type 1 responsible for Gi and Gq coupling by mutagenesis study. Biochem Biophys Res Commun 1996; 218:383–389.
17. Schieffer B, Paxton WG, Marrero MB, et al. Importance of tyrosine phosphorylation in angiotensin II type 1 receptor signalling. Hypertension 1996; 27:476–480.
18. Tsuzuki S, Ichiki T, Nakakubo H, et al. Molecular cloning and expression of the gene encoding human angiotensin II type 2 receptor. Biochem Biophys Res Commun 1994; 200:1449–1454.
19. Nahmias C, Strosberg AD. The angiotensin AT_2 receptor: searching for signal-transduction pathways and physiological function. Trends Pharmacol Sci 1995; 16:223–225.
20. Wright JW, Harding JW. Brain angiotensin receptor subtypes AT_1, AT_2, and AT_4 and their functions. Regul Pept 1995; 59:269–295.
21. Hall KL, Venkateswaran S, Hanesworth JM, et al. Characterization of a functional angiotensin IV receptor on coronary microvascular endothelial cells. Regul Pept 1995; 58:107–115.
22. Benter IF, Ferrario CM, Morris M, et al. Antihypertensive actions of angiotensin-(1–7) in spontaneously hypertensive rats. Am J Physiol (Heart) 1995; 269:H313–H319.
23. Paul M, Wagner J, Dzau VJ. Gene expression of the renin-angiotensin system in human tissues: Quantitative analysis by the polymerase chain reaction. J Clin Invest 1993; 91:2058–2064.
24. Chiou C-Y, Williams GH, Kifor I. Study of the rat adrenal renin-angiotensin system at a cellular level. J Clin Invest 1995; 96:1375–1381.
25. Harp JB, DiGirolamo M. Components of the renin-angiotensin system in adipose tissue: changes with maturation and adipose mass enlargement. J Gerontol A Biol Sci Med Sci 1995; 50:B270–B276.
26. Tian Y, Balla T, Baukal AJ, et al. Growth responses to angiotensin II in bovine adrenal glomerulosa cells. Am J Physiol (Endocrinol) 1995; 268:E135–E144.
27. Cox BE, Word RA, Rosenfeld CR. Angiotensin II receptor characteristics and subtype expression in uterine arteries and myometrium during pregnancy. Endocrinology 1996; 81:49–58.
28. Vinson GP. The adrenal renin-angiotensin system. Adv Exp Med Biol 1995; 377:237–251.
29. Ganong WF. Reproduction and the renin-angiotensin system. Neurosci Biobehav Rev 1995; 19:241–250.
30. Hollenberg NK, Chenitz WR, Adams DF, et al. Reciprocal influence of salt intake on adrenal glomerulosa and renal vascular responses to angiotensin II in normal man. J Clin Invest 1974; 54:34–42.
31. Williams GH, Hollenberg NK. "Sodium sensitive" essential hypertension: emerging insights into pathogenesis and therapeutic implications. In: Klahr S, Massry SG, eds. Contemporary Nephrology. 3rd ed. New York: Plenum, 1985: 303–331.
32. Laragh JH, Sealey JE, Niarchos AP, et al. The vasoconstrictor volume spectrum in normotension and in the pathogenesis of hypertension. Fed Proc 1982; 41:2415–2423.
33. Safar ME, London GM, Simon AC, et al. Volume factors, total exchangeable sodium, and potassium in hypertensive disease. In: Genest J, Kuchel O, Hamet P, et al, eds. Hypertension: Pathophysiology and Treatment. New York: McGraw-Hill, 1983: 42–53.
34. Vaughan ED, Laragh JH, Gavras I, et al. Volume factor in low and normal renin essential hypertension: treatment with either spironolactone or chlorthalidone. Am J Cardiol 1973; 32:522–532.
35. Woods JW, Liddle GW, Michelakis AM, et al. Effect of an adrenal inhibitor in hypertensive patients with suppressed renin. Arch Intern Med 1969; 123:366–370.
36. Wisgerhof M, Brown RD. Increased adrenal sensitivity to angiotensin II in low renin essential hypertension. J Clin Invest 1979; 63:1456–1462.
37. Marks AD, Marks DB, Kanefsky TM, et al. Enhanced adrenal responsiveness to angiotensin II in patients with low renin essential hypertension. J Clin Endocrinol Metab 1979; 48:266–270.
38. Kisch ES, Dluhy RG, Williams GH. Enhanced aldosterone response to angiotensin II in human hypertension. Circ Res 1976; 38:502–505.
39. Shoback DM, Williams GH, Moore TJ, et al. Defect in the sodium-modulated tissue responsiveness to angiotensin II in essential hypertension. J Clin Invest 1983; 72:2115–2124.
40. Williams GH, Dluhy RG, Lifton RP, et al. Non-modulation as an intermediate phenotype in essential hypertension. Hypertension 1992; 20:788–796.
41. Beretta-Piccoli C, Pusterla C, Stadler P, et al. Blunted aldosterone responsiveness to angiotensin II in normotensive subjects with familial predisposition to essential hypertension. J Hypertens 1988; 6:57–61.
42. Leonetti Luparini R, Ferri C, Santucci A, et al. Atrial natriuretic peptide in non-modulating essential hypertension. Hypertension 1993; 21:803–809.
43. Hollenberg NK, Williams GH. Abnormal renal function, sodium-volume homeostasis and renin system behavior in normal-renin essential hypertension: the evolution of the non-modulator concept. In: Laragh JH, Brenner BM, eds. Hypertension: Pathophysiology, Diagnosis, and Management. 2nd edition. New York: Raven, 1995: 1837–1856.
44. Gaboury CL, Hollenberg NK, Hopkins PN, et al. Metabolic derangements in non-modulating hypertension. Am J Hypertens 1995; 8:870–875.
45. Ferri C, Bellini C, Desideri G, et al. Metabolic features of non-modulating essential hypertension: insulin resistance, dyslipidemia, and salt sensitivity. 1997 (in press).
46. Taylor TT, Moore TJ, Hollenberg NK, et al. Converting enzyme inhibition corrects the altered adrenal response to angiotensin II in essential hypertension. Hypertension 1984; 6:92–99.
47. Redgrave JE, Rabinowe SL, Hollenberg NK, et al. Correction of abnormal renal blood flow response to angiotensin II by converting enzyme inhibition in essential hypertensives. J Clin Invest 1985; 75:1285–1290.
48. Hollenberg NK, Moore TJ, Shoback DM, et al. Abnormal renal sodium handling in essential hypertension: relation to failure of renal and adrenal modulation of responses to angiotensin II. Am J Med 1986; 81:412–418.
49. Lifton RP, Hopkins PN, Williams RR, et al. Evidence for heritability of non-modulating essential hypertension. Hypertension 1989; 13:884–889.
50. Hopkins PN, Lifton RP, Hollenberg NK, et al. Blunted renal vascular response to angiotensin II is associated with a common variant of the angiotensinogen gene and obesity. J Hypertens 1996; 14:199–207.
51. Hopkins PN, Hunt SC, Wu LL, et al. Hypertension, dyslipidemia, and insulin resistance: links in a chain or spokes on a wheel? Curr Opin Metab 1996; 7:241–253.
52. DeFronzo RA, Ferrannini E. Insulin resistance: a multifaceted syndrome responsible for NIDDM, obesity, hypertension, dyslipidemia, and atherosclerotic cardiovascular disease. Diabetes Care 1991; 14:173–194.
53. Reaven GM, Hofman BB. Hypertension as a disease of carbohydrate and lipoprotein metabolism. Am J Med 1989; 8:S2–S6.
54. Saad MF, Lillioja S, Nyomba BL, et al. Racial differences in the relation between blood pressure and insulin resistance. New Engl J Med 1991; 324:733–739.
55. Modan M, Halkin H, Halmog S, et al. Hyperinsulinemia: a link between hypertension, obesity and glucose intolerance. J Clin Invest 1985; 75:809–816.
56. Ferrannini E, Buzzigoli G, Bonadonna R, et al. Insulin resistance in essential hypertension. New Engl J Med 1987; 317:350–357.
57. DeFronzo RA. Insulin resistance, hyperinsulinemia, and coronary artery disease: a complex metabolic web. J Cardiovasc Pharmacol 1992; 20:S1–S15.
58. Levy J, Gavin JR III, Hammerman MR, et al. Ca^{2+} + Mg^{2+} ATPase activity in kidney basolateral membrane in non-insulin dependent diabetic rats: effect of insulin. Diabetes 1986; 35:899–905.
59. Draznin B, Lewis D, Houlder N, et al. Mechanism of insulin resistance induced by sustained levels of cytosolic free calcium in rat adipocytes. Endocrinology 1989; 125:2341–2349.
60. Draznin B, Sussman KE, Eckel RH, et al. Possible role of cytosolic free

calcium concentrations in mediating insulin resistance of obesity and hyperinsulinemia. J Clin Invest 1988; 28:1848–1852.

61. Anderson EA, Hoffman RP, Balon TW, et al. Hyperinsulinemia produces both sympathetic neural activation and vasodilation in normal humans. J Clin Invest 1991; 84:2246–2252.

62. DeFronzo RA, Cooke CR, Adres R, et al. The effect of insulin on renal handling of sodium, potassium, calcium and phosphate in man. J Clin Invest 1975; 55:845–855.

63. Sharma AM, Rutland K, Spies KP, et al. Salt sensitivity in young normotensive subjects is associated with a hyperinsulinemic response to oral glucose. J Hypertens 1991; 9:329–335.

64. Sharma AM, Schorr U, Distler A. Insulin resistance in young, salt-sensitive normotensive subjects. Hypertension 1993; 22:273–279.

65. Bigazzi R, Bianchi S, Baldari D, et al. Microalbuminuria in salt-sensitive patients: a marker for renal and cardiovascular risk factors. Hypertension 1994; 23:195–199.

66. Townsend RA, Zhao H. Plasma renin activity and insulin sensitivity in normotensive subjects. Am J Hypertens 1994; 7:894–898.

67. Egan BM, Stepniakowski K, Goodfriend TL. Renin and aldosterone are higher and the hyperlipidemic effect of salt restriction greater in subjects with risk factor clustering. Am J Hypertens 1994; 7:886–893.

68. McCarron DA, Morris CD, Cole C. Dietary calcium in human hypertension. Science 1982; 217:267–269.

69. Witteman JC, Willett WC, Stampfer MJ, et al. A prospective study of nutritional factors and hypertension among US women. Circulation 1989; 80:1320–1327.

70. McCarron DA, Morris CD, Henry HJ, et al. Blood pressure and nutrient intake in the United States. Science 1984; 224:1392–1398.

71. Morris CD, Reusser ME. Calcium intake and blood pressure: epidemiology revisited. Semin Nephrol 1995; 15:490–495.

72. Bucher HC, Cook RJ, Guyatt GH, et al. Effects of dietary calcium supplementation in blood pressure: a meta-analysis of randomized controlled trials. JAMA 1996; 275:1016–1022.

73. Allender PS, Cutler JA, Follmann D, et al. Dietary calcium and blood pressure: a meta-analysis of randomized clinical trials. Ann Intern Med 1996; 124:825–831.

74. Bukoski RD, Ishibashi K, Bian K. Vascular actions of the calcium regulating hormones. Semin Nephrol 1995; 15:536–549.

75. Wang R, Wu L, Karpinski E, et al. The changes in contractile status of single vascular smooth muscle cells and ventricular cells induced by bPTH-(1–34). Life Sci 1993; 52:793–801.

76. Pang PKT, Lewanczuk RZ. Parathyroid origin of a new hypertensive factor in spontaneously hypertensive rats. Am J Hypertens 1989; 2:898–902.

77. Shan J, Benishin CG, Lewanczuk RZ, et al. Mechanism of the vascular action of parathyroid hypertensive factor. J Cardiovasc Pharmacol 1994; 23:S1–S8.

78. Lewanczuk RZ, Pang PKT. Expression of parathyroid hypertensive factor in hypertensive primary hyperparathyroid patients. Blood Pressure 1993; 2:22–27.

79. Takahashi K, Inoue D, Ando K, et al. Parathyroid hormone–related peptide as a locally produced vasorelaxant: regulation of its mRNA by hypertension in rats. Biochem Biophys Res Commun 1995; 208:447–455.

80. Ishibashi K, Evans A, Shingi T, et al. Differential expression and effect of calcitriol on myosin in the arterial tree. Am J Physiol 1995; 269:C443–C450.

81. Goldblatt H, Lynch J, Hanzel R. Studies on experimental hypertension. J Exp Med 1934; 59:347.

82. Leadbetter WF, Burkland CE. Hypertension in unilateral renal disease. J Urol 1938; 39:611.

83. Albers FJ. Clinical characteristics of atherosclerotic renovascular disease. Am J Kidney Dis 1994; 24:636–641.

84. Dustan HP, Humphries AW, deWolfe VG, et al. Normal arterial pressures in patients with renal artery stenosis. JAMA 1964; 187:1028.

85. Rimmer JM, Gennari FJ. Atherosclerotic renovascular disease and progressive renal failure. Ann Intern Med 1993; 118:712–719.

86. Canzanello VJ, Textor SC. Noninvasive diagnosis of renovascular disease. Mayo Clin Proc 1994; 69:1172–1181.

87. Johnson G. Renovascular hypertension: new diagnostic and therapeutic procedures. Scand J Urol Nephrol Suppl 1995; 170:1–78.

88. Sfakianakis GN, Bourgoignie JJ, Georgiou M, et al. Diagnosis of renovascular hypertension with ACE inhibition scintigraphy. Radiol Clin North Am 1993; 31:831–848.

89. Nally JV Jr. Provocative captopril testing in the diagnosis of renovascular hypertension. Urol Clin North Am 1994; 21:227–234.

90. King BF Jr. Diagnostic imaging evaluation of renovascular hypertension. Abdom Imaging 1995; 20:395–405.

91. Nally VJ Jr, Olin JW, Lammert GK. Advances in noninvasive screening for renovascular disease. Cleve Clin J Med 1994; 61:328–336.

92. Ram CV, Clagett GP, Radford LR. Renovascular hypertension. Semin Nephrol 1995; 15:152–174.

93. Textor SC. Renovascular hypertension. Endocrinol Metab Clin North Am 1994; 23:235–253.

94. Rosenthal T. Drug therapy in renovascular hypertension. Drugs 1993; 45:895–909.

95. Conn JW, Cohen EL, Lucas CP, et al. Primary reninism: hypertension, hyperreninemia, and secondary aldosteronism due to renin-producing juxtaglomerular cell tumors. Arch Intern Med 1972; 130:682–696.

96. Hollenberg NK, Raij L. Angiotensin-converting enzyme inhibition and renal protection: an assessment of implications for therapy. Arch Intern Med 1993; 153:2426–2435.

97. Lewis EJ, Hunsicker LG, Bain RP, et al. The effect of angiotensin-converting enzyme inhibition in diabetic nephropathy. The Collaborative Study Group. New Engl J Med 1993; 329:1456–1462.

98. Maschio C, Alberti D, Janin G, et al. Effect of the angiotensin converting enzyme inhibitor benazepril on the progression of chronic renal insufficiency. The Angiotensin-Converting-Enzyme Inhibition in Progressive Renal Insufficiency Study Group. N Engl J Med 1996; 334:939–945.

99. Kalra PA, Mamtora H, Holmes AM, et al. Renovascular disease and renal complications of angiotensin converting enzyme inhibitor therapy. Q J Med 1990; 77:1013–1018.

100. National High Blood Pressure Education Working Group Report on High Blood Pressure in Pregnancy. Am J Obstet Gynecol 1990; 163:1689–1712.

101. Guzick DS, Klein VR, Tyson JE, et al. Risk factors for the occurrence of pregnancy-induced hypertension. Clin Exp Hypertens 1987; B6:281–297.

102. de Swiet M. The physiology of normal pregnancy. In: Rubin PC, ed. Hypertension in Pregnancy (Birkhenager WH, Reid JC, eds. Handbook of Hypertension. Vol 10). Amsterdam: Elsevier, 1988: 1–9.

103. Chesley LC, Lindheimer MD. Renal hemodynamics and intravascular volume in normal and hypertensive pregnancy. In: Rubin PC, ed. Hypertension in Pregnancy (Birkhenager WH, Reid JC, eds. Handbook of Hypertension, Vol 10). Amsterdam: Elsevier, 1988: 38–65.

104. Graves SW, Moore TJ, Seely EW. Increased platelet angiotensin II receptor number in pregnancy-induced hypertension. Hypertension 1992; 20:627–632.

105. Chelsley LC. Plasma and red cell volumes during pregnancy. Am J Obstet Gynecol 1972; 112:440–450.

106. Hays PM, Cruikshank DP, Dunn LJ. Plasma volume determination in normal and preeclamptic pregnancies. Am J Obstet Gynecol 1985; 151:958–966.

107. Brown MA, Zammit VC, Mitar DM. Extracellular fluid volumes in pregnancy-induced hypertension. J Hypertens 1992; 10:61–68.

108. Groenendijk R, Trimbos MJ, Wallenburg HCS. Hemodynamics measurements in preeclampsia: preliminary observations. Am J Obstet Gynecol 1984; 150:232–236.

109. Wallenburg HCS. Hemodynamics in hypertensive pregnancy. In: Rubin PC, ed. Hypertension in Pregnancy (Birkhenager WH, Reid JC, eds. Handbook of Hypertension. Vol 10). Amsterdam: Elsevier, 1988: 66–101.

110. Seely EW, Williams GH, Graves SW. Markers of sodium and volume homeostasis in pregnancy-induced hypertension. J Clin Endocrinol Metab 1992; 74:150–156.

111. Miyamoto S, Shimokawa H, Sumioki H, et al. Physiologic role of endogenous human atrial natriuretic peptide in preeclamptic pregnancies. Am J Obstet Gynecol 1989; 160:155–159.

112. Lowe SA, Zammit VC, Mitar D, et al. Atrial natriuretic peptide and plasma volume in pregnancy-induced hypertension. Am J Hypertens 1991; 4:897–903.

113. Graves SW, Williams GH. Endogenous digitalis-like factors. Annu Rev Med 1987; 38:433–444.

114. Sowers JR, Zemel MB, Bronsteen RA, et al. Erythrocyte cation metabolism in preeclampsia. Am J Obstet Gynecol 1989; 161:441–445.

115. Testa I, Rabini RA, Danieli G, et al. Abnormal membrane cation transport in pregnancy-induced hypertension. Scand J Clin Lab Invest 1988; 48:7–13.

116. Friedman SA. Preeclampsia: a review of the role of prostaglandins. Obstet Gynecol 1988; 71:122–137.

117. Fitzgerald DJ, Entman SS, Mulloy K, et al. Decreased prostacyclin biosynthesis preceding the clinical manifestation of pregnancy-induced hypertension. Circulation 1987; 75:956–963.

118. Zemel MB, Zemel PC, Berry S, et al. Altered platelet calcium metabolism as an early predictor of increased peripheral vascular resistance and preeclampsia in urban black women. N Engl J Med 1990; 323:434–438.

119. Bower D. The influence of dietary salt intake on pre-eclampsia. J Obstet Gynaecol Brit Comm 1964; 71:123–125.

120. Gallery EDM, Mitchell MDM, Redman CWG. Fall in blood pressure in response to volume expansion in pregnancy-associated hypertension (preeclampsia): Why does it occur? J Hypertens 1984; 2:177–182.

121. Beaufils M, Uzan S, Donsimoni R, et al. Prevention of preeclampisa by early antiplatelet therapy. Lancet 1985; 1:840–842.

122. Schiff E, Peleg E, Goldenberg M, et al. The use of aspirin to prevent pregnancy-induced hypertension and lower the ratio of thromboxane A$_2$ to prostacyclin in relatively high risk pregnancies. N Engl J Med 1989; 321:351–356.

123. Conn JW. Presidential address: Part I. Painting background. Part II. Primary aldosteronism, a new clinical syndrome. J Lab Clin Med 1955; 45:3–17.

124. Gregoire JR. Adjustment of the osmostat in primary aldosteronism. Mayo Clin Proc 1994; 69:1108–1110.

125. Young WF Jr, Klee GG. Primary aldosteronism: diagnostic evaluation. 1988; 17:367–395.

126. Blumenfeld JD, Sealey JE, Schlussel Y, et al. Diagnosis and treatment of primary hyperaldosteronism. Ann Intern Med 1994; 121:877–885.

127. Campbell SE, Diaz-Arias AA, Weber KT. Fibrosis of the human heart and systemic organs in adrenal adenoma. Blood Pressure 1992; 1:149–156.

128. Torres VE, Young WF Jr, Offord KP, et al. Association of hypokalemia, hypoaldosteronism, and renal cysts. N Engl J Med 1990; 322:345–351.

129. Hypokalemia, aldosteronism, and renal cysts. N Engl J Med 1990; 323:29–31 (letter).

130. Ganguly A. Cellular origin of aldosteronomas. J Clin Invest 1992; 70:392–395.

131. Melby JC. Diagnosis of hyperaldosteronism. Endocrinol Clin North Am 1991; 20:247–255.

132. Wisgerhof M, Brown RD, Hogan MJ, et al. The plasma aldosterone response to angiotensin II infusion in aldosterone-producing adenoma and idiopathic hyperaldosteronism. J Clin Endocrinol Metab 1981; 52:195–198.

133. Dluhy RG, Lifton RP. Glucocorticoid-remediable aldosteronism. Endocrinol Clin North Am 1994; 23:285–297.

134. Ganguly A, Melada GA, Luetscher JA, et al. Control of plasma aldosterone in primary aldosteronism: distinction between adenoma and hyperplasia. J Clin Endocrinol Metab 1973; 37:765–775.

135. Lifton RP, Dluhy RG, Powers M, et al. A chimaeric 11-hydroxylase/aldosterone synthase gene causes glucocorticoid-remediable aldosteronism and human hypertension. Nature 1992; 355:262–265.

136. Rich GM, Ulick S, Cook S, et al. Glucocorticoid-remediable aldosteronism in a large kindred: clinical spectrum and diagnosis using a characteristic biochemical phenotype. Ann Intern Med 1992; 116:813–820.

137. Young WF Jr, Hogan MJ, Klee GG, et al. Primary aldosteronism: diagnosis and treatment. Mayo Clin Proc 1990; 65:96–110.

138. McKenna TJ, Sequeira SJ, Heffernan A, et al. Diagnosis under random conditions of AII disorders of the renin-angiotensin-aldosterone axis, including primary hyperaldosteronism. J Clin Endocrinol Metab 1991; 73:952–957.

139. Lyons DF, Kem DC, Brown RD, et al. Single dose captopril as a diagnostic test for primary aldosteronism. J Clin Endocrinol Metab 1983; 57:892–896.

140. Naomi S, Iwaoka T, Umeda T, et al. Clinical evaluation of the captopril screening test for primary aldosteronism. Jpn Heart J 1985; 26:549–556.

141. Bravo EL, Tarazi RC, Dustan HP, et al. The changing clinical spectrum of primary aldosteronism. Am J Med 1983; 74:641–651.

142. Holland OB, Brown H, Kuhnert L, et al. Further evaluation of saline infusion for the diagnosis of primary aldosteronism. Hypertension 1984; 6:717–723.

143. Kem DC, Weinberger MH, Mayes DM, et al. Saline suppression of plasma aldosterone in hypertension. Arch Intern Med 1971; 128:380–386.

144. Fontes RG, Kater CE, Biglieri EG, et al. Reassessment of the predictive value of the postural stimulation test in primary aldosteronism. Am J Hypertens 1991; 4:786–791.

145. Ganguly A, Dowdy AJ, Luetscher JA, et al. Anomalous postural response of plasma aldosterone concentration in patients with aldosterone-producing adrenal adenoma. J Clin Endocrinol Metab 1973; 36:401–404.

146. Fraser R, Lantos CP. 18-Hydroxycorticosterone: a review. J Steroid Biochem 1978; 9:273–286.

147. Ulick S, Blumenfield JD, Atlas SA, et al. The unique steroidogenesis of the aldosteronoma in the differential diagnosis of primary aldosteronism. J Clin Endocrinol Metab 1993; 76:873–878.

148. Chu MD, Ulick S. Isolation and identification of 18-hydroxycortisol from the urine of patients with primary aldosteronism. J Biol Chem 1982; 258:2218–2224.

149. Banks WA, Kastin AJ, Biglieri EG, et al. Primary adrenal hyperplasia: a new subset of primary aldosteronism. J Clin Endocrinol Metab 1984; 58:783–785.

150. Irony I, Kater CE, Biglieri EG, et al. Correctable subsets of primary aldosteronism: primary adrenal hyperplasia and renin responsive adenoma. Am J Hypertens 1990; 3:576–582.

151. Lifton RP, Dluhy RG, Powers M, et al. Hereditary hypertension caused by chimaeric gene duplications and ectopic expression of aldosterone synthase. Nature Genet 1992; 2:66–74.

152. Hsueth WA. New insights into the medical management of primary aldosteronism. Hypertension 1986; 8:76–82.

153. Nadler JL, Hseuth W, Horton R. Therapeutic effect of calcium channel blockade in primary aldosteronism. J Clin Endocrinol Metab 1985; 60:896–899.

154. Freed MI, Rastegar A, Bia MJ. Effects of calcium channel blockers on potassium homeostasis. Yale J Biol Med 1991; 64:177–186.

155. Bravo EL, Fouad FM, Tarazi RC. Calcium channel blockade with nifedipine in primary aldosteronism. Hypertension 1986; 8(Suppl I):191–194.

156. Laidlaw JC. Dexamethasone-suppressible hyperaldosteronism: patients JS and LS 20 years later. In: New MI, Borrelli P, eds. Dexamethasone-suppressible hyperaldosteronism. (Rome, Serono Symposia Review No. 10) New York: Raven, 1986: 133–137.

157. Lieberman E. Pediatric hypertension: clinical perspective. Mayo Clin Proc 1994; 69:1098–1107.

158. Morgenstern BZ. Hypertension in pediatric patients: current issues. Mayo Clin Proc 1994; 69:1089–1097.

159. White PC, Dupont J, New M, et al. A mutation in CYP11B1 (Arg488His) associated with steroid 11-hydroxylase deficiency in Jews of Moroccan origin. J Clin Invest 1991; 87:1664–1667.

160. Biason A, Mantero F, Scaroni C, et al. Deletion within the CYP17 gene together with insertion of foreign DNA is the cause of combined complete 17-hydroxylase/17,20 lyase deficiency in an Italian patient. Mol Endocrinol 1991; 5:2037–2045.

161. Fardella CE, Hum DW, Homoki J, et al. Point mutation of Arg440 to His in cytochrome P450c17 causes severe 17-hydroxylase deficiency. J Clin Endocrinol Metab 1994; 79:160–164.

162. Funder JW. 11-Hydroxysteroid dehydrogenase and the meaning of life. Mol Cell Endocrinol 1990; 68:C3–C5.

163. Stewart PM, Corrie JET, Shackleton CHL. Syndrome of apparent mineralocorticoid excess: a defect in the cortisol-cortisone shuttle. J Clin Invest 1988; 82:340–349.

164. Stewart PM, Shackelton CHL, Edwards CRW. The cortisol-cortisone shuttle and the genesis of hypertension. In: Mantero F, Vecse P, eds. Corticosteroids and Peptide Hormones in Hypertension (Serono Symposia Publications). New York: Raven, 1987: 163.

165. Funder JW, Pearce PT, Smith R, et al. Mineralocorticoid action: target-tissue specificity is enzyme, not receptor, mediated. Science 1988; 242:583–585.

166. Arriza JL, Simerly RB, Swanson LW, et al. The neuronal mineralocorticoid receptor as a mediator of glucocorticoid response. Neuron 1988; 1:887–900.

167. Lakshmi V, Monder C. Purification and characterization of the corticosteroid 11-dehydrogenase component of the rat liver 11-hydroxysteroid dehydrogenase complex. Endocrinology 1989; 123:2390–2398.

168. Albiston A, Obeyesekere V, Smith R, et al. Cloning and tissue distribution of the human 11-beta hydroxysteroid dehydrogenase type II enzyme. Mol Cell Endocrinol 1994; 105:R11–R17.

169. Liddle GW, Blesdoe T, Coppage WS Jr. A familial renal disorder simulating primary aldosteronism but with negligible aldosterone sectetion. Trans Assoc Am Physicians 1963; 76:199–213.

170. Shimkets RA, Warnock DG, Bositis CM, et al. Liddle's syndrome: heritable human hypertension caused by mutations in the subunit of the epithelial sodium channel. Cell 1994; 79:407–414.

171. Hansson JH, Nelson-Williams C, Suzuki H, et al. Hypertension caused by a truncated epithelial sodium channel subunit: genetic heterogeneity of Liddle syndrome. Nature Genet 1995; 11:76–82.

172. Ross EJ, Marshall-Jones P, Friedman M. Cushing's syndrome: diagnostic criteria. Q J Med 1966; 35:149.

173. Plotz CM, Knowlton AI, Ragan C. The natural history of Cushing's syndrome. Am J Med 1952; 13:597–614.

174. Gomez-Sanchez CE. Cushing's syndrome and hypertension. Hypertension 1986; 8:258–264.

175. Mantero F, Boscardo M. Glucocorticoid-dependent hypertension. J Steroid Biochem Mol Biol 1992; 43:409–413.

176. Cassar J, Loizou S, Kelly WF, et al. Deoxycorticosterone and aldosterone excretion in Cushing's syndrome. Metabolism 1980; 29:115–119.

177. Krakoff L, Nicolis G, Amsel B. Pathogenesis of hypertension in Cushing's syndrome. Am J Med 1975; 58:216–220.

178. Pirpiris M, Yeung S, Dewar E, et al. Hydrocortisone-induced hypertension in man: the role of cardiac output. Am J Hypertens 1993; 6:287–294.

179. Sato A, Suzuki H, Murakami M, et al. Glucocorticoid increases angiotensin II type 1 receptor and its gene expression. Hypertension 1994; 23:25–30.

180. Kornel L, Manisundaram B, Nelson W. Glucocorticoids regulate transport in vascular smooth muscle through the glucocorticoid receptor–mediated mechanism. Am J Hypertens 1993; 6:736–744.

181. Sutton MG, Sheps SG, Lie JT. Prevalence of clinically unsuspected pheochromocytoma: review of a 50-year autopsy series. Mayo Clin Proc 1981; 56:354–360.

182. Stenstrom G, Svardsudd K. Pheochromocytoma in Sweden 1958–1981: an analysis of the National Cancer Registry Data. Acta Med Scand 1986; 220:225–232.

183. Bravo EL. Evolving concepts in the pathophysiology, diagnosis, and treatment of pheochromocytoma. Endocr Rev 1994; 15:356–368.

184. Bravo EL, Gifford RW Jr. Pheochromocytoma: diagnosis, localization and management. N Engl J Med 1984; 311:1298–1303.

185. Oishi S, Sasaki M, Ohno M, et al. Urinary normetanephrine and metanephrine measured by radioimmunoassay for the diagnosis of pheochromocytoma: utility of 24-hour and random 1-hour urine determinations. J Clin Endocrinol Metab 1988; 67:614–618.

186. Glazer GM, Francis IR, Quint LE. Imaging of the adrenal glands. Invest Radiol 1988; 23:3–11.

187. Doppman JL, Reinig JW, Dwyer AJ, et al. Differentiation of adrenal masses by magnetic resonance imaging. Surgery 1987; 102:1018–1026.

188. Van Gils APG, Falke THM, van Erkel AR, et al. MR imaging and MIBG scintigraphy of pheochromocytomas and extraadrenal functioning paragangliomas. Radiograph 1991; 11:37–57.

189. Sisson JC, Frager MS, Valk TW, et al. Scintigraphic localization of pheochromocytoma. N Engl J Med 1981; 305:12–17.

190. Lamberts SWJ, Bakker WH, Reubi JC. Somatostatin-receptor imaging in the localization of endocrine tumors. N Engl J Med 1990; 323:1246–1249.

191. Desmonts JM, Marty J. An anesthetic management of patients with pheochromocytoma. Br J Anesth 1984; 56:781–789.

192. Nicholson JP Jr, Vaughn ED Jr, Pickering TG, et al. Pheochromocytoma and prazosin. Ann Intern Med 1983; 99:477–479.

193. Anderson GH Jr, Blakeman N, Streeten DHP. The effect of age on prevalence of secondary forms of hypertension in 4429 consecutively referred patients. J Hypertens 1994; 12:609–615.

194. Streeten DHP, Anderson GH Jr, Howland T, et al. Effects of thyroid function on blood pressure: recognition of hypothyroid hypertension. Hypertension 1988; 11:78–83.

195. Klein I. Thyroid hormone and the cardiovascular system. Am J Med 1990; 88:631–637.

196. Woeber KA. Thyrotoxicosis and the heart. N Engl J Med 1992; 327:94–98.

197. Falkheden T, Sjögren B. Extracellular fluid volume and renal function in pituitary insufficiency and acromegaly. Acta Endocrinol (Copenh) 1964; 46:80–88.

198. Strauch G, Vallotton MB, Touitou Y, et al. The renin-angiotensin-aldosterone system in normotensive and hypertensive patients with acromegaly. N Engl J Med 1972; 287:795–799.

199. Cain JP, Williams GH, Dluhy RG. Plasma renin activity and aldosterone secretion in patients with acromegaly. J Clin Endocrinol Metab 1972; 34:73–81.

200. Lind L, Wengle B, Wide L, et al. Hypertension in primary hyperparathyroidism: reduction of blood pressure by long-term treatment with vitamin D (alpha-calcidiol): double-blind, placebo-controlled study. Am J Hypertens 1988; 1:397–402.

201. Diamond TW, Botha JR, Wing J, et al. Parathyroid hypertension: a reversible disorder. Arch Intern Med 1986; 146:1709–1712.

202. Broulik PD, Horky K, Pacovsky V. Blood pressure in patients with primary hyperparathyroidism before and after parathyroidectomy. Exp Clin Endocrinol 1985; 86:346–352.

203. Jones DB, Jones JH, Lloyd HJ, et al. Changes in blood pressure and renal function after parathyroidectomy in primary hyperparathyroidism. Postgrad Med J 1983; 59:350–353.

204. Sancho JJ, Rouco J, Riera-Vida R, et al. Long-term effects of parathyroidectomy for primary hyperparathyroidism on arterial hypertension. World J Surg 1992; 16:732–736.

205. Consensus Development Conference Panel. Diagnosis and management of asymptomatic primary hyperparathyroidism: Consensus Development Conference Statement. Ann Intern Med 1991; 114:593–597.

206. Stefenelli T, Mayr H, Bergler-Klein J, et al. Primary hyperparathyroidism: incidence of cardiac abnormalities and partial reversibility after successful parathyroidectomy. Am J Med 1993; 95:197–202.

207. Palmer M, Adami H-O, Bergstrom R, et al. Survival and renal function in persons with untreated hypercalcemia: a population-based cohort study with 13 years of follow-up. Lancet 1987; 1:59–62.

208. Knopp RH. The effect of postmenopausal estrogen therapy on the incidence of arteriosclerotic vascular disease. Obstet Gynecol 1988; 72:23S–30S.

209. Bretza JA, Novey HS, Vaziri ND, et al. Hypertension: a complication of danazol therapy. Arch Intern Med 1980; 140:1379–1380.

15

DISORDERS OF THE OVARIES AND FEMALE REPRODUCTIVE TRACT

Bruce R. Carr

INTRODUCTION

The ovaries are the source of ova and of the hormones that regulate female sexual life. These two functions are under precise but complex feedback control by the hypothalamic-pituitary axis. The rapid growth of a single follicle that will become dominant and release an ovum and the regularity of this process for an average of 38 y are remarkable phenomena. The complex regulation and compartmentalization in the ovary that control follicular growth appear to be governed by factors produced within the ovary itself. Estrogens, the principal hormones secreted by the ovary, promote growth and differentiation of the uterus, fallopian tubes, and vagina and induce other aspects of sexual maturation. Disorders of the ovary can give rise to sexual precocity, abnormalities of the menstrual cycle, androgen excess, and infertility. With aging, most remaining follicles undergo atresia so that by age 50 few follicles remain, estrogen levels decline, secondary sexual characteristics regress, and menopause ensues.

NORMAL OVARY AND OVARIAN FUNCTION

Early Development of the Ovary

Fetal Ovary

Genetic sex is determined at conception, and the development of the gonads takes place early in fetal development. The bipotential gonadal anlagen, which give rise to either the ovaries or the testes, can be identified in human embryos by 30 d after fertilization, and the ovary can be identified histologically by about day 70.[1] The ovary is composed of three principal cell types: (1) coelomic epithelial cells, which are derived from the gonadal ridge and later differentiate into granulosa cells; (2) mesenchymal cells of the gonadal ridge, which give rise to the ovarian stroma; and (3) primordial germ cells, which arise from the endoderm of the yolk sac and migrate into the gonadal ridge before differenting into ova.

During the third week of gestation the primordial germ cells can be identified in the yolk sac at the caudal end of the ovary. The sex of the migrating primordial cells can be determined by analysis of sex chromatin. In female germ cells, one X chromosome is inactivated during migration to the gonadal ridge.[2] As formulated by Lyon,[3] X chromosome inactivation prevents the expression of more than one X chromosome in a given cell line. Primordial cell migration can be traced by cytochemical demonstration of high alkaline phosphatase activity. The mechanisms that stimulate and direct the amoeboid movement of primordial cells to the gonadal ridge are poorly understood. Fibronectin has been identified in the migratory pathway and can stimulate primordial cell movement in vitro.[4] Chemotactic substances secreted by the gonadal anlagen may also play a role in regulating the migratory process.[5] During migration the number of germ cells increases by replication. In the human embryo, 700 to 1300 germ cells are present at 5 wk, and by 8 wk 600,000 germ cells can be identified in the developing ovary.[6, 7]

Early in fetal development, the ovary is near the mesonephros (a temporarily functioning kidney). The mesonephros influences gonadal differentiation and is essential for complete ovarian development in mammals (Fig. 15–1).[8] Whereas the ovary is not histologically distinguishable until about 10 to 11 wk of fetal life, the fetal testis can be identified by about the seventh week (see Chapter 29). After the primordial cells reach the fetal ovary, they continue to proliferate by successive mitotic division and reach the maximal number of 6 to 7 million oogonia by the 20th week of gestation (Fig. 15–2).[7] Afterward, the number of germ cells decreases (a process known as *atresia*), so that only 1 million are present at birth, 400,000 are present at menarche, and only a few remain by the menopause (Fig. 15–3). Two X chromosomes are required for normal development of the ovary. In people with a 45,X karyotype, ovarian development occurs and primordial germ cells appear in the gonad, but follicular development is incomplete and the rate of atresia is accelerated so that only a fibrous streak remains at birth.[9] As discussed later, gonadotropin is required for complete maturation of ovarian follicles. Follicular development is reduced in anencephalic human fetuses and after fetal hypophysectomy in monkeys.[10, 11]

The ovary-mesonephros association persists during early ovarian differentiation, and the mesonephros regresses slowly. In the human the ovary is invaded by mesonephric cells that form the medulla and force the germ cells to occupy the periphery or ovarian cortex.[12] The oogonia continue to undergo mitosis until they are converted to primary oocytes,

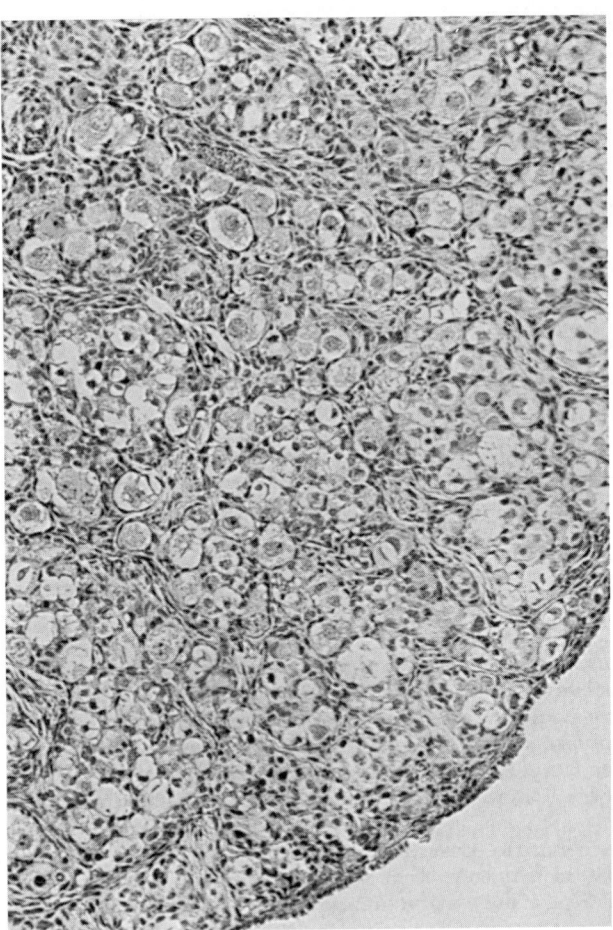

Figure 15–2. Histologic section of an ovary from a 16-week-old human fetus. (Courtesy of Dr. W. E. Rainey.)

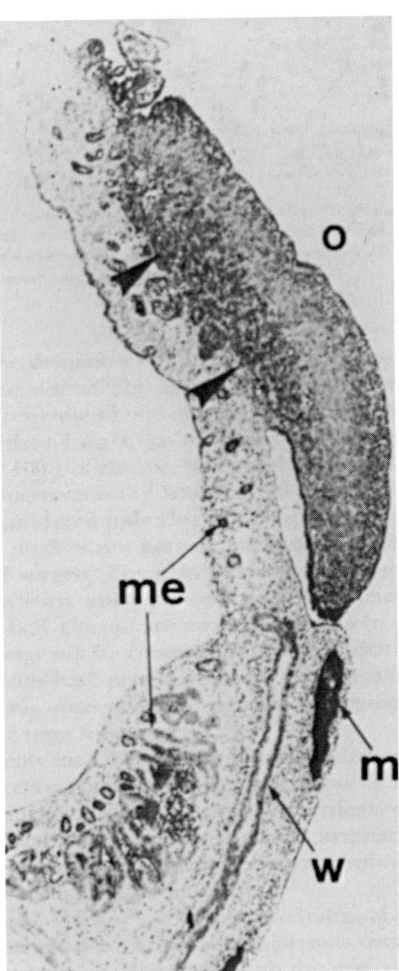

Figure 15–1. Ovary-mesonephros complex of an 11-week-old human fetus. The ovary (o) is attached to the cranial part of the mesonephros (*arrowheads*). Other features include the mesonephric tubules (me), wolffian duct (w), and müllerian duct (m). Magnification × 200. (From Byskov AG, Hoyer PE. Embryology of mammalian gonads. In: Knobil E, Neill J, eds. The Physiology of Reproduction. New York: Raven, 1988: 267, with permission.)

beginning as early as the 8th to the 12th weeks of gestation.[2, 13] The primary oocytes begin meiosis, but the process is arrested in the diplotene, or resting, stage of the first meiotic division, where the cells remain until puberty. With the onset of ovulation the first meiotic phase is completed (Fig. 15–4). The second meiotic phase occurs after ovulation and is completed after fertilization. Meiosis appears to be regulated by autocrine factors produced locally in the ovary. Meiosis-preventing substance, or oocyte maturation inhibitor, is produced by granulosa cells and arrests the oocyte in the diplotene stage. Later, meiosis is triggered by a small molecule (<2 kd) termed *meiosis-inducing substance*.[14, 15]

After the primary oocyte is arrested at the diplotene stage it becomes surrounded by a layer of primitive granulosa cells; together these make up the primordial follicle, the morphologic marker of fetal ovarian differentiation.[10] A basement membrane separates the primordial follicle from the surrounding stromal (interstitial) tissues. The conversion of oogonia into primary oocytes and subsequent formation of primordial follicles are not completed until 6 mo after birth. Oocytes that are not incorporated into follicles undergo degeneration and account for the majority of oocytes that have disappeared by birth.[7, 16] The first primordial follicles are found at the inner part of the cortex near the medulla. Follicle formation depends on adequate numbers of mesonephros-derived granulosa cells, as discussed previously.[12] The surface of the ovary, which is derived from coelomic epithelium and is inappropriately named the *germinal epithelium*, is not involved in the formation of germ cells or follicles.[12] At approximately 20 wk of fetal life, follicles begin to grow under the influence of gonadotropins (Fig. 15–5). By the seventh month of gestation, follicle maturation reaches the antrum stage.

At 8 wk of gestation the human ovary has the capacity to produce estrogens from androgens but secretes only small amounts of steroids in vitro.[17, 18] Binding sites for luteinizing hormone (LH) and human chorionic gonadotropin (hCG) are not detectable in human fetal ovaries, and LH, follicle-stimulating hormone (FSH), and hCG do not stimulate steroidogenesis in vitro, which suggests independence of gonadotropin control.[19, 20] Human fetal ovaries possess most of the enzymes required for de novo synthesis of steroid hormones from cholesterol as demonstrated in vitro, but there is no convincing evidence that they secrete significant quantities of steroid hormones in vivo.[21]

The primordial genital ducts, namely the wolffian ducts (male) and the müllerian ducts (female), do not arise simultaneously. The wolffian duct develops first from the mesonephros and may participate in the formation of the müllerian ducts.[12] During normal female fetal development, the wolffian duct degenerates as a result of the lack of locally produced androgen. Degeneration of the wolffian duct begins soon after gonadal differentiation but is not complete until the beginning of the third trimester of pregnancy.[22] In the female the müllerian duct forms the fallopian tubes, the uterus, and the upper third of the vagina. At about 10 wk the uterus differentiates into an upper corpus and a lower cervix.[22] Although the cervix and corpus are initially the same length, the cervix is two thirds of the total length by the time of birth.[12] The development of the müllerian duct requires neither the gonads nor hormonal secretion, because it has been shown to develop normally in fetuses without gonads.[12]

Childhood and Premenarchal Ovary

After birth, the mean ovarian weight increases from about 250 mg to approximately 4000 mg by menarche.[23] Histologic evidence obtained from postmortem examination indicates that active follicular growth and atresia occur during infancy and childhood.[16, 24] The increase in size and weight of the ovaries is caused by increases in the amount of stroma, the

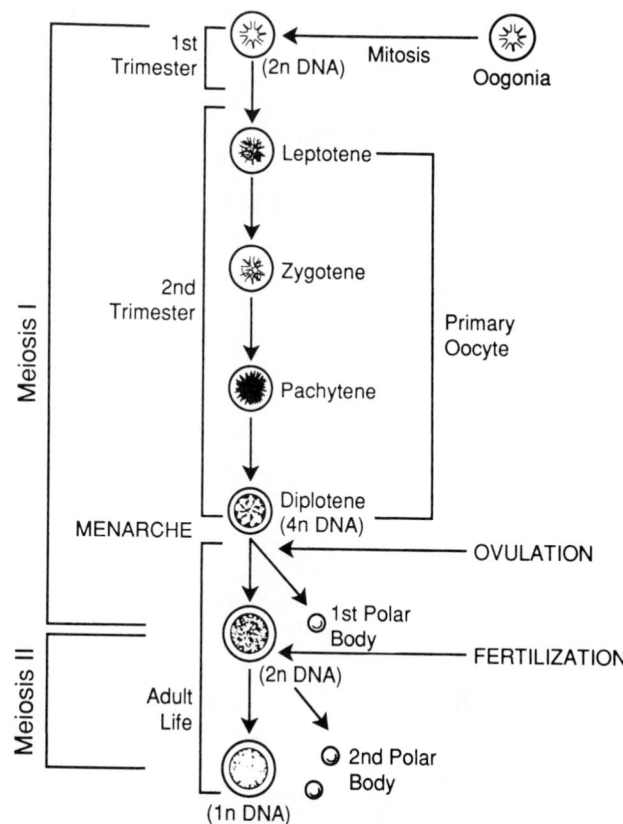

Figure 15–4. The life cycle of the oocyte. During the first trimester of fetal life the oogonium undergoes mitosis. Meiosis I is initiated during the second trimester but is arrested at the diplotene stage (4n DNA). After menarche, at the time of ovulation, meiosis resumes in one ovum with the formation of the first polar body (2n DNA). Meiosis II is initiated at the time of fertilization and is completed with the formation of the second polar body (1n DNA). Fusion with the male pronucleus restores the nuclear content to 2n DNA.

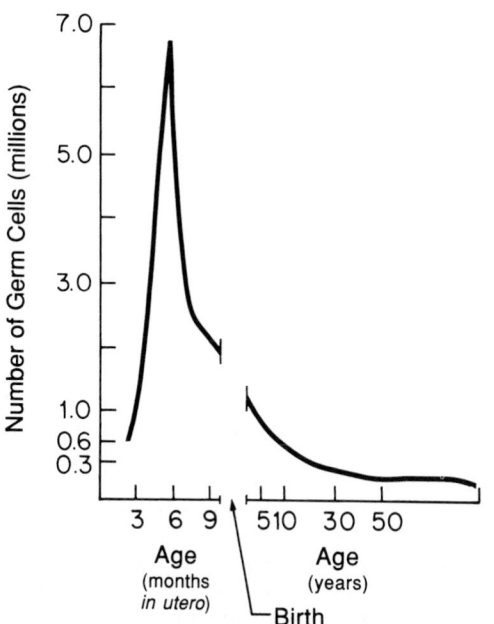

Figure 15–3. Changes in germ cell number in the human ovary with increasing age. (From Baker TG. A quantitative and cytological study of germ cells in the human ovaries. Proc R Soc Lond B Biol Sci 1963; 158:417–433, with permission.)

size of individual follicles, and the number of follicles (Fig. 15–6).[16] The final maturation of the ovarian follicles at puberty occurs in response to increasing levels of FSH and LH.

Levels of gonadotropin vary significantly during the different stages of life in the female (Fig. 15–7). Plasma gonadotropins rise during the second trimester of fetal development, reaching levels equivalent to those observed in the menopause.[25] This peak in gonadotropin levels may be causally related to maximal development of follicles. During the later part of the second trimester, the hypothalamic-pituitary axis (the so-called gonadostat) undergoes maturation and becomes more sensitive to the suppressive effects of high levels of estrogen and progesterone secreted by the placenta, so that fetal plasma concentrations of gonadotropins decrease and become virtually undetectable at birth.[26, 27]

After birth, gonadotropin levels rise abruptly because of the decrease in estrogen and progestagen levels that occurs with separation of the placenta.[28] Elevated levels of gonadotropins persist for the first few months of life, decreasing again to low levels by 1 to 3 y.[28] Low levels of gonadotropins during the childhood years are thought to result from exquisite sensitivity of the hypothalamic-pituitary axis, which remains suppressed despite extremely low levels of circulating gonadal steroids.[26] In keeping with this hypothesis is the fact that gonadotropin levels are elevated in children with gonadal dysgenesis and in children who have been castrated during the first 4 y of life (Fig. 15–8).[29] The prepubertal hypothalamic-pituitary axis (in normal children) is 6 to 15 times more sensitive to estrogen than is the adult feedback mechanism.[27]

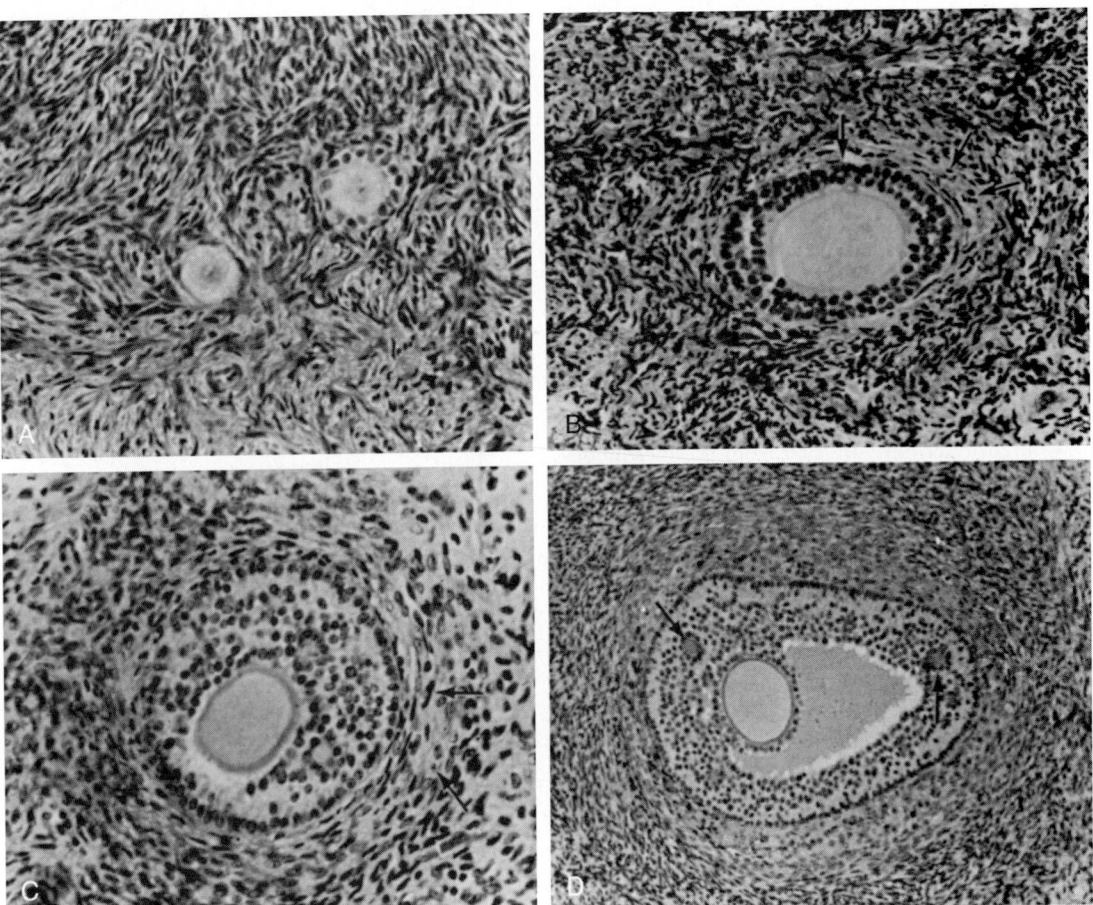

Figure 15–5. *A,* Primordial follicle *(lower left)* and primary follicle *(upper right)* in human ovary. *B,* Primary follicle with three layers of granulosa cells and incipient differentiation of theca *(arrows)* from surrounding stroma. *C,* Primary follicle with multiple layers of granulosa cells and beginning epithelioid transformation of theca *(arrows). D,* Graafian follicle. Note the epithelioid character of the theca cells and the Call-Exner bodies *(arrows)* among the granulosa cells.

In addition to the highly sensitive gonadal steroid–dependent negative-feedback system, a steroid-independent mechanism for inhibitory control of central nervous system (CNS) responses is also operative, because gonadotropin levels also fall in the absence of a gonad (see Fig. 15–8) and in children with gonadal dysgenesis between ages 5 and 11.[27]

To date, no physiological inhibitors of the secretion of luteinizing hormone–releasing hormone (LHRH, also called gonadotropin-releasing hormone [GnRH]) have been identified in humans or other primates.[30] The infusion of LHRH stimulates additional release of gonadotropins in agonadal children, substantiating the concept of a steroid hormone–independent mechanism of inhibition of the hypothalamic-pituitary axis.[31] Although the pineal gland has been proposed to be an inhibitor of gonadotropin secretion, in the human neither the pineal gland nor melatonin has a major inhibitory effect on the hypothalamic-pituitary axis.[27]

Although basal gonadotropin secretion is low in prepubertal girls, small but detectable pulses are observed at 2- to 3-h intervals, as in adults.[32] During puberty the pituitary becomes more sensitive to infusions of LHRH, and the LH and FSH responses to LHRH increase in age-dependent increments.[33] As puberty approaches, three major developments can be delineated: (1) adrenarche, the onset of adrenal androgen secretion; (2) decreased sensitivity of the gonadostat to feedback control by gonadal steroids, leading to activation or disinhibition of the LHRH neurosecretory neurons in the medial basal hypothalamus, with a consequent increase in pituitary gonadotropin release; and (3) gonadarche, the enhancement of estrogen secretion by the ovary and the onset of ovulatory cycles.

An increase in secretion of adrenal androgens occurs before maturation of gonadotropin secretion. The levels of androstenedione, dehydroepiandrosterone (DHEA), and dehydroepiandrosterone sulfate (DHEAS) increase in children beginning at approximately age 6 to 8. In association with the rise in adrenal androgen secretion, the expression of 3β-hydroxysteroid dehydrogenase (3β-HSD) in the reticularis zone of the human adrenal declines after age 5.[34] This increased secretion by the adrenal cortex is probably under the control of corticotropin (also called ACTH or adrenocorticotropin).[34–36] A variety of other peptide or protein hormones have been proposed as adrenal androgen–stimulating factors for the initiation of adrenarche, but evidence for the role of a hormone other than corticotropin remains elusive.[36]

Adrenal androgens must be converted to more potent androgens to exert androgenic effects, but they are believed to be involved in the initial spurt in skeletal growth and the development of axillary and pubic hair. Because of the close relation between the onset of adrenarche and the initiation of gonadarche, it has been proposed that the increased secretion of LHRH and gonadotropin by the hypothalamic-pituitary axis is influenced by adrenal activation. However, evidence of several types suggests that the control mechanisms for adrenarche and gonadarche are independent. Adrenarche occurs normally in patients with Kallmann's syndrome (hypogonadotropic hypogonadism) and in those with gonadal dysgenesis (hypergonadotropic hypogonadism). Premature pubarche

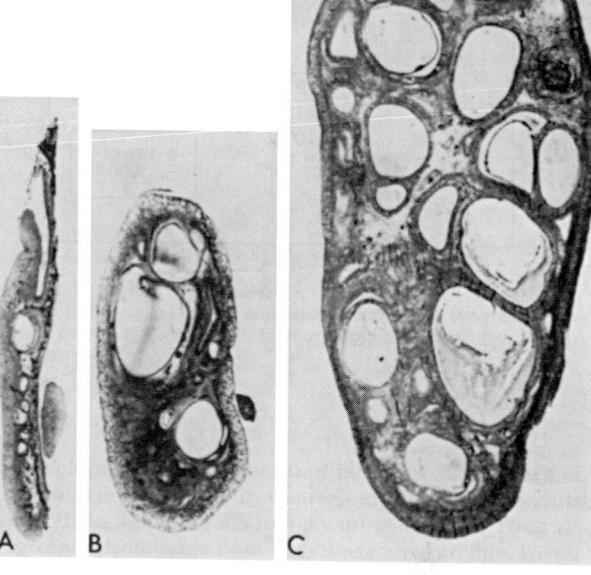

Figure 15–6. Ovaries of *(A)* a newborn, *(B)* a 10-month-old infant, and *(C)* a 9-year-old girl. Magnification of all × 6.5. (From Peters H, Byskov AG, Grinsted J. Follicular growth in fetal and prepubertal ovaries in humans and other primates. Clin Endocrinol Metab 1978; 7:469–485, with permission.)

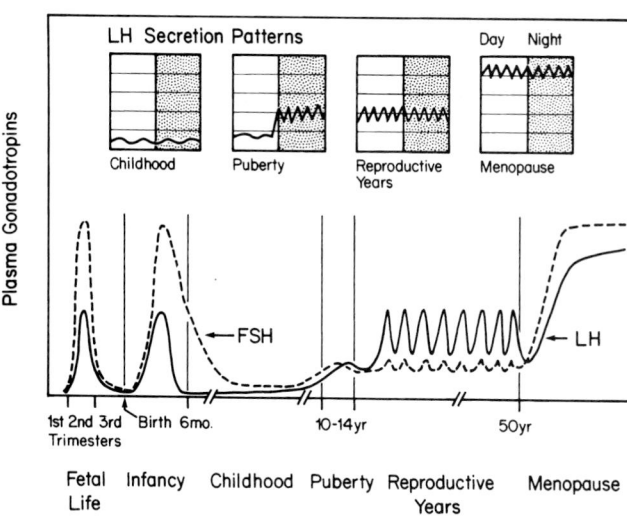

Figure 15–7. Pattern of gonadotropin secretion during different stages of life in women. The secretory patterns of LH during the waking hours *(clear area)* and at night *(stippled area)* for each stage are indicated in the upper insets. (From Carr BR, Wilson JD. Disorders of the ovary and female reproductive tract. In: Braunwald E, Isselbacher KJ, Petersdorf RG, et al., eds. Harrison's Principles of Internal Medicine. 11th ed. New York: McGraw-Hill, 1987: 1818–1837. Reproduced with permission of McGraw-Hill, Inc. As modified from Yen SCC. In: Ferin M, ed. Biorhythms and Human Reproduction. New York: John Wiley & Sons, 1974; 219–238. Copyright © 1974, John Wiley & Sons, Inc.)

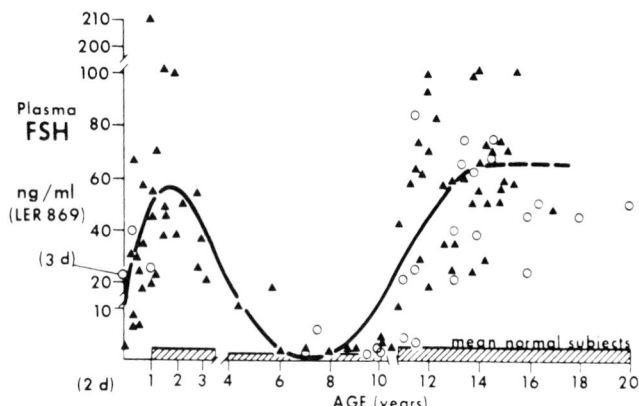

Figure 15–8. Pattern of plasma FSH concentration in relation to age in 58 patients with gonadal dysgenesis. Solid triangles indicate patients with 45,X karyotype; open circles indicate patients with structural abnormalities of the X chromosome and mosaics. The hatched area indicates the mean range for FSH values in normal females. To convert FSH values to international units per liter, multiply by 8.4. (From Conte FA, Grumbach MM, Kaplan SL. A diphasic pattern of gonadotropin secretion in patients with the syndrome of gonadal dysgenesis. J Clin Endocrinol Metab 1975; 40:670–674. Copyright © 1975, by The Endocrine Society.)

TABLE 15–2. Stages of Female Puberty

Stage	Breast	Pubic Hair
1	Preadolescent; only papillae are elevated.	Preadolescent; vellus hair only and hair is similar to development over anterior abdominal wall (i.e., no pubic hair).
2	Breast bud and papilla are elevated and a small mount is present; areola diameter is enlarged.	There is sparse growth of long, slightly pigmented, downy hair or only slightly curled hair, appearing along labia.
3	Further enlargement of breast mound; increased palpable glandular tissue.	Hair is darker, coarser, more curled, and spreads to the pubic junction.
4	Areola and papilla are elevated to form a second mound above the level of the rest of the breast.	Adult-type hair; area covered is less than that in most adults; there is no spread to the medial surface of thighs.
5	Adult mature breast; recession of areola to the mound of breast tissue, rounding of the breast mound, and projection of only the papilla are evident.	Adult-type hair with increased spread to medial surface of thighs; distribution is as an inverse triangle.

Adapted from Marshall WA, Tanner JM. Variations in pattern of pubertal changes in girls. Arch Dis Child 1969: 44:2291–303.

area of attachment of the ovary to the mesovarium. The anatomic components and function of the adult ovary are illustrated schematically in Figure 15–13.

GERMINAL EPITHELIUM. The germinal epithelium consists of coelomic epithelial cells. Its function is incompletely understood, but it is likely that germ cell number is fixed prenatally in all mammals, including humans.[57] The germinal epithelium undergoes decidualization in response to the hormones of pregnancy. With aging, the ovary becomes convoluted, giving rise to crypts lined with germinal epithelium. At times the continuity between the germinal epithelium in these crypts and the remaining epithelium is disrupted, giving rise to isolated rests or nests of germinal epithelium cells. After the menopause, these nests can develop into inclusion cysts or solid nests of metaplastic epithelial cells.[58]

FOLLICLES. The follicles are embedded in loose connective tissue of the ovarian cortex and can be subdivided into two functional types: nongrowing, or primordial, and growing. The majority of follicles (90 to 95%) are nongrowing throughout reproductive life (Fig. 15–14; see Fig. 15–5A). Recruitment of a primordial follicle initiates dramatic changes in growth,

structure, and function. The growing follicles are divided into five stages: primary, secondary, tertiary, graafian, and atretic. The first three stages of growth can occur in the absence of the pituitary and therefore appear to be controlled by intraovarian mechanisms. One hypothesis suggests that the early stages of follicular development occur over several menstrual cycles, so that the total time to attain a preovulatory status averages 85 days.[59] However, most researchers believe that a group of primary follicles are recruited in the luteal phase of the previous menstrual cycle.[37] After a follicle enters the tertiary stage, continued growth and steroidogenesis depend on the presence of gonadotropins.[60]

The primordial follicle is composed of a single layer of granulosa cells and a single immature oocyte arrested in the diplotene stage of the first meiotic division. The primordial follicle is separated from the surrounding stroma by a thin basal lamina (basement membrane). The oocyte is enclosed by a single layer of spindle-shaped cells with protoplasmic processes that reach the basal lamina, providing a route for transfer of nutrients. The oocyte and granulosa cells do not have a direct blood supply and therefore exist in a microenvi-

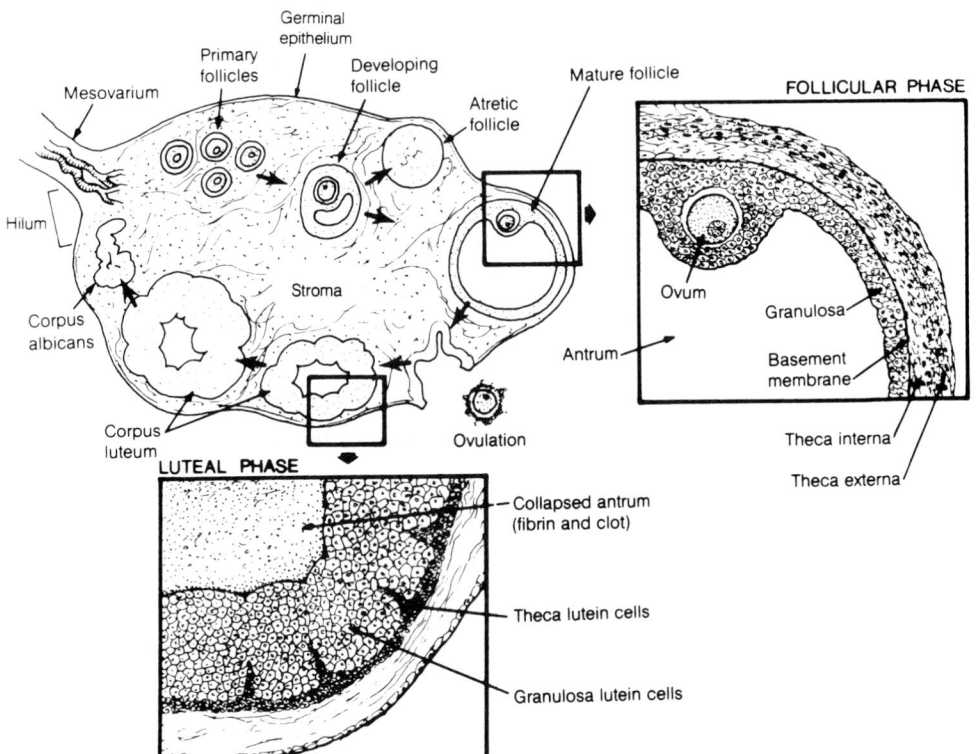

Figure 15–13. Developmental changes in the adult ovary during a complete menstrual cycle. (From Carr BR, Wilson JD. Disorders of the ovary and female reproductive tract. In: Braunwald E, Isselbacher KJ, Petersdorf RG, et al, eds. Harrison's Principles of Internal Medicine. 11th ed. New York: McGraw-Hill, 1987: 1818–1837. Reproduced with permission of McGraw-Hill, Inc.)

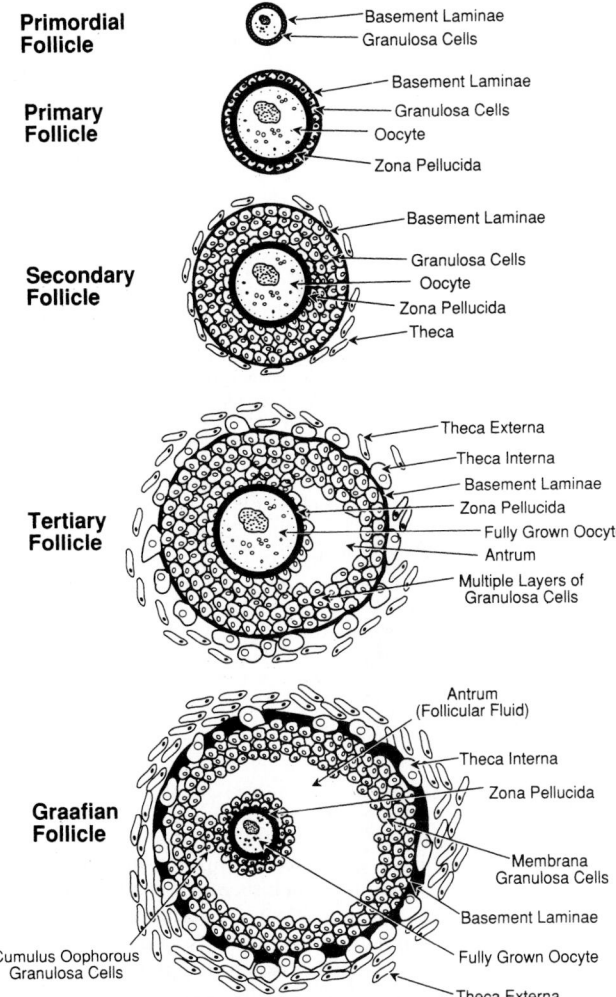

Figure 15–14. The structure and classification of the ovarian follicle during growth and development. (Adapted from Erickson GF, Magoffin DA, Dyer CA. The ovarian androgen producing cells: a review of structure/function relations. Endocr Rev 1985; 6:371–379. Copyright © 1985 by The Endocrine Society.)

ronment separated from contact with other cells by the basal lamina.[61]

The first sign of follicular recruitment is cuboidal differentiation in the spindle-shaped cells inside the basal lamina, which then undergo successive mitotic divisions to form a multilayered stratum granulosa or zona granulosa. The oocyte enlarges and secretes a glycoprotein-containing mucoid substance called the *zona pellucida*, which surrounds the oocyte and separates the granulosa cells from the oocyte (see Figs. 15–5B and C and 15–14).[62, 63] This structure is a primary follicle.

The secondary follicle is formed by further proliferation of granulosa cells and by the final phase of oocyte growth, in which the oocyte reaches 120 μm in diameter. Coincident with proliferation of granulosa cells, stromal cells outside the basal lamina differentiate and become arranged in concentric perifollicular layers of cells to constitute the theca (see Figs. 15–5B and C and 15–14). The portion of the theca adjacent to the basal lamina is termed the *theca interna*. Thecal cells that merge with the surrounding stroma are designated the *theca externa*. The secondary follicle acquires an independent blood supply consisting of one or more arterioles that terminate in a capillary bed at the basal lamina. Capillaries do not penetrate the basement membrane, and the granulosa and oocyte remain avascular. A distinct morphologic feature of the

granulosa cells consists of a basal lamina attached to granulosa cells associated with a cavity filled with basal lamina and a flocculent, protein-like material. These *Call-Exner bodies* appear during development of the secondary follicle (see Fig. 15–5D). Little is known about their formation or physiological significance.

The tertiary follicle is characterized by further hypertrophy of the theca and the appearance of a fluid-filled space among the granulosa cells, named the antrum (see Figs. 15–5D and 15–14). The fluid in the antrum consists of a plasma transudate and secretory products of granulosa cells, some of which (estrogens) are found there in higher concentrations than in peripheral blood.[64] In association with the formation of the antrum, the granulosa and thecal cells develop specialized contacts between cells known as *gap junctions*.[65, 66] Gap junctions allow small molecules to pass from one cell to another, thereby permitting cell-cell communication and synchronized coordination of follicular function (Fig. 15–15).

At this stage the follicle rapidly increases in size under the influence of gonadotropins to form the mature or graafian follicle (see Fig. 15–14). During this stage the granulosa and oocyte remain encased by the basal lamina and are devoid of direct vascularization. The antral fluid increases in volume, and the oocyte, surrounded by an accumulation of granulosa cells (the cumulus oophorus), occupies a polar, eccentric position within the follicle.[67] The mature graafian follicle is ready to release the ovum by the process of ovulation (see later discussion). Based on findings in women with natural cycles and in women with hypogonadotropic hypogonadism treated with gonadotropins, the average time for development of a primary follicle to the point of ovulation is 10 to 14 d.[68]

Recruited primordial follicles either develop into dominant, mature graafian follicles destined to ovulate or degenerate as a result of atresia.[64] During atresia, the oocyte and granulosa cells within the basal lamina die and are replaced by fibrous tissue. In contrast, the thecal cells outside the basal lamina do not die but dedifferentiate and return to the pool of cells consisting of ovarian interstitial or stromal cells.[56] The process of atresia is generally thought to result from lack of the hormones or growth factors that are formed by the mature dominant follicle through intrinsic intraovarian mechanisms. There is general agreement that atresia of follicles is due to apoptosis (programmed cell death).[69]

STROMA. The ovarian stroma consists of three major cell types: connective tissue cells similar to those of other tissues, contractile cells, and several types of interstitial cells.[58] The interstitial cells are the most important because they secrete steroid hormones (principally androgens) and undergo morphologic changes in response to LH and hCG.[56] Interstitial cells are derived from mesenchymal cells of the ovarian stroma.[70] The human ovary contains four major categories of interstitial cells: primary, secondary, thecal, and hilar.

The primary interstitial cells are the first to develop and are identifiable in the fetal ovary only between weeks 12 and 20 of fetal life.[71] They closely resemble early Leydig cells of the fetal testis and have the ultrastructural features of steroid-secreting cells.[71]

Secondary interstitial cells are derived from the thecal cells of atretic follicles.[70, 72] These large epithelial cells hypertrophy and maintain the active steroidogenic features of the thecal interstitial cells from which they are derived. Secondary cells retain responsiveness to LH[71] but differ in that they are innervated and respond to catecholamines, which stimulate structural changes and hormone secretion.[73]

Thecal interstitial cells in tertiary follicles are the active site of androgen secretion.[74] They develop from mesenchymal cells that differentiate when secondary follicles form. Thecal interstitial cells contain LH receptors and the steroidogenic enzymes 3β-HSD and Δ^{4,5}-isomerase. The transformation from

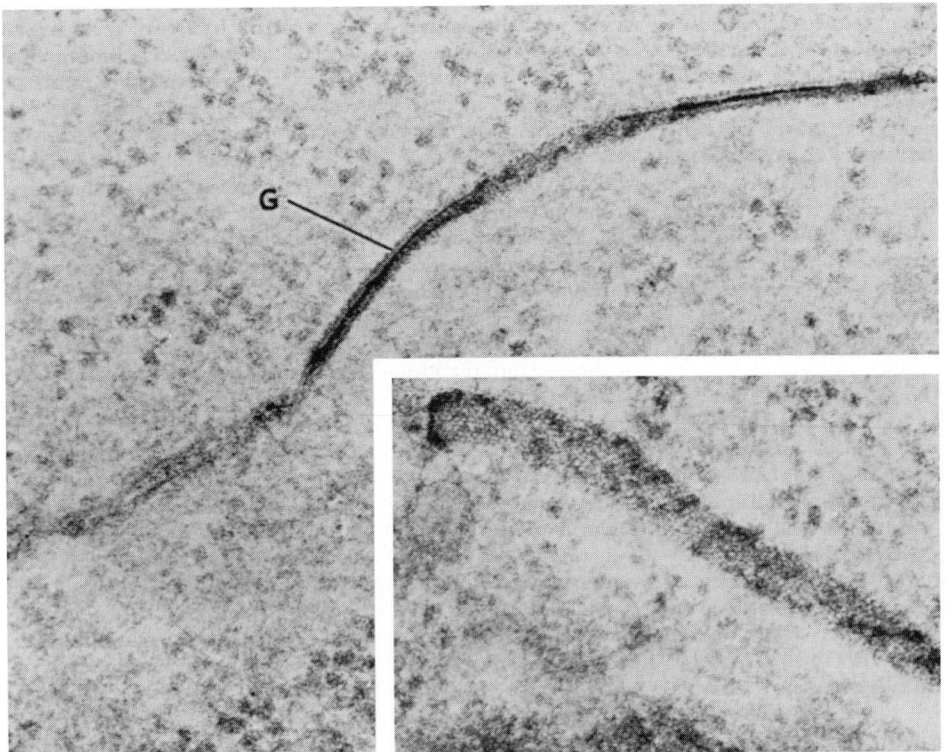

Figure 15–15. The gap junction (G) of an early antral follicle. Magnification × 139,800. Inset is an en face section of the junction revealing the quasihexagonal ordering of subunits. Magnification × 139,800. (From Albertini DF, Anderson E. The appearance and structure of intracellular connections during the ontogeny of the rabbit ovarian follicle with particular reference to gap junctions. Reproduced from the Journal of Cell Biology, 1974, vol 63, pp 234–250 by copyright permission of the Rockefeller University Press.)

stromal cells is influenced locally by the secondary follicle but appears to depend on gonadotropin stimulation.[75] These cells markedly increase in size and develop ultrastructural changes characteristic of steroid-secreting cells. Thecal interstitial cells give rise to secondary interstitial cells after follicular atresia, as stated previously.

The hilum, where the blood vessels, lymphatics, and nerves enter the ovary, is the locus of specific interstitial cells termed *hilar cells*. These cells contain crystalloids of Reinke and are morphologically indistinguishable from Leydig cells of the testes.[56, 76] Hilar cells, which are difficult to identify before puberty, synthesize and secrete testosterone in response to LH. Occasionally, hyperplastic or neoplastic changes in hilar cells result in virilization associated with excessive testosterone secretion.[70] The physiological function of hilar cells is obscure but because of their intimate association with nerve fibers and blood vessels, they may influence ovarian function.

OVUM. In the mature dominant follicle, oocyte growth occurs and meiosis is completed. During growth, the oocyte increases in diameter from 20 to 120 μm. The growth period is associated with accumulation of nutritional stores. Oocyte growth is linear until the follicle reaches the tertiary stage and thereafter ceases.[77]

The presence of granulosa cells is an absolute requirement for growth of the oocyte.[78] The oocyte is surrounded by a collection of granulosa cells termed the *corona radiata* that interact with the oocyte by gap junctions, as described previously. The zona pellucida that forms between the corona radiata and the oocyte during formation of the primary follicle contains species-specific receptors for sperm, prevents polyspermy, and promotes movement of the fertilized ovum from the fallopian tube to the uterus.[79] The zona pellucida consists of three glycoproteins secreted by the growing oocyte.[80]

As depicted in Figure 15–4, meiosis resumes at the time of ovulation. The roles of oocyte maturation inhibitor and meiosis-inducing substance in the resumption of meiosis were described previously. The resumption of meiosis occurs after the preovulatory surge of LH.[81] The oocytes of mature follicles

undergo meiosis when placed in culture, supporting the concept that an inhibitory influence suppresses meiosis before ovulation. The progression of meiosis in the mature oocyte is associated with loss of the nuclear or germinal membrane, condensation of chromatin into bivalents, separation of homologous chromosomes, and arrest at metaphase II.[82] Meiosis is completed with the release of the second polar body at the time of fertilization. High concentrations of estradiol in follicular fluid are required for normal meiotic maturation.[83]

CORPUS LUTEUM. At the time of the preovulatory surge of LH, a series of biochemical and morphologic changes occurs in the cells of the granulosa and theca interna. This process is called luteinization. During luteinization these cells undergo hypertrophy and exhibit increased RNA and protein synthesis under the influence of LH.[84] After ovulation the basement membrane separating the granulosa from the theca breaks down, and blood vessels and capillaries invade the granulosa cells. The growth of new vessels and invading fibroblasts is believed to be caused by an angiogenic factor or factors secreted by the ovary after ovulation.[85]

The morphology of the developing corpus luteum (yellow body) has been well characterized.[86, 87] In brief, proliferation of the granulosa cells occurs during the day after ovulation. Capillary invasion of the granulosa cells begins on day 2 after ovulation and reaches the central cavity by day 4. Hemorrhage into the cavity can occur on any day, with the formation of a fibrin clot, and fibroblasts appear in the central cavity by day 5 (Fig. 15–16; see Fig. 15–13). Maximal capillary dilation is attained by days 7 to 8, a time that corresponds to maximal progesterone secretion. The human corpus luteum secretes as much as 40 mg of progesterone per day during the midluteal phase of the ovarian cycle.[88] In view of the small size of the corpus luteum, it is the most active steroidogenic tissue in humans. The cells of the corpus luteum are derived from cells that make up the follicle, namely the granulosa and the theca. The granulosa cells become granulosa-lutein cells (large cells), and the theca cells are transformed into theca-lutein cells (small cells; see Fig. 15–16).[89] The so-called K cells, scattered throughout the corpus luteum, are believed to be macrophages.[90]

In the absence of pregnancy, the corpus luteum undergoes degeneration. This process, termed *luteolysis,* and is first apparent on the eighth day after ovulation.[86] During luteolysis the granulosa-lutein cells shrink, and the thecal cells appear to be more prominent. Later both types of cells undergo cell death, possibly involving the process of apoptosis in some species.[91] The remaining corpus luteum is composed of dense connective tissue and is termed the *corpus albicans.*

Physiology of Ovarian Function

HYPOTHALAMIC-PITUITARY-OVARIAN AXIS: AN OVERVIEW. The hypothalamus plays an important role in the hormonal regulation of female reproductive function (Fig. 15–17). Understanding of the hormonal control of reproduction has progressed from the identification of ovarian steroids and pituitary gonadotropins to the discovery of hypothalamic releasing factors and the identification of a host of ovarian hormones and growth factors that modulate gonadotropin secretion and intraovarian regulation.[92] It is now believed that the follicle destined to ovulate initiates the sequence of coordinated events that control the menstrual cycle by way of the hypothalamic-pituitary system.

The hypothalamus is connected to the pituitary by a portal vascular system that serves as a conduit for transport of hormones from the brain to the pituitary. The primary direction of blood flow is from the hypothalamus to the pituitary, and interruption of this connection leads to a decline in gonadotropin levels and eventually to atrophy of the ovaries

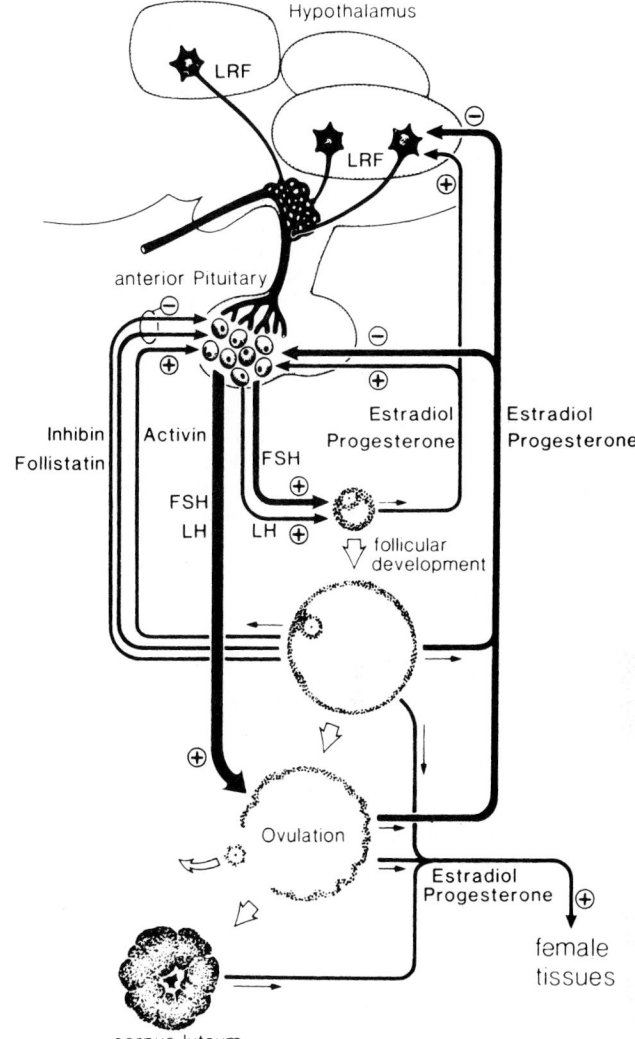

Figure 15–17. A diagrammatic representation of the hypothalamic-pituitary-ovarian axis. LRF, luteinizing-releasing factor. (From Ying SY. Inhibins, activins, and follistatins: gonadal proteins modulating the secretion of follicle-stimulating hormone. Endocr Rev 1988; 9:267–293. Copyright © 1988, by The Endocrine Society.)

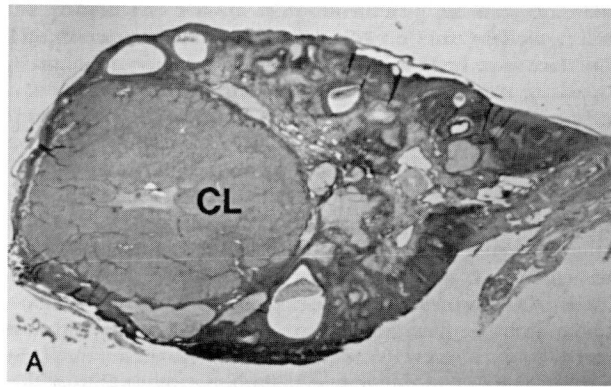

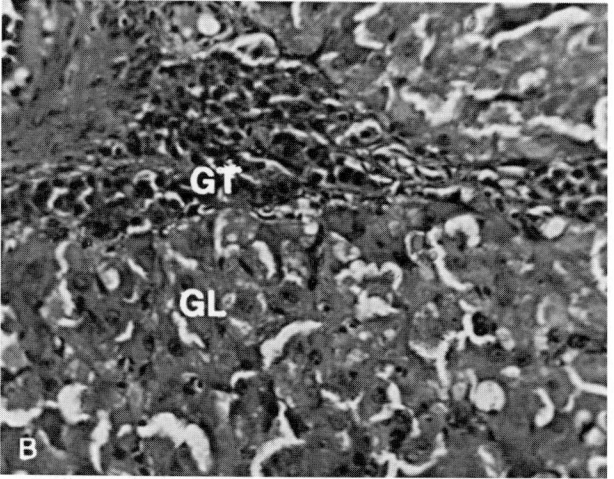

Figure 15–16. *A,* Photomicrograph of a human corpus luteum (CL). *B,* The larger, pale-staining granulosa-lutein cells (GL) can readily be distinguished from the smaller, dark-staining theca-lutein cells (GT).

with failure of hormone secretion. Retrograde flow also occurs in the portal vessels, providing a short feedback loop from pituitary to hypothalamus.[93]

The principal hypothalamic releasing factor regulating reproductive function is LHRH, a decapeptide. Although separate releasing hormones were originally believed to exist for LH and FSH, the current predominant view is that LHRH is the only gonadotropin-releasing hormone.[92, 94] A large number of LHRH analogues have been developed.[95] All inhibit release of both LH and FSH; none selectively inhibits LH or FSH. The variations in response of LH and FSH after infusion of LHRH are believed to be caused by feedback effects of ovarian hormones on the hypothalamic-pituitary axis.

The hypothalamic release of LHRH is influenced by neurons from other regions of the brain whose terminals end in the arcuate nucleus. Epinephrine and norepinephrine increase LHRH release, whereas dopamine, serotonin, and endogenous opioid peptides are inhibitory.[96] Other hormones, in particular gut-related peptide hormones, also modulate LHRH release.[96]

The half-life of LHRH is short (2 to 4 min), and its metabolic clearance rate averages 800 L/m² body surface area/d.[97] The fact that LH and FSH are secreted in short pulsatile bursts led to the assumption that LHRH release is also pulsatile. This conclusion was confirmed by measurements in hypothalamic-pituitary portal venous blood from monkeys and sheep showing that LHRH is secreted in a pulsatile fashion at intervals of 70 to 90 min.[40, 98–100]

Knobil showed in the rhesus monkey that the area of the brain responsible for the LHRH pulse generator is in the arcuate nucleus of the medial basal hypothalamus.[40] Pulsatile LHRH secretion by the arcuate nucleus is a prerequisite for normal secretion of pituitary gonadotropins.[40] This conclusion is based on studies of reactivation of gonadotropin secretion after destruction of the arcuate nucleus in the rhesus monkey, in which it was shown that normal LH and FSH release requires the pulsatile infusion of LHRH at intervals of approximately 1 h.[101] LHRH pulses of a lesser or greater frequency or administration of LHRH by continuous infusion failed to stimulate the release of LH and FSH (Fig. 15–18).[101, 102] The pulsatile release of LHRH is required for the midcycle surge of gonadotropins, which is regulated primarily by ovarian hormone feedback at the level of the pituitary, but its role appears to be permissive.[101] These observations have been confirmed in humans by showing that the pulsatile administration of LHRH to women with isolated LHRH deficiency can reproduce the hormonal changes seen during the menstrual cycle and can result in ovulation and fertility.[103]

LHRH acts on the gonadotropic cells of the pituitary to stimulate the release of LH and FSH. The initial step involves binding of LHRH to high-affinity receptor sites on the plasma membranes of these cells.[104, 105] LHRH-induced release of gonadotropins after binding to the receptor appears to be independent of cyclic AMP and instead requires calcium and activation of protein kinase C.[104, 105]

Three types of secretory patterns can be distinguished for gonadotropin in women:

1. *Trigintan* or *circatrigintan patterns* are low-frequency changes in gonadotropin secretion that occur approximately every 30 d during the normal menstrual cycle.[106]

2. *Diurnal patterns* are intermittent-frequency changes in gonadotropin secretion that recur every 24 h. These changes are minimal in adult women but are marked during sleep at the initiation of puberty in girls, as discussed previously.[39]

3. *Circhoral patterns* are high-frequency changes in gona-

dotropin secretion characterized by pulses approximately every hour.[40]

LHRH regulates (1) synthesis and storage of gonadotropins, (2) activation or movement of gonadotropins from reserve to a pool ready for secretion, and (3) immediate release of gonadotropins. LH and FSH, like thyrotropin and hCG, are glycoproteins composed of two polypeptide chains designated alpha and beta. A single gene appears to be responsible for the expression of the alpha subunit, which is similar for all four glycoproteins and contains 92 amino acids.[107] The beta chains for the glycoprotein hormones are unique, ensuring specific biologic activity for each hormone. Both subunits are required for full expression of biologic activity.[108] The beta subunit of hCG (β-hCG), the largest subunit, is similar to the beta subunit of LH except for an additional 30-amino-acid residue and a large carbohydrate moiety at the COOH terminus.[108] The half-life of hCG is the longest, followed by that of FSH and then LH, and is determined in part by the sialic content of the hormones.[109, 110]

FSH and LH are secreted in a coordinated fashion to regulate follicle growth, ovulation, and maintenance of the corpus luteum (see later discussion). As mentioned previously, the release of FSH and LH requires the constant pulsatile release of LHRH from the hypothalamus. In addition, the release of LH and FSH is affected both positively and negatively by estrogen and progesterone. Whether estrogen and progesterone stimulate or inhibit gonadotropin release depends on concentration and duration of exposure of the pituitary to the steroids.[111] In addition to steroid hormones, at least three gonadal protein hormones modulate FSH release. Activin appears to stimulate FSH, whereas inhibin and folliculostatin suppress FSH (see Fig. 15–17).[92]

Negative Feedback. Estrogen exerts its inhibitory effect on both the hypothalamus and the pituitary. Negative feedback is evidenced by the increase in LH and FSH that occurs when ovarian secretion of estrogen decreases after menopause or castration.[112] Inhibition of FSH and LH secretion occurs at low levels of estrogen but is more complete at high levels. Progesterone at high concentrations inhibits FSH and LH primarily at the level of the hypothalamus.[113] As noted, both inhibin and folliculostatin selectively inhibit FSH secretion.[92]

Positive Feedback. In addition to a negative feedback, gonadal hormones exert a positive effect on gonadotropin secretion. The positive feedback is paramount in the promotion of the LH surge required to initiate ovulation and is triggered by a sharply rising plasma level of estrogen. Two features are essential for this mechanism: (1) an estradiol concentration of more than 700 pmol/L (200 pg/mL) and (2) persistence of the elevated level of estradiol for at least 48 to 50 h.[114] Progesterone is reportedly responsible for the midcycle FSH surge.[115] Progesterone at low concentrations stimulates LH release, but only after previous prolonged exposure of the pituitary to estrogen.[116] In addition, secretion of activin by granulosa cells serves to augment FSH release (see Fig. 15–17).[92]

Ovarian Hormones

STEROID HORMONES

CLASSIFICATION. The ovarian steroids are classified on the basis of chemical structure and principal biologic function and consist of three major types: estrogens, progestagens, and androgens (Fig. 15–19).[117]

Estrogens. The naturally occurring estrogens are C_{18}-steroids characterized by the presence of an aromatic A ring, a phenolic hydroxyl group at C-3, and either a hydroxyl group (estradiol) or a ketone group (estrone). The principal and most important, as well as most potent, estrogen secreted by

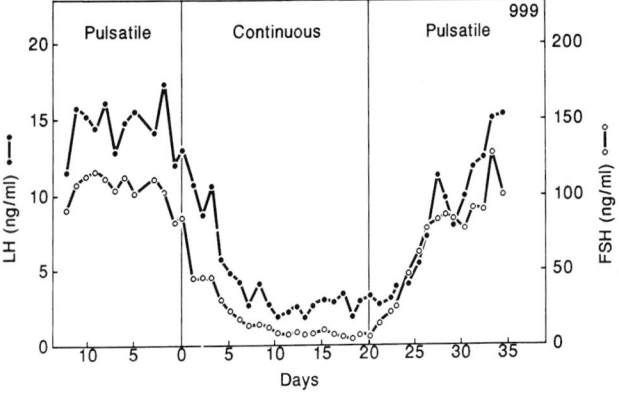

Figure 15–18. The effect of pulsatile or continuous administration of LHRH to ovariectomized monkeys rendered LHRH deficient by placement of a lesion in the hypothalamus. LH and FSH release was restored by hourly LHRH infusion, inhibited during a continuous LHRH infusion, and again restored after reinstitution of pulsatile LHRH administration. (Adapted from Belchetz PE, Plant TM, Nakai Y, et al. Hypophysial responses to continuous and intermittent delivery of hypothalamic gonadotropin-releasing hormone. Science 1978; 202:631–633. Copyright © 1978, by the American Association for the Advancement of Science.)

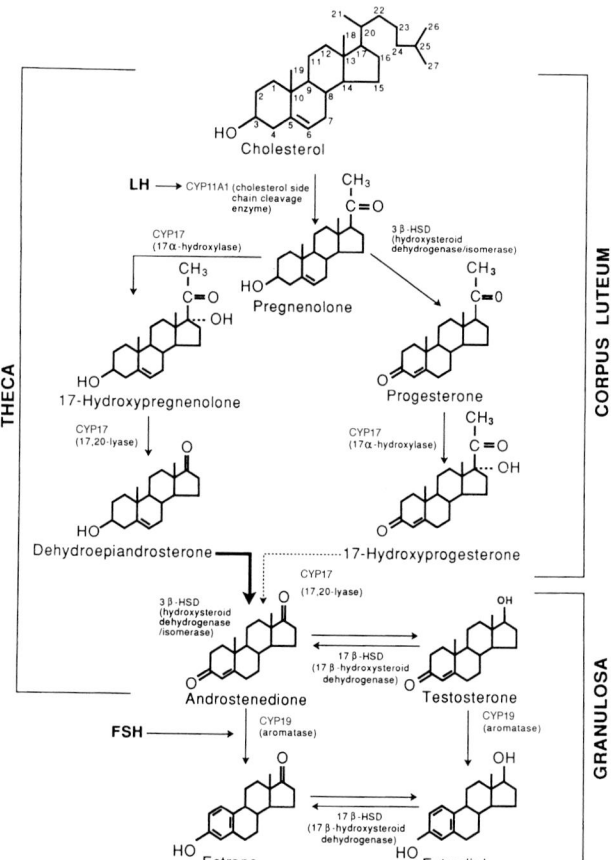

Figure 15–19. Principal pathways of steroid hormone biosynthesis in the human ovary. Although each cell type of the ovary contains the complete enzyme complement required for the formation of estradiol from cholesterol, the amounts of the various enzymes and consequently the predominant hormones formed differ among the cell types. The major enzyme complements for the corpus luteum, theca, and granulosa cells are shown in brackets; these cells produce predominantly progesterone and 17-hydroxyprogesterone (corpus luteum), androgen (theca), and estrogen (granulosa). The major sites of actions of LH and FSH in mediating this pathway are shown by the horizontal arrows. The dotted line emphasizes that the metabolism of 17-hydroxyprogesterone is limited in the human ovary.

ity in the endometrium of the estrogen-primed uterus). Progesterone is required for implantation of the fertilized ovum and maintenance of pregnancy. It also induces decidualization of the endometrium, inhibits uterine contractions, increases the viscosity of cervical mucus, promotes glandular development of the breast, and increases basal body temperature. However, 17-OHP, also secreted by the corpus luteum, has little, if any, biologic activity.[122]

Androgens. The ovary secretes a variety of C_{19}-steroids, including DHEA, androstenedione, testosterone, and dihydrotestosterone. They are produced by the thecal cells and to a lesser degree by the ovarian stroma. The major C_{19}-steroid is androstenedione (see Fig. 15–19), part of which is secreted directly into plasma, with the remainder converted to estrogen by the granulosa cells (see later discussion). Androstenedione can be converted to estrogen or testosterone in the ovary and in extraglandular tissues. Only testosterone and dihydrotestosterone are true androgens with the capacity of interacting with the androgen receptor. Excessive production of androgens by the ovary or adrenal can cause sexual ambiguity in the newborn or hirsutism or virilization in women.[122]

BIOGENESIS OF STEROID HORMONES. All the steroids of the ovary, as well as those produced by the testes, adrenal, and placenta, are derived from cholesterol. Cholesterol can be obtained from three sources: (1) preformed cholesterol circulating in blood in the form of lipoproteins, (2) cholesterol synthesized de novo within the ovary from two-carbon units (acetylcoenzyme A), and (3) cholesterol liberated from cholesterol esters stored within lipid droplets (Fig. 15–20). The cholesterol used by the human ovary for steroidogenesis is derived primarily from the uptake of plasma low-density-lipoprotein (LDL) cholesterol.[88, 123]

In the ovary, LH stimulates the activity of adenylate cyclase, which releases cyclic AMP, which in turn serves as a second messenger to stimulate an increase in the messenger RNA (mRNA) for the LDL receptor, thereby increasing binding and uptake of LDL cholesterol as well as the formation of cholesterol esters.[123, 124] Cholesterol is then transported to the inner mitochondrial membrane by cyclic AMP–activated steroidogenic acute regulatory (StAR) protein, a 30-kd mitochondrial protein that is believed to be the key mediator of the acute induction of steroidogenesis.[125] The conversion of cholesterol to pregnenolone is the rate-limiting step in ovarian steroidogenesis; it is catalyzed by a cholesterol side-chain cleavage enzyme complex consisting of cytochrome P450 side-chain cleavage enzyme (CYP11A1), adrenodoxin, and flavoprotein (see Fig. 15–19).[126]

The principal steroid-producing cells of the ovary— namely the granulosa, theca, and corpus luteum cells—possess the complete enzymatic complement required for steroid hormone formation. The main pathway of steroid synthesis in the human corpus luteum is the Δ^4-pathway, which involves conversion of pregnenolone to progesterone (see Fig. 15–19). In the ovarian follicle the Δ^5-pathway is preferred for the formation of androgens and estrogens, because thecal cells of the human ovary metabolize 17-hydroxypregnenolone more efficiently than 17-OHP.[127] The predominant steroid produced differs among the cell types: the corpus luteum primarily forms progesterone and 17-OHP, the thecal and stromal cells secrete androgen, and the granulosa cells produce mainly estrogen. The factors that determine which steroid is secreted by each cell type include the levels of gonadotropin and gonadotropin receptors, the expression of steroidogenic enzymes, and the availability of LDL cholesterol.

The rate of steroid production during the menstrual cycle is a function of the content of four key enzymes: CYP11A1, 3β-HSD, steroid 17α-hydroxylase (CYP17) and aromatase (CYP19).[128–131] These enzymes catalyze, respectively, the conversion of cholesterol to pregnenolone, pregnenolone to pro-

the ovary is estradiol-17β. Although estrone is also secreted by the ovary, the principal source of estrone is extraglandular conversion of androstenedione in peripheral tissues.[118] Estriol (16-hydroxyestradiol) is the most abundant estrogen in urine and is produced by the metabolism of estrone and estradiol. Obesity and hypothyroidism are associated with an increase in estriol formation.[119, 120] Catechol estrogens are formed by hydroxylation of estrogens at the C-2 or C-4 position. The physiological role of catechol estrogen, if any, is unclear. Low body weight and hyperthyroidism are associated with increased formation of catechol estrogens.[121] Estrone sulfate, formed by peripheral conversion of estradiol and estrone, is the most abundant estrogen in blood but is not physiologically active.[122] Estrogens promote development of the secondary sexual characteristics of women, uterine growth, thickening of the vaginal mucosa, thinning of the cervical mucus, and development of the ductal system of the breast.

Progestagens. The principal progestagens are C_{21}-steroids (see Fig. 15–19) and include pregnenolone, progesterone, and 17-hydroxyprogesterone (17-OHP). Pregnenolone is of primary importance in the ovary because of its key position as precursor of all steroid hormones. Progesterone is the principal secretory product of the corpus luteum and is responsible for the progestational effects (i.e., induction of secretory activ-

trone) and of estrone sulfotransferase. The net effect of these actions of progesterone is to decrease the biologic action of estradiol on the endometrium during the luteal phase.[254-256]

On cycle day 17, the glands become more tortuous and dilated. By day 18, the vacuoles in the epithelium are smaller and are often located beside the nuclei. At this time, glycogen is present in the apex of the cells. On day 19, intraluminal secretion is present, and pseudostratification and vacuolation have almost disappeared. On days 21 and 22, the endometrial stroma becomes edematous. On day 23, stromal cells surrounding the spiral arterioles begin to enlarge, and stromal mitoses become apparent. Cycle day 24 is characterized by the appearance of predecidual cells around the spiral arterioles and numerous stromal mitoses. By day 25, the predecidua begins to differentiate under the surface epithelium. By day 27, the upper portion of the endometrial stroma appears as a solid sheet of well-developed decidua-like cells. Differentiation of the decidua is accompanied by a marked increase in lymphocytic infiltration. Menstruation begins on cycle day 28.

In the absence of conception, the breakdown of the endometrium begins after the decline of the corpus luteum results in a decrease of plasma estrogens and progestagens. These hormonal changes cause endometrial effects, including vascular changes, tissue death, and finally menstruation. With a reduction and shrinkage in the height of the endometrium, blood flow through the spiral vessels decreases and vasodilation ensues. The spiral vessels feeding the endometrium then undergo rhythmic vasoconstriction and vasodilation. These responses lead to disruption of the blood vessels and eventually to endometrial ischemia and cell death.[257, 258] Menstruation ensues, with the menstrual fluid consisting of blood and desquamated superficial endometrial tissues. The average duration of menstrual flow is 4 to 6 d, and the average amount of menstrual blood loss is 30 mL.[259]

After the resumption of estrogen secretion by the ovarian follicles, endometrial healing leads to prolonged vasoconstriction and formation of a clot over the denuded endometrial vessels.[260] Necrosis of the endometrium and vasospasm of the spiral vessels are thought to be caused by prostaglandins. Prostaglandins are present in large amounts in secretory endometrium and menstrual blood.[261-263] Infusions of prostaglandin $F_{2\alpha}$ to women during the luteal phase induce endometrial necrosis and bleeding.[264] The release of prostaglandins is believed to be secondary to a decrease in stability of the lysosomal membranes in the endometrial cell.[265, 266] This results in the liberation of phospholipids, with a subsequent synthesis of prostaglandin $F_{2\alpha}$. Prostaglandin synthetase inhibitors decrease the amount of menstrual bleeding in normal women and in women using contraceptive devices (see Chapter 18). The noncoagulability of menstrual blood may be a result of the presence of fibrinolytic activity.[267]

The glands of the endocervix undergo cyclic changes more closely related to those of the vaginal epithelium than of the endometrium.[268] The glands of the endocervix secrete mucus. After the menses, the amount of mucus is limited and viscous. In response to increasing levels of estrogen secreted by the follicle during the later half of the follicular phase, the quantity of mucus increases up to 30-fold.[269] The mucus also changes in quality to become watery and elastic, and a fine thread can be demonstrated when a drop of mucus is stretched (spinnbarkeit). In addition, a characteristic ferning or palm-leaf arborization is observed when the mucus is spread on a glass slide.[269] Progesterone reverses the effects of estrogen on cervical mucus.

Vaginal epithelial cells are also influenced by estrogen and progesterone. During the early follicular phase, exfoliated vaginal epithelial cells are basophilic and have vesicular nuclei. In response to increasing levels of estrogen in the latter half of the follicular phase, acidophilic cells with pyknotic nuclei

predominate.[270] During the luteal phase, in the presence of increasing levels of progesterone, the percentage of acidophilic cells decreases and the number of leukocytes increases.[269, 270] Several indices for characterization of vaginal cytology are available.[269]

Fertilization and Early Implantation of the Ovum

A complex and coordinated set of events leads to maturation of the sperm and egg, transport in the female reproductive tract, fertilization, and implantation.

SPERM TRANSPORT AND CAPACITATION. After ejaculation, sperm leave the vagina and pass through the cervix, the entire length of the uterine cavity, and the uterotubal junction to arrive at the ampullary-isthmic junction of the fallopian tube, where fertilization occurs. Transport of sperm is aided by intrinsic flagellar beating, uterine contractions, and the actions of uterine and tubal cilia.[271] The process of sperm transport is rapid, and sperm have been found at the distal end of the fallopian tube 5 min after vaginal insemination.[272] However, the rate of attrition of sperm in the female reproductive tract is high. Of an estimated 250 million sperm deposited in the vagina, only 50 to 200 reach the end of the oviduct and achieve proximity to the egg (Fig. 15–34).[273] The major loss of sperm occurs through retention in the vagina and expulsion from the introitus.

In most species sperm must reside in or be exposed to the female reproductive tract before they are capable of fertilizing the ovum. A process called *capacitation*,[274] which is not well understood, prepares the sperm to undergo the acrosomal reaction that involves breakdown and merging of the plasma membrane with the acrosomal membrane of the sperm head.[271] The process of capacitation is followed by a release of enzymes that are thought to play a role in penetration of the ovum. Whether the process of capacitation in the female reproductive tract is required in humans is unclear, because human sperm are capable of fertilization in vitro after a short incubation in defined culture media.[275]

OVUM AND ZYGOTE TRANSPORTATION. At the time of ovulation, the fimbriated end of the fallopian tube sweeps across the surface of the ovary, and the extruded ovum and adherent granulosa cells (cumulus oophorus) are collected by the adhesive fimbriae. The transport of the egg into the tube is aided by ciliary action and tubal contractions.[271] Removal of the granulosa cells before the egg is picked up impairs egg transport. Cells of the cumulus are able to communicate by paracrine mechanisms over a network of intracellular bridges through the zona to the perivitelline space[276] and may play a role in nutrition of the egg.

The ovum and zygote pass through the fallopian tube in three stages. The first stage encompasses the period from ovum pickup at the fimbriated end of the tube until the egg reaches the ampullary-isthmic junction; the egg is retained at this junction for 1 to 2 d, during which time fertilization occurs.[271, 277] The block at the ampullary-isthmic junction is functional, because the junction is not a clearly defined anatomic entity. The second stage of transport begins soon after fertilization. The fertilized egg traverses the isthmic portion of the tube, where it is again retained for 1 to 2 d at another functional block, the isthmic-utero or uterotubal junction. The period from ovulation until the egg enters the uterine cavity is species dependent and averages 3 to 4 d in women. Detention of the egg at the areas of functional block within the fallopian tube appears to be influenced by estrogen and progesterone.[278] By the time the fertilized egg arrives in the uterine cavity during the final stage of transport (3 to 4 d after ovulation), it has entered the morula stage (see Fig. 15–34).[279]

FERTILIZATION. After ovulation the fertilizable life span

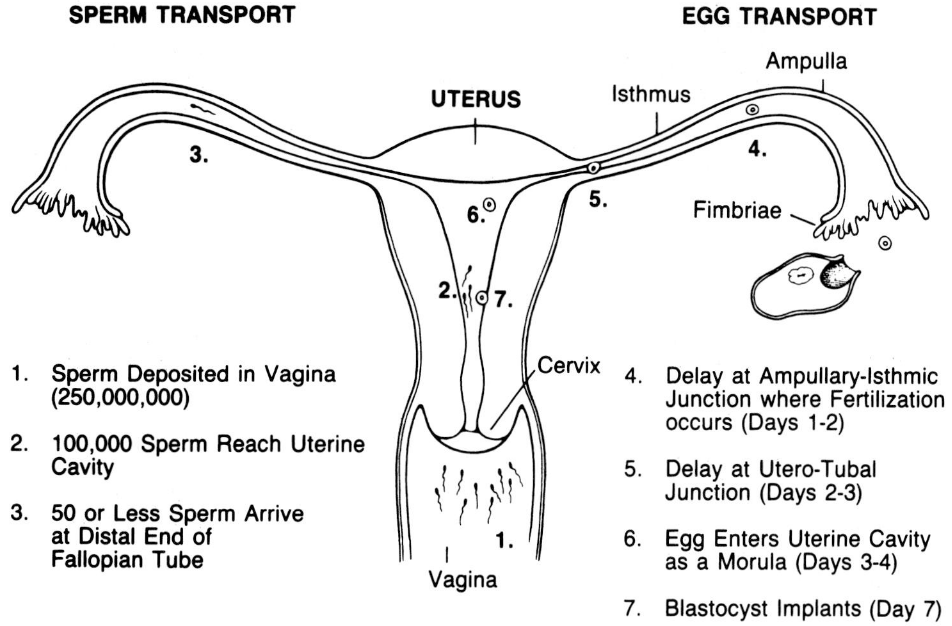

SPERM TRANSPORT

EGG TRANSPORT

UTERUS

Ampulla

Isthmus

Fimbriae

Cervix

Vagina

Figure 15–34. Transport of the sperm and the egg in the female reproductive tract. (From Carr BR. Fertilization, implantation and endocrinology of pregnancy. In: Griffin JE, Ojeda SR, eds. Textbook of Endocrine Physiology. New York: Oxford University Press, 1988: 186–203, with permission.)

1. Sperm Deposited in Vagina (250,000,000)

2. 100,000 Sperm Reach Uterine Cavity

3. 50 or Less Sperm Arrive at Distal End of Fallopian Tube

4. Delay at Ampullary-Isthmic Junction where Fertilization occurs (Days 1-2)

5. Delay at Utero-Tubal Junction (Days 2-3)

6. Egg Enters Uterine Cavity as a Morula (Days 3-4)

7. Blastocyst Implants (Day 7)

of the human ovum is thought to be less than 24 h, and the estimated life span for human sperm after ejaculation is 48 to 72 h.[275, 276] The first step of fertilization involves adherence of the sperm head to the zona pellucida surrounding the egg (Fig. 15–35). The sperm then penetrates the zona, which requires 15 to 25 min. After passage through the zona pellucida, the sperm moves rapidly across the perivitelline space and attaches to and penetrates the perivitelline membrane; this step takes less than 1 min.[276, 280] After the sperm has reached this point, the male pronucleus is formed.

The penetration of the vitelline membrane initiates two critical events. The first is the release of cortical granules into the perivitelline space, which blocks other sperm from penetrating the perivitelline membrane and prevents polyspermia.[281] These granules contain various hydrolytic enzymes that induce the zona reaction and inactivate sperm receptors. The second event is the triggering of the final stage of meiosis of the oocyte. The second polar body is extruded from the egg, leaving a haploid complement of chromosomes in the egg pronucleus just before fertilization.[276]

The male and female pronuclei are visible about 2 to 3 h after the sperm has penetrated the vitelline membrane. By 4 h, the sperm tail is incorporated within the egg.[279] The two pronuclei move toward the center of the egg, their respective haploid chromosomes replicate, a mitotic spindle forms, and the first division occurs with the formation of two blastomeres.

The initial cleavage of the egg occurs in the fallopian tube. The rate of cleavage is remarkably constant in various mammalian species.[276] The timing in fertilized human eggs, determined from studies of in vitro fertilization, is as follows: two cells, 28 h; four cells, 46 to 48 h; eight cells, 51 to 62 h; morula formation, 111 to 135 h; and formation of a blastocyst, 123 to 147 h.[282]

IMPLANTATION. In women the fertilized egg enters the uterine cavity as a morula on the third to fourth day after ovulation.[283, 284] The morula is transformed into a blastocyst by the fifth to sixth day after ovulation. At this stage of development the embryo is a hollow sphere with two cell types: the outer trophectoderm cells, which will form the placenta, and the inner cell mass, from which the fetus will develop.[283] On the seventh day after ovulation, the blastocyst implants on the endometrial lining of the uterine cavity and penetrates the

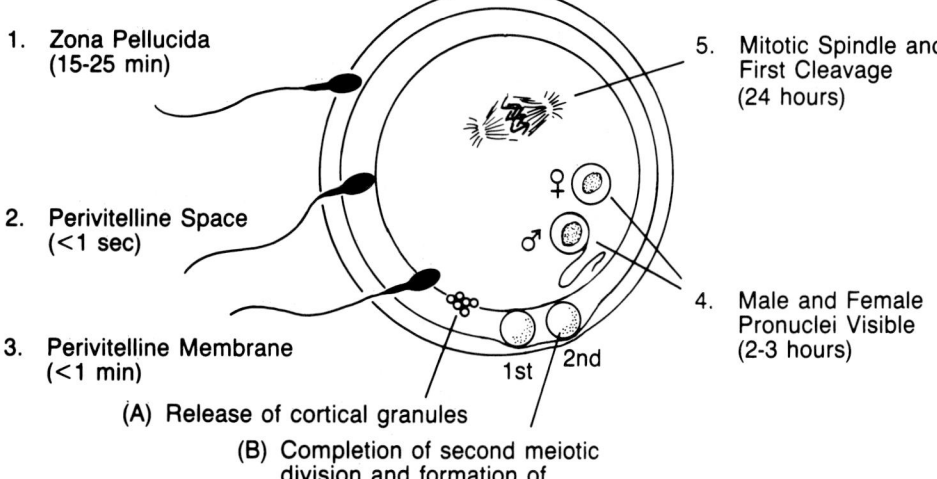

Figure 15–35. The process of fertilization of the human egg. (From Carr BR. Fertilization, implantation and endocrinology of pregnancy. In: Griffin JE, Ojeda SR, eds. Textbook of Endocrine Physiology. New York: Oxford University Press, 1988: 186–203, with permission.)

1. Zona Pellucida (15-25 min)

2. Perivitelline Space (<1 sec)

3. Perivitelline Membrane (<1 min)

(A) Release of cortical granules

(B) Completion of second meiotic division and formation of polar body.

5. Mitotic Spindle and First Cleavage (24 hours)

4. Male and Female Pronuclei Visible (2-3 hours)

Estrogens

The presence of normal secondary sexual characteristics (e.g., breast development) implies that estrogen production was adequate in the past. Indications of the current estrogen status can be obtained from the pelvic examination. The presence of a moist, rugated vagina with copious, clear, thin cervical mucus that can be stretched and exhibits arborization or ferning when spread on a slide is strong evidence of adequate estrogen production. As discussed previously, vaginal squamous epithelial cells can be graded by various techniques, and the presence of mature epithelial cells and abundant cornified squamous epithelial cells with pyknotic nuclei confirms the presence of adequate estrogen levels.[269]

The progestagen withdrawal test provides a useful functional assessment of estrogen status in women with a normal outflow tract. If menstruation occurs within 7 to 10 d after the end of a trial of medroxyprogesterone acetate (10 mg by mouth, once or twice daily, for 5 d) or after an intramuscular injection of progesterone (100 to 200 mg), then the prior estrogen level was adequate to allow withdrawal bleeding.[326]

Plasma estradiol levels can be determined by radioimmunoassay, chemiluminescent assay, FIA, or ELISA, and the values fluctuate throughout the normal cycle (see Table 15–3 and Fig. 15–27). There is little indication for measurement of estradiol levels in women with disorders of ovarian hormone secretion, because the clinical assessment and the response to a progestagen challenge are usually adequate to indicate the status of estrogen production. However, a determination of plasma estradiol levels is helpful in monitoring anovulatory women during attempts to induce ovulation with human menopausal gonadotropins (hMG) and in women undergoing in vitro fertilization. Ultrasonography is used in conjunction with this technique to assess adequate follicular growth.[327]

Progesterone

Spontaneous, cyclic, predictable menses imply that the patient is ovulating and that progesterone is secreted during the luteal phase. Progesterone levels in blood may be measured by radioimmunoassay, chemiluminescent assay, FIA, or ELISA (for normal values, see Table 15–3). Progesterone measurements are used to document ovulation or adequacy of the luteal phase in infertile women and to aid in the diagnosis of women with müllerian agenesis and testicular feminization.[328, 329] The determination of 17-OHP is useful in evaluation of women with adult-onset adrenal hyperplasia resulting from 21-hydroxylase deficiency.[330]

Progesterone secretion can also be assessed more simply. The simplest test is the measurement of basal body temperature throughout a cycle. Because of the thermogenic properties of progesterone, documentation of a monthly biphasic curve with an elevated temperature for approximately 13 to 14 d after ovulation indicates ovulation and suggests normal progesterone secretion during the luteal phase (see Fig. 15–27). The presence of viscous cervical mucus that does not stretch or fern, the finding of predominant intermediate cells on vaginal cytology, and the demonstration of a properly dated secretory endometrium after endometrial biopsy during the luteal phase (see Fig. 15–27) provide additional evidence of adequate progesterone secretion.[269]

Androgens

The presence of abnormal hair growth (hirsutism) or masculinization (virilization) implies excessive levels of androgens, principally testosterone. The rate of production of testosterone parallels the degree of clinical androgen excess.[331, 332] Excessive testosterone may result from increased secretion by the adrenal or ovary or from increased extraglandular production from androstenedione secreted by the ovary or adrenal. Serum androgens (testosterone) and other C_{19}-steroids (DHEA, DHEAS, androstenedione) are measured by radioimmunoassay, chemiluminescent assay, ELISA, or FIA. Normal serum levels in ovulatory women are summarized in Table 15–3. The presence of elevated urinary 17-ketosteroids (derived principally from DHEA) is sometimes a useful finding in the diagnosis of adrenal virilizing tumors.[333]

Prediction of Ovulation

Rapid assays for urinary LH make it possible to predict the time of ovulation in infertile women.[334] Ultrasonography of follicles can also be used to predict the adequacy and time of ovulation.[327] These tests are widely used in evaluation and treatment of infertile women.

Specific Diagnostic Tests

IMAGING TECHNIQUES. As mentioned, ultrasonography using a vaginal probe is useful in evaluating infertility and for following follicular and endometrial growth during treatment of anovulatory women.[327] Ultrasonography or magnetic resonance imaging (MRI) can establish the presence of a uterus, a uterine developmental anomaly, or a vaginal septum.[335] Hysterosalpingography, in which radiopaque dye is injected into the uterus during fluoroscopy, is helpful for delineating the uterine cavity and patency of the fallopian tubes.[336] MRI and computed tomographic (CT) scans are routinely used in the diagnosis of pituitary, hypothalamic, adrenal, uterine, and ovarian masses.[337]

CHROMOSOMAL ANALYSIS. The use of buccal smears to evaluate the chromosomal sex is not of sufficient accuracy to be clinically useful. Karyotypic analysis of peripheral blood leukocytes should be done instead.[338, 339] Cells are treated with phytohemagglutinin to stimulate cell division, which is arrested at metaphase with colchicine. The cells are then harvested, stained, and examined. The determination of a chromosomal karyotype is particularly useful in women with sexual ambiguity (see Chapter 29) and in women with ovarian failure to determine the presence of a Y chromosome.[340] To rule out mosaicism, evaluation of a large number of cells or assessment of the chromosomal complement of other tissues may be required.

OPERATIVE PROCEDURES. Diagnostic hysteroscopy is useful to evaluate the uterine cavity in women with abnormal uterine development or with infertility.[341] Diagnostic laparoscopy may be indicated in women with abnormal uterine development before a planned surgical procedure or during evaluation for infertility.[342]

Diagnosis of Pregnancy

The diagnosis of pregnancy is usually suspected on the basis of the history and physical examination. For example, a woman with previous cyclic menses who complains of amenorrhea accompanied by breast tenderness, malaise, lassitude, and nausea and who on physical examination exhibits a softening and enlargement of the uterus is probably pregnant. Because of the secretion of hCG by the placenta into the maternal circulation and its excretion in urine, pregnancy can be diagnosed before clinical signs appear. Modern immunoassays utilizing monoclonal antibodies directed against β-hCG have improved the ability to measure small quantities of hCG in blood and urine and minimize cross-reactivity with serum LH.[343] It is now possible to detect pregnancy 8 to 10 d after ovulation and before the first missed menstrual period. β-hCG assay kits can detect concentrations of 20 IU/L or higher in urine in only 5 min. Quantitative β-hCG immunoassays are helpful in the diagnosis of ectopic pregnancy, hydatidiform mole, and choriocarcinoma.

DISORDERS OF OVARIAN FUNCTION

Disorders of ovarian function cause different clinical presentations depending on the phase of reproductive life during which they first manifest. No classification can encompass all the nuances associated with ovarian dysfunction. The developmental classification chosen here provides a rational approach by classifying disorders of ovarian function as fetal or neonatal, prepubertal, or reproductive. The menopause is not considered a disorder of ovarian function, because it is a natural process in all women. Diagnosis and classification of these disorders have improved as a result of the ability to measure small amounts of hormones in blood and the development of better imaging techniques.

Disorders During Fetal and Neonatal Life

Disturbances in female sexual differentiation during embryogenesis can arise from a variety of mechanisms and may be expressed as ambiguous genitalia at birth, delayed puberty, amenorrhea, or a combination of these conditions. For example, gonadal dysgenesis, müllerian agenesis, and complete androgen resistance (testicular feminization) are all compatible with an apparently normal female phenotype but cause amenorrhea at the expected time of puberty. In the absence of sexual ambiguity, most of these disorders are not diagnosed during the neonatal period unless a palpable gonad is discovered in an inguinal hernia (testicular feminization) or absence of the vagina and uterus (e.g., müllerian agenesis) is noted during the physical examination of the newborn; these disorders are discussed in the section on amenorrhea. Sexual ambiguity at birth may be caused by mixed gonadal dysgenesis, true hermaphroditism, female pseudohermaphroditism, congenital adrenal hyperplasia, masculinizing syndromes in the mother, or incomplete masculinization of male infants (male pseudohermaphroditism). All may cause significant health risks and psychological trauma if not properly diagnosed. Sexual ambiguity and its management are described in Chapter 29.

During fetal life, ovarian cysts may undergo torsion, which can be diagnosed by ultrasonographic studies.[344] Most of these cysts appear to be functional but regress during the neonatal period. Ovarian tumors such as embryonal cell carcinoma may also develop during infancy.

Disorders During the Prepubertal Years

In girls puberty is said to be precocious when the onset of breast budding occurs before age 8 or menarche commences before age 9.[51, 345] This definition is based on statistical and practical considerations. Precocious puberty is about eight times more common in girls than in boys, and 90% of cases are idiopathic.[346] Those disorders in which the premature sexual characteristics are appropriate for the genetic and gonadal sex (i.e., feminization in girls or virilization in boys) are termed isosexual precocity. Heterosexual precocity occurs when sexual characteristics are inappropriate for the genetic sex (e.g., feminizing syndromes in boys or virilizing syndromes in girls). Disorders of pubertal development in boys are described in Chapters 16 and 31.

Isosexual Precocity

Isosexual precocity can be divided into three categories (Table 15–6); differentiation of these categories is clinically

TABLE 15–6. Classification of Sexual Precocity

I. Isosexual precocity
   A. True precocious puberty
      1. Constitutional
      2. Organic brain disease
      3. Congenital adrenal hyperplasia (delayed treatment)
   B. Precocious pseudopuberty
      1. Ovarian tumors
      2. Adrenal tumors
      3. McCune-Albright syndrome
      4. Hypothyroidism
      5. Russell-Silver syndrome
      6. Estrogen-containing medications
   C. Isolated forms of pubertal development
      1. Premature thelarche
      2. Premature adrenarche
      3. Premature pubarche
II. Heterosexual precocity
   A. Ovarian tumors
   B. Adrenal tumors
   C. Congenital adrenal hyperplasia

important for two reasons. First, true precocious puberty is idiopathic in most cases but is not ovarian in origin, whereas a primary ovarian disorder is often the basis for precocious pseudopuberty. Making this distinction therefore helps the clinician design appropriate therapy. Second, the cause, seriousness, and treatment of these two disorders differ. The clinical course in most girls with true precocious puberty is benign, whereas precocious pseudopuberty may be life-threatening.[27, 345–347]

Determination of the type of isosexual precocity is complicated by the fact that the early signs are similar, and separation may be feasible only late in the course. Diagnostic procedures may also be inconclusive early, making it necessary to temporize or to use additional diagnostic procedures. If the possibility of a life-threatening disorder can be excluded, observation is justified and is unlikely to increase morbidity or affect prognosis adversely.

TRUE PRECOCIOUS PUBERTY. True precocious puberty, also known as complete isosexual precocity (premature activation of the hypothalamic-pituitary axis), is characterized by an early but otherwise normal female pubertal development. Although puberty occurs at an early age (sometimes even in infancy), the endocrine events are normal in that the cyclic function of the hypothalamic-pituitary-ovarian axis leads to gonadotropin secretion, follicular maturation, and ovulation. Cyclic, predictable menses and ovulatory cycles are the hallmarks of true precocious puberty.[27]

Constitutional or idiopathic precocious puberty is responsible for 90% of cases. In these young women, no cause for the premature maturation of the hypothalamic-pituitary axis can be identified, and the diagnosis is one of exclusion. About half of these patients have abnormal electroencephalograms.[348] The basal levels of gonadotropins and gonadal steroids are increased, and the LH pulse frequency and amplitude, as well as the response of LH to the administration of LHRH, are in the normal pubertal range.[349, 350] The early appearance of secondary sexual characteristics and of ovulatory cycles with the accompanying risk of fertility may cause significant emotional disturbances. Therefore, prompt diagnosis and treatment are imperative.

About 10% of girls with true precocious puberty have organic brain disease. About half of these cases are caused by CNS tumors, including hamartomas, gliomas, neurofibromas, astrocytomas, ependymomas, germinomas, and, rarely, craniopharyngiomas or pinealomas.[351–357] Other CNS disorders that can give rise to true precocious puberty include encephalitis, meningitis, hydrocephalus, head injury, brain abscess, and tuberous sclerosis.[27]

It is essential to separate patients with CNS causes from those with the idiopathic disorder, recognizing that some patients initially diagnosed as idiopathic may prove later to have organic brain disease. However, most patients with organic brain disease have other neurologic signs and symptoms before the appearance of precocious puberty. Evaluation of patients with isosexual precocity must include imaging of the head with either CT or MRI. The location of CNS tumors that cause precocious puberty makes both surgical and radiation treatment difficult. For example, deaths have occurred after operative removal of hypothalamic hamartomas. Surgical extirpation is not recommended if the tumor is slow-growing and can be monitored by imaging techniques and if precocious sexual development can be controlled by medical therapy.[27, 358]

A rare cause of isosexual precocity is virilizing adrenal hyperplasia resulting from 21-hydroxylase deficiency in girls in whom treatment is delayed until age 4 to 8. After initiation of glucocorticoid replacement, such patients may undergo true isosexual precocious puberty.[27]

PRECOCIOUS PSEUDOPUBERTY. Isosexual precocious pseudopuberty, or incomplete isosexual precocity, occurs when girls feminize as a consequence of endogenous estrogen production or exogenous estrogen exposure but do not ovulate or have cyclic menses. Ovarian cysts or tumors that secrete estrogen (granulosa or thecal cell tumors) are the most frequent cause.[359–362] The Peutz-Jeghers syndrome of intestinal polyps and mucocutaneous pigmentation is associated with ovarian tumors that secrete estrogen (or androgen that is converted to estrogen at extraglandular sites) and cause precocious pseudopuberty.[363] Most ovarian tumors can be diagnosed by rectoabdominal examination, but ultrasonography, CT, or laparoscopy may also be of help.

Most tumors are unilateral and benign and can be cured by oophorectomy. Gonadotropin levels are suppressed, and the LH response to LHRH is blunted.[361] The presence of ovarian cysts can cause problems in diagnosis. Ultrasonography may be helpful to differentiate a benign cyst from a cystic-solid ovarian tumor, but exploratory laparotomy is ultimately necessary in most cases, with the recognition that unnecessary removal of a benign cyst may lead to adhesions and infertility later in life. Follicular growth of up to 3 cm may occur in patients with true precocious puberty as a consequence of increased gonadotropin secretion and is not an indication for exploration. Ovarian teratomas, choriocarcinomas or germinomas, and hepatoblastomas that secrete pure hCG do not appear to cause precocious puberty in girls unless estrogen is secreted concomitantly by the tumor (i.e., hCG or LH in the absence of FSH does not stimulate ovarian estrogen secretion).[27, 364] Rarely, feminizing tumors of the adrenal can cause isosexual precocious puberty, either by formation of estrogen directly or by secretion of androgens that are aromatized to estrogens in extraglandular sites.[365]

Other types of isosexual precocious pseudopuberty include two disorders occasionally associated with increased gonadotropin secretion. The first is the McCune-Albright syndrome, which consists of the triad of café au lait spots, polyostotic fibrous dysplasia, and precocious puberty.[366, 367] This disorder is more common in girls. It is caused by a somatic mutation of the $G_{\alpha s}$ subunit of the G-protein complex which renders it constitutively active even in the absence of LH.[368] Consequently, the disorder falls into the category of gonadotropin-independent precocious puberty.[346, 368–371] Increased estrogen secretion by the autonomous functioning cysts may spontaneously regress and recur but is not suppressed by LHRH analogues that lower plasma LH.[369] However, patients may respond to aromatase inhibitors.[371] McCune-Albright syndrome is also associated with other endocrinopathies, including excessive secretion of growth hormone, prolactin, thyroid hormone, or cortisol.[372]

The second type of incomplete isosexual precocity that may be associated with increased gonadotropin secretion is hypothyroidism. Hypothyroidism usually is associated with delayed pubertal development and amenorrhea, but occasionally patients present with precocious puberty, galactorrhea, and ovarian cysts.[373] In addition to increased levels of thyrotropin, gonadotropin and prolactin levels are also increased; the cause for the enhanced gonadotropin secretion is unknown.[374–376] In most cases bone age is retarded, and pituitary hypersecretion and retardation of bone development respond to thyroid hormone replacement.

Another rare disease that may be associated with precocious pseudopuberty is the Russell-Silver syndrome, which is characterized by short stature, craniofacial dysostosis, and asymmetrical development of extremities.[377] Estrogen-containing medications, including oral contraceptives, and estrogen-contaminated meat or poultry are also rare causes of incomplete precocious pseudopuberty.[378, 379]

ISOLATED FORMS OF PUBERTAL DEVELOPMENT. In some cases of isosexual precocity, an isolated premature pubertal event may occur, such as premature breast budding (premature thelarche) or premature development of axillary or pubic hair (so-called premature adrenarche or pubarche). Premature thelarche is the development of breast budding before the age of 8 y without other evidence of estrogen effect or advanced bone age.[380] This disorder is thought to be caused by a transient increase in estrogen secretion or a temporary increase in end-organ sensitivity to the low levels of circulating estrogens that are present before puberty. It occurs most frequently by age 2 and rarely after age 4. Girls with premature thelarche exhibit increased FSH secretion after treatment with LHRH, whereas LH levels do not increase.[380] Premature thelarche is self-limited and resolves spontaneously.

Premature adrenarche (pubarche) is the appearance of axillary hair, pubic hair, or both, without other signs of pubertal development or virilization. It is caused by an increased secretion of adrenal androgens, usually after age 6. Rare cases associated with transient ovarian androgen secretion resulting from ovarian cysts have also been reported.[381] In most cases of premature adrenarche the disorder is nonprogressive and requires no treatment. Patients enter puberty at the appropriate time.[27]

Heterosexual Precocity

Virilization in a prepubertal female is usually caused by congenital adrenal hyperplasia or testosterone secretion by an adrenal or ovarian tumor. Virilization in girls with congenital adrenal hyperplasia usually is associated with a history of sexual ambiguity at birth.

Evaluation and Treatment of Sexual Precocity*

The evaluation of sexual precocity requires a careful history and physical examination, including a rectoabdominal examination, which may often suggest the correct diagnosis. Other tests include ultrasonographic study or CT scan of ovaries and adrenals, determination of bone age, and measurement of plasma thyrotropin, gonadotropins (including hCG), and levels of androgen and estrogen, if appropriate. A CT or MRI scan of the head is required to rule out a CNS tumor.

Treatment of CNS tumors may include surgery or radiation therapy; treatment of ovarian tumors is surgical.[27] LHRH analogues are the most effective treatment for most forms of gonadotropin-dependent (idiopathic) sexual precocity. Other

---

*Also see Chapter 31.

agents that have been used include medroxyprogesterone acetate, danazol, and cyproterone acetate.[27] LHRH analogues are preferred, because they cause prompt regression of breast development and vaginal bleeding and cessation of bone maturation.[382–385] McCune-Albright syndrome may respond to administration of aromatase inhibitors such as testolactone.[371] Hypothyroidism is treated by thyroid hormone replacement. Diagnostic tests and treatment of sexual precocity are summarized in Table 15–7.

Disorders During the Reproductive Years

Disorders of the Menstrual Cycle

DYSMENORRHEA. Dysmenorrhea, or painful menstruation, is common, affecting about 50% of women at some time in life.[37] The disorder may be primary or secondary. Primary dysmenorrhea is associated with ovulatory cycles and is caused by uterine smooth muscle contractions induced by prostaglandins formed in secretory endometrium.[386] Patients with primary dysmenorrhea often have additional symptoms, including nausea, diarrhea, headaches, and emotional disorders. This form of dysmenorrhea can be treated by prevention of ovulation with oral contraceptives (if fertility control is desired) or by use of prostaglandin synthetase inhibitors. If either therapy fails to relieve symptoms after an adequate trial of 3 to 6 mo, diagnostic laparoscopy may be indicated.

Secondary dysmenorrhea is associated with a variety of conditions such as endometriosis, pelvic inflammatory disease, congenital defects in uterine development, uterine leiomyoma, and presence of intrauterine devices. Secondary dysmenorrhea usually requires surgical or medical therapy. However, about 80% of women who experience either primary or secondary dysmenorrhea have some relief with the use of prostaglandin inhibitors.[387]

PREMENSTRUAL SYNDROME. Almost all women experience a variety of cyclic premenstrual symptoms that occur after ovulation and disappear after menstruation. These symptoms include breast tenderness, abdominal bloating, headache, weight gain, behavioral changes, and many other occasional complaints. In some women, the combination of symptoms, known as premenstrual syndrome (PMS), is more severe for unknown reasons.[388] Although the cause is not known, prevention of ovulation by use of oral contraceptives or LHRH analogues is often helpful. Removal of the ovaries and uterus cures the disorder. However, castration is rarely indicated because of the sequelae of estrogen deprivation.

Short of removal of the ovaries, no single form of therapy is completely effective. Other treatments that may relieve some symptoms include drug therapy with bromocriptine, prostaglandin synthetase inhibitors, mild diuretics, fluoxetine, or alprazolam (if depression is severe), change in lifestyle, diet, and exercise.[37, 388–390]

ABNORMAL UTERINE BLEEDING. Between menarche and the menopause, almost every woman experiences one or more episodes of abnormal uterine bleeding, defined as any bleeding pattern that differs in frequency, duration, or amount from the pattern observed during a normal menstrual cycle.[37, 391, 392] A variety of descriptive terms (e.g., menometrorrhagia) have been used to characterize patterns of abnormal bleeding. A more logical approach is to divide abnormal bleeding patterns into those associated with ovulatory cycles and those associated with anovulatory cycles.

Abnormal Bleeding Associated with Ovulatory Cycles. Normal menstrual bleeding begins on average after the 28th day of an ovulatory cycle and is spontaneous, regular, cyclic, and predictable. The amount and duration of bleeding are also predictable and constant, and dysmenorrhea is frequently present. The average duration of bleeding is 4 to 6 d, and the average blood loss is 30 mL.[259] Regular ovulatory cycles in which the length or amount of uterine bleeding deviates from normal are often associated with pathologic abnormalities of the reproductive tract or bleeding dyscrasias. For instance, regular but excessive and prolonged bleeding episodes can result from abnormalities of the uterus, including leiomyomas, adenomyosis, endometrial polyps, or coagulation defects (e.g., von Willebrand's disease). Regular ovulatory cycles characterized by only spotting, light bleeding, or no bleeding at all (amenorrhea) may be caused by obstructive pathologic conditions of the reproductive tract, such as intrauterine adhesions (synechiae) or scarring of the cervix.

Intermenstrual bleeding, or spotting between episodes of regular, ovulatory menses, is often caused by cervical or endometrial lesions and requires surgical evaluation and treatment.

Abnormal Bleeding Associated with Anovulatory Cycles. Uterine bleeding during anovulatory cycles is unpredictable with respect to amount, onset, and duration and is known as dysfunctional uterine bleeding (DUB). DUB is usually painless because of the absence of ovulation. This disorder is caused not by primary abnormalities of the uterus but rather by interruption of normal maturation and development of the endometrium. In the absence of ovulation and with failure of luteal progesterone support of the endometrium, bleeding is irregular and unpredictable. In contrast, the bleeding in normal ovulatory cycles is cyclic and predictable as a result of the orderly development of the endometrium induced by estrogen priming during the proliferative phase and progesterone support followed by decline of corpus luteum function during the luteal phase. In the absence of estrogen priming, as when a castrate or a postmenopausal woman is given progesterone, withdrawal bleeding usually does not occur. The exposure of endometrium to estrogen unopposed by progesterone (i.e., anovulatory bleeding, or DUB) causes a hyperplastic or proliferative endometrium.[393] Both types of endometrium have a reduced capacity to synthesize prostaglandin $F_{2\alpha}$, which explains in part the absence of painful menses.[394]

DUB occurs in normal women at the extremes of reproductive life, normally in the early postmenarcheal and late perimenopausal years.[183–185] Most causes are associated with

---

TABLE 15–7. Diagnostic Tests and Treatment of Sexual Precocity

Diagnostic Tests

  History and physical examination
  Bone age
  CNS imaging
  Sonography of ovaries
  CT scan of adrenal (if virilized)
  Thyroid function tests
  Estradiol
  FSH, LH, hCG
  Testosterone, DHEAS, 17α-hydroxyprogesterone (if virilized)

Treatment

  Isosexual precocity
    True precocious puberty
      Constitutional: LHRH analogues/progestagens
      Organic brain disease: Surgery, radiation, LHRH analogues/progestagens
      Congenital adrenal hyperplasia (delayed treatment): LHRH analogues/progestagens
    Precocious pseudopuberty
      Ovarian tumors: Surgery
      Adrenal tumors: Surgery
      McCune-Albright syndrome: Testolactone, ketoconazole
      Russell-Silver syndrome: ? LHRH analogues/progestagens
      Estrogen-containing medications: Discontinue use
    Isolated forms of pubertal development: Observation
  Heterosexual precocity
    Ovarian tumors: Surgery
    Adrenal tumors: Surgery
    Congenital adrenal hyperplasia: glucocorticoids

chronic anovulation (e.g., PCOS). Anovulatory bleeding can result from several mechanisms, including estrogen breakthrough bleeding and progesterone breakthrough bleeding.

Estrogen Breakthrough Bleeding. Estrogen breakthrough bleeding occurs when continuous estrogen stimulation of the endometrium is not interrupted by cyclic progesterone exposure. This is the most common type of DUB, and it is caused by anovulation associated with chronic acyclic estrogen production (PCOS). Women with this disorder have histories of irregular, unpredictable menses, oligomenorrhea, or amenorrhea (see later discussion). Estrogen breakthrough bleeding can also occur in women with hypogonadotropic hypogonadism, in postmenopausal women given continuous estrogen therapy, and in women with estrogen-secreting tumors of the ovary or adrenal gland. In some women estrogen breakthrough bleeding may be profuse and prolonged. When bleeding is prolonged, the endometrium is typically thin and fragile because of incomplete or absent repair between episodes of bleeding.[395]

Progesterone Breakthrough Bleeding. Progesterone breakthrough bleeding is a pharmacologically induced anovulatory bleeding that occurs in the presence of high ratios of progesterone to estrogen. This type of bleeding occurs in women treated with continuous progestagens (levonorgestrel implants or depo medroxyprogesterone acetate used for contraception) or with continuous or cyclic low-dose oral contraceptives. In these instances the endometrium is thin and atrophic (see Chapter 18).

Diagnosis and Treatment. The approach to a patient with abnormal uterine bleeding begins with a history of menstrual patterns and prior hormonal therapy and a careful physical examination of the reproductive tract. Because not all bleeding from the urogenital tract is from the uterus, rectal and bladder sources should also be considered and evaluated. If the bleeding is from the uterus, pregnancy-related disorders such as threatened or incomplete abortion or ectopic pregnancy must be excluded.

The severity and frequency of bleeding dictate the extent of laboratory evaluation before therapy. After visible or palpable lesions of the reproductive tract are ruled out, the following studies are indicated: cervical cytology, measurement of β-hCG, endometrial biopsy, and a complete blood cell count. If severe bleeding is associated with ovulatory cycles, coagulation studies are also indicated.

The diagnosis of ovulatory bleeding episodes associated with organic disease of the reproductive tract is usually established by the history and physical examination, although occasionally hysteroscopy or hysterosalpingography may be re-

---

TABLE 15–8. Classification of Amenorrhea (Not Including Disorders of Congenital Sexual Ambiguity)

I. Anatomical defects (outflow tract)
  A. Labial agglutination/fusion
  B. Imperforate hymen
  C. Transverse vaginal septum
  D. Cervical agenesis—isolated
  E. Cervical stenosis—iatrogenic
  F. Vaginal agenesis—isolated
  G. Müllerian agenesis (Mayer-Rokitansky-Küster-Hauser syndrome)
  H. Complete androgen resistance (testicular feminization)
  I. Endometrial hypoplasia or aplasia—congenital
  J. Asherman's syndrome (uterine synechiae)
II. Ovarian failure (hypergonadotropic hypogonadism)
  A. Gonadal agenesis
  B. Gonadal dysgenesis
    1. Abnormal karyotype
      a. Gonadal dysgenesis 45,X
      b. Mosaicism
    2. Normal karyotype
      a. Pure gonadal dysgenesis
        i. 46,XX
        ii. 46,XY (Swyer's syndrome)
  C. Ovarian enzymatic deficiency
    1. 17α-Hydroxylase deficiency
    2. 17,20-Lyase deficiency
  D. Premature ovarian failure
    1. Idiopathic—premature aging
    2. Injury
      a. Mumps oophoritis
      b. Radiation
      c. Chemotherapy
    3. Resistant ovary (Savage's syndrome)
    4. Autoimmune disease
    5. Galactosemia
III. Chronic anovulation with estrogen present
  A. PCOS
    1. Hyperthecosis
  B. Adrenal disease
    1. Cushing's syndrome
    2. Adult-onset adrenal hyperplasia
  C. Thyroid disease
    1. Hypothyroidism
    2. Hyperthyroidism
  D. Ovarian tumors
    1. Granulosa-theca cell tumors
    2. Brenner tumors
    3. Cystic teratomas
    4. Mucinous/serous cystadenomas
    5. Krukenberg's tumor

IV. Chronic anovulation with estrogen absent (hypogonadotropic hypogonadism)
  A. Hypothalamic
    1. Tumors
      a. Craniopharyngioma
      b. Germinoma
      c. Hamartoma
      d. Hand-Schüller-Christian disease
      e. Teratoma
      f. Endodermal sinus tumors
      g. Metastatic carcinoma
    2. Infection and other disorders
      a. Tuberculosis
      b. Syphilis
      c. Encephalitis/meningitis
      d. Sarcoidosis
      e. Kallman's syndrome
      f. Idiopathic hypogonadotropic hypogonadism
      g. Chronic debilitating disease
    3. Functional
      a. Stress
      b. Weight loss/diet
      c. Malnutrition
      d. Psychological (anorexia nervosa, bulimia)
      e. Exercise
  B. Pituitary
    1. Tumors
      a. Prolactinomas
      b. Other hormone-secreting pituitary tumors (corticotropin, thyrotropin, growth hormone)
      c. Nonfunctional tumors (craniopharyngioma)
      d. Metastatic carcinoma
    2. Space-occupying lesions
      a. Empty sella syndrome
      b. Arterial aneurysm
    3. Necrosis
      a. Sheehan's syndrome
      b. Panhypopituitarism
    4. Inflammatory/infiltrative
      a. Sarcoidosis
      b. Hemachromatosis

quired to confirm the source of uterine bleeding. In some instances, prolonged or excessive ovulatory bleeding can be reduced by half with prostaglandin synthetase inhibitors; this form of treatment can be helpful in benign types of uterine disease if future fertility is desired.[396]

The diagnosis of anovulatory bleeding is one of exclusion and is supported by the history of the bleeding episodes. Once the diagnosis of anovulatory uterine bleeding or DUB is established, a rational approach to management is as follows. During a first episode of anovulatory bleeding the patient can simply be observed, provided the bleeding is not copious and the patient is not anemic. Recurrent bleeding that is moderately severe and not too prolonged may be treated with progestagens such as medroxyprogesterone acetate (10 mg/d for 10 d). The patient should be informed that withdrawal bleeding will occur after cessation of progestagen therapy. If this therapy is successful and the patient does not desire contraception, progestagens may be taken for 10 d of each month.[37] Progestagen therapy is most often used in women in the early premenopausal or postmenopausal years. However, if symptoms of estrogen deficiency are present or if the bleeding does not respond to progestagen alone, then estrogen plus cyclic progestagen therapy is indicated (see discussion in the section on hormonal therapy).

With severe and prolonged anovulatory bleeding, the endometrial lining of the uterus becomes thin and fragile and unresponsive to progestagens alone. In these instances bleeding can be controlled with a combined low-dose oral contraceptive regimen of two to three tablets per day (for a total daily dose of about 105 μg estrogen and up to 3 mg progestagen) for 1 wk, followed by tapering of the dose over 1 mo. If the bleeding is severe enough to cause anemia or hypovolemia, hospitalization and fluid and blood replacement may be needed. In these instances, high doses of oral, intramuscular, or intravenous estrogens may be necessary.[397] Parenteral estrogen is no more effective than oral estrogen, but high doses of the latter may induce gastrointestinal side effects such as nausea or vomiting. In either case progestagen therapy (medroxyprogesterone acetate, 10 mg/d by mouth) should be started as soon as the bleeding is controlled.

If hormonal therapy does not control bleeding or if the woman is at risk for endometrial cancer (e.g., a woman approaching the age of menopause or a massively obese woman), a dilatation and curettage may be required for diagnosis and therapy. This procedure by itself is not curative in most cases of chronic anovulatory bleeding, and DUB may recur. In women in the reproductive age group, long-term therapy with cyclic low-dose oral contraceptives provides adequate control of bleeding as well as effective contraception (see Chapter 18). When pregnancy is desired, contraceptive therapy is discontinued, and ovulation is stimulated (see discussion in the section on infertility).

Hysterectomy or uterine endometrial ablation by laser or cautery is the last resort for treatment of abnormal bleeding when fertility is no longer desired or significant pelvic pathologic abnormality is present.

AMENORRHEA. Amenorrhea is defined as the absence or cessation of menstrual bleeding, and it is a manifestation of a variety of pathophysiological disorders. The criteria used to determine which women require evaluation and diagnosis are not uniform. Most investigators agree that failure of menarche by age 16, regardless of the presence or absence of secondary sexual characteristics, or absence of menstruation in a woman with previous periodic menses merits evaluation. However, a patient who does not meet these criteria should be evaluated if she or her family members are greatly concerned, if secondary sexual characteristics (e.g., breast enlargement) have not developed by age 14, or if ambiguous external genitalia or virilization is present.[398]

Women with delayed puberty by definition also have amenorrhea and need not be considered separately. Women with sexual ambiguity or virilization may also present with amenorrhea, but in these cases the primary complaint is not amenorrhea. Women with sexual ambiguity should be evaluated as for a disorder of sexual differentiation (see Chapter 29). Women with hirsutism and virilization should also be evaluated differently, as discussed later in this chapter. These distinctions simplify the diagnosis, evaluation, and treatment of amenorrhea.

Amenorrhea is traditionally categorized as either primary (no history of menstruation) or secondary (cessation of menses after a variable time). Although this distinction is useful, some disorders can cause either primary or secondary amenorrhea. For example, most women with gonadal dysgenesis have primary amenorrhea, but some patients have residual follicles and ovulate, and in these women some menstruation and rare pregnancies may occur.[399–401] Patients with chronic anovulation (PCOS) usually have secondary amenorrhea but occasionally have primary amenorrhea.[150] For these reasons, categorization of amenorrhea into primary or secondary types is less helpful than a classification based on the underlying pathophysiological disorder: anatomic defect, ovarian failure, or chronic anovulation with or without current estrogen production (Table 15–8).

Amenorrhea Associated with Anatomic Defect. A variety of anatomic defects of the female reproductive outflow tract preclude menstrual bleeding. Some are iatrogenic or caused by infection (Fig. 15–39). Women with amenorrhea caused by anatomic defects of the outflow track have normal ovarian function; they ovulate and have normal secondary sexual characteristics.

Beginning at the caudal end of the female genital tract, labial agglutination secondary to infection may obstruct menstrual flow.[402] Idiopathic labial fusion may occur in the absence of other clinical findings associated with sexual ambiguity (i.e., clitoral enlargement).[403] Imperforate hymen, transverse vaginal septum, or isolated absence of the vagina or cervix can also cause amenorrhea.[404, 405] Women with these defects frequently have an accumulation of blood behind the obstruction and present with cyclic, predictable episodes of pain in the absence of menses (see Fig. 15–39).[404] If undiagnosed, these disorders can lead to endometriosis, adhesions, and later infertility. More severe müllerian anomalies include müllerian agenesis (the Mayer-Rokitansky-Küster-Hauser syndrome) and defects in lateral or vertical müllerian fusion in which the caudal portion of the müllerian duct fails to fuse normally

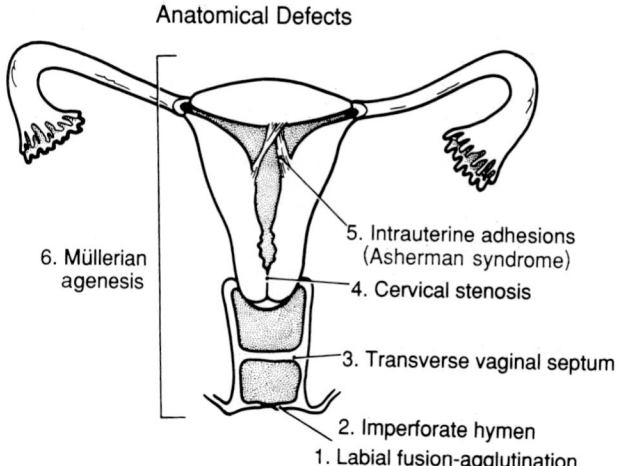

Anatomical Defects

6. Müllerian agenesis

5. Intrauterine adhesions (Asherman syndrome)

4. Cervical stenosis

3. Transverse vaginal septum

2. Imperforate hymen

1. Labial fusion-agglutination

Figure 15–39. Diagrammatic representation of causes of amenorrhea resulting from disorders of the female reproductive (outflow) tract.

with the urogenital sinus.[406] Defects in lateral fusion include double uterus (uterus didelphys), half uterus (uterus unicornis), partial duplication (uterus bicornis), and partial or complete uterine septum. In those patients with complete obstruction (e.g., a blind uterine horn), amenorrhea and cyclic pain are the presenting symptoms, whereas those with communicating uterine defects characteristically present with dysmenorrhea.[406, 407]

Müllerian agenesis is the second most common cause of primary amenorrhea, after gonadal dysgenesis.[408] Women with müllerian agenesis have a 46,XX karyotype, female secondary sexual characteristics, and normal ovarian function, including ovulation, but have absence of the vagina and either absence or severe hypoplasia of the uterus.[328] The uterus, when present, usually consists of only rudimentary bicornuate cords. If the uterus contains endometrium, cyclic abdominal pain and accumulation of blood may occur, as with other disorders of vertical and lateral obstruction of the outflow tract. Women with müllerian agenesis often have associated abnormalities of the urogenital tract (15 to 40%), including a pelvic kidney or unilateral absence of a kidney.[409] About 12% have skeletal anomalies, usually involving the spine.[328]

The major diagnostic problem is differentiation of müllerian agenesis from complete androgen resistance (testicular feminization), in which 46,XY genetic men with testes also have female breast development, a blind-ending vaginal pouch, and an absent uterus (Table 15–9). The latter disorder is caused by defects in the androgen receptor that cause profound resistance to the action of testosterone during embryogenesis and in postnatal life[329, 410, 411] (see Chapter 29). Testicular feminization is suspected if pubic and axillary hair is absent or deficient and an inguinal hernia is present. The diagnosis of testicular feminization is confirmed by demonstration of a male level of serum testosterone and a 46,XY karyotype, whereas the diagnosis of müllerian agenesis can be established by documentation of the presence of biphasic basal body temperatures characteristic of ovulatory women, elevated progesterone levels during the luteal phase, and a 46,XX karyotype. Subjects with testicular feminization should have the testes removed after breast development because of the risk of malignant transformation.[340]

In other instances women lack a uterus, do not feminize at the time of expected puberty, and have infantile female external genitalia. In these women who have a 46,XY karyotype and androgen deficiency, causes include deficiency of CYP17, 17β-hydroxysteroid dehydrogenase 3, and 5α-reductase 2; testicular regression syndrome; and gonadal agenesis (see Chapter 29). Those patients with a 46,XX karyotype have müllerian agenesis along with another disorder such as ovarian failure or gonadotropin insufficiency.[412]

Other abnormalities of the uterus that cause amenorrhea include congenital absence of the cervix and obstruction of

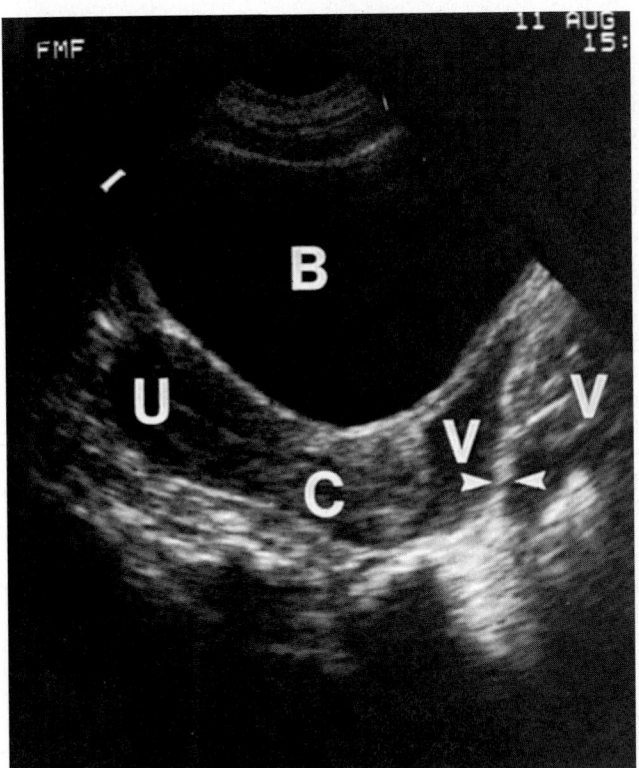

Figure 15–40. Transabdominal ultrasonographic study demonstrating a transverse vaginal septum. Arrowheads denote the location and width of the transverse septum. B, bladder; U, uterus; C, cervix; V, vagina. Menstrual blood is located between the septum and the cervix. (From Doody KM, Carr BR. Amenorrhea. Obstet Gynecol Clin North Am 1990; 17:361–387, with permission.)

the cervix caused by scarring or stenosis. The latter usually results from dilatation and curettage or from treatment of cervical dysplasia or cervical intraepithelial neoplasia by laser, electrocautery, or cryosurgery. In rare instances amenorrhea is caused by endometrial hypoplasia or aplasia.[404] Destruction of the endometrium (Asherman's syndrome) can follow vigorous curettage in association with postpartum hemorrhage, therapeutic abortion complicated by infection, or a missed abortion and is associated with endometrial adhesions or synechiae.[413] Asherman's syndrome can also occur after uterine surgery such as a metroplasty, myomectomy, or cesarean section and can result from tuberculosis or schistosomiasis.[413] Women with Asherman's syndrome may have amenorrhea in severe cases or scant menses at regular predictable intervals.

Diagnosis and Treatment. The diagnosis of a defect of the outflow tract is usually established by history and physical examination. In women with primary amenorrhea and no history of prior surgery of the reproductive tract, the pelvic examination may be diagnostic. Labial agglutination, labial fusion, imperforate hymen, and transverse vaginal septum are easily recognized. In cases of transverse vaginal septum, ultrasonography is helpful in determining the location and length of the septum before surgical repair is undertaken (Fig. 15–40).[414] If the vaginal opening is patent and a cervix is visualized by a speculum examination, a sound or probe can confirm the presence or absence of cervical stenosis or scarring. If a uterus is not palpated during a bimanual pelvic examination, an ultrasonographic study or MRI scan is useful to document whether a uterus is present and whether it contains an endometrial cavity.[335, 336] These studies are also helpful in the diagnosis of other uterine anomalies such as double uterus or blind uterine horns. Finally, hysterosalpingography, hysteroscopy, and occasionally laparoscopy may be required for diag-

TABLE 15–9. Differential Diagnosis of a Phenotypic Female with Secondary Sexual Development and No Uterus

Feature	Müllerian	Complete Androgen Resistance (Testicular Feminization)
Hereditary pattern	Sporadic	X-linked recessive
Gonad	Ovary	Testis
Chromosomes	46,XX	46,XY
Serum testosterone	Low	Male
Serum LH	Normal	Increased
Breasts	+ +	+ +
Pubic/axillary hair	+ +	−
Other anomalies	+ +	−

From Doody KM, Carr BR. Amenorrhea. Obstet Gynecol Clin North Am 1990; 17:361–387.

nosis of Asherman's syndrome or other abnormalities of uterine development.[336, 341, 342]

Most disorders of the outflow tract are successfully treated by surgery. Incision or excision in cases of labial fusion, imperforate hymen, or vaginal septum often leads to normal menstruation and later fertility.[415] Labial adhesions in children have been treated successfully with estrogen cream.[416] A functional vagina in women with müllerian agenesis or testicular feminization can be created either by nonsurgical dilatation of a blind-ending pouch or perineal dimple or, if needed, by surgical construction with the use of skin grafts.[417–419] Asherman's syndrome is best treated by direct hysteroscopic resection.[420, 421]

Ovarian Failure. Ovarian failure, or hypergonadotropic hypogonadism, is the occurrence of amenorrhea, hypoestrogenism, and elevated gonadotropin levels before age 40. Cessation of ovarian function can occur at any age, even in utero. If it occurs before puberty the presentation is as primary amenorrhea; after pubertal development and menarche the presentation is as secondary amenorrhea. Ovarian failure can result from multiple causes (see Table 15–8). Gonadal agenesis, the most severe form, is most often associated with a 46,XY karyotype and sexual infantilism. Rare cases have been associated with a 46,XX karyotype.[422]

Gonadal dysgenesis results when the germ cells are lacking and the ovary is replaced by a fibrous streak[423] (see Chapter 29). Women with gonadal dysgenesis can be divided into two broad groups on the basis of karyotype. The first group has an abnormal chromosomal karyotype; deletion of genetic material in the X chromosome accounts for about two thirds of cases.[424] A 45,X karyotype is found in about half, and most of these women have somatic defects, including short stature, webbed neck, shield chest, short metacarpals, increased carrying angle of the arms, cardiovascular defects, and sexual infantilism, collectively termed Turner syndrome (Fig. 15–41).[425]

The remainder of patients with identifiable abnormalities of the X chromosome have chromosomal mosaicism with or without structural abnormalities of the X chromosome. Short stature is seen in patients with gonadal dysgenesis who have monosomy of the short arm of the X chromosome. Genes on both the long and short arms of the X chromosome are involved in ovarian development.[426] The most common form

of mosaicism in gonadal dysgenesis is 45,X/46,XX.[424] Trisomy for the X chromosome (46,XXX) is also associated with ovarian failure or premature menopause.[427]

Gonadal tumors are rare in patients with the 45,X karyotype, but those with chromosome mosaicism involving the Y chromosome have a 25% risk for development of gonadal malignancy.[423] Therefore, a chromosomal analysis should be obtained in all cases of ovarian failure in patients younger than 30 y, and the streak gonad should be removed if a Y chromosome is present. Although patients with gonadal dysgenesis appear to have a normal complement of oocytes during early fetal development, the gonad is usually devoid of follicles by birth.[9] For this reason, more than 90% of women with gonadal dysgenesis resulting from deletion of genetic material in the X chromosome never have menstrual bleeding. A few patients have sufficient residual follicles to experience menses and, rarely, fertility.[423, 424, 428]

The second form of gonadal dysgenesis is associated with a normal 46,XX or 46,XY karyotype and is termed *pure gonadal dysgenesis*.[399, 429, 430] These patients have normal or above average stature as a result of failure of estrogen-mediated epiphyseal closure in the presence of a normal chromosomal constitution. In most cases the cause of pure gonadal dysgenesis is unknown, but it may result from single-gene defects or destruction of germinal tissue in utero by environmental or infectious processes.[430] Approximately 10% of patients with a 46,XY karyotype develop signs of virilization, including clitorimegaly, and have an increased incidence of tumors in the gonadal streaks; therefore gonadal streaks should be removed prophylactically by laparoscopic techniques, as described previously, if a Y chromosome is present.[430] Although signs of virilization are rare in women with 46,XX gonadal dysgenesis, the gonadal streak should be removed if the source of androgen excess is thought to be gonadal.[431] Approximately two thirds of patients with 46,XX gonadal dysgenesis experience no menses, and the remainder have one or more menstrual episodes and are occasionally fertile.[423]

Other causes of ovarian failure include deficiency of 17α-hydroxylase or of 17,20-lyase, resistant ovary syndrome, galactosemia, autoimmune disorders, and physical trauma (e.g., chemotherapy and radiation therapy for malignancy or infection). 17α-Hydroxylase deficiency is characterized by primary amenorrhea, sexual infantilism, and hypertension resulting

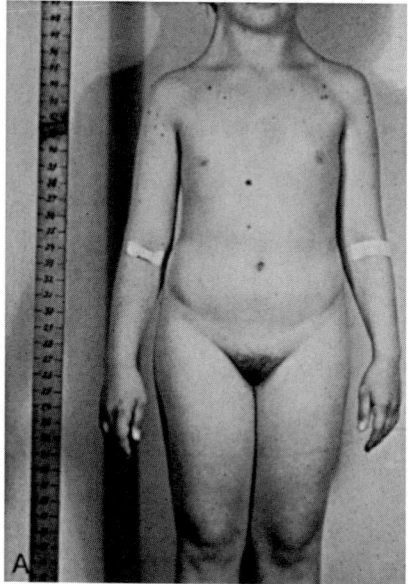
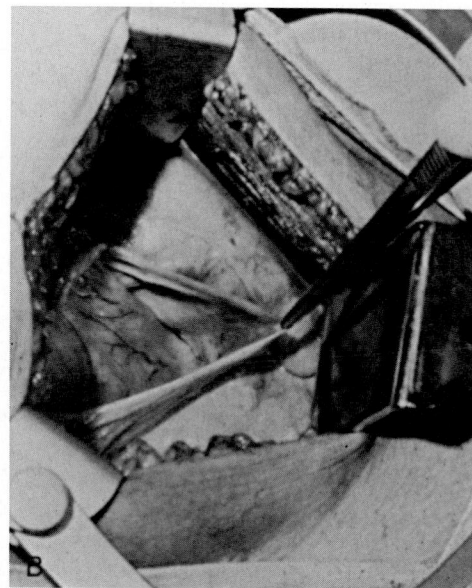
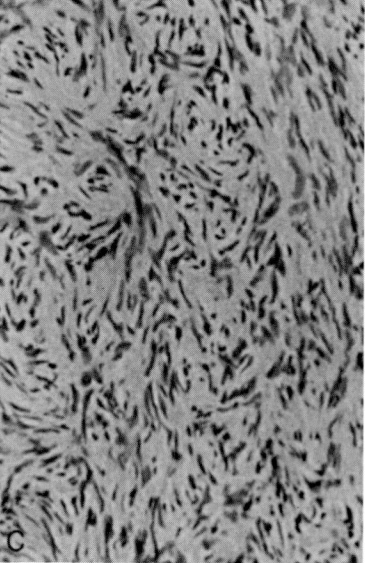

Figure 15–41. Turner syndrome. *A,* Patient with stigmata of gonadal dysgenesis, including short stature, sexual infantilism, webbed neck, and broadly spaced nipples. *B,* Streak ovary (held by forceps). *C,* Microscopic section of a streak ovary demonstrating fibrous replacement of ovarian structures and absence of germ cells and follicles.

from increased production of deoxycorticosterone, whereas women with 17,20-lyase deficiency have primary amenorrhea and sexual infantilism with normal blood pressure.[432, 433] The diagnosis of these enzyme deficiencies can be established by measuring levels of progesterone and 17-OHP.

The resistant ovary syndrome is a rare disorder in which the ovaries contain follicles arrested in development before the antral stage, possibly because of an abnormality or deficiency of the FSH receptor.[143, 434] To differentiate this disorder from the 46,XX variety of pure gonadal dysgenesis, both of which are associated with amenorrhea and sexual infantilism, it is necessary to perform an ovarian biopsy. However, such a distinction is not clinically useful, because the treatment of infertility in both conditions is usually unsuccessful (see later discussion).

The ovarian failure of galactosemia is caused by deficiency of galactose-containing compounds or excessive accumulation of galactose 1-phosphate in the ovary.[435] Premature ovarian failure may also occur as an isolated autoimmune disorder or in association with hypothyroidism, hypoadrenalism, hypoparathyroidism, or systemic lupus erythematosus (also see Chapter 33).[436] In some of these cases antibodies to the ovary can be identified. Because premature ovarian failure may be associated with polyglandular failure, which may be life-threatening, a thorough evaluation is indicated to rule out other endocrine failure. Ovarian failure may be caused by radiation therapy and chemotherapy for treatment of malignancy.[437, 438] A dose of more than 8 Gy (800 rad) directed to the ovary usually causes permanent ovarian failure.[438] Infection can also cause ovarian failure and infertility.[439]

Diagnosis and Treatment. The diagnosis of ovarian failure is suspected in all cases of primary amenorrhea and sexual infantilism and in women with secondary amenorrhea who have hot flushes and other signs of estrogen deficiency. It is confirmed by documentation of FSH levels in the menopausal range (i.e., >40 IU/L). In women younger than age 30, a chromosomal karyotype should be obtained. If indicated, other assays may be helpful in confirming the diagnosis: progesterone, deoxycorticosterone, and 17-OHP (17α-hydroxylase and 17,20-lyase deficiency); galactose 1-phosphate (galactosemia); serum levels of calcium, phosphorus, cortisol, and thyroxine; and antibodies to thyroid, adrenal, and ovary (autoimmune disorders).

Because ovarian failure is usually permanent, all patients should be treated with estrogen and progestagen replacement or with oral contraceptives. Estrogen therapy promotes and maintains secondary sexual characteristics and prevents premature osteoporosis and coronary heart disease. In girls with gonadal dysgenesis and short stature whose epiphyses are not closed, growth hormone or growth hormone plus oxandrolone may be administered to accelerate growth (Fig. 15–42).[440, 441] Some studies have reported greater than predicted adult height after such treatment.[440] After growth hormone therapy (if any) and closure of the epiphyses in all subjects, lowdose estrogen therapy is indicated.[442] In gonadal dysgenesis, estrogen is usually taken in a cyclic fashion, with an initial dose of 0.3 mg/d of conjugated estrogens until growth ceases, at which time the daily estrogen dose is increased to between 0.625 and 1.25 mg to augment breast development. It is necessary to initiate and continue progestagen therapy to induce regular withdrawal bleeding and reduce the risk of endometrial carcinoma.

Patients with 17α-hydroxylase deficiency should be treated with glucocorticoids as well as oral contraceptives or estrogen and progestagen replacement. Women with autoimmune ovarian failure have been treated with short courses of glucocorticoids or plasmapheresis, with only temporary improvement in most cases.[437] Occasionally, prophylactic repositioning of the ovary (oophoropexy) may prevent ovarian failure in women who are to receive ionizing radiation.[443]

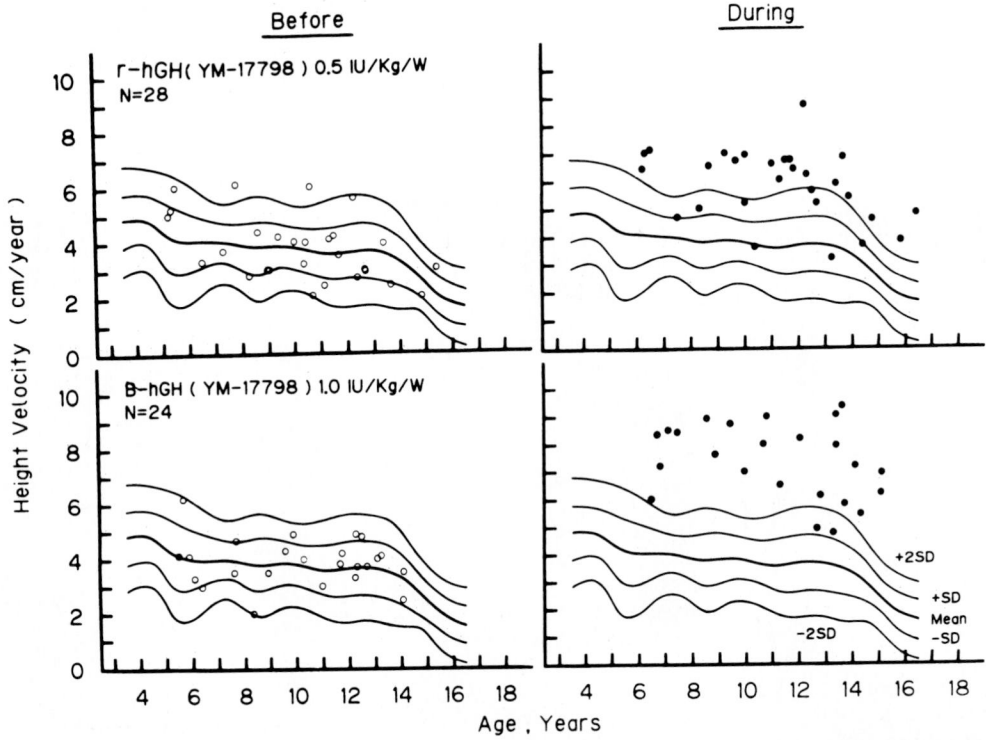

Figure 15–42. Growth rates of girls with gonadal dysgenesis before *(open circles)* and during *(solid circles)* treatment with two levels of methionine-free recombinant human growth hormone (hGH) compared with curves indicating the natural growth rate of girls with gonadal dysgenesis (mean ± 1 or 2 SDs). (From Takano K, Shizume K, Hibi I, et al. Turner's syndrome: treatment of 203 patients with recombinant human growth hormone for one year. A multicentre study. Acta Endocrinol 1989; 120:559–568, with permission.)

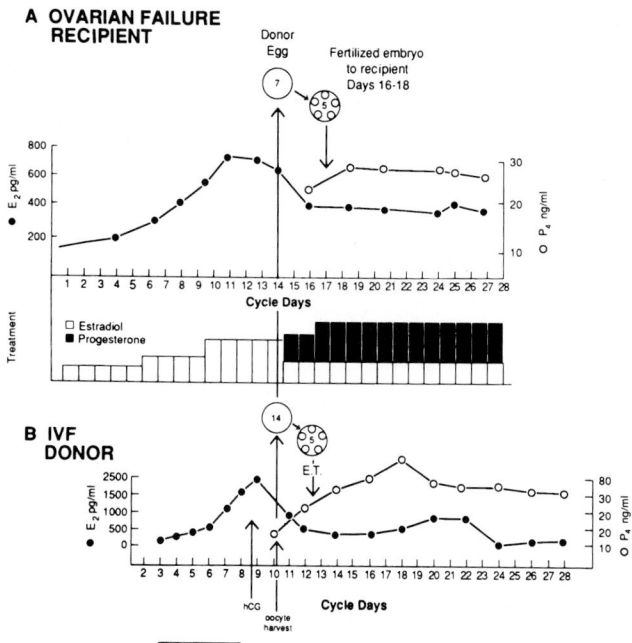

A OVARIAN FAILURE RECIPIENT

B IVF DONOR

Figure 15–43. Diagrammatic representation of donation of excess oocytes by a woman undergoing in vitro fertilization (IVF) to a woman with ovarian failure treated with exogenous estrogen and progesterone. *A*, Woman with ovarian failure treated with increasing doses of estrogen during days 1 through 14 of the cycle. Exogenous progesterone was added to the estrogen treatment on days 15 through 28 and continued if pregnancy was diagnosed. Seven donor eggs were fertilized with sperm from the recipient's husband, and five embryos were transferred to the uterus between days 16 and 18. *B*, The IVF patient-donor was treated with human menopausal gonadotropin (hMG) until day 8, when hCG was given, and oocytes were harvested 32 to 36 h later. Half of the eggs were donated to the ovarian failure recipient, and the other half were fertilized with sperm from the donor's husband; the five fertilized eggs were transferred to the uterus of the IVF donor. E$_2$ (estradiol) and P$_4$ (progesterone) plasma levels in both women are shown. To convert estradiol values to picomoles per liter, multiply by 3.671. To convert progesterone values to nanomoles per liter, multiply by 3.180. (Adapted from Rosenwaks Z. Donor eggs: their application in modern reproductive technologies. Fertil Steril 1987; 47:895–909, with permission.)

Pretreatment with LHRH analogues, antiestrogens, or oral contraceptives before chemotherapy may be successful in maintaining ovarian function.[438]

In a few cases ovarian follicular depletion may not be complete, and occasional spontaneous ovulatory cycles and even pregnancy may occur.[444] Various stimulation protocols, including high-dose estrogens plus progestagens (either alone or combined with gonadotropins) or pretreatment with LHRH analogues followed by gonadotropins, have been used for women with premature menopause who desire pregnancy.[445–447] Most women with secondary ovarian failure who subsequently conceive have been treated with estrogen replacement. Estrogen is believed to suppress gonadotropins and either stimulate formation of new FSH receptors or prevent down-regulation of FSH receptors. Sporadic pregnancies have been reported with and without therapy, but because the number of reported patients is small, no definite conclusion can be drawn about the efficacy of treatment. It is difficult to predict which patients with ovarian failure will respond. An ovarian biopsy includes only a small part of the ovary, and pregnancies have occurred despite the fact that a biopsy was devoid of follicles. For this reason ovarian biopsy is not indicated. Women with small follicles demonstrated by ultrasonographic studies may be more likely to ovulate. Use of donor oocytes and ovum transfer combined with in vitro fertilization and synchronization of the endometrium with cyclic exogenous estrogen and progestagen has also been used to achieve pregnancies (Fig. 15–43).[234]

Chronic Anovulation. The most common cause of amenorrhea is chronic anovulation. Women with chronic anovulation do not ovulate spontaneously but have ovaries with follicles and may ovulate with appropriate therapy. The ovaries of such women do not secrete estrogen in a normal cyclic pattern. It is useful to differentiate those women who produce sufficient estrogen to have withdrawal bleeding after progestagen therapy from those with hypogonadotropic hypogonadism who fail to produce enough estrogen to have withdrawal bleeding. Although this distinction is useful, some women with chronic anovulation caused by stress, weight loss, exercise, or hyperprolactinemia have reduced estrogen production but still experience withdrawal bleeding after a progestagen challenge. This result simply indicates that some estrogen is being produced.

Chronic Anovulation with Estrogen Present. Women with chronic anovulation who experience withdrawal bleeding after progesterone administration are said to be in a state of "estrus" because of the acyclic production of estrogen (largely estrone) by extraglandular aromatization of circulating androstenedione. This condition may be caused by altered feedback loops. It has been proposed that the ovary is initially normal but that the hypothalamic-pituitary unit is regulated by signals that do not originate in the ovary.[150] Support for this concept is provided by animal models in which the administration of androgens to newborns before maturation of the hypothalamic-pituitary axis permanently modifies feedback relations. Such animals do not begin cyclic ovarian function at puberty but enter into a state of continuous estrus in which the ovaries contain many cystic follicles and overproduce androgens.[448]

The most common cause of chronic anovulation with estrogen present is PCOS, a complex disorder characterized by infertility, hirsutism, obesity, and various menstrual disturbances: amenorrhea, oligomenorrhea, or DUB (Table 15–10). The symptoms and features are variable even when the diagnosis is based on the presence of polycystic ovaries as determined by histologic or ultrasonographic studies.[449, 450] There appears to be a strong familial component, and autosomal dominant or X-linked genetic transmission has been suggested.[451–454]

Classic PCOS as described by Stein and Leventhal[455] is characterized by enlarged, polycystic ovaries, but the syndrome and its characteristic endocrine abnormalities are associated with a variety of pathologic findings in the ovaries, only some of which result in their enlargement and none of which is pathognomonic.[455–459] The term *polycystic ovaries* itself is misleading, because the ovaries are studded with atretic follicles, not with cysts. The most common pathologic finding is a white, smooth, sclerotic ovary with a thickened capsule, multi-

TABLE 15–10. Incidence of Symptoms Associated with Polycystic Ovarian Syndrome*

	Incidence (%)		
Symptom	**Mean**	**Range**	**No. of Usable Cases**
Infertility	74	35–95	596
Hirsutism	69	17–83	819
Amenorrhea	51	15–77	640
Obesity	41	16–49	600
Functional bleeding	29	6–65	547
Dysmenorrhea	23		75
Corpus luteum at surgery	22	0–71	391
Virilization	21	0–28	431
Biphasic body temperature	15	12–40	288
Cyclic menses	12	7–28	395

*Tabulated from 187 references with a total of 1079 cases. The number of usable cases indicates how many of the 1079 total cases could be evaluated for the presence or absence of a particular symptom.

Adapted from Goldzieher JW, Axelrod LR. Clinical and biochemical features of polycystic ovarian disease. Fertil Steril 1963; 14:631–653.

ple follicles in various stages of atresia, a hyperplastic theca and stroma, and rare or absent corpora albicans (Fig. 15–44).[457–459] Further confusion is caused by the fact that polycystic ovaries as defined by ultrasonographic studies (at least 10 follicles and increased ovarian stroma) may be present in normal women with ovulatory cycles and no hirsutism.[460]

Some investigators have attempted to define PCOS in terms of endocrine levels. Because plasma LH levels are often elevated and plasma FSH levels are normal or low, it has been suggested that an LH/FSH ratio higher than 2 to 3 may serve as a useful laboratory definition of PCOS.[461, 462] An exaggerated release of LH may occur in women with PCOS after administration of an intravenous bolus of LHRH.[463, 464] Increases in both pulse amplitude and frequency of LH pulses suggest an abnormality of the LHRH pulse generator located in the hypothalamus.[465, 466] The most plausible explanation is that the increased secretion of LH occurs as a result of disturbances in steroid feedback in the hypothalamic-pituitary unit.[467] For clinical purposes, the interpretation of a single sample of gonadotropins is rarely useful for confirming the diagnosis. Even with frequent sampling or measurement after LHRH administration, gonadotropin levels are normal in 10 to 20%

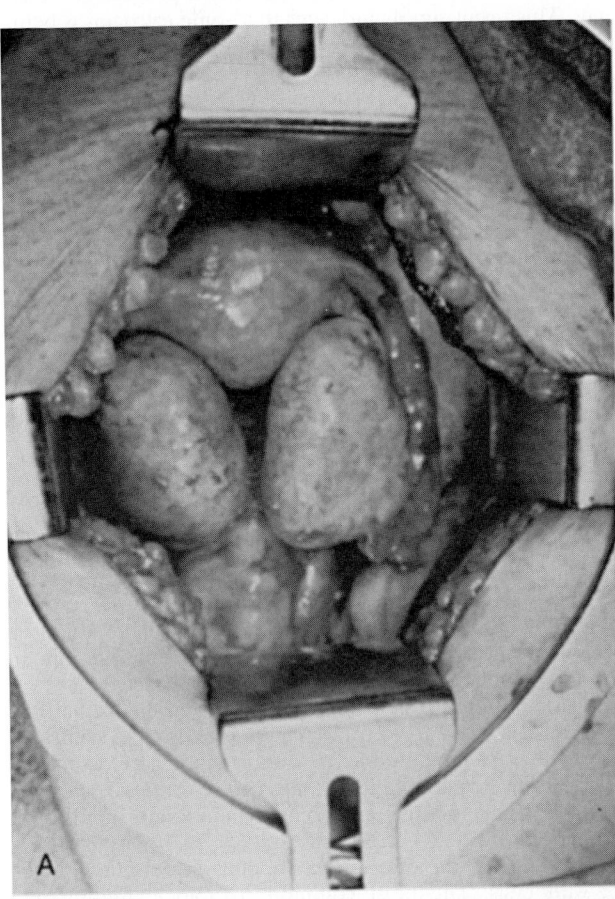

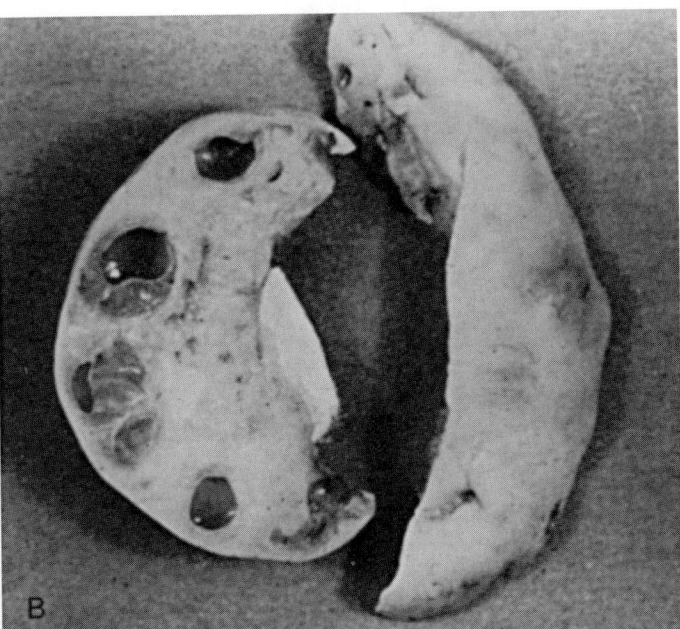

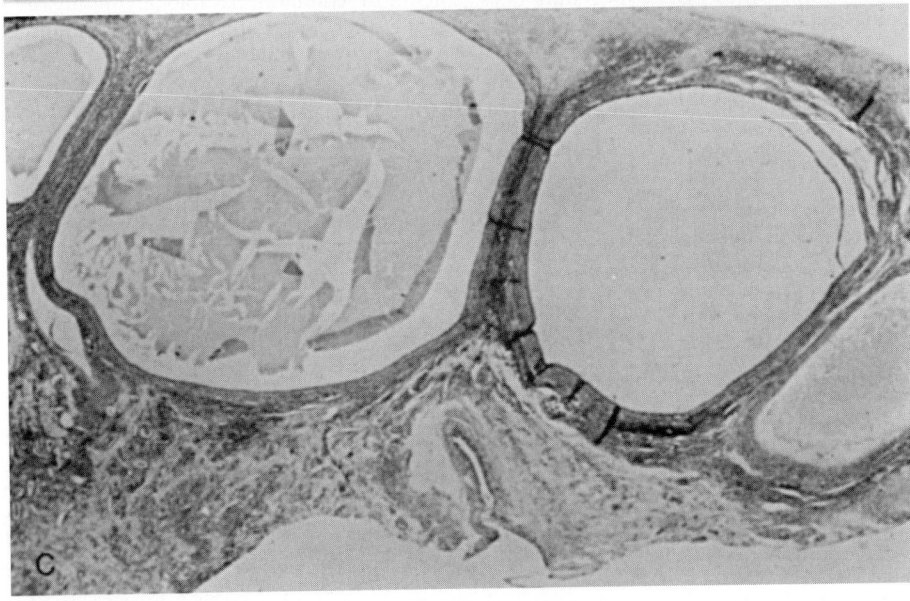

Figure 15–44. Polycystic ovaries. *A,* Operative findings of classic enlarged polycystic ovaries. The uterus is located superior to the ovaries. *B,* Sectioned polycystic ovary with numerous follicles. *C,* Histologic section of polycystic ovaries demonstrating cystic follicles with reduced number of granulosa cells and increased ovarian theca and stroma. Magnification × 33.

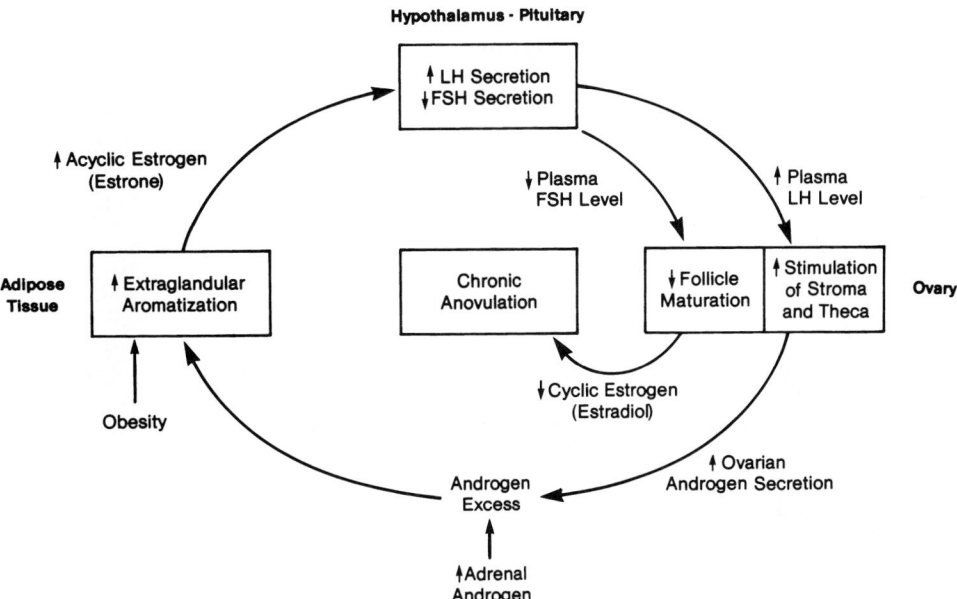

Figure 15–45. Proposed mechanism for the initiation and perpetuation of chronic anovulation in women with polycystic ovary syndrome (PCOS). The cycle may be entered or initiated by adrenal androgen excess or obesity, both of which result in enhanced extraglandular formation of estrogens. The therapy for this disease involves interruption of the cycle. (Adapted from Yen SSC. Chronic anovulation caused by peripheral endocrine disorders. In: Yen SSC, Jaffe RB. Reproductive Endocrinology: Physiology, Pathophysiology and Clinical Management. 2nd ed. Philadelphia: WB Saunders, 1986: 441–499; and from Carr BR, Wilson JD. Disorders of the ovary and female reproductive tract. In: Braunwald E, Isselbacher KJ, Petersdorf RG, et al, eds. Harrison's Principles of Internal Medicine. 11th ed. New York: McGraw-Hill, 1987: 1818–1837, with permission.)

of women with PCOS.[450, 463] Some have suggested that bioactive LH (as contrasted to immunoreactive LH) is elevated in these women and that assay of bioactive LH may help in the diagnosis.[468]

In more than half of women with PCOS, plasma androstenedione and testosterone levels (total or free) are increased.[461] The principal source of androgen is the ovary. Treatment with LHRH analogues lowers gonadotropins and reduces androstenedione and testosterone to castrate levels, whereas levels of adrenal androgens such as DHEAS remained unchanged.[469] Although some women with PCOS have elevated plasma DHEAS levels, levels of 11β-hydroxyandrostenedione (an adrenal metabolite of androstenedione) are similar to those found in control subjects.[470] About 15 to 20% of women with PCOS have mild elevations of plasma prolactin.[471, 472] Increased prolactin secretion may be caused by chronic exposure to estrogen or by deficiency of hypothalamic dopamine.[467]

The diagnosis of PCOS is not based primarily on pathologic changes in the ovaries or on plasma hormone disturbances but is instead a clinical diagnosis based on the coexistence of chronic anovulation and varying degrees of hirsutism. In most women with PCOS, menarche occurs at the expected time, but uterine bleeding is dysfunctional and is unpredictable in onset, duration, and amount. Oligomenorrhea or amenorrhea ensues after a variable time. Five to 10% of patients present with primary amenorrhea.[473] The signs of androgen excess usually become evident at about the expected time of menarche.

One theory suggests that this disorder originates as an exaggerated adrenarche in obese girls who also have insulin resistance (Fig. 15–45).[150] The combination of elevated adrenal androgens, insulin resistance, and obesity would result in increased formation of extraglandular estrogen. In women with PCOS, levels of estrone are elevated, but so are levels of free estradiol, resulting in part from reduced levels of TeBG.[474, 475] The acyclic production of extraglandular estrogen would lead to a positive feedback on LH secretion and a negative feedback on FSH secretion, resulting in the characteristic LH/FSH ratio in plasma. The elevated LH leads to hyperplasia of the ovarian stroma and thecal cells, further increasing androgen production and in turn providing more substrate for extraglandular aromatization and perpetuation of chronic anovulation. In obese women this sequence of events is en-

hanced, because adipose tissue stromal cells aromatize androgens to estrogens, exaggerating inappropriate LH release.[300, 476]

Therefore the fundamental defect in the PCOS is viewed as one of inappropriate signals to the hypothalamus and pituitary. Others have proposed that a hypothalamic disorder independent of abnormal steroid feedback is the primary defect in PCOS.[477] However, most believe that abnormal steroid feedback signals are the primary alteration, that the hypothalamic-pituitary axis responds appropriately to high levels of estrogen, and that ovulation can be induced with antiestrogens such as clomiphene citrate.[37, 450] The concept that the fundamental defect is one of inappropriate signals is supported by the findings in the ovary itself. Ovarian follicles from women with PCOS have low CYP19 activity, but CYP19 can be induced if the follicles are treated in vitro with FSH (Fig. 15–46).[478] Also, women with PCOS can be induced to ovulate by administration of FSH.[479, 480] In short, the anovulation does not appear to be caused by an intrinsic abnormality in the ovary but rather by FSH deficiency and LH excess.

Other theories of the origin of PCOS include anomalies of dopamine, endorphin, and inhibin secretion.[473, 481-483] An association of hyperandrogenemia and PCOS with insulin resistance has been documented in both obese and nonobese women.[484-486] Insulin stimulates androgen secretion in ovarian stroma in vitro,[487] and, in women with PCOS who also have insulin resistance, insulin or IGFs may act on the ovary by means of IGF receptors (Fig. 15–47).[171, 484, 488]

Chronic anovulation with estrogen present, obesity, hirsutism, and polycystic ovaries may also occur in a variety of endocrine disorders. Most such patients have PCOS, but the functional abnormalities also may be seen in women with Cushing's syndrome, hyperthyroidism, hypothyroidism, or late-onset adrenal hyperplasia resulting from 21-hydroxylase or 11β-hydroxylase deficiency.[150, 461, 489-491] Chronic anovulation with estrogen present may also result from tumors of the ovary, including granulosa-theca cell tumors, Brenner tumors, cystic teratomas, mucinous cystadenomas, and Krukenberg's tumors (see discussion in the section on hirsutism and virilization). Such tumors can either secrete excess estrogen or produce androgens that are aromatized in extraglandular sites.[492] As a result, clinical features of PCOS are produced. Occasionally, areas of the ovary not involved with tumor demonstrate characteristic histologic features of polycystic ovaries.

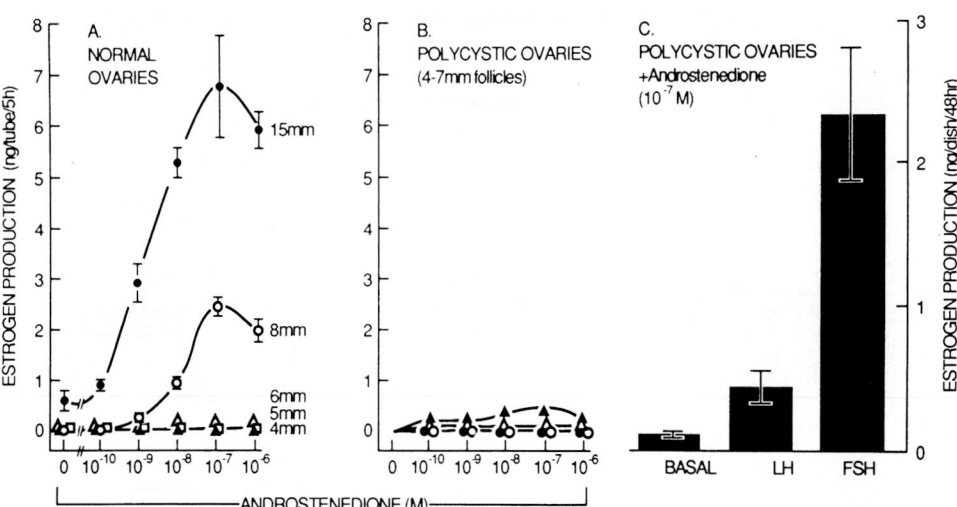

Figure 15–46. Estrogen production by granulosa cells from normal (control) and polycystic ovaries. *A,* Estrogen production from follicles of various sizes obtained from normal ovaries. *B,* Estrogen production from follicles of polycystic ovaries. *C,* Estrogen production from follicles of polycystic ovaries treated with androstenedione plus LH or FSH. (Adapted from Erickson GF, Hsueh AJW, Quigley ME, et al. Functional studies of aromatase activity in human granulosa cells from normal and polycystic ovaries. J Clin Endocrinol Metab 1979; 49:514–519. Copyright © 1979, by The Endocrine Society.)

Treatment of PCOS is directed toward interruption of the self-perpetuating hormonal cycle and can be accomplished in several ways. Ovarian androgen secretion can be decreased directly by laparoscopic ovarian drilling (wedge resection) or indirectly by lowering LH levels (oral contraceptive pills and LHRH analogues). Other approaches include weight reduction and enhancement of FSH secretion (with clomiphene, hMG, urofollitropin [pure FSH], or pulsatile LHRH therapy).[461, 467, 473, 493–501] LHRH analogue therapy has been combined with hMG, FSH, or pulsatile LHRH therapy in attempts to increase pregnancy rates and to reduce hyperstimulation.

The choice of therapy depends on the clinical picture as well as the wishes of the patient. Weight reduction is appropriate in all patients who are obese, because it reduces androgen levels and decreases insulin resistance. Weight loss may cause ovulation to return to normal in some women.[495, 501] If the woman is not hirsute and does not desire pregnancy, monthly withdrawal menses should be induced by progestage therapy or oral contraceptives to reduce the risk of endometrial neoplasia.[502, 503] If the woman is hirsute but does not desire pregnancy, excess androgen production can be suppressed with oral contraceptives, glucocorticoids, LHRH analogues, or antiandrogens (e.g., spironolactone). Oral contraceptives are also indicated if prolonged or excessive menstrual bleeding is present. If pregnancy is desired, ovulation must be induced. The initial drug of choice is clomiphene citrate, which induces ovulation in about three fourths of patients.[473]

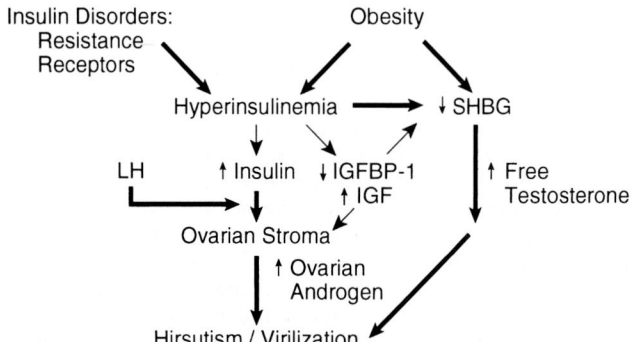

Figure 15–47. Proposed relation between insulin resistance and androgen excess. IGF, insulin-like growth factor; IGFBP-1, insulin-like growth factor–binding protein-1; LH, luteinizing hormone; SHBG, sex hormone–binding globulin (testosterone-binding globulin [TeBG]). (Adapted from Poretsky L. On the paradox of insulin-induced hyperandrogenism in insulin resistant states. Endocr Rev 1991; 12:3–13. © 1991, by The Endocrine Society.)

In those women who do not ovulate or do not conceive after 6 to 12 mo of therapy, clomiphene combinations (clomiphene plus glucocorticoids, hCG, or bromocriptine), hMG, pure FSH, pulsatile LHRH by itself, pulsatile LHRH combined with an LHRH analogue, or cautery or wedge resection of the ovaries may be successful (see discussion in the section on drugs to induce ovulation).

Chronic Anovulation with Estrogen Absent. Women with chronic anovulation and low or absent estrogen production do not experience withdrawal bleeding or have only minimal spotting after progestagen treatment. This disorder is the result of hypogonadotropic hypogonadism secondary to organic or functional disorders of the CNS-hypothalamic-pituitary axis (see Table 15–8).

A defect in the formation and migration of LHRH neurons is called isolated hypothalamic hypogonadism (IHH) or congenital isolated LHRH deficiency; when associated with anosmia and agenesis of the olfactory bulbs, this condition is termed *Kallmann's syndrome.*[504, 505] Affected women are sexually infantile with an eunuchoid habitus and have low levels of gonadotropins as a result of defects in the release of LHRH. Kallmann's syndrome, a familial disorder usually inherited in women as an autosomal dominant trait, is more commonly symptomatic in men and is frequently associated with anosmia, color blindness, and occasionally midline defects such as cleft lip and palate.[506] The X-linked form of the disorder is caused by mutations in the *KAL* gene that impair migration of neurons into the olfactory bulb.[507] MRI scans often demonstrate a defect in development of the olfactory bulbs and sulci of the rhinencephalon (Fig. 15–48).[508]

Additional syndromes associated with hypogonadotropic hypogonadism include the Prader-Willi and Bardet-Biedl syndromes.[346] Rare hypothalamic lesions or developmental defects that can also impair LHRH production and cause hypogonadotropic hypogonadism include craniopharyngioma, germinoma, eosinophilic granuloma (Hand-Schüller-Christian syndrome), teratomas, endodermal sinus tumors, tuberculosis, syphilis, sarcoidosis, hamartomas, and metastatic tumors.[509] These disorders can usually be identified by radiographs or CT or MRI scans of the head. Trauma or radiation to the CNS can also cause hypothalamic amenorrhea, sometimes associated with deficiencies of other pituitary hormones.

More commonly, gonadotropin deficiency leading to chronic anovulation arises from functional disorders of the hypothalamus or higher centers in the absence of defects identifiable on MRI or CT scans. The diagnosis of a functional cause of chronic anovulation in the absence of estrogen production is one of exclusion. A history of a stressful event is

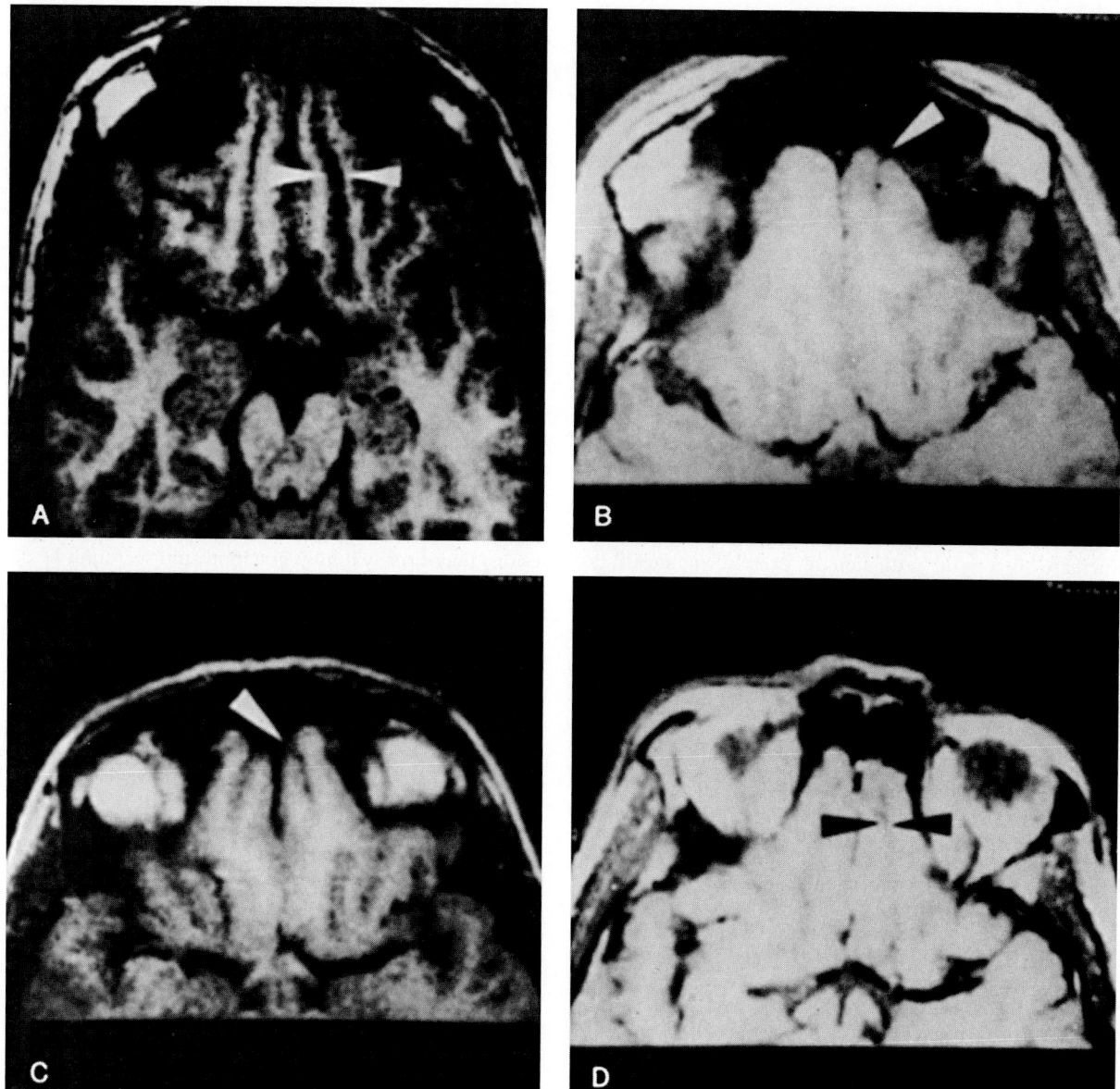

Figure 15–48. Transverse MRI images through the rhinencephalon comparing the normal anatomy of olfactory sulci *(A)* with the findings in three patients with Kallmann's syndrome *(B through D)*. Rudimentary sulci *(B and C)* and hypoplastic sulci *(D)* are denoted by arrowheads. (Adapted from Klingmuller D, Dewes W, Krahe T, et al. Magnetic resonance imaging of the brain in patient with anosmia and hypothalamic hypogonadism [Kallmann's syndrome]. J Clin Endocrinol Metab 1987; 65:581–584. Copyright © 1987, by The Endocrine Society.)

frequently obtained. For example, chronic anovulation can begin suddenly in a woman who leaves home for the first time, enters college, or experiences the death of a loved one. Gonadotropin and estrogen levels are low or in the low-normal range compared with those of ovulatory women in the early follicular phase. In more severe cases the frequency and amplitude of LH pulses are markedly reduced (Fig. 15–49).[510] Alterations in LHRH secretion and subsequent decreased gonadotropin levels may be caused by increased levels of dopamine or β-endorphin. Administration of naloxone, an opioid antagonist, enhances LH levels in women with functional hypogonadotropic amenorrhea.[511]

In Western societies a common cause of chronic anovulation is weight loss associated with dieting.[512, 513] The extreme form is anorexia nervosa (see Chapter 22). Anorexia nervosa is characterized by the development in a young woman of weight loss with associated amenorrhea, disoriented attitudes

toward eating and weight gain, self-induced vomiting, extreme emaciation, and distorted body image.[513–515] Amenorrhea in anorexia nervosa can precede, follow, or appear coincidentally with weight loss. Women with anorexia also exhibit disturbances of thyroid hormone and vasopressin secretion.[515] Rigorous exercise such as marathon running, ballet, or swimming can also result in weight loss and lead to chronic anovulation or amenorrhea, particularly in women with a history of menstrual irregularity.[516–520] The cause of amenorrhea associated with exercise is complex. Because it may develop in women who exercise strenuously without weight loss or change in body composition,[521, 522] other factors, including the stress of competition, fuel expenditure, and neuroendocrine disturbances, may contribute to amenorrhea.[509]

Women who have amenorrhea associated with stress, exercise, or dieting exhibit alterations that progress from the normal cycle through luteal phase dysfunction and anovulatory

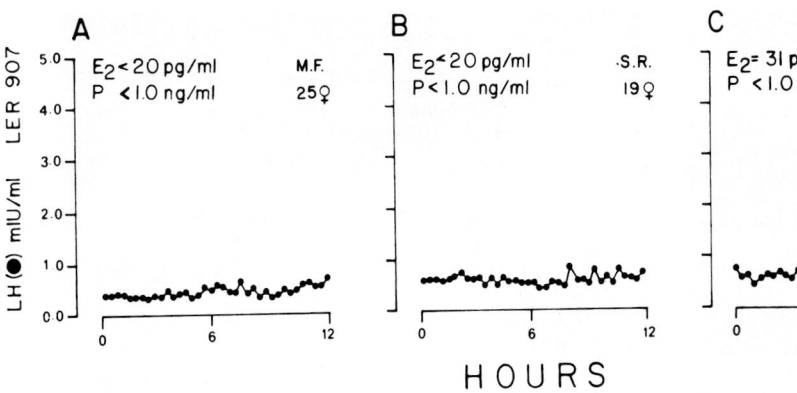

Figure 15–49. Demonstration of apulsatile secretion of LH levels in three women with hypothalamic amenorrhea. Note the complete absence of detectable LH pulses coupled with low levels of estradiol (E$_2$) and progesterone (P). To convert LH values to international units per liter, multiply by 1.0. To convert E$_2$ values to picomoles per liter, multiply by 3.671. To convert P values to nanomoles per liter, multiply by 3.180. (From Crowley WF Jr, Filicori M, Spratt DI, et al. The physiology of gonadotropin-releasing hormone [GnRH] secretion in men and women. Recent Prog Horm Res 1985; 41:473–531, with permission.)

cycles to oligomenorrhea and, finally, amenorrhea. Withdrawal bleeding after progestagen challenge occurs in the anovulatory phase if some estrogen is produced but does not occur if estrogen deficiency becomes severe (Fig. 15–50).[215, 520, 523] After the primary cause of amenorrhea is corrected (i.e., increase in weight, reduction in exercise or stress), a progressive reversal from amenorrhea to ovulatory menstrual cycles occurs. In addition, chronic debilitating diseases such as end-stage kidney disease, malignancy, acquired immunodeficiency syndrome, or malabsorption may lead to hypogonadotropic hypogonadism by a central mechanism.

The diagnosis of CNS-hypothalamic disorders that cause chronic anovulation with estrogen absent is suggested by the history but requires some form of imaging of the brain (CT or MRI) to rule out a tumor, because the diagnosis of functional disorders is made by exclusion. CNS imaging is especially important if amenorrhea develops suddenly or is associated with neurologic signs.

Treatment of chronic anovulation resulting from CNS-hypothalamic disorders should be directed at reversal of the primary cause (i.e., reversal of stress, reduction of exercise, or correction of weight loss). Successful treatment of this disorder is of particular importance, because these women are susceptible to the development of osteoporosis.[524–529] Cyclic estrogen-progestagen replacement therapy (see discussion in the section on hormonal therapy) or oral contraceptives are indicated if amenorrhea persists or if reversal of the primary cause is not possible; such therapy prevents further bone loss and induces or maintains normal secondary sexual characteristics. If pregnancy is desired, body weight and nutritional status must be returned to normal, because the risk of a low-birth-weight infant is greater in underweight women.[530] If normal body weight and nutrition are attained but amenorrhea persists, gonadotropin or pulsatile LHRH therapy is often successful in inducing ovulatory cycles.[531, 532]

Several disorders of the pituitary can lead to the estrogen-deficient form of chronic anovulation: (1) space-occupying lesions that directly inhibit gonadotropin secretion by destruction of gonadotropin-producing cells or that indirectly inhibit gonadotropin release by blocking delivery or secretion of LHRH (metastatic cancer); (2) spontaneous necrosis of the pituitary (Sheehan's syndrome); and (3) alterations in other CNS-hypothalamic peptides that influence LHRH neurons (prolactinomas).

Pituitary tumors make up approximately 10% of all intracranial tumors. Such tumors were previously considered to be nonfunctional, but most are now known to secrete hormones.[509] Pituitary cells of all types can be transformed into adenomatous lesions, and pituitary tumors may secrete one or more hormones, including prolactin, FSH, LH, growth hormone, corticotropin, and thyrotropin (see Chapter 9).[533] Pituitary tumors usually grow slowly; when they enlarge they may impinge on the optic chiasm, leading to blurred vision and field defects.

Prolactin-secreting adenomas are the most common pituitary tumors. Prolactinomas can be divided into microadenomas (<10 mm in diameter) and macroadenomas (>10 mm). Hyperprolactinemia is often associated with low levels of gonadotropin, and women with hyperprolactinemia commonly have amenorrhea and galactorrhea. Hyperprolactinemia from inappropriate prolactin secretion may occur in a number of disorders in addition to prolactin-secreting adenomas (Table 15–11).

Because about 10% of women with amenorrhea have elevated prolactin levels, serum prolactin should be measured in all cases of amenorrhea.[509] Most women with increased levels of prolactin have normal pubertal development followed by secondary amenorrhea, but prolactinomas have been reported in girls with primary amenorrhea and delayed pubertal development.[534] The most common clinical feature associated with elevated levels of prolactin is galactorrhea. However, some women with hyperprolactinemia do not exhibit galactorrhea, probably because of concomitant estrogen deficiency associated with the hypogonadotropic form of amenorrhea.[535] More than half of women with amenorrhea and galactorrhea have elevated prolactin levels. Occasionally such patients experience withdrawal bleeding after treatment with progestagens. In other women with mild elevation of prolactin, ovulatory cycles or luteal phase–deficient cycles may occur (see Fig. 15–50). Some women with hyperprolactinemia and ovulatory menses secrete high-molecular-weight forms of prolactin that are immunoreactive but lack bioactivity.[536]

Most prolactin-secreting adenomas grow slowly, and studies of their natural history suggest that significant tumor

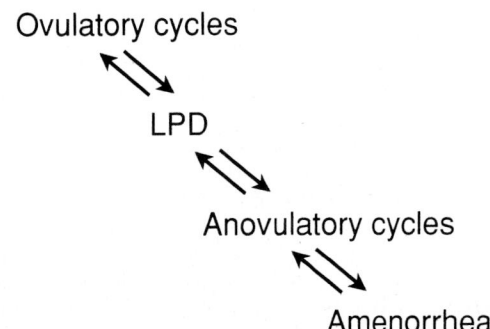

Figure 15–50. Transition from ovulatory cycles to amenorrhea that may be associated with stress, exercise, weight loss, dieting, anorexia, or hyperprolactinemia. During the development of these disorders luteal-phase defects (LPD) may occur, followed by oligoanovulatory cycles and finally amenorrhea. During the time of weight gain, the reverse may occur, and amenorrhea may progress to anovulatory or LPD cycles until normal ovulatory cycles are re-established.

TABLE 15–11. Conditions Associated with Inappropriate Prolactin Secretion

Pharmacologic Causes	Pathologic Causes
Estrogen therapy	*Hypothalamic lesions*
Anesthesia	Craniopharyngioma
DA receptor blocking agents	Glioma
Phenothiazines	Granulomas
Haloperidol	Histiocytosis disease
Metoclopramide	Sarcoid
Domperidone	Tuberculosis
Pimozide	Stalk transection
Sulpiride	Postsurgical or head injury
DA re-uptake blocker	Irradiation damage of the
Nomifensine	hypothalamus
CNS-DA depleting agents	Pseudocyesis (functional)
Reserpine	*Pituitary tumors*
α-Methyldopa	Cushing disease
Monoamine oxidase inhibitor	Acromegaly
Inhibition of DA turnover	Prolactinoma
Opiates	Mixed GH, or ACTH- and PRL-
Stimulation of serotoninergic system	secreting adenomas
Amphetamines	"Nonfunctional" adenomas
Hallucinogens	*Reflex causes*
Histamine H₂-receptor antagonists	Chest wall injury and herpes zoster
Cimetidine	neuritis
	Upper abdominal surgery
	Hypothyroidism
	Renal failure
	Ectopic production
	Bronchogenic carcinoma
	Hypernephroma

From Yen SSC. Prolactin in human reproduction. In: Yen SSC, Jaffe RB, eds. Reproductive Endocrinology. 3rd ed. Philadelphia: WB Saunders, 1991: 357–388.

growth is unlikely to occur in most women; many patients show clinical and radiographic improvement, and some experience spontaneous resolution of tumor.[537–540] The increased frequency of diagnosis of prolactin-secreting tumors during the past two decades is probably a result of several factors, including increased awareness, improved radiographic detection methods, and availability of prolactin assays. Attempts to link the increased incidence of prolactinomas with the use of oral contraceptives have not been successful.[541] However, because prolactinomas occur more frequently in women and because exogenous estrogen use increases prolactin levels, estrogen may play a role in prolactinoma development.[542] The

exact incidence of prolactinomas and hyperprolactinemia is unknown, but the prevalence of microprolactinomas in autopsy series varies from 9 to 27%.[543]

If hyperprolactinemia is present, a careful history may reveal the cause (see Table 15–11). A woman with persistent hyperprolactinemia, especially if it is associated with amenorrhea, should undergo radiographic evaluation.[544] At what level of plasma prolactin elevation radiographic investigation should be initiated in the absence of amenorrhea is not clear.[545] Some physicians recommend radiographic evaluation of all women with elevated levels of prolactin (>20 to 30 μg/ L), whereas others evaluate when levels exceed a specific maximal concentration, such as 50 or 100 μg/L. Women with prolactin levels greater than 50 μg/L have a 20% frequency of harboring a prolactinoma, those with 100 μg/L have a 50% frequency, and those with levels of 100 to 300 μg/L have a high frequency of at least a small macroadenoma.[544, 545] The choice of radiographic techniques with which to evaluate pituitary tumors varies in different institutions. In general, MRI is superior to CT in clarity of definition of the soft tissues, optic chiasm, and vasculature. It also avoids exposure to radiation (Fig. 15–51).[546]

The management of prolactinomas includes surgery, radiation, and pharmacologic therapy with dopamine analogues (see Chapter 9). Initially, transsphenoidal surgery was recommended as primary therapy for prolactin-secreting microadenomas and macroadenomas. Because of the inability to achieve a complete long-term cure with a surgical approach, the high incidence of recurrence (30% for microadenomas and 90% for macroadenomas), and the chance of surgical complications, most physicians now recommend long-term pharmacologic therapy.[545, 547, 548] Results with radiation therapy are less satisfactory than those with surgical therapy, because response is slow and the incidence of panhypopituitarism is greater.[545]

Microadenomas respond to bromocriptine therapy with shrinkage of tumor, and ovulatory menses resume in most women.[549–552] Bromocriptine is also successful in reducing tumor size and causing resumption of menses in women with macroadenomas, but a complete cure may require a combination of surgery or radiation (or both) plus bromocriptine.[545] Discontinuation of bromocriptine is usually followed by rapid regrowth of prolactin-secreting adenomas and recurrence of amenorrhea and galactorrhea, so long-term therapy is often

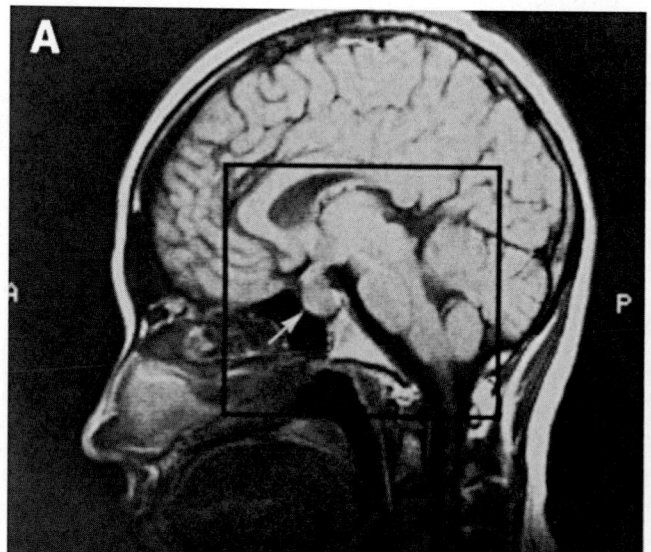
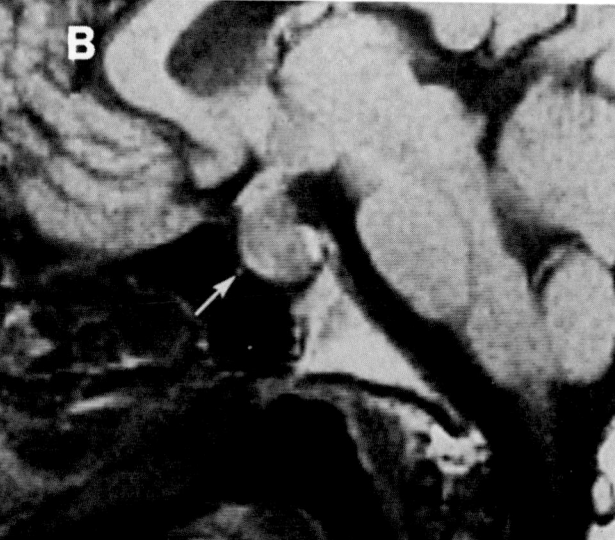

Figure 15–51. *A,* MRI scan of a woman with amenorrhea, galactorrhea, and hyperprolactinoma who had a 3-cm macroprolactinoma *(arrow). B,* Enlargement of *A* demonstrating the macroprolactinoma *(arrow).* (From Doody KM, Carr BR. Amenorrhea. Obstet Gynecol Clin North Am 1990; 17:361–387, with permission.)

required. Because the natural course of most microprolactinomas is benign, treatment may be discontinued after a few years, in some cases with resumption of spontaneous ovulatory cycles.[553]

In women desiring pregnancy, the risk of tumor expansion and development of visual disturbances during pregnancy should be considered. Only about 7% of women with microadenomas treated with bromocriptine to induce ovulatory cycles experience tumor growth during pregnancy.[554-556] Between 15 and 35% of women with macroadenomas experience worsening of symptoms during the course of pregnancy if bromocriptine has been discontinued.[557] If signs of visual impairment or tumor expansion occur during pregnancy, bromocriptine can be reinstituted without an effect on the pregnancy or the fetus.[557-559] Some investigators have suggested that bromocriptine should be used continuously in pregnancies associated with macroadenomas, but most physicians discontinue therapy after the diagnosis of pregnancy.[538]

Galactorrhea and elevated prolactin levels may occur in association with other endocrine-secreting tumors of the pituitary (e.g., acromegaly, Cushing's disease).[509, 560] Craniopharyngiomas account for 30% of pituitary tumors and consist of stratified squamous epithelium containing solid and cystic components.[561] These tumors arise from remnants of Rathke's pouch and can expand to fill the pituitary sella (see Chapter 9). The degree of hypopituitarism and resultant decreased gonadotropin secretion and the degree of decreased secretion of thyrotropin, corticotropin, growth hormone, and vasopressin depend on the size of the tumor and the extent of compression of the pituitary stalk.[562] Patients with craniopharyngiomas may present with sexual infantilism, delayed puberty, and primary amenorrhea if the tumor produces symptoms before puberty, or with secondary amenorrhea if it produces symptoms after puberty. Craniopharyngiomas often calcify, and the diagnosis may be suspected by conventional skull radiographic films. Occasionally prolactin levels are elevated. In those instances in which bromocriptine fails to shrink a suspected prolactinoma, other pituitary tumors such as craniopharyngiomas or growth hormone–secreting adenomas must

be considered, because surgical treatment may be indicated.[560-563]

Panhypopituitarism may occur spontaneously, develop after surgery or radiation of pituitary adenomas, or develop after severe postpartum hemorrhage (Sheehan's syndrome). Women with Sheehan's syndrome exhibit characteristic manifestations, including failure to lactate or resume menses, loss of genital and axillary hair, and, in severe cases, evidence of panhypopituitarism.[509]

The empty sella syndrome is an enlargement of the pituitary sella caused by a congenital defect in the diaphragma sellae, with expansion of the sella and flattening of the anterior pituitary caused by transmittal of cerebrospinal fluid pressure. This disorder may produce amenorrhea or galactorrhea with elevated prolactin levels. The condition is readily detected by CT or MRI scans.[564, 565]

Evaluation of Amenorrhea. A schema for the evaluation of women with amenorrhea is presented in Figure 15–52. In the physical examination, special attention should be given to three features: (1) degree of maturation of the breasts, pubic and axillary hair, and external genitalia; (2) current estrogen status; and (3) presence or absence of a uterus. As previously discussed, amenorrhea may coexist with disorders of sexual development, and if sexual ambiguity is present the patient should be evaluated as discussed in Chapter 29. If virilization is present, the diagnosis of a tumor of the adrenal or ovary must be considered (see discussion on evaluation of hirsutism and virilization). All reproductive-age women with amenorrhea should be assumed to be pregnant until proved otherwise. Except when pubertal development is absent (sexual infantilism), pregnancy should be excluded by urine or serum β-hCG testing even if the history and physical examination are not suggestive. After this is done, the cause of amenorrhea can frequently be diagnosed by history or physical examination. For example, Asherman's syndrome is suggested by a history of curettage in a woman who had previously menstruated; in women with primary amenorrhea, sexual infantilism, and a uterus, the differential diagnosis is between ovarian failure (most often gonadal dysgenesis) and hypogonado-

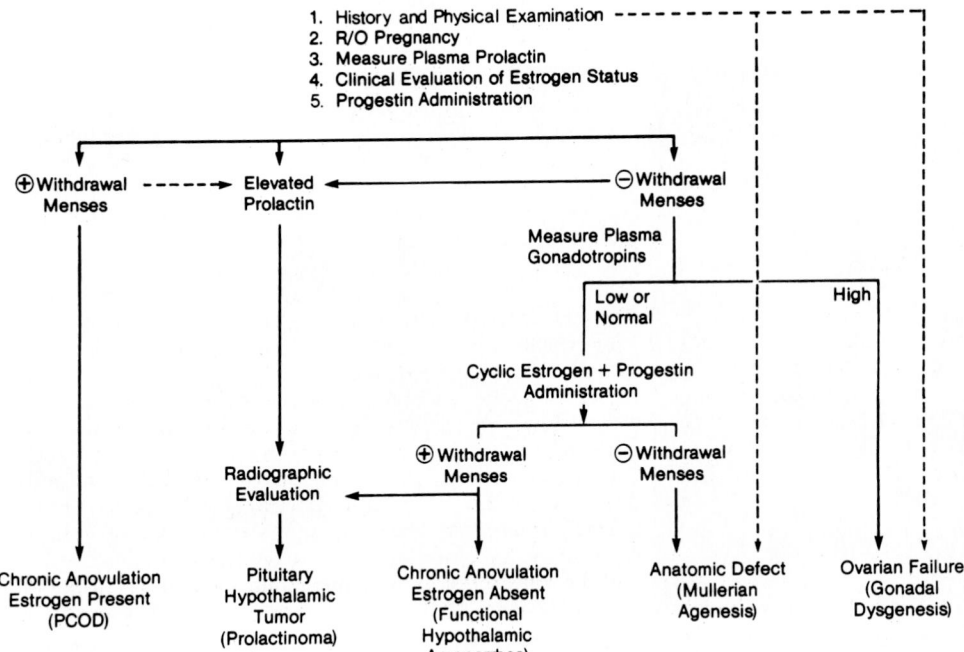

EVALUATION OF AMENORRHEA

1. History and Physical Examination
2. R/O Pregnancy
3. Measure Plasma Prolactin
4. Clinical Evaluation of Estrogen Status
5. Progestin Administration

Figure 15–52. Flow diagram for the evaluation of women with amenorrhea. The most common diagnosis for each category is shown in parentheses. The dotted lines indicate that in some instances a correct diagnosis can be reached on the basis of history and physical examination alone. (From Carr BR, Wilson JD. Disorders of the ovary and female reproductive tract. In: Braunwald E, Isselbacher KJ, Petersdorf RG, et al, eds. Harrison's Principles of Internal Medicine. 11th ed. New York: McGraw-Hill, 1987: 1818–1837. Reproduced with permission of McGraw-Hill, Inc.)

tropic hypogonadism. Gonadal dysgenesis or an anatomic defect of the outflow tract (müllerian agenesis, testicular feminization, vaginal septum, or cervical stenosis) can usually be recognized on physical examination. If a specific diagnosis is suspected, it is appropriate to proceed directly to confirmation (e.g., by obtaining a chromosomal karyotype or by measuring plasma gonadotropin levels).

After the initial examination a plasma prolactin level should be obtained. A measurement of plasma thyrotropin can be ordered if the prolactin level is elevated or if symptoms suggest the diagnosis of hypothyroidism (see Chapter 11). Estrogen status is evaluated by determining whether the vaginal mucosa is moist and rugated and whether the cervical mucus can be stretched and shown to fern after drying.

The woman's estrogen status can be evaluated further by a progestagen challenge, most often administration of 10 mg of medroxyprogesterone acetate by mouth once or twice daily for 5 d or 100 to 200 mg of progesterone in oil intramuscularly. If estrogen levels are adequate (and the outflow tract is intact), menstrual bleeding should occur within 1 wk of cessation of the progestagen treatment. Women who bleed after a progestagen challenge have a plasma estradiol level greater than 150 pmol/L (40 pg/mL), which makes a diagnosis of hypogonadotropic hypogonadism or ovarian failure unlikely.[566] The progestagen challenge test is preferable to obtaining plasma levels of estrogen for the following reasons: (1) it serves as a bioassay of current mean estrogen production, whereas estrogen levels fluctuate throughout the day and during the cycle; (2) plasma estradiol assays are expensive; and (3) the challenge test provides insight as to the drug of choice to induce ovulation in women with amenorrhea (see discussion in the section on drugs to induce ovulation).

If withdrawal bleeding occurs after a progestagen challenge, the diagnosis is chronic anovulation with estrogen present (usually PCOS). If no withdrawal bleeding occurs, the subsequent work-up depends on the initial prolactin assay. If plasma prolactin is elevated, imaging of the pituitary by MRI or CT scan is indicated. If plasma prolactin is normal in a woman with amenorrhea and failure to bleed after a progestagen challenge, plasma gonadotropin levels should be measured. Gonadotropins should also be measured if the patient experiences minimal bleeding or spotting in the withdrawal phase or if ovarian failure is suspected. If the gonadotropin levels are elevated, the diagnosis is ovarian failure. If the gonadotropin levels are in the low or normal range, the diagnosis is either hypothalamic-pituitary disorder or an anatomic defect of the outflow tract.

As discussed previously, the diagnosis of outflow tract disorders is usually established on the basis of the history and physical findings. If the physical findings are not diagnostic, it may be useful to administer cyclic estrogen plus progestagen in the form of a 1-mo package of oral contraceptives or 1.25 mg of oral conjugated estrogens daily for 4 wk plus 10 mg of medroxyprogesterone acetate for the last 10 d of treatment. If no bleeding occurs and a uterus is present, the diagnosis of Asherman's syndrome is suspected and can be confirmed by hysterosalpingography or hysteroscopy. If withdrawal bleeding occurs after use of the estrogen-progestagen combination, the diagnosis of chronic anovulation with estrogen absent (functional hypothalamic amenorrhea) is suggested. Imaging of the CNS to evaluate for lesions of the pituitary or hypothalamus may be indicated, because the diagnosis of functional hypothalamic amenorrhea is one of exclusion.

Hirsutism and Virilization

Hirsutism is defined as the presence of excessive growth of hair in locations where hair growth in women is normally minimal or absent (Table 15–12). Although it may be the

TABLE 15–12. Clinical Findings in Women with Hirsutism and Virilization

Hirsutism: An excessive growth of hair in women that occurs in specific androgen-sensitive areas of the body:
  Face
  Chest
  Areola
  Linea alba
  Lower back
  Buttock
  Inner thigh
  External genitalia

Virilization: The combination of hirsutism plus:
  Clitoral enlargement
  Deepening of voice
  Temporal hair loss
  Loss of female body contour

initial sign of a serious underlying disorder, hirsutism by itself is usually benign and is frequently associated with PCOS. In contrast, virilization is the combination of hirsutism plus other signs of masculinization, such as clitorimegaly, deepening of the voice, temporal balding, decreased breast size, and loss of female body contour (Fig. 15–53). Virilization is less common than hirsutism and is more often associated with a potentially serious disorder such as an ovarian or adrenal tumor. Hirsutism is usually associated with normal or slightly elevated levels of serum androgens, whereas virilization is associated with markedly increased androgen production by the ovary or adrenal (or both) and markedly increased plasma androgens.

The number of hairs per unit area of skin is determined by genetic factors and is the same for both sexes of a similar ethnic background. For example, women and men of Mediterranean descent tend to have more body hairs per unit area than do Asians.[567] In both women and men, hair follicles cover the body except for the lips, palms of the hands, and soles of the feet. Hair follicles are of two types: vellus and terminal.[568] In women, excess androgen production stimulates vellus hairs to develop into long, coarse, pigmented terminal hairs in most areas of the body except the scalp, where terminal hairs are converted to vellus hairs, eventually resulting in temporal balding.[569] Androgens stimulate, whereas estrogens inhibit hair growth in women.[569]

The primary mechanism leading to the development of hirsutism and virilization is increased secretion of androgens by the ovary or adrenal. The principal sources of circulating androgens in normal women are summarized in Figure 15–54. Under normal circumstances the circulating testosterone level is derived from direct secretion by the ovary and by extraglandular conversion of androstenedione secreted by the ovary and the adrenal. Little, if any, testosterone is released by the adrenal,[570] but the adrenal is the major source of DHEA and DHEAS in the circulation.[571]

In women with isolated hirsutism, 75% of circulating testosterone is from ovarian secretion. In the presence of increased levels of testosterone, TeBG levels are reduced, leading to increased free testosterone and an increased metabolic clearance rate for testosterone.[572] In women with mild hirsutism who have ovulatory menstrual cycles and normal levels of testosterone, androstenedione, and adrenal androgens (i.e., idiopathic or simple hirsutism), the excessive body hair has been explained by increased sensitivity of the pilosebaceous unit to normal plasma levels of androgen. These women have been reported to have an increased number of androgen receptors, increased 5α-reductase activity, and increased levels of the dihydrotestosterone metabolite, 5α-androstane-3αβ-diol glucuronide.[573, 574]

A classification for hirsutism is presented in Table 15–13. A frequent cause is ovarian dysfunction, and in this category

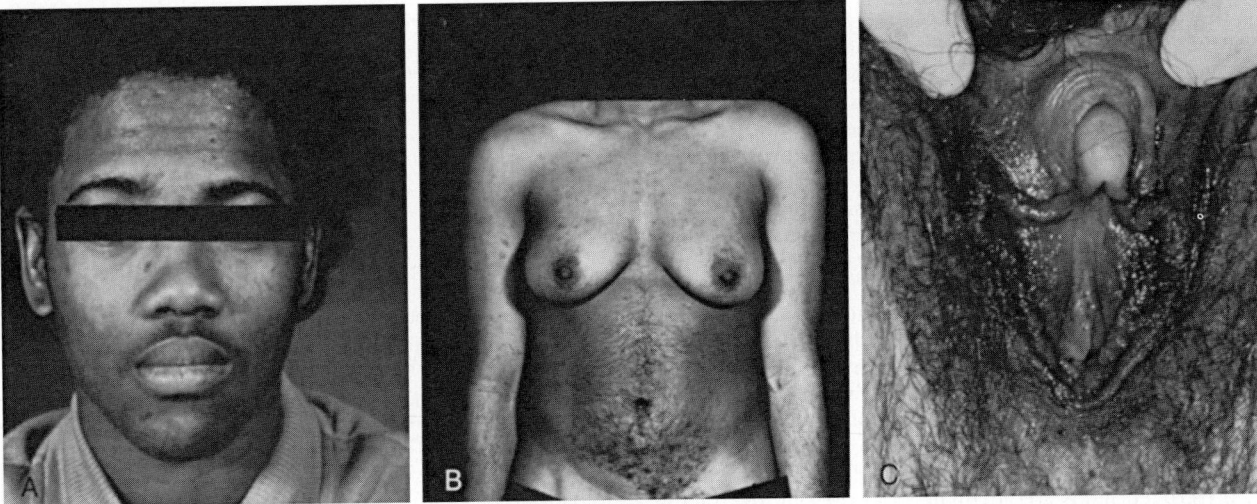

Figure 15–53. Clinical features of hirsutism and virilization in a woman with a virilizing adrenal adenoma. *A,* Photograph demonstrating facial hair and temporal balding. *B,* Photograph of the trunk and abdomen demonstrating muscle development and male escutcheon. *C,* Clitorimegaly. (Courtesy of Dr. Karen D. Bradshaw.)

the most common cause is PCOS.[575] As discussed earlier, PCOS is diagnosed on clinical grounds, and the onset of hirsutism and other symptoms associated with the syndrome usually occurs at about the time of menarche. In most cases, the rate of progression of hirsutism is constant but slow. On rare occasion signs of virilization (e.g., clitorimegaly) may develop in women with PCOS; this usually occurs as a result of particularly high rates of testosterone secretion in women with stromal hyperthecosis,[571, 576] a condition in which islands of luteinized thecal cells are present in the ovarian stroma distant from ovarian follicles. Hyperthecosis is probably not a distinct entity but rather an exaggerated manifestation of PCOS. Women with hyperthecosis are more likely to have an LH/FSH ratio less than 2 and to fail to ovulate after treatment with clomiphene citrate. They are also more likely to exhibit insulin resistance than women with PCOS alone.[576–578] The diagnosis is suspected from the history and the presence of bilateral enlarged ovaries. It may be confirmed by histologic section of the ovaries at the time of wedge resection or oophorectomy, but only if these surgical procedures are indicated for other reasons.

The association of hyperandrogenism, insulin resistance, and acanthosis nigricans (so-called HAIR-AN syndrome) constitutes a specific subset of PCOS or hyperthecosis.[570] A number of syndromes are associated with this triad of manifestations (Table 15–14 and Fig. 15–55).[579] In women with type A insulin resistance resulting from intrinsic defects in the insulin receptor, the hirsutism is severe and is usually associated with hyperthecosis. The structure of the insulin receptor in women

with type A insulin resistance and PCOS is usually normal, however.[580]

Rare androgen-secreting ovarian tumors can cause virilization (Table 15–15; see Table 15–13). The onset of hirsutism and virilization is more abrupt than in women with PCOS or hyperthecosis and can occur at any age. In most cases (>80%) a unilateral adnexal mass is palpable.[575] Ovarian tumors that cause virilization are derived from sex cord or stromal cells and include Sertoli-Leydig cell tumors (arrhenoblastomas), hilar cell tumors, lipoid cell tumors, and adrenal rest tumors.[581] Occasionally virilization occurs in association with other tumors of the ovary (Brenner tumors, cystadenomas, and cystadenocarcinomas) because the tumor stimulates androgen secretion by the surrounding ovarian stroma.

TABLE 15–13. Classification of Hirsutism and Virilization

Ovarian
 PCOS
 Hyperthecosis
 Neoplasms
  Sex cord tumors
  Germ cell tumors
  Hilar cell tumors
  Adrenal rest tumors
  Mixed germ cell and gonadal tumors
  Tumors with functioning stroma
 Pregnancy associated
  Luteoma
  Hyperreactio luteinalis
Adrenal
 Congenital adrenal hyperplasia/adult-onset adrenal hyperplasia
  21-Hydroxylase deficiency
  11β-Hydroxylase deficiency
  3β-Hydroxysteroid dehydrogenase deficiency
 Neoplasms
  Adenomas
  Carcinomas
Cushing's syndrome
Drugs
 Phenytoin
 Diazoxide
 Anabolic steroids
 Progestagens (19-norsteroid derivatives)
 Danazol
Idiopathic
Miscellaneous
 Hyperprolactinemia
 Acromegaly
 Menopause

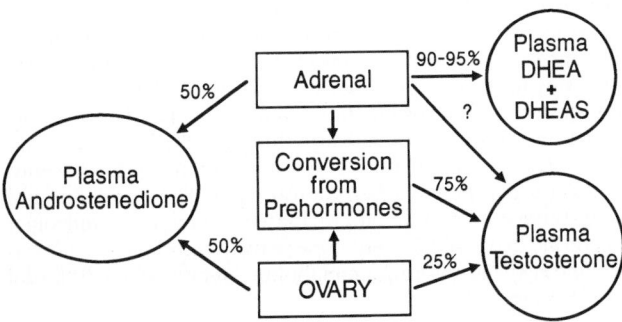

Figure 15–54. Sources of circulating androgens in normal women.

Table 15–14. Syndromes of Hyperandrogenism and Hyperinsulinemia

Condition	Prevalence	Age of Onset	Clinical Signs/ Symptoms	Hyperandrogenism	Insulin Levels	Etiology
Leprechaunism	Rare	Congenital	Growth retardation, elfin facies	Gonadal enlargement	+ + + +	Mutations in insulin receptor gene/ other genetic defects in insulin action
Rabson-Mendenhall syndrome	Rare	Congenital	Dental precocity, thickened nails	Gonadal enlargement	+ + + +	
Lipoatrophy	Rare	Congenital; adolescence, adulthood	Loss of subcutaneous fat, hepatomegaly	+ + +	+ + + +	
Type A syndrome	Rare	Adolescence	True virilization	+ + + +	+ + + +	
Type B syndrome	Rare	Adulthood	Autoimmune disease	+ + +	+ + + +	Antibodies to insulin receptor
PCOS	Common	Adolescence	Obese and lean PCOS; anovulation; IGT, 3rd–4th decades	+ +	NL-+ +	? Primary defect in insulin receptor signaling, ? secondary glucose transporter defect, other (unknown)

From Dunaif A. Hyperinsulinemia-hyperandrogenism. In: Adashi E, Rock JA, et al, eds. Reproductive Endocrinology, Surgery and Technology. Philadelphia: Lippincott-Raven, 1996: 1522–1573.
IGT, impaired glucose tolerance; NL, normal.

Ovarian tumors may secrete a variety of hormones in addition to androgens, including estrogens, hCG, serotonin, and thyroxine (see Table 15–15). All choriocarcinomas, some dysgerminomas, and a few malignant ovarian teratomas secrete hCG.[582, 583] Primary ovarian carcinoids may produce serotonin in quantities sufficient to increase secretion of 5-hydroxyindoleacetic acid and produce the carcinoid syndrome (see Chapter 37).[584–586] Teratomas that contain thyroid tissue (struma ovarii) may secrete thyroxine, although rarely in sufficient quantities to cause hyperthyroidism (see Chapter 11).[587, 588]

Adrenal virilization is most commonly caused by congenital adrenal hyperplasia (21-hydroxylase deficiency). In women the diagnosis is usually made at birth because of sexual ambiguity (see Chapter 29).[589] Less severe forms are caused by mutations that impair the function of the gene less severely and are variously termed *late-onset, acquired, partial, attenuated, nonclassic,* or *cryptic 21-hydroxylase deficiency.*[589, 590] In women with late-onset 21-hydroxylase deficiency, hirsutism begins at about the expected time of puberty. The frequency of this disorder in hirsute women has been estimated to be between 1 and 20% and probably is less than 5%.[590, 591] Hirsutism, amenorrhea, and polycystic ovaries may develop in women with Cushing's syndrome caused by excessive production of corticotropin by a pituitary tumor, adrenal adenoma, or adrenal carcinoma or by ectopic secretion of corticotropin.[571] Women with acromegaly or hyperprolactinemia may also have mild hirsutism.

Virilizing adrenal tumors are a rare cause of androgen excess in women. The symptoms and clinical signs have an abrupt onset and progress rapidly, features that aid in making the diagnosis. The diagnosis is also suspected if the serum level of DHEAS is higher than 22 μmol/L (8000 ng/mL) or if urinary 17-ketosteroid levels are higher than 100 μmol/d (30 mg/d). Adrenal tumors can readily be detected by CT or MRI scan (Fig. 15–56).[571]

Iatrogenic hirsutism may result from drug therapy. One cause of hirsutism, amenorrhea, and signs of virilization is the use of androgens for the purpose of body-building or in treatment of diminished libido or menopause.[592] Other drugs that cause hirsutism include danazol, metyrapone, phenothiazines, phenytoin, diazoxide, and minoxidil.[592] Menopausal

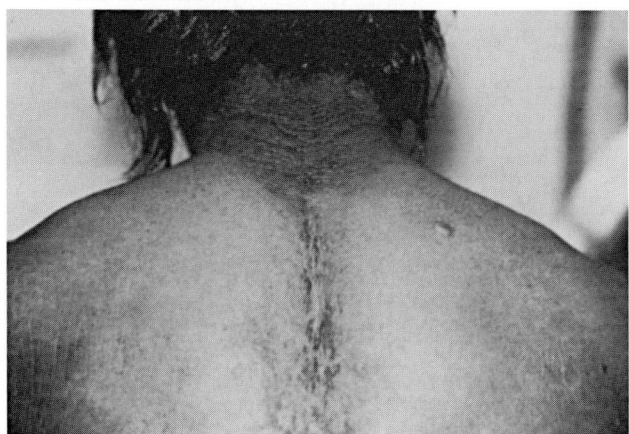

Figure 15–55. Acanthosis nigricans in a woman with insulin resistance and hyperandrogenism. Note the increased pigmentation of the neck. (Courtesy of Dr. R. Ann Word.)

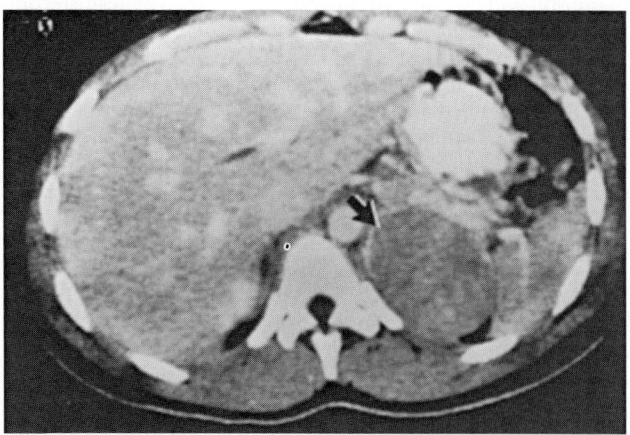

Figure 15–56. CT scan demonstrating an adrenal adenoma (*arrow*) of the woman with virilization pictured in Figure 15–53. (Courtesy of Dr. Karen D. Bradshaw.)

TABLE 15–15. Clinical Features of Hormone-Producing Ovarian Tumors

Tumor	Hormones Produced	Age in Years		Incidence of		Size in cm	Miscellaneous
		Peak	Range	Malignancy (%)	Bilaterality (%)		
Sex cord–stromal tumors							
Granulosa-theca cell tumors	Estrogen, androgens, progestagens	30–70	≤1–92	10–20	10–15	≤1–≥30	Most common functioning ovarian neoplasms
Androblastomas (Sertoli-Leydig cell tumors)	Androgens, estrogens	20–40	4–84	20	Rare	≥5–≤25	Most common virilizing tumors
Lipid cell tumors							
Hilar cell type	Androgens	45–75	4–86	Rare	Rare	0.5–15	—
Adrenal cell type	Estrogens	20–25	6–78	20	Rare	0.5–30	Often associated with diabetes
Germ cell tumors							
Dysgerminomas	Chorionic gonadotropin	10–30	4–76	100	5–10	3–50	—
Teratomas							
Carcinoids	Serotonin	50–70	36–79	Rare	Rare	≤1–15	Carcinoid syndrome may occur
Stuma ovarii	Thyroxine	30–60	21–69	Rare	Rare	≤5–20	
Mixed carcinoid and struma	Serotonin, thyroxine	40–60	21–77	Rare	None	≤1–26	May be clinically hyperthyroid (rare)
Choriocarcinomas	Chorionic gonadotropin	6–15	6–42	100	Rare	>5	—
Gonadoblastomas	Androgens, chorionic gonadotropin	10–30	6–36	50	40	≤1–≥30	Usually occur in male pseudohermaphrodites

women also often complain of increased facial hirsutism, but this is physiological because of the change in the ratio of estrogens and androgens.

The diagnosis and evaluation of hirsutism require a careful history and physical examination as well as laboratory testing. Familial occurrence, age at onset, severity, and rate of progression are important. Hirsutism that begins at the expected time of puberty may be caused by PCOS or hyperthecosis, simple hirsutism, or late-onset adrenal hyperplasia. In contrast, sudden onset of hirsutism suggests an iatrogenic cause or, if associated with virilization, a tumor of the ovary or adrenal. The presence of acanthosis nigricans suggests the diagnosis of the HAIR-AN syndrome in association with PCOS or hyperthecosis. Clitorimegaly, as defined by a clitoral index (equal to the product of the sagittal and transverse diameters of the glans) greater than 35 mm^2, male-pattern baldness, and other virilizing signs suggest an ovarian or adrenal tumor.[593]

Useful laboratory tests in the diagnosis and management of androgen excess include measurement of serum testosterone and DHEAS levels. Serum testosterone is usually markedly elevated in ovarian causes of virilization, and DHEAS, which is derived primarily from the adrenal, is elevated in cases of virilization of adrenal origin. If mild to moderate hirsutism and normal or near-normal levels of testosterone and DHEAS are present, more extensive testing is not usually indicated if the history suggests PCOS. If there is a family history of adrenal hyperplasia or if the symptoms of hirsutism are more severe, basal 17-OHP should be measured. Levels greater than 9 nmol/L (3 μg/L) suggest late-onset adrenal hyperplasia.[594] In some instances corticotropin stimulation should be performed; the change in the level of 17-OHP before and after injection of corticotropin is measured.[571, 589, 595] A useful laboratory approach to the evaluation of androgen excess is presented in Figure 15–57.

The treatment of hirsutism is not ideal, in that cures are rarely possible. The therapeutic approach is directed first at decreasing the rate of androgen secretion or inhibiting androgen action in the pilosebaceous unit itself. Oral contraceptives are commonly used to treat ovarian causes of hirsutism. Other drugs that may be useful include LHRH analogues, antiandrogens (e.g., spironolactone), and cyproterone acetate. Glucocorticoids are indicated if an adrenal enzyme defect such as

21-hydroxylase deficiency is present. (For a detailed discussion see the section on drugs to treat hirsutism.)

After androgen secretion or androgen action is reduced, additional physical methods to remove hair may be instituted. These include temporary methods, such as shaving, depilatories, waxing, or tweezing, and permanent methods of hair removal (electrolysis). Hormonal control requires 6 mo to 1 y to produce even partial clinical improvement in most cases.

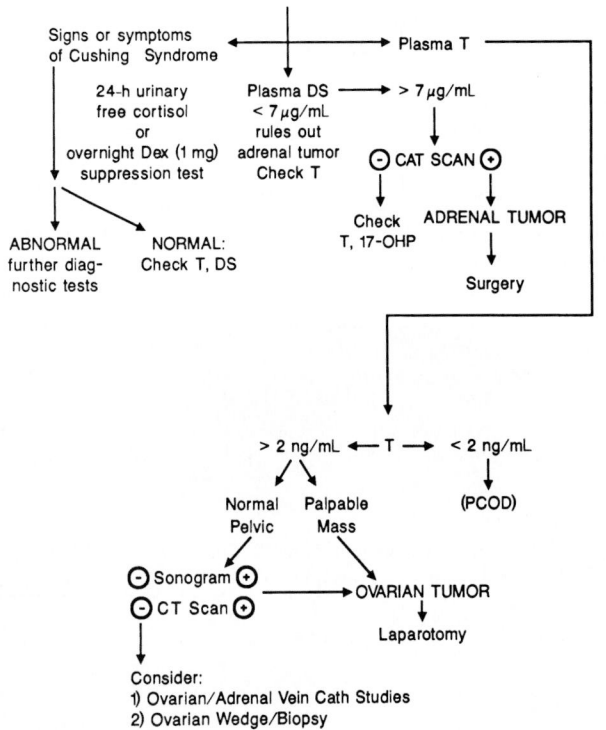

Figure 15–57. Laboratory tests and interpretations used in the evaluation of hirsutism and virilization. T, testosterone; 17-OHP, 17-hydroxyprogesterone; PCOD, polycystic ovary disease; Dex, dexamethasone; DS, dehydroepiandrosterone sulfate.

Surgical removal of the ovaries may be indicated in women with hyperthecosis in whom childbearing is no longer desired and in whom severe hirsutism is unresponsive to standard therapy.

Infertility

Infertility, the failure to conceive after 1 y of unprotected intercourse, affects approximately 10 to 15% of couples and is one of the common complaints for which women seek gynecologic care.[596] Male factors, which include decreased production and motility of spermatozoa, increased production of abnormal spermatozoa, ductal obstruction, abnormal or absent ejaculatory processes, and immunologic factors, account for 40% of infertility problems (see Chapter 16). In women, ovulatory disorders account for 30%, pelvic factors (including tubal disease, uterine or cervical disease, and endometriosis) account for 50%, and immunologic factors are implicated in 5% of infertility evaluations.[597] In 10 to 15% of women no cause is found, and in about 20 to 30% of couples both male and female factors account for the infertility. The incidence of infertility increases with age, particularly in women (Table 15–16).[598]

The initial step in evaluation of the infertile couple is to determine whether the man or the woman is the infertile partner, ordinarily by obtaining a semen analysis in the man and documentation of presumed ovulation in the woman. A woman who has a history of regular, spontaneous, and cyclic menses is considered to be ovulatory. The presumptive diagnosis of ovulation is most easily and economically obtained by daily measurement of basal body temperatures throughout the month. A biphasic increase of 0.22°C (0.4°F) during a luteal phase of at least 11 d is presumptive evidence of ovulation and a normal luteal phase. Occasionally, accurate basal body temperature records are not obtained, and other methods to evaluate ovulation are required. These methods include measurement of serum progesterone levels during the luteal phase, documentation of a secretory endometrium by biopsy, serial ultrasonographic studies to document follicular growth and subsequent rupture of a dominant follicle, and documentation of the LH surge by home urinary dipstick assay.[597] Measurement of FSH levels on day 3 of the menstrual cycle may be useful in predicting ovarian reserve in women 30 to 35 years of age or older; a value greater than 25 IU/L is associated with poor chances of conception in cycles in which in vitro fertilization with embryo transfer (IVF-ET) is used.[599]

If the infertility is associated with amenorrhea, then the work-up is the same as that described in Figure 15–52. If infertility is the result of anovulation caused by PCOS, ovulation can be induced, most commonly by administration of clomiphene citrate. If ovulation is not induced with clomiphene citrate alone, combined treatment with clomiphene citrate and glucocorticoids (if serum androgen levels are elevated) or bromocriptine (if prolactin levels are slightly elevated) may be successful.[600] Other agents to induce ovulation

include hMG, urofollitropin, or pulsatile LHRH with or without concomitant LHRH analogues.[461, 467, 473, 496–498] Women with chronic anovulation with estrogen absent as a result of hypothalamic causes can be treated with hMG or pulsatile LHRH.[498, 531, 532] Bromocriptine is the treatment of choice to induce ovulation in women with amenorrhea and hyperprolactinemia[545]; on occasion, surgical removal or radiation therapy may be required for treatment of prolactinomas, as described previously.

Infertility may also be caused by more subtle defects in folliculogenesis, including luteinized unruptured follicle syndrome, in which a mature follicle fails to rupture and the ovum is entrapped but the granulosa cells undergo luteinization.[601] This abnormality is usually diagnosed by serial ultrasonography. A spontaneous luteinized unruptured follicle may occur in as many as 10% of ovulations in normal fertile women.[216] The incidence appears to be similar in fertile and infertile women, and at present this defect is not considered by all to be a syndrome or a cause of infertility, because most women do not exhibit repetitive luteinized unruptured follicle cycles.[601] Rupture of a follicle without release of an oocyte may also occur.

Ovulation with inadequate luteinization and reduced progesterone secretion during the luteal phase has been termed *luteal-phase dysfunction*.[215] Luteal-phase dysfunction is manifested by a short luteal phase, in which the interval between the LH peak and subsequent onset of the menses is less than 10 d, or an inadequate luteal phase, in which the luteal phase is of normal length but is associated with reduced progesterone secretion.[602, 603] These types of luteal dysfunction are believed to cause infertility in about 5% of infertile women. Infertility in this disorder is caused by failure of implantation of fertilized ova as a result of an incompletely developed endometrium. Luteal-phase dysfunction is believed to result from disorders of gonadotropin secretion that cause poor follicular development and reduced granulosa cell growth. This leads to reduced numbers of granulosa-lutein cells, low progesterone secretion, and reduced endometrial maturation during the luteal phase.[215, 222, 223] Luteal-phase dysfunction may occur sporadically in normally ovulating, fertile women, but it is more common in women with hyperprolactinemia and in women who have experienced excessive exercise or weight loss and are at the extremes of reproductive life.

The diagnosis of the short luteal phase can be made by the basal body temperature chart, whereas the inadequate luteal phase is diagnosed by endometrial biopsy or measurement of serum progesterone. Although the interpretation of a single midluteal-phase serum progesterone determination is fraught with difficulty, an inadequate luteal phase is rare in cycles in which the value is greater than 50 nmol/L (15 μg/L).[222] Endometrial biopsy samples obtained from the uterine fundus in the late luteal phase should show results at least 2 d out of phase from those expected from the cycle length (as determined by the onset of the subsequent cycle or, more accurately, by the onset of the LH surge in at least two cycles).[253, 602]

Treatment of luteal-phase dysfunction varies depending on the cause and may include reduction of serum prolactin by bromocriptine, decrease in exercise, or weight gain regimens. Otherwise, follicular development may be stimulated with clomiphene citrate, gonadotropins, or progesterone replacement, usually by administration of 25 mg of progesterone by vaginal suppository twice daily.[215, 602]

The primary diagnostic test to evaluate tubal patency and the uterine cavity is the hysterosalpingogram.[336, 604] Further evaluation of tubal and ovarian disease can be obtained by the demonstration at diagnostic laparoscopy of dye spillage from the fimbria after transcervical injection.[342] Adhesions, filling defects, or abnormal shape of the uterus can be further evalu-

TABLE 15–16. Percentage of Couples Conceiving in 12 Mo of Unprotected Intercourse Related to the Age of the Woman

Woman's Age (y)	% Conceiving in 12 Mo
20–24	86
25–29	78
30–34	63
35–39	52

Adapted from Hendershot GE, Mosher WD, Pratt WF. Infertility and age: an unresolved issue. Family Planning Perspectives. Volume 14: Number 5 (September/October 1982), p. 288. © The Alan Guttmacher Institute.

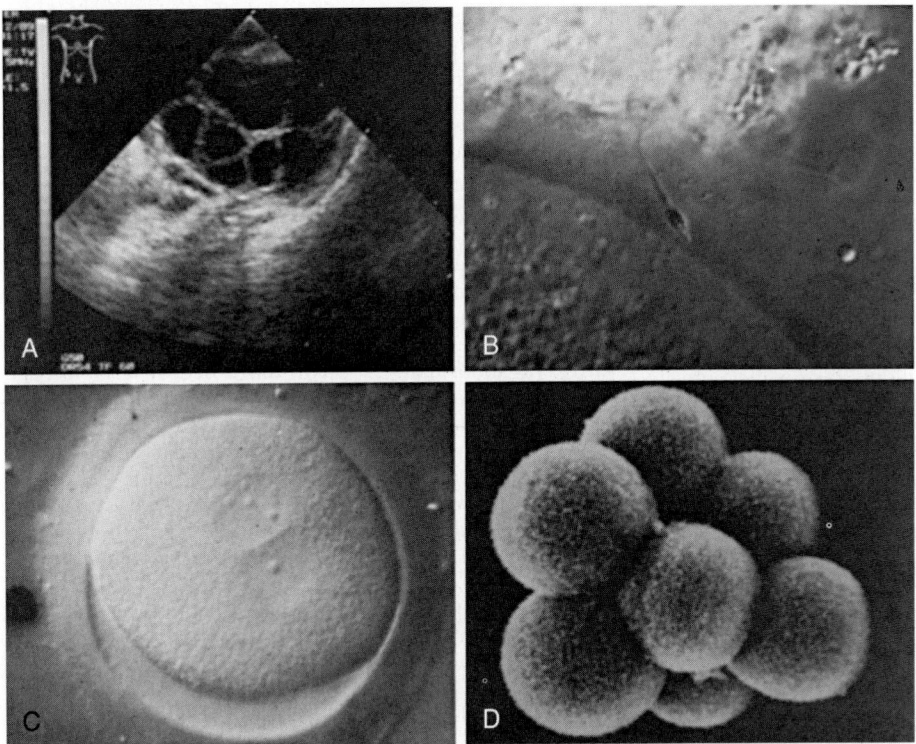

Figure 15–58. In vitro fertilization of a human oocyte. *A,* Ultrasonographic study of a gonadotropin-stimulated ovary demonstrating seven follicles. *B,* After aspiration of the follicles, ova are mixed with sperm; this figure demonstrates the attachment of sperm to the zona pellucida. *C,* The male and female pronuclei are present. *D,* A fertilized embryo ready for transfer to the uterus. (Courtesy of Dr. Karen D. Bradshaw and Dr. William Byrd.)

ated and treated by operative hysteroscopy.[341] Treatment of occluded fallopian tubes or tubal ovarian adhesions by microsurgical techniques has resulted in improved pregnancy rates compared with standard macrosurgical approaches.[605, 606] If possible, adhesive disease and tubal occlusion are treated by operative laparoscopy, also called pelviscopic surgery, which requires multiple puncture sites and use of a variety of surgical instruments, cautery, or laser.[607–610]

Endometriosis is defined by the presence and proliferation of endometrial tissue (glands and stroma) outside the endometrial cavity. The clinical manifestations are variable, but the diagnosis is often made at the time of diagnostic laparoscopy during an evaluation for infertility. Although endometriosis is not always associated with infertility, the fertility rate of women with moderate to severe endometriosis is reduced.[611, 612] Treatment of endometriosis associated with infertility includes operative laparoscopy with resection or ablation of endometriotic implants by cautery or laser; laparotomy with resection for more advanced disease; and temporary gonadal suppression by danazol (400 to 800 mg orally in divided doses), progestagens (medroxyprogesterone acetate, 10 to 20 mg/d by mouth), continuous oral contraceptive tablets (no placebo or pill-free intervals), or LHRH agonists (leuprolide acetate, 3.75 mg given intramuscularly; goserelin, 3.6 mg subcutaneous depot implant once a month for a period usually up to 6 mo; or nafarelin acetate, 200 μg nasally twice a day).[612]

Infertility may be caused by congenital anatomic defects or postsurgical scarring of the cervix. An additional problem is insufficient cervical mucus. Cervical mucus should be evaluated after coitus. The test is preferably performed at or near the time of ovulation (as determined by a rise in urinary LH), when the cervical mucus is thin. The aim is to evaluate penetration and survival of the sperm in the female reproductive tract. Standards of abnormality are not well defined, but a reduced number of motile sperm has been associated with a lower fertility rate in some but not all studies.[613, 614] If a cervical factor is suspected, the problem can be treated by intrauterine insemination using the husband's sperm.[615, 616]

The role of antibodies in relation to sperm in the female genital tract is controversial. The presence of antisperm antibodies attached to sperm, as detected by immunobead testing, is associated with infertility in men. Treatment of sperm antibodies with glucocorticoids or other therapy is usually unsuccessful.[617, 618]

If standard treatment modalities for infertility caused by tubal obstructive disease, cervical factors, endometriosis, male factors, or unexplained infertility are unsuccessful, various assisted reproductive technologies including IVF-ET have been successful.[619] In IVF-ET, multiple follicles are stimulated by gonadotropin treatment and are subsequently aspirated under guidance by transvaginal ultrasonography (Fig. 15–58). After fertilization and cleavage in vitro, embryos are transferred to the uterine cavity by means of an intrauterine catheter. Although pregnancy rates vary, successful pregnancy has been reported to be as high as 40% per transfer. Term pregnancy at most centers averages 15%.[620]

In women with patent fallopian tubes and infertility caused by male factors or unexplained reasons, gamete intrafallopian transfer (GIFT) or intrauterine insemination with washed sperm after stimulation with gonadotropins has resulted in pregnancy rates of 20% per cycle.[620, 621] Other technologies include zygote intrafallopian transfer (ZIFT) and pronuclear stage tubal transfer (PROST). The specific advantages of these procedures and their pregnancy rates compared with those of IVF-ET and GIFT are not known.[622, 623] Cryopreservation of embryos is now integrated into many IVF-ET programs, because often more than four to five eggs can be retrieved and fertilized. Because of the risk of multiple pregnancy no more than four to five embryos should be transferred to the uterus in one cycle. Frozen embryos may be transferred in subsequent cycles.[624] Oocyte donation using fresh or thawed embryos has been successful even in women who have ovarian failure as a result of gonadal dysgenesis or premature menopause, providing they are cycled with estrogen and progesterone before transfer.[234] In couples with repeated failure of fertilization with standard IVF-ET techniques or male factor infertility, the use of intracytoplasmic sperm injection (ICSI) has resulted in pregnancy rates of greater than 30% per cycle.[625]

HORMONAL THERAPY

Gonadal Steroids

Progestagens

The primary use of progestagens is in conjunction with estrogen in the form of oral contraceptives (see Chapter 18). In addition, progestagens plus estrogens are used to promote the full maturation of the endometrium in postmenopausal and hypogonadal premenopausal women. In certain instances progestagen therapy is appropriate by itself. Indications include (1) induction of withdrawal bleeding in the diagnosis of amenorrhea, (2) fertility control (progestagen-only birth control pill), (3) inhibition of gonadotropin secretion in girls with precocious puberty or in the treatment of endometriosis, (4) treatment and prophylaxis of DUB and endometrial hyperplasia (PCOS), (5) treatment of infertility caused by luteal-phase dysfunction, and (6) palliative therapy for endometrial carcinoma.

Therapeutically useful progestagens include progesterone and synthetic progestagens. The routes of administration and doses of commonly used preparations are presented in Table 15–17. The potency of progestagens is determined from their ability to alter an estrogen-primed endometrium in animals or to induce withdrawal bleeding in women (see Chapter 18).[626] Progesterone is poorly absorbed by mouth but is well absorbed when given as a vaginal or rectal suppository (Fig. 15–59).[215] A micronized form of progesterone is absorbed orally.[627] Progesterone in oil given by injection results in higher peak plasma concentrations than those achieved by vaginal or rectal administration (see Fig. 15–59).[626]

TABLE 15–17. Routes of Administration and Dosages of Commonly Used Progestagens

Progestagen	Route	Dosage per Day* (D) or Week (W)
Progesterone		
Progesterone suppositories	Vaginal	25–200 mg (D)
	Rectal	25–200 mg (D)
Progesterone in oil	Intramuscular	50–200 mg (D)
Micronized	Oral	100–300 mg (D)
17α-Hydroxy derivatives		
Medroxyprogesterone acetate	Oral	2.5–10 mg (D)
	Intramuscular	250–1000 mg (D,W)
Megestrol acetate	Oral	20–320 mg (D)
17α-Hydroxyprogesterone caproate	Intramuscular	125–250 mg (W)
19-Nortestosterone derivatives		
Ethynodiol diacetate	Oral	1 mg (D)
Norethindrone	Oral	0.35–10 mg (D)
Norethindrone acetate	Oral	1.0–10 mg (D)
Norethynodrel	Oral	2.5–5 mg (D)
Norgesterel	Oral	0.3–0.5 mg (D)
Levonorgesterel	Oral	0.075–0.5 mg (D)
Halogenated progesterone		
Cyproterone acetate	Oral	10–50 mg (D)
Retroprogesterone		
Dydrogesterone	Oral	5–20 mg (D)

*See Physicians' Desk Reference (Oradell, NJ: Medical Economics Company, 1991) for specific dose per indication.

The dosage of progestagens depends on the indication. For example, medroxyprogesterone acetate is given in a dose of 2.5 to 10 mg/d to menopausal women, 5 to 10 mg/d for a progestagen challenge, or 100 to 1000 mg/d for treatment of endometrial hyperplasia or carcinoma (see Table 15–17). Synthetic progestagens can be administered orally, intramuscularly, or transdermally.

The side effects of progestational therapy include amenorrhea, irregular bleeding or spotting, malaise, mild weight gain and edema, depression, hirsutism, acne, and adverse

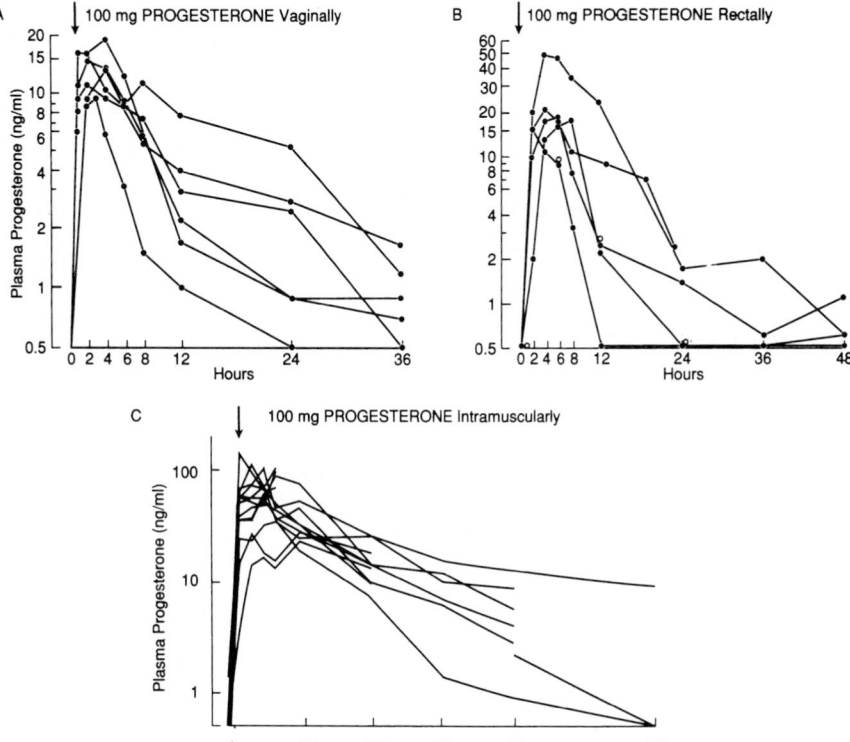

Figure 15–59. Plasma levels of progesterone after administration of 100 mg progesterone by vaginal suppository (A), by rectal suppository (B), or by intramuscular injection in oil (C). Arrows denote time of institution of therapy. (Adapted from Nillius SJ, Johansson EDB. Plasma levels of progesterone after vaginal, rectal or intramuscular administration of progesterone. Am J Obstet Gynecol 1971; 110:470–477, with permission.)

effects on lipoproteins (decreased HDL cholesterol and increased LDL cholesterol levels).[626] If side effects are severe, the dose may be decreased, or a different progestagen may be prescribed (see Table 15–17). Some synthetic progestagens (e.g., nortestosterone derivatives) are not recommended during pregnancy because of the potential risk of virilization of female embryos, but there is little evidence that progesterone itself is harmful.[628]

Estrogens

The primary use of estrogens in conjunction with progestagens is for fertility control in the form of oral contraceptives (see Chapter 18). Estrogens are also indicated for treatment of gonadal failure, for induction and maintenance of secondary sexual characteristics in hypogonadotropic premenopausal women, for hormone replacement therapy in postmenopausal women, for the management of DUB, for preparation of the endometrium before donor egg and embryo transfer in hypogonadal women, and for treatment of carcinoma of the breast (see Chapter 35).

As with progestagens, therapeutically useful estrogens include naturally derived and synthetic forms (Table 15–18). Natural estrogens include estrone, estradiol, and conjugated equine estrogens. Estrogens are most often administered by mouth, but they can also be administered effectively by vaginal, intranasal, intramuscular, intravenous, and transdermal routes.[629]

When given by mouth, estrone sulfate, estradiol valerate, and micronized estradiol result in higher plasma levels of estrone than of estradiol (Fig. 15–60).[630,631] This feature results from the fact that estradiol is converted to estrone in the intestinal mucosa.[632] Further metabolism of estrogen occurs in the liver.[633] In contrast, the administration of estradiol vaginally or by transdermal or intramuscular injection results in higher levels in plasma of estradiol than estrone, because the intestinal metabolism of orally administered estrogens is bypassed.[634–636] Maximal serum estrogen levels after oral ingestion are reached in 4 to 6 h.[637] Oral intake of 0.625 mg conjugated equine estrogens, 1.25 mg estrone sulfate, or 1.0 mg of micronized estradiol results in similar peak levels of estrogens: estradiol, 110 to 150 pmol/L (30 to 40 pg/mL), and estrone, 550 to 920 pmol/L (150 to 250 pg/mL).[638] Circulating levels of estrogen after vaginal administration are about

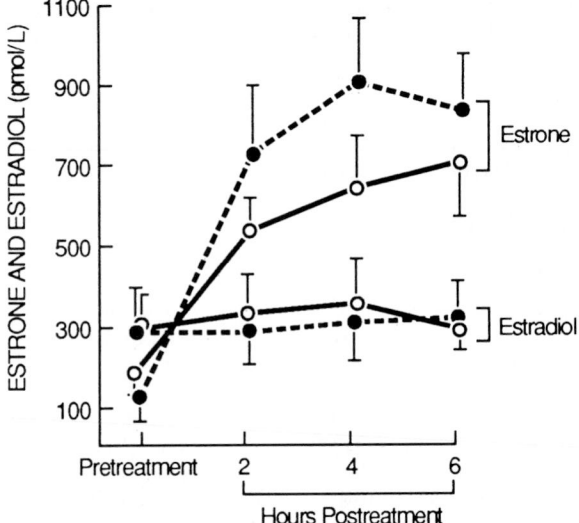

Figure 15–60. Mean serum concentrations of estradiol and estrone 2 to 6 h after oral administration of estradiol valerate (*solid circles*) or piperazine estrone sulfate (*open circles*). (Adapted from Anderson ABM, Sklovsky E, Sayers L, et al. Comparison of serum oestrogen concentrations in post-menopausal women taking oestrone sulphate and oestradiol. Br Med J 1978; 1:140–142, with permission.)

one fourth those observed with equivalent doses given by mouth.[639] Transdermal administration of estradiol with a patch applied every 3 to 4 d provides controlled and constant levels of estradiol (Fig. 15–61).[634] A transdermal patch that lasts for a week is also available.

The only estrogens used in contraceptives are synthetic (see Chapter 18). The insertion of an ethinyl group at the α position at C-17 or a methyl group at C-3 of estradiol (to create ethinyl estradiol or mestranol, respectively) allows estrogen to be absorbed efficiently and inhibits intestinal and hepatic metabolism. The most commonly used nonsteroidal estrogen is diethylstilbestrol, an inexpensive and potent estrogen. All

TABLE 15–18. Routes of Administration and Dosages of Commonly Used Estrogens

Estrogens	Route	Dosage per Day* (D) or Month (M)
Natural and equine estrogens		
Conjugated equine estrogens	Oral	0.3–2.5 mg (D)
	Intramuscular	25 mg (D)
	Intravenous	25 mg (D)
	Vaginal	2–4 g (D)
Piperazine estrone sulfate	Oral	0.625–2.5 mg (D)
	Vaginal	2–4 g (D)
Estradiol	Patch	0.05–0.1 mg†
	Vaginal	1–4 g (D)
Micronized, valerate	Oral	1–2 mg (D)
Valerate	Intramuscular	10 mg (M)
Cypionate	Intramuscular	1–5 mg (M)
Synthetic estrogens		
Ethinyl estradiol	Oral	20–50 μg (D)
Mestranol	Oral	50–100 μg (D)
Diethylstilbestrol	Oral	1–5 mg (D)
Quinestrol	Oral	0.1 mg (D)

*See Physicians' Desk Reference (Oradell, NJ: Medical Economics Company, 1991) for specific dose per indication.
†Every 3 to 4 days.

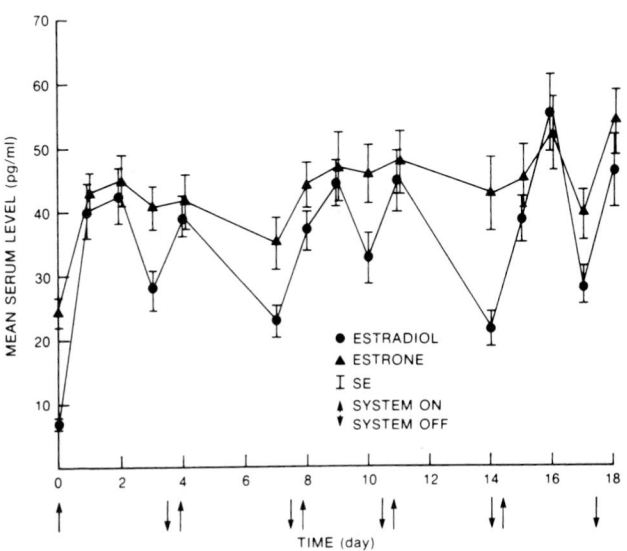

Figure 15–61. Plasma levels of estradiol and estrone in women during continuous use of an estradiol patch (0.05 mg). Arrows designate initiation and replacement of estradiol patches. To convert estrogen values to picomoles per liter, multiply by 3.671. To convert estrone values to picomoles per liter, multiply by 3.699. (From Powers MS, Schenkel L, Darley PE, et al. Pharmacokinetics and pharmacodynamics of transdermal dosage forms of 17β-estradiol: comparison with conventional oral estrogens used for hormone replacement. Am J Obstet Gynecol 1985; 152:1099–1106, with permission.)

TABLE 15–19. Relative Potency of Drugs According to Four Specific Measures of Estrogenicity

Estrogen Preparation	Serum FSH	Serum CBG-BC*	Serum SHBG-BC‡	Serum Angiotensinogen
Piperazine estrone sulfate	1.0	1.0	1.0	1.0
Conjugated estrogens	1.4	2.5	3.2	3.5
Micronized estradiol	1.3	1.9	1.0	0.7
Diethylstilbestrol	3.8	7.9	2.8	13
Ethinyl estradiol	80–200	1000	624	232

*Corticosteroid-binding globulin–binding capacity.
†Sex hormone–binding globulin–binding capacity.
From Mashchak CA, Lobo RA, Dozono-Takano R, et al. Comparison of pharmacodynamic properties of various estrogen formulations. Am J Obstet Gynecol 1982; 144:511–518.

synthetic estrogens are more potent than natural estrogens, as demonstrated in Table 15–19.

The contraindications to estrogen therapy are similar to those for oral contraceptives (see Chapter 18). Minor side effects include breast tenderness, nausea, vomiting, and mild weight gain. In these instances, the dose of estrogen may be lowered or, for gastrointestinal symptoms, alternative (vaginal or transdermal) routes may be tried.

Androgens

There are no clearly defined indications for androgen therapy in women. A few investigators have advocated use of androgens for treatment of menopausal symptoms and decreased libido, but in view of the side effects (e.g., hirsutism, male-pattern baldness) and the potential for increasing the risk of heart disease, such therapy is of limited value.

Indications for Gonadal Steroids

HYPOESTROGENEMIA. In women with decreased estrogen production, whether caused by disease of the ovaries (gonadal dysgenesis) or by hypogonadotropic hypogonadism, treatment with cyclic estrogen plus a progestagen should be instituted at the expected time of puberty for the promotion and maintenance of female sexual characteristics and to help prevent osteoporosis and premature atherosclerotic heart disease.[640] The most commonly used medications are conjugated estrogens (0.625 mg to 1.25 mg/d by mouth), ethinyl estradiol (0.02 to 0.1 mg/d by mouth), micronized estradiol (1 mg/d by mouth), and transdermal estrogen (0.05 to 0.1 mg by patch every 3 to 4 d). The addition of a progestagen (medroxyprogesterone acetate, 5 to 10 mg) is recommended during the last 10 to 14 d of estrogen treatment each month to prevent development of endometrial hyperplasia. Women treated with such regimens experience withdrawal bleeding after cessation of hormone therapy at the end of each month. In women receiving these forms of hormone replacement, abnormal uterine bleeding at other times during the cycle requires histologic evaluation of the endometrium. If the endometrial biopsy reveals proliferative changes or hyperplasia, the dose of progestagen is increased, and the endometrium is rebiopsied in a subsequent cycle.

An alternative form of therapy for treatment of hypoestrogenemia is oral contraceptives. Oral contraceptives are useful in the treatment of PCOS to control abnormal bleeding and in the treatment of hirsutism to suppress ovarian androgen secretion (Fig. 15–62).

Temporary administration of estrogens in larger quantities (up to two times the usual dosage) may be necessary in pubertal girls to induce full development of secondary sexual characteristics and in older women for the control of menopausal symptoms. Occasionally, high doses of oral contracep-

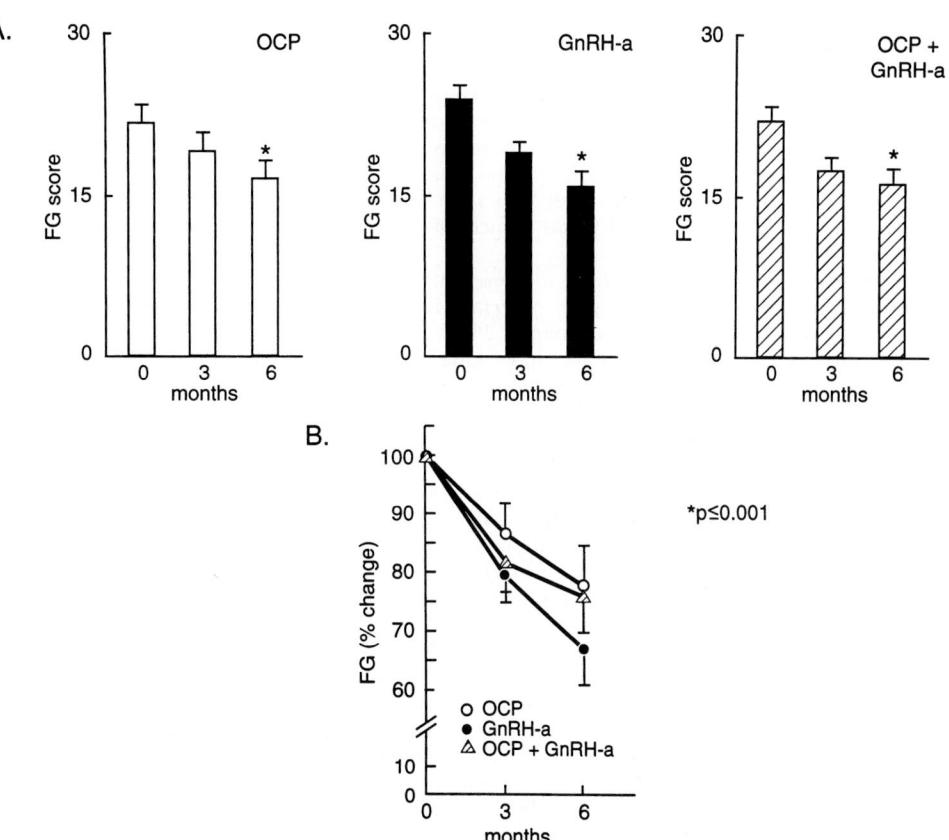

Figure 15–62. Comparison of the effects of oral contraceptives (OCP), gonadotropin-releasing hormone agonists (GnRH-a), and the combination (OCP + GnRH-a) on Ferriman-Gallway score as a function of time (A) and as percentage change from baseline (B). Results are presented as mean ± SE. *p ≤ 0.001 compared with baseline. (From Carr BR, Breslau NA, Givens C, et al. Oral contraceptives, gonadotropin-releasing hormone agonists, or use in combination for treatment of hirsutism: a Clinical Research Center study. J Clin Endocrinol Metab 1995; 80:1169–1178. Copyright © 1995, by The Endocrine Society.)

tives or parenteral estrogens may be required for brief periods in the treatment of DUB, as discussed previously. In contrast, low doses of estrogen (100 ng/kg body weight) may stimulate bone growth in women with gonadal dysgenesis.[442]

MENOPAUSE. Estrogen replacement is successful in treating the symptoms of menopause (vasomotor symptoms and vaginal atrophic) and in reducing the risk of osteoporosis and atherosclerotic heart disease. In postmenopausal women who have undergone a hysterectomy, therapy should be with estrogen alone. The major problem is how to treat the postmenopausal woman with a uterus. The addition of a progestagen, either cyclically or continuously, to concomitant estrogen therapy reduces the risk of estrogen-induced hyperplasia or carcinoma but poses additional problems (namely, withdrawal bleeding in up to 80% of women treated with cyclic therapy or irregular spotting in women treated with continuous estrogen plus progestagen). Furthermore, progestagens appear to negate, in part, the beneficial effects of estrogen in preventing atherosclerotic heart disease (i.e., decreased HDL cholesterol and increased LDL cholesterol). Approaches to these problems and indications for endometrial biopsy are discussed later.

The menopause is not associated with a simple state of estrogen deprivation, because some estrogens continue to be produced, especially in obese women. The predominant estrogen is estrone, which is formed by extraglandular conversion of adrenal androgens. Because estrone is a weak estrogen, most menopausal women are biologically hypoestrogenic. As is true for all estrogen therapy, treatment of the menopause, whether by replacement of estradiol or by replacement of other estrogens, does not duplicate the changes in plasma estrogen observed in the normal menstrual cycle. Estrogens recommended for replacement therapy in postmenopausal women are the natural estrogens, including estradiol itself, conjugated equine estrogens, and estrone sulfate; they are given orally or in estrogen-containing vaginal creams or transdermal estradiol patches.[636]

The most common indications for estrogen therapy in the menopause, and the symptoms for which benefit is most proven, are relief of vasomotor symptoms (hot flushes) and prevention or treatment of atrophy of the urogenital epithelium and skin.[304, 641] Estrogen therapy usually ameliorates these symptoms. Estrogen therapy that is designed to treat hot flushes alone should be continued for a few years only, because hot flushes tend to diminish after 2 to 5 y in untreated women.[308] Estrogen therapy of all forms is successful in treating vaginal atrophy and dryness.

Estrogen therapy is also beneficial in preventing the complications of osteoporosis (Fig. 15–63), especially in high-risk women (i.e., thin white women; see Chapter 25).[305, 311–314] This is especially true in women who have undergone premature menopause, women with gonadal dysgenesis, and those with premenopausal hypogonadotropic hypogonadism, in all of whom the incidence and complications of osteoporosis are increased. In normal menopause, estrogen therapy also prevents the loss of bone, slows the progress of osteoporosis, and reduces the risk of fractures of the hip, radius, and vertebrae.[641] To be effective for the prevention of osteoporosis, lifelong therapy is indicated. The minimal effective doses of oral estrogen that reduce the loss of bone and the incidence of fracture are 0.625 mg/d of conjugated equine estrogens, 1.25 mg/d of estrone sulfate, or 0.02 mg/d of ethinyl estradiol.[640] The effective doses of other oral estrogens, transdermal estrogen, and vaginal estrogens to prevent osteoporosis have not been clearly determined.

Estrogen replacement therapy changes the lipid profiles of older women (Table 15–20).[307, 642] The raising of HDL cholesterol and the lowering of LDL cholesterol levels may be beneficial in prevention of atherosclerotic heart disease. The

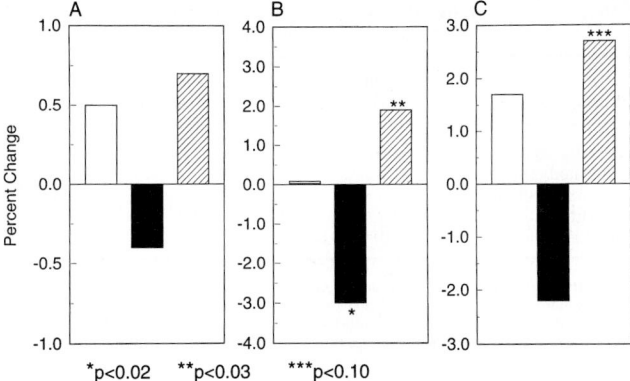

*p<0.02 **p<0.03 ***p<0.10

Figure 15–63. Changes in bone density at specific sites in women treated with oral contraceptives (OCP, *open bar*), gonadotropin-releasing hormone agonists (GnRH-a, *solid bar*), or the combination (OCP + GnRH-a, *hatched bar*). *A*, Radius. *B*, Spine. *C*, Femoral neck. Data are presented as percentage change from baseline. (From Carr BR, Breslau NA, Givens C, et al. Oral contraceptives, gonadotropin-releasing hormone agonists, or use in combination for treatment of hirsutism: a Clinical Research Center study. J Clin Endocrinol Metab 1995; 80:1169–1178. Copyright © 1995, by The Endocrine Society.)

risk of coronary heart disease appears to be less in estrogen-treated postmenopausal women as reported in both retrospective and prospective studies.[306, 307, 643] However, progestagens have effects opposite to those of estrogen on the lipid profiles (see Table 15–20), and consequently progestagens should be prescribed at the lowest doses required to prevent endometrial hyperplasia. The risk of heart disease in women treated with estrogen plus progestagen is not known.

Of the potential deleterious side effects of estrogen therapy, the possibility of endometrial adenocarcinoma is the most worrisome. The relative risk for development of endometrial carcinoma in women using estrogen alone is between 6 and 8, but the actual incidence of endometrial cancer in estrogen users is low (100 to 200 per 100,000 woman-years).[644, 645] The risk is increased with duration and dosage of estrogen and is decreased in women given estrogen plus progestagen.[626] Women treated with estrogens alone who contract endometrial carcinoma have longer life expectancies than women with endometrial carcinoma who never received estrogen therapy.[646]

Worsening of hypertension and thromboembolic disease has been reported in association with the use of estrogen-progestagen oral contraceptives, but this does not appear to occur with estrogen use in menopausal women. There is no evidence that estrogen therapy in menopausal women increases the risk of hypertension; estrogen therapy may be administered to postmenopausal women with well-controlled

TABLE 15–20. One-Year Prospective Study of the Effect of Estrogen and Cyclic Progestogen on Serum Lipids in Postmenopausal Women

Lipids	% Change from Pretreatment at 12 Mo			
	0.625 mg CEE, 5 mg MPA	0.625 mg CEE, Placebo	1.25 mg CEE, 5 mg MPA	1.25 mg CEE, Placebo
Triglycerides	↑ 39.0	↑ 34.0	↑ 42.0	↑ 19.0
Cholesterol	↓ 2.0	↑ 5.5	↓ 0.1	↓ 5.0
HDL	↑ 4.3	↑ 13.7	↑ 13.4	↑ 19.0
LDL	↓ 3.4	↓ 0.3	↓ 8.3	↓ 17.6
HDL/LDL	↑ 7.3	↑ 13.6	↑ 24.0	↑ 43.0

CEE, conjugated equine estrogens; MPA, medroxyprogesterone acetate.

Adapted from Sherwin BB, Gelfand MM. A prospective one-year study of estrogen and progestogen in postmenopausal women: effects on clinical symptoms and lipoprotein lipids. Reprinted with permission from The American College of Obstetricians and Gynecologists Obstetrics and Gynecology, vol. 73, 1989, pp. 759–766.

hypertension.[647] Low-dose estrogen therapy also does not increase the incidence of thrombophlebitis, pulmonary embolism, or stroke in menopausal women. There is a slightly increased risk for development of gallbladder disease with estrogen use during the menopause.[648]

The breast is a major target organ for estrogen, and some breast tumors are estrogen responsive (see Chapter 35). There is evidence both for and against a relation between dose and duration of estrogen therapy and development of breast cancer.[649–655] Based on all available data, however, long-term administration of estrogen in the doses commonly used in menopausal women does not appear to increase the risk of breast cancer substantially. Nevertheless, estrogen therapy should not be instituted if breast disease is present and should be discontinued if malignant breast disease develops.

Whether estrogens should be given routinely to all postmenopausal women is unsettled, but evidence is accumulating that the benefits of estrogen for the prevention of complications of osteoporosis and probably for reduction in the risk of heart disease significantly outweigh the risks. Therefore, all women without contraindications to estrogen therapy should be considered as candidates for treatment. For long-term use estrogens should be given in the minimally effective dose (0.625 mg conjugated estrogen, 1.25 mg estrone sulfate, or 1 mg of micronized estradiol). Vaginal and transdermal estrogens are probably equally effective in reducing fractures and preventing coronary heart disease, but these benefits have not been demonstrated directly. Recommended regimens of estrogen therapy include continuous daily use or cyclic replacement (estrogens for 25 d each month followed by a 5- to 6-d period of rest). For a woman with an intact uterus, the addition of a progestagen in cyclic fashion (medroxyprogesterone acetate, 5 to 10 mg for the last 10 to 14 d of estrogen therapy) or continuous low-dose progestagen (medroxyprogesterone acetate, 2.5 mg given daily) is usually prescribed to prevent endometrial hyperplasia. The continuous therapy has the potential benefit of reduced bleeding and amenorrhea but is occasionally complicated by breakthrough bleeding. Similar therapy is indicated in women with premature menopause. In women who have had a hysterectomy, progestagens are not recommended because they have adverse effects on serum lipids.

Every woman receiving estrogen alone or in combination with progestagens must be monitored indefinitely, at a minimum of yearly intervals. Endometrial sampling is required before initiation of therapy, at yearly intervals, and when any uterine bleeding occurs in women who refuse progestagens or who experience unacceptable side effects of progestagens and are treated with estrogens alone. Sampling is also required in women treated with estrogen plus a progestagen given cyclically (10 to 14 d/mo) or if bleeding occurs at times other than those expected (i.e., after cessation of progestagen). In women treated with estrogen plus continuous progestagen, a biopsy should be obtained if irregular bleeding occurs. If no unexpected bleeding occurs in women treated with estrogen plus a progestagen given cyclically or continuously, a consensus has not been reached as to the frequency of endometrial sampling needed. An option to endometrial biopsy is measurement of endometrial thickness by transvaginal ultrasound; if the endometrial width is less than 6 mm, the incidence of endometrial hyperplasia or cancer is about 5%.[656]

Drugs to Induce Ovulation

Clomiphene citrate has replaced ovarian wedge resection as the initial therapy to induce ovulation in women with chronic anovulation with estrogen present (PCOS) who experience withdrawal menstrual bleeding after a progestagen challenge.

Clomiphene citrate is an antiestrogen that acts by binding to estrogen receptors and blocking estrogen action in the hypothalamus. The drug causes a rise of plasma FSH, stimulation of follicular development, and ovulation.[600] Clomiphene citrate therapy is usually initiated in a dose of 50 mg by mouth daily for 5 d commencing on the fifth day of progestagen-induced uterine bleeding. Presumptive evidence for ovulation is obtained by documentation of a rise in basal body temperature, elevated progesterone levels in the luteal phase, secretory endometrium by biopsy, or ultrasonographic demonstration of collapse of a dominant follicle. If ovulation does not occur, the dose of clomiphene is serially increased by 50-mg increments up to 150 mg/d for 5 d. Some have suggested increasing the dose up to 250 mg or extending the length of therapy, but results are often unsuccessful.[600] Such therapy results in ovulation in 60 to 80% of anovulatory women and pregnancy rates of 30 to 50%.[473, 600] If ovulation does not occur on the 150-mg dose, a variety of clomiphene combinations or other treatments may be used (Table 15–21). Most women with PCOS ovulate on one or more of the regimens listed, but the percentage of women who conceive is variable. In women with PCOS who fail to ovulate with these methods, laparoscopic ovarian drilling (wedge resection) may improve pregnancy rates, but it is associated with an increased incidence of adhesions.[657]

If a woman successfully ovulates but does not conceive while taking clomiphene citrate, other factors for infertility should be evaluated. Side effects of clomiphene citrate include multiple pregnancy (5 to 7%), persistent ovarian cysts, vasomotor symptoms, and occasionally visual symptoms. If these symptoms occur, the dose of clomiphene citrate should be lowered or other drugs should be tried to induce ovulation.

The hormones hMG and hCG are used for women who fail to ovulate while taking clomiphene citrate and for women with hypogonadotropic hypogonadism who do not bleed after a progestagen challenge.[531, 532] Urofollitropin may be used in place of hMG in women with PCOS.[497] The usual regimen is a schedule requiring 150 to 450 IU of hMG (1 to 3 ampules) or urofollitropin per day given intramuscularly over an 8- to 12-d period to achieve adequate follicular development and growth, followed by a single injection of 5000 to 10,000 U of hCG 12 to 24 h after the last injection of hMG or urofollitropin. Ovulation is successful in 90% of hypogonadotropic women, and pregnancy rates exceed 50 to 60%.[497, 600] Daily measurement of estrogen levels and frequent evaluation of follicular development are required. Side effects of gonadotropin therapy include the ovarian hyperstimulation syndrome, in which excessive stimulation of ovarian follicles with resultant enlargement of the ovaries may progress to ascites, hypotension, and shock.[658] Gonadotropin therapy also carries a 20% risk of multiple pregnancies.[659]

Bromocriptine is a dopamine antagonist that is effective in inducing ovulation in women with elevated prolactin levels, including women with known pituitary prolactinomas. Treatment is instituted at an oral dose of 2.5 mg daily, with a

TABLE 15–21. Drugs for Inducing Ovulation in Women with PCOS Who Fail to Ovulate When Given Clomiphene Citrate Alone

Clomiphene citrate combinations
  Clomiphene citrate + hCG
  Clomiphene citrate + estrogen
  Clomiphene citrate + glucocorticoids
  Clomiphene citrate + hMG + hCG
  Bromocriptine + clomiphene citrate
hMG + hCG
Gonadorelin (pulsatile LHRH)
Urofollitropin (pure FSH) + hCG
LHRH agonist + hMG, FSH, or pulsatile LHRH + hCG

gradual increase to 2.5 mg three times daily. Each dose should be taken with a meal. Dosage should be increased until prolactin is in the normal range. Treatment is discontinued as soon as pregnancy is diagnosed. The risk of pituitary growth during pregnancy in women with microadenomas is low, but neurologic symptoms develop in up to 30% of women with macroadenomas.[557] If pituitary enlargement occurs during pregnancy in a woman with a pre-existing macroadenoma, bromocriptine therapy may be reinstituted and is often successful. Because of the high rate of development of symptoms in women with macroadenomas, some have advocated either surgical or radiation treatment before pregnancy is attempted or maintenance of bromocriptine treatment throughout pregnancy (also see Chapter 9).[554-557] There is no increase in complications of pregnancy or birth defects in children of women treated with bromocriptine either before or during pregnancy.[660] Long-term follow-up of children exposed to bromocriptine during pregnancy has revealed normal growth and development.[661, 662] Side effects of bromocriptine include nausea and hypotension. In women with severe nausea, bromocriptine may be given vaginally in doses of 2.5 mg three times per day.[663]

Gonadorelin (LHRH) has been used successfully to induce ovulation in hypogonadotropic women. Gonadorelin is infused subcutaneously or intravenously by a portable infusion pump that administers pulses in doses of 5 to 25 mg at 90- to 120-min intervals for 10 to 20 d. Gonadorelin promotes a physiologic cycle in that usually only one follicle develops and the risk of multiple pregnancy is rare.[498, 664] Side effects are minimal, but inflammation or infection may occur at the site of infusion. Rates of ovulation approximate 90%, and the rate of successful pregnancy is equivalent to that observed for gonadotropins (50 to 60%).[498]

Drugs to Treat Hirsutism

Because abnormal hair growth can be caused either by excess androgen secretion or by increased sensitivity to androgens, treatment is aimed at lowering plasma levels of androgens or inhibiting androgen action in the hair follicle.

Oral Contraceptives

The most commonly used therapy for hirsutism is the oral contraceptive pill.[499] Oral contraceptives lower androgen levels primarily by inhibiting LH release (see Chapter 18).[249, 499] They also increase the level of TeBG, resulting in a disproportionate decrease in free testosterone.[665, 666] In addition, oral contraceptives suppress adrenal androgens (DHEAS), possibly by reducing secretion of plasma corticotropin.[249, 667-672]

High-dose oral contraceptive pills containing mestranol (75 μg) plus norethynodrel (5 mg) are effective in treating hirsutism; however, because of the potential risks and side effects of this medication, this form of therapy is no longer recommended. Low-dose oral contraceptives containing norethindrone or norgestimate are effective in lowering total and free testosterone and DHEAS.[666, 670, 673] For this reason, low-dose oral contraceptives containing 35 μg or less of ethinyl estradiol are recommended for treatment of hirsutism caused by ovarian or combined ovarian and adrenal hyperandrogenism. Patients should be cautioned that therapy must be continued indefinitely and that 6 mo to 1 y may be required before any observable decrease in hair growth occurs.[500, 674] Oral contraceptives appear to be as effective as LHRH analogues in the treatment of hirsutism[675] (see Fig. 15–62). The goal of oral contraceptive treatment is to arrest further hair growth. Existing hairs do not disappear with hormone suppression alone, and physical methods such as electrolysis or shaving are required to remove existing hair. Treatment should be started at the earliest possible time.

Antiandrogens

The most widely used antiandrogens for the treatment of hirsutism are spironolactone (100 to 200 mg/d by mouth) and cyproterone acetate (50 to 100 mg/d by mouth). Both act primarily to block androgen effects at the pilosebaceous unit by competing with testosterone for the androgen receptor.[674, 676-678] Cyproterone acetate also inhibits LH levels, whereas spironolactone inhibits CYP enzymes involved in ovarian and adrenal steroidogenesis.[677] Cyproterone acetate is not available for use in the United States but is used extensively in other countries in doses of 2 to 100 mg/d combined with low-dose oral contraceptives.[677, 678] Side effects of spironolactone include cramping and diarrhea, drowsiness, rash, and gastritis. Side effects of cyproterone acetate include weight gain, fatigue, nausea, headaches, mastodynia, and the possibility of adrenal suppression. The androgen receptor antagonist flutamide in doses of 375 to 500 mg/d and the 5α-reductase inhibitor finasteride in doses of 5 mg/d are reported to be effective for treatment of hirsutism but are not approved for this purpose.[679, 680] Flutamide can cause liver damage, and all antiandrogens must be used in conjunction with a contraceptive because they can potentially cross the placenta and impair virilization of the male embryo.

Glucocorticoids

Two glucocorticoids, dexamethasone (0.25 to 0.5 mg) and prednisone (2.5 mg), have been used for treatment of hirsutism of adrenal origin; either is given as an oral dose at bedtime.[674] These doses are effective in women with adult-onset congenital adrenal hyperplasia, but higher doses may be required in women with severe hirsutism. The risks of glucocorticoid therapy include overdosage (Cushing's syndrome) and adrenal suppression.

Other Treatments

LHRH analogues are potentially useful for treatment of hirsutism.[674] Nasal, subcutaneous, and depot forms are available (see later discussion). Ketoconazole, an imidazole derivative, inhibits production of CYP–linked steroidogenic enzymes (principally 17α-hydroxylase) and lowers serum androgen levels in hirsute women.[678-680] A dose of 400 mg/d given orally is effective in women with PCOS, whereas 1000 mg/d may be required for those with hyperthecosis.[679, 680] Because of side effects that include gastrointestinal complaints, pruritus, and alterations in hepatic function, widespread use of ketoconazole for the treatment of hirsute women will probably be limited.

LHRH Analogues

Inhibition of gonadotropin release to the point of hypogonadism may be produced by LHRH agonists or antagonists. The agonist gonadorelin requires continuous infusion, whereas long-acting agonists such as leuprolide acetate or antagonists can be given once daily. These agents have been used for fertility control and for treatment of precocious puberty, endometriosis, leiomyomas, and hirsutism. They may be combined with gonadotropins to induce ovulation or for in vitro fertilization stimulation protocols.[681] Leuprolide can be administered subcutaneously daily or monthly in long-acting depot forms.[682] Goserelin is available as a subcutaneous implant, and nafarelin is available in a nasal spray that is used two or three times daily.[683] Side effects of such therapy are those expected for hypogonadism, including hot flushes, vaginal dryness and atrophy, negative calcium balance with potential risk of bone loss, and possible alteration in lipid profiles.[684] Because of these side effects, treatment is limited to a maximum of 6 mo, unless add-back therapy with estrogen is utilized to prevent bone loss (see Fig. 15–63).[675]

REFERENCES

1. Gillman J. The development of the gonads in man, with a consideration of the whole fetal endocrines and the histogenesis of ovarian tumors. Contrib Embryol Carnegie Inst Wash 1948; 32:67–80.
2. Ohno S, Klinger HP, Atkin WB. Human oogenesis. Cytogenetics 1962; 1:42–51.
3. Lyon MF. Gene action in the X-chromosome of the mouse (Mus musculus). Nature 1961; 190:372–373.
4. Alvarez-Buylla A, Merchant-Larios H. Mouse primordial germ cells use fibronectin as a substrate for migration. Exp Cell Res 1986; 165:362–368.
5. Kuwana T, Maeda-Suga H, Fujimoto T. Attraction of chick primordial germ cells by gonadal anlage in vitro. Anat Rec 1986; 215:403–406.
6. Witschi E. Migration of the germ cells of human embryos from the yolksac to the primitive gonadal fold. Contrib Embryol 1948; 32:67–80.
7. Baker TG. A quantitative and cytological study of germ cells in the human ovaries. Proc R Soc Lond B [Biol] 1963; 158:417–433.
8. Wartenberg H. Development of the early human ovary and the role of the mesonephrose in the differentiation of the cortex. Anat Embryol 1982; 165:253–280.
9. Singh RP, Carr DH. The anatomy and histology of XO human embryos and fetuses. Anat Rec 1966; 155:369–375.
10. Baker TG, Scrimgeous JB. Development of the gonad in normal and anencephalic human fetuses. J Reprod Fertil 1980; 60:193–199.
11. Guylas BJ, Hodgen GD, Tullner WW, et al. Effects of fetal and maternal hypophysectomy on endocrine organs and body weight in infant monkey (Macaca mulatta) with particular emphasis on oogenesis. Biol Reprod 1977; 16:216–227.
12. Byskov AG, Hoyer PE. Embryology of mammalian gonads and ducts. In: Knobil E, Neill JD, eds. The Physiology of Reproduction. 2nd ed, Vol 1. New York: Raven, 1994: 487–540.
13. Baker TG, Franchi LL. The fine structure of oogonia and oocytes in human ovaries. J Cell Sci 1967; 2:213–224.
14. Byskov AG. Regulation of meiosis in mammals. Ann Biol Anim Biochim Biophys 1979; 19:1251–1261.
15. Tsafriri A, Dekel N, Bar-Ami S. The role of oocyte maturation inhibitor in follicular regulation of oocyte maturation. J Reprod Fertil 1982; 64:541–551.
16. Peters H, Byskov AG, Grinsted J. Follicular growth in fetal and prepubertal ovaries in humans and other primates. Clin Endocrinol Metab 1978; 7:469–485.
17. George FW, Wilson JD. Conversion of androgen to estrogen by the human fetal ovary. J Clin Endocrinol Metab 1978; 47:550–555.
18. Jungman RA, Schweppe JS. Biosynthesis of steroids and steroids from acetate-14C by human fetal ovaries. J Clin Endocrinol Metab 1968; 28:1599–1604.
19. Molsberry RL, Carr BR, Mendelson CR, et al. Human chorionic gonadotropin binding to human fetal testes as a function of gestational age. J Clin Endocrinol Metab 1982; 55:791–794.
20. Wilson EA, Jawad MJ. The effect of trophic agents on fetal ovarian steroidogenesis in organ culture. Fertil Steril 1979; 32:73–79.
21. Miller W. Molecular biology of steroid hormone synthesis. Endocr Rev 1988; 9:295–311.
22. O'Rahilly R. The embryology and anatomy of the uterus. In: Norris HJ, Hertig AT, Abell MR, eds. The Uterus. Baltimore: Williams & Wilkins, 1973: 17–39.
23. Wehefritz E. Systematische Gewichtsuntersuchungen am Ovarien mit Berucksichtigung anderen Drusen mit inner Sekretion. Z Gest Anat 1923; 9:161.
24. Peters H, McNatty KP. The Ovary. Berkeley: University of California Press, 1980: 12–34.
25. Faiman C, Winter JSD, Reyes FI. Patterns of gonadotropins and gonadal steroids throughout life. Clin Obstet Gynecol 1976; 3:467–483.
26. Kaplan SL, Grumbach MM, Aubert ML. The ontogenesis of pituitary hormones and hypothalamic factors in the human fetus: maturation of the central nervous system regulation of anterior pituitary function. Recent Prog Horm Res 1976; 32:161–243.
27. Styne DM, Grumbach MM. Disorders of puberty in the male and female. In: Yen SSC, Jaffe RB, eds. Reproductive Endocrinology: Physiology, Pathophysiology and Clinical Management. 3rd ed. Philadelphia: WB Saunders, 1991: 511–554.
28. Winter JSD, Hughes IA, Reyes FI, et al. Pituitary-gonadal steroid concentrations in man from birth to two years of age. J Clin Endocrinol Metab 1976; 42:679–686.
29. Conte FA, Grumbach MM, Kaplan SL. A diphasic pattern of gonadotropin secretion in patients with the syndrome of gonadal dysgenesis. J Clin Endocrinol Metab 1975; 40:670–674.
30. Yanovski JA, Cutler GB. The reproductive axis: pubertal activation. In: Adashi EY, Rock JA, Rosenwaks Z, eds. Reproductive Endocrinology, Surgery and Technology. Philadelphia: Lippincott-Raven, 1996: 76–101.
31. Roth JC, Kelch RP, Kaplan SL, et al. FSH and LH response to luteinizing hormone–releasing factor in prepubertal and pubertal children, adult males and patients with hypogonadotropic and hypergonadotropic hypogonadism. J Clin Endocrinol Metab 1973; 37:680–686.
32. Jakacki RI, Kelch RP, Sauder SE, et al. Pulsatile secretion of luteinizing hormone in children. J Clin Endocrinol Metab 1982; 55:453–458.
33. Grumbach MM, Roth JC, Kaplan SL, et al. Hypothalamic-pituitary regulation of puberty in man: evidence and concepts derived from clinical research. In: Grumbach MM, Grave GD, Mayer FE, eds. Control of the Onset of Puberty. New York: John Wiley & Sons, 1974: 115–166.
34. Gill JS, Atkins B, Margrof L, et al. Adrenarche is associated with alterations in adrenal reticulosis expression of 3β-hydroxysteroid dehydrogenase. I Soc Gynecol Invest 1996; 3(Suppl):140A.
35. Kelnar CJH, Brook CGD. A mixed longitudinal study of adrenal steroid excretion in childhood and the mechanism of adrenarche. Clin Endocrinol 1983; 19:117–129.
36. Parker L, Odell WD. Control of adrenal androgen secretion. Endocr Rev 1980; 1:392–410.
37. Speroff L, Glass RH, Kase NG. Clinical Gynecologic Endocrinology and Infertility. 5th ed. Baltimore: Williams & Wilkins, 1994: 1–989.
38. Plant TM, Gay VL, Marshall GR, et al. Puberty in monkeys is triggered by chemical stimulation of the hypothalamus. Proc Natl Acad Sci USA 1989; 86:2506–2510.
39. Kapen S, Boyer RM, Hellman L, et al. Twenty-four-hour patterns of luteinizing hormone secretion in humans: ontogenic and sexual considerations. Prog Brain Res 1975; 42:103–113.
40. Knobil E. The neuroendocrine control of the menstrual cycle. Recent Prog Horm Res 1980; 36:53–78.
41. Crowley WF, McArthur JW. Stimulation of the normal menstrual cycle in Kallmann's syndrome by pulsatile administration of luteinizing hormone–releasing hormone (LHRH). J Clin Endocrinol Metab 1980; 51:173–175.
42. Crowley WF Jr, Comite F, Vale W, et al. Therapeutic use of pituitary desensitization with a long-acting LHRH agonist: a potential new treatment for idiopathic precocious puberty. J Clin Endocrinol Metab 1981; 53:370–372.
43. Mansfield MJ, Beardsworth DE, Loughlin JS, et al. Long-term treatment of central precocious puberty with a long-acting analogue of luteinizing hormone–releasing hormone. N Engl J Med 1983; 309:1286–1290.
44. Comite F, Cutler GB Jr, Rivier J, et al. Short-term treatment of idiopathic precocious puberty with a long-acting analogue of luteinizing hormone–releasing hormone: a preliminary report. N Engl J Med 1981; 305:1546–1550.
45. Winter JSD, Faiman C, Reyes FI, et al. Gonadotropins and steroid hormones in the blood and urine of prepubertal girls and other primates. Clin Endocrinol Metab 1978; 7:513–530.
46. Burstein S, Schoff-Blass E, Blass J, et al. Changing ratio of bioactive to immunoactive LH through puberty. J Clin Endocrinol Metab 1985; 61:508–513.
47. Burger HG, McLachlan RI, Bangah M, et al. Serum inhibin concentrations rise throughout normal male and female puberty. J Clin Endocrinol Metab 1988; 67:689–694.
48. Merimee TJ, Zapf J, Hewlett B, et al. Insulin-like growth factors in pygmies. N Engl J Med 1987; 316:906–911.
49. Mansfield MJ, Rudlin CR, Crigler JF, et al. Changes in growth and serum growth hormone and plasma somatomedin-C levels during suppression of gonadal sex steroid secretion in girls with central precocious puberty. J Clin Endocrinol Metab 1988; 66:3–9.
50. Dawson-Hughes B, Stern D, Goldman J, et al. Regulation of growth hormone and somatomedin-C secretion in postmenopausal women: effect of physiologic estrogen replacement. J Clin Endocrinol Metab 1986; 63:424–432.
51. Marshall WA, Tanner JM. Variations in pattern of pubertal changes in girls. Arch Dis Child 1969; 44:291–303.
52. Frisch RE, McArthur JW. Menstrual cycles: fatness as a determinant of minimum weight for height necessary for their maintenance at onset. Science 1974; 185:949–951.
53. Frisch RE. Fatness, puberty, menstrual periodicity and fertility. In: Vaitukaitis JL, ed. Clinical Reproductive Neuroendocrinology. New York: Elsevier Biomedical, 1982: 105–135.
54. Zacharias L, Rand WM, Wurtman RJ. A prospective study of sexual development and growth in American girls: the statistics of menarche. Obstet Gynecol Surv 1976; 31:325–337.
55. Woodburne RT. Essentials of Human Anatomy. New York: Oxford University Press, 1965: 527–528.
56. Mossman HW, Duke KL. Comparative Morphology of the Mammalian Ovary. Madison, WI: University of Wisconsin Press, 1973.
57. Franchi LL, Mandl AM, Zuckerman S. The development of the ovary and the process of oogenesis. In: Zuckerman S, Mandl AM, Eckstein P, eds. The Ovary. London: Academic, 1961: 1–88.
58. Ross GT, Schreiber JR. The ovary. In: Yen SSC, Jaffe RB, eds. Reproductive Endocrinology: Physiology, Pathophysiology and Clinical Management. 2nd ed. Philadelphia: WB Saunders, 1986: 115–139.
59. Gougeon A. Dynamics of follicular growth in the human: a model from preliminary results. Hum Reprod 1986; 1:1–87.

60. Adashi EY. The ovarian follicular apparatus. In: Adashi EY, Rock JA, Rosenwaks Z, eds. Reproductive Endocrinology, Surgery and Technology. Philadelphia: Lippincott-Raven, 1996: 18–40.

61. Zamboni L. Fine morphology of ovarian follicle maturation. In: Tozziniri RI, Reeves G, Pineda RL, eds. Endocrine Physiopathology of the Ovary. Amsterdam: Elsevier/North-Holland Biomedical, 1980: 63–99.

62. Greve JM, Salzman GS, Roller RS, et al. Biosynthesis of the major zona pellucida glycoprotein secreted by oocytes during mammalian oogenesis. Cell 1982; 31:749–759.

63. Dunbar BS. Morphological, biochemical and immunochemical characterization of the mammalian zona pellucida. In: Hartmann J, ed. Mechanism and Control of Animal Fertilization. London: Academic, 1983: 140–175.

64. Peters H, McNatty KP. The Ovary. Berkeley: University of California Press, 1980: 12–34.

65. Albertini DF, Anderson E. The appearance and structure of intracellular connections during the ontogeny of the rabbit ovarian follicle with particular reference to gap junctions. J Cell Biol 1974; 63:234–250.

66. Burghardt RC, Anderson E. Hormonal modulation of ovarian interstitial cells with particular reference to gap junctions. J Cell Biol 1979; 81:104–114.

67. Adashi EY. Endocrinology of the ovary. Hum Reprod 1994; 9:815–827.

68. Santen RJ, Paulsen CA. Hypogonadotropic eunuchoidism. II: Gonadal responsiveness to exogenous gonadotropin. J Clin Endocrinol Metab 1973; 36:55–63.

69. Tilly JL, Kowalski KJ, Johnson AL, et al. Involvement of apoptosis in ovarian follicular atresia and postovulatory regression. Endocrinology 1991; 129:2799–2801.

70. Erickson FG, Magoffen D, Dyer CA, et al. The ovarian androgen-producing cells: a review of structure/function relationships. Endocr Rev 1985; 6:371–399.

71. Gondos B, Hobel CG. Interstitial cells in the human fetal ovary. Endocrinology 1976; 93:736–739.

72. Dawson AB, McCabe M. The interstitial tissue of the ovary in infantile and juvenile rats. J Morphol 1951; 88:543–571.

73. Dyer CA, Erickson FG. Norepinephrine amplifies hCG-stimulated androgen biosynthesis by ovarian thecal-interstitial cells. Endocrinology 1985; 116:1645–1652.

74. McNatty KP, Makris A, DeGrazia C, et al. The production of progesterone, androgens and estrogens by granulosa cells, thecal tissue and stromal tissue from human ovaries in vitro. J Clin Endocrinol Metab 1979; 49:687–699.

75. Eshkal A, Lunenfeld B. Gonadotropic regulation of ovarian development in mice during infancy. In: Saxena BB, Gandy HM, Billing CG, eds. Gonadotropins. New York: John Wiley & Sons, 1972: 335–346.

76. Upadhyay S, Zamboni L. Ectopic germ cells: natural model for the study of germ cell sexual differentiation. Proc Natl Acad Sci USA 1982; 79:6584–6588.

77. Green SH, Zuckerman S. Quantitative aspects of the growth of the human ovum and follicle. J Anat 1951; 85:373–375.

78. Eppig JJ. A comparison between oocyte growth in coculture with granulosa cells and oocytes with granulosa cell–oocyte junctional contact maintained in vitro. J Exp Zool 1979; 209:345–353.

79. Austin CR. The Mammalian Egg. Springfield, IL: Charles C Thomas, 1961.

80. Bleil JD, Wassarman PM. Structure and function of the zona pellucida: identification and characterization of the proteins of the mouse oocyte's zona pellucida. Dev Biol 1980; 76:185–202.

81. Dekel N, Hillensjo T, Kraicer PF. Maturational effects of gonadotropins on the cumulus-oocyte complex of the rat. Biol Reprod 1979; 20:191–197.

82. Erickson GF. The ovary: basic principles and concepts. A: Physiology. In: Felig P, Baxter JD, Broders AG, et al, eds. Endocrinology and Metabolism. 3rd ed. New York: McGraw-Hill, 1995: 973–1015.

83. Moor RM. Role of steroids in the maturation of ovine oocytes. Ann Biol Anim Biochim Biophys 1978; 18:477–482.

84. Patton PE, Stouffer RL. Current understanding of the corpus luteum in women and nonhuman primates. Clin Obstet Gynecol 1991; 34:127–143.

85. Koos RD, LeMaire WJ. Factors that may regulate the growth and regression of blood vessels in the ovary. Semin Reprod Endocrinol 1983; 1:295–307.

86. Corner GW Jr. Histological dating of human corpus luteum of menstruation. Am J Anat 1956; 98:377–401.

87. Crisp TM, Dessouky DA, Denys FR. The fine structure of the human corpus luteum of early pregnancy and during the progestational phase of the menstrual cycle. Am J Anat 1970; 127:37–69.

88. Carr BR, MacDonald PC, Simpson ER. The role of lipoproteins in the regulation of progesterone secretion by the human corpus luteum. Fertil Steril 1982; 38:303–311.

89. Ohara A, Mori T, Taii S, et al. Functional differentiation in steroidogenesis of two types of luteal cells isolated from mature human corpora lutea of menstrual cycle. J Clin Endocrinol Metab 1987; 65:1192–1200.

90. Gillim SW, Christensen AK, McLennon CE. Fine structure of the human menstrual corpus luteum at its stage of maximum secretory activity. Am J Anat 1970; 126:409–415.

91. Juengel JL, Garverick HA, Johnson AL, et al. Apoptosis during luteal cell regression in cattle. Endocrinology 1993; 132:249–254.

92. Ying SY. Inhibins, activins, and follistatins: gonadal proteins modulating the secretion of follicle-stimulating hormone. Endocr Rev 1988; 9:267–293.

93. Oliver C, Mical RS, Porter JC. Hypothalamic-pituitary vasculature: evidence for retrograde blood flow in the pituitary stalk. Endocrinology 1977; 101:598–604.

94. McCann SM, Snyder GD, Ojeda SR, et al. Roles of peptides in the control of gonadotropin secretion. In: McKerns KW, Naoro Z, eds. Hormone Control of the Hypothalamic-Pituitary-Gonadal Axis. New York: Plenum, 1984: 3–13.

95. Karten MJ, Rivier JE. Gonadotropin-releasing hormone analog design. Structure-function studies toward the development of agonists and antagonists: rationale and perspective. Endocr Rev 1986; 7:44–66.

96. Marshall JC. Regulation of gonadotropin secretion. In: DeGroot LJ, Besser GM, Cahill GF Jr, et al, eds. Endocrinology. 2nd ed. Philadelphia: WB Saunders, 1989: 1903–1914.

97. Huseman CA, Kelch RP. Gonadotropin response and metabolism of synthetic gonadotropin-releasing hormone (GnRH) during constant infusion of GnRH in men and boys with delayed adolescence. J Clin Endocrinol Metab 1978; 47:1325–1331.

98. Evans WS, Griffins ML, Yankov VI. The pituitary gonadotroph: dynamics of gonadotropin release. In: Adashi EY, Rock JA, Rosenwaks Z, eds. Reproductive Endocrinology, Surgery and Technology. Philadelphia: Lippincott-Raven, 1996: 182–210.

99. Carmel PW, Araki S, Ferin M. Pituitary stalk portal blood collection in rhesus monkeys: evidence of pulsatile release of gonadotropin releasing hormone (GnRH). Endocrinology 1976; 99:243–248.

100. Clarke IJ, Cummins JT. The temporal relationship between gonadotropin releasing hormone (GnRH) and luteinizing hormone (LH) secretion in ovariectomized ewes. Endocrinology 1982; 111:1737–1739.

101. Knobil E, Plan TM, Wildt TL, et al. Control of the rhesus monkey menstrual cycle: permissive role of hypothalamic gonadotropin releasing hormone. Science 1980; 207:1371–1373.

102. Belchetz PE, Plant TM, Nakai Y, et al. Hypophysial responses to continuous and intermittent delivery of hypothalamic gonadotropin-releasing hormone. Science 1978; 202:631–638.

103. Leyendecker G, Wildt L, Hansmen M. Pregnancies following chronic intermittent pulsatile administration of GnRH. J Clin Endocrinol Metab 1980; 51:1214–1216.

104. Conn PM. The molecular basis of gonadotropin-releasing hormone action. Endocr Rev 1986; 7:3–11.

105. Conn PM, Crowley WF Jr. Gonadotropin-releasing hormone and its analogs. N Engl J Med 1991; 324:93–103.

106. Yen SSC, Rebar RW. Endocrine rhythms in gonadotropins and ovarian steroids with reference to reproductive processes. In: Kreiger DT, ed. Endocrine Rhythms. New York: Raven, 1979: 259–298.

107. Fiddes JC, Talmadge K. Structure, expression, and evolution of the genes for human glycoprotein hormones. Recent Prog Horm Res 1984; 40:43–78.

108. Vaitukaitis JL, Ross GT, Bourstein GD, et al. Gonadotropins and their subunits: basic and clinical studies. Recent Prog Horm Res 1976; 32:289–331.

109. Kholer PO, Ross GT, Odell WD. Metabolic clearance and production rates of human luteinizing hormone in pre- and postmenopausal women. J Clin Invest 1968; 47:38–47.

110. Keller PJ. The renal clearance of follicle-stimulating and luteinizing hormone in postmenopausal women. Acta Endocrinol 1966; 53:225–233.

111. Fink G. Gonadotropin secretion and its control. In: Knobil E, Neill JD, eds. The Physiology of Reproduction. Vol 1. New York: Raven, 1988: 1349–1377.

112. Chappel SC, Resko JA, Norman RL, et al. Studies on rhesus monkeys on the site where estrogen inhibits gonadotropins: delivery of 17β-estradiol to the hypothalamus and pituitary gland. J Clin Endocrinol Metab 1981; 52:1–8.

113. Wildt L, Hutchinson JS, Marshall G, et al. On the site of action of progesterone in the blockade of the estradiol-induced gonadotropin discharge in the rhesus monkey. Endocrinology 1981; 109:1293–1294.

114. Filicori M, Butler JP, Crowley WF. Neuroendocrine regulation of the corpus luteum in the human. J Clin Invest 1984; 73:1638–1647.

115. Liu JH, Yen SSC. Induction of midcycle gonadotropin surge by ovarian steroids in women: a critical evaluation. J Clin Endocrinol Metab 1983; 57:797–802.

116. Batista MC, Cartledge TP, Zellmer W, et al. Evidence for a critical role of progesterone in the regulation of the midcycle gonadotropin surge and ovulation. J Clin Endocrin Metab 1992; 74:565–570.

117. Gore-Langton RE, Armstrong DT. Follicular steroidogenesis and its control. In: Knobil E, Neill JD, eds. The Physiology of Reproduction. 2nd ed, Vol 1. New York: Raven, 1994: 571–628.

118. Siiteri PK, MacDonald PC. Role of extraglandular estrogen in human endocrinology. In: Greep RO, Astwood EB, eds. Handbook of Physiology. Sect 7: Endocrinology. Vol II. Female Reproductive System. Washington, DC: American Physiological Society, 1973: 615–630.

119. Brown JB, Matthew GD. The application of urinary estrogen methods to problems in gynecology. Recent Prog Horm Res 1962; 18:337–385.

120. Fishman J, Hellman L, Zumoff B, et al. Influence of thyroid hormone on estrogen metabolism in man. J Clin Endocrinol Metab 1962; 22:389–392.

121. Merriam GR, Lipsett MB. Catechol Estrogens. New York: Raven, 1983.

122. Lipsett M. Steroid hormones. In: Yen SSC, Jaffe RB, eds. Reproductive Endocrinology: Physiology, Pathophysiology and Clinical Management. 2nd ed. Philadelphia: WB Saunders, 1986: 140–153.

123. Gwynne JT, Strauss JF. The role of lipoproteins in steroidogenesis and cholesterol metabolism in steroidogenic glands. Endocr Rev 1982; 3:299–329.

124. Golos TG, Strauss JF III, Miller WL. Regulation of low density lipoprotein

receptor and cytochrome P-450$_{scc}$ mRNA levels in human granulosa cells. J Steroid Biochem 1987; 27:767–773.

125. Clark BJ, Soo SC, Caron KM. Hormonal and developmental regulation of the steroidogenic acute regulatory protein. Mol Cell Endocrinol 1995; 9:1346–1355.

126. Waterman MR, Simpson ER. Regulation of the biosynthesis of cytochrome P-450 involved in steroid hormone synthesis. Mol Cell Endocrinol 1985; 39:81–89.

127. McAllister JM, Kerin JFP, Trant JM, et al. Regulation of cholesterol side-chain cleavage and 17α-hydroxylase/lyase activities in proliferating human theca interna cells in long term monolayer culture. Endocrinology 1989; 125:1959–1966.

128. Doody KJ, Lorence MC, Mason IJ, et al. Expression of messenger ribonucleic acid species encoding steroidogenic enzymes in human follicles and corpora lutea throughout the menstrual cycle. J Clin Endocrinol Metab 1990; 70:1041–1045.

129. Suzuki T, Sasano H, Kimura N, et al. Immunohistochemical distribution of progesterone, androgen and oestrogen receptors in the human ovary during the menstrual cycle: relationship to expression of steroidogenic enzymes. Hum Reprod 1994; 9:1589–1595.

130. Sano Y, Suzuki K, Arai K, et al. Changes in enzyme activities related to steroidogenesis in human ovaries during the menstrual cycle. J Clin Endocrinol Metab 1981; 52:994–1001.

131. Suzuki T, Sasano H, Tamura M, et al. Temporal and spatial localization of steroidogenic enzymes in premenopausal human ovaries: in situ hybridization and immunohistochemical study. Mol Cell Endocrinol 1993; 97:135–143.

132. McNatty KP, Makris A, DeGrazia C, et al. The production of progesterone, androgens, and estrogens by granulosa cells, theca tissue and stroma tissue from human ovaries in vitro. J Clin Endocrinol Metab 1979; 49:687–699.

133. Steinkampf MP, Mendelson CR, Simpson ER. Effects of epidermal growth factor and insulin-like growth factor I on the levels of mRNA encoding aromatase cytochrome P-450 of human ovarian granulosa cells. Mol Cell Endocrinol 1988; 59:93–99.

134. Zhang Y, Word A, Fesmire S, et al. Human ovarian expression of 17β-hydroxysteroid dehydrogenase Types 1, 2, and 3. J Clin Endocrinol Metab 1996; 81:3594–3598.

135. Carr BR, Sadler RK, Rochelle DB, et al. Plasma lipoprotein regulation of progesterone biosynthesis by human corpus luteum tissue in organ culture. J Clin Endocrinol Metab 1981; 52:875–881.

136. Ohashi M, Carr BR, Simpson ER. Lipoprotein binding sites in human corpus luteum membrane fractions. Endocrinology 1982; 110:1477–1482.

137. Yeko TR, Shan-Dawood FS, Dawood MY. Human corpus luteum: luteinizing hormone and chorionic gonadotropin receptors during the menstrual cycle. J Clin Endocrinol Metab 1989; 68:529–534.

138. Illingworth DR, Corbin DK, Kemp ED, et al. Hormone changes during the menstrual cycle in abetalipoproteinemia: reduced luteal phase progesterone in a patient with homozygous hypobetalipoproteinemia. Proc Natl Acad Sci USA 1982; 79:6685–6689.

139. Reiter EO, Goldenberg RL, Vaitukaitis JL, et al. Evidence for a role of estrogen in the ovarian augmentation reaction. Endocrinology 1972; 91:1518–1522.

140. Hsueh AJW, Adashi EY, Jones PBC, et al. Hormonal regulation of the differentiation of culture ovarian granulosa cells. Endocr Rev 1984; 5:76–127.

141. Tilly JL, LaPolt PS, Hsueh AJ. Hormonal regulation of follicle-stimulating hormone receptor messenger ribonucleic acid levels in cultured rat granulosa cells. Endocrinology 1992; 130:1296–1302.

142. Hsueh AJW. Ovarian hormone synthesis, circulation, and mechanism of action. In: DeGroot LJ, Besser GM, Cahill GF Jr, et al, eds. Endocrinology. 2nd ed. Philadelphia: WB Saunders, 1989: 1929–1939.

143. Glasier AF, Baird DT, Hillier SG. FSH and the control of follicular growth. J Steroid Biochem 1989; 32:167–170.

144. Seegar-Jones G, DeMoraes-Ruehsen M. A new syndrome of amenorrhea in association with hypergonadotropism and apparently normal ovarian follicular apparatus. Am J Obstet Gynecol 1969; 104:597–600.

145. Baird DT, Horton R, Longcope C, et al. Steroid dynamics under steady state conditions. Recent Prog Horm Res 1969; 25:611–663.

146. Baird DT, Horton R, Longcope C, et al. Steroid prehormones. Perspect Biol Med 1968; 11:384–421.

147. Tait JF. Review: the use of isotopic steroids for the measurement of production rates in vivo. J Clin Endocrinol Metab 1963; 23:1285–1297.

148. Gurpide E, Gandy H. Dynamics of hormone production. In: Fuchs F, Klopper A, eds. Endocrinology of Pregnancy. New York: Harper & Row, 1971: 1–14.

149. Siiteri PK, MacDonald PC. Placental estrogen biosynthesis during human pregnancy. J Clin Endocrinol Metab 1966; 26:751–761.

150. Yen SSC. Chronic anovulation caused by peripheral endocrine disorders. In: Yen SSC, Jaffe RB, eds. Reproductive Endocrinology: Physiology, Pathophysiology and Clinical Management. 3rd ed. Philadelphia: WB Saunders, 1991: 576–630.

151. Rosner W. Sex steroid transport: binding proteins. In: Adashi EY, Rock JA, Rosenwaks Z, eds. Reproductive Endocrinology, Surgery and Technology. Philadelphia: Lippincott-Raven, 1996: 605–626.

152. Mendel CM. The free hormone hypothesis: distinction from the free hormone transport hypothesis. J Androl 1992; 13:107–116.

153. Ekins R. The free hormone concept. In: Hennemann G, ed. Thyroid Hormone Metabolism. New York: Marcel Dekker, 1986: 77–106.

154. Pardridge WM, Landaw EM. Tracer kinetic model of blood-brain barrier transport of plasma protein-bound ligands: empiric testing of the free hormone hypothesis. J Clin Invest 1984; 74:745–752.

155. Iqbal MJ, Johnson MW. Purification and characterization of human sex hormone–binding globulin. J Steroid Biochem 1979; 10:535–540.

156. Anderson DC. Sex hormone–binding globulin. Clin Endocrinol 1974; 3:69–96.

157. Barnea A, Gorsic J. Estrogen-induced protein: time course of synthesis. Biochemistry 1970; 9:1899–1904.

158. Clark JH, Shailaja KM. Actions of ovarian steroid hormones. In: Knobil E, Neill JD, eds. The Physiology of Reproduction. 2nd ed, Vol 1. New York: Raven, 1994: 1011–1059.

159. Welshoun WV, Lieberman MS, Gorski J. Nuclear localization of unoccupied estrogen receptors. Nature 1984; 307:745–749.

160. Simpson ER, Mendelson CR. The molecular basis of hormone action. In: Carr BR, Blackwell RE, eds. Textbook of Reproductive Medicine. Norwalk, CT: Appleton & Lange, 1993: 121–140.

161. Kumar V, Green S, Stack G, et al. Functional domains of the human estrogen receptor. Cell 1987; 51:941–951.

162. Scholl S, Lippman ME. The estrogen receptor in MCF-7 cells: evidence from dense amino acid labelling for rapid turnover and a dimeric model of activated nucleic acid receptor. Endocrinology 1984; 115:1295–1301.

163. DeSombre ER, Kuivanen PC. Progestin modulation of estrogen-dependent marker protein synthesis in the endometrium. Semin Oncol 1985; 12:6–11.

164. Adashi EY. The ovarian follicle: life cycle of a pelvic clock. In: Adashi EY, Rock JA, Rosenwaks Z, eds. Reproductive Endocrinology, Surgery and Technology. Philadelphia: Lippincott-Raven, 1996: 211–234.

165. Adashi EY, Leung PCK, eds. The Ovary. New York: Raven Press, 1993: 1–687.

166. Tsafriri A. Local nonsteroidal regulators of ovarian function. In: Knobil E, Neill JD, eds. The Physiology of Reproduction. 2nd ed, Vol 1. New York: Raven, 1994: 817–860.

167. Sawetawan C, Carr BR, McGee E, et al. Inhibin and activin differentially regulate androgen production and 17α-hydroxylase expression in human ovarian thecal-like tumor cells. J Endocrinol 1996; 148:213–221.

168. Koos RD. Potential relevance of angiogenic factors to ovarian physiology. Semin Reprod Endocrinol 1989; 7:29–40.

169. Fukuoka M, Vasuda K, Emi N, et al. Cytokine modulation of progesterone and estradiol secretion in cultures of luteinized human granulosa cells. J Clin Endocrinol Metab 1992; 75:254–258.

170. Li CH, Ramasharma K, Yamashiro D, et al. Gonadotropin-releasing peptide from human follicular fluid: isolation, characterization and chemical synthesis. Proc Natl Acad Sci USA 1987; 84:959–963.

171. Guidice LC. Insulin-like growth factors and ovarian follicular development. Endocr Rev 1992; 13:641–699.

172. McGee EA, Sawetawan C, Bird I, et al. The effect of insulin and insulin-like growth factors on the expression of steroidogenic enzymes in a human ovarian theca-like tumor model. Fertil Steril 1996; 65:87–93.

173. Carr BR, McGee EA, Sawetawan C, et al. The effect of transforming growth factor beta on steroidogenesis and expression of key steroidogenic enzymes using a human ovarian theca-like tumor cell model. Am J Obstet Gynecol 1996 (in press).

174. Ueno S, Takahashi M, Manganaro TF, et al. Cellular localization of mullerian inhibiting substance in the developing rat ovary. Endocrinology 1989; 124:1000–1006.

175. Khan-Dawood FS, Goldsmith LT, Weiss G, et al. Human corpus luteum secretion of relaxin, oxytocin and progesterone. J Clin Endocrinol Metab 1989; 68:627–631.

176. Sherwood OD. Relaxin. In: Knobil E, Neill JD, eds. The Physiology of Reproduction. 2nd ed Vol 1. New York: Raven, 1994: 861–1009.

177. Lightman A, Palumbo A, DeCherney AH, et al. The ovarian renin-angiotensin system. Semin Reprod Endocrinol 1989; 7:79–93.

178. Rainey WE, Bird IM, Byrd W, Carr BR. Effect of angiotensin II on human luteinized granulosa cells. Fertil Steril 1993; 59:143–147.

179. Trzeciak WH, Ahmed CE, Simpson ER, et al. Vasoactive intestinal peptide induces the synthesis of the cholesterol side-chain cleavage enzyme complex in cultured rat ovarian granulosa cells. Proc Natl Acad Sci USA 1986; 83:7490–7494.

180. Treloar AE, Boynton BE, Behn BG, et al. Variations of the human menstrual cycle through reproductive life. Int J Fertil 1967; 12:77–126.

181. Vollman RF. The Menstrual Cycle. Philadelphia: WB Saunders, 1977.

182. Presser HB. Temporal data relating to the human menstrual cycle. In: Ferin M, Halber F, Richart RM, et al, eds. Biorhythms and Human Reproduction. New York: John Wiley & Sons, 1974: 145–160.

183. Apter D, Raisanen I, Ylostalo P, et al. Follicular growth in relation to serum hormonal patterns in adolescence compared with adult menstrual cycles. Fertil Steril 1987; 47:82–88.

184. Fraser IS, Michie EA, Wide L, et al. Pituitary gonadotropin and ovarian function in adolescent dysfunctional uterine bleeding. J Clin Endocrinol Metab 1973; 37:407–414.

185. Sherman BM, West JH, Korenman SG. The menopausal tradition: analysis of LH, FSH, estradiol, and progesterone concentrations during menstrual cycles of older women. J Clin Endocrinol Metab 1976; 42:629–636.

186. Hodgen GD. The dominant ovarian follicle. Fertil Steril 1982; 38:281–300.

187. Goodman AL, Hodgen GD. The ovarian triad of the primate menstrual cycle. Recent Prog Horm Res 1983; 39:1–73.

188. Groom MP, Illengworth PJ, O'Brian M, et al. Measure of dimeric inhibin throughout the human menstrual cycle. J Clin Endocrinol Metab 1996; 81:1401–1405.

189. Baird DT. A model for follicular selection and ovulation: lessons from superovulation. J Steroid Biochem 1987; 27:15–23.

190. Dorrington JH, Armstrong DT. Effects of FSH on gonadal functions. Recent Prog Horm Res 1979; 39:301–342.

191. Nimrod A, Erickson GF, Ryan KJ. A specific FSH receptor in rat granulosa cells: properties of binding in vitro. Endocrinology 1976; 98:56–64.

192. Amsterdam A, Rotmensch S. Structure-function relationships during granulosa cell differentiation. Endocr Rev 1987; 8:309–337.

193. Zeleznik AJ, Midgley AR Jr, Reichert LE Jr. Granulosa cell maturation in the rat: increased binding of human chorionic gonadotropin following treatment with follicle-stimulating hormone in vivo. Endocrinology 1974; 95:818–825.

194. Erickson GF, Wang C, Hsueh AJW. FSH induction of functional LH receptors in granulosa cells cultured in a chemically defined medium. Nature 1979; 279:336–338.

195. McNatty KP, Markis A, Reinhold VN, et al. Metabolism of androstenedione by human ovarian tissue in vitro with particular reference to reductase and aromatase activity. Steroids 1979; 34:429–443.

196. Hillier SG, Van den Boogard AMJ, Reichert LE, et al. Intraovarian sex steroid hormone interactions and the regulation of follicular maturation: aromatization of androgens by human granulosa cells in vitro. J Clin Endocrinol Metab 1980; 50:640–647.

197. McNatty KP. Cyclic changes in antral fluid hormone concentrations in humans. Clin Endocrinol Metab 1978; 7:577–600.

198. McNatty KP, Smith DM, Makris A, et al. The microenvironment of the human antral follicle: interrelationships among the steroid levels in antral fluid, the population of granulosa cells, and the status of the oocyte in vivo and in vitro. J Clin Endocrinol Metab 1979; 49:851–860.

199. Sanyal MK, Berger MJ, Thompson IE, et al. Development of graafian follicles in adult human ovary. I. Correlation of estrogen and progesterone concentration in antral fluid with growth of follicles. J Clin Endocrinol Metab 1974; 38:828–835.

200. Brailly S, Gourgeon A, Milgrom E, et al. Androgens and progestins in human ovarian follicle: differences in the evolution of preovulatory, healthy nonovulatory and atretic follicles. J Clin Endocrinol Metab 1981; 53:128–134.

201. Bomsel-Helmreich O. The preovulatory human oocyte and its microenvironment. In: Beier HM, Lindner HR, eds. Fertilization of the Human Egg In Vitro. Berlin: Springer-Verlag, 1983: 10–34.

202. Wang CF, Lasley BL, Lein A, et al. The functional changes of the pituitary gonadotropins during the menstrual cycle. J Clin Endocrinol Metab 1986; 42:718–728.

203. Ream N, Saunder SE, Kelch RP, et al. Pulsatile gonadotropin secretion during the menstrual cycle: evidence for altered frequency of gonadotropin-releasing hormone secretion. J Clin Endocrinol Metab 1984; 59:328–337.

204. Hoff JD, Quigley ME, Yen SSC. Hormonal dynamics at midcycle: a reevaluation. J Clin Endocrinol Metab 1983; 57:792–796.

205. Pauerstein CJ, Eddy CA, Croxatto HD, et al. Temporal relationships of estrogen, progesterone and luteinizing hormone levels to ovulation in women and infrahuman primates. Am J Obstet Gynecol 1978; 130:876–886.

206. Weiss TJ, Seamark RF, McIntosh JEA, et al. Cyclic AMP in sheep ovarian follicles: site of production and response to gonadotropins. J Reprod Fertil 1976; 46:347–353.

207. Channing CP, Schaerf FW, Anderson LD, et al. Ovarian follicular and luteal physiology. In: Greep RO, ed. International Review of Physiology. Vol 22. Baltimore: University Park Press, 1980: 117–201.

208. Espey LL, Lipner H. Ovulation. In: Knobil E, Neill JD, eds. The Physiology of Reproduction. 2nd ed, Vol 1. New York: Raven, 1994: 725–780.

209. Espey LL. Ovarian proteolytic enzymes and ovulation. Biol Reprod 1974; 10:216–235.

210. Piquelte GN, Crabtree ME, El-Danasouri I, et al. Regulation of plasminogen activator inhibitor-1 and -2 messenger ribonucleic acid levels in human cumulus and granulosa luteal cells. J Clin Endocrinol Metab 1993; 76:518–523.

211. Priddy AR, Killick SR, Elstein M. The effect of prostaglandin synthetase inhibitors on human preovulatory follicular fluid prostaglandin, thromboxane and leukotriene concentrations. J Clin Endocrinol Metab 1990; 71:235–242.

212. Tsafriri A, Chun SY. Ovulation. In: Adashi EY, Rock JA, Rosenwaks Z, eds. Reproductive Endocrinology, Surgery and Technology. Philadelphia: Lippincott-Raven, 1996: 236–249.

213. Lumsden MA, Kelly RW, Templeton AA, et al. Changes in the concentrations of prostaglandins in preovulatory human follicles after administration of hCG. J Reprod Fertil 1986; 77:119–124.

214. Yoshimura Y, Wallach EE. Studies on the mechanisms of mammalian ovulation. Fertil Steril 1987; 47:22–34.

215. Doody KJ, Carr BR. Diagnosis and treatment of luteal dysfunction. In: Hillier SG, ed. Ovarian Endocrinology. London: Blackwell Scientific, 1991: 260–318.

216. Killick S, Elstein M. Pharmacologic production of luteinized unruptured follicles by prostaglandin synthetase inhibitors. Fertil Steril 1987; 47:773–777.

217. Murdoch WJ, Cavender JL. Effect of indomethacin on the vascular architecture of preovulatory ovine follicles: possible implication in the luteinized unruptured follicle syndrome. Fertil Steril 1989; 51:153–155.

218. Yen SSC. The human menstrual cycle. In: Yen SSC, Jaffe RB, eds. Reproductive Endocrinology: Physiology, Pathophysiology and Clinical Management. 2nd ed. Philadelphia: WB Saunders, 1986: 200–236.

219. Niswender GD, Nett TM. The corpus luteum and its control in infraprimate species. In: Knobil E, Neill JD, eds. The Physiology of Reproduction. 2nd ed, Vol 1. New York: Raven, 1994: 781–816.

220. Vande Wiele RL, Bogumil J, Dyrenfurth I, et al. Mechanisms regulating the menstrual cycle in women. Recent Prog Horm Res 1970; 26:63–103.

221. Segaloff A, Sternberg WH, Gaskill CJ. Effects of luteotrophic doses of chorionic gonadotropin in women. J Clin Endocrinol Metab 1951; 11:936–944.

222. McNeely MJ, Soules MR. The diagnosis of luteal phase deficiency. Fertil Steril 1988; 50:1–15.

223. Stouffer RL, Hodgen GD. Induction of luteal phase defects in rhesus monkeys by follicular fluid administration at the onset of the menstrual cycle. J Clin Endocrinol Metab 1980; 51:669–671.

224. Sheehan KL, Casper RF, Yen SSC. Luteal phase defects induced by an agonist of luteinizing hormone releasing factor: a model for fertility control. Science 1982; 215:170–172.

225. Keyes PL, Wiltbank MC. Endocrine regulation of the corpus luteum. Annu Rev Physiol 1988; 50:465–482.

226. Cooke ID. The corpus luteum. Hum Reprod 1988; 3:153–156.

227. Hutchison JS, Zeleznik AJ. The corpus luteum of the primate menstrual cycle is capable of recovering from a transient withdrawal of pituitary gonadotropin support. Endocrinology 1985; 117:1043–1049.

228. Rojas FJ, Moretti-Rojas I, Balmaceda JP, et al. Regulation of gonadotropin-stimulable adenylyl cyclase of the primate corpus luteum. J Steroid Biochem 1989; 32:175–182.

229. Auletta FJ, Flint APF. Mechanisms controlling corpus luteum function in sheep, cows, nonhuman primates, and women especially in relation to the time of luteolysis. Endocr Rev 1988; 9:88–105.

230. Schulz KD, Geiger W, Del Poso E, et al. Pattern of sexual steroids, prolactin and gonadotropic hormones during prolactin inhibition in normally cycling women. Am J Obstet Gynecol 1978; 132:561–566.

231. Bohnet HG, McNeilly AS. Prolactin: assessment of its role in the human female. Horm Metab Res 1979; 11:533–546.

232. Hahlin M, Dennefors B, Johanson C, et al. Luteotropic effects of prostaglandin E₂ on the human corpus luteum of the menstrual cycle and early pregnancy. J Clin Endocrinol Metab 1988; 66:909–914.

233. Hodgen GD. Surrogate embryo transfer combined with estrogen-progesterone therapy in monkeys. Implantation, gestation, and delivery without ovaries. JAMA 1983; 250:2167–2171.

234. Lutjen P, Trounson A, Leeton J, et al. The establishment and maintenance of pregnancy using in vitro fertilization and embryo donation in a patient with primary ovarian failure. Nature 1984; 307:174–175.

235. Auletta FJ. The role of prostaglandin F₂α in human luteolysis. Contemp Obstet Gynecol 1987; 30:119–129.

236. Wentz AC, Jones GS. Transient luteolytic effect of prostaglandin F₂α in the human. Obstet Gynecol 1973; 42:172–181.

237. Schoonmaker JN, Bergman KS, Steiner RA, et al. Estradiol-induced luteal regression in the rhesus monkey: evidence of an extra-ovarian site of action. Endocrinology 1984; 110:1708–1715.

238. Karsch FJ, Krey LC, Weick RF, et al. Functional luteolysis in the rhesus monkey: role of estrogens. Endocrinology 1973; 92:1148–1152.

239. Johansson EDB, Gemzell C. Plasma levels of progesterone during the luteal phase in normal women treated with synthetic estrogens (RS 2874, F 6103, and ethinyloestradiol). Acta Endocrinol 1971; 68:551–560.

240. Westfahl PK, Resko JA. Effects of clomiphene on luteal function in the nonpregnant cynomolgus macaque. Biol Reprod 1983; 29:963–969.

241. Ellinwood WE, Resko JA. Effect on inhibition of estrogen synthesis during the luteal phase on function of the corpus luteum in rhesus monkeys. Biol Reprod 1983; 28:636–644.

242. Iwai T, Nanbu Y, Iwai M, et al. Immunohistochemical localization of oestrogen receptors and progesterone receptors in the human ovary throughout the menstrual cycle. Virchows Arch A 1990; 417:319–357.

243. Khan-Dawood FS, Huang JC, Dawood MY. Baboon corpus luteum oxytocin: an intragonadal peptide modulator on luteal function. Am J Obstet Gynecol 1988; 158:882–891.

244. Givens JR, Andersen RN, Ragland JB, et al. Adrenal function in hirsutism. I: Diurnal change and response of plasma androstenedione, testosterone, 17-hydroxyprogesterone, cortisol, LH and FSH to dexamethasone and 1/2 unit of ACTH. J Clin Endocrinol Metab 1975; 40:988–1000.

245. Judd HL, Yen SSC. Serum androstenedione and testosterone levels during the menstrual cycle. J Clin Endocrinol Metab 1973; 36:475–481.

246. Abraham GE, Chakmakjian AH. Serum steroid levels during the menstrual cycle in a bilaterally adrenalectomized woman. J Clin Endocrinol Metab 1973; 37:581–587.

247. Dyrenfurth I, Jewelewica R, Warren M, et al. Temporal relationships of hormonal variables in the menstrual cycle. In: Ferin M, Halberg F, Richart RM, et al, eds. Biorhythms and Reproduction. New York: John Wiley & Sons, 1974: 171–201.

248. Genazzani AR, Lemarchand-Beraud TH, Aubert ML, et al. Pattern of plasma ACTH, hGH and cortisol during menstrual cycle. J Clin Endocrinol Metab 1975; 41:431–437.

249. Carr BR, Parker Jr CR, Madden JD, et al. Plasma levels of adrenocorticotropin (ACTH) and cortisol in women receiving oral contraceptive treatment. J Clin Endocrinol Metab 1979; 49:346–349.

250. Carr BR, Wilson JD. Disorders of the ovary and female reproductive tract. In: Braunwald E, Isselbacher KJ, Petersdorf RG, et al, eds. Harrison's Principles of Internal Medicine. 11th ed. New York: McGraw-Hill, 1987: 1818–1837.

251. Casey ML, MacDonald PC. Extraadrenal formation of a mineralocorticosteroid: deoxycorticosterone and deoxycorticosterone sulfate biosynthesis and metabolism. Endocr Rev 1982; 3:396–403.

252. Parker Jr CR, Winkel CA, Rush AJ, et al. Plasma concentrations of 11-deoxycorticosterone in women during the menstrual cycle. Obstet Gynecol 1981; 58:26–30.

253. Noyes RW, Hertig AW, Rock J. Dating the endometrial biopsy. Fertil Steril 1950; 1:3–25.

254. Tseng L, Gurpide E. Effects of progestins on estradiol receptor levels in human endometrium. J Clin Endocrinol Metab 1975; 41:402–404.

255. Lessy BA, Killman AP, Metzger DA, et al. Immunohistochemical analyses of human uterine estrogen and progesterone receptors throughout the menstrual cycle. J Clin Endocrinol Metab 1988; 69:334–340.

256. Tseng L, Liu HC. Stimulation of arylsulfotransferase activity by progestins in human endometrium in vitro. J Clin Endocrinol Metab 1981; 53:418–421.

257. Sixma JJ, Cristiens GCML, Hospels AS. The sequence of hemostatic events in the endometrium during normal menstruation. In: Dicefalusy E, Fraser IS, Webb FTG, eds. WHO Symposium on Steroid Contraception and Endometrial Bleeding. 1980: 86.

258. Wilborn WH, Flowers CE Jr. Cellular mechanisms for endometrial conservation during menstrual bleeding. Semin Reprod Endocrinol 1984; 2:307–341.

259. Hallberg L, Hogdahl A, Nilsson L, et al. Menstrual blood loss: a population study. Acta Obstet Gynecol Scand 1966; 45:320–351.

260. Edman CD. The effects of steroids on the endometrium. Semin Reprod Endocrinol 1983; 1:79–187.

261. Pickles VR, Hall WJ, Best FA, et al. Prostaglandins in endometrium and menstrual fluid from normal and dysmenorrheic subjects. J Obstet Gynaecol Br Commonw 1965; 72:185–192.

262. Willman EA, Collins WP, Clayton SG. Studies in the involvement of prostaglandins in uterine symptomatology and pathology. Br J Obstet Gynaecol 1976; 83:337–341.

263. Schwarz BE. The production and biologic effects of uterine prostaglandins. Semin Reprod Endocrinol 1983; 1:189–195.

264. Turksoy RN, Safaii HS. Immediate effect of prostaglandin F$_{2\alpha}$ during the luteal phase of the menstrual cycle. Fertil Steril 1975; 26:634–637.

265. Henzl MR, Smith RE, Boost G, et al. Lysosomal concept of menstrual bleeding in humans. J Clin Endocrinol Metab 1972; 34:860–875.

266. Ferency A, Guralnick M. Endometrial microstructure: structure-function relationships throughout the menstrual cycle. Semin Reprod Endocrinol 1983; 1:205–219.

267. Todd AS. Localization of fibrinolytic activity in tissues. Br Med Bull 1964; 20:210–212.

268. Papanicolaou GN, Traut HF, Marchetti AA. The Epithelia of Women's Reproductive Organs: A Correlative Study of Cyclic Changes. New York: Commonwealth, 1948.

269. Rebar RE. Practical evaluation of hormonal status. In: Yen SSC, Jaffe RB, eds. Reproductive Endocrinology: Physiology, Pathophysiology and Clinical Management. 3rd ed. Philadelphia: WB Saunders, 1991: 830–886.

270. Gaudefoy M. Cytologic criteria of estrogen effect. Acta Cytol 1958; 2:347–362.

271. Harper MJK. Gamete and zygote transport. In: Knobil E, Neill JD, eds. The Physiology of Reproduction. 2nd ed, Vol 1. New York: Raven, 1994: 123–187.

272. Settlage DSF, Motoshima M, Tredway DR. Sperm transport from the external cervical os to the fallopian tubes in women: a time and quantitation study. Fertil Steril 1973; 24:655–661.

273. Ahlgren M. Sperm transport to and survival in the human fallopian tube. Gynecol Invest 1975; 6:206–214.

274. Byrd W. Fertilization, embryogenesis and implantation. In: Carr BR, Blackwell RE, eds. Textbook of Reproductive Medicine. Norwalk, CT: Appleton & Lange, 1993: 1–15.

275. Wassarman PM. Fertilization in mammals. Sci Am 1988; 259:78–84.

276. Yanagimachi R. Mammalian fertilization. In: Knobil E, Neill JD, eds. The Physiology of Reproduction. 2nd ed, Vol 1. New York: Raven, 1994: 189–317.

277. Croxatto HB, Ortiz MS. Egg transport in the fallopian tube. Gynecol Invest 1975; 6:215–225.

278. Pauerstein CJ, Eddy CA. The role of the oviduct in reproduction: our knowledge and our ignorance. J Reprod Fertil 1979; 55:223–229.

279. Blandau RJ. Gamete transport in the female mammal. In: Greep RO, Astwood EB, eds. Handbook of Physiology. Sect 7: Endocrinology. Vol II. Female Reproductive System. Washington, DC: American Physiological Society, 1973: 153–167.

280. Wassarman PM. The biology and chemistry of fertilization. Science 1987; 235:553–560.

281. Zaneveld LJD, Polakoski KL, Williams WL. Properties of a proteolytic enzyme from rabbit sperm acrosomes. Biol Reprod 1972; 6:30–39.

282. Veech LI. Atlas of the Human Oocyte and Early Conceptus. Baltimore: Williams & Wilkins, 1986: 1–331.

283. Pederson RA, Burdsal CH. Early mammalian embryogenesis. In: Knobil E, Neill JD, eds. The Physiology of Reproduction. 2nd ed, Vol 1. New York: Raven, 1994: 187–230.

284. Hertig AT, Rock J, Adams EC, et al. Thirty-four fertilized ova, good, bad and indifferent from 210 women of known fertility. Pediatrics 1959; 23:202–211.

285. Weitauf HM. Biology of implantation. In: Knobil E, Neill JD, eds. The Physiology of Reproduction. 2nd ed, Vol 1. New York: Raven, 1994: 391–440.

286. Chan CLK, Cameron IT, Findlay JK, et al. Oocyte donation and in vitro fertilization for hypergonadotropic hypogonadism: clinical state of the art. Obstet Gynecol Surv 1987; 42:350–362.

287. Dey SK. Implantation. In: Adashi EY, Rock JA, Rosenwaks Z, eds. Reproductive Endocrinology, Surgery and Technology. Philadelphia: Lippincott-Raven, 1996: 422–434.

288. Shelesnyak MC. Inhibition of decidual cell formation in the pseudopregnant rat by histamine antagonists. Am J Physiol 1952; 170:522–527.

289. Heap RB, Flint AP, Gadsby JE. Role of embryonic signals in the establishment of pregnancy. Br Med Bull 1979; 35:129–135.

290. Kennedy TG. Evidence for a role for prostaglandins in the initiation of blastocyst implantation in the rat. Biol Reprod 1977; 16:286–291.

291. Harper MJK. Platelet-activating factor: a paracrine factor in preimplantation stages of reproduction? Biol Reprod 1989; 40:907–913.

292. A Statistical Portrait of Women in the U.S. Publication No. 58. Current Population Report, Special Studies Series. Washington, DC: US Dept of Commerce, Bureau of the Census, 1976: 23.

293. Utian WH. Menopause in Modern Perspective. New York: Appleton-Century-Crofts, 1980.

294. Linquist O, Bengtsson C. Menopausal age in relation to smoking. Acta Med Scand 1979; 205:73–77.

295. Sauramo H. Histology, histopathology and function of the senile ovary. Ann Chir Gynaecol Fenn 1952; 4(Suppl):1–66.

296. Nagamani M, Stuart CA, Doherty NG. Increased steroid production by ovarian stromal tissue of postmenopausal women with endometrial cancer. J Clin Endocrinol Metab 1992; 74:172–176.

297. Scaglia H, Medina M, Pinto-Ferriera AL, et al. Pituitary LH and FSH secretion and responsiveness in women of old age. Acta Endocrinol 1976; 81:673–679.

298. Chakravarti S, Collins WP, Forecast JD, et al. Hormonal profiles after the menopause. Br Med J 1976; 2:784–787.

299. Judd JL. Hormonal dynamics associated with the menopause. Clin Obstet Gynecol 1976; 19:775–788.

300. Edman CD, MacDonald PC. Effect of obesity on conversion of plasma androstenedione to estrone in ovulatory and anovulatory young women. Am J Obstet Gynecol 1978; 130:456–461.

301. Hemsell DL, Grodin JM, Brenner PF, et al. Plasma precursors of estrogen. II. Correlation of the extent of conversion of plasma androstenedione to estrone with age. J Clin Endocrinol Metab 1974; 38:476–479.

302. Tataryn IV, Lomax P, Bajorek JG, et al. Postmenopausal hot flushes: a disorder of thermoregulation. Maturitas 1980; 2:101–107.

303. Walsh BW, Schiff I. Physiology of the climacteric. In: Carr BR, Blackwell RE, eds. Textbook of Reproductive Medicine. Norwalk, CT: Appleton & Lange, 1993: 587–600.

304. Brincat M, Moniz CJ, Studd JW, et al. Long-term effects of the menopause and sex hormones on skin thickness. Br J Obstet Gynaecol 1985; 92:256–259.

305. Weiss NS, Ure CL, Ballard JH, et al. Decreased risk of fractures of the hip and lower forearm with postmenopausal use of estrogen. N Engl J Med 1980; 303:1195–1198.

306. Barrett-Conner E, Brown WV, Turner J, et al. Heart disease risk factors and hormone use in postmenopausal women. JAMA 1979; 241:2167–2169.

307. Ross RK, Paganini-Hill A, Mack TM, et al. Estrogen use and cardiovascular disease. In: Mishell DR, ed. Menopause: Physiology and Pharmacology. Chicago: Year Book Medical, 1987: 209–223.

308. Jaszmann L, Van Lith ND, Zoat JCA. The perimenopausal symptoms. Med Gynecol Sociol 1969; 4:268–277.

309. Meldrum DR. The pathophysiology of postmenopausal symptoms. Semin Reprod Endocrinol 1983; 1:11–17.

310. Riggs BL, Wahner HW, Melton LJ III, et al. Rates of bone loss in the appendicular and axial skeletons of women. J Clin Invest 1986; 77:1487–1491.

311. Alderman BW, Weiss NS, Daling JR, et al. Reproductive history and postmenopausal risk of hip and forearm fracture. Am J Epidemiol 1986; 124:262–267.

312. Beals RK. Survival following hip fracture: long term follow-up of 607 patients. J Chronic Dis 1972; 25:235–244.

313. Nilas L, Christiansen C. Bone mass and its relationship to age and the menopause. J Clin Endocrinol Metab 1987; 65:697–702.

314. Lindsay R, Herrington BS. Estrogens and osteoporosis. Semin Reprod Endocrinol 1983; 1:55–67.

315. Henderson BE, Ross RK, Paganini-Hill A, et al. Estrogen use and cardiovascular disease. Am J Obstet Gynecol 1986; 154:1181–1186.

316. Matthews KA, Meilahn E, Kuller LH, et al. Menopause and risk factors for coronary heart disease. N Engl J Med 1989; 321:641–646.

317. Colditz GA, Willett WC, Stampfer MJ, et al. Menopause and the risk of coronary heart disease in women. N Engl J Med 1987; 316:1105–1110.

318. Bush TL, Barrett-Connor E, Cowan DK, et al. Cardiovascular mortality and noncontraceptive use of estrogen in women: results from the Lipid Research Clinics Program Follow-Up Study. Circulation 1987; 75:1102–1109.

319. Stampfer MJ, Willett WC, Colditz GA, et al. Postmenopausal estrogen therapy and coronary heart disease: ten-year follow-up from the Nurses' Health Study. N Engl J Med 1991; 325:756–762.

320. Santen RJ, Bardin CW. Episodic luteinizing hormone secretion in man: pulse analysis, clinical interpretation, physiologic mechanism. J Clin Invest 1973; 52:2617–2628.

321. Goldenberg RL, Grodin JM, Rodbard D, et al. Gonadotropins in women with amenorrhea. Am J Obstet Gynecol 1973; 116:1003–1012.

322. Yen SSC, Vela P, Rankin J. Inappropriate secretion of follicle-stimulating hormone and luteinizing hormone in polycystic ovarian disease. J Clin Endocrinol Metab 1970; 30:435–442.

323. Yen SSC, VandenBerg G, Rebar R, et al. Variation of pituitary responsiveness to synthetic LRF during different phases of the menstrual cycle. J Clin Endocrinol Metab 1972; 35:931–937.

324. Rebar R, Yen SSC, VandenBerg G, et al. Gonadotropin responses to synthetic LRF: dose-response relationship in men. J Clin Endocrinol Metab 1973; 36:10–16.

325. Yen SSC, Rebar R, Vandenberg G, et al. Hypothalamic amenorrhea and hypogonadism: responses to LRF. J Clin Endocrinol Metab 1973; 36:811–816.

326. Kletzky OA, Davajan V, Nakamura RM, et al. Clinical categorization of patients with secondary amenorrhea using progesterone-induced uterine bleeding and measurement of serum gonadotropin levels. Am J Obstet Gynecol 1975; 121:695–703.

327. Ritchie WGM. Ultrasound in the evaluation of normal and induced ovulation. Fertil Steril 1985; 43:167–181.

328. Griffin JE, Edwards C, Madden JD, et al. Congenital absence of the vagina. Ann Intern Med 1976; 85:224–236.

329. Griffin JE, Wilson JD. The syndromes of androgen resistance. N Engl J Med 1980; 302:198–209.

330. New MI, Dupont B, Pang S, et al. An update of congenital adrenal hyperplasia. Recent Prog Horm Res 1981; 37:105–181.

331. Ferriman D, Gallwey JD. Clinical assessment of body hair growth in women. J Clin Endocrinol Metab 1961; 21:1440–1447.

332. Bardin CW, Lipsett MB. Testosterone and androstenedione blood production rates in normal women and women with idiopathic hirsutism or polycystic ovaries. J Clin Invest 1967; 46:891–902.

333. Lipsett MB. Clinical considerations of 17-ketosteroid and testosterone measurements. In: Sunderman FW, Sunderman Jr FW, eds. Laboratory Diagnosis of Endocrine Disease. St Louis: Warren H Green, 1971: 555.

334. Vermesh M, Kletzky OA, Davajan V, et al. Monitoring techniques to predict and detect ovulation. Fertil Steril 1987; 47:259–264.

335. Hricak H. MRI of the female pelvis: a review. Am J Radiol 1986; 146:1115–1122.

336. Winfield AC, Wentz AC. Diagnostic Imaging of Infertility. Baltimore: Williams & Wilkins, 1987.

337. Bradshaw JR. Magnetic resonance imaging of the CNS. Br J Hosp Med 1989; 42:472–479.

338. Tjio JH, Levan A. The chromosome number in man. Hereditas 1956; 42:1–6.

339. Seabright M. A rapid banding technique for human chromosomes. Lancet 1971; 2:971–972.

340. Manuel M, Katayama KP, Jones HW Jr. The age of occurrence of gonadal tumors in intersex patients with a Y chromosome. Am J Obstet Gynecol 1976; 124:293–300.

341. Baggish MS, Barbot J, Valle RF. Diagnostic and Operative Hysteroscopy: A Text and Atlas. Chicago: Year Book, 1989.

342. Nordenskjold F, Ahlgreen M. Laparoscopy in female infertility. Acta Obstet Gynecol Scand 1983; 62:609–615.

343. Buster JE, Simon JA. Placental hormones, hormone preparation for and control of parturition, and hormonal diagnosis of pregnancy. In: DeGroot LJ, Besser GM, Cahill GF Jr, et al, eds. Endocrinology. 2nd ed. Philadelphia: WB Saunders, 1989: 2043–2073.

344. Gaudin J, Le Treguilly C, Parent P, et al. Neonatal ovarian cysts: twelve cysts with antenatal diagnosis. Pediatr Surg Int 1988; 3:158–164.

345. Brenner PF. Precocious puberty in the female. In: Mishell DR Jr, Davajan V, eds. Infertility, Contraception and Reproductive Endocrinology. Oradell, NJ: Medical Economics Books, 1986: 223–236.

346. Dean HJ, Winter JSD. Abnormalities of pubertal development. In: Collu R, Ducharme JD, Guyda HJ, eds. Pediatric Endocrinology. 2nd ed. New York: Raven, 1989: 331–366.

347. Thamdrup E. Precocious sexual development: a clinical study of 100 children. Dan Med Bull 1961; 8:140–142.

348. Liu N, Grumbach MM, de Napoli RA, et al. Prevalence of electroencephalographic abnormalities in idiopathic precocious puberty and premature pubarche: bearing on pathogenesis and neuroendocrine regulation of puberty. J Clin Endocrinol Metab 1965; 25:1296–1308.

349. Jenner MR, Kelch RP, Kaplan SL, et al. Hormonal changes in puberty. IV. Plasma estradiol, LH and FSH in prepubertal children, pubertal females,

and in precocious puberty, premature thelarche, hypogonadism, and in a child with a feminizing ovarian tumor. J Clin Endocrinol Metab 1972; 34:521–530.

350. Reiter EO, Kaplan SL, Conte FA, et al. Responsivity of pituitary gonadotropes to luteinizing hormone–releasing factor in idiopathic precocious puberty, precocious thelarche, precocious adrenarche, and in patients treated with medroxyprogesterone acetate. Pediatr Res 1975; 9:111–116.

351. Sigurjonsdottir TH, Hayles AB. Precocious puberty: a report of 96 cases. Am J Dis Child 1968; 115:309–321.

352. Saxena KM. Endocrine manifestations of neurofibromatosis in children. Am J Dis Child 1970; 120:265–271.

353. Fienman NL, Yakovac WC. Neurofibromatosis in childhood. J Pediatr 1970; 76:339–346.

354. Mahachoklertwaltana P, Kaplan SL, Grumbach MM. The luteinizing hormone–releasing hormone–secreting hypothalamic hamartoma is a congenital malformation: natural history. J Clin Endocrinol Metab 1993; 77:118–124.

355. Cabezudo JM, Perez C, Vaquera J, et al. Pubertas praecox in craniopharyngioma. J Neurosurg 1981; 55:127–131.

356. Zuniga OF, Tanner SM, Wild WO, et al. Hamartoma of CNS associated with precocious puberty. Am J Dis Child 1983; 137:127–133.

357. Kubo O, Yamasaki N, Kamijo Y, et al. Human chorionic gonadotropin produced by ectopic pinealoma in a girl with precocious puberty. J Neurosurg 1977; 47:101–105.

358. Styne DM. Precocious puberty. Compr Ther 1987; 13:14–19.

359. Towne BH, Mahour GH, Woolley MM, et al. Ovarian cysts and tumors in infancy and childhood. J Pediatr Surg 1975; 10:311–320.

360. Young RH, Dickerson GR, Scully RE. Juvenile granulosa cell tumor of the ovary. A clinicopathological analysis of 125 cases. Am J Surg Pathol 1984; 8:575–596.

361. Thompson JP, Dockerty MB, Symonds RE, et al. Ovarian and parovarian tumors in infants and children. Am J Obstet Gynecol 1967; 97:1059–1065.

362. Eberlein WR, Bongiovanni AM, Jones IT, et al. Ovarian tumors and cysts associated with sexual precocity. J Pediatr 1960; 57:484–497.

363. Solh HM, Azoury RS, Najjar SS. Peutz-Jeghers syndrome associated with precocious puberty. J Pediatr 1983; 103:593–595.

364. England AT, Geffner ME, Nagel RA, et al. Pediatric germ cell and human chorionic gonadotropin-producing tumors, clinical and laboratory features. Am J Dis Child 1991; 145:1294–1297.

365. Drop SLS, Bruining GJ, Visser HKA, et al. Prolonged galactorrhea in a 6-year-old girl with isosexual precocious puberty due to a feminizing adrenal tumor. Clin Endocrinol 1981; 15:37–43.

366. McCune DJ. Osteitis fibrosa cystica: the case of a nine-year-old girl who also exhibits precocious puberty, multiple pigmentation of the skin and hyperthyroidism. Am J Dis Child 1936; 52:743–747.

367. Albright F, Butler AM, Hampton AO, et al. Syndrome characterized by osteitis fibrosa disseminata, areas of pigmentation and endocrine dysfunction, with precocious puberty in females. N Engl J Med 1937; 216:726–746.

368. Shenker A, Weinstein LS, Sweet DE, et al. An activating G$_s$α mutation is present in fibrous dysplasia of bone in the McCune-Albright syndrome. J Clin Endocrinol Metab 1994; 79:750–755.

369. Comite F, Shawker TH, Pescovitz OH, et al. Cyclical ovarian function resistant to treatment with an analogue of luteinizing hormone–releasing hormone in McCune-Albright syndrome. N Engl J Med 1984; 311:1032–1036.

370. D'Armiento RM, Camagna G, Tardella L. McCune-Albright syndrome: evidence for autonomous multiendocrine hyperfunction. J Pediatr 1983; 102:584–586.

371. Feuillan PP, Foster CM, Pescovitz OH, et al. Treatment of precocious puberty in the McCune-Albright syndrome with the aromatase inhibitor testolactone. N Engl J Med 1986; 315:1115–1119.

372. Cuttler L, Jackson JA, uz-Zafar MS, et al. Hypersecretion of growth hormone and prolactin in McCune-Albright syndrome. J Clin Endocrinol Metab 1989; 68:1148–1154.

373. Van Wyk JJ, Grumbach MM. Syndrome of precocious menstruation and galactorrhea in juvenile hypothyroidism: an example of hormonal overlap in pituitary feedback. J Pediatr 1960; 57:416–435.

374. Pringle PJ, Stanhope R, Hindmarsh P, et al. Abnormal pubertal development in primary hypothyroidism. Clin Endocrinol 1988; 28:479–486.

375. Hemady ZS, Siler-Khodr TM, Najjar S. Precocious puberty in juvenile hypothyroidism. J Pediatr 1978; 92:55–59.

376. Castro-Magana M, Angula M, Canas A, et al. Hypothalamic-pituitary gonadal axis in boys with primary hypothyroidism and macroorchidism. J Pediatr 1988; 112:397–402.

377. Silver HK. Asymmetry, short stature and variations in sexual development: syndrome of genital malformation. Am J Dis Child 1964; 107:495–515.

378. Hertz R. Accidental ingestion of estrogens by children. Pediatrics 1958; 21:203–206.

379. Saenz de Rodriguez CA, Bongiovanni AM, Conde de Borrego L. An epidemic of precocious development in Puerto Rican children. J Pediatr 1985; 107:393–396.

380. Pescovitz OH, Hench KD, Barnes KM, et al. Premature thelarche and central precocious puberty: the relationship between clinical presentation and the gonadotropin response to luteinizing hormone–releasing hormone. J Clin Endocrinol Metab 1988; 67:474–479.

381. Muritano M, Zachmann M, Manella B, et al. Transient ovarian testosterone

and androstenedione hypersecretion: a cause of virilization or premature pubarche in prepubertal girls. Horm Res 1987; 28:37–41.

382. Mansfield MJ, Beardsworth DE, Loughlin JS, et al. Long term treatment of central precocious puberty with a long acting analogue of luteinizing hormone–releasing hormone. N Engl J Med 1983; 309:1286–1290.

383. Comite F, Rescovitz OH, Rieth KG, et al. Luteinizing hormone–releasing hormone analog treatment of boys with hypothalamic hamartoma and true precocious puberty. J Clin Endocrinol Metab 1984; 59:888–892.

384. Rescovitz OH, Comite F, Hench K, et al. The NIH experience with precocious puberty: diagnostic subgroups and response to short-term luteinizing hormone–releasing hormone analogue therapy. J Pediatr 1986; 108:47–54.

385. Paul D, Conte FA, Gumbach MM, et al. Long-term effect of gonadotropin-releasing hormone agonist therapy on final and near-final height in 26 children with true precocious puberty treated at a median age of less than five years. J Clin Endocrinol Metab 1995; 80:546–551.

386. Dawood MY, ed. Dysmenorrhea. Baltimore: Williams & Wilkins, 1981.

387. Owen PR. Prostaglandin synthetase inhibitors in the treatment of primary dysmenorrhea: outcome trials reviewed. Am J Obstet Gynecol 1984; 148:96–103.

388. Mortola JF. The premenstrual syndrome. In: Adashi EY, Rock JA, Rosenwaks Z, eds. Reproductive Endocrinology, Surgery and Technology. Philadelphia: Lippincott-Raven, 1996: 1635–1647.

389. Wood SH, Mortola JF, Chan Y-F, et al. Treatment of premenstrual syndrome with fluoxetine: a double-blind, placebo-controlled, crossover study. Obstet Gynecol 1992; 80:339–344.

390. Bancroft J, Backstrom T. Premenstrual syndrome. Clin Endocrinol 1985; 22:313–336.

391. March CM, Hoffman DI, Lobo RA. Dysfunctional uterine bleeding. In: Mishell DR Jr, Davajan V, eds. Infertility, Contraception and Reproductive Endocrinology. Oradell, NJ: Medical Economics Books, 1986: 337–351.

392. Smith SK, Abel MT, Kelly RW, et al. Synthesis of prostaglandins from persistent proliferative endometrium. J Clin Endocrinol Metab 1982; 55:284–289.

393. Kurman RJ, Kaminski PT, Norris HJ. The behavior of endometrial hyperplasia: a long-term study of "untreated" hyperplasia in 170 patients. Cancer 1985; 56:403–412.

394. Van Eijkeren MA, Christiaens GCML, Sixma JJ, et al. Menorrhagia: a review. Obstet Gynecol Surv 1989; 44:421–429.

395. Ferenczy A. Studies on the cytodynamics of human endometrial regeneration: I. Scanning electron microscopy. Am J Obstet Gynecol 1976; 124:64–74.

396. van Eijkeren MA, Christiaens GCML, Geuze JH, et al. Effects of mefenamic acid on menstrual hemostasis in essential menorrhagia. Am J Obstet Gynecol 1992; 166:1419–1428.

397. DeVore GR, Owens O, Kase N. Use of intravenous premarin in the treatment of dysfunctional uterine bleeding: a double-blind randomized control study. Obstet Gynecol 1982; 59:285–291.

398. Carr BR. Current Evaluation and Treatment of Amenorrhea. The American Fertility Society: Guidelines for Practice. 1994: 1–11.

399. Simpson JL, Christakos AC, Horwith M, et al. Gonadal dysgenesis in individuals with apparently normal chromosomal complements: tabulation of cases and compilation of genetic data. Birth Defects 1971; 8:215–228.

400. Rosen GF, Kaplan B, Lobo RA. Menstrual function and hirsutism in patients with gonadal dysgenesis. Obstet Gynecol 1988; 71:677–680.

401. Hague WM, Adams J, Reeders ST, et al. 45,X Turner's syndrome in association with polycystic ovaries: case report. Br J Obstet Gynaecol 1989; 96:613–618.

402. Capraro VJ, Greenberg H. Adhesions of the labia minora: a study of 50 patients. Obstet Gynecol 1972; 39:65–69.

403. Klein VR, Willman SP, Carr BR. Familial posterior labial fusion. Obstet Gynecol 1989; 73:500–503.

404. Soules MR. Adolescent amenorrhea. Pediatr Clin North Am 1987; 43:1083–1103.

405. Baird DT. Amenorrhea, anovulation, and dysfunctional uterine bleeding. In: DeGroot LJ, Besser GM, Cahill GF Jr, et al, eds. Endocrinology. 2nd ed. Philadelphia: WB Saunders, 1989: 1950–1968.

406. Rock JA. Anomalous development of the vagina. Semin Reprod Endocrinol 1986; 4:13–31.

407. Rock JA, James HW Jr. The double uterus associated with an obstructed hemivagina and ipsilateral renal agenesis. Am J Obstet Gynecol 1980; 138:339–342.

408. Reindollar RH, Byrd JR, McDonough PG. Delayed sexual development: a study of 252 patients. Am J Obstet Gynecol 1981; 140:371–380.

409. Fore SR, Hammond CB, Parker RT, et al. Urologic and genital anomalies in patients with congenital absence of the vagina. Obstet Gynecol 1975; 46:410–416.

410. Griffin JE, Wilson JD. The androgen resistance syndromes: 5α-reductase deficiency, testicular feminization, and related syndromes. In: Scriver CR, Beaudet AL, Sly WS, et al, eds. The Metabolic Basis of Inherited Disease. 6th ed. New York: McGraw-Hill, 1989: 1919–1944.

411. Perez-Palacios G, Chavez B, Mendez JP, et al. The syndromes of androgen resistance revisited. J Steroid Biochem 1987; 27:1101–1108.

412. Joshi NP, Sortrel G. Diagnostic laparoscopy in apparent uterine agenesis. J Adolesc Health Care 1988; 9:403–406.

413. Schenker JG, Margalioth EJ. Intrauterine adhesions: an updated appraisal. Fertil Steril 1992; 37:593–610.

414. Rock JA, Zacur HA, Dlugi AM, et al. Pregnancy success following surgical correction of imperforate hymen and complete transverse vaginal septum. Obstet Gynecol 1982; 59:448–451.

415. Wheeless CR Jr. Excision of transverse vaginal septum. In: Wheeless CR Jr, ed. Atlas of Pelvic Surgery. 2nd ed. Philadelphia: Lea & Febiger, 1988: 74–75.

416. Aribarg A. Topical oestrogen therapy for labial adhesions in children. Br J Obstet Gynaecol 1975; 82:424–425.

417. Frank RT. The formation of an artificial vagina. Am J Obstet Gynecol 1938; 35:1053–1057.

418. Ingram JM. The bicycle seat stool in the treatment of vaginal agenesis and stenosis: a preliminary report. Am J Obstet Gynecol 1981; 140:867–873.

419. McIndoe A. The treatment of congenital absence and obliterative conditions of the vagina. Br J Plast Surg 1950; 2:254–273.

420. Levine RU, Neuwirth RS. Simultaneous laparoscopy and hysteroscopy for intrauterine adhesions. Obstet Gynecol 1973; 42:441–445.

421. March CM, Israel R. Gestational outcome following hysteroscopic lysis of adhesions. Fertil Steril 1981; 36:455–459.

422. Levinson G, Zarate A, Guzman-Toledano R, et al. An XX female with sexual infantilism, absent gonads, and lack of müllerian ducts. J Med Genet 1976; 13:68–69.

423. Simpson JL. Gonadal dysgenesis and abnormalities of the human sex chromosomes: current status of phenotypic-karyotypic correlations. Birth Defects 1975; 11:23–59.

424. Tho PT, McDonough PG. Gonadal dysgenesis and its variants. Pediatr Clin North Am 1981; 28:309–329.

425. Turner HH. A syndrome of infantilism, congenital webbed neck, and cubitus valgus. Endocrinology 1938; 23:566–574.

426. Jaffe RB. Disorders of sexual development. In: Yen SSC, Jaffe RB, eds. Reproductive Endocrinology: Physiology, Pathophysiology and Clinical Management. 2nd ed. Philadelphia: WB Saunders, 1986: 283–312.

427. Michalak DP, Zacur HA, Rock JA, et al. Autoimmunity in a patient with 47,XXX karyotype. Obstet Gynecol 1983; 62:667–669.

428. Kaneko N, Kawagoe S, Hiroi M. Turner's syndrome—review of the literature with references to a successful pregnancy outcome. Gynecol Obstet Invest 1990; 29:81–87.

429. Simpson JL. Genetic forms of gonadal dysgenesis in 46,XY individuals. Semin Reprod Endocrinol 1983; 1:93–100.

430. Wilson EE, Vuitch F, Carr BR. Laparoscopic removal of dysgenetic gonads containing a gonadoblastoma in a patient with Swyer's syndrome. Obstet Gynecol 1992; 79:842–844.

431. Carr BR, Aiman J. Steroid production in a woman with gonadal dysgenesis, breast development, and clitoral hypertrophy. Obstet Gynecol 1980; 56:492–498.

432. Biglieri EG, Herron MA, Brust N. 17-Hydroxylation deficiency in man. J Clin Invest 1966; 45:1946–1954.

433. Larrea F, Lisker R, Banuelos R, et al. Hypergonadotrophic hypogonadism in an XX female subject due to 17,20 steroid desmolase deficiency. Acta Endocrinol 1983; 103:400–405.

434. Maxon WS, Wentz AC. The gonadotropin-resistant ovary syndrome. Semin Reprod Endocrinol 1983; 1:147–160.

435. Kaufman FR, Xu YK, Ng WG, et al. Gonadal function and ovarian galactose metabolism in classic galactosemia. Acta Endocrinol 1989; 120:129–133.

436. LaBarbera AR, Miller MM, Ober C, et al. Autoimmune etiology in premature ovarian failure. Am J Reprod Immunol Microbiol 1988; 16:115–122.

437. Verp MS. Environmental causes of ovarian failure. Semin Reprod Endocrinol 1983; 1:101–111.

438. Ash P. The influence of radiation on fertility in man. Br J Radiol 1980; 53:271–278.

439. Morrison JC, Givens JR, Wiser WL, et al. Mumps oophoritis: a cause of premature menopause. Fertil Steril 1975; 26:655–659.

440. Takano K, Shizume K, Hibi I, et al. Turner's syndrome: treatment of 203 patients with recombinant human growth hormone for one year. A multicentre study. Acta Endocrinol 1989; 120:559–568.

441. Neely EK, Rosenfeld RG. Growth in Turner syndrome. Endocrinologist 1991; 1:313–322.

442. Ross JL, Cutler GB. The optimal use of estrogen in the treatment of Turner's syndrome. Endocrinologist 1992; 2:119–121.

443. Horning SJ, Hoppe RT, Kaplan HS, et al. Female reproductive potential after treatment for Hodgkin's disease. N Engl J Med 1981; 304:1377–1382.

444. Alper MM, Jolly EE, Garner PR. Pregnancies after premature ovarian failure. Obstet Gynecol 1986; 67(Suppl):59S–62S.

445. Check JH, Wu CH, Check ML. The effect of leuprolide acetate in aiding induction of ovulation in hypergonadotropic hypogonadism: a case report. Fertil Steril 1988; 49:542–543.

446. Amos WL Jr. Pregnancy in patient with gonadotropin-resistant ovary syndrome. Am J Obstet Gynecol 1985; 153:154–155.

447. Surrey ES, Cedars MI. The effect of gonadotropin suppression on the induction of ovulation in premature ovarian failure patients. Fertil Steril 1989; 52:36–41.

448. Barraclough CA. Steroid regulation of reproductive neuroendocrine processes. In: Greep RO, Astwood EB, eds. Handbook of Physiology. Sect 7: Endocrinology. Vol II. Female Reproductive System. Washington, DC: American Physiological Society, 1973: 29–56.

449. Goldzieher JW, Axelrod LR. Clinical and biochemical features of polycystic ovarian disease. Fertil Steril 1963; 14:631–653.

450. Franks S. Polycystic ovary syndrome: a changing perspective. Clin Endocrinol 1989; 31:87–120.

451. Hauge WM, Adams J, Reeders ST, et al. Familial polycystic ovaries: a genetic disease? Clin Endocrinol 1988; 29:593–605.

452. Cooper HE, Spellacy WN, Prem KA, et al. Hereditary factors in the Stein-Leventhal syndrome. Am J Obstet Gynecol 1968; 100:371–387.

453. Wilroy RS, Givens JR, Wiser WL, et al. Hyperthecosis: an inheritable form of polycystic ovarian disease. Birth Defects 1975; 17:81–85.

454. Mandel FP, Chang RJ, Dupont B, et al. HLA genotyping in family members and patients with familial polycystic ovarian disease. J Clin Endocrinol Metab 1983; 56:862–864.

455. Stein IF, Leventhal ML. Amenorrhoea associated with bilateral polycystic ovaries. Am J Obstet Gynecol 1935; 29:181–191.

456. Smith KO, Steinberger E, Perloff WH. Polycystic ovarian disease: a report of 301 patients. Am J Obstet Gynecol 1965; 93:994–1001.

457. Shearman RP, Cox RI. The enigmatic polycystic ovary. Obstet Gynecol Surv 1966; 21:1–33.

458. Raj SG, Thompson IE, Berger MJ, et al. Clinical aspects of the polycystic ovary syndrome. Obstet Gynecol 1977; 49:552–556.

459. Seibel MM, Taymor ML. Polycystic ovarian syndrome: new insights into pathophysiology and treatment. In: Taymor ML, Nelson JH Jr, eds. Progress in Gynecology. Vol 7. New York: Grune & Stratton, 1983: 101–128.

460. Polson DW, Franks S, Reed MJ, et al. The distribution of oestradiol in plasma in relation to uterine cross-sectional area in women with polycystic or multifollicular ovaries. Clin Endocrinol 1987; 26:581–588.

461. Lobo RA. Polycystic ovary syndrome. In: Mishell DR Jr, Davajan V, eds. Infertility, Contraception and Reproductive Endocrinology. Oradell, NJ: Medical Economics Books, 1986: 223–236.

462. Barnes R, Rosenfield RL. The polycystic ovary syndrome: pathogenesis and treatment. Ann Intern Med 1989; 110:386–399.

463. Rebar R, Judd HL, Yen SSC, et al. Characterization of the inappropriate gonadotropin secretion in polycystic ovary syndrome. J Clin Invest 1976; 57:1320–1329.

464. Aono T, Minagawa J, Kinugasa T, et al. The diagnostic significance of LH-releasing hormone test in patients with amenorrhea. Am J Obstet Gynecol 1974; 119:740–748.

465. Kazer RR, Kessel B, Yen SSC. Circulating luteinizing hormone pulse frequency in women with polycystic ovary syndrome. J Clin Endocrinol Metab 1987; 65:233–236.

466. Waldstreicher J, Santoro NF, Hall JE, et al. Hyperfunction of the hypothalamic-pituitary axis in women with polycystic ovarian disease: indirect evidence for partial gonadotroph desensitization. J Clin Endocrinol Metab 1988; 66:165–172.

467. McKenna TJ. Pathogenesis and treatment of polycystic ovary syndrome. N Engl J Med 1988; 318:558–562.

468. Fauser BCJM, Pache TD, Hop WCJ, et al. The significance of serum LH measurements in women with cycle disturbances: discrepancies between immunoreactive and bioactive hormone estimates. Clin Endocrinol 1992; 37:445–452.

469. Chang RJ, Laufer LR, Meldrum DR, et al. Steroid secretion in polycystic ovarian disease after ovarian suppression by a long-acting gonadotropin-releasing hormone agonist. J Clin Endocrinol Metab 1983; 56:897–903.

470. Polson DW, Reed MJ, Franks S, et al. Serum 11-hydroxyandrostenedione as an indicator of the source of excess androgen production in women with polycystic ovaries. J Clin Endocrinol Metab 1988; 66:946–950.

471. Futterweit W. Pituitary tumours and polycystic ovarian disease. Obstet Gynecol 1983; 62(Suppl):74S–79S.

472. Luciano AA, Chapler FK, Sherman BM. Hyperprolactinemia in polycystic ovary syndrome. Fertil Steril 1968; 41:719–725.

473. Futterweit W. Polycystic Ovarian Disease. New York: Springer-Verlag, 1984: 1–210.

474. Lobo RA, Granger L, Goeblesmann U, et al. Elevation in unbound serum estradiol as a possible mechanism for inappropriate gonadotropin secretion in women with PCO. J Clin Endocrinol Metab 1981; 52:156–158.

475. Lobo RA, Goeblesmann U. Effect of androgen excess on inappropriate gonadotropin secretion as found in the polycystic ovary syndrome. Am J Obstet Gynecol 1982; 142:394–401.

476. Ackerman GE, Smith ME, Mendelson CR, et al. Aromatization of androstenedione by human adipose stromal cells in monolayer culture. J Clin Endocrinol Metab 1981; 53:412–417.

477. Zumoff B, Freeman R, Coupey S, et al. A chronobiologic abnormality in luteinizing hormone secretion in teenage girls with the polycystic ovary syndrome. N Engl J Med 1983; 309:1206–1209.

478. Erickson GF, Hsueh AJ, Quiglen ME, et al. Functional studies of aromatase activity in human granulosa cells from normal and polycystic ovaries. J Clin Endocrinol Metab 1979; 49:514–519.

479. Seibel MM, McArdle C, Smith D, et al. Ovulation induction in polycystic ovary syndrome with urinary follicle-stimulating hormone or human menopausal gonadotropin. Fertil Steril 1985; 43:703–708.

480. Claman P, Seibel MM, McArdle C, et al. Comparison of intermediate-dose purified urinary follicle-stimulating hormone with and without human chorionic gonadotropin for ovulation induction in polycystic ovarian disease. Fertil Steril 1986; 46:528–521.

481. Quigley ME, Rakoff JS, Yen SS. Increased luteinizing hormone sensitivity to dopamine inhibition in polycystic ovary syndrome. J Clin Endocrinol Metab 1981; 52:231–234.

482. Cumming DC, Reid RL, Quigley ME, et al. Evidence for decreased endogenous dopamine and opioid inhibitory influences on LH secretion in polycystic ovary syndrome. Clin Endocrinol 1984; 20:643–648.

483. Buckler HM, McLachlan RI, Maclachlan VB, et al. Serum inhibin levels in polycystic ovary syndrome: basal levels and response to luteinizing hormone–releasing hormone agonist and exogenous gonadotrophin administration. J Clin Endocrinol Metab 1988; 66:798–803.

484. Poretsky L. On the paradox of insulin-induced hyperandrogenism in insulin-resistant states. Endoc Rev 1991; 12:3–13.

485. Dunaif A, Segal KR, Shelly DR, et al. Evidence for distinctive and intrinsic defects in insulin action in polycystic ovary syndrome. Diabetes 1992; 41:1257–1266.

486. Ciaraldi TP, el-Roeiy A, Madar Z, et al. Cellular mechanisms of insulin resistance in polycystic ovarian syndrome. J Clin Endocrinol Metab 1992; 75:577–583.

487. Barbieri RL, Makris A, Randall RW, et al. Insulin stimulates androgen accumulation in incubations of ovarian stroma obtained from women with hyperandrogenism. J Clin Endocrinol Metab 1986; 62:904–910.

488. Adashi EY, Resnick CE, D'Ercole AJ, et al. Insulin-like growth factors as intraovarian regulators of granulosa cell growth and function. Endocr Rev 1985; 6:400–420.

489. Goldzieher JW, Green JA. The polycystic ovary. I. Clinical and histologic features. J Clin Endocrinol Metab 1962; 22:325–338.

490. Newmark S, Dluhy RG, Williams GH, et al. Partial 11- and 21-hydroxylase deficiencies in hirsute women. Am J Obstet Gynecol 1977; 127:594–598.

491. Cathelineau G, Brerault JL, Fiet J, et al. Adrenocortical 11β-hydroxylation defect in adult women with postmenarcheal onset of symptoms. J Clin Endocrinol Metab 1980; 51:287–291.

492. Aiman EJ, Nalick RH, Jacobs A, et al. The origin of androgen and estrogen in a virilized postmenopausal woman with bilateral benign cystic teratomas. Obstet Gynecol 1977; 49:695–704.

493. Donesky BW, Adashi EY. Surgically induced ovulation in the polycystic ovary syndrome: wedge resection revisited in the age of laparoscopy. Fertil Steril 1995; 63:439–463.

494. Dunaif A, Mandeli J, Fluhr H, et al. The impact of obesity and chronic hyperinsulinemia on gonadotropin release and gonadal steroid secretion in the polycystic ovary syndrome. J Clin Endocrinol Metab 1988; 66:131–139.

495. Pasquali R, Antenucci D, Casimirri F, et al. Clinical and hormonal characteristics of obese amenorrheic hyperandrogenic women before and after weight loss. J Clin Endocrinol Metab 1989; 68:173–179.

496. Filicori M, Flamigni C, Merrigiola MC, et al. Endocrine response determines the clinical outcomes of pulsatile gonadotropin-releasing hormone ovulation induction in different ovulatory disorders. J Clin Endocrinol Metab 1991; 72:965–972.

497. Sagle MA, Hamilton-Fairley D, Kiddy DS, Froness A. A comparative randomized study of low-dose human menopausal gonadotropin and follicle-stimulating hormone in women with polycystic ovarian syndrome. Fertil Steril 1991; 55:56–60.

498. Filicori M, Flamigni C, Dellai P, et al. Treatment of anovulation with pulsatile gonadotropin-releasing hormone: prognostic factors and clinical values in 600 cycles. J Clin Endocrinol Metab 1994; 79:1215–1220.

499. Givens JR. Role of oral contraceptives in the treatment of hyperandrogenism of hirsute women. In: Mahesh VB, Greenblatt RB, eds. Hirsutism and Virilism: Pathogenesis, Diagnosis and Management. Boston: John Wright PSG, 1983: 351–367.

500. Gambrell RD Jr. Hormonal therapy. In: Greenblatt RB, Mahesh VB, Gambrell RD, eds. The Cause and Management of Hirsutism. Park Ridge, NJ: Parthenon, 1987: 137–146.

501. Bates GW, Whitworth NS. Effect of body weight reduction on plasma androgens in obese, infertile women. Fertil Steril 1982; 38:406–409.

502. Chamlian DL, Taylor HB. Endometrial hyperplasia in young women. Obstet Gynecol 1970; 36:659–666.

503. Jackson RL, Dockerty MB. The Stein-Leventhal syndrome: analysis of 43 cases with special reference to association with endometrial carcinoma. Am J Obstet Gynecol 1950; 73:161–173.

504. Kallmann FJ, Schoenfeld WA, Barrera SE. The genetic aspects of primary eunuchoidism. Am J Ment Defic 1944; 48:203–236.

505. Schwanzel-Fukuda M, Pfaff DW. Origin of luteinizing hormone–releasing hormone neurons. Nature 1989; 338:161–164.

506. Lieblich JM, Rogol AD, White BJ, et al. Syndrome of anosmia with hypogonadotropic hypogonadism (Kallmann syndrome). Am J Med 1982; 73:506–519.

507. Merriam GR. Congenital isolated gonadotropin-releasing hormone deficiency. In: Adashi EY, Rock JA, Rosenwaks Z, eds. Reproductive Endocrinology, Surgery and Technology. Philadelphia: Lippincott-Raven, 1996: 1018–1037.

508. Klingmuller D, Dewes W, Krahe T, et al. Magnetic resonance imaging of the brain in patients with anosmia and hypothalamic hypogonadism (Kallmann's syndrome). J Clin Endocrinol Metab 1987; 65:581–584.

509. Yen SSC. Chronic anovulation due to CNS-hypothalamic-pituitary dysfunction. In: Yen SSC, Jaffe RB, eds. Reproductive Endocrinology: Physiology, Pathophysiology and Clinical Management. 3rd ed. Philadelphia: WB Saunders, 1991: 631–688.

510. Santoro N, Filicori M, Crowley WF Jr. Hypogonadotropic disorders in men and women: diagnosis and therapy with pulsatile gonadotropin-releasing hormone. Endocr Rev 1986; 7:11–23.

511. Quigley ME, Sheehan KL, Casper RF, et al. Evidence for increased dopaminergic and opioid activity in patients with hypothalamic hypogonadotropic amenorrhea. J Clin Endocrinol Metab 1980; 50:949–954.

512. Warren MP, Holderness CC, Lesabre V. Hypothalamic amenorrhea: a hidden nutritional insult. Obstet Gynecol 1993; 81:669–674.

513. Gadpaille WJ, Sanborn CF, Wagner WW. Athletic amenorrhea, major affective disorders, and eating disorders. Am J Psychiatry 1987; 144:939–942.

514. Herzog DB, Coopeland PM. Eating disorders. N Engl J Med 1985; 313:295–303.

515. Warren MP, Vande Wiele RL. Clinical and metabolic features of anorexia nervosa. Am J Obstet Gynecol 1973; 117:435–449.

516. Warren MP. Amenorrhea in endurance runners. J Clin Endocrinol Metab 1992; 75:1393–1397.

517. Prior JC, Vigna YM. Ovulation disturbance and exercise training. Clin Obstet Gynecol 1991; 24:180–190.

518. Cumming DC, Rebar RW. Hormonal changes with acute exercise and with training in women. Semin Reprod Endocrinol 1985; 3:55–64.

519. Howlett TA, Tomlin S, Ngahfoong L, et al. Release of beta-endorphin and met-enkephalin during exercise in normal women: response to training. Br Med J 1984; 288:1950–1952.

520. Bullen BA, Skriinar GS, Beitins IZ, et al. Induction of menstrual disorders by strenuous exercise in untrained women. N Engl J Med 1985; 312:1349–1353.

521. McArthur JW, Bullen BA, Bertins IZ, et al. Hypothalamic amenorrhea in runners of normal body composition. Endocrinol Res Commun 1980; 7:13–25.

522. Abraham SF, Beumont PJV, Fraser IS, et al. Body weight, exercise and menstrual status among ballet dancers in training. Br J Obstet Gynaecol 1982; 89:507–510.

523. Shangold M, Freeman R, Thysen B, et al. The relationship between long-distance running, plasma progesterone and luteal phase length. Fertil Steril 1979; 31:130–133.

524. Drinkwater BL, Nilson K, Chestnut CH, et al. Bone mineral content of amenorrheic and eumenorrheic athletes. N Engl J Med 1984; 311:277–281.

525. Drinkwater BL, Nilson K, Ott S, et al. Bone mineral density after resumption of menses in amenorrheic athletes. JAMA 1986; 256:380–382.

526. Fisher EC, Nelson ME, Frontera WR, et al. Bone mineral content and levels of gonadotropins and estrogens in amenorrheic running women. J Clin Endocrinol Metab 1986; 62:1232–1236.

527. Lindberg JS, Fears WB, Hunt MM, et al. Exercise-induced amenorrhea and bone density. Ann Intern Med 1984; 101:647–648.

528. Marcus R, Cann CE, Madvig P, et al. Menstrual function and bone mass in elite women distance runners. Ann Intern Med 1985; 102:158–163.

529. Lloyd T, Triantafyllou SJ, Baker ER, et al. Women athletes with menstrual irregularity have increased musculoskeletal injuries. Med Sci Sports Exerc 1986; 18:374–379.

530. Van Der Spuy ZM, Steer PJ, McCusker M, et al. Outcome of pregnancy in underweight women after spontaneous and induced ovulation. Br Med J 1988; 296:962–965.

531. Gindoff PR, Jewelewicz R. Use of gonadotropin in ovulation induction. NY State J Med 1985; 85:580–584.

532. Archer DF. Use of luteinizing hormone–releasing hormone for ovulation induction. Semin Reprod Endocrinol 1986; 4:285–291.

533. Snyder PJ. Extensive personal experience: gonadotropin adenomas. J Clin Endocrinol Metab 1995; 4:1059–1061.

534. Howlett TA, Wass JAH, Grossman A, et al. Prolactinomas presenting as primary amenorrhoea and delayed or arrested puberty: response to medical therapy. Clin Endocrinol 1989; 30:131–140.

535. Schlechte J, Sherman B, Halmi N, et al. Prolactin-secreting pituitary tumors. Endocr Rev 1980; 1:295–308.

536. Jackson RD, Wortsman J, Malarkey WB. Characterization of a large molecular weight prolactin in women with idiopathic hyperprolactinemia and normal menses. J Clin Endocrinol Metab 1985; 61:258–264.

537. Schlechte J, Dolan K, Sherman B, et al. The natural history of untreated hypoprolactinemia: a prospective analysis. J Clin Endocrinol Metab 1989; 68:412–418.

538. Molitch ME. Pathologic hyperprolactinemia. Endocrinol Metab Clin North Am 1992; 21:877–901.

539. Sisam DA, Sheehan JP, Sheeler LR. The natural history of untreated microprolactinomas. Fertil Steril 1987; 48:67–71.

540. Martin TL, Kim M, Malarkey WB. The natural history of idiopathic hyperprolactinemia. J Clin Endocrinol Metab 1985; 60:855–858.

541. Pituitary Adenoma Study Group. Pituitary adenomas and oral contraceptives: a multicenter case-control study. Fertil Steril 1983; 39:753–760.

542. Yen SSC. Prolactin in human reproduction. In: Yen SSC, Jaffe RB, eds. Reproductive Endocrinology: Physiology, Pathophysiology and Clinical Management. 3rd ed. Philadelphia: WB Saunders, 1991: 357–388.

543. Burrow GN, Wortzman G, Rewcastle NB, et al. Microadenomas of the pituitary and abnormal sellar tomograms in an unselected autopsy series. N Engl J Med 1981; 304:156–158.

544. Blackwell RE, Boots LR, Goldenberg RL, et al. Assessment of pituitary function in patients with serum prolactin levels greater than 100 ng/ml. Fertil Steril 1979; 32:177–182.

545. Chang RJ. Anovulation of CNS origin: anatomic causes. In: Carr BR, Blackwell RE, eds. Textbook of Reproductive Medicine. Norwalk, CT: Appleton & Lange, 1993: 265–295.

546. Stein AL, Levenick MN, Kletzky OA. Computed tomography versus magnetic resonance imaging for the evaluation of suspected pituitary adenomas. Obstet Gynecol 1989; 73:996–999.

547. Schlechte JA, Sherman BM, Chapler FK, et al. Long-term follow-up of women with surgically treated prolactin-secreting pituitary tumors. J Clin Endocrinol Metab 1986; 62:1296–1301.

548. Parl FF, Cruz VE, Cobb CA, et al. Late recurrence of surgically removed prolactinomas. Cancer 1986; 57:2422–2426.

549. Wang C, Lam KSL, Ma JTC, et al. Long-term treatment of hyperprolactinemia with bromocriptine: effect of drug withdrawal. Clin Endocrinol 1987; 27:363–371.

550. McGregor AM, Scanlon MF, Hall R, et al. Effects of bromocriptine on pituitary tumour size. Br Med J 1979; 2:700–703.

551. Molitch ME, Elton RL, Blackwell RE, et al. Bromocriptine as primary therapy for prolactin-secreting macroadenomas: results of a prospective multicenter study. J Clin Endocrinol Metab 1985; 60:698–705.

552. Thorner MO, Martin WH, Rogol AD, et al. Rapid regression of pituitary prolactinomas during bromocriptine treatment. J Clin Endocrinol Metab 1980; 51:438–445.

553. Koppelman MCS, Jaffe MJ, Rieth KG, et al. Hyperprolactinemia, amenorrhea, and galactorrhea: a retrospective assessment of twenty-five cases. Ann Intern Med 1984; 100:115–121.

554. Corenblum B. Successful outcome of ergocryptine-induced pregnancies in twenty-one women with prolactin-secreting pituitary adenomas. Fertil Steril 1979; 32:183–186.

555. Divers WA, Yen SSC: Prolactin-producing microadenomas in pregnancy. Obstet Gynecol 1983; 62:425–429.

556. Magyar DM, Marshall JR. Pituitary tumors and pregnancy. Am J Obstet Gynecol 1978; 132:739–751.

557. Molitch ME. Pregnancy and the hyperprolactinemic woman. N Engl J Med 1985; 312:1364–1370.

558. DeWit W, Coelingh Bennink HJT, Gerards LJ. Prophylactic bromocriptine treatment during pregnancy in women with macroprolactinomas: report of 13 pregnancies. Br J Obstet Gynaecol 1984; 91:1059–1069.

559. Holmgren U, Bergstrand G, Hagenfeldt K, et al. Women with prolactinoma: effect of pregnancy and lactation on serum prolactin and on tumour growth. Acta Endocrinol 1986; 111:452–459.

560. Bohler HCL, Jones EE, Brines ML. Marginally elevated prolactin levels require magnetic resonance imagery and evaluation for acromegaly. Fertil Steril 1994; 61:1168–1170.

561. Banna M. Craniopharyngioma: based on 160 cases. Br J Radiol 1976; 49:206–223.

562. Petito CK, DeGirolami U, Earle KM. Craniopharyngiomas: a clinical and pathological review. Cancer 1976; 37:1944–1952.

563. Bevan JS, Burke CW, Esiri MM, et al. Misinterpretation of prolactin levels leading to management errors in patients with sellar enlargement. Am J Med 1987; 82:29–32.

564. Kaufman B. The "empty" sella turcica: a manifestation of the intrasellar subarachnoid space. Radiology 1968; 90:931–941.

565. Neelon FA, Goree JA, Lebovitz HE. The primary empty sella: clinical and radiographic characteristics and endocrine function. Medicine (Baltimore) 1973; 52:73–92.

566. Kletzky OA, Davajan V, Nakamura RM, et al. Clinical categorization of patients with secondary amenorrhea using progesterone-induced uterine bleeding and measurement of serum gonadotropin levels. Am J Obstet Gynecol 1975; 121:695–703.

567. Greenblatt RB. Hirsutism: ancestral curse on endocrinopathy. In: Greenblatt RB, Mahesh VB, Gambrell RD, eds. The Cause and Management of Hirsutism. Park Ridge, NJ: Parthenon, 1987: 17–29.

568. Hamilton JB. Effect of castration in adolescent and young males upon further changes in the proportions of bare and hairy scalp. J Clin Endocrinol Metab 1960; 20:1309–1318.

569. Uno H. Biology of hair growth. Semin Reprod Endocrinol 1986; 4:131–141.

570. Barbieri RL, Smith S, Ryan KJ. The role of hyperinsulinemia in the pathogenesis of ovarian hyperandrogenism. Fertil Steril 1988; 50:197–212.

571. Lobo RA. Hirsutism and virilism. In: Adashi EY, Rock JA, Rosenwaks Z, eds. Reproductive Endocrinology, Surgery and Technology. Philadelphia: Lippincott-Raven, 1996: 1257–1269.

572. Chang RJ. Ovarian steroid secretion in polycystic ovarian disease. Semin Reprod Endocrinol 1984; 2:244–250.

573. Horton R, Hawks D, Lobo RA. 3α,17β-Androstanediol glucuronide in plasma: a marker of androgen action in idiopathic hirsutism. J Clin Invest 1982; 82:1203–1207.

574. Serafini P, Ablan R, Lobo RA. 5α-Reductase activity in the genital skin of hirsute women. J Clin Endocrinol Metab 1985; 60:349–355.

575. Rebar RW. Hirsutism, hyperandrogenism, and polycystic ovarian syndrome. In: DeGroot LJ, Besser GM, Cahill GF Jr, et al, eds. Endocrinology. 2nd ed. Philadelphia: WB Saunders, 1989: 1982–1993.

576. Judd HL, Scully RE, Herbst AL, et al. Familial hyperthecosis: comparison of endocrinologic and histologic findings with polycystic ovarian disease. Am J Obstet Gynecol 1973; 117:976–982.

577. Nagamani M. Polycystic ovary syndrome variants: hyperthecosis. In: Adashi EY, Rock JA, Rosenwaks Z, eds. Reproductive Endocrinology, Surgery and Technology. Philadelphia: Lippincott-Raven, 1996: 1257–1269.

578. Nagamani M, Dinh TV, Kelver ME. Hyperinsulinemia in hyperthecosis of the ovaries. Am J Obstet Gynecol 1986; 154:384–389.

and consequently cause decreased androgen production and defective spermatogenesis, either as an isolated defect or as part of more complex pituitary insufficiency (see Chapter 9). Thus destructive lesions of the pituitary such as infarction, pituitary macroadenomas, metastatic or suprasellar tumors, infections, or granulomatous processes can cause panhypopituitarism and lead to a secondary testicular defect.

Primary isolated gonadotropin deficiency (Kallmann's syndrome) occurs in both sporadic and familial forms. The incidence of the disorder has not been established but in most centers it is second only to Klinefelter's syndrome as a cause of hypogonadism in men. The disorder was originally described by Kallmann as a familial syndrome associated with anosmia.[375] The term *Kallmann's syndrome* is now used to refer to both the sporadic and familial forms with and without anosmia, although the syndrome encompasses more than one entity. Affected individuals can sometimes be identified in childhood because of the presence of microphallus or cryptorchidism, or both.[376–379] Male urethral development is usually complete. Because major growth of the penis occurs during the latter two thirds of gestation, the presence of microphallus in this disorder has been interpreted as evidence for a role of pituitary gonadotropin in regulating testosterone production only during the later portion of gestation. The growth pattern in childhood is normal although bone age is usually retarded.

Most affected individuals are identified because of a failure to undergo puberty.[380] A subset of individuals, particularly familial cases, has associated congenital defects, commonly anomalies involving the midline facial and head structures, and partial deficiencies of other pituitary hormones.[381, 382] At the opposite end of the spectrum less severely affected individuals have only partial defects in the production of FSH or LH, or both. This variant, which was originally known as the fertile eunuch syndrome, is even harder to separate from delayed puberty than is the typical disorder.[383–386] Isolated gonadotropin deficiency, of both sporadic and familial types, is less common in women than in men but when present is usually manifested as primary amenorrhea and sexual infantilism associated with disturbances of smell.[387–389]

The pattern of inheritance in most families is compatible either with X-linkage or autosomal transmission with primary manifestations in males.[375, 390, 391] More than one mutant gene may be responsible for the phenotype because certain familial cases that are associated with midline abnormalities appear to be due to an autosomal recessive mutation[381] and because mutations in the *DAX1* gene on the X chromosome cause combined X-linked congenital adrenal hypoplasia and hypogonadism.[392] Half or more of patients have a negative family history, which suggests that new mutations may be common. The underlying defect in most patients is at the hypothalamic level; after short-term administration of LHRH, plasma LH and FSH levels increase in about half of individuals.[393–396] After repetitive treatment for 5 d or longer plasma gonadotropin levels rise to the normal range in most individuals with Kallmann's syndrome but not in individuals with panhypopituitarism.[330, 397, 398] The more severe the deficiency the longer LHRH must be administered to correct gonadotropin secretion.[399]

Santoro and colleagues showed that the disorder encompasses defects in the pulsatile release of LHRH, including total absence of LH secretion, defects in the amplitude and frequency of LH secretion, and altered bioactivity of the gonadotropin released.[400] Consequently it is most appropriate to view the disorder as a spectrum of defects of LH secretion that includes the typical Kallmann's syndrome, the fertile eunuch syndrome, and even less severe defects. The common defect involves neurogenic control mechanisms that regulate LHRH release.[401] The neurons that secrete LHRH originate in the olfactory placode of the fetus and migrate into the brain with the olfactory, terminalis, and vomeronasal nerves; the defect in this disorder is believed to impair the migration of these nerves thus accounting for the LHRH deficiency, the olfactory disturbance, and the hypoplasia of the olfactory bulbs. The genetic locus for X-linked Kallmann's syndrome has been assigned to Xp23.3, and the gene has been cloned and predicts a protein with homology to neural cell adhesion molecules.[402] Of 19 patients with X-linked Kallmann's syndrome, different point mutations in the coding sequence were identified in 9 patients.[403]

In the presence of olfactory disturbances, other midline defects, a positive family history, or a combination of these factors, the diagnosis is not difficult to establish either in an infant with microphallus or an undervirilized adult. In patients with anosmia or hyposomia defects of the rhinencephalon may be demonstrated by magnetic resonance imaging.[404] In older individuals without midline abnormalities or anosmia and with uninformative family histories, the diagnosis can be made (after the presence of a pituitary tumor is excluded) by documenting a normal acute response to LHRH administration after a week of LHRH treatment. This technique is rarely performed in practice. The separation in the middle teen years of individuals with hypogonadotropic hypogonadism from those with delayed puberty may require prolonged observation (see Chapter 31).

Three forms of therapy can be used: androgen replacement to virilize, gonadotropin therapy to induce fertility, and administration of LHRH analogues to replace the deficit in the most physiological way possible. In the infant or the young child with microphallus the administration of testosterone for limited periods (3 mo) may cause enlargement of the penis to the normal range without affecting linear growth or causing other significant virilization.[272, 405] In the older child or the adult, long-acting testosterone esters are administered parenterally, as for other forms of hypogonadism.[286] Also, as in other forms of androgen deficiency, the nearer the time of onset of normal puberty that replacement therapy is begun, the more effective the promotion of normal virilization. Administration of hCG over the long term also causes serum testosterone levels to increase to normal adult male levels,[406–408] but in individuals with severe (prepubertal) hypogonadotropic hypogonadism the induction of fertility usually requires the administration of FSH, in the form of human menopausal gonadotropin, in addition to hCG.[409] The response to gonadotropin therapy in this disorder is not influenced by prior testosterone therapy[410] but is a function of the initial testis size, men with testes less than 4 mL in volume responding less favorably.[411] After a normal sperm count is achieved it may be maintained by use of hCG or, occasionally, testosterone esters.[412] In occasional patients with partial defects in gonadotropin secretion spermatogenesis can be promoted by testosterone therapy alone.[413] The long-term administration of LHRH in a pulsatile manner to men with hypogonadotropic hypogonadism results in normal plasma testosterone levels, normal pulsatile secretion of LH, normal mean levels of plasma LH and FSH and, in most, mature sperm in the ejaculate.[414, 415] After the induction of spermatogenesis by such treatment normal spermatogenesis in one study was maintained by nasal administration of LHRH.[416]

Another syndrome associated with hypogonadotropic hypogonadism is the Prader-Willi syndrome of obesity, short stature, mental retardation, and hypotonia caused by deletions or uniparenteral disomy of chromosome 15.[417]

Acquired gonadotropin deficiency can be caused by factors other than pathologic conditions of the hypothalamus or pituitary. For example elevated plasma cortisol levels, as in Cushing's syndrome, can depress LH secretion independently of a space-occupying lesion of the pituitary.[392, 418–420] The serum LH level in these men, as in other forms of secondary testicular dysfunction, is usually in the normal range and only occasionally decreased. However it is inappropriately low for the depressed serum testosterone level. Even when Cushing's syndrome is due to a pituitary adenoma the hypogonadotropic hypogonadism appears to be secondary to the hypercortisolism because treatment by bilateral adrenalectomy or mitotane results in return of testosterone levels to normal.[418, 419] Chronic administration of exogenous glucocorticoids can also lower testosterone levels by inhibiting LHRH secretion.[420]

Hyperprolactinemia also causes secondary testicular dysfunction. Hyperprolactinemia can be produced by either microadenomas or macroadenomas of the pituitary. Macroadenomas may give rise to hyperprolactinema either because of direct secretion by the tumor (prolactinomas) or because of interference with the delivery of normal inhibitory influences from the hypothalamus to the pituitary by the mass effect of a nonsecretory tumor. Hypogonadism can result from hyperprolactinemia itself, destruction of the normal pituitary, or a combination of these effects. Prolactin excess by itself can cause both underandrogenization and infertility and lead to impotence,[421–423] probably by impairing LHRH release. Most men with hyperprolactinemia respond to administration of LHRH with a normal increase in plasma LH level.[421–423] The administration of low doses of bromocriptine to some patients with microadenomas causes an initial increase in plasma LH level and a subsequent increase in serum testosterone level.[424] Impotence associated with hyperprolactinemia is not always due to a decreased serum testosterone level because some hyperprolactinemic men given testosterone replacement do not have return of potency until the prolactin levels are corrected by the administration of bromocriptine.[423] In part because of delays in seeking evaluation, men with prolactin-secreting pituitary adenomas usually have macroadenomas at the time of diagnosis.[421–423] When a macroadenoma is present it is critical to document that deficiencies of other pituitary hormones do not coexist with the hyperprolactinemia (see Chapter 9). After surgery for macroadenomas the plasma prolactin level does not usually return to normal[425] but may respond to bromocriptine.[426]

Idiopathic hemochromatosis causes iron deposition in the pituitary and testes[427] and about half of affected men have hypogonadism, usually accompanied by testicular atrophy. The abnormalities of testicular function in this disorder may in part result from the associated liver disease[427] but most testicular dysfunction is due to hypogonadotropic hypogonadism.[428–432] The pituitary nature of the hypogonadism was recognized because of the lack of response of LH to LHRH stimulation[429, 431, 432] and the normal response of plasma testosterone to hCG.[431, 432] However occasionally men with hemochromatosis have an elevated LH level associated with low testosterone levels, suggesting that a primary testicular abnormality may also occur.[430] Acquired transfusional iron overload can cause similar abnormalities of the pituitary-testicular axis.[433]

Hypothalamic or pituitary injury can occur after head trauma even in the absence of fracture, and the most common manifestation is deficiency of gonadotropins and human growth hormone, although multiple deficiencies can be present. Clinical evidence of hormone deficiency may be apparent immediately after injury or not until years later.[434]

In several other conditions the testosterone levels may be decreased in association with normal LH levels and the mechanism is less clear. Men with massive obesity have decreased TeBG levels and decreased levels of total and bioavailable testosterone that return toward normal with weight loss.[435] In men with a body mass index greater than 40, the free testosterone levels, LH levels, and LH pulse amplitude are decreased, implying malfunction of the hypothalamic-pituitary system.[436] Obesity may be the cause of decreased testosterone levels in the pickwickian syndrome.[437] Some men with tempo-

ral lobe seizures have hormonal findings consistent with hypogonadotropic hypogonadism.[438] Finally, hypogonadotropic hypogonadism may occur as an acquired idiopathic disorder.[439, 440]

Testicular Disorders. Abnormalities of testicular function in the adult can be grouped into several categories: developmental and structural defects of the testes, acquired testicular defects, abnormalities associated with systemic or neurologic diseases, and androgen resistance.

Developmental and Structural Defects. The most common developmental defect of the testis is Klinefelter's syndrome (see also Chapter 29). The disorder is characterized by small, firm testes; various degrees of impaired sexual maturation; azoospermia; gynecomastia; and elevated gonadotropin levels.[441] The underlying defect is the presence of an extra X chromosome,[442–444] the usual chromosomal karyotype being either 47,XXY (classic form) or 46,XY/47,XXY (mosaic form). The incidence is approximately 1 in 500 males.[445]

Prepubertal boys with Klinefelter's syndrome have small testes with a decreased number of spermatogonia but are otherwise normal.[446] The diagnosis is usually made after the time of expected puberty because of the development of gynecomastia or underandrogenization, or both, and later by infertility (Table 16–5). Damage to the seminiferous tubules and azoospermia are consistent features of the 47,XXY variety. The small, firm testes are usually less than 2 cm and always less than 3.5 cm in length (corresponding to 2 and 12 mL volumes, respectively).[447, 448] Typical histologic changes in the testes include hyalinization of the tubules, absence of spermatogenesis, and an apparent increase in the number of Leydig cells (see Fig. 16–17C).[449]

The increased mean body height is the result of a longer lower body segment; the fact that this feature is present before puberty suggests that it is not secondary to androgen deficiency but is probably related to the underlying chromosomal abnormality.[450] Gynecomastia occurs in about 85% of patients[442]; it develops during adolescence, is usually bilateral and painless, and may become disfiguring.[442] Obesity and varicose veins occur in a third to a half of individuals,[45] and mild mental deficiency or social maladjustment, or both,[452, 453] subtle abnormalities of thyroid function,[454] diabetes mellitus,[446] and restrictive pulmonary disease[455] are more common. The risk of breast cancer is 20 times that of normal men, although the incidence is only about a fifth of that for women.[456, 457] Most individuals have a male psychosexual orientation and function sexually as men.

46,XY/47,XXY mosaicism is the cause of about 10% of cases of Klinefelter's syndrome, as estimated by chromosomal karyotypes of peripheral blood leukocytes. The true prevalence may be underestimated because chromosomal mosa-

TABLE 16–5. Characteristics of Patients with Classic Versus Mosaic Klinefelter's Syndrome*

Characteristic	47,XXY (%)	47,XY/47,XXY (%)
Abnormal testicular histologic features	100	94†
Decreased length of testis	99	73†
Azoospermia	93	50†
Decreased testosterone level	79	33
Decreased facial hair	77	64†
Increased gonadotropin level	75	33
Decreased sexual function	68	56
Gynecomastia	55	33†
Decreased axillary hair	49	46
Decreased length of penis	41	21

*Table based on 519 47,XXY patients and 51 46,XY/47,XXY patients.
†Significantly different at $P < .05$ or better.
Data from Gordon DL, Krmpotic E, Thomas W, et al. Pathologic testicular findings in Klinefelter's syndrome. 47,XXY vs. 46,XY-47,XXY. Arch Intern Med 1972; 130:720–729.

icism can be present in the testes in individuals in whom the chromosomal karyotype of peripheral leukocytes is normal.[442, 443] As summarized in Table 16–5 the manifestations of the mosaic form are usually less severe than with the 47,XXY variety and the testes may be normal in size.[443] The endocrine abnormalities are also less severe and gynecomastia and azoospermia are less common. Occasional patients with the mosaic form may even be fertile.[458] In some individuals the diagnosis may not be suspected because of the minor degree of the associated abnormalities.

Approximately 30 additional karyotypic varieties of Klinefelter's syndrome have been described, including those with uniform cell lines (such as 48,XXYY, 48,XXXY, and 49,XXXXY) and a number of mosaicisms of the X chromosome with or without associated structural abnormalities of the X chromosome. 48,XXYY individuals have a more severe degree of mental retardation and antisocial behavior,[459] and 49,XXXXY individuals may have cryptorchidism and bone abnormalities.[460]

The 47,XXY form of Klinefelter's syndrome is due to meiotic nondisjunction of the chromosomes during gametogenesis. About 40% of the responsible meiotic nondisjunctions occur in the father and 60% occur in the mother. Advanced maternal age is a predisposing factor in the latter cases.[461] The mosaic form of the disorder, in contrast, results from chromosomal mitotic nondisjunction after fertilization of the zygote and can arise either in a 46,XY zygote or a 47,XXY zygote. The latter situation (double nondisjunction, meiotic and mitotic) may be the usual cause of the mosaic form and thus explain why the mosaic form is less common than the 47,XXY disorder.[462]

Characteristic endocrine changes include elevation of plasma FSH and LH levels. FSH shows the best discrimination and little overlap occurs with normal individuals, a consequence of the consistent damage to the seminiferous tubules.[444] In the late teens the plasma testosterone level may be normal.[463, 464] By the middle 20s the plasma testosterone level averages half the normal value but the range is broad and overlaps the normal range.[442, 444, 463, 464] Mean plasma estradiol levels are elevated[465] and TeBG levels are about twice normal.[466] The reasons for the elevated plasma estradiol level (and the development of gynecomastia) are complex. In adolescence the plasma testosterone level is kept in the normal range at the expense of an elevated plasma LH value, and estradiol secretion by the testes is increased. As testicular function becomes more impaired testicular secretion of both testosterone and estradiol decreases. Eventually estrogen in these men is almost exclusively derived from extraglandular aromatization of adrenal androgen; at this point estrogen formation, although low, is high relative to that of testosterone. The net result both early and late is a variable degree of feminization and insufficient androgenization. The feminization, including the development of gynecomastia, is thought to depend on the ratio of circulating estrogen to androgen (see Chapter 17). The lower the plasma testosterone and the higher the plasma estradiol levels, the more likely the development of gynecomastia. After the age of expected puberty the increase in plasma gonadotropin after LHRH administration is exaggerated[467] and the feedback inhibition of testosterone on pituitary LH secretion is diminished.[468] Older men with untreated Klinefelter's syndrome may have an enlarged or an abnormal sella turcica, presumably secondary to the impairment of gonadal steroid feedback and gonadotrope hyperplasia.[469]

No method is available for reversing the infertility if no germ cells are present, and mastectomy is the only satisfactory treatment for gynecomastia. Some underandrogenized patients benefit from supplemental androgen,[451, 470] but such treatment may paradoxically worsen the gynecomastia, pre-

sumably by providing increased substrate for the conversion to estrogens in peripheral tissues. Androgen treatment in the form of testosterone cypionate or testosterone enanthate usually causes plasma LH levels to return to normal but only after several months.[468]

The XX male syndrome, a variant of Klinefelter's syndrome, occurs in approximately 1 in 20,000 to 1 in 24,000 male births.[471] More than 150 XX males have been described.[472] The findings resemble those in Klinefelter's syndrome: the testes are small and firm, generally less than 2 cm long; gynecomastia is usual; the penis is normal to small in size; and azoospermia and hyalinization of the seminiferous tubules are present. Affected individuals have male psychosexual identification and an absence of female internal genitalia. The mean plasma testosterone concentration is low and levels of plasma estradiol and gonadotropins are high.[473, 474] Affected individuals differ from typical patients with Klinefelter's syndrome in that the average height is less than that of normal men,[466] the incidence of mental deficiency is not increased,[466] and hypospadias is common.[475]

Four theories have been proposed to explain male development in the absence of a Y chromosome: (1) mosaicism in some tissues for a Y chromosome–containing cell line; (2) a gain of function mutation for some autosomal gene; (3) deletion or inactivation of some gene or genes that normally suppress testicular development; and (4) interchange of a portion of the Y chromosome with the X chromosome.[467] Evidence has now been obtained for the presence of mechanisms 1 and 4 in 46,XX sex reversal. Y chromosome sequences are detectable in approximately two thirds of 46,XX men and are present in the distal region of the X chromosome.[476–478] Thus in most XX males the cause is presumably analogous to that in the sxr mouse, in which a critical fragment of the Y chromosome has been translocated to the X chromosome.[479] The other third of 46,XX men are "Y-negative" and lack sequences for SRY. Clinically the two groups differ in that the Y-negative group is more likely to have ambiguity of the external genitalia, whereas the Y-positive group has the Klinefelter phenotype.[476–478] The translocated region of the Y can be quite small and involve only the SRY gene itself. In one study of 10 46,XX men, 6 had the SRY gene on the distal end of the X chromosome, 1 had mosaicism so that an intact Y chromosome was present in 1% of cells, and 3 lacked Y sequences by both Southern blotting and polymerase chain reaction (PCR) analysis; the cause of the disorder in the latter group is unknown.[480] These findings document the heterogeneity of the disorder. The management is similar to that for Klinefelter's syndrome.

Acquired Defects. The most common cause of acquired testicular failure in the adult is viral orchitis.[481] Mumps virus is most frequent, followed by echovirus, lymphocytic choriomeningitis virus, and group B arboviruses.[482] The orchitis is due to actual invasion of the tissue by the virus rather than to indirect effects of infection.[483] Orchitis is a common complication of mumps, occurring in as many as a fourth of adult men with the disease.[484] In about two thirds of cases it is unilateral. It usually develops a few days after the onset of parotitis but occasionally precedes it. During acute orchitis the plasma LH and FSH levels are elevated and the plasma testosterone level is decreased.[484] After the acute inflammatory phase the testis gradually decreases in size, although swelling can persist for months. The testis may return to normal size and function or undergo atrophy. The atrophy results from both the direct effects of the virus and ischemia caused by pressure and edema within the taut tunica albuginea. The histologic features of the atrophic testis include progressive tubular sclerosis and hyalinization; the findings are sometimes similar to those in Klinefelter's syndrome. Even when only one testis is involved clinically degenerative changes can occur in the other.

The degree of atrophy is not necessarily proportional to the severity of the orchitis. It is usually apparent within 1 to 6 mo after the orchitis subsides, but the full extent of damage may not be evident for many years. Atrophy occurs in approximately one third of men who acquire orchitis and is bilateral in about a tenth.[481] The hormonal changes associated with gynecomastia due to mumps orchitis include normal extraglandular estrogen formation from adrenal androgens and a profound decrease in testosterone production.[485] The frequency with which mumps results in infertility is not known.[486] Almost half of men with unilateral mumps orchitis have sperm densities of less than 10 million/mL in the first 3 mo, but within 1 to 2 y the sperm count returns to normal in about three fourths of individuals.[487] In contrast semen parameters return to normal in less than a third of men with bilateral orchitis.[487] The initial treatment of mumps orchitis is bed rest and scrotal support. If severe pain is present the administration of prednisone often results in prompt defervescence and reduction of swelling and pain.[488] Glucocorticoid therapy does not appear to have a beneficial effect on the return of the sperm count to normal.[487]

Trauma is second to viral orchitis as a cause of testicular atrophy in the adult. The exposed position of the testis in the scrotum renders it uniquely susceptible to both thermal and physical damage.

Both spermatogenesis and testosterone production are sensitive to *radiation;* the diminished secretion of testosterone appears to be a consequence of diminished testicular blood flow.[489] Although doses of radiation as low as 0.2 Gy (20 rad) result in temporary increases of both LH and FSH levels and damage to spermatogonia, a permanent decrease in testosterone production is uncommon.[490] However a tenth of patients receiving approximately 8 Gy (800 rad) of scattered radiation to the testes during childhood[491] and most boys receiving 24 to 30 Gy (2400 to 3000 rad) of direct testicular radiation for acute lymphoblastic leukemia[492] have permanently low plasma testosterone levels (see the section later on infertility with normal virilization.)

Drugs can cause underandrogenization and infertility in several ways: direct inhibition of testosterone synthesis, blockade of the peripheral actions of androgen, and enhancement of estrogen levels. In addition, agents such as propranolol and guanethidine can impair erectile function in men whose hypothalamic-pituitary-testicular axis is normal.[493]

Two drugs that in high doses block testosterone synthesis are spironolactone and cyproterone, both of which interfere with the late reactions in testosterone biosynthesis.[494, 495] Spironolactone appears to impair 17α-hydroxylase and 17,20-lyase activities.[494] Plasma testosterone levels do not change appreciably, however, during usual therapeutic regimens.[494] The antifungal agent ketoconazole blocks testosterone synthesis,[301] also by inhibiting the 17,20-lyase and 17α-hydroxylase reactions.[496] The decrease in testosterone after a single dose of ketoconazole is transient, with the nadir occurring 4 to 8 h after administration and returning to baseline by 24 h as ketoconazole concentrations fall. However with doses of ketoconazole greater than 400 mg/d, depression of plasma testosterone levels may be sustained.[497] The agent also inhibits the cortisol response to corticotropin.[497] Tetracycline has been reported to lower testosterone levels about 20% during short-term administration.[498] Impairment of libido is common in men with epilepsy, partly as a consequence of medication.[499, 500] Enzyme-inducing antiepileptic drugs such as phenytoin and carbamazepine lower bioavailable testosterone, raise plasma TeBG and LH levels, and decrease the metabolic clearance of testosterone.[501] The effect is more pronounced with multiple-drug regimens.[499, 500] Valproic acid does not appear to have as severe an adverse effect in this regard.[500]

Independent of its effects on the liver ethanol ingestion

reduces testosterone levels acutely and chronically,[502] the result of inhibition of testosterone synthesis.[503–507] In men without liver disease who are given 40% of food intake as alcohol, a 25 to 50% decrease in the plasma testosterone level and production rate is demonstrable within 5 d after starting the regimen and these effects last as long as 3 wk.[503] In alcohol-fed rats the decrease in plasma testosterone level is accompanied by testicular atrophy.[504] Smaller amounts of ethanol decrease only the testicular response to gonadotropin.[505] The inhibition of steroidogenesis appears to occur at the 3β-hydroxysteroid dehydrogenase reaction as the result of a decrease in the concentration or availability, or both, of the pyridine nucleotide cofactors for the reaction,[506] probably mediated by the ethanol metabolite acetaldehyde.[507] The fact that the lower testosterone levels in most men given alcohol are not accompanied by appropriate elevations of plasma LH suggests that hypothalamic-pituitary function is also impaired.[502, 503] Ethanol may also interfere with the capacitation of sperm[508] and increase the number of morphologic abnormalities in epididymal sperm.[509]

Antineoplastic and chemotherapeutic agents, especially cyclophosphamide, commonly induce infertility (see later). Combination chemotherapy for acute leukemia, Hodgkin's disease, and other malignancies may also impair Leydig cell function.[510–512] In pubertal boys this effect is manifested by decreased serum testosterone levels, elevated plasma LH, and marked gynecomastia.[510, 511] In adult men the testosterone levels do not decline, and the impaired Leydig cell function is detectable only by an exaggerated LH response to LHRH.[512] This toxic effect on the Leydig cell seems to be produced primarily by alkylating agents such as cyclophosphamide because pubertal boys given other regimens for acute lymphoblastic leukemia may not develop testicular dysfunction.[513] Treatment with alkylating agents during the prepubertal years does not interfere with testicular function in later life.[510] High-dose interleukin-2 therapy for metastatic cancer causes a transient reduction in serum testosterone levels.[514]

Plasma testosterone levels may be low in men ingesting large amounts of marihuana, heroin, or methadone.[515–517] In general, elevations of plasma LH do not occur, suggesting a combined hypothalamic-pituitary and testicular abnormality. Studies of the effects of marihuana on the pituitary-testicular axis in animals also suggest a dual inhibition.[518–520] Testosterone synthesis by mouse testes in vitro is reduced more than 80% by addition of the marihuana component tetrahydrocannabinol,[518] and plasma LH levels in mice decline after administration of a single oral dose of tetrahydrocannabinol.[519] In addition marihuana may have a direct inhibitory effect on sperm motility.[521]

Elevated plasma estradiol levels and decreased plasma testosterone levels may be present in men taking digitalis preparations, the mechanism being unclear.[522] Drugs can interfere with gonadotropin production either as the result of a direct inhibition[523, 524] (as in medroxyprogesterone acetate administration) or as a secondary consequence of enhanced prolactin secretion.[525] Medroxyprogesterone acetate also seems to decrease testosterone secretion at the testicular level.[526]

Several drugs inhibit androgen action by competition at the receptor level. Although spironolactone can inhibit testosterone synthesis, in the usual dosage regimens it acts primarily by antagonizing androgen binding to the androgen receptor, which leads to gynecomastia and impotence.[494] Cyproterone also acts as an androgen antagonist.[495] The most commonly administered drug that is an androgen antagonist is cimetidine,[527–529] which binds to androgen receptors in vitro.[528] Gynecomastia can occur in men who are treated with the drug, and decreased sperm density and elevated basal testosterone levels are accompanied by a slight diminution of the LH response to LHRH.[527] Ranitidine appears to be a less potent antiandrogen.[529] Omeprazole can also cause gynecomastia or impotence, or both.[530]

Prolonged exposure of men to lead as an *environmental toxin* results in direct testicular toxicity, with an impaired pituitary response as indicated by a slight plasma LH elevation.[531] Similar hormonal changes have been documented in an animal model of lead toxicity.[532]

Testicular failure can occur as part of a generalized *autoimmune* disorder in which multiple primary endocrine deficiencies coexist and in which circulating antibodies to the basement membrane of the testes can be documented (see Chapter 33).[533, 534]

The testis can also be a site of involvement in *granulomatous disease*. Testicular atrophy occurs in 10 to 20% of men with lepromatous leprosy as the result of direct invasion of the tissue (and in some instances the paratesticular structures as well) by the bacilli. The tubules are involved initially, followed by endarteritis and destruction of Leydig cells. The result is a decreased plasma testosterone level and elevated plasma LH and FSH levels.[535] Destruction of the testis is less common in other systemic granulomatous diseases.

Defects Associated with Systemic Diseases. Abnormalities of the hypothalamic-pituitary-testicular axis occur in a number of systemic diseases. Given the chronic ill health and generalized wasting that may occur with these disorders, it is often difficult to distinguish effects specifically caused by the underlying condition (e.g., renal failure) from those attributable to malnutrition.

About half of men undergoing dialysis for *renal failure* experience decreased libido and impotence associated with impairments in both spermatogenesis and testosterone biosynthesis.[536] The defect in spermatogenesis varies from partial to total destruction of the germ cells.[537, 538] The plasma testosterone level is decreased and plasma LH and FSH levels are increased, indicating a defect at the testicular level.[538-540] However, hypothalamic function may be impaired, as suggested by reduced pulsatile secretion of LH and a subnormal increase in gonadotropin levels in response to the low testosterone.[541] Plasma testosterone production rates are decreased[539] and the response of plasma testosterone to hCG is subnormal.[538, 542] In Leydig cells that are isolated from uremic rats, impaired responsiveness to hCG correlates with a diminished number of LH-hCG receptors. The addition of cAMP, however, does not completely repair the defect in testosterone synthesis, suggesting an impairment distal to cAMP production as well.[543] After dialysis plasma testosterone levels and testosterone production rates improve but usually not to the normal range.[538, 539, 542, 543] One potential mechanism for the testicular abnormalities in renal failure is estrogen excess. Androgen-estrogen dynamics have not been examined in detail but the low testosterone levels coupled with normal or increased plasma estrogen levels[544] probably account for the development of gynecomastia in about half of men undergoing chronic hemodialysis. Hyperprolactinemia occurs in a fourth of men receiving long-term dialysis,[545] and treatment with bromocriptine to lower prolactin levels may raise testosterone levels and restore potency in some.[546] There does not appear to be much difference in most parameters of testicular function before and after dialysis.[538] By contrast, successful renal transplantation causes a return of testosterone and prolactin levels to normal and a slight decrease in LH and FSH levels.[547, 548] Most men experience improved sexual function after transplantation, and half have sperm densities of more than 10 million/mL.[547]

The effects of *cirrhosis of the liver* on testicular function occur independent of the direct toxic effects of ethanol. Gynecomastia and testicular atrophy are present in half of men with cirrhosis, and three fourths of men with hepatic cirrhosis are impotent.[549] Histologic evidence of decreased spermatogenesis and peritubular fibrosis are present in about half of patients. The plasma estradiol level is usually elevated and the plasma testosterone level is decreased.[549, 550] The net result is a ratio in serum of unbound estradiol to unbound testosterone of about 10 times normal.[550] Levels of TeBG are about twice normal. The metabolic clearance and production rates of testosterone are decreased and estradiol production is increased.[549] Extraglandular conversion of androgens, primarily adrenal androgens, to estradiol and estrone is increased about threefold, presumably because of decreased hepatic extraction of androgens.[551] Basal levels of LH and FSH range from normal to moderately elevated.[549, 552] In men with low testosterone levels pulsatile LH secretion is impaired, implying a defect at the level of the hypothalamus-pituitary,[553] whereas dynamic tests of the pituitary-testicular axis and hCG responsiveness tests point to a testicular defect.[549, 552] The increase in plasma LH after the administration of LHRH is normal in most men with cirrhosis, but in men with testicular atrophy the plasma FSH response is enhanced; the degree of LH responsiveness correlates inversely with the response of testosterone to hCG.[554] Thus modest elevation of basal LH and FSH levels, coupled with the lack of hyperresponsiveness to LHRH, suggests that the hypothalamic-pituitary response to the diminished testosterone levels is blunted. The reason for abnormality in testicular function and in the hypothalamic-pituitary response is uncertain. Elevated estrogen levels could cause both defects. Alternatively, basal prolactin levels are elevated on average fourfold in men with cirrhosis,[555] and the increased prolactin could also have an effect on the pituitary-testicular axis.

Testosterone therapy has been tried.[556] Although estradiol levels increased (in direct correlation with the severity of the cirrhosis) after administration of testosterone enanthate, the estrogen/androgen ratio became normal.[556] Whether such therapy is beneficial in the long term is not known, but treatment of 24 cirrhotic men for 4 wk did not cause worsening of gynecomastia or liver function.[557] Men with alcoholic cirrhosis may have spontaneous recovery of sexual function when they abstain from alcohol, despite the persistence of liver abnormalities.[558] However men with alcoholic cirrhosis and testicular atrophy are less likely to experience improvement in sexual function with abstinence from alcohol.[558] Sexual function and testosterone levels are also decreased in men with other forms of liver disease.[559] The hormonal abnormalities in the pituitary-testicular axis can be reversed by liver transplantation.[560]

Boys with *sickle cell anemia* have impaired sexual maturation in adolescence.[561-563] Furthermore in 32 adult men with sickle cell anemia, secondary sexual characteristics were subnormal in all but 2 men and testicular atrophy was noted in about a third.[562] Testicular biopsy in two men revealed maturation arrest of spermatogenesis. The defect may be either testicular[562] or hypothalamic.[563]

Abnormalities in Leydig cell function, which are frequently accompanied by decreased sperm counts, occur in a variety of chronic systemic diseases including *protein-calorie malnutrition*,[564] advanced *Hodgkin's disease* and *cancer* before chemotherapy,[565, 566] *cystic fibrosis*,[577] and *amyloidosis*.[568] Except for amyloidosis these disorders cause a lowered plasma testosterone level and either a normal or slightly increased plasma LH level, suggesting combined hypothalamic-pituitary and testicular defects. The low plasma testosterone level is not the result of inhibitors that interfere with the binding to TeBG and hence is not analogous to the euthyroid sick syndrome.[569] Indeed because the mean plasma TeBG is elevated, the bioavailable testosterone may be even lower than the total testosterone.[570] The previously mentioned pattern of changes in testosterone and LH may be nonspecific effects of illness because similar changes occur after *surgery*,[571, 572] *myocardial infarction*,[573] and *severe burns*.[574, 575] Severe illness has less effect on Sertoli cell function as assessed by measurement of serum inhibin.[576]

The changes in the hypothalamic-pituitary-testicular axis in *thyrotoxicosis* may be secondary to increased estrogen levels and include decreased sperm count and semen volume, increased plasma total testosterone level, and normal levels of unbound testosterone.[577] The testosterone response to hCG is blunted and basal LH levels are increased.[577]

Immune disease may cause testicular dysfunction and laboratory evidence of primary or secondary hypogonadism is common in men with acquired immunodeficiency syndrome (AIDS), about half of whom have low testosterone levels without an appropriate increase in plasma LH.[578] Although the disease may involve the testes directly, the hormonal changes are suggestive of a nonspecific response to systemic illness. The central question in regard to the testosterone deficiency in this illness is whether it contributes to the weight loss and muscle wasting. Although AIDS patients with wasting have lower testosterone levels than do those without weight loss, it is unclear whether hypogonadism is causal in this regard because coexisting factors such as medications, infections, and stage of illness could contribute to the low testosterone.[579] The current practice is to prescribe androgen replacement in AIDS patients with testosterone deficiency and clinical evidence of hypogonadism.[578] Additional studies will have to be performed to assess the benefits of androgen therapy for weight loss in these patients. Men with rheumatoid arthritis may have low serum testosterone, particularly during disease flares. Testosterone levels are usually normal in men with long-standing, stable rheumatoid arthritis, except those receiving glucocorticoid therapy, in whom testosterone may be low.[580]

Neurologic disease can cause testicular abnormalities. Men with myotonic dystrophy usually have small testes, low plasma testosterone levels, and elevated plasma LH and FSH levels.[581-584] Spinal bulbar muscular atrophy is a form of adult-onset degenerative motor neuropathy associated with gynecomastia, testicular atrophy, a hormonal profile suggestive of androgen resistance (see later) and an expansion of the homopolymeric glutamine repeat region in the amino-terminal end of the androgen receptor gene.[585] Although the effects are variable, spinal cord lesions that cause quadriplegia or paraplegia initially cause diminished plasma testosterone levels that generally return toward normal, but defective spermatogenesis appears to persist.[586, 587] Some patients retain the capacity to obtain erections and ejaculate, depending on the extent of involvement of the lumbosacral spinal cord.[588]

Men with trisomy 21 have impairment of both germinal and Leydig cell function. Plasma FSH and LH levels are elevated.[589]

Androgen Resistance. A limited form of androgen resistance results in underandrogenization and infertility in men with normal external genitalia.[590] Some men from a family with Reifenstein's syndrome were noticed to have gynecomastia and infertility without the usual hypospadias, but associated with the same abnormality in the androgen receptor as more severely affected members of the same family.[182] Subsequently men with a negative family history and apparent idiopathic infertility were found to have androgen resistance, as characterized by increased testosterone production, elevations of plasma LH levels in some, and abnormal androgen receptors in cultured genital skin fibroblasts.[590] Only one of the initial three men had gynecomastia, and virilization was normal in the other two. Subsequently in a study of unselected men with idiopathic infertility, 40% of those with idiopathic azoospermia had androgen receptor deficiency.[591] The presence of elevated testosterone or LH levels, or both, is not a reliable predictor of which men have a receptor defect. Testicular biopsy results for five affected men showed maturation arrests or germinal cell aplasia similar to that shown in Figure 16–17D and E.[591]

Another severe manifestation of androgen receptor mutations has been observed in men with gynecomastia, undervirilization and, in some, fertility.[592, 593] Point mutations have been identified in the hormone-binding domain of the androgen receptor in men with the isolated infertility and undervirilized, fertile male phenotypes.[594, 595]

INFERTILITY WITH NORMAL VIRILIZATION. Some conditions lead to isolated infertility and thus a separate group of diagnoses should be considered in the evaluation of infertile men with normal Leydig cell function. Isolated infertility can be due to defects in the hypothalamic-pituitary system, the testis, or the sperm transport system (see Table 16–4).

Hypothalamic-Pituitary Disorders. Isolated FSH deficiency has been reported in men in whom virilization, plasma LH levels, and plasma testosterone levels were normal but the plasma FSH level was persistently low.[596] Plasma FSH levels in such men increase after LHRH stimulation.[596] Hyperprolactinemia occasionally leads to infertility alone but more commonly also causes impotence and low testosterone levels (see earlier). In occasional patients with infertility as the sole manifestation bromocriptine treatment that corrects the hyperprolactinemia returns the sperm count to normal.[597] In some men with chronic untreated or undertreated congenital adrenal hyperplasia due to 21-hydroxylase deficiency, gonadotropin secretion is suppressed as the result of overproduction of adrenal androgens, and infertility is a consequence.[598] This diagnosis is suggested by the presence of small testes, normal to elevated levels of testosterone, and suppressed levels of gonadotropins and is confirmed by finding elevated plasma levels of 17-hydroxyprogesterone and androstenedione (see Chapters 12 and 29).[598]

When androgens are administered in pharmacologic doses to normal men, gonadotropins are suppressed and about half of men experience azoospermia (see Chapter 18). Although men who present with isolated infertility are unlikely to be receiving testosterone replacement therapy the use of androgens by weightlifters and bodybuilders is common. Self-prescribed regimens may include parenteral testosterone esters and a variety of oral and parenteral substituted androgens, often termed *anabolic steroids* (see later). Anabolic steroids can cause reversible azoospermia in normal men.[599]

Testicular Disorders

Developmental and Structural Defects. *Germinal cell aplasia* is a poorly understood defect of the testis (the Sertoli-cell–only syndrome). This term encompasses histologic features that can result from several causes. In some instances the disorder appears to be due to a single-gene defect. Other patients with the typical histologic and clinical features have a history of viral orchitis, cryptorchidism,[600, 601] alcoholism,[602] or androgen resistance.[591] The distinguishing feature of the testicular biopsy is complete absence of germinal elements (see Fig. 16–17E). The clinical features include azoospermia, normal virilization, absence of gynecomastia, normal to small testes, and normal chromosomal complement. Plasma testosterone and LH values are usually normal and plasma FSH values are high.[603] This disorder (or histologic entity) apparently accounts for a tenth to a third of men with azoospermia.[601, 604]

The concept of germinal cell aplasia became even more complex with the recognition that a Y chromosome determinant other than the *SRY* gene is essential for spermatogenesis.[605] Six men were found to have a deletion of the long arm of the Y chromosome. This region was postulated to encode an azoospermia factor (AZF) and was subsequently mapped to Yq11.23.[606] As many as 18% of men with azoospermia (occasionally severe oligospermia) have microdeletions in this region.[607] The testicular histologic features in such men have varied from germinal cell aplasia to maturation arrest, and the plasma FSH is elevated. Two candidate genes for AZF have been identified by positional cloning; the first is a family of genes termed Y-located RNA recognition motif *(YRRM)* genes,[608] which are members of a larger family of genes that encode RNA-binding proteins. The *YRRM* genes are expressed in germ cells but the fact that there are multiple genes in this family makes it hard to assess their function. The second AZF candidate termed *DAZ* (for deleted in azoospermia) also encodes an RNA recognition motif that is testis specific.[609] In one study 12 of 89 azoospermic men had Yq deletions that included the *DAZ* gene, making *DAZ* a strong candidate for an AZF gene but not excluding a role for *YRRM.*[609]

Azoospermia is also compatible with testis histologic characteristics of hypospermatogenesis, spermatogenic arrest (see Fig.16–17*F)* or, in men with obstruction of the vas deferens, a normal germinal epithelium.[610] Familial male infertility with hypospermatogenesis or maturation arrest has been reported.[611, 612] In one family the inheritance pattern suggested X-linkage,[611] whereas in other families parental consanguinity suggested an autosomal recessive transmission.[612] In both familial and sporadic cases meiosis is defective because of desynapsis, lack of chiasmata, and degeneration of spermatocytes. The majority of men with defective meiosis do not have a positive family history[612] and in most cases the cause of this type of infertility is unknown.

Unilateral *cryptorchidism,* even when corrected before puberty, is associated with abnormal semen in many individuals (see earlier). This finding suggests that the testicular abnormality is bilateral even in unilateral cryptorchidism.

Varicocele is believed by some to be the most common treatable cause of male infertility; it may be of causative importance in as many as a third of infertile men.[613] Varicocele is caused by retrograde flow of blood into the internal spermatic vein that eventuates in a progressive, often palpable, dilation of the peritesticular pampiniform plexus of veins. It is thought to result from incompetence of the valve between the internal spermatic vein and the renal vein and is more common (85%) on the left.[614] The incidence of varicocele is about 10 to 15% in the general population and 20 to 40% in men with infertility. The findings on semen analysis are usually nonspecific. Decreased sperm density is often seen with medium or large varicoceles.[615, 616]

The mechanism by which varicocele leads to infertility is an enigma.[614] Not all men with varicocele are infertile and most do not have a detectable abnormality of the hypothalamic-pituitary-testicular axis. The occurrence of infertility with unilateral varicocele might result from anastomoses of the venous system between the two testes but extensive anastomoses have not been demonstrated convincingly in humans.[614] The leading theory for the adverse effect is that varicocele leads to an increased scrotal temperature, but in two studies the scrotal temperatures of infertile men were higher than those of fertile men regardless of the presence of varicocele.[617, 618] Presumably an increased scrotal (and testicular) temperature would cause poor quality semen and infertility. Studies of the effects of surgically induced unilateral varicocele in rats and dogs support the concept that obstructed venous return leads to increased testicular blood flow and increased temperature bilaterally.[619]

On average, semen quality improves in patients who have had surgical repair of varicoceles but the effect on fertility is unclear. The impregnation rate after varicocele repair is probably less than 50%. One large retrospective, uncontrolled study of almost 1000 men reported an association between subsequent fertility and preoperative sperm density.[620] Patients who had preoperative sperm densities of more than 10 million/mL (about 40% of the men in this study) had a 70% impregnation rate after repair.[620]

The *immotile cilia syndrome* is a hereditary disorder characterized by defective motility of the cilia in the airways and either immotile or poorly motile spermatozoa.[210] The disorder is usually inherited as an autosomal recessive trait. In the airways the defective cilia cause chronic sinusitis and bronchiectasis, and the immotile sperm cannot fertilize. Kartagener's syndrome is a subcategory of the immotile cilia syndrome associated with situs inversus. The structural abnormalities that impair motility of cilia can be defined by electron microscopy and include missing or abnormally short dynein arms, short spokes with no central sheath, missing central microtubules, and displacement of one of the microtubule doublets (see Fig. 16–14). Cilia from epithelia and sperm from the same individual exhibit the same defects. Other less well understood mutations can apparently lead to immotile sperm without involvement of cilia in the lung.[621] In evaluating sperm for structural abnormalities care should be taken to examine a number of axonemes and to confirm the structural defect because variations in axonemal structure occur frequently in normal functional respiratory cilia and sperm.[339] The infertility should (at least theoretically) be treatable by empirical methods (see later).

Acquired Defects. Acquired testicular causes of isolated infertility include *Mycoplasma* infection, radiation, drugs, environmental toxins, and autoimmunity. A role for *Mycoplasma (Ureaplasma urealyticum)* in infertility has been long suspected; mycoplasmal infection occurs with increased frequency in women whose infertility is associated with a "male factor," which suggests that genital tract mycoplasmal infection may cause male infertility.[622] Furthermore when the infection is successfully eradicated the pregnancy rate is increased, although the presence of mycoplasmal infection in the male cannot be correlated with any specific alteration in sperm density or morphologic features.[623]

Radiation can cause isolated infertility. Spermatogonia are exquisitely sensitive to radiation, damage being demonstrable after only 0.15 Gy (15 rad).[490] With doses higher than 1 Gy (100 rad) extreme oligospermia or azoospermia develops. Higher doses also damage spermatids and cause more rapid decreases in sperm counts. Recovery occurs in a dose-dependent fashion. Return to preirradiation sperm densities requires 9 to 18 mo after doses of 1 Gy (100 rad) or less, 30 mo for doses of 2 to 3 Gy (200 to 300 rad), and 5 y or more for doses of 4 to 6 Gy (400 to 600 rad).[624] Fractionated radiation may have a more profound effect on the testes than that of single-dose radiation.[625] In a study of 27 men with variable radiation exposure of the testes (0.01 to 25 Gy [1 to 2500 rad]) to scatter radiation for treatment of soft tissue sarcoma, there was a dose-dependent increase in serum FSH levels with the maximal change at 6 mo. Only patients receiving less than 0.5 Gy (50 rad) recovered completely within 12 mo of therapy. Patients receiving greater than 2 Gy (200 rad) had elevations in plasma LH and FSH levels but the testosterone value did not change.[625] Permanent infertility may occur after radiation for malignant lymphoma of the abdomen in spite of shielding.[626] Men given radioactive iodine for thyroid cancer may also have impairment of spermatogenesis and elevation of plasma FSH levels. The threshold for this effect appears to be a cumulative iodine ^{131}I dose of more than 3.7 × 10^3 mBq (100 mCi); recovery occurs in about 2 y.[627]

The principal *drugs* that cause isolated infertility are alkylating agents such as cyclophosphamide. The primary pathologic lesion produced by the drugs is depletion of the germinal epithelium.[628] Spermatocytes and spermatogonia may disappear completely, resulting in germinal cell aplasia with only Sertoli cells lining the tubular lumen. The serum FSH level rises about fivefold and serves as a marker for germ cell loss. The serum LH and testosterone levels usually remain within normal limits in the presence of germinal cell depletion. However in men treated in childhood with cyclophosphamide for nephrotic syndrome[629] and in men treated as adults with combination chemotherapy for Hodgkin's disease,[630] the serum LH level was elevated in those with severe damage to the germinal epithelium. Other chemotherapeutic agents can cause germ cell depletion. Chlorambucil in doses up to 400 mg causes reversible oligospermia, and cumulative doses greater than 400 mg can cause azoospermia and germinal aplasia. Similarly germinal aplasia can occur in men receiving more than 6 to 10 g of cyclophosphamide. Cessation of cyclophosphamide therapy is followed by return of spermatogenesis within 3 y in about half of azoospermic patients.[631] Vinblastine, doxorubicin, procarbazine, and cisplatin are toxic to the germinal epithelium of animals and humans, although specific dose-toxicity relationships have not been established.

Combination drug regimens have an even more profound impact on spermatogenesis. The combination of mechlorethamine HCl, vincristine, procarbazine, and prednisone (MOPP) causes azoospermia, germinal aplasia, testicular atrophy, and elevated FSH levels in more than 80% of men.[511, 628] The combination of doxorubicin (Adriamycin), bleomycin, vinblastine, and dacarbazine results in azoospermia only one third as often, and spermatogenesis usually recovers in these patients.[632] Combination chemotherapy also causes azoospermia in about half of prepubertal boys so treated.[633-635] Chemotherapy-induced azoospermia after treatment with vinblastine, bleomycin, and cisplatin for testicular cancer is usually reversible within 2 y of stopping treatment.[636] Sulfasalazine, methotrexate, and colchicine may also cause oligospermia and infertility.[637-639]

Because of the potential toxic effects of physical and chemical agents on spermatogenesis, the occupational and recreational history should be carefully evaluated in all men with infertility. Known *environmental toxins* include chemicals such as nematocide dibromochloropropane and related compounds,[640] ethylene glycol,[641] cadmium,[642] lead,[643] microwaves,[644] and ultrasound.[645] Men who had been exposed to sulfur mustard chemical warfare 1 to 3 y previously had a 30% incidence of oligospermia.[646]

In a large meta-analysis of studies in normal men sperm density was said to have declined from 113 million/mL in 1940 to 66 million/mL in 1990.[647] This report has subsequently been supported[648, 649] and refuted.[650] Enviromental toxins that might act as estrogens or antiandrogens have been proposed as possible causes,[651] and the increasing incidence of gynecomastia in men is in keeping with the possibility of estrogen exposure (see Chapter 17). Cigarette smoking has also been suggested as a cause for decreasing sperm density.[652]

Although *autoimmunity* may cause combined underandrogenization and infertility it usually causes isolated infertility. Antibodies to the basement membrane of the seminiferous tubules[653] or, more commonly, to the sperm themselves may cause a significant fraction of male infertility.[654] There is no correlation between the presence of sperm-associated antibodies and specific abnormalities in the semen analysis.[655] Not all men with antisperm antibodies are infertile and a decrease in antibody titers is not always associated with improved fertility. Thus the exact role of antisperm antibodies in infertility is uncertain. Although immunosuppression of men with antisperm antibodies by administration of prednisone is reported to improve fertility,[656] such therapy has been replaced by in vitro fertilization techniques (see later). The occurrence of antisperm antibodies is not always a primary phenomenon because they have been identified in men with both bilateral[657] and unilateral[658] obstruction of the vas deferens and after vasectomy.[659]

Defects Associated with Systemic Disease. Infertility alone may also occur in association with systemic diseases. Perhaps the most common alteration of seminiferous tubule function is the temporary decrease in semen quality, particularly decreased sperm density, that often follows an acute febrile illness. This is one of the reasons that several semen analyses must be obtained for men with suspected infertility to be confident that true basal parameters have been determined (see earlier). Men with celiac disease have a distinct testicular abnormality, namely the hormonal pattern is typical of androgen resistance with elevated plasma testosterone and LH levels.[660-662] Because men with regional enteritis do not have this hormonal pattern, gluten enteropathy may cause a reversible androgen resistance–like state.[660-662] As discussed earlier, the neurologic disorder that causes isolated infertility is spinal cord injury.[586, 587]

Androgen Resistance. Androgen resistance may cause infertility without underandrogenization and may be the cause in as many as 20% of men with apparent idiopathic azoospermia (see earlier).[591, 663]

Impairment of Sperm Transport. Disorders of sperm transport may be responsible for as much as 6% of male infertility.[613] Such disorders may be unilateral or bilateral, congenital or acquired. In men with unilateral obstruction infertility may be due to antisperm antibodies.[658] Obstructive azoospermia at the level of the epididymis also occurs in association with chronic infections of the paranasal sinuses and lungs[664]; it is possible that this syndrome may be due to unsuspected mercury poisoning.[665] In polycystic kidney disease dilated cysts of the seminal vesicles may cause obstruction to semen transport.[666] Tuberculosis, leprosy, and gonorrhea can cause obstruction of the wolffian duct structures. Acquired bilateral obstruction of sperm transport has also been reported in men with deep midline müllerian duct cysts.[667] Congenital defects of the vas deferens that result in azoospermia or oligospermia may be present in sons of women given diethylstibestrol during pregnancy.[668] Congenital bilateral absence of the vas deferens is common in men with cystic fibrosis, and mutations in the gene responsible for cystic fibrosis, the transmembrane conductor regulator (*CFTR*) gene, can cause congenital bilateral absence of the vas deferens without causing the other manifestations of cystic fibrosis.[669-671] Congenital unilateral absence of the vas deferens may be an incomplete form of congenital bilateral absence of the vas deferens.[671] Thus congenital bilateral absence of the vas deferens and cystic fibrosis are extreme forms of a spectrum of mutations of a common gene. Magnetic resonance imaging may be useful for visualizing the seminal vesicles in the evaluation of obstructive azoospermia.[672] In one study of the success of surgical therapy for suspected obstructive azoospermia, obstruction of the epididymis was more common than absence or obstruction of the vas deferens.[673] Vasoepididymostomy resulted in sperm densities of more than 10 million/mL in almost half and impregnation of the patient's partner in a fifth. Successful impregnation was more likely in the absence of antisperm antibodies.[673]

Idiopathic Infertility. The known conditions associated with male infertility do not explain all cases of infertility. In large series of consecutive patients known causes or associated conditions account for only about 60% and the remainder are classified as having *idiopathic infertility* (Table 16–6).[613, 674] Because at best only about half of infertile men with a varicocele achieve fertility after surgical repair, it is probably more appropriate to consider 60% of infertile men as having idiopathic infertility. The causes of the idiopathic disorder are no doubt heterogeneous. Some may have androgen resistance, and many may have disorders involving the *AZF* gene (see earlier). Others have oligospermia or azoospermia with normal plasma LH and testosterone levels but an elevated FSH level in the absence of cryptorchidism, radiation, or drug exposure. Studies of small groups of such men indicate that the isolated FSH elevation may be associated with a decreased LHRH pulse frequency[675] and that pulsatile LHRH administration to such men may lower FSH levels.[676, 677] Men with oligospermia and normal FSH levels may also have altered pulsatile

TABLE 16–6. Relative Frequency of Causes and Associated Conditions in Men Who Present with Infertility

Cause or Condition	% in Study of Greenberg et al.[613] (n = 425)	% in Study of Baker et al.[674] (n = 1041)
Hypogonadotropic hypogonadism	0.9	0.6
Klinefelter's syndrome	1.6	1.9
Cryptorchidism	6.1	6.4
Varicocele	37.4	40.3
Immotile sperm	0.5	0.6
Viral orchitis	1.9	1.6
Radiation-chemotherapy	—	0.5
Obstruction of epididymis or vas deferens	6.1	4.1
Androgen resistance	—	0.1
Coital disorders	4.0	0.5
Idiopathic disorders	41.5*	43.4†

*Includes miscellaneous semen abnormalities, 10.2% and undiagnosed primary testicular failure, 5.9.%

†Includes possible obstruction, 4.5%.

secretion of gonadotropins and testosterone[678] and testosterone production rates are said to be low in selected infertile men with isolated FSH elevations and normal total serum testosterone levels.[679] Whether these abnormalities are of causative significance is not known.

MANAGEMENT OF INFERTILITY. The management of infertility has generally been unsatisfactory because the number of potentially correctable causes of male infertility is relatively small (see Table 16–6). However when appropriate, associated hormonal disorders and coexisting medical conditions may be treated; likewise, offending drugs may be discontinued in appropriate circumstances. In addition men with hypogonadotropic hypogonadism may be given gonadotropins or LHRH (see later).

Men with infertility with no known cause or those who have a varicocele, or both, have been treated empirically. Although claims of success have been made for a variety of empirical therapies for infertilty with oligospermia, most such claims fail to take into account the spontaneous fertility rate in untreated oligospermic men (25% in 1 y).[338] Treatment-independent pregnancy among infertile couples occurs in all forms of human infertility (male and female factors) and it is consequently necessary for all therapies to be evaluated by randomized clinical trials.[680] When several forms of conventional empirical therapy—including testosterone rebound, nonaromatizable androgen (mesterolone), gonadotropin, anti-estrogen (clomiphene), antibiotics, bromocriptine, varicocele repair, artificial insemination, and no therapy—were compared in one large retrospective analysis of oligospermic men, no improvement in the relative pregnancy rate was demonstrated for any empirical therapy.[681]

The only effective empirical therapy for male infertility is in vitro fertilization. Using standard techniques in vitro fertilization requires as few as 500,000 motile sperm/mL of ejaculate. Although the fertilizing capacity of sperm from men with abnormal sperm parameters is diminished, conventional techniques can obtain 10% or more live births per attempt in men with mild to moderate abnormalities.[682] Such rates are three- to fivefold higher than natural impregnation rates in such men. However standard in vitro fertilization does not produce good results in men with more severe defects in spermatogenesis. In the Melbourne experience in men with sperm counts less than 5 million/mL, poor motility, and increased numbers of abnormal forms, standard in vitro fertilization had low fertilization rates.[683]

Better results have been obtained with the development of intracytoplasmic sperm injection, namely fertility rates of 50 to 70% using poor quality semen,[684] including men with different sperm abnormalities (e.g., decreased numbers, impaired motility, increased abnormal forms, and combinations of defects).[685] Even in men with obstructive azoospermia, in whom sperm must be aspirated from the epididymis, fertilization rates are near normal.[686]

In the past men with nonobstructive azoospermia, typically with elevated plasma FSH levels, were not treatable; such patients include men with maturation arrest, postcryptorchidism tubular atrophy, mumps orchitis, and Klinefelter's syndrome. However, when minute amounts of sperm can be identified by testicular biopsy, successful fertilization and impregnation have been achieved with rare spermatozoa or spermatids retrieved from such biopsies using intracytoplasmic sperm injection.[687, 688]

Intracytoplasmic sperm injection should not be undertaken until men with abnormal semen undergo a complete work-up, so that hypogonadotropic hypogonadism or some other treatable condition is not missed. Furthermore intracytoplasmic sperm injection may increase the chances of transmitting mutations to offspring.

Old Age

The decrease in total and bioavailable testosterone and the increase in estradiol with aging probably have no direct consequences for male sexual function. However this changing hormonal milieu may be involved in the pathogenesis of breast enlargement in elderly men (see Chapter 17) and in the development of prostatic hyperplasia.

PROSTATIC HYPERPLASIA. Enlargement of the prostate to the extent that it produces obstruction to urethral outflow is common in elderly men.[689] The gland weighs only a few grams at birth; at puberty it undergoes androgen-mediated growth and reaches the adult size of approximately 20 g by age 20. This maturation is accompanied by transformation of the cuboidal epithelium of the acinar units of the gland to a columnar, secretory epithelium and initiation of secretion of the prostatic component of the ejaculate. The weight of the gland remains stable for about 25 y. Commencing in the fifth decade of life a second growth spurt occurs in the majority of men. This second growth phase, unlike the earlier growth that involves the gland diffusely, typically begins in the periurethral region as a localized proliferation involving both glandular and stromal elements. This hyperplasia may remain limited in scope but in many men the growth continues and eventually compresses the remaining normal portion of the prostate. The progressive increase in gland size is associated with development of urinary tract obstruction and sometimes with constipation. Indeed men can acquire hyperplasia primarily of the periurethral region and hence experience obstruction to urine outflow in the absence of gross prostatic enlargement.

The second growth spurt, like the growth at puberty, requires a functioning testis. Dihydrotestosterone that is formed within the prostate from testosterone is the androgen that mediates the embryonic development, pubertal growth, and hyperplastic growth of the prostate.[690, 691] The administration to animals of a 5α-reductase inhibitor to block dihydrotestosterone formation causes involution of the gland in the face of an elevated concentration of prostatic testosterone.[692–694] Furthermore although the plasma testosterone level declines with age, the level of dihydrotestosterone in the hyperplastic gland either remains constant or increases.[695–697]

The dog is the major species other than the human in which prostatic hyperplasia develops, and most research work on the pathogenesis of the disorder has been done in that species. The administration to the castrated dog of androgens that cause an increase in the prostatic dihydrotestosterone concentration results in prostatic enlargement that is comparable to that seen in naturally occurring canine prostatic hyperplasia.[698] Estrogen acts synergistically with dihydrotestosterone to enhance prostatic growth in the dog[698, 699] and this synergism appears to be due to the fact that estrogen increases the amount of androgen receptor in the tissue.[142] Thus two hormones participate in the development of prostatic hyperplasia in the dog: dihydrotestosterone is responsible for prostate growth and estradiol enhances the action of dihydrotestosterone.

Three types of evidence suggest that dihydrotestosterone and estradiol are also involved in human prostatic hyperplasia. First, estradiol levels increase with age.[141] Second, either surgical or pharmacologic castration[700–702] or inhibition of androgen action by antiandrogens[703, 704] causes a decrease in the size of the hyperplastic prostate, clearly indicating that continuing androgen action is essential for maintaining the hyperplastic state. Third, inhibition of prostatic 5α-reductase with agents such as finasteride causes a profound decrease in prostatic dihydrotestosterone levels[705] and a 20 to 30% decrease in prostate volume after 3 to 6 mo of therapy,[706] an effect that is maintained for up to 4 y and is associated with few and minor side effects.[707] Furthermore urinary flow rates improve in many men so treated.[708]

The exact therapeutic role of 5α-reductase inhibitors is not established because there is a strong placebo effect on urinary symptomatology, there is no clearcut relation between symptoms and urine flow, and the natural history of the disorder (particularly how to predict which subset of men will experience significant obstruction) is not well understood. As a consequence the indications for either surgical or medical management are sometimes unclear. Nevertheless many men given finasteride for symptomatic disease either have improvement or stabilization of symptoms. Consequently although surgery provides more prompt relief of symptoms, medical therapy may play an increasingly important role in the routine management of moderate symptomatic disease[708] and in the treatment of severe symptoms in men who are poor surgical risks.[709–711]

Documentation of a hormonal role in prostatic hyperplasia does not necessarily provide insight into its pathogenesis. Androgens may be involved only in a permissive sense rather than acting as true initiators of the hyperplasia, and the reason that the disorder is limited to only a few species is unclear.

PROSTATIC CANCER. The endocrine aspects of prostatic cancer are discussed in Chapter 35.

Disorders of All Ages

TESTICULAR TUMORS. Tumors of the testes occur with an incidence of 2 to 3 per 100,000 men/y in the United States and account for about 1% of cancer deaths in men.[712–714] These tumors are the second most common malignancy (after leukemia) in men between ages 20 and 35. The frequency shows a trimodal curve, with peaks in childhood (embryonal carcinomas and teratocarcinomas), young adulthood, and old age (seminomas). The incidence increased between 1970 and 1985, particularly in adults, but mortality rates declined because of improved treatment.[715, 716] The tumors are commonly bilateral (either simultaneous or sequential, e.g., a seminoma developing in one testis many years after the removal of the other).[717] The incidence in black persons is a sixth or less that in whites. Reports of familial occurrence are numerous, including occasional concordance in monozygotic twins.[718] In most germ cell tumors an isochromosome of the short arm of chromosome 12 can be identified.[719]

Several factors predispose individuals to testicular tumor development. Men with cryptorchidism have a fivefold increased risk of developing testicular tumors, intra-abdominal testes being more at risk than high inguinal testes.[720] In one series, however, only 10 of 131 men with testicular cancer had antecedent maldescent.[721] Three fourths of tumors that are associated with maldescent are seminomas, the remainder being other germ cell tumors. Early orchiopexy facilitates detection, but whether it reduces the incidence of tumor development is not clear.[722] The incidence of gonadal malignancy may be higher in testes of patients with abnormal sexual development (i.e., 45,X/46,XY mixed gonadal dysgenesis or testicular feminization) than in patients with other forms of testicular maldescent.[723–726] Occupational exposure to extreme high or low temperature may increase the risk of testicular cancer.[727] Estrogen administration to pregnant women may also predispose male offspring to the development of testicular tumors,[721] and both the Klinefelter's syndrome[728] and HIV infection[729] may be associated with an increased incidence of germ cell tumors.

The relation between congenital adrenal hyperplasia due to steroid 21-hydroxylase (CYP21) deficiency and testicular tumors is complex; most testicular tumors that occur in patients with this disorder consist of adrenal cell rests, are dependent on corticotropin for growth and secretion, and develop in patients who are inadequately treated and hence have incomplete suppression of plasma corticotropin concentrations.[730, 731] However on histologic grounds the tumors are difficult to separate from interstitial cell tumors and on occasion act like malignant tumors.[732]

Diagnosis. Most testicular cancers produce symptoms related to the testes, but significant delay in making a diagnosis is common because of oversights by both physicians and patients. Most testicular cancers occur in men younger than age 45, and men should be educated about the need to seek prompt medical advice for any change in a previously normal testis, including the development of a mass, a feeling of heaviness, pain, swelling, or other unusual findings.[733] To reduce delay physicians should consider any testicular mass to be a tumor until proved otherwise. Pain occurs in half of men with testicular neoplasms and thus does not rule out cancer. If testicular symptoms or signs do not promptly regress a surgical consultation should be obtained.[734]

Classification. The most widely used classification is that of Mostofi[735] (Table 16–7). This classification is based on the cell type from which the tumor originates, i.e., germ cells (spermatogonia), stromal cells (Leydig and Sertoli cells), and rete cells at the site of attachment of the testis and epididymis. Lymphomas[736] and carcinoid tumors[737] of the testis are rare.

Germ cell tumors are the most common and are presumed to be derived from primordial germ cells. Seminomas are characterized by large cells with clear cytoplasm in a delicate fibrovascular stroma infiltrated with lymphocytes; the granulomatous reaction around the tumor can be so intense as to suggest the presence of a graft-versus-host reaction.[738] These tumors account for at least half of all testicular neo-

TABLE 16–7. Classification of Testicular Tumors

I. Germ cell tumors (95%)
A. Single-cell–type tumors (60%)
Seminomas
Yolk sac tumors (embryonal cell tumors)
Teratomas
Choriocarcinoma
B. Combination tumors (40%)
II. Tumors of gonadal stroma (1–2%)
Leydig cell
Sertoli cell
Primitive gonadal structures
III. Gonadoblastomas
Germ cell + stroma cell

Data from Mostofi FK. Pathology of germ cell tumors of testis: a progress report. Cancer 1980; 45:1735–1754.

plasms and can be subdivided into spermatocytic and anaplastic varieties. Spermatocytic seminomas in older men are associated with a 90 to 95% 5-y survival, whereas the anaplastic type has a poor prognosis. Unlike other seminomas spermatocytic seminoma is believed not to evolve from carcinoma in situ.[739] Embryonal carcinomas are the most frequent testicular tumors in children, resemble embryonal carcinomas of the ovary, and have 5-y survivals of around 70% in infants and 25% in adults. Choriocarcinomas contain syncytiotrophoblastic cells and occur most commonly in the second and third decades of life; prognosis is poor. Teratomas contain at least two germ cell layers and may be either benign or malignant; they are second in frequency to embryonal carcinomas in childhood but occur as only a tenth of adult tumors. Tumors that contain combinations of germ cell types account for 40% of germ cell tumors; the biology of such tumors is usually determined by the least differentiated (most malignant) element. Of the mixed tumors that contain cells of germinal and stromal origin perhaps the most distinctive is the gonadoblastoma, which consists of germ cells, sex cords and, usually, Leydig cells. Gonadoblastomas commonly originate from dysgenetic testes containing a Y chromosome and usually synthesize androgen.[655]

Germ cell tumors of all types can also originate in extragonadal sites as well, including the mediastinum[741-745] and the brain.[746-750] These extragonadal tumors are presumed to arise from aberrant migration of germ cells early in embryogenesis or, alternatively, from some common precursor stem cell line that normally gives rise to germ cells and cells of the thymus and the pineal gland.[5]

The usual presentation of a testicular germ cell tumor is a nodule or painless swelling of the testis. Occasionally the tumors are identified as the result of metastases or because of the peripheral manifestations of hCG secretion by the tumor. After the tumors are diagnosed staging is performed either by surgical exploration or by computed tomographic scanning or magnetic resonance imaging. Stage I is limited to the testes, stage II involves metastases to infradiaphragmatic lymph nodes but not beyond, stage III involves supradiaphragmatic lymph nodes, and stage IV involves extralymphatic metastases.

Germinomas may secrete several distinct tumor cell markers into plasma, of which the most important is hCG both because of its value as a tumor marker and because of its endocrine effects. Normal testes synthesize hCG but in such small amounts that only trace quantities reach the circulation.[751] Virtually all germ cell tumors also secrete hCG and its subunits,[752] but the hormone is secreted into the circulation in large amounts only by subsets of nonseminoma germ cell tumors (all choriocarcinomas and a third of teratocarcinomas and yolk sac tumors).[753, 754] Tumors containing yolk sac elements may also produce α-fetoprotein and teratomas on occasion secrete carcinoembryonic antigen.[755-761] An elevated level of one of these tumor markers in the plasma of a patient whose tumor has been classified as a pure seminoma usually indicates that the tumor is actually a combination tumor. These markers are particularly useful for following the response to therapy.[750, 762, 763] The secreted hCG may be endocrinologically active and cause enhanced formation of testosterone[764] and, more importantly, of estradiol[765] by the testes. The net result can be a feminizing syndrome, with consequent inhibition of the secretion of LH and FSH by the pituitary (also see Chapter 17).[766]

The treatment of germ cell tumors constitutes a major triumph of cancer therapy. Appropriate therapeutic strategies include debulking of the tumor mass, resection of involved lymph nodes, administration of chemotherapy (usually combinations of cisplatin, vinblastine, etoposide, and bleomycin), radiation, and the monitoring of tumor cell markers.[714, 750, 767-772] The surgical cure rates for patients with seminomas approximate 90% for stage I disease, and individuals with stage III nonseminoma tumors, which were previously uni-

formly lethal, now have good survival rates.[684] Because young men with germ cell tumors may have infertility due to castration, radiation, chemotherapy, or a combination, cryopreservation of semen before treatment has been advocated as a means of preserving fertility[773]; however most men have adequate sperm production after chemotherapy.[774] Treatment is associated with a small risk for secondary solid tumors and leukemia.[775]

Stromal tumors account for only 1 to 2% of testicular tumors. Such malignancies usually involve Leydig or Sertoli cells and both cell types may coexist within the same tumor. Rarely adrenal rest tumors may occur in the testes.[731, 776] As would be expected interstitial cell tumors commonly secrete testosterone and thus may cause virilization in prepubertal boys (precocious pseudopuberty). Leydig cell tumors are usually benign. Approximately a fourth of these tumors secrete estradiol as well as testosterone and thus cause mixed signs of feminization and virilization during the prepubertal years and feminizing signs in adult men. Endocrinologically active tumors cause suppression of endogenous gonadotropins, azoospermia, and decreased size of the contralateral testis. Estrogen secretion can inhibit LH production and suppress plasma testosterone.[777] Because the tumors may be small and sometimes can be recognized only by ultrasonography, documenting that the testis is the site of increased estrogen production may require selective catheterization of the testicular veins. After removal of the involved testis, gynecomastia regresses and the high estradiol, low testosterone, and low sperm count return to normal.[778]

Sertoli cell tumors show a bimodal age distribution, with most patients being younger than 1 y or between ages 20 and 45. The tumors are frequently bilateral and may be associated with the Peutz-Jeghers syndrome.[779, 780] Gynecomastia occurs in about a fourth of patients. Decreased spermatogenesis and atrophy of the contralateral testis are common in the estrogen-secreting group. Leydig cell hyperplasia can occur in the area around the tumor, which implies either that the tumor is of mixed cell origin or that Sertoli cells secrete some factor that stimulates Leydig cell differentiation.[781] The usual course is for complete cure and regression of any feminizing signs after surgical resection. The secretion of estrogen by Sertoli cell and Leydig cell tumors is consistent with the view that estrogen synthesis in the normal testis takes place in both cell types.[72] The treatment of these tumors is surgical. Approximately a tenth of stromal tumors are malignant and follow an aggressive course[778, 781, 782]; occasionally such patients respond to mitotane.[776] Adenocarcinoma of the rete testes is rare but tends to be highly malignant.[783, 784]

In summary testicular tumors can cause enhanced production of estradiol and testosterone by more than one mechanism. When production of steroid hormones by the tumor is autonomous, plasma gonadotropin levels and androgen secretion by uninvolved portions of the testes are depressed and azoospermia is common. When hCG is secreted by the tumor the gonadotropin acts to increase estradiol and testosterone production in unaffected areas of the testes and azoospermia is uncommon. Furthermore occasional choriocarcinomas that cannot synthesize steroids de novo nevertheless convert circulating androgens to estrogens. When androgens or estrogens, or both, are formed directly or indirectly by the tumors the response varies depending on the pattern of hormones produced and the age of the subject. Some patients are clinically normal, whereas others experience feminization or virilization.

HORMONAL THERAPY

Androgen Therapy

Testosterone administered by mouth is absorbed into the portal blood and degraded promptly by the liver so that only a small portion reaches the systemic circulation. Parenterally injected testosterone is also rapidly absorbed and degraded so that maintenance of physiological levels in plasma is difficult. As a consequence effective androgen therapy requires either the administration of testosterone in a slowly absorbed form (dermal patches or a micronized oral preparation) or the administration of chemically modified analogues. Such chemical modifications either retard the rate of absorption or catabolism to maintain effective blood levels or enhance the androgenic potency of each molecule so that hormonal effects can be achieved at a lower plasma level of drug. Three general types of modification of testosterone are clinically useful: esterification of the 17β-hydroxyl group (type A), alkylation at the 17α-position (type B), and modification of the A, B, or C rings, particularly substitutions at the 1, 2, 9, and 11 carbons (type C) (Fig. 16–19). Most agents actually contain combinations of ring structure alterations and either 17α-alkylation or esterification of the 17β-hydroxyl.

Esterification of testosterone with various carboxylic acids decreases the polarity of the steroid, makes it more soluble in the fat vehicles that are used for injection, and hence slows release of the injected steroid into the circulation.[785–787] The esters of 19-nortestosterone appear to have particularly slow release and turnover.[599] The longer the carbon chain in the ester, the more fat soluble the steroid becomes and hence the more prolonged the action. For example testosterone propionate must be injected daily, whereas testosterone cypionate and testosterone enanthate can be administered every 2 or 3 wk. Even more slowly hydrolyzed esters are under investigation, such as testosterone buciclate, which is administered every 12 wk.[792] Testosterone cypionate or enanthate was for many years the treatment of choice for male hypogonadism.[286, 468, 788–791] Although the esters can be detected in plasma they must be hydrolyzed before the hormone acts so that effectiveness of therapy can be monitored by assaying the plasma level of testosterone after administration. Most esters cannot be administered by mouth and must be injected. However, two esters—methenolone acetate and testosterone undecanoate—have special features that make administration by mouth possible. Testosterone undecanoate is absorbed via the lymphatic system into the systemic circulation, so that physiological blood levels of testosterone can be achieved at doses of approximately 120 mg/d.[793–797] Because of rapid turnover in plasma, however, testosterone undecanoate must be administered twice daily.[798, 799] The reason for the oral effectiveness of methenolone acetate (and of mesterolone) is not entirely clear; the methyl group in the 1 position may slow the rate of hepatic inactivation and allow effective blood levels to be maintained.[800–802]

The use of a transdermal therapeutic preparation of testosterone in which a testosterone-loaded film is applied each day to either the scrotum or the back in the form of a patch makes it possible to sustain serum testosterone levels in the normal male range.[803–806] When the scrotal patch is applied in the morning the serum testosterone level increases to reach a peak within 2 to 3 h and maintains a level that is 60 to 80% of the peak value throughout the day, thus avoiding the wide swings in serum testosterone values that are characteristic of therapy with parenterally administered testosterone esters.[804] The nonscrotal formulation uses two patches and is applied at bedtime to provide peak levels in the morning.[806] These systems therefore offer advantages over other modalities for administering testosterone in that they both replace the missing molecule and avoid the necessity for parenteral administration. The scrotal preparation causes a disproportionate increase in plasma dihydrotestosterone to a level that is 30 to 40% that of testosterone, presumably because of the high level of 5α-reductase in scrotal skin.[807, 808] Such increases in serum dihydrotestosterone level have also been reported after treatment with the extremely long-acting parenteral testosterone ester testosterone buciclate[809] and with the oral ester testosterone undecanoate.[810] As long as the total androgen level in serum is maintained within the normal range dihydrotestosterone acts similarly to testosterone as an effective androgen and does not appear to have any deleterious side effects. Indeed after the percutaneous administration of therapeutic preparations of dihydrotestosterone for as long as 3 mo, no change occurred in the ratio of HDL cholesterol to LDL cholesterol, and no deleterious side effects were observed.[811, 812]

17α-Alkylated androgens, such as methyltestosterone and methandrostenolone, are effective when given by mouth because alkylated steroids are absorbed into the portal circulation but are slowly catabolized by the liver and reach the systemic circulation in effective amounts. For this reason 17α-methyl or 17α-ethyl substitution is a common feature of most orally active androgens. Because all 17α-alkylated steroids are believed to act within the cell as such (i.e., the alkyl groups are not removed), because they may cause abnormalities of liver function, and because assays are not routinely available for monitoring blood levels, these steroids have a limited role in medicine.[813, 814]

Other alterations of the ring structure have been adopted empirically; in some instances the effect is to slow the rate of inactivation, whereas in others the alteration enhances the potency of a given molecule or alters its metabolism. For example the potency of fluoxymesterone, 19-nortestosterone, or 1-methyl–substituted steroids, or a combination, may be due in part to the fact that they are poor precursors for estrogen formation in extraglandular tissues.[815] In contrast 19-nortestosterone is a more potent androgen than testosterone because its more planar ring structure, like that of dihydrotestosterone, fits more tightly into the binding site of the androgen receptor.[816] The 5α-reduced metabolites of 19-nortestosterone and 7α-methyl-19-nortestosterone bind less well to the androgen receptor and hence are less effective androgens than the parent compounds.[817] As is true for 17α-alkylated steroids, androgens with ring alterations are usually not con-

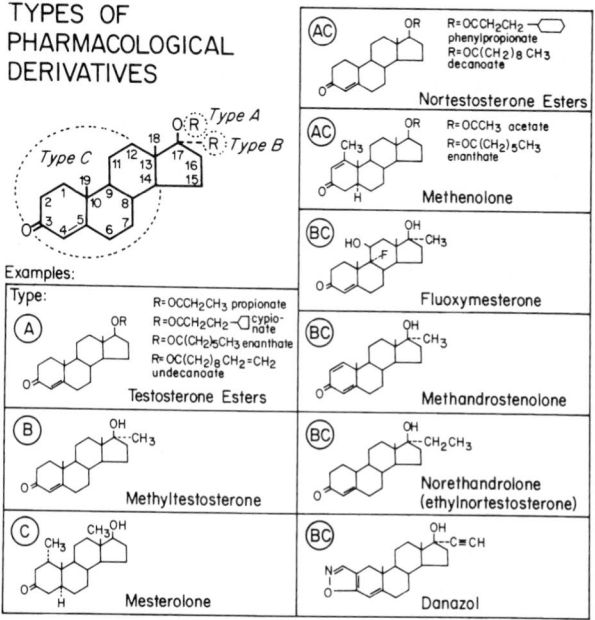

Figure 16–19. Some of the androgen preparations available for clinical use, classified into three types. Type A derivatives are esterified in the 17β-position. Type B steroids have alkyl groups in a 17α-position. Type C derivatives include a variety of additional alterations of ring structure that enhance activity, impede catabolism, or influence both functions. Most androgen preparations involve combinations of type AC or type BC changes.

verted to testosterone in vivo and hence specific assays for each must be used to monitor blood levels. Because most steroids with altered ring structures also contain 17α-substitutions they also have the same deleterious effects on liver function as methyltestosterone and thus have little clinical usefulness. One orally effective androgen, mesterolone, is neither esterified nor alkylated in the 17α-position. In addition the molecule cannot be aromatized to estrogens in peripheral tissues, so effective androgen replacement can be achieved by oral administration without causing abnormalities of liver function; unfortunately the steroid has no effective feedback regulation of gonadotropin secretion and consequently is a poor agent for routine androgen replacement therapy.[800–802]

Other means of administering testosterone have been proposed. It can be administered sublingually as testosterone cyclodextrin, in which the steroid is surrounded by a carbohydrate ring that facilitates testosterone absorption through the oral mucosa; the short half-life requires administration three times a day.[818] After subcutaneous implantation of testosterone-filled silicone elastomer (Silastic) capsules the hormone is released slowly for long periods into the plasma,[819] but this mode may not be practical in humans because of the large size of such capsules. When oral testosterone in microparticulate form is administered in large amounts (200 to 400 mg/d) physiological blood levels can be achieved, but the preparation has to be taken several times a day.[820–822] Furthermore this dosage level of hormone induces hepatic drug-metabolizing enzymes, the long-term effects of which are uncertain.[823] Topical administration of testosterone that is suspended in creams appears to be effective insofar as the hormone can be absorbed from skin into the bloodstream and thus act systemically.[824, 825] The use of topical testosterone cream for lichen sclerosis of the vulva can cause profound virilization in women.[826, 827] Administration of testosterone via rectal suppository[828] or nasal drops[829] also results in only short-term elevation of plasma levels. Because of the frequency of administration that is necessary to sustain effective blood levels none of these other techniques appears to be clinically useful.

ADMINISTRATION OF ANDROGENS TO NORMAL MEN. The administration of testosterone esters to normal men in amounts sufficient to replace the normal daily testicular secretion (equivalent to 5 to 10 mg/d) has little physiological effect.[468] When the plasma testosterone level is raised above the normal range both the basal levels of LH and FSH and the peak response after LHRH administration are diminished. As a consequence the testicular volume is decreased about 20%, sperm production is uniformly decreased by 90% or more, and the volume of the ejaculate remains unchanged.[789, 830–832] The administration of comparable amounts of 17α-alkylated androgens by mouth results in decreases in the plasma testosterone level but similar changes in gonadotropin level and sperm count.[833, 834] These properties are the basis for trials of the agents as male contraceptives in the hope that sperm production could be effectively inhibited but androgen action maintained. Unfortunately the inhibition of sperm production is not usually complete when androgens are administered in doses low enough not to cause significant side effects (see Chapter 18). When plasma testosterone is increased significantly above control levels body weight increases about 3% (largely because of an increase in extracellular fluid volume), the hemoglobin level rises by about 10 g/L (1 g/dL), acne is common, and the serum estradiol concentration doubles.[830]

ADMINISTRATION OF ANDROGENS TO HYPOGONADAL MEN. The aim of androgen therapy in hypogonadal men is to restore or bring to normal male secondary sexual characteristics (beard, body hair, external genitalia) and male sexual behavior and to promote normal male somatic development (hemoglobin, voice, muscle mass, nitrogen balance, and epiphyseal closure). Because a reliable assay for plasma testos-

terone is widely available for monitoring therapy, the treatment of androgen deficiency is straightforward and almost universally successful. The parenteral administration of a long-acting testosterone ester such as 100 to 300 mg of testosterone enanthate at 1- to 3-wk intervals results in a sustained increase in plasma testosterone concentration to the normal male range or slightly above.[286, 468, 788, 789, 835] The usual replacement regimen is 200 mg every 2 wk.[788] Similar effects are obtained with the percutaneous administration of testosterone.[803–809] In most individuals such regimens reduce the plasma LH level and maintain serum testosterone within the normal range.[788] If the hypogonadism is primary and of long duration (as in Klinefelter's syndrome) suppression of the plasma LH value to the normal range may not occur for many weeks, if at all.[468, 836–839] There is considerable variability in the relation between plasma testosterone and male sexual behavior but in postpubertal testicular failure, even of many years' duration, resumption of normal sexual activity is usual after adequate replacement.[840, 841] The major effects of androgen appear to be on libido[842] and on the frequency of erections.[843, 844] Androgen therapy does not ordinarily restore spermatogenesis to normal in hypogonadal states, but the volume of the ejaculate, which is derived largely from the prostate and seminal vesicles, and other secondary sexual characteristics return to normal. Treatment of hypogonadal men with testosterone causes growth of the prostate to the same degree as that of age-matched controls.[845] The somatic effects of endogenous androgen, including effects on hemoglobin, nitrogen balance, and skeletal development, are also reproduced.[289] In a subset of hypogonadal men androgen treatment increases blood volume significantly.[846]

During normal puberty androgens promote epiphyseal fusion and increase bone mass. In men with incomplete puberty due to primary or secondary testicular failure, androgen therapy may increase bone density, although the degree of improvement decreases with age.[847–849] Acquired androgen deficiency is associated with bone loss that is similar to the bone loss of estrogen deficiency in women and that may be mediated by derepression of interleukin-6 production.[850] The epiphyseal fusion associated with normal puberty or androgen administration appears to be mediated by the estrogenic metabolites of testosterone.[83, 84]

In men of all ages in whom hypogonadism develops before expected puberty (such as individuals with hypogonadotropic hypogonadism), it is appropriate to bring plasma testosterone into the adult range slowly. When therapy is begun at the time of expected puberty in such patients the normal events of male puberty proceed in the usual fashion. If therapy is delayed until long after the time of usual puberty the degree to which normal virilization will occur is variable. Many such patients undergo a late but relatively complete anatomic and functional male maturation. Intermittent androgen therapy is sometimes administered to prepubertal hypogonadal boys with microphallus to stimulate the growth of the external genitalia[272, 405] (Fig. 16–20) and is useful for some boys with hypospadias and microphallus before surgical repair,[851, 852] although the long-term consequences of such therapy are unclear.[853] If patients are monitored closely and androgen is given for only short periods, such therapy probably has no adverse effects on somatic growth.

In boys of pubertal age with either isolated hypogonadotropic hypogonadism or primary testicular deficiency, the initial administration of small doses of testosterone esters followed by a gradual increase to doses of 100 to 150 mg/m² of body surface area/mo results in the development of a normal pubertal growth spurt.[854] Penile growth, deepening of the voice, and appearance of other secondary sexual characteristics usually commence during the first year of treatment. Puberty in normal boys extends over several years, and treatment

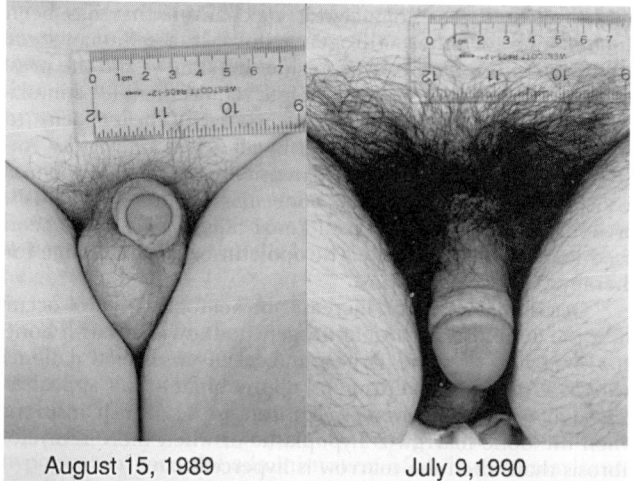

August 15, 1989   July 9,1990

Figure 16–20. Effect on penile size of 200 mg testosterone cypionate intramuscularly every 2 wk for 11 mo in a previously untreated 22-year-old man with microphallus due to hypogonadotropic hypogonadism. (From Griffin JE, Wilson JD. Disorders of sexual differentiation. In: Walsh PC, Retik AB, Stamey TA, et al, eds. Campbell's Urology. 6th ed. Philadelphia: WB Saunders, 1992: 1509–1542, with permission.)

that is designed to replicate normal development cannot shorten the process greatly. The usual practice is to institute androgen therapy in hypogonadal boys between the ages of 12 and 14, depending on their subjective need for sexual development. Testosterone exerts its full action only in the presence of a balanced hormonal environment and particularly in the presence of adequate levels of hCG. Consequently prepubertal boys with coexisting deficiency of hCG exhibit a diminished response to androgens in regard to both growth and the development of secondary sexual characteristics unless hCG is given simultaneously.[854–857] As noted earlier testosterone may promote growth in pubertal boys by enhancing the secretion of human growth hormone and IGF1.[291, 292, 858]

USE OF ANDROGENS FOR PURPOSES OTHER THAN REPLACEMENT THERAPY

Enhanced Nitrogen Balance and Muscle Development.
Soon after the identification of testosterone as the principal androgen produced by the testis it was recognized that the administration of the hormone to hypogonadal or castrated men has systemic effects in addition to those on the male urogenital tract. These effects include reduction in the urinary excretion of nitrogen, sodium, potassium, and chloride and induction of a gain in weight.[286] In contrast in normal men who are given pharmacologic amounts of androgen, nitrogen retention is only about half that of hypogonadal men, and when food intake is constant, normal men gain little or no weight. In all situations other than hypogonadism, the positive nitrogen balance is short-lived (probably lasting no more than 1 to 2 mo).

A major component of androgen-induced weight gain and nitrogen retention in hypogonadal men is due to an increase in skeletal and muscle mass. In several species, including humans, the skeletal muscles that support the forelimbs, namely the muscles of the pectoral and shoulder region, show the greatest response, but most muscles probably have some degree of response to androgen administration.[289] The enlargement of responsive muscles is due to the formation of new myofilaments along the myofibrils and to division of the enlarging myofibrils; the net consequence is an increase in the diameter of muscle fibers and fibrils.[859]

Because androgens have significant effects on muscle mass and body weight when administered to hypogonadal men it was initially assumed that androgens in pharmacologic

amounts could promote growth of muscle mass to greater levels than those produced by the normal testicular secretion. The anabolic and androgenic actions of androgens were believed to be distinct and independent hormone actions, so a concerted effort was made to devise pure anabolic steroids with no androgenic effects. In fact, however, androgenic and anabolic effects do not result from different actions of the same hormone but represent the same action in different tissues. Krieg and Voigt showed that androgen-responsive muscle contains the same androgen receptor system that is known to mediate the action of the hormone in other androgen target tissues.[860] It is theoretically possible that a steroid might be devised that would be taken up by or retained selectively by muscle,[861] but no anabolic hormone devoid of androgenic effects has been found.[862, 863]

Indeed all anabolic agents tested in humans so far are also androgens and in appropriate doses can be used for androgen replacement.[864–866] For example methandrostenolone, which has a greater effect on nitrogen balance per unit weight than does methyltestosterone, is a potent androgen and can be used for replacement therapy in hypogonadal men.[864] 19-Nortestosterone derivatives come closest to being selective anabolic agents because the parent compounds are fully active in muscle (and other tissues), whereas the 5α-reduced metabolites that form in the male urogenital tract are less active; however all such agents tested to date can be used for androgen replacement in hypogonadal animals.[817] For these reasons, because the effects of androgens on nitrogen balance are of limited magnitude and of short duration in normal men, and because no beneficial effects of ordinary doses of androgen have been documented on muscle development in normal postpubertal men, the likelihood of developing a specific anabolic steroid seems remote. However androgens have been tried in a variety of clinical situations other than hypogonadism with the hope that improvement in nitrogen balance and muscle development could outweigh any deleterious side effects.

Attempts to Improve Nitrogen Balance in Catabolic States. After injury, infection, or surgery, body protein is broken down more rapidly than it is formed and as a consequence excess nitrogen is excreted in the urine. During the subsequent recovery phase nitrogen deficits are replaced. Anabolic steroids can improve the nitrogen balance during the first few days after relatively minor operations in well-nourished individuals,[867] but the diminution in nitrogen loss is minimal and does not appear to be of therapeutic benefit.[867] Likewise any effect of androgens on weight in undernourished, debilitated, or elderly individuals is complicated by the fact that many such men, including some men with AIDS, also have secondary testosterone deficiency.[868] In appropriately controlled studies no consistent effects on weight or strength have been documented after androgen treatment.[869, 870] These negative results are probably the consequence of several factors, including the dependence of anabolic effects on adequate nutrition and health, the paucity of androgenic effects in men when androgen levels are normal, and the temporary nature of any positive nitrogen balance when it does occur. In short androgens are disappointing as therapeutic aids to promote anabolism in acute illness, continuing trauma, and protein depletion associated with chronic illness.

Androgens are also of no proven value in the management of nitrogen accumulation in chronic renal failure; at best they induce a transient improvement in nitrogen balance but this effect is of doubtful benefit.[871] In one study of boys receiving chronic hemodialysis in whom growth velocity was low, low-dose testosterone therapy stimulated growth in the short term.[872] In acute renal failure androgens cause a decrease in the rate of urea production and a consequent de-

136. Terasaka T, Nowlin DM, Pardridge WM. Differential binding of testosterone and estradiol to isoforms of sex hormone–binding globulin: selective alteration of estradiol binding in cirrhosis. J Clin Endocrinol Metab 1988; 67:639–643.

137. Plymate SR, Leonard JM, Paulsen CA, et al. Sex hormone–binding globulin changes with androgen replacement. J Clin Endocrinol Metab 1983; 57:645–648.

138. Pardridge WM. Transport of protein-bound hormone into tissues in vivo. Endocr Rev 1981; 2:103–123.

139. Anderson DC. Sex-hormone–binding globulin. Clin Endocrinol Metab 1974; 3:69–96.

140. Wilson JD. Metabolism of testicular androgens. In: Greep RO, Astwood EB, eds. Handbook of Physiology. Sect 7: Endocrinology. Vol V. Male Reproductive System. Washington, DC: American Physiological Society, 1975: 491–508.

141. Siiteri PK, MacDonald PC. Role of extraglandular estrogen in human endocrinology. In: Greep RO, Astwood EB, eds. Handbook of Physiology. Sect 7: Endocrinology. Vol II. Female Reproductive System. Part I. Washington, DC: American Physiological Society, 1973: 615–629.

142. Moore RJ, Gazak JM, Wilson JD. Regulation of cytoplasmic dihydrotestosterone binding in dog prostate by 17β-estradiol. J Clin Invest 1979; 63:351–357.

143. Wilson JD, Aiman J, MacDonald PC. The pathogenesis of gynecomastia. Adv Intern Med 1980; 25:1–32.

144. MacDonald PC, Madden JD, Brenner PF, et al. Origin of estrogen in normal men and in women with testicular feminization. J Clin Endocrinol Metab 1979; 49:905–916.

145. Ito T, Horton R. The source of plasma dihydrotestosterone in man. J Clin Invest 1971; 50:1621–1627.

146. Bruchovsky N, Wilson JD. The conversion of testosterone to 5α-androstan-17β-ol-3-one by rat prostate in vivo and in vitro. J Biol Chem 1968; 243:2012–2021.

147. Anderson KM, Liao S. Selective retention of dihydrotestosterone by prostatic nuclei. Nature 1968; 219:277–279.

148. Labrie C, Belanger A, Labrie F. Androgenic activity of dehydroepiandrosterone and androstenedione in the rat ventral prostate. Endocrinology 1988; 123:1412–1417.

149. Dorfman RI, Shipley RA. Androgens: Biochemistry, Physiology, and Clinical Significance. New York: John Wiley & Sons, 1956.

150. Thigpen AE, Davis DL, Milatovich A, et al. Molecular genetics of steroid 5α-reductase 2 deficiency. J Clin Invest 1992; 90:799–809.

151. Wilson JD, Griffin JE, Russell DW. Steroid 5α-reductase 2 deficiency. Endocr Rev 1993; 14:577–593.

152. Moore RJ, Wilson JD. Steroid 5α-reductase in cultured human fibroblasts: biochemical and genetic evidence for two enzyme activities. J Biol Chem 1976; 251:5895–5900.

153. Russell DW, Wilson JD. Steroid 5α-reductase: two genes/two enzymes. Annu Rev Biochem 1994; 63:25–61.

154. George FW, Peterson K. 5-Dihydrotestosterone formation is necessary for embryogenesis of the rat prostate. Endocrinology 1988; 122:1159–1164.

155. Moore RJ, Wilson JD. The effect of androgenic hormones on the reduced nicotinamide adenine dinucleotide phosphate: Δ⁴-3-ketosteroid 5 alpha-oxidoreductase of rat ventral prostate. Endocrinology 1973; 93:581–592.

156. George FW, Russell DW, Wilson JD. Feed-forward control of prostate growth: dihydrotestosterone induces expression of its own biosynthetic enzyme, steroid 5α-reductase. Proc Natl Acad Sci USA 1991; 88:8044–8047.

157. Kato R, Onoda K, Omori Y. Mechanism of thyroxine-induced increase in steroid Δ⁴-reductase activity in male rats. Endocrinol Jpn 1970; 17:215–219.

158. Hellman L, Bradlow HL, Zumoff B, et al. Thyroid androgen interrelations and the hypocholesterolemic effect of androsterone. J Clin Endocrinol Metab 1959; 19:936–948.

159. Horton R, Pasupuletti V, Antonipillai I. Androgen induction of steroid 5α-reductase may be mediated via insulin-like growth factor-I. Endocrinology 1993; 133:447–451.

160. Wilson JD, Lasnitzki I. Dihydrotestosterone formation in fetal tissues of the rabbit and rat. Endocrinology 1971; 89:659–668.

161. Thigpen AE, Davis DL, Milatovich A, et al. Molecular genetics of steroid 5α-reductase 2 deficiency. J Clin Invest 1992; 90:799–809.

162. Frederiksen DW, Wilson JD. Partial characterization of the nuclear reduced nicotinamide adenine dinucleotide phosphate: Δ⁴-3-ketosteroid 5 alpha-oxidoreductase of rat prostate. J Biol Chem 1971; 246:2584–2593.

163. Corbin CJ, Graham-Lorence S, McPhaul MJ, et al. Isolation of a full-length cDNA insert encoding human aromatase system cytochrome P-450 and its expression in nonsteroidogenic cells. Proc Natl Acad Sci USA 1988; 85:8948–8952.

164. Mahendroo MS, Mendelson CR, Simpson ER. Tissue-specific and hormonally controlled alternative promoters regulate aromatase cytochrome P450 gene expression in human adipose tissue. J Biol Chem 1993; 268:19463–19470; 4:503–520.

165. Brooks RV. Androgens. Clin Endocrinol Metab 1975; 4:503–520.

166. Williams-Ashman HG. Metabolic effects of testicular androgens. In: Greep RO, Astwood EB, eds. Handbook of Physiology. Sect 7: Endocrinology. Vol V. Male Reproductive System. Washington, DC: American Physiological Society, 1975: 473–490.

167. Evans RM. The steroid and thyroid hormone receptor superfamily. Science 1988; 240:889–895.

168. George FW, Wilson JD. Sex determination and differentiation. In: Knobil E, Neill JD, eds. The Physiology of Reproduction. 2nd ed. New York: Raven Press 1994: 3–28.

169. Baker HWG, Bailey DJ, Feil PD, et al. Nuclear accumulation of androgens in perfused rat accessory sex organs and testes. Endocrinology 1977; 100:709–721.

170. Payne AH, Kawano A, Jaffe RB. Formation of dihydrotestosterone and other 5α-reduced metabolites by isolated seminiferous tubules and suspensions of interstitial cells in a human testis. J Clin Endocrinol Metab 1973; 37:448–453.

171. Price P, Wass JAH, Griffin JE, et al. High dose androgen therapy in male pseudohermaphrodism due to 5α-reductase deficiency and disorders of the androgen receptor. J Clin Invest 1984; 74:1496–1508.

172. Wilson EM, French FS. Binding properties of androgen receptors: evidence for identical receptors in rat testes, epididymis, and prostate. J Biol Chem 1976; 251:5620–5629.

173. Verhoeven G. Androgen binding proteins in mouse submandibular gland. J Steroid Biochem 1979; 10:129–138.

174. Snochowski M, Dahlberg E, Gustafsson J-A. Characterization and quantification of the androgen and glucocorticoid receptors in cytosol from rat skeletal muscle. Eur J Biochem 1980; 111:603–616.

175. McGill HC Jr, Anselmo VC, Buchanan JM, et al. The heart is a target organ for androgen. Science 1980; 207:775–777.

176. McCormick PD, Razel AJ, Spelsberg TC, et al. Evidence for an androgen receptor in the human placenta. Am J Obstet Gynecol 1981; 140:8–13.

177. Tsai Y-H, Sanborn BM, Steinberger A, et al. Sertoli cell chromatin acceptor sites for androgen-receptor complexes. J Steroid Biochem 1980; 13:711–718.

178. Verhoeven G. Androgen receptor in cultured interstitial cells derived from immature rat testis. J Steroid Biochem 1980; 13:469–474.

179. Menon M, Tananis CE, Hicks LL, et al. Characterization of the binding of a potent synthetic androgen, methyltrienolone, to human tissues. J Clin Invest 1978; 61:150–162.

180. Blondeau J-P, Baulieu E-E, Robel P. Androgen-dependent regulation of androgen nuclear receptor in the rat ventral prostate. Endocrinology 1982; 110:1926–1932.

181. Rajfer J, Namkung PC, Petral PH. Identification, partial characterization and age-related changes of a cytoplasmic androgen receptor in the rat penis. J Steroid Biochem 1980; 13:1489–1492.

182. McPhaul MJ, Marcelli M, Zoppi S, et al. The spectrum of mutations in the androgen receptor gene that causes androgen resistance. J Clin Endocrinol Metab 1993; 76:17–23.

183. Griffin JE, Punyashthiti K, Wilson JD. Dihydrotestosterone binding by cultured human fibroblasts: comparison of cells from control subjects and from patients with hereditary male pseudohermaphroditism due to androgen resistance. J Clin Invest 1976; 57:1342–1351.

184. Grino PB, Griffin JE, Wilson JD. Testosterone at high concentrations interacts with the human androgen receptor similarly to dihydrotestosterone. Endocrinology 1990; 126:1165–1172.

185. Migeon BR, Brown TR, Axelman J, et al. Studies of the locus for androgen receptor: localization on the human X chromosome and evidence for homology with the Tfm locus in the mouse. Proc Natl Acad Sci USA 1981; 78:6339–6343.

186. Lubahn DB, Joseph DR, Sullivan PM, et al. Cloning of human androgen receptor complementary DNA and localization to the X chromosome. Science 1988; 240:327–330.

187. Chang C, Kokontis CJ, Liao S. Molecular cloning of human and rat complementary DNA encoding androgen receptors. Science 1988; 240:324–326.

188. Trapman J, Klaassen P, Kuiper GGJM, et al. Cloning, structure and expression of a cDNA encoding the human androgen receptor. Biochem Biophys Res Commun 1988; 153:241–248.

189. Tilley WD, Marcelli M, Wilson JD, et al. Characterization and expression of a cDNA encoding the human androgen receptor. Proc Natl Acad Sci USA 1989; 86:327–331.

190. Maes M, Sulta C, Zerhourni N, et al. Role of testosterone binding to the androgen receptor in male sexual differentiation of patients with 5α-reductase deficiency. J Steroid Biochem 1979; 11:1385–1390.

191. Kaufman M, Pinsky L. The dissociation of testosterone- and 5-dihydrotestosterone-receptor complexes formed within cultured human genital skin fibroblasts. J Steroid Biochem 1983; 18:121–125.

192. Kovacs WJ, Griffin JE, Weaver DD, et al. A mutation that causes lability of the androgen receptor under conditions that normally promote transformation to the DNA-binding state. J Clin Invest 1984; 73:1095–1104.

193. Deslypere J-P, Young M, Wilson JD, et al. Testosterone and 5-dihydrotestosterone interact differently with the androgen receptor to enhance transcription of the MMTV-CAT reporter gene. Mol Cell Endocrinol 1992; 88:15–22.

194. Zhou ZX, Wong CI, Sar M, et al. The androgen receptor: an overview. Recent Prog Horm Res 1994; 49:249–274.

195. Rundlett SE, Miesfeld RL. Quantitative differences in androgen and glucocorticoid receptor DNA binding properties contribute to receptor-selective transcriptional regulation. Mol Cell Endocrinol 1995; 109:1–10.

196. Celis L, Claessens F, Peeters B, et al. Proteins interacting with an andro-

gen-responsive unit in the C3(1) gene intron. Mol Cell Endocrinol 1993; 94:165–172.

197. Roehrborn CG, Lange JL, George FW, et al. Changes in amount and intracellular distribution of androgen receptor in human foreskin as a function of age. J Clin Invest 1987; 79:44–47.

198. Johnson L, Petty CS, Neaves WB. Further quantification of human spermatogenesis. Germ cell loss during postprophase of meiosis and its relationship to daily sperm production. Biol Reprod 1983; 29:207–215.

199. Clermont Y. The cycle of the seminiferous epithelium in man. Am J Anat 1963; 112:35–45.

200. Nikkanen V, Söderström K-O, Parvinen M. Identification of the spermatogenic stages in living seminiferous tubules of man. J Reprod Fertil 1978; 53:255–257.

201. Johnson L. A new approach to study the architectural arrangement of spermatogenic stages revealed little evidence of a partial wave along the length of human seminiferous tubules. J Androl 1994; 15:435–441.

202. Fawcett DW. The Cell. 2nd ed. Philadelphia: WB Saunders, 1981: 604–617.

203. Heller CG, Clermont Y. Spermatogenesis in man: an estimate of its duration. Science 1963; 140:184–186.

204. Rowley MJ, Teshima F, Heller CG. Duration of transit of spermatozoa through the human male ductular system. Fertil Steril 1970; 21:390–396.

205. Bedford JM. Maturation, transport, and fate of spermatozoa in the epididymis. In: Greep RO, Astwood EB. Handbook of Physiology. Sect 7: Endocrinology. Vol V. Male Reproductive System. Washington, DC: American Physiological Society, 1975: 303–317.

206. Hinrichsen MJ, Blaquier JA. Evidence supporting the existence of sperm maturation in the human epididymis. J Reprod Fertil 1980; 60:291–294.

207. Satir R. Basis of flagellar motility in spermatozoa: current status. In: Fawcett DW, Bedford JM, eds. The Spermatozoon. Baltimore: Urban and Schwarzenberg, 1979: 81–90.

208. Linck RW. Advances in the ultrastructural analysis of the sperm flagellar axoneme. In: Fawcett DW, Bedford JM, eds. The Spermatozoon. Baltimore: Urban and Schwarzenberg, 1979: 99–115.

209. Gibbons BH. Studies on the mechanism of flagellar movement. In: Fawcett DW, Bedford JM, eds. The Spermatozoon. Baltimore: Urban and Schwarzenberg, 1979: 91–97.

210. Afzelius BA, Mossberg B. Immotile-cilia syndrome (primary ciliary dyskinesia), including Kartagener syndrome. In: Scriver CR, Beaudet AL, Sly WS, Valle D, eds. The Metabolic and Molecular Bases of Inherited Disease. New York: McGraw-Hill, 1995: 3943–3954.

211. Setchell BP. Regulation of spermatogenesis and possible sites for contraceptive action. In: Jeffcoate SL, Sandler M, eds. Progress Towards a Male Contraceptive. New York: John Wiley & Sons, 1982: 1–18.

212. Heckert L, Griswold MD. Expression of the FSH receptor in the testis. Recent Prog Horm Res 1993; 48:61–77.

213. Vornberger W, Prins G, Musto NA, et al. Androgen receptor distribution in rat testis: new implications for androgen regulation of spermatogenesis. Endocrinology 1994; 134:2307–2316.

214. Bremner WJ, Millar MR, Sharpe RM, et al. Immunohistochemical localization of androgen receptors in the rat testis: evidence for stage-dependent expression and regulation by androgens. Endocrinology 1994; 135:1227–1234.

215. Lyon MF, Glenister PH, Lamoreux ML. Normal spermatozoa from androgen-resistant germ cells of chimeric mice and the role of androgen in spermatogenesis. Nature 1975; 258:620–622.

216. Pescovitz OH, Srivastava CH, Breyer PR, et al. Paracrine control of spermatogenesis. Trends Endocrinol Metab 1994; 5:125–131.

217. Huang HFS, Li MT, Pogach LM, et al. Messenger ribonucleic acid of rat testicular retinoic acid receptors: developmental pattern, cellular distribution, and testosterone effect. Biol Reprod 1994; 51:541–550.

218. Johnson RS, Spiegelman BM, Papaioannou V. Pleiotropic effects of a null mutation in the c-fos proto-oncogene. Cell 1992; 71:577–586.

219. Zsebo KM, Williams DA, Geissler EN, et al. Stem cell factor is encoded at the Sl locus of the mouse and is the ligand for the c-kit tyrosine kinase receptor. Cell 1990; 63:213–224.

220. Morrison-Graham K, Takahashi Y. Steel factor and c-kit receptor: from mutants to a growth factor system. Bioessays 1993; 15:77–83.

221. Nantel F, Monaco L, Foulkes NS, et al. Spermiogenesis deficiency and germ-cell apoptosis in CREM-mutant mice. Nature 1996; 159–162.

222. Blendy JA, Kaestner KH, Weinbauer GF, et al. Severe impairment of spermatogenesis in mice lacking the CREM gene. Nature 1996; 162–165.

223. Skinner MK. Cell-cell interactions in the testis. Endocr Rev 1991; 45–77.

224. Verhoeven G. Local control systems within the testis. Baillieres Clin Endocrinol Metab 1992; 6:313–333.

225. Mayo KE. Inhibin and activin. Molecular aspects of regulation and function. Trends Endocrinol Metab 1994; 5:407–415.

226. Hakovirta H, Kaipia A, Söder O, et al. Effects of activin-A, inhibin-A, and transforming growth factor-1 on stage-specific deoxyribonucleic acid synthesis during rat seminiferous epithelial cycle. Endocrinology 1993; 133:1664–1668.

227. Parvinen M, Pelto-Huikko M, Söder O, et al. Expression of beta-nerve growth factor and its receptor in rat seminiferous epithelium: specific function at the onset of meiosis. J Cell Biol 1992; 117:629–641.

228. Spiteri-Grech J, Nieschlag E. The role of growth hormone and insulin-like growth factor I in the regulation of male reproductive function. Horm Res 1992; 38(Suppl 1):22–27.

229. Söder O, Syed V, Callard GV, et al. Production and secretion of an interleukin-1-like factor is stage-dependent and correlates with spermatogonial DNA synthesis in the rat seminiferous epithelium. Int J Androl 1991; 14:223–231.

230. Matsumoto AM, Paulsen CA, Bremner WJ. Stimulation of sperm production by human luteinizing hormone in gonadotropin-suppressed normal men. J Clin Endocrinol Metab 1984; 59:882–887.

231. Matsumoto AM, Karpas AE, Bremner WJ. Chronic human chorionic gonadotropin administration in normal men: evidence that follicle-stimulating hormone is necessary for the maintenance of quantitatively normal spermatogenesis in man. J Clin Endocrinol Metab 1986; 62:1184–1192.

232. McLachlan RI, Wreford NG, O'Donnell L, et al. The endocrine regulation of spermatogenesis: independent roles for testosterone and FSH. J Endocrinol 1996; 148:1–9.

233. Tarin JJ, Trounson AO. Inducers of the acrosome reaction. Reprod Fertil Dev 1994; 6:33–35.

234. Perreault SD, Rogers BJ. Capacitation pattern of human spermatozoa. Fertil Steril 1982; 38:258–260.

235. Gorus FK, Finsy R, Pipeleers DG. Effect of temperature, nutrients, calcium, and cAMP on motility of human spermatozoa. Am J Physiol 1982; 242:C304–C311.

236. Blandau RJ. In vitro fertilization and embryo transfer. Fertil Steril 1980; 33:3–11.

237. Evans MI, Mukherjee AB, Schulman JD. Human in vitro fertilization. Obstet Gynecol Surv 1980; 35:71–81.

238. Siiteri PK, Wilson JD. Testosterone formation and metabolism during male sexual differentiation in the human embryo. J Clin Endocrinol Metab 1974; 38:113–125.

239. Reyes FI, Bordoditsky RS, Winter JSD, et al. Studies on human sexual development. II: Fetal and maternal serum gonadotropin and sex steroid concentrations. J Clin Endocrinol Metab 1974; 38:612–617.

240. Forest MG, Sizonenko PC, Cathiard AM, et al. Hypophyso-gonadal function in humans during the first year of life. I: Evidence for testicular activity in early infancy. J Clin Invest 1974; 53:819–828.

241. Forest MG, Cathiard AM. Pattern of plasma testosterone and Δ^4-androstenedione in normal newborns: evidence for testicular activity at birth. J Clin Endocrinol Metab 1975; 41:977–984.

242. Bidlingmaier F, Dörr HG, Eisenmenger W, et al. Testosterone and androstenedione concentrations in human testis and epididymis during first two years of life. J Clin Endocrinol Metab 1983; 57:311–315.

243. Winter JSD, Hughes IA, Reyes FI, et al. Pituitary-gonadal relations in infancy. 2: Patterns of serum gonadal steroid concentrations in man from birth to two years of age. J Clin Endocrinol Metab 1976; 42:679–686.

244. Frasier SD, Gafford F, Horton R. Plasma androgens in childhood and adolescence. J Clin Endocrinol Metab 1969; 29:1404–1408.

245. August GP, Grumbach MM, Crapo L, et al. Hormonal changes in puberty. III: Correlation of plasma testosterone, LH, FSH, testicular size, and bone age with male pubertal development. J Clin Endocrinol Metab 1972; 34:319–326.

246. Vermeulen A, Reubens R, Verdonck L. Testosterone secretion and metabolism in male senescence. J Clin Endocrinol Metab 1972; 34:730–735.

247. Stearns EL, MacDonnell JA, Kaufman BJ, et al. Declining testicular function with age: hormonal and clinical correlates. Am J Med 1974; 57:761–766.

248. Pirke KM, Doerr P. Age related changes in free plasma testosterone, dihydrotestosterone and oestradiol. Acta Endocrinol 1975; 80:171–178.

249. Bremner WJ, Vitiello MV, Prinz PM. Loss of circadian rhythmicity in blood testosterone levels with aging in normal men. J Clin Endocrinol Metab 1983; 56:1278–1281.

250. Davidson JM, Chen JJ, Crapo L, et al. Hormonal changes and sexual function in aging men. J Clin Endocrinol Metab 1983; 57:71–77.

251. Jost A. The role of fetal hormones in prenatal development. Harvey Lect 1961; 55:201–226.

252. Jost A. A new look at the mechanism controlling sex differentiation in mammals. Johns Hopkins Med J 1972; 130:38–53.

253. George FW, Wilson JD. Embryology of the genital tract. In: Walsh PC, Retik AB, Stamey TA, et al, eds. Campbell's Urology. 6th ed. Philadelphia: WB Saunders, 1992: 1496–1508.

254. Donahoe PK, Cate RL, MacLaughlin DT, et al. Mullerian inhibiting substance: gene structure and mechanism of action of a fetal regressor. Recent Prog Horm Res 1987; 43:431–468.

255. George FW, Wilson JD. Sexual differentiation. In: Beard RW, Nathanielsz PW, eds. Fetal Physiology and Medicine. The Basis of Perinatology. 2nd ed. New York: Marcel Dekker, 1984: 57–79.

256. George FW, Noble JF. Androgen receptors are similar in fetal and in adult rabbits. Endocrinology 1984; 115:1451–1458.

257. Kaplan SL, Grumbach MM. The ontogenesis of human foetal hormones. II: Luteinizing hormone (LH) and follicle stimulating hormone (FSH). Acta Endocrinol 1976; 81:808–829.

258. Molsberry RL, Carr BR, Mendelson CR, et al. Human chorionic gonadotropin binding to human fetal testis as a function of gestational age. J Clin Endocrinol Metab 1982; 55:791–794.

259. Tapanainen J, Kellokumpu-Lehtinen P, Pelliniemi L, et al. Age-related changes in endogenous steroids of human fetal testis during early and midpregnancy. J Clin Endocrinol Metab 1981; 52:98–102.

260. Reyes FI, Faiman C, Winter JSD. Development of the regulatory mecha-

nisms of the hypothalamic-pituitary-gonadal system in the human fetus: the chorionic-hypothalamic-pituitary-gonadal axis. In: Novy MJ, Resko JA, eds. Fetal Endocrinology. New York: Academic, 1981: 283–302.

261. Ellinwood WE, Baughman WL, Resko JA. The effects of gonadectomy and testosterone treatment on luteinizing hormone secretion in fetal rhesus monkeys. Endocrinology 1982; 110:183–189.

262. Zondek LH, Zondek T. Observations on the testis in anencephaly with special reference to the Leydig cells. Biol Neonate 1965; 8:329–347.

263. George FW, Simpson ER, Milewich L, et al. Studies on the regulation of the onset of steroid hormone biosynthesis in fetal rabbit gonads. Endocrinology 1979; 105:1100–1106.

264. Reinisch JM. Effects of prenatal hormone exposure on physical and psychological development in humans and animals: with a note on the state of the field. In: Sachar EJ, ed. Hormones, Behavior, and Psychopathology. New York: Raven, 1976: 69–94.

265. Wilson JD. Gonadal hormones and sexual behavior. In: Besser GM, Martini L, eds. Clinical Neuroendocrinology. Vol II. New York: Academic, 1982: 1–29.

266. Burger HG, Yamada Y, Bangah ML, et al. Serum gonadotrophin, sex steroid, and immunoreactive inhibin levels in the first two years of life. J Clin Endocrinol Metab 1991; 72:682–686.

267. Davidson JM, Levine S. Endocrine regulation of behavior. Annu Rev Physiol 1972; 34:375–408.

268. De Moor P, Verhoeven G, Heyns W. Permanent effects of fetal and neonatal testosterone secretion on steroid metabolism and binding. Differentiation 1973; 1:241–253.

269. Gustafsson J-A, Stenberg A. Neonatal programming of androgen responsiveness of liver of adult rats. J Biol Chem 1974; 249:719–723.

270. Mann DR, Gould KG, Collins DC, et al. Blockade of neonatal activation of the pituitary-testicular axis: effect on peripubertal luteinizing hormone and testosterone secretion and on testicular development in male monkeys. J Clin Endocrinol Metab 1989; 68:600–607.

271. Reiter EO, Grumbach MM, Kaplan SL, et al. The response of pituitary gonadotropes to synthetic LRF in children with glucocorticoid-treated congenital adrenal hyperplasia: lack of effect of intrauterine and neonatal androgen excess. J Clin Endocrinol Metab 1975; 40:318–325.

272. Guthrie RD, Smith DW, Graham CB. Testosterone treatment for micropenis during early childhood. J Pediatr 1973; 83:247–252.

273. Ducharme JR, Collu R. Pubertal development: normal, precocious and delayed. Clin Endocrinol Metab 1982; 11:57–87.

274. Wierman ME, Beardsworth DE, Crawford JD, et al. Adrenarche and skeletal maturation during luteinizing hormone releasing hormone analogue suppression of gonadarche. J Clin Invest 1986; 77:121–126.

275. Forti G, Santoro S, Grisolia GA, et al. Spermatic and peripheral plasma concentrations of testosterone and androstenedione in prepubertal boys. J Clin Endocrinol Metab 1981; 53:883–886.

276. Winter JSD, Faiman C. Serum gonadotropin concentrations in agonadal children and adults. J Clin Endocrinol Metab 1972; 35:561–564.

277. Jakacki RI, Kelch RP, Sauder SE, et al. Pulsatile secretion of luteinizing hormone in children. J Clin Endocrinol Metab 1982; 55:453–458.

278. Boyar RM, Rosenfeld RS, Kapen S, et al. Human puberty: simultaneous augmented secretion of luteinizing hormone and testosterone during sleep. J Clin Invest 1974; 54:609–618.

279. Lucky AW, Rich BH, Rosenfield RL, et al. LH bioactivity increases more than immunoreactivity during puberty. J Pediatr 1980; 97:205–213.

280. Mauras N, Veldhuis JD, Rogol AD. Role of endogenous opiates in pubertal maturation: opposing actions of naltrexone in prepubertal and late pubertal boys. J Clin Endocrinol Metab 1986; 62:1256–1263.

281. Ulloa-Aguirre A, Mendez JP, Gonzalez-Castillo A, et al. Changes in the responsiveness of luteinizing hormone secretion to infusion of the opioid antagonist naloxone throughout male sexual maturation. Clin Endocrinol 1988; 29:17–28.

282. Parra A, Cervantes C, Sanchez M, et al. The relationship of plasma gonadotrophins and androgen concentrations to body growth in boys. Acta Endocrinol 1981; 98:137–147.

283. Katz SH, Hediger ML, Zemel BS, et al. Adrenal androgens, body fat and advanced skeletal age in puberty: new evidence for the relations of adrenarche and gonadarche in males. Hum Biol 1985; 57:401–413.

284. Burger HG, McLachlan RI, Bangah M, et al. Serum inhibin concentrations rise throughout normal male and female puberty. J Clin Endocrinol Metab 1988; 67:689–694.

285. Nielsen CT, Skakkebaek NE, Richardson DW, et al. Onset of the release of spermatozoa (spermarche) in boys in relation to age, testicular growth, pubic hair, and height. J Clin Endocrinol Metab 1986; 62:532–535.

286. Wilson JD, Griffin JE. The use and misuse of androgens. Metabolism 1980; 29:1278–1295.

287. Scow RO, Hagan SN. Effect of testosterone propionate on myosin, collagen and other protein fractions in striated muscle of gonadectomized rats. Endocrinology 1957; 60:273–276.

288. Finkelstein JS, Klibanski A, Neer RM, et al. Osteoporosis in men with idiopathic hypogonadotropic hypogonadism. Ann Intern Med 1987; 106:354–361.

289. Hamilton JB. The role of testicular secretions as indicated by the effects of castration in man and by studies of pathological conditions and the short lifespan associated with maleness. Recent Prog Horm Res 1948; 3:257–322.

290. Kirkland RT, Keenan BS, Probstfield JL, et al. Decrease in plasma high-density lipoprotein cholesterol levels at puberty in boys with delayed adolescence. Correlation with plasma testosterone levels. JAMA 1987; 257:502–507.

291. Mauras N, Blizzard RM, Link K, et al. Augmentation of growth hormone secretion during puberty: evidence for a pulse amplitude–modulated phenomenon. J Clin Endocrinol Metab 1987; 64:596–601.

292. Merimee TJ, Zapf J, Hewlett B, et al. Insulin-like growth factors in pygmies. The role of puberty in determining final stature. N Engl J Med 1987; 316:906–911.

293. Marshall WA, Tanner JM. Variations in the pattern of pubertal changes in boys. Arch Dis Child 1970; 45:13–23.

294. Lee PA, Jaffe RB, Midgley AR Jr. Serum gonadotropin, testosterone and prolactin concentrations throughout puberty in boys: a longitudinal study. J Clin Endocrinol Metab 1974; 39:664–672.

295. Schonfeld WA. Primary and secondary sexual characteristics. Study of their development in males from birth through maturity, with biometric study of penis and testes. Am J Dis Child 1943; 65:535–549.

296. Takihara H, Sakatoku J, Fujii M, et al. Significance of testicular size measurement in andrology. I: A new orchiometer and its clinical application. Fertil Steril 1983; 39:836–840.

297. Harlan WR, Grillo GP, Cornoni-Huntley J, et al. Secondary sex characteristics of boys 12 to 17 years of age: the U.S. Health Examination Survey. J Pediatr 1979; 95:293–297.

298. Zachmann M, Prader A, Kind HP, et al. Testicular volume during adolescence. Cross-sectional and longitudinal studies. Helv Paediatr Acta 1974; 29:61–72.

299. Karling P, Hammar M, Varenhorst E. Prevalence and duration of hot flushes after surgical or medical castration in men with prostatic carcinoma. J Urol 1994; 152:1170–1173.

300. Harrison RG. Effect of temperature on the mammalian testis. In: Greep RO, Astwood EB, eds. Handbook of Physiology. Sect 7: Endocrinology. Vol V. Male Reproductive System. Washington, DC: American Physiological Society, 1975: 219–223.

301. Leatham JH. Nutritional influences on testicular composition and function in mammals. In: Greep RO, Astwood EB, eds. Handbook of Physiology. Sect 7: Endocrinology. Vol V. Male Reproductive System. Washington, DC: American Physiological Society, 1975: 225–232.

302. Masters WH, Johnson VE. Sex and the aging process. J Am Geriatr Soc 1981; 29:385–390.

303. Martin CE. Factors affecting sexual functioning in 60- to 79-year-old married males. Arch Sex Behav 1981; 10:399–420.

304. Tsitouras PD, Martin CE, Harman SM. Relationship of serum testosterone to sexual activity in healthy elderly men. J Gerontol 1982; 37:288–293.

305. Harman SM, Tsitouras PD. Reproductive hormones in aging men. I: Measurement of sex steroids, basal luteinizing hormone, and Leydig cell response to human chorionic gonadotropin. J Clin Endocrinol Metab 1980; 51:35–40.

306. Tsitouras PD, Hagen TC. Testosterone, LH, FSH, prolactin and sperm in aging healthy men. 7th International Congress of Endocrinology, Quebec City, Canada. 1984: 1236 (abstract).

307. Deslypere JP, Vermeulen A. Leydig cell function in normal men: effect of age, life-style, residence, diet, and activity. J Clin Endocrinol Metab 1984; 59:955–962.

308. Nankin HR, Calkins JH. Decreased bioavailable testosterone in aging normal and impotent men. J Clin Endocrinol Metab 1986; 63:1418–1420.

309. Tenover JS, Matsumoto AM, Plymate SR, et al. The effects of aging in normal men on bioavailable testosterone and luteinizing hormone secretion: response to clomiphene citrate. J Clin Endocrinol Metab 1987; 65:1118–1126.

310. Gray A, Feldman HA, McKinley JB, et al. Age, disease, and changing sex hormone levels in middle-aged men: results of the Massachusetts male aging study. J Clin Endocrinol Metab 1991; 73:1016–1025.

311. Pirke KM, Sintermann R, Vogt HJ. Testosterone and testosterone precursors in the spermatic vein and in the testicular tissue of old men. Gerontology 1980; 26:221–230.

312. Takahashi J, Higashi Y, LaNasa JA, et al. Studies of the human testis. XVIII: Simultaneous measurement of nine intratesticular steroids: evidence for reduced mitochondrial function in testis of elderly men. J Clin Endocrinol Metab 1983; 56:1178–1187.

313. Vermeulen A, Deslypere JP. Intratesticular unconjugated steroids in elderly men. J Steroid Biochem 1986; 24:1079–1083.

314. Neaves WH, Johnson L, Petty CS. Seminiferous tubules and daily sperm production in older adult men with varied numbers of Leydig cells. Biol Reprod 1987; 36:301–308.

315. McLachlan R, Tenover J, Matsumoto A, et al. Decreased serum inhibin levels in normal elderly men: evidence for decreased Sertoli cell function with aging. Clin Res 1988; 36:125A.

316. Harman SM, Tsitouras PD, Costa PT, et al. Reproductive hormones in aging men. II: Basal pituitary gonadotropins and gonadotropin responses to luteinizing hormone–releasing hormone. J Clin Endocrinol Metab 1982; 54:547–551.

317. Deslypere JP, Kaufman JM, Vermeulen T, et al. Influence of age on pulsatile luteinizing hormone release and responsiveness of the gonadotrophs to sex hormone feedback in men. J Clin Endocrinol Metab 1987; 64:68–73.

318. Urban RJ, Veldhuis JD, Blizzard RM, et al. Attenuated release of biologically active luteinizing hormone in healthy aging men. J Clin Invest 1988; 81:1020–1029.

319. Tenover JS, Dahl KD, Hsueh AJW, et al. Serum bioactive and immunoreactive follicle-stimulating hormone levels and the response to clomiphene in healthy young and elderly men. J Clin Endocrinol Metab 1987; 64:1103–1107.

320. Slag MF, Morley JE, Elson MK, et al. Impotence in medical clinic outpatients. JAMA 1983; 249:1735–1740.

321. Goldzieher JW, Dozier TS, Smith KD, et al. Improving the diagnostic reliability of rapidly fluctuating plasma hormone levels by optimized multiple-sampling techniques. J Clin Endocrinol Metab 1976; 43:824–830.

322. Rich BH, Rosenfield RL, Moll GW Jr, et al. Bioactive luteinizing hormone pituitary reserves during normal and abnormal male puberty. J Clin Endocrinol Metab 1982; 55:140–146.

323. Vermeulen A, Verdonck G. Representativeness of a single point plasma testosterone level for the long term hormonal milieu in men. J Clin Endocrinol Metab 1992; 74:939–942.

324. Horton R, Hsieh P, Barberia J, et al. Altered blood androgens in elderly men with prostate hyperplasia. J Clin Endocrinol Metab 1975; 41:793–796.

325. Cooke RR, McIntosh RP, McIntosh JGA, et al. Serum forms of testosterone in men after an hCG stimulation: relative increase in non-protein bound forms. Clin Endocrinol 1990; 32:165–175.

326. Walsh PC, Curry N, Mills RC, et al. Plasma androgen response to hCG stimulation in prepubertal boys with hypospadias and cryptorchidism. J Clin Endocrinol Metab 1976; 42:52–59.

327. Grant DB, Laurance BM, Atherden SM, et al. hCG stimulation test in children with abnormal sexual development. Arch Dis Child 1976; 51:596–601.

328. Wollesen F, Swerdloff RS, Odell WD. LH and FSH responses to luteinizing-releasing hormone in normal, adult, human males. Metabolism 1976; 28:845–863.

329. Harman SM, Tsitouras PD, Costa PT, et al. Evaluation of pituitary gonadotropic function in men: value of luteinizing hormone–releasing hormone response versus basal luteinizing hormone level for discrimination of diagnosis. J Clin Endocrinol Metab 1982; 54:196–200.

330. Synder PJ, Rudenstein RS, Gardner DF, et al. Repetitive infusion of gonadotropin-releasing hormone distinguishes hypothalamic from pituitary hypogonadism. J Clin Endocrinol Metab 1979; 48:864–868.

331. Lubs HA Jr. Testicular size in Klinefelter's syndrome in men over fifty. Report of a case with XXY/XY mosaicism. N Engl J Med 1962; 267:326–331.

332. Diamond JM. Variation in human testis size. Nature 1986; 320:488–489.

333. Rivkees SA, Hall DA, Boepple PA, et al. Accuracy and reproducibility of clinical measures of testicular volume. J Pediatr 1987; 110:914–917.

334. Donohue RE, Fauver HE. Unilateral absence of the vas deferens. A useful clinical sign. JAMA 1989; 261:1180–1182.

335. Sigman M, Howards SS. Male infertility. In: Walsh PC, Retik AB, Stamey TA, et al, eds. Campbell's Urology. 6th ed. Philadelphia: WB Saunders, 1992: 661–705.

336. Gordon DL, Herrigel JE, Moore DJ, et al. Efficacy of Coulter counter in determining low sperm concentrations. Am J Clin Pathol 1967; 47:226–228.

337. Johnson L. A re-evaluation of daily sperm output of men. Fertil Steril 1982; 37:811–816.

338. Sherins RJ, Brightwell D, Sternthal PM. Longitudinal analysis of semen of fertile and infertile men. In: Troen P, Nankin HR, eds. The Testis in Normal and Infertile Men. New York: Raven, 1977: 473–488.

339. Wilton LJ, Teichtahl H, Temple-Smith PD, et al. Structural heterogeneity of the axonemes of respiratory cilia and sperm flagella in normal men. J Clin Invest 1985; 75:825–831.

340. Alexander NJ. Male evaluation and semen analysis. Clin Obstet Gynecol 1982; 25:463–482.

341. Amelar RD, Dubin L. Semen analysis. In: Amelar RD, Dubin L, Walsh PC, eds. Male Infertility. Philadelphia: WB Saunders, 1977: 105–140.

342. Coburn M, Wheeler T, Lipshultz LI. Testicular biopsy. Its use and limitations. Urol Clin North Am 1987; 14:551–561.

343. Mallidis C, Baker HW. Fine needle tissue aspiration biopsy of the testis. Fertil Steril 1994; 61:367–375.

344. Scott RS, Burger HG. An inverse relationship exists between seminal plasma inhibin and serum follicle-stimulating hormone in man. J Clin Endocrinol Metab 1981; 52:796–803.

345. Illingworth PJ, Groome NP, Byrd W, et al. Inhibin-B: a likely candidate for the physiologically important form of inhibin in men. J Clin Endocrinol Metab 1996; 81:1321–1325.

346. Wang C. Bioassay of follicle stimulating hormone. Endocr Rev 1988; 9:374–377.

347. Weinstein RL, Kelch RP, Jenner MR, et al. Secretion of unconjugated androgens and estrogens by the normal and abnormal human testis before and after human chorionic gonadotropin. J Clin Invest 1974; 53:1–6.

348. Klein KO, Baron J, Colli MJ, et al. Estrogen levels in childhood determined by an ultrasensitive recombinant cell bioassay. J Clin Invest 1994; 94:2475–2480.

349. Wilson JD, Goldstein JL. Classification of hereditary disorders of sexual development. Birth Defects 1975; 11:1–16.

350. Rafjer J. Congenital anomalies of the testes. In: Walsh PC, Retik AB, Stamey TA, et al, eds. Campbell's Urology. 6th ed. Philadelphia: WB Saunders, 1992: 1543–1562.

351. Cendron M, Huff DS, Keating MA, et al. Anatomical, morphological and volumetric analysis: a review of 759 cases of testicular descent. J Urol 1993; 149:570–573.

352. Buyse M, Feingold M. Syndromes associated with abnormal external genitalia. In: Vallet HL, Porter IH, eds. Genetic Mechanisms of Sexual Development. New York: Academic, 1979: 425–435.

353. Andersen H, Andreassen M, Quaade F. Testicular biopsies in cryptorchidism. Acta Endocrinol 1955; 18:567–569.

354. Saito S, Kumamoto Y. The number of spermatogonia in various congenital testicular disorders. J Urol 1989; 141:1166–1168.

355. Diamond DA, Caldamone AA, Elder JS. Prevalence of the vanishing testis in boys with a unilateral impalpable testis: is the side of presentation significant? J Urol 1994; 152:502–503.

356. Cortes D, Thorup JM, Lenz K, et al. Laparoscopy in 100 consecutive patients with 128 impalpable testes. Br J Urol 1995; 75:281–287.

357. Huff DS, Snyder HM III, Hadziselimovic F, et al. An absent testis is associated with contralateral testicular hypertrophy. J Urol 1992; 148:627–628.

358. Koff SA. Does compensatory testicular enlargement predict monorchism? J Urol 1991; 146:632–633.

359. Maghnie M, Del Maschio A, Severi F. The accuracy of magnetic resonance imaging and ultrasonography compared with surgical findings in the localization of the undescended testis. Arch Pediatr Adolesc Med 1994; 148:699–703.

360. Jones C, Kern I. Laparoscopy for the non-palpable testis: a review of twenty-eight patients. Aust NZ J Surg 1993; 63:451–453.

361. Krabbe S, Berthelsen JG, Volsted P, et al. High incidence of undetected neoplasia in maldescended testis. Lancet 1979; 1:999–1000.

362. Fonger JD, Filler RM, Rider WD, et al. Testicular tumours in maldescended testes. Can J Surg 1981; 24:353–355.

363. Eik-Nes K. Secretion of testosterone by the ectopic and the cryptorchid testes in the same dog. Can J Physiol Pharmacol 1966; 44:629–633.

364. Farrer JH, Sikka SC, Xie HW, et al. Impaired testosterone biosynthesis in cryptorchidism. Fertil Steril 1985; 44:125–132.

365. Lipshultz LI, Caminos-Torres R, Greenspan CS, et al. Testicular function after orchiopexy for unilaterally undescended testis. N Engl J Med 1976; 295:15–18.

366. Hezmall HP, Lipshultz LI. Cryptorchidism and infertility. Urol Clin North Am 1982; 9:361–369.

367. Lee PA, Bellinger MF, Songer NJ, et al. An epidemiologic study of paternity after cryptorchidism: initial results. Eur J Pediatr 1993; 152(Suppl 2):S25–S27.

368. Alpert PF, Klein RS. Spermatogenesis in the unilateral cryptorchid testis after orchiopexy. J Urol 1983; 129:301–302.

369. Urry RL, Carrell DT, Starr NT, et al. The incidence of antisperm antibodies in infertility patients with a history of cryptorchidism. J Urol 1994; 151:381–383.

370. Christiansen P, Müller J, Buhl S, et al. Hormonal treatment of cryptorchidism—hCG or CnRH—a multicentre study. Acta Paediatr 1992; 81:605–608.

371. Waldschmidt J, Doede T, Vygen I. The results of 9 years of experience with a combined treatment with LH-RH and HCG for cryptorchidism. Eur J Pediatr 1993; 152(Suppl 2):S34–S36.

372. Bica DTG, Hadziselimovic F. Buserelin treatment of cryptorchidism: a randomized, double-blind, placebo-controlled study. J Urol 1992; 148:617–621.

373. Hoorweg-Nijman JJG, Havers HM, Delemarre-van de Waal HA. Effect of human chorionic gonadotrophin (hCG)/follicle-stimulating hormone treatment versus hCG treatment alone on testicular descent: a double-blind placebo-controlled study. Eur J Endocrinol 1994; 130:60–64.

374. Pyörälä S, Huttunen N-P, Uhari M. A review and meta-analysis of hormonal treatment of cryptorchidism. J Clin Endocrinol Metab 1995; 80:2795–2799.

375. Kallmann FJ, Schoenfeld WA, Barrerra SE. The genetic aspects of primary eunuchoidism. Am J Ment Defic 1944; 48:203–236.

376. Turner RC, Bobrow M, Bobrow LB, et al. Cryptorchidism in a family with Kallmann's syndrome. Proc R Soc Med 1974; 67:33–35.

377. Walsh PC, Wilson JD, Allen TD, et al. Clinical and endocrinological evaluation of patients with congenital microphallus. J Urol 1978; 120:90–95.

378. Laron Z, Kaushanski A, Josefsberg Z. Penile size and growth in children and adolescents with isolated gonadotropin deficiency (IGnD). Clin Endocrinol 1977; 6:265–270.

379. Danish RK, Lee PA, Mazur T, et al. Micropenis. II: Hypogonadotropic hypogonadism. Johns Hopkins Med J 1980; 146:177–184.

380. Kaushanski A, Laron Z. Growth pattern of boys with isolated gonadotropin deficiency. Isr J Med Sci 1979; 15:518–521.

381. Lieblich JM, Rogol AD, White BJ, et al. Syndrome of anosmia with hypogonadotropic hypogonadism (Kallmann syndrome). Clinical and laboratory studies in 23 cases. Am J Med 1982; 73:506–519.

382. Boyar RM, Finkelstein JW, Witkin M, et al. Studies of endocrine function in "isolated" gonadotropin deficiency. J Clin Endocrinol Metab 1973; 36:64–72.

383. Faiman C, Hoffman DL, Ryan RJ, et al. The "fertile eunuch" syndrome: demonstration of isolated luteinizing hormone deficiency by radioimmunoassay technique. Mayo Clin Proc 1968; 43:661–667.

384. Del Pozo E, Bolte E, Very M. Suprasellar disturbance in the syndrome of fertile eunuchoidism: case report. Acta Endocrinol 1975; 80:165–170.

385. Boyar RM, Wu RHK, Kapen S, et al. Clinical and laboratory heterogeneity in idiopathic hypogonadotropic hypogonadism. J Clin Endocrinol Metab 1976; 43:1268–1275.

386. Smals AGH, Kloppenborg PWC, Van Haelst UJG, et al. Fertile eunuch syndrome versus classic hypogonadotrophic hypogonadism. Acta Endocrinol 1978; 87:389–399.

387. Tagatz G, Fialkow PJ, Smith D, et al. Hypogonadotropic hypogonadism associated with anosmia in the female. N Engl J Med 1970; 283:1326–1329.

388. Soules MR, Hammond CB. Female Kallmann's syndrome: evidence for a hypothalamic luteinizing hormone–releasing hormone deficiency. Fertil Steril 1980; 33:82–85.

389. Kemmann E, Conrad P, Jones JR. Cardiac abnormalities in female hypogonadotropic hypogonadism with anosmia. Am J Obstet Gynecol 1980; 136:964–966.

390. Nowakowski H, Lenz W. Genetic aspects of male hypogonadism. Recent Prog Horm Res 1961; 17:53–95.

391. Santen RJ, Paulsen CA. Hypogonadotropic eunuchoidism. I: Clinical study of the mode of inheritance. J Clin Endocrinol Metab 1973; 36:47–54.

392. Yuanase T, Takayanagi R, Oba K, et al. New mutations of DAX-1 genes in two Japanese patients with X-linked congenital adrenal hypoplasia and hypogonadotropic hypogonadism. J Clin Endocrinol Metab 1996; 81:530–535.

393. Marshall JC, Harsoulis P, Anderson DC, et al. Isolated pituitary gonadotrophin deficiency: gonadotrophin secretion after synthetic luteinizing hormone and follicle stimulating hormone–releasing hormone. Br Med J 1972; 4:643–645.

394. Mortimer CH, Besser GM, McNeilly AS, et al. Luteinizing hormone and follicle stimulating hormone–releasing hormone test in patients with hypothalamic-pituitary-gonadal dysfunction. Br Med J 1973; 4:73–77.

395. Bell J, Spitz I, Slonim A, et al. Heterogeneity of gonadotropin response to LHRH in hypogonadotropic hypogonadism. J Clin Endocrinol Metab 1973; 36:791–794.

396. Oettinger M, Bruneteau DW, Psaoudakis A, et al. FSH and LH response to LHRF in Kallmann's syndrome. Obstet Gynecol 1976; 47:233–236.

397. Reitano JF, Caminos-Torres R, Snyder PJ. Serum LH and FSH responses to the repetitive administration of gonadotropin-releasing hormone in patients with idiopathic hypogonadotropic hypogonadism. J Clin Endocrinol Metab 1975; 41:1035–1042.

398. Dickerman Z, Prager-Lewin R, Laron Z. The effect of repeated injections of synthetic luteinizing hormone–releasing hormone on the response of plasma luteinizing hormone and follicle-stimulating hormone in young hypogonadotropic-hypogonadal patients. Fertil Steril 1976; 27:162–166.

399. Barkan AL, Reame NE, Kelch RP, et al. Idiopathic hypogonadotropin hypogonadism in men: dependence of the hormone responses to gonadotropin-releasing hormone (GnRH) on the magnitude of the endogenous GnRH secretory defect. J Clin Endocrinol Metab 1985; 61:1118–1125.

400. Santoro N, Filicori M, Crowley WF Jr. Hypogonadotropic disorders in men and women: diagnosis and therapy with pulsatile gonadotropin-releasing hormone. Endocr Rev 1976; 7:11–23.

401. Quigley ME, Sheehan KL, Casper RF, et al. Evidence for increased dopaminergic and opioid activity in patients with hypothalamic hypogonadotropic amenorrhea. J Clin Endocrinol Metab 1980; 50:949–954.

402. Franco B, Guilo S, Pragliola A, et al. A gene deleted in Kallmann's syndrome shares homology with neural cell adhesion and axonal pathfinding molecules. Nature 1991; 353:529–536.

403. Hardelin JP, Levilliers J, Blanchard S, et al. Heterogeneity in the mutations responsible for X chromosome–linked Kallmann syndrome. Hum Mol Genet 1993; 2:373–377.

404. Klingmüller D, Dewes W, Krahe T, et al. Magnetic resonance imaging of the brain in patients with anosmia and hypothalamic hypogonadism (Kallmann's syndrome). J Clin Endocrinol Metab 1987; 65:581–584.

405. Burstein S, Grumbach MM, Kaplan SL. Early determination of androgen-responsiveness is important in the management of microphallus. Lancet 1979; 2:983–986.

406. Smals AGH, Pieters GFFM, Kloppenborg PW, et al. Lack of a biphasic steroid response to single human chorionic gonadotropin administration in patients with isolated gonadotropin deficiency. J Clin Endocrinol Metab 1980; 50:879–881.

407. Santen RJ, Paulsen CA. Hypogonadotropic eunuchoidism. II: Gonadal responsiveness to exogenous gonadotropins. J Clin Endocrinol Metab 1973; 36:55–63.

408. Wang C, Paulsen CA, Hopper BR, et al. Acute steroidogenic responsiveness to human luteinizing hormone in hypogonadotropic hypogonadism. J Clin Endocrinol Metab 1980; 51:1269–1273.

409. Finkel DM, Phillips JL, Snyder PJ. Stimulation of spermatogenesis by gonadotropins in men with hypogonadotropic hypogonadism. N Engl J Med 1985; 313:651–655.

410. Ley SB, Leonard JM. Male hypogonadotropic hypogonadism: factors influencing response to human chorionic gonadotropin and human meno-

411. Burris AS, Rodbard HW, Winters SJ, et al. Gonadotropin therapy in men with isolated hypogonadotropic hypogonadism: the response to human chorionic gonadotropin is predicted by initial testicular size. J Clin Endocrinol Metab 1986; 66:1144–1151.

412. Baranetsky NG, Carlson HE. Persistence of spermatogenesis in hypogonadotropic hypogonadism treated with testosterone. Fertil Steril 1980; 34:477–482.

413. Rowe RC, Schroeder M-L, Faiman C. Testosterone-induced fertility in a patient with previously untreated Kallmann's syndrome. Fertil Steril 1983; 40:400–401.

414. Spratt DI, Finkelstein JS, Odea LSTL, et al. Long-term administration of gonadotropin-releasing hormone in men with idiopathic hypogonadotropic hypogonadism. Ann Intern Med 1986; 105:848–855.

415. Shargil AA. Treatment of idiopathic hypogonadotropic hypogonadism in men with luteinizing hormone–releasing hormone: a comparison of treatment with daily injections and with the pulsatile infusion pump. Fertil Steril 1987; 47:492–501.

416. Klingmüller D, Schweikert H-U. Maintenance of spermatogenesis by intranasal administration of gonadotropin-releasing hormone in patients with hypothalamic hypogonadism. J Clin Endocrinol Metab 1985; 61:868–872.

417. Nicholls RD. Genomic imprinting and uniparental disomy in Angelman and Prader-Willi syndromes: a review. Am J Med Genet 1993; 46:16–25.

418. Luton J-P, Thieblot P, Valcke J-C, et al. Reversible gonadotropin deficiency in male Cushing's disease. J Clin Endocrinol Metab 1977; 45:488–495.

419. Nicholls RD. McKenna TJ, Lorber D, Lacroix A, et al. Testicular activity in Cushing's disease. Acta Endocrinol 1979; 91:501–510.

420. MacAdams MR, White RH, Chipps BE. Reduction of serum testosterone levels during chronic glucocorticoid therapy. Ann Intern Med 1986; 104:648–651.

421. Carter JN, Tyson JE, Tolis G, et al. Prolactin-secreting tumors and hypogonadism in 22 men. N Engl J Med 1978; 299:847–852.

422. Thorner MO, Besser GM. Bromocriptine treatment of hyperprolactinaemic hypogonadism. Acta Endocrinol (Suppl) 1978; 88:131–146.

423. Franks S, Jacobs HS, Marti N, et al. Hyperprolactinaemia and impotence. Clin Endocrinol 1978; 8:277–287.

424. Davis JL. Lowering prolactin level in a hyperprolactinemic man. Responses of luteinizing hormone, follicle-stimulating hormone, and testosterone. Arch Intern Med 1982; 142:146–148.

425. Randall RV, Laws ER Jr, Abboud CF, et al. Transsphenoidal microsurgical treatment of prolactin-producing pituitary adenomas. Results in 100 patients. Mayo Clin Proc 1983; 58:108–121.

426. Prescott RWG, Johnston DG, Kendall-Taylor P, et al. Hyperprolactinaemia in men—response to bromocriptine therapy. Lancet 1982; 1:245–248.

427. MacDonald RA, Mallory GK. Hemochromatosis and hemosiderosis. Study of 211 autopsied cases. Arch Intern Med 1960; 105:686–700.

428. Stocks AE, Powell LW. Pituitary function in idiopathic haemochromatosis and cirrhosis of the liver. Lancet 1972; 2:298–301.

429. Leonard JM, Milder MS. Pituitary origin of hypogonadism in idiopathic hemochromatosis (I.H.). Clin Res 1978; 26:106A.

430. Edwards CQ, Cartwright GE, Skolnick MH, et al. Homozygosity for hemochromatosis: clinical manifestations. Ann Intern Med 1980; 93:519–525.

431. Charbonnel B, Chupin M, Le Grand A, et al. Pituitary function in idiopathic haemochromatosis: hormonal study in 36 male patients. Acta Endocrinol 1981; 98:178–183.

432. Iyer R, Duckworth WC, Solomon SS. Hypogonadism in idiopathic hemochromatosis. Arch Intern Med 1981; 141:517–518.

433. Schafer AI, Cheron RG, Dluhy R, et al. Clinical consequence of acquired transfusional iron overload in adults. N Engl J Med 1981; 304:319–324.

434. Edwards OM, Clark JDA. Post-traumatic hypopituitarism. Six cases and a review of the literature. Medicine 1986; 65:281–290.

435. Strain GW, Zumoff B, Miller LK, et al. Effect of massive weight loss on hypothalamic-pituitary-gonadal function in obese men. J Clin Endocrinol Metab 1988; 66:1019–1023.

436. Giagulli VA, Kaufman JM, Vermeulen A. Pathogenesis of the decreased androgen levels in obese men. J Clin Endocrinol Metab 1994; 79:997–1000.

437. Semple PA, Graham A, Malcolm Y, et al. Hypoxia, depression of testosterone, and impotence in pickwickian syndrome reversed by weight reduction. Br Med J 1984; 29:801–802.

438. Herzog AG, Seibel MM, Schomer DL, et al. Reproductive endocrine disorders in men with partial seizures of temporal lobe origin. Arch Neurol 1986; 43:347–350.

439. Cunningham GR. Idiopathic post-pubertal LH deficiency. Clin Res 1983; 31:896A.

440. Korenman SG, Stanik-Avis S, Mooradian A, et al. Evidence for a high prevalence of hypogonadotropic hypogonadism. Clin Res 1987; 35:182A.

441. Klinefelter HF Jr, Reifenstein EC Jr, Albright F. Syndrome characterized by gynecomastia, aspermatogenesis without A-Leydigism, and increased excretion of follicle-stimulating hormone. J Clin Endocrinol Metab 1942; 2:615–627.

442. Paulsen CA, Gordon DL, Carpenter KW, et al. Klinefelter's syndrome and its variants: a hormonal and chromosomal study. Recent Prog Horm Res 1968; 24:321–363.

443. Gordon DL, Krmpotic E, Thomas W, et al. Pathologic testicular findings

in Klinefelter's syndrome, 47,XXY vs 46,XY/47,XXY. Arch Intern Med 1972; 130:726–729.

444. Leonard JM, Paulsen CA, Ospina LF, et al. The classification of Klinefelter's syndrome. In: Vallet HL, Porter IH, eds. Genetic Mechanisms of Sexual Development. New York: Academic, 1979: 407–423.

445. Court-Brown WM. Human Population Cytogenetics. New York: John Wiley & Sons, 1967.

446. Mikamo K, Aguercif M, Hazeghi P, et al. Chromatin-positive Klinefelter's syndrome. A quantitative analysis of spermatogonial deficiency at 3, 4, and 12 months of age. Fertil Steril 1968; 19:731–739.

447. Laron Z, Hochman IH. Small testes in prepubertal boys with Klinefelter's syndrome. J Clin Endocrinol Metab 1971; 32:671–672.

448. Caldwell PD, Smith DW. The XXY Klinefelter's syndrome in childhood: detection and treatment. J Pediatr 1972; 80:250–258.

449. Ahmad KN, Dykes JRW, Ferguson-Smith MA, et al. Leydig cell volume in chromatin-positive Klinefelter's syndrome. J Clin Endocrinol Metab 1971; 33:517–520.

450. Schibler D, Brook CGD, Kind HP, et al. Growth and body proportions in 54 boys and men with Klinefelter's syndrome. Helv Paediatr Acta 1974; 29:325–333.

451. Becker KL. Clinical and therapeutic experience with Klinefelter's syndrome. Fertil Steril 1972; 23:568–578.

452. Ratcliffe SG, Bancroft J, Axworthy D, et al. Klinefelter's syndrome in adolescence. Arch Dis Child 1982; 57:6–12.

453. Nielsen J, Pelsen B. Follow-up 20 years later of 34 Klinefelter males with karyotype 47,XXY and 16 hypogonadal males with karyotype 46,XY. Hum Genet 1987; 77:188–192.

454. Smals AGH, Kloppenborg PWC, Lequin RL, et al. The pituitary-thyroid axis in Klinefelter's syndrome. Acta Endocrinol 1977; 84:72–79.

455. Huseby JS, Petersen D. Pulmonary function in Klinefelter's syndrome. Chest 1981; 80:31–33.

456. Scheike O, Visfeldt J, Petersen B. Male breast cancer. 3: Breast carcinoma in association with the Klinefelter syndrome. Acta Pathol Microbiol Scand A 1973; 81:352–358.

457. Griesemer DA. Klinefelter syndrome and breast cancer. Johns Hopkins Med J 1976; 138:102–108.

458. Laron Z, Dickerman Z, Zamir R, et al. Paternity in Klinefelter's syndrome–a case report. Arch Androl 1982; 8:149–151.

459. Bloomgarden ZT, Delozier CD, Cohen MP, et al. Genetic and endocrine findings in a 48,XXYY male. J Clin Endocrinol Metab 1980; 50:740–743.

460. Day RW, Levinson J, Larson W, et al. An XXXXY male. J Pediatr 1963; 63:589–598.

461. Ferguson-Smith MA. Sex chromatin, Klinefelter's syndrome and mental deficiency. In: Moore KL, ed. The Sex Chromatin. Philadelphia: WB Saunders, 1966: 277–315.

462. Sanger R, Tippett P, Gavin J. Xg groups and sex abnormalities in people of northern European ancestry. J Med Genet 1971; 8:417–426.

463. Gabrilove JL, Freiberg EK, Thornton JC, et al. Effect of age on testicular function in patients with Klinefelter's syndrome. Clin Endocrinol 1979; 11:343–347.

464. Gabrilove JL, Freiberg EK, Nicholis GL. Testicular function in Klinefelter's syndrome. J Urol 1980; 124:825–826.

465. Wang C, Baker HWG, Burger HG, et al. Hormonal studies in Klinefelter's syndrome. Clin Endocrinol 1975; 4:399–411.

466. Wieland RG, Zorn EM, Johnson MW. Elevated testosterone-binding globulin in Klinefelter's syndrome. J Clin Endocrinol Metab 1980; 51:1199–1200.

467. de Behar BR, Mendilaharzu H, Rivarola MA, et al. Gonadotropin secretion in prepubertal and pubertal primary hypogonadism: response to LHRH. J Clin Endocrinol Metab 1975; 41:1070–1075.

468. Caminos-Torres R, Ma L, Snyder PJ. Testosterone-induced inhibition of the LH and FSH responses to gonadotropin-releasing hormone occurs slowly. J Clin Endocrinol Metab 1977; 44:1142–1153.

469. Samaan NA, Stepanas AV, Danziger J, et al. Reactive pituitary abnormalities in patients with Klinefelter's and Turner's syndromes. Arch Intern Med 1979; 139:198–201.

470. Myhre SA, Ruvalcaba RHA, Johnson HR, et al. The effects of testosterone treatment in Klinefelter's syndrome. J Pediatr 1970; 76:267–276.

471. de la Chapelle A. Analytic review: nature and origin of males with XX sex chromosomes. Am J Hum Genet 1972; 24:71–105.

472. de la Chapelle A. The etiology of maleness in XX men. Hum Genet 1981; 58:105–116.

473. Perez-Palacios G, Medina M, Ullao-Aguirre A, et al. Gonadotropin dynamics in XX males. J Clin Endocrinol Metab 1981; 53:254–257.

474. Schweikert HU, Weissbach L, Leyendecker G, et al. Clinical, endocrinological, and cytological characterization of two 46,XX males. J Clin Endocrinol Metab 1982; 54:745–752.

475. Roe TF, Alfi OS. Ambiguous genitalia in XX male children: report of two infants. Pediatrics 1977; 60:55–59.

476. Ferguson-Smith MA, Cooke A, Affara NA, et al. Genotype-phenotype correlations in XX males and their bearing on current theories of sex determination. Hum Genet 1990; 84:198–202.

477. Auwera BV, VanRoy N, De Paepe A, et al. Molecular cytogenetic analysis of XX males using Y-specific DNA sequences, including SRY. Hum Genet 1992; 89:23–28.

478. Boucekkine C, Toublanc JE, Abbas N, et al. Clinical and anatomical

479. Mardon G, Mosher R, Disteche CM, et al. Duplication, deletion, and polymorphism in the sex-determining region of the mouse Y chromosome. Science 1989; 243:78–80.

480. Fukutani K, Kajiwara T, Nagafuchi S, et al. Detection of the testis determining factor in an XX man. J Urol 1993; 149:126–128.

481. Werner CA. Mumps orchitis and testicular atrophy. I: Occurrence. Ann Intern Med 1950; 32:1066–1074.

482. Riggs S, Sanford JP. Viral orchitis. N Engl J Med 1962; 266:990–993.

483. Bjorvatn B. Mumps virus recovered from testicles by fine-needle aspiration biopsy in cases of mumps orchitis. Scand J Infect Dis 1973; 5:3–5.

484. Adamopoulos DA, Lawrence DM, Vassilopoulos P, et al. Pituitary testicular interrelationships in mumps orchitis and other viral infections. Br Med J 1978; 1:1177–1180.

485. Aiman J, Brenner PF, MacDonald PC. Androgen and estrogen production in elderly men with gynecomastia and testicular atrophy after mumps orchitis. J Clin Endocrinol Metab 1980; 50:380–386.

486. Werner CA. Mumps orchitis and testicular atrophy. II: A factor in male sterility. Ann Intern Med 1950; 32:1075–1086.

487. Bartak V, Skalova E, Nevarilova A. Spermiogram changes in adults and youngsters after parotitic orchitis. Int J Fertil 1968; 13:226–232.

488. Petersdorf RG, Bennett IL Jr. Treatment of mumps orchitis with adrenal hormones. Report of twenty-three cases with a note on hepatic involvement in mumps. Arch Intern Med 1957; 99:222–233.

489. Wang J, Galil KAA, Setchell BP. Changes in testicular blood flow and testosterone production during aspermatogenesis after irradiation. J Endocrinol 1983; 98:35–46.

490. Oakberg EF. Effects of radiation on the testis. In: Greep RO, Astwood EB, eds. Handbook of Physiology. Sect 7: Endocrinology. Vol V. Male Reproductive System. Washington, DC: American Physiological Society, 1975: 233–243.

491. Shalet SM, Beardwell CG, Jacobs HS, et al. Testicular function following irradiation of the human prepubertal testis. Clin Endocrinol 1978; 9:483–490.

492. Brauner R, Czernichow P, Cramer P, et al. Leydig-cell function in children after direct testicular irradiation for acute lymphoblastic leukemia. N Engl J Med 1983; 309:25–28.

493. Smith CG. Drug effects on male sexual function. Clin Obstet Gynecol 1982; 25:525–531.

494. Lorioux DL, Menard R, Taylor A, et al. Spironolactone and endocrine dysfunction. Ann Intern Med 1976; 85:630–636.

495. Neumann F, van Berswordt-Wallrabe R, Elger W, et al. Aspects of androgen-dependent events as studied by antiandrogens. Recent Prog Horm Res 1970; 26:337–410.

496. Rajfer J, Sikka SC, Rivera F, et al. Mechanism of inhibition of human testicular steroidogenesis by oral ketoconazole. J Clin Endocrinol Metab 1986; 63:1193–1198.

497. Pont A, Graybill Jr, Craven PC, et al. High-dose ketoconazole therapy and adrenal and testicular function in humans. Arch Intern Med 1984; 144:2150–2153.

498. Pulkkinen MO, Mäenpää J. Decrease in serum testosterone concentration during treatment with tetracycline. Acta Endocrinol 1983; 103:269–272.

499. Brunet M, Rodamilans M, Martinez-Osaba MJ, et al. Effects of long-term antiepileptic therapy on the catabolism of testosterone. Pharmacol Toxicol 1995; 76:371–375.

500. Macphee GJA, Larkin JG, Butler E, et al. Circulating hormones and pituitary responsiveness in young epileptic men receiving long-term antiepileptic medication. Epilepsia 1988; 29:468–475.

501. Wheeler MJ, Toone BK, Dannatt A, et al. Metabolic clearance rate of testosterone in male epileptic patients on anti-convulsant therapy. J Endocrinol 1991; 129:465–468.

502. Cicero TJ. Alcohol-induced deficits in the hypothalamic-pituitary-luteinizing hormone axis in the male. Alcoholism Clin Exp Res (NY) 1982; 6:207–215.

503. Gordon GG, Altman K, Southern AL, et al. Effect of alcohol (ethanol) administration on sex-hormone metabolism in normal men. N Engl J Med 1976; 295:793–797.

504. Van Thiel DH, Gavaler JS, Lester R, et al. Alcohol-induced testicular atrophy. An experimental model for hypogonadism occurring in chronic alcoholic men. Gastroenterology 1975; 69:326–332.

505. Boyden TW, Silvert MA, Pamenter RW. Chronic ethanol feeding impairs human chorionic gonadotropin–stimulated testicular testosterone responses of dogs. Biol Reprod 1982; 27:652–657.

506. Gordon GG, Vittek J, Southern AL, et al. Effect of chronic alcohol ingestion on the biosynthesis of steroids in rat testicular homogenate in vitro. Endocrinology 1980; 106:1880–1885.

507. Van Thiel DH, Cobb CF, Herman GB, et al. An examination of various mechanisms for ethanol-induced testicular injury: studies utilizing the isolated perfused rat testes. Endocrinology 1981; 109:2009–2015.

508. Anderson RA Jr, Reddy JM, Joyce C, et al. Inhibition of mouse sperm capacitation by ethanol. Biol Reprod 1982; 27:833–840.

509. Anderson RA Jr, Willis BR, Oswald C, et al. Ethanol-induced male infertility: impairment of spermatozoa. J Pharmacol Exp Ther 1983; 225:479–486.

510. Sherins RJ, Olweny CLM, Med M, et al. Gynecomastia and gonadal

dysfunction in adolescent boys treated with combination chemotherapy for Hodgkin's disease. N Engl J Med 1978; 229:12–16.

511. Whitehead E, Shalet M, Blackledge G, et al. The effects of Hodgkin's disease and combination chemotherapy on gonadal function of the adult male. Cancer 1982; 49:418–422.

512. Chapman RM, Rees LH, Sutcliff SB, et al. Cyclical combination chemotherapy and gonadal function. Lancet 1979; 1:285–289.

513. Blatt J, Poplack DG, Sherins RJ. Testicular function in boys after chemotherapy for acute lymphoblastic leukemia. N Engl J Med 1981; 304:1121–1124.

514. Meikle AW, Cardoso de Sousa JC, Ward JH, et al. Reduction of testosterone synthesis after high dose interleukin-2 therapy of metastatic cancer. J Clin Endocrinol Metab 1991; 73:931–935.

515. Kolodny RC, Masters WH, Kolodner RM, et al. Depression of plasma testosterone levels after chronic intensive marihuana use. N Engl J Med 1974; 290:872–874.

516. Wang C, Chan V, Yeung RTT. The effect of heroin addiction on pituitary-testicular function. Clin Endocrinol 1978; 9:455–461.

517. Mendelson JH, Mendelson JE, Patch VD. Plasma testosterone levels in heroin addiction and during methadone maintenance. J Pharmacol Exp Ther 1975; 192:211–217.

518. Dalterio S, Bartke A, Burstein S. Cannabinoids inhibit tetosterone secretion by mouse testes in vitro. Science 1977; 196:1472–1473.

519. Dalterio S, Bartke A, Roberson C, et al. Direct and pituitary-mediated effects of Δ⁹-THC and cannabinol on the testis. Pharmacol Biochem Behav 1977; 8:673–678.

520. Tyrey L. Δ⁹-Tetrahydrocannabinol: a potent inhibitor of episodic luteinizing hormone secretion. J Pharmacol Exp Ther 1980; 213:306–308.

521. Hong CY, Chaput de Saintonge DM, Turner P. Δ⁹-Tetrahydrocannabinol inhibits human sperm motility. J Pharm Pharmacol 1981; 33:746–747.

522. Stoffer SS, Mynes KM, Jiang N-S, et al. Digoxin and abnormal serum hormone levels. JAMA 1973; 225:1643–1644.

523. Geller J, Fruchtman B, Meyer C, et al. Effect of progestational agents on gonadal and adrenal cortical function in patients with benign prostatic hypertrophy and carcinoma of the prostate. J Clin Endocrinol Metab 1967; 27:556–560.

524. Blumer D, Migeon C. Hormone and hormonal agents in the treatment of aggression. J Nerv Ment Dis 1975; 160:127–137.

525. Bixler EO, Santen RJ, Kales A, et al. Inverse effects of thioridazine (Mellaril) on serum prolactin and testosterone concentrations in normal men. In: Troen P, Nankin HR, eds. The Testis in Normal and Infertile Men. New York: Raven, 1977: 403–408.

526. Rosenthal SM, Grumbach MM. Gonadotropin-independent familial sexual precocity with premature Leydig and germinal cell maturation (familial testotoxicosis): effects of a potent luteinizing hormone–releasing factor agonist and medroxyprogesterone acetate therapy in four cases. J Clin Endocrinol Metab 1983; 57:571–579.

527. Van Thiel DH, Gavaler JS, Smith WI Jr, et al. Hypothalamic-pituitary-gonadal dysfunction in men using cimetidine. N Engl J Med 1979; 300:1012–1015.

528. Funder JW, Mercer JE. Cimetidine, a histamine H2 receptor antagonist, occupies androgen receptors. J Clin Endocrinol Metab 1979; 48:189–191.

529. Peden NR, Boyd EJS, Browning MCK, et al. Effects of two histamine H2-receptor blocking drugs on basal levels of gonadotrophins, prolactin, testosterone and oestradiol-17β during treatment of duodenal ulcer in male patients. Acta Endocrinol 1981; 96:564–568.

530. Lindquist M, Edwards IR. Endocrine adverse effects of omeprazole. Br Med J 1992; 305:451–452.

531. Rodamilans M, Osaba MJM, To-Figueras J, et al. Lead toxicity on endocrine testicular function in an occupationally exposed population. Hum Toxicol 1988; 7:125–128.

532. Sokol RZ, Mading CE, Swerdloff R. Lead toxicity and the hypothalamic-pituitary-testicular axis. Biol Reprod 1985; 33:722–728.

533. Murthy GG, Peress NS, Khan SA. Demonstration of antibodies to testicular basement membrane by immunofluorescence in a patient with multiple primary endocrine deficiencies. J Clin Endocrinol Metab 1976; 42:637–641.

534. Elder M, Maclaren N, Riley W. Gonadal autoantibodies in patients with hypogonadism and/or Addison's disease. J Clin Endocrinol Metab 1981; 52:1137–1142.

535. Saporta L, Yuksel A. Androgenic status in patients with lepromatous leprosy. Br J Urol 1994; 74:221–224.

536. Sherman FP. Impotence in patients with chronic renal failure on dialysis: its frequency and etiology. Fertil Steril 1975; 26:221–223.

537. de Kretser DM, Atkins RC, Hudson B, et al. Disordered spermatogenesis in patients with chronic renal failure undergoing maintenance haemodialysis. Aust NZ J Med 1974; 4:178–181.

538. Holdsworth S, Atkins RC, de Kretser D. The pituitary-testicular axis in men with chronic renal failure. N Engl J Med 1977; 296:1245–1249.

539. Stewart-Bentley M, Gans D, Horton R. Regulation of gonadal function in uremia. Metabolism 1974; 23:1065–1072.

540. Lim VS, Fang VS. Gonadal dysfunction in uremic men. A study of the hypothalamo-pituitary-testicular axis before and after renal transplantation. Am J Med 1975; 58:655–662.

541. Handelsman DJ, Dong Q. Hypothalamo-pituitary gonadal axis in chronic renal failure. Neuroendocrinology 1993; 22:145–161.

542. Rager K, Bundschu H, Gupta D. The effect of hCG on testicular androgen production in adult men with chronic renal failure. J Reprod Fertil 1975; 42:113–120.

543. Briefel GR, Tsitouras PD, Kowatch MA, et al. Decreased in vitro testosterone production by isolated Leydig cells from uremic rats. Endocrinology 1982; 110:976–981.

544. Lim VS, Fang VS. Restoration of plasma testosterone levels in uremic men with clomiphene citrate. J Clin Endocrinol Metab 1976; 43:1370–1377.

545. Gomez F, de la Cueva R, Wauters J-P, et al. Endocrine abnormalities in patients undergoing long-term hemodialysis. The role of prolactin. Am J Med 1980; 68:522–530.

546. Vircburger MI, Prelevic GM, Peric LA, et al. Testosterone levels after bromocriptine treatment in patients undergoing long-term hemodialysis. J Androl 1985; 6:113–116.

547. Holdsworth SR, de Kretser DM, Atkins RC. A comparison of hemodialysis and transplantation in reversing the uremic disturbance of male reproductive function. Clin Nephrol 1978; 10:146–150.

548. Chopp RT, Mendez R. Sexual function and hormonal abnormalities in uremic men on chronic dialysis and after renal transplantation. Fertil Steril 1978; 29:661–666.

549. Baker HWG, Burger HG, de Kretser DM, et al. A study of the endocrine manifestations of hepatic cirrhosis. Q J Med 1976; 45:145–178.

550. Chopra IJ, Tulchinsky D, Greenway FL. Estrogen-androgen imbalance in hepatic cirrhosis. Studies in 13 male patients. Ann Intern Med 1973; 79:198–203.

551. Gordon GG, Olivo J, Rafii F, et al. Conversion of androgens to estrogens in cirrhosis of the liver. J Clin Endocrinol Metab 1975; 40:1018–1026.

552. Van Thiel DH, Lester R, Sherins RJ. Hypogonadism in alcoholic liver disease: evidence for a double defect. Gastroenterology 1974; 67:1188–1199.

553. Bannister P, Handley T, Chapman C, et al. Hypogonadism in chronic liver disease: impaired release of luteinising hormone. Br Med J 1986; 293:1191–1193.

554. Distiller LA, Sagel J, Dubowitz B, et al. Pituitary-gonadal function in men with alcoholic cirrhosis of the liver. Horm Metab Res 1976; 8:461–465.

535. Van Thiel DH, McClain CJ, Elson MK, et al. Evidence for autonomous secretion of prolactin in some alcoholic men with cirrhosis and gynecomastia. Metabolism 1978; 27:1778–1784.

556. Kley HK, Strohmeyer G, Krüskemper HL. Effect of testosterone application on hormone concentrations of androgens and estrogens in male patients with cirrhosis of the liver. Gastroenterology 1979; 76:235–241.

557. Gluud C, Bennett P, Dietrichson O, et al. Short-term parenteral and peroral testosterone administration in men with alcoholic cirrhosis. Scand J Gastroenterol 1981; 16:749–755.

558. Van Thiel DH, Gavaler JS, Sanghvi A. Recovery of sexual function in abstinent alcoholic men. Gastroenterology 1982; 84:677–682.

559. Zifroni A, Schlavi RC, Schaffner F. Sexual function and testosterone levels in men with nonalcoholic liver disease. Hepatology 1991; 14:479–482.

560. Van Thiel DH, Kumar S, Gavaler JS, et al. Effect of liver transplantation on the hypothalamic-pituitary-gonadal axis of chronic alcoholic men with advanced liver disease. Alcohol Clin Exp Res 1990; 14:478–481.

561. Olambiwonnu NO, Penny R, Frasier SD. Sexual maturation in subjects with sickle cell anemia: studies of serum gonadotropin concentration, height, weight, and skeletal age. J Pediatr 1975; 87:459–464.

562. Abbasi AA, Prasad AS, Ortega J, et al. Gonadal function abnormalities in sickle cell anemia. Studies in adult male patients. Ann Intern Med 1976; 85:601–605.

563. Landefeld CS, Schambelan M, Kaplan SL, et al. Clomiphene-responsive hypogonadism in sickle cell anemia. Ann Intern Med 1983; 99:480–483.

564. Smith SR, Chhetri MK, Johanson AJ, et al. The pituitary-gonadal axis in men with protein-calorie malnutrition. J Clin Endocrinol Metab 1975; 41:60–69.

565. Vigersky RA, Chapman RM, Berenberg J, et al. Testicular dysfunction in untreated Hodgkin's disease. Am J Med 1982; 73:482–486.

566. Chlebowski RT, Heber D. Hypogonadism in male patients with metastatic cancer prior to chemotherapy. Cancer Res 1982; 42:2495–2498.

567. Landon C, Rosenfeld RG. Short stature and pubertal delay in male adolescents with cystic fibrosis. Androgen treatment. Am J Dis Child 1984; 138:388–391.

568. Handelsman DJ, Yue DK, Turtle JR. Hypogonadism and massive testicular infiltration due to amyloidosis. J Urol 1983; 129:610–612.

569. Chopra IJ, Hershman JM, Pardridge WM, et al. Thyroid function in nonthyroidal illnesses. Ann Intern Med 1983; 98:946–957.

570. Goussis OS, Pardridge WM, Judd HL. Critical illness and low testosterone: effects of human serum on testosterone transport into rat brain and liver. J Clin Endocrinol Metab 1983; 56:710–714.

571. Glass AR, Smith CE, Kidd GS, et al. Response of the hypothalamic-pituitary-testicular axis to surgery. Fertil Steril 1978; 30:560–563.

572. Wang C, Chan V, Yeung RTT. Effect of surgical stress on pituitary-testicular function. Clin Endocrinol 1978; 9:255–266.

573. Wang C, Chan V, Tse TF, et al. Effect of acute myocardial infarction on pituitary-testicular function. Clin Endocrinol 1978; 9:249–253.

574. Vogel AV, Peake GT, Rada RT. Pituitary-testicular axis dysfunction in burned men. J Clin Endocrinol Metab 1985; 60:658–664.

575. Lephart ED, Baxter CR, Parker CR Jr. Effect of burn trauma on adrenal and testicular steroid hormone production. J Clin Endocrinol Metab 1987; 64:842–848.

576. Dong Q, Hawker F, McWilliam D, et al. Circulating immunoreactive inhibin and testosterone levels in men with critical illness. Clin Endocrinol 1992; 36:399–404.

577. Kidd GS, Glass AR, Vigersky RA. The hypothalamic-pituitary-testicular axis in thyrotoxicosis. J Clin Endocrinol Metab 1979; 48:798–802.

578. Poretsky L, Can S, Zumoff B. Testicular dysfunction in human immunodeficiency virus-infected men. Metabolism 1995; 44:946–953.

579. Wagner G, Rabkin JG, Tabkin R. Illness stage, concurrent medications, and other correlates of low testosterone in men with HIV illness. J Acquir Immune Defic Syndr Hum Retrovir 1995; 8:204–207.

580. Martens HF, Sheets PK, Tenover JS, et al. Decreased testosterone levels in men with rheumatoid arthritis: effect of low dose prednisone therapy. J Rheumatol 1994; 21:1427–1431.

581. Sagel J, Distiller LA, Morley JE, et al. Myotonia dystrophica: studies on gonadal function using luteinizing hormone–releasing hormone (LRH). J Clin Endocrinol Metab 1975; 40:1110–1113.

582. Febres F, Scaglia H, Lisker R, et al. Hypothalamic-pituitary-gonadal function in patients with myotonic dystrophy. J Clin Endocrinol Metab 1975; 41:833–840.

583. Takeda R, Ueda M. Pituitary-gonadal function in male patients with myotonic dystrophy–serum luteinizing hormone, follicle stimulating hormone and testosterone levels and histological damage of the testis. Acta Endocrinol 1977; 84:382–389.

584. Vazquez JA, Pinies JA, Martul P, et al. Hypothalamic-pituitary-testicular function in 70 patients with myotonic dystrophy. J Endocrinol Invest 1990; 13:375–379.

585. Trifiro MA, Kazemi-Esfarjani P, Pinsky L. X-linked muscular atrophy and the androgen receptor. Trends Endocrinol Metab 1994; 5:416–421.

586. Claus-Walker J, Scurry M, Carter RE, et al. Steady state hormonal secretion in traumatic quadriplegia. J Clin Endocrinol Metab 1977; 44:530–535.

587. Cortes-Gallegos V, Castaneda G, Alonso R, et al. Diurnal variations of pituitary and testicular hormones in paraplegic men. Arch Androl 1982; 8:221–226.

588. Piera JB. The establishment of a prognosis for genito-sexual function in the paraplegic and tetraplegic male. Paraplegia 1973; 10:271–278.

589. Hasen J, Boyar RM, Shapiro LR. Gonadal function in trisomy 21. Horm Res 1980; 12:345–350.

590. Aiman J, Griffin JE, Gazak JM, et al. Androgen insensitivity as a cause of infertility in otherwise normal men. N Engl J Med 1979; 330:223–227.

591. Aiman J, Griffin JE. The frequency of androgen receptor deficiency in infertile men. J Clin Endocrinol Metab 1982; 54:725–732.

592. Grino PB, Griffin JE, Cushard WG, et al. A mutation of the androgen receptor associated with partial androgen resistance, familial gynecomastia, and fertility. J Clin Endocrinol Metab 1988; 66:754–761.

593. Pinsky L, Kaufman M, Killinger DW. Impaired spermatogenesis is not an obligate expression of receptor-defective androgen resistance. J Med Genet 1989; 32:100–104.

594. Yong EL, NG SC, Roy AC, et al. Pregnancy after hormonal correction of severe spermatogenic defect due to mutation in androgen receptor gene. Lancet 1994; 344:826–827.

595. Tsukada T, Inoue M, Tachibana S, et al. An androgen receptor mutation causing androgen resistance in undervirilized male syndrome. J Clin Endocrinol Metab 1994; 79:1202–1207.

596. Mozaffarian GA, Higley M, Paulsen CA. Clinical studies in an adult male patient with "isolated follicle stimulating hormone (FSH) deficiency." J Androl 1983; 4:393–398.

597. Segal S, Polishuk WZ, Ben-David M. Hyperprolactinemic male infertility. Fertil Steril 1976; 27:1425–1427.

598. Bonaccorsi AC, Adler I, Figueiredo JG. Male infertility due to congenital adrenal hyperplasia: testicular biopsy findings, hormonal evaluation, and theapeutic results in three patients. Fertil Steril 1987; 47:664–670.

599. Schürmeyer T, Belkien L, Knuth UA, et al. Reversible azoospermia induced by the anabolic steroid 19-nortestosterone. Lancet 1984; 1:417–420.

600. Rothman CM, Sims CA, Stotts CL. Sertoli cell only syndrome 1982. Fertil Steril 1982; 38:388–390.

601. Ishida H, Isurugi K, Aso Y, et al. Endocrine studies in Sertoli-cell-only syndrome. J Urol 1976; 116:56–58.

602. Pajarinen JT, Karhunen PJ. Spermatogenic arrest and "Sertoli cell–only" syndrome—common alcohol-induced disorders of the human testis. Int J Androl 1994; 17:292–299.

603. Edwards JA, Bannerman RM. Familial gynecomastia. Birth Defects 1971; 7:193–195.

604. de Kretser DM, Burger HG, Fortune D, et al. Hormonal, histological and chromosomal studies in adult males with testicular disorders. J Clin Endocrinol Metab 1972; 35:392–401.

605. Tiepolo L, Zuffardi O. Localization of factors controlling spermatogenesis in the nonfluorescent portion of the human Y chromosome long arm. Hum Genet 1976; 34:119–124.

606. Chandley AC, Cooke HJ. Human male fertility—Y-linked genes and spermatogenesis. Hum Mol Genet 1994; 3:1449–1452.

607. Najmabadi H, Huant V, Yen P, et al. Substantial prevalence of microdeletions of the Y-chromosome in infertile men with idiopathic azoospermia and oligozoospermia detected using a sequence-tagged site-based mapping strategy. J Clin Endocrinol Metab 1996; 81:1347–1352.

608. Ma K, Inglis JD, Sharkey A, et al. A Y chromosome gene family with RNA-binding protein homology: candidates for the azoospermia factor AZF controlling human spermatogenesis. Cell 1993; 75:1287–1295.

609. Reijo R, Lee T-Y, Alagappan R, et al. Diverse spermatogenic defects in humans caused by Y chromosome deletions encompassing a novel RNA-binding protein gene. Nature Genet 1995; 10:383–393.

610. Foresta C, Ferlin A, Rossato M, et al. Diagnostic and clinical features in azoospermia. Clin Endocrinol 1995; 43:537–543.

611. Chaganti RSK, German J. Human male infertility, probably genetically determined, due to defective meiosis and spermatogenic arrest. Am J Hum Genet 1979; 31:634–641.

612. Chaganti RSK, Jhanwar SC, German J. Genetically determined asynapsis, spermatogenic degeneration, and infertility in men. Am J Hum Genet 1980; 32:833–848.

613. Greenberg SH, Lipshultz LI, Wein AJ. Experience with 425 subfertile male patients. J Urol 1978; 119:507–510.

614. Turner TT. Varicocele: still an enigma. J Urol 1983; 129:695–699.

615. Rodriguez-Rigau LJ, Steinberger E. Varicocele and the morphology of spermatozoa. Fertil Steril 1981; 35:54–57.

616. Fariss BL, Fenner DK, Plymate SR, et al. Seminal characteristics in the presence of a varicocele as compared with those of expectant fathers and prevasectomy men. Fertil Steril 1981; 35:325–327.

617. Mieusset R, Bujan L, Mondinat C, et al. Association of scrotal hyperthermia with impaired spermatogenesis in infertile men. Fertil Steril 1987; 48:1006–1011.

618. Zorgniotti AW, Sealfon AI. Measurement of intrascrotal temperature in normal and subfertile men. J Reprod Fertil 1988; 82:563–566.

619. Saypol DC, Howards SS, Turner TT, et al. Influence of surgically induced varicocele on testicular blood flow, temperature, and histology in adult rats and dogs. J Clin Invest 1981; 68:39–45.

620. Dubin L, Amelar RD. Varicocelectomy: 986 cases in a twelve-year study. Urology 1977; 10:446–449.

621. Pedersen H, Hammen R. Ultrastructure of human spermatozoa with complete subcellular derangement. Arch Androl 1982; 9:251–259.

622. Cassell GH, Younger JB, Brown MB, et al. Microbiologic study of infertile women at the time of diagnostic laparoscopy. N Engl J Med 1983; 308:502–505.

623. Toth A, Lesser ML, Brooks C, et al. Subsequent pregnancies among 161 couples treated for T-mycoplasma genital-tract infection. N Engl J Med 1983; 308:505–507.

624. Hahn EW, Feingold SM, Nisce L. Aspermia and recovery of spermatogenesis in cancer patients following incidental gonadal irradiation during treatment: a progress report. Radiology 1976; 119:223–225.

625. Shapiro E, Kinsella TJ, Makuch RW, et al. Effects of fractionated irradiation on endocrine aspects of testicular function. J Clin Oncol 1985; 3:1232–1239.

626. Asbjornsen G, Molne K, Klepp O, et al. Testicular function after radiotherapy to inverted "Y" field for malignant lymphoma. Scand J Haematol 1976; 17:96–100.

627. Handelsman DJ, Turtle JR. Testicular damage after radioactive iodine (I-131) therapy for thyroid cancer. Clin Endocrinol 1983; 18:465–472.

628. Schilsky RL, Sherins RJ. Gonadal dysfunction. In: DeVita VT Jr, Hellman S, Rosenberg SA, eds. Cancer: Principles and Practice of Oncology. Vol 2. Philadelphia: JB Lippincott, 1985: 2032–2039.

629. Watson AR, Rance CP, Bain J. Long term effects of cyclophosphamide on testicular function. Br Med J 1985; 291:1457–1460.

630. Tsatsoulis A, Whitehead E, St. John J, et al. The pituitary–Leydig cell axis in men with severe damage to the germinal epithelium. Clin Endocrinol 1987; 27:683–689.

631. Buchanan JD, Fairley KF, Barrie JU. Return of spermatogenesis after stopping cyclophosphamide therapy. Lancet 1975; 2:156–157.

632. Santoro A, Viviani S, Zucali R, et al. Comparative results and toxicity of MOPP vs ABVD combined with radiotherapy in PS IIB, III Hodgkin's disease. Proc Am Soc Clin Oncol 1983; 2:223 (abstract).

633. Rautonen J, Koskimies AI, Siimes MA. Vincristine is associated with the risk of azoospermia in adult male survivors of childhood malignancies. Eur J Cancer 1992; 28A:1837–1841.

634. Shafford EA, Kingston JE, Malpas JS, et al. Testicular function following the treatment of Hodgkin's disease in childhood. Br J Cancer 1993; 68:1199–1204.

635. Mustieles C, Munoz A, Alonso M, et al. Male gonadal function after chemotherapy in survivors of childhood malignancy. Med Pediatr Oncol 1995; 24:347–351.

636. Drasga RE, Einhorn LH, Williams SD, et al. Fertility after chemotherapy for testicular cancer. J Clin Oncol 1983; 1:179–183.

637. Birnie GG, McLeod TIF, Watkinson G. Incidence of sulphasalazine-induced male infertility. Gut 1981; 22:452–455.

638. Morris LF, Harrod MJ, Menter MA, et al. Methotrexate and reproduction in men: case report and recommendations. J Am Acad Dermatol 1993; 29:913–916.

639. Sarica K, Silzer O, Gürler A, et al. Urological evaluation of Behçet patients and the effect of colchicine on fertility. Eur Urol 1995; 27:39–42.

640. Whorton MD. Male occupational reproductive hazards. West J Med 1982; 137:521–524.

641. Veulemans H, Steeno O, Masschelein R, et al. Exposure to ethylene glycol ethers and spermatogenic disorders in man: a case-control study. Br J Industr Med 1993; 50:71–78.

642. Dwivedi C. Cadmium-induced sterility: possible involvement of the cholinergic system. Arch Environ Contam Toxicol 1983; 12:151–156.

643. Assennato G, Paci C, Baser ME, et al. Sperm count suppression without endocrine dysfunction in lead-exposed men. Arch Environ Health 1986; 41:387–390.

644. Lancranjan I, Maicanescu M, Rafaila E, et al. Gonadic function in workmen with long-term exposure to microwaves. Health Phys 1975; 29:381–383.

645. Fahim MS, Fahim Z, Harman J, et al. Ultrasound as a new method of male contraception. Fertil Steril 1977; 28:823–831.

646. Azizi F, Keshavarz A, Roshanzamir F, et al. Reproductive function in men following exposure to chemical warfare with sulphur mustard. Medicine 1995; 11:34–44.

647. Carlsen E, Giwercman A, Keiding N, et al. Evidence for decreasing quality of semen during past 50 years. Br Med J 1992; 305:609–613.

648. Auger J, Kunstmann JM, Czyglik F, et al. Decline in semen quality among fertile men in Paris during the past 20 years. N Engl J Med 1995; 332:281–285.

649. Irvine S, Cawood E, Richardson D, et al. Evidence of deteriorating semen quality in the United Kingdom: birth cohort study in 577 men in Scotland over 11 years. Br Med J 1996; 312:467–471.

650. Bujan L, Mansat A, Pontonnier F, et al. Time series analysis of sperm concentration in fertile men in Toulouse, France between 1977 and 1992. BMJ 1996; 312:471–472.

651. DeKretser DM. Declining sperm counts. Br Med J 1996; 312:457–458.

652. Vine MF. Worldwide decline in semen quality might be due to smoking. Br Med J 1996; 312:506.

653. Salomon F, Saremaslani P, Jakob M, et al. Immune complex orchitis in infertile men. Immunoelectron microscopy of abnormal basement membrane structures. Lab Invest 1982; 47:555–567.

654. Bronson R, Cooper G, Rosenfeld D. Sperm antibodies: their role in infertility. Fertil Steril 1984; 42:171–183.

655. Haas GG Jr. Antibody-mediated causes of male infertility. Urol Clin North Am 1987; 14:539–550.

656. Turek PJ, Lipshultz LI. Immunologic infertility. Urol Clin North Am 1994; 21:447–468.

657. Phadke AM, Padukone K. Presence and significance of autoantibodies against spermatozoa in the blood of men with obstructed vas deferens. J Reprod Fertil 1964; 7:163–170.

658. Hendry WF, Parslow JM, Stedronska J, et al. The diagnosis of unilateral testicular obstruction in subfertile males. Br J Urol 1982; 54:774–779.

659. Ansbacher R. Vasectomy: sperm antibodies. Fertil Steril 1973; 24:788–792.

660. Green JRB, Goble HL, Edwards CRW, et al. Reversible insensitivity to androgens in men with untreated gluten enteropathy. Lancet 1977; 1:280–282.

661. Farthing MJG, Edwards CRW, Rees LH, et al. Male gonadal function in coeliac disease. 1: Sexual dysfunction, infertility, and semen quality. Gut 1982; 23:608–614.

662. Farthing MJG, Rees LH, Boylan LM, et al. Male gonadal function in coeliac disease. 2: Sex hormones. Gut 1983; 24:127–135.

663. Morrow AF, Gyorki S, Warne GL, et al. Variable androgen receptor levels in infertile men. J Clin Endocrinol Metab 1987; 64:1115–1121.

664. Handelsman DJ, Conway AJ, Boylan LM, et al. Young's syndrome. Obstructive azoospermia and chronic sinopulmonary infections. N Engl J Med 1984; 310:3–9.

665. Hendry WF, A'Hern RP, Cole PJ. Was Young's syndrome caused by exposure to mercury in childhood? Br Med J 1993; 307:1579–1582.

666. Van der Linden EFH, Bartelink AKM, Ike BW, et al. Polycystic kidney disease and infertility. Fertil Steril 1995; 64:202–203.

667. Sharlip ID. Obstructive azoospermia or oligozoospermia due to müllerian duct cyst. Fertil Steril 1983; 39:435–436.

668. Gill WB, Schumacher FGB, Bibbo M. Pathological semen and anatomical abnormalities of the genital tract in human male subjects exposed to diethylstilbestrol in utero. J Urol 1977; 117:477–480.

669. Anguiano A, Oates RD, Amos JA, et al. Congenital bilateral absence of the vas deferens. A primarily genital form of cystic fibrosis. JAMA 1992; 267:1794–1797.

670. Culard JF, Desgeorges M, Costa P, et al. Analysis of the whole CFTR coding regions and splice junctions in azoospermic men with congenital bilateral aplasia of epididymis or vas deferens. Hum Genet 1994; 93:467–470.

671. Chillón M, Casals T, Mercier B, et al. Mutations in the cystic fibrosis gene in patients with congenital absence of the vas deferens. N Engl J Med 1995; 332:1475–1480.

672. McClure RD, Hricak H. Magnetic resonance imaging: its application to male infertility. Urology 1986; 27:91–98.

673. Hendry WF, Parslow JM, Stedronska J. Exploratory scrototomy in 168 azoospermic males. Br J Urol 1983; 55:785–791.

674. Baker HWG, Burger HG, de Kretser DM, et al. Relative incidence of etiological disorders in male infertility. In: Santen RJ, Swerdloff RS, eds. Male Reproductive Dysfunction: Diagnosis and Management of Hypogonadism, Infertility and Impotence. New York: Marcel Dekker, 1986: 341–372.

675. Gross KM, Matsumoto AM, Southworth MB, et al. Evidence for decreased luteinizing hormone–releasing hormone pulse frequency in men with selective elevations of follicle-stimulating hormone. J Clin Endocrinol Metab 1985; 60:197–202.

676. Gross KM, Matsumoto AM, Berger RE, et al. Increased frequency of

677. pulsatile luteinizing hormone–releasing hormone administration selectively decreases follicle-stimulating hormone levels in men with idiopathic azoospermia. Fertil Steril 1986; 45:392–396.

677. Hönigl W, Knuth UA, Nieschlag E. Selective reduction of elevated FSH levels in infertile men by pulsatile LHRH treatment. Clin Endocrinol 1986; 24:177–182.

678. Reyes-Fuentes A, Chavarria ME, Carrera A, et al. Alterations in pulsatile luteinizing hormone and follicle-stimulating hormone secretion in idiopathic oligoasthenospermic men: assessment by deconvolution analysis—a clinical research center study. J Clin Endocrinol Metab 1996; 81:524–529.

679. Booth JD, Merriam GR, Clark RV, et al. Evidence for Leydig cell dysfunction in infertile men with a selective increase in plasma follicle-stimulating hormone. J Clin Endocrinol Metab 1987; 64:1194–1198.

680. Collins JA, Wrixon W, Janes LB, et al. Treatment-independent pregnancy among infertile couples. N Engl J Med 1983; 309:1201–1205.

681. Baker HWG. Male infertility of undetermined etiology. In: Krieger DT, Bardin CW, eds. Current Therapy in Endocrinology 1983–1984. Philadelphia: BC Decker, 1983: 366–371.

682. Bhasin S, de Kretser DM, Baker HWG. Pathophysiology and natural history of male infertility. J Clin Endocrinol Metab 1994; 79:1525–1529.

683. Baker HWG, Liu DY, Bourne H, et al. Diagnosis of sperm defects in selecting patients for assisted fertilization. Hum Reprod 1993; 8:1779–1780.

684. Palermo G, Joris H, Devroey P, et al. Pregnancies after intracytoplasmic injection of single spermatozoon into an oocyte. Lancet 1992; 340:17–18.

685. Harari O, Bourne H, McDonald M, et al. Intracytoplasmic sperm injection: a major advance in the management of severe male subfertility. Fertil Steril 1995; 64:360–368.

686. Silber SJ, Nagy ZP, Liu J, et al. Conventional in-vitro fertilization versus intracytoplasmic sperm injection for patients requiring microsurgical sperm aspiration. Hum Reprod 1994; 9:1705–1709.

687. Yemini M, Vanderzwalmen P, Mukaida T, et al. Intracytoplasmic sperm injection, fertilization, and embryo transfer after retrieval of spermatozoa by testicular biopsy from an azoospermic male with testicular tubular atrophy. Fertil Steril 1995; 63:1118–1120.

688. Fishel S, Green S, Thornton S, et al. Pregnancy after intracytoplasmic injection of spermatid. Lancet 1995; 345:1641–1642.

689. Walsh PC. Benign prostatic hyperplasia. In: Walsh PC, Retik AB, Stamey TA, et al, eds. Campbell's Urology. 6th ed. Philadelphia: WB Saunders, 1992: 1009–1027.

690. Wilson JD. The pathogenesis of benign prostatic hyperplasia. Am J Med 1980; 68:745–756.

691. Schroder FH. Medical treatment of benign prostatic hyperplasia: the effect of surgical or medical castration. Prog Clin Biol Res 1994; 386:191–196.

692. Wenderoth UK, George FW, Wilson JD. The effect of a 5α-reductase inhibitor on androgen-mediated growth of the dog prostate. Endocrinology 1983; 113:569–573.

693. Liang T, Hiss CE. Inhibition of 5α-reductase, receptor binding, and nuclear uptake of androgens in the prostate by a 4-methyl-4-aza-steroid. J Biol Chem 1981; 256:7998–8005.

694. Brooks JR, Berman C, Glitzer MS, et al. Effect of a new 5α-reductase inhibitor on size, histological characteristics and androgen concentrations of the canine prostate. Prostate 1982; 3:35–44.

695. Siiteri PK, Wilson JD. Dihydrotestosterone in prostatic hypertrophy. I: The formation and content of dihydrotestosterone in the hypertrophic prostate of man. J Clin Invest 1970; 49:1737–1745.

696. Hammond GL. Endogenous steroid levels in the human prostate from birth to old age: a comparison of normal and diseased tissues. J Endocrinol 1978; 78:7–19.

697. Walsh PC, Hutchins GM, Ewing LL. Tissue content of dihydrotestosterone in human prostatic hyperplasia is not supranormal. J Clin Invest 1983; 72:1772–1777.

698. Walsh PC, Wilson JD. The induction of prostatic hypertrophy in the dog with androstanediol. J Clin Invest 1976; 57:1093–1097.

699. Aumüller G, Funke PJ, Hahn A, et al. Phenotypic modulation of the canine prostate after long-term treatment with androgens and estrogens. Prostate 1982; 3:361–373.

700. Peters CA, Walsh PC. The effect of nafarelin acetate, a luteinizing hormone–releasing hormone agonist, on benign prostatic hyperplasia. N Engl J Med 1987; 317:599–604.

701. Gabrilove JL, Levine AC, Kirschenbaum A, et al. Effect of a GnRH analogue (leuprolide) on benign prostatic hypertrophy. J Clin Endocrinol Metab 1987; 64:1331–1333.

702. Matzkin H, Chen J, Lewysohn O, et al. Treatment of benign prostatic hypertrophy by a long-acting gonadotropin-releasing hormone analogue: 1-year experience. J Urol 1991; 145:309–312.

703. Eri LM, Haug E, Tveter KJ. Effects on the endocrine system of long-term treatment with the non-steroidal anti-androgen Casodex in patients with benign prostatic hyperplasia. Br J Urol 1995; 75:335–340.

704. Eri LM, Tveter KJ. Safety, side effects and patient acceptance of the antiandrogen Casodex in the treatment of benign prostatic hyperplasia. Eur Urol 1994; 26:219–226.

705. McConnell JD, Wilson JD, George FW, et al. Finasteride, an inhibitor of 5α-reductase, suppresses prostatic dihydrotestosterone in men with benign prostatic hyperplasia. J Clin Endocrinol Metab 1992; 74:505–508.

706. Gormley GJ, Stoner E, Bruskewitz RC, et al. The effect of finasteride in men with benign prostatic hyperplasia. The Finasteride Study Group. N Engl J Med 1992; 327:1185–1191.

707. Stoner E. Three-year safety and efficacy data on the use of finasteride in the treatment of benign prostatic hyperplasia. Urology 1994; 43:284–292.

708. Kirby RS, Vale J, Bryan J, et al. Long-term urodynamic effects of finasteride in benign prostatic hyperplasia: a pilot study. Eur Urol 1993; 24:20–26.

709. McConnell JD. Benign prostatic hyperplasia. Hormonal treatment. Urol Clin North Am 1995; 22:387–400.

710. Geller J, Albert J, Geller S. Acute therapy with megestrol acetate decreases nuclear and cytosol androgen receptors in human BPH tissue. Prostate 1982; 3:11–15.

711. Petrangeli E, Sciarra F, Di Silverio F, et al. Effects of two different medical treatments on dihydrotestosterone content and androgen receptors in human benign prostatic hyperplasia. J Steroid Biochem 1988; 30:395–399.

712. Kaplan JH, Kudish HG, Sacks SA. Testicular tumors of germ cell origin. I: Epidemiology, pathogenesis, clinical presentation, and diagnosis. Postgrad Med 1981; 70:114–121.

713. Morse MJ, Whitmore WF. Neoplasms of the testis. In: Walsh PC, Gittes RF, Perlmutter AD, et al, eds. Campbell's Urology. 5th ed. Philadelphia: WB Saunders, 1986: 1535–1582.

714. Hainsworth JD, Greco FA. Testicular germ cell neoplasms. Am J Med 1983; 75:817–832.

715. Forman D, Moller H. Testicular cancer. Cancer Surv 1994; 19-20:323–341.

716. Moller H, Jorgensen N, Forman D. Trends in incidence of testicular cancer in boys and adolescent men. Int J Cancer 1995; 61:761–764.

717. Lefevre RE, Levin HS, Banowsky LH, et al. Bilateral testicular tumors of germ cell origin. J Urol 1975; 114:556–559.

718. Nicholson PW, Harland SJ. Inheritance and testicular cancer. Br J Cancer 1995; 71:421–426.

719. Heimdal K, Fossa SD. Genetic factors in malignant germ-cell tumors. World J Urol 1994; 12:178–181.

720. Fonger JD, Filler RM, Rider WD, et al. Testicular tumors in maldescended testes. Can J Surg 1981; 24:353–355.

721. Henderson BE, Benton B, Jing J, et al. Risk factors for cancer of the testis in young men. Int J Cancer 1979; 23:598–602.

722. Raina V, Shukla NK, Gupta NP, et al. Germ cell tumours in uncorrected cryptorchid testis at Institute Rotary Cancer Hospital, New Delhi. Br J Cancer 1995; 71:380–382.

723. Schellhas HF. Malignant potential of the dysgenetic gonad. Part I. Obstet Gynecol 1974; 44:298–309.

724. Shellhas HF. Malignant potential of the dysgenetic gonad. Part II. Obstet Gynecol 1974; 44:455–462.

725. Manuel M, Katayama KP, Jones HW Jr. The age of occurrence of gonadal tumors in intersex patients with a Y chromosome. Am J Obstet Gynecol 1976; 24:293–300.

726. Simpson JL, Photopulos G. The relationship of neoplasia to disorders of abnormal sexual differentiation. Birth Defects 1976; 12:15–50.

727. Zhang ZF, Vena JE, Zielezny M, et al. Occupational exposure to extreme temperature and risk of testicular cancer. Arch Environ Health 1995; 50:13–18.

728. Carroll PR, Morse J, Koduru PPK, et al. Testicular germ cell tumor in patient with Klinefelter syndrome. Urology 1988; 31:72–74.

729. Buzelin F, Karam G, Moreau A, et al. Testicular tumor and the acquired immunodeficiency syndrome. Eur Urol 1994; 26:71–76.

730. Kirkland RT, Kirkland JL, Keenan BS. Bilateral testicular tumors in congenital adrenal hyperplasia. J Clin Endocrinol Metab 1977; 44:369–378.

731. Srikanth MS, West BR, Ishitani M, et al. Benign testicular tumors in children with congenital adrenal hyperplasia. J Pediatr Surg 1992; 27:639–641.

732. Davis JM, Woodroof J, Sadasivan R, et al. Case report: congenital adrenal hyperplasia and malignant Leydig cell tumor. Am J Med Sci 1995; 309:63–65.

733. Turner D. Testicular cancer and the value of self-examination. Nurs Times 1995; 91:30–31.

734. Bosl GJ, Vogelzang NJ, Goldman A, et al. Impact of delay in diagnosis on clinical stage of testicular cancer. Lancet 1981; 2:970–973.

725. Mostofi FK. Pathology of germ cell tumors of testis: a progress report. Cancer 1980; 45:1735–1754.

736. Moller MB, d'Amore F, Christensen BE. Testicular lymphoma: a population-based study of incidence, clinicopathological correlations and prognosis. The Danish Lymphoma Study Group, LYFO. Eur J Cancer 1994; 30A:1760–1764.

737. Zavala-Pompa A, Ro JY, el-Naggar A, et al. Primary carcinoid tumor of testis. Immunohistochemical, ultrastructural, and DNA flow cytometric study of three cases with a review of the literature. Cancer 1993; 72:1726–1732.

738. Marshall AHE, Dayan AD. An immune reaction in man against seminomas, dysgerminomas, pinealomas, and the mediastinal tumours of similar histological appearance? Lancet 1964; 2:1102–1104.

739. Grigor KM. A new classification of germ cell tumors of the testis. Eur Urol 1993; 23:93–100.

740. Scully RE. Gonadoblastoma: a review of 74 cases. Cancer 1970; 25:1340–1356.

741. Besznyak I, Sebesteny M, Kuchar F. Primary mediastinal seminoma. A case report and review of literature. J Thorac Cardiovasc Surg 1973; 65:930–934.

742. Luna MA, Valenzuela-Tamariz J. Germ-cell tumors of the mediastinum, postmortem findings. Am J Clin Pathol 1976; 65:450–454.

743. Bush SE, Martinez A, Bagshaw MA. Primary mediastinal seminoma. Cancer 1981; 48:1877–1882.

744. Raghavan D, Barrett A. Mediastinal seminomas. Cancer 1980; 46:1187–1191.

745. Mukai K, Adams WR. Yolk sac tumor of the anterior mediastinum. Am J Surg Pathol 1979; 3:77–83.

746. Chang CG, Kageyama N, Kobayashi T, et al. Pineal tumors: clinical diagnosis, with special emphasis on the significance of pineal calcification. Neurosurgery 1981; 8:656–668.

747. Kirshner JJ, Ginsberg SJ, Fitzpatrick AV, et al. Treatment of a primary intracranial germ cell tumor with systemic chemotherapy. Med Pediatr Oncol 1981; 9:361–365.

748. Kobayashi T, Kageyama N, Kida Y, et al. Unilateral germinomas involving the basal ganglia and thalamus. J Neurosurg 1981; 55:55–62.

749. Koide O, Iwai S. An ultrastructural study on germinoma cells. Acta Pathol Jpn 1981; 31:755–766.

750. Ellis M, Sikora K. The current management of testicular cancer. Br J Urol 1987; 59:2–9.

751. Braunstein GD, Rasor J, Wade ME. Presence in normal human testes of a chorionic-gonadotropin-like substance distinct from human luteinizing hormone. N Engl J Med 1975; 293:1339–1343.

752. Madersbacher S, Kratzik C, Gerth R, et al. Human chorionic gonadotropin (hCG) and its free subunits in hydrocele fluids and neoplastic tissue of testicular cancer patients: insights into the in vivo hCG-secretion pattern. Cancer Res 1994; 54:5096–5100.

753. Keogh B, Hreshchyshyn MM, Moore RH, et al. Urinary gonadotropins in management and prognosis of testicular tumor. Urology 1975; 5:496–503.

754. Cochran JS, Walsh PC, Porter JC, et al. The endocrinology of human chorionic gonadotropin–secreting testicular tumors: new methods in diagnosis. J Urol 1975; 114:549–555.

755. Masopust J, Kithier K, Radl J, et al. Occurrence of fetoprotein in patients with neoplasms and non-neoplastic diseases. Int J Cancer 1968; 3:364–373.

756. Talerman A. Endodermal sinus (yolk sac) tumor elements in testicular germ-cell tumors in adults. Cancer 1980; 46:1213–1217.

757. Javadpour N. The role of biologic tumor markers in testicular cancer. Cancer 1980; 45:1755–1761.

758. Szymendera JJ, Zborzil J, Sikorowa L, et al. Value of five tumor markers (AFP, CEA, hCG, hPL, and SP1) in diagnosis and staging of testicular germ cell tumors. Oncology 1981; 38:222–229.

759. Willemse PHB, Sleijfer DT, Schraffordt Koops H, et al. Tumor markers in patients with non-seminomatous germ cell tumors of the testis. Oncodev Biol Med 1981; 2:117–128.

760. Willemse PHB, Sleijfer DT, Schraffordt Koops H, et al. The value of AFP and hCG half-lives in predicting the efficacy of combination chemotherapy in patients with non-seminomatous germ cell tumors of the testis. Oncodev Biol Med 1981; 2:129–134.

761. Lange PH, McIntire KR, Waldmann TA, et al. Serum alpha fetoprotein and human chorionic gonadotropin in the diagnosis and management of non-seminomatous germ-cell testicular cancer. N Engl J Med 1976; 295:1237–1240.

762. Bosl GJ, Geller NL, Cirrincione C, et al. Serum tumor markers in patients with metastatic germ cell tumors of the testis. Am J Med 1983; 75:29–35.

763. Bosl GJ, Geller N, Cirrincione C, et al. Interrelationships of histopathology and other clinical variables in patients with germ cell tumors of the testis. Cancer 1983; 51:2121–2125.

764. Fung LC, Honey RJ, Gardiner GW. Testicular seminoma presenting with features of androgen excess. Urology 1994; 44:927–929.

765. Aiginger P, Kolbe H, Kühböck J, et al. The endocrinology of testicular germinal cell tumors. Acta Endocrinol 1981; 97:419–426.

766. Reznik Y, Rieu M, Kuhn JM, et al. Luteinizing hormone regulation by sex steroids in men with germinal and Leydig cell tumours. Clin Endocrinol 1993; 38:487–493.

767. Bergmann KA. Current concepts in clinical therapeutics: testicular cancer. Clin Pharm 1987; 6:693–706.

768. Bey P, Guillemin F, Malissard L, et al. Testicular seminomas: study of relapses and causes of death in a series of 86 patients. In: Khoury S, Kuss R, Murphy GP, et al, eds. Testicular Cancer. New York: Alan R Liss, 1985: 493–498.

769. Fraley EE, Lange PH, Kennedy BJ. Germ-cell testicular cancer in adults. N Engl J Med 1979; 301:1370–1377.

770. Leibovitch I, Foster RS, Ulbright TM, et al. Adult primary pure teratoma of the testis. The Indiana experience. Cancer 1995; 75:2244–2250.

771. Price BA, Shepherd AF, Peters NH. 12 year review of testicular tumour treatment by the army medical services. J R Army Med Corps 1993; 139:89–93.

772. Ondrus D, Hornak M, Matoska J, et al. Chemotherapy of testicular cancer: 10-year experience. Neoplasma 1993; 40:247–253.

773. Reed E, Sanger WG, Armitage JO. Results of semen cryopreservation in young men with testicular carcinoma and lymphoma. J Clin Oncol 1986; 4:537–539.

774. Fossa SD, Lehne G, Heimdal K, et al. Clinical and biochemical long-term toxicity after low-stage testicular cancer. Oncology 1995; 52:300–305.

775. Bokemeyer C, Schmoll HJ. Treatment of testicular cancer and the development of secondary malignancies. J Clin Oncol 1995; 13:283–292.

776. Freeman DA. Steroid hormone–producing tumors in man. Endocr Rev 1986; 7:204–220.

777. Masumori N, Kumamoto Y, Itoh N, et al. Leydig cell tumor: a case report with reference to its endocrinological features. Eur Urol 1993; 24:302–304.

778. Gabrilove JL, Nicolis GL, Mitty HA, et al. Feminizing interstitial cell tumor of the testis: personal observations and a review of the literature. Cancer 1975; 35:1184–1202.

779. Niewenhuis JC, Wolf MC, Kass EJ. Bilateral asynchronous Sertoli cell tumor in a boy with the Peutz-Jeghers syndrome. J Urol 1994; 152:1246–1248.

780. Dreyer L, Jacyk WK, du Plessis DJ. Bilateral large-cell calcifying Sertoli cell tumor of the testes with Peutz-Jeghers syndrome: a case report. Pediatr Dermatol 1994; 11:335–337.

781. Gabrilove JL, Freiberg EK, Leiter E, et al. Feminizing and non-feminizing Sertoli cell tumors. J Urol 1980; 124:757–767.

782. Nogales FF, Andujar M, Zulauga A, et al. Malignant large cel calcifying Sertoli cell tumor of the testis. J Urol 1995; 153:1935–1937.

783. Stein JP, Freeman JA, Esrig D, et al. Papillary adenocarcinoma of the rete testis: a case report and review of the literature. Urology 1994; 44:588–594.

784. Burns MW, Chandler WL, Krieger JN. Adenocarcinoma of rete testis. Role of inguinal orchiectomy plus retroperitoneal lymph node dissection. Urology 1991; 37:571–573.

785. Junkmann K. Long-acting steroids in reproduction. Recent Prog Horm Res 1957; 13:389–419.

786. James KC, Nicholls PJ, Roberts M. Biological half-lives of [4-14C]testosterone and some of its esters after injection into the rat. J Pharm Pharmacol 1969; 21:24–27.

787. Honrath WL, Wolff A, Meli A. The influence of the amount of solvent (sesame oil) on the degree and duration of action of subcutaneously administered testosterone and its propionate. Steroids 1963; 2:425–428.

788. Snyder PJ, Lawrence DA. Treatment of male hypogonadism with testosterone enanthate. J Clin Endocrinol Metab 1980; 51:1335–1339.

789. Mauss J, Borsch G, Bormacher K, et al. Effect of long-term testosterone oenanthate administration on male reproductive function: clinical evaluation, serum FSH, LH, testosterone, and seminal fluid analyses in normal men. Acta Endocrinol 1975; 78:373–384.

790. Nieschlag E. Current status of testosterone substitution therapy. Int J Androl 1982; 5:225–228.

791. Sokol RZ, Saul C, Campfield LA, et al. Testosterone enanthate kinetics: compartmental modeling. Fertil Steril 1981; 36:428 (abstract).

792. Behre HM, Nieschlag E. Testosterone buciclate (20 Aet-1) in hypogonadal men: pharmacokinetics and pharmacodynamics of the new long-acting androgen ester. J Clin Endocrinol Metab 1992; 75:1204–1210.

793. Gooren LJG. Long-term safety of the oral androgen testosterone undecanoate. Int J Androl 1986; 9:21–26.

794. Davidson DW, O'Carroll R, Bancroft J. Increasing circulating androgens with oral testosterone undecanoate in eugonadal men. J Steroid Biochem 1987; 26:713–715.

795. Nieschlag E, Mauss J, Coert A, et al. Plasma androgen levels in men after oral administration of testosterone or testosterone undecanoate. Acta Endocrinol 1975; 79:366–374.

796. Franchimont P, Kocovic PM, Mattei A, et al. Effects of oral testosterone undecanoate in hypogonadal male patients. Clin Endocrinol 1978; 9:313–320.

797. Gooren LJ. A ten-year safety study of the oral androgen testosterone undecanoate. J Androl 1994; 15:212–215.

798. Maisey NM, Bingham J, Marks V, et al. Clinical efficacy of testosterone undecanoate in male hypogonadism. Clin Endocrinol 1981; 14:625–629.

799. Schürmeyer TH, Wickings EJ, Freischem CW, et al. Saliva and serum testosterone following oral testosterone undecanoate administration in normal and hypogonadal men. Acta Endocrinol 1983; 102:456–462.

800. Petry R, Rausch-Stroomann J-G, Hienz HA, et al. Androgen treatment without inhibiting effect on hypophysis and male gonads. Acta Endocrinol 1968; 59:497–507.

801. Aakvaag A, Stromme SB. The effect of mesterolone administration to normal men on the pituitary-testicular function. Acta Endocrinol 1974; 77:380–386.

802. Luisi M, Franchi F. Double-blind group comparative study of testosterone undecanoate and mesterolone in hypogonadal male patients. J Endocrinol Invest 1980; 3:305–308.

803. Findlay JC, Place V, Snyder PJ. Treatment of primary hypogonadism in men by the transdermal administration of testosterone. J Clin Endocrinol Metab 1989; 68:369–373.

804. Place VA, Atkinson L, Prather DA, et al. Transdermal testosterone replacement through genital skin. In: Nieschlag S, Behre HM, eds. Testosterone: Action, Deficiency, Substitution. Berlin: Springer-Verlag, 1990; 165–180.

805. Cunningham GR, Cordero E, Thornby JI. Testosterone replacement with transdermal therapeutic systems. JAMA 1989; 261:2525–2530.

806. Meikle AW, Mazer NA, Moellmer JF, et al. Enhanced transdermal delivery of testosterone across nonscrotal skin produces physiological concentrations of testosterone and its metabolites in hypogonadal men. J Clin Endocrinol Metab 1992; 74:623–628.

807. Bals-Pratsch M, Langer K, Place VA, et al. Substitution therapy of hypogonadal men with transdermal testosterone over one year. Acta Endocrinol 1988; 118:7–13.

808. Ahmed SR, Boucher AE, Manni A, et al. Transdermal testosterone therapy in the treatment of male hypogonadism. J Clin Endocrinol Metab 1988; 66:546–551.

809. Weinbauer GF, Marshall GR, Nieschlag E. New injectable testosterone ester maintains serum testosterone of castrated monkeys in the normal range for four months. Acta Endocrinol 1986; 113:128–132.

810. Gooren LJG. Long-term safety of the oral androgen testosterone undecanoate. Int J Androl 1986; 9:21–26.

811. Kuhn JM, Rieu M, Laudat MH, et al. Effects of 10 days administration of percutaneous dihydrotestosterone on the pituitary-testicular axis in normal men. J Clin Endocrinol Metab 1984; 58:231–235.

812. Vermeulen A, Deslypere JP. Long-term transdermal dihydrotestosterone therapy: effects on pituitary gonadal axis and plasma lipoproteins. Maturitas 1985; 7:281–287.

813. Mosbach EH, Shefer S, Abell LL. Identification of the fecal metabolites of 17α-methyltestosterone in the dog. J Lipid Res 1968; 9:93–97.

814. Alkalay D, Khemani L, Bartlett MF. Spectrophotofluorometric determination of methyltestosterone in plasma or serum. J Pharm Sci 1972; 61:1746–1749.

815. Doerr P, Pirke KM. Regulation of plasma oestrogens in normal adult males. Acta Endocrinol 1974; 75:617–624.

816. Liao S, Liang T, Fang S, et al. Steroid structure and androgenic activity. Specificity involved in the receptor binding and nuclear retention of various androgens. J Biol Chem 1973; 248:6154–6162.

817. Sundaram K, Kumar N, Bardin CW. 7-Methyl-19-nortestosterone: an ideal androgen for replacement therapy. Recent Prog Horm Res 1994; 49:373–376.

818. Salehian B, Wang C, Alexander G, et al. Pharmacokinetics, bioefficacy, and safety of sublingual testosterone cyclodextrin in hypogonadal men: comparison to testosterone enanthate—a clinical research center study. J Clin Endocrinol Metab 1995; 80:3567–3575.

819. Marberger H. Hormonal therapy with steroid-filled Silastic rubber implants. Br J Urol 1976; 48:153–154.

820. Johnsen SG, Bennett EP, Jensen VG. Therapeutic effectiveness of oral testosterone. Lancet 1974; 2:1473–1475.

821. Daggett PR, Wheeler MJ, Nabarro JDN. Oral testosterone, a reappraisal. Horm Res 1978; 9:121–129.

822. Fogh M, Corker CS, McLean H, et al. Serum-testosterone during oral administration of testosterone in hypogonadal men and transsexual women. Acta Endocrinol 1978; 87:643–649.

823. Johnsen SG, Kampmann JP, Bennett EP, et al. Enzyme induction by oral testosterone. Clin Pharmacol Ther 1976; 20:233–237.

824. Jacobs SC, Kaplan GW, Gittes RF. Topical testosterone therapy for penile growth. Urology 1975; 6:708–710.

825. Ben-Galim E, Hillman RE, Weldon VV. Topically applied testosterone and phallic growth. Am J Dis Child 1980; 134:296–298.

826. Parker LU, Bergfeld WF. Virilization secondary to topical testosterone. Cleve Clin J Med 1991; 58:43–46.

827. Kapelrud H, Johannesen O, Oftebro H. Testosterone/epitestosterone ratio in urine: a possible diagnostic tool in the disclosure of exogenous testosterone administration. J Intern Med 1992; 232:453–455.

828. Aakvaag A, Vogt JH. Plasma testosterone values in different forms of testosterone treatment. Acta Endocrinol 1969; 60:537–542.

829. Danner CH, Frick J. Androgen substitution with testosterone containing nasal drops. Int J Androl 1980; 3:429–435.

830. Cunningham GR, Silverman VE, Thornby J, et al. The potential for an androgen male contraceptive. J Clin Endocrinol Metab 1979; 49:520–526.

831. Swerdloff RS, Palacios A, McClure RD, et al. Male contraception: clinical assessment of chronic administration of testosterone enanthate. Int J Androl 1978; 2:731–747.

832. Palacios A, McClure RD, Campfield A, et al. Effect of testosterone enanthate on testis size. J Urol 1981; 126:46–48.

833. Vigersky RA, Easley RB, Loriaux DL. Effect of fluoxymesterone on the pituitary-gonadal axis: the role of testosterone-estradiol-binding globulin. J Clin Endocrinol Metab 1976; 43:1–9.

834. Jones TM, Fang VS, Landau RL, et al. The effect of fluoxymesterone administration on testicular function. J Clin Endocrinol Metab 1977; 44:121–129.

835. Aakvaag A, Vogt JH. Plasma testosterone values in different forms of testosterone treatment. Acta Endocrinol 1969; 60:537–542.

836. Scaglia HE, Ramirez AM, Gaytan JR, et al. Gonadotropin dynamics in Klinefelter's syndrome. Reproduction 1975; 2:7–12.

837. Smals AGH, Kloppenborg PWC, Pieters GFE, et al. Modulation of the gonadotropin response to constant luteinizing hormone–releasing hormone infusion by acute and chronic testosterone administration in Klinefelter's syndrome. J Clin Endocrinol Metab 1979; 48:148–152.

838. Fukutani K, Isurugi K, Takayasu H, et al. Effects of depot testosterone therapy on serum levels of luteinizing hormone and follicle-stimulating hormone in patients with Klinefelter's syndrome and hypogonadotropic eunuchoidism. J Clin Endocrinol Metab 1974; 39:856–864.

839. Capell PT, Paulsen CA, Derleth D, et al. The effect of short-term testosterone administration on serum FSH, LH and testosterone levels: evidence for selective abnormality in LH control in patients with Klinefelter's syndrome. J Clin Endocrinol Metab 1973; 37:752–759.

840. Davidson JM, Camargo CA, Smith ER. Effects of androgen on sexual behavior in hypogonadal men. J Clin Endocrinol Metab 1979; 48:955–958.

841. Salmimies P, Kockott G, Pirke KM, et al. Effects of testosterone replacement on sexual behavior in hypogonadal men. Arch Sex Behav 1982; 11:345–353.

842. Kwan M, Greenleaf WJ, Mann J, et al. The nature of androgen action on male sexuality: a combined laboratory–self-report study on hypogonadal men. J Clin Endocrinol Metab 1983; 57:557–562.

843. O'Carroll R, Shapiro C, Bancroft J. Androgens, behaviour and nocturnal erection in hypogonadal men: the effects of varying the replacement dose. Clin Endocrinol 1985; 23:527–538.

844. Greenstein A, Plymate SR, Katz PG. Visually stimulated erection in castrated men. J Urol 1995; 153:650–652.

845. Behre HM, Bohmeyer J, Nieschlag E. Prostate volume in testosterone-treated and untreated hypogonadal men in comparison to age-matched normal controls. Clin Endocrinol 1994; 40:341–349.

846. Krauss DJ, Taub HA, Lantinga LJ, et al. Risks of blood volume changes in hypogonadal men treated with testosterone enanthate for erectile impotence. J Urol 1991; 146:1566–1570.

847. Arisaka O, Arisaka M, Nakayama Y, et al. Effect of testosterone on bone density and bone metabolism in adolescent male hypogonadism. Metabolism 1995; 44:419–423.

848. Kübler A, Schulz G, Cordes U, et al. The influence of testosterone substitution on bone mineral density in patients with Klinefelter's syndrome. Exp Clin Endocrinol 1992; 100:129–132.

849. Wong FHW, Pun KK, Wang C. Loss of bone mass in patients with Klinefelter's syndrome despite sufficient testosterone replacement. Osteoporosis Int 1993; 3:3–7.

850. Bellido T, Jilka RL, Boyce BF, et al. Regulation of interleukin-6, osteoclastogenesis, and bone mass by androgens. The role of the androgen receptor. J Clin Invest 1995; 95:2886–2895.

851. Gearhart JP, Jeffs RD. The use of parenteral testosterone therapy in genital reconstructive surgery. J Urol 1987; 138:1077–1078.

852. Davits RJ, van den Aker ES, Scholtmeijer RJ, et al. Effect of parenteral testosterone therapy on penile development in boys with hypospadias. Br J Urol 1993; 71:593–595.

853. McMahon DR, Kramer SA, Husmann DA. Micropenis: does early treatment with testosterone do more harm than good? J Urol 1995; 154:825–829.

854. Zachmann M, Prader A. Anabolic and androgenic effect of testosterone in sexually immature boys and its dependency on growth hormone. J Clin Endocrinol 1970; 30:85–95.

855. Aynsley-Green A, Zachmann M, Prader A. Interrelation of the therapeutic effects of growth hormone and testosterone on growth in hypopituitarism. J Pediatr 1976; 89:992–999.

856. Tanner JM, Whitehouse RH, Hughes PCR, et al. Relative importance of growth hormone and sex steroids for the growth at puberty of trunk length, limb length, and muscle width in growth hormone–deficient children. J Pediatr 1976; 89:1000–1008.

857. Pertzelan A, Blum I, Grunebaum M, et al. The combined effect of growth hormone and methandrostenolone on the linear growth of patients with multiple pituitary hormone deficiencies. Clin Endocrinol 1977; 6:271–276.

858. Parker MW, Johanson AJ, Rogol AD, et al. Effect of testosterone on somatomedin-C concentrations in prepubertal boys. J Clin Endocrinol Metab 1984; 58:87–90.

859. Venable JH. Morphology of the cells of normal, testosterone-deprived and testosterone-stimulated levator ani muscles. Am J Anat 1966; 119:271–301.

860. Krieg M, Voigt KD. Biochemical substrate of androgenic actions at cellular levels in prostate, bulbocavernosus/levator ani and skeletal muscle. In: Symposium on Developments in Endocrinology in Honour of Dr. G. A. Overbeek. The Netherlands: Organon International Oss, 1976: 43–89.

861. Toth M. Relative androgenic and myotropic activity plots of 19-nortestosterone. J Steroid Biochem 1981; 14:1085–1090.

862. Wynn V. The anabolic steroids. Practitioner 1968; 200:509–518.

863. Overbeek GA, van der Vies J, de Visser J. The so-called "pure" anabolic agents. J Am Med Wom Assoc 1969; 24:54–59.

864. Liddle GW, Burke HA Jr. Anabolic steroids in clinical medicine. Helv Med Acta 1960; 27:504–513.

865. Nowakowski H. Metabolic studies with anabolic steroids. Acta Endocrinol 1961; 39(Suppl 63):37–53.

866. van Wayjen RGA, Buyze G. Clinical-pharmacological evaluation of certain anabolic steroids. Acta Endocrinol 1961; 39(Suppl 63):18–36.

867. Tweedle D, Walton C, Johnston IDA. The effect of an anabolic steroid on postoperative nitrogen balance. Br J Clin Pract 1972; 27:130–132.

868. Rabkin JG, Rabkin R, Wagner G. Testosterone replacement therapy in HIV illness. Gen Hosp Psychiatry 1995; 17:37–42.

869. Watson RN, Bradley MH, Callahan R, et al. A six month evaluation of an anabolic drug, norethandrolone, in underweight persons. Am J Med 1959; 26:238–242.

870. Kalliomaki JL, Pirila AM, Ruikka I. A therapeutic trial with ethyl-estrenol in geriatric patients. Acta Endocrinol 1961; 39(Suppl 63):124–131.

871. Thaysen JH. Anabolic steroids in the treatment of renal failure. In: Gross F, ed. Protein Metabolism. Berlin: Springer-Verlag, 1962: 450–478.

872. Kassmann K, Rappaport R, Broyer M. The short-term effect of testosterone on growth in boys on hemodialysis. Clin Nephrol 1992; 37:148–154.

873. Blagg CR, Parsons FM, Young GA. Effect of dietary glucose and protein in acute renal failure. Lancet 1962; 1:608–612.

874. Wilson JD. Androgen abuse by athletes. Endocr Rev 1988; 9:181–199.

875. Elashoff JD, Jacknow AD, Shain SG, et al. Effects of anabolic-androgenic steroids on muscular strength. Ann Intern Med 1991; 115:387.

876. Forbes GB. The effect of anabolic steroids on lean body mass: the dose response curve. Metabolism 1985; 115:387.

877. Griggs RC, Kingston W, Jozefowicz RF, et al. Effects of testosterone on muscle mass and muscle protein synthesis. J Appl Physiol 1989; 66:498.

878. Bhasin S, Storer TW, Berman N, et al. The androgenic/anabolic steroid controversy: do supraphysiological doses of testosterone increase fat-free mass, muscle size and strength in eugonadal men? N Engl J Med 1996; 335:1–7.

879. Kennedy BJ, Gilbertsen AS. Increased erythropoiesis induced by androgenic-hormone therapy. N Engl J Med 1957; 256:719–726.

880. Shahidi NT. Androgens and erythropoiesis. N Engl J Med 1973; 289:72–80.

881. Evens RP, Amerson AB. Androgens and erythropoiesis. J Clin Pharmacol 1974; 14:94–101.

882. Hengstum V, Steenbergen J, Haanen C. Clinical course in 28 unselected patients with aplastic anaemia treated with anabolic steroids. Br J Haematol 1979; 41:323–333.

883. Najean Y. Long-term follow-up in patients with aplastic anemia. A study of 137 androgen-treated patients surviving more than two years. Am J Med 1981; 71:543–551.

884. Branda RF, Amsden TW, Jacob HS. Randomized study of nandrolone therapy of anemias due to bone marrow failure. Arch Intern Med 1977; 137:65–69.

885. Camitta BM, Thomas ED, Nathan DG, et al. A prospective study of androgens and bone marrow transplantation for treatment of severe aplastic anemia. Blood 1979; 53:504–514.

886. French Cooperative Group for the Study of Aplastic and Refractory Anaemias. Androgen therapy in aplastic anaemia: a comparative study of high and low doses and of 4 different androgens. Scand J Haematol 1986; 36:346–352.

887. Mirand EA, Murphy GP. Erythropoietin activity in anephric humans given prolonged androgen treatment. J Surg Oncol 1971; 3:59–65.

888. Eschbach JW, Funk D, Adamson J, et al. Erythropoiesis in patients with renal failure undergoing chronic dialysis. N Engl J Med 1967; 276:653–658.

889. Eschbach JW, Adamson JW. Improvement in the anemia of chronic renal failure with fluoxymesterone. Ann Intern Med 1973; 78:527–532.

890. Hendler ED, Goffinet JA, Ross S, et al. Controlled study of androgen therapy in anemia of patients on maintenance hemodialysis. N Engl J Med 1974; 291:1046–1051.

891. Koch KM, Patyna WD, Shaldon S, et al. Anemia of the regular hemodialysis patient and its treatment. Nephron 1974; 12:405–419.

892. Williams S, Stein JH, Ferris TF. Nandrolone decanoate therapy for patients receiving hemodialysis. Arch Intern Med 1974; 134:289–292.

893. Cattran DC, Fenton SSA, Wilson DR, et al. A controlled trial of nandrolone decanoate in the treatment of uremic anemia. Kidney Int 1977; 12:430–437.

894. von Hartitzsch B, Kerr DNS, Morley G, et al. Androgens in the anemia of chronic renal failure. Nephron 1977; 18:13–20.

895. Besa EC. Hematologic effects of androgens revisited: an alternative therapy in various hematologic conditions. Semin Hematol 1994; 31:134–145.

896. Spaulding WB. Methyltestosterone therapy for hereditary episodic edema (hereditary angioneurotic edema). Ann Intern Med 1960; 53:739–745.

897. Blohme G, Ysander L, Korsan-Bengtsen K, et al. Hereditary angioneurotic oedema in three families. Acta Med Scand 1972; 91:209–219.

898. Rosse WF, Logue GL, Silberman HR. The effect of synthetic androgens in hereditary angioneurotic edema: alteration of C1 inhibitor and C4 levels. Trans Assoc Am Phys 1976; 89:122–132.

899. Frank MM, Gelfand JA, Atkinson JP. Hereditary angioedema: the clinical syndrome and its management. Ann Intern Med 1976; 84:580–593.

900. Gelford JA, Sherins RJ, Alling DW, et al. Treatment of hereditary angioedema with danazol. Reversal of clinical and biochemical abnormalities. N Engl J Med 1976; 295:1444–1448.

901. Sheffer AL, Fearon DT, Austen KF. Methyltestosterone therapy in hereditary angioedema. Ann Intern Med 1977; 86:306–308.

902. Saihan EM, Warin RP. Treatment of hereditary angioneurotic oedema with methandienone. Br Med J 1978; 1:367.

903. Gould DJ, Cunliffe WJ, Smiddy EG. Anabolic steroids in hereditary angioedema. Lancet 1978; 1:770–771.

904. Agostoni A, Cicardi M, Cugno M, et al. Clinical problems in the C1-inhibitor deficient patient. Behring Inst Mitt 1993; 93:306–312.

905. Barbosa J, Seal US, Doe RP. Effects of anabolic steroids on haptoglobin, orosomucoid, plasminogen, fibrinogen, transferrin, ceruloplasmin, α1-antitrypsin, β-glucuronidase and total serum proteins. J Clin Endocrinol 1971; 33:388–398.

906. Carl-Bertil L, Rannevik G. A comparison of plasma protein changes induced by danazol, pregnancy, and estrogens. J Clin Endocrinol Metab 1979; 49:719–725.

907. Madanes AE, Farber M. Danazol. Ann Intern Med 1982; 96:625–630.

908. Gralnick HR, Rick ME. Danazol increases factor VIII and factor IX in classic hemophilia and Christmas disease. N Engl J Med 1983; 308:1393–1395.

909. Ahn YS, Harrington WJ, Simon SR, et al. Danazol for the treatment of

idiopathic thrombocytopenic purpura. N Engl J Med 1983; 308:1396–1399.

910. Limbeck GA, Ruvalcaba RHA, Mahoney CP, et al. Studies on anabolic steroids. IV: The effects of oxandrolone on height and skeletal maturation in uncomplicated growth retardation. Clin Pharmacol Ther 1971; 12:798–805.

911. Bettman HK, Goldman HS, Abramowicz M, et al. Oxandrolone treatment of short stature: effect on predicted mature height. J Pediatr 1971; 79:1018–1023.

912. Moore DC, Tattoni DS, Limbeck GA, et al. Studies of anabolic steroids. V: Effect of prolonged oxandrolone administration on growth in children and adolescents with uncomplicated short stature. Pediatrics 1976; 58:412–422.

913. Clayton PE, Shalet SM, Price DA, et al. Growth and growth hormone responses to oxandrolone in boys with constitutional delay of growth and puberty (CDGP). Clin Endocrinol 1988; 29:123–130.

914. Wilson DM, Kei J, Hintz RL, et al. Effects of testosterone therapy for pubertal delay. Am J Dis Child 1988; 142:96–99.

915. Albanese A, Stanhope R. Predictive factors in the determination of final height in boys with constitutional delay of growth and puberty. J Pediatr 1995; 126:545–550.

916. Adan L, Souberbielle JC, Brauner R. Management of the short stature due to pubertal delay in boys. J Clin Endocrinol Metab 1994; 78:478–482.

917. Jackson JA, Waxman J, Spiekerman AM. Prostatic complications of testosterone replacement therapy. Arch Intern Med 1989; 149:2365–2366.

918. Kennedy BJ, Nathanson IT. Effects of intensive sex steroid hormone therapy in advanced breast cancer. JAMA 1953; 152:1135–1141.

919. Fruehan HE, Frawley TH. Current use of anabolic steroids. JAMA 1963; 184:527–532.

920. Fyrand O, Fiskaadal HJ, Trygstad O. Acne in pubertal boys undergoing treatment with androgens. Acta Derm Venereol 1992; 72:148–149.

921. Kearns WM. Oral therapy of testicular deficiency. J Clin Endocrinol 1941; 1:126–130.

922. Laron Z. Effectiveness of fluoxymesterone on linear growth and weight in children with growth retardation and underweight. Acta Endocrinol 1961; 36:541–548.

923. Foss GL, Simpson SL. Oral methyltestosterone and jaundice. Br Med J 1959; 1:259–263.

924. Kory RC, Bradley MH, Watson RN, et al. A six-month evaluation of an anabolic drug, norethandrolone, in underweight persons. II: BSP retention and liver function. Am J Med 1959; 26:243–248.

925. Arias IM. The effects of anabolic steroids on liver function. In: Gross F, ed. Protein Metabolism. Berlin: Springer-Verlag, 1962: 434–445.

926. deLorimier AA, Gordan GS, Lowe RC, et al. Methyltestosterone, related steroids, and liver function. Arch Intern Med 1965; 116:289–294.

927. Yoshida EM, Erb SR, Scudamore CH, et al. Severe cholestasis and jaundice secondary to an esterified testosterone, a non-C17 alkylated anabolic steroid. J Clin Gastroenterol 1994; 18:268–270.

928. Muller AF, Valatlan M, Manning EL. Effet de la 17-ethyl-19-nor-testosterone sur la secretion du cortisol. Helv Med Acta 1960; 27:678–682.

929. Sweeney EC, Evans DJ. Hepatic lesions in patients treated with synthetic anabolic steroids. J Clin Pathol 1976; 29:626–633.

930. Shapiro P, Ikeda RM, Ruebner BH, et al. Multiple hepatic tumors and peliosis hepatis in Fanconi's anemia treated with androgens. Am J Dis Child 1977; 131:1104–1106.

931. McDonald EC, Speicher CE. Peliosis hepatis associated with administration of oxymetholone. JAMA 1978; 240:243–244.

932. Arnold GL, Kaplan MM. Peliosis hepatis due to oxymetholone—a clinically benign disorder. Am J Gastroenterol 1979; 71:213–216.

933. Farrell GC, Uren RF, Perkins KW, et al. Androgen-induced hepatoma. Lancet 1975; 1:430–431.

934. Goldfarb S. Sex hormones and hepatic neoplasia. Cancer Res 1976; 36:2584–2588.

935. Hernandez-Nieto L, Bruguera M, Bombi JA, et al. Benign liver-cell adenoma associated with long-term administration of an androgenic-anabolic steroid (methandienone). Cancer 1977; 40:1761–1764.

936. Antunes CMF, Stolley PD. Cancer induction by exogenous hormones. Cancer 1977; 39:1896–1898.

937. Goodman MA, Laden AMJ. Hepatocellular carcinoma in association with androgen therapy. Med J Aust 1977; 1:220–221.

938. Westaby D, Paradinas FJ, Ogle SJ, et al. Liver damage from long-term methyltestosterone. Lancet 1977; 2:261–263.

939. Boyd PR, Mark GJ. Multiple hepatic adenomas and a hepatocellular carcinoma in a man on oral methyl testosterone for eleven years. Cancer 1977; 40:1765–1770.

940. Coombes GB, Reiser J, Paradinas EJ, et al. An androgen-associated hepatic adenoma in a trans-sexual. Br J Surg 1978; 65:869–870.

941. Balazs M. Primary hepatocellular tumours during long-term androgenic steroid therapy. A light and electron microscopic study of 11 cases with emphasis on microvasculature of the tumours. Acta Morphol Hungarica 1991; 39:201–216.

942. Shephard RJ, Killinger D, Fried T. Response to sustained use of anabolic steroid. Br J Sports Med 1977; 11:170–173.

943. Thompson PD, Cullinane EM, Sady SP, et al. Contrasting effects of testosterone and stanozolol on serum lipoprotein levels. JAMA 1989; 261:1165–1168.

944. Zmuda JM, Fahrenbach MC, Younkin BT, et al. The effect of testosterone aromatization on high-density lipoprotein cholesterol level and postheparin lipolytic activity. Metabolism 1993; 42:446–450.

945. Asscheman H, Gooren LJ, Megens JA, et al. Serum testosterone level is the major determinant of the male-female differences in serum levels of high-density lipoprotein (HDL) cholesterol and HDL2 cholesterol. Metabolism 1994; 43:935–939.

946. Bagatell CJ, Bremner WJ. Androgen and progestagen effects on plasma lipids. Prog Cardiovasc Dis 1995; 38:255–271.

947. Matsumoto AM, Sandblom RE, Schoene RB, et al. Testosterone replacement in hypogonadal men: effects on obstructive sleep apnea, respiratory drives, and sleep. Clin Endocrinol 1985; 22:713–721.

948. Cistulli PA, Grunstein RR, Sullivan CE. Effect of testosterone administration on upper airway collapsibility during sleep. Am J Respir Crit Care Med 1994; 149:530–532.

949. Zelissen PMJ, Stricker BHC. Severe priapism as a complication of testosterone substitution therapy. Am J Med 1988; 85:273–274.

950. Sokol RZ, McClure RD, Peterson M, et al. Gonadotropin therapy failure secondary to human chorionic gonadotropin-induced antibodies. J Clin Endocrinol Metab 1981; 52:929–933.

951. Burger HG, de Kretser DM, Hudson B, et al. Effects of preceding androgen therapy on testicular response to human pituitary gonadotropin in hypogonadotropic hypogonadism: a study of three patients. Fertil Steril 1981; 35:64–68.

952. Rosemberg E. Gonadotropin therapy of male infertility. In: Hafez ESE, ed. Human Semen and Fertility Regulation in Men. St. Louis: CV Mosby, 1976: 464–475.

953. Saal W, Happ J, Cordes U, et al. Subcutaneous gonadotropin therapy in male patients with hypogonadotropic hypogonadism. Fertil Steril 1991; 56:319–324.

954. Kung AW, Zhong YY, Lam KS, et al. Induction of spermatogenesis with gonadotrophins in Chinese men with hypogonadotrophic hypogonadism. Int J Androl 1994; 17:214–247.

955. Kirk JM, Savage MO, Grant DB, et al. Gonadal function and response to human chorionic and menopausal gonadotrophin therapy in male patients with idiopathic hypogonadotrophic hypogonadism. Clin Endocrinol 1994; 41:57–63.

956. van de Berk D, Wijnberg M, van Dop PA. Initiation of spermatogenesis and successful in vitro fertilization in an infertile male with panhypopituitarism; superiority of pulsatile LH-RH over gonadotrophins? A case report. Eur J Obstet Gynecol Reprod Biol 1991; 40:153–157.

957. Claustrat B, David L, Faure A, et al. Development of antihuman chorionic gonadotropin antibodies in patients with hypogonadotropic hypogonadism. A study of four patients. J Clin Endocrinol Metab 1983; 57:1041–1047.

958. Gabrilove JL, George AC, Kirschenbaum A, et al. Effect of a GnRH analogue (leuprolide) on benign prostatic hypertrophy. J Clin Endocrinol Metab 1987; 64:1331–1333.

959. Peters CA, Walsh PC. The effect of nafarelin acetate, a luteinizing hormone–releasing hormone agonist, on benign prostatic hyperplasia. N Engl J Med 1987; 317:599–604.

960. Vickery BH. Comparison of the potential for therapeutic utilities with gonadotropin-releasing hormone agonists and antagonists. Endocr Rev 1986; 7:115–124.

961. Santoro N, Filicori M, Crowley WF Jr. Hypogonadotropic disorders in men and women: diagnosis and therapy with pulsatile gonadotropin-releasing hormone. Endocr Rev 1986; 7:11–23.

962. Delemarre-Van de Wall HA, Odink RJ. Pulsatile GnRH treatment in boys and girls with idiopathic hypogonadotrophic hypogonadism. Hum Reprod 1993; 8(Suppl 2):180–183.

963. Delemarre-Van de Wall HA. Induction of testicular growth and spermatogenesis by pulsatile, intravenous administration of gonadotrophin-releasing hormone in patients with hypogonadotrophic hypogonadism. Clin Endocrinol 1993; 38:473–480.

964. Simoni M, Montanini V, Fustini MF, et al. Circadian rhythm of plasma testosterone in men with idiopathic hypogonadotrophic hypogonadism before and during pulsatile administration of gonadotrophin-releasing hormone. Clin Endocrinol 1992; 36:29–34.

965. Klingmuller D, Schweikert H-U. Maintenance of spermatogenesis by intranasal administration of gonadotropin-releasing hormone in patients with hypothalamic hypogonadism. J Clin Endocrinol Metab 1985; 61:868–872.

966. Liu L, Chaudhari N, Corle D, et al. Comparison of pulsatile subcutaneous gonadotropin-releasing hormone and exogenous gonadotropins in the treatment of men with isolated hypogonadotropic hypogonadism. Fertil Steril 1988; 49:302–308.

967. Schopohl J. Pulsatile gonadotrophin releasing hormone versus gonadotrophin treatment of hypothalamic hypogonadism in males. Hum Reprod 1993; 8(Suppl 2):175–179.

968. Cacciari E, Frejaville E, Becca A. Treatment of cryptorchidism by intranasal synthetic LH-RH and its analogue D-Ser(TBU)6-LHRH-EA10. Eur J Pediatr 1982; 139:280–284.

969. Hagberg S, Westphal O. Treatment of undescended testes with intranasal application of synthetic LH-RH. Eur J Pediatr 1982; 139:285–288.

970. Frick J. Cryptorchidism. In: Krieger DT, Bardin CW, eds. Current Therapy in Endocrinology 1983–1984. Philadelphia: BC Decker, 1983: 371–374.

971. Santen RJ. Endocrine treatment of prostate cancer. J Clin Endocrinol Metab 1992; 75:685–689.

972. Crawford ED, DeAntoni EP. Current status of combined androgen blockade: optimal therapy for advanced prostate cancer. J Clin Endocrinol Metab 1995; 80:1062–1066.

973. Neely EK, Hintz RL, Parker B, et al. Two-year results of treatment with depot leuprolide acetate for central precocious puberty. J Pediatr 1992; 121:634–640.

974. Carel JC, Lahlou N, Guazzarotti L, et al. Treatment of central precocious puberty with depot leuprorelin. French Leuprorelin Trial Group. Eur J Endocrinol 1995; 132:699–704.

975. Dickey R. The management of a case of treatment-resistant paraphilia with a long-acting LHRh agonist. Can J Psychiatr 1992; 37:567–569.

976. Cooper AJ, Cernovsky ZZ. Comparison of cyproterone acetate (CPA) and leuprolide acetate (LHRH agonist) in a chronic pedophile: a clinical case study. Biol Psychiatr 1994; 36:269–271.

977. Thibaut F, Cordier B, Kuhn JM. Effect of a long-lasting gonadotrophin hormone–releasing hormone agonist in six cases of severe male paraphilia. Acta Psychiatr Scand 1993; 87:445–450.

978. Richer M, Crismon ML. Pharmacotherapy of sexual offenders. Ann Pharmacother 1993; 27:316–320.

979. Gonzalez-Barcena D, Vadillo-Buenfil M, Gomez-Orta F, et al. Responses to the antagonistic analog of LH-RH (SB-75, Cetrorelix) in patients with benign prostatic hyperplasia and prostatic cancer. Prostate 1994; 24:84–92.

980. Loprinzi CL, Michalak JC, Quella SK, et al. Megestrol acetate for the prevention of hot flashes. N Engl J Med 1994; 331:347–352.

981. Barbieri RL, Ryan KJ. Direct effects of medroxyprogesterone acetate (MPA) and megestrol acetate (MGA) on rat testicular steroidogenesis. Acta Endocrinol 1980; 94:419–425.

982. Meyer WJ, Walker PA, Emory LE, et al. Physical, metabolic, and hormonal effects on men of long-term therapy with medroxyprogesterone acetate. Fertil Steril 1985; 43:102–109.

983. Feldman D. Ketoconazole and other imidazole derivatives as inhibitors of steroidogenesis. Endocr Rev 1986; 7:409–420.

984. Mahler C, Verhelst J, Denis L. Ketoconazole and liarozole in the treatment of advanced prostatic cancer. Cancer 1993; 71(Suppl 3):1068–1073.

985. Dorrington-Ware P, McCartney ACE, Holland S, et al. The effect of spironolactone on hirsutism and female androgen metabolism. Clin Endocrinol 1985; 23:161–167.

986. Helfer EL, Miller JL, Rose LI. Side effects of spironolactone therapy in women. J Clin Endocrinol Metab 1988; 40:208–211.

987. Cusan L, Dupont A, Gomez J-L, et al. Comparison of flutamide and spironolactone in the treatment of hirsutism: a randomized controlled trial. Fertil Steril 1994; 61:281–287.

988. Rittmaster RS. Finasteride. N Engl J Med 1994; 330:120–125.

989. Vermeulen A, Giagulli VA, De Schepper P, et al. Hormonal effects of an orally active 4-azasteroid inhibitor of 5α-reductase in humans. Prostate 1989; 14:45–53.

990. McConnell JD, Wilson JD, George FW, et al. Finasteride, an inhibitor of 5α-reductase, suppresses prostatic dihydrotestosterone in men with benign prostatic hyperplasia. J Clin Endocrinol Metab 1992; 74:505–508.

991. Cunningham GR, Hirshkowitz M. Inhibition of steroid 5α-reductase with finasteride: sleep-related erections, potency, and libido in healthy men. J Clin Endocrinol Metab 1995; 80:1934–1940.

992. Stoner E. The clinical effects of a 5α-reductase inhibitor, finasteride, on benign prostatic hyperplasia: The Finasteride Study Group. J Urol 1992; 147:1298–1302.

993. Barradell LB, Faulds D. Cyproterone. A review of its pharmacology and therapeutic efficacy in prostate cancer. Drugs Aging 1994; 5:59–80.

994. Neumann F. The antiandrogen cyproterone acetate: discovery, chemistry, basic pharmacology, clinical use and tool in basic research. Exp Clin Endocrinol 1994; 102:1–32.

995. Knuth UA, Hano R, Nieschlag E. Effect of flutamide or cyproterone acetate on pituitary and testicular hormones in normal men. J Clin Endocrinol Metab 1984; 59:963–969.

996. Cooper AJ, Cernovovsky Z. The effects of cyproterone acetate on sleeping and waking penile erections in pedophiles: possible implications for treatment. Can J Psychiatr 1992; 37:33–39.

997. Bradford JM, Pawlak A. Effects of cyproterone acetate on sexual arousal patterns of pedophiles. Arch Sex Behav 1993; 22:629–641.

998. Bradford JM, Pawlak A. Double-blind placebo crossover study of cyproterone acetate in the treatment of the paraphilias. Arch Sex Behav 1993; 22:383–402.

999. Parys BT, Hamid S, Thomson RG. Severe hepatocellular dysfunction following cyproterone acetate therapy. Br J Urol 1991; 67:312–313.

1000. Watanabe S, Yamasaki S, Tanae A, et al. Three cases of hepatocellular carcinoma among cyproterone users. Ad hoc committee on Androcur users. Lancet 1994; 344:1567–1568.

1001. Neri RO. Antiandrogens. Adv Sex Horm 1976; 2:233–262.

1002. Marchetti B, Labrie F. Characteristics of flutamide action on prostatic and testicular functions in the rat. J Steroid Biochem 1988; 29:691–698.

1003. Stone NN, Clejan SJ. Response of prostate volume, prostate-specific antigen, and testosterone to flutamide in men with benign prostatic hyperplasia. J Androl 1991; 12:376–380.

1004. Wysowski DK, Freiman JP, Tourtelox JB, et al. Fatal and nonfatal hepatotoxicity associated with flutamide. Ann Intern Med 1993; 118:860–864.

1005. Dankoff JS. Near fatal liver dysfunction secondary to administration of flutamide for prostate cancer. J Urol 1992; 148:1914.

1006. Gomez JL, Dupont A, Cusan L, et al. Incidence of liver toxicity associated with the use of flutamide in prostate cancer patients. Am J Med 1992; 92:465–470.

1007. Eri LM, Tveter KJ. Safety, side effects and patient acceptance of the antiandrogen Casodex in the treatment of benign prostatic hyperplasia. Eur Urol 1994; 26:219–226.

1008. Schellhammer P, Sharifi R, Block N, et al. A controlled trial of bicalutamide versus flutamide, each in combination with luteinizing hormone-releasing hormone analogue therapy, in patients with advanced prostate cancer. Casodex Combination Study Group. Urology 1995; 45:745–752.

1009. Iversen P. Update of monotherapy trials with the new anti-androgen, Casodex (ICI 176,334). International Casodex Investigators. Eur Urol 1994; 26(Suppl 1):5–9.

1010. Bertagna C, De Gery A, Hucher M, et al. Efficacy of the combination of nilutamide plus orchidectomy in patients with metastatic prostatic cancer. A meta-analysis of seven randomized double-blind trials (1056 patients). Br J Urol 1994; 73:396–402.

1011. Gomez JL, Dupont A, Cusan L, et al. Simultaneous liver and lung toxicity related to the nonsteroidal antiandrogen nilutamide (Anandron): a case report. Am J Med 1992; 92:563–566.

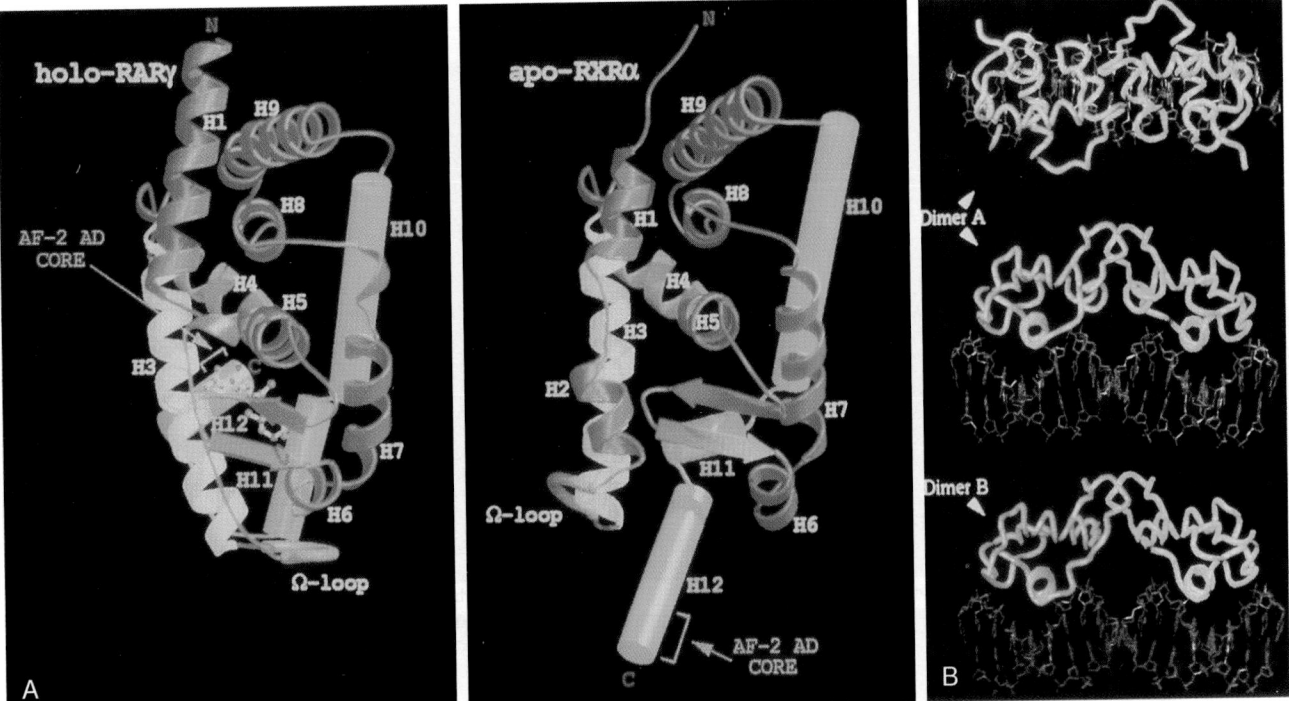

Figure 4–15. *A*, Structure of the ligand-binding domain of RAR bound to its ligand and RXR (without ligand). *B*, Crystal structure of the DNA-binding domain of ER binding to its response element. (*A* reprinted with permission from Renaud JP, Rochel M, Ruff V, et al. Crystal structure of the RAR-gamma ligand-binding domain bound to all-trans retinoic acid. Nature 1995; 378:681–689. Copyright 1995 Macmillan Magazines Ltd. *B* from Schwabe JWR, Chapman L, Finch JT, et al. The crystal structure of the estrogen receptor DNA-binding domain bound to DNA: how receptors discriminate between their response elements. Cell 1993; 75:567–578. Copyright 1993, Cell Press.)

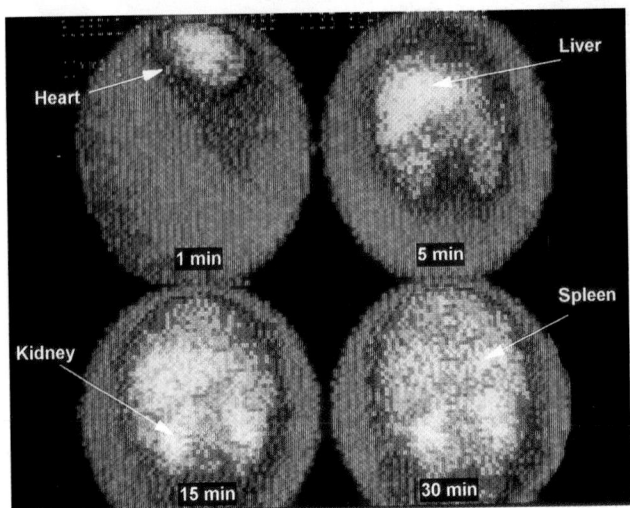

Figure 5–2. Scintiscans obtained 3 min *(upper left)*, 10 min *(upper right)*, 20 min *(lower left)*, and 30 min *(lower right)* after antecubital vein injection of 0.84 mCi of labeled insulin into a normal female volunteer (age 25, weight 63 kg, height 168 cm). Studies of insulin receptors in vivo using ^{131}I-insulin and scintillation scanning.

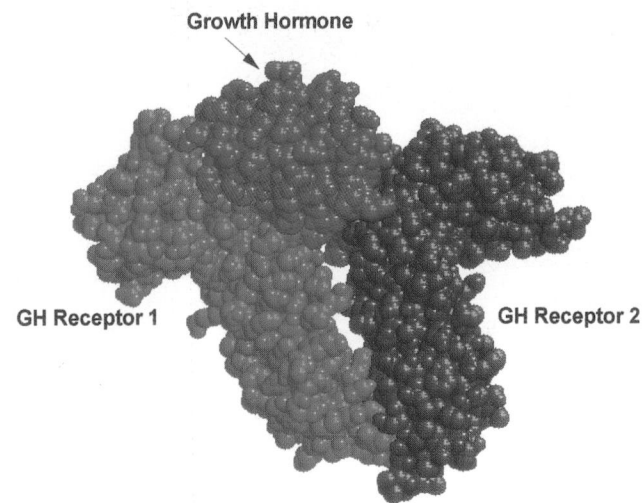

Figure 5–9. *C*, X-ray crystallographic model of a single GH molecule binding to the extracellular domain of two adjacent GH receptors. (Data from Chen D, Van Horn DJ, White MF, et al. Mol Cell Biol 1995; 15:4711–4717.)

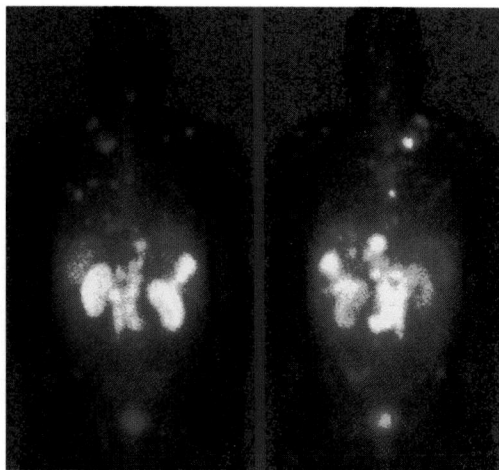

Figure 37–2. Posterior and anterior planar images following the IV injection of 6 mCi ^{111}In pentetreotide in a 53-year-old man with carcinoid syndrome. Areas of increased uptake are noted in the thoracic and abdominal regions, demonstrating metastases in the lymph nodes and liver.

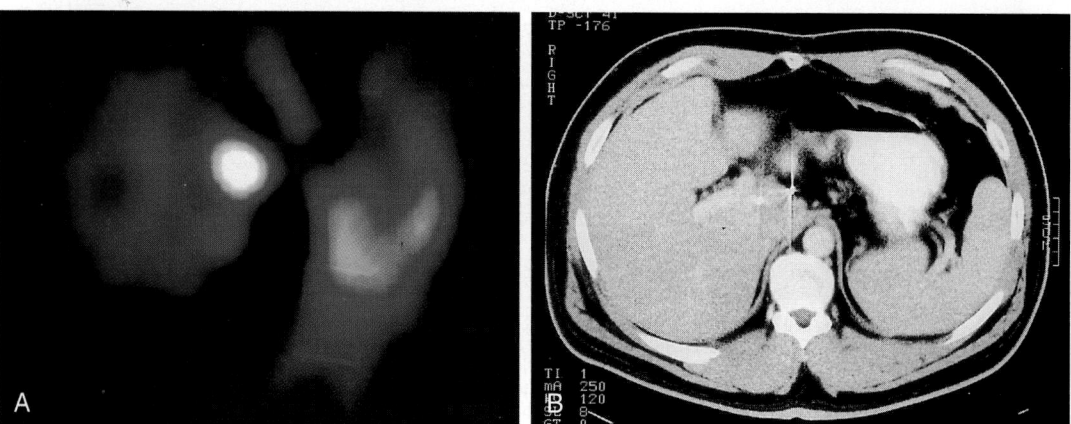

Figure 37–3. [111]In pentetreotide scan A, in a patient with a history of a previously resected midgut carcinoid tumor and negative serial spiral abdominal CT scans and biochemical markers (5-HIAA and chromogranin A). The abdominal CT scan B, was obtained concomitantly with the ^{111}In pentetreotide scan. Laparotomy with partial hepatectomy revealed a single hepatic site of involvement and histologically confirmed the presence of recurrent disease.

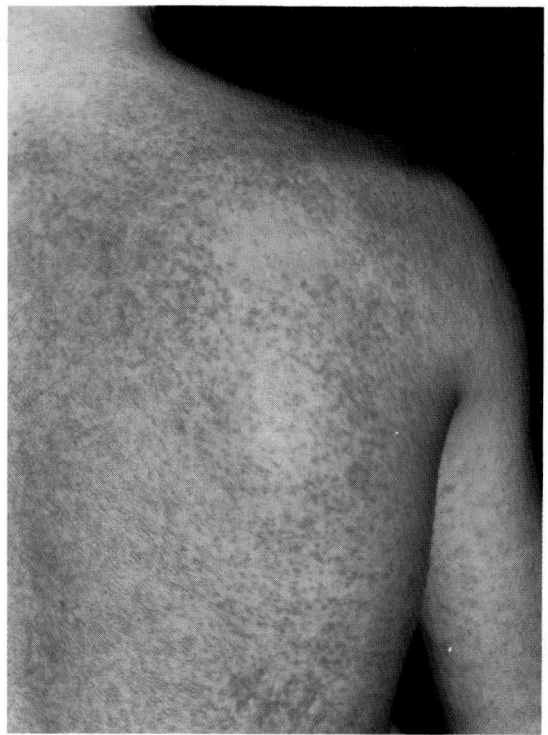

Figure 37–5. Cutaneous lesions of urticaria pigmentosa.

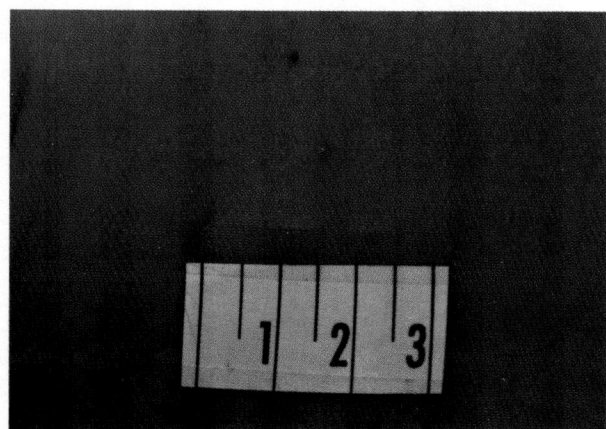

Figure 37–6. Acneiform cutaneous lesions found in some patients with mastocytosis and the syndrome of systemic mast cell activation.

17

ENDOCRINE DISORDERS OF THE BREAST

Andrew G. Frantz and Jean D. Wilson

NORMAL DEVELOPMENT

Fetal Life Through Adolescence

Early in fetal life epithelial cells, derived from the epidermis in the area that will later become the areola, proliferate into the underlying mesenchyme. In the human, 20 or so short cords are formed and eventually develop lumina to become ducts that are connected to the nipple and open to the surface. Surrounding the ducts is a network of myoepithelial cells, destined ultimately to serve in the expulsion of milk. In the later stages of gestation the blind ends of the ducts bud to form alveolar structures, and a small amount of secretory activity occurs.[1-4] This results in the formation of so-called witch's milk, which can be expressed from the breasts of most full-term infants by the fifth to seventh day after birth and which persists for 1 to 7 wk thereafter.[5, 6] Subsequently, with the decline in circulating fetal prolactin and in the absence in the infant of estrogen and progesterone of placental origin, the breast regresses to a resting stage composed of a small number of scattered ducts. Such regression may not be complete until many months after birth.[7]

In several species there is sexual dimorphism in the embryogenesis of the excretory duct system. For example, in the male rodent the excretory ducts regress during the later phases of embryogenesis (as a result of androgen action), and the breast remnant becomes an isolated island in the subcutaneous tissue.[8-11] However, such dimorphism has never been documented in the human embryo, and there does not appear to be any histologic or functional difference in the breasts of girls and boys before the onset of puberty.[12] Shortly before human menarche, with increased secretion of ovarian estrogen, lengthening and branching of the ducts begin in the female breast, accompanied by budding of the terminal ends and increased formation of underlying fat and connective tissue. With the onset of menses, further growth takes place in a cyclic fashion, some regression occurring at the end of each cycle.[13-15]

Pregnancy

During pregnancy the maternal breast is exposed to high levels of estrogen, progesterone, and prolactin (also see Chapter 27). Prolactin increases in concentration steadily throughout gestation, presumably as a consequence of estrogenic stimulation. Levels of human placental lactogen also increase, particularly during the terminal phase. Under these conditions breast growth is stimulated dramatically and is characterized by additional branching of ducts and differentiation of the end buds to form alveoli; the alveoli group in clusters known as lobules. Toward the end of pregnancy, secretory vacuoles are seen within the epithelial cells, and some secretions may be present in the ducts, although actual lactation does not occur until after parturition. The secretions contain many components, including fat, protein (casein, lactalbumin, lactoglobulin), and lactose.[16-21]

HORMONAL REGULATION OF BREAST DEVELOPMENT

Development of the breast involves the coordinated action of many hormones, including prolactin, estrogen, progesterone, glucocorticoids, insulin, growth hormone, and thyroid hormone.[22] In simplified terms, duct growth is promoted by estrogen, alveolar development is controlled by prolactin and progesterone, and lactation is mediated by prolactin. Despite an enormous amount of work, however, the precise roles of each hormone are difficult to delineate because a given hormone, besides acting directly on the breast, may also influence the secretion and activity of other hormones. In vitro findings do not always parallel those in intact animals, and species differences make uncertain the application of some observations to humans, who have been less studied than other species.

Prolactin

Prolactin is critical to breast control.[23, 24] Its importance in all phases of breast development was established by the careful studies of Lyons and co-workers.[25] In hypophysectomized, adrenalectomized, gonadectomized rats, estrogen alone is ineffective in inducing ductal or other mammary growth. If administered together with prolactin and growth hormone, however, or if administered to animals with intact pituitaries, estrogen promotes ductal growth. Estrogen is similarly ineffective in the hypophysectomized goat in the absence of pituitary hormones.[26] In the triply operated rat prolactin causes some ductal and lobuloalveolar growth,[27] but prolactin stimulates epithelial cell proliferation only in the presence of estrogen and fosters lobuloalveolar development only in the presence of progesterone. Prolactin also controls many steps in lactogenesis, including the synthesis of the milk proteins casein and α-lactalbumin. The measurement of these and other secretory products can be used as a specific and quantitative index of prolactin activity both in vitro and in vivo.[17, 28]

Prolactin receptors in mammary tissues appear to increase in number during gestation and after parturition.[24, 29–33] They are also present in certain other tissues such as rat liver.[34] Ovine prolactin increases the level of prolactin receptors in the rabbit mammary gland, and progesterone can block this effect.[35] Prolactin receptors in rat mammary tumors decrease after estrogen treatment.[36] Antibodies to prolactin receptors block prolactin-mediated events such as the incorporation of tritiated leucine into casein.[37] The human prolactin receptor is a protein of 598 amino acids, whereas the prolactin receptor of the rat consists of multiple isoforms.[38] These receptors contain a single transmembrane domain and have about 30% homology with the growth hormone receptor. These two receptors, together with receptors for granulocyte colony-stimulating factor, erythropoietin, macrophage colony-stimulating factor, and some interleukins, constitute a family of single membrane-spanning receptors[38] (see Chapter 5).

Placental lactogen also circulates in large amounts in maternal blood during human pregnancy. Although of slightly less potency than prolactin on a weight basis,[39] human placental lactogen is present at higher levels and therefore must contribute, along with prolactin, to breast growth during pregnancy. However, placental lactogen cannot be essential for lactation, because women with deletions of the genes that encode the hormone can undergo successful pregnancy and lactation.[40]

Estrogen

The role of estrogen in breast physiology is complex. Although a highly potent mammogen, it is ineffective in the absence of anterior pituitary hormones.[25, 26] Administration of estrogen to intact animals promotes the formation of lactotropic cells in the pituitary and increases the secretion of prolactin[39] and growth hormone.[41] In the presence of these two hormones, estrogen acts to promote ductal development in the breast. Although estrogen prepares the breast for eventual milk formation, it also acts to inhibit lactation and in this respect acts as a prolactin antagonist.[42] It is largely because of the high levels of circulating estrogen and progesterone that women do not lactate during pregnancy, and it is the abrupt withdrawal of these two hormones with the termination of pregnancy that triggers the onset of lactation. As noted previously, estrogen also acts to regulate the number of prolactin receptors in breast tissue.

Breast adipocytes, like adipose tissue elsewhere, have the capacity to form estrogens by aromatization of the circulating androgens, androstenedione and testosterone.[43–46] Cortisol, platelet-derived growth factor (PDGF), and basic fibroblast growth factor (bFGF) appear to play roles in the regulation of aromatase activity in human breast tissue.[47] The importance of local estrogen production in breast physiology is unknown.

Estrogen receptors, both cytoplasmic and nuclear, are present in normal and in tumorous breast tissue[48–51] (see Chapter 4). Concentrations of receptor in breast vary with the menstrual cycle[49, 51] and increase during later pregnancy and the first part of lactation. Both estrogen and progesterone are capable of stimulating estrogen receptor synthesis.[52, 53]

Progesterone

Like estrogens, progesterone has no effect on the breast in the absence of anterior pituitary hormones.[25, 26] Even in the presence of prolactin, progesterone may be ineffective unless there is concomitant or preceding estrogen stimulation. Under optimal conditions progesterone acts synergistically with prolactin in promoting lobuloalveolar development.[54] Some actions of progesterone on the breast, like those on the uterus, appear to be antiestrogenic.[55] Like estrogen, progesterone inhibits lactation,[56, 57] but exogenously administered progesterone is less effective than estrogen in stopping lactation once the process is established.[58] Progesterone receptors in breast are regulated primarily by estrogens, although prolactin is probably also involved.[52, 53, 59, 60]

Growth Hormone

Growth hormone appears to synergize with prolactin and may be able to substitute for prolactin in promoting certain aspects of breast growth such as ductal development.[25, 26] Growth hormones from different species possess varying degrees of prolactin-like activity in homologous and heterologous species, human growth hormone (hGH) having strong lactogenic activity. A variant form, hGH-V, which is synthesized in the placenta and increases in concentration in maternal blood as pregnancy progresses,[61, 62] has activity similar to that of pituitary growth hormone but less lactogenic potency.[63] Growth hormone appears to enhance the degree of breast growth in hypophysectomized animals by acting through its own receptor,[64] but many of its actions appear to be mediated through the actions of insulin-like growth factor I (IGF1; see next section). Growth hormone is probably not essential for breast growth in humans, because dwarfs who lack pituitary growth hormone develop breasts and lactate normally after parturition.[65]

Insulin and Insulin-Like Growth Factors

Insulin action is necessary for prolactin to act on breast tissue in vitro, and insulin or IGFs are probably necessary in vivo as well.[17, 66] IGF1, also called somatomedin-C, can mimic most if not all of the effects of insulin on breast tissue.[67] Receptors for insulin and for IGF1 are present in breast tissues.[68–70] The extent to which these two hormones act through their own receptors, as opposed to each other's, is not clear;

the mitogenic action of insulin on long-term cultures of human breast cells may be mediated largely through the IGF1 receptor.[68] In mouse breast tissue in organ culture, IGF1 cannot substitute for the effects of growth hormone,[71] but in hypophysectomized rats some effects of growth hormone may result from local or systemic generation of IGF1.[72]

Other Growth Factors

Epidermal growth factor can stimulate growth of both mammary and pigeon crop-sac epithelia,[73-75] but whether it plays a role in breast growth is unclear.[76] Nicoll and his colleagues have reported that prolactin acts on the liver to stimulate secretion of synlactin, which synergizes with prolactin to enhance growth of mammary epithelium and the pigeon crop sac (similar to the effects of IGF1).[77-79] Another substance that partially mimics the actions of prolactin is present in the livers of lactating rats,[80] and the human pituitary contains a substance, different from prolactin, growth hormone, or other known breast stimulants, that is capable of promoting breast growth in both monkeys and rats.[81] Additional factors, including members of the transforming growth factor β (TGF β) family, appear to stimulate breast growth by local or paracrine mechanisms.[82-84]

Glucocorticoids

Glucocorticoids appear to be necessary for breast growth and secretion in vitro and in vivo.[17] Glucocorticoid receptors are present in lactating mammary tissue.[85] As with insulin, glucocorticoids probably play a permissive rather than a regulatory role.

Thyroid Hormone

Thyroid hormone does not appear to be essential for breast development or lactation, although both processes may be abnormal in states of thyroid hormone deficiency or excess.[4]

LACTATION

Lactation begins when the maternal breast, primed by long exposure to high levels of prolactin, estrogen, and pro-gesterone, is subjected to sudden withdrawal of the latter two hormones. Lactation then continues in an environment of relatively high (declining) prolactin levels and low estrogen and progesterone levels. Suckling provides an essential stimulus for the release of both oxytocin and prolactin.

Oxytocin

Expulsion of milk from the alveoli and ducts, a necessary component of effective lactation, is caused by contraction of the surrounding myoepithelial cells under the influence of oxytocin. The secretion of oxytocin by the posterior pituitary can be enhanced by purely psychological factors, such as anticipation of nursing, or by sensory stimuli arising from the nipple during the act of nursing.[86] Enhanced oxytocin secretion is experienced by the mother as a sensation of milk let-down and as the appearance of milk, sometimes spontaneously ejected at the nipple. Uterine cramps may also occur during nursing. Indeed, in the later stages of pregnancy nipple stimulation can be used to produce uterine contractions as part of a standardized contraction test.[87-90] Oxytocin secretion can be inhibited (with marked impairment of milk yield) by stress and by fright, both of which appear to cause activation of the sympathetic nervous system and release of norepinephrine and epinephrine.

Prolactin

Suckling is a powerful stimulus in women post partum for the release of prolactin. Unlike oxytocin, which is also released by neurogenic impulses transmitted from the nipples by dorsal nerve roots to the hypothalamus, prolactin is not secreted in response to anticipatory psychological stimuli. Oxytocin and prolactin are released independently and one may be liberated without the other (Fig. 17–1).[86, 91, 92] In the first few weeks after delivery, maternal serum prolactin levels are continuously high and undergo further elevation (5- to 10-fold) with each nursing episode. Between 3 and 7 wk after parturition, concentrations of prolactin fall to the normal range between nursing episodes (< 20 to 25 μg/L) most of the time. However, in most women, some rise in prolactin levels continues during each suckling episode for many months (Fig. 17–2). This rise in prolactin levels in response to suckling is probably important in maintaining the breast in the lactating state,[91, 92] but is not demonstrable in all women

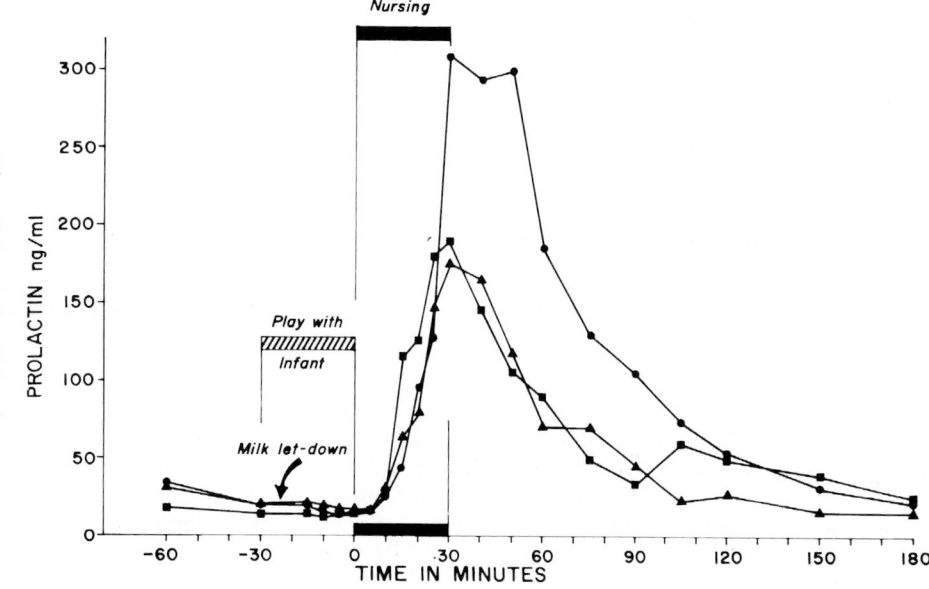

Figure 17–1. Plasma prolactin concentrations during anticipation of nursing and course of nursing in three women 22 to 26 d post partum. The women played with their infants for 30 min before suckling began. Milk let-down, an oxytocin-mediated phenomenon, occurred in each case approximately 25 min before suckling. Prolactin levels did not rise until there was contact with the breast itself. (Noel GL, Suh HK, Frantz AG. Prolactin release during nursing and breast stimulation in postpartum and non-postpartum subjects. J Clin Endocrinol Metab 1974; 38:413–423. Copyright © 1974, by The Endocrine Society.)

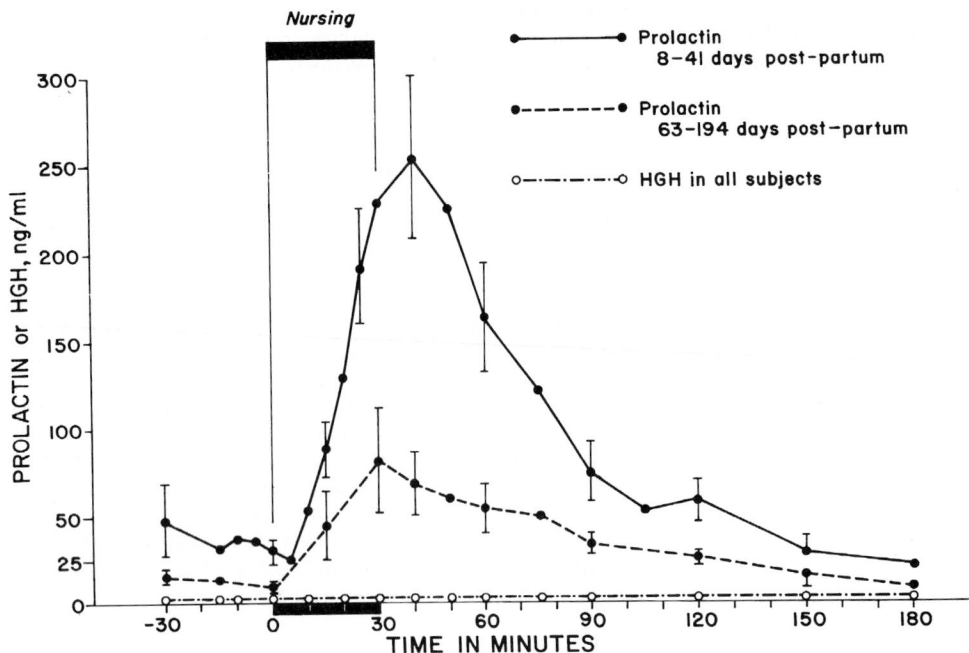

PROLACTIN AND GROWTH HORMONE DURING NURSING
Effect of Time Post-Partum

Figure 17–2. Plasma prolactin and growth hormone concentrations during nursing in postpartum women. Eight women were studied at 8 to 41 d after delivery and six at 63 to 194 d after delivery. Prenursing prolactin levels in the latter group are within the normal range. Plasma growth hormone showed no change in any of the subjects during nursing. (Noel GL, Suh HK, Frantz AG. Prolactin release during nursing and breast stimulation in postpartum and nonpostpartum subjects. J Clin Endocrinol Metab 1974; 38:413–423. Copyright © 1974, by The Endocrine Society.)

who continue to lactate for long periods.[93] Therefore, high levels of prolactin appear to be necessary for the initiation of lactation, but once breast enzyme systems are activated lactation can continue with mean prolactin concentrations that are normal or only modestly elevated. Even at these low levels, however, prolactin is essential for maintenance of lactation, and lactation ceases if prolactin levels are further lowered by dopamine agonists.

Growth Hormone

The facts that the level of growth hormone is low throughout lactation and does not rise with nursing (see Fig. 17–2)[91] and that growth hormone–deficient dwarfs lactate normally suggest that growth hormone does not play a critical role in lactation. Nevertheless, the administration of supplemental hGH to normal nursing mothers enhances milk yields (without changing milk composition).[94] This effect is similar to the enhancement of milk yields in cows after treatment with bovine growth hormone.[95] Growth hormone also stimulates lactation in the rat.[96] Growth hormone may produce these effects by enhancing IGF1 production, by effecting changes in growth hormone binding proteins, or by increasing blood flow to the breast.[97]

Parathyroid Hormone–Related Protein

Parathyroid hormone–related protein (PTH-rP), which has sequence homology with PTH and binds to the PTH receptor, is secreted by a variety of tumors associated with the humoral hypercalcemia of malignancy (see Chapter 24). The hormone is also present in normal tissues, including breast[98] and lactating breast,[99] and in milk.[100, 101] PTH-rP has PTH-like actions and activity resembling that of TGF β.[102] The facts that suckling in the rat increases expression of PTH-rP mRNA,[103] that PTH-rP can be detected in the blood of nursing women but not in controls,[104] and that the concentration of PTH-rP in milk is 10,000 to 100,000 times higher than in blood suggest that the hormone plays a physiological role in lactation, possi-

bly in the mobilization of calcium for milk.[104, 105] Hypercalcemia during pregnancy and lactation correlates with high levels of circulating PTH-rP,[106] and in one instance hypercalcemia of pregnancy associated with elevated PTH-rP levels and massive hyperplasia of the breasts resolved after bilateral mastectomy.[107]

Other Hormones

Thyrotropin, though originally reported to be unaffected by suckling,[108] is in fact increased (along with prolactin and oxytocin) after suckling in the early postpartum period.[86] Thyrotropin-releasing hormone stimulates oxytocin release in vivo[109] and may participate in the release of all three of these pituitary hormones by nursing.

Breast Stimulation in Normal Subjects

Manual stimulation of the breast and nipple causes a twofold or greater increase in prolactin levels in about one third[91] or more[110] of normally menstruating, nonpostpartum women. The factors that separate women who respond from those who do not are unclear, and men consistently have no prolactin response to breast stimulation. The reflex for this type of response appears to be present in latent form in women and is somehow turned on or enhanced by the hormonal events of pregnancy and parturition.

Induction of Lactation in the Absence of Pregnancy

The induction of lactation in nonpostpartum women for the purpose of breast-feeding adopted infants has received little attention in the scientific literature. Anecdotal accounts exist of women, sometimes postmenopausal and usually in primitive tribes, who are able to initiate lactation when placed in contact with an infant to be nursed. Only 13 such instances were documented in the literature between 1900 and 1970.[111] We were unsuccessful in inducing either galactorrhea or any breast engorgement in two normal young women who underwent self-stimulation of the breast for four 30-min periods each day for 2 wk.[91] However, a study by questionnaire of 240 women who had tried adoptive nursing[112] suggests that successful induction of lactation may be more common. After applying breast and nipple stimulation for several weeks beforehand, half of the women were able to induce some breast secretion before the arrival of the infant. This secretion was milky, as opposed to clear or colostrum-like, in 43% of the women who had previously nursed biologic offspring. Milky secretions were obtained in only 14% of those who had never been pregnant and in 12% of those who had had a previous pregnancy but had not nursed previously.[112] The amount of milk obtained after the infant began to nurse regularly was not documented, and all but two of the women supplemented their own milk with external sources during part or all of the nursing period. Eleven percent of the women noted a change in menstrual cycling after initiation of breast-feeding, and 4% reported amenorrhea. Six percent had used hormone preparations of some kind before the infant's arrival, usually an oxytocin nasal spray to enhance milk ejection. No hormone measurements were made. Despite the limitations of this uncontrolled study, the findings emphasize the importance of breast and nipple stimulation in the induction of lactation. The effectiveness of such techniques in inducing lactation would probably be enhanced by pretreatment with estrogen and progesterone designed to simulate the hormonal changes of pregnancy, followed by abrupt withdrawal of these agents.[113]

A course of chlorpromazine or metoclopramide, preceded in some cases by a single intramuscular injection of medroxyprogesterone acetate, was successful in inducing lactation is 24 of 27 nonpueperal women.[114]

Clinical Aspects of Postpartum Lactation

SUPPRESSION OF LACTATION. If a woman does not nurse or empty the breasts post partum, lactation usually stops spontaneously in a week or two, accompanied by involution of much of the recently differentiated lobuloalveolar structure of the breast. Stasis of milk in the ducts and alveoli and a rise in intraductal pressure lead to alveolar rupture and cell death and are major factors in the cessation of lactation, but the mechanisms are not understood in detail.[58] Prolactin levels return promptly to normal, and menses usually resume within 4 to 12 wk (mean, 8 wk), although the menstrual cycle may not return to normal for 6 mo or longer.[115]

In women who do not nurse, there is a variable amount of discomfort during the first week or two post partum that is caused by breast engorgement and can usually be treated by simple measures such as ice packs, a tight binder, and analgesics. To minimize discomfort in women who do not nurse it was previously the practice to administer drugs for the suppression of lactation, such as oral estrogens or a single intramuscular injection during labor of a long-acting estrogen-androgen combination.[58] The hormones are less effective if administered after lactation has begun. Because of the potential toxicity of estrogen therapy, however, the administration of steroids to suppress lactation has greatly declined.[116] For several years bromocriptine, an ergot derivative that suppresses prolactin secretion by virtue of its long-acting dopamine agonist properties, was considered the agent of choice for suppression of lactation.[117, 118] However, in 1995, because of the occurrence of some cases of hypertension, stroke, seizures, and myocardial infarction in persons on bromocriptine, primarily nursing mothers, the manufacturer withdrew the recommendation for its use for suppression of postpartum lactation.[119] It seems inadvisable to use any drugs to suppress lactation in the postpartum period.

FAILURE OF LACTATION. The first endocrine disorder known to be associated with failure of lactation was Sheehan's syndrome (see Chapter 9). This disorder is due to infarction of the pituitary during labor and delivery and may be first manifest by lack of postpartum milk production, presumably because of low circulating prolactin, followed by failure of resumption of menses, sparse regrowth of shaved pubic hair, and development of hypothyroidism or adrenal insufficiency, or both. The pattern of hormone deficiencies in Sheehan's syndrome is variable, and spontaneous amelioration may occur.[120, 121] Lymphocytic hypophysitis, a condition that occurs post partum and mimics Sheehan's syndrome, can also cause hypoprolactinemia and failure of lactation.[90, 122, 123] Hypoprolactinoma also can occur as an isolated hormone deficiency associated with alactogenesis[124] or in association with other pituitary diseases.

Diminished milk production, particularly in mothers of premature infants, has been treated with metoclopramide, an agent that stimulates prolactin release.[125, 126] However, milk production is not a simple function of serum prolactin levels. Many instances of insufficient lactation are believed to be caused by emotional factors, which could operate through noradrenergic pathways to inhibit oxytocin secretion.

LACTATION-ASSOCIATED INFERTILITY. If postpartum nursing is prolonged, amenorrhea usually continues for at least 4 to 6 mo, but menses resume in half of women by 6 mo[127] and in two thirds of women by 9 mo after parturition[115] despite continued lactation. Lactation-associated amenorrhea in the early postpartum period is primarily a result of the inhibition of gonadotropin secretion by hyperprolactinemia. Factors such as the suckling stimulus, which may suppress ovulation independently of prolactin, may also be involved, particularly in the later postpartum period when serum prolactin levels are normal much of the time.[128]

Amenorrhea does not guarantee infertility, and conception can occur post partum without an intervening menstrual period. Therefore, contraception, if desired, should be begun soon after delivery, at least before the fifth week, whether or not the mother nurses her child (see Chapter 18). If oral contraceptives are used in a nursing mother, a low-dose estrogen preparation should be chosen to minimize inhibitory effects on milk yield.[115] Another possible side effect of maternal estrogen use is enlargement of the child's breast because of secretion of the steroid into the milk.[129] In many species other than primates, prolonged lactation is no barrier to rapid resumption of ovulatory cycles. Insemination of domestic cows is frequently undertaken 3 mo or less post partum despite copious lactation, which proceeds, if milking continues, throughout the ensuing gestation.[4]

DISORDERS OF BREASTS IN WOMEN

Galactorrhea

Galactorrhea may be defined as any persistent discharge of milk or milk-like secretions from the breast in the absence of parturition or beyond 6 mo post partum in a non-nursing mother. Formerly regarded as rare, galactorrhea is now often diagnosed, particularly if one includes minimal degrees of secretion that may be evident only by squeezing of the breast. Doubt as to whether the secretion represents milk may be resolved by doing fat stains or, for greater specificity, analysis of specific milk products such as α-lactalbumin, casein, or lactose. Clinically, such tests are rarely necessary. Nonmilky nipple discharges (serous, purulent, sanguineous) are rarely reflective of an endocrine disturbance. Most nonbloody secretions are associated not with malignancy but with fibrocystic disease.[130–134] A careful search for breast nodules should nevertheless be made if such discharges are detected. True galactorrhea is not associated with an increased incidence of cancer.

Causes

Galactorrhea occurs in a wide variety of endocrine disorders and nonendocrine disorders. The largest series (235 patients) reported is that of Kleinberg and colleagues[135]; the discussion in this section is based on this series, the findings of which are in general agreement with those of other observers.[136-138]

GALACTORRHEA WITH PITUITARY TUMORS. The most important diagnostic consideration in galactorrhea is pituitary tumor. Twenty percent of our patients with galactorrhea and 34% of those with both galactorrhea and amenorrhea had pituitary tumors. The true prevalence of tumors is undoubtedly higher than these figures indicate because of failure to detect some small microadenomas before the availability of computed tomographic (CT) scans and magnetic resonance imaging (MRI). The histologic appearance is almost always that of a prolactinoma. A minority of patients have associated acromegaly with elevated levels of both prolactin and growth hormone. As a group, patients with tumors have the highest serum prolactin values (Fig. 17–3), and the likelihood of finding a tumor is proportional to the level of serum prolactin. In our experience all patients with concentrations higher than 300 µg/L have had tumors, and any value higher than 75 to 100 µg/L should be regarded with great suspicion. Of the few patients with tumors who had normal serum prolactin values, all but two had acromegaly or had received treatment for acromegaly. Amenorrhea occurs in more than 80% of patients with galactorrhea and tumors and was the primary complaint in 10% of these patients. Menses, if present, are apt to be abnormal; only 3 of 48 patients with tumors in our series had regular periods.

IDIOPATHIC GALACTORRHEA WITH MENSES. The largest category of patients with galactorrhea are those with regular menses and no associated endocrine disease. Galactorrhea is often overlooked because patients may not think it worth reporting. In more than half of patients the galactorrhea represents a residue of postpartum lactation that has never altogether disappeared despite resumption of menses. Most of these patients have prolactin levels within the normal range (see Fig. 17–3), and fertility is usually normal. In these women the abnormality probably is not primarily hormonal but rather an excessive sensitivity of the breast to normal levels of circulating prolactin. From a clinical standpoint, the combination of regular menses and normal serum prolactin is strong evidence against the presence of pituitary tumor. It is probably unnecessary to do MRI or CT scans in these patients, although the serum prolactin level should be redetermined on one or more occasions.

IDIOPATHIC GALACTORRHEA WITH AMENORRHEA. A minority of women with galactorrhea have associated amenorrhea, no history of drug ingestion, and a normal sella turcica by conventional radiographs. Most such women have hyperprolactinemia (see Fig. 17–3). Many have small sellar abnormalities on MRI or CT scans. In the absence of definitive radiographic changes, the likelihood of a pituitary tumor increases directly with the level of the serum prolactin. It is probable that the hyperprolactinemia causes the amenorrhea, because any treatment that lowers prolactin to near or within the normal range is likely to restore menses. Possible mechanisms of amenorrhea include interference by prolactin at the hypothalamic level with the release of luteinizing hormone–releasing hormone (LHRH), alteration of pituitary sensitivity to the action of LHRH, and interference with gonadotropin action at the ovarian level. Defective production of LHRH appears to be the predominant factor.[139, 140]

CHIARI-FROMMEL SYNDROME. The so-called Chiari-Frommel syndrome is defined as galactorrhea and amenorrhea persisting more than 6 mo post partum in the absence of nursing and without evident pituitary tumor. Some of these patients probably harbor occult microadenomas that later may become radiologically evident, but in about half menses return

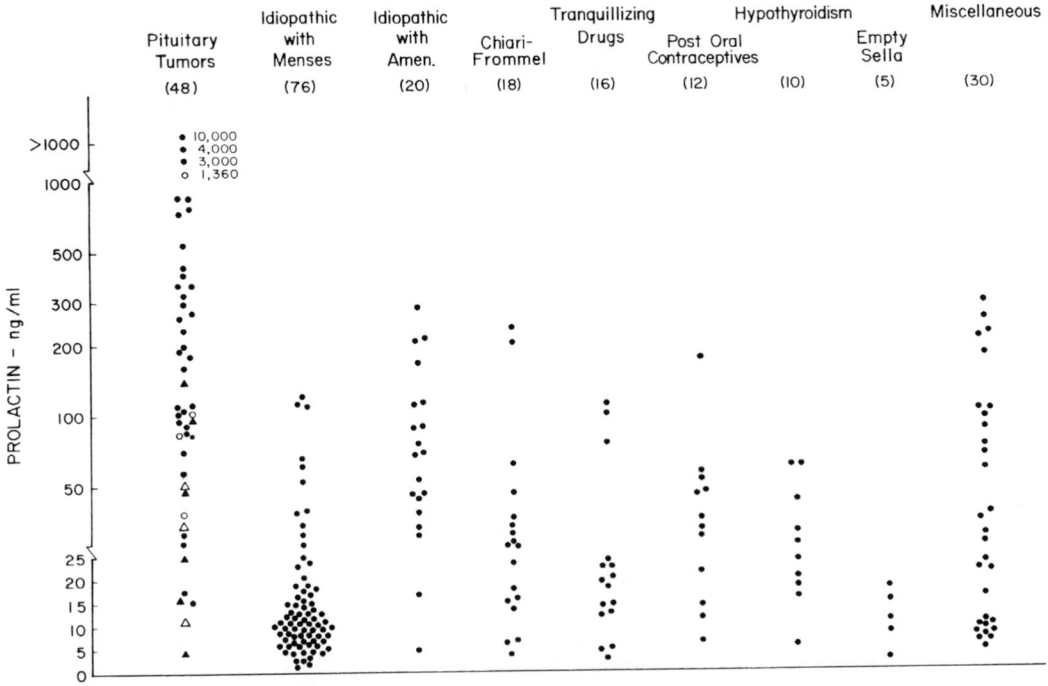

Figure 17–3. Plasma prolactin in 235 patients with galactorrhea of varying causes. Among the patients with tumor, triangles denote patients with acromegaly. Open circles or triangles denote patients studied only after radiotherapy or surgical resection. Normal female levels of prolactin are considered to be less than 25 ng/mL. (Kleinberg DL, Noel GL, Frantz AG. Galactorrhea: a study of 235 cases including 48 with pituitary tumors. Reprinted by permission of the New England Journal of Medicine, 296;589–600, 1977.)

over a period of months or years.[135] The serum prolactin level is elevated in some but not all patients (see Fig. 17–3).

POST–ORAL CONTRACEPTIVE GALACTORRHEA. Galactorrhea is less common after discontinuation of oral contraceptives than is amenorrhea, with which it is usually associated. Both sequelae are relatively infrequent. As with the Chiari-Frommel syndrome, some patients eventually develop radiologically evident tumors. As in the postpartum state, milk production in this syndrome is triggered by the withdrawal of estrogen and progesterone after a period of stimulation by these hormones (and also in part by estrogen-enhanced prolactin secretion).

HYPOTHYROIDISM. Galactorrhea is a rare accompaniment of primary hypothyroidism both in children in whom it may be associated with precocious puberty[141] (see Chapter 22) and in adults.[142] Among adults with primary hypothyroidism, prolactin levels are usually within the normal range or only slightly elevated (see Fig. 17–3).[135, 143, 144] Enlargement of the sella turcica may occur in primary hypothyroidism, and if hyperprolactinemia is present the condition may mimic a prolactinoma.[145] Administration of thyroid hormone lowers the prolactin somewhat and usually stops the galactorrhea. In children thyroid hormone may also cause precocious menses to cease until the normal time of menarche. The underlying mechanisms may involve complex alterations of prolactin and gonadotropin production and degradation or changes in breast tissue sensitivity. Administration of thyroid hormone to euthyroid patients with other forms of galactorrhea does not stop milk production.[146]

THYROTOXICOSIS. Galactorrhea was present in a high percentage of women with thyrotoxicosis in one report.[147] The serum prolactin level was normal in all women, and the mechanisms are obscure.

DRUG ADMINISTRATION. Galactorrhea is associated with a wide variety of drugs that raise serum prolactin levels,[135–137] including phenothiazines, butyrophenones, reserpine, methyldopa, tricyclic antidepressants, estrogens, opiates, metoclopramide, verapamil,[148] cimetidine,[149] and cocaine.[150] Many of these appear to act as antidopaminergic agents, decreasing dopamine-mediated inhibition of prolactin secretion at the level of the pituitary or hypothalamus, or both.

MAJOR SURGERY AND DISORDERS OF THE CHEST WALL. Galactorrhea occurs occasionally after major surgery such as cholecystectomy, and its likelihood may be greater after oophorectomy.[135] Presumably, the mechanisms involve in part the acute release of prolactin[151] plus the effect of acute estrogen withdrawal when the ovaries are removed. Galactorrhea also occurs in diseases affecting the chest wall, such as herpes zoster, after thoracotomy,[111, 152] and occasionally after augmentation mammoplasty.[153] This has led to speculation that increased prolactin secretion can result from stimulation of nerves originating in the breast and areola; however, sustained hyperprolactinemia does not occur in all patients after chest wall surgery, and it is not clear that galactorrhea is more likely after thoracotomy than after other major surgical procedures.[152]

MISCELLANEOUS. Conditions occasionally associated with galactorrhea include various hypothalamic and pituitary diseases (sarcoidosis, Schüller-Christian disease, craniopharyngioma, Cushing's disease, and head trauma) in which alteration of normal hypothalamic-pituitary connections may lead to reduced hypothalamic inhibition and consequent hyperprolactinemia. Refeeding after starvation can also cause galactorrhea.[135] Hyperprolactinemia, with or without accompanying galactorrhea, is present in some patients with renal failure[154] and hepatic cirrhosis.[155] Self-manipulation of the breasts in an attempt to reduce gynecomastia has been associated with galactorrhea in adolescent boys.[156]

Role of Prolactin in Galactorrhea

Serum prolactin concentrations were within the normal range in 46% of our patients. Therefore galactorrhea can be present without hyperprolactinemia. Likewise, hyperprolactinemia can exist without galactorrhea. In the latter case the absence of galactorrhea may result from inadequacy of estrogenic and progestational priming (as in most men) or lack of a suitable triggering event involving estrogen withdrawal (oophorectomy, abortion, cessation of estrogen, or oral contraceptive medication). In many cases of galactorrhea, however, no triggering event is evident from the history. In patients with galactorrhea and normal serum prolactin levels, an earlier transient period of hyperprolactinemia may have existed at the time of onset of the galactorrhea, analogous to the situation in nursing mothers in whom milk secretion, once established, can continue for many months with what appear to be normal prolactin levels. Galactorrhea remains prolactin-dependent, however, because lowering of serum prolactin concentrations with dopamine agonists usually stops the galactorrhea. In summary, although prolactin is essential for milk production, the serum levels of the hormone do not correlate with the magnitude of milk production in patients with galactorrhea.

Clinical Considerations in Galactorrhea

DIAGNOSIS. A careful history is essential, with attention to menses, drug ingestion, and symptoms suggestive of pituitary or hypothalamic disease (e.g., headaches; visual disturbances; abnormalities of temperature, thirst, or appetite regulation), thyroid disease, or adrenal dysfunction. Visual fields should be assessed, and evidence of endocrine disease should be sought, such as abnormal skin texture, pigmentation, or hirsutism and signs of acromegaly, hypothyroidism, Cushing's syndrome, or hyperthyroidism. The breast should be examined for nodules and gently but firmly compressed by the physician or patient to assess the degree of galactorrhea. Serum prolactin and serum gonadotropin levels should be measured in patients with amenorrhea. Thyroid function should be assessed, but other hormonal assays, e.g., for growth hormone and adrenal steroids, are not necessary in the absence of specific indications. MRI or CT scans should be performed if the serum prolactin level is even slightly elevated or if there are other signs suggestive of a pituitary tumor; such scans are not mandatory in cases of minimal galactorrhea if the serum prolactin value is within the normal range and menses are regular. Prolactin stimulation and suppression tests, involving the assessment of response to such agents as levodopa, phenothiazines, thyrotropin-releasing hormone, and metoclopramide, are too variable in their results to be useful.[157] The diagnosis of pituitary tumor rests essentially on the results of the serum prolactin determination and on radiographic evidence.[158]

TREATMENT. In most cases the galactorrhea does not require treatment for its own sake. If fertility is not desired and if there is no evidence of pituitary tumor, treatment for elevated prolactin alone is not necessary, because there is no evidence that prolonged hyperprolactinemia in the absence of associated amenorrhea is deleterious. If amenorrhea accompanies hyperprolactinemia, as is often the case, then patients are at increased risk for development of osteoporosis[159–162] (see Chapters 15 and 25). Although hypoestrogenism undoubtedly accounts for most of the increased risk of osteoporosis in such patients, hyperprolactinemia itself may contribute independently.[160] Such observations provide a rationale for treating hyperprolactinemia in amenorrheic women, but to date the effects that lowering prolactin levels have on bone mineral content are not wholly clear.[160, 162, 163] The rate of bone loss in hyperprolactinemic subjects may be affected by factors in addition to estrogen status.[164-166]

If MRI or CT scanning discloses the presence of a pituitary tumor but fertility is not desired, the choice of therapy depends chiefly on the size of the tumor (see Chapter 9). If the tumor is a microadenoma, i.e., less than 1 cm in diameter, and if the risks of osteoporosis do not appear to necessitate treatment, it may be appropriate to observe such patients without specific therapy. Most of these tumors do not progress to macroadenomas.[167-169] Furthermore, a gradual reduction of serum prolactin may take place over a period of years, sometimes accompanied by spontaneous resumption of menses and cessation of galactorrhea.[168] The serum prolactin level should be assessed at 6- to 12-mo intervals, with MRI or CT scanning performed less frequently (e.g., at 2- to 5-y intervals). For macroadenomas some form of therapy—surgery, radiotherapy, or prolactin-lowering pharmacotherapy—is usually considered advisable to prevent further growth and to shrink the tumor if local pressure symptoms (e.g., visual field defects) are present.

Transsphenoidal surgery in experienced hands is a safe procedure, with mortality rates averaging 0.9% for macroadenomas and 0.27% for microadenomas.[170] Return of the serum prolactin level to normal after surgery depends both on the initial level of serum prolactin and on the size of the tumor. With initial serum prolactin values of less than 200 to 250 µg/L and with microadenomas, the immediate postoperative cure rates may be as high as 83 to 86%; with higher serum prolactin values and macroadenomas generally, the cure rate is less than 50%.[170-174] Enthusiasm for surgery as primary therapy for prolactinomas has declined because recurrence rates in patients originally considered cured are higher than originally anticipated.[174-181] These recurrence rates range from 17%[175, 176] to 91%[179] after several years.

Radiotherapy alone is usually effective in arresting tumor growth and shrinking existing tumors and is followed by a progressive decrease in serum prolactin levels over a period of many years.[182-184] Because of the slowness of the decline in prolactin levels, the availability of drug therapy, and the possibility of inducing late-developing hypopituitarism (which has ranged from 13%[184] to 100%[183]), radiotherapy is usually reserved as an adjunct to surgical treatment of larger tumors or for use in patients considered unacceptable risks for surgery. With either surgery or radiotherapy, restoration of menses and cessation of galactorrhea require that the serum prolactin level be lowered to near or within the normal range.

The dopamine agonists such as bromocriptine are more effective than other forms of treatment in lowering serum prolactin, stopping galactorrhea, and restoring ovulatory menses in patients with hyperprolactinemia, whether related to tumor or other causes.[117, 135, 185] The usual dose of bromocriptine is 2.5 mg/d for 1 wk, increased to 2.5 mg twice or three times a day thereafter. Initial nausea is experienced by many patients but usually disappears with time. Postural hypotension and nasal stuffiness may occur. In most cases hyperprolactinemia and the associated abnormalities recur after the agent is withdrawn. Complications related to tumor growth during pregnancy are comparatively few and are easily managed.[186, 187]

In addition to lowering serum prolactin levels, ergot derivatives shrink prolactin-secreting pituitary tumors. Pergolide is as effective as bromocriptine both for tumor shrinkage and lowering of serum prolactin and requires only once-daily therapy.[188, 189] Although tumor shrinkage has approached 100% in some series of patients treated with dopamine agonists,[190] a meta-analysis of several published series indicated that some degree of shrinkage occurs in 89% and that 79% experience reduction in tumor volume of more than 25%.[191] Tumor shrinkage can be rapid, beginning within hours or days after administration of bromocriptine. The degree of tumor shrinkage does not correlate with serum prolactin re-

duction. Rarely, tumor growth may occur despite continued prolactin suppression.[192] The serum prolactin level remains suppressed as long as ergot drugs are given but usually rises after they are stopped. With continued therapy (2 y or more) dose reduction may be possible,[193] and the serum prolactin level may not rise fully to its original levels on withdrawal of the drug. Some degree of tumor re-expansion must also be anticipated after withdrawal of ergot drugs, but this may not occur for many months if therapy has been prolonged.[190, 194-197]

Despite the need for indefinite treatment, the success of these agents in lowering serum prolactin values and shrinking tumors has led to their use as first-line therapy instead of surgery for macroadenomas.[190] A long-acting injectable form of bromocriptine may have particular advantages in achieving rapid results with tumors.[198-202] Cabergoline, an oral derivative with long duration of action, has been effective in preliminary trials,[203] and a nonergot dopamine agonist is effective in some patients who are resistant to bromocriptine.[204-207] Dopamine agonists may on occasion effect dramatic size reductions in some giant invasive prolactinomas.[188, 208] Short-term therapy with these agents may also be useful before surgery to shrink the tumor and thereby facilitate transsphenoidal resection.[209]

Hypoplasia

Hypoplasia or aplasia of the breast caused by delayed or absent sexual maturation, as in gonadal dysgenesis, usually responds to cyclic estrogen-progesterone therapy. The same is true of the breast atrophy that follows premature menopause. Occasionally, partial or total failure of breast development, sometimes only one-sided,[210] occurs in women with regular menses and who appear to be endocrinologically normal. Hypomastia is linked in some cases with mitral valve prolapse.[211] The problem in hypomastia may be either a deficiency of breast tissue related to a developmental defect or an insensitivity of breast tissue to normal hormonal stimulation. Estrogen or other hormone therapy should not be used to augment breast size in these patients. Estrogens are unlikely to have any significant effect in doses close to the physiological range, and the pharmacologic doses that could conceivably produce slight improvement carry unacceptable risks. If treatment appears necessary for psychological reasons, mammoplasty is indicated.[210, 212]

Macromastia

Macromastia, usually defined as massive breast enlargement in women, is an uncommon but unsolved problem.[213] As is the case with breast enlargement in men, breast enlargement in women is compounded by problems of definition. To separate macromastia from cases of moderate or minimal breast enlargement, the usual practice is to limit the diagnosis to women in whom the weight bearing itself is uncomfortable or in whom stretching of the overlying skin causes ulceration. If the variant associated with extreme obesity is excluded, the disorder is most commonly classified into three types: pubertal macromastia (approximately 83%), macromastia during pregnancy (about 13%), and macromastia in adult women in whom no initiating cause is identified (about 4%).[214] In addition, the disorder may be associated with penicillamine therapy. In each of these variants the enlargement can be grossly asymmetrical and can be associated with simultaneous development of ancillary breast masses in the axillae.

Macromastia of puberty can commence before or after the onset of menses, may recur after reduction mammoplasty has reduced the size of the breasts by 3 to 8 kg of weight, and may on occasion be associated with hypothyroidism.[215-219] When associated with pregnancy, macromastia usually has its onset in the first or second trimester; it may begin during the first pregnancy or after uneventful previous pregnancies. It may subside minimally or completely after termination of pregnancy and may worsen with subsequent pregnancies.[220–229] Hypercalcemia has been reported in association with pregnancy-related macromastia, apparently as a result of the formation of PTH-rP by the breast tissue.[107] Penicillamine-induced macromastia has been reported in several women between the ages of 25 and 45 years who were receiving relatively modest amounts of the drug, and it may not regress after the drug is discontinued.[230–235]

On biopsy, the histologic characteristics of the breast tissue in all these various disorders are appropriate for the physiological state. Hormonal studies in women with macromastia are usually unremarkable, including normal levels of gonadal steroids, plasma prolactin, and placental lactogen.[233] It is assumed that the disorder results from some type of enhanced end-organ response to physiological amounts of hormone.

Reduction mammoplasty is the most common treatment,[236, 237] but recurrence may make total mastectomy necessary.[218, 228, 238] Various empirical therapies have been tried, including bromocriptine,[227, 229] tamoxifen,[217, 227, 228] dydrogesterone,[213, 219, 228] medroxyprogesterone,[217] and danazol,[233–235] but the experience is too small to allow assessment of efficacy with any of these agents.

Mastalgia

Many women complain at times of pain in the breast.[239–241] In the large series studied by Preece and colleagues,[239] the pain was commonly diffuse and subject to cyclic premenstrual induction or exacerbation. A smaller group had localized pain ascribed to ductal ectasia and periductal mastitis. Tietze's syndrome, trauma, and cancer were diagnoses in a smaller number of cases. The response to placebo therapy among these patients tends to be so high that careful double-blind studies are necessary to document the effect of hormonal or other therapy. Evening primrose oil, a plant extract with few side effects, and bromocriptine were about equally effective, and both were more effective than placebo in relieving pain in patients with cyclic, as opposed to noncyclic, mastalgia.[242] Danazol, an antigonadotropic agent, is more effective than either of these drugs.[242–244] In view of the menstrual irregularities, weight gain, and occasional androgenic effects that may occur with danazol, however, this drug should be used, if at all, only in severe cases after other measures have failed and then only for short periods.[245] Tamoxifen, an antiestrogen, may be as effective as danazol with fewer side effects, although its use is still experimental.[246] Because of the chronicity of symptoms and the likely need for long-term therapy, any hormonal treatment should be undertaken with caution.[247]

DISORDERS OF BREASTS IN MEN

Gynecomastia

Clinical Features

The consideration of gynecomastia is complicated by formidable problems of definition. The general view has been that any palpable breast tissue in men is abnormal except for three situations: the transient gynecomastia of the newborn, the breast enlargement at puberty in boys, and the gynecomastia that occasionally occurs in elderly men.[248] However, this view has been challenged by Nuttall and his colleagues, who reported that 36% of normal men between the ages of 17 and 80 years have palpable breast tissue and that the overall prevalence in hospitalized men is 65%.[249, 250] In another study

Ley and colleagues reported a prevalence of 34% in normal men.[251]

A confounding problem in the ascertainment of gynecomastia is that it may be difficult to distinguish true enlargement of breast tissue from lipomastia, in which the enlargement is caused by adipose tissue.[252] The false-positive rate for the estimation of gynecomastia by physical examination has never been established by performance of biopsies for all subjects.[253] Differentiating gynecomastia from lipomastia is particularly difficult in overweight men, and in this regard it is important to remember that the bulk of breast tissue in normal women and in most men is adipose tissue. The endocrine cause (or causes) for the local proliferation of adipose tissue in the breasts has never been defined, and most work on the endocrine control of the tissue has focused on breast tissue per se.

The available pathologic data are not of much help in establishing the true prevalence of gynecomastia. In three large unselected autopsy series the incidence of active gynecomastia (epithelial hyperplasia and periductal stromal hyperplasia) was 9%,[248] 7%,[254] and 5%[255]; in these reports gynecomastia was most common in the young and the elderly. Evidence of inactive or burned-out gynecomastia was more common, 32%[248] and 48%.[254] The autopsy data do not provide insight into what fraction of gynecomastia—active or inactive—is theoretically palpable. In summary, major uncertainties exist. Although it was previously believed that gynecomastia (in contrast to lipomastia) may be unusual, gynecomastia may be so common as to be a normal variant in the absence of an obvious underlying endocrinopathy. It is also possible that an increase in the prevalence of gynecomastia may have occurred in the recent past related to some unrecognized cause. True gynecomastia can be separated from lipomastia by mammography[256, 257] or by sonography.[258, 259]

For the purposes of this discussion, we shall assume that any palpable breast tissue in men (other than in the three so-called physiological states) may be indicative of an underlying endocrinopathy and deserves at least a limited evaluation.

Histopathology and Etiology

Gross asymmetry in the development of gynecomastia is frequent; furthermore, unilateral gynecomastia may be a temporary phenomenon in that one breast may enlarge or become painful for years or months before the other. The histologic features of gynecomastia have been studied in detail in subjects with diethylstilbestrol-induced breast enlargement, but the histology in all forms of gynecomastia correlates better with the duration rather than with the cause, suggesting a common pathogenesis.[260–262] Initially, the disorder is characterized by proliferation of the fibroblastic stroma and of the duct system, which elongates, buds, and duplicates. In gynecomastia of longer duration (even when the stimulation is continued, as in prolonged diethylstilbestrol therapy), progressive fibrosis and hyalinization occur in association with regression of epithelial proliferation. Eventually, the ducts decrease in number. Mononuclear cell infiltration is common.

On correction of the cause, resolution occurs by reduction in size and cell content of the ductular epithelia followed by gradual disappearance of the ducts, leaving hyaline bands that may eventually disappear. However, if the gynecomastia is of long duration, fibrosis and hyalinization may be so extensive that complete resolution never occurs even after the underlying cause is corrected.

Because estradiol is a normal male hormone, because estradiol is a growth hormone for the breast in women, and because the administration of diethylstilbestrol and other estrogens to men causes breast enlargement that is histologically indistinguishable from other forms of gynecomastia, gynecomastia has generally been viewed as a disturbance of estrogen physiology.

Lewin was apparently the first to suggest that all gynecomastia is caused either by increased estrogen secretion or by a decreased androgen/estrogen ratio,[263] a formulation that has been further developed by Gabrilove[264] and has been used in some[265-267] but not all[268] subsequent attempts to classify the causes of gynecomastia.

Estrogen Production in Men

A basic knowledge of androgen physiology is essential to understanding estrogen physiology in normal men (see Chapter 16). In brief, testosterone secretion by the Leydig cells of the testis is regulated largely by luteinizing hormone (LH) from the pituitary. Follicle-stimulating hormone (FSH) may augment testosterone secretion, possibly by regulating the number of LH receptors on the plasma membrane of the Leydig cells. Testosterone feeds back on the pituitary to alter the sensitivity of the gland to the hypothalamic LHRH. The molecular mechanism by which testosterone regulates LH production is thought (on the basis of studies of subjects with single gene defects that impair the function of the androgen receptor) to be identical to that by which the hormone acts in other target cells: androgen combines with a specific cytoplasmic receptor protein to form a hormone-receptor complex that activates specific genes within the nuclei of target cells.

Plasma testosterone serves as a circulating precursor or prohormone for the formation of two other types of active hormones, which in turn mediate many of the physiological processes involved in androgen action.[269] Testosterone can undergo 5α-reduction to dihydrotestosterone, which performs many of the differentiative, growth, and functional actions involved in male sexual differentiation and virilization. Alternatively, circulating androgens can be converted (aromatized) in extraglandular tissues of both sexes to estrogens. The physiological consequences of testosterone represent the combined effects of testosterone plus estrogen and dihydrotestosterone. The two active androgens (testosterone and dihydrotestosterone) are responsible for virilization of the male. The potent estrogen (estradiol) acts in the male to effect closure of the epiphyses,[270, 271] enhances the secretion of growth hormone at male puberty,[272] mediates the inhibition of gonadotropin secretion in the pituitary by testosterone,[273, 274] and may regulate the levels of high-density lipoproteins in men.[275] There is no naturally occurring syndrome of androgen excess in men, but estrogen in excess acts principally in opposition to androgen to feminize.

Urinary production rates for the estrogens estrone and estradiol average about 220 and 160 nmol/d (60 and 45 µg/d) in normal men (Fig. 17–4). Therefore, under ordinary circumstances, men produce approximately 100 times more testosterone than estradiol. All of estrone and about 85% of estradiol production can be accounted for by formation from androstenedione and testosterone in extraglandular sites. However, about 22 nmol (6 µg) of estradiol is normally secreted directly into the circulation by the testes each day.[276, 277] When pharmacologic amounts of human chorionic gonadotropin (hCG) are administered to normal men, however, direct secretion of estradiol by the testis increases in proportion to the enhancement of testosterone secretion.[278] This phenomenon explains why estradiol secretion by the testis is usually elevated when the plasma LH level is increased (as in Klinefelter's syndrome, testicular feminization, or chronic hCG administration). In brief, testicular secretion of estradiol is of minor significance in the normal man but may be profound in pathological states. Within the testes, estrogen is

formed principally within Leydig cells but also by Sertoli cells.[279] Extraglandular estrogen formation from testosterone and androstenedione occurs in many tissues, including the breast itself,[280] and it is possible that locally formed estrogen may act by autocrine/paracrine mechanisms within the breast to promote growth. Whether derived from the plasma or synthesized locally, estradiol exerts its growth-promoting properties in the breast and other estrogen target tissues through the same high-affinity receptor protein that binds the hormone to the nuclear acceptor sites in other estrogen target tissues[281-284] (see Chapters 4 and 35). Despite abundant indirect evidence that gynecomastia is a disorder of relative or absolute estrogen excess, plasma estrogen levels correlate poorly with feminizing states in men. This is almost certainly because conventional estadiol assays are not sensitive enough to measure normal male plasma levels accurately. Development of an ultrasensitive (100 times more sensitive) bioassay[285] will make it possible to re-examine the relation between plasma estradiol and gynecomastia.

Classification of Gynecomastia (Table 17–1)

PHYSIOLOGICAL GYNECOMASTIA

During three phases of male life, breast enlargement can be regarded as a physiological rather than a pathological event.

GYNECOMASTIA IN THE NEWBORN. The enlargement of the neonatal breast that is present in many normal newborns probably results from the action of maternal and/or placental estrogens. The swelling may or may not be associated with witch's milk (see previous discussion), and it ordinarily

---

TABLE 17–1. Classification of Endocrine Gynecomastia

Physiological Gynecomastia

Gynecomastia in the newborn
Adolescent gynecomastia
Gynecomastia of aging

Pathologic Gynecomastia

Testosterone deficiency
  Congenital defects
    Congenital anorchia
    Klinefelter's syndrome
    Androgen resistance (testicular feminization and Reifenstein's syndrome)
    Defects in testosterone synthesis
  Secondary testicular failure (viral orchitis, trauma, castration, neurologic and granulomatous diseases, renal failure)
Increased estrogen production
  Increased testicular estrogen secretion
    Testicular tumors
    Bronchogenic carcinoma and other tumors producing hCG
    True hermaphroditism
  Increased substrate for extraglandular aromatase
    Adrenal disease
    Liver disease
    Starvation
    Thyrotoxicosis
  Increase in extraglandular aromatase
Drugs
  Estrogens or drugs that act like estrogens (diethylstilbestrol, estrogen-containing cosmetics, birth control pills, digitalis, estrogen-contaminated foods, phytoestrogens)
  Drugs that enhance endogenous estrogen formation (gonadotropins, clomiphene)
  Drugs that inhibit testosterone synthesis and/or action (ketoconazole, metronidazole, cimetidine, etomidate, alkylating agents, cisplatin, flutamide, spironolactone)
  Drugs that act by unknown mechanisms (busulfan, isoniazid, methyldopa, calcium channel–blocking agents, captopril, tricyclic antidepressants, penicillamine, diazepam, marijuana, heroin)

Idiopathic Gynecomastia

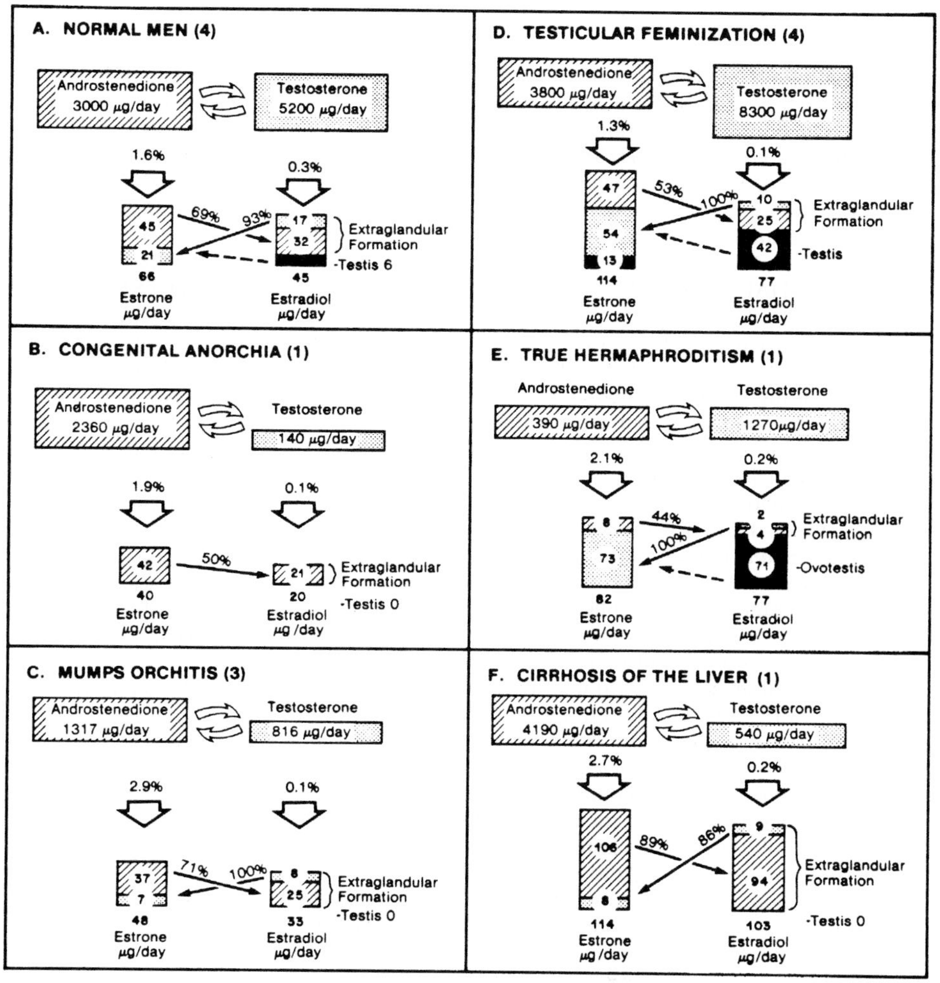

Figure 17–4. Dynamics of androgen and estrogen production in normal men and in patients with gynecomastia. Average production rates of androgen are indicated in upper boxes, and production rates of estrogen are shown at bottom of each vertical bar. The extent of conversion of plasma testosterone and androstenedione to estradiol and estrone is shown by vertical arrows, and interconversions of estradiol and estrone and of testosterone and androstenedione are indicated by horizontal arrows. Sources of estradiol and estrone are indicated by vertical bars. Black bars indicate estrogen secreted directly by the testis. Estradiol arises from plasma testosterone, from estrone, and from direct secretion by the testis; estrone arises from plasma androstenedione, from estradiol, and in some instances from direct secretion by the testis. (A and D, data from MacDonald PC, et al. J Clin Endocrinol Metab 1979; 49:905–916; B, data from Edman CD, et al. Obstet Gynecol 1977; 49:209–217; C, data from Aiman J, et al. J Clin Endocrinol Metab 1980; 50:380–386; E, data from Aiman J, et al. Am J Obstet Gynecol 1978; 132:401–409; F, data courtesy of Dr. C. D. Edman.)

disappears in a few weeks, although it may persist longer in exceptional cases.[286]

ADOLESCENT GYNECOMASTIA. Transient enlargement of the breast is a normal occurrence in male adolescence. Of 1855 adolescent boys of different ages examined at one Boy Scout camp, 39% had gynecomastia,[287] whereas in another population survey the condition was somewhat less common.[288] The median age at onset is 14 years. In many boys the breasts are grossly asymmetrical and may be tender. By age 20 only a small number of men have palpable vestiges of gynecomastia in one or both breasts. The most severe form of this disorder, termed pubertal macromastia, may persist to adulthood.[289] This is almost certainly a pathological subset of adolescent gynecomastia and may be caused by partial abnormalities in the 17β-hydroxysteroid dehydrogenase system.[290]

The cause of ordinary pubertal breast enlargement is uncertain. In boys the plasma estradiol value reaches the adult level before the adult level of plasma testosterone is attained.[291, 292] Furthermore, average plasma estradiol levels have been reported to be slightly higher in boys with gynecomastia.[293] As a result, in boys with pubertal gynecomastia the plasma ratios of testosterone to estradiol[294] and of adrenal androgens to estrone[295] tend to be low. This is presumably because the aromatase in the testis completes maturation before testosterone synthesis reaches the adult level or because extraglandular aromatase matures and converts adrenal androgen (androstenedione) efficiently to estrogen before testosterone formation by the testes reaches its maximum. In either case the ratio of estrogen (formed in the testes or in

extraglandular tissues) to testosterone is temporarily high.[276] Local formation of estrogen within the breast may also play a role in the gynecomastia of puberty.[296]

GYNECOMASTIA OF AGING. The fact that gynecomastia may occur in otherwise healthy elderly men has been known for many years; because gynecomastia can also be an indication of underlying pathology, the diagnosis of involutional gynecomastia is one of exclusion. What is remarkable is the frequency of this disorder; Williams reported that 40% of elderly men at autopsy have true gynecomastia,[248] and Niewoehner and Nuttall described a prevalence of 72% in hospitalized men aged 50 to 69.[250] However, many elderly patients receive multiple medications and have concurrent disorders of cardiovascular and liver function, and gynecomastia of aging, if it exists, may be caused by the increased incidence of a variety of medical problems with age rather than by age itself.[297]

Nevertheless, changes in estrogen and androgen metabolism have been characterized in men older than 70 years of age, including decrease in mean levels of plasma testosterone, decrease in plasma levels of bioavailable testosterone, elevation of plasma testosterone-binding globulin, increase in the rate of peripheral aromatization, decrease in the ratio of androgen to estrogen, increase in levels of plasma LH and FSH, and diminution or loss of the circadian rhythmicity of plasma testosterone levels (see Chapter 16). Such changes in elderly men may result in a sufficient alteration of the ratio of testosterone to estradiol within breast cells to feminize and therefore may be causal in breast enlargement in the absence of other diseases.

hyperplasia. The feminization in boys with congenital adrenal hyperplasia related to 21-hydroxylase deficiency may be complicated because it can be associated with benign testicular tumors. However, in most boys with congenital adrenal hyperplasia, enhanced estrogen production is thought to be the consequence of increased production of androstenedione and hence of increased availability of substrate for peripheral aromatase.[358-362] In 3β-hydroxysteroid dehydrogenase deficiency, feminization is believed to result from a combination of decreased testosterone levels and increased availability of adrenal androgens for extraglandular aromatization.[315, 363] As noted previously, increased availability of adrenal androgen for extraglandular aromatization also contributes to the feminization in patients with 17β-hydroxysteroid dehydrogenase deficiency.[290, 314]

TESTOSTERONE ADMINISTRATION. The administration of testosterone to children commonly causes gynecomastia, correlating with an increase in urinary estrogens,[364] whereas treatment of adult men with conventional replacement doses of testosterone esters causes an increase in plasma estradiol but only rarely results in gynecomastia.[365] In contrast, testosterone administration to men with cirrhosis of the liver causes a profound increase in plasma estrogen levels.[366] Furthermore, when supraphysiological amounts of aromatizable androgens are taken by body builders, weight lifters, and athletes in hope of improving muscle strength, plasma estradiol levels can rise as much as seven-fold,[367] and gynecomastia is common with such regimens.[368, 369] In probing the history for possible causes of gynecomastia it should be remembered that some androgenic agents (dihydrotestosterone, fluoxymesterone, 19-nor-testosterone analogues) are either not aromatizable or are weak substrates for the enzyme.

LIVER DISEASE. Liver disease, in particular cirrhosis of the liver, is a common cause of feminization. Because both plasma concentrations and urinary excretion rates of estrogens are elevated, gynecomastia is thought to be largely a result of overproduction of estrogen. However, the liver is not the direct source of the estrogens. Gordon and colleagues[370] reported that the extraglandular aromatization of plasma androgens to estrogen is increased in cirrhosis, and Edman and colleagues[371] showed that the increased extraglandular formation is mainly the consequence of decreased hepatic extraction of androstenedione (7% of the normal rate) and a secondary increased availability of androstenedione for extrasplanchnic metabolism, including aromatization. However, the development of gynecomastia in subjects with liver disease does not correlate closely with the measurable endocrine abnormalities,[372, 373] and administration of testosterone to men with alcoholic cirrhosis may cause a decreased prevalence of gynecomastia[374] despite a rise in plasma estradiol.[366] These findings imply that androgen deficiency, possibly among other factors, plays a role in the gynecomastia of liver disease. In carcinoma of the liver feminization can be the consequence of increased aromatase activity in the tumor itself.[375, 376]

STARVATION. Starvation is also associated with feminizing signs. Approximately 15% of American prisoners of war in Japanese prison camps developed gynecomastia.[377, 378] Three fourths of cases were bilateral, and most regressed within 5 to 7 mo. About a third of the cases occurred during refeeding after release, and other instances were associated with temporary improvements in the food supply during imprisonment. Infectious hepatitis and liver disease may have played a role in the pathogenesis, because some of the men affected also had spider angiomata and fatty infiltration of the liver. The exact cause of starvation gynecomastia has never been clarified, but the pathogenesis may be similar to that of liver disease, namely, diminished hepatic clearance of androgens and consequent shunting of androgens to the extraglandular sites of aromatization.

THYROTOXICOSIS. Thyrotoxicosis can cause gynecomastia in hyperthyroid men, and as many as 80% may have histologic evidence of gynecomastia.[379-381] Such men have elevated plasma estradiol levels,[382-385] probably because of elevated androstenedione production rates and the consequent increased formation of estrogen in extraglandular sites (despite a normal rate constant for the reaction).[386] Therefore, the mechanism of increased estrogen production is probably similar to that in liver disease: increased availability of substrate for extraglandular aromatization.

Increase in Extraglandular Aromatase

Increased extraglandular estrogen production can also arise from increased activity of aromatase enzymes in peripheral tissues. Hemsell and co-workers[387] described an 8-year-old boy who developed a striking feminization syndrome; he converted half of circulating androstenedione to estrone each day, for an estrogen production rate of 780 μg/d, more than 50 times the normal rate of extraglandular aromatase activity. The genetic basis of the disorder in the index case is not clear, but two brothers with a similar condition have been described by Berkowitz and colleagues,[388] implying that it is caused by a single gene mutation. A characteristic feature in the three reported cases is that the onset of the gynecomastia corresponded with the onset of adrenarche and therefore occurred before the time of normal puberty. A similar trait is present in the Sebright bantam chicken, in which an autosomal dominant gene causes an increase of more than 100-fold in extraglandular aromatization.[389]

DRUGS

Drugs can cause gynecomastia by direct action as estrogens, by enhancement of testicular production of estrogens, by inhibition of testosterone synthesis or action, or by unknown mechanisms.

ESTROGENS AND DRUGS THAT ACT LIKE ESTROGENS. Estrogens given to men in any form can result in severe gynecomastia. That which occurs in diethylstilbestrol-treated men[390] and transsexual men given estrogens[391] is best characterized. In some instances estrogens may be taken for other therapeutic reasons.[392] Young men and boys are particularly sensitive to estrogens and may develop gynecomastia from industrial exposure or from exposure to dermal ointments containing estrogens.[393-402] Unraveling the source of estrogen exposure may require a high index of suspicion, as in the case of a barber who massaged the scalps of customers with an antibaldness nostrum containing estrogen,[397] workers in factories where oral contraceptives are manufactured,[394] and children of workers in a diethylstilbestrol manufacturing plant who absorbed the drug from the clothing of their fathers.[402] Sufficient estrogen to induce gynecomastia can be absorbed by men during sexual intercourse with partners who use vaginal creams containing estrogen.[403, 404] In the United States no federal regulation governs the use of estrogens in cosmetics provided no therapeutic claims are made; estradiol concentrations may be as high as 18 ng/g in cosmetic creams and as high as 50 mg/dL in some lotions.[405]

Epidemics of gynecomastia among children in Bahrain and in Italy have been described in which the estrogen source was the ingestion of milk or meat from estrogen-injected cows.[406, 407] These reports are of particular interest because they raise the possibility that long-term exposure to small amounts of estrogenic agents may be the cause of idiopathic gynecomastia. Such agents may be derived from meat and dairy products from animals treated with estrogenic implants other than diethylstilbestrol,[408] from endogenous estrogens in animal tissues,[409] or from fungal or plant estrogens in foods.[410-413]

Although an association between digitalis administration and gynecomastia is well known, the pathophysiology is unclear. About 10% of men who have been given digitalis for a year develop gynecomastia,[414, 415] However, LeWinn pointed out that many patients with digitalis-induced gynecomastia also have abnormal liver function,[414] and in one study of patients with heart disease gynecomastia correlated better with the presence of right- or left-sided heart failure than with administration of the drugs.[416] Nevertheless, the same digitalis preparations that are associated with gynecomastia also have an estrogenic effect on the squamous epithelium of the vagina in postmenopausal women.[417] Digitalis has no identifiable effect on plasma estrogens[418] but itself binds to the human estrogen receptor and may promote breast growth directly.[419] Alternatively, Ricken has suggested that digitalis glycosides act to enhance the action of endogenous estrogens.[420]

DRUGS THAT ENHANCE ENDOGENOUS ESTROGEN FORMATION. The administration of hCG to boys or men may result in gynecomastia,[421] as would be predicted because it causes an increase in estradiol secretion by the testes.[277] Clomiphene citrate (both a weak estrogen and an antiestrogen) has been used to treat gynecomastia in boys, but paradoxically it can cause gynecomastia on withdrawal, presumably by increasing LH secretion and consequently increasing estradiol secretion by the testes.[422]

DRUGS THAT INHIBIT TESTOSTERONE SYNTHESIS OR ACTION. The antifungal drug ketoconazole blocks steroid hormone synthesis in Leydig cells; the principal step appears to be at the 17,20-desmolase reaction.[423] A similar effect occurs with other imidazole drugs, including metronidazole and etomidate.[423, 424] The inhibition of synthesis by ketoconazole is transient, and plasma testosterone returns to normal after blood levels of the drug fall. Gynecomastia occurs only if the dosage and administration schedule are such as to cause prolonged lowering of plasma androgen levels.[425] In this situation, inhibition of testosterone synthesis presumably causes feminization by mechanisms similar to that in testicular failure, namely, by altering the ratio of estradiol to testosterone.[426, 427]

Antineoplastic agents may cause a long-lasting impairment of testosterone synthesis, presumably through toxic effects on the Leydig cells; such damage may occur when the therapy is directed either toward systemic neoplasms (e.g., alkylating agents for treatment of Hodgkin's disease) or toward testicular cancers.[428–431] The precise mechanism of the gynecomastia has not been elucidated, but elevation in plasma gonadotropin levels secondary to the testicular damage may enhance testicular estrogen synthesis.[431]

Approximately half of men who receive 150 mg spironolactone/d develop gynecomastia.[432] Spironolactone has at least two effects on androgen metabolism: it inhibits testosterone biosynthesis by inhibiting the 17,20-desmolase reaction, and it prevents the binding of androgen to its receptor.[433–435] The incidence of gynecomastia is dose related,[436] but spironolactone may cause gynecomastia in doses as low as 50 mg/d—an amount that apparently does not impair testosterone synthesis. At these low doses the drug is thought to cause gynecomastia by inhibiting androgen binding to the receptor. At higher doses, testosterone synthesis is also inhibited, and plasma testosterone levels fall as a consequence. Spironolactone-induced gynecomastia may disappear when the active metabolite of the drug canrenoate is substituted for spironolactone.[437]

Several antiandrogens that have been tried for the treatment of prostatic disease, including cyproterone, flutamide, zanoterone, and bicalutamide, inhibit testosterone binding to the receptor and cause gynecomastia.[438–441] Gynecomastia is a common side effect of cimetidine therapy.[442–446] The drug has the capacity to block the binding of androgen to the androgen receptor and to block the binding of histamine to the H₂ receptor; in addition, it may inhibit the catabolism of estradiol.[447] Gynecomastia is less common in subjects receiving ranitidine than in those receiving cimetidine.[445, 448, 449] Suggestive evidence for induction of gynecomastia by an antiandrogen has come from studies of an epidemic of temporary gynecomastia that affected about one tenth of male Haitian refugees in five detention centers set up by the United States government in 1981.[450] The delousing agent used in these centers, which has an affinity for the androgen receptor similar to that of the synthetic androgen methyltrienolone and acts as an antiandrogen in rats, has been suggested as the cause of the gynecomastia.[451] From this cumulative experience it can be concluded that antiandrogens can cause gynecomastia and that unidentified antiandrogens may cause some of the cases now designated as idiopathic.

DRUGS THAT ACT BY UNKNOWN MECHANISMS. A variety of drugs cause gynecomastia by unknown mechanisms. For example, gynecomastia occurs in both prepubertal boys and elderly men given hGH,[452, 453] possibly by mediation through a direct effect of IGF1. A long list of drugs appears to be associated with gynecomastia with a frequency that is probably not coincidental; these include busulfan, calcium channel–blocking agents, converting enzyme inhibitors, diazepam, isoniazid, methyldopa, omeprozole, penicillamine, and tricyclic antidepressants, some of which may act by altering liver function.[454–460] The problem with interpreting such reports is that many patients receiving such agents have other conditions, such as congestive heart failure, that may predispose to gynecomastia.[416]

Both marijuana and heroin are suspected causes of gynecomastia, but the available data make it impossible to establish a direct causal relation.[461–464]

IDIOPATHIC GYNECOMASTIA

In all published series half or more of subjects evaluated for gynecomastia do not have an underlying endocrinopathy that is diagnosable at autopsy[465, 466] or by careful endocrine work-up.[467] If one adds those instances in all large series in which the designated cause is tenuous, the idiopathic category accounts for approximately three fourths of cases. At present it is not known whether men with gynecomastia of unknown origin are in fact normal (as proposed by Nuttall[249]), whether they had a feminizing factor that was transient and was not present at the time of work-up, whether their gynecomastia results from widespread exposure to small amounts of one or more environmental estrogens or antiandrogens, or whether the gynecomastia is the consequence of subtle, unrecognized endocrinopathies. Endocrinopathies that are known to cause breast enlargement are associated with severe gynecomastia, and the extent to which minor endocrine disorders are not recognized with current methodologies is uncertain. The fact that gynecomastia can develop as the result of subtle environmental exposure to estrogens or to antiandrogens raises the possibility that some gynecomastia may be be caused by long-term, unrecognized exposure to endocrine substances.[402, 406–413, 451] The problem of gynecomastia is analogous to that of the pathogenesis of euthyroid goiter in that the cause has been explained in only a fraction of cases. The critical clinical point, however, is that whatever the cause, the diagnosis of idiopathic gynecomastia carries no known import as to health.

PROLACTIN DOES NOT PLAY A DIRECT ROLE IN GYNECOMASTIA

Plasma prolactin levels are usually normal in men with gynecomastia of diverse causes, and men who have prolonged elevation in plasma prolactin secondary to use of psychotropic drugs do not commonly develop gynecomastia.[468–471] As a consequence, prolactin is not believed to play a direct role in the disorder. This conclusion is in keeping with the fact that prolactin is not a growth hormone for the breast. Furthermore, when gynecomastia develops in men with prolactin-secreting tumors of the pituitary and high plasma prolactin levels,[472–474] the gynecomastia is probably the consequence of secondary testicular failure as a result of either the effects of the tumor mass or direct inhibition by prolactin of gonadotropin secretion. In other instances of gynecomastia in which the prolactin level is elevated, the elevation may be a secondary consequence of hyperestrogenemia.[475, 476]

Diagnosis

The dilemma is to separate men with underlying endocrinopathies from those in the larger category of idiopathic disorders. In general, only men whose gynecomastia is symptomatic are evaluated, but if there is a serious question as to whether the gynecomastia is real the issue can probably best be solved by mammography or ultrasonography, or both.[256–259]

The routine measurement of androgen and estrogen kinetics is impractical, but most of the known causes of gynecomastia can be identified by a work-up that includes (1) a careful drug history that encompasses potential environmental and indirect exposures to endocrinologically active substances; (2) a detailed physical examination including the testes (the finding of small testes bilaterally suggests testicular insufficiency, and asymmetrical testes raise the possibility of testicular tumors); (3) evaluation of liver function; and (4) a limited endocrine work-up including measurement of plasma dehydroepiandrosterone or urinary 17-ketosteroids (usually elevated in adrenal feminizing states), measurement of plasma estradiol (helpful if elevated but usually normal), and measurement of plasma LH and testosterone (high LH and normal or low testosterone levels suggest testicular insufficiency; low LH and low testosterone levels suggest hypopituitarism, estrogen secretion from a tumor, or an exogenous source of estrogen; and high LH and high testosterone levels suggest androgen resistance). If these parameters are normal, as is frequently the case, the usual recourse is to observe the patient without treatment. If the symptoms persist or worsen and if the enlargement is progressive, a more extensive work-up may have to be undertaken.

Treatment

The difficulty in treating gynecomastia is inherent in its natural history; if the feminizing process persists for a long period, the initial glandular hyperplasia is replaced by a progressive fibrosis and hyalinization that does not regress after the source of excess estrogen is corrected.[260] Consequently, surgery remains the mainstay of therapy and is frequently indicated for psychological and cosmetic reasons. Such surgery is usually accomplished through a circumareolar approach.[477–481]

Medical management is most successful when it is addressed to gynecomastia of recent onset or to prevention of its development. Testosterone administration has inconsistent effects in the Klinefelter's syndrome but can cause dramatic improvement in subjects with other forms of testicular failure (e.g., anorchia, viral orchitis). The uncertain element in testosterone therapy results from the fact that it can serve as substrate for extraglandular estrogen formation, and under some circumstances (e.g., liver disease) androgen therapy can cause a disproportionate increase in plasma estrogen levels. Various drug regimens have been tried for gynecomastia with varying degrees of success, including the antiestrogens tamoxifen[482–484] and clomiphene,[485, 486] the aromatase inhibitor testolactone,[487]

and danazol,[488, 489] a weak androgen that acts by inhibiting gonadotropin secretion and causing a fall in plasma testosterone. Treatment with dihydrotestosterone (which cannot be aromatized to estrogen) is also reported to cause significant symptomatic improvement in gynecomastia.[490–492] However, no prospective controlled studies have been performed with any of these regimens, and their clinical usefulness is not established.

Perhaps the most effective form of therapy for gynecomastia is prevention of its development by breast radiation before the institution of stilbestrol therapy in men who have carcinoma of the prostate.[493–495] This treatment approaches 90% effectiveness, and the complication rate is low in the age group affected with prostatic cancer.

Conclusion

The clinical problem of gynecomastia is clouded by questions of definition and incidence. After the diagnosis is made, the disorder must be separated into the idiopathic type (of uncertain significance as well as cause), which may account for three fourths of cases, and endocrine gynecomastia, which can arise from any of several disturbances in androgen and estrogen physiology. It is useful to consider the endocrine causes in terms of the androgen/estrogen ratio, namely, disturbances that arise from decreases in androgen production (or action) and those that result from increases in estrogen formation. The latter, in turn, can arise from estrogen secretion by tumors or increase in extraglandular estrogen formation. Most drugs that cause gynecomastia also act to alter the ratio of androgen to estrogen. It is rational in most instances of gynecomastia to perform only a limited endocrine work-up and to monitor the course of this disorder before undertaking more extensive diagnostic evaluation.

Galactorrhea in Men

Men account for about 5% of galactorrheic patients. The relative infrequency of this disorder in men is presumably a consequence of the fact that appropriate estrogen priming of the breast is less common in men who have elevations in plasma prolactin. When galactorrhea does occur in men it is appropriate to evaluate the patients both for feminizing syndromes and for prolactin excess. Prolactin-secreting pituitary tumors are a common cause of prolactin excess in men as well as women.

Carcinoma of the Male Breast

Gynecomastia is a risk factor for malignancy in that men with gynecomastia have breast cancer with a greater frequency and at a younger age than men without gynecomastia.[496–500] It is probably gynecomastia itself rather than mutations in the androgen receptor gene that is responsible for the apparent increased risk for breast cancer in men with the Reifenstein's syndrome.[501, 502] Nevertheless, the increased risk in men with gynecomastia is small, and of 228 patients with gynecomastia followed for up to 10 y none developed breast cancer.[503] It is of interest that the *BRCA2* hereditary breast cancer mutation carries an increased risk of breast cancer in both men and women.[504] In most families the *BRCA1* mutation is associated with an increased risk of ovarian and breast cancer in women but an increased incidence of prostate rather than breast cancer in men.[504] However, a *BRCA1* mutation has been described in a man with both breast and prostate cancer.[505] If cancer is suspected, mammography is helpful in establishing the diagnosis. In one study, 11 of 60 men who underwent surgery for unilateral gynecomastia proved to have breast cancer.[506] Although the frequency of breast cancer in men with gynecomastia is less than that in normal women, when it occurs in men it appears to have a worse prognosis.[498]

REFERENCES

1. Rosen JM, Humphreys R, Krnacik S, et al. The regulation of mammary gland development by hormones, growth factors, and oncogenes. Prog Clin Biol Res 1994; 387:95–111.
2. Anbazhagan R, Bartek J, Monaghan P, et al. Growth and development of the human infant breast. Am J Anat 1991; 192:407–417.
3. Laurence DJ, Monaghan P, Gusterson BA. The development of the normal human breast. Oxf Rev Reprod Biol 1991; 13:149–174.
4. Cowie AT, Forsyth IA, Hart IC. Hormonal Control of Lactation. Berlin: Springer-Verlag, 1980.
5. McKiernan JF, Hull D. Breast development in the newborn. Arch Dis Child 1981; 56:525–529.
6. McKiernan JF, Hull D. Prolactin, maternal oestrogens, and breast development in the newborn. Arch Dis Child 1981; 56:770–774.
7. McKiernan J, Coyne J, Cahalane S. Histology of breast development in early life. Arch Dis Child 1988; 63:136–139.
8. Raynaud A. Morphogenesis of the mammary gland. In: Kon SK, Cowie HT, eds. Milk: The Mammary Gland and Its Secretions. Vol 1. New York: Academic Press, 1961: 3–46.
9. Kratochwil K. In vitro analysis of the hormonal basis for the sexual dimorphism in the embryonic development of the mouse mammary gland. J Embryol Exp Morphol 1971; 25:141–153.
10. Kratochwil K, Schwartz P. Tissue interaction in androgen response of embryonic mammary rudiment of the mouse: identification of the target tissue for testosterone. Proc Natl Acad Sci USA 1976; 73:4041–4044.
11. Cardy RH. Sexual dimorphism of the normal rat mammary gland. Vet Pathol 1991; 28:139–145.
12. Pfaltz CR. Das embryonale und postnatale Verhalten den Mannlichen brustdruse beim Menschen. II. Das Mammanorgan in Kindes-, Junglings-, Mannes-, and Greisenaltern. Acta Anat 1949; 8:293–328.
13. Vogel PM, Georgiade NG, Fetter BF, et al. The correlation of histologic changes in the human breast with the menstrual cycle. Am J Pathol 1981; 104:23–34.
14. Longacre TA, Bartow SA. A correlative morphologic study of human breast and endometrium in the menstrual cycle. Am J Surg Pathol 1986; 10:382–393.
15. Going JJ, Anderson TJ, Battersby S, et al. Proliferative and secretory activity in human breast during natural and artificial menstrual cycles. Am J Pathol 1988; 130:193–204.
16. Anderson RR. Endocrinological control. In: Larson BL, Smith VR, eds. Lactation: A Comprehensive Treatise. New York: Academic Press, 1974: 97–140.
17. Topper YJ, Oka T. Some aspects of mammary gland development in the mature mouse. In: Larson BL, Smith VR, eds. Lactation: A Comprehensive Treatise. New York: Academic, 1974: 327–348
18. Vorherr H. Hormonal and biochemical changes of pituitary and breast during pregnancy. Semin Perinatol 1979; 3:193–198.
19. Tucker HA. Endocrinology of lactation. Semin Perinatol 1979; 3:199–223.
20. Knight CH, Peaker M. Development of the mammary gland. J Reprod Fertil 1982; 65:521–536.
21. Battersby S, Anderson TJ. Proliferative and secretory activity in the pregnant and lactating human breast. Virchows Arch [A] 1988; 413:189–196.
22. Topper YJ, Freeman CS. Multiple hormone interactions in the developmental biology of the mammary gland. Physiol Rev 1980; 60:1049–1105.
23. Nicoll CS. Physiological actions of prolactin. In: Greep RO, Astwood EB, Knobil E, et al, eds. Handbook of Physiology. Sect 7: Endocrinology. Vol IV. The Pituitary Gland and Its Neuroendocrine Control. Part 2. Washington, DC: American Physiological Society, 1974; 23:253–292.
24. Shiu RPC, Friesen HG. Mechanism of action of prolactin in the control of mammary gland function. Annu Rev Physiol 1980; 42:83–96.
25. Lyons WR, Li CH, Johnson RE. The hormonal control of mammary growth and lactation. Recent Prog Horm Res 1958; 14:219–254.
26. Cowie AT, Tindal JS, Yokoyama A. The induction of mammary growth in the hypophysectomized goat. J Endocrinol 1966; 34:185–195.
27. Talwalker PK, Meites J. Mammary lobulo-alveolar growth induced by anterior pituitary hormones in adreno-ovariectomized and adreno-ovariectomized-hypophysectomized rats. Proc Soc Exp Biol Med 1961; 107:880–883.
28. Kleinberg DL, Todd J, Niemann W. Prolactin stimulation of α-lactalbumin in normal primate mammary gland. J Clin Endocrinol Metab 1978; 47:435–441.
29. Holdaway IM, Friesen HG. Hormone binding by human mammary carcinoma. Cancer Res 1977; 37:1946–1952.
30. Djiane J, Durand P, Kelly PA. Evolution of prolactin receptors in rabbit mammary gland during pregnancy and lactation. Endocrinology 1977; 100:1348–1356.
31. Hayden TJ, Bonney RC, Forsyth IA. Ontogeny and control of prolactin receptors in the mammary gland and liver of virgin, pregnant and lactating rats. J Endocrinol 1979; 80:259–269.
32. Dhadly MS, Walker RA. The localization of prolactin binding sites in human breast tissue. Int J Cancer 1983; 31:433–437.
33. Jahn GA, Edery M, Belair L, et al. Prolactin receptor gene expression in rat mammary gland and liver during pregnancy and lactation. Endocrinology 1991; 128:2976–2984.
34. Posner BI, Kelly PA, Friesen HG. Prolactin receptors in rat liver: possible induction by prolactin. Science 1975; 188:57–59.
35. Djiane J, Durand P. Prolactin-progesterone antagonism in self-regulation of prolactin receptors in the mammary gland. Nature 1977; 266:614–643.
36. Kledzik GS, Bradley CJ, Marshall S, et al. Effects of high doses of estrogen on prolactin-binding activity and growth of carcinogen-induced mammary cancers in rats. Cancer Res 1976; 36:3265–3268.
37. Shiu RPC, Friesen HG. Blockade of prolactin action by an antiserum to its receptors. Science 1976; 192:259–261.
38. Kelly PA, Djiane J, Postel-Vinay M-C, et al. The prolactin/growth hormone receptor family. Endocr Rev 1991; 12:235–251.
39. Frantz AG, Kleinberg DL, Noel GL. Studies on prolactin in man. Recent Prog Horm Res 1972; 28:527–590.
40. Wurzel JM, Parks JS, Herd JE, et al. A gene deletion is responsible for absence of human chorionic somatomammotropin. DNA 1982; 1:251–257.
41. Frantz AG, Rabkin MT. Effects of estrogen and sex difference on secretion of human growth hormone. J Clin Endocrinol Metab 1965; 25:1470–1480.
42. Kleinberg DL, Todd J, Babitsky G, et al. Estradiol inhibits prolactin induced α-lactalbumin production in normal primate mammary tissue in vitro. Endocrinology 1982; 110:279–281.
43. Perel E, Wilkins D, Killinger DW. The conversion of androstenedione to estrone, estradiol, and testosterone in breast tissue. J Steroid Biochem 1980; 13:89–94.
44. Perel E, Davis S, Killinger DW. Androgen metabolism in male and female breast tissue. Steroids 1981; 37:345–352.
45. Perel E, Killinger DW. The metabolism of androstenedionë and testosterone to C₁₉ metabolites in normal breast, breast carcinoma and benign prostatic hypertrophy tissue. J Steroid Biochem 1983; 19:1135–1139.
46. James VHT, McNeill JM, Lai LC, et al. Aromatase activity in normal breast and breast tumor tissues: in vivo and in vitro studies. Steroids 1987; 50:269–279.
47. Schmidt M, Löffler G. Induction of aromatase in stromal vascular cells from human breast adipose tissue depends on cortisol and growth factors. FEBS Lett 1994; 341:177–181.
48. Wagner RK, Jungblut PW. Oestradiol- and dihydrotestosterone receptors in normal and neoplastic human mammary tissue. Acta Endocrinol 1976; 82:105–120.
49. Silva JS, Georgiade GS, Dilley WG, et al. Menstrual cycle–dependent variations of breast cyst proteins and sex steroid receptors in the normal human breast. Cancer 1983; 51:1297–1302.
50. Ricketts D, Turnbull L, Ryall G, et al. Estrogen and progesterone receptors in the normal female breast. Cancer Res 1991; 51:1817–1822.
51. Söderqvist G, von Schoultz B, Tani E, et al. Estrogen and progesterone receptor content in breast epithelial cells from healthy women during the menstrual cycle. Am J Obstet Gynecol 1993; 168:874–879.
52. Edery M, Imagawa W, Larson L, et al. Regulation of estrogen and progesterone receptor levels in mouse mammary epithelial cells grown in serum-free collagen gel cultures. Endocrinology 1985; 116:105–112.
53. Muldoon TG. Prolactin mediation of estrogen-induced changes in mammary tissue estrogen and progesterone receptors. Endocrinology 1987; 121:141–149.
54. Freeman CS, Topper YJ. Progesterone is not essential to the differentiative potential of mammary epithelium in the male mouse. Endocrinology 1978; 103:186–192.
55. Mauvais-Jarvis P, Kuttenn F, Gompel A. Antiestrogen action of progesterone in breast tissue. Horm Res 1987; 28:212–218.
56. Davis JW, Wikman-Coffelt J, Eddington CL. The effect of progesterone on biosynthetic pathways in mammary tissue. Endocrinology 1972; 91:1011–1019.
57. Shamay A, Zeelon E, Ghez Z, et al. Inhibition of casein and fat synthesis and α-lactalbumin secretion by progesterone in explants from bovine lactating mammary glands. J Endocrinol 1987; 113:81–88.
58. Vorherr H, ed. Suppression of lactation. In: The Breast: Morphology and Lactation. New York: Academic, 1974: 198–217.
59. Haslam SZ, Shyamala G. Progesterone receptors in normal mammary glands of mice: characterization and relationship to stage of development. Endocrinology 1979; 105:786–795.
60. Shyamala G, Schneider W, Schott D. Developmental regulation of murine mammary progesterone receptor gene expression. Endocrinology 1990; 126:2882–2889.
61. Frankenne F, Closset J, Gomez F, et al. The physiology of growth hormones (GHs) in pregnant women and partial characterization of the placental GH variant. J Clin Endocrinol Metab 1988; 66:1171–1180.
62. Daughaday WH, Trivedi B, Winn HN, et al. Hypersomatotropism in pregnant women, as measured by a human liver radioreceptor assay. J Clin Endocrinol Metab 1990; 70:215–221.
63. MacLeod JN, Worsley I, Ray J, et al. Human growth hormone-variant is a biologically active somatogen and lactogen. Endocrinology 1991; 128:1298–1302.
64. Feldman M, Ruan W, Cunningham BC, et al. Evidence that the growth hormone receptor mediates differentiation and development of the mammary gland. Endocrinology 1993; 133:1602–1608.
65. Rimoin DL, Holzman GB, Merimee TJ, et al. Lactation in the absence of human growth hormone. J Clin Endocrinol Metab 1968; 28:1183–1188.

66. Topper YJ, Nicholas KR, Sankaran L, et al. Insulin as a developmental hormone. Prog Clin Biol Res 1984; 142:63–77.

67. Prosser CG, Sankaran L, Hennighausen L, et al. Comparison of the roles of insulin and insulin-like growth factor I in casein gene expression and in the development of α-lactalbumin and glucose transport activities in the mouse mammary epithelial cell. Endocrinology 1987; 120:1411–1416.

68. Furlanetto RW, DiCarlo JN. Somatomedin-C receptors and growth effects in human breast cells maintained in long-term tissue culture. Cancer Res 1984; 44:2122–2128.

69. Peyrat JP, Bonneterre J, Laurent JC, et al. Presence and characterization of insulin-like growth factor I receptors in human benign breast disease. Eur J Cancer Clin Oncol 1988; 24:1425–1431.

70. Duclos M, Houdebine L-M, Djiane J. Comparison of insulin-like growth factor 1 and insulin effects on prolactin-induced lactogenesis in the rabbit mammary gland in vitro. Mol Cell Endocrinol 1989; 65:129–134.

71. Plaut K, Ikeda M, Vonderhaar BK. Role of growth hormone and insulin-like growth factor-I in mammary development. Endocrinology 1993; 133:1843–1848.

72. Ruan W, Catanese V, Wieczorek R, et al. Estradiol enhances the stimulatory effect of insulin-like growth factor-I (IGF1) on mammary development and growth hormone–induced IGF1 messenger ribonucleic acid. Endocrinology 1995; 136:1296–1302.

73. Tonelli QJ, Sorof S. Epidermal growth factor requirement for development of cultured mammary gland. Nature 1980; 285:250–252.

74. Imagawa W, Tomooka Y, Hamamoto S, et al. Stimulation of mammary epithelial cell growth in vitro: interaction of epidermal growth factor and mammogenic hormones. Endocrinology 1985; 116:1514–1524.

75. Anderson TR, Mayer GL, Hebert N, et al. Interactions among prolactin, epidermal growth factor, and proinsulin on the growth and morphology of the pigeon crop-sac mucosal epithelium in vivo. Endocrinology 1987; 120:1258–1264.

76. Nishikawa S, Moore RC, Nonomura N, et al. Progesterone and EGF inhibit mouse mammary gland prolactin receptor and β-casein gene expression. Am J Physiol 1994; 267(Suppl 1):C1467–C1472.

77. Nicoll CS, Anderson TR, Hebert NJ, et al. Comparative aspects of the growth-promoting actions of prolactin on its target organs: evidence for synergism with an insulin-like growth factor. In: MacLeod RM, Thorner MO, Scapagnini U, eds. Prolactin: Basic and Clinical Correlates. New York: Springer-Verlag, 1985:393–410.

78. Nicoll CS, Hebert NJ, Russell SM. Lactogenic hormones stimulate the liver to secrete a factor that acts synergistically with prolactin to promote growth of the pigeon crop-sac mucosal epithelium in vivo. Endocrinology 1985; 116:1449–1453.

79. English DE, Russell SM, Katz LS, et al. Evidence for a role of the liver in the mammotrophic action of prolactin. Endocrinology 1990; 126:2252–2256.

80. Hoeffler JP, Frawley LS. Liver tissue produces a potent lactogen that partially mimics the actions of prolactin. Endocrinology 1987; 120:1679–1681.

81. Newman CB, Cosby H, Friesen HG, et al. Evidence for a nonprolactin, non-growth-hormone mammary mitogen in the human pituitary gland. Proc Natl Acad Sci USA 1987; 84:8110–8114.

82. Robinson SD, Silberstein GB, Roberts AB, et al. Regulated expression and growth inhibitory effects of transforming growth factor-β isoforms in mouse mammary gland development. Development 1991; 113:867–878.

83. Silberstein GB, Flanders KC, Roberts AB, et al. Regulation of mammary morphogenesis: evidence for extracellular matrix-mediated inhibition of ductal budding by transforming growth factor-β1. Dev Biol 1992; 152:354–362.

84. Oka T, Yoshimura M, Lavandero S, et al. Control of growth and differentiation of the mammary gland by growth factors. J Dairy Sci 1991; 74:2788–2800.

85. Shyamala G. Specific cytoplasmic glucocorticoid hormone receptors in lactating mammary glands. Biochemistry 1973; 12:3085–3090.

86. Dawood MY, Khan-Dawood FS, Wahi RS, et al. Oxytocin release and plasma anterior pituitary and gonadal hormones in women during lactation. J Clin Endocrinol Metab 1981; 52:678–683.

87. Huddleston JF, Sutliff G, Robinson D. Contraction stress test by intermittent nipple stimulation. Obstet Gynecol 1984; 63:669–673.

88. Finley BE, Amico J, Castillo M, et al. Oxytocin and prolactin responses associated with nipple stimulation contraction stress tests. Obstet Gynecol 1986; 67:836–839.

89. Keegan KA Jr, Helm DA, Porto M, et al. A prospective evaluation of nipple stimulation techniques for contraction stress testing. Am J Obstet Gynecol 1987; 157:121–125.

90. Curtis P, Evens J, Resnick J, et al. Patterns of uterine contractions and prolonged uterine activity using three methods of breast stimulation for contraction stress tests. Obstet Gynecol 1989; 73:631–638.

91. Noel GL, Suh HK, Frantz AG. Prolactin release during nursing and breast stimulation in postpartum and nonpostpartum subjects. J Clin Endocrinol Metab 1974; 38:413–423.

92. Johnston JM, Amico JA. A prospective longitudinal study of the release of oxytocin and prolactin in response to infant suckling in long-term lactation. J Clin Endocrinol Metab 1986; 62:653–657.

93. Tyson JE, Friesen HG, Anderson MS. Human lactational and ovarian response to endogenous prolactin release. Science 1972; 177:897–900.

94. Milsom SR, Breier BH, Gallaher BW, et al. Growth hormone stimulates galactopoiesis in healthy lactating women. Acta Endocrinol 1992; 127:337–343.

95. Breier BH, Gluckman PD, McCutcheon SN, et al. Physiological responses to somatotropin in the ruminant. J Dairy Sci 1991; 74(Suppl 2):20–34.

96. Flint DJ, Gardner M. Evidence that growth hormone stimulates milk synthesis by direct action on the mammary gland and that prolactin exerts effects on milk secretion by maintenance of mammary deoxyribonucleic acid content and tight junction status. Endocrinology 1994; 135:1119–1124.

97. Breier BH, Milsom SR, Blum WF, et al. Insulin-like growth factors and their binding proteins in plasma and milk after growth hormone–stimulated galactopoiesis in normally lactating women. Acta Endocrinol 1993; 129:427–435.

98. Liapis H, Crouch EC, Grosso LE, et al. Expression of parathyroidlike protein in normal, proliferative, and neoplastic human breast tissues. Am J Pathol 1993; 143:1169–1178.

99. Thiede MA, Rodan GA. Expression of a calcium-mobilizing parathyroid hormone–like peptide in lactating mammary tissue. Science 1988; 242:278–280.

100. Budayr AA, Halloran BP, King JC, et al. High levels of a parathyroid hormone–like protein in milk. Proc Natl Acad Sci USA 1989; 86:7183–7185.

101. Thurston AW, Cole JA, Hillman LS, et al. Purification and properties of parathyroid hormone–related peptide isolated from milk. Endocrinology 1990; 126:1183–1190.

102. Insogna KL, Stewart AF, Morris CA, et al. Native and a synthetic analogue of the malignancy-associated parathyroid hormone–like protein have in vitro transforming growth factor-like properties. J Clin Invest 1989; 83:1057–1060.

103. Thiede MA. The mRNA encoding a parathyroid hormone–like peptide is produced in mammary tissue in response to elevations in serum prolactin. Mol Endocrinol 1989; 3:1443–1447.

104. Grill V, Hillary J, Ho PMW, et al. Parathyroid hormone–related protein: a possible endocrine function in lactation. Clin Endocrinol 1992; 37:405–410.

105. Ratcliffe WA. Role of parathyroid hormone–related protein in lactation. Clin Endocrinol 1992; 37:402–404.

106. Lepre F, Grill V, Ho PWM, et al. Hypercalcemia in pregnancy and lactation associated with parathyroid hormone–related protein. N Engl J Med 1993; 328:666–667.

107. Khosla S, van Heerden JA, Gharib H, et al. Parathyroid hormone–related protein and hypercalcemia secondary to massive mammary hyperplasia. N Engl J Med 1990; 322:1157.

108. Gautvik KM, Weintraub BD, Graeber CT, et al. Serum prolactin and TSH: effects of nursing and pyroGlu-His-ProNH₂ administration in postpartum women. J Clin Endocrinol Metab 1973; 37:135–139.

109. Weitzman RE, Firemark HM, Glatz TH, et al. Thyrotropin-releasing hormone stimulates release of arginine-vasopressin and oxytocin in vivo. Endocrinology 1979; 104:904–907.

110. Kolodny RC, Jacobs LS, Daughaday WH. Mammary stimulation causes prolactin secretion in non-lactating women. Nature 1972; 238:284–286.

111. Richardson GS. Reflex lactation (thoracotomy) and reflex ovulation (intercostal block): case report, review of the literature, and discussion of mechanisms. Obstet Gynecol Surv 1970; 25:1021–1036

112. Auerbach KG, Avery JL. Induced lactation. Am J Dis Child 1981; 135:340–343.

113. Thearle MJ, Weissenberger R. Induced lactation in adoptive mothers. Aust NZ J Obstet Gynaecol 1984; 24:283–286.

114. Nemba K. Induced lactation: a study of 37 non-puerperal mothers. J Trop Pediatr 1994; 40:240–242.

115. Vorherr H, ed. Lactation and reproductive function. In: The Breast: Morphology and Lactation. New York: Academic, 1974: 184–197.

116. Wong S, Stepp-Gilbert E. Lactation suppression: nonpharmaceutical versus pharmaceutical method. J Obstet Gynecol Neonatal Nursing 1985; 14:302–310.

117. Vance ML, Evans WS, Thorner MO. Bromocriptine. Ann Intern Med 1984; 100:78–91.

118. Duchesne C, Leke R. Bromocriptine mesylate for prevention of postpartum lactation. Obstet Gynecol 1981; 57:464–467.

119. Sandoz Pharmaceuticals Corp. Parlodel. In: Physicians Desk Reference. 50th ed. Montvale, NJ: Medical Economics Co, 1996: 2281–2284.

120. Sheehan HL. Atypical hypopituitarism. Proc R Soc Med 1961; 54:43–48.

121. Sheehan HL, Davis JC. Pituitary necrosis. Br Med Bull 1968; 24:59–70.

122. Cosman F, Post KD, Holub DA, et al. Lymphocytic hypophysitis: report of 3 new cases and review of the literature. Medicine 1989; 68:240–256.

123. Thodou E, Asa SL, Kontogeorgos G, et al. Clinical case seminar: lymphocytic hypophysitis—clinicopathological findings. J Clin Endocrinol Metab 1995; 80:2302–2311.

124. Kauppila A, Chatelain P, Kirkinen P, et al. Isolated prolactin deficiency in a woman with puerperal alactogenesis. J Clin Endocrinol Metab 1987; 64:309–312.

125. Gupta AP, Gupta PK. Metoclopramide as a lactogogue. Clin Pediatr 1985; 24:269–272.

126. Ehrenkranz RA, Ackerman BA. Metoclopramide effect on faltering milk production by mothers of premature infants. Pediatrics 1986; 78:614–620.

127. Diaz S, Cárdenas H, Brandeis A, et al. Early difference in the endocrine profile of long and short lactational amenorrhea. J Clin Endocrinol Metab 1991; 72:196–201.

128. McNeilly AS. Lactational amenorrhea. Endocr Metab Clin North Am 1993; 22:59–73.

129. Madhavapeddi R, Ramachandran P. Side effects of oral contraceptive use in lactating women: enlargement of breast in a breast-fed child. Contraception 1985; 32:437–443.

130. Rimsten A, Skoog B, Stenkvist B. On the significance of nipple discharge in the diagnosis of breast disease. Acta Chir Scand 1976; 142:513–518.

131. Urban JA, Egeli RA. Non-lactational nipple discharge. CA 1978; 28:130–140.

132. Murad TM, Contesso G, Mouriesse H. Nipple discharge from the breast. Ann Surg 1982; 195:259–264.

133. Leis HP Jr. Management of nipple discharge. World J Surg 1989; 13:736–742.

134. Fiorica JV. Nipple discharge. Obstet Gynecol Clin North Am 1994; 21:453–460.

135. Kleinberg DL, Noel GL, Frantz AG. Galactorrhea: a study of 235 cases, including 48 with pituitary tumors. N Engl J Med 1977; 296:589–600.

136. Tolis G, Somma M, Van Campenhout J, et al. Prolactin secretion in 65 patients with galactorrhea. Am J Obstet Gynecol 1974; 118:91–101.

137. Boyd AE III, Reichlin S, Tuskoy RN. Galactorrhea-amenorrhea syndrome: diagnosis and therapy. Ann Intern Med 1977; 87:165–175.

138. Gomez F, Reyes FI, Faiman C. Nonpuerperal galactorrhea and hyperprolactinemia: clinical findings, endocrine features, and therapeutic responses in 56 cases. Am J Med 1977; 62:648–660.

139. Evans WS, Thorner MO. Mechanisms for hypogonadism in hyperprolactinemia. Semin Reprod Endocrinol 1984; 2:9–22.

140. McNeilly AS. Prolactin and the control of gonadotrophin secretion. J Endocrinol 1987; 115:1–5.

141. Van Wyk JJ, Grumbach MM. Syndrome of precocious menstruation and galactorrhea in juvenile hypothyroidism: an example of hormonal overlap in pituitary feedback. J Pediatr 1960; 57:416–435.

142. Edwards CRW, Forsyth IA, Besser GM. Amenorrhoea, glactorrhoea, and primary hypothyroidism with high circulating levels of prolactin. Br Med J 1971; 3:462–464.

143. Bigos ST, Ridgway EC, Kourides IA, et al. Spectrum of pituitary alterations with mild and severe thyroid impairment. J Clin Endocrinol Metab 1978; 46:317–325.

144. Honbo KS, Van Herle AJ, Kellett KA. Serum prolactin levels in untreated primary hypothyroidism. Am J Med 1978; 64:782–787.

145. Grubb MR, Chakeres D, Malarkey WB. Patients with primary hypothyroidism presenting as prolactinomas. Am J Med 1987; 83:765–769.

146. Malarkey WB, Beck P. 24-hour prolactin profiles in normal and disease states: failure of thyroxine to modify prolactin secretion. J Clin Endocrinol Metab 1975; 40:708–712.

147. Kapcala LP. Galactorrhea and thyrotoxicosis. Arch Intern Med 1984; 144:2349–2350.

148. Gluskin LE, Strasberg B, Shah JH. Verapamil-induced hyperprolactinemia and galactorrhea. Ann Intern Med 1981; 95:66–67.

149. Ehrinpreis MN, Dhar R, Narula A. Cimetidine-induced galactorrhea. Am J Gastroenterol 1989; 84:563–565.

150. Mendelson JH, Mello NK, Teoh SK, et al. Cocaine effects on pulsatile secretion of anterior pituitary, gonadal, and adrenal hormones. J Clin Endocrinol Metab 1989; 69:1256–1260.

151. Noel GL, Suh HK, Stone G, et al. Human prolactin and growth hormone release during surgery and other conditions of stress. J Clin Endocrinol Metab 1972; 35:840–851.

152. MacFarlane IA, Rosin MD. Galactorrhoea following surgical procedures to the chest wall: the role of prolactin. Postgrad Med J 1980; 56:23–25.

153. Caputy GG, Flowers RS. Copious lactation following augmentation mammaplasty: an uncommon but not rare condition. Aesthetic Plast Surg 1994; 18:393–397.

154. Lim VS, Kathpalia SC, Frohman LA. Hyperprolactinemia and impaired pituitary response to suppression and stimulation in chronic renal failure: reversal after transplantation. J Clin Endocrinol Metab 1979; 48:101–107.

155. Van Thiel DH, McClain CJ, Elson MK, et al. Evidence for autonomous secretion of prolactin in some alcoholic men with cirrhosis and gynecomastia. Metabolism 1978; 27:1778–1784.

156. Rohn RD. Benign galactorrhea/breast discharge in adolescent males probably due to breast self-manipulation. J Adolesc Health Care 1984; 5:210–212.

157. Frantz AG. Endocrine diagnosis of prolactin-secreting pituitary tumors. In: Black PM, Zervas NT, Ridgway EC, et al, eds. Secretory Tumors of the Pituitary Gland. New York: Raven, 1984: 45–52.

158. Burrow GN, Wortzman G, Rewcastle NB, et al. Microadenomas of the pituitary and abnormal sellar tomograms in an unselected autopsy series. N Engl J Med 1981; 304:156–158.

159. Klibanski A, Neer RM, Beitins IZ, et al. Decreased bone density in hyperprolactinemic women. N Engl J Med 1980; 303:1511–1514.

160. Schlechte JA, Sherman B, Martin R. Bone density in amenorrheic women with and without hyperprolactinemia. J Clin Endocrinol Metab 1983; 56:1120–1123.

161. Koppelman MCS, Kurtz DW, Morrish KA, et al. Vertebral body bone mineral content in hyperprolactinemic women. J Clin Endocrinol Metab 1984; 59:1050–1053.

162. Schlechte J, El-Khoury G, Kathol M, et al. Forearm and vertebral bone mineral in treated and untreated hyperprolactinemic amenorrhea. J Clin Endocrinol Metab 1987; 64:1021–1026.

163. Klibanski A, Greenspan SL. Increase in bone mass after treatment of hyperprolactinemic amenorrhea. N Engl J Med 1986; 315:542–546.

164. Biller BMK, Baum HBA, Rosenthal DI, et al. Progressive trabecular osteopenia in women with hyperprolactinemic amenorrhea. J Clin Endocrinol Metab 1992; 75:692–697.

165. Schlechte J, Walkner L, Kathol M. A longitudinal analysis of premenopausal bone loss in healthy women and women with hyperprolactinemia. J Clin Endocrinol Metab 1992; 75:698–703.

166. Wardlaw SL, Bilezikian JP. Hyperprolactinemia and osteopenia. J Clin Endocrinol Metab 1992; 75:690–691.

167. Schlechte J, Dolan K, Sherman B, et al. The natural history of untreated hyperprolactinemia: a prospective analysis. J Clin Endocrinol Metab 1989; 68:412–418.

168. Koppelman MCS, Jaffe MJ, Rieth KG, et al. Hyperprolactinemia, amenorrhea, and galactorrhea: a retrospective assessment of 25 cases. Ann Intern Med 1984; 100:115–121.

169. Sisam DA, Sheehan JP, Sheeler LR. The natural history of untreated microadenomas. Fertil Steril 1987; 48:67–71.

170. Zervas NT. Surgical results for pituitary adenomas: results of an international survey. In: Black PM, Zervas NT, Ridgway EC, et al, eds. Secretory Tumors of the Pituitary Gland. New York: Raven, 1984: 377–385.

171. Tucker HStG, Grubb SR, Wigand JP, et al. Galactorrhea-amenorrhea syndrome: follow-up of 45 patients after pituitary tumor removal. Ann Intern Med 1981; 94:302–307.

172. Faria MA Jr, Tindall GT. Transsphenoidal microsurgery for prolactin-secreting pituitary adenomas: results in 100 women with the amenorrhea-galactorrhea syndrome. J Neurosurg 1982; 56:33–43.

173. Hardy J. Transsphenoidal microsurgery of prolactinomas. In: Black PM, Zervas NT, Ridgway EC, et al, eds. Secretory Tumors of the Pituitary Gland. New York: Raven, 1984: 73–81.

174. Laws ER Jr, Ebersold MJ, Piepgras DG, et al. The role of surgery in the management of prolactinoma. In: MacLeod PM, Thorner MO, Scapagnini U, eds. Prolactin: Basic and Clinical Correlates. New York: Springer-Verlag, 1985: 849–853.

175. Webster J, Page MD, Bevan JS, et al. Low recurrence rate after partial hypophysectomy for prolactinoma: the predictive value of dynamic prolactin function tests. Clin Endocrinol 1992; 36:35–44.

176. Thomson JA, Davies DL, McLaren EH, et al. Ten-year follow-up of microprolactinoma treated by transsphenoidal surgery. BMJ 1994; 309:1409–1410.

177. Rodman EF, Molitch ME, Post KD, et al. Long-term follow-up of transsphenoidal selective adenomectomy for prolactinoma. JAMA 1984; 252:921–924.

178. Serri O, Rasio E, Beauregard H, et al. Recurrence of hyperprolactinemia after selective transsphenoidal adenomectomy in women with prolactinomas. N Engl J Med 1983; 309:280–283.

179. Parl FF, Cruz VE, Cobb CA, et al. Late recurrence of surgically removed prolactinomas. Cancer 1986; 57:2422–2426.

180. Schlechte JA, Sherman BM, Chapler FK, et al. Long-term follow-up of women with surgically treated prolactin-secreting pituitary tumors. J Clin Endocrinol Metab 1986; 62:1296–1301.

181. Ciccarelli E, Ghigo E, Miola C, et al. Long-term follow-up of "cured" prolactinoma patients after successful adenomectomy. Clin Endocrinol 1990; 32:583–592.

182. Frantz AG, Cogen PH, Chang CH, et al. Long-term evaluation of the results of transsphenoidal surgery and radiotherapy in patients with prolactinoma. In: Crosignani PG, Rubin BL, eds. Endocrinology of Human Infertility: New Aspects. New York: Grune & Stratton, 1981: 161–170.

183. Johnston DG, Hall K, Kendall-Taylor P, et al. The long-term effects of megavoltage radiotherapy as sole or combined therapy for large prolactinomas: studies with high definition computerized tomography. Clin Endocrinol 1986; 24:675–685.

184. Mehta AE, Reyes FI, Faiman C. Primary radiotherapy of prolactinomas: eight- to 15-year follow-up. Am J Med 1987; 83:49–58.

185. Friesen HG, Tolis G. The use of bromocriptine in the galactorrhea-amenorrhea syndromes: the Canadian cooperative study. Clin Endocrinol (Oxf) 1977; 6(Suppl):91s–99s.

186. Gemzell C, Wang CF. Outcome of pregnancy in women with pituitary adenoma. Fertil Steril 1979; 31:363–372.

187. Molitch ME. Pregnancy and the hyperprolactinemic woman. N Engl J Med 1985; 312:1364–1370.

188. Kleinberg DL, Boyd AE III, Wardlaw S, et al. Pergolide for the treatment of pituitary tumors secreting prolactin or growth hormone. N Engl J Med 1983; 309:704–709.

189. Lamberts SWJ, Quik RFP. A comparison of the efficacy and safety of pergolide and bromocriptine in the treatment of hyperprolactinemia. J Clin Endocrinol Metab 1991; 72:635–641.

190. Molitch ME, Elton RL, Blackwell RE et al. Bromocriptine as primary therapy for prolactin-secreting macroadenomas: results of a prospective multicenter study. J Clin Endocrinol Metab 1985; 60:698–705.

191. Bevan JS, Webster J, Burke CW, Scanlon MF. Dopamine agonists and pituitary tumor shrinkage. Endocr Rev 1992; 13:220–240.

192. Kupersmith MJ, Kleinberg D, Warren FA, et al. Growth of prolactinoma despite lowering of serum prolactin by bromocriptine. Neurosurgery 1989; 24:417–423.

193. Liuzzi A, Dalabonzana D, Oppizzi G, et al. Low doses of dopamine agonists

in the long-term treatment of macroprolactinomas. N Engl J Med 1985; 313:656–659.

194. Johnston DG, Hall K, Kendall-Taylor P, et al. Effect of dopamine agonist withdrawal after long-term therapy in prolactinomas. Lancet 1984; 2:187–192.

195. Moriondo P, Travaglini P, Nissim M, et al. Bromocriptine treatment of microprolactinomas: evidence of stable prolactin decrease after drug withdrawal. J Clin Endocrinol Metab 1985; 60:762–772.

196. van't Verlaat JW, Croughs RJM. Withdrawal of bromocriptine after long-term therapy for macroprolactinomas; effect on plasma prolactin and tumour size. Clin Endocrinol 1991; 34:175–178.

197. Faglia G. Should dopamine agonist treatment for prolactinomas be lifelong? Clin Endocrinol 1991; 34:173–174.

198. Montini M, Pagani G, Giànola D, et al. Long-lasting suppression of prolactin secretion and rapid shrinkage of prolactinomas after a long-acting, injectable form of bromocriptine. J Clin Endocrinol Metab 1986; 63:266–268.

199. Grossman A, Ross R, Wass JAH, et al. Depot-bromocriptine treatment for prolactinomas and acromegaly. Clin Endocrinol 1986; 24:231–238.

200. Benker G, Gieshoff B, Freundlieb O, et al. Parenteral bromocriptine in the treatment of hormonally active pituitary tumours. Clin Endocrinol 1986; 24:505–513.

201. Schettini G, Lombardi G, Merola B, et al. Rapid and long-lasting suppression of prolactin secretion and shrinkage of prolactinomas after injection of long-acting repeatable form of bromocriptine (Parlodel LAR). Clin Endocrinol 1990; 33:161–169.

202. Pagani MD, Tengattini F, Montini M, et al. Efficacy of a new long-acting injectable form of bromocriptine in hyperprolactinaemic patients. Clin Endocrinol 1992; 36:369–374.

203. Webster J, Piscitelli G, Polli A, et al. Dose-dependent suppression of serum prolactin by cabergoline in hyperprolactinaemia: a placebo controlled, double blind, multicentre study. Clin Endocrinol 1992; 37:534–541.

204. Serri O, Beauregard H, Lesage J, et al. Long term treatment with CV 205-502 in patients with prolactin-secreting pituitary macroadenomas. J Clin Endocrinol Metab 1990; 71:682–687.

205. Duranteau L, Chanson P, Lavoinne A, et al. Effect of the new dopaminergic agonist CV 205-502 on plasma prolactin levels and tumour size in bromocriptine-resistant prolactinomas. Clin Endocrinol 1991; 34:25–29.

206. Shoham Z, Homburg R, Jacobs HS. CV 205-502: effectiveness, tolerability, and safety over 24-month study. Fertil Steril 1991; 55:501–506.

207. van der Lely AJ, Brownell J, Lamberts SWJ. The efficacy and tolerability of CV 205-502 (a nonergot dopaminergic drug) in macroprolactinoma patients and in prolactinoma patients intolerant to bromocriptine. J Clin Endocrinol Metab 1991; 72:1136–1141.

208. Murphy FY, Vesely DL, Jordan RM, et al. Giant invasive prolactinomas. Am J Med 1987; 83:995–1002.

209. Fahlbusch R, Buchfelder M, Schrell U. Short-term preoperative treatment of macroprolactinomas by dopamine agonists. J Neurosurg 1987; 67:807–815.

210. Juri J. Mammary asymmetry: A brief classification. Aesth Plast Surg 1989; 13:47–53.

211. Rosenberg CA, Derman GH, Grabb WC, et al. Hypomastia and mitral-valve prolapse: evidence of a linked embryologic and mesenchymal dysplasia. N Engl J Med 1983; 309:1230–1232.

212. Pierre ML, Jouglard J-P. Treatment of unilateral congenital hypoplasia or absence of the breast. Plast Reconstr Surg 1975; 56:146–151.

213. Mayl N, Vasconez LO, Jurkiewicz MJ. Treatment of macromastia in the actively enlarging breast. Plast Reconstr Surg 1974; 54:6–12.

214. Strombeck JO. Types of macromastia. Acta Chir Scand Suppl 1964; 341:37–39.

215. Fisher W, Smith JW. Macromastia during puberty. Plast Reconstr Surg 1971; 47:445–451.

216. Hollingsworth DR, Archer R. Massive virginal breast hypertrophy at puberty. Am J Dis Child 1973; 125:293–295.

217. Sperling RL, Gold JJ. Use of an anti-estrogen after a reduction mammaplasty to prevent recurrence of virginal hypertrophy of breasts. Plast Reconstr Surg 1973; 52:439–442.

218. de Castro CC, Subcutaneous mastectomy for gigantomastia in an adolescent girl. Plast Reconstr Surg 1977; 59:575–578.

219. Gliosci A, Presutti F. Virginal gigantomastia: validity of combined surgical and hormonal treatments. Aesth Plast Surg 1993; 17:61–65.

220. Burslem RW, Dewhurst CJ. Massive hypertrophy of the breasts in pregnancy. J Obstet Gynaecol Br Emp 1952; 59:380–381.

221. Williams PC. Massive hypertrophy of the breasts and axillary breasts in successive pregnancies. Am J Obstet Gynecol 1957; 74:1326–1329.

222. Blaydes RM, Kinnebrew CA. Massive breast hyperplasia complicating pregnancy. Obstet Gynecol 1958; 12:601–602.

223. Lewison EF, Jones GS, Trimble FH, et al. Gigantomastia complicating pregnancy. Surg Gynecol Obstet 1960; 110:215–223.

224. Nolan JJ. Gigantomastia. Obstet Gynecol 1962; 19:526–529.

225. Greeley PW, Robertson LE, Curtin JW. Mastoplasty for massive bilateral benign breast hypertrophy associated with pregnancy. Ann Surg 1965; 162:1081–1083.

226. Miller CJ, Becker DW Jr. Management of first trimester breast enlargement with necrosis. Plast Reconstr Surg 1979; 63:383–386.

227. Lafreniere R, Temple W, Ketcham A. Gestational macromastia. Am J Surg 1984; 148:413–418.

228. Ryan RF, Pernoll ML. Virginal hypertrophy. Plast Reconstr Surg 1985; 75:737–742.

229. Eben F, Cameron MD, Lowy C. Successful treatment of mammary hyperplasia in pregnancy with bromocriptine. Br J Obstet Gynecol 1993; 100:95–98.

230. Desai SN. Sudden gigantism of breasts: drug induced? Br J Plast Surg 1973; 26:371–372.

231. Passas C, Weinstein A. Breast gigantism with penicillamine therapy. Arthritis Rheum 1978; 21:167–168.

232. Thew DCN, Stewart IM. DPenicillamine and breast enlargement. Ann Rheum Dis 1980; 39:200.

233. Taylor PJ, Cumming DC, Corenblum B. Successful treatment of D-penicillamine-induced breast gigantism with danazol. Br Med J 1981; 282:362–363.

234. Rooney PJ, Cleland J. Successful treatment of D-penicillamine-induced breast gigantism with danazol. Br Med J 1981; 282:1627–1628.

235. Finer N, Emery P, Hicks BH. Mammary gigantism and D-penicillamine. Clin Endocrinol 1984; 21:219–222.

236. Versaci AD. Reduction mammaplasty for moderate macromastia. Ann Plast Surg 1981; 6:253–260.

237. Ariyan S. Reduction mammaplasty with the nipple-areola carried on a single, narrow inferior pedicle. Ann Plast Surg 1980; 5:167–177.

238. Boyce SW, Hoffman PG Jr, Mathes SJ. Recurrent macromastia after subcutaneous mastectomy. Ann Plast Surg 1984; 13:511–518.

239. Preece PE, Mansel RE, Bolton PM, et al. Clinical syndromes of mastalgia. Lancet 1976; 2:670–673.

240. Dowle CS. Breast pain: Classification, aetiology and management. Aust NZ J Surg 1987; 57:423–428.

241. Wetzig NR. Mastalgia: a 3 year Australian study. Aust NZ J Surg 1994; 64:329–331.

242. Pye JK, Mansel RE, Hughes LE. Clinical experience of drug treatments for mastalgia. Lancet 1985; 2:373–377.

243. Mansel RE, Dogliotti L. European multicentre trial of bromocriptine in cyclical mastalgia. Lancet 1990; 335:190–193.

244. Hinton CP, Bishop HM, Holliday HW, et al. A double-blind controlled trial of danazol and bromocriptine in the management of severe cyclical breast pain. Br J Clin Pract 1986; 40:326–330.

245. Mansel RE, Wisbey JR, Hughes LE. Controlled trial of the antigonadotropin danazol in painful nodular benign breast disease. Lancet 1982; 1:928–930.

246. Fentiman IS, Caleffi M, Hamed H, et al. Dosage and duration of tamoxifen treatment for mastalgia: a controlled trial. Br J Surg 1988; 75:845–846.

247. Maddox PR. The management of mastalgia in the UK. Horm Res 1989; 32(suppl 1):21–27.

248. Williams MJ. Gynecomastia: its incidence, recognition and host characterization in 447 autopsy cases. Am J Med 1963; 34:103–112.

249. Nuttall FQ. Gynecomastia as a physical finding in normal men. J Clin Endocrinol Metab 1979; 48:338–340.

250. Niewoehner CB, Nuttall FQ. Gynecomastia in a hospitalized male population. Am J Med 1984; 77:633–638.

251. Ley SB, Mozaffarian GA, Leonard JM, et al. Palpable breast tissue versus gynecomastia as a normal physical finding. Clin Res 1980; 28:24A.

252. Georgiadis E, Papandreou L, Evangelopoulou C, et al. Incidence of gynaecomastia in 954 young males and its relationship to somatometric parameters. Ann Hum Biol 1994; 21:579–587.

253. Friedman PJ. Gynecomastia in a hospitalized male population. Am J Med 1985; 78:A40–A43.

254. Andersen JA, Gram JB. Male breast at autopsy. Acta Pathol Microbiol Immunol Scand A 1982; 90:191–197.

255. Sandison AT. An autopsy study of the adult human breast. Natl Cancer Inst Monogr 1962; 8:77–80.

256. Cooper RA, Gunter BA, Ramamurthy L. Mammography in men. Radiology 1994; 191:651–656.

257. Chantra PK, So GJ, Wollman JS, et al. Mammography of the male breast. AJR 1995; 164:853–858.

258. Wigley KD, Thomas JL, Bernardino ME, et al. Sonography of gynecomastia. AJR 1981; 136:927–930.

259. Jackson VP, Gilmore RL. Male breast carcinoma and gynecomastia: comparison of mammography with sonography. Radiology 1986; 149:533–536.

260. Nicolis GL, Modlinger RS, Gabrilove JL. A study of the histopathology of human gynecomastia. J Clin Endocrinol Metab 1971; 32:173–178.

261. Bannayan GA, Hajdu SI. Gynecomastia: clinicopathologic study of 351 cases. Am J Clin Pathol 1972; 57:431–437.

262. Anderson JA, Gram JB. Gynecomastia: histological aspects in a surgical material. Acta Pathol Microbiol Immunol Scand A 1982; 90:185–190.

263. Lewin ML. Gynecomastia: the hypertrophy of the male breast. J Clin Endocrinol Metab 1941; 1:511–514.

264. Gabrilove JL. Some recent advances in virilizing and feminizing syndromes and hirsutism. Mt Sinai J Med 1974; 41:636–654.

265. Wilson JD, Aiman J, MacDonald PC. The pathogenesis of gynecomastia. Adv Intern Med 1980; 25:1–32.

266. Bercovici JP, Maudelonde T. Physiologie et physiopathologie du développement mammaire chez l'homme. Ann Endocrinol (Paris) 1982; 43:221–245.

267. von Werder K. Diagnostisches vorgehen bei Gynakomastie. Dtsch Med Wochenschr 1988; 113:776–778.

268. Carlson JE. Gynecomastia. N Engl J Med 1980; 303:795–799.

269. Wilson JD. Metabolism of testicular androgens. In: Greep RO, Astwood

EB, eds. Handbook of Physiology. Sect. 7: Endocrinology. Vol V. Male Reproductive System. Washington, DC: American Physiological Society, 1975: 491–508.

270. Smith EP, Boyd J, Frank GR, et al. Estrogen resistance caused by a mutation in the estrogen-receptor gene in a man. N Engl J Med 1994; 331:1056–1061.

271. Morishima A, Grumbach MM, Simpson ER, et al. Aromatase deficiency in male and female siblings caused by a novel mutation and the physiological role of estrogens. J Clin Endocrinol Metab 1995; 80:3689–3698.

272. Keenas BS, Richards GE, Ponder SW, et al. Androgen-stimulated pubertal growth: the effects of testosterone and dihydrotestosterone on growth hormone and insulin-like growth factor-I in the treatment of short stature and delayed puberty. J Clin Endocrinol Metab 1993; 76:996–1001.

273. Bagatell CJ, Dahl KD, Bremner WJ. The direct pituitary effect of testosterone to inhibit gonadotropin secretion in men is partially mediated by aromatization to estradiol. J Androl 1994; 15:15–21.

274. Bhatnagar AS, Muller P, Schenkel L, et al. Inhibition of estrogen biosynthesis and its consequences on gonadotrophin secretion in the male. J Steroid Biochem Mol Biol 1992; 41:437–443.

275. Bagatell CJ, Knopp RH, Rivier JE, et al. Physiological levels of estradiol stimulate plasma high density lipoprotein$_2$ cholesterol levels in normal men. J Clin Endocrinol Metab 1994; 78:855–861.

276. Siiteri PK, MacDonald PC. Role of extraglandular estrogen in human endocrinology. In: Greep RO, Astwood EB, eds. Handbook of Physiology. Sect. 7: Endocrinology. Vol II. Female Reproductive System. Part 1. Washington, DC: American Physiological Society, 1975: 615–629.

277. Kelch RP, Jenner MR, Weinstein R, et al. Estradiol and testosterone secretion by human, simian and canine testes in males with hypogonadism and in male pseudohermaphrodites with the feminizing testis syndrome. J Clin Invest 1972; 51:824–830.

278. Weinstein RL, Kelch RP, Jenner MR, et al. Secretion of unconjugated androgens and estrogens by the normal and abnormal human testis before and after human chorionic gonadotropin. J Clin Invest 1974; 53:1–6.

279. Payne AH, Kelch RP, Musich SS, et al. Intratesticular site of aromatization in the human. J Clin Endocrinol Metab 1976; 42:1081–1087.

280. Simpson ER, Mahendroo MS, Nichols JE, et al. Aromatase gene expression in adipose tissue: relationship to breast cancer. Int J Fertil Menopausal Stud 1994; 39(Suppl 2):75–83.

281. Rajendran KG, Shah PN, Bagli NP, et al. Oestradiol receptors in non-neoplastic gynaecomastic tissue of phenotypic males. Horm Res 1976; 7:193–200.

282. Poulsen HS, Hermansen C, Andersen A, et al. Gynecomasty: estrogen and androgen receptors. A clinical-pathological investigation. Acta Pathol Microbiol Immunol Scand A 1985; 93:229–233.

283. Pacheco MM, Oshima CF, Lopes MP, et al. Steroid hormone receptors in male breast diseases. Anticancer Res 1986; 6:1013–1018.

284. Andersen J, Orntoft TF, Andersen JA, et al. Gynecomastia. Immunohistochemical demonstration of estrogen receptors. Acta Pathol Microbiol Immunol Scand A 1987; 95:263–267.

285. Klein KO, Baron J, Colli MJ, et al. Estrogen levels in childhood determined by an ulterasensitive recombinant cell bioassay. J Clin Invest 1994; 94:2475–2480.

286. McKiernan JF, Hudd D. Breast development in the newborn. Arch Dis Child 1981; 56:525–529.

287. Nydick M, Bustos J, Dale JD Jr, et al. Gynecomastia in adolescent boys. JAMA 1961; 178:449–454.

288. Harlan WR, Grillo GP, Cornoni-Huntley J, et al. Secondary sex characteristics of boys 12 to 17 years of age: the U.S. health examination survey. J Pediatr 1979; 95:293–297.

289. Marynick SP, Nisula BC, Pita JC Jr, et al. Persistent pubertal macromastia. J Clin Endocrinol Metab 1980; 50:128–130.

290. Castro-Magana M, Angulo M, Uy J. Male hypogonadism with gynecomastia caused by late-onset deficiency of testicular 17-ketosteroid reductase. N Engl J Med 1993; 328:1297–1301.

291. Bidlingmaier F, Knorr D. Plasma testosterone and estrogens in pubertal gynecomastia. Z Kinderheilkd 1973; 115:89–94.

292. Lee PA. The relationship of concentrations of serum hormones to pubertal gynecomastia. J Pediatr 1975; 86:212–215.

293. LaFranchi SH, Parlow AF, Lippe BM, et al. Pubertal gynecomastia and transient elevation of serum estradiol level. Am J Dis Child 1975; 129:927–931.

294. Eversmann T, Moito J, von Werder K. Testosteron- und Ostradiolspiegel bei der Gynäkomastie des Mannes. Klinische und endokrine Befunde bei Behandlung mit Tamoxifen. Dtsch Med Wochenschr 1984; 109:1678–1682.

295. Moore DC, Schlaepfer LV, Paunier L, et al. Hormonal changes during puberty: V. Transient pubertal gynecomastia: abnormal androgen-estrogen ratios. J Clin Endocrinol Metab 1984; 58:492–499.

296. Bulard J, Mowszkowicz I, Schaison G. Increased aromatase activity in pubic skin fibroblasts from patients with isolated gynecomastia. J Clin Endocrinol Metab 1987; 64:618–623.

297. Eversmann T, Buchner A, Bock L, et al. Diagnosis and medical treatment of gynecomastia in different endocrine and metabolic diseases. Acta Endocrinol 1983; 102:139–140.

298. Kirschner MA, Jacobs JB, Fraley EE. Bilateral anorchia with persistent testosterone production. N Engl J Med 1970; 289:240–244.

299. Edman CD, Winters AJ, Porter JC, et al. Embryonic testicular regression: a clinical spectrum of XY agonadal individuals. Obstet Gynecol 1977; 49:209–217.

300. Casey RW, Wilson JD. Antiestrogenic action of dihydrotestosterone in mouse breast: competition with estradiol for binding to the estrogen receptor. J Clin Invest 1984; 74:2272–2278.

301. Gordon DL, Krompotic E, Thomas W, et al. Pathological testicular findings in Klinefelter's syndrome: 47,XXY vs 46,XY/47,XXY. Arch Intern Med 1972; 130:726–729.

302. Paulsen CA, Gordon DL, Carpenter RW, et al. Klinefelter's syndrome and its variants: a hormonal and chromosomal study. Recent Prog Horm Res 1968; 24:321–363.

303. Becker KL, Hoffman DL, Albert A, et al. Klinefelter's syndrome: clinical and laboratory findings in 50 patients. Arch Intern Med 1966; 118:314–321.

304. Wang C, Baker HWG, Burger HG, et al. Hormonal studies in Klinefelter's syndrome. Clin Endocrinol 1975; 4:399–411.

305. Aiman J, Hemsell DL, Brenner PF, et al. Origin of estrogen in adolescents with Klinefelter syndrome and gynecomastia. J Androl 1981; 2:6.

306. Gabrilove JL, Freiberg EK, Thornton JC, et al. Effect of age on testicular function in patients with Klinefelter's syndrome. Clin Endocrinol 1979; 11:343–347.

307. Gabrilove JL, Freiberg EK, Nicolis GL. Testicular function in Klinefelter's syndrome. J Urol 1980; 124:825–826.

308. Salbenblatt JA, Bender BG, Puck MH, et al. Pituitary-gonadal function in Klinefelter syndrome before and during puberty. Pediatr Res 1985; 19:82–86.

309. Griffin JE, McPhaul MJ, Russell DW, et al. The androgen resistance syndromes: 5α-reductase 2 deficiency, testicular feminization, and related disorders. In: Scriver CR, Beaudet AL, Sly WS, et al., eds. The Metabolic and Molecular Bases of Inherited Disease. 7th ed. New York: McGraw-Hill, 1995: 2967–2998.

310. MacDonald PC, Madden JD, Brenner PF, et al. Origin of estrogen in normal men and in women with testicular feminization. J Clin Endocrinol Metab 1979; 49:905–916.

311. Wilson JD, Harrod MJ, Goldstein JL, et al. Familial incomplete male pseudohermaphroditism, type I: evidence for androgen resistance and variable clinical manifestations in a family with the Reifenstein syndrome. N Engl J Med 1974; 290:1097–1103.

312. Madden JD, Walsh PC, MacDonald PC, et al. Clinical and endocrinologic characterization of a patient with the syndrome of incomplete testicular feminization. J Clin Endocrinol Metab 1975; 40:751–760.

313. Martin F, Perheentupa J, Adlercreutz H. Plasma and urinary androgens and oestrogens in a pubertal boy with 3-β-hydroxysteroid dehydrogenase deficiency. J Steroid Biochem 1980; 13:197–201.

314. Imperato-McGinley J, Peterson RE, Stoller R, et al. Male pseudohermaphroditism secondary to 17β-hydroxysteroid dehydrogenase deficiency: gender role change with puberty. J Clin Endocrinol Metab 1979; 49:391–395.

315. Cavanah SF, Dons RF. Partial 3 beta-hydroxysteroid dehydrogenase deficiency presenting as new-onset gynecomastia in a eugonadal adult male. Metabolism 1993; 42:65–68.

316. Werner CA. Mumps orchitis and testicular atrophy: I. Occurrence. Ann Intern Med 1950; 32:1066–1074.

317. Riggs S, Sanford JP. Viral orchitis. N Engl J Med 1962; 266:990–993.

318. Werner CA. Mumps orchitis and testicular atrophy: II. A factor in male sterility. Ann Intern Med 1950; 32:1075–1086.

319. Petersdorf RF, Bennett IL Jr. Treatment of mumps orchitis with adrenal hormones: report of twenty-three cases with a note on hepatic involvement in mumps. Arch Intern Med 1957; 99:222–233.

320. Aiman J, Brenner PF, MacDonald PC. Androgen and estrogen production in elderly men with gynecomastia and testicular atrophy after mumps orchitis. J Clin Endocrinol Metab 1980; 50:380–386.

321. Nolten WE, Viosca SP, Korenman SG, et al. Association of elevated estradiol with remote testicular trauma in young fertile men. Fertil Steril 1994; 62:143–149.

322. Clarke BG, Shapiro S, Monroe RG. Myotonia atrophia with testicular atrophy. J Clin Endocrinol 1956; 16:1235–1244.

323. Cooper IS, Ryanson EA, Bailey AA, et al. The relation of spinal cord disease to gynecomastia and testicular atrophy. Staff Proc Mayo Clin 1950; 25:320–326.

324. Morely JE, Distiller LA, Sagel J, et al. Hormonal changes associated with testicular atrophy and gynaecomastia in patients with leprosy. Clin Endocrinol 1977; 6:299–303.

325. Rolston R, Mathews M, Taylor PM, et al. Hormone profile in lepromatous leprosy: a preliminary study. Int J Lepr 1981; 49:31–36.

326. Kannan V, Vijaya G. Endocrine testicular functions in leprosy. Horm Metab Res 1984; 16:146–150.

327. Nagel TC, Freinkel N, Bell RH, et al. Gynecomastia, prolactin, and other peptide hormones in patients undergoing chronic hemodialysis. J Clin Endocrinol Metab 1973; 36:428–432.

328. Sawin CT, Longcope C, Schmitt GW, et al. Blood levels of gonadotropins and gonadal hormones in gynecomastia associated with chronic hemodialysis. J Clin Endocrinol Metab 1973; 36:988–990.

329. Holdsworth S, Atkins RC, de Kretser DM. The pituitary testicular axis in men with chronic renal failure. N Engl J Med 1977; 296:1245–1249.

330. Schmitt GW, Shehadeh I, Sawin CT. Transient gynecomastia in chronic renal failure during chronic intermittent hemodialysis. Ann Intern Med 1968; 69:73–79.

331. Gupta D, Burdschu HD. Testosterone and its binding in the plasma of male subjects with chronic renal failure. Clin Chim Acta 1972; 36:479–484.

332. Maywood BT, Krumlowsky F, Hugh NE. Gynecomastia in the chronic renal dialysis patient: beware. Plast Reconstr Surg 1982; 69:41–44.

333. Vircburger MI, Prelevic GM, Peric LA, et al. Testosterone levels after bromocriptine treatment in patients undergoing long-term hemodialysis. J Androl 1985; 6:113–116.

334. Cochran JS, Walsh PC, Porter JC, et al. The endocrinology of human chorionic gonadotropin-secreting testicular tumors: new methods in diagnosis. J Urol 1975; 114:549–555.

335. Reznik Y, Rieu M, Kuhn JM, et al. Luteinizing hormone regulation by sex steroids in men with germinal and Leydig cell tumours. Clin Endocrinol 1993; 38:487–493.

336. Gabrilove JL, Nicholis GL, Mitty HA, et al. Feminizing interstitial cell tumor of the testis: personal observations and a review of the literature. Cancer 1975; 38:1184–1202.

337. Gabrilove JL, Freiberg EK, Leiter E, et al. Feminizing and non-feminizing Sertoli cell tumors. J Urol 1980; 123:757–767.

338. Perez C, Novoa J, Alcaniz J, et al. Leydig cell tumour of the testis with gynaecomastia and elevated oestrogen, progesterone and prolactin levels: case report. Clin Endocrinol 1980; 13:409–412.

339. Bercovici JP, Nahoul K, Tate D, et al. Hormonal profile of Leydig cell tumors with gynecomastia. J Clin Endocrinol Metab 1984; 59:625–630.

340. Siegel SW, Thomas AJ Jr. Gynecomastia and Leydig cell tumors in the adult. Cleve Clin Q 1984; 51:395–399.

341. Mineur P, de Cooman S, Hustin J, et al. Feminizing testicular Leydig cell tumor: hormonal profile before and after unilateral orchidectomy. J Clin Endocrinol Metab 1987; 64:686–691.

342. Hendry WS, Garvie WHH, Ah-See AK, et al. Ultrasonic detection of occult testicular neoplasms in patients with gynaecomastia. Br J Radiol 1984; 57:571–572.

343. Mellor SG, McCutchan JDS. Gynaecomastia and occult Leydig cell tumour of the testis. Br J Urol 1989; 63:420–422.

344. Coen P, Kulin H, Ballantine T, et al. An aromatase-producing sex-cord tumor resulting in prepubertal gynecomastia. N Engl J Med 1991; 324:317–322.

345. Kuhn JM, Mahoudeau JA, Billaud L, et al. Evaluation of diagnostic criteria for Leydig cell tumours in adult men revealed by gynaecomastia. Clin Endocrinol 1987; 26:407–416.

346. Berenszstein E, Belgorosky A, de Davila MT, et al. Testicular steroid biosynthesis in a boy with a large cell calcifying Sertoli cell tumor producing prepubertal gynecomastia. Steroids 1995; 60:220–225.

347. Whitcomb RW, Schimke RN, Kyner JL, et al. Endocrine studies in a male patient with choriocarcinoma and gynecomastia. Am J Med 1986; 81:917–920.

348. Forst T, Beyer J, Cordes U, et al. Gynaecomastia in a patient with a hCG producing giant cell carcinoma of the lung: case report. Exp Clin Endocrinol Diabetes 1995; 103:28–32.

349. Fairlamb D, Boesen E. Gynaecomastia associated with gonadotrophin-secreting carcinoma of the lung. Postgrad Med J 1977; 53:269–271.

350. Wurzel RS, Yamase HT, Nieh PT. Ectopic production of human chorionic gonadotropin by poorly differentiated transitional cell tumors of the urinary tract. J Urol 1987; 137:502–504.

351. Aiman J, Hemsell DL, MacDonald PC. Production and origin of estrogen in two true hermaphrodites. Am J Obstet Gynecol 1978; 132:401–409.

352. Bacon GE, Lowrey GH. Feminizing adrenal tumor in a six year old boy. J Clin Endocrinol 1965; 25:1403–1406.

353. Gabrilove JL, Nicolis GL, Hardsknecht RU, et al. Feminizing adrenocortical carcinoma in a man. Cancer 1975; 35:153–160.

354. Bhettay E, Bonnici F. Pure oestrogen-secreting feminizing adrenocortical adenoma. Arch Dis Child 1977; 52:241–243.

355. Gabrilove JL, Sharma DC, Wotiz HH, et al. Feminizing adrenocortical tumors in the male. Medicine (Baltimore) 1965; 44:37–79.

356. Desai MB, Kapadia SN. Feminizing adrenocortical tumors in male patients: adenoma versus carcinoma. J Urol 1988; 139:101–103.

357. Zayed A, Stock JL, Liepman MK, et al. Feminization as a result of both peripheral conversion of androgens and direct estrogen production from an adrenocortical carcinoma. J Endocrinol Invest 1994; 17:275–278.

358. Maclaren NK, Migeon CJ, Raiti S. Gynecomastia with congenital virilizing adrenal hyperplasia (11-β-hydroxylase deficiency). J Pediatr 1975; 86:579–581.

359. Kadair RG, Block MB, Katz FH, et al. "Masked" 21-hydroxylase deficiency of the adrenal presenting with gynecomastia and bilateral testicular masses. Am J Med 1977; 62:278–282.

360. Gabrilove JL, Nicolis GL, Sohval AR. Non-tumorous feminizing adrenogenital syndrome in the male subject. J Urol 1973; 110:710–713.

361. Boyar RM, Hellman L. Syndrome of benign nodular adrenal hyperplasia associated with feminization and hyperprolactinemia. Ann Intern Med 1974; 80:389–394.

362. Durand A, Roger M, Chaussain JL, et al. L'hyperplasie congénitale virilisante des surrenales par déficit en 11 beta-hydroxylase. Semin Hop Paris 1981; 57:1392–1397.

363. Frank-Raue K, Raue F, Korth-Schutz S, et al. Clinical features and diagnosis of mild 3-beta-hydroxysteroid dehydrogenase deficiency in men. Dtsch Med Wochenschr 1989; 114:331–334.

364. Kearns WM. Oral therapy of testicular deficiency. J Clin Endocrinol 1941; 1:126.

365. Cunningham GR, Silverman VE, Thornby J, et al. The potential for an androgen male contraceptive. J Clin Endocrinol Metab 1979; 49:520–526.

366. Huggins C. Endocrine substances in the treatment of cancers. JAMA 1949; 141:750.

367. Alen M, Reinila M, Vihko R. Response of serum hormones to androgen administration in power athletes. Med Sci Sports Exerc 1985; 17:354.

368. Alen M, Hakkinen K. Physical health and fitness of an elite bodybuilder during 1 year of self-administration of testosterone and anabolic steroids: a case study. Int J Sports Med 1985; 6:24.

369. Reyes RJ, Zicchi S, Hamed H, et al. Surgical correction of gynaecomastia in bodybuilders. Br J Clin Pract 1995; 49:177–179.

370. Gordon GG, Olivo J, Rafii F, et al. Conversion of androgens to estrogens in cirrhosis of the liver. J Clin Endocrinol Metab 1975; 40:1018–1026.

371. Edman DC, Hemsell DL, Brenner PF, et al. Extraglandular estrogen formation in subjects with cirrhosis. Gastroenterology 1975; 69:819.

372. Bahnsen M, Gluud C, Johnsen SG, et al. Pituitary-testicular function in patients with alcoholic cirrhosis of the liver. Eur J Clin Invest 1981; 11:473–479.

373. Olivo J, Gordon GG, Rafii F, et al. Estrogen metabolism in hyperthyroidism and in cirrhosis of the liver. Steroids 1975; 26:47–56.

374. Copenhagen Study Group for Liver Diseases. Testosterone treatment of men with alcoholic cirrhosis: a double-blind study. Hepatology 1986; 6:807–813.

375. Kew MC, Kirschner MA, Abrahams GE, et al. Mechanism of feminization in primary liver cancer. N Engl J Med 1977; 296:1084–1088.

376. Aabo K, Dimitro NV. Feminization in hepatocellular carcinoma corrected by chemotherapy: a case report. Med Pediatr Oncol 1980; 8:275–280.

377. Klatskin G, Saltin WT, Humm FD. Gynecomastia due to malnutrition. Am J Med Sci 1947; 213:19–30.

378. Zurbiran S, Gomez-Mont F. Endocrine disturbances in chronic human malnutrition. Vitam Horm 1953; 11:97–132.

379. Ashkar FW, Smoak WM, Gilson AJ, et al. Gynecomastia and mastoplasia in Graves' disease. Metabolism 1970; 19:946–951.

380. Becker KL, Winnacker JL, Matthews MJ, et al. Gynecomastia and hyperthyroidism: an endocrine and histological investigation. J Clin Endocrinol 1968; 28:227–285.

381. Becker KL, Matthews MJ, Higgins GA Jr, et al. Histologic evidence of gynecomastia in hyperthyroidism. Arch Pathol 1974; 98:257–260.

382. Chopra IJ, Tulchinsky D. States of estrogen-androgen balance in hyperthyroid men with Graves' disease. J Clin Endocrinol Metab 1974; 38:269–277.

383. Chopra IJ. Gonadal steroids and gonadotropins in hyperthyroidism. Med Clin North Am 1975; 59:1109–1121.

384. Bercovici JP, Mauvais-Jarvis P. Hyperthyroidism and gynecomastia: metabolic studies. J Clin Endocrinol Metab 1972; 35:671–677.

385. Chopra IJ, Abraham GE, Chopra N, et al. Alterations in circulating estradiol-17 in male patients with Graves' disease. N Engl J Med 1972; 286:124–129.

386. Southren AL, Olivo J, Gordon GG, et al. The conversion of androgens to estrogens in hyperthyroidism. J Clin Endocrinol Metab 1974; 38:207–214.

387. Hemsell DL, Edman CD, Marks JF, et al. Massive extraglandular aromatization of plasma androstenedione resulting in feminization of a prepubertal boy. J Clin Invest 1977; 60:455–464.

388. Berkowitz GD, Gerami A, Brown TR, et al. Familial gynecomastia with increased extraglandular aromatization of plasma carbon 19-steroid. J Clin Invest 1985; 75:1763–1769.

389. Wilson JD, Leshin M, George FW. The Sebright bantam chicken and the genetic control of extraglandular aromatase. Endocr Rev 1987; 8:363–376.

390. Hendrickson DA, Anderson WR. Diethylstilbesterol therapy: gynecomastia. JAMA 1970; 213:468.

391. Orentreich N, Durr NP. Mammogenesis in transsexuals. J Invest Dermatol 1974; 63:142–146.

392. Brandt NJ, Cohn J, Hiller M. Controlled trial of oral contraceptives in haemophilia. Scand J Haematol 1973; 11:225–229.

393. Beas F, Vargas L, Spada RP, et al. Pseudoprecocious puberty in infants caused by a dermal ointment containing estrogens. J Pediatr 1969; 75:127–130.

394. Landolt R, Murset G. Premature signs of puberty as late sequelae of unintentional estrogen administration. Schweiz Med Wochenschr 1968; 98:638–641.

395. Edidin DV, Levitsky LL. Prepubertal gynecomastia associated with estrogen-containing hair cream. Am J Dis Child 1982; 136:587–588.

396. Gabrilove JL, Luria M. Persistent gynecomastia resulting from scalp inunction of estradiol. Arch Dermatol 1978; 117:1672–1673.

397. Cimorra FA, Gonzalez-Peirona E, Ferrandez A. Percutaneous oestrogen-induced gynaecomastia: a case report. Br J Plast Surg 1982; 35:209–210.

398. Halperin DK, Sizonenko PC. Prepubertal gynecomastia following topical inunction of estrogen containing ointment. Helv Paediat Acta 1983; 38:361–366.

399. Gottswinter JM, Korth-Schutz S, Ziegler R. Gynecomastia caused by estrogen containing hair lotion. J Endocrinol Invest 1984; 7:383–386.

400. Schmidt KU, Wagner G, Mensing H. Ostrogen-induzierte gynakomastie nach anwendung ostrogenhaltiger lokaltherapeutika. Dtsch Med Wochenschr 1987; 112:926–928.

401. Harrington JM, Stein GF, Rivera RO, et al. The occupational hazards of formulating oral contraceptives: a survey of plant employees. Arch Environ Health 1978; 33:12–15.

402. Pacynski A, Budzynska A, Przylecki S. Hiperestrogenizm v pracownikow zakladow farmaceutyczaych i ich dzieci jako choroba zawodowa. Endokrynol Pol 1971; 22:149–154.

403. DeRaimondo CV, Roach AC, Meador CK. Gynecomastia from exposure to vaginal estrogen cream. N Engl J Med 1980; 302:1089–1090.

404. Moore N, Paux G, Noblet C, et al. Spouse-related drug side-effects. Lancet 1988; 1:137.

405. Abramowicz M. Estrogens in cosmetics. Med Lett 1985; 27:54–55.

406. Kimball AM, Hamadeh R, Mahmood RAH, et al. Gynaecomastia among children in Bahrain. Lancet 1981; 1:671–672.

407. Fara GM, Del Vorvo G, Bernuzzi S, et al. Epidemic of breast enlargement in an Italian school. Lancet 1979; 2:295–297.

408. Sundlof SF, Strickland C. Zearalenone and zeranol: potential residue problems in livestock. Vet Hum Toxicol 1986; 28:242–250.

409. Henricks DM, Gray SL, Hoover JLB. Residue levels of endogenous estrogens in beef tissues. J Anim Sci 1983; 57:247–255.

410. Verdeal K, Ryan DS. Naturally-occurring estrogens in plant foodstuffs: a review. J Food Protect 1979; 42:577–583.

411. Katzenellenbogen BS, Katzenellenbogen JA, Fordecai D. Zearalenones: characterization of the estrogenic potencies and receptor interactions of a series of fungal β-resorcylic acid lactones. Endocrinology 1979; 105:33–40.

412. Herman C, Adlercreutz T, Goldin BR, et al. Soybean phytoestrogen intake and cancer risk. J Nutr 1995; 757S–770S.

413. Adlercreutz H, Markkanen H, Watanabe S. Plasma concentrations of phytooestrogens in Japanese men. Lancet 1993; 342:1209–1210.

414. LeWinn EB. Gynecomastia during digitalis therapy. N Engl J Med 1953; 248:316–320.

415. Wolfe CJ. Gynecomastia following digitalis administration. J Fla Med Assoc 1975; 62:54–55.

416. Murray NP, Daly MJ. Gynaecomastia and heart failure: adverse drug reaction or disease process? J Clin Pharm Ther 1991; 16:275–279.

417. Navab A, Koss LG, LaDue JS. Estrogen-like activity of digitalis: its effect on the squamous epithelium of the female genital tract. JAMA 1965; 194:30–32.

418. Kley HK, Abendroth H, Hehrmann R, et al. Kein Einfluss von Digitalis auf Sexual- und Nebennierenrindenhormone bei gesunden Probanden und bein Patienten mit Herzinsuffizienz. Klin Wochenschr 1984; 62:65–73.

419. Rifka SM, Pita JC, Vigersky RA, et al. Interaction of digitalis and spironolactone with human sex steroid receptors. J Clin Endocrinol Metab 1977; 46:338–344.

420. Ricken K. The estrogenic potency of digitalis glycosides. Naunyn Schmiedebergs Arch Pharmacol 1975; 287(Suppl):25.

421. Maddock WO, Nelson WO. The effects of chorionic gonadotropin in adult men: increased estrogen and 17-ketosteroid excretion, gynecomastia, Leydig cell stimulation and seminiferous tubule damage. J Clin Endocrinol Metab 1952; 12:985–1014.

422. Lee PA. The occurrence of gynecomastia upon withdrawal of clomiphene citrate treatment for idiopathic oligospermia. Fertil Steril 1980; 34:285–286.

423. Feldman D. Ketoconazole and other imidazole derivatives as inhibitors of steroidogenesis. Endocr Rev 1986; 7:409–420.

424. Grosso DS, Boyden TW, Parmenter RW, et al. Ketoconazole inhibition of testicular secretion of testosterone and displacement of steroid hormones from serum transport proteins. Antimicrob Agents Chemother 1983; 23:207–212.

425. Fagan TC, Johnson DG, Grosso DS. Metronidazole-induced gynecomastia. JAMA 1985; 254:3217.

426. DeFelice R, Johnson DG, Galgiani JN. Gynecomastia with ketoconazole. Antimicrob Agents Chemother 1981; 19:1073–1074.

427. Pont A, Goldman ES, Sugar AM, et al. Ketoconazole-induced increase in estradiol-testosterone ratio. Arch Intern Med 1985; 145:1429–1431.

428. Whitehead E, Shalet SM, Blackledge G, et al. The effects of Hodgkin's disease and combination chemotherapy on gonadal function in the adult male. Cancer 1982; 49:418–422.

429. Trump DK, Pavy MD, Staal S. Gynecomastia in men following antineoplastic therapy. Arch Intern Med 1982; 142:511–513.

430. Turner AR, Morrish DW, Berry J, et al. Gynecomastia after cytotoxic therapy for metastatic testicular cancer. Arch Intern Med 1982; 142:896–897.

431. Saeter G, Fossa DK, Norman N. Gynaecomastia following cytotoxic therapy for testicular cancer. Br J Urol 1987; 59:348–352.

432. Jeunemaitre X, Chatellier G, Kreft-Jais C, et al. Efficacy and tolerance of spironolactone in essential hypertension. Am J Cardiol 1987; 60:820–825.

433. Loriaux DL, Menard R, Taylor A, et al. Spironolactone and endocrine dysfunction. Ann Intern Med 1976; 85:630–636.

434. Caminos-Torres R, Ma L, Snyder PJ. Gynecomastia and semen abnormalities induced by spironolactone in normal men. J Clin Endocrinol Metab 1977; 5:255–260.

435. Clark E. Spironolactone therapy and gynecomastia. JAMA 1965; 193:163–164.

436. De Gasparo M, Whitebread SE, Preiswerk G, et al. Antialdosterones: incidence and prevention of sexual side-effects. J Steroid Biochem 1989; 32:223–227.

437. DuPont A. Disappearance of spironolactone-induced gynaecomastia during treatment with potassium canrenoate. Lancet 1985; 2:731.

438. Geller J, Vazakas G, Fruchtman B, et al. The effect of cyproterone acetate on advanced carcinoma of the prostate. Surg Gynecol Obstet 1968; 127:748–758.

439. Caine M, Perlberg S, Gordon R. The treatment of benign prostatic hypertrophy with flutamide (SCH 13521): a placebo controlled study. J Urol 1975; 114:564–568.

440. Berger BM, Naadimuthu A, Boddy A, et al. The effect of zanoterone, a steroidal androgen receptor antagonist, in men with benign prostatic hyperplasia: the Zanoterone Study Group. J Urol 1995; 154:1060–1064.

441. Verhelst J, Denis L, Van Vliet P, et al. Endocrine profiles during administration of the new non-steroidal anti-androgen Casodex in prostate cancer. Clin Endocrinol 1994; 41:525–530.

442. Hall WH. Breast changes in males on cimetidine. N Engl J Med 1976; 295:841.

443. Funder JW, Mercer JE. Cimetidine occupies androgen receptors. J Clin Endocrinol Metab 1979; 48:189–191.

444. Sultan C, Terraza A, Descomps B, et al. Cimetidine competition with androgens for binding to human sex skin fibroblast androgen receptors. J Steroid Biochem 1980; 13:839–840.

445. Rodriguez LAG, Jick H. Risk of gynaecomastia associated with cimetidine, omeprazole, and other iantiulcer drugs. Br Med J 1994; 308:503–506.

446. Jensen RT, Collen MJ, Pandol SJ, et al. Cimetidine-induced impotence and breast changes in patients with gastric hypersecretory states. N Engl J Med 1983; 308:883–887.

447. Galbraith RA, Michnovicz JJ. The effects of cimetidine on the oxidative metabolism of estradiol. N Engl J Med 1989; 321:269–274.

448. Mignon M, Vallor TH, Mayeur S, et al. Ranitidine and cimetidine in Zollinger-Ellison syndrome. Br J Clin Pharmacol 1980; 10:173–174.

449. Allende HD, Collen MJ, Pandol SJ, et al. Cimetidine-induced impotence and gynecomastia: reversal with ranitidine. Gastroenterology 1982; 82:1007.

450. CDC. Gynecomastia in Haitians: Puerto Rico, Florida, Texas, New York. MMWR Morb Mortal Wkly Rep 1982; 31:205–206.

451. Brody SA, Winters J, Down MA, et al. An epidemic of gynecomastia among Haitian refugees: possible exposure to anti-androgen. Endocr Soc Abstr 1983; 724.

452. Malozowski S, Stadel BV. Prepubertal gynecomastia during growth hormone therapy. J Pediatr 1995; 126:659–661.

453. Cohn L, Feller AG, Draper MW, et al. Carpal tunnel syndrome and gynecomastia during growth hormone treatment of elderly men with low circulating IGF-I concentrations. Clin Endocrinol 1993; 39:417–425.

454. Markusse HM, Meyboom RHB. Gynaecomastia associated with captopril. Br Med J 1988; 296:1262–1263.

455. Tanner LA, Bosco LA. Gynecomastia associated with calcium channel blocker therapy. Arch Intern Med 1988; 148:379–380.

456. Bergman D, Futterweit W, Segal R, et al. Increased oestradiol in diazepam related gynaecomastia. Lancet 1981; 1:1225–1226.

457. Reid DM, Martynoga AG, Nuki G. Reversible gynaecomastia associated with D-penicillamine in a man with rheumatoid arthritis. Br Med J 1982; 285:1083–1084.

458. Lindquist M, Edwards IR. Endocrine adverse effects of ameprazole. Br Med J 1992; 305:451–452.

459. Boyd IW. Gynaecomastia in association with calcium antagonists. Med J Aust 1994; 161:328.

460. Llop R, Gomez-Farran F, Figueras A, et al. Gynecomastia associated with enalapril and diazepam. Ann Pharmacother 1994; 28:671–672.

461. Mendelson JH, Kuehnle J, Ellingboe J, et al. Plasma testosterone levels before, during and after chronic marijuana smoking. N Engl J Med 1974; 291:1051–1055.

462. Harmon JW, Aliapoulios MA. Marijuana-induced gynecomastia: clinical and laboratory experience. Surg Forum 1974; 25:423–425.

463. Cicero TJ, Bell RD, Wiest WG, et al. Function of the male sex organs in heroin and methadone users. N Engl J Med 1975; 292:882–887.

464. Mendelson JH, Mendelson JE, Patch VD. Plasma testosterone levels in heroin addiction and during methadone maintenance. J Pharmacol Exp Ther 1975; 192:211–217.

465. Sirtori C, Veronesi U. Gynecomastia: a review of 218 cases. Cancer 1957; 10:645–654.

466. Bannayan GA, Hajdu SI. Gynecomastia: clinicopathologic study of 351 cases. Am J Clin Pathol 1972; 57:431–437.

467. McFadyen IJ, Bolton AE, Camerson EHD, et al. Gonadal-pituitary hormone levels in gynaecomastia. Clin Endocrinol 1980; 13:77–86.

468. Turkington RW. Serum prolactin levels in patients with gynecomastia. J Clin Endocrinol 1972; 34:62–66.

469. Frantz AG, Kleinberg DL, Noel GL. Studies on prolactin in man. Recent Prog Horm Res 1972; 82:527–590.

470. Large DM, Anderson DC, Laing I. Twenty-four hour profiles of serum prolactin during male puberty with and without gynaecomastia. Clin Endocrinol 1980; 12:293–302.

471. Beck W. Normoprolactinemia in boys with marked gynecomastia. Eur J Pediatr 1981; 137:41–44.

472. Besser GM, Parke L, Edwards CRW, et al. Galactorrhoea: successful treatment with reduction of plasma prolactin levels by brom-ergocriptine. Br Med J 1972; 3:669–672.

473. Thorner MO, McNeilly AS, Hagan C, et al. Long-term treatment of galactorrhoea and hypogonadism with bromocriptine. Br Med J 1974; 2:419–422.

TABLE 18–1. Estimated Number of Couples Using Birth Control, Worldwide, by Method, 1970, 1977, and 1984

Method	1970 (Millions)	1977 (Millions)	1984 (Millions)
Voluntary sterilization	20	80	137
Oral contraception	30	55	55
Condom	25	35	37
Intrauterine device (IUD)	12	15	70
Other methods*	60	65	26
Total	147	250	325
Abortion (annual incidence)	40	40	—

* Barrier and natural family-planning methods.
Adapted from Hammerstein J. Contraception: an overview. Am J Obstet Gynecol 1987; 57:1020–1023, with permission.

ization; 26% used oral contraceptives; 13% used condoms; 8% used intrauterine devices (IUDs) or diaphragms; and 21% used other methods (Fig. 18–2).[4]

FERTILITY CONTROL IN WOMEN

The various methods of fertility control for women and their primary targets in the body are depicted in Figure 18–3. These methods include (1) hormonal contraceptives, (2) intrauterine devices (IUDs), (3) barrier methods, (4) natural family-planning methods, (5) immunologic techniques, (6) sterilization, and (7) abortion.

Hormonal Contraceptives

Steroidal Contraceptives

ORAL CONTRACEPTIVES

Background

In 1928 Fellner demonstrated that estrogen extracts were effective contraceptives in rodents.[5] Further development of steroids as contraceptive agents awaited the purification and crystallization of estrogen[6, 7] and progesterone.[8]

Sturgis and Albright[9] observed that the injection of estradiol benzoate caused improvement in dysmenorrhea by inhibiting ovulation. Subsequently, chemical modifications of estrogens resulted in the production of orally active estrogens—ethinyl estradiol and the 3-methyl ether of ethinyl estradiol,

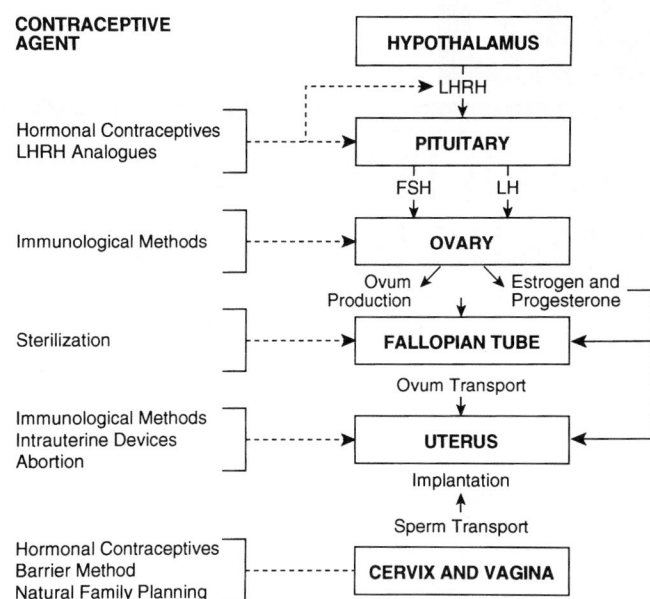

Figure 18–3. Principal sites of action of various contraceptives on the female reproductive tract.

mestranol. Removal of the C-19 methyl group from testosterone (19-nortestosterone) reduces its androgenicity, and the orally active derivative of this compound with an ethinyl group at C-17 was shown to be a potent progestagen. These discoveries led to the first clinical trials of oral contraceptives by Pincus and colleagues.[10]

Pharmacology

STRUCTURE. The two estrogens in oral contraceptive agents are ethinyl estradiol and mestranol. In addition, seven synthetic progestagens are utilized in oral contraceptives in the United States: norethindrone, norethynodrel, norethindrone acetate, ethynodiol diacetate, norgestrel (D,L-norgestrel or D-levonorgestrel), desogestrel, and norgestimate (Fig. 18–4).[11] Additional progestagens (gestodene, lynestrenol, and cyproterone acetate) are used in oral contraceptives marketed in Western Europe.

FORMULATIONS. At present, four types of oral contraceptive preparations are available in the United States (Table 18–2). These include fixed-combination oral contraceptive pills in which the estrogen and progestagen composition remains constant throughout therapy; biphasic and triphasic oral contraceptive pills in which the estrogen composition remains constant or varies slightly but the progestagen composition varies markedly during the cycle; and progestagen-only contraceptive pills. The fixed-combination pills are the most widely utilized form of oral contraceptives and are the principal source of information regarding side effects. Because of potential dose-related side effects the hormonal content of oral contraceptives has declined since their introduction. At present the maximal dose of estrogen in oral contraceptives is 50 μg, and the maximal dose of progestagen is 1.0 mg. The effectiveness of all combination oral contraceptives is similar (theoretically greater than 99%) but is somewhat less for the progestagen-only (mini) pills.[12] The biphasic and triphasic oral contraceptives allow for lower doses of progestagen during the early part of the cycle, thus reducing the total dose compared with fixed-combination oral contraceptives. The progestagen-only pill is used by relatively few women. The three brands available contain either 0.35 mg of norethindrone or 0.075 mg of norgestrel per tablet and are taken daily on a continual

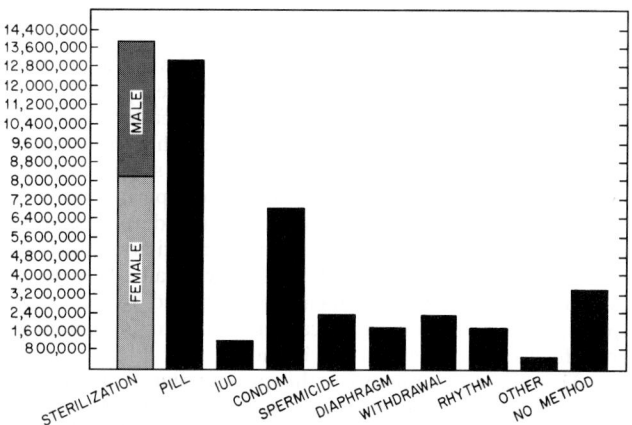

Figure 18–2. Contraceptive choices of U.S. couples aged 15 to 44 in 1988. (From Cunningham FG, Gant NF, MacDonald PC, eds. Contraceptive choices of U.S. couples aged 15 to 44 in 1988. Williams Obstetrics. 18th ed. Norwalk, CT: Appleton & Lange, 1989: 922, with permission.)

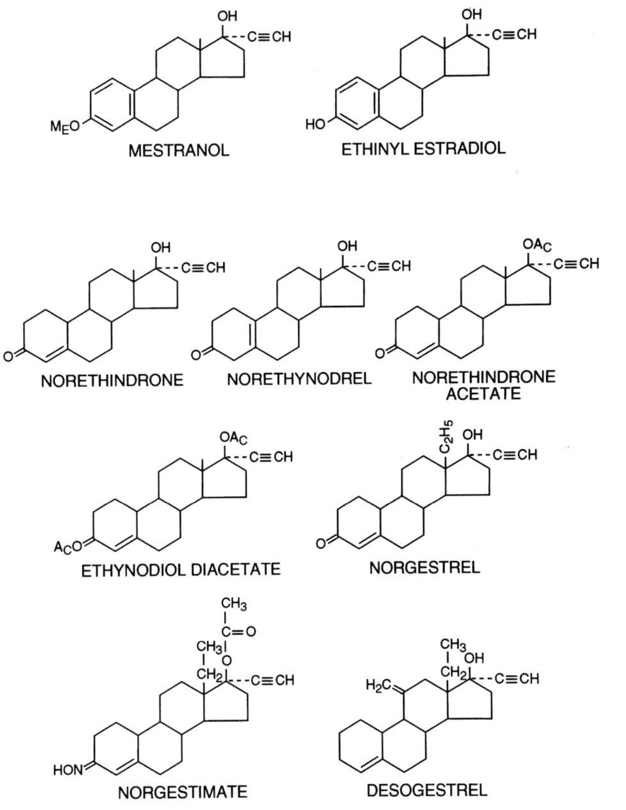

Figure 18–4. Structure of estrogens (A) and progestagens (B) that are available in oral contraceptive pills.

basis. The progestagen-only pill was developed in hopes of decreasing the risk of side effects that are thought to be due to the estrogen component of fixed-combination oral contraceptives.[13] Some workers have recommended that the progestagen-only pill should be the contraceptive agent of choice for women older than age 35; for women with headaches, hypertension, or varicose veins; and for lactating women.[14] However, the risk of hypertension, myocardial infarction, and stroke may be increased by the progestagen component of oral contraceptives rather than by the estrogen component.[15] Thus the absolute contraindications for the use of fixed-combination oral contraceptives may also pertain to the progestagen-only pill. However, the risk of developing significant side effects in women utilizing the progestagen-only pill is not known because of the lack of adequate long-term studies. The use of progestagen-only pills is associated with a slightly higher pregnancy rate owing to occasional failure to suppress ovulation.[14]

Sequential oral contraceptive pills involving the administration of estrogen alone for 2 wk followed by a combination of estrogen and a progestagen for 1 wk were previously available but were banned by the Food and Drug Administration after reports that these agents caused endometrial atypical hyperplasia and endometrial carcinoma.[16] Although no definite causal relationship between endometrial carcinoma and sequential oral contraceptives could be established, the morphologic changes in the endometrium associated with their use were believed to be due to the relatively low progestational activity; i.e., the progestational activity in sequential contraceptives was ineffective in protecting against the induction of hyperplasia by the estrogen component. In addition, sequential contraceptives were not as effective as the other oral contraceptive agents in preventing pregnancy.[17]

POTENCY. The biologic effects of the various synthetic

estrogens and progestagens alone and in combination oral contraceptive agents have been assessed in animal and human studies. Ethinyl estradiol is twice as potent as mestranol in its ability to produce vaginal keratinization in rats,[18] but in women there is little difference in potency between the two hormones.[19–21] Ethinyl estradiol is the estrogen in all estrogen-containing oral contraceptive agents that contain less than 50 µg of estrogen.

The progestagens in oral contraceptive agents do not possess all the properties of progesterone, and in addition they exhibit varying estrogenic and androgenic side effects. The most widely used means of assessing progestational potency of steroids is the Clauberg test,[22] in which immature female rabbits are primed with estrogen for 6 d and receive a test compound for 5 d; the uterus is then removed and evaluated by histologic grading. In this assay, norgestrel is the most potent progestagen.[23] These results, however, may not apply to humans. Attempts to assess progestational potency in women, including assessment of the delay of menses and histologic analysis of the glycogen deposition in endometrial glands, are difficult to interpret because of the use of different estrogens preceding progestagen administration and the failure to achieve parallel dose-response curves.[22–25]

Potency tables, which are based on delay of menses and glycogen deposition data, have been developed to aid in selecting the appropriate oral contraceptive pill for a particular patient.[26, 27] However, the interpretation of various progestational tests is difficult,[22, 25] and there does not appear to be a good correlation between potency scales and side effects.[28] A more rational approach to drug selection takes into account data from clinical trials of the incidence of specific serious adverse side effects with specific combinations of ethinyl estradiol and progestagens.

Metabolism

Mestranol and ethinyl estradiol are absorbed efficiently in the gastrointestinal tract, and up to 60% of an oral dose is excreted in urine after 24 h.[24] Mestranol is not physiologically active until it is converted to ethinyl estradiol. The latter is metabolized principally to glucuronides and sulfates. Peak levels of ethinyl estradiol in plasma are reached 1 h after oral administration, followed by an initial rapid decline and a second slower phase of decline. Approximately 3% of ethinyl estradiol remains in plasma 24 h after administration.[29] Norethindrone, norethynodrel, and norgestrel are rapidly absorbed, peak concentrations being reached 1 to 3 h after administration; peak levels of ethynodiol diacetate and norethindrone acetate are achieved somewhat later, because they may undergo deacylation in the gastrointestinal tract before absorption. Progestagen metabolism is more complex than that of estrogens, and more than 30 metabolites have been identified.[24] Small amounts of some progestagens may be metabolized to estrogens, but it is not known whether this is important clinically.[30]

Mechanism of Action

Steroid hormones in oral contraceptive pills act both within the central nervous system and in tissues of the urogenital tract to inhibit reproductive function. The principal site of action is at the level of the hypothalamus and pituitary to prevent the midcycle surge of luteinizing hormone (LH), and hence to prevent ovulation. The basal concentrations of LH and follicle-stimulating hormone (FSH) and plasma levels of estradiol and progesterone are suppressed in users of oral contraceptives, as shown in Figure 18–5.[31] This effect on basal concentrations of plasma gonadotropins is related to dose and time.[32, 33] The increase in plasma levels of gonadotropins after

TABLE 18–2. Composition of Oral Contraceptives

Name	Estrogen	µg	Progestagen	mg
Combination Type				
		Estrogen Content = 50 µg		
Ortho-Novum 1/50	Mestranol	50	Norethindrone	1.0
Norinyl 1 + 50	Mestranol	50	Norethindrone	1.0
Norethin 1/50M	Mestranol	50	Norethindrone	1.0
Ovcon-50	Ethinyl estradiol	50	Norethindrone	1.0
Ovral	Ethinyl estradiol	50	Norgestrel	0.5
Demulen 1/50	Ethinyl estradiol	50	Ethynodiol diacetate	1.0
		Estrogen Content < 50 µg		
Ortho-Novum 1/35	Ethinyl estradiol	35	Norethindrone	1.0
Norinyl 1 + 35	Ethinyl estradiol	35	Norethindrone	1.0
Norethin 1/35E	Ethinyl estradiol	35	Norethindrone	1.0
Modicon	Ethinyl estradiol	35	Norethindrone	0.5
Brevicon	Ethinyl estradiol	35	Norethindrone	0.5
Ovcon-35	Ethinyl estradiol	35	Norethindrone	0.4
Demulen 1/35	Ethinyl estradiol	35	Ethynodiol diacetate	1.0
Loestrin 1.5/30*	Ethinyl estradiol	30	Norethindrone acetate	1.5
Loestrin 1/20*	Ethinyl estradiol	20	Norethindrone acetate	1.0
Nordette	Ethinyl estradiol	30	Levonorgestrel	0.15
Levlen	Ethinyl estradiol	30	Levonorgestrel	0.15
Lo/Ovral	Ethinyl estradiol	30	Norgestrel	0.3
Desogen	Ethinyl estradiol	30	Desogestrel	0.15
Ortho-Cept	Ethinyl estradiol	30	Desogestrel	0.15
Ortho-Cyclen	Ethinyl estradiol	35	Norgestimate	0.25
Biphasic Type				
Ortho-Novum 10/11				
First 10 d	Ethinyl estradiol	35	Norethindrone	0.5
Next 11 d	Ethinyl estradiol	35	Norethindrone	1.0
Jenest-28				
First 7 d	Ethinyl estradiol	35	Norethindrone	0.5
Next 14 d	Ethinyl estradiol	35	Norethindrone	1.0
Triphasic Type				
Ortho-Novum 7/7/7				
First 7 d	Ethinyl estradiol	35	Norethindrone	0.5
Second 7 d	Ethinyl estradiol	35	Norethindrone	0.75
Third 7 d	Ethinyl estradiol	35	Norethindrone	1.0
Tri-Norinyl				
First 7 d	Ethinyl estradiol	35	Norethindrone	0.5
Next 9 d	Ethinyl estradiol	35	Norethindrone	1.0
Next 5 d	Ethinyl estradiol	35	Norethindrone	0.5
Ortho Tri-Cyclen				
First 7 d	Ethinyl estradiol	35	Norgestimate	0.18
Next 7 d	Ethinyl estradiol	35	Norgestimate	0.215
Next 7 d	Ethinyl estradiol	35	Norgestimate	0.25
Tri-Levlen				
First 6 d	Ethinyl estradiol	30	Levonorgestrel	0.05
Next 5 d	Ethinyl estradiol	40	Levonorgestrel	0.075
Next 10 d	Ethinyl estradiol	30	Levonorgestrel	0.125
Triphasil				
First 6 d	Ethinyl estradiol	30	Levonorgestrel	0.05
Next 5 d	Ethinyl estradiol	40	Levonorgestrel	0.075
Next 10 d	Ethinyl estradiol	30	Levonorgestrel	0.125
Progestagen Only				
Micronor	None		Norethindrone	0.35
Nor-Q.D.	None		Norethindrone	0.35
Ovrette	None		Norgestrel	0.075

* Also available with iron (Loestrin 1/20 Fe, Loestrin 1.5/30 Fe).

the administration of luteinizing hormone–releasing hormone (LHRH) is either normal[34] or slightly decreased.[35]

Follicular growth is inhibited, although the number of primary follicles is similar to that in control subjects.[32] Whether follicular atresia is increased by oral contraceptive pills is unclear, but the age at which menopause begins is not affected by previous oral contraceptive use.[32] Motility of the fallopian tubes, a process that is essential for the transport of the gametes before and after fertilization, is affected by estrogen and progestagen treatment in vitro.[36] The role of these effects on tubal motility in fertility control is unclear. Oral contraceptive agents cause glandular atrophy in uterine endometrium, induce a pseudodecidual reaction in the endometrial stroma, and cause formation of subnuclear vacuoles in

the endometrial endothelium throughout the menstrual cycle.[37] The hormonal effects on the endometrium may inhibit implantation of the blastocyst. In addition, oral contraceptives cause the formation of a thick cervical mucus that inhibits sperm motility and migration.[33]

Metabolic Effects

POTENTIAL RISKS. No contraceptive is 100% effective, and none is without risk. Oral contraceptives are usually effective, and their actions are usually reversible when treatment is stopped (Table 18–3). Furthermore, the incidence of potentially lethal side effects in oral contraceptive users (Table 18–4) may be less than the mortality risk resulting from preg-

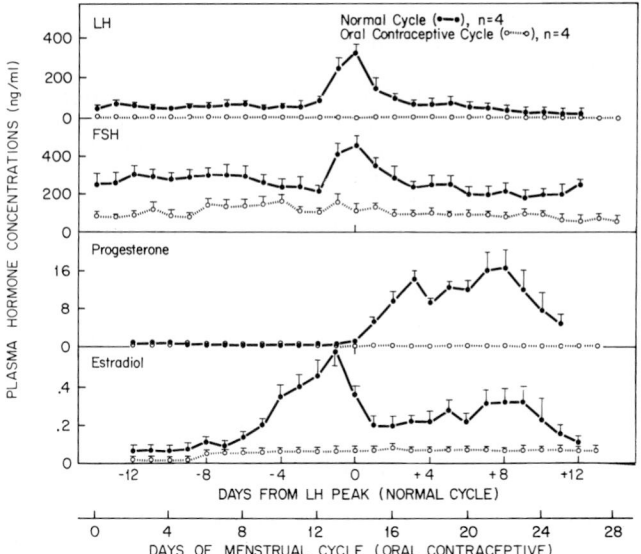

Figure 18–5. Plasma levels of gonadotropins, estradiol-17β, and progesterone during the ovarian cycles of four ovulatory women and four women treated with Norinyl 1 + 80. (From Carr BR, Parker CR Jr, Madden JD, et al. Plasma levels of adrenocorticotropin and cortisol in women receiving oral contraceptive steroid treatment. J Clin Endocrinol Metab 1979; 49:346–349. © 1979, by The Endocrine Society.)

nancy. The death rates from surgical procedures such as tubal sterilization (8 per 100,000 procedures) and hysterectomy (100 per 100,000 procedures) are higher than are death rates in young, nonsmoking oral contraceptive users.[38, 39]

Soon after the introduction of oral contraceptives, it was suggested that the use of these agents might be associated with serious cardiovascular side effects such as ischemic heart disease (myocardial infarction), thromboembolic disease, stroke, and hypertension. This issue has been analyzed in both retrospective, case-controlled studies and prospective, cohort studies. Such data are commonly expressed either as a relative risk (the ratio of the incidence of a disease among users to that among nonusers) or attributive risk (the difference in the incidence of disease between users and nonusers). The characteristics of three major cohort studies that began in 1968 are given in Table 18–5. The mortality rates for oral contraceptive users compared with those for nonusers may have declined in recent years.[12] For example, in the Royal College of General Practitioners Oral Contraceptive Study, the relative risk of mortality in current users was 4.7 in 1977[40] and 4.0 in 1981.[41] In the Oxford study the relative risk of mortality in 140,000 woman-years of observation was 2.5, which is not significantly different from that in nonusers.[42] In the Walnut Creek study involving more than 127,000 woman-years of observation, the relative risk of mortality from oral contraceptive use was 2.1, which again is not statistically significant.[43] In a prospective study by the Group Health Cooperative of Puget Sound, no deaths from cardiovascular disease were reported among oral contraceptive users between 1977 and 1988.[44] The apparent decrease in mortality rates for oral contraceptive users appears to be the consequence of (1) larger studies and more exact estimates, (2) increased use of agents that contain smaller amounts of estrogens, and (3) more extensive use of other methods of birth control in women in high-risk categories.[12] In the United States, the United Kingdom, Sweden, and Taiwan the overall death rates do not appear to reflect any deleterious effects of contraceptive use.[12]

Circulatory System

Ischemic Heart Disease (Myocardial Infarction). The incidence of myocardial infarction is rare in young women, in-

TABLE 18–3. Percentage of Women Experiencing a Contraceptive Failure During the First Year of Typical Use and the First Year of Perfect Use and the Percentage Continuing Use at the End of the First Year, United States

Method	% of Women Experiencing an Accidental Pregnancy within the First Year of Use		% of Women Continuing Use at One Year
	Typical Use	Perfect Use	
Chance[4]	85	85	
Spermicides[5]	21	6	43
Periodic abstinence	20		67
Calendar		9	
Ovulation method		3	
Symptothermal[6]		2	
Postovulation		1	
Withdrawal	19	4	
Cap[7]			
Parous women	36	26	45
Nulliparous women	18	9	58
Sponge			
Parous women	36	20	45
Nulliparous women	18	9	58
Diaphragm[7]	18	6	58
Condom[8]			
Female (Reality)	21	5	56
Male	12	3	63
Pill	3		72
Progestin only		0.5	
Combined		0.1	
Intrauterine device (IUD)			
Progesterone T	2.0	1.5	81
Copper T 380A	0.8	0.6	78
LNg 20	0.1	0.1	81
Depo-Provera	0.3	0.3	70
Norplant (6 capsules)	0.09	0.09	85
Female sterilization	0.4	0.4	100
Male sterilization	0.15	0.10	100

From Hatcher RA, Trussell J, Steward F, et al. Contraception Technology. Irvington: New York 1994: 113; and Trussell J, Hatcher RA, Cates W, et al. Contraceptive failure in the United States: an update. Stud Fam Plann 1990; 21:51–54.

creases with age, and is increased further by other risk factors such as smoking, hypertension, hypercholesterolemia, and diabetes mellitus.[45, 46] In the United States in 1976, the death rate from myocardial infarction was 1.9 per 100,000 in women aged 25 to 34 and 14.6 per 100,000 in women aged 35 to 44.[47] The relative risk of myocardial infarction in women who smoke varies with the number of cigarettes used. For example, the relative risk of myocardial infarction is 3.4 in women who smoke 1 to 24 cigarettes a day compared with 7.8 in women who smoke more than 25 cigarettes a day.[48]

In 1968 Inman and Vessey[49] suggested that the incidence of ischemic heart disease was increased in oral contraceptive users, and additional studies of the relationship between oral

TABLE 18–4. Annual Death Rates Associated with Fertility Control per 100,000 Nonsterile Women

Contraceptive Technique	Death Rate for Age Group of					
	15–19	20–24	25–29	30–34	35–39	40–44
None (birth related)	7.0	7.4	9.1	14.8	25.7	28.2
Oral contraceptives						
Smokers	2.4	3.6	6.8	13.7	51.4	117.6
Nonsmokers	0.5	0.7	1.1	2.1	14.1	32.0
Intrauterine device (IUD)	1.3	1.1	1.3	1.3	1.9	2.1
Abortion	0.5	1.1	1.3	1.9	1.8	1.1
Barrier methods (birth related)	1.5	1.4	1.0	0.8	1.3	7.6

Adapted from HW Ory, Mortality associated with fertility and fertility control: 1983. Family Planning Perspectives. Vol 15: Number 2 (March/April 1983), pp 57–63. © The Alan Guttmacher Institute.

TABLE 18–5. Characteristics of Sample Populations of Major Cohort Studies of Oral Contraceptives

Study and Population	Number in Sample
Royal College of General Practitioners, 1968–present	
Oral contraceptive users	23,611
Never users	22,766
Oxford/Family Planning Association Study, 1968–present	
Oral contraceptive users	9,653
Diaphragm users	4,217
Intrauterine device (IUD) users	3,162
Walnut Creek/Kaiser Permanente Study, 1968–1977	
Oral contraceptive users	6,107
Former users	4,217
Never users	6,503

Adapted from Lettenmaier C, Liskin L, Church CA, et al. Mothers' lives matter: maternal health in the community. Population Reports, Series L, No. 7. Baltimore: The Johns Hopkins University, Population Information Program, September 1988, with permission.

contraceptives and myocardial infarction have reported a relative risk between 2 and 6.[12] In one large cohort study Slone and colleagues[50] reported that in addition to a threefold increase in the risk of myocardial infarction in current oral contraceptive users, there is also an increased risk in previous long-term users of the agents (5 y or more). That study suggests that previous oral contraceptive use is associated with a greater risk of myocardial infarction, even when the agents have been discontinued for up to 10 y. Stampfer and colleagues[51] reported the results of a large prospective study (Nurses' Health Study Cohort) of 484,096 person-years. They observed no increase of cardiovascular risk, including coronary disease, among previous users of oral contraceptives, even with prolonged use, and the risk of death from circulatory disease, principally myocardial infarction and stroke, appears to be related to age and smoking (Table 18–6).[12, 41, 51] Analysis of these data suggests that (1) smokers have a greater risk than nonsmokers regardless of age, (2) the deleterious effects of oral contraceptives and smoking increase with age, and (3) smokers older than age 35 should not use oral contraceptives but an alternative form of fertility control. The Walnut Creek cohort study, which was somewhat small in scope, did not find an increased mortality in users of oral contraceptives who smoked compared with smokers alone.[43]

Although the mechanisms by which oral contraceptives

TABLE 18–6. Circulatory Disease Mortality Rates (Deaths per 100,000 Woman-Years) and Risks by Age, Smoking Status, and Oral Contraceptive Use: Royal College of General Practitioners Oral Contraceptive Study, 1981

Age and Smoking Status	Ever Users	Never Users	Relative Risk	Excess Risk per 100,000 Woman-Years
15–24 y				
Nonsmokers	0.0	0.0	—	0.0
Smokers	10.5	0.0	—	10.5
25–34 y				
Nonsmokers	4.4	2.7	1.6	1.7
Smokers	14.2	4.2	3.4	10.0
35–44 y				
Nonsmokers	21.5	6.4	3.3	15.1
Smokers	63.4	15.2	4.2*	48.2*
≥45 y				
Nonsmokers	52.4	11.4	4.6*	40.9*
Smokers	206.7	27.9	7.4*	178.8*

*Statistically significant differences in risk ($P < .05$).
Adapted from Royal College of General Practitioners. Further analyses of mortality in oral-contraceptive users. Lancet 1981; 1:541–546; with permission.

result in an increased incidence of ischemic heart disease are not fully understood, changes in serum lipoprotein levels may be involved. The effects of oral contraceptive use on plasma lipoprotein levels and, in particular, high-density lipoprotein (HDL) cholesterol levels have been assessed because of the purported inverse relationship between the serum HDL level and the development of myocardial infarction.[46, 52] Pills containing 50 μg or more of estrogen increase levels of low-density lipoprotein and very-low-density lipoprotein, but the levels of HDL may be raised or lowered depending on the type and amount of progestagen.[15, 53–56] Women using the progestagen-only or minipill have lower levels of HDL,[57, 58] and oral contraceptive pills containing a progestagen with high progestational activity,[27] such as norgestrel in combination with a low dose of estrogen, tend to produce more profound lowering of HDL levels than do other preparations.[55] Oral contraceptives containing desogestrel, norgestimate and gestodene are said to increase HDL levels.[56] It is not known whether these changes are of clinical importance.

The Royal College of General Practitioners Oral Contraceptive Study noted a positive correlation and increasing rates of myocardial infarction with increasing doses of progestagens in oral contraceptive agents.[59, 60] Some progestagens may be more deleterious than others with respect to altering lipoprotein patterns and causing disease of the circulatory system.[55, 56] However, the use of low-dose combination pills containing 30 to 35 μg of ethinyl estradiol does not appear to be associated with ischemic heart disease and exerts minimal effects on lipoprotein profiles.[55, 60] Indeed one study has reported a decrease in the risk of myocardial infarction and stroke in women younger than age 40 who use low-dose combination pills.[61]

Thromboembolic Disease. During the 1960s several retrospective studies suggested a relative risk of developing thromboembolism of 3 to 11 in users of oral contraceptives.[12] These studies were based largely on the clinical diagnosis of deep vein thrombosis, a diagnosis fraught with difficulty, and these results have been challenged.[62] However, it now appears that the risk of developing thromboembolism, frequently subclinical, is increased in pill users.[63–65]

Three large cohort studies have observed lower relative risk rates of thromboembolism (2 to 5) than those reported in the retrospective studies.[12] The lower incidence may be due to more careful screening and elimination of women with high-risk factors before oral contraceptives are prescribed. Although the incidence of thromboembolism is increased, the risk of death from venous thromboembolism is rare (5 per 450,000 woman-years).[45] Moreover, the risk of development of thromboembolism may be related to the dose of estrogen in the pill. For example the incidence of thromboembolic disease in the Royal College study in 1974 was 112 per 100,000 woman-years with agents containing more than 50 μg estrogen, and 81 per 100,000 woman-years with lower-dose pills.[66] However, in the follow-up study by the Royal College of General Practitioners in 1978, a dose relationship could be demonstrated only for superficial thromboembolism; the incidence of deep vein thrombosis was unrelated to the dose of estrogen or to the progestagen component.[67] In Sweden, where all users were changed from high- to low-dose estrogen pills, a decrease in the incidence of thromboembolism from 25 to 9 per 100,000 woman-years occurred, unassociated with a change in mortality from thromboembolism, cardiovascular disease, or cerebrovascular accident.[68] Meade and co-workers[59] reported relatively low death rates from both arterial and venous thromboembolism with pills containing 30 μg of estrogen or less compared with those containing more than that amount. Two studies confirmed a relationship between current oral contraceptive use and venous thromboembolism but no relationship for previous use. However, the Oxford-Family Planning Association Contraceptive Study[69] observed a lower incidence with agents containing less than 50 μg of estrogen, whereas Helmrich and associates[70] reported no relation to estrogen dose. These discrepancies may be due to methodologic differences.[71] The risk of developing thromboembolism in oral contraceptive users does not appear to be related to the duration of use, and any risk disappears soon after discontinuance of the pills.[45] Possible mechanisms whereby oral contraceptives predispose to venous thromboembolic disease include (1) endothelial proliferation, (2) decrease in the rate of venous blood flow, and (3) increase in coagulability of blood because of changes in platelets, coagulation factors, and the fibrinolytic system.[45] Women with antiphospholipid antibodies and subclinical lupus erythematosus may be at more risk for developing venous thrombosis while on oral contraceptives; however, the use of screening tests (measurements of antithrombin III, phospholipid antibodies, and factor V Leiden) are not cost effective as screening tools in all women who are given oral contraceptives. In summary, with the current use of low-dose contraceptive pills the risk of developing serious thromboembolic disease is probably low.

Cerebrovascular Accident. Smoking, hypertension, and age increase the risk of developing cerebrovascular accidents (stroke).[12] As with myocardial infarction, the risk of stroke is highest in older, hypertensive women who smoke. Case-control studies suggest a relative risk of 3 to 14 for development of stroke in oral contraceptive users.[12] Two cohort studies (Royal College of General Practitioners and Walnut Creek) reported higher incidences of subarachnoid hemorrhage (but not other types of stroke) in contraceptive users than in nonusers.[41, 72] Death from stroke is rare and is confined to older women. The risk increases in relation to the dose of estrogen and possibly of progestagen.[60, 73] Because of the seriousness of stroke, users of oral contraceptives who develop severe visual symptoms or vascular headaches should discontinue the agent and use another form of fertility control.

Hypertension. Most women have small elevations in blood pressure (1 to 2 mm Hg diastolic and 5 mm Hg systolic) while taking oral contraceptives.[12] The mechanism for the development of hypertension involves the renin-angiotensin-aldosterone system and is principally due to an increase in renin substrate (angiotensinogen), with a secondary increase in angiotensin.[74] Significant hypertension, i.e., higher than 140 mm Hg systolic or 90 mm Hg diastolic, develops in a small fraction of patients; the relative risk was about 2.6 times greater in users in the Royal College study.[66] The development of hypertension appears to be related to the duration of oral contraceptive use and, in particular, to the type and dose of progestagen.[74, 75] Some of the third-generation progestagens may reduce the risk of hypertension.[76] Hypertension that develops with use of oral contraceptives usually returns to normal after discontinuation of the medication. There appears to be no significant relation between pregnancy-associated hypertension and the development of sustained hypertension with subsequent oral contraceptive use.[4] As with myocardial infarction and stroke, the risk of development of hypertension in contraceptive users increases with age.[46]

Carbohydrate Intolerance. Some women who take oral contraceptives develop impairment of glucose tolerance as manifested by elevated plasma glucose and elevated plasma insulin levels after a glucose load, which suggests the development of insulin resistance. These levels usually return to normal after the drug is stopped.[77] This impairment is apparently due to progestagen, because elevations in insulin levels occur in women using the progestagen-only pills.[78, 79] The use of oral contraceptives is also associated with a decrease in the number and affinity of insulin receptors on monocytes.[80, 81] The new low-dose oral contraceptives do not appear to affect insulin or glucose responses to a glucose load.[15, 82] Given the propensity

to induce glucose intolerance and insulin resistance and the increased risk of cardiovascular disease in diabetics, it is probably prudent to recommend other forms of birth control in women with diabetes mellitus.

Neoplasia. Because some malignancies of the female reproductive tract respond to steroid hormones, a possible association with oral contraceptives and the development of neoplasia has been a major concern. No convincing evidence exists of a role for these agents in the development of cancers of the endometrium or ovary.[12, 83–88] In fact, the agents may provide beneficial, protective effects against the development of neoplasia.[83–86] The majority of the studies suggest that the incidence of breast cancer is not increased in present or past users of oral contraceptives.[89–91] A few studies reported an increase in the incidence of breast cancer in previous users,[92] but there is no consensus regarding oral contraceptive use and the development of breast cancer.

The question of cervical cancer is also unsettled. This is due to the difficulty in controlling the risk factors for cervical neoplasia, such as sexual behavior (age at first intercourse and the number of sexual partners), and to exposure to sexually transmitted diseases. When sexual behavior is taken into account, a small risk factor of 1.3 to 3.4 for the development of cervical dysplasia was found in oral contraceptive users.[93]

An infrequent but serious association exists between the development of benign liver tumors (hepatocellular adenomas and peliosis hepatis) and the use of oral contraceptive agents.[12] These tumors may cause death because of spontaneous rupture and sudden massive hemorrhage. The risk apparently increases with duration of use,[94] but overall is low (1.2 per 100,000 woman-years), so that no liver tumors have been detected in the cohort studies to date.[95] However, the risk of developing hepatocellular carcinoma is reported to increase with duration of use.[96] Oral contraceptives should not be used by women with liver function abnormalities or by women with known acute or chronic liver disease. Oral contraceptives may induce jaundice in women predisposed to the development of recurrent jaundice of pregnancy.

In a follow-up of the Walnut Creek study a suggestion of significant increased risk of development of malignant melanomas was reported, but the study was not controlled for the effect of exposure to sunlight, which is a major risk factor in the development of this malignancy.[97] Other studies have not demonstrated any relationship between oral contraceptives and melanomas.[98, 99]

Other Potential Side Effects. Oral contraceptives produce an increase in the concentration of cholesterol in bile, which is probably the cause of the observed twofold increase in cholecystitis and cholelithiasis in women taking these agents.[100] Users are also at risk for developing pigmentation of the face (chloasma), which is augmented by exposure to sunlight. This effect appears to be related to the dose of estrogen and is unusual with the lower-dose agents currently in use.[13] Minor side effects attributed to oral contraceptives include dyspepsia, breast discomfort, weight gain, psychological changes, and changes in libido. Whether such symptoms are in fact due to contraceptive use is doubtful on the basis of double-blind crossover studies.[101]

Breakthrough Bleeding. Women taking very-low-dose estrogen-containing combination oral contraceptives or the progestagen-only pills may develop breakthrough bleeding, which gives rise to concern and fear; consequently, prior to initiating therapy the patient should be told that this may occur. If the amount of estrogen is lowered beyond some critical point, the progestagen-stimulated endometrium tends to be fragile and prone to breakdown, which results in asynchronous bleeding of two types. The initial bleed is associated with the first few months of oral contraceptive use. The recommended treatment is observation and reassurance because it usually resolves by the third month. Possible causes include incorrect use or failure to take the drug consistently, concurrent drug therapy, or poor absorption because of vomiting.[13] Late breakthrough bleeding may occur at any time after the first few months of contraceptive use and is thought to be a consequence of induction of a thin, atrophic endometrium. Originally, doubling of the pill dosage was recommended, but because this measure increases the intake of both estrogen and progestagen, the atrophic endometrium is unchanged.[13] Therefore when the bleeding is excessive or bothersome, a pill containing a higher estrogen content may be instituted for one to two cycles, or conjugated estrogens or ethinyl estradiol may be added to the oral contraceptive. In most cases the latter solution appears to be sufficient because the problem is usually self-limited. When bleeding is not controlled by these methods, a thorough re-examination must be performed, and other causes of bleeding (cervical, uterine, or pregnancy complications) must be excluded.

Amenorrhea. The use of low-dose oral contraceptive agents and the progestagen-only pills may also be associated with an absence of withdrawal bleeding. The incidence of this is thought to be low (around 1%).[14] The mechanism for the amenorrhea is similar to that for breakthrough bleeding, i.e., atrophy of the endometrium. Such amenorrhea is reversible and hence does not result in future problems after the agents are discontinued, but it causes anxiety in the patient because of the possibility of pregnancy. A careful history and physical examination are indicated when amenorrhea occurs in oral contraceptive users, and a diagnostic test for pregnancy (such as the radioimmunoassay for the β subunit of human chorionic gonadotropin) may be indicated. After pregnancy has been excluded, the patient can be reassured of the benign nature of the amenorrhea, and, if indicated, a pill containing a higher estrogen content can be instituted.

Postpill Amenorrhea. Eighty percent of women resume normal menstrual function 3 mo after discontinuing oral contraceptives, and 95 to 98% are ovulatory within a year. The incidence of failure of the menses to resume after discontinuation of the pill is similar to that of the development of spontaneous secondary amenorrhea in the population as a whole. Thus, subsequent fertility is probably not impaired by previous use of oral contraceptives, as had been suggested by some earlier studies.[102, 103]

Birth Defects. Some, but not all, retrospective studies suggested that oral contraceptive use during pregnancy is associated with cardiovascular and limb defects in the fetus.[12, 104] In most studies the incidence of birth defects is not increased after discontinuation of the pill.[12, 105]

Galactorrhea-Prolactinoma. A slight increase in basal prolactin levels may occur, and galactorrhea may be detected in up to one tenth of women who take oral contraceptives.[106] The reported increased incidence of prolactinomas in men and women may be due to (1) greater physician awareness, (2) availability of prolactin assays and improved radiologic testing, or (3) the use of oral contraceptives. Most studies refute the oral contraceptive theory.[107-111] For example a careful multicenter retrospective study reported no association between their use and the development of prolactinoma.[112]

Effect on Laboratory Values. Changes in values for a number of clinical laboratory tests occur in women taking oral contraceptive pills and need to be taken into consideration when laboratory data are evaluated (Table 18–7).

Drug Interactions. Several drugs may interfere with the efficacy of oral contraceptives. Some act by enhancing the activity of liver enzymes and thus accelerate the clearance of estrogens by the liver.[113] Particular attention has been directed to the effect of antibiotics, in particular rifampin, because an increased incidence of pregnancy has been reported when rifampin is used concurrently with oral contraceptives.[114, 115]

TABLE 18–7. Effects of Oral Contraceptives on Laboratory Tests

	Increased	Decreased
Hematological		
	Erythrocyte sedimentation rate	Prothrombin time
	Plasmin, plasminogen	Antithrombin III
	Euglobulin lysis	
	Clotting factors I, II, VII, VIII, IX, X, XII	
	Platelet count, aggregation, adhesiveness	
	Cryofibrinogen	
	Partial thromboplastin time	
	Serum iron concentration	
Liver		
	Alkaline phosphatase	Haptoglobin
	Bilirubin	Urobilinogen
	Glutamic-oxaloacetic transaminase, glutamic-pyruvic transaminase	
	Leucine aminopeptidase	
	Sulfobromophthalein retention	
Serum Proteins		
	α_1-, α_2-globulin	Immunoglobulins G, A, M
	Ceruloplasmin	Albumin
	Iron-binding capacity	
	Corticosteroid-binding globulin	
	Transferrin	
	Thyroid-binding globulin	
	Testosterone-binding globulin	
Vitamins		
	A	B_2, B_6, B_{12}
		C
		Folate
Hormones		
	Insulin	Triiodothyronine uptake (resin)
	Triiodothyronine, thyroxine, protein-bound iodine	Estradiol
	Aldosterone	Progesterone
	Angiotensinogen	Follicle-stimulating hormone, luteinizing hormone
	Angiotensin I and II	Renin
	Cortisol	Corticotropin
	Growth hormone	
	Prolactin	
	Testosterone	
Others		
	Glucose	Magnesium
	Cholesterol	Zinc
	Triglycerides	Calcium
	Lipoproteins	Complement-reactive protein

Data from Hatcher RA, Trussel J, Stewart F, et al. Contraceptive Technology. 16th ed (revised). New York: Irvington, 1994 and Effects of oral contraceptives on laboratory test results. Med Lett 1979; 21:54–56, with permission.

Other medications that may alter the efficacy of oral contraceptives include phenobarbitol, phenytoin, primidone, and carbamazepine. Consequently in women taking these medications nonhormonal contraceptives should be used. There is little evidence to suggest that antibiotics such as ampicillin and tetracycline interfere with oral contraceptives.

POTENTIAL BENEFITS. Unanticipated benefits of contraceptive use include control of dysmenorrhea and anovulatory dysfunctional uterine bleeding, which results in a decrease in uterine blood loss.[12] Oral contraceptives have also been beneficial in preventing certain types of sexually transmitted diseases. For example the incidence of pelvic inflammatory disease is decreased in pill users, possibly owing to changes in cervical mucus.[116] The incidence of ectopic pregnancies is also decreased,[12] and women who take oral contraceptives appear to have a reduced risk of developing uterine leiomyomas.[117]

Oral contraceptive use may decrease the incidence of endometrial and ovarian carcinoma[83-86] and of functional ovarian cysts.[118, 119] The incidence of fibroadenomas and of fibrocystic disease of the breast is decreased.[12] Oral contraceptives may reduce the risk of development of endometriosis, and they are one of the treatment regimens for this disorder. Hirsutism and acne in women with polycystic ovarian disease are also effectively treated by oral contraceptive agents.[120] Contraceptive use may reduce the incidence of rheumatoid arthritis.[121]

Selection and Prescription of Oral Contraceptives: Recommendations. A thorough history and physical examination must be performed before oral contraceptive therapy is initiated. The absolute and relative contraindications to oral contraceptives should be considered before such therapy is prescribed (Table 18–8). The physical examination should include an evaluation of blood pressure, the breasts, the abdomen (with particular attention to the liver), and the pelvis, including a Papanicolaou smear. Follow-up examinations should be performed at 6 mo to 1 y. When oral contraceptives are prescribed, the woman should be told to notify her physician of the development of serious side effects, including leg swelling or pain, headache, visual disturbances, speech defects, sensory or motor impairment, and chest or abdominal pain.

The need for laboratory testing before prescribing oral contraceptives is controversial. A family history of cardiovascular disease, hormone-dependent cancer, and diabetes mellitus may be an indication for evaluations performed more frequently and at an earlier age. In women younger than age 30, screening for sexually transmitted disease, hematocrit, urinalysis, plasma lipid levels, and sickle cell testing (in black women) are sufficient. In women between ages 30 and 35, plasma glucose and a mammogram are obtained if the history suggests diabetes mellitus or breast disease. All of these tests are recommended for women older than age 35 if oral contraceptives are to be prescribed.[122] If the plasma cholesterol level is higher than 8 mmol/L (300 mg/dL) or plasma triglyceride level is higher than 5.5 mmol/L (500 mg/dL), another form of contraception is indicated.[123]

The use of oral contraceptives by women of older reproductive age (ages 35 to 50) remains controversial. Sterilization, IUDs, barrier contraceptives, and natural family planning are usually recommended for these women. However, some believe that if women of this age are healthy, without risk factors, and have negative laboratory screening test results, low-dose oral contraceptives may be safe.[124]

An additional consideration when beginning oral contraceptive use is when in the menstrual cycle to initiate therapy. Most commonly, the pill is started on the fifth day or the first Sunday after the beginning of menstruation. In women with chronic anovulation (such as in polycystic ovarian disease) who are amenorrheic, oral contraceptives can be started after a negative screening test result for pregnancy followed by a progestagen-induced withdrawal bleed. After a full-term pregnancy, oral contraceptives should be initiated on or after the fourth postpartum week, or 2 wk after delivery in women who are treated with bromocriptine to prevent lactation. After a spontaneous or an induced abortion, oral contraceptives are usually started within 5 d because ovulation may occur within 2 wk in these situations.[122]

A preparation should be recommended that offers effective contraception with the greatest margin of safety and fewest side effects. Safety is probably greater with pills containing less than 35 µg of estrogen. Most physicians recommend a combination pill containing 20 to 35 µg of estrogen, although the lowest doses may produce more breakthrough bleeding.[13] Older data regarding potency and serious side effects may not apply to the low-dose pills, which have a reduced incidence of side effects.

Postcoital Contraception (Interception). The risk of pregnancy from unprotected midcycle intercourse ranges up to 30%, and a postcoital contraceptive or interception pill is occasionally indicated,[125] for example after rape. Historically, women have used a variety of agents to avoid pregnancy after unprotected midcycle intercourse. Modern posthormonal interception, often called the morning-after pill, involves administration of high-dose estrogens.[126] Although these agents are effective, their use is associated with nausea, vomiting, and menstrual disturbances. The use of 50 µg of ethinyl estradiol and 0.5 mg of norgestrel is equally effective and results in fewer side effects. The recommended dosage is two tablets within 72 h of exposure and two more tablets 12 h later.[127] Mifepristone as a 600-mg oral dose appears to be effective as a postcoital contraceptive but was not approved for this use in the United States as of 1996.[128]

Long-Acting Contraceptive Steroids. A variety of long-acting steroid contraceptives have been developed as alternatives to oral agents. Some of these methods are being utilized extensively in developing countries. Originally they were developed to eliminate the estrogen component of the oral contraceptives; however, agents containing only progestagen cause significant amenorrhea, breakthrough bleeding, and other deleterious side effects, as discussed earlier.

Injectable Steroids. The principal long-acting injectable contraceptives are medroxyprogesterone acetate (150 mg IM every 3 mo) and norethindrone enanthate (200 mg IM every 8 wk for 6 mo, then every 12 wk).[129] Slightly higher pregnancy rates occur with norethindrone enanthate than with medroxyprogesterone acetate, and the pregnancy rates with both treatment methods are higher shortly after the first injection. The mechanism of action of long-acting progestational agents includes inhibition of ovulation; production of a thick, unfavorable cervical mucus; induction of a decidual reaction, which results in an unfavorable endometrium, and possibly delayed ovum transport. Depot medroxyprogesterone acetate is the only injectable contraceptive approved for use in the United States. Its benefits include better compliance and reduced incidence of endometrial cancer; side effects include irregular uterine bleeding and spotting, weight gain, depression, decrease in HDL cholesterol levels, and possibly breast cancer.[130, 131] A number of new progestagens are being tested as long-activating injectable agents in the form of microspheres or microcapsules that release hormones slowly at a constant rate and are effective for 1 to 6 mo.[129] To reduce vaginal spotting and bleeding problems with pure progestagens, monthly estrogen-progestagen formulations are used in some developing countries.[129]

Implants. Subdermal implantation of polydimethylsiloxone (Silastic) capsules or rods containing a variety of progestagens have been used for contraception.[129, 132] Such an implant containing levonorgestrel is available in the United States. The capsules are implanted through a small incision on the forearm or inguinal or gluteal surfaces and must be removed after

---

TABLE 18–8. Contraindications for Oral Contraceptive Use

Absolute Contraindications

Known or suspected estrogen-dependent neoplasia
Thrombophlebitis or thromboembolic disease (or history thereof)
Cerebrovascular or coronary artery disease (or history thereof)
Active liver disease or adenoma
Undiagnosed vaginal bleeding
Known or suspected pregnancy
Smokers older than age 35 y

Relative Contraindications

Severe headaches or migraines
Hypertension
Diabetes mellitus
Gallbladder disease
Sickle cell disease (hemoglobin SS or SC)
Elective surgery
Leg injury or cast
Hyperlipemia

the steroid has been released. The levonorgestrel is released in a constant fashion, and the implant is effective for 5 y.[129] Thus, a major advantage of this contraceptive is compliance. Although implants are effective, they require removal and are associated with breakthrough bleeding and amenorrhea similar to that seen when the agents are injected. Progestagen implants may be less effective in the obese. Biodegradable implants containing progestagens that do not require removal are in the developmental phase, as are biodegradable pellets.[129]

Vaginal Rings. Steroids may also be administered in Silastic vaginal rings that are impregnated with hormone.[129, 133] Most of these rings contain a progestagen, but a few contain an estrogen and a progestagen. They are fitted as a diaphragm in the vagina, kept in place for 3 wk, removed for 1 wk to allow for withdrawal bleeding, and then reinserted. These rings are undergoing trials. Problems include vaginitis, expulsion, interference with coitus, difficulty of insertion, and occasional breakthrough bleeding.[133]

Steroid-Releasing Intrauterine Devices. The Progestasert IUD is the only hormonal IUD available in the United States (see later). Its main advantage is that its use results in decreased bleeding during menstruation (a common cause of discontinuation of the IUD) and decreased menstrual cramping.[134] The disadvantages are breakthrough bleeding and the requirement for yearly replacement. IUDs are being tested that contain norgestrel and require replacement every 3 to 5 y.

Progesterone Antagonists. The development of a synthetic competitive progesterone antagonist, mifepristone (RU 486), has opened new approaches to fertility control. Mifepristone prevents ovulation in women, induces luteolysis and premature menstruation,[135, 136] and is used as a postcoital contraceptive.[128] This form of medication is not associated with any major side effects and may be used in the future as a contraceptive until women reach menopause.[137] Its use as an abortifacient is described later in this chapter.

Nonsteroidal Contraceptives

A variety of luteinizing hormone–releasing hormone (LHRH) analogues have been synthesized in an attempt to prolong the activity of the hormone. Paradoxically, prolonged continuous administration of LHRH and its agonists results in the lowering of gonadotropin levels.[138] Consequently, the use of LHRH as a contraceptive has been attempted in men and women. Its primary site of action is the pituitary. During long-term continuous administration of LHRH and its agonists, the rate of gonadotropin secretion increases during the first week and then decreases.[138] Potential mechanisms whereby LHRH analogues may act as contraceptives include (1) inhibition of ovulation, (2) induction of luteal-phase defects, and (3) enhancement of luteolysis.[138] Daily administration of the agonists by injection[139] or intranasally[140] inhibits ovulation and provides effective contraception. Most of the reports utilized either buserelin or nafarelin by daily intranasal administration.[140, 141] In these studies there were no pregnancies, but some women developed oligomenorrhea, irregular bleeding, or amenorrhea. To achieve regular withdrawal bleeding patterns and to prevent the possible development of endometrial hyperplasia, other investigators administered LHRH analogues for 21 d with added progestagen during days 17 to 21 and no therapy for 7 d each month.[142] This regimen results in regular withdrawal bleeding but is also associated with intermenstrual spotting. Because continous or prolonged intermittent therapy induces a pseudomenopause or low-estrogen state and increases the risk of bone loss, the use of LHRH analogues for female contraception is not an acceptable alternative to other forms of hormonal contraception.

The effects of smaller doses of LHRH agonists on luteal function have been investigated in hopes of preventing the low-estrogen state that accompanies the inhibition of ovulation. Administration of 50 μg of LHRH agonists by subcutaneous injection daily during the first 3 d of the menstrual cycle is followed by a significant decrease in FSH level, with prolongation of the follicular phase, shortening of the luteal phase, and decreased progesterone secretion.[143] Other investigators using similar regimens found delayed ovulation but no effect on the length of the luteal phase.[138]

Attempts have also been made to induce luteolysis by injection of LHRH analogues at the time of expected ovulation,[138] and to induce luteal-phase insufficiency by administering the analogues by injection or intranasally between the fifth and eighth days of the luteal phase.[144, 145] A major problem with these alternative schedules is the accurate timing of ovulation.

Intrauterine Device

Approximately 85 million women worldwide use the IUD, including more than 59 million women in China.[146] The IUD was first used in antiquity, but modern use was initiated with the development of intrauterine rings. Two types of IUD are now used worldwide: (1) unmedicated (Lippes loop, single-coil stainless steel ring) and (2) medicated, containing copper (Copper-7, TCu-200B, TCu-380A) or hormone (Progestasert). Because of economic reasons and the inability of the manufacturers to obtain liability insurance, the only devices currently marketed in the United States are Progestasert and a copper-containing IUD (TCu-380A). The TCu-380A contains 380 mm² of exposed copper wrapped around the vertical stem and arms of the plastic device to enhance contraceptive effectiveness.[146] Progestasert, also a T-shaped plastic device, contains 38 mg of progesterone, which is released at a daily rate of 65 μg.[134] IUDs may be inserted at any time of the menstrual cycle but are usually inserted at the time of menstrual bleeding to enhance the ease of insertion and to diminish the chance of pregnancy.

All devices used worldwide are roughly equal in contraceptive effectiveness, with failure rates ranging from 1.4 to 4 per 100 women at 1 y after insertion.[146] The major advantages of the copper-containing IUDs are (1) a smaller increase in menstrual blood flow than with the unmedicated IUDs, (2) a lower expulsion rate, and (3) less pain after insertion. The progesterone-containing IUD is associated with a decrease in both menstrual bleeding and dysmenorrhea.[146] The drawbacks of the progesterone-containing IUDs compared with the TCu-380A IUD is the necessity for yearly replacement.

The precise mechanism by which the IUD acts as a contraceptive is unclear. The devices may prevent fertilization by impairing sperm transport and by damaging sperm directly.[147, 148] Another action is thought to result from an induction of an endometrial inflammatory response, so that the endometrium is unfavorable for implantation. Plasma cells and macrophages in the inflammatory response may phagocytose spermatozoa or possibly the fertilized ovum.[149-150] Copper appears to increase the inflammatory action, and the progesterone-containing IUD interferes with the hormonal response of the endometrium.[146, 151] Complications of IUD use include excessive bleeding, infection, and expulsion. Approximately 5 to 15% of women discontinue its use within the first year because of bleeding and pain.[146] The increased loss of blood rarely results in significant anemia, but intermittent iron replacement or use of nonsteroidal anti-inflammatory drugs may be appropriate. The increased bleeding is thought to be due to vascular disruption, increased fibrinolytic activity, or increased activity of mast cells with local release of heparin.[146, 152]

A potentially serious complication of IUD use is the development of pelvic inflammatory disease, which usually occurs soon after insertion.[146] To minimize the risk of infection most physicians administer prophylactic antibiotics (500 mg tetracycline by mouth) prior to insertion of the IUD. This issue is important both because of the acute morbidity and because of an increased risk of infertility related to tubal obstruction. Current IUD users are 1.6 times more likely to be hospitalized with pelvic inflammatory disease than women utilizing no forms of contraception, and 4.5 times more likely than oral contraceptive users.[153] Indeed, the incidence of pelvic inflammatory disease may actually be reduced in women using barrier contraceptives or oral contraceptives. Potential mechanisms for the increased incidence of pelvic inflammatory disease include the entry of bacteria into the endometrium at the time of or shortly after insertion, and promotion of bacterial growth by the increased volume and duration of menstrual bleeding.[146] The highest rates of pelvic inflammatory disease occurred with the Dalkon Shield device. Retrospective and prospective studies suggest a lower but still significant risk of pelvic inflammatory disease in women using currently available IUDs compared with nonusers, but it should be emphasized that the risk of infection in IUD users is related to the number of sexual partners. There does not appear to be an increased risk of infection in IUD users who are monogamous.[154] Occasionally, the infection may be so severe that it results in bilateral tubo-ovarian abscesses. Prompt recognition and treatment of pelvic inflammatory disease are critical for maintaining tubal function. Therapy includes removal of the IUD, prompt initiation of antibiotics, and hospitalization if indicated. Responsible organisms include *Neisseria gonorrhoeae*, *Chlamydia*, *Escherichia coli*, *Bacteroides*, *Peptostreptococcus*, and rarely *Actinomyces*.[155]

If pregnancy occurs, the IUD should be removed (if the string is visible) to reduce the incidence of spontaneous abortion, severe infection, and occasional maternal death in IUD users.[156] If the IUD string is not visible, the choice of abortion is offered, and if abortion is not acceptable, the patient should be observed for signs of infection. Such pregnancy is more likely to be extrauterine than intrauterine, because the IUD reduces the incidence of intrauterine pregnancies more efficiently than that of ectopic pregnancies.[146]

The effects of IUD use on subsequent fertility have not been fully evaluated. Most women who discontinue IUD use conceive as rapidly as nonusers.[146] Because IUDs increase the risk of developing pelvic infection, women who have pelvic inflammatory disease may develop tubal obstruction. Until this issue is settled, women who are nulligravid should use other forms of contraception. In addition, women with a history of pelvic inflammatory disease or who have multiple sex partners run an increased risk of developing pelvic inflammatory disease and also should use an alternative form of contraception. There is no evidence that IUD users develop cancer of the reproductive tract more often than do nonusers.[157] A rare complication is perforation at the time of insertion, which is an indication for surgical removal. Absolute contraindications for IUD use include active or previous pelvic infection, abnormalities or distortion of the uterine cavity, undiagnosed genital bleeding, uterine or cervical malignancy, history of ectopic pregnancy, increased susceptibility to infection (leukemias, diabetes, valvular heart disease, acquired immunodeficiency syndrome, and long-term glucocorticoid therapy), genital actinomycosis, allergies to copper or Wilson disease (for copper-containing IUDs), and known or suspected pregnancy.[146, 158]

Barrier Methods

Barrier methods of contraception circumvent many of the potential risks that accompany the use of oral contraceptives and IUDs. These methods are among the oldest, safest, and most widely used forms of birth control.

Originally, the term barrier implied a physical barrier that prevents the sperm from reaching the fertilizable egg. More recently, the definition has broadened to include biologic, chemical, and physical means of preventing fertilization. Barrier contraceptives are often underutilized, but if they are used correctly and continuously they provide adequate contraception. In addition, they are simple to use and provide some protection against sexually transmitted diseases.[159] All barrier methods of contraception require prior planning and motivation.

The vaginal diaphragm is one of the most commonly utilized forms of female barrier contraception. The diaphragm consists of a shallow rubber cup that is stabilized by a circumscribing, rubber-covered steel spring. The three types of diaphragms (the coil spring, the flat spring, and the arching spring) are designed for various vaginal shapes. The efficacy of the diaphragm depends on selection of the appropriate type and size, proper placement, and continued usage. Proper use requires the placement of a spermicidal cream or jelly inside the dome of the diaphragm before insertion prior to intercourse. For maximal effectiveness, the diaphragm must be left in place for at least 6 h after intercourse. Failure rates vary from 2.4 to 17 per 100 women per year of usage.[14] The effectiveness, as with all forms of barrier contraception, depends primarily on continued use. Complications include occasional allergic reactions to latex or to the spermicidal agent. In addition, improperly fitted diaphragms may cause vaginal irritation or pain. A profuse, foul-smelling vaginal discharge may occur if a diaphragm is left in place too long; for this reason, it is recommended that it be removed and washed once every 24 h.[14, 159]

The cervical cap is a smaller version of the diaphragm that fits directly over the cervix and is used in conjunction with a spermicidal jelly.[159] The cervical cap requires fitting by a trained physician. Some women cannot be fitted properly because of a developmental or a surgical deformity of the cervix. The effectiveness and side effects of the cervical cap and the recommendations for time of insertion and removal are similar to those for the vaginal diaphragm.

The female condom (Reality) is a barrier device made of polyurethane. It is appropriate for couples with latex allergies and is stronger than latex condoms. Failure rates appear to be similar to those for other barrier methods in women.[160]

Chemical or spermicidal agents can be used by themselves or as a supplement to other barrier contraceptive methods. Such agents are available in jellies, creams, suppositories, aerosol foams, film, and sponges and comprise two components: a relatively inert base that physically blocks the passage of sperm and any of several chemical spermicides.[159, 161] The active ingredients in some commonly available spermicidal agents are given in Table 18–9. The majority utilize nonoxynol 9 (nonylphenoxypolyethoxyethanol).

Toxic shock syndrome has been reported rarely in users of diaphragms and sponges.[162] Women who use cervical caps may also be at risk for the development of toxic shock syndrome.

Failure rates of spermicidal agents that are used alone range from 2 to 29 pregnancies per 100 woman-years of use.[14] Like mechanical barriers, they provide some protection against sexually transmitted diseases including syphilis, gonorrhea, and disorders caused by *Chlamydia*, *Trichomonas*, *Candida*, human immunodeficiency virus, and papillomavirus.[159, 161, 163] There are relatively few complications associated with spermicidal agents other than infrequent allergic reactions or irritation.[159] In some studies a slightly increased risk of congenital abnormalities has been reported in the offspring of women

TABLE 18–9. Some Available Spermicidal Agents

Type	Product	Active Ingredient
Cream	Conceptrol	Nonoxynol 9 (5%)
	Ortho-Creme	Nonoxynol 9 (2%)
	Koromex II	Octoxynol (3%)
	Milex Cream	Glyceryl ricinoleate (0.36%)
Jelly	Koromex II	Octoxynol (1%)
	Ortho-Gynol	p-Diisobutylphenoxypolyethoxyethanol
	Preceptin	p-Diisobutylphenoxypolyethoxyethanol
	Ramses "10-hour"	Dodecaethylene glycol monolaurate (5%)
Suppository	Encare	Nonoxynol 9 (2.5%)
	Ortho-forms	Nonoxynol 9 (2%)
	Semicid	Nonoxynol 9 (6.6%)
	S-Positive	Nonoxynol 9 (10%)
Foam	Delfen	Nonoxynol 9 (12.5%)
	Koromex	Nonoxynol 9 (12.5%)
	Emko	Nonoxynol 9 (8%)
	Because	Nonoxynol 9 (8%)
Sponge	Today	Nonoxynol 9 (1 g)
Film	VCF	Nonoxynol 9 (72 mg)

who used spermicides vaginally.[164] A number of larger studies have failed to demonstrate such an association.[159, 165–167]

Natural Family-Planning Methods

Natural family planning is one of the most widely used methods of fertility regulation, particularly by those who for religious, financial, or cultural reasons do not use drugs or devices for contraception. Such methods are based on periodic abstinence from sexual relations during the fertile period surrounding the time of ovulation, which usually occurs about 14 d before the next expected menstrual period. Techniques for identifying the fertile period, commonly termed rhythm methods, include the calendar method, basal body temperature method, cervical mucus method, and symptothermal method. Successful application of these techniques requires both training and motivation.[168, 169]

The calendar method is based on the work of Ogino[170] and Knaus.[171] Calculation of the fertile period rests on three assumptions: (1) ovulation occurs on day 14 before the onset of the next menses, (2) sperm remain viable for only 48 to 72 h, and (3) the unfertilized ovum survives for only 12 to 24 h.[168] This method requires the use of a menstrual calendar on which the woman records the length of her menstrual cycles for at least 6 and preferably 12 cycles. The first day of the potential fertile period is the shortest cycle minus 18 d, and the last day of the potential fertile period is the longest cycle minus 11 d. As an example, in a woman whose menstrual cycles vary from 26 to 31 d, application of the calendar method would mean a potential fertility period as follows: the first day of potential fertility, 26 − 18 = 8; the last day of potential fertility, 31 − 11 = 20. This would mean that the period of fertility would range from the 8th to the 20th days of the cycle, so that the safe days during which intercourse would be allowed, with the calendar method, would be from the first day of menstrual flow through the 7th day of the cycle and from the 20th day until the onset of the next menses. Women with grossly irregular cycles cannot use this method.

The basal body temperature method depends on identification of the rise in basal body temperature from a relatively low level during the follicular phase to the higher level during the luteal phase of the menstrual cycle in response to the thermogenic effect of progesterone.[169] The rise in temperature is small (between 0.2 and 0.5°C), occurs abruptly over a 24-h period, and is sometimes preceded by a small drop in temperature. To use this method, a woman records her basal temperature each day for 3 consecutive months. The elevated tempera-tures begin 1 to 2 d after ovulation and correspond to the rising levels of progesterone. Intercourse is not permitted between the end of menses and 3 d after the temperature rise. Problems with this method include difficulty in interpreting temperature charts and the fact that abstinence is necessary for the entire preovulatory period.[168]

Changes in the character and appearance of cervical secretions occur just before ovulation in most women and are the basis of the mucus method.[168] To practice this method the woman must differentiate between sensations of dryness, moistness, and wetness of the secretions at the vaginal opening during the different phases of the menstrual cycle. The viscous mucus that is present during the preovulatory and postovulatory phases must be differentiated from the slippery, clear, and copious mucus that appears just before ovulation. It is necessary to identify the time at which the change in character of the mucus occurs; mucus is removed from the vagina to determine whether it possesses increased stretchiness (spinnbarkeit). By this method, abstinence must start the first day after such a change in mucus is observed and continue until the fourth day after the maximal amount of cervical mucus is observed. All other days until menstruation are considered infertile days. Care must be taken to differentiate cervical mucus from lubricants and semen.

The symptothermal method combines the previously described techniques for identifying the fertile period including changes in cervical mucus, calendar calculations to estimate the onset of the fertile period, and basal body temperature charts. In addition, symptoms such as ovulatory abdominal pain (mittelschmerz); midcycle ovulatory bleeding; self-observed changes in the position, texture, moistness, and dilation of the cervix; breast tenderness; edema; and mood changes can be used to identify the fertile period.

Natural family-planning methods can be used during the fertile days in conjunction with other forms of contraception such as condoms, diaphragms, and spermicidal agents. The major complication with all these methods is a high rate of unplanned pregnancies. The overall effectiveness is a function of the degree of patient education and dedication, and it varies from as high as 99% to an average of around 70%.[168, 169] In a prospective study, there was no difference in birth defects between the offspring of women using natural family planning and the offspring of women using other methods.[172]

The development of home urinary or blood assay kits to determine and predict precisely the time of the initial rise of estrogen before ovulation and the rise of progesterone to detect the postovulatory state is under investigation. Current assays are not sensitive enough to predict ovulation until about 5 d prior to ovulation. It is hoped that improved methods will increase the reliability and effectiveness of natural family planning.[173, 174]

Other types of natural family planning include abstinence after pregnancy in certain societies in which intercourse is taboo during this period; coitus interruptus; or the withdrawal method. The last-named requires no devices, no chemicals, and little education; the failure rate is around 16 pregnancies per 100 women per year of usage.[14] Coitus interruptus may also be used with other natural family-planning methods during the period of expected fertility to enhance their effectiveness.

Breast-feeding has been advocated as a physiological mechanism for spacing births, but reliance on this form of birth control in certain parts of the world has probably been responsible, in part, for the exponential increase in the birth rate. The basis for this method is that breast-feeding inhibits ovulation after delivery, presumably as a consequence of the amount of prolactin that is secreted during breast stimulation. The effectiveness of this method depends on the frequency and continued use of breast-feeding, but most investigators consider it unreliable as a means of birth control.[14, 175] Even the associated amenorrhea that occurs is unreliable as an indication of a safe period of infertility, because nearly 80% of women who breast-feed ovulate unpredictably before their first menstrual period.[176] After menstruation resumes, the risk of pregnancy is similar in women who continue to breast-feed and in non–breast-feeding women. Because of the high risk of pregnancy in breast-feeding women, contraceptive counseling should begin early in the postpartum period. The preferred methods of birth control in such women include abstinence, barrier methods, and IUDs. Whereas some of the higher-dosage oral contraceptives reduce the volume of breast milk, the new low-dose estrogen and progestagen-only contraceptives have no effect or may slightly increase milk volume.[175] Small quantities of orally ingested steroid hormones are secreted in milk and are thus transmitted to the newborn infant. Because of the possible long-term effects of steroid hormones on the infant, oral contraceptives probably should not be given to nursing mothers.

Immunologic Techniques

Contraceptive vaccines are under investigation as an effective method of fertility control. Hormones and proteins of the female reproductive tract or of early pregnancy are not in themselves antigenic and must be linked to other proteins such as serum albumin or tetanus toxoid to induce an antibody response.[177, 178] Anti-LHRH antibodies, anti-LH antibodies,[178] anti-FSH antibodies,[179] and antibodies against zona pellucida antigens have been used to induce infertility in experimental animals.[177–179] Anti–human chorionic gonadotropin vaccines are now being subjected to phase I clinical trials in women. No significant complications have been observed to date in women so immunized, and in most cases a variable period of temporary infertility results.[179]

Sterilization

Sterilization is now the most widely used form of birth control worldwide; by 1984 a total of 94 million women had undergone some form of sterilization procedure.[180] Between 1970 and 1980 approximately 5 million women in the United States underwent surgical sterilization procedures.[14] The increased use of such procedures during the recent past is due to improvement in surgical techniques and dissatisfaction with the complications of other contraceptive methods (Table 18–10).[14]

Surgical Sterilization

Simple ligation of the fallopian tubes through a standard abdominal or minilaparotomy incision is one of the oldest

TABLE 18–10. Methods of Sterilization in Women

Surgical	Chemical
Fallopian tube	Liquid installation
Ligation, resection	Quinicrine
Abdominal	Methyl-2-cyanoacrylate (MCA)
Minilaparotomy	Silicone elastomers (Silastic)
Vaginal	Gelatin-resorcinol-formaldehyde (GRF)
Laparoscopy	Phenol (carbolic acid) compounds
Fulguration, division	Solid plugs
Clips	Silicone elastomers
Bands	Polyethylene
Uterus	Dacron
Hysteroscopic fulguration of tubal ostia	Teflon
Hysterectomy	

Data from Population Reports. Minilaparotomy and laparoscopy: safe, effective, and widely used. Series C, No. 9. Female Sterilization. Baltimore: The Johns Hopkins University, 1985, with permission.

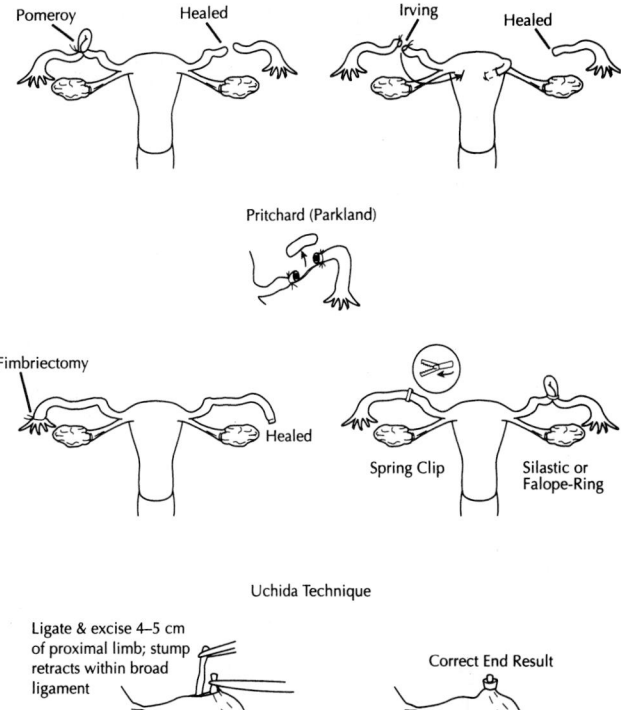

Figure 18–6. Illustration of various methods used for tubal sterilization. (From Hatcher RA, Trussl J, Stewart F, et al. Contraceptive Technology. 16th ed, revised. New York, Irvington, 1994, with permission.)

forms of tubal sterilization and one of the most common surgical procedures performed today. Other methods to interrupt fallopian tubes include ligation and crushing, ligation and resection, and resection of a midportion of the tube followed by insertion of the tubal stumps into the mesosalpinx or the wall of the uterus (Irving procedure). The procedure can be performed during the puerperal period, usually through a small periumbilical incision. In the nonpuerperal woman, techniques for ligation and resection of the fallopian tube include a minilaparotomy incision and conventional colpotomy incision through the posterior vagina, followed by ligation and partial resection of the fallopian tubes or fimbriectomy (Fig. 18–6).

Various laparoscopic techniques have been devised to reduce the duration of the hospital stay and the length of the abdominal incision. These include fulguration by hot cautery (unipolar or bipolar) and the application of clips (silicone-titanium and spring-loaded clips) or bands (Silastic rings).[180]

Surgical techniques involving the uterus include hysterectomy and fulguration of tubal ostia by hysteroscopic examination. In the latter the tubal ostium is visualized through the hysteroscope, an electrode is placed in the tubal ostium, and an electrical current is applied. The principal problem is the high failure rate because of incomplete fulguration. Hysterectomy for sterilization may be indicated if other uterine disorders or pelvic diseases are present, such as leiomyomata, menorrhagia, pelvic pain, uterine prolapse, stress urinary incontinence, or cervical intraepithelial neoplasia.

The mortality rate for tubal sterilization procedures in the United States is approximately 8 per 100,000.[39] Complications of the abdominal and minilaparotomy procedures are similar to those of other surgical procedures involving the abdomen and include anesthetic-related complications, wound infection, hemorrhage, and bowel or bladder injury. The vaginal approach is associated with an increased inci-

TABLE 18–11. Pregnancy Rates After Sterilization Procedures

Method	Pregnancy Rate (per 100 Procedures)
Ligation, resection	
Puerperal abdominal	0.2*
Interval abdominal	0.6*
Vaginal	0.3*
Laparoscopic	
Coagulation and cutting	0.8†
Spring clip	2.3†
Silicone elastomer band	0.8†
Hysteroscopic procedures	2.3*

*Data from Shepherd MK. Female contraceptive sterilization. Obstet Gynecol Surv 1974; 29:739.
†Data from Brenner WE. Evaluation of contemporary sterilization methods. J Reprod Med 1981; 26:439–453.

dence of infection. The failure rates of the various abdominal and vaginal sterilization procedures, defined as the number of pregnancies, range between 0.2 and 0.6 per 100 procedures (Table 18–11).[181, 182]

Complications of laparoscopic procedures include perforation of the uterus by the uterine manipulator and complications resulting from the carbon dioxide introduced into the abdomen to produce pneumoperitoneum. These complications include creation of cutaneous emphysema and the injection of carbon dioxide into the intestine or into the intravascular spaces. In addition, perforation of the intestine or vessels can occur during insertion of the trocar. These severe complications are rare; their occurrence appears to be related to the skill and experience of the surgeon.[180–183] Coagulation with a unipolar cautery, which is the original method for laparoscopic sterilization, may cause bowel burns. Bipolar cautery causes this complication less often but does not completely alleviate the danger.[180] Consequently, spring clips and Silastic band techniques were introduced. The spring clip method has a higher rate of technical failure.[184] The failure rates for the various laparoscopic methods of sterilization are summarized in Table 18–11. Although the failure rates for hysterectomy are essentially zero, the postoperative course, morbidity, and mortality are 10- to 100-fold greater than those for a tubal ligation.[38] The problems that are associated with hysteroscopic fulguration include thermal injury to the bowel and a high pregnancy rate.[180]

Chemical Sterilization

Several chemical methods of sterilization are under investigation (see Table 18–10). The most extensive experience is with quinacrine, which is injected into the uterus near the tubal ostia and produces sclerosis of the tubal lumen. Complications, although relatively rare, include seizures, intrauterine adhesions, and abdominal pain; the failure rate is around 30%.[180] Adhesive substances such as Silastic (a silicone polymer), methyl-2-cyanoacrylate, and gelatin-resorcinol-formaldehyde have been instilled experimentally into the uterotubal junction to form a plug. These compounds are viscous when instilled and solidify when in place. Although morbidity is low, failure rates are significant.[180]

Various types of solid plugs have been devised that can be inserted into the uterine or fimbrial ends of the tubes. These plugs include Silastic, polyethylene, ceramic, Dacron, and Teflon devices. Preliminary results indicate that these methods of contraception are reversible when the plugs are removed.[180]

The number of women seeking sterilization continues to increase, particularly young women with relatively small families. An increasing number of these young women may later desire reversal of the sterilization procedure. As many as 1 or 2 per 1000 sterilized women may be candidates for tubal reanastomosis.[185] Before a decision is made on a reanastomosis procedure, the couple must be carefully screened for other infertility factors and coexisting medical disorders, and the woman must be evaluated for distal tubal disease and for adequacy of tubal length. Those procedures in which clips or ligation involve only a small portion of the fallopian tubes have a greater chance of successful reversal. Laparoscopic fulguration often causes severe damage to a greater length of the fallopian tube, and thus successful reversals are less frequent. Improved pregnancy rates have been reported with surgical techniques utilizing operative microscopes.[185] If the length of the remaining tubes is insufficient or the patient fails to conceive after a surgical reversal, then in vitro fertilization and embryo transfer may be offered.

Abortion

Between 30 and 50 million abortions are performed worldwide each year, primarily as a means of fertility control. In the United States a pregnant woman and her physician can make the decision to abort for fertility control through 24 to 26 wk.[186, 187] However, state governments may regulate abortions particularly during the time between the first trimester and 24 to 26 wk of gestation (now considered to be the age of fetal viability). Since abortions became legal in 1973, deaths from illegal abortions have declined markedly.[188]

The choice of method of abortion depends primarily on the stage of pregnancy, on whether associated uterine diseases are present, and on whether sterilization is desired.

Surgical Abortion

Menstrual extraction by suction can be performed in the first few weeks after a missed menstrual period. A small, flexible plastic cannula is inserted and the uterine contents are evacuated by suction applied to the cannula. The main problem with this technique is occasional failure to abort the pregnancy. The traditional dilatation and curettage procedure circumvents this difficulty but requires greater dilation of the cervix and is associated with more pain and blood loss.[4]

Suction or vacuum curettage is the most widely used method of abortion in the United States.[4] A laminaria tent, which is made from stems of the seaweed *Laminaria digitata* or *L. japonica* or from synthetic osmotic dilators, is usually placed in the cervix 6 to 24 h before the procedure and slowly dilates the cervix by osmotic swelling. A small plastic cannula is then inserted into the uterus, and the contents are evacuated by utilizing an electrically powered vacuum source.

Surgical methods of abortion during the second trimester include dilation by *Laminaria* and extraction of the products of conception by suction curettage and/or forceps. Other surgical procedures include hysterotomy (which is analogous to a small cesarean section) or hysterectomy when another clear indication for such a procedure is present. Morbidity and mortality rates after these last two procedures are high, and they are therefore used infrequently for abortion.

Chemical Abortion

Midtrimester abortions (more than 14 to 16 wk of gestational age) can be induced by the intrauterine instillation of solutions such as dinoprost (prostaglandin $F_{2\alpha}$), hypertonic saline, or hypertonic urea.[14, 189] In addition, dinoprostone (prostaglandin E_2) vaginal suppositories are available for termination of pregnancy in the second trimester in cases of fetal death in utero up to 28 wk. To shorten the abortion time and blood loss, *Laminaria* and oxytocin are used in conjunction with these methods. Because of the potential complications of the intrauterine installation of chemicals, this approach has been replaced by dilation and extraction, which are safer, faster, and less expensive.

Progesterone antagonists, such as mifepristone (RU 486), have been used to induce abortions in early human gestation either alone or in combination with oral prostaglandins.[190, 191] This agent is used for early termination of pregnancy in China, France, and other countries but has not been approved in the United States.

Complications from chemical methods include hemorrhage, infection, retention of the products of conception, and cervical injury. The risk of death from abortions is low, but when death occurs it is more likely associated with pregnancies of more than 8 wk gestation.

FERTILITY CONTROL IN MEN

Fertility control in men involves either use of the condom or vasectomy. A major attempt has been made to develop reversible contraceptives for men, but that objective still remains an unfulfilled promise. Because of the importance of such an agent, we review briefly the sites at which contraceptives might act: e.g., the hypothalamic-pituitary level, the testis, the epididymis, or the vas deferens (Fig. 18–7).

Condom

The condom is the oldest form of barrier contraception, and use of the latex rubber condom is a major method of male contraception. In Japan almost 80% of couples practicing contraception rely on the condom.[192] Condoms are safe and effective; when used properly and consistently, their effectiveness is greater than 97%.[192] Like other forms of barrier contraceptives, condoms offer significant protection against sexually transmitted diseases. The only complication of condom use is allergic reaction to, or irritation from, latex rubber or the lubricant used.[192] A plastic condom has been developed that overcomes this problem and is less subject to breakage despite being thinner.[192]

Vasectomy

Background and Current Use

Surgical sterilization procedures have gained widespread acceptance since the 1950s.[193] In the United States, almost

TABLE 18–12. Characteristics of Two Groups of Vasectomy Patients in Montreal

Group	Age <35 y	No. of Children 1 or 2	Married <10 y
1968–1971	26%	31%	23%
1974–1978	55%	58%	61%
	P<.01	P<.01	P<.01

Adapted from Ramos-Cordero RA, Ackman CFD, Naftolin F. Changing profiles in vasectomy subjects in the past decade. Fertil Steril 1979; 31:410–412. Reproduced with permission of the publisher, The American Fertility Society.

50% of couples choose surgical interruption of the vas deferens (vasectomy), and about 500,000 vasectomy procedures are performed each year.[194–196] The profile of men undergoing vasectomy has changed in that the average age, length of marriage, and number of living children were greater in 1968 to 1971 than in 1974 to 1978 (Table 18–12).[197] These figures indicate that sterilization of men has gained social acceptance in North America.

Vasectomy has also been utilized extensively as a method of fertility control in India and China. The use of vasectomy in India has declined so that it accounted for only 42% of surgical sterilizations in 1992.[198] In contrast, vasectomy is still widely used in China where more than 30 million men have undergone the procedure since 1970 and where more than 80% of couples who choose sterilization utilize vasectomy.[199]

Methods, Success Rate, and Acute Complications

Bilateral partial vasectomy is a relatively simple operative procedure and is usually performed with local anesthesia. Common incisions and the surgical techniques are illustrated in Figure 18–8.[194] The dorsal lithotomy position allows the weight of the testes to elongate and stretch the vasa, which facilitates entrapment of the vas between the thumb and forefinger of the surgeon and allows infiltration of local anesthetic both in the skin and around the isolated vas. The skin is

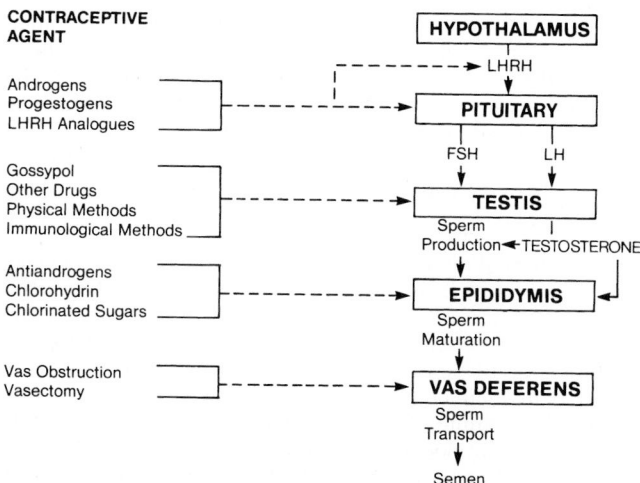

Figure 18–7. Principal sites of action of contraceptive agents on the male reproductive tract.

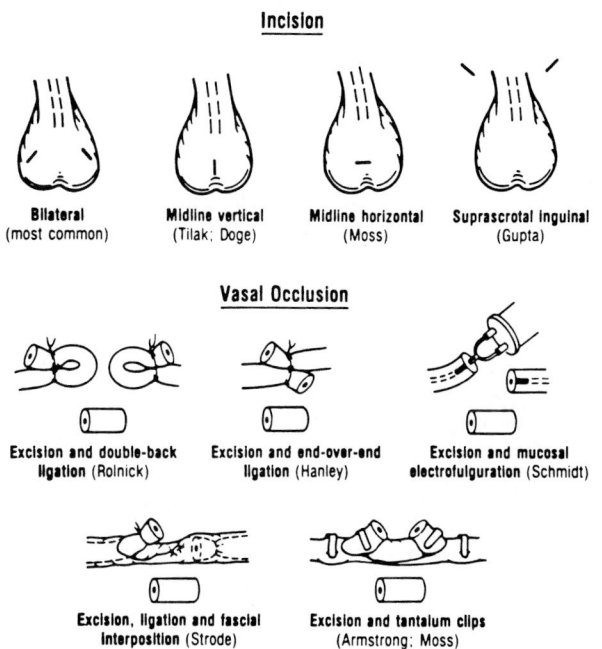

Figure 18–8. Diagram depicting common incisions for and methods of vasal occlusion. (From Lipshultz LI, Benson GS. Vasectomy—1980. Urol Clin North Am 1980; 7:89–105, with permission.)

incised, the vas is separated from its surrounding sheath, and a minimum of 1 cm is excised. With all techniques for permanent closure of the remaining vasal stumps (see Fig. 18–8), the rare possibility of spontaneous recanalization is always present (see later). Usually the skin edges are only loosely approximated, and an ice pack is recommended for 12 h and scrotal support for an additional 72 h.

A rapid "nonsurgical" method of male sterilization (less than 10 min) is used in China in which the spermatic ducts are injected with a sclerosing agent, phenol.[200] This method was reported to be successful in 91% of 50,000 men and to involve a smaller incidence of hematoma and infection than that after vasectomy. The Chinese have also developed a no-scalpel surgical vasectomy,[201, 202] in which a loop of vas deferens is fixed by a clamp and delivered through the skin for resection by sharp dissecting forceps; this procedure is said to cause less tissue injury, less swelling and pain, and a lower complication rate.[203]

Intravasal devices are aimed at producing a reversible vasectomy.[193] These methods appear to be effective in animals but have not been tried in humans.

Common causes of failure include division or ligation of some cord-like structure other than the vas (hence the need for pathologic examination of the resected tissue) and spontaneous postsurgical recanalization. In two large series the failure rates related to recanalization were 0.3%[204] and 1.2%.[205] The greater the length of the vas resected, the less likely was recanalization to occur.[205]

Vasectomy is considered to be successful when sperm cannot be demonstrated in direct wet mounts of the semen on two consecutive specimens. The median time for development of azoospermia after vasectomy is 24 ejaculations, and conception caused by the presence of residual sperm has been reported 6 wk after a technically successful vasectomy.[206] Thus most patients are evaluated at 3 mo, although some physicians recommend initial examination at 1 mo with search only for motile sperm.[207] When recanalization occurs, it develops at a median time of 6 mo.[204]

The acute complications of vasectomy include swelling, hematoma formation, inflammation, and recanalization. The frequency of complications in three large series is shown in Table 18–13.[204, 208, 209] Vasitis, funiculitis, and epididymitis are not the result of infection but rather are due to extravasation of sperm into the interstitium.[208] The overall complication rate is about 6%.

Development of sperm granuloma is the most common serious postoperative complication of vasectomy.[194] It is apparently less common when a double-back ligation technique or electrofulguration is used than after simple vasal excision and ligation.[208] Immediately after vasectomy, induration and swelling develop in the stumps, probably because of compromise in the blood supply to the vas by the ligature. In most cases a scar forms and the ends of the vas become sealed off. However, necrosis of the ligated stump may occur, resulting in a leak and formation of a sperm granuloma. Sperm granulomas are painful and may initiate a spontaneous reanastomosis, thus causing the vasectomy to fail. This anastomosis is thought to occur because islands of mucosal cells in the inflammatory tissue of the granuloma can proliferate to form irregular narrow canals that finally connect the two ends.

Effects on Testicular Histologic Features and Endocrine Function

The changes in the testis after occlusion of the vas have been extensively studied in animals.[210] They vary from species to species and with the site and type of operative vasal occlusion. Occlusion of the vas deferens in the primate is compatible with continued spermatogenesis in the testis. The sperm may be resorbed or stored in distended ducts and cysts. Testicular volume in men does not change after vasectomy.[211] The transient degeneration of the germinal epithelium that occurs in the immediate postoperative period is not demonstrable several years after vasectomy. Quantitative morphometric studies of the testis of men undergoing vasectomy reversal disclosed increased thickness of the seminiferous tubule walls and reduction in the mean number of Sertoli cells.[212] Focal interstitial fibrosis was present in 23% and was associated with an increased likelihood of subsequent infertility in spite of a technically successful vasectomy reversal.[212] Changes in the epididymis may be permanent owing to rupture and fibrosis.[213]

Small amounts of steroid hormones are present in the seminal fluid. It has been generally believed that testicular hormones are present in the fluid that enters the epididymis and that these hormones are passed through the epididymis and the ejaculatory system to the seminal fluid. However, the content of several of these hormones in seminal fluid decreases only slightly after vasectomy, which suggests that they are derived in large part from the seminal vesicle and prostate rather than directly from the testes.[214] The fact that some (but not all) prostatic contributions to the ejaculate decrease after vasectomy suggests that prostatic function may also diminish.[215]

There appear to be no significant systemic endocrine sequelae of vasectomy. In five representative studies, levels of plasma testosterone, LH, and FSH did not change after vasectomy.[216–220] These studies include prospective trials[217, 218, 220] and follow-ups for as long as 5 y after surgery.[217, 220] In addition, Leydig cell reserve, as assessed by response to human chorionic gonadotropin, is normal 4 y after vasectomy.[220]

Antibodies and Atherosclerosis After Vasectomy

Sperm-agglutinating antibodies in the sera of vasectomized men were first reported in 1959.[221] Shortly thereafter, complement-dependent sperm-immobilizing antibodies were detected.[222] Approximately 2% of control men have sperm-agglutinating titers, whereas no immobilizing antibody can be detected in men before vasectomy.[223] Sperm antibodies are detectable beginning 7 to 11 d after vasectomy.[223] In general, 40% of men develop significant agglutinating antibody titers within a year after vasectomy, and 20% have sperm-immobilizing antibodies.[195, 223, 224]

The development of antibodies to sperm after vasectomy

TABLE 18–13. Postoperative Complications of Vasectomy in Three Large Series

Complication	% for Series		
	A (Total No. 2711)	B (Total No. 1000)	C (Total No. 843)
Epididymitis	1.0	1.8	1.8
Abscess formation	0.7		1.5
Vasitis and funiculitis	0.4	3.2	
Hematoma	0.5	0.3	0.5
Hydrocele	0.1		0.4
Sperm granuloma	<0.1	1.2	
Vas cutaneous adhesion	0.7		
Vas cutaneous fistula	0.5		
Cellulitis and other	1.2		1.1
Recanalization	0.3	0.8	0.2
	5.5	7.3	5.5

Data for column A from Leader AJ, Axelrad SD, Frankowski R, et al. Complications of 2,711 vasectomies. J Urol 1974; 111:365–369. Data for column B from Klapproth HJ, Young IS. Vasectomy, vas ligation and vas occlusion. Urology 1973; 1:292–300. Data for column C from Penna RM, Potash J, Penna SM. Elective vasectomy: a study of 843 patients. J Fam Pract 1979; 8:857–858.

raised the question whether other forms of autoimmune reactions might occur in such men. In two studies involving more than 1000 vasectomized men, there was no increased incidence of antibodies directed to antigens other than sperm.[225, 226] In addition, there was no increased incidence of autoimmune disease in the vasectomized men.[230] However, in 1978 Alexander and Clarkson reported that vasectomy increases both the extent and the severity of diet-induced atherosclerosis in cynomolgus monkeys.[227] Studies involving several thousand subjects evaluated the incidence of nonfatal myocardial infarction, coronary artery disease, and outcome in vasectomized and control men.[228–231] No increased prevalence of complications or mortality from atherosclerotic cardiovascular disease or in overall mortality rates was found in the vasectomized group in any of the studies, even after 10 y or more.[228–231] It must be concluded, therefore, that there is no association between vasectomy and atherosclerosis in men.

Prostate Cancer

Although there does not appear to be any change in overall mortality, death from cancer is said to be increased in men 20 y or more after vasectomy.[231] Furthermore in both prospective[232] and retrospective[233] cohort studies the relative risk for prostate cancer was found to be 1.66 and 1.56, respectively, after vasectomy. The proposed mechanism for facilitating prostate cancer is that the reduction in prostate secretion might favor carcinogen exposure.[233] However, there is no evidence to support such a mechanism, and the weak association might be due to chance or unmeasured confounding bias.[234] In another study, vasectomy increased the risk for prostate cancer only in men who had had the procedure more than 20 y previously or before age 35.[235] Conflicting or negative results have been reported in other studies,[236–238] and additional studies may be required to determine whether or not there is a risk.[239, 240] Because of the uncertainty, the possibility must be included in presterilization counseling.

Psychosexual Effects

Most men who undergo vasectomy are satisfied with the procedure and would, in retrospect, have it done again.[241–243] Increased sexual enjoyment and increased frequency of intercourse are common, probably related to decreased anxiety about unwanted pregnancies. Vasectomy has no deleterious effect on potency or sexual performance, and marital harmony usually improves or remains unchanged after vasectomy.

Reversal of Vasectomy

Vasectomy should be recommended only to men who desire permanent sterilization. However, it is inevitable that some will change their minds and request reversal. Reasons for such requests include the death of children, an improved economic situation, and remarriage after divorce or death of the wife. Two vasovasostomy techniques (single-layer and double-layer microscopic closure) have been developed for such reanastomoses.[244] With both techniques the success rate for reappearance of sperm in the ejaculate is 80 to 90%. However, the associated pregnancy rate is only 30 to 50%.[245–249] A number of technical issues influence the anatomic success of the reanastomosis procedure, but the functional success is probably determined by whether antisperm antibodies are present (Table 18–14).[250–253] In some, but not all, studies, men who are able to father a child after vasovasostomy are less likely to have antisperm antibodies than those who remain infertile.[254] The relationship is not absolute, but the antisperm antibodies presumably interfere with sperm function. Isolated immuno-

TABLE 18–14. Percentage of Vasovasostomy Subjects with Positive Antisperm Antibody in Relation to Achieving Pregnancy

| Variable | % for Series* | | | |
	A (45 Couples)	B (51 Couples)	C (20 Couples)	D (51 Couples)
Pregnancy	48	18	8	15
No pregnancy	94	69	75	71

* A, ref. 250; B, ref 251; C, ref. 252; D, ref. 253.

globulin G and Fab antibodies from vasectomized guinea pigs inhibit fertilization in vitro.[255]

Conclusion

Vasectomy is a relatively simple procedure that is more than 99% effective in producing permanent infertility. Postoperative complications are minor. No adverse effects on the testis or its endocrine function have been detected. Although acceleration of atherosclerosis associated with immune complex formation occurs in vasectomized monkeys, there is no evidence that a similar phenomenon occurs in humans. Whether there is an increased risk of prostate cancer is unclear. Surgical reanastomosis can restore fertility in 30 to 50% of vasectomized men.

Search for a Male Contraceptive
Drugs That Inhibit Hypothalamic-Pituitary Function

Because spermatogenesis requires normal gonadotropin levels, inhibition of the production of LH and FSH, either directly through an effect on the pituitary or indirectly through suppression of LHRH, will decrease sperm production.

ANDROGENS ALONE. The administration of exogenous testosterone to normal men suppresses gonadotropin secretion and inhibits spermatogenesis; it simultaneously prevents the deficiency in testosterone production that would otherwise follow gonadotropin suppression and consequently avoids the adverse effects on libido and potency. The preparations that are available for administering pharmacologic doses of testosterone safely are long-acting esters, testosterone cypionate and testosterone enanthate, both of which must be given intramuscularly. The optimal replacement dose is about 200 mg every 2 wk.[256] Patches for the transdermal administration of testosterone are useful only for replacement therapy (see Chapter 16). Most oral androgen preparations have 17α-alkyl substitutions in the steroid molecule to prevent inactivation by the liver. These preparations are not safe for testosterone replacement because of the risk of hepatotoxicity (see Chapter 16).

Administration of 200 mg of testosterone enanthate every 2 wk causes azoospermia in less than one fourth of men after a year, whereas a regimen of 200 mg of testosterone enanthate every 7 to 10 d causes asoospermia in about one half (Table 18–15).[257–260] The weekly regimen causes an average 50% increase in plasma testosterone levels and suppression of plasma LH and FSH levels by 60 to 80%.[256, 259, 260]

Maximal suppression of sperm density was achieved within 8 to 10 wk, and recovery of sperm density to control levels occurred within 20 to 28 wk after cessation of therapy.[259] The side effects of weekly 200-mg testosterone enanthate injections for 18 mo were evaluated in a multicenter contraceptive efficacy study involving 271 healthy men, including 82 Chinese and 189 other men.[261] Azoospermia was achieved in 58% of the men during the 6 mo suppression phase, and

TABLE 18–15. Effect of Weekly Injections of 200 mg of Testosterone Enanthate on Sperm Density in Normal Men

Investigators	No. of Men	Duration of Treatment (wk)	% of Men with Azoospermia
Steinberger and Smith[257]	5	42	100
Paulsen et al.[258]	42	26	48
Cunningham et al.[259]	20	12	25
Swerdloff et al.[260]	17	16	59

these men entered the 12 mo efficacy study; during the efficacy phase 24% of the men discontinued therapy for a variety of reasons. Almost 30% developed acne, and 9 subjects discontinued for this reason. Twenty-two men developed fatigue, weight gain (3 to 4 kg) occurred in 12, and testicular volume uniformly decreased about 20%. Seven men reported increased aggressiveness, and nine subjects developed gynecomastia. The hematocrit increased by an average of 6.4%, and in two men the hematocrit was greater than 550 g/L. Serum triglyceride and LDL cholesterol levels did not change. In the non-Chinese men HDL cholesterol decreased 18%. All changes were reversed during the recovery phase.

The efficacy phase of the study involved only the 70% of men who achieved consistent azoospermia during the suppression phase; the pregnancy rate during the efficacy phase was 0.8 per 100 person-years.[262] The same group subsequently extended the contraceptive efficacy trial to 399 men in nine countries who were rendered either azoospermic or profoundly oligospermic (sperm density <3 million/mL) during the suppression phase.[263] In the efficacy phase four pregnancies occurred during 50 person-years involving men with oligospermia (0.1 to 3 million/mL), and none occurred during 230 person-years in the azoospermic men for overall pregnancy rates of 1.4 per 100 person-years. This result compares favorably with the typical first year with oral contraceptives in women. The reason that some men became oligospermic and some developed azoospermia is not clear,[264] although the conversion of testosterone to dihydrotestosterone was greater in the oligospermic subset.[265] In summary, weekly injection of testosterone enanthate is not a practical regimen for long-term use. Longer acting preparations such as testosterone buciclate (see Chapter 16) or testosterone implants[266] might be more effective.

PROGESTATIONAL AGENTS. Progestational agents inhibit pituitary gonadotropin secretion in both women and men and have been considered as a potential means of fertility control in men. Because the suppression of plasma LH results in a lowering of testosterone levels, progestagens are used in conjunction with androgens. The most extensively studied combination is 150 to 200 mg of medroxyprogesterone acetate and 200 to 500 mg of testosterone enanthate by injection,[267–269] usually on a monthly basis. Azoospermia is achieved on average in about half of the men, usually within 2 to 3 mo.[267] Escape from the suppression of spermatogenesis may occur after several months.[267]

Side effects of the combination therapy include mild acne and occasional gynecomastia. Most subjects gained weight; in one study the average weight gain was 6 kg.[269] Some men reported decreased libido, possibly because the plasma testosterone value was only 10 to 30% of baseline one month after the injection.[269] Medroxyprogesterone acetate has a longer duration of action and results in chronic gonadotropin suppression after exogenous testosterone has been depleted.[270] Levonorgestrel is a progestagen that in combination with a replacement dose of testosterone enanthate (l00 mg/wk) induces a more rapid suppression of spermatogenesis than testosterone alone,[271] but the percentage of men achieving a

sperm density of less than 3 million/mL is no greater than with testosterone cypionate alone at 200 mg/wk.[263]

Cyproterone acetate, a progestational agent with potent antiandrogenic properties, has been tried as an antifertility agent. In animals the drug causes both gonadotropin suppression and impairment of androgen action at the level of the testis or epididymis. However, the drug is ineffective in lowering sperm density below the normal range in most men, and only rarely do men develop azoospermia. Cyproterone acetate (50 or 100 mg/d) has also been tried for fertility control in combination with 100 mg/wk of testosterone enanthate.[275] All 10 men given the combination regimen achieved azoospermia within 6 wk. No change in lipoprotein levels was detected, sexual function remained normal, and there was a small decrease in the hematocrit. The changes reverted to normal during the recovery phase.

LUTEINIZING HORMONE–RELEASING HORMONE ANALOGUES. As discussed earlier, a family of LHRH analogues (both agonists and antagonists) has been synthesized. When the LHRH agonists are modified at positions 6 and 10, they are more potent than the native hormone.[276] Prolonged administration of these agonists causes a paradoxical inhibition of gonadotropin secretion,[277] possibly because of decreases in the number of LHRH receptors and inhibiting postreceptor events involved in the secretion of gonadotropin.[278]

Daily administration of the agonist D-Trp[6]-Pro[9]-N-ethylamide-LHRH by subcutaneous injections to eight normal men resulted in a 90% decrease in plasma testosterone levels and a 50% decrease in plasma gonadotropin levels.[279] It is of interest that levels of bioactive LH decrease to a greater extent than levels of immunoreactive LH after treatment with this analogue.[280] The pulsatile pattern of LH release was diminished, and the gonadotropin response to pulsatile administration of LHRH was lost, but the Leydig cell remained responsive to exogenous human LH during treatment with the agonist.[281] Thus the locus of action of the analogue in humans appears to be at the level of the pituitary.[281] In contrast to the decreasing ratio of bioactive LH to immunoactive LH during treatment with this agonist, the ratio of bioactive to immunoactive FSH was normal.[282] Although treatment was discontinued in most men after 6 or 7 wk because of impotence, one subject developed azoospermia after 10 wk of therapy. Recovery of spermatogenesis occurred by 14 wk after cessation of therapy in all subjects.[279]

Initial trials suggested that LHRH analogues and testosterone were synergistic in inhibiting gonadotropins,[283] but daily injection of LHRH analogues combined with biweekly testosterone injections were no more successful than LHRH analogues alone in producing azoospermia in men.[284] When the agonist was given by constant infusion and in conjunction with biweekly testosterone injections, three of seven men developed azoospermia.[285] In one study the administration of the agonist blocked the antifertility effects of androgens.[286]

Because the combination of LHRH agonist and testosterone had not consistently induced azoospermia in normal men, clinical trials of LHRH antagonists have been performed. One antagonist, Nal-Glu (Ac D[2]NaL[1], D4Cl Phe[2], D3Pal[3], Arg[5], DGlu[6] (AA) DAla[10]-LHRH) has been studied by several groups.[287, 288] LHRH antagonists compete with endogenous LHRH for binding to receptors in pituitary gonadotrophs and thereby inhibit gonadotropin secretion. Prolonged administration of the Nal-Glu LHRH antagonist by daily injection lowers the levels of inhibin, LH, and FSH and the ratio of bioactive to immunoactive LH and decreases the serum testosterone level by 70 to 78%.[287, 288] The combination of weekly testosterone injection plus Nal-Glu LHRH was more effective in suppressing serum LH, FSH, and inhibin levels than either Nal-Glu alone or testosterone alone.[288] There have been three human contraceptive trials of antagonist plus testosterone.[289–291] A total of 7 of 8 men in each of the first two trials achieved azoospermia, and 7 of 10 men became azoospermic in the third.

In summary, the control of fertility in men with drugs that inhibit the hypothalamic-pituitary system is limited by the need for frequent injections of androgens. A method of delivering testosterone to cause sustained levels in the physiological range coupled with either a depot LHRH antagonist (or nonpeptidyl oral mimic) or cyproterone acetate seems most promising. Weekly testosterone injections and the adverse effects of pharmacologic doses of testosterone on HDL cholesterol levels are probably unacceptable.

Drugs and Other Agents That Affect the Testis Directly

A number of antineoplastic drugs and other relatively toxic compounds impair sperm production by direct effects on the testes. Most of these compounds produce additional unacceptable side effects. This section deals with the oral agent gossypol and other plant extracts, reviews studies with other drugs, and describes physical and immunologic attempts to inhibit spermatogenesis.

GOSSYPOL AND OTHER PLANT EXTRACTS. In the late 1950s an increased frequency of infertility was noted in areas of the People's Republic of China where crude cottonseed oil was used in cooking. It was found that the antifertility agent in cottonseed oil is gossypol (Fig. 18–9), a naphthalphenol present in various parts of the cotton plant.

Clinical trials of gossypol as an antifertility agent in the People's Republic of China involved almost 10,000 men over a decade.[292, 293] Gossypol affects the spermatogenic tubules predominantly, with little change in Leydig cells. The administration of 20 mg by mouth daily for 60 d (loading period) causes the sperm in the ejaculate to become immotile and to decrease in number or disappear. A sperm density of less than 4 million/mL was achieved in 99.9% of men. Because gossypol affects sperm motility as well as sperm number, azoospermia may not be necessary to ensure consistent infertility, as in the case of drugs that inhibit pituitary function. The actual assessment of fertility has not been described in men receiving gossypol.[292, 293] After a low sperm count is achieved (usually 60 d), the maintenance dose is decreased to one third the original dose.

Short-term side effects included fatigue, decreased libido, and decreased appetite. During chronic therapy the incidence of symptomatic hypokalemia varied from as high as 4.7% to an undetectable amount among groups,[294] and hypokalemic paralysis occurred in a few subjects; the hypokalemia is due to renal postassium wasting.[294] Attempts to decrease the dose of gossypol to prevent hypokalemia were unsuccessful.[295] Supplemental potassium salts and triamterine were also ineffective in preventing hypokalemia.[296]

The drug impairs both spermatogenesis and sperm maturation, with the result that motility is impaired.[293] In long-term studies, male sexual function appears not to be affected after the loading period. The factor that is likely to prevent further clinical trials of gossypol is the failure of sperm density to return to normal after cessation of therapy.[293, 297] In a study at two centers, about 40% of azoospermic men at cessation of gossypol therapy did not recover normal sperm density by 2 y, and half remained azoospermic.[297]

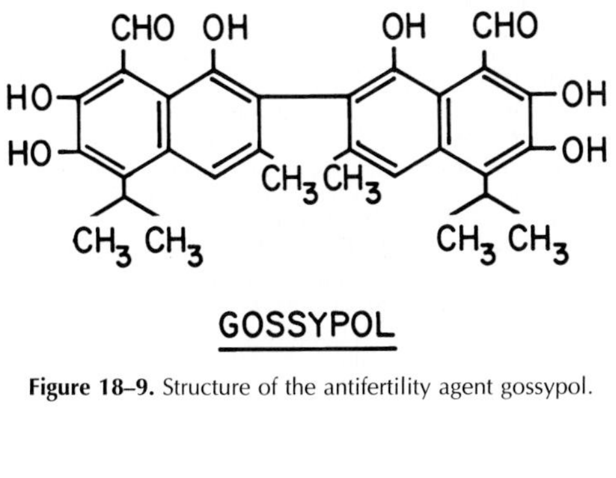

An extract of *Tripterygium wilfordii* (GWT), which is used to treat rheumatoid arthritis in China, was found to cause azoospermia.[289–299] The active ingredients are thought to be a series of diterpene oxides. An oral dose of 20 mg/d causes oligospermia and impairment of sperm motility within 2 mo.[299] Within 2 mo of discontinuing therapy semen parameters return to normal, and there appears to be no significant side effects. Animal studies suggest that the drug affects both spermatogenesis and epididymal function. At dosages five or more times those needed for the antifertility effects, GWT causes immunosuppression. Future development of components of this plant for use in the control of male fertility will require demonstration of safety and separation of contraceptive effects from immunosuppression.[299]

A subcapsular intratesticular assay has been developed for the preliminary screening of male antifertility agents in animals.[300] This method compares favorably with the standard WHO oral screening assay for male contraceptives.[300]

OTHER DRUGS. Sulfasalazine is a drug that is used for the management of inflammatory bowel disease. Like gossypol, sulfasalazine appears to impair spermatogenesis and inhibit sperm motility, presumably related to effects on the epididymis.[301] The incomplete inhibition of spermatogenesis and the frequency of side effects make it unacceptable as a male contraceptive.

Other drugs with antispermatogenic activity in animals include nitrofurans, thiophenes, dinitropyrroles, and bis-(dichloroacetyl)-diamines.[302] Of these, the diamines appear to be sufficiently free from severe toxic effects for human trials to be undertaken. However, the trials were abandoned when an antabuse-like effect was discovered after the use of the drugs was combined with alcohol ingestion.[302]

Indazole carboxylic acids such as tolnidamine may have potential for fertility control in men.[303] These chemicals have a selective action on the testicular germinal epithelium in rats, rabbits, and rhesus monkeys and have a paucity of side effects. Spermatogenesis returns to normal when the drug is discontinued. The site of action of tolnidamine appears to be the Sertoli cells.[303]

PHYSICAL METHODS. The suppressive effect of heat on spermatogenesis is manifested by the temporary decreases in sperm density that follow acute febrile illnesses or hot baths. The 2°C higher temperature of the abdomen than that of the scrotum is thought to account for the infertility of cryptorchidism. The thermal effect of hot water, infrared heat, microwaves, and ultrasound has been evaluated in rats as a potential antifertility therapy.[304] Electronic means of heat induction appear to be more effective than the other thermal methods in causing infertility, and ultrasound is more effective at a lower temperature than microwaves.[304]

Ultrasound as a physical means of inhibiting spermatogenesis has been investigated in several species.[304] Spermatogenesis can be suppressed in cats, dogs, and monkeys without causing histologic damage to Leydig cells and without altering plasma testosterone levels. This effect is believed to be temporary. Pilot studies of ultrasound treatment in men with prostate cancer before orchiectomy demonstrated reductions in spermatogenesis without an effect on Leydig cell morphology or plasma testosterone level.[304]

IMMUNOLOGIC METHODS. Immunologic approaches to fertility control in men have utilized the production of antibodies to hormones or the induction of autoimmune reactions to some component of the testes, sex accessory organs,

Figure 18–9. Structure of the antifertility agent gossypol.

or spermatozoa.[305] The ideal target hormone would appear to be FSH, which is required for the induction of spermatogenesis. When FSH is neutralized with anti-FSH antibodies in monkeys, spermatogenesis is severely impaired in mature animals without a reduction in plasma LH or testosterone levels.[306, 307] The effect of neutralization of FSH in humans is not known. Passive immunization with anti-FSH antibodies is impractical in the long term. Active immunization of male rhesus monkeys with purified FSH was ineffective for fertility control in a long-term study.[308]

Induction of an immunologic reaction to some component of the testis may result in either the induction of an autoimmune orchitis or the elicitation of a specific antibody response to a specific sperm antigen. The injection of testicular homogenates induces allergic orchitis in at least eight mammalian species. In the guinea pig at least four different antigens have been identified in testicular homogenates when Freund complete adjuvant and repeated subcutaneous injections are used. Talwar and colleagues[309, 310] have described a technique in which intratesticular injection of bacille Calmette-Guérin vaccine alone was used to achieve aspermatogenesis. Oligospermia can be achieved within 6 wk in dogs and monkeys, whereas both basal testosterone levels and the testosterone response to human chorionic gonadotropin administration are normal.[309] These effects are reversible in some animals.[310]

A specific isozyme of lactate dehydrogenase (LDH-X), which is expressed only in the testis and spermatozoa, is a potential candidate for induction of the immune response for fertility control in men. Immunization with this antigen does not result in aspermatogenesis or orchitis but does impair sperm motility in rabbits.[311] The resulting infertility is reversible in rabbits and mice.

In summary, gossypol does not appear to be a suitable oral contraceptive for men, and the long-term effects of extracts of *Tripterygium wilfordii* are unknown. The indazole carboxylic acids, other chemicals with promise, have been studied only in animals. Ultrasound may be effective and safe but is associated with an uncertain duration of effect. Most active immunization methods have an indeterminate duration of action and involve repeated injections of Freund adjuvant. Passive immunization may cause acute allergic reactions and immune complex disease.

Drugs That Affect the Epididymis

Selective inhibition of epididymal function that would cause impairment of sperm maturation would theoretically control fertility without the risk of impaired testicular function. The time required to achieve an effect on fertility with such agents should also be less than the 2 to 3 mo necessary for agents affecting the pituitary or testis.

ANTIANDROGENS. Because normal androgen action is necessary for epididymal function, antiandrogens are logical candidates to inhibit sperm maturation in the epididymis. Cyproterone acetate, an antiandrogen, does inhibit gonadotropin secretion. Both cyproterone (the free alcohol) and the nonsteroidal antiandrogen flutamide appear to be ineffective in inhibiting epididymal function. These agents inhibit the negative feedback of endogenous androgens and cause an increased LH and testosterone synthesis, thus overcoming any inhibitory effect of the antiandrogen in the epididymis.[312, 313]

α-CHLOROHYDRIN. α-Chlorohydrin, a monochloro derivative of glycerol (3-chloro-1,2-propanediol), is commercially available as a racemic mixture of $S(+)$ and $R(-)$ forms. The $S(+)$-3-chlorohydrin form is active in inducing infertility and has less toxicity than the mixture, whereas the $R(-)$ isomer is ineffective for fertility control.[314] These observations suggest that any antifertility properties are due to a specific metabolic action and not to their random action as alkylating agents. The compound induces temporary infertility in rats, guinea pigs, and monkeys without causing loss of libido and without alterations in ejaculation or in the morphology of ejaculated spermatozoa. α-Chlorohydrin may inhibit oxidative phosphorylation, glycolysis, and glycerol metabolism.[315] The toxicity of the agent appears to be its limiting factor. The compound causes bone marrow depression in monkeys and hepatotoxicity or nephrotoxicity in other species.[316] A better understanding of the specific mechanism of action of this drug on sperm metabolism might lead to the development of other less toxic compounds.

CHLORINATED SUGARS. The 6-chloro-6-deoxy sugars have been investigated as potential inhibitors of the glycolytic pathway in spermatozoa.[317] Like α-chlorohydrin, these compounds produce reversible infertility in male rats with a paucity of toxic side effects. No direct inhibitory effect of 6-chloro-6-deoxyglucose has been demonstrated in spermatozoa, so the compounds are probably converted to another active metabolite in the body. Rats made infertile with 6-chloro-6-deoxyglucose continue to produce normal numbers of spermatozoa and to mate with females as frequently as control subjects. However, spermatozoa from treated animals are unable to oxidize glucose, and they quickly become immotile after removal from the epididymis and incubation with glucose as an energy source. Unfortunately, neurotoxicity has been detected in marmoset monkeys and mice that were given high doses of 6-chloro-6-deoxyglucose.[318]

In summary, antiandrogens are ineffective. α-Chlorohydrin and chlorinated sugars are effective in animals but have significant toxicity.

REFERENCES

1. Population Reports. Migration, population growth, and development. Series M, No. 7. Demographics. Baltimore: The Johns Hopkins University, 1983: M20–M92.
2. Pannenborg CO. Contraceptive needs in the Third World: the present paradox of a future planning-technology nexus. Excerpta Med Int Congr Ser 1987; 759:21–44.
3. Segal AJ. Contraceptive research: a male chauvinist plot? Fam Plann Perspect 1972; 4:21–25.
4. Cunningham FA, MacDonald PC, Gant NF, et al. Williams Obstetrics. 19th ed. Norwalk, CT: Appleton & Lange, 1993: 1321–1360.
5. Goldzieher JW. Estrogens in oral contraceptives: historical perspectives. Johns Hopkins Med J 1982; 150:165–169.
6. Doisy EA, Veler CD, Tayer S. Folliculin from urine of pregnant women. Am J Physiol 1929; 90:329–330.
7. Butenandt A. Progynon, a crystalline female sexual hormone. Naturwissenchafen 1929; 17:879.
8. Butenandt A, Westphal V. Zur Isolierung und Charakterisierung des Corpus-Luteum-Hormones. Berl Dtsch Chem Ges 1934; 67:1440–1442.
9. Sturgis SH, Albright R. Mechanism of estrin therapy in the relief of dysmenorrhea. Endocrinology 1940; 26:68–72.
10. Pincus G, Roch J, Garcia CR. Effects of certain 19-nor steroids upon the reproductive process. Ann NY Acad Sci 1958; 71:677–690.
11. Chez RA. Three new progestins for OCs: do they offer benefits? Contemp OB/GYN 1988; 32:51–60.
12. Population Reports. Oral contraceptives in the 1980s. Series A, No. 6. Oral Contraceptives. Baltimore: The Johns Hopkins University, 1982: A190–A222.
13. Speroff L. The formulation of oral contraceptives: does the amount of estrogen make any clinical difference? Johns Hopkins Med J 1982; 150:170–176.
14. Hatcher RA, Trussel J, Stewart F, et al. Contraceptive Technology. 16th ed, revised. New York: Irvington, 1994.
15. Gaspard UJ. Metabolic effects of oral contraceptives. Am J Obstet Gynecol 1987; 157:1029–1041.
16. Silverberg S, Makowski E. Endometrial carcinoma in young women taking oral contraceptive agents. Obstet Gynecol 1975; 46:503–506.
17. Liggins GC. The effect of variation in estrogen dosage on the pregnancy rate during sequential oral contraception. Fertil Steril 1967; 18:191–197.
18. Jones RC, Edgren RA. The effects of various steroids on the vaginal histology in the rat. Fertil Steril 1973; 24:284–291.
19. Goldzieher JW, Maqueo M, Chenault CB, et al. Comparative studies of the ethinyl estrogens used in oral contraceptives. I: Endometrial response. Am J Obstet Gynecol 1975; 122:615–618.

20. Goldzieher JW, de la Pena A, Chenault CB, et al. Comparative studies of the ethinyl estrogens used in oral contraceptives. II: Anovulatory potency. Am J Obstet Gynecol 1975; 122:619–624.

21. Goldzieher JW, de la Pena A, Chenault CB, et al. Comparative studies of the ethinyl estrogens used in oral contraceptives. III: Effect on plasma gonadotropins. Am J Obstet Gynecol 1975; 122:625–636.

22. Edgren RA. Relative potencies of oral contraceptives. In: Moghissi KS, ed. Controversies in Contraception. Baltimore: Williams & Wilkins, 1979: 1–18.

23. Dorflinger LJ. Relative potency of progestins used in oral contraceptives. Contraception 1985; 31:557–570.

24. Fotherby K. Pharmacokinetics and metabolism of progestins in humans. In: Goldzieher JW, Fotherby K, eds. Pharmacology of the Contraceptive Steroids. New York: Raven Press, 1994: 99–126.

25. Edgren RA, Sturtevant FM. Potencies of oral contraceptives. Am J Obstet Gynecol 1976; 125:1029–1038.

26. Dickey RP, Stone SC. Progestational potency of oral contraceptives. Obstet Gynecol 1976; 47:106–112.

27. Dickey RP. Initial pill selection and managing the contraceptive pill patient. Int J Gynaecol Obstet 1979; 16:547–555.

28. Berger GS, Talwar PP. Oral contraceptive potencies and side effects. Obstet Gynecol 1978; 51:545–547.

29. Goldzieher JW. Pharmacokinetics and metabolism of ethinyl estrogens. In: Goldzhier JW, Fotherby K, eds. Pharmacology of the Contraceptive Steroids. New York: Raven Press. 1994: 127–151.

30. Barbieri RL, Petro Z, Canick JA, et al. Aromatization of norethindrone to ethinyl estradiol by human placental microsomes. J Clin Endocrinol Metab 1983; 57:299–303.

31. Carr BR, Parker CR Jr, Madden JD, et al. Plasma levels of adrenocorticotropin and cortisol in women receiving oral contraceptive steroid treatment. J Clin Endocrinol Metab 1979; 49:346–349.

32. Bronson RA. Oral contraception: mechanisms of action. Clin Obstet Gynecol 1981; 24:869–877.

33. Baird DT, Glasier AF. Hormonal contraception. N Engl J Med 1993; 328:1543–1549.

34. Vandenberg G, DeVane G, Yen SSC. Effects of exogenous estrogen and oral progestin on pituitary responsiveness to synthetic luteinizing hormone–releasing factor. J Clin Invest 1974; 53:1750–1754.

35. Spellacy WN, Kalra PS, Buhi WR, et al. Pituitary and ovarian responsiveness to a graded gonadotropin releasing factor stimulation test in women using a low estrogen on a regular type of oral contraceptive. Am J Obstet Gynecol 1980; 137:109–115.

36. Greenwald GS. In vivo recording of intraluminal pressure changes in the rabbit oviduct. Fertil Steril 1963; 14:666–674.

37. Hillard GD, Norris HJ. Pathological effects of oral contraceptives. Recent Results Cancer Res 1979; 66:49–71.

38. Gray MJ, Grimes DA. Birth control, abortion and sterilization. In: Romney SC, Gray MJ, Little AB, et al, eds. Gynecology and Obstetrics: The Health Care of Women. New York: McGraw-Hill, 1981: 817–852.

39. Peterson HB, DeStefano F, Greenspan JR, et al. Mortality risk associated with tubal sterilization in United States hospitals. Am J Obstet Gynecol 1982; 143:125–129.

40. Royal College of General Practitioners Oral Contraceptive Study. Mortality among oral contraceptive users. Lancet 1977; 2:727–733.

41. Royal College of General Practitioners Oral Contraceptive Study. Further analyses of mortality in oral contraceptive users. Lancet 1981; 1:541–546.

42. Vessey MP, McPherson K, Yeates D. Mortality in oral contraceptive users. Lancet 1981; 1:549–550.

43. Ramcharan S, Pelligrin FA, Ray R, et al. Mortality. In: Ramcharan S, Pelligrin FA, Ray R, et al, eds. The Walnut Creek Contraceptive Drug Study: A Prospective Study of the Side Effects of Oral Contraceptives. Vol 3: An Interim Report—A Comparison of Disease Occurrence Leading to Hospitalization or Death in Users and Nonusers of Oral Contraceptives. Bethesda: Center for Population Research, 1981: 189–210.

44. Porter JB, Jick H, Walker AM. Mortality among oral contraceptive users. Obstet Gynecol 1987; 70:29–32.

45. Stadel BV. Oral contraceptives and cardiovascular disease (first of two parts). N Engl J Med 1981; 305:612–618.

46. Stadel BV. Oral contraceptives and cardiovascular disease (second of two parts). N Engl J Med 1981; 305:672–677.

47. World Health Organization. The world's main health problems. From WHO's sixth report on the world health situation. World Health Forum 1981; 2:264–280.

48. Shapiro S, Slone D, Rosenberg L, et al. Oral-contraceptive use in relation to myocardial infarction. Lancet 1979; 1:743–747.

49. Inman WHW, Vessey MP. Investigation of deaths from pulmonary, coronary, and cerebral thrombosis and embolism in women of childbearing age. Br Med J 1968; 2:193–199.

50. Slone D, Shapiro S, Kaufman DW, et al. Risk of myocardial infarction in relation to current and discontinued use of oral contraceptives. N Engl J Med 1981; 305:420–424.

51. Stampfer MJ, Willett WC, Colditz GA, et al. A prospective study of past use of oral contraceptive agents and risk of cardiovascular disease. N Engl J Med 1988; 319:1313–1317.

52. Castelli WP. Cardiovascular disease in women. Am J Obstet Gynecol 1988; 158:1553–1560.

53. Wallace RB, Hoover J, Barrett-Connor E, et al. Altered plasma lipid and lipoprotein levels associated with oral contraceptive and oestrogen use: report from the Medications Working Group of the Lipid Research Clinics Program. Lancet 1979; 2:111–115.

54. Heiss G, Tamir I, Davis CE, et al. Lipoprotein-cholesterol distributions in selected North American populations: The Lipid Research Clinics Program Prevalence Study. Circulation 1980; 61:302–315.

55. La Rosa JC. The varying effects of progestins on lipid levels and cardiovascular disease. Am J Obstet Gynecol 1988; 158:1621–1629.

56. Speroff L, DeCherney A. Evaluation of a new generation of oral contraceptives. The advisory board for the new progestins. Obstet Gynecol 1993; 81:1034–1047.

57. Bradley DD, Wingerd J, Petitti DB, et al. Serum high-density-lipoprotein cholesterol in women using oral contraceptives, estrogens and progestins. N Engl J Med 1978; 299:17–20.

58. Krauss RM, Lindgren FT, Silvers A, et al. Changes in serum high density lipoproteins in women on oral contraceptive drugs. Clin Chim Acta 1977; 80:465–470.

59. Meade TW, Greenberg G, Thompson SC. Progestogens and cardiovascular reactions associated with oral contraceptives and a comparison of the safety of 50- and 30-µg oestrogen preparations. Br Med J 1980; 280:1157–1161.

60. Meade TW. Effects of progestogens on the cardiovascular system. Am J Obstet Gynecol 1982; 142:776–780.

61. Hirronen E, Heikkila-Idanpen J. Cardiovascular death among women under 40 years of age using low-estrogen oral contraceptives and intrauterine devices in Finland from 1975 to 1984. Am J Obstet Gynecol 1990; 163:281–284.

62. Barnes RW, Krapf T, Hoak JC. Erroneous clinical diagnosis of leg vein thrombosis in women on oral contraceptives. Obstet Gynecol 1978; 51:556–558.

63. Sagar S, Stamatakis JD, Thomas DP, et al. Oral contraceptives, antithrombin-III activity, and postoperative deep-vein thrombosis. Lancet 1976; 1:509–511.

64. Stamatakis JD, Lawrence D, Kakkar VV. Surgery, venous thrombosis and anti-Xa. Br J Surg 1977; 64:709–711.

65. Alkjaersig N, Fletcher A, Burstein R. Association between oral contraceptive use and thromboembolism: a new approach to its investigation based on plasma fibrinogen chromatography. Am J Obstet Gynecol 1975; 122:199–211.

66. Royal College of General Practitioners. Oral Contraceptives and Health. New York: Pittman, 1974.

67. Royal College of General Practitioners Oral Contraceptive Study. Oral contraceptives, venous thrombosis, and varicose veins. J R Coll Gen Pract 1978; 28:393–399.

68. Bottinger LE, Boman G, Eklund G, et al. Oral contraceptives and thromboembolic disease: effects of lowering oestrogen content. Lancet 1980; 1:1097–1101.

69. Oxford-Family Planning Association Contraceptive Study. Oral contraceptives and venous thromboembolism: findings in a large prospective study. Br Med J 1986; 292:526.

70. Helmrich SP, Rosenberg L, Kaufman DW, et al. Venous thromboembolism in relation to oral contraceptive use. Obstet Gynecol 1987; 69:91–95.

71. Realini JP, Goldzieher JW. Oral contraceptives and cardiovascular disease: a critique of the epidemiologic studies. Am J Obstet Gynecol 1985; 152:729–798.

72. Ramcharan S, Pelligrin FA, Ray R, et al. Diseases of the circulatory system. In: Ramcharan S, Pelligrin FA, Ray R, et al, eds. The Walnut Creek Contraceptive Drug Study: A Prospective Study of the Side Effects of Oral Contraceptives. Vol 3: An Interim Report—A Comparison of Disease Occurrence Leading to Hospitalization or Death in Users and Nonusers of Oral Contraceptives. Bethesda: Center for Population Research, 1981: 130–132.

73. Meade TW. Risks and mechanisms of cardiovascular events in users of oral contraceptives. Am J Obstet Gynecol 1988; 158:1646–1652.

74. Woods JW. Oral contraceptives and hypertension. Hypertension 1988; 11(Suppl II):III1–III5.

75. Royal College of General Practitioners Oral Contraceptive Study. Effect on hypertension and benign breast disease of progestogen component in combined oral contraceptives. Lancet 1977; 1:624.

76. Rebar RW, Zerson K. Characteristics of the new progestogens used in contraceptives. Contraception 1991; 44:1–10.

77. Sondheimer S. Metabolic effects of the birth control pill. Clin Obstet Gynecol 1981; 24:927–941.

78. Spellacy WN, Buhi WC, Birk SA. The effect of the progestogen ethynodiol diacetate on glucose, insulin and growth hormone after six-month treatment. Acta Endocrinol 1972; 70:373–384.

79. Spellacy WN, Buhi WC, Birk SA. Effects of norethindrone on carbohydrate and lipid metabolism. Obstet Gynecol 1975; 46:560–563.

80. Depirro R, Forte F, Bertoli A, et al. Changes in insulin receptors during oral contraception. J Clin Endocrinol Metab 1981; 52:29–33.

81. Seed M, Godsland IF, Wyn V, et al. The effects of cyproterone acetate and ethinyl estradiol on carbohydrate metabolism. Clin Endocrinol 1984; 21:689–699.

82. der Vang NV, Kloosterboer HJ, Haspels AA. Effect of seven low-dose combined oral contraceptive preparations on carbohydrate metabolism. Am J Obstet Gynecol 1987; 156:918–922.

83. Centers for Disease Control Cancer and Steroid Hormone Study. Oral

contraceptive use and the risk of ovarian cancer. JAMA 1983; 249:1596–1599.

84. Cramer DW, Hutchinson GB, Welch WR, et al. Factors affecting the association of oral contraceptives and ovarian cancer. N Engl Med J 1982; 307:1047–1051.

85. Rosenberg L, Shapiro S, Slone D, et al. Epithelial ovarian cancer and combination oral contraceptives. JAMA 1982; 247:3210–3212.

86. Centers for Disease Control Cancer and Steroid Hormone Study. Oral contraceptive use and the risk of endometrial cancer. JAMA 1983; 249: 1600–1604.

87. Cancer and Steroid Hormone Study of the Centers for Disease Control and the National Institute of Child Health and Human Development. Combined oral contraceptive use and the risk of endometrial cancer. JAMA 1987; 257:796–800.

88. Cancer and Steroid Hormone Study of the Centers for Disease Control and the National Institute of Child Health and Human Development. The reduction in risk associated with oral-contraceptive use. N Engl J Med 1987; 316:650–655.

89. Romieu I, Berlin JA, Colditz G. Oral contraceptives and breast cancer: review and meta-analysis. Cancer 1990; 66:2253–2263.

90. Centers for Disease Control Cancer and Steroid Hormone Study. Long-term oral contraceptive use and the risk of breast cancer. JAMA 1983; 249:1591–1595.

91. Schlesselman JJ, Stadel BV, Murray P, et al. Breast cancer in relation to early use of oral contraceptives. JAMA 1988; 259:1828–1833.

92. Population Reports. Oral contraceptives. Lower dose pills. Series A, No. 7. Oral Contraceptives. Baltimore: The Johns Hopkins University, 1988.

93. Harris RW, Brinton LA, Cowdell RH, et al. Characteristics of women with dysplasia or carcinoma in situ of the cervix uteri. Br J Cancer 1980; 42:359–369.

94. Jick H, Herman R. Oral-contraceptive–induced benign liver tumors—the magnitude of the problem. JAMA 1978; 240:828–829 (letter).

95. Rooks JB, Ory HW, Ishak KG, et al. Cooperative Liver Tumor Study Group. Epidemiology of hepatocellular adenoma: the role of oral contraceptive use. JAMA 1979; 242:644–648.

96. Oral contraceptives and neoplasia. WHO Tech Rep Ser 1992; 817:22–26.

97. Ramcharan S, Pelligrin FA, Ray R, et al. Infective parasitic diseases: malignant neoplasms; benign neoplasms. In: Ramcharan S, Pelligrin FA, Ray R, et al, eds. The Walnut Creek Contraceptive Drug Study: A Prospective Study of the Side Effects of Oral Contraceptives. Vol 3: An Interim Report—A Comparison of Disease Occurrence Leading to Hospitalization or Death in Users and Nonusers of Oral Contraceptives. Bethesda: Center for Population Research, 1981: 43–78.

98. Adams SA, Sheaves JK, Wright NH, et al. A case-control study of the possible association between oral contraceptives and malignant melanoma. Br J Cancer 1981; 44:45–50.

99. Kay CR. Malignant melanoma and oral contraceptives. Br J Cancer 1981; 44:479 (letter).

100. Boston Collaborative Drug Surveillance Program. Oral contraceptives and venous thromboembolic disease, surgically confirmed gall-bladder disease, and breast tumours. Lancet 1973; 1:1399–1404.

101. Goldzieher JW, Moses LE, Averkin E, et al. A placebo-controlled double-blind crossover investigation of the side effects attributed to oral contraceptives. Fertil Steril 1971; 22:609–623.

102. Archer DF, Thomas RL. The fallacy of the postpill amenorrhea syndrome. Clin Obstet Gynecol 1981; 24:943–950.

103. Hull MG, Bromham DR, Savage PE, et al. Normal fertility in women with post-pill amenorrhoea. Lancet 1981; 1:1329–1332.

104. Heinonen OP, Slone D, Monson RR, et al. Cardiovascular birth defects and antenatal exposure to female sex hormones. N Engl J Med 1977; 296:67–70.

105. Bracken MB. Oral contraception and congenital malformations in offspring: a review and meta-analysis of the population studies. Obstet Gynecol 1990; 76:552–557.

106. Holtz G. Galactorrhea in oral contraceptive users. J Reprod Med 1982; 27:210–212.

107. Vaisrub S. Pituitary prolactinoma and estrogen contraceptives. JAMA 1979; 242:177–178.

108. Sherman BM, Schlechte J, Halmi NS, et al. Pathogenesis of prolactin-secreting pituitary adenomas. Lancet 1978; 2:1019–1021.

109. Coulam CB, Annegers JF, Abboud CF, et al. Pituitary adenoma and oral contraceptives: a case-control study. Fertil Steril 1979; 31:25–28.

110. Wingrave SJ, Kay CR, Vessey MP. Oral contraceptives and pituitary adenomas. Br Med J 1980; 280:685–686.

111. Shy KK, McTiernan AM, Daling JR, et al. Oral contraceptive use and the occurrence of pituitary prolactinoma. JAMA 1983; 249:2204–2207.

112. Pituitary Adenoma Study Group. Pituitary adenomas and oral contraceptives: a multicenter case-control study. Fertil Steril 1983; 39:753–760.

113. Szoka PR, Edgren RA. Drug interactions with oral contraceptives: compilation and analysis of an adverse experience report data base. Fertil Steril 1988; 49(Suppl):31S–38S.

114. Bolt HM, Bolt M, Kappus H. Interaction of rifampicin treatment with pharmacokinetics and metabolism of ethinyloestradiol in man. Acta Endocrinol 1977; 85:189–197.

115. Back DJ, Breckenridge AM, Crawford F, et al. The effect of rifampicin on norethisterone pharmacokinetics. Eur J Clin Pharmacol 1979; 15:193–197.

116. Rubin GL, Ory HW, Layde PM. Oral contraceptives and pelvic inflammatory disease. Am J Obstet Gynecol 1982; 144:630–635.

117. Ross RK, Pike MC, Vesse MP, et al. Risk factors for uterine fibroids: reduced risk associated with oral contraceptives. Br Med J 1986; 293:359–362.

118. Ory H. Functional ovarian cysts and oral contraceptives: negative association confirmed surgically. JAMA 1974; 228:68–69.

119. Vessey M, Metcalfe A, Wells C, et al. Ovarian neoplasms, functional ovarian cysts and oral contraceptives. Br Med J 1987; 294:1518–1520.

120. Carr BR, Breslau NA, Givens C. Oral contraceptive pills, gonadotropin-releasing hormone agonists, or use in combination for treatment of hirsutism: a clinical research center study. J Clin Endocrinol Metab 1995; 80:1169–1178.

121. Royal College of General Practitioners Oral Contraceptive Study. Reduction in incidence of rheumatoid arthritis associated with oral contraceptives. Lancet 1978; 1:569–571.

122. Carr BR. Starting the new patient on oral contraceptives. Int J Fertil 1988; 33(Suppl):21–26.

123. Prevention and management of cardiovascular risk in women. Am J Obstet Gynecol 1988; 158(Suppl):1659–1661.

124. Mishell DR. Use of oral contraceptives in women of older reproductive age. Am J Obstet Gynecol 1988; 158:1652–1657.

125. Glasier A, Baird DT. Post-ovulatory contraception. Baillieres Clin Obstet Gynecol 1990; 4:283–291.

126. Silvestre L, Bouali Y, Ulmann A. Postcoital contraception: myth or reality? Lancet 1991; 338:39–41.

127. Yuzpe AA, Smith RP, Rademaker AW. A multicenter clinical investigation employing ethinyl estradiol combined with DL-norgestrel as a postcoital contraceptive agent. Fertil Steril 1982; 37:508–513.

128. Glasier A, Thong KJ, Dewar M, et al. Mifepristone (RU 486) compared with high-dose estrogen and progestogen for emergency postcoital contraception. N Engl J Med 1992; 327:1041–1044.

129. Population Reports. Hormonal contraception: new long-acting methods. Series K, No. 3. Injectables and Implants. Baltimore: The Johns Hopkins University, 1987: K57–K87.

130. Garza-Flores J, De la Cruz DL, Valles de Gourges V, et al. Long term effects of depot-medroxyprogesterone acetate on lipoprotein metabolism. Contraception 119; 44:61–71

131. Skegg DCG, Noonan EA, Paul C. Depot medroxyprogesterone acetate and breast cancer. JAMA 1995; 273:799–804.

132. Segal SJ. Contraceptive implants. In: Mishell DR, ed. Advances in Infertility Research. Vol 1. New York: Raven, 1982:117–127.

133. Nash HA, Jackonicz TM. Vaginal rings. In: Mishell DR, ed. Advances in Infertility Research. Vol 1. New York: Raven, 1982: 129–144.

134. ALZA Corporation. The Progestasert: Progesterone Uterine Therapeutic System. Palo Alto, CA, 1976.

135. Luukkainen T, Heikinhemio O, Hasukkamaa M, et al. Inhibition of folliculogenesis and ovulation by the antiprogesterone RU 486. Fertil Steril 1988; 49:961–963.

136. Baulieu EE, Ulman A. Antiprogesterone activity of RU 486 and its contragestive and other applications. Hum Reprod 1986; 1:107–110.

137. Hodgen GD. Progesterone antagonists: useful for contraception. Contemp OB/GYN 1988; 32:65–66.

138. Andreyko JL, Marshall LA, Dumesic DA, et al. Therapeutic uses of gonadotropin-releasing hormone analogs. Obstet Gynecol Surv 1987; 42:1–21.

139. Nillius SJ, Bergquist C, Wide L. Inhibition of ovulation in women by chronic treatment with a stimulating LHRH analogue—a new approach to birth control? Contraception 1978; 17:537–545.

140. Monroe SE, Blumenfeld Z, Andreyko J, et al. Dose dependent inhibition of pituitary-ovarian function during administration of GnRH agonistic analog (nafarelin). J Clin Endocrinol Metab 1986; 63:1334–1341.

141. Bergquist C, Nillius SJ, Wide L. Peptide contraception in women. Inhibition of ovulation by chronic intranasal LRH agonist therapy. Ups J Med Sci 1984; 89:99–106.

142. Lemay A, Faure N, Labrie F, et al. Inhibition of ovulation during discontinuous intranasal luteinizing hormone–releasing hormone agonist dosing in combination with gestagen. Fertil Steril 1985; 43:868–877.

143. Sheehan KL, Casper RF, Yen SSC. Luteal phase defects induced by an agonist of luteinizing hormone–releasing hormone factor: a model for fertility control. Science 1982; 215:170–172.

144. Sheehan KL, Casper RF, Yen SSC. Induction of luteolysis by luteinizing hormone–releasing hormone factor (LRF) agonist: sensitivity, reproducibility, and reversibility. Fertil Steril 1982; 37:209–212.

145. Lemay A, Faure N, Labrie F. Sensitivity of pituitary and corpus luteum responses to single intranasal administration of (D-Ser[TBU]6-des-gly-NH210) luteinizing hormone–releasing hormone ethylamide (Buserelin) in normal women. Fertil Steril 1982; 37:193–200.

146. Population Reports. IUDs: a new look. Series B, No. 5. Intrauterine Devices. Baltimore: The Johns Hopkins University, 1988: 1–31.

147. Alvarez F, Branche V, Fernadez E, et al. New insights on the mode of action of intrauterine contraceptive devices in women. Fertil Steril 1988; 49:768–773.

148. World Health Organization. Mechanism of action, safety and efficacy of intrauterine devices. WHO Tech Rep Ser 1987; 753:12–17.

149. Gupta PK, Malkani PK, Bhasin K. Cellular responses in the uterine cavity after IUD insertion and structural changes of the IUD. Contraception 1971; 4:375–384.

150. Moyer DL, Mishell DR Jr. Reactions of human endometrium to the intrauterine foreign body. 2: Long-term effects on the endometrial histology and cytology. Am J Obstet Gynecol 1971; 111:66–80.

151. Newton J, Tacchi D. Long-term use of copper intrauterine devices. Lancet 1990; 335:1322–1323.

152. Toppozada T. Treatment of increased menstrual blood loss in IUD users. Contraception 1987; 36:145–157.

153. Burkman RT. The Women's Health Study. Association between intrauterine device and pelvic inflammatory disease. Obstet Gynecol 1981; 57:269–276.

154. Kronmal RA, Whitney CW, Mumford SD. The intrauterine device and pelvic inflammatory disease; the women's health study reanalyzed. J Clin Epidemiol 1991; 44:109–122.

155. Weström L. Pelvic inflammatory disease: bacteriology and sequelae. Contraception 1987; 36:111–128.

156. Cates W Jr, Ory HW, Rochat RW, et al. The intrauterine device and deaths from spontaneous abortion. N Engl J Med 1976; 295:1155–1159.

157. Tatum HJ. A reassessment of intrauterine contraception. In: Mishell DR, ed. Advances in Infertility Research. Vol 1. New York: Raven, 1982: 47–74.

158. The intrauterine device. ACOG Technical Bulletin. No. 104. Washington, DC: American College of Obstetricians and Gynecologists, 1987.

159. Population Reports. New developments in vaginal contraception. Series H, No. 7. Barrier Devices. Baltimore: The Johns Hopkins University, 1984: H157–H190.

160. Trussell J, Sturgen K, Strickler J, et al. Comparative efficacy of the female condom and other barrier methods. Fam Plann Perspect 1994; 26:66-72.

161. Niruthisard S, Roddy RE, Chutivongse S. Use of nonoxynol-9 and reduction in rate of gonococcal and chlamydial cervical infections. Lancet 1992; 339:1371–1375.

162. Baehler EA, Dillon WP, Cumb TJ, et al. Prolonged use of a diaphragm and toxic shock syndrome. Fertil Steril 1982; 38:248–250.

163. Feldblum PJ, Fortney JA. Condoms, spermicides, and the transmission of human immunodeficiency virus: a review of the literature. Am J Public Health 1988; 78:52–54.

164. Jick H, Walker AM, Rothman KJ, et al. Vaginal spermicides and congenital disorders. JAMA 1981; 245:1329–1332.

165. Louik C, Mitchell AA, Werler MM, et al. Maternal exposure to spermicides in relation to certain birth defects. N Engl J Med 1987; 317:474–478.

166. Warburton D, Neugut RH, Lustenberger A, et al. Lack of association between spermicide use and trisomy. N Engl J Med 1987; 317:478–482.

167. Bracken MB. Spermicidal contraceptives and poor reproductive outcomes: the epidemiologic evidence against an association. Am J Obstet Gynecol 1988; 151:552–556.

168. Population Reports. Periodic abstinence: how well do new approaches work? Series I, No. 3. Periodic Abstinence. Baltimore: The Johns Hopkins University, 1981; I34–I71.

169. Bonnar J. Natural family planning including breast feeding. In: Mishell DR, ed. Advances in Infertility Research. Vol 1. New York: Raven, 1982: 1–18.

170. Ogino K. Ovulationstermin und Konzeptionstermin. Zentralbl Gynaekol 1930; 54:464–479.

171. Knaus H. Die periodische Frucht und Unfruchtbarkeit des Weibes. Zentralbl Gynaekol 1933; 57:1393.

172. Oechsli FW. Studies of the consequences of contraceptive failure: final report. Berkeley, CA: University of California, Berkeley, Apr 8, 1976 (Contract N01-HD–5–2816): 20.

173. Brown JB, Blackwell LF, Billing JJ, et al. Natural family planning. Am J Obstet Gynecol 1987; 157:1082–1089.

174. Queenan JT, Moghiss NS. Natural family planning: looking ahead. Am J Obstet Gynecol 1991; 165:1972–1980.

175. Population Reports. Breast-feeding, fertility, and family planning. Series J, No. 24. Breast-Feeding. Baltimore: The Johns Hopkins University, 1981: J526–J575.

176. Kennedy KI, Visness CM. Contraceptive efficacy of lactational amenorrhea. Lancet 1992; 339:227–230.

177. Talwae GP, ed. Immunologic Approaches to Contraception and Infertility. New York: Plenum, 1986.

178. Anderson DJ, Alexander NJ. A new look at antifertility vaccines. Fertil Steril 1983; 40:557–571.

179. Aitken RJ, Paterson M, Koothan PT: Contraceptive vaccines. Br Med Bull 1993; 49:88–99.

180. Population Reports. Mini laparotomy and laparoscopy: safe, effective and widely used sterilization. Series C, No. 9. Sterilization. Baltimore: The Johns Hopkins University, 1985: C125–C167.

181. Shepherd MK. Female contraceptive sterilization. Obstet Gynecol Surv 1974; 29:739–787.

182. Sterilization. ACOG Technical Bulletin. No. 113. Washington, DC: American College of Obstetricians and Gynecologists, 1988.

183. Hulka JF, Peterson HB, Phillips JM. American Association of Gynecologic Laparoscopists' 1988 membership survey on laparoscopy sterilization. J Reprod Med 1990; 35:584–586.

184. Brenner WE. Evaluation of contemporary female sterilization methods. J Reprod Med 1981; 26:439–453.

185. Population Reports. Reversing female sterilization. Series C, No. 8. Female Sterilization. Baltimore: The Johns Hopkins University, 1980: C97–C123.

186. *Jane Roe et al. v. Henry Wade.* Supreme Court of the United States. Opinion No. 70-18, Jan 22, 1973.

187. *Doe et al. v. Bolton. Attorney General of Georgia et al.* Supreme Court of the United States. Opinion No. 74-1151 and 74-1419, July 1, 1976.

188. Atrash HK, Mackay T, Binkin NJ, et al. Legal abortion mortality in the United States: 1972 to 1982. Am J Obstet Gynecol 1987; 156:605–612.

189. Population Reports. The use of PGs in human reproduction. Series G, No. 8. Prostaglandins. Baltimore: The Johns Hopkins University, 1980: G77–G119.

190. Grimes DA, Mishell DR, Shoupe D. Early abortion with a single dose of the antiprogestin RU 486. Am J Obstet Gynecol 1988; 158:1307–1312.

191. Cameron IT, Baird DT. Early pregnancy termination: a comparison between vacuum aspiration and medical abortion using prostaglandin (16,16 dimethyl-trans-Δ²-PGE₁ methyl ester) or the antiprogestogen RU 486. Br J Obstet Gynaecol 1988; 95:271–276.

192. Contraceptive technology update 1995; 16:17–28.

193. Hackett RE, Waterhouse K. Vasectomy—reviewed. Am J Obstet Gynecol 1973; 116:438–455.

194. Lipschultz LI, Benson GS. Vasectomy—1980. Urol Clin North Am 1980; 7:89–105.

195. Forste R, Tanfer K, Tedrow L. Sterilization among currently married men in the United States, 1991. Fam Plann Perspect 1995; 27:100–107, 122.

196. Marquette CM, Koonin LM, Antarsh L, et al. Vasectomy in the United States, 1991. Am J Public Health 1995; 85:644–649.

197. Ramos-Cordero RA, Ackman CFD, Naftolin F. Changing profiles in vasectomy subjects in the past decade. Fertil Steril 1979; 31:410–412.

198. Tripathy SP, Ramachandran CR, Ramachandran P. Health consequences of vasectomy in India. Bull World Health Organ 1994; 72:779–782.

199. Liu X, Li S. Vasal sterilization in China. Contraception 1993; 48:255–265.

200. Anonymous. New method of male sterilization. Chin Med J (Engl) 1980; 93:205–206.

201. Li S, Goldstein M, Zhu J, et al. The no-scapel vasectomy. J Urol 1991; 145:341–344.

202. Schlegel PN, Goldstein M. No-Scapel Vasectomy. Semin Urol 1992; 10:252–256.

203. Reynolds RD. Vas deferens occlusion during no-scalpel vasectomy. J Fam Pract 1994; 39:577–582.

204. Leader AJ, Axelrad SD, Frankowski R, et al. Complications of 2,711 vasectomies. J Urol 1974; 111:365–369.

205. Kaplan KA, Heuther CA. A clinical study of vasectomy failure and recanalization. J Urol 1975; 113:71–74.

206. Lo CN, Mumford SD, Atwood RJ. Postvasectomy residual sperm pregnancy. Fertil Steril 1980; 33:668–669.

207. Edwards IS. Postvasectomy testing: reducing the delay. Med J Aust 1981; 1:649.

208. Klapproth HJ, Young IS. Vasectomy, vas ligation and vas occlusion. Urology 1973; 1:292–300.

209. Penna RM, Potash J, Penna SM. Elective vasectomy: a study of 843 patients. J Fam Pract 1979; 8:857–858.

210. Neaves WB. Biological aspects of vasectomy. In: Greep RO, Astwood EB, eds. Handbook of Physiology. Sect 7: Endocrinology. Vol V. Male Reproductive System. Washington, DC: American Physiological Society, 1975: 383–404.

211. Gupta AS, Kothari LK, Dhruva A, et al. Surgical sterilization by vasectomy and its effect on the structure and function of the testis in man. Br J Surg 1975; 62:59–63.

212. Jarow JP, Buden RE, Dym M, et al. Quantitative pathologic changes in the human testis after vasectomy: a controlled study. N Engl J Med 1985; 313:1252–1256.

213. Horan AH. When and why does occlusion of the vas deferens affect the testis? Fertil Steril 1975; 62:59–63.

214. Ying W, Hedman M, de la Torre B, et al. Effect of vasectomy on the steroid profile of human seminal plasma. Int J Androl 1983; 6:116–124.

215. Naik VK, Joshi UM, Sheth AR. Long-term effects of vasectomy on prostatic function in men. J Reprod Fertil 1980; 58:289–293.

216. Varma MM, Varma RR, Johanson AJ, et al. Long-term effects of vasectomy on pituitary-gonadal function in man. J Clin Endocrinol Metab 1975; 40:868–871.

217. Purvis K, Saksena SK, Cekan Z, et al. Endocrine effects of vasectomy. Clin Endocrinol 1976; 5:263–272.

218. Smith KD, Tcholakian K, Chowdhury M, et al. An investigation of plasma hormone levels before and after vasectomy. Fertil Steril 1976; 27:145–151.

219. Skegg DCG, Mathews JD, Guillevaud J, et al. Hormonal assessment before and after vasectomy. Br Med J 1976; 1:621–622.

220. Whitby RM, Gordon RD, Blair BR. The endocrine effects of vasectomy: a prospective five-year study. Fertil Steril 1979; 31:518–520.

221. Rumke P, Hellinga G. Autoantibodies against spermatozoa in sterile men. Am J Clin Pathol 1959; 32:357–363.

222. Ansbacher R, Keung-Yeung K, Wurster JC. Sperm antibodies in vasectomized men. Fertil Steril 1972; 23:640–643.

223. Ansbacher R. Vasectomy: sperm antibodies. Fertil Steril 1973; 24:788–792.

224. Alexander NJ, Schmidt SS, Free MJ, et al. Sperm antibodies after vasectomy with fulguration. J Urol 1976; 115:77–78.

225. Mathews JD, Skegg DCG, Vessey MP, et al. Weak antibody reactions to antigens other than sperm after vasectomy. Br Med J 1976; 2:1359–1360.

226. Bullock JY, Gilmore LL, Wilson JD. Autoantibodies following vasectomy. J Urol 1977; 118:604–606.

227. Alexander NJ, Clarkson TB. Vasectomy increases the severity of diet-induced atherosclerosis in *Macaca fascicularis.* Science 1978; 201:538–541.

228. Goldacre MJ, Holford TR, Vessey MP. Cardiovascular disease and vasec-

tomy: findings from two epidemiologic studies. N Engl J Med 1983; 308:805–808.

229. Massey FJ, Bernstein GN, O'Fallon WM, et al. Vasectomy and health: results from a large cohort study. JAMA 1984; 252:1023–1029.

230. Rosenberg L, Schwingl PJ, Kaufman DW, et al. The risk of myocardial infarction 10 or more years after vasectomy in men under 55 years of age. Am J Epidemiol 1986; 123:1049–1056.

231. Giovannucci MD, Tosteson TD, Speizer FE et al. A long-term study of mortality in men who have undergone vasectomy. N Engl J Med 1992; 326:1392–1398.

232. Giovannucci E, Ascherio A, Rimm EB, et al. A prospective cohort study of vasectomy and prostate cancer in US men. JAMA 1993; 269:873–877.

233. Giovannucci E, Tosteson TD, Speizer FE, et al. A retrospective cohort study of vasectomy and prostate cancer in US men. JAMA 1993; 269:878–882.

234. Howards SS, Peterson HB. Vasectomy, and prostate cancer. Chance, bias, or a causal relationship? JAMA 1993; 269:913–914.

235. Hayes RB, Pottern LM, Greenberg R, et al. Vasectomy and prostate cancer in US blacks and whites. Am J Epidemiol 1993; 137:263–269.

236. Rosenberg L, Palmer JR, Zauber AG. Vasectomy and the risk of prostate cancer. Am J Epidemiol 1990; 132:1051–1055.

237. Rosenberg L, Palmer JR, Zauber AG, et al. The relation of vasectomy to the risk of cancer. Am J Epidemiol 1994; 140:431–438.

238. John EM, Whittemore AS, Wu AH, et al. Vasectomy and prostate cancer: results from a multiethnic case-control study. J Natl Cancer Inst 1995; 87:662–669.

239. DerSimonian R, Clemens J, Spiritas R, et al. Vasectomy and prostate cancer risk: methodological review of the evidence. J Clin Epidemiol 1993; 46:163–172.

240. Guess HA. Is vasectomy a risk factor for prostate cancer? Eur J Cancer 1993; 29a:1055–1060.

241. Doty FO. Emotional aspects of vasectomy: a review. J Reprod Med 1973; 10:156–161.

242. Kohli KL, Sobrero AJ. Vasectomy: a study of psychosexual and general reactions. Soc Biol 1973; 20:298–302.

243. Vaughn RL. Behavioral response to vasectomy. Arch Gen Psychiatry 1979; 36:815–821.

244. Lipshultz LI, Benson GS. Vasectomy: an anatomical, physiologic, and surgical review. In: Cunningham GR, Schill W-B, Hafez ESE, eds. Regulation of Male Fertility. The Hague: Martinus Nijhoff, 1980: 169–186.

245. Lee HY. Observations of the results of 300 vasectomies. J Androl 1980; 1:11–15.

246. Mehrotra ML, Gupta RL, Nagar AM, et al. Fertility status of men following vaso-vasostomy. Indian J Med Res 1981; 73:33–40.

247. Martin DC. Microsurgical reversal of vasectomy. Am J Surg 1981; 142:48–50.

248. Lee HY. A 20-year experience with vasovasostomy. J Urol 1986; 136:413–415.

249. Yarbro ES, Howards SS. Vasovasostomy. Urol Clin North Am 1987; 14:515–526.

250. Sullivan MJ, Howe GE. Correlation of circulating antisperm antibodies to functional success in vasovasostomy. J Urol 1977; 117:189–191.

251. Bagshaw HA, Masters JRW, Pryor JP. Factors influencing the outcome of vasectomy reversal. Br J Urol 1980; 52:57–60.

252. Linnet L, Hjort T, Fogh-Andersen P. Association between failure to impregnate after vasovasostomy and sperm agglutinins in semen. Lancet 1981; 1:117–119.

253. Royle MG, Parslow JM, Kingscott MMB, et al. Reversal of vasectomy: the effects of sperm antibodies on subsequent fertility. Br J Urol 1981; 53:644–659.

254. Thomas AJ Jr, Pontes JE, Rose NR, et al. Microsurgical vasovasostomy: immunologic consequences and subsequent fertility. Fertil Steril 1981; 35:447–450.

255. Huang TTF Jr, Tung KSK, Yanagimachi R. Autoantibodies from vasectomized guinea pigs inhibit fertilization in vitro. Science 1981; 213:1267–1269.

256. Snyder PJ, Lawrence DA. Treatment of male hypogonadism with testosterone enanthate. J Clin Endocrinol Metab 1980; 51:1335–1339.

257. Steinberger E, Smith KD. Effect of chronic administration of testosterone enanthate on sperm production and plasma testosterone, follicle-stimulating hormone, and luteinizing hormone levels: a preliminary evaluation of a possible male contraceptive. Fertil Steril 1977; 28:1320–1328.

258. Paulsen CA, Leonard JM, Burgess EC, et al. Male contraceptive development: re-examination of testosterone enanthate as an effective single entity agent. In: Patanelli DJ, ed. Proceedings of Hormonal Control of Male Fertility. Washington, DC: Government Printing Office, 1978: 17–36.

259. Cunningham GR, Silverman VE, Thornby J, et al. The potential for an androgen male contraceptive. J Clin Endocrinol Metab 1979; 49:520–526.

260. Swerdloff RS, Campfield LA, Palacios A, et al. Suppression of human spermatogenesis by depot androgen: potential for male contraception. J Steroid Biochem 1979; 11:663–670.

261. Wu FCW, Farley TMM, Pergoudov A, et al. Effects of testosterone enanthate in normal men: experience from a multicenter contraceptive efficacy study. Fertil Steril 1996; 65:626–636.

262. World Health Organization Task Force on Methods for the Regulation of Male Fertility. Contraceptive efficacy of testosterone-induced azoospermia in normal men. Lancet 1990; 336:955–959.

263. World Health Organization Task Force on Methods for the Regulation of Male Fertility. Contraceptive efficacy of testosterone-induced azoospermia and oligospermia in normal men. Fertil Steril 1996; 65:821–829.

264. Anderson RA, Wu FCC. Comparison between testosterone enanthate–induced asoospermia and oligospermia in a male contraceptive study. II: Pharmacokinetics and pharmacodynamics of once weekly administration of testosterone enanthate. J Clin Endocrinol Metab 1996; 81:896–901.

265. Anderson RA, Wallace AM, Wu FCC. Comparison between testosterone enanthate–induced azoospermia and oligospermia in a male contraceptive study. III: Higher 5-reductase activity in oligospermic men administered supraphysiological doses of testosterone. J Clin Endocrinol Metab 1996; 81:902–908.

266. Handelsman DJ, Conway AJ, Boylan LM. Suppression of human spermatogenesis by testosterone implants. J Clin Endocrinol Metab 1992; 175:1326–1332.

267. Alvarez-Sanchez F, Faundes A, Brache V, et al. Attainment and maintenance of azoospermia with combined monthly injections of depo medroxyprogesterone acetate and testosterone enanthate. Contraception 1977; 15:635–648.

268. Brenner PF, Mishell DR Jr, Bernstein GS, et al. Study of medroxyprogesterone acetate and testosterone enanthate as a male contraceptive. Contraception 1977; 15:679–691.

269. Faundes A, Brache V, Leon P, et al. Sperm suppression with monthly injections of medroxyprogesterone acetate combined with testosterone enanthate at a high dose (500 mg). Int J Androl 1981; 4:235–245.

270. Hedman M, Gottlieb C, Svanborg K, et al. Endocrine, seminal and peripheral effects of depo medroxyprogesterone acetate and testosterone enanthate in men. Int J Androl 1988; 11:265–276.

271. Bebb RA, Anawalt BD, Christensen RB, et al. Combined administration of levonorgestrel and testosterone induces more rapid and effective suppression of spermatogenesis than testosterone alone: A promising male contraceptive approach. J Clin Endocrinol Metab 1996; 81:757–762.

272. Fogh M, Corker CS, Hunter WM, et al. The effects of low doses of cyproterone acetate on some functions of the reproduction system in normal men. Acta Endocrinol 1979; 91:545–552.

273. Wang C, Yeung KK. Use of low-dosage oral cyproterone acetate as a male contraceptive. Contraception 1980; 21:245–272.

274. Moltz L, Rommler A, Post K, et al. Medium dose cyproterone acetate (CPA): effects on hormone secretion and on spermatogenesis in men. Contraception 1980; 21:393–413.

275. Meriggiola MC, Bremner WJ, Paulsen CA, et al. A combined regimen of cyproterone acetate and testosterone enanthate as a potentially highly effective male contraceptive. J Clin Endocrinol Metab 1996; 81:3018–3023.

276. Crowley WF, Beitins IZ, Vale W, et al. The biologic activity of a potent analogue of gonadotropin-releasing hormone in normal and hypogonadotropic men. N Engl J Med 1980; 302:1052–1057.

277. Labrie F, Belanger A, Cusan L, et al. Antifertility effects of LHRH agonists in the male. J Androl 1980; 1:209–228.

278. Marchetti B, Reeves JJ, Pelletier G, et al. Modulation of pituitary luteinizing hormone–releasing hormone receptors by sex steroids and luteinizing hormone–releasing hormone in the rat. Biol Reprod 1982; 27:133–145.

279. Linde R, Doelle GC, Alexander N, et al. Reversible inhibition of testicular steroidogenesis and spermatogenesis by a potent gonadotropin-releasing hormone agonist in normal men. N Engl J Med 1981; 305:663–667.

280. Evans RM, Doelle GC, Lindner J, et al. A luteinizing hormone–releasing hormone agonist decreases biological activity and modifies chromatographic behavior of luteinizing hormone in man. J Clin Invest 1984; 73:262–266.

281. Evans RM, Doelle GC, Alexander AN, et al. Gonadotropin and steroid secretory patterns during chronic treatment with a luteinizing hormone–releasing hormone agonist analog in men. J Clin Endocrinol Metab 1984; 58:862–867.

282. Pavlou SN, Dahl KD, Wakefield G, et al. Maintenance of the ratio of bioactive to immunoactive follicle-stimulating hormone in normal men during chronic luteinizing hormone–releasing hormone agonist administration. J Clin Endocrinol Metab 1988; 66:1005–1009.

283. Bhasin S, Heber O, Steiner B, et al. Hormonal effects of GnRH agonist in the human male. II: Testosterone enhances gonadotropin suppression induced by GnRH agonist. Clin Endocrinol 1984; 20:119–128.

284. Bhasin S, Heber D, Steiner BS, et al. Hormonal effects of gonadotropin-releasing hormone (GnRH) agonist in the human male. III: Effects of long term combined treatment with GnRH agonist and androgen. J Clin Endocrinol Metab 1985; 60:998–1003.

285. Bhasin S, Yuan QX, Steiner BS, et al. Hormonal effects of gonadotropin releasing hormone (GnRH) agonist in men: effects of long term treatment with GnRH agonist infusion and androgen. J Clin Endocrinol Metab 1987; 65:568–574.

286. Behre HM, Nashan D, Hubert W, et al. Depot gonadotropin-releasing hormone agonist blunts the androgen-induced suppression of spermatogenesis in a clinical trial of male contraception. J Clin Endocrinol Metab 1992; 74:84–90.

287. Pavlou SN, Wakefield G, Schlechter NL, et al. Mode of suppression of pituitary and gonadal function after acute or prolonged administration of a luteinizing hormone–releasing hormone antagonist in normal men. J Clin Endocrinol Metab 1989; 68:446–454.

288. Bagatell CJ, McLachlan RI, de Krester DM, et al. A comparison of the

suppressive effect of testosterone and a potent new gonadotropin-releasing hormone antagonist on gonadotropin and inhibin levels in normal men. J Clin Endocrinol Metab 1989; 69:43–48.

289. Pavlou SN, Brewer K, Farley MG, et al. Combined administration of a gonadotropin-releasing hormone antagonist and testosterone in men induces reversible asoospermia without loss of libido. J Clin Endocrinol Metab 1991; 73:1360–1369.

290. Tom L, Bhasin S, Salmeh W, et al. Induction of azoospermia in normal men with combined Nal-Glu gonadotropin-releasing hormone antagonist and testosterone enanthate. J Clin Endocrinol Metab 1992; 75:476–483.

291. Bagatell CJ, Matsumoto AM, Christensen RB, et al. Comparison of a gonadotropin-releasing hormone antagonist plus testosterone (T) versus T alone as potential male contraceptive regimens. J Clin Endocrinol Metab 1993; 77:427–432.

292. National Coordinating Group on Male Antifertility Agents. Gossypol—a new antifertility agent for males. Chin Med J 1978; 4:417–428.

293. Liu GZ. Clinical study of gossypol as a male contraceptive. Reproduccion 1981; 5:189–193.

294. Shaozhen Q, Guangwei J, Ziaoyun W, et al. Gossypol related hypokalemia. Clinicopharmacologic studies. Chin Med J 1980; 93:477–482.

295. Liu GZ, Lyle KC, Cao J. Experiences with gossypol as a male pill. Am J Obstet Gynecol 1987; 157:1079–1082.

296. Liu GZ, Chiu-Hinton K, Cao J, et al. Effects of K salt or a potassium blocker on gossypol-related hypokalemia. Contraception 1988; 37:111–117.

297. Meng G-D, Zhu J-C, Chen Z-W, et al. Recovery of sperm production following the cessation of gossypol treatment: a two-centre study in China. Int J Androl 1988; 11:1–11.

298. Qian SZ. *Tripterygium wilfordii*, a Chinese herb effective in male fertility regulation. Contraception 1987; 36:335–345.

299. Qian SZ, Xu Y, Zhang JW. Recent progress in research on *Tripterygium*: a male antifertility plant. Contraception 1995; 51:121–129.

300. Xu YE, Want YI, Lin N, et al. Subcapsular intratesticular assay: a preliminary screening method for putative male antifertility drugs. Int J Androl 1995; 18(Suppl 1):53–57.

301. Giwercman A, Skakkebaek NE. The effect of salicylazosulphapyridine (sulphasalazine) on male fertility. A review. Int J Androl 1986; 9:38–52.

302. Jackson H. Antispermatogenic agents. Br Med Bull 1970; 26:79–86.

303. Spitz IM, Gunsalus GL, Mather JP, et al. The effects of the indazole carboxylic acid derivative, tolnidamine, on testicular function. I: Early changes in androgen binding protein secretion in the rat. J Androl 1985; 6:171–178.

304. Kandeel FR, Swerdloff RS. Role of temperature in regulation of spermatogenesis and the use of heating as a method for contraception. Fertil Steril 1988; 49:1–23.

305. Madhwa Raj HG, Sairam MR, Hieschlag E. Immunologic approach to regulation of fertility in the male. In: Cunningham GR, Schill W-B, Hafez ESE, eds. Regulation of Male Fertility. The Hague: Martinus Nijhoff, 1980: 209–218.

306. Sheela Rani CS, Murty GSRC, Moudgal NR. Effect of chronic neutralization of endogenous FSH on testicular function in the adult male bonnet monkey—assessment using biochemical parameters. Int J Androl 1978; 1:489–500.

307. Murty GSRC, Sheela Rani CS, Moudgal NR, et al. Effect of passive immunization with specific antiserum to FSH on the spermatogenic process and fertility of adult male bonnet monkeys. J Reprod Fertil 1979; 26:147–163.

308. Srinath BR, Wickings EJ, Witting C, et al. Active immunization with follicle-stimulating hormone for fertility control: a 4½-year study in male rhesus monkeys. Fertil Steril 1983; 40:110–117.

309. Talwar GP, Naz RK, Das C, et al. A practicable immunological approach to block spermatogenesis without loss of androgens. Proc Natl Acad Sci USA 1979; 76:5882–5885.

310. Talwar GP, Naz RK. Immunological control of male fertility. Arch Androl 1981; 7:177–185.

311. Goldberg E, Wheat TE. Induction of infertility in male rabbits by immunization with LDH-X. In: Spilman CH, Lobl TJ, Kirton KT, et al, eds. Regulatory Mechanisms of Male Reproductive Physiology. Amsterdam: Excerpta Medica, 1976: 133–139.

312. Setty BS. Regulation of epididymal function and sperm maturation—endocrine approach to fertility control in male. Endokrinologie 1979; 74:100–117.

313. Neumann F, Schenck B. Antiandrogens: basic concepts and clinical trials. In: Cunningham GR, Schill W-B, Hafez ESE, eds. Regulation of Male Fertility. The Hague: Martinus Nijhoff, 1980: 93–104.

314. Lobl TJ. α-Chlorohydrin: review of a model posttesticular antifertility agent. In: Cunningham GR, Schill W-B, Hafez ESE, eds. Regulation of Male Fertility. The Hague: Martinus Nijhoff, 1980: 109–122.

315. Ford WCL, Harrison A. Effect of α-chlorohydrin on glucose metabolism by spermatozoa from the cauda epididymis of the rhesus monkey (*Macaca mulatta*). J Reprod Fertil 1980; 60:59–64.

316. Morris ID, Williams LM. Some preliminary observations of the nephrotoxicity of the male antifertility drug (±)α-chlorohydrin. J Pharm Pharmacol 1980; 32:35–38.

317. Ford WCL. The contraceptive effect of 6-chloro-6-deoxysugars in the male. In: Cunningham GR, Schill W-B, Hafez ESE, eds. Regulation of Male Fertility. The Hague: Martinus Nijhoff, 1980: 123–126.

318. Jacobs JM, Ford WCL. The neurotoxicity and antifertility properties of 6-chloro-6-deoxyglucose in the mouse. Neurotoxicology 1981; 2:405–417.

hibiting calcium uptake and reducing myofibrillar calcium.[11, 12] Nitric oxide synthase is an oxygen-dependent enzyme. At the low PO_2 values of the flaccid penis, this enzyme has weak activity. With neurogenic vascular relaxation, as arterial inflow increases, regional oxygen tension increases, activating the enzyme in the nerve endings and in the endothelium and propagating the erectile impulse.[13] Situations that cause a decrease in NO synthase, such as ischemic smooth muscle degeneration, impair erectile function. The pelvic sympathetic plexus emerging from T10-12 sends fibers to innervate the smooth muscles of the arterioles and sinusoids of the penis. These fibers maintain penile flaccidity by tonic α_2-adrenergic discharges that sustain high levels of intracellular calcium, and inhibition of these discharges contributes to cavernosal sinusoidal and vascular smooth muscle relaxation, thus promoting erection.[14]

A variety of receptors are present in corporeal tissues, so that in different species relaxation may be produced in vitro by nicotine, vasoactive intestinal peptide, isoproterenol, phenoxybenzamine, phentolamine, rimiterol, acetylcholine, carbachol, methacholine, prostaglandin E_1, prostaglandin E_2, and adenosine. On the other hand, norepinephrine, epinephrine, dopamine, serotonin, histamine, prostaglandin $F_{2\alpha}$, bradykinin, vasopressin, angiotensin II, substance P, ATP, phenylephrine, and prostaglandin I_2 (prostacyclin) all cause corporeal smooth muscle contraction.[15]

There are five phases of erection (Fig. 19–1).[16] In the latent phase, immediately after the onset of stimulation, resistance of the penile arterioles and cavernosal sinusoids is reduced, followed promptly by a two- to threefold increase in flow without an increase of intracavernosal pressure, engorging the corporal sinusoids. Cavernosal pressure begins to rise; as a full erection approaches, cavernosal diastolic blood pressure remains near zero, and systolic pressure approaches the systemic level. During the rigid erection phase, contraction of the ischiocavernous muscles as a result of pudendal nerve stimulation produces intracavernosal pressures higher than the systemic blood pressure as the engorged cavernosal sinusoids are compressed against the unyielding tunica albuginea.[17, 18] This is the phase of maximal erectile strength. Detumescence is associated with loss of the relaxation stimulus and α_2-sympathetic vasoconstrictor activity.

Development of an erection depends on inhibition of penile venous return as well as increased arterial inflow. The corporal sinusoids drain into a subtunical venous plexus that coalesces into a number of penetrating veins that course at an angle through the tunica albuginea into a series of circumfer-ential veins that empty largely into the dorsal vein of the penis. When an erection begins, dilatation of the corporal sinusoids compresses the subtunical venous plexus and the penetrating veins against the tunica albuginea, profoundly inhibiting venous return. In rabbits it takes only a small increase in penile pressure to shut off venous outflow.[19]

Emission, Ejaculation, and Orgasm

Emission, ejaculation, and orgasm are controlled principally by sympathetic nerves and, under appropriate circumstances, may be separable from each other.[20] Emission refers to the secretion of seminal fluid into the posterior urethra. It is initiated by stimulation of the genitalia, which activates a specific center between T-12 and L-2, and is also under voluntary control. Emission results from peristalsis of the vas deferens and the ampulla, rhythmic contractions of the seminal vesicle, and constriction of prostatic smooth muscle. The proximal vesicle sphincter (bladder neck) and the distal vesicle sphincter contract actively, resulting in a sensation of ejaculatory inevitability. Ejaculation, the expulsion of semen from the urethra, is a reflex response to the entry of semen into the bulbous urethra from the posterior urethra and does not require cerebral input. Ejaculation results from three to seven contractions of the muscles of the pelvic floor. Normal antegrade ejaculation requires firm closure of the proximal vesicle sphincter and a functioning distal sphincter. Disorders of the distal sphincter cause a seeping ejaculation, and impairment of the proximal sphincter causes retrograde ejaculation.

Orgasm is the subjective sensation of pleasure initiated at about the time of emission and continuing through the ejaculatory process. Although orgasm is associated with and enhanced by the various events of the emission and ejaculatory process, it is separable from them in that it may occur without ejaculation, as in prepubertal children, and with markedly attenuated sensation, as in anesthetic ejaculation.[9]

Ejaculate volume is androgen dependent and decreases with age. Profound reduction in ejaculatory volume is associated with reduced sexual pleasure. Retrograde ejaculation can occur after impairment of the function of the proximal vesicle sphincter by transurethral prostatectomy or with autonomic nervous system neuropathy (e.g., in diabetes mellitus). Painful ejaculation may reflect injury to the ejaculatory ducts. A variety of surgical procedures, neurologic disorders, and spinal cord injuries that interfere with the pelvic sympathetic nerves impair emission, as do drugs that impair the sympathetic nervous system, particularly α_2-adrenergic blockers and ganglionic blockers.[7, 8, 21]

Premature ejaculation remains an etiologic puzzle, but its therapy has received a great deal of attention since Masters and Johnson reported a high cure rate with the use of education and simple techniques for developing voluntary control by delaying initiation of emission through desensitization to stimulatory impulses.[22] Their success rate has been difficult to duplicate. Reduced time to ejaculation is a common early manifestation of secondary ED, however, and its onset should be taken seriously.

Pudendal nerve afferents stimulate nocturnal penile tumescence (NPT) and reflex erections that are maintained even with spinal cord injury. NPT occurs throughout life, primarily during rapid eye movement sleep, and results in the adult in two to eight full erections per night that last up to 40 min each. The number and quality of nocturnal erections decrease with age, in association with the decline in rapid eye movement sleep.[23]

Normal sexual function depends on the interaction of libido and potency. Androgens are required for normal seminal fluid content and volume and play an important role in libido and in the frequency of nonerotic or reflex erections,

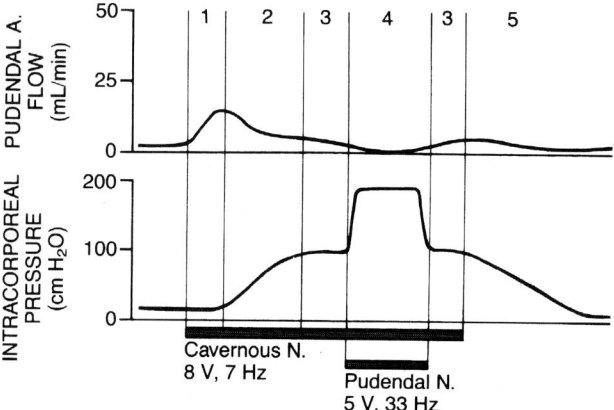

Figure 19–1. The five phases of erection, as delineated by sequential electrostimulation of the cavernosal and pudendal nerves in the monkey. 1, latent phase; 2, tumescence phase; 3, full erection phase; 4, rigid erection phase; 5, detumescence phase. (From Lue TF. The mechanism of penile erection in the monkey. Semin Urol 1986; 4:217–224, with permission.)

including NPT.[24] In aging men the frequency of NPT correlates with the level of bioavailable testosterone.[25] Androgens do not seem to be involved acutely in erections associated with erotic stimuli,[5] but in rats testosterone acts to facilitate apomorphine-induced central erection and yawning (a sexual response).[26] While the mechanism of androgen action is not known, androgens have many central nervous system effects, including stimulation of certain sexually dimorphic nuclei and increasing the size and dendritic length in the spinal cord of motor neurons that innervate the ischiocavernosus and bulbospongiosus muscles.[27] Androgens also enhance the augmentation of corpus cavernosal pressure by electrical stimulation of the pelvic ganglion in castrated rats.[28] Dihydrotestosterone is responsible for the maintenance of NO synthase activity in the corpus cavernosum of castrated rats, and this activity is tightly linked to electric field–stimulated smooth muscle contraction.[29] Thus androgens condition both nervous and vascular responsivity to erotic stimuli.

Sexual Dysfunction

Pathophysiological Mechanisms

Based on a consideration of the mechanisms of erection, ED can be due to a variety of pathophysiological mechanisms (Table 19–1), namely arterial and veno-occlusive insufficiency, loss of neuronal integrity, psychogenic inhibition of the erotic response, endocrinopathy, and cavernosal factors. These mechanisms are not independent and often act together to produce erectile insufficiency.

Population studies provide prevalence risks for ED for individuals with various conditions (Table 19–2),[4] whereas men who present to sexual dysfunction clinics demonstrate somewhat different prevalence rates (Table 19–3).[30-33]

TABLE 19–2. Epidemiologic Correlates of Erectile Dysfunction (ED)

Correlation with ED	No Correlation with ED	Inverse Correlation with ED
Age	Ulcer disease	Dominant personality
Heart disease, hypertension, diabetes mellitus	Arthritis Allergies Alcohol intake	High plasma HDL cholesterol level
Associated medications	Schizophrenia	High plasma DHEAS level
Cigarette smoking Depression Indices of anger	Plasma cortisol or dihydrotestosterone level	

Adapted from Feldman HA, Goldstein I, Hatzichristou DG, et al. Impotence and its medical and psychosocial correlates: results of the Massachusetts Male Aging Study. J Urol 1994; 151:54–61.

Epidemiology

Sexual activity in men progressively declines with age,[34] as evidenced by reduced interest and involvement in sexual matters, difficulty in achieving erections, and reduced satisfaction from sex. The decline in sexual activity is accelerated in the presence of other underlying health conditions. With age, erotogenic stimuli must be of greater intensity to produce a response, and episodes of spontaneous erections decrease in frequency or disappear.[22] The duration of the latent phase increases, penile filling slows, and there is less complete venous occlusion, which results in a less firm maximal erection. Paradoxically, the time to ejaculation may be prolonged, enhancing the quality of coitus. The time required to attain the next erection is prolonged, and in some men penile sensation declines substantially.

In the Massachusetts Male Aging Study of men 40 to 70 years of age, 48% were potent, and 17.2, 25.2, and 9.6% had minimal, moderate, and complete ED, respectively.[4] The clinical correlates of ED in this study are given in Table 19–2. As one might expect, age, depression, diabetes mellitus, and heart disease relate to ED, but, surprisingly, hypertension and alcohol consumption per se were not associated with ED. The protective effects of dominance, a high-density lipoprotein (HDL) level, and a high dehydroepiandrosterone (DHEA) are intriguing, but they should not be overinterpreted.

Disease Associations

HYPOGONADISM. Severe hypogonadism causes loss of libido and of erectile function and reduction in ejaculate volume,[5, 24] although there are reports of retained erectile capability in adult castrates.[35] Lesser degrees of hypogonadism are common with aging.[33, 36] Testosterone plays an important

TABLE 19–1. Mechanisms Contributing to Erectile Dysfunction

Type of Condition	Disorder
Vascular	
Aortoiliac arterial obstruction	Aorto-occlusive disease
Hypogastric-penile arterial obstruction	Atherosclerosis
Arterial dysplasia	Primary impotence in young men
Veno-occlusive incompetence	Age, diabetes mellitus, Peyronie's disease
Neurogenic	
Central nervous system and spinal neuronal loss	Cerebrovascular accident (stroke), multiple sclerosis, epilepsy
Peripheral autonomic neuronal loss	Surgery, Shy-Drager syndrome, diabetes mellitus
Disordered signal transmission	Drugs
Psychogenic inhibition of the erotic response	Depression (psychogenic)
Endocrine	
Deficient androgen availability	
Testicular failure	Castration, radiation, chemotherapy
Hypothalamic-pituitary disease	Age, pituitary adenoma, ethanol
Prolactin excess	Prolactinoma, uremia, drugs
Estrogen excess	Alcoholism, cirrhosis, drugs
Inhibition of androgen action	Spironolactone, cimetidine, ranitidine, flutamide, ketoconazole, ethanol
Secondary hyperparathyroidism	Uremia
Hypothyroidism and hyperthyroidism	
Local	
Peyronie's disease	
Intersinusoidal fibrosis	Diabetes mellitus, aging
Penile trauma	
Pudendal nerve trauma	Bicycle rider's palsy
Penile carcinoma	

TABLE 19–3. Clinical Characteristics of 301 Patients Presenting to a Sexual Dysfunction Clinic*

Disorder	% of Patients with Disorder
Hypertension	45.8
Diabetes mellitus	30.0
Atherosclerosis	33.6
Myocardial infarction	16.3
Stroke	9.6
Occlusive vascular disease	7.0
Angina	9.6
Coronary bypass graft	5.3
Transurethral prostate resection	16.9
Arthritis	22.2

*Patients with active alcoholism, progressive systemic illness, psychosis, or established hypogonadism were not admitted to the study. Mean duration of impotence was 4.8 y. Ponderal index (kg/m²) was 27.3.

role in nocturnal erections but is not so acutely involved in erections due to erotic stimuli.[37] While testosterone and bioavailable testosterone levels decrease with age,[36] they are identical in potent and impotent men in the presence or absence of a medical illness.[38] Because of reduced production and increased protein binding of testosterone, the bioavailable testosterone level is below the normal range for young men in 40% of older men. Almost all such older men have values consistent with hypogonadotropic hypogonadism, and many have reduced responsiveness to luteinizing hormone–releasing hormone (LHRH). Perhaps the more important measure is tissue availability of androgens, which is reduced with aging,[39] but tissue levels of androgens have not been compared in potent and impotent men.

VASCULAR DISEASE. The majority of cases of secondary ED appear to be the result of atherosclerosis. Occlusive vascular disease was associated with a 51% rate of ED in 367 patients.[40–43] ED was most likely to occur with the most severe arterial lesions (by angiographic visualization), and relief of major vessel obstruction did not alleviate the ED in most cases,[41] suggesting that distal arteries and intrinsic penile tissues are involved.

Myocardial infarction was associated with a pre-existing rate of ED of 44% and an overall sexual dysfunction rate of 64% in one large series.[44] A similar prevalence was seen in a control group under medical treatment.[45] Other studies reported comparable results.

DIABETES MELLITUS. Several large series suggest a prevalence of ED of about 50% in unselected patients with diabetes mellitus,[46] increasing steadily with age. The onset of ED is inversely related to age at diagnosis of diabetes (Fig. 19–2).[47] NPT is almost invariably abnormal in diabetics with ED, as compared with either normal subjects or potent diabetics.[48]

Hypogonadism plays a minor role in ED associated with diabetes mellitus because the prevalence of primary and secondary hypogonadism is similar in men with diabetes and in nondiabetic men of the same age with ED[46, 47] and in healthy control subjects.[38] Androgens are ineffective as therapy for diabetic ED.

Both vascular and neurogenic factors play a prominent role in diabetic ED. Neurogenic factors appear more common in insulin-dependent diabetes mellitus (IDDM),[49] and vascular factors predominate in non–insulin-dependent diabetes mellitus (NIDDM).[50] Borderline or low penile blood pressure is more frequent in NIDDM (79%) than in IDDM (47%),[47] and the incidence of vascular lesions demonstrated by Doppler ultrasound was high in a group of patients with NIDDM.[51] By contrast, patients with IDDM have a higher prevalence of neurologic defects than do potent IDDM patients or nondiabetic patients with ED.[49]

HYPERTENSION. Hypertension has long been thought to be associated with an increased incidence of ED. In one large study 20% of hypertensive men were impotent before initiation of therapy, and ED rates higher than 30% were reported in drug-treated groups.[52] However, the age-specific incidence of ED in hypertensive men probably does not differ from that in the general population receiving medical care.[4, 53]

The onset of ED is often associated with initiation of antihypertensive therapy. Central and peripheral autonomic agents have been especially implicated, but all antihypertensive agents, including diuretics, angiotensin-converting enzyme inhibitors, and calcium channel blockers, can cause ED.[8, 21, 54] None of the published studies relate the degree of blood pressure control to sexual dysfunction. Reduction of arterial blood pressure and reduced resistance in nonpenile vascular beds may accentuate the reduction in flow rate associated with an obstructive lesion in the hypogastric-penile arterial tree, so adequate control of blood pressure might reduce maximal penile-filling capacity.[55]

UREMIA. Nearly half of uremic men have ED.[56–60] Possible contributing elements include levels of elevated prolactin; elevated levels of LH and estradiol; and low levels of plasma testosterone. Both an increased secretion rate of prolactin and a reduced metabolic clearance of prolactin are seen. Secondary hyperparathyroidism, zinc depletion, and autonomic neuropathy have also been proposed as factors contributing to the ED of uremia. Vascular disease, therapy for hypertension, and volume depletion during dialysis may reduce the penile filling rate. Bromocriptine, clomiphene, and androgens are of little use in treating ED in subjects on dialysis. Erythropoietin (EPO) has been reported to improve sexual function, concomitant with reduction of the serum prolactin level and increased gonadotropin pulse amplitude.[61, 62] The nonendocrine roles of EPO in increasing blood volume and pressure and in increasing oxygen delivery to corpora cavernosa have not been explored.

NEUROLOGIC DISEASE. Multiple sclerosis was considered to produce a high degree of sexual dysfunction in both sexes; however, in a community-based survey 80% of the respondents reported no sexual dysfunction, and most of those with problems were women.[63] Temporal lobe epilepsy can cause sexual dysfunction in both men and women, probably the consequence of impairment of arousal and worsened by antiepileptic medications.[64] Cerebrovascular accidents[65] are associated with a high prevalence of ED, presumably by impairing central or peripheral erectile centers or pathways. Pelvic surgery impairs erectile function by interrupting the autonomic fibers of the nervi erigentes that control the erectile process[10] or by decreasing the penile blood supply.[66] Pelvic irradiation causes ED because of both impairment of arterial flow and damage to the pelvic autonomic nervous system.

NEOPLASTIC DISEASE. Patients with cancer frequently

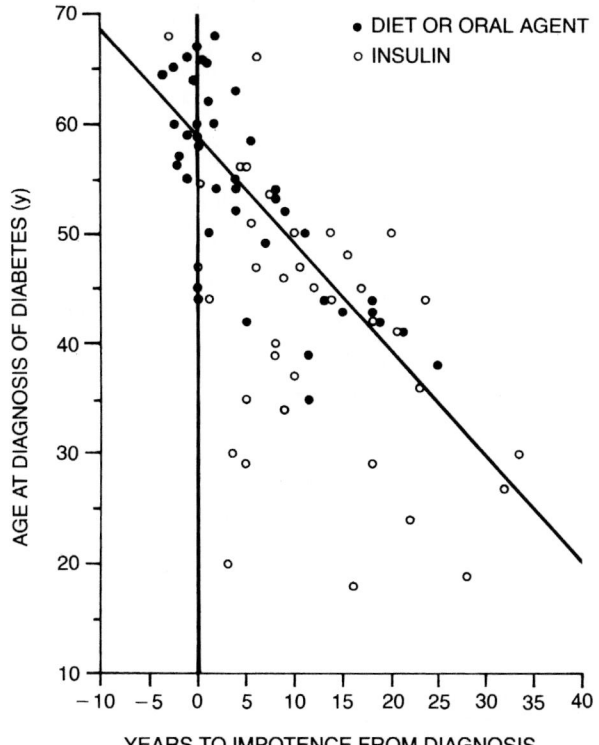

$$y = 58.844 - 0.965x \quad R = 0.75$$

- ● DIET OR ORAL AGENT
- ○ INSULIN

Figure 19–2. The relationship between the onset of diabetes mellitus and the onset of ED was assessed in 64 consecutive diabetics seen in an ED clinic.[47]

have a diminution in the quality of their sexual life.[67, 68] Among patients with pelvic tumors, including prostatic cancer, about 20% before and 80% after surgery had ED.[69, 70] Walsh and Schlegl[70] developed an improved technique for radical prostatectomy and cystoprostatectomy that has resulted in acceptable recurrence rates and potency rates above 75% in younger patients.[71] In some cases of failure to retain erectile function, vascular factors rather than nerve injury may be causal.[72]

Surgery for rectal cancer results in a 60 to 80% ED rate after abdominal-perineal resection and a 40% rate after a low resection.[73, 74] Radiation therapy for pelvic tumors also produces a high rate of ED,[75] with severe sexual dysfunction common after radiation therapy for prostate carcinoma.[76] Treatment of neoplastic diseases may also cause sexual dysfunction. For example, 24% of male survivors of bone marrow transplantation reported ED, and 13% had ejaculatory problems.[77]

OTHER CHRONIC DISEASES. High rates of ED and of impairment of libido and sexual activity have been reported in men with chronic back pain,[78, 79] chronic obstructive pulmonary disease,[80] pulmonary fibrosis,[81] hyperthyroidism,[82] celiac disease,[83] arthritis,[84, 85] scleroderma,[86, 87] hemochromatosis,[88] acromegaly, and prolactinoma.

DRUG-RELATED CAUSES. Sexual dysfunction, including loss of libido, ED, and ejaculatory insufficiency, has been reported with a wide variety of drugs, but most studies of the phenomenon are anecdotal and uncontrolled (see references 7, 8, 21, and 52 for discussion of individual therapeutic agents). The principal culprits are neurotransmitter agonists or antagonists used for the treatment of hypertension, angina, and afterload reduction or for alleviation of psychosis, anxiety, and depression. They may act by inhibiting the parasympathetic erectile mechanism, stimulating α-adrenergic vasoconstrictor tone, interfering with central erotic responsiveness, or blocking the dopaminergic inhibition of prolactin secretion. Prolactin hypersecretion both affects central nervous system control of sexual responsiveness and inhibits gonadotropin secretion. Agents that reduce androgen availability or act directly as estrogens include digitalis, cimetidine, ranitidine, spironolactone, ketoconazole, progestagens, LHRH agonists or antagonists, and estrogens themselves. The 5α-reductase 2 inhibitor finasteride appears to have little or no effect on sexual function in normal men.[89] The sexual effects of narcotics, cocaine, and marijuana are predominantly depressive, although cocaine has a reputation for enhancing sexual pleasure.

Excessive alcohol consumption per se does not appear to affect erectile function,[4, 90] but chronic alcoholism with liver damage is associated with a high prevalence of ED.[91, 92] Alcoholism can also cause hypogonadism, feminization,[93] (Table 19–4) and neuropathy, and vascular disease is worsened by the smoking that commonly accompanies alcohol excess.

Alcoholics may respond to high doses of nonaromatizable androgens, which suggests that a form of hypogonadism is common.[94] Long-term rehabilitation resulted in return of sexual function in only 25% of alcoholics in one study,[94] indicating that ED should be addressed as early as possible in the treatment of alcoholism.

Cigarette smoking is considered a risk factor for ED.[4, 95, 96] Cigarette smoking is increased in men with ED compared with matched control subjects, with a high prevalence of heavy smokers among the sexually dysfunctional group. Among nonsmokers with ED, a history of previous smoking was common. In dogs, electrically stimulated erections are inhibited by passive inhalation of smoke from two cigarettes per hour or by intravenous nicotine injection.[96] The inhibitory effect of nicotine is due to a reduction in corporeal blood flow and in cavernosal venoconstriction in the absence of effects on systemic blood pressure. This finding suggests that nicotine, and

perhaps other cigarette volatiles, either inhibit erectile nerve vasodilator activity or stimulate α-adrenergic vasoconstrictor activity or both. Thus cigarette smoking may contribute to vascular ED both by its chronic enhancement of the development of peripheral vascular disease and by inhibiting vasodilatation acutely.

PSYCHOGENIC CAUSES. The cause and prevalence of psychogenic ED are unclear. The results of any study of ED depend on the sources of patients, the age distribution, the extent of the work-up, and the criteria for assignment of cases to one or another diagnostic category. Most studies attribute less than a third of ED to psychogenic causes. Some researchers[31, 33] identify organic etiologic factors in more than 90% of men older than age 50 with ED. The author and others prefer a risk factor approach to the diagnosis of ED and doubt the relevance of the distinction between organic and psychogenic ED.[97] Complete vascular, neurologic, and psychological assessments are difficult to make and may be uninterpretable if not performed in the actual erotic setting. Furthermore, assessment of NPT is not a valid means of distinguishing among causes of ED.

In primary psychiatric disease, ambulatory schizophrenics do not appear to have a high prevalence of ED,[98] whereas depression is associated with sexual dysfunction, ED, and abnormal NPT.[4, 99, 100] However, in one study of depressed men in the unmedicated state sexual activity was normal, and treatment with benzodiazepines was associated with a high degree of ED.[101] Patients presenting with ED do not appear to have a greater prevalence of psychopathology than potent men.

PEYRONIE'S DISEASE. Peyronie's disease is a scarring disorder of the tunica albuginea that is a local cause of ED. Depletion of elastic fiber characterizes Peyronie's disease.[102] The greatly stiffened tunica albuginea makes it difficult to achieve veno-occlusion, and extensive plaque may interfere with arterial inflow, both impairing normal erectile function. Plaque may be found at the periphery of the penis or in the midline, where the corpora meet. In the early stages the disorder seems to be an inflammatory process with cellular infiltrates followed by collagen deposition. The scars distort the erect penis and often cause ED. Careful examination of the stretched penis throughout its length may be required to detect plaque, and the disorder may first be noted as a bent penis at the time of vasodilator-induced erections.

Diagnostic Evaluation

History and Physical Examination

The diagnostic evaluation for ED requires a careful history, an appropriate physical examination, and special diag-

TABLE 19–4. Chronic Reproductive-Endocrine Consequences of Ethanol Abuse

Cell or System	Effect
Leydig cells	Increased gonadotropin receptors
	Reduced cyclic AMP concentration
	Increased sensitivity to estrogens
	Acetaldehyde toxicity
	Reduced NAD$^+$/NADH inhibits steroidogenesis
	Reduced 3β-hydroxysteroid dehydrogenase
	Injures mitochondria
	Increased presence of testicular autoantibodies
Enhanced testosterone metabolism	Induction of 5α-reductase activity with acute or short-term exposure
Estrogen metabolism	Chronically increased aromatase activity
	Probably increased estrogen receptors in tissues (including testis and liver)
	Reduced intracellular estrogen metabolism
	Phytoestrogens in alcohol-containing beverages

nostic procedures. The sexual history should record the extent of the dysfunction, its duration, its progression, and its characteristics. A self-administered form can be utilized for documenting such a record.[97] Appropriate questions concern current sexual activities; partner availability; the presence of spontaneous morning erections; the quality, duration, and usability of the best erections; and the ejaculatory capacity. A substantial decrease in sexual interest or responsiveness suggests the possibilities of hypogonadism, an effect of drugs, or clinical depression. The impact of ED on self-image and interpersonal relations provides insight into the urgency of diagnostic and therapeutic approaches.

It is important to involve the partner early in the discussion of sexual function and of the various therapeutic alternatives. Successful therapy depends to a great degree on the availability, interest, health, and psychological state of the partner. Some women, particularly in the geriatric age group, may not desire or be prepared for resumption of an active sex life.

A complete medical evaluation should be performed because ED may be the presenting complaint in serious medical illness, including diabetes mellitus (see Fig. 19–2), occlusive vascular disease, or pituitary tumor.

The physical examination should emphasize evidence of hypogonadism, including reduced testicular size and density, loss of scrotal rugation, diminution of body hair, and development of fine facial wrinkles. Penile size and shape, the presence of Peyronie's plaque or fibrous tissue, and the size, firmness, symmetry, and nodularity of the prostate should also be assessed. Autonomic nervous system function may be tested by evaluating for postural hypotension and assessment of heart rate responses to deep breathing.

LABORATORY TESTS

The author believes that the endocrine tests should include a measurement of bioavailable testosterone (BT) and ultrasensitive thyrotropin. Both hyperthyroidism and hypothyroidism may be associated with ED and may be difficult to diagnose on clinical grounds, particularly in older men. The diagnosis of hypogonadism by hormone assay may be difficult. The author considers a BT value of less than 2.3 nmol/L (67 ng/dL) to be below the lower limit of normal.[38] Men with a low BT should have assessment of LH and prolactin. Most such men have normal LH values, and pituitary adenomas are rarely present. Unless the prolactin level is elevated, magnetic resonance imaging (MRI) of the pituitary should not be obtained.

SPECIAL DIAGNOSTIC TESTS. The advent of simple therapies for ED that do not depend on a specific etiology eliminates much of the rationale for the performance of complex, invasive, and expensive diagnostic tests. This fact is particularly true of older men who experience ED after many years of normal sexual function.

Diagnostic Intracorporeal Injection. The author employs intracorporeal vasodilator injection to determine erectile capability directly, to determine the extent of penile distortion due to Peyronie's disease, and to demonstrate the procedure to the patient and estimate the therapeutic dose in case they should elect self-injection as treatment.[103] It is also employed during angiography and cavernosography to ensure adequate visualization of the penile vessels and during duplex ultrasonographic assessment of arterial reactivity.

Intracorporeal injections of papaverine or papaverine-phentolamine combinations were used initially, but alprostadil (prostaglandin E_1) or various combinations of alprostadil, phentolamine, and/or papaverine are now employed (see the section on therapy). Patients with neurologic disorders may have denervation hypersensitivity to these drugs. Prostaglan-

din E_1 occasionally causes painful erections.[104] In some studies, drug effectiveness depends on dose.[103–105]

Initial intracavernosal injections carry a risk of priapism, hematoma, infection, local pain, and systemic hypotension (rare). The quality of the erection attained helps determine the degree of vascular insufficiency. The author employs a five-point scale: 5 = rigid; 4 = firm, usable; 3 = maximum diameter but soft, nonusable; 2 = partially erect; 1 = some tumescence. A strong, persistent erection excludes significant arterial or venous insufficiency as the cause of ED, whereas a weak erection supports the diagnosis of arterial disease or impaired venous occlusion if a sufficient dose of vasodilator has been given.

Nocturnal Penile Tumescence. The author does not believe that monitoring of NPT is a useful test for evaluating ED. NPT testing by continuous monitoring of penile diameter and sleep stage and visually assessing the rigidity of erection can determine whether the reflex erectile mechanism is intact.[23] This assessment requires at least two nights of observation in a sleep laboratory. Alternatively the Rigiscan portable NPT monitor (Dacomed, Minneapolis, MN) can be utilized at home by the patient. It records the number and quality of erectile episodes throughout the night, but the normal range of response has never been established.

Simple inexpensive tests for determining whether NPT has occurred include the stamp test, in which a ring of postage stamps is placed around the flaccid penis at bedtime and a break indicates an episode of diameter increase, and the Dacomed Snap Gauge.[106]

Men with normal vasculature may have abnormal NPT because of disturbed sleep, and NPT can be normal with organic ED associated with a pelvic steal syndrome.[107] In potent men both the frequency and the quality of NPT episodes decrease with age. Davis and colleagues[31] found that more than 90% of men older than age 50 with secondary ED had abnormal NPT.

Penile-Brachial Blood Pressure Index (PBPI). This index compares the penile and the brachial systolic pressures. The test is of limited specificity and sensitivity but can be used to determine the presence of a pelvic steal syndrome.[108] Pelvic steal occurs when obstructive lesions of the iliac or hypogastric arterial system permit adequate flow for erection at rest (or during NPT) but cause shunting of blood away from the penis during exercise. The PBPI is difficult to do well. The author does not use it as a diagnostic test.

Duplex Scanning. Duplex scanning of penile arteries before and after papaverine-induced erection determines whether corporeal arterial diameters are reduced and whether they dilate after exposure to vasodilatation.[15] Failure of erection despite good arterial flow is diagnostic of veno-occlusive insufficiency. Duplex scanning does not provide information as to whether a pelvic steal syndrome is present, does not assist in characterizing intrapenile lesions, and has lost favor as a diagnostic test because it does not distinguish between psychogenic and organic causes.[109] It is most effective in distinguishing veno-occlusive from arterial disease.

Penile arteriography, cavernosography, cavernosometry, and electromyographic recording to assess nerve damage are not indicated in the usual case of ED and should be reserved for centers expert in penile surgery and for ED in young men or after trauma.[3]

Therapy

Therapy for ED should follow thorough discussion of the benefits and risks of the alternatives with the couple. Management should be based on a risk factor approach, because the presence of hypogonadism does not rule out vascular ED, combined arterial and veno-occlusive incompetence is common, and psychological factors are always present to some degree. Age itself is not barrier to therapy.

INTRACORPOREAL PHARMACOTHERAPY. ED may be treated quite effectively in most cases by self-administration of intracorporeal vasodilators, including alprostadil, papaverine, and alprostadil–papaverine–phentolamine combinations.[110] Alprostadil is used more frequently than are papaverine-based solutions because it is effective, rapidly metabolized (never measurable in the circulation), causes less penile induration, and does not affect liver function.[111] It does, however, cause penile burning and discomfort in many men, which impairs its acceptance and effectiveness, and may sometimes cause prolonged erections.

Contraindications to intracavernosal pharmacotherapy include sickle cell anemia and, possibly, severe vascular disease, for which it is unlikely to be effective. Intracavernosal pharmacotherapy is not for everyone. Only about one half of men who begin intracavernosal pharmacotherapy continue long-term treatment (see the review by Linet and Neff[112]). Intracavernosal alprostadil has a high degree of effectiveness and, provided that the dose is kept to a minimum, an acceptable level of side effects. The agent comes as a powder in doses of 10 or 20 μg, which the patient must mix with the use of a prefilled syringe. The author recommends a diagnostic dose of 5 μg, and if a stage IV or V erection is achieved in the examining room and lasts no more than 1 h, the dose should be utilized at home. If such an erection is not achieved, a higher dose can be tried. If a firm, long-lasting erection is achieved (usually in men with a major neurologic disorder), the dose should be decreased to 2.5 μg. The author usually recommends that the patients keep a supply of pseudoephedrine at home, and if an erection lasts longer than desired the ingestion of 30 mg by mouth usually causes detumescence within 15 to 20 min.

An intraurethral alprostadil delivery device (MUSE [Vivus, Palo Alto, CA]) may offer a more acceptable method of administration of the drug.[112a]

EXTERNAL VACUUM TUMESCENCE DEVICES. A variety of external vacuum devices are marketed, most of which feature a large plastic cylinder enclosing the penis, a vacuum pump, and an obstructing band.[113] Application of the vacuum causes blood to flow into the penis, and when a sufficient erection is attained an obstructing band is applied to the base of the penis to retain the accumulated blood in the corpora. After the patient learns how to use them, the devices are usually a satisfactory and cost-effective solution for ED. Tissues are not adversely affected. A normal coital pattern may be restored with 2 to 10 episodes per month, and erectile duration is satisfactory, lasting an average of 16 min.[113] Some couples find the loss of spontaneity inhibiting. In patients with normal sensation, excessive negative pressure is prevented by pain. The erection is not completely normal in that the engorged penis may become reddened and sometimes cyanotic because of the filling of the superficial penile vessels as well as the corpora and because the base of the penis is not engorged. The glans penis is normally distended.

The principal complications are occasional reversible hematomas, discomfort from the bands, and cold temperature of the erect penis, which can be treated by warming. Occasionally the tightness of the band results in an inability to ejaculate; more frequently, the ejaculate has little force and simply seeps from the urethra.

This approach can also be useful in the management of patients with an unsatisfactory result from a penile prosthesis either after its removal or with it in place. It is also effective in patients who have experienced a spinal cord injury or who have had major pelvic surgery.

OTHER MEDICAL THERAPIES. No medical therapy is effective for unselected patients with ED, but some therapies may be useful in carefully selected patients.

Androgens. When there is coexisting hypogonadism, especially with severe hypogonadism in young persons, erectile function may be restored with testosterone replacement therapy. In older men who have a high prevalence of coexisting vascular disease, androgen therapy may not return erectile function to normal even when hypogonadism is present; such men should receive other therapy for erectile impotence. However, androgens in such men may improve energy, mood, and the sense of well-being and will protect the bones from osteopenia. Such therapy should be in the form of either long-acting testosterone esters or testosterone skin patches (see Chapter 16).

Other Hormone-Directed Therapies. Unsuccessful agents include bromocriptine, clomiphene, periodic administration of LHRH agonists, and yohimbine (an α_2-adrenergic blocker). In contrast, erythropoietin therapy in men with uremia may improve ED, although the mechanism is not clear.[61, 62] The use of this agent merits further study in uremic men who do not have penile vascular insufficiency.

Vascular Surgery. Vascular surgery is rarely indicated in the treatment of ED. Surgical ligation of the superficial and deep dorsal veins draining the penis is a relatively simple procedure that may give a 60% initially excellent or good result in restoring erectile function but is rarely a permanent solution.[114] Arterialization of the dorsal penile vein by using the inferior epigastric artery has been reported to be associated with a 60% success rate. Major vascular complications occurred in 6% of patients. The technique should be performed in only a few centers.

PENILE PROSTHESES. Penile prostheses are devices that when inserted into the corpora cavernosa confer rigidity, either continuously as in the semirigid varieties or on demand, as in the inflatable types. These are now considered to be second-line therapies,[3] and the frequency of their use has declined. They are expensive and invasive and, depending on the type, have high complication rates, produce poor erections, and undergo frequent mechanical failure. None of the devices allow swelling of the glans penis, which is therefore susceptible to trauma during intercourse. Anecdotal reports suggest that men with diabetes mellitus have an increased incidence of infection and externalization of the prostheses.

SEX THERAPY. New insight into the pathogenesis of ED and the availability of effective therapies have led to changing views as to the value of sex therapy in the management of ED.[115, 116] In older men with secondary ED, the author anticipates an organic cause and treats the patients accordingly. However, depression may interfere with sexual performance, and loss of a mate often leads to depression and social isolation. Men may lose confidence in their sexual abilities, which creates anxieties that contribute greatly to failure to initiate new relationships. The physician who treats ED may have the opportunity to identify and treat depression and to refer the patients for further support.

Sex therapy techniques may allow improvement of sexual attitudes and capacity in organic as well as psychogenic ED. Sex therapy should focus on the couple. Unrealistic expectations and marital discord must be addressed, and the characteristics of a more satisfactory sex life defined. Behavioral changes that may assist include eliminating exposure to nicotine, arranging an appropriate time and environment for sexual intercourse, and encouraging intimacy, mutual pleasuring, experimentation, and communication. The effectiveness of sex therapy has never been fully evaluated. Although it has been reported that an improvement in erectile function is common with sex therapy,[117, 118] the level of improvement is not always sufficient for coitus.[119]

SEXUAL FUNCTION AND DYSFUNCTION IN WOMEN

Anatomic, physiological, and psychosocial differences between women and men cause differences in patterns of sexual dysfunction, but the underlying themes are similar, just as the anatomic elements and the physiological responses to arousal are analogous. Women experience disturbances of the desire (libido), arousal (proceptivity), and orgasmic phases of the sexual response cycle, as well as painful intercourse (dyspareunia). Vaginismus, severe contractions of the vaginal musculature that prevent penile entry, is rare.

Female Sexual Response Mechanism

Women have periodic nocturnal increases in vaginal blood flow and pulse amplitude. The parasympathetic and sympathetic neural elements supporting the female sexual response are similar to those for men, and a degree of dysfunction may follow pelvic or genital surgery. After somatosensory stimulation, orgasm is an adrenergic response.

The female response cycle consists of desire, arousal, plateau, orgasm, and resolution. Desire begins in the brain, with perception of erotogenic stimuli via the special senses or through fantasy. On arousal the clitoris becomes erect. The labia minora becomes engorged. Blood flow in the entire vaginal vault triples. The upper two thirds of the vagina dilates. "Sweating" of lubricant from the vaginal surface occurs, followed by thickening and dilatation of the lower third of the vagina, forming the "orgasmic platform." The clitoris and vagina have dense somatosensory innervation, providing intense sensory responsiveness. At orgasm, rhythmic vaginal smooth muscle and pelvic contractions take place. Women can experience multiple orgasms without a refractory period. Intense vaginal and sometimes clitoral stimulation may be required for orgasm in some women.

The role of hormones in influencing sexual function is of practical as well as theoretical interest because women receive nonphysiological amounts and proportions of estrogens and progestagens in oral contraceptives and as therapy for the postmenopausal state. They also frequently undergo surgery on fallopian tubes, uterus, and ovaries, with uncertain consequences for sexual behavior.

Estrogens, progestagens, and androgens influence sexual behavior in animals. Responsiveness results from central nervous system–mediated autonomic nervous system signals. Estrogens are responsible for the development and maintenance of the female sexual tissues.

The menopause is associated with cessation of ovarian estrogen secretion (see Chapter 15). As a result of aromatization of adrenal precursors, postmenopausal women continue to produce some estrone and estradiol. A variable decrease in sexual behavior characterizes the perimenopausal period.[120–122]

Estrogen replacement therapy appears to restore sexual desire and responsiveness in symptomatic postmenopausal women.[123]

As a result of studies in primates,[124] it has been proposed that androgens control libido in women as in men. There are anecdotal reports of increased libido in women with breast cancer who are treated with large doses of androgens, but in the author's experience and in that of others,[125] young women with androgen excess syndromes do not have increased libido or altered sexual behavior. Finally, in controlled trials androgens do not seem to enhance the effects of estrogens in women with menopausal hyposexuality.[126, 127]

Sexual Dysfunction in Women

Epidemiology

There have been few objective, population-based, detailed analyses of female sexual dysfunction, and available reports have utilized varying diagnostic criteria. During the adult reproductive years, the principal dysfunctions reported by women in several surveys[120, 121, 128–130] are low desire (18%), low arousal (25%), global orgasmic difficulty (9%), situational orgasmic difficulty (27%), and dyspareunia (8%) (Table 19–5). The relative consistency of the reports suggests that these average values are correct. Unfortunately, there is little information on sexual dysfunction in young women.

Osborn and colleagues,[129] in a community-based study in Great Britain that evaluated the changing physiological status of women as they go through menopause, demonstrated that substantial increases in operationally defined sexual dysfunctions occur in women with age (Table 19–6). The principal problem seems to be a decrease in sexual interest and arousability in a subset of women and an increased incidence of anorgasmic episodes of coitus. These findings were related not to gynecologic problems or menopausal state but rather to age itself. The subjects perceived themselves to be much less sexually dysfunctional than did the investigators. In this cross-sectional study, cohorts played an important role in sexual expectations. Only 4% of the women were interested in pursuing the "problem."

Similar findings, but with a higher rate of perception of dysfunction, were noted in a clinic, where 85% of patients admitted having a sexual problem and 22% of the problems were attributed to the partner.[130] A decrease in sexual activity with advancing age was considered to be normal,[122] but in a study of healthy men and women ranging in age from 80 to 102, Bretschneider and McCoy[121] found considerable sexual activity in both sexes. Touching and caressing without coitus were reported by 64% of women, masturbation by 40%, and sexual intercourse by 30%. Bretschneider and McCoy comment that the principal decrease in sexual activity and enjoyment occurs during the early postmenopausal years and that in healthy women, sexual interest and activity remain relatively constant thereafter, although coital opportunity and frequency decrease precipitously with age. A recent review of

TABLE 19–5. Sexual Dysfunction in Healthy Women with a Regular Partner

Author	Schover	Jensen	Frank et al.	Schover et al.	Osborn et al.
Reference	118	46	119	128	129
Year	1981	1981	1978	1987	1988
Number of patients	92	40	100	76	436
Mean age (y)	30	38	35	41	
Low sexual desire (%)	10	23	35	10	17
Low arousal (%)	14	24	48	10	50
Orgasmic difficulty					
Global (%)	9	7	15	4	
Situational (%)	18	30	33	26	
Total (%)	27	37	48	30	16
Dyspareunia (%)	8	8		10	8

TABLE 19–6. Sexual Dysfunction in Women According to Age

Dysfunction	%					
	Ages 35–39	Ages 40–44	Ages 45–49	Ages 50–54	Ages 55–59	All Ages
Low sexual desire	4	8	6	29	28	17
Frequency of orgasm	5	8	14	22	35	16
Dyspareunia	0	1	9	17	17	8
Vaginal dryness	8	12	16	26	22	17
Any of above	14	19	32	51	48	33

geriatric sexuality in women emphasizes the potential to retain sexual activity and enjoyment when health is sustained and, in most cases, when a partner is available.[122]

Specific Types of Dysfunction

The four principal sexual dysfunctions in women are lack of interest, failure of arousal, anorgasmia, and dyspareunia. One important factor that has not been studied in "normal" populations is the effect of childhood sexual abuse and of rape on lifelong sexual behavior. With as many as 15 to 38% of girls being abused before the age of 18 and a high incidence of rape, mostly not reported,[131] such experiences could have a grave impact on lifelong sexual enjoyment. A study of 371 self-referred, previously assaulted women indicated that 59% had remaining sexual problems, most of which were attributed to the assault.[132] The extremely high prevalence of prior abuse in women with the unexplained pelvic pain syndrome[133] suggests that careful study of traumatic sexual experiences may shed light on the high prevalence of low desire and arousal reported for some populations (see Table 19–5). In women with regular menstrual cycles, sexuality does not seem to relate well to reproductive hormone levels,[134] and administration of either androgens or estrogens has little effect on sexuality.[135] However, one study focused on the effects of androgen deficiency (testosterone values <0.4 nmol/L [<0.1 ng/mL]) as a result of surgery or chemotherapy on libido in comparison to treated women (testosterone values >1 nmol/L [>0.3 ng/mL]) and demonstrated a virtually complete loss of sexual interest and responsiveness, leading to the suggestion that androgen therapy may be of use in this situation.[136] Hypothalamic-pituitary disease was associated with reduced or absent sexual desire and function.[137]

Local factors play an important role in the sexuality of women. Median episiotomy at delivery produced greater sexual dysfunction than that in women who did not undergo episiotomy.[138] Pelvic surgery and ostomy placement also have the potential for serious impairment of sexual function,[139] but many such patients do quite well. Relaxed vaginal outlet as a result of multiple vaginal deliveries commonly causes reduced sexual enjoyment of both partners owing to a feeling of "looseness" and a lack of feeling of penile containment. Treatment with Kegel exercises to improve pelvic muscle tone is of dubious help.[140] In the presence of stress incontinence or uterine descensus, surgical correction may be indicated.

A variety of gynecologic disorders cause dyspareunia, including vaginitis resulting from infection with trichomonads, yeasts, and bacteria; pelvic infections; endometriosis; and postmenopausal atrophy of urogenital tissues. Other factors include infections of Skene's or Bartholin's glands, vulvitis, and hymenal obstruction. A similar syndrome may result from episiotomy scarring and postradiation vaginal atrophy.

The impact of medical illness on sexual interest and arousal in women is difficult to assess because of the high prevalence of subjective dysfunction in healthy women (see Table 19–5) and because of the difficulty of distinguishing between the effects of illness and the effects of drugs. Pelvic and breast neoplasms cause highly variable degrees of sexual dysfunction.[128, 141, 142] Multiple sclerosis,[143] scleroderma,[144] uremia,[145] and myocardial infarction[146] cause a decrease in sexual activity. The irritable bowel syndrome appears to be associated with more disordered sexual function than either inflammatory bowel disease or peptic ulcer disease.[147]

Diabetes mellitus in women results in far fewer sexual consequences than it does in men[148, 149] and may have no effect,[46] perhaps because diabetic women have less atherosclerotic disease than diabetic men of comparable age. Arthritis[150] also has minimal sexual consequences, as does hysterectomy.[151] The effects of hypertension and its therapy on the sexual function of women are probably minimal.[152]

There are reports of adverse effects of α- and β-adrenergic inhibitors, narcotics, and mood-altering drugs on libido and orgasm in women.[8] Chronic alcoholism is associated with reduced sexual satisfaction,[153] and acute ethanol ingestion inhibits orgasmic response.[154]

Diagnostic Evaluation

A complete medical assessment should include a sensitive inquiry about sexual dysfunction. If the patient seeks help or gives a positive response to questioning, inquiry should be made into the nature of the problem (interest, arousability, orgasm, or dyspareunia), its duration and progression, and the expectations of the patient regarding sexual activity and enjoyment. Does the dysfunction represent a lifelong pattern, or is it secondary to some event or illness? Is there general and sexual marital compatibility? Is there a history of sexual abuse? The medical evaluation should include detailing of medical illnesses and use of drugs, surgical interventions, and psychiatric background. The physical examination should include careful assessment of the pelvis, and abnormal findings must be pursued because sexual dysfunction may be a presenting complaint in serious conditions.

Endocrine diagnostic testing is pointless in a woman with regular menstrual cycles, and all postmenopausal women are hypogonadal. Perimenopausal hormone changes and abnormal or absent cycles warrant more study. When androgen therapy in hypogonadal or hypopituitary women is being considered, measurement of BT and total testosterone is useful.

Investigators have measured sexual arousal in response to erotic stimuli or during sleep by assessment of vaginal temperature or blood flow. These techniques do not provide clinically useful information because subjective arousal and objective arousal are not correlated and because the techniques have not been applied systematically to older women, in whom alterations may be expected to occur.[155]

Treatment

Treatment of sexual dysfunction in women requires evaluation of the couple and therapy for both partners, individually and together. Education of the couple about the basis of the problem and establishment of communication by the couple are of great help. Identified organic problems should be treated appropriately. Postmenopausal loss of desire and atrophy of urogenital tissues should be treated with estrogens and progestagens. Restoration of vaginal tissue integrity and of sexual interest may require several months, and tissue integrity may be incomplete. For women who cannot or will not take systemic estrogens, low-dose vaginal suppositories may be helpful for local symptoms.

Sex therapy, as described earlier, may have some value for improving general sexual and marital satisfaction in women who have inhibited desire or arousal, but the results are not spectacular.[118] The ability to achieve orgasm by various means can also be helped in some women with a program of education and training in masturbation. Coital orgasm is less frequently achieved.[156]

CONCLUSION

Advances in understanding and appreciation of the importance and frequency of sexual dysfunction, insight into the pathophysiology of ED, and development of new therapeutic alternatives have made it possible to improve and restore an active sexual life for many dysfunctional couples, thus enhancing their overall quality of life.

REFERENCES

1. Krane RJ, Goldstein I, Saenz de Tejada I. Impotence. N Engl J Med 1989; 321:1648–1659.
2. Korenman SG. Sexual dysfunction. In: Wilson JD, Foster DW, eds. Williams Textbook of Endocrinology. 8th ed. Philadelphia: WB Saunders, 1992: 1033–1048.
3. Impotence. National Institutes of Health Consensus Statement. 1992; 10:1.
4. Feldman HA, Goldstein I, Hatzichristou DG, et al. Impotence and its medical and psychosocial correlates: results of the Massachusetts Male Aging Study. J Urol 1994; 151:54–61.
5. Davidson JM, Camargo CA, Smith ER. Effects of androgen on sexual behavior in hypogonadal men. J Clin Endocrinol Metab 1979; 48:955–958.
6. Salmimies P, Kockett G, Pirke KM, et al. Effects of testosterone replacement on sexual behavior in hypogonadal men. Arch Sex Behav 1982; 11:345–353.
7. Wein AJ, Van Arsdale KN. Drug-induced male sexual dysfunction. Urol Clin North Am 1988; 15:23–31.
8. Buffum J. Pharmacosexology: the effects of drugs on sexual function—a review. J Psychoactive Drugs 1982; 14:5–44.
9. Williams W. Anaesthetic ejaculation. J Sex Marital Ther 1985; 11:19–29.
10. Lue TF, Zeinah SJ, Schmidt RA, et al. Neuroanatomy of penile erection: its relevance to iatrogenic impotence. J Urol 1984; 131:273–280.
11. Saenz de Tejada I, Goldstein I, Azadzoi K, et al. Impaired neurogenic and endothelium-mediated relaxation of penile smooth muscle from diabetic men with impotence. N Engl J Med 1989; 320:1025–1030.
12. Ignarro LJ, Bush PA, Buga JM, et al. Nitric oxide and cyclic GMP formation upon electric field stimulation cause relaxation of corpus cavernosum smooth muscle. Biochem Biophys Res Commun 1990; 170:843–850.
13. Kim N, Vardi Y, Padma-Nathan H, et al. Oxygen tension regulates the nitric oxide pathway. J Clin Invest 1993; 91:437–442.
14. Wagner G, Gerstenberg T, Levin RJ. Electrical activity of corpus cavernosum during flaccidity, and erection of the human penis: a new diagnostic method. J Urol 1989; 142:723–725.
15. Lue TF, Tanagho EA. Physiology of erection and pharmacological management of impotence. J Urol 1987; 137:829–836.
16. Lue TF, Takamura T, Umraiya M, et al. Hemodynamics of canine corpora cavernosa during erection. Urology 1984; 24:347–352.
17. Schmidt MH, Schmidt HS. The ischiocavernosus and bulbospongiosus muscles in mammalian penile rigidity. Sleep 1993; 16:171–183.
18. Aboseif SR, Lue TF. Hemodynamics of penile erection. Urol Clin North Am 1988; 15:1–7.
19. Saenz de Tejada I, Maroukian P, Tessier J, et al. Trabecular smooth muscle modulates the capacitor function of the penis: studies on a rabbit model. Am J Physiol 1991; 260:H150–H159.
20. Newman HF, Reiss H, Northrup JD. Physical basis of emission, ejaculation, and orgasm in the male. Urology 1982; 19:341–350.
21. Drugs that cause sexual dysfunction. Med Lett 1987; 29:65–70.
22. Masters WH, Johnson VE. Human Sexual Inadequacy. Boston: Little, Brown, 1970.
23. Karacan I, Williams RL, Thornby JI, et al. Sleep-related tumescence as a function of age. Am J Psychiatry 1975; 132:932–937.
24. Kwan M, Greenleaf WJ, Mann J, et al. The nature of androgen action on male sexuality: a combined laboratory-self-report study on hypogonadal men. J Clin Endocrinol Metab 1983; 57:557–562.
25. Schiavi RC, White D, Mandeli J, et al. Hormones and nocturnal penile tumescence in healthy aging men. Arch Sex Behavior 1992; 22:207–215.
26. Heaton JPW, Varrin SJ. Effects of castration and exogenous testosterone supplementation in an animal model of penile erection. J Urol 1994; 151:797–800.
27. Kurz EM, Sengelaub DR, Arnold AP. Androgens regulate the dendritic length of mammalian motoneurons in adulthood. Science 1986; 232:395–396.
28. Mills TM, Stopper VS, Wiedmeier VT. Effects of castration on the hemodynamics of penile erection in the rat. Biol Rep 1994; 51:234–238.
29. Lugg JA, Rajfer J, Gonzalez-Cadavid NF. Dihydrotestosterone is the active androgen in the maintenance of nitric oxide–mediated penile erection in the rat. Endocrinology 1995; 136:1495–1501.
30. Kaiser FE, Korenman SG. Impotence in diabetic men. Am J Med 1988; 85:147–152.
31. Davis SS, Viosca S, Guralnik M, et al. Evaluation of impotence in older men. West J Med 1985; 142:499–505.
32. Slag MF, Morley JE, Elson MK, et al. Impotence in medical clinic outpatients. JAMA 1983; 249:1736–1740.
33. Kaiser FE, Viosca SP, Morley JE, et al. Impotence and aging: clinical and hormonal factors. J Am Geriatr Soc 1988; 36:511–519.
34. McKinlay JB, Feldman HA. In: Sexuality Across the Life Course. Chicago: University of Chicago Press, 1994: 261–285.
35. Bremer J. Asexualization: A Follow-Up Study of 244 Cases. Oslo, Norway: Oslo University Press, 1958.
36. Tenover JS, Matsumoto AM, Plymate SR, et al. The effects of aging in normal men on bioavailable testosterone and luteinizing hormone secretion: response to clomiphene citrate. J Clin Endocrinol Metab 1987; 65:1118–1126.
37. Carani C, Bancroft J, Granata A, et al. Testosterone and erectile function, nocturnal penile tumescence and rigidity and erectile response to visual erotic stimuli in hypogonadal and eugonadal men. Psychoneuroendocrinology 1992; 17:647–654.
38. Korenman SG, Morley JE, Mooradian AD, et al. Secondary hypogonadism in older men: its relation to impotence. J Clin Endocrinol Metab 1990; 71:963–969.
39. Deslypere JP, Vermeulen A. Influence of age on steroid concentrations in skin and striated muscle in women and in cardiac muscle and lung tissue in men. J Clin Endocrinol Metab 1985; 61:648–653.
40. Metz P. Erectile function in men with occlusive disease in the legs. Dan Med Bull 1983; 30:185–189.
41. Dewar ML, Blundell PE, Lidstone D, et al. Effects of abdominal aneurysmectomy, aortoiliac bypass grafting and angioplasty on male sexual potency: a prospective study. Can J Surg 1985; 28:154–159.
42. Forsberg L, Olsson AM, Neglen P. Erectile function before and after aortoiliac reconstruction: a comparison between measurements of Doppler acceleration ratio, blood pressure and angiography. J Urol 1982; 127:379–382.
43. Queral L, Whitehouse W, Flinn W, et al. Pelvic hemodynamics after aortoiliac reconstruction. Surgery 1979; 86:799–809.
44. Wabrek AJ, Burchell RC. Male sexual dysfunction associated with coronary heart disease. Arch Sex Behav 1980; 9:69–75.
45. Dhabuwala CB, Kumar A, Pierce JM. Myocardial infarction and its influence on male sexual function. Arch Sex Behav 1986; 15:499–504.
46. Jensen SB. Diabetic sexual dysfunction: a comparative study of 160 insulin-treated diabetic men and women and an age-matched control group. Arch Sex Behav 1981; 10:493–504.
47. Kaiser FE, Korenman SG. Impotence in diabetic men. Am J Med 1988; 85:147–152.
48. Schiavi RC, Fisher C, Quadland M, et al. Nocturnal penile tumescence evaluation of erectile function in insulin-dependent diabetic men. Diabetologia 1985; 28:90–94.
49. Bemelmans BLH, Meuleman EJH, Doesburg WH, et al. Erectile dysfunction in diabetic men: the neurological factor revisited. J Urol 1994; 151:884–889.
50. Jevtich MJ, Edson M, Jarmon WD, et al. Vascular factor in erectile failure among diabetics. Urology 1982; 19:163–168.
51. Benvenuti F, Boncinelli L, Vignoli GC. Male sexual impotence in diabetes mellitus: vasculogenic versus neurogenic factors. Neuroneurol Urodynamics 1993;12:145–152.
52. Bulpitt CJ, Dollery CT. Side effects of hypotensive agents evaluated by a self-administered questionnaire. Br Med J 1973; 3:485–490.
53. Newman HF, Marcus H. Erectile dysfunction in diabetes and hypertension. Urology 1985; 26:135–137.
54. Moss HB, Procci WR. Sexual dysfunction associated with oral antihypertensive medications: a critical survey of the literature. Gen Hosp Psychiatry 1982; 4:121–129.
55. Lue TF, Hricak H, Marich KW, et al. Vasculogenic impotence evaluated by high-resolution ultrasonography and pulsed Doppler spectrum analysis. Radiology 1985; 155:778–782.
56. Rodger RCS, Fletcher K, Dewar J, et al. Prevalence and pathogenesis of impotence in one hundred uremic men. Uremia Invest 1984–85; 8:89–96.

57. Nghiem D, Corry R, Picon-Mendez G, et al. Factors influencing male sexual impotence after renal transplantation. Urology 1983; 21:49–52.
58. Procci WR, Martin DJ. Effect of maintenance hemodialysis on male sexual performance. J Nerv Ment Dis 1985; 173:366–372.
59. Weizman R, Weizman A, Levi J, et al. Sexual dysfunction associated with hyperprolactinemia in males and females undergoing hemodialysis. Psychosom Med 1983; 45:259–269.
60. Foulks CJ, Cushner HM. Sexual dysfunction in the male dialysis patient: pathogenesis, evaluation and therapy. Am J Kidney Dis 1986; 8:211–222.
61. Steffenson G, Aunsholt AA. Does erythropoietin cause hormonal changes in haemodialysis patients? Nephrol Dial Transplant 1993; 8:1215–1218.
62. Schaefer F, van Kaick B, Veldhuis JD, et al. Changes in the kinetics and biopotency of luteinizing hormone in hemodialyzed men during treatment with recombinant human erythropoietin. J Am Soc Nephrol 1994; 5:1208–1215.
63. Rodriguez M, Siva A, Ward J, et al. Impairment, disability, and handicap in multiple sclerosis: a population-based study in Olmsted County, Minnesota. Neurology 1994; 44:28–33.
64. Morrell MJ, Sperling MR, Stecker M, et al. Sexual dysfunction in partial epilepsy: a deficit in physiologic sexual arousal. Neurology 1994; 44:243–247.
65. Sjogren K, Damber J-E, Liliequist B. Sexuality after stroke with hemiplegia: aspects of sexual function. Scand J Rehabil Med 1983; 15:55–61.
66. Melman A. Iatrogenic causes of impotence. Urol Clin North Am 1988; 15:33–39.
67. Schover LR, Evans RB, von Eschenbach AC. Sexual rehabilitation in a cancer center: diagnosis and outcome in 384 consultations. Arch Sex Behav 1987; 16:445–461.
68. Andersen BL. Sexual functioning morbidity among cancer survivors. Cancer 1985; 55:1835–1842.
69. Pontes JE, Huben RP, Wolf R. Sexual function after radical prostatectomy. Prostate 1986; 8:123–126.
70. Walsh PC, Schlegl PN. Radical pelvic surgery with preservation of sexual function. Ann Surg 1988; 208:391–400.
71. Surya BV, Provet S, Dalbogni G, et al. Experience with potency preservation during radical prostatectomy. Urology 1988; 32:498–501.
72. Aboseif S, Shinohara K, Breza J, et al. Role of penile vascular injury in erectile dysfunction after radical prostatectomy. Br J Urol 1994; 73:75–82.
73. Fegiz G, Trenti A, Bezzi M, et al. Sexual and bladder dysfunction following surgery for rectal carcinoma. Ital J Surg Sci 1986; 16:103–109.
74. Kinn A, Oman U. Bladder and sexual function after surgery for rectal cancer. Dis Colon Rectum 1986; 29:43–48.
75. Goldstein I, Feldman MI, Deckers PJ, et al. Radiation-associated impotence: a clinical study of its mechanism. JAMA 1984; 25:903–910.
76. Helgason AR, Fredrikson M, Adolfsson J, et al. Decreased sexual capacity after external radiation therapy for prostate cancer impairs quality of life. Int J Radiat Oncol Biol Phys 1995; 32:33–39.
77. Wingard JR, Curbow B, Baker F, et al. Sexual satisfaction in survivors of bone marrow transplantation. Bone Marrow Transplant 1992; 9:185–190.
78. Sjogren K, Fugl-Meyer AR. Chronic back pain and sexuality: sexuality and disablement. Int Rehabil Med 1981; 3:19–25.
79. Maruta T, Osborne D, Swanson DW, et al. Chronic pain patients and spouses, marital and sexual adjustment. Mayo Clin Proc 1981; 56:307–310.
80. Fletcher E, Martin R. Sexual dysfunction and erectile impotence in chronic obstructive pulmonary disease. Chest 1982; 81:413–421.
81. Semple PDA, Beastall GH, Brown TM, et al. Sex hormone suppression and sexual impotence in hypoxic pulmonary fibrosis. Thorax 1984; 39:46–51.
82. Kidd GS, Glass AR, Vigersky RA. The hypothalamic-pituitary-testicular axis in thyrotoxicosis. J Clin Endocrinol Metab 1979; 48:798–802.
83. Farthing MJG, Edwards CRW, Rees L, et al. Male gonadal function in coeliac disease: sexual dysfunction, infertility, and semen quality. Gut 1982; 23:608–614.
84. Todd RC, Lightowler CDR, Harris J. Low-friction arthroplasty of the hip and sexual activity. Acta Orthop Scand 1973; 44:690–693.
85. Currey HLF. Osteoarthritis of the hip joint and sexual activity. Ann Rheum Dis 1970; 29:488–493.
86. Lally E, Jimenez S. Impotence in progressive systemic sclerosis. Ann Intern Med 1981; 95:150–153.
87. Nowlin NS, Brick JE, Weaver DJ, et al. Impotence in scleroderma. Ann Intern Med 1986; 104:794–798.
88. Stremmel W, Niederau C, Berger M, et al. Abnormalities in estrogen, androgen, and insulin metabolism in idiopathic hemochromatosis. Ann NY Acad Sci 1988; 526:209–223.
89. Cunningham GR, Hirshkowitz M. Inhibition of steroid 5α-reductase with finasteride: sleep-related erections, potency, and libido in healthy men. J Clin Endocrinol Metab 1995; 80:1934–1940.
90. Schiavi RC, Stimmel BB, Mandeli J, et al. Chronic alcoholism and male sexual function. Am J Psychiatry 1995; 152:1045–1051.
91. Fahrner EM. Sexual dysfunction in male alcohol addicts: prevalence and treatment. Arch Sex Behav 1987; 16:247–257.
92. Jensen SB. Sexual function and dysfunction in younger married alcoholics. Acta Psychiatr Scand 1984; 69:543–549.
93. Van Thiel DH, Gavaler JS. Hypothalamic-pituitary-gonadal function in liver disease with particular attention to the endocrine effects of chronic alcohol abuse. Prog Liver Dis 1986; 8:273–282.
94. Van Thiel DH, Gavaler JS, Sanghvi A. Recovery of sexual function in abstinent alcoholic men. Gastroenterology 1982; 84:677–682.
95. Condra M, Surridge DH, Morales A, et al. Prevalence and significance of tobacco smoking in impotence. Urology 1986; 27:495–498.
96. Juenemann K, Lue TF, Luo J, et al. The effect of cigarette smoking on penile erection. J Urol 1987; 138:438–441.
97. Schover LR, Jenson SB. Sexuality and Chronic Illness. New York: Guilford, 1988.
98. Verhulst J, Schneidman B. Schizophrenia and sexual functioning. Hosp Community Psychiatry 1981; 34:259–262.
99. Matthew RJ, Weinman ML. Sexual dysfunctions in depression. Arch Sex Behav 1982; 11:323–328.
100. Nofzinger EA, Thase ME, Reynolds CF III, et al. Sexual function in depressed men: assessment by self-report, behavioral, and nocturnal penile tumescence measures before and after treatment with cognitive behavior therapy. Arch Gen Psychiatry 1993; 50:24–30.
101. Ghadirian AM, Annable L, Belanger MC. Lithium, benzodiazepines, and sexual function in bi-polar patients. Am J Psychiatry 1992; 149:801–805.
102. Iacono F, Barra S, De Rosa G, et al. Microstructural disorders of tunica albuginea in patients affected by Peyronie's disease with or without erection dysfunction. J Urol 1993; 150:1806–1809.
103. Waldhauser M, Schramek P. Efficiency and side effects of prostaglandin E$_1$ in the treatment of impotence. J Urol 1988; 140:525–527.
104. Porst H. Value of prostaglandin E$_1$ in the diagnosis of impotence in comparison with papaverine and papaverine/phentolamine in 61 patients with impotence. Urologe [A] 1988; 27:22–26.
105. Gutierrez P, Pye S, Bancroft J. What does duplex ultrasound add to sexual history, nocturnal penile tumescence and intracavernosal injection of smooth muscle relaxant, in the diagnosis of erectile dysfunction? Int J Impot Res 1993; 5:123–132.
106. Anders EK, Bradley WE, Krane RJ. Nocturnal penile rigidity measured by the Snap Gauge band. J Urol 1983; 130:964–966.
107. Schiavi RC, Schreiner-Engel P. Nocturnal penile tumescence in healthy aging men. J Gerontol 1988; 43:146–150.
108. Goldstein I, Siroky MB, Nath RL, et al. Vasculogenic impotence: role of the pelvic steal test. J Urol 1982; 128:300–306.
109. Pescatori ES, Hatzichristou DG, Namburi S, et al. A positive intracavernous injection test implies normal veno-occlusive but not necessarily normal arterial function: a hemodynamic study. J Urol 1994; 151:1209–1216.
110. van Ahlen H, Peskar BA, Sticht G, et al. Pharmacokinetics of vasoactive substances administered into the human corpus cavernosum. J Urol 1994; 151:1227–1230.
111. Sidi AA, Reddy PK, Chen KK. Patient acceptance of and satisfaction with vasoactive intracavernous pharmacotherapy for impotence. J Urol 1988; 140:293–294.
112. Linet OI, Neff LL. Intracavernous prostaglandin E$_1$ in erectile dysfunction. Clin Investig 1994; 72:139–149.
112a. Padma-Nathan H, Hellstrom WJG, Kaiser FE, et al. Treatment of men with erectile dysfunction with transurethral alprostadil. N Engl J Med 1997; 336:1–7.
113. Korenman SG, Viosca SP, Kaiser FE, et al. Use of a vacuum tumescence device in the management of impotence. J Am Geriatr Soc 1990; 38:217–220.
114. Lewis RW. Venous surgery for impotence. Urol Clin North Am 1988; 15:115–121.
115. Zilbergeld B. Alternatives to couples counseling for sex problems: group and individual therapy. J Sex Marital Ther 1980; 6:3–18.
116. LoPiccolo JL, Heiman JR, Hogan DR, et al. Effectiveness of single therapists versus cotherapy teams in sex therapy. J Consult Clin Psychol 1985; 53:287–294.
117. De Amicis LA, Goldberg DC, LoPiccolo J, et al. Three-year follow-up of couples evaluated for sexual dysfunction. J Sex Marital Ther 1984; 10:215–227.
118. Schover LR. Male and female therapists' responses to male and female client sexual material: an analogue study. Arch Sex Behav 1981; 10:477–491.
119. Frank E, Anderson C, Rubinstein D. Frequency of sexual dysfunction in "normal couples." N Engl J Med 1978; 299:111–115.
120. Pfeiffer E, Davis GC. Determinants of sexual behavior in middle and old age. J Am Geriatr Soc 1972; 20:151–158.
121. Bretschneider JG, McCoy NL. Sexual interest and behavior in healthy 80 to 102 year olds. Arch Sex Behav 1988; 17:109–129.
122. Roughan PA, Kaiser FE, Morley JE. Sexuality and the older woman. Clin Geriatr Med 1993; 9:87–106.
123. Dennerstein L, Burrows GD, Wood C, et al. Hormones and sexuality: effect of estrogen and progestogen. Obstet Gynecol 1980; 56:316–322.
124. Herbert J. The neuroendocrine basis of sexual behavior in primates. In: Money J, Musaph H, eds. Handbook of Sexology. Amsterdam: Elsevier/North-Holland, 1978: 449–457.
125. Raboch J, Kobilková J, Raboch J, et al. Sexual life of women with the Stein-Leventhal syndrome. Arch Sex Behav 1985; 14:263–270.
126. Mathews A, Whitehead A, Kellett J. Psychological and hormonal factors in the treatment of female sexual dysfunction. Psychol Med 1983; 13:83–92.
127. Dow MGT, Hart DM, Forrest CA. Hormonal treatments of sexual unresponsiveness in postmenopausal women: a comparative study. Br J Obstet Gynaecol 1983; 90:361–366.
128. Schover LR, Evans RB, von Eschenbach AC. Sexual rehabilitation in a cancer center: diagnosis and outcome in 384 cases. Arch Sex Behav 1987; 16:445–461.

129. Osborn M, Hawton K, Gath D. Sexual dysfunction among middle-aged women in the community. Br Med J 1988; 296:959–962.

130. Sarrell P, Whitehead MI. Sex and menopause: defining the issues. Maturitas 1985; 7:217–224.

131. Bachmann GA, Moeller TP, Benett J. Childhood sexual abuse and the consequences in adult women. Obstet Gynecol 1988; 71:631–642.

132. Becker JV, Skinner LJ, Abel GG, et al. Sexual problems of sexual assault survivors. Women Health 1984; 9:5–20.

133. Walker E, Katon W, Harrop-Griffiths J, et al. Relationship of chronic pelvic pain to psychiatric diagnoses and childhood sexual abuse. Am J Psychiatry 1988; 145:75–80.

134. Bancroft J. Hormones and human sexual behavior. J Sex Marital Ther 1984; 10:3–21.

135. Sanders D, Bancroft J. Hormones and the sexuality of women—the menstrual cycle. Clin Endocrinol Metab 1982; 11:639–657.

136. Kaplan HS, Owett T. The Female Androgen Deficiency Syndrome. J Sex Marital Ther 1993; 19:3–24.

137. Hulter B, Lundberg PO. Sexual function in women with hypothalamic-pituitary disorders. Arch Sex Behav 1994; 23:171–182.

138. Klein MC, Gautier RJ, Robbins JM, et al. Relationship of episiotomy to perineal trauma and morbidity, sexual dysfunction and pelvic floor relaxation. Am J Obstet Gynecol 1994; 171:591–598.

139. Neale K, Phillips R. Living with a stoma. Br Med J 1988; 297:310–311.

140. Freese MP, Levitt EE. Relationships among intravaginal pressure, orgasmic function, parity factors and urinary leakage. Arch Sex Behav 1984; 13:261–268.

141. Anderson BL, Lachenbruch PA, Anderson B, et al. Sexual dysfunction and signs of gynecologic cancer. Cancer 1986; 57:1880–1886.

142. Thranov I, Klee M. Sexuality among gynecologic cancer patients. Gynecol Oncol 1994; 52:14–19.

143. Minderhoud JM, Leemhuis JG, Kremer J, et al. Sexual disturbances arising from multiple sclerosis. Acta Neurol Scand 1984; 70:299–306.

144. Bhaduria S, Moser D, Clements PJ, et al. Genital tract abnormalities and female sexual function impairment in systemic sclerosis. Am J Obstet Gynecol 1995; 172:580–587.

145. Schaefer RM, Kokot F, Wernze H, et al. Improved sexual function in hemodialysis patients on recombinant erythropoietin: a possible role for prolactin. Clin Nephrol 1989; 31:1–5.

146. Papadopoulos C, Beaumont C, Shelley SI, et al. Myocardial infarction and sexual activity of the female patient. Arch Intern Med 1983; 143:1528–1530.

147. Guthrie E, Creed FH. Severe sexual dysfunction in women with the irritable bowel syndrome: comparison with inflammatory bowel disease and duodenal ulceration. Br Med J 1987; 295:577–578.

148. Schreiner-Engel P, Schiavi RC, Vietorisz D, et al. The differential impact of diabetes type on female sexuality. J Psychosom Res 1987; 31:23–33.

149. Newman AS, Bertelson AD. Sexual dysfunction in the diabetic woman. J Behav Med 1986; 9:261–270.

150. Blake DJ, Maisaik R, Koplan A, et al. Sexual dysfunction among subjects with arthritis. Clin Rheumatol 1988; 7:50–60.

151. Coppen A, Bishop M, Beard RJ, et al. Hysterectomy, hormones, and behaviour: a prospective study. Lancet 1981; 1:126–128.

152. Duncan L, Bateman DN. Sexual function in women: do antihypertensive drugs have an impact? Drug Safety 1993; 8:225–234.

153. Peterson JS, Hartsock N, Lawson G. Sexual dissatisfaction of female alcoholics. Psychol Rep 1984; 55:744–746.

154. Malatesta VJ, Pollack RH, Crotty TD, et al. Acute alcohol intoxication and female orgasmic response. J Sex Res 1982; 18:1–17.

155. Rogers GS, Van de Castle RL, Evans WS, et al. Vaginal pulse amplitude response patterns during erotic conditions and sleep. Arch Sex Behav 1985; 14:327–342.

156. LoPiccolo J, Stock WE. Treatment of sexual dysfunction. J Consult Clin Psychol 1986; 54:158–167.

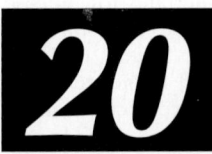

20

GLUCOSE HOMEOSTASIS AND HYPOGLYCEMIA

Philip E. Cryer and Kenneth S. Polonsky

INTRODUCTION

Maintenance of the plasma glucose concentration is critical to survival because plasma glucose is the predominant fuel used by the central nervous system under most conditions. The central nervous system cannot synthesize glucose or store more than a few minutes' supply as glycogen. Thus brief hypoglycemia can cause profound brain dysfunction, and prolonged severe hypoglycemia causes brain death.

The plasma glucose concentration is normally maintained within a relatively narrow range, roughly 3.9 to 8.3 mmol/L (70 to 150 mg/dL), despite wide variations in glucose influx and efflux such as those that occur after meals and during exercise. Glucoregulatory failure due to insulin deficiency and resulting in hyperglycemia (diabetes mellitus) is common (see Chapter 21). In contrast, hypoglycemia is uncommon, except when produced as a side effect of diabetes treatment. Because severe hypoglycemia is incompatible with life, glucoregulatory mechanisms have evolved to protect against low glucose levels. These mechanisms include feedback inhibition of insulin secretion and activation of glucose counterregulatory systems (including stimulation of glucagon and epinephrine secretion) as the plasma glucose concentration falls.

Elucidation of the physiology of glucoregulation and of glucose counterregulation has provided major insights into the pathophysiology of hypoglycemia in humans. Nevertheless there are major gaps in our understanding of the causes, mechanisms, and management of many hypoglycemic states. Hypoglycemia, particularly hypoglycemia in diabetes, has been reviewed in detail.[1-5]

PHYSIOLOGY OF SYSTEMIC GLUCOREGULATION

Cellular and molecular glucoregulation is discussed in Chapter 21. Glucose metabolism and systemic glucose balance and their regulation are summarized here, with emphasis on the aspects relevant to glucose counterregulation. The physiology of human glucose counterregulation is then discussed in greater detail.

Glucose Metabolism

Origin and Fate of Glucose

Glucose is derived from three sources: intestinal *absorption* that follows digestion of dietary carbohydrates; *glycogenolysis,* the breakdown of glycogen, which is the polymerized storage form of glucose; and *gluconeogenesis,* the formation of glucose from precursors, including lactate (and pyruvate), amino acids (especially alanine and glutamine) and, to a lesser extent, glycerol (Fig. 20–1).

Although most tissues express the enzyme systems required to synthesize (glycogen synthase) and hydrolyze (phosphorylase) glycogen, only the liver and kidneys express glucose-6-phosphatase, the enzyme necessary for the release of glucose into the circulation. The liver and kidneys also contain the enzymes necessary for gluconeogenesis (including the crit-ical gluconeogenic enzymes pyruvate carboxylase, phosphoenolpyruvate carboxykinase, and fructose-1,6-bisphosphatase).

There are multiple potential metabolic fates for glucose that is transported into cells (external losses are normally negligible). It may be stored as glycogen. It may undergo glycolysis to pyruvate, which can be reduced to lactate, transaminated to form alanine, or converted to acetyl coenzyme A (CoA), which in turn can be oxidized to carbon dioxide and water via the tricarboxylic acid cycle, converted to fatty acids (and stored as triglycerides), or utilized for ketone body (acetoacetate, β-hydroxybutyrate) or cholesterol synthesis. Finally glucose may be released into the circulation. As summarized in the following paragraphs, these outcomes differ in different organs.

Hepatic Glucose Metabolism

The liver is remarkably flexible in its role in glucose homeostasis and is the major source of net endogenous glucose production. Under conditions of high glucose output (e.g., fasting) the energy needs of the liver are largely provided by the beta oxidation of fatty acids. Conversely the liver can also be an organ of net glucose uptake, with glucose stored as glycogen, oxidized for energy, or converted to fat, which can either remain in the liver or be transported to other tissues as very-low-density lipoproteins.

Glucose Utilization

Muscle can store glucose as glycogen or metabolize glucose through glycolysis to pyruvate, which either is reduced to lactate or transaminated to form alanine or is oxidized. Lactate (and pyruvate) released from muscle is transported to the liver where it serves as a gluconeogenic precursor (the Cori or glucose-lactate cycle). However, to the extent that lactate and pyruvate carbons are derived from glucose, they cannot result in net new glucose formation. Alanine, glutamine, and other amino acids may also flow from muscle to liver where

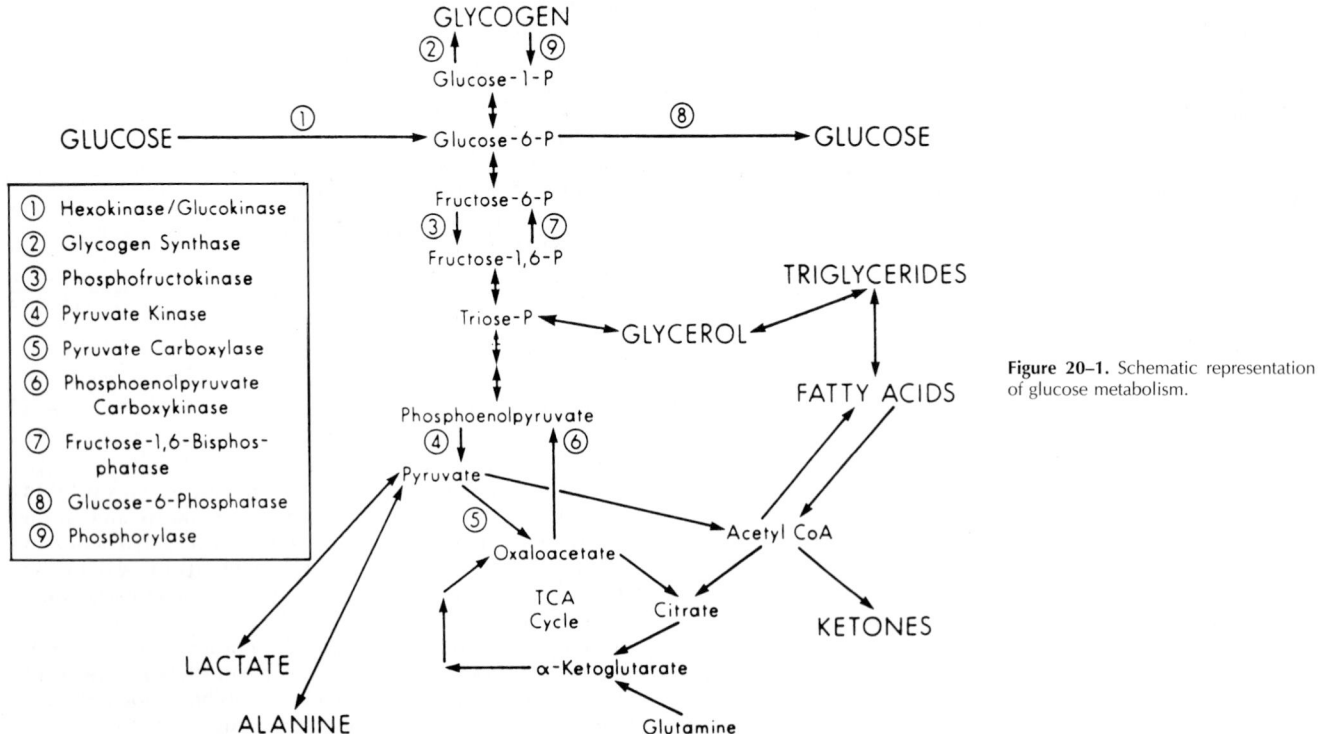

Figure 20–1. Schematic representation of glucose metabolism.

they too serve as gluconeogenic precursors. Circulating alanine is also largely derived from glucose (glucose-alanine cycle). Glutamine is a major precursor for new glucose formation, although it too is partially derived from glucose (glucose-glutamine cycle).[6] During a fast, muscle can reduce its glucose uptake virtually to zero, oxidize fatty acids for its energy needs, and, through proteolysis, mobilize amino acids for transport to the liver to serve as gluconeogenic precursors for net glucose formation.

Although quantitatively less important than muscle, adipose tissue can also use glucose for fatty acid synthesis or formation of glycerol-3-phosphate, which can then esterify fatty acids (derived largely from circulating very-low-density lipoproteins) to form triglycerides. During a fast, adipocytes decrease their glucose utilization and satisfy energy needs from the beta oxidation of fatty acids. Other tissues, such as the formed elements of the blood and the renal medullae, do not have the capacity to decrease glucose utilization during fasting and therefore produce lactate at relatively fixed rates.

As mentioned earlier, glucose is the predominant metabolic fuel used by the brain under most conditions. Glucose undergoes terminal oxidation to carbon dioxide and water in the brain. When ketones are plentiful in the circulation, as during prolonged fasting, they can support the majority of the energy needs of the brain and thus reduce its glucose utilization.

Systemic Glucose Balance

Maintenance of the normal plasma glucose concentration requires precise matching of glucose utilization and endogenous glucose production or dietary glucose delivery.

Fasting

The postabsorptive state is the interdigestive period that begins approximately 5 to 6 h after a meal. However, the term is most commonly used in reference to data obtained after a 10- to 14-h overnight fast. In the postabsorptive state plasma glucose concentrations are stable; thus glucose production and utilization rates are equal. They average 12 μmol/kg/min (2.2 mg/kg/min) and range from about 10 to 14 μmol/kg/min (1.8 to 2.6 mg/kg/min) in normal adults after an overnight fast.[7] Approximately 60% of basal glucose utilization is accounted for by the brain. The remainder is used by glycolyzing tissues, such as the formed elements of the blood and the renal medullae and to some extent muscle and fat. Hepatic glucose production results from both glycogenolysis and gluconeogenesis even after an overnight fast. Glycogenolysis may be the predominant source after a typical overnight fast, but gluconeogenesis becomes the predominant source within the first 24 h of fasting.[8]

The liver is the predominant source of net endogenous glucose production after an overnight fast. The kidneys, which both use and produce glucose, contribute only about 5%.[9] However, renal and hepatic glucose production is regulated. For example, renal glucose release (largely if not entirely via gluconeogenesis rather than glycogenolysis) accounts for about 40% of the initial increase in epinephrine-stimulated glucose production and virtually all of the increase after 2.5 to 3 h.[9] Thus the common practice of equating endogenous glucose production with hepatic glucose production is not appropriate under some conditions.

The importance of gluconeogenesis in providing new glucose and supporting hepatic glycogen stores after an overnight fast becomes apparent when one considers the limited availability of preformed glucose. The glucose pool, namely free glucose in the extracellular fluid and in the cells of certain tissues (primarily in the liver but also small amounts in the

kidneys, intestinal mucosa, pancreatic islet cells, brain, and blood cells), is about 83 to 111 mmol (15 to 20 g) in the normal adult. Glycogen that can be mobilized to provide circulating glucose (e.g., hepatic glycogen) contains approximately 390 mmol glucose (70 g), with a range of about 135 to 722 mmol (25 to 130 g). Thus in an adult of average size preformed glucose can provide as little as a 3-h supply of glucose and less than an 8-h supply on average, even at the diminished rate of glucose utilization that occurs during the postabsorptive state. Clearly, therefore, gluconeogenesis is important for maintenance of the plasma glucose concentration even during an overnight fast.

If fasting is prolonged to 24 to 48 h the plasma glucose level declines and then stabilizes, hepatic glycogen content falls to less than 55 mmol (10 g), and gluconeogenesis becomes the sole source of glucose production.[8] Because amino acids are the main gluconeogenic precursors that result in net glucose formation, muscle protein is degraded. Glucose utilization by muscle and fat virtually ceases. As lipolysis and ketogenesis accelerate and circulating ketone levels rise, ketones become a major source of fuel for the brain. Thus glucose utilization by the brain declines by about half, resulting in a decrease in the rate of gluconeogenesis required to maintain the plasma glucose concentration and hence in diminished protein wasting. After prolonged fasting (40 d) ketones provide an estimated 80 to 90% of the energy used by the brain, and renal gluconeogenesis provides up to half of the endogenous glucose production.[10]

Feeding

After a meal, glucose absorption into the circulation is more than twice the rate of postabsorptive endogenous glucose production, depending on the carbohydrate content of the meal and the rate of its digestion and absorption. As glucose is absorbed endogenous glucose production is suppressed and glucose utilization by liver, muscle, and fat accelerates.[11] Thus exogenous glucose is assimilated and the plasma glucose concentration returns to the postabsorptive level.

Exercise

Exercise increases glucose utilization (by muscle) to rates that can be severalfold greater than those of the postabsorptive state. Endogenous glucose production normally accelerates to match the utilization so that the plasma glucose concentration is maintained.

From these examples it is clear that the plasma glucose concentration is normally maintained within a narrow range despite wide variations in glucose flux, a homeostatic feat accomplished by hormonal, neural, and substrate glucoregulatory factors.[1–5, 12, 13] From a mechanistic perspective hypoglycemia could result from decreased glucose production or increased glucose utilization, or both.

Glucoregulatory Factors
Hormonal Glucoregulatory Factors

Hormones are the most important glucoregulatory factors, and the regulation of their secretion is complex. Glucose, specifically the plasma glucose concentration, is the most important determinant of the secretion of glucoregulatory hormones, including insulin, glucagon, epinephrine, growth hormone, and cortisol.

INSULIN. This hormone, which is the dominant glucose-lowering hormone,[1–5, 12, 13] suppresses endogenous glucose production and stimulates glucose utilization, thereby lowering the plasma glucose concentration. Insulin is secreted from the beta cells of the pancreatic islets into the hepatic portal circulation and acts on the liver and peripheral tissues. It inhibits hepatic glycogenolysis and gluconeogenesis and, in concert with other factors (including hyperglycemia and hypoglucagonemia), converts the liver into an organ of net glucose uptake and fuel storage (glycogen and triglycerides). It also stimulates glucose uptake, storage, and utilization by other tissues such as muscle and fat. In the postabsorptive state insulin regulates the plasma glucose concentration primarily by restraining hepatic glucose production.[14] Higher levels, such as those that occur after meals, are required to stimulate glucose utilization.[14]

Conversely, decreased insulin secretion causes increased glucose production and decreased glucose utilization by insulin-sensitive tissues and thus tends to raise the plasma glucose concentration. Insulin is therefore both a glucose lowering (regulatory) and a glucose raising (counterregulatory) hormone. The rate of insulin secretion is regulated by a number of factors, the most important of which is glucose. A fall in the plasma glucose concentration has an immediate inhibitory effect on insulin secretion, thereby limiting a further fall in the plasma glucose level. Insulin is a potent and critical hormone. Either profound insulin deficiency or marked insulin excess can be lethal, but it is not the only glucoregulatory hormone.

COUNTERREGULATORY HORMONES. Glucose-raising or counterregulatory hormones include glucagon, epinephrine, growth hormone, and cortisol. In response to falling plasma glucose levels glucagon is secreted from the alpha cells of the pancreatic islets into the hepatic portal circulation and is believed to act exclusively on the liver under physiological conditions.[15] It activates glycogenolysis and gluconeogenesis and increases hepatic glucose production within minutes. This increase is transient. Despite ongoing hyperglucagonemia, glucose production returns toward basal rates over about 90 min, although the hormone continues to support glucose production (i.e., withdrawal of glucagon causes a further decrease in glucose production thereafter).[16] Glucagon-induced hyperglycemia is also transient because the glucagon-induced increase in glycogenolysis does not persist; during sustained hyperglucagonemia gluconeogenesis increases progressively, over at least 4 h in dogs.[17] The transient nature of the glycogenolytic response to sustained hyperglucagonemia is not the result of glycogen depletion, as a further increase in glucagon causes a further increase in glucose release, but is instead the result of glucose-induced insulin secretion and the autoregulatory effect of hyperglycemia (see later), although other factors may be involved.

The hyperglycemic effect of the adrenal hormone epinephrine (Fig. 20–2) is more complex.[18] The hormone is secreted in response to falling plasma glucose levels and both stimulates hepatic glucose production and limits glucose utilization. The actions of epinephrine are both direct and indirect and are mediated through both α- and β-adrenergic receptors.[18–20] α-Adrenergic limitation of insulin secretion, an important indirect hyperglycemic action of epinephrine, allows the hyperglycemic response to occur, although the increase in insulin secretion as plasma glucose rises limits the magnitude of the glycemic response.[18, 20] β-Adrenergic stimulation of glucagon secretion also occurs,[21, 22] but its contribution to the hyperglycemic effect of epinephrine appears to be minor under physiological conditions.[18, 20] Epinephrine also acts directly (i.e., independent of changes in other hormones) to increase hepatic glycogenolysis and gluconeogenesis. In humans the hepatic effect is mediated predominantly through β2-adrenergic mechanisms,[18, 19, 23] although a small direct α-adrenergic stimulation of hepatic glucose production has been reported.[24] Epinephrine also mobilizes gluconeogenic precursors (e.g., lactate, alanine, and glycerol) and, like glucagon,

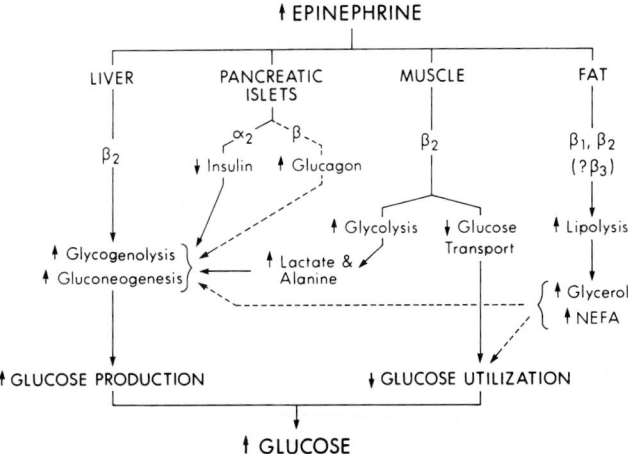

Figure 20–2. Schematic representation of the mechanisms of the hyperglycemic effect of epinephrine. (From Cryer PE. Catecholamines, pheochromocytoma and diabetes. Diabetes Rev 1993; 1:309-317. © Copyright 1993, American Diabetes Association, Alexandria, Virginia.)

acts within minutes to produce a transient increase in glucose production and basal rates of glucose production thereafter. In contrast to glucagon, however, epinephrine also limits glucose utilization by insulin-sensitive tissues such as skeletal muscle, predominantly through direct β2-adrenergic mechanisms.[18–20] Because of the persistent effect on glucose utilization, sustained hyperepinephrinemia results in persistent hyperglycemia.

Long-term elevations of growth hormone and of cortisol limit glucose utilization and stimulate glucose production. Initially, however, growth hormone has a plasma glucose–lowering (insulin-like) effect; its hyperglycemic effect does not appear for several hours.[25] Similarly cortisol causes an increase in the plasma glucose level after 2 to 3 h.[26] The hyperglycemic effect of the combination of glucagon, epinephrine, and cortisol is greater than the sum effect of each hormone individually.[26] These synergistic interactions are potentially relevant to glucose counterregulation.

Neural Glucoregulatory Factors

The sympathetic neurotransmitter norepinephrine exerts hyperglycemic actions by mechanisms assumed to be similar to those of epinephrine, except that norepinephrine is released primarily from terminals of sympathetic postganglionic neurons. These terminals are adjacent to adrenergic receptors on target cells within the innervated tissues. Electrical stimulation of hepatic sympathetic nerves decreases glycogen content, increases glucose release, and causes hyperglycemia in animals[27] and in humans.[28] Parasympathetic stimulation increases hepatic glycogen content and decreases hepatic glucose release.[27, 29] It is reasonable to anticipate that peptide neurotransmitters and neuromodulators also affect glucose metabolism.

Substrate Glucoregulatory Factors

Glucose per se shifts hepatic metabolism in favor of glycogen storage.[30] Hepatic glucose autoregulation (namely the fact that the rate of hepatic glucose production is an inverse function of the plasma glucose concentration independent of hormonal and neural regulatory factors) is an important glucose counterregulatory factor in dogs[31, 32] and in humans.[33–35] Fatty acids support glucose production and limit glucose oxidation.

Control of Glucoregulatory Factors

Hypoglycemia suppresses the secretion of insulin and stimulates the secretion of glucagon, epinephrine, cortisol, and growth hormone, among other hormones.[7, 12, 13] It also stimulates the release of norepinephrine and acetylcholine from sympathetic and parasympathetic postganglionic neurons, respectively. The insulin and glucagon secretory responses to hypoglycemia appear to be independent of the central nervous system in humans. Reciprocal changes occur in insulin and glucagon release from pancreatic islet cells in vitro and from the perfused pancreas in response to changes in medium glucose concentrations, and neither sympathetic nor parasympathetic neural connections are required for the glucagon secretory response to hypoglycemia in vivo.[36–39] In contrast, the response of the adrenal medulla is mediated through the central nervous system. Although sympathetic reflexes at the spinal cord level can be elicited by various stimuli in persons with cervical spinal cord transections,[40] sympathochromaffin responses to hypoglycemia[36] or to cellular glucopenia produced by 2-deoxyglucose[41] do not occur in these individuals. Thus brain centers are required to mediate the sympathochromaffin response to signals initiated by sensors in the brain or in the peripheral organs such as the liver, or both. Parenthetically the response of plasma norepinephrine, as well as epinephrine, to hypoglycemia is derived largely from the adrenal medullae.[42, 43] The secretory responses of growth hormone and cortisol (via corticotropin, also called adrenocorticotropic hormone [ACTH, or adrenocorticotropin]) to hypoglycemia are also mediated through the brain.

Glucose Counterregulation

The simplest model of glucoregulation would be regulation of the plasma glucose concentration by insulin alone: as the plasma glucose level increases, insulin secretion increases, causing the glucose level to decrease. As the plasma glucose level decreases, insulin secretion decreases, causing the glucose level to increase. With respect to defense against increasing glucose levels this model is sufficient. The absence of an increase in insulin results in hyperglycemia. With respect to decreasing glucose levels, however, the model is too simple. The prevention and correction of hypoglycemia involves a more complex model: suppression of insulin secretion and activation of a hierarchic array of redundant glucose counterregulatory systems.[6, 7, 12, 24, 44–54] The physiology of the prevention and correction of hypoglycemia in humans has been reviewed.[2, 13] For this discussion glucose counterregulation is divided into two categories: the correction of hypoglycemia and the prevention of hypoglycemia. This distinction is admittedly arbitrary because the principles are the same.

Correction of Hypoglycemia

The temporal relationships between the kinetics of glucose counterregulation and the activation of glucose counterregulatory systems during insulin-induced hypoglycemia were defined in humans by Garber and colleagues[7] (Fig. 20–3). The rapid intravenous injection of insulin causes prompt suppression of hepatic glucose production and stimulation of glucose utilization, which causes a fall in plasma glucose level. Subsequently glucose utilization declines to baseline, and glucose production rises above baseline to cause plasma glucose levels to rise. The burst of glucose production that restores euglycemia after short-term hypoglycemia is largely the result of glycogenolysis, although gluconeogenesis is accelerated as well[7, 44] (see Fig. 20–3). The onset of the glucose counterregulatory process is marked by a decline in (insulin-stimulated) glucose utilization and an increase in (insulin-suppressed)

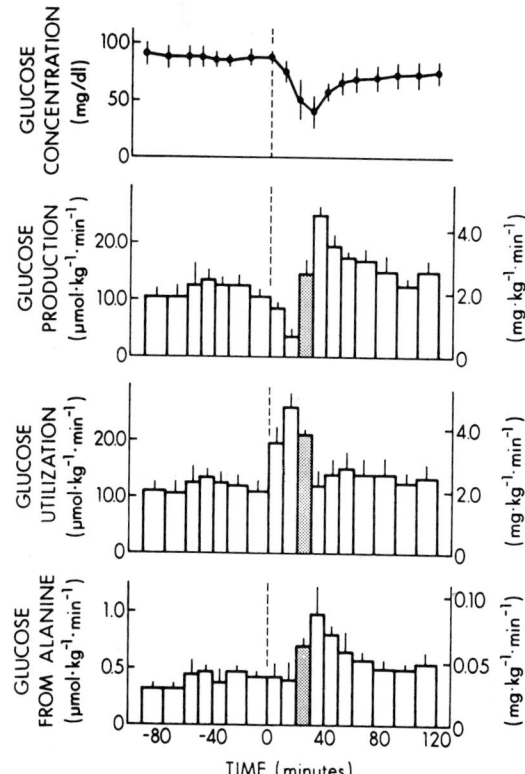

Figure 20–3. Mean ($\pm$SE), plasma glucose concentrations, glucose production and utilizaton rates, and estimated rates of glucose formation from alanine (via gluconeogenesis) before and after rapid intravenous injection of insulin (0.05 U/kg) *(vertical dashed line)* in normal humans. Shaded columns mark the time frame of the onset of the glucose counterregulatory process. Data from Clarke WL, Santiago JV, Thomas L, et al.[44] (From Cryer PE. The sympathoadrenal system in human glucose counterregulation and diabetes mellitus. In: Ziegler MG, Lake CR, eds. Norepinephrine. Baltimore: Williams & Wilkins, 1984: 471. Copyright 1984, Alan R. Liss, New York.)

glucose production from its nadir (see shaded columns in Fig. 20–3). Clearly any model of glucose counterregulation must include a component that acts within this time frame, generally less than 30 min after intravenous insulin injection.[7, 44] Plasma insulin concentrations continue to be increased at least 10-fold over baseline levels at the onset of the glucose counterregulatory process (Fig. 20–4).[7, 44] Thus dissipation of insulin cannot be the sole explanation for recovery from hypoglycemia. An additional counterregulatory factor or factors overcomes the effects of elevated insulin levels and must be involved in the correction of hypoglycemia.

Insulin-induced hypoglycemia causes increases in plasma glucagon and epinephrine and norepinephrine levels at the onset of the glucose counterregulatory process (Fig. 20–5).[7, 44] Increases in plasma growth hormone and cortisol levels occur somewhat later in the counterregulatory process (Fig. 20–6).[7, 44] However, growth hormone and cortisol are not likely to be rapid glucose counterregulatory factors because of the delayed onset of their hyperglycemic actions, as discussed earlier.

The effects of selective deficiencies of the secretion or action of the potentially important glucose counterregulatory factors, alone and in combination, on glucose recovery from short-term hypoglycemia[42, 44, 45] are summarized in Figure 20–7. Glucose recovery is impaired (by approximately 40%) during somatostatin-induced suppression of glucagon and growth hormone secretion. The impaired glucose recovery is due to suppression of glucagon rather than growth hormone, as evidenced by the fact that the defect is corrected by replace-

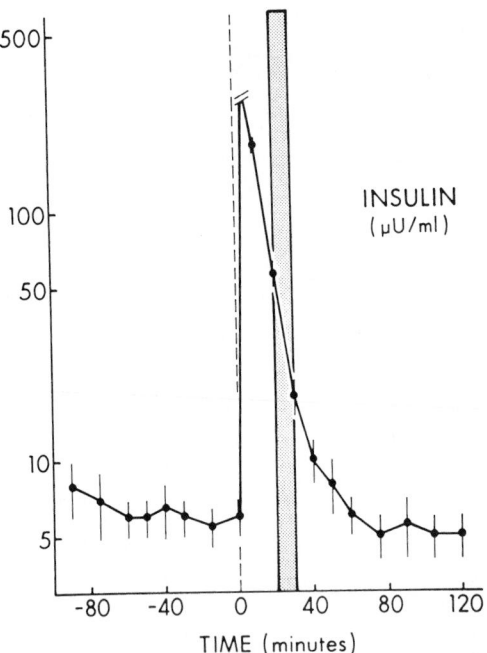

Figure 20–4. Mean (±SE) plasma insulin concentrations in the study shown in Figure 20–3. Regular insulin (0.05 U/kg) was injected intravenously *(vertical dashed line)* into normal humans. The shaded column marks the time frame of the onset of the glucose counterregulatory process (see Fig. 20–3). Data from Clarke WL, Santiago JV, Thomas L, et al.[44] To convert insulin values to pmol/L multiply by 6.0. (From Cryer PE. The sympathoadrenal system in human glucose counterregulation and diabetes mellitus. In: Ziegler MG, Lake CR, eds. Norepinephrine. Baltimore: Williams & Wilkins, 1984: 471. Copyright 1984, Alan R. Liss, New York.)

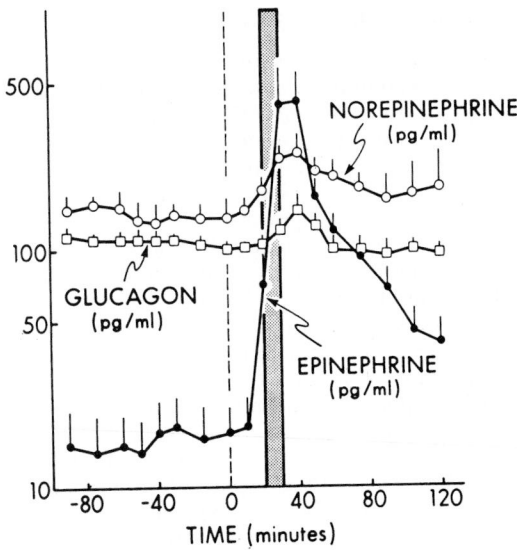

Figure 20–5. Mean (±SE) plasma glucagon, epinephrine and norepinephrine concentrations in the study shown in Figure 20–3. Regular insulin (0.05 U/kg) was injected intravenously *(vertical dashed line)* into normal humans. The shaded column marks the time frame of the onset of the glucose counterregulatory process (see Fig. 20–3). Data from Clarke WL, Santiago JV, Thomas L, et al.[44] To covert to SI units: epinephrine (pmol/L), multiply by 5.458; glucagon (pmol/L), multiply by 0.287; norepinephrine (nmol/L), multiply by 0.005911. (From Cryer PE. The sympathoadrenal system in human glucose counterregulation and diabetes mellitus. In: Ziegler MG, Lake CR, eds. Norepinephrine. Baltimore: Williams & Wilkins, 1984: 471. Copyright 1984, Alan R. Liss, New York.)

ment of the former during somatostatin infusion. Thus glucagon plays an important role in glucose counterregulation. However, substantial glucose recovery (approximately 60% of normal) occurs in the absence of glucagon secretion (see Fig. 20–7). Thus an additional factor must be involved, at least when glucagon secretion is deficient. Epinephrine is the likely candidate because of its rapid and substantial secretion in response to hypoglycemia, its rapid hyperglycemic actions, and its enhanced secretion during the impaired glucose recovery produced by deficient glucagon secretion.[42]

Recovery from short-term insulin-induced hypoglycemia is affected little by pharmacologic adrenergic blockade[44, 46] or epinephrine deficiency (bilateral adrenalectomy).[42] However, the combination of adrenergic blockade and inhibition of glucagon secretion markedly impairs recovery from hypoglycemia (see Fig. 20–7). Furthermore, with combined deficiencies of glucagon and epinephrine (the bilaterally adrenalectomized human given somatostatin) glucose recovery fails to occur (see Fig. 20–7). This total disruption of hypoglycemic glucose counterregulation occurs despite dissipation of insulin.

The foregoing data indicate that in concert with decreasing insulin levels, glucagon plays a primary role in promoting glucose recovery from hypoglycemia; epinephrine is not normally critical but compensates partially when glucagon secretion is deficient; and recovery from insulin-induced hypoglycemia fails to occur only in the absence of both glucagon and epinephrine. Secretion of growth hormone and cortisol is not critical to recovery from short-term hypoglycemia.[42, 44, 45]

Impairment of glucagon secretory responses to hypoglycemia is common in patients with insulin-dependent diabetes mellitus (IDDM).[55] Such patients are dependent on epinephrine to promote recovery from hypoglycemia,[46] providing further support for the role of glucagon in normal glucose coun-

terregulation. The fact that patients with deficiencies of both glucagon and epinephrine are at risk for severe hypoglycemia during intensive insulin therapy[47] provides further support for the critical roles of these two hormones. These pathophysiological findings provide independent confirmation of the physiological construct. The power of the counterregulatory systems is attested to by the fact that partial glucose counter-

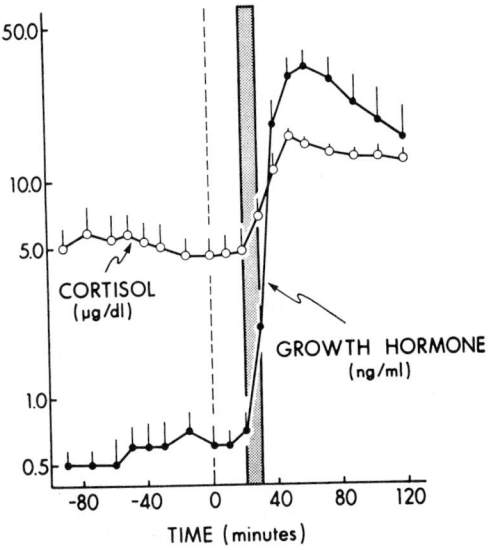

Figure 20–6. Mean (±SE) plasma cortisol and growth hormone concentrations in the study shown in Figure 20–3. Regular insulin (0.05 U/kg) was injected intravenously *(vertical dashed line)* into normal humans. The shaded column marks the time frame of the onset of the glucose counterregulatory process (see Fig. 20–3). Data from Clarke WL, Santiago JV, Thomas L, et al.[44] (From Cryer PE. The sympathoadrenal system in human glucose counterregulation and diabetes mellitus. In: Ziegler MG, Lake CR, eds. Norepinephrine. Baltimore: Williams & Wilkins, 1984: 471. Copyright 1984, Alan R. Liss, New York.)

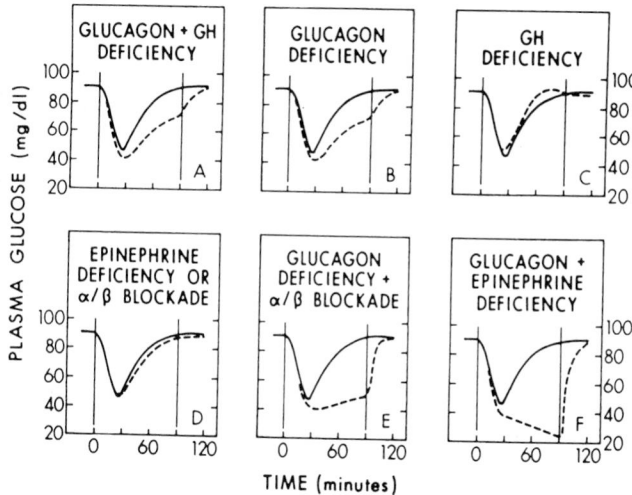

Figure 20–7. Summary of studies of the mechanisms of the correction of hypoglycemia. Plasma glucose curves during insulin-induced hypoglycemia in normal humans during control studies *(solid curves, same in all panels)* and as modified *(dashed curves)* by somatostatin infusion (glucagon + growth hormone [GH] deficiency) *(A);* somatostatin + growth hormone replacement (glucagon deficiency) *(B);* somatostatin + glucagon replacement (GH deficiency) *(C);* phentolamine and propranolol infusion (combined alpha- and beta-adrenergic blockade) or studies performed in bilaterally adrenalectomized individuals (epinephrine deficiency) *(D);* somatostatin + phentolamine and propranolol (glucagon deficiency + alpha- and beta-adrenergic blockade) *(E);* F. somatostatin infusion in bilaterally adrenalectomized individuals (glucagon + epinephrine deficiency) *(F).* Insulin was injected intravenously at time 0 min. Interventions were started at time 0 min and stopped at time 90 min. (i.e., between the vertical lines in each panel). Curves derived from data in Gerich J, Davis J, Lorenzi M, et al.[42]; Clarke WL, Santiago JV, Thomas L, et al.[44]; and Rizza RA, Cryer PE, Gerich JE.[45](From Cryer PE. Glucose counterregulation in man. Diabetes 1981; 30:261–264. Copyright 1981, American Diabetes Association, Alexandria, Virginia.)

regulation, sufficient to prevent symptomatic central nervous system glucose deprivation, occurs in nondiabetic subjects subjected to sustained fivefold elevations of the plasma insulin level.[47]

Growth hormone and cortisol also play roles in the defense against prolonged hypoglycemia.[57, 59] However, growth hormone and cortisol are not critical to recovery from prolonged hypoglycemia (or to prevention of hypoglycemia after an overnight fast), at least in adults.[59] Furthermore, glucose autoregulation is operative in humans, albeit only during severe hypoglycemia.[60, 61] Nonetheless the fact that glucose counterregulation is disrupted, resulting in progressive hypoglycemia, when glucagon and epinephrine are deficient and insulin is present despite normal growth hormone and cortisol secretion and intact autoregulatory mechanisms indicates that the latter factors stand low in the hierarchy of redundant glucose counterregulatory factors.

Insulin is the dominant glucose regulatory factor and a decrease in insulin is an important glucose counterregulatory factor. Glucose recovery from hypoglycemia does not occur when hyperinsulinemia sufficient to induce hypoglycemia is sustained despite substantial increments in the levels of the glucose counterregulatory hormones.[12] Nonetheless biologic glucose recovery from hypoglycemia, sufficient to disengage the counterregulatory systems, can occur despite maintenance of approximately twofold peripheral hyperinsulinemia.[12] Clearly, therefore, glucose recovery from hypoglycemia is not solely due to dissipation of insulin. The data just summarized indicate that glucagon plays a primary counterregulatory role and that epinephrine becomes critical to the correction of hypoglycemia when glucagon is deficient.

Prevention of Hypoglycemia

If the counterregulatory hormones are involved in the prevention and correction of hypoglycemia, they must be re-

leased as the plasma glucose concentration falls at glucose levels higher than those that produce symptoms and impair brain function. That prerequisite has been met[62, 64] as illustrated in Figure 20–8. Insulin secretion decreases as the plasma glucose level falls within the physiological range, and secretion of both glucagon and epinephrine increases as the plasma glucose level falls to just below the physiological range at higher glucose concentrations than those that produce symptoms of hypoglycemia and impair cognitive function.

The findings that the glycemic thresholds for decreased insulin secretion lie within the physiological range and those for increased glucagon and epinephrine secretion lie just below that range[60–62] are consistent with, but do not prove, the hypothesis that these hormones are critically involved in the prevention as well as the correction of hypoglycemia. However, that hypothesis has been supported by studies conducted in the overnight[49] and 3-d[50] fasted state, in the postprandial state,[51, 52] and during physical exercise[53, 54] (Fig. 20–9). Under all these conditions, when glucagon secretion was suppressed and insulin levels were held constant, plasma glucose concentrations were reduced, but the levels plateaued and hypoglycemia did not develop[49, 50, 52, 54]; glucose concentrations were affected little[54] or not at all[49, 50, 52] when epinephrine was deficient or its actions blocked; and hypoglycemia developed when glucagon was suppressed and epinephrine was deficient or its actions were blocked.[49, 50, 52, 55] Thus, as in the correction of hypoglycemia, glucagon plays a primary role in the prevention of hypoglycemia, and epinephrine becomes critical when glucagon is deficient.

Principles of Glucose Counterregulation

Glucose counterregulation[13] involves two distinct principles: (1) the prevention or correction of hypoglycemia requires both dissipation of insulin and activation of glucose counterregulatory systems and (2) although insulin is the dominant plasma glucose–lowering (regulatory) factor, the (counterregulatory) factors are redundant and hierarchic. In other words the multiple counterregulatory factors constitute a fail-safe system that prevents failure of counterregulation when one or more of the components fails, and some of those factors are more important than others.

Decreased insulin secretion is the first defense against falling plasma glucose levels (Fig. 20–10), and glucagon is the primary counterregulatory hormone. Epinephrine is not normally critical but becomes essential when glucagon is deficient. Hypoglycemia develops or progresses when both glucagon and epinephrine are deficient and insulin is present despite the actions of other hormones, neurotransmitters, and substrates. Thus insulin, glucagon, and epinephrine stand high in the hierarchy of redundant glucoregulatory factors. Growth hormone,[57] cortisol,[58] glucagon,[65] and epinephrine[66] are all involved in the defense against prolonged, as opposed to short-term, hypoglycemia, but neither growth hormone nor cortisol is critical to the correction of even prolonged hypoglycemia or to the prevention of hypoglycemia after an overnight fast in adults.[59] Thus growth hormone and cortisol are lower in the hierarchy. Glucose autoregulation is also operative in humans but only during severe hypoglycemia.[60, 61] Other hormones, neurotransmitters, and substrates other than glucose may be involved, but their quantitative contribution is minor.[13]

The redundant defenses against hypoglycemia account for the rarity of hypoglycemia in nondiabetic individuals and the capacity of many persons with intensively treated IDDM to maintain plasma glucose at levels sufficient for normal cerebral function despite hyperinsulinemia and deficient glucagon responses. The susceptibility to hypoglycemia of many patients with IDDM is largely the result of deficient glucagon and epinephrine secretion.[47]

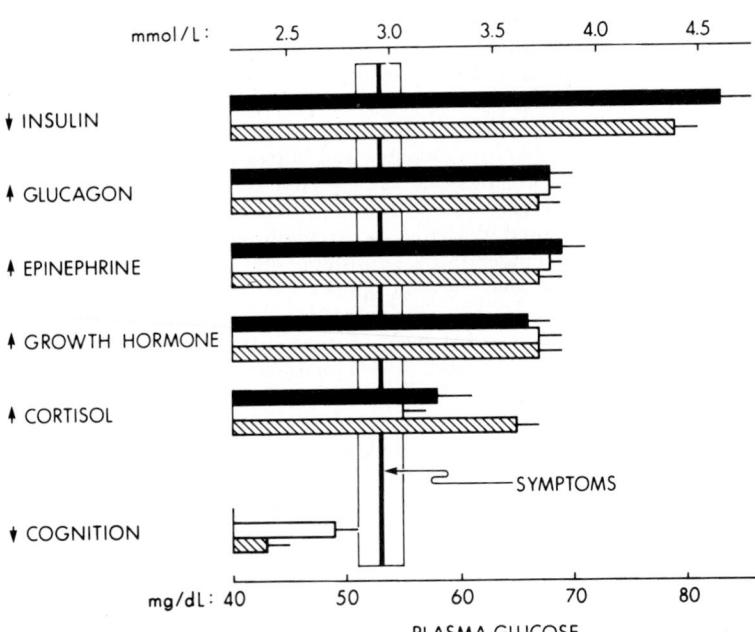

Figure 20–8. Mean (±SE) arterialized venous glycemic thresholds for decrements in insulin secretion (determined by measurement of C-peptide concentrations), increments in plasma glucagon, epinephrine, growth hormone and cortisol concentrations, symptoms and hypoglycemic cognitive dysfunction during decrements in the plasma glucose concentration in normal humans. (Data for solid columns from Schwartz NS, Clutter WE, Shah SD, et al. J Clin Invest 1987; 79:777–781. Data for open columns from Mitrakou A, Ryan C, Veneman T, et al. Am J Physiol 1991; 260:E67–E74. Data for cross-hatched columns from Fanelli C, Pampanelli S, Epifano L, et al. Diabetologia 1994; 37:797–807.)

Figure 20–9. Composite of studies of the mechanisms of the prevention of hypoglycemia. Mean (±SE) plasma glucose concentrations are shown. *A,* Glucose levels during infusion of somatostatin (SRIF) with partial insulin replacement alone *(closed symbols)* and with combined β- and α-adrenergic blockade with propranolol (PRP) and phentolamine (PTL) *(open symbols)* after an overnight fast in normal humans. *B,* Glucose levels after overnight *(closed symbols)* and 3-d *(open symbols)* fasts during insulin replacement in a dose estimated to produce portal insulin levels after the 3-d fast comparable to those after the overnight fast (Ins alone), continued insulin replacement plus somatostatin infusion to produce glucagon deficiency (↓G), combined α- and β-adrenergic blockade alone (↓α/β), and adrenergic blockade plus glucagon deficiency produced by insulin replacement and somatostatin infusion (↓α/β/↓G) in normal humans. *C,* Glucose levels before and after oral glucose (75 g) ingestion in normal humans (between the continuous lines) and bilaterally adrenalectomized humans without intervention *(open symbols),* (Epinephrine Deficient) and with somatostatin infusion with partial insulin replacement (both starting at 220 min) to produce glucagon deficiency *(closed symbols),* (Epinephrine + Glucagon Deficient). *D,* Glucose levels before *(open columns)* and after *(closed columns)* 60 min of moderate (60% of peak VO₂) cycle exercise in normal humans with no intervention (control), somatostatin infusion with insulin and glucagon replacement at fixed, basal rates throughout (Clamp [No Δ Insulin or Glucagon]), somatostatin infusion with insulin and glucagon replacement in altered doses during exercise to approximate the decrements in insulin and increments in glucagon that occurred during the control study (Clamp with ↓ Insulin and ↑ Glucagon), α- and β-adrenergic blockade alone (Adrenergic Blockade), and somatostatin infusion with insulin and glucagon replacement at fixed, basal rates plus adrenergic blockade (Clamp, No Δ Insulin or Glucagon + Adrenergic Blockade). Data from refs. 53 and 54. Data for *A* from Rosen SG, Clutter WE, Berk MA, et al[49]; data for *B* from Rosen SG, Clutter WE, Berk MA, et al[50]; data for *C* from Tse TF, Clutter WE, Shah SD, et al[52]; and data for *D* from Hirsch IB, Marker JC, Smith L, et al[53]; and Marker JC, Hirsch IB, Smith L, et al.[54] (From Cryer PE. Hypoglycemia: the limiting factor in the homeostasis and management of IDDM. Diabetes 1994; 43:1378–1389. Copyright 1994, American Diabetes Association, Alexandria, Virginia.)

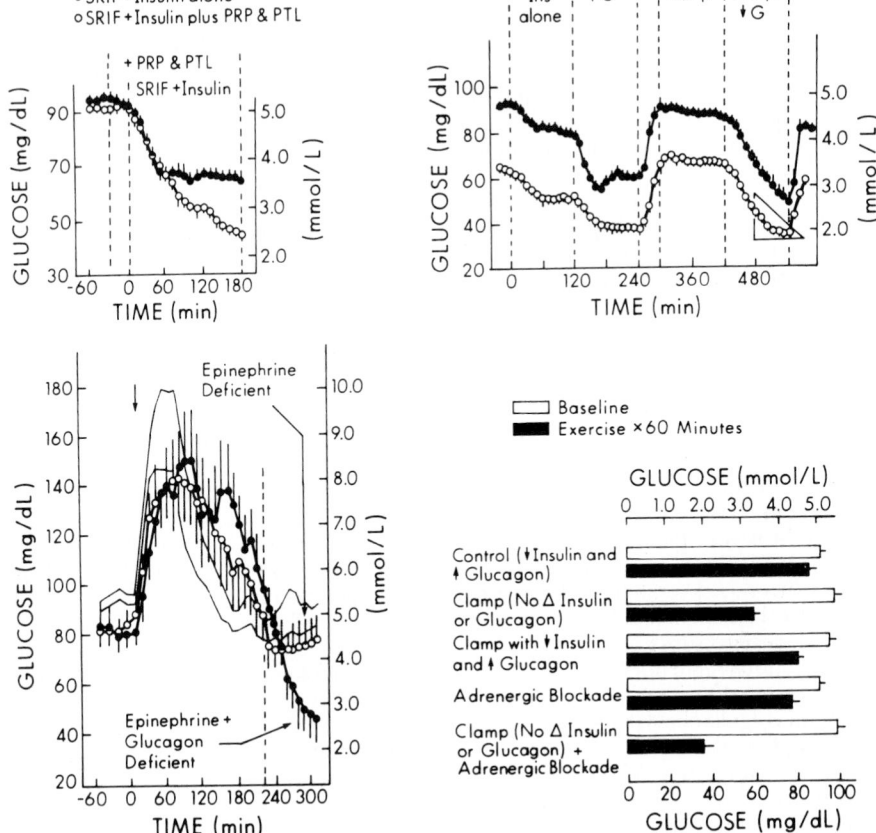

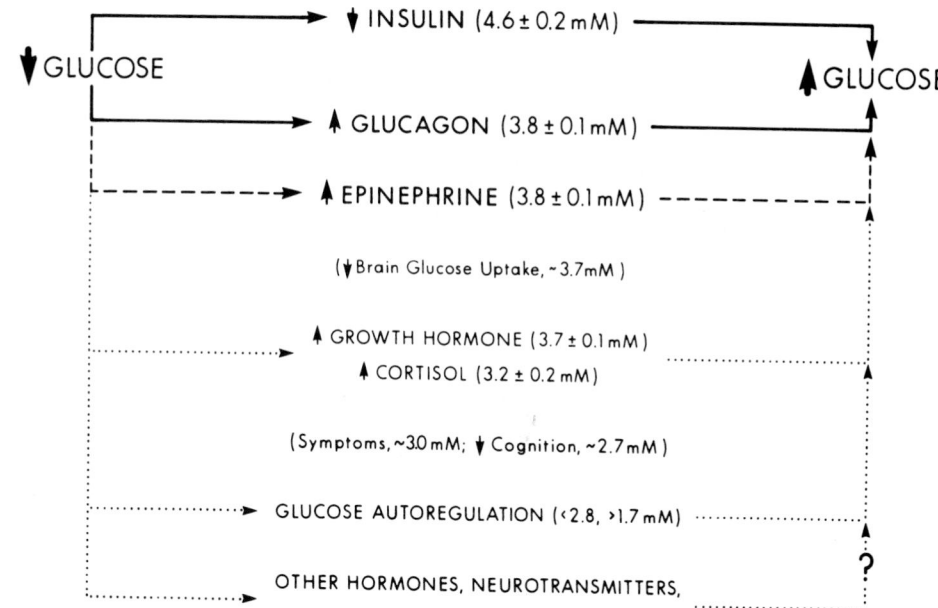

Figure 20–10. Schematic representation of the physiology of normal glucose counterregulation in humans. Mean (±SE) arterialized glycemic thresholds for the various responses to falling plasma glucose concentrations are also shown. See text for discussion. (From Cryer PE. Glucose counterregulation: the prevention and correction of hypoglycemia in humans. Am J Physiol 1993; 264:E149–E155. Copyright 1993, American Physiological Society, Bethesda, Maryland.)

PATHOPHYSIOLOGY OF HYPOGLYCEMIA

Clinical Manifestations of Hypoglycemia

The clinical manifestations of hypoglycemia are conventionally divided into two categories: neurogenic (or autonomic) and neuroglycopenic. Each is the result of central nervous system fuel (glucose) deprivation, but their mechanisms differ.

Neurogenic manifestations of hypoglycemia are the result of the expression and perception of central nervous system–mediated autonomic nervous system discharge triggered by hypoglycemia.[39] That discharge includes activation of the adrenal medullae and the sympathetic nervous system (which together compose the sympathochromaffin, or sympathoadrenal, system) and the parasympathetic nervous system.[67] The adrenal medullae release epinephrine primarily but also release norepinephrine and several peptides. Most sympathetic postganglionic neurons release norepinephrine, but a subset release acetylcholine. Parasympathetic postganglionic neurons release acetylcholine.

Neurogenic symptoms and signs of hypoglycemia (Fig. 20–11) include sweating, hunger, and paresthesias. These are cholinergic symptoms (mediated by acetylcholine), and the diaphoretic response is caused by release of acetylcholine from sympathetic postganglionic neurons.[39, 68] Tremor, palpitations, anxiety, increased heart rate, and elevation of systolic blood pressure are adrenergic symptoms (mediated by catecholamines). The extent to which adrenergic manifestations are mediated by adrenomedullary epinephrine or sympathetic neural norepinephrine, or both, is not clear. However, some symptoms (e.g., palpitations) do not occur when the adrenal medullae are absent.

Neuroglycopenic manifestations of hypoglycemia (see Fig. 20–11) are the result of central nervous system glucose deprivation per se[69] and range from subtle impairment of mentation to seizures, coma, and even death. Between these extremes other manifestations include sensations of warmth (despite cool, moist skin) or weakness; difficulty in thinking or confusion; feelings of tiredness, drowsiness, faintness, or dizziness; difficulty in speaking; blurred vision; and, rarely, focal neuro-

logic deficits (e.g., diplopia, hemiparesis). Hypothermia is often present and hyperthermia may follow hypoglycemia.

The magnitude of the responses to hypoglycemia is an inverse function of the glucose concentration at nadir.[56] The rate of the fall in plasma glucose is not a determinant of the magnitude.[56, 70, 71] As summarized in Figure 20–8, the arterialized venous blood glucose thresholds for activation of several glucose counterregulatory systems during falls in plasma glucose normally lie just below the range of physiological plasma glucose concentration, which is greater than the glucose levels that produce symptoms of hypoglycemia.[62–65, 72] Glucose counterregulatory systems are activated at glucose levels of about 3.6 to 3.9 mmol/L (65 to 70 mg/dL), whereas symptoms develop at glucose concentrations of about 2.8 to 3 mmol/L (50 to 55 mg/dL), and cognitive dysfunction occurs initially at glucose levels of about 2.5 to 2.8 mmol/L (45 to 50 mg/dL).

Glucose metabolism, not transport, normally determines the rate of glucose utilization by the brain. The plasma glucose

NEUROGENIC

SWEATY
HUNGRY
TINGLING
SHAKY/TREMULOUS
HEART POUNDING
NERVOUS/ANXIOUS

NEUROGLYCOPENIC

WARM
WEAK
DIFFICULTY THINKING/
    CONFUSED
TIRED/DROWSY
FAINT
DIZZY
DIFFICULTY SPEAKING
BLURRED VISION

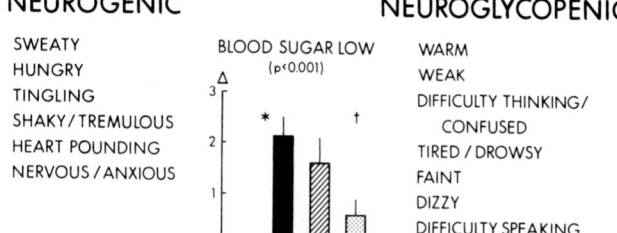

Figure 20–11. Neurogenic (autonomic) and neuroglycopenic symptoms of hypoglycemia in normal humans. Among the neurogenic symptoms "sweaty," "hungry," and "tingling" are cholinergic while "shaky/tremulous," "heart pounding" and "nervous/anxious" are adrenergic. See text for discussion. Mean (±SE) subject scores for awareness of hypoglycemia (BLOOD SUGAR LOW) during euglycemia (EU) and hypoglycemia (HYPO) alone *(closed column)*, with combined α- and β-adrenergic blockade (ADB, *cross-hatched column)* and with panautonomic blockade (PAB, *stippled column)* with both adrenergic and cholinergic antagonists are also shown. Data from Towler DA, Havlin CE, Craft S, et al.[39] (From Cryer PE. Hypoglycemia: the limiting factor in the management of IDDM. Diabetes 1994; 43:1378–1389. Copyright, 1994, American Diabetes Association, Alexandria, Virginia.)

concentration at which the rate of glucose transport across the blood-brain barrier is half-maximal approximates normal plasma glucose concentrations, and the rate of blood-to-brain glucose transport is about twice that of brain glucose metabolism at normal plasma glucose levels.[73] Glucose transport becomes rate-limiting when the plasma glucose concentration falls to low levels—namely at arterial plasma glucose concentrations of about 3.6 to 3.9 mmol/L (65 to 70 mg/dL),[74] the same levels at which central nervous system–mediated neuroendocrine responses are first demonstrable in normal humans[62–65, 72] (see Fig. 20–8).

These glycemic thresholds for neuroendocrine (including counterregulatory hormone) manifestations are reproducible in normal humans when similar experimental designs are used,[62–65, 71] although other designs result in somewhat different calculated thresholds.[13] Nonetheless the glycemic thresholds, at least those for neuroendocrine and symptomatic responses, are dynamic rather than static[2, 3] and can differ among individuals in relation to previous plasma glucose levels. For example, individuals with poorly controlled IDDM have some hormonal (e.g., epinephrine) responses and suffer symptoms of hypoglycemia at higher plasma glucose concentrations than do nondiabetic individuals, whereas patients with well-controlled IDDM require lower plasma glucose levels to elicit hormonal and symptomatic responses to hypoglycemia.[75–77] Similar tolerance of hypoglycemia occurs in other recurrent hypoglycemic states, such as that resulting from an insulin-secreting tumor of the pancreatic islet cells.[78] Indeed, as discussed later, as little as one episode of hypoglycemia can cause decreased neuroendocrine levels and symptomatic hypoglycemia the following day in normal humans.[79] The mechanisms of these shifts in glycemic thresholds are not known. Based on the findings of decreased extraction of glucose by the brain in hyperglycemic rats[80, 81] and increased extraction in chronically hypoglycemic rats,[82] it appears that increased blood-to-brain glucose transport with tight glycemic control shifts the glycemic thresholds to lower plasma glucose levels in IDDM.[83] The finding of increased glucose transporter (GLUT-1) mRNA and protein in the brains (presumably in the microvessels that include the blood-brain barrier) of rats after 3 d of hypoglycemia,[84, 85] the finding that 56 h of hypoglycemia between meals is associated with increased brain glucose uptake at a given level of hypoglycemia in nondiabetic humans,[74] and the finding that brain glucose uptake during hypoglycemia is preserved in patients with well-controlled IDDM are all consistent with that notion.[86]

Diagnosis of Hypoglycemia

The manifestations of hypoglycemia are nonspecific, vary among individuals, and may change from time to time in the same individual. They are also typically episodic. Thus, although the history is of fundamental importance in suggesting the possibility of hypoglycemia, the diagnosis cannot be made solely on the basis of symptoms and signs.

The diagnosis of hypoglycemia should also not be made solely on the basis of plasma glucose measurements unless they are unequivocally subnormal. It is not possible to define a plasma glucose concentration below which neuroglycopenia invariably occurs and above which neuroglycopenia never occurs. Although neuroglycopenia commonly occurs with plasma glucose levels of less than 3 mmol/L (54 mg/dL),[62–65, 71] it can occur at higher plasma glucose levels in poorly controlled IDDM[75, 77] and only at lower glucose levels in well-controlled IDDM.[75, 76] In addition, venous plasma glucose concentrations substantially less than 3 mmol/L (54 mg/dL) may occur in normal individuals late after glucose ingestion (arterial glucose levels are higher) and in some women and children during fasting without producing recognizable symptoms. This is not to say that distinctly low plasma glucose measurements should be ignored. Some patients with endogenous hyperinsulinism[78] or intensively treated diabetes[75, 76] tolerate glucose levels that are unequivocally subnormal much of the time, as mentioned earlier. Since these patients can have neuroglycopenic symptoms at other times (presumably when glucose levels are even lower), it would be inappropriate to deny that they have hypoglycemia.

In general, venous plasma glucose concentrations of greater than 3.9 mmol/L (70 mg/dL) after an overnight fast are normal, those between 2.8 and 3.9 mmol/L (50 and 70 mg/dL) are suggestive of hypoglycemia, and those less than 2.8 mmol/L (50 mg/dL) indicate postabsorptive hypoglycemia. Since substantial glucose extraction occurs across the forearm under hyperinsulinemic conditions, arterial glucose concentrations (those relevant to brain function) are as much as 30% higher than venous glucose concentrations after an oral glucose load. Artifactually low measured glucose levels can result from glycolysis in vitro (pseudohypoglycemia), particularly in the presence of leukocytosis or polycythemia, or both, or if separation of plasma from the formed elements of the blood is delayed. The diagnosis of hypoglycemia is most convincingly established when it is based on Whipple's triad[87]: symptoms consistent with hypoglycemia, a low plasma glucose concentration, and relief of symptoms when the plasma glucose concentration is raised to normal levels.

Postabsorptive Versus Postprandial Hypoglycemia

Reproducible hypoglycemia in the postabsorptive state implies the presence of disease and requires diagnostic explanation and therapy. This condition is commonly referred to as postabsorptive or fasting hypoglycemia. However, it need not be apparent initially or exclusively during prolonged fasting or after an overnight fast, but it may become symptomatic during the latter portion of any interdigestive period or with exercise. In contrast, postprandial (reactive, stimulative) hypoglycemia usually does not imply a serious underlying disorder. Thus the distinction between postabsorptive and postprandial hypoglycemia is useful.

Mechanisms of Hypoglycemia

Hypoglycemia indicates that the rate of glucose efflux from the circulation exceeds that of glucose influx into the circulation and can result from excessive glucose efflux (excessive utilization, external losses) or deficient glucose influx (deficient endogenous production in the absence of exogenous glucose delivery), or both. Conditions in which glucose utilization is increased include exercise, pregnancy, and sepsis; renal losses can occur at physiological plasma glucose concentrations (e.g., renal glycosuria, pregnancy). However, because of the capacity of the normal liver to increase glucose production severalfold, as discussed earlier, clinical hypoglycemia rarely results solely from excessive glucose efflux. Rather it is commonly the result of inappropriately low glucose production relative to the rate of glucose utilization.

Hypoglycemia can be caused by regulatory, enzymatic, or substrate defects. Glucoregulatory defects include excessive secretion of insulin or deficient secretion of glucose counterregulatory hormones. Enzymatic defects in glucose production may be primary or may result from hepatic disease. Substrate defects include failure to mobilize or utilize gluconeogenic substrates.

Clinical Classification of Hypoglycemia

Hypoglycemia can be classified on the basis of glucose kinetic patterns, pathogenic mechanisms, or disease groups.

TABLE 20–1. Clinical Classification of Hypoglycemia

Postabsorptive (fasting) hypoglycemia
  Drugs
    Especially insulin, sulfonylureas, alcohol
    Also pentamidine, quinine
    Rarely, salicylates, sulfonamides
    ? Others
  Critical illnesses
    Hepatic disease
    Cardiac disease
    Renal disease
    Sepsis
    Inanition
  Hormonal deficiencies
    Cortisol or growth hormone, or both
    Glucagon and epinephrine
  Non–beta cell tumors
  Endogenous hyperinsulinism
    Pancreatic beta cell disorders
      Tumor (insulinoma)
      Nontumor
    Beta cell secretagogue (e.g., sulfonylureas)
    Autoimmune hypoglycemia
      Insulin antibodies
      Insulin receptor antibodies
      ? Beta cell antibodies
    ? Ectopic insulin secretion
  Hypoglycemias of infancy and childhood
Postprandial (reactive) hypoglycemia
  Congenital deficiencies of enzymes of carbohydrate metabolism
    Hereditary fructose intolerance
    Galactosemia
  Alimentary hypoglycemia
  Idiopathic (functional) postprandial hypoglycemia

The latter approach is used in this chapter (Table 20–1). Postabsorptive, or fasting, hypoglycemia can be the result of drugs, critical illnesses including hepatic or renal failure, hormonal deficiencies, non–beta cell tumors, endogenous hyperinsulinism (including that caused by pancreatic beta cell tumors), or metabolic disorders of infancy and childhood. Postprandial, or reactive, hypoglycemia is rarely caused by congenital enzyme defects but can follow gastric surgery and even more rarely as an idiopathic disorder.

Most episodes of hypoglycemia result from drugs, particularly insulin, sulfonylureas, or alcohol. In one series of patients treated in an emergency room for hypoglycemia, two thirds had diabetes mellitus and two thirds had been drinking alcohol.[88] Clearly the combination of drug-treated diabetes and alcohol ingestion can be devastating. Nearly one fourth of the patients were septic, but diabetes or alcohol ingestion were common even in those patients. Drugs are also a common cause of hypoglycemia in inpatients.[89] In this case, however, critical illnesses—renal or hepatic failure, sepsis, and inanition—are common. Hypoglycemia resulting from hormonal deficiencies is uncommon but often treatable by hormone replacement. Hypoglycemia due to non–beta cell tumors or caused by endogenous hyperinsulinism is rare.

HYPOGLYCEMIA IN DIABETES MELLITUS

Insulin-Dependent Diabetes Mellitus

Hypoglycemia is the limiting factor in the management of diabetes. Were it not for the devastating effects of hypoglycemia, particularly on the brain, diabetes would be rather easy to treat. One would simply administer enough insulin (or enough sulfonylurea in appropriate patients) to lower plasma glucose concentrations to or below the nondiabetic range. Such therapy would alleviate hyperglycemia, prevent acute complications of diabetes, almost assuredly prevent the chronic complications (retinopathy, nephropathy, and neuropathy), and likely reduce the risk of atherosclerosis. However, because of the effects of hypoglycemia, the management of diabetes is much more complex.

Because of the imperfections of insulin replacement regimens and the compromised glucose counterregulatory defenses against the hyperinsulinemia that results from those imperfect regimens, iatrogenic hypoglycemia prevents the achievement and maintenance of euglycemia in most individuals with IDDM.[1–5, 90–92] Those receiving conventional therapy experience an average of one episode of symptomatic hypoglycemia per week, and those receiving intensive therapy have an average of two such episodes per week. At a minimum, a tenth of patients receiving conventional therapy and a fourth of those receiving intensive therapy have one episode of severe, temporarily disabling hypoglycemia, often with seizure or coma, each year. In retrospective series approximately 4% of deaths in individuals with IDDM resulted from hypoglycemia. In addition to physical morbidity and some mortality, hypoglycemia can also cause recurrent or persistent psychosocial morbidity. Clearly for many individuals with IDDM iatrogenic hypoglycemia is a major unsolved problem.[2–5]

Frequency

The continuum of iatrogenic hypoglycemia can be divided into three categories[3]: (1) asymptomatic (biochemical) hypoglycemia, (2) mild to moderate symptomatic hypoglycemia, and (3) severe hypoglycemia, most often defined as sufficiently disabling to require the assistance of another individual.[90–92] Asymptomatic hypoglycemia probably occurs in all persons with IDDM. The vast majority of these individuals have many episodes of symptomatic hypoglycemia, and most experience some episodes of severe hypoglycemia.

The true frequency of asymptomatic (biochemical) hypoglycemia in IDDM is not known but it is common.[3] In one study of patients treated to a median daytime blood glucose concentration of 5 mmol/L (90 mg/dL), 10% of serial daytime blood glucose values were less than 3 mmol/L (54 mg/dL).[93] Similarly in 9 of 10 patients treated to a mean plasma glucose concentration of 5.6 mmol/L (100 mg/dL) plasma glucose levels were less than 2.8 mmol/L (50 mg/dL) 10% of the time during continuous 24-h glucose measurements.[94] Only one fourth of the 23 detected episodes were recognized by the patients. Hypoglycemia is particularly common during the night, typically the longest interprandial period. Based on hourly sampling through the night Pramming and colleagues[95] estimated that if the bedtime blood glucose level was less than 6 mmol/L (108 mg/dL), the likelihood of nocturnal hypoglycemia was 80%. Again most of the detected episodes were asymptomatic.

An array of symptoms idiosyncratic in nature[96] have been attributed to hypoglycemia.[3] A given symptom or symptom complex may be meaningful to one patient but not to another and may be both neurogenic and neuroglycopenic in nature. Because awareness of hypoglycemia is based largely on the perception of neurogenic symptoms,[39] these are most often used to recognize developing hypoglycemia. The extent to which neuroglycopenic symptoms are also recognizable is unclear. Both the absence of symptoms (hypoglycemia unawareness, discussed later) and the failure of the patient to interpret symptoms as indicative of hypoglycemia are major contributing factors to the development of severe hypoglycemia.[90]

In a study of 441 patients with IDDM (75% using intermediate and regular insulin twice daily, i.e., a conventional therapy regimen), an average of 1.8 episodes of mild to moderate symptomatic hypoglycemia occurred per week,[97] a rate similar to the one to two episodes per week in the Diabetes Control and Complications Trial (DCCT) noted earlier. Thus the average patient experiences thousands of episodes of symptomatic hypoglycemia over a lifetime of IDDM.

A total of 1441 patients were followed an average of 6.5 y in the DCCT.[91] Thirty-five percent of those in the conventional therapy group (n = 730) and 65% of those in the intensive therapy group (n = 711) had episodes of severe hypoglycemia[92] (Fig. 20–12). Nineteen percent and 38%, respectively, had severe hypoglycemia with seizure or coma so that the incidence of severe hypoglycemia was twofold higher during attempts to achieve near-normal plasma glucose levels. Nineteen and 61 episodes of severe hypoglycemia per 100 patient-years occurred in the conventional and intensive therapy groups, respectively, more than a threefold increased risk for severe hypoglycemia during attempts to achieve near-normal plasma glucose concentrations[92] (see Fig. 20–12). Although the increase in the event rates (more than threefold) was greater than the increase in the proportion of patients affected (approximately twofold), both were increased during intensive therapy.

For several reasons the DCCT data provide *minimum* estimates of the frequency of iatrogenic hypoglycemia. First, the DCCT patients were highly selected and probably represented the most physically and emotionally healthy and highly motivated individuals with IDDM. Second, patients with a history of severe hypoglycemia, a strong predictor of subsequent severe hypoglycemia,[90] were excluded from the DCCT. Third, the DCCT patients received extensive education and professional support throughout the trial. Therefore the higher rates of severe hypoglycemia reported in other studies[3] may be more representative of the true experience with IDDM.

Impact

Iatrogenic hypoglycemia causes physical morbidity, psychosocial morbidity, and some mortality.[3] The physical morbidity from an episode of hypoglycemia ranges from unpleasant symptoms to neurologic manifestations such as behavioral changes, cognitive impairment, seizures, and coma. Focal neurologic defects and decerebrate posturing are rare. The magnitude of permanent neurologic damage is a function of both the depth and duration of hypoglycemia. For example plasma glucose levels less than 1.1 mmol/L (20 mg/dL) for 5 to 6 h are required to produce consistent neurologic damage in monkeys.[98] The incidence of permanent neuropsychological damage was not increased in the intensive therapy group in the DCCT.[99]

Largely because the post mortem diagnosis of hypoglycemia is difficult if not impossible,[100] the true hypoglycemic mortality rate in IDDM is unknown.[3] A commonly cited estimate is that 4% of deaths in individuals with IDDM are caused by hypoglycemia.[101, 102] Although the causal relationship was clear in only one case, 3 (9%) of 35 deaths in patients receiving intensive therapy were attributed to hypoglycemia in one study.[103] Based on historical controls the authors concluded that intensive therapy does not confer excessive risk of death from iatrogenic hypoglycemia. The relationship, if any, of hypoglycemia to the deaths of patients who appeared well on retiring but were found dead in their beds[104] is unknown. Few deaths occurred in the DCCT. The relative risk of death (1.7) was not increased significantly in the intensive therapy group.[92] One death was attributed to hypoglycemia in each group.

At the least an episode of hypoglycemia is a nuisance and a distraction. It can be embarrassing and lead to social ostracism or employment discrimination, it can be mistaken for alcohol intoxication or illicit drug use, and the aberrant behavior and impaired judgment can lead to abusive or illegal acts. The psychological morbidity of iatrogenic hypoglycemia[3] includes fear of an episode, guilt about that rational fear, anxiety, and lower levels of overall happiness.[97, 105–107] The performance of critical tasks is impaired. For example motor vehicle driving skills are impaired[108] and accidents have been documented.[3, 92] Nonetheless, with one exception,[109] accident rates do not appear to be excessive in persons with diabetes.[3] Finally the management of IDDM can intrude on all aspects of daily life.

Risk Factors and Pathophysiology

Relative or absolute hyperinsulinemia occurs from time to time in all individuals with IDDM because of the imperfections of current insulin replacement regimens. Conventional risk factors for iatrogenic hypoglycemia[2–5] are based on the premise that insulin excess is the sole determinant of risk. Relative or absolute insulin excess occurs when (1) insulin doses are excessive, ill-timed, or of the wrong type; (2) the influx of exogenous glucose is decreased, as during an overnight fast or after a missed meal or snack; (3) insulin-independent glucose utilization is increased, as during physical exercise; (4) endogenous glucose production is decreased, as after alcohol ingestion; (5) sensitivity to insulin is increased, as during effective intensive therapy, in the middle of the night, after exercise, or after weight loss; or (6) insulin clearance is decreased, as with renal failure. However, these risk factors explained a minority of episodes of severe hypoglycemia in the DCCT.[90] Thus we must look beyond the conventional risk factors to understand most episodes of hypoglycemia in individuals with IDDM.

An alternative view is that iatrogenic hypoglycemia is the result of the interplay of relative or absolute insulin excess and compromised glucose counterregulation in IDDM.[2, 3, 5] In other words, although insulin excess of sufficient magnitude will cause hypoglycemia regardless of the actions of the glucose counterregulatory factors, the integrity of the glucose counterregulatory systems determines whether the less marked hyperinsulinemia that occurs commonly in the treatment of IDDM results in hypoglycemia. Causes of compromised glucose counterregulation in IDDM include defective glucose counterregulation, hypoglycemia unawareness, elevated glycemic thresholds during intensive therapy and after hypoglycemia, and administration of a β-adrenergic antagonist.

As discussed earlier, insulin, glucagon, and epinephrine normally are redundant glucoregulatory factors critical to the prevention or correction of hypoglycemia[13] (see Fig. 20–10),

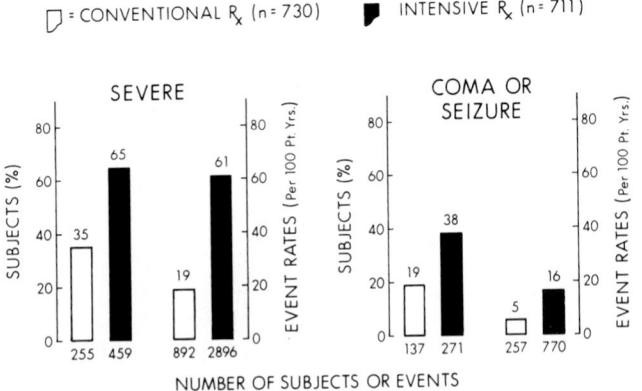

Figure 20–12. Proportion of patients affected and event rates for severe hypoglycemia (*left*) and severe hypoglycemia with seizure or coma (*right*) in the Diabetes Control and Complications Trial (DCCT). Data from The Diabetes Control and Complications Trial Research Group.[92]

ALTERED GLUCOSE COUNTERREGULATION IN IDDM

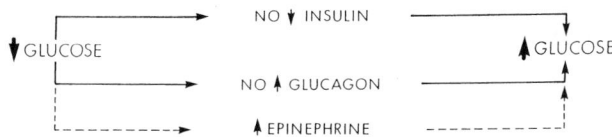

DEFECTIVE GLUCOSE COUNTERREGULATION IN IDDM

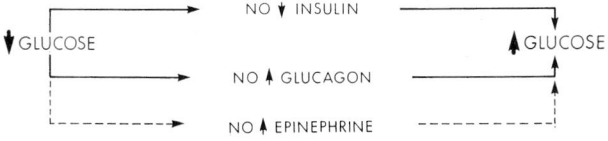

Figure 20–13. Schematic representation of the pathophysiology of glucose counterregulation in people with IDDM: altered and ultimately defective glucose counterregulation.

and all three are compromised with fully established IDDM.[2, 3, 5] First, because insulin is passively absorbed from subcutaneous injection sites in patients with IDDM, plasma insulin levels do not decrease as the plasma glucose concentrations fall. Second, the glucagon secretory response to hypoglycemia is lost over the first few years of IDDM.[55, 110, 111] Albeit acquired, this defect (specific for the stimulus of hypoglycemia) develops early in the course of IDDM,[110] is the rule in established IDDM, and is tightly linked to absolute insulin deficiency.[111] Thus in established IDDM the plasma insulin level does not decrease, and the plasma glucagon level does not increase as the plasma glucose concentration falls (Fig. 20–13). Nonetheless glucose counterregulation is generally adequate, probably because epinephrine compensates for the deficient glucagon response. Third, somewhat later in the course of IDDM the epinephrine response to hypoglycemia becomes impaired[110, 112, 113] (Fig. 20–14). Like the deficient glucagon response, the reduced epinephrine response is specific for the stimulus of hypoglycemia; glucagon and epinephrine responses to other stimuli are generally preserved. Unlike the deficient glucagon response, however, the reduced epinephrine response appears to be a threshold abnormality; an epinephrine response is elicited but at a lower plasma glucose concentration.[113] The reduced epinephrine response is not the result of classic diabetic autonomic neuropathy[113] (see Fig. 20–14). The role of recent antecedent hypoglycemia is discussed later in this section. Thus in fully established IDDM the insulin level does not decrease, the plasma glucagon level does not increase, and the plasma epinephrine level increases little as the plasma glucose concentration falls. All three components of this pattern are readily demonstrable in patients with an average duration of IDDM of less than 10 y.[114]

DEFECTIVE GLUCOSE COUNTERREGULATION. Glucose counterregulation is compromised by the deficient epinephrine responses and impaired glucagon responses in individuals with IDDM (see Fig. 20–13). Patients with combined deficiencies of the glucagon and epinephrine responses are at a 25-

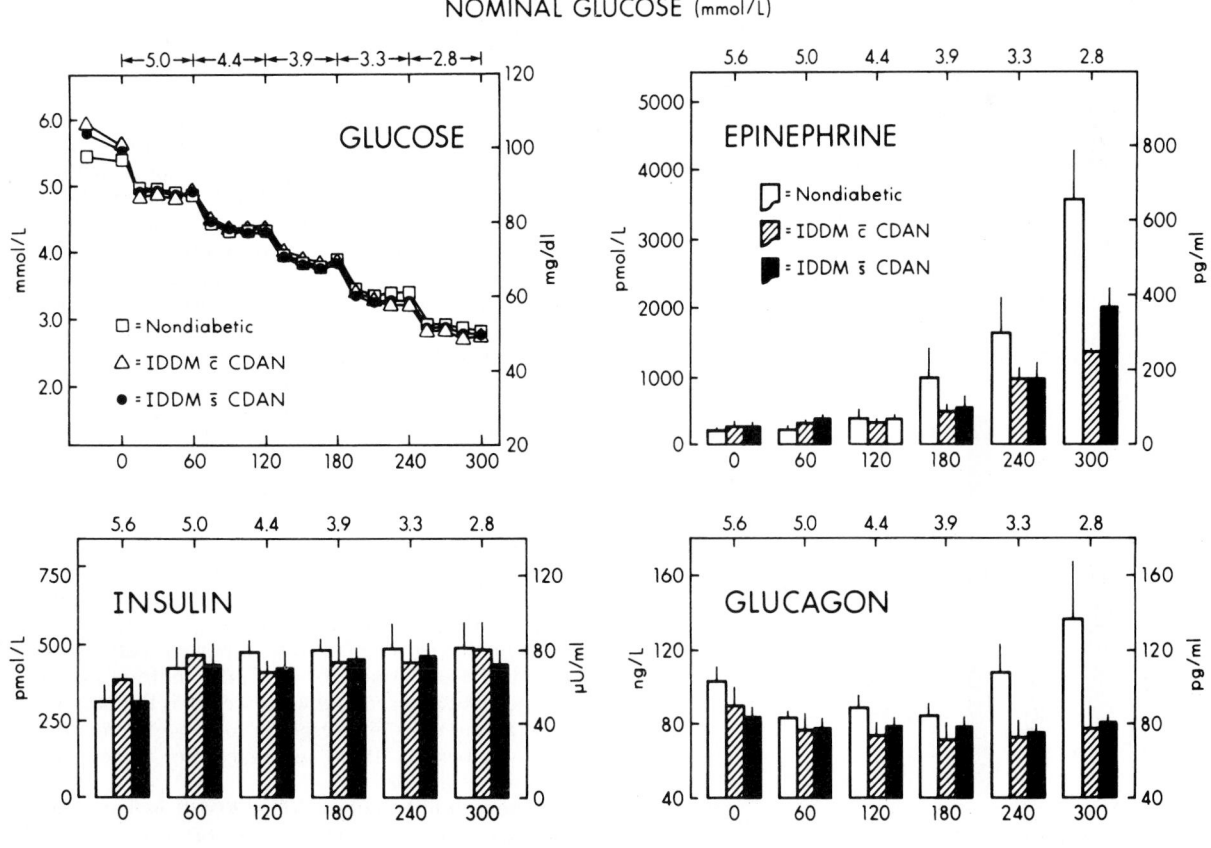

Figure 20–14. Mean (±SE) plasma glucose, insulin, epinephrine and glucagon concentrations during hyperinsulinemic stepped hypoglycemic glucose clamps in nondiabetic subjects *(open squares and columns)*, people with IDDM with classical diabetic autonomic neuropathy (CDAN, *open triangles and cross-hatched columns*) and people with IDDM without CDAN *(closed circles and columns)*. (From Dagogo-Jack SE, Craft S, Cryer PE. Hypoglycemia-associated autonomic failure in insulin dependent diabetes mellitus. J Clin Invest 1993; 91:819–828. Copyright, 1994, American Society for Clinical Investigation, New York.)

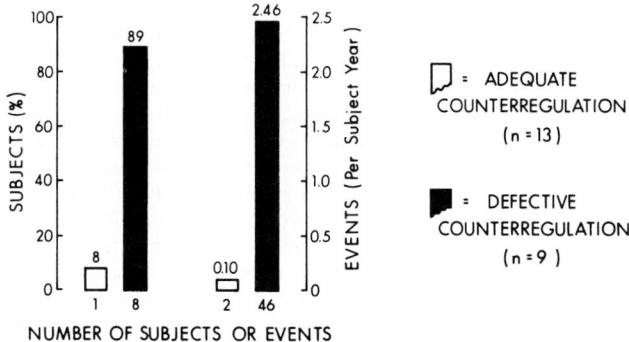

Figure 20–15. Proportion of patients affected and event rates for severe hypoglycemia during intensive therapy of patients with IDDM and adequate (altered) and defective glucose counterregulation. Data from White NH, Skor DA, Cryer PE, et al.[47] (From Cryer PE, Fisher JN, Shamoon H. Hypoglycemia. Diabetes Care 1994; 17:734–755. Copyright, 1994, American Diabetes Association, Alexandria, Virginia.)

fold or greater increased risk for the development of severe iatrogenic hypoglycemia than are those with absent glucagon but intact epinephrine responses[47, 115] (Fig. 20–15). Furthermore the combination of deficient glucagon and epinephrine responses to hypoglycemia characterizes patients with recurrent severe hypoglycemia.[116] Such patients have the syndrome of defective glucose counterregulation[2, 3, 5] (see Fig. 20–13).

HYPOGLYCEMIA UNAWARENESS. Hypoglycemia unawareness[97, 117–121] is the loss of the warning symptoms of hypoglycemia that previously prompted the patient to act (e.g., eat) to prevent progression to severe hypoglycemia. Because awareness of hypoglycemia normally involves the perception of neurogenic symptoms,[39] hypoglycemia unawareness is primarily due to the loss of neurogenic symptoms of developing hypoglycemia. Thus the first clinical manifestation is neuroglycopenia, and it is often too late at this point to abort the episode with self-treatment. Affected patients are at about a sixfold increased risk for severe iatrogenic hypoglycemia[122] (Fig. 20–16). Like those with defective glucose counterregulation, patients with hypoglycemia unawareness require lower plasma glucose concentrations to elicit autonomic and symptomatic responses to hypoglycemia.[120, 123, 124] The role of recent

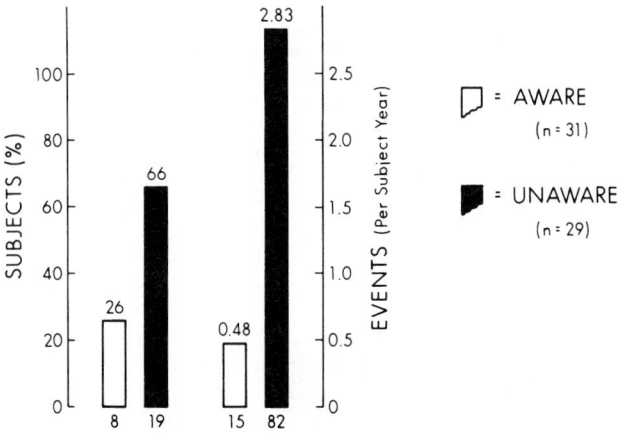

Figure 20–16. Proportion of patients affected and event rates for severe hypoglycemia in people with IDDM and normal or reduced awareness of hypoglycemia. Data from Gold AE, MacLeod KM, Frier BM.[122] (From Cryer PE, Fisher JN, Shamoon H. Hypoglycemia. Diabetes Care 1994; 17:734–755. Copyright, 1994, American Diabetes Association, Alexandria, Virginia.)

antecedent hypoglycemia in the pathogenesis of this syndrome is discussed later.

ELEVATED GLYCEMIC THRESHOLDS DURING INTENSIVE THERAPY. Lower plasma glucose concentrations are also required to elicit autonomic and symptomatic responses to hypoglycemia during intensive therapy in IDDM.[75, 76] Because a more intense hypoglycemic stimulus (a lower plasma glucose concentration) is required to elicit these responses, such patients have elevated thresholds for autonomic and symptomatic responses to hypoglycemia. Whether the glycemic thresholds for hypoglycemic cognitive dysfunction are[125–127] or are not[127–130] elevated as well is unclear. Conversely glycemic thresholds for autonomic, at least epinephrine, and symptomatic responses to hypoglycemia are reduced in patients with poorly controlled IDDM.[76, 77]

ELEVATED GLYCEMIC THRESHOLDS AFTER RECENT HYPOGLYCEMIA. As little as one 2-h episode of hypoglycemia causes reduced autonomic responses, including epinephrine, and symptomatic responses to subsequent hypoglycemia in healthy individuals[79, 131–133] and in individuals with IDDM[113, 134, 135] (Figs. 20–17 and 20–18). This phenomenon probably explains, in part, the fact that intensive therapy of IDDM (just discussed) produces similar elevation of glycemic thresholds for the response to hypoglycemia.

ELEVATED GLYCEMIC THRESHOLDS DURING β-ADRENERGIC BLOCKADE. In the setting of absent glucagon responses, the administration of β-adrenergic antagonists impairs glucose recovery from hypoglycemia in IDDM.[46] This is the result of antagonism of the β_2-adrenergic actions of epinephrine. β_1-Adrenergic antagonists do not have this effect, but the β-adrenergic selectivity of "cardioselective" drugs, such as metoprolol and atenolol, is only relative. These agents also produce some β_2-adrenergic antagonism at least in the higher dose ranges. β_2-Adrenergic antagonism also elevates glycemic thresholds for symptoms of hypoglycemia in IDDM.[136] It is not clear whether use of β-adrenergic antagonists increases the frequency of iatrogenic hypoglycemia in patients with IDDM, but this issue has not been examined critically in the setting of intensive therapy of IDDM.

HYPOGLYCEMIA-ASSOCIATED AUTONOMIC FAILURE. Defective glucose counterregulation, hypoglycemia unawareness, and elevated glycemic thresholds during intensive therapy and after hypoglycemia have much in common.[137] They are all associated with a high frequency of iatrogenic hypoglycemia, they tend to segregate together clinically, and they share several features including elevated glycemic thresholds (lower plasma glucose concentrations required) for autonomic and symptomatic responses to hypoglycemia. Affected patients have reduced adrenomedullary (epinephrine), parasympathetic neural (pancreatic polypeptide) and, perhaps, sympathetic neural (neurogenic symptoms) responses to a given level of hypoglycemia. Therefore these syndromes can be conceptualized as examples of *hypoglycemia-associated autonomic failure in IDDM*.[137] The pathogenesis is not fully understood, may not be the same in all the syndromes, and may be multifactorial in a given syndrome. Nonetheless, antecedent iatrogenic hypoglycemia is one important pathogenetic factor but not the only one. For example, there is no compelling evidence that antecedent hypoglycemia is the proximate cause of the absent glucagon response to hypoglycemia that characterizes established IDDM and that is key to defective glucose counterregulation.

The overall hypothesis (Fig. 20–19) is that recent antecedent hypoglycemia is a major cause of hypoglycemia-associated autonomic failure in IDDM and that hypoglycemia-associated autonomic failure, by reducing both the physiological defense against hypoglycemia (i.e., reduced epinephrine response together with absent glucagon response) and the symptoms of hypoglycemia (i.e., reduced awareness), results in recurrent

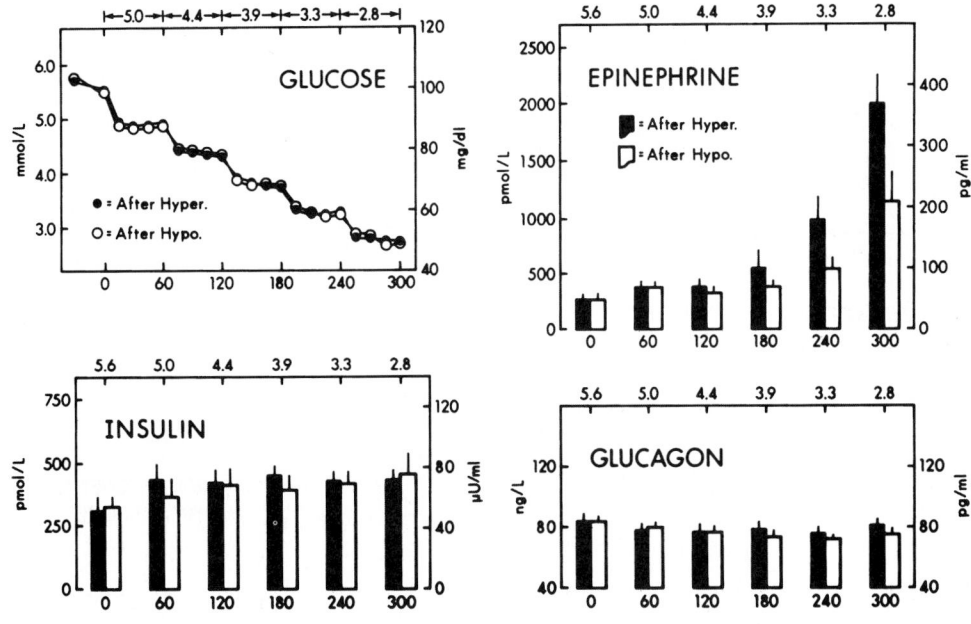

Figure 20–17. Mean (±SE) plasma glucose, insulin, epinephrine and glucagon concentrations during hyperinsulinemic, stepped hypoglycemic glucose clamps in patients with IDDM without classical diabetic autonomic neuropathy on mornings following afternoon hyperglycemia *(closed circles and columns)* and on mornings following afternoon hypoglycemia *(open circles and columns)*. (From Dagogo-Jack SE, Craft S, Cryer PE. Hypoglycemia-associated autonomic failure in insulin dependent diabetes mellitus. J Clin Invest 1993; 91:819–828. Copyright, 1993, American Society for Clinical Investigation, New York.)

episodes of hypoglycemia and creates a perpetuating cycle.[137] Antecedent hypoglycemia elevates glycemic thresholds for autonomic and symptomatic responses to subsequent hypoglycemia in healthy individuals[79, 131–133] and in individuals with IDDM[113, 134, 135] (see Figs. 20–17 and 20–18) and impairs the physiological defense against hyperinsulinemia in patients with IDDM[113] (Fig. 20–20). This phenomenon is demonstrable in well-controlled IDDM (and is thus clinically generalizable), is specific for the stimulus of hypoglycemia (autonomic responses to other stimuli are not reduced), and is not simply the result of prior activation of the system.[138]

The syndrome of hypoglycemia unawareness in IDDM is reversible by short-term avoidance of iatrogenic hypoglycemia.[139–142] As illustrated in Figure 20–21, in the syndrome

of hypoglycemia unawareness symptoms of hypoglycemia are virtually absent at baseline, increase after 3 d of prevention of hypoglycemia, and are indistinguishable from normal responses after about 3 wk of scrupulous avoidance of iatrogenic hypoglycemia.[142] Symptomatic responses consistently return to normal in as little as 2 wk.[139, 142] Increased but not normal plasma epinephrine responses to hypoglycemia have been found in most studies.[139–141] Absent glucagon responses to hypoglycemia are unaffected by avoidance of hypoglycemia.[139–142] Glycemic thresholds for a battery of cognitive function test responses were reduced toward normal in the studies of Fanelli and colleagues[139, 141] but not in other studies.[142]

These findings[111, 138–142] provide strong support for hypoglycemia-associated autonomic failure in IDDM[137] (see Fig.

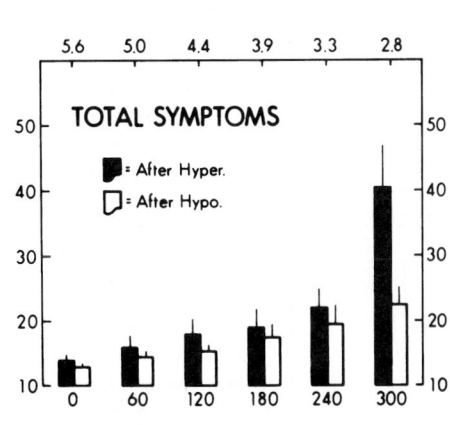

Figure 20–18. Mean (±SE) total, neurogenic, and neuroglycopenic symptom scores during hyperinsulinemic, stepped hypoglycemic glucose clamps in patients with IDDM without classical diabetic autonomic neuropathy on mornings following afternoon hyperglycemia *(closed columns)* and on mornings following afternoon hypoglycemia *(open columns)*. (From Dagogo-Jack SE, Craft S, Cryer PE. Hypoglycemia-associated autonomic failure in insulin dependent diabetes mellitus. J Clin Invest 1993; 91:819–828. Copyright, 1993, American Society for Clinical Investigation, New York.)

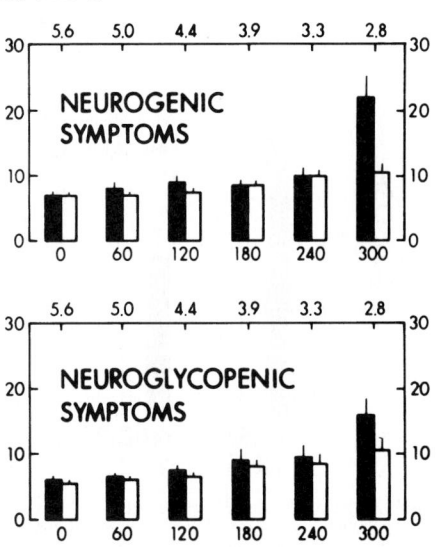

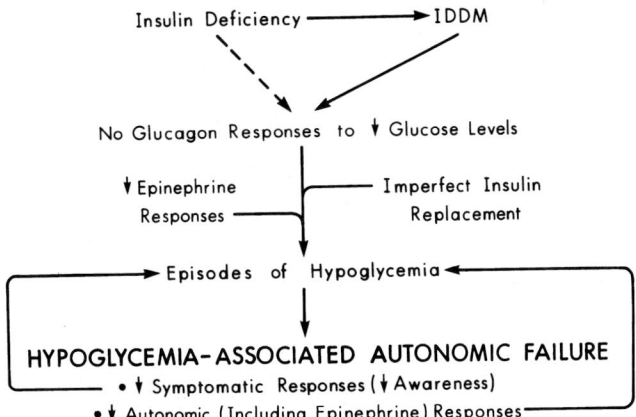

Figure 20–19. Schematic diagram of the concept of hypoglycemia-associated autonomic failure in IDDM. See text for discussion. Modified from Cryer PE.[137] (From Cryer PE, Fisher JN, Shamoon H. Hypoglycemia. Diabetes Care 1994; 17:734–755. Copyright, 1994, American Diabetes Association, Alexandria, Virginia.)

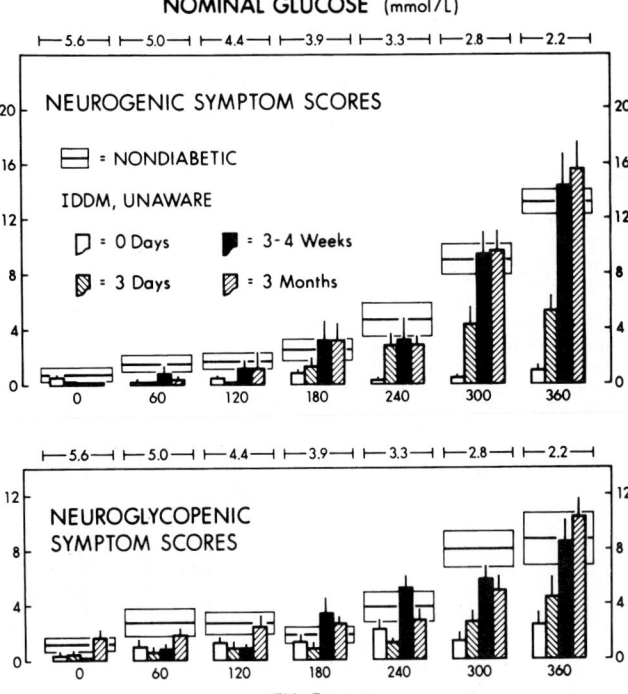

Figure 20–21. Mean (±SE) neurogenic and neuroglycopenic symptom scores during hyperinsulinemic stepped hypoglycemic glucose clamps in nondiabetic subjects *(rectangles)* and people with IDDM and hypoglycemia unawareness at baseline before (0 d, *open columns*), and after 3 d *(first set of cross-hatched columns)*, 3 to 4 wk *(closed columns)*, and 3 mo *(second set of cross-hatched columns)* of scrupulous avoidance of iatrogenic hypoglycemia. (From Dagogo-Jack SE, Rattarasarn C, Cryer PE. Reversal of hypoglycemia unawareness, but not defective glucose counterregulation, in IDDM. Diabetes 1994; 43:1426–1434. Copyright, 1994, American Diabetes Association, Alexandria, Virginia.)

20–20). Recent antecedent iatrogenic hypoglycemia causes the syndrome of hypoglycemia unawareness, probably causes elevated glycemic thresholds during effective intensive therapy, and contributes (by reducing the epinephrine response) to the pathogenesis of defective glucose counterregulation. However, other factors, as yet unknown, play a critical role in the pathogenesis of the key component (the absent glucagon response) of the syndrome of defective glucose counterregulation. Another as yet unanswered critical question is whether glycemic thresholds for hypoglycemic cognitive dysfunction also shift to lower plasma glucose concentrations after recent antecedent hypoglycemia.[72, 113, 133] This is a key question from both clinical and mechanistic perspectives. If the thresholds for cognitive dysfunction do not shift to lower glucose levels, whereas those for autonomic and symptomatic responses do change, clinical neuroglycopenia could cause devastating clinical consequences before counterregulatory activation. Dissociation of the glycemic thresholds for cognitive dysfunction from those for autonomic and symptomatic responses is inconsistent with a simple unifying mechanism such as a hypoglycemia-induced generalized increase in blood-to-brain glucose transport.[74, 80–86] The mechanism or mechanisms of these hypo-

glycemia-induced shifts in glycemic thresholds remain to be clarified.

The possibility that treatment with human (as contrasted to animal) insulin might enhance hypoglycemia unawareness was raised,[143, 144] but the evidence does not support that possibility.[145–147] For example in a prospective, randomized, double-blind crossover comparison of human and porcine insulin in individuals with IDDM, Colagiuri and colleagues[146] found no difference in the frequency of iatrogenic hypoglycemia or of hypoglycemia with reduced or absent symptoms.

Prevention

We must learn to administer insulin in a more physiological fashion, to prevent, correct, or compensate for compromised glucose counterregulation, if we are to eliminate hypoglycemia in individuals with IDDM. In the meantime we must make every effort to minimize the frequency of iatrogenic hypoglycemia.

The first step in the prevention of hypoglycemia is the selection and ongoing reassessment of prudent, individual glycemic goals. In this way the application of the principles of modern treatment of IDDM—patient education and professional support, frequent self–blood glucose monitoring, and flexible insulin replacement regimens—can minimize the frequency of hypoglycemia without compromising glycemic control.[139–142, 148] The higher frequency of hypoglycemia in the intensive therapy group in the DCCT[90–92] was a function of the glycemic goals in the two groups, not of intensive therapy per se.

The management of IDDM is of course empirical. Barring

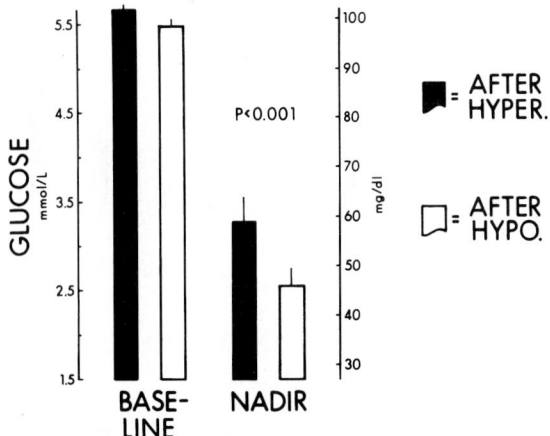

Figure 20–20. Mean (±SE) baseline and nadir plasma glucose concentrations during morning insulin infusion tests following afternoon hyperglycemia *(closed columns)* and following afternoon hypoglycemia *(open columns)* in people with IDDM without classical diabetic autonomic neuropathy. Data from Dagogo-Jack SE, Craft S, Cryer PE.[113]

a contraindication to aggressive therapy the DCCT findings provide further impetus to attempt to provide plasma glucose levels as close to the nondiabetic range as can be achieved safely, i.e., with infrequent symptomatic hypoglycemia and no severe hypoglycemia. In practice one tightens control until the patient hits the barrier of hypoglycemia. Measures to limit hypoglycemia include consideration of the conventional risk factors as they relate to insulin dose, timing, and type; the meal plan; exercise; drug interactions, including alcohol; sensitivity to insulin; and insulin clearance. However, they also include consideration of the more recently recognized risk factors discussed in the preceding paragraphs. Although the key component of defective glucose counterregulation—an absent glucagon response to a falling plasma glucose concentration—cannot as yet be reversed, scrupulous avoidance of iatrogenic hypoglycemia for a short period can reverse hypoglycemia unawareness and partially restore the critical (in the absence of a glucagon response) epinephrine response.[139–142]

Treatment

Most episodes of asymptomatic and mild to moderate symptomatic hypoglycemia are effectively self-treated by ingestion of glucose or carbohydrate in the form of juices, soft drinks, milk, crackers, candy, or a meal.[114, 149, 150] A commonly recommended dose of glucose is 20 g (0.3 g/kg in children). However, the glycemic response to oral glucose is transient, usually less than 2 h in insulin-induced hypoglycemia in IDDM[114] (Fig. 20–22). Thus ingestion of a more substantial mixed snack or meal shortly after the plasma glucose level is raised is generally advisable.

Parenteral treatment is necessary when a hypoglycemic subject is unable or unwilling (because of neuroglycopenia) to take carbohydrate orally. Glucagon is commonly injected subcutaneously or intramuscularly by a spouse or family member.[114, 149, 151–153] The standard dose, 1 mg (15 μg/kg in children), can cause substantial but transient hyperglycemia[114] (see Fig. 20–22). Therefore the dose should not be reduced to produce less hyperglycemia. Intranasal administration of

glucagon causes a glycemic response similar to that of injected glucagon.[154–156] Although glucagon can be administered intravenously by medical personnel,[151] intravenous glucose, 25 g initially, is the standard intravenous therapy. Because the glycemic response is transient, a subsequent glucose infusion is often needed and food should be provided orally as soon as the patient is able to take it safely.

Experimental approaches to the prevention and treatment of hypoglycemia include oral administration of the amino acid alanine (which stimulates glucagon secretion) and parenteral or oral administration of the β2-adrenergic agonist terbutaline (which exerts epinephrine-like actions on glucose production and utilization and stimulates neural norepinephrine release).[114, 157] These regimens produce a more sustained glycemic response than does glucagon or glucose. Indeed bedtime administration of alanine or terbutaline prevents nocturnal hypoglycemia more effectively than does a conventional bedtime snack in individuals with IDDM.[158]

Non–Insulin-Dependent Diabetes Mellitus

Hypoglycemia also occurs in individuals with non–insulin-dependent diabetes mellitus (NIDDM) treated with a sulfonylurea or insulin. Metformin and acarbose should not cause hypoglycemia. The reported frequency of severe sulfonylurea-induced hypoglycemia in patients with NIDDM is low, about two episodes per 100 patient-years.[159] Glyburide and chlorpropamide produce the highest rates of hypoglycemia. Risk factors include advanced age, poor nutrition, drug interactions with sulfonylureas, and hepatic or renal disease leading to reduced metabolism or excretion of the drugs.[160] Sulfonylurea-induced severe hypoglycemia has a mortality rate of around 10%, and about 5% of survivors have permanent neurologic damage.[160]

Severe iatrogenic hypoglycemia is more common in insulin-treated NIDDM. Indeed the rates are similar in insulin-treated NIDDM and insulin-treated IDDM matched for duration of insulin therapy.[161]

The pathophysiology of glucose counterregulation in NIDDM[162, 163] has been studied less extensively than has that in IDDM. The glucagon response to hypoglycemia produced by subcutaneous insulin in patients with NIDDM is reduced but not absent.[163] This reduction is associated with a decreased burst of glucose production in early hypoglycemia, but recovery from hypoglycemia is only slightly impaired, perhaps because of a normal epinephrine response. Nonetheless the finding of similar frequencies of severe hypoglycemia in insulin-treated NIDDM and IDDM[161] raises the possibility that glucose counterregulation might be more substantially compromised in patients at the insulin-deficient end of the spectrum of NIDDM.

Because sulfonylurea-induced hypoglycemia can be prolonged and may recur after initial treatment, hospitalization is generally recommended. Glucagon probably should not be used to treat sulfonylurea-induced hypoglycemia because it stimulates insulin secretion in patients with NIDDM. Drugs that inhibit insulin secretion, such as diazoxide[164] or octreotide,[165] might be used in conjunction with glucose infusion.

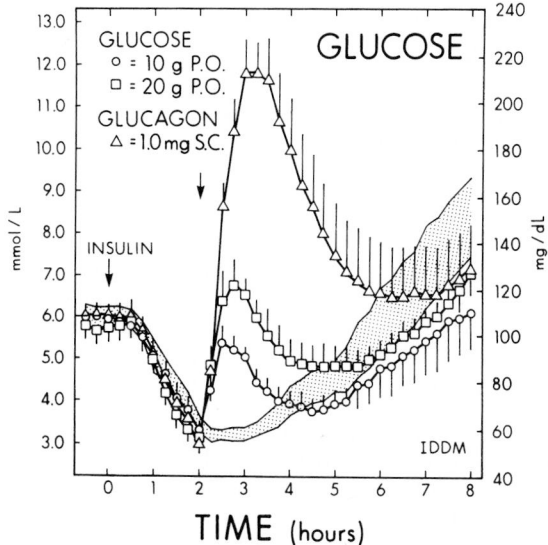

Figure 20–22. Mean (±SE) plasma glucose concentrations, in a model of hypoglycemia produced by subcutaneous insulin administration to people with IDDM, in response to 10 g (circles) and 20 g (squares) of oral glucose and 1.0 mg of subcutaneous glucagon (triangles) compared with placebo. (From Wiethop BV, Cryer PE. Alanine and terbutaline in the treatment of hypoglycemia in IDDM. Diabetes Care 1993; 16:1131–1136. Copyright, 1993, American Diabetes Association, Alexandria, Virginia.)

POSTABSORPTIVE (FASTING) HYPOGLYCEMIAS

The differential diagnosis of postabsorptive (fasting) hypoglycemia is outlined in Table 20–1. In most instances (e.g., drug-treated diabetes) the cause of hypoglycemia is apparent clinically. When the cause is not apparent measurement of plasma glucose, insulin, C peptide, and sulfonylurea levels permits classification of the hypoglycemic mechanism as hypoinsulinemic or hyperinsulinemic (absolute or relative)[166] and often provides diagnostic information.[1, 167, 168]

Drugs

Drugs, particularly insulin or a sulfonylurea, are the most common cause of hypoglycemia.[85, 86, 166] Other drugs that cause hypoglycemia include alcohol, pentamidine, quinine, and, rarely, salicylates and sulfonamides. Insulin and particularly sulfonylureas are possible causative agents even when there is no history of diabetes because both are sometimes taken surreptitiously or as a result of a pharmacy or other error.[169] Many other drugs have been associated with hypoglycemia, often under complex clinical conditions in which a causative relationship cannot be established. Known and putative hypoglycemia-causing drugs are listed in Table 20–2.

Ethanol inhibits gluconeogenesis[170] because its metabolism to acetaldehyde and acetate depletes hepatic nicotinamide-adenine dinucleotide, a cofactor critical to the entry of most precursors into the gluconeogenic pathway (see Fig. 20–1). It does not inhibit glycogenolysis. Ethanol also inhibits cortisol[170, 171] and growth hormone[170–172] responses and delays the epinephrine[170, 173] response to hypoglycemia. Glucagon responses are normal[170] or delayed.[173]

In normal humans ethanol administration does not cause postabsorptive hypoglycemia[174] or impair recovery from short-term hypoglycemia,[173] presumably because of intact glucagon secretion and responsive hepatic glycogenolysis, perhaps coupled with decreased sensitivity to insulin.[173–176] However, because gluconeogenesis is the dominant source of hepatic glucose production during prolonged hypoglycemia,[170] ethanol can contribute to the progression of hypoglycemia in insulin-treated patients with diabetes.

Alcohol-induced hypoglycemia in nondiabetic individuals typically follows (by 6 to 24 h) a binge of moderate to heavy alcohol consumption during which the person eats little food (i.e., in the setting of glycogen depletion).[171] Hypoglycemia can be profound and mortality rates may be as high as 10%. Children appear to be particularly susceptible to hypoglycemia after the accidental ingestion of alcohol. Ethanol is usually still measurable in the blood at the time the patient presents with hypoglycemia, but the levels may be moderately elevated and correlate poorly with the plasma glucose concentration.[171]

Salicylates in relatively large doses (4 to 6 g/d) can lower the plasma glucose concentration[177] and produce hypoglycemia in children and, rarely, in adults.[178, 179] The mechanism or mechanisms of salicylate-induced hypoglycemia are not known. Sulfonamides also rarely produce hypoglycemia through an unknown mechanism.[180]

Pentamidine, a beta cell toxin, produces hypoglycemia by causing insulin release.[181, 182] In one series of 128 immunocompromised patients with pneumocystis pneumonia treated with pentamidine 7% experienced hypoglycemia, 14% experienced hypoglycemia followed by diabetes, and 18% experienced diabetes without hypoglycemia being detected.[182] Risk factors for hypoglycemia include pentamidine therapy of longer duration and increased dose, previous pentamidine therapy, and renal insufficiency.[181, 182]

Hypoglycemia occurs commonly with severe malaria.[183, 187] Although associated with relative hyperinsulinemia attributed to quinine-induced insulin release in some patients,[183, 184] hypoglycemia can occur in the absence of quinine therapy[185] and in the absence of hyperinsulinemia in quinine-treated patients.[186] It is possible that the frequency of hypoglycemia in malaria is no higher than in other serious illnesses.[187]

Hypoglycemia has been attributed rarely to many other drugs (see Table 20–2). In many of the reported cases other potential causes of hypoglycemia have been present. The β-adrenergic antagonists, such as propranolol, are prominent examples. Although hypoglycemia attributed to propranolol has been reported in otherwise healthy children,[188, 189] most of the reported incidents occurred in individuals with diabetes who used insulin. As discussed earlier, epinephrine-mediated β-adrenergic mechanisms are not normally critical to glucose counterregulation, at least in adults, but become critical in glucagon-deficient patients with IDDM. Thus propranolol increases the risk of hypoglycemia in such patients but has little effect on glucoregulation when islet cell hormone secretion is normal.

Critical Illnesses

Among hospitalized patients drugs, particularly insulin, are the most common cause of hypoglycemia,[89] and serious diseases are the second most common,[89] including hepatic, cardiac, and renal failure; sepsis; and inanition.[89]

Hepatic Disease

In addition to appropriate regulatory signals and sufficient precursors, maintenance of the postabsorptive plasma glucose concentration requires a functionally and structurally intact liver, the major source of endogenous glucose production via glycogenolysis and gluconeogenesis. Total hepatectomy results in profound hypoglycemia.[190] Specific enzyme deficiencies that cause hypoglycemia are discussed in the section on hypoglycemias of infancy and childhood. Hypoglycemia due to generalized hepatic damage is discussed here.

Because the normal liver can increase the production of glucose severalfold, extensive liver disease is required to produce hypoglycemia in the absence of accelerated glucose utilization.[191] Hepatogenous hypoglycemia is most common when destruction of the liver is rapid and massive (e.g., in toxic hepatitis) and has been reported in fulminant viral hepatitis,[192] in fatty liver attributed to starvation or alcohol ingestion, and in cholangitis and biliary obstruction. It is unusual in the common forms of cirrhosis and hepatitis, although glucose metabolism is demonstrably altered (with lower postabsorptive plasma glucose concentrations, diminished glycemic responses to glucagon, and reduced hepatic glycogen) in uncomplicated viral hepatitis.[193] Hypoglycemia is common with primary malignant hepatic tumors but is the result of a glucoregulatory abnormality in such patients (see the section on non–beta

TABLE 20–2. Established and Putative Hypoglycemia-Causing Drugs

| Established | Agents Causing Hypoglycemia | |
	Commonly	Rarely
Used commonly	Insulin Sulfonylureas Alcohol	Salicylates Sulfonamides
Used rarely	Pentamidine Quinine	

Putative

Antihypertensives: β-adrenergic antagonists (nonselective > β₁-selective); enalapril
Other analgesic and anti-inflammatory drugs: indomethacin, acetaminophen, propoxyphene, phenylbutazone, penicillamine
Antigout drugs: colchicine, sulfinpyrazone
Lipid-lowering drugs: clofibrate, bezafibrate
Antibiotics: chloramphenicol, ketoconazole, para-aminosalicylic acid, ethionamide
Antipsychotic agents: haloperidol
Antianginal agents: perhexilene
Others: monoamine oxidase inhibitors, thalidomide, orphenadrine, selegiline

cell tumors). It is unusual in metastatic liver disease despite extensive hepatic replacement.[194]

Hypoglycemia in hepatic failure is the result of parenchymal dysfunction despite normal regulatory signals. In this construct, relative peripheral hyperinsulinemia can result from shunting of blood from the portal to the peripheral circulation (i.e., decreased clearance of insulin by the diseased liver),[195] and one would expect that C peptide levels, an index of insulin secretion, would be appropriately suppressed. However, in a study of five patients with acute liver failure, Vilstrup and co-workers[196] found markedly elevated plasma C peptide and insulin levels under both euglycemic and hyperglycemic conditions; the patients were demonstrably resistant to insulin (and had elevated glucagon levels) under those conditions and were not studied during hypoglycemia.

Cardiac Disease

Hypoglycemia occurs in occasional patients with severe cardiac failure of diverse causes. The pathogenesis of hypoglycemia is not known; possibilities include hepatic congestion, inanition, gluconeogenic substrate limitation, and hepatic hypoxia. The finding of elevated blood lactate levels associated with hypoglycemia[197] raises the possibility of inhibited gluconeogenesis.

Renal Disease

Postabsorptive hypoglycemia occurs in some patients with renal failure,[198–202] and the finding of a high frequency of renal insufficiency among hospitalized patients with low plasma glucose levels[89] suggests that compromised glucose counterregulation is a common feature of renal failure. However, the pathogenesis of hypoglycemia in such patients is not known and may involve multiple mechanisms.

Most patients with hypoglycemia attributed to renal failure are cachectic. One such patient had reduced glucose turnover, diminished gluconeogenesis from alanine, and reduced alanine turnover.[200] During fasting, plasma glucose levels declined, blood lactate levels did not increase, and blood alanine concentrations fell to low levels. Hypoglycemia was attributed to substrate limitation of gluconeogenesis. However, at least one patient did not respond to substrate (glycerol, alanine) administration,[202] and patients have been reported with normal blood alanine concentrations and elevated blood lactate levels, suggesting inhibited gluconeogenesis.[202] Furthermore glycemic responses to exogenous glucagon are reported to be decreased in some[202, 203] but not all studies.[204] Some patients with hypoglycemia attributed to renal failure also have diabetes mellitus.[198, 200] Presumably because of decreased renal metabolism of insulin, insulin requirements decrease with advancing renal failure in diabetes, enhancing the risk of insulin-induced hypoglycemia. Hypoglycemia can also occur during and after dialysis.[205] The extent to which reduced renal glucose production[9] might contribute to the hypoglycemia in end-stage renal disease is unknown.

Sepsis

Sepsis is associated with hypoglycemia,[88, 89, 206] and the pathogenesis of hypoglycemia has been studied in septic animals. Increased glucose utilization and, initially, glucose production characterize experimental sepsis[207–209]; hypoglycemia develops when hepatic glucose production decreases.[209, 210] Increased glucose utilization by skeletal muscle accounts for about 25% of the increase in glucose utilization[211]; increased glucose utilization by macrophage-rich tissues such as liver, spleen, and ileum appears to be responsible for most of the increase in glucose utilization.[212, 213]

The factors responsible for increased glucose turnover and failure of glucose production to keep pace with increased glucose utilization in septic patients are not entirely clear. Cytokines such as tumor necrosis factor α and interleukin-6 are thought to increase glucose utilization.[214–216] The initial increase in glucose production is, at least in part, mediated by increased glucagon[217] and catecholamine[216, 218, 219] release triggered by cytokines.[220] The later decline in glucose production, which results in hypoglycemia, is not the result of a glucose counterregulatory failure. Rather it appears to be caused by decreased hepatic responsiveness to the counterregulatory hormones.[221]

Inanition

Hypoglycemia from prolonged starvation[222] is thought to be rare in developed countries but has been reported in the United States.[223] Based on the fact that hypoglycemia can persist despite high rates of intravenous glucose infusion, these patients must have had high rates of glucose utilization. Beyond this the pathogenesis of the hypoglycemia is unknown; it is likely that glucose becomes the sole metabolic fuel in the setting of total body fat depletion. Postabsorptive hypoglycemia (with low blood alanine levels) can also occur with profound muscle atrophy,[224] perhaps the result of an insufficient availability of amino acids from muscle to support hepatic gluconeogenesis.

Hormonal Deficiencies

Except in patients with IDDM, hormonal glucoregulatory abnormalities resulting in hypoglycemia are not common, a testimony to the effectiveness of those systems under normal conditions and of the presence of redundant glucose counterregulatory mechanisms.

Cortisol and Growth Hormone Deficiency

Most adults with deficient levels of cortisol or growth hormone, or both, do not experience hypoglycemia. Indeed plasma glucose concentrations (and hepatic glucose production) after an overnight fast are indistinguishable from normal in glucocorticoid-withdrawn patients with primary adrenocortical failure[225] and in glucocorticoid-withdrawn patients with panhypopituitarism never treated with growth hormone.[59] However, important postabsorptive hypoglycemia can occur in young children with chronic deficiencies of these hormones, particularly in the neonatal period and in children less than 5 y of age.[226, 227] This observation suggests that cortisol or growth hormone, or both, play a more important role in the physiology of glucose counterregulation in early life than they do in adults. Indeed severely glucocorticoid-deficient (corticotropin-releasing hormone knockout) newborn male mice become more hypoglycemic than do normal mice during fasting.[228]

Hypoglycemia in children with cortisol deficiency or growth hormone deficiency, or both, is generally preceded by caloric deprivation, consistent with the observation that hypoglycemia can sometimes be provoked by 24 to 30 h of fasting in children with hypopituitarism who do not exhibit hypoglycemia after an overnight fast.[229, 230] This intolerance to fasting is largely corrected by glucocorticoid replacement, whereas human growth hormone replacement has little effect.[229, 230] These findings suggest that a defect in gluconeogenesis causes hypoglycemia when hepatic glycogen stores are depleted. Cortisol tends to increase gluconeogenesis both by direct effects on hepatic gluconeogenic enzyme activities and by mobilizing gluconeogenic precursors to the liver.[231, 232] Postabsorptive hypoglycemia is associated with low levels of circulating gluconeogenic precursors,[209, 233] suggesting a substrate limitation mechanism, but oral alanine administration does not reverse hypoglycemia completely.[233] Finally, in view of the fact that cortisol deficiency causes reduced epinephrine secretion,[234] presumably because adrenomedullary phenylethanolamine-N-methyltransferase is regulated by cortisol, epinephrine deficiency might contribute to the pathogenesis of hypoglycemia. Glucagon secretion is not reduced in such patients. Thus it is not surprising that glucose recovery, at least from short-term hypoglycemia, is generally normal in children with deficient secretion of cortisol or growth hormone, or both.[235]

Adults with hypopituitarism can acquire hypoglycemia when glucose utilization or loss is increased, as during exercise or pregnancy,[236] or when glucose production is impaired, as during alcohol ingestion.[237]

Glucagon and Epinephrine Deficiency

Postabsorptive hypoglycemia occurs when both glucagon and epinephrine are deficient in the setting of therapeutic insulin excess in individuals with IDDM as discussed earlier. This combination of hormonal deficiencies has not been demonstrated convincingly in other conditions. Hypoglycemia is not a feature of the epinephrine-deficient state that results from bilateral adrenalectomy when glucocorticoid replacement is adequate,[43, 45, 52] and hypoglycemia does not occur during pharmacologic blockade of catecholamine action when other systems are intact[24, 44, 45, 49, 52, 54]

Urinary[238, 239] and plasma[240] epinephrine responses to insulin-induced hypoglycemia are decreased in ketotic hypoglycemia of childhood. Therapeutic responses to ephedrine, a catecholamine-releasing drug, have been reported in uncontrolled studies of such patients.[241, 242] Some patients have diminished glycemic responses to glucagon during fasting.[241–243] Hypoglycemia has been attributed to epinephrine deficiency in one member of each of three sets of twins.[244, 245] Compared with their unaffected twins the hypoglycemic children had reduced, but not absent, urinary epinephrine responses to infused 2-deoxyglucose and to hypoglycemia induced by fasting. However the glucagon secretory status was not evaluated, and the affected infants had inappropriately high insulin levels while they were hypoglycemic.[244] Finally, reduced epinephrine excretion in infants of diabetic mothers is associated with the occurrence of neonatal hypoglycemia.[246]

Isolated glucagon deficiency would be expected to result in lowered postabsorptive plasma glucose concentrations but not hypoglycemia if epinephrine secretion were intact and insulin secretion were suppressed appropriately.[13] Postabsorptive hypoglycemia has been attributed to isolated glucagon deficiency in an adult reported in abstract[247]; a young man in whom insulinopenic hypoglycemia occurred after 18 h of fasting had plasma glucagon concentrations that were low during hypoglycemia and after arginine infusion. Glucagon infusion in a supraphysiological dose of 1 μg/min prevented hypoglycemia after 20 h of fasting.[42] The status of the sympathochromaffin system in this patient is unknown. Postabsorptive hypoglycemia has been reported in another glucagon-deficient adult, but growth hormone and cortisol secretion were also deficient.[248] Neonatal hypoglycemia has also been attributed to glucagon deficiency.[249, 250] In one such patient hypoglycemia became refractory to conventional therapy but responded to glucagon (0.4 mg of zinc protamine glucagon twice daily) when the patient was 3 mo old.[249] In this infant plasma glucagon levels were low during hypoglycemia and did not rise in response to intravenous insulin, and glucose formation from [U-14C] alanine, an index of gluconeogenesis, was decreased. Urinary catecholamine excretion was normal. However plasma insulin concentrations averaged 60 pmol/L (10 U/mL) dur-

ing hypoglycemia, and blood lactate, alanine, and ketone levels were low or in the low-normal range. Thus the hypoglycemia might have been the result of hyperinsulinism. Findings were similar in another patient with neonatal hypoglycemia attributed to glucagon deficiency.[250]

As a first step in the assessment of glucoregulatory hormone secretion, plasma counterregulatory hormone levels can be measured during spontaneous hypoglycemia. Elevated values exclude deficient secretion (although impairment of action remains a theoretical possibility). Random values that are not elevated during clinical hypoglycemic episodes do not definitively document deficient secretion but provide a clue that requires specific testing. One can measure the plasma cortisol response to injected corticotropin or the plasma 11-deoxycortisol response to metyrapone and the plasma growth hormone response to oral levodopa or clonidine or intravenous arginine (see Chapter 9). Conversely if the clinical situation permits, the most relevant information is gained by systematic assessment of the response of the counterregulatory hormones to rapid insulin-induced decrements in the plasma glucose concentration.

Non–Beta Cell Tumors

Postabsorptive hypoglycemia occurs in association with rare non–beta cell tumors. The majority are large mesenchymal tumors: fibrosarcoma, mesothelioma, rhabdomyosarcoma, leiomyosarcoma, liposarcoma, hemangiopericytoma, neurofibroma, and lymphosarcoma. More than a third are retroperitoneal, about a third are intra-abdominal, and the remainder are in the thorax. In general they are slow-growing, although many are malignant, and even partial tumor resection can cause prolonged remission of hypoglycemia.

Epithelial non–beta cell tumors that are occasionally associated with postabsorptive hypoglycemia include hepatomas, adrenocortical tumors (usually malignant), and carcinoid tumors. More than 25% of 142 patients with hepatomas reported from Hong Kong experienced hypoglycemia, and in 10% hypoglycemia was a major, recurrent problem.[251] Adrenocortical tumors that cause hypoglycemia are also generally large and may or may not secrete excessive quantities of steroid hormones. Carcinoid tumors associated with hypoglycemia can be located in the ileum, bronchus, or pancreas. Common carcinomas, including those of the stomach, colon, lung, breast, prostate, kidney, testis, and acinar pancreas, are rarely associated with hypoglycemia. Patients with leukemia, lymphoma, multiple myeloma, melanoma, teratoma, or pseudomyxoma experience hypoglycemia occasionally. In patients with leukemias, pseudohypoglycemia (low glucose levels resulting from the metabolism of glucose in vitro by the large number of leukocytes present) is more common than true hypoglycemia. Pseudohypoglycemia also occurs with benign forms of leukocytosis.[252] It is suspected because of the absence of symptoms and documented by finding normal levels of glucose in plasma promptly separated from the formed elements of the blood. Hypoglycemia also occurs rarely with neuroblastoma or paraganglioma, including pheochromocytoma.

The pathogenesis of non–beta cell tumor hypoglycemia may differ among patients and can be multifactorial in a given patient. High rates of glucose turnover are common,[253–255] and the administration of large amounts of intravenous glucose may be required to prevent recurrent hypoglycemia.[256] However the liver normally has the capacity to increase glucose production severalfold, and increased glucose utilization per se should not cause hypoglycemia if hepatic glucoregulatory, enzymatic, and substrate supply mechanisms are intact. It is thus likely that reduced or inappropriately low hepatic glucose production plays an important role in the development of non–beta cell tumor hypoglycemia.[253, 255, 257]

Insulin and related peptides have been studied most extensively in this disorder. Ectopic insulin secretion has not been demonstrated convincingly, although relative hyperinsulinemia may be present with fibrosarcomas,[258, 259] carcinoma of the cervix,[260] and carcinoid tumors.[261–263] However, insulin secretion is suppressed appropriately during hypoglycemia in most instances of non–beta cell tumor hypoglycemia. Similarly, plasma levels of insulin-like growth factor I (IGF-I or somatomedin-C), the peptide that mediates the growth-promoting effects of growth hormone and that can lower plasma glucose levels, are normal in such patients.

Instead overproduction of IGF-II, specifically an incompletely processed form ("big" IGF-II), is the cause of hypoglycemia in most patients with non–beta cell tumors.[264–274] The 150-kd complex (IGF-II, insulin-like growth factor binding protein 3 [IGFBP-3], and an acid-labile subunit) that normally transports most of the IGF-II in the circulation is greatly decreased in affected patients. As a result most of the IGF-II is transported in a smaller complex that enters target tissues more readily, and serum free IGF-II concentrations are elevated. Hypoglycemia may be the result of direct insulin-like actions of IGF-II, but IGF-II also suppresses glucagon and growth hormone levels, and these indirect effects may contribute to the pathogenesis of hypoglycemia. Finally, a radioimmunoassay of a portion of pro-IGF-II has been used to diagnose the disorder.[274]

Endogenous Hyperinsulinism

General

Hypoglycemia due to excess endogenous insulin[1, 275] can be caused by (1) a primary pancreatic islet beta cell disorder, typically a beta cell tumor (insulinoma), sometimes multiple insulinomas or microadenomatosis or, especially in young children, a functional beta cell disorder without a well-defined anatomic correlate; (2) a beta cell secretagogue, typically a sulfonylurea, at least theoretically a beta cell–stimulating autoantibody; or (3) an autoantibody to insulin. The critical feature of each disorder is failure of the plasma insulin concentration to fall to very low levels as the plasma glucose concentration declines below the physiological range. Thus although insulin levels may or may not be elevated absolutely, they are inappropriately high relative to the low plasma glucose concentration, i.e., there is relative hyperinsulinism. In a patient with unequivocal postabsorptive hypoglycemia (plasma glucose <2.5 mmol/L, [<45 mg/dL]), a plasma insulin concentration greater than 36 pmol/L (6 μU/mL) is diagnostic of endogenous hyperinsulinism.[1] In primary beta cell disorders (e.g., insulinoma) this pattern is accompanied by a plasma C peptide concentration greater than 0.2 nmol/L (0.6 ng/mL).[1] (C peptide levels are low in exogenous hyperinsulinism.[275]) Proinsulin concentrations are also elevated[1, 276–280] (>5 pmol/L [>20% of the insulin value]) in insulinoma patients. Sulfonylureas produce an indistinguishable plasma glucose, insulin, and C peptide pattern, but sulfonylureas are measurable in serum or urine, and proinsulin levels are not elevated disproportionately.[278] Antibodies to insulin[281–288] produce a similar glucose and insulin pattern, but insulin antibodies are measurable in the serum. Free C peptide levels are low, but total C peptide concentrations may not be low because of the cross-reactivity of antibodies with the C peptide portion of proinsulin.[284] Hypoglycemia can also be caused, rarely, by insulin receptor–stimulating autoantibodies.[289–294] Plasma glucose and C peptide levels are low but insulin levels can be high, presumably because receptor-bound antibodies impede the clearance of insulin.[292] Antibodies that stimulate beta cell insulin secre-

tion in vitro have been found in sera from patients with hypoglycemia,[295–297] but a corresponding clinical syndrome has not been clearly defined. Finally, although it is a theoretical possibility, ectopic insulin secretion[258–263] has not been demonstrated convincingly.

In a patient with suspected or previously documented postabsorptive hypoglycemia that is not adequately explained, it is essential to obtain plasma samples for glucose, insulin, C peptide, and proinsulin determinations and serum (or urine) for a sulfonylurea screen at a time when the patient is unequivocally hypoglycemic in the postabsorptive state, preferably with symptoms of hypoglycemia.[1, 276] (As mentioned earlier, these measurements should be obtained anytime a patient presents with hypoglycemia of obscure origin, but often this is not done.) The simplest initial approach is to measure the plasma glucose concentration (and the other parameters if the glucose level is unequivocally low) after an overnight fast and repeat the procedure if necessary. If the overnight fasted plasma glucose concentration is unequivocally low (<2.5 mmol/L [45 mg/dL]) and insulin, C peptide, proinsulin, and sulfonylurea levels are determined, the requisite diagnostic information is nearly complete. The additional measurement needed is an estimate of the serum insulin antibody titer, which need not be obtained when the patient is hypoglycemic; antibodies to insulin produce artifactually high insulin values in the double-antibody radioimmunoassays of insulin, and a negative result excludes the possibility that hypoglycemia is caused by an autoantibody to insulin.

If the overnight fasting plasma glucose concentration is normal (e.g., >5 mmol/L [90 mg/dL]) on several occasions, a judgment has to be made based on the degree of clinical suspicion of postabsorptive hypoglycemia. If it is determined that the diagnosis should be pursued or if the overnight fasting plasma glucose level is equivocally low, a prolonged fast is indicated. Intermediate attempts can be made by extending the overnight fast on an outpatient basis, but a full 72-h fast requires hospitalization. Although there are rare exceptions, the absence of hypoglycemia during a 72-h fast excludes a diagnosis of endogenous hyperinsulinism caused by a primary beta cell disorder.[1, 276] It does not exclude sulfonylurea-induced hypoglycemia at other times or hypoglycemia caused by an autoantibody to insulin, which is thought to result from dissociation of antibody-bound insulin that accumulated after the previous meal so that hypoglycemia typically occurs during the transition from the postprandial to the postabsorptive state. Other tests have been used to diagnose insulinoma,[1, 276] including the tolbutamide tolerance test[298] and the C peptide suppression test.[299]

Insulinoma

An insulinoma is the most common cause of hypoglycemia resulting from endogenous hyperinsulinism.[1, 276, 300–302] In adults, solitary insulinomas are most common, although multiple adenomas or microadenomatosis also occurs. The majority of small children and some adults do not have discrete tumors and are thought to have beta cell hyperplasia,[303] including a histologic pattern termed *nesidioblastosis*—clusters of beta cells that appear to bud from pancreatic ducts. However, the specificity of the latter is open to serious question,[304, 305] and there may be no specific histopathologic findings in patients with endogenous hyperinsulinism who do not have insulinomas.

Insulinomas are rare, the estimated incidence being one case per 250,000 patient-years,[306] but it is a curable cause of potentially lethal hypoglycemia. Insulinomas occur in both sexes (approximately 60% in women) and at all ages. In the Mayo Clinic series[306] the median age at diagnosis was 50 y in sporadic cases but 23 y in patients with multiple endocrine neoplasia, type 1[300, 301] (see Chapter 32). Insulinomas occur within the substance of the pancreas in more than 99% of patients; ectopic insulinomas have been found in areas of pancreatic heterotopia, including the wall of the duodenum, the porta hepatis, and the vicinity of the pancreas. Isulinomas are generally small, averaging 1 to 2 cm in diameter but ranging up to 15 cm. They almost always come to clinical attention because of hypoglycemia. Five to 10% of insulinomas are malignant, a diagnosis that can be made with confidence only when metastases are present. In addition to insulin these tumors can secrete human chorionic gonadotropin, corticotropin, serotonin, gastrin, glucagon, somatostatin, and pancreatic polypeptide.[300] Indeed somatostatin, glucagon, and insulin genes were expressed in four insulinomas in one report.[307] Overproduction of one hormone, such as insulin, may predominate at one time, but that of another hormone may predominate later in the course of the disease.[300, 308]

The most consistent insulin secretory abnormality with insulinoma is failure of a normal decrease in insulin secretion as the plasma glucose level declines in the postabsorptive state. This results in relative hyperinsulinism, i.e., plasma insulin levels that are inappropriately high for the ambient plasma glucose concentration, and documentation of relative hyperinsulinism is fundamental to the diagnosis. Hyperinsulinism in the portal and peripheral circulations results in low rates of glucose production and rates of glucose utilization that are inappropriately high relative to the plasma glucose concentration so that the plasma glucose concentration declines progressively in the postabsorptive state.[309]

The common symptoms of hypoglycemia with insulinomas are summarized in Table 20–3.[310] Neuroglycopenic symptoms usually predominate, but neurogenic symptoms also occur. Because the overnight fast is generally the longest interdigestive period, symptomatic episodes occur commonly in the morning before breakfast but may also occur at other postabsorptive times, especially in the late afternoon, and are often associated with exercise. Symptoms referable to mass effects are unusual even when metastases are present.

Rarely insulinomas cause postprandial (reactive) hypoglycemia without readily demonstrable postabsorptive hypoglycemia.[311] However most insulinoma patients with postprandial hypoglycemia also have postabsorptive hypoglycemia. When both forms of hypoglycemia are present the differential diagnosis is that of postabsorptive hypoglycemia.

Autoimmune Hypoglycemias

Autoantibodies to insulin can develop in the absence of insulin administration and result in postabsorptive or late postprandial hypoglycemia with relative hyperinsulinemia.[281–288] Clinically apparent autoimmune diseases are the rule in such patients. This disorder is rare in North America and Europe but is more common in Japan. Hypoglycemia attributable to an autoantibody to the insulin receptor is quite rare.[289–294] In such patients postabsorptive hypoglycemia is due to the insulin-like agonist action of the receptor antibodies. The presence of acanthosis nigricans and autoimmune phenomena may provide clues to the presence of antireceptor antibodies. Some patients have a history of glucose intolerance or diabetes mellitus. Finally, the presence of islet-stimulating antibodies in the sera of patients with hypoglycemia[295, 296] suggests the possibility of a new form of autoimmune hypoglycemia.

Management of Insulinoma

LOCALIZATION. Once a diagnosis of endogenous hyperinsulinism is established and sulfonylurea ingestion and autoimmune mechanisms are excluded, a pancreatic beta cell lesion is presumed to be present. The extent to which one should attempt to define the nature and anatomy of the beta cell lesion before surgery is a matter of judgment.[1, 276, 300, 301, 312] Computed tomography or magnetic resonance imaging of the upper abdomen should be performed initially, although a normal study does not exclude insulinoma, as the tumors are often small. Detection rates of approximately 45 to 75% have been reported.[313, 314] Most malignant insulinomas are detected and staged with computed tomographic scans.[313] Preoperative ultrasonography is of relatively little value,[313, 314] but intraoperative ultrasonography has high sensitivity and specificity, can detect tumors that are not palpable by the surgeon, and helps define the relationship of the tumor to vital structures within the pancreas such as the pancreatic duct and the great vessels.[301, 314, 315] Selective arteriography has been used widely to localize insulinomas; reported sensitivities range from 30 to 85%, but false-positive results occur.[313] Because it is invasive, arteriography is not indicated if the tumor is localized with computed tomography or magnetic resonance imaging scans. Octreotide scanning localizes about half of insulinomas.[316] Given convincing clinical and biochemical evidence of the presence of an insulinoma, surgical exploration may be indicated in patients with normal computed tomography or magnetic resonance imaging scans, particularly in view of the utility of intraoperative ultrasonography.[312]

Pancreatic venous sampling for insulin, via the percutaneous transhepatic route, has successfully localized insulinomas.[313, 314, 315, 317] However, false-positive localizations do occur and can sometimes be recognized if other pancreatic hormones (e.g., glucagon) are also measured.[317] Selective arterial injection of calcium into arteries supplying the pancreatic head (gastroduodenal and superior mesenteric arteries) and the body and tail (splenic artery) of the pancreas with measurements of hepatic venous insulin concentrations has been used successfully to localize insulinomas.[318] These invasive techniques should be reserved for difficult cases (e.g., patients in whom exploration has yielded negative findings) and can be performed in a limited number of centers.

SURGICAL TREATMENT. Because most patients with endogenous hyperinsulinism have solitary benign insulinomas, surgical therapy is generally effective.[301] For solitary insulinomas enucleation is sufficient. More extensive pancreatectomy is warranted for multiple adenomas or microadenomatosis. Even when total resection is not practical, reduction of the tumor mass often alleviates hypoglycemia, at least temporarily. When lesions are not apparent despite intraoperative ultrasonography, sequential resection starting with the tail of the pancreas is often performed. Total pancreatectomy is not advisable because of its morbidity and mortality, because partial pancreatectomy is often beneficial, and because of the availability of medical therapy for hypoglycemia. Postoperative complications include pancreatitis, peritonitis, pancreatic fistulae, abscesses, and intestinal obstruction. In a large series surgical mortality was 10%,[319] although the figure was lower in subsequent reports.[301] Hyperglycemia commonly follows effective surgery but is usually transient over a few days. Permanent diabetes mellitus occurs in about 10% of patients.

MEDICAL TREATMENT. Medical therapy is indicated in

TABLE 20–3. Symptoms of Hypoglycemia in Patients with Insulinomas

Symptom	Incidence (%)
Various combinations of diplopia, blurred vision, sweating, palpitations, or weakness	85
Confusion or abnormal behavior	80
Unconsciousness or amnesia	53
Grand mal seizures	12

From Service FJ, Dale AJD, Elveback LR, et al. Insulinoma. Clinical and diagnostic features of 60 consecutive cases. Mayo Clin Proc 1976; 51:417–429, with permission.

patients with malignant insulinomas and in those who will not, or cannot, undergo surgery. This therapy consists of measures designed to prevent hypoglycemia and, in patients with malignant tumors, to reduce the tumor burden. Diazoxide, which inhibits insulin secretion and may have additional hyperglycemic actions, is often effective in preventing hypoglycemia in patients with endogenous hyperinsulinism.[320-323] The somatostatin analogue octreotide is effective in some patients.[324-328] Available chemotherapeutic regimens are not effective in the treatment of malignant insulinomas. Streptozotocin, alone or in combination with fluorouracil, has been tried.[329, 330] Hepatic artery embolization can be used to palliate metastatic islet cell carcinomas.[331]

Hypoglycemia in Infancy and Childhood

Some causes of hypoglycemia are unique to infancy or childhood. Others persist throughout life but begin shortly after birth or in childhood. The differential diagnosis and features of postabsorptive hypoglycemia in infancy and childhood are outlined in Table 20-1.[332, 333] Drugs and particularly non–beta cell tumors are infrequent causes of hypoglycemia; critical illnesses and hormonal deficiencies are occasionally responsible; and endogenous hyperinsulinemia is more common than discrete insulinomas, at least in infants.

The fetus relies on a continuous supply of glucose from the maternal circulation, and after birth the infant must make a transition to endogenous glucose production with only intermittent exogenous glucose delivery. Perhaps because of their relatively large brains, infants have relatively high rates of glucose utilization (approximately three times higher than adults per unit of body weight[335]). Correspondingly high rates of glucose production are required to maintain the plasma glucose concentrations. Because glycogen stores are limited and feeding is intermittent, the newborn is dependent on gluconeogenesis for survival during the first 4 to 6 h after birth.[332] Therefore the appropriate glucoregulatory signals (especially low insulin and high glucagon, epinephrine, and other glucose counterregulatory hormone levels),[332, 334] structural and enzymatic integrity of the liver, and availability of sufficient gluconeogenic precursors are essential. The combination of relatively low glucose levels, hypoinsulinemia, and activated glucose counterregulatory systems also favors lipolysis, and high levels of nonesterified fatty acids and glycerol provide alternative fuels for tissues other than the brain, support glucose production, and limit glucose utilization by muscle and fat. Impairment of any of these adaptations to extrauterine life can result in transient neonatal hypoglycemia, and persistent defects at any of the steps can cause recurrent or persistent hypoglycemia. The hypoglycemias of infancy and childhood result from transient intolerance of fasting, hyperinsulinism, or a deficiency of a critical enzyme.

Transient Intolerance of Fasting

Neonatal hypoglycemia (developing in the first 72 h after birth) is usually transient.[333] It is particularly common in preterm or small-for-gestational age infants and is thought to result from incomplete development of gluconeogenic mechanisms,[336] although glucose counterregulatory responses may be impaired.[337] Congenital hypopituitarism, adrenal hypoplasia, or adrenal hyperplasia (e.g., C_{21}-hydroxylase deficiency) can cause hypoglycemia early in life.

In general, children tolerate fasting less well than do adults, and hypoglycemia is usual after 24 to 48 h of fasting in normal children.[338] The syndrome of ketotic hypoglycemia of childhood may constitute that fraction of young persons who are the least tolerant of fasting.[339] Hypoglycemia occurs when feeding is interrupted, typically during an intercurrent illness.

This syndrome has its onset between ages 2 and 5 and typically remits spontaneously before age 10. It appears to involve diminished provision of alanine (a major gluconeogenic substrate) to the liver from muscle.[340, 341] Blood alanine levels are low during hypoglycemia, and alanine infusion increases the plasma glucose level. Glycogenolytic and gluconeogenic mechanisms appear to be intact and, aside from low epinephrine levels,[238-243] glucoregulatory signals are appropriate. Deficient epinephrine secretion may impair alanine mobilization, as epinephrine accelerates alanine turnover in humans.[342] In contrast, epinephrine deficiency per se does not cause hypoglycemia in adults, as discussed earlier.

Hyperinsulinism

The most common cause of hyperinsulinemic neonatal hypoglycemia is maternal diabetes.[333] Infants of diabetic mothers are hyperglycemic (in proportion to the mother's hyperglycemia) and correspondingly hyperinsulinemic. Presumably reflecting chronic stimulation of fetal insulin secretion in utero and the failure of this stimulation to become suppressed normally shortly after birth, transient neonatal hypoglycemia occurs. Transient hyperinsulinemia also underlies neonatal hypoglycemia in infants with Rh factor incompatibility or the Beckwith-Wiedemann syndrome (macroglossia, omphalocele, and visceromegaly). The mechanism or mechanisms of hyperinsulinemia in these disorders is unknown. Hypoglycemia can also follow exchange transfusion, resulting from hyperinsulinemia stimulated by the glucose administered during the procedure. Hypoglycemia can also be caused by drugs given to the mother, including agents that stimulate fetal insulin secretion (e.g., a sulfonylurea) or that produce maternal and fetal hyperglycemia and thus fetal hyperinsulinemia (e.g., a β_2-adrenergic agonist used to delay labor). Accidental or malicious administration of sulfonylureas or insulin and the development of autoantibodies to insulin are rare causes of hypoglycemia with absolute or relative hyperinsulinemia in children.

Postabsorptive hypoglycemia caused by otherwise unexplained endogenous hyperinsulinism may persist from the neonatal period or may develop in the first year of life.[333, 343] Such patients rarely have discrete insulinomas and are usually treated initially with diazoxide, with or without octreotide; near-total pancreatectomy may be indicated.[343] Conversely, hyperinsulinemic hypoglycemia that develops after the first year of life is more likely to be caused by an insulinoma.

Persistent hyperinsulinemic hypoglycemia of infancy is an autosomal recessive disorder that is the most common cause of nontransient hypoglycemia developing in the neonatal period.[344, 345] Excessive insulin secretion in this disorder appears to be caused by mutations in the sulfonylurea receptor gene on chromosome 11.[346] The sulfonylurea receptor is functionally linked to a beta cell adenosine triphosphate–sensitive potassium channel, and closure of the channel triggers insulin secretion.[347] Two splice mutations in the sulfonylurea receptor gene that segregated with the persistent hyperinsulinemic hypoglycemia of infancy phenotype were found in affected individuals from nine families.[346]

Enzymatic Defects

Mutations of a gene that encodes a transcription factor (C/EBPα) that *trans*-activates several energy-related genes cause fatal neonatal hypoglycemia in mice.[348] Comparable disorders have not been documented in humans, but several enzyme deficiencies, generally inherited as autosomal recessive traits, cause hypoglycemia in humans. If the disorder can be treated to minimize the impact of recurrent hypoglycemia, hypoglycemia persists into adult life. These disorders are typically diagnosed in infancy or childhood, but mild forms are sometimes first recognized in adults.[349, 350] Clinical features and biochemical patterns suggest a subset of diagnostic possibilities, but definitive diagnosis generally requires documentation of deficient enzyme activity in affected tissues. Given the increasing number of defined underlying mutations and rapidly advancing technology, molecular diagnosis will undoubtedly become possible for these disorders. Although glucose metabolism is ultimately affected, the primary enzymatic defect can involve a step in the metabolism of carbohydrate, protein, or fat outlined in Figure 20–1.

Enzymatic defects in carbohydrate metabolism[332, 333] that cause postabsorptive hypoglycemia include several of the glycogen storage diseases,[351] glycogen synthase deficiency,[351] and fructose-1,6-bisphosphatase deficiency.[352] Fructose-1-phosphate aldolase deficiency (hereditary fructose intolerance)[352] and galactose-1-phosphate uridyl transferase deficiency (galactosemia)[353] can cause postprandial hypoglycemia. Glycogen storage diseases that cause postabsorptive hypoglycemia include type I glycogen storage disease (glucose-6-phosphatase deficiency, von Gierke's disease), type III glycogen storage disease (debrancher deficiency, limit dextrinosis, Cori's or Forbes' disease), and type VI glycogen storage disease (liver phosphorylase deficiency, Hers' disease, and phosphorylase kinase deficiency).[351]

As first documented by Cori and Cori[354] in 1952, deficient glucose-6-phosphatase activity causes type I glycogen storage disease. Glucose-6-phosphatase normally is highly expressed only in liver, kidneys, and pancreatic beta cells. The active site of the enzyme is inside the lumen of the endoplasmic reticulum, and its substrates and products must cross the endoplasmic reticulum membrane.[351] Deficient glucose-6-phosphatase activity can be caused by deficiency of the catalytic subunit of the enzyme (type Ia), deficiency of the glucose-6-phosphatase regulatory protein (IaSP), deficiency of the hepatic microsomal glucose-6-phosphate transport system termed *T1* (type Ib), deficiency of the microsomal phosphate transport system termed *T2β* (type Ic), or a defect in microsomal glucose transport caused by deficiency of the GLUT-7 glucose transporter (type Id). Several mutations have been described.[351, 355] Type I glycogen storage disease is the prototype glycogen storage disease.[351] Because hydrolysis of glucose-6-phosphate to glucose is the common pathway for glucose production from either glycogenolysis or gluconeogenesis, glucose-6-phosphatase deficiency causes profound postabsorptive hypoglycemia with hypoinsulinemia; activated glucose counterregulatory systems; elevated lactate, alanine, and ketone body levels; metabolic acidosis with hyperuricemia; and elevated triglyceride levels. It can present in the neonatal period or at 3 to 4 mo of age with hepatomegaly or hypoglycemic seizures, or both. Hepatomegaly (caused by hepatocyte accumulation of fat and glycogen) is a universal finding. With the exception of hepatomegaly the abnormalities can be reversed by the prevention of hypoglycemia with frequent feedings during waking hours and continuous intragastric glucose infusion during sleep[356] or with bedtime administration of uncooked cornstarch.[357] Liver transplantation corrects hypoglycemia and the associated metabolic abnormalities.[358] Adults with (presumably inadequately treated) type I glycogen storage disease have a high incidence of hepatic adenomas and renal disease, including focal glomerulosclerosis.[350] Interestingly, renal transplantation does not correct hypoglycemia.[351] The mechanism by which patients with type I glycogen storage disease maintain some level, albeit subnormal, of hepatic glucose production is unclear.[359]

Type III glycogen storage disease resembles the type I disorder in infancy and childhood, but most affected adults are asymptomatic. Hypoglycemia, if present, is mild in type VI glycogen storage disease.[351] Glycogen synthase deficiency, which causes hypoglycemia without hepatomegaly in early infancy, is rare.[351] Because it blocks gluconeogenesis, fructose-1,6-bisphosphatase deficiency causes postabsorptive hypoglycemia with lactic acidosis, ketosis, and elevated alanine levels that if unrecognized can be fatal in the neonatal period.[352, 360] Hyperlipidemia, hyperuricemia, and hepatomegaly (due to fat accumulation) occur as in type I glycogen storage disease.

Postprandial rather than postabsorptive hypoglycemia can be a feature of hereditary fructose intolerance[352] and, rarely, galactosemia.[353] Fructose-1-phosphate aldolase deficiency, the enzymatic defect in hereditary fructose intolerance, causes severe hypoglycemia and vomiting after fructose ingestion. Fructose-1-phosphate accumulates and inhibits glycogenolysis (at the phosphorylase level) and gluconeogenesis (at the mutant aldolase level). The patients are asymptomatic when fructose is eliminated from the diet. Galactose uridyl transferase deficiency, one of the causes of galactosemia, can also cause postprandial hypoglycemia that has been attributed to inhibition of glycogenolysis.[353, 361]

Deficiencies of enzymes of amino acid metabolism can also cause postabsorptive hypoglycemia. Maple syrup urine disease, or branched chain ketoaciduria, is caused by a deficiency of the branched chain α-keto acid dehydrogenase complex.[362] The levels of the branched chain amino acids (leucine, isoleucine, and valine), particularly leucine, are elevated in plasma and urine. The pathogenesis of hypoglycemia is not entirely clear, although it results from defective gluconeogenesis.[363, 364] Hypoglycemia due to impaired gluconeogenesis also occurs in methylmalonic aciduria.[365]

Several defects that ultimately impair fatty acid oxidation result in postabsorptive hypoglycemia with *hypo*ketonemia.[366–370] They include defects of the carnitine cycle (carnitine transport defect, carnitine palmitoyltransferase I [CPT-I]) deficiency, carnitine-acylcarnitine translocase deficiency, carnitine palmitoyltransferase II [CPT-II] deficiency), defects of the beta oxidation spiral (long chain acyl-CoA dehydrogenase deficiency, long chain L-3-hydroxyacyl-CoA dehydrogenase deficiency, short chain L-3-hydroxyacyl-CoA dehydrogenase deficiency, 2,4-dienoyl-CoA reductase deficiency, medium chain acyl-CoA dehydrogenase deficiency, short chain acyl-CoA dehydrogenase deficiency), several defects of electron transfer, and defects in ketogenesis (HMG-CoA lyase deficiency).

Normally, low insulin and high glucagon (and catecholamine) states such as fasting favor the mobilization of fatty acids from fat (lipolysis) and their transport to the liver. These regulatory conditions also favor fatty acid oxidation with adenosine triphosphate formation and ketogenesis over the synthesis of triglycerides, phospholipids, and cholesterol esters or peroxisomal oxidation. Mitochondrial fatty acid oxidation (especially in skeletal muscle) or ketogenesis (especially in liver) requires transport of fatty acids across the plasma membrane, formation of fatty acyl-CoA derivatives, and transport of the latter into mitochondria. Since the inner mitochondrial membranes are not permeable to long chain (as opposed to medium and short chain) fatty acyl-CoA esters, the former are transesterified to fatty acylcarnitines at the outer surface of the membranes (CPT-I), translocated across the membranes (translocase), and reconverted to the fatty acyl-CoA esters, which can then be oxidized or converted to ketones, at the inner surface of the membranes (CPT-II). Insulin decreases fat oxidation and ketogenesis both by decreasing lipolysis, and therefore decreasing fatty acid levels, and by increasing lipogenesis and the formation of malonyl-CoA, which inhibits CPT-I activity. Catecholamines favor fatty acid oxidation and ketogenesis by stimulating lipolysis. Glucagon does so by decreasing malonyl-CoA levels. Any enzymatic defect in the carnitine cycle, the beta oxidation spiral, or electron transport decreases fatty acid oxidation and reciprocally increases glucose metabolism and postabsorptive hypoglycemia with hypoketonemia.[371] Reduced plasma carnitine levels (20 to 50% of normal) are the rule in these disorders, but extremely low plasma carnitine levels characterize the carnitine transport defect, a true carnitine deficiency state that is responsive to carnitine supplementation.[366] Specific enzymatic defects are suggested by specific acylcarnitine and organic acid profiles.[366]

Medium chain acyl-CoA dehydrogenase deficiency is the most commonly diagnosed disorder of fatty acid oxidation.[366, 370] The affected child typically presents with postabsorptive hypoglycemia without ketosis; intravenous glucose generally causes prompt improvement. Some have presented with Reye's syndrome. All are at risk for sudden death, presumably from cardiac causes. Although hypoglycemia is common, coma may be caused by other factors, perhaps toxic effects of accumulated fatty acids or their metabolites, since coma can occur without hypoglycemia.[366] Treatment includes provision of adequate caloric intake, avoidance of fasting, and support of the blood glucose level during intercurrent illnesses.

POSTPRANDIAL (REACTIVE) HYPOGLYCEMIAS

Postprandial (reactive, stimulative) hypoglycemia occurs exclusively after meals, typically within 4 h after food ingestion. All disorders that cause postabsorptive hypoglycemia can also result in hypoglycemia detected after a meal. However the diagnostic and therapeutic approach is that of postabsorptive hypoglycemia in such a patient.

Congenital deficiencies of enzymes of carbohydrate metabolism, such as hereditary fructose intolerance[352] and galactosemia,[353] mentioned earlier, are rare causes of the postprandial hypoglycemia that becomes apparent early in life. Postprandial hypoglycemia can occur in patients who have undergone gastric surgery that causes rapid movement of ingested food into the small intestine (e.g., gastrectomy, gastroenterostomy, pyloroplasty, gastric bypass).[372, 373] This type of postprandial hypoglycemia, termed *alimentary hypoglycemia*, is thought to be the result of marked early hyperinsulinemia caused by rapid absorption of ingested nutrients or the enhanced secretion of insulinotropic gut factors, or both. Hypoglycemia occurs early after food ingestion, typically within 1.5 to 3 h. Symptoms of hypoglycemia must be distinguished from those of the dumping syndrome—abdominal fullness, nausea, weakness—which occur less than 1 h after meals.

The frequency and even the existence of clinically relevant idiopathic (or functional) postprandial hypoglycemia is a matter of debate.[1] Idiopathic postprandial hypoglycemia is often erroneously diagnosed by patients and by physicians. For example, only 16 of 118 patients evaluated for suspected postprandial hypoglycemia in one series had both a plasma glucose concentration lower than the 10th percentile of asymptomatic individuals and typical symptoms after an oral glucose load; only 5 of those 16 patients had similar symptoms after their regular meals.[374] Furthermore most patients thought to have hypoglycemic symptoms and low glucose levels after glucose ingestion have normal glucose levels after a mixed meal.[375–377] In one series in which blood glucose was measured during symptomatic episodes, only 5% of 132 episodes were associated with blood glucose levels of 2.8 mmol/L (50 mg/dL) or less.[377]

A diagnosis of postprandial hypoglycemia should *not* be made on the basis of plasma glucose concentrations during an oral glucose tolerance test. The lower limits of normal for plasma glucose concentrations late after glucose ingestion can be defined in statistical terms. For example, in 650 individuals who remained asymptomatic after ingestion of 100 g of glucose, glucose concentrations at nadir were as follows: lower

2.5th percentile, 2.2 mmol/L (40 mg/dL); 5th percentile, 2.4 mmol/L (43 mg/dL); 10th percentile, 2.6 mmol/L (47 mg/dL); and 25th percentile, 3 mmol/L (54 mg/dL).[375] However, because the lowest glucose levels in these individuals cause no recognizable symptoms, are self-limited, have no known long-term ill effects, and do not imply the presence of disease, there is no reason to arbitrarily classify 2.5 or 5% of the population as abnormal. Thus the diagnosis of reactive hypoglycemia requires appropriate symptoms temporally related to a low plasma glucose concentration after a mixed meal and relief of symptoms as the plasma glucose concentration rises (Whipple's triad).[1] The diagnosis cannot be made on the basis of an oral glucose tolerance test.

The pathogenesis of true idiopathic postprandial hypoglycemia (fulfilling Whipple's triad) is unknown. There is no evidence that insulin secretion is excessive. Increased sensitivity to insulin[378, 379] and normal monocyte insulin receptors[378] have been reported. These data are consistent with either increased cellular responsiveness to insulin at a site or sites of action distal to the insulin receptors or with decreased counterregulatory hormone secretion or action. As discussed earlier, glucagon, in concert with dissipation of insulin, normally regulates the transition from exogenous glucose delivery to endogenous glucose production late after glucose ingestion.[52] Epinephrine normally is not critical but compensates partially and becomes critical when glucagon secretion is deficient. Thus, deficient glucagon secretion would plausibly explain the pathogenesis of the postprandial syndrome, including compensatory enhancement of epinephrine secretion, the production of symptoms attributable to the sympathochromaffin response, and the prevention of severe hypoglycemia and restoration of euglycemia. In accord with this possibility, lower plasma glucagon levels have been reported in persons with glucose nadirs less than 2.8 mmol/L (50 mg/dL) as compared with those with higher glucose nadirs after glucose ingestion.[380] However, glucagon levels were lower at baseline as well and were not discernibly lower in two patients with "severe" hypoglycemia (nadirs of 1.5 and 1.3 mmol/L [27 and 23 mg/dL]).[380] Whether those with lower glucose nadirs had symptoms was not stated. Moreover in another study, similarly selected patients (glucose nadir less than 2.8 mmol/L [50 mg/dL]) had elevated glucagon-like immunoreactivity and normal pancreatic glucagon levels after glucose ingestion.[381] Enhanced, and presumably compensatory, epinephrine responses have been reported in patients with sweating, tremor, and increased heart rate temporally related to the low glucose nadir late after glucose ingestion.[382]

Diets low in carbohydrate and high in protein are commonly recommended to patients designated as having reactive hypoglycemia. Their efficacy has not been established by controlled trials. Frequent feedings and avoidance of simple sugars are also advised. Anticholinergic drugs have been reported to be beneficial in patients with idiopathic reactive hypoglycemia but may cause undesirable side effects.[383] Propranolol reduces symptoms (except diaphoresis) in patients with postgastrectomy hypoglycemia, and pectin is said to decrease postprandial hypoglycemia after gastric surgery.[384] Such patients have also been treated surgically with reversal of a segment of proximal jejunum.[385]

TREATMENT OF POSTABSORPTIVE HYPOGLYCEMIA

In view of the vulnerability of the brain to prolonged hypoglycemia, the plasma glucose concentration must be raised at least to normal levels as rapidly as possible, and recurrence of hypoglycemia must be prevented. Because it is self-limited, postprandial hypoglycemia rarely requires emergent treatment. In contrast, postabsorptive hypoglycemias are typically persistent or progressive and require short- and long-term therapy.

The urgent treatment of iatrogenic hypoglycemia in individuals with IDDM or NIDDM—with oral carbohydrate or glucose per se or with parenteral glucagon or glucose—was discussed earlier in the section on hypoglycemia in diabetes mellitus. Clinical improvement should occur within about 15 min after the plasma glucose level is raised and maintained provided that brain damage has not occurred. Whenever possible the presence of hypoglycemia should be documented before therapy, and the response of plasma glucose to therapy should be followed by frequent measurements of the plasma glucose level. If these are not available and there is no clinical response within 15 min, the initial therapy should be repeated and access to plasma glucose monitoring and intravenous glucose infusion should be obtained as soon as possible. Even if there is a response to initial therapy, glucose monitoring is essential to ensure maintenance of the plasma glucose concentration.

Although central nervous system function usually recovers promptly after restoration of the plasma glucose level, recovery may be delayed, perhaps because of cerebral edema. Unconsciousness lasting more than 30 min after the plasma glucose concentration has been raised to normal and maintained is referred to as *posthypoglycemic coma*[386] and is treated with intravenous mannitol (40 g as a 20% solution over 20 min) or glucocorticoids (e.g., dexamethasone, 10 mg), or both,[386–388] along with maintenance of normal plasma glucose levels.

Definitive treatment of the postabsorptive hypoglycemias requires correction of the underlying defect whenever possible. When that is not possible attempts must be made to increase exogenous or endogenous glucose delivery and to limit glucose utilization. Although the judicious use of snacks is a useful component of therapy for individuals with IDDM, frequent feedings are less than ideal for the long-term treatment of chronic hypoglycemia. One problem is weight gain. However, frequent feedings, even overnight gastric infusions, are sometimes necessary when other measures are inadequate.

Hypoglycemia caused by drugs is limited to the duration of action of the offending drug. The management is straightforward: discontinuation of the drug (at least temporarily), maintenance of the plasma glucose level while drug action continues, and adjustment of subsequent drug regimens to avoid recurrent hypoglycemia—if the causative drug is known. Therapy is more difficult if the drug is used surreptitiously.

As discussed earlier, postabsorptive hypoglycemia due to endogenous hyperinsulinism is often curable by the surgical removal of an insulinoma. If this is not possible because of multiple or metastatic tumors or the absence of a definable lesion, diazoxide is sometimes effective.[320–323] Diazoxide (100 to 800 mg/d in adults and 5 to 30 mg/kg/d in infants) raises the plasma glucose concentration in large part by suppressing insulin secretion. The finding of an exaggerated insulin secretory response to tolbutamide during diazoxide administration[389] suggests that diazoxide inhibits insulin release. Diazoxide is bound tightly to albumin and has a plasma half-time of 20 to 30 h.[390] When given by rapid intravenous injection it is a potent hypotensive drug, but when given orally or by slow intravenous infusion it has little hypotensive action; indeed hypertensive responses may occur. Although chemically related to the thiazide diuretics, diazoxide causes sodium retention. Coadministration of a thiazide diuretic both limits sodium retention and potentiates the hyperglycemic action of diazoxide.[322, 323] Both edema formation and gastrointestinal side effects (anorexia, nausea, sometimes vomiting) are dose-related. Generalized growth of lanugo hair (hypertrichosis

lanuginosa) may occur during prolonged therapy. Allergic reactions, including skin rashes and agranulocytosis, are rare.

The treatment of hypoglycemia associated with non–beta cell tumors involves short-term measures pending effective medical, surgical, or radiotherapeutic treatment of the tumor. Administration of a glucocorticoid or human growth hormone sometimes alleviates hypoglycemia. The former, but not the latter, has been reported to reduce IGF-II levels.[391] Hypoglycemia resulting from glucocorticoid deficiency is corrected by replacement therapy. Hypoglycemia is rarely an indication for human growth hormone replacement. Remissions of autoimmune hypoglycemias have been associated with immunosuppressive therapy, including glucocorticoids, but controlled trials are lacking. The treatment of hypoglycemia due to inanition, hepatic or renal disease, cardiac failure, or sepsis includes short-term measures and, when possible, treatment or management of the underlying disease process. The treatment of the hypoglycemias of infancy and childhood, and that of postprandial hypoglycemia, were already discussed.

APPROACH TO THE PATIENT WITH HYPOGLYCEMIA

The first step in the care of a patient with suspected hypoglycemia is clear documentation that an abnormally low plasma glucose concentration is in fact present. Establishment of the relationship between documented hypoglycemia and symptoms and signs attributable to hypoglycemia is fundamental, as is the distinction between postprandial and postabsorptive hypoglycemic states. As emphasized throughout this chapter, the presence of postabsorptive hypoglycemia raises the distinct possibility of a potentially fatal disorder and demands conclusive diagnostic assessment, treatment, and follow-up. The presence of postprandial hypoglycemia is diagnostically irrelevant in a patient with postabsorptive hypoglycemia. In contrast, isolated postprandial hypoglycemia is self-limited, rarely produces ominous symptoms, and is not progressive.

Hypoglycemia is often suspected on the basis of symptoms that are nonspecific and is more often suspected than diagnosed. In some patients plasma drawn for reasons other than suspected hypoglycemia is reported to have a low glucose concentration. Although artifact (e.g., glycolysis in vitro) is reasonably suspected under these conditions, true hypoglycemia must be considered. Occasionally patients are found to be hypoglycemic at the time of presentation to a hospital. This represents a frequently missed diagnostic opportunity; samples should be saved for subsequent measurements of insulin, C peptide, proinsulin, and sulfonylureas should the hypoglycemia be persistent or recurrent and its cause not apparent.

If hypoglycemia is documented in the absence of an obvious cause, three questions need to be addressed: Is hypoglycemia a recurrent phenomenon? Are there associated symptoms that are relieved when the plasma glucose concentration is raised to normal (Whipple's triad)? Is this postabsorptive hypoglycemia? These questions are approached initially by measurement of the plasma glucose concentration after an overnight fast, which is repeated if necessary. The same procedure is appropriate in suspected hypoglycemia. If this measurement answers all three questions in the affirmative, the hypoglycemic mechanism must be defined. If the plasma glucose concentration is normal after an overnight fast, a judgment must be made regarding the need for a more prolonged diagnostic fast. Once postabsorptive hypoglycemia is excluded the physician must decide whether postprandial hypoglycemia is likely enough to warrant further testing by frequent plasma glucose measurements after meals.

A conservative approach in patients with affirmative answers to the foregoing questions is as follows: if a plausible hypoglycemic mechanism (e.g., drugs, adrenocortical insufficiency) is apparent and treatable or self-limited, further diagnostic evaluation should not be undertaken with the expectation that hypoglycemia will not be a continuing problem. This approach requires documentation that hypoglycemia resolves. Rarely two different causes for hypoglycemia coexist. Obviously it would be a serious error to assume an untreatable hypoglycemic mechanism and miss a treatable one.

If a plausible hypoglycemic mechanism is not apparent after the initial history, physical examination, and routine laboratory determinations in a patient with documented postabsorptive hypoglycemia, the initial diagnostic considerations should include hyperinsulinism caused by an insulinoma or related beta cell disorder or the surreptitious use of sulfonylureas or insulin. Clinically occult hormonal deficiencies or a non–beta cell tumor, the surreptitious use of alcohol, autoimmune hypoglycemias, and occult defects in glucogenic enzyme systems are less likely possibilities.

This chapter has emphasized that hypoglycemia is an uncommon clinical event except when produced as a side effect of the treatment of diabetes. Because of its danger, however, it is a tragedy to miss the diagnosis or to treat the condition improperly.

REFERENCES

1. Service FJ. Hypoglycemic disorders. N Engl J Med 1995; 332:1144–1152.
2. Cryer PE: Hypoglycemia: the limiting factor in the management of IDDM. Diabetes 1994; 43:1378–1389.
3. Cryer PE, Fisher JN, Shamoon H: Hypoglycemia. Diabetes Care 1994; 17:734–755.
4. Frier BM, Fisher BM (eds): Hypoglycemia and Diabetes. London: Edward Arnold, 1993.
5. Cryer PE, Gerich JE. Hypoglycemia in insulin dependent diabetes mellitus: interplay of insulin excess and compromised glucose counterregulation. In: Porte D, Sherwin R, Rifkin H, eds. Ellenberg and Rifkin's Diabetes Mellitus, Theory and Practice. 5th ed. New York: Elsevier Science Publishing, in press.
6. Perriello G, Jorde R, Nurjhan N, et al. Estimation of glucose-alanine-lactate-glutamine cycles in postabsorptive humans: role of skeletal muscle. Am J Physiol 1995; 269:E443–E450.
7. Garber AJ, Cryer PE, Santiago JV, et al. The role of adrenergic mechanisms in the substrate and hormonal response to insulin induced hypoglycemia in man. J Clin Invest 1976; 58:7–15.
8. Rothman DL, Magnusson I, Katz LD, et al. Quantitation of hepatic glycogenolysis and gluconeogenesis in fasting humans with ^{13}C NMR. Science 1991; 254:573–576.
9. Stumvoll M, Chintalapudi U, Perriello G, et al. Uptake and release of glucose by the human kidney. J Clin Invest 1995; 96:2528–2533.
10. Owen OE, Felig P, Morgan AP, et al. Liver and kidney metabolism during prolonged starvation. J Clin Invest 1969; 48:574–583.
11. Radziuk J, McFonald TJ, Ruenstein D, et al. Initial splanchnic extraction of ingested glucose in normal man. Metabolism 1978; 27:657–669.
12. Heller SR, Cryer PE. Hypoinsulinemia is not critical to glucose recovery from hypoglycemia in humans. Am J Physiol 1991; 261:E41–E48.
13. Cryer PE. Glucose counterregulation: the prevention and correction of hypoglycemia in humans. Am J Physiol 1993; 264:E149–E155.
14. Rizza RA, Mandarino L, Gerich JE. Dose-response characteristics for the effects of insulin on production and utilization of glucose in man. Am J Physiol 1981; 240:630–639.
15. Cryer PE. Glucagon and glucose counterregulation. In: Lefebvre P, ed. Glucagon. Vol 3. Berlin: Springer-Verlag, 1996: 149–158.
16. Rizza RA, Gerich JE. Persistent effect of sustained hyperglucagonemia on glucose production in man. J Clin Endocrinol Metab 1979; 48:352–353.
17. Cherrington AD, Williams PE, Shulman GI, et al. Differential time course of glucagon's effect on glycogenolysis and gluconeogenesis in the conscious dog. Diabetes 1981; 30:180–187.
18. Cryer PE. Catecholamines, pheochromocytoma and diabetes. Diabetes Rev 1993; 1:309–317.
19. Rizza RA, Cryer PE, Haymond MW, et al. Adrenergic mechanisms for the effect of epinephrine on glucose production and clearance in man. J Clin Invest 1980; 65:682–689.
20. Berk MA, Clutter WE, Skor D, et al. Enhanced glycemic responsiveness to epinephrine in insulin dependent diabetes mellitus is the result of the inability to secrete insulin. J Clin Invest 1985; 75:1842–1851.
21. Gerich JE, Lorenzi M, Tsalikian E, et al. Studies on the mechanisms of epinephrine induced hyperglycemia in man. Diabetes 1976; 25:65–71.
22. Gray DE, Lickley HLA, Vranic M. Physiologic effects of epinephrine on glucose turnover and plasma free fatty acid concentrations mediated independently of glucagon. Diabetes 1980; 29:600–608.
23. Deibert DC, DeFronzo RA. Epinephrine induced insulin resistance in man. J Clin Invest 1980; 65:717–721.
24. Rosen SG, Clutter WE, Shah SD, et al. Direct, α-adrenergic stimulation of hepatic glucose production in postabsorptive man. Am J Physiol 1983; 245:E616–E626.
25. MacGorman LR, Rizza RA, Gerich JE. Physiological concentrations of growth hormone exert insulin-like and insulin antagonist effects on both hepatic and extrahepatic tissues in man. J Clin Endocrinol Metab 1981; 53:556–559.
26. Shamoon H, Hendler R, Sherwin RS. Synergistic interactions among antiinsulin hormones in the pathogenesis of stress hyperglycemia in humans. J Clin Endocrinol Metab 1981; 52:1235–1241.
27. Lautt WW. Hepatic nerves: a review of their functions and effects. Can J Physiol Pharmacol 1980; 58:105–123.
28. Nobin ABF, Ingemansson S, Jarhult J, et al. Organization and function of the sympathetic innervation of the human liver. Acta Physiol Scand 1977; 452(Suppl):103–106.
29. Boyle PJ, Liggett SB, Shah SD, et al. Direct muscarinic cholinergic inhibition of hepatic glucose production in humans. J Clin Invest 1988; 82:445–449.
30. Hers HG. The control of glycogen metabolism in the liver. Annu Rev Biochem 1976; 45:167–189.
31. Shulman GI, Liljenquist JE, Williams PE, et al. Glucose disposal during insulinopenia in somatostatin-treated dogs. The roles of glucose and glucagon. J Clin Invest 1978; 62:487–491.
32. Sacca L, Cryer PE, Sherwin RS. Blood glucose regulates the effects of insulin and counterregulatory hormones on glucose production in vivo. Diabetes 1979; 28:533–536.
33. Sacca L, Hendler R, Sherwin RS. Hyperglycemia inhibits glucose production in man independent of changes in glucoregulatory hormones. J Clin Endocrinol Metab 1979; 47:1160–1163.
34. Liljenquist JE, Mueller GL, Cherrington AD, et al. Hyperglycemia per se (insulin and glucagon withdrawn) can inhibit hepatic glucose production in man. J Clin Endocrinol Metab 1979; 48:171–174.
35. Sacca L, Sherwin R, Hendler R, et al. Influence of continuous physiologic hyperinsulinemia on glucose kinetics and counterregulatory hormones in normal and diabetic humans. J Clin Invest 1979; 63:849–857.
36. Palmer JP, Henry DP, Benson JW, et al. Glucagon response to hypoglycemia in sympathectomized man. J Clin Invest 1976; 57:522–525.
37. Palmer JP, Werner PL, Hollander P, et al. Evaluation of the control of glucagon secretion by the parasympathetic nervous system in man. Metabolism 1979; 28:549–552.
38. Werner PL, Benson JW, Brodsky JB, et al. Comparison of glucagon response to 2-deoxy-D-glucose and hypoglycemia in man. Am J Physiol 1980; 239:E227–E231.
39. Towler DA, Havlin CE, Craft S, et al. Mechanisms of awareness of hypoglycemia: perception of neurogenic (predominantly cholinergic) rather than neuroglycopenic symptoms. Diabetes 1993; 42:1791–1798.
40. Mathias CJ, Christensen NJ, Corbett JL, et al. Plasma catecholamines during paroxysmal neurogenic hypertension in quadriplegic man. Circ Res 1976; 39:204–208.
41. Brodows RG, Pi-Sunyer FX, Campbell RG. Neural control of counterregulatory events during glucopenia in man. J Clin Invest 1973; 52:1841–1844.
42. Gerich J, Davis J, Lorenzi M, et al. Hormonal mechanisms of recovery from insulin-induced hypoglycemia in man. Am J Physiol 1979; 236:E380–E385.
43. Shah SD, Tse TF, Clutter WE, et al. The human sympathochromaffin system. Am J Physiol 1984; 247:E380–E384.
44. Clarke WL, Santiago JV, Thomas L, et al. Adrenergic mechanisms in recovery from hypoglycemia in man: adrenergic blockade. Am J Physiol 1979; 236:E147–E152.
45. Rizza RA, Cryer PE, Gerich JE. Role of glucagon, epinephrine and growth hormone in human glucose counterregulation: effects of somatostatin and adrenergic blockade on plasma glucose recovery and glucose flux rates following insulin induced hypoglycemia. J Clin Invest 1979; 64:62–71.
46. Popp DA, Shah SD, Cryer PE. The role of epinephrine mediated β-adrenergic mechanisms in hypoglycemic glucose counterregulation and posthypoglycemic hyperglycemia in insulin-dependent diabetes mellitus. J Clin Invest 1982; 69:315–326.
47. White NH, Skor DA, Cryer PE, et al. Identification of type 1 diabetic patients at increased risk for hypoglycemia during intensive therapy. N Engl J Med 1983; 308:485–491.
48. Gray RS, Scarlett JA, Criffin J, et al. In vivo deactivation of peripheral, hepatic and pancreatic insulin action in man. Diabetes 1983; 31:929–936.
49. Rosen SG, Clutter WE, Berk MA, et al. Epinephrine supports the postabsorptive plasma glucose concentration, and prevents hypoglycemia, when glucagon secretion is deficient in man. J Clin Invest 1984; 73:405–411.
50. Rosen SG, Clutter WE, Berk MA, et al.. Insulin, glucagon and catecholamines in the prevention of hypoglycemia during fasting in humans. Am J Physiol 1989; 256:E651–E661.
51. Tse TF, Clutter WE, Shah SD, et al. Neuroendocrine responses to glucose ingestion in man: specificity, temporal relationships and quantitative aspects. J Clin Invest 1983; 721:270–277.
52. Tse TF, Clutter WE, Shah SD, et al. Mechanisms of postprandial glucose counterregulation in man: physiologic roles of glucagon and epinephrine

vis-a-vis insulin in the prevention of hypoglycemia late after glucose ingestion. J Clin Invest 1983; 72:278–286.

53. Hirsch IB, Marker JC, Smith L, et al. Insulin and glucagon in the prevention of hypoglycemia during exercise in humans. Am J Physiol 1991; 260:E695–E704.

54. Marker JC, Hirsch IB, Smith L, et al. Catecholamines in the prevention of hypoglycemia during exercise in humans. Am J Physiol 1991; 260:E705–E712.

55. Gerich JE, Langlois M, Noacco C, et al. Lack of glucagon response to hypoglycemia in diabetes: evidence for an intrinsic pancreatic alpha-cell defect. Science 1973; 182:171–173.

56. Santiago JV, Clarke WL, Shah SD, et al. Epinephrine, norepinephrine, glucagon and growth hormone release in association with physiologic decrements in the plasma glucose concentration in normal and diabetic man. J Clin Endocrinol Metab 1980; 51:877–883.

57. DeFeo P, Preiello G, Torlone E, et al. Demonstration of a role for growth hormone in glucose counterregulation. Am J Physiol 1989; 256:E835–E843.

58. DeFeo P, Periello G, Torlone E, et al. Contribution of cortisol to glucose counterregulation. Am J Physiol 1989; 257:E35–E42.

59. Boyle PJ, Cryer PE. Growth hormone, cortisol, or both are involved in defense against, but are not critical to recovery from prolonged hypoglycemia in humans. Am J Physiol 1991; 260:E395–E402.

60. Bolli G, DeFeo P, Periello G, et al. Role of hepatic autoregulation in defense against hypoglycemia in humans. J Clin Invest 1985; 75:1623–1631.

61. Hansen I, Firth R, Haymond M, et al. The role of autoregulation of hepatic glucose production in man. Diabetes 1986; 35:186–191.

62. Schwartz NS, Clutter WE, Shah SD, et al. The glycemic thresholds for activation of glucose counterregulatory systems are higher than the threshold for symptoms. J Clin Invest 1987; 79:777–781.

63. Mitrakou A, Ryan C, Veneman T, et al. Hierarchy of glycemic thresholds for activation of counterregulatory hormone secretion, initiation of symptoms and onset of cerebral dysfunction in normal humans. Am J Physiol 1991; 260:E67–E74.

64. Fanelli C, Pampanelli S, Epifano L, et al. Relative roles of insulin and hypoglycaemia on induction of neuroendocrine responses to, symptoms of and deterioration of cognitive function in hypoglycaemia in male and female humans. Diabetologia 1994; 37:797–807.

65. DeFeo P, Perriello G, Torlone E, et al. Evidence against important catecholamine compensation for absent glucagon counterregulation. Am J Physiol 1991; 260:E203–E212.

66. DeFeo P, Perriello G, Torlone E, et al. Contribution of adrenergic mechanisms to glucose counterregulation in humans. Am J Physiol 1991; 261:E725–E736.

67. Cryer PE. Diseases of the sympathochromaffin system. In: Felig P, Baxter J, Frohman L, eds. Endocrinology and Metabolism. 3rd ed. New York: McGraw-Hill, 1995: 713–714.

68. Robertshaw D. Hyperhidrosis and the sympathoadrenal system. Med Hypotheses 1979; 5:317–322.

69. Marks V, Marrack D, Rose FC. Hyperinsulinism in the pathogenesis of neuroglycopenic syndromes. Proc R Soc Med 1961; 54:747–749.

70. Amiel SA, Simonson DC, Tamborlane WV, et al. Rate of glucose fall does not affect counterregulatory hormone responses to hypoglycemia in normal and diabetic humans. Diabetes 1987; 36:518–522.

71. Mitrakou A, Mokan M, Ryan C, et al. Influence of plasma glucose rate of decrease on hierarchy of responses to hypoglycemia. J Clin Endocrinol Metab 1993; 76:462–465.

72. Hvidberg A, Fanelli CB, Hershey TG, et al. Impact of recent antecedent hypoglycemia on hypoglycemic cognitive dysfunction in nondiabetic humans. Diabetes 1996; 45:1030–1036.

73. Blomqvist G, Gjedde A, Gutniak M, et al. Facilitated transport of glucose from blood to brain in man and the effect of moderate hypoglycaemia on cerebral glucose utilization. Eur J Nucl Med 1991; 18:834–837.

74. Boyle PJ, Nagy R, O'Connor AM, et al. Adaptation in brain glucose uptake following recurrent hypoglycemia. Proc Natl Acad Sci USA 1994; 91:9352–9356.

75. Amiel SA, Sherwin RS, Simonson DC, et al. Effect of intensive insulin therapy on glycemic thresholds for counterregulatory hormone release. Diabetes 1988; 37:901–907.

76. Amiel SA, Tamborlane WV, Simonson DC, et al. Defective glucose counterregulation after strict glycemic control of insulin dependent diabetes mellitus. N Engl J Med 1987; 316:1376–1383.

77. Boyle PJ, Schwartz NS, Shah SD, et al. Plasma glucose concentrations at the onset of hypoglycemic symptoms in patients with poorly controlled diabetes and nondiabetics. N Engl J Med 1988; 318:1487–1492.

78. Mitrakou A, Fanelli C, Veneman T, et al. Reversibility of hypoglycemia unawareness. N Engl J Med 1993; 329:834–839.

79. Heller SA, Cryer PE. Reduced neuroendocrine and symptomatic response to subsequent hypoglycemia after one episode of hypoglycemia in nondiabetic humans. Diabetes 1991; 40:223–226.

80. Gjedde A, Crone A. Blood-brain glucose transfer: repression in chronic hyperglycemia. Science 1981; 214:456–457.

81. McCall AL, Millington WR, Wurtman RJ. Metabolic fuel and amino acid transport into the brain in experimental diabetes mellitus. Proc Natl Acad Sci USA 1982; 79:5406–5410.

82. McCall AL, Fixman LB, Fleming N, et al. Chronic hypoglycemia increases brain glucose transport. Am J Physiol 1986; 251:E442–E447.

83. Cryer PE. Does central nervous system adaptation to antecedent glycemia occur in patients with insulin dependent diabetes mellitus? Ann Intern Med 1985; 103:284–286.

84. Koranyi L, Bourey RE, James D, et al. Glucose transporter gene expression in rat brain: pretranslational changes associated with chronic insulin-induced hypoglycemia, fasting and diabetes. Mol Cell Neurosci 1991; 2:244–252.

85. Kumagai AK, Kang YS, Boado RJ, et al. Up regulation of blood-brain barrier GLUT-1 glucose transporter protein and mRNA in experimental chronic hypoglycemia. Diabetes 1995; 44:1399–1404.

86. Boyle PJ, Kempers SF, O'Connor AM, et al. Brain glucose uptake and unawareness of hypoglycemia in patients with insulin dependent diabetes mellitus. N Engl J Med 1995; 333:1726–1731.

87. Whipple AO. The surgical therapy of hyperinsulinism. J Int Chir 1938; 3:237–276.

88. Malouf R, Brust JCM. Hypoglycemia: causes, neurological manifestations, and outcome. Ann Neurol 1985; 17:421–430.

89. Fischer KF, Lees JA, Newman JH. Hypoglycemia in hospitalized patients. Causes and outcomes. N Engl J Med 1986; 315:1245–1250.

90. The Diabetes Control and Complications Trial Research Group. Epidemiology of severe hypoglycemia in the Diabetes Control and Complications Trial. Am J Med 1991; 90:450–459.

91. The Diabetes Control and Complications Trial Research Group. The effect of intensive treatment of diabetes on the development and progression of long-term complications in insulin-dependent diabetes mellitus. N Engl J Med 1993; 329:977–986.

92. The Diabetes Control and Complications Trial Research Group. Adverse events and their association with treatment regimens in the Diabetes Control and Complications Trial. Diabetes Care 1995; 18:1415–1427.

93. Thorsteinsson B, Pramming S, Lauritzen T, et al. Frequency of daytime biochemical hypoglycaemia in insulin-treated diabetics: relationship to daily median blood glucose concentration. Diabetic Med 1986; 3:147–151.

94. Arias P, Kerner W, Zier H, et al. Incidence of hypoglycemic episodes in diabetic patients under continuous subcutaneous insulin infusion and intensified conventional insulin treatment: assessment by means of continuous blood glucose monitoring. Diabetes Care 1985; 8:134–140.

95. Pramming S, Thorsteinsson B, Bendtson I, et al. Nocturnal hypoglycaemia in patients receiving conventional treatment with insulin. Br Med J 1985; 291:376–379.

96. Cox DJ, Clarke WL, Gonder-Frederick L, et al. Accuracy of perceiving blood glucose in IDDM. Diabetes Care 1985; 8:529–536.

97. Pramming S, Thorsteinsson B, Bendtson I, et al. Symptomatic hypoglycaemia in 411 type I diabetic patients. Diabetic Med 1991; 8:217–222.

98. Kahn KJ, Myers RE. Insulin-induced hypoglycaemia in the non-human primate. I: Clinical consequences. In: Brain Hypoxia, Clinics in Developmental Medicine. London: Heineman, 1971: 185–193.

99. The Diabetes Control and Complications Trial Research Group. Effects of intensive diabetes therapy on neuropsychological function in adults in the Diabetes Control and Complications Trial. Ann Intern Med 1996; 124:379–388.

100. Tattersall RB, Gale EAM. Mortality. In: Frier BM, Fisher BM, eds. Diabetes and Hypoglycaemia. London: Edward Arnold, 1993: 190–198.

101. Deckert T, Poulsen JE, Larsen M. Prognosis of diabetics with diabetes before the age of thirty-one. I: Survival, cause of deaths and complications. Diabetologia 1978; 14:363–370.

102. Turnbridge WMG. Factors contributing to deaths of diabetics under 50 years of age. Lancet 1981; 2:569–572.

103. Teutsch SM, Herman WH, Dwyer DM, et al. Mortality among diabetic patients using continuous subcutaneous insulin infusions pumps. N Engl J Med 1984; 310:361–368.

104. Tattersall RB, Gill GV. Unexplained deaths of type I diabetic patients. Diabetic Med 1991; 8:49–58.

105. Cox DJ, Irvine A, Gonder-Frederick L, et al. Fear of hypoglycemia: quantification, validation and utilization. Diabetes Care 1987; 10:617–621.

106. Wredling RAM, Theorell PGT, Roll HM, et al. Psychosocial state of patients with IDDM prone to recurrent episodes of severe hypoglycaemia. Diabetes Care 1992; 15:518–520.

107. Gill G. Socioeconomic problems of hypoglycemia. In: Frier BM, Fisher BM, eds. London: Edward Arnold, 1993: 362–370.

108. Cox DJ, Gonder-Frederick L, Clarke WL. Driving decrements in type 1 diabetes during moderate hypoglycemia. Diabetes 1993; 42:239–473.

109. Hansotia P, Broste SK. The effect of epilepsy or diabetes mellitus on the risk of automobile accidents. N Engl J Med 1991; 324:22–26.

110. Bolli G, DeFeo P, Compagnucci P, et al. Abnormal glucose counterregulation in insulin-dependent diabetes mellitus: interaction of anti-insulin antibodies and impaired glucagon and epinephrine secretion. Diabetes 1983; 32:134–141.

111. Fukuda M, Tanaka A, Tahara Y, et al. Correlation between minimal secretory capacity of pancreatic β-cells and stability of diabetic control. Diabetes 1988; 37:81–88.

112. Hirsch BR, Shamoon H. Defective epinephrine and growth hormone responses in type 1 diabetes are stimulus specific. Diabetes 1987; 36:20–26.

113. Dagogo-Jack SE, Craft S, Cryer PE. Hypoglycemia-associated autonomic failure in insulin dependent diabetes mellitus. J Clin Invest 1993; 91:819–828.

114. Wiethop BV, Cryer PE. Alanine and terbutaline in the treatment of hypoglycemia in IDDM. Diabetes Care 1993; 16:1131–1136.

115. Bolli GB, DeFeo P, DeCosmo S, et al. A reliable and reproducible test for adequate glucose counterregulation in type I diabetes mellitus. Diabetes 1984; 33:732–737.

116. Sjöbom NC, Adamson U, Lins PE: The prevalence of impaired glucose counterregulation during an insulin infusion test in insulin-treated patients prone to severe hypoglycaemia. Diabetologia 1989; 32:818–825.

117. Heller SR, Herbert M, Macdonald IA, et al: Influence of sympathetic nervous system on hypoglycemic warning symptoms. Lancet 1987; 2:359–363.

118. Hepburn DA, Patrick AW, Eadington DW, et al. Unawareness of hypoglycaemia in insulin-treated diabetic patients: prevalence and relationship to autonomic neuropathy. Diabetic Med 1990; 7:711–717.

119. Ryder REJ, Owens DR, Hayes TM, et al. Unawareness of hypoglycaemia and inadequate glucose counterregulation: no causal relationship with diabetic autonomic neuropathy. Br Med J 1990; 301:783–787.

120. Grimaldi A, Bosquet F, Davidoff P, et al. Unawareness of hypoglycemia by insulin-dependent diabetics. Horm Metab Res 1990; 22:90–95.

121. Gerich JE, Mokan M, Veneman T, et al. Hypoglycemia unawareness. Endocr Rev 1991; 12:356–371.

122. Gold AE, MacLeod KM, Frier BM. Frequency of severe hypoglycemia in patients with type I diabetes with impaired awareness of hypoglycemia. Diabetes Care 1994; 17:697–703.

123. Clarke WL, Gonder-Frederick LA, Richards FE, et al. Multifactorial origin of hypoglycemic symptom awareness in insulin dependent diabetes mellitus. Diabetes 1991; 40:680–685.

124. Hepburn DA, Patrick AW, Brash HM, et al. Hypoglycaemia unawareness in type I diabetes: a lower plasma glucose is required to stimulate sympathoadrenal activation. Diabetic Med 1991; 8:934–945.

125. Ziegler D, Hübinger A, Mühlen H, et al. Effects of previous glycemic control on the onset and magnitude of cognitive dysfunction during hypoglycaemia in type 1 (insulin-dependent) diabetic patients. Diabetologia 1992; 35:828–834.

126. Jones TW, McCarthy G, Tamborlane WV, et al. Resistance to neuroglycopenia: an adaptive response during intensive insulin treatment of diabetes. Diabetes 1991; 40:557A (abstract).

127. Widom B, Simonson DC. Glycemic control and neuropsychologic function during hypoglycemia in patients with insulin-dependent diabetes mellitus. Ann Intern Med 1990; 112:904–912.

128. Blackman JD, Towle VL, Sturis J, et al. Hypoglycemic thresholds for cognitive dysfunction in IDDM. Diabetes 1992; 41:392–399.

129. Maran A, Lomas J, Macdonald I, et al. Lack of preservation of higher brain function during hypoglycaemia in patients with intensively-treated IDDM. Diabetologia 1995; 38:1412–1418.

130. Draelos MT, Jacobson AM, Weinger K, et al. Cognitive function in patients with insulin-dependent diabetes mellitus during hyperglycemia and hypoglycemia. Am J Med 1995; 98:135–143.

131. Davis M, Shamoon H. Counterregulatory adaptation to recurrent hypoglycemia in normal humans. J Clin Endocrinol Metab 1991; 73:995–1001.

132. Widom B, Simonson DC. Intermittent hypoglycemia impairs glucose counterregulation. Diabetes 1992; 41:1597–1602.

133. Veneman T, Mitrakou A, Mokan M, et al. Induction of hypoglycemia unawareness by asymptomatic nocturnal hypoglycemia. Diabetes 1993; 42:1233–1237.

134. Davis MR, Mellman M, Shamoon H. Further defects in counterregulatory responses induced by recurrent hypoglycemia in type I diabetes. Diabetes 1992; 41:1335–1340.

135. Lingenfelser T, Renn W, Sommerwerck U, et al. Compromised hormonal counterregulation, symptom awareness, and neurophysiological function after recurrent short-term episodes for insulin-induced hypoglycemia in IDDM patients. Diabetes 1993; 42:610–618.

136. Hirsch IB, Boyle PJ, Craft S, et al. Higher glycemic thresholds for symptoms during β-adrenergic blockade in IDDM. Diabetes 1991; 40:1177–1186.

137. Cryer PE. Iatrogenic hypoglycemia as a cause of hypoglycemia-associated autonomic failure in IDDM: a vicious cycle. Diabetes 1992; 41:255–260.

138. Rattarasarn C, Dagogo-Jack SE, Zachwieja JJ, et al. Hypoglycemia-induced autonomic failure in IDDM is specific for the stimulus of hypoglycemia and is not attributable to prior autonomic activation per se. Diabetes 1994; 43:809–818.

139. Fanelli CG, Epifano L, Rambotti AM, et al. Meticulous prevention of hypoglycemia normalizes the glycemic thresholds and magnitude of most neuroendocrine responses to, symptoms of and cognitive function during hypoglycemia in intensively treated patients with short-term IDDM. Diabetes 1993; 42:1683–1689.

140. Cranston I, Lomas J, Maran A, et al. Restoration of hypoglycaemia unawareness in patients with long duration insulin-dependent diabetes mellitus. Lancet 1994; 344:283–287.

141. Fanelli C, Pampanelli S, Epifano L, et al. Long-term recovery from unawareness, deficient counterregulation and lack of cognitive dysfunction during hypoglycemia following institution of rational intensive therapy in IDDM. Diabetologia 1994; 37:1265–1276.

142. Dagogo-Jack SE, Rattarasarn C, Cryer PE. Reversal of hypoglycemia unawareness, but not defective glucose counterregulation, in IDDM. Diabetes 1994; 43:1426–1434.

143. Egger M, Smith GD, Teuscher AU, et al. Influence of human insulin on symptoms and awareness of hypoglycaemia: a randomized double blind crossover trial. Br Med J 1991; 303:622–626.

144. Egger M, Smith GD, Imhoof H, et al. Risk of severe hypoglycaemia in insulin treated diabetic patients transferred to human insulin: a case control study. Br Med J 1991; 303:617–621.

145. Hepburn DA, Eadington DW, Patrick AW, et al. Symptomatic awareness of hypoglycaemia: does it change on transfer from animal to human insulin? Diabetic Med 1989; 6:585–690.

146. Colagiuri S, Miller JJ, Petocz P. Double blind crossover comparison of human and porcine insulins in patients reporting lack of hypoglycaemia awareness. Lancet 1992; 339:1432–1435.

147. Cryer PE. Hypoglycemia unawareness in IDDM. Diabetes Care 1993; 16(Suppl 3):40–47.

148. Hirsch IB, Farkas-Hirsch R, Cryer PE. Continuous subcutaneous insulin infusion for the treatment of diabetic patients with hypoglycemia unawareness. Diabetes Metab Nutr 1991; 4:41–43.

149. MacCuish AC. Treatment of hypoglycemia. In: Frier BM, Fisher BM, eds. Diabetes and Hypoglycaemia. London: Edward Arnold, 1993: 212–221.

150. Brodows RG, Williams C, Amatruda JM. Treatment of insulin reactions in diabetics. JAMA 1984; 252:3378–3381.

151. Collier A, Steedman DJ, Patrick AW, et al. Comparison of intravenous glucagon and dextrose in treatment of severe hypoglycemia in an accident and emergency department. Diabetes Care 1987; 10:712–715.

152. Namba M, Hanafusa T, Kono N, et al. Clinical evaluation of biosynthetic glucagon treatment for recovery from hypoglycemia developed in diabetic patients. Diabetes Res Clin Pract 1993; 19:133–138.

153. Hvidberg AM, Jørgensen S, Hilsted J. The effect of genetically engineered glucagon on glucose recovery after hypoglycaemia in man. Br J Clin Pharmacol 1992; 34:547–550.

154. Pontiroli AE, Pozza G. Intranasal administration of peptide hormones: factors affecting transmucosal absorption. Diabetic Med 1990; 7:770–774.

155. Slama G, Alamowitch C, Desplanque N, et al. A new non-invasive method for treating insulin-reaction: intranasal lyophilized glucagon. Diabetologia 1990; 33:671–674.

156. Rosenfalck AM, Bendtson I, Jørgensen S, et al. Nasal glucagon in the treatment of hypoglycaemia in type I (insulin-dependent) diabetic patients. Diabetes Res Clin Pract 1992; 17:43–50.

157. Wiethop BV, Cryer PE. Glycemic actions of alanine and terbutaline in IDDM. Diabetes Care 1993; 16:1124–1130.

158. Saleh T, Cryer PE. Alanine and terbutaline in the prevention of nocturnal hypoglycemia in IDDM. Diabetes 1996; 45:56A (abstract).

159. Campbell IW. Hypoglycaemia and type 2 diabetes: sulfonylureas. In: Frier BM, Fisher BM, eds. Hypoglycaemia and Diabetes. London: Edward Arnold, 1993: 387–392.

160. Gerich JE. Oral hypoglycemic agents. N Engl J Med 1989; 34:1231–1245.

161. Hepburn DA, MacLeod KM, Pell ACH, et al. Frequency and symptoms of hypoglycemia experienced by patients with type 2 diabetes treated with insulin. Diabetic Med 1993; 10:231–237.

162. Heller SR. Hypoglycaemia and type 2 diabetes: insulin therapy. In: Frier BM, Fisher BM, eds. Hypoglycaemia and Diabetes. London: Edward Arnold, 1993: 393–400.

163. Bolli GB, Tsalikian E, Haymond MW, et al. Defective glucose counterregulation after subcutaneous insulin in noninsulin dependent diabetes mellitus. J Clin Invest 1984; 73:1532–1541.

164. Palatnick W, Meatherall RC, Tenebein M. Clinical spectrum of sulfonylurea overdose and experience with diazoxide therapy. Arch Intern Med 1991; 151:1859–1862.

165. Boyle PJ, Justice K, Krentz AJ, et al. Octreotide reverses hyperinsulinemia and prevents hypoglycemia induced by sulfonylurea overdoses. J Clin Endocrinol Metab 1993; 76:752–756.

166. Bailey CJ, Flatt PR, Marks V. Drugs inducing hypoglycaemia. Pharmacol Ther 1989; 42:361–384.

167. Polonsky KS. A practical approach to fasting hypoglycemia. N Engl J Med 1992; 326:1020–1021.

168. Marks V. Recognition and differential diagnosis of spontaneous hypoglycaemia. Clin Endocrinol 1992; 37:309–316.

169. Klonoff DC, Barrett BJ, Nolte MS, et al. Hypoglycemia following inadvertent or factitious sulfonylurea overdosages. Diabetes Care 1995; 18:563–567.

170. Lecavalier L, Bolli G, Cryer P, et al. Contributions of gluconeogenesis and glycogenolysis during glucose counterregulation in normal humans. Am J Physiol 1989; 256:E844–E851.

171. Marks V. Alcohol and carbohydrate metabolism. Clin Endocrinol Metab 1978; 7:33–41.

172. Wilson N, Brown P, Juil S, et al. Glucose turnover and metabolic and hormonal changes in ethanol induced hypoglycemia. Br Med J 1982; 282:849–853.

173. Kolaczynski JW, Ylikahri R, Härkonen M, et al. The acute effect of ethanol on counterregulatory response and recovery from insulin induced hypoglycemia. J Clin Endocrinol Metab 1988; 67:384–388.

174. Yki-Järvinen H, Koivisto VA, Ylikahri R, et al. Acute effects of ethanol and acetate on glucose kinetics in normal subjects. Am J Physiol 1988; 254:E175–E180.

175. Shelmet JJ, Reichard GA, Skutches CL, et al. Ethanol causes acute inhibition of carbohydrate, fat and protein oxidation and insulin resistance. J Clin Invest 1988; 81:1137–1145.

176. Shah JH. Alcohol decreases insulin sensitivity in healthy subjects. Alcohol Alcoholism 1988; 23:103–109.

177. Fang V, Foyle WO, Robinson SM, et al. Hypoglycemic activity and chemical structure of salicylates. J Pharm Sci 1968; 57:2111–2116.

178. Arena FP, Dugowson C, Saudek CD: Salicylate-induced hypoglycemia and ketoacidosis in a nondiabetic adult. Arch Intern Med 1978; 138:1153–1156.

179. Raschke R, Arnold-Capell PA, Richeson R, et al. Refractory hypoglycemia secondary to topical salicylate intoxication. Arch Intern Med 1991; 151:591–593.

180. Poretsky L, Moses AC. Hypoglycemia associated with trimethoprim/sulfa-methoxazole therapy. Diabetes Care 1984; 7:508–509.

181. Waskin H, Stehr-Green JK, Helmick CG, et al. Risk factors for hypoglycemia associated with pentamidine therapy for pneumocystis pneumonia. JAMA 1988; 260:345–347.

182. Assan R, Perronne C, Assan D, et al. Pentamidine-induced derangements of glucose metabolism. Diabetes Care 1995; 18:47–55.

183. White NJ, Warrell DA, Chanthavanich P, et al. Severe hypoglycemia and hyperinsulinemia in falciparum malaria. N Engl J Med 1983; 309:61–66.

184. Phillips RE, Looareesuwan S, Molyneux ME, et al. Hypoglycaemia and counterregulatory hormone responses in severe falciparum malaria: treatment with sandostatin. Q J Med 1993; 86:223–240.

185. White NJ, Miller KD, Marsh K, et al. Hypoglycaemia in African children with severe malaria. Lancet 1987; 1:708–711.

186. Taylor TE, Molyneux ME, Wirima JJ, et al. Blood glucose levels in Malawian children before and during the administration of intravenous quinine for severe falciparum malaria. N Engl J Med 1988; 319:1040–1047.

187. Kawo NG, Msengi AE, Swai ABM, et al. Specificity of hypoglycaemia for cerebral malaria in children. Lancet 1990; 336:458–461.

188. Hesse B, Pedersen JT. Hypoglycemia after propranolol in children. Acta Med Scand 1973; 193:551–552.

189. McBride JT, McBride MC, Vites PH. Hypoglycemia associated with propranolol. Pediatrics 1973; 51:1085–1087.

190. Mann FC, Magath TB. Studies on the physiology of the liver. II: The effect of the removal of the liver on the blood sugar level. Arch Intern Med 1922; 30:73–84.

191. Zimmerman HJ, Thomas LJ, Scherrr EH. Fasting blood sugar in hepatic disease with reference to infrequency of hypoglycemia. Arch Intern Med 1953; 91:577–584.

192. Samson RL, Trey C, Timme AH, et al. Fulminaint hepatitis with recurrent hypoglycemia and hemorrhage. Gastroenterology 1967; 53:291–300.

193. Felig P, Brown WV, Levine RA, et al. Glucose homeostasis in viral hepatitis. N Engl J Med 1970; 283:1436–1440.

194. Younus S, Soterakis J, Sosi AJ, et al. Hypoglycemia secondary to metastases to the liver. Gastroenterology 1977; 72:334–337.

195. Johnston DG, Alberti KGMM. Hyperinsulinism of hepatic cirrhosis: diminished degradation or hypersecretion. Lancet 1977; 1:10–13.

196. Vilstrup H, Iversen J, Tygstrup N. Glucoregulation in acute liver failure. Eur J Clin Invest 1986; 16:193–197.

197. Medalle R, Webb R, Waterhouse C. Lactic acidosis and hypoglycemia. Arch Intern Med 1971; 128:273–278.

198. Block MB, Rubenstein AH. Spontaneous hypoglycemia in diabetic patients with renal insufficiency. JAMA 1970; 213:1863–1866.

199. Frizell M, Larsen PR, Field JB. Spontaneous hypoglycemia associated with chronic renal failure. Diabetes 1973; 22:493–498.

200. Garber AJ, Bier DM, Cryer PE, et al. Hypoglycemia in compensated chronic renal insufficiency. Diabetes 1974; 23:982–986.

201. Peitzman SJ, Agarwal BN. Spontaneous hypoglycemia in end-stage renal disease. Nephron 1977; 19:131–139.

202. Rutsky EA, McDaniel HG, Tarpe DL, et al. Spontaneous hypoglycemia in chronic renal failure. Arch Intern Med 1978; 138:1364–1368.

203. Schmitz O. Peripheral and hepatic resistance to insulin and hepatic resistance to glucagon in uraemic patients. Acta Endocrinol 1988; 118:125–134.

204. Baylor P, Shilo S, Zonszein J, et al. β-Adrenergic contribution to glucagon-induced glucose production and insulin secretion in uremia. Am J Physiol 1986; 251:E322–E327.

205. Greenblatt DJ. Fatal hypoglycaemia occurring after peritoneal dialysis. Br Med J 1972; 2:270–271.

206. Miller SI, Wallace RJ Jr, Musher DM, et al. Hypoglycemia as a manifestation of sepsis. Am J Med 1980; 68:649–653.

207. Hargrove DM, Bagby GJ, Lang CH, et al. Adrenergic blockade does not abolish elevated glucose turnover during bacterial infection. Am J Physiol 1988; 254:E16–E22.

208. Hargrove DM, Bagby GJ, Lang CH, et al. Adrenergic blockade prevents endotoxin-induced increases in glucose metabolism. Am J Physiol 1988; 255:E629–E635.

209. Naylor JM, Kronfeld DS. In vivo studies of hypoglycemia and lactic acidosis in endotoxic shock. Am J Physiol 1985; 248:E309–E316.

210. Lang CH, Spolarics Z, Ohlakan A, et al. Effect of high dose endotoxin on glucose production and utilization. Metabolism 1993; 42:1351–1358.

211. Meszaros K, Bagby GJ, Lang CH, et al. Increased uptake and phosphorylation of 2-deoxyglucose by skeletal muscles in endotoxin-treated rats. Am J Physiol 1987; 253:E33–E39.

212. Meszaros K, Lang CH, Bagby GJ, et al. In vivo glucose utilization by individual tissues during nonlethal hypermetabolic sepsis. FASEB J 1988; 2:3083–3086.

213. Lang CH, Dobrescu C. Sepsis-induced increases in glucose uptake by macrophage-rich tissues persist during hypoglycemia. Metabolism 1991; 40:585–593.

214. Lee MD, Zentella A, Pekala PH, et al. Effect of endotoxin-induced monokines on glucose metabolism in the muscle cell line L6. Proc Natl Acad Sci USA 1987; 84:2590–2594.

215. Wolfe RR, Elahi D, Spitzer JJ. Glucose and lactate kinetics after endotoxin administration in dogs. Am J Physiol 1977; 232:E180–E185.

216. Mathison JC, Wolfson E, Ulevitch RJ. Participation of tumor necrosis factor in the mediation of gram negative bacterial lipopolysaccharide-induced injury in rabbits. J Clin Invest 1988; 81:1925–1937.

217. Lang CH, Bagby GJ, Blakesley HL, et al. Importance of hyperglucagonemia in eliciting the sepsis-induced increase in glucose production. Circulatory Shock 1989; 29:181–191.

218. McKechnie K, Dean HG, Furman BL, et al. Plasma catecholamines during endotoxin infusion in conscious unrestrained rats: effects of adrenal demedullation and/or guanethidine treatment. Circulatory Shock 1985; 17:85–94.

219. Bagby GJ, Lang CH, Skrepnik N, et al. Attenuation of glucose metabolic changes resulting from TNF administration by adrenergic blockade. Am J Physiol 1992; 262:R628–R635.

220. Stouthard JML, Romijn JA, van der Poll T, et al. Endocrinologic and metabolic effects of interleukin-6 in humans. Am J Physiol 1995; 268:E813–E819.

221. Hargrove DM, Lang CH, Bagby GJ, et al. Epinephrine-induced increase in glucose turnover is diminished during sepsis. Metabolism 1989; 38:1070–1076.

222. Wharton B. Hypoglycemia in children with kwashiorkor. Lancet 1970; 1:171–173.

223. Elias AN, Gwinup G. Glucose-resistant hypoglycemia in inanition. Arch Intern Med 1982; 142:743–746.

224. Bruce AK, Jacobsen E, Dossing H, et al. Hypoglycaemia in spinal muscular atrophy. Lancet 1995; 346:609–610.

225. Maleribi D, Liberman B, Guirno-Filho A, et al. Glucocorticoids and glucose metabolism: hepatic glucose production in untreated Addisonian patients and on two different levels of glucocorticoid administration. Clin Endocrinol 1988; 28:415–422.

226. Artavia-Loria E, Chaussian JL, Bougneres PF, et al. Frequency of hypoglycemia in children with adrenal insufficiency. Acta Endocrinol 1986; S279:275–277.

227. Goodman HG, Grumbach MM, Kaplan SL. Growth and growth hormone. II: A comparison of isolated growth hormone deficiency and multiple pituitary hormone deficiencies in 35 patients with idiopathic hypopituitary dwarfism. N Engl J Med 1968; 278:57–68.

228. Muglia L, Jacobsen L, Dikkies P, et al. Corticotropin-releasing hormone deficiency reveals major fetal but not adult glucocorticoid need. Nature 1995; 373:427–432.

229. Haymond MW, Karl I, Weldon VV, et al. The role of growth hormone and cortisone in glucose and gluconeogenic substrate regulation in fasted hypopituitary children. J Clin Endocrinol Metab 1976; 42:846–856.

230. Wolfsdorf JI, Sadeghi-Nejad A, Senior B. Hypoketonemia and age-related fasting hypoglycemia in growth hormone deficiency. Metabolism 1983; 32:457–462.

231. Frizell RT, Campbell PJ, Cherrington AD. Gluconeogenesis and hypoglycemia. Diabetes Metab Rev 1988; 4:51–70.

232. Rizza RA, Mandarino L, Gerich JE. Cortisol induced insulin resistance in man: impaired suppression of glucose production and stimulation of glucose utilization due to a postreceptor defect of insulin action. J Clin Endocrinol Metab 1981; 54:131–138.

233. Aynsley-Green A, Moncrieff MW, Ratter S, et al. Isolated ACTH deficiency. Arch Dis Child 1978; 53:499–502.

234. Rudman D, Moffitt SD, Fernhoff PM, et al. Epinephrine deficiency in hypocorticotropic hypopituitary children. J Clin Endocrinol Metab 1981; 53:722–729.

235. Voorhees ML, Jakubowski AF, MacGillivray MH. The adrenomedullary and glucagon responses of hypopituitary children to insulin induced hypoglycemia. Pediatr Res 1981; 15:912–915.

236. Smallridge RC, Corrigan DF, Thomason AM, et al. Hypoglycemia in pregnancy. Occurrence due to adrenocorticotropic hormone and growth hormone deficiency. Arch Intern Med 1980; 140:564–565.

237. Steer P, Marnell R, Werk EE Jr. Clinical alcohol hypoglycemia and isolated adrenocorticotropic hormone deficiency. Ann Intern Med 1969; 71:343–348.

238. Broberger O, Jungner I, Zetterstrom R. Studies in spontaneous hypoglycemia in childhood. Failure to increase epinephrine secretion in insulin-induced hypoglycemia. J Pediatr 1959; 55:713–719.

239. Tietze HU, Zurbrug RP, Zuppinger KA, et al. Occurrence of impaired cortisol regulation to children with hypoglycemia associated with adrenal medullary hyporesponsiveness. J Clin Endocrinol Metab 1972; 34:948–958.

240. Christensen NJ. Hypoadrenalinemia during insulin hypoglycemia in children with ketotic hypoglycemia. J Clin Endocrinol Metab 1974; 38:107–112.

241. Rosenbloom AL, Tiwary CM. Ketotic (idiopathic glucagon unresponsive) hypoglycemia. Catecholamine excretion and effects of ephedrine therapy. Arch Dis Child 1972; 47:924–926.

242. Court JM, Dunlop ME, Boulton TJC. Effect of ephedrine in ketotic hypoglycemia. Arch Dis Child 1974; 49:63–65.

243. Sizonenko PC, Paunier L, Vallotton MB, et al. Response to 2-deoxy-glucose and to glucagon in "ketotic hypoglycemia" of childhood: evidence for epinephrine deficiency and altered alanine availability. Pediatr Res 1973; 7:983–993.

244. Kerr DS, Brooke OG, Robinson HM. Fasting energy utilization in the smaller of twins with epinephrine-deficient hypoglycemia. Metabolism 1981; 30:6–17.

245. Kerr DS, Picou DIM. Fasting glucose production in the smaller of twins with epinephrine-deficient hypoglycemia. Metabolism 1981; 30:18–26.

246. Light IJ, Sutherland JM, Loggie JM, et al. Impaired epinephrine release in hypoglycemic infants of diabetic mothers. N Engl J Med 1967; 277:394–398.

247. Bleicher SJ, Levy LJ, Zarowitz H, et al. Glucagon deficiency hypoglycemia: a new syndrome? Clin Res 1970; 19:355 (abstract).

248. Starke AAR, Valverde I, Botazzo GF, et al. Glucagon deficiency associated with hypoglycaemia and the absence of islet cell antibodies in the polyglandular failure syndrome before the onset of insulin-dependent diabetes mellitus: a case report. Diabetologia 1983; 25:336–339.

249. Vidnes J, Oyaseater S. Glucagon deficiency causing severe neonatal hypoglycemia in a patient with normal insulin secretion. Pediatr Res 1977; 11:943–949.

250. Kollee LA, Monnens LA, Cejka V, et al. Persistent neonatal hypoglycemia due to glucagon deficiency. Arch Dis Child 1978; 53:422–424.

251. McFadzean AJS, Yeung RTT. Further observations of hypoglycaemia in hepato-cellular carcinoma. Am J Med 1969; 47:220–235.

252. Arem R, Jeang MK, Blevens TC, et al. Polycythemia rubra vera and artifactual hypoglycemia. Arch Intern Med 1982; 142:2199–2201.

253. Benn JJ, Firth RGR, Sönksen PH. Metabolic effects of an insulin-like factor causing hypoglycaemia in a patient with a hemangiopericytoma. Clin Endocrinol 1990; 32:769–780.

254. Møller N, Blum WF, Mengel A, et al. Basal and insulin stimulated substrate metabolism in tumor induced hypoglycaemia: evidence for increased muscle glucose uptake. Diabetologia 1991; 34:17–20.

255. Eastman RC, Carson RE, Orloff DG, et al. Glucose utilization in a patient with hepatoma and hypoglycemia. J Clin Invest 1992; 89:1958–1963.

256. Crawford WH. Hypoglycemia with coma in a case of primary carcinoma of the liver. Am J Med Sci 1931; 181:496–502.

257. Silbert C, Rossini AA, Ghazvinian S, et al. Tumor hypoglycemia: deficient splanchnic glucose output and deficient glucagon secretion. Diabetes 1976; 25:202–206.

258. Olefsky S, Bailey L, Samols E, et al. A fibrosarcoma with hypoglycemia and high serum insulin levels. Lancet 1962; 2:378–380.

259. Lyall SS, Marieb MJ, Wise JK, et al. Hyperinsulinemic hypoglycemia associated with a neurofibrosarcoma. Arch Intern Med 1975; 135:865–867.

260. Kiang DT, Bauer GE, Kennedy BJ. Immunoassayable insulin in carcinoma of the cervix associated with hypoglycemia. Cancer 1973; 31:801–805.

261. Shames JM, Dhurandhar NE, Blackard WG. Insulin-secreting bronchial carcinoid tumor with widespread metastases. Am J Med 1968; 44:632–636.

262. Appleyard TN, Losowsky MD. A pancreatic tumor with carcinoid syndrome and hypoglycemia. Postgrad Med J 1970; 46:159–171.

263. Marks V, Samols E. Hypoglycemia of nonendocrine origin. Proc R Soc Med 1966; 59:338–340.

264. Daughaday WH, Trivedi B, Kapadia M. Measurement of insulin-like growth factor II by a specific radioreceptor assay in serum of normal individuals, patients with abnormal growth hormone secretion, and patients with tumor-associated hypoglycemia. J Clin Endocrinol Metab 1981; 53:289–294.

265. Daughaday WH, Emanuelle MA, Brooks MH, et al. Synthesis and secretion of insulin-like growth factor II by a leiomyosarcoma with associated hypoglycemia. N Engl J Med 1988; 319:1434–1440.

266. Ron D, Powers AC, Pandian MR, et al. Increased insulin-like growth factor II production and consequent suppression of growth hormone secretion: a dual mechanism of tumor-induced hypoglycemia. J Clin Endocrinol Metab 1989; 68:701–706.

267. Lowe WL, Roberts CT, LeRoith D, et al. Insulin-like growth factor-II in nonislet cell tumors associated with hypoglycemia: increased levels of messenger ribonucleic acid. J Clin Endocrinol Metab 1989; 69:1153–1159.

268. Merimee TJ. Insulin-like growth factors in patients with nonislet cell tumors and hypoglycemia. Metabolism 1986; 35:360–363.

269. Wu J-C, Daughaday WH, Lee S-D, et al. Radioimmunoassay of serum IGF-I and IGF-II in patients with chronic liver diseases and hepatocellular carcinoma with or without hypoglycemia. J Lab Clin Med 1988; 112:589–594.

270. Daughaday WH, Kapadia M. Significance of abnormal serum binding of insulin-like growth factor II in the development of hypoglycemia in patients with non-islet-cell tumors. Proc Natl Acad Sci USA 1989; 86:6778–6782.

271. Zapf J, Futo E, Peter M, et al. Can "big" insulin-like growth factor II in serum of tumor patients account for the development of extrapancreatic tumor hypoglycemia? J Clin Invest 1992; 90:2574–2584.

272. Daughaday Wh, Trivedi B, Baxter RC. Serum "big insulin-like growth factor II" from patients with tumor hypoglycemia lacks normal E-domain O-linked glycosylation, a possible determinant of normal propeptide processing. Proc Natl Acad Sci USA 1993; 90:5823–5827.

273. Fukuda I, Hizuka N, Takano K, et al. Circulating forms of insulin-like growth factor II (IGF-II) in patients with non–islet cell tumor hypoglycemia. Endocrinol Metab 1994; 1:89–95.

274. Daughaday WH. The pathophysiology of IGF-II hypersecretion in non-islet tumor hypoglycemia. Diabetes Rev 1995; 3:62–72.

275. Grunberger G, Weiner-JL, Silverman R, et al. Factitious hypoglycemia due to surreptitious administration of insulin. Ann Intern Med 1988; 108:252–257.

276. Marks V. Recognition and differential diagnosis of spontaneous hypoglycaemia. Clin Endocrinol 1992; 37:309–316.

277. Cohen RM, Given BD, Licinio-Paixo J, et al. Proinsulin radioimmunoassay in the evaluation of insulinomas and familial hyperproinsulinemia. Metabolism 1986; 36:1137–1146.

278. Hamptom SM, Beyzavi K, Teale D, et al. A direct assay for proinsulin in plasma and its application in hypoglycaemia. Clin Endocrinol 1988; 29:9–16.

279. Hale PJ, Djurup R, Baddeley RM, et al. Insulin and proinsulin concentrations in patients with insulinoma before and after surgical treatment. Diabetes Nutr Metab 1991; 4:113–116.

280. Kao PC, Taylor RL, Service FJ. Proinsulin by immunochemiluminometric assay for the diagnosis of insulinoma. J Clin Endocrinol Metab 1994; 78:1048–1051.

281. Hirata Y, Tominaga M, Ito JI, et al. Spontaneous hypoglycemia with insulin autoimmunity in Graves' disease. Ann Intern Med 1974; 81:214–218.

282. Ichihara K, Shima K, Saito Y, et al. Mechanism of hypoglycemia observed in a patient with autoimmune syndrome. Diabetes 1977; 26:500–506.

283. Anderson JH, Blackard WG, Goldman J, et al. Diabetes and hypoglycemia due to insulin antibodies. Am J Med 1978; 64:868–872.

284. Goldman J, Baldwin D, Rubenstein AH. Characterization of circulating insulin and proinsulin binding antibodies in autoimmune hypoglycemia. J Clin Invest 1979; 63:1050–1059.

285. Redmon B, Pyzdrowski KL, Elson MK, et al. Brief report, hypoglycemia due to a monoclonal insulin-binding antibody in multiple myeloma. N Engl J Med 1992; 326:994–998.

286. Burch HB, Clement S, Sokol MS, et al. Reactive hypoglycemic coma due to insulin autoimmune syndrome: case report and literature review. Am J Med 1992; 92:681–685.

287. Uchigata Y, Tokunaga K, Nepom G, et al. Differential immunogenetic determinants of polyclonal insulin autoimmune syndrome (Hirata's disease) and monoclonal insulin autoimmune syndrome. Diabetes 1995; 44:1227–1232.

288. Arnqvist HJ, Halban PA, Mathiesen UL, et al. Hypoglycaemia caused by a typical insulin antibodies in a patient with benign monoclonal gammopathy. J Intern Med 1993; 234:421–427.

289. Taylor SI, Barbetti F, Accili D, et al. Syndromes of autoimmunity and hypoglycemia. Endocrinol Metab Clin North Am 1989; 18:123–143.

290. Moller DE, Ratner RE, Borenstein DG, et al. Autoantibodies to the insulin receptor as a cause of autoimmune hypoglycemia in systemic lupus erythematosus. Am J Med 1988; 84:334–338.

291. Rocket N, Blanche S, Carel JC, et al. Hypoglycemia induced by antibodies to insulin receptor following a bone marrow transplantation in a immunodeficient child. Diabetologia 1989; 32:167–172.

292. Kiyokawa H, Kono N, Hamaguchi T, et al. Hyperinsulinemia due to impaired insulin clearance associated with fasting hypoglycemia and postprandial hyperglycemia: an analysis of a patient with antiinsulin antibodies. J Clin Endocrinol Metab 1989; 69:616–621.

293. De Pirro R, Borboni P, Marini MA, et al. Antibodies directed to the insulin receptor. Clinical aspects and applications to the study of insulin action. J Endocrinol Invest 1990; 13:951–968.

294. Di Paolo S, Giogrino R. Insulin resistance and hypoglycemia in a patient with systemic lupus erythematosus: description of antiinsulin receptor antibodies that enhance insulin binding and inhibit insulin actions. J Clin Endocrinol Metab 1991; 73:650–657.

295. Wilkin TJ, Hammonds P, Mirza JH, et al. Graves' disease of the β-cell: glucose dysregulation due to islet-cell stimulating antibodies. Lancet 1988; 2:1155–1158.

296. Wilkin TJ. Receptor autoimmunity in endocrine disorders. N Engl J Med 1990; 323:1318–1324.

297. Foggensteiner L, Bone AJ, Webster KA, et al. Increased preproinsulin mRNA in pancreatic islets incubated with islet cell–stimulating antibodies from serums of type I diabetic patients. Diabetes 1990; 39:1165–1169.

298. McMahon MM, O'Brien PC, Service FJ. Diagnostic interpretation of the intravenous tolbutamide test for insulinoma. Mayo Clin Proc 1989; 64:1481–1488.

299. Service FJ, O'Brien PC, Kao PC, et al. C-peptide suppression test: effects of gender, age and body mass index and implications for diagnosis of insulinoma. J Clin Endocrinol Metab 1992; 74:204–210.

300. Perry RR, Vinik AI. Diagnosis and management of functioning islet cell tumors. J Clin Endocrinol Metab 1995; 80:2273–2278.

301. Norton JA, Whitman ED. Insulinoma. Endocrinologist 1995; 3:258–267.

302. Spitz L, Bhargava RK, Grant DB, et al. Surgical treatment of hyperinsulinaemic hypoglycaemia in infancy and childhood. Arch Dis Child 1992; 67:201–205.

303. Brennan MD, Service FJ, Carpenter A-M, et al. Diagnosis of pancreatic islet hyperplasia causing hypoglycemia in a patient with portocaval anastomosis. Am J Med 1980; 68:941–948.

304. Witte DP, Greider MH, DeSchryver-Kecskemeti K, et al. The juvenile human endocrine pancreas: normal v. idiopathic hyperinsulinemic hypoglycemia. Semin Diagn Pathol 1984; 1:30–42.

305. Rahier J. Relevance of endocrine pancreas nesidioblastosis to hyperinsulinemic hypoglycemia. Diabetes Care 1989; 12:164–166.

306. Service FJ, McMahon MM, O'Brien PC, et al. Functioning insulinoma–incidence, recurrence, and long-term survival of patients. Mayo Clin Proc 1991; 66:711–719.

307. Philippe J, Powers AC, Mojsov S, et al. Expression of peptide hormone genes in human islet cell tumors. Diabetes 1988; 37:647–651.

308. D'Arcangues CM, Awoke S, Lawrence GD. Metastatic insulinoma with long survival and glucagonoma syndrome. Ann Intern Med 1984; 100:233–235.

309. Rizza RA, Haymond MW, Verdonk CA, et al. Pathogenesis of hypoglycemia in insulinoma patients. Suppression of hepatic glucose production by insulin. Diabetes 1981; 30:377–381.

310. Service FJ, Dale AJD, Elveback LR, et al. Insulinoma: clinical and diagnostic features of 60 consecutive cases. Mayo Clinic Proc 1976; 51:417–429.

311. Rayfield EJ, Pulini M, Golub A, et al. Nonautonomous function of a pancreatic insulinoma. J Clin Endocrinol Metab 1976; 43:1307–1310.

312. Axelrod L. Insulinoma: cost-effective care in patients with rare disease. Ann Intern Med 1995; 123:311–312.

313. Clarke LR, Jaffe MH, Choyke PL, et al. Pancreatic imaging. Radiol Clin North Am 1985; 23:489–501.

314. Fraker DL, Norton JA. Localization and resection of insulinomas and gastrinomas. JAMA 1988; 259:3601–3605.

315. Norton JA, Shawker TH, Doppman JH, et al. Localization and surgical treatment of occult insulinomas. Ann Surg 1990; 212:615–620.

316. Lamberts SWJ, Bakker WH, Reubi J-C, et al. Somatostatin-receptor imaging in the localization of endocrine tumors. N Engl J Med 1990; 323:1246–1249.

317. Kinoshita Y, Nonaka H, Suzuki S, et al. Accurate localization of insulinomas using percutaneous transhepatic portal venous sampling—usefulness of simultaneous measurement of plasma insulin and glucagon levels. Clin Endocrinol 1985; 23:587–593.

318. Doppman JL, Chang R, Fraker DL, et al. Localization of insulinomas to regions of the pancreas by intra-arterial stimulation with calcium. Ann Intern Med 1995; 123:269–273.

319. Stefanini P, Carboni M, Patrassi N, et al. Beta-islet tumors of the pancreas: results of a study on 1,067 cases. Surgery 1974; 75:597–609.

320. Marks V, Rose FC, Samols E. Hyperinsulinism due to metastasizing insulinoma: treatment with diazoxide. Proc R Soc Med 1965; 58:577–578.

321. Graber AL, Porte D Jr, Williams RH. Clinical use of diazoxide and mechanism for its hyperglycemic effects. Diabetes 1966; 15:143–148.

322. Fajans SS, Flogel JC Jr, Thiffault CA, et al. Further studies on diazoxide suppression of insulin release from abnormal and normal islet tissue in man. Ann NY Acad Sci 1968; 150:261–280.

323. Marks V, Samols E. Diazoxide therapy of intractable hypoglycemia. Ann NY Acad Sci 1968; 150:442–454.

324. Osei K, O'Dorisio TM. Malignant insulinoma: effects of a somatostatin analog (compound 201-995) on serum glucose, growth and gastro-entero-pancreatic hormones. Ann Intern Med 1985; 103:223–225.

325. Kvols LK, Buck M, Moertel CG, et al. Treatment of metastatic islet cell carcinoma with a somatostatin analogue (SMS 201-995). Ann Intern Med 1987; 107:162–168.

326. Alberts AS, Falkson G. Rapid reversal of life-threatening hypoglycaemia with a somatostatin analogue (octreotide). S Afr Med J 1988; 74:75–76.

327. Hearn PR, Ahmed M, Woodhouse NJY. The use of SMS 201-995 (somatostatin analogue) in insulinomas. Horm Res 1988; 29:211–213.

328. Boden G, Ryan IG, Shuman CR. Ineffectiveness of SMS 201-995 in severe hyperinsulinemia. Diabetes Care 1988; 11:664–668.

329. Broder LE, Carter SK. Pancreatic islet cell carcinoma. II: Results of therapy with streptozotocin in 52 patients. Ann Intern Med 1973; 79:108–118.

330. Moertel CG, Hanley JA, Johnson LA. Streptozotocin alone compared with streptozotocin plus fluorouracil in the treatment of advanced islet cell carcinoma. N Engl J Med 1980; 303:1189–1195.

331. Ajani JA, Carrasco H, Charnsangavej C, et al. Islet cell tumors metastatic to the liver: effective palliation by sequential hepatic artery embolization. Ann Intern Med 1988; 108:340–344.

332. Cowett RM. Pathophysiology, diagnosis and management of glucose homeostasis in the neonate. In: Lockhardt JD, ed. Current Problems in Pediatrics. Vol 15. Chicago: Year Book Medical, 1985: 1–47.

333. Gregory JW, Aynsley-Green A. Hypoglycaemia in the infant and child. Bailleres Clin Endocrinol Metab 1993; 7:683–704.

334. Sperling MA, Garguli S, Leslie N, et al. Fetal-perinatal catecholamine secretion: role in perinatal glucose homeostasis. Am J Physiol 1984; 247:E69–E74.

335. Bier DM, Leake RD, Haymond MW, et al. Measurement of "true" glucose production rates with 6,6-dideutero-glucose. Diabetes 1977; 26:1016–1023.

336. Haymond MW, Karl IE, Pagliara AS. Increased gluconeogenic substrates in small for gestational age infants. N Engl J Med 1974; 291:332–328.

337. Hawdon JM, Weddell A, Aynsley-Green A, et al. Hormonal and metabolic response to hypoglycaemia in small for gestational age infants. Arch Dis Child 1993; 68:269–273.

338. Haymond MW, Karl IE, Clarke WL, et al. Differences in circulating gluconeogenic substrates during short term fasting in men, women and children. Metabolism 1982; 31:33–42.

339. Senior B. Ketotic hypoglycemia. J Pediatr 1973; 82:555–556.

340. Pagliara AS, Karl IE, DeVivo DC, et al. Hypoalaninemia: a concomitant of ketotic hypoglycemia. J Clin Invest 1972; 51:1440–1449.

341. Haymond MW, Karl IE, Pagliara AS. Ketotic hypoglycemia: an amino acid substrate limited disorder. J Clin Endocrinol Metab 1974; 38:521–530.

342. Miles JM, Nissen S, Gerich J, et al. Effects of epinephrine infusion on leucine and alanine kinetics in humans. Am J Physiol 1984; 247:E166–E172.

343. Worden FP, Freidenberg G, Pescovitz OH. The diagnosis and management of neonatal hyperinsulinism. Endocrinologist 1994; 4:196–204.

344. Leibowitz G, Glaser B, Higazi AA, et al. Hyperinsulinemic hypoglycemia of infancy (nesidioblastosis) in clinical remission: high incidence of diabetes mellitus and persistent β-cell dysfunction at long-term follow-up. J Clin Endocrinol Metab 1995; 80:386–392.

345. Aparicio L, Carpenter MW, Schwartz R, et al. Prenatal diagnosis of familial neonatated hyperinsulinemia. Acta Paediatr 1993; 82:683–686.

346. Thomas PM, Cote GJ, Wohllk N, et al. Mutations in the sulfonylurea receptor gene in familial persistent hyperinsulinemic hypoglycemia of infancy. Science 1995; 268:426–429.

347. Aguilar-Bryan L, Nichols C, Wechsler SW, et al. Cloning of the β cell high affinity sulfonylurea receptor: a regulator of insulin secretion. Science 1995; 268:423–426.

348. Wang N, Finegold MJ, Bradley A, et al. Impaired energy homeostasis in C/EBP knockout mice. Science 1995; 269:1108–1112.

349. Pears JS, Jung RT, Hopwood D, et al. Glycogen storage disease diagnosed in adults. Q J Med 1992; 82:207–222.

350. Talente GM, Coleman RA, Alter C, et al. Glycogen storage disease in adults. Ann Intern Med 1994; 120:218–226.

351. Chen YT, Burchell A. Glycogen storage diseases. In: Scriver CR, Beaudet AL, Sly WS, et al, eds. The Metabolic and Molecular Bases of Inherited Disease. 7th ed. New York: McGraw-Hill, 1995: 935–965.

352. Gitzelmann R, Steinmann B, Van den Berghe G. Disorders of fructose metabolism. In: Scriver CR, Beaudet AL, Sly WS, et al, eds. The Metabolic and Molecular Bases of Inherited Disease. 7th ed. New York: McGraw-Hill, 1995: 905–934.

353. Segal S, Berry GT. Disorders of galactose metabolism. In: Scriver CR, Beaudet AL, Sly WS, et al, eds. The Metabolic and Molecular Bases of Inherited Disease. 7th ed. New York: McGraw-Hill, 1995: 967–1000.

354. Cori GT, Cori CF. Glucose-6-phosphatase of the liver in glycogen storage disease. J Biol Chem 1952; 199:661–667.

355. Lei K-J, Shelly LL, Lin B, et al. Mutations in the glucose-6-phosphatase gene are associated with glycogen storage disease types Ia and IaSP but not Ib and Ic. J Clin Invest 1995; 95:234–240.

356. Greene HL, Slonim AE, Burr IM, et al. Type 1 glycogen storage disease. Five years of management with nocturnal intragastric feeding. J Pediatr 1989; 96:590–595.

357. Wolfsdorf JI, Ehrlich S, Landy HS, et al. Optimal daytime feeding regimen to prevent postprandial hypoglycemia in type 1 glycogen storage disease. Am J Clin Nutr 1992; 56:587–592.

358. Kirschner BS, Baker AL, Thorpe FK. Growth in adulthood after liver transplantation for glycogen storage disease type I. Gastroenterology 1991; 101:238–241.

359. Rother KI, Schwenk WF. Glucose production in glycogen storage disease I is not associated with increased cycling through hepatic glycogen. Am J Physiol 1995; 269:E774–E778.

360. Pagliara AS, Karl IE, Keating JP, et al. Hepatic fructose-1,6-diphosphatase deficiency: a cause of lactic acidosis and hypoglycemia in infancy. J Clin Invest 1972; 51:2115–2123.

361. Kaufman U, Froesch ER. Inhibition of phosphorylase-a by fructose-1-phosphate, alpha-glycerophosphate and fructose-1,6-diphosphate: explanation for fructose-induced hypoglycemia in hereditary fructose intolerance and fructose-1,6-diphosphatase deficiency. Eur J Clin Invest 1973; 3:407–413.

362. Chuang DT, Shih VE. Disorders of branched chain amino acid and keto acid metabolism. In: Scriver CR, Beaudet AL, Sly WS, et al, eds. The Metabolic and molecular Bases of Inherited Disease. 7th ed. New York: McGraw-Hill, 1995: 1239–1277.

363. Haymond MW, Ben-Galim E, Strobel KE. Glucose and alanine metabolism in children with maple syrup urine disease. J Clin Invest 1978; 62:398–405.

364. Nobukuni Y, Mitsubuchi H, Endo F, et al. Maple syrup urine disease. J Clin Invest 1990; 869:242–247.

365. Cheema-Dhadli S, Lernoff CC, Halperin ML. Effect of 2-methylcitrate on citrate metabolism: implications for the management of patients with propionic acidemia and methylmalonic aciduria. Pediatr Res 1975; 9:905–908.

366. Roe CR, Coates PM. Mitochondrial fatty acid oxidation disorders. In: Scriver CR, Beaudet AL, Sly WS, et al, eds. The Metabolic and Molecular Bases of Inherited Disease. 7th ed. New York: McGraw-Hill, 1995: 1501–1533.

367. Vockley J. The changing face of disorders of fatty acid oxidation. Mayo Clin Proc 1994; 69:249–257.

368. Taroni F, Verderio E, Fiorucci S, et al. Molecular characterization of inherited carnitine palmitoyltransferase II deficiency. Proc Natl Acad Sci USA 1992; 89:8429–8433.

369. Pandi SV, Brivet M, Slama A, et al. Carnitine-acylcarnitine translocase deficiency with severe hypoglycemia and auriculoventricular block. J Clin Invest 1993; 91:1247–1252.

370. Brackett JC, Sims HF, Steiner RD, et al. A novel mutation in medium chain acyl-CoA dehydrogenase causes sudden neonatal death. J Clin Invest 1994; 94:1477–1483.

371. Glasgow AM, Engel AG, Bier DM, et al. Hypoglycemia, hepatic dysfunction, muscle weakness, cardiomyopathy, free carnitine deficiency and long chain acylcarnitine excess responsive to medium chain triglyceride diet. Pediatr Res 1983; 17:319–326.

372. Leichter SB, Permutt MA. Effect of adrenergic agents on postgastrectomy hypoglycemia. Diabetes 1975; 24:1005–1010.

373. Shultz KT, Neelon FA, Nilsen LB, et al. Mechanism of postgastrectomy hypoglycemia. Arch Intern Med 1971; 128:240–246.

374. Charles MA, Hofeldt F, Shackelford A, et al. Comparison of oral glucose tolerance tests and mixed meals in patients with apparent idiopathic post-absorptive hypoglycemia. Diabetes 1981; 30:465–470.

375. Lev-Ran A, Anderson RW. The diagnosis of postprandial hypoglycemia. Diabetes 1981; 30:996–999.

376. Betteridge DJ. Reactive hypoglycemia. Br Med J 1987; 295:286–287.

377. Palardy J, Havrankova J, Lepage R, et al. Blood glucose measurements during symptomatic episodes in patients with suspected postprandial hypoglycemia. N Engl J Med 1989; 321:1421–1425.

378. Goldman J. Pathogenesis of functional or idiopathic reactive hypoglycemia: hyperresponsiveness to insulin and increased receptor effector coupling. In: Andreani D, DePirro R, Lauro R, et al, eds. Current Views on Insulin Receptors. New York: Academic, 1981: 499–505.

379. Tamburrano G, Leonetti F, Sbraccia P, et al. Increased insulin sensitivity in patients with idiopathic reactive hypoglycemia. J Clin Endocrinol Metab 1989; 69:885–890.

380. Foa PP, Dunbar JC, Klein SP, et al. Reactive hypoglycemia and A-cell ("pancreatic") glucagon deficiency in the adult. JAMA 1980; 244:2281–2285.

381. Shima K, Tabata M, Tanaka A, et al. Exaggerated response of plasma glucagon-like immunoreactivity to oral glucose in patients with reactive hypoglycemia. Endocrol Jpn 1981; 28:249–256.

382. Chalew SA, McLaughlin JV, Mersey J, et al. The use of the plasma epinephrine response in the diagnosis of idiopathic postprandial syndrome. JAMA 1984; 251:612–615.

383. Permutt MA, Keller D, Santiago JV. Cholinergic blockade in reactive hypoglycemia. Diabetes 1977; 26:121–127.

384. Jenkins DJA, Bloom SR, Albuquerque RH, et al. Pectin and complications after gastric surgery: normalization of postprandial glucose and endocrine responses. Gut 1980; 21:574–579.

385. Fink WJ, Hucke ST, Gray TW, et al. Treatment of postoperative reactive hypoglycemia by a reversed intestinal segment. Am J Surg 1976; 131:19–22.

386. Kay WW. The treatment of prolonged insulin coma. J Ment Sci 1961; 107:194–238.

387. MacCuish AC, Munro JF, Duncan LJP. Treatment of hypoglycaemic coma with glucagon, intravenous dextrose, and mannitol infusion in a hundred diabetics. Lancet 1970; 2:946–949.

388. Hoffbrand BI, Sevitt LH. Use of mannitol in prolonged coma due to insulin overdosage. Lancet 1966; 1:402.

389. Anderson JH, Byrd GW, Blackard WG. Hyperresponsiveness to tolbutamide of dogs pretreated with diazoxide. Metabolism 1971; 20:1023–1030.

390. Koch-Weser J. Diazoxide. N Engl J Med 1976; 294:1271–1273.

391. Baxter RC, Holman SR, Corbould A, et al. Regulation of the insulin-like growth factors and their binding proteins by glucocorticoid and growth hormone in nonislet cell tumor hypoglycemia. J Clin Endocrinol Metab 1995; 80:2700–2708.

21

DIABETES MELLITUS

Roger H. Unger and Daniel W. Foster

Diabetes mellitus comprises a heterogeneous group of hyperglycemic disorders. The hyperglycemia is the consequence of a relative or absolute deficiency of insulin and a relative or absolute excess of glucagon. If the insulin deficiency is extreme, these hormonal abnormalities cause ketoacidosis and other manifestations of accelerated catabolism. Diabetes is associated with late complications involving the eyes, kidneys, nerves, and blood vessels. It is a leading cause of adult blindness in the United States and a major cause of renal failure, gangrene, myocardial infarction, and stroke.[1]

DIAGNOSIS OF DIABETES

Fasting Plasma Glucose

The "gold standard" for the diagnosis of diabetes is an elevated plasma glucose level after an overnight fast. The diagnostic value usually cited is 7.8 mmol/L (140 mg/dL) or higher on at least two occasions.[2] In 1997 the American Diabetes Association recommended lowering the diagnostic level to 7.0 mmol/L (126 mg/dL)[3] (Table 21–1).

Oral Glucose Tolerance Test

Because the distribution curve of oral glucose tolerance tests (OGTTs) in the general population is unimodal, no single set of glucose values separates all nondiabetics from all diabetics. Various diagnostic standards for diabetes have been recommended. The most sensitive, those of Mosenthal and Barry,[4] gave positive results in 40% of a random population,[5] making them too nonspecific for diagnosis (Table 21–2). However, the fact that fewer than 1% of persons who are classified as normal by these criteria develop overt diabetes within 10 y indicates that postglucose values of less than 8.3 mmol/L (150 mg/dL) make future development of diabetes unlikely. The

TABLE 21–1. Criteria for Diagnosis of Diabetes in Nonpregnant Adults

I. *In a clinical setting.* Any one of the following is considered diagnostic of diabetes. In each case, measurement of glucose concentration should be repeated on a second occasion to confirm the diagnosis.

A. Presence of the classic symptoms of diabetes, such as polyuria, polydipsia, ketonuria, and rapid weight loss, together with gross and unequivocal elevation of plasma glucose, e.g., postprandial or random plasma glucose concentration ≥ 11.1 mmol/L (200 mg/dL).

B. Elevated fasting glucose concentration on more than one occasion: venous plasma ≥ 7.8 mmol/L (140 mg/dL), venous whole blood ≥ 6.7 mmol/L (120 mg/dL), or capillary whole blood ≥ 6.7 mmol/L (120 mg/dL). If the fasting glucose concentration meets these criteria, it is considered diagnostic of diabetes, and the OGTT is not required. Virtually all persons with FPG ≥ 7.8 mmol/L (140 mg/dL) will exhibit an OGTT that meets or exceeds the secondary criteria (see I.C.).

C. Fasting glucose concentration less than that which is diagnostic of diabetes (see I.B.), but sustained elevated glucose concentration during the OGTT. The NDDG requires that both the 2-h sample and some other sample taken between administration of the 75-g glucose dose and 2 h later meet the following criteria; the WHO requires only that the 2-h sample meet these criteria: venous plasma ≥ 11.1 mmol/L (200 mg/dL), venous whole blood ≥ 10.0 mmol/L (180 mg/dL), or capillary whole blood ≥ 11.1 mmol/L (200 mg/dL).

II. *In an epidemiologic setting.* In epidemiologic research or during screening for diabetes, it is usually impossible to conduct careful plasma glucose measurements. Any one of the following criteria, which are compromises, is considered sufficient to denote diabetes in these circumstances:

A. Medical history of diabetes diagnosed by a physician.

B. A single elevated fasting glucose concentration: venous plasma ≥ 7.8 mmol/L (140 mg/dL), venous whole blood ≥ 6.7 mmol/L (120 mg/dL), or capillary whole blood ≥ 6.7 mmol/L (120 mg/dL).

C. A single elevated glucose concentration 2 hours after ingestion of a 75-g glucose dose: venous plasma ≥ 11.1 mmol/L (200 mg/dL), venous whole blood ≥ 10.0 mmol/L (180 mg/dL), or capillary whole blood ≥ 11.1 mmol/L (200 mg/dL).

FPG, fasting plasma glucose; OGTT, oral glucose tolerance test; NDDG, National Diabetes Data Group; WHO, World Health Organization.

National Diabetes Data Group: Classification and diagnosis of diabetes mellitus and other categories of glucose intolerance. Diabetes 1979;28:1039–1057; World Health Organization: Second Report of the Expert Committee on Diabetes Mellitus. WHO Technical Report Series, No. 646. Geneva, Switzerland. World Health Organization, 1980. See ref. 3 for modified criteria for diagnosis recommended by the American Diabetes Association.

most specific diagnostic criteria are those of the National Diabetes Data Group (see Table 21–2), which selected 11.1 mmol/L (200 mg/dL) at either 1 or 2 h as the diagnostic OGTT value. This choice is consistent with the separation point between nondiabetic and diabetic OGTT modes in the Pima Indians, a population with a bimodal distribution of OGTT values.[6] Its diagnostic validity is supported by the fact that microaneurysms almost never develop in subjects whose glucose levels are below this value after a glucose load.[7]

The OGTT is influenced by many factors other than diabetes, including age, diet, state of health, gastrointestinal function, medications, and emotional state. When it is used for screening in large populations, the test overestimates the prevalence of diabetes. After age 50 glucose tolerance declines as a consequence of changes in insulin sensitivity of target tissues.[8, 9] Therefore, in a middle-aged or elderly person, a diagnosis of diabetes based on the Mosenthal-Barry or Fajans-Conn standards for oral glucose tolerance (see Table 21–2) serves no useful clinical purpose and needlessly jeopardizes employability and insurability. By contrast, the same abnormality in a child usually indicates early diabetes.

Standards for the OGTT were derived from studies in normal populations; their application to patients who are ill, carbohydrate-restricted, physically inactive, or taking certain medications produces many false-positive results. Therefore, an OGTT should be performed only in well persons who have been consuming a normal diet with adequate carbohydrates for 3 days before the test. Because abnormal glucose tolerance in an ill person may reflect stress hyperglycemia rather than diabetes, the test should be deferred until after the patient has fully recovered. The OGTT is not necessary if the fasting plasma glucose level is consistently elevated.

Intravenous Glucose Tolerance Test (K Value)

The intravenous glucose tolerance test is not sensitive for the diagnosis of diabetes, but it is useful for the assessment of glucose disposal. Results are reported as K values, a reflection of the time required for glucose to clear the circulation. ($K = 0.69/T_{1/2} \times 100$, where $T_{1/2}$ is the time required for plasma glucose to reach one half of the calculated zero-time concentration.) The normal value for K is 1.2 or greater.

The insulin response to intravenously injected glucose provides a useful index of residual beta-cell function during the development of diabetes, and an abbreviated test is used to estimate insulin reserve in prediabetic subjects at risk for the disease. Glucose is infused as a 25% solution for 3 min at a total load of 0.5 g/kg body weight. Plasma insulin is measured at 1 and 3 min, and the values above baseline are added. Sums below 340 pmol/L (48 μU/mL) are predictive of diabetes, especially if the subject is islet cell cytoplasmic antibody (ICA) positive.[10]

Glycosylated Hemoglobin (Hemoglobin A$_{1c}$)

An increased level of hemoglobin A$_{1c}$ (HbA$_{1c}$) constitutes presumptive evidence of diabetes, although verification by standard procedures is required. A normal HbA$_{1c}$ level does not exclude impaired glucose tolerance or mild diabetes, but HbA$_{1c}$ determinations correlate with the fasting plasma glucose level.[11, 12] Although values vary from laboratory to laboratory, the distributions of HbA$_{1c}$ concentrations in normal persons and in diabetic patients do not overlap.[12] The HbA$_{1c}$ levels of patients with normal fasting plasma glucose concentrations but impaired glucose tolerance are intermediate between those of normal persons and those of diabetics. A value greater than 3 standard deviations above the normal mean is more than 99% specific for diabetes. Measurement of HbA$_{1c}$ provides an integrated assessment of antecedent glycemia over an extended period.

Muscle Capillary Basement Membrane Thickening

Thickening of the capillary basement membranes occurs in tissues throughout the body, but it is most conveniently measured in specimens of quadriceps muscle. A muscle capillary basement membrane width greater than 180 nm (1800 Å) is diagnostic of diabetes provided vascular disease such as lupus erythematosus is not present. Although originally proposed as a marker of diabetes that was independent of hyperglycemia,[13] basement membrane thickening is now regarded as a consequence of the metabolic disorder.[14–16] Muscle

TABLE 21–2. Glucose Levels Recommended as Diagnostic for Diabetes by Oral Glucose Tolerance Testing

Time After Ingestion	Mosenthal-Barry	Fajans-Conn	National Diabetes Data Group
1 h*	9.2 mmol/L (165 mg/dL)	10.3 mmol/L (185 mg/dL)	11.1 mmol/L (200 mg/dL)
2 h	6.4 mmol/L (115 mg/dL)	7.8 mmol/L (140 mg/dL)	11.1 mmol/L (200 mg/dL)

*"True glucose" measurements in plasma (measurements in whole blood are 15% lower). Results of the Hoffman ferricyanide method used in autoanalyzers are approximately 0.3 mmol/L (5 mg/dL) above the true glucose value.

TABLE 21–3. Classification of the Types of Diabetes

Insulin-dependent diabetes mellitus (IDDM)	Low or absent levels of circulating endogenous insulin; dependent on injected insulin to prevent ketosis and sustain life
	Onset predominantly in youth but can occur at any age
	Associated with certain HLA and GAD antigens
	Abnormal immune response; islet cell antibodies are frequently present at diagnosis
	Cause probably only partially genetic; only about 35% of monozygotic twins are concordant for IDDM
Non–insulin-dependent diabetes mellitus (NIDDM)	Insulin levels may be normal, elevated, or depressed; hyperinsulinemia and insulin resistance characterize most patients; insulinopenia may develop as the disease progresses
	Not insulin dependent or ketosis prone under normal circumstances, but may require insulin for treatment of hyperglycemia
	Onset predominantly after age 40 years but can occur at any age
	Approximately 50% of men and 70% of women are obese
	Cause probably strongly genetic; 60–90% of monozygotic twins are concordant for NIDDM
Gestational diabetes	Glucose intolerance that has its onset or recognition during pregnancy
	Associated with older age, obesity, family history of diabetes
	Conveys increased risk for the woman for subsequent progression to NIDDM
	Associated with increased risk of macrosomia
Other types of diabetes*	In addition to the presence of the specific condition, hyperglycemia at a level diagnostic of diabetes is also present
	Causes of hyperglycemia are known for some conditions (e.g., pancreatic disease); for others, an etiologic relation between diabetes and the condition is suspected

*Includes diabetes secondary to or associated with pancreatic disease, hormonal disease, drug or chemical exposure, insulin receptor abnormalities, and certain genetic syndromes.

capillary basement membrane thickness appears to recede within 2 y after return of the plasma glucose level to near normal by aggressive insulin therapy.[17, 18]

NOMENCLATURE AND DEFINITIONS

Diabetes mellitus can be divided into two major categories depending on whether endogenous insulin secretion is sufficient to prevent diabetic ketoacidosis. In most classifications, including that of the National Diabetes Data Group[2] (Table 21–3), the terms *insulin-dependent diabetes mellitus* (IDDM) and *type I diabetes* are used synonymously.[19, 20] In this chapter the designation IDDM is applied to all forms of diabetes in which exogenous insulin is required to prevent diabetic ketoacidosis, regardless of etiologic cause. The term type I diabetes is applied only to diabetes resulting from autoimmune destruction of beta cells, regardless of whether the destruction is sufficiently complete to result in ketoacidosis-prone IDDM.

Similarly, the terms *non–insulin-dependent diabetes mellitus* (NIDDM) and *type II diabetes* are usually used synonymously. In this chapter, the designation NIDDM is applied to any form of diabetes, regardless of origin, in which endogenous insulin production is sufficient to prevent diabetic ketoacidosis. The term type II diabetes is restricted to patients with NIDDM who do not have autoimmune destruction of beta cells (type I disease), pancreatic disease, or other rare causes of hyperglycemia. In this formulation IDDM and NIDDM indicate only the absence or presence of beta-cell function, whereas type I and type II distinguish between autoimmune and nonautoimmune forms of diabetes. For example, if a patient with autoimmune diabetes were to pass through a transient non–insulin-dependent period during which beta-cell destruction is incomplete, he or she would be classified as having type I NIDDM until such time as insulin dependence appeared, whereupon the classification would change to type I IDDM. This classification is useful but sometimes breaks down in practice. For example, ketoacidosis occasionally occurs in patients previously classified as having NIDDM.[21]

INSULIN-DEPENDENT DIABETES MELLITUS

Demography
Prevalence

Type I IDDM is predominantly a disease of whites and of populations with a substantial white genetic admixture,

including African Americans. It is rare in Japanese, Chinese, Filipinos, Asiatic Indians, Native Americans, African blacks, Polynesians, Eskimos, Micronesians, and Melanesians (Table 21–4).[22–25] In Israeli children of European parentage the prevalence of IDDM is almost three times that in Israeli children of Asiatic or African parentage.[26]

These differences may not be entirely racial, because there may be regional differences in prevalence within the same country.[27] An environmental impact is also suggested by seasonal variations in rate of appearance[28, 29] and by the fact that fewer than half of identical twins are concordant for IDDM.[30]

The prevalence of type I IDDM in the United States is about 260 per 100,000 (0.26%) by age 20,[31] and an equal number develop the disease after age 20.[32] In England the prevalence of type I IDDM is 220 per 100,000 (0.22%) by age 20,[33] and the disease seems to be manifesting itself at an earlier age.[34]

Incidence

In countries in which the population is predominantly white, the reported yearly appearance rate of IDDM ranges from 3.7 to 20.0 per 100,000.[31] In midwestern Poland the incidence almost doubled, from 3.5 new cases per 100,000 in the period from 1970 to 1981 to 6.6 per 100,000 from 1982 to 1984,[35] an increase largely in younger children. The Pittsburgh registry in the United States showed an incidence ranging from 10 per 100,000 per year for nonwhite males to 16 per

TABLE 21–4. Prevalence of Insulin-Dependent Diabetes in General Populations (1970–1980)*

Country	Age Group (y)	Method of Ascertainment	Prevalence/1000
Australia	20 (men)	Interview and screening for national service	3.7
Cuba	0–14	National registry	0.13
France	0–19	Central registry	0.3
Japan	6–15	Urine tests on 25,000 persons	0.12
Sweden	0–15	Known cases	2.2
United States	0–15	Household interviews	0.38
United States	0–16	Known cases	1.3
United States	6–18	School records	1.9

*As evidenced by the three studies in the United States, estimates of prevalence vary depending on method of ascertainment; if the criteria of Table 21–2 were applied, different prevalence values would be found.

Adapted from West KM. Epidemiology of Diabetes and Its Vascular Lesions. New York: Elsevier, 1978: 292–293.

100,000 per year for white males. Rates for women were intermediate between those for nonwhite and white males.[31] The incidence in Rochester, Minnesota, is 8.4 per 100,000 per year.[36] In Denmark the incidence is about 13.2 per 100,000 per year up to 29 y of age.[29, 37] In Finland the incidence between 1987 and 1989 was 38.4 per 100,000 per year in boys and 32.2 in girls, the highest in the world.[38] By contrast, the incidence is only 0.6 per 100,000 per year in Korea and Mexico. In Europe the incidence is highest in the northern regions and lowest in the south,[39] with Greece having an incidence of 4.6 per 100,000 per year (Fig. 21–1). There are exceptions, however; in Sardinia the incidence is virtually the same as in Finland, and in Iceland the incidence is one third that in Finland.[40] The reasons for these differences are obscure, although the introduction of dairy products at less than 2 months of age is said to be associated with an increased risk for IDDM.[41] In both the United States and Denmark the peak age of onset is between 10 and 14 y.[31, 33]

Some[34, 35, 37] but not all[24, 31] researchers think that the incidence of type I diabetes has increased during the last several decades. The incidence of IDDM may have increased in the Netherlands[41] and in Scandinavia,[42, 43] but not in Iceland.[40]

Family Studies

Familial aggregation of type I IDDM is uncommon.[44–46] The concordance rate of 50% or less for IDDM in monozygotic twins contrasts with the familial aggregation and the almost 100% concordance in monozygotic twins in type II NIDDM.[47] In 493 families studied after identification of a proband with IDDM,[48] the risk of IDDM in siblings was higher (8.5%) if the proband had been diagnosed before age 10 than if he or she had been diagnosed after age 10 (4.6%). Only 79 (16%) of the families had one or more siblings or parents with IDDM. An evaluation of seven studies involving 9000 families revealed a mean risk for diabetes of 1.3% in parents, 4.2% in siblings, and 1.9% in offspring.[49] Although slightly higher estimates have come from other studies,[50] familial transmission of IDDM is not common. Offspring of type I diabetic fathers with the DR4 allele (see next section) are at higher risk for diabetes than offspring of type I diabetic mothers.[51, 52]

Genetics

Major Histocompatibility Complex

The major histocompatibility complex (MHC) is important in diabetes, both because susceptibility to type I IDDM appears to be linked to certain human leukocyte antigen (HLA) alleles and because the region controls immune response.

The MHC is located on the short arm of the sixth chromosome. The products of the MHC genes include glycoprotein molecules in the plasma membranes of cells (Fig. 21–2),[53–55] the C2 and C4 components of the classic complement pathway, and factor Bf of the alternative complement pathway. The genes for tumor necrosis factors α and β (TNF α, TNF β) and for steroid 21-hydroxylase (CYP21, formerly called P450$_{c21}$) are located within the MHC region, and because the region is large in genetic terms, additional proteins are probably encoded there. HLA loci are designated by the letters A, B, C, and D (Fig. 21–3). Alleles are identified by arabic numerals (e.g., HLA-B8). The addition of a lowercase w indicates that identification of the antigen is provisional (e.g., Dw2). The D region has three distinct loci, DP, DQ, and DR.[56, 57] Gene products of the MHC are classified according to their function. Class I molecules include gene products of the HLA-

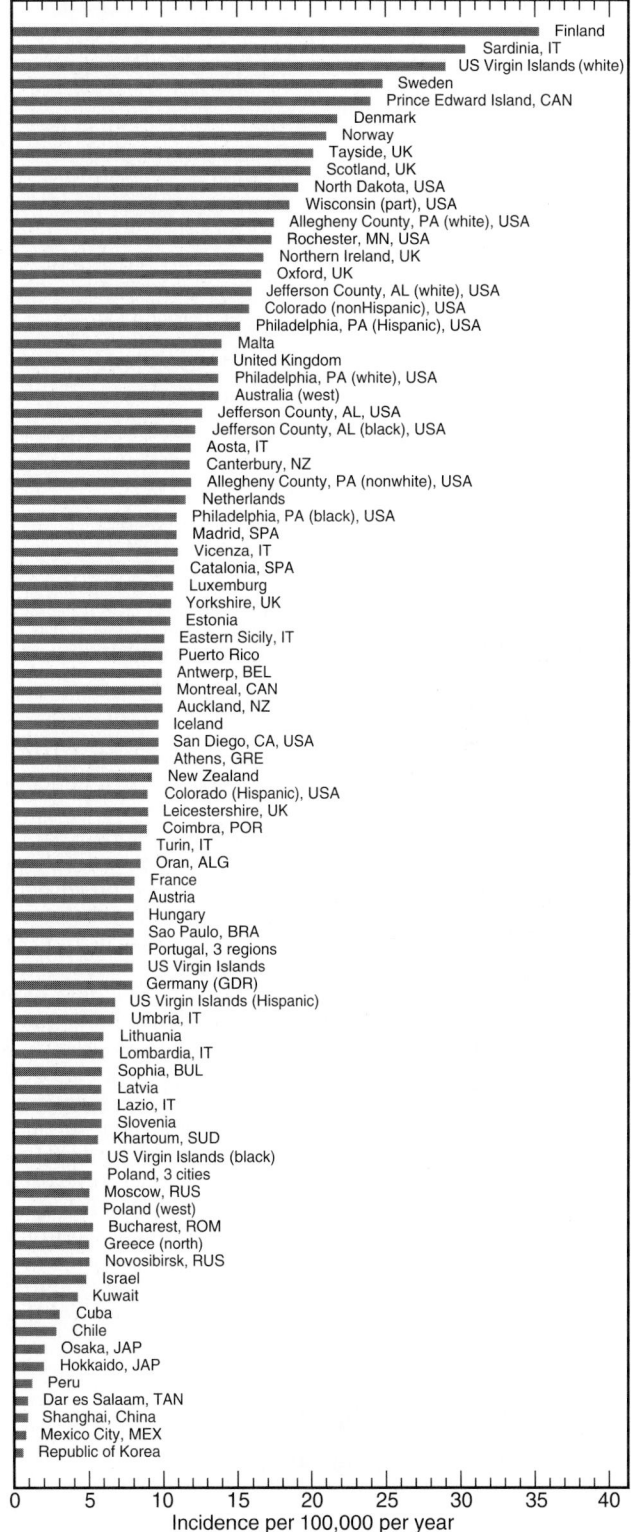

Figure 21–1. Geographic variations in IDDM incidence. (Redrawn and modified from King H, Rewers M, WHO Ad Hoc Diabetes Reporting Group: Global estimates for prevalence of diabetes mellitus and impaired glucose tolerance in adults. Diabetes Care 1993; 16:157–177.)

A, -B, and -C loci; class II molecules are encoded at D (and D-related) sites; and class III molecules are the complement-related proteins.

CLASS I MOLECULES. Class I antigens, expressed on all nucleated cells, are equivalent to the gene products that are

Class I   **Class II**

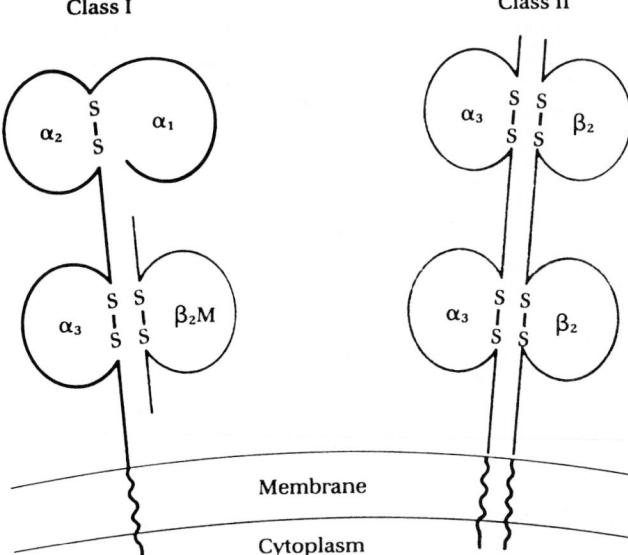

Figure 21–2. Structure of class I and class II MHC molecules. In class I the alpha chain is variable but β₂-microglobulin (β₂M) is invariant. In class II the alpha chain is largely invariant, while beta chains are variable. (From Golub ES. Immunology: A Synthesis. Sunderland, MA: Sinauer Associates, 1987: 222–233.)

encoded in mice at the K and D sites of the H-2 locus (MHC). The antigens consist of two chains that are associated noncovalently (see Fig. 21–2). The larger chain, a glycosylated polypeptide with an apparent molecular mass of about 43 kd, is encoded on chromosome 6; the smaller chain, β₂-microglobulin (apparent molecular mass, 12 kd), is encoded on chromosome 15. Genetic variability is accounted for by the larger chain. Class I molecules are involved in cell-mediated immunity and are required for recognition and rejection of all foreign (nonself) cells and of intrinsic (self) cells that have been altered by viral infection or malignant disease.[53] Quiescent T lymphocytes become capable of inducing cell lysis (cytotoxic T cells or killer [K] cells) by exposure to antigen-presenting cells, which are macrophages that process antigens such as viral proteins and present peptide fragments of such antigens in association with the class I molecule expressed on the cell surface. Only the subset of T lymphocytes with receptors for both the viral antigen and the class I molecule (i.e., the "neoantigen" formed by a viral protein complexed to the class I antigen) become activated.[58] This obligate requirement for class I molecules in the recognition of and response to foreign antigens, the so-called MHC restriction, ensures that

only cells bearing the processed foreign antigen–class I molecule complex are lysed by the activated cytotoxic T cell.

CLASS II MOLECULES. Class II molecules are equivalent to Ia antigens in the murine system and are often so designated. Figure 21–3 shows the orientation of the human HLA-D region on the short arm of chromosome 6, and Figure 21–4 provides a map of the class II loci of this region. DR specificities can be determined by mixed lymphocyte culture and serologic testing or DNA sequencing, DQ by immunologic assay or DNA sequencing. However, the polymerase chain reaction is now routinely employed to obtain the most complete and pertinent analysis for genetic screening. Class II molecules normally are expressed only on B lymphocytes, tissue and circulating macrophages, endothelial cells, and some activated T lymphocytes; they are not normally present on connective tissue cells or epithelial cells. This limited expression protects against inappropriate T-cell activation and autoimmunity.[59] Class II antigens (see Fig. 21–2) consist of a heavy alpha chain with an apparent molecular mass of 33 kd (range, 29 to 34 kd) and a lighter beta chain with an apparent molecular mass of 28 kd (range, 25 to 28 kd). The alpha chain is largely invariant, whereas the beta chain is highly polymorphic. In a manner analogous to activation of cytotoxic T cells, helper T cells are activated by exposure to cells presenting a foreign antigen or an autoantigen in association with the class II molecule; in other words, helper T-lymphocyte activation is also MHC restricted. The activation of helper-inducer T lymphocytes involves a receptor complex composed of a monomeric antigen designated T3 and a heterodimer called Ti to which antigen-presenting cells bind[60] (Fig. 21–5). Activated helper T cells then interact with B lymphocytes and with plasma cells expressing the same antigen–class II complex expressed by the activating macrophage and enhance antibody formation.

How helper T cells interact with cytotoxic T cells in rejection of transplanted allografts is not completely understood, although survival is prolonged by antibodies directed against class II molecules on the antigen-presenting cell.[61, 62]

Both class I and class II molecules could be important in the immune reactions that characterize development of type I IDDM, although the mechanism is unknown. It may be speculated, for example, that high-risk class I or class II molecules (or both) confer susceptibility for IDDM through more effective presentation of antigen.

Associations Between HLA Antigens and Type I IDDM

Approximately 95% of white patients with type I IDDM have either DR3 or DR4 antigens,[63–66] and 55 to 60% have

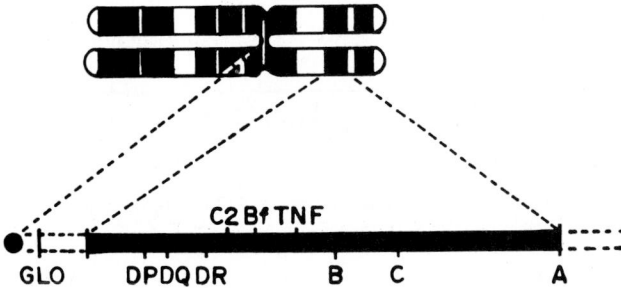

Figure 21–3. Schematic representation of the major histocompatibility complex in humans. Loci are approximate. C2 and Bf are complement-related sites, and TNF is the tumor necrosis factor gene. (Adapted from Irvine WJ. Immunological aspects of diabetes mellitus: a review [including the salient points of the NDDG report on the classification of diabetes]. In: Irvine WJ, ed. Immunology of Diabetes. Edinburgh: Teviot Scientific Publications, 1980: 1–53.)

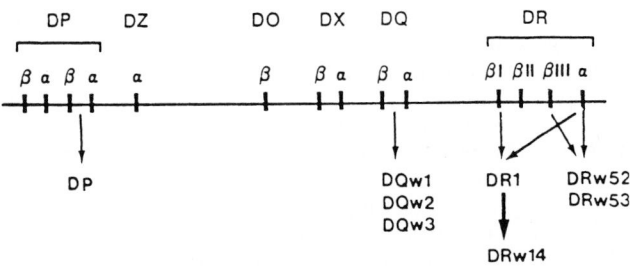

Figure 21–4. Map of the class II loci of the human HLA-D region on the short arm of chromosome 6. The DRβI and DRα gene products associate to form a cell-surface heterodimeric glycoprotein. The resulting molecule reacts with the alloantisera that define the major DR allotypes. The relatively nonpolymorphic DRβIII gene products are utilized in several DR allotypes. DRβII is a pseudogene. The DQα and DQβ genes encode the DQ serologic specificities (DQw1, DQw2, and DQw3). Only one DPα and DPβ gene is expressed. The second DPα and DPβ and DXα and DXβ genes are not expressed. DOβ and DZα are expressed only in very small amounts. (From Todd JA, Bell JI, McDevitt HO. HLA-DQβ gene contributes to susceptibility and resistance to insulin-dependent diabetes mellitus. Reprinted by permission from Nature, Vol. 329, pp. 599–604. Copyright © 1987, by Macmillan Magazines Limited.)

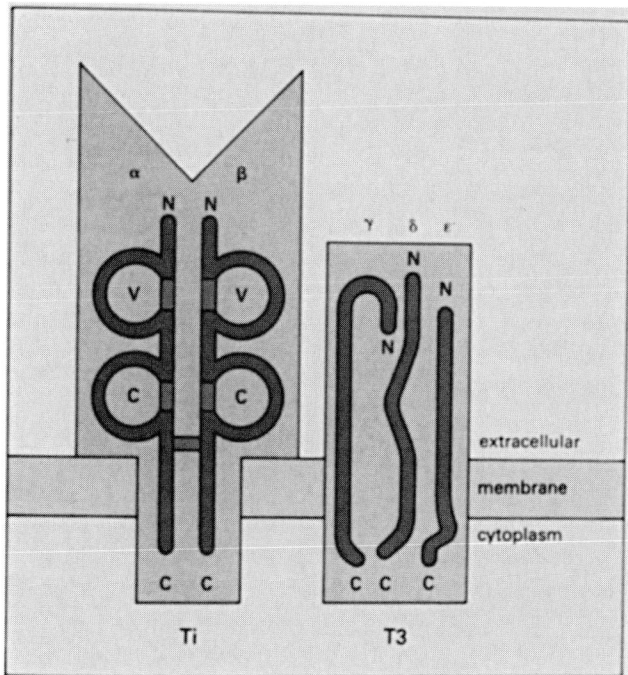

Figure 21–5. Structure of the human T-cell receptor. The T-cell receptor is a complex of the Ti molecule, which binds antigen/MHC and the T3 molecular complex. Ti consists of a disulfide-linked heterodimer formed of alpha and beta chains. Each of these chains consists of variable (V) and constant (C) domains stabilized by intrachain disulfide bonds, a short hinge-like segment, and transmembrane and intracytoplasmic portions. The Ti portion of the molecule is polymorphic and carries the T-cell idiotype. The T3 complex consists of three noncovalently associated peptides, each of which probably traverses the cell membrane. They are monomorphic and appear to transduce the activation signal from Ti to the cell itself. The monoclonal antibody CD3 recognizes primarily the delta chain of T3. (From Male D, Champion B, Cooke A. The T cell antigen receptor. In: Advanced Immunology. London: Gower Medical Publishing, 1987: 7.1–7.7. Courtesy of Male D, Champion B, and Cooke A and Gower Medical Publishing.)

both DR3 and DR4. In other ethnic groups HLA-linked susceptibility to diabetes may involve different alleles.[67]

It was previously thought that a susceptibility gene was linked to the DR3 and DR4 loci, but it is now believed that HLA-DQ beta-chain alleles primarily determine susceptibility and resistance to autoimmune destruction of beta cells. If an aspartic acid residue occupies position 57 in both alleles of that chain, autoimmune diabetes ordinarily does not occur. Full susceptibility requires that both alleles be Asp-57–negative[68] (Table 21–5). However, Asp-57 does not appear to be protective in DR4/DR4 individuals,[69] suggesting that additional amino acids are involved in susceptibility.

Terminology changes frequently in the HLA area. For example, the allele currently designated DQB1*0301 was formerly called DQw7 or DQw3.1. Similarly, DQB1*0302 was

TABLE 21–5. Predicted Susceptibility for Autoimmune Diabetes of DR3 and/or DR4 Subjects in General Population Based on DNA Sequence of DQ Beta Chain Gene

Asp-57*	Susceptibility
Neg/neg	Full
Neg/pos	10%
Pos/pos	0

*Asp-57, presence of aspartic acid residue at position 57 in the two alleles.
From Todd JA, Bell JI, McDevitt HO. HLA-DQβ gene contributes to susceptibility and resistance to insulin-dependent diabetes mellitus. Reprinted by permission from Nature, Vol. 329, pp. 599–604. Copyright © 1987, by Macmillan Magazines Limited.

previously designated DQw8 or DQw3.2. HLA haplotypes can be separated using probes for DQB alleles. DR4-containing haplotypes can be divided into DQB1*0301 or DQB1*0302. DQB1*0201 segregates with DR3-containing haplotypes; DQB1*0602 is associated with DR2 haplotypes, as is DQB1*0502. Primary susceptibility alleles are DQB1*0302 and DQB1*0201, the DQB1*0302/DQB1*0201 haplotype being at especially high risk. DQB1*0602 is found rarely in persons with IDDM and is considered a dominant protective gene; i.e., its presence overrides a susceptibility gene like DQB1*0302.[70] HLA identity in ICA-positive siblings of IDDM children is associated with a lower first-phase insulin response to intravenous glucose if the patient carries a high-risk genotype (DQB1*0302/DQB1*0201).[71] Although certain DR4 and DR3 haplotypes predict susceptibility, DR2/DR2 homozygotes rarely get diabetes. When the disease does occur in such persons, it is caused by a recombination that associates DR2 with a DQB1 susceptibility gene such as *0302.[72] The same is probably true for the DR2 association with diabetes in the IDDM of Wolfram syndrome.

Association of IDDM with TAP and LMP Alleles

Because of their participation in antigen processing, *TAP* (transporter associated with antigen processing) and *LMP* (large multifunctional protease) genes have been examined, but neither is thought to contribute to the susceptibility to IDDM.[73]

IDDM Susceptibility Genes

A current view is that genetic susceptibility to IDDM involves several, perhaps many, genes. With the use of positional cloning and other techniques, candidate loci for susceptibility genes have been identified on chromosomes 2q, 6q, 15q, and 11q.[74–77] In nonobese diabetic (NOD) mice 16 potential susceptibility genes (now called *IDD1*, *IDD2*, and so on) have been identified. Because the primary genetic susceptibility is linked to the MHC, other genes probably have lesser, modulating effects.

Is There Heterogeneity Within IDDM?

It would be useful to subclassify type I IDDM according to HLA haplotype if there were, in fact, clinical and etiologic distinctions between DR3/DR3-associated diabetes and DR4/DR4-associated disease. It has been postulated that homozygous DR3 results in a primary autoimmune form of IDDM and that IDDM in homozygous DR4 patients is caused by a primary environmental insult with a secondary autoimmune response.[78–80] Subjects in the DR3 subgroup may have an increased prevalence of other autoimmune diseases (e.g., adrenal insufficiency, Hashimoto's thyroiditis), a female preponderance, an older age at onset, and a low capacity for forming antibodies to insulin. By contrast, subjects with the DR4 alleles supposedly have little immune endocrine disease but exhibit a younger onset and a high capacity to form insulin antibodies.[78, 81] An analysis of 745 patients with type I diabetes that began between 1 and 19 y of age revealed that those with HLA-DR3 had milder, more slowly progressive disease with less ketonuria at diagnosis and a tendency for partial remissions.[81] Non-DR3/non-DR4 genotypes are more prevalent in type I patients presenting after age 15.[32] These patients have a lower frequency of ICAs at the time of diagnosis and less severe initial insulin deficiency.

Inheritance

The mode of inheritance of type I IDDM is unknown. A dominant mode of inheritance has been suggested,[82, 83] but the rarity of IDDM in parents, siblings, and offspring of affected subjects excludes simple dominant inheritance.[45, 48, 84]

Recessive inheritance is suggested by the high frequency of HLA identity (two shared haplotypes) in concordant siblings with type I IDDM,[85, 86] but against the recessive theory is the fact that homozygosity for the HLA-DR3 or -DR4 allele does not increase the risk for diabetes, whereas a specific heterozygosity, now known as DQB1*0302/DQB1*0201, does.[87–89]

The observation that heterozygosity for DR3/DR4 increases the risk for diabetes as compared with homozygosity for other high-risk alleles suggests a polygenic mode of inheritance. Susceptibility to autoimmune diabetes in NOD mice is under the control of at least 10 separate genes,[90] and perhaps as many as 16.[74] A diabetogenic MHC haplotype appears to be necessary for IDDM susceptibility but may be influenced positively or negatively by genes not linked to the MHC. Two non–MHC-linked loci on chromosome 3, IDD3 and IDD10, protect NOD mice from diabetes.[91]

In human type I diabetes, susceptibility is under the control of the HLA locus on chromosome 6p21 called IDDM1, and of at least 11 other loci on nine chromosomes. The HLA-DQB1 and HLA-DRB1 class II immune response genes of the IDDM1 locus account for about 35% of familial clustering. IDDM2, a minisatellite repeat sequence in the 5' regulatory region of the insulin gene on chromosome 11p15, interacts with IDDM1. IDDM4 is on chromosome 11q, and IDDM5 is on chromosome 6q.[90] The identification of the other loci requires linkage disequilibrium mapping and sequencing of the candidate genes in the regions of linkage.[92–94]

The autoimmune process requires recognition of the class II molecule–antigen complex by the T-cell receptor (TcR), and subsets of T lymphocytes may be recruited to pancreatic islets preferentially,[95] in response to the same or similar antigens.[96] The TcR may be important in susceptibility to or protection from autoimmune diabetes.

Other gene markers may also play a role in IDDM. It has been reported that increased expression of memory helper T lymphocytes bearing the CD45RO marker seems to define protection against diabetes in the discordant partner of the twin with the disease.[97]

Analysis of various genes involved in type I IDDM is difficult because of the interaction of environmental factors with the susceptibility genes (see next section). Relative risk and prevalence of autoimmune diabetes in siblings of diabetic probands are shown in Table 21–6.

Environmental-Genetic Interactions

The contributions of genetics and environment to the pathogenesis of individual cases of type I diabetes vary (see Fig. 21–11; see review by Cahill and McDevitt[98]). Anecdotal reports, such as the development of diabetes in two haplo-

nonidentical siblings within 1 wk after mumps infection, raise the possibility of primary environmental input. A case of massive beta-cell necrosis also seems to bypass genetic requirements and fit this category.[99] This type of disorder would be comparable to the nonautoimmune destruction of beta cells by streptozocin or alloxan in animals or by the poison Vacor in humans.[100] The maternal ingestion of N-nitroso compounds used in curing mutton has been linked to autoimmune diabetes in boys in Iceland.[101] Because patients with newly diagnosed IDDM may have antibodies to bovine serum albumin (BSA) and to a 17-amino-acid bovine albumin peptide called ABBOS,[102] it has been hypothesized that such antibodies act through the ABBOS domain common to BSA and a 69-kd pancreatic beta-cell protein to cause beta-cell destruction.[103] Aside from a Finnish report that introduction of dairy products in infants younger than 2 months of age increases the risk of IDDM,[104] there is skepticism concerning an etiologic role of these antibodies.[105]

At the other end of the spectrum of environmental-genetic interaction is the spontaneous diabetes that develops in the BioBreeding/Worcester (BB/W) rat[106] and the NOD mouse.[107] In these forms of autoimmune diabetes no environmental factor has been identified, and the syndrome is regarded as primary (first-degree) autoimmunity. Except for rare instances of fulminating destruction of beta cells by viruses or chemicals, human type I diabetes requires a genetic background of susceptibility. The concept that environmental factors are involved in precipitating autoimmunity to beta cells in genetically susceptible persons is based on inheritance and concordance patterns in identical twins and on family studies, as discussed previously. From such studies it has been postulated that type I IDDM results when an environmental insult to the beta cells exceeds the individual's tolerance to beta-cell injury. Stated differently, the genetic contribution is necessary but insufficient and requires an environmental factor to trigger its initiation. It follows that discordance for diabetes in monozygotic twins is caused by differences in environmental factors. Possible environmental triggers are listed in Table 21–7.

Viruses

Viruses could trigger beta-cell destruction (see review by Szopa and colleagues[108]) through any of three mechanisms: (1) direct cellular destruction by a betacytotropic virus; (2) generation of cytokines that damage beta cells; or (3) molecular mimicry. The viral hypothesis would explain the increased incidence of onset of IDDM in autumn and winter and in colder climates.

The onset of type I IDDM sometimes coincides with or follows viral infection, such as mumps, rubella, cytomegalovirus measles, influenza, encephalitis, poliovirus, or Epstein-Barr virus infection.[109] Congenital rubella appears to induce diabetes in about 20% of affected persons in the United States and Australia (but not in England).[109] If the affected child is DR3 or DR4, the prevalence may increase to 40%.[110] Congeni-

TABLE 21–6. Prevalence of and Relative Risk for Autoimmune Diabetes in 16-Year-Old Siblings of Diabetic Probands*

Relationship	Prevalence (%)	Relative Risk
HLA-identical siblings	14	118
Haplo-identical siblings	4	31
Nonidentical siblings	1	NS
All siblings	5	36

*Many studies show that the prevalence (concordance rate) in identical twins is less than 50%.
NS, not significant.
Adapted with permission from Gorsuch AN, Spencer KM, Lister J, et al. Can future type 1 diabetes be predicted? Diabetes 1982; 31:862–866. Copyright 1982 by the American Diabetes Association.

TABLE 21–7. Possible Environmental Triggers for Diabetes Mellitus

Viruses	Betacytotoxins
Mumps virus	N-Nitroso compounds
Rubella virus	Vacor
Cytomegalovirus	Others?
Coxsackieviruses B4 and B5	
Retroviruses with type C	
particles	
Reoviruses	
Encephalomyocarditis virus	

tal infection with rubella is a bona fide instance of the initiation of autoimmune diabetes by a viral infection.

COXSACKIEVIRUSES

Two thirds of children with new-onset diabetes in Sweden had immunoglobulin M (IgM) antibodies against coxsackievirus B, compared with 12% of control children.[111] However, differences in antiviral antibody titers are not always demonstrable in identical twins discordant for diabetes,[112] and IDDM is not always associated with viral epidemics or with increased virus antibody titers.[113]

Coxsackievirus B4 was isolated from a patient who died in ketoacidosis with apparent postinfectious diabetes,[114] probably the consequence of fulminating beta-cell destruction rather than a virally triggered autoimmune disorder. Beta-cell destruction with acute and chronic inflammation of the islets was observed in 4 of 7 cases of fatal coxsackievirus B infection, 20 of 45 cases of cytomegalovirus infection, 2 of 14 cases of varicella-zoster infection, and 2 of 45 cases of congenital rubella.[115] However, viruses were not isolated from tissues, and it was not clear whether autoimmune diabetes would have supervened if the patients had lived. A report that cytomegalovirus is incorporated in the genome of 22% of type I diabetics[116] has not been confirmed.

In a prospective study of coxsackievirus B and other enterovirus infections in Finland, enterovirus antibodies were elevated in pregnant mothers whose children subsequently developed IDDM before 3 years of age, and enteroviral infection was almost twice as prevalent in siblings who developed IDDM as in nondiabetic siblings.[117]

MOLECULAR MIMICRY

Molecular mimicry refers to an immune response to a viral protein that has an amino acid sequence homology with a beta-cell protein and that could theoretically induce antiviral CD8 lymphocytes to react with beta cells. For example, a 24-amino-acid epitope of the glutamic acid decarboxylase of beta cells (GAD65) is highly homologous to a domain in the P2C protein of the diabetogenic coxsackievirus B4.[118] A viral infection can induce autoimmune diabetes in mice in which a protein of that virus has been transgenically expressed,[119, 120] so a coxsackievirus infection theoretically could trigger anti-GAD65 autoimmunity.

Because there are marked differences in susceptibility to diabetes after viral infection in different strains of mice,[121] susceptibility appears to be genetically determined.[122] Suscepti-

bility could derive from sensitivity of beta cells to a particular dose of virus or from a propensity to develop an autoimmune response to a viral antigen expressed in beta cells or to autoantigens exposed by beta-cell damage. Viruses that attack the pancreas vary in virulence, and virulence can be increased by serial passage through islet tissue.[123] The genetic basis of viral diabetogenicity has been studied by analysis of the nucleotide sequences of viral genomes, and codon differences between the nondiabetogenic and diabetogenic variants of Coxsackievirus B4 have been identified.[108, 124] Concomitant exposure to nonviral islet toxins enhances host susceptibility to viral damage and may represent another variable.[125] Retrovirus-like particles in NOD mice are presumed to be vertically transmitted,[126] and antibodies to the particles are detectable before the decline in beta-cell function.[127] Diabetes can be induced by a viral infection in previously tolerant transgenic mice that express a gene for a protein of that virus in their beta cells and express the relevant TcR in their repertoire,[119, 128] Therefore, it seems reasonable that viral genes in normal human beta cells could be triggered by some minor insult or by viral mutation to produce viral proteins.

In summary, viruses appear to be the environmental agents most likely to induce diabetes in susceptible persons. However, because exposure to certain viruses may actually protect susceptible individuals from autoimmune diabetes,[129] discordance between twins may result from viral protection rather than viral damage.

Is Type I IDDM an Immune-Mediated Disease?

The evidence that type I IDDM is an immune-mediated disease is summarized in Table 21–8. (1) IDDM is linked with class II (D-region) antigens known to be associated with autoimmune disease.[62–72] (2) Type I IDDM may occur with other forms of immune endocrinopathy, such as Hashimoto's thyroiditis or adrenal insufficiency, and with pernicious anemia, myasthenia gravis, and vitiligo.[130] (3) The coupling of diabetes with immune endocrinopathy may cluster in families.[130] (4) An early lesion in diabetes in both animals[131] and humans[132–134] is lymphocytic infiltration of the islets of Langerhans (insulitis or isletitis) that resembles lymphocytic infiltrations in other autoimmune diseases. (5) Antibodies directed against both cytoplasmic and cell-surface determinants on islet cells are present in many type I diabetic subjects at diagnosis.[78, 98] Such antibodies are also found in survivors of Vacor poisoning who develop diabetes[134] and in rats made diabetic with streptozotocin[135] or infected with diabetogenic viruses.[136]

TABLE 21–8. Islet Cell Autoantigens of Insulin-Dependent Diabetes Mellitus

Autoantigen	Characteristics
Sialoglycolipid	Target of islet antibodies in humans, GM2-1, non–beta-cell specific
Glutamate decarboxylase (GAD)	Target of 64-kd antigen/GAD antibody in humans and animal models of IDDM, two forms (GAD65 and GAD67), cellular immune antigen, synaptic-like microvesicle protein, disease-modifying antigen
Insulin	Target of insulin autoantibody (IAA) in humans and nonobese diabetic (NOD) mice, cellular immune antigen, disease-modifying antigen
Insulin receptor	Target of autoantibodies in humans, determined by bioassay
38-kd autoantigen	Target of 38-kd antigen in humans, induced by cytomegalovirus, localized to insulin secretory granules, cellular immune antigen, multiple antigens of this molecular mass?
Bovine serum albumin (BSA)	Target of BSA antibody in humans and animal models of IDDM, contains ABBOS peptide, has molecular mimic in beta-cell p69 protein (PM-1), disease-modifying antigen
Glucose transporter	Target of autoantibodies in humans, inhibits glucose stimulation, GLUT-2–directed?
Heat shock protein 65	Target of autoantibodies and cellular immunity in NOD mice, disease-modifying antigen, contains p277 peptide
Carboxypeptidase H	Target of autoantibodies in humans, identified by immunoscreening of islet cDNA, insulin secretory granule protein
52-kd autoantigen	Target of autoantibodies in humans and NOD mice, molecular mimic with rubella virus
Islet cell antigens 12 and 512	Target of autoantibodies in humans, identified by immunoscreening of islet cDNA, 512 homology to CD45
150-kd autoantigen	Target of autoantibodies in humans, beta-cell specific, membrane-associated
RIN polar	Target of autoantibodies in humans and NOD mice present on insulinoma cells

From Atkinson MA, Maclaren NK: Islet cell autoantigens in insulin-dependent diabetes. J Clin Invest 1993; 92:1608–1616. Copyright ©, by The American Society for Clinical Investigation.

(6) The fact that overt diabetes in the low-dose streptozotocin model[131] and in the spontaneously diabetic BB/W rat[137] can be prevented by immunotherapy suggests that autoimmunity plays a role in these forms of diabetes and that they are not simply a consequence of islet cell injury. Further evidence in support of this thesis is the fact that diabetes can be induced in prediabetic BB rats by the administration of splenic lymphocytes from diabetic BB animals activated with concanavalin A.[138] Diabetes can also be induced in strains of BB/W rats that are normally resistant to diabetes by pretreatment with cyclophosphamide, partial thymectomy, or injections of anti-lymphocyte antibodies.[139, 140] These maneuvers apparently eliminate a class of T lymphocytes that restrain those T lymphocytes responsible for beta-cell destruction. Conversely, treatment with whole blood from a diabetes-resistant BB strain prevents diabetes in a susceptible strain,[141] the blood presumably containing suppressor T lymphocytes. Activated T lymphocytes from type I diabetic patients include both helper (CD4) and cytotoxic (CD8) cells, consistent with a role for both humoral and cell-mediated immunity in the induction of type I diabetes.[142] In addition, remissions in human type I diabetes can be induced for as long as 1 y by altering the immune response with cyclosporine.[143] (7) Perhaps the most compelling evidence is that rapid development of isletitis and destruction of beta cells occur in pancreases transplanted from unaffected monozygotic twins into the twins with diabetes.[144]

An increased helper/suppressor T-lymphocyte ratio could augment the immune response on exposure to self-antigens. Early reports suggested deficiencies of suppressor T cells,[145] but in other studies the decrease in cells expressing CD4 was greater than in those expressing CD8.[146, 147] Failure to find an elevated helper/suppressor ratio may reflect the time of testing, because the ratio tends to be elevated early after diagnosis, returning toward normal with time.[148] Although this theory is conceptionally attractive, the problem has become much more complicated with the demonstration that CD4/CD8 ratios are genetically determined and vary from family to family.[149]

To summarize, type I IDDM is an autoimmune disease,[150, 151] and several aspects of the immune response appear to be important.

Islet Antibodies

Cytoplasmic Islet Cell Antibodies

In sections of fresh human pancreas, cytoplasmic islet cell antibodies (ICAs) are present in the serum of 60 to 90% of newly diagnosed patients with type I diabetes, compared with 0.5% of nondiabetic controls.[152] The antigen that induces these antibodies may be a pancreatic sialoglycolipid.[153] The antibodies generally react with all four types of islet cells—those that secrete glucagon (alpha cells), insulin (beta cells), somatostatin (delta cells), and pancreatic polypeptides (PP or F cells)—although in some patients antibodies are specific for beta cells.[154] Antibodies that react only with beta cells are said to be less predictive of future IDDM than are those that react with both beta and alpha cells,[154] even though only beta cells are destroyed in this disease, the non beta islet cells being normal or increased in number.[155, 156] The infiltrating lymphocytes in isletitis are confined to islets containing beta cells, further implying a killing specificity for the insulin-producing sites.[133, 157] Alpha, delta, and pancreatic polypeptide cells are also spared in diabetes produced by streptozocin[158] or viruses.[159]

ICAs disappear in most type I patients within 2 to 3 y after onset of IDDM.[160, 161] The 10 to 15% of patients in whom these antibodies persist for longer than 2 to 3 y exhibit (1) a high prevalence of thyroid and gastric autoantibodies; (2) frequent coexistence of autoimmune endocrinopathy; (3) a strong family history of other autoimmune disorders; (4) a female preponderance; (5) a strong association with HLA-DR3/B8, the HLA axis associated with other organ-specific antibodies; and (6) reduced levels of IgG antibodies to exogenous insulin.[162–164] Heterogeneity of type I IDDM has long been suspected[165] (Table 21–9; see previous section on heterogeneity within IDDM).

Why patients with type I diabetes sometimes exhibit disease in other endocrine glands is not known (see Chapter 33), but ICAs cross-react with a common antigenic determinant in different tissues.[166] Such interaction suggests a pathogenetic role for these antibodies, but the weight of evidence suggests that they are simply markers of beta-cell damage. The growing list of islet antibodies observed at the onset of IDDM now includes, in addition to ICAs,[167] antibodies to insulin,[168] GAD,[169] proinsulin,[170] immunoglobulins,[171] insulin receptors,[172] carboxypeptidase H (52-kd autoantigens),[173, 174] 37- and 38-kd peptides (tryptic fragments of 64-kd antigen),[175] islet cell antigen 69,[175] and islet cell antigen 512[176, 177] (Table 21–9; see Table 21–8).

In the general population ICA-positivity is uncommon. ICAs were positive ($\geq$40 Juvenile Diabetes Foundation [JDF] units) in 1.05% of school children in southern Germany[178] and in 3% of Swedish children 0 to 14 years of age.[179]

The islet cell antigens with which ICAs react have not been clearly identified and are probably heterogeneous. Particular interest has focused on GAD, because anti-GAD antibodies are predictive of subsequent diabetes. Preabsorption of ICA-positive antisera with recombinant human GAD reduces or blocks ICA reactivity in 27% of new-onset IDDM patients and 39% of prediabetics.[180] Beta-cell–selective ICA, but not diffusely staining ICA, can be absorbed out of ICA-positive antisera by rat brain homogenates, probably because brain expresses GAD.

The ICA test is widely used despite its several shortcomings. These include the requirement for fresh pancreas, preferably human, the relatively cumbersome technology of immunostaining, the subjective nature of the readout, poor reproducibility, and intralaboratory variability.[181]

Glutamic Acid Decarboxylase Antibodies

GAD, the rate-limiting enzyme for biosynthesis of the inhibitory neurotransmitter γ-aminobutyric acid (GABA), is expressed in several extraneural tissues, including beta cells. GAD antibodies were first reported in stiff man syndrome (SMS), in which IDDM sometimes occurs.[182] In 1990 GAD, previously known as the 64-kd protein, was identified as a major autoantigen in type I diabetes.[183, 184] However, there is at least one 64-kd pancreatic islet antigen distinct from GAD.[184]

There are two human GAD isoenzymes, a 65-kd polypeptide and a 67-kd form (see Atkinson and Maclaren[50] for review). They differ in their NH_2-terminal regions and subcellular distributions; GAD65 appears to be expressed in punctate fashion in the Golgi region, and GAD67 is diffusely distributed

TABLE 21–9. Prevalence of Islet Cell Cytoplasmic Antibodies (ICA)*

Population	% Positive
Normal	0.5
New-onset type I IDDM	60–90
New-onset nonobese NIDDM	20
Gestational diabetes	10
First-degree relatives of patients with type I IDDM	3

*Approximate percentage from a variety of studies.

in the cytoplasm. The gene for GAD65 maps to chromosome 2q31, and that for GAD67 maps to chromosome 10q11.23. Antibodies to the 65-kd isoform are more common in IDDM.

Measurement of GAD antibodies may be the procedure of choice for screening for prediabetes and for confirming the diagnosis of autoimmunity as the cause of diabetes (Fig. 21–6). The test may be positive 10 y before the onset of clinical diabetes.[185] It is more reproducible and fluctuates less with time than measurements of other autoantibodies and is simpler to perform. Paradoxically, high levels of GAD antibody are associated with a slower conversion rate to IDDM (10% in 4 y) than are low levels (50% at 4 y),[186] possibly because high levels of anti-GAD antibodies indicate preferential activation of humoral immunity and less activation of cell-mediated immunity. IDDM is due primarily to cell-mediated destruction of beta cells by cytotoxic T lymphocytes.

Insulin Autoantibodies

Insulin autoantibodies (IAA) may be present in up to 50% of patients with new-onset IDDM developing before age

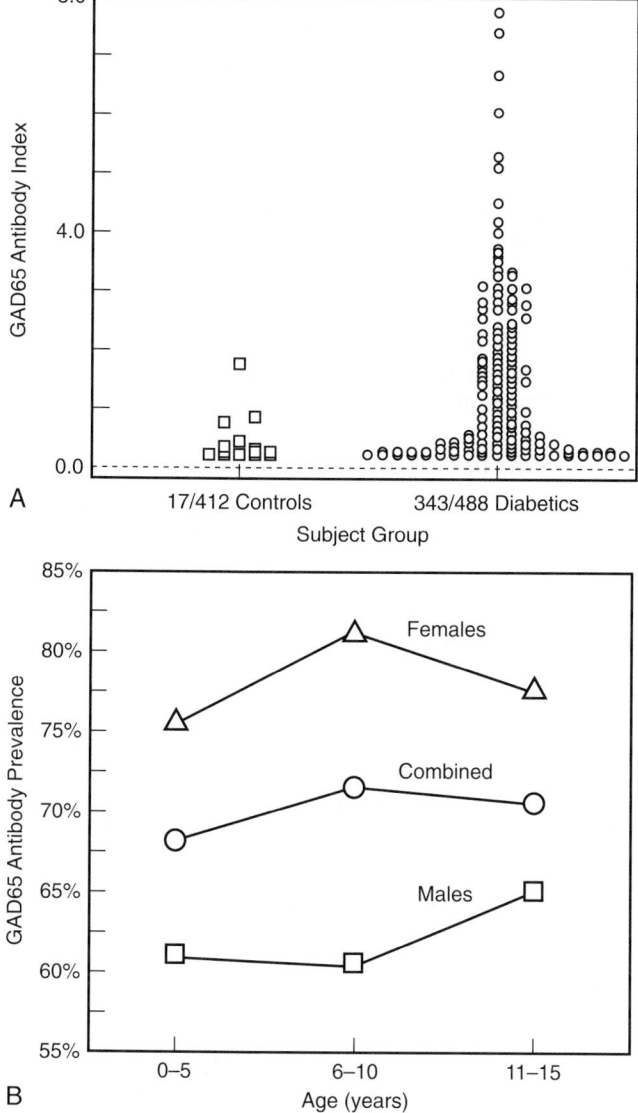

Figure 21–6. *A,* GAD65 antibody index in 343 of 488 diabetic children with GAD65 antibody *(right)* and in 17 of 412 control children with GAD65 antibody *(left). B,* GAD65 antibody prevalence versus age in diabetic children. (△) females, (□) males. For the entire cohort, $P \le .0001$ for GAD65 antibody versus gender. For specific age groups, $P \le .05$.

5. IAA titers decline with age, in contrast to ICA.[10] In Belgian children with the high-risk HLA haplotype DQA1*0301/DQB1*0302, IAAs were present in 90% and ICAs in 92%. This relationship is less striking after 10 years of age.[187] In one series of IDDM patients, 34% had proinsulin autoantibodies and 23% had IAAs before insulin therapy.[188] With sensitive techniques, about 50% of new-onset patients, particularly those with an HLA-DR4 phenotype,[189] are positive for IAA. Other autoantigens in beta cells include carboxypeptide H, the enzyme that converts proinsulin to insulin,[173] heat shock protein 65,[190, 191] and peripherin, a cytoskeletal protein.[192] Antibodies to GLUT2, the high-K_m facilitative glucose transporter expressed in beta cells, are present in many patients with new-onset IDDM[193, 194]; they have not been observed in prediabetic sera and appear to have no predictive value. IDDM is not associated with autoimmunity to heat shock proteins.[195]

P69/ABBOS Antibodies

Another candidate autoantibody is directed against a 69-kd beta-cell membrane protein, called P69, with a domain that shares a limited homology with a 17-amino-acid sequence in BSA known as ABBOS.[102, 103] However, the specificity of the IDDM immunity toward BSA is unconfirmed, and the evidence of cellular immunity against BSA in IDDM patients is not compelling.[105] The possible role of albumin in cow's milk as an environmental factor in IDDM is based on circumstantial evidence. Finnish children with diabetes have increased levels of IgA antibodies to bovine milk proteins and both IgA and IgG antibodies to β-lactoglobulin when compared with healthy age-matched controls.[196] The duration of breast-feeding is inversely related to the level of β-lactoglobulin and bovine milk protein IgA antibodies.[197]

Do Autoantigens Induce Cellular Immunity?

If any of the autoantigens that elicit an antibody response have a pathogenic role in beta-cell destruction, they must also elicit cellular immunity. GAD is the leading candidate, because it can induce both humoral and cellular immunity. Cytotoxic T cells for GAD have been detected in patients with preclinical and recent-onset IDDM carrying the HLA-A*0201 allele[198] and in 4-week-old NOD mice, a murine model of autoimmune diabetes.[199] The diabetes and the T-cell proliferative response can be delayed by intraperitoneal or intrathymic[200] injections of GAD65, perhaps explaining the prevention of diabetes in NOD mice by intrathymic islet transplantation.[201]

In first-degree relatives of patients with IDDM, GAD autoimmunity is either predominantly humoral or predominantly cellular. The foregoing observations could be related to alteration in the relative activities of type I helper T lymphocytes (Th1), which enhance cellular immunity, and type II helper T lymphocytes (Th2), which enhance humoral immunity. As noted, destruction of the beta cell in IDDM is primarily cell mediated. Th1 and Th2 cells regulate each other through cytokine release. Stimulation of Th1 cells enhances cellular immunity through release of interferon γ (IFN-γ), interleukin-2 (IL-2), and IL-12, these cytokines simultaneously inhibiting Th2 activity.[202] Activation of Th2 cells augments humoral immunity and inhibits Th1-mediated cellular immunity by release of IL-4.[203]

A role for GAD-induced cellular immunity in the pathogenesis of IDDM is attractive but is not proved.

Superantigens

In contrast to conventional antigens that activate only a small fraction of T cells, superantigens are products of viruses and bacteria or of endogenous or integrated viral genes[204] that can activate up to 20% of T cells. One superantigen is a product of the mouse mammary tumor virus that causes clonal deletion of $V_\beta 14$-expressing T cells.[205] It has been proposed that exposure to a superantigen could activate many T-cell clones and thereby initiate the destructive process in beta cells. The other cytoplasmic antigens discussed previously, such as GAD, would become accessible to T and B lymphocytes, and a destructive cascade would ensue.[206]

Predicting IDDM by Means of Islet Antibodies: Practicality of Pre-IDDM Screening in Children

In anticipation of preventive interventions before the onset of the disease, the risk for overt IDDM in persons with antibodies to various islet antigens has been studied carefully. In people with a high titer of ICA the risk is about 9 to 10% per year,[207] and in one study the risk of IDDM was 45% within 7 y of a positive ICA test.[208] In a Swedish study the predictive value of positivity for ICA or IAA (or both) was only 7%[179]; the addition of GAD65 antibody positivity to the other two improved sensitivity but not sufficiently to justify early immunointervention in the general population.[209] It was concluded that ICA screening of the general population is not practical, but the presence of GAD65 antibodies predicted IDDM in 5 of 7 children who developed the disease.[210]

Islet Antibodies in NIDDM

The approximate prevalences of ICA and anti-GAD positivity in different types of diabetes are shown in Tables 21–9 and 21–10, respectively. The highest prevalence is in newly diagnosed type I patients, followed by patients with NIDDM and gestational diabetes.[152] The prevalence of ICA in first-degree relatives of subjects with type I diabetes is six times that in nondiabetic persons. The prevalence of ICA positivity[211] and of antibodies to GAD65[185, 212] patients with NIDDM raises the possibility that some adult-onset diabetic patients with supposed NIDDM actually have a variant of autoimmune diabetes that does not cause complete destruction.

Natural History of Type I Diabetes

Type I diabetes usually proceeds through an ordered sequence: prediabetes, impaired glucose tolerance, NIDDM, and finally IDDM (Fig. 21–7).[213] The development of diabetes in discordant monozygotic twins or triplets after long latent periods is in accord with this scheme.[214, 215] As mentioned previously, progression from ICA positivity to overt diabetes is not inevitable, especially in adults.[216] Patients with apparent

TABLE 21–10. Proportion of Anti-GAD–Positive Subjects During the Prediabetic Period Among Diabetic Women and in a Random Sample of Young Women

Type of Diabetes	Number of Women Studied	Cases Positive for Anti-GAD		Age (y)	
		Number	%	Mean	Range
Insulin-dependent	28	23	82	30	23–39
Non–insulin-dependent	11	4	34	32	22–39
Gestational: insulin-treated	32	5	15	32	22–40
Gestational: diet-treated	80	1	1	32	20–45
Random population sample	100	0	0	36	25–45

From Tuomilehto J, Zimmet P, Mackay IR, et al. Antibodies to glutamic acid decarboxylase as predictors of insulin-dependent diabetes mellitus before clinical onset. Lancet 1994; 343:1383–1385. Copyright © 1994, by The Lancet Ltd.

NIDDM who are ICA positive are believed to have type I diabetes in slow evolution (subtotal beta-cell damage).

Cell-Mediated Immunity

The early evidence favoring cell-mediated immune mechanisms in the pathogenesis of type I diabetes includes the following: (1) Lymphocytes from children with IDDM adhere to insulinoma cells in co-culture, forming rosettes, and kill insulinoma cells.[217] (2) Levels of killer T lymphocytes and antibody-dependent cytotoxicity are increased in newly diagnosed type I diabetic subjects and in ICA-positive unaffected siblings of diabetic children.[218] (3) Isletitis is present in islets of patients with acute diabetes of recent onset[133, 157]; defective suppressor T-lymphocyte function may play a role.[219]

In the BB rat, RT6[+] cells play a role in preventing isletitis and diabetes.[140] Isletitis and diabetes can be transferred to radiated, diabetes-resistant nonobese normal (NON) mice through transfusion of cells from bone marrow,[220] spleen,[221, 222] and lymph nodes.[223] The transfused cells migrate to the spleen and to immature lymph nodes within 24 h[224] and proliferate and mature before beginning the autoimmune process in the islets on about the fifth day after the transfusion. Adoptive transfer of L3T4[+] cells (the murine equivalent of CD4[+] helper T cells in humans) and Lyt2[+] T cells (the equivalent of CD8[+] cytotoxic T cells in humans) is required for transfer of isletitis and diabetes.[223–226]

The nature of the cells that destroy beta cells is unclear. In BB rats cytotoxic T cells are virtually absent, suggesting that natural killer (NK) cells are cytotoxic in this model,[227] and the number and activity of NK cells are increased in diabetes-prone BB rats.[227, 228] These cells can be activated by IL-2.[229] IL-4 inhibits IL-2–driven responses of T cells[230] and can prevent progression to diabetes in NOD mice in which splenocytes underproduce IL-4.[231] In humans the DR3 haplotype causes underproduction of IL-4, which may account for its link to diabetes susceptibility.[232] In humans the predominant cytotoxic cell type in isletitis is the CD8[+] T lymphocyte.[233, 234]

Mechanisms of Cellular Killing

Killing of beta cells by cytotoxic lymphocytes can be separated into three phases: (1) effector cell–target cell interaction involving recognition and cell-cell contact between immunocytes and beta cells; (2) effector-cell preparation for delivery of the lethal blow; and (3) direct and indirect K-cell destruction of target cells.[235, 236]

Cytotoxic T cells and enlarged granular lymphocytes that do not bear the classic T and B cell markers are involved in killing. The latter, called K cells, constitute 10% of total lymphocytes; they may also kill by antibody-mediated cytotoxicity.[233, 234]

Most T cells recognize antigens associated with class I molecules on the target cell by means of the TcR (Fig. 21–8); a few recognize target cells through an unidentified mechanism. K cells recognize targets through binding of Fc receptors to IgG antibodies coating the target cells.

After conjugation with target cells, lymphocytes undergo changes that culminate in the secretion of cytolysins (Fig. 21–9). The granules congregate at the pole of the lymphocyte that is in contact with the target cell and are released by exocytosis. These granules contain pore-forming proteins called *perforins*, which bind to cell membranes and polymerize to *polyperforins*. Polyperforins are inserted into the membrane, creating transmembrane channels. At this point incompletely identified mediators kill the cells. Killing by this mechanism differs from that caused by complement. The attack complex of complement induces reversible and then irreversible cell swelling, and cytotoxicity occurs through apoptosis. Mitochon-

Stages in the Development of Diabetes Mellitus

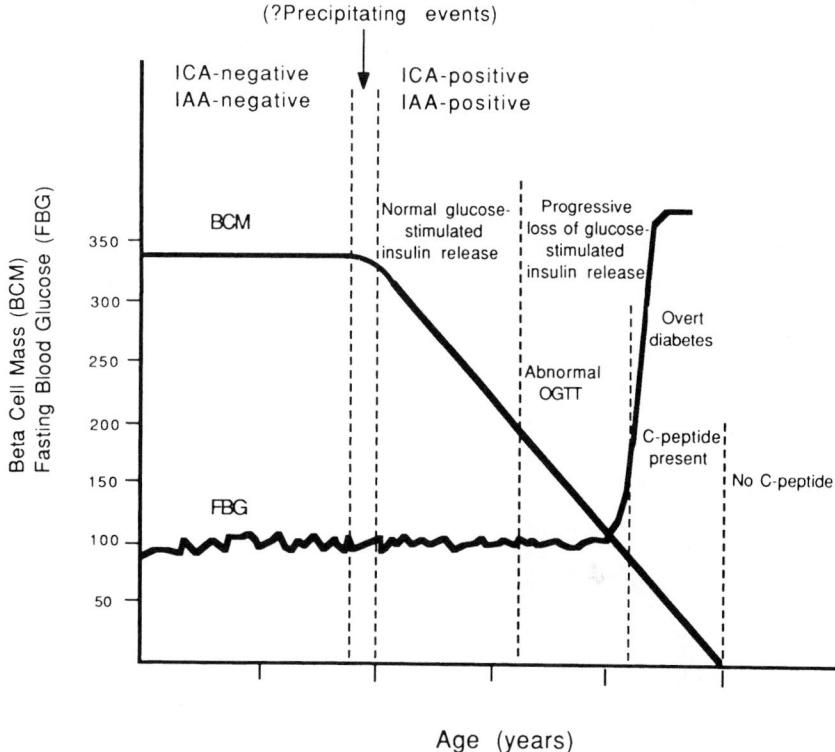

Figure 21–7. Hypothetical depiction of the natural history of autoimmune diabetes. Genetically susceptible people begin their lives without any detectable abnormality. A precipitating event (e.g., viral infection) causing minimal destruction of beta cells is followed by autoimmunity. This is reflected by positive tests for islet cell antibodies (ICA) and insulin autoantibodies (IAA). Although beta-cell mass decreases, the functional reserve of beta cells is more than enough to maintain normal glucose levels. Continued injury results in sufficient loss of beta-cell mass and causes diminution in glucose-stimulated insulin release and ultimately an abnormal OGTT. As the destruction of beta cells continues, fasting glucose levels rise above normal but the patient may remain asymptomatic. In the strict sense this is NIDDM, a state that may be relatively short-lived. Then the classic manifestations of IDDM may appear with marked hyperglycemia, glycosuria, and ketonemia, which culminate in ketoacidosis unless treated. At the onset of this overt phase of the diabetes, C peptide is still present, indicating that some beta cells have survived. Ultimately these disappear and C peptide levels become unmeasurable. (Modified from Eisenbarth GS. Type 1 diabetes mellitus: a chronic autoimmune disease. Modified with permission from the New England Journal of Medicine, 314: 1360–1368, 1986.)

drial structure is preserved, but the cell produces blebs and ultimately becomes fragmented to form so-called apoptotic bodies that have intact plasma membranes. These bodies undergo secondary necrosis.[235, 236]

In addition, indirect killing can be caused by cytotoxic substances released from lymphocytes and macrophages. Resident macrophages normally surround rat islets, but these cells are only weakly responsive to immunogenic stimuli. A few weeks before the onset of diabetes, additional macrophages are recruited and aggregate at periductal and perivascular locations adjacent to noninfiltrated islets.[237] At least two macrophage-produced cytokines, IL-1 and TNF α, have destructive effects on beta cells. IL-1 is a selective beta-cell cytotoxin that is effective in picomolar concentrations[238, 239] and is potentiated by TNF α.[240] The effects of IL-1 on isolated islets in vitro are bimodal. At low concentrations IL-1 stimulates preproinsulin messenger RNA (mRNA) production and proinsulin biosynthesis and potentiates glucose-induced insulin secre-

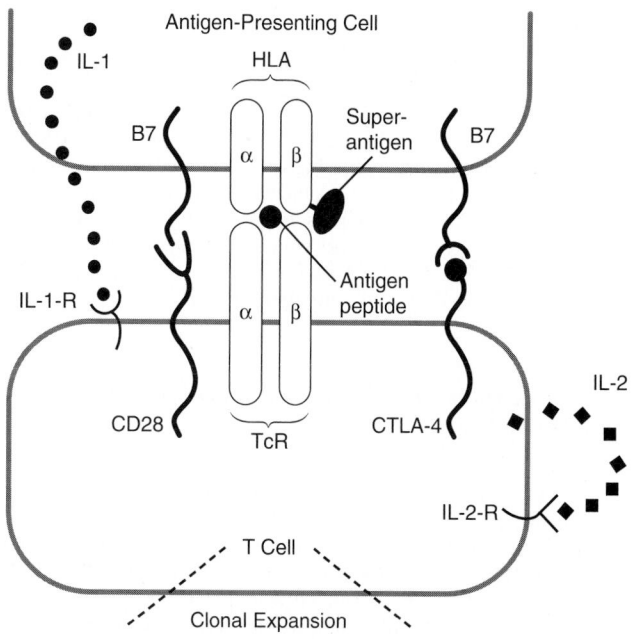

Figure 21–8. A model depicting the interaction between the T-cell receptor (TcR) and the antigen/MHC. Binding activates the T cells and causes them to differentiate to effector cells. Antigen binds to both HLA chains and interacts with the T-cell receptor (TcR). The other signal is antigen independent and is mediated by the engagement of the T-cell surface molecules CD28 with members of the B7 family on the antigen-presenting cell. The precise role of the CD28 homologue cytotoxic lymphocyte antigen 4 (CTLA-4) is controversial. The superantigens are products of ubiquitous viruses or bacteria or integrated viral genes that can activate up to 20% of T cells.

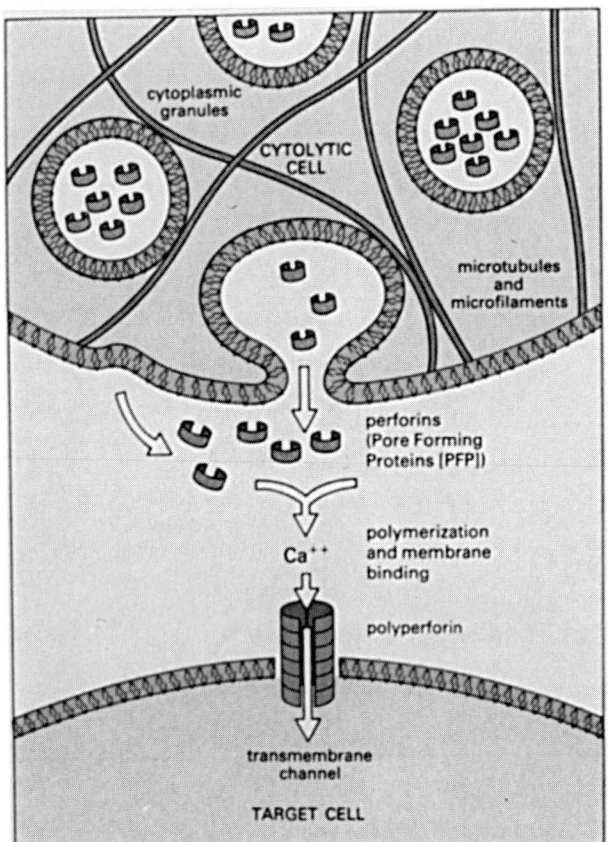

Figure 21–9. Exocytosis of perforins leads to transmembrane channel formation in target cells. Killing of target cells by cytolytic lymphocytes involves the secretion of granule contents into the intercellular environment between the closely apposed effector and target cells. Perforins, monomeric pore-forming proteins, are one of the major constituents of granules; in the presence of Ca^{2+} they bind to the target cell membrane and polymerize to form polyperforins, which are inserted into the membrane to create transmembrane channels. This process appears to be essential, although not sufficient, for target cell killing by cytotoxic effector cells. The nature of other mediators is not yet known. (From Male D, Champion B, Cooke A. Cytotoxic cells. In: Advanced Immunology. London: Gower Medical Publishing, 1987: 7.1–7.7. Courtesy of Male D, Champion B, and Cooke A and Gower Medical Publishing.)

tion (GSIS).[241, 242] At higher concentrations these functions are inhibited, and cytotoxicity occurs.[242]

The IL-1 effects on beta cells may be mediated by oxygen-derived free radicals.[243] Beta cells are exquisitely sensitive to free radicals,[244–250] including superoxide anions, hydrogen peroxide, and hydroxyl radicals. Normally, free radicals are scavenged by antioxidant mechanisms; their accumulation causes disorganization of intracellular enzymes and membranes.

Another potential toxin is nitric oxide (NO), which is synthesized in rat islets[251] and which may be involved in the isletitis in BB rats.[252, 253] However, NO does not appear to mediate cytokine-induced impairment of human beta-cell function.[254]

Aberrant Expression of Class II Molecules as a Cause of Type I Diabetes

It has been suggested that aberrant HLA-DR expression and antigen presentation by beta cells is a factor in endocrine autoimmunity.[59, 255] However, DR-expressing, insulin-containing cells in the diabetic pancreas are not beta cells but are macrophages that have engulfed insulin granules.[256, 257] Transgenic technology employed to express class II molecules on mouse beta cells failed to produce evidence of isletitis or

autoimmune destruction of beta cells, suggesting that aberrant expression of DR molecules is not the cause of autoimmune destruction of beta cells.[258, 259] Nor does expression of class II molecules on beta cells endow them with an antigen-presenting function that could be responsible for autoimmunity.[260] On the other hand, transgenic mice that express IFN-γ on beta cells develop an isletitis that culminates in diabetes.[258] The mechanism by which IFN-γ works is unknown.[261, 262]

Addressins constitute a unique endothelial cell recognition system of homing receptors that control lymphocyte traffic into inflamed tissues.[263] Addressin α4 may play a role in the isletitis in murine IDDM.[264, 265]

Summary of Immunologic Information

1. Autoimmune diabetes develops almost exclusively in persons expressing DR3 or DR4 molecules, or both. Susceptibility is closely linked with DQ beta chain. Primary susceptibility alleles are DQB1*0302 and DQB1*0201, whereas DQB1*0602 is dominantly protective.

2. Susceptibility phenotypes are necessary but not sufficient to cause the disease.

3. Even a trivial injury to a small minority of beta cells, whether caused by viruses or by betacytotoxic substances, can initiate a progressive autoimmune isletitis that ultimately destroys beta cells.

4. Although viruses and betacytotoxins are triggers of autoimmune diabetes in humans, no clear-cut associations have been established to explain most cases of autoimmune diabetes mellitus.

5. Autoimmune diabetes in humans is a slowly progressive disorder that becomes clinically overt only after more than 90% of beta cells are destroyed. Antibodies to various proteins can be demonstrated in the cytoplasm and on the cell surface of beta cells before this stage is reached.

6. Antibodies are generally regarded as markers of the destructive process rather than its cause.

7. The destructive isletitis is cell-mediated rather than antibody-mediated, and NK cells may play a role. Macrophages, helper T lymphocytes, and cytotoxic/suppressor T lymphocytes are present in isletitis, and both helper and cytotoxic/suppressor subsets are required for adoptive transfer of the disease in animals.[266]

8. IL-1 in picomolar concentrations can damage and destroy beta cells in isolated islets without destroying alpha or delta cells. Its effects are greatly potentiated by TNF α and INF-γ and by stimulation of beta-cell secretory activity.

9. Beta cells are exquisitely sensitive to free radicals. Antioxidant depletion enhances and antioxidant supplementation decreases beta cell destruction in both experimental and spontaneous diabetes of animals.

Working Hypothesis for the Pathogenesis of Autoimmune Diabetes

A working hypothesis for autoimmune diabetes (Fig. 21–10) focuses on a cytokine-mediated final common pathway of beta-cell destruction that could be activated by molecular mimicry or repeated inflammatory challenge. The intensity of the immune response, powerful or weak, would be determined by HLA genes that confer susceptibility or protection[267] and by varying levels of cytokine response, which also may be genetically determined. For example, genes for TNF α and TNF β are linked to the human MHC complex.[268] It may be significant that monocytes from an HLA DR2–positive patient that were resistant to IDDM were low secretors of TNF α when challenged with endotoxin.[269]

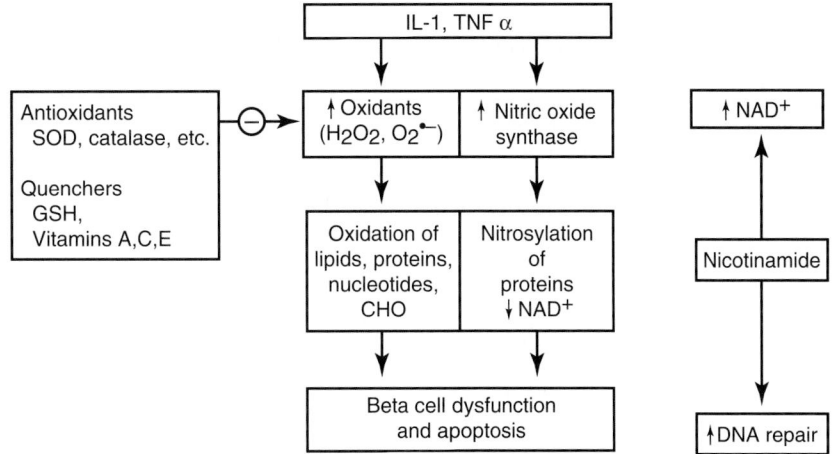

Figure 21–10. The lymphokine hypothesis for the pathogenesis of type I diabetes. In response to nonspecific infections macrophages release IL-1 and TNF α, which exert a streptozocin-like action on beta cells. The resulting destruction of beta cells is slight and is followed in the normal population by complete recovery without any evidence of impaired beta-cell function. In genetically susceptible persons, an autoimmune process is initiated. The final common pathway involved in beta-cell death is thought by some to be the generation of toxic oxygen radicals. Beta-cell death presumably can be prevented by the activity of superoxide dismutase, chemical antioxidants, scavenging molecules, or stimulation of DNA repair with nicotinamide, which reflects NAD+, among other effects (see Fig. 21–11). Antioxidants and nicotinamide are capable of preventing beta-cell damage that results from the administration of streptozocin or alloxan to animals. Oxidants are thought to mediate damage to cells resulting from autoimmunity and rejection. (see also Fig. 21–5). Nicotinamide is thought to protect beta cells by replenishing NAD+, which is reduced by the increased poly(ADP ribose) synthetase activity required for repair of DNA breakage caused by the free radicals, and also by reducing formation of nitric oxide.

PREVENTION OF TYPE I (AUTOIMMUNE) DIABETES

The prevention of autoimmune diabetes is a realistic possibility. Type I diabetes is an autoimmune disorder, and the autoimmune process begins years before beta-cell destruction becomes complete, thereby providing a window of opportunity for intervention. HLA susceptibility markers have been identified, and autoantibody tests make possible the identification of persons at high risk for the disease.

It is essential that intervention in otherwise healthy prediabetic children be free of significant risks and toxicity and simple enough to avoid significant intrusion on the quality of life. Several strategic approaches are currently under investigation.

Potential Prophylactic Agents

Oral Insulin

Oral administration of autoantigens suppresses autoimmunity in animals with autoimmune encephalitis[270–272] or collagen-induced arthritis.[273–275] Oral insulin is reported to reduce the severity of lymphocytic infiltration in the pancreatic islets of NOD mice.[276] The mechanism by which oral antigens induce tolerance has not been elucidated.[277] There is no evidence that oral insulin can prevent IDDM in humans.

Parenteral Insulin

Aggressive insulin treatment of new-onset type I diabetes in humans increases the frequency and duration of insulin-free remissions,[278] and prophylactic insulin treatment of diabetes-prone BBW rats[279] and NOD mice reduces both destructive isletitis and overt diabetes.[280, 281] In a study of the prophylactic value of 5-day courses of intravenous insulin given to ICA-positive children at risk for type I diabetes every 9 mo combined with daily low-dose subcutaneous insulin therapy, 1 of 5 treated children and all 7 untreated controls developed clinical diabetes over a 2- to 3-y period.[282] The efficacy of this intervention is being studied further.[283] One possible explanation for the prophylactic effect of parenteral insulin is a reduc-

tion in beta-cell secretory activity. Insulin-induced hypoglycemia reduces biosynthesis of insulin,[284] GLUT2,[285] and other putative autoantigens.[286, 287] On the other hand, the preventive effects of insulin in NOD mice may operate by an immunologic mechanism rather than by beta-cell "rest," because intermittent immunization with insulin or with the metabolically inactive insulin beta chain prevents diabetes in NOD mice.[281] Alternatively, insulin may act on T cells as a cytokine and play a role in regulating the Th2/IL-4–mediated response pathway.[288] A final hypothesis is based on insulin's capacity to block apoptosis.[288]

Immunomodulation in Autoimmune Diabetes

CYCLOSPORINE

In some patients with diabetes of 2 mo duration or less, cyclosporine may induce a remission such that insulin treatment may no longer be required.[289] For example, in a group with a mean age of 15.4 y and a duration of diabetes of 39 y, cyclosporine induced a 12-mo remission in 45%. Patients older than 16 y of age benefited more frequently than younger patients, and those who began the drug within 3 wk of initiation of insulin treatment benefited more often than those who started later.[289] When remission occurred, levels of glycosylated hemoglobin decreased to normal, and glucagon-stimulated C peptide response approached normal. When cyclosporine was discontinued, relapse invariably occurred within weeks. Initial remissions in up to two thirds of patients and year-long remissions in almost half have been reported in another study.[143] In randomized controlled trials, remissions of 12 mo duration occurred in 24%[290] and 32%[291] of treated patients, compared with 10%[290] and 3%[291] of controls. Fifty percent of children between 7 and 15 y of age experienced insulin-free remissions for up to 1 y with cyclosporine,[292] in contrast to 25% of children aged 1 to 2.5 y.[293] Nephrotoxicity may make it necessary to decrease the dose, but, even at full dosage, insulin dependence ultimately reappears in many patients.[294] Because of limited efficacy and unacceptable toxicity, trials have been discontinued.

The cyclosporine studies provide powerful support for the autoimmune nature of type I diabetes and demonstrate that a complement of beta cells is intact or at least viable at the onset of metabolic decompensation. This is consistent with findings in BB rats, in which 20% of the normal complement of insulin-containing cells are present when overt diabetes develops.[295] Patients in remission induced by cyclosporine have a diminished insulin response to glucose but a normal insulin response to nonglucose nutrients.[296]

NICOTINAMIDE PROPHYLAXIS

Nicotinamide, the amide of nicotinic acid, is a component of NAD^+ and $NADP^+$ and is an essential dietary constituent, the recommended daily requirement being approximately 5 to 20 mg in adults.

Intravenous administration of nicotinamide before administration of a diabetogenic dose of alloxan prevents diabetes in 60% of rats,[297] and nicotinamide prevents diabetes and reduces the severity of isletitis in young NOD mice.[298] The multiple actions of nicotinamide make it difficult to determine the specific mechanism of this dramatic finding,[245] but nicotinamide increases intracellular NAD^+ content both by serving as a precursor for its synthesis and by reducing poly- or mono-ADP ribosylation, or both.

Nicotinamide may stimulate beta-cell regeneration in 90% of depancreatized rats,[246] possibly acting through the REG ("regenerating") gene.[299, 300] Injection of REG protein in rodents enhances beta-cell replication.[301]

In vitro exposure of isolated mouse pancreatic islets to nicotinamide increases DNA synthesis in beta cells[302] but not in cultured human islets.[303]

Among 14 prediabetic children treated with nicotinamide, only 1 developed IDDM, compared with 8 cases among 8 untreated controls.[304] A 20-nation international clinical trial, the European Nicotinamide Diabetes Intervention Trial (ENDIT), is underway, and the initial results[304] suggest that the onset of human type I diabetes can be delayed by nicotinamide, particularly if it is begun early enough.

Additional Strategies for Preventing Autoimmune Diabetes (Table 21–11)

PREVENTION OF THE INITIAL INJURY TO BETA CELLS. Intervention at the level of the external environment to prevent beta-cell injury is not realistic because of the uncertainty that any single chemical, virus, or other biologic agent is an important factor in most human diabetes. However, even though a relation between bovine milk and IDDM is unproven, the epidemiologic data from Finland[196, 197] justify encouragement of breast-feeding in families at risk.

PREVENTION OF ANTIGEN PRESENTATION. Intervention at the level of antigen presentation could be accomplished either by eliminating the macrophages[305, 306] or by administering antibodies directed against the class II molecules that present antigens.[307] Alternatively, a nonimmunogenic peptide that is homologous with a portion of the beta-cell antigen could be administered to compete with the natural antigen for binding in the cleft of the class II molecule.[308] However, the antigen or antigens responsible for type I diabetes have not been identified, although candidates include GAD65[169] and islet cell antigen 512.[176, 177]

PREVENTION OF AUTOIMMUNE EFFECTOR FUNCTION. Inhibition of macrophage function with silica can prevent antigen presentation and initiation of the autoimmune process,[309] but a safe and effective means of doing this in humans is not known. Antibodies against cytotoxic T cells or NK cells[310, 311] and an antibody that depletes NK cell activity[312] protect against diabetes in rodents. Blockade of the activation of NK cells could also block effector function.[313] Infection of NOD mice with lymphocytic choriomeningitis virus reduces

TABLE 21–11. Potential Strategies for Preventing Type I Diabetes

Prevention of the initial injury	Not practical
Prevention of antigen presentation	
Elimination of macrophages	Impractical and harmful
Anti–class II monoclonal antibodies	Impractical
Nonimmunogenic competitive inhibitor of antigen binding to class II molecule 3	Not yet practical
Blockade of effector cells	
Monoclonal antibody versus cytotoxic T cells or NK cells; IL-1β and/or IFN γ blockade	Not yet practical
Prevention of antigen recognition or effector function	Not practical in humans
Anti-TCRXβ	
Anti-CD3	
Anti-CD4	
Anti-CD8	
Protective viral infection	
Blockade of final common pathway	Nicotinamide clinical trials ongoing
Antioxidants (nicotinamide)	(European Nicotinamide Diabetes
NAD^+ repletion (nicotinamide)	Intervention Trial [ENDIT])
Nitric oxide synthase inhibitor (aminoguanidine)	
Interventions of uncertain mechanisms	Ongoing clinical trials
Oral insulin	
Parenteral insulin	
Immunosuppression	
Cyclosporin A	No longer used

the incidence of diabetes by attacking the helper T-lymphocyte subset of $L3T4^+$ cells.[129, 314]

PREVENTION OF ANTIGEN RECOGNITION OR AUTOIMMUNE EFFECTOR FUNCTION. Administration of monoclonal antibodies (mAbs) that target any of the components of the antigen recognition triad (the antigen itself, the MHC molecules into which it is processed, and the CD3/TcR complex and its coreceptors) can prevent IDDM in rodents.[314–320] Antibody therapy can be discontinued without the subsequent appearance of diabetes.

BLOCKADE OF FINAL COMMON PATHWAY (see Fig. 21–11). IL-1 and TNF α may damage beta cells both by generation of lethal levels of oxygen radicals[321] and by enhancement of NO secretion from macrophages infiltrating the islets and from intraislet endothelial cells.[322] The cytotoxicity of IL-1 was abolished by monomethyl-L-arginine inhibition of NO synthase,[323] and the onset of diabetes can be delayed in NOD

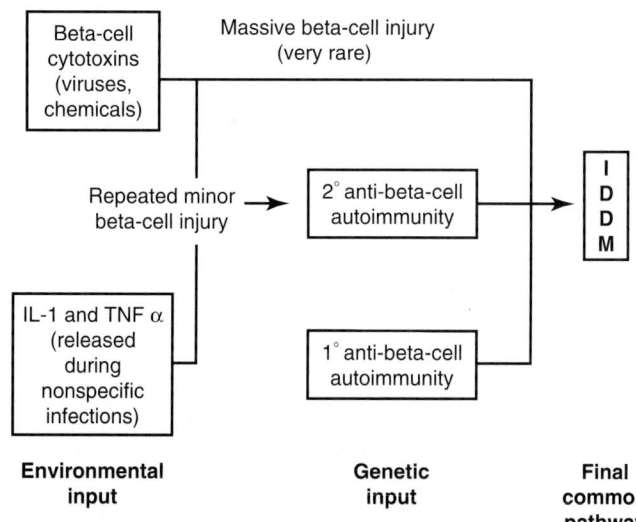

Figure 21–11. A scheme depicting the interactions of environment and heredity in the pathogenesis of IDDM.

mice by administration of the NO synthase inhibitor amino-guanidine.[324]

Pathology of the Islets of Langerhans in Type I IDDM

Early Pathology

Infiltration of the pancreatic islets of patients with type I IDDM by lymphocytes and macrophages is termed isletitis[325]; it is present in two thirds of diabetics studied at autopsy within 6 mo after the initial symptoms.[133] Lymphocytic infiltration of the pancreas in type I IDDM can also be demonstrated with the use of radiolabeled lymphocytes and scanning techniques.[326] Isletitis may be a result of subtotal islet injury rather than its cause.[327–328] Focal regeneration of beta cells occurs soon after the onset of diabetes[157] but less frequently as the disease progresses.

Late Pathology

The reduction in pancreatic weight in subjects with type I diabetes at autopsy (Table 21–12)[329] is caused by atrophy of exocrine tissue, which constitutes about 98% of pancreatic volume. The atrophy may result from loss of the high levels of insulin that perfuse the acinar tissue through the pancreatic vasculature and that may exert a trophic effect on acini.[330, 331]

The islets in IDDM are fewer and often smaller than normal, averaging less than one third of the volume in nondiabetic controls or in patients with type II NIDDM.[329] Beta cells are virtually absent, and the islets consist almost entirely of alpha and delta cells and, in the dorsal part of the head of the pancreas, PP or F cells (Fig. 21–12). The normal islet architecture, with its nonrandom arrangement of islet cell types, is lost.[156] Because insulin, glucagon, and somatostatin exert major effects on various islet cells (Table 21–13), the structural changes may have profound functional consequences. The number of alpha and delta cells per islet is normal or increased,[156] and the total alpha- and delta-cell mass per pancreas is within the normal range.[332]

HORMONAL PATHOPHYSIOLOGY OF IDDM

Insulin

A decrease in insulin secretion or diminished activity of insulin in relation to glucagon in target tissues is critical to the development of symptomatic diabetes. In uncontrolled diabetes insulin deficiency causes a rise in glucagon concentrations; the decreased insulin/glucagon ratio increases production of glucose by the liver, and insulin deficiency impairs glucose utilization by insulin-requiring tissues, activates lipolysis in adipose tissue, enhances proteolysis in muscle, and inten-

sifies the effects of glucagon on liver (Table 21–14).[333] Insulin deficiency therefore enhances the delivery to the liver of the substrates for glucose and ketone production (amino acids and free fatty acids [FFAs], respectively), and glucagon activates glycogenolysis, gluconeogenesis, and ketosis in the liver.

Glucagon and Other Counterregulatory Hormones

Increased secretion of epinephrine, norepinephrine, cortisol, growth hormone, β-endorphin, angiotensin, and vasopressin may play an auxiliary role in development of diabetic ketoacidosis (Table 21–15).[334] The hyperglycemic impact of these factors is exaggerated by the insulin deficiency. Extreme hyperglucagonemia may occur with infection,[335] myocardial infarction,[336] trauma,[337] or burns,[338] and also with diabetic ketoacidosis itself.[339] Even in nondiabetic patients these disorders may cause stress hyperglycemia. Epinephrine causes a marked decrease in sensitivity of peripheral tissues to insulin and inhibits insulin-mediated reduction in glucose production by the liver, both by direct action and by stimulation of glucagon secretion.[340] Finally, epinephrine may block release of any residual insulin still present in patients with IDDM.

Alpha-Cell Dysfunction

Insulin-dependent diabetes mellitus can be defined as a state in which insulin deficiency prevents normal suppression of glucagon secretion and in which hepatic glucose and ketone production are increased. Insulin deficiency in IDDM is always associated with relative or absolute hyperglucagonemia,[341, 342] resulting from loss of the restraining influence of insulin on the alpha cell[343, 344] (Fig. 21–13). Glucagon response to a protein meal[341] (Fig. 21–14) or to an arginine infusion[342] is increased in IDDM and is not blunted by hyperglycemia, although both responses are corrected by insulin.[345, 346] The return of the plasma glucose to near-normal levels with insulin therapy corrects basal hyperglucagonemia[347] and the exaggerated glucagon response to an arginine infusion or a protein meal. The suppressive effect of insulin on alpha cells is the result of both an immediate block of glucagon release[348] (Fig. 21–15) and inhibition (within hours) of glucagon gene expression in alpha cells[349] (Fig. 21–16B and C; see color section between pages 875 and 877).

Disordered Insulin-Glucagon Relations in IDDM

Major overproduction of glucose and ketones by the liver cannot occur unless glucagon is present (see Fig. 21–13a through d).[350] In normal fasting subjects at rest, hepatic glucose production and steady-state glucose utilization by peripheral tissues are equal—about 10 g/h (see Fig. 21–13a).[351, 352] The brain requires about 6 g of glucose per hour if ketosis is insignificant.[353] Glucose metabolism in the brain is insulin

TABLE 21–12. Comparison of Pancreatic Weight and Mass of Endocrine Cells at Autopsy

| | Total Pancreatic Weight (Mean and Range, g) | Weight of Pancreatic Endocrine Component (mg) | Total Mass of Endocrine Cells (mg) | | | | Alpha/Beta Ratio |
			Beta	Alpha	Delta	Pancreatic Polypeptide	
Normals	82 (67–110)	1395	850	225	125	190	0.26
Type I IDDM	40 (26–51)	413	0	150	90	185	—
Type II NIDDM	73 (55–100)	1449	825	375	100	180	0.45

Data from Rahier J, Goebbels RM, Henquin JC. Cellular composition of the human diabetic pancreas. Diabetologia 1983;24:366–371. Mass of endocrine cells was estimated from Figure 3 of the cited reference and should be considered approximate.

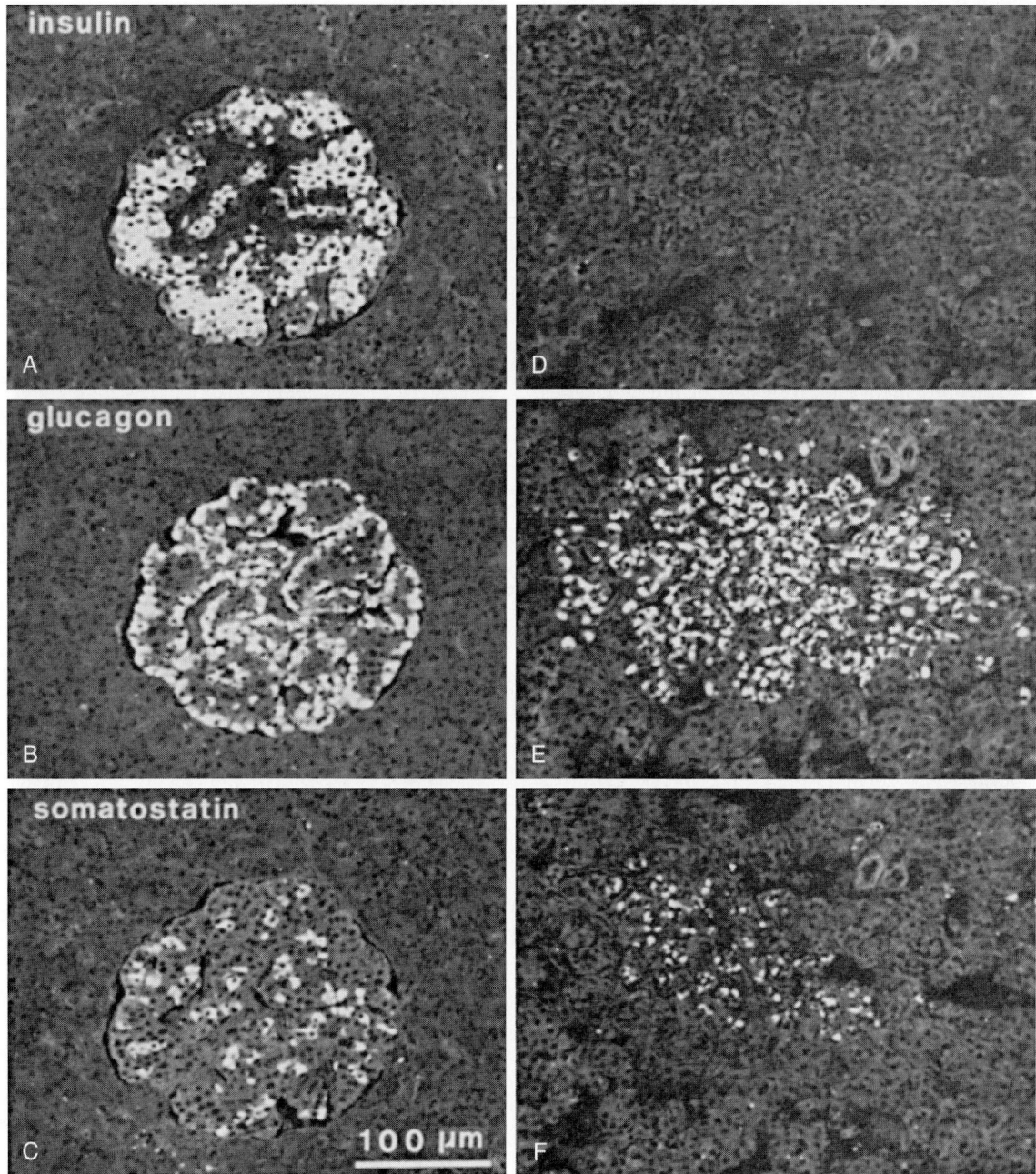

Figure 21–12. Consecutive serial sections of an islet from the tail of the normal human pancreas *(A to C)* and an islet from the tail of the pancreas of a patient with type I diabetes mellitus of 5 y duration *(D to F)* stained for immunofluorescence with anti-insulin, antiglucagon, and antisomatostatin antisera. In the diabetic islet there are no insulin-containing cells but there are numerous glucagon- and somatostatin-containing cells, which have lost their normal distribution pattern and appear scattered throughout the islets. (Courtesy of L. Orci.)

TABLE 21–13. Effects of Islet Hormones on Secretion by Islet Cells

Hormone	Alpha Cells	Beta Cells	Delta Cells	Pancreatic Polypeptide Cells
Glucagon	—	↑	↑	?
Insulin	↓	↓	↓ ?	↓ ?
Somatostatin	↓	↓	↓	↓

↑, increase; ↓, decrease; —, no effect.

TABLE 21–14. Contribution of Hormonal Abnormalities to Metabolic Derangements of Severe Diabetes*

Derangement	Insulin Deficiency	Glucagon Excess
Underutilization of glucose	+ + + +	0
Overproduction of glucose	+	+ + + +
Increased glycogenolysis	+	+ + + +
Increased gluconeogenesis	+	+ + + +
Increased release of amino acids	+ + + +	0
Increased lipolysis	+ + + +	+ (?)
Increased hepatic ketogenesis	+ (?)	+ + + +

*The pluses are semiquantitative indices of the magnitude of effect, from minor (+) to major (+ + + +); 0 is no effect; ? is uncertain.

independent. In humans about 75% of hepatic glucose production is mediated by glucagon,[354] and about 40% of total glucose utilization is mediated by insulin. Therefore, if both insulin and glucagon were absent (Fig. 21–17), glucose production would decrease by 75% to approximately 2.5 to 4 g/h, and utilization would decrease by 40% to approximately 6 g/h.[355] Instead of the hyperglycemia that occurs with insulin deficiency in the presence of glucagon (see Fig. 21–13*f*), glucose levels would remain constant or fall.[356-358] Indeed, the syndrome of congenital glucagon deficiency is associated with intractable hypoglycemia.[358] In the absence of glucagon, ketone production is limited despite insulin deficiency.[359, 360]

Five types of bihormonal deficiency of insulin and glucagon have provided insight into this relation: (1) somatostatin-induced glucagon suppression in insulin-deprived type I diabetes[361]; (2) somatostatin-secreting tumors[362]; (3) hypophysectomized, depancreatized (Houssay) dogs[363]; (4) surgically induced bihormonal deficiency in humans,[364] (Fig. 21–18) and in dogs[350]; and (5) administration of a glucagon receptor antagonist that blocks glucagon action to diabetic rats.[365]

Glucagon suppression by somatostatin prevents both the hyperglycemia and the hyperketonemia that otherwise occur in insulin-deprived IDDM patients, in a sense transforming IDDM into a mild (ketoacidosis-resistant) NIDDM for the duration of the glucagon suppression.[359] This effect can be sustained for up to 48 h.[361] When glucagon is infused, hyperglycemia and ketonemia rapidly appear (Fig. 21–19). In subjects with a somatostatinoma, suppression of the secretion of both insulin and glucagon by somatostatin causes mild iabetes without overproduction of glucose or ketones.[362] Similarly, in dogs after hypophysectomy, which causes a profound deficiency of glucagon,[363] total pancreatectomy results in mild fasting hyperglycemia or normoglycemia and postprandial hyperglycemia without ketoacidosis; administration of glucagon causes severe IDDM.[363]

Pancreatectomized humans have variable plasma glucagon concentrations depending on the adequacy of insulin replacement and the state of metabolic control.[364, 366-368] If such patients are deprived of exogenous insulin, levels of glucagon rise to increase hepatic glucose and ketone production, but more slowly than in patients with type I IDDM.[367] The biologic potency of glucagon, demonstrable in hepatocytes in vitro at concentrations as low as 10^{-13} mol/L,[369] is enhanced by the absence of insulin. Glucagon deficiency in pancreatec-

tomized individuals is rarely complete, but in one such patient levels of immunoreactive pancreatic glucagon, gut glucagon-like immunoreactivity, and insulin were unmeasurable (see Fig. 21–18). When this patient was deprived of insulin, blood glucose levels were normal during a 12-h study.[364] In other depancreatectomized persons plasma glucagon[368] may be derived from extrapancreatic sites.

The explanation for the modest metabolic consequences of insulin deficiency in the absence of glucagon is that the major direct effect of insulin on the liver is to oppose the effects of glucagon[333]; i.e., insulin has a minimal effect on hepatic glucose and ketone metabolism when glucagon is not present. The biochemical mechanisms of these interactions are discussed later in this chapter.

NON–INSULIN-DEPENDENT DIABETES MELLITUS

Demography

Prevalence of Diagnosed NIDDM

NIDDM is the most common of the hyperglycemic states. The disease exists in all populations, but prevalence varies greatly[370] (Fig. 21–20); the highest rates ever reported were 34% in the Micronesians of Nauru[23, 371] and 40% in the Pima Indians of Arizona.[6] In American whites the figure in 1976 was between 1 and 2%, using modern criteria for the definition of diabetes,[372] but the prevalence has risen as the population ages and becomes more obese, and more than 10% of the older population now suffer from the disease.[373, 374] Epidemiologic studies based on a single OGTT may overestimate the prevalence somewhat.[375, 376]

The high prevalence of NIDDM among Nauruans and Pimas is a result of a change in the pattern of food intake from one of chronic caloric deprivation, in which both obesity and diabetes were rare, to one of caloric abundance, in which both abnormalities are common. A similar phenomenon (usually called urbanization) has occurred in other Native Ameri-

TABLE 21–15. Effects of Stress-Related Hormones on Secretion of Islet Hormones and on Metabolism of Liver and Other Tissues

Hormone	Islets		Extrapancreatic Tissues		
	Insulin Secretion	*Glucagon Secretion*	*Adipocytes: Lipolysis*	*Muscle: Glucose Utilization*	*Liver: Glucose Production*
Catecholamines	↓	↑	↑	↓	↑
Corticotropin	—	—	↑	—	—
Cortisol	±	↑	↑	↓	↑
Growth hormone	↑	↑	↑	↓	↑
β-Endorphin	↑	↑	—	—	—
Vasopressin	—	↑	—	—	↓

↑, increase; ↓, decrease; —, no effect or not known.

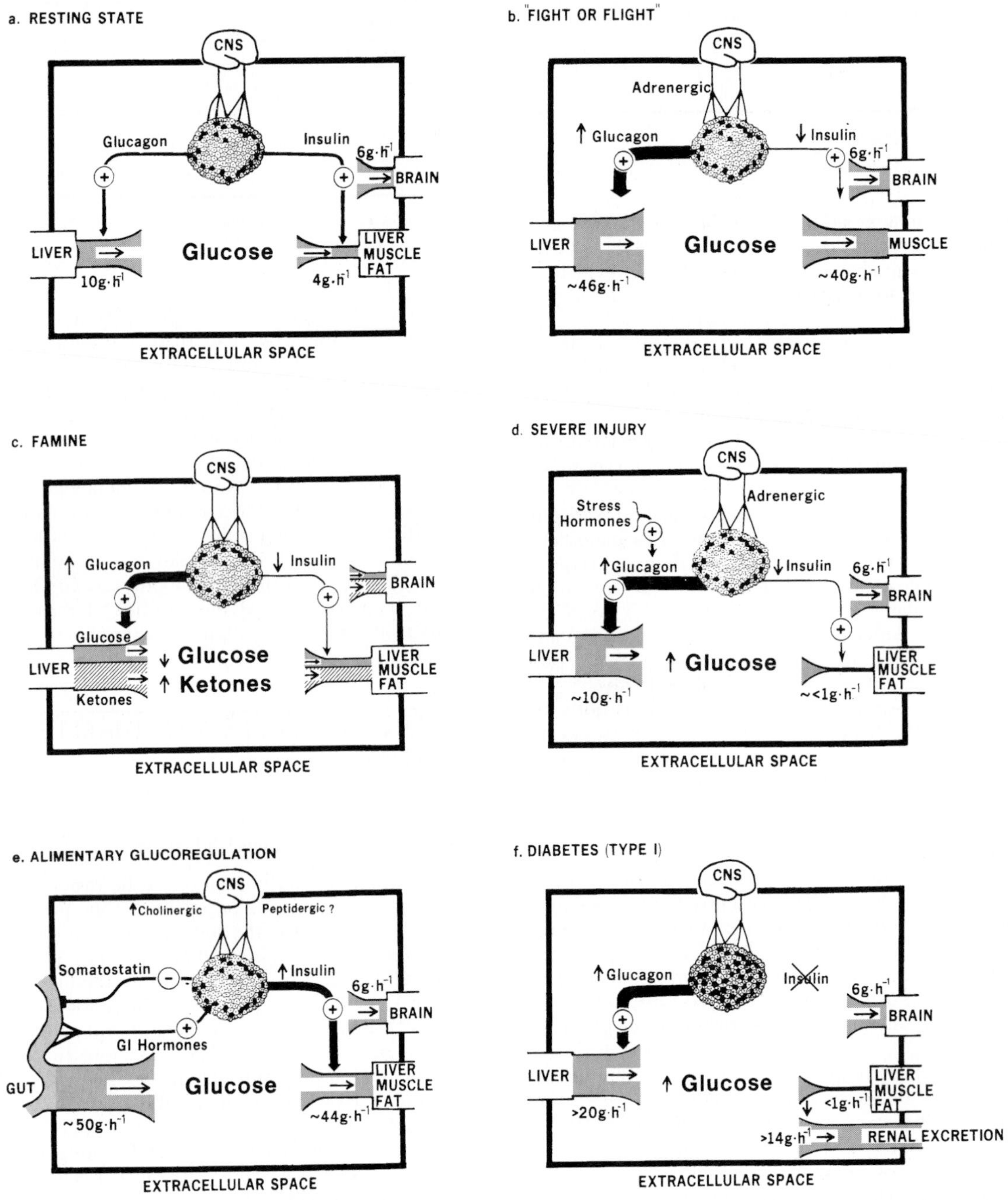

Figure 21-13. Regulation of glucose by insulin and glucagon under various conditions of fuel need and availability. The islet of Langerhans is depicted with neural connections to the central nervous system (CNS). The extracellular space is indicated by a box (heavy border) into which glucose flows from the liver or gut and from which it flows, independent of insulin action, to the brain and, under insulin mediation, into other tissues. Values given for rates of glucose utilization and production are estimates. In the resting state (a), insulin and glucagon maintain equality between the rate of glucose utilization and that of hepatic glucose production. Approximately 75% of basal glucose production is estimated to be glucagon-mediated. In "fight or flight" (b), the huge increase in glucose utilization by muscle would cause hypoglycemia if the liver did not replace this glucose precisely—in large part through an adrenergically mediated increase in glucagon level and a decrease in insulin level. The latter minimizes the uptake of endogenously produced glucose by tissues other than exercising muscles and brain. In famine (starvation) (c), the rise in glucagon level, coupled with a decrease in insulin level, promotes glycogenolysis and gluconeogenesis; within 1 wk, a shift to ketone production occurs (hatched area). This shift is required for continued survival. In severe injury (d), an adrenergically mediated increase in glucagon level and a decrease in insulin secretion stimulate hepatic glucose production and minimize glucose utilization by insulin-responsive tissues. The stress hormones—growth hormone, β-endorphin, epinephrine, and cortisol—all increase glucagon secretion. In alimentary glucoregulation (e), signals arising in the gastrointestinal tract immediately after a meal (gastrointestinal hormones, cholinergic and perhaps peptidergic neurotransmitters) reach the islets of Langerhans and elicit an anticipatory response of insulin secretion, thereby avoiding major perturbations in the concentration of glucose and other ingested nutrients. Ambient glucose concentration is the major determinant of the magnitude of insulin response to these signals. In type I diabetes (f), islets consist primarily of cells secreting glucagon and somatostatin but little or no insulin. In insulin deprivation there is marked hyperglucagonemia and overproduction of glucose and ketones (not shown) by the liver. Unrestrained secretion and and unopposed actions of glucagon are unbuffered by an insulin-mediated increase in glucose uptake into insulin-sensitive tissues. Consequently, the rise in plasma glucose is limited only by glucose excretion and glucose utilization by insulin-independent tissues such as brain. If glucagon is absent, the lack of insulin does not generate massive hepatic overproduction of ketones and glucose. (From Unger RH, Orci L. Glucagon and the A cell: physiology and pathophysiology. Reprinted by permission of The New England Journal of Medicine 1981, 304: 1518–1524.)

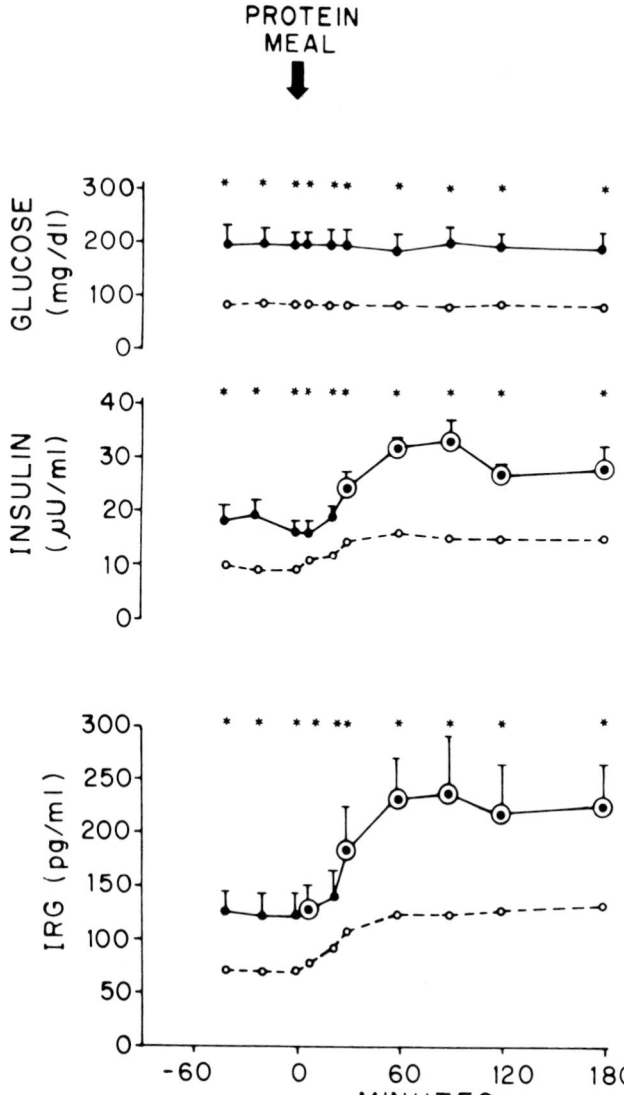

PROTEIN MEAL

Figure 21–14. The plasma glucose, insulin, and immunoreactive glucagon (IRG) responses to a protein meal in 10 subjects with adult-onset diabetes and 12 subjects who received constant infusion of insulin at 1 U/h. ●, diabetic subjects; ○, nondiabetic subjects; *, P < .05 diabetic versus nondiabetic subjects; ⊙, P < 0.05 versus baseline. (From Raskin P, Aydin I, Yamamoto T, et al. Abnormal alpha cell function in human diabetes: the response to oral protein. Am J Med 1978; 64:988–997.)

can tribes,[20] Pacific Islanders,[23] Australian aboriginals,[377] and Asiatic Indian groups.[378] Presumably the same changes in lifestyle have occurred in the US population, facilitating expression of a predisposition for NIDDM.[23] The urbanization phenomenon has been most carefully studied in nonwhite groups but is probably ethnically and racially nonspecific.

Incidence

According to the 1990–1992 National Health Interview Survey, approximately 625,000 cases of diabetes are diagnosed in the United States each year.[379] The US estimated incidence in 1990–1992 was 6.4 times the 1935–1936 rate.[373] Pima Indians have an appearance rate of 2650 cases per 100,000 population per year, the highest in the world.[380]

Familial Aggregation

In contrast to type I IDDM, 38% of siblings and one third of the offspring of persons with NIDDM have diabetes or

abnormal glucose tolerance.[381, 382] The percentage of affected siblings varies inversely with the obesity of the proband.[381] Concordance in identical twins of type II NIDDM in some studies approaches 100%,[47, 383] compared with 50% or less in type I IDDM (Table 21–16). In one study, 58% of twins of type II diabetic patients were diabetic, but most of the originally discordant co-twins became diabetic during the next 10 y.[384] A realistic estimate for concordance in monozygotic twins may be 70 to 80%.[385]

HLA and Type II NIDDM

There is no association between HLA and true type II NIDDM. However, the putative variant of autoimmune diabetes that results in subtotal beta-cell destruction and phenotypic "non–insulin-dependent diabetes" (usually transient) presumably has MHC linkages comparable to those seen in ordinary IDDM. Autoantibodies to beta-cell antigens are present in 10 to 33% of NIDDM patients,[211–213] raising the possibility of an autoimmune subtype of NIDDM ("type I NIDDM"). As mentioned previously, some patients with apparent NIDDM develop transient insulin dependence.[21]

Genetics of NIDDM

Phenotype

NIDDM involves two defects, peripheral insulin resistance and hyperinsulinemia, in the prediabetic phase, which is followed by subsequent failure of insulin secretion to compensate for the insulin resistance, with resultant hyperglycemia and overt diabetes. Insulin resistance and hyperinsulinemia de-

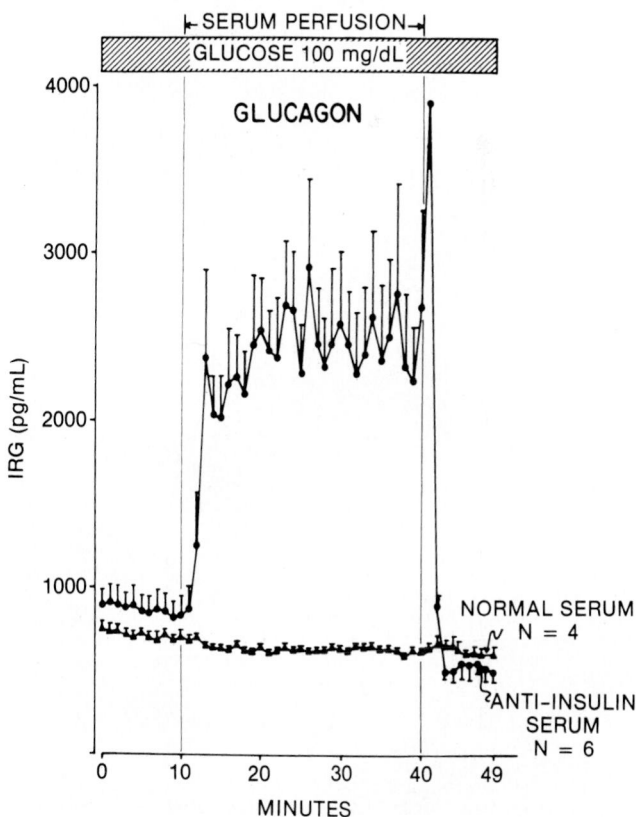

Figure 21–15. The effect of anti-insulin serum (●) on glucagon secretion (mean ± SEM) in the isolated perfused rat pancreas. Normal guinea pig serum (▲) was used as a control. The rapid rise in glucagon during perfusion of the antiserum is consistent with intravascular neutralization of newly secreted insulin as it passes through the islet from beta cells to alpha cells.

INSULIN   GLUCAGON

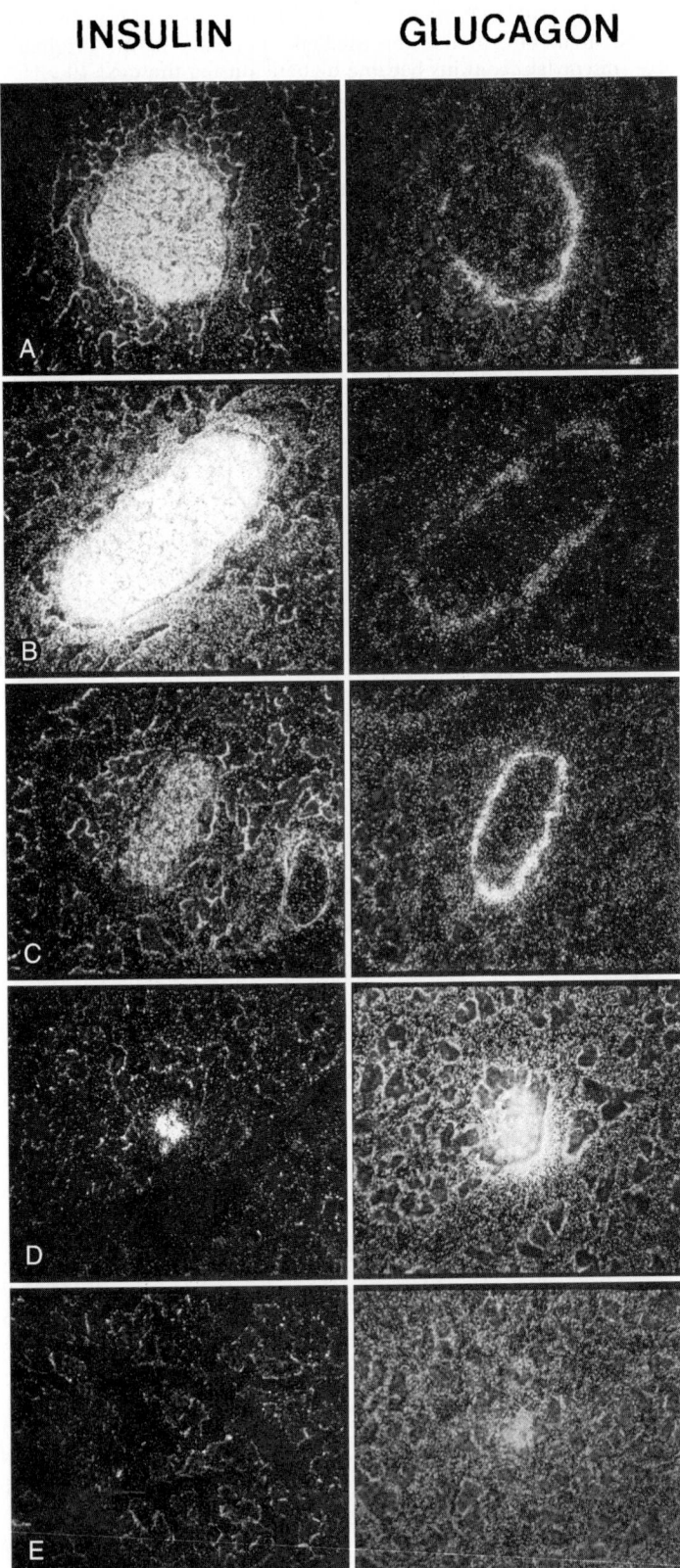

Figure 21–16. In situ hybridization for proinsulin mRNA and proglucagon mRNA of islets from normal rats *(A)* and of islets from normal rats after 5 d of continuous intravenous infusion of 50% glucose *(B)*, after chronic hypoglycemia induced by infusion of insulin *(C)*, with severe streptozocin-induced IDDM after 2 d of insulin deprivation *(D)*, and after 2 d of insulin deprivation followed by injection of regular insulin 1 h before sacrifice *(E)*. *B,* Chronic hyperglycemia induced by glucose infusion causes an increase in insulin and a decrease in glucagon gene expression. *C,* Chronic hypoglycemia causes a decrease in insulin and an increase in glucagon gene expression. *D,* Insulin deprivation in severe streptozocin-induced IDDM causes a marked increase in glucagon gene expression, which at 1 h after insulin administration is profoundly reduced *(E)*. (See color section between pages 875 and 877.)

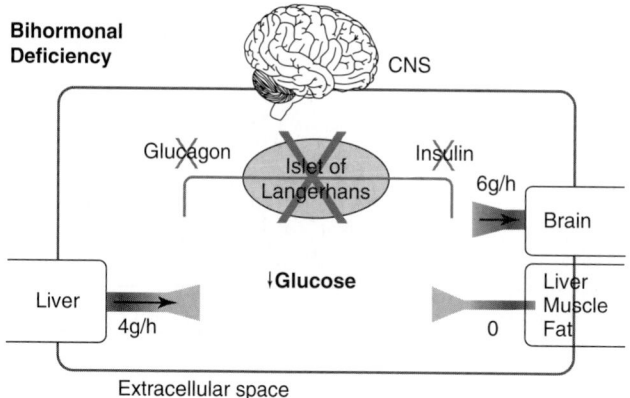

Figure 21–17. Schematic representation of combined insulin and glucagon deficiency. In the absence of both hormones, hepatic glucose production is low (about 4 g/h) after an overnight fast. Plasma glucose concentration is normal or below normal because, despite low insulin-mediated glucose utilization, non–insulin-mediated uptake in the brain continues (about 6 g/h). Replacement of glucagon would cause hyperglycemia (see Fig. 21–18).

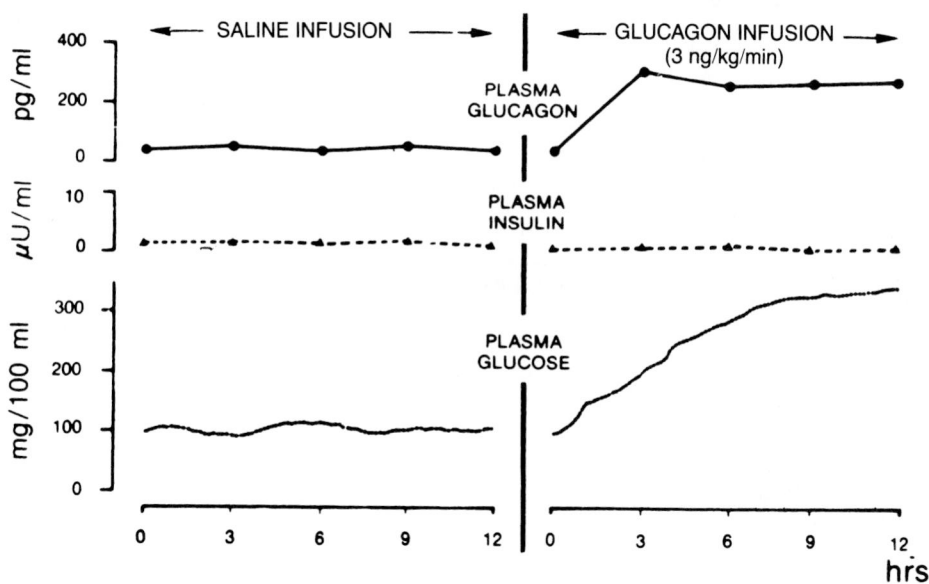

Figure 21–18. Bihormonal deficiency state in humans produced by total pancreatectomy. Note lack of hyperglycemia despite absence of measurable free insulin *(left)*. Infusion of glucagon causes hyperglycemia *(right)*. (From Santeusanio F, Massi-Benedetti M, Angeletti G, et al. Glucagon and carbohydrate disorder in a totally pancreatectomized man [a study with the aid of an artificial endocrine pancreas]. J Endocrinol Invest 1981; 4:93–96.)

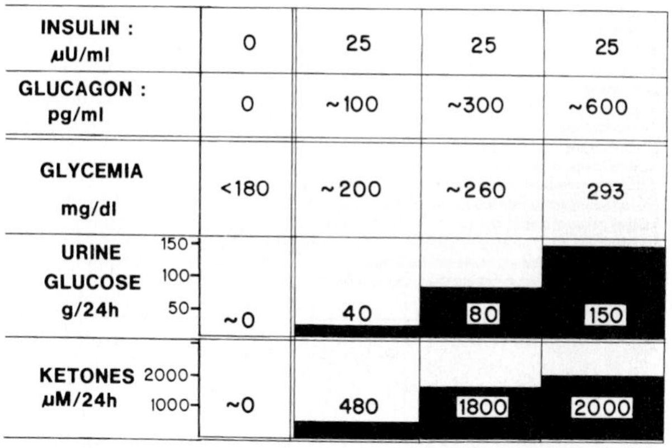

Figure 21–19. Roles of insulin and glucagon in hepatic fuel overproduction in IDDM. When both insulin and glucagon are absent, the massive hyperglycemia and hyperketonemia observed in the presence of glucagon do not occur. In patients in whom insulin was clamped at approximately 25 μU/mL for 3 d, hyperglycemia, glycosuria, and ketonuria increased progressively as glucagon levels rose consequent to glucagon infusion. Therefore, deficiency of insulin does not result in massive overproduction of fuels by the liver unless glucagon is present. (From Unger RH. The milieu interieur and the islets of Langerhans. Diabetologia 1981; 20:1–11.)

INSULIN : μU/ml	0	25	25	25
GLUCAGON : pg/ml	0	~100	~300	~600
GLYCEMIA mg/dl	<180	~200	~260	293
URINE GLUCOSE g/24h	~0	40	80	150
KETONES μM/24h	~0	480	1800	2000

TABLE 21–16. Summary of Twin Studies and NIDDM

Ref.	Type of Twins	No. of Pairs	Concordance (%)	Comments
63	MZ	35	100	Ascertainment uncertain, criteria for diabetes diagnosis not current
64	MZ	47	55	Ascertainment from the Danish twin register; diabetes defined as "maturity onset"
65	MZ	10	70	Diabetes diagnosed at age >40 years in one twin; ascertainment possibly biased
63, 66, 67	MZ	113	69	Ascertainment biased by referral of one twin with NIDDM
68	MZ	34	58	Ascertained unbiased, from the Veterans Twin Study after two examinations; diabetes
	DZ	42	17	defined with 50-g glucose load as 1-h glucose ≥13.8 mmol/L (≥250 mg/dL); discordant MZ twins had higher glucose levels than controls; maximum proband concordance rate for MZ twins = 65%
69	MZ	46	80	Ascertainment biased by referral of one or more twins with diabetes; diagnosis
	DZ	10	40	using WHO criteria
70	MZ	140	34	Ascertainment unbiased, from the Finnish Twin Registry; diabetes diagnosed only
	DZ	303	16	from hospital discharge registry, drug registry, and death certificates; likely to underestimate prevalence

MZ, monozygotic; DZ, dizygotic; WHO, World Health Organization.
From Diabetes in America, 2nd Edition, Chapter 9: Risk factors for non–insulin-dependent diabetes, p. 183. References noted in table are listed in the referenced chapter.

velop years before impairment of glucose tolerance and may not result in beta-cell failure and NIDDM. The failure of insulin secretion, by contrast, correlates with the impairment of glucose tolerance and is presumed to be its cause. Glucose-stimulated insulin secretion (GSIS) is an excellent marker for the decline in beta-cell function. GSIS disappears as fasting hyperglycemia appears.[386] Insulin resistance, beta-cell defects, and NIDDM all exhibit familial clustering. Although most authorities consider insulin resistance to be the primary lesion, others believe that it is secondary to primary hyperinsulinemia, which causes compensatory insulin resistance to prevent hypoglycemia. A third possibility is that a common defect causes both hyperinsulinemia and insulin resistance.[387]

Environmental-Genetic Interactions

NIDDM has a genetic component that is subject to major influence from the environment.[385] NIDDM may not become manifest unless the environment permits a generous dietary intake and a degree of adiposity. Conversely, the clinical phenotype may appear in the absence of a complete NIDDM genotype in persons who develop massive obesity.

It is not clear whether NIDDM is a collection of similar diseases with major and minor forms or a single disease with multiple variations caused by varying genetic interactions. The authors favor the view that NIDDM is a polygenic disease in which one or two major genes interact with a number of other loci. This is referred to as a mixed or "multiplicative" pattern. Because insulin resistance and beta-cell dysfunction could be caused by a defect in one or more of at least 100 proteins, the unraveling of the pathophysiology is a daunting task.[388, 389]

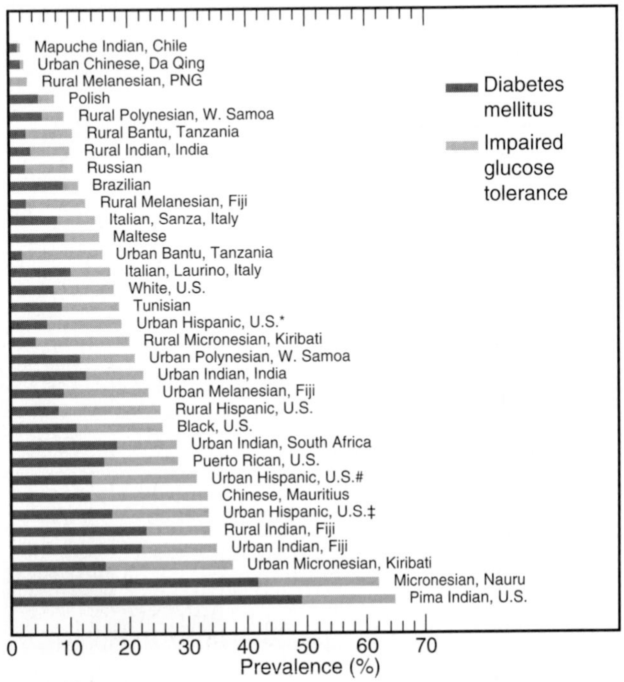

MOLECULAR GENETICS OF NIDDM

Some of the genes and gene defects involved in NIDDM are shown in Table 21–17.

TABLE 21–17. Genetic Classification of NIDDM

I. Genetically characterized forms of NIDDM
 A. Maturity-onset diabetes of the young (MODY)
  1. *MODY1*—linked to chromosome 20q
  2. *MODY2*—linked to glucokinase (7p13-15)
  3. *MODY3*—linked to chromosome 12q
  4. Others
 B. Defects in the insulin gene (11p15)
  1. Familial hyperproinsulinemia
  2. Mutant insulin molecules
 C. Defects in the insulin receptor (10p13)
  1. Leprechaunism
  2. Type A syndrome of insulin resistance
  3. Rabson-Mendenhall syndrome
 D. Mutation in mitochondrial gene for tRNA[Leu]
  1. Maternally inherited diabetes with neurosensory deafness
  2. MELAS syndrome
 E. Mutation in *GLUT2* glucose transporter (3q26) (one case only)
II. Genes involved in ordinary NIDDM
 A. Genes with some evidence for involvement
  1. HLA locus-DR4 (6p21-23)—in elderly persons with NIDDM only
  2. Glucagon receptor gene (17q25)
  3. Insulin receptor substrate-1 (2q76)
  4. Glycogen synthase (19q13)
  5. Intestinal fatty acid–binding proteins (4q)
  6. *RAD* (2q3637)
 B. Genes for which significant involvement has been ruled out
  1. Insulin gene (11p15)
  2. MODY genes (20q, 7p, 12q)
  3. ATP-sensitive K+ channel (21q22)
  4. Glucagon-like peptide-1 (GLP-1) receptor (6p21)
  5. *GLUT2* (3q36)
  6. *GLUT4* (17p13)
  7. Insulin receptor (19p13)

Figure 21–20. Prevalence of NIDDM in various populations. *, upper income; #, middle income; ‡, low income; PNG, Papua New Guinea. Data are age standardized to the world population for ages 30 to 64 y, both sexes combined. (Redrawn and modified from King H, Rewers M, WHO Ad Hoc Diabetes Reporting Group. Global estimates for prevalence of diabetes mellitus and impaired glucose tolerance in adults. Diabetes Care 1993; 16:157–177.)

Mutations in Genes Involved in Insulin Resistance

Insulin Receptor Gene

The insulin receptor consists of two α subunits that bind the insulin and two β subunits that form a β-α-α-β heterotetramer (Fig. 21–21).[390, 391] As of 1996 more than 40 mutations of the insulin receptor gene are known to cause insulin resistance,[392] most of these in rare disorders such as leprechaunism, Rabson-Mendenhall syndrome, or type A insulin resistance.[393–399] The insulin resistance in these syndromes is more severe than in NIDDM, plasma insulin levels ranging from 359 to 2153 pmol/L (50 to 300 μU/mL) in the fasting state and from 2870 to 17,938 pmol/L (400 to 2500 μU/mL) after a glucose load.[392] Mutations may involve the insulin-binding α subunit, the tyrosine kinase domain of the β subunit, or the intracellular processing site between the subunits[392] (see Fig. 21–21). The most severe manifestation is leprechaunism with severe growth retardation, other developmental defects, and death in infancy. The disorder is caused by homozygous or compound heterozygous mutations in the insulin receptor gene. In type A and Rabson-Mendenhall syndromes, heterozygosity of the mutations is the rule. The major features in these two conditions are insulin resistance, acanthosis nigricans, hyperandrogenism, and polycystic ovary syndrome. Mutations also have been described in obese women with NIDDM and hyperandrogenism, acanthosis nigricans, and menstrual disorders (HAIR-AN syndrome).[400] Insulin resistance in ordinary NIDDM is not usually caused by defects in the insulin receptor,[401, 402] despite rare heterozygous mutations.[403] An example of the latter is the substitution of alanine for threonine in position 831 of the β subunit (Thr[831] → Ala) in a Japanese family with NIDDM.[403]

The expression of two normal variant insulin receptor isoforms does not differ in lean, obese, and NIDDM subjects.[404, 405] These isoforms are generated by alternative splicing of the 36-base-pair exon 11 and differ by the presence or absence of 12 amino acids at the COOH terminus of the α subunit. The isoform that lacks exon 11 has twice the insulin-binding affinity and a higher internalization rate than the exon 11–containing isoform.[406]

A restriction fragment length polymorphism in the insulin receptor gene was reported in 12 of 51 NIDDM subjects compared with 4 of 52 nondiabetic control subjects.[407] Even nondiabetic subjects with the polymorphism had hyperinsulinemia or a nondiagnostic impairment of glucose tolerance, or both, implying an association between the polymorphism and insulin resistance.[407] However, the role of these polymorphisms in the pathogenesis of NIDDM has not been established. It has also been reported that upstream regulatory regions for the insulin receptor gene were defective in their capacity to bind DNA-binding proteins in patients with NIDDM, with the result that insulin receptor transcription was decreased.[408] A comparable defect in the promoter sequence of the human apolipoprotein CIII gene abolishes insulin regulation of that gene,[409] and a similar mutation causes transcriptional silencing

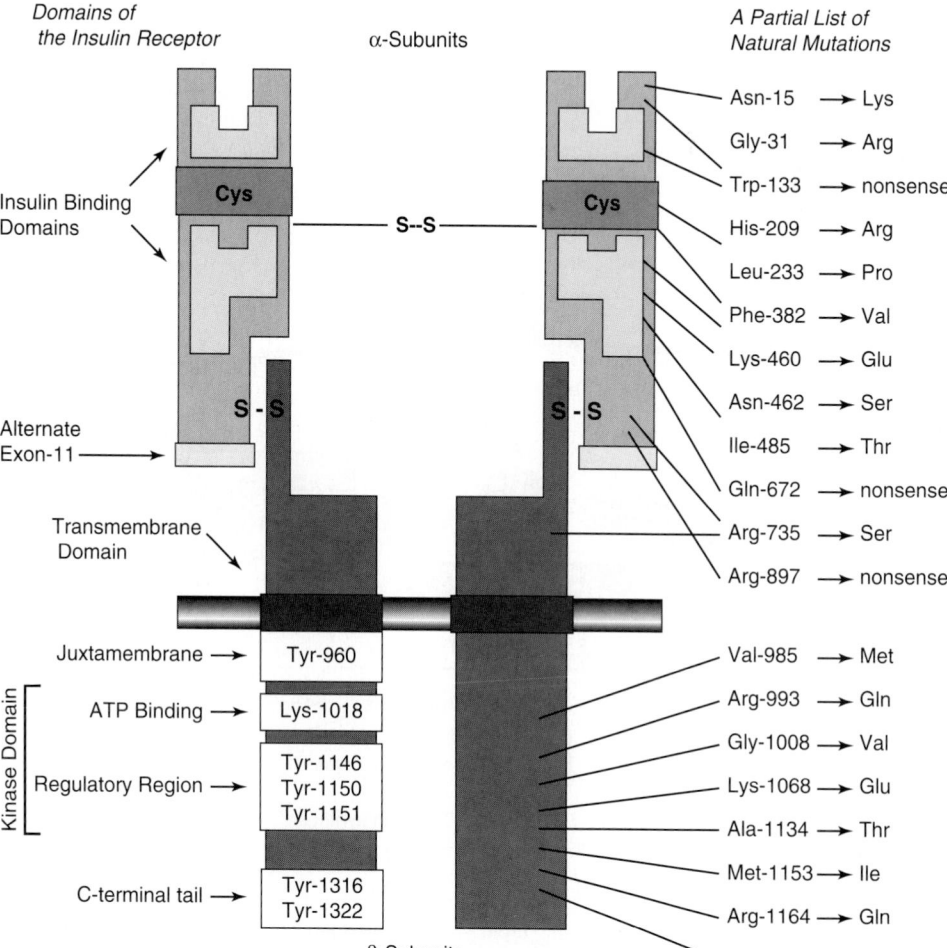

Figure 21–21. Schematic representation of the insulin receptor tyrosine kinase. The labeling on the left indicates the functional domains of the receptor. The labeling on the right gives a partial list of the naturally occurring mutations. (Redrawn from Kahn CR, Vicent D, Doria A. Genetics of non–insulin-dependent (type II) diabetes mellitus. Annu Rev Med 1996; 47:509–531. © 1996, by Annual Reviews Inc.)

of the tumor suppressor gene product p16.[410] In all these cases the sequence that encodes receptor structure is not mutated, but transcription is altered.

To summarize, mutations in the structural sequence of the insulin receptor gene are not believed to cause the insulin resistance in ordinary NIDDM (see complete review by Taylor and co-workers[411]).

Insulin Receptor Substrate-1

Insulin receptor substrate-1 (IRS-1) is the major substrate of the insulin-receptor and insulin-like growth factor (IGF)–receptor tyrosine kinases,[412] and the IRS-1 gene is thus a candidate gene in NIDDM (Fig. 21–22).[413] Although mutations in this gene have been identified in patients with NIDDM, they are common in nondiabetic control subjects as well. For example, in 40 Finnish people with typical NIDDM, three variants, $Gly^{818} \rightarrow Arg$, $Ser^{892} \rightarrow Gly$, and $Gly^{971} \rightarrow Arg$, were identified.[414] The third variant was found in 9.8% of 112 NIDDM patients and in 8.7% of controls. $Ser^{892} \rightarrow Gly$ is of interest because it abolishes a potential serine phosphorylation site and could alter insulin-mediated signal transduction.[414] A $Gly^{971} \rightarrow Arg$ substitution was identified in 10 Danish patients with NIDDM, 7 of 31 Italian patients with NIDDM, and 4 of 32 normal controls.[415]

It seems unlikely that mutations in the IRS-1 gene are major contributors to the pathogenesis of IDDM,[413] although a variant of IRS-1 may reinforce the negative effect of obesity on insulin sensitivity.[416] On the other hand, mice with IRS-1 deficiency are resistant to both insulin and IGF-1 but do not develop fasting hyperglycemia despite reduced glucose tolerance, possibly because of the alternative insulin-signaling pathway involving IRS-2, a larger insulin receptor kinase substrate.[417]

GLUT4

As the "insulin-responsive" facilitative glucose transporter in skeletal muscle and adipocytes, GLUT4 was considered a prime candidate for a role in the insulin resistance of NIDDM. However, GLUT4 polymorphisms occur with approximately equal frequency in controls and in subjects with NIDDM,[418, 419] indicating that GLUT4 mutations are not involved in the pathogenesis of NIDDM. Furthermore, ablation of the GLUT4 gene causes little impairment of glucose tolerance.[420]

Hexokinase II

Missence mutations in the hexokinase II gene that encodes the principal hexokinase isoenzyme occur with equal frequency in NIDDM patients and in controls.[421] Hexokinase II activity has been reported to be decreased in muscle of patients with NIDDM.[422]

Glycogen Synthase

Glycogen synthesis and glycogen synthase are reduced in NIDDM.[423–425] The gene that encodes glycogen synthase has two alleles, A1 and A2. The A2 allele is said to be present in 30% of Finnish patients with NIDDM, compared with 8% of normal controls,[426] but an association between the A1 allele and NIDDM has been reported in France. A Japanese study reported no A2 alleles in 98 NIDDM patients, but a simple tandem repeat DNA allele was identified in 17.7% of NIDDM patients as opposed to 8.7% of controls.[427] It is not clear whether the different findings in these reports reflect ethnic differences.

A $Gly^{464} \rightarrow Ser$ mutation in the glycogen synthase gene was found in 2 of 228 Finnish NIDDM patients but in none of 154 controls; both patients had severe insulin resistance and premature atherosclerosis.[428] In most Finnish NIDDM patients glycogen synthase protein in skeletal muscle was increased.[429] Although glycogen synthase mutations probably do not play a major role in NIDDM, a modifying role in some subsets of patients with NIDDM cannot be excluded.

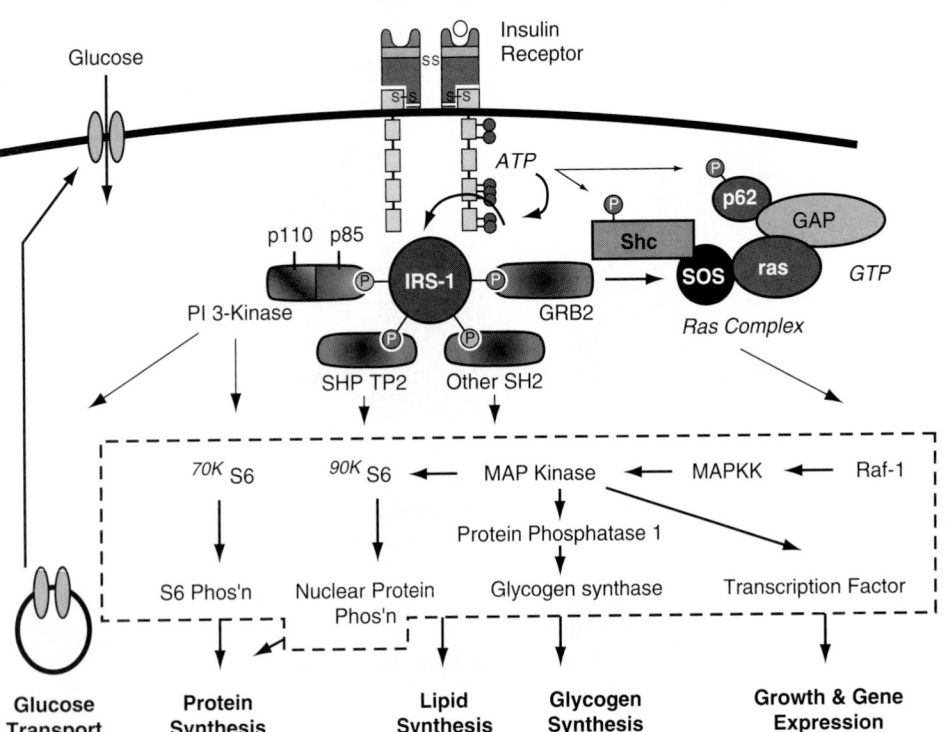

Figure 21–22. Downstream effects insulin/insulin receptor interaction. The initial phosphorylation substrate is IRS-1. See text for details. (Redrawn from Kahn CR. Banting Lecture: Insulin action, diabetogenesis, and the cause of type II diabetes. Diabetes 1994; 43:1066–1084.)

Mutations in Genes Encoding Beta-Cell Proteins Involved in the Quality and Quantity of Secreted Insulin (Fig. 21–23)

Proinsulin and Insulin

Since 1979, six mutations have been reported in the structural gene for proinsulin.[430, 431] Three consist of alterations in the alpha and beta chains that impair binding of the peptide to its receptor; the other mutations impair the processing of proinsulin. All affected subjects are heterozygotes with hyperinsulinemia or hyperproinsulinemia and little impairment of glucose homeostasis until age and/or obesity alter the balance between insulin production and insulin requirements.[392]

A polymorphism in the 5′ flanking region of the insulin gene is present in obese British women,[432] and a variant insulin promoter with reduced promoter activity may contribute to diabetes in 5 to 6% of black patients with NIDDM.[433] However, insulin gene mutations do not appear to play a role in common forms of NIDDM.[434]

GLUT2

GLUT2, the high-K_m glucose transporter,[435] is a candidate gene in NIDDM.[436–438] All animal models of spontaneous NIDDM thus far studied exhibit loss of GSIS accompanied by a reduction in GLUT2 mRNA and protein.[439] Reduction of GLUT2 by means of transgenic expression of GLUT2 antisense mRNA causes impaired GSIS and diabetes in mice.[440]

Nevertheless, GLUT2 mutations are not common in NIDDM,[441, 442] although, rarely, they may contribute. In a study of 48 African American women who developed postpartum NIDDM after gestational diabetes, two mutations were found, a Val[197] → Ile and a Thr[110] → Ile, both in the membrane-spanning regions of the protein (Fig. 21–24). The Val[197] → Ile mutation abolished glucose transport activity when the mutant cDNA was expressed in Xenopus oocytes.[443]

Glucokinase

Because it encodes the rate-limiting enzyme in the high-K_m glucose metabolism pathway,[444] the glucokinase gene is

another candidate gene for the beta-cell dysfunction of NIDDM.[444] Glucokinase gene mutations occur in the mild disorder known as maturity-onset diabetes of the young (MODY) together with partial impairment in the beta-cell response to intravenous glucose.[445–448] However, structural mutations in the glucokinase gene do not appear to play a role in the common forms of NIDDM observed in Caucasians[449, 450] or in Japanese,[451] although one Japanese patient with late-onset NIDDM had a nonsense mutation in codon 186 that abolished the activity of the enzyme.[452]

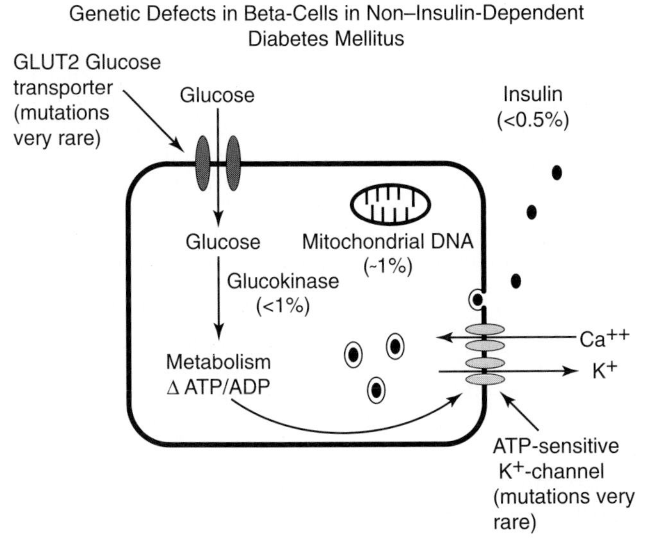

ATP-Sensitive Potassium Channel Subunit

Closure of ATP-Sensitive potassium (K^+) channels by ATP depolarizes the beta-cell plasma membrane and activates voltage-dependent calcium (Ca^{2+}) channels; the influx of Ca^{2+} initiates exocytosis of insulin-containing granules.[453, 454] Studies in 1237 unselected Caucasian patients with NIDDM, in Mexican American sib pairs with NIDDM,[455] in MODY families, and in patients with gestational diabetes suggest that mutations in the ATP-sensitive K^+ channel do not play a significant role in any of these forms of diabetes.[456, 457]

Sulfonylurea Receptor

Mutations in the sulfonylurea receptor gene on chromosome 11 cause familial persistent hyperinsulinemic hypoglycemia of infancy.[458] Because this receptor regulates insulin secretion and its natural ligand has not been identified,[459] it warrants consideration as a candidate gene in NIDDM.

Mitochondrial Genes

Mitochondrial DNA is a circular molecule of 16,569 base pairs containing 37 genes encoding 22 transfer RNAs (tRNAs) and 13 enzymes of oxidative phosphorylation. It is maternally determined. A syndrome of maternally transmitted NIDDM and deafness is caused by substitution of guanine for adenine at position 3243 of leucyl tRNA.[460] This substitution impairs tRNA[Leu] and the binding of the transcription termination factor, thereby leading to defective synthesis of mitochondrial proteins. Two of 100 Japanese NIDDM patients with a family history of diabetes had this mutation, and 60% of patients with both NIDDM and deafness had the mutation; 3 of 55 Japanese IDDM patients had the mutation as well.[461] This mutation also is associated with the syndrome of mitochondrial myopathy, encephalopathy, lactic acidosis, and stroke-like episodes (MELAS), with or without diabetes. The same genetic defect can cause the complete MELAS syndrome in some patients and relatively mild NIDDM and an incomplete MELAS syndrome in others.[461] This variability may be caused by heteroplasmy, the unequal separation of mitochondrial populations during mitosis.[462]

Deafness may be absent or may appear before or after the onset of diabetes. The diabetes may initially respond to diet alone but ultimately requires sulfonylurea therapy or even insulin. For example, one Japanese patient became hyperglycemic at age 19 and required insulin treatment at age 27. As mentioned, this mutation may induce autoimmunity to beta cells and cause ICA-positive IDDM.[461] Awareness that on rare occasions NIDDM is maternally inherited and may be the result of a mitochondrial mutation is of importance for purposes of genetic counseling.[462]

Mutations in Genes Involved in Lipid Metabolism and Obesity

Connection of Lipid Metabolism and NIDDM

The relation between alterations of lipid metabolism, obesity, and diabetes has been recognized for decades (see review

Genetic Defects in Beta-Cells in Non–Insulin-Dependent Diabetes Mellitus

Figure 21–23. Schematic representation of a pancreatic beta cell. The numbers in parentheses indicate the approximate frequency of genetic mutation in NIDDM. (Redrawn from Kahn CR, Vicent D, Doria A. Genetics of non–insulin-dependent (type II) diabetes mellitus. Annu Rev Med 47:509–531. 1996. © 1996, by Annual Reviews Inc.)

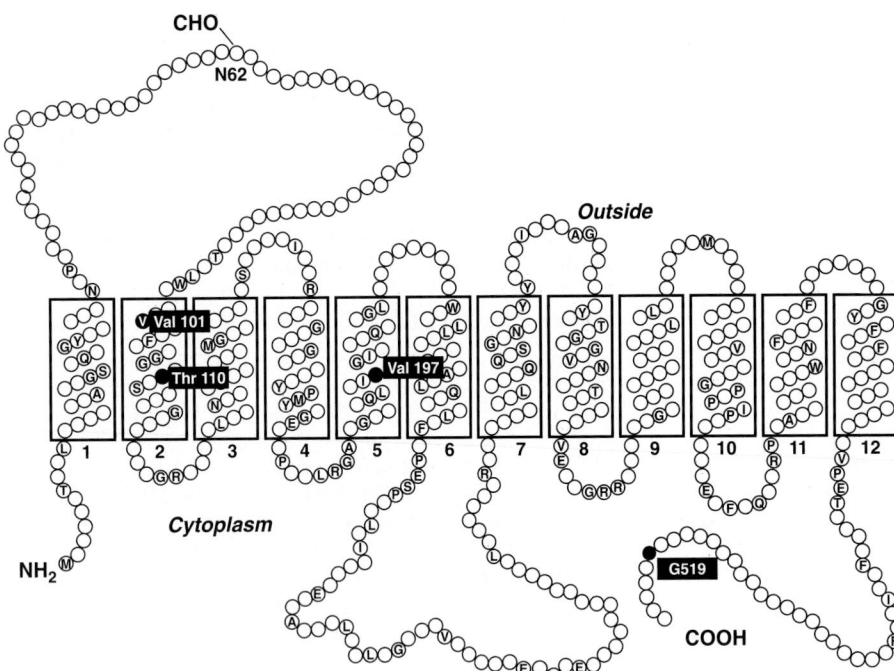

Figure 21-24. A model of the high-K$_m$ glucose transporter, GLUT2, expressed in beta cells, hepatocytes, and intestinal and renal epithelium with mutations described thus far.

by McGarry[463]). Increases in long-chain fatty acyl–CoA may interfere with glucose metabolism in peripheral tissues[464–468] and in islets,[469–472] causing insulin resistance in muscle and impairment of insulin secretory function. Because this combination of insulin resistance and failure of beta-cell compensation is characteristic of NIDDM, a number of candidate genes involved in lipid metabolism have been studied.

Lipoprotein Lipase

Lipoprotein lipase (LPL) gene mutations may cause high levels of triglycerides and reduced levels of high-density lipoproteins (HDLs), common occurrences in NIDDM. Although polymorphic enzymes were detected in 36 members of NIDDM families in Utah, they were not considered to explain the abnormalities in lipid metabolism in patients.[473]

Apolipoprotein D

An association between apolipoprotein D polymorphism and NIDDM has been reported in Nauruan and South Indian patients but not in Finns.[474]

Fatty Acid–Binding Protein

Pima Indians have a polymorphism at codon 54 of the gene that encodes the intestinal fatty acid–binding protein (FABP).[475] An Ala[54] → Thr substitution doubles the affinity of the protein for long-chain fatty acids and could increase the rate of uptake and oxidation of fatty acids, suppressing glucose utilization. Individuals who were heterozygous or homozygous for the Thr[54] allele had greater insulin resistance and hyperinsulinemia than Ala[54]-homozygotes.[475] Nevertheless, there was no linkage to NIDDM in a survey of 760 Pimas or in three European NIDDM groups with a similar frequency of the Thr[54] allele.[476] It is surprising that this form of insulin resistance does not appear to enhance susceptibility to diabetes.

Obesity-Related Gene Defects

β₃-ADRENORECEPTOR GENE

In humans the β₃-adrenoreceptor gene is expressed in visceral adipose tissue surrounding the gastrointestinal tract

and is believed to influence both resting metabolic rate and lipolysis.[477, 478] A missense mutation, Trp[64] → Arg, occurs with similar frequency in obese and nonobese French populations, but heterozygotes for the allele have a somewhat increased tendency to gain weight.[479] In Pima Indians, most of whom are obese, the frequency of the allele is 0.3, compared with 0.13 in Mexican Americans, 0.12 in African Americans, and 0.08 in Caucasians.[480] Although there is no increase in the prevalence of NIDDM, the age of onset of NIDDM may be earlier in homozygotes for the Arg[64] allele. The role of this receptor in human obesity is uncertain.[481]

LEPTIN AND LEPTIN RECEPTOR GENES

The product of the *ob* gene is a 167-amino-acid peptide called leptin that is expressed in and secreted by adipocytes.[482] Mutation or deletion of the leptin gene causes massive obesity and NIDDM in *ob/ob* mice. In *db/db* mice with obesity and diabetes the leptin gene is normal, but the leptin receptor[483] in the hypothalamus is abnormally spliced,[484, 485] so that the long intracellular domain is missing. This alteration interferes with the capacity to inhibit neuropeptide Y, a hypothalamic neuropeptide that stimulates food intake and increases thermogenesis in brown adipose tissue. The fatty Zucker rat also has a mutation of the leptin receptor.[486] These findings validate and supplement the concepts of Coleman.[487]

No leptin or leptin receptor mutations have been detected in obese humans, and it appears unlikely that such mutations can account for more than a small fraction of human obesity. Nevertheless, the hyperleptinemia of obese humans (31.3 ± 24.1 ng/mL) compared with lean controls (7.5 ± 9.3 ng/mL) suggests that insensitivity to endogenous leptin[488] is the prevailing defect in this condition.

Mutations in Genes Relevant to Insulin Action (Fig. 21–25)

Tumor Necrosis Factor α

The cytokine TNF α is synthesized by adipocytes and by macrophages[489] and may affect the response to insulin in target tissues.[490–494] In adipose tissue from obese subjects, the

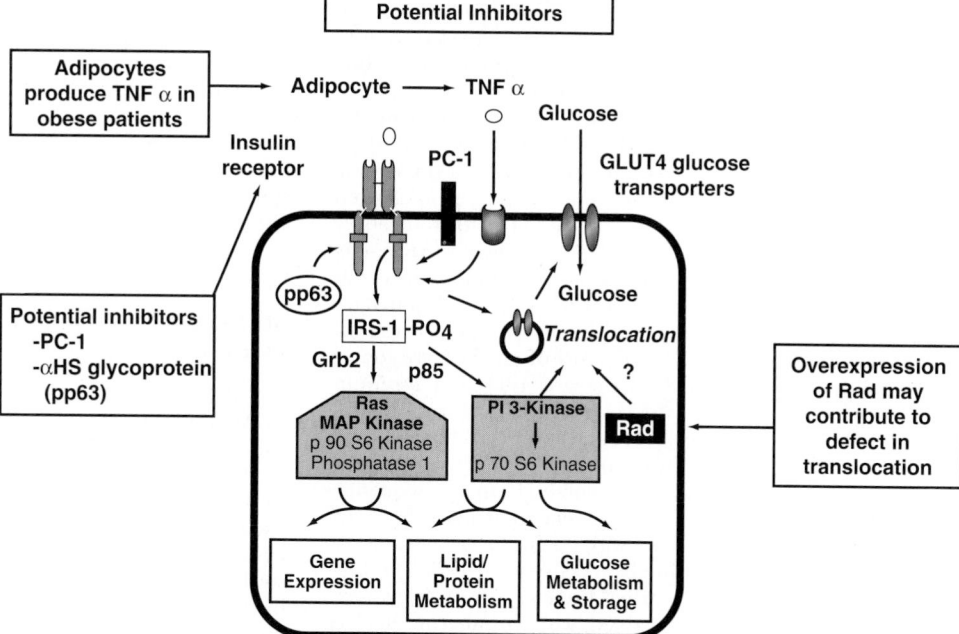

Figure 21–25. Models of insulin action and sites of insulin resistance: potential inhibitors of insulin action. (Redrawn from Kahn CR, Vicent D, Doria A. Genetics of non–insulin-dependent (Type II) diabetes mellitus. Annu Rev Med 1996, 47:509–531. © 1996, by Annual Reviews Inc.)

level of TNF α mRNA was 2.5 times higher than in lean controls and was correlated with the level of hyperinsulinemia; with weight loss TNF α mRNA expression declined.[490] However, no associations between percent body fat and polymorphisms in the promoter of the TNF α gene have been demonstrated.[495]

Other Candidate Diabetogenes: RAD, PC1, and PP63

RAD (*RAS*-related protein associated with diabetes) is a novel member of the *RAS* gene superfamily.[496] In about 20% of NIDDM patients *RAD* is overexpressed an average of 8.6-fold in muscle. *RAD* can inhibit insulin-stimulated glucose uptake in vitro,[392] but no mutations have yet been identified in the *RAD* gene.[497]

The activity of PC1, a cellular glycoprotein that inhibits insulin action at the insulin receptor kinase level, was increased in 7 of 9 patients with NIDDM.[498] No mutations have as yet been identified.

A glycoprotein called PP63 or α-HS glycoprotein inhibits insulin receptor tyrosine kinase and insulin-stimulated DNA synthesis.[499] No abnormalities in expression, secretion, or action of this protein have been reported.

Miscellaneous Mutations in Genes Without Known Diabetogenicity

Glucagon Receptor

A Gly[40] → Ser missense mutation is found in about 5% of French patients with NIDDM, compared with about 1% of controls.[500] Because this mutation reduces affinity for glucagon, it is difficult to ascribe to it any pathophysiological role in NIDDM. A Japanese population was found not to contain such a mutation.[501]

Adenine Deaminase

In one large family with MODY a polymorphism in the adenine deaminase gene (ADA) cosegregated with the disorder.[502]

Current Status of Candidate Genes

No consistent genetic abnormality has been implicated in the common form of NIDDM,[503] and it seems unlikely that a single gene is responsible.[504]

Inheritance of NIDDM

The mode of inheritance of type II NIDDM is unknown. Recessive inheritance with low penetrance is unlikely,[505, 506] and inheritance is probably multifactorial.[506]

One form of NIDDM, MODY, is inherited as an autosomal dominant defect.[507, 508] The manifestations are usually mild, and many affected persons are asymptomatic.[508] Most are not obese. Late degenerative complications may be less common than in other forms of diabetes.[509] There are no associations with HLA[510] or with polymorphic DNA sequences linked to the insulin gene.[511] MODY may be heterogeneous, because the insulin response to glucose is low in some patients and high in others.[509] Moreover, a noted MODY was associated in one family with a polymorphism in *ADA*[512] rather than in the glucokinase gene with which it is most commonly associated.[445–448]

Is There an Autoimmune Type II NIDDM?

Some lean NIDDM patients appear to resemble patients with type I IDDM (see Table 21–10).[152, 185, 211, 212] This subset of patients tends to be hypoinsulinemic rather than hyperinsulinemic and probably represents a slowly developing form of autoimmune diabetes.

PATHOLOGY OF THE ISLETS OF LANGERHANS IN NIDDM

Endocrine Cell Composition

The islet cell mass is normal in patients with new-onset NIDDM (see Table 21–12),[329] although late in the disease beta cells may be reduced in association with amyloid deposition in islets.[513] The proportion of alpha cells is increased slightly, and the beta-cell mass is normal in size,[332] so the ratio of alpha to beta cells in type II patients is twice normal.

BETA-CELL GLUT2. Beta-cell GLUT2 is reduced in the spontaneously occurring NIDDM of the ZDF rat,[514] the GK rat,[515] and the *db/db* mouse[516] and in the NIDDM of the neonatal streptozotocin-treated rat[517] and the glucocorticoid-treated rat.[518] The percentage of GLUT2-positive beta cells is inversely correlated with the level of hyperglycemia and directly correlated with GSIS.[514] However, because normal human beta cells have not been shown to display GLUT2,[519] the GLUT2 changes of rodent NIDDM do not appear to occur in human NIDDM.

AMYLOID AND AMYLIN. Deposits of amyloid are found frequently in type II diabetic pancreatic islets but rarely in islets of controls.[520] The amyloid is composed of a 37-amino-acid peptide, known variously as diabetes-associated peptide, islet-amyloid polypeptide (IAPP), or amylin. Amylin, which is derived from an 89-amino-acid precursor,[521] shares sequence homology with the calcitonin gene–related peptide.[513, 522] In normal islets amylin is packaged with insulin in beta-cell granules, but it is deposited outside beta cells in NIDDM. The fact that amylin is expressed in normal human and rat islets (see Fig. 21–12)[521, 522] and is cosecreted with insulin in the rat pancreas suggests that it may have a hormonal role. Impairment of amylin secretion accompanies beta-cell damage or depletion, but the effects of amylin on insulin action and insulin secretion remain controversial. Amylin secretion is enhanced in obesity and in NIDDM.[523] Overexpression of a transgene encoding amylin in mice does not cause hyperglycemia, hyperinsulinemia, or obesity, arguing against an inhibitory role in insulin secretion or action.[524] However, amyloid fibrils form in cultured islets of transgenic mice that express human but not rat amylin.[524] Human amylin fibers induce apoptosis in vitro in adult rat and human beta cells on direct contact with the cell surface,[525] raising the possibility that chronic beta-cell hypersecretion in compensation for insulin resistance may ultimately lead to self-destruction of the beta cell.

Normal Islet Cell Function

Molecular Basis of Insulin Action

Insulin inhibits lipolysis, stimulates lipogenesis, stimulates DNA and protein biosynthesis, inhibits protein breakdown, activates transport of glucose, amino acids, and ions, and promotes glycogen synthesis and glycolysis. Insulin inhibits catabolism by suppressing secretion of glucagon, the primary catabolic hormone, and by blocking the hepatic effects of glucagon through enhancement of hepatic phosphodiesterase activity, which inhibits cyclic AMP–dependent protein kinase (see later discussion) and thereby inhibits glycogenolysis and gluconeogenesis. The anabolic/catabolic state of the organism therefore can be smoothly regulated by the relative concentration of these two antagonistic hormones.

MOLECULAR EVENTS IN INSULIN ACTION: LEVEL 1 EVENTS (see Fig. 21–11*J*)

INSULIN–INSULIN RECEPTOR INTERACTIONS AND TYROSINE KINASE. Insulin action begins when it binds to the α subunit of the insulin receptor (see Fig. 21–22). The β subunit of the insulin receptor is a tyrosine kinase that is activated by insulin binding and that phosphorylates the insulin receptor itself and other substrates, thereby initiating the signaling cascade.[526, 527] The α subunit is a regulatory subunit that restrains the activity of the tyrosine kinase moiety: if a portion of the α subunit is removed by tryptic digestion or by in vitro mutagenesis, its inhibitory effect on the β subunit disappears, and tyrosine kinase is permanently activated.[528] Binding of insulin to the α subunit achieves the same effect. Cysteine[647] appears to transmit the signal from the insulin-bound α subunit to the β subunit; insulin receptors that lack the Cys[647] site cannot be activated by insulin.[529] Insulin-stimulated autophosphorylation is largely asymmetrical, with one β subunit phosphorylating its neighboring β subunit within the same heterodimer.[530]

DOWNSTREAM PROPAGATION OF SIGNALS: INSULIN RECEPTOR SUBSTRATE-1. Within seconds after insulin binds to its receptor, a high-molecular-weight tyrosylphosphorylated protein known as IRS-1 becomes detectable. IRS-1 exhibits high sequence conservation among species, including 20 to 22 potential tyrosine phosphorylation sites. IRS-1 is also a substrate for the IGF-1 receptor.[531]

IRS-1 stimulates phosphatidylinositol 3-kinase (PI 3-kinase), the enzyme that catalyzes the phosphorylation of PI, PI-4-P, and PI-4,5-P2 and ultimately enhances protein synthesis and glucose transport (Fig. 21–26). Phosphorylated IRS-1 acts as a docking protein that binds to and stimulates the p21^{ras} signaling pathway[532] through its association with GRB2, which

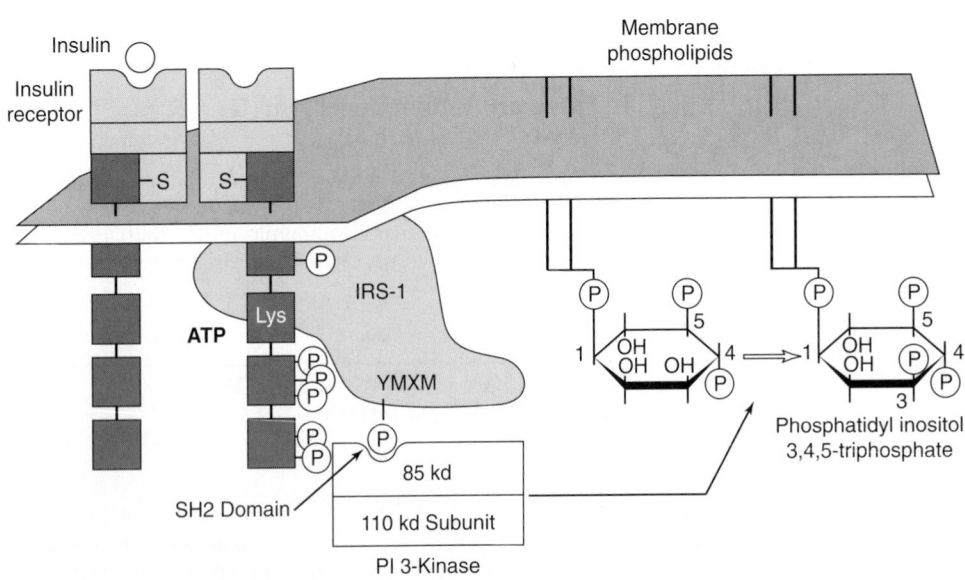

Figure 21–26. Insulin and phosphatidylinositol 3-kinase (PI 3-kinase). Phosphorylated insulin receptor substrate-1 (IRS-1) interacts with the SH2 domain of PI 3-kinase, which has the capacity to phosphorylate several phosphatidylinositol derivatives. Shown here is the phosphorylation of phosphatidylinositol-4,5-diphosphate to phosphatidylinositol-3,4,5-triphosphate. YMXM, the phosphorylation site (Y, tyrosine; M, methionine; X, any amino acid).

interacts with the mammalian homologue to the *Drosophila* protein, son-of-sevenless (SOS) in the *RAS* complex (see Fig. 21–22).

Molecular Events in Insulin Action: Level 2 Events

The *RAS* complex plays a role in cell growth and metabolism and modulates glycogen synthesis in a pathway that activates raf-1 kinase, which in turn phosphorylates and activates mitogen-activated protein kinase–kinase (MAPKK). MAPKK then phosphorylates and activates MAPK, which phosphorylates and activates pp90S6 kinase, which activates the glycogen-associated protein phosphatase-1, which in turn activates glycogen synthase and inactivates phosphorylase kinase and glycogen phosphorylase. An alternative p21^ras activation is depicted in Figure 21–22. (For a more complete review see Cheatum and Kahn[533]).

Molecular Basis of Glucagon Action

Glucagon Receptor

The glucagon receptor appears to transduce signals that lead to the accumulation of cyclic AMP and calcium, probably through the same stimulatory guanine nucleotide–binding regulatory protein, $G\alpha_s$.[534, 535]

The effects of glucagon on hepatic glucose metabolism, mediated by its second messengers, cyclic AMP and Ca^{2+}, are to activate the cyclic AMP–dependent protein kinase A and the Ca^{2+}-dependent protein kinase C, respectively. These in turn affect a broad spectrum of enzymatic processes, including glycogenolysis, gluconeogenesis, ketogenesis, and ureagenesis. In addition, transcriptional control of the formation of certain enzymes, perhaps through cyclic AMP–dependent response elements, also plays a role in glucagon action.

Adenylyl Cyclase Activation

The action of glucagon is mediated in large part by activation of adenylyl cyclase. When the hormone binds to the glucagon receptor on the cell surface, the receptor interacts within the membrane with G_s to release the α subunit of G_s, thereby disaggregating and activating the enzyme.[536–538] The inhibitory G protein, G_i, inhibits adenylyl cyclase.[539] Adenylyl cyclase catalyzes the conversion of ATP to cyclic AMP, causing the intracellular cyclic AMP to rise within a few seconds of glucagon binding. Phosphodiesterase lowers the level of cyclic AMP by degrading it to AMP.

Cyclic AMP binds to and activates cyclic AMP–dependent protein kinase A in a dose-dependent manner by dissociating its regulatory subunits, thereby freeing its catalytic subunits.[540] Insulin opposes this dissociation and thereby reduces the activity of cyclic AMP.[540, 541]

Inositol Phospholipid Breakdown

Glucagon and/or its 19-29 fragment[535] also acts through a cyclic AMP–independent pathway to elevate cytosolic Ca^{2+} by enhancing the breakdown of inositol phospholipid.[542] The rapid breakdown of phosphatidylinositol 4,5-bisphosphate (PIP_2) causes release of 1,4,5-triphosphate (IP_3) and 1,2-diacylglycerol (DAG). IP_3 induces release of Ca^{2+} from endoplasmic reticulum. Blockade of calcium influx from outside the cells inhibits glycogenolysis and gluconeogenesis in rat hepatocytes.[543] Whatever its source, an increase in cytosolic Ca^{2+} together with DAG activates protein kinase C, and the actions of glucagon are thought to depend on the phosphorylation cascades initiated by protein kinase C.[544, 545]

Effects of Phosphorylation on Glycogenolysis and Glycogenesis

Protein kinase A and protein kinase C increase glycogenolysis by phosphorylating phosphorylase *b* kinase, which converts inactive phosphorylase *b* to active phosphorylase *a*, the rate-limiting enzyme for glycogenolysis in the liver. The simultaneous phosphorylation of glycogen synthase *a* converts it to the active *b* form, thereby preventing glycogen formation (Fig. 21–27).

How Glucagon Causes Hyperglycemia and Ketogenesis when Insulin Action is Absent or Impaired

GLUCONEOGENESIS AND GLYCOLYSIS. Glucagon enhances hepatic gluconeogenesis and inhibits glycolysis by cyclic AMP–mediated increase in protein kinase A activity (see Fig. 21–27, *top*). The key step in glycolysis is the conversion of fructose 6-phosphate to fructose 1,6-bisphosphate by 6-phosphofructo-1-kinase; the equivalent regulatory step in gluconeogenesis is the conversion of fructose 1,6-bisphosphate to fructose 6-phosphate by fructose-1,6-bisphosphatase. The activity of 6-phosphofructo-1-kinase is allosterically increased by fructose 2,6-bisphosphate, and the activity of fructose-1,6-bisphosphatase is reciprocally inhibited.[546–549] Thus, fructose 2,6-bisphosphate promotes glycolysis and inhibits gluconeogenesis by controlling the key steps in the two opposing pathways. Fructose 2,6-bisphosphate is formed from fructose 6-phosphate by 6-phosphofructo-2-kinase/fructose-2,6-bisphosphatase. This unusual enzyme is bifunctional, the activity being determined by the phosphorylation state.[548, 550] The dephosphorylated form is a kinase, and the phosphorylated form is a phosphatase. Glucagon therefore works by the sequence: ↑ cyclic AMP → ↑ cyclic AMP–dependent protein kinase → ↑ phosphorylation of 6-phosphofructo-2-kinase/fructose-2,6-bisphosphatase → ↓ fructose 2,6-bisphosphate → ↓ glycolysis and ↑ gluconeogenesis (Fig. 21–28A). Insulin presumably reverses the sequence by reducing the level of cyclic AMP and deactivating cyclic AMP–dependent kinase, thereby increasing the level of fructose 2,6-bisphosphate (see Fig. 21–28B). The effects of glucagon occur within minutes in vitro,[551] but the reversal of action is slower. This is important because glycogen resynthesis after a fast occurs primarily from gluconeogenesis, newly synthesized glucose 6-phosphate being diverted into glycogen and away from release as glucose into the blood by inhibition of glucose-6-phosphatase.[552] The slower reversal of glucagon-induced changes in fructose 2,6-bisphosphate allows continued gluconeogenesis after refeeding. Although phosphorylation-dephosphorylation is the primary short-term control mechanism, insulin and glucagon exert long-term control by controlling the synthesis of various enzymes.[553]

KETOGENESIS AND LIPOGENESIS. Glucagon induces ketogenesis and blocks hepatic lipogenesis (see Figs. 21–27 and 21–28),[554] events orchestrated by a fall in intrahepatic levels of the first product in the pathway of fatty acid synthesis, malonyl-CoA.[555] This decrease results from a block in substrate flow from glucose to acetyl-CoA caused by the inhibition of glycolysis just described and by inhibition of acetyl-CoA carboxylase[556] through a phosphorylation mechanism.[557] Malonyl-CoA inhibits carnitine palmitoyltransferase (CPT-I),[558] which transesterifies fatty acyl–CoA to fatty acyl carnitine, enabling it to traverse the mitochondrial membrane and undergo beta oxidation to ketones (Fig. 21–29).[558] By reducing malonyl-CoA levels, glucagon disinhibits the enzyme, thereby accelerating the synthesis of acetoacetate and β-hydroxybutyrate when fatty acid and fatty acyl–CoA levels increase in the liver secondary to increased lipolysis resulting from the insulin deficiency.[559] Glucagon also increases hepatic carnitine levels by an unknown

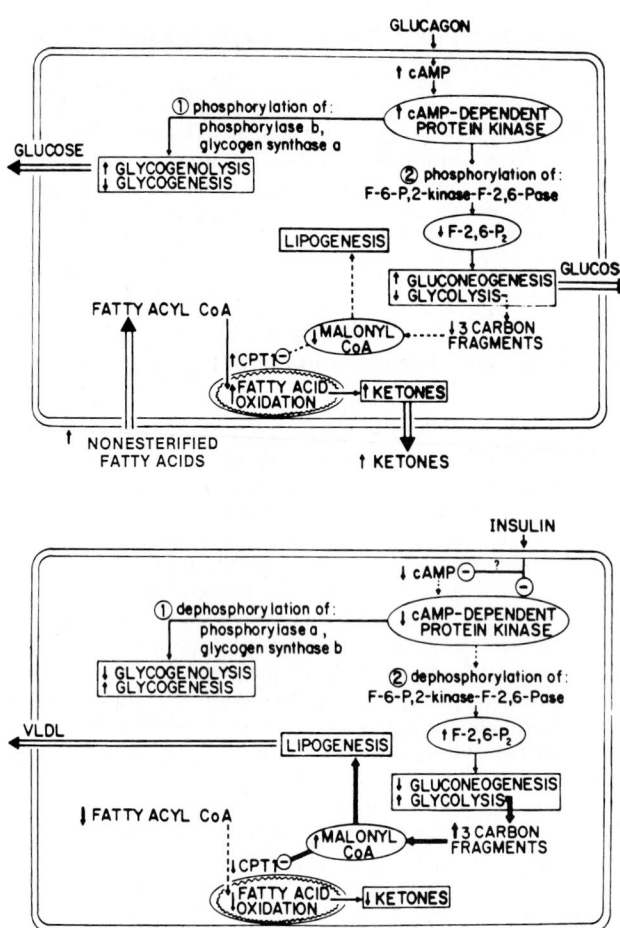

Figure 21–27. *Top,* Glucagon-induced catabolic cascade in hepatocytes. Binding of glucagon to the regulatory subunit of its receptor activates adenylate cyclase to increase cyclic AMP levels. This activates cyclic AMP–dependent protein kinase, which initiates all the known actions of glucagon by phosphorylating certain key enzymes, thereby redirecting their activities toward catabolism. Phosphorylation of inactive phosphorylase *b* ① converts it to the active *a* form, thereby promoting glycogenolysis and enhanced glucose production. Phosphorylation of glycogen synthase *a* inactivates it to the *b* form and reduces glycogen formation. Phosphorylation of the bifunctional enzyme ② that regulates fructose 2,6-bisphosphate (F-2,6-P$_2$) synthesis and degradation, 6-phosphofructo-2-kinase/fructose-2,6-bisphosphatase (F-6,P,2-kinase-F-2,6-Pase), lowers its kinase activity and increases its phosphatase action. This depletes F-2,6-P$_2$, a stimulator of glycolysis and an inhibitor of gluconeogenesis. The result of F-2,6-P$_2$ depletion is enhanced glucose production from nonglucose precursors and diminished formation of pyruvate, the substrate for lipogenesis. Consequently, levels of malonyl-CoA, the product of the first committed step in lipogenesis, are reduced. This abolishes the inhibitory action of malonyl-CoA on carnitine palmitoyltransferase I (CPT I), the enzyme responsible for transesterification of fatty acyl–CoA to fatty acyl carnitine, allowing fatty acids to enter into the mitochondria, the site of beta oxidation to ketones. The level of fatty acyl–CoA derived from free fatty acids delivered to the liver from adipocytes is increased as the consequence of deficiency of insulin, an antilipolytic hormone. Therefore, the high glucagon–low insulin mixture induces the full catabolic syndrome of increased glucose production and accelerated ketogenesis. *Bottom,* Insulin-induced anabolic cascade. Insulin, when present in sufficient concentration, lowers glucagon release and reverses the glucagon-mediated catabolic cascade. The cyclic AMP concentration is lowered, probably by an insulin-mediated increase in phosphodiesterase activity. The major effect of insulin may be to inactivate the cyclic AMP–dependent protein kinase. Dephosphorylation of enzymes at ① and ② promotes glycogen formation and increases F-2,6-P$_2$ levels, thereby stimulating glycolysis and inhibiting gluconeogenesis. Pyruvate becomes available for lipogenesis, increasing malonyl-CoA levels and inhibiting CPT I. Ketone formation slows and fatty acid synthesis increases. Fatty acids are esterified to triglycerides, which are then packaged and released as VLDL. Plasma free fatty acid levels are much lower but continue to contribute to triglyceride and VLDL formation.

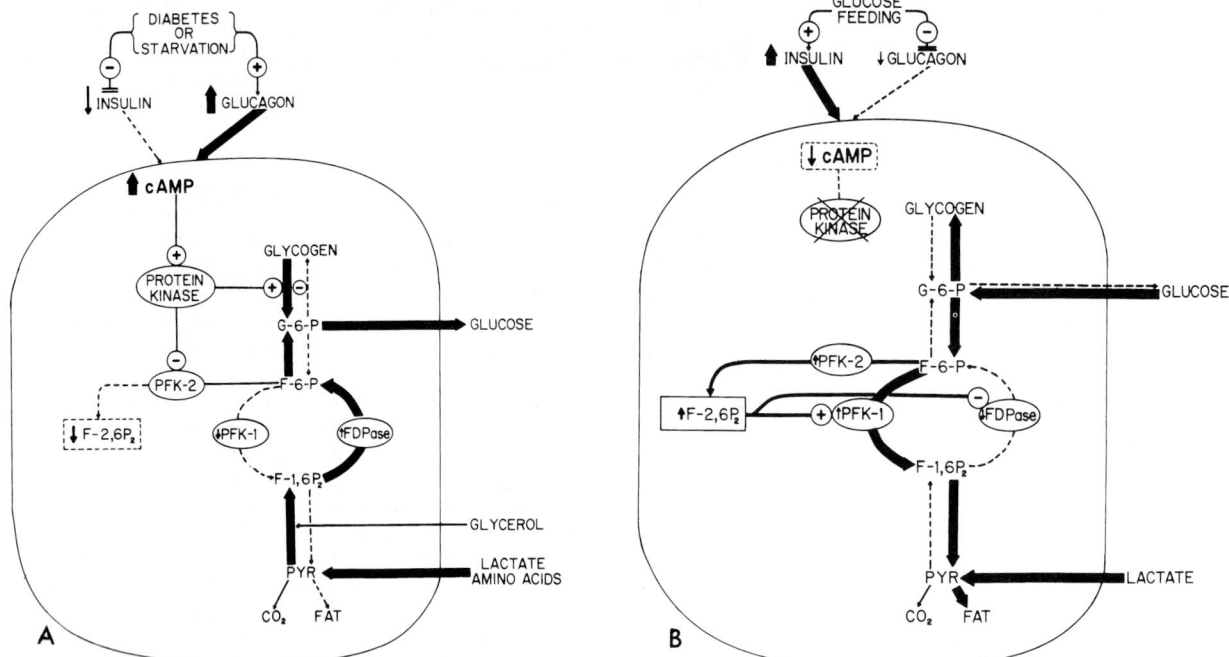

Figure 21–28. *A,* Enhancement of gluconeogenesis and glycogenolysis by glucagon in diabetes and starvation. Both processes are activated by an increase in cyclic AMP concentration in the hepatocyte. Phosphofructokinase 1 (PFK-1) catalyzes the formation of fructose 1,6-bisphosphate (F-1,6P$_2$) in the glycolytic pathway, and PFK-2 synthesizes fructose 2,6-bisphosphate (F-2,6P$_2$), a regulator of PFK-1 activity. PFK-2 and fructose-2,6-bisphosphatase activities are contained in the same protein. Cyclic AMP–induced phosphorylation of the enzyme decreases the former and increases the latter. Decreased levels of F-2,6P$_2$ result in decreased glycolysis and increased gluconeogenesis. *B,* Inhibition of gluconeogenesis and activation of glycogen synthesis, glycolysis, and lipogenesis by insulin. Insulin decreases the level of cyclic AMP, deactivates protein kinase, and reverses changes in F-2,6P$_2$ and substrate flux over the glycolytic-gluconeogenic pathway produced by glucagon. Glycogen synthesis and lipogenesis are also increased.

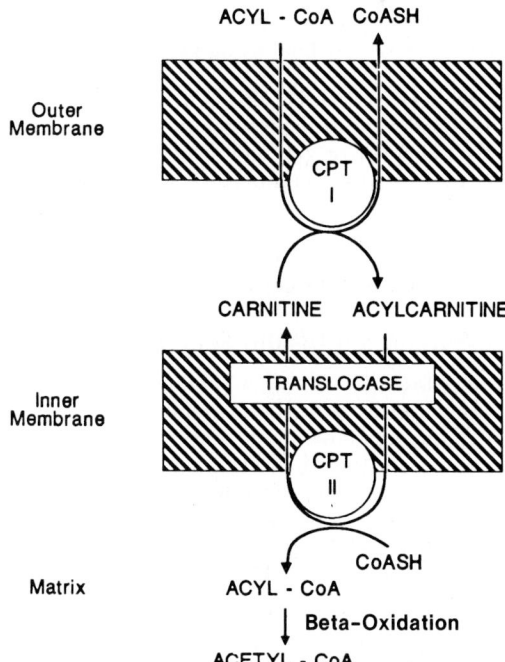

Figure 21–29. Fatty acid oxidation system in liver. The inner mitochondrial membrane is impermeable to long-chain fatty acyl–CoA but permeable to fatty acyl carnitine. Formation of the carnitine ester is catalyzed by CPT I, the rate-limiting step in the sequence. This enzyme is inhibited by malonyl-CoA. The transesterification reaction is reversed inside mitochondria by CPT II. Most of the fatty acid molecules entering the mitochondria are converted to ketones, only a small amount of the acetyl-CoA generated being oxidized in the tricarboxylic acid cycle.

mechanism.[560] The combination of increased fatty acyl–CoA and carnitine levels and activated CPT-I ensures brisk rates of ketogenesis.

INTERACTIONS OF ISLET CELL HORMONES

Normally, glucagon secretion is suppressed by relatively small increases in insulin levels,[561] and insulin secretion is stimulated by small increases in the concentration of glucagon.[343] Minute increments of somatostatin suppress release of both insulin and glucagon in vitro[562] and in vivo,[563] whereas a modest increase of glucagon is required to stimulate somatostatin.[562] These facts and the nonrandom arrangement of the three major types of cells[564] within the normal islets have led to the concept of a paracrine system by which the three peptides influence neighboring cells through the intervening interstitium[565] and through intercellular channels called gap junctions that connect the cytosol of contiguous cells to one another to form syncytial domains[566, 567] (Figs. 21–30 and 21–31). However, the major route of within-islet communication between cells is probably not the interstitium or gap junctions but the local circulation, which (in the rat at least) flows from the beta-cell–rich medulla of the islet to the alpha-cell–rich cortex (Fig. 21–32).[568] This arrangement exposes alpha cells (and delta cells) to the highest circulating insulin concentrations in the body and facilitates the action of insulin as an inhibitor of glucagon release (see Fig. 21–15).[344, 569] The beta cell, on the other hand, receives systemic blood and is therefore exposed to lower concentrations of glucagon than would be the case if there were direct flow from alpha cell to beta cell.

ISLET CELL HORMONE RESPONSES IN FUEL REGULATION

GLUCOSE NEED. The responses of alpha and beta cells to various stimuli are influenced by plasma glucose levels.

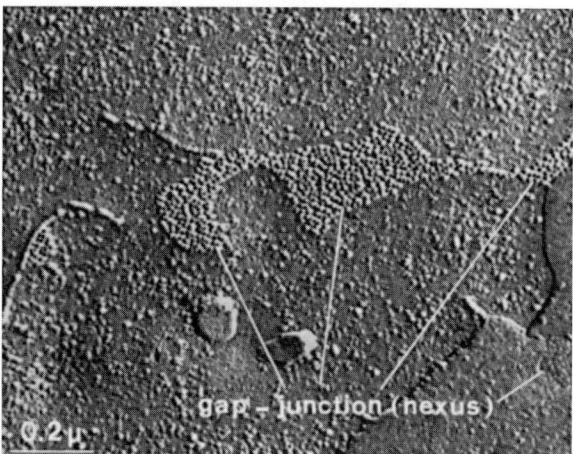

Figure 21–30. A freeze-fracture electron photomicrograph showing a gap junction, an aggregation of intramembranous particles or connexons (see also Fig. 21–31). (Courtesy of L. Orci.)

Coordinated secretion of insulin and glucagon vigorously defends against glycemic fluctuations below or above the normal range (for a review, see Unger[570]). Maintenance of glucose constancy is a vital function of the islets, with defense against hypoglycemia its most critical mission, because the energy needs of the brain can be met only by glucose. A fall in glucose concentration toward the lower level of normal causes a prompt fall in insulin level and a rise in glucagon secretion (Fig. 21–33). An increase in glucose utilization from the resting state (see Fig. 21–13a), as in exercise, results in the following: (1) glucagon (and catecholamine) levels increase and enhance hepatic glucose production, primarily through glycogen breakdown; (2) insulin secretion decreases concomitantly, contributing to the rise in glucagon concentration; and (3) decreased insulin concentration reduces peripheral glucose utilization, potentiates the hepatic action of glucagon, and enhances release of FFAs from adipocytes.[571] Hypoglycemia is thereby prevented, and glucose delivery is maintained to the brain and to exercising muscles. A similar decrease in insulin and rise in glucagon occurs during starvation (see Fig. 21–13a),[572] with a resulting increase in glycogenolysis and gluconeogenesis; again the fall in insulin reduces nonessential glucose utilization and enhances FFA release from adipocytes, thereby providing an alternative source of fuel. Conversion of FFAs to the ketone bodies (acetoacetate and β-hydroxybutyrate) provides a back-up substrate that can substitute for glucose in the brain.[373] In prolonged starvation the shift of the body to a lipid-based energy supply (FFAs and ketones) mini-

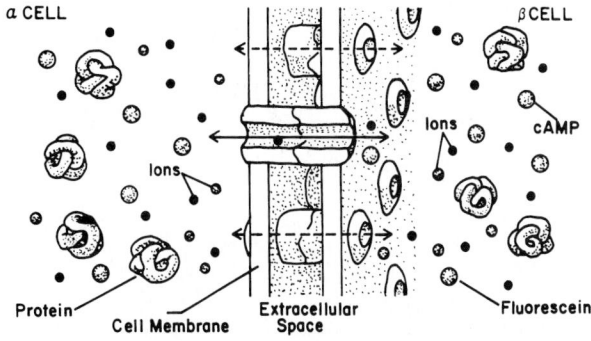

Figure 21–31. Schematic representation of gap junctions. Conduits through which small molecules such as ions, nucleotides, or fluorescein pass from the cytosol of one cell to that of a contiguous cell without entering the intercellular space are called connexons. The gap junction is an aggregation of connexons in a differentiated portion of the cell membranes. (Courtesy of L. Orci.)

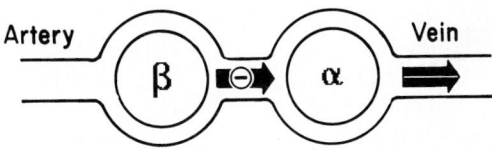

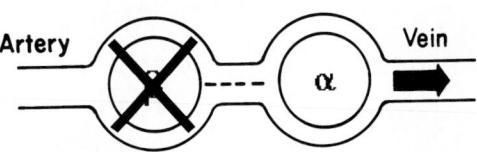

Figure 21–32. Schematic representation of blood flow from beta cell to alpha cell. Locally secreted insulin restrains glucagon release, as indicated by the minus sign *(top)*. The effluent therefore contains an appropriate mixture of insulin and glucagon. Glucagon is presumed to reach the beta cell only through the systemic (not local) circulation. In IDDM, absent beta cells *(bottom)* remove this restraint, accounting for hyperglucagonemia. The effluent consists, therefore, almost entirely of glucagon.

mizes protein wastage by reducing the need for protein-derived gluconeogenesis.[573]

To summarize, in circumstances of glucose need, the fall in insulin and rise in glucagon levels increase glycogen breakdown, enhance gluconeogenesis, and induce a shift to the use of fat for energy by providing increased levels of FFAs and ketone bodies.

GLUCOSE ABUNDANCE. Infusion of glucose (see Fig. 21–33) or ingestion of carbohydrate (see Fig. 21–19) elicits a rise in insulin level and a decrease in glucagon concentration (see Fig. 21–13e).[341] Because the increase in insulin level during a meal occurs before the rise in arterial glucose levels,[574] the enhancement of insulin secretion is thought to be mediated by hormonal[575] and parasympathetic[576] signals arising in the gastrointestinal tract, the so-called enteroinsular axis.[577] A key signal in the axis may be glucagon-like peptide I (GLP-I).[578] Elimination of the action of GLP-I impairs the handling of a glucose meal because of decreased early insulin response

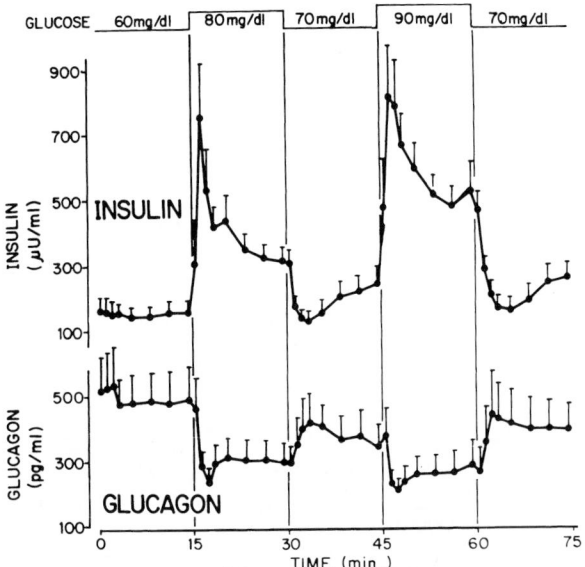

Figure 21–33. Response of insulin and glucagon to modest changes in glucose concentration in the isolated perfused dog pancreas. Note the reciprocal changes in glucagon and insulin release. (Unpublished work of K. Kawai and R. H. Unger.)

and higher blood glucose levels. The early anticipatory insulin release allows increased glucose disposal during absorption and prevents hyperglycemia. When a carbohydrate-free protein meal is ingested (see Fig. 21–14), insulin concentrations rise slightly to promote incorporation of amino acids into protein; a parallel rise in glucagon concentration[341] caused by protein-induced insulin secretion prevents hypoglycemia.[579]

ISLET CELL FUNCTION IN NIDDM

Glucose-Stimulated Insulin Secretion

Selective loss of GSIS when fasting hyperglycemia first appears characterizes both NIDDM and IDDM. The inability to return elevated glucose levels to normal after an overnight fast, the abnormality on which the diagnosis of overt diabetes is based, is invariably accompanied by impaired or absent GSIS, even though nonglucose secretagogues may still elicit an insulin response.[580–582] A more subtle abnormality in patients with NIDDM is lack of the normal secretion of insulin in 12- to 15-min bursts.[583, 584]

Normal Pathways for Glucose "Signaling" and Glucose "Fueling"

Like all cells, beta cells have intrinsic fuel requirements. Because low-K_m glucose metabolism and the low-K_m enzyme hexokinase I are present in islets, basal glucose needs for fuel may be satisfied through metabolic pathways that are separate from the specialized glucose-signaling pathway for response of beta cells to the rise in plasma glucose after a carbohydrate-containing meal. The postprandial signaling function correlates with expression in beta cells of the high-K_m facilitative glucose transporter, GLUT2.[582] GLUT2 is expressed only in beta cells, hepatocytes, and intestinal and renal epithelium.[435] High-K_m GLUT2 is coexpressed in beta cells and hepatocytes with the high-K_m enzyme glucokinase, both of which appear to be necessary for the beta cells to "sense" a rising blood glucose level.[585] It therefore appears that this specialized signaling pathway for glucose is functionally, if not anatomically, separate from the low-K_m pathway of glucose metabolism of beta cells.

Although the glucose-signaling apparatus may begin with and require both the high-K_m glucose transporter and the high-K_m kinase,[585] the influx of Ca^{2+} through voltage-dependent calcium channels triggers insulin secretion.[453, 454] Ca^{2+} influx results from depolarization of the beta-cell membrane as a consequence of closure of ATP-sensitive K^+ channels caused by the enhanced glucose metabolism, as described previously. The pathway for high-K_m glucose metabolism is depicted in Figure 21–34.

Glucose Signaling Pathway in NIDDM

GLUT2 AND GLUCOKINASE. Beta-cell GLUT2 is reduced in rodent models of NIDDM[439, 582]; glucose transport is not rate-limiting in normal islets,[436] but full activity of glucokinase, the rate-limiting enzyme in the pathway, may require the presence of GLUT2.[585] Reduction of GLUT2 by infection with a transgene that expresses GLUT2 antisense mRNA impairs GSIS and causes diabetes.[440] In rodent forms of NIDDM glucokinase activity is not reduced, but GSIS is impaired. A 70% reduction in glucokinase protein and activity in mice reduces GSIS but does not cause hyperglycemia.[586] Taken together, these findings suggest that the GLUT2/glucokinase couple is the primary transducer for GSIS in rodents.

GLYCEROL-3-PHOSPHATE SHUTTLE. A third possible

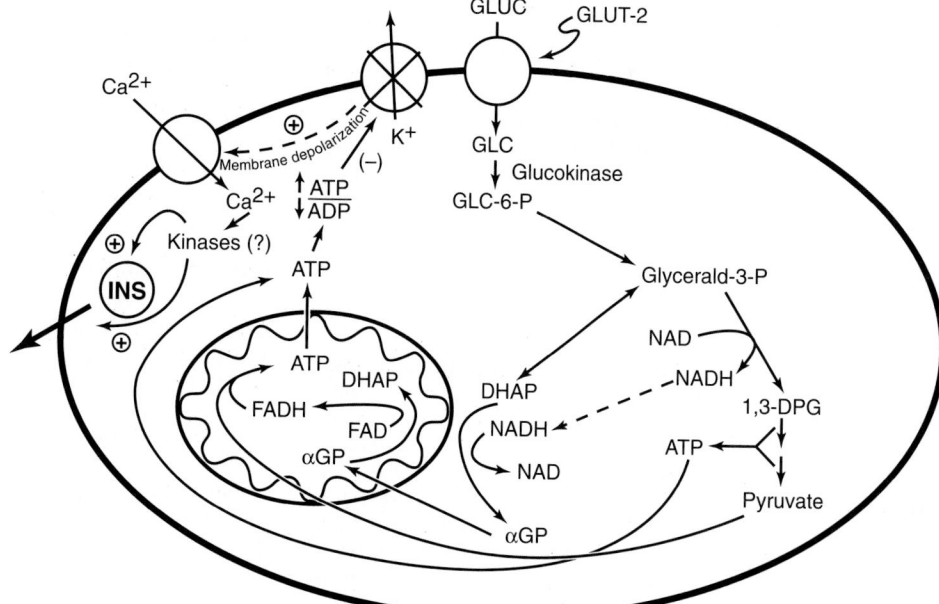

Figure 21–34. Schematic summary of signals for insulin release generated by glucose metabolism. (Redrawn from Newgard CB, McGarry JD. Metabolic coupling factors in pancreatic beta-cell signal transduction. Annu Rev Biochem 1995; 64:689–717. Courtesy of Dr. Christopher Newgard.)

site of disrupted glucose signaling is the FAD^+-linked glycerol-3-phosphate shuttle, which may generate the ATP that closes the ATP-sensitive K^+ channels in beta cells.[587–589] With the onset of diabetes in Zucker rats GSIS declines by 90%, and monomethyl succinate–induced secretion falls by 44%, suggesting that the defect in GSIS is caused by both glycolytic and postglycolytic mitochondrial abnormalities.[590]

GLUCOSE-6-PHOSPHATASE. Finally, enhanced glucose-6-phosphatase activity in beta cells could cause a futile cycle in which phosphorylated glucose leaves the islet in the form of glucose, escaping metabolism and thereby impairing GSIS. Islets from ob/ob mice reportedly have 19 times more glucose-6-phosphatase activity than their lean littermates.[591]

GLUCOSE-STIMULATED INSULIN SECRETION AND LIPIDS. GSIS may be mediated by acyl-CoA esters such as diacylglycerol.[592–595] Acetyl-CoA derived from glucose or lipid metabolism enters the lipogenic pathway to form malonyl-CoA, an

inhibitor of CPT-I,[559] thereby blocking fatty acid oxidation. The long-chain fatty acyl–CoA thus rescued from oxidation can be esterified to form diacylglycerol, which stimulates protein kinase C activity (Fig. 21–35).

INSULIN RESISTANCE

Genetics and Environment

The sensitivity of target tissues to the glucoregulatory action of insulin is thought to be genetically determined, and future risk for development of NIDDM is inversely related to the level of insulin sensitivity.[596–598] An acquired pathogenic factor is obesity, particularly abdominal obesity.[599–601] The effect of obesity on insulin resistance is greater in members of

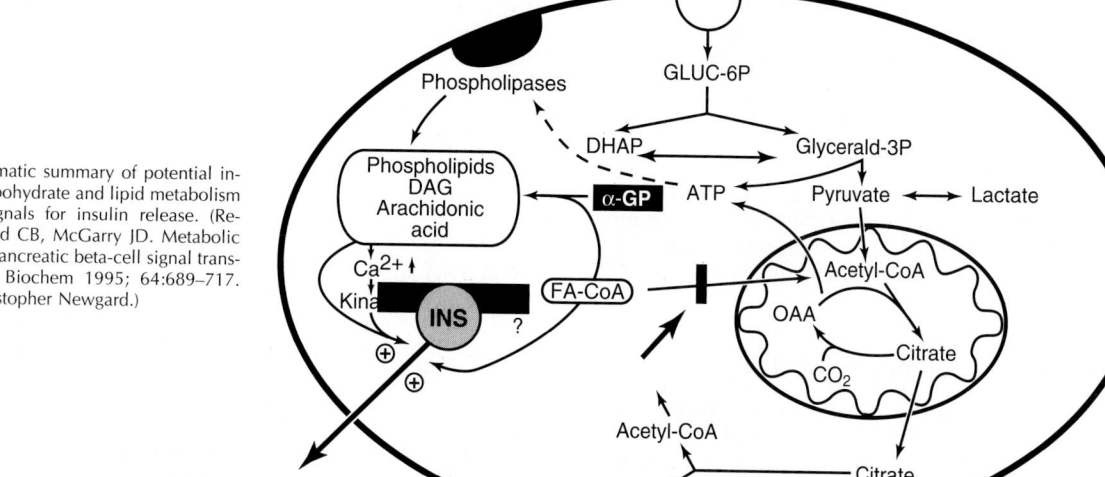

Figure 21–35. Schematic summary of potential interplay between carbohydrate and lipid metabolism in generation of signals for insulin release. (Redrawn from Newgard CB, McGarry JD. Metabolic coupling factors in pancreatic beta-cell signal transduction. Annu Rev Biochem 1995; 64:689–717. Courtesy of Dr. Christopher Newgard.)

diabetic families than in persons with no family history of diabetes.[596]

Relatives of patients with NIDDM may be insulin resistant even if they are young, nonobese, and tolerant to glucose.[596, 597] About 50% of first-degree relatives of NIDDM patients are insulin resistant three to four decades before they develop NIDDM.[598] The evidence that insulin resistance is an inherited defect predicting the development of overt NIDDM now seems compelling,[598] but it is not sufficient to cause the disease.[602, 603]

Contribution of Hepatic Insulin Resistance

In NIDDM patients with moderate fasting hyperglycemia, the liver production of glucose is increased by about 0.5 mg/kg/min, or about 50 g/d above normal.[603] This modest increase is the consequence of reduced suppression of hepatic glucose production by insulin[604] and could be nullified by reducing dietary carbohydrate by 50 g/d. The increased hepatic glucose production in NIDDM is probably caused by lack of an insulin-mediated reduction in glucagon secretion[341] rather than hepatic resistance to insulin action. The importance of increased hepatic gluconeogenesis is underlined by the fact that when phosphoenolpyruvate carboxykinase (PEPCK), a regulatory enzyme of gluconeogenesis, is overexpressed in mice carrying a transgene expressing the protein hyperglycemia results.[605] However, it is unlikely that increased hepatic glucose production plays a primary role in the pathogenesis of human NIDDM.

Contribution of Insulin Resistance in Skeletal Muscle

In normal persons 75% of the glucose in a carbohydrate meal is taken up by muscle, and it is mainly stored as glycogen. In insulin-resistant patients given supraphysiologic insulin infusions, glycogen synthesis in skeletal muscle is reduced more than oxidative metabolism. When physiologic insulin levels are maintained, both muscle glycogen storage and glucose oxidation are impaired.[606] The fact that knockout of *GLUT4* gene expression does not cause hyperglycemia in mice[420] indicates that total loss of insulin-stimulated glucose transport is not sufficient to cause NIDDM. Insulin directs the translocation of GLUT4 to the plasma membrane. Microinjection of H-ras into cardiac myocytes mimics this action of insulin.[607]

Linkage analysis of 19 candidate loci with potential for causing insulin resistance has excluded GLUT4, hexokinase II, glucagon, growth hormone, phosphoenolpyruvate, carboxykinase, pyruvate kinase, hepatic phosphofructokinase, apolipoproteins B and A₂, LDL, very-low-density lipoprotein receptor, IRS-1, RAD, FABP2, and the Pima insulin resistance locus.[608]

Abnormal Inhibitors

Insulin resistance in NIDDM may be the result of inhibitors of insulin action. A putative inhibitor of insulin receptor tyrosine kinase, a membrane glycoprotein called PC-1,[498] was increased in fibroblasts of 7 of 9 patients with typical NIDDM, as mentioned previously.

Insulin Resistance in Adipocytes

Insulin resistance in adipose tissue may play a role in the obese diabetic. The cellular content of GLUT4, the facilitative glucose transporter of adipocytes and skeletal muscles, is reduced by 40% in obese persons without NIDDM and by 85% in obese persons with NIDDM.[609]

The increased fat cell mass of obesity, in addition to being intrinsically insulin resistant, may export insulin resistance to muscle, both by releasing FFAs into the general circulation and by infiltrating muscle with adipocytes (marbleization of muscle). The concentrations of glycerol in the interstitial fluid of muscle are 42 times higher than in plasma (3710 versus 87μmol/L),[610] making it likely that marbleized muscle of obese individuals is exposed to high levels of substances released from adipocytes such as nonesterified or FFAs and TNFα.

Free Fatty Acids

Elevated plasma FFAs in obesity[611] can cause insulin resistance,[612–616] probably by inhibiting muscle glucose metabolism and inducing hyperinsulinemia through upregulation of low-K_m glucose metabolism in islets[472, 617] (Fig. 21–36).

Fat cells store fuel in the form of triglycerides in time of nutritional abundance and release FFAs and glycerol when food is not available. FFA release conserves the dwindling supply of glucose, the essential fuel for the central nervous system, by substituting for glucose as a fuel and thereby limiting glucose utilization in tissues for which it is not essential, i.e., skeletal muscle.[618–620] Because glucose is spared in time of glucose need, the increase in fatty acyl–CoA in tissues prolongs the survival time of starving organisms. The insulin resistance of obesity resembles the survival strategy for starvation except that the normal glucose-sparing effect of FFAs takes place even in the fed state, when glucose sparing is harmful.

Tumor Necrosis Factor α

TNF α has important effects on whole-body lipid and glucose metabolism.[491–493] Production and expression of TNF

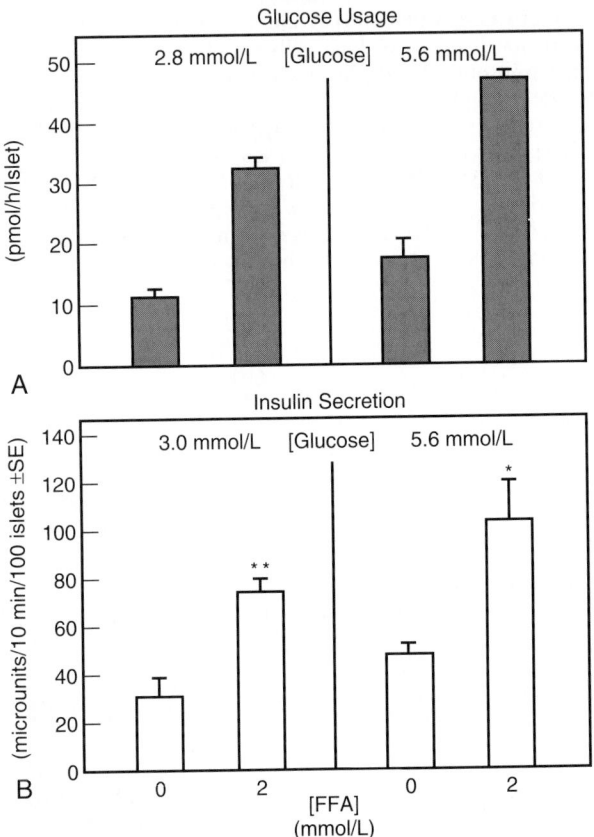

Figure 21–36. The effect of administration of 2 mmol/L long-chain fatty acid (FFA) on glucose usage and insulin secretion in normal islets cultured for 7 d. The exposure to FFA appears to increase glucose metabolism in islets and enhance the output of insulin. This effect may explain how normal beta cells compensate for the insulin resistance caused by the high FFA levels that occur in obesity.

α in adipose tissue are increased in most models of rodent obesity,[489, 621] and TNF α can cause many of the changes seen in the insulin-resistant state.[492, 494] For example, TNF α down-regulates GLUT4 mRNA levels in preadipocyte cultures,[493] inhibits glucose transport, impairs the tyrosine kinase activity of the insulin receptor by lowering its autophosphorylation, and decreases the phosphorylation of IRS-1[492] through activation of a phosphotyrosine phosphatase.[622] Neutralization of TNF α increases tyrosine phosphorylation in Zucker fatty rats,[492] suggesting that the overexpression of TNF α in adipocytes of obese animals is partly responsible for the insulin resistance.[623] Because the plasma levels of TNF α are too low to detect, an endocrine role of TNF α in the pathogenesis of insulin resistance and NIDDM cannot be established. However, given the abundance of adipocytes that marbleize the muscle of obese animals, TNF α released from these cells may produce interstitial levels that exceed those in plasma, as has been demonstrated to be the case with glycerol and FFA, two other adipocyte products.[610]

In summary, the insulin resistance associated with obesity can be accounted for, in part, by increased tissue levels of FFA and perhaps TNF α. However, insulin resistance in lean, glucose-tolerant relatives of NIDDM patients cannot be ex-plained on this basis and probably involves a primary defect in skeletal muscle.

How Obesity Affects Beta-Cell Function: The Lipotoxicity Hypothesis

Obesity-induced hyperinsulinemia results both from expansion of beta-cell mass and from an increase in low-K_m glucose metabolism in the enlarged islets[617] (Fig. 21–36). A hyperinsulinemic obese person becomes overtly diabetic only if the beta cells do not maintain the hyperinsulinemia at a level sufficient to counteract the insulin resistance. Increased insulin secretion and increased low-K_m glucose metabolism can be induced in normal islets in vitro by culture for 7 days in medium containing FFAs in concentrations comparable to those in obese prediabetic animals.[617]

At the onset of diabetes in animals hyperinsulinemia declines slightly, insulin response to glucose disappears, and expression of the facilitative glucose transporter of beta cells, GLUT2, is reduced.[514] In prediabetic obese Zucker diabetic fatty rats a rise in plasma FFA begins approximately 2 weeks before the onset of the hyperglycemia[624] (Fig. 21–37). By the time hyperglycemia appears, the islet triglyceride content has

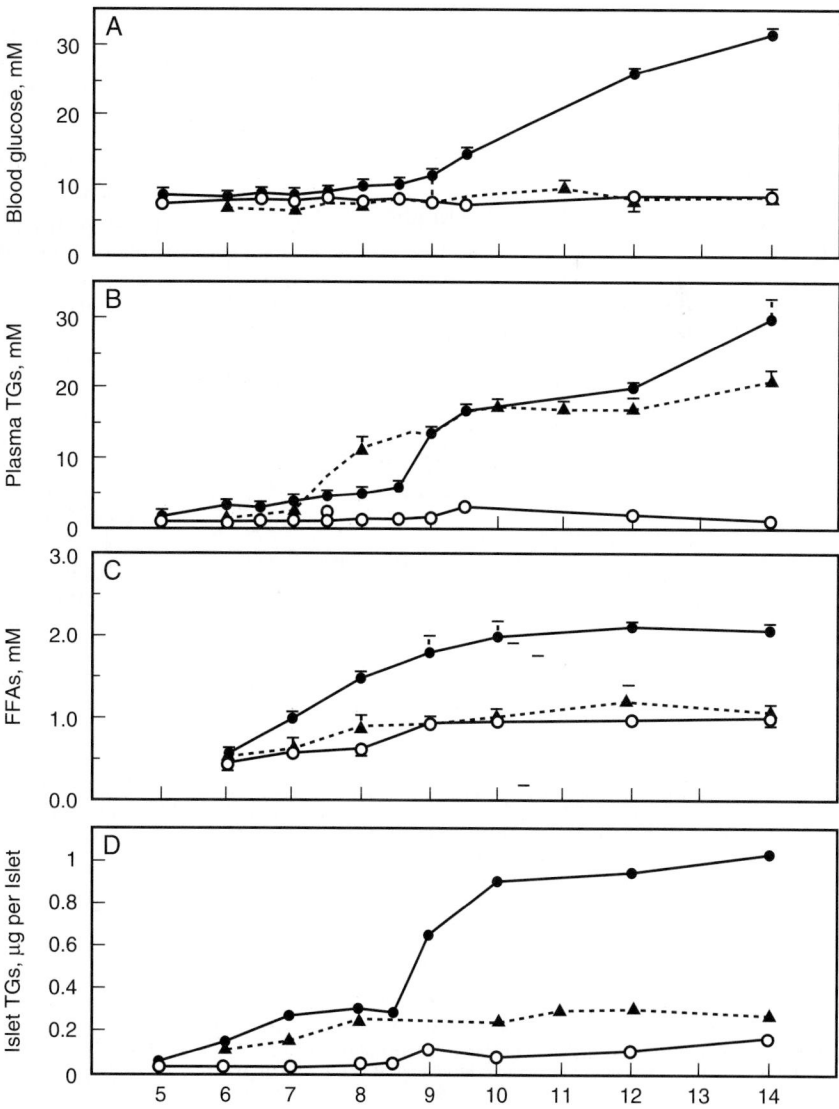

Figure 21–37. Longitudinal studies of levels of plasma glucose (A), plasma TG (B), plasma FFA (C) and islet triglyceride content (D) in lean male ZDF rats (fa/+) (○); obese female ZDF rats (fa/fa) (▲), which do not develop diabetes; and obese male ZDF rats (fa/fa) (●), which develop diabetes between the ages of 8 and 10 weeks. (Redrawn from Lee Y, Hirose H, Ohneda M, et al. β-cell lipotoxicity in the pathogenesis of non–insulin-dependent diabetes mellitus of obese rats: impairment in adipocyte–β-cell relationships. Proc Natl Acad Sci USA 1994; 91:10878–10882.)

risen 10-fold[624] (see Fig. 21–37), indicating that intracellular levels of fatty acyl–CoA have exceeded the oxidative capacity of the cells and have been re-esterified to triglycerides. The FFA-mediated blockade of glucose metabolism in islets could account for the selective loss of beta-cell glucose responsiveness[625-628]; this is known as the lipotoxicity hypothesis (Fig. 21–38).[472] Measures that reduce FFA, such as caloric restriction[629] and nicotinamide treatment,[472] reduce the basal hyperinsulinemia and prevent the loss of GSIS, the loss of beta-cell GLUT2, and the fasting hyperglycemia in the ZDF rat.

Relation Between Beta-Cell Dysfunction and Peripheral Insulin Resistance in NIDDM

Islet dysfunction and peripheral insulin resistance coexist in overt NIDDM, as noted previously. Some have argued that insulin resistance (primary or secondary to obesity) is the primary lesion and causes a secondary defect in the beta cell through "exhaustion."[629] Alternatively, hyperinsulinemia could be the initial lesion, and the insulin resistance a secondary defense against the hyperinsulinemia.

A third possibility is that both the insulin resistance and the beta-cell changes could be secondary to a common abnormality, such as high levels of FFA.[472] The coexistence of high FFAs and hyperinsulinemia is prima facie evidence of resistance in adipocytes to the antilipolytic action of insulin, suggesting that a primary antilipolytic insulin resistance in adipocytes causes a secondary glucoregulatory insulin resistance in muscle.

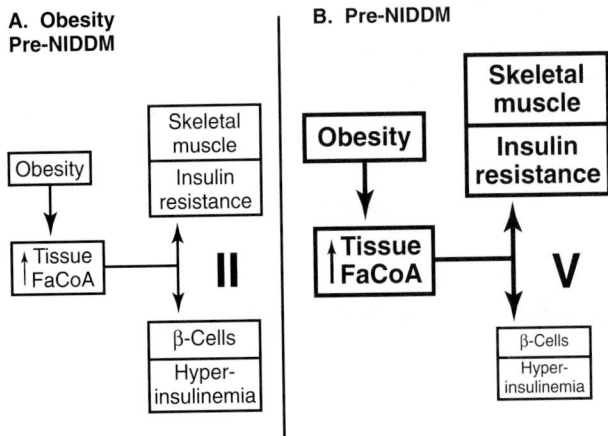

Figure 21–38. The lipotoxic hypothesis. *A,* In obese rats without diabetes there is a relative increase in plasma FFA levels (>0.5 to <1.5 mmol/L) and presumably in the tissue levels of fatty acyl–CoA (FACoA). This hyperlipacidemia may be a consequence of the expanded adipocyte mass or of insensitivity of adipocytes to the antilipolytic action of insulin, or both. The presumed increase in tissue FFA levels throughout the body interferes with normal glucose metabolism at multiple levels. In target tissues of insulin, such as muscle, this interference is referred to as insulin resistance. In islets, the increased FFA levels stimulate insulin secretion and induce beta-cell proliferation and expansion of low-K_m glucose metabolism, which increases basal insulin secretion and potentiates insulin responses to all stimuli. Because FFA-induced changes in tissues are proportional to the levels of FFAs, the insulin resistance and the insulin hypersecretion are perfectly matched, and glucose tolerance remains normal. *B,* In obese rats that become diabetic, FFAs rise to still higher levels (>1.5 mmol/L) and "marbelization" of tissues occurs as FACoA is increasingly esterified to TGs. In muscle this intensifies insulin resistance, but the islets, which have already responded fully to more moderate FFA overload, are incapable of further increases in insulin secretion to match insulin resistance. The FFA overload interferes with glucose metabolism and impairs the capacity of beta cells to respond to postprandial hyperglycemia. Hyperinsulinemia at this point no longer matches the increases in insulin resistance and NIDDM begins. (Redrawn from Unger RH. Lipotoxicity in the pathogenesis of obesity-dependent NIDDM: genetic and clinical implications. Diabetes 1995; 44:863–870.)

HORMONAL PATHOPHYSIOLOGY IN NIDDM

The absence of a profound reduction in insulin/glucagon ratio in NIDDM comparable to that of IDDM accounts for the fact that a severe catabolic state is usually absent.

CLINICAL FEATURES

Type I IDDM

Uncomplicated Onset

Weight loss despite polyphagia reflects the severe catabolic state. Protein catabolism provides substrate for hepatic gluconeogenesis, and increased lipolysis augments delivery of FFA, the ketogenic substrate, to the liver. Hyperglycemia usually reaches a plateau in the range of 17 to 28 mmol/L (300 to 500 mg/dL), at which point glucose excretion approximates the rate of hepatic glucose overproduction.

In children the onset of symptoms often occurs over a short period. Families can sometimes give the precise time the illness appears, even if the onset is not heralded by ketoacidosis. This does not mean that the pathologic process leading to overt diabetes is brief.[213-215] As discussed previously, destruction of beta cells usually occurs over a period now estimated to average 3 y. The diagnosis in children can often be established in the non–insulin-requiring phase of the disease.

Acute Decompensation: Diabetic Ketoacidosis

Diabetic ketoacidosis may be the presenting event in IDDM, or it may occur at any time after diagnosis (see review by Foster and McGarry[630]). It is precipitated by stress, other illness, or omission of insulin. It may also develop slowly after a protracted period of poor control. As mentioned, catecholamines released during stress not only oppose insulin action but also stimulate glucagon release. Catecholamines both potentiate and mimic glucagon's actions (see Table 21–15). Hypovolemia caused by the osmotic diuresis enhances the secretion of glucagon,[339] catecholamines, and other hormones of stress[631] and, by decreasing renal blood flow, reduces glucagon degradation by the kidney. The result is extreme and unopposed hyperglucagonemia, with profound overproduction of glucose and ketones by the liver (Fig. 21–39).[630]

If the osmotic diuresis is prolonged, decreased glomerular filtration curtails renal excretion of glucose to a rate less than that of hepatic glucose production, and plasma glucose levels then rise above the previous 17- to 28-mmol/L plateau (see Fig. 21–39). Hyperosmolality removes water from cells; sodium, potassium, magnesium, bicarbonate, and chloride are lost in the urine; and hyperketonemia increases the hydrogen ion concentration of the body fluids. Disruption of the extracellular milieu places the function of all cells at jeopardy. Central nervous system dysfunction, for example, is primarily a result of intracellular dehydration.[631] Death is inevitable without appropriate intervention.

Admission Findings

The history usually reveals polyuria, polydipsia, polyphagia, and weight loss for a variable period. Abdominal pain, nausea, and vomiting are common and may be caused by the ketoacidosis, but associated disorders such as pyelonephritis, pancreatitis, or an acute abdomen must always be suspected. The mental status can vary from slight drowsiness to profound lethargy, but deep coma is rare. The rapid, deep respirations

DIABETIC KETOACIDOSIS

NONKETOTIC HYPEROSMOLAR COMA

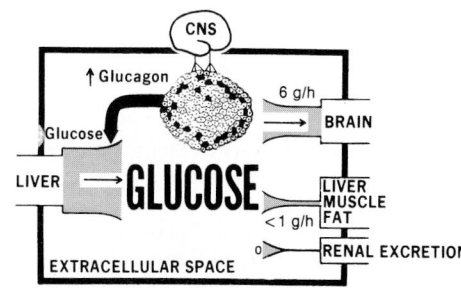

Figure 21–39. Acute decompensation in diabetes mellitus. Diabetic ketoacidosis is usually associated with unmeasurable insulin levels and extremely high glucagon levels. The resulting overproduction of glucose, coupled with negligible glucose utilization by tissues other than brain, causes hyperglycemia, which reaches a plateau when glucose excretion plus cerebral glucose uptake equals hepatic glucose production. Ketone production rises sharply to produce a metabolic acidosis. In nonketotic hyperosmolar coma, insulin levels may also be quite low, although the islets may contain functioning beta cells in patients with NIDDM. A stressful precipitating illness with a prolonged osmotic diuresis reduces the effective extracellular space, thereby increasing discharge of insulin-inhibiting and glucagon-stimulating hormones (see also Table 21–13). Glucose utilization is reduced, and glucose production is increased. In contrast to the situation early in the development of diabetic ketoacidosis, renal excretion of glucose is reduced because of more severe volume depletion, thereby permitting a rapid increase in plasma concentration to extreme levels. Why ketone production does not increase to ketoacidosis levels is not known.

of Kussmaul partially compensate for the metabolic acidosis by disposing of carbon dioxide; respiration may be depressed if central nervous system impairment is severe and the pH is very low.[632] A high plasma acetone level imparts a fruity odor to the breath. Skin turgor is decreased, and mucous membranes are dry. Tachycardia and hypotension may be present. Fever strongly suggests infection, but leukocytosis may be present without infection. The initial examination usually suggests the diagnosis, but documentation of hyperglycemia and ketosis is required.

Typical admission laboratory findings in diabetic ketoacidosis are shown in Table 21–18. The metabolic acidosis results primarily from increased levels of acetoacetic and β-hydroxybutyric acids, with FFAs, lactate, and organic acids playing a minor role. Serum osmolality is almost always high when consciousness is impaired. Although sodium losses in the urine and vomitus may be substantial, the relative or absolute hyponatremia in large part reflects a shift of intracellular water into the extracellular space in response to hyperglycemia. Hypertriglyceridemia, manifested by milkiness of serum or lipemia retinalis, can cause spurious hyponatremia if serum sodium is not measured in water. A sodium value lower than 120 mmol/L usually is caused by hyperlipemia, although occasionally it results from acute dilution caused by vomiting with continued water intake. Despite urinary potassium loss, hyper-

kalemia on admission is a common consequence of the metabolic acidosis. A normal or low potassium level before treatment suggests a severe total body deficit of potassium. Increased serum levels of myoglobin and creatine kinase consistent with nontraumatic rhabdomyolysis may be present in seriously ill patients.[633]

DIFFERENTIAL DIAGNOSIS

Altered consciousness with ketoacidosis is usually easily differentiated from hypoglycemia in diabetic subjects on clinical grounds. Measurement of urinary ketones and plasma glucose in capillary blood by a reflectance meter or chemical strip should provide adequate guidelines pending formal laboratory confirmation. Rarely, cerebrovascular accidents lead to glycosuria and ketonuria, but the initial diagnostic confusion in such cases is rapidly resolved by the clinical course.

Diabetic ketoacidosis is an anion gap acidosis, meaning that the unmeasured anion fraction is greater than 16 mmol/L (calculated by subtracting the plasma concentration of chloride plus bicarbonate from that of sodium plus potassium). There are five major causes of anion gap acidosis: diabetic ketoacidosis, alcoholic ketoacidosis,[634] lactic acidosis, renal failure, and certain poisonings (e.g., ethylene glycol, methyl alcohol).[630] Starvation in late pregnancy or during lactation may rarely cause ketosis sufficient to result in an anion gap acidosis of the ketoacidosis type. Ketoacidosis can be differentiated from other forms of metabolic acidosis accompanied by fasting ketosis (positive urinary ketones) by semiquantitative measurement of ketones in serial dilutions of plasma with reagent sticks that detect acetone and acetoacetate. Because even prolonged starvation rarely causes total ketone concentrations greater than 4 to 6 mmol/L,[353, 573] a moderate to large response in any diluted sample suggests ketoacidosis (moderate to large readings on diagnostic sticks indicate a level of acetone plus acetoacetate of 4 mmol/L or greater). Alcohol- and pregnancy-associated ketoacidosis can be differentiated by the history and by the fact that hyperglycemia and glycosuria are ordinarily absent, although some alcoholics with ketoacidosis may be hyperglycemic.[634] The ketoacidosis in the latter conditions represents an exaggerated response to fasting and is rapidly reversed by glucose or glucose plus a small amount of insulin (5 to 10 U), a response that rules out diabetic ketoacidosis. The diagnosis of lactic acidosis requires the measurement of lactate in the plasma, but the initial clue is severe

TABLE 21–18. Initial Laboratory Findings in Severe Diabetic Decompensation

	Diabetic Ketoacidosis*	Hyperosmolar Coma†
Glucose (mmol/L [mg/dL])	216 (475)	65 (1166)
Sodium (mmol/L)	132	144
Potassium (mmol/L)	4.8	5
Bicarbonate (mmol/L)	<10.0	17
Blood urea nitrogen (mmol/L [mg/dL])	9 (25)	31 (87)
Acetoacetate (mmol/L)	4.8	ND
β-Hydroxybutyrate (mmol/L)	13.7	ND
Free fatty acids (mmol/L)	2.1	0.73
Lactate (mmol/L)	4.6	ND
Osmolarity (mmol/kg)	310	384

ND, not done.
*Based on 88 consecutive episodes of diabetic ketoacidosis at Parkland Memorial Hospital (D. W. Foster, unpublished study).
†Arieff AT, Carroll HJ. Nonketotic hyperosmolar coma with hyperglycemia. Medicine 1972; 51:73–74. Copyright © 1972, by Williams & Wilkins, Baltimore.

metabolic acidosis with absent urinary ketones or a plasma ketone result that is positive only in the undiluted state despite a large urinary acetone content. Tests for urinary ketones may be positive in lactic acidosis because nausea and vomiting induce starvation ketosis.

Type II NIDDM
Uncomplicated Onset

Type II NIDDM varies in severity. Many patients are asymptomatic, and the diagnosis is made by the detection of hyperglycemia or glycosuria on routine examination. In such subjects the mean level of glucose in the plasma throughout the day is below the renal threshold, and glycosuria is absent or intermittent, so that symptomatic osmotic diuresis does not supervene. Even if frank hyperglycemia develops, the onset is often so gradual that diagnosis is delayed for weeks or months. Rarely, the onset of symptoms is as acute as in IDDM, usually as a result of the stress of an acute intercurrent illness. Occasionally, the presenting symptom is a diabetic complication such as peripheral neuropathy, gangrene, or a vascular event that leads the physician to test for hyperglycemia or to perform a glucose tolerance test.

Acute Decompensation: Nonketotic Hyperosmolar Coma

The characteristic acute catabolic complication of type II NIDDM, analogous to diabetic ketoacidosis in type I IDDM, is nonketotic hyperosmolar coma, a syndrome of extreme hyperglycemia and dehydration. The pathophysiology involves an imbalance between glucose production and its excretion in the urine. As noted previously, maximal hepatic production of glucose results in a plasma glucose plateau of 17 to 28 mmol/L (300 to 500 mg/dL) so long as urinary output is maintained and glucose excretion keeps pace with hepatic glucose production. Hyperosmolar coma results when the sum of glucose excretion plus utilization is less than the rate at which glucose enters the extracellular space (see Fig. 21–39). Hyperosmolar coma most often occurs in older patients when an intercurrent illness increases glucose production secondary to elevated production of stress hormones and impairs the capacity to ingest fluids. As the extracellular fluid and plasma volumes shrink, the capacity to excrete glucose decreases or disappears as urine volume falls, while hepatic glucose production pours glucose into a shrinking plasma space from which glucose clearance is impaired. As the plasma glucose level rises, central nervous system dysfunction appears (presumably the consequence of intracellular dehydration), water intake is further impaired, urine flow decreases further, and the blood glucose level continues to rise (see Fig. 21–39), causing monumental hyperglycemia, hyperosmolality, and a high mortality.[635, 636] In patients younger than 50 years of age, mortality rates may be lower.[637]

Although usually a complication of NIDDM, nonketotic hyperosmolar coma can occur in any type of diabetes and at any age, even in children, provided that insulin therapy has prevented ketone overproduction but has not corrected the hyperglycemia, thus allowing a prolonged osmotic diuresis. Restoration of normal fluid balance is crucial in both diabetic ketoacidosis[638] and hyperosmolar coma.[639]

The mechanism by which ketoacidosis is suppressed in NIDDM with extreme hyperglycemia is not known. Hyperosmolality inhibits lipolysis in vitro,[639] and FFA levels in hyperosmolar coma average 0.7 mmol/L,[635, 636] compared with 2.0 mmol/L in diabetic ketoacidosis,[640] presumably providing less substrate for ketogenesis in the liver. However, hyperosmolar coma can occur in diabetic patients with FFA levels of 1.4 to 4.0 mmol/L.[640] Nor can the absence of serious ketosis in

hyperosmolar coma be attributed to lower concentrations of glucagon, because the concentrations equal or surpass those seen in ketoacidosis,[641] suggesting that extreme hyperglycemia somehow breaks through the glucagon-mediated blockade of lipogenesis and permits synthesis of sufficient malonyl-CoA (perhaps from glucose-derived lactate) to inhibit CPT-I activity and to restrain the production of acetoacetate and β-hydroxybutyrate.

ADMISSION FINDINGS

The precipitating event may color or dominate the clinical presentation; conversely, the precipitating event may be camouflaged by the metabolic crisis. Stroke, myocardial infarction, pneumonia and other infections, burns, and heat stroke are typical precipitating events. Acute pancreatitis is common, although it is not always clear whether it initiates the syndrome or is a consequence of it. Pancreatitis impairs residual insulin release and sequesters large amounts of extracellular fluid in the "third space"—the inflammatory bed surrounding the pancreas. Abdominal pain may be a transient accompaniment of the metabolic disturbance, or it may reflect important precipitating intra-abdominal disease.

On examination, patients with hyperosmolar coma exhibit extreme dehydration and may have supine or orthostatic hypotension and hypothermia. Kussmaul respiration is usually absent, an important clinical clue in differentiating the disorder from diabetic ketoacidosis. Hyperpnea, if present, suggests lactic acidosis. Gastric distention, ileus, and even hematemesis may occur and may recede with treatment.[642] Impairment of the central nervous system ranges from confusion to coma. Seizures are common and may be either focal or generalized.[643] Other neurologic findings may include rapidly reversible hemiplegia. Neurologic signs may recede with treatment, or, if they result from underlying central nervous system disease worsened by the metabolic insult, they may not be reversible. Pleural and/or pericardial friction rubs and electrocardiographic changes may result from metabolic alterations and disappear with rehydration, or they may indicate infection or pulmonary infarction.[642]

Lactic acidosis occurs when fluid deficits lead to hypotension and decreased tissue perfusion. Because the patients frequently have starved for hours to days before admission, the urine may be positive for ketones, causing confusion with ketoacidosis. Differentiation between the two entities can usually be made by semiquantitative analysis of ketones in dilute plasma, as already described, but plasma should be drawn for the quantitative measurement of lactate (and ketones, if available) to confirm the clinical diagnosis.

Typical laboratory findings are shown in Table 21–18. Plasma osmolality is elevated. Although the plasma glucose level is, on average, about 67 mmol/L (1200 mg/dL), values as high as 267 mmol/L (4800 mg/dL) have been reported.[644] If plasma osmolality cannot be measured directly, a close estimate may be obtained from routine analyses (all values in mmol/L):

$$\text{Plasma osmolality} = 2[Na^+ + K^+] + \text{glucose} + \text{blood urea nitrogen}$$

Virtually all patients have elevated levels of blood urea nitrogen (average, 31 mmol/L [87 mg/dL]) and creatinine (average, 486 μmol/L [5.5 mg/dL]).[636]

DIFFERENTIAL DIAGNOSIS

The differential diagnosis of nonketotic hyperosmolar coma is not a problem once extreme hyperglycemia is documented. The diagnostic challenge consists in the elucidation of the pathophysiology and precipitating mechanism. The range of possibilities is large because of the broad spectrum of complicating illnesses. Occasionally, the disorder occurs solely because of insufficient insulin or sulfonylureas, particularly if the patient replaces the fluid loss with sugar-containing soft drinks.[642] The syndrome may be caused iatrogenically by the administration of drugs[645–647] (phenytoin, glucocorticoids, thiazide diuretics, cimetidine, or furosemide) or by high-calorie tube feedings, intravenous hyperalimentation, intravenous infusion of hypertonic glucose, or peritoneal dialysis with glucose-containing solutions.

In hyperosmolar coma without apparent precipitating illness the differential diagnosis is that of altered central nervous system function, usually stroke, head injury, or brain tumor. For this reason imaging of the brain is useful, especially if the neurologic deficit fails to improve as the metabolic disorder recedes.

COMPLICATIONS OF DIABETES

Since the availability of insulin and antibiotics, the number of deaths from acute metabolic complications has decreased, and disability and death in both IDDM and NIDDM usually result from the degenerative complications of the disease. A study in Denmark of 2930 patients showed a 30 to 40% decrease in mortality for subjects diagnosed after 1956 compared with those diagnosed between 1933 and 1946,[648] suggesting a decrease in death rates from both acute and chronic complications.

Traditionally, retinopathy, neuropathy, and nephropathy have been designated *microvascular* complications, whereas atherosclerosis and its sequelae (stroke, myocardial infarction, gangrene) are termed *macrovascular* complications.

Role of Metabolic Control

The relation between diabetic complications and the metabolic derangements of diabetes has been established unequivocally by the Diabetes Control and Complications Trial (DCCT).[649–651] The evidence supporting a relation between metabolic abnormalities of diabetes and its microangiopathic complications has long been impressive. The 98% of people who are normoglycemic are untouched by the microvascular complications of diabetes. Nodular glomerulosclerosis, which is present in 55% of hyperglycemic Pima Indians, has never been demonstrated in a normoglycemic member of the tribe.[652] The 6-year incidence of diabetic retinopathy is negligible in Pima Indians with a 2-h OGTT glucose level lower than 11 mmol/L (200 mg/dL), but it is 20% in those with 2-h glucose levels above that value.[7] A similar relation between retinopathy and 2-h blood glucose levels has been observed in London,[653] Athens,[654] and Oxford, Massachusetts.[655]

The facts that glomerular basement membranes are normal at the onset of both primary type I IDDM and secondary acquired diabetes but become thickened within 3.5 to 5 y[656, 657] and that diabetic nephropathy develops in normal kidneys transplanted from nondiabetic donors into diabetic recipients[658] support a pathogenic influence of the metabolic milieu. Nevertheless, a genetic contribution to hyperglycemia-induced microvascular complications is suggested by the report that 83% of diabetic siblings of IDDM probands with diabetic nephropathy also had evidence of nephropathy, compared with only 17% of diabetic siblings of IDDM probands without apparent nephropathy.[659]

Can Meticulous Control Prevent the Complications of Diabetes?

Evidence that diabetic complications occur only in the presence of diabetes mellitus does not necessarily prove that such complications can be prevented by meticulous control of glycemia. Until 1993 none of the studies designed to test this critical question had provided a conclusive answer.

DIABETES CONTROL AND COMPLICATIONS TRIAL

The DCCT, a large multicenter prospective trial sponsored by the National Institutes of Health, was designed to test the effect of meticulous blood glucose control on development of diabetic complications in the United States. Of 1441 patients with IDDM, 726 had no retinopathy and 715 had mild retinopathy on entering the study. They were randomly assigned to one of two intensive insulin therapy regimens or to conventional therapy. Intensive therapy was delivered either by continuous subcutaneous insulin infusion (CSII) using an external insulin pump or by three or more daily injections guided by frequent blood glucose monitoring. The conventional therapy program consisted of one or two daily insulin injections. After a mean of 6.5 y of follow-up in the retinopathy-free patients, the appearance of retinopathy was reduced by 76% in the intensively treated group compared with the group treated conventionally. Among those patients who entered the study with mild retinopathy, intensive therapy slowed the progression by 54% and reduced proliferative or severe nonproliferative retinopathy by 47%. Intensive therapy also reduced the occurrence of microalbuminuria by 39% and of gross albuminuria by 54%. Clinical neuropathy was lowered by 60%.[649, 650] Similar results were obtained in a Swedish study.[651]

In the American study the median HbA$_{1c}$ levels of intensively treated patients ranged between 7.0 and 7.2%, and the mean daily plasma glucose levels during the years of the study ranged between 8.0 ± 2.8 mmol/L (145 ± 50 mg/dL) and 8.7 ± 2.5 mmol/L (157 ± 45 mg/dL). By contrast, HbA$_{1c}$ levels in the conventional therapy group ranged between 8.8 and 9.3%, and the mean of seven daily plasma glucose measurements fluctuated between 12.7 ± 4.1 mmol/L (229 ± 74 mg/dL) and 13.0 ± 4.7 mmol/L (235 ± 85 mg/dL). Clearly, either the reduction of hyperglycemia or some unidentified metabolic improvement associated with the amelioration of hyperglycemia prevented or slowed the progression of the microvascular complications of IDDM.[649, 650]

COMPLICATIONS OF METICULOUS CONTROL

In the DCCT intensive treatment was accompanied by a threefold increase in severe hypoglycemia. A disproportionate number of such episodes occurred during sleep, and one third of daytime hypoglycemic episodes were unaccompanied by warning symptoms. Frequency of severe hypoglycemia decreased with time.

Intensively managed patients experienced greater weight gain than those on conventional therapy, and by the end of the DCCT study 33.6% were considered overweight, compared with 17.5% in the conventionally-treated group.[649, 650] Insulin resistance caused by obesity may have accounted for the reduction in hypoglycemic events in the later part of the study.

Can Meticulous Control Reverse Established Microangiopathic Complications?

In muscle, a tissue in which capillaries are constantly being replaced, good control can reduce the width of thickened capillary basement membranes.[18] In tissues in which capillaries are not replaced, such as retina and glomeruli, diabetic microvascular disease does not appear to be reversible.[660] Occasionally, diabetic retinopathy worsens after a period of intensive therapy for unknown reasons.[661] Perhaps retinal glucopenia in ischemic areas of the glucose-dependent retina may stimulate vascular endothelial growth factor

(VEGF). VEGF receptors are present in retinal endothelial cells and in the endothelial cells of major vessels.[662, 663]

The manifestation of diabetic nephropathy may also progress despite meticulous control (P. Raskin, A. O. Pietri, R. H. Unger, et al., unpublished). Motor nerve conduction velocity may improve,[664] but improvement in symptoms is minimal. Vibration sense is unimproved.

In summary, meticulous control of the blood sugar prevents or retards the development of complications but does not reverse established microangiopathy; progression of diabetic retinopathy may be accelerated, at least in the initial period of meticulous control.

Potential Mechanisms in the Pathogenesis of Complications

The various diabetic complications do not necessarily have the same pathogenic mechanisms. Three possible mechanisms have been implicated in these tissue changes: (1) overglycation of proteins, (2) increase in polyol pathway activity, and (3) hemodynamic abnormalities.

Glycation of Proteins

Post-translational enzymatic glycosylation expands the structural and functional repertoire of proteins that can be synthesized from only 20 amino acids.[665] Basement membrane protein, α_2-macroglobulin, collagen, some cell-surface receptors, HLA antigens, immunoglobulins, and glycoprotein hormones are but a few of the important glycoproteins formed enzymatically. In the presence of a high glucose concentration, glucose can be incorporated nonenzymatically into proteins by an unregulated glycation reaction. The reaction involves the formation of a Schiff base (aldimine), followed by a much slower internal shift (Amadori rearrangement; Fig. 21–40).[666] Lysine and valine residues are the primary sites of glucose addition. Such unregulated glycation may change protein structure and impair function. Nondiabetics are protected by the tight control of blood glucose within normal limits.

In the case of hemoglobin, the most extensively studied of the nonenzymatically glycated proteins, glycation of the terminal valine of the beta chain alters the surface charge and converts it to fast-moving HbA_{1c} on electrophoresis.[667] The level of HbA_{1c} provides an index of integrated glucose concentration over the life span of the red blood cell, which normally is about 100 to 120 d. The measurement of glycated albumin, which turns over more rapidly than hemoglobin, provides a short-term clinical index of diabetic control.[668] If plasma glucose is normal for a week, levels of glycated serum proteins decrease by approximately 40%, while the HbA_{1c} level drops only 10%.[669]

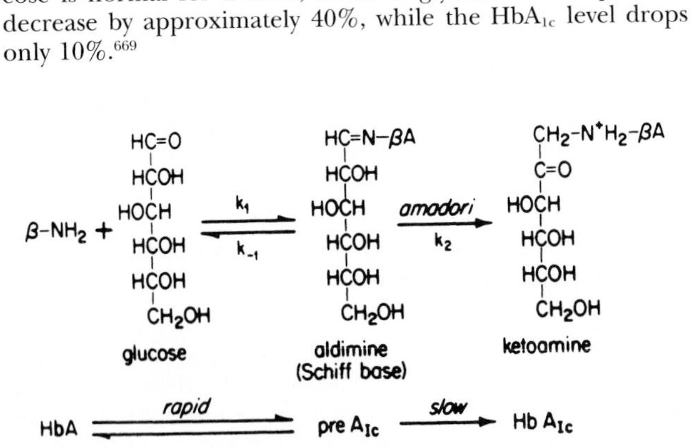

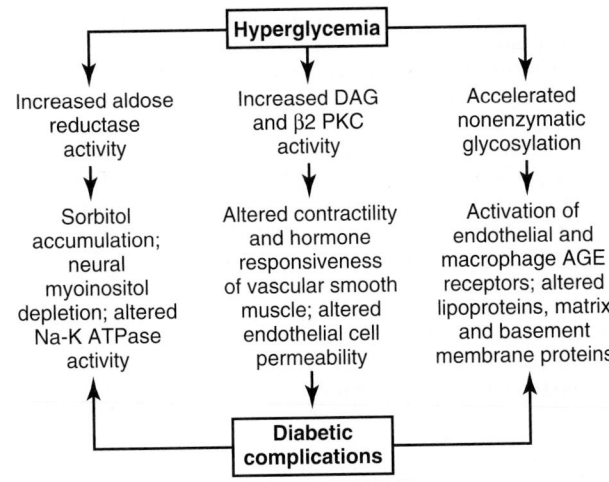

Figure 21–41. How too much glucose may lead to the long-term complications of diabetes. AGE, advanced glycosylation end products; DAG, diacylglycerol; PKC, protein kinase C. (Redrawn from Porte D Jr, Schwartz MW. Diabetes complications: why is glucose potentially toxic? Science 1996; 272:699–700. Copyright © 1996, by American Association for the Advancement of Science.)

It is likely that all proteins in the body can undergo glycation if exposed to elevated glucose or glucose 6-phosphate concentrations. Intracellular proteins in insulin-requiring tissues of the diabetic subject may be partially protected from glycation despite extracellular hyperglycemia, because glucose is excluded from entering the cell by deficiency of or resistance to insulin.[670] Nevertheless, at autopsy, tissues from diabetic subjects exhibit a generalized increase in glycation.[671]

ADVANCED GLYCATION END PRODUCTS (Fig. 21–41)

Nonenzymatically glycated proteins slowly form fluorescent cross-linked protein adducts called *a*dvanced *g*lycation *e*nd products, or AGEs. This process, known as "browning" or the Maillard reaction, is accelerated by elevation of the ambient glucose concentration and by age. Browning can be assayed by measurement of collagen-linked fluorescence in skin biopsy specimens. Patients with long-standing diabetes have levels at least twice those of normal subjects.[672] Fluorescence is increased in patients with severe retinopathy and nephropathy.

AGEs are believed to cause tissue damage because of their reactivity and protein cross-linking. A prime cross-linking intermediate is 3-deoxyglucosone, which can be derived from glucose or fructose.[673] Not all AGEs exhibit fluorescence, and more specific assays may provide a truer picture of their effects.[674]

One of the AGEs that results from the reaction of pentoses with proteins is pentosidine, a marker of accelerated tissue modification that is enhanced in diabetic patients with severe complications.[675] There is an association between fluorescence and retinopathy and between pentosidine levels and nephropathy. Auto-oxidation of these compounds plays a major role in the cross-linking of collagen by glucose.[676–679] The availability of AGE-specific antibodies has allowed identification of an AGE-modified form of human hemoglobin termed hemoglobin-AGE (HbAGE), which accounts for 0.42% of circulating hemoglobin in normal persons but increases to 0.75% in people with hyperglycemia.[680]

AGEs can cause disrupting and damaging tissue changes. Receptors for AGE proteins are expressed on endothelial cells, fibroblasts, mesangial cells, and macrophages.[676] A macrophage-monocyte receptor for AGEs mediates the uptake of AGE-modified proteins and the release of TNF α, IL-1, IGF-1,

Figure 21–40. Nonenzymatic glycosylation of hemoglobin to form hemoglobin A_{1c}. This reaction is prototypical for glycosylation of proteins. Amino acids primarily glycosylated are lysine and valine. (From Higgins PJ, Bunn HF. Kinetic analysis of the nonenzymatic glycosylation of hemoglobin. J Biol Chem 1981; 256:5204–5208.)

and platelet-derived growth factor (PDGF).[676] Endothelial cell AGE receptors internalize AGEs to the subepithelium, thereby enhancing permeability and endothelium-dependent coagulant activity.[681] AGE receptors in the renal mesangium mediate the production of PDGF-dependent extracellular matrix protein, and AGE receptors on fibroblasts may enhance cellular proliferation by epithelial growth factor (EGF). Advanced glycation end products also induce expression of vascular cell adhesion molecule-1.[682]

AGEs on the surface of diabetic erythrocytes may enhance their interaction with endothelial cells, causing binding and oxidant stress,[678] which are important for the development of vascular complications.[683] The AGE inhibitor, aminoguanidine, prevents some complications of diabetes in animals[678] and prevents macrophage activation, stimulation of cytokine/growth factor secretion, and increased endothelial cell permeability.[681]

AGEs can react directly with plasma lipoproteins to prevent their recognition by tissue low-density lipoprotein (LDL) receptors.[684] The administration of aminoguanidine to diabetic patients resulted in a 28% decrease in circulating LDL, probably because of modification of apolipoprotein B100.[684] Finally, subendothelial AGEs chemically inactivate NO, the endothelial-derived relaxing factor, possibly contributing to the defective vasodilatory responsiveness. Therefore, the AGE system may play a broad role in the complications of diabetes.

FUNCTIONAL CONSEQUENCES OF OVERGLYCATION

For interference with function of a protein by glycation to occur, either the affected intrachain lysines must be close to the active site or sites of the molecule or the protein structure must be distorted. The function of some proteins is known to be altered by glycation, and in other cases the possibility is suspected but unproved. In the former category are hemoglobin, albumin, lens protein, fibrin, collagen, lipoproteins, the glycoprotein recognition system of hepatic endothelial cells,[685] and antithrombin.[686] In the latter category are IgG, red blood cell membranes, circulating leukocytes, myelin, and von Willebrand's factor.

Glycation of hemoglobin causes a clinically insignificant increase in oxygen affinity.[687, 688] Glycated albumin inhibits the hepatic uptake of glycoproteins[687] and is taken up into the walls of small blood vessels more rapidly than native albumin. AGE-modified albumin can induce features of diabetic glomerulosclerosis[689] (see later discussion). Glycated fibrin is less susceptible to digestion by plasmin,[690] which may cause its accumulation in diabetic tissues.[691] Glycation of the lens proteins may promote cataract formation by enhancement of disulfide links between protein molecules.[692]

It is not known whether glycation of collagen in glomerular basement membranes contributes to their thickening in diabetes, which is associated with a generalized increase in basement membrane synthesis.[693] Glycated collagen is more insoluble and more resistant to digestion by collagenase.[694, 695] It has also been postulated that decreased proteoglycan synthesis may cause increased permeability of basement membranes and that thickening is a compensatory response.[696] Glycation is probably responsible for changes such as the tight waxy skin and limited joint mobility that are said to indicate an increased risk of late complications.[697]

Glycation of the red cell membrane could play a role in the reduction in erythrocyte survival time[698] and perhaps in the loss of the normal red blood cell deformability in poorly controlled diabetes,[699, 700] which in turn could cause sludging of blood and lead to retinal and renal ischemia.[700] Glycation of myelin protein[701] may contribute to the impairment in nerve conduction. Membrane glycation in leukocytes may cause the impairments in chemotaxis, diapedesis, phagocyto-

sis, bactericidal activity, and cell-mediated immunity that are reported.[702–706] The defective response of T cells and B cells to mitogens can be restored by the return of glucose levels to normal.[707] Overglycation of von Willebrand's factor could contribute to the increased platelet aggregation reported in poorly controlled diabetes.[708] AGE products may contribute to the macrovascular complications.[709]

Polyol Pathway

A second potential cause of diabetic complications is activation of the polyol pathway (see Fig. 21–41).[710] In this pathway glucose is reduced to sorbitol by aldose reductase (D-aldose:NADP$^+$ 1-oxidoreductase). Sorbitol can be oxidized to fructose by sorbitol dehydrogenase (L-iditol dehydrogenase). Aldose reductase is present in the retina, kidney papillae, lens, Schwann cells, and aorta. Polyols have been implicated in the pathogenesis of cataracts,[711] retinopathy,[712] neuropathy,[713] and aortic disease.[714] In the lens, sorbitol may cause osmotic swelling, which is initially reversible, but subsequently Na$^+$,K$^+$-ATPase activity falls.[711] How the latter phenomena interact with the postulated role of glycated lens proteins in the genesis of cataracts[692, 715] is not known. In nerves polyols inhibit Na$^+$,K$^+$-ATPase,[716, 717] which is also reduced in the myo-inositol deficiency of diabetic neuropathy in animals[713, 716–718] but not in humans.[719] Retinopathy,[712] cataracts,[711] nephropathy,[710] and peripheral neuropathy[713, 717] in animals can be prevented by inhibition of the polyol pathway. Sorbinil, an aldose reductase inhibitor tested in human trials, may relieve symptoms in painful diabetic neuropathy,[720] and may enhance nerve regeneration in diabetic humans.[721] In diabetic animals the second half of the polyol pathway, namely the formation of fructose, may be more important in inducing complications than the synthesis of sorbitol. An inhibitor of sorbitol dehydrogenase increased levels of sorbitol in tissues but improved vascular and nerve function.[722]

The polyol pathway may contribute to nonenzymatic glycation of proteins, because fructose can bind nonenzymatically to protein (so-called fructation), and fluorescence of collagen from diabetic animals is decreased by inhibitors of aldol reductase.[723]

Hemodynamic Hypothesis

A third postulated general mechanism of tissue injury is based on the observation that blood flow is increased in patients studied shortly after the onset of IDDM (for a review, see Parving and colleagues[724]). Because the blood pressure is usually normal, arteriolar resistance is probably decreased. The increased hydrostatic pressure in the capillary beds is thought to increase filtration of potentially damaging proteins and other macromolecules (including immune complexes) into the walls of blood vessels and mesangium, secondarily stimulating synthesis of mesangial and basement membrane components. The latter step is presumed to enhance capillary "leakiness." The hemodynamic hypothesis has received the most attention in connection with diabetic renal disease.[725]

Atherosclerosis

Diabetes is a risk factor for atherosclerosis, particularly in women.[726] Macrovascular complications account for 80% of the deaths in NIDDM, 60% being attributable to ischemic heart disease. The atherosclerotic risk is greatest in poorly controlled patients, possibly because of associated hypercholesterolemia and hypertriglyceridemia. Involvement of coronary, cerebral, and peripheral vessels increases the incidence of myocardial infarction, stroke, and lower-extremity gangrene. The atherosclerotic syndromes in diabetes are not dis-

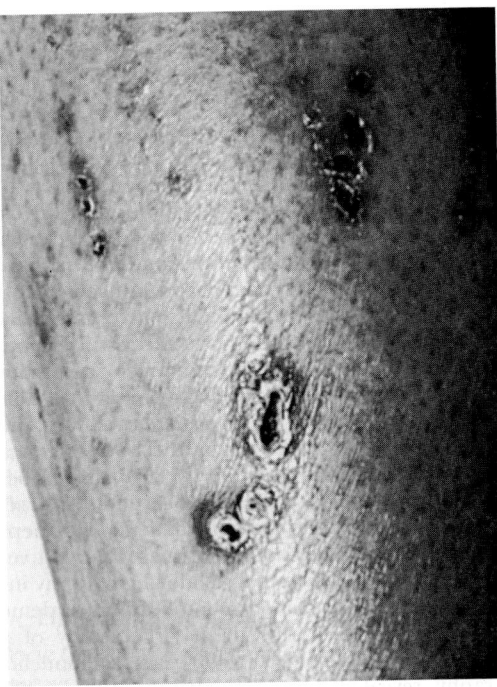

Figure 21–43. Early lesions of dermopathy showing central crusting; in this patient the lesions appear in a somewhat linear arrangement. (From Binkley GW. Dermopathy in the diabetic syndrome. Arch Dermatol 1965; 92:625. Copyright 1965, American Medical Association.)

may not occur, permitting continuing trauma and leading to the breakdown of skin. This defect may be present even though routine sensory examination is normal. If the capacity to sweat is lost because of autonomic neuropathy, the resulting dryness of the skin leads to cracking, superficial inflammation, and chronic dermatitis.[779] The normal increase in blood flow required for healing after trivial trauma or infection may be impaired by vascular disease. Callus formation secondary to abnormal distribution of pressure because of the proprioceptive defect predisposes to pressure ischemia, and microthrombi contribute to ulcer development or gangrene. A prospective study of 86 diabetic patients for 15 to 34 months indicated that plantar ulcerations occurred in 35% of those with elevated foot pressure measured by plethysmography; no ulcers occurred in patients with normal foot pressures.[782]

The most important aspect of management for the diabetic foot syndrome is prophylaxis. Diabetic patients should inspect their feet daily, searching for redness and other signs of trauma, which may not be symptomatic. Soaking the feet for 20 min in warm water followed by an application of oil-based lotions may help keep the skin soft. Well-fitting shoes are imperative, and, if possible, a different pair of shoes should be worn each half-day to minimize pressure in the same areas. Jogging shoes are ideal. Calluses should be treated by sanding with paper or an emery board or trimmed by a podiatrist, physician, or specially trained nurse. After an ulcer develops, the most important treatment is bed rest to remove pressure, coupled with débridement, soaks, and antibiotics if infection is present. Some physicians treat ulcers by placing a well-fitting orthopedic walking cast to redistribute pressure. The advantage is that the patient can continue to work. X-ray examination of the foot is indicated in every patient with an ulcer, because foreign bodies (pins, tacks, glass, nails) are commonly present and are often unrecognized because of impaired pain sensation. A corollary is that diabetic subjects should never go barefoot.

The diabetic foot is perhaps the most preventable of all

diabetic complications, using the relatively simple measures just mentioned. Unfortunately, such measures do not always receive adequate attention.

Nephropathy

Diabetic nephropathy accounts for about half of the patients receiving long-term renal dialysis in the United States, but estimates of the prevalence of end-stage diabetic nephropathy vary widely. In the United States one study reported that 50% of people with childhood-onset IDDM and 30% of those with IDDM beginning before age 31 developed nephropathy.[783] Yet, a 40-y follow-up of IDDM patients indicated that the majority did not develop proteinuria and only 8% developed end-stage nephropathy.[784] In Sweden the cumulative incidence of persistent albuminuria after 25 y of IDDM decreased from 30% in patients whose diabetes commenced between 1961 and 1965 to 8.9% in those whose diabetes was diagnosed between 1966 and 1976,[785] a decline attributed to better glycemic control. The DCCT provided clear evidence that meticulous control significantly reduces the incidence of albuminuria in patients with IDDM. The risk of micoalbuminuria is higher in patients with an HbA_{1c} level higher than 8.9%.[786] Death from renal disease is less common in type II diabetes, perhaps because of the shorter duration of disease and the higher cardiovascular mortality.

In Japan renal disease was the cause of death in 11.9% of

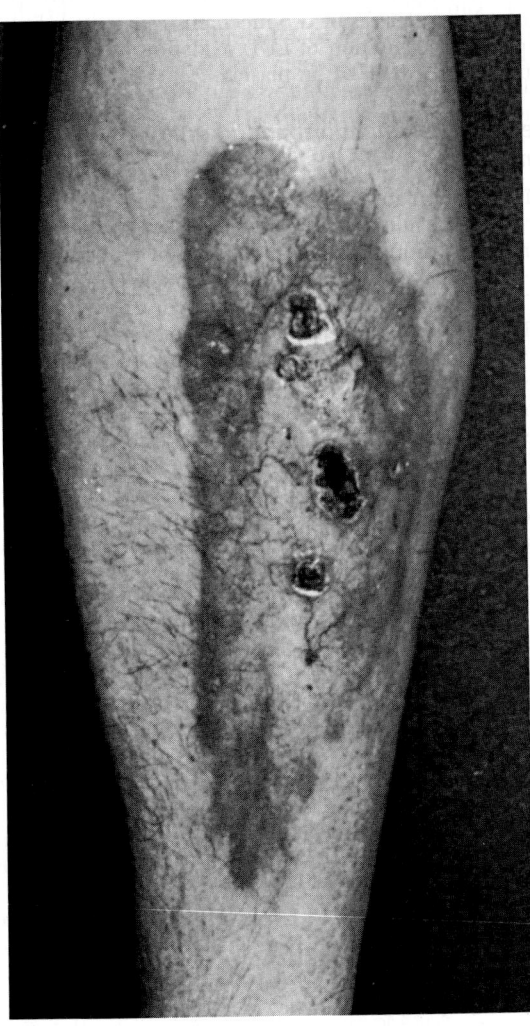

Figure 21–44. Extensive dry ulcerative plaque of necrobiosis lipoidica diabeticorum. (Courtesy of Dr. George Odland.)

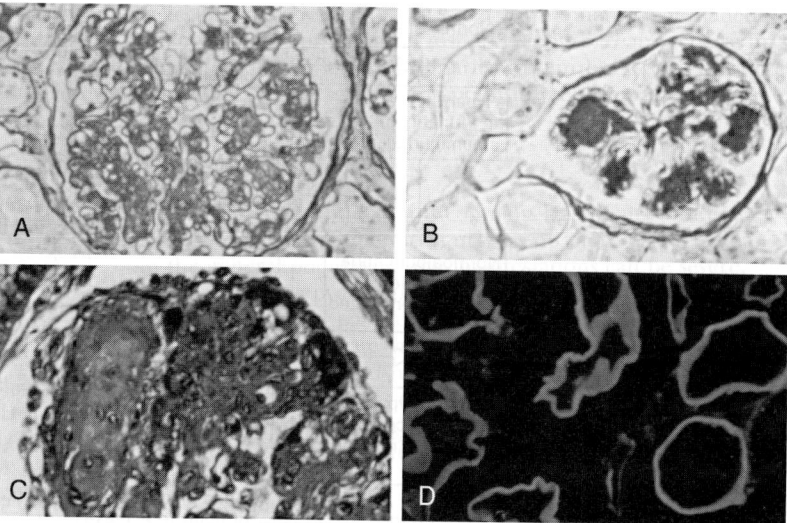

Figure 21–45. Representative lesions of diabetic nephropathy. *A,* Glomerulus showing diffuse diabetic glomerulosclerosis. There is diffuse thickening of all mesangial areas by a moderate increase in mesangial matrix. PAS, light microscopy. Magnification × 400. *B,* Glomerulus showing nodular diabetic glomerulosclerosis. There is focal accentuation of the mesangial matrix into rounded nodules (Kimmelstiel-Wilson nodules). PAS, light microscopy. Magnification × 400. *C,* Portion of glomerulus showing mesangial nodule of Kimmelstiel-Wilson at the left and regions of fuchsinophilic "fibrin caps." Trichrome stain. Magnification × 600. *D,* Small segment of renal cortex from a diabetic patient showing diffuse intense linear staining along all tubular basement membranes with antisera to human albumin. Immunofluorescence microscopy. Magnification × 600. (Photomicrographs courtesy of Drs. Fred G. Silva, Conrad L. Pirani, and Edwin H. Elgenbrodt.)

subjects who died during a 20-y follow-up of 1221 diabetic patients,[787] but nephropathy appears to be rare in Japanese American men with diabetes.[788] Although end-stage renal disease is uncommon in type II diabetes, 65% of diabetic Pima Indians, all with NIDDM, had histologic evidence of diabetic glomerulosclerosis at autopsy.[789]

The differing prevalence rates of nephropathy in different populations may be a consequence of genetic factors. Some families with multiple members afflicted with diabetes rarely exhibit nephropathy, whereas in other multiplex families more than 80% of affected siblings have renal disease.[790] A genetic predisposition to diabetic nephropathy has been ascribed to DNA sequence differences in the gene for ACE,[791, 792] which activates angiotensin I to the vasoconstrictor angiotensin II and inactivates the vasodilator bradykinin.[793] However, the relation between ACE gene polymorphism and the predisposition to diabetic nephropathy is controversial.

Pathology

Diabetic glomerulosclerosis is ordinarily divided into two forms, a diffuse form and a nodular form that represents accelerated disease (Fig. 21–45).[794] In the diffuse form the entire mesangium is thickened. The nodular form consists of capsular drops, fibrin caps, and adhesions in the glomeruli, microaneurysms, and large spherical accumulations of PAS-positive material in the mesangium at the periphery of the glomerular tufts (the glomerular nodules of Kimmelstiel and Wilson).[794]

Diabetic nephropathy begins with thickening of the glomerular basement membrane, an increase in the mesangial matrix (a forerunner of diffuse glomerulosclerosis), and subintimal hyaline thickening of both afferent and efferent arterioles. These changes begin to appear 1.5 to 5.0 y after the metabolic abnormality is recognized.[656–658] The mesangial matrix between the glomerular capillaries, which together with the afferent and efferent glomerular vessels form the glomerular hilum, contains nerve endings, smooth muscle, and angiotensin II receptors. Normally the mesangium takes up and processes macromolecules from the circulation.[795] In rodents such molecules move from the periphery of the mesangium to the hilum of the glomerulus and leave the area through the distal tubular cells.[796] The capacity to clear macromolecules is impaired in diabetes.[795] Accumulation of albumin and larger proteins within the glomerular wall and in the mesangium may stimulate mesangial matrix production and lead to the diffuse and nodular changes of diabetic nephropathy.[795] In humans, plasma proteins, particularly albumin, are deposited along the tubular basement membrane and Bowman's capsule

in the kidney (see Fig. 21–35*D*)[797] and in basement membranes of muscle and skin.[798] Five years after the onset of diabetes, hyalinosis of the efferent glomerular arterioles and early Kimmelstiel-Wilson nodules may be detectable.[799] Normal kidneys transplanted into diabetic recipients develop these changes within 4 y,[800] suggesting that an abnormal metabolic environment is causal. Conversely, transplantation of kidneys with established diabetic nephropathy into nondiabetic recipients is said to correct the thickened mesangial matrix and glomerular capillary basement membranes and to cause disappearance of arteriolar subintimal deposits.[801] This unique report has not been confirmed.

Natural History

The natural history of diabetic nephropathy is summarized in Table 21–19 and Figure 21–46. At the onset of diabetes the kidneys are usually enlarged[802] owing to increased glomerular and tubular size.[656, 657] When metabolic control is poor, the glomerular filtration rate is high.[802, 803] Microproteinuria (<550 mg protein/24 h), mainly albumin of glomerular origin, is present in suboptimally controlled patients and recedes after 72 h of intensive insulin treatment,[804] although the glomerular size remains above normal. Microproteinuria is not detected by reagent strips for urinary protein and requires immunoassay. The reversible component of microproteinuria is attributed to the hemodynamic abnormalities and to loss of charge selectivity of the glomerular membranes.[805, 806]

At first, microalbuminuria is present only after a provocative exercise test.[807] However, if microproteinuria exceeds 50

TABLE 21–19. Typical Clinical Course of Diabetic Nephropathy

Years After Onset of Diabetes	Clinical Course
0	Enlarged kidneys, supernormal function, microalbuminuria reversed by meticulous insulin treatment
2	Thickening of glomerular basement membrane and increase in mesangial matrix
10–15	Silent period: no overt proteinuria; microalbuminuria may be present, especially after exercise (>30 μg/min indicative of future proteinuria)
10–20	Proteinuric period intermittent at first, then persistent (>0.5 g/24 h), indicating that a relentless decline in glomerular function has begun
>15	Azotemic period begins on average 17 y after onset
20	Uremic period: diabetic retinopathy, hypertension, and nephrotic syndrome may be present

TABLE 21–20. Effects of Intervention Modalities

Test Parameter	Insulin (Insulin Pumps)	Antihypertensive: ACE Inhibition	Antihypertensive: Non-ACE Inhibition	Low-Protein Diet
Hyperfiltration (an elevated filtration fraction)	Long-term GFR ↓ ~5% (Aarhus)	Filtration fraction ↓ by ACE	No studies	↓ Hyperfiltration (Aarhus)
Borderline elevated UAE	Total normalization in a 4-y follow-up study (Oslo)	No studies	No studies	No studies
Persistent microalbuminuria (30–300 mg/24 h)	Stabilization (Gentofte)	Microalbuminuria somewhat ↓ (Paris)	Long-term regression of microalbuminuria (Aarhus)	Reduced in a small series on a short-term basis
Proteinuria without ↑ BP, possibly with ↓ GFR	No studies	Studies ongoing	No studies	Reduction of fall rate in GFR and reduced proteinuria according to preliminary studies (London, Dallas)
Proteinuria, ↑ BP, ↓ GFR	No effect seen in a small series (does not rule out an effect) (London)	In patients conventionally treated; additional ACE inhibitor may reduce progression (Goteborg)	Long-term treatment with cardioselective beta-blockers, diuretics, and vasodilators considerably reduces decline in GFR (Aarhus, Copenhagen)	

ACE, angiotensin-converting enzyme; UAE, urinary albumin excretion; BP, blood pressure; GFR, glomerular filtration rate; ↑, increased; ↓, decreased.
From Mogensen CE. Therapeutic interventions in nephropathy of IDDM. Diabetes Care 1988; 11(Suppl 1):10–15. Reproduced with permission of the American Diabetes Association, Inc.

day and serum creatinine of 2.5 mg/dL or less.[851] The prophylactic use of ACE inhibitors is under study.

Unless renal insufficiency is present, the goal of antihypertensive therapy should be a blood pressure of 120/80 mm Hg (standing). Side effects of antihypertensive drugs may be a greater problem in diabetic than in nondiabetic subjects. Hyperglycemia and impotence may be aggravated by thiazides and other antihypertensives, and the impairment of counterregulatory response to hypoglycemia by β-adrenergic blockade may predispose to serious episodes of hypoglycemia. Potassium must always be administered with caution in diabetic patients, because tolerance to exogenous potassium is impaired when potassium-stimulated increase in insulin secretion is reduced.[837] Hyporeninemic hypoaldosteronism, which may precede serious renal failure, accentuates this problem. A low-protein diet may reduce diabetic hyperfiltration,[852] diminish proteinuria,[853] and slow the rate of disease progression,[854] but low-protein diets are difficult to follow. The effects of various interventions are summarized in Table 21–20.

When the creatinine clearance rate falls below 20 mL/min, planning for the treatment of uremia by dialysis or kidney transplantation must begin. Hemodialysis is a widely used form of treatment with survival rates of approximately 50% at 3 y, 30% at 5 y, and 10% at 9 y.[855, 856] Some diabetic patients tolerate dialysis well, but for many the quality of life is compromised by cardiac, peripheral vascular, and ophthalmologic complications.[856, 857] Continuous ambulatory peritoneal dialysis is used by a subset of patients.[858]

Renal transplantation results in 5-y survival rates in some centers as high as 65% and 10-y rates approaching 45%.[856] Related-donor transplants and transplants between HLA-matched donors are even more successful.[856, 859] Retinopathy is said to be arrested or improved after successful renal transplantation in 80% of the recipients.[860] Meticulous postoperative control of diabetes is indicated in the hope of retarding the development of nephropathy in the transplanted kidney.

Hyporeninemic hypoaldosteronism with hyperchloremic acidosis should be treated with Shohl's solution (sodium citrate–citric acid) or sodium bicarbonate titrated to bring the bicarbonate concentration of plasma to about 22 mmol/L. In some cases fludrocortisone is required to control hyperkalemia.[833]

Pyelonephritis is an absolute indication for hospitalization in diabetic subjects. Treatment requires the intravenous administration of antibiotics.

Retinopathy

Although diabetes is a leading cause of adult blindness in the United States, the risk of blindness in an individual patient is low, probably less than 10%.[861, 862] Nevertheless, it is an ever-present fear for those with the disease. The retinopathy is usually categorized as background (simple) or proliferative (Table 21–21); these forms presumably represent different stages of the same pathophysiological process.

Background Retinopathy

Background retinopathy is present in 3% of diabetic Pima Indians at the time of diagnosis.[7] The prevalence increases with age, and after 25 to 30 y of disease at least 90% of patients have retinal lesions[863]; 99.5% of IDDM patients have some type of retinopathy after 15 y of disease, and 67% have proliferative retinopathy after 35 y of IDDM.[864]

Background or simple retinopathy includes dilation, constriction, and tortuosity of vessels; microaneurysms, dot-shaped inner retinal hemorrhages; dot-blot, linear, or flame-shaped preretinal hemorrhages; and hard or soft exudates. Hard exudates are caused by leakage of proteins and lipids from hyperpermeable capillaries and tend to form rings, often in the macular area. Cotton-wool exudates represent microinfarctions. A sudden increase in cotton-wool spots usually heralds a rapid progression of retinopathy. Hard exudates may coalesce into yellow patches and impair vision if they extend into the macular region. Microaneurysms of retinal capillaries, which are thought to develop subsequent to loss of supporting pericytes around the capillary wall, are transient, lasting from months to years (Fig. 21–47); they frequently become hyalin-

TABLE 21–21. Lesions of Diabetic Retinopathy

Background	Proliferative
Increased capillary permeability	New vessels
Capillary closure and dilation	Scar (retinitis proliferans)
Microaneurysms	Vitreal hemorrhage
Arteriovenous shunts	Retinal detachment
Dilated veins	
Hemorrhages (dot-blot)	
Cotton-wool spots	
Hard exudates	

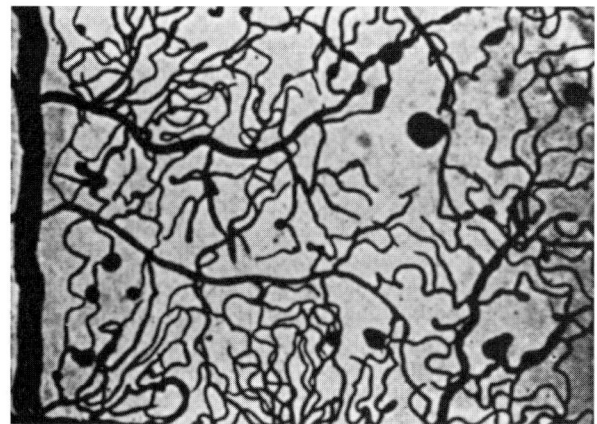

Figure 21–47. Capillary microaneurysms in diabetic retinopathy. India ink perfusion of retinal vessels. (From Ashton N. Arteriolar involvement in diabetic retinopathy. Br J Ophthalmol 1953; 37:282–292.)

ized and appear as whitish spots. Macular edema can lead to serious loss of vision.

Proliferative Retinopathy

Proliferative retinopathy, the most serious complication of diabetic ophthalmopathy, carries a high risk of vitreous hemorrhage, scarring, retinal detachment, and blindness (see Table 21–21).[863, 865] Although estimates vary widely, up to 10% of patients with IDDM develop proliferative retinopathy within 15 y, and more than 25% are affected after 20 to 50 y. Blindness develops in 40% of IDDM patients and in 60% of NIDDM patients within 5 y after the onset of proliferative retinopathy.[863] Because of associated nephropathy and coronary artery disease, proliferative retinopathy indicates poor prognosis for life as well as for vision. The initiating event in proliferative disease is new vessel formation. The new vessels radiate out from the optic disc or peripheral vessels, initially on the retinal surface unsupported by connective tissue, and may rupture and bleed into the vitreoretinal space. Ultimately they become encased in connective tissue, forming adhesions between the vitreal gel and the retina. Traction from the vitreous humor caused by glial proliferation may result in either hemorrhage or retinal detachment. Vitreal hemorrhage itself may stimulate contraction, leading to a lifting of the retina attached to it. Glial proliferation from the disc may also occur independently of vascularization and, if it covers the macula, may cause blindness.

Pathogenesis

Capillary vasodilation and hyperpermeability, basement membrane thickening, loss of endothelial cells and pericytes, focal occlusion of capillaries, and formation of arteriovenous shunts are thought to combine with abnormalities in the blood to cause retinal ischemia, the presumed first step in the pathogenesis of retinopathy (Fig. 21–48).[866] Factors leading to decreased blood flow in the retina are identical to those previously postulated to play a role in renal disease. These include increased blood viscosity,[867, 868] red blood cell sludging and aggregation,[699, 700] increased levels of fibrinogen, and diminished fibrinolysis related to inhibition of plasmin by increased concentrations of α_2-globulin[698, 869, 870] or increased activity of tPA inhibitor type 1.[728, 763] High levels of von Willebrand factor,[755] increased production of thromboxane A_2 by platelets,[753] and reduced prostacyclin production by endothelial cells[757] favor platelet aggregation. Other evidence,[758] discussed previously, argues against this provocative formulation.

Impaired release of oxygen from hemoglobin,[687, 817] resulting from the combined effect of increased HbA_{1c} and reduced 2,3-diphosphoglycerate levels, may contribute to local hypoxia. Increased vascular permeability is a very early lesion in the pathogenetic sequence[862]; osmotic stress or increased vesicular transport may play a role.[871, 872]

Ischemia probably stimulates compensatory new vessel formation, because similar neovascularization occurs in other conditions in which retinal oxygen content is diminished, such as sickle cell–hemoglobin C disease, polycythemia vera, and central retinal vein occlusion.[873] Capillary closure, the first step in neovascularization,[874, 875] causes fragmentation of the vascular basement membrane followed by migration of endothelial cells from the wall of the vessel into the interstitium to form capillary sprouts.[876] A local capillary growth factor may be involved, because fluid samples from eyes of patients with ocular neovascularization stimulate vascular endothelial cell migration and proliferation.[876] IGF-1 appears to be elevated in type I diabetic patients with proliferative and exudative retinopathy,[877] but VEGF is a candidate angiogenic factor released in response to retinal hypoxia.[878]

Diabetic retinopathy is thought to be caused by the altered metabolic state accompanying insulin deficiency, because background retinopathy appears in secondary diabetes caused by cystic fibrosis,[879] chronic pancreatitis, or total pancreatectomy.[880] The possibility that polyol pathway activity is involved is suggested by studies in galactose-fed animals. Such animals develop basement membrane thickening[712] and capillary microaneurysms[881] identical to the lesions in diabetes; the lesions can be prevented by treatment with an aldose reductase inhibitor.[712] Capillary leakage may result from a dysfunctional endothelium caused by AGE, because blockade of the receptor for AGE reverses vascular hyperpermeability in diabetic rats.[882]

The enzymes for sorbitol formation are present in the retina,[883] and support for a causal role of the polyol pathway in diabetic retinopathy comes from studies indicating that retinopathy in animals[713] and alteration of the blood-retina barrier in humans[884] can be prevented or reversed by inhibitors of aldose reductase.

Genetic determinants may also be operative.[885] IDDM patients with HLA-DR4 who are negative for DR3 are five times more likely to develop proliferative retinopathy than those negative for both DR4 and DR3.[86] In one study an allele (Z-2) of the aldose reductase gene was associated with early-onset retinopathy.[864]

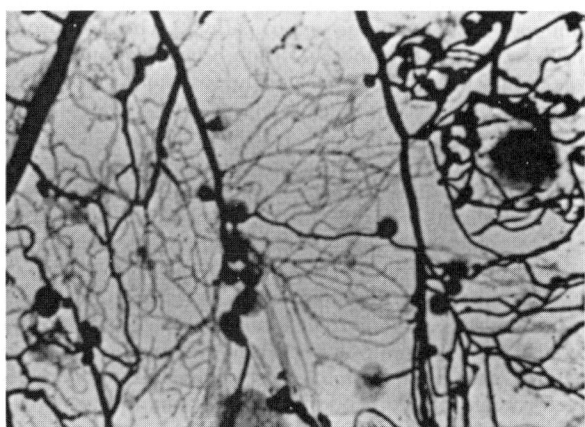

Figure 21–48. Retinal nonperfusion in diabetic retinopathy. Combined India ink perfusion and trypsin digestion. Note central area of nonperfusion with remaining acellular capillaries. (Photograph by N. Ashton. From Bresnick GH, Segal P, Mattson D. Fluorescein angiographic and clinicopathologic findings. In: Little HL, Jack RL, Patz A, et al., eds. Diabetic Retinopathy. New York: Thieme-Stratton, 1983: 37–71.)

electrocardiogram running and marked at inspiratory and expiratory points. Maximal and minimal R-R intervals are measured and converted to heart rate. Immediate heart rate response to standing is tested by measuring the R-R interval at the 15th and 30th beats after the patient rises from a supine to an upright posture. The result is reported as the 30:15 ratio.

Blood pressure response to standing is determined by using the fall in systolic blood pressure on standing as the test marker. Blood pressure response to static exercise is tested with a hand grip dynamometer. Maximal effort is determined first, and the blood pressure is assessed after 5 min of exertion at 30% of maximum. The blood pressure normally rises during isometric exercise. Three basal diastolic pressures are compared with the highest diastolic pressure developed during hand grip.

Although normal values for these tests must be established for each laboratory,[928] standard interpretations are given in Table 21–22. An alternative test is a "squat test" (SqT), which compares favorably with other tests of cardiovascular autonomic neuropathy in diabetes. The squat test is said to be more sensitive than other single tests in identifying mild autonomic involvement, and it provides information on both parasympathetic and sympathetic function.[941] The patient stands still for 3 min, squats for 1 min, and then stands up again during an inspiratory phase. The ratio of the R-R interval mean before squatting and the longest R-R interval after squatting is the SqT vagal (SqTv). The ratio of the basal R-R interval and the shortest R-R interval at standing is the SqT sympathetic (SqTs). Forty-two percent of diabetic patients had an SqTv outside the 99% confidence interval, and 40% had an abnormal SqTs.[941]

Cause of Neuropathy

There are three major hypotheses about the cause of diabetic neuropathy: the vascular hypothesis, the axonal hypothesis, and the metabolic hypothesis.[894, 942, 943] Ischemic disease of arterioles is generally acknowledged as a primary cause of mononeuropathy, but microvascular disease also contributes to other forms of neuropathy.[943] The axonal hypothesis supposes that early slow axonal transport is followed by structural degeneration.[944]

The metabolic abnormalities have been studied in diabetic rats, in which the *myo*-inositol content of nerves and motor conduction velocity decrease in parallel.[718] However, the *myo*-inositol content in sural nerves is not decreased in human diabetic patients either with or without neuropathy.[718] Mean endoneural glucose, fructose, and sorbitol values are elevated in diabetic patients, and the sorbitol content of nerves is inversely related to the number of myelinated fibers. In animals both defects can be repaired by meticulous control of diabetes or by feeding *myo*-inositol. Hyperglycemia lowers the *myo*-inositol content of Schwann cells and axons, probably

by the following sequence: hyperglycemia → increased sorbitol-fructose → decreased *myo*-inositol in Schwann cells and axons → decreased phosphoinositol turnover → decreased Na$^+$,K$^+$-ATPase activity → abnormal energy metabolism → nerve dysfunction → structural damage.[710, 713, 894, 942] Treatment of affected animals with a polyol pathway inhibitor prevents the fall in *myo*-inositol content and the decrease in ATPase activity, thereby reversing the functional abnormalities. Inhibition of aldol reductase partially restores structural defects in sural nerves of patients with diabetic neuropathy[514] but produces only minor improvement in nerve function. In established neuropathy, structural changes may be so advanced that it is too late to correct metabolic abnormalities. The role of glycosylated myelin, if any, is not known.[701]

Treatment of Diabetic Neuropathy

There is no specific therapy for diabetic neuropathy. Tight regulation of blood glucose may improve nerve conduction, but vibratory sense does not change and clinical benefit is limited. In 13 diabetic patients with normoglycemia for 2 y after combined pancreatic and renal transplantation, sensory neuropathy and autonomic dysfunction were not reversed even though nerve conduction improved.[945] Because there was little difference in clinical improvement between this group and a group of diabetic patients who received only a kidney graft, it was the correction of uremia rather than "cure" of hyperglycemia that played an ameliorating role. Although successful pancreas transplantation can halt the progression of diabetic polyneuropathy, improvement in the manifestations of neuropathy is minor even after sustained metabolic normalization.[946] Painful neuropathy should be treated first with mild analgesics, followed by nonsteroidal anti-inflammatory drugs. Although phenytoin[947] and carbamazepine[948] have been recommended, the authors do not find them helpful. In severe cases a trial of amitriptyline, 75 mg at bedtime, with or without fluphenazine, 1 mg three times daily, may be of benefit.[949] Desipramine appears to be as effective as amitriptyline, but fluoxetine, a serotonin uptake inhibitor, is not more effective than placebo.[950]

Aldol reductase inhibitors are used to inhibit polyol accumulation in tissues in the hope of preventing diabetic complications such as neuropathy despite hyperglycemia. The reduced nerve conduction velocity associated with experimental diabetes in rats can be reversed by correction of hyperglycemia with insulin,[718] by supplementation of the diet with *myo*-inositol,[718, 949, 951] or by administration of an aldose reductase inhibitor[952] such as sorbinil[953] or epalrestat.[954] As noted, sorbinil prevents fluorescence of collagen in diabetic rats,[515] suggesting a link between the polyol pathway and nonenzymatic glycosylation.

Because of complications[955] and because the benefits have been marginal[956, 957] sorbinil is no longer undergoing trials.[958] However, epalrestat and tolrestat reportedly improved motor nerve conduction, pain, and numbness.[959, 960] No aldose inductase inhibitors are on the market in the United States, but epalrestat and tolrestat are available in Europe.

Peripheral Vascular Disease

Peripheral atherosclerosis in diabetic patients is similar to that found in control subjects, but it begins at an earlier age, advances more rapidly, and is more common.[961, 962] Leg and foot amputations are five times more common in diabetic patients.[963] Bilateral lesions and distal arterial occlusions of small and medium-sized arteries below the knee are common,[961, 964] and, together with microvascular disease and neuropathic lesions, cause the increase in gangrene. Lipid abnor-

TABLE 21–22. Normal and Abnormal Values in Tests of Autonomic Function

Test	Normal	Borderline	Abnormal
Parasympathetic (heart rate response)			
Valsalva (Valsalva ratio)	≥1.21	1.11–1.20	≤1.10
Deep breathing (max:min HR)	≥15 beats/min	11–14 beats/min	≤10 beats/min
Standing (30:15 ratio R-R)	≥1.04	1.01–1.03	≤1.00
Sympathetic (blood pressure response)			
Standing (↓ systolic)	≤10 mm Hg	11–29 mm Hg	≥30 mm Hg
Exercise (↑ diastolic)	≥16 mm Hg	11–15 mm Hg	≤10 mm Hg

Adapted from Dyrberg T, Benn J, Christiansen JS, et al. Prevalence of diabetic autonomic neuropathy measured by simple bedside tests. Diabetologia 1981;20:190–194.

malities, smoking, and hypertension are added risk factors for gangrene.[965]

Intermittent claudication can occur in the calf, thigh, or buttocks. Pain at rest can result from diabetic neuropathy or ischemia; it tends to be relieved by dependency of the lower extremities. The need to sleep in a chair may lead to the development of dependent edema. The skin of the leg may be atrophic, hairless, and cold with thickened toenails caused by fungal infection. There is pallor and a delayed refilling after elevation and subsequent lowering of the leg. Despite vascular insufficiency, the dorsalis pedis and posterior tibial pulses may be palpable.

Noninvasive evaluation of peripheral vascular disease has traditionally utilized Doppler-assisted blood pressure measurements, but these may not be accurate in diabetic subjects.[558] Measurement of the transcutaneous oxygen tension appears to be a better technique.[966, 967] Definitive study requires arteriography, but there is a significant risk.

Treatment of peripheral vascular disease is unsatisfactory. Vasodilators may be harmful because of reduced collateral blood flow to an ischemic area.[968] Sympathectomy is ineffective, perhaps because autonomic neuropathy has already produced an "autosympathectomy."[969] Vascular surgery is the only option, but the risks of arteriography are high. After intravenous pyelography, for example, exacerbation of renal disease occurs in about three fourths of patients whose creatinine levels exceed 180 μmol/L (2 mg/dL).[970] Indications for arteriography include nocturnal or rest pain, ulcerations that fail to respond to optimal medical treatment, and gangrene. Obstructions of the aorta and iliac arteries can be treated by endarterectomy. For obstructions below the inguinal ligament, saphenous vein bypass graft may be helpful. Most such grafts lose function within a decade, and reoperation is usually unsuccessful.[971] Angioplasty to fracture obstructing plaques is under study.[972, 973]

Although conservative amputation should be attempted for gangrene, failure rates for distal amputations are high when macrovascular disease is a major contributor (50% for digits and >30% for transmetatarsal amputation), requiring more proximal amputations. Arteriography and segmental pressure and pulse measurements have poor predictability for stump healing, but measurements of blood flow have been helpful. In one study amputations at sites with a blood flow of more than 2.6 mL/100 g of tissue per minute invariably healed, but healing did not occur if the flow was less than 2.0 mL/100 g tissue/min.[971]

PREGNANCY IN DIABETES

Maternal Fuel-Hormone Physiology in Normal Pregnancy

In the first trimester of a nondiabetic pregnancy the action of insulin is enhanced by estrogens and progesterone, and glucose levels tend to decrease[974] (see Chapter 27). By contrast, in late pregnancy glucose tolerance is slightly reduced, and insulin levels increase,[975] suggesting insulin resistance.[976] This resistance is in part related to human placental lactogen, an insulin antagonist that increases in concentration in proportion to the placental mass.[975, 977] The insulin resistance of pregnancy appears to be a postreceptor phenomenon.[978] Because delivery of the fuels required for the growth and oxidative needs of the fetus is a function of the maternal fuel concentration and placental blood flow, resistance to insulin action in the maternal circulation raises the mean levels of glucose and other nutrients in the maternal circulation, thereby shunting a larger amount of glucose and amino

acids from the mother to the fetus in the last half of pregnancy, the time of maximal fetal growth.[979]

The maternal adjustment to fetal needs has been characterized as "accelerated starvation." Fasting during pregnancy in animals elicits higher rates of lipolysis,[980] ketogenesis,[981] and gluconeogenesis[982] than in the nonpregnant state, and it is assumed that similar changes occur in women. Therefore, the omission of a single meal, which is a routine procedure before laboratory tests, may have a significant metabolic impact on the pregnant woman and could be dangerous if ketone bodies are teratogenic, as has been reported.[975, 983]

In a mother with borderline beta-cell function the metabolic changes of pregnancy cause gestational diabetes. With pre-existing diabetes an increased insulin dosage is needed.

Infant of the Diabetic Mother

In the United States there are more than 400,000 diabetic women of reproductive age, and approximately 1 in 100 pregnant nondiabetic women has carbohydrate intolerance.[984] Despite attempts to treat diabetes aggressively during pregnancy, the fetal and neonatal death rates of infants of diabetic mothers are higher than normal.[985] Table 21–23 lists some of the disorders encountered in such infants. Infants of mothers with gestational diabetes experience fewer perinatal problems than those of overtly diabetic mothers.

Macrosomia (oversized fetus) is the most common neonatal abnormality. Because insulin does not cross the placenta, the metabolism of maternal substrates by the fetus depends on fetal insulin. In a normal pregnancy the postprandial maternal nutrients that cross to the fetus, particularly amino acids, stimulate the secretion of fetal insulin and other growth factors. The fetal glucose concentration parallels the narrow range of blood glucose levels of the nondiabetic mother. In a diabetic pregnancy fetal nutrient levels reflect the elevated maternal levels. If the diabetes in the mother is poorly controlled, hyperglycemia and hyperaminoacidemia cause fetal hyperinsulinemia and hyperplasia of beta cells in the fetal pancreas. Whereas in normal pregnancy the fetal beta cells are stimulated predominantly by amino acids rather than by glucose,[986] in a poorly controlled diabetic pregnancy the fetal beta cells respond to elevated glucose levels as vigorously as in the adult.[987, 988] The resulting hyperinsulinemia stimulates fetal growth, which from the 30th week of gestation onward correlates with amniotic fluid insulin level[989] and the maternal concentration of HbA$_{1c}$.[990] The birth weight and length of infants of diabetic mothers with poorly controlled disease average 550 g and 1.5 cm greater than normal, respectively.[991] Subcutaneous adipose tissue is increased, and most organs, including the liver, are enlarged.[989] The size of the brain is not increased. Because of hyperinsulinemia, infants of diabetic mothers should be monitored for hypoglycemia during the first hours and days of life.

Fetal hyperglycemia causes delay in lung maturation, and the incidence of respiratory distress syndrome is increased

TABLE 21–23. Abnormalities Encountered in Infants of Diabetic Mothers

Macrosomia	Renal vein thrombosis
Hypoglycemia	Persistence of fetal circulation
Hypocalcemia	Cardiomyopathy
Respiratory distress syndrome	Congenital heart disease
Polycythemia	Caudal regression syndrome
Hyperbilirubinemia	Miscellaneous congenital anomalies

Adapted by permission of Elsevier Science Publishing Co., Inc., from Fleischman AR, Finberg L. The infant of the diabetic mother and diabetes in infancy. In: Ellenburg M, Rifkin H, eds. Diabetes Mellitus. Theory and Practice. 3rd ed. New Hyde Park, NY: Medical Examination Publishing, 1983: 715–725. Copyright 1983 by Medical Examination Publishing Company, Inc.

should be observed for at least 2 or 3 d before making another increase. However, if unexplained hypoglycemia occurs (not accounted for by a skipped meal or unusual exercise), an immediate reduction in insulin dose is required.

In most patients with IDDM, control of symptoms is achieved with relative ease with conventional regimens. However, although the catabolic state is eliminated and glycosuria is minimized, postprandial hyperglycemia and levels of glycosylated hemoglobin are not normal. For other patients, life is a series of dose readjustments that never succeed in eliminating either hyperglycemic or hypoglycemic fluctuations.[1032] The reasons for this brittleness are not understood. Dietary inconsistency may play a role, and stress or tension, acting through counterregulatory hormone release, probably is important in many. Variations in the absorption of insulin and fluctuating insulin antibody levels may contribute in others.[1032, 1033] The maintenance of even minimal secretory capacity of residual beta cells is an important factor in glycemic stability in IDDM patients.[1034] The C peptide response to glucose (a measure of endogenous insulin secretion) correlates with stability in that patients with little or no response tend to be unstable. Intravenous glucagon testing may stimulate a rise in C peptide levels in diabetics previously considered to have no residual beta-cell function.[1034] C peptide nonresponders are more apt to develop neuroglucopenia during insulin clamping tests and are less able to increase endogenous glucagon secretion with hypoglycemia than are C peptide responders. Alterations in gastric emptying may contribute to instability. Usually the precise problem is never identified. The presence of brittle diabetes is an indication for attempts at meticulous control. In some patients a chronic catabolic state leaves the liver depleted of glycogen, thereby removing the primary substrate for defense against hypoglycemia; if so, a period of a high-carbohydrate feeding and increased insulin may be useful to replenish glycogen stores.

Patients who monitor metabolic control solely by urine testing should obtain the prebreakfast specimen 30 min after voiding the overnight contents of the bladder. They should be taught that 4+ glycosuria in a small volume of urine does not signify as much glucose loss as 4+ glycosuria in a large volume of urine. If home glucose monitoring is not possible, measurement of the glycosylated hemoglobin level provides a more accurate picture of control than do random glucose determinations in the physician's office.[1035, 1036] Glycosylated hemoglobin values are useful in all patients because the test provides a check on the accuracy of home monitoring of capillary blood glucose levels.

Meticulous Control

Maintenance of the plasma glucose level in the normal range throughout the day reduces long-term complications of diabetes. To achieve meticulous control the patient must be willing and able to make a formidable commitment of time, effort, and money, and the physician must determine whether the clinical situation justifies the effort before advising such a course. First, the competence and willingness of the patient to assume the role of physician's assistant must be determined. Second, the potential clinical benefit must justify the venture. For example, pregnancy and renal transplantation in diabetic patients *demand* meticulous control. In most patients with complication-free IDDM the proven advantages of meticulous control in preventing complications make it a reasonable but not obligatory therapeutic option. For persons whose life expectancy is limited by advanced age, by the presence of established diabetic complications, by cardiovascular or cerebrovascular disease, or by any life-shortening condition, a rigorous program is rarely justified on the basis of potential benefits.[845] Even successful pancreatic transplantation that results in per-

manent normoglycemia fails to reverse or even to stem the progression of early or advanced proliferative retinopathy[1037] or neuropathy.[945] Put simply, aggressive insulin therapy with a goal of achieving normoglycemia should be considered mandatory in pregnancy and renal transplantation, highly desirable in all IDDM patients at the onset of their disease, and desirable for any patient with established IDDM in whom no absolute or relative contraindication exists (see later discussion).

REGIMENS OF METICULOUS CONTROL

Regimens intended to achieve meticulous control must attempt to mimic the normal diurnal profile of endogenous insulin release. In nondiabetic subjects insulin levels rise spontaneously in response to an increase in glucose concentrations in plasma. In IDDM the normal glucose-sensing system and the endogenous insulin source are missing, so the patient must be trained to substitute for both. Plasma glucose levels must be measured several times each day (up to seven times daily), and appropriate doses of insulin must be given. This can be accomplished in two ways: intensified multiple subcutaneous injections or use of a CSII device.

The glycemic goals of intensive therapy in the DCCT program were 3.9 to 6.7 mmol/L (70 to 120 mg/dL) fasting and preprandial and less than 10 mmol/L (<180 mg/dL) postprandially with glucose less than 3.6 mmol/L (<65 mg/dL) at 3 AM. The HbA$_{1c}$ goal was to remain within 2 standard deviations of the nondiabetic mean level.[652] Figure 21–49 shows that these goals are attainable.

INTENSIFIED MULTIPLE SUBCUTANEOUS INSULIN INJECTIONS. Several doses of insulin are administered throughout the day, the amounts based on self-monitoring of glucose by a reflectance meter or chemical strip. Various programs are available, and the physician custom designs a system for each patient (Table 21–24). In general, regular insulin is given before each meal.[1038–1040] Basal coverage is provided either by intermediate-acting insulin (NPH or Lente) given before bedtime or by long-acting insulin (PZI or Ultralente) given together with regular insulin before the evening meal. In the former schedule, four injections a day are required: evening intermediate insulin and regular insulin before each meal. With long-acting insulin, only three injections are needed: regular before breakfast and lunch, and long-acting plus regular before supper. For patients who object to multiple injections, a button infuser permits injections through a nee-

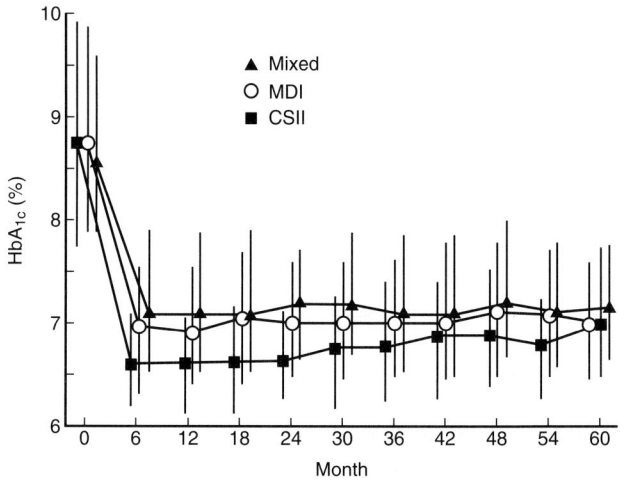

Figure 21–49. Comparison of HbA$_{1c}$ in patients with IDDM treated with continuous subcutaneous insulin infusion (CSII), multiple daily injections of insulin (MDI), or a mixture of both (mixed).

TABLE 21–24. Intensified Multiple Subcutaneous Insulin Injections: Typical Schedule*

	Plasma Glucose, mmol/L (mg/dL)		Appropriate Change in Insulin Dosage	
	Fasting	*Pre- or Postprandial*	*Intermediate Units*	*Regular Units*
Initiation or readjustment of therapy	>5 (>90) <3.3 (<60)	>7.8 (>140) <3.3 (<60)	+2 −2	+2 −2
Daily therapy		<3.3 (<60)		−2
		3.3–5 (60–90)		No change
		5–6.7 (90–120)		+1
		6.7–8.3 (120–150)		+2
		8.3–11.1 (150–200)		+3
		11.1–13.9 (200–250)		+4
		>13.9 (250)		+6

*For initial therapy 0.6–0.7 U/kg/d is given, 25% NPH or Lente, 75% regular. Intermediate insulin is given at 2100 h and is changed every 48 h solely on the basis of the fasting plasma glucose level. In the initiation phase the regular insulin dose for each meal is based on the postprandial glucose value from the previous day. Once the therapeutic plan is developed, alterations in the daily insulin dose are based on immediate preprandial glucose values. If seven- or eight-point glucose testing shows the overall pattern of glycemia to have changed, readjustment can be carried out in a fashion similar to initiation. This plan should be considered only a guide. Responses vary, so that treatment in each patient must be custom designed.
Data from Schiffrin A, Belmonte MM. Comparison between continuous subcutaneous insulin infusion and multiple injections of insulin. Diabetes 1982;31:255–264. Copyright © 1982, by the American Diabetes Association.

dle port that is inserted once daily. Alternatively, a 23- or 25-gauge butterfly needle may be inserted into the abdominal wall and replaced every 5 d.[1041, 1042]

For the initiation of therapy in a person not previously treated with insulin, 0.6 to 0.7 U/kg/d is a reasonable starting dose.[1038] For persons already taking insulin, a slight reduction of 20 to 30% is suggested if the daily dose is greater than 1.0 U/kg. In the four-dose schedule, about 25% of the daily insulin is given as NPH before bedtime (9 to 10 PM), and the remaining 75% is given as regular insulin distributed so that a slightly larger amount is given before breakfast—e.g., 30% breakfast, 22.5% lunch, 22.5% supper. Adjustment of intermediate insulin is based on the fasting plasma glucose level, changes being made at 2-d intervals. Similarly, the regular insulin dosage is altered, depending on the postprandial values during the previous day (see Table 21–24). After a reasonable pattern has been obtained, a sliding scale is prescribed to guide daily dosage adjustments. Capillary glucose measurement can be limited to fasting and premeal measurements during stable periods, with periodic resumption of a full seven- or eight-point schedule to confirm that the shorter profile is accurate. Three-dose insulin schedules using Ultralente can be handled according to the same general scheme, although a higher percentage of the total daily dose is given as Ultralente, usually 40 to 60%.

Intensive multiple injection regimens can be effective and

yield results equivalent to those obtained with insulin infusion pumps.[1038, 1043] However, such therapy requires never-ending surveillance, which only the patient can provide. Consequently, intensive training in blood glucose measurement, insulin therapy, and meal composition is essential. Simple lectures and films are not sufficient. After a training program the patient's competence should be tested to certify the capability for self-care.

CONTINUOUS SUBCUTANEOUS INSULIN INFUSION.
Meticulous regulation of blood glucose and a greater flexibility of lifestyle can be achieved by CSII with a portable insulin infusion device.[1044–1047] The available instruments vary in cost and sophistication. Insulin is delivered through an indwelling 25-gauge scalp vein needle that is positioned under the abdominal skin and connected to the pump by a catheter. The needle site is changed at least every other day to avoid infection and needle blockage.

Insulin is infused at a constant basal rate (usually 0.5 to 2.0 U/h), with a bolus given before meals. The basal rate can be programmed for automatic delivery of up to four different basal rates in a 24-h period.[1048] Most patients require only one or two basal rates per day, the lower rate to supply low nocturnal requirements and the higher rate to cope with early-morning hyperglycemia, the so-called dawn phenomenon. The pump is programmed to deliver boluses 30 min before meals. Conversion to pump therapy requires 3 to 5 d of inpatient training to obtain good results. One may begin with the same total daily dose of insulin that was being given with conventional treatment or decrease it by 20 to 30% if large amounts (>1 U/kg/d) are being used. For first-time therapy, 0.6 to 0.7 U/kg/d is reasonable. From 40 to 50% of the dose is administered basally at a constant rate, and the remainder is given before the three meals in burst fashion over a 30-min period. For example, a 60-kg patient who had been receiving 24 U of intermediate insulin per day with conventional therapy would begin with a basal rate of 12 U/d (0.5 U/h), which would be adjusted downward if the 3 AM glucose level were lower than 4.4 mmol/L (80 mg/dL) or upward if the 7 AM value were higher than 7.8 mmol/L (140 mg/dL). The remaining 50% of the previous dose would be used to mimic normal meal-induced insulin release. A typical preprandial variable insulin dose schedule appears in Table 21–25. Despite its lower caloric content, breakfast requires a larger bolus than the evening meal. CSII can result in return of diurnal glucose to near-normal levels, at least in an ideal setting. Such results may not be achievable when large groups of patients are followed in a busy clinical practice. For example, in a group of 100 patients cared for in a private clinic, the mean fasting glucose value decreased from 11 mmol/L (200 mg/dL) during conventional therapy to 8.8 mmol/L (158 mg/dL) during pump therapy. Equivalent figures for nonfasting values were 11.8 mmol/L (213 mg/dL) and 8 mmol/L (145 mg/dL), respectively.[1048] Children have more difficulty in attaining good

TABLE 21–25. Typical Variable Insulin Schedule for a Patient Receiving CSII*

Capillary Blood Glucose		Units of Insulin Before					
mmol/L	*mg/dL*	*Breakfast*	*Snack*	*Lunch*	*Snack*	*Dinner*	*Snack*
<2.8	<50	5	0	3	0	3	0
2.8–5.6	51–100	6	0.5	4	0.5	5	0
5.6–8.3	101–150	7	1	5	1	6	1
8.3–11.1	151–200	8	1.5	6	1.5	7	1.5
11.1–13.9	201–250	9	2	7	2	8	2
13.9–16.7	251–300	10	2.5	8	2.5	9	2.5
>16.7	>300			Call health care team			

* About 50% of the daily insulin dose is given at a constant basal rate, the remainder being administered as a bolus 15 to 30 min before meals, depending on preprandial glucose value; e.g., if blood glucose is 230 before dinner, 7 U of insulin is given. Basal rate adjustments are usually made from the 3 AM glucose level and are decreased for any value lower than 80 mg/dL.
Adapted from Raskin P. Treatment of insulin-dependent diabetes mellitus with portable insulin infusion device. Med Clin North Am 1982; 66:1269–1283.

control than adults do.[1048] The requirements for education and training of patients for CSII are even more stringent than those recommended for intensive conventional therapy.

Specific complications of pump therapy include cutaneous abscesses that can be serious (in one case fatal sepsis resulted), subcutaneous lumps, severe diabetic decompensation (including ketoacidosis) caused by undetected interruption of insulin delivery, hypoglycemia, and death.[1049]

IMPLANTABLE INTRAPERITONEAL PUMPS. Despite its success, the DCCT study achieved only near-normoglycemia when insulin was administered by CSII or by multiple injection and caused an increased frequency of severe hypoglycemia.[652] A study of implantable intraperitoneal pumps programmed to permit variable insulin delivery rates in 224 IDDM patients followed for 353 patient-years reported better glycemic control (HbA$_{1c}$ 6.8% versus 7.4%) and fewer hypoglycemic episodes (2.5 versus 15.2 per 100 patient-years) than with intensive subcutaneous insulin therapy.[1050] These pumps (made by Merrumed, Sylman, USA, by Infusaid, Boston, USA, and by Siemens, Solna, Sweden) are implanted in the subcutaneous fat of the lower left abdomen, and the catheter tip is inserted into the peritoneal cavity. They are refilled at 1- to 3-month intervals. Infection is rare, but catheter blockages frequently require surgical intervention.

BENEFITS OF METICULOUS CONTROL

In addition to the delay or prevention of diabetic complications, other benefits include near-normal levels of amino acids, plasma glycoproteins, FFAs, triglycerides, LDL and HDL cholesterol, lactate, and pyruvate.[1051, 1052] Plasma glucagon levels and the responses of growth hormone and catecholamine to exercise become normal. Rapid healing of recalcitrant foot ulcers has been reported after 6 to 8 wk of CSII, and, if confirmed, would become a cautious indication for its use in patients with advanced complications.[1053] Neuropathic components of the diabetic syndrome, such as gastroparesis, may improve with enhanced diabetic control.[925]

As stated previously, good control without hypoglycemia is obligatory in every diabetic pregnancy and should be started before conception to protect the fetus from congenital disease. The same applies to the recipient of a renal transplant, the goal of meticulous control being protection of the transplanted kidney from the microvascular disease that afflicts the recipient.

RISKS OF METICULOUS CONTROL

ACCELERATION OF RETINOPATHY. Acceleration of retinopathy is not a common complication,[660, 1049, 1054–1056] but amelioration of severe retinopathy cannot be expected. Although deterioration is always a matter of concern when patients with this complication are subjected to meticulous control, the progression of early retinopathy slowed in the DCCT study.[649] Established proliferative retinopathy does not appear to improve or to stabilize after "cure" of diabetes by pancreas transplantation.[1037] In dogs with alloxan-caused diabetes, microaneurysms and other lesions that develop during 60 mo of hyperglycemia can be inhibited by good control beginning at the onset of the diabetes. However, if 30 mo of poor control precedes 30 mo of good control, retinopathy develops during the period of good control,[1057] suggesting that, after the process has begun, good glycemic control is not necessarily beneficial.

Although there are exceptions, pump therapy and intensive conventional therapy are usually contraindicated in patients with severe coronary artery disease, cerebrovascular disease, renal failure, proliferative retinopathy, or advanced autonomic neuropathy.[845] Background retinopathy is not a

contraindication, but frequent ophthalmologic surveillance is required to detect accelerated neovascularization.[660, 661] Although frank renal failure is a strong contraindication, proteinuria with or without mild azotemia does not preclude aggressive insulin therapy. Such therapy may reverse microproteinuria[804] but has not been documented to reverse renal failure.[1058]

SEVERE NEUROGLUCOPENIA. Thirty-five mostly unexpected deaths were reported in North America early after the introduction of CSII therapy.[1059] Many occurred at night during sleep, suggesting hypoglycemia as the cause. There was little evidence of deliberate or inadvertent overdosing of insulin, and pumps did not malfunction. Furthermore, the death rate in patients given CSII was not excessive for IDDM,[1059] and some of the deaths occurred in patients with contraindications for meticulous control as outlined. Incompetence, psychiatric problems, or motivational defects made others unsuitable for a self-care regimen.[845] More recent studies report no excess deaths.[649–651] Had stringent criteria for selection of patients been applied, most of these early mishaps might have been avoided. Recommended criteria for selection of patients for meticulous control by multiple subcutaneous injections or by CSII are listed in Table 21–26. Despite these difficulties, CSII is now a commonly used means of obtaining superior glycemic control in IDDM patients.[1060] Furthermore, it appears that intensified insulin therapy carried out in the setting of a university diabetes center can safely and effectively be transferred to a general medicine clinic.[1061]

Nocturnal hypoglycemia is a danger for any patient being treated by intensive conventional or pump therapy, and that danger is enhanced if counterregulatory defenses are impaired. In many patients given intensive treatment regimens, glucose levels reach a nadir at 3 AM and rise by 1 to 6 mmol/L (20 to 100 mg/dL) at 7 AM. This early morning rise, known as the dawn phenomenon, is thought to be caused by nocturnal surges of the counterregulatory hormones, glucagon, epinephrine, cortisol, and growth hormone.[941] The rise in glucose level is a result of increased hepatic glucose production and decreased glucose clearance.

A normal 7 AM glucose level may signify that the glucose concentration was dangerously low at 3 AM; only a glucose determination in the early morning hours can exclude this possibility. In pumps with programming capabilities it is possible to reduce the basal rate after midnight and increase it before 7 AM. Alternatively, one can accept a slightly elevated 7 AM glucose level and, by reducing the breakfast and raising the prebreakfast insulin bolus, achieve near-normal glucose levels by midmorning. The dawn phenomenon occurs in approximately 89% of patients with IDDM. The longer the duration of the diabetes, the smaller the dawn phenomenon, be-

TABLE 21–26. Criteria for Selection of Patients for Meticulous Control in Diabetes

Indications	Contraindications
Absolute	Absolute
Pregnancy	Counterregulatory failure
Postrenal transplantation	Unwillingness or inability for any reason to assume full responsibility for acceptable implementation of a diabetes self-care program
Relative	Relative
Otherwise healthy patient unable to normalize hemoglobin A$_{1c}$ or achieve other therapeutic objectives*	Life expectancy <10 y
	Diabetic retinopathy or nephropathy
	Cerebrovascular disease
	Cardiovascular disease

* Other objectives could include greater well-being, greater resistance to infection, improved healing of foot ulcers, normalization of lipid profile, improvement in gastroparesis.

cause of attenuation in the response of counterregulatory hormones to predawn hypoglycemia.[1062]

Exercise-induced hypoglycemia tends to be less dangerous than nocturnal hypoglycemia because the patient is awake and can usually take appropriate measures or obtain help. Counterregulatory hormone release does not appear to be significantly impaired in type II NIDDM.[1063]

Avoidance of hypoglycemia should have an even higher priority than avoidance of hyperglycemia. It is probable that if the criteria for selection of patients listed in Table 21–26 were stringently applied and a strategy were designed for avoidance of hypoglycemia, meticulous control would be as safe as conventional therapy. Some investigators have suggested that all patients considered for intensive insulin therapy should be tested for counterregulatory response beforehand.[1064]

Complications of Conventional Insulin Therapy

HYPOGLYCEMIA

Clinical manifestations of hypoglycemia are caused by epinephrine release or central nervous system manifestations. The epinephrine symptoms (perspiration, tachycardia, tremor, pallor, and a subjective feeling of uneasiness) occur early, before the hypoglycemia becomes profound. The central nervous system manifestations (changes in personality or behavior, confusion, obtundation, convulsions, and coma) develop after the arterial glucose level has fallen too low to meet cerebral needs. Nocturnal hypoglycemia may be manifested by nightmares, night sweats, and morning headache. Occasionally, patients with cerebrovascular disease develop focal neurologic signs as a result of reduced delivery of glucose to hypoperfused areas of the brain, sometimes in the absence of serious systemic hypoglycemia. In such patients, meticulous control carries a high risk of further neurologic damage.

If the patient is conscious, a sweet drink, sugar, or candy should be ingested. All insulin-treated patients should carry carbohydrate and identification that indicates that they have diabetes. In unconscious subjects glucose must be administered intravenously, or 1 mg glucagon can be injected intramuscularly. Glucagon availability is particularly important for insulin-treated diabetics who live in rural areas without quick access to medical facilities, but any hypoglycemia-prone, insulin-requiring diabetic patient should have a vial of glucagon on hand.

WHY THE VULNERABILITY FOR HYPOGLYCEMIA IN IDDM? During exercise or prolonged fasting, normal persons are protected from hypoglycemia by a decrease in insulin level and a rise in levels of glucagon and catecholamines, which themselves modulate changes in islet hormone secretion. The decrease in insulin reduces glucose utilization by insulin-requiring tissues, enhances the release of FFAs from adipocytes, and disinhibits glucagon secretion, thereby increasing hepatic glucose production sufficiently to maintain normal glucose levels and ensure fuel for the brain. In the patient with insulin-treated IDDM, insulin levels cannot decrease with exercise or fasting. Therefore, glucose utilization does not decrease, and FFA release continues to be inhibited. Moreover, continuing suppression of glucagon secretion by insulin eliminates glucagon's opposition to the hepatic effects of insulin on hepatic glucose and ketone production. The diabetic patient is vulnerable to hypoglycemia under conditions that do not impose risks for normal persons.

COUNTERREGULATORY FAILURE. An impaired ability to prevent hypoglycemia is probably characteristic of IDDM, but correction usually occurs through secretion of counterregulatory hormones (see Table 21–15).[1065–1069] However, in some patients with long-standing IDDM this ability wanes.[1067–1069] In normal subjects insulin-induced hypoglycemia elicits an increase in the levels of glucagon, catecholamines, cortisol, and growth hormone, the first two being of major importance in the acute defense response, which requires glycogen breakdown.[1065] If the glucagon response is blocked during insulin-induced hypoglycemia, the catecholamine response restores blood glucose; if catecholamine action in response to hypoglycemia is blocked, the glucagon response restores glucose levels. However, if both are blocked, hypoglycemia persists.[1065, 1068] In IDDM of more than 2 y duration, the glucagon response to insulin-induced hypoglycemia is usually reduced,[1067, 1068] but a normal catecholamine response provides adequate protection. After about 15 y of diabetes, the catecholamine response may wane, leaving the patient defenseless against hypoglycemia.[1069, 1070] The defect in catecholamine secretion appears to be specific for hypoglycemia because catecholamine release in response to other stimuli is intact.[1069] Counterregulatory failure in diabetes carries a high risk of prolonged hypoglycemia, permanent brain damage, and death. It may not be associated with other evidence of autonomic neuropathy, and its cause is uncertain.

HYPOGLYCEMIA UNAWARENESS. The impaired hormonal defense against hypoglycemia just described can occur in patients undergoing intensive insulin therapy with or without recent hypoglycemia,[1071] and it may be accompanied by "hypoglycemia unawareness," the absence of warning symptoms of impending hypoglycemia such as anxiety, sweating, palpitations, and other neurogenic symptoms.[1072] Normally, symptoms of hypoglycemia appear at plasma glucose concentrations of about 3.0 mmol/L (55 mg/dL), before the hypoglycemic level necessary to impair central nervous system function is reached. Hypoglycemia and intensive insulin therapy appear to reset thresholds so that release of counterregulatory hormones does not occur at the expected glucose level. Consequently, the patient has no warning signal, and serious symptoms can include coma and convulsions. Hormonal unresponsiveness to hypoglycemia and hypoglycemia unawareness are separate entities; avoidance of hypoglycemia can improve hypoglycemia unawareness but may not correct hormonal unresponsiveness.[1071] One possible mechanism for hypoglycemia unawareness is that a compensatory increase in glucose uptake into the brain during hypoglycemia in IDDM patients may blunt the signals for counterregulatory hormone release,[1072] depriving the ventromedial hypothalamus of the glucopenia required to elicit a full counterregulatory response.[1073] Such a mechanism would not seem reasonable when a single episode of afternoon hypoglycemia produces the syndrome the next day.[1074] Hypoglycemia unawareness is treated by avoidance of hypoglycemia.

REBOUND HYPERGLYCEMIA. The term *Somogyi phenomenon* designates rebound hyperglycemia that occurs after an episode of undetected hypoglycemia.[1075] Rebound hyperglycemia is reduced by decreasing the dose of insulin.[1076] Although this phenomenon does exist, it is less common than was previously thought. Deliberate induction of nocturnal hypoglycemia by infusion of insulin in insulin-dependent diabetic patients failed to cause fasting hyperglycemia.[1077] The phenomenon may be more common in children; in one study, 6 of 34 children had asymptomatic nocturnal hypoglycemia with hyperglycemic rebound.[1078] If glycosuria and hyperglycemia persist throughout the day, it is unlikely that this represents overinsulinization and rebound hyperglycemia.

INSULIN LIPODYSTROPHY AND LIPOATROPHY

Atrophy or hypertrophy of subcutaneous tissue may occur at insulin injection sites. The problem is usually seen with impure animal insulins and has almost disappeared with the use of synthetic insulins. Hypoesthetic masses may develop and become tempting sites for insulin injections. The absorption of insulin from such areas is unpredictable and may cause erratic or poor control. The patient should be taught to rotate injection sites and to avoid such areas. Lipoatrophy tends to develop during the first year of insulin therapy and to regress thereafter. It is prevalent in children and women and may involve an immune reaction to some contaminant of the older insulins, because it improves when purified or synthetic insulin is injected into the affected region. Occasionally, lipoatrophy develops at sites never used for insulin injection.

INSULIN ALLERGY

Cutaneous reactions to insulin occur in up to 5% of patients treated with the hormone.[1079] The reactions are mediated primarily by IgE antibodies, although IgG may participate. Allergy may develop with initiation of insulin therapy, usually within the first month, but severe reactions usually occur in patients who resume therapy after an insulin-free period. Many patients with insulin allergy have histories of sensitivity to other drugs as well. Local insulin allergy is characterized by erythema, pruritus, and induration at the injection site, whereas systemic allergy is manifested by generalized urticaria, angioneurotic edema, or frank anaphylaxis. In a study of 117 patients with insulin allergy, 87 had cutaneous reactions only, 18 had both cutaneous and systemic manifestations, and 12 had only systemic reactions.[1080]

Local insulin reactions should be treated with an antihistamine, and if animal insulins are used, a switch to biosynthetic human insulin should be made. If the patient does not respond to these measures, desensitization is required. Desensitization is mandatory if systemic reactions occur.[1081] After this is accomplished, insulin therapy should not be stopped for any reason.

INSULIN RESISTANCE

As noted previously, insulin resistance plays a prominent role in NIDDM and is mediated primarily by obesity. Modest insulin resistance is also present in the absence of obesity in type I IDDM[1082] and recedes with good control.[1083] The rare syndromes of insulin resistance have been reviewed.[1084] The defect can be at the prereceptor level (e.g., antibodies to the insulin molecule), at the level of binding to the receptor (e.g., type A binding defects or type B insulin resistance with anti-insulin receptor antibodies), or at a postbinding site (e.g., obesity, leprechaunism). Many insulin-resistant states are associated with acanthosis nigricans. Diabetes caused by a primary state of insulin resistance is considered at the end of this chapter.

IMMUNOLOGIC RESISTANCE. Insulin resistance in which antibodies are directed against insulin occurs in only about 0.01% of insulin-treated subjects, even though essentially all patients have detectable levels of insulin antibodies after 3 mo of therapy. True resistance, arbitrarily defined as an insulin requirement of at least 200 U/d,[1085] can be attributed to insulin antibodies only if the titer is high enough to bind large amounts of insulin.[1086] Anti-insulin antibodies are usually the consequence of insulin therapy but may develop spontaneously in patients without diabetes who have unrelated monoclonal gammopathy[1087] or autoimmune endocrinopathy such as thyroid disease.[1088] Autoantibodies against insulin can cause either insulin-resistant hyperglycemia or, if they release bound insulin inappropriately, hypoglycemia.[1088]

Insulin requirements may be extremely high in patients with antibodies against insulin.[1079, 1085] The use of human insulin usually does not prevent or reverse the syndrome. Concentrated insulin (U-500) is effective in some cases,[1089] as is sul-

fated insulin, presumably because it has a higher affinity for the insulin receptor than for the insulin antibody.[1090] If the foregoing maneuvers are unsuccessful, high-dose glucocorticoids (80 to 100 mg prednisone/d) should be given, with rapid tapering after the response is obtained, sometimes as early as 48 h after initiation of the therapy. About three fourths of patients respond to such treatment.[1085, 1079]

SUBCUTANEOUS DEGRADATION OR MALABSORPTION OF INSULIN. Insulin resistance can result from abnormal absorption or enhanced degradation of injected hormone.[1086–1088] The diagnosis of subcutaneous destruction is usually based on the observation that large amounts of insulin given subcutaneously are ineffective but intravenous insulin works normally.[1089] In one patient 5000 U given subcutaneously was required for adequate control.[1086] Increased degradation of insulin can also occur in the plasma.[1090] Addition of aprotinin, a protease inhibitor, to the insulin solution may provide improvement,[1089] although its effects may be caused by local enhancement of blood flow rather than inhibition of insulin degradation.[1091] Alterations in subcutaneous blood flow may be involved in the brittle diabetes syndrome, even in persons not characterized as resistant.[1092] Anaphylactic reactions to aprotinin have been reported, and only about one third of patients presumed to have subcutaneous insulin resistance respond to the drug.[1032, 1033] This syndrome appears to come and go spontaneously.

Treatment is difficult. Large amounts of insulin can be given subcutaneously with or without aprotinin, using intravenously administered insulin for acute complications such as ketoacidosis, or insulin can be administered into the peritoneal cavity.[1093] The latter approach has been recommended, but the authors are aware of one patient who failed to respond to intraperitoneal insulin. Therefore, the syndrome of non–antibody-mediated insulin resistance must be considered an unsolved problem.

Diet Therapy

In normal persons the postprandial influx of nutrients causes a rise in insulin secretion to prevent or minimize change in nutrient concentration, particularly that of glucose. The early phase of insulin response seems to be triggered primarily by hormones released from the gut[577] or by parasympathetic signals (or both), inasmuch as it occurs before the rise in glucose levels.[574] Regimens designed to provide meticulous control with pump therapy or multiple insulin injections attempt to duplicate this pattern by providing an anticipatory premeal dose of insulin given early enough to minimize postprandial hyperglycemia. The timing of meals must be carefully matched with that of insulin injections if normoglycemia is to be achieved.

For many years the American Diabetes Association recommended standard diets in the treatment of diabetes.[1094] Nutritional recommendations have been updated and modified, with standard diets no longer recommended.[1095] It is now thought advantageous to have diets as normal as possible without the need to calculate exchange values of foods as was previously done. Even sucrose in moderation is not proscribed.

Normal weight persons with diabetes usually require about 35 kcal/kg body weight/d and 0.8 to 1.0 g protein/kg body weight/d. The amounts of carbohydrate and fat that should be eaten are not entirely clear. A standard recommendation is for fat to be 30% or less of total calories and for saturated fat to be in the range of 7 to 10%. On the other hand, increased intake of monounsaturated fatty acids also has been recommended. A diet containing 35% carbohydrate and 50% fat, 33% of which was monounsaturated, lowered mean plasma glucose levels, reduced insulin requirements, lowered plasma levels of VLDL triglycerides, and increased HDL cholesterol levels; LDL concentrations were not affected.[1096] If LDL cholesterol is elevated and cannot be lowered without pharmacologic intervention, HMG–CoA reductase inhibitors appear to be as effective in diabetics as in nondiabetics and are devoid of any serious side effects. There is no question that lower cholesterol levels save lives in persons with coronary artery disease. Some authorities believe that total cholesterol levels should be reduced below the currently defined acceptable range of 200 to 210 mg/dL, a goal that would require much wider use of the HMG–CoA reductase inhibitors.[1097]

Many clinicians prefer to divide food intake into three meals and three snacks, with 20% of the calories at breakfast, 20% at lunch, and 30% at dinner time. Midmorning, midafternoon, and bedtime snacks make up the remaining 30%. In patients who do not take a midmorning snack, 10% can be added to the bedtime snack to provide additional protection against nocturnal hypoglycemia. Because blood glucose levels and insulin requirements are highest between breakfast and lunch, it is reasonable to shift much of the carbohydrate from breakfast to the evening meal and bedtime snack. The caloric intake should be appropriately adjusted if the weight increases or decreases. Ordinarily sweets and refined sugar are not permitted, although this proscription need not be absolute.[1098, 1099]

Despite the importance of diet, few physicians or patients are truly knowledgeable in this area. The distribution of pamphlets and food exchange lists does little to promote dietary adherence. The most effective way to manage the diabetic diet is to provide the patient with practical training in meal preparation under the supervision of a nutritionist. If this approach is not available, the physician and patient must follow written guidelines to diet therapy.[1100]

Exercise in IDDM

Exercise can be either helpful or harmful.[1101] Presumably, as in normal persons, regular exercise is of benefit for the cardiovascular system. Exercise may also lower plasma glucose levels. On the other hand, exercise may cause hypoglycemia. In normal persons the plasma glucose level rises slightly with vigorous exercise and decreases if exercise is prolonged (>90 min). Moderate exercise for short periods does not change glucose levels because enhanced glucose utilization in skeletal muscle is matched by increased hepatic production.[1102] If a poorly controlled diabetic patient exercises, plasma glucose concentrations may rise because insulin is inadequate to allow a maximal increase in its utilization in muscle in the presence of elevated production of glucose.[1102] Conversely, in the well-controlled patient, hypoglycemia may supervene because hepatic glucose production remains restrained by the undiminished circulating insulin levels and glucose utilization in muscle is increased because of the exercise.[1103, 1104] This problem is in part the result of injection of insulin subcutaneously in an area where exercise may increase the absorption rate of the hormone.[1104] However, hypoglycemia can occur independently of increased insulin absorption because additional capillaries open up in the exercising muscle, enhancing glucose utilization in previously inactive fibers.[1101–1105] To prevent exercise-induced hypoglycemia in patients treated with insulin infusion pumps, the premeal insulin bolus may be reduced or omitted.[1106, 1107] All diabetic patients requiring insulin must be warned of the danger of exercise-induced hypoglycemia. Self-testing of the plasma glucose response to exercise may be valuable for those who exercise regularly so as to formulate a program for appropriate modification of the insulin dose on exercise days. This is even more important if meticulous control is being attempted.

Treatment of NIDDM

Metabolic Goals

The therapeutic objectives in NIDDM do not differ from those in IDDM: return of metabolic abnormalities to normal in the hope of maintaining health and extending life. In contrast to IDDM, insulin is not an obligatory form of therapy in NIDDM. There is within the NIDDM category a broad clinical spectrum of islet cell function, body weight, and insulin resistance that requires a careful choice of therapeutic options. The older age of the patients and the greater frequency of other clinical problems make it necessary to devise individual therapeutic regimens.

Therapeutic Options

Patients can be divided into three therapeutic categories according to beta-cell function relative to insulin sensitivity: (1) those with sufficient islet cell reserve and insulin sensitivity to maintain relatively normal glucose levels provided the intake of calories and carbohydrate is restricted, (2) those in whom dietary restriction is not adhered to or is not effective and in whom oral antihyperglycemic drugs are needed, and (3) those in whom hyperglycemia is not controlled by the foregoing therapy.

Patients must also be separated for therapeutic purposes into obese and nonobese groups, inasmuch as beta-cell function and sensitivity can be improved in the former by weight reduction.[1108] Pima Indians with obese type II NIDDM experienced improvement in beta-cell function and glucose intolerance after 3 wk of caloric restriction and improved sensitivity of target tissues after 18 wk.[1109] Such remissions occurred only in patients with fasting glucose levels below 14 mmol/L (250 mg/dL) and diabetes of less than 5 y duration. Unfortunately, in the United States dietary adherence and weight reduction are seldom achieved in the obese patient with NIDDM.

Diet Therapy in NIDDM

Every diabetic, regardless of type, requires a diet that allows an optimal quality of life and minimizes the dietary contribution to hyperglycemia. Because the sine qua non of diabetes is inability to correct postprandial hyperglycemia, the dietary prescription seeks to minimize hyperglycemia after meals. The use of agents such as acarbose and dietary fiber, both of which may minimize postprandial hyperglycemia (see later discussion), simply substitutes for the willpower required to reduce carbohydrate intake.

In NIDDM there are two distinct objectives of caloric restriction that are often confused: one objective is to reduce postprandial hyperglycemia at each meal, and the other is to prevent or correct obesity. Because postprandial hyperglycemia may last many hours, its elimination reduces morning blood glucose values and converts a patient with seemingly recalcitrant hyperglycemia into a model of good diabetic control.

The second objective of dietary treatment in NIDDM is directed toward reduction of obesity. As discussed previously, there is a close correlation between obesity and NIDDM.[1110] Relatively modest reductions in weight can dramatically improve glycemic control in obese patients with poorly controlled NIDDM and in obese rats.[1112] Dietary restriction reduces insulin resistance, perhaps by reducing the release of adipocyte products such as FFA and TNF α, which are believed to contribute to both insulin resistance and loss of GSIS.

Oral Antihyperglycemic Drugs

In principle, oral antihyperglycemics should be used only for the treatment of hyperglycemia that persists despite full adherence to an optimal diabetic diet. In practice, obesity is rarely corrected, and dietary prescriptions are usually ignored. The antihyperglycemic drugs are therefore often employed, albeit inappropriately, as initial therapy rather than as adjuvants to a dietary regimen.

SULFONYLUREAS. The pharmacologic characteristics of sulfonylurea drugs are summarized in Table 21–27. The mechanism of action is still debated. Acute administration of a sulfonylurea stimulates insulin release by means of a beta-cell sulfonylurea receptor.[458] These drugs may act to lower the glycemic threshold required for a given beta-cell secretory response.[1113] During long-term administration, insulin levels tend to decrease as hyperglycemia recedes, suggesting increased beta-cell sensitivity to hyperglycemia or improvement of insulin resistance in target tissues. Sulfonylureas have been reported to cause increased insulin binding to fibroblasts[1114] and hepatocytes,[1115] but this finding has been disputed.[1116] Sulfonylureas also potentiate insulin action in the absence of increased insulin binding[1115, 1117] by enhancing glucose disposal.[1118] They also appear to decrease hepatic glucose production.[1119] The use of sulfonylureas together with a single evening dose of NPH insulin in NIDDM is said to be as effective as two doses of insulin in some patients,[1120] but, in practice, control is only rarely improved with combined sulfonylurea and insulin therapy.

Because sulfonylureas are ineffective in type I IDDM or pancreatectomized animals, it has been assumed that their major mechanism of action is to enhance beta-cell function. However, the sulfonylureas glipizide and glyburide enhance glucose uptake in cultured skeletal muscle cells by increasing the level of the facilitative glucose transporter GLUT1, but not GLUT4, in plasma membranes.[1121] In a similar study, glimepiride increased glucose transport and increased GLUT1 and GLUT4 expression in cultured cardiac cells.[1122]

Therapeutic Efficacy of Sulfonylureas. Most patients with fasting glucose levels higher than 16.7 mmol/L (300 mg/dL) do not respond to sulfonylureas, whereas most of those with levels lower than 14 mmol/L (250 mg/dL) exhibit at least a partial response. Overall, about 85% of unselected patients with NIDDM respond initially to the drugs, but secondary failure occurs in about 25%.[1123] Transient failures may result from intercurrent infection, surgery, or other stress, with a return of responsiveness after removal of the stress. Failure to adhere to diet and continued weight gain play a role in many secondary failures. In other instances unresponsiveness to sulfonylureas may reflect the progression of what in reality was type I autoimmune insulinopathy rather than type II NIDDM.[79] Finally, bona fide type II NIDDM may be a progressive disorder, despite conventional assumptions to the contrary.

Most studies have failed to show that sulfonylurea therapy of glucose-intolerant patients can slow progression to overt diabetes or slow development of cardiovascular disease. However, one long-term study revealed remarkable improvement in both categories in glucose-intolerant men given tolbutamide at 1.5 g/d over a 10-y follow-up period.[1124] This result remains to be confirmed.

Toxicity of Sulfonylureas. Toxic side effects of sulfonylureas occur in about 3% of treated patients[1123] and include bone marrow depression, hemolytic anemia, rash (including the Stevens-Johnson syndrome), nausea and vomiting, abnormal liver function (especially increased levels of alkaline phosphatase), vasomotor flushing with alcohol, and antidiuresis, which can cause hyponatremia. The antidiuretic effect, most commonly seen with chlorpropamide, is caused by increased release of vasopressin. Concern that sulfonylureas predispose to coronary artery disease has dissipated.[1123]

BIGUANIDES. The biguanide phenformin was withdrawn from use in the United States because of an enhanced risk of lactic acidosis,[1125] the mechanism being uncertain.[1126] The risk of lactic acidosis with metformin is much lower than with phenformin.[1126] Metformin has been used widely in Europe and Canada for decades and is now approved for use in the United States.[1127] Metformin lowers blood glucose by 13 to 37% in 80 to 90% of obese and nonobese NIDDM patients, mainly through diminished hepatic gluconeogenesis. It is far more effective when combined with sulfonylureas.[1128] Metformin should not be used in patients with renal insufficiency and should be withdrawn during intercurrent illnesses.

INSULIN

In contrast to IDDM, in which insulin is essential for maintaining life, insulin in NIDDM is reserved for patients who do not respond to combinations of diet and treatment with sulfonylurea or metformin, or both. The efficacy of insulin treatment in NIDDM is determined both by the compliance of the patient with dietary restrictions and by the degree of insulin resistance. The greater the insulin resistance, the less efficacious is insulin treatment. In obesity the combination of insulin resistance and poor dietary compliance makes insulin treatment a frustrating exercise in which daily insulin doses greater than 100 U/d do not control hyperglycemia. At the other extreme of the NIDDM spectrum, nonobese patients with a mild deficiency of endogenous insulin and little insulin resistance are very responsive to insulin treatment.

Experimental Drugs

AGENTS THAT REDUCE POSTPRANDIAL HYPERGLYCEMIA

ACARBOSE. This drug, which is not available for general use in the United States, is an α-glucosidase inhibitor that interferes with the intestinal absorption of carbohydrates[1129] and thereby reduces postprandial hyperglycemia.[1130] A 12-mo multicenter clinical trial reported improvement in postprandial glycemia and in HbA$_{1c}$ and no serious side effects. How-

TABLE 21–27. Sulfonylureas

Agent	Daily Dose (mg)	Dose/Day	Duration of Hyperglycemic Action (h)	Metabolism/Excretion
Acetohexamide	250–1500	1 or 2	12–18	Liver/kidney
Chlorpropamide	100–500	1	60	Kidney
Tolazamide	100–1000	1 or 2	12–14	Liver
Tolbutamide	500–3000	2 or 3	6–12	Liver
Glyburide* (glybenclamide)	1.25–20	1 or 2	Up to 24	Liver/kidney
Glipizide	2.5–40	1 or 2	Up to 24	Liver/kidney
Glibornuride	12.5–100	1 or 2	Up to 24	Liver/kidney

* Glyburide is the generic name in the United States; glybenclamide is the international nonproprietary name.
Adapted by permission of Elsevier Science Publishing Co., Inc. from Lebovitz HE, Feinglos MN. The oral hypoglycemic agents. In: Ellenberg M, Rifkin H, eds. Diabetes Mellitus: Theory and Practice. 3rd ed. New Hyde Park, NY: Medical Examination Publishing, 1983: 591–610. Copyright © 1983, by Medical Examination Publishing Company, Inc.

ever, flatulence occurred in 73% of treated patients, compared with 39% of controls, and diarrhea and abdominal discomfort were reported in a substantial minority.[1131]

AGENTS THAT REDUCE INSULIN RESISTANCE

THIAZOLIDINEDIONES. The thiazolidinediones include ciglitazone, troglitazone, pioglitazone, and englitazone. Cigli-tozone lowers blood glucose levels in *ob/ob* and *db/db* mice, increasing the basal rate of glucose metabolism, lipogenesis, insulin receptor number, and postreceptor response to insulin.[1132, 1133] These drugs may block the autocrine inhibitory effect of TNF α on the lipogenic and antilipolytic actions of insulin on adipocytes.[1134] This blockade appears to be at the level of the insulin receptor kinase, which is inhibited by TNF α.[492] Pioglitazone increases autophosphorylation of the insulin receptor.[1135]

Troglitazone has been used in patients with NIDDM and reportedly improves insulin action on liver, skeletal muscle, and adipose tissue by direct action; it reduces both fasting and postprandial hyperglycemia and hyperinsulinemia,[1135–1137] increasing insulin-mediated glucose disposal by 40 to 60%.[1138] It also increases expression of GLUT1 and GLUT4 in undifferentiated preadipocytes by stabilization of GLUT1 and GLUT4 mRNA.[1138] Troglitazone not only prevents the inhibitory effect of TNF α on adipogenesis, antilipolysis, and GLUT4 expression but also blocks the inhibitory effects of IL-1, IL-6, and TNF α on preadipocyte differentiation.[1136] Thioglitazone corrects the abnormally high phosphoenolpyruvate carboxykinase (PEPCK) level of poorly controlled diabetes and lowers its mRNA to normal, meanwhile reducing hepatic gluconeogenesis despite the concomitant reduction in insulin levels.[1137] Pioglitazone appears to restore insulin sensitivity at the hepatic level.[1138] Troglitazone enhances GSIS in both isolated rat islets and a hamster beta-cell line, possibly through an increase in glucose uptake.[1139] Englitazone prevents the defect in glucose transport caused by a high-fat diet.[1140]

AGENTS THAT MIMIC INSULIN

Vanadate ions mimic physiological actions of insulin.[1141] The actions of vanadate include stimulation of glucose uptake and metabolism, activation of glycogen synthase, inhibition of lipolysis, stimulation of potassium uptake and calcium influx, and increase in L-type pyruvate kinase gene expression. When given orally to streptozotocin diabetic rats or db/db and ob/ob mice, it lowered blood glucose levels and restored hepatic glycogen levels.[1142–1146] Although the mechanism of vanadate action is complex, an important effect involves inhibition of the elevated tyrosine phosphatase activity in the hepatocytes of ob/ob and db/db mice.[1146, 1147]

MODIFIERS OF FATTY ACID METABOLISM

FFA levels are increased in the plasma and tissues of obese patients with NIDDM, and elevations of plasma FFA cause insulin resistance in skeletal muscle.[612, 614–616] Acipimox (5-methyl-pyrazine carboxylic acid 4-oxide), a potent and long-acting antilipolytic derivative of nicotinic acid, lowers FFA levels and produces a 30% reduction in hyperglycemia, but plasma glucose does not fall below 8.5 mmol/L.[1148] FFA levels tend to escape the marked suppression observed on the first day, and the long-term efficacy of the agent remains to be determined. Acipimox may reduce insulin resistance but does not by itself result in blood glucose control.[1148]

Treatment of Diabetic Ketoacidosis

Reviews of this subject have been published by Foster and McGarry,[630] Alberti and Hockaday,[1149] and Clements and Vourganti.[1150]

Replacement of Fluid and Electrolytes

Hypovolemia and vascular collapse are the cause of death in uncomplicated ketoacidosis, and correction of the volume deficit is the most urgent therapeutic priority.[1151] Volume repletion alone (without insulin administration) can lower plasma glucose levels[638] and decrease counterregulatory hormone concentrations but does not reverse the acidosis. For this reason, insulin is always required.[115]

The average fluid deficit in adults is 3 to 5 L, and the rate of volume replacement is determined by clinical assessment. Usually 1 or 2 L of isotonic saline is administered rapidly during the first 2 h, but if hypotension, extreme hyperglycemia, and oliguria are present, more should be given. If hypernatremia develops, 0.45% sodium chloride can be substituted for isotonic saline, but this usually is not necessary. Free water is ordinarily provided by the infusion of 5% dextrose begun as the plasma glucose level falls below 16.7 mmol/L (300 mg/dL). Correction of the extracellular fluid volume deficit takes precedence over correction of the free water deficit. Lactated Ringer's solution can be used in lieu of saline to minimize the chloride load. Large amounts of sodium chloride contribute to the hyperchloremic acidosis that commonly occurs during and after therapy. Long-standing disagreement concerning which fluid to use probably reflects the fact that sodium chloride and balanced electrolyte solutions are equally effective, particularly if underlying renal function is normal.

The hyperkalemia that is usually present on admission recedes after insulin action begins and potassium moves back into cells. Potassium replacement is required at this point to prevent hypokalemia. Potassium given before insulin has begun to act is potentially lethal if initial plasma concentrations are high. At times the potassium level is initially low (or low-normal) because of vomiting or diarrhea; this requires reversal of the usual strategy. Potassium movement into cells is one of insulin's most powerful effects, and respiratory arrest or fatal arrhythmias may develop if potassium replacement is not begun before administration of insulin. Normally, insulin should be delayed for approximately 1 h, during which time intravenous potassium is given at rates of 20 to 40 mmol/h. Serum potassium levels should at first be measured every hour if hypokalemia is present at entry or every 2 h in the more common hyperkalemic state. The total amount of potassium required ordinarily does not exceed 160 mmol in the first 24 h. Potassium should be given with extreme care, if at all, in the anuric patient.

Phosphate deficits usually range from 0.5 to 1.5 mmol/kg body weight but may be larger,[1152, 1153] becoming apparent only when insulin action shifts phosphate back into cells with restoration of glucose metabolism. Rhabdomyolysis, impaired cardiac function, hemolysis, and respiratory failure are rare consequences of phosphate deficiency. Reduced levels of red blood cell 2,3-diphosphoglycerate lower tissue oxygenation by no more than 20%, but even this may be significant if associated microvascular disease, autonomic neuropathy, or hypovolemia prevents a compensatory increase in capillary blood flow. Phosphate depletion is usually silent clinically, and phosphate replacement has little effect on the course of diabetic ketoacidosis.[1152, 1153] If initial phosphate values are low, the potassium can be administered in the form of potassium phosphate to provide 40 to 60 mmol of the anion.

The matter of bicarbonate administration is unsettled.[1154] Severe acidosis impairs myocardial contractility and, if coupled with volume depletion, may cause shock.[630] If the pH is lower than 7.0 or the bicarbonate level is less than 5 mmol/L, it is prudent to infuse sodium bicarbonate (100 mmol NaHCO₃ per liter of 0.45% saline) as initial therapy,[1155] although in one retrospective study this failed to produce clinical benefit.[1156] Opposition to bicarbonate therapy is based on the fact that when the red blood cell 2,3-diphosphoglycerate level is low, a sudden rise in pH may reduce oxygen release to tissues by shifting the oxygen dissociation curve to the left, thereby predisposing to lactic acidosis. One study in a small number of patients suggested that bicarbonate produced a delay in reversal of ketoacidosis compared with the rate in control subjects not receiving it.[1157] Based on studies in perfused rat liver, this was thought to be caused by increased ketone production. Bicarbonate may induce paradoxical intracellular acidification, especially in the heart, thereby decreasing left ventricular function. If given, bicarbonate administration should be halted when the pH reaches 7.2.

Insulin Therapy

All patients in diabetic ketoacidosis require regular insulin administered by vein or, in the absence of venous access, by intramuscular injection. At one time insulin was recommended in doses of 50 to 100 U/h,[630] but low-dose treatment (6 to 10 U/h) is now recognized as equally effective.[1155] The advantage of the low-dose regimen is its simplicity. Its disadvantage is delayed recovery from acidosis in the patient with significant insulin resistance caused by a high titer of insulin antibodies or other factors. The authors believe that an initial bolus of 50 U followed by a constant infusion of 10 to 20 U/h is a reasonable approach. Larger doses of insulin are required if acidosis does not begin to respond over a 3- to 4-h period as indicated by a rise in pH or a reduction in the anion gap. Insulin must be given until the urine is free of ketones because continued ketosis, even in the absence of acidosis, indicates that the enzymes mediating hepatic fatty acid oxidation and synthesis of acetoacetate and β-hydroxybutyrate have not been deactivated. Under these circumstances any rise in FFA concentration can cause recurrent ketoacidosis. Occasionally, the anion gap does not narrow despite a blood pH that returns to normal with clearance of urine ketones. Presumably caused by exchange of unmeasured anions from tissue buffers, this "pseudo–insulin resistance" is easily differentiated from true insulin resistance because acidosis and ketones persist in the latter.

Glucose Administration

After insulin has restored glucose uptake by the insulin-requiring tissues and reversed hyperglucagonemia,[630] hypoglycemia occurs unless exogenous glucose is provided. Because glucose levels almost always fall before ketone levels decrease, exogenous glucose must be provided to cover the insulin needed to reverse the ketosis. Infusions are ordinarily begun when the plasma glucose level reaches 14 to 17 mmol/L (250 to 300 mg/dL) to minimize the risk of cerebral edema. Hypoglycemia is never a problem if glucose is started early.

Mechanisms by Which Appropriate Therapy Reverses Diabetic Ketoacidosis

Replacement of fluid and electrolyte deficits restores perfusion of tissues to normal, corrects or prevents hypoxia, and lowers the high levels of counterregulatory hormones. Suppression of glucagon lowers the hepatic cyclic AMP level and the activity of cyclic AMP–dependent protein kinases; this re-establishes hepatic glycogenesis, stops glycogenolysis, and raises fructose 2,6-bisphosphate levels (see Fig. 21–27, bottom). The increase in fructose 2,6-bisphosphate blocks gluconeogenesis and activates hepatic glycolysis, thereby providing substrate for lipogenesis. The rise in malonyl-CoA concentration inhibits CPT-I activity and blocks ketogenesis. The levels of ketones fall as a consequence of continued catabolism in the face of inhibited synthesis. In adipocytes, insulin inhibits

lipolysis and reduces FFA delivery to the liver. Simultaneously, insulin action in the periphery increases glucose uptake by muscle and lowers the level of blood glucose. Anabolic processes are thereby re-established, and catabolism is inhibited.

Complications of Diabetic Ketoacidosis

Death is rare in patients with properly treated diabetic ketoacidosis. Precipitating or complicating illness, such as myocardial infarction, sepsis, or acute pancreatitis, accounts for most of the mortality.[1150] Death also can result from shock (caused by volume depletion, reduced myocardial contractility, and diminished responsiveness of the arteries to catecholamines) or from therapeutic errors.

INFECTION. Although leukocytosis often occurs in diabetic ketoacidosis in the absence of infection, fever usually indicates infection and demands a careful hunt for pneumonia, pyelonephritis, or septicemia. Infections that are ordinarily trivial (e.g., apical tooth abscess, furunculosis) can sometimes precipitate diabetic ketoacidosis. The rare mucormycosis of the paranasal sinuses is a unique ketoacidosis-associated infection manifested by facial pain, bloody nasal discharge, orbital swelling, proptosis, blurred vision, and impairment of consciousness. This ubiquitous fungus is believed to become a pathogen in diabetic ketoacidosis as the result of an acidosis-induced block in the binding of iron to transferrin, which provides the pathogen with free iron, an obligatory growth factor.[1158]

VASCULAR THROMBOSIS. A thrombotic event may occur during or after apparently successful management of hyperosmolar coma or ketoacidosis. Both disorders predispose to thrombosis as a consequence of volume contraction, low cardiac output, increased viscosity of the blood, underlying atherosclerosis, direct damage to endothelium by the hyperosmolal milieu, and changes in clotting factors and platelet function.[1159] Factor VIII activity is increased, partial thromboplastin time is shortened, and the level of antithrombin III is reduced. As previously noted, patients with uncontrolled diabetes are in a procoagulant state. In addition to increases in factor VIII and von Willebrand factor, fibrinolysis is impaired, and endothelial dysfunction predisposes to platelet aggregation and loss of NO-induced basal dilation.[1160–1164]

Platelets from patients with ketoacidosis exhibit increased in vivo aggregation.[754] The spontaneous aggregation of platelets and disseminated intravascular coagulation in uncontrolled diabetes can be reversed by improvement in the metabolic state.

CEREBRAL EDEMA. Cerebral edema may develop during the course of treatment of ketoacidosis in children and adolescents but is rare in adults.[1165] The complication should be suspected when a patient with ketoacidosis who had no underlying neurologic illness begins to develop increasing stupor or coma coupled with signs of increased intracranial pressure 3 to 10 h into treatment. Papilledema, pupillary dysfunction, hyperpyrexia, and other neurologic manifestations may be present. The treatment involves administration of hypertonic mannitol and dexamethasone[1166] and induction of respiratory alkalosis using a respirator under the direction of an anesthesiologist or pulmonologist to decrease cerebral blood flow. The cause of the cerebral edema is not known, although osmotic disequilibrium between intracellular and extracellular fluids probably plays a role. A rapid fall in the plasma oncotic pressure during treatment may be contributory.[1167]

RESPIRATORY DISTRESS SYNDROME. Another complication of both ketoacidosis and hyperosmolar coma is the adult respiratory distress syndrome.[1168] The picture is heralded by unexplained hypoxemia and dyspnea in the absence of pneumonia or underlying pulmonary or cardiac disease. Physical findings may be absent early, although rales are heard later.

The x-ray findings resemble those in pulmonary edema, but, in contrast to cardiogenic pulmonary edema, the capillary wedge pressure is normal or low as determined by Swan-Ganz catheter. Mortality is high despite treatment with positive end-expiratory pressure and careful fluid management.

Clinical Errors

Clinical errors contribute importantly to the mortality in diabetic ketoacidosis (Table 21–28). The erroneous administration of hypertonic glucose at the outset increases intracellular dehydration. The administration of insulin without sufficient fluids to patients with major volume depletion may shift extracellular water into cells, further shrinking the extracellular fluid volume and impairing blood flow to critical vascular beds or precipitating vascular collapse. The premature administration of potassium before insulin has begun to act may cause fatal hyperkalemia early, whereas failure to administer potassium may lead to fatal hypokalemia in potassium-depleted patients, as discussed.

Common nonlethal conditions resulting from therapeutic errors include recurrent ketoacidosis. This may be caused by failure to maintain glucose and insulin treatment until ketones have been cleared and depleted glycogen stores restocked. Hypoglycemia may be caused by insufficient glucose administration.

Treatment of Nonketotic Hyperosmolar Coma

Fluid repletion is the most important aspect of treatment. The deficit, which may reach 10 L or more, exceeds that of diabetic ketoacidosis.[636, 637] The first 2 or 3 L should be given rapidly, even in elderly patients with uncertain cardiac function. Careful monitoring of the central venous pressure permits rapid repletion of volume without a risk of overexpansion. The initial serum sodium level may be high, normal, or low, depending on the relative losses of sodium and water in the urine caused by a shift of water out of cells secondary to hyperglycemia. Treatment should begin with normal saline at a rate that will replenish at least half of the estimated fluid deficit within 6 h, after which 0.45% saline can be given to complete volume replacement. Re-expansion of the extracellular fluid volume reduces the levels of glucagon, catecholamines, and the other hormones of stress and re-establishes glucose excretion if renal function is intact.[630]

Although fluids reduce hyperglycemia, insulin should also be given. A low-dose schedule consisting of a 10-U bolus and 5 to 10 U/h thereafter is appropriate.

Insulin can precipitate vascular collapse if it causes a major shift of extracellular fluid into cells or causes a capillary leak syndrome. Insulin therapy should always be preceded or accompanied by appropriate administration of fluids. Because of the high rate of infection, particularly with gram-negative organisms, antibiotics should be given empirically to any pa-

tient with fever pending the outcome of blood, urine, or sputum (transtracheal aspirate) cultures. Although mortality rates are generally high in hyperosmolar coma (>50%), lower rates (14%) are reported by some.[637] Fatalities are highest in older patients.

Prevention and Treatment of Vascular Complications

Macrovascular Disease

Macrovascular disease accounts for much of the morbidity and mortality in diabetic patients. Risk factors such as hypertension and cigarette smoking contribute to the morbidity, and attempts to correct hyperglycemia without also eliminating the other risk factors may be futile.

Management of hypercholesterolemia represents a special problem. The most appropriate diet is one in which monounsaturated or polyunsaturated fats are substituted for unsaturated fats and carbohydrate intake is limited.[1096] If dietary management fails to control hypercholesterolemia or hypertriglyceridemia, medications such as HMG-CoA reductase inhibitors, bile salt–binding resins, nicotinic acid, probucol, and gemfibrozil can be employed as in nondiabetic patients[1097, 1169] (see Chapter 23). HMG-CoA reductase inhibitors are most important. Gemfibrozil and HMG-CoA reductase inhibitors should be used together with caution because of the danger of induction of myositis. Early attention to atherogenic risk factors is more effective than intervention after these complications are advanced.

More specific treatment for complications of diabetes is not available. Aminoguanidine, an agent that prevents cross-linking between arterial wall proteins in experimental diabetes, is under study.[1170]

Microvascular Disease

At present, microvascular disease is untreatable. As noted previously, aldose reductase inhibitors prevent microvascular complications in experimental diabetes, but their effects in established complications in humans are minimal. A means of inhibiting new vessel formation would be helpful in diabetic retinopathy approaching the proliferative stage; a heparin analogue, β-cyclodextrin tetradecasulfate, is a powerful inhibitor of neovascularization in the rabbit cornea.[1171] Other factors that regulate angiogenesis could also be exploited.[1172]

ACE inhibitors appear to slow progress of diabetic nephropathy and should be included in treatment for hypertension. Some physicians believe they should be used at the earliest sign of renal disease.

Pancreas Transplantation

According to the International Pancreas Transplant Registry, 1839 pancreases were transplanted in the United States between 1987 and 1992. The overall 1-y patient survival rate

TABLE 21–28. Errors in the Therapy of Diabetic Ketoacidosis

Time	Therapeutic Error	Consequences
Initial 4 h	Hypertonic glucose administered because of erroneous diagnosis of hypoglycemia	Further increase in hyperosmolality and intracellular dehydration
	Inappropriate potassium administration	Hyperkalemic cardiotoxicity
	Overly rapid correction of hyperglycemia	Cerebral edema
	Insufficient saline solution	Hypotension
	Too much insulin without enough fluid	Decreased blood pressure caused by a shift of volume from extracellular to intracellular space
After 6–12 h	Insufficient potassium	Hypokalemic cardiotoxicity
	Insufficient glucose	Hypoglycemia; reappearance of ketosis

for 1986 to 1990 was 89%, and 62% of grafts were functioning after 1 y.[1173] Graft failure was attributed to rejection, recurrence of disease, infection, bleeding, or unknown causes.[1174] More than 6% of patients died with a functioning graft. In a Swedish series patient survival at 1 y was 95%, and graft survival was 83%.[1175] Most successfully transplanted patients reported an improved emotional and mental state and a sense of well-being.[1176-1179]

The effects of pancreas transplantation on established complications of diabetes are disappointing, even when metabolic control is excellent. Although occasionally a pancreas graft may slow or halt the progress of autonomic neuropathy, it does not correct the cardiorespiratory reflexes, which are believed to be a cause of sudden death in such patients. Usually, nerve conduction velocity increases without clear-cut improvement in autonomic neuropathy.[1180-1184] Much of the improvement in combined pancreas-kidney transplantation may be the result of the elimination of uremia.

The effect of successful pancreas transplantation on diabetic retinopathy is similarly disappointing. No difference between combined kidney-pancreas transplantation and transplantation of a kidney alone can be demonstrated.[1185-1187] In an Austrian study, retinopathy appeared to be stabilized in more than 73% of successful pancreas transplant recipients, improvement occurred in only 8.8%, and deterioration took place in 17.7%. In a control group deterioration occurred in 46%, suggesting that successful pancreas transplantation has a stabilizing influence.[1188] Interpretations are difficult because many subjects had end-stage retinopathy and pretransplantation treatments varied. Whatever the effects on established retinopathy, however, the previously cited DCCT studies indicate beyond question that strict control prevents or retards development of diabetic retinopathy.[649]

In summary, pancreas transplantation does not reverse established complications. Retinal and glomerular blood vessels cannot be replaced, and damage to small blood vessels resulting from decades of hyperglycemia cannot be reversed by correction of hyperglycemia.

Furthermore, because pancreas transplants require ongoing immunosuppression, they are usually done at the time of kidney replacement in patients with renal failure, who will receive immunosuppression in any case.[1189] As surgical techniques have been improved, pancreas transplantation has been undertaken in some patients with early renal disease.[1190]

Although the risks of the procedure and the rates of graft failure have declined, the dangers of prolonged immunosuppression limit the use of this procedure to a fraction of patients with IDDM.[1174]

Islet Transplantation

Islet transplantation has several advantages over pancreas transplantation: implantation can be done without major surgery, and islets can be microencapsulated in permselective membrane devices and implanted without the need for immunosuppression. Successful islet transplantation in rodents and dogs (see Lanza and associates[1191] for review) has been accomplished with biohybrid devices such as disc-shaped diffusion chambers,[1192-1196] millipore cellulose membranes,[1192-1194] tubular membrane chambers,[1197-1199] and microcapsules.[1200-1202] Favorable results were reported in diabetic rats receiving canine, bovine, and porcine islets in permselective acrylic membranes.[1202,1203] The implants appeared to be morphologically and functionally intact 30 to 130 days after transplantation, thereby proving the protective value of the membranes.

Several humans have received islet transplantation. One patient with IDDM of 25 y duration and renal failure received fresh islets and a kidney from one donor and cryopreserved islets from four other donors. More than 10,000 islets were infused into the left portal vein through an indwelling Silastic catheter inserted through the umbilical vein after completion of the kidney transplant. Immunosuppression was induced by antilymphocyte globulin and maintained with azothioprine, prednisone, and cyclosporin A.[1204] Insulin treatment was stopped during the ninth postoperative week, after which fasting glucose levels averaged 4.7 mmol/L (85 mg/dL) and the 24-h mean glucose levels averaged 6.6 mmol/L (119 mg/dL). However, not all patients have been able to discontinue exogenous insulin treatment.[1205] Although there are reports of successful islet transplantation with insulin independence and euglycemia lasting for longer than 6 months,[1206] this procedure is still in its infancy. Even if such problems as variable viability of donor islets and standards of quantity and quality of islets required to confer insulin independence are solved, the availability of human islets is a limiting factor. For this reason efforts have been made to bypass the need for human islets. One strategy has been the use of islets from other species (islet xenografts).

The porcine fetal pancreas provides a source of islet-like cell clusters that reverse diabetes when transplanted into experimental animals. A few porcine islet-like cell clusters have been transplanted into 10 IDDM patients who were receiving standard immunosuppression after renal transplantation; the functional and morphologic integrity of these islets persisted for 200 to 400 days,[1207] but there have been no reports of a therapeutically successful xenograft in a human patient with IDDM.

REFERENCES

1. National Diabetes Advisory Board. Diabetes in the 1980's: challenges for the future. US Department of Health and Human Services, Public Health Service. NIH Publication No. 82-2143. Washington, DC: Government Printing Office, 1982.
2. National Diabetes Data Group. Classification and diagnosis of diabetes mellitus and other categories of glucose intolerance. Diabetes 1979; 28:1039–1057.
3. Report of the expert committee on the diagnosis and classification of diabetes mellitus. Diabetes Care 1997; 20:1183–1197.
4. Mosenthal HO, Barry E. Criteria for and interpretation of normal glucose tolerance tests. Ann Intern Med 1950; 33:1175–1194.
5. Unger RH. The standard two-hour oral glucose tolerance test in the diagnosis of diabetes mellitus in subjects without fasting hyperglycemia. Ann Intern Med 1957; 47:1138–1153.
6. Bennett PH, Rushforth NB, Miller M, et al. Epidemiologic studies of diabetes in the Pima Indians. Recent Prog Horm Res 1976; 32:333–376.
7. Pettitt DG, Knowler WC, Lisse JR, et al. Development of retinopathy and proteinuria in relation to plasma-glucose concentrations in Pima Indians. Lancet 1980; 2:1050–1052.
8. Fink RI, Kolterman OG, Griffin J, et al. Mechanisms of insulin resistance in aging. J Clin Invest 1983; 71:1523–1535.
9. Rowe JW, Minaker KL, Pallotta JA, et al. Characterization of the insulin resistance of aging. J Clin Invest 1983; 71:1581–1587.
10. Thai A-C, Eisenbarth GS. Natural history of IDDM. Diabetes Reviews 1993; 1:1–14.
11. Dunn PJ, Cole RA, Soeldner JS, et al. Temporal relationship of glycosylated haemoglobin concentrations to glucose control in diabetics. Diabetologia 1979; 17:213–220.
12. Singer DE, Coley CM, Sarnat JH, et al. Tests of glycemia in diabetes mellitus: their use in establishing a diagnosis and in treatment. Ann Intern Med 1989; 110:125–137.
13. Siperstein MD, Unger RH, Madison LL. Studies of muscle capillary basement membranes in normal subjects, diabetic, and prediabetic patients. J Clin Invest 1968; 47:1973–1999.
14. Karam JH, Rosenthal M, O'Donnell JJ, et al. Discordance of diabetic microangiopathy in identical twins. Diabetes 1976; 25:24–28.
15. Ganda OP, Williamson JR, Soeldner JS, et al. Muscle capillary basement membrane width and its relationship to diabetes mellitus in monozygotic twins. Diabetes 1983; 32:549–556.
16. Barnett AH, Spiliopoulos AJ, Pyke DA, et al. Muscle capillary basement membrane in identical twins discordant for insulin-dependent diabetes. Diabetes 1983; 32:557–560.
17. Peterson CM, Jones RL, Esterly JA, et al. Changes in basement membrane thickening and pulse volume concomitant with improved glucose control and exercise in patients with insulin-dependent diabetes mellitus. Diabetes Care 1980; 3:586–589.
18. Raskin P, Pietri A, Unger RH, et al. The effect of diabetic control on

skeletal muscle capillary basement membrane width in patients with type I diabetes mellitus. N Engl J Med 1983; 309:1546–1550.

19. Bennett PH. Classification of diabetes. In: Ellenberg M, Rifkin H, eds. Diabetes Mellitus: Theory and Practice. 3rd ed. New Hyde Park, NY: Medical Examination Publishing, 1983:409–414.

20. Keen H. Problems in the definition of diabetes mellitus and its subtypes. In: Köbberling J, Tattersall R, eds. The Genetics of Diabetes Mellitus. Proceedings of the Serono Symposia. Vol 47. London: Academic, 1982: 1–11.

21. Aizawa T, Katakura M, Taguchi N, et al. Ketoacidosis-onset noninsulin dependent diabetes in Japanese subjects. Am J Med 1995; 310:198–201.

22. West KM. Epidemiology of Diabetes and Its Vascular Lesions. New York: Elsevier, 1978: 292–293.

23. Zimmet P. Epidemiology of diabetes and its macrovascular manifestations in Pacific populations: the medical effects of social progress. Diabetes Care 1979; 2:144–153.

24. Gamble DR. The epidemiology of insulin dependent diabetes, with particular reference to the relationship of virus infection to its etiology. Epidemiol Rev 1980; 2:49–70.

25. Holmgren G, Samuelson G, Hermansson B. The prevalence of diabetes mellitus: a study of children and their relatives in a northern Swedish county. Clin Genet 1974; 5:465–468.

26. Cohen T. Juvenile diabetes in Israel. Isr J Med Sci 1971; 7:1558–1561.

27. Teuscher A, Zuppinger K, Lüschner R, et al. Häufigkeit des jugendlichen Diabetes mellitus in Kanton Bern (Schweiz). Schweiz Med Wochenschr 1975; 105:1218–1223.

28. Bloom A, Hayes TM, Gamble DR. Register of newly diagnosed diabetic children. Br Med J 1975; 3:580–583.

29. Christau B, Kromann H, Andersen OO, et al. Incidence, seasonal and geographical patterns of juvenile-onset insulin-dependent diabetes mellitus in Denmark. Diabetologia 1977; 13:281–284.

30. Tattersall RB, Pyke DA. Diabetes in identical twins. Lancet 1972; 2:1120–1125.

31. LaPorte RE, Fishbein HA, Drash AL, et al. The Pittsburgh insulin-dependent diabetes mellitus (IDDM) registry: the incidence of insulin-dependent diabetes mellitus in Allegheny County, Pennsylvania (1965–1976). Diabetes 1981; 30:279–284.

32. Caillat-Zucman S, Garchon HJ, Timsit J, et al. Age-dependent HLA genetic heterogeneity of type I insulin-dependent diabetes mellitus. J Clin Invest 1992; 90:2242–2250.

33. Green A, Andersen PK. Epidemiological studies of diabetes mellitus in Denmark. 3: Clinical characteristics and incidence of diabetes among males aged 0 to 19 years. Diabetologia 1983; 25:226–230.

34. Kurtz Z, Peckham CS, Ades AE. Changing prevalence of juvenile-onset diabetes mellitus. Lancet 1988; 2:88–90.

35. Rewers M, LaPorte RE, Walczak M, et al. Apparent epidemic of insulin-dependent diabetes mellitus in midwestern Poland. Diabetes 1987; 36:106–113.

36. Melton LJ III, Palumbo PJ, Chu C-P. Incidence of diabetes mellitus by clinical type. Diabetes Care 1983; 6:75–86.

37. Christau B, Kromann H, Christy M, et al. Incidence of insulin-dependent diabetes mellitus (0–29 years at onset) in Denmark. Acta Med Scand (Suppl) 1979; 624:54–60.

38. Tuomilehto J, Louamaa R, Tuomilehto-Wolf E, et al. Epidemiology of childhood diabetes mellitus in Finland: background of a nationwide study of type 1 (insulin-dependent) diabetes mellitus. Diabetologia 1992; 35:70–76.

39. Karvonen M, Tuomilehto J, Libman I, et al. A review of the recent epidemiological data on the worldwide incidence of type 1 (insulin-dependent) diabetes mellitus. Diabetologia 1993; 35:883–892.

40. Helgason T, Danielsen R, Thorsson AV. Incidence and prevalence of type 1 (insulin-dependent) diabetes mellitus in Icelandic children 1970–1989. Diabetologia 1992; 35:880–883.

41. Drykoningen CEM, Mulder ALM, Vaandrager GJ, et al. The incidence of male childhood type 1 (insulin-dependent) diabetes mellitus is rising rapidly in the Netherlands. Diabetologia 1992; 35:139–142.

42. Green A, Andersen PK, Svendsen AJ, et al. Increasing incidence of early onset type 1 (insulin-dependent) diabetes mellitus: a study of Danish male birth cohorts. Diabetologia 1992; 35:178–182.

43. Akerblom HK, Reunanen A. The epidemiology of insulin-dependent diabetes mellitus (IDDM) in Finland and in northern Europe. Diabetes Care 1985; 8(Suppl 1):10–16.

44. Simpson NE. The genetics of diabetes: a study of 233 families of juvenile diabetics. Ann Hum Genet 1962; 26:1–21.

45. Tattersall RB, Fajans SS. A difference between the inheritance of classical juvenile-onset and maturity-onset type diabetes of young people. Diabetes 1975; 24:44–53.

46. Pociot E, Norgaard K, Hobolth N, et al. A nationwide population-based study of the familial aggregation of type 1 (insulin-dependent) diabetes mellitus in Denmark. Diabetologia 1993; 36:870–875.

47. Barnett AH, Eff C, Leslie RDG, et al. Diabetes in identical twins: a study of 200 pairs. Diabetologia 1981; 20:87–93.

48. Chern MM, Anderson VE, Barbosa J. Empirical risk for insulin-dependent diabetes (IDD) in sibs: further definition of genetic heterogeneity. Diabetes 1982; 31:1115–1118.

49. Wagener DK, Sacks JM, LaPorte RE, et al. The Pittsburgh study of insulin-dependent diabetes mellitus: risk for diabetes among relatives of IDDM. Diabetes 1982; 31:136–144.

50. Atkinson MA, Maclaren NK. Islet cell autoantigens in insulin-dependent diabetes. J Clin Invest 1993; 92:1608–1616.

51. Warram JH, Krowlewski AS, Gottlieb MS, et al. Differences in risk of insulin-dependent diabetes in offspring of diabetic mothers and diabetic fathers. N Engl J Med 1984; 311:149–152.

52. Vadheim CM, Rotter JI, Maclaren NK, et al. Preferential transmission of diabetic alleles within the HLA gene complex. N Engl J Med 1986; 315:1314–1318.

53. Benacerraf B. Role of MHC gene products in immune regulation. Science 1981; 212:1229–1238.

54. Steinmetz M, Hood L. Genes of the major histocompatibility complex in mouse and man. Science 1983; 222:727–733.

55. Shackelford DA, Kaufman JF, Korman AJ, et al. HLA-DR antigens: structure, separation of subpopulations, gene cloning and function. Immunol Rev 1982; 66:133–187.

56. Corte G, Calabi F, Damiani G, et al. Human Ia molecules carrying DC1 determinants differ in both α- and β-subunits from Ia molecules carrying DR determinants. Nature 1981; 292:357–360.

57. Strominger JL. Biology of the human histocompatibility leukocyte antigen system and a hypothesis regarding the generation of autoimmune diseases. J Clin Invest 1986; 77:1411–1415.

58. Kämpe O, Bellgrau D, Hammerling U, et al. Complex formation of class I transplantation antigens and a viral glycoprotein. J Biol Chem 1983; 258:10594–10598.

59. Bottazzo GF, Pujol-Borrell R, Hanafusa T, et al. Role of aberrant HLA-DR expression and antigen presentation in induction of endocrine autoimmunity. Lancet 1983; 2:1115–1119.

60. Acuto O, Reinherz EL. The human T-cell receptor: structure and function. N Engl J Med 1985; 312:1100–1111.

61. Faustman D, Hauptfeld V, Lacy P, et al. Prolongation of murine islet allograft survival by pretreatment of islets with antibody directed to Ia determinants. Proc Natl Acad Sci USA 1981; 78:5156–5159.

62. Bach FH, Sachs DH. Current concepts: immunology. Transplantation immunology. N Engl J Med 1987; 317:489–492.

63. Barbosa J, King R, Noreen H, et al. The histocompatibility system in juvenile, insulin-dependent diabetic multiplex kindreds. J Clin Invest 1977; 60:989–998.

64. Spielman RS, Baker L, Zmijewski CM. Gene dosage and susceptibility to insulin-dependent diabetes. Ann Hum Genet 1980; 44:135–150.

65. Walker A, Cudworth AG. Type I (insulin-dependent) diabetic multiplex families: mode of genetic transmission. Diabetes 1980; 29:1036–1039.

66. Nerup J, Mandrup-Poulsen T, Molvig J. The HLA-IDDM association: implications for etiology and pathogenesis of IDDM. Diabetes Metab Rev 1987; 3:779–802.

67. Sakurami T, Ueno Y, Nagaoka K, et al. HLA-DR specifications in Japanese with juvenile-onset insulin-dependent diabetes mellitus. Diabetes 1982; 31:105–116.

68. Todd JA, Bell JI, McDevitt HO. HLA-DQβ gene contributes to susceptibility and resistance to insulin-dependent diabetes mellitus. Nature 1987; 329:599–603.

69. Kwok WW, Lotshaw C, Milner ECB, et al. Mutational analysis of the HLA-DQ3.2 insulin-dependent diabetes mellitus susceptibility gene. Proc Natl Acad Sci USA 1989; 86:1027–1030.

70. Pugliese A, Gianani R, Moromisato R, et al. HLA-DQB1*0602 is associated with dominant protection from diabetes even among islet cell antibody-positive first-degree relatives of patients with IDDM. Diabetes 1995; 44:608–613.

71. Veijola R, Vahasalo P, Tuomilehto-Wolf E, et al. Human leukocyte antigen identity and DQ risk alleles in autoantibody-positive siblings of children with IDDM are associated with reduced early insulin response. Diabetes 1995; 44:1021–1028.

72. Cohen N, Brantbar C, Font MP, et al. HLA-DR2-associated DW-subtypes correlate with RFLP clusters: most DR2 IDDM patients belong to one of these clusters. Immunogenetics 1986; 23:47–51.

73. Van Endert P, Liblau RS, Patel SD, et al. Major histocompatibility complex-encoded antigen processing gene polymorphism in IDDM. Diabetes 1994; 43:110–117.

74. Rich SS. Positional cloning works! Identification of genes that cause IDDM. Diabetes 1995; 44:139–140.

75. Owerbach D, Gabbay KH. Localization of a type I diabetes susceptibility locus to the variable tandem repeat region flanking the insulin gene. Diabetes 1993; 42:1708–14.

76. Owerbach D, Gabbay KH. The HOSXD8 locus (2q31) is linked to type I diabetes: interaction with chromosome 6 and 11 disease susceptibility genes. Diabetes 1995; 44:132–136.

77. Ikegami H, Makino S, Yamato E, et al. Identification of a new susceptibility locus for insulin-dependent diabetes mellitus by ancestral haplotype congenic mapping. J Clin Invest 1995; 96:1936–1942.

78. Bottazzo GF, Doniach D. Pancreatic autoimmunity and HLA antigens. Lancet 1976; 2:800.

79. Irvine WJ. Classification of idiopathic diabetes. Lancet 1977; 1:638–642.

80. Rotter JI, Rimoin DL. Heterogeneity in diabetes mellitus—update, 1978: Evidence for further genetic heterogeneity within juvenile-onset insulin-dependent diabetes mellitus. Diabetes 1978; 27:599–608.

81. Ludvigsson J, Samuelsson U, Beuforts C, et al. HLA-DR3 is associated with a more slowly progressive form of type 1 (insulin-dependent) diabetes. Diabetologia 1986; 29:207–210.

82. MacDonald MJ. Hypothesis: the frequencies of juvenile diabetes in American blacks and Caucasians are consistent with dominant inheritance. Diabetes 1980; 29:110–114.

83. MacDonald MJ, Gottschall J, Hunter JB, et al. HLA-DR4 in insulin-dependent diabetic parents and their diabetic offspring: a clue to dominant inheritance. Proc Natl Acad Sci USA 1986; 83:7049–7053.

84. Barbosa J, Chern MM, Anderson VE, et al. Linkage analysis between the major histocompatibility system and insulin-dependent diabetes in families with patients in two consecutive generations. J Clin Invest 1980; 65:592–601.

85. Rubinstein P, Suciu-Foca N, Nicholson JF. Genetics of juvenile diabetes mellitus: a recessive gene closely linked to HLA D and with 50 per cent penetrance. N Engl J Med 1977; 297:1036–1040.

86. Pyke DA. Diabetes: the genetic connections. Diabetologia 1979; 17:333–343.

87. Nerup J. HLA studies in diabetes mellitus: a review. Adv Metab Disord 1978; 9:263–277.

88. Rotter JI, Anderson CE, Rubin R, et al. HLA genotypic study of insulin-dependent diabetes: the excess of DR3/DR4 heterozygotes allows rejection of the recessive hypothesis. Diabetes 1983; 32:169–174.

89. Williams RC. Has the recessive hypothesis for susceptibility to insulin-dependent diabetes mellitus been firmly and unequivocally rejected? Diabetes 1983; 32:774–776.

90. Todd JA. Genetic analysis of type I diabetes using whole genome approaches. Proc Natl Acad Sci USA 1995; 93:8560–8565.

91. Wicker LS, Todd JA, Prins JB, et al. Resistance alleles at two non-major histocompatibility complex-linked insulin-dependent diabetes loci on chromosome 3, Idd3 and Idd10, protect nonobese diabetic mice from diabetes. J Exp Med 1994; 180:1705–13.

92. Rowe RE, Wapelhorst B, Bell GI, et al. Linkage and association between insulin-dependent diabetes mellitus (IDDM) susceptibility and markers near the glucokinase gene on chromosome 7. Nat Genet 1995; 10:240–242.

93. Copeman JB, Cucca F, Hearne CM, et al. Linkage disequilibrium mapping of a type I diabetes susceptibility gene (IDDM7) to chromosome 2q31-q33. Nature Genetics 1995; 9:80–85.

94. Todd JA, Bennett ST. Diabetes genes: mutatis mutandis. Nature 1995; 374:601–602.

95. Santamaria P, Lewis C, Jessurun J, et al. Skewed T-cell receptor usage and junctional heterogeneity among isletitis αβ and γδ T-cells in human IDDM. Diabetes 1994; 43:599–606.

96. Durinovic-Bello I, Steinle A, Ziegler AG, et al. HLA-DQ–restricted islet-specific T-cell clones of a type 1 diabetic patient: T-cell receptor sequence similarities to insulitis-inducing T-cells of nonobese diabetic mice. Diabetes 1994; 43:1318–1325.

97. Peakman M, Alviggi L, Hussain MJ, et al. Increased expression of T-cell markers of immunological memory associated with protection from type 1 diabetes: a study of identical twins. Diabetes 1994; 43:712–717.

98. Cahill GF Jr, McDevitt HO. Insulin-dependent diabetes mellitus: the initial lesion. N Engl J Med 1981; 304:1454–1465.

99. Foulis AK, Francis ND, Farquharson MA, et al. Massive synchronous B-cell necrosis causing type 1 (insulin-dependent) diabetes: a unique histopathological case report. Diabetologia 1988; 31:46–50.

100. Karam JH, Lewitt PA, Young CW, et al. Insulinopenic diabetes after rodenticide (Vacor) ingestion: a unique model of acquired diabetes in man. Diabetes 1980; 29:971–978.

101. Helgason T, Jonasson MR. Evidence for food additive as a cause of ketosis prone diabetes. Lancet 1981; 2:716–720.

102. Karjalainen J, Martin JM, Knip M, et al. A bovine albumin peptide as a possible trigger of insulin-dependent diabetes mellitus. N Engl J Med 1992; 327:302–307.

103. Pietropaolo M, Castrane L, Babu S, et al. Cell antigen 69 kD (ICA 69): molecular cloning and characterization of a novel diabetes-associated autoantigen. J Clin Invest 1993; 92:359–371.

104. Virtanen SM, Rasanen A, Aro J, et al. Infant feeding in Finnish children less than 7 yrs of age with newly diagnosed IDDM: childhood diabetes in Finland study group. Diabetes Care 1991; 14:415–417.

105. Atkinson MA, Bowman MA, Kao K-J, et al. Lack of bovine responsiveness to bovine serum albumin in insulin-dependent diabetes. N Engl J Med 1993; 329:1853–1858.

106. Mordes JP, Desemone J, Rossini AA. The BB rat. Diabetes Metab Rev 1987; 3:725–750.

107. Kataoka S, Satoh J, Fujiya H, et al. Immunologic aspects of the nonobese diabetic (NOD) mouse: abnormalities of cellular immunity. Diabetes 1983; 32:247–253.

108. Szopa TM, Tichener PA, Portwood ND, et al. Diabetes mellitus due to viruses-some recent developments. Diabetologia 1993; 36:687–695.

109. Yoon J-W, Ray UR. Perspectives on the role of viruses in insulin-dependent diabetes. Diabetes Care 1985; 8(Suppl 1): 39–44.

110. Menser MA, Forrest JM, Bransby RD. Rubella infection and diabetes mellitus. Lancet 1978; 1:57–60.

111. Frisk G, Fohlman J, Kobbah M, et al. High frequency of Coxsackie-B-virus–specific IgM in children developing type 1 diabetes during a period of high-diabetes morbidity. J Med Virol 1985; 17:219–227.

112. Nelson PG, Pyke DA, Gamble DR. Viruses and the aetiology of diabetes: a study in identical twins. Br Med J 1975; 4:249–251.

113. An epidemic of childhood diabetes in the United States? Evidence from Allegheny County, Pennsylvania. Diabetes Care 1993; 16:1606–1611.

114. Yoon J-W, Austin M, Onodera T, et al. Virus-induced diabetes mellitus: isolation of a virus from the pancreas of a child with diabetic ketoacidosis. N Engl J Med 1979; 300:1173–1179.

115. Jenson AB, Rosenberg HS, Notkins AL. Pancreatic islet-cell damage in children with fatal viral infections. Lancet 1980; 2:354–358.

116. Pak CY, Eun H-M, McArthur RG, et al. Association of cytomegalovirus infection with autoimmune type 1 diabetes. Lancet 1988; 2:1–4.

117. Hyoty H, Hiltunen M, Knip M, et al. A prospective study of the role of Coxsackie B and other enterovirus infections in the pathogenesis of IDDM. Diabetes 1995; 44:652–657.

118. Hou J, Said C, Franchi D, et al. Antibodies to glutamic acid decarboxylase and P2-C peptides in sera from Coxsackie virus B4-infected mice and IDDM patients. Diabetes 1994; 43:1260–1266.

119. Kaufman DL, Erlander MG, Clare-Salzler M, et al. Autoimmunity to two forms of glutamic acid decarboxylase in insulin-dependent diabetes mellitus. J Clin Invest 1992; 89:283–292.

120. Oldstone MB, Nerenberg M, Southern P, et al. Virus infection triggers insulin-dependent diabetes mellitus in a transgenic model: role of anti-self (virus) immune response. Cell 1991; 65:319–331.

121. Yoon J-W, Onodera T, Notkins AL. Virus-induced diabetes mellitus. XV: Beta cell damage and insulin-dependent hyperglycemia in mice infected with coxsackie virus B4. J Exp Med 1978; 148:1068–1080.

122. Yoon J-W, Notkins AL. Virus-induced diabetes mellitus. VI: Genetically determined host differences in the replication of encephalomyocarditis virus in pancreatic beta cells. J Exp Med 1976; 143:1170–1185.

123. Yoon J-W, Onodera T, Notkins AL. Virus-induced diabetes mellitus. VIII: Passage of encephalomyocarditis virus and severity of diabetes in susceptible and resistant strains of mice. J Gen Virol 1977; 37:225–232.

124. Jenkins O, Booth JO, Minor PD, et al. The complete nucleotide sequence of Coxsackie virus B4 and its comparison to other members of the Picornaviridae. J Gen Virol 1987; 68:1835–1848.

125. Toniolo A, Takashi O, Yoon J-W, et al. Induction of diabetes by cumulative environmental insults from viruses and chemicals. Nature 1980; 288:383–385.

126. Fujita H. Retrovirus-like particles in pancreatic β-cells of NOD mice. Biomed Res 1984; 5:67–70.

127. Leiter EL, Fewell JW, Kuff EL. Glucose induces type A retroviral gene transcription and translation in pancreatic beta cells. J Exp Med 1986; 163:87–100.

128. Jones DB, McLaughlin PJ, Armstrong N, et al. Does Coxsackie B4 virus infection induce GAD and HSP65 autoreactivity in type 1 diabetes? Diabetic Med 1992; 9(Suppl 2):524 (abstract).

129. Oldstone MB. Viruses as therapeutic agents: treatment of nonobese insulin-dependent diabetic mice with virus prevents insulin-dependent diabetes while maintaining general immune competence. J Exp Med 1990; 171:2077–2089.

130. Nerup J, Cathelineau C, Seignalet J, et al. HLA and endocrine disease. In: Dausset J, Svejgaard A, eds. HLA and Disease. Copenhagen: Munksgaard, 1977: 149–167.

131. Rossini AA, Like AA, Chick WL, et al. Studies of streptozotocin-induced insulitis and diabetes. Proc Natl Acad Sci USA 1977; 74:2485–2489.

132. Bottazo GF. β-cell damage in diabetic insulitis: are we approaching a solution? Diabetologia 1984; 26:241–249.

133. Gepts W, In't Veld P. Islet morphologic changes. Diabetes Metab Rev 1987; 3:859–872.

134. Karam JH, Prosser PR, LeWitt PA. Islet-cell surface antibodies in a patient with diabetes mellitus after a rodenticide ingestion. N Engl J Med 1978; 299:1191.

135. Like AA, Rossini AA. Streptozotocin-induced pancreatic insulitis: new model of diabetes mellitus. Science 1976; 193:415–417.

136. Craighead JE. The role of viruses in the pathogenesis of pancreatic disease and diabetes mellitus. Prog Med Virol 1975; 19:161–214.

137. Like AA, Rossini AA, Guberski DL, et al. Spontaneous diabetes mellitus: reversal and prevention in the BB/W rat with antiserum to rat lymphocytes. Science 1979; 206:1421–1423.

138. Koevary S, Rossini A, Stoller W, et al. Passive transfer of diabetes in the BB/W rat. Science 1983; 220:727–728.

139. Like AA, Weringer EJ, Holdash A, et al. Nature of resistance to autoimmune diabetes in BioBreeding/Worcester control rats. Diabetologia 1983; 25:175.

140. Greiner DL, Mordes JP, Handler ES, et al. Depletion of RT6.1+ T-lymphocytes induces diabetes in resistant BioBreeding/Worcester (BB/W) rats. J Exp Med 1987; 166:461–475.

141. Rossini AA, Mordes JP, Pelletier AM, et al. Transfusions of whole blood prevent spontaneous diabetes mellitus in the BB/W rat. Science 1983; 219:975–977.

142. Jackson RA, Morris MA, Haynes BF, et al. Increased circulating Ia-antigen–bearing T cells in type I diabetes mellitus. N Engl J Med 1982; 306:785–788.

143. Bougneres PF, Carel JC, Castino L, et al. Factors associated with early remission of type 1 diabetes in children treated with cyclosporine. N Engl J Med 1988; 318:663–670.

144. Sibley RK, Sutherland DER, Groetz F, et al. Recurrent diabetes mellitus in the pancreas iso- and allograft: a light and electron microscopic and immunohistochemical analysis of four cases. Lab Invest 1985; 53:132–144.

145. Pozzilli P, Zuccarini O, Iavicoli M, et al. Monoclonal antibodies defined abnormalities of T-lymphocytes in type 1 (insulin-dependent) diabetes. Diabetes 1983; 32:91–94.

146. Quinion-Debrie MC, Debray-Sachs M, Dardenne M, et al. Anti-islet cellular and humoral immunity. T-cell subsets and thymic function in type 1 diabetes. Diabetes 1985; 34:373–379.

147. Hitchcock CL, Riley WJ, Alamo A, et al. Lymphocyte subsets and activation in prediabetes. Diabetes 1986; 35:1416–1422.

148. Buschard K, Röpke C, Madsbad S, et al. T lymphocyte subsets in patients with newly diagnosed type 1 (insulin-dependent) diabetes: a prospective study. Diabetologia 1983; 25:247–251.

149. Amadori A, Zamarchi R, De Silvestro G, et al. Genetic control of the CD4/CD8 T-cell ratio in humans. Nat Med 1995; 1:1279–1283.

150. Lernmark Å, Li S, Baekkeskov S, et al. Islet-specific immune mechanisms. Diabetes Metab Rev 1987; 3:959–980.

151. Barbosa J, Bach FH. Cell-mediated autoimmunity in type 1 diabetes. Diabetes Metab Rev 1987; 3:981–1004.

152. Irvine WJ, Gray RS, Steel JM. Islet cell antibody as a marker for early stage type 1 diabetes mellitus. In: Irvine WJ, ed. Immunology of Diabetes. Edinburgh: Teviot Scientific Publications, 1980: 117–154.

153. Nayak RC, Omar MAK, Rabizadeh A, et al. "Cytoplasmic" islet cell antibodies: evidence that the target antigen is a sialogycogonjugate. Diabetes 1985; 34:617–619.

154. Bottazzo GF, Landrum R. Separate autoantibodies to human pancreatic glucagon and somatostatin cells. Lancet 1976; 2:873–876.

155. Orci L, Baetens D, Rufener C, et al. Hypertrophy and hyperplasia of somatostatin-containing D-cells in diabetes. Proc Natl Acad Sci USA 1976; 73:1338–1342.

156. Volk BW, Wellmann KF. The pathology of the diabetic pancreas. In: Ellenberg M, Rifkin H, eds. Diabetes Mellitus: Theory and Practice. 3rd ed. New Hyde Park, NY: Medical Examination Publishing, 1983: 309–321.

157. Gepts W, LeCompte PM. The pancreatic islets in diabetes. Am J Med 1981; 70:105–115.

158. Orci L. The microanatomy of the islets of Langerhans. Metabolism 1976; 25(Suppl 1):1303–1313.

159. Stefan Y, Malaisse-Lagae F, Yoon J-W, et al. Virus-induced diabetes in mice: a quantitative evaluation of islet cell population by immunofluorescence technique. Diabetologia 1978; 15:395–401.

160. Irvine WJ, McCallum CJ, Gray RS, et al. Pancreatic islet-cell antibodies in diabetes mellitus correlated with the duration and type of diabetes, coexistent autoimmune disease, and HLA type. Diabetes 1977; 26:138–147.

161. Kolb H, Dannehl K, Grüneklee D, et al. Prospective analysis of islet cell antibodies in children with type 1 (insulin-dependent) diabetes. Diabetologia 1988; 31:189–194.

162. Bottazzo GF, Cudworth AG, Moul DJ, et al. Evidence for a primary autoimmune type of diabetes mellitus. Br Med J 1978; 2:1253–1255.

163. Cudworth AG, Spencer KM, Gorsuch AN, et al. Immunogenetic heterogeneity in insulin-dependent diabetes. In: Köbberling FJ, Tattersall R, eds. The Genetics of Diabetes Mellitus. Proceedings of the Serono Symposia. Vol 47. London: Academic, 1982: 63–78.

164. Schernthaner G, Ludwig H, Mayr WR. Immunoglobulin G-insulin antibodies and immune region-associated alloantigens in insulin-dependent diabetes mellitus. J Clin Endocrinol Metab 1979; 48:403–407.

165. Rotter JI, Rimoin DL. Genetics of insulin-dependent diabetes. In: Martin JM, Ehrlich RM, Holland FJ, eds. Etiology and Pathogenesis of Insulin-Dependent Diabetes Mellitus. New York: Raven, 1981: 37–59.

166. Satoh J, Prabhakar BS, Haspel MV, et al. Human monoclonal autoantibodies that react with multiple endocrine organs. N Engl J Med 1983; 309:217–220.

167. Lernmark A. Islet cell antibodies. Diabet Med 1982; 4:285–292.

168. Srikanta S, Ricker AT, McCulloch DK, et al. Autoimmunity to insulin, beta cell dysfunction, and development of insulin-dependent diabetes mellitus. Diabetes 1986; 35:139–142.

169. Baekkeskov S, Aanstoot H-J, Christgan S, et al. Identification of the 64K autoantigen in insulin-dependent diabetes as the GABA-synthesizing enzyme glutamic acid decarboxylase. Nature 1990; 347:151–156.

170. Kuglin B, Gries FA, Kolb H. Evidence of IgG autoantibodies against human proinsulin in patients with IDDM before insulin treatment. Diabetes 1988; 37:130–132.

171. Di Mario U, Dotta F, Crisa L, et al. Circulating anti-immunoglobulin antibodies in recent-onset type I diabetic patients. Diabetes 1988; 37:462–466.

172. Ludwig SM, Faiman C, Dean HJ. Insulin and insulin-receptor autoantibodies in children with newly diagnosed IDDM before insulin therapy. Diabetes 1987; 36:420–425.

173. Castano L, Russo E, Zhou L, et al. Identification on cloning of a granule autoantigen (carboxypeptides H) associated with type 1 diabetes. J Clin Endocrinol Metab 1991; 73:1197–1201.

174. Powers A, Bowen S, West S. Carboxypeptidase-H is an autoantigen of the ICA and is expressed on the cell surface of islet cells. Diabetes 1991; 40:1a (abstract).

175. Roep BD, Arden SD, DeVries RR, et al. T-cell clones from a type 1 diabetic patient respond to insulin secretory granule proteins. Nature 1990; 345:632–634.

176. Gianani R, Rabin DU, Verge CF, et al. ICA512 autoantibody radioassay. Diabetes 1995; 44:1340–1344.

177. Myers MA, Rabin DU, Rowley MJ. Pancreatic islet cell cytoplasmic antibody in diabetes is represented by antibodies to islet cell antigen 512 and glutamic acid decarboxylase. Diabetes 1995; 44:1290–1295.

178. Boehn BO, Manifras B, Seibler J, et al. Epidemiology and immune-genetic background of islet cell antibody-positive nondiabetic school children. Diabetes 1991; 40:1435–1439.

179. Landin-Olsson M, Palmer JP, Lernmark Å, et al. Predictive value of islet cell and insulin autoantibodies for type 1 (insulin-dependent) diabetes mellitus in a population-based study of newly-diagnosed diabetic and matched control children. Diabetologia 1992: 1068–1073.

180. Yu L, Gianni R, Eisenbarth GS. Quantitation of glutamic acid decarboxylase autoantibody levels in prospectively evaluated relatives of patients with type 1 diabetes. Diabetes 1994; 33:1229–1233.

181. Lernmärk Å, Molenaar JL, van Beers, WAM, et al. The Fourth International Serum Exchange Workshop to standardize cytoplasmic islet cell antibodies. Diabetologia 1991; 34:534–535.

182. Solimena M, Folli F, Aparisi R, et al. Autoantibodies to GABA-nergic neurons and pancreatic beta cells in stiff-man syndrome. N Engl J Med 1990; 322:1555–1560.

183. Baekkeskov S, Nielsen JH, Warner J, et al. Autoantibodies in newly diagnosed diabetic children immunoprecipitate human islet cell proteins. Nature 1982; 298:167–169.

184. Baekkeskov S, Jan-Aanstoot H, Christgan S, et al. Identification of the 64K autoantigen in insulin-dependent diabetes as the GABA-synthesizing enzyme glutamic acid decarboxylase. Nature 1990; 151–156.

185. Tuomilehto J, Zimmet P, Mackay IR, et al. Antibodies to glutamic acid decarboxylase as predictors of insulin-dependent diabetes mellitus before clinical onset. Lancet 1994; 343:1383–1385.

186. Harrison LC, Honeyman MC, DeAizpurua, HJ, et al. Inverse relationship between humoral and cellular immunity to glutamic acid decarboxylase in subjects at risk of insulin-dependent diabetes. Lancet 1993; 341:1365–1369.

187. Vandewalk CL, Decraene T, Schuit FC, et al. Insulin autoantibodies and high titre islet cell antibodies are preferentially associated with the HLA DQA1*0301-DQB1*0302 haplotype at clinical onset of type 1 (insulin-dependent) diabetes mellitus before age 10 years but not at onset between age 10 and 40 years. Diabetologia 1993; 36:1155–1162.

188. Böhmer K, Keilackes H, Kuglin B, et al. Proinsulin autoantibodies are more closely associated with type 1 (insulin-dependent) diabetes mellitus than insulin antibodies. Diabetologia 1991; 34:830–834.

189. Vardi P, Ziegler AG, Matthews JH, et al. Concentration of insulin autoantibodies at onset of type 1 diabetes: inverse log-linear correlation with age. Diabetes Care 1988; 11:736–740.

190. Elias D, Markevitz D, Reshef T, et al. Induction and therapy of autoimmune diabetes in the non-obese diabetic mouse by a 65-kDa heat shock protein. Proc Natl Acad Sci USA 1990; 87:1576–1580.

191. Jones DB, Hunter NR, Duff GW. Heat shock protein 65 as a β cell antigen of insulin-dependent diabetes. Lancet 1990; 335:583–585.

192. Boitard C, Villa MC, Becourt C, et al. Peripherin: an islet antigen that is cross-reactive with nonobese diabetic mouse class II gene products. Proc Natl Acad Sci USA 1992; 89:172–176.

193. Johnson JH, Crider BP, McCorkle K, et al. Inhibition of glucose transport into rat islet cells by immunoglobulins from patients with new-onset insulin-dependent diabetes mellitus. N Engl J Med 1990; 322:653–659.

194. Inman LR, McAllister CT, Chen L, et al. Autoantibodies to GLUT-2 in new onset insulin-dependent diabetes mellitus. Proc Natl Acad Sci USA 1993; 90:1281–1286.

195. Atkinson MA, Holmes LA, Sharp DW, et al. No evidence for serological autoimmunity toward islet cell heat shock protein in insulin-dependent diabetes. J Clin Invest 1991; 87:721–724.

196. Savilahti E, Akerblom HK, Koskimies S. Children with newly diagnosed insulin-dependent diabetes have increased levels of cows' milk antibodies. Diabetes Res 1988; 7:137–140.

197. Borch-Johnsen K, Joner G, Mandrup-Poulsen T, et al. Relation between breast-feeding and incidence rates of insulin-dependent diabetes mellitus: a hypothesis. Lancet 1984; 2(8411):1083–1086.

198. Atkinson M, Kaufman DL, Campbell KA, et al. Response of peripheral-blood mononuclear cells to glutamate decarboxylase in insulin-dependent diabetes. Lancet 1992; 339:458–459.

199. McDevitt HO. Autoimmune diabetes and its antigenic triggers. Hosp Pract 1995; 30:55–62.

200. Elliott JF, Qin H-Y, Bhatti S, et al. Immunization with the larger isoforms of mouse glutamic acid decarboxylase (GAD67) prevents autoimmune diabetes in NOD mice. Diabetes 1994; 43:1494–1499.

201. Posselt AM, Barker CF, Friedman AL, et al. Prevention of autoimmune diabetes by intrathymic islet transplantation at birth. Science 1992; 256:1321–1324.

202. Clerici M, Shearer G. The Th1-Th2 hypothesis of HIV infection: new insights. Immunol Today 1994; 15:375–381.

203. Rabinovitch A. Immunoregulatory and cytokine imbalances in the pathogenesis of IDDM: therapeutic intervention by immunostimulation? Diabetes 1994; 43:613–621.

204. MacDonald HR, Acha-Orbea H. Superantigen as suspect. Nature 1994; 371:283–284.

205. Scherer MT, Ignatowicz F, Pullen A, et al. The use of mammary tumor virus (Mtv)-negative and single-Mtv mice to evaluate the effects of superantigens on the T cell repertoire. J Exp Med 1995; 182:1493–1504.
206. Gurad B, Weldmann E, Truccoi G, et al. Evidence for superantigen involvement in insulin-dependent diabetes mellitus etiology. Nature 1994; 371:351–355.
207. Ziegler AG, Herskowitz RD, Jackson RA, et al. Predicting type 1 diabetes. Diabetes Care 1990; 13:762–775.
208. Schatz D, Krischer J, Horne G, et al. Islet cell antibodies predict insulin-dependent diabetes in United States school children as powerfully as in unaffected relatives. J Clin Invest 1994; 93:2403–2407.
209. Hagopian WA, Sanjeevi CB, Kockum I, et al. Glutamate decarboxylase-, insulin-, and islet cell-antibodies and HL typing to detect diabetes in a general population-based study of Swedish children. J Clin Invest 1995; 95:1505–1511.
210. Aanstoot H-J, Sigurdsson E, Jaffe M, et al. Value of antibodies to GAD65 combined with islet cytoplasmic antibodies for predicting IDDM in a childhood population. Diabetologia 1994; 37:917–924.
211. Niskanen L, Karjalainen J, Sarlund H, et al. Five-year follow-up of islet cell antibodies in type 2 (non–insulin-dependent) diabetes mellitus. Diabetologia 1991; 34:402–408.
212. Tuomi T, Groop LC, Zimmet PZ, et al. Antibodies to glutamic acid decarboxylase reveal latent autoimmune diabetes mellitus in adults with a non–insulin-dependent onset of diabetes. Diabetes 1993; 42:359–362.
213. Eisenbarth GS, Connelly J, Soeldner JS. The "natural" history of type 1 diabetes. Diabetes Metab Rev 1987; 3:873–891.
214. Srikanta S, Ganda OP, Jackson RA, et al. Type I diabetes mellitus in monozygotic twins: chronic progressive beta cell dysfunction. Ann Intern Med 1983; 99:320–326.
215. Srikanta S, Ganda OP, Eisenbarth GS, et al. Islet-cell antibodies and beta-cell function in monozygotic triplets and twins initially discordant for type I diabetes mellitus. N Engl J Med 1983; 308:322–325.
216. Maclaren NK. Perspectives in diabetes: how, when and why to predict IDDM. Diabetes 1988; 37:1591–1594.
217. Huang S-W, Maclaren NK. Insulin-dependent diabetes: a disease of autoaggression. Science 1976; 192:64–66.
218. Pozzilli P, Sensi M, Gorsuch A, et al. Evidence for raised K-cell levels in type-1 diabetes. Lancet 1979; 2:173–175.
219. Rossini AA. Immunotherapy for insulin-dependent diabetics? N Engl J Med 1983; 308:333–335.
220. Serreze DV, Leiter EH, Worthen SM, et al. NOD marrow stem cells adoptively transfer diabetes to resistant (NOD × NON) F1 mice. Diabetes 1988; 37:252–255.
221. Bendelac A, Carnand C, Boitard C, et al. Syngeneic transfer of autoimmune diabetes from diabetic NOD mice to healthy neonates. Requirement for both L3T4+ and Lyt-2+ T cells. J Exp Med 1987; 166:823–832.
222. Wicker LS, Miller BJ, Mullen Y. Transfer of autoimmune diabetes mellitus with splenocytes from nonobese diabetic (NOD) mice. Diabetes 1986; 35:855–860.
223. Hanafusa T, Sugihara S, Fujina-Kurihara H, et al. Induction of insulitis by adoptive transfer with L3T4+ Lyt2− lymphocytes in T-lymphocyte-depleted NOD mice. Diabetes 1988; 37:204–208.
224. Logothetopoulos J, Valiquette N, MacGregor I, et al. Adoptive transfer of insulitis and diabetes in neonates of diabetes-prone and -resistant rats: tissue localization of injected blasts. Diabetes 1987; 36:1116–1123.
225. Miller BJ, Appel MC, O'Neill JJ, et al. Both Lyt-2+ and L3T4+ T cell subsets are required for the transfer of diabetes in nonobese diabetic mice. J Immunol 1988; 440:52–58.
226. Charlton B, Mandel TE. Progression from insulitis to beta-cell destruction requires L3T4+ T-lymphocytes. Diabetes 1988; 37:1108–1112.
227. Woda BA, Biron CA. Natural killer cell number and function in the spontaneously diabetic BB/W rat. J Immunol 1986; 137:1860–1866.
228. Woda BA, Padden C. BioBreeding/Worcester (BB/Wor) rats are deficient in the generation of functional cytotoxic T cells. J Immunol 1987; 139:1514–1517.
229. Pukel C, Baquerizo H, Rabinovitch A. Interleukin 2 activates BB/W diabetic rat lymphoid cells cytotoxic to islet cells. Diabetes 1987; 36:1217–1222.
230. Kawakami Y, Custer MC, Rosenberg SA, et al. IL-4 regulates IL-2 induction of lymphokine-activated killer activity from human lymphocytes. J Immunol 1989; 142:3452–3461.
231. Rapoport MJ, Jaramillo A, Zipris D, et al. Interleukin-4 reverses T-cell proliferative unresponsiveness and prevents the onset of diabetes in nonobese diabetic mice. J Exp Med 1993; 178:87–99.
232. Gladstone P, Nepom GT. Prevention of IDDM: injecting insulin into the cytokine network. Diabetes 1995; 44:859–862.
233. Atkinson MA, MacLaren NK. The pathogenesis of insulin-dependent diabetes mellitus. N Engl J Med 1994; 331:1428–1436.
234. Santamari P, Lewis C, Jessurun J, et al. Skewed T-cell receptor usage and junctional heterogeneity among isletitis αβ and γδ T-cells in human IDDM. Diabetes 1994; 48:599–606.
235. Male D, Champion B, Cooke S. Cytotoxic lymphocytes. In: Advanced Immunology. London: Gower Medical, 1987: 7.1–7.7.
236. Podack ER. The molecular mechanism of lymphocyte-mediated tumour cell lysis. Immunol Today 1985; 6:21–27.
237. Walker R, Bone AJ, Cooke A, et al. Distinct macrophage subpopulations in pancreas of BB/E rats: possible role for macrophages in the pathogenesis of IDDM. Diabetes 1988; 37:1301–1304.
238. Bendtzen K, Mandrup-Poulsen T, Nerup J, et al. Cytotoxicity of human pI 7 interleukin-1 for pancreatic islets of Langerhans. Science 1986; 232:1545–1547.
239. Nerup J, Mandrup-Poulsen T, Mølvig J, et al. Mechanisms of pancreatic β-cell destruction in type I diabetes. Diabetes Care 1988; 11(Suppl 1):16–23.
240. Mandrup-Poulsen T, Bendtzen K, Dinarello CA, et al. Human tumor necrosis factor potentiates human interleukin-1 mediated rat pancreatic β-cell toxicity. J Immunol 1987; 139:4077–4082.
241. McDaniel ML, Hughes JH, Wolf BA, et al. Descriptive and mechanistic considerations of interleukin 1 and insulin secretion. Diabetes 1988; 37:1311–1315.
242. Sandler S, Andersson H, Hellerström C. Inhibitory effects of interleukin 1 on insulin secretion, insulin biosynthesis, and oxidative metabolism of isolated rat pancreatic islets. Endocrinology 1987; 121:1424–1431.
243. Nerup J, Mandrup-Poulsen J, Mølvig J, et al. Immune interactions with islet cells: implications for the pathogenesis of insulin-dependent diabetes mellitus. In: Pipeleers D, ed. Pathology of the Endocrine Pancreas in Diabetes. Berlin: Springer-Verlag, 1988: 71–84.
244. Dulin WE, Wyse BM. Reversal of streptozotocin diabetes with nicotinamide. Proc Soc Exp Biol Med 1969; 130:992–994.
245. Yamada K, Nonaka K, Hanafusa T, et al. Preventive and therapeutic effects of large dose nicotinamide injections on diabetes associated with insulitis: an observation in nonobese diabetic (NOD) mice. Diabetes 1982; 31:749–753.
246. Okamoto H. The role of poly(ADP-ribose) synthetase in the development of insulin-dependent diabetes and islet β-cell regeneration. Biomed Biochim Acta 1985; 44:15–20.
247. Asayama K, Kooy NW, Burn IM. Effect of vitamin E deficiency and selenium deficiency on insulin secretory reserve and free radical scavenging systems in islets: decrease of islet manganosuperoxide dismutase. J Lab Clin Med 1986; 107:459–464.
248. Halliwell B, ed. Oxygen Radicals and Tissue Injury. Proceedings of a Brook Lodge Symposium, April 27–29, 1987. Bethesda: FASEB (for Upjohn), 1988.
249. Heikkila RE, Winston B, Cohen G, et al. Alloxan-induced diabetes: evidence for the hydroxyl radical as a cytotoxic intermediate. Biochem Pharmacol 1976; 25:1085–1092.
250. Yan SD, Yan SF, Chen X, et al. Non-enzymatically glycated tau in Alzheimer's disease induces neuronal oxidant stress resulting in cytokine gene expression and release of amyloid β-peptide. Nat Med 1995; 1:693–699.
251. Karlsen AE, Andersen HU, Vising H, et al. Cloning and expression of cytokine-inducible nitric oxide synthase: cDNA from rat islets of Langerhans. Diabetes 1995; 44:753–758.
252. Lindsay RM, Smith W, Rossiter SP, et al. N-Nitro-L-arginine methyl ester reduces the incidence of IDDM in BB/E rats. Diabetes 1995; 44:365–368.
253. Kröncke KD, Kolb-Bachofer V, Berschick, et al. Activated macrophages kill pancreatic syngeneic islet cells via arginine-dependent nitric oxide generation. Biochem Biophys Res Commun 1991; 175:752–758.
254. Eizirik DL, Sandler S, Welsh N, et al. Cytokines suppress human islet function irrespective of their effects on nitric oxide generation. J Clin Invest 1994; 93:1968–1974.
255. Bottazzo GF, Dean BM, McNally JM, et al. In situ characterization of autoimmune phenomena and expression of HLA molecules in the pancreas in diabetic insulitis. N Engl J Med 1985; 313:353–360.
256. Signore A, Cooke A, Pozzilli P, et al. Class-II and IL2 receptor positive cells in the pancreas of NOD mice. Diabetologia 1987; 30:902–905.
257. In't Veld PA, Pipellers DG. In situ analysis of pancreatic islets in rats developing diabetes: appearance of nonendocrine cells with surface MHC class II antigens and cytoplasmic insulin immunoreactivity. J Clin Invest 1988; 82:1123–1128.
258. Sarvetnick N, Liggitt D, Pitts SL, et al. Insulin-dependent diabetes mellitus induced in transgenic mice by ectopic expression of class II MHC and interferon-gamma. Cell 1988; 52:773–782.
259. Lo D, Burkely LC, Widora G, et al. Diabetes and tolerance in transgenic mice expressing class II MHC molecules in pancreatic beta cells. Cell 1988; 53:159–168.
260. Markmann J, Lo D, Naji A, et al. Antigen presenting function of class II MHC expressing pancreatic β-cells. Nature 1988; 336:475–479.
261. Yagi N, Yokono K, Amano K, et al. Expression of intercellular adhesion molecule 1 on pancreatic β-cells accelerates β-cell destruction by cytotoxic T-cells in murine autoimmune diabetes. Diabetes 1995; 44:744–752.
262. Itoh N, Hanafusa T, Miyazaki A, et al. Mononuclear cell infiltration and its relation to expression of major histocompatibility antigens and adhesion molecules in pancreas biopsy specimens from newly diagnosed insulin-dependent diabetes mellitus patients. J Clin Invest 1993; 92:2313–2322.
263. Hänninen A, Taylor C, Streeter PR, et al. Vascular addressins are induced on islet vessels during insulitis in nonobese diabetic mice and are involved in lymphoid cell binding to islet endothelium. J Clin Invest 1993; 92:2509–2515.
264. Baron JL, Reich E-P, Visintin I, et al. The pathogenesis of adoptive murine autoimmune diabetes requires an interaction between α4-integrins and vascular cell adhesion molecule-1. J Clin Invest 1994; 93:1700–1708.
265. Yang X-D, Michie SA, Fisch R, et al. A predominant role of integrin α4

in the spontaneous development of autoimmune diabetes in nonobese diabetic mice. Proc Natl Acad Sci USA 1994; 91:12604–12608.

266. Buschard K, Rygaard J. Passive transfer of streptozotocin induced diabetes with spleen cells. Acta Pathol Microbiol Scand 1977; 85:469.

267. Rieux-Laucat F, Le Deist F, Hivroz C, et al. Mutations in *Fas* associated with human lymphoproliferative syndrome and autoimmunity. Science 1995; 268:1347–1349.

268. Spies T, Morton CC, Nedospasov SA, et al. Genes for the tumor necrosis factors α and β are linked to the human histocompatibility complex. Proc Natl Acad Sci USA 1986; 83:8699–8702.

269. Molvig J, Baek L, Christensen P, et al. Endotoxin stimulated human monocyte secretion of interleukin 1, tumor necrosis factor alpha and protoglandin E2 shows stable interindividual differences. Scand J Immunol 1988; 27:705–716.

270. Higgins PJ, Weiner HL. Suppression of experimental autoimmune encephalomyelitis by oral administration of myelin basic protein and its fragments. J Immunol 1988; 140:450–455.

271. Lider O, Santos LMB, Lee CSY, et al. Suppression of experimental autoimmune encephalomyelitis by oral administration of myelin basic protein II: suppression of disease and in vitro immune response is mediated by antigen specific CD8 + T lymphocytes. J Immunol 1989; 142:748–752.

272. Bitar DM, Whitacre CC. Suppression of experimental autoimmune encephalomyelitis by the oral administration of myelin basic protein. Cell Immunol 1988; 112:364–370.

273. Zhang JZ, Lee CSY, Lider O, et al. Suppression of adjuvant arthritis in Lewis rats by oral administration of Type II collagen. J Immunol 1990; 145:2489–2493.

274. Nagler-Anderson C, Bober LA, Robinson ME, et al. Suppression of type II collagen-induced arthritis by introgastric administration of soluble type II collagen. Proc Natl Acad Sci USA 1986; 83:7443–7446.

275. Thompson HSG, Staines NA. Gastric administration of type II collagen delays the onset and severity of collagen-induced arthritis in rats. Clin Exp Immunol 1986; 64:581–586.

276. Zhang ZJ, Davidson L, Eisenbarth GS, et al. Suppression of diabetes in nonobese diabetic mice by oral administration of porcine insulin. Proc Natl Acad Sci USA 1991; 88:10252–10256.

277. Miller A, Lider O, Roberts AB, et al. Suppressor T cells generated by oral tolerization to myelin basic protein suppress both in vitro and in vivo immune responses by the release of transferring growth factor beta after antigen-specific triggering. Proc Natl Acad Sci USA 1992; 89:421–425.

278. Mirouze J, Selam J-L, Pham TC, et al. The external artificial pancreas: an instrument to induce remissions in severe recent juvenile diabetes. Comparison with a preprogrammed insulin infusion system. Horm Metab Res Suppl 1978; 8:141–145.

279. Gotfredsen CF, Buschard K, Frandsen EK. Reduction of diabetes incidence of BB Wistar rats by early prophylactic insulin treatment. Diabetologia 1985; 28:933–955.

280. Atkinson MA, Maclaren NK, Luchetta R. Insulitis and diabetes in NOD mice reduced by prophylactic insulin therapy. Diabetes 1990; 39:927–928.

281. Muir A, Ped A, Clare-Salzler MC, et al. Insulin immunization induces a protective insulitis characterized by diminished intraislet interferon α transcription. J Clin Invest 1995; 95:628–634.

282. Keller RJ, Eisenbarth GS, Jackson RA. Insulin prophylaxis in individuals at high risk of type 1 diabetes. Lancet 1993; 341:927–928.

283. Eisenbarth GS, Verge CF, Allen H, et al. Design of trials for the prevention of IDDM. Diabetes 1993; 42:941–947.

284. Chen L, Komiya I, Inman L, et al. Effects of hypoglycemia and prolonged fasting on insulin and glucagon gene expression: studies with in situ hybridization. J Clin Invest 1989; 84:711–714.

285. Chen L, Alam T, Johnson JH, et al. Regulation of β-cell glucose transporter gene expression. Proc Natl Acad Sci USA 1990; 87:4088–4092.

286. Aaen KJ, Rygaard K, Josefsen H, et al. Dependence of antigen expression functional state of beta-cells. Diabetes 1990; 39:697–701.

287. Björk E, Kämpe J, Grawe A, et al. Modulation of beta-cell activity and its influence on islet cell antibody (ICA) and islet cell surface antibody (ICSA) reactivity. Autoimmunity 1993; 16:181–188.

288. Gladstone P, Nepom GT. The prevention of IDDM: injecting insulin into the cytokine network. Diabetes 1995; 44:859–862.

289. Stiller CR, Dupré J, Gent M, et al. Effects of cyclosporine immunosuppression in insulin-dependent diabetes mellitus of recent onset. Science 1984; 223:1362–1367.

290. Assan R, Bach JF, DuRostu H, et al. Metabolic and immunological effect of cyclosporine in recently diagnosed type I diabetes mellitus. Lancet 1985; 1:67–71.

291. Report of the Canadian-European Randomized Control Trial: cyclosporin in insulin-dependent diabetes mellitus (IDDM). Clin Invest Med 1987; 10:1365 (abstract).

292. Martin S, Schernthaner G, Nerup J, et al. Follow-up of cyclosporin A treatment in type 1 (insulin-dependent) diabetes mellitus: lack of long-term effects. Diabetologia 1991; 34:429–434.

293. Jenner M, Gradish A, Stiller C, et al. Cyclosporin A treatment of young children with newly-diagnosed type 1 (insulin-dependent) diabetes mellitus. Diabetologia 1992; 35:884–888.

294. Filippe G, Carel JC, Boitard C, et al. Long-term results of early cyclosporin therapy in juvenile IDDM. Diabetes 1996; 45:101–104.

295. Tominaga M, Komiya I, Johnson JH, et al. Loss of insulin response to

296. Dupré J, Stiller CR, Jenner M, et al. Responses to nutrients in non–insulin-requiring (NIR) remission of type I diabetes during administration of cyclosporin. Diabetes 1987; 36(Suppl 1):74A (abstract).

297. Lazarow A, Lambies L, Tausch AJ. Protection against diabetes with nicotinamide. J Lab Clin Med 1950; 38:249–258.

298. Tamada K, Nonaka K, Hanafusa T, et al. Preventive and therapeutic effects of large-dose nicotinamide injections on diabetes associated with insulitis. Diabetes 1982; 31:749–753.

299. Terazona K, Yamamoto H, Takasawa S, et al. A novel gene activated in regenerating islets. J Biol Chem 1988; 263:2111–2114.

300. Miyaura C, Chen L, Appel M, et al. Expression of reg/PSP, a pancreatic exocrine gene: relationship to changes in islet β-cell mass. Mol Endocrinol 1991; 5:226–234.

301. Watanabe T, Yonemura Y, Yonekura H, et al. Pancreatic beta-cell replication and amelioration of surgical diabetes by Reg protein. Proc Natl Acad Sci 1994; 91:3589–3592.

302. Sandler S, Andersson A. Long-term effects of exposure of pancreatic islets to nicotinamide in vitro on DNA synthesis, metabolism and B-cell function. Diabetologia 1986; 29:199–202.

303. Sandler S, Hellerström C, Eizirik DL. Effects of nicotinamide supplementation on human pancreatic islet function tissue culture. J Clin Endocrinol Metab 1993; 77:1574–1576.

304. Elliot RB, Chase HP. Prevention or delay of type 1 (insulin dependent) diabetes mellitus in children using nicotinamide. Diabetologia 1991; 34:362–365.

305. Lee K-U, Pak CY, Yoon J-W. Prevention of lymphocytic thyroiditis and insulitis in diabetes-prone BB rats by depletion of macrophages. Diabetologia 1988; 31:400–402.

306. Lee KU, Amano K, Yoon J-W. Evidence for initial involvement of macrophage in development of insulitis in NOD mice. Diabetes 1988; 37:989–991.

307. Baitard C, Michie S, Serrurier P, et al. In vivo prevention of thyroid and pancreatic autoimmunity in the BB rat by antibody to class II major histocompatibility complex gene products. Proc Natl Acad Sci USA 1985; 82:6627–6631.

308. Adorini L, Muller S, Cardinaux F, et al. In vivo competition between self peptides and foreign antigens in T-cell activation. Nature 1988; 334:623–625.

309. Charlton B, Bacelj A, Mandel TE. Administration of silica particles or anti-Lyt2 antibody prevents beta-cell destruction in NOD mice given cyclophosphamide. Diabetes 1988; 37:930–935.

310. Herold KC, Montac AG, Fitch FW. Treatment with anti-T-lymphocyte antibodies prevents induction of insulitis in mice given multiple doses of streptozotocin. Diabetes 1987; 36:796–801.

311. Like AA, Biron CA, Weringer EJ, et al. Prevention of diabetes with monoclonal antibodies that recognize T lymphocytes or natural killer cells. J Exp Med 1986; 164:1145–1159.

312. Jacobson JD, Markmann JF, Brayman KL, et al. Prevention of recurrent autoimmune diabetes in BB rats by anti–asialo-GM2 antibody. Diabetes 1988; 37:838–841.

313. Nair MP, Lewis EW, Schwartz SA. Immunoregulatory dysfunctions in type I diabetes: natural and antibody-dependent cellular cytotoxic activities. J Clin Immunol 1986; 6:363–372.

314. Oldstone MB. Prevention of type I diabetes in nonobese diabetic mice by virus infection. Science 1988; 239:500–502.

315. Koike T, Itoh Y, Ishii T, et al. Preventive effect of monoclonal anti L3T4 antibody on development of diabetes in NOD mice. Diabetes 1987; 36:534–541.

316. Shizuru JA, Taylor-Edwards C, Banks BA, et al. Immunotherapy of the nonobese diabetic mouse: treatment with an antibody to T-helper cells. Science 1988; 240:659–662.

317. Hayward AR, Shreiber M. Neonatal injection of CD3 antibody into nonobese diabetic mice reduces the incidence of insulitis and diabetes. J Immunol 1989; 143:1555–1559.

318. Boitard C, Yasunami R, Cardenne M, et al. T-cell–mediated inhibition of the transfer of autoimmune diabetes in NOD mice. J Exp Med 1989; 169:1669–1680.

319. Sempé P, Bedossa P, Richard MF, et al. Anti-alpha/beta T cell receptor provides an efficient therapy for autoimmune diabetes in nonobese diabetic (NOD) mice. Eur J Immunol 1991; 21:1163–1190.

320. Chatenoud L, Thervet E, Primo J, et al. Anti-CD3 antibody induces long-term remission of overt autoimmunity in nonobese diabetic mice. Proc Natl Acad Sci USA 1994; 91:123–127.

321. Nerup J, Mandrup-Poulson T, Molvig J, et al. Mechanism of pancreatic β-cell destruction in type I diabetes. Diabetes Care 1988; 11:16–23.

322. Kröncke KD, Kolb-Bachofen V, Berschick B, et al. Activated macrophages kill pancreatic syngeneic islet cells via arginine-dependent nitric oxide generation. Biochem Biophys Res Commun 1991; 175:752–758.

323. Bergmann L, Kröncke KD, Suschek C, et al. Cytotoxic action of IL-1 beta against pancreatic islets is mediated via nitric oxide formation and is inhibited via NG-monomethyl-L-arginine. FEBS Lett 1992; 299:103–106.

324. Corbett JA, Mikhael A, Shimizu J, et al. Nitric oxide production in islets from nonobese diabetic mice: aminoguanidine-sensitive and -resistant

stages in the immunological diabetic process. Proc Natl Acad Sci USA 1993; 90:8992–8995.

325. Weichselbaum A. Uber dei Veränderungen des Pankreas bei Diabetes Mellitus. Sitzungsber Kais Akad Wiss Wien Math Naturwiss Kl Abt 1 1910; 119:73–281.

326. Kaldany A, Hill T, Wentworth S, et al. Trapping of peripheral blood lymphocytes in the pancreas of patients with acute-onset insulin-dependent diabetes mellitus. Diabetes 1982; 31:463–466.

327. Bonnevie-Nielsen V, Steffes MW, Lernmark Å. A major loss in islet mass and B-cell function precedes hyperglycemia in mice given multiple low doses of streptozotocin. Diabetes 1981; 30:424–429.

328. Leiter EH, Beamer WG, Shultz LD. The effect of immunosuppression on streptozotocin-induced diabetes in C57BL/KsJ mice. Diabetes 1983; 32:148–155.

329. Rahier J, Goebbels RM, Henquin JC. Cellular composition of the human diabetic pancreas. Diabetologia 1983; 24:366–371.

330. Korc M, Owerback D, Quinto C, et al. Pancreatic islet–acinar cell interaction: amylase messenger RNA levels are determined by insulin. Science 1981; 213:351–353.

331. Kawai K, Orci L, Unger RH. High somatostatin uptake by the isolated perfused dog pancreas consistent with an "insuloacinar" axis. Endocrinology 1982; 110:660–662.

332. Stefan Y, Orci L, Malaisse-Lagae F, et al. Quantitation of endocrine cell content in the pancreas of nondiabetic and diabetic humans. Diabetes 1982; 31:694–700.

333. Boyd ME, Albright EB, Foster DW, et al. In vitro reversal of the fasting state of liver metabolism in the rat. J Clin Invest 1981; 68:142–152.

334. Shamoon H, Hendler R, Sherwin RS. Altered responsiveness to cortisol, epinephrine, and glucagon in insulin-infused juvenile-onset diabetics. Diabetes 1980; 29:284–291.

335. Rocha DM, Santeusanio F, Faloona GR, et al. Abnormal pancreatic alpha-cell function in bacterial infections. N Engl J Med 1973; 288:700–703.

336. Willerson JT, Hutcheson DR, Leshin SJ, et al. Serum glucagon and insulin levels and their relationship to blood glucose values in patients with acute myocardial infarction and acute coronary insufficiency. Am J Med 1974; 57:747–753.

337. Lindsey CA, Faloona GR, Unger RH. Glucagon and the insulin:glucagon ratio in severe trauma. Trans Assoc Am Physicians 1973; 86:264–271.

338. Wilmore DW, Moylan JA, Pruitt BA, et al. Hyperglucagonaemia after burns. Lancet 1974; 1:73–75.

339. Müller WA, Faloona GR, Unger RH. Hyperglucagonemia in diabetic ketoacidosis: its prevalence and significance. Am J Med 1973; 54:52–57.

340. Diebert DC, DeFronzo RA. Epinephrine-induced insulin resistance in man. J Clin Invest 1980; 65:717–721.

341. Müller WA, Faloona GR, Aguilar-Parada E, et al. Abnormal alpha-cell function in diabetes: response to carbohydrate and protein ingestion. N Engl J Med 1970; 283:109–115.

342. Unger RH, Aguilar-Parada E, Müller WA, et al. Studies of pancreatic alpha cell function in normal and diabetic subjects. J Clin Invest 1970; 49:837–848.

343. Samols E, Marri G, Marks V. Promotion of insulin secretion by glucagon. Lancet 1965; 2:415–416.

344. Samols E, Weir GC, Bonner-Weir S. Intraislet insulin-glucagon-somatostatin relationships. In: Lefebvre PJ, ed. Glucagon II. Berlin: Springer-Verlag, 1983: 133–173.

345. Raskin P, Aydin I, Unger RH. Effect of insulin on the exaggerated glucagon response to arginine stimulation in diabetes mellitus. Diabetes 1976; 25:227–229.

346. Raskin P, Aydin I, Yamamoto T, et al. Abnormal alpha cell function in human diabetes: the response to oral protein. Am J Med 1978; 64:988–997.

347. Raskin P, Pietri A, Unger RH. Changes in glucagon levels after four to five weeks of glucoregulation by portable insulin infusion pumps. Diabetes 1979; 28:1033–1035.

348. Starke A, Imamura T, Unger RH: Relationship of glucagon suppression by insulin and somatostatin to the ambient glucose concentration: implications for the etiology of diabetic hyperglucagonemia. J Clin Invest 1987; 79:20–24.

349. Chen L, Komiya I, Inman L, et al. Molecular and cellular responses of islets during perturbations of glucose homeostasis determined by in situ hybridization histochemistry. Proc Natl Acad Sci USA 1989; 86:1367–1371.

350. Dobbs R, Sakurai H, Sasaki H, et al. Glucagon: role in the hyperglycemia of diabetes mellitus. Science 1975; 187:544–547.

351. Wahren J, Felig P, Cerasi E, et al. Splanchnic and peripheral glucose and amino acid metabolism in diabetes mellitus. J Clin Invest 1972; 51:1870–1878.

352. Owen OE, Reichle FA, Mozzoli MA, et al. Hepatic, gut, and renal substrate flux rates in patients with hepatic cirrhosis. J Clin Invest 1981; 68:240–252.

353. Owen OE, Morgan AP, Kemp HG, et al. Brain metabolism during fasting. J Clin Invest 1967; 46:1589–1595.

354. Liljenquist JE, Mueller GL, Cherrington AD, et al. Evidence for an important role of glucagon in the regulation of hepatic glucose production in normal man. J Clin Invest 1977; 59:369–374.

355. Unger RH, Orci L. Glucagon and the A cell: physiology and pathophysiology. N Engl J Med 1981; 304:1518–1524, 1575–1580.

356. Koerker DJ, Ruch W, Chideckel E, et al. Somatostatin: hypothalamic inhibitor of the endocrine pancreas. Science 1974; 184:482–484.

357. Sakurai H, Dobbs R, Unger RH. Somatostatin-induced changes in insulin and glucagon secretion in normal and diabetic dogs. J Clin Invest 1974; 54:1395–1402.

358. Vidnes J, Oyasaeter S. Glucagon deficiency causing severe neonatal hypoglycemia in a patient with normal insulin secretion. Pediatr Res 1977; 11:943–949.

359. Gerich JE, Lorenzi M, Bier DM, et al. Prevention of human diabetic ketoacidosis by somatostatin: evidence for an essential role of glucagon. N Engl J Med 1975; 292:985–989.

360. Scheen AJ, Krzentowski G, Castillo M, et al. A 6-hour nocturnal interruption of a continuous subcutaneous insulin infusion. 2: Marked attenuation of the metabolic deterioration by somatostatin. Diabetologia 1983; 24:319–325.

361. Raskin P, Unger RH. Hyperglucagonemia and its suppression: importance in the metabolic control of diabetes. N Engl J Med 1978; 299:433–436.

362. Unger RH. Somatostatinoma. N Engl J Med 1977; 296:998–1000.

363. Nakabayashi H, Dobbs RE, Unger RH. The role of glucagon deficiency in the Houssay phenomenon of dogs. J Clin Invest 1978; 61:1355–1362.

364. Santeusanio F, Massi-Benedetti M, Angeletti G, et al. Glucagon and carbohydrate disorder in a totally pancreatectomized man (a study with the aid of an artificial endocrine pancreas). J Endocrinol Invest 1981; 4:93–96.

365. Johnson DG, Goebel CU, Hruby VJ, et al. Hyperglycemia of diabetic rat decreased by a glucagon receptor antagonist. Science 1982; 215:1115–1116.

366. Boden G, Master RW, Rezvani I, et al. Glucagon deficiency and hyperaminoacidemia after total pancreatectomy. J Clin Invest 1980; 65:706–716.

367. Barnes AJ, Bloom SR. Pancreatectomised man: a model for diabetes without glucagon. Lancet 1976; 1:219–221.

368. Holst JJ, Pedersen JH, Baldissera F, et al. Circulating glucagon after total pancreatectomy in man. Diabetologia 1983; 25:396–399.

369. Richards CS, Furuya E, Uyeda K. Regulation of fructose-2,6-P2 concentration in isolated hepatocytes. Biochem Biophys Res Commun 1981; 100:1673–1679.

370. King H, Rewers M, World Health Organization Ad Hoc Diabetes Reporting Group. Global estimates for prevalence of diabetes mellitus and impaired glucose tolerance in adults. Diabetes Care 1993; 16:157–177.

371. Zimmet P, Taft P, Guinea A, et al. The high prevalence of diabetes mellitus on a Central Pacific island. Diabetologia 1977; 13:111–115.

372. Genuth SM, Houser HB, Carter JR Jr, et al. Community screening for diabetes by blood glucose measurement: results of a five year experience. Diabetes 1976; 25:1110–1117.

373. National Center for Health Statistics. Current estimates from the National Health Interview Survey in the United States: 1992. Vital and Health Statistics Series 10, No. 189, 1994.

374. American Diabetes Association on Statistics: Standardization of the oral glucose tolerance test. Diabetes 1969; 18:299–307.

375. Stern MP, Valdez RA, Haffner SM, et al. Stability over time of modern diagnostic criteria for type II diabetes. Diabetes Care 1993; 16:978–983.

376. Genuth SM, Houser HB, Carter JR, et al. Observations on the value of mass indiscriminate screening for diabetes mellitus based on a five-year follow up. Diabetes 1978; 44:377–383.

377. Wise PH, Edwards FM, Craig RJ, et al. Diabetes and associated variables in the south Australian aboriginal. Aust NZ J Med 1976; 6:191–196.

378. Zimmet P, Kirk R, Serjeantson S, et al. Diabetes in Pacific populations: genetic and environmental interactions. In: Melish JS, Hanna J, Baba S, eds. Genetic-Environmental Interaction in Diabetes Mellitus. Amsterdam: Excerpta Medica, 1982: 9–17.

379. Kenny SJ, Aubert RE, Geiss LS. Prevalence and incidence of non-insulin dependent diabetes. In: National Diabetes Data Group. Diabetes in America. NIH Publication No. 95-1468; 1995: 47–67.

380. Knowler WC, Bennett PH, Hamman RF, et al. Diabetes incidence and prevalence in Pima Indians: a 19-fold greater incidence than in Rochester, Minnesota. Am J Epidemiol 1978; 108:497–505.

381. Köbberling J. Studies on the genetic heterogeneity of diabetes mellitus. Diabetologia 1971; 7:46–49.

382. Köbberling J, Tillil H. Empirical risk figures for first degree relatives of non-insulin dependent diabetics. In: Köbberling J, Tattersall R, eds. The Genetics of Diabetes Mellitus. Proceedings of the Serono Symposia. Vol 47. London: Academic, 1982: 201–209.

383. Barnett AH, Spiliopoulos AJ, Pyke DA, et al. Metabolic studies in unaffected co-twins of non–insulin-dependent diabetics. Br Med J 1981; 282:1656–1658.

384. Newman B, Selby JV, King MC, et al. Concordance for type 2 (non–insulin-dependent) diabetes in male twins. Diabetologia 1987; 30:763–768.

385. Ghosh S, Schork NJ. Genetic analysis of NIDDM: the study of quantitative traits. Diabetes 1996; 45:1–14.

386. Pfeiffer MA, Halter JB, Porte D Jr. Insulin secretion in diabetes mellitus. Am J Med 1981; 70:579–588.

387. Unger RH. Lipotoxicity in the pathogenesis of obesity-dependent NIDDM. Diabetes 1995; 44:863–870.

388. Rich SS. Mapping genes in diabetes: genetic epidemiologic perspective. Diabetes 1990; 39:1315–1319.

389. McCarty MI, Froguel P, Hitman GA. The genetics of non–insulin-dependent diabetes: tools and aims. Diabetologia 1994; 37:959–968.

390. Ulrich A, Gray A, Tam AW, et al. Human insulin receptor and its relation-

ship to the tyrosine kinase family of oncogenes. Nature 1985; 313:756–761.

391. Ekina Y, Ellis L, Jarnagin K, et al. The human insulin receptor cDNA: the structural basis for hormone-activated transmembrane signaling. Cell 1985; 40:747–758.

392. Kahn CR, Vicent D, Doria A. Genetics of non–insulin-dependent (type II) diabetes mellitus. Annu Rev Med 1996; 47:509–531.

393. Taylor SI, Wertheimer E, Acilli D, et al. Mutations in the insulin receptor gene: update 1994. Endocr Rev 1994; 2:58–65.

394. Flier JS. Syndromes of insulin resistance: from patient to gene and back again. Lilly Lecture. Diabetes 1992; 41:1207–1219.

395. Nozaki O, Suzuki Y, Shimada F, et al. A glycine-1008 to valine mutation in the insulin receptor in a woman with type A insulin resistance. J Clin Endocrin Metab 1993; 77:169–172.

396. Roach P, Zick Y, Formisano P, et al. A novel human insulin receptor gene mutation uniquely inhibits insulin binding without impairing post-translational processing. Diabetes 1994; 43:1096–1102.

397. Krook A, Kumar S, Laing I, et al. Molecular scanning of the insulin receptor gene in syndromes of insulin resistance. Diabetes 1994; 43:357–368.

398. Cama A, Sierra ML, Kadowaki T, et al. Two mutant alleles of the insulin receptor gene in a family with a genetic form of insulin resistance: a 10 base pair deletion in exon 1 and a mutation substituting serine for asparagine-462. Hum Genet 1995; 95:174–182.

399. O'Rahilly S, Choi WH, Patel P, et al. Detection of mutation in insulin-receptor gene in NIDDM by analysis of single-stranded conformation polymorphisms. Diabetes 1991; 40:777–782.

400. Kadawaki H, Kadewaki T. HAIR-AN syndrome. Nippon Rinsho 1994; 52:2648–2652.

401. Moller DE, Yokota A, Flier JS. Normal insulin receptor cDNA sequence in Pima Indians with NIDDM. Diabetes 1989; 38:1496–1500.

402. Kusari J, Verma US, Buse JB, et al. Analysis of gene sequence of the insulin receptor and the insulin-sensitive glucose transporter (GLUT-4) in patients with common type non–insulin-dependent diabetes mellitus. J Clin Invest 1991; 88:1323–1330.

403. Kan M, Kanai F, Iida M, et al. Frequency of mutations of insulin receptor gene in Japanese patients with NIDDM. Diabetes 1995; 44:1081–1086.

404. Anderson CM, Henry RR, Knudsen PE, et al. Relative expression of insulin receptor isoforms does not differ in lean, obese and noninsulin-dependent diabetes mellitus subjects. J Clin Endocrinol Metab 1993; 76:1380–1382.

405. Mosthaf L, Eriksson J, Haring HU, et al. Insulin receptor isotype expression correlates with risk of non–insulin-dependent diabetes. Proc Natl Acad Sci USA 1993; 90:2633–2635.

406. Yamaguchi Y, Flier JS, Benecke H, et al. Ligand-binding properties of the two isoforms of the human insulin receptor. Endocrinology 1993; 132:1132–1138.

407. McClain DA, Henry RR, Ulrich A, et al. Restriction-fragment-length polymorphism in insulin-receptor gene and insulin resistance in NIDDM. Diabetes 1988; 37:1071–1075.

408. Brunetti A, Brunetti L, Foti D, et al. Human diabetes associated with defects in nuclear regulatory proteins for the insulin receptor gene. J Clin Invest 1996; 97:258–262.

409. Li WW, Dammerman MM, Smith JD, et al. Common genetic variation in the promoter of the human apo CIII gene abolishes regulation by insulin and may contribute to hypertriglyceridemia. J Clin Invest 1995; 96:2601–2605.

410. Merlo A, Herman JG, Mao L, et al. 5′ CpG island methylation is associated with transcriptional silencing of the tumor suppressor p16/CDKN2/MTS1 in human cancers. Nat Med 1995; 1:686–692.

411. Taylor SI, Wertheimer E, Accili D, et al. Mutations in the insulin receptor gene: update 1994. Endocr Rev 1994; 2:58–65.

412. White MF, Maron R, Kahn CR. Insulin rapidly stimulates tyrosine phosphorylation of a Mr-185,000 protein in intact cells. Nature 1985; 318:183–186.

413. Imai Y, Fusco A, Suzuki Y, et al. Variant sequences of insulin receptor substrate-1 in patients with noninsulin-dependent diabetes mellitus. J Clin Endocrinol Metab 1994; 79:1655–1658.

414. Laakso M, Malkki M, Kekäläinen P, et al. Insulin receptor substrate-1 variants in non–insulin-dependent diabetes. J Clin Invest 1994; 94:1141–1146.

415. Almind K, Bjørbaek C, Vestergaard H, et al. Aminoacid polymorphisms of insulin receptor substrate-1 in non–insulin-dependent diabetes mellitus. Lancet 1993; 342:828–832.

416. Clausen JO, Hansen T, Bjorbaek C, et al. Insulin resistance: interactions between obesity and a common variant of insulin receptor substrate-1. Lancet 1995; 346:397–402.

417. Tamemota N, Kadowaki T, Tobe K, et al. Insulin resistance and growth retardation in mice lacking insulin receptor substrate-1. Nature 1994; 372:182–186.

418. Kusari J, Verma US, Buse JB. Analysis of the gene sequences of the insulin receptor and the insulin-sensitive glucose transporter (GLUT-4) in patients with common type non–insulin-dependent diabetes mellitus. J Clin Invest 1991; 88:1323–1330.

419. Choi WH, O'Rahilly S, Buse JB, et al. Molecular scanning of insulin-responsive glucose transporter (GLUT4) gene in NIDDM subjects. Diabetes 1991; 40:1712–1718.

420. Katz EB, Sfenbit AE, Halton K, et al. Cardiac and adipose tissue abnormalities but not diabetes in mice deficient in GLUT-4. Nature 1995; 377:151–155.

421. Echward SM, Bjorbaek C, Hansen T, et al. Identification of four amino acid substitutions in hexokinase II and studies of relationships to NIDDM, glucose effectiveness and insulin sensitivity. Diabetes 1995; 44:347–353.

422. Vestergaard H, Bjorbaek C, Hansen T, et al. Impaired activity and gene expression of hexokinase II in muscle from non–insulin-dependent diabetes mellitus patients. J Clin Invest 1995; 96:2639–2645.

423. Thorburm AW, Gumbiner B, Bulacan F, et al. Multiple defects in muscle glycogen synthase activity contribute to reduced glycogen synthesis in non–insulin-dependent diabetes mellitus. J Clin Invest 1991; 87:489–495.

424. Vaag A, Henriksen JE, Beck-Nielsen H. Decreased insulin activation of glycogen synthase in skeletal muscles in young nonobese Caucasian first-degree relatives of patients with non–insulin-dependent diabetes mellitus. J Clin Invest 1992; 89:782–788.

425. Schalin-Jantti C, Harkonen M, Groop LC. Impaired activation of glycogen synthase in people at increased risk for developing NIDDM. Diabetes 1992; 41:598–604.

426. Groop LC, Kankuri M, Schalin-Jantti C, et al. Association between polymorphism of the glycogen synthase gene and non–insulin-dependent diabetes mellitus. N Engl J Med 1993; 328:10–14.

427. Kuroyama H, Sanke T, Ohagi S, et al. Simple tandem repeat DNA polymorphism in the human glycogen synthase gene is associated with NIDDM in Japanese subjects. Diabetologia 1994; 37:536–539.

428. Orho M, Nikula-ljas P, Schalin-Jantti C, et al. Isolation and characterization of the human muscle glycogen synthase gene. Diabetes 1995; 44:1099–1105.

429. Lofman M, Yki-Jarvinen H, Parkkonen M, et al. Increased concentration of glycogen synthase protein in skeletal muscle of patient with NIDDM. Am J Physiol 1995; 269:E27–E32.

430. Tager H, Given B, Baldwin D, et al. A structurally abnormal insulin causing human diabetes. Nature 1979; 281:121–125.

431. Steiner DF, Tager HS, Chan SJ, et al. Lessons learned from molecular biology of insulin-gene mutations. Diabetes Care 1990; 13:600–609.

432. Weaver JU, Kopelman PG, Hitman GA. Central obesity and hyperinsulineamia in women are associated with polymorphism in the 5′ flanking region of the human insulin gene. Euro J Clin Invest 1992; 22:265–270.

433. Olanski L, Welling C, Giddings S, et al. A variant insulin promoter in non-insulin dependent diabetes mellitus. J Clin Invest 1992; 98:1596–1602.

434. Elbein SC, Corsetti L, Goldgar L, et al. Insulin gene in familial NIDDM:lack of linkage in Utah Mormon pedigrees. Diabetes 1988; 37:569–576.

435. Thorens B, Sarkar HK, Kaback HR, et al. Cloning and functional expression cDNA in bacteria of a novel glucose transporter present in liver, intestine, kidney and pancreatic β-cells. Cell 1988; 55:281–290.

436. Tal M, Liang Y, Najfji H, et al. Expression and function of GLUT-1 and GLUT-2 glucose transporter isoforms in cells of cultured rat pancreatic islets. J Biol Chem 1992; 267:17241–17247.

437. Newgard CB, Quaade C, Hughes SD, et al. Glucokinase and glucose transporter expression in liver and islets: implications for control of glucose homeostasis. Biochem Soc Trans 1990; 18:851–853.

438. Hughes SD, Quaade C, Johnson JH, et al. Transfection of AtT-20ins cells with GLUT-2 but not GLUT-1 confers glucose-stimulated insulin secretion: relationship to glucose metabolism. J Biol Chem 1993; 268:15205–15212.

439. Unger RH. Diabetic hyperglycemia: link to impaired glucose transport in pancreatic β cell. Science 1991; 251:1200–1205.

440. Valera A, Solanes G, Fernandez-Alvarez J, et al. Expression of GLUT-2 antisense RNA in β cells of transgenic mice leads to diabetes. J Biol Chem 1994; 45:28543–28546.

441. Janssen RC, Bogardus C, Takeda J, et al. Linkage analysis of acute insulin secretion with GLUT2 and glucokinase in Pima indians and the indentification of a missense mutation in GLUT2. Diabetes 1994; 43:558–563.

442. Patel P, Bell GI, Cook JTE, et al. Multiple restriction fragment length polymorphisms at the GLUT2 locus: GLUT 2 haplotypes for genetic analysis of type 2 (non–insulin-dependent) diabetes mellitus. Diabetologia 1991; 34:817–821.

443. Mueckler M, Kruse M, Strube M, et al. A mutation in the GLUT2 glucose transporter gene of a diabetic patient abolished transport activity. J Biol Chem 1994; 27:17765–17767.

444. Matschinsky F, Liang Y, Kesavan P, et al. Glucokinase as pancreatic β cell glucose sensor and diabetes gene. J Clin Invest 1993; 92:2092–2098.

445. Froguel P, Zouali H, Vionnet N, et al. Familial hyperglycemia due to mutations in glucokinase. N Engl J Med 1993; 328:696–702.

446. Pilkis S, Weber IR, Harrison RW, et al. Glucokinase: structural analysis of a protein involved in susceptibility to diabetes. J Biol Chem 1994; 269:21925–21928.

447. Vionnet N, Stoffel M, Takeda J, et al. Nonsense mutation in the glucokinase gene causes early-onset non–insulin-dependent diabetes mellitus. Nature 1992; 356:721–722.

448. Sun F, Knebelmann B, Pueyo ME, et al. Deletion of the donor splice site of intron 4 in the glucokinase gene causes maturity-onset diabetes of the young. J Clin Invest 1993; 92:1174–1180.

449. Elbein SC, Hoffman M, Qin H, et al. Molecular screening of the glucokinase gene in familial type 2 (non–insulin-dependent) diabetes mellitus. Diabetologia 1994; 37:182–187.

450. Elbein SC, Hoffman M, Chiu K, et al. Linkage analysis of the glucokinase

957. Fagins J, Brattberg A, Jameson S, et al. Limited benefit of treatment of diabetic polyneuropathy with an aldose reductase inhibitor: a 24 week controlled trial. Diabetologia 1985; 28:323–329.

958. Martyn CN, Reid W, Young RJ, et al. Six-month treatment with sorbinil in asymptomatic diabetic neuropathy: failure to improve abnormal nerve function. Diabetes 1987; 36:987–990.

959. Hotta N, Kakuta H, Kimura M, et al. Experimental and clinical trial of aldose reductase inhibitor in diabetic neuropathy. Diabetes 1985; 34(Suppl 1):98A (abstract).

960. Koglan L, Clark C, Ryder S, et al. The results of long-term open-label administration of ALREDASE in the treatment of diabetic neuropathy. Diabetes 1985; 34(Suppl 1):202A (abstract).

961. Warren S, LeCompte PM, Legg MA. Pathology of Diabetes Mellitus. Philadelphia: Lea & Febiger, 1966: 284–294.

962. Brownlee M, Cahill GF Jr. Diabetic control and vascular complications. In: Paoletti R, Gotto AM Jr, eds. Atherosclerosis Reviews. Vol 4. New York: Raven, 1979: 29–70.

963. Report of the National Commission on Diabetes to the Congress of the United States. DHEW Publication No. (NIH) 76-1022, Vol 3, Part 2. Washington, DC: Government Printing Office, 1976: 64.

964. Strandness DE Jr, Priest RE, Gibbons GE. Combined clinical and pathologic study of diabetic and nondiabetic peripheral arterial disease. Diabetes 1964; 13:1366–1372.

965. Beach KW, Strandness DE Jr. Arteriosclerosis obliterans and associated risk factors in insulin-dependent and non–insulin-dependent diabetes. Diabetes 1980; 29:882–888.

966. White RA, Nolan L, Harley D, et al. Noninvasive evaluation of peripheral vascular disease using transcutaneous oxygen tension. Am J Surg 1982; 144:68–75.

967. Railton R, Newman P, Hislop J, et al. Reduced transcutaneous oxygen tension and impaired vascular response in type 1 (insulin-dependent) diabetes. Diabetologia 1983; 25:340–342.

968. Coffman JD. Vasodilator drugs in peripheral vascular disease. N Engl J Med 1979; 300:713–717.

969. Smith RB III, Dratz AF, Coberly JC, et al. Effect of lumbar sympathectomy on muscle blood flow in advanced occlusive vascular disease. Am Surg 1971; 37:247–251.

970. Harkonen S, Kjellstrand CM. Exacerbation of diabetic renal failure following intravenous pyelography. Am J Med 1977; 63:939–946.

971. Levin ME, O'Neal LW. Peripheral vascular disease. In: Ellenberg M, Rifkin H, eds. Diabetes Mellitus: Theory and Practice. 3rd ed. New Hyde Park, NY: Medical Examination Publishing, 1983: 803–828.

972. Abbott WM. Percutaneous transluminal angioplasty: surgeon's view. AJR 1980; 135:917–920.

973. Greenfield AJ. Femoral, popliteal, and tibial arteries: percutaneous transluminal angioplasty. AJR 1980; 135:927–935.

974. Kalkhoff RK, Kissebah AH, Kim H-J. Carbohydrate and lipid metabolism during normal pregnancy: relationship to gestational hormone action. Semin Perinatol 1978; 2:291–307.

975. Freinkel N. Of pregnancy and progeny. Diabetes 1980; 29:1023–1035.

976. Tsibris JCM, Raynor LO, Buhi WC, et al. Insulin receptors in circulating erythrocytes and monocytes from women on oral contraceptives or pregnant women near term. J Clin Endocrinol Metab 1980; 51:711–717.

977. Gewolb IH, Warshaw JB. Influences on fetal growth. In: Warshaw JB, ed. The Biological Basis of Reproductive and Developmental Medicine. New York: Elsevier Biomedical, 1983: 365–389.

978. Moore P, Kolterman O, Weyant J, et al. Insulin binding in human pregnancy: comparisons to the postpartum, luteal, and follicular states. J Clin Endocrinol Metab 1981; 52:937–941.

979. Kimura RE, Warshaw JB. Metabolism during development. In: Warshaw JB, ed. The Biological Basis of Reproductive and Developmental Medicine. New York: Elsevier Biomedical, 1983: 337–364.

980. Knopp RH, Herrera E, Freinkel N. Metabolism of adipose tissue isolated from fed and fasted pregnant rats during late gestation. J Clin Invest 1970; 49:1438–1446.

981. Herrera E, Knopp RH, Freinkel N. Plasma fuels, insulin, liver composition, gluconeogenesis, and nitrogen metabolism during late gestation in the fed and fasted rat. J Clin Invest 1969; 48:2260–2272.

982. Freinkel N, Metzger BE. Some considerations of fuel economy in the fed state during late human pregnancy. In: Camerini-Davalos RA, Cole HS, eds. Early Diabetes in Early Life. New York: Academic, 1975: 289–301.

983. Horton WE Jr, Sadler TW. Effects of maternal diabetes on early embryogenesis: alterations in morphogenesis produced by the ketone body, β-hydroxybutyrate. Diabetes 1983; 32:610–616.

984. Health Interview Survey. Washington, DC: National Center for Health Statistics, 1973.

985. Fleischman AR, Finberg L. The infant of the diabetic mother and diabetes in infancy. In: Ellenberg M, Rifkin H, eds. Diabetes Mellitus: Theory and Practice. 3rd ed. New Hyde Park, NY: Medical Examination Publishing, 1983: 715–725.

986. Chez RA, Mintz DH, Horger EO III, et al. Factors affecting the response to insulin in the normal subhuman pregnant primate. J Clin Invest 1970; 49:1517–1527.

987. Mintz DH, Chez RA, Hutchinson DL. Subhuman primate pregnancy complicated by streptozotocin-induced diabetes mellitus. J Clin Invest 1972; 51:837–847.

988. Obenshain SS, Adam PAJ, King KC, et al. Human fetal insulin response to sustained maternal hyperglycemia. N Engl J Med 1970; 283:566–570.

989. Ogata ES, Sabbagha R, Metzger BE, et al. Serial ultrasonography to assess evolving fetal macrosomia: studies in 23 pregnant diabetic women. JAMA 1980; 243:2405–2408.

990. Widness JA, Schwartz HC, Thompson D, et al. Glycohemoglobin (HbA$_{1c}$): a predictor of birth weight in infants of diabetic mothers. J Pediatr 1978; 92:8–12.

991. Osler M, Pedersen J. The body composition of newborn infants of diabetic mothers. Pediatrics 1960; 26:985–992.

992. Robert MF, Neff RK, Hubbell JP, et al. Association between maternal diabetes and the respiratory-distress syndrome in the newborn. N Engl J Med 1976; 294:357–360.

993. Gewolb IH, Barrett C, Wilson CM, et al. Delay in pulmonary glycogen degradation in fetuses of streptozotocin diabetic rats. Pediatr Res 1982; 16:869–873.

994. Warburton D. Chronic hyperglycemia reduces surface active material flux in tracheal fluid of fetal lambs. J Clin Invest 1983; 71:550–555.

995. Oski FA, Naiman JL. Polycythemia and hyperviscosity in the neonatal period. In: Oski FA, Naiman JL, eds. Hematologic Problems in the Newborn. 3rd ed. Philadelphia: WB Saunders, 1982: 87–96.

996. Avery ME, Oppenheimer EH, Gordon HH. Renal-vein thrombosis in newborn infants of diabetic mothers: report of two cases. N Engl J Med 1957; 256:1134–1138.

997. Gersony WM. Persistence of the fetal circulation: a commentary. J Pediatr 1973; 82:1103–1106.

998. Taylor PM, Wofson JH, Bright NH, et al. Hyperbilirubinemia in infants of diabetic mothers. Biol Neonate 1963; 5:289–298.

999. Gabbe SG. Diabetes mellitus in pregnancy: have all the problems been solved? Am J Med 1981; 70:613–618.

1000. Rusnak SL, Driscoll SG. Congenital spinal anomalies in infants of diabetic mothers. Pediatrics 1965; 35:989–995.

1001. Rowland TW, Hubbell JP Jr, Nadas AS. Congenital heart disease in infants of diabetic mothers. J Pediatr 1973; 83:815–820.

1002. Garner P. Type 1 diabetes mellitus and pregnancy. Lancet 1995; 346:157–161.

1003. Metzger BE. Overview of GDM: Accomplishments of the last decade, challenges for the future. Diabetes 1993; 341:1306–1309.

1004. Ratner RE. Gestational diabetes mellitus. After three international workshops do we know how to dispose and manage it yet. Clinical review 47. J Clin Endocrinol Metab 1993; 77:1–4.

1005. Gabbe SG, Mestman JH, Freeman RK, et al. Management and outcome of pregnancy in diabetes mellitus, classes B to R. Am J Obstet Gynecol 1977; 129:723–732.

1006. Whittle MJ, Anderson D, Lowensohn RI, et al. Estriol in pregnancy. VI: Experience with unconjugated plasma estriol assays and antepartum fetal heart rate testing in diabetic pregnancies. Am J Obstet Gynecol 1979; 135:764–772.

1007. Visser GH, Huisjes HJ. Diagnostic value of the unstressed antepartum cardiotocogram. Br J Obstet Gynaecol 1977; 84:321–326.

1008. Landon MB, Gabbe SG. Diabetes and pregnancy. Med Clin North Am 1988; 72:1493–1511.

1009. Eriksson UJ, Dahlstrom E, Hellerstrom C. Diabetes in pregnancy: skeletal malformations in the offspring of diabetic rats after intermittent withdrawal of insulin in early gestation. Diabetes 1983; 32:1141–1145.

1010. Mills JL, Baker L, Goldman AS. Malformations in infants of diabetic mothers occur before the seventh gestational week: implications for treatment. Diabetes 1979; 28:292–293.

1011. Pedersen JF, Molsted-Pederson L. Early fetal growth delay detected by ultrasound marks increased risk of congenital malformation in diabetic pregnancy. Br Med J 1981; 283:269–271.

1012. Pedersen JF, Molsted-Pederson L. Early growth delay predisposes the fetus in diabetic pregnancy to congenital malformation. Lancet 1982; 1:737.

1013. Pedersen J, Molsted-Pederson L. Congenital malformations: the possible role of diabetes care outside pregnancy. CIBA Found Symp 1979; 63:265–271.

1014. Mills JF, Knaff RH, Simpson JL, et al. Lack of relation of increased malformation rates in infants of mothers to glycemic control during organogenesis. N Engl J Med 1988; 318:671–676.

1015. Karlsson K, Kjellmer I. The outcome of diabetic pregnancies in relation to the mother's blood sugar level. Am J Obstet Gynecol 1972; 112:213–220.

1016. Dobbing J. Prenatal nutrition and neurological development. In : Craviots J, Hambraeus L, Vahlquist B, eds. Symposia of the Swedish Nutrition Foundation XII: Early Malnutrition and Mental Development. Uppsala: Almquist and Wiksell, 1974: 96–110.

1017. O'Sullivan JB, Charles D, Mahan CM, et al. Gestational diabetes and perinatal mortality rate. Am J Obstet Gynecol 1973; 116:901–904.

1018. Roversi GD, Gargiulo M, Nicolini U, et al. Maximal tolerated insulin therapy in gestational diabetes. Diabetes Care 1980; 3:489–494.

1019. McEvoy RC, Franklin B, Ginsberg-Fellner. Gestational diabetes mellitus: evidence for autoimmunity against the pancreatic beta cells. Diabetologia 1991; 34:507–510.

1020. Damm P, Kuhl C, Bertelsen A, et al. Predictive factors for the development of diabetes in women with previous gestational diabetes mellitus. Am J Obst Gynecol 1992; 40(Suppl 2):131–135.

1021. Schade DS. Surgery and diabetes. Med Clin North Am 1988; 72:1531–1543.

1022. Roy B, Chou MCY, Field JB. Time-action characteristics of regular and NPH insulin in insulin-treated diabetics. J Clin Endocrinol Metab 1980; 50:475–479.

1023. Nolte MS, Poon V, Grodsky GM, et al. Reduced solubility of short-acting soluble insulins when mixed with longer-acting insulin. Diabetes 1983; 32:1177–1181.

1024. Skyler JS. Insulin pharmacology. Med Clin North Am 1988; 72:1337–1354.

1025. Zinman B. The physiologic replacement of insulin: an elusive goal. N Engl J Med 1989; 321:363–370.

1026. Sonnenberg GE, Chantelau E, Sundermann S, et al. Human and porcine regular insulins are equally effective in subcutaneous replacement therapy: results of a double-blind crossover study in type I diabetic patients with continuous subcutaneous insulin infusion. Diabetes 1982; 31:600–602.

1027. Home PD, Massi-Benedetti M, Shepherd GAA, et al. A comparison of the activity and disposal of semi-synthetic human insulin and porcine insulin in normal man by the glucose clamp technique. Diabetologia 1982; 22:41–45.

1028. Heding LG, Marshall MO, Persson B, et al. Immunogenicity of monocomponent human and porcine insulin in newly diagnosed type I (insulin-dependent) diabetic children. Diabetologia 1984; 27(Suppl):96–98.

1029. Skyler JS, Pfeiffer EF, Raptis S, et al. Biosynthetic human insulin: progress and prospects. Diabetes Care 1981; 4:140–143.

1030. Zuppinger K, Aebi C, Fankhauser S, et al. Comparison of human and porcine insulin therapies in children with newly diagnosed diabetes mellitus. Diabetologia 1987; 30:912–915.

1031. Teuscher A, Berger WG. Hypoglycemia unawareness in diabetics transferred from beef/pork insulin to human insulin. Lancet 1987; 2:382–385.

1032. Schade DS. Brittle diabetes: strategies, diagnosis, and treatment. Diabetes Metab Rev 1988; 4:371–390.

1033. Schade DS, Santiago JV, Skyler JS, et al. Unstable diabetes and insulin resistance. In: Schade DS, Santiago JV, Skyler JS, et al., eds. Intensive Insulin Therapy. Princeton: Excerpta Medica, 1983: 264–283.

1034. Fukuda M, Tanaka A, Tahara Y, et al. Correlation between minimal secretory capacity of pancreatic beta-cells and stability of diabetic control. Diabetes 1988; 37:81–88.

1035. Nathan DM, Singer DE, Hurxthal K, et al. The clinical information value of the glycosylated hemoglobin assay. N Engl J Med 1984; 310:341–346.

1036. Goldstein DE. Is glycosylated hemoglobin clinically useful? N Engl J Med 1984; 310:384–385.

1037. Ramsay RC, Goetz FC, Sutherland DER, et al. Progression of diabetic retinopathy after pancreas transplantation for insulin-dependent diabetes mellitus. N Engl J Med 1988; 318:208–214.

1038. Schiffrin A, Belmonte MM. Comparison between continuous subcutaneous insulin infusion and multiple injections of insulin: a one-year prospective study. Diabetes 1982; 31:255–264.

1039. Skyler JS, Skyler DL, Seigler DE, et al. Algorithms for adjustment of insulin dosage by patients who monitor blood glucose. Diabetes Care 1981; 4:311–318.

1040. Rizza RA, Gerich JE, Haymond MW, et al. Control of blood sugar in insulin-dependent diabetes: comparison of an artificial endocrine pancreas, continuous subcutaneous insulin infusion, and intensive conventional insulin therapy. N Engl J Med 1980; 303:1313–1318.

1041. Raskin P. Open and closed insulin infusion systems: newer methods of insulin delivery. In: Ellenberg M, Rifkin H, eds. Diabetes Mellitus: Theory and Practice. 3rd ed. New Hyde Park, NY: Medical Examination Publishing, 1983: 941–957.

1042. Slama G, Garrel D, Tchobroutsky G. Multiple daily insulin injections through subcutaneously implanted needle. Lancet 1980; 1:1078.

1043. Reeves ML, Seigler DE, Ryan EA, et al. Glycemic control in insulin-dependent diabetes mellitus: comparison of outpatient intensified conventional therapy with continuous subcutaneous insulin infusion. Am J Med 1982; 72:673–680.

1044. Pickup JC, Keen H, Parsons JA, et al. Continuous subcutaneous insulin infusion: improved blood-glucose and intermediary-metabolite control in diabetics. Lancet 1979; 1:1255–1258.

1045. Tamborlane WV, Sherwin RS, Genel M, et al. Reduction to normal of plasma glucose in juvenile diabetes by subcutaneous administration of insulin with a portable infusion pump. N Engl J Med 1979; 300:573–578.

1046. Felig P, Bergman M. Intensive ambulatory treatment of insulin-dependent diabetes. Ann Intern Med 1982; 97:225–230.

1047. Kitabchi AE, Fisher JN, Matteri R, et al. The use of continuous insulin delivery systems in treatment of diabetes mellitus. Adv Intern Med 1983; 28:449–490.

1048. Mecklenburg RS, Benson JW Jr, Becker NM, et al. Clinical use of the insulin infusion pump in 100 patients with type I diabetes. N Engl J Med 1982; 307:513–518. '

1049. Schade DS, Santiago JV, Skyler JS, et al. Hazards of intensive insulin therapy. In: Schade DS, Santiago JV, Skyler JS, et al., eds. Intensive Insulin Therapy. Princeton: Excerpta Medica, 1983: 287–301.

1050. Broussolle C, Jeandidler N, Hanaire-Broutin H, et al. French multicentre experience of implantable insulin pumps. Lancet 1994; 343:514–515.

1051. Schade DS, Santiago JV, Skyler JS, et al. Effects of intensive treatment on substrate and hormonal abnormalities. In: Schade DS, Santiago JV, Skyler JS, et al., eds. Intensive Insulin Therapy. Princeton: Excerpta Medica, 1983: 71–87.

1052. Rosenstock J, Vega GL, Raskin P. Effect of intensive diabetes treatment on low-density lipoprotein apolipoprotein β kinetics in type I diabetics. Diabetes 1988; 37:393–397.

1053. Rubinstein A, Pierce CE Jr II, Bloomgarden Z. Rapid healing of diabetic foot ulcers with continuous subcutaneous insulin infusion. Am J Med 1983; 75:161–165.

1054. Lauritzen T, Frost-Larsen K, Larsen H-W, et al. The effect of near-normal blood glucose levels upon retinopathy: two-year follow-up. Diabetologia 1983; 25:174 (abstract).

1055. Lauritzen T, Frost-Larsen K, Larsen HW, et al. Two-year experience with continuous subcutaneous insulin infusion in relation to retinopathy and neuropathy. Diabetes 1985; 34(Suppl 3):74–79.

1056. Holman RR, Mayon-White V, Orde-Peackar C, et al. Prevention of deterioration of renal and sensory-nerve function by more intensive management of insulin-dependent diabetic patients: a two-year randomised prospective study. Lancet 1983; 1:204–208.

1057. Engerman RL, Kern TS. Progression of incipient diabetic retinopathy during good glycemic control. Diabetes 1987; 36:808–812.

1058. Rosenstock J, Friberg T, Raskin P. Effect of glycemic control on microvascular complications in patients with type I diabetes mellitus. Am J Med 1986; 81:1012–1018.

1059. Teutsch SM, Herman WH, Dwyer DM, et al. Mortality among diabetic patients using continuous subcutaneous insulin-infusion pumps. N Engl J Med 1984; 310:361–368.

1060. Mecklenburg RS, Benson JW Jr, Blumenstein BA, et al. Long-term metabolic control with insulin pump therapy: Report of experience with 127 patients. N Engl J Med 1985; 313:464–468.

1061. Jorgens V, Gruber M, Bott U, et al. Effective and safe translation of intensified insulin therapy to general internal medicine departments. Diabetologia 1993; 36:99–105.

1062. Perriello G, De Feo P, Torlone E, et al. The dawn phenomenon in type 1 (insulin-dependent) diabetes mellitus: magnitude, frequency, variability, and dependency on glucose counterregulation and insulin sensitivity. Diabetologia 1991; 34:21–28.

1063. Boden G, Soriano M, Hoeldtke RD, et al. Counterregulatory hormone release and glucose recovery after hypoglycemia in noninsulin-dependent diabetic patients. Diabetes 1983; 32:1055–1059.

1064. White NH, Skor DA, Cryer PE, et al. Identification of type 1 diabetic patients at increased risk for hypoglycemia during intensive therapy. N Engl J Med 1983; 308:485–491.

1065. Cryer PE. Glucose counterregulation in man. Diabetes 1981; 30:261–264.

1066. Gerich J, Davis J, Lorenzi M, et al. Hormonal mechanisms of recovery from insulin-induced hypoglycemia in man. Am J Physiol 1979; 236:E380–E385.

1067. Bolli G, De Feo P, Compagnucci P, et al. Important role of adrenergic mechanisms in acute glucose counterregulation following insulin-induced hypoglycemia in type I diabetes: evidence for an effect mediated by beta-adrenoreceptors. Diabetes 1982; 31:641–647.

1068. De Feo P, Bolli G, Perriello G, et al. The adrenergic contribution to glucose counterregulation in type I diabetes mellitus: dependency on A-cell function and mediation through beta2-adrenergic receptors. Diabetes 1983; 32:887–893.

1069. Boden G, Reichard GA Jr, Hoeldtke RD, et al. Severe insulin-induced hypoglycemia associated with deficiencies in the release of counter-regulatory hormones. N Engl J Med 1981; 305:1200–1205.

1070. Cryer PE. Decreased sympathochromaffin activity in IDDM. Diabetes 1989; 38:405–409.

1071. Dagogo-Jack S, Rattersarn C, Cryer PE, et al. Reversal of hypoglycemia unawareness, but not defective glucose counterregulation, in IDDM. Diabetes 1994; 43:1426–1434.

1072. Boyle PJ, Kempers SF, O'Connor AM, et al. Brain glucose uptake and unawareness of hypoglycemia in patients with insulin-dependent diabetes mellitus. N Engl J Med 1995; 333:1726–1731.

1073. Borg WP, Sherwin RS, During MJ, et al. Local ventromedial hypothalamus glucopenia triggers counterregulatory hormone release. Diabetes 1995; 44:180–184.

1074. Bolli GB, Fanelli CG. Unawareness of hypoglycemia. N Engl J Med 1995; 333:1771–1772.

1075. Somogyi M. Exacerbation of diabetes by excess insulin action. Am J Med 1959; 26:169–191.

1076. Wilson DE. Excessive insulin therapy: biochemical effects and clinical repercussions. Current concepts of counterregulation in type I diabetes. Ann Intern Med 1983; 98:219–227.

1077. Tordjman KM, Havlin CE, Levandoski LA, et al. Failure of nocturnal hypoglycemia to cause fasting hyperglycemia in patients with insulin-dependent diabetes mellitus. N Engl J Med 1987; 317:1552–1559.

1078. Winter RJ. Profiles of metabolic control in diabetic children: frequency of asymptomatic nocturnal hypoglycemia. Metabolism 1981; 30:666–672.

1079. Kahn CR, Rosenthal AS. Immunologic reactions to insulin: insulin allergy, insulin resistance, and the autoimmune insulin syndrome. Diabetes Care 1979; 2:283–295.

1080. Kahn CR, Mann D, Rosenthal AS, et al. The immune response to insulin in man: interaction of HLA alloantigens and the development of the immune response. Diabetes 1982; 31:716–723.

1081. Galloway JA, Bressler R. Insulin treatment in diabetes. Med Clin North Am 1978; 62:663–680.

1082. DeFronzo RA, Hendler R, Simonson D. Insulin resistance is a prominent feature of insulin-dependent diabetes. Diabetes 1982; 31:795–801.

1083. Bonora E, Coscelli C, Butturini U. Residual B cell function and insulin sensitivity in type I (insulin-dependent) diabetes mellitus. Diabetologia 1983; 25:298.

1084. Kahn CR. Role of insulin receptors in insulin-resistant states. Metabolism 1980; 29:455–466.

1085. Shipp JC, Cunninham RW, Russell RO, et al. Insulin resistance: clinical features, natural course and effects of adrenal steroid treatment. Medicine 1965; 44:165–186.

1086. Kurtz AB, Nabarro JDN. Circulating insulin-binding antibodies. Diabetologia 1980; 19:329–334.

1087. Rhie FH, Ganda OP, Bern MM, et al. Insulin resistance and monoclonal gammopathy. Metabolism 1971; 30:41–45.

1088. Goldman J, Baldwin D, Rubenstein AH, et al. Characterization of circulating insulin and proinsulin-binding antibodies in autoimmune hypoglycemia. J Clin Invest 1979; 63:1050–1059.

1089. Nathan DM, Axelrod L, Flier JS, et al. U-500 insulin in the treatment of antibody-mediated insulin resistance. Ann Intern Med 1971; 94:653–656.

1090. Davidson JK, DeBra DW. Immunologic insulin resistance. Diabetes 1978; 27:307–318.

1091. Paulsen EP, Courtney JW III, Duckworth WC. Insulin resistance caused by massive degradation of subcutaneous insulin. Diabetes 1979; 28:640–645.

1092. Kitabchi AE, Stentz FB, Cole C, et al. Accelerated insulin degradation: an alternate mechanism for insulin resistance. Diabetes Care 1979; 2:414–417.

1093. Schade DS, Eaton RP, Warhol RM, et al. Subcutaneous peritoneal access device for type I diabetic patients nonresponsive to subcutaneous insulin. Diabetes 1982; 31:470–473.

1094. Franz MJ, Horton ES, Bantle JP, et al. Nutrition principles for the management of diabetes and related complications. Diabetes Care 1994; 17:490–518 (technical review).

1095. Position statement: nutrition recommendations and principles for people with diabetes mellitus. Diabetes Care 1996; 19(suppl 1):S16–S19.

1096. Garg A, Bonanome A, Grundy SM, et al. Comparison of a high-carbohydrate diet in patients with non–insulin-dependent diabetes mellitus. N Engl J Med 1988; 319:829–834.

1097. Brown MS, Goldstein JL. Heart attacks: gone with the century? Science 1996; 272:629.

1098. Bantle JP, Laine DC, Castle GW, et al. Postprandial glucose and insulin responses to meals containing different carbohydrates in normal and diabetic subjects. N Engl J Med 1983; 309:7–12.

1099. Crapo PA, Olefsky JM. Food fallacies and blood sugar. N Engl J Med 1983; 309:44–45.

1100. Arky RA. Nutritional management of the diabetic. In: Ellenberg M, Rifkin H, eds. Diabetes Mellitus: Theory and Practice. 3rd ed. New Hyde Park, NY: Medical Examination Publishing, 1983: 539–566.

1101. Kemmer FW, Berger M. Therapy and better quality of life: the dichotomous role of exercise in diabetes mellitus. Diabetes Metab Rev 1986; 2:53–68.

1102. Wahren J, Felig P, Hagenfeldt L. Physical exercise and fuel homeostasis in diabetes mellitus. Diabetologia 1978; 14:213–222.

1103. DeFronzo RA, Ferrannini E, Sato Y, et al. Synergistic interaction between exercise and insulin on peripheral glucose uptake. J Clin Invest 1981; 68:1468–1474.

1104. Zinman B, Murray FT, Vranic M, et al. Glucoregulation during moderate exercise in insulin-treated diabetics. J Clin Endocrinol Metab 1977; 45:641–652.

1105. Kemmer FW, Berchtold P, Berger M, et al. Exercise-induced fall of blood glucose in insulin-treated diabetics unrelated to alteration of insulin mobilization. Diabetes 1979; 28:1131–1137.

1106. Martin MJ, Robbins DC, Bergenstal R, et al. Absence of exercise-induced hypoglycaemia in type I (insulin-dependent) diabetic patients during maintenance of normoglycaemia by short-term, open-loop insulin infusion. Diabetologia 1982; 23:337–342.

1107. Poussier P, Zinman B, Marliss EB, et al. Open-loop intravenous insulin waveforms for postprandial exercise in type I diabetes. Diabetes Care 1983; 6:129–134.

1108. Savage PJ, Bennion LJ, Flock EV, et al. Diet-induced improvement of abnormalities in insulin and glucagon secretion and in insulin receptor binding in diabetes mellitus. J Clin Endocrinol Metab 1979; 48:999–1007.

1109. Andrews WJ, Vasquez B, Nagulesparan M, et al. Insulin therapy in obese noninsulin-dependent diabetes induces improvements in insulin action and secretion which are maintained for two weeks after insulin withdrawal. Diabetes 1984; 33:634–642.

1110. Knowler WC, Pettitt DJ, Saad MF, et al. Obesity in the Pima Indians: its magnitude and relationship with diabetes. Am J Clin Nutr 1991; 53:1543S–1551S.

1111. Hanson RL, Narayan KMV, McCance Dr, et al. Rate of weight gain, weight fluctuation, and incidence of NIDDM. Diabetes 1995; 43:261–266.

1112. Ohneda M, Inman L, Unger RH. Caloric restriction in obese prediabetic rats prevents beta cell depletion, loss of beta cell GLUT-2 and glucose incompetence. Diabetologia 1995; 38:173–179.

1113. Pfeifer MA, Halter JB, Porte D Jr. Insulin secretion in diabetes mellitus. Am J Med 1981; 70:579–588.

1114. Prince MJ, Olefsky JM. Direct in vitro effect of a sulfonylurea to increase human fibroblast insulin receptors. J Clin Invest 1980; 66:608–611.

1115. Salhanick AI, Konowitz P, Amatruda JM. Potentiation of insulin action by a sulfonylurea in primary cultures of hepatocytes from normal and diabetic rats. Diabetes 1983; 32:206–212.

1116. Vigneri R, Pezzino V, Wong KY, et al. Comparison of the in vitro effect of biguanides and sulfonylureas on insulin binding to its receptors in target cells. J Clin Endocrinol Metab 1982; 54:95–100.

1117. Maloff BL, Lockwood DH. In vitro effects of a sulfonylurea on insulin action in adipocytes: Potentiation of insulin-stimulated hexose transport. J Clin Invest 1981; 68:85–90.

1118. Putnam WS, Andersen DK, Jones RS, et al. Selective potentiation of insulin-mediated glucose disposal in normal dogs by the sulfonylurea glipizide. J Clin Invest 1981; 67:1016–1023.

1119. Groop L, Luzi L, Melander A, et al. Different effects of glyburide and glipizide on insulin secretion and hepatic glucose production in normal and NIDDM subjects. Diabetes 1987; 36:1320–1328.

1120. Yki-Jarvinen H, Kauppila M, Kujansuu E, et al. Comparison of insulin regimens in patients with non–insulin-dependent diabetes mellitus. N Engl J Med 1992; 327:1426–1433.

1121. Tsiani E, Ramial R, Leiter L, et al. Stimulation of glucose uptake and increased plasma membrane content of glucose transporters in L6 skeletal muscle cells by the sulfonylureas gliciazide and glyburide. Endocrinology 1995; 136:2505–2512.

1122. Bahr T, Holtey MV, Muller G, et al. Direct stimulation of myocardial glucose transport and glucose transporter-1 (GLUT1) and GLUT4 protein expression by the sulfonylurea glimepiride. Endocrinology 1995; 136:2547–2553.

1123. Lebovitz HE, Feinglos MN. The oral hypoglycemic agents. In: Ellenberg M, Rifkin H, eds. Diabetes Mellitus: Theory and Practice. 3rd ed. New Hyde Park, NY: Medical Examination Publishing, 1983: 591–610.

1124. Sartor G, Schersten B, Carlström S, et al. Ten-year follow-up of subjects with impaired glucose tolerance: prevention of diabetes by tolbutamide and diet regulation. Diabetes 1980; 29:41–49.

1125. Misbin RI. Phenformin-associated lactic acidosis: pathogenesis and treatment. Ann Intern Med 1977; 87:591–595.

1126. Cohen RD, Woods HF. Lactic acidosis revisited. Diabetes 1983; 32:181–191.

1127. Bailey CJ. Biguanidines and NIDDM. Diabetes Care 1992; 15:755–772.

1128. Unger RH, Madison LL, Carter NW. Tolbutamide-phenform in ketoacidosis-resistant patients. JAMA 1960; 174:2132–2136.

1129. Caspary WF. Sucrose malabsorption in man after ingestion of α-glucosidehydrolase inhibitor. Lancet 1978; 1:1231–1233.

1130. Taylor RH, Jenkins DJA, Barker HM, et al. Effect of acarbose on the 24-hour blood glucose profile and pattern of carbohydrate absorption. Diabetes Care 1982; 5:92–96.

1131. Chiasson JL, Josse RG, Hunt JA, et al. The efficacy of acarbose in the treatment of patients with non–insulin-dependent diabetes mellitus. Ann Intern Med 1994; 121:928–935.

1132. Chang AY, Wyse BM, Gilchrist BJ, et al. Ciglitazone: a new hypoglycemic agent. I: Studies in ob/ob and db/db mice, diabetic Chinese hamsters, and normal and streptozotocin-diabetic rats. Diabetes 1983; 32:830–838.

1133. Chang AY, Wyse BM, Gilchrist BJ. Ciglitazone: a new hypoglycemic agent. II: Effect on glucose and lipid metabolisms and insulin binding in the adipose tissue of C57BL/6J-ob/ob and ±/? mice. Diabetes 1983; 32:839–845.

1134. Szalkowski D, White-Carrington S, Berger J, et al. Antidiabetic thiazolidinediones block the inhibitory effect of tumor necrosis factor-alpha on differentiation, insulin-stimulated glucose uptake, and gene expression in 3T3-L1 cells. Endocrinology 1995; 136:1474–1481.

1135. Kobayashi M, Iwanishi M, Egawa K, et al. Pioglitazone increases insulin sensitivity by activating insulin receptor kinase. Diabetes 1992; 41:476–483.

1136. Ohsumi J, Sakakibara S, Yamaguchi J, et al. Troglitazone prevents the inhibitory effects of inflammatory cytokines on insulin-induced adipocyte differentiation in 3T3-L1 cells. Endocrinology 1994; 135:2279.

1137. Hoffmann CA, Edwards CW, Hillman RA, et al. Treatment of insulin-resistant mice with the oral antidiabetic agent pioglitazone: evaluation of liver GLUT2 and phosphoenolpyruvate carboxykinase expression. Endocrinology 1992; 130:735–740.

1138. Sandouk T, Reda D, Hofmann AC. The antidiabetic agent pioglitazone increases expression of glucose transporters in 3T3-F442A cells by increasing messenger ribonucleic acid transcript stability. Endocrinology 1993; 133:352–359.

1139. Masuda K, Okamoto Y, Tsuura Y, et al. Effects of troglitazone (CS-043) on insulin secretion in isolated rat pancreatic islets and HIT cells: an insulinotropic mechanism distinct from glibenclamide. Diabetologia 1995; 38:24–30.

1140. Stevenson RW, McPherson RK, Persson LM, et al. The antihyperglycemic agent englitazone prevents the defect in glucose transport in rats fed a high-fat diet. Diabetes 1996; 45:60–66.

1141. Shechter Y. Perspective in diabetes: insulin-mimetic effects of vanadate. Possible implications for future treatment of diabetes. Diabetes 1990; 39:1–5.

1142. Helliger CE, Tahiliani AG, McNeill JH. Effect of vanadate on elevated blood glucose and depressed cardiac performance of diabetic rats. Science 1985; 227:1474–1476.

1143. Gil J, Mirapelx M, Carreras J, et al. Insulin-like effects of vanadate on glucokinase activity and fructose 2,6-bisphosphate levels in the liver of diabetic rats. J Biol Chem 1988; 263:1868–1871.

1144. Strout HV, Vacario PP, Biswas C, et al. Vanadate treatment of streptozotocin diabetic rats restores expression of the insulin-responsive glucose transporter in skeletal muscle. Endocrinology 1990; 126:2728–2732.

1145. Rossetti L, Laughlin MR. Correction of chronic hyperglycaemia with vanadate, but not with phlorizin, normalises in vivo glycogen repletion and in vitro glycogen synthase activity in diabetic skeletal muscle. J Clin Invest 1989; 84:892–899.

1146. Meyerovitch J, Rothenberg P, Shechter Y, et al. Vanadate normalises hyperglycaemia in two mouse models of non–insulin-dependent diabetes mellitus. J Clin Invest 1991; 87:1286–1294.

1147. Robertson RP, Klein DJ. Treatment of diabetes mellitus. Diabetologia 1992; 35(Suppl 2):S8–S17.

1148. Worm D, Henriksen JE, Vaag A, et al. Pronounced blood glucose-lowering effect of the antilipolytic drug acipimox in noninsulin-dependent diabetes mellitus patients during a 3-day intensified treatment period. J Clin Endocrinol Metab 1994; 78:717–721.

1149. Alberti KGMM, Hockaday TDR. Diabetic coma: a reappraisal after five years. Clin Endocrinol Metab 1977; 6:421–455.

1150. Clements RS Jr, Vourganti B. Fatal diabetic ketoacidosis: major causes and approaches to their prevention. Diabetes Care 1978; 1:314–325.

1151. Foster DW, McGarry JD. Diabetes mellitus: acute complications, ketoacidosis, hyperosmolar coma, lactic acidosis. In: DeGroot LJ, et al, eds. Endocrinology. Vol 2, 3rd ed. Philadelphia: WB Saunders, 1995: 1506–1521.

1152. Wilson HK, Keuer SP, Lea AS, et al. Phosphate therapy in diabetic ketoacidosis. Arch Intern Med 1982; 142:517–520.

1153. Keller U, Berger W. Prevention of hypophosphatemia by phosphate infusion during treatment of diabetic ketoacidosis and hyperosmolar coma. Diabetes 1980; 29:87–95.

1154. Matz R. Diabetic acidosis. Rationale for not using bicarbonate. NY State J Med 1976; 76:1299–1303.

1155. Kitabichi AE. Low-dose insulin therapy in diabetic ketoacidosis: fact or fiction? Diabetes Metab Rev 1989; 5:337–363.

1156. Lever E, Jaspan JB. Sodium bicarbonate therapy in severe diabetic ketoacidosis. Am J Med 1983; 75:263–268.

1157. Okuda Y, Adrogue HJ, Field JB, et al. Counterproductive effects of sodium bicarbonate in diabetic ketoacidosis. J Clin Endocrinol Metab 1996; 81:314–320.

1158. Artis WM, Fountain JA, Delcher KH, et al. A mechanism of susceptibility to mucormycosis in diabetic ketoacidosis: transferrin and iron availability. Diabetes 1982; 31:1109–1114.

1159. Paton RC. Haemostatic changes in diabetic coma. Diabetologia 1981; 21:172–177.

1160. McGill JB, Schneider DJ, Artken CL, et al. Factors responsible for impaired fibrinolysis in obese subjects and NIDDM patients. Diabetes 1994; 43:104–109.

1161. Leurs PB, van Oerle R, Hamulyak K, et al. Tissue factor pathway inhibitor activity in patients with IDDM. Diabetes 1995; 44:80–84.

1162. Lukala R, Tracy KJ, Surami A. Advanced glycosylation products quench nitric oxide and mediate defective endothelium-dependent vasodilation in experimental diabetes. J Clin Invest 1991; 87:432–438.

1163. Ting HH, Timimi FK, Boles KS. Vitamin C improves endothelium-dependent vasodilation in patients with non–insulin-dependent diabetes mellitus. J Clin Invest 1996; 97:22–28.

1164. Ceriello A, Giacomello R, Stel G, et al. Hyperglycemia-induced thrombin formation in diabetes: the possible role of oxidative stress. Diabetes 1995; 44:924–928.

1165. Rosenbloom AL, Riley WJ, Weber FT, et al. Cerebral edema complicating diabetic ketoacidosis in childhood. J Pediatr 1980; 96:357–361.

1166. Franklin B, Liu J, Ginsberg-Fellner F. Cerebral edema and ophthalmoplegia reversed by mannitol in a new case of insulin-dependent diabetes mellitus. Pediatrics 1982; 69:87–90.

1167. Fein IA, Rackow EC, Sprung CL, et al. Relation of colloid osmotic pressure to arterial hypoxemia and cerebral edema during crystalloid volume loading of patients with diabetic ketoacidosis. Ann Intern Med 1982; 96:570–575.

1168. Carroll P, Matz R. Adult respiratory distress syndrome complicating severely uncontrolled diabetes mellitus: report of nine cases and a review of the literature. Diabetes Care 1982; 5:574–580.

1169. Grundy SM. Drug therapy: HMG-CoA reductase inhibitors for treatment of hypercholesterolemia. N Engl J Med 1988; 319:24–32.

1170. Brownlee M, Vlassara H, Kooney A, et al. Aminoguanidine prevents diabetes-induced arterial wall cross-linking. Science 1986; 232:1629–1632.

1171. Folkman J, Weisz PB, Joullié MM, et al. Control of angiogenesis with synthetic heparin substitutes. Science 1989; 243:1490–1493.

1172. Folkman J. Successful treatment of an angiogenic disease. N Engl J Med 1989; 320:1211–1212.

1173. Sutherland DER. Report from the International Pancreas Transplant Registry. Diabetologia 1991; 34:S28–S39.

1174. Remuzzi G, Ruggenenti P, Mauer SM. Pancreas and kidney/pancreas transplants: experimental medicine or real improvement? Lancet 1991; 343:27–31.

1175. Olausson M, Nyberg G, Norden G, et al. Outcome of pancreas transplantations in Goteborg, Sweden 1985–1990. Diabetologia 1991; 34:S1–S3.

1176. Zehr PS, Milde FK, Hart LK, et al. Pancreas transplantation: assessing secondary complications and life quality. Diabetologia 1991; 34:S138–S140.

1177. Secchi A, Di Carlo V, Martinenghi S, et al. Effect of pancrease transplanta-

1178. Zehrer I, Gross CR. Quality of life of pancreas transplant recipients. Diabetologia 1991; 34:S145–S149.

1179. Piehlmeier W, Bullinger M, Nusser J, et al. Quality of life in type I (insulin-dependent) diabetic patients prior to and after pancreas and kidney transplantation in relation to organ function. Diabetologia 1991; 34:S150–S157.

1180. Navarro X, Kennedy R, Sutherland DER. Autonomic neuropathy and survival in diabetes mellitus: effects of pancreas transplantation. Diabetologia 1991; 34:S108–S112.

1181. Comi G, Galardi G, Amadio S, et al. Neurophysiological study of the effect of combined kidney and pancreas transplantation on diabetic neuropathy: a 2-year follow-up evaluation. Diabetologia 1991; 34:S103–S107.

1182. Muller-Felber W, Landgraf R, Wagner ST, et al. Follow-up study sensory-motor polyneuropathy in type I (insulin-dependent) diabetic subjects after simultaneous pancreas and kidney transplantation and afgter graft rejection. Diabetologia 1991; 34:S113–S117.

1183. Boucek P, Bartos V, Vanek I, et al. Diabetic autonomic neuropathy after pancreas and kidney transplantation. Diabetologia 1991; 34:S121–S124.

1184. Solders G, Tyden G, Persson A, et al. Improvement in diabetic neuropathy 4 years after successful pancreatic and renal transplantation. Diabetologia 1991; 34:S125–S127.

1185. Bandello F, Vigano C, Secchi A, et al. Effect of pancreas transplantation on diabetic retinopathy: a 20-case report. Diabetologia 1991; 34:S92–S94.

1186. Scheider A, Meyer-Schwickerath E, Nusser J, et al. Diabetic retinopathy and pancreas tranplantation: a 3-year follow-up. Diabetologia 1991; 34:S95–S99.

1187. Zech JC, Trepsat D, Grain-Gueugnon M, Lefrancois N, et al. Ophthalmological follow-up of type 1 (insulin-dependent) diabetic patients after kidney and pancreas transplantation. Diabetologia 1991; 34:S89–S91.

1188. Konigrainer A, Miller K, Steurer W, et al. Does pancreas transplantation influence the course of diabetic retinopathy? Diabetologia 1991; 34:S86–S88.

1189. Sutherland DER. Who should get a pancreas transplant? Diabetes Care 1988; 11:681–685.

1190. The University of Michigan Pancreas Transplant Committee. Pancreatic transplantation as treatment for IDDM: proposed candidate criteria before end-stage diabetic nephropathy. Diabetes Care 1988; 11:669–675.

1191. Lanza RP, Sullivan SJ, Chick WL. Islet transplantation with immunoisolation. Diabetes 1992; 41:1503–1510.

1192. Algire GH, Legallais FY. Recent developments in the transplantation-chamber technique as adapted to the mouse. J Natl Cancer Inst 1949; 10:225–253.

1193. Algire GH, Weaver JM, Prehn RT. Growth of cells in vivo in diffusion chambers. 1: Survival of homografts in immunized mice. J Natl Cancer Inst 1954; 15:493–507.

1194. Prehn RT, Weaver JM, Algire GH. The diffusion-chamber technique applied to a study of the nature of homograft resistance. J Natl Cancer Inst 1954; 15:509–517.

1195. Gates RJ, Lazarus NR. Reversal of streptozotocin-induced diabetes in rats by intraperitoneal implantation of encapsulated neonatal rabbit pancreatic tissue. Lancet 1979; 1:972–972.

1196. Theodorou NA, Vrbova H, Tyhurst M, et al. Problems in the use of polycarbonate diffusion chambers for syngeneic pancreatic islet transplantation in rats. Diabetologia 1980; 18:313–317.

1197. Lanza RP, Butler DH, Borland KM, et al. Xenotransplantation of canine, bovine, and porcine islets in diabetic rats without immunosuppression. Proc Natl Acad Sci USA 1991; 88:11100–11104.

1198. Lanza RP, Butler DH, Borland KM, et al. Successful xenotransplantation of a diffusion-based biohybrid artificial pancreas: a study using canine, bovine, and porcine islets. Transplant Proc 1992; 24:669–671.

1199. Lanza RP, Borland KM, Lodge P, et al. Treatment of severely diabetic, pancreatectomized dogs using a diffusion-based hybrid pancreas. Diabetes 1992; 41:886–889.

1200. Lim F, Sun AM. Microencapsulated islets as bioartificial endocrine pancreas. Science 1980; 210:908–910.

1201. Norton J, Weber C, Reemtsma K. Microencapsulation: prevention of islet graft rejection. In: Van Schilgaarde R, Hardy M, eds. Transplantation of the Endocrine Pancreas in Diabetes Mellitus. Amsterdam, Elsevier, 1988.

1202. Lanza RP, Soon-Shiong P. Experimental xenotransplantation of encapsulated islets. In: Cooper DKC, Kemp E, Reemtsa K, et al., eds. Xenotransplantation: The Transplantation of Organs and Tissues Between Species. Heidelberg, Germany: Springer-Verlag, 1991: 299–312.

1203. Lanza RP, Butler DH, Borland KM, et al. Xenotransplantation of canine, bovine, and porcine islets in diabetic rats without immunosuppression. Proc Natl Acad Sci USA 1991; 88:11100–11104.

1204. Warnock GL, Kneteman NM, Ryan E, et al. Normoglycaemia after transplantation of freshly isolated and cryopreserved pancreatic islets in type I (insulin-dependent) diabetes mellitus. Diabetologia 1991; 34:55–58.

1205. Warnock GL, Kneteman NM, Ryan EA, et al. Long-term follow-up after transplantation of insulin-producing pancreatic islets into patients with type I (insulin-dependent) diabetes mellitus. Diabetologia 1992; 35:89–95.

1206. Gores PF, Najarian JS, Stephanian E, et al. Insulin independence in type I diabetes after transplantation of unpurified islets from single donor with 15-deoxyspergualin. Lancet 1993; 341:19–21.

1207. Groth CG, Korsgren O, Tibell A, et al. Transplantation of porcine fetal pancreas to diabetic patients. Lancet 1994; 344:1402–1404.

The first uses techniques designed to assess the amount of fat in the body. Values are established for persons presumed to be normal, and obesity is defined by a value greater than the normal range in statistical terms. This approach may involve direct measures of body fat or indirect estimates using methods that correlate with the direct measurements. A second technique is to define obesity in terms of risk to life, i.e., significant obesity is the level of overweight that causes excess mortality relative to an idealized normal weight. This approach makes sense but is complex in practice because the risk of any degree of excess adiposity can differ among individuals based on the variable presence of susceptibility to complications such as diabetes mellitus, hypertension, or hyperlipidemia. Finally, fatness can be defined visually: a person who looks fat probably is fat.[2] This technique is the only one that is not based on statistics; only two groups are identified—fat and nonfat. Unfortunately the various methods for evaluating fatness do not give the same answers when compared directly.[3, 4] Therefore it is not easy to make the diagnosis precisely.

DIRECT TECHNIQUES FOR ESTIMATING BODY FAT. A number of procedures are available for the measurement of body fat; some are applicable clinically and others are research tools. They include densitometry, estimates of total body water, measurement of total body potassium, neutron activation techniques, computed tomography (CT) and magnetic resonance imaging scans, electrical methods measuring impedance and conductivity, and dual-energy x-ray absorptiometry.[4, 5] All have limitations because they require assumptions that may not hold true for the individual under study.

Densitometry. This technique is generally considered to be the "gold standard" for estimating body fat, and underwater weighing is the usual method for the assessment of body volume. It is assumed that fat-free tissue and fat have different densities, which are fixed. Standard formulas also assume that hydration of tissues is constant and that bone mineral content is fixed. The data supporting these assumptions are minuscule. One widely used "reference body" was based on measurements from only three cadavers. Formulas in the literature vary considerably in their constants.[3, 4] Four examples follow:

$$\% \text{ fat} = 100 \left(\frac{5.053}{\text{density}} - 4.164 \right) \quad (1)$$

$$\% \text{ fat} = 100 \left(\frac{4.201}{\text{density}} - 3.813 \right) \quad (2)$$

$$\% \text{ fat} = 100 \left(\frac{4.570}{\text{density}} - 5.142 \right) \quad (3)$$

$$\% \text{ fat} = 100 \left(\frac{4.950}{\text{density}} - 4.50 \right) \quad (4)$$

All give roughly the same answers, the error usually not exceeding 4%.[6] In the four formulas listed, a measured body density of 1.06 would give percent fat values of 15, 15, 17, and 17%, respectively.

Total Body Water Estimates. Total body water is usually measured with tritiated or deuterated water. Isotope dilution is allowed to reach the steady state, usually 2 to 3 h after administration, and water in the body is assumed to be limited to fat-free mass. The lean body mass is calculated from the assumption of a fixed percentage of water in lean tissue, usually 70 to 72%. Body fat is then taken as the difference between weight and calculated lean body mass, with a correction for the weight of the skeleton. Even if total water content is measured accurately, the percentage of water in the tissues varies in individuals from 69.3 to 77.5%.[3] The effects of such differences can be dramatic; a change of constant from 70 to 77% can result in a 10-kg difference in estimated body fat content.

Total Body Potassium Measurements. Estimates of lean body weight can also be made via measurement of total potassium in the body, if it is assumed that potassium is essentially limited to the fat-free compartment.[7] Potassium can be measured either by isotope dilution using potassium 42 or by assessing total body potassium 40 in a whole body counter. Various constants have been suggested.[4] Once again the assumption of a fixed constant renders estimated values suspect because the potassium content per kilogram of intracellular water in lean tissue can vary from individual to individual.

Other Methods.[4, 8] Other methods for estimation of fat content have been reported, but experience with them is limited. Neutron activation appears to be accurate, although constants are based on data from animals. It is reported that the technique can give values for body water, ash, lean tissue, and fat mass. Expense precludes wide use. Regional fat content can be assessed by CT or magnetic resonance imaging but the application of the values to the whole body is problematic. Measurement of electrical impedance is inexpensive and appears to be fairly accurate. Dual-photon beam absorptiometry also has promise.[5]

In summary, methods for directly estimating body fat often use constants based on minimal data. They are probably adequate for broad comparisons of groups of patients and for longitudinal study of individual subjects, but absolute values may not be accurate. Validation by chemical measurement of total fat in the body obviously is not possible in humans. The upper limit of normality for percent fat has been listed as 19% for men and 22% for women,[9] but other studies have shown higher values in nonobese individuals.[7]

INDIRECT TECHNIQUES FOR ESTIMATING BODY FAT

Skinfold Measurements. The percentage of body fat can be estimated by measuring the width of subcutaneous skinfolds with calibrated calipers.[3, 10] The best estimates appear to require four skinfold measurements (biceps, triceps, subscapular, and suprailiac), but acceptable values can be obtained with two measurements.[11, 12] Equations and nomograms are available for conversion of skinfold thickness to body fat.[11, 12] Although there are some technical problems, such as the amount of pressure that should be applied to the calipers, the main difficulty is that fat distribution can differ in individuals with the same amount of total adipose tissue. Thus in some forms of obesity the fat distribution is generalized, whereas in others the fat is largely abdominal.[13, 14] Estimates of percent fat are inaccurate insofar as distribution is skewed. In addition to these anatomic variations, the ratio of subcutaneous fat to deep fat also varies, values being reported to range from 0.1 to 0.7.[10] This variation is important because in some patients the bulk of new fat may be deposited in the abdomen and not accurately reflected by skinfold measurement. For example, body fat increases with aging, whereas skinfold thickness does not.[8] Despite these potential difficulties, skinfold measurements are adequate for longitudinal study of body composition in individuals and appear to provide useful information in cross-sectional studies of the population.[15]

Obesity is usually delineated by comparison of skinfold measurements in the test subject with values obtained in young men and nonpregnant women. Data from the Health and Nutrition Examination Survey 1971–1974 in the United States were used to define severe obesity as a combined skinfold measurement (triceps and subscapular) above the 95th percentile for ages 20 to 29.[16] The absolute value for the upper limits of normal was 51 mm in men and 70 mm in women. In the Ten State Nutritional Survey any value above the 85th percentile (triceps measurement alone) was considered abnormal.[1] Thus attention to definitions of obesity is imperative when comparing the results of surveys.

Weight/Height Ratios. The most widely used clinical tool for the assessment of obesity is the body mass index (BMI), defined as weight in kilograms divided by the square of the height in meters (W/H²). Correlation with body fat measured directly by densitometry is good.[17] Although the denominator in the BMI is H² in adults, a different formula is preferable in children.[17] A BMI of 25 has generally been considered the upper limit of normal, with 25 to 29.9 considered overweight and 30 or greater obese.[17] However, since both morbidity and mortality begin to increase as BMIs rise above 19 to 20,[18] albeit with a shallow slope, BMIs within what is generally viewed as the "normal range" may confer significant risk,[19] whether or not we describe the individual at risk as being obese. Formulas have been derived for calculating percent fat in the body from the BMI:

$$\text{(1) for men: } \% \text{ fat} = 1.218(W/H^2) - 10.13;$$
$$\text{(2) for women, } \% \text{ fat} = 1.48(W/H^2) - 7.17$$

Morbidity and mortality can be predicted from BMI values,[18, 20] but the precise relationship between BMI and morbidity is debated. The mortality associated with severe or "morbid" obesity, defined as greater than 45 kg greater than ideal weight or BMI greater than 40, is unquestioned[21]; however, the health consequences of mild to moderate overweight have been controversial, and leanness has itself been linked to increased mortality by a number of studies.[22, 23] A publication from the Nurses Health Study shows that the increased mortality associated with a low BMI is not seen when women who smoked and the results of the first 4 y are excluded, suggesting that the apparent risk of leanness is the result of smoking per se, morbidity associated with smoking, or other pre-existing disease and illness-associated weight loss.[18] When only nonsmokers are included, the relationship between all causes of mortality and the BMI is direct. Small, insignificant increases in mortality are seen at BMIs within the normal range, with the lowest risk seen with BMIs less than 19 (Fig. 22–1).[18] In analyses of disease-specific mortality among women who never smoked, BMI was positively related to the risk of death from cardiovascular disease, cancer, and other causes.[18] For death due to coronary disease, the relative risks for the increasing levels of BMI were 1 (BMI <19), 1 (BMI 19 to 21.9), 1.4 (BMI 22 to 24.9), 1.7 (BMI 25 to 26.9), 3.1 (BMI 27 to 28.9), 4.6 (BMI 29 to 31.9), and 5.8 (BMI >32). Rates of cancer among obese women were double those of the leanest women.

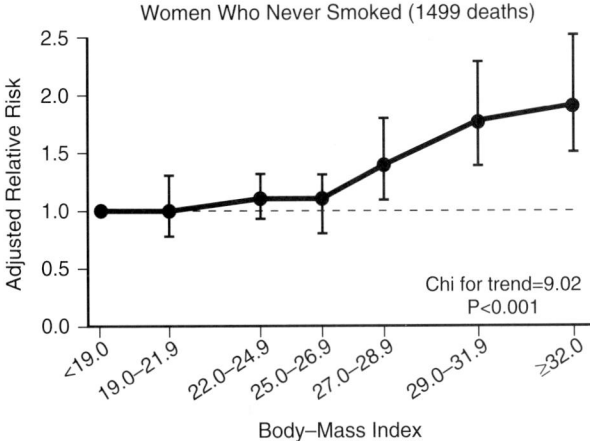

Figure 22–1. Relative risk of death from all causes, 1976–1992, according to body mass index, for women who never smoked. All relative risks are adjusted for age in 5-y categories. The bars represent 95% confidence intervals, and the reference category is women with a body mass index (BMI) less than 19. (Redrawn from Manson JE, Willett WC, Stampfer MJ, et al. Body weight and mortality among women. N Engl J Med 1995; 333:677–685. Copyright 1995, Massachusetts Medical Society. All rights reserved.)

Waist/Hip Ratios. All fat is not equal. Complications of obesity correlate best with abdominal fat and less well with lower body fat (buttocks and legs).[13, 14] The term *android* is sometimes used for central ("beer belly") obesity; *gynoid* is the adjective chosen for obesity of the lower body often seen in women. The distal localization of fat in some women may be so extreme as to suggest a forme fruste of partial lipodystrophy—the ribs are easily visible and the waist is not enlarged, but the buttocks and legs are significantly, even massively, obese. Distribution is assessed clinically by measuring the circumference of the waist and hips and expressing the values as a ratio. The waist is measured at the narrowest point between the rib cage and iliac crests; the hips are measured at the maximal point for the buttocks. Although values higher than 0.72 are considered abnormal,[8] complication rates increase substantially at ratios higher than 1 for men and 0.9 for women,[20] suggesting that these values are threshold levels for assignment of clinical risk. The impact of fat distribution is not minor. For example, although obesity imparted a relative risk for diabetes of 3.7 in a group of white women, central obesity in the same group increased the risk to 10.3.[24] (It is not that obesity of the lower body has no risk, only that the risks are lower.) Some studies have suggested that deep abdominal fat is more detrimental than is abdominal subcutaneous fat,[25] whereas others suggest that both deep and subcutaneous abdominal fat contribute to the insulin resistance that has been linked to many adverse consequences of obesity.[26] Deep and superficial fat can be differentiated by CT, but clinically this is unnecessary. The larger the abdominal girth the greater the amount of deep fat.

STANDARD TABLES. The most widely used standards for acceptable weight of adults in the United States have been those provided by the Metropolitan Life Insurance Company. These tables base the definition of acceptable weights on mortality experience in age- and sex-ranked weights per height at the time of entry into the life insurance system; i.e., the acceptable ranges were those encompassing the lowest mortality of the insured in each height-weight category. Separate ranges were established for small, medium, and large frames, although no definitions for these categories were provided. For this reason the Fogarty Conference on Obesity in America suggested a modification in which "average weight" was considered to be the median value for medium frame at each height, and the acceptable range was bracketed by the lowest weight for a small frame and the highest weight for a large frame.[27] One little-recognized alteration was that the original heights and weights from the Metropolitan tables were obtained with individuals wearing clothes and shoes, whereas the Fogarty tables list acceptable weights and heights obtained without clothes or shoes. It has been recommended that 2.54 cm (1 inch) be added to the heights and 2.3 and 1.4 kg (5 and 3 lb) be added to the weights of men and women, respectively, in the Fogarty tables when making comparisons with the data from the 1979 Build Study.[9] The convention of using an acceptable range of weights without referral to frame size is widely accepted.[17]

New tables of desirable weight were published in 1983 based on the 1979 Build Study of the Society of Actuaries and Association of Life Insurance Medical Directors of America.[9] The new standards, modified to conform to the Fogarty Conference style, are shown in Table 22–1. The interpretation of these data is complicated by several factors. First, the data are based on a preselected sample of the population defined by willingness or ability to purchase life insurance; presumably, those of lower socioeconomic status are underrepresented. Second, the data are not broken down by age or race. Third, persons accepted for insurance probably had no obvious major illness, which suggests that the individuals composing the sample were healthier at the start than the population as

living animals tend to be relatively stable over long periods, and periods of caloric restriction or overfeeding are met with compensatory physiological changes that resist the effects of these perturbations (Fig. 22–4).[47, 48] Specifically, in response to periods of food restriction or overfeeding, food intake and energy expenditure are altered to maintain energy stores constant. In response to overfeeding, as by gavage feeding of rodents or voluntary overfeeding of humans, spontaneous food intake is decreased and energy expenditure is increased, the net effect being a return to the previous weight once overfeeding ceases. In contrast, during a period of food restriction energy expenditure decreases, and when access to food is resumed spontaneous food intake increases until body energy stores are regained. Kennedy proposed that a homeostatic mechanism is based on a putative signal that reflects the size of adipose energy stores.[49] The existence of such a signal was indirectly supported by parabiosis experiments using mice with single-gene mutations that caused severe obesity (ob/ob, db/db).[50] These experiments suggested that one strain of mice (ob/ob) failed to produce a "satiety factor" to which the other strain (db/db) was unable to respond. The molecular identity and even the existence of a responsible factor was not evident until the *ob* gene was cloned in 1994.[51] This landmark study revealed the existence of a secretory product of the adipocyte, now referred to as leptin, that is capable of reversing the syndrome of ob/ob but not db/db mice.[52–54] The biology of leptin and the mechanism by which it influences body weight and energy stores through actions on the brain to regulate food intake and energy expenditure are now under investigation.[55] The discovery of leptin has invigorated the area of regulated energy balance.

Regulation of Food Intake and Energy Homeostasis by the Brain

The brain plays a critical role in the regulation of energy homeostasis through at least three physiological actions: control of hunger and satiety, influence of the rate of energy expenditure, and regulation of the secretion of hormones involved in disposition of energy stores. The hypothalamus, the site most centrally involved in the control of energy metabolism, integrates an array of internal and external signals pertinent to energy homeostasis and produces efferent signals that promote changes appropriate for energy homeostasis. Broadly speaking, these signals may be viewed as anabolic or catabolic, the former favoring ingestion of nutrients and energy storage and the latter favoring limitation of nutrient intake and dissipation of energy. A diagrammatic illustration of the factors involved in energy homeostasis is seen in Figure 22–5.

Inputs to the brain centers that regulate energy homeostasis can be divided into two categories. Short-term, situational, and meal-related signals may arise from internal sites such as the gut, external sites such as food cues in the environment, and higher brain centers involved in cognitive and emotional aspects of food ingestion; these signals mainly influence the size and timing of individual meals. Long-term signals, represented by the fat-derived hormone leptin, reflect the state of energy balance. This type of signal also acts on the brain to ensure that food intake and energy expenditure are coupled to the state of energy stores over the "long term." The molecular details of the mechanisms whereby peripheral signals regulate central nervous system outputs are beginning to be understood.

ROLE OF THE HYPOTHALAMUS: HISTORICAL PERSPECTIVE. Studies of electrical stimulation of discrete brain regions or of lesions induced by physical, chemical, or electrical means produced the idea that the hypothalamus plays a central role in energy homeostasis. Stimulation of the ventromedial hypothalamic (VMH) nucleus inhibited food intake, and destruction of this nucleus caused hyperphagia and obesity,[56] whereas similar manipulation of the lateral hypothalamic (LHA) nucleus produced opposite effects.[57] This led to the theory that the VMH and LHA are "satiety" and "hunger" centers.[58] Since glucose has opposite effects on the rate of neural firing in VMH and LHA neurons, it was proposed that the fall of glucose level with food deprivation might regulate ingestive behavior by effects on these sites.[59] Additional sites in the brain must also be involved because lesions of the VMH or LHA do not prevent compensatory feeding responses to starvation.[60] In addition a fall in the blood glucose level is no longer regarded as being a primary signal that triggers feeding responses at these sites.

HYPOTHALAMIC NEUROTRANSMITTERS AND NEUROPEPTIDES INVOLVED IN ENERGY BALANCE. One approach to defining the role of the hypothalamus in regulation of energy balance has been to identify molecular mediators of such events and to establish the neural circuitry involved. A list of the major factors known to participate in the regulation of food intake is seen in Table 22–2. Two categories of neurotransmitters that may be involved have been defined. The first are classic neurotransmitters such as norepinephrine, dopamine, and acetylcholine. Studies with microinjection of these agents and with pharmacologic manipulation using agonists, antagonists, and other means of changing local levels indicate that these neurotransmitters play a role in regulation of en-

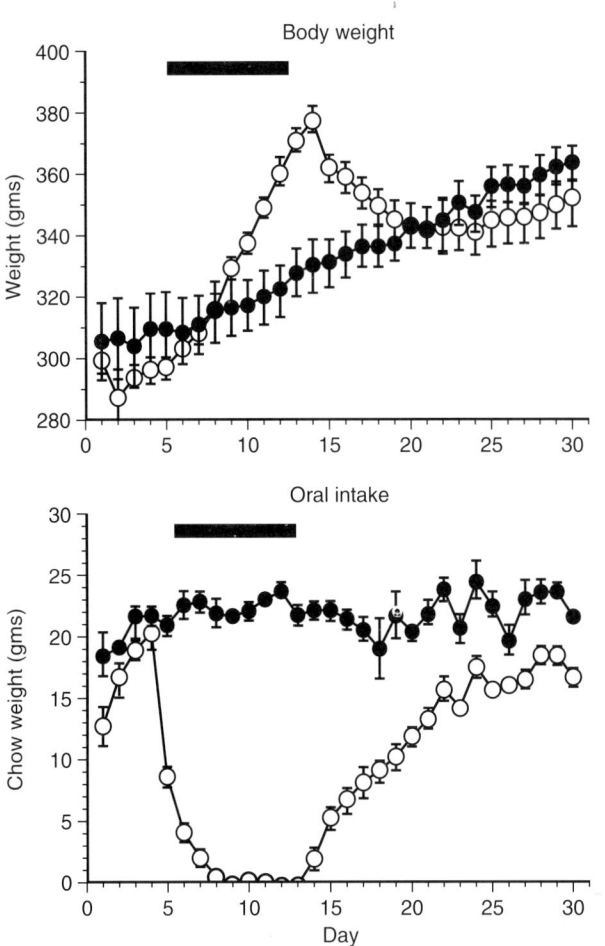

Figure 22–4. Daily body weight and weight of chow consumed spontaneously during 8 h in a group of seven gavage overfed *(open symbols)* and five control *(closed symbols)* rats. Solid bar represents the period of gavage overfeeding. (Redrawn from Weigle DS. Appetite and the regulation of body composition. FASEB J 1994; 8:302–310, with permission.)

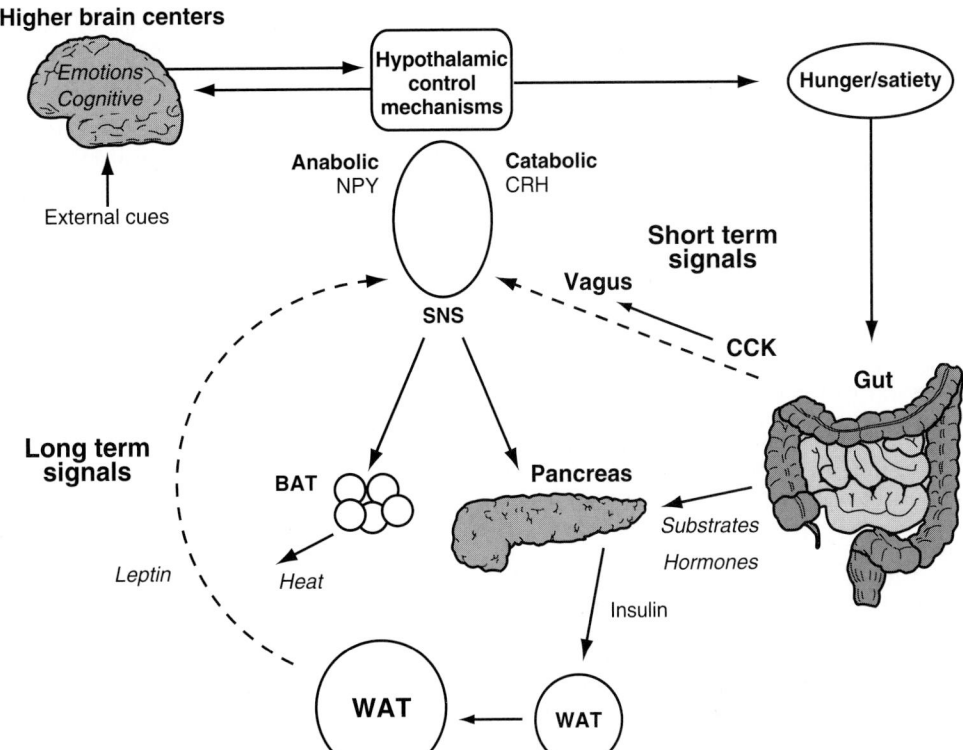

Figure 22–5. Physiological signals involved in the regulation of energy balance. NPY, neuropeptide Y; CRH, corticotropin-releasing hormone; CCK, cholecystokinin; SNS, sympathetic nervous system; BAT, brown adipose tissue; WAT, white adipose tissue.

ergy homeostasis. The role of serotonin has also received much attention, as serotonergic neurons in the brain are thought to participate in the regulation of food intake and appetite.[61] Direct injection of serotonin into the hypothalamus suppresses food intake,[62] and drugs that release serotonin from nerve endings (fenfluramine) or block its reuptake (fluoxetine) decrease food intake and body weight.[63, 64] The identity of the serotonin receptor subtype or subtypes that underlie these effects is not yet clear,[65] although transgenic

mice with knockout of the type 2c serotonin receptors experience mild obesity with disordered regulation of food intake.[66] In addition to serotonin affecting appetite, serotonin levels in the brain are influenced by nutritional factors. Changes in brain levels of the serotonin precursor tryptophan cause changes in brain serotonin levels, and changes in the ratio of carbohydrate to protein in the diet affect serum tryptophan levels and brain tryptophan uptake.[67] The hypothesis that serotonin specifically regulates carbohydrate appetite and that defects in this pathway underlie "carbohydrate craving" in humans[68] is unproved.[69, 70]

Many neuropeptides and peripheral hormones influence food intake in experimental systems and might participate in the control of feeding behavior.[71] These hypothalamic neuropeptides include neuropeptide Y (NPY),[72] melanin-concentrating hormone,[73] corticotropin-releasing hormone (CRH),[74] urocortin,[75] glucagon-like peptide I,[76] bombesin, galanin, and somatostatin. NPY and CRH, the most intensively studied, are concentrated in the paraventricular nuclei, dorsal and rostral to the VMH, and lesions of this area indicate that it is important for compensatory feeding in response to changes in energy homeostasis.[77]

NPY is believed to play a role in the physiological response to starvation and the promotion of obesity. NPY, a 36-amino-acid peptide, is a member of the pancreatic polypeptide gene family and is present in both the peripheral and central nervous systems.[78] Expression of NPY mRNA increases with starvation,[79] primarily in the arcuate nucleus, and NPYergic neurons project to the paraventricular nuclei, where increased NPY content is seen with food restriction. Injection of NPY into cerebral ventricles or specific brain regions enhances food intake in rodents,[72] and immunoneutralization of hypothalamic NPY reduces the hyperphagic response to starvation, suggesting that NPY modulates the normal physiological response to energy deprivation. Importantly, central NPY administration also promotes other responses that favor energy storage, including reduced sympathetic nervous system outflow to

TABLE 22–2. Molecules That Regulate Food Intake

Factors That Decrease Food Intake	Effect on Energy Expenditure
Neurotransmitters	
Norepinephrine—β-receptor	Increase
Dopamine	—
Serotonin	—
Hypothalamic Peptides	
Corticotropin-releasing factor (CRF)	Increase
Urocortin	?
Glucagon-like peptide I (GLP-I)	?
Cholecystokinin (CCK)	?
Peripheral Factors	
Leptin—long-term signal	Increase
CCK—meal-related signal	?
Insulin—effect observed after central administration	?
Factors That Increase Food Intake	
Central Factors	
Norepinephrine—α-receptor	Decrease
Neuropeptide Y (NPY)	Decrease
Melanin-concentrating hormone (MCH)	?
Galanin	?
Growth hormone–releasing hormone (GHRH)	?
Opioid peptides	?
Peripheral Factors	
Hypoglycemia	

brown adipose tissue (BAT)[80] (thereby reducing thermogenesis), stimulation of insulin secretion independent of increased food intake, and stimulation of adipose tissue lipoprotein lipase activity.[81] A role for NPY in the promotion of anabolism is also supported by observations that NPY expression is increased in the hypothalamus of ob/ob mice[78] and by the fact that NPY expression in the hypothalamus is diminished by treatment of ob/ob mice with recombinant leptin,[82] the fat protein that is mutated in these animals.[83] Nevertheless mice with targeted disruption of the *NPY* gene appear to regulate body weight normally,[84] suggesting that systems for regulating energy balance are redundant. Conversely, ob/ob mice with targeted disruption of the *NPY* gene have a major reduction in all aspects of the obesity syndrome,[84a] indicating that increases in NPY expression may be necessary for a full obesity syndrome to develop. A role for NPY in the pathogenesis of human obesity has not been explored because of the difficulty of obtaining relevant tissue for analysis. NPY acts through a family of receptors, and one receptor species (Y5) appears to mediate its actions in relation to energy homeostasis in the brain.[85]

The identity of central effectors of catabolic responses is less clear. CRH, a 41-amino-acid peptide that is the main regulator of the hypothalamic-pituitary-adrenal axis (see Chapters 5 and 6), has also been proposed to function as a central effector of catabolism.[74] When administered into its main site of biosynthesis in the paraventricular nuclei, CRH causes reduced food intake,[86] increased sympathetic outflow,[87] and hyperglycemia with less than the expected rise in insulin level. CRH excess can inhibit NPY expression with starvation.[88] Thus CRH may function to promote catabolic responses in opposition to the anabolic effects of NPY. Urocortin, a homologue of CRH in the hypothalamus, may be a more potent inhibitor of food intake than CRH.[75]

PERIPHERAL SATIETY SIGNALS. As discussed earlier, at least two types of signals are believed to regulate hunger and satiety: short-term factors related to the size and duration of individual meals and long-term factors that regulate overall energy stores and energy balance.

Short-term satiety factors can be divided into metabolic factors and gastrointestinal peptides. A venerable theory in obesity research is the glucostatic theory[89] in which the body assesses energy needs via glucosensitive neurons in the brain that respond to the rate of glucose utilization and are capable of regulating food intake by actions on the VMH and LHA. Although acute hypoglycemia produces hunger, whether plasma glucose is an important physiological trigger of hunger is unproved.

The fact that enteric hormones are key regulators of the assimilation of nutrients led to the view that one or more of these hormones might provide a satiety signal to the brain. Although glucagon, bombesin, and somatostatin reduce meal size after peripheral administration, the most compelling evidence for a physiological role is for cholecystokinin (CCK). Peripheral administration of CCK reduces meal size.[90] Since intraperitoneal administration is more potent than intravenous administration, and since an intact vagus nerve is required for the effect, vagal afferents must transmit the CCK signal to the hypothalamus.[91] Since repeated administration of CCK reduces meal size but is associated with more frequent food ingestion and maintenance of body weight,[92] CCK does not appear to be a major component of the system for long-term regulation of body weight.

PERIPHERAL SIGNALS INVOLVED IN THE LONG-TERM REGULATION OF ADIPOSITY. Studies in rodents of the changes in food intake that follow weight gain from forced feeding or weight loss from food restriction support the idea that the brain can sense a signal that reflects total body energy stores.[48] The existence of a peripheral factor that reflects

energy stores and is capable of regulating the brain centers involved in energy homeostasis is also supported by results of lipectomy experiments[93] and of parabiosis experiments wherein distinct strains of genetically obese animals are surgically joined to lean animals.[50] One molecule proposed to play such a role was insulin,[94] based on the fact that insulin levels in the periphery tend to reflect the extent of adiposity and the fact that injections of insulin into the central nervous system inhibit NPY expression and limit food intake.[95] In addition, insulin can be transported across the blood-brain barrier to sites where it may exert these effects.[96] However, it has not been possible to ascribe to peripheral insulin a role in the normal regulation of adiposity.

LEPTIN. The hypothesis that a peripheral factor reflective of total adipose mass could serve as a signal to the brain of energy stores received powerful support from the identification of a genetic locus responsible for obesity in ob/ob mice. The *ob* gene was identified by positional cloning[83] and was found to produce a novel mRNA encoding a fat-specific protein with characteristics of a secreted protein.[83] Obese ob/ob mice have two mutant alleles that harbor missense mutations that prevent synthesis of intact protein, suggesting that this molecule is the long-sought peripheral signal of adipose stores, total deficiency of which results in massive obesity with both hyperphagia and decreased energy expenditure. Indeed treatment of ob/ob mice with recombinant leptin by a peripheral route appears to correct all features of the disorder, including hyperphagia, decreased thermogenesis, and insulin resistance.[52, 53] The fact that much lower doses administered centrally have the same effects suggests that its predominant site of action is in the brain. Administration of the ob gene product, now termed *leptin*, from the Greek root *leptos* (thin), reduces NPY expression in the hypothalamus.[82] The fact that db/db mice are resistant to leptin is consistent with the idea proposed by Coleman and Hammel on the basis of parabiosis experiments[50] that these mice become obese because of an inherited inability to respond to the peripheral signal, now known to be leptin. Receptors for leptin have been identified through an expression cloning approach[97]; db/db mice have a mutation of this gene that deletes a critical domain of the receptor.[98]

When normal and obese animals are studied across a broad range of body fat contents in the fed state, circulating leptin levels correlate closely with body fat content.[99] In contrast, with food restriction leptin levels fall acutely (i.e., over hours) in rodents[99] and humans.[100] It thus appears that leptin levels in the fed state reflect adipose stores, whereas leptin levels respond acutely to changes in energy balance out of proportion to the state of energy stores. This is probably related to the fact that a central role of leptin in physiology is to signal a state of starvation to the brain.[101] The identity of the intracellular and extracellular factors that participate in the acute and chronic regulation of leptin expression is the subject of much study. Leptin expression is positively regulated by insulin[102] and by several cytokines[103] and is negatively regulated by agents such as β-adrenergic agonists that increase cellular cAMP.[104]

Regulation of Energy Expenditure

Because the tendency to gain or lose body fat is determined by the long-term balance between energy intake and expenditure, it is important to understand the factors that compose and regulate energy expenditure under normal conditions.

COMPONENTS OF ENERGY EXPENDITURE. In simple terms heat generation, or thermogenesis, can be divided into several categories (Fig. 22–6).[105] The basal metabolic rate is the energy produced by a subject resting in bed in the morn-

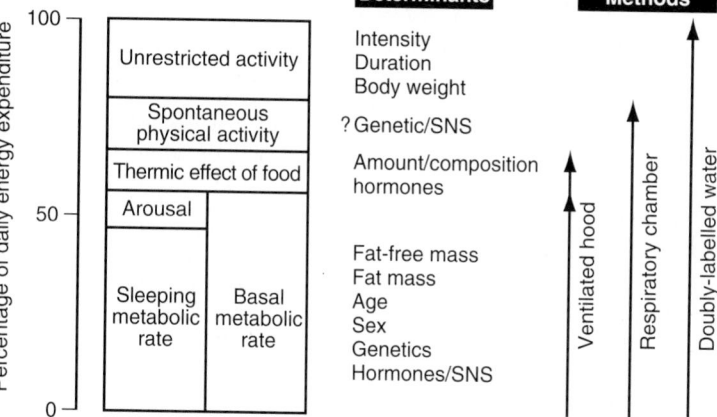

Figure 22–6. The determinants of energy expenditure. SNS, sympathetic nervous system. (Redrawn from Ravussin E, Swinburn BA. Pathophysiology of obesity. Lancet 1992; 340:404–408. Copyright 1992, The Lancet.)

ing in the fasting state and includes the cost of maintaining body systems and the homeothermic temperature at rest. The basal metabolic rate accounts for 50 to 70% of daily energy expenditure in most sedentary adults. The thermic effect of food or diet-induced thermogenesis is the increase in heat production in response to food ingestion. This represents the energy cost of digesting, absorbing, and storing nutrients and accounts for about 10% of daily energy expenditure. Physical activity is the most variable component of energy expenditure and is influenced by the amount and the energy cost of activity. A final category of thermogenesis is referred to as adaptive (or regulatory) thermogenesis. This thermogenesis functions to produce additional heat as opposed to work or energy storage and serves to protect the body temperature at times of environmental cold stress and to provide a buffer against obesity. In addition to shivering, which generates heat through muscle activity, rodents use a specialized BAT to produce heat by uncoupling the usually tight relationship between substrate oxidation and energy needs of the cell.[106] The role of BAT in adult humans is unclear.

CELLULAR BASIS FOR THERMOGENESIS. The energy released by the oxidation of substrates is for the most part captured in high-energy nucleotides, especially adenosine triphosphate (ATP) which are then used to drive thermodynamically unfavorable reactions in the body such as contraction of muscles and synthesis of fat. Even in the most efficient systems some energy is lost as heat, e.g., heat wastage is 30 to 50% in contracting skeletal muscles. For regulatory purposes, such as generating heat in the cold or minimizing weight gain from excess calories, several ATP-utilizing, heat-releasing reactions are not coupled to useful ends.[107]

Brown Fat. BAT is a specialized type of adipose tissue, the function of which is energy expenditure[106] rather than energy storage, which is the primary function of white adipose tissue. In rodents, BAT is present in the interscapular area and around the kidneys and large vessels. BAT is present in human infants but diminishes with age, and the amount of functional BAT in adult humans is uncertain. In rodents BAT is regulated mainly through input from the sympathetic nervous system, which increases BAT activity in response to environmental cold or increased food ingestion.[106] Sympathetic outflow to BAT, acting through β-adrenergic receptors that include the β₃ subtype found almost exclusively on white and brown adipose cells, causes marked changes in the structure and function of this tissue to promote heat generation.

The biochemical mechanism through which brown adipose cells generate heat involves a unique, BAT-specific protein named *thermogenin*,[108] a 32-kd protein that makes up 10 to 15% of the inner mitochondrial membrane in brown fat. Thermogenin, also known as uncoupling protein, is a proton

channel that has the capacity to dissipate proton gradients across the inner mitochondrial membrane. In coupled electron transport oxidation of NADH (the reduced form of NAD) is linked to ATP synthesis, and protons are pumped from the mitochondrial matrix across the inner mitochondrial membrane to the inner membrane space, which is in equilibrium with the cytoplasm by the action of electron-transporting respiratory enzymes. The protons then re-enter the matrix through a complex ATP synthase consisting of a transmembrane proton channel (Fo) and a larger matrix subunit of multiple chains (F1) that function as an ATPase when detached from the membrane. The energy of re-entrant protons provides the energy for ATP synthesis. Thermogenin effectively bypasses the proton-translocating ATP synthase by allowing proton entry through its own channel. This allows fatty acid oxidation to proceed in unimpeded (uncoupled) fashion with concomitant release of heat.

Heat generation in brown fat is regulated by both acute and adaptive mechanisms. The acute effects follow the generation of cAMP, resulting from occupancy of β-adrenergic receptors by norepinephrine released from sympathetic nerve terminals. The "unmasking" of pre-existing thermogenin, possibly by increased levels of free fatty acids in the cell, uncouples respiration.[109–111] More prolonged stimulation of BAT by sympathetic activity over hours to days stimulates increased transcription of thermogenin,[112] increases BAT blood flow, and causes an actual hyperplasia of BAT.[113]

The role of BAT in energy homeostasis in rodents has been clarified by studies of transgenic mice that were engineered to be BAT deficient through the expression of a BAT-specific toxigene.[114] These mice experience obesity, initially without hyperphagia, suggesting efficient metabolism,[114] but eventually they acquire more severe obesity and increased food intake, suggesting that BAT may play a role in regulation of food intake. Since these animals are hyperphagic despite high levels of circulating leptin,[115] BAT may influence the function of the hypothalamus in some as yet unclear way. The transgenic mice are also susceptible to the development of non–insulin-dependent diabetes mellitus (NIDDM) and extreme obesity when exposed to high-fat diets, suggesting that BAT plays a role as a physiological buffer against both obesity and diabetes mellitus.[116]

The function of BAT is impaired in several types of rodent obesity, including the Zucker obese rat, the ob/ob mouse, and mice with VMH lesions. This functional impairment in BAT is probably responsible for the defect in thermogenesis in these animals. The defect appears not to reside in BAT itself but is a consequence of reduced input to BAT from the sympathetic nervous system. In the ob/ob mouse this thermogenic defect may be corrected by treatment with leptin, possibly through the lowering of levels of hypothalamic NPY, which increases BAT activity.[117]

No direct information is available on the functional status of BAT in normal or obese humans. Studies of variants of the human β_3-adrenergic receptor gene raise the possibility that BAT function may exist in humans and that variants in that function might contribute to obesity and its complications.[118–120] The β_3-adrenergic receptor is a subtype of β-receptor initially identified as mediating BAT function and thermogenesis in rodents.[121, 122] These receptors are present on brown and white adipose cells and couple to cAMP generation. Specific agonists for β_3-receptors[123] stimulate lipolysis in white adipocytes and hyperfunction of brown adipocytes, including increased in vivo thermogenesis, and diminish obesity and diabetes mellitus in animals.[123–126] Mice with targeted deletion of the β_3-adrenergic receptor gene have mild obesity.[127] A β_3-adrenergic receptor variant is present in approximately 10% of both European and American populations, and in several studies the abnormal allele correlates with decreased energy expenditure,[118] early onset of diabetes mellitus,[118, 119] central adiposity,[119] insulin resistance, or a combination of these factors.[119] Whether these associations indicate defective function of BAT or white adipose tissue is unknown.

The possibility that mitochondrial uncoupling may occur outside of BAT has been raised by the discovery of another member of the uncoupling protein family. This "uncoupling protein 2" is found in many tissues, including skeletal muscle, and provides an additional mechanism for regulated thermogenesis in health and disease.[126a]

Other potential mechanisms for heat generation and inefficient metabolism include futile metabolic cycles. An example is the coupled reactions catalyzed by phosphofructokinase and fructose-bisphosphatase, which are key enzymes regulating reciprocal flow over glycolytic and gluconeogenic pathways in liver. Under normal circumstances these reactions do not operate simultaneously.[128] Should they do so, ATP would be broken down and release heat in the absence of a change of substrate levels, thus fulfilling the definition of a futile cycle. Substrate cycling with ATP breakdown has been directly demonstrated at this step in humans,[129] but whether diminished energy dissipation via such mechanisms contributes to obesity is unknown. A second possible site for inefficient metabolism is the plasma membrane Na^+,K^+-ATPase responsible for extrusion of intracellular sodium against a concentration gradient at the expense of ATP. Two observations focused attention on this ATPase. First, it was suggested that the thermogenic effects of thyroid hormone in rodents were in large part mediated by induced activity of this enzyme.[130] Second, activity of this enzyme is diminished in livers of mice with genetic obesity.[131] Subsequently some[132–134] but not all[135, 136] authors reported reduced expression or activity of Na^+,K^+-ATPase in erythrocytes of obese humans. Results in different populations have been variable, and the role of this enzyme in the etiology of human obesity remains uncertain. A genetic linkage of obesity to the locus encoding the Na^+,K^+-ATPase has been reported.[137]

Adipose Tissue and the Adipose Cell

Adipocytes are highly differentiated cells that have three major roles: storage of excess metabolic energy in the form of triglyceride; release of energy from triglyceride stores under neural, endocrine, and metabolic control; and signaling to local and distant sites through the release of specific transmitter molecules. The role of the adipocyte in regard to storage and release of energy is well known, whereas the role of the adipocyte as an endocrine organ has been more recently identified.[138] To accommodate lipid storage, adipocytes are capable of changing their diameters 20-fold and changing their volumes by several 1000–fold. A normal individual has

between 10 and 20 kg of body fat, representing storage of 90,000 to 180,000 calories in the subcutaneous and intraperitoneal depots. Obesity may be associated with 40 to 100 kg of body fat or more.

CELL BIOLOGY OF THE ADIPOCYTE. Histologic studies and studies of adipocyte development in tissue culture indicate that adipocytes derive from precursor cells or adipoblasts that are visibly indistinguishable from fibroblasts.[139] Adipocytes are distinguished by the specific array of genes and the encoded proteins they express.[140, 141] By identifying adipose-specific genes such as the fatty acid binding protein aP-2 it has been possible to dissect the molecular events that underlie adipose differentiation. Specific DNA sequences in the promoter regions of adipocyte-specific genes are capable of driving their expression.[142] Nuclear proteins act through such DNA elements to cause fat cells to express the correct array of specific genes. One such factor is CEBPα, which, although not specific for adipocytes, drives the expression of many fat-specific genes.[143] Targeted deletion of this gene in mice produces animals devoid of adipose tissue.[144] Another key factor is the PPARγ transcription factor, which is relatively fat specific and is capable of causing undifferentiated fibroblasts to differentiate into adipocytes in culture.[145] The PPARγ transcription factor acts in synchrony with other factors and can be activated by binding to an intracellular member of the prostaglandin family.[146] PPARγ is also activated by the antidiabetic thiazolidinedione class of drugs.[147]

DEVELOPMENT OF ADIPOSE TISSUE. Adipose tissue grows through an increase in both size and number of cells. Adipocytes first appear at the 15th week of gestation, continue to develop until 23 weeks of gestation, and then accumulate more slowly during the remainder of gestation. Both adipose cell number and size increase during the first 2 y of life. Adipose mass is then relatively stable until a substantial increase occurs at puberty through an increase in cell number. In individuals who remain lean, cell size and number remain stable throughout adult life.

Studies of adipocyte size and number in individuals with obesity of varying severity and age of onset led to the concepts of hyperplastic vs. hypertrophic obesity[148]; in the former the number and size of adipocytes is increased, and in the latter only cell size is increased. The general concept has been that early-onset obesity is hyperplastic, whereas adult-onset obesity is hypertrophic.[41, 149] It has also been suggested that adipocyte number does not decline with weight loss[149] and that this might predispose the individual to regaining weight, although a mechanism for this idea has not been advanced. Adult-onset obesity, if massive, is also associated with increased adipocyte cell number.[148] Preadipocytes from obese individuals are said to replicate more rapidly in culture than do similar cells from lean controls.[150]

ADIPOCYTE SECRETED PRODUCTS. Adipocytes release the products of lipolysis, glycerol, and free fatty acids to serve as substrates and fuels in other tissues, although free fatty acids can also play a role in the regulation of metabolism through various effects that include influencing the expression of several genes.[151] Adipocytes also release other molecules, including some peptides not previously known to be expressed in fat cells. This list includes complement factors, cytokines, hormone precursors, and other regulators, but the physiological role of their expression in adipocytes has not been defined. The protein product of the *ob* gene leptin was discussed earlier. This peptide is apparently the afferent limb of a feedback loop from adipose mass to the central nervous system, the purpose of which is to regulate energy balance in the long term and to signal the central nervous system whether energy stores are sufficient.[101] Adipocytes produce and secrete the alternative complement factor D, also known as adipsin, and expression of this protein is reduced in adipocytes of several forms of rodent obesity[152] but not in human obesity.[153] The function of adipsin is not known. Adipocytes also synthesize and secrete tumor necrosis factor α (TNF α), the expression level of which is increased in enlarged adipocytes from obese animals and men.[154] As discussed later, the overproduction of TNF has been implicated in promoting the insulin resistance of obesity.[155] Adipocytes also produce angiotensinogen whose expression is increased in obesity and decreased with starvation.[156] A possible connection to the alterations in blood flow in fat with nutritional perturbations has been hypothesized.

Adipocytes also secrete lipoprotein lipase, the enzyme responsible for hydrolyzing triglycerides in chylomicrons and circulating very-low-density lipoproteins (VLDLs) to free fatty acids for uptake into adipocytes.[157] The level of adipose tissue lipoprotein lipase activity is greater in obese individuals than in lean ones[158] and this activity does not diminish, and may actually increase after weight reduction in obese subjects.[159-161] It has therefore been hypothesized that these changes might predispose an individual to weight gain by enhancing the filling of adipocytes. If increased adipose tissue lipoprotein lipase precedes obesity and promotes adipose cell lipid storage, it is necessary to determine whether and by what mechanism this expression could lead to chronic alterations of energy balance productive of obesity.

REGIONAL HETEROGENEITY OF ADIPOSE CELLS. Adipocytes in different anatomic regions display biochemical and functional differences. Subcutaneous adipocytes from the thigh are smaller than adipocytes obtained simultaneously from abdominal subcutaneous tissue and are less responsive to epinephrine-induced lipolysis.[162] Triglyceride turnover and catecholamine-induced lipolysis are higher in intra-abdominal and abdominal subcutaneous sites than in subcutaneous fat from other regions,[162-164] possibly because of a preponderance of stimulatory β-receptors over inhibitory α_2-receptors.[165] The state of insulin-mediated antilipolysis in adipocytes from different regions is less clear, but the antilipolytic effect of insulin may be reduced in intra-abdominal cells as a result of both receptor and postreceptor effects.[164] Studies of the differentiation of preadipocytes derived from different anatomic regions to adipocytes in culture suggest that some of the regional differences may be inherent to the cells from different regions.[166] The fact that intra-abdominal and abdominal subcutaneous adipocytes have greater lipid turnover and therefore are more lipolytically active may explain the fact that fat accumulation in these sites is tightly linked to the metabolic complications of obesity, such as insulin resistance, NIDDM, and hypertension,[13] since free fatty acids are important mediators of insulin resistance. It has not been demonstrated that individuals with ordinary obesity have an altered balance between catecholamine-induced lipolysis and insulin-induced antilipolysis that might promote energy storage in fat.[167]

What Causes Obesity?

OVERVIEW. The pathophysiology of obesity is in one sense clear: energy intake is chronically greater than energy expenditure. What causes this disturbance in energy balance is less clear. In theory the imbalance could be due to an increase in energy intake, a decrease in energy expenditure, or a combination of the two. The definition of the state of energy intake and expenditure in obesity has been difficult for two major reasons. First, accurate measurement of energy intake and expenditure is difficult in free-living humans. Second, the two parameters are functionally linked so that chronic increases in nutrient intake cause increased energy expenditure and vice versa.[168] Obese animals are somewhat more tractable, and important work has made use of rodents with single-gene defects that impair both energy intake and

expenditure.[169] The fact that weight in most individuals is relatively stable over the long term and the fact that single-gene defects can impair energy intake and expenditure suggest the existence in both animals and humans of a physiological system for the long-term regulation of energy balance.[48] Identification of the *ob* gene, discussed earlier, is a major advance.[83] Its product, the circulating protein termed *leptin*, is capable of regulating both food intake and energy expenditure in rodents primarily through actions in the brain.[52, 53]

Although leptin is a useful tool for understanding the operation of this system, body weight is affected by many additional factors. For example, one reason that individuals overeat is because food tastes good and is readily available. The higher fat content of Western diets is also important. No study has failed to show greater energy expenditure in established obesity than in the lean; thus, absolute levels of food intake are always greater in obese than in lean subjects. Animal studies clearly show that obesity can be produced simply by exposure to unlimited amounts of a tasty diet, although different strains differ in their susceptibility.[170] Other factors undoubtedly play a role. Strong genetic influences are evident, and these have so far been demonstrated primarily in energy expenditure.[171] If metabolic efficiency in the population represents a bell-shaped curve, persons generating the least amount of heat under basal conditions or after eating, exercise, or exposure to cold may be more vulnerable to the threat of attractive or inexpensive food than those who are less efficiently coupled. Indeed, a low relative resting metabolic rate over 24 h (i.e., low for body size and composition) is a risk factor for subsequent weight gain.[172] It is likely, however, that there is not a single-gene defect leading to metabolic efficiency in most individuals but simply movement down a normal distribution curve created through the impact of several genes. Although disturbances in body image, differences in perinatally determined fat cell number, and diminished exercise may play a role, these effects have been difficult to prove. A diminished response to a satiety signal or signals would appear to be reasonable and is supported by studies of the effects of leptin. A major problem is separating primary and secondary events. For example, physical activity always decreases with massive obesity, but this does not imply its presence during the genesis of obesity. What can be said with certainty is that obesity involves a dysregulation of the long-term system for maintenance of normal energy balance, and excess weight, once established, essentially always involves excessive levels of food intake.[171]

LEVEL OF ENERGY INTAKE IN OBESE INDIVIDUALS. Obese individuals commonly believe that they ingest fewer calories than many lean individuals. Accurate quantitation of food intake over time in free-living individuals is difficult to obtain, and investigators of energy intake based on food recall information and body weight have often come to the conclusion that the relationship between these two parameters is inverse,[173] supporting the belief of many obese individuals that they have a primary defect in efficiency of metabolism. Conversely, measurements of energy expenditure reveal a positive relationship between this parameter and body weight (Fig. 22–7).[171] Since at stable body weight, energy intake equals energy expenditure, energy intake must also be increased, not decreased, in comparison to lean individuals. How can these findings be reconciled? It appears that obese individuals are more likely than lean individuals to underreport their food intake. In studies of free-living individuals in which energy expenditure is measured with double-labeled water and energy intake is estimated by food diaries, it was found that the obese underreported food intake by 34 to 54%, whereas lean subjects underreported by 0 to 20%.[174-176] The psychological or biochemical basis for what appears to be an inability to

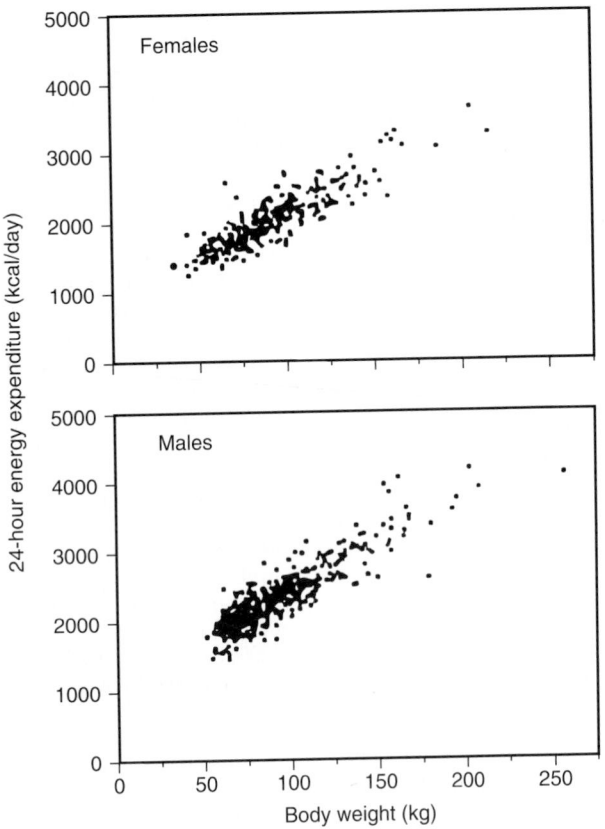

Figure 22–7. Relation between 24-h energy expenditure and body weight in 297 females and 402 males after at least 3 d on a weight-maintaining diet, as measured in a respiratory chamber. (Redrawn from Ravussin E, Swinburn BA. Pathophysiology of obesity. Lancet 1992; 340:404–408. Copyright 1992, The Lancet.)

perceive the level of energy intake in obese individuals is unknown and is an important subject for further study.

As indicated earlier, caloric intake in most individuals with obesity at steady weight exceeds that of their lean counterparts. Thus by either absolute or relative criteria, increased food intake is a feature of most cases of human obesity. The basis for this dysregulation of food intake is not yet defined and is likely to be complex. The dysregulation of food intake in obesity has been explored from the perspectives of psychology, sociology, neurobiology, and endocrinology. Ultimately the insights obtained from each of these disciplines have to be combined to provide a coherent picture of this disorder.

Food intake is regulated by both external and internal signals. The former refers to things such as the availability and attractiveness of food; the latter reflects the physiological indicators of hunger and satiety. The two types of signals are not independent because metabolic events may alter emotional responses, and emotional factors may trigger or modulate physiological control of food intake.[177]

One theory regarding eating in obesity suggests that the sequence begins with overfeeding in infancy so that the infant learns to eat nonphysiologically; i.e., because the mother supplies breast or bottle in response to crying or irritation, even if it is not the normal feeding time, a learning disorder is induced in which emotions such as anger or tension are interpreted as hunger.[178] This might lead to a tendency to eat primarily in response to external signals, especially the availability of food. Both of these interpretations have been questioned. For example, obese mothers, who tend to have obese children,[1] underfeed their infants in comparison to nonobese controls.[179] Similarly although considerable evidence suggests that obese subjects respond preferentially to external cues for eating, significant overlap exists between obese and lean subjects, rendering the externality theory nondecisive.[180] It is possible, however, that a greater percentage of obese individuals than lean ones are influenced strongly by external cues.

Cultural factors may also contribute to the trend toward fatness in the United States and other developed countries. When both parents work there is increasing dependence on fast-food meals obtained outside the home and on microwave preparations with short cooking times.[181] Such foods tend to be high in fat. Adiposity in humans and animals correlates positively with fat content of the diet,[182] although different inbred strains of mice have differing susceptibilities to this effect.[170] Whether the effect of fat content is due to the higher caloric density of fat relative to carbohydrate and protein or the consequence of regulatory effects of differing fat/carbohydrate ratios[183] is not clear.

Until recently, investigation of the peripheral and central factors (such as gut peptides, neuropeptides, and neurotransmitters) that are capable of influencing food intake and energy balance, had not led to major insight into the dysregulated food intake of human obesity. For example, no difference in the expression or action of molecules such as CCK or NPY has been demonstrated in obese vs. lean individuals. The discovery of leptin provided a new mechanism for evaluation of molecular dysfunction in obesity. In the ob/ob mouse total deficiency of this protein caused by missense mutation in the *ob* gene causes a syndrome of severe obesity accompanied by hyperphagia, decreased energy expenditure, and insulin resistance.[184] In contrast, many other forms of obesity in mice—including those associated with the *db* gene,[38] chemical[185] or mechanical[38] disruption of the hypothalamus, brown fat deficiency,[185] and high-fat diet[115]—are associated with increased expression of leptin mRNA or circulating leptin protein, or both,[38, 185] which in the context of obesity and hyperphagia suggests a state of "leptin resistance." Understanding the molecular basis of leptin resistance will require information on its state of transport in association with binding proteins in the blood,[186] its method for gaining access to sites of action in the central nervous system,[187] the method of signaling through the leptin receptor,[188] and the identity of the molecular targets that it regulates.

Mutations in the coding sequence of the leptin[189] and leptin receptor[190] mRNAs have been sought in a limited group of individuals with morbid obesity, and no defects have been found, indicating that morbid obesity in humans is not equivalent to obesity in ob/ob or db/db mice. Virtually all obese humans have increased levels of immunoreactive leptin in the circulation, and these levels correlate positively with their degree of adiposity (Fig. 22–8).[191] With chronic weight loss levels decline.[191] Thus as in rodents[99] leptin levels in the circulation generally reflect the size of adipose stores. Since such obese individuals nearly always exhibit hyperphagia while obese, it may be concluded that physiological resistance to leptin exists in most obese individuals or that the physiological role of leptin in humans differs from that in the rodent, where leptin limits food intake and increases energy expenditure.[52, 53] The ability of leptin to gain access to sites of action in the central nervous system may be reduced in obesity as suggested by the fact that leptin levels in the cerebrospinal fluid are not proportional to the increased serum levels in obesity.[192] In addition, despite the robust correlations between body fat and leptin levels mentioned previously, different individuals with the same BMI may have different leptin levels.[191] It is important to determine whether individuals with similar degrees of obesity but varying leptin levels are physiologically or clinically distinguishable.

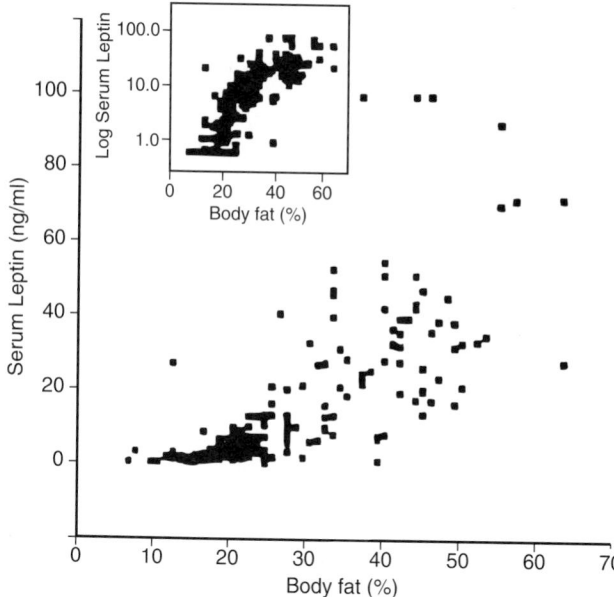

Figure 22–8. The relation between the percentage of body fat and the serum leptin concentration in 136 normal-weight and 139 obese subjects. The inset shows the natural log of the serum leptin concentration plotted against the percentage of body fat. (Redrawn from Considine RV, Sinha M, Heiman M, et al. Serum immunoreactive leptin concentrations in normal weight and obese humans. N Engl J Med 1995; 334:292–295, with permission.)

STATE OF ENERGY EXPENDITURE IN HUMAN OBESITY.

Obese patients frequently believe that they gain weight on amounts of food that do not cause obesity in other persons, implying a more efficient use of calories in obese than in lean individuals. This issue has been studied by measurements of metabolic rate using (1) indirect calorimetry in which oxygen uptake and carbon dioxide production are monitored over short intervals; (2) direct calorimetry, in which heat production is directly measured[193]; and (3) the double labeled water technique, which allows estimates of energy expenditure under free-living conditions.[194, 195] All these techniques indicate that in absolute terms obese individuals expend more energy than do lean individuals so that obesity cannot be attributed to a low absolute metabolic rate.[196] The dominant reason for the positive correlation between body weight and energy expenditure is the fact that obesity is also associated with an increase in lean body mass,[7] which accounts for approximately 81% of the variance among individuals.[197] Indeed obese individuals may have increased resting energy expenditure even when corrected for a given amount of fat-free mass.[198]

The possibility of differences in postprandial thermogenesis between obese and normal subjects is unsettled. In more than 40 studies examining the thermic effect of various foods about 60% found a reduced thermic effect of food, and the remainder found no difference.[171] If present, any differences may be secondary to obesity rather than primary,[199] and the small differences in postprandial energy expenditure are not likely to be important in the pathogenesis of obesity.[200] Could differences in the amount of or energy cost of physical activity play a role in the pathogenesis of obesity? The increased prevalence of obesity parallels the increase in sedentary lifestyles, and studies of Pima Indians using respiratory chambers and double-labeled water suggest that physical activity is inversely related to both age and adiposity.[201] Conversely, exercise-induced thermogenesis is not impaired in established obesity,[200, 202] doubtless because more energy is required to move an increased body mass.

IMPACT OF CHANGES IN BODY WEIGHT ON ENERGY

EXPENDITURE. Although measurements of energy expenditure in lean vs. obese individuals show that established obesity is associated with increased energy expenditure and therefore, by necessity, increased absolute levels of food intake, chronic changes in the level of food intake can have effects on the level of energy expenditure, and these effects exert an influence on the ability to regulate body weight. When an individual chronically increases caloric intake, the increase in energy balance causes both obesity and increased lean body mass. The increase in body weight, in particular the increased amount of lean body mass, increases 24-h energy expenditure. This increased energy expenditure changes the energy balance equation to resist subsequent weight gain. Instead of a continuous increase in body energy stores (and body weight), body weight tends to come into balance despite continued higher energy intake at a slightly higher level of energy intake, energy expenditure, and energy stores.

The effect of differences in the amount of lean body mass (typically reflecting changes in body fat) on the energy balance equation and the susceptibility to weight gain or loss on a given caloric intake is well established. Careful studies of energy metabolism have been carried out in lean and obese individuals at their initial weights and after stable increases or decreases of 10% of body weight,[198] and maintenance of reduced or elevated body weight is associated with compensatory changes in energy expenditure that oppose the maintenance of the altered body weight (Fig. 22–9).[198] Thus a 10% loss in body weight caused a 15% decrease in total daily energy expenditure, which was due to both a fall in fat-free mass and a fall in energy expenditure per fat-free mass.[198] Likewise a 10% weight gain caused a 16% increase in total energy expenditure, due to both increased lean body mass and increased energy expenditure per unit of lean body mass.[198] The cellular and biochemical basis for the changes in energy expenditure in lean body mass that follow alterations in body weight is not yet defined. Given the fact that levels of the fat-derived hormone leptin fall with weight loss[191] and rise with overfeeding[115] in both rodents and humans,[100] a role for this hormone in the changes in energy expenditure is possible. Other mechanisms for changes might increase modification of sympathetic nervous system activity or the function of BAT, or both. The possible contribution of changes in levels of thyroid hormone has received little attention, but formerly obese individuals at stable reduced weight are said to have reduced levels of free triiodothyronine (T_3).[203]

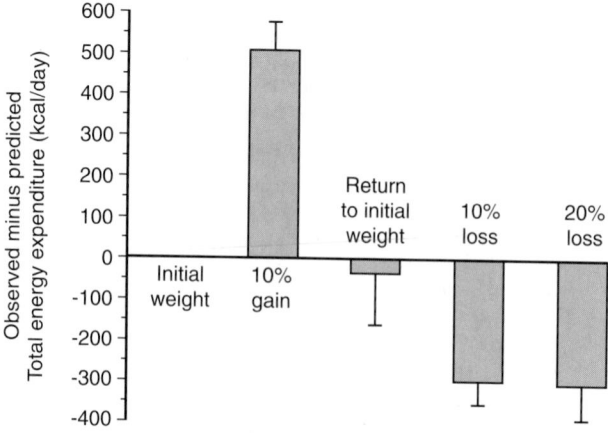

Figure 22–9. Observed minus predicted total energy expenditure in individuals after 10% weight gain, 10 or 20% weight loss, or return to previous weight after weight gain, all compared with values in same subjects at their initial weights. (Redrawn from Leibel R, Rosenbaum M, Hirsch J. Changes in energy expenditure resulting from altered body weight. N Engl J Med 1995; 332:621–628. Copyright 1995, Massachusetts Medical Society.)

Whatever the mechanism, changes in energy expenditure accompanying diet-induced weight changes have important implications for the management of obesity. In an individual who ingests 2500 kcal at weight stability, a 15% fall in energy expenditure caused by a 10% fall in body weight would produce an initial positive energy balance of 375 kcal/d at the new lower weight if caloric intake was not reduced. Furthermore, if the decrease in leptin level brought about by weight loss caused an increase in hunger, such an unfavorable development would tend to promote regaining of the lost weight. In addition, examination of data on energy expenditure of lean and obese individuals at original (natural) body weight and after stable weight loss is revealing. The mean energy expenditure in nonobese individuals at initial weight was 2481 kcal/d or 47 kcal/kg fat-free mass.[198] The mean value for obese individuals was 3162 kcal/d or 51 kcal/kg fat-free mass. Importantly when food was restricted in the obese group to the point at which they were 20% less than initial weight but were still markedly obese (obese, 95 kg; controls, 66 kg), their energy expenditure was 2243 kcal/d or 39 kcal/kg fat-free mass, both values less than the mean values for lean individuals at normal weight. These data suggest that after substantial weight loss but persistent obesity many obese individuals might gain weight, or at least fail to lose weight, on levels of energy intake that support normal weight in lean individuals.

GENETICS OF OBESITY. A substantial number of monogenic disorders cause severe obesity in rodents (Table 22–3), implying that specific genes and their encoded proteins play critical roles in the regulation of body weight. The genes responsible for the obesity of ob/ob and db/db mice were discussed earlier. The syndrome in these two disorders is similar when expressed on the same genetic background and includes early-onset severe obesity, hyperphagia, decreased thermogenesis, and severe insulin resistance with diabetes mellitus. In addition both ob/ob and db/db mice have defects in hypothalamic function, including hypothalamic amenorrhea and increased activity of the hypothalamic-pituitary-adrenal axis. All these defects are reversed by treatment with recombinant leptin in totally leptin-deficient ob/ob mice, but no effect is seen in leptin-resistant db/db mice.[98] Zucker fa/fa rats also have a mutation in the leptin receptor gene that impairs but does not disrupt leptin signal transduction.[204]

Two other monogenic syndromes of rodent obesity are due to mutations at the tub and agouti loci. The tub locus encodes a protein of unknown function that is expressed in the hypothalamus, and disruption of this gene causes an autosomal recessive obesity of later onset, retinal degeneration, and neurosensory hearing loss.[205] The Ay mouse has autosomal dominant obesity due to ectopic expression of the agouti protein, which is normally expressed solely in skin during hair growth.[206] The mechanism by which widespread ectopic expression of this protein causes obesity is uncertain.[207] The fat locus is associated with an autosomal recessive syndrome of obesity due to mutation of the gene encoding carboxypeptidase E.[208] As a result of this mutation a number of hormones and neurotransmitters are not processed normally, but the mechanism by which this defect produces obesity is unknown. These mice have high levels of an incompletely processed and biologically less active form of insulin in the circulation as a consequence of the mutation.

Although genetic forms of obesity occur in humans, they are so far associated with specific phenotypes that led to their identification. The genes responsible for the Prader-Willi, Alström, Bardet-Biedl, and Cohen syndromes have been mapped but not yet identified and do not appear to be the human equivalents of any of the identified mouse obesity genes. The Prader-Willi syndrome is characterized by infantile hypotonia, early childhood obesity, mental deficiency, short stature, small hands and feet, and hypogonadism.[209] In 70% of patients there is a deletion of variable length on chromosome 15 at 15q11-q13.[210] The Alström syndrome is manifested by childhood blindness related to retinal degeneration, infantile obesity (which may disappear in adulthood), nerve deafness, diabetes mellitus with insulin resistance, acanthosis nigricans, chronic nephropathy, and hypogonadism in males but not females.[211] The testicular failure appears to be primary because the testes are small, testosterone levels in plasma are low, and gonadotropin levels are high. Patients with the Bardet-Biedl syndrome exhibit retinitis pigmentosa, mental retardation, obesity, polydactyly, and hypogonadism.[211] The last is associated with low gonadotropin levels in contrast to the Alström syndrome. Diabetes mellitus, deafness, and renal disease may occur. The Carpenter syndrome is characterized by obesity, mental retardation, male hypogonadism, acrocephaly, polydactyly, and syndactyly. Patients with the Cohen syndrome have microcephaly, severe mental retardation, short stature, facial abnormalities, and modest obesity.[212] Blount disease consists of bowed legs, tibial torsion, and obesity.[213] Although obesity is common, it may not be intrinsic to the disorder.

Ordinary obesity is not inherited by simple mendelian patterns, but obese children tend to have obese parents. In four studies covering 2002 children, one or both parents were obese 72% of the time.[214] Mothers appeared to be more obese on average than fathers. First-degree relatives of individuals with childhood-onset obesity were twice as likely to be obese as were relatives of those with adult-onset obesity.[215] However, clustering of obesity in families does not distinguish between genetic and shared environmental influences. The best evidence for genetic influence comes from studies of adoptees in Denmark[216] and twins who were reared apart in Sweden.[217] The BMI of adoptees is more closely related to their biologic parents than to their adopted parents (Fig. 22–10).[216] Monozygotic twins resemble each other more than do dizygotic twins whether they are reared together or apart.[214, 217] In 93 pairs of

TABLE 22–3. Monogenic Rodent Obesities

Gene	Chromosome-Inheritance	Site of Production	Gene Product	Action
ob	6/AR	White adipose tissue (WAT)	Leptin	Food intake Energy expenditure Neuroendocrine effect
db	4/AR	Hypothalamus and elsewhere (choroid plexus, lung, kidney)	Leptin receptor	Mediates leptin signal
tub	7/AR	Hypothalamus	Protein of unknown function	?
fat	8/AR	Endocrine, neuroendocrine tissues (beta cells, hypothalamus)	Carboxypeptidase E	Prohormone processing
Ay	2/AD	Ubiquitous (skin in wild-type)	Agouti protein	Melanocortin antagonist

AR, autosomal recessive; AD, autosomal dominant.

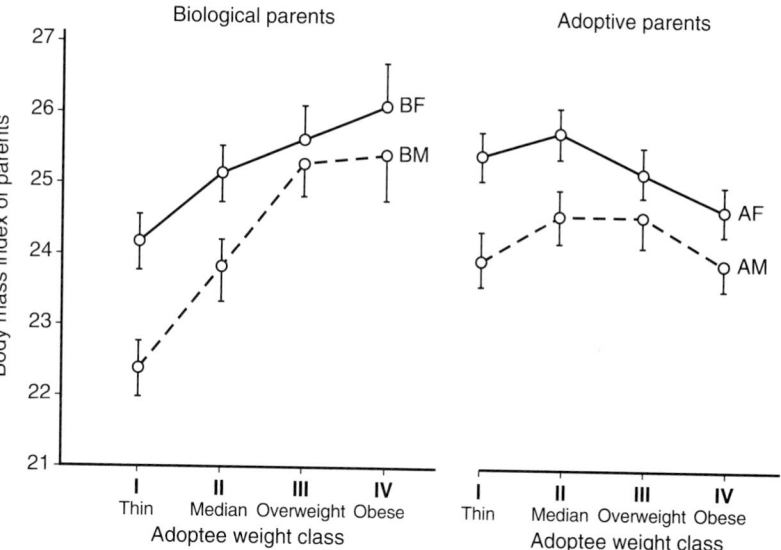

Figure 22–10. Mean body mass index (BMI) (+/− SEM) of biologic fathers (BF), biologic mothers (BM), adoptive fathers (AF), and adoptive mothers (AM) as a function of the weight class (class I = thin with BMI in lowest 25%; class II = medium with BMI in the 26th through 91st percentile; class III = overweight with BMI in the 92nd to 96th percentile; class IV = obese with BMI above the 96th percentile). (Redrawn from Stunkard AJ, Sorensen TI, Hanis C, et al. An adoption study of human obesity. N Engl J Med 1986; 314[4]:193–198. Copyright 1986, Massachusetts Medical Society. All rights reserved.)

identical twins reared apart the intrapair correlation for BMI was 0.70 for men and 0.66 for women. It is also possible that inheritance of fat in different regions may be different. Genetic contribution to subcutaneous fat is reported to be low, whereas genes may contribute 30% of the variance in the level of visceral fat.[218, 219]

A genetic predisposition to obesity could result from inheritance of high metabolic efficiency, a tendency to hyperphagia, or defects in both parameters. The level of the resting metabolic rate appears to have an important genetic component (Fig. 22–11).[220, 221] After adjustment of the metabolic rate for fat-free mass, age, and gender, 40% of the remaining variance may be explained by genetic factors.[221] When monozygotic twins are overfed, weight gain is closer within pairs than among pairs.[222] Although the level of food intake tracks with families as well, the role of environmental vs. genetic factors in bringing this about is uncertain.[223]

It is likely that most cases of obesity are due to interactions between multiple genes and the environment. So far the evaluation of possible candidate genes for obesity has been limited. The coding regions of leptin[189] and the leptin receptor[190] have been evaluated in persons with morbid obesity, and no mutations or variations have been found. Linkages to the leptin locus have been reported in some populations, possibly resulting from variations in the promoter sequence of the gene or differences in other linked genes.[224] A polymorphic variant in the gene encoding the β_3-adrenergic receptor is a common variant in several ethnic groups. The variant sequence changes a single amino acid in the first intracellular loop of this receptor, and this variant has been reported to be associated with slight lowering of metabolic rate in Pima Indians,[118] an earlier age at onset of diabetes mellitus in obese Pima Indians and Finns,[118, 119] and central obesity with insulin resistance in Finns.[119] Because this variant allele may be present in more than 10% of the population, its possible association with obesity and obesity-related complications is important, but additional work is needed to confirm and extend this finding, especially given the fact that association with obesity is not observed in several other large cohorts.[225] It will be important to evaluate other genes involved in energy homeostasis as they emerge, including genes encoding regulators of energy balance and adipocyte function.

Some types of obesity may result from genetic variation that at one point provided a favorable adaptation to chronically limited food supplies. Thus the ability to survive famine would be greater in individuals with efficient energy storage. However, the same trait that would promote survival in the context of famine might promote obesity in the presence of abundant food supplies and a limited necessity for physical exertion.

ENVIRONMENTAL INFLUENCES. Even individuals predisposed to obesity by genetic endowment do not become obese in the face of severely limited food supplies. The influence of exercise was discussed previously. Cultural factors also influ-

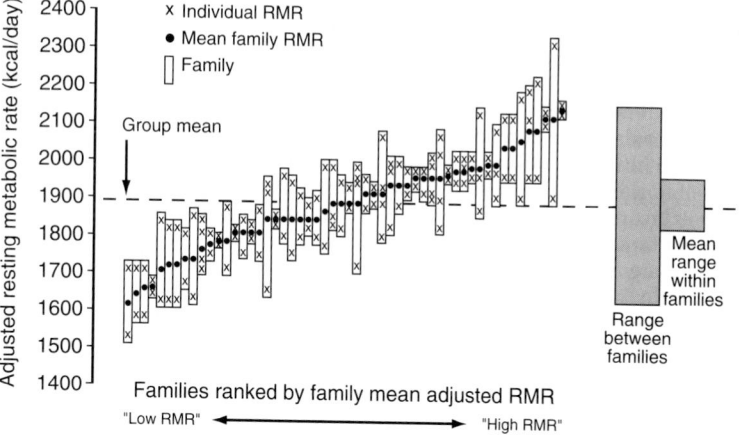

Figure 22–11. Mean family and individual resting metabolic rates (RMR) in Pima Indians adjusted for the covariances of fat free mass, age, and sex. (Redrawn from Bogardus C, Lillioja S, Ravussin E. Genetic effect in resting metabolic rate. N Engl J Med 1986; 315:96–99, with permission.)

Obesity imposes circulatory changes because of the necessity to perfuse the increased mass of tissue (lean and fat). Pulmonary and systemic blood volumes are increased and stroke volume and cardiac output are high.[282] The increased workload on the heart leads to dilatation and hypertrophy, particularly if systemic resistance is elevated by hypertension. Simultaneously myocardial oxygen demand is increased. These circulatory adjustments predispose the individual to congestive heart failure and, if coronary atherosclerosis is present, may lead to infarction and death as oxygen demand exceeds supply. Weight reduction decreases ventricular mass.[283]

HYPERTENSION. Obesity is associated with hypertension,[15, 17, 239, 274] which improves or reverses with weight reduction.[274, 284] Obesity appears to exert this adverse effect on blood pressure even in students of high school age.[285] The cause is uncertain. Increased plasma volume and increased peripheral resistance appear to be coupled to a high cardiac output.[286] Obese persons also have increased basal and stimulated levels of norepinephrine.[287] This increase could conceivably play an important role in raising peripheral resistance. Norepinephrine values,[287] plasma renin levels, and aldosterone levels decline with weight loss.[284, 287]

The mechanisms by which these changes occur remain obscure. Enhanced sympathetic nervous system activity appears to be mediated by diet, with carbohydrate playing the major stimulatory role,[288, 289] and sensitivity to salt may also be a problem in the hypertension of obesity.[290] Considerable attention has been paid to the possibility that insulin resistance causes the development of hypertension in obesity[291, 292] and in nonobese persons as well.[293] Insulin increases sodium absorption in the proximal and distal tubules[294] and increases the activity of the sympathetic nervous system.[288] Although possible, a causal role for insulin resistance in the hypertension of obesity is unproved.

PULMONARY DYSFUNCTION. Abnormalities in pulmonary function in obesity range from quantitative abnormalities in pulmonary function tests with no clinical significance to major dysfunction with symptomatic and morbid consequences. Pulmonary dysfunction is common in severe obesity, especially in the supine position.[282, 286, 295] Chest wall mechanics are altered, with reduced respiratory compliance and impaired respiratory muscle function due to deposition of subcutaneous fat and increased work of breathing. Obese patients tend to take rapid, shallow breaths. Functional residual capacity and expiratory reserve volume of the lung are low. Maximal expiratory flow rates are low in obese men (but not in women), even if they have never smoked.[296] Ventilation takes place predominantly in the upper lobes, whereas perfusion occurs primarily in the lower segments, resulting in a ventilation-perfusion mismatch and hypoxemia.[296] Seriously overweight patients are also at risk for hypoventilation, the presence of which is defined by an elevated PCO_2. Hypoxemia alone may occur in simple obesity, but the combination of hypoxemia and carbon dioxide retention together justify the diagnosis of obesity-hypoventilation (pickwickian) syndrome. The cause of the hypoventilation appears to be a diminished ventilatory response to both hypoxia and hypercapnia, although mechanical factors and respiratory muscle weakness doubtless also play a role. Sleep apnea is common in obese patients with alveolar hypoventilation. What is not clear is whether the prevalence is more common in obese individuals than in a normal-weight population.[296] However, sleep apnea in obesity has more severe consequences because of the coexisting pulmonary dysfunction. Apnea in this syndrome may be central (no respiratory movements), obstructive (no airflow despite respiratory movements), or mixed (initial absence of respiratory muscle activity followed by ineffective activity). The obstructive form is probably more common in obesity and

may require tracheostomy.[297] Sleep studies are required to differentiate central from obstructive apnea. In obese patients with obstructive sleep apnea, the first line treatment is weight loss. The patient should sleep in the lateral position and should avoid sedatives and ethanol. Sleep apnea can improve with relatively small amounts (i.e., 10 to 20 kg) of weight loss.[298] Central apnea may respond to medroxyprogesterone therapy,[299] and even if obstructive apnea is present a trial of medroxyprogesterone may be indicated because an element of primary hypoventilation may coexist with predominant obstruction. Continuous positive airway pressure is frequently effective. Surgical procedures that have been tried with claims of success include tracheostomy,[300] uvulopalatopharyngoplasty, and, in patients with morbid obesity, gastric restriction or bypass surgery.[301]

Pulmonary hypertension, polycythemia, and cor pulmonale may result from combined respiratory dysfunction. Morbidly obese persons with compromised pulmonary function are at risk during anesthesia and may die suddenly (presumably from arrhythmias) during surgery or in the immediate postoperative period.[282]

GALLSTONES. Gallstones are more common in obese than in normal individuals,[17] with persons 50% above ideal body weight having a sixfold increase in the incidence of symptomatic cholelithiasis.[302] The reason for gallstone formation is that the bile of obese individuals is supersaturated because of enhanced biliary secretion of cholesterol.[297] Saturability further increases in the fasting state because the concentration of solubilizing phospholipids falls while cholesterol output remains high. Low-calorie diets, in contrast, do not produce this change. From the standpoint of cholelithiasis, fasting, especially prolonged fasting, is not an optimal therapeutic regimen.

ENDOCRINE ABNORMALITIES. A number of endocrine changes accompany the obese state, but most are secondary because they can be induced by overfeeding previously normal persons and reversed by weight loss.[303, 304] The obesity-associated changes in endocrine function are summarized in Table 22–3.[305]

Endocrine Pancreas. The fact that obesity is associated with insulin resistance and hyperinsulinism was discussed earlier. The only syndrome of obesity in which insulin excess causes the weight gain is that related to ventromedial hypothalamic lesions in animals[306]; removal of the pancreatic islets from neural (vagal) control by autotransplantation reverses hyperinsulinemia, diminishes food intake, and restores weight gain to control levels. Hyperinsulinism is also present in humans with hypothalamic obesity,[307] but it is not known whether the increased levels are primary, as in rodents with ventromedial hypothalamic damage, or secondary, as in simple human obesity.[160, 299]

As noted earlier, elevated insulin concentrations in ordinary obesity are primarily due to pancreatic hypersecretion.[272] Abnormal feedback of insulin on its own secretion may play a role in the overproduction of insulin,[308] but this theory may reflect only the higher starting levels of insulin in the obese because percent decreases in C peptide (a marker of endogenous insulin secretion) following insulin infusion are similar in lean and obese individuals.

In summary, hyperinsulinism is common in obesity, and insulin resistance is characteristic when major weight gain occurs. Insulin resistance is probably due to obesity, but several factors may contribute.

Less information is available for the other pancreatic hormones. The glucagon level has been reported to be normal, elevated, or decreased in obesity, but pancreatic glucagon (as opposed to total glucagon) is elevated in at least some persons.[309] Whether this elevation is a manifestation of relative insulin resistance or of some other mechanism is not known.

Glucagon resistance has been reported in obese animals[310] and could conceivably play a role in humans. Basal pancreatic polypeptide levels are low in human obesity, and the response to a protein meal is blunted. These low concentrations are of potential importance because pancreatic polypeptide, as noted earlier, functions as a satiety factor in rodents.[311] Release of somatostatin from the pancreas of obese Zucker rats is increased after stimulation by amino acids,[312] although elevation of the somatostatin content of gastrointestinal tissue consequent to starvation appears no different in lean and obese animals.[313] Metabolism of somatostatin has not been fully evaluated in human obesity, but plasma levels appear to be normal in the basal state and after glucose stimulation in obese Pima Indians.[314]

Thyroid Gland. Because of the possibility that obesity is related to a metabolic defect, there has been extensive study of thyroid function in overweight humans.[305, 315, 316] Basically, thyroid hormone concentrations are normal in obesity, although some persons have an elevated T_3 level, probably due to carbohydrate overfeeding.[317] With caloric restriction the T_3 level falls, and the reverse T_3 concentration rises in both obese and normal persons.[305, 318, 319] In one group of formerly obese women at stable reduced weight, concentrations of free T_3 were lower than in weight-stable controls, and this decrease was accompanied by a lower level of resting metabolic rate adjusted for fat-free mass, suggesting that the obese state might be associated with reduced thyroid thermogenesis.[203] This study needs to be confirmed. The thyrotropin (also called thyroid-stimulating hormone) response to thyrotropin-releasing hormone (TRH) is normal in obesity.[318–320] A small percentage of patients have low radioactive iodine uptake that is unresponsive to thyrotropin,[305] probably the consequence of subclinical thyroiditis rather than of obesity. Receptors for T_3 are reported to be low in nuclear extracts of monocytes from patients with obesity.[321] Nuclear T_3 receptors are low in the liver and lung of ob/ob mice, which may be the cause of decreased activity of Na^+,K^+-ATPase in these tissues.[322]

Adrenal Gland. Since excess glucocorticoids promote accumulation of adipose mass, a possible role of adrenal steroids in the genesis of obesity has been considered. In addition, glucocorticoids are commonly increased in obese animals, and adrenalectomy can prevent obesity in such models. These effects of glucocorticoids are most likely the consequence of actions directly on peripheral tissues, but glucocorticoids may also affect energy balance through reciprocal changes in the hypothalamic expression of CRH, which promotes catabolism through actions that include suppression of NPY.[77] Whatever the role for glucocorticoid in the etiology, a common problem in differential diagnosis is to separate Cushing's syndrome from simple obesity, since glucose intolerance and hypertension are common in both. Simple obesity may be accompanied by a central distribution of fat and striae. The latter are ordinarily white but occasionally purplish, so as to resemble those in adrenocortical hyperfunction. Although cortisol production rates and 24-h urinary 17-hydroxysteroid values are often elevated in obesity, basal plasma cortisol and urinary free cortisol values tend to be normal.[305, 323] However, 5% of patients with obesity have increased urinary free cortisol, and some patients with early Cushing's syndrome have normal levels.[324, 325] Overnight dexamethasone suppression is normal in about 90% of obese controls but in only 2% of subjects with Cushing's syndrome.[323] Thus about 10% of obese patients in whom Cushing's syndrome is in question will need the standard (long) dexamethasone suppression test. Obese individuals almost invariably show suppression in the standard test.[323, 326] Other tests for Cushing's syndrome, such as continuous 7-h dexamethasone infusion,[327] have not been applied to large numbers of obese individuals but have given normal results in small series.[328] Although most obese patients do not have

Cushing's syndrome, some investigators continue to explore the possibility that subtle increases in cortisol production may contribute to the pathophysiology of "simple obesity," especially that variety with predominance of abdominal fat.[329] Given the fact that the adipocyte hormone leptin has been shown to inhibit the activity of the hypothalamic-pituitary-adrenal axis in rodents,[101] the possible relationship of leptin resistance to mild hyperactivity of the adrenal gland must be considered.

The adrenal steroid dehydroepiandrosterone is said to have an antiobesity effect in animals,[330] and obese persons have been noted to have a negative correlation between excess body weight and dehydroepiandrosterone production.[331] Nevertheless, dehydroepiandrosterone levels are normal in human obesity,[332] and administration of large doses to obese men produced no change in body weight.[333]

Catecholamines are thermogenic hormones, and reduced sympathetic nervous system activity could cause reduced energy expenditure. Norepinephrine turnover is decreased in several forms of animal obesity,[334] and reduced sympathetic innervation of BAT may account for reduced BAT activity in these models. In obese humans basal norepinephrine concentrations are normal, decrease appropriately with diminished caloric intake, and increase with upright posture.[335, 336] Epinephrine response to isometric exercise is deficient in obese women but normal in obese men.[336] Thermogenic response to infused norepinephrine is blunted in the obese,[335] possibly accounting for the fact that in some studies the rise in oxygen uptake after a meal is less in obese than in normal individuals.[337] Insulin produces equivalent rises in plasma norepinephrine values in lean and obese persons.[337]

Testis. The concentration of testosterone in plasma of massively obese men is low.[305, 338] Levels of testosterone-binding globulin (also called sex hormone–binding globulin) are decreased, and the percentage of free testosterone is elevated, resulting in normal levels of free testosterone in most individuals. Low levels of testosterone-binding globulin may be an effect of high levels of insulin on hepatic expression of this protein.[339] Some massively obese men have low free testosterone levels.[338] Plasma levels of androstenedione and dihydrotestosterone are normal.[305] The hypothalamic-pituitary-testicular axis is grossly intact.[305, 338, 340] Thus the administration of clomiphene citrate results in appropriate rises in levels of follicle-stimulating hormone, luteinizing hormone (LH), and testosterone.[340] However, gonadotropin secretion in individuals with low free testosterone fails to increase in compensation, suggesting a mild state of hypogonadotropic hypogonadism.[341] Concentrations of estradiol and estrone are both increased in obese men, and estrogen production rates are high.[340, 342] Most of the increase comes from extraglandular conversion of androgen precursors to estrogen, but there may be some increase in estradiol secretion from the testis.[340] The increased estrogen levels in obese men usually are clinically silent; gynecomastia, impotence, and feminization are rare.[342] The abnormal gonadal steroid concentrations are reversible by weight loss.[342]

Ovary. Obese women have a higher incidence of menstrual disturbances and hirsutism,[343] and the endocrine profile is somewhat different in women with a predominance of upper body vs. lower body obesity.[344] Upper body obesity is associated with increased testosterone production, decreased testosterone-binding globulin,[345] and increased free plasma testosterone levels. This constellation of endocrine changes is probably the cause of the amenorrhea not infrequently seen in morbidly obese women and probably part of the spectrum of polycystic ovarian disease. Androgen excess and amenorrhea are reversible with weight loss.[346, 347] Upper body obesity is associated with insulin resistance and hyperinsulinemia, findings consistent with the possibility that insulin plays a role

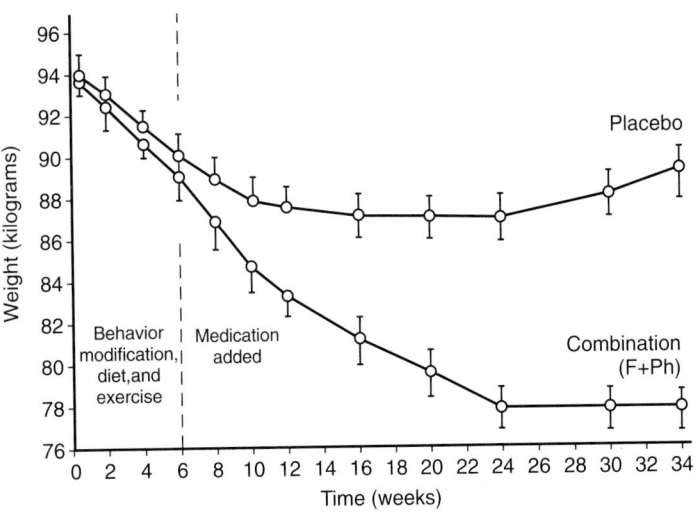

Figure 22–13. Body weight by week (mean +/− SEM) in placebo group (n = 54) and group treated with phentermine plus fenfluramine (n = 58). (Redrawn from Weintraub M, Sundaresan PR, Madan M, et al. Long-term weight control study I (weeks 0–34). Clin Pharmacol Ther 1992; 51:586–594, with permission.)

activation of BAT is unclear, and whether they will have beneficial effects in human obesity must await the results of clinical trials.

The addition of liothyronine to very-low-calorie diets to counteract the fall in plasma concentrations of T_3 with semistarvation causes modest increases in the rate of weight loss in the short term.[318, 319] However, nitrogen loss is accelerated by such therapy so that three fourths of the extra loss comes from the lean body mass, not adipose tissue.[319, 404] Liothyronine therapy therefore is not appropriate. A variety of other drugs have been tested in weight loss programs, including human chorionic gonadotropin, levodopa, bromocriptine, opioid antagonists, and γ-linolenic acid.[368, 395] There is no evidence that any are of benefit. Sucrose polyester, a nonabsorbable mixture of six- to eight-carbon fatty acids in ester linkage with sucrose, has been used as a caloric diluent and causes modest decreases in total caloric intake (about 25%).[405, 406] A beneficial side effect is a slight lowering of LDL cholesterol and triglyceride levels in plasma. Sucrose polyester appears to be safe, although prolonged use may produce deficiencies of fat-soluble vitamins.[405] Thus far only short-term studies have been carried out, leaving the question of clinical usefulness unresolved.[405, 406] Some reports suggest that GH injections may enhance the loss of body fat[407, 408]; such fat loss was accompanied by an increase in lean body mass in elderly men.[408] The effects of GH treatment in ordinary obesity have not been extensively evaluated, although a modest decrease in fat mass and an increase in lean body mass have been reported in a group of women treated for 5 wk.[409] Potential side effects have not been evaluated.

SURGERY. Because of the lack of success in medical therapy for massive obesity, attempts have been made to reverse the condition by surgery. For a number of years the most widely used procedure was the jejunoileal bypass.[365] The first two forms of jejunoileal bypass were the Payne procedure (35 cm of jejunum anastomosed end-to-side to 10 cm of ileum) and the Scott operation (30 cm of jejunum anastomosed end-to-end with 15 cm of ileum, the proximal cut portion of the latter being inserted into the transverse colon).[410] Operative mortality was ordinarily about 4% but was often higher.[365] Large, sustained weight loss after surgery is due to both decreased food intake and malabsorption. The loss of appetite may be related to bacterial overgrowth in the bypassed segment.[411] However, significant complications after both procedures[412] include diarrhea (essentially universal); vitamin D deficiency with osteomalacia; diminished plasma levels of vitamin B_{12}, vitamin A, and folic acid; arthritis; renal calculi (oxalate); hyperuricemia; deficiencies of magnesium, calcium, and potassium; and liver disease, which in some cases progresses to cirrhosis and hepatic coma. Because of these complications, jejunoileal bypass is no longer performed in most centers.[365, 412, 413] Variants have been tried, including biliopancreatic and biliointestinal bypass operations.[368, 414] In the former, drainage from the stomach is divided so that the fundus is isolated from the antrum, which is drained along with pancreatic and biliary ducts. In the latter the bypassed loop is attached to the gallbladder, which allows bile salt reabsorption in the ileum. The patient must have a functioning gallbladder for this procedure.

The two operative procedures recognized by the 1991 National Institutes of Health Conference are the vertical banded gastroplasty and the gastric bypass procedure.[415] The vertical banded gastroplasty restricts food intake by limiting gastric volume. A 15-mL gastric reservoir is created by one of several stapling techniques. The gastric reservoir empties through a narrow channel that is reinforced with prosthetic material into the residual stomach. Gastrointestinal continuity is preserved and malabsorption does not occur. A second procedure is the gastric bypass, which appears to be effective in producing weight loss without the late complications seen with the jejunoileal procedure.[416–419] In controlled studies gastric bypass appears slightly more effective than gastroplasty.

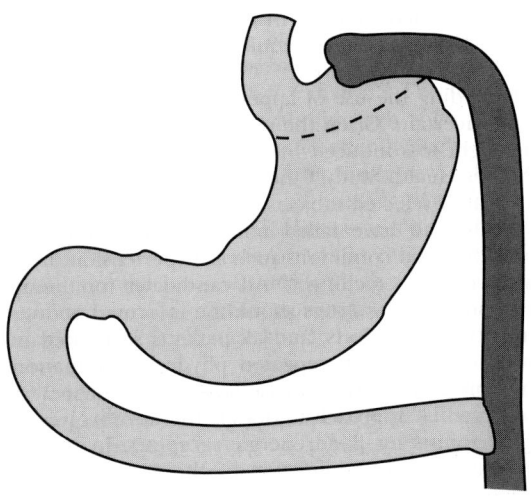

Figure 22–14. Gastric bypass operation for morbid obesity.

Although usually initially successful in almost all patients, long-term success is variable. Indeed the failure rate for both procedures has been as high as 50% in some studies.[366] However, some studies suggest excellent long-term results with the gastric bypass procedure,[420] namely, a mean stable weight loss of 45 kg over 14 y of follow-up and dramatic reversal of most comorbid conditions. It is clear that gastric stapling or bypass surgery may be reasonable options in patients with morbid obesity (e.g., BMI >40 or 45 kg more than ideal weight) who have not responded to conventional nonsurgical therapies. Of course it is critical that the surgeon be experienced in this area and function as part of an integrated health care team. Operative mortality is usually less than 1%, but iron, vitamin B$_{12}$, and thiamine deficiencies may complicate gastric bypass.[368]

Other procedures include jaw wiring and the placement of gastric balloons.[8, 368, 414] The former causes weight loss, but the latter is no more effective than a sham operation in controlled trials.[368] Liposuction is useful for cosmetic purposes only.

SUMMARY. The results of therapy for obesity are poor. The initial approach should be moderate dietary restriction with emphasis on long-term weight loss. Fasting or very-low-calorie, high-protein diets should be used only for initiation of therapy or for circumstances in which rapid weight loss is required because of a serious complication: diabetes mellitus, cardiac disease, pulmonary distress, or the need for elective surgery. Exercise should be added both for an improved sense of well-being and for its effect on caloric balance, with recognition that the limitation of caloric intake is more important. The use of drugs as a supplement to diet and exercise is debated; currently available drugs have modest efficacy but are effective only if administered chronically. Gastric bypass surgery or plication should probably be reserved for patients with major medical complications of obesity, although the presence of such complications may increase the operative risk. Conceivably surgery may be justified in patients with uncomplicated obesity whose illness has precluded employment or otherwise ruined the patient's personal life. Physicians who deal with obese patients should have extensive experience with ministers, teachers, and police officers who have been discriminated against because of a weight problem. It should be remembered that surgery is expensive and not always reimbursable by insurance.

The patient with serious obesity should be seen regularly by the professionals directing care: the nutritionist in every case, the behavioral therapist if such services are available, and the physician. Occasionally it may be worthwhile for those who can afford it to enter a special resident program as a form of shock treatment to reinforce the seriousness of the problem.[274]

The conclusion is inescapable that obesity is an unsolved therapeutic problem.

ANOREXIA NERVOSA–BULIMIA NERVOSA

Anorexia nervosa and bulimia nervosa are common syndromes characterized by bizarre eating patterns that become the central focus of the patient's life. Occurring primarily in young women, they represent life-disrupting illnesses for the afflicted and their families, and they lead to death in a significant number of cases. In this discussion anorexia and bulimia will be considered variant expressions of the same underlying disorder. Although the clinical manifestations and outcome of the two syndromes are distinctive, overlapping features suggest that the root disorder is the same: an obsessive fear of being fat. In anorexic patients the primary reactive mechanism is

the rigid restriction of food intake; with bulimia a loss of control in the drive to eat is compensated for by induced vomiting and laxative use.

History and Prevalence

Anorexia nervosa was described by Richard Morton in 1689, who reported the case of a girl age 17 who was "like a skeleton only clad with skin."[421] He concluded that she had "a nervous consumption." The name *anorexia nervosa* appears to have been coined by Sir William Gull. Gull and Charles Lasègue, a French contemporary, both published accurate descriptions of the clinical manifestations. Anorexia nervosa became confused with pituitary apoplexy for a number of decades because of Simmonds' report of death by "emaciation" in a woman with pituitary destruction, but the issue was reclarified in 1930 when Berkman published his experience with 117 patients and emphasized that the physiological abnormalities were due to a psychic disturbance.[421, 422]

The true prevalence of anorexia and bulimia is unknown. Anorexia has been estimated to be present in 1% of upper-class adolescent girls in the United Kingdom[423] and in 2.9% of South African schoolgirls.[424] In the epidemiologic archives of disease in Rochester, Minnesota, the incidence was 7.3/100,000 patient-years, with an overall prevalence of 0.1% (0.2% in women, 0.02% in men).[425] Discrepancies in prevalence doubtless derive from different criteria for diagnosis and different methods of ascertainment. Although subclinical disease may be present in up to 5% of the population,[426] most authorities accept a value of about 1% in whites. Similar figures have been found for bulimia,[427] although estimates of 1 to 4% have been cited.[428]

Diagnosis

The diagnosis of anorexia nervosa or bulimia nervosa usually is not difficult. In 1972 Feighner and colleagues[429] outlined diagnostic criteria that were used for many years and were fairly restrictive. Since that time the diagnostic standards of the American Psychiatric Association have changed so that the prevalence of eating disorders has increased. Current criteria are shown in Tables 22–4 and 22–5. For anorexia nervosa the weight loss requirement is 85% of expected weight (not defined). Presumably standard tables should be used (see

---

TABLE 22–4. Diagnostic Criteria for Anorexia Nervosa

A. Refusal to maintain body weight at or above a minimally normal weight for age and height (e.g., weight loss leading to maintenance of body weight less than 85% of that expected; or failure to make expected weight gain during period of growth, leading to body weight less than 85% of that expected).

B. Intense fear of gaining weight or becoming fat, even though underweight.

C. Disturbance in the way in which one's body weight or shape is experienced, undue influence of body weight or shape on self-evaluation, or denial of the seriousness of the current body weight.

D. In postmenarchal females, amenorrhea, i.e., the absence of at least three consecutive menstrual cycles. (A woman is considered to have amenorrhea if her periods occur only following hormone [e.g., estrogen] administration.)

Specify Type:

Restricting type: During the episode of anorexia nervosa the person does not regularly engage in binge-eating or purging behavior (i.e., self-induced vomiting or the misuse of laxatives, diuretics, or enemas).

Binge eating/purging type: During the episode of anorexia nervosa, the person regularly engages in binge-eating or purging behavior (i.e., self-induced vomiting or the misuse of laxatives, diuretics, or enemas).

Reprinted with permission from the Diagnostic and Statistical Manual of Mental Disorders, Fourth Edition. Washington, DC: American Psychiatric Association, 1994: 544–555. Copyright 1994, American Psychiatric Association.

TABLE 22–5. Diagnostic Criteria for Bulimia Nervosa

A. Recurrent episodes of binge-eating. An episode of binge-eating is characterized by both of the following:
1. Eating, in a discrete period of time (e.g., within any 2-h period), an amount of food that is definitely larger than most people would eat during a similar period of time and under similar circumstances.
2. A sense of lack of control over eating during the episode (e.g., a feeling that one cannot stop eating or control what or how much one is eating).
B. Recurrent inappropriate compensatory behavior to prevent weight gain, such as self-induced vomiting, misuse of laxatives, diuretics, or other medications; fasting; or excessive exercise.
C. The binge-eating and inappropriate compensatory behaviors both occur, on average, at least twice a week for 3 mos.
D. Self-evaluation is unduly influenced by body shape and weight.
E. The disturbance does not occur exclusively during episodes of anorexia nervosa.

Specify Type:
Purging type: the person regularly engages in self-induced vomiting or the misuse of laxatives or diuretics.
Nonpurging type: the person uses other inappropriate compensatory behaviors, such as fasting or excessive exercise, but does not regularly engage in self-induced vomiting or the misuse of laxatives or diuretics.

Reprinted with permission from the Diagnostic and Statistical Manual of Mental Disorders, Fourth Edition. Washington, DC: American Psychiatric Association, 1994: 549–550. Copyright 1994, American Psychiatric Association.

Table 22–1). Some authorities favor the use of an absolute weight standard rather than a percent, with a BMI of 18 (weight [kg]/height [m²]) required for diagnosis.[430] Amenorrhea, an intense fear of becoming fat, and a disturbance of body perception are essential criteria. Patients are further divided into restricting and binge-eating–purging types. Movement between subtypes is possible; a given individual may have bulimic behavior before a typical restricting pattern develops.

The criteria for diagnosis of bulimia nervosa include recurrent binge-eating coupled with a sense that food intake is out of control. In addition other measures to combat weight gain must be present; e.g., self-induced vomiting (most common); use of laxatives or diuretics, or both; fasting; or excessive exercise. Binges cannot occur exclusively during episodes of anorexia nervosa. Two subtypes are recognized: purging and nonpurging.

Care must be taken not to overlook other illnesses that may cause weight loss, vomiting, or increased food intake. Occult malignancy, diabetes mellitus, renal failure, and inflammatory bowel disease must be considered. At times a classic eating disorder may coexist with organic illness, such as anorexia nervosa in individuals with insulin-dependent diabetes mellitus.

Clinical Picture

ANOREXIA NERVOSA. The clinical features of anorexia nervosa are well delineated in reviews that provide access to the literature on this subject.[430-436]

Demographic Features. Anorexia nervosa is primarily a disease of women; only 4 to 6% of affected individuals are males. The age at onset ranges from prepuberty to the early 30s. The most common time of appearance is 4 to 5 y after menarche.[433] Originally the disorder was diagnosed primarily in whites, usually in families from the middle or upper class, but Hispanic and Native American females are equally affected. It is less common in women of African and Asian American origin.[437] There is an increased prevalence of anorexia in parents and siblings of index cases.[438] In one study, 29 of 102 patients had a primary family member who was at least 20% below the mean weight of a matched population.[433] Only 10 family members were as much as 20% overweight.

Because the prevalence of obesity in the general population is much greater than 10%, it can be concluded that fatness in families of subjects with anorexia is not excessive. This conclusion is important because in the past it was considered that the disorder might have something to do with a reaction to obesity in a parent. Onset of disease frequently follows a stressful event in the subject's life.

Behavioral Characteristics. The term *anorexia* is really inappropriate because true loss of appetite does not occur until late in the course of disease, if at all. Patients are not free of hunger; rather they are obsessed with the fear of being fat so that hunger sensations are ignored or denied. An intense preoccupation with food is usually discernible. Although anorexic patients drastically restrict their own food intake, it is not unusual for them to enjoy preparing elaborate meals for others and to collect recipes and hoard food in the home. Most subjects appear knowledgeable about nutritional matters, particularly the caloric content of food, although some show lesser insight than matched controls.[439] It is usually stated that carbohydrates are avoided, but this is not always the case. Fat intake tends to be low and protein intake is high. Sporadic dieting usually begins about a year before the start of the disease proper, often at the point at which maximal weight was reached.[433]

To assist weight loss it is common for patients to exercise excessively, often in ritualistic fashion. A significant percentage induce vomiting and use laxatives or diuretics. Periodic gorging of the type seen in the bulimic variant of the disease may also occur in classic anorexia nervosa.

Perceptual Abnormalities. Patients with anorexia nervosa characteristically deny illness, at least until the disease is far advanced. Resistance to treatment is profound. They deny hunger, fatigue, and change in physical appearance. Affected persons may have a disturbance of body image that makes them see themselves as continually fat.[440, 441] Several types of objective evaluation show the propensity of anorexic patients to overestimate true body size, whereas the capacity to assess other objects accurately is maintained. However, there are doubts about the specificity of distorted body image in anorexia nervosa.[442-445] Similar distortions can be seen in control populations. The tendency to overestimate body size is usual in adolescence and tends to ameliorate or disappear with age or maturation.

Symptoms. The denials that characterize anorexia nervosa tend to minimize spontaneous revelation of symptoms, although almost all patients will discuss amenorrhea when asked. Sleep disturbances are fairly common.[433, 438, 446] Constipation is not unusual, although diarrhea may occur with laxative use.[434] Complaints of early satiety and abdominal pain are frequent. The cause of these gastrointestinal symptoms is not known, although abnormally slow gastric emptying has been reported.[447] Gastric rupture can occur, usually in bulimic patients, but it may be seen with classic anorexia nervosa during refeeding.[448] Cold intolerance is often acknowledged, and true hypothermia has been reported.[431] Traditionally cold intolerance has been attributed to "functional hypothyroidism," but abnormality of the hypothalamic temperature-regulating centers may be a more likely explanation.[449] Patients with anorexia nervosa do not defend well against either heat or cold challenge. Heat production in muscle, measured directly by microcalorimetry, is diminished about 50% per unit muscle mass in anorexia nervosa compared with normal controls.[450] Heat generation in platelets is not impaired, nor is the defect in muscle seen in bulimic persons. Whether this defect is regulated locally or by the central nervous system is not known. Anorexic patients may also experience excessive vasoconstriction, cyanosis, and numbness of the extremities on exposure to cold, which reflects an abnormal sensitivity of the vessels to low temperatures.[451] Raynaud's phenomenon has been noted.

Finally CT studies show that subcutaneous fat loss is greater than deep fat loss in anorexia.[452] Subcutaneous fat provides thermal insulation and its absence allows greater heat loss.

Physical Findings. The physical examination in classic anorexia nervosa is characterized pre-eminently by cachexia so severe as to be reminiscent of concentration camp victims in World War II. In the fully dressed state the degree of weight loss may not be appreciated because the victims tend to wear masking clothes (long sleeves, long skirts, slacks). Parotid enlargement related to malnutrition may soften the angularity of the face expected with this degree of weight loss. As in other forms of semistarvation, the pulse rate is slow and blood pressure is on the low side. Cardiac abnormalities may include mitral valve prolapse associated with reduced left ventricular mass.[453, 454] The basal metabolic rate is decreased consequent to diminished body mass. Peripheral edema is common. It usually results not from hypoalbuminemia but from a failure to mobilize the normal extracellular fluid volume with starvation. Muscle weakness occurs in approximately half of patients, and peripheral neuropathy has been reported.[455] An increase in body hair, usually quite fine, may be present. A yellow cast to the skin related to carotenemia is a helpful clue because carotene levels are characteristically low in other forms of malnutrition. A summary of the physical findings in 65 anorexic patients is shown in Table 22–6.[456]

BULIMIA NERVOSA. The term *bulimia* means literally "ox hunger" or a voracious appetite. It has come to stand for a syndrome of astonishing food intake during short periods in young women who usually have a previous or current picture of anorexia nervosa. The gorging is then followed by induced vomiting and often by the use of laxatives in large amounts. Two fundamental features characterize the syndrome: (1) an irresistible urge to overeat and (2) a marked fear of becoming fat. The former predominates in this form of the illness, but other features distinguish it from anorexia nervosa. In simple terms patients with nonbulimic anorexia nervosa deal with the fear of being fat by restricting food intake (restrictors). Their phobia of being fat appears to be so powerful that control over eating is not lost. In contrast, bulimic patients lose such control and thus become gorgers. They control weight gain only by vomiting and using laxatives. Laxative abuse in bulimic subjects is nearly four times more common than in the community at large (14.9 versus 4.2%).[457] A careful study of 30 patients illustrates the ontogeny of the bulimic syndrome.[458] Eleven of 30 patients began bulimic behavior after a period of weight gain, whereas 19 started during a period of weight loss. Eventually all patients began to gain weight. At the time treatment was sought, 24 persons were still underweight, 2 persons were of normal weight, and 4 individuals were above healthy weight. In every case, however, bulimia was interpreted to be a signal of actual or anticipated failure in control of food intake.

Demographic Features. As with anorexia nervosa, most patients are women. Occasionally the disease develops in men. There appears to be little difference in the family background of bulimic subjects relative to those with anorexia nervosa. Mothers of bulimic patients may have a higher prevalence of obesity, but the difference is not great.

Behavioral Characteristics. The drive to eat in bulimic patients is overwhelming. Thoughts are constantly on food and even dreams may focus on eating. The drive is not from hunger. One patient described it as follows: "It is not hunger. Hunger is a feeling of a gap inside you. You eat something small to stop that feeling. I go on eating after I've satisfied that hunger. I want to keep on eating until I feel full—it's the final limit—you can then eat no more."[458] The amount of food ingested can be enormous, up to 50,000/kcal/d. In a series of 40 patients, the mean duration of binge-eating episodes was 1.2 h, but an episode could last as long as 8 h.[459] On average gorging occurred 12 times a week, but the range was from as few as 1 to as many as 46 times. The mean number of calories ingested per episode was 3415, but the number could reach 11,500 at one sitting. In these 40 patients the major foods eaten, in descending order of frequency, were ice cream, bread or toast, candy, doughnuts, soft drinks, and other foods. Usually more than one food was used in an episode. Overeating is ordinarily carried out secretly and alone, generally in the afternoon and evening.[458, 459] Often the episodes appear to be precipitated by ingestion of a "forbidden" high-carbohydrate food, which sets up an unstoppable chain reaction. If the urge to eat the first morsel can be controlled, binges do not occur. (Some have likened this situation to the "first drink" phenomenon in alcoholics.) There may thus be an all-or-none pattern to the eating. The term *dietary chaos* has been coined to describe the eating behavior in bulimic individuals,[460] and it is an accurate description.

After gorging, essentially all patients with bulimia induce vomiting,[458, 459] most often by activating the gag reflex with the fingers or a toothbrush, although some subjects learn to regurgitate spontaneously. Ipecac may be used by as many as 20% of patients and may cause myopathy and, possibly, cardiomyopathy.[461] Vomiting may become ritualistic, with a fixed number of retchings required to allow satisfaction that all food has been removed. As noted before, laxative use is common. Other forms of weight control, such as excessive exercise and use of diuretics, probably occur to a similar extent in both anorexic and bulimic syndromes.

A striking feature of bulimia is the propensity to carry out antisocial behavior.[458, 462, 463] Twelve to 14% of patients with bulimia admit stealing (most often food); the actual percentage may be higher. Stealing is not a feature of anorexia nervosa with major weight loss.[462] Patients in the bulimic phase use both street drugs and alcohol to a greater extent than do anorexic individuals.[435] Self-mutilation and suicide attempts are three to four times more common in bulimia than in anorexia (Table 22–7). Although most patients with eating disorders are uninterested in sex, sexual promiscuity can occur.[458]

Perceptual Abnormalities. Formal testing of body image perception in the bulimic subset has not been reported, although it has been stated that overestimation of body size was greater in bulimics than in a control group. There is probably no major difference from classic anorexia.

Symptoms. In contrast to classic anorexia nervosa, amenorrhea was present in only 11 of 28 individuals when cessation of menses was not used as part of the selection criteria.[458] This difference is probably because weight loss was less severe in the bulimic group. Although amenorrhea is not frequently seen, irregular menses and oligomenorrhea are common.[464] As might be expected from repetitive binge-eating, vomiting, and purging, gastrointestinal symptoms are common; bloating,

TABLE 22–6. Physical Findings in 65 Patients with Anorexia Nervosa

Abnormality	% Affected
Skin (e.g., hairiness, dryness)	88
Hypothermia (<35.9°C [96.6°F], rectal)	85
Bradycardia (<60 beats/min)	80
Cachexia	72
Bradypnea (<15 breaths/min)	66
Hypotension (<70 mm Hg systolic)	52
Heart murmur	38
Edema	23

Adapted from Silverman JA. Anorexia nervosa: clinical and metabolic observations in a successful treatment plan. In: Vigersky RA, ed. Anorexia Nervosa. New York: Raven, 1977: 331–339.

TABLE 22–7. Behavioral Patterns in Anorexia Nervosa and Bulimia Nervosa

	% of Patients	
Behavior	Anorexia Nervosa	Bulimia Nervosa
Use of alcohol	4.8	20.4
Use of illicit drugs	11.6	28.6
Stealing	0	12.1
Self-mutilation	1.5	9.2
Suicide attempts	7.1	23.1

Adapted from Garfinkel PE, Moldofsky H, Garner DM. The heterogeneity of anorexia nervosa. Bulimia as a distinct subgroup. Arch Gen Psychiatry 1980; 37:1036–1040. Copyright 1980, American Medical Association.

flatulence, constipation, abdominal pain, borborygmi, and nausea are present in half to two thirds of patients.[465] Despite frequent vomiting hypokalemia is rare in bulimia, and muscle weakness is unusual.[466] Rarely tetany and convulsions may appear, possibly as a consequence of metabolic alkalosis. Depression and obsessive-compulsive disorder are common in bulimia.[467, 468]

Physical Findings. Bulimic patients usually are not emaciated and as a consequence do not exhibit bradycardia, relative hypotension, or hypothermia. Parotid enlargement may follow binges. They may have scars from self-mutilation or suicide attempts. Dental erosion is frequent in vomiters.[469]

Laboratory Abnormalities

Although many systems of the body are affected in severe anorexia nervosa, most of the laboratory changes are of little consequence and not unique because they occur in other forms of semistarvation. Laboratory abnormalities in bulimia are less common. Unless specified otherwise, the changes described in this section are for anorexia. Hematologic findings include anemia, leukopenia (relative neutropenia, lymphocytosis), thrombocytopenia, low erythrocyte sedimentation rate, and decreased fibrinogen levels in plasma.[431, 432, 434, 435, 470] The anemia and occasional pancytopenia appear to be due to hypoplasia of the bone marrow, which is filled with a gelatinous mucopolysaccharide. Peripheral blood smears may show acanthosis. Hypokalemia may occur in both anorexia and bulimia secondary to vomiting or laxative use, as noted earlier, but it is not common.

Plasma protein levels tend to be normal, although hypoalbuminemia may be seen.[432, 434] Essential amino acid values are not low, in contrast to kwashiorkor, probably because of the relatively high protein intake of anorexic persons.

β-Carotene levels in plasma are high, together with vitamin A and its derivatives.[434] The mechanism of this elevation is not clear. However, the fact that anorexic individuals who vomit have serum carotene levels only one half those of nonvomiters suggests that dietary intake plays a major role.[471]

Mild hypercholesterolemia is frequent in anorexia nervosa. The cholesterol elevation is in the LDL fraction; both HDL and VLDL levels are normal.[472, 473] Plasma triglyceride concentrations are normal despite low values for hepatic lipase and LPL activities. The cause of the hypercholesterolemia is not known, although neutral sterol and bile acid secretion appears to be low.[473] The failure of ovulation and amenorrhea that is almost universal in anorexia doubtless plays a major role. The ritualized exercise of anorexia would be expected to lower LDL and increase HDL levels, but this beneficial effect is neutralized in amenorrheic women.[474] It is presumed that estrogen deficiency is the primary cause, probably acting through a diminution in hepatic LDL receptor number.

In view of the known relationship between malnutrition and depressed immune function (variable effect on humoral immune function; profound effect on cellular immunity), there has been considerable interest in the immune response in anorexia nervosa. In a series of five patients,[475] mean levels of immunoglobulin G, immunoglobulin M, and transferrin were low before hyperalimentation. The deficiencies were reversed by feeding. A number of alternative complement pathway proteins were also low. The mechanism was thought to be decreased synthesis. When 22 consecutively admitted patients were studied by an anergy panel to test delayed hypersensitivity, only 6 showed defective responses.[476] This number is in accord with the view that most patients with anorexia nervosa are surprisingly free of infection.[476–478] Occasionally infection does occur, as indicated by a death from herpes simplex encephalitis.[477]

Other abnormalities have been reported, but none is of major clinical significance. The glomerular filtration rate is generally slightly low, and prerenal azotemia with blood urea nitrogen levels as high as 21 to 25 mM (60 to 70 mg/dL) may be seen.[456] Renal concentrating ability is impaired and polyuria may occur.[479] Arginine vasopressin is not released normally in response to an osmotic stimulus, and its action in the kidney may be impaired.[432, 479, 480] Levels of vasopressin in the cerebrospinal fluid are elevated relative to those in plasma.[479] Nonspecific ST-T changes may be seen on electrocardiographic examination. Serum amylase levels may be elevated in the absence of clinical signs of pancreatitis. High levels of amylase are more common in bulimia than in anorexia.[461, 481] In 30 hospitalized patients with anorexia nervosa, plasma zinc and copper values were low, although the content of these metals in hair was normal.[482] Iron-binding capacity was decreased, but plasma iron and ceruloplasmin levels were normal. Hypogeusia (taste impairment) was noted and was most marked for bitter and sour stimuli.

Endocrine Findings

Considerable interest has focused on the endocrine system in anorexia nervosa for two reasons. First, the earlier period of confusion between pituitary insufficiency and anorexia nervosa needed to be clarified. Second, amenorrhea is an almost constant feature in the typical form of the disease. It now seems clear that the endocrine changes are all secondary; i.e., there is no evidence for primary dysfunction in the pituitary gland, gonads, thyroid, or adrenal glands. A summary of endocrine changes in anorexia and bulimia is shown in Table 22–8. For reviews, see references 483 and 495.

AMENORRHEA. About one half of patients with anorexia nervosa experience secondary amenorrhea concomitant with the onset of dieting, whereas one fifth cease menses before the onset of overt disease. The remaining patients undergo secondary failure of menses only after weight loss is significant.[434, 484] Presumably, early amenorrhea is due to psychological stress antedating clinical illness.[485] It is now generally accepted that the primary defect is localized in the hypothalamus and operates via impaired release of LHRH. Baseline LH and FSH values are low, and the 24-h LH profile regresses to either a prepubertal pattern (all values low) or a pubertal pattern (sleep-dependent LH release only).[486] The prepubertal pattern is most common.[487] With weight gain, reversal of the abnormalities occurs, the pubertal pattern appearing at about 70% ideal body weight and the adult pattern near 80% ideal body weight. The pituitary response to LHRH is abnormal with severe weight loss but reverses to normal with weight gain.[488] Pituitary responsiveness to LHRH can be restored either by low-dose LHRH treatment (given by infusion) or by pulsatile injection.[488, 489] Characteristically FSH responds first and then LH, the pattern mirroring the events that take place during normal puberty. Presumably, the lack

TABLE 22–8. Endocrine Changes in Anorexia Nervosa
and Bulimia Nervosa

Anorexia Nervosa	Bulimia Nervosa
Hypothalamus and Pituitary Gland	
↓ LH (↓ response to LHRH)	→ or ↓ LH (↑ response to LHRH)
↓ FSH	→ or ↓ FSH
↑ or → growth hormone (↓ IGF1)	↑ or → growth hormone (↓ IGF1)
→ thyrotropin (delayed response to TRH)	→ thyrotropin (delayed response to TRH)
→ corticotropin (↓ response to CRH)	→ corticotropin (↓ or → response to CRH)
→ or ↓ prolactin (↓ response to TRH)	→ or ↓ prolactin (↑ response to TRH)
Abnormal regulation vasopressin	? vasopressin regulation
Thyroid Gland	
↓ thyroxine	→ thyroxine
↓ T₃	→ or ↓ T₃
↑ reverse T₃	? reverse T₃
Adrenal Gland	
→ or ↑ cortisol	→ or ↑ cortisol
↑ urinary free cortisol	→ urinary free cortisol
Abnormal dexamethasone suppression	Abnormal dexamethasone suppression
↓ dehydroepiandrosterone and its sulfate	
Ovary	
↓ estradiol	→ or ↓ estradiol
↓ estrone	→ or ↓ estrone
↓ progesterone	→ or ↓ progesterone
Testis	
↓ testosterone	

Symbols: ↓, decreased; ↑, increased; →, normal; LH, luteinizing hormone; LHRH, luteinizing hormone–releasing hormone; FSH, follicle-stimulating hormone; IGF1, insulin-like growth factor 1; TRH, thyrotropin-releasing hormone.

of pituitary responsiveness to acute stimulation by LHRH represents removal of a trophic effect of LHRH with prolonged semistarvation. Why the hypothalamus is unable to release LHRH in anorexia nervosa is not known, although abnormalities in norepinephrine and dopamine metabolism in the central nervous system have been postulated.[434, 464] Bromocriptine, a dopaminergic agonist, has no effect on the abnormalities, however.[488] The hypothalamic-pituitary axis is likewise unresponsive to clomiphene.[490]

Low estrogen levels and failure to ovulate in anorexia appear to be solely due to gonadotropin deficiency, because ovulation can be induced by either exogenous gonadotropins or LHRH administration for prolonged periods.[491, 492] Although menses usually return with weight gain, this is not invariably so because psychological factors can continue to override the reversal of cachexia. It has been claimed that after secondary amenorrhea a body weight about 10% greater than that needed for menarche is required.[493]

Men with anorexia nervosa appear to have the same abnormalities in gonadotropins seen in females, and in consequence testosterone levels are low.[494]

As noted earlier, amenorrhea is not as common in bulimia as in anorexia. Studies of gonadotropic function in bulimia are not in agreement. Part of the problem may be that menstruating and anovulatory patients were pooled. It is likely that basal LH levels are low in bulimic women with menstrual irregularities and that as a consequence estradiol and progesterone concentrations are also low.[483] It has been reported that in bulimic women the LH response to LHRH was enhanced, in contrast to the diminished response characteristic of anorexia nervosa with weight loss.[483, 495]

OTHER PITUITARY HORMONES. Basal GH values are elevated in some patients with both anorexia nervosa and bulimia.[449, 464, 483] Overall about one third to one half of patients have elevated basal levels.[464, 483, 496] GH response to provocative stimuli is also impaired; e.g., no increase occurs after

dexamethasone challenge.[497] IGF1 levels are low in both anorexia nervosa and bulimia nervosa.[464, 483, 498] It is possible that elevated GH levels are the consequence of diminished feedback activity by IGF1. IGF1 levels are probably low because of both decreased synthesis and the presence of inhibitors of somatomedins in plasma, features characteristic of malnutrition and weight loss of any cause. Plasma prolactin levels are usually normal in anorexia.[449, 499, 500] Prolactin levels have been reported as both normal and low in bulimia.[483] Prolactin response to TRH is said to be blunted in anorexia,[501] whereas some individuals have a paradoxical rise after LHRH.[502] Bulimic patients are said to have an increased release of prolactin after TRH. Abnormal control of vasopressin was cited earlier.[479] Thyrotropin and corticotropin (adrenocorticotropic hormone) will be discussed later.

THYROID GLAND. Despite the slow pulse and low basal metabolic rate that characterize anorexia nervosa and other forms of weight loss, there is no evidence of hypothyroidism.[503, 504] The usual picture is low-normal thyroxine (T₄), low T₃, and increased reverse T₃ levels. There are two forms of the euthyroid sick syndrome: one in which the T₃ value is low and both T₄ and reverse T₃ levels are elevated,[505] and the other in which both T₄ and T₃ levels are low.[506] The former mimics hyperthyroidism, the latter hypothyroidism. The low-normal T₄ syndrome is thought to be due to an inhibitor that blocks binding of T₄ to thyroid-binding globulin.[506] The thyrotropin response to TRH may be abnormal in the low T₄, T₃ syndrome.[506] A common pattern is delay in the peak response to TRH, although absolutely blunted responses are also seen.[464] Reversal of the thyroid abnormalities occurs with weight gain. Some patients have an overshoot of T₃ accompanied by symptoms of mild hyperthyroidism in the recovery phase.[507] Thyroid function is essentially normal in bulimia nervosa.[483, 508] Thyrotropin levels are normal, but a delayed time to peak release after TRH is seen, as in anorexia.

ADRENAL GLAND. Adrenal function has been extensively studied in the eating disorders but is still not completely understood.[464] Chemical findings suggest hypercortisolism, but no clinical features of cortisol excess are noted.[509] Plasma cortisol levels are high-normal or elevated. Urinary free cortisol is also elevated. The half-life of plasma cortisol is prolonged, and urinary metabolites are decreased.[510] Cortisol production rates are normal or slightly elevated, particularly if body mass is considered.[464, 511] Many explanations for elevated cortisol levels have been offered, including peripheral resistance to the hormone.[509] Cortisol binding in plasma is normal. The consensus is that the primary defect is localized in the hypothalamus, but the mechanism is unknown. Dexamethasone suppression is abnormal in anorexia, and the corticotropin response to CRH is blunted.[497, 509, 512] CRH levels in the cerebrospinal fluid are elevated,[512, 513] whereas corticotropin levels are low.[514] The presumption is that the initial lesion is hypersecretion of CRH, hypersecretion of corticotropin overproduction of cortisol, and hyperplasia of the adrenals, with subsequent feedback of cortisol on the pituitary so that corticotropin levels fall into the normal range.[509] It is assumed that feedback on the hypothalamus is impaired, which would account for the elevated CRH levels. Although the corticotropin response to synthetic CRH is blunted, the cortisol response expected from a given rise in corticotropin is increased.[509]

Bulimic individuals without weight loss have normal urinary free cortisol levels, with high-normal concentrations in plasma. Failure of dexamethasone suppression is common.[483] The corticotropin response to CRH has been reported to be both normal[509] and impaired.[515]

Levels of dehydroepiandrosterone and its sulfate are low in anorexia.[516] A number of enzyme defects have been reported (e.g., 5α-reductase deficiency), but their significance is unknown.[431, 434, 517]

The abnormalities in hypothalamic-pituitary-adrenal function are restored by weight gain.

MISCELLANEOUS. Melatonin levels have generally been found to be increased with higher than normal day/night ratios,[518, 519] although night concentrations were not increased in one study.[520] The response of glucagon to hypoglycemia is impaired, whereas release after administration of arginine is normal.[521]

Positron emission tomography shows global hypometabolism of glucose in the brains of anorexic patients.[522] Differing patterns of cerebral blood flow in anorexia nervosa compared with bulimia nervosa have been reported, but the significance is uncertain.[523] Insulin function is normal in bulimia nervosa despite the fact that polycystic ovarian disease is common and may be accompanied by insulin resistance.[524] The regulation of atrial natriuretic peptide is impaired in anorexia nervosa.[525]

Complications of Anorexia Nervosa and Bulimia Nervosa

Serious complications may develop when the eating disorders are severe or prolonged. Osteoporosis in anorexia nervosa can involve both the spine and peripheral bones.[526–530] Osteopenia progresses most rapidly if dieting begins before the peak bone mass has been attained and if amenorrhea is primary or begins early.[530] The primary mechanism appears to be estrogen deficiency, but dietary calcium or vitamin D deficiency and hypercortisolism may play ancillary roles.

Atrophy of the brain with dilated ventricles was found by CT in both anorexia[531] and bulimia.[532] Because the bulimic patients studied were not underweight, the explanation for the atrophy is not forthcoming. It is claimed that an inverse relationship exists between plasma concentrations of T_3 and ventricular size in both types of eating disorders,[532] but the meaning of this negative correlation is not clear. Electroencephalographic abnormalities have also been seen, predominantly in binge eaters.[461] Some consider the changes to be nonspecific.

Heart disease is a potentially fatal complication of anorexia nervosa and may cause sudden death.[533] Ventricular tachyarrhythmias are the major mechanism, similar to the deaths occurring with liquid protein diets. All patients should be followed with electrocardiograms, a prolonged Q-T interval being a distinct sign of danger. In addition severe weight loss leads to both systolic and diastolic dysfunction of the ventricles, with the possibility of congestive heart failure, especially on refeeding.[534] Heart rate and blood pressure responses to exercise are routinely blunted. Mitral valve prolapse is common in women with anorexia nervosa and resolves with weight gain.[453, 454] The mechanism is thought to be a valvuloventricular mismatch; i.e., decreased left ventricular volume caused by starvation leaves the normal leaflets too long. Heart disease is relatively rare in normal-weight bulimic subjects, although hypokalemia related to vomiting may cause arrhythmias.[461] As mentioned earlier, heavy use of ipecac can potentially cause cardiomyopathy.

The serious complications of bulimia nervosa are the consequence of binge eating and vomiting. Tears or ruptures of the esophagus may result in pneumomediastinum or pneumoperitoneum.[461] Spontaneous rupture of the stomach may follow gorging or may occur with refeeding in anorexic patients.[448, 461] If vomiting is severe, hypotension related to volume depletion and metabolic acidosis may ensue. Finally, fatal pulmonary aspiration with asphyxiation may follow giant gorges.

Etiology

The cause of anorexia nervosa is not known. It has been argued[535] that hypothalamic dysfunction is primary, but the evidence appears persuasive that the disorder is a psychiatric one. The psychodynamics are not clear and in fact may not be fixed. Whatever other factors operate in the genesis of the disease, the families tend to be "enmeshed": there are blurred generational boundaries so that parents and children are constantly involved in each other's problems.[434, 536] Some workers suggest that both major eating disorders—the anorexia nervosa and bulimia nervosa syndromes and obesity—have as a fundamental characteristic a paralyzing sense of ineffectiveness induced by early events in family life.[537] Subjects experience themselves as acting only in response to demands coming from others and as not doing anything because they want to. This has been colorfully stated as follows: "The development of anorexia may be conceived as a shouting and unrelenting 'No' which extends to every area of living, though most conspicuous in the food refusal. Uncontrolled obesity, on the other hand, is the manifest expression of despair, of having given up all efforts to establish a sense of inner control and independent identity."[537] The family members of bulimic persons have a higher prevalence of affective disorders, alcoholism, and drug use than is the case with classic anorexia nervosa.[538] Some have thought that traditional explanations of enmeshed families are oversimplified,[539, 540] but others continue to favor the classic view.[541] Some investigators have suggested that sexual abuse plays a role, but the evidence is not persuasive.[542, 543]

Although family structure appears to play a primary role in the genesis of anorexia nervosa, culture is also important.[435, 544] In contemporary Western society the ideal female figure is that of a slender prepubertal girl bearing the secondary sexual characteristics of a mature woman. Preoccupation with diets and weight loss is common in normal teen-age girls in these societies: up to 70% in the 12th grade.[545] The prevalence of anorexia nervosa in dancers is 10 times that in the general population, which suggests that even occupation may play a role. Anorexia-like syndromes have been seen with increasing frequency in athletes who want to reduce their fat to 5 to 7% of body weight.[546, 547] Thus if there is a rising prevalence of anorexia nervosa, it may be due to relentless cultural pressures to diet, stay slim, and exercise, this pressure selecting those predisposed to develop the illness. There appears to be a genetic contribution to both anorexia nervosa and bulimia nervosa, but its nature is not clear.[548, 549]

How the psychodynamic dysfunction is translated into biologic disease remains a mystery. Although neurotransmitters may be involved, only future research can provide answers.[550–553]

Treatment

Eating disorders are serious illnesses, especially anorexia nervosa, which is associated with significant mortality rates.[554, 555] In a meta-analysis of 42 studies, the mortality was estimated to be 0.56% per y.[555] Firm mortality rates are not available for bulimia nervosa, but fewer deaths have been reported.[556] There is no specific treatment for anorexia or bulimia, although multiple approaches have been tried. Most experts in the field agree that there is no one way to approach what is an incredibly difficult problem. However, certain general principles can be developed.[557–559]

First, some attempt must be made to provide insight to the patient about the problem. Second, behavior has to be modified. Third, families must be involved. In general, both individual and group psychotherapy is required. Drug therapy is now standard in bulimia nervosa and many cases of anorexia nervosa.[553] Tricyclic antidepressants have been used for years, and some feel that fluoxetine, a serotonin reuptake inhibitor, is the drug of choice.

Most therapy is received on an outpatient basis. It may be

preferable to initiate treatment in the hospital when weight loss is extreme.[557, 558] Hospitalization is always indicated with complications such as arrhythmias, aspiration, or rupture of the gastrointestinal tract. The immediate aim of hospitalization is weight gain. Every attempt should be made to accomplish this by having the patient eat. Tube feeding or intravenous hyperalimentation should be undertaken only as a last resort. Care must be taken to keep electrolyte values within normal limits. Phosphate depletion is especially dangerous and may lead to cardiac or respiratory failure.[534, 560] The patient must be encouraged to eat and must be repeatedly assured of the "safety" of eating. It may be useful for the physician to state specifically: "I will not let you get fat" and set up a contractual relationship as a guarantee, e.g., "If you gain x pounds, which is necessary for your safety, we will stop there for several months before proceeding." During the initial phases of therapy, whether as an inpatient or an outpatient, every effort should be made to keep the patient from eating alone.

To summarize, there is no definitive therapy for the eating disorders. Patience is an absolute requirement for the health care team, who must be thought trustworthy by the patient. Many patients are followed in special clinics for eating disorders, but many are managed by nonpsychiatrists.[561] The long-term outlook in anorexia and bulimia is difficult to ascertain and impossible to relate to treatment programs. Although some individuals improve, the eating disorders are usually lifelong illnesses. Full recovery is rare.[554]

REFERENCES

Obesity

1. Garn SM, Clark DC. Trends in fatness and the origins of obesity. Pediatrics 1976; 57:443–456.
2. Coll M, Meyer A, Stunkard AJ. Obesity and food choices in public places. Arch Gen Psychiatry 1979; 36:795–797.
3. Grande F. Assessment of body fat in man. In: Bray GA, ed. Obesity in Perspective. Washington DC: DHEW, 1975: 189–203.
4. Lukaski HC. Methods for the assessment of human body composition: traditional and new. Am J Clin Nutr 1987; 46:537–556.
5. Van Loan MD, Mayclin PL. Body composition assessment: dual energy x-ray absorptiometry (DEXA) compared to reference methods. Eur J Clin Nutr 1992; 46:125–130.
6. Pearson AM, Purchas RW, Reineke EP. Theory and potential usefulness of body density as a predictor of body composition. In: Body Composition in Animals and Man. Washington, DC: National Academy of Sciences, 1968: 169.
7. Forbes GB, Welle SL. Lean body mass in obesity. Int J Obes 1983; 7:99–107.
8. Bray GA. Obesity: basic consideration and clinical approaches. Dis Mon 1989; 35:449–537.
9. Build study. Society of Actuaries and Association of Life Insurance Medical Directors of America, 1979.
10. Durnin JVGA, Womersley J. Body fat assessed from total body density and its estimation from skinfold thickness: measurement on 481 men and women age 16 to 72 years. Br J Nutr 1974; 32:77–97.
11. Lohman TG. Skinfolds and body density and their relation to body fatness: a review. Hum Biol 1981; 53:181–225.
12. Sloan AW, Weir JB. Nomograms for prediction of body density and total body fat from skinfold measurements. J Appl Physiol 1970; 28:221–222.
13. Kissebah AH, Vvdelingum N, Murray R. Relation of body fat distribution to metabolic complications of obesity. J Clin Endocrinol Metab 1982; 54:254–260.
14. Kissebah AH, Krakower GR. Regional adiposity and morbidity. Physiol Rev 1994; 74:761–811.
15. Hubert HB, Feinleib M, McNamara PM, et al. Obesity as an independent risk factor for cardiovascular disease: a 26-year follow-up of participants in the Framingham Heart Study. Circulation 1983; 67:968–977.
16. Abraham S, Johnson CL. Prevalence of severe obesity in adults in the United States. Am J Clin Nutr 1980; 33:364–369.
17. Black D, James WPI, Besser GM. Obesity. J R Coll Physicians Lond 1983; 17:5–65.
18. Manson JE, Willett WC, Stampfer MJ, et al. Body weight and mortality among women. N Engl J Med 1995; 333:677–685.
19. Willett WC, Manson JE, Stampfer MJ, et al. Weight, weight change, and coronary heart disease in women: risk within the normal range. JAMA 1995; 273:461–465.
20. Bray GA. Overweight is risking fate: definition, classification, prevalence, and risks. Ann NY Acad Sci 1987; 499:14–28.
21. Van Itallie TB. Obesity: adverse effects on health and longevity. Am J Clin Nutr 1979; 2723–2733.
22. Society of Actuaries and Association of Life Insurance Medical Directors of America. 1980.
23. Waaler HT. Height, weight and mortality: the Norwegian experience. Acta Med Scand 1984; 679(Suppl):1–56.
24. Kissebah AH, Peiris AN. Biology of regional body fat distribution and relationship to non–insulin-dependent diabetes mellitus. Diabetes Metab Rev 1989; 5:83–109.
25. Despres N, Nadeau A, Tremblay A, et al. Role of deep abdominal fat in the association between regional adipose tissue distribution and glucose tolerance in obese women. Diabetes 1989; 38:304–309.
26. Abate N, Garg A, Peshock RM. Relationship of generalized and regional adiposity to insulin sensitivity in men. J Clin Invest 1995; 96:88–98.
27. Bray GA, ed. Obesity in America. DHEW Publication No (NIH) 79-359. Washington DC: Government Printing Office, 1979: 1–19.
28. Colditz GA, Willett WC, Rotnitsky A, et al. Weight gain as risk factor for clinical diabetes mellitus in women. Ann Intern Med 1995; 122:481–486.
29. Willett WC, Stampfer M, Manson J. New weight guidelines for Americans: justified or injudicious? Am J Clin Nutr 1991; 53:1102–1103.
30. Nutrition and your health: dietary guidelines for Americans. 3rd ed. US Department of Agriculture, US Department of Health and Human Services, 1990.
31. Meritt RJ. Obesity. Curr Probl Pediatr 1982; 12:1–58.
32. Ginsberg-Fellner F, Jagendorf LA, Carmel H. Overweight and obesity in preschool children in New York City. Am J Clin Nutr 1981; 34:2236–2241.
33. Health, United States. DHEW Publication No. (PHS) 78-1322. Washington, DC. Government Printing Office 1978: 215.
34. Van Itallie TB. Health implications of overweight and obesity in the United States. Ann Intern Med 1985; 103:983–988.
35. Kuczmarski RJ, Flegal KM, Campbell SM, et al. Increasing prevalence of overweight among US adults: the national health and nutrition examination surveys. JAMA 1994; 272:205–211.
36. Eid EE. Follow-up study of physical growth of children who had excessive weight gain in first six months of life. Br Med J 1970; 2:74–76.
37. Charney E, Goodman HC, McBride M. Childhood antecedents of adult obesity: do chubby infants become obese adults? N Engl J Med 1976; 295:6–9.
38. Maffei M, Halaas J, Ravussin E, et al. Leptin levels in human and rodent: measurement of plasma leptin and ob RNA in obese and weight-reduced subjects. Nat Med 1995; 1:1155–1161.
39. Poskitt EMF, Cole IJ. Do fat babies stay fat? Br Med J 1977; 1:7–9.
40. Stark O, Atkins F, Wolff OH. Longitudinal study of obesity in the National Survey of Health and Development. Br Med J 1981; 283:13–17.
41. Knittle JL, Jimmers K, Ginsberg-Fellner F. The growth of adipose tissue in children and adolescents: cross-sectional and longitudinal studies of adipose cell number and size. J Clin Invest 1979; 63:239–246.
42. Dietz WH. Critical periods in childhood for the development of obesity. Am J Clin Nutr 1994; 59:955–959.
43. Braddon FEM, Rodgers B, Wadsworth MEJ. Onset of obesity in a 36 year birth cohort. Br Med J 1996; 293:299–303.
44. Mossberg HO. 40 year follow-up of overweight children. Lancet 1989; 2:491–493.
45. Ravelli GP, Stein ZA, Susser MW. Obesity in young men after famine exposure in utero and early infancy. N Engl J Med 1976; 295:349–353.
46. Pettitt DJ, Baird HR, Aleck KA, et al. Excessive obesity in offspring of Pima Indian women with diabetes during pregnancy. N Engl J Med 1983; 308:242–245.
47. Wilson BE, Meyer GE, Cleveland JC Jr, et al. Identification of candidate genes for a factor regulating body weight in primates. Am J Physiol 1990; 259:R1148–R1155.
48. Weigle DS. Appetite and the regulation of body composition. FASEB J 1994; 8:302–310.
49. Kennedy GL. The role of depot fat in the hypothalamic control of food intake in the rat. Proc R Soc Lond 1953; 140:579–592.
50. Coleman DL, Hummel KP. Effects of parabiosis of normal with genetically diabetic mice. Am J Physiol 1969; 217:1298–1304.
51. Zhang E, Graziano MP, Doebber TW, et al. Down-regulation of the expression of the obese gene by an antidiabetic thiazolidinedione in Zucker diabetic fatty rats and db/db mice. J Biol Chem 1996; 271:9455–9459.
52. Halaas J, Gajiwala K, Maffei M, et al. Weight-reducing effect of the plasma protein encoded by the obese gene. Science 1995; 269:543–546.
53. Campfield L, Smith F, Guisez Y, et al. Recombinant mouse OB protein: evidence for a peripheral signal linking adiposity and central neural networks. Science 1995; 269:546–548.
54. Pellymounter M, Cullen M, Baker M, et al. Effects of the obese gene product on body weight regulation in ob/ob mice. Science 1995; 269:540–543.
55. Spiegelman BM, Flier JS. Adipogenesis and obesity: rounding out the big picture. Cell 1996; 87:377–389.
56. Hetherington A, Ranson SW. Hypothalamic lesions and obesity in the rat. Anat Rec 1940; 78:149–172.
57. Anand BK, Brobeck JR. Localization of a "feeding center" in the hypothalamus of the rat. Proc Soc Exp Biol Med 1951; 77:323–324.
58. Mayer J. Genetic, traumatic and environmental factors in the etiology of obesity. Physiol Rev 1953; 33:472–508.

59. Smith GP, Epstein AN. Increased feeding in response to decreased glucose utilization in rat and monkey. Am J Physiol 1969; 217:1083–1087.
60. Lareu-Achagiotis C, Le Magnen J. Effects of short-term nocturnal and diurnal food depravation on subsequent feeding in intact and VMH lesioned rats: relation to blood glucose levels. Physiol Behav 1982; 28:245–248.
61. Silverstone T, Goodall E. Serotonergic mechanisms in human feeding: the pharmacologic evidence. Appetite 1986; 7(Suppl):85–97.
62. Kruk ZL. Dopamine and 5-hydroxytryptamine inhibit feeding in rats. Nature 1973; 246:52–53.
63. Levine LR, Rosenblatt S, Bosomworth J. Use of a serotonin reuptake inhibitor, fluoxetine, in the treatment of obesity. Int J Obes 1987; 11(Suppl)3:185–190.
64. Blundell JE. Serotonin and appetite. Neuropharmacology 1984; 23:1537–1551.
65. Dourish CT. Multiple serotonin receptors: opportunities for new treatments for obesity? Obes Res 1995; 4:449S–462S.
66. Tecott LH, Sun LM, Akana SF. Eating disorder and epilepsy in mice lacking 5-HT2c serotonin receptors. Nature 1995; 374:542–546.
67. Fernstrom JD. Role of precursor availability in the control of monoamine biosynthesis in brain. Physiol Rev 1983; 63:484–546.
68. Wurtman JJ, Wurtman RJ, Growden JH. Carbohydrate craving in obese people: suppressions by treatments affecting serotonergic transmission. Int Eat Disord 1981; 1:2.
69. Blundell JE. Serotonin and the biology of feeding. Am J Clin Nutr 1992; 55:155S–159S.
70. Blundell JE, Hill AJ. Nutrition, serotonin and appetite: case study in the evolution of a scientific idea. Appetite 1987; 8:183–194.
71. Morley JE. Neuropeptide regulation of appetite and weight. Endocr Rev 1987; 8:256–287.
72. Stanley BG, Kyrkouli SE, Lampert S, et al. Neuropeptide Y chronically injected into the hypothalamus: a powerful neurochemical inducer of hyperphagia and obesity. Peptides 1986; 7:1189–1192.
73. Qu D, Ludwig D, Gammeltoft S, et al. A role for melanin-concentrating hormone in the central regulation of feeding behavior. Nature 1996; 380:243–247.
74. Arase K, York DA, Shimizu H. Effect of corticotropin releasing factor on food intake and brown adipose tissue thermogenesis in rats. Am J Physiol 1988; 255:E255–E259.
75. Spina M, Merlo-Pich E, Chan RK, et al. Appetite-suppressing effects of urocortin, a CRF-related neuropeptide. Science 1996; 273:1561–1564.
76. Turton MD, O'Shea D, Gunn I, et al. A role for glucagon-like peptide-1 in the central regulation of feeding. Nature 1996; 379:69–72.
77. Schwartz MW, Dallman MF, Woods SC. Hypothalamic response to starvation: implications for the study of wasting disorders. Am J Physiol 1995; 269:R949–R957.
78. Dryden S, Frankish H, Wang Q, et al. Neuropeptide Y and energy balance: one way ahead for the treatment of obesity? Eur J Clin Invest 1994; 24:293–308.
79. Marks JL, Schwartz M, Porte DJ. Effect of fasting on regional levels of neuropeptide Y mRNA and insulin in the rat hypothalamus: an autoradiographic study. Mol Cell Neurol 1992; 3:199–205.
80. Billington CJ, Briggs JE, Grace M, et al. Effects of intracerebroventricular injection of neuropeptide Y on energy metabolism. Am J Physiol 1991; 260:R321–R327.
81. Zarjevski N, Cusin I, Vetter F, et al. Chronic intracerebroventricular neuropeptide Y administration to normal rats mimics hormonal and metabolic changes of obesity. Endocrinology 1993; 133:1753–1758.
82. Stephens TW, Basinski M, Bristow PK, et al. A role for neuropeptide Y in the antiobesity action of the obese gene product. Nature 1995; 377:530–532.
83. Zhang Y, Proenca R, Maffei M, et al. Positional cloning of the mouse *ob* gene and its human homologue. Nature 1994; 372:425–432.
84. Erickson J, Clegg K, Palmiter R. Sensitivity to leptin and susceptibility to seizures of mice lacking neuropeptide Y. Nature 1996; 381:415–418.
84a. Erickson JC, Ahima RS, Hallopeter G, et al. Regulatory Peptides (in press).
85. Gerald C, Walker M, Criscione L, et al. A receptor subtype involved in neuropeptide-Y–induced food intake. Nature 1996; 382:168–170.
86. Krahn DD, Gosnell BA. Behavioral effects of corticotrophin releasing factor: localization and characterization of central effects. Brain Res 1988; 443:63–69.
87. Rothwell N. Central effects of CRF on metabolism and energy balance. Neurosci Biobehav Rev 1989; 14:263–271.
88. Van Huijsduijnen OB, Rohner-Jeanrenaud HF, Jeanrenaud B. Hypothalamic neuropeptide Y mRNA levels in pre-obese and genetically obese (fa/fa) rats: potential regulation thereof by corticotropin releasing factor. J Neuroendocrinol 1993; 5:381–386.
89. Van Itallie T. The glucostatic theory 1953–1988: root and branches. Int J Obes 1990; 14:1–10.
90. Gibbs J, Young RC, Smith GP. Cholecystokinin decreases food intake in rats. J Comp Physiol Psychol 1973; 84:488–495.
91. Garlicki J, Konturek PK, Majka J, et al. Cholecystokinin receptors and vagal nerves in control of food intake in rats. Am J Physiol 1990; 258:E40–E45.
92. West DB, Fey D, Woods SC. Cholecystokinin persistently suppresses meal size but not food intake in free-feeding rats. Am J Physiol 1984; 246:R776–R787.
93. Faust IM, Johnson PR, Hirsch J. Adipose tissue regeneration following lipectomy. Science 1977; 197:391–393.
94. Schwartz MW, Figlewicz DP, Baskin DG. Insulin and the central regulation of energy balance: update 1994. Endocr Rev 1994; 2:109–113.
95. Schwartz MW, Sipols AJ, Marks JL, et al. Inhibition of hypothalamic neuropeptide Y gene expression by insulin. Endocrinology 1992; 130:3608–3616.
96. Baura GD, Foster DM, Porte DJ, et al. Saturable transport of insulin from plasma into the central nervous system of dogs in vivo. J Clin Invest 1993; 92:1824–1830.
97. Tartaglia LA, Dembrski M, Weng X, et al. Identification and expression cloning of a leptin receptor. Cell 1995; 83:1263–1271.
98. Lee GH, Proenca R, Montez JM, et al. Abnormal splicing of the leptin receptor in diabetic mice. Nature 1996; 379:632–635.
99. Frederich RC, Hamann A, Anderson S, et al. Leptin levels reflect body lipid content in mice: evidence for diet-induced resistance to leptin action. Nature Med 1995; 1:1311–1314.
100. Kolaczynski JW, Considine RV, Ohannesian J, et al. Responses of leptin to short-term fasting and refeeding in humans. Diabetes 1996; 45:1511–1515.
101. Ahima RS, Prabarkarian D, Mantzoros C, et al. Role of leptin in the neuroendocrine response to fasting. Nature 1996; 382:250–252.
102. MacDougald OA, Hwang CS, Fan H, et al. Regulated expression of the obese gene product (leptin) in white adipose tissue and 3T3-L1 adipocytes. Proc Natl Acad USA 1995; 92:9034–9037.
103. Grunfeld C, Zhao C, Fuller J. Endotoxin and cytokines induce expression of leptin, the *ob* gene product, in hamsters. J Clin Invest 1996; 97:2151–2157.
104. Mantzoros CS, Qu D, Frederich RC, et al. Activation of β3-adrenergic receptors suppresses leptin expression and mediates a leptin-independent inhibition of food intake in mice. Diabetes 1996; 45:909–914.
105. James WPT, Trayhurn P. Thermogenesis and obesity. Br Med Bull 1981; 37:43–48.
106. Himms-Hagen J. Brown adipose tissue thermogenesis and obesity. Prog Lipid Res 1989; 28:67–115.
107. Newsholme EA. A possible metabolic basis for the control of body weight. N Engl J Med 1980; 302:400–405.
108. Nicholls DG, Locke RM. Thermogeneic mechanisms in brown fat. Physiol Rev 1984; 64:1–64.
109. Bukowiecki LJ, Follea N, Lupien J, et al. Metabolic relationships between lipolysis and respiration in rat brown adipocytes. J Biol Chem 1981; 256:12840–12848.
110. Locke RM, Rial E, Scott ID, et al. Fatty acids as acute regulators of the proton conductance of hamster brown-fat mitochondria. Eur J Biochem 1982; 129:373–380.
111. Strieleman PJ, Schalinske KL, Shrago E. Fatty acid activation of the reconstituted brown adipose tissue mitochondria uncoupling protein. J Biol Chem 1985; 260:13402–13405.
112. Ricquier D, Bouillaud F, Toumelin P. Expression of uncoupling protein mRNA in thermogenic or weakly thermogenic brown adipose tissue. J Biol Chem 1986; 261:13905–13910.
113. Himms-Hagen J. Brown adipose tissue thermogenesis: interdisciplinary studies. FASEB J 1990; 4:2890–2898.
114. Lowell BB, Susulic VS, Hamann A, et al. Development of obesity in transgenic mice after genetic ablation of brown adipose tissue. Nature 1993; 366:740–742.
115. Frederich RC, Hamann A, Anderson S. Leptin levels reflect lipid content in mice: evidence for diet-induced resistance to leptin action. Nature Med 1995; 1:1311–1314.
116. Hamann A, Flier JS, Lowell BB. Decreased brown fat markedly enhances susceptibility to diet-induced obesity, diabetes and hyperlipidemia. Endocrinology 1996; 137:21–29.
117. Collins S, Kuhn CM, Petro AE, et al. Role of leptin in fat regulation (letter). Nature 1996; 380:677.
118. Walston J, Silver K, Bogardus C, et al. Time of onset of non–insulin-dependent diabetes mellitus and genetic variation in the β3-adrenergic receptor gene. N Engl J Med 1995; 333:343–347.
119. Widen E, Lehto M, Kanninen T, et al. Association of a polymorphism in the β3-adrenergic receptor gene with features of the insulin resistance syndrome in Finns. N Engl J Med 1995; 333:348–351.
120. Clement K, Vaisse C, Manning BSJ, et al. Genetic variation in the β3-adrenergic receptor and an increased capacity to gain weight in patients with morbid obesity. N Engl J Med 1995; 333:352–354.
121. Emorine LJ, Marullo S, Briend-Sutren MM, et al. Molecular characterization of the human β3-adrenergic receptor. Science 1989; 245:1118–1121.
122. Granneman JG, Lahners KN, Chaudhry A. Molecular cloning and expressions of the rat β3-adrenergic receptor. Mol Pharmacol 1991; 40:895–899.
123. Bloom JD, Dutia MD, Johnson BD. CL316, 243, a potent beta-adrenergic agonist virtually specific for beta-3 receptors: a promising antidiabetic and antiobesity agent. J Med Chem 1992; 35:3081–3084.
124. Cawthorne MA, Sennitt MV, Arch JRS, et al. BRL 35135, a potent and selective atypical beta adrenoceptor agonist. Am J Clin Nutr 1992; 55:2525–2575.
125. Holloway BR, Howe R, Rao BS, et al. ICI D7114: a novel selective adrenoceptor agonist of brown fat and thermogenesis. Am J Clin Nutr 1992; 55:2625–2645.
126. Himms-Hagen J, Danforth E. The potential role of β3-adrenoceptor agonists in the treatment of obesity and diabetes. Curr Opin Endocr Diabetes 1996; 3:59–65.

126a. Fleury C, Neverova M, Collins S, et al. Uncoupling protein-2: a novel gene linked to obesity and hyperinsulinemia. Nat Genet 1997; 15:269–272.

127. Susulic VS, Frederich RC, Lawitts J, et al. Targeted disruption of the β$_3$-adrenergic receptor gene. J Biol Chem 1995; 270:29483–29492.

128. Hers HG, Hue L. Gluconeogenesis and related aspects of glycolysis. Annu Rev Biochem 1983; 52:617–653.

129. Shulman GI, Landenson PW, Wolfe MH. Substrate cycling between gluconeogenesis and glycolysis in euthyroid, hypothyroid and hyperthyroid man. J Clin Invest 1985; 76:757–764.

130. Edelman IS. Thyroid thermogenesis. N Engl J Med 1974; 290:1303–1308.

131. Bray GA, York DA, Yukimura Y. Activity of (Na$^+$ + K$^+$)-ATPase in the liver of animals with experimental obesity. Life Sci 1978; 22:1637–1642.

132. DeLuise M, Blackburn GL, Flier JS. Reduced activity of the red-cell sodium-potassium pump in human obesity. N Engl J Med 1980; 303:1017–1022.

133. DeLuise M, Rappaport E, Flier JS. Altered erythrocyte Na$^+$ + K$^+$ pump in adolescent obesity. Metabolism 1982; 31:1153–1158.

134. Klimes I, Nagulesparan M, Unger RH. Reduced Na$^+$,K$^+$-ATPase activity in intact red cells and isolated membranes from obese man. J Clin Endocrinol Metab 1982; 54:721–724.

135. Mir MA, Charalambous BM, Morgan K. Erythrocyte sodium-potassium-ATPase and sodium transport in obesity. N Engl J Med 1981; 305:1264–1268.

136. Simat BM, Mayrand RR, From AHL. Is the erythrocyte sodium pump altered in human obesity? J Clin Endocrinol Metab 1983; 56:925–929.

137. Deriaz O, Dionne F, Perusse L, et al. DNA variation in the genes of the Na, K-adenosine triphosphatase and its relation with resting metabolic rate, respiratory quotient, and body fat. J Clin Invest 1994; 93:838–843.

138. Flier JS. The adipocyte: storage depot or node on the energy information superhighway? Cell 1995; 80:15–18.

139. Greene H, Kehinde O. Sublines of mouse 3T3 cells that accumulate lipid. Cell 1974; 1:113–116.

140. Ailhaud G, Grimaldi P, Negrel R. Cellular and molecular aspects of adipose tissue development. Annu Rev Nutr 1992; 12:207–233.

141. MacDonald OA, Lane MD. Transcriptional regulation of gene expression during adipocyte differentiation. Annu Rev Biochem 1995; 64:345–373.

142. Graves RA, Tontonoz P, Spiegelman BM. Analysis of a tissue-specific enhancer: ARF-6 regulates adipogenic gene expression. Mol Cell Biol 1992; 12:1202–1208.

143. Christy RJ, Przbla AE, MacDonald RJ. Differentiation-induced gene expression in 3T3 L1 preadipocytes: CCAAT/enhancer binding protein interacts with and activates the promoters of two adipocyte specific genes. Genes Dev 1989; 3:1323–1335.

144. Wang ND, Finegold MJ, Bradley A, et al. Impaired energy homeostasis in C/EBP alpha knockout mice. Science 1995; 269:1108–1112.

145. Tontonoz P, Hu E, Spiegelman BM. Stimulation of adipogenesis in fibroblasts by PPARγ2, a lipid-activated transcription factor. Cell 1994; 79:1147–1156.

146. Forman BM, Tontonoz P, Chen J, et al. 15-Deoxy-Δ12-14-prostaglandin J2 is a ligand for the adipocyte determination factor PPARγ. Cell 1995; 83:803–812.

147. Willson TM, Cobb JE, Cowan DJ. The structure-activity relationship between PPARγ agonism and the antihyperglycemic activity of thiazolidinedione. J Med Chem 1996; 39:665–668.

148. Hirsch J, Batchelor B. Adipose tissue cellularity in human obesity. Clin Endocrinol Metab 1976; 299–311.

149. Ginsberg-Fellner F, Knittle JL. Weight reduction in young obese children. I. Effects on adipose tissue cellularity and metabolism. Pediatr Res 1981; 15:1381–1389.

150. Roncari DAK, Lau DCW, Kindler S. Exaggerated replication in culture of adipocyte precursors from massively obese persons. Metabolism 1981; 30:425–427.

151. Auwerx J. Regulation of gene expression by fatty acids and fibric acid derivatives: an integrative role for peroxisomal proliferator activated receptors. Horm Res 1992; 38:269–277.

152. Flier JS, Cook KS, Usher P, et al. Severely impaired adipsin expression in genetic and acquired obesity. Science 1987; 237:405–408.

153. Napolitano A, Lowell BB, Damm D, et al. Concentrations of adipsin in blood and rates of adipsin secretion by adipose tissue in humans with normal, elevated, diminished adipose tissue mass. Int J Obes Relat Metab Disord 1994; 18:213–218.

154. Hotamisligil GS, Peraldi P, Spiegelman BM. The molecular link between obesity and diabetes. Curr Opin Endocr Diabetes 1996; 3:16–23.

155. Hotamisligil GS, Spiegelman BM. Tumor necrosis factor alpha: a key component of the obesity-diabetes link. Diabetes 1994; 43:1271–1278.

156. Frederich RC, Kahn BB, Peach MJ, et al. Tissue-specific nutritional regulation of angiotensinogen in adipose tissue. Hypertension 1992; 19:339–344.

157. Eckel RH. Lipoprotein lipase: a multifunctional enzyme relevant to common metabolic diseases. N Engl J Med 1989; 320:1060–1068.

158. Ong JM, Kern PA. Effect of feeding and obesity on lipoprotein lipase activity, immunoreactive protein, and messenger RNA levels in human adipose tissue. J Clin Invest 1989; 84:305–311.

159. Schwartz RS, Brunzell JD. Increased adipose-tissue lipoprotein-lipase activity in moderately obese men after weight reduction. Lancet 1978; 1:1230–1231.

160. Maruhama Y, Abe R. A familial form of obesity without hyperinsulinism at the outset. Diabetes 1981; 30:14–18.

161. Kern PA, Ong JM, Saffari B. The effects of weight loss on the activity and expression of adipose-tissue lipoprotein lipase in very obese humans. N Engl J Med 1990; 322:1053–1059.

162. Lafontan M, Dang-Tran L, Berlan M. Alpha-adrenergic antilipolytic effect of adrenaline in human fat cells of the thigh: comparison with adrenaline responsiveness of different fat deposits. Eur J Clin Invest 1979; 9:261–266.

163. Ostman J, Arner P, Engfeldt P. Regional differences in the control of lipolysis in human adipose tissue. Metabolism 1979; 28:1198–1205.

164. Bolinder J, Kager L, Ostman J, et al. Differences at the receptor and postreceptor levels between human omental and subcutaneous adipose tissue in the action of insulin on lipolysis. Diabetes 1983; 32:117–123.

165. Wahrenberg H, Lonnqvist F, Arner P. Mechanisms underlying regional differences in lipolysis in human adipose tissue. J Clin Invest 1989; 84:458–467.

166. Sztalryd C, Azhar S, Reaven GM. Difference in insulin action as a function of original anatomical site of newly differentiated adipocytes obtained in primary culture. J Clin Invest 1991; 88:1629–1635.

167. Arner P. Control of lipolysis and its relevance to development of obesity in man. Diabetes 1988; 4:507–515.

168. Leibel RL, Rosenbaum M, Hirsch J. Change in energy expenditure resulting from altered body weight. N Engl J Med 1995; 332:621–628.

169. Friedman JM, Leibel RL. Tackling a weighty problem. Cell 1992; 69:217–220.

170. West DB, Boozer CN, Moody DL, et al. Dietary obesity in nine inbred mouse strains. Am J Physiol 1992; 262:R1025–R1032.

171. Ravussin E, Swinburn BA. Pathophysiology of obesity. Lancet 1992; 340:404–408.

172. Ravussin E, Lillioja A, Knowler WC, et al. Reduced rate of energy expenditure as a risk factor for body weight gain. N Engl J Med 1988; 318:467–472.

173. Romieu I, Willett WC, Stampfer MJ, et al. Energy intake and other determinants of relative weight. Am J Clin Nutr 1988; 47:406–412.

174. Livingstone MB. Assessment of food intakes: are we measuring what people eat? Br J Biomed Sci 1995; 52:58–67.

175. Bandini LG, Schoeller DA, Cyr H, et al. Validity of reported intake in obese and non-obese adolescents. Am J Clin Nutr 1990; 52:421–425.

176. Prentice AM, Black AE, Coward WA. High levels of energy expenditure in obese women. BMJ 1986; 292:983–987.

177. Sahakian BJ. The interaction of psychological and metabolic factors in the control of eating and obesity. Hum Nutr Appl Nutr 1982; 36A:262–271.

178. Bruch H. Developmental considerations of anorexia nervosa and obesity. Can J Psychiatry 1981; 26:212–217.

179. Rodin J. Recent Advances in Obesity Research: In: Bjorntorp P, Cairella M, Howard AN, eds. Recent Advances in Obesity Research. London: John Libby, 1981: 106–123.

180. Rodin J, Schank D, Striegel-Moore R. Psychological features of obesity. Med Clin North Am 1989; 73:47–66.

181. Cassell JA. Commentary: American food habits in the 1980s. Top Clin Nutr 1989; 4:47–58.

182. Dreon DM, Frev-Hewitt B, Ellsworth N. Dietary fat:carbohydrate ratio and obesity in middle-aged men. Am J Clin Nutr 1988; 47:995–1000.

183. Flatt JP. Importance of nutrient balance in body weight regulation. Diabetes Metab Rev 1988; 571–581.

184. Fiedorek FT. Rodent genetic models for obesity and non-insulin dependent diabetes mellitus. In: Taylor SI, Olefsky JM, eds. Diabetes Mellitus. Philadelphia: Lippincott-Raven, 1996: 604–618.

185. Frederich RC, Lollmann B, Hamann A, et al. Expression of ob mRNA and its encoded protein in rodents: impact of nutrition and obesity. J Clin Invest 1995; 96:1658–1663.

186. Houseknecht KL, Mantzoros CS, Kuliawat R, et al. Evidence for leptin binding to proteins in serum of rodents and humans: modulation with obesity. Diabetes 1996; 45:1638–1643.

187. Banks WA, Kastin AJ, Huang W, et al. Leptin enters the brain by a saturable system independent of insulin. Peptides 1996; 17:305–311.

188. Ghilardi N, Ziegler S, Wiestner A, et al. Defective STAT signalling by the leptin receptor in diabetic mice. Proc Natl Acad Sci USA 1996; 93:6231–6235.

189. Considine R, Considine E, Williams C, et al. Evidence against either a premature stop codon or the absence of obese gene mRNA in human obesity. J Clin Invest 1995; 95:2986–2988.

190. Considine RV, Considine EL, Williams CJ, et al. The hypothalamic leptin receptor in humans. Diabetes 1996; 19:992–994.

191. Considine RV, Sinha M, Heiman M, et al. Serum immunoreactive leptin concentrations in normal weight and obese humans. N Engl J Med 1995; 334:292–295.

192. Caro JF, Kolaczynski JW, Nyce MR, et al. Decreased cerebrospinal-fluid/serum leptin ratio in obesity: a possible mechanism for leptin resistance. Lancet 1996; 348:159–161.

193. Ravussin E, Burnard B, Schutz Y, et al. Twenty-four-hour energy expenditure and resting metabolic rate in obese, moderately obese, and control subjects. Am J Clin Nutr 1982; 35:566–573.

194. Schoeller DA, Ravussin E, Schutz Y, et al. Energy expenditure by doubly labeled water: validation in humans and proposed calculation. Am J Physiol 1986; 250:R823–R830.

195. Welle S, Forbes GB, Statt M, et al. Energy expenditure under free-living conditions in normal-weight and overweight women. Am J Clin Nutr 1992; 14:14–21.

196. Ravussin E. Metabolism differences and the development of obesity. Metabolism 1995; 44:12–14.

197. Ravussin E, Lillioja S, Anderson TE. Determinants of 24-hour energy expenditure in man: methods and results using a respiratory chamber. J Clin Invest 1986; 78:1568–1578.

198. Leibel R, Rosenbaum M, Hirsch J. Changes in energy expenditure resulting from altered body weight. N Engl J Med 1995; 332:621–628.

199. Thorne A. Diet-induced thermogenesis: an experimental study in healthy and obese individuals. Acta Chir Scand 1990; 558:6–59.

200. Blaza S, Garrow JS. Thermogenic response to temperature, exercise and food stimuli in lean and obese women, studied by 24-h direct calorimetry. Br J Nutr 1983; 49:171–180.

201. Ravussin E, Harper I, Rising R, et al. Human obesity is associated with lower levels of physical activity: results from doubly-labelled water and gas exchanges. FASEB J 1991; 5:554A.

202. Segal KR, Gutin B. Thermic effects of food and exercise in lean and obese women. Metabolism 1983; 32:581–589.

203. Astrup A, Buemann B, Toubro S, et al. Low resting metabolic rate in subjects predisposed to obesity: a role for thyroid status. Am J Clin Nutr 1996; 63:879–883.

204. Chua SJ, White D, Wu-Penz Z. Phenotype of fatty due to Gn269 Pro mutation of the leptin receptor. Diabetes 1996; 45:1141–1143.

205. Noben-Trauth K, Naggert J, North M, et al. A candidate for the mouse mutation tubby. Nature 1996; 380:534–538.

206. Bultman S, Michaud E, Woychik R. Molecular characterization of the mouse agouti locus. Cell 1992; 71:1195–1204.

207. Lu D, Willard D, Patel IR, et al. Agouti protein is an antagonist of the melanocyte-stimulating hormone receptor. Nature 1994; 371:799–802.

208. Naggert JK, Fricker LD, Varlamov O, et al. Hyperproinsulinaemia in obese fat/fat mice associated with a carboxypeptidase E mutation which reduces enzyme activity. Nature Genet 1995; 10:134–142.

209. Rimoin DL, Schimke RN. Genetic Disorders of the Endocrine Glands. St. Louis: CV Mosby 1971.

210. Webb T, Clarke D, Hardy CA. A clinical, cytogenetic and molecular study of 40 adults with the Prader Willi syndrome. J Med Genet 1995; 32:181–185.

211. Goldstein JL, Fialkow PJ. The Alström syndrome: report of three cases with further delineation of the clinical, pathophysiological, and genetic aspects of the disorder. Medicine 1973; 52:53–71.

212. Goecke T, Majewski F, Kauther KD, et al. Mental retardation, hypotonia, obesity, ocular, facial, dental, and limb abnormalities (Cohen syndrome): report of three patients. Eur J Pediatr 1982; 138:338–340.

213. Dietz WH Jr, Gross WL, Kirkpatrick JA Jr. Blount disease (tibia vara): another skeletal disorder associated with childhood obesity. J Pediatr 1982; 101:735–737.

214. Gray GA. The inheritance of corpulence. In: Cioffi LA, James WPT, Van Itallie TB, eds. The Body Weight Regulatory System: Normal and Disturbed Mechanisms. New York: Raven; 1981: 185–195.

215. Price RA, Stunkard AJ, Ness R. Childhood onset (age <10) obesity has high familial risk. Int J Obes 1989; 14:185–188.

216. Stunkard AJ, Sorensen TIA, Hanis C, et al. An adoption study of human obesity. N Engl J Med 1986; 314:193–198.

217. Stunkard AJ, Harris JR, Pedersen NL, et al. The body-mass index of twins who have been reared apart. N Engl J Med 1990; 322:1483–1487.

218. Mallick MJ. Health hazards of obesity and weight control in children: a review of the literature. Am J Public Health 1983; 73:78–82.

219. Bouchard O. Genetic factors in obesity. Med Clin North Am 1989; 73:67–81.

220. Bogardus C, Lillioja S, Ravussin E. Genetic effect in resting metabolic rate. N Engl J Med 1986; 315:96–99.

221. Bouchard C, Tremblay A, Nadeau T, et al. Genetic effect in resting and exercise metabolic rates. Metabolism 1989; 38:364–368.

222. Bouchard O, Tremblay A, Despres JP. The response to long-term overfeeding in identical twins. N Engl J Med 1990; 322:1477–1482.

223. Perusse L, Tremblay A, LeBlanc A, et al. Familial resemblance in energy intake: contribution of genetic and environmental factors. Am J Clin Nutr 1988; 47:629–630.

224. Clement K, Garner C, Hager J, et al. Indication for linkage of the human *ob* gene region with extreme obesity. Diabetes 1996; 45:687–690.

225. Gagnon J, Mauriége P, Roy S, et al. The Trp64Arg mutation of the β3-adrenergic receptor gene has no effect on obesity phenotypes in the Québec Family Study and Swedish obese subjects cohorts. J Clin Invest 1996; 98:2086–2093.

226. Sobal J, Stunkard AJ. Socioeconomic status and obesity: a review of the literature. Psychol Bull 1989; 105:260–262.

227. Dietz WH, Gortmaker SL. Do we fatten our children at the television set? Obesity and viewing in children and adolescents. Pediatrics 1985; 75:807–809.

228. Hill JO, Peters JC, Reed GW. Nutrient balance in humans: effects of diet composition. Am J Clin Nutr 1991; 54:10–17.

229. Hill JO, Drougas H, Peters JC. Obesity treatment: can diet composition play a role? Ann Intern Med 1993; 119:694–697.

230. Horton TJ, Drougas H, Brachey A. Fat and carbohydrate overfeeding in humans: different effects on energy storage. Am J Clin Nutr 1995; 62:19–29.

231. Hill JO, Lin D, Yakubu F. Development of dietary obesity in rats: influence of amount and composition of dietary fat. Int J Obes 1992; 16:321–333.

232. Thomas CD, Peters JC, Reed GW. Nutrient balance and energy expenditure during ad libitum feeding of high fat and high carbohydrate diets in humans. Am J Clin Nutr 1992; 55:934–942.

233. Allon N. The stigma of overweight in everyday life. In: Bray GA, ed. Obesity in Perspective. Washington DC: DHEW, 1975: 83–102.

234. Dwyer J, Mayer J. The dismal condition: problems faced by obese adolescent girls in American society. In: Bray GA, ed. Obesity in Perspective. Washington DC: DHEW, 1975: 75–708.

235. Charles SO, Blumberg P. Assessment of psychiatric status among the morbidly obese. Obes Bariatr Med 1982; 11:71–78.

236. McGinnis JM, Foege WH. Actual causes of death in the United States. JAMA 1993; 270:2207–2212.

237. Drenick EJ, Bale GS, Seltzer F. Excessive mortality and causes of death in morbidly obese men. JAMA 1980; 243:443–446.

238. Heald FP. The natural history of obesity. Adv Psychosom Med 1972; 7:102–115.

239. Larsson B, Bjorntorp P, Tibblin G. The health consequences of moderate obesity. Int J Obes 1981; 5:97–116.

240. Walker ARP, Segal I. The puzzle of obesity in the African black female (letter). Lancet 1980; 1:263.

241. Rabinowitz D, Zierler KL. Forearm metabolism in obesity and its response to intraarterial insulin: characterization of insulin resistance and evidence for adaptive hyperinsulinism. J Clin Invest 1962; 41:2173–2176.

242. Kolterman OG, Insel J, Saekow T, et al. Mechanisms of insulin resistance in human obesity: evidence for receptor and postreceptor defects. J Clin Invest 1980; 65:1272–1273.

243. Peiris A, Struve MF, Mueller RA, et al. Glucose metabolism in obesity: influence of body fat distribution. J Clin Endocrinol Metab 1988; 67:760–763.

244. National Diabetes Data Group. Classification and diagnosis of diabetes mellitus and other categories of glucose intolerance. Diabetes 1979; 28:1039–1057.

245. Olefsky JM. Insulin resistance and insulin action: an in vitro and in vivo perspective. Diabetes 1981; 30:148–162.

246. Polonsky KS, Sturis J, Bell GI. Seminars in Medicine of the Beth Israel Hospital, Boston. Non-insulin-dependent diabetes mellitus—a genetically programmed failure of the beta cell to compensate for insulin resistance. N Engl J Med 1996; 334:777–783.

247. Lillioja S, Bogardus C. Obesity and insulin resistance: lessons learned from the Pima Indians. Diabetes Metab Rev 1988; 4:517–540.

248. Ludvik B, Nolan JJ, Baloga J, et al. Effect of obesity on insulin resistance in normal subjects and patients with NIDDM. Diabetes 1995; 44:1121–1125.

249. Campbell PJ, Gerich JE. Impact of obesity on insulin action in volunteers with normal glucose tolerance: demonstration of a threshold for the adverse effect of obesity. J Clin Endocrinol Metab 1990; 70:1114–1118.

250. Kahn CR, White MF. The insulin receptor and the molecular mechanism of insulin action. J Clin Invest 1988; 82:151–156.

251. Cheatham B, Kahn CR. Insulin action and the insulin signaling network. Endocr Rev 1995; 16:117–142.

252. Ciaraldi TP, Kolterman OG, Olefsky JM. Mechanism of the postreceptor defect in insulin action in human obesity: decrease in glucose transport system activity. J Clin Invest 1981; 68:875–880.

253. Hissin PJ, Karnieli E, Simpson IA. A possible mechanism of insulin resistance in the rat adipose cell with high-fat/low-carbohydrate feeding: depletion of intracellular glucose transport systems. Diabetes 1982; 31:589–592.

254. Kahn BB. Glucose transport: pivotal step in insulin action. Diabetes 1996; 45:1644–1654.

255. Prager R, Wallace P, Olefsky JM. In vivo kinetics of insulin action on peripheral glucose disposal and hepatic glucose output in normal and obese subjects. J Clin Invest 1986; 78:472–481.

256. Bougneres PF, Artavia-Loria E, Henry S. Increased basal glucose production and utilization in children with recent obesity versus adults with long-term obesity. Diabetes 1989; 38:477–483.

257. Ferrannini E, Barrett EJ, Bevilacqua S. Effect of fatty acids on glucose production and utilization in man. J Clin Invest 1983; 72:1737–1740.

258. Bjorntorp P. Metabolic implications of body fat distribution. Diabetes Care 1991; 14:1132–1143.

259. Randle PJ, Kerbey AL, Espinal J. Mechanisms decreasing glucose oxidation in diabetes and starvation: role of lipid fuels and hormones. Diabetes Metab Rev 1988; 4:623–638.

260. Rebrin K, Steil GM, Mittelman SD, et al. Causal linkage between insulin suppression of lipolysis and suppression of liver glucose output in dogs. J Clin Invest 1996; 98:741–749.

261. Bevilacqua S, Bonadonna R, Buzzigoli G. Acute elevation of free fatty acid levels leads to hepatic insulin resistance in obese subjects. Metabolism 1987; 36:502–506.

262. Meylan M, Henny C, Temier E. Metabolic factors in the insulin resistance in human obesity. Metabolism 1987; 36:256–260.

263. Hotamisligil GS, Shargill NS, Spiegelman BM. Adipose expression of tumor necrosis factor-alpha: direct role in obesity-linked insulin resistance. Science 1993; 259:87–91.

264. Hotamisligil GS, Peraldi P, Budavari A, et al. IRS-1–mediated inhibition of insulin receptor tyrosine kinase activity in TNF-alpha–and obesity-induced insulin resistance. Science 1996; 271:665–668.

265. Hotamisligil GS, Budavari A, Murray D, et al. Reduced tyrosine kinase activity of the insulin receptor in obesity-diabetes: central role of tumor necrosis factor-alpha. J Clin Invest 1994; 94:1543–1549.

266. Hotamisligil GS, Arner P, Caro JF, et al. Increased adipose tissue expression of tumor necrosis factor-alpha in human obesity and insulin resistance. J Clin Invest 1995; 95:2409–2415.

267. Hotamisligil GS, Murray DL, Choy LN, et al. Tumor necrosis factor alpha inhibits signaling from the insulin receptor. Proc Natl Acad Sci USA 1994; 91:4854–4858.

268. Baron AD, Steinberg HO, Chaker H, et al. Insulin-mediated skeletal muscle vasodilation contributes to both insulin sensitivity and responsiveness in lean humans. J Clin Invest 1995; 96:786–792.

269. Baron AD. The coupling of glucose metabolism and perfusion in human skeletal muscle: the potential role of endothelium-derived nitric oxide. Diabetes 1996; 45:S105–S109.

270. Laakso M, Edelman SV, Brechtel G, et al. Decreased effect of insulin to stimulate skeletal muscle blood flow in obese man. J Clin Invest 1990; 85:1844–1852.

271. Steinberg HO, Chaker H, Leaming R, et al. Obesity/insulin resistance is associated with endothelial dysfunction: implications for the syndrome of insulin resistance. J Clin Invest 1996; 97:2601–2610.

272. Polonsky KS, Given BD, Hirsch L, et al. Quantitative study of insulin secretion and clearance in normal and obese subjects. J Clin Invest 1988; 81:435–441.

273. Polonsky KS, Given BD, Van Cauter E. Twenty-four–hour profiles and pulsatile patterns of insulin secretion in normal and obese subjects. J Clin Invest 1988; 81:442–448.

274. Nehus SJ, Heyden S, Hansen JP. Lipoprotein and blood pressure changes during weight reduction at Duke's Dietary Rehabilitation Clinic. Ann Nutr Metab 1982; 26:384–392.

275. Wolf RN, Grundy SM. Influence of weight reduction on plasma lipoproteins in obese patients. Arteriosclerosis 1983; 3:160–169.

276. Grundy SM, Mok HYI, Zech L. Transport of very low density lipoprotein triglycerides in varying degrees of obesity and hypertriglyceridemia. J Clin Invest 1979; 63:1274–1276.

277. Equsa G, Beltz WF, Grundy SM. Influence of obesity on metabolism of apolipoprotein B in humans. J Clin Invest 1985; 76:596–600.

278. Jackson TK, Sahalnick AI, Elovson J, et al. Insulin regulates apolipoprotein B turnover and phosphorylation in rat hepatocytes. J Clin Invest 1990; 86:1746–1750.

279. Peeples LH, Carpenter JW, Israel RG. Alterations in low-density lipoproteins in subjects with abdominal adiposity. Metabolism 1989; 38:1029–1036.

280. Ostlund REJ, Staten M, Kohrt WM. The ratio of waist-to-hip circumference, plasma insulin level, and glucose intolerance as independent predictors of the HDL2 cholesterol level in older adults. N Engl J Med 1990; 322:229–234.

281. Vague P, Juhan-Vague I, Chabert V. Fat distribution and plasminogen activator inhibitor activity in nondiabetic obese women. Metabolism 1989; 38:913–915.

282. Vaughan RW, Conahan TJ. Cardiopulmonary consequences of morbid obesity. Life Sci 1980; 26:2119–2127.

283. MacMahon SW, Wilcken DEL, MacDonald GJ. The effect of weight reduction on left ventricular mass: a randomized controlled trial in young overweight hypertensive patients. N Engl J Med 1986; 314:334–339.

284. Tuck ML, Sowers J, Dornfeld L. The effect of weight reduction on blood pressure, plasma renin activity and plasma aldosterone levels in obese patients. N Engl J Med 1981; 304:930–933.

285. Goldring D, Hernandez A, Choi S. Blood pressure in a high school population. II: Clinical profile of the juvenile hypertensive. J Pediatr 1979; 95:298–304.

286. Messerli FH, Ventura HO, Reisin E. Borderline hypertension and obesity: two prehypertensive states with elevated cardiac output. Circulation 1982; 66:55–60.

287. Sowers JR, Whitfield LA, Beck FW. Role of enhanced sympathetic nervous system activity and reduced Na⁺,K⁺-dependent adenosine triphosphatase activity in maintenance of elevated blood pressure in obesity: effects of weight loss. Clin Sci 1982; 63:121s–124s.

288. Landsberg L, Krieger DR. Obesity, metabolism, and the sympathetic nervous system. Am J Hypertens 1989; 2:125S–132S.

289. Reaven GM, Lithell H, Landsberg L. Hypertension and associated metabolic abnormalities—the role of insulin resistance and the sympathoadrenal system. N Engl J Med 1996; 334:374–381.

290. Rocchini AP, Key J, Bondie D. The effect of weight loss on the sensitivity of blood pressure to sodium in obese adolescents. N Engl J Med 1989; 321:580–585.

291. Kaplan NM. The deadly quartet: upper-body obesity, glucose intolerance, hypertriglyceridemia, and hypertension. Arch Intern Med 1989; 149:1514–1520.

292. DeFronzo RA, Ferrannini E. Insulin resistance: a multifaceted syndrome responsible for NIDDM, obesity, hypertension, dyslipidemia, and atherosclerotic cardiovascular disease. Diabetes Care 1991; 14:173–176.

293. Reaven GM. Insulin resistance, hyperinsulinemia, hypertriglyceridemia and hypertension: parallels between human disease and rodent models. Diabetes Care 1991; 14:195–200.

294. Skott P, Hother-Nielsen O, Bruun NE. Effect of insulin on kidney function and sodium excretion in healthy subjects. Diabetologia 1989; 32:694–700.

295. Luce JM. Respiratory complications of obesity. Chest 1980; 78:626–631.

296. Block AJ, Boysen PG, Wynne JW. Sleep apnea, hypopnea and oxygen desaturation in normal subjects: a strong male predominance. N Engl J Med 1979; 300:513–517.

297. Grundy SM. Mechanism of cholesterol gallstones formation. Semin Liver Dis 1983; 3:97–111.

298. Smith PL, Gold AR, Meyers DA. Weight loss in mildly to moderately obese patients with obstructive sleep apnea. Ann Intern Med 1985; 103:850–855.

299. Horton ES, Danforth EJ, Sims EAH. Endocrine and metabolic alterations in spontaneous and experimental obesity. In: Bray GA, ed. Obesity in Perspective. Washington DC: DHEW, 1975; 323–334.

300. Prowse K, Allen MB. Sleep apnea. Br J Dis Chest 1989; 82:329–331.

301. Charuzi I, Ovnat A, Peiser J. The effect of surgical weight reduction on sleep quality in obesity-related sleep apnea syndrome. Surgery 1985; 97:535–540.

302. Maclure KM, Hayes KC, Colditz GA, et al. Weight, diet, and the risk of symptomatic gallstones in middle-aged women. N Engl J Med 1989; 321:563–567.

303. Sims EAH. Experimental obesity, dietary-induced thermogenesis, and their clinical implications. J Clin Endocrinol Metab 1976; 5:377–395.

304. Sims EAH, Danforth EJ, Horton ES. Endocrine and metabolic effects of experimental obesity in man. Recent Prog Horm Res 1973; 29:457–496.

305. Glass AR. Endocrine aspects of obesity. Med Clin North Am 1989; 73:139–160.

306. Inoue S, Bray GA, Mullen YS. Transplantation of pancreatic B-cells prevents development of hypothalamic obesity in rats. Am J Physiol 1978; 235:E266–E271.

307. Bray GA, Gallagher TF. Manifestations of hypothalamic obesity in man: a comprehensive investigation of eight patients and a review of the literature. Medicine 1975; 54:301–330.

308. Elahi D, Nagulesparan M, Hershcopf RJ, et al. Feedback inhibition of insulin secretion by insulin: relation to the hyperinsulinemia of obesity. N Engl J Med 1982; 306:1196–1202.

309. Stark AAR, Erhardt G, Berger M. Elevated pancreatic glucagon in obesity. Diabetes 1984; 33:277–280.

310. Malewiak MI, Griglio S, Kalopissis AD. Oleate metabolism in isolated hepatocytes from lean and obese Zucker rats: influence of a high fat diet and in vivo response to glucagon. Metabolism 1983; 32:661–668.

311. Lassmann V, Vague P, Vialettes B. Low plasma levels of pancreatic polypeptide in obesity. Diabetes 1980; 29:428–430.

312. Boden G, Baile CA, McLaughlin CL. Effects of starvation and obesity on somatostatin, insulin, and glucagon release from an isolated perfused organ system. Am J Physiol 1981; 241:E215–E220.

313. Voyles NR, Awoke S, Wade A, et al. Starvation increases gastrointestinal somatostatin in normal and obese Zucker rats: a possible regulatory mechanism. Horm Metab Res 1982; 14:392–395.

314. Sasaki H, Nagulesparan M, Dubois A, et al. Hyperinsulinemia in obesity: lack of relation to gastric emptying of glucose solution or to plasma somatostatin levels. Metabolism 1983; 32:701–705.

315. Jung RT, Shetty PS, James WPT. Nutritional effects on thyroid and catecholamine metabolism. Clin Sci 1980; 58:183–191.

316. Glass AR, Kushner J. Obesity, nutrition, and the thyroid. Endocrinologist 1996; 6:392–403.

317. Danforth EJ, Horton ES, O'Connell M. Dietary-induced alterations in thyroid hormone metabolism during overnutrition. J Clin Invest 1979; 64:1336–1347.

318. Azizi F. Effect of dietary composition on fasting-induced changes in serum thyroid hormones and thyrotropin. Metabolism 1978; 27:935–942.

319. Carlson HF, Drenick EJ, Chopra IJ. Alterations in basal and TRH-stimulated serum levels of thyrotropin, prolactin, and thyroid hormones in starved obese men. J Clin Endocrinol Metab 1977; 45:707–713.

320. Wilcox RG. Triiodothyronine, TSH, and prolactin in obese women. Lancet 1977; 1:1027–1029.

321. Burman KD, Latham KR, Djuh YY. Solubilized nuclear thyroid hormone receptors in circulating human mononuclear cells. J Clin Endocrinol Metab 1980; 51:106–116.

322. Guernsey DI, Morishige WK. Na⁺ pump activity and nuclear T₃ receptors in tissues of genetically obese (ob/ob) mice. Metabolism 1979; 28:629–632.

323. Crapo I. Cushing's syndrome: a review of diagnostic tests. Metabolism 1979; 28:955–977.

324. Zelissen PM, Koppeschaar HP, Erkelens DW. Beta-endorphin and adrenocortical function in obesity. Clin Endocrinol (Oxf) 1991; 35:369–372.

325. Reincke M, Nieke J, Krestin GP, et al. Preclinical Cushing's syndrome in adrenal "incidentalomas": comparison with adrenal Cushing's syndrome. J Clin Endocrinol Metab 1992; 75:826–832.

326. Eddy RI, Jones AL, Gilliland PF, et al. Cushing's syndrome: a prospective study of diagnostic methods. Am J Med 1973; 55:621–630.

327. Biemond P, de Jong FH, Lamberts SWJ. Continuous dexamethasone infusion for seven hours in patients with the Cushing syndrome: a superior differential diagnostic test. Ann Intern Med 1990; 112:738–742.

328. Abou Samra AB, Dechaud H, Estour B, et al. Lipotropin and cortisol response to an intravenous infusion dexamethasone suppression test in Cushing syndrome and obesity. J Clin Endocrinol Metab 1985; 61:116–119.

329. Pasquali R, Cantobelli S, Casimirri F, et al. The hypothalamic-pituitary-adrenal axis in obese women with different patterns of body fat distribution. J Clin Endocrinol Metab 1993; 77:341–346.

330. Clearly MP. Antiobesity effect of dehydroepiandrosterone in the Zucker rat, hormones, thermogenesis, and obesity. In: Lardy H, Stratman F, eds. New York: Elsevier, 1989: 365–370.

331. Lopez SA, Krehl WA. A possible interrelation between glucose-6-phosphate

dehydrogenase and dehydroepiandrosterone in obesity. Lancet 1967; 2:485–490.

332. Kurtz BR, Givens JR, Komindr S. Maintenance of normal circulating levels of 4-androstenedione and dehydroepidandrosterone in simple obesity despite increased metabolic clearance rates: evidence for a servo-control mechanism. J Clin Endocrinol Metab 1987; 64:1261–1265.

333. Usiskin KS, Butterworth S, Clore JN, et al. Lack of effect of dehydroepiandrosterone in obese men. Int J Obes 1990; 14:457–460.

334. Yoshida T, Kemnitz JW, Bray GA. Lateral hypothalamic lesions and norepinephrine turnover in rats. J Clin Invest 1983; 79:919–927.

335. Jung RT, Shetty PS, James WPT. Plasma catecholamines and autonomic responsiveness in obesity. Int J Obes 1982; 6:131–141.

336. Gustafson AB, Kalkhoff RK. Influence of sex and obesity on plasma catecholamine response to isometric exercise. J Clin Endocrinol Metab 1982; 55:703–708.

337. O'Hare JA, Minaker KL, Meneilly GS, et al. Effect of insulin on plasma norepinephrine and 3,4-dihydroxyphenylalanine in obese men. Metabolism 1989; 38:322–329.

338. Glass AR, Swerdloff RS, Bray GA. Low serum testosterone and sex-hormone-binding-globulin in massively obese men. J Clin Endocrinol Metab 1977; 45:1211–1219.

339. Plymate SR, Matej LA, Jones RE, et al. Inhibition of sex hormone–binding globulin production in the human hepatoma (Hep G2) cell line by insulin and prolactin. J Clin Endocrinol Metab 1988; 67:460–464.

340. Schneider G, Kirschner MA, Berkowitz R. Increased estrogen production in obese men. J Clin Endocrinol Metab 1979; 48:633–638.

341. Strain GW, Zumoff B, Kream J. Mild hyogonadotropic hypogonadism in obese men. Metabolism 1982; 21:871–875.

342. Stanik S, Dornfeld LP, Maxwell MH. The effect of weight loss on reproductive hormones in obese men. J Clin Endocrinol Metab 1981; 53:828–832.

343. Hartz AJ, Barboriak PN, Wong A. The association of obesity with infertility and related menstrual abnormalities in women. Int J Obes 1979; 3:57–60.

344. Kirschner MA, Samojlik E, Drejka M. Androgen-estrogen metabolism in women with upper body versus lower body obesity. J Clin Endocrinol Metab 1990; 70:473–479.

345. Kopelman PG, Pilkington TRE, White N. Abnormal sex steroid secretion and binding in massively obese women. Clin Endocrinol 1980; 12:363–369.

346. Glass AR, Dahms WT, Abraham G. Secondary amenorrhea in obesity: etiologic role of weight-related androgen excess. Fertil Steril 1978; 30:243–244.

347. Clark AM, Ledger W, Galletly C, et al. Weight loss results in significant improvement in pregnancy and ovulation rates in anovulatory obese women. Hum Reprod 1995; 10:2705–2712.

348. Dunaif A, Xia J, Book CB, et al. Excessive insulin receptor serine phosphorylation in cultured fibroblasts and in skeletal muscle: a potential mechanism for insulin resistance in the polycystic ovary syndrome. J Clin Invest 1995; 96:801–810.

349. Dunaif A, Scott D, Finegood D, et al. The insulin-sensitizing agent troglitazone improves metabolic and reproductive abnormalities in the polycystic ovary syndrome. J Clin Endocrinol Metab 1996; 81:3299–3306.

350. Dunaif A, Green G, Phelps RG, et al. Acanthosis nigricans, insulin action, and hyperandrogenism: clinical, histological, and biochemical findings. J Clin Endocrinol Metab 1991; 73:590–595.

351. Evans DJ, Hoffman RG, Kalkhoff RK. Relationship of androgenic activity to body fat topography, fat cell morphology, and metabolic aberrations in premenopausal women. J Clin Endocrinol Metab 1983; 57:304–308.

352. O'Dea JPK, Wieland RG, Hallberg MC. Effect of dietary weight loss on sex steroid binding, sex steroids, and gonadotropins in obese postmenopausal women. J Lab Clin Med 1979; 93:1004–1008.

353. Zumoff B, Strain GW, Kream J. Obese young men have elevated plasma estrogen levels but obese premenopausal women do not. Metabolism 1981; 30:1011–1014.

354. Edman CD, MacDonald PC. Effect of obesity on conversion of plasma androstenedione to estrone in ovulatory and anovulatory young women. Am J Obstet Gynecol 1978; 130:456–461.

355. Cooper SC, Roncari DA. 17-Beta-estradiol increases mitogenic activity of medium from cultured preadipocytes of massively obese persons. J Clin Invest 1989; 83:1925–1929.

356. Meistas MT, Foster GV, Margolis S. Integrated concentrations of growth hormone, insulin, C-peptide and prolactin in human obesity. Metabolism 1982; 31:1224–1228.

357. Phillips LS, Vassilopoulou-Sellin R. Somatomedins. N Engl J Med 1980; 302:371–380, 438–446.

358. Frystyk J, Vestbo E, Skjaerbaek C, et al. Free insulin-like growth factors in human obesity. Metabolism 1995; 44:37–44.

359. Cordido F, Casanueva FF, Dieguez C. Cholinergic receptor activation by pyridostigmine restores growth hormone (GH) responsiveness to GH-releasing hormone administration in obese subjects: evidence for hypothalamic somatostatinergic participation in the blunted GH release of obesity. J Clin Endocrinol Metab 1989; 68:290–293.

360. Procopio M, Maccario M, Grottoli S, et al. Short-term fasting in obesity fails to restore the blunted GH responsiveness to GH-releasing hormone alone or combined with arginine. Clin Endocrinol 1995; 43:665–669.

361. Jung RT, Campbell RG, James WPT. Altered hypothalamic and sympathetic responses to hypoglycemia in familial obesity. Lancet 1982; 1:1043–1046.

362. Drenick EJ, Carlson HE, Robertson GL. The role of vasopressin and prolactin in abnormal salt and water metabolism of obese patients before and after fasting and during refeeding. Metabolism 1977; 26:309–317.

363. Drenick EJ. The prognosis of conventional treatment in severe obesity. In: Bjorntorp P, Cairella M, Howard AN, eds. Recent Advances in Obesity Research: III. London: John Libbey, 1981: 80–84.

364. Bray GA. Effect of caloric restriction on energy expenditure in obese patients. Lancet 1969; 2:397–398.

365. Joffe SN. Surgical management of morbid obesity. Gut 1981; 22:242–254.

366. Freeman JB, Burchett H. Failure rate with gastric partitioning for morbid obesity. Am J Surg 1983; 145:113–119.

367. Atkinson RL. Low and very low calorie diets. Med Clin North Am 1989; 73:203–215.

368. Bray GA, Gray DS. Treatment of obesity: an overview. Diabetes Metab Rev 1988; 4:653–679.

369. Runcie J, Hilditch TE. Energy provision, tissue utilization, and weight loss in prolonged starvation. Br Med J 1974; 2:352–356.

370. Yang MU, Van Itallie TB. Composition of weight lost during short-term weight reduction: metabolic responses of obese subjects to starvation and low-calorie ketogenic and nonketogenic diets. J Clin Invest 1976; 58:722–730.

371. Passmore R, Strong JA, Ritchie FJ. The chemical composition of the tissue lost by obese patients on a reducing regimen. Br J Nutr 1958; 12:113–122.

372. Drenick EJ, Johnson D. Weight reduction by fasting and semistarvation in morbid obesity: long-term follow-up. Int J Obes 1978; 2:123–132.

373. Amatruda JM. Very low calorie diets for the treatment of simple and complicated obesity. Endocrinologist 1991; 1:171–175.

374. Bogardus C, LaGrange BM, Horton ES. Comparison of carbohydrate-containing and carbohydrate-restricted hypocaloric diets in the treatment of obesity: endurance and metabolic fuel homeostasis during strenuous exercise. J Clin Invest 1981; 63:399–404.

375. Howard AN. The historical development, efficacy and safety of very low calorie diets. Int J Obes 1981; 5:195–208.

376. Isner JM, Sours HE, Paris AL. Sudden, unexpected death in avid dieters using the liquid-protein-modified-fast diet: observations in 17 patients and the role of the prolonged QT interval. Circulation 1979; 60:1401–1412.

377. Sours HE, Frattali VP, Brand CD. Sudden death associated with very low calorie weight reduction regimens. Am J Clin Nutr 1981; 34:453–461.

378. Latigua RA, Amatruda JM, Biddle TL. Cardiac arrhythmias associated with a liquid protein diet for the treatment of obesity. N Engl J Med 1980; 303:735–738.

379. Vertes V, Genuth SM, Hazelton IM. Supplemented fasting as a large-scale outpatient program. JAMA 1977; 238:2151–2153.

380. Genuth SM, Vertes V, Hazelton IM. Supplemented fasting in the treatment of obesity. In: Bray GA, ed. Recent Advances in Obesity Research. II. Westport, CT: Food and Nutrition Press, 1978: 370–378.

381. Broomfield PH, Chopra R, Sheinbaum RC. Effects of ursodeoxycholic acid and aspirin on the formation of lithogenic bile and gallstone during loss of weight. N Engl J Med 1988; 319:1567–1570.

382. Pavloe KN, Krey S, Steffee WP. Exercise as an adjunct to weight loss and maintenance in moderately obese subjects. Am J Clin Nutr 1989; 49:1115–1120.

383. Rodin J, Wing RR. Behavioral factors in obesity. Diabetes Metab Rev 1988; 4:701–725.

384. Brownell KD, Kramer FM. Behavioral management of obesity. Med Clin North Am 1989; 73:185–201.

385. Stunkard AJ, Penick SB. Behavioral modification in the treatment of obesity: the problem of maintaining weight loss. Arch Gen Psychiatry 1979; 36:801–806.

386. Stunkard AJ, Craighead LW, O'Brien R. Controlled trial of behaviour therapy, pharmacotherapy, and their combination in the treatment of obesity. Lancet 1980; 2:1045–1047.

387. Passmore R, Durnin JVGA. Human energy expenditure. Physiol Rev 1955; 35:801–840.

388. Hanefeld M, Zschornack M, Weck M. Physical training in obese subjects: selection, motivation, organization and follow-up problems. In: Bjorntorp P, Cairella M, Howard AN, eds. Recent Advances in Obesity Research. III. London: John Libbey, 1981: 290–294.

389. Foss ML. Exercise prescription and training programs for obese subjects. In: Bjorntorp P, Cairella M, Howard AN, eds. Recent Advances in Obesity Research. III. London: John Libbey, 1981: 307–314.

390. Phinney SF, La Grange BM, O'Connell M. Effects of aerobic exercise on energy expenditure and nitrogen balance during very low calorie dieting. Metabolism 1988; 37:758–764.

391. Kukkonen K, Rauramaa R, Siitonen O. Physical training of obese middle-aged persons. Ann Clin Res 1982; 14:80–85.

392. Krotkiewski M, Mandroukas K, Sjostrom L. Effects of long-term physical training on body fat, metabolism, and blood pressure in obesity. Metabolism 1979; 28:650–658.

393. Segal KR, Pi-Sunyer FX. Exercise and obesity. Med Clin North Am 1989; 73:217–236.

394. Bray GA. Barriers to the treatment of obesity. Ann Intern Med 1991; 115:152–153.

395. Munroe JF. General principles of drug therapy in obesity. In: Bjorntorp P, Cairella M, Howard AN, eds. Recent Advances in Obesity Research III. London: John Libbey, 1981: 180–183.

396. Guy-Grand B. Clinical studies with dexfenfluramine: from past to future. Obes Res 1995; 4:491S–496S.

397. Garattini S. Biological actions of drugs affecting serotonin and eating. Obes Res 1995; 4:463S–470S.
398. Atkinson RL, Hubbard VS. Report on the NIH workshop on pharmacologic treatment of obesity. Am J Clin Nutr 1994; 60:153–156.
399. Weintraub M, Sundaresan PR, Madan M, et al. Long-term weight control study I (weeks 0–34). Clin Pharmacol Ther 1992; 51:586–594.
400. Weintraub M, Sundaresan PR, Shuster B, et al. Long-term weight control study II (weeks 34–104). Clin Pharmacol Ther 1992; 51:595–601.
401. Connolly HM, Crary JL, McGoon MD, et al. Valvular heart disease associated with fenfluramine-phentermine. N Engl J Med 1997; 337:581–588.
402. Abenhaim L, Moride Y, Brenot F, et al. Appetite-suppressant drugs and the risk of primary pulmonary hypertension. N Engl J Med 1996; 1121:609–616.
403. Manson JE, Faich GA. Pharmacotherapy for obesity—do the benefits outweigh the risks? N Engl J Med 1996; 335:609–616.
404. Koppeschaar HP, Meinders AE, Schwarz F. Metabolic responses in grossly obese subjects treated with a very-low-calorie diet with and without triiodothyronine treatment. Int J Obes 1983; 7:133–141.
405. Glueck CJ, Hastings MM, Allen C. Sucrose polyester and covert caloric dilution. Am J Clin Nutr 1982; 1352–1359.
406. DeGraaf C, Hulshof T, Weststrate JA, et al. Nonabsorbable fat (sucrose polyester) and the regulation of energy intake and body weight. Am J Physiol 1996; 270:R1386–R1393.
407. Snyder DK, Clemmons DR, Underwood LE. Dietary carbohydrate content determines responsiveness to growth in energy-restricted humans. J Clin Endocrinol Metab 1989; 69:745–752.
408. Rudman D, Feller AG, Nagraj HS. Effects of human growth hormone in men over 60 years old. N Engl J Med 1990; 323:1–6.
409. Richelsen B, Pedersen SB, Borglum JD, et al. Growth hormone treatment of obese women for 5 wk: effect on body composition and adipose tissue LPL activity. Am J Physiol 1994; 266:E211–E216.
410. Gaspar MR, Movus HJH, Rosental JJ. Comparison of Payne and Scott operations for morbid obesity. Ann Surg 1976; 184:507–515.
411. Maxwell JD, McGouran RC. Jejuno-ileal bypass: clinical and experimental aspects. Scand J Gastroenterol 1982; 17:129–147.
412. Halverson JD, Wise I, Wazna MF. Jejunoileal bypass for morbid obesity: a critical appraisal. Am J Med 1978; 64:461–475.
413. Hocking MP, Duerson MC, O'Leary JP. Jejunoileal bypass for morbid obesity: late follow-up in 100 cases. N Engl J Med 1983; 308:995–999.
414. Kral JG. Surgical treatment of obesity. Med Clin North Am 1989; 73:251–264.
415. NIH Consensus Development Panel. National Institutes of Health Consensus Development Conference Statement. Gastrointestinal Surgery for Severe Obesity. Ann Intern Med 1991; 115:956–961.
416. Mason EE, Printen KJ, Hartford CE. Optimizing results of gastric bypass. Ann Surg 1975; 182:405–414.
417. Griffen WO, Young VS, Stevenson CC. A prospective comparison of gastric and jejunoileal by pass procedures for morbid obesity. Ann Surg 1977; 186:500–509.
418. Alden JF. Gastric and jejunoileal by pass: a comparison in the treatment of morbid obesity. Arch Surg 1977; 112:799–806.
419. Benotti PN, Forse RA. The role of gastric surgery in the multidisciplinary management of severe obesity. Am J Surg 1995; 169:361–367.
420. Pories WJ, Swanson MS, MacDonald KG, et al. Who would have thought it? An operation proves to be the most effective therapy for adult-onset diabetes mellitus. Ann Surg 1995; 222:350–352.

Anorexia Nervosa–Bulimia Nervosa

421. Lucas AR. Toward the understanding of anorexia nervosa as a disease entity. Mayo Clin Proc 1981; 56:254–264.
422. Berkman JM. Anorexia nervosa, anorexia, inanition, and low basal metabolic rate. Am J Med Sci 1930; 180:411–424.
423. Crisp AH, Palmer RL, Kalucy RS. How common is anorexia nervosa? A prevalence study. Br J Psychiatry 1976; 128:549–554.
424. Ballot NS, Delaney NE, Erskine PJ, et al. Anorexia nervosa—a prevalence study. S Afr Med J 1981; 59:992–993.
425. Lucas AR, Beard CM, O'Fallon WM, et al. Anorexia nervosa in Rochester, Minnesota: a 45-year study. Mayo Clin Proc 1988; 63:433–442.
426. Button EJ, Whitehouse A. Subclinical anorexia nervosa. Psychol Med 1981; 11:509–516.
427. Ben-Tovim DI, Subbiah N, Scheutz B, et al. Bulimia: symptoms and syndromes in an urban population. Aust NZ J Psychiatry 1989; 23:73–80.
428. Herzog DB, Copeland PM. Bulimia nervosa—psyche and satiety. N Engl J Med 1988; 319:716–718.
429. Feighner JP, Robins E, Guze SB, et al. Diagnostic criteria for use in psychiatric research. Arch Gen Psychiatry 1972; 26:57–63.
430. Woodside DB. A review of anorexia nervosa and bulimia nervosa. Curr Probl Pediatr 1995; 25:67–89.
431. Halmi KA. Anorexia nervosa: recent investigations. Annu Rev Med 1978; 29:137–148.
432. Drossman DA, Ontjes DA, Heizer WD. Anorexia nervosa. Gastroenterology 1979; 77:1115–1131.
433. Crisp AH, Hsu LKG, Harding B, et al. Clinical features of anorexia nervosa. A study of a consecutive series of 102 female patients. J Psychosom Res 1980; 24:179–191.
434. Schwabe AD, Lippe BM, Chang RJ, et al. Anorexia nervosa. Ann Intern Med 1981; 94:371–381.
435. Herzog DB, Copeland PM. Eating disorders. N Engl J Med 1985; 313:295–303.
436. Zerbe KJ. Anorexia nervosa and bulimia nervosa: when pursuit of bodily 'perfection' becomes a killer. Postgrad Med 1996; 99:161–164; 167–169.
437. Crago M, Shisslak CM, Estes LS. Eating disturbances among American minority groups: a review. Int J Eat Disord 1996; 19:239–248.
438. Halmi KA. Anorexia nervosa: demographic and clinical features in 94 cases. Psychosom Med 1974; 36:18–26.
439. Beumont PJV, Chambers TL, Rouse L, et al. The diet composition and nutritional knowledge of patients with anorexia nervosa. J Hum Nutr 1981; 35:265–273.
440. Hsu LKG. Is there a disturbance in body image in anorexia nervosa? J Nerv Ment Dis 1982; 170:305–307.
441. Rosen JC, Reiter J, Orosan P. Assessment of body image in eating disorders with the body dysmorphic disorder examination. Behav Res Ther 1995; 33:77–84.
442. Strober M, Goldenberg I, Green J, et al. Body image disturbance in anorexia nervosa during the acute and recuperative phase. Psychol Med 1979; 9:695–701.
443. Ben-Tovim DI, Whitehead J, Crisp AH. A controlled study of the perception of body width in anorexia nervosa. J Psychosom Res 1979; 23:267–272.
444. Garfinkel PE, Moldofsky H, Garner DM. The stability of perceptual disturbances in anorexia nervosa. Psychol Med 1979; 9:703–708.
445. Garner DM. Body image in anorexia nervosa. Can J Psychiatry 1981; 26:224–227.
446. Halmi KA, Goldberg SC, Eckert E, et al. Pretreatment evaluation in anorexia nervosa. In: Vigersky RA, ed. Anorexia Nervosa. New York: Raven, 1977: 43–54.
447. Holt S, Ford MJ, Grant S, et al. Abnormal gastric emptying in primary anorexia nervosa. Br J Psychiatry 1981; 139:550–552.
448. Saul SH, Dekker A, Watson CG. Acute gastric dilatation with infarction and perforation. Report of fatal outcome in patient with anorexia nervosa. Gut 1981; 22:978–983.
449. Vigersky RA, Loriaux DL. Anorexia nervosa as a model of hypothalamic dysfunction. In: Vigersky RA, ed. Anorexia Nervosa. New York: Raven, 1977: 109–121.
450. Fagher B, Monti M, Theander S. Microcalorimetric study of muscle and platelet thermogenesis in anorexia nervosa and bulimia. Am J Clin Nutr 1989; 49:476–481.
451. Luck P, Wakeling A. Increased cutaneous vasoreactivity to cold in anorexia nervosa. Clin Sci 1981; 61:559–567.
452. Mayo-Smith W, Hayes CW, Biller BM, et al. Body fat distribution measured with CT: correlations in healthy subjects, patients with anorexia nervosa, and patients with Cushing syndrome. Radiology 1989; 170:515–518.
453. Meyers DG, Starke H, Pearson PH, et al. Leaflet to left ventricular size disproportion and prolapse of a structurally normal mitral valve in anorexia nervosa. Am J Cardiol 1987; 60:911–914.
454. de Simone G, Scalfi L, Galderisi M, et al. Cardiac abnormalities in young women with anorexia nervosa. Br Heart J 1994; 71:287–292.
455. Patchell RA, Fellows HA, Humphries LL. Neurologic complications of anorexia nervosa. Acta Neurol Scand 1994; 89:111–116.
456. Silverman JA. Anorexia nervosa: clinical and metabolic observations in a successful treatment plan. In: Vigersky RA, ed. Anorexia Nervosa. New York: Raven, 1977: 331–339.
457. Neims DM, McNeil J, Giles TR, et al. Incidence of laxative abuse in community and bulimic populations: a descriptive review. Int J Eat Disord 1995; 17:211–228.
458. Russell G. Bulimia nervosa: an ominous variant of anorexia nervosa. Psychol Med 1979; 9:429–448.
459. Mitchell JE, Pyle RL, Eckert ED. Frequency and duration of binge-eating episodes in patients with bulimia. Am J Psychiatry 1981; 138:835–836.
460. Palmer RL. The dietary chaos syndrome: a useful new term? Br J Med Psychol 1979; 52:187–190.
461. Mitchell JE, Seim HC, Colon E, et al. Medical complications and medical management of bulimia. Ann Intern Med 1987; 107:71–77.
462. Crisp AH, Hsu LKG, Harding B. The starving hoarder and voracious spender: stealing in anorexia nervosa. J Psychosom Res 1980; 24:225–231.
463. Herzog DB. Bulimia: the secretive syndrome. Psychosomatics 1982; 23:481–487.
464. Newman MM, Halmi KA. The endocrinology of anorexia nervosa and bulimia nervosa. Endocrinol Metab Clin North Am 1988; 17:195–212.
465. Chami TN, Andersen AE, Crowell MD, et al. Gastrointestinal symptoms in bulimia nervosa: effects of treatment. Am J Gastroenterol 1995; 90:88–92.
466. Greenfield D, Mickley D, Quinlan DM, et al. Hypokalemia in outpatients with eating disorders. Am J Psychiatry 1995; 152:60–63.
467. Levy AB, Dixon KN, Stern SL. How are depression and bulimia related? Am J Psychiatry 1989; 146:162–169.
468. Thiel A, Broocks A, Ohlmeier M, et al. Obsessive-compulsive disorder among patients with anorexia nervosa and bulimia nervosa. Am J Psychiatry 1995; 152:72–75.
469. Robb ND, Smith BG, Geidrys-Leeper E. The distribution of erosion in the dentitions of patients with eating disorders. Br Dent J 1995; 178:171–175.
470. Myers TJ, Perkerson MD, Witter BA, et al. Hematologic findings in anorexia nervosa. Conn Med 1981; 45:14–17.

471. Bhanji S, Mattingly D. Anorexia nervosa: some observations on "dieters" and "vomiters," cholesterol and carotene. Br J Psychiatry 1981; 139:238–241.

472. Mordasini R, Klose G, Greten H. Secondary type II hyperlipoproteinemia in patients with anorexia nervosa. Metabolism 1978; 27:71–79.

473. Nestel PJ. Cholesterol metabolism in anorexia nervosa and hypercholesterolemia. J Clin Endocrinol Metab 1974; 38:325–328.

474. Lamon-Fava S, Fisher EC, Nelson ME, et al. Effect of exercise and menstrual cycle status on plasma lipids, low density lipoprotein particle size, and apolipoproteins. J Clin Endocrinol Metab 1989; 68:17–21.

475. Wyatt RJ, Farrell M, Berry PL, et al. Reduced alternative complement pathway control protein levels in anorexia nervosa: response to parenteral alimentation. Am J Clin Nutr 1982; 35:973–980.

476. Pertschuk MJ, Crosby LO, Barot L, et al. Immunocompetency in anorexia nervosa. Am J Clin Nutr 1982; 35:968–972.

477. George GCW. Anorexia nervosa with herpes simplex encephalitis. Postgrad Med J 1981; 57:366–367.

478. Bowers TK, Eckert E. Leukopenia in anorexia nervosa. Lack of increased risk of infection. Arch Intern Med 1978; 138:1520–1523.

479. Gold PW, Kaye W, Robertson GL, et al. Abnormalities in plasma and cerebrospinal-fluid arginine vasopressin in patients with anorexia nervosa. N Engl J Med 1983; 308:1117–1123.

480. Nishita JK, Ellinwood EH Jr, Rockwell WJ, et al. Abnormalities in the response of plasma arginine vasopressin during hypertonic saline infusion in patients with eating disorders. Biol Psychiatry 1989; 26:73–86.

481. Gwirtsman HE, Kaye WH, George DT, et al. Hypermylasemia and its relationship to binge-purge episodes: development of a clinically relevant laboratory test. J Clin Psychiatry 1989; 50:196–204.

482. Casper RC, Kirschner B, Sandstead HH, et al. An evaluation of trace metals, vitamins, and taste function in anorexia nervosa. Am J Clin Nutr 1980; 33:1801–1808.

483. Levy AB. Neuroendocrine profile in bulimia nervosa. Biol Psychiatry 1989; 25:98–109.

484. Fries H. Studies on secondary amenorrhea, anorectic behavior, and body-image perception: importance for the early recognition of anorexia nervosa. In: Vigersky RA, ed. Anorexia Nervosa. New York: Raven, 1977: 163–176.

485. Lachelin GCL, Yen SSC. Hypothalamic chronic anovulation. Am J Obstet Gynecol 1978; 130:825–831.

486. Boyar RM, Katz J. Twenty-four hour gonadotropin secretory patterns in anorexia nervosa. In: Vigersky RA, ed. Anorexia Nervosa. New York: Raven, 1977: 177–187.

487. Pirke KM, Fichter MM, Lund R, et al. Twenty-four hour sleep-wake pattern of plasma LH in patients with anorexia nervosa. Acta Endocrinol 1979; 92:193–204.

488. Beumont PJV, Abraham SF. Continuous infusion of luteinizing hormone releasing hormone (LHRH) in patients with anorexia nervosa. Psychol Med 1981; 11:477–484.

489. Marshall JC, Kelch RP. Low dose pulsatile gonadotropin-releasing hormone in anorexia nervosa: a model of human pubertal development. J Clin Endocrinol Metab 1979; 49:712–718.

490. Wakeling A, Marshall JC, Beardwood CJ, et al. The effects of clomiphene citrate on the hypothalamic-pituitary-gonadal axis in anorexia nervosa. Psychol Med 1976; 6:371–380.

491. Espinosa-Campos J, Robles C, Gual C, et al. Hypothalamic, pituitary, and ovarian function assessment in a patient with anorexia nervosa. Fertil Steril 1974; 25:453–458.

492. Nillius SJ, Fries H, Wide L. Successful induction of follicular maturation and ovulation by prolonged treatment with LH-releasing hormone in women with anorexia nervosa. Am J Obstet Gynecol 1975; 122:921–928.

493. Frisch RE. Food intake, fatness, and reproductive ability. In: Vigersky RA, ed. Anorexia Nervosa. New York: Raven, 1977: 149–161.

494. McNab D, Hawton K. Disturbances of sex hormones in anorexia nervosa in the male. Postgrad Med J 1981; 57:254–256.

495. Devlin MJ, Walsh BT, Katz JL, et al. Hypothalamic-pituitary-gonadal function in anorexia nervosa and bulimia. Psychiatry Res 1989; 28:11–24.

496. Brambilla F, Ferrari E, Cavagnini F, et al. Alpha 2-adrenoceptor sensitivity in anorexia nervosa: GH response to clonidine or GHRH stimulation. Biol Psychiatry 1989; 25:256–264.

497. Scacchi M, Invitti C, Pincelli AI, et al. Lack of growth hormone response to acute administration of dexamethasone in anorexia nervosa. Eur J Endocrinol 1995; 132:152–158.

498. Rappaport R, Prevot C, Czernichow P. Somatomedin activity and growth hormone secretion. I. Changes related to body weight in anorexia nervosa. Acta Paediatr Scand 1980; 69:37–41.

499. Issacs AJ, Leslie RDG, Gomez J, et al. The effect of weight gain on gonadotrophins and prolactin in anorexia nervosa. Acta Endocrinol 1980; 94:145–150.

500. Skrabanek P, Devlin J, McDonald D, et al. Plasma prolactin and gonadotrophins in anorexia nervosa and amenorrhoea due to weight loss. Acta Endocrinol 1981; 97:433–435.

501. Waldhauser F, Toifel K, Spona J, et al. Diminished prolactin response to thyrotropin and insulin in anorexia nervosa. J Clin Endocrinol Metab 1984; 59:538–541.

502. Beumont PJV, Abraham SF, Turtle J. Paradoxical prolactin response to gonadotropin-releasing hormone during weight gain in patients with anorexia nervosa. J Clin Endocrinol Metab 1980; 51:1283–1285.

503. Burman KD, Vigersky RA, Loriaux DL, et al. Investigations concerning thyroxine deiodinative pathways in patients with anorexia nervosa. In: Vigersky RA, ed. Anorexia Nervosa. New York: Raven 1977: 255–261.

504. Moshang T Jr, Utiger RD. Low triiodothyronine euthyroidism in anorexia nervosa. In: Vigersky RA, ed. Anorexia Nervosa. New York: Raven, 1977: 263–270.

505. Schimmel M, Utiger RD. Thyroidal and peripheral production of thyroid hormones. Review of recent findings and their clinical implications. Ann Intern Med 1977; 87:760–768.

506. Kaptein EM, Grieb DA, Spencer CA, et al. Thyroxine metabolism in the low thyroxine state of critical nonthyroidal illnesses. J Clin Endocrinol Metab 1981; 53:764–771.

507. Moore R, Mills IH. Serum T₃ and T₄ levels in patients with anorexia nervosa showing transient hyperthyroidism during weight gain. Clin Endocrinol 1979; 10:443–449.

508. Spalter AR, Gwirtsman HE, Demitrock MA, et al. Thyroid function in bulimia nervosa. Biol Psychiatry 1993; 33:408–414.

509. Gold PW, Gwirtsman H, Avgerinos PC, et al. Abnormal hypothalamic-pituitary-adrenal function in anorexia nervosa. Pathophysiologic mechanisms in underweight and weight-corrected patients. N Engl J Med 1986; 314:1335–1342.

510. Boyar RM, Hellman LD, Roffwarg H, et al. Cortisol secretion and metabolism in anorexia nervosa. N Engl J Med 1977; 296:190–193.

511. Walsh BT, Katz JL, Levin J, et al. The production rate of cortisol declines during recovery from anorexia nervosa. J Clin Endocrinol Metab 1981; 53:203–205.

512. Hotta M, Shibasaki T, Masuda A, et al. The responses of plasma adrenocorticotropin and cortisol to corticotropin-releasing hormone (CRH) and cerebrospinal fluid immunoreactive CRH in anorexia nervosa patients. J Clin Endocrinol Metab 1986; 62:319–324.

513. Kaye WH, Gwirtsman HE, George DT, et al. Elevated cerebrospinal fluid levels of immunoreactive corticotropin-releasing hormone in anorexia nervosa: relation to state of nutrition, adrenal function, and intensity of depression. J Clin Endocrinol Metab 1987; 64:203–208.

514. Gwirtsman HE, Kaye WH, George DT, et al. Central and peripheral ACTH and cortisol levels in anorexia nervosa and bulimia. Arch Gen Psychiatry 1989; 46:61–69.

515. Mortola JF, Rasmussen DD, Yen SSC. Alterations of the adrenocorticotropin-cortisol axis in normal weight bulimic women: evidence for a central mechanism. J Clin Endocrinol Metab 1989; 68:517–522.

516. Zumoff B, Walsh BT, Katz JL, et al. Subnormal plasma dehydroisoandrosterone to cortisol ratio in anorexia nervosa: a second hormonal parameter of ontogenic regression. J Clin Endocrinol Metab 1983; 56:668–672.

517. Doerr P, Fichter M, Pirke KM, et al. Relationship between weight gain and hypothalamic pituitary adrenal function in patients with anorexia nervosa. J Steroid Biochem 1980; 13:529–537.

518. Ferrari E, Foppa S, Bossolo PA, et al. Melatonin and pituitary-gonadal function in disorders of eating behavior. J Pineal Res 1989; 7:115–124.

519. Tortosa F, Puig-Domingo M, Peinado MA, et al. Enhanced circadian rhythm of melatonin in anorexia nervosa. Acta Endocrinol 1989; 120:574–578.

520. Kennedy SH, Garfinkel PE, Parienti V, et al. Changes in melatonin levels but not cortisol levels are associated with depression in patients with eating disorders. Arch Gen Psychiatry 1989; 46:73–78.

521. Fujii S, Tamai H, Kumai M, et al. Impaired glucagon secretion to insulin-induced hypoglycemia in anorexia nervosa. Acta Endocrinol 1989; 120:610–615.

522. Delvenne V, Lotstra F, Goldman S, et al. Brain hypometabolism of glucose in anorexia nervosa: a PET scan study. Biol Psychiatry 1995; 37:161–169.

523. Nozoe S, Narno T, Yanekura R, et al. Comparison of regional cerebral blood flow in patients with eating disorders. Brain Res Bull 1995; 36:251–255.

524. Nussey SS, Lacey JH. Ovarian morphology and insulin sensitivity in women with bulimia nervosa. Clin Endocrinol 1995; 43:451–455.

525. Baranowska B, Wasilewska-Dzinbinska E, Radzikowska M, et al. Impaired response of atrial natriuretic peptide to acute water load in obesity and in anorexia nervosa. Eur J Endocrinol 1995; 132:147–151.

526. Newman MM, Halmi KA. Relationship of bone density to estradiol and cortisol in anorexia nervosa and bulimia. Psychiatry Res 1989; 29:105–112.

527. Hay PJ, Hall A, Delahunt JW, et al. Investigation of osteopaenia in anorexia nervosa. Aust NZ J Psychiatry 1989; 23:261–268.

528. Carmichael KA, Carmichael DH. Bone metabolism and osteopenia in eating disorders. Medicine 1995; 74:254–267.

529. Biller BM, Saxe V, Herzog DB, et al. Mechanisms of osteoporosis in adult and adolescent women with anorexia nervosa. J Clin Endocrinol Metab 1989; 68:548–554.

530. Klibanski A, Biller BMK, Rosenthal DI, et al. Effects of prolactin and estrogen deficiency in amenorrheic bone loss. J Clin Endocrinol Metab 1988; 67:124–130.

531. Krieg JC, Lauer C, Leinsinger G, et al. Brain morphology and regional cerebral blood flow in anorexia nervosa. Biol Psychiatry 1989; 25:1041–1048.

532. Krieg JC, Lauer C, Pirke KM. Structural brain abnormalities in patients with bulimia nervosa. Psychiatry Res 1989; 27:39–48.

533. Issner JM, Roberts WC, Heymsfield SB, et al. Anorexia nervosa and sudden death. Ann Intern Med 1985; 102:49–52.

534. Schocken DD, Holloway JD, Powers PS. Weight loss and the heart. Effects of anorexia nervosa and starvation. Arch Intern Med 1989; 149:877–881.

535. Vande Wiele RL. Anorexia nervosa and the hypothalamus. Hosp Pract 1977; 12:45–51.

536. Norris DL. Clinical diagnostic criteria for primary anorexia nervosa. An analysis of 54 consecutive admissions. S Afr Med J 1979; 56:987–993.

537. Bruch H. Developmental considerations of anorexia nervosa and obesity. Can J Psychiatry 1981; 26:212–217.

538. Strober M, Salkin B, Burroughs J, et al. Validity of the bulimia-restricter distinction in anorexia nervosa. Parental personality characteristics and family psychiatric morbidity. J Nerv Ment Dis 1982; 170:345–351.

539. Marcus D, Wiener M. Anorexia nervosa reconceptualized from a psychosocial transactional perspective. Am J Orthopsychiatry 1989; 59:346–354.

540. Woodside DB, Shekter-Wolfson LF, Garfinkel PE, et al. Familial interactions in bulimia nervosa. II: Complex intrafamily comparisons and clinical significance. Int J Eat Disord 1995; 17:117–126.

541. Humphrey LL. Observed family interactions among subtypes of eating disorders using structural analysis of social behavior. J Consult Clin Psychol 1989; 57:206–214.

542. Fullerton DT, Wonderlich SA, Gosnell BA. Clinical characteristics of eating disorder patients who report sexual or physical abuse. Int J Eat Disord 1995; 17:243–249.

543. Andrews B, Valentine ER, Valentine JD. Depression and eating disorders following abuse in childhood in two generations of women. Br J Clin Psychol 1995; 34:37–52.

544. Garfinkel PE. Some recent observations on the pathogenesis of anorexia nervosa. Can J Psychiatry 1981; 26:218–223.

545. Huenemann RL, Shapiro LR, Hampton MC, et al. A longitudinal study of gross body composition and body conformation and their association with food and activity in a teen-age population. Views of teen-age subjects on body conformation, food and activity. Am J Clin Nutr 1966; 18:325–338.

546. Smith NJ. Excessive weight loss and food aversion in athletes simulating anorexia nervosa. Pediatrics 1980; 66:139–142.

547. Yates A, Leehey K, Shisslak CM. Running—an analogue of anorexia? N Engl J Med 1983; 308:251–255.

548. Hebebrand J, Remschmidt H. Anorexia nervosa viewed as an extreme weight condition: genetic implications. Hum Genet 1995; 95:1–11.

549. Greenfield O, Mickley D, Quinlan DM, et al. The structure of the genetic and environmental risk factors for six major psychiatric disorders in women: phobia, generalized anxiety disorder, panic disorder, bulimia, major depression, and alcoholism. Arch Gen Psychiatry 1995; 52:374–383.

550. Halmi K. Eating disorder research in the past decade. Ann NY Acad Sci 1996; 789:67–77.

551. Jarry JL, Vaccarino FJ. Eating disorder and obsessive-compulsive disorder: neurochemical and phenomenological commonalities. J Psychiatry Neurosci 1996; 21:36–48.

552. Fava M, Copeland PM, Schweiger U, et al. Neurochemical abnormalities of anorexia nervosa and bulimia nervosa. Am J Psychiatry 1989; 146:963–971.

553. Advokat C, Kutlesic V. Pharmacotherapy of the eating disorders: a commentary. Neurosci Biobehav Rev 1995; 19:59–66.

554. Eckert ED, Halmi KA, Grove W, et al. Ten-year follow-up of anorexia nervosa: clinical course and outcome. Psychol Med 1995; 25:143–156.

555. Sullivan PF. Mortality in anorexia nervosa. Am J Psychiatry 1995; 152:1073–1074.

556. Herzog DB, Keller MB, Lavori PW. Outcome in anorexia nervosa and bulimia nervosa. A review of the literature. J Nerv Ment Dis 1988; 176:131–143.

557. Piazza E, Piazza N, Rollins N. Anorexia nervosa: controversial aspects of therapy. Compr Psychiatry 1980; 21:177–189.

558. Russell G. The current treatment of anorexia nervosa. Br J Psychiatry 1981; 138:164–166.

559. Balaa MA, Drossman DA. Anorexia nervosa and bulimia: the eating disorders. Dis Mon 1985; 31:1–52.

560. Gustavsson CG, Eriksson L. Acute respiratory failure in anorexia nervosa with hypophosphataemia. J Intern Med 1989; 225:63–64.

561. Health and Public Policy Committee, American College of Physicians. Position paper. Eating disorders: anorexia nervosa and bulimia. Ann Intern Med 1986; 105:790–794.

DISORDERS OF LIPID METABOLISM

Robert W. Mahley, Karl H. Weisgraber, and Robert V. Farese, Jr.

LIPID BIOCHEMISTRY AND CHOLESTEROL METABOLISM

Lipids are hydrophobic molecules that are insoluble or minimally soluble. They are found in membranes, which maintain the integrity of cells and allow the compartmentalization of the cytoplasm into specific organelles. Lipids function as a major form of stored nutrients (triglycerides), as precursors for adrenal and gonadal steroids and bile acids (cholesterol), and as extracellular and intracellular messengers (e.g., prosta-

glandins, phosphatidylinositol). Lipoproteins provide a vehicle for transporting the complex lipids in the blood as water-soluble complexes and deliver lipids to cells throughout the body.

Classes of Lipids: Structure and Function

FATTY ACIDS

Fatty acids vary in length and in the number and position of double bonds (Fig. 23–1). Saturated fatty acids lack double

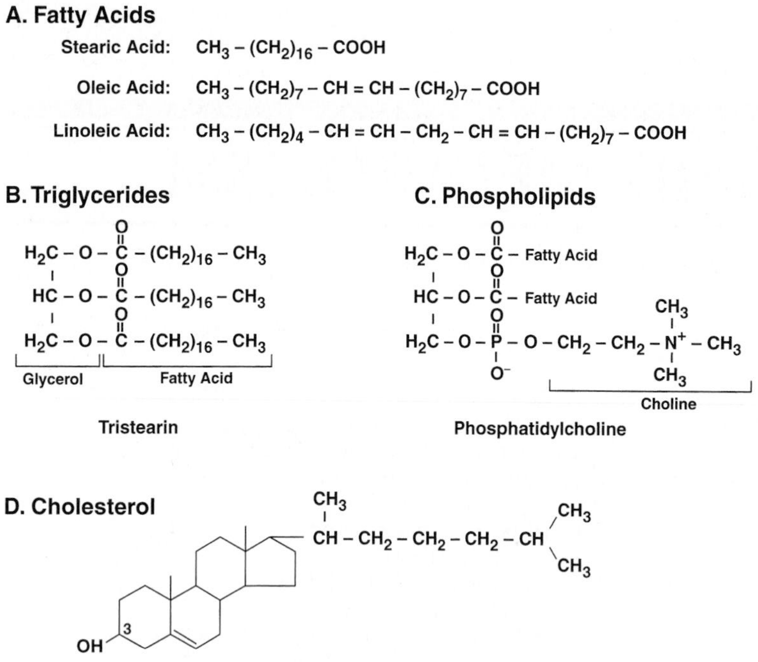

A. Fatty Acids

Stearic Acid: $CH_3 - (CH_2)_{16} - COOH$

Oleic Acid: $CH_3 - (CH_2)_7 - CH = CH - (CH_2)_7 - COOH$

Linoleic Acid: $CH_3 - (CH_2)_4 - CH = CH - CH_2 - CH = CH - (CH_2)_7 - COOH$

B. Triglycerides

Glycerol Fatty Acid

Tristearin

C. Phospholipids

Choline

Phosphatidylcholine

Figure 23–1. Structures of the common lipids.

D. Cholesterol

bonds (all carbon atoms have a full complement of hydrogen), and unsaturated fatty acids have one or more double bonds. Monounsaturated fatty acids have one double bond, and polyunsaturated fatty acids have two or more. The common fatty acids and their sources in foods are listed in Table 23–1.

Fatty acids are a readily available source of energy, and in tissues they can be esterified to other organic molecules to form complex lipids (e.g., triglycerides). In the blood they may be transported on lipoproteins as complex lipids, or they may be transported in the nonesterified state as free fatty acids bound to albumin.

CHOLESTEROL

Cholesterol is a four-ring hydrocarbon with an eight-carbon side chain (see Fig. 23–1). It serves a critical role as a major component of cell membranes and as a precursor of steroid hormones (adrenal and gonadal hormones). Cholesterol is also a precursor of bile acids, which are formed in the liver, stored in the gall bladder, and secreted in the intestine to participate in the absorption of fat. In the blood, about two

thirds of the cholesterol is esterified (i.e., has a fatty acid esterified to the hydroxyl group at position 3).

COMPLEX LIPIDS

TRIGLYCERIDES (TRIACYLGLYCEROL). Triglycerides consist of three fatty acid molecules esterified to a glycerol molecule (see Fig. 23–1). Diglycerides (diacylglycerols) contain two fatty acids, and monoglycerides have only one fatty acid per glycerol molecule. Triglycerides serve to store fatty acids and form large lipid droplets in adipose tissue. They are also transported as a component of certain lipoproteins. When triglycerides are hydrolyzed in adipocytes or on lipoprotein particles, free fatty acid molecules are released to be used as a source of energy.

PHOSPHOLIPIDS. Phospholipids have fatty acids esterified at two of the three hydroxyl groups of glycerol (see Fig. 23–1). The third hydroxyl group is esterified to phosphate (this complex lipid is referred to as phosphatidic acid). Typically, in mammalian tissue, the phosphatidic acid is esterified to the hydroxyl group of a hydrophilic molecule, such as

TABLE 23–1. Major Fatty Acids

Chemical Designation*	Common Name	Common Food Sources
Saturated fatty acids (no double bonds)		
C-12:0	Lauric	Coconut oil
C-14:0	Myristic	Coconut oil, butter fat
C-16:0	Palmitic	Butter, cheese, meat
C-18:0	Stearic	Beef, chocolate
Monounsaturated fatty acids (one double bond)		
C-18:1 Δ^9	Oleic	Olive oil, canola oil
Polyunsaturated fatty acids (two or more double bonds)		
Omega-6 fatty acids		
C-18:2ω6 Δ^9, Δ^{12}	Linoleic	Sunflower, corn, soybean, and safflower oils
C-20:4ω6 Δ^5, Δ^8, Δ^{11}, Δ^{14}	Arachidonic	
Omega-3 fatty acids		
C-20:5ω3	Eicosapentaenoic (EPA)	Salmon, cod, mackerel, tuna
C-22:6ω3	Docosahexaenoic (DHA)	Salmon, cod, mackerel, tuna

*The numeral after the C indicates the number of carbon atoms; the numeral after the colon indicates the number of double bonds. Carbon number 1 is the carboxylic acid carbon, and the ω carbon atom is the carbon most distant from the carboxyl group. The placement of the double bonds is shown by the Δ designations (e.g., Δ^9 indicates a double bond between carbons 9 and 10). In omega-6 fatty acids the first double bond occurs after the sixth carbon atom from the ω carbon atom (indicated by ω6), and in omega-3 fatty acids it occurs after the third carbon atom from the ω carbon atom (ω3).

choline, serine, or ethanolamine, to form phosphatidylcholine (commonly called lecithin), phosphatidylserine, or phosphatidylethanolamine, respectively. Lysolecithin is phosphatidylcholine from which one of the fatty acids has been removed. The combination of hydrophobic and hydrophilic regions in phospholipids enables them to be miscible at the water-lipid interface and makes them ideal components of membranes and of surface coats of lipoproteins. They are the most hydrophilic of the complex lipids.

Cholesterol Biosynthesis and the Low-Density Lipoprotein Receptor Pathway

Cholesterol is either absorbed from the diet or synthesized by cells in the body. All dietary cholesterol is of animal origin, i.e., from meats, dairy products, and eggs. Plants do not produce cholesterol; plant membranes contain sitosterol, which, except in a rare genetic disease, is not absorbed. Cholesterol is produced in many tissues (e.g., liver, skin, adrenals, gonads, brain, intestine). In most mammals, including humans, about 10 to 20% of the total synthesis of cholesterol occurs in the liver.[1-8]

CHOLESTEROL BIOSYNTHESIS

Cholesterol synthesis, illustrated schematically in Figure 23–2A, begins with acetate. Three molecules of acetate are condensed to form 3-hydroxy-3-methylglutaryl–coenzyme A (HMG-CoA), which is then converted to mevalonic acid by the enzyme HMG-CoA reductase. Through a series of steps, mevalonic acid is converted to cholesterol. The key (rate-limiting) step regulating cholesterol biosynthesis involves HMG-CoA reductase. Competitive inhibitors of this enzyme (the statins) reduce cholesterol biosynthesis and lower plasma cholesterol levels. Increased cholesterol content of cells feeds back on the HMG-CoA reductase, decreases its activity, and thereby decreases cholesterol biosynthesis. Conversely, a deficiency of intracellular cholesterol increases reductase activity and increases cholesterol biosynthesis[1-8] (see later discussion).

Cholesterol cannot be eliminated by catabolism to carbon dioxide and water; it must be either excreted as free choles-

terol in the bile or converted to bile acids and secreted into the intestine.[9] About 50% of the cholesterol entering the intestine is reabsorbed and recirculates to the liver; the remainder is eliminated in the feces. Almost all of the secreted bile acids (97%) are reabsorbed from the intestine and transported back to the liver. This recirculation of cholesterol and bile acids from the intestine to the liver is called the *enterohepatic circulation* (Fig. 23–2B). The reabsorbed cholesterol and bile acids regulate de novo cholesterol and bile acid synthesis in the liver. For example, if the amount of bile acids returning to the liver is decreased (as occurs in the intestine during treatment with bile acid–binding resins), then bile acid synthesis is increased, enhancing the amount of cholesterol being converted to bile acids.

CHOLESTEROL 7α-HYDROXYLASE

This enzyme of about 57 kd (503 amino acids), known as CYP7 (formerly P450$_{7\alpha}$), converts free cholesterol to 7α-hydroxycholesterol. This is the rate-limiting step in bile acid synthesis, and it is under feedback regulation by recirculated bile acids. The interruption of bile acid recirculation increases cholesterol 7α-hydroxylase activity. This enzyme and HMG-CoA reductase are closely coupled, and their activities usually change in parallel (for a review see references 3, 5, and 10 to 12). In this way, the intracellular cholesterol level for bile acid production remains rather constant.

LOW-DENSITY LIPOPROTEIN RECEPTOR

Cholesterol levels in the blood are controlled primarily through the low-density lipoprotein (LDL) receptor pathway.[4, 13] This receptor is present on the surface of all cells throughout the body, including hepatocytes, and mediates the uptake of cholesterol-rich lipoproteins (e.g., LDL) from the blood. Specific proteins on the surface of certain lipoproteins (apolipoprotein B100 and apolipoprotein E) interact with the LDL receptor and facilitate lipoprotein internalization by cells. By this mechanism, cells that require cholesterol can obtain the preformed sterol. The LDL receptor also allows the liver (the principal site for LDL catabolism) to take up LDL and eliminate cholesterol from the body (discussed under section on lipoprotein receptors controlling lipoprotein metabolism).

The number of LDL receptors on the cell surface is tightly regulated.[4, 13] If the cholesterol content of a cell is elevated, there is a decrease in the number of receptors synthesized (i.e., a down-regulation in receptor expression). On the other hand, if a cell requires cholesterol, expression of LDL receptors is up-regulated, and the number of receptors on the cell surface increases. This system keeps the intracellular cholesterol concentration relatively constant and prevents excessive and possibly toxic accumulation. Within the cell cholesterol can be esterified by the enzyme acyl-coenzyme A:cholesterol acyltransferase (ACAT).

ACYL-COENZYME A:CHOLESTEROL ACYLTRANSFERASE

ACAT is an enzyme of the endoplasmic reticulum (about 65 kd, 550 amino acids) that catalyzes the formation of cholesteryl esters by transferring a long-chain fatty acid (oleic acid is the preferred substrate) to free cholesterol.[14-18] When lipoproteins enter the cell by receptor-mediated endocytosis and are degraded within the lysosomes, free cholesterol is generated, esterified by ACAT, and stored in droplets. Cholesteryl ester hydrolysis by cholesteryl ester hydroxylase generates free cholesterol again for efflux from the cells or to serve as a biosynthetic substrate (e.g., for steroid hormones, cell

A. Cholesterol Biosynthesis

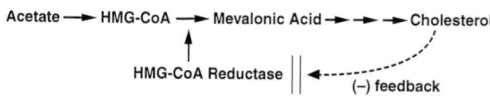

B. Enterohepatic Circulation

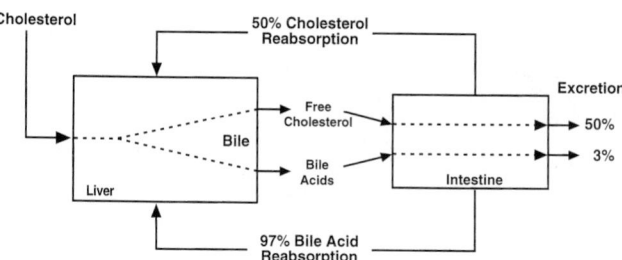

Figure 23–2. *A,* Cholesterol biosynthesis. HMG-CoA reductase is a rate-limiting enzyme regulating cholesterol biosynthesis. The enzyme is down-regulated by excess cholesterol in the cell. *B,* Enterohepatic circulation of cholesterol and bile acids. About 50% of cholesterol and 97% of bile acids are reabsorbed from the intestine and recirculated to the liver. (*A* Modified from Brown MS, Goldstein JL. A receptor-mediated pathway for cholesterol homeostasis. Science 1986; 232:34–47.)

membranes) within the cells. The pool of intracellular cholesterol and cholesteryl esters is dynamic.

In the intestine, ACAT may promote the uptake of free cholesterol from the lumen by esterifying the free cholesterol in the cell and thereby creating and maintaining a transmembrane free cholesterol gradient.[16, 17] Agents that inhibit intestinal ACAT are said to decrease cholesterol absorption by the intestine.[18]

Metabolism of Dietary Lipids

The digestion of dietary fats begins in the stomach and continues in the proximal small intestine.[19–23] Triglycerides are hydrolyzed to free fatty acids and small amounts of monoglycerides and diglycerides; cholesteryl esters are hydrolyzed to free cholesterol; phospholipids are converted primarily to lysolecithin. Bile salt micelles disperse and partially solubilize water-insoluble lipids; this facilitates the intestinal transport and delivery of lipids to the unstirred water layer of intestinal epithelial cells, from which they can be taken up by the cells. Bile acids also activate pancreatic lipase, which participates in the hydrolysis of triglycerides. Long-chain fatty acids are taken up primarily by the enterocytes of the duodenum and proximal jejunum, re-esterified into triglycerides, and used in the biosynthesis of intestinal lipoproteins (chylomicrons), which are delivered to the mesenteric lymph and enter the general circulation with the thoracic duct lymph. Medium-chain fatty acids (≤10 carbons) are absorbed into the portal blood without being esterified and are cleared directly from the blood by the liver. Bile acids are reabsorbed primarily from the ileum, enter the portal blood, and are taken up by the liver.

Triglyceride and Free Fatty Acid Metabolism

STORAGE AND USE

Free fatty acids are released from triglycerides of chylomicrons and very-low-density lipoproteins (VLDL) through the action of lipoprotein lipase (LPL). As discussed later, LPL is bound to the capillary endothelial cells adjacent to adipose, muscle, and breast tissue, where it liberates free fatty acids from lipoprotein triglyceride. The level of LPL in tissues differs under different physiological circumstances[24] so that free fatty acids are directed to tissues requiring them as substrates or energy sources. For example, during fasting LPL activity decreases in adipose tissue and increases in heart muscle. In the breast LPL levels are low until parturition, when they increase 10-fold to promote milk formation.

In adipose tissue high levels of glucose and insulin promote the conversion of free fatty acids to triglyceride for storage. Insulin stimulates LPL activity and fatty acid esterification through formation of glycerol phosphate and decreases free fatty acid release through inhibition of hormone-sensitive lipase.[25] Insulin deficiency, as in diabetes mellitus, is associated with decreased LPL activity. Insulin and glucose also stimulate the biosynthesis of free fatty acids in the liver and, to a lesser degree, in adipocytes when dietary fat is replaced by carbohydrates. As a result, hepatic free fatty acids are converted to triglyceride and packaged into VLDL particles (discussed under section on plasma lipoproteins).

FATTY ACID RELEASE FROM ADIPOSE TISSUE

The net release of free fatty acids and glycerol from adipose triglyceride stores occurs during various physiological conditions, including stress, exercise, fasting, and uncontrolled diabetes mellitus. This release occurs in response to hormones (Table 23–2), most of which act by means of cyclic

TABLE 23–2. Hormones That Affect Lipolysis In Vitro

Rapid Stimulation	Slow Stimulation
Catecholamines (β-1 agonists)	Glucocorticoids
Corticotropin	Growth hormone
Glucagon	**Suppression**
Placental lactogen	Insulin
Prolactin	Gastric inhibitory polypeptide
Secretin	Oxytocin
Thyrotropin	Prostaglandin
Vasoactive intestinal peptide	Somatomedins
Vasopressin	

Modified from Bierman EL, Glomset JA. Disorders of lipid metabolism. In: Wilson JD, Foster DW, eds. Williams Textbook of Endocrinology. 8th ed. Philadelphia: WB Saunders, 1992: 1367–1395.

AMP to activate a hormone receptor–coupled protein kinase that in turn activates a hormone-sensitive lipase (Fig. 23–3).[25] In contrast to numerous hormones that stimulate adipose tissue hormone-sensitive lipase, insulin inhibits this process. Growth hormone liberates free fatty acids by a different mechanism, which requires enhancement of the synthesis of hormone-sensitive lipase.

After triglyceride hydrolysis in adipose tissue, the released free fatty acids bind to albumin and circulate in the plasma. Released glycerol is taken up by the liver and kidney for triglyceride synthesis or for gluconeogenesis. The fate of the free fatty acid–albumin complexes is determined in part by blood flow. With intense exercise and diminished blood flow to the splanchnic bed, free fatty acids are targeted to muscle. Depending on the metabolic state, free fatty acids taken up by the liver are reused for triglyceride or phospholipid synthesis (exported on VLDL), oxidized to carbon dioxide, or converted to ketone bodies.

FATTY ACID OXIDATION AND KETOGENESIS

Both oxidation of fatty acids and ketogenesis take place in the mitochondria, except for very-long-chain fatty acids (C-24 and C-26), which are oxidized in peroxisomes. Because free fatty acids and their CoA derivatives can penetrate only the outer leaflet of the mitochondrial membrane, they are converted to carnitine derivatives within the mitochondrial membrane to allow for transmembrane transport. Once inside the mitochondria, they are reconverted to CoA derivatives and oxidized by beta oxidation, which produces acetyl-CoA and the reduced forms of nicotinamide-adenine dinucleotide (NADH) and flavin-adenine dinucleotide (FADH).

With a normal flux of free fatty acids, the NADH and

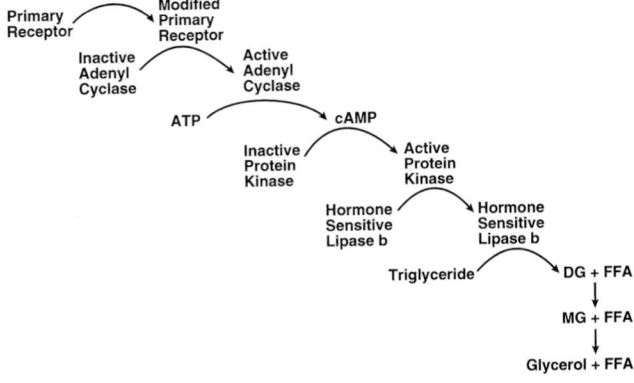

Figure 23–3. Cascade of reactions involved in activation of hormone-sensitive lipase. FFA, free fatty acid. (From Steinberg D, Huttunen JK. The role of cyclic AMP in activation of hormone-sensitive lipase of adipose tissue. Adv Cyclic Nucleotide Res 1972; 1:47–62, with permission.)

FADH enter the electron transport system, resulting in formation of ATP and water. The condensation of acetyl-CoA with oxaloacetic acid yields citrate, which can enter the citric acid cycle, where it is oxidized to carbon dioxide or is transported out of the mitochondria and converted again to free fatty acids. If free fatty acid flux to the liver is massively increased, as in insulin-deficient states such as prolonged fasting or uncontrolled diabetes mellitus, the production of VLDL-triglyceride from free fatty acids is limited. As a result, NADH, FADH, and acetyl-CoA accumulate in the mitochondria and give rise to the products of ketogenesis: acetoacetate, β-hydroxybutyrate, and acetone.

Ketogenesis occurs in several steps. Initially, acetyl-CoA condenses in two steps to form acetoacetyl-CoA and then HMG-CoA. The latter is cleaved to acetoacetate and acetyl-CoA, which leads to the liberation of CoA and its use in beta oxidation of free fatty acids. Acetoacetate can be reduced by NADH to form β-hydroxybutyrate; the NAD produced can be used for continued beta oxidation of fatty acids. Alternatively, the acetoacetate can decompose to form acetone. The ketones are released into the plasma and, if they accumulate, cause ketoacidosis.

FATTY ACID BIOSYNTHESIS

Under normal conditions the diet supplies sufficient fatty acids through the ingestion of fat. However, increases in the ratio of carbohydrate to fat in the diet stimulate fatty acid synthesis by the liver and adipose tissue. Fatty acids are synthesized from two carbon units of acetyl-CoA. Because acetyl-CoA is produced in the mitochondria, it must first be converted to citrate by condensation with oxaloacetate and then transported into the cytosol, where it is reconverted to acetyl-CoA and oxaloacetate. Eight acetyl-CoA units are condensed to form palmitic acid (16 carbon atoms) in a series of reactions involving the enzymes fatty acid synthase and acetyl-CoA carboxylase. Longer fatty acids, such as stearic acid (18 carbon atoms) or oleic acid (18 carbon atoms with a single double bond), are synthesized from palmitic acid by chain extension. In this way fatty acid synthesis can meet most of the body's requirements.

Certain essential polyunsaturated fatty acids cannot be synthesized in humans and must be supplied in the diet. These include linoleic acid (18 carbon atoms with two double bonds) and linolenic acid (18 carbon atoms with three double bonds). Essential fatty acids are required for a number of special functions, including prostaglandin synthesis.[26-28]

PLASMA LIPOPROTEINS: APOLIPOPROTEINS, RECEPTORS, AND ENZYMES

General Structure and Major Classes of Lipoproteins

Lipoproteins function as vehicles to transport lipids in the blood in the form of soluble complexes of lipids and proteins. The lipids include triglycerides, cholesteryl esters, free cholesterol, and phospholipids. About 10 different protein moieties, called apolipoproteins, are associated with various lipoproteins and are given letter designations (Table 23–3).[4, 8, 29-32] Lipoproteins also transport fat-soluble vitamins (A, D, and E), drugs (e.g., probucol, cyclosporine), some viruses, and certain antioxidant enzymes (e.g., paraoxonase[33] and platelet-derived activating factor hydrolase[34]).

Lipoproteins are spherical particles with a core of mostly hydrophobic lipids (triglycerides and cholesteryl esters) and a surface layer of more hydrophilic constituents, namely protein, free cholesterol, and phospholipids (Fig. 23–4). Six major classes of lipoproteins serve different roles in lipid transport (see Table 23–3), and the specific apolipoproteins on the surface determine the fate of the lipoproteins. To understand lipoprotein metabolism and the disease states associated with lipid abnormalities, it is necessary to consider the roles of the individual apolipoproteins in regulating lipid metabolism. Some of their properties are summarized in Table 23–4 and Fig. 23–5.[8, 31, 32]

Major Apolipoproteins Regulating Lipoprotein Metabolism

Apolipoprotein B

In human plasma, apolipoprotein B (apo-B) occurs in two forms, apo-B100 and apo-B48, which are derived from a single gene[35-39] on the short arm of chromosome 2. The human apo-B gene comprises 29 exons and 28 introns and is approximately 45 kb in length. A unique RNA-editing mechanism is responsible for the synthesis of apo-B100 and apo-B48

TABLE 23–3. Major Classes of Plasma Lipoproteins

Type	Density (g/mL)	Electrophoretic Mobility	Site of Origin	Major Lipids	Major Apolipoproteins
Chylomicrons	<0.95	Origin	Intestine	85% Triglyceride	B48, AI, AIV (E, CI, CII, CIII—by transfer from HDL)
Chylomicron remnants	<1.006	Origin	Intestine	60% Triglyceride, 20% cholesterol	B48, E
VLDL*	<1.006	Pre-β	Liver	55% Triglyceride, 20% cholesterol	B100, E, CI, CII, CIII
IDL*	1.006–1.019	β	Derived from VLDL	35% Cholesterol, 25% triglyceride	B100, E
LDL	1.019–1.063	β	Derived from IDL	60% Cholesterol, 5% triglyceride	B100
HDL	1.063–1.21	α	Liver, intestine, plasma	25% Phospholipid, 20% cholesterol, 5% triglyceride (50% protein)	AI, AII, CI, CII, CIII, E
HDL₂	1.063–1.125	α			
HDL₃	1.125–1.21	α			

*The term VLDL remnants often refers to small, partially lipolyzed VLDL and IDL.

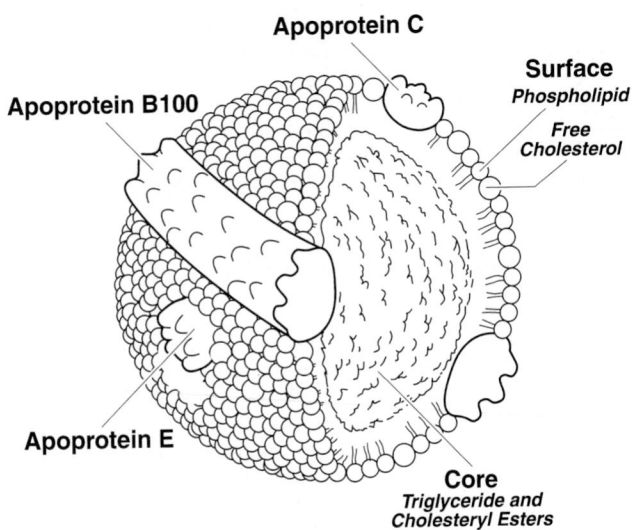

Figure 23–4. General structure of lipoproteins (a schematic representation of VLDL).

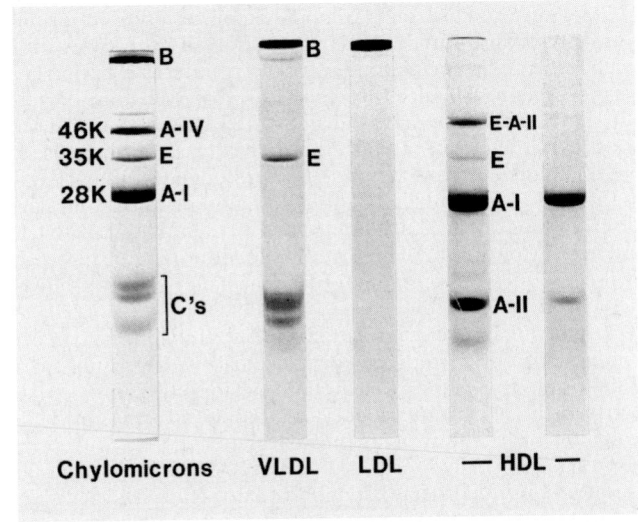

Figure 23–5. Polyacrylamide gel showing the various apolipoproteins characteristic of each type of plasma lipoprotein particle. (Modified from Mahley RW, Innerarity TL. Lipoprotein receptors and cholesterol homeostasis. Biochim Biophys Acta 1983; 737:197–222. With permission from Elsevier Science–NL, Sara Burgerhartstraat 25, 1055 KV Amsterdam, The Netherlands.)

from the apo-B mRNA (Fig. 23–6) (for a review see references 37, 40, and 41). An editing protein (or proteins) interacts with the apo-B mRNA in the human intestine to change a single nucleotide so that the modified mRNA directs the synthesis of a truncated form of apo-B (apo-B48). In humans this modification of the apo-B mRNA occurs only in the intestine and not in the liver; therefore the liver produces the full-length apo-B100. Apo-B100 (but not apo-B48) is also expressed in the yolk sac of mammals.

The editing of apo-B mRNA results in the change of a cytosine at nucleotide 6666 in the apo-B100 mRNA to a uracil.[42–44] This cytosine is part of the codon CAA, which encodes for glutamine at amino acid residue 2153 in apo-B100, whereas the codon UAA is a stop codon and terminates translation of the protein chain (see Fig. 23–6). Therefore, apo-B48 possesses 2152 amino acids, compared with the 4536 residues in apo-B100. Apo-B100, a 513-kd protein, is synthesized in the liver; it serves as a structural protein of VLDL and of intermediate-density lipoproteins (IDL) and is the exclusive protein

constituent of LDL. Each VLDL, IDL, and LDL particle contains one molecule of apo-B100. The primary structure of apo-B contains many hydrophobic and amphipathic sequences, forming alpha-helices and beta-strands, that occur throughout the molecule and appear to function as lipid-binding domains. In addition to its structural role, apo-B100 functions as a ligand for the LDL receptor.

Apo-B48, a 241-kd protein, is a structural constituent of chylomicrons.[35–37] Each chylomicron appears to possess one molecule of apo-B48. Because it lacks the carboxyl-terminal domain of apo-B100, apo-B48 cannot bind to the LDL receptor. The carboxyl-terminal domain of apo-B100 in the region of amino acid residues 3000 to 3700 is critical for the binding of apo-B100 to the LDL receptor (Fig. 23–7).[45, 46] Selective chemical modification of the apo-B100 of LDL demonstrated that the positively charged (basic) amino acids arginine and lysine are important in the interaction of LDL with its recep-

TABLE 23–4. Characterization of Human Apolipoproteins

Apolipoprotein	Average Plasma Concentration (mg/dL)	Chromosome	Gene (bases)	Molecular Weight (×1000)	Mature Protein (amino acids)	Major Sites of Synthesis	Major Functions
AI	130	11	1,863	~29	243	Liver, intestine	Structural protein/HDL. Cofactor for LCAT. Ligand for putative HDL receptor.
AII	40	1	1,330	~17 (dimer)	77	Liver	Inhibits apo-E binding to receptors (through the E–AII complex).
AIV	40	11	2,600	~45	376	Intestine	May facilitate cholesterol efflux from cells. Activator of LCAT. Possible role in triglyceride metabolism.
B100	85	2	43,000	~513	4536	Liver	Structural protein/VLDL and LDL. Ligand for LDL receptor.
B48	Variable			~241	2152	Intestine	Structural protein/chylomicrons.
CI	6	19	4,653	~6.6	57	Liver	Modulates remnant binding to receptors. Activates LCAT.
CII	3	19	3,320	8.9	79	Liver	Cofactor for LPL.
CIII	12	11	3,133	8.8	79	Liver	Modulates remnant binding to receptors.
E	5	19	3,597	~34	299	Liver, brain, skin, testes, spleen	Ligand for LDL and remnant receptors. Local lipid redistribution. Reverse cholesterol transport (HDL with apo-E).
apo(a)	Variable	6	Variable	~400–800	4000–6000	Liver	Modulates thrombosis/fibrinolysis.
D	10	3	12,000	~20	169	Liver, intestine	Activator of LCAT(?)

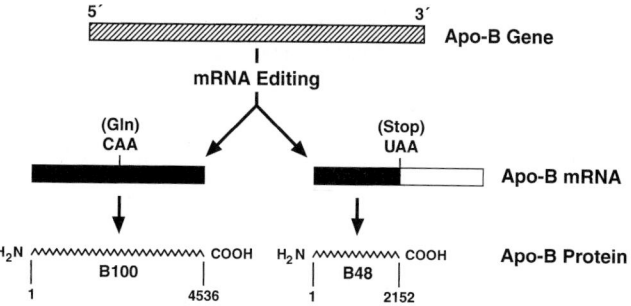

Figure 23–6. Synthesis of apo-B100 and apo-B48 by a unique mRNA-editing mechanism. In the human intestine, a specific cytosine (C) is changed to a uracil (U) in the apo-B mRNA. This change results in a stop codon and the formation of apo-B48, which contains only the first 2152 amino acids of the full-length apo-B100 (4536 amino acids).

tor, and when apo-B100 was sequenced, several regions enriched in arginine and lysine residues became candidates for receptor binding, including residues 3147 to 3157, residues 3357 to 3367, and amino acids in the vicinity of residue 3500.[35, 38, 45–47] Although the critical binding domain remains to be identified, the fact that a single amino acid substitution in the carboxyl-terminal region of apo-B100 markedly disrupts the normal binding of LDL to the LDL receptor substantiates the critical role of this region of apo-B. Patients expressing defective apo-B have hypercholesterolemia and high HDL levels. This genetic disorder, familial defective apo-B100 (see later discussion), is caused by the substitution of glutamine for arginine at amino acid residue 3500 of apo-B100.[48]

ROLE OF APOLIPOPROTEIN B IN LIPID METABOLISM

Apo-B100 and apo-B48 play critical roles in the biosynthesis of apo-B–containing lipoproteins (for a review see references 8, 30 to 32, 35, 36, 47, and 49). In addition, as discussed, the apo-B100 in LDL interacts with the LDL receptor. Although apo-B100 is also a constituent of VLDL and IDL, it does not play a major role in the binding of these lipoproteins

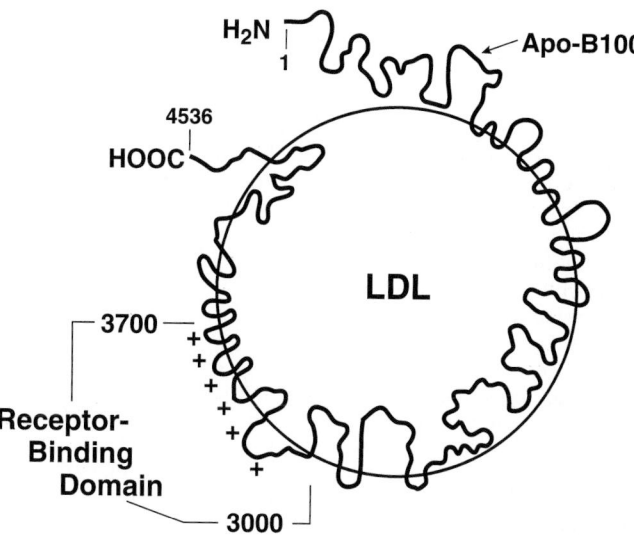

Figure 23–7. Schematic representation of apo-B100 on the surface of an LDL particle. The receptor-binding domain may form a cluster of positively charged arginine and lysine residues (a basic patch) capable of interacting with critical negatively charged glutamic and aspartic acid residues in the ligand-binding domain of the LDL receptor. (Adapted from Yang C-Y, et al. Structure of apolipoprotein B-100 of human low density lipoproteins. Arteriosclerosis 1989; 9:96–108.)

to LDL receptors. Apo-E is responsible for most of the receptor-mediated clearance of VLDL and IDL; presumably the lipid or apolipoprotein content of the VLDL and IDL masks or alters the conformation of the receptor-binding domain of the apo-B100 on these particles. Apo-B100 is, however, the major (or exclusive) protein moiety of LDL and is responsible for directing the clearance of these lipoproteins via the LDL receptor pathway.

Overexpression of apo-B in transgenic mice causes an increase in the levels of LDL and other apo-B–containing lipoproteins[50–53] and an increased susceptibility to diet-induced atherosclerosis.[54] Knockout of the apo-B gene in mice is embryonically lethal.[55, 56] Production of apo-B in the yolk sac appears to play an essential role in the delivery of lipids to the developing mouse embryo; delivery of α-tocopherol may be particularly important to embryonic tissues.[57]

Apolipoprotein E

Apo-E[58–60] mediates the interaction of apo-E–containing lipoproteins with the LDL receptor and with the chylomicron remnant (apo-E) receptor, presumably the LDL receptor–related protein (LRP). As a consequence, apo-E plays a critical role in determining the metabolic fate of several classes of lipoproteins and plays a central role in cholesterol metabolism. In addition, apo-E appears to be involved in cholesterol transport to cells undergoing proliferation and repair and may modulate lymphocyte response and smooth muscle cell proliferation (for a review see references 58 and 59).

Apo-E, a 34-kd protein composed of 299 amino acids,[58] circulates in the plasma both as a constituent of chylomicrons, chylomicron remnants, VLDL, and IDL and as a component of a minor subclass of high-density lipoproteins (HDL), referred to as HDL with apo-E, or HDL$_1$ (Fig. 23–5). Normal plasma apo-E levels range from 30 to 70 µg/mL, approximately half of which is associated with HDL and serves as a reservoir of apo-E for redistribution to chylomicrons and VLDLs as they enter the plasma. In lymph and interstitial fluid apo-E is associated with lipid complexes (phospholipid–apo-E disks) or with HDL.

Approximately 75% of plasma apo-E is synthesized by hepatocytes, and the remainder is synthesized in a variety of tissues. Macrophages can synthesize and secrete the protein, especially when they are loaded with cholesterol, and are responsible for a portion of the apo-E found in interstitial fluid. Smooth muscle cells of arteries and keratinocytes in the skin are additional sites of apo-E synthesis (see Table 23–4). The tissue with the second highest level of apo-E mRNA (after the liver) is the brain, where apo-E is synthesized by astrocytes. Cerebrospinal fluid contains apo-E derived from the brain (approximately 0.3 mg/dL, or 5 to 10% of plasma apo-E levels). Apo-E appears to play a key role in cholesterol transport in both the central and peripheral nervous systems and may be involved in the pathogenesis of Alzheimer's disease (for review, see references 58 and 61 to 63).

The apo-E gene is located on chromosome 19 and is part of a gene cluster that includes the genes for apo-CI and apo-CII. The apo-E gene locus has multiple alleles that give rise to a common genetic protein polymorphism.[58–60, 63–65] The three major forms of apo-E—apo-E2, apo-E3, and apo-E4—arise from three alleles, referred to as ε2, ε3, and ε4, that occur in several populations with a frequency of about 8, 77, and 15%, respectively (Fig. 23–8). There are three homozygous (E2/2, E3/3, and E4/4) and three heterozygous (E3/2, E4/2, and E4/3) phenotypes. About 60% of individuals are homozygous for apo-E3.

These genetic polymorphisms are caused by single amino acid substitutions at one of two sites in the protein (see Fig. 23–8).[32, 47, 58, 59, 63, 65, 66] Apo-E2 differs from apo-E3 at residue

158, where cysteine is substituted for arginine, and apo-E4 differs from apo-E3 at residue 112, where arginine is substituted for cysteine. In addition, apo-E displays a second type of polymorphism, post-translational glycosylation. Carbohydrate attachment at threonine-194 and the presence of multiple sialic acid residues give rise to minor acidic isoforms.

Apo-E functions in both receptor binding and lipid binding, and the different isoforms have different activities. Apo-E3 and apo-E4 are equally capable of interacting with LDL receptors, but the binding of apo-E2 to LDL receptors is impaired and is associated with the development of type III hyperlipoproteinemia.[65] Apo-E isoforms also bind differently to specific types of lipids and lipoproteins.[59] Apo-E4 interacts preferentially with large, triglyceride-rich lipoprotein (e.g., VLDL), whereas apo-E3 and apo-E2 bind preferentially to smaller, phospholipid-rich HDL.

The apo-E primary translational product is a 317–amino acid protein with an 18–amino acid signal peptide that is cleaved before the mature protein (299 amino acids, $M_r \cong$ 34,000) is secreted into plasma. The molecule contains two domains (Fig. 23–9).[58, 59] The amino-terminal domain (residues 1 to 191) contains the receptor-binding region, and the carboxyl-terminal domain (residues 192 to 299) appears to have three amphipathic alpha-helices (one face being hydrophilic and the other hydrophobic) and is responsible for lipid binding. Residues 242 to 272 are key in the binding of apo-E to lipoproteins.[67] Paradoxically, the lipid-binding region of apo-E resides in the carboxyl-terminal domain, but the amino acid differences that distinguish the three major apo-E isoforms are in the amino-terminal domain (residue 112 or 158). The fact that the isoforms display different specificities for different types of lipoproteins (i.e., apo-E4 for VLDL and apo-E3 and apo-E2 for HDL) suggests that the amino- and car-

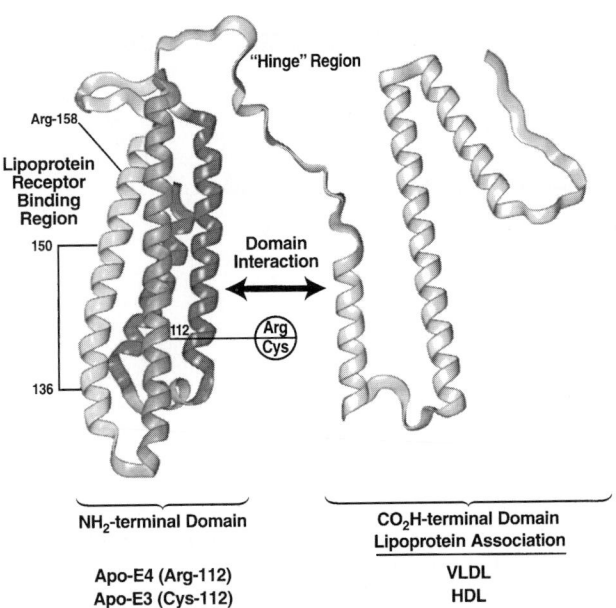

Figure 23–9. Predicted secondary structure of apo-E. The majority of the structure is composed of alpha-helices, beta-sheet structures, and beta-turns. A region of random structure encompassing residues 165 to 200 appears to form a boundary or hinge region between the two functional domains.

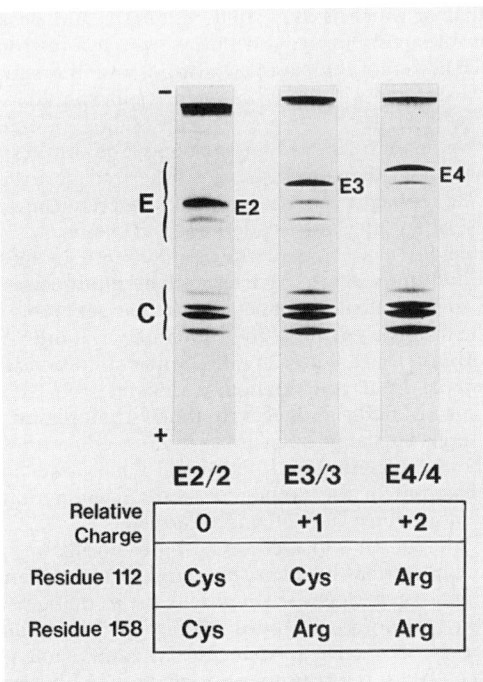

Figure 23–8. Isoelectric focusing gels of VLDL apolipoproteins from three individuals homozygous for the common apo-E phenotypes. The relative charge differences among the different apo-E isoforms are accounted for by the specific amino acid substitutions that are responsible for the three isoforms. The minor, more acidic apo-E isoforms represent sialylated forms of the protein. (From Mahley RW, Rall SC, Jr. Type III hyperlipoproteinemia (dysbetalipoproteinemia): the role of apolipoprotein E in normal and abnormal lipoprotein metabolism. In: Scriver CR, Beaudet AL, Sly WS, et al., eds. The Metabolic and Molecular Bases of Inherited Disease. 7th ed. New York: McGraw-Hill, 1995:1953–1980.)

boxyl-terminal domains interact so that specific residues in the amino terminus alter the conformation and specificity of the lipid-binding domain in the carboxyl terminus for certain types of lipoproteins (for a more complete discussion see references 59, 63, and 67 to 69).

The critical amino acids that mediate the binding of apo-E to the LDL receptor are in the vicinity of residues 134 to 160 (Fig. 23–10).[58, 59, 65, 66] Positively charged arginine and lysine in the sequence 136 to 150 may interact with the negatively charged glutamic and aspartic acids in the ligand-binding region of the LDL receptor. The amino-terminal domain of apo-E (residues 1 to 191) has been shown by x-ray crystallography (Fig. 23–11) to form a four-helix bundle.[67–69] The fourth helix encompasses residues 130 to 165, the area envisioned to be the receptor-binding region. The basic residues in the vicinity of amino acids 134 to 150 are oriented away from the surface of the molecule and are probably involved in the direct interaction of apo-E with the LDL receptor.[68, 69]

The identification of naturally occurring mutants of apo-E that are defective in receptor binding has provided key insights into the specific residues involved (see Fig. 23–10). The most common variant that is defective in binding is apo-E2 (Arg-158 → Cys). This substitution appears to alter receptor binding secondarily by altering the conformation of residues in the 136 to 150 region of apo-E. Other variants that are defective in binding involve single amino acid substitutions: Arg-136→Ser, Arg-142→Cys, Arg-145→Cys, and Lys-146→Gln or Glu. Site-directed mutagenesis showed that Arg-150 also plays a key role in receptor binding. A rare apo-E mutation, apo-E Leiden, involves a duplication of seven amino acids (residues 121 to 127) inserted in tandem at the junction between helices 3 and 4. This insertion probably disrupts receptor binding by altering the conformation of the 136 to 150 receptor-binding region.

Apo-E also binds to heparin and to heparan sulfate proteoglycans (HSPG).[63, 70] As discussed later, binding of apo-E to HSPG is important in the clearance of remnant lipoproteins by the LRP pathway. Residues in the 136 to 150 region of apo-E are responsible for the ionic interaction with the sulfate groups of heparin-like molecules and for binding to the LRP.

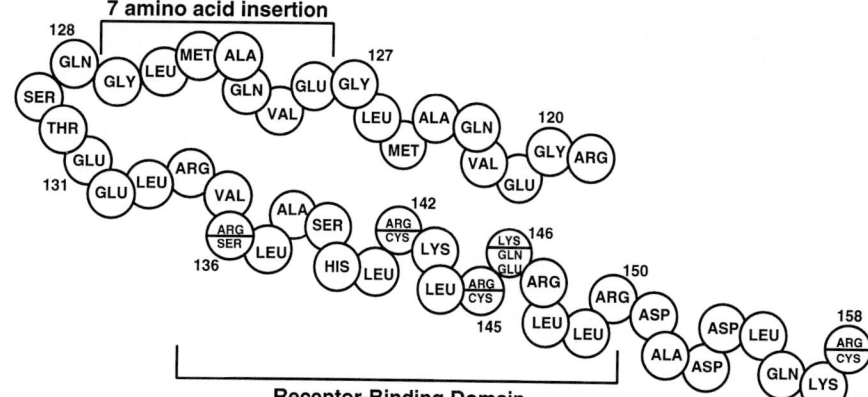

Figure 23–10. Schematic representation of the receptor-binding domain of apo-E, indicating the location and identity of naturally occurring amino acid substitutions that lead to type III hyperlipoproteinemia. In each substitution, the bottom amino acid represents the mutant.

ROLES OF APOLIPOPROTEIN E IN LIPID METABOLISM

Apo-E functions in two aspects of lipid and cholesterol transport.[58] The first, involving chylomicron and VLDL metabolism, provides a global transport role for apo-E. The knockout of apo-E by gene targeting in mice results in marked hyperlipidemia and the development of severe atherosclerosis, confirming the importance of this protein in cholesterol homeostasis and lipid transport.[71, 72] In the second pathway, apo-E facilitates the redistribution of lipids (including cholesterol) among cells within a tissue or organ. This local transport role redistributes lipids from cells with excess cholesterol to those requiring cholesterol, phospholipids, and other lipids for repair, proliferation, or other purposes. This pathway may involve lipid-laden HDL and apo-E that can acquire tissue lipids or apo-E–lipid complexes formed in the interstitial fluid. As stated previously, apo-E is synthesized and secreted by a variety of cells and is available in interstitial fluid to transport lipids.

Cells requiring cholesterol up-regulate their LDL receptors, and apo-E targets the apo-E–containing HDL or lipid complexes to cells deficient in necessary lipids. For example, the local transport pathway for apo-E is involved in lipid redistribution within a nerve after injury and during regeneration.[58, 61, 63]

Apolipoprotein AI

Apo-AI is a 29-kd protein encoded by a gene on the long arm of chromosome 11, part of a cluster that includes genes for apo-CIII and apo-AIV.[31, 73–76] The apo-AI gene is 1863 base pairs in length, and its mRNA encodes a 267–amino acid protein that includes an 18–amino acid prepeptide and a 6–amino acid propeptide. The propeptide is cleaved extracellularly to yield the mature circulating protein of 243 amino acids (see Table 23–3).

Apo-AI is synthesized by the human intestine and liver and is a constituent of chylomicrons and HDL. It binds to lipids of these lipoproteins, mainly through a series of 22–amino acid amphipathic alpha-helices separated by helix-breaking proline residues.[73] The polar face of the amphipathic helix is exposed to the aqueous environment, whereas the nonpolar face binds to the lipid (primarily phospholipid) on the surface of the particle. There are eight complete 22–amino acid amphipathic helices and two 11–amino acid repeats in apo-AI.

In addition to its role as a structural protein in HDL, apo-AI activates lecithin:cholesterol acyltransferase (LCAT), which esterifies free cholesterol on HDL particles. It may facilitate the interaction of LCAT with phosphatidylcholine, the substrate of LCAT, but the LCAT activation site has not been identified. Several regions may serve this function. Other apolipoproteins, such as apo-AIV and apo-CI, which have similar lipid-binding properties, can also activate LCAT (discussed in detail in a later section).

Apo-AI–associated particles, either HDL or a phospholipid-rich precursor of HDL (referred to as pre-β HDL), serve as acceptors for cholesterol released from cells.[30, 73, 74] The efflux of cholesterol to HDL represents part of the so-called reverse cholesterol transport pathway (discussed under section on metabolic pathways involving HDL).[77–79] Apo-AI also may serve as the recognition protein for the binding of HDL to the postulated HDL receptor that mediates cholesterol uptake by cells. A candidate HDL receptor has been described.[80]

Mutations that give rise to apo-AI deficiency are characterized by absent or low levels of HDL (discussed under section on primary disorders of HDL metabolism).[73, 76] Apo-AI synthesis is required for HDL production. Apo-AI deficiency causes a variety of manifestations: planar xanthomas, corneal clouding, and sometimes premature coronary heart disease (CHD). Apo-AI is often described as an antiatherogenic apolipopro-

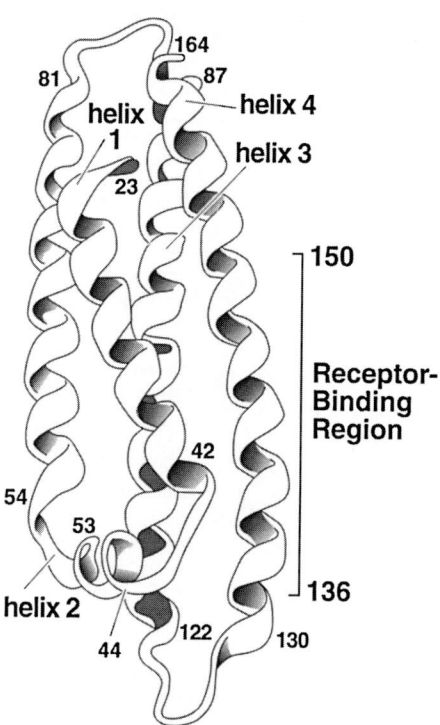

Figure 23–11. Three-dimensional structure of the amino-terminal region (residues 1–191) of apo-E, which forms a four-helix bundle. The receptor-binding domain resides in helix 4. (Modified from Wilson C, Wardell MR, Weisgraber KH, et al. Three-dimensional structure of the LDL receptor-binding domain of human apolipoprotein E. Science 1991; 252:1817–1822, with permission.)

tein. Although apo-E–deficient mice typically develop very extensive atherosclerosis,[71, 72] the overexpression of human apo-AI in these mice causes an increase in HDL and a significant decrease in atherosclerosis.[81, 82]

Apolipoprotein AII

The apo-AII gene is on the long arm of chromosome 1.[31, 73–75] The mRNA encodes a 100–amino acid protein, but the mature circulating form of apo-AII is 77 amino acids in length. In the plasma, human apo-AII exists primarily as a homodimer. A cysteine at residue 6 of apo-AII forms a disulfide bond with a second apo-AII molecule. Heterodimers of apo-AII and apo-E only occur in persons with apo-E2 and apo-E3, which possess free cysteine residues. Heterodimer formation interferes with the ability of apo-E to bind to the LDL receptor.

Apo-AII is synthesized primarily in the liver.[31, 73, 75] It is found together with apo-AI on a subfraction of HDL referred to as Lp-AI/AII particles. Apo-AII may play a role in the activation of hepatic lipase and the inhibition of LCAT. The genetic absence of apo-AII in two sisters did not produce any obvious phenotypic effects and did not cause low HDL levels.

The overexpression of apo-AII in mice leads to an increased susceptibility to atherosclerosis,[83] possibly because apo-AII displaces apo-AI from HDL. This could interfere with the normal ability of apo-AI–containing HDL to transport cellular cholesterol to the liver for excretion. Therefore, apo-AII is considered a proatherogenic apolipoprotein.

C Apolipoproteins

The genes for apo-CI and apo-CII reside on chromosome 19 near the gene that encodes apo-E, whereas the apo-CIII gene is part of the apo-AI and apo-AIV gene cluster on chromosome 11 (for a review see references 8 and 30 to 32). The C apolipoproteins (see Table 23–4 and Fig. 23–5) readily exchange among various lipoproteins and are synthesized primarily by the liver (apo-CI is also produced by macrophages, and small amounts of apo-CII are synthesized by the intestine). HDL appears to serve as a reservoir for the C apolipoproteins, which can then be transferred to triglyceride-rich lipoproteins. The C apolipoproteins appear to regulate triglyceride metabolism and to influence the inverse relation between triglyceride levels and HDL cholesterol. Apo-CI (6.6 kd) modulates the uptake of triglyceride-rich lipoprotein (chylomicron remnants, VLDL, and IDL) by interfering with the ability of apo-E to mediate binding to lipoprotein receptor pathways. Apo-CIII (8.8 kd) may have a similar function in preventing the normal interaction of triglyceride-rich, apo-E–containing lipoproteins with receptors and cell-surface HSPG. Apo-CI and apo-CIII may displace apo-E from the particles. Apo-CII (8.9 kd) is a cofactor for LPL, and mutations in the apo-CII gene result in a marked hypertriglyceridemia (discussed later).

The overexpression of apo-CI, apo-CII, or apo-CIII in transgenic mice results in hypertriglyceridemia (for a review see references 31 and 84). In the case of apo-CI and apo-CIII, the resulting hyperlipidemia appears to be caused by displacement of apo-E from triglyceride-rich particles, which results in impaired receptor-mediated uptake, displacement of apo-CII, and impaired lipolytic processing. A polymorphism of the apo-CIII gene promoter region in mice is also associated with increased levels of apo-CIII and hypertriglyceridemia.[85]

The hypertriglyceridemia that follows the overexpression of apo-CII was initially puzzling,[31] because apo-CII is a cofactor activating LPL-mediated hydrolysis of triglycerides. However, the triglyceride-rich lipoproteins that accumulate in the plasma are poor in apo-E and do not interact well with cell-surface HSPG to allow lipase activity to occur or with receptors

in the proteoglycan-rich matrices of the cell surface for uptake. Therefore, either the overproduction or the underproduction of apo-CII can cause hypertriglyceridemia.

Lipoprotein Receptors Controlling Lipoprotein Metabolism

LDL Receptor Gene Family

Members of this gene family, in addition to the LDL receptor itself, include the LRP, the gp330 receptor, and the VLDL receptor. These receptors share common structural motifs but perform different functions.[86, 87]

LDL RECEPTOR

The LDL receptor, a glycoprotein with an apparent molecular weight of 160,000, is expressed on the surface of most cells and especially in liver. It functions in the uptake of apo-B– and apo-E–containing lipoproteins, including LDL, chylomicron remnants, VLDL, VLDL remnants, IDL, and HDL$_1$.[32, 47, 58] Most HDL particles lack apo-E and do not interact with the LDL receptor. Cells can acquire cholesterol from the plasma by the uptake of these lipoproteins through the LDL receptors. The LDL receptor was first identified in 1973, and its gene was characterized in 1985 in the laboratory of Joseph L. Goldstein and Michael S. Brown.[13, 88–90] Two proteins on the lipoprotein surface, apo-B100 and apo-E, bind to the LDL receptor, which for this reason is sometimes referred to as the apo-B100, apo-E receptor.

After the lipoprotein binds to the LDL receptor, the complex becomes localized to a specialized area of the cell membrane called a coated pit. The "coat" contains a protein complex called clathrin, which clusters the receptors in a region of the cell membrane that can invaginate and form an intracellular vesicle to contain the lipoprotein. As these internalized vesicles, or endosomes, move into the cytoplasm, the internal environment becomes progressively more acidic, causing the receptor and the lipoprotein to dissociate. The lipoproteins are degraded in the lysosomes, and the unoccupied receptors recycle to the cell surface (Fig. 23–12).

The LDL receptor is synthesized in the endoplasmic reticulum as a protein of 839 amino acids[88–90] with an apparent

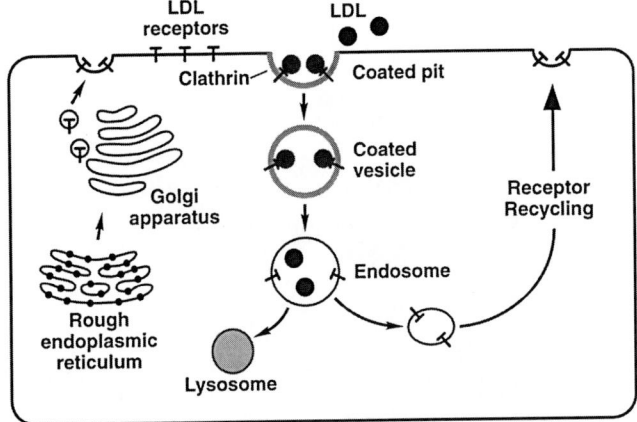

Figure 23–12. LDL receptor pathway. The LDLs interact with their receptors on the cell surface. The complex enters the coated pit and is internalized. The coated vesicle loses its clathrin coat and becomes an endosome, the site of lipoprotein and receptor dissociation. The receptors recycle to the cell surface, and the lipoproteins are degraded. Alternatively, new receptors are synthesized in the rough endoplasmic reticulum and transported to the cell surface. (Modified from Brown MS, Goldstein JL. A receptor-mediated pathway for cholesterol homeostasis. Science 1986; 232:34–47; and Myant NB. Cholesterol Metabolism, LDL, and the LDL Receptor. San Diego: Academic Press, 1990, with permission.)

molecular weight of 120,000. Glycosylation of the protein in the endoplasmic reticulum and in the Golgi apparatus increases its weight to about 160,000. The LDL receptor has five distinct structural and functional domains[90] (Fig. 23–13). Mutations within these domains disrupt the normal function of the receptor in lipoprotein metabolism and cause the genetic disorder familial hypercholesterolemia (FH)[90] (discussed later).

LIGAND-BINDING DOMAIN. The ligand-binding domain consists of the 292 amino acids at the amino terminus (see Fig. 23–13). This region of the molecule is rich in cysteines and contains glutamic and aspartic acid residues that are critical in mediating the binding to apo-B and apo-E. It is composed of seven repeats of approximately 40 amino acids each. Each repeat contains six cysteines that form three intrarepeat disulfide bonds, resulting in a very stable structure. In addition, each repeat contains a Ser-Asp-Glu triplet that mediates the interaction of apo-B– and apo-E–containing lipoproteins with the LDL receptor. The ligand-receptor binding is an ionic interaction between positively charged arginines and lysines in apo-B100 and apo-E and negatively charged aspartic and glutamic acids in the ligand-binding domain of the LDL receptor.

The application of site-directed mutagenesis and the analysis of naturally occurring mutants of the LDL receptor associated with FH have provided insights into the roles of specific repeats and residues in ligand binding.[90] Ligand-binding domain repeat 1 does not play a major role in the binding of either apo-B–containing (LDL) or apo-E–containing (β-VLDL) lipoproteins. The deletion of repeats 2 through 7, however, markedly impairs the binding of LDL. Binding of β-VLDL is mediated by apo-E and is impaired only if repeat 5 is deleted. Therefore, the requirements for binding of LDL are more stringent than those for the binding of β-VLDL.

Single amino acid substitutions of critical residues in the ligand-binding repeats also impair binding activity. For example, in patients with FH Puerto Rico, in which the serine of the ligand-binding triplet (Ser-Asp-Glu) in repeat 4 is changed to a leucine, the LDL fails to bind, although apo-E–containing β-VLDL binds with near-normal affinity. In FH Mexico, in which lysine is substituted for the glutamic acid of the ligand-binding triplet of repeat 5, neither LDL nor β-VLDL binds normally.

The defect in the Watanabe heritable hyperlipidemic (WHHL) rabbit with hypercholesterolemia and accelerated atherosclerosis involves a deletion of four amino acids in repeat 4. Although this defect is associated with a reduced number of receptors reaching the cell surface, those that do reach the surface retain the ability to bind β-VLDL (apo-E) but not LDL (apo-B).[90]

As demonstrated in the WHHL rabbit, mutations in the ligand-binding domain also can disrupt the normal transport of the LDL receptor to the cell surface. The decreased transport of the mutant receptor from the endoplasmic reticulum to the Golgi apparatus and to the cell surface is undoubtedly caused by the improper folding of the molecule and increased intracellular degradation. For example, FH Afrikaner, with a glutamic acid substituted for the aspartic acid in the triplet of repeat 5, results in defective transport and the lack of normal expression of the receptor on the cell surface.

EPIDERMAL GROWTH FACTOR PRECURSOR HOMOLOGY DOMAIN. This region is composed of 400 amino acids and is about 33% identical to the sequence of the human epidermal growth factor (EGF) precursor.[88–90] It contains three cysteine-rich repeats (A, B, and C), each of which is approximately 40 amino acids in length. The repeats are not homologous to the 40–amino acid repeats of the ligand-binding domain but are related to the EGF. Repeat A is involved in the binding of LDL, and if repeat A is deleted LDL binding is markedly inhibited (β-VLDL binding is retained). The EGF precursor domain also plays a role in allowing the LDL receptor or receptors to dissociate from the lipoproteins and recycle to the cell surface. Deletion of the EGF precursor homology domain allows normal binding and internalization of β-VLDL but prevents dissociation of the ligand and receptor, as a result of which receptors do not recycle to the cell surface. The role of the EGF precursor domain was established with the use of site-directed mutagenesis, and FH Osaka was subsequently found to have the same deletion.

O-LINKED SUGAR DOMAIN. This domain is composed of 58 amino acids.[88–90] Serine and threonine are its major amino acids, and many of these residues serve as sites for the attachment of O-linked carbohydrate chains. No functional role for this domain has been described, and its deletion has no functional consequences.

MEMBRANE-SPANNING DOMAIN. The 22 amino acids in this domain are hydrophobic and function to anchor the receptor within the plasma membrane (see Fig. 23–13).[88–90] Truncation mutations that exclude this region are characterized by secretion of the receptor from the cell so that lipoproteins are not internalized.

CYTOPLASMIC DOMAIN. The carboxyl-terminal region of the LDL receptor is composed of 50 amino acids[88–90] and contains the sequence "NPXY" (N, asparagine; P, proline; X, any amino acid; Y, tyrosine), which is responsible for clustering the receptors in coated pits and mediating internalization of the receptors by the cells. One of the early mutations associated with FH (J.D. allele, FH Bari) provided insights into the role of a critical residue for directing internalization. In the mutant form of the receptor, the tyrosine at residue 807 is changed to a cysteine. Site-directed mutagenesis demonstrated that this position must be occupied by an aromatic amino acid (tyrosine, phenylalanine, or tryptophan) for normal internalization. The tetrameric sequence Asn-Pro-Val-Tyr, in which tyrosine-807 occurs, is the signal directing the receptors to the coated pit.

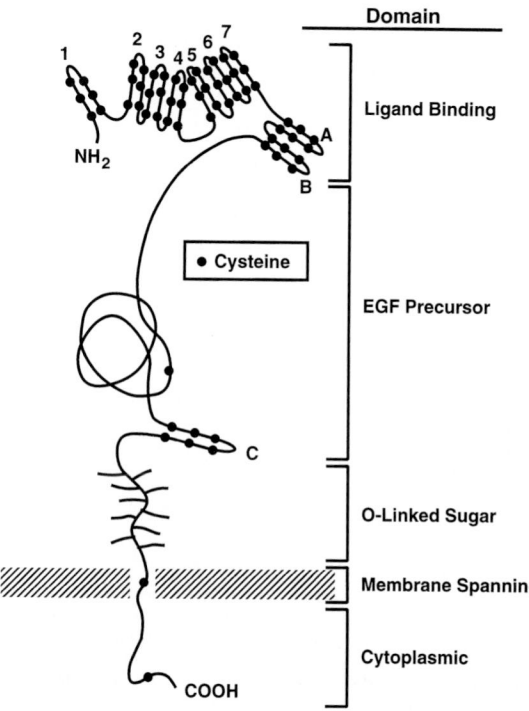

Figure 23–13. Functional domains of the LDL receptor. See text for complete description.

LDL Receptor Gene Regulation

The LDL receptor gene is 45 kb in length and is located on the distal portion of the short arm of chromosome 19. Synthesis of the LDL receptor is regulated by DNA sequences in the 5′-flanking region of the LDL receptor gene (Fig. 23–14).[91–93] A sequence of approximately 10 bases in this region, called the sterol regulatory element (SRE), and two other repeats that bind the transcription factor Sp1 are necessary for the regulation of the LDL receptor mRNA levels. If intracellular sterol levels are high, LDL receptor mRNA is not transcribed. When the sterol content of the cells decreases, the expression of LDL receptors on the cell surface increases, causing an increased uptake of apo-B– and apo-E–containing lipoproteins and increased delivery of cholesterol to the cells. The LDL receptor gene "senses" the sterol level of the cell and appropriately controls receptor mRNA production and protein biosynthesis to meet the needs of the cell.

The mechanism of control of LDL receptor expression has been elucidated in considerable detail.[91–93] Two related (approximately 50% identical) transcription factors, the sterol regulatory element–binding proteins SREBP-1a and SREBP-2, regulate the level of LDL receptors. The intact 125-kd SREBP is an integral membrane protein containing two membrane-spanning regions (see Fig. 23–14). The full-length protein is present in the nuclear membrane and endoplasmic reticulum. To become an active transcription factor and to be translocated to the nucleus to interact with the SRE of the LDL receptor gene, the intact SREBP must be cleaved by a protease to liberate a fragment (approximately 68 kd) representing the active amino-terminal half of the protein. The carboxyl-terminal domain of the SREBP remains membrane bound. It is postulated that, when sterols are present in the cells, the SREBP assumes a conformation within the membrane that prevents the protease from releasing the active component. Absence or deficiency of sterols may allow the SREBP to be present in a conformation that allows proteolysis and liberation of the active component, which is transported to the nucleus, where it induces expression of the LDL receptor and of the other genes involved in cholesterol biosynthesis.

LDL Receptor–Related Protein

The LRP is an integral membrane receptor composed of two components: a 515-kd amino-terminal extracellular domain and an 85-kd cytoplasmic and membrane-spanning domain (the precursor protein, composed of 4525 amino acids, is cleaved after synthesis).[94, 95] This large protein is equivalent structurally to approximately four LDL receptors and possesses 31 ligand-binding domains. The LRP contains the four structural motifs characteristic of other members of the LDL receptor gene family: multiple ligand-binding repeats, EGF repeats and EGF precursor homology domains, a single membrane-spanning region, and two NPXY internalization signals. The LRP is expressed primarily in liver (parenchymal cells), brain (neurons), and placenta (syncytiotrophoblast cells).[86, 87, 96]

The LRP interacts with approximately 18 ligands and has several functions. With respect to lipoprotein metabolism, the LRP binds apo-E–enriched chylomicron remnants and VLDL remnants with high affinity and internalizes these particles. Interaction of these lipoproteins with the LRP requires the addition of multiple apo-E molecules per particle, which serve

Absence of Sterol: Generation of Active SREBP

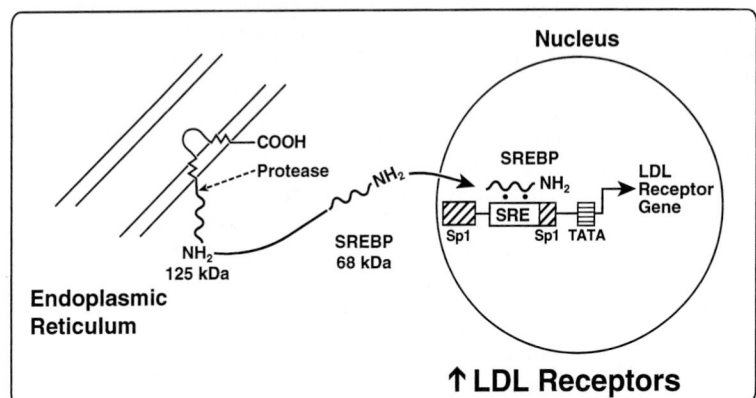

Figure 23–14. LDL receptor gene regulation.

Presence of Sterol: No Generation of Active SREBP

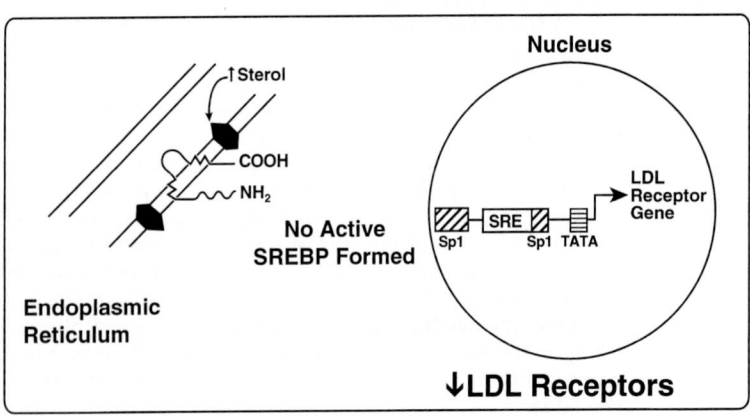

as ligands. An initial binding of the lipoprotein to cell-surface HSPG is necessary to facilitate the interaction or transfer of the apo-E–enriched remnants to the LRP[70] (discussed further under section on chylomicron remnant (apo-E) receptors in remnant catabolism). The LRP does not bind LDL.

The LRP can also interact with LPL[97] and hepatic lipase.[98] This interaction could mediate the hepatic binding and uptake of remnant lipoproteins possessing these enzymes on their surface. Other ligands for the LRP, unrelated directly to lipid metabolism, include α_2-macroglobulin, plasminogen activators and inhibitors, and bacterial toxins.[86, 87] Knockout of the LRP in mice is lethal, demonstrating its critical importance,[99] but the reason for the lethality remains to be elucidated.

A receptor-associated protein (RAP) of 39 kd can be isolated along with purified LRP and effectively competes with all the ligands for the LRP binding. This protein also binds to the gp330 and VLDL receptors (described later) and blocks ligand binding to these receptors as well. However, RAP does not appear to be secreted from the cells, and it may serve as an intracellular chaperone that occupies the ligand-binding sites for transport of the LRP to the cell surface. The knockout of RAP by gene targeting in mice causes a marked reduction in the expression of LRP in both liver and brain, further suggesting an intracellular transport role for this protein.[100] Alternatively, it may play a role in the intracellular recycling of the receptors. Regardless of its physiological role, RAP is an inhibitor of the interaction of LRP and its ligands both in cultured cells and in intact animals.

GP330

The gp330 receptor, also referred to as the major Heymann nephritis antigen, is a large protein (about 600 kd) that possesses many of the structural motifs of the LDL receptor.[86, 87] It is expressed in the proximal tubules of the kidney and the ependymal cells in the brain and is not present in liver. Although gp330 binds apo-E–containing lipoproteins and LDL, its role in lipoprotein metabolism is unknown. The knockout of gp330 by gene targeting does not have an obvious effect on lipoprotein metabolism, but these animals have developmental abnormalities of the central nervous system (holoprosencephaly).[101]

VLDL Receptor

The VLDL receptor closely resembles the LDL receptor except that it possesses an eighth ligand-binding repeat.[102] The VLDL receptor (about 130 kd) binds apo-E–containing lipoproteins and is present primarily in muscle, fat, and brain. In the nervous system it is present in the choroid plexus and in some neurons. It is absent from liver, and its role in lipoprotein metabolism remains to be determined.

Scavenger Receptor

The scavenger receptor, also known as the acetyl LDL receptor, interacts with chemically modified LDL but not with native LDL. LDL that had been modified by acetylation, acetoacetylation, or malondialdehyde were taken up by high-affinity cell-surface receptors on macrophages, resulting in marked cholesterol accumulation. It is now known that this receptor also serves to mediate the uptake of oxidized LDL, the postulated atherogenic form of LDL that causes foam cell formation. Two forms of the scavenger receptor (type I and type II) are generated by alternative splicing of the mRNA encoded by a gene on chromosome 8.[86]

In addition to macrophages, the scavenger receptor is present on endothelial cells in the liver and smooth muscle

cells of the artery wall in some species. The predicted structure is that of a trimer (approximately 220 kd) composed of three identical subunits (each about 77 kd). The type I receptor contains six domains: the cytoplasmic, amino-terminal domain (50 amino acids), a transmembrane domain (26 amino acids), a spacer (74 amino acids), an alpha-helical coiled-coil domain (121 amino acids), a collagen-like domain (72 amino acids with a Gly-X-Tyr repeat), and a cysteine-rich domain (110 amino acids). The type II scavenger receptor is identical to the type I receptor except that it lacks the carboxyl-terminal cysteine-rich domain. The collagen-like domain is responsible for ligand binding. Clusters of positively charged residues (lysines) appear to mediate the interaction with the chemically modified lipoproteins (see section on the LDL paradox and oxidized lipids for a discussion of the role of the scavenger receptor in atherogenesis).

Other receptors that bind oxidized LDL but not chemically modified LDL have been described,[103, 104] but it is unclear how many and what types of receptors mediate the uptake of oxidized LDL.

HDL Receptor

An HDL receptor, envisioned to mediate the interaction of HDL with cells to facilitate the efflux of intracellular cholesterol, has been postulated. Many cell types loaded with cholesterol exhibit specific HDL binding, and several different candidate proteins have been isolated. The most likely HDL receptor has been identified by Krieger and associates; it is an 82-kd protein, a member of the CD36 family that binds HDL and is expressed in liver, adrenals, ovaries, and testes. HDL that bind to this receptor are not degraded, but cholesterol can be transferred to the cells from the HDL.[80]

Enzymes and Transfer Proteins Involved in Lipid and Lipoprotein Metabolism

LIPOPROTEIN LIPASE

Human LPL is a protein composed of 448 amino acids (approximately 50 kd). It is synthesized by adipocytes, by myocytes in skeletal and cardiac muscle, and by macrophages but is not produced by hepatocytes. After secretion from adipocytes and myocytes, LPL is transported to the surface of capillary endothelial cells of these tissues and attaches to cell-surface HSPG. Here, the endothelial cell–attached LPL interacts with the chylomicrons and VLDL in the circulation and mediates the hydrolysis of the triglycerides from these particles to release free fatty acids for use by the tissues. The fatty acids are stored as triglyceride in adipocytes and used as a source of energy in muscle and for triglyceride synthesis in the formation of hepatic VLDL.[105–109]

The active form of LPL is a dimer. Although the crystal structure is not known, LPL has a high degree of homology with another serine esterase, pancreatic lipase, whose structure is known. Based on similarities between LPL and pancreatic lipase, a model for LPL function has been suggested (Fig. 23–15), and five functional domains have been identified in LPL on the basis of structural and mutational studies.[105, 109]

HEPARIN-BINDING SITE. The heparin-binding site mediates the interaction of LPL with HSPG on endothelial cells. Clusters of positively charged arginine and lysine residues on one face of the LPL appear to mediate this interaction, particularly the charged residues in the carboxyl terminus of the molecule.

LIPID-BINDING SITE. The domain of the protein that allows the enzyme to interact with the surface of the chylomicron is in the carboxyl terminus, particularly around residues 245 to 253.

the space of Disse on chylomicron remnants, and hepatic lipase may be localized there. These lipases facilitate binding and uptake of remnants by interacting with the LRP.

The actual hepatocyte uptake of the particles may involve two or more receptors (see Fig. 23–17), the *LDL receptor*, which interacts with apo-B100 and apo-E–containing lipoproteins,[119] possibly a unique apo-E or chylomicron remnant receptor. The previously mentioned LRP is a good candidate receptor for this function.[86, 87, 96, 120]

Whereas remnant particles with LPL or hepatic lipase on their surfaces may interact by means of these molecules with the HSPG in the space of Disse and facilitate binding and uptake by the LRP,[97, 98] apo-E–mediated interactions with HSPG and the LRP are critical in remnant metabolism. Patients with apo-E mutations that prevent interaction with HSPG or lipoprotein receptors develop hyperlipidemia characterized by remnant lipoprotein accumulation, despite having normal lipase activity.[65] In addition, knockout of apo-E by gene targeting in mice causes a profound accumulation of remnant lipoproteins.[72, 73]

ROLE OF THE *LDL* RECEPTOR IN REMNANT CATABOLISM

The LDL receptor is also believed to play a role in chylomicron remnant uptake by the liver.[87, 119] The lack of accumulation of chylomicrons or chylomicron remnants in patients with absent or defective LDL receptors could reflect the fact that remnant clearance requires several steps, as described. For example, sequestration of the particles in the space of Disse (HSPG binding) is normal in patients with defective LDL receptors and could prevent accumulation of remnants in plasma. It is also likely that the chylomicron or apo-E receptor could compensate for deficiency of LDL receptors. Both receptors probably function in the uptake of the remnants, and in the absence of one the other continues to function, possibly with less efficiency. At present, it is impossible to ascertain the relative importance of LDL receptors compared with other receptors in the uptake of remnant lipoproteins by hepatocytes.

CHYLOMICRON REMNANT (APO-E) RECEPTORS IN REMNANT CATABOLISM

Evidence suggests that the LRP is a good candidate to be the chylomicron remnant (apo-E) receptor. This protein is a member of the LDL receptor gene family (discussed previously).[86, 87]

As noted earlier, LRP binds with high affinity to apo-E–enriched lipoproteins but does not bind LDL to a significant extent. Apo-E must be added to remnant lipoproteins before they bind to the LRP with high affinity. Apo-E exists in the space of Disse in high concentration, probably because it is secreted by hepatocytes and binds to HSPG in the space of Disse. The HSPG could then serve as a reservoir for apo-E, allowing enrichment of the remnants with this apolipoprotein (Fig. 23–18).[65, 70, 87, 96]

These and other observations have led to the hypothesis that apo-E functions in a process called *secretion-capture*.[120–122] It is envisioned that apo-E combines with lipids or lipoproteins and directs them to cells expressing LDL receptors or the LRP. In the liver, the LRP and apo-E could interact in this way to capture chylomicron remnants (see Fig. 23–18). The LRP is also present in other tissues, including brain, and may function locally in the uptake of lipids. The secretion-recapture role of apo-E functions in peripheral nerve injury and repair and in the normal maintenance of neurons.[58, 61–63]

As already stated, LRP-mediated uptake of remnants requires the initial interaction of apo-E–containing lipoproteins with cell-surface HSPG (see Fig. 23–18). If HSPG are hydrolyzed by treatment of cells with heparinase in vitro or by infusion of heparinase into the portal vein of mice, apo-E–enriched remnants do not bind to the cell surface and do not interact with the LRP even though the receptor is present. After the lipoproteins interact with HSPG, the remnants may be transferred to the LRP for internalization by the cells, or the HSPG/LRP complex may be internalized. This type of two-step process involving cell-surface proteoglycans and receptors has also been described for growth factors, the process being referred to as the HSPG/LRP pathway.[63, 70, 122–124] It is also possible that HSPG alone can mediate remnant uptake directly without the LRP.

The LRP interacts not only with apo-E–containing lipoproteins but also with an unrelated protein, α_2-macroglobulin, a broad-spectrum endopeptidase inhibitor that is involved in clearing of proteases from the plasma by the liver. The binding of protease activates α_2-macroglobulin, which then binds to the LRP. Activated α_2-macroglobulin competes with remnants for binding to the LRP.[96] Radiolabeled chylomicron remnants are rapidly cleared from the plasma of mice, but the injection of α_2-macroglobulin along with the chylomicron remnants impairs remnant clearance. This finding indicates that α_2-macroglobulin and the remnants are binding to the same receptor, the LRP.

Herz and colleagues demonstrated that the LRP is probably the chylomicron remnant (apo-E) receptor and docu-

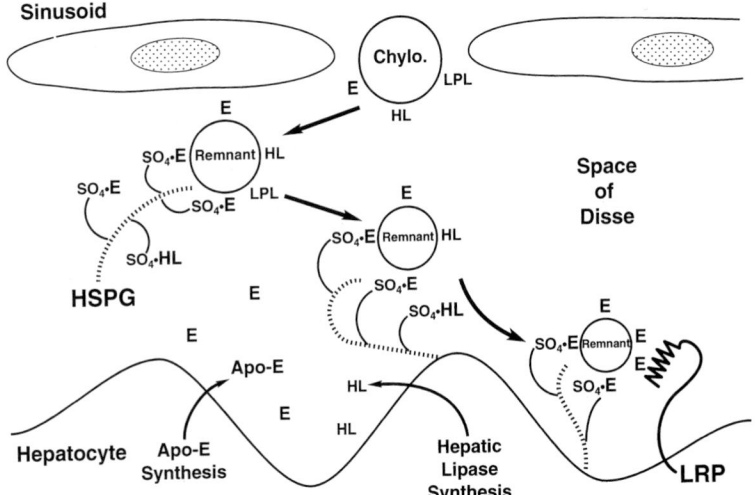

Figure 23–18. Heparan sulfate proteoglycan (HSPG)/LDL receptor–related protein (LRP) pathway.

mented its importance in remnant catabolism.[87] These studies used RAP, which blocks the interaction of all ligands with the LRP, to demonstrate the role of the LRP in remnant clearance in mice. Knockout of RAP in mice results in a loss of LRP expression in the liver. Double-knockout mice, in which both RAP and LDL receptor are missing, develop hyperlipidemia characterized by accumulation of remnant lipoproteins in the plasma.[100]

In summary, the catabolism of chylomicron remnants involves several steps and several components: sequestration, further lipolytic processing, and receptor-mediated endocytosis utilizing both the LDL receptor pathway and the HSPG/LRP pathway.

Very-Low-Density Lipoproteins

CHARACTERISTICS

VLDL are particles 300 to 700 Å in diameter that float on ultracentrifugation at plasma density of less than 1.006 g/mL (see Table 23–3). They are composed of 85 to 90% lipid (about 55% triglyceride, 20% cholesterol, and 15% phospholipid) and 10 to 15% protein. The distinctive apolipoprotein is apo-B100, the hepatic form of apo-B. VLDL also contain apo-E and apo-Cs (see Fig. 23–5). VLDL have pre-β– or α₂-electrophoretic mobility and were previously called pre-β lipoproteins.[4, 8, 30, 32]

ORIGIN

VLDL are synthesized by the liver, and their production is stimulated by increased delivery of free fatty acids to the hepatocytes, either from a high intake of dietary fat or from the mobilization of fatty acids from adipose tissue with fasting or uncontrolled diabetes mellitus. Triglycerides and phospholipids to be used in the formation of VLDL are synthesized in the liver, whereas VLDL cholesterol can be synthesized de novo or reutilized from LDL cholesterol. The VLDL particles are first visible at the rough endoplasmic reticulum–smooth endoplasmic reticulum junction (transitional elements) before they enter the Golgi apparatus.[125] Within the Golgi apparatus, the carbohydrate processing of several of the apolipoproteins occurs. Large Golgi secretory vesicles migrate to the brush border surface of the hepatocytes, fuse with the plasma membrane, and release the VLDL particles into the space of Disse, from which they enter the plasma (Fig. 23–19). The major protein constituents of the newly synthesized VLDL are apo-B100, apo-E, and small amounts of the C apolipoproteins. In plasma, VLDL acquire additional C apolipoproteins and apo-E, primarily from HDLs.

CONTROL OF VLDL SECRETION RATE

The quantity of VLDL secreted from the liver is not controlled by changes in apo-B100 mRNA levels. Apo-B100 is constitutively expressed and is not highly variable.[126–129] Newly synthesized apo-B100 is subject to two fates: (1) it can be combined with lipid to form VLDL particles, or (2) it can be degraded, in which case a VLDL particle is not secreted.[130] If there is a stimulus for VLDL production, such as the delivery of free fatty acids to the liver, the balance is shifted away from apo-B100 degradation to formation and secretion of apo-B100–containing VLDL.

VLDL BIOSYNTHESIS

Newly synthesized apo-B100 first binds to the membrane of the rough endoplasmic reticulum and then is translocated across the membrane. If not significantly lipidated, it is des-

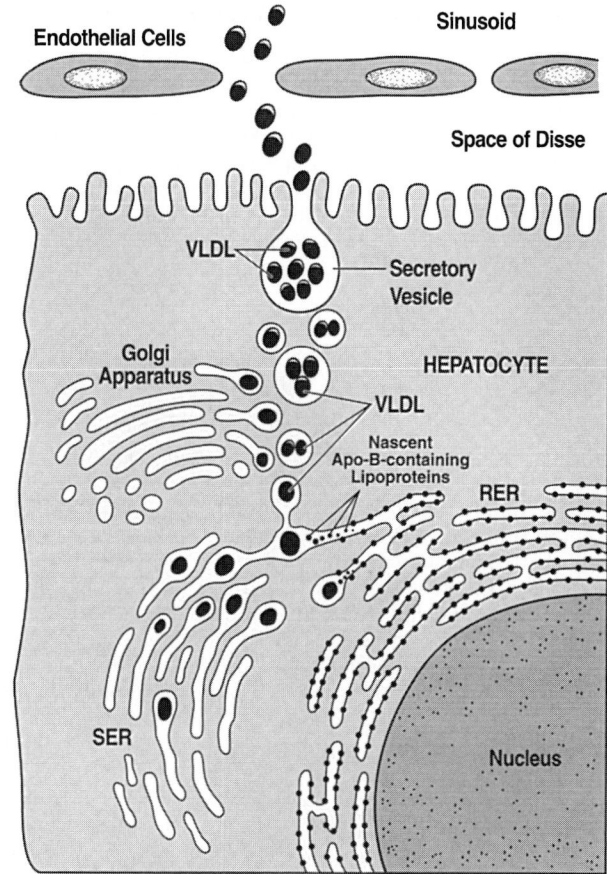

Figure 23–19. VLDL biosynthesis by hepatocytes. The nascent apo-B–containing apolipoproteins synthesized by the rough endoplasmic reticulum (RER) apparently combine with the lipids in the smooth endoplasmic reticulum (SER). The VLDLs are processed in the Golgi apparatus and accumulate in large secretory vesicles. They are then released into the space of Disse, from which they enter the plasma. (Modified from Alexander CA, Hamilton RL, Havel RJ. Subcellular localization of B apoprotein of plasma lipoproteins in rat liver. J Cell Biol 1976; 69:241–263; by copyright permission of The Rockefeller University Press.)

tined to be degraded. If there is significant lipid available, the apo-B100 binds the lipid as it enters the endoplasmic reticulum and forms triglyceride-rich particles which can increase in size, enter the secretory pathway, and exit from the cell as mature VLDL.[128, 129]

The lipidation of apo-B100 to form a particle may begin with the formation of a protein-phospholipid in the lumen as the nascent apo-B100 polypeptide is translocated across the membrane. The newly synthesized apo-B100 could associate with the inner leaflet of the endoplasmic reticulum and serve as a lipid nucleation site capable of accepting triglycerides to form a central core for the VLDL particles. Triglycerides and possibly cholesteryl esters and phospholipids are transferred into the particle by the microsomal triglyceride transfer protein (MTP),[131, 132] and additional triglyceride, cholesterol, and phospholipid may be added in passage through the rough endoplasmic reticulum. At the junction of the rough and smooth endoplasmic reticulum, lipid-rich particles lacking apo-B have been identified in rat liver, and these particles may fuse with the apo-B–containing VLDL precursors to form the mature particle.[125] However, because rat liver synthesizes both apo-B100– and apo-B48–containing VLDL, the postulated fusion step may apply only to apo-B48–VLDL and may be more relevant to apo-B48–containing chylomicron synthesis by the intestine (see Fig. 23–19).

MICROSOMAL TRIGLYCERIDE TRANSFER PROTEIN

MTP is produced in the liver and intestine at the sites of synthesis of apo-B100–containing VLDL and apo-B48–containing chylomicrons, respectively. MTP (97 kd) occurs as a heterodimer complex with the 58-kd protein disulfide isomerase (PDI), an association required for MTP activity. PDI reshuffles disulfide bonds of cysteine residues and therefore may play a role in altering the conformation of apo-B for lipidation. In addition to transferring triglycerides to nascent VLDL, MTP also transfers cholesteryl esters and phospholipids.[131, 132]

More than a dozen mutations of MTP are known to interfere with its activity. Defective MTP is responsible for the lipid disorder abetalipoproteinemia, a condition in which patients essentially lack apo-B–containing lipoproteins in plasma.[132] Therefore, MTP is critical for the biosynthesis of both apo-B100 VLDL in the liver and apo-B48 chylomicrons in the intestine.

The luminal surfaces of the hepatocytes express LDL receptors and the LRP, and VLDL possess both apo-B100 and apo-E that can react with the receptors. How do VLDL traverse the space of Disse and enter the blood? First, lipids such as phosphatidylethanolamine on the surface of the newly secreted VLDL may alter the reactivity of the lipoproteins with the receptors. Newly secreted VLDL are rich in phosphatidylethanolamine, but VLDL in the circulation are poor in phosphatidylethanolamine. This phospholipid may prevent the particle from interacting with the receptors, i.e., specific lipids may mask the receptor-binding domains of apo-B100 and apo-E.

Second, other apolipoproteins may mask the receptor-binding domains of the VLDL apo-B100 and apo-E. Although the amount of C apolipoproteins on newly secreted VLDL is small, they may alter the conformation or availability of the apolipoproteins capable of interacting with the lipoprotein receptors. Specifically, when the VLDL are formed in the liver and apo-E becomes associated, the C apolipoproteins may be positioned so as to mask the apo-E and thereby block its reactivity with the receptor or with proteoglycans in the space of Disse. Alternatively, apo-E associated with the particles intracellularly may not be available to bind to the receptors; only newly acquired apo-E obtained from HDL may possess the appropriate conformation for receptor binding.

METABOLIC FATE

VLDL triglycerides are hydrolyzed by the actions of LPL and hepatic lipase. They are converted to smaller and smaller particles that become increasingly rich in cholesterol (see Fig. 23–16). The products of VLDL catabolism are IDL ($d = 1.006$ to 1.019 g/mL). IDL retain apo-B100 and apo-E but have lost most of the C apolipoproteins. IDL are processed to LDL ($d = 1.019$–1.063 g/mL) by LPL with final processing by hepatic lipase. LDL are the major cholesterol-carrying lipoproteins in the plasma and contain only apo-B100.

Approximately half of VLDL are converted to LDL, and the remainder are cleared directly by the liver as VLDL remnants (small VLDL) and IDL (see Fig. 23–16). The uptake of VLDL remnants and IDL by liver parenchymal cells is mediated by apo-E, and the uptake of LDL by the LDL receptor is mediated by apo-B100.[4, 30]

Intermediate-Density Lipoproteins

IDL ($d = 1.006$ to 1.019 g/mL) are normally present in low concentrations in the plasma and are intermediate in size and composition between VLDL and LDL (see Table 23–3). Their primary proteins are apo-B100 and apo-E.[4, 8, 30] The IDL are precursors of LDL and represent metabolic products of VLDL catabolism in the plasma by the action of lipases. As shown in Figure 23–16, IDL may be further processed by hepatic lipase or removed from the plasma by the LDL receptor. IDL are often considered to be VLDL remnants and to be atherogenic.

Low-Density Lipoproteins

CHARACTERISTICS

LDL ($d = 1.019$ to 1.063 g/mL) are the major cholesterol-carrying lipoproteins in the plasma; about 70% of total plasma cholesterol is in LDL, which are about 200 Å in diameter. The LDL are composed of approximately 75% lipid (about 35% cholesteryl ester, 10% free cholesterol, 10% triglyceride, and 20% phospholipid) and 25% protein (see Table 23–3). Apo-B100 is the principal protein in these particles, along with trace amounts of apo-E (see Fig. 23–5). LDL have β-electrophoretic mobility and were previously referred to as β lipoproteins.[1, 4, 8, 30]

ORIGIN

LDL are the end products of lipase-mediated hydrolysis of VLDL (see Fig. 23–16). Moreover, as the triglyceride-rich core of the larger VLDL particles is removed, the surface lipids and proteins are remodeled, and excess surface constituents are transferred to HDL, the result being formation of a small, cholesterol-rich LDL devoid of almost all apolipoproteins except apo-B100.

METABOLIC FATE

About 75% of LDL is taken up by hepatocytes. Other tissues take up smaller amounts of LDL. Approximately two thirds of uptake is mediated by the LDL receptor, and the remainder is mediated by a poorly defined process that does not involve receptors. LDL are considered to be atherogenic.

APOLIPOPROTEINS B AND E DETERMINE RATE OF PLASMA LIPOPROTEIN CLEARANCE

The rate of clearance of lipoproteins from the plasma is determined by the apolipoprotein that mediates the interaction with the receptor and by the number of receptors expressed on the cell surface (primarily in the liver). VLDL and IDL are rapidly cleared from the plasma (their half-lives are measured in minutes to a few hours). Apo-E mediates their binding to the LDL receptors. Multiple apo-E molecules per lipoprotein can interact with more than one receptor or with multiple sites on a receptor. Multiple interactions cause an enhanced affinity of binding and increased clearance of these particles from the plasma. The clearance of LDL is mediated by apo-B100. The affinity of apo-B100 for the LDL receptor is lower than that of apo-E, and clearance of LDL is much slower (with a half-life of 2 to 3 d). Apo-E–containing lipoproteins have a 20-fold greater affinity for the LDL receptor than apo-B100–containing LDL.[8, 32, 47]

This difference in affinity may affect the circulating levels of apo-B100– and apo-E–containing lipoproteins. In the presence of high levels of apo-E associated with remnants, VLDL, and IDL, these lipoproteins effectively compete with LDL for binding to the LDL receptor, and LDL levels could rise. Conversely, apo-E at low levels and apo-E that is defective in receptor-binding activity (apo-E2 associated with type III hyperlipoproteinemia) do not compete effectively with LDL for the LDL receptor; as a result, the LDL concentrations are lower. Thus, the difference in the affinities of apo-B100 and apo-E plays a role in plasma cholesterol homeostasis.

All cells have the capability of synthesizing cholesterol de novo.[1, 2, 4–6] However, LDL is used as a source of cholesterol for many cells. Cholesterol taken up by the liver has several fates: membrane biosynthesis, VLDL biosynthesis, excretion as cholesterol in the bile, and conversion to bile acids. Cholesterol is used as a precursor for steroid hormone production in the adrenals, ovaries, and testes. In other peripheral tissues, cholesterol is used in membrane biosynthesis for cell repair and proliferation.

FACTORS AFFECTING LDL LEVELS IN THE BLOOD

Plasma LDL levels can be increased through two primary mechanisms: (1) increased VLDL biosynthesis and secretion, secondary to increased flux of free fatty acids to the liver from dietary fats or from mobilization from adipose tissue and (2) decreased LDL catabolism. Decreased catabolism can result from (1) decreased LDL receptor levels in hepatic and extrahepatic tissues (down-regulation of LDL receptor expression occurs when cells possess an adequate cholesterol content for their metabolic needs or when diets are high in saturated fat and cholesterol), (2) increased numbers of high-affinity apo-E–containing lipoproteins that compete with LDL for receptor interaction (as discussed previously), (3) defective LDL receptors incapable of normal interaction with apo-B100, and (4) defective apo-B100 incapable of normal interaction with the LDL receptors.

High-Density Lipoproteins

CHARACTERISTICS

HDL are small particles (70 to 120 Å in diameter) that float at densities of 1.063 to 1.21 g/mL. They are somewhat arbitrarily divided into two major subclasses: HDL_2 ($d = 1.063$ to 1.125 g/mL) and HDL_3 ($d = 1.125$ to 1.21 g/mL). HDL contain about 50% lipid (25% phospholipid, 15% cholesteryl ester, 5% free cholesterol, and 5% triglyceride) and 50% protein (see Table 23–3). Their major apolipoproteins are apo-AI (65%), apo-AII (25%), and smaller amounts of the C apolipoproteins and apo-E (see Fig. 23–5). Apo-E is a minor component of a subclass of HDL referred to as HDL_1, but about 50% of total plasma apo-E is in this HDL fraction. The major classes of HDL lack apo-E and therefore do not interact with the LDL receptor. HDL serves as a reservoir for apo-E and the C apolipoproteins to be distributed to other lipoproteins when they enter the plasma (e.g., chylomicrons, VLDL). Subclasses of HDL may contain only apo-AI (called Lp-AI) or apo-AI and apo-AII (called Lp-AI/AII). The HDL as a class have α-electrophoretic mobility and previously were referred to as α lipoproteins.[8, 30, 31, 73–75]

ORIGIN

HDL originate from three major sources (Fig. 23–20). First, the liver secretes an apo-AI–phospholipid disc called nascent HDL. Second, the intestine directly synthesizes a small apo-AI–containing HDL particle. Third, HDL are derived from surface material (primarily apo-AI and phospholipid) that comes from chylomicrons and VLDL during lipolysis. As chylomicrons and VLDL are acted on by LPL and the triglyceride-rich core is hydrolyzed, excess material is shed from the surface in combination with apo-AI to form small HDL discs.

MATURATION OF HDL

The nascent or precursor HDL particles exist as apo-AI–phospholipid disks. They are designated Lp-AI pre-$β_1$, pre-

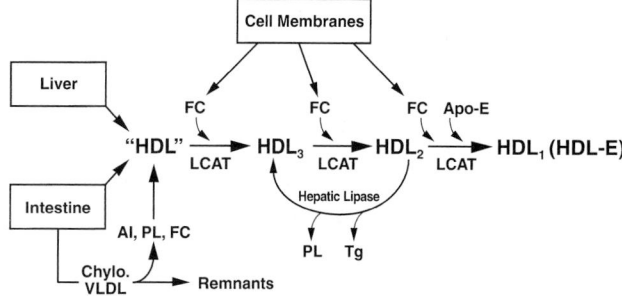

Figure 23–20. Origin of HDL from liver, intestine, and surface material from chylomicrons and VLDL. AI, apo-AI; FC, free cholesterol; HDL-E, HDL-with apo-E; LCAT, lecithin:cholesterol acyltransferase; PL, phospholipid; Tg, triglyceride.

$β_2$, and pre-$β_3$.[30, 73] They are excellent acceptors of free cholesterol from cell membranes with excess cholesterol or from other lipoproteins. Only a limited amount of free cholesterol can be accommodated by the pre-β phospholipid discs. However, esterification of the cholesterol with a long-chain fatty acid decreases its hydrophilicity, and the newly formed cholesteryl ester moves away from the surface of the disc, beginning the process of forming a cholesteryl ester–rich core and converting the disc to a sphere. The enzyme in the plasma that converts free cholesterol to cholesteryl ester is LCAT.

The small, spherical mature HDL particles (Lp-AI, HDL_3) also serve as acceptors for free cholesterol, and as more free cholesterol is acquired and esterified the particles increase in size, forming HDL_2. These HDL subclasses can include Lp-AI, or they can be converted to Lp-AI/AII particles by the addition of apo-AII.

In some animals and to a lesser extent in humans, HDL_2 can be further enriched in cholesteryl ester and at the same time acquire apo-E (Fig. 23–21). HDL_1 is a minor but metabolically active subclass of HDL.[8, 32, 47] The presence of apo-E targets the HDL_1 to cells expressing the LDL receptor. Typical HDL lack apo-E and do not interact with the LDL receptor. The HDL_1 represent a major HDL class in many lower species and in humans with abetalipoproteinemia or CETP deficiency.

HDL_1 appears to arise from a precursor particle that displays γ-electrophoretic mobility and is called γLp-E.[133] This particle is approximately 80% protein and 20% lipid (primarily sphingomyelin and phosphatidylcholine, with some free

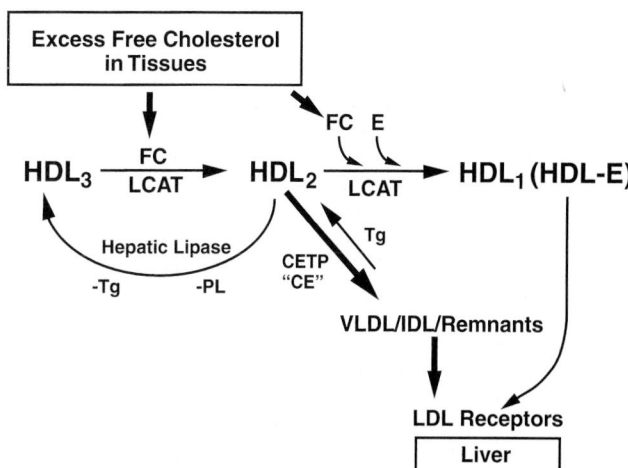

Figure 23–21. Role of HDL in the redistribution of lipids from cells with excess cholesterol to cells requiring cholesterol or to the liver for excretion. The reverse cholesterol transport pathway is indicated by bold arrows (net transfer of cholesterol from cells → HDL → LDL → liver). FC, free cholesterol; HDL-E, HDL-with apo-E.

cholesterol). The γLp-E is a good acceptor of free cholesterol from cells and appears to be converted to the larger HDL₁ by the action of LCAT. HDL₁ also contains apo-AI and sometimes apo-AI/AII. It is difficult to fractionate these various subclasses of HDL, but the major HDL subclasses are believed to be Lp-AI and Lp-AI/AII.

HDL ACQUISITION OF CHOLESTEROL

HDL, especially HDL₃ and precursors of mature HDL, can acquire cholesterol from cells by two different mechanisms.

AQUEOUS TRANSFER FROM CELLS. The HDL come in close contact with cells having excess cholesterol and acquire free cholesterol (not cholesteryl ester) from the cell surface. Free cholesterol follows a physicochemical concentration gradient from the cell to the HDL particle, from a high concentration of free cholesterol in the membranes of cells with excess cholesterol to a low concentration at the surface of the HDL. This process is referred to as passive desorption.[134]

FACILITATED TRANSPORT BY A CELL-SURFACE–BINDING PROTEIN. HDL particles bind to sites on the membranes of cells that have an increased cholesterol content. HDL are believed to bind to a specific protein (referred to as the HDL receptor, as discussed previously), but could bind to a lipid patch or even to the carbohydrate cell coat. The binding does not lead to uptake and degradation of the HDL but facilitates the acquisition of free cholesterol by the HDL.[73]

ENZYME INVOLVED IN HDL METABOLISM: LCAT

LCAT (47 kd, 416 amino acids) is synthesized as a glycoprotein (25% of total mass is carbohydrate) primarily by the liver and to a lesser extent in the brain and testes.[111, 116, 135, 136] It is associated in the plasma primarily with Lp-AI or pre-β₃ and small mature HDL and to a lesser extent with LDL. Apo-AI activates LCAT. Apo-CI and apo-AIV also can activate the enzyme. In humans, LCAT is responsible for the production of most cholesteryl esters in plasma lipoproteins. Although HDL is the preferred substrate for LCAT, a small proportion of free cholesterol is esterified on LDL; LCAT possesses both α-LCAT activity (acting on HDL) and β-LCAT activity (acting on LDL). In the human disorder called fish-eye disease, a single amino acid substitution of threonine for isoleucine-123 blocks the ability of LCAT to esterify cholesterol in HDL, but the mutated protein still catalyzes the esterification of cholesterol on LDL. Therefore, this form of LCAT deficiency is less severe than complete LCAT deficiency.

LCAT has two different enzymatic activities. In *lecithin cleavage (phospholipase activity)*, the ester bond of the fatty acid in position 2 of lecithin, which is usually linoleic acid (C18:2), is hydrolyzed to yield lysolecithin and the fatty acid. The fatty acid becomes covalently linked to serine at amino acid residue 181 in the LCAT molecule. In *transesterification (transacylase activity)*, the fatty acid attached to LCAT is transferred to the 3β-hydroxyl position of cholesterol, forming a cholesteryl ester that enters the core of the lipoprotein particle. The mechanism for the transfer of the fatty acid to cholesterol has not been defined.

Much has been learned about the normal function of LCAT in lipoprotein metabolism by studying patients who have low or undetectable activity of this enzyme in plasma. This disorder can be caused by mutations that affect the structure of LCAT or of apo-AI. LCAT deficiency is manifested by low levels of cholesteryl esters, low levels of HDL, and clinical features ranging from mild symptoms such as corneal clouding (caused by free cholesterol accumulation in the cornea) to severe disorders such as renal failure.

METABOLIC PATHWAYS INVOLVING HDL

HDL function in the redistribution of lipids among lipoproteins and cells by a process called *reverse cholesterol transport.* The HDL acquire cholesterol from cells and transport it to the liver for excretion or to other cells that require cholesterol. The scheme is shown in Figure 23–21.[8, 73, 116]

HDL₃ particles are converted to HDL₂ and then to HDL₁, as previously described. Apo-E, which is associated with HDL₁, targets this minor HDL subclass to cells expressing LDL receptors.[32, 47] In this way, cholesterol can be redistributed from cells with excess cholesterol to cells that require cholesterol. This apo-E–mediated pathway may also deliver cholesterol to the liver for excretion. HDL₁ does not represent a major transport pathway for cholesteryl ester delivery to the liver in humans but is a major route in some species.

A second pathway of cholesterol redistribution involves the action of CETP (Fig. 23–21)[77–79, 112, 118] CETP transfers cholesteryl ester from HDL₂ to VLDL, IDL, and remnants. The cholesterol is thus delivered indirectly to the liver through VLDL and chylomicron remnant pathways. In exchange for transfer of the cholesteryl ester, CETP transfers triglyceride to HDL₂, which becomes enriched with triglycerides. The CETP pathway is the major route for the transport and delivery of cholesteryl esters from HDL to the liver in humans, nonhuman primates, and rabbits that possess CETP.

HDL₂ IS RECONVERTED TO HDL₃ TO ACT AS A CHOLESTEROL ACCEPTOR

As stated previously, HDL₂ particles are depleted in cholesteryl ester and enriched in triglycerides by the action of CETP. Hepatic lipase can then act on the large, triglyceride-enriched HDL₂ to hydrolyze the triglycerides (and possibly also excess phospholipids), converting the HDL₂ to HDL₃. HDL₃ serves as an acceptor for free cholesterol, thus perpetuating the HDL₂–HDL₃ cycle (see Fig. 23–21).[8, 30, 73]

The catabolism of HDL is not entirely understood. The specific lipid moieties of the HDL can be taken up by cells without removal of the intact HDL particle from the plasma compartment. For example, cholesteryl esters are removed from the particle by selective uptake and preferentially delivered to liver, adrenal glands, and gonads.[137] Hepatic lipase may be involved in the selective uptake of cholesterol from the HDL by hydrolyzing the phospholipids on the particles and creating a chemical gradient that promotes transfer of the cholesterol from the particle to the cell. In the kidneys, apo-AI is removed in preference to cholesterol; this apo-AI may be dissociated from the HDL particle, filtered, and degraded. Ultimately, intact HDL can be taken up by hepatocytes and degraded. Although HDL₁ represents a small fraction of total HDL, it is taken up directly by LDL receptors and degraded in the liver through the LDL pathway.

SELECTIVE UPTAKE OF CHOLESTEROL BY STEROIDOGENIC CELLS

HDL is more efficient than LDL in delivering cholesterol to steroidogenic cells of the adrenal, ovary, and testis. In these organs, the lipoproteins concentrate on the surface of the cells in microvillar channels.[138, 139] The channels represent flaps of cell-surface membrane that form a 150- to 250-Å wide cleft in which the lipoproteins are trapped at least transiently. Within these channels, cholesteryl ester and free cholesterol can be extracted from the HDL without the particles' being endocytosed or degraded. Recall that hepatic lipase is selectively localized to these same organs and is believed to modify HDL in such a way as to facilitate the selective uptake of cholesterol. Presumably the particles are released to re-enter the circulation after some cholesterol is extracted.

The importance of HDL and specifically apo-AI–containing HDL for delivery of cholesterol to steroidogenic cells has been shown in apo-AI knockout mice.[139] In the adrenal glands the reticularis and fasiculata cells are usually loaded with lipid droplets. In knockout mice, however, there is no lipid in these cells, lipoproteins are absent from the microvillar channels, and luteal cells of the ovary and Leydig's cells of the testis have markedly reduced levels of lipid. The absence of lipid and cell-surface lipoprotein particles is not observed in the adrenal gland, ovary, or testis of mice in which apo-AII or apo-E have been knocked out. Therefore, apo-AI appears to play an important role, possibly by targeting the particles to the channels or by providing particles with the proper composition to allow entry into the channels for selective delivery of cholesterol to the cells.

The importance of the apo-AI–HDL pathway in delivering cholesterol to the adrenal is further shown by the blunted synthesis and secretion of glucocorticoids in apo-AI knockout mice that are acutely stressed.

CHOLESTERYL ESTER TRANSFER PROTEIN

As discussed previously, CETP facilitates the transfer of cholesteryl esters from HDL to the lower-density, triglyceride-rich lipoproteins (primarily VLDL, IDL, and remnants).[117] CETP plays a pivotal role in lipid metabolism and may affect susceptibility or resistance to the development of atherosclerosis.[140] For example, humans, monkeys, and rabbits have significant amounts of CETP activity in their plasma. As a consequence, they form only small amounts of HDL₁; they dispose of most of their HDL cholesteryl esters by delivering them to lower-density lipoproteins (see Fig. 23–21). Ultimately, most of the cholesteryl esters leave the plasma by the LDL pathway. These species are susceptible to atherosclerosis and tend to have higher levels of LDL. On the other hand, rats, mice, and dogs have no CETP activity, readily form HDL₁, and can deliver the cholesterol directly to the liver by the apo-E–mediated pathway. These animals have very low levels of LDL and are resistant to the development of atherosclerosis. These observations have led to the postulate that high levels of CETP activity accelerate atherogenesis and that inhibition of CETP may be beneficial in treating certain types of hyperlipidemia.

However, this concept has recently been brought into question by the observation that Japanese Americans with a deficiency of CETP have increased HDL but nevertheless develop CHD.[117, 141] The HDL in these individuals tends to be the large HDL₁, and levels of the smaller HDL₃ are decreased. If these data concerning the atherogenicity of low CETP activity are confirmed, it may mean that low levels of HDL₃, which serves as the most potent acceptor of cellular cholesterol, are a major risk factor for CHD in these individuals.

Data obtained from overexpression of CETP in transgenic mice do not clarify whether high levels are protective or detrimental.[31, 75, 117] In one study, overexpression of CETP led to accelerated atherogenesis,[142] but in a study in which CETP was overexpressed in hypertriglyceridemic mice expressing high levels of apo-CIII, there was less atherosclerosis even though the mice were hyperlipidemic and had low HDL levels.[117] The potential therapeutic value of lowering CETP to retard atherogenesis must be questioned until these inconsistencies are sorted out.

HDL AS ANTIATHEROGENIC LIPOPROTEINS

Numerous studies have demonstrated that high levels of HDL cholesterol are associated with a lower incidence of CHD. Conversely, low levels of HDL cholesterol are associated with a higher incidence of CHD. The protective mechanism involving HDL may relate to its role in reverse cholesterol transport, which results in redistribution of cholesterol away from the artery wall. It is also possible that a low level of HDL may be only a marker for some other metabolic event that has a direct effect on atherogenesis. For example, HDL levels are inversely related to VLDL and triglyceride levels, and a low HDL level may be a marker for an increase in a specific subclass of triglyceride-rich lipoproteins that are particularly atherogenic. In addition, it must be kept in mind that the HDL are a heterogeneous group of molecules having different metabolic roles. Some may be protective (e.g., small Lp-AI, HDL₃), and others may not be (e.g., Lp-AI/AII). As the complex nature of HDL is unraveled, it may be possible to define an antiatherogenic spectrum of HDL particles and determine the metabolic and therapeutic measures needed to alter these HDL selectively.

LIPIDS AND ATHEROSCLEROSIS

Atherosclerosis is a disease that causes a reduction of blood flow and insufficient delivery of oxygen and nutrients to affected organs. With insufficient oxygen, ischemia or infarction results, leading to angina or myocardial infarction in the case of restricted blood flow to the heart muscle, to stroke with reduced blood flow to the brain, or to intermittent claudication with restricted blood flow to the lower extremities. CHD is the leading cause of death in the United States (about 35% of all deaths) and in Western Europe.

The restricted arterial blood flow in atherosclerosis is caused by changes in the vessel wall characterized by lipid deposition and cell proliferation. Narrowing of the vessel lumen may lead to obstruction.[143] The deposited lipids are derived from plasma lipoproteins, and elevated plasma cholesterol represents a major risk factor. Other important risk factors include low HDL levels, cigarette smoking, hypertension, male sex, diabetes mellitus, obesity, stress, and lack of exercise.[9, 144] The discussion here focuses on plasma lipoproteins and the cholesterol-diet-heart hypothesis.

Cholesterol-Diet-Heart Hypothesis

For the last 40 years, evidence linking high plasma cholesterol concentrations with an increased risk for CHD has been accumulating,[9, 20–22, 145, 146] and the evidence is now overwhelming and indisputable. The cholesterol-diet-heart hypothesis states that (1) increased plasma cholesterol concentrations increase the risk of CHD, (2) diets high in fat (especially saturated fat) and cholesterol result in increased levels of plasma cholesterol, and (3) lowering plasma cholesterol levels results in a decreased risk of CHD.

ANIMAL MODELS

Numerous animal models demonstrate that diets enriched in cholesterol and saturated fat elevate plasma cholesterol levels and lead to the development of atherosclerosis with many of the features of the human disease.[147–150] Studies in monkeys are particularly relevant.[149, 150] Feeding monkeys a diet that approximates the typical Western diet (500 mg cholesterol/d and 20% of calories as saturated fat) results in elevation of plasma LDL concentrations and atherosclerotic lesions that are almost identical to those seen in humans.[149] The LDL levels can be reduced and the lesions can be made to regress by elimination of the saturated fat and cholesterol from the diet. In addition to elevations in LDL concentrations, cholesterol-fat feeding in animals causes accumulation of β-VLDL. These cholesterol-enriched remnant lipoproteins are derived from lipoproteins secreted by the intestine and liver and also accumulate in type III hyperlipoproteinemia[32, 65, 147, 148] (discussed later).

Single-gene mutation in animals also have demonstrated the link between hypercholesterolemia and atherosclerosis. The WHHL rabbit is a model of familial hypercholesterolemia in which the LDL receptors are defective; elevated LDL concentrations result from retarded clearance rates.[151] Another model of familial hypercholesterolemia is the LDL receptor–deficient mouse in which functional receptors have been eliminated by gene targeting.[152] As discussed previously, apo-E–deficient mice represent another model of defective remnant lipoprotein clearance.[71, 72] As a result of high levels of remnant accumulation, these animals develop severe spontaneous atherosclerosis, even when fed a low-fat diet.

EPIDEMIOLOGIC EVIDENCE

Several epidemiologic studies have demonstrated a relation between plasma cholesterol and an increased incidence of CHD. For example, the Multiple Risk Factor Intervention Trial (Fig. 23–22) showed that there is increased risk at levels above 5.2 mmol/L (200 mg/dL).[153] The Seven Countries Study also demonstrated a relation between an increased incidence of CHD and high plasma cholesterol levels (Fig. 23–23).[22, 146]

The causal relationship between elevated plasma cholesterol levels and accelerated atherosclerosis is established. Epidemiological studies have linked the intake of high levels of dietary fat, especially saturated fats, with increased plasma cholesterol levels.[9, 19–22] Likewise, diets high in cholesterol also tend to increase plasma cholesterol levels.[19–21] Therefore, restriction of saturated fat and cholesterol is the backbone of dietary therapy for elevated blood cholesterol levels.

FAMILIAL HYPERCHOLESTEROLEMIA

Some of the most compelling evidence for a causative effect of plasma cholesterol has come from studies of familial hypercholesterolemia.[13, 90] This genetic disorder results from a series of mutations in the LDL receptor that cause the accumulation of LDL in the plasma as a result of defective clearance of LDL by the receptors. These studies conclusively demonstrate that increased plasma concentrations of LDL cause atherosclerosis.

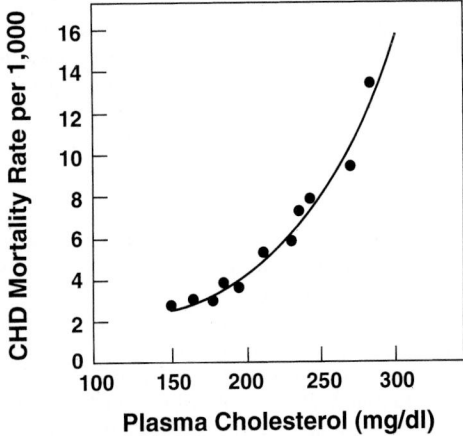

Figure 23–22. Relation between plasma cholesterol levels and coronary heart disease mortality in the Multiple Risk Factor Intervention Trial. (Modified from Stamler J, Wentworth, D, Neaton JD. Is relationship between serum cholesterol and risk of premature death from coronary heart disease continuous and graded? Findings in 356,222 primary screenees of the Multiple Risk Factor Intervention Trial (MRFIT). J Am Med Assoc 1986; 256:2823–2828; Copyright © 1986, by the American Medical Association.)

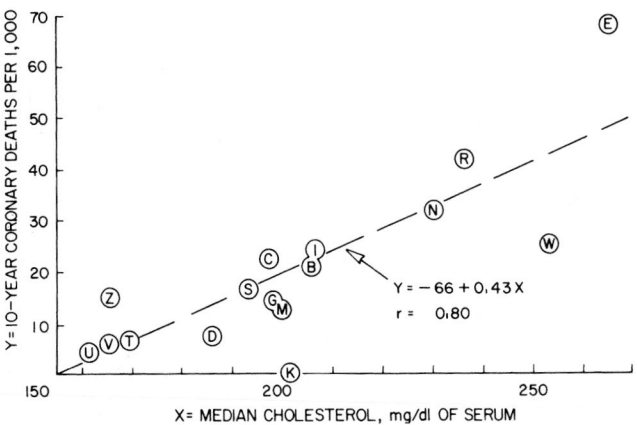

Figure 23–23. Coronary heart disease mortality (10-y death rates) versus median serum cholesterol (mg/dL). All men were free of heart disease at the beginning of the study. B = Belgrade, Serbia; C = Crevalcore, Italy; D = Dalmatia, Croatia; E = East Finland; G = Corfu, Greece; I = Italian railroad workers (Rome division); K = Crete, Greece; M = Montegiorgio, Italy; N = Zutphen, The Netherlands; R = American railroad workers (Greenbay, WI; San Francisco, CA; Seattle, WA); S = Slavonia, Croatia; T = Tanushimaru, Japan; U = Ushibuka, Japan; W = West Finland; Z = Zrenjanin, Serbia. (From Keys A. Seven Countries: A Multivariate Analysis of Death and Coronary Heart Disease. Cambridge, Massachusetts: Harvard University Press, 1980, with permission.)

EXPERIMENTAL EVIDENCE IN HUMANS

An additional line of evidence supporting the cholesterol-diet-heart hypothesis showed that lowering plasma cholesterol levels reduces the risk of CHD. The Lipid Research Clinics Coronary Primary Prevention Trial followed approximately 3800 men (ages 35 to 59) with plasma cholesterol concentrations higher than 6.7 mmol/L (260 mg/dL) and with no prior evidence of CHD.[154] The men were divided into two groups: a control group given a placebo and minimal dietary advice and an experimental group given the lipid-lowering drug cholestyramine and dietary management. Over the 7-year study, reductions of 19%, 19%, and about 25% were seen in total and LDL cholesterol concentrations, in the incidence of fatal and nonfatal myocardial infarction, and in the incidence of angina, respectively. At high doses of cholestyramine, the results were even more dramatic, with 35% and 50% reductions in LDL cholesterol levels and in the incidence of symptomatic CHD, respectively.

The Familial Atherosclerosis Treatment Study took the cholesterol-diet-heart hypothesis a step further.[155] In this study, 120 high-risk men were treated aggressively with lipid-lowering protocols for 2.5 y. All subjects had plasma cholesterol and LDL concentrations higher than 7.0 mmol/L (270 mg/dL) and 4.7 mmol/L (180 mg/dL), respectively, and all had angiographic documentation of CHD. Digitized quantitative coronary arteriography was used for documentation. Men receiving either drug treatment (lovastatin and colestipol or niacin and colestipol) displayed dramatic reductions in plasma LDL concentrations and in the progression of coronary atherosclerosis. More importantly, established atherosclerotic lesions actually regressed.

In spite of the impressive results of these intervention trials, critics continued to question recommendations for diet and drug therapy to reduce the risk of CHD,[156, 157] based on the fact that the trials, although they clearly demonstrated a marked reduction in CHD-related events, did not conclusively prove that lowering cholesterol prolonged life. Concern was expressed that an increased risk of death from other causes could result from the treatment. Two important prospective studies have addressed these concerns: the Scandinavian Simvastatin Survival Study Group (4S), conducted in high-risk patients with preexisting coronary disease (a so-called secondary prevention study),[158] and the West of Scotland Coronary Prevention Study Group, conducted in men without preexisting coronary disease (a so-called primary prevention study).[159]

The 4S trial included 4444 patients, of which 19% were women, with angina pectoris or a previously documented myocardial infarction and with elevated plasma cholesterol concentrations (5.5 to 8.0 mmol/L [214 to 311 mg/dL]). The subjects, who were previously on a lipid-lowering diet, were randomly divided into placebo and treatment groups; the drug tested was simvastatin, an HMG-CoA reductase inhibitor. The groups were observed for an average of 5.4 y (the time interval at which 10% of the study participants died). The mean changes in total plasma cholesterol, LDL cholesterol, and HDL cholesterol in the drug group compared with the placebo group were −25%, −35%, and +8%, respectively. The placebo group had 256 (12%) deaths, and the simvastatin group had 182 (8%), for a relative risk of death of .70. Deaths from CHD-related events were 189 in the placebo group and 111 in the simvastatin group, for a relative risk of death in the drug group of .58. There were no differences in noncardiovascular deaths between the two groups (49 versus 46, respectively). In addition, the relative risk for one or more coronary events was .66 for the drug group, and there was a 37% reduction in the need for myocardial procedures.[158] In this study cholesterol lowering prolonged life in persons with established CHD.

The results from the West of Scotland study were equally impressive.[159] This trial was designed to test the effect of another HMG-CoA reductase inhibitor (pravastatin) in men (6595 subjects, 45 to 65 years old) with elevated plasma cholesterol concentrations (average 7.0 ± 0.6 mmol/L [272 ± 23 mg/dL]) but with no prior history of cardiac disease. The dosage of pravastatin was 40 mg/d, and the subjects were followed for an average of 4.9 y. Drug treatment lowered plasma cholesterol and LDL cholesterol concentrations by 20% and 26%, respectively, while the placebo group had no changes in these levels. The placebo group had 248 documented coronary events (either nonfatal myocardial infarction or death from CHD), compared with 174 for the drug group. This represents a 31% reduction in risk with treatment. The drug group had a 32% reduction in death from all cardiovascular causes and a 22% reduction in the risk of death from any cause. Furthermore, reduction in clinical cardiac events was evident within 6 to 12 mo. Again, cholesterol lowering in men at high risk for CHD reduced death from cardiovascular events without increasing the risk of noncardiovascular death.

In summary, the current evidence overwhelmingly supports the cholesterol-diet-heart hypothesis. The unanimous conclusion of the participants of the Consensus Conference on Lowering Blood Cholesterol to Prevent Coronary Heart Disease organized by the National Heart, Lung, and Blood Institute was that the cause-and-effect relation between cholesterol and CHD is established.[160] Recommended guidelines for patient treatment established by the National Cholesterol Education Program (NCEP) are discussed in a later section.[144]

Atherogenic Lipoproteins

In addition to LDL, almost all classes of lipoproteins that contain apo-B—VLDL, β-VLDL, IDL, Lp(a), and oxidized LDL—are considered to be atherogenic. A common feature of these atherogenic lipoproteins is that they contain various amounts of cholesteryl esters and either apo-B100 or apo-B48. In addition, Lp(a) contains apo(a), a protein that is disulfide-linked to apo-B and is homologous to plasminogen; apo(a) may contribute to atherogenesis by mechanisms related to thrombosis.[161, 162] Finally, the atherogenic potential of LDL

differs among the various LDL size and density subclasses, with the small, dense LDL subclass being the most atherogenic.[163]

Apo-B–containing remnant lipoproteins may also be atherogenic[147, 148, 164] based on the fact that β-VLDL, which accumulate in the plasma of cholesterol-fed animals and in patients with type III hyperlipoproteinemia, are associated with accelerated formation of atherosclerotic lesions. These particles, representing chylomicron remnants and VLDL remnants (IDL), are taken up by macrophages, including presumably macrophages in the artery wall, in a nonsaturable manner. This results in massive intracellular accumulation of cholesteryl esters in the form of lipid droplets. The lipid-engorged macrophages resemble the foam cells of the early fatty streak (discussed below).

Another related class of atherogenic apo-B–containing lipoproteins is triglyceride-rich lipoproteins, which are associated with postprandial lipemia after ingestion of a fatty meal.[165] Whereas chylomicrons and large, triglyceride-rich VLDL are not believed to be atherogenic, remnants derived from these particles may be.

The LDL Paradox and Oxidized Lipids

Because LDL cholesterol levels are a strong predictor of CHD and atherosclerosis, it was expected that LDL would be taken up avidly by macrophages, leading to the formation of foam cells. However, in vitro experiments showed that only low levels of LDL are taken up by macrophages. This low uptake presumably occurred because of the highly regulated LDL receptor pathway: the delivery of LDL cholesterol to macrophages causes down-regulation of LDL receptor expression, which protects the cells from the overaccumulation of LDL cholesterol. These results led to the so-called LDL paradox (i.e., how do LDL contribute to atherosclerosis if only limited quantities are taken up by macrophages?).[166] The explanation may be that LDL that have been modified (i.e., by acetylation) are taken up by macrophages in an unregulated manner through receptors unrelated to the LDL receptor.[167] These receptors for modified LDL were originally referred to as acetyl-LDL receptors[167] but are now commonly referred to as scavenger receptors.[166]

In vitro experiments have demonstrated that a number of chemical modifications, including acetylation, acetoacetylation, and reaction with malondialdehyde,[168] circumvent the LDL receptor pathway and cause massive amounts of modified LDL to enter macrophages by means of the scavenger receptor.[167] Furthermore, macrophages are capable of altering LDL so that they can be taken up by macrophages in an unregulated manner.[169] Other cells, including smooth muscle cells and macrophages, are also capable of LDL modification.[166, 170, 171]

The important LDL modification involves oxidation and results in lipid peroxidation. The oxidized LDL hypothesis proposes that unsaturated lipids on the particle undergo oxidative modification, which subsequently leads to oxidation of apo-B, which alters the protein's affinity for cell-surface receptors. As a corollary, antioxidant vitamins (such as A, C, and E), drugs (such a probucol), and enzymes (such as paraoxonase) may limit these oxidative processes. It appears that production of reactive oxygen species (i.e., free radicals) is an integral part of the modification and may be related to the general aging process, in which lipid peroxidation may be a component.[172, 173] Two products of lipid peroxidation, 4-hydroxynonenal and malondialdehyde, modify amino acids of apo-B100, resulting in its fragmentation. Modification is inhibited by antioxidants. Phospholipase and lipoxigenases also have been implicated in LDL modification.[170, 171] In addition to macrophage uptake, oxidized LDL may participate directly in atherogenesis because they are cytotoxic,[174] they serve as chemoattractants for circulating monocyte/macrophages,[175] and they are immunogenic.[176]

The role of oxidized LDL as a major contributor to atherosclerosis remains to be proved in vivo. However, what appear to be oxidatively modified forms of LDL have been identified in atherosclerotic lesions and inflammatory fluid.[176, 177] Also, epitopes of malondialdehyde- and 4-hydroxynonenal–modified apo-B100 have been observed in lesions.[176] Therefore, the formation of oxidized LDL, which may participate in the pathogenesis of atherosclerosis in a number of ways, is an attractive solution to the LDL paradox.

Overview of the Atherosclerotic Process

Until the last several years, two theories of atherogenesis prevailed. The first, referred to initially as the lipid infiltration hypothesis, proposed that excess blood lipids in the form of lipoproteins infiltrated into the arterial wall. This theory was supported by epidemiologic evidence and the identification of atherogenic lipoproteins. The second theory was the endothelial injury hypothesis, which proposed that injury to the endothelial surface is required and results in removal of these cells, exposing a thrombogenic surface to which platelets adhere. Adherence of platelets was suggested to result in the release of platelet-derived growth factor, which would stimulate the smooth muscle cell proliferation and migration that are characteristic of early lesion formation. Endothelial denudation also would remove the endothelial barrier, allowing lipoproteins to enter the vessel wall. The current view of atherosclerosis development combines features from both theories.[178–180] However, the loss of endothelial cells is not a necessary event for the development of an atherosclerotic lesion, and atherogenic lipoproteins can and do penetrate intact endothelium to enter the artery wall.

Atherosclerotic lesions share many features with wound healing or inflammation: (1) proliferation of smooth muscle cells and accumulation of macrophages; (2) formation, by smooth muscle cells, of a connective tissue matrix composed of elastic fibers, collagen, and proteoglycans; and (3) deposition of lipid, primarily cholesterol, both intracellularly and extracellularly. The pattern of lesion formation does not occur randomly within the arterial tree but is focal in nature. Susceptible regions are more permeable to plasma components, and endothelial cell turnover is greater, although the endothelial surface appears to be intact. The focal nature of atherosclerosis suggests that local hemodynamic factors are involved.

Normally, the endothelium forms a nonadherent and relatively impermeable barrier. The endothelial cells and the relatively narrow region beneath them (subintimal space), which contains an occasional smooth muscle cell, constitutes the intima of the artery wall (Fig. 23–24A). Beneath the intima is a layer of many smooth muscle cells, the media, which constitutes the bulk of the artery wall. The adventitia is the outermost layer of the artery wall and is composed of loose connective tissue.

A current model of atherogenesis is depicted in Fig. 23–24 B through E. The major cell types involved include endothelial cells, smooth muscle cells, and inflammatory mononuclear cells, such as macrophages and possibly lymphocytes. One of the initial events is the focal attachment of circulating monocytes to the endothelial surface (Fig. 23–24B). It is not clear which factors are responsible for the adherence of monocytes, although oxidized LDL or other atherogenic lipoproteins may be an initiating factor; areas of microinjury may contribute as well. The monocytes modify the endothelial surface and induce the expression of leukocyte adhesion molecules such as vascular adhesion molecule 1.[181] Once adhered, the monocytes migrate between the endothelial cells, enter the subendothelial space, and differentiate

to macrophages (Fig. 23–24B). In addition, LDL and other atherogenic lipoproteins can enter this space. Within the wall LDL may become entrapped in the matrix and undergo oxidation or further chemical modifications. The macrophages take up the oxidized or modified LDL and begin to take on the appearance of foam cells as lipid accumulates. These initial steps set in motion a chain of events that includes the expression of growth factors (mediators of cell proliferation and chemotaxis) and cytokines (mediators involved in inflammation and immunity).

The monocyte chemoattractant protein 1, produced by endothelial and smooth muscle cells, likely plays a role in further monocyte recruitment into lesions and may be induced by the presence of oxidized LDL. Other growth factors that have been implicated include platelet-derived growth factor, basic fibroblast growth factor, insulin-like growth factors, interleukin-1, tumor necrosis factor, and transforming growth factor β.[178, 179] These factors, which can stimulate smooth muscle cell proliferation, are not expressed in the normal artery wall but are present in areas of lesion development. Several of these mitogens are also chemoattractants with specificity for endothelial cells, smooth muscle cells, or monocyte/macrophages. Inflammatory response cytokines include interleukin-1, gamma interferon, tissue necrosis factor α, interleukin-2, and the colony-stimulating factors. It is unlikely that the various factors act in isolation from each other, but they probably act through a network of cellular interactions operating in a paracrine or autocrine manner.[178]

The first grossly visible lesion is referred to as a fatty streak (Fig. 23–24C). Macrophages accumulate in abundance in the subintimal space and are converted to foam cells, presumably caused by the uptake of oxidized LDLs or remnant lipoproteins. The recruitment of monocytes continues, and smooth muscle cells begin to migrate into the intima. Fatty streaks probably come and go depending on the local stimuli present in the artery wall.

As the cycle of interactions continues, the plaque matures from the fatty streak to a proliferative or fibrous lesion, which is raised and begins to extend into the lumen of the vessel (Fig. 23–24D). The foam cells begin to necrose, probably because of the cytotoxicity of the accumulated lipid; as the lesion progresses, crystals of cholesterol develop. Foam cell death leads to extracellular lipid deposition, accompanied by collagen synthesis and smooth muscle cell migration and proliferation. In the continued presence of factors that promote atherogenesis (e.g., high plasma concentrations of atherogenic lipoproteins), the plaque continues to progress to the complicated lesion stage (Fig. 23–24E). The surfaces of complicated lesions may become thrombogenic as endothelial cells are lost and the subendothelial space is exposed. Platelets can adhere to this exposed surface, promoting thrombus formation. At late stages in complicated lesions, T lymphocytes infiltrate the lesion, and there is evidence of an autoimmune response characterized by lymphocyte infiltration of the adventitia. Calcification is also a feature of late lesions. Advanced lesions can weaken the elasticity and integrity of the artery wall, with the potential to lead to an aneurysm of the vessel. As experiments in humans have shown, the removal or reduction of the atherogenic stimulus can result in plaque regression, leaving a remnant devoid of lipid that resembles a wound scar.

HYPERLIPIDEMIA: DEFINITIONS AND OVERVIEW

Plasma lipid levels vary among individuals of different populations owing to genetic and dietary factors. For example,

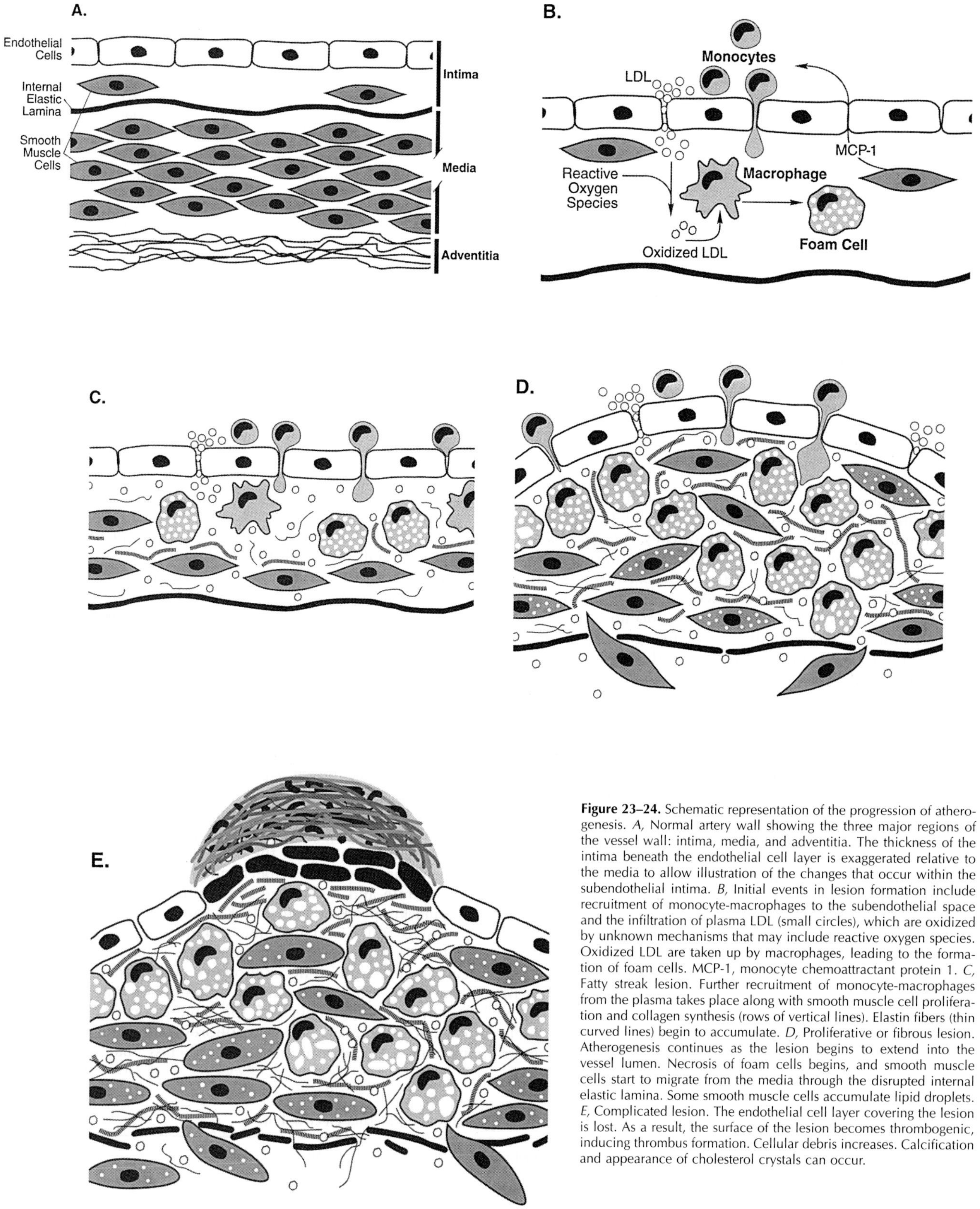

A.

Endothelial Cells

Internal Elastic Lamina

Smooth Muscle Cells

Intima

Media

Adventitia

B.

Monocytes

LDL

MCP-1

Reactive Oxygen Species

Macrophage

Oxidized LDL

Foam Cell

C.

D.

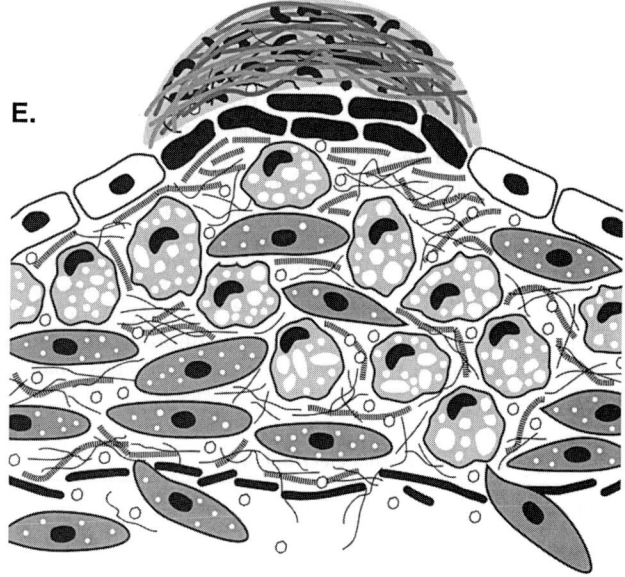

E.

Figure 23–24. Schematic representation of the progression of atherogenesis. *A*, Normal artery wall showing the three major regions of the vessel wall: intima, media, and adventitia. The thickness of the intima beneath the endothelial cell layer is exaggerated relative to the media to allow illustration of the changes that occur within the subendothelial intima. *B*, Initial events in lesion formation include recruitment of monocyte-macrophages to the subendothelial space and the infiltration of plasma LDL (small circles), which are oxidized by unknown mechanisms that may include reactive oxygen species. Oxidized LDL are taken up by macrophages, leading to the formation of foam cells. MCP-1, monocyte chemoattractant protein 1. *C*, Fatty streak lesion. Further recruitment of monocyte-macrophages from the plasma takes place along with smooth muscle cell proliferation and collagen synthesis (rows of vertical lines). Elastin fibers (thin curved lines) begin to accumulate. *D*, Proliferative or fibrous lesion. Atherogenesis continues as the lesion begins to extend into the vessel lumen. Necrosis of foam cells begins, and smooth muscle cells start to migrate from the media through the disrupted internal elastic lamina. Some smooth muscle cells accumulate lipid droplets. *E*, Complicated lesion. The endothelial cell layer covering the lesion is lost. As a result, the surface of the lesion becomes thrombogenic, inducing thrombus formation. Cellular debris increases. Calcification and appearance of cholesterol crystals can occur.

TABLE 23–9. Clinical Disorders Associated with Secondary Hyperlipidemia

Disorder	Lipoprotein Type	Elevated Plasma Lipoprotein	Proposed Mechanism	References*
ENDOCRINE/METABOLIC				
Diabetes mellitus	IV, V	VLDL, chylomicrons	Increased VLDL production; decreased VLDL catabolism	(see text)
Hypothyroidism	IIa (rarely III)	LDL (rarely β-VLDL)	Decreased LDL clearance	(see text)
Estrogen therapy	IV (rarely V)	VLDL	Increased VLDL production (especially in genetically predisposed persons)	(see text)
Glucocorticoid therapy	IIa or IIb	VLDL, LDL	Increased VLDL production with conversion to LDL	189–191
Hypopituitarism (ateliotic dwarfism)	IIb	VLDL, LDL	Increased VLDL production with conversion to LDL	192
Acromegaly	IV	VLDL	Increased VLDL production	193
Anorexia nervosa	IIa	LDL	Decreased biliary excretion of cholesterol and bile acids	194, 195
Lipodystrophy (congenital or acquired)	IV	VLDL	Increased VLDL production	196
Werner syndrome	IIa	LDL	Unknown	197
Acute intermittent porphyria	IIa	LDL	Unknown	198
Glycogen storage disease	IV (rarely V)	VLDL	Increased VLDL production; decreased VLDL catabolism	199, 200
NONENDOCRINE				
Alcohol	IV (rarely V)	VLDL (rarely chylomicrons)	Increased VLDL production (especially in genetically predisposed persons)	(see text)
Nephrotic syndrome	IIa or IIb	VLDL, LDL	Increased VLDL production	(see text)
Uremia	IV	VLDL	Decreased VLDL clearance	201
Biliary obstruction/cholestasis	—	LP-X	Diversion of biliary cholesterol and phospholipid into circulation	202
Hepatitis	IV	VLDL	Decreased LCAT	203, 204
Systemic lupus erythematosis	I	Chylomicrons	Antibodies bind heparin and thereby decrease LPL activity	205
Monoclonal gammopathy	IIa, III, IV	VLDL, IDL, LDL	Antibodies bind lipoproteins and interfere with catabolism	206, 207

*References are given for those disorders not discussed in the text. For a thorough review of the metabolism associated with many of the secondary hyperlipidemic disorders, see Havel RJ, Goldstein JL, Brown MS. Lipoproteins and lipid transport. In: Bondy PK, Rosenberg LE, eds. Metabolic Control and Disease. 8th ed. Philadelphia: WB Saunders, 1980: 393–494.

concentrations range from 14.2 mmol/L (550 mg/dL) to 24.6 mmol/L (950 mg/dL). In addition to the xanthelasma and tendon xanthomas found in heterozygotes, homozygous individuals also frequently have planar xanthomas, which are almost unique to this disorder and almost always noticed by age 6. These xanthomas are raised plaques of cholesterol deposits that occur in the skin at areas of trauma, such as the elbows and knees. Symptoms of CHD may occur before age 10,[213] and, if not treated, these homozygous individuals usually die from myocardial infarction by age 20. Myocardial infarction has been reported as early as age 18 months.[214] Homozygotes are also susceptible to both valvular and supravalvular aortic stenosis.[215]

ORIGIN AND PATHOGENESIS

FH is an autosomal dominant disorder caused by mutations in the LDL receptor gene.[208, 216] Many different types of mutations have been described, including null mutations or nonsense mutations that affect the production of a functional protein, mutations that affect the ability of the receptor to bind to its ligands on lipoproteins, and mutations in which receptors bind LDL normally but are unable to internalize the lipoprotein.[88] A milder phenotype occurs when the ability to bind LDL is impaired but not absent. Different LDL receptor mutations occur in different ethnic groups; for example, there is an increased prevalence (about 60%) of a large deletion mutation in French-Canadians with heterozygous FH.[217] Lack of LDL receptors impairs the clearance of lipoproteins that rely on the LDL receptor for this purpose; these include LDL, in which apo-B100 is the ligand, and remnant lipoproteins (IDL) that are cleared by apo-E. In the heterozygous state, this results in a two- to threefold increase in the plasma cholesterol concentration and in the homozygous state a three- to sixfold increase. The high levels of LDL in the plasma

are taken up by scavenger receptors on macrophages in a nonsaturable manner, possibly after the LDL undergoes oxidative modification.[170, 218, 219] As a consequence, cholesterol accumulates in tissue macrophages in the arterial wall, tendons, and skin and causes the pathological processes observed in these tissues.

DIAGNOSIS

The diagnosis of heterozygous FH is suggested by the presence of high plasma levels of total and LDL cholesterol, normal plasma triglycerides, tendon xanthomas, and a family history of premature CHD. Up to 25% of subjects do not have xanthomas. Heterozygous FH should be suspected in any individual with premature heart disease. In one study, heterozygous FH accounted for 4% of men who survived myocardial infarction before age 60.[220] The differential diagnosis includes familial defective apo-B100,[221] which shares many of the same phenotypical characteristics, including tendon xanthomas. The pattern of isolated high LDL cholesterol also occurs in the more common disorder of polygenic hypercholesterolemia, but tendon xanthomas are not usually a feature of the latter. The diagnosis of FH is primarily a clinical diagnosis because tests to detect one of the many LDL receptor gene mutations or to demonstrate diminished LDL receptor function are performed only in specialized research laboratories. The diagnosis can be confirmed in the laboratory by culturing skin fibroblasts and demonstrating a reduced ability of LDL to bind to receptors on the cells.[222] The diagnosis of FH is important not only for proper treatment of the affected individual but also for identification of other family members that may be at high risk of developing CHD.

The diagnosis of homozygous FH should be suspected in any child with extremely high plasma cholesterol (typically >12.9 mmol/L [500 mg/dL]) or xanthomas. Both parents

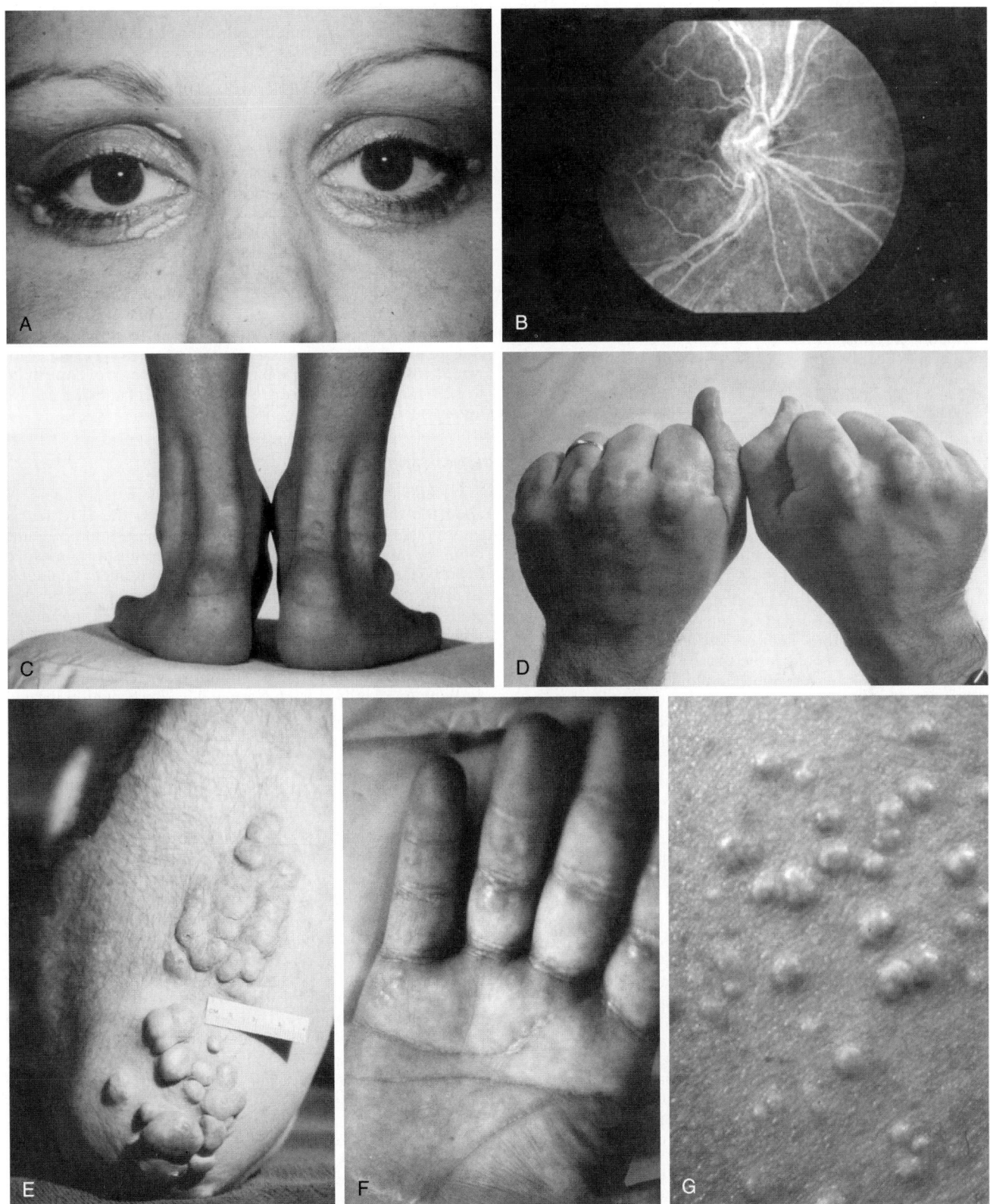

Figure 23–25. Physical examination findings associated with hyperlipidemia (see color section between pages 875 and 877). *A,* Xanthelasma. *B,* Lipemia retinalis. *C,* Achilles tendon xanthomas. Note the marked thickening of the tendons. *D,* Tendon xanthomas. *E,* Tuberous xanthomas. *F,* Palmar xanthomas. *G,* Eruptive xanthomas. (*A* and *B,* Courtesy of Dr. Mark Dresner and Hospital Practice [May 1990, p 15]. *C, D, E,* and *F,* Courtesy of Dr. Tom Bersot. *G,* Courtesy of Dr. Alan Chait.)

will be obligate heterozygotes and should manifest the phenotype of heterozygous FH.

TREATMENT

Treatment of heterozygous FH[223] consists of a diet low in total and saturated fat (approximately 20% and 6% of calories, respectively) and low in cholesterol (<2.6 mmol/day [100 mg/day])[224] and, in most cases, combined drug therapy. Dietary modifications usually result in only minor decreases in the plasma cholesterol levels (5 to 15%). Adequate cholesterol lowering in these patients is rarely achieved by a single therapeutic drug, but combinations of two or three drugs can return plasma cholesterol levels to normal.[225] Effective drug combinations usually include low doses of bile acid sequestrants together with HMG-CoA reductase inhibitors[226] or niacin[227, 228] or all three agents combined.[229] Bile acid sequestrants and HMG-CoA reductase inhibitors both work by depleting cholesterol from hepatic cells (see later discussion), thereby causing increased expression of functional LDL receptors (from the normal allele) on cells, which in turn lowers the plasma cholesterol.[230] Because high Lp(a) concentrations appear to be an adverse risk factor for patients with heterozygous FH,[231] the plasma Lp(a) level should be determined; if it is elevated, niacin should be considered in the drug regimen because this agent can lower plasma Lp(a) levels.[232] Based on studies using animal models of FH,[233, 234] antioxidant agents may be of therapeutic benefit for preventing CHD, but this has not been demonstrated directly in humans. Probucol treatment has resulted in xanthoma regression.[235] Ileal bypass surgery,[236] which, like bile acid sequestrants, causes decreased reabsorption of bile acids from the gut, may be considered in those patients who cannot tolerate medicines.

The age at which treatment should begin in heterozygous FH is somewhat controversial. On the one hand, development of atherosclerosis in these subjects is a long process that begins early in life, and one could argue that treatment should begin during the early stages of lesion development. On the other hand, CHD is usually not symptomatic until the third or fourth decade of life in men and ten years later in women. Because established CHD is reversible,[155, 237] one could argue that medicines can be withheld until after age 25 in men or age 35 in women. A rational approach may be to use diet therapy and bile acid sequestrants, which do not have systemic toxicity, in the early years and to add more potent drug combinations later. The presence of additional risk factors (e.g., high plasma Lp(a) levels, low plasma HDL cholesterol levels, smoking) in an affected individual is an indication for more aggressive treatment at a young age.

Unless the causative mutation is such that there is some residual LDL binding, drug therapy in FH homozygotes is usually ineffective for lowering plasma cholesterol. The most effective means of therapy in these patients is selective removal of LDL from the plasma by extracorporeal pheresis combined with LDL immunoadsorption[238, 239] performed every 1 to 3 wk. Experimental therapies include liver transplantation,[240, 241] which provides functional LDL receptors, portacaval shunting,[242, 243] and gene therapy.[244, 245]

Familial Defective Apolipoprotein B100

Familial defective apo-B100 is a relatively common disorder caused by a mutation in apo-B100, the ligand for the LDL receptor, that results in high plasma LDL and total cholesterol levels and increased susceptibility to CHD. It is phenotypically similar to FH.

CLINICAL FEATURES

This disorder occurs with a frequency of 1 in 500 to 1 in 750 in Caucasian persons with hypercholesterolemia.[48, 246, 247]

The prevalence of familial defective apo-B100 was 0.08% in an ethnically diverse, unselected population.[248] Familial defective apo-B100 had not been described in non-Caucasian populations until 1993, when it was detected in an individual of Chinese ancestry.[249] The clinical features of heterozygous familial defective apo-B100 overlap extensively with those of heterozygous FH and include isolated elevations of plasma LDL cholesterol (type IIa pattern), tendon xanthomas, xanthelasmas, and premature CHD.[221, 246, 250, 251] Although there is extensive overlap, familial defective apo-B100 is usually milder in its manifestations, than FH.[48, 251] Subjects who are homozygous for the familial defective apo-B100 mutation also appear to have a milder clinical phenotype than FH homozygotes.[252-254] In one report, a 66-year-old man and his 69-year-old sister with homozygous familial defective apo-B100 had total plasma cholesterol levels of 9.6 mmol/L (370 mg/dL) and 11.9 mmol/L (460 mg/dL), respectively, and only the man had evidence of CHD.[253] Presumably, the less severe phenotype relates to the fact that, in familial defective apo-B100, the binding of apo-B to LDL receptors is defective but not totally absent, whereas the apo-E–mediated clearance of remnant particles, which is impaired in FH and can contribute to LDL formation, is normal in persons with familial defective apo-B100.

ORIGIN AND PATHOGENESIS

Familial defective apo-B100 is caused by a mutation in apo-B100 that impairs its ability to bind to the LDL receptor.[255-257] To date, a single mutation, the substitution of glutamine for arginine at amino acid 3500, accounts for almost all cases of familial defective apo-B100.[48] Apo-B allele haplotype analysis of DNA from affected individuals has indicated that almost all cases can be traced back to an original founder.[248] Only after extensive screening has this mutation been detected in persons with a different apo-B haplotype for the allele carrying the mutation, one of whom was of Chinese ancestry[249] and one in a kindred from Germany.[258] The mutation located at apo-B amino acid 3500 disrupts the conformation of the protein in the receptor-binding domain[259] and reduces receptor binding of LDL from heterozygotes to levels that are about one third of normal in tissue culture assays.[255] Isolation of the binding-defective LDL from affected individuals demonstrated that it binds with 4 to 9% of normal activity to LDL receptors.[260] Decreased affinity of the defective apo-B100 for its receptor leads to a delay in the clearance of LDL from the plasma (about 50% of normal)[257] and elevation of plasma LDL cholesterol levels. Defective LDL particles accumulate in the plasma in increased proportions relative to normal LDL. A second mutation at amino acid 3500 (tryptophan for arginine) has been reported.[261]

Another mutation located near the receptor-binding region of the apo-B molecule (a substitution of cysteine for arginine at amino acid 3531) also impairs binding of apo-B to the LDL receptor.[262] This mutation decreases LDL binding to LDL receptors by 35 to 40% in tissue culture assays and is associated with moderate elevations in plasma LDL cholesterol levels.

DIAGNOSIS

As in heterozygous FH, the diagnosis of familial defective apo-B100 is suggested by the presence of increased plasma LDL cholesterol and normal triglyceride levels, especially in the presence of tendon xanthomas and a family history of premature CHD. Without specialized testing, however, familial defective apo-B100 is clinically indistinguishable from FH. Because familial defective apo-B100 is caused primarily by one mutation, in contrast to the many mutations that cause FH,[88] it is possible to screen easily for the familial defective apo-B100 mutation using a polymerase chain reaction–based assay of genomic DNA isolated from blood.[263] At present this test is available only in specialized laboratories.

TREATMENT

Treatment of familial defective apo-B100 is similar to that of heterozygous FH and consists of a low-fat, low-cholesterol diet and a combination drug regimen.[221] Drugs that either decrease LDL production (e.g., niacin[264]) or increase the expression of LDL receptors to facilitate the clearance of the normal apo-B100–containing particles are effective in lowering the plasma LDL cholesterol level.[221, 265] Treatment of two individuals with homozygous familial defective apo-B100, whose LDL had receptor-binding affinities 10 to 20% of normal, with HMG-CoA reductase inhibitors markedly reduced plasma cholesterol levels.[253] Family members at risk should be screened as well for the presence of the dominant mutation.

Familial Combined Hyperlipidemia

Originally described in 1973,[220, 266, 267] familial combined hyperlipidemia is a common disorder of unknown genetic cause associated with elevations of plasma cholesterol and triglyceride levels and increased susceptibility to CHD and is inherited as an autosomal dominant trait. The phenotype of familial combined hyperlipidemia overlaps with and may be the same as that observed in familial hyperapobetalipoproteinemia,[268] in subjects with plasma elevations of small, dense LDL particles,[269] and in subjects with "syndrome X," a disorder that includes insulin resistance, increased plasma levels of small, dense LDL, elevated plasma triglycerides, and low plasma HDL levels.[270]

CLINICAL FEATURES

The features of familial combined hyperlipidemia include moderate elevations of plasma cholesterol, triglycerides, or both within individuals of an affected kindred. This corresponds to lipoprotein pattern types IIa, IV, or IIb on plasma electrophoresis. The predominant lipid abnormality may vary in a single person over time or among affected family members[220]; the variable phenotype in this disorder led in part to the decreased utility of pattern typing of hyperlipoproteinemia by plasma electrophoresis in the clinical evaluation.[188] Levels of HDL cholesterol are often moderately decreased,[271] especially in the setting of increased plasma triglycerides. Although it was originally thought that lipid abnormalities usually develop after puberty, it is now known that the phenotype can be detected in children.[220, 272] Neither xanthomas nor xanthelasma is a feature of familial combined hyperlipidemia. Associated metabolic disturbances may include glucose intolerance, obesity, and hyperuricemia. Premature CHD is a common feature: in one study of male survivors of myocardial infarction, familial combined hyperlipidemia was found in 11.3% of those younger than 60 years of age.[220] CHD often is present in men by age 50.

ORIGIN AND PATHOGENESIS

Although familial combined hyperlipidemia is a common disorder (estimated prevalence, 0.5 to 2.0%),[220, 273] neither its genetic cause nor its metabolic pathogenesis is clear. Given the dominant pattern of inheritance, it is presumed that familial combined hyperlipidemia is caused by a single gene defect,[220] but the responsible gene or genes remain obscure. The phenotype of this disorder has been mapped to loci on chromosomes 11[274] and 19,[275] and several different loci may underlie the expression of the phenotype.[276] The heterozygous state for

LPL deficiency may constitute a subset of familial combined hyperlipidemia.[277] A significant problem with mapping this disorder is the difficult task of assigning phenotypes to individuals given the fluctuating and indistinct clinical features. Familial hyperapobetalipoproteinemia, a disorder characterized by high plasma levels of apo-B in association with normal plasma cholesterol levels,[268] overlaps with the phenotype of familial combined hyperlipidemia,[273] as does the familial syndrome characterized by small, dense LDL[269] and the "syndrome X" characterized by insulin resistance and other metabolic abnormalities.[270] The metabolic defect that leads to the hypercholesterolemia and/or hypertriglyceridemia is also unclear, but overproduction of apo-B may be a contributing factor[278, 279]; apo-B overproduction can result in elevations in plasma VLDL, LDL, or both.[280] Similarly, the pathogenesis of the low HDL in this disorder remains unclear. The finding of low HDL cholesterol in association with hypertriglyceridemia is common and could relate to either decreased substrate for HDL formation because of impaired catabolism of the apo-B–containing lipoproteins or to enhanced CETP-mediated cholesteryl ester transfer from HDL to the apo-B–containing lipoproteins.

DIAGNOSIS

Familial combined hyperlipidemia should be suspected in subjects with moderate hypertriglyceridemia and/or moderate hypercholesterolemia (lipoprotein types IIa, IIb, or IV), especially in the setting of a family history of premature CHD. Xanthomas are not a feature of this disorder. Low plasma HDL cholesterol, obesity, insulin resistance, and hyperuricemia are often present. The diagnosis is a clinical one; it requires demonstration of the clinical phenotype in the affected individual and family members and exclusion of other primary or secondary disorders. Secondary disorders that produce a similar phenotype include diabetes mellitus, nephrotic syndrome, and occasionally hypothyroidism. Many patients with diabetes mellitus and combined hyperlipidemia may have a genetic susceptibility due to inheritance of familial combined hyperlipidemia.

TREATMENT

Weight reduction and dietary treatment can help correct metabolic abnormalities such as obesity and insulin resistance that contribute to the hyperlipidemia. Drug therapy should be directed at the predominant lipid abnormality. For example, plasma elevations of total and LDL cholesterol can be treated with HMG-CoA reductase inhibitors, niacin, or bile acid sequestrants. Of these, HMG-CoA reductase inhibitors may be preferable, because niacin can cause or worsen glucose intolerance and hyperuricemia, and bile acid sequestrants can cause hypertriglyceridemia.[281] Gemfibrozil can lower triglyceride and raise HDL cholesterol levels; this drug reduced the incidence of coronary events in the Helsinki Heart Study.[282] Low HDL cholesterol levels can be treated by niacin, gemfibrozil, or HMG-CoA reductase inhibitors.[283] Because familial combined hyperlipidemia is associated with premature CHD, affected family members should be identified.

Type III Hyperlipoproteinemia (Familial Dysbetalipoproteinemia)

Type III hyperlipoproteinemia, or familial dysbetalipoproteinemia, is an uncommon disorder of lipoprotein metabolism characterized by moderate to severe hypertriglyceridemia and hypercholesterolemia caused by the accumulation of cholesterol-rich remnant particles in the plasma.[65, 284] Premature peripheral vascular disease and coronary artery disease are common. The cause is mutations in apo-E that result in defective binding to lipoprotein receptors. In most instances the disorder, which is associated with the apo-E2 isoform (described previously), is inherited as an autosomal recessive trait that requires a secondary exacerbating metabolic factor (either genetic or environmental) for expression of the phenotype. Several rare apo-E mutations result in the dominant expression of the disorder.

CLINICAL FEATURES

Type III hyperlipoproteinemia usually is diagnosed in adulthood and is only rarely detected in individuals younger than 20 years of age, with the exception of those with the rare autosomal dominant apo-E mutations.[65] The disorder is more common in men and is usually not manifested in women until after menopause. The disorder is characterized by moderately severe elevations in plasma triglyceride and cholesterol levels; typically these values range from 3.4 to 4.5 mmol/L (300 to 400 mg/dL) and 7.8 to 10.3 mmol/L (300 to 400 mg/dL), respectively. Concentrations of HDL cholesterol are normal, and LDL cholesterol is almost always reduced. Xanthomas are present in more than half of affected individuals.[284] The presence of palmar xanthomas, which are planar xanthomas in the palmar creases (see Fig. 23–25F; see color section between pages 875 and 877), is virtually pathognomonic for this disorder. Tuberous or tuberoeruptive xanthomas (Fig. 23–25E; see color section) are also common but are less specific for this disorder. Tendon xanthomas and xanthelasma occur in some patients. Premature vascular disease is common, and peripheral vascular disease occurs in addition to premature CHD.[65] Type III hyperlipoproteinemia accounts for 0.2 to 1.0% of lipid disorders associated with myocardial infarction in persons younger than 60 years of age. Coexisting metabolic conditions that exacerbate the phenotype of type III hyperlipoproteinemia, such as obesity, alcohol consumption, diabetes mellitus, and hypothyroidism, are often present.

ORIGIN AND PATHOGENESIS

Type III hyperlipoproteinemia is caused by the plasma accumulation of cholesterol-rich remnants of VLDL, IDL, and chylomicron particles. The clearance defect arises from mutations in the apo-E protein that lead to defective binding of apo-E to remnant receptors, including LDL receptors (discussed under section on roles of apo-E in lipid metabolism). The remnants that accumulate have lost much of their triglyceride through LPL-mediated triglyceride hydrolysis and therefore are cholesterol-rich. The predominant remnant particles are termed β-VLDL and can be isolated in the VLDL ultracentrifugation density range (<1.006 g/mL). In contrast to normal VLDL that migrate as pre-β particles, these remnants are characterized by β-migration on agarose gel electrophoresis.

Homozygosity for the apo-E2 isoform occurs at a frequency of about 1 in 100 in the general population. Despite this high frequency, the type III hyperlipoproteinemia phenotype is relatively rare; only about 1 in 10 to 1 in 100 subjects with apo-E2 homozygosity develop the dyslipidemia (overall prevalence of 1 in 10,000). The manifestation of the dyslipidemia appears to require the presence of a secondary factor, such as a metabolic condition that contributes to the phenotype of impaired remnant clearance. Such conditions can be caused by lipoprotein overproduction syndromes, such as obesity, diabetes mellitus, or alcohol consumption, or by conditions that further impair lipoprotein clearance, such as hypothyroidism. In conditions characterized by VLDL overproduction, the increased generation of remnant particles through catabolism of VLDL overwhelms the ability to clear these remnants from the plasma. Because the manifestations are so sensitive to condi-

tions that increase hepatic lipoprotein production, this disorder is also one of the most sensitive to therapeutic modalities directed at decreasing hepatic lipoprotein production, such as dietary modifications, weight loss, or alcohol cessation.

In addition to homozygosity for the apo-E2 isoform, six mutations in the apo-E gene are known to lead to the type III hyperlipoproteinemia phenotype in an autosomal dominant fashion.[65, 285, 286] In these dominant disorders, the phenotype is present at an early age and does not require a coexisting metabolic condition as an exacerbating factor. These rare dominant disorders are of great interest because they illustrate how different mutations in a single protein can give rise to either recessively or dominantly inherited phenotypes. How a given apo-E mutation interacts with the HSPG/LRP pathway is believed to determine whether the mutation gives rise to a dominant or recessive phenotype. For example, in recessive expression of the disorder, as occurs with apo-E2 homozygosity, apo-E2 interacts very poorly with the LDL receptor but almost normally with the HSPG/LRP pathway so that in the absence of exacerbating secondary factors remnant lipoproteins are cleared effectively. However, in the presence of a secondary factor that overwhelms or impairs even slightly the normal pathways, the apo-E2 is unable to clear remnants in an efficient manner. The dominant apo-E mutations interact poorly with both the LDL receptor and the HSPG/LRP pathway, and remnant lipoprotein clearance is impaired even in the heterozygous state. Another contributing factor is the particular lipoprotein fractions with which the apo-E molecule preferentially associates[65] (discussed under section on roles of apo-E in lipid metabolism).

The accumulation of cholesterol-rich remnant lipoproteins in the plasma leads to the deposition of cholesterol in tissue macrophages, which avidly bind and take up β-VLDL.[287] The deposition of β-VLDL–derived cholesterol in macrophages leads to foam cell formation and accumulation, manifested as skin xanthomas and as atherosclerotic vascular disease.[65] In addition to the frequent occurrence of CHD, β-VLDL hyperlipidemia appears to cause a disproportionately high incidence of peripheral vascular disease. The onset of premature CHD in men occurs at ~40 y of age and in women at ~50 y of age.[288]

DIAGNOSIS

The diagnosis of type III hyperlipoproteinemia should be suspected in patients with moderately severe elevations in both the plasma triglyceride and cholesterol concentrations. Typically the cholesterol and triglyceride levels are in the range of 3.4 to 4.5 mmol/L (300 to 400 mg/dL) and 7.8 to 10.3 mmol/L (300 to 400 mg/dL), respectively. Because this disorder is most commonly recessive in nature, there is often no family history of hyperlipidemia or premature CHD. The presence of palmar or tuberous xanthomas makes the diagnosis highly likely.

In the absence of palmar or tuberous xanthomas, the specific diagnosis is more difficult and requires specialized testing. If available, a measurement of the VLDL cholesterol level allows detection of cholesterol-rich remnant particles. The VLDL cholesterol/triglyceride ratio is a useful screen: in type III hyperlipoproteinemia, the VLDL cholesterol/triglyceride ratio is usually greater than 0.3 (when hyperlipidemia is present). In contrast, the normal VLDL cholesterol/triglyceride ratio is typically around 0.2 (i.e., the VLDL cholesterol concentration is about 20% of the plasma triglyceride level, as estimated by the Friedewald formula; see later discussion). The elevated ratio occurs because β-VLDL remnants are rich in cholesterol and cause the VLDL fraction to be cholesterol-rich. The electrophoresis of plasma samples on agarose gels typically demonstrates the presence of a broad band in the β-migrating lipoprotein region (type III pattern), hence the names broad-β disease, dysbetalipoproteinemia, or type III hyperlipoproteinemia. Patients suspected of having type III hyperlipoproteinemia can be evaluated for apo-E2 homozygosity either by the isoelectric focusing of plasma (see Fig. 23–8), or by apo-E genotyping of DNA obtained from leukocytes.[289] The diagnosis of other rare dominant mutations in apo-E is performed only in specialized laboratories.

TREATMENT

Because type III hyperlipoproteinemia is greatly influenced by coexisting metabolic conditions, a vigorous search should be made to identify and treat obesity, alcohol consumption, diabetes mellitus, and hypothyroidism. If such conditions can be identified and successfully treated, often the lipid abnormalities can be resolved and plasma lipids returned to normal without the use of drug therapies. Type III hyperlipoproteinemia associated with hypothyroidism, in particular, responds dramatically to thyroid hormone replacement therapy.[290] Dietary therapy should be aimed at restriction of total fat, saturated fat and cholesterol (step 1 or step 2 American Heart Association Diet) and at caloric restriction to reduce weight if appropriate. Treatment with estrogen should be considered in postmenopausal women because it can dramatically diminish the hyperlipidemia,[291] probably by stimulating LDL receptor–mediated remnant particle clearance.

If dietary therapy and treatment of coexisting metabolic conditions are unsatisfactory, drug therapy should be initiated using either niacin, fibric acid derivatives, or HMG-CoA reductase inhibitors, all of which are effective in the treatment of this disorder.[65] Through its effects on decreasing VLDL synthesis and secretion, niacin lowers triglyceride and VLDL cholesterol levels by about 40% and LDL cholesterol levels by 20% and can raise HDL cholesterol concentrations by 20%.[292, 293] The fibric acid derivatives, gemfibrozil or clofibrate, can also lower triglyceride and VLDL cholesterol levels.[294] The HMG-CoA reductase inhibitors, through their ability to increase LDL receptor levels, can also lower the plasma cholesterol levels.[295, 296] Those cases that are refractory to treatment with individual drugs can be treated with combinations of fibric acid derivatives and HMG-CoA reductase inhibitors, although this combination should be used cautiously because of the risk of myopathy.[297, 298] Because of the premature vascular disease in this disorder, screening of first-degree relatives such as siblings (or offspring if the affected individual's spouse has an apo-E2 allele) should be performed.

Lipoprotein Lipase Deficiency

LPL deficiency is a rare, recessive disorder that results from mutations in the LPL gene. These abnormalities cause LPL deficiency and severe hypertriglyceridemia by blocking the clearance of triglyceride-rich lipoproteins from the plasma. Massive accumulations of these proteins in the plasma, known as the *chylomicronemia* syndrome,[299, 300] can be accompanied by severe clinical manifestations including pancreatitis.

CLINICAL FEATURES

LPL deficiency usually is recognized in infancy or childhood as a chylomicronemia syndrome,[299–301] marked hypertriglyceridemia associated with recurrent abdominal pain or pancreatitis, which can be life-threatening. A syndrome of recurrent abdominal pain and severe hypertriglyceridemia but without overt pancreatitis or elevated serum amylase concentrations also exists.[299] The pain syndrome is associated with triglyceride levels of more than 22.6 mmol/L (2000 mg/dL) and abates with triglyceride lowering. When plasma triglycer-

ide levels exceed 22.6 mmol/L (2000 mg/dL), findings include eruptive xanthomas (Fig. 23–25G; see color section between pages 875 and 877) and lipemia retinalis (Fig. 23–25B; see color section). The plasma may be visibly lipemic; the overnight refrigeration of plasma (see Table 23–6) can demonstrate chylomicrons (type I pattern) with a cream layer on the top, VLDL (type IV pattern) with a turbid plasma infranatant, or both (type V pattern). Chylomicrons can be assumed to be present if the fasting triglyceride concentration is greater than 11.3 mmol/L (1000 mg/dL).[301] The degree of fasting chylomicronemia is, in large part, determined by the dietary fat intake. In addition to eruptive xanthomas, the accumulation of triglycerides in tissue reticuloendothelial cells can lead to hepatomegaly and splenomegaly. Chylomicronemia can also cause neurologic manifestations[302–304] and dyspnea.[302] CHD is not a prominent feature. Massive triglyceride elevations can occupy significant plasma volume and lead to artifactually low measurements of serum electrolytes such as sodium (pseudohyponatremia) if the electrolyte measurements are not corrected for serum water.[305]

Subjects who are heterozygous for LPL deficiency may have reduced LPL activity and often have mild to moderate hypertriglyceridemia, increased VLDL cholesterol levels, and decreased HDL cholesterol levels.[277, 306] This phenotype, which may constitute a subset of familial combined hyperlipidemia,[277] is exacerbated by age and obesity.

ORIGIN AND PATHOGENESIS

Complete LPL deficiency results from homozygous or compound heterozygous mutations in the LPL gene that lead to absence or inactivation of the LPL protein.[107, 307] A variety of mutations have been described. The frequency of homozygotes and compound heterozygotes for these mutations is approximately 1 in 10^6 persons. Heterozygotes for LPL deficiency, who have half-normal LPL activities[277] and may develop hypertriglyceridemia in the presence of secondary factors,[306] occur at a frequency of 1 in 500 persons in the general population but as high as 1 in 40 in areas of Quebec.[308] The absence of functional LPL[109, 309] causes the accumulation of triglyceride-rich lipoproteins in the plasma. Because of the impaired clearance of these lipoproteins, plasma triglyceride levels are especially sensitive to dietary fat intake. Whereas chylomicrons normally are cleared from the plasma within 8 h after eating, clearance in patients with this disorder may take days. The triglyceride-rich particles infiltrate organs, where they are taken up by reticuloendothelial cells. The accumulation of these lipoproteins in the pancreas can cause pancreatitis, presumably from chemical irritation of the pancreas by fatty acids and lysolecithin liberated by the action of pancreatic lipases.[299]

DIAGNOSIS

The diagnosis of LPL deficiency should be suspected in children with pancreatitis or recurrent abdominal pain. Eruptive xanthomas are often present. LPL deficiency should also be suspected in any individual in whom lipemic serum is present despite a 12-h fast. Plasma triglyceride levels are usually higher than 11.3 mmol/L (1000 mg/dL) and may be considerably higher, depending on the dietary fat intake. Eruptive xanthomas, lipemia retinalis, and pancreatitis usually are apparent only when triglycerides are greater than 22.6 mmol/L (2000 mg/dL). Because LPL deficiency is a recessive disease, family history is usually uninformative except in siblings.

The definitive diagnosis is established by demonstration of the absence of lipase activity in plasma after heparin administration.[307] Heparin, when infused intravenously, displaces

LPL from its binding sites on HSPG in capillary endothelium and releases it into plasma, which can be assayed for lipase activity. LPL deficiency must be distinguished from deficiency of apo-CII, a cofactor for LPL, which is another cause of chylomicronemia. Because multiple mutations can result in LPL deficiency, the identification of specific mutations is performed only by specialized laboratories.

TREATMENT

During the initial stages of treatment, a fat-free diet is given until plasma triglycerides reach a safe level (e.g., <11.3 mmol/L [1000 mg/dL]). After the acute chylomicronemia syndrome has resolved, the mainstay of treatment is a diet that contains very small amounts of fat (e.g., <10% of calories or 20 to 25 g/d). Because medium-chain triglycerides, in contrast to long-chain triglycerides, are absorbed directly into the portal circulation and do not rely on chylomicron formation for hepatic uptake, they can provide a source of fat in the diet; however, these agents may cause hepatic toxicity.[310, 311] Fat-soluble vitamins should be supplemented. The goal of therapy is to maintain the plasma triglyceride level at less than 11.3 mmol/L (1000 mg/dL), which will prevent further episodes of pancreatitis.[299]

Drug therapy for primary LPL deficiency is largely ineffective; however, clofibrate, gemfibrozil, or niacin may lower VLDL production and prevent severe hypertriglyceridemia.[301] Secondary causes of hypertriglyceridemia, such as diabetes mellitus or hypothyroidism, should be screened for and treated if present.

Apolipoprotein CII Deficiency

The rare autosomal recessive disorder of apo-CII deficiency occurs in fewer than 1 in 10^6 persons and causes a chylomicronemia syndrome similar to that in LPL deficiency.[299, 307] As in LPL deficiency, the features include pancreatitis or recurrent bouts of abdominal pain in children or young adults and lipemic serum after a 12-h fast. Plasma triglyceride levels are usually severely elevated (>11.3 mmol/L [1000 mg/dL]) and are the result of the accumulation of chylomicrons (type I pattern), VLDL (type IV pattern), or both lipoproteins (type V pattern) in the plasma. This hyperlipoproteinemia results from the lack of apo-CII, an activating cofactor for LPL, which causes a functional LPL deficiency. More then 10 mutations are known to cause apo-CII deficiency.[307] The accumulation of triglyceride-rich particles results in a pathophysiological process that is nearly identical to that described for LPL deficiency. Heterozygotes may have slightly elevated triglyceride concentrations, but they do not develop pancreatitis. The diagnosis requires specialized testing in which either apo-CII is demonstrated to be absent on the electrophoresis of the plasma apolipoproteins or the plasma is shown to be incapable of activating LPL in vitro.[300, 312] The treatment of apo-CII deficiency is identical to that of primary LPL deficiency with the exception that severe hypertriglyceridemia and pancreatitis can be treated with transfusions of plasma.

Familial Hypertriglyceridemia

Familial hypertriglyceridemia, a relatively common autosomal dominant disorder, is characterized by increased plasma concentrations of triglyceride-rich VLDL, which cause elevations of plasma triglycerides but not plasma cholesterol levels.

CLINICAL FEATURES

Subjects with familial hypertriglyceridemia typically have plasma triglyceride levels in the range of 2.3 to 5.6 mmol/L (200 to 500 mg/dL). The hypertriglyceridemia is often associated with low plasma HDL cholesterol levels.[313] The elevated triglyceride levels usually are not evident until adulthood[220] and may be exacerbated by secondary factors, including hypothyroidism, estrogen therapy, or alcohol ingestion. Such exacerbations can be associated with severe elevations of triglycerides (>11.3 mmol/L [1000 mg/dL]), placing subjects at risk for eruptive xanthomas and pancreatitis. However, xanthomas usually are not present. Obesity and insulin resistance are common. Although familial hypertriglyceridemia was originally thought to be associated with increased risk for CHD,[220] this relation has been questioned.[314] The association of decreased HDL cholesterol levels with hypertriglyceridemia may contribute to increased CHD risk.[313]

ORIGIN AND PATHOGENESIS

Familial hypertriglyceridemia appears to be caused by overproduction of VLDL triglycerides in the presence of near-normal apo-B production,[278, 279, 315] which leads to the secretion of large, triglyceride-rich VLDL. Secondary disorders (e.g., insulin resistance) that lead to VLDL overproduction, can exacerbate the syndrome. The low plasma HDL levels commonly found in hypertriglyceridemia are associated with enhanced apo-AI fractional catabolism.[316, 317] The genetic defect in familial hypertriglyceridemia is unknown, but its inheritance as an autosomal dominant defect suggests a monogenic cause. Whether the large, triglyceride-rich VLDL are atherogenic is unclear; an enhanced risk for premature CHD may relate to whether concomitant decreases in HDL cholesterol occur.

DIAGNOSIS

Familial hypertriglyceridemia should be suspected in individuals with increased plasma triglyceride levels and normal plasma cholesterol. The disorder can be diagnosed only if hypertriglyceridemia is found in half of the first-degree relatives at risk, and it can be difficult to distinguish from familial combined hyperlipidemia, which also may present as isolated hypertriglyceridemia from increased plasma VLDL (type IV pattern). Measurement of plasma lipid levels in children does not help to distinguish these disorders because lipid abnormalities usually are not present until after puberty in either disorder. The elevated VLDL levels can be observed as a cloudy appearance of the plasma after overnight refrigeration.

TREATMENT

In addition to dietary fat restriction, secondary disorders such as diabetes mellitus, estrogen administration, or alcohol intake should be screened for and treated. Drugs that lower triglyceride levels (e.g., niacin, gemfibrozil) may be useful. Because niacin can impair glucose tolerance, it should be used cautiously in patients with underlying insulin resistance.

Elevated Plasma Lp(a)

This disorder consists of elevations of modified LDL particles in the plasma, in which the apo-B protein of LDL is covalently bonded to apo(a).[318–321] Apo(a) is a protein of unknown function that shares high sequence homology with plasminogen but is not catalytically active.[322] Some[271, 323–325] but not all[326–330] studies suggest that elevated plasma Lp(a) concentrations are associated with an increased risk for CHD.

CLINICAL FEATURES

There are no characteristic physical findings or lipoprotein patterns to suggest elevated plasma Lp(a) levels. Elevated

Lp(a) (>30 mg/dL) may be suspected, however, in patients with premature CHD. Plasma Lp(a) concentrations are influenced by heredity[331–333] and vary among different ethnic populations.[334] For example, levels are higher in African populations.[319] Some data suggest that elevations of plasma Lp(a) may be atherogenic only in the presence of high concentrations of LDL.[335] In support of this, elevated Lp(a) concentrations are a risk factor for development of CHD in subjects with FH.[231]

ORIGIN AND PATHOGENESIS

Apo(a) is found only in humans, primates, and hedgehogs.[319] Its function from an evolutionary perspective is unclear. Nevertheless, the presence of high plasma levels of apo(a) appears to have been selected for in certain populations.[334] Apo(a) is attached by disulfide bonds to the apo-B protein of LDL.[336] Plasma Lp(a) levels are in large part determined by heredity and appear to be related to the number of repeats of a motif termed "kringles" in the protein.[331] The larger isoforms that contain more kringle repeats are found in lower concentrations in the plasma,[337] possibly relating to impaired processing of these large forms for secretion by hepatocytes. The factors that control the production and clearance of Lp(a) are largely unknown. An increased susceptibility to atherosclerosis from high plasma levels of Lp(a) could relate to impaired fibrinolysis caused by competition for plasminogen receptors,[338, 339] to effects on smooth muscle proliferation,[340] or to unknown factors.

DIAGNOSIS

The diagnosis of high plasma Lp(a) levels is made by specific assays of plasma for apo(a) or intact Lp(a) particles; care should be taken to ensure that samples are collected and stored appropriately and that the assay does not detect plasminogen. Levels of Lp(a) of more than 30 mg/dL are considered high.

TREATMENT

Of the drugs currently available, only niacin appears to lower plasma Lp(a) levels.[232] Treatment with 4 g/d of niacin lowers Lp(a) levels by 35 to 40%.

Polygenic Hypercholesterolemia

By definition, 5% of individuals have cholesterol values that exceed the 95th percentile for the population and therefore have hypercholesterolemia. A study by Goldstein and coworkers[220] suggested that about 10% of these individuals have familial combined hyperlipidemia and about 5% have familial hypercholesterolemia. In a large proportion of the remaining 85% the cause of the hypercholesterolemia is unknown but probably results largely from combinations of genetic and environmental factors. Other genetic factors that contribute to hypercholesterolemia may involve physiological processes that influence cholesterol absorption, bile acid metabolism, or intracellular cholesterol metabolism. The diagnosis of polygenic hypercholesterolemia is made by excluding other primary genetic causes, by the absence of tendon xanthomas, and by demonstration that hypercholesterolemia is present in no more than 10% of first-degree relatives.[220] The hypercholesterolemia is treated according to NCEP guidelines (described later).

Sporadic Hypertriglyceridemia

As with high plasma cholesterol, unknown genetic and environmental factors can result in elevated plasma triglyceride levels.[220] Such sporadic cases of hypertriglyceridemia can be distinguished from familial syndromes by the absence of hypertriglyceridemia in relatives. Treatment of sporadic hypertriglyceridemia includes dietary fat restriction, treatment of secondary conditions that exacerbate hypertriglyceridemia, and administration of drugs that lower triglyceride levels, such as niacin or gemfibrozil.

PRIMARY DISORDERS OF HDL METABOLISM

Several genetic disorders can result in decreased or increased plasma levels of HDL cholesterol (Table 23–10).

Familial Hypoalphalipoproteinemia

The autosomal dominant disorder familial hypoalphalipoproteinemia is manifested by low plasma HDL cholesterol levels and an increased risk for premature CHD.[271, 341, 342] The diagnosis is suggested by HDL cholesterol levels that are less than the 10th percentile (<0.8 mmol/L [30 mg/dL] in men or 1.0 mmol/L [40 mg/dL] in premenopausal women). There are no characteristic physical findings, but there often is a family history of low HDL cholesterol levels and premature CHD. The genetic and metabolic defects that lead to low plasma HDL levels are unknown, but it appears that up to 50% of low HDL cholesterol levels can be linked to the hepatic lipase or the apo-AI/apo-CIII/apo-AIV gene locus.[343] The lack of HDL in the plasma accelerates development of atherosclerosis, presumably because of impairment of reverse cholesterol transport or other protective effects of HDL.[344, 345] Drug ther-

TABLE 23–10. Genetic Disorders of HDL Metabolism

Disorder	Mutant Gene	Inheritance	Population Frequency	Typical Plasma HDL Cholesterol (mmol/L [mg/dL])	Typical Clinical Manifestations	
					Corneal Opacifications	Premature Vascular Disease
Familial hypoalphalipoproteinemia	Unknown	Autosomal dominant	~1/400	0.5–0.8 (20–30)	—	+
Familial apo-AI and apo-CIII deficiency	Apo-AI or apo-AI/apo-CIII	Autosomal recessive	Rare	<0.1 (5)	+	+
Apo-AI_Milano	Apo-AI	Autosomal dominant	Rare	~0.3 (10)	—	—
LCAT deficiency	LCAT	Autosomal recessive	Rare	<0.3 (10)	+	+
Fisheye disease	LCAT	Autosomal recessive	Rare	<0.3 (10)	+	—
Tangier disease*	Unknown	Autosomal recessive	Rare	<0.1 (5)	+	+
CETP deficiency	CETP	Autosomal recessive	Rare	>2.6 (100)	—	—

*Clinical manifestations also include orange tonsils.
CETP, cholesteryl ester transfer protein; LCAT, lecithin:cholesterol acyltransferase.

apy should be aimed at raising the plasma HDL concentration or lowering the plasma LDL concentration or both.[283, 346] Treatments aimed at raising HDL levels include estrogen therapy for postmenopausal women,[347–349] aerobic exercise,[350] and the drugs niacin or gemfibrozil.[282, 283] Because increasing HDL cholesterol is difficult with current therapies, lowering of the LDL cholesterol concentration may be the most effective therapy, with the premise that the lowering of atherogenic LDL particles can overcome some, if not all, of the effects of low HDL.[283]

APOLIPOPROTEIN AI MUTATIONS

Mutations in the apo-AI gene[351, 352] can cause a decrease in HDL formation and low plasma HDL cholesterol levels. Apo-AI deficiency can be caused by point mutations in the apo-AI gene or by deletions or gene rearrangements at the apo-AI/apo-CIII/apo-AIV gene locus.[351] Apo-AI deficiency typically results in plasma HDL cholesterol levels less than 0.3 mmol/L (10 mg/dL).[352] Manifestations include a predisposition to premature CHD, xanthomas, and corneal opacities.[352] The molecular diagnosis can be made only by specialized analysis, including electrophoresis of the plasma apolipoproteins and DNA analysis to determine the mutation. Inasmuch as it is difficult to raise the plasma apo-AI or HDL cholesterol levels in these disorders, the treatment should be directed toward lowering the levels of plasma non-HDL cholesterol.

Other rare variants of apo-AI exist,[351] including apo-AI Milano,[353] which is caused by a substitution of cysteine for arginine at amino acid 173 and results in a lowering of plasma HDL cholesterol levels. This mutation is inherited as an autosomal dominant trait and has not been associated with premature CHD. Whether the mutation is protective against development of atherosclerosis or whether this kindred has mitigating genetic or environmental factors is not known. Other apo-AI variants are associated with amyloidosis.[354–356]

Cholesteryl Ester Transfer Protein Deficiency

This hereditary syndrome results in increased plasma HDL cholesterol levels because of diminished activity of plasma CETP.[118, 357, 358] Once thought to be rare, the disorder is not uncommon in the Japanese population.[141] Features include marked elevations of plasma HDL cholesterol in homozygotes (usually >2.6 mmol/L [100 mg/dL]) and a possible protection against development of CHD.[357] Heterozygotes have moderately elevated HDL cholesterol levels. The diminished activity of CETP results in diminished transport of cholesteryl esters from HDL to the apo-B–containing lipoproteins. As a result, more cholesteryl esters are found in HDL, and the ratio of total cholesterol to HDL cholesterol is markedly reduced. Presumably, the combination of reduced amounts of atherogenic LDL and increased antiatherogenic HDL results in decreased atherosclerosis susceptibility. Studies in transgenic mice have confirmed this relation between CETP and atherosclerosis. Although mice normally do not have significant plasma CETP activity and have high plasma HDL cholesterol levels, transgenic mice that express CETP have increased plasma LDL cholesterol, decreased HDL cholesterol, and increased susceptibility to atherosclerosis.[142, 359, 360] However, CETP expression may be antiatherogenic in the setting of hypertriglyceridemia.[361] The molecular diagnosis of subjects with CETP deficiency requires the measurement of plasma CETP activity in vitro or the determination of the DNA mutation. At present, no treatment is available.

Lecithin:Cholesterol Acyltransferase Deficiency

The very rare autosomal recessive disorder LCAT deficiency causes corneal opacities,[211] normochromic anemia, and renal failure in young adults.[362] About 30 kindreds of LCAT deficiency and a number of mutations have been described.[362, 363] The deficiency of LCAT results in decreased esterification of cholesterol to cholesteryl esters on HDL particles.[364] This, in turn, leads to an accumulation of free cholesterol on lipoprotein particles and in peripheral tissues, presumably because of impaired reverse cholesterol transport. Cholesterol deposits accumulate in tissues such as the cornea, red blood cell membranes, and renal glomeruli. Plasma cholesterol levels in LCAT deficiency are variable, HDL cholesterol levels are reduced, and the ratio of free cholesterol to esterified cholesterol in the plasma is increased.[363] Normally, free cholesterol accounts for about one third of the total cholesterol in the plasma; in LCAT deficiency, free cholesterol accounts for most of the plasma cholesterol. The accumulation of free cholesterol in vascular tissues can lead to premature CHD. At present, there is no means to increase the plasma activity of LCAT; therefore, the treatment is preventive (by dietary fat restriction) and symptomatic (e.g., renal transplant).

A variant of LCAT deficiency is called fish-eye disease.[362, 365] Although this disorder is also caused by mutations of the LCAT gene,[366–368] the phenotype is less severe than that seen in complete LCAT deficiency. Fish-eye disease is characterized by low plasma HDL cholesterol levels and corneal opacities; anemia, renal disease, and premature atherosclerosis are not present. The phenotypic differences between LCAT deficiency and fish-eye disease have been attributed to whether LCAT activity is absent from both HDL and apo-B–containing lipoproteins (LCAT deficiency) or from HDL only (fish-eye disease);[369] however, one subject with phenotypic fish-eye disease had normal HDL-associated LCAT activity.[370]

Tangier Disease

Tangier disease is a rare autosomal recessive disorder associated with hypolipidemia, including decreases in both plasma HDL and LDL cholesterol levels, and the presence of orange tonsils.[76, 371] Other features include corneal opacities,[211] hepatosplenomegaly, peripheral neuropathy, and premature CHD.[372] Although the underlying mutation is unknown, metabolic studies have demonstrated that the disorder is associated with an enhanced catabolism of plasma HDL.[373] The molecular defect may involve impaired efflux of cholesterol from cells.[374–376] Whatever the mechanism, massive amounts of cholesteryl esters accumulate in macrophages of the reticuloendothelial system. Cholesterol deposits in the tonsils give rise to the orange tonsils observed in this disorder. There is no specific treatment.

PRIMARY GENETIC HYPOLIPIDEMIAS

Familial Hypobetalipoproteinemia

Familial hypobetalipoproteinemia, an autosomal dominant disorder of apo-B metabolism, is associated with plasma cholesterol and LDL cholesterol levels that are less than one-half normal in heterozygotes and with marked hypocholesterolemia (<1.3 mmol/L [50 mg/dL]) in homozygotes.[377]

CLINICAL FEATURES

Heterozygous subjects, about 1 in 500 persons, are usually asymptomatic but come to attention from the detection of low plasma cholesterol levels. Typically, the total plasma cholesterol level is less than the 5th percentile, and it may be less than 2.6 mmol/L (100 mg/dL). Plasma LDL cholesterol levels are also reduced by one half or more, and HDL cholesterol levels are normal or slightly increased.[378] Plasma triglyceride levels are reduced in some kindreds. Although heterozygotes are usually asymptomatic, fat malabsorption has been reported.[379, 380] The syndrome is associated with longevity,[381] probably the result of a low risk for CHD.

Subjects who are homozygotes or compound heterozygotes for these apo-B mutations are rare, occurring in about 1 in 10[6] persons. Homozygotes may be detected at a young age because of fat malabsorption and decreased plasma cholesterol levels. Fat malabsorption is caused by an inability to form chylomicrons in the intestine and a subsequent failure to absorb fats and fat-soluble vitamins. Fat malabsorption may be accompanied by a progressive neurologic degenerative disease resulting from vitamin E deficiency, retinitis pigmentosa, and acanthocytosis. The latter is caused by alterations in red blood cell membrane lipids. Despite the low plasma cholesterol levels, steroidogenesis appears to be normal except when demands are quite high.[382, 383] Homozygotes who produce enough of a truncated isoform of apo-B to facilitate some fat absorption may have a milder phenotype.

ORIGIN AND PATHOGENESIS

Most cases of known origin result from mutations in the apo-B gene.[377] More than 30 mutations have been described; most are either nonsense or frameshift mutations that lead to the formation of truncated apo-B proteins.[384] Metabolic turnover studies indicate that these apo-B gene mutations result in impaired synthesis of apo-B–containing lipoproteins in some cases[385] and enhanced clearance of apo-B–containing lipoproteins from the plasma in others.[386] The decreased levels of apo-B–containing lipoproteins in the plasma cause low plasma cholesterol and triglyceride levels. Although most known cases of hypobetalipoproteinemia involve apo-B mutations, additional undefined genetic factors can result in low cholesterol levels.[387–389]

In the homozygous state, the absence of apo-B leads to impaired intestinal chylomicron formation, which in turn leads to the impaired absorption of fats and fat-soluble vitamins. Cholesterol absorption is probably also impaired, as demonstrated by a transgenic mouse that lacks intestinal apo-B expression and chylomicron formation.[390] As noted, vitamin E malabsorption results in low tissue stores of tocopherol and a degenerative neurologic disease. Retinal degeneration may also be related to deficiencies of fat-soluble vitamins.[391]

DIAGNOSIS

The diagnosis is suggested by the presence of low plasma total and LDL cholesterol levels inherited as an autosomal dominant trait. The homozygous condition is suggested by the presence of extremely low plasma cholesterol and triglyceride levels in an infant or child with fat malabsorption. The differential diagnosis of the homozygous state includes abetalipoproteinemia (see later discussion) and Anderson's disease (chylomicron retention disease).[342, 392, 393] The molecular diagnosis of hypobetalipoproteinemia can be performed only in specialized laboratories by the examination of the plasma apo-B by gel electrophoresis or analysis of DNA to identify specific mutations.

TREATMENT AND PROGNOSIS

Because heterozygotes are almost always asymptomatic, no specific treatment is indicated, but dietary supplementation of fat-soluble vitamins (especially vitamin E) in heterozygous subjects is reasonable. Heterozygotes should be informed that if their spouse also has a very low plasma cholesterol level, the possibility exists that offspring could have homozygous or compound heterozygous hypobetalipoproteinemia; in this scenario, subjects should be referred to a lipid clinic for genetic counseling.

Subjects with homozygous hypobetalipoproteinemia (phenotypic abetalipoproteinemia) should be treated with very large doses of vitamin E orally (100 to 300 mg/kg/d), which can raise the tissue vitamin E concentrations and prevent the neurologic complications.[310, 394] It is imperative to make the diagnosis and begin treatment at an early age to prevent nutritional deficiencies. Fat should be provided in the diet up to a level that symptoms allow (usually 15 to 20% of calories). Supplementation with medium-chain triglycerides is probably contraindicated because of reports of liver toxicity.[311]

Abetalipoproteinemia

Abetalipoproteinemia is a rare autosomal recessive disorder caused by a deficiency in MTP, which results in a virtual absence of the apo-B–containing lipoproteins in the plasma.[131, 395–397]

CLINICAL FEATURES

Abetalipoproteinemia is rare, occurring in fewer than 1 in 10[6] persons and has the same phenotype as homozygous hypobetalipoproteinemia (described previously), including malabsorption of fat and fat-soluble vitamins from the intestine, which can lead to neurologic disease related to vitamin E deficiency. The disorder is frequently detected in infancy because of fat malabsorption associated with marked decreases in the levels of plasma cholesterol and triglycerides.

ORIGIN AND PATHOGENESIS

Abetalipoproteinemia is caused by a deficiency of MTP,[395] a protein that transfers triglycerides or phospholipids onto nascent apo-B–containing lipoproteins during their formation in the ER. Insufficient lipidation of nascent particles impairs the synthesis and secretion of these particles by the intestine and the liver, and little if any apo-B is found in the plasma. Several mutations in the MTP gene have been described.[131, 397] The lack of MTP in the intestine leads to impaired chylomicron formation and malabsorption of fats and fat-soluble vitamins.

DIAGNOSIS

The diagnosis is suggested by the presence of fat malabsorption associated with extremely low levels of plasma cholesterol (usually <1.3 mmol/L [50 mg/dL]) and of triglyceride in an infant or young child.[396] Cholesterol levels in the parents, who are obligate heterozygotes, are normal. The demonstration of the molecular defect requires a specialized laboratory for detection of low or absent MTP in intestinal biopsy specimens or DNA analysis to identify specific mutations. The differential diagnosis of abetalipoproteinemia includes homozygous hypobetalipoproteinemia, in which the obligate heterozygote parents have low plasma lipid levels, and Anderson's disease.[342, 392, 393] The latter disorder, which is also called chylomicron retention syndrome, is a very rare condition that is phenotypically similar to abetalipoproteinemia. Individuals with Anderson's disease have an inability to secrete chylomicrons from the intestine owing to an as yet undefined recessive mutation.

TREATMENT

Subjects with abetalipoproteinemia are treated as described previously for subjects with homozygous hypobetalipoproteinemia. Very large doses of vitamin E are given by mouth to prevent the neurologic sequelae of vitamin E deficiency.

OTHER RARE PRIMARY LIPID DISORDERS

Hepatic Lipase Deficiency

Hepatic lipase deficiency is a disorder associated with the lack of hepatic lipase activity in the plasma.[398–403] The features include combined hyperlipidemia, with elevated levels of plasma cholesterol (6.5 to 38.8 mmol/L [250 to 1500 mg/dL]) and triglyceride (4.5 to 92.6 mmol/L [395 to 8200 mg/dL]), palmar and tuboeruptive xanthomas, and premature arcus corneae. Levels of β-VLDL are increased (however, the VLDL-cholesterol/triglyceride ratio is <0.3, in contrast to type III hyperlipoproteinemia), and there is a threefold to fivefold enrichment of triglyceride in the LDL and HDL fractions. Levels of HDL cholesterol are normal or slightly increased. Susceptibility to atherosclerosis is thought to be increased. The demonstration of hepatic lipase deficiency requires specialized in vitro hepatic lipase activity assays of the subject's plasma or specific DNA analysis to identify mutations. Dietary restriction of fat and cholesterol can lower the plasma lipid levels.

Sitosterolemia

In this rare disorder, dietary sitosterol and other plant sterols, which are not normally absorbed in significant quantities in the intestine, are absorbed in large amounts, resulting in their accumulation in the plasma and in peripheral tissues.[404] The precise molecular defect is unknown. Clinically, affected children have tendon xanthomas and normal to high plasma levels of LDL cholesterol; the differential diagnosis includes familial hypercholesterolemia and cerebrotendinous xanthomatosis. The diagnosis can be confirmed by gas-liquid chromatography of plasma lipids to demonstrate the abnormal sterols. Treatment consists of restriction of plant sterols in the diet.

Cerebrotendinous Xanthomatosis

Cerebrotendinous xanthomatosis[404, 405] is a rare disorder of sterol metabolism associated with neurologic disease, tendon xanthomas, and cataracts in young adults. Neurologic manifestations include cerebellar ataxia, dementia, spinal cord paresis, and subnormal intelligence. Premature atherosclerosis is common.[406] Osteoporosis has been reported and is presumably caused by alterations in vitamin D metabolism.[407] The disorder results from mutations that cause deficiencies of 27-hydroxylase, a key enzyme in cholesterol oxidation and bile acid synthesis.[408] As a result, high levels of cholesterol and cholestanol, a 5α-dihydro derivative of cholesterol, accumulate in the plasma, tendons, and tissues of the nervous system. Treatment is with chenodeoxycholic acid,[409] often in combination with an HMG-CoA reductase inhibitor.[410, 411]

Acid Cholesteryl Ester Hydrolase Deficiency

This autosomal recessive disorder is caused by deficiency of a lysosomal esterase, which results in the massive accumula-

tion of cholesteryl esters and triglycerides in lysosomes.[412–414] In the variant called Wolman's disease, which is usually fatal in the first year of life, there is a complete deficiency of the lysosomal esterase. Cholesteryl ester storage disease is a milder variant in which there may be some residual esterase activity; affected individuals can survive past childhood but may develop premature CHD.

Familial Isolated Vitamin E Deficiency

This rare disorder of vitamin E metabolism is characterized by low plasma levels of vitamin E in association with progressive neurologic degenerative disease.[415, 416] It is caused by a lack of hepatic α-tocopherol transfer protein,[417] which is postulated to facilitate the incorporation of α-tocopherol onto nascent VLDL during their formation in the liver. When the protein is lacking, there is a lack of vitamin E on VLDL, which is a major transport mechanism for delivery of vitamin E to peripheral tissues. Treatment consists of daily supplementation with high doses of oral vitamin E.

SECONDARY DISORDERS OF LIPID METABOLISM

A number of metabolic diseases and drug therapies influence plasma lipids.[196, 418, 419] The secondary disorders of hyperlipidemia are listed in Table 23–9. Factors that affect HDL levels are listed in Table 23–11.

Diabetes Mellitus

Of the common disease states, diabetes mellitus exerts some of the most profound effects on plasma lipid metabolism.[420–423] Hypertriglyceridemia is found in up to one third of all diabetic patients and is related to the critical role that insulin plays in the production and clearance of triglyceride-rich lipoproteins from the plasma.[420] In addition, diabetics frequently have high plasma levels of atherogenic lipoproteins and low plasma HDL, predisposing them to premature CHD, a leading cause of death in diabetics.

It is useful to consider type I and type II diabetes separately with regard to their effects on plasma lipids and response to treatment. In type I diabetes, insulin deficiency and poor glycemic control are associated with increases in plasma levels of triglycerides and the apo-B–containing lipoproteins because of effects on plasma lipid metabolism in peripheral tissues and the liver. In peripheral tissues, insulin deficiency results in impaired LPL activity and diminished clearance of triglyceride-rich particles,[424] insulin deficiency also causes enhanced lipolysis, which results in increased free fatty acid flux to the liver. In the liver, increased free fatty acid flux drives triglyceride synthesis and VLDL synthesis and secretion. Plasma LDL cholesterol levels may also be increased, possibly

---

TABLE 23–11. Factors Affecting Plasma HDL Levels

Factors That Increase HDL
Estrogens
Exercise
Alcohol
Drugs: nicotinic acid, fibrates, HMG-CoA reductase inhibitors
Factors That Decrease HDL
Androgens
Progestins
Cigarette smoking
Obesity
Low-fat diet
Drugs: probucol, β-blockers

because insulin stimulates LDL receptor–mediated LDL degradation.[425]

In its most severe form, insulin deficiency can cause a chylomicronemia syndrome known as *diabetic lipemia*.[424, 426] In this disorder, massive increases in plasma triglyceride levels (>22.6 mmol/L [2000 mg/dL]) can result in lipemia retinalis, eruptive xanthomas, fatty liver, and pancreatitis. This disorder arises from an acquired LPL deficiency[424] and is relatively rare in the modern era of insulin therapy. The acquired lack of LPL activity results in an accumulation of chylomicrons in the plasma (type I pattern), similar to that seen in primary genetic LPL deficiency. The disorder may result from the occurrence of diabetes mellitus in combination with some underlying disorder of triglyceride metabolism.[427] The hyperlipidemia due to insulin deficiency and type I diabetes is reversible with intensive insulin therapy. Persistent lipid abnormalities in type I diabetics with excellent glycemic control suggest that another disorder of lipid metabolism is present.

In type II diabetes, which accounts for more than 90% of cases, the metabolic defect relates to insulin resistance and relative insulin deficiency. The insulin resistance appears to be caused by both genetic and acquired factors; metabolic abnormalities that accompany the insulin resistance include obesity, hyperglycemia, hypertension, plasma lipid abnormalities, and hyperuricemia, which are referred to as syndrome X.[270] One of the most common lipid abnormalities in type II diabetes is a moderate hyperlipidemia characterized by an increase in VLDL (type IV pattern), which can be accompanied by various degrees of chylomicronemia (type V pattern), depending on the dietary fat intake.[270] This disorder is characterized by the accumulation in the plasma of apo-B–containing lipoproteins, which are likely to be proatherogenic. The plasma triglyceride and cholesterol levels are often moderately elevated, the HDL cholesterol concentration may be low,[428, 429] and IDL, or remnants, which are probably atherogenic, are also often increased.[430] Increased plasma levels of LDL are found in some but not all subjects. However, the hyperlipidemia in type II diabetics is often characterized by an increase in the small, dense LDL (LDL subclass pattern B),[431] which are particularly atherogenic; this increase occurs even in the absence of hyperlipidemia.[431] In addition, a portion of the plasma LDL undergo glycosylation, which may make them more susceptible to oxidation.[432] Xanthomas are usually absent in this disorder.

Contributing factors to the lipoprotein abnormalities that occur with type II diabetes include decreased LPL activity in muscle and adipose tissue and increased free fatty acid flux to the liver from peripheral adipose tissue stores.[421] When insulin levels are high, this free fatty acid flux can drive triglyceride synthesis and VLDL production in the liver.[433] The lipid abnormalities associated with the VLDL overproduction state may be worse if a primary genetic disorder of lipid metabolism coexists.[427, 434]

The mainstay of therapy for type II diabetics with hyperlipidemia is glycemic control through diet, oral hypoglycemic agents, or insulin therapy. Periodic monitoring of the glycosylated hemoglobin is helpful in assessing the glycemic control. However, in contrast to the situation in type I diabetes, the hyperlipidemia in type II diabetes may be difficult to eradicate even with excellent glycemic control, because these subjects have accompanying genetic and acquired metabolic abnormalities that are not resolved by returning blood sugar levels to normal. Decreasing insulin resistance through weight loss can, however, have dramatic effects on both the hyperglycemia and the hyperlipidemia. Metformin, a hypoglycemic agent, may lower plasma glucose levels and produce a modest lowering of plasma lipid levels.[435] In addition to glycemic control, drugs for diabetic hyperlipidemia include gemfibrozil and HMG-CoA reductase inhibitors. Niacin should be used with caution

as it can impair or worsen glucose tolerance. Treatment with insulin can lower plasma LDL cholesterol levels in both type I[436] and type II[437] diabetes mellitus.

Hypothyroidism

Alterations in thyroid function can have profound effects on plasma lipids,[418, 438, 439] and all patients with significant hyperlipidemia should be screened for hypothyroidism. The classic manifestation of hypothyroidism is an elevation of the plasma LDL cholesterol level (6.5 to 15.5 mmol/L [250 to 600 mg/dL]), but this disorder also can be associated with high plasma triglyceride levels.[438, 440] Levels of HDL cholesterol are usually unchanged or slightly lower in hypothyroidism and may be reduced in hyperthyroidism[441, 442]; the latter effect may relate to alterations in hepatic lipase activity.[441, 443] The elevations of plasma LDL cholesterol in hypothyroidism are associated with impaired clearance of LDL,[444–446] probably the result of decreased LDL receptor expression.[447] The high LDL cholesterol levels in hypothyroidism are associated with an increased risk for atherosclerosis,[448] but risk for myocardial infarction is not necessarily increased,[448, 449] perhaps because there is decreased myocardial oxygen demand in hypothyroidism. Subclinical hypothyroidism, in which metabolic abnormalities are present without symptoms, can also cause hypercholesterolemia that responds to treatment with thyroid hormone.[450] Hypothyroidism is also associated with low LPL activity,[438, 451] thereby predisposing to increased plasma triglyceride levels. Hyperlipidemia with hypothyroidism may be more marked in those with underlying genetic susceptibility,[290, 440] but it responds dramatically to thyroid hormone replacement. In elderly patients with CHD or significant risk factors thyroid hormone should be replaced cautiously, because rapid replacement can aggravate underlying ischemic heart disease.

Estrogen Therapy

Estrogen therapy causes increases in plasma triglyceride levels[182, 452] and can occasionally cause marked hypertriglyceridemia, especially in predisposed individuals.[453] The hypertriglyceridemia appears to be dose-related.[347] Although most women taking either oral contraceptives or postmenopausal estrogens maintain triglyceride levels in the normal range, massive hypertriglyceridemia can on occasion cause pancreatitis.[453] For this reason, triglyceride levels should be measured in women before estrogen therapy is initiated. Estrogens appear to cause hypertriglyceridemia through increased production of VLDL.[454] Adipose tissue LPL activity is not altered.

Estrogen therapy also enhances the clearance of LDL from the circulation[452] and lowers plasma LDL cholesterol. Enhanced LDL clearance likely results from increased hepatic LDL receptor expression.[455] Treatment of postmenopausal women with estrogen can lower LDL cholesterol by 15%.[349, 452] Estrogens can also reduce the hyperlipidemia of type III hyperlipoproteinemia.[291]

Estrogens have significant effects on HDL metabolism, increasing HDL cholesterol in postmenopausal women by more than 15%,[349, 452] primarily by increasing the HDL$_2$ subfraction. Women have higher HDL cholesterol levels than men at all ages after puberty. This presumably is a result of the effects of androgens, because HDL cholesterol levels decrease at puberty in men but remain constant in women.[185] The mechanism for alterations in the HDL cholesterol levels from gonadal hormones is uncertain but may reflect differences in hepatic lipase activity. The effects of estrogen to raise HDL and lower LDL cholesterol levels can be offset if estrogens are combined with progestational agents, which lower HDL and raise LDL cholesterol levels.[456] Because estrogens tend to lower LDL and raise HDL cholesterol, the net result is that estrogen therapy in postmenopausal women appears to decrease significantly the risk for CHD.[457, 458]

Alcohol Consumption

The regular consumption of large amounts of alcohol can significantly affect plasma triglyceride metabolism.[459] Alcohol inhibits fatty acid oxidation in the liver and enhances fatty acid synthesis. These alterations lead to increased triglyceride synthesis, fatty liver, and enhanced VLDL production.[460] The enhanced VLDL production raises plasma triglycerides and occasionally causes massive hypertriglyceridemia and pancreatitis, especially in persons with an underlying genetic susceptibility.[299] Plasma electrophoresis reveals an accumulation of VLDL in the plasma (type IV pattern) and occasionally a superimposed chylomicronemia (type V pattern) as these particles compete for saturable clearance mechanisms.[461] Individuals with type III hyperlipoproteinemia are particularly sensitive to the effects of alcohol consumption, because the alcohol-induced overproduction of VLDL and associated remnant particles occurs in the setting of impaired remnant clearance. Hypertriglyceridemia can be an important contributor to pancreatitis associated with alcohol consumption.

Alcohol consumption is also associated with higher plasma levels of HDL cholesterol,[462] which in turn may explain why alcohol consumption may protect against CHD.[460, 463, 464] Indeed, alcohol consumption in the form of wine may be inversely correlated with CHD mortality.[465]

Nephrotic Syndrome

Hyperlipidemia, which almost always accompanies the nephrotic syndrome, is caused predominantly by elevation of LDL (type IIa pattern) but also can be caused by high VLDL levels (type IV pattern). Total, VLDL, and LDL cholesterol; total triglycerides; and plasma apo-B are all elevated.[466] The ratio of total to HDL cholesterol is increased, consistent with an atherogenic phenotype. Plasma Lp(a) levels can also be elevated.[467] The pathogenesis of the hyperlipidemia appears to be related to increased production rates of LDL or VLDL, or both.[466, 468, 469] The cause of VLDL overproduction is unclear but may relate to a generalized hypersecretion phenomenon in the liver. Because myocardial infarction ranks second only to renal failure as the cause of death in individuals with nephrotic syndrome, the hyperlipidemia should be treated vigorously. HMG-CoA reductase inhibitors appear to be particularly effective.[470]

Other Drugs

In addition to estrogens, other therapeutic agents can cause hyperlipidemia.[443] These agents include glucocorticoids[189–191] and antihypertensive agents such as thiazide diuretics and β-adrenergic blockers.[443, 471–473] Exogenous androgens can reduce HDL cholesterol levels.[474, 475]

TREATMENT OF LIPID DISORDERS

Approach to the Hyperlipidemic Patient

Individuals come to attention for evaluation for a lipid disorder because of the presence of atherosclerotic vascular disease, pancreatitis, xanthomas or xanthelasma or because of detection of a high plasma cholesterol or triglyceride level. The initial evaluation of these patients includes a history and physical examination, including assessments of CHD risk factors, and the measurement of plasma lipids.

RISK FACTORS

The initial examination should include an assessment of risk factors for development of atherosclerotic CHD. Table 23–12 lists the current risk factors, as specified by the NCEP.[184] Particular emphasis should be placed on obtaining a detailed history of all first-degree relatives for cholesterol disorders or premature CHD.

PHYSICAL EXAMINATION

A thorough physical examination should be performed with emphasis on the cardiovascular system and the manifestations of hyperlipidemia. Elevated plasma lipids (cholesterol or triglycerides) can accumulate in macrophage reticuloendothelial cells in certain tissues, particularly the skin, tendons, eyes, liver, and spleen. Deposits in the skin or tendons are manifested as xanthomas or xanthelasmas. In almost all cases, these tissue lipid deposits are reversible with lipid-lowering therapy. Several of the clinical findings are illustrated in Fig. 23–25.

Xanthelasmas (see Fig. 23–25A) are small, raised, yellowish macules that typically appear on or near the eyelids above and around the medial canthus. They are seen in familial hypercholesterolemia, familial defective apo-B100, and type III hyperlipoproteinemia. Xanthelasmas occasionally occur in patients with normal plasma cholesterol levels, possibly as the result of enhanced uptake of oxidized or modified lipoproteins by tissue macrophages. Xanthelasmas typically regress with cholesterol lowering and can also often be effectively treated in the setting of normal cholesterol levels with low doses of probucol, an antioxidant drug. *Lipemia retinalis* (Fig. 23–25B), a condition in which lipemic plasma can be visualized by routine ophthalmologic examination of the fundi, is typically seen only when the triglyceride levels are 22.6 mmol/L (2000 mg/dL) or higher. *Tendon xanthomas* (Figs. 23–25C and 23–25D) are nodular deposits of cholesterol that accumulate in tissue macrophages in the Achilles and other tendons, including the extensor tendons in the hands, knees and elbows. Tendon xanthomas are often present in familial hypercholesterolemia (approximately 75% of subjects), in familial defective apo-B100, and sometimes in type III hyperlipoproteinemia. Small tendon xanthomas can be overlooked if not specifically searched for. The examination of the Achilles tendon should include an assessment for thickness and for irregularities of contour (Fig. 23–25C). Achilles tendon xanthomas can also be detected by xeroradiography. *Tuberous* or *tuboeruptive xanthomas* (Fig. 23–25E) are subcutaneous nodules that develop in the skin over areas susceptible to trauma such as the elbows or the knees. They may be singular or multiple and may range from pea-sized to lemon-sized. Tuberous xanthomas are most often seen in type III hyperlipoproteinemia and also occur in familial hypercholesterolemia. *Palmar xantho-*

TABLE 23–12. Major Risk Factors for Coronary Heart Disease

Positive
1. Age (men ≥45 y; women ≥55 y or premature menopause without hormone treatment)
2. Family history of premature coronary heart disease (male parent or sibling <55 y, female parent or sibling <65 y)
3. Current cigarette smoking
4. Hypertension
5. Diabetes mellitus
6. Low HDL cholesterol (<0.9 mmol/L [<35 mg/dL])
7. High LDL cholesterol

Negative
1. High HDL cholesterol (≥1.6 mmol/L [≥60 mg/dL])

Adapted from The Expert Panel. Summary of the second report of the National Cholesterol Education Program (NCEP) Expert Panel on Detection, Evaluation, and Treatment of High Blood Cholesterol in Adults (Adult Treatment Panel II). J Am Med Assoc 1993; 269:3015–3023.

mas (Fig. 23–25*F*) are cutaneous deposits in the palmar and digital creases of the hands. This type of xanthoma is almost pathognomonic for the presence of high plasma levels of β-VLDL and type III hyperlipoproteinemia. *Eruptive xanthomas* (Fig. 23–25*G*) are cutaneous xanthomas that appear as small, yellowish, round papules that contain a pale center and an erythematous base. They are similar in appearance to, and can be mistaken for, acne. The distribution of eruptive xanthomas includes the abdominal wall, the back, the buttocks, and other pressure contact areas. They are caused by an accumulation of triglyceride in dermal histiocytes and generally occur when plasma triglyceride is 11.3–22.6 mmol/L (1000–2000 mg/dL) or more. They can disappear rapidly with lowering of the plasma triglyceride level.

SCREENING FOR SECONDARY DISORDERS

The history and physical examination should be directed toward uncovering any secondary disorders of lipid metabolism, such as diabetes mellitus, hypothyroidism, or the nephrotic syndrome, and toward identification of any agents that could cause hyperlipidemia, such as estrogens, alcohol, or β-adrenergic blockers. In addition to a historical assessment for secondary disorders, a screening laboratory evaluation should include determination of fasting blood sugar or glycosylated hemoglobin, or both; serum chemistry analyses to assess renal and hepatic function; a urinalysis to assess for urinary protein; and a plasma TSH level to screen for hypothyroidism, as the prevalence of hypothyroidism is increased in dyslipidemic individuals.[476]

MEASUREMENT OF PLASMA LIPIDS

Ideally, plasma lipids should be measured at least twice in fasting steady-state conditions before therapeutic decisions are made that might be indefinite. Although it is usual to measure plasma lipids after a 12-h fast, the plasma lipid response in the postabsorptive state, which may include significant elevations in atherogenic remnant lipoproteins, may be important in atherogenesis. Because cholesterol is a minor component of chylomicrons, plasma cholesterol can be measured in either the fasting or nonfasting state. Of note, plasma lipids can be decreased in the setting of acute myocardial infarction,[477] and follow-up measurements are essential in these patients.

Most clinical laboratories measure plasma levels of total triglycerides, total cholesterol, and HDL cholesterol; the latter analysis is performed after the precipitation of apo-B–containing lipoproteins from the plasma with an agent such as heparin. The plasma LDL cholesterol concentration is then calculated from these measurements by the Friedewald formula[478]:

LDL cholesterol = total cholesterol −
    HDL cholesterol − triglycerides ÷ 5.

This formula relies on an estimate of the VLDL cholesterol that is about 20% of the plasma triglyceride level and is reliable for triglyceride levels of 4.5 mmol/L (400 mg/dL) or less. Plasma LDL concentrations calculated by this formula may be inaccurate in the setting of severe hypertriglyceridemia. Specialized lipid laboratories separate the plasma into different density fractions (e.g., VLDL, LDL, and HDL) by sequential ultracentrifugation of the plasma and then measure the lipid concentrations directly in each fraction. The main advantage of the latter technique is that VLDL cholesterol, which can reflect atherogenic remnant lipoproteins, is directly measured.

Because the plasma lipids can be divided roughly into the *proatherogenic* apo-B–containing lipoproteins and the *antiath-erogenic* HDL, assessment of the relative proportions of cholesterol in these two fractions can be valuable in the individual lipid profile. One method is to assess absolute levels of HDL and non-HDL cholesterol.[479] Another method is to calculate and assess the ratio of total cholesterol to HDL cholesterol[480–482]; it is desirable for the ratio to be about 4.5 or lower (i.e., to have at least 25% of the plasma cholesterol in the HDL fraction). Both methods allow for incorporation of the potentially atherogenic apo-B–containing lipoproteins into the assessment of cardiovascular risk from hyperlipidemia by including VLDL cholesterol levels in the assessment.

Several caveats for interpretation of the plasma triglyceride level deserve mention. First, a triglyceride level higher than 11.3 mmol/L (1000 mg/dL) usually signifies the presence of two or more disorders of lipid metabolism (e.g., estrogen therapy in the presence of underlying familial hypertriglyceridemia).[483] Second, elevated plasma triglyceride levels can fluctuate markedly in a single person over short periods. This occurs because the LPL-mediated clearance mechanisms for triglyceride-rich particles become saturated at plasma triglyceride concentrations of ~5.6 mmol/L (500 mg/dL), and above this level plasma triglyceride levels largely reflect dietary influences. In this range the plasma triglyceride levels may rise precipitously with high dietary fat intake and fall rapidly with dietary fat restriction.[299]

In some instances, the inspection of the plasma after its overnight refrigeration can be helpful in understanding a disorder of lipoprotein metabolism. To accomplish this, plasma should be collected in an EDTA-containing tube and refrigerated overnight. The presence of a creamy layer on the top signifies the presence of chylomicrons (type I hyperlipidemia), which are less dense than plasma and float to the surface. A turbid plasma infranatant signifies high levels of VLDL (type IV hyperlipidemia). The combination of a creamy top layer and turbid plasma indicates the presence of both chylomicrons and VLDL (type V hyperlipidemia). In addition to visual inspection, plasma can be analyzed by electrophoresis on paper or agarose gels and stained for neutral lipids to analyze the amount of lipids in the various lipoprotein classes.[187] This type of analysis is now rarely used because it has little utility in the classification or treatment of lipid disorders.[188] Nevertheless, much of the terminology used to describe lipoprotein disorders is derived from the originally described patterns (see Table 23–6).

Specialized tests used in assessment of plasma lipid disorders include measurements of plasma Lp(a) levels and plasma apolipoproteins and screening of genomic DNA for mutations. Plasma Lp(a) levels can be determined by enzyme-linked immunoabsorbent assays if warranted. The Lp(a) assay must distinguish the apo(a) protein from plasminogen, which is highly homologous. Plasma Lp(a) measurement may be helpful in assessing CHD risk, and high levels of Lp(a) may suggest the use of niacin as a therapeutic agent.[232] Plasma apo-B and apo-AI levels may be of great value in predicting CHD risk[484]; however, because the assays for these apolipoproteins are difficult to perform and add minimal information to that obtained from plasma cholesterol measurements, they are not routinely used. Specialized tests such as in vitro assays for enzyme activities (e.g., LPL, CETP) or DNA screening for mutation analysis (e.g., the familial defective apo-B100 mutation) are, currently performed in specialized laboratories.

SELECTION OF PATIENTS FOR PLASMA LIPID MEASUREMENTS

In addition to patients suspected of a plasma lipid disorder, guidelines published by the NCEP recommend that the plasma total cholesterol should be measured in all adults 20 years of age and older at least once every 5 y.[184] In addition,

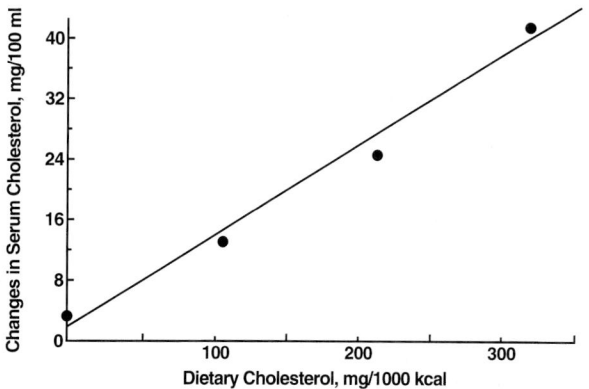

Figure 23–26. Relation between cholesterol intake and change in serum cholesterol after 21 d on a cholesterol-free formula diet of constant fatty acid composition. (Adapted from Mattson FH, Erickson BA, Kligman AM. Effect of dietary cholesterol on serum cholesterol in man. Am J Clin Nutr 1972; 25:589–594. Copyright © 1972, by American Society for Clinical Nutrition.)

Drug Treatment

Categories of drugs for treatment of lipid abnormalities[479, 522] are listed in Table 23–16. These include drugs that interfere with bile acid absorption from the gut, such as bile acid sequestrants, or with cholesterol biosynthesis in cells, such as HMG-CoA reductase inhibitors. These agents deplete cholesterol levels and increase LDL receptor expression in cells, thereby lowering plasma LDL concentrations. Other agents, including niacin and gemfibrozil, either inhibit VLDL synthesis and secretion or enhance the clearance of triglyceride-rich particles by enhancing LDL-mediated catabolism. Finally, drugs that work primarily as antioxidants are being tested. The choice of drug for treatment of hyperlipidemia depends primarily on the type of disorder needing treatment (Table 23–17) and on the side effects of each drug. In cases of severe hypercholesterolemia (e.g., familial hypercholesterolemia) combinations of agents may act additively or synergistically and reduce plasma cholesterol concentrations with great efficacy.

HMG-CoA REDUCTASE INHIBITORS

Several potent inhibitors of HMG-CoA reductase, the rate-limiting enzymatic step in cholesterol biosynthesis are available.[522] The inhibition of cholesterol biosynthesis results in up-regulation of cellular LDL receptors and enhanced clearance of LDL from the plasma into cells.[230] The inhibitors differ in their side chains, which can affect their relative hydrophobicity.[523] For example, lovastatin and simvastatin are relatively hydrophobic and lipophilic, compared with pravastatin, which is more hydrophilic; these properties appear to be of little significance with respect to the ability to lower LDL levels. Therapeutic doses of these agents reduce total cholesterol levels by 15 to 30% and LDL cholesterol levels by 20 to 40%,[524, 525] frequently reduce plasma triglyceride levels by 10 to 20%, and cause small increases in plasma HDL cholesterol levels (5 to 10%). Atorvastatin, appears to be a more potent cholesterol-lowering agent with significant triglyceride-lowering ability (20 to 45%).[526] These agents are best taken at night, when maximal cholesterol biosynthesis occurs. The reductase inhibitors are well tolerated and cause few side effects. The most serious potential side effect is myopathy, which occurs in fewer than 1% of persons taking lovastatin[524] but which can cause myoglobinuria and renal failure.[527] Patients taking HMG-CoA reductase inhibitors who develop myalgias should have serum creatine phosphokinase (CPK) measurements, and the drug should be stopped immediately if evidence of myositis is found. The risk of myopathy is increased

been evaluated for the treatment of hyperlipidemia and the prevention of CHD.[511] Although they lower VLDL levels and are effective for the treatment of hypertriglyceridemia, fish oils appear to have little effect on total cholesterol levels, and many patients with hypertriglyceridemia develop increased LDL levels with fish oil therapy.[511, 512] Fish oils may have beneficial effects on cardiovascular disease by means other than their effects on lipoproteins, such as the inhibition of platelet aggregation,[513] but a prospective study of male health professionals found no protective effects of increased dietary fish oil intake on the development of CHD.[514] In addition, fish oil supplementation can worsen glycemic control in persons with type II diabetes.[515]

Of all the types of fatty acids, monounsaturated fats may have the least deleterious effects on plasma lipoprotein metabolism.[21, 500, 516] Monounsaturated fats, such as oleic acid, are found in high quantities in olive oil and canola oil. When substituted for saturated fats, monounsaturated fats lowered total plasma cholesterol levels without lowering the plasma HDL cholesterol levels.[516]

Other dietary components may influence plasma lipid levels. For example, soluble fibers such as psyllium or oat bran, which may bind bile acids in the gut and promote net cholesterol excretion, can result in modest (<10%) decreases in LDL cholesterol levels.[517–519] Garlic[520] and walnuts[521] are reported to result in modest decreases in plasma cholesterol levels.

TABLE 23–16. Drugs Commonly Used for Treating Hyperlipidemia

Class	Drugs Available	Dosage	Major Lipoprotein Decreased	Mechanism	Common Side Effects
Bile acid sequestrants	Cholestyramine Colestipol	4–12 g bid 5–15 g bid	LDL	Increases sterol excretion; increases LDL receptor–mediated removal of LDL	Gastrointestinal symptoms; can increase triglycerides; binds other drugs
Nicotinic acid	Niacin	1–2 g tid	VLDL (LDL)	Decreases VLDL production	Flushing; hyperglycemia; hepatic dysfunction; gout
Fibric acid derivatives	Gemfibrozil Clofibrate	600 mg bid 1 g bid	VLDL (LDL)	Decreases VLDL production; enhances LPL action	Gallstones; myopathy
HMG-CoA reductase inhibitors	Lovastatin Pravastatin Simvastatin Fluvastatin Atorvastatin	10–80 mg qd 10–40 mg qd 5–40 mg qd 20–40 mg qd 10–80 mg qd	LDL	Decreases cholesterol synthesis; increases LDL receptor–mediated removal of LDL	Hepatic dysfunction; myopathy
Probucol	Probucol	500 mg bid	LDL, HDL	Weak hypolipidemic agent; potent antioxidant	Diarrhea; QT interval prolongation

TABLE 23–17. Drug Selection Based on Major Lipid Abnormality

Major Elevated Plasma Lipid(s)	Drugs
Cholesterol	Bile acid sequestrants
	Niacin
	HMG-CoA reductase inhibitor
	Probucol
Cholesterol and triglyceride	Niacin
	Fibric acid derivative
	HMG-CoA reductase inhibitor
Triglyceride	Niacin
	Fibric acid derivative
	Fish oils
Lp(a)	Niacin

if an HMG-CoA reductase inhibitor is used in combination with niacin,[528] gemfibrozil,[527] erythromycin, or cyclosporine.[529] These drug combinations should be avoided if possible, and the plasma CPK level probably should be monitored if the combinations are used. Serum transaminase elevations (>three times normal) occur in 2 to 3% of patients.[524] The long-term side effects of HMG-CoA reductase inhibitor therapy are not known, but no significant long-term toxicities have been observed with lovastatin, which has now been in use for more than 10 y.

BILE ACID SEQUESTRANTS

Bile acid sequestrants are anion-exchange resins that exchange chloride for negatively charged bile acids. The bound bile acids are then excreted in the feces.[530] The increased excretion of bile acids causes increased oxidation of cholesterol to form bile acids in hepatocytes, and the resultant upregulation of hepatic LDL receptors in turn lowers plasma LDL concentrations.[531] Because bile acid sequestrants act in the intestine, the side effects are limited to local effects in the gastrointestinal system (e.g., bloating, gas, constipation). At therapeutic doses, these agents can lower plasma cholesterol level by 15 to 25%. These agents must be used with caution in patients predisposed to hypertriglyceridemia, because they can result in increases in plasma triglyceride levels.[532] In addition, because they bind negatively charged molecules in the intestine, they can interfere with the absorption of other medications, including levothyroxine, digoxin, warfarin, and thiazide diuretics. Therefore, resins are given at least 4 h before or 1 h after other medications.

NIACIN

The most inexpensive drug for treating hyperlipidemia is the B vitamin niacin. Therapeutic doses of niacin (typically 2.0 to 4.5 g/d) lower both total and LDL cholesterol by 15 to 30%, lower triglyceride levels by 30 to 40%, and raise HDL cholesterol levels by 15 to 25%.[533] Maximal HDL increases usually occur with therapeutic doses of 1.5 to 2.0 g/d. Niacin also lowers plasma Lp(a) concentrations by up to 40%.[232, 534] The preparation must be niacin and not niacinamide, which has no efficacy. The mechanism whereby niacin affects plasma lipids is unclear but seems to be associated with decreased hepatic VLDL production. The most troublesome side effect of niacin therapy is a flushing syndrome that occurs shortly after taking the medicine. This side effect can be minimized by initiating therapy with small doses (e.g., 100 mg) and gradually increasing the dosage to the therapeutic range over weeks to months. Repeated dosing is associated with a gradual tolerance to the flushing syndrome. In addition, taking an aspirin about 1 h before the niacin can diminish the flushing side effects, possibly by inhibiting prostaglandin-mediated side effects. The most serious side effect associated with niacin

therapy is hepatotoxicity, and therapy should be accompanied by monitoring of serum liver function tests. Mild increases in serum transaminases are common when doses are increased rapidly; however, therapy should be discontinued, if transaminases reach highly elevated levels (e.g., >10 times normal). Because hepatotoxicity appears to be more common with sustained-release preparations of niacin,[535] the immediate-release crystalline form is preferred. Other prominent side effects of niacin therapy include impairment or worsening of glucose tolerance and hyperuricemia. For this reason, niacin should be used with great caution in patients with glucose intolerance or a history of gout. Niacin is contraindicated in patients with active peptic ulcer disease.

FIBRIC ACID DERIVATIVES

The fibric acid derivatives, clofibrate and gemfibrozil, lower plasma triglycerides (by about 40%) and increase HDL cholesterol levels (by about 10%)[282] but have only minor effects on LDL cholesterol. These agents act by uncertain mechanisms to decrease VLDL triglyceride production and to increase the LPL-mediated catabolism of triglyceride-rich lipoproteins.[536] They are given twice a day and are well tolerated. Side effects include gastrointestinal discomfort and possibly an increased incidence of cholesterol gallstones. Clofibrate received adverse publicity from a large clinical trial in which slightly more cancer deaths were noted in the clofibrate-treated group,[537] but there is no firm evidence that it is carcinogenic in humans. Fibric acid derivatives should be used with great caution in the setting of renal insufficiency because there is an increased propensity to developing myopathy in this setting.[538]

PROBUCOL AND OTHER ANTIOXIDANTS

Probucol is an agent that has minimal effects on lowering plasma LDL cholesterol but also lowers HDL cholesterol levels.[539] Probucol is transported on lipoproteins and is a potent antioxidant. Animal studies using probucol have suggested that despite its tendency to lower HDL, probucol therapy protects against the development of atherosclerotic lesions.[233, 234] In a trial in humans,[540] probucol treatment failed to result in benefits in patients with established peripheral vascular disease. The suggestion that the antioxidant effects of probucol may be more beneficial at early stages of atherosclerosis[541] remains to be tested. Probucol is given twice daily and is generally well tolerated. Because QT interval prolongation has been observed with probucol treatment, the QT interval should be monitored in patients treated with this drug.

There is interest in the use of other antioxidants, including the antioxidant vitamins (the fat-soluble vitamins E and A and the water-soluble vitamin C), in the treatment or prevention of atherosclerosis. Evidence to support this approach currently comes from population studies in which the high intake of antioxidants, such as β-carotene, is associated with decreased coronary events.[542] Prospective data demonstrating that supplemental antioxidant vitamin therapy can prevent atherosclerosis or CHD events in humans are lacking.

COMBINATION THERAPY

For patients with severe elevations of plasma cholesterol (e.g., >7.8 mmol/L [300 mg/dL]), in whom treatment goals are to reduce the plasma and LDL cholesterol levels by 50% or more, combination drug therapy is usually required.[522] Often this can be achieved with combinations that employ lower doses than needed when these agents are used as single agents. For example, combined therapy with an HMG-CoA reductase inhibitor and niacin[227, 228] or with an HMG-CoA

receptor suggest a physiological role as lipoprotein receptor. EMBO J 1988; 7:4119–4127.

95. Strickland DK, Ashcom JD, Williams S, et al. Sequence identity between the α₂-macroglobulin receptor and low density lipoprotein receptor-related protein suggests that this molecule is a multifunctional receptor. J Biol Chem 1990; 265:17401–17404.

96. Mahley RW, Hussain MM. Chylomicron and chylomicron remnant catabolism. Curr Opin Lipidol 1991; 2:170–176.

97. Beisiegel U, Weber W, Bengtsson-Olivecrona G. Lipoprotein lipase enhances the binding of chylomicrons to low density lipoprotein receptor-related protein. Proc Natl Acad Sci USA 1991; 88:8342–8346.

98. Ji Z-S, Lauer SJ, Fazio S, et al. Enhanced binding and uptake of remnant lipoproteins by hepatic lipase-secreting hepatoma cells in culture. J Biol Chem 1994; 269:13429–13436.

99. Herz J, Clouthier DE, Hammer RE. LDL receptor–related protein internalizes and degrades uPA–PAI-1 complexes and is essential for embryo implantation. Cell 1992; 71:411–421.

100. Willnow TE, Armstrong SA, Hammer RE, et al. Functional expression of low density lipoprotein receptor-related protein is controlled by receptor-associated protein *in vivo*. Proc Natl Acad Sci USA 1995; 92:4537–4541.

101. Willnow TE, Hilpert J, Armstrong SA, et al. Defective forebrain development in mice lacking gp330/megalin. Proc Natl Acad Sci USA 1996; 93:8460–8464.

102. Jingami H, Yamamoto T. The VLDL receptor: wayward brother of the LDL receptor. Curr Opin Lipidol 1995; 6:104–108.

103. Ramprasad MP, Fischer W, Witztum JL, et al. The 94- to 97-kDa mouse macrophage membrane protein that recognizes oxidized low density lipoprotein and phosphatidylserine-rich liposomes is identical to macrosialin, the mouse homologue of human CD68. Proc Natl Acad Sci USA 1995; 92:9580–9584.

104. Sambrano GR, Steinberg D. Recognition of oxidatively damaged and apoptotic cells by an oxidized low density lipoprotein receptor on mouse peritoneal macrophages: role of membrane phosphatidylserine. Proc Natl Acad Sci USA 1995; 92:1396–1400.

105. Olivecrona T, Bengtsson-Olivecrona G. Lipases involved in lipoprotein metabolism. Curr Opin Lipidol 1990; 1:116–121.

106. Lalouel J-M, Wilson DE, Iverius P-H. Lipoprotein lipase and hepatic triglyceride lipase: molecular and genetic aspects. Curr Opin Lipidol 1992; 3:86–95.

107. Hayden MR, Ma Y, Brunzell J, et al. Genetic variants affecting human lipoprotein and hepatic lipases. Curr Opin Lipidol 1991; 2:104–109.

108. Brunzell JD. Familial lipoprotein lipase deficiency and other causes of the chylomicronemia syndrome. In: Scriver CR, Beaudet AL, Sly WS, et al., eds. The Metabolic and Molecular Bases of Inherited Disease. 7th ed, Vol 2. New York: McGraw-Hill, 1995: 1913–1932.

109. Santamarina-Fojo S, Dugi KA. Structure, function and role of lipoprotein lipase in lipoprotein metabolism. Curr Opin Lipidol 1994; 5:117–125.

110. Kern PA. Lipoprotein lipase and hepatic lipase. Curr Opin Lipidol 1991; 2:162–169.

111. Applebaum-Bowden D. Lipases and lecithin:cholesterol acyltransferase in the control of lipoprotein metabolism. Curr Opin Lipidol 1995; 6:130–135.

112. Thuren T, Weisgraber KH, Sisson P, et al. Role of apolipoprotein E in hepatic lipase catalyzed hydrolysis of phospholipid in high-density lipoproteins. Biochemistry 1992; 31:2332–2338.

113. Homanics GE, de Silva HV, Osada J, et al. Mild dyslipidemia in mice following targeted inactivation of the hepatic lipase gene. J Biol Chem 1995; 270:2974–2980.

114. Busch SJ, Barnhart RL, Martin GA, et al. Human hepatic triglyceride lipase expression reduces high density lipoprotein and aortic cholesterol in cholesterol-fed transgenic mice. J Biol Chem 1994; 269:16376–16382.

115. Fan J, Wang J, Bensadoun A, et al. Overexpression of hepatic lipase in transgenic rabbits leads to a marked reduction of plasma high density lipoproteins and intermediate density lipoproteins. Proc Natl Acad Sci USA 1994; 91:8724–8728.

116. Glomset JA, Assmann G, Gjone E, et al. Lecithin:cholesterol acyltransferase deficiency and fish eye disease. In: Scriver CR, Beaudet AL, Sly WS, et al., eds. The Metabolic and Molecular Bases of Inherited Disease. 7th ed, Vol 2. New York: McGraw-Hill, 1995: 1933–1951.

117. Tall A. Plasma lipid transfer proteins. Annu Rev Biochem 1995; 64:235–257.

118. Tall AR. Plasma cholesteryl ester transfer protein. J Lipid Res 1993; 34:1255–1274.

119. Choi SY, Fong LG, Kirven MJ, et al. Use of an anti–low density lipoprotein receptor antibody to quantify the role of the LDL receptor in the removal of chylomicron remnants in the mouse in vivo. J Clin Invest 1991; 88:1173–1181.

120. Brown MS, Herz J, Kowal RC, et al. The low-density lipoprotein receptor-related protein: double agent or decoy? Curr Opin Lipidol 1991; 2:65–72.

121. Ji Z-S, Fazio S, Lee Y-L, et al. Secretion-capture role for apolipoprotein E in remnant lipoprotein metabolism involving cell surface heparan sulfate proteoglycans. J Biol Chem 1994; 269:2764–2772.

122. Shimano H, Namba Y, Ohsuga J, et al. Secretion-recapture process of apolipoprotein E in hepatic uptake of chylomicron remnants in transgenic mice. J Clin Invest 1994; 93:2215–2223.

123. Ji Z-S, Brecht WJ, Miranda RD, et al. Role of heparan sulfate proteoglycans in the binding and uptake of apolipoprotein E–enriched remnant lipoproteins by cultured cells. J Biol Chem 1993; 268:10160–10167.

124. Ji Z-S, Brecht WJ, Miranda RD, et al. Intravenous heparinase hydrolysis of hepatic heparan sulfate proteoglycans inhibits remnant lipoprotein clearance *in vivo*. Circulation 1994; 90:I-290 (abstract).

125. Alexander CA, Hamilton RL, Havel RJ. Subcellular localization of B apoprotein of plasma lipoproteins in rat liver. J Cell Biol 1976; 69:241–263.

126. Pullinger CR, North JD, Teng B-B, et al. The apolipoprotein B gene is constitutively expressed in HepG2 cells: regulation of secretion by oleic acid, albumin, and insulin, and measurement of the mRNA half-life. J Lipid Res 1989; 30:1065–1077.

127. Sorci-Thomas M, Wilson MD, Johnson FL, et al. Studies on the expression of genes encoding apolipoproteins B100 and B48 and the low density lipoprotein receptor in nonhuman primates: comparison of dietary fat and cholesterol. J Biol Chem 1989; 264:9039–9045.

128. Boström K, Borén J, Wettesten M, et al. Studies on the assembly of apo B-100-containing lipoproteins in HepG2 cells. J Biol Chem 1988; 263:4434–4442.

129. Borén J, Rustaeus S, Wettesten M, et al. Influence of triacylglycerol biosynthesis rate on the assembly of apoB-100-containing lipoproteins in Hep G2 cells. Arterioscler Thromb 1993; 13:1743–1754.

130. Ginsberg HN. Synthesis and secretion of apolipoprotein B from cultured liver cells. Curr Opin Lipidol 1995; 6:275–280.

131. Sharp D, Blinderman L, Combs KA, et al. Cloning and gene defects in microsomal triglyceride transfer protein associated with abetalipoproteinaemia. Nature 1993; 365:65–69.

132. Gregg RE, Wetterau JR. The molecular basis of abetalipoproteinemia. Curr Opin Lipidol 1994; 5:81–86.

133. Huang Y, von Eckardstein A, Wu S, et al. A plasma lipoprotein containing only apolipoprotein E and with γ mobility on electrophoresis releases cholesterol from cells. Proc Natl Acad Sci USA 1994; 91:1834–1838.

134. Johnson WJ, Mahlberg FH, Rothblat GH, et al. Cholesterol transport between cells and high-density lipoproteins. Biochim Biophys Acta 1991; 1085:273–298.

135. Assmann G, von Eckardstein A, Funke H. Lecithin:cholesterol acyltransferase deficiency and fish-eye disease. Curr Opin Lipidol 1991; 2:110–117.

136. Yang C-Y, Manoogian D, Pao Q, et al. Lecithin:cholesterol acyltransferase: functional regions and a structural model of the enzyme. J Biol Chem 1987; 262:3086–3091.

137. Glass C, Pittman RC, Weinstein DB, et al. Dissociation of tissue uptake of cholesterol ester from that of apoprotein A-I of rat plasma high density lipoprotein: selective delivery of cholesterol ester to liver, adrenal, and gonad. Proc Natl Acad Sci USA 1983; 80:5435–5439.

138. Reaven E, Tsai L, Azhar S. Cholesterol uptake by the 'selective' pathway of ovarian granulosa cells: early intracellular events. J Lipid Res 1995; 36:1602–1617.

139. Williams DL. Selective uptake of lipoprotein cholesteryl ester: past, present, and future. J Lipid Res (in press).

140. Ha YC, Barter PJ. Differences in plasma cholesteryl ester transfer activity in sixteen vertebrate species. Comp Biochem Physiol [B] Comp Biochem 1982; 71:265–269.

141. Inazu A, Jiang X-C, Haraki T, et al. Genetic cholesteryl ester transfer protein deficiency caused by two prevalent mutations as a major determinant of increased levels of high density lipoprotein cholesterol. J Clin Invest 1994; 94:1872–1882.

142. Marotti KR, Castle CK, Boyle TP, et al. Severe atherosclerosis in transgenic mice expressing simian cholesteryl ester transfer protein. Nature 1993; 364:73–75.

143. Stary HC. The sequence of cell and matrix changes in atherosclerotic lesions of coronary arteries in the first forty years of life. Eur Heart J 1990; 11(Suppl E):3–19.

144. National Cholesterol Education Program. Second report of the Expert Panel on Detection, Evaluation, and Treatment of High Blood Cholesterol in Adults (Adult Treatment Panel II). Circulation 1994; 89:1329–1445.

145. Keys A. Coronary heart disease: the global picture. Atherosclerosis 1975; 22:149–192.

146. Keys A: Seven Countries: A Multivariate Analysis of Death and Coronary Heart Disease. Cambridge, Massachusetts: Harvard University Press, 1980.

147. Mahley RW. Development of accelerated atherosclerosis: concepts derived from cell biology and animal model studies. Arch Pathol Lab Med 1983; 107:393–399.

148. Mahley RW. Atherogenic lipoproteins and coronary artery disease: concepts derived from recent advances in cellular and molecular biology. Circulation 1985; 72:943–948.

149. Vesselinovitch D. Animal models and the study of atherosclerosis. Arch Pathol Lab Med 1988; 112:1011–1017.

150. Faggiotto A, Ross R, Harker L. Studies of hypercholesterolemia in the nonhuman primate. I. Changes that lead to fatty streak formation. Arteriosclerosis 1984; 4:323–340.

151. Buja LM, Clubb FJ Jr., Bilheimer DW, et al. Pathobiology of human familial hypercholesterolaemia and a related animal model, the Watanabe heritable hyperlipidaemic rabbit. Eur Heart J 1990; 11(Suppl E):41–52.

152. Ishibashi S, Goldstein JL, Brown MS, et al. Massive xanthomatosis and atherosclerosis in cholesterol-fed low density lipoprotein receptor–negative mice. J Clin Invest 1994; 93:1885–1893.

153. The Multiple Risk Factor Intervention Trial Research Group. Mortality rates after 10.5 years for participants in the Multiple Risk Factor Intervention Trial: findings related to a priori hypotheses of the trial. J Am Med Assoc 1990; 263:1795–1801.

154. Lipid Research Clinics Program. The Lipid Research Clinics Coronary Primary Prevention Trial results. II: The relationship of reduction in incidence of coronary heart disease to cholesterol lowering. J Am Med Assoc 1984; 251:365–374.

155. Brown G, Albers JJ, Fisher LD, et al. Regression of coronary artery disease as a result of intensive lipid-lowering therapy in men with high levels of apolipoprotein B. N Engl J Med 1990; 323:1289–1298.

156. Oliver MF. Doubts about preventing coronary heart disease: multiple interventions in middle aged men may do more harm than good. Br Med J 1992; 304:393–394.

157. Smith GD, Pekkanen J. Should there be a moratorium on the use of cholesterol lowering drugs? Br Med J 1992; 304:431–434.

158. Scandinavian Simvastatin Survival Study Group. Randomised trial of cholesterol lowering in 4444 patients with coronary heart disease: the Scandinavian Simvastatin Survival Study (4S). Lancet 1994; 344:1383–1389.

159. Shepherd J, Cobbe SM, Ford I, et al. Prevention of coronary heart disease with pravastatin in men with hypercholesterolemia. N Engl J Med 1995; 333:1301–1307.

160. Consensus Conference. Lowering blood cholesterol to prevent heart disease. J Am Med Assoc 1985; 253:2080–2086.

161. Scanu AM. Lipoprotein(a): a genetic risk factor for premature coronary heart disease. J Am Med Assoc 1992; 267:3326–3329.

162. Berg K. Lp(a) lipoprotein: an overview. Chem Phys Lipids 1994; 67/68:9–16.

163. Krauss RM. Low-density lipoprotein subclasses and risk of coronary artery disease. Curr Opin Lipidol 1991; 2:248–252.

164. Mahley RW, Weisgraber KH, Innerarity TL, et al. Genetic defects in lipoprotein metabolism: elevation of atherogenic lipoproteins caused by impaired catabolism. J Am Med Assoc 1991; 265:78–83.

165. Havel R. McCollum Award Lecture, 1993: Triglyceride-rich lipoproteins and atherosclerosis—new perspectives. Am J Clin Nutr 1994; 59:795–799.

166. Steinberg D. Lipoproteins and the pathogenesis of atherosclerosis. Circulation 1987; 76:508–514.

167. Brown MS, Goldstein JL. Lipoprotein metabolism in the macrophage: implications for cholesterol deposition in atherosclerosis. Annu Rev Biochem 1983; 52:223–261.

168. Haberland ME, Fless GM, Scanu AM, et al. Malondialdehyde modification of lipoprotein(a) produces avid uptake by human monocyte-macrophages. J Biol Chem 1992; 267:4143–4151.

169. Henriksen T, Mahoney EM, Steinberg D. Enhanced macrophage degradation of low density lipoprotein previously incubated with cultured endothelial cells: recognition by receptors for acetylated low density lipoproteins. Proc Natl Acad Sci USA 1981; 78:6499–6503.

170. Steinberg D, Parthasarathy S, Carew TE, et al. Beyond cholesterol: modifications of low-density lipoprotein that increase its atherogenicity. N Engl J Med 1989; 320:915–924.

171. Witztum JL. The oxidation hypothesis of atherosclerosis. Lancet 1994; 344:793–795.

172. Stadtman ER. Protein oxidation and aging. Science 1992; 257:1220–1224.

173. Harman D. Free radical theory of aging: role of free radicals in the origination and evolution of life, aging, and disease processes. In: Johnson JE Jr., Walford R, Harman D, et al., eds. Free Radicals, Aging, and Degenerative Diseases. New York: Alan R Liss, 1986: 3–49.

174. Chisolm GM. Cytotoxicity of oxidized lipoproteins. Curr Opin Lipidol 1991; 2:311–316.

175. Quinn MT, Parthasarathy S, Fong LG, et al. Oxidatively modified low density lipoproteins: a potential role in recruitment and retention of monocyte/macrophages during atherogenesis. Proc Natl Acad Sci USA 1987; 84:2995–2998.

176. Palinski W, Ylä-Herttuala S, Rosenfeld ME, et al. Antisera and monoclonal antibodies specific for epitopes generated during oxidative modification of low density lipoprotein. Arteriosclerosis 1990; 10:325–335.

177. Haberland ME, Fong D, Cheng L. Malondialdehyde-altered protein occurs in atheroma of Watanabe heritable hyperlipidemic rabbits. Science 1988; 241:215–218.

178. Ross R. The pathogenesis of atherosclerosis: a perspective for the 1990s. Nature 1993; 362:801–809.

179. Schwartz CJ, Valente AJ, Sprague EA. A modern view of atherogenesis. Am J Cardiol 1993; 71:9B–14B.

180. Gimbrone MA Jr.: Vascular endothelium: nature's blood container. In: Vascular Endothelium in Hemostasis and Thrombosis. Edinburgh: Churchill Livingstone, 1986: 1–13.

181. Cybulsky MI, Gimbrone MA Jr. Endothelial expression of a mononuclear leukocyte adhesion molecule during atherogenesis. Science 1991; 251:788–791.

182. Wallace RB, Hoover J, Sandler D, et al. Altered plasma-lipids associated with oral contraceptive or œstrogen consumption: the Lipid Research Clinic program. Lancet 1977; 2:11–14.

183. Verschuren WMM, Jacobs DR, Bloemberg BPM, et al. Serum total cholesterol and long-term coronary heart disease mortality in different cultures: twenty-five-year follow-up of the Seven Countries Study. J Am Med Assoc 1995; 274:131–136.

184. The Expert Panel. Summary of the second report of the National Cholesterol Education Program (NCEP) Expert Panel on Detection, Evaluation, and Treatment of High Blood Cholesterol in Adults (Adult Treatment Panel II). J Am Med Assoc 1993; 269:3015–3023.

185. Heiss G, Tamir I, Davis CE, et al. Lipoprotein-cholesterol distributions in selected North American populations: the Lipid Research Clinics Program Prevalence Study. Circulation 1980; 61:302–315.

186. Martin MJ, Hulley SB, Browner WS, et al. Serum cholesterol, blood pressure, and mortality: implications from a cohort of 361 662 men. Lancet 1986; 2:933–936.

187. Beaumont JL, Carlson LA, Cooper GR, et al. Classification of hyperlipidaemias and hyperlipoproteinaemias. Bull World Health Organ 1970; 43:891–907.

188. Fredrickson DS. It's time to be practical. Circulation 1975; 51:209–211.

189. Bagdade JD, Porte D Jr., Bierman EL. Steroid-induced lipemia: a complication of high-dosage corticosteroid therapy. Arch Intern Med 1970; 125:129–134.

190. Taskinen M-R, Nikkilä EA, Pelkonen R, et al. Plasma lipoproteins, lipolytic enzymes, and very low density lipoprotein triglyceride turnover in Cushing's syndrome. J Clin Endocrinol Metab 1983; 57:619–626.

191. Ettinger WH Jr., Hazzard WR. Prednisone increases very low density lipoprotein and high density lipoprotein in healthy men. Metabolism 1988; 37:1055–1058.

192. Merimee TJ, Hollander W, Fineberg SE. Studies of hyperlipidemia in the HGH-deficient state. Metabolism 1972; 21:1053–1061.

193. Nikkilä EA, Pelkonen R. Serum lipids in acromegaly. Metabolism 1975; 24:829–838.

194. Klinefelter HF. Hypercholesterolemia in anorexia nervosa. J Clin Endocrinol Metab 1965; 25:1520–1521.

195. Crisp AH, Blendis LM, Pawan GLS. Aspects of fat metabolism in anorexia nervosa. Metabolism 1968; 17:1109–1118.

196. Havel RJ, Goldstein JL, Brown MS. Lipoproteins and lipid transport. In: Bondy PK, Rosenberg LE, eds. Metabolic Control and Disease. 8th ed. Philadelphia, WB Saunders, 1980: 393–494.

197. Epstein CJ, Martin GM, Schultz AL, et al. Werner's syndrome: a review of its symptomatology, natural history, pathologic features, genetics and relationship to the natural aging process. Medicine 1966; 45:177–221.

198. Lees RS, Song CS, Levere RD, et al. Hyperbeta-lipoproteinemia in acute intermittent porphyria. N Engl J Med 1970; 282:432–433.

199. Hülsmann WC, Eijkenboom WHM, Koster JF, et al. Glucose-6-phosphatase deficiency and hyperlipaemia. Clin Chim Acta 1970; 30:775–778.

200. Jakovcic S, Khachadurian AK, Hsia DY-Y. The hyperlipidemia in glycogen storage disease. J Lab Clin Med 1966; 68:769–779.

201. Goldberg A, Sherrard DJ, Brunzell JD. Adipose tissue lipoprotein lipase in chronic hemodialysis: role in plasma triglyceride metabolism. J Clin Endocrinol Metab 1978; 47:1173–1182.

202. McIntyre N, Harry DS, Pearson AJG. The hypercholesterolaemia of obstructive jaundice. Gut 1975; 16:379–391.

203. Simon JB. Lecithin:cholesterol acyltransferase in human liver disease. Scand J Clin Lab Invest 1974; 33(Suppl 137):107–113.

204. Sabesin SM, Hawkins HL, Kuiken L, et al. Abnormal plasma lipoproteins and lecithin-cholesterol acyltransferase deficiency in alcoholic liver disease. Gastroenterology 1977; 72:510–518.

205. Glueck CJ, Kaplan AP, Levy RI, et al. A new mechanism of exogenous hyperglyceridemia. Ann Intern Med 1969; 71:1051–1062.

206. Taylor JS, Lewis LA, Battle JD Jr., et al. Plane xanthoma and multiple myeloma with lipoprotein–paraprotein complexing. Arch Dermatol 1978; 114:425–431.

207. Kihara S, Matsuzawa Y, Kubo M, et al. Autoimmune hyperchylomicronemia. N Engl J Med 1989; 320:1255–1259.

208. Goldstein JL, Brown MS. Familial hypercholesterolemia. In: Stanbury JB, Wyngaarden JB, Fredrickson DS, et al., eds. The Metabolic Basis of Inherited Disease. 5th ed. New York: McGraw-Hill, 1983: 672–712.

209. Goldstein JL, Brown MS. The LDL receptor locus and the genetics of familial hypercholesterolemia. Annu Rev Genet 1979; 13:259–289.

210. Shapiro JR, Fallat RW, Tsang RC, et al. Achilles tendinitis and tenosynovitis: a diagnostic manifestation of familial type II hyperlipoproteinemia in children. Am J Dis Child 1974; 128:486–490.

211. Barchiesi BJ, Eckel RH, Ellis PP. The cornea and disorders of lipid metabolism. Surv Ophthalmol 1991; 36:1–22.

212. Stone NJ, Levy RI, Fredrickson DS, et al. Coronary artery disease in 116 kindred with familial type II hyperlipoproteinemia. Circulation 1974; 49:476–488.

213. Sprecher DL, Schaefer EJ, Kent KM, et al. Cardiovascular features of homozygous familial hypercholesterolemia: analysis of 16 patients. Am J Cardiol 1984; 54:20–30.

214. Coetzee GA, van der Westhuyzen DR, Berger GMB, et al. Low density lipoprotein metabolism in cultured fibroblasts from a new group of patients presenting clinically with homozygous familial hypercholesterolemia. Arteriosclerosis 1982; 2:303–311.

215. Allen JM, Thompson GR, Myant NB, et al. Cardiovascular complications of homozygous familial hypercholesterolaemia. Br Heart J 1980; 44:361–368.

216. Lehrman MA, Goldstein JL, Brown MS, et al. Internalization-defective LDL receptors produced by genes with nonsense and frameshift mutations that truncate the cytoplasmic domain. Cell 1985; 41:735–743.

217. Hobbs HH, Brown MS, Russell DW, et al. Deletion in the gene for the low-density-lipoprotein receptor in a majority of French Canadians with familial hypercholesterolemia. N Engl J Med 1987; 317:734–737.

218. Goldstein JL, Ho YK, Basu SK, et al. Binding site on macrophages that mediates uptake and degradation of acetylated low density lipoprotein,

producing massive cholesterol deposition. Proc Natl Acad Sci USA 1979; 76:333–337.

219. Brown MS, Deuel TF, Basu SK, et al. Inhibition of the binding of low-density lipoprotein to its cell surface receptor in human fibroblasts by positively charged proteins. J Supramol Struct 1978; 8:223–234.

220. Goldstein JL, Schrott HG, Hazzard WR, et al. Hyperlipidemia in coronary heart disease. II: Genetic analysis of lipid levels in 176 families and delineation of a new inherited disorder, combined hyperlipidemia. J Clin Invest 1973; 52:1544–1568.

221. Myant NB. Familial defective apolipoprotein B-100: a review, including some comparisons with familial hypercholesterolaemia. Atherosclerosis 1993; 104:1–18.

222. Brown MS, Goldstein JL. Familial hypercholesterolemia: defective binding of lipoproteins to cultured fibroblasts associated with impaired regulation of 3-hydroxy-3-methylglutaryl coenzyme A reductase activity. Proc Natl Acad Sci USA 1974; 71:788–792.

223. Packard CJ, Shepherd J. Current concepts in the treatment of familial hypercholesterolaemia. Curr Opin Lipidol 1995; 6:57–61.

224. Connor WE, Connor SL. Importance of diet in the treatment of familial hypercholesterolaemia. Am J Cardiol 1993; 72:42D–53D.

225. Illingworth DR. How effective is drug therapy in heterozygous familial hypercholesterolemia? Am J Cardiol 1993; 72:54D–58D.

226. Mabuchi H, Sakai T, Sakai Y, et al. Reduction of serum cholesterol in heterozygous patients with familial hypercholesterolemia. Additive effects of compactin and cholestyramine. N Engl J Med 1983; 308:609–613.

227. Kane JP, Malloy MJ, Tun P, et al. Normalization of low-density-lipoprotein levels in heterozygous familial hypercholesterolemia with a combined drug regimen. N Engl J Med 1981; 304:251–258.

228. Illingworth DR, Phillipson BE, Rapp JH, et al. Colestipol plus nicotinic acid in treatment of heterozygous familial hypercholesterolaemia. Lancet 1981; 1:296–298.

229. Malloy MJ, Kane JP, Kunitake ST, et al. Complementarity of colestipol, niacin, and lovastatin in treatment of severe familial hypercholesterolemia. Ann Intern Med 1987; 107:616–623.

230. Bilheimer DW, Grundy SM, Brown MS, et al. Mevinolin and colestipol stimulate receptor-mediated clearance of low density lipoprotein from plasma in familial hypercholesterolemia heterozygotes. Proc Natl Acad Sci USA 1983; 80:4124–4128.

231. Seed M, Hoppichler F, Reaveley D, et al. Relation of serum lipoprotein(a) concentration and apolipoprotein(a) phenotype to coronary heart disease in patients with familial hypercholesterolemia. N Engl J Med 1990; 322:1494–1499.

232. Carlson LA, Hamsten A, Asplund A. Pronounced lowering of serum levels of lipoprotein Lp(a) in hyperlipidaemic subjects treated with nicotinic acid. J Intern Med 1989; 226:271–276.

233. Carew TE, Schwenke DC, Steinberg D. Antiatherogenic effect of probucol unrelated to its hypocholesterolemic effect: evidence that antioxidants in vivo can selectively inhibit low density lipoprotein degradation in macrophage-rich fatty streaks and slow the progression of atherosclerosis in the Watanabe heritable hyperlipidemic rabbit. Proc Natl Acad Sci USA 1987; 84:7725–7729.

234. Kita T, Nagano Y, Yokode M, et al. Probucol prevents the progression of atherosclerosis in Watanabe heritable hyperlipidemic rabbit, an animal model for familial hypercholesterolemia. Proc Natl Acad Sci USA 1987; 84:5928–5931.

235. Yamamoto A, Matsuzawa Y, Yokoyama S, et al. Effects of probucol on xanthomata regression in familial hypercholesterolemia. Am J Cardiol 1986; 57:29H–35H.

236. Buchwald H, Varco RL, Matts JP, et al. Effect of partial ileal bypass surgery on mortality and morbidity from coronary heart disease in patients with hypercholesterolemia: report of the Program on the Surgical Control of the Hyperlipidemias (POSCH). N Engl J Med 1990; 323:946–955.

237. Kane JP, Malloy MJ, Ports TA, et al. Regression of coronary atherosclerosis during treatment of familial hypercholesterolemia with combined drug regimens. JAMA 1990; 264:3007–3012.

238. Stoffel W, Borberg H, Greve V. Application of specific extracorporeal removal of low density lipoprotein in familial hypercholesterolaemia. Lancet 1981; 2:1005–1007.

239. Gordon BR, Saal SD. Advances in LDL-apheresis for the treatment of severe hypercholesterolemia. Curr Opin Lipidol 1994; 5:69–73.

240. Bilheimer DW, Goldstein JL, Grundy SM, et al. Liver transplantation to provide low-density-lipoprotein receptors and lower plasma cholesterol in a child with homozygous familial hypercholesterolemia. N Engl J Med 1984; 311:1658–1664.

241. Valdivielso P, Escolar JL, Cuervas-Mons V, et al. Lipids and lipoprotein changes after heart and liver transplantation in a patient with homozygous familial hypercholesterolemia. Ann Intern Med 1988; 108:204–206.

242. Forman MB, Baker SG, Mieny CJ, et al. Treatment of homozygous familial hypercholesterolaemia with portacaval shunt. Atherosclerosis 1982; 41:349–361.

243. McNamara DJ, Ahrens EH Jr., Kolb R, et al. Treatment of familial hypercholesterolemia by portacaval anastomosis: effect on cholesterol metabolism and pool sizes. Proc Natl Acad Sci USA 1983; 80:564–568.

244. Brown MS, Goldstein JL, Havel RJ, et al. Gene therapy for cholesterol. Nat Genet 1994; 7:349–350.

245. Grossman M, Raper SE, Kozarsky K, et al. Successful ex vivo gene therapy directed to liver in a patient with familial hypercholesterolaemia. Nat Genet 1994; 6:335–341.

246. Schuster H, Rauh G, Kormann B, et al. Familial defective apolipoprotein B-100: comparison with familial hypercholesterolemia in 18 cases detected in Munich. Arteriosclerosis 1990; 10:577–581.

247. Tybjærg-Hansen A, Gallagher J, Vincent J, et al. Familial defective apolipoprotein B-100: detection in the United Kingdom and Scandinavia, and clinical characteristics of ten cases. Atherosclerosis 1990; 80:235–242.

248. Ludwig EH, McCarthy BJ. Haplotype analysis of the human apolipoprotein B mutation associated with familial defective apolipoprotein B100. Am J Hum Genet 1990; 47:712–720.

249. Bersot TP, Russell SJ, Thatcher SR, et al. A unique haplotype of the apolipoprotein B-100 allele associated with familial defective apolipoprotein B-100 in a Chinese man discovered during a study of the prevalence of this disorder. J Lipid Res 1993; 34:1149–1154.

250. Rauh G, Keller C, Kormann B, et al. Familial defective apolipoprotein B$_{100}$: clinical characteristics of 54 cases. Atherosclerosis 1992; 92:233–241.

251. Miserez AR, Keller U. Differences in the phenotypic characteristics of subjects with familial defective apolipoprotein B-100 and familial hypercholesterolemia. Arterioscler Thromb Vasc Biol 1995; 15:1719–1729.

252. März W, Baumstark MW, Scharnagl H, et al. Accumulation of "small dense" low density lipoproteins (LDL) in a homozygous patient with familial defective apolipoprotein B-100 results from heterogenous interaction of LDL subfractions with the LDL receptor. J Clin Invest 1993; 92:2922–2933.

253. Gallagher JJ, Myant NB. The affinity of low-density lipoproteins and of very-low-density lipoprotein remnants for the low-density lipoprotein receptor in homozygous familial defective apolipoprotein B-100. Atherosclerosis 1995; 115:263–272.

254. Funke H, Rust S, Seedorf U, et al. Homozygosity for familial defective apolipoprotein B-100 (FDB) is associated with lower plasma cholesterol concentrations than homozygosity for familial hypercholesterolemia (FH). Circulation 1992; 86:I-691 (abstract).

255. Innerarity TL, Weisgraber KH, Arnold KS, et al. Familial defective apolipoprotein B-100: low density lipoproteins with abnormal receptor binding. Proc Natl Acad Sci USA 1987; 84:6919–6923.

256. Soria LF, Ludwig EH, Clarke HRG, et al. Association between a specific apolipoprotein B mutation and familial defective apolipoprotein B-100. Proc Natl Acad Sci USA 1989; 86:587–591.

257. Vega GL, Grundy SM. In vivo evidence for reduced binding of low density lipoproteins to receptors as a cause of primary moderate hypercholesterolemia. J Clin Invest 1986; 78:1410–1414.

258. Rauh G, Schuster H, Schewe CK, et al. Independent mutation of arginine$_{(3500)}$→glutamine associated with familial defective apolipoprotein B-100. J Lipid Res 1993; 34:799–805.

259. Lund-Katz S, Innerarity TL, Arnold KS, et al. ^{13}C NMR evidence that substitution of glutamine for arginine 3500 in familial defective apolipoprotein B-100 disrupts the conformation of the receptor-binding domain. J Biol Chem 1991; 266:2701–2704.

260. Arnold KS, Balestra ME, Krauss RM, et al. Isolation of allele-specific, receptor-binding-defective low density lipoproteins from familial defective apolipoprotein B-100 subjects. J Lipid Res 1994; 35:1469–1476.

261. Gaffney D, Reid JM, Cameron IM, et al. Independent mutations at codon 3500 of the apolipoprotein B gene are associated with hyperlipidemia. Arterioscler Thromb Vasc Biol 1995; 15:1025–1029.

262. Pullinger CR, Hennessy LK, Chatterton JE, et al. Familial ligand-defective apolipoprotein B. Identification of a new mutation that decreases LDL receptor binding affinity. J Clin Invest 1995; 95:1225–1234.

263. Hansen PS, Rüdiger N, Tybjærg-Hansen A, et al. Detection of the apoB-3500 mutation (glutamine for arginine) by gene amplification and cleavage with MspI. J Lipid Res 1991; 32:1229–1233.

264. Schmidt EB, Illingworth DR, Bacon S, et al. Hypolipidemic effects of nicotinic acid in patients with familial defective apolipoprotein B-100. Metabolism 1993; 42:137–139.

265. Schmidt EB, Illingworth DR, Bacon S, et al. Hypocholesterolemic effects of cholestyramine and colestipol in patients with familial defective apolipoprotein B-100. Atherosclerosis 1993; 98:213–217.

266. Rose HG, Kranz P, Weinstock M, et al. Inheritance of combined hyperlipoproteinemia: evidence for a new lipoprotein phenotype. Am J Med 1973; 54:148–160.

267. Nikkilä EA, Aro A. Family study of serum lipids and lipoproteins in coronary heart disease. Lancet 1973; 1:954–959.

268. Sniderman A, Shapiro S, Marpole D, et al. Association of coronary atherosclerosis with hyperapobetalipoproteinemia (increased protein but normal cholesterol levels in human plasma low density [β] lipoproteins). Proc Natl Acad Sci USA 1980; 77:604–608.

269. Krauss RM. Dense low density lipoproteins and coronary artery disease. Am J Cardiol 1995; 75:53B–57B.

270. Reaven GM. Pathophysiology of insulin resistance in human disease. Physiol Rev 1995; 75:473–486.

271. Genest JJ Jr., Martin-Munley SS, McNamara JR, et al. Familial lipoprotein disorders in patients with premature coronary artery disease. Circulation 1992; 85:2025–2033.

272. Cortner JA, Coates PM, Gallagher PR. Prevalence and expression of familial combined hyperlipidemia in childhood. J Pediatr 1990; 116:514–519.

273. Grundy SM, Chait A, Brunzell JD. Familial combined hyperlipidemia workshop. Arteriosclerosis 1987; 7:203–207.

274. Wojciechowski AP, Farrall M, Cullen P, et al. Familial combined hyperlipidemia linked to the apolipoprotein AI-CIII-AIV gene cluster on chromosome 11q23–q24. Nature 1991; 349:161–164.

275. Nishina PM, Johnson JP, Naggert JK, et al. Linkage of atherogenic lipoprotein phenotype to the low density lipoprotein receptor locus on the short arm of chromosome 19. Proc Natl Acad Sci USA 1992; 89:708–712.

276. Rotter JI, Bu X, Cantor R, et al. Multilocus genetic determination of LDL particle size in coronary artery disease families. Clin. Res. 1994; 42:16A (abstract).

277. Babirak SP, Iverius P-H, Fujimoto WY, et al. Detection and characterization of the heterozygote state for lipoprotein lipase deficiency. Arteriosclerosis 1989; 9:326–334.

278. Chait A, Albers JJ, Brunzell JD. Very low density lipoprotein overproduction in genetic forms of hypertriglyceridaemia. Eur J Clin Invest 1980; 10:17–22.

279. Janus ED, Nicoll AM, Turner PR, et al. Kinetic bases of the primary hyperlipidaemias: studies of apolipoprotein B turnover in genetically defined subjects. Eur J Clin Invest 1980; 10:161–172.

280. Brunzell JD, Albers JJ, Chait A, et al. Plasma lipoproteins in familial combined hyperlipidemia and monogenic familial hypertriglyceridemia. J Lipid Res 1983; 24:147–155.

281. Crouse JR III. Hypertriglyceridemia: a contraindication to the use of bile acid binding resins. Am J Med 1987; 83:243–248.

282. Frick MH, Elo O, Haapa K, et al. Helsinki Heart Study: primary-prevention trial with gemfibrozil in middle-aged men with dyslipidemia. Safety of treatment, changes in risk factors, and incidence of coronary heart disease. N Engl J Med 1987; 317:1237–1245.

283. Vega GL, Grundy SM. Lipoprotein responses to treatment with lovastatin, gemfibrozil, and nicotinic acid in normolipidemic patients with hypo-alphalipoproteinemia. Arch Intern Med 1994; 154:73–82.

284. Brewer HB Jr., Zech LA, Gregg RE, et al. Type III hyperlipoproteinemia: diagnosis, molecular defects, pathology, and treatment. Ann Intern Med 1983; 98:623–640.

285. Havel RJ, Kotite L, Kane JP, et al. Atypical familial dysbetalipoproteinemia associated with apolipoprotein phenotype E3/3. J Clin Invest 1983; 72:379–387.

286. Rall SC Jr., Newhouse YM, Clarke HRG, et al. Type III hyperlipoproteinemia associated with apolipoprotein E phenotype E3/3: structure and genetics of an apolipoprotein E3 variant. J Clin Invest 1989; 83:1095–1101.

287. Koo C, Wernette-Hammond ME, Innerarity TL. Uptake of canine β-very low density lipoproteins by mouse peritoneal macrophages is mediated by a low density lipoprotein receptor. J Biol Chem 1986; 261:11194–11201.

288. Morganroth J, Levy RI, Fredrickson DS. The biochemical, clinical, and genetic features of type III hyperlipoproteinemia. Ann Intern Med 1975; 82:158–174.

289. Hixson JE, Vernier DT. Restriction isotyping of human apolipoprotein E by gene amplification and cleavage with HhaI. J Lipid Res 1990; 31:545–548.

290. Hazzard WR, Bierman EL. Aggravation of broad-β disease (type 3 hyperlipoproteinemia) by hypothyroidism. Arch Intern Med 1972; 130:822–828.

291. Kushwaha RS, Hazzard WR, Gagne C, et al. Type III hyperlipoproteinemia: paradoxical hypolipidemic response to estrogen. Ann Intern Med 1977; 87:517–525.

292. Hoogwerf BJ, Bantle JP, Kuba K, et al. Treatment of type III hyperlipoproteinemia with four different treatment regimens. Atherosclerosis 1984; 51:251–259.

293. Schaefer EJ. Type III hyperlipoproteinemia: diagnosis, molecular defects, pathology, and treatment. Dietary and drug treatment. Ann Intern Med 1983; 98:633–640.

294. Hoogwerf BJ, Peters JR, Frantz ID Jr., et al. Effect of clofibrate and colestipol singly and in combination on plasma lipids and lipoproteins in type III hyperlipoproteinemia. Metabolism 1985; 34:978–981.

295. Illingworth DR, O'Malley JP. The hypolipidemic effects of lovastatin and clofibrate alone and in combination in patients with type III hyperlipoproteinemia. Metabolism 1990; 39:403–409.

296. Stuyt PMJ, Mol MJTM, Stalenhoef AFH. Long-term effects of simvastatin in familial dysbetalipoproteinaemia. J Intern Med 1991; 230:151–155.

297. Feussner G, Eichinger M, Ziegler R. The influence of simvastatin alone or in combination with gemfibrozil on plasma lipids and lipoproteins in patients with type III hyperlipoproteinemia. Clin Invest 1992; 70:1027–1035.

298. Wiklund O, Angelin B, Bergman M, et al. Pravastatin and gemfibrozil alone and in combination for the treatment of hypercholesterolemia. Am J Med 1993; 94:13–20.

299. Chait A, Brunzell JD. Chylomicronemia syndrome. Adv Intern Med 1991; 37:249–273.

300. Santamarina-Fojo S, Brewer HB Jr. The familial hyperchylomicronemia syndrome: new insights into underlying genetic defects. J Am Med Assoc 1991; 265:904–908.

301. Brunzell JD, Bierman EL. Chylomicronemia syndrome: interaction of genetic and acquired hypertriglyceridemia. Med Clin North Am 1982; 66:455–468.

302. Chait A, Robertson HT, Brunzell JD. Chylomicronemia syndrome in diabetes mellitus. Diabetes Care 1981; 4:343–348.

303. Heilman KM, Fisher WR. Hyperlipidemic dementia. Arch Neurol 1974; 31:67–68.

304. Mathew NT, Meyer JS, Achari AN, et al. Hyperlipidemic neuropathy and dementia. Eur Neurol 1976; 14:370–382.

305. Steffes MW, Freier EF. A simple and precise method of determining true sodium, potassium, and chloride concentrations in hyperlipemia. J Lab Clin Med 1976; 88:683–688.

306. Wilson DE, Emi M, Iverius P-H, et al. Phenotypic expression of heterozygous lipoprotein lipase deficiency in the extended pedigree of a proband homozygous for a missense mutation. J Clin Invest 1990; 86:735–750.

307. Fojo SS, Brewer HB. Hypertriglyceridaemia due to genetic defects in lipoprotein lipase and apolipoprotein C-II. J Intern Med 1992; 231:669–677.

308. Gagné C, Brun L-D, Julien P, et al. Primary lipoprotein-lipase-activity deficiency: clinical investigation of a French Canadian population. Can Med Assoc J 1989; 140:405–411.

309. Eckel RH. Lipoprotein lipase: a multifunctional enzyme relevant to common metabolic diseases. N Engl J Med 1989; 320:1060–1068.

310. Illingworth DR, Connor WE, Miller RG. Abetalipoproteinemia: report of two cases and review of therapy. Arch Neurol 1980; 37:659–662.

311. Partin JS, Partin JC, Schubert WK, et al. Liver ultrastructure in abetalipoproteinemia: evolution of micronodular cirrhosis. Gastroenterology 1974; 67:107–118.

312. Brunzell JD. Familial lipoprotein lipase deficiency and other causes of the chylomicronemia syndrome. In: Scriver CR, Beaudet AL, Sly WS, et al., eds. The Metabolic Basis of Inherited Disease. 6th ed. New York: McGraw-Hill, 1989: 1165–1180.

313. Schaefer EJ. Familial lipoprotein disorders and premature coronary artery disease. Med Clin North Am 1994; 78:21–39.

314. Brunzell JD, Schrott HG, Motulsky AG, et al. Myocardial infarction in the familial forms of hypertriglyceridemia. Metabolism 1976; 25:313–320.

315. Chuntharapai A, Lee J, Burnier J, et al. Neutralizing monoclonal antibodies to human IL-8 receptor A map to the NH$_2$-terminal region of the receptor. J Immunol 1994; 152:1783–1789.

316. Schaefer EJ, Zech LA, Jenkins LL, et al. Human apolipoprotein A-I and A-II metabolism. J Lipid Res 1982; 23:850–862.

317. Brinton EA, Eisenberg S, Breslow JL. Increased apo A-I and apo A-II fractional catabolic rate in patients with low high density lipoprotein–cholesterol levels with or without hypertriglyceridemia. J Clin Invest 1991; 87:536–544.

318. Berg K. A new serum type system in man: the Lp system. Acta Pathol Microbiol Scand 1963; 59:369–382.

319. Utermann G. The mysteries of lipoprotein(a). Science 1989; 246:904–910.

320. Scanu AM, Fless GM. Lipoprotein (a): heterogeneity and biological relevance. J Clin Invest 1990; 85:1709–1715.

321. Gaw A, Hobbs HH. Molecular genetics of lipoprotein (a): new pieces to the puzzle. Curr Opin Lipidol 1994; 5:149–155.

322. McLean JW, Tomlinson JE, Kuang W-J, et al. cDNA sequence of human apolipoprotein(a) is homologous to plasminogen. Nature 1987; 330:132–137.

323. Dahlen GH, Guyton JR, Attar M, et al. Association of levels of lipoprotein Lp(a), plasma lipids, and other lipoproteins with coronary artery disease documented by angiography. Circulation 1986; 74:758–765.

324. Sandkamp M, Funke H, Schulte H, et al. Lipoprotein(a) is an independent risk factor for myocardial infarction at a young age. Clin Chem 1990; 36:20–23.

325. Genest J Jr., Jenner JL, McNamara JR, et al. Prevalence of lipoprotein (a) [Lp(a)] excess in coronary artery disease. Am J Cardiol 1991; 67:1039–1045.

326. Gurewich V, Mittleman M. Lipoprotein(a) in coronary heart disease: is it a risk factor after all? J Am Med Assoc 1994; 271:1025–1026.

327. Ridker PM, Hennekens CH, Stampfer MJ. A prospective study of lipoprotein(a) and the risk of myocardial infarction. J Am Med Assoc 1993; 270:2195–2199.

328. Jauhiainen M, Koskinen P, Ehnholm C, et al. Lipoprotein (a) and coronary heart disease risk: a nested case-control study of the Helsinki Heart Study participants. Atherosclerosis 1991; 89:59–67.

329. Schaefer EJ, Lamon-Fava S, Jenner JL, et al. Lipoprotein(a) levels and risk of coronary heart disease in men: the Lipid Research Clinics Coronary Primary Prevention Trial. J Am Med Assoc 1994; 271:999–1003.

330. Rosengren A, Wilhelmsen L, Eriksson E, et al. Lipoprotein (a) and coronary heart disease: a prospective case-control study in a general population sample of middle aged men. Br Med J 1990; 301:1248–1251.

331. Boerwinkle E, Leffert CC, Lin J, et al. Apolipoprotein(a) gene accounts for greater than 90% of the variation in plasma lipoprotein(a) concentrations. J Clin Invest 1992; 90:52–60.

332. Lamon-Fava S, Jimenez D, Christian JC, et al. The NHLBI Twin Study: heritability of apolipoprotein A-I, B, and low density lipoprotein subclasses and concordance for lipoprotein(a). Atherosclerosis 1991; 91:97–106.

333. Berg K. Twin research in coronary heart disease. Prog Clin Biol Res 1981; 69C:117–130.

334. Sandholzer C, Hallman DM, Saha N, et al. Effects of the apolipoprotein(a) size polymorphism on the lipoprotein(a) concentration in 7 ethnic groups. Hum Genet 1991; 86:607–614.

335. Maher VMG, Brown BG, Marcovina SM, et al. Effects of lowering elevated LDL cholesterol on the cardiovascular risk of lipoprotein(a). J Am Med Assoc 1995; 274:1771–1774.

336. McCormick SPA, Ng JK, Taylor S, et al. Mutagenesis of the human apolipoprotein B gene in a yeast artificial chromosome reveals the site of attachment for apolipoprotein(a). Proc Natl Acad Sci USA 1995; 92:10147–10151.

337. Gavish D, Azrolan N, Breslow JL. Plasma Lp(a) concentration is inversely correlated with the ratio of Kringle IV/Kringle V encoding domains in the apo(a) gene. J Clin Invest 1989; 84:2021–2027.

338. Hajjar KA, Gavish D, Breslow JL, et al. Lipoprotein(a) modulation of endothelial cell surface fibrinolysis and its potential role in atherosclerosis. Nature 1989; 339:303–305.

339. Miles LA, Fless GM, Levin EG, et al. A potential basis for the thrombotic risks associated with lipoprotein(a). Nature 1989; 339:301–303.

340. Grainger DJ, Kirschenlohr HL, Metcalfe JC, et al. Proliferation of human smooth muscle cells promoted by lipoprotein(a). Science 1993; 260:1655–1658.

341. Third JLHC, Montag J, Flynn M, et al. Primary and familial hypoalphalipoproteinemia. Metabolism 1984; 33:136–146.

342. Vergani C, Bettale G. Familial hypo-alpha-lipoproteinemia. Clin Chim Acta 1981; 114:45–52.

343. Cohen JC, Wang Z, Grundy SM, et al. Variation at the hepatic lipase and apolipoprotein AI/CIII/AIV loci is a major cause of genetically determined variation in plasma HDL cholesterol levels. J Clin Invest 1994; 94:2377–2384.

344. Eisenberg S. High density lipoprotein metabolism. J Lipid Res 1984; 25:1017–1058.

345. Tall AR. Plasma high density lipoproteins: metabolism and relationship to atherogenesis. J Clin Invest 1990; 86:379–384.

346. Rosenson RS. Low levels of high-density lipoprotein cholesterol (hypoalphalipoproteinemia): an approach to management. Arch Intern Med 1993; 153:1528–1538.

347. Knopp RH, Walden CE, Wahl PW, et al. Oral contraceptive and postmenopausal estrogen effects on lipoprotein triglyceride and cholesterol in an adult female population: relationships to estrogen and progestin potency. J Clin Endocrinol Metab 1981; 53:1123–1132.

348. Bradley DD, Wingerd J, Petitti DB, et al. Serum high-density-lipoprotein cholesterol in women using oral contraceptives, estrogens and progestins. N Engl J Med 1978; 299:17–20.

349. Tikkanen MJ, Nikkilä EA, Vartiainen E. Natural œstrogen as an effective treatment for type-II hyperlipoproteinæmia in postmenopausal women. Lancet 1978; 2:490–491.

350. Gordon DJ, Witztum JL, Hunninghake D, et al. Habitual physical activity and high-density lipoprotein cholesterol in men with primary hypercholesterolemia: the Lipid Research Clinics Coronary Primary Prevention Trial. Circulation 1983; 67:512–520.

351. Assmann G, von Eckardstein A, Funke H. High density lipoproteins, reverse transport of cholesterol, and coronary artery disease. Insights from mutations. Circulation 1993; 87:III-28–III-34.

352. Schaefer EJ. Clinical, biochemical, and genetic features in familial disorders of high density lipoprotein deficiency. Arteriosclerosis 1984; 4:303–322.

353. Franceschini G, Sirtori CR, Capurso A, et al. A-I_{Milano} apoprotein: decreased high density lipoprotein cholesterol levels with significant lipoprotein modifications and without clinical atherosclerosis in an Italian family. J Clin Invest 1980; 66:892–900.

354. Soutar AK, Hawkins PN, Vigushin DM, et al. Apolipoprotein AI mutation Arg-60 causes autosomal dominant amyloidosis. Proc Natl Acad Sci USA 1992; 89:7389–7393.

355. Nichols WC, Dwulet FE, Liepnieks J, et al. Variant apolipoprotein AI as a major constituent of a human hereditary amyloid. Biochem Biophys Res Commun 1988; 156:762–768.

356. Nichols WC, Gregg RE, Brewer HB Jr., et al. A mutation in apolipoprotein A-I in the Iowa type of familial amyloidotic polyneuropathy. Genomics 1990; 8:318–323.

357. Inazu A, Brown ML, Hesler CB, et al. Increased high-density lipoprotein levels caused by a common cholesteryl-ester transfer protein gene mutation. N Engl J Med 1990; 323:1234–1238.

358. Tall AR. Plasma cholesteryl ester transfer protein and high-density lipoproteins: new insights from molecular genetic studies. J Intern Med 1995; 237:5–12.

359. Marotti KR, Castle CK, Murray RW, et al. The role of cholesteryl ester transfer protein in primate apolipoprotein A-I metabolism: insights from studies with transgenic mice. Arterioscler Thromb 1992; 12:736–744.

360. Jiang XC, Masucci-Magoulas L, Mar J, et al. Down-regulation of mRNA for the low density lipoprotein receptor in transgenic mice containing the gene for human cholesteryl ester transfer protein: mechanism to explain accumulation of lipoprotein B particles. J Biol Chem 1993; 268:27406–27412.

361. Hayek T, Masucci-Magoulas L, Jiang X, et al. Decreased early atherosclerotic lesions in hypertriglyceridemic mice expressing cholesteryl ester transfer protein transgene. J Clin Invest 1995; 96:2071–2074.

362. Norum KR, Gjone E, Glomset JA. Familial lecithin:cholesterol acyltransferase deficiency, including fish eye disease. In: Scriver CR, Beaudet AL, Sly WS, et al., eds. The Metabolic Basis of Inherited Disease. 6th ed, Vol 1. New York: McGraw-Hill, 1989: 1181–1194.

363. Funke H, von Eckardstein A, Pritchard PH, et al. Genetic and phenotypic heterogeneity in familial lecithin:cholesterol acyltransferase (LCAT) deficiency: six newly identified defective alleles further contribute to the structural heterogeneity of this disease. J Clin Invest 1993; 91:677–683.

364. Glomset JA. The plasma lecithin:cholesterol acyltransferase reaction. J Lipid Res 1968; 9:155–167.

365. Carlson LA, Philipson B. Fish-eye disease: a new familial condition with massive corneal opacities and dyslipoproteinæmia. Lancet 1979; 2:921–924.

366. Klein H-G, Lohse P, Pritchard PH, et al. Two different allelic mutations in the lecithin-cholesterol acyltransferase gene associated with the fish eye syndrome. Lecithin-cholesterol acyltransferase (Thr_{123} → Ile) and lecithin-cholesterol acyltransferase (Thr_{347} → Met). J Clin Invest 1992; 89:499–506.

367. Funke H, von Eckardstein A, Pritchard PH, et al. A molecular defect causing fish eye disease: an amino acid exchange in lecithin–cholesterol acyltransferase (LCAT) leads to the selective loss of α-LCAT activity. Proc Natl Acad Sci USA 1991; 88:4855–4859.

368. Skretting G, Prydz H. An amino acid exchange in exon I of the human lecithin:cholesterol acyltransferase (LCAT) gene is associated with fish eye disease. Biochem Biophys Res Commun 1992; 182:583–587.

369. Carlson LA, Holmquist L. Evidence for the presence in human plasma of lecithin:cholesterol acyltransferase activity (β-LCAT) specifically esterifying free cholesterol of combined pre-β- and β-lipoproteins. Studies of fish eye disease patients and control subjects. Acta Med Scand 1985; 218:197–205.

370. Klein H-G, Santamarina-Fojo S, Duverger N, et al. Fish eye syndrome: a molecular defect in the lecithin-cholesterol acyltransferase (LCAT) gene associated with normal α-LCAT-specific activity. Implications for classification and prognosis. J Clin Invest 1993; 92:479–485.

371. Fredrickson DS, Altrocchi PH, Avioli LV, et al. Tangier disease: combined clinical staff conference at the National Institutes of Health. Ann Intern Med 1961; 55:1016–1031.

372. Serfaty-Lacrosniere C, Civeira F, Lanzberg A, et al. Homozygous Tangier disease and cardiovascular disease. Atherosclerosis 1994; 107:85–98.

373. Bojanovski D, Gregg RE, Zech LA, In vivo metabolism of proapolipoprotein A-I in Tangier disease. J Clin Invest 1987; 80:1742–1747.

374. Schmitz G, Assmann G, Robenek H, et al. Tangier disease: a disorder of intracellular membrane traffic. Proc Natl Acad Sci USA 1985; 82:6305–6309.

375. Francis GA, Knopp RH, Oram JF. Defective removal of cellular cholesterol and phospholipids by apolipoprotein A-I in Tangier disease. J Clin Invest 1995; 96:78–87.

376. Walter M, Gerdes U, Seedorf U, et al. The high density lipoprotein– and apolipoprotein A-I–induced mobilization of cellular cholesterol is impaired in fibroblasts from Tangier disease subjects. Biochem Biophys Res Commun 1994; 205:850–856.

377. Linton MF, Farese RV Jr., Young SG. Familial hypobetalipoproteinemia. J Lipid Res 1993; 34:521–541.

378. Welty FK, Hubl ST, Pierotti VR, et al. A truncated species of apolipoprotein B (B67) in a kindred with familial hypobetalipoproteinemia. J Clin Invest 1991; 87:1748–1754.

379. Mars H, Lewis LA, Robertson AL Jr., et al. Familial hypo-β-lipoproteinemia: a genetic disorder of lipid metabolism with nervous system involvement. Am J Med 1969; 46:886–900.

380. Levy E, Roy CC, Thibault L, et al. Variable expression of familial heterozygous hypobetalipoproteinemia: transient malabsorption during infancy. J Lipid Res 1994; 35:2170–2177.

381. Glueck CJ, Gartside PS, Mellies MJ, et al. Familial hypobeta-lipoproteinemia: studies in 13 kindreds. Trans Assoc Am Physicians 1977; 90:184–203.

382. Illingworth DR, Kenny TA, Orwoll ES. Adrenal function in heterozygous and homozygous hypobetalipoproteinemia. J Clin Endocrinol Metab 1982; 54:27–33.

383. Parker CR Jr., Illingworth DR, Bissonnette J, et al. Endocrine changes during pregnancy in a patient with homozygous familial hypobetalipoproteinemia. N Engl J Med 1986; 314:557–560.

384. Farese RV Jr., Linton MF, Young SG. Apolipoprotein B gene mutations affecting cholesterol levels. J Intern Med 1992; 231:643–652.

385. Aguilar-Salinas CA, Barrett PHR, Parhofer KG, et al. Apoprotein B-100 production is decreased in subjects heterozygous for truncations of apoprotein B. Arterioscler Thromb Vasc Biol 1995; 15:71–80.

386. Parhofer KG, Daugherty A, Kinoshita M, et al. Enhanced clearance from plasma of low density lipoproteins containing a truncated apolipoprotein, apoB-89. J Lipid Res 1990; 31:2001–2007.

387. Fazio S, Sidoli A, Vivenzio A, et al. A form of familial hypobetalipoproteinaemia not due to a mutation in the apolipoprotein B gene. J Intern Med 1991; 229:41–47.

388. Hobbs HH, Leitersdorf E, Leffert CC, et al. Evidence for a dominant gene that suppresses hypercholesterolemia in a family with defective low density lipoprotein receptors. J Clin Invest 1989; 84:656–664.

389. Vega GL, von Bergmann K, Grundy SM, et al. Increased catabolism of VLDL-apolipoprotein B and synthesis of bile acids in a case of hypobetalipoproteinemia. Metabolism 1987; 36:262–269.

390. Young SG, Cham CM, Pitas RE, et al. A genetic model for absent chylomicron formation: mice producing apolipoprotein B in the liver, but not in the intestine. J Clin Invest 1995; 96:2932–2946.

391. Runge P, Muller DPR, McAllister J, et al. Oral vitamin E supplements can prevent the retinopathy of abetalipoproteinaemia. Br J Ophthalmol 1986; 70:166–173.

392. Bouma M-E, Beucler I, Aggerbeck L-P, et al. Hypobetalipoproteinemia with accumulation of an apoprotein B-like protein in intestinal cells: immunoenzymatic and biochemical characterization of seven cases of Anderson's disease. J Clin Invest 1986; 78:398–410.

393. Roy CC, Levy E, Green PHR, et al. Malabsorption, hypocholesterolemia, and fat-filled enterocytes with increased intestinal apoprotein B: chylomicron retention disease. Gastroenterology 1987; 92:390–399.

394. Kayden HJ, Traber MG. Clinical, nutritional and biochemical consequences of apolipoprotein B deficiency. Adv Exp Med Biol 1986; 201:67–81.

395. Wetterau JR, Aggerbeck LP, Bouma M-E, et al. Absence of microsomal triglyceride transfer protein in individuals with abetalipoproteinemia. Science 1992; 258:999–1001.

396. Rader DJ, Brewer HB Jr. Abetalipoproteinemia. New insights into lipoprotein assembly and vitamin E metabolism from a rare genetic disease. J Am Med Assoc 1993; 270:865–869.

397. Shoulders CC, Brett DJ, Bayliss JD, et al. Abetalipoproteinemia is caused by defects of the gene encoding the 97 kDa subunit of a microsomal triglyceride transfer protein. Hum Mol Genet 1993; 2:2109–2116.

398. Ameis D, Greten H, Schotz MC. Hepatic and plasma lipases. Semin Liver Dis 1992; 12:397–402.

399. Breckenridge WC, Little JA, Alaupovic P, et al. Lipoprotein abnormalities associated with a familial deficiency of hepatic lipase. Atherosclerosis 1982; 45:161–179.

400. Connelly PW, Maguire GF, Lee M, et al. Plasma lipoproteins in familial hepatic lipase deficiency. Arteriosclerosis 1990; 10:40–48.

401. Auwerx JH, Babirak SP, Hokanson JE, et al. Coexistence of abnormalities of hepatic lipase and lipoprotein lipase in a large family. Am J Hum Genet 1990; 46:470–477.

402. Carlson LA, Holmquist L, Nilsson-Ehle P. Deficiency of hepatic lipase activity in post-heparin plasma in familial hyper-α-triglyceridemia. Acta Med Scand 1986; 219:435–447.

403. Hegele RA, Vezina C, Moorjani S, et al. A hepatic lipase gene mutation associated with heritable lipolytic deficiency. J Clin Endocrinol Metab 1991; 72:730–732.

404. Björkhem I, Skrede S. Familial diseases with storage of sterols other than cholesterol: cerebrotendinous xanthomatosis and phytosterolemia. In: Scriver CR, Beaudet AL, Sly WS, et al., eds. The Metabolic Basis of Inherited Disease. 6th ed, Vol 1. New York: McGraw-Hill, 1989: 1283–1302.

405. Leitersdorf E, Meiner V. Cerebrotendinous xanthomatosis. Curr Opin Lipidol 1994; 5:138–142.

406. Fujiyama J, Kuriyama M, Arima S, et al. Atherogenic risk factors in cerebrotendinous xanthomatosis. Clin Chim Acta 1991; 200:1–11.

407. Berginer VM, Shany S, Alkalay D, et al. Osteoporosis and increased bone fractures in cerebrotendinous xanthomatosis. Metabolism 1993; 42:69–74.

408. Leitersdorf E, Reshef A, Meiner V, et al. Frameshift and splice-junction mutations in the sterol 27-hydroxylase gene cause cerebrotendinous xanthomatosis in Jews of Moroccan origin. J Clin Invest 1993; 91:2488–2496.

409. Berginer VM, Salen G, Shefer S. Long-term treatment of cerebrotendinous xanthomatosis with chenodeoxycholic acid. N Engl J Med 1984; 311:1649–1652.

410. Nakamura T, Matsuzawa Y, Takemura K, et al. Combined treatment with chenodeoxycholic acid and pravastatin improves plasma cholestanol levels associated with marked regression of tendon xanthomas in cerebrotendinous xanthomatosis. Metabolism 1991; 40:741–746.

411. Peynet J, Laurent A, De Liege P, et al. Cerebrotendinous xanthomatosis: treatments with simvastatin, lovastatin, and chenodeoxycholic acid in 3 siblings. Neurology 1991; 41:434–436.

412. Klima H, Ullrich K, Aslanidis C, et al. A splice junction mutation causes deletion of a 72-base exon from the mRNA for lysosomal acid lipase in a patient with cholesteryl ester storage disease. J Clin Invest 1993; 92:2713–2718.

413. Schmitz G, Assmann G. Acid lipase deficiency: Wolman disease and cholesteryl ester storage disease. In: Scriver CR, Beaudet AL, Sly WS, et al., eds. The Metabolic Basis of Inherited Disease. 6th ed, Vol 2. New York: McGraw-Hill, 1989: 1623–1644.

414. Anderson RA, Byrum RS, Coates PM, et al. Mutations at the lysosomal acid cholesteryl ester hydrolase gene locus in Wolman disease. Proc Natl Acad Sci USA 1994; 91:2718–2722.

415. Sokol RJ, Kayden HJ, Bettis DB, et al. Isolated vitamin E deficiency in the absence of fat malabsorption—familial and sporadic cases: characterization and investigation of causes. J Lab Clin Med 1988; 111:548–559.

416. Kayden HJ. The neurologic syndrome of vitamin E deficiency: a significant cause of ataxia. Neurology 1993; 43:2167–2169.

417. Ouahchi K, Arita M, Kayden H, et al. Ataxia with isolated vitamin E deficiency is caused by mutations in the α-tocopherol transfer protein. Nat Genet 1995; 9:141–145.

418. Koppers LE, Palumbo PJ. Lipid disturbances in endocrine disorders. Med Clin North Am 1972; 56:1013–1020.

419. Stone NJ. Secondary causes of hyperlipidemia. Med Clin North Am 1994; 78:117–141.

420. Bierman EL. Insulin and hypertriglyceridemia. Isr J Med Sci 1972; 8:303–308.

421. Howard BV. Lipoprotein metabolism in diabetes mellitus. J Lipid Res 1987; 28:613–628.

422. Reaven GM, Greenfield MS. Diabetic hypertriglyceridemia: evidence for three clinical syndromes. Diabetes 1981; 30(Suppl 2):66–75.

423. Tomkin GH, Owens D. Insulin and lipoprotein metabolism with special reference to the diabetic state. Diabetes Metab Rev 1994; 10:225–252.

424. Bagdade JD, Porte D Jr., Bierman EL. Acute insulin withdrawal and the regulation of plasma triglyceride removal in diabetic subjects. Diabetes 1968; 17:127–132.

425. Chait A, Bierman EL, Albers JJ. Low-density lipoprotein receptor activity in cultured human skin fibroblasts: mechanism of insulin-induced stimulation. J Clin Invest 1979; 64:1309–1319.

426. Bagdade JD, Porte D Jr., Bierman EL. Diabetic lipemia: a form of acquired fat-induced lipemia. N Engl J Med 1967; 276:427–433.

427. Brunzell JD, Hazzard WR, Motulsky AG, et al. Evidence for diabetes mellitus and genetic forms of hypertriglyceridemia as independent entities. Metabolism 1975; 24:1115–1121.

428. Laakso M, Pyörälä K, Sarlund H, et al. Lipid and lipoprotein abnormalities associated with coronary heart disease in patients with insulin-dependent diabetes mellitus. Arteriosclerosis 1986; 6:679–684.

429. Manzato E, Crepaldi G. Dyslipoproteinaemia in manifest diabetes. J Intern Med 1994; 236(Suppl 736):27–31.

430. Joven J, Vilella E, Costa B, et al. Concentrations of lipids and apolipoproteins in patients with clinically well-controlled insulin-dependent and non–insulin-dependent diabetes. Clin Chem 1989; 35:813–816.

431. Feingold KR, Grunfeld C, Pang M, et al. LDL subclass phenotypes and triglyceride metabolism in non-insulin-dependent diabetes. Arterioscler Thromb 1992; 12:1496–1502.

432. Bowie A, Owens D, Collins P, et al. Glycosylated low density lipoprotein is more sensitive to oxidation: implications for the diabetic patient? Atherosclerosis 1993; 102:63–67.

433. Tobey TA, Greenfield M, Kraemer F, et al. Relationship between insulin resistance, insulin secretion, very low density lipoprotein kinetics, and plasma triglyceride levels in normotriglyceridemic man. Metabolism 1981; 30:165–171.

434. Eto M, Watanabe K, Sato T, et al. Apolipoprotein-E2 and hyperlipoproteinemia in noninsulin-dependent diabetes mellitus. J Clin Endocrinol Metab 1989; 69:1207–1212.

435. DeFronzo RA, Goodman AM, the Multicenter Metformin Study Group. Efficacy of metformin in patients with non–insulin-dependent diabetes mellitus. N Engl J Med 1995; 333:541–549.

436. Rosenstock J, Vega GL, Raskin P. Effect of intensive diabetes treatment on low-density lipoprotein apolipoprotein B kinetics in type I diabetes. Diabetes 1988; 37:393–397.

437. Taskinen M-R, Kuusi T, Helve E, et al. Insulin therapy induces antiatherogenic changes of serum lipoproteins in noninsulin-dependent diabetes. Arteriosclerosis 1988; 8:168–177.

438. Valdemarsson S, Hansson P, Hedner P, et al. Relations between thyroid function, hepatic and lipoprotein lipase activities, and plasma lipoprotein concentrations. Acta Endocrinol 1983; 104:50–56.

439. Kinlaw WB III. Atherosclerosis and the thyroid. Thyroid Today 1991; 14:1–8.

440. Abrams JJ, Grundy SM, Ginsberg H. Metabolism of plasma triglycerides in hypothyroidism and hyperthyroidism in man. J Lipid Res 1981; 22:307–322.

441. Hansson P, Valdemarsson S, Nilsson-Ehle P. Experimental hyperthyroidism in man: effects on plasma lipoproteins, lipoprotein lipase and hepatic lipase. Horm Metab Res 1983; 15:449–452.

442. Agdeppa D, Macaron C, Mallik T, et al. Plasma high density lipoprotein cholesterol in thyroid disease. J Clin Endocrinol Metab 1979; 49:726–729.

443. Henkin Y, Como JA, Oberman A. Secondary dyslipidemia. Inadvertent effects of drugs in clinical practice. J Am Med Assoc 1992; 267:961–968.

444. Thompson GR, Soutar AK, Spengel FA, et al. Defects of receptor-mediated low density lipoprotein catabolism in homozygous familial hypercholesterolemia and hypothyroidism in vivo. Proc Natl Acad Sci USA 1981; 78:2591–2595.

445. Scarabottolo L, Trezzi E, Roma P, et al. Experimental hypothyroidism modulates the expression of the low density lipoprotein receptor by the liver. Atherosclerosis 1986; 59:329–333.

446. Sykes M, Cnoop-Koopmans WM, Julien P, et al. The effects of hypothyroidism, age, and nutrition on LDL catabolism in the rat. Metabolism 1981; 30:733–738.

447. Chait A, Bierman EL, Albers JJ. Regulatory role of triiodothyronine in the degradation of low density lipoprotein by cultured human skin fibroblasts. J Clin Endocrinol Metab 1979; 48:887–889.

448. Vanhaelst L, Neve P, Chailly P, et al. Coronary-artery disease in hypothyroidism: observations in clinical myxoedema. Lancet 1967; 2:800–802.

449. Steinberg AD. Myxedema and coronary artery disease: a comparative autopsy study. Ann Intern Med 1968; 68:338–344.

450. Arem R, Patsch W. Lipoprotein and apolipoprotein levels in subclinical hypothyroidism: effect of levothyroxine therapy. Arch Intern Med 1990; 150:2097–2100.

451. Pykälistö O, Goldberg AP, Brunzell JD. Reversal of decreased human adipose tissue lipoprotein lipase and hypertriglyceridemia after treatment of hypothyroidism. J Clin Endocrinol Metab 1976; 43:591–600.

452. Walsh BW, Schiff I, Rosner B, et al. Effects of postmenopausal estrogen replacement on the concentrations and metabolism of plasma lipoproteins. N Engl J Med 1991; 325:1196–1204.

453. Davidoff F, Tishler S, Rosoff C. Marked hyperlipidemia and pancreatitis associated with oral contraceptive therapy. N Engl J Med 1973; 289:552–555.

454. Glueck CJ, Fallat RW, Scheel D. Effects of estrogenic compounds on triglyceride kinetics. Metabolism 1975; 24:537–545.

455. Windler EET, Kovanen PT, Chao Y-S, et al. The estradiol-stimulated lipoprotein receptor of rat liver: a binding site that mediates the uptake of rat lipoproteins containing apoproteins B and E. J Biol Chem 1980; 255:10464–10471.

456. Wahl P, Walden C, Knopp R, et al. Effect of estrogen/progestin potency on lipid/lipoprotein cholesterol. N Engl J Med 1983; 308:862–867.

457. Psaty BM, Heckbert SR, Atkins D, et al. A review of the association of estrogens and progestins with cardiovascular disease in postmenopausal women. Arch Intern Med 1993; 153:1421–1427.

458. Stampfer MJ, Colditz GA, Willett WC, et al. Postmenopausal estrogen therapy and cardiovascular disease: ten-year follow-up from the Nurses' Health Study. N Engl J Med 1991; 325:756–762.

459. Janus ED, Lewis B. Alcohol and abnormalities of lipid metabolism. Clin Endocrinol Metab 1978; 7:321–332.

460. Steinberg D, Pearson TA, Kuller LH. Alcohol and atherosclerosis. Ann Intern Med 1991; 114:967–976.

461. Brunzell JD, Hazzard WR, Porte D Jr., et al. Evidence for a common, saturable, triglyceride removal mechanism for chylomicrons and very low density lipoproteins in man. J Clin Invest 1973; 52:1578–1585.

462. Hulley SB, Gordon S. Alcohol and high-density lipoprotein cholesterol: causal inference from diverse study designs. Circulation 1981; 64:III-57–III-63.

463. Gaziano JM, Buring JE, Breslow JL, et al. Moderate alcohol intake, increased levels of high-density lipoprotein and its subfractions, and decreased risk of myocardial infarction. N Engl J Med 1993; 329:1829–1834.

464. Suh I, Shaten BJ, Cutler JA, et al. Alcohol use and mortality from coronary heart disease: the role of high-density lipoprotein cholesterol. Ann Intern Med 1992; 116:881–887.

465. Criqui MH, Ringel BL. Does diet or alcohol explain the French paradox? Lancet 1994; 344:1719–1723.

466. Joven J, Villabona C, Vilella E, et al. Abnormalities of lipoprotein metabolism in patients with the nephrotic syndrome. N Engl J Med 1990; 323:579–584.

467. Wanner C, Rader D, Bartens W, et al. Elevated plasma lipoprotein(a) in patients with the nephrotic syndrome. Ann Intern Med 1993; 119:263–269.

468. Kekki M, Nikkilä EA. Plasma triglyceride metabolism in the adult nephrotic syndrome. Eur J Clin Invest 1971; 1:345–351.

469. Warwick GL, Caslake MJ, Boulton-Jones JM, et al. Low-density lipoprotein metabolism in the nephrotic syndrome. Metabolism 1990; 39:187–192.

470. Grundy SM. Management of hyperlipidemia of kidney disease. Kidney Int 1990; 37:847–853.

471. Lardinois CK, Neuman SL. The effects of antihypertensive agents on serum lipids and lipoproteins. Arch Intern Med 1988; 148:1280–1288.

472. Pollare T, Lithell H, Berne C. A comparison of the effects of hydrochlorothiazide and captopril on glucose and lipid metabolism in patients with hypertension. N Engl J Med 1989; 321:868–873.

473. Rohlfing JJ, Brunzell JD. The effects of diuretics and adrenergic-blocking agents on plasma lipids. West J Med 1986; 145:210–218.

474. Haffner SM, Kushwaha RS, Foster DM, et al. Studies on the metabolic mechanism of reduced high density lipoproteins during anabolic steroid therapy. Metabolism 1983; 32:413–420.

475. Webb OL, Laskarzewski PM, Glueck CJ. Severe depression of high-density lipoprotein cholesterol levels in weight lifters and body builders by self-administered exogenous testosterone and anabolic-androgenic steroids. Metabolism 1984; 33:971–975.

476. Diekman T, Lansberg PJ, Kastelein JJP, et al. Prevalence and correction on hypothyroidism in a large cohort of patients referred for dyslipidemia. Arch Intern Med 1995; 155:1490–1495.

477. Watson WC, Buchanan KD, Dickson C. Serum cholesterol levels after myocardial infarction. Br Med J 1963; 2:709–712.

478. Friedewald WT, Levy RI, Fredrickson DS. Estimation of the concentration of low-density lipoprotein cholesterol in plasma, without use of the preparative ultracentrifuge. Clin Chem 1972; 18:499–502.

479. Havel RJ, Rapaport E. Management of primary hyperlipidemia. N Engl J Med 1995; 332:1491–1498.

480. Castelli WP, Garrison RJ, Wilson PWF, et al. Incidence of coronary heart disease and lipoprotein cholesterol levels: the Framingham Study. J Am Med Assoc 1986; 256:2835–2838.

481. Castelli WP, Abbott RD, McNamara PM. Summary estimates of cholesterol used to predict coronary heart disease. Circulation 1983; 67:730–734.

482. Arntzenius AC, Kromhout D, Barth JD, et al. Diet, lipoproteins, and the progression of coronary atherosclerosis: the Leiden Intervention Trial. N Engl J Med 1985; 312:805–811.

483. Chait A, Brunzell JD. Severe hypertriglyceridemia: role of familial and acquired disorders. Metabolism 1983; 32:209–214.

484. Stampfer MJ, Sacks FM, Salvini S, et al. A prospective study of cholesterol, apolipoproteins, and the risk of myocardial infarction. N Engl J Med 1991; 325:373–381.

485. Hulley SB, Newman TB, Grady D, et al. Should we be measuring blood cholesterol levels in young adults? J Am Med Assoc 1993; 269:1416–1419.

486. American College of Physicians. Guidelines for using serum cholesterol, high-density lipoprotein cholesterol, and triglyceride levels as screening tests for preventing coronary heart disease in adults. Ann Intern Med 1996; 124:515–517.

487. Salt WB, II, Schenker S. Amylase—its clinical significance: a review of the literature. Medicine 1976; 55:269–289.

488. Carlson LA, Rosenhamer G. Reduction of mortality in the Stockholm Ischaemic Heart Disease Secondary Prevention Study by combined treatment with clofibrate and nicotinic acid. Acta Med Scand 1988; 223:405–418.

489. Canner PL, Berge KG, Wenger NK, et al. Fifteen year mortality in Coronary Drug Project patients: long-term benefit with niacin. J Am Coll Cardiol 1986; 8:1245–1255.

490. Trial of clofibrate in the treatment of ischaemic heart disease: five-year study by a group of physicians of the Newcastle upon Tyne region. Br Med J 1971; 4:767–775.

491. Leren P. The effect of plasma cholesterol lowering diet in male survivors of myocardial infarction: a controlled clinical trial. Acta Med Scand Suppl 1966; 466:1–92.

492. Rossouw JE, Lewis B, Rifkind BM. The value of lowering cholesterol after myocardial infarction. N Engl J Med 1990; 323:1112–1119.

493. Blankenhorn DH, Nessim SA, Johnson RL, et al. Beneficial effects of combined colestipol-niacin therapy on coronary atherosclerosis and coronary venous bypass grafts. J Am Med Assoc 1987; 257:3233–3240.

494. Ornish D, Brown SE, Scherwitz LW, et al. Can lifestyle changes reverse coronary heart disease? The Lifestyle Heart Trial. Lancet 1990; 336:129–133.

495. Brown BG, Zhao X-Q, Sacco DE, et al. Lipid lowering and plaque regression: new insights into prevention of plaque disruption and clinical events in coronary disease. Circulation 1993; 87:1781–1791.

496. Criqui MH. Cholesterol, primary and secondary prevention, and all-cause mortality. Ann Intern Med 1991; 115:973–976.

497. Muldoon MF, Manuck SB, Matthews KA. Lowering cholesterol concentrations and mortality: a quantitative review of primary prevention trials. Br Med J 1990; 301:309–314.

498. MacMahon S. Lowering cholesterol: effects on trauma death, cancer death and total mortality. Aust N Z J Med 1992; 22:580–582.

499. Connor WE, Connor SL. The dietary treatment of hyperlipidemia: rationale, technique and efficacy. Med Clin North Am 1982; 66:485–518.

500. Nutrition Committee, American Heart Association. 1988 Dietary guidelines for healthy American adults: a statement for physicians and health professionals. Circulation 77:721A–723A.

501. Denke MA, Grundy SM. Individual responses to a cholesterol-lowering diet in 50 men with moderate hypercholesterolemia. Arch Intern Med 1994; 154:317–325.

502. Ginsberg HN, Barr SL, Gilbert A, et al. Reduction of plasma cholesterol levels in normal men on an American Heart Association step 1 diet or a step 1 diet with added monounsaturated fat. N Engl J Med 1990; 322:574–579.

503. Hunninghake DB, Stein EA, Dujovne CA, et al. The efficacy of intensive dietary therapy alone or combined with lovastatin in outpatients with hypercholesterolemia. N Engl J Med 1993; 328:1213–1219.

504. Cobb MM, Teitelbaum HS, Breslow JL. Lovastatin efficacy in reducing low-density lipoprotein cholesterol levels on high- vs low-fat diets. J Am Med Assoc 1991; 265:997–1001.

505. Willett WC. Diet and health: What should we eat? Science 1994; 264:532–537.

506. Spady DK, Dietschy JM. Dietary saturated triacylglycerols suppress hepatic low density lipoprotein receptor activity in the hamster. Proc Natl Acad Sci USA 1985; 82:4526–4530.

507. Packard CJ, McKinney L, Carr K, et al. Cholesterol feeding increases low density lipoprotein synthesis. J Clin Invest 1983; 72:45–51.

508. Mensink RP, Katan MB. Effect of a diet enriched with monounsaturated or polyunsaturated fatty acids on levels of low-density and high-density lipoprotein cholesterol in healthy women and men. N Engl J Med 1989; 321:436–441.

509. Mensink RP, Katan MB. Effect of dietary trans fatty acids on high-density and low-density lipoprotein cholesterol levels in healthy subjects. N Engl J Med 1990; 323:439–445.

510. Kromhout D, Bosschieter EB, de Lezenne Coulander C. The inverse relation between fish consumption and 20-year mortality from coronary heart disease. N Engl J Med 1985; 312:1205–1209.

511. Harris WS. Fish oils and plasma lipid and lipoprotein metabolism in humans: a critical review. J Lipid Res 1989; 30:785–807.

512. Sullivan DR, Sanders TAB, Trayner IM, et al. Paradoxical elevation of LDL apoprotein B levels in hypertriglyceridaemic patients and normal subjects ingesting fish oil. Atherosclerosis 1986; 61:129–134.

513. Leaf A, Weber PC. Cardiovascular effects of n-3 fatty acids. N Engl J Med 1988; 318:549–556.

514. Ascherio A, Rimm EB, Stampfer MJ, et al. Dietary intake of marine n-3 fatty acids, fish intake, and the risk of coronary disease among men. N Engl J Med 1995; 332:977–982.

515. Friday KE, Childs MT, Tsunehara CH, et al. Elevated plasma glucose and lowered triglyceride levels from omega-3 fatty acid supplementation in type II diabetes. Diabetes Care 1989; 12:276–281.

516. Grundy SM. Comparison of monounsaturated fatty acids and carbohydrates for lowering plasma cholesterol. N Engl J Med 1986; 314:745–748.

517. Connor WE. Dietary fiber: nostrum or critical nutrient? N Engl J Med 1990; 322:193–195.

518. Jenkins DJA, Wolever TMS, Rao AV, et al. Effect on blood lipids of very high intakes of fiber in diets low in saturated fat and cholesterol. N Engl J Med 1993; 329:21–26.

519. Sprecher DL, Harris BV, Goldberg AC, et al. Efficacy of psyllium in reducing serum cholesterol levels in hypercholesterolemic patients on high- or low-fat diets. Ann Intern Med 1993; 119:545–554.

520. Warshafsky S, Kamer RS, Sivak SL. Effect of garlic on total serum cholesterol: a meta-analysis. Ann Intern Med 1993; 119:599–605.

521. Sabaté J, Fraser GE, Burke K, et al. Effects of walnuts on serum lipid levels and blood pressure in normal men. N Engl J Med 1993; 328:603–607.

522. Ginsberg HN. Update on the treatment of hypercholesterolemia, with a focus on HMG-CoA reductase inhibitors and combination regimens. Clin Cardiol 1995; 18:307–315.

523. Grundy SM. HMG-CoA reductase inhibitors for treatment of hypercholesterolemia. N Engl J Med 1988; 319:24–33.

524. Bradford RH, Shear CL, Chremos AN, et al. Expanded Clinical Evaluation of Lovastatin (EXCEL) Study results. I: Efficacy in modifying plasma lipoproteins and adverse event profile in 8245 patients with moderate hypercholesterolemia. Arch Intern Med 1991; 151:43–49.

525. Vega GL, Grundy SM. Treatment of primary moderate hypercholesterolemia with lovastatin (mevinolin) and colestipol. J Am Med Assoc 1987; 257:33–38.

526. Bakker-Arkema RG, Davidson MH, Goldstein RJ, et al. Efficacy and safety of a new HMG-CoA reductase inhibitor, atorvastatin, in patients with hypertriglyceridemia. J Am Med Assoc 1996; 275:128–133.

527. Marais GE, Larson KK. Rhabdomyolysis and acute renal failure induced by combination lovastatin and gemfibrozil therapy. Ann Intern Med 1990; 112:228–230.

528. Reaven P, Witztum JL. Lovastatin, nicotinic acid, and rhabdomyolysis. Ann Intern Med 1988; 109:597–598.

529. East C, Alivizatos PA, Grundy SM, et al. Rhabdomyolysis in patients receiving lovastatin after cardiac transplantation. N Engl J Med 1988; 318:47–48.

530. Ast M, Frishman WH. Bile acid sequestrants. J Clin Pharmacol 1990; 30:99–106.

531. Shepherd J, Packard CJ, Bicker S, et al. Cholestyramine promotes receptor-mediated low-density-lipoprotein catabolism. N Engl J Med 1980; 302:1219–1222.

532. Beil U, Crouse JR, Einarsson K, et al. Effects of interruption of the enterohepatic circulation of bile acids on the transport of very low density-lipoprotein triglycerides. Metabolism 1982; 31:438–444.

533. Packard CJ, Stewart JM, Third JLHC, et al. Effects of nicotinic acid therapy on high-density lipoprotein metabolism in type II and type IV hyperlipoproteinaemia. Biochim Biophys Acta 1980; 618:53–62.

534. Gurakar A, Hoeg JM, Kostner G, et al. Levels of lipoprotein Lp(a) decline with neomycin and niacin treatment. Atherosclerosis 1985; 57:293–301.

535. McKenney JM, Proctor JD, Harris S, et al. A comparison of the efficacy and toxic effects of sustained- vs immediate-release niacin in hypercholesterolemic patients. J Am Med Assoc 1994; 271:672–677.

536. Kissebah AH, Adams PW, Harrigan P, et al. The mechanism of action of clofibrate and tetranicotinoylfructose (bradilan) on the kinetics of plasma free fatty acid and triglyceride transport in type IV and type V hypertriglyceridaemia. Eur J Clin Invest 1974; 4:163–174.

537. Oliver MF, Heady JA, Morris JN, et al. A co-operative trial in the primary prevention of ischaemic heart disease using clofibrate: report from the Committee of Principal Investigators. Br Heart J 1978; 40:1069–1118.

538. Pierides AM, Alvarez-Ude F, Kerr DNS, et al. Clofibrate-induced muscle damage in patients with chronic renal failure. Lancet 1975; 2:1279–1282.

539. Buckley MM-T, Goa KL, Price AH, et al. Probucol: a reappraisal of its pharmacological properties and therapeutic use in hypercholesterolaemia. Drugs 1989; 37:761–800.

540. Walldius G, Erikson U, Olsson AG, et al. The effect of *probucol* on femoral atherosclerosis: the Probucol Quantitative Regression Swedish Trial (PQRST). Am J Cardiol 1994; 74:875–883.

541. Steinberg D. Clinical trials of antioxidants in atherosclerosis: are we doing the right thing? Lancet 1995; 346:36–38.

542. Gaziano JM, Manson JE, Ridker PM, et al. Beta carotene therapy for chronic stable angina. Circulation 1990; 82:III-201 (abstract).

543. Sanderson SL, Iverius P-H, Wilson DE. Successful hyperlipemic pregnancy. J Am Med Assoc 1991; 265:1858–1860.

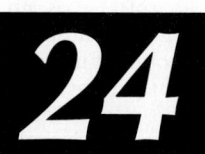

HORMONES AND DISORDERS OF MINERAL METABOLISM

F. Richard Bringhurst, Marie B. Demay, and Henry M. Kronenberg

BASIC BIOLOGY OF MINERAL METABOLISM

Introduction: Roles of the Mineral Ions

Calcium and phosphorus are the principal constituents of bone, and together they constitute 65% of its weight. Bone, in turn, contains nearly all of the calcium and phosphorus and more than half of the magnesium in the body. However, the quantitatively minor amounts of each of these ions in the extracellular fluid and within cells play crucial roles in normal physiology (Fig. 24–1).

Ninety-nine percent of total body calcium resides in bone, of which 99% is located within the crystal structure of the mineral phase. The remaining 1% of bone calcium is rapidly exchangeable with the nonosseous extracellular calcium pool, which is in equilibrium with intracellular calcium. Extracellular calcium is the principal substrate for the mineralization of cartilage and bone and also serves as a cofactor for many extracellular enzymes, most notably the enzymes of the coagulation cascade, and as a source of calcium ions for many cellular processes. These processes include automaticity of nerve and muscle; contraction of cardiac, skeletal, and smooth muscle; neurotransmitter release; and various forms of endocrine and exocrine secretion.

In blood, approximately 50% of total calcium is bound to proteins, mainly albumin and globulins. The ionized calcium concentration in serum is approximately 1.2 mmol/L (5 mg/dL), and this fraction is biologically active and tightly controlled by hormonal mechanisms. As intracellular cytosolic free calcium concentrations typically are in the range of only 100 nmol/L, a large (i.e., 10,000:1) chemical gradient, augmented by the large negative electrical potential, favors calcium entry into cells through calcium channels. This gradient is maintained by the limited conductance of resting calcium channels and by the energy-dependent extrusion of calcium into the extracellular fluid via high-affinity Ca^{2+},H^+-ATPases and low-affinity Na^+/Ca^{2+} exchangers.

	Calcium ions	Phosphate ions
Extracellular		
Concentration		
total, in serum	2.5×10^{-3} M	1.00×10^{-3} M
free	1.2×10^{-3} M	0.85×10^{-3} M
Functions	bone mineral	bone mineral
	blood coagulation	
	membrane excitability	
Intracellular		
Concentration	10^{-7} M	$1\text{-}2 \times 10^{-3}$ M
Functions	signal for:	• structural role
	• neuronal activation	• high energy bonds
	• hormone secretion	• regulation of proteins
	• muscle contraction	by phosphorylation

Figure 24–1. Distribution and function of calcium and phosphate. Note the dramatic differences between intracellular and extracellular concentrations of calcium ion and the dramatically different functions of calcium and phosphate inside cells.

More than 99% of intracellular calcium exists in the form of complexes within the mitochondrial compartment, bound to the inner plasma membrane, or associated with the inner membranes of the endoplasmic reticulum and other compartments. Release of calcium from membrane-bound compartments transduces cellular signals and is tightly regulated. The mechanisms responsible for translocations of intracellular calcium between the cytosol and these sequestered regions are becoming better understood with the identification of specific receptors for calcitropic signaling molecules, such as the inositol 1,4,5-trisphosphate and ryanodine receptors.

Phosphate is more widely distributed in nonosseous tissues than is calcium. Eighty-five percent of body phosphate is in the mineral phase of bone, and the remainder is located in inorganic or organic form throughout the extracellular and intracellular compartments. In human serum, inorganic phosphate is present at a concentration of approximately 1 mmol/L (3 mg/dL) and exists almost entirely in ionized form as either $H_2PO_4^-$ or HPO_4^{2-}. Only 12% of serum phosphate is protein-bound, and an additional fraction is loosely complexed with calcium, magnesium, and other cations. Intracellular free phosphate concentrations generally are comparable to those in the extracellular fluid (i.e., 1 to 2 mmol/L), although the inside-negative electrical potential of the cell creates a significant energy requirement for translocation of phosphate into cells. This translocation generally is accomplished through sodium-phosphate cotransport driven by the transmembrane sodium gradient. A number of sodium-phosphate cotransporters have been cloned; various cells and tissues employ different species of such transporters with distinct regulatory characteristics.

Organic phosphate is a key component of virtually all classes of structural, informational, and effector molecules essential for normal genetic, developmental, and physiological processes. Phosphate is an integral constituent of nucleic acids; phospholipids; complex carbohydrates; glycolytic intermediates; structural, signaling, and enzymatic phosphoproteins; nucleotide cofactors for enzymes and G proteins; and a large number of organic glycolytic intermediates. Of particular importance are the high-energy phosphate ester bonds present in molecules such as ATP, diphosphoglycerate, and creatine phosphate that store chemical energy. Phosphate plays a particularly prominent role as the key substrate or recognition site in numerous kinase and phosphatase regulatory cascades. Cytosolic phosphate per se also directly regulates a number of critical intracellular reactions, including those involved in glucose transport, lactate production, and synthesis of ATP. In light of these diverse roles, it is not surprising that severe depletion of intracellular phosphate leads to profound and global impairment of organ function.

Magnesium is the fourth most abundant cation in the body. Roughly half is found in bone, and half is in muscle and other soft tissues. As much as half of the magnesium in bone is not sequestered in the mineral phase but is freely exchangeable with the extracellular fluid and therefore may serve as a buffer against changes in extracellular magnesium level. Less than 1% of magnesium in the body is present in the extracellular fluid, where the magnesium concentration is approximately 0.5 mmol/L (1.2 mg/dL).[1, 2] The concentration of magnesium in serum normally is 0.7 to 1.0 mmol/L (1.7 to 2.4 mg/dL), of which roughly one third is protein bound, 15% is loosely complexed with phosphate or other anions, and 55% is present as the free ion.[1] More than 95% of intracellular magnesium is bound to other molecules, most notably ATP, the concentration of which is approximately 5 mmol/L. The intracellular cytosolic free magnesium concentration is approximately 0.5 mmol/L—i.e. 1000-fold higher than that of calcium—and is maintained by an active sodium-magnesium antiporter. The mechanism or mechanisms by which magnesium enters cells, presumably down a favorable electrochemical gradient, is unknown, although regulated channels may be present.[3]

Intracellular magnesium, like phosphate, is necessary for a wide range of cellular functions. It is an essential cofactor in enzymatic reactions, including most of the same glycolytic, kinase, and phosphatase pathways that also involve phosphate. Magnesium stabilizes the structures of a variety of macromolecules and complexes, including DNA, RNA, and ribosomes, activates many of the ATPase-coupled ion transporters, and plays a direct role in mitochondrial oxidative metabolism.[2] As a result, magnesium is critical for energy metabolism and the maintenance of a normal intracellular environment. Extracellular magnesium is crucial for normal neuromuscular excitability and nerve conduction, and many of the clinical consequences of magnesium deficiency or excess reflect abnormalities in this sphere.

The importance of the mineral ions for normal cellular physiology as well as skeletal integrity is reflected in the powerful endocrine control mechanisms that have evolved to maintain their extracellular concentrations within relatively narrow limits. The following sections describe the structures, secretory controls, actions, and interactions of parathyroid hormone, calcitonin, and 1,25-dihydroxyvitamin D ($1,25(OH)_2D$)—the major hormones involved in mineral ion homeostasis. Subsequent sections detail the wide variety of clinical disorders that accompany abnormalities in this hormonal network.

Parathyroid Hormone

Parathyroid hormone (PTH) is a peptide hormone that controls the minute-to-minute level of ionized calcium in the blood and extracellular fluids. PTH binds to cell surface receptors in bone and kidney and thereby triggers responses that increase blood calcium (Fig. 24–2). The increase in blood calcium feeds back on the parathyroid gland to decrease the secretion of PTH. The parathyroid gland, bones, and kidney thus are the crucial organs that control PTH-mediated calcium homeostasis.

Parathyroid Gland Biology

Parathyroid chief cells have three properties vital for their homestatic function: they rapidly secrete stored hormone in response to changes in blood calcium; they can synthesize,

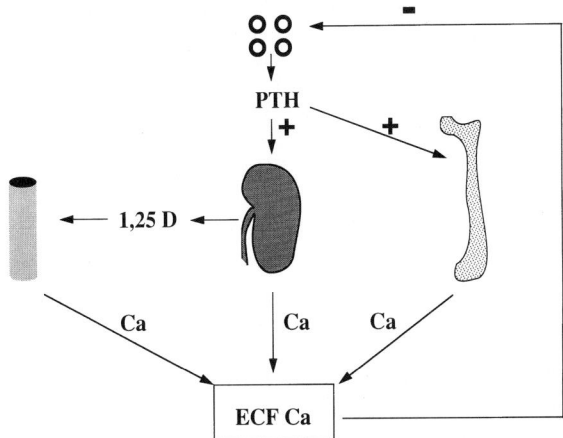

Figure 24–2. PTH-calcium feedback loop that controls calcium homeostasis. Four organs—the parathyroid glands, intestine, kidneys, and bone—together determine the parameters of calcium homeostasis. Plus signs indicate positive effects; minus sign indicates negative effect.

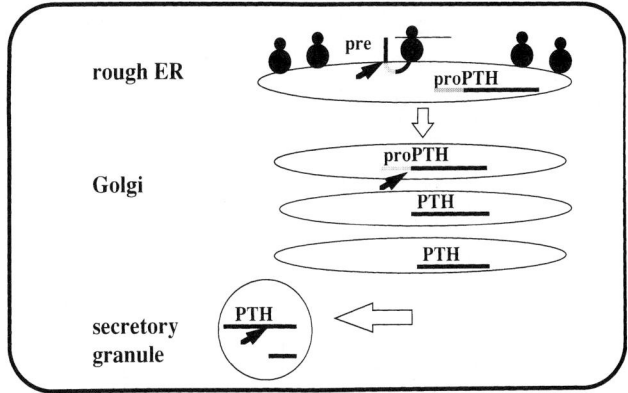

Figure 24–4. Intracellular processing of pre-pro-PTH. Diagonal arrows indicate sites of cleavage by enzymes that generate pro-PTH in the endoplasmic reticulum, PTH in the Golgi apparatus, carboxyl-terminal fragments of PTH in the secretory granule.

process, and store large amounts of PTH in a regulated manner; and they replicate when chronically stimulated. These functional attributes allow for short-, intermediate- and long-term adaptation, respectively, to changes in calcium availability.

PARATHYROID HORMONE BIOSYNTHESIS

PTH, a protein of 84 amino acids, is synthesized as a larger precursor, pre-proparathyroid hormone (Fig. 24–3). These pre-pro-PTH sequences share a 25-residue "pre" or signal sequence, and a 6-residue "pro" sequence.[4–11] The signal sequence, along with the short "pro" sequence, directs the protein into the secretory pathway (Fig. 24–4). During transit across the membrane of the endoplasmic reticulum, the signal sequence is cleaved and rapidly degraded. The importance of the signal sequence for normal processing of

PTH is illustrated by the finding that a mutation in the signal sequence of pre-pro-PTH causes hypoparathyroidism.[12, 13]

The role of the short pro sequence is not completely understood; it may help the signal sequence work efficiently and ensure accurate cleavage of the precursor.[14] After cleavage of the pro sequence, the mature PTH(1–84) is concentrated in secretory vesicles and granules. One morphologically distinct subtype of granule contains both PTH and the proteases, cathepsins B and H.[15, 16] This co-localization of proteases and PTH in secretory granules probably explains the observation that a portion of the PTH secreted from parathyroid glands consists of carboxy-terminal PTH fragments.[17] No amino-terminal fragments of PTH are secreted. Since carboxy-terminal fragments of PTH are unlikely to play an important role in calcium homeostasis (see later), the intracellular fragmentation of PTH probably represents an inactivating pathway. The intracellular degradation of newly synthesized PTH provides an important regulatory mechanism. Under conditions of hypercalcemia, the secretion of PTH is substantially decreased, and most of what is secreted consists of inactive carboxy-terminal fragments.[18–21]

PARATHYROID HORMONE SECRETION

Although catecholamines, magnesium, and other stimuli can affect PTH secretion,[22] the major regulator of PTH secretion is the concentration of ionized calcium in blood. Increased serum ionized calcium decreases PTH secretion (Fig. 24–5A). The shape of the dose-response curve is sigmoidal. Such a curve can be defined by four parameters—the maximal secretory rate (A in Fig. 24–5B), the slope of the curve at its midpoint (B), the level of calcium at the midpoint, often called the set point (C), and the minimal secretory rate (D).[23]

Properties of the parathyroid cell determine the shape of the sigmoidal curve but do not alone determine the point on the curve that represents a physiological steady state for an individual. This point, usually between the midpoint and the bottom of the curve, is determined by the response of target organs to PTH.[24] Figure 24–5C (solid line) shows how serum calcium rises in response to increases in PTH; the parathyroid gland's sigmoidal curve is the dotted line. In the steady state, the blood levels of PTH and calcium in a given individual represent the intersection of the two lines.

The sigmoidal curve illustrates several physiological properties of the parathyroid gland. The minimal secretory rate is low but not zero. The maximal secretory rate represents the reserve of the parathyroid with which to respond to hypocalcemia. Since the steady state in normal individuals occurs in

	PRE	↓ PRO ↓	PTH
	-31	-6 +1	+10
human	MIPAKDMAKVMIVMLAICFLTKSDG	KSVKKR	SVSEIQLMHN
bovine	MMSAKDMVKVMIVMLAICFLARSDG	KSVKKR	AVSEIQFMHN
porcine	MMSAKDTVKVMVVMLAICFLARSDG	KPIKKR	SVSEIQLMHN
rat	MMSASTMAKVMILMLAVCLLTQADG	KPVKKR	AVSEIQLMHN
canine	MMSAKDMVKVMIVMFAICFLAKSDG	KPVKKR	SVSEIQFMHN
chicken	MTSTKNLAKAIVILYAICFFTNSDG	RPMMKR	SVSEMQLMHN

	+20	+30	+40	+50
human	LGKHLNSMERVEWLRKKLQDVHNFVALGAPLAPRDAGSQRPRK
bovine	LGKHLSSMERVEWLRKKLQDVHNFVALGASIAYRDGSSQRPRK
porcine	LGKHLSSLERVEWLRKKLQDVHNFVALGASIVHRDGGSQRPRK
rat	LGKHLASVERMQWLRKKLQDVHNFVSLGVQMAAREGSYQRPTK
canine	LGKHLSSMERVEWLRKKLQDVHNFVALGAPIAHRDGSSQRPLK
chicken	LGEHRHTVERQDWLQMKLQDVH..SALE.....DARTQRPRN

	+60	+70	+80
human	KEDNVLVE...SHEKSLGEA.........DKADVNVLTKAKSQ
bovine	KEDNVLVE...SHQKSLGEA.........DKADVDVLIKAKPQ
porcine	KEDNVLVE...SHQKSLGEA.........DKAAVDVLIKAKPQ
rat	KEENVLVD...GNSKSLGEG.........DKADVDVLVKAKSQ
canine	KEDNVLVE...SYQKSLGEA.........DKADVDVLTKAKSQ
chicken	KEDIVLGEIRNRRLLPEHLRAAVQKKSIDLDKAYMNVLFKTKP.

Figure 24–3. Sequences of pre-proparathyroid hormone from six species. Completely conserved residues are in boldface. Arrows indicate the sites of signal sequence ("pre") and "pro" sequence cleavage. Numbers start at residue +1 of mature parathyroid hormone; because of gaps, the numbers correspond only to the mammalian, and not the chicken, sequence. Amino acids are indicated by the single letter code: A, Ala; R, Arg; N, Asn; D, Asp; C, Cys; Q, Gln; E, Glu; G, Gly; H, His; I, Ile; L, Leu; K, Lys; M, Met; F, Phe; P, Pro; S, Ser; T, Thr; W, Trp; Y, Tyr; V, Val.

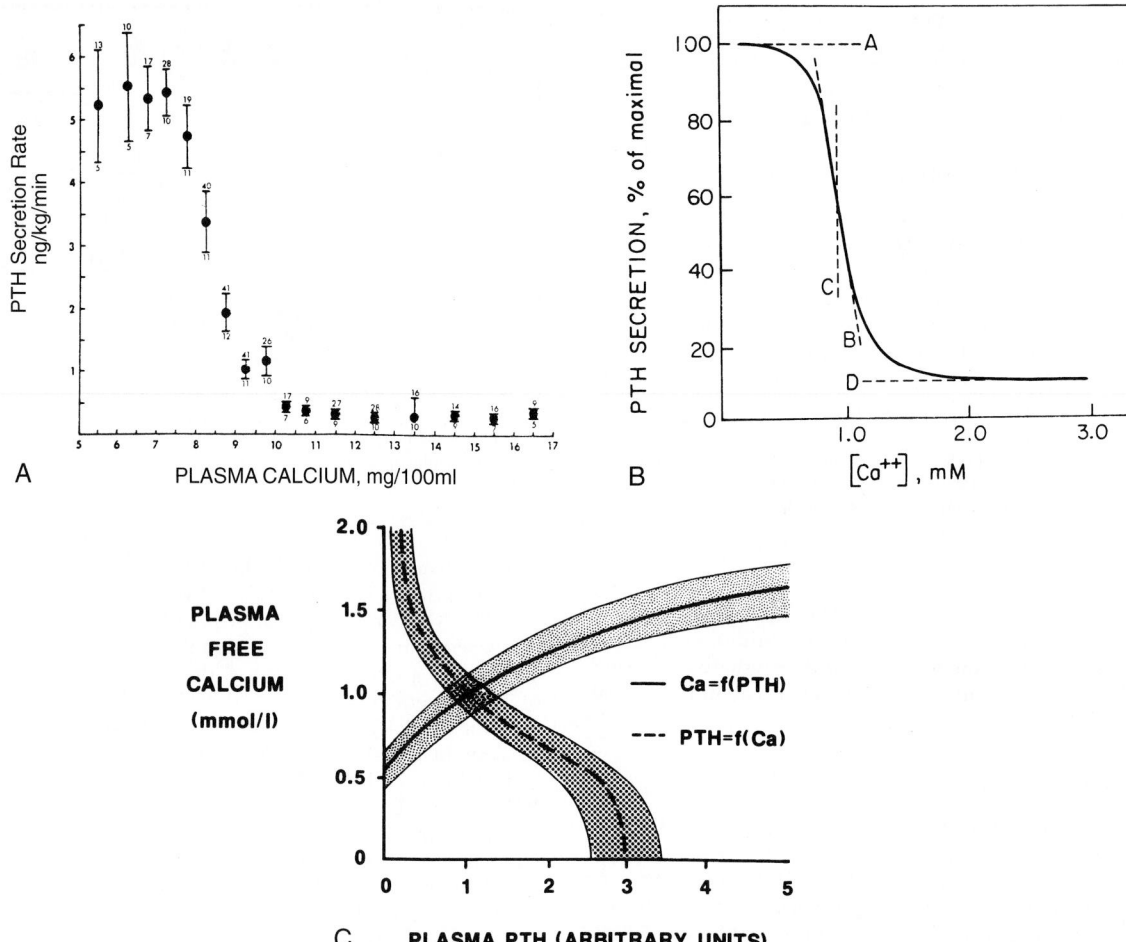

Figure 24–5. *A,* Secretory response of bovine parathyroid glands to induced alterations of plasma calcium concentration. Calves were infused with calcium chloride or EDTA, and PTH secretion was assessed by measuring PTH levels in the parathyroid venous effluent. The symbols and vertical bars indicate the secretory rate (mean ± SE) in calcium concentration ranges of 1.0 or 0.5 mg/100 mL. The number of calves and samples are indicated, respectively, by numbers below and above the bars.

B, Sigmoidal curve generated by the equation, $Y = \{[A - D]/[1 + (X/C)^B]\} + D$; the significance of A, B, C, and D are described in the text.

C, Relationships between calcium and PTH levels when each, in turn, is treated as an independent variable. The dashed line represents the sigmoidal relationship between calcium and PTH, when calcium is the independent variable. This curve is the same as that in Figure 24–5*A* and *B* but is turned on its side, because the axes are reversed. The solid line represents the relationship between calcium and PTH when PTH is considered the independent variable; values for this curve result from measurements made during PTH infusions in parathyroidectomized animals. Actual data are limited, so the curves should be viewed as illustrative. (*A* from Mayer GP, Hurst JG. Sigmoidal relationship between parathyroid hormone secretion rate and plasma calcium concentration in calves. Endocrinology 1978; 10:1037–1042. © The Endocrine Society. *B* from Brown EM. Four-parameter model of the sigmoidal relationship between parathyroid hormone release and extracellular calcium concentration in normal and abnormal parathyroid tissue. J Clin Endocrinol Metab 1983; 56:572–581. © The Endocrine Society. *C* from Parfitt AM. In: Mundy GR, Martin TJ, eds. Physiology and Pharmacology of Bone. New York: Springer-Verlag, 1993, with permission.)

the lower portion of the sigmoidal curve, the system responds more dramatically to hypocalcemia than to hypercalcemia.

Studies in humans confirmed this sigmoidal relationship and showed that the parathyroid cell responds both to the absolute level of blood calcium and to the rate of change of calcium.[25] Thus, PTH levels briefly increase more during a sudden drop in blood calcium than during a more gradual fall in calcium. This property of the parathyroid cell offers an additional protection against sudden hypocalcemia.

The biochemical and cellular determinants of the sigmoidal response curve of the parathyroid gland have been defined in some detail. The calcium sensor[26, 27] on the parathyroid cell surface has been cloned and shown to be a member of the G protein–coupled family of receptors. The sequence of the receptor suggests that it spans the plasma membrane seven times, like other receptors in the G protein–linked receptor family (Fig. 24–6). A large extracellular domain, presumed to bind calcium, resembles similar domains in brain metabotropic glutamate receptors and in bacterial periplasmic proteins designed to bind small ligands, including cations. The receptor has been expressed in a number of cell types where

it activates phospholipase C and blocks stimulation of cyclic AMP production, as it does in normal parathyroid cells.[28]

Convincing proof of the identity of the parathyroid calcium sensor came with the finding that most patients with familial hypocalciuric hypercalcemia, a disease of defective calcium sensing (see later), have inactivating mutations in the calcium sensor gene.[29] Mice genetically engineered to have only one functioning copy of the calcium sensor gene also have defects in parathyroid calcium sensing.[30] Further, calcimimetic compounds that activate the cloned calcium sensor inhibit PTH secretion in humans.[31] Such compounds may prove useful in the treatment of primary and secondary hyperparathyroidism.

The properties of the calcium sensor explain one of the most unusual features of the parathyroid cell. Most cells maintain a constant and very low level of intracellular calcium despite fluctuations in extracellular calcium. The parathyroid cell is exceptional, in that modest changes in extracellular calcium lead to corresponding changes in intracellular calcium. When calcium activates the cell surface calcium sensor, intracellular calcium rises because of release of calcium from intracellular stores and of opening of plasma membrane calcium channels. This increase in intracellular calcium then leads to a decrease in PTH secretion by mechanisms that remain to be clarified.

REGULATION OF THE PARATHYROID HORMONE GENE

Whereas PTH blood levels are regulated on a minute-to-minute basis by the two mechanisms already discussed—control of PTH secretion by the calcium sensor and amplification of this regulation by intracellular degradation of stored hormone—over a longer time frame the parathyroid cell also regulates the expression of the *PTH* gene.[6, 11, 32–34]

Although 1,25-dihydroxyvitamin D (1,25(OH)$_2$D), the active form of vitamin D, has no direct effect on PTH secretion, it dramatically suppresses *PTH* gene transcription.[35–40] This suppression of transcription does not occur when 1,25(OH)$_2$D is administered to chronically hypocalcemic animals, however, perhaps because hypocalcemia causes a fall in parathyroid cell vitamin D receptors.[41, 42] The ability of hypocalcemia to override the effects of high levels of 1,25(OH)$_2$D represents an important defense, since it provides a way of making large amounts of PTH and 1,25(OH)$_2$D at the same time, when both are needed.

Calcium also regulates the biosynthesis of PTH. Acute hypocalcemia in rats leads, within an hour, to an increase in PTH messenger RNA.[43, 44] In contrast, hypercalcemia leads to little[44] or no[43] change in PTH mRNA. Thus, under normal conditions the inhibition of PTH biosynthesis by calcium is nearly maximal, just as it is for PTH secretion. The parathyroid gland is poised to respond to a fall in calcium much more than it is to a rise. The mechanism for the increase in PTH mRNA in response to hypocalcemia is uncertain; differing experimental paradigms suggest regulation at the levels of gene transcription,[40] mRNA stability,[45] and mRNA translation.[46]

The regulation of expression of the *PTH* gene has particular relevance in patients with renal failure in whom hypocalcemia, low levels of 1,25(OH)$_2$D, and, possibly, uremic toxins disrupt normal calcium homeostasis. Therapy with 1,25(OH)$_2$D and calcium increases calcium absorption and also inhibits PTH synthesis by direct effects on the parathyroid gland.

REGULATION OF PARATHYROID CELL NUMBER

Parathyroid cells divide during growth but replicate little in adulthood.[47] Parathyroid cell number can dramatically increase, however, in the setting of hypocalcemia or low levels of 1,25(OH)$_2$D and during neoplastic growth.

Calcium, acting through the parathyroid calcium sensor, appears to restrain parathyroid proliferation. This phenomenon has been difficult to demonstrate consistently in experiments[48–53] but is evident in neonates who lack both copies of the calcium sensor gene. These neonates have severe primary hyperparathyroidism with large, diffusely hyperplastic glands, presumably because of insufficient activation by extracellular calcium of the parathyroid calcium sensor.

The role of 1,25(OH)$_2$D, independently of blood calcium, in the regulation of parathyroid cell proliferation is less well established than is that of calcium. That 1,25(OH)$_2$D can dramatically affect parathyroid cell number has been shown in vivo in many settings,[48, 54] but such studies cannot rigorously eliminate the effects of transient changes in blood calcium. Nevertheless the dramatic suppression of proliferation of cultured parathyroid cells by 1,25(OH)$_2$D[53, 55] suggests that the metabolite directly inhibits parathyroid cell replication.

Although the ability to increase parathyroid cell number in response to physiological challenge is an important defense against hypocalcemia, the response is slow and not easily re-

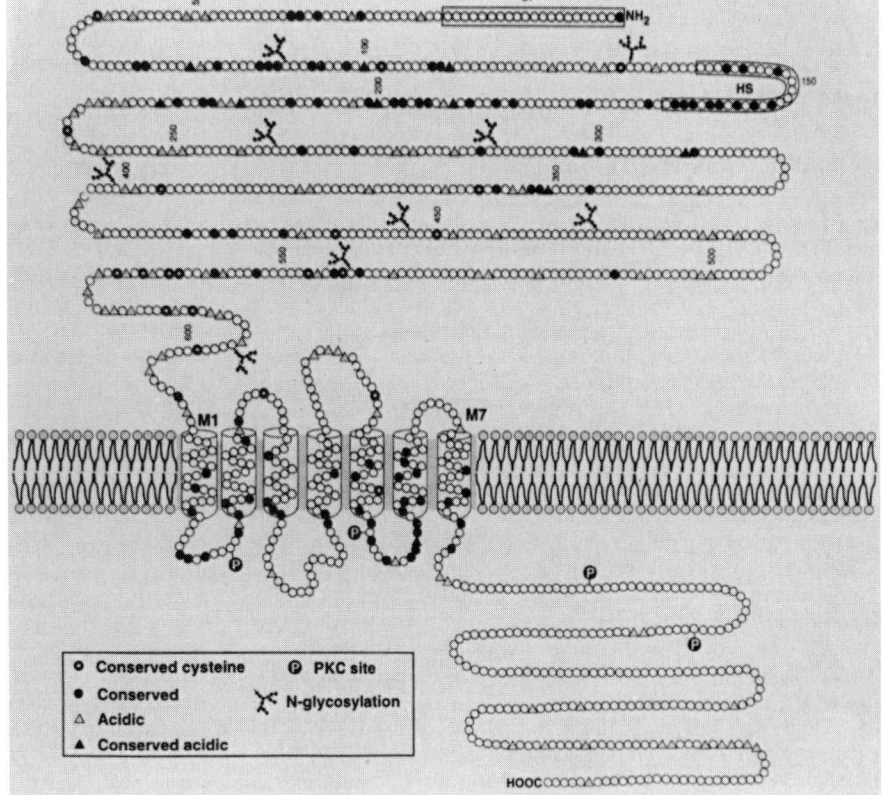

Figure 24–6. Structural model of parathyroid cell calcium-sensing receptor predicted from its amino acid sequence. The large amino-terminal domain is extracellular. Conserved residues among the metabotropic glutamate receptors and the bovine parathyroid calcium-sensing receptor are indicated by symbols noted in the box. The figure also indicates potential glycosylation and protein kinase C phosphorylation sites. (From Brown EM, Gamba G, Riccardi D, et al. Cloning and characterization of an extracellular Ca^{2+}-sensing receptor from bovine parathyroid. Nature 1993; 366:575–580. Copyright 1993, Macmillan Magazines Ltd.)

versible. When the need for an increased number of parathyroid cells disappears, for example after renal transplantation for uremia, persistent hyperparathyroidism can cause vexing clinical problems for months and years thereafter. The mechanisms for decreasing parathyroid cell number, if they exist, are unknown.

Peripheral Metabolism of Parathyroid Hormone

The earliest radioimmunoassays for PTH demonstrated that the forms of PTH in the circulation differ from those in the parathyroid gland.[56] As noted earlier, both PTH(1–84) and carboxy-terminal fragments of PTH are secreted from the parathyroid gland;[17] the ratio of inactive-to-active PTH secretion increases with increasing blood calcium. Secreted PTH(1–84) is rapidly metabolized by the liver (70%) and the kidneys (20%) and disappears from the circulation with a half-life of 2 min. This rapid peripheral metabolism of PTH is unaffected by widely varying levels of blood calcium or $1,25(OH)_2D$.[57] Less than 1% of the secreted hormone finds its way to PTH receptors on target organs.[58] These features of PTH metabolism ensure that the blood level of PTH is determined principally by the rate of PTH secretion and that blood levels respond rapidly to changes in the rate of secretion of the hormone.

In the liver, a small amount of PTH binds to PTH receptors, but most of the intact PTH is cleaved, initially after residues 33 and 36, probably by cathepsins.[59] In the kidney, a small amount of intact PTH binds to PTH receptors, but most is filtered at the glomerulus and is subsequently degraded in tubules.[60] Carboxy-terminal fragments are also cleared efficiently by glomerular filtration. In fact, the kidney is the only known site of clearance of carboxy-terminal PTH fragments, so that these fragments accumulate when the glomerular filtration rate falls. Even in the presence of normal renal function, the half-life of carboxyl-terminal fragments of PTH is several-fold increased compared with that of PTH(1–84). Consequently the concentration of carboxyl-terminal fragments in the circulation exceeds that of intact PTH, even though intact PTH is the major form of PTH secreted from the parathyroid gland.

Actions of Parathyroid Hormone

Actions on the Kidney

STIMULATION OF CALCIUM REABSORPTION. Almost all of the calcium in the glomerular filtrate is reabsorbed, 65% by the proximal convoluted and straight tubules. Most reabsorption occurs by a passive, paracellular route.[61, 62] Changes in the transepithelial voltage gradient, determined largely by the rate of sodium reabsorption, control the rate of calcium transport. PTH does little to affect calcium flux in the proximal tubules. Twenty percent of the calcium is reabsorbed in the thick ascending limb of Henle's loop, and another 10% is reabsorbed in the distal convoluted and connecting tubules. Half of the calcium reabsorption in the thick ascending limb is by a passive paracellular route. Like proximal calcium reabsorption, this process is sensitive to the lumen-positive voltage gradient and therefore is decreased by loop diuretics such as furosemide. The remaining half of calcium reabsorption in the thick ascending limb and virtually all of the reabsorption in the distal tubular segments occur by a transcellular route under the control of PTH.

Figure 24–7 depicts the transcellular pathway taken by calcium in the distal tubular segments. The intracellular level of calcium is extremely low, about 150 nmol/L, compared to the millimolar levels in the glomerular filtrate and the blood.

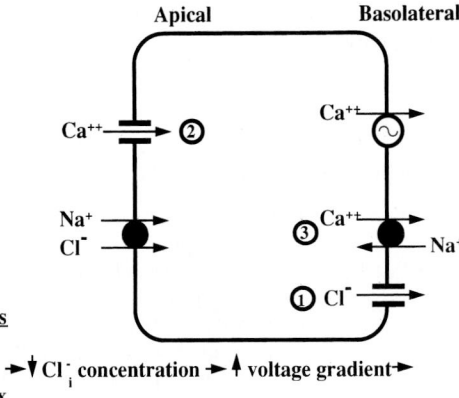

PTH actions

① ▲ Cl⁻ efflux → ▼ Cl$_i$ concentration → ▲ voltage gradient →

② ▲ Ca⁺⁺ influx

③ ▲ Ca⁺⁺-Na⁺ exchange

Figure 24–7. Effects of PTH on distal tubular calcium transport. PTH acts to increase chloride efflux through channels in the basolateral membrane. As indicated, this increase leads to calcium influx through apical calcium channels. PTH also increases basolateral Ca^{2+}/Na^+ exchange. The apical Na^+,Cl^- cotransporter allows chloride to enter the cell and is the target of thiazide diuretics. (Adapted from Friedman PA, Gesek FA. Calcium transport in renal epithelial cells. Am J Physiol 1993; 264:F181–F198, with permission.)

Calcium enters the cell from the tubular lumen through voltage-sensitive calcium channels. This conductance is passive but is regulated by the electrochemical gradient across the apical membrane. PTH increases the conductance (2 in Fig. 24–7) by increasing the transmembrane voltage gradient,[63, 64] probably by increasing chloride exit through basolateral chloride channels (1 in Fig. 24–7). Calcium then leaves the cell at the basolateral membrane through active processes involving sodium-calcium exchange and an ATP-driven calcium pump. Sodium-calcium exchange is increased by PTH (3 in Fig. 24–7).[65]

The amount of calcium in the urine reflects all of the tubular reabsorption processes just enumerated and the filtered load of calcium. PTH acts to raise blood calcium, so that the filtered load of calcium is high in states of PTH excess. In that setting, even though the distal tubular resorption of calcium is increased by PTH, the total amount of calcium in the final urine is likely to be high.

INHIBITION OF PHOSPHATE TRANSPORT. Phosphate reabsorption occurs mainly in the proximal tubules, which reclaim roughly 80% of the filtered load. Some additional phosphate (8 to 10%) is reabsorbed in the distal tubule but not in Henle's loop, leaving about 10 to 12% for excretion in the urine. The normal overall tubular reabsorption of phosphate (or "TRP") therefore is about 88%, although a more reliable measure of renal phosphate handling is the "phosphate threshold" or T_mP/GFR, which can be derived from the TRP through the use of a nomogram (Fig. 24–8) based on studies of experimental phosphate infusions in normal subjects and patients with a variety of diseases that affect phosphate excretion.[66]

Phosphate reabsorption in both proximal and distal tubules is strongly inhibited by PTH, although the proximal effect is quantitatively most important. Phosphate is reabsorbed by a transepithelial route, and transport from the glomerular filtrate into the cell is mediated by sodium-phosphate cotransporters;[67] cDNAs encoding these transporters have been cloned.[68] The low level of sodium within the cell drives the cotransport of sodium and phosphate, even though the phosphate travels against an electrochemical gradient. In response to PTH, the V_{max} for sodium-phosphate cotransport decreases. PTH decreases the amount of transporter protein in the plasma membrane,[69] probably by blocking the fusion of

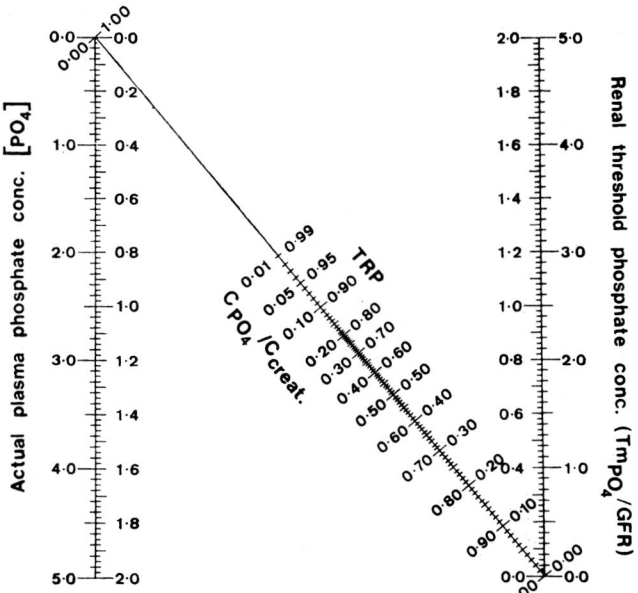

Figure 24–8. Nomogram for determining renal threshold phosphate concentration (T_mPO_4/GFR) from the plasma phosphate concentration and the fractional reabsorption of filtered phosphate (TRP) or fractional excretion of filtered phosphate ($1 - $ TRP or Clearance$_{PO_4}$/Clearance$_{creat}$). Because the blood level of phosphate influences the renal handling of phosphate, the renal threshold phosphate concentration best separates normal from abnormal renal phosphate handling. (From Walton RJ, Bijvoet OLM. Nomogram of derivation of renal threshold phosphate concentration. Lancet 1975; 2:309–310, with permission.)

vesicles containing the transporter with the plasma membrane.[70] To a lesser extent, PTH also decreases the levels of transporter mRNA.

Dietary intake of phosphate, perhaps through changes in the level of phosphate in the blood, also regulates the activity of sodium-phosphate transporters and thus the proximal tubular absorption of phosphate by a mechanism that is independent of PTH. Dietary deprivation of phosphate leads to a stimulation of phosphate reabsorption that can override the effects of PTH on the proximal tubule.

OTHER RENAL EFFECTS OF PTH. PTH stimulates the synthesis of $1,25(OH)_2D$ in the proximal tubule by activating the $25(OH)D$ 1α-hydroxylase[71, 72] and decreasing the activity of the renal 24-hydroxylase[73] (see section on metabolism of cholecalciferol). PTH inhibits sodium, water, and bicarbonate reabsorption[74] and stimulates gluconeogenesis in the proximal tubule. PTH also acts directly on the glomerulus to decrease both the single-nephron and whole-kidney glomerular filtration rates.[75]

ACTIONS OF PTH ON BONE

PTH stimulates bone resorption by increasing the activity and number of osteoclasts by several mechanisms (Fig. 24–9). Osteoclasts are the only cells in bone with the capacity to release calcium from the mineral phase into the bloodstream. In response to the administration of PTH, the activity of individual mature osteoclasts is increased. However, despite the clear connection between PTH and osteoclastic bone resorption, isolated mature osteoclasts cannot respond to PTH[76, 77] and do not harbor receptors that bind PTH with high affinity. The addition of osteoblasts to isolated osteoclasts restores the ability of the osteoclasts to resorb bone in response to PTH.[76] These findings suggest that PTH activates osteoclasts by stimulating osteoblasts and perhaps osteoblast precursors, which then activate osteoclasts (1 in Fig. 24–9). The mechanism of this activation has not been defined.

Because osteoclasts may not resorb bone easily through its overlying unmineralized osteoid,[78] PTH-stimulated osteoblasts may prepare the way for osteoclasts by digesting the underlying osteoid (3 in Fig. 24–9).[79]

Sustained PTH administration also increases the number of mature osteoclasts in bone by increasing the number of mononuclear, late committed precursors of osteoclasts.[80] PTH may activate osteoclast precursors directly;[81] alternatively, PTH may stimulate osteoclast development through signals from osteoblasts or stromal cells[82, 83] (2 in Fig. 24–9).

The actions of PTH on bone include several effects on cells of the osteoblast lineage. PTH binds to osteoblasts that are actively laying down bone matrix and to a subset of stromal cells away from the bone surface.[84] PTH inhibits a number of activities of isolated osteoblasts, including the synthesis of type I collagen, the major protein of bone matrix (4 in Fig. 24–9),[85] and inhibits the conversion of osteoblast precursors to mature osteoblasts (5 in Fig. 24–9).[86] Nevertheless in intact bone PTH increases the rate of bone formation. Much of this increase is an indirect response to growth factors, such as insulin-like growth factor I (IGF-I), IGF-II, and transforming growth factor β (TGF β) that are released during osteoclastic bone resorption (6 in Fig. 24–9). PTH can also, however, stimulate the release of IGF-I from osteoblasts themselves (7 in Fig. 24–9).[87] Thus, through an autocrine loop PTH may increase bone formation under certain conditions, such as intermittent, pharmacologic administration. The net effect of PTH on bone formation in vivo varies, depending on the dose, manner of administration (intermittent or continuous), and type of bone.[87] These complexities presumably explain the complicated responses of bone in hyperparathyroidism (see later) and the attempts to utilize the anabolic effects of intermittently administered PTH in the experimental treatment of osteoporosis (see next chapter).

MOLECULAR BASIS OF PTH ACTION

Ever since the discovery that PTH stimulates the excretion of cyclic AMP in the urine,[88] PTH has been thought to act by triggering a cascade of intracellular second messengers. This guiding hypothesis postulates that all the actions of PTH result from the binding of the hormone to transmembrane receptors on target tissues. These receptors are members of a large

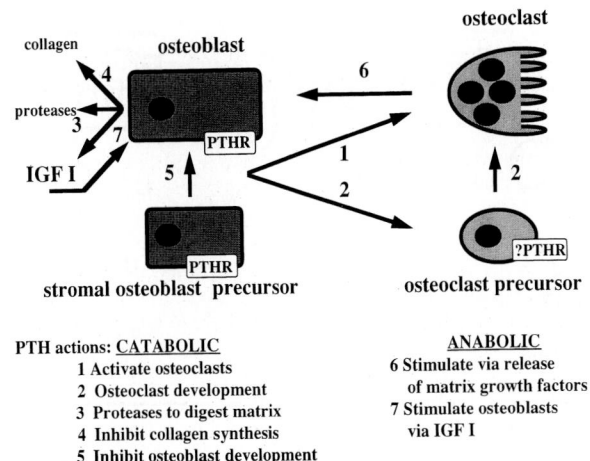

Figure 24–9. Actions of PTH on bone. PTH receptors (PTHR) are found on osteoblasts and osteoblast precursors. Since not all osteoclast precursors have been identified and characterized, the possible presence of PTH receptors on osteoclast precursors cannot be eliminated. PTH can have catabolic effects (stimulation of bone resorption or inhibition of bone formation) or anabolic effects (stimulation of bone formation) through both direct and indirect actions, depending on the dose and pattern of delivery of PTH.

family of G protein–linked receptors that span the plasma membrane seven times (Fig. 24–10). The binding of hormone on the outside of the membrane causes conformational changes in the receptor molecule that activate the receptor's ability to release GDP from the α subunit of a G protein bound to the receptor. The G protein then binds GTP in place of GDP. The GTP-binding α subunit of the G protein then separates from the βγ subunits, and the separate subunits of the G protein then modulate the activity of enzymes and channels. The activity of these enzymes and channels affect downstream proteins, eventually leading to the physiological responses of bone and kidney cells.

PTH AND PTH-RELATED PROTEIN RECEPTORS. DNA encoding a receptor that mediates the action of PTH and of PTH-related protein (PTHrP) has been isolated from rat, opossum, human, pig, and *Xenopus* (toad) cells and tissues.[89–95] The predicted amino acid sequence of the receptor suggests that the receptor spans the plasma membrane seven times, but the sequence does not closely resemble the sequences of most known G protein–linked receptors and is instead a member of a subfamily of closely related receptors. These receptors all bind peptides 30 to 40 amino acids in length. Known members include receptors for the secretin family of peptides (secretin, vasoactive intestinal peptide, glucagon, glucagon-like peptide, growth hormone–releasing hormone, pituitary adenylyl cyclase–activating peptide, gastrin inhibitory peptide), corticotropin-releasing hormone, calcitonin, and insect diuretic hormones related to corticotropin-releasing hormone.[96–98] The PTH/PTHrP receptor most closely resembles those of the secretin group. The gene encoding the PTH/PTHrP receptor has a complicated structure, with 13 introns interrupting the coding sequence.[99, 100] A downstream promoter is used in all tissues that express the gene, including bone,[100, 101] and an upstream promoter is used primarily in kidney and to some extent in liver.

The cloned PTH/PTHrP receptor binds amino-terminal fragments of PTH and PTHrP with equal affinity. The receptor is expressed at high levels in kidney and in osteoblasts of bone and is also expressed in tissues such as smooth muscle, brain, and fetal tissues that are thought to be target tissues more for PTHrP than for PTH.[92, 102, 103] In response to binding of PTH or PTHrP, the receptor activates G proteins, including G_s, G_q, and its close relatives, G_i, and perhaps others.[104–106] The G proteins then activate cascades of effectors (see Fig. 24–10).

The PTH/PTHrP receptor is believed to mediate many of the actions of both PTH and PTHrP. The ligand binding and signaling properties of the receptor, its pattern of expression, and the consequences of mutation of the receptor sequence (see later) are persuasive in this regard. Nevertheless the scheme of PTH action illustrated in Figure 24–10 should be considered as a simplified outline. It is unlikely that all the actions of PTH can be explained by interactions with the cloned PTH/PTHrP receptor: Fragments of PTH that do not bind the receptor may have biologic actions;[107–109] some cells respond to PTH in ways not mimicked by the cloned receptor;[110–113] the carboxyl-terminal portion of PTH(1–84) binds a cell surface protein distinct from the PTH/PTHrP receptor;[114] and a second PTH receptor has been cloned.[115] This receptor is expressed in brain, pancreas, testis, and placenta but not in bone or kidney. The functional role of this receptor and the identity of the physiologically relevant ligand need to be established.

FUNCTIONAL IMPLICATIONS OF PTH STRUCTURE. Amino-terminal fragments of PTH as short as PTH(1–34) have potency at least as great as the full-length PTH(1–84).[116] Full-length PTH(1–84) does not bind the cloned PTH/PTHrP receptor better than PTH(1–34), and carboxyl-terminal fragments do not bind at all.[117] For these reasons most studies of PTH structure-function relationships have used amino-terminal PTH fragments.

Several discrete portions of the PTH(1–34) peptide interact with the receptor.[118] The first 13 residues of PTH trigger the conformational change in the receptor that results in the transmembrane activation of G_S and adenylate cyclase,[119–122] and these residues are highly conserved between PTH and PTHrP. This activation domain interacts with the transmembrane domains and extracellular loops.[123–125]

The more carboxyl-terminal portions of PTH(1–34) contribute to the specificity and affinity of binding of PTH to the PTH/PTHrP receptor, through interactions with the amino-terminal extracellular domain of the receptor.[126] Studies of the structure of PTH by nuclear magnetic resonance spectroscopy[127] suggest that the activation domain and the carboxyl-terminal domain of PTH(1–34) are discrete entities separated by a flexible loop that allows the two domains to fold near each other (Fig. 24–11).

ACTIVATION OF SECOND MESSENGERS. Precisely how binding of PTH to the extracellular domains of the PTH/PTHrP receptor leads to activation of G_S is not understood. The similarity of the PTH/PTHrP receptor to other receptors[128, 129] and the behavior of certain mutant PTH/PTHrP receptors[125] suggest that the seven transmembrane domains of the PTH/PTHrP receptors form a ring, with the seventh transmembrane domain adjacent to the first and second. Presumably, binding of PTH to the receptor[130] changes the relationships of the transmembrane domains so as to alter the interaction of the three intracellular loops and carboxyl-terminal tail with G proteins.

Receptors with certain point mutations in the second[131] and sixth[132] transmembrane domains can activate G_S even without stimulation by hormone. These mutant receptors were discovered by analyzing the PTH/PTHrP receptors in Jansen's metaphyseal chondrodystrophy.[133, 134] Individuals with this disorder have signs of parathyroid overactivity (hypercalcemia, hypophosphatemia, and high levels of 1,25(OH)$_2$D and urinary cyclic AMP) but have low PTH and PTHrP levels. The mutations must change the conformation of the intracellular face of the receptor in a way that resembles the effect of binding of PTH to the normal receptor. The observation that inappropriate activation of the PTH/PTHrP receptor in Jansen's chondrodystrophy leads to all of the metabolic abnormalities found in primary hyperparathyroidism is one of the most persuasive pieces of evidence that the cloned PTH/

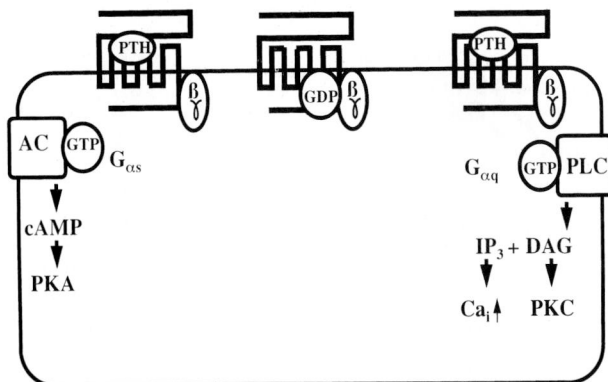

Figure 24–10. PTH/PTHrP receptors act as nucleotide exchangers. PTH binding to the receptor leads to the exchange of GTP for GDP bound to Gα subunits. Gα subunits bound to GTP are released from the receptor and from the βγ subunits and then activate effectors. G$_s$ activates adenylate cyclase; this leads to the formation of cyclic AMP, which then activates protein kinase A (PKA). G$_q$ and related α subunits activate phospholipase C (PLC). PLC hydrolyzes phosphatidyl-inositol 1,4,5-trisphosphate to generate diacyl glycerol (DAG) and inositol 1,4,5-trisphosphate (IP$_3$). The DAG then activates protein kinase C (PKC), and the IP$_3$ activates a receptor on microsomal vesicles that directs the movement of calcium from microsomal vesicles into the cytosol.

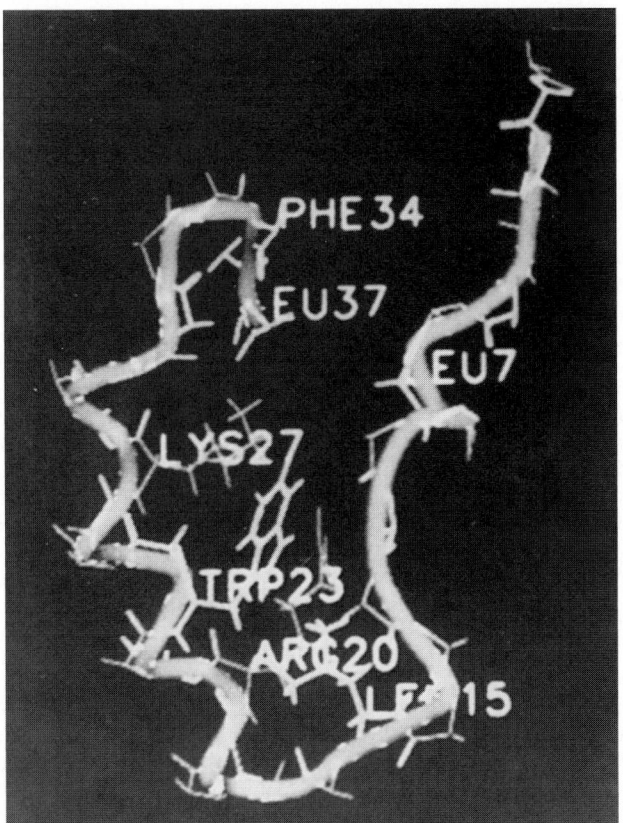

Figure 24–11. Structure of the peptide backbone of human PTH(1–37) determined by magnetic resonance spectroscopy. The activation domain of PTH consists of a short alpha helix (residues 5–10) flanked by a disordered amino-terminal region (residues 1–4) and a flexible link (residues 11–13) joined to a well-defined turn (residues 14–17). Residues 17–28 form an alpha helix that interacts with the turn in such a way that the two helices are folded near each other. (From Marx UC, Austermann S, Bayer P, et al. Structure of human parathyroid hormone 1–37 in solution. J Biol Chem 1995; 270:15194–15202, with permission.)

PTHrP receptor does, in fact, mediate the actions of PTH in bone and kidney.

SECOND MESSENGERS AND DISTAL EFFECTS OF PTH. The activation of multiple G proteins by PTH[104–106] raises questions about the individual roles of each second messenger and their possible interactions. The importance of cyclic AMP as a mediator of the physiological actions of PTH has been demonstrated by studies in vivo[88, 135–137] and in vitro.[138–141] Further, patients with pseudohypoparathyroidism type 1, who fail to increase urinary cyclic AMP levels in response to PTH, exhibit renal resistance to PTH (see later).

Phospholipase C, with concomitant activation of protein kinase C and synthesis of IP$_3$, may mediate physiological actions of PTH as well,[142] such as inhibition of sodium-phosphate cotransport[143] and stimulation of the renal 25(OH)D 1α-hydroxylase.[144] Some actions of PTH may require activation of both adenylate cyclase and phospholipase C for optimal effects.

TARGET CELL RESPONSIVENESS TO PTH. Physiological responses depend on the concentration of PTH in blood and on the responsiveness of target cells to PTH. This responsiveness can be modified by prior exposure to PTH or by exposure to other hormones and paracrine factors. Responsiveness can be changed by alterations at virtually every step in the cellular response to PTH.

Major regulators of PTH/PTHrP receptor gene expression include, not surprisingly, PTH and 1,25(OH)$_2$D, both of which can decrease PTH/PTHrP receptor mRNA in certain

target cells.[145–148] In some settings, PTH decreases the amount of immunoreactive and functional receptor on the cell surface without changing the levels of PTH/PTHrP mRNA.[149, 150] Presumably, this decrease reflects ligand-induced internalization and degradation of receptors. Internalization of receptor is stimulated by PTH binding[151] and is modulated by sequences found in the membrane-proximal portion of the receptor's cytoplasmic tail.[152] Even without change in receptor number, prior exposure to PTH leads to inefficient triggering of G proteins (desensitization).[150]

Parathyroid Hormone–Related Protein

PTHrP was discovered because the secretion of PTHrP by a wide variety of tumors contributes to the humoral hypercalcemia of malignancy. For this reason the initial studies of PTHrP in humans and animals stressed the PTH-like structure and properties of the molecule. Subsequent studies soon showed, however, that PTHrP, unlike PTH, is made by a wide variety of normal tissues, in which it acts locally in ways that may have little relevance to the control of blood calcium.

Gene and Protein Structure

PTHrP sequences from human, rat, mouse, dog, and chicken have been cloned[10, 153–158] (Fig. 24–12). In humans, alternative RNA splicing yields transcripts that encode three distinct proteins of 139, 141, and 173 residues that differ only after residue 139. Inspection of these sequences suggests that PTHrP has several functionally distinct domains. Eight or nine of the first 13 residues of PTHrP are identical to those in known mammalian PTH sequences. These sequences encompass the known "activation" domain of PTH (see earlier) and are instrumental in the ability of PTHrP to activate PTH/PTHrP receptors. The conserved histidine at position 5 of all

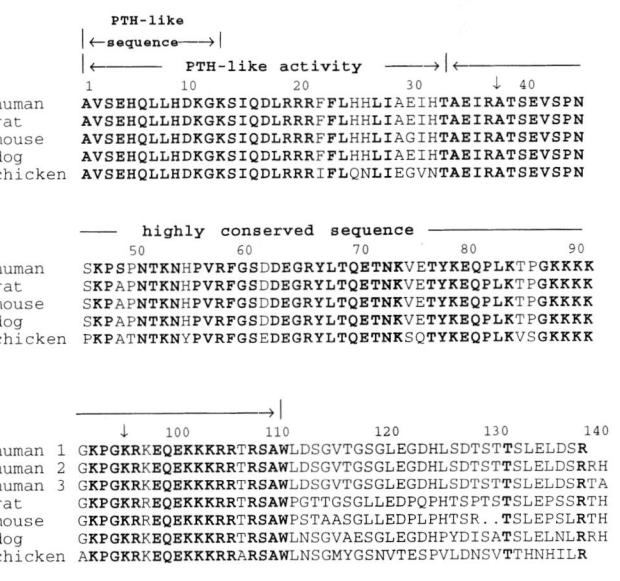

Figure 24–12. Sequences of parathyroid hormone–related protein from five species. Completely conserved residues are in boldface; note the high level of conservation through residue 111. Arrows indicate sites of internal cleavage after residues 37 and 95, which lead to generation of PTHrP(38–94) amide and PTHrP(38–95). Another site of cleavage, generating PTHrP(38–101) and perhaps PTHrP(107–139), is not shown in the figure.[165] The three human sequences represent proteins synthesized from alternatively spliced mRNAs and differ only after residue 139. Amino acids are indicated by the single letter code (see the legend to Figure 24–3 for code).

PTHrP molecules, which differ from the hydrophobic residue found at the corresponding position in all PTHs, allows PTHrP to activate the PTH/PTHrP receptor but not the PTH-specific PTH2 receptor.[159]

The sequences in PTHrP(14–34) are also highly conserved. Although these sequences have little resemblance to the corresponding region of PTH, they can displace PTH from the PTH/PTHrP receptor.[160, 161] Studies of the secondary and tertiary structures of PTHrP(1–34) and PTH(1–37) suggest that a flexible region at the end of the common activation domain of each peptide allows the carboxyl-terminal structures to fold back on and contact the amino-terminal domains.[127, 162]

The remaining portion of the PTHrP molecule bears no resemblance to corresponding sequences in PTH. Nevertheless, residues 35–111 of PTHrP are highly conserved, with only 9 residues varying among known mammalian and chicken PTHrP sequences. This sequence conservation is greater than that in the carboxyl-terminal portion of PTH and suggests that this region of PTHrP has unique and important functions. After residue 111, the PTHrP sequences vary considerably from species to species.

Interspersed within the PTHrP sequences are multiple sites containing one or several basic residues that might serve as post-translational cleavage sites (see Fig. 24–12), and analyses of PTHrP fragments in tumors, cell lines, and transfected cells have shown that several of these sites are, in fact, functional cleavage signals.[163] Cleavage of PTHrP after the arginine at residue 37,[164] followed by carboxyl-peptidase cleavage, generates a PTH-like 1–36 fragment and the fragments PTHrP(38–94)amide, PTHrP(38–95), and PTHrP(38–101).[165] Additional carboxyl-terminal fragments of PTHrP have also been detected in cells.

In the blood of patients with humoral hypercalcemia of malignancy, multiple immunoreactive species of PTHrP may correspond to the fragments of PTHrP found in cells and tissue culture media, although precise characterization of these various species is incomplete (see later).[166–168] Full-length PTHrP may not circulate, since an amino-terminal–specific immunoaffinity column was unable to extract carboxyl-terminal immunoreactivity from the serum of patients with malignant hypercalcemia.[168]

Functions of PTHrP

The first actions of PTHrP to be defined were the PTH-like actions associated with the humoral hypercalcemia of malignancy. In this circumstance PTHrP functions as a hormone; it is secreted from the tumor into the bloodstream and then acts on bone and kidney to raise calcium levels[169–171] (see the section on malignant hypercalcemia). Whether PTHrP circulates at high enough levels in normal adults to contribute to normal calcium homeostasis is an unanswered question.

However, PTHrP acts as a calciotropic hormone during fetal life and during lactation. PTHrP secreted from the fetal parathyroid gland stimulates transport of calcium across the placenta in sheep,[172, 173] whereas PTH has no effect on placental calcium transport. Further, fetal mice missing the PTHrP gene transport ^{45}Ca across the placenta inefficiently.[174]

A second humoral action of PTHrP is in lactation. Secretion of PTHrP from the breast into the bloodstream may promote the movement of calcium from maternal bone into breast milk.[175–180] An exaggeration of the lactational role of PTHrP may explain the rare development of hypercalcemia and high PTHrP levels in pregnant and lactating women.[181–183] Large amounts of PTHrP are also secreted into breast milk, although its role in milk is unknown.

Most of the actions of PTHrP are likely to be paracrine or autocrine.[184] During fetal life PTHrP is synthesized at one time or another in virtually every tissue. Its role in the development of fetal bone has been established by showing that genetically engineered mice missing the PTHrP gene have striking bone defects.[185] These findings suggest that PTHrP normally delays the differentiation of growth plate chondrocytes and allows them to proliferate and form orderly columns of cells. The role of PTHrP in many other fetal tissues may similarly involve regulation of proliferation and differentiation. The widespread expression of the PTHrP in fetal life may explain the expression of PTHrP in a wide variety of malignancies. As is often the case in malignancy, the expression of PTHrP represents the reinitiation of a fetal pattern of gene expression.

PTHrP is also synthesized by many adult tissues.[184] In tissues such as skin and hair, PTHrP may regulate cell proliferation and differentiation.[186, 187] PTHrP is also synthesized in response to stretching the smooth muscle of blood vessels, the gastrointestinal tract, uterus, and bladder and acts in an autocrine fashion to relax smooth muscle. PTHrP is also widely expressed in neurons of the central nervous system; its function in the brain is unknown.

Calcitonin

Calcitonin functions to regulate blood calcium in fish and has a demonstrable role in rodents, but the role of calcitonin in human calcium homeostasis is uncertain. The existence of a second calcium-regulating hormone, in addition to PTH, was first demonstrated during perfusion studies of the thyroid and parathyroid glands of dogs.[188] High calcium perfusion resulted in a rapid decrease in plasma calcium, even more rapid than that after parathyroidectomy. This finding suggested that calcium had stimulated the secretion of a hormone that lowered blood calcium. It was subsequently demonstrated that this hormone, named calcitonin for its role in regulating the "tone" or level of calcium, was elaborated by the thyroid gland, not the parathyroids.[189] Calcitonin is found in nonfollicular cells of the thyroid, called C cells, which have an embryologic origin from the neural crest.[190, 191] In fish, the location of the C cells in distinct organs called the ultimobranchial bodies led to the rapid isolation of calcitonin from the ultimobranchial bodies of dogfish,[192] salmon,[193] and several other species for sequence analysis[194, 195] and studies of its structure and biologic function.

Synthesis and Secretion

Calcitonin is a 32-amino-acid polypeptide with an intrachain disulfide bond provided by the cysteines at positions 1 and 7 (Fig. 24–13). These two cysteine residues, along with the carboxyl-terminal proline amide and six additional residues, are the only amino acids conserved among the calcitonins from various species.[196] The disulfide linkage and proline amide residues are important for the function of the molecule, although biologically active analogues lacking disulfide bonds have been developed. Interestingly, fish calcitonin is more potent in mammals than is the mammalian hormone. The mature peptide is derived from a 136-amino-acid precursor.[197] The human calcitonin gene on the short arm of chromosome 11[198] contains six exons that are alternatively spliced in a tissue-specific manner to yield the mRNAs encoding calcitonin or calcitonin gene-related peptide (CGRP; Fig. 24–14). The mRNA encoding calcitonin is derived by splicing together the first four exons[199] and represents more than 95% of mature transcripts in the thyroid C cells. The splicing of the first three exons to exons five and six results in an mRNA that encodes the 37-amino-acid α-CGRP peptide. The mRNA encoding α-CGRP is expressed in multiple tissues and is the only mature transcript of the calcitonin gene in neural tissue. A

Figure 24–13. The amino acid sequences of calcitonin, CGRP, and amylin and adrenomedullin (ADM) from selected species. The bold Cs represent the cysteine residues that form the disulfide linkages critical for the secondary structure of these peptides. The other residues conserved among species are indicated by a dashed line. The single letter amino acid code is indicated in the legend to Figure 24–3.

Peptide	Species	Sequence
Calcitonin	human	**C**GNLST**C**MLGTYTQDFNKFHTFPQTAIGVGAP -NH₂
	Salmon-1	**C**S----**C**V--KLS-ELH-LQTY-R-NT-SGT- -NH₂
	Salmon-2	**C**S----**C**V--KLS-DLH-LQTF-R-NT-AGV- -NH₂
	Salmon-3	**C**S----**C**M--KLS-DLH-LQTF-R-NT-AGV- -NH₂
CGRP	Human-α	A**C**DTAT**C**VTHRLAGLLSRSGGVVKNNFVPTNVGSKAF -NH₂
	Human-β	-**C**N---**C**------GL-S-----VKS----------- -NH₂
	Salmon	-**C**N---**C**------DF-N-----GNS----------- -NH₂
Amylin	Human	A**C**DTAT**C**VTHRLAGLLSRSGGVVKNNFVPTNVGSKAF -NH₂
ADM	Human	YRQSMNNFQGLRSFG**C**RFGTC**C**TVQKLAHQIYQFTDKDKDNVAPRSKISPQGY -NH₂

second CGRP gene encodes the closely related β-CGRP. In humans, the predicted sequence of β-CGRP differs from that of α-CGRP by only three amino acids (see Fig. 24–13). The β-CGRP gene is also located on chromosome 11[198] and is expressed in essentially the same tissues as α-CGRP.

The synthesis and secretion of calcitonin are tightly regulated, and in the pig there is a linear relationship between the secretion of calcitonin and ambient calcium levels.[200] Cell culture studies with calcium ionophores and calcium channel blockers demonstrate that the calcium ion concentration within the C cell determines this secretion rate.[201, 202] The calcium sensor expressed in parathyroid cells is also found in C cells;[203] this receptor may therefore regulate the secretion of calcitonin as well. Other calcitonin secretagogues include glucocorticoids, CGRP, glucagon, enteroglucagon, gastrin, pentagastrin, pancreozymin, and β-adrenergic agents.[204, 205] The physiological role of the gastrointestinal hormones in regulating calcitonin remains unclear, although they may play a role in the regulation of postprandial hypercalcemia. The secretion of calcitonin is inhibited by somatostatin, which is also secreted by the thyroidal C cells.[206, 207] In vivo[208] and in vitro[209, 210] studies have demonstrated that 1,25(OH)₂D de-

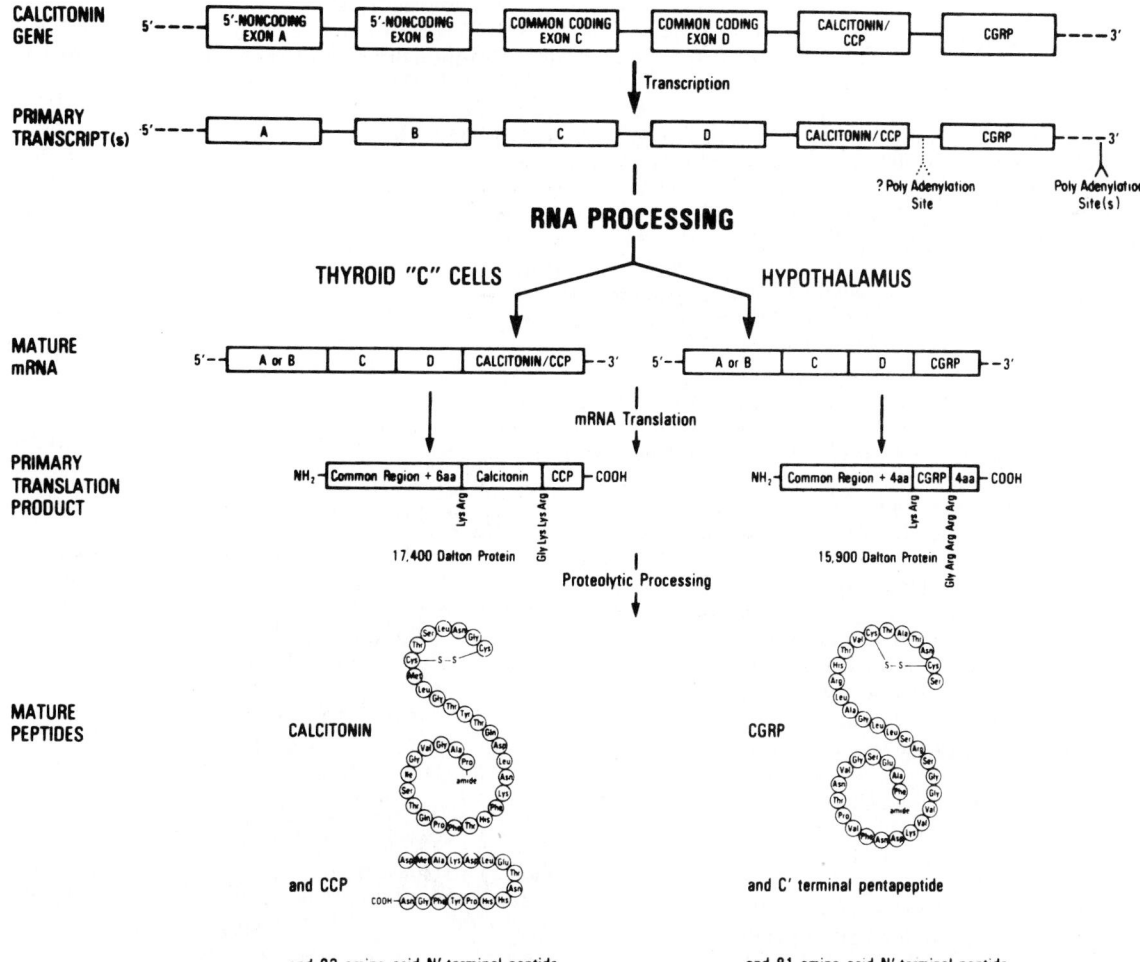

Figure 24–14. Tissue-specific expression of the calcitonin gene. Splicing of alternative exons leads to two different mRNAs. The mRNA encoding calcitonin is found predominantly in the thyroid C cell; the mRNA encoding CGRP is found predominantly in the hypothalamus and other nervous tissue. (From Amara SG, Jonas V, Rosenfeld MG, et al. Alternative RNA processing in calcitonin gene expression generates mRNAs encoding different polypeptide products. Nature 1982; 298:240–244. Copyright 1982, Macmillan Magazines Ltd.)

creases calcitonin mRNA levels by inhibiting transcription of the gene.

Calcitonin has several effects on calcium handling by the kidney[211] and impairs osteoclast-mediated bone resorption by a direct action on osteoclasts.[212] In rodents, calcitonin plays a role in the regulation of postprandial hypercalcemia.[213] The physiological role of calcitonin in humans, however, remains elusive. The effect of calcitonin on bone density was examined in patients with long-term hypercalcitoninemia secondary to medullary carcinoma of the thyroid (MCT) and in patients with subtotal thyroidectomy resulting in lack of calcitonin secretory reserve;[214] bone density at the lumbar spine and distal radius were not influenced by calcitonin levels. Furthermore, no physiological abnormalities have been reported with long-term, high-dose administration of exogenous calcitonin.[215]

Calcitonin acts by binding to a G protein–coupled cell surface receptor of the PTH-secretin receptor family.[216] The mRNA encoding this receptor is present in many tissues, including kidney, brain, and osteoclasts. The coupling of this receptor to different G proteins results in the activation of either adenylate cyclase or phospholipase C; in some settings, the choice of second messenger pathway is cell cycle dependent.[217] Several isoforms of the calcitonin receptor have been described,[218–222] the functional significance of which is not known. The receptor is widely expressed[223, 224] and binds CGRP and amylin as well.

Calcitonin Family: CGRP, Amylin, and Adrenomedullin

CGRP is thought to act as a neurotransmitter rather than as a hormone. Immunohistochemical studies in the brain and peripheral nervous system suggest that CGRP plays an important role in sensory and integrative motor functions.[225] CGRP is also a potent vasodilator. CGRP receptors have been identified by radioligand binding assays in the nervous system,[226] and one CGRP receptor has been cloned.[227]

Amylin, also known as IAPP (islet amyloid polypeptide), binds to the cloned porcine calcitonin receptor and stimulates the production of cAMP.[228] The physiological significance of the interaction of amylin with the calcitonin receptor is unclear. Amylin is highly homologous to CGRP and calcitonin (see Fig. 24–13). The increased amylin in the pancreas of patients with type II diabetes mellitus suggests an etiologic role for this peptide in this disorder.[229, 230]

Adrenomedullin (see Fig. 24–13) has vasodilatory effects similar to those of CGRP. In addition to activating CGRP receptors, adrenomedullin binds to specific receptors in the heart and lungs.[231] The physiological roles of CGRP, amylin, and adrenomedullin and the functional correlates of their receptor interactions have not yet been established.[231]

Calcitonin in Human Disease

Calcitonin is secreted by several endocrine malignancies and therefore can serve as a tumor marker. The measurement of basal and pentagastrin-stimulated calcitonin levels has been used to identify and follow those at risk or affected by medullary carcinoma of the thyroid (see Chapter 32), although basal and stimulated levels may also be high in patients on chronic hemodialysis.[232] Calcitonin can be secreted ectopically by other tumors, including insulinomas,[233] VIPomas,[234] and lung cancers.[235] Severely ill patients, including those with burn inhalation injury,[236] toxic shock syndrome,[237] and pancreatitis,[238] may also have elevated calcitonin levels.

Therapeutic Uses

The fact that calcitonin inhibits osteoclastic bone resorption has led to its therapeutic use for the treatment of several disorders associated with excess bone resorption, including osteoporosis and Paget's disease (see Chapter 25). Calcitonin has an analgesic effect in patients with vertebral crush fractures, osteolytic metastases, or phantom limb.[239, 240]

Vitamin D (Calciferols)

Metabolism of Vitamin D

Vitamin D is not a true vitamin, since nutritional supplementation is not required in humans who have adequate exposure to sunlight. When exposed to ultraviolet irradiation, the cutaneous precursor of vitamin D, 7-dehydrocholesterol, undergoes photochemical cleavage of the carbon bond between carbons 9 and 10 of the steroid ring (Fig. 24–15). The resultant product, previtamin D, is thermally labile and over a period of 48 h undergoes a temperature-dependent molecular rearrangement that results in the production of vitamin D.[241] Alternatively, this product can isomerize to two biologically inert products, lumisterol and tachysterol. This alternative photoisomerization may prevent production of excessive amounts of vitamin D with prolonged sun exposure. In addition, the degree of skin pigmentation, which increases in response to solar exposure, regulates the conversion of 7-dehydrocholesterol to vitamin D by influencing the penetration of ultraviolet rays.

The alternative source of vitamin D is dietary. The elderly, the institutionalized, and those living in northern climates

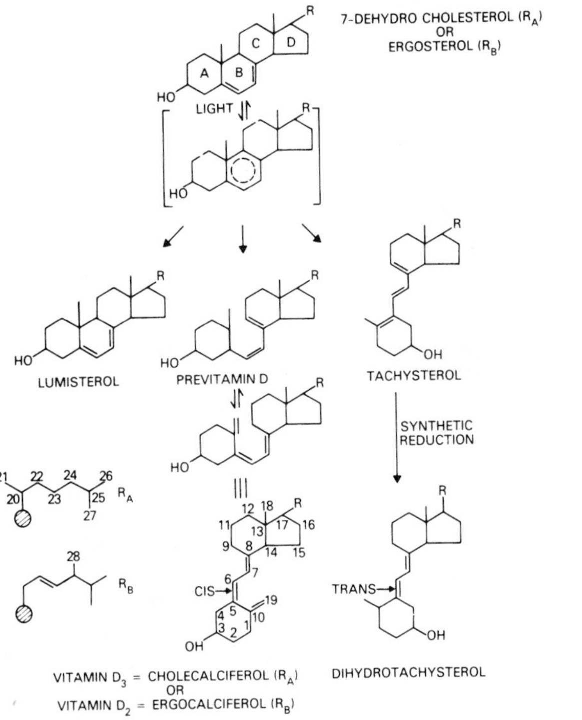

Figure 24–15. Vitamin D precursors and alternative reaction products. The numbering system for vitamin D carbons and the distinct structures of vitamin D_2 and D_3 are noted, as is the structure of dihydrotachysterol, a synthetic product not produced in vivo. Note that the 3-hydroxyl group of dihydrotachysterol is in a pseudo-1-hydroxyl configuration. This configuration may explain the relatively high potency of dihydrotachysterol in conditions associated with low 1-hydroxylase activity. (From Aurbach GD, Marx SJ, Spiegel AM. Parathyroid hormone, calcitonin, and the calciferols. In: Wilson JD, Foster DW, eds. Williams Textbook of Endocrinology. 8th ed. Philadelphia: WB Saunders, 1992: 1421, with permission.)

probably obtain most of their vitamin D from dietary sources. However, with the increasing use of sunscreens, dietary sources of vitamin D have become a more important source for the general population as well. The principal dietary sources of vitamin D are fortified dairy products, although the lack of monitoring of supplementation results in marked variation in the amount of vitamin D provided.[242] Other dietary sources include egg yolks, fish oils, and fortified cereal products. Vitamin D provided by plant sources is in the form of vitamin D_2, which has the side chain of plant sterols, whereas that provided by animal sources is in the form of vitamin D_3, which has the cholesterol side chain. These two forms have equivalent biologic potencies and are activated equally efficiently by the hydroxylases in humans, and the term *vitamin D* is used in this chapter to indicate either or both vitamins D_2 and D_3.

Vitamin D is absorbed into the lymphatics and enters the circulation bound primarily to vitamin D–binding protein, although a fraction of vitamin D circulates bound to albumin. The vitamin D–binding protein is an α-globulin, with a molecular mass of approximately 52 kd, that is synthesized in the liver. The protein has a high affinity for 25-hydroxyvitamin D (25(OH)D) but also binds vitamin D and 1,25-dihydroxyvitamin D (1,25(OH)$_2$D). Approximately 88% of 25(OH)D circulates bound to the vitamin D–binding protein, 0.03% is free, and the rest circulates bound to albumin.[243] Similarly 85% of the circulating 1,25(OH)$_2$D binds to the vitamin D–binding protein, 0.4% is free, and the rest binds to albumin.[244]

In the liver vitamin D undergoes 25-hydroxylation by a cytochrome P450 (CYP) enzyme in the mitochondria and microsomes. The half-life of 25(OH)D is approximately 2 to 3 wk. The 25-hydroxylation of vitamin D is not tightly regulated, and the blood levels of 25(OH)D reflect the amount of vitamin D entering the circulation. When levels of the vitamin D–binding protein are low, such as in nephrotic syndrome, circulating levels of 25(OH)D are also reduced. The half-life of 25(OH)D is shortened by increases in levels of its active metabolite, 1,25(OH)$_2$D.

The final step in the production of the active hormone is the 1α-hydroxylation of 25(OH)D to 1,25(OH)$_2$D in the kidney. The half-life of this hormone is approximately 6 to 8 h. Like the 25-hydroxylase, the 1α-hydroxylase in the proximal convoluted tubule is a CYP mixed-function oxidase, but unlike the 25-hydroxylase, the 1α-hydroxylase is tightly regulated. PTH and hypophosphatemia are the major inducers of this microsomal enzyme,[245] whereas calcium and the enzyme product 1,25(OH)$_2$D repress its activity. In animal models and in vitro studies, other hormones, such as estrogen, calcitonin,

growth hormone, and prolactin, increase 1α-hydroxylase activity, but the clinical importance of these observations has not been established. Ketoconazole decreases levels of 1,25(OH)$_2$D in a dose-dependent manner, presumably by interfering with 1α-hydroxylase activity.[246]

1α-hydroxylase activity is also found in the trophoblastic layer of the placenta,[247] some lymphomas,[248] and sarcoidosis and other granulomata.[249] In malignant and granulomatous tissue, the 1α-hydroxylase is not regulated by PTH, phosphate, calcium, or vitamin D metabolites. Activation of macrophages with interferon γ, however, stimulates the production of 1,25(OH)$_2$D, whereas treatment of sarcoidosis-associated hypercalcemia with glucocorticoids, ketoconazole,[250] or chloroquine[251] lowers serum 1,25(OH)$_2$D levels.

25(OH)D and 1,25(OH)$_2$D can also be hydroxylated by the vitamin D 24-hydroxylase in most tissues including kidney, cartilage, and intestine.[252] 1,24,25-trihydroxyvitamin D is not thought to play major biologic roles other than inactivation of 1,25(OH)$_2$D.[253] While 24,25(OH)$_2$D has actions in a number of biologic systems,[254, 255] no receptor for this metabolite has been identified, and its role in human physiology remains unclear. 1,25(OH)$_2$D increases the activity of the 24-hydroxylase, thereby inducing its own metabolism.

1,25(OH)$_2$D is also metabolized to several inactive products by 23- or 26-hydroxylation and by side-chain oxidation and cleavage. Side-chain cleavage that results in the formation of calcitroic acid occurs in the liver and intestine, whereas inactivation of 1,25(OH)$_2$D in many target tissues occurs by 24-hydroxylation. Polar metabolites of 1,25(OH)$_2$D are excreted in the bile, and some of these metabolites are deconjugated in the intestine and reabsorbed into the enterohepatic recirculation.[256]

Actions of Vitamin D

VITAMIN D RECEPTORS

1,25(OH)$_2$D accomplishes its biologic functions by binding to a nuclear receptor,[257] which then regulates transcription of RNA. The vitamin D receptor most closely resembles the retinoic acid, triiodothyronine, and retinoid-X (RXR) receptors (see Chapter 4). The affinity of the receptor for 1,25(OH)$_2$D is approximately three orders of magnitude higher than that for other vitamin D metabolites. Although 25(OH)D is less potent on a molar basis, its concentration in the serum is approximately three orders of magnitude higher than that of 1,25(OH)$_2$D (Fig. 24–16) and its free concentration is two orders of magnitude greater than that of

Figure 24–16. Relative potency of analogues of 1,25(OH)$_2$D$_3$ in competitive binding to vitamin D receptors of chick intestinal mucosa. (From Proscal DA, Okamura WH, Norman AW. Structural requirements for the interaction of 1α,25-(OH)$_2$-vitamin D$_3$ with its chick intestinal system. J Biol Chem 1975; 250:8382–8388, with permission.)

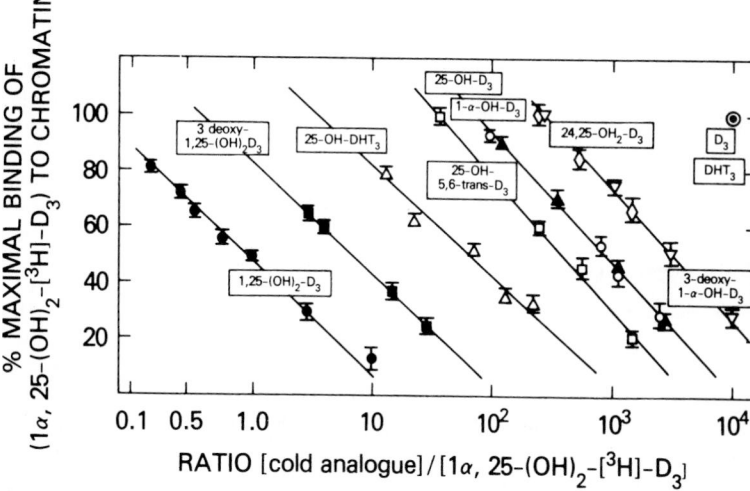

1,25(OH)$_2$D. Therefore, in normal circumstances it is unlikely that 25(OH)D makes any important contribution to calcium homeostasis. In vitamin D intoxication, however, 25(OH)D may well have direct hypercalcemic actions. Furthermore, because the affinity of the vitamin D–binding protein in serum for 25(OH)D is greater than for 1,25(OH)$_2$D, the free levels of 1,25(OH)$_2$D may increase in states of vitamin D intoxication[258] because 25(OH)D displaces it from the vitamin D–binding protein. 25(OH)D may therefore play a role in the clinical syndrome of vitamin D intoxication both by its direct biologic effects, when present at toxic levels, and by increasing free levels of 1,25(OH)$_2$D.

The vitamin D receptor forms a heterodimer with the retinoid-X receptor, and the heterodimer binds to specific DNA sequences in the 5′-regulatory region of target genes to control 1,25(OH)$_2$D-dependent RNA transcription.[259] The up-regulatory response elements for vitamin D contain hexameric repeats separated by three bases[260–264] (Fig. 24–17). In contrast, the mechanism of transcriptional repression by vitamin D remains poorly understood.

In addition to binding 1,25(OH)$_2$D, DNA, and the RXR receptor, the vitamin D receptor also undergoes a ligand-dependent phosphorylation that is thought to be necessary for its biologic activity.[265] The carboxyl-terminal region of the vitamin D receptor interacts with the basal transcription apparatus by directly contacting the transcription factor, TFIIB,[266] presumably an interaction that leads to initiation of gene transcription.

Glucocorticoids[267] decrease the expression of the vitamin D receptor gene in osteosarcoma cell lines, whereas 1,25(OH)$_2$D increases its expression in many cells. In the renal proximal convoluted tubule, however, 1,25(OH)$_2$D decreases the level of vitamin D receptors. This decrease has been postulated to decrease activation of the renal 24-hydroxylase by 1,25(OH)$_2$D and thereby protect newly synthesized 1,25(OH)$_2$D from local inactivation.[268]

1,25(OH)$_2$D also has some biologic effects that occur too rapidly to involve transcriptional mechanisms. These "nongenomic actions" include the rapid increase in intracellular calcium, activation of phospholipase C, and opening of calcium channels observed in several cell types within minutes of exposure to 1,25(OH)$_2$D.[269] Additional evidence for nongenomic actions that do not involve the classic receptor include the identification of specific binding sites for 1,25(OH)$_2$D on the antiluminal surface of intestinal cells[270] and a disparity between the affinity of the various vitamin D analogues for the nuclear receptor and their potency in these nongenomic actions.[271] At least one of the nongenomic actions, the rapid intracellular accumulation of cGMP in association with the vitamin D receptor, is dependent on the presence of an intact intracellular receptor, since this effect does not occur in cells from patients with vitamin D receptor mutations.[272] The physiological importance of the nongenomic actions of vitamin D metabolites is not established.

The vitamin D receptor is expressed in most tissues and regulates cellular differentiation and function in many cell types. However, the most dramatic physiological effects of vitamin D, acting through the vitamin D receptor, involve regulation of intestinal calcium transport. This is most clearly demonstrated by the phenotype of patients with mutant vitamin D receptors (vitamin D–dependent rickets type II).[273] In these patients, profound abnormalities in bone mineralization can be reversed by administration of intravenous calcium.

INTESTINAL CALCIUM ABSORPTION

Under normal dietary conditions, calcium intake is in the range of 700 to 900 mg/d, about 30 to 35% of which is absorbed; however, because of losses from intestinal secretion of calcium, net daily uptake is approximately 200 mg.[274] Although vitamin D is the major hormonal determinant of intestinal calcium absorption, the bioavailability of mineral ions in the intestinal lumen is also affected by local factors and dietary constituents. Absorption of calcium and magnesium is impaired by bile salt deficiency, unabsorbed free fatty acids in malabsorption states, and high dietary content of fiber or phytate, each of which alters the relation between total and ionized intraluminal calcium. Gastric acid is needed to promote dissociation of calcium from anionic components of food or therapeutic preparations of calcium salts. Administration of calcium salts with meals, especially in achlorhydrics, and use of divided doses or more soluble salts such as calcium citrate may increase calcium bioavailability.

Calcium is absorbed by three pathways: the transcellular route, vesicular calcium transport, and paracellular transport. The first two pathways are dependent on 1,25(OH)$_2$D. Although the necessity of vitamin D for paracellular calcium absorption remains controversial, the hormone probably enhances this pathway as well.[275, 276] The vesicular pathway is thought to involve the nongenomic actions of 1,25(OH)$_2$D.[277, 278] However, this rapid transport, referred to as transcaltachia, occurs only in vitamin D–replete animals. The relative contribution of vesicular calcium transport to intestinal calcium absorption and the specific mediators are unknown.

The most extensively studied mechanism of intestinal calcium absorption is the transcellular route, which involves three steps: entry of calcium into the enterocyte, transport across the cell, and extrusion across the basolateral membrane.

ENTRY INTO THE ENTEROCYTE. A number of brush border proteins, including the intestinal membrane calcium-binding protein, brush border alkaline phosphatase, and low affinity Ca, Mg ATPase are induced by 1,25(OH)$_2$D. The activity of these proteins correlates with active calcium transport, but a causal relationship remains to be established.[279] On entering the enterocyte, presumably through calcium channels, calcium binds to components of the brush border complex adjacent to the plasma membrane.[280] Calmodulin is redistributed to the brush border in response to 1,25(OH)$_2$D and may play a role in this process, as may the 1,25(OH)$_2$D-inducible calcium-binding protein, calbindin.[281]

TRANSCELLULAR TRANSPORT. The best studied effect of vitamin D on the enterocyte is induction of the synthesis of the intestinal calcium-binding protein, calbindin$_{9K}$. This protein binds two calcium ions per molecule.[282] The affinity of calbindin for calcium is approximately four times that of the brush border calcium-binding components,[280] so that calcium is preferentially transferred to calbindin. Calbindin buffers the intracellular free calcium concentration during calcium absorption. It is found in association with microtubules and may play a role in the transport of calcium across the enterocyte. In states of high dietary calcium intake, organelles such as the mitochondria, Golgi apparatus, and endoplasmic reticulum also serve as repositories for intracellular calcium.

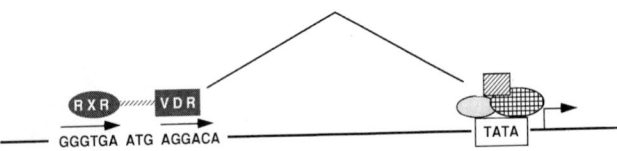

Figure 24–17. Transcriptional activation by 1,25(OH)$_2$D. A heterodimer of retinoid X receptor (RXR) and vitamin D receptor (VDR) binds to a pair of hexameric sequences separated by three intervening bases (ATG). The arrows indicate that the hexamers, found in the up-regulated rat osteocalcin gene, are variants of a consensus sequence repeated here with identical orientations (direct repeats). On binding to DNA, the RXR-VDR heterodimer facilitates formation of a transcription initiation complex, which binds to DNA at and near the TATA sequence.

EXIT FROM THE ENTEROCYTE. The transport of calcium across the antiluminal surface of the enterocyte, the final process involved in intestinal calcium absorption, is dependent on 1,25(OH)$_2$D. The main mechanism of calcium extrusion is the 1,25(OH)$_2$D inducible ATP-dependent Ca^{2+} pump.[283] The affinity of the pump for calcium is approximately 2.5 times that of calbindin.[280] With high calcium intake, a 1,25(OH)$_2$D-independent Na$^+$/Ca^{2+} exchanger may also play a role in the transfer of calcium across the basolateral membrane.[284]

ACTIONS ON THE PARATHYROID GLAND

1,25(OH)$_2$D inhibits the proliferation of dispersed parathyroid cells in culture, although the relative contribution of calcium and 1,25(OH)$_2$D in the regulation of parathyroid cell proliferation in vivo has not been established. 1,25(OH)$_2$D has been shown to decrease the transcription of the PTH gene both in vivo and in vitro.[35-37] This action has been exploited in the use of 1,25(OH)$_2$D in the treatment of the secondary hyperparathyroidism associated with chronic renal failure (see the sections on parathyroid hormone biosynthesis and vitamin D deficiency).

ACTIONS ON BONE

The effects of 1,25(OH)$_2$D on bone are numerous. 1,25(OH)$_2$D is a major transcriptional regulator of the two most abundant bone matrix proteins: it represses the synthesis of type I collagen[285] and induces the synthesis of osteocalcin.[286] 1,25(OH)$_2$D stimulates the differentiation of osteoclasts from monocyte-macrophage stem cell precursors in vitro. Vitamin D also increases osteoclastic bone resorption independently of PTH in vitro and in vivo[287, 288] and up-regulates the expression of the osteoclast $\alpha_v\beta_3$ integrin gene.[289] Despite the multiple effects of 1,25(OH)$_2$D on the biology of bone in vitro, in vivo studies in 1,25(OH)$_2$D-deficient rats suggest that the major osseous consequences of 1,25(OH)$_2$D deficiency can be reversed when mineral ion homeostasis is corrected with parenteral calcium and phosphate infusions.[290, 291] In addition, parenteral calcium infusions heal the osteomalacia in children with mutant vitamin D receptors.[292] These observations suggest that the major role of 1,25(OH)$_2$D in bone is to provide the proper microenvironment for bone mineralization through stimulation of the intestinal absorption of calcium and phosphate. Nevertheless the actions of 1,25(OH)$_2$D on bone cells in vitro suggest that there may be subtle changes in the bone matrix composition or in the biomechanical properties of bone in vitamin D deficiency that have not yet been characterized in vivo.

OTHER ACTIONS OF VITAMIN D

The effects of 1,25(OH)$_2$D on phosphate transport are less well studied than those on calcium transport; however, vitamin D does promote the already efficient intestinal phosphate absorption.[293]

An unexplained feature of profound vitamin D deficiency is the severe proximal myopathy.[294] Muscle cells have vitamin D receptors, and 1,25(OH)$_2$D also has nongenomic effects on muscle.[295] Furthermore 1,25(OH)$_2$D increases amino acid uptake and alters phospholipid metabolism in vitro in muscle cells.[294] Vitamin D administration increases the concentration of troponin C, a calcium-binding protein that plays a role in excitation coupling and increases the rate of uptake of calcium by the sarcoplasmic reticulum.[296] However, little is known regarding the direct role of vitamin D in normal muscle physiology. The myopathy of vitamin D deficiency is characterized by normal creatine phosphokinase (CPK) levels, a myopathic electromyogram, and biopsy findings of loss of myofibrils, fatty infiltration, and interstitial fibrosis. The myopathy resolves within days to weeks of vitamin D replacement and is not related to return of mineral ion homeostasis to normal.

VITAMIN D ANALOGUES

The recognition that 1,25(OH)$_2$D promotes cellular differentiation and inhibits cellular proliferation has led to attempts to synthesize analogues that retain these effects but do not cause hypercalcemia. Several analogues exhibit antiproliferative effects in normal cells, in malignant cells in vitro, and in xenografts in immunosuppressed mice.[297-300] In addition, analogues of vitamin D synergized with cyclosporine in preventing rejection of transplanted islet cells in a murine model.[301] One "nonhypercalcemic" analogue, 22-oxacalcitriol, suppresses PTH synthesis and secretion in rats[302] at doses that stimulate intestinal calcium absorption less than 1,25(OH)$_2$D. This suggests that such analogues may be useful in the prevention and treatment of hyperparathyroidism. The antiproliferative effects of vitamin D have been utilized for the treatment of psoriasis.[303] Although analogues with reduced calcemic activity are predominantly used, hypercalcemic crisis can occur after topical use of such compounds.[304]

The physiology underlying the differential biologic effects of these analogues is not completely understood. Altered affinity for the vitamin D–binding protein, metabolism by target tissues,[305] and effects on vitamin D receptor[306-308] may contribute to the unique properties of vitamin D analogues.

Calcium and Phosphate Homeostasis

The cytosolic concentrations of intracellular calcium, phosphorus, and magnesium differ markedly, as reviewed earlier, and their physiological roles within cells are diverse and largely unrelated (see Fig. 24–1). In contrast, the concentrations of these minerals in extracellular fluid are comparable (i.e., 1 to 2 mmol/L), and it is here that they exert effects with cells and with one another that are critical for bone mineralization, neuromuscular function, and normal mineral ion homeostasis. Extracellular calcium and phosphate, in particular, exist so close to the limits of their mutual solubility that stringent regulation of their concentrations is required to avoid diffuse precipitation of calcium phosphate crystals in tissues.

Serum concentrations and total body balances of the mineral ions are maintained within narrow limits by powerful, interactive homeostatic mechanisms. PTH and 1,25(OH)$_2$D regulate mineral ion levels; mineral ion levels regulate PTH and 1,25(OH)$_2$D secretion; and the hormones regulate the production of each other. The operation of these homeostatic mechanisms can be illustrated by considering the following examples of how the organism adapts to changes in calcium loads (Fig. 24–18).

Dietary calcium restriction, for example, causes an increase in the efficiency of intestinal calcium absorption. This results from a sequence of responses in which lowered blood ionized calcium activates secretion of PTH, PTH augments synthesis of 1,25(OH)$_2$D by the proximal tubules of the kidney, and 1,25(OH)$_2$D then acts directly on enterocytes to increase calcium absorption. Enhanced calcium absorption is the most important response to calcium deprivation, but other homeostatic events limit the impact of this stress. Renal tubular calcium reabsorption is increased by PTH and perhaps by hypocalcemia (which deactivates distal tubular calcium sensors), and approximately 15% of the impact of dietary calcium

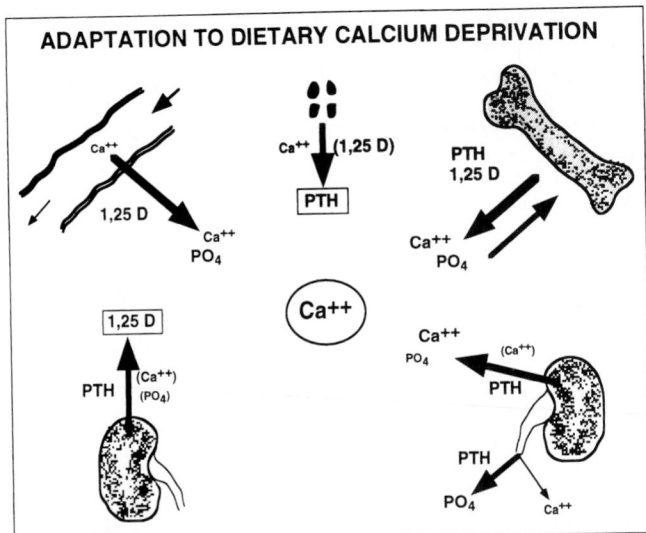

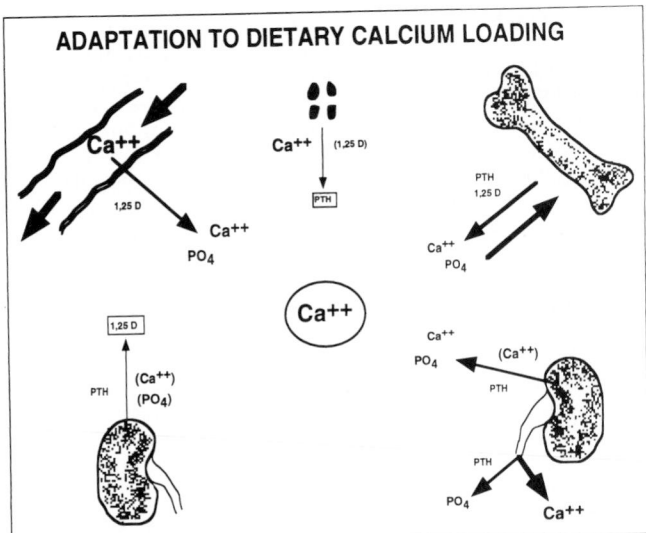

Figure 24–18. Homeostatic responses to variations in dietary calcium content. Major homeostatic responses to dietary calcium deprivation or loading are depicted. Arrow thickness indicates relative activity of transport or secretory mechanisms, whereas amounts of hormones or transported ions are related to the size of their notations. Parentheses indicate an inhibitory regulation. Note that the extracellular calcium concentration is well maintained, although different underlying mechanisms are involved in the two circumstances (see text for details).

deprivation is buffered by release of calcium from bone in response to PTH.

The increase in net bone resorption releases phosphate as well as calcium into the extracellular fluid. Intestinal phosphate absorption also is increased by $1,25(OH)_2D$. The consequences of increased phosphate loads are problematic, because phosphate lowers ionized calcium in extracellular fluid, suppresses renal synthesis of $1,25(OH)_2D$, and inhibits bone resorption. These potentially negative effects of phosphate are mitigated by the powerful phosphaturic action of PTH.

Finally, unrestrained secretion of PTH, leading to excessive bone resorption and severe hypophosphatemia, is prevented by the effects of calcium on PTH secretion and by the direct suppressive effect of $1,25(OH)_2D$ on the synthesis of PTH and of PTH receptors. As a result of these homeostatic responses, calcium-deprived subjects maintain nearly normal serum calcium and phosphate levels but have increased intestinal calcium absorption, increased bone resorption and progressive osteopenia, increased renal tubular calcium reabsorption, decreased renal tubular phosphate reabsorption, low urinary calcium excretion, elevated urinary phosphate excretion, and high serum levels of PTH and $1,25(OH)_2D$.

Calcium loads induce an opposite series of adaptations: parathyroid suppression, inhibition of renal synthesis of $1,25(OH)_2D$, decreased intestinal active transport of calcium, increased renal excretion of calcium and decreased excretion of phosphate (secondary consequences of functional hypoparathyroidism), and a decrease in bone resorption sufficient to allow positive skeletal calcium balance. The decline in intestinal calcium absorption is the major safeguard against calcium overload, although this mechanism may be overridden at extraordinarily high intakes of calcium because of the passive, non–vitamin D–dependent mode of calcium absorption. Moreover, nonenteral sources of calcium, such as intravenous calcium infusion or excessive net bone resorption (e.g., from immobilization, malignancy), may overwhelm the homeostatic adaptations that remain once suppressed intestinal calcium absorption is bypassed. In such situations the kidney, rather than the intestine, is the principal defense against hypercalcemia, and calcium homeostasis is critically dependent on adequate renal function. If renal function is impaired in these

settings, severe hypercalcemia and pathologic calcium deposition in extraskeletal sites may ensue.

Laboratory Assessment of Mineral Metabolism

Parathyroid Hormone

The major challenges in the measurement of blood PTH have been the low levels of circulating PTH and the presence of inactive PTH fragments in far greater abundance than the intact, biologically active PTH molecule. The measurement of inactive fragments would not be a concern if the ratio of inactive to active PTH molecules were constant. However, this ratio changes in response to changes in glomerular filtration rate and parathyroid gland secretory activity (see section on parathyroid hormone secretion and peripheral metabolism of parathyroid hormone, above). Consequently, radioimmunoassays of PTH have suffered from a lack of sensitivity and from the inability to measure the biologically active hormone directly.

For these reasons, two-site assays that require the presence of amino-terminal and carboxyl-terminal sequences of full-length PTH(1–84) on the same molecule have replaced older radioimmunoassays.[309] Reassuringly, assays of this type have very similar normal ranges for blood PTH and are sensitive enough to detect PTH in normal individuals. There is a modest circadian variation in PTH levels and some pulsatility in PTH secretion, but these variations do not interfere with the diagnostic usefulness of randomly drawn PTH measurements. Some studies have reported modest increases of PTH levels with age, although others have not. Unlike older radioimmunoassays, the two-site assays demonstrate virtually no overlap in PTH levels between patients with primary hyperparathyroidism and those with nonparathyroid hypercalcemia (Fig. 24–19). Since this distinction is the most important challenge in the clinical setting, the use of the two-site assay has been particularly useful for establishing the cause of hypercalcemia.

Parathyroid Hormone–Related Protein

The development of clinically useful assays for PTHrP is more difficult than for PTH. The concentration of PTHrP in

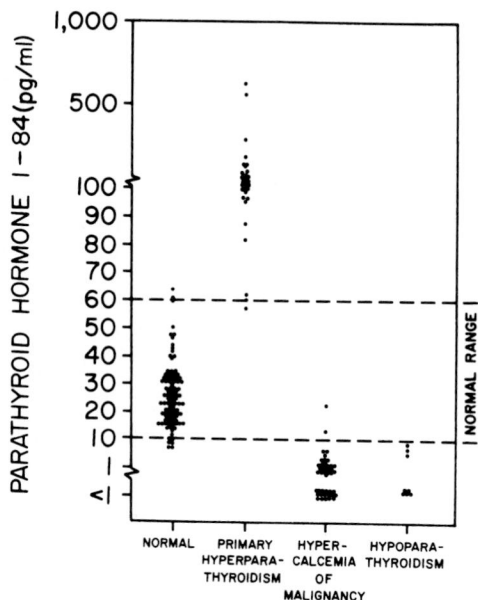

Figure 24–19. Intact immunoreactive PTH determined using a two-site immunoradiometric assay in normal subjects and patient groups. Note some overlap between the normal subjects and the patients with primary hyperparathyroidism, but no overlap between hypercalcemic patients with primary hyperparathyroidism and hypercalcemia of malignancy. (From GV Segre. Advances in techniques for measurement of parathyroid hormone: current applications in clinical medicine and directions for future research. Trends Endocrinol Metab 1990; 1:243–247. Copyright 1990 by Elsevier Science Inc.)

the bloodstream, even in some patients with PTHrP-mediated malignant hypercalcemia, is not high, and the characterization of biologically active fragments is incomplete. Despite these problems, assays for PTHrP can be helpful in the evaluation of a subset of hypercalcemic patients.[310] Radioimmunoassays for amino-terminal portions of PTHrP[311, 312] and two-site assays

for amino-terminal and midregion PTHrP[167, 168, 313] separate normal subjects and patients with nonmalignant hypercalcemia from most patients with the humoral hypercalcemia of malignancy (Fig. 24–20). With the use of the most recent assays, PTHrP levels are elevated in most patients with malignant hypercalcemia without bone metastases and in the majority with hypercalcemia and bony metastases. In occasional patients, the PTHrP assay has helped distinguish occult malignancy from other causes of non-PTH–dependent hypercalcemia.[177] Nevertheless, since the diagnosis of malignancy as the cause of hypercalcemia is usually clinically obvious and since the PTH assay can be used to diagnose primary hyperparathyroidism, the role of PTHrP assays in clinical practice is likely to be limited. Further improvement in assay sensitivity and further insight into the normal functions of circulating PTHrP fragments may change this assessment.

Calcitonin

Assays for measuring serum calcitonin are based on single- or double-antibody radioimmunoassays, several of which are sufficiently sensitive to detect calcitonin deficiency.[314] The calcitonin monomer is thought to be the biologically active molecule; therefore, some investigators believe that extraction of the multimeric forms prior to radioimmunoassay[315] provides a more sensitive and specific measurement of serum calcitonin levels. However, the double-antibody radioimmunoassay is thought by others to provide the same information with less sample manipulation.[316] The only clinical use of the calcitonin assay is as a tumor marker, primarily in medullary carcinoma of the thyroid.

Vitamin D Metabolites

Radioligand assays for determining the levels of vitamin D metabolites require fractionation and extraction of the hormone from serum proteins by high-pressure liquid chromatography (HPLC) or silica cartridges. These assays are sufficiently

Figure 24–20. Plasma PTHrP(1–74) determined by two-site immunoradiometric assay in selected patient groups and normal subjects. Also shown are concentrations of PTHrP in milk (solid circles, human; open circles, bovine). Two normocalcemic patients with cancer (solid filled triangles) subsequently became hypercalcemic. Hatched area denotes levels too low to detect with this assay. (Adapted from Burtis WJ, Brady TG, Orloff JJ, et al. Immunochemical characterization of circulating parathyroid hormone–related protein in patients with humoral hypercalcemia of cancer. N Engl J Med 1990; 322:1106–1112. Copyright 1990. Massachusetts Medical Society. All rights reserved.)

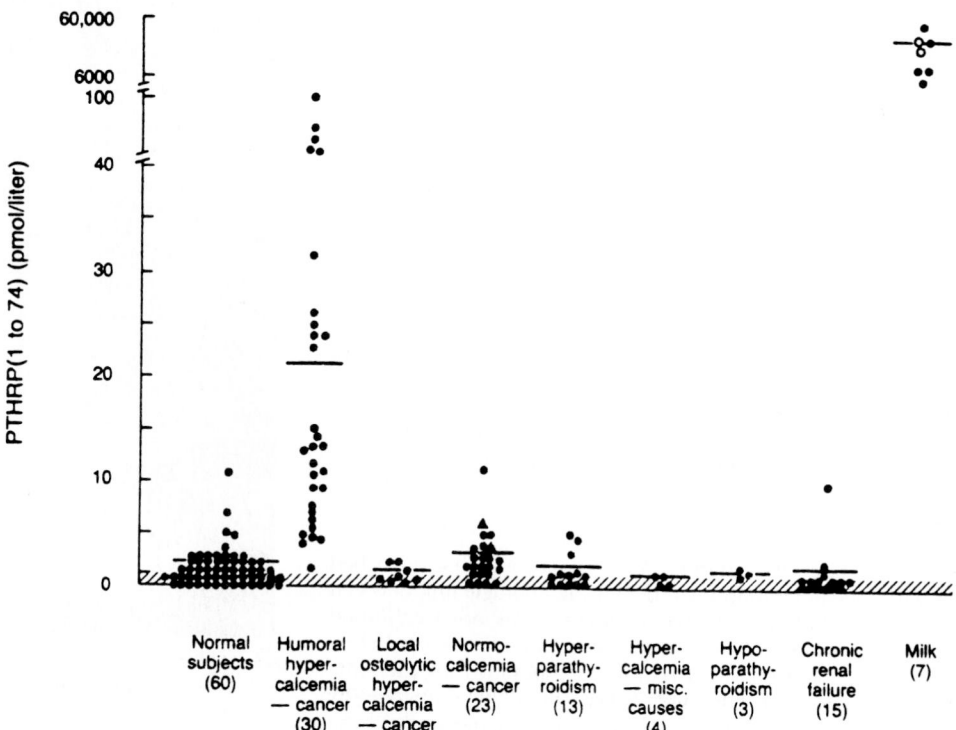

sensitive to detect subnormal values, but because the assays measure both protein-bound and unbound vitamin D metabolites, results may not always reflect the levels of biologically relevant ("free") metabolites. This limitation may lead to misleading results in patients with nephrotic syndrome and vitamin D intoxication.

The levels of 25(OH)D correlate better with the clinical signs and symptoms of vitamin D deficiency than do the levels of 1,25(OH)$_2$D. Because the 25-hydroxylation of vitamin D is not tightly regulated, measurements of 25(OH)D more accurately reflect body stores of vitamin D. Measurement of this metabolite should, therefore, be performed when vitamin D deficiency is suspected.

Measurements of 1,25(OH)$_2$D should be reserved for cases when excessive or impaired 1α-hydroxylation is suspected. High 1,25(OH)$_2$D levels can be seen in sarcoidosis, lymphomas, Williams syndrome, and intoxication with 1α-hydroxylated metabolites (see section on hypercalcemia). Impaired 1α-hydroxylation can contribute to the hypocalcemia of patients with renal dysfunction, oncogenic osteomalacia, and hereditary defects of vitamin D metabolism (see section on hypocalcemia).

CLINICAL DISORDERS

Hypercalcemic Disorders

Parathyroid-Dependent Hypercalcemia

It is useful to distinguish two categories of hypercalcemia: that associated with dysfunction of the parathyroid cell and that in which hypercalcemia occurs despite appropriate parathyroid suppression. This distinction is useful clinically because it emphasizes the centrality of the PTH assay in the diagnostic approach to the hypercalcemic patient. Abnormal parathyroid glands are associated with hypercalcemia in three settings—primary hyperparathyroidism, familial hypocalciuric hypercalcemia, and lithium-induced hypercalcemia.

PRIMARY HYPERPARATHYROIDISM

In primary hyperparathyroidism, a primary abnormality of the parathyroid glands leads to inappropriate secretion of PTH. In contrast, increased secretion of PTH that is an appropriate response to hypocalcemia is called secondary hyperparathyroidism. The inappropriately high serum PTH level in primary hyperparathyroidism, in turn, causes excessive renal calcium reabsorption, phosphaturia, and 1,25(OH)$_2$D synthesis, and increased bone resorption. These actions of PTH produce the characteristic biochemical phenotype of hypercalcemia and hypophosphatemia, loss of cortical bone, hypercalciuria, and the various clinical sequelae of chronic hypercalcemia. Primary hyperparathyroidism results most often (75 to 80%) from the occurrence of one or more adenomas in previously normal parathyroid glands; in 20% of cases all parathyroid glands may be hyperplastic, and rarely parathyroid carcinoma may be found (fewer than 1 to 2%).[317–320]

Classic Primary Hyperparathyroidism

The bone disease *osteitis fibrosa cystica* was first described by von Recklinghausen in 1891, but the etiologic link between this disease and parathyroid neoplasms was not established until 1925, when the Viennese surgeon Mandl observed clinical improvement following removal of a parathyroid adenoma from a 39-year-old male with severe bone disease. In early clinical descriptions of primary hyperparathyroidism[321–324] the disease was considered to be an uncommon disorder with

significant morbidity and mortality, in which most patients manifested radiographically significant or symptomatic skeletal or renal involvement or both. Although occasional cases were recognized in which symptoms were mild or absent, only the widespread application of multichannel serum chemistry screening to clinical medicine in the 1960s and 1970s made it clear that mild or asymptomatic primary hyperparathyroidism is a much more common disorder.

The skeletal involvement in classic primary hyperparathyroidism is due to a generalized increase in osteoclastic bone resorption, accompanied by fibrovascular marrow replacement and increased osteoblastic activity. The radiographic features (Fig. 24–21) include *generalized demineralization of bone*, with coarsening of the trabecular pattern (due to osteoclastic resorption of the smaller trabeculae); characteristic *subperiosteal resorption*, often most evident in the phalanges of the hands, which gives an irregular, serrated appearance to the outer, subperiosteal cortex and which may progress to extensive cortical resorption; *bone cysts*, usually multiple, which contain a brownish serous or mucoid fluid, tend to occur in the central medullary portions of the shafts of the metacarpals, ribs or pelvis, and may expand into and disrupt the overlying cortex; *osteoclastomas* or *"brown tumors,"* composed of numerous multinucleated osteoclasts ("giant cells") admixed with stromal cells and matrix, which are found most often in trabecular portions of the jaw, the long bones, and ribs; and *pathologic fractures*. The skull may exhibit a finely mottled, ground-glass appearance, with loss of definition of the inner and outer cortices. Dental radiographs typically show erosion or

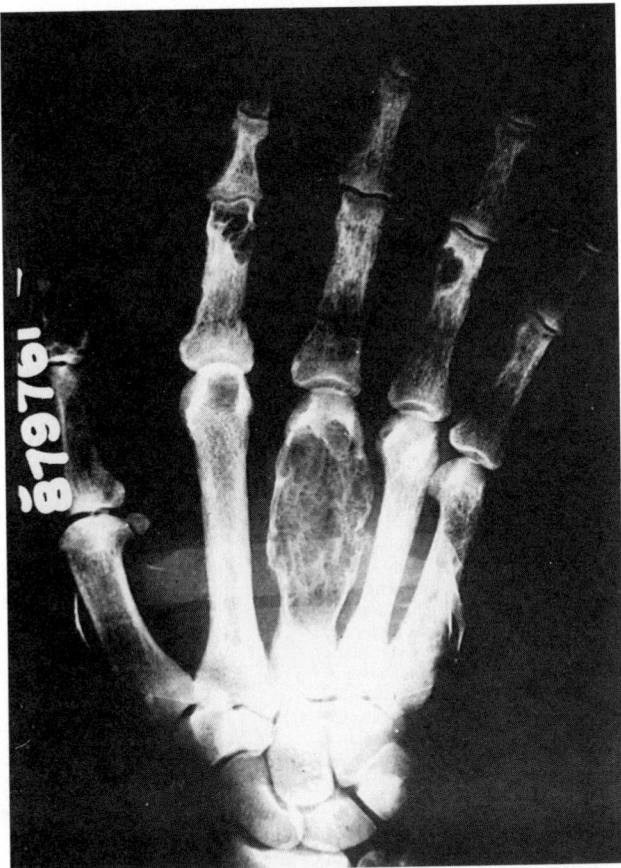

Figure 24–21. Radiograph of hand from patient with severe primary hyperparathyroidism. Note the dramatic remodeling associated with the intense region of high bone turnover in the third metacarpal, in addition to widespread evidence of subperiosteal, endosteal, and trabecular resorption. (From the collection of Fuller Albright, Massachusetts General Hospital.)

disappearance of the lamina dura due to subperiosteal resorption, often with extension into the adjacent mandibular bone. The erosion and demineralization of cortical bone may lead to radiographic disappearance of some bones, most notably the tufts of the distal phalanges of the hands, the inferolateral cortex of the distal third of the clavicles, the distal ulna, the inferior margin of the femoral neck and pubis, and the medial aspect of the proximal tibia. The clinical correlates of these changes may include bone pain and tenderness, "bowing" of the shoulders, kyphosis and loss of height, and collapse of lateral ribs or pelvis with "pigeon-breast" and triradiate deformities, respectively.

The renal manifestations of severe primary hyperparathyroidism include recurrent calcium nephrolithiasis, nephrocalcinosis, and functional abnormalities that range from impaired concentrating ability to end-stage renal failure. Associated symptoms include recurrent flank pain, polyuria, and polydipsia. No unique features of the nephrolithiasis in primary hyperparathyroidism serve to distinguish it from that associated with other, more common causes of calcium kidney stones (see Chapter 26). The nephrolithiasis may be recurrent and severe, and in some patients the stones may be composed entirely of calcium phosphate, instead of the pure oxalate or the mixtures of oxalate and phosphate encountered in other disorders. In patients with conditions diagnosed prior to 1965, the frequency with which nephrolithiasis complicated primary hyperparathyroidism was as high as 60 to 80% (currently less than 25%), but in studies of unselected patients over the past 50 y primary hyperparathyroidism accounted for less than 5% of all calcium kidney stones.

Nephrocalcinosis refers to the presence of bilateral, extensive, but minute calcifications evident on plain abdominal radiographs, usually in the renal pyramids and medullary regions and which correlate with deposits of calcium in the epithelium of the renal tubules. In classic severe primary hyperparathyroidism, nephrocalcinosis occurs with about one third the frequency of symptomatic nephrolithiasis, although it may occur in the absence of stones.

Other features of classic severe primary hyperparathyroidism were conjunctival calcifications, band keratopathy, hypertension (50%), gastrointestinal symptoms (anorexia, nausea, vomiting, constipation, or abdominal pain), peptic ulcer disease, and acute or chronic pancreatitis. Whether primary hyperparathyroidism increases the risk of peptic ulcer disease and pancreatitis remains controversial. Although hyperparathyroidism is associated with a higher risk of hypertension, successful parathyroidectomy does not correct the hypertension.

Symptoms may result from the involvement of bone or kidneys, peptic ulcer disease, pancreatitis, or hypercalcemia per se. Patients may experience a variety of neuropsychiatric symptoms, ranging from weakness, fatigue, apathy, or difficulty in concentrating to depression, dementia, psychosis, or coma. Irritability, memory loss, and emotional lability may occur. The presence and severity of neuropsychiatric symptoms, in particular, correlate poorly with the serum calcium level, although few patients with severe hypercalcemia are entirely asymptomatic. Elderly subjects are more likely to exhibit such symptoms. A peculiar neuromuscular syndrome associated with hyperparathyroidism was first described in 1949 and subsides with successful surgical cure of the disease. This rarely encountered syndrome includes symmetrical proximal weakness and gait disturbance, muscle atrophy, characteristic electromyographic abnormalities, generalized hyperreflexia, and tongue fasciculations.[325]

Modern Primary Hyperparathyroidism

Few patients diagnosed after the introduction of multichannel autoanalyzers have the symptoms of classic primary hyperparathyroidism. In recent years the reported prevalence of hypercalcemia detected during screening of large populations, both ambulatory and hospitalized, has ranged from 0.1 to 1%, and the annual incidence of primary hyperparathyroidism in the United States and Britain overall is about 0.3 per 1000 of population, although the incidence rises more than 10-fold (to 0.7 to 1.5 per 1000) between the ages of 15 and 65. The disease is rare in persons younger than age 15, and among those younger than 45 the annual incidence in Rochester, Minnesota, was only 0.03 per 1000. Women are affected at least twice as often as men, and the incidence appears to peak in the sixth decade of life. The appearance of primary hyperparathyroidism in women often seems related to the onset of menopause, and one report suggests that women with the disease have more body fat than age-matched control subjects.[326]

The natural history of untreated primary hyperparathyroidism, as currently detected, appears to be relatively benign. Although some surgical reports suggest a high incidence of symptoms, most unselected patients probably are asymptomatic,[327] have mild hypercalcemia that fluctuates by no more than 2 to 5%, and do not progress to severe hypercalcemia or other significant complications. Extended follow-up of large cohorts of patients with hypercalcemia (and presumed primary hyperparathyroidism) in Sweden suggests a 40 to 60% higher incidence of malignancies and a 10% reduction in survival, due mostly to cardiovascular disease, when such patients are observed for a decade or more.[328, 329] These provocative findings need further exploration.

Abnormalities of bone in mild primary hyperparathyroidism are more subtle than in the classic disease. Histologically the rate at which new bone remodeling cycles are activated is increased. Because restorative bone formation at each remodeling site takes much more time than the initial resorptive phase, such an increase in remodeling rate inevitably increases the ambient volume of the "remodeling space" and thus the porosity of bone. Depending on the rate and extent of the accompanying increase in osteoblastic activity and the local balance between net bone formation and resorption, mineralized bone volume may decrease further, remain stable, or even increase (despite an increased remodeling space). For reasons not yet understood, the balance between increased resorption and formation of bone in primary hyperparathyroidism depends both on the severity of the hyperparathyroidism and location within the skeleton. Net resorption of endosteal bone may predominate in cortical sites, whereas net accretion of mineral may occur in trabecular bone (Fig. 24–22).[330, 331]

In mild primary hyperparathyroidism osteopenia generally is not evident radiographically, although bone mineral density may be reduced, particularly at sites of predominantly cortical bone, such as the midradius, by as much as 10 to 20%.[331-335] The mass of trabecular or cancellous bone, however, as represented in the vertebral bodies, is typically normal or even increased in patients with asymptomatic primary hyperparathyroidism. This preservation of trabecular bone may explain why vertebral fractures are not more common in these patients. On the other hand, the reduction in cortical bone mineral density in primary hyperparathyroidism may be associated with the same high risk of fractures of the wrist, hip, and other appendicular bones as in otherwise normal subjects with reduced bone density,[336] although an increased risk of such fractures has not yet been demonstrated in patients with the mild, asymptomatic primary hyperparathyroidism.

Kidney stones are now reported in only 10 to 25% of patients with primary hyperparathyroidism, although some degree of renal dysfunction, either a significant reduction in creatinine clearance or impaired concentrating or acidifying ability, may be found in about one third of those with asymptomatic disease.[337] As with the reduction in cortical bone min-

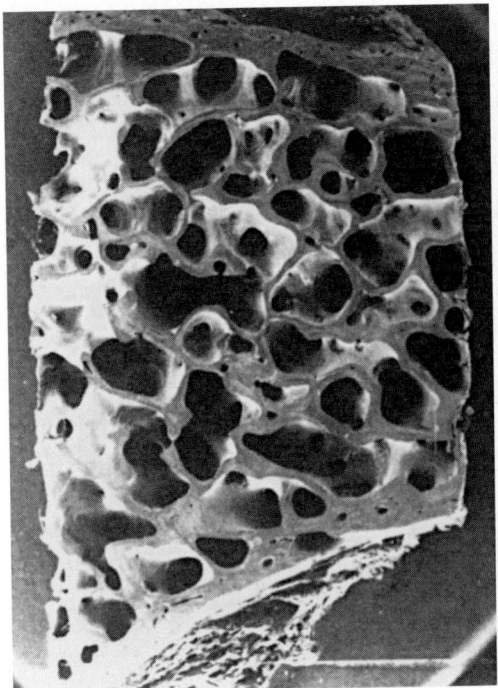
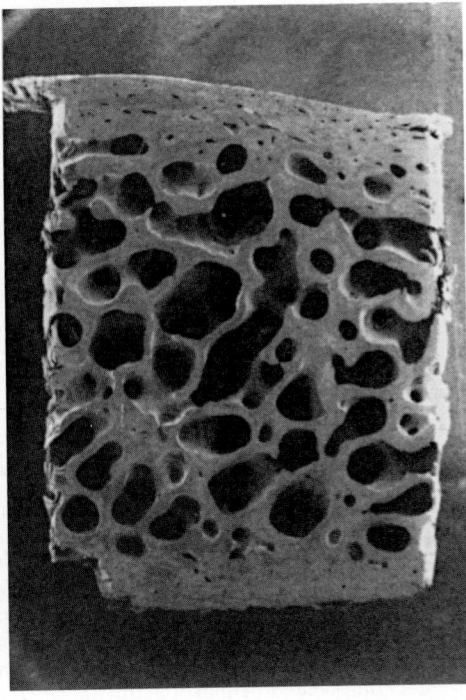

Figure 24–22. Iliac crest biopsies of a patient with primary hyperparathyroidism *(left)* and a normal control *(right)*, viewed by scanning electron microscopy. Note the thin cortices and contrasting maintenance of trabecular bone in the patient. (From Parisien M, Silverberg SJ, Shane E, et al. The histomorphometry of bone in primary hyperparathyroidism: preservation of cancellous bone structure. J Clin Endocrinol Metab 1990; 70:930–938. © The Endocrine Society.)

eral density, these renal abnormalities are usually not progressive.[333, 338] The association of kidney stones with primary hyperparathyroidism generally is viewed as an indication for parathyroidectomy, however, because successful surgery usually prevents further stone disease. The reasons that a subset of patients with primary hyperparathyroidism develop nephrolithiasis is unknown.[339]

Etiology and Pathogenesis

Parathyroid adenomas are caused by somatic mutations in parathyroid cells that confer a proliferative or survival advantage over normal cells.[340, 341] As a consequence, the descendants of one particular parathyroid cell (a clone of cells) undergo clonal expansion to produce an adenoma.

Multiple chromosomal regions have been shown to be missing in the parathyroid cells of individual parathyroid adenomas, probably reflecting the deletion of tumor suppressor genes. These chromosomal loci include portions of chromosome 1p-pter (in 40% of adenomas),[342] 6q (in 32% of adenomas),[343] 15q (in 30% of adenomas),[343] and 11q (in 25 to 30% of adenomas).[344, 345] The 11q deletion may involve the tumor suppressor gene also mutated in the inherited disorder, multiple endocrine neoplasia type 1 (MEN 1; see Chapter 32). The widespread presence of somatic mutations in sporadic parathyroid adenomas, which are detectable only because large numbers of cells in any one tumor contain the same deletion, constitutes the strongest evidence that parathyroid adenomas are due to clonal expansions of mutant cells.

One parathyroid proto-oncogene, the PRAD1 or cyclin D1 gene, was discovered at the breakpoint of an inversion on chromosome 11 in a parathyroid adenoma.[346] This inversion led to the juxtaposition of the regulatory region of the *PTH* gene and the DNA encoding cyclin D1, and as a consequence the cyclin D1 gene was overexpressed. Cyclin D1 regulates the transition from the G_1 phase of the cell cycle, which follows mitosis, to the S phase, associated with DNA synthesis, and is mutated or amplified in a wide variety of malignancies.[341] Cyclin D1 is overexpressed in about 20% of parathyroid adenomas,[347] although cyclin D1 gene rearrangements have been documented in only 5% of adenomas.

As might be expected for a disease caused by mutations in DNA, parathyroid adenomas occur more frequently in patients exposed to neck irradiation decades earlier, with greater radiation exposure leading to higher risk.[348] Most patients have no obvious exposure to specific mutagens, however. The possibility that abnormalities of vitamin D physiology might predispose to primary hyperparathyroidism is suggested by the observation that patients with parathyroid adenomas are more likely than others to inherit a particular allele of the vitamin D receptor gene.[349]

The cause of sporadic primary parathyroid *hyperplasia* is unknown. The known stimuli for parathyroid cell proliferation (low levels of blood calcium or $1,25(OH)_2D$) are not present in this disease. Presumably some other stimulus outside the parathyroid glands or a genetic defect in all four parathyroid glands leads to inappropriate cell proliferation. Such abnormalities have been found in several inherited forms of parathyroid hyperplasia (see later), but most cases of parathyroid hyperplasia are not familial.

The theoretical distinction between adenoma as a clonal proliferation and hyperplasia as a polyclonal growth is a clear one. In some settings, however, clonal expansion can occur in the context of pre-existing polyclonal proliferation. The clearest example of this sequence is in the large parathyroid glands associated with severe renal failure. In many such glands removed surgically, evidence of clonal proliferation complicating secondary hyperplasia has been found.[350, 351] Analogous mechanisms may be operative in other disorders associated with stimuli to parathyroid cell proliferation, such as X-linked hypophosphatemia[352] and long-term lithium therapy.[353, 354] Further, just as clonal tumors can arise in the setting of *secondary* parathyroid hyperplasia, they can also arise in the setting of sporadic *primary* parathyroid hyperplasia[353] and in MEN 1.[344, 355]

The distinction between adenoma and hyperplasia is important because parathyroid adenomas can be cured by removal of the one abnormal gland, whereas removal of multiple glands is required to cure parathyroid hyperplasia. Unfortunately the ability to distinguish pathologically between adenoma, hyperplasia, and normal parathyroid tissue is not straightforward. Pathologists distinguish normal from abnormal parathyroid glands by the increased size and paucity of fat in abnormal glands. Attempts have been made to distinguish the morphology of an adenoma from that of an individual hyperplastic gland, but no criteria have proved completely reliable.[318] The formation of clonal neoplasms in originally hyperplastic tumors may explain the difficulty of pathologic diagnosis.

An increase in cell number is not the only abnormality in primary hyperparathyroidism. A normal ability of the parathyroid cell to suppress PTH secretion in response to hypercalcemia should protect the individual from sustained hypercalcemia, even if the number of parathyroid cells were moderately increased. Unfortunately parathyroid cells in parathyroid adenomas usually have abnormal responsiveness to calcium, with a shift of the set point to the right (Fig. 24–23).[356] This shift, combined with the nonsuppressible component of PTH secretion, leads to a new steady state in which both the PTH level and the blood calcium level are higher than normal. The molecular underpinning of the abnormal parathyroid cell responsiveness is beginning to be understood. Parathyroid cells from adenomas respond to changes in extracellular calcium with smaller than normal increases in intracellular calcium,[357] and the amount of calcium-sensor protein on the cell surface may be reduced.[358]

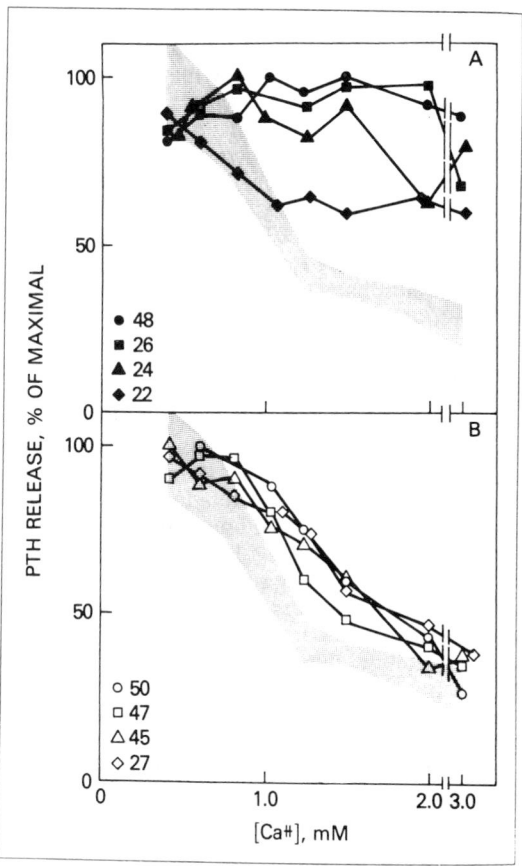

Figure 24–23. Abnormal patterns of PTH secretion from cells prepared from adenomatous glands and stimulated with varying levels of calcium in tissue culture. The shaded area shows the pattern of PTH release (± 1 SD) from normal human parathyroid cells. *Panel A* illustrates the pattern from four patients with little suppression of PTH secretion by calcium. *Panel B* illustrates the pattern from four patients with relatively intact suppression of PTH secretion by calcium. Even in this group the set point for calcium suppression is shifted to the right. (From Brown EM. Calcium-regulated parathyroid hormone release in primary hyperparathyroidism: studies in vitro with dispersed parathyroid cells. Am J Med 1979; 66:923–931. Copyright 1979 by Excerpta Medica Inc.)

Inherited Primary Hyperparathyroidism (see also Chapter 32)

Although uncommon, inherited forms of primary hyperparathyroidism are important primarily because of the insight they provide into pathogenesis. Furthermore the management of the parathyroid tumors in familial parathyroid syndromes often differs from that of sporadic primary hyperparathyroidism. In addition, extraparathyroidal manifestations of inherited syndromes may need treatment, and awareness of familial clustering should prompt systematic family screening.

MULTIPLE ENDOCRINE NEOPLASIA TYPE 1 (MEN 1). Although MEN 1 includes tumors of the parathyroid, anterior pituitary, and pancreatic islets, the parathyroid tumors are the most common; 95% of these patients eventually develop hyperparathyroidism. The onset of hypercalcemia occurs in the second and third decades of life, occasionally in the first decade. Hypercalcemia never presents at birth or during infancy. The disease involves all four parathyroid glands, although the involvement can be asymmetrical and apparently asynchronous. Apart from the earlier age at diagnosis, the features resemble those of sporadic primary hyperparathyroidism. One complicating feature is that hypercalcemia can increase the gastrin levels and increase the symptomatology of patients who also have gastrinomas. Treatment of the parathyroid disease in this setting may simplify the management of the gastric hyperacidity. After parathyroid surgery, hypoparathyroidism and recurrent hyperparathyroidism are more common than in other forms of hyperparathyroidism.[359, 360] The timing and type of surgery are therefore more complicated issues than in sporadic primary hyperparathyroidism. All series agree that parathyroid disease recurs if fewer than three glands are removed. Some surgeons prefer subtotal parathyroidectomy, while others prefer total parathyroidectomy with forearm implantation of a small amount of parathyroid tissue.

MULTIPLE ENDOCRINE NEOPLASIA, TYPE 2A (MEN 2A). Parathyroid disease is a late and infrequent (5 to 20%) occurrence in MEN 2A, a disease defined by the clustering of medullary carcinoma of the thyroid, pheochromocytoma, and hyperparathyroidism. Both parathyroid hyperplasia and adenoma have been noted at surgery. Since asymptomatic parathyroid hyperplasia may be present at the time of thyroid surgery, hyperplasia may progress to adenoma in MEN 2A. The approach to diagnosis and treatment of hyperparathyroidism is similar to that of sporadic primary hyperparathyroidism but with an increased frequency of hyperplasia as the underlying disorder. Hyperparathyroidism does not occur in MEN 2B, the variant associated with mucosal neuromas. The pathogenesis of the hyperparathyroidism is uncertain; however, the *RET* gene, which is mutated in virtually all cases of MEN 2A,[361, 362] is expressed in parathyroid cells,[363] and abnormal *RET* expression in parathyroid cells may directly cause parathyroid tumorigenesis.

OTHER INHERITED SYNDROMES. Two other distinct autosomal dominant forms of primary hyperparathyroidism have been characterized. Hereditary isolated primary hyperparathyroidism[364] is characterized by parathyroid tumors that can be multiple and occasionally malignant. No other endocrine glands are abnormal in these families, and the disease does not map to either the *MEN1* or *MEN2A* locus. Hereditary hyperparathyroidism–jaw tumor syndrome[365] presents with parathyroid adenomas that are usually cystic and with fibrous jaw tumors that are unrelated to the hyperparathyroidism. Parathyroid cancer and Wilms' tumor may occur in these families. This disorder maps to chromosome 1q21–q31.

Management of Primary Hyperparathyroidism

The strategy for management of primary hyperparathyroidism has changed in parallel with the changing presenta-

tablishing the success of the surgery and monitoring the patient for symptomatic hypocalcemia and for uncommon complications, such as bleeding, vocal cord paralysis, and laryngospasm. After successful resection of a parathyroid adenoma, serum intact PTH levels decline rapidly, often to undetectable concentrations, with a disappearance half-time of about 20 min, whereas serum calcium typically reaches a nadir between 24 and 36 h. Serum PTH returns to the normal range within 30 h, although the parathyroid secretory response to hypocalcemia may not return to normal for weeks.[394, 395] Patients generally are maintained on a low-calcium diet until serum calcium is normal, ampules of injectable calcium and other seizure precautions are maintained at the bedside, serum calcium is measured at least every 12 h until stable, and symptomatic hypocalcemia is promptly treated with calcium, either intravenously (90-mg bolus, 50 to 100 mg/h) or orally (1.5 to 3.0 g/d). Patients with large adenomas and severe hyperparathyroidism or elevated alkaline phosphatase may exhibit an increased calcium requirement for many weeks postoperatively as they remineralize their skeletons. This "hungry bone" syndrome is associated with hypocalcemia, hypophosphatemia, and low urinary calcium excretion. In such cases, treatment with oral $1,25(OH)_2D$ (0.5 to 1.5 μg/d) and larger doses of oral calcium (2 to 4 g of elemental calcium) may be needed to maintain even a low-normal serum calcium concentration. Serum PTH should be measured in such circumstances (but at least 48 h after surgery) to exclude the possibility of concurrent postoperative hypoparathyroidism, and serum magnesium should be checked as well. Outpatient monitoring of serum and urinary calcium at frequent intervals may be necessary initially to avoid progressive hypocalcemia or hypercalcemia and to guide adjustment of calcium and vitamin D therapy. Since bone mineral density increases for at least 1 y after successful parathyroidectomy, it is prudent to continue calcium supplementation for at least that long.

The approach to patients with persistent or recurrent hyperparathyroidism is colored by the fact that parathyroid hyperplasia or carcinoma, ectopic or supernumerary parathyroid tissue, and postoperative hypoparathyroidism and other complications of further surgery are more common in this population.[317, 380, 381, 391, 393] The first issue is whether surgery is indicated. When a presumed adenoma is not identified initially, the original indications for surgery generally still exist. However, some patients may not be suitable candidates for more extensive surgery, such as median sternotomy, because of concurrent medical illness. Patients with parathyroid hyperplasia may have experienced significant clinical improvement, even after incomplete parathyroidectomy, although those with MEN 1 are very likely to have further progression of disease.[359]

Preoperative localization studies, though unnecessary for initial neck exploration, are justified in patients who have failed to respond to surgery or have a recurrence after a first operation. A variety of noninvasive techniques have been employed in the past to localize parathyroid tissue, including ultrasonography, computed tomography (CT), magnetic resonance imaging and technetium-thallium subtraction scanning. The sensitivity of these approaches is between 25% and 85%, depending on the center where they were performed, the patient population, and the location of the lesion or lesions. False-positive rates approach 15%.[379] Ultrasonography can be useful in identifying parathyroid enlargement in the lower neck—but not in the mediastinum or locations deeper in the neck, where many ectopic parathyroids reside. Computed tomography or MRI may provide visualization of mediastinal adenomas.[379, 381] ^{99m}Tc-sestamibi scanning has been reported to offer excellent sensitivity (approximately 90%) and can be employed with ^{123}I scanning to improve distinction from thyroid nodules and with single-photon emission CT (SPECT) to achieve an accuracy in localization not possible with planar

imaging or the technetium-thallium subtraction technique[381, 396–398] (Fig. 24–25). However, sestamibi scanning may not reveal small glands or demonstrate multiple abnormal glands in cases of parathyroid hyperplasia, the most common cause of persistent postoperative hyperparathyroidism. Furthermore, uptake of sestamibi is not specific for parathyroid tissue but occurs also in thyroid adenomas, which may accompany parathyroid disease in 20 to 40% of patients.[399, 400] More invasive techniques have been employed as well, including angiography and selective venous sampling for measurement of PTH, although the sensitivity of these procedures for detection of residual abnormal parathyroid glands is only 50 to 65%.[381, 401] Angiography does offer the opportunity to attempt angioablation of any identified tissue, although this procedure is not routinely successful.[401, 402] In addition, when all other parathyroid tissue has been previously removed, angioablation precludes the opportunity to avoid hypoparathyroidism by autotransplantation of parathyroid fragments at surgery. Ultrasonography or CT-guided fine-needle aspiration of suspected parathyroid tissue may be used to obtain cytologic or immunoassay confirmation prior to surgery,[403] and intraoperative ultrasonography has been useful in some cases in locating cervical or intrathyroidal glands.[381] Thoracoscopic resection of documented mediastinal lesions[404, 405] offers a new therapeutic approach to this type of persistent hyperparathyroidism.

The need for these procedures depends on the experience of the original surgeon and the confidence that the neck was adequately explored initially. For example, among reoperations at one center, more than half of the "missed" hyperplastic parathyroid glands in those cases previously explored by a highly experienced parathyroid surgeon were found in the mediastinum or another ectopic location, whereas more than 90% of the "missed" glands in patients

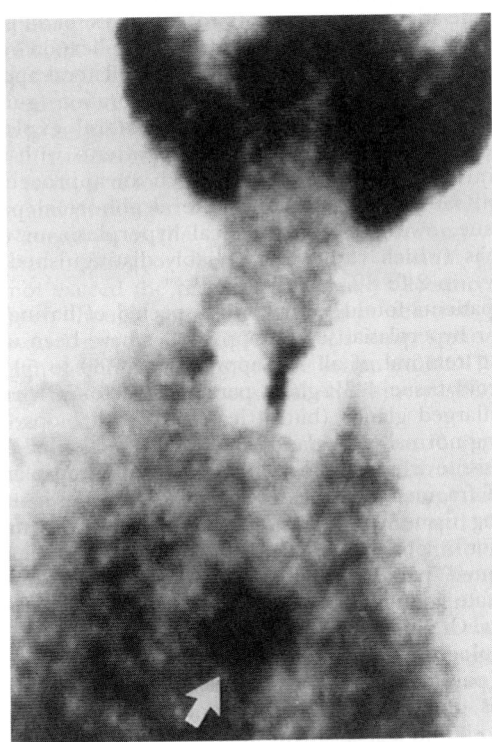

Figure 24–25. Tc-99m sestamibi ^{123}I subtraction scanning of a patient with persistent hyperparathyroidism after two prior unsuccessful operations. Arrow points to parathyroid adenoma, shown as increased tracer uptake in the aortopulmonary window. (From Thule P, Thakore K, Vansant J, et al. Preoperative localization of parathyroid tissue with technetium-99m sestamibi ^{123}I subtraction scanning. J Clin Endocrinol Metab 1994; 78:77–82. © The Endocrine Society.)

referred by less experienced surgeons were discovered in the neck.[317]

Following successful surgery for primary hyperparathyroidism, bone mass generally improves by as much as 6 to 10% in the first year, although normal bone mineral density may not be achieved.[332, 334, 335] This improvement, which is most apparent in patients with the greatest preoperative reductions in bone mass, may be related in part to rapid remineralization of the previously enlarged bone-remodeling volume.[334, 335, 406] The fact that improvement in bone mass may continue over several years, however, particularly at sites enriched in trabecular bone (i.e., vertebrae), suggests that cure of primary hyperparathyroidism causes a sustained increase in net bone formation and total bone volume.[335]

Other benefits of surgery, apart from cure of hypercalcemia per se and symptoms directly attributable to it, are more difficult to demonstrate. The incidence of recurrent kidney stones appears to be reduced, although this has only been examined retrospectively in patients with relatively severe disease and over relatively short intervals of follow-up.[407–409] As noted earlier, hypertension is not improved by parathyroidectomy. Other abnormalities, such as subtle muscle weakness, may improve,[407] although the clinical significance of such changes is not known. Limited unconfirmed evidence suggests an improvement in mortality in patients who underwent surgery,[328] but other data do not indicate a reduction in the risk of cardiovascular or malignant disease.[410]

FAMILIAL HYPOCALCIURIC HYPERCALCEMIA

Familial hypocalciuric hypercalcemia (FHH), also appropriately called familial benign hypercalcemia, is, in most families, an autosomally dominant disorder caused by mutations of the calcium-sensor gene found in the parathyroid glands, kidney, and other organs[29] (see earlier discussion of calcium sensing). Mutations that cause complete or partial loss of function of the calcium sensor lead to a shift in the parathyroid cell's set point for calcium.[411] As a consequence, higher than normal levels of blood calcium are needed to suppress PTH secretion. Furthermore abnormal calcium-sensor function in the thick ascending limb of the renal tubule leads to increased, PTH-independent calcium reabsorption and consequent hypocalciuria. The presence of one abnormal sensor gene usually leads to a mild clinical disorder. In contrast, rarely patients who inherit mutant calcium-sensor genes from both parents have severe, life-threatening primary hyperparathyroidism at birth and almost always require immediate parathyroid surgery.

Familial hypocalciuric hypercalcemia is manifest at birth by hypercalcemia. Most observers believe that the condition is asymptomatic and that apparent symptoms represent ascertainment bias.[31] Possible exceptions include the chondrocalcinosis and perhaps pancreatitis. Blood calcium is usually less than 3 mmol/L (<12 mg/dL) but can be higher. Phosphate levels are low, as in primary hyperparathyroidism. Blood magnesium levels are high-normal or slightly elevated. PTH levels are inappropriately normal for the degree of hypercalcemia and are occasionally modestly elevated. Urine calcium is usually low.

When patients present as adults, the distinction from mild primary hyperparathyroidism can be difficult (but is very important). Patients with primary hyperparathyroidism who are treated surgically are cured, whereas hypercalcemia always recurs after surgery for FHH, unless the patient is rendered hypoparathyroid by the removal of all parathyroid tissue. Therefore, surgery is contraindicated for FHH. No blood or urine measurements are completely reliable for distinguishing the two conditions, although the ratio of calcium clearance to creatinine clearance distinguishes most patients with FHH

from those with primary hyperparathyroidism[412] (Fig. 24–26). The most helpful diagnostic information is the presence of hypercalcemia in an infant relative; such early hypercalcemia does not occur in MEN 1. Furthermore a past history of a documented normal blood calcium level, considerably lower than current measurements, makes FHH unlikely, if no other reason for a change in blood calcium level exists.

LITHIUM TOXICITY

Treatment of patients with bipolar affective disorders with lithium commonly leads to mild, persistent increases in blood calcium,[353, 354, 413] occasionally out of the normal range. After several years of therapy, clear elevations of PTH levels and modest increases in parathyroid gland size may occur.[353] Usually, when lithium therapy is stopped the blood calcium and PTH return to normal within several months, but substantial hypercalcemia and clear hyperparathyroidism may ensue. At surgery, parathyroid hyperplasia and, occasionally, parathyroid adenomas have been found.

The management of patients with mild, lithium-induced hypercalcemia is somewhat complicated. Like patients with mild primary hyperparathyroidism, patients taking lithium usually tolerate mild hypercalcemia without obvious symptoms. These patients can be followed with protocols similar to those for patients with asymptomatic primary hyperparathyroidism. Close attention must be paid to urine-concentrating ability because the nephrogenic diabetes insipidus associated with lithium therapy can cause dehydration and sudden worsening of hypercalcemia. Substantial hypercalcemia should lead to withdrawal of lithium therapy, if possible, and trial of newer psychopharmacologic agents. If hypercalcemia persists after withdrawal of lithium, the decisions about surgery follow the same guidelines as those for patients with primary hyperparathyroidism.

Lithium increases the set point for PTH secretion when

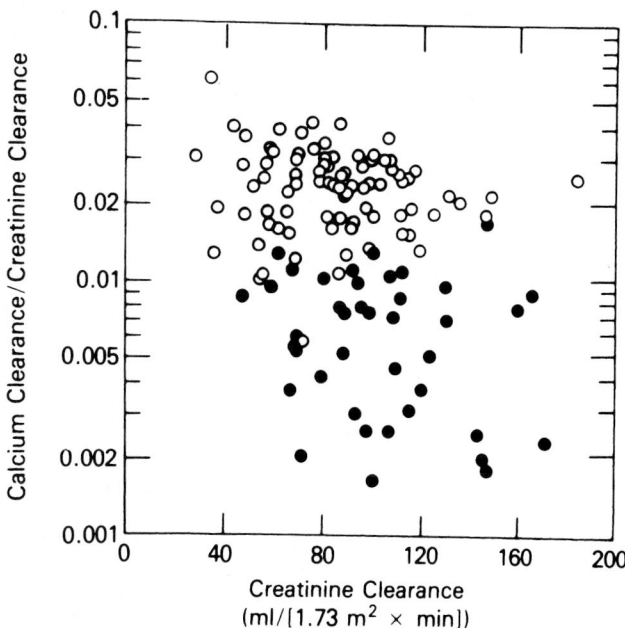

Figure 24–26. Index of urinary excretion rate for calcium as a function of creatinine clearance. Each point represents the mean of multiple determinations of a hypercalcemic patient with familial hypocalciuric hypercalcemia (*solid circles*) or with typical primary hyperparathyroidism (*open circles*). The data are based on average 24-h urinary excretion values and average fasting serum samples. (From Marx SJ, Attie MF, Levine M, et al. The hypocalciuric or benign variant of familial hypercalcemia: clinical and biochemical features in fifteen kindreds. Medicine 1981; 60:397–412, with permission.)

it is added to isolated parathyroid cells in culture.[414] A corresponding shift in the concentration of extracellular calcium needed to raise intracellular calcium levels[415] suggests that lithium interferes with the action of the parathyroid calcium sensor, perhaps by interfering with inositol phosphate metabolism.

Parathyroid-Independent Hypercalcemia

In parathyroid-independent hypercalcemia, PTH secretion is appropriately suppressed. PTH levels, measured using two-site assays, are invariably lower than 25 pg/mL and are usually lower than normal or undectable. Most such patients have malignant hypercalcemia, although parathyroid-independent hypercalcemia occurs in a number of other settings as well.

HYPERCALCEMIA OF MALIGNANCY

The diagnosis of malignant hypercalcemia is seldom a subtle one. Most malignancies produce hypercalcemia only when they are far advanced and the diagnosis is evident after routine studies, guided by the history and physical examination. Patients with malignant hypercalcemia usually die in the first or second month after hypercalcemia is discovered.[416] Manifestations include the classic symptoms of hypercalcemia: confusion, polydipsia, polyuria, constipation, nausea, and vomiting. Perhaps because of the acuteness of the hypercalcemia and the elderly patient population involved, dramatic changes in mental status may culminate in coma. The diagnosis can be missed because the symptoms overlap those of the underlying malignancy and because low blood albumin may lead to an apparently normal total blood calcium, despite an elevated blood ionized calcium. Even though the prognosis is grim, the diagnosis of malignant hypercalcemia is important to make. Treatment is usually simple and effective in the short term; such treatment may reverse the symptoms for several weeks and provide time for a fundamental attack on the underlying tumor, if it is treatable. Only effective treatment of the underlying neoplasm can influence the long-term prognosis of patients with malignant hypercalcemia.

Even though mechanisms in a given patient may be complex, it is useful to distinguish hypercalcemia associated with local involvement of bone from that caused by humoral mechanisms. In all cases resorption of bone plays a pivotal role in the pathogenesis.

Local Osteolytic Hypercalcemia

Hypercalcemia from invasion of tumors into bone occurs most commonly in multiple myeloma and in some patients with breast cancer. Little evidence exists that the tumor cells themselves resorb bone. Instead, active osteoclasts found near the tumor cells are thought to be the proximate mediators of bone resorption.[417] Myeloma cells and marrow cells associated with myeloma cells secrete numerous cytokines capable of stimulating bone resorption, including lymphotoxin (tumor necrosis factor β), interleukin-1β (IL-1β), and IL-6.[418, 419] Treatment of myeloma patients with intermittent intravenous pamidronate (a bisphosphonate) inhibits this resorption and reduces the incidence of bone pain, fracture, and hypercalcemia.[420]

The pathogenesis of hypercalcemia in breast cancer is not completely understood. Extensive metastases to bone are found in most patients with hypercalcemia and breast cancer, suggesting that factors produced by the metastatic cells may be important. Breast cancer cells make a host of cytokines capable of resorbing bone, including PTHrP.[417] The majority of breast cancer patients with hypercalcemia have elevated blood levels of PTHrP,[311, 313, 421] and this circulating PTHrP and

PTHrP produced in bone by metastatic cells may generate the hypercalcemia. Primary breast tumors that stain for PTHrP are more likely to result in bony metastases than those that do not stain for PTHrP;[421] thus PTHrP may be involved in the establishment of lytic metastases.[422]

Humoral Hypercalcemia of Malignancy

Albright proposed in 1941 that a PTH-like humoral factor caused the hypercalcemia in patients with malignancy but with few or no bony metastases. Four decades later it was demonstrated that such patients have high blood calcium, low blood phosphate, and high urinary cyclic AMP but no elevation in immunoreactive PTH levels.[423] The stimulation of cyclic AMP production was used as an assay to purify PTHrP from human tumors associated with the humoral hypercalcemia of malignancy.[153–155, 157, 424]

The evidence that PTHrP mediates the humoral hypercalcemia of malignancy in most patients is substantial. As noted earlier PTHrP binds to the PTH/PTHrP receptor and mimics all of the actions of amino-terminal fragments of PTH.[169–171] Blood levels of PTHrP are elevated in most patients with solid tumors and hypercalcemia,[168, 177, 313] and in animal models of the humoral hypercalcemia of malignancy antibodies against PTHrP can reverse the hypercalcemia.[312, 425]

However, the acute actions of PTHrP cannot explain all of the findings in patients with the hypercalcemia of malignancy. Acute administration of PTHrP, like that of PTH, increases blood levels of $1,25(OH)_2D$ by stimulating the renal 1α-hydroxylase. Nevertheless patients with the humoral hypercalcemia of malignancy usually have low levels of $1,25(OH)_2D$.[423] This finding is puzzling because human tumors associated with low $1,25(OH)_2D$ levels stimulate $1,25(OH)_2D$ synthesis after they are transplanted into nude mice.[426] Possible explanations for the low $1,25(OH)_2D$ levels in patients include inhibition of the 1α-hydroxylase by hypercalcemia[427] or by tumor products.[428]

A second disparity between the acute actions of PTHrP and the findings in patients with malignant hypercalcemia involves the rate of bone formation. Acutely PTHrP, like PTH, increases bone formation. Nevertheless in patients with malignant hypercalcemia bone formation is low. The explanation for this effect could well lie in the action of other cytokines, immobilization, or particular fragments of PTHrP with novel properties.

The tumors most commonly associated with humoral hypercalcemia include squamous cell cancers of the lung, head and neck, esophagus, cervix, vulva, and skin; breast cancer; renal cell cancer; and bladder cancer. Benign or malignant pheochromocytomas, islet cell tumors, and carcinoids can overproduce PTHrP and cause hypercalcemia as well. The aggressive T-cell lymphoma associated with human T-cell leukemia/lymphoma virus (HTLV-I) infection is the only hematologic malignancy commonly associated with PTHrP overproduction and hypercalcemia.

It is unlikely that PTHrP is the sole cause of the humoral hypercalcemia of malignancy. As noted earlier, many cytokines produced by tumors can stimulate bone resorption, and the actions of these cytokines synergize with those of PTHrP in some experimental models.[429] Furthermore in hypercalcemic patients with non-Hodgkin's lymphoma blood levels of $1,25(OH)_2D$ are higher than expected.[430] In these patients the relative importance of $1,25(OH)_2D$, cytokines (like those implicated in multiple myeloma), PTHrP, and immobilization needs to be clarified.

In a few instances malignant tumors secrete PTH, and not PTHrP.[431–434] Although this phenomenon is well documented, concurrent primary hyperparathyroidism, not ectopic PTH production, is the cause of the hyperparathyroidism in most patients with cancer and high PTH levels.

VITAMIN D INTOXICATION

Because the synthesis of $1,25(OH)_2D$ is tightly regulated, large doses of vitamin D, on the order of 100,000 U/d, are required to cause hypercalcemia. Such doses are only available in the United States by prescription, so most cases of vitamin D intoxication are iatrogenic. Inadvertent ingestion occasionally occurs.[258, 435] Patients present with nausea, vomiting, weakness, and altered state of consciousness. Hypercalcemia can be severe and prolonged, because of the storage of vitamin D in fat. As expected, PTH levels are suppressed, and levels of $25(OH)D$, which are poorly regulated and reflect vitamin D levels, are dramatically elevated. In contrast, the levels of $1,25(OH)_2D$ are only modestly elevated and may be normal or low. The modest changes in $1,25(OH)_2D$ levels result from the down-regulation of the renal 1α-hydroxylase by low levels of PTH and high levels of phosphate, calcium, and $1,25(OH)_2D$ itself. The cause of the hypercalcemia, when it occurs in the setting of normal levels of $1,25(OH)_2D$, is uncertain but may reflect the direct action of $25(OH)D$ and possibly other vitamin D metabolites, which are capable of binding the $1,25(OH)_2D$ receptor weakly. Also, the weaker vitamin D metabolites may displace $1,25(OH)_2D$ from the circulating vitamin D–binding protein and increase the concentration of active, free $1,25(OH)_2D$.[258]

The hypercalcemia of vitamin D intoxication results from both increased intestinal absorption of calcium and the increased resorption of bone. In severe cases therefore glucocorticoid therapy, which counters the action of $1,25(OH)_2D$ on both bone and intestine, should be added to the therapeutic regimen of hydration and omission of dietary calcium.[436]

SARCOIDOSIS AND OTHER GRANULOMATOUS DISEASES

Sarcoidosis may cause hypercalcemia and even more commonly hypercalciuria. Hypercalcemic patients have high levels of $1,25(OH)_2D$,[437] which probably cause the hypercalcemia. As expected in $1,25(OH)_2D$-dependent hypercalcemia, intestinal absorption of calcium is increased, and PTH levels are suppressed. Furthermore the hypercalcemia and high levels of $1,25(OH)_2D$ decrease with glucocorticoid therapy. The unregulated synthesis of $1,25(OH)_2D$, found in even an anephric patient,[249] occurs not in the kidney but in the sarcoid granulomas. Removal of a large amount of granulomatous tissue can reverse hypercalcemia.[438] Furthermore isolated sarcoid macrophages can synthesize $1,25(OH)_2D$ from $25(OH)D$, as can normal macrophages stimulated with interferon γ.[439, 440]

The unregulated synthesis of $1,25(OH)_2D$ by activated macrophages explains many of the features of hypercalcemia in sarcoidosis. These patients have unusual sensitivity to vitamin D and can become hypercalcemic in response to ultraviolet irradiation or oral vitamin D intake.[437, 441] Abnormalities in calcium metabolism usually occur only in patients with active disease and large, obvious, total-body burdens of granulomas. Nevertheless hypercalcemia can present in patients who do not have obvious pulmonary disease. Furthermore subtle abnormalities of vitamin D metabolism can be demonstrated even in patients with mild sarcoidosis. For example, patients with normal levels of angiotensin-converting enzyme in their blood have normal levels of $1,25(OH)_2D$, but these levels do not fall normally in response to an oral calcium challenge.[442]

Hypercalcemia is also associated with other granulomatous diseases, such as tuberculosis, fungal infections, and berylliosis, and has been reported in Wegener's granulomatosis,[443] in *Pneumocystis carinii* infection related to acquired immunodeficiency syndrome (AIDS),[444] and in association with extensive granulomatous foreign body reactions.

HYPERTHYROIDISM

Mild hypercalcemia can result from hyperthyroidism.[445] Blood calcium levels seldom exceed 2.7 mmol/L (11 mg/dL), but mild elevations are found in a fourth of hyperthyroid patients.[446] Patients have low PTH levels, low $1,25(OH)_2D$ levels, and hypercalciuria. The hypercalcemia is caused by a direct stimulation of bone resorption by thyroid hormones.[447] β-Adrenergic blocking agents can reverse the hypercalcemia.[448]

VITAMIN A INTOXICATION

Excess ingestion of vitamin A (retinol) causes a syndrome of dry skin, pruritus, headache from pseudotumor cerebri, bone pain, and occasionally hypercalcemia. Hypercalcemia occurs only with the ingestion of 10 times the recommended daily allowance vitamin A (5000 IU/d) or from ingestion of the vitamin A derivatives isotretinoin (13-*cis*-retinoic acid) or tretinoin (all-*trans*-retinoic acid), used to treat acne.[449] Bones can show characteristic periosteal calcification on radiographs.[450] Hypercalcemia is probably caused by direct stimulation of bone resorption by retinoids. The diagnosis is made by the association of a history of excess ingestion of retinoids with the characteristic syndrome and abnormal liver function tests; elevated vitamin A levels confirm the diagnosis. Treatment involves hydration, cessation of vitamin A ingestion, and if necessary glucocorticoids.

ADRENAL INSUFFICIENCY

Hypercalcemia occurs in the setting of adrenal insufficiency. The blood calcium level is elevated partly as a result of hemoconcentration and increased albumin levels,[451] but the level of ionized calcium can be increased as well.[452] The hypercalcemia in one well-studied case[452] resulted from a combination of an influx of calcium into the vascular space, probably from bone, and low renal clearance.

THIAZIDE DIURETICS

Thiazide diuretics do not cause hypercalcemia alone but can exacerbate the hypercalcemia of primary hyperparathyroidism. The mechanism of the hypercalcemia may involve increased distal tubular calcium reabsorption.[61] Thiazides block sodium-chloride cotransport into these cells (see Fig. 24–7), and the fall in intracellular chloride hyperpolarizes the cell and thereby increases calcium influx through voltage-sensitive channels.[211] Decreased renal clearance of calcium alone raises blood calcium levels in the normal human only transiently, because hypercalcemia suppresses PTH secretion and returns the blood calcium to normal. As predicted by this model, thiazide administration leads to chronic hypercalcemia only in patients with abnormal parathyroid physiology.[453] In primary hyperparathyroidism, thiazide administration exacerbates the hypercalcemia, and in hypoparathyroidism thiazide administration facilitates the maintenance of normal blood calcium levels when given in conjunction with calcitriol and calcium.[454]

MILK-ALKALI SYNDROME

The triad of hypercalcemia, metabolic alkalosis, and renal failure can be the consequence of massive ingestion of calcium and absorbable alkali.[455] This syndrome was first described when milk and sodium bicarbonate were used in large amounts to treat peptic ulcer disease. With the change in ulcer treatment to nonabsorbable antacids and suppression of acid secretion, milk-alkali syndrome became rare. In the last several years, however, the increased use of calcium carbonate to treat dyspepsia and osteoporosis has led to the reappearance of milk-alkali syndrome.[456, 457] In most cases there is a history of ingestion of several grams per day of calcium in the form of calcium carbonate. The pathogenesis of the syndrome is not understood in detail but may involve a perpetuating sequence in which alkalosis decreases renal calcium clearance and hypercalcemia helps maintain alkalosis. Nephrocalcinosis, nephrogenic diabetes insipidus, decrease in glomerular filtration rate associated with hypercalcemia, and hypovolemia from vomiting all lead to volume depletion and renal failure, which can be severe. PTH levels, measured with current two-site assays, are invariably low,[456, 457] as are levels of $1,25(OH)_2D$. After clearance of the calcium by hydration or dialysis, if necessary, renal function generally returns to normal, unless the disorder is severe and long-standing.

IMMOBILIZATION

Immobilization can cause bone resorption sufficient to cause hypercalcemia. The immobilization is usually caused by spinal cord injury or extensive casting after fractures. Hypercalcemia of immobilization occurs predominantly in the young or in patients with other reasons for high bone turnover, such as Paget's disease or extensive fractures. Hypercalciuria and substantial bone loss are more common than hypercalcemia. After spinal cord injury hypercalciuria is maximal at 4 mo and can persist for more than a year.[458] PTH and $1,25(OH)_2D$ levels are low;[459] bone biopsies show increased resorption and decreased formation of bone.[460] The combination of calcitonin and bisphosphonates has been used to reverse the hypercalcemia and hypercalciuria of spinal cord injury.[461]

RENAL FAILURE

Following rhabdomyolysis, during the oliguric phase of acute renal failure, severe hypocalcemia can result from acute hyperphosphatemia and calcium deposition in muscle.[462, 463] PTH levels are high. In the diuretic phase that follows, hypercalcemia can occur. The hypercalcemia results from high levels of $1,25(OH)_2D$ in some patients and from mobilization of the calcium deposits.[464]

In chronic renal failure hypercalcemia can result from tertiary hyperparathyroidism or may appear during therapy in patients with aplastic bone disease associated with low PTH levels and sometimes with aluminum toxicity.[465]

WILLIAMS SYNDROME

Williams syndrome is a developmental disorder in which supravalvular aortic stenosis is associated with elfin facies and mental retardation.[466, 467] Hypercalcemia may occur transiently in the first 4 y of life. Affected hypercalcemic infants have been found to have increased intestinal absorption of calcium and elevated levels of $1,25(OH)_2D$ that fall to normal as the blood calcium returns to normal.[468] Levels of $25(OH)D$ are normal. The hypercalcemia can generally be controlled by restriction of dietary calcium and vitamin D.

Molecular analysis has clarified the origin of the connective tissue component of Williams syndrome.[469, 470] Isolated supravalvular aortic stenosis is associated with deletion or translocation of the distal portion of the elastin gene. Williams syndrome, with more protean connective tissue abnormalities and mental retardation, is associated with large deletions that include the elastin gene and a gene encoding the protein

kinase LIM-kinase 1.[471] The subgroup of patients with infantile hypercalcemia may have deletion of another gene near the elastin locus. This possible genetic heterogeneity may explain the conflicting literature, which has found no consistent abnormality of calcium metabolism in patients with Williams syndrome.[472]

JANSEN'S METAPHYSEAL CHONDRODYSPLASIA

Jansen's metaphyseal chondrodysplasia is a rare disease that presents in childhood with short stature and hypercalcemia[133] (Fig. 24–27). Blood chemistries suggest hyperparathyroidism, with high calcium, low normal phosphate, high $1,25(OH)_2D$, and high alkaline phosphatase and urinary hydroxyproline but low PTH levels.[134] A generalized defect in endochondral bone formation results from growth plates with abnormally organized chondrocytes. Metaphyses appear disordered and rachitic on radiographs. The bones may show signs of osteitis fibrosa cystica. Constitutive activation of the PTH/PTHrP receptor is caused by point mutations in the transmembrane domains of the receptor.[131, 132] The abnormal serum chemistries result from PTH-like actions of the receptor in bone and kidney, and the growth plate disorder results from PTHrP-like actions of the receptor on the growth plate.[473]

APPROACH TO THE HYPERCALCEMIC PATIENT

The diagnostic approach to hypercalcemia is influenced by the clinical setting and the knowledge that primary hyperparathyroidism is at least twice as common as all other causes combined (Table 24–2). This is particularly true of the patient who seems otherwise well and in whom the hypercalcemia is detected incidentally or is mild, stable, or known to be of long duration (i.e., years). Among outpatients referred to endocrinologists for evaluation of hypercalcemia, for example, more than 90% have primary hyperparathyroidism. In ill or hospitalized patients, malignant disease is the cause of more than 50% of cases. The differential diagnosis is seldom complicated, however, because malignant hypercalcemia usually presents in the context of advanced, clinically obvious disease. Nevertheless this straightforward picture is complicated by the

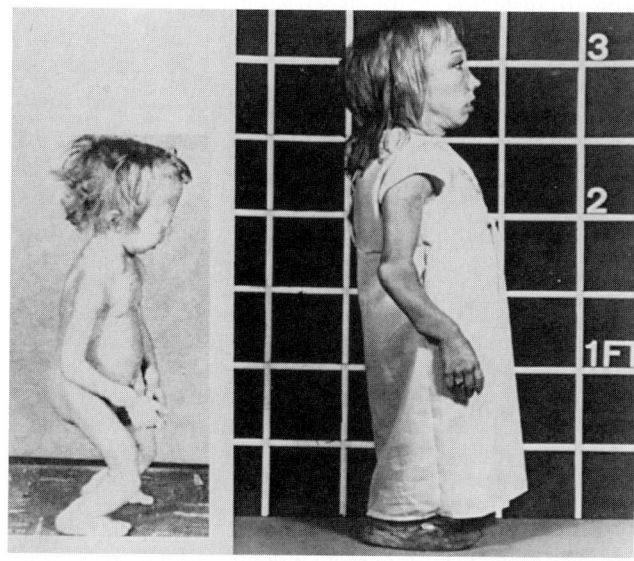

Figure 24–27. A patient with Jansen's metaphyseal chondrodysplasia at ages 5 and 22. Note the short stature, characteristic facies, and misshapen metaphyseal regions of the long bones. (From Frame B, Poznanski AK. Conditions that may be confused with rickets. In: DeLuca HF, Anastas CS, eds. Pediatric Diseases Related to Calcium. New York: Elsevier, 1980: 269–289, with permission.)

TABLE 24–2. Causes of Hypercalcemia

Parathyroid-Dependent Hypercalcemia

Primary hyperparathyroidism
Tertiary hyperparathyroidism
Familial hypocalciuric hypercalcemia
Lithium-associated hypercalcemia

Parathyroid-Independent Hypercalcemia

Neoplasms
  PTHrP-dependent
  Other humoral syndromes
  Osteolytic metastases and multiple myeloma
Excess vitamin D/1,25(OH)$_2$D
  Vitamin D ingestion
  Calcitriol intoxication
  Topical vitamin D analogues
  Granulomatous disease
  Williams syndrome
Thyrotoxicosis
Adrenal insufficiency
Renal failure
  Acute renal failure
  Chronic renal failure with aplastic bone disease
Immobilization
Jansen's disease
Drugs
  Vitamin A intoxication
  Milk-alkali syndrome
  Thiazide diuretics
  Theophylline

observation that as many as 10% of patients with malignancy and hypercalcemia have concurrent primary hyperparathyroidism, presumably the coincidence of two common disorders.

As hypercalcemia is usually first detected as an elevation of total serum calcium, it is important to distinguish hemoconcentration or rare instances of calcium-binding paraproteinemia from a true increase in serum ionized calcium by concurrent measurement of serum albumin and globulin or direct determination of ionized calcium. Especially when hypercalcemia is mild, it is prudent to repeat the measurement of serum total or ionized calcium at least twice, preferably fasting and without venous occlusion, before proceeding with more costly diagnostic studies. A careful history and physical examination, combined with efforts to recover prior results of routine multichannel serum chemistry determinations, most often will point to the probable diagnosis. Serum phosphate is often low in hyperparathyroidism but is also low with PTHrP-secreting malignancies. The presence of hypophosphatemia therefore is not helpful in distinguishing these possibilities. When serum phosphate is normal or high despite correction of dehydration, the possibility of PTH- or PTHrP-independent hypercalcemia should be considered more strongly. Serum chloride and alkaline phosphatase levels are often elevated in primary hyperparathyroidism, but these findings are not useful in the differential diagnosis of hypercalcemia. Important elements of the medical history of hypercalcemic patients include inquiries about kidney stones or fractures; weight loss; back or bone pain; fatigue or weakness; cough or dyspnea; ulcer disease or pancreatitis; ingestion of vitamins, calcium preparations, lithium or thiazides; dates of most recent mammograms and chest radiographs; and a family history of hypercalcemia, kidney stones, ulcer disease, endocrinopathy, or tumors of the head or neck.

The single most important test in the differential diagnosis of hypercalcemia is the measurement of serum PTH, preferably in a two-site assay specific for the intact, biologically active molecule (Fig. 24–19). A consistently elevated serum PTH in the presence of true hypercalcemia is always abnormal and usually indicates the diagnosis of primary hyperparathyroidism. The exceptions are familial hypocalciuric hypercalce-

mia, autonomous parathyroid secretion complicating secondary hyperparathyroidism ("tertiary" hyperparathyroidism), and rarely ectopic PTH secretion by a malignant neoplasm. Although as many as 10% of patients with primary hyperparathyroidism may exhibit PTH levels within the (high) normal range with current PTH assays, such levels are inappropriate in the setting of ambient hypercalcemia and therefore establish the diagnosis of PTH-dependent hypercalcemia. Many such patients manifest elevated serum PTH levels if retested, especially if dietary calcium is restricted beforehand. Mild hypercalcemia or hyperparathyroidism, or both, occur in a significant fraction of patients treated with lithium.

When a patient with primary hyperparathyroidism is young (<40 years of age), has a serum PTH within or only slightly above the normal range, or has a family history suggestive of hypercalcemia or elements of an MEN syndrome, screening of family members for hypercalcemia should be undertaken to search for FHH, familial hyperparathyroidism, or an MEN syndrome (usually MEN 1). In such patients, 24-h urine collections should also be performed to determine the clearance of calcium relative to that of creatinine (a ratio of less than 0.01 suggests FHH).

A low or undetectable serum PTH signifies the presence of nonparathyroid hypercalcemia and therefore should prompt a detailed evaluation for malignancy or other causes of PTH-independent hypercalcemia. Breast and lung cancer alone account for more than 50% of malignancy-associated hypercalcemia. Mammography, chest radiograph with or without CT, abdominal CT, and serum and urinary immunoelectrophoresis are among the more useful procedures for detecting the cause of nonparathyroid hypercalcemia. Although humoral mechanisms, especially secretion of PTHrP, are implicated in the pathogenesis of most cancer-associated hypercalcemias, bone metastases are also common, particularly in breast cancer. Technetium-99m bone scanning therefore is useful for detecting this syndrome and identifying bones vulnerable to fracture. The utility of serum PTHrP measurements is limited to the unusual situation in which serum PTH is suppressed but an underlying malignancy cannot be readily demonstrated.

In the absence of evident malignancy, unusual causes of hypercalcemia should be sought. Vitamin D and vitamin A intoxication can be excluded by measurement of serum 25(OH)D and retinoids, respectively. Elevated 1,25(OH)$_2$D levels and hypercalcemia may occur in several settings, including sarcoidosis and other granulomatous diseases, B- and T-cell lymphomas (including AIDS-associated lymphomas), and uncommonly in epithelial neoplasms such as lung cancer. Rarely, patients with severe idiopathic hypercalciuria and excessive absorption of dietary calcium may manifest mild, dietary-dependent hypercalcemia. Overtreatment of hypoparathyroidism or other conditions with calcitriol or topical use of analogues of the active vitamin D metabolites in psoriasis should be obvious from the history. Because hypercalcemia and hypercalciuria occur in up to 10 and 30%, respectively, of patients with thyrotoxicosis, measurement of serum thyroid-stimulating hormone (TSH) may be helpful especially in older patients, who may be less overtly symptomatic. Adrenal insufficiency and pheochromocytoma are usually accompanied by characteristic clinical features but may be diagnosed with appropriate studies. Granulomatous diseases are among the more common disorders that underlie initially unexplained hypercalcemia.

THERAPY FOR SEVERE HYPERCALCEMIA

Causes of Severe Hypercalcemia

Acute, severe hypercalcemia, usually defined as a serum calcium concentration greater than 3.5 mmol/L (14 mg/dL), is unusual because most patients with hypercalcemia have primary hyperparathyroidism, in which hypercalcemia is typically chronic and mild. Episodes of acute, severe hypercalcemia may occur occasionally in primary hyperparathyroidism ("parathyroid crisis"), however. These patients typically have large parathyroid adenomas and very high PTH levels. The severe hypercalcemia develops in the setting of dehydration due to diarrheal illness, protracted vomiting, or diuretics; recovery from major surgery; immobilization; ingestion of large amounts of oral calcium salts; or parathyroid carcinoma.

Most often, acute severe hypercalcemia occurs in patients with underlying malignancy, in whom accelerated bone resorption increases the filtered load of calcium. The ensuing hypercalciuria impairs renal tubular sodium reabsorption, which induces progressive extracellular volume depletion, reduces glomerular filtration, impairs renal calcium clearance, and aggravates the hypercalcemia. In many such patients, elevated levels of serum PTHrP compound the problem by mimicking the action of PTH to enhance renal tubular calcium reabsorption.

Clinical Features of Severe Hypercalcemia

The indications for urgent therapy of hypercalcemia usually relate more to the presence of clinical manifestations than to the absolute level of serum calcium, although few clinicians would hesitate to treat patients in whom total serum calcium exceeded 3.5 mmol/L (14 mg/dL). Many patients with previously mild hypercalcemia become symptomatic when serum calcium concentrations exceed 3 mmol/L (12 mg/dL). It is important to remember that hypoalbuminemia may mask elevations of ionized calcium. The most common symptoms of severe hypercalcemia are those referable to disturbances of nervous system and gastrointestinal function—fatigue, weakness, lethargy, confusion, coma (rarely), anorexia, nausea, abdominal pain (rarely due to pancreatitis), and constipation.[474] Polyuria, nocturia, and polydipsia are common. Bone pain may be due to underlying metastatic disease. Cardiac arrhythmias may include bradyarrhythmias or heart block, and digitalis toxicity may be potentiated. Coma, hypotension, acute pancreatitis, acute renal failure, widespread soft tissue calcification, heart failure, or venous thrombosis, particularly of the renal veins, may lead to a fatal outcome in acute severe hypercalcemia.

Management of Severe Hypercalcemia

The first decision to be made in the management of acute, severe hypercalcemia is whether or not to treat the problem. This decision may be an issue for the patient with an incurable, widely disseminated malignancy, when other approaches to controlling the neoplasm are exhausted and the patient has chosen not to have complications treated. Otherwise, as noted earlier patients with serum calcium above 3.5 mmol/L (14 mg/dL) should be treated aggressively. Treatment most often entails rehydration and administration of a bisphosphonate intravenously, and calcitonin can be useful early in therapy. Gallium nitrate, plicamycin, and intravenous phosphate are little used because of toxicity.

REHYDRATION. The first priority is to correct the extracellular volume depletion that invariably is present, usually by infusing isotonic saline at a rate of 2 to 4 L/d. The aggressiveness with which the individual patient is rehydrated must be considered in relation to both the volume status and the risk of precipitating congestive heart failure. Diuretics, particularly thiazides, should be discontinued. The conventional use of furosemide or other potent "loop" diuretics to promote calciuresis may exacerbate extracellular volume depletion if used early in the course of treatment.[475] In light of the current availability of effective alternatives for the treatment of hypercalcemia, diuretics probably are best avoided, except in circumstances in which vigorous rehydration fails to improve severe hypercalcemia or might precipitate congestive heart failure. In any case the prolonged use of saline-induced calciuresis without an effective antiresorptive agent should be avoided.

BISPHOSPHONATES. Several drugs are available for treatment of acute hypercalcemia (Table 24–3). Each inhibits osteoclastic bone resorption, although efficacy and toxicity vary substantially. The antiresorptive drug of first choice in most situations is an intravenous bisphosphonate. Of the two currently available in the United States, pamidronate more reliably returns serum calcium to normal, frequently after a single intravenous infusion, although the therapy can be repeated in refractory cases. The drug is generally well tolerated, although local pain or swelling at the infusion site, low-grade fever 1 to 2 d after the infusion, transient lymphopenia, and mild hypophosphatemia or hypomagnesemia may occur. Serum calcium usually declines rapidly, reaching the normal range within 2 to 3 days in more than 80% of cases and occasionally falling below normal at the nadir.[474] The duration of the response to pamidronate varies from a week to several months and cannot be predicted in an individual patient.[476] Use of intravenous etidronate in this setting has waned, not only because of its lower efficacy but also because of concern that it may induce a mineralization defect in bone, as has been observed in patients treated for Paget's disease with higher doses of oral etidronate. Oral alendronate, or other bisphosphonates currently being evaluated, may prove useful in preventing recurrence once severe hypercalcemia has been controlled.

CALCITONIN. Calcitonin, which directly inhibits osteoclast function, is frequently administered with other antiresorptive agents to achieve more rapid control of hypercalcemia.[474, 477, 478] Calcitonin rarely produces a decline in serum calcium of more than 0.5 mmol/L (2 mg/dL), and its efficacy is usually limited to a few days at most, possibly because of receptor down-regulation in target cells of bone and kidney.[477] Its major advantages are rapid onset of action (several hours) and its potential to augment renal calcium excretion directly. Calcitonin may produce a significant analgesic effect in patients with fracture or metastatic bone disease. Calcitonin is generally well tolerated, although transient nausea, vomiting, abdominal cramps, flushing, and local skin reactions may occur.[474]

GALLIUM NITRATE. Gallium nitrate restores serum calcium to normal and reduces urinary calcium and hydroxyproline within 5 to 7 days in most patients after a 5-d infusion of 200 mg/m².[479] Because of nephrotoxicity and less frequent adverse effects such as hypotension, nausea, vomiting, hypophosphatemia, and anemia, however, gallium generally is less widely used than are bisphosphonates.

PLICAMYCIN. Plicamycin (formerly "mithramycin") is an antiresorptive drug that for many years was the first-line agent

TABLE 24–3. Therapy for Severe Hypercalcemia

Therapy	Usual Dose	Frequency
Rehydration	2–4 L/d of 0.9% NaCl IV	qd × 1–5 d
Pamidronate	60–90 mg IV over 4–24 h	qd × 1 d
Etidronate	7.5 mg/kg IV over 4 h	qd × 3–7 d
Calcitonin	4 IU/kg SC	q6–12 h (salmon)
	0.5 mg SC	q12–24 h (human)
Gallium nitrate	200 mg/m² body surface area IV	qd × 5 d
Plicamycin	15–25 μg/kg IV over 4–6 h	qd or qod × 1–5 d
Glucocorticoids	200–300 mg hydrocortisone IV	qd × 3–5 d
Dialysis		

for treatment of severe hypercalcemia. Plicamycin causes a broad range of hepatic, renal, and hematologic side effects after repeated use. When plicamycin is administered, serum calcium typically begins to decline within 12 h and reaches a nadir at 48 to 72 h. The duration of action is unpredictable, however, ranging from a few days to several weeks.[474]

PHOSPHATE. Intravenous phosphate infusion was employed in the past to control hypercalcemia in patients with concomitant hypophosphatemia, but the mechanism of action, which may partly depend on direct inhibition of osteoclasts, almost certainly also involves generalized precipitation of calcium:phosphate salts in soft tissues, notably in the kidneys, pancreas, heart, lungs, stomach, and vessels. For this reason, and also because intravenous phosphate administration may produce severe, life-threatening hypocalcemia or hypotension, this therapy can no longer be considered standard for severe hypercalcemia.[474, 480] Oral phosphate in doses up to 2000 mg/d has been advocated for therapy of hypercalcemia in hypophosphatemic patients with normal renal function, but its efficacy is limited, it is not effective for urgent therapy of severe hypercalcemia, and its use is accompanied by frequent nausea, abdominal cramps, and diarrhea.

OTHER APPROACHES. Other strategies for control of severe hypercalcemia may be applicable in specific circumstances. High-dose glucocorticoids, for example, may be very helpful in vitamin D intoxication, granulomatous diseases such as sarcoidosis, and hematologic malignancies known or likely to be glucocorticoid-responsive. Because the effects of antiresorptive agents are somewhat delayed (i.e., days) and because acute reduction of serum calcium during the first 12 to 24 h depends mainly on inducing calciuresis through adequate rehydration, peritoneal or (preferably) hemodialysis may be required early in the management of life-threatening hypercalcemia. In this case, it is desirable to employ low- or zero-calcium dialysate.

Hypocalcemic Disorders

Clinical Presentation

The predominant manifestations of hypocalcemia are those of neuromuscular irritability, including perioral paresthesias, tingling of the fingers and toes, and spontaneous or latent tetany. Tetany can be elicited by percussion of the facial nerve below the zygoma, resulting in ispilateral contractions of the facial muscle (Chvostek's sign), or by 3 min of occlusive pressure with a blood pressure cuff, resulting in carpal spasm that on occasion can be painful (Trousseau's sign; Fig. 24–28). The usefulness of these signs in diagnosing hypocalcemia and following therapeutic responses cannot be overemphasized. Electrocardiographic abnormalities also result from hypocalcemia, including prolonged Q-T intervals[481] and marked QRS and ST changes that may mimic acute myocardial infarction or conduction abnormalities.[482] Ventricular arrhythmias are a rare complication of hypocalcemia, although congestive heart failure corrected by return of serum calcium to normal has been reported.[483] In profound or acute hypocalcemia grand mal seizures or laryngeal spasm may occur. Chronic hypocalcemia is associated with mild neuromuscular irritability and may be asymptomatic. Long-standing hypocalcemia associated with hyperphosphatemia (observed with PTH deficiency or resistance) can lead to calcification of the basal ganglia and occasional extrapyramidal disorders.[484] In addition, mineral deposits in the lens may lead to cataract formation. Chronic hypocalcemia, particularly when associated with hypophosphatemia, as in vitamin D deficiency, causes growth plate abnormalities in children (rickets) and defects in the mineralization of new bone (osteomalacia; see Chapter 25). Severe symptomatic hypocalcemia is an emergency that requires im-

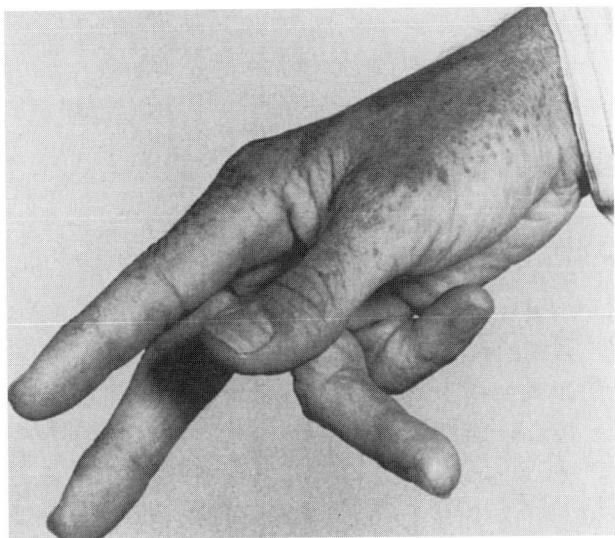

Figure 24–28. Trousseau's sign. (From Burnside JW, McGlynn TJ. Physical Diagnosis. 17th ed. Baltimore: Williams & Wilkins, 1987: 63, with permission.)

mediate therapy to prevent seizures and death from laryngeal spasm or cardiac causes.

Total calcium in serum includes both the free (biologically active) and protein-bound components; the major binding protein is albumin (see the introduction to this chapter). Therefore measurements of total calcium cannot be interpreted without concurrent measurement of albumin. Studies of hypoalbuminemic patients with cirrhosis have led to a formula for correction of total calcium based on concurrent albumin levels (a decrease in calcium of 0.2 mmol/L (0.8 mg/dL) for every 10 g/L (1 g/dL) decrease in albumin). No formula has proved accurate, however, for assessment of calcium in acutely ill patients, probably because of the variety of factors that can increase protein binding and decrease the free calcium, including alkalosis, elevated circulating free fatty acids, and lipid infusions.[485] Consequently ionized calcium should be measured when the diagnosis of hypocalcemia is considered in the setting of acute illness and/or severe hypoalbuminemia.

Chronic hypocalcemia is due most often to deficiency of parathyroid hormone or $1,25(OH)_2D$ or to resistance to the biologic effects of these calcium-regulating hormones (Table 24–4).

Parathyroid-Related Disorders

Hypocalcemia due to parathyroid disease can be differentiated from other causes by routine laboratory tests. Serum calcium is low owing to lack of PTH-mediated bone resorption and calcium reabsorption by the kidney. Serum phosphate is elevated owing to impaired renal clearance. Levels of $1,25(OH)_2D$ are low because PTH and hypophosphatemia stimulate the renal $25(OH)D$ 1α-hydroxylase. Consequently, $1,25(OH)_2D$–mediated intestinal calcium absorption is decreased, further exacerbating the hypocalcemia. PTH levels, using sensitive two-site PTH assays (see Fig. 24–19) are usually low or undetectable but may be inappropriately normal, if some degree of PTH production is preserved. Levels of PTH are elevated in syndromes associated with resistance to the action of PTH.

CONGENITAL OR INHERITED PARATHYROID DISORDERS

Several rare syndromes associated with congenital or inherited hypoparathyroidism appear sporadically or in a variety

TABLE 24–4. Causes of Hypocalcemia

Parathyroid-Related Disorders

Absence of the Parathyroid Glands or of PTH

Congenital
  DiGeorge syndrome
  X-linked or autosomally inherited hypoparathyroidism
  Autoimmune polyglandular syndrome type I
  PTH gene mutations
Postsurgical hypoparathyroidism
Infiltrative disorders
  Hemochromatosis
  Wilson's disease
  Metastases
Hypoparathyroidism after radioactive iodine thyroid ablation

Impaired Secretion of PTH

Hypomagnesemia
Respiratory alkalosis
Activating mutations of the calcium sensor

Target-Organ Resistance

Hypomagnesemia
Pseudohypoparathyroidism
  Type I
  Type II

Vitamin D–Related Disorders

Vitamin D Deficiency
Dietary absence
Malabsorption

Accelerated Loss

Impaired enterohepatic recirculation
Anticonvulsant medications

Impaired 25-Hydroxylation

Liver disease
Isoniazid

Impaired 1α-Hydroxylation

Renal failure
Vitamin D–dependent rickets type I
Oncogenic osteomalacia

Target-Organ Resistance

Vitamin D–dependent rickets type II
Phenytoin

Other Causes

Excessive Deposition in the Skeleton
Osteoblastic malignancies
Hungry bone syndrome

Chelation

Foscarnet
Phosphate infusion
Infusion of citrated blood products
Infusion of EDTA containing contrast reagents
Fluoride

Neonatal Hypocalcemia

Prematurity
Asphyxia
Diabetic mother
Hyperparathyroid mother

Critical Illness

Pancreatitis
Toxic shock syndrome
Intensive care unit patients

of inheritance patterns, suggesting multiple etiologies. Di-George syndrome occurs sporadically and is associated with an embryologic defect in the formation of the third, fourth, and fifth branchial pouches, resulting in the absence of parathyroid glands. Complete DiGeorge syndrome is also associated with cardiac defects and immunodeficiency due to concomitant thymic aplasia. Microdeletion of 22q11.21-q11.23[486] and a t(2;22)(q14;q11) balanced translocation suggest that a gene at chromosome 22q11 may be the cause of this syndrome.[487] Hypoparathyroidism also has been reported in two patients with a 22q11 deletion.[488]

DiGeorge syndrome may, in fact, be a neurocrestopathy, since ablation of the premigratory cephalic neural crest in chick embryos produces a similar phenotype.[489] The contribution of homeobox genes to parathyroid development and their potential relationship to DiGeorge syndrome are suggested by the absence of thymic and parathyroid tissue, accompanied by cardiac and craniofacial abnormalities, in mice lacking the homeobox gene hox-1.5.[490] Multiple genetic loci play an important role in the development of the parathyroid glands; for example, the gene responsible for X-linked, recessive hypoparathyroidism is located on Xq26-Xq27.[491]

Familial hypoparathyroidism is seen in conjunction with mucocutaneous candidiasis, Addison's disease, and other immune disorders in autosomal recessive autoimmune polyglandular syndrome type I (see Chapter 33). Other inherited forms of hypoparathyroidism may occur as isolated defects[492] or present with other features, such as lymphedema, dysmorphism, hearing impairment, and renal and cardiac abnormalities.[493–495]

ABNORMALITIES IN THE *PTH* GENE

Specific defects in the *PTH* gene have been found in a small number of kindreds affected by congenital hypoparathyroidism. These defects include point mutations in the signal peptide[12] and in an intron border, leading to aberrant splicing.[496] No abnormalities in the sequences encoding PTH(1–84) have been discovered in familial hypoparathyroidism.

DESTRUCTION OF THE PARATHYROID GLANDS

The most common cause of chronic hypocalcemia is postsurgical hypoparathyroidism. This condition may occur after removal of all parathyroid tissue during thyroidectomy and radical neck dissection for malignancies or after inadvertent interruption of the blood supply to the parathyroid glands during head and neck surgery. Transient hypoparathyroidism, attributed to chronic suppression of the remaining normal glands, is common after parathyroidectomy; permanent hypoparathyroidism occasionally may be due to vascular or surgical injury or inadvertent removal of all parathyroid tissue. Rarely, transient hypoparathyroidism may follow spontaneous infarction of autonomous tissue in primary hyperparathyroidism.[497, 498] Hypoparathyroidism is a rare complication of radioactive iodine ablation of the thyroid gland for Graves' disease.[499]

Hypoparathyroidism can also occur as a result of infiltrative diseases of the parathyroids. This is seen in diseases of iron overload such as in hemochromatosis and in patients with thalassemia major who have been heavily transfused.[500] Copper deposition in Wilson's disease[501] may cause parathyroid dysfunction. Metastatic disease to the parathyroids is a rare cause of hypoparathyroidism, presumably because all four glands must be involved before significant hypoparathyroidism occurs.

IMPAIRED PTH SECRETION

Impaired secretion of PTH from the parathyroid glands can lead to functional hypoparathyroidism, as in profound hypomagnesemia,[502] in which target-organ resistance to PTH can also occur. Both of these abnormalities are reversible on magnesium repletion[503, 504] (see the section on magnesium disorders).

Chronic respiratory alkalosis leads to hyperphosphatemia and decreased ionized calcium levels accompanied by impaired renal calcium resorption and inappropriately normal PTH levels.[505] This biochemical phenotype suggests both an abnormality of PTH secretion and renal resistance to PTH.

TABLE 24–5. Types of Pseudohypoparathyroidism

Disorder	Response of Urinary cAMP to PTH	Response of Urinary PO₄ to PTH	Other Hormonal Resistance	AHO	Pathophysiology
Pseudohypoparathyroidism type IA	Decreased	Decreased	Yes	Yes	$G_{\alpha s}$ mutation
Pseudopseudohypoparathyroidism	Normal	Normal	No	Yes	$G_{\alpha s}$ mutation
Pseudohypoparathyroidism type IB	Decreased	Decreased	No	No	?PTH receptor regulation defect
Pseudohypoparathyroidism type IC	Decreased	Decreased	Yes	Yes	$G_{\alpha s}$ function normal
Pseudohypoparathyroidism type II	Normal	Decreased	No	No	Vitamin D deficiency in some cases

AHO, Albright's hereditary osteodystrophy.

Activating mutations in the calcium-sensing receptor cause autosomal dominant hypocalcemia associated with inappropriately normal PTH levels. The mutation in the sensor causes augmented signal transduction, such that the gland appears to sense a higher serum calcium than is actually present.[506, 507]

PSEUDOHYPOPARATHYROIDISM

The idiopathic and inherited forms of PTH resistance are referred to as pseudohypoparathyroidism (PHP). The first cases of documented PTH resistance were described by Albright and colleagues in 1942.[508] These patients were hypocalcemic and hyperphosphatemic and exhibited a number of features now called Albright's hereditary osteodystrophy (AHO). These features include short stature, rounded face, foreshortened fourth metacarpals and other bones of the hands and feet, obesity, and subcutaneous calcifications (Figs. 24–29 and 24–30). The administration of PTH to these patients failed to provoke a phosphate diuresis or an increase in serum calcium, and it was subsequently shown that these patients have elevated PTH levels and that PTH infusions fail to stimulate renal production of cAMP. This measurement proved a more reliable diagnostic test than measurements of phosphate clearance, and the measurement of cAMP in the urine following an infusion of synthetic PTH(1–34) is now used to establish the diagnosis of PTH resistance.[509] Failure of stimulation of cAMP production suggests a defect in the PTH receptor or in its cAMP-mediated signal transduction.[510, 511]

The variable presence of AHO and renal resistance to PTH has led to the subclassification of PHP (Table 24–5). Type IA is characterized by autosomal dominant inheritance, AHO, and diminished $G_{\alpha s}$ activity (approximately 50% of normal). The diminished $G_{\alpha s}$ activity has been demonstrated in several tissues, including kidney, fibroblasts, transformed lymphocytes, platelets, and erythrocytes. Decreased amounts of $G_{\alpha s}$ mRNA (50%) are present in fibroblasts of many patients with PHP type IA,[512, 513] and mutations in the $G_{\alpha s}$ gene have been identified in several kindreds.[514, 515] Mentation is impaired in approximately half of the patients with PHP type IA and appears to be related to the $G_{\alpha s}$ deficiency rather than to chronic hypocalcemia, since patients with other forms of PHP and hypocalcemia have normal mentation.[516] The $G_{\alpha s}$ deficiency in PHP type IA may cause not only PTH resistance but also resistance to TSH, glucagon, and gonadotropins, resulting in thyroid and gonadal dysfunction.

Two central features of PHP type IA that remain unexplained are (1) the dominant phenotype of heterozygous patients, whose one normal G_S allele might be expected to support normal G_S function, and (2) the disproportionate effect of the mutations on the growth plate, leading to AHO, and on renal PTH responsiveness.

Paradoxically, two unrelated males with both PHP type IA and gonadotropin-independent precocious puberty have been

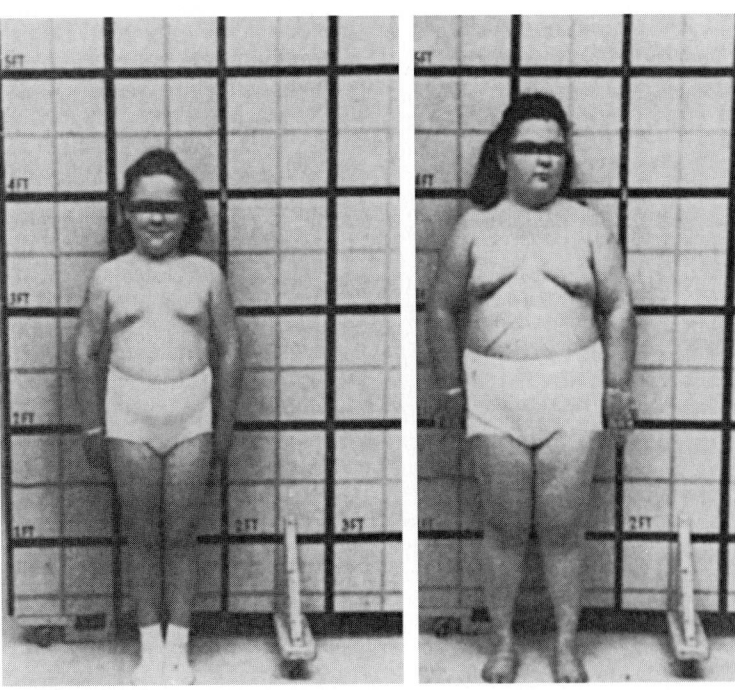

Figure 24–29. Daughter *(left)* and mother *(right)* with pseudohypoparathyroidism and Albright's hereditary osteodystrophy. (From Aurbach GD, Marx SJ, Spiegel AM: Parathyroid hormone, calcitonin, and the calciferols. In: Wilson JD, Foster DW, eds. Williams Textbook of Endocrinology. 8th ed. Philadelphia: WB Saunders, 1992: 1460, with permission.)

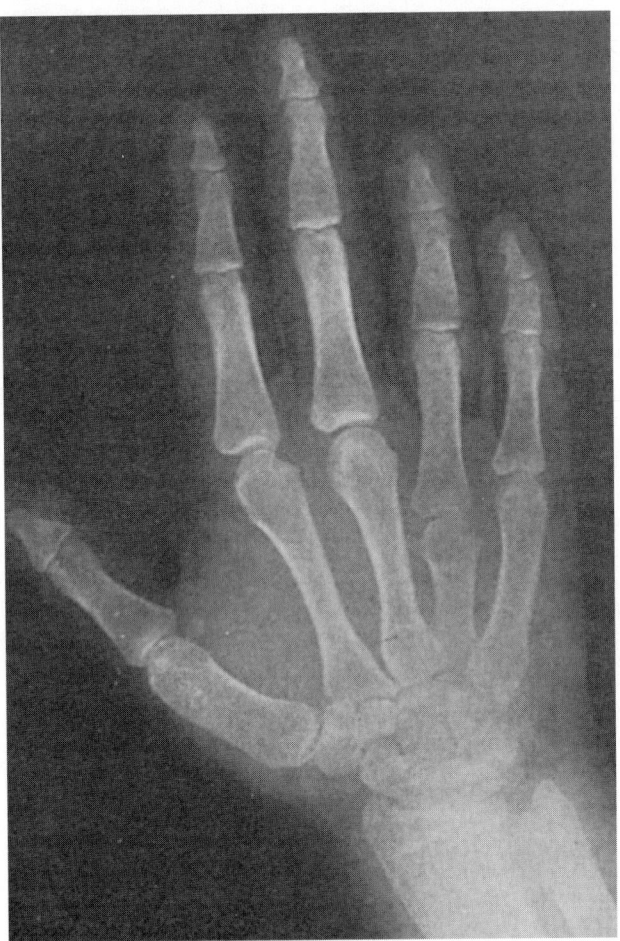

Figure 24–30. Radiograph of hand of patient with pseudohypoparathyroidism and Albright's hereditary osteodystrophy. Note shortened fourth metacarpal. (From Aurbach GD, Marx SJ, Spiegel AM. Parathyroid hormone, calcitonin, and the calciferols. In: Wilson JD, Foster DW, eds. Williams Textbook of Endocrinology. 8th ed. Philadelphia: WB Saunders, 1992: 1461, with permission.)

described. The $G_{\alpha S}$ point mutation in these individuals is thought to lead to a protein that is unstable at 37°C and therefore to confer renal resistance to PTH. At the lower temperature of the testes, however, the protein is not degraded. In this setting, the stable but mutated protein is constitutively active and stimulates the Leydig cell, in the same way that the G_S mutations act constitutively in McCune-Albright syndrome (see Chapter 25).[517]

Pseudopseudohypoparathyroidism (pseudo-PHP) is a term used to refer to individuals with the phenotype of AHO but with normal biochemical parameters. Patients with pseudo-PHP often are found in the same kindreds as those with PHP type IA and invariably inherit the abnormal $G_{\alpha S}$ gene found in their PTH-resistant relatives.[518] When the abnormality is maternally transmitted, the children inheriting the abnormal $G_{\alpha S}$ gene exhibit PTH resistance, whereas when it is paternally transmitted, AHO may occur in isolation. This suggests that in addition to autosomal dominant inheritance of the AHO phenotype genetic imprinting may play a role in the inheritance of PTH resistance.[519, 520] Several patients with AHO and PTH resistance have had normal $G_{\alpha S}$ activity; this subgroup has been designated PHP type IC. Biochemical characterization in one case[521] revealed a significant decrease in the manganese-stimulated adenylate cyclase activity in fibroblast membranes of the affected individual, raising the possibility that a second defect in the cAMP pathway may lead to a phenotype resembling that of PHP type IA.

PHP type IB presents with hypocalcemia and failure of PTH infusions to increase urinary cAMP production. However, it is not accompanied by AHO, and it is not associated with abnormal $G_{\alpha S}$ levels. Renal resistance to PTH is the only consistent feature of type IB; therefore several investigators have postulated that this syndrome is due to an isolated abnormality of the PTH receptor. However, a search for mutations in the coding exons of the receptor gene in 17 affected patients revealed only three silent polymorphisms and one missense mutation that had no effect on receptor function in vitro.[522] The target-organ manifestations of PHP type IB are variable, with some affected individuals having manifestations of PTH overactivity in bone and PTH resistance in kidney. Cultured osteoblast-like cells from a patient with this disorder demonstrated normal cAMP responsiveness to PTH, despite the lack of renal responsiveness.[523] This finding suggests that differential tissue-specific regulation of expression or splicing of the receptor or differences in signal transduction pathways in different tissues may be responsible. Dexamethasone pretreatment of cultured fibroblasts from some patients with PHP type IB restores normal PTH-stimulated cAMP production[524] and returns PTH/PTHrP receptor mRNA levels in fibroblasts to normal.[525] These results support the hypothesis that regulatory abnormalities in the expression of the receptor may be the underlying defect.

In PHP type II, PTH infusions increase urinary cAMP normally but do not elicit a phosphaturic response.[526] This syndrome, like PHP type IB, lacks signs of AHO or resistance to other hormones but unlike PHP type IB is not familial in origin. The age at onset is variable, ranging from infancy to senescence, suggesting that it is an acquired defect or that the biochemical phenotype may be unmasked by intercurrent abnormalities. A similar biochemical phenotype can be observed in vitamin D deficiency, and some authors have suggested that PHP type II is a manifestation of vitamin D deficiency rather than a distinct clinical entity.[527] Minagawa and colleagues reported cases of three neonates with no signs of rickets and with normal levels of vitamin D who presented with transient PHP type II that resolved at about 6 months of age.[528] They postulated that PTH responsiveness is subject to maturation during fetal and neonatal development. PHP type II therefore seems to constitute a heterogeneous clinical disorder associated with defects in PTH responsiveness distal to cAMP or involving a separate signal transduction pathway.[529]

The resistance to PTH in PHP has not been documented in bone cells; rather, several patients with PHP type IB have had skeletal changes consistent with hyperparathyroidism.[530–533] Patients with PHP have lower bone density than normal and hypoparathyroid control subjects. Basal urinary hydroxyproline excretion in patients with PHP is twice that of hypoparathyroid control subjects, and the two groups have similar increases in response to parathyroid extract.[534] Because the markers of bone turnover in patients with PHP are not as high as those of hyperparathyroid patients with similar or lower PTH levels, the PTH resistance in bone may be relative.[532] However, normal cAMP response to PTH has been documented in osteoblasts isolated from patients with PHP type IA[535] and PHP type IB,[523] suggesting that the hypocalcemia in PHP is not secondary to skeletal resistance but a consequence of the renal resistance to PTH that results in both increased urinary calcium losses and impaired 25(OH)D 1α-hydroxylation. The lack of activation of vitamin D decreases intestinal calcium absorption and causes osteomalacia, both of which exacerbate the hypocalcemia. Deficiency of 1,25(OH)$_2$D and the resultant hypocalcemia can, in turn, impair the phosphaturic, but not the urinary, cAMP responses to PTH;[536] therefore it is imperative that studies to confirm the diagnosis of PHP type II be performed in normocalcemic patients who have normal vitamin D status.

Vitamin D–Related Disorders

Hypocalcemia secondary to vitamin D deficiency or resistance to the biologic effects of $1,25(OH)_2D$ is easily differentiated from hypoparathyroidism by routine clinical and laboratory evaluation. The primary cause of hypocalcemia in vitamin D deficiency is decreased intestinal absorption of calcium. In the setting of normal renal function, the hypocalcemia of vitamin D deficiency, unlike that of hypoparathyroidism, is accompanied by hypophosphatemia and increased renal phosphate clearance. This increase in phosphate clearance is a result of compensatory (secondary) hyperparathyroidism, which is a direct result of the hypocalcemic stimulus to PTH secretion and of stimulation of *PTH* gene expression and parathyroid cell proliferation by hypocalcemia and low levels of $1,25(OH)_2D$ (see the section on parathyroid hormone biosynthesis). Therefore measurement of serum phosphate and PTH are very useful in distinguishing these disorders from hypoparathyroidism. The secondary hyperparathyroidism results in increased calcium mobilization from the skeleton, increased renal reabsorption of calcium and increased renal 1α-hydroxylation of $25(OH)D$. In severe vitamin D deficiency, the increased levels of PTH no longer lead to increased bone resorption, perhaps because osteoclasts cannot resorb unmineralized osteoid.

In severe vitamin D deficiency the level of $1,25(OH)_2D$ is usually low, but in moderate vitamin D deficiency the stimulation of the renal 1α-hydroxylase by PTH can result in a normal or even an elevated $1,25(OH)_2D$ level. These high levels of $1,25(OH)_2D$ reflect the action of PTH on the renal 1α-hydroxylase. The ineffectiveness of the high levels of total $1,25(OH)_2D$ may be due to a high degree of binding to the vitamin D–binding protein in the absence of $25(OH)D$, which normally binds to the same site on the binding protein.

VITAMIN D DEFICIENCY

Because the two sources of vitamin D are the diet and cutaneous synthesis after ultraviolet irradiation, lack of solar irradiation and decreased intake or impaired absorption of vitamin D can lead to vitamin D deficiency. As the population has become increasingly educated about the risks of skin cancer from solar irradiation, the avoidance of long periods of intense sun exposure and the use of high SPF (solar protective factor) sunblocks have resulted in increased reliance on dietary sources of vitamin D. The recommended daily allowance for vitamin D is 200 IU; however, in the absence of solar exposure, this amount is two to three times lower than that required to prevent vitamin D deficiency.[537] Vitamin D is present in many food sources, both vegetable and animal, and many prepared foods, especially cereal products, are fortified with vitamin D. Although dairy products have been fortified with vitamin D as well, the actual amount of vitamin D provided does not correlate well with the purported content.[242] The vitamin D derived from vegetable sources is vitamin D_2 (ergocalciferol) and that from animal sources is vitamin D_3 (cholecalciferol). These two forms of vitamin D are metabolized identically and have equivalent biologic potency in humans. Both forms have been used to fortify foods.

Early vitamin D deficiency can be detected when the serum level of $25(OH)D$ falls below 37 nmol/L (15 ng/mL), since this level is associated with the development of secondary hyperparathyroidism. Owing to the presence of vitamin D in many food products, true dietary vitamin D deficiency is rare in the normal ambulatory population, but is a problem among elderly homebound individuals.[538] The clinical relevance of vitamin D deficiency in the elderly has been confirmed by a study demonstrating that vitamin D administration (800 IU/d) to an ambulatory elderly population decreases serum PTH levels and the incidence of hip fracture.[539] Malabsorption, however, can cause vitamin D deficiency in all age groups. Because vitamin D is a fat-soluble vitamin, its absorption is dependent on emulsification by bile acids. Any cause of fat malabsorption or short bowel syndrome can result in vitamin D deficiency; therefore, malabsorption should be ruled out in patients with low $25(OH)D$ levels (<19 nmol/L [<8 ng/mL]).

ACCELERATED LOSS OF VITAMIN D

$25(OH)D$ and $1,25(OH)_2D$ are secreted into the bile and undergo enterohepatic circulation;[540] therefore intestinal disease may also cause vitamin D deficiency due to excessive losses. Increased metabolism of vitamin D can lead to low blood levels of $25(OH)D$ in individuals given anticonvulsant medications and antituberculous therapy. Phenobarbital, primidone, phenytoin,[541] rifampin, and glutethimide[542] accelerate the hepatic inactivation of vitamin D.

IMPAIRED 25-HYDROXYLATION OF VITAMIN D

The vitamin D that is absorbed undergoes 25-hydroxylation in the liver; therefore hepatic parenchymal disease can cause $25(OH)D$ deficiency. Clinically $25(OH)D$ deficiency as a consequence of liver disease is rare, since the degree of hepatic destruction necessary to impair 25-hydroxylation is incompatible with long-term survival. However, isoniazid decreases the 25-hydroxylation of vitamin D.[543] Two kindreds have been described in whom the clinical and biochemical features and therapeutic responses suggest an inherited 25-hydroxylation defect.[544]

IMPAIRED 1α-HYDROXYLATION OF 25-HYDROXYVITAMIN D

The final step in the activation of vitamin D is the hydroxylation of $25(OH)D$ by the renal 1α-hydroxylase to yield $1,25(OH)_2D$. Renal parenchymal damage therefore can result in deficiency of the active metabolite of vitamin D once creatinine clearance decreases to approximately 30 to 40 mL/min. Unlike liver failure, dialysis permits long-term survival of patients with renal failure; therefore deficiency of $1,25(OH)_2D$ due to impaired renal 1α-hydroxylation is a common and important entity. The metabolic consequences of chronic renal failure on the parathyroid glands and the skeleton are complex (see Chapter 25). Impaired renal 1α-hydroxylation decreases intestinal absorption of calcium, resulting in hypocalcemia. The diminished phosphate clearance associated with renal failure leads to elevated levels of blood phosphate; this, in turn, further lowers levels of calcium and $1,25(OH)_2D$. The resulting secondary hyperparathyroidism increases release of calcium and phosphate from bone, but because of the renal insufficiency, PTH does not have a phosphaturic effect. As a result serum phosphate rises even further. Oral phosphate binders are used to lower blood phosphate. Currently calcium-containing antacids are used as oral phosphate binders, in preference to the more toxic aluminum-containing antacids (see Chapter 25). Calcium administration also attenuates the hypocalcemic stimulus to parathyroid secretion. Calcitriol $(1,25(OH)_2D)$ is critical for the absorption of calcium and should be administered early in the course of renal failure (when the creatinine clearance falls below 30 to 40 mL/min) to avoid the development of secondary hyperparathyroidism, with careful monitoring to prevent the development of hypercalcemia. Once secondary hyperparathyroidism has developed, the administration of pharmacologic doses of calcitriol intravenously[545] or by mouth[546–549] may be required to suppress *PTH* gene transcription and parathyroid cellular proliferation.

Efforts are currently underway to develop nonhypercalcemic analogues of $1,25(OH)_2D$ that maintain the PTH suppressing and antiproliferative effects. Such analogues would be invaluable for the prevention and treatment of secondary hyperparathyroidism in the setting of chronic renal failure and perhaps in the treatment of malignancies whose proliferation is inhibited by pharmacologic doses of calcitriol. Decreased levels of $1,25(OH)_2D$ may also be observed in patients taking ketoconazole[246] and in oncogenic osteomalacia (see Chapter 25).[550]

A rare autosomal recessive defect of vitamin D activation has been described in several kindreds. Biochemically, vitamin D–dependent rickets type I is characterized by hypocalcemia and secondary hyperparathyroidism. The only metabolic abnormalities that differentiate it from dietary vitamin D deficiency are the presence of normal or elevated levels of vitamin D and $25(OH)D$ accompanied by low levels of $1,25(OH)_2D$.[551, 552] The disease presents in infancy with rickets, osteomalacia, and seizures.[553] Because of the high levels of vitamin D and $25(OH)D$ and low levels of $1,25(OH)_2D$, it has been postulated that this disease represents an inherited form of impaired renal 1α-hydroxylation. Although the precise biochemical defect has not been elucidated, the therapeutic response to physiological replacement doses of 1α-hydroxylated metabolites of vitamin D such as calcitriol supports the hypothesis of a defect in 1α-hydroxylation as the underlying abnormality.[554, 555]

TARGET-ORGAN RESISTANCE TO 1,25(OH)₂D

A second rare autosomal recessive disorder, characterized by resistance to the biologic actions of $1,25(OH)_2D$, is referred to as vitamin D–dependent rickets type II. Its features of hypocalcemia, hypophosphatemia, and secondary hyperparathyroidism resemble those of vitamin D deficiency, but it is accompanied by elevated levels of $1,25(OH)_2D$. The molecular basis for this disease is mutation of the vitamin D receptor gene, resulting in impaired target-organ responsiveness. Most of the described mutations involve the DNA binding domain of the receptor[556–561] and decrease the affinity of the receptor for binding to its response elements on target genes,[559, 560] leading to impaired regulation of these genes. Mutations in the hormone binding domain[562] of the receptor have also been described in kindreds with vitamin D–dependent rickets type II. The clinical presentation of vitamin D–dependent rickets type II is variable; most patients present in infancy with rickets, hypophosphatemia, and seizures, although presentation in late adolescence has also been described.[563] Alopecia totalis develops in the first 2 y of life in some kindreds.[564]

Because of the target-organ resistance to the active metabolite of vitamin D, there is no ideal treatment for vitamin D–dependent rickets type II. Pharmacologic doses of vitamin D calcifediol ($25(OH)D$), $24,25(OH)D$, and calcitriol have been administered in an attempt to overcome this target-organ resistance,[565, 566] with variable effects. In the patients in whom the hypocalcemia and osteomalacia are resistant to such therapeutic interventions, parenteral calcium infusions may heal osteomalacic lesions.[292] Lifelong therapy is usually required, although spontaneous remissions have been described.[564, 565, 567–569] The pathophysiology of the spontaneous remissions is not understood, since the underlying genetic defect still exists. It is likely that these "remissions" reflect compensated calcium homeostasis once the needs of the growing skeleton are met. In support of this hypothesis is a report of a relapse in a pregnant woman, followed by a postpartum remission.[570]

Phenytoin causes target-organ resistance to the biologic effects of $1,25(OH)_2D$ in addition to its acceleration of the hepatic catabolism of vitamin D metabolites. Phenytoin also impairs intestinal calcium absorption in rats[571] and impairs PTH and $1,25(OH)_2D$–mediated bone resorption in vitro.

Other Causes of Hypocalcemia

EXCESSIVE DEPOSITION OF CALCIUM INTO THE SKELETON

Excessive deposition of calcium into the skeleton can occur in association with osteoblastic metastases, with chondrosarcomas,[572] and in the hungry bone syndrome. This syndrome presents as prolonged hypocalcemia, hypocalciuria, and hypophosphatemia after parathyroidectomy for primary hyperparathyroidism (see the section on primary hyperparathyroidism). Hungry bone syndrome is a consequence of remineralization of a skeleton that has been subjected to the bone-resorbing effects of PTH over a prolonged period. The syndrome can also be observed after treatment of other diseases associated with excessive bone resorption and has been described following radioactive iodine treatment of a patient with Graves' disease.[573]

CHELATION

Decreases in ionized calcium have been reported with foscarnet, a pyrophosphate analogue that is used as an antiviral agent,[574] perhaps because of complex formation between ionized calcium and the drug.

Hyperphosphatemia, due to phosphate administration or rapid destruction of soft tissue (i.e., rhabdomyolysis, chemotherapy of hematologic malignancies), may cause profound hypocalcemia by complexing and precipitating calcium in bone or soft tissues, by inhibiting bone resorption, and by blocking renal synthesis of $1,25(OH)_2D$ (see section on phosphate disorders).

Massive infusions of citrated blood products can cause hypocalcemia, presumably because citrate complexes calcium in the recipient's plasma.[575] Large doses of EDTA-containing radiographic contrast dyes may also cause hypocalcemia. Hypocalcemia due to formation of complexes of calcium and fluoride has been reported with hydrofluoric acid burns.[576]

NEONATAL HYPOCALCEMIA

Neonatal hypocalcemia is seen in infants of hyperparathyroid mothers, infants of mothers with diabetes mellitus, premature infants, and infants with birth asphyxia. The cause of hypocalcemia in infants of diabetic mothers is likely multifactorial,[577] but the response of premature infants and infants of mothers with diabetes mellitus to exogenous PTH suggests that functional hypoparathyroidism may in part account for the increased hypocalcemia in these two groups.[577, 578] The hypocalcemia in infants of hyperparathyroid mothers is presumably secondary to the maternal hypercalcemia, which in turn suppresses fetal parathyroid function.[579]

CRITICAL ILLNESS

Severe acute pancreatitis is often associated with hypocalcemia, and this association is a negative prognostic indicator. The hypocalcemia occurs shortly after the onset of the pancreatitis and is associated with an increase in PTH levels, suggesting that parathyroid function is normal. It has long been thought that this hypocalcemia is secondary to deposition of "calcium soaps" consisting of calcium and fatty acids; supporting this hypothesis, studies in a patient with a pancreatic fistula have demonstrated hypocalcemia (1.1 mmol/L [4.3 mg/dL]) in the setting of high levels of calcium (6.5 mmol/L [26 mg/dL]) and fatty acids in ascitic fluid.[580] Subsequent studies in a rat model have supported this finding and demonstrated that oleate has a high binding capacity for calcium.[581] However, in a porcine model of experimental pancreatitis hypocalcemia did not occur when the animals were subjected to thyroidectomy prior to the induction of pancreatitis,[582] suggesting a role for calcitonin in the development of hypocalcemia with acute pancreatitis, although calcitonin levels are normal in hypocalcemic individuals with pancreatitis.[583] Severe hypocalcemia with hypercalcitoninemia and hypophosphatemia occurs in the toxic shock syndrome,[237] in sepsis, and in critically ill patients.[584] As in acute pancreatitis, this hypocalcemia is usually accompanied by increases in serum levels of PTH, and the degree of hypocalcemia is a negative prognostic indicator. The mechanism of hypocalcemia in these patients is likely to be heterogeneous and has not been clearly defined.

Treatment of Hypocalcemia

Acute hypocalcemia is an emergency that requires prompt attention. If symptoms of neuromuscular irritability are present and carpopedal spasm is elicited on physical examination, treatment with intravenous calcium is indicated until the signs and symptoms of hypocalcemia subside. Approximately 100 mg of elemental calcium should be infused over a period of 10 to 20 min (Table 24–6). If this does not alleviate the clinical manifestations, an infusion of 100 mg/h can be given to adults for several hours, with close monitoring of calcium levels. In hypocalcemia associated with hypomagnesemia, magnesium replacement also is required. Magnesium should be given intravenously, 50 mmol over 24 h in the acute setting. Because most of the parenteral magnesium is excreted in the urine, oral magnesium oxide should be administered as soon as possible to replenish body stores. Special caution and reduced doses are necessary when administering magnesium to patients with renal failure (see section on magnesium disorders).

The treatment of hypocalcemia should be directed at the underlying disorder. In all cases, replacement with exogenous calcium (1 to 3 g daily) should be instituted. Calcium carbonate is the least expensive formulation but requires acidification for efficient absorption. This is an important consideration in patients with achlorhydria and in those in whom gastric acid production is being suppressed with pharmacologic agents. Because of the acid buffering capacity of calcium carbonate, patients should take calcium carbonate in divided doses of 1 g or less with food or citrus drinks to promote maximal absorption.

In cases of vitamin D deficiency or resistance, the metabolite of vitamin D chosen depends on the underlying disorder. If renal 1α-hydroxylation is impaired, as in renal failure, hypoparathyroidism (or PTH resistance), or the vitamin D–dependent rickets, metabolites that do not require this modification should be administered (calcitriol 0.25 to 1 μg/d or dihydrotachysterol, 0.2 to 1 mg/d). If decreased intake or increased losses are the problem, vitamin D should be administered, and treatment should be directed at the underlying disorder. Initial repletion of stores can be undertaken with 50,000 IU of vitamin D daily for 1 to 2 wk, followed by weekly or bimonthly administration until the underlying disorder is corrected. In patients with resistance to vitamin D, such as those on phenytoin, high doses (50,000 IU one to three times weekly) should be administered as maintenance therapy. In other patients, once treatment of the underlying disorder and repletion of body stores have been addressed, two multivitamins (800 IU/d) should provide sufficient maintenance therapy. In cases of severe malabsorption, vitamin D can be administered parenterally (in hyperalimentation or up to 500,000 IU intramuscularly twice a year).

Patients should be monitored closely to assess response to therapy and prevent therapeutic complications. Serum calcium should be monitored frequently (daily with profound hypocalcemia, weekly with moderate hypocalcemia) for the first month of therapy. Concomitant with resolution of hypocalcemia, serum PTH level should decline as the secondary hyperparathyroidism resolves. Measurement of serum PTH and assessment of 24-h urinary calcium excretion should be performed within 2 to 4 wk of institution of therapy. The urinary calcium measurement reflects the effect of therapy on calcium absorption. In addition, it provides important information on which to base therapeutic modifications to avoid nephrolithiasis. Once serum and urinary calcium levels are normal and PTH levels are decreased, aggressive replacement therapy should be changed to maintenance therapy to prevent hypercalcemia and nephrolithiasis. These same parameters

TABLE 24–6. Therapeutic Mineral Ion Preparations

Compound	MW*	Mineral Ion Content mg/g	Mineral Ion Content mmol/g	Oral Preparations COMPOUND	Oral Preparations ION CONTENT		Parenteral Preparations COMPOUND	Parenteral Preparations ION CONTENT	
Calcium									
Ca carbonate	100	400	10.0	1250 mg‡	500 mg	12.5 mmol			
Ca phosphate	310	383	9.6	1565 mg	600 mg	15.0 mmol			
Ca acetate	158	253	6.3	668 mg‡	167 mg	4.2 mmol			
Ca citrate	498	210	6.0	950 mg‡	200 mg	5.0 mmol			
Ca lactate	218	130	4.6	650 mg‡	84 mg	2.1 mmol			
Ca glubionate		64	1.7	5 mL	115 mg	2.0 mmol			
Ca gluconate	430	93	2.3	1000 mg‡	93 mg	2.3 mmol	10% soln	93 mg/10 mL	2.3 mmol/10 mL
Ca glucoptate	488	82	2.0				22% soln	90 mg/5 mL	2.3 mmol/10 mL
Ca chloride	147	273	6.8				10% soln	273 mg/10 mL	11.2 mmol/10 mL
Magnesium									
Mg oxide	40	603	24.8	400 mg‡	241 mg	9.9 mmol			
Mg gluconate	450	54	2.2	500 mg	27 mg	1.1 mmol			
Mg chloride	203	120	4.9	535 mg	64 mg	2.6 mmol	20% soln	24 mg/mL	1.0 mmol/mL
Mg sulfate	246	99	4.1				50% soln‡	49 mg/mL	2.0 mmol/mL
Phosphorus†									
Na/K phosphate (neutral)				Capsule	250 mg	8.1 mmol			
K phosphate (neutral)				Capsule	250 mg	8.1 mmol	Solution	94 mg/mL	3.0 mmol/mL
Na phosphate (neutral)							Solution	94 mg/mL	3.0 mmol/mL

*Molecular weights (MW) of compounds shown are for usual chemical forms, including water molecules (i.e., $MgSO_4$, 7 H_2O).
†Phosphate preparations contain buffered mixtures of monobasic (H_2PO_4) and dibasic (HPO_4) ions; the P content therefore is specified in millimoles. Oral phosphates contain 7 mEq Na and K per capsule (Na/K form) or 14 mEq K/capsule (K form). Parenteral solutions typically contain 4 mEq of Na or K per mL.
‡Other formulations exist. Those shown are among those approved in the United States.
Data from Drug Facts and Comparisons. 49th ed. St. Louis: Facts and Comparisons, 1995.

and $1,25(OH)_2D$ is inappropriately normal. The bone disease dominates the clinical picture (see Chapter 25).

Rapid entry of extracellular phosphate into cells is the cause of hypophosphatemia during administration of intravenous glucose, insulin therapy for hyperglycemia, administration of catecholamines (pressors or bronchodilators), profound respiratory alkalosis, or leukemic blast crisis. Hypophosphatemia in these situations is most pronounced when there is underlying phosphate depletion, as in hyperparathyroidism or vitamin D deficiency or with prolonged malnutrition, alcoholism, or glycosuria. Accelerated uptake of phosphate into cells, principally into muscle and bone in postsurgical or trauma patients may be promoted by high levels of circulating catecholamines and exacerbated by concurrent respiratory alkalosis, fever, volume expansion, sepsis, or hypokalemia. Similar mechanisms may pertain in nonsurgical illnesses, such as acute myocardial infarction. Hypophosphatemia with administration of hematopoietic growth factors such as erythropoietin is due to the high demand for new intracellular phosphate imposed by rapid cellular proliferation in the bone marrow.

CLINICAL FEATURES OF HYPOPHOSPHATEMIA

The significance of hypophosphatemia probably depends on the presence and severity of underlying phosphate depletion. Unfortunately the status of the total-body phosphorus pool is reflected only indirectly by the concentration of phosphate in the extracellular fluid, which contains less than 5% of body phosphorus. Thus although serum phosphate concentrations generally are used to characterize hypophosphatemia as severe (<0.3 to 0.5 mmol/L [<1 to 1.5 mg/dL]), moderate (0.5 to 0.7 mmol/L [1.5 to 2.2 mg/dL]), or mild (0.75 to 1.0 mmol/L [2.2 to 3.0 mg/dL]), serum phosphate may be normal or even high (depending on renal function) in the presence of profound intracellular phosphate deficiency. Conversely, serum phosphate may be low when intracellular phosphate is relatively normal, as following a sudden movement of extracellular phosphate into cells.

The prevalence of severe hypophosphatemia among hospitalized patients is less than 1%, whereas mild or moderate hypophosphatemia may be present in 2 to 5%.[617-619] Hypophosphatemia is recognized most often in critically ill patients, alcoholics or other malnourished individuals, subjects with decompensated diabetes mellitus, and those with acute infectious or pulmonary disease.[617-620]

The manifestations of severe hypophosphatemia are protean and include neuromuscular symptoms, ranging from progressive lethargy, muscle weakness, and paresthesias to paralysis, coma, and even death, depending on the severity of the phosphate depletion. Confusion, profound weakness, paralysis, seizures, and other major sequelae generally are limited to those with serum phosphate concentrations below 0.25 to 0.32 mmol/L (0.8 to 1.0 mg/dL).[610, 621-624] Biochemical evidence of muscle injury is observed within 1 to 2 d in more than one third of patients whose serum phosphate concentrations fall to less than 0.6 mmol/L (2 mg/dL).[625] Rhabdomyolysis may also be overt, especially in the setting of chronic alcoholism with underlying malnutrition and phosphate depletion.[626, 627] However, by the time rhabdomyolysis is recognized the serum phosphate may be raised by the release of cellular phosphate from the damaged muscle. Respiratory failure due to respiratory muscle weakness may preclude successful weaning from ventilatory support.[628-630] Left ventricular dysfunction, heart failure, and ventricular arrhythmias may result from profound hypophosphatemia, especially when serum phosphate is below 0.5 mmol/L (1.5 mg/dL).[605, 631-634] Correction of moderate hypophosphatemia (<0.6 mmol/L [<2 mg/dL]) in patients with septic shock increases blood pressure and improves ventricular function and arterial pH.[632] Hematologic sequelae of hypophosphatemia include hemolysis, platelet dysfunction with bleeding, and impaired leukocyte function (phagocytosis and killing).[635-637] Erythrocytes demonstrate increased fragility; altered membrane composition, rigidity and microspherocytosis; and reduced levels of ATP and 2,3-diphosphoglycerate (2,3-DPG).[635] The reduction in erythrocyte 2,3-DPG impairs oxyhemoglobin dissociation and thereby may reduce oxygen delivery to tissues, which together with accelerated hemolysis may cause a substantial increase in cardiac output. The blockade in cellular glycolysis is demonstrable at levels of serum phosphate between 0.3 and 0.6 mmol/L (1 and 2 mg/dL).[638] Glucose intolerance and insulin resistance may be present in these patients.[639]

TREATMENT OF HYPOPHOSPHATEMIA

Hypophosphatemia occurs most often in acutely or critically ill individuals. Accordingly it is often difficult to discern whether hypophosphatemia is responsible for the multiple organ dysfunction encountered in such patients. For example although intracellular high-energy organophosphates may be decreased during treatment of diabetic ketoacidosis and although phosphate repletion leads to more rapid recovery of erythrocyte 2,3-DPG concentrations, opinion is divided as to whether phosphate therapy in diabetic ketoacidosis hastens recovery, prevents complications, or improves mortality.[640-642] Nevertheless because severe hypophosphatemia can cause serious neuromuscular, cardiovascular, and hematologic dysfunction that is at least partially reversible with phosphate repletion, most now agree that treatment is appropriate for moderate or severe hypophosphatemia.[605, 629, 632]

The decision to correct hypophosphatemia urgently should be guided by the estimated severity of the cellular phosphate deficit, the presence of signs or symptoms suggestive of phosphate depletion, and the overall clinical status of the patient. The presence of renal insufficiency (a risk for iatrogenic hyperphosphatemia), concomitant administration of intravenous glucose (alone or as a component of hyperalimentation solutions), and the potential for aggravating coexistent hypocalcemia also should be considered.

Limited data are available from clinical trials to predict the appropriate dose and rate of phosphate administration. In patients without severe renal insufficiency or hypocalcemia, administration of intravenous elemental phosphorus at rates of 2 to 8 mmol/h over 4 to 8 h frequently corrects hypophosphatemia without provoking hyperphosphatemia or hypocalcemia.[618, 643-645] Suggested guidelines based on serum phosphate are shown in Table 24–9. It is essential that serum calcium and phosphate be monitored every 6 to 12 h during and after phosphate therapy, both to detect untoward conse-

---

TABLE 24–9. Acute Therapy for Hypophosphatemia

Consider:
  Severity of hypophosphatemia
  Likelihood of underlying phosphate depletion
  Clinical condition of the patient
  Renal function
  Serum calcium
  Concurrent parenteral therapy (glucose, hyperalimentation)

Guidelines:

mmol/L	Serum PO$_4$ (mg/dL)	Rate of Infusion (mmol/h)	Duration (h)	Total PO$_4$ (mmol)
<0.8	(<2.5)	2.0	6	12
<0.5	(<1.5)	4.0	6	24
<0.3	(<1.0)	8.0	6	48

Rates shown are for a 70-kg person. Most formulations available in the United States provide 3 mmol/mL of sodium or potassium phosphate.

quences and because additional infusions may be required for recurrent hypophosphatemia within 24 to 48 h of apparently successful repletion. Less acute or severe hypophosphatemia should be managed with oral (or enteral) phosphate supplements if possible, generally given as a total of 1.0 to 2.0 g/d (as elemental phosphate) of neutral sodium or potassium phosphate in divided doses three to four times a day (see Table 24–6). In many patients, however, the effectiveness of oral phosphate therapy is limited by nausea or diarrhea.

Disorders of Magnesium Metabolism

The fourth most abundant extracellular cation, magnesium, like calcium, plays a critical physiological role, particularly in neuromuscular function.[2] The role of intracellular magnesium in energy metabolism, as a cofactor for ATP and a wide variety of enzymes and transporters, is reflected in the global effects that accompany disorders of magnesium homeostasis. Hypomagnesemia and hypermagnesemia are among the most common electrolyte disturbances; one or the other of these abnormalities is present in as many as 20% of hospitalized patients and 30 to 40% of patients admitted to intensive care units.[646, 647]

Hypermagnesemia

Magnesium homeostasis is achieved mainly through highly efficient regulation of tubular magnesium reabsorption in the loop of Henle.[3] As normal kidneys can readily excrete large amounts of magnesium (i.e., 250 mmol/d), high filtered loads of magnesium rarely cause hypermagnesemia except in patients with renal failure.[648, 649] Increased magnesium loads may arise from ingestion of large amounts of oral magnesium salts, typically given as cathartics or antacids, or from extensive soft-tissue ischemia or necrosis in patients with trauma, sepsis, cardiopulmonary arrest, burns, or shock[648] (Table 24–10). Hypermagnesemia can also result from parenteral administration of magnesium salts, as in the treatment of preeclampsia.[650, 651] The infants of such hypermagnesemic mothers may develop transient hypermagnesemia, which causes parathyroid suppression and neurobehavioral symptoms.[652, 653] The use of oral magnesium preparations as laxatives may lead to hypermagnesemia if absorption is increased by ileus, obstruction, or perforation of the intestine.[654, 655]

Manifestations of hypermagnesemia include vasodilation and neuromuscular blockade, which may involve both presynaptic and postsynaptic inhibition of neuromuscular

TABLE 24–10. Causes of Hypermagnesemia

Excessive Magnesium Intake

  Cathartics, antacids, enemas
  Dead Sea drowning
  Parenteral magnesium administration
  Magnesium-rich urologic irrigants
  Intestinal obstruction or perforation
    following magnesium ingestion

Rapid Mobilization from Soft Tissues

  Trauma
  Shock, sepsis
  Cardiac arrest
  Burns

Impaired Magnesium Excretion

  Renal failure
  Familial hypocalciuric hypercalcemia

Other

  Adrenal insufficiency
  Hypothyroidism
  Hypothermia

transmission.[656–658] Signs and symptoms generally do not appear unless the serum magnesium exceeds 2 mmol/L (5 mg/dL).[2, 648] Hypotension, often refractory to pressors and volume expansion, may be one of the earliest signs of hypermagnesemia.[657–659] Lethargy, nausea, and weakness, accompanied by reduction or loss of deep tendon reflexes, may progress to stupor or coma with respiratory insufficiency or quadriparesis at serum concentrations in excess of 4 to 5 mmol/L (10 to 12 mg/dL). Gastrointestinal hypomotility or ileus is common. Facial flushing and pupillary dilatation may be observed. Hypotension may be complicated by a paradoxical relative bradycardia, and other cardiac manifestations include prolongation of the PR, QRS, and QTc intervals, heart block, and, ultimately, asystole as serum concentrations approach 10 mmol/L (24 mg/dL).

Hypermagnesemia also causes hypocalcemia and increased urinary calcium excretion, the result of both a direct suppression of PTH secretion and a PTH-independent inhibition of renal tubular calcium reabsorption.[650, 660–662] Severe hypocalcemia blocks the effect of hypermagnesemia on PTH secretion, so that serum PTH is usually within the normal range but still inappropriate for the level of serum calcium.[663, 664]

Successful treatment of hypermagnesemia requires identification and interruption of the source of magnesium and measures to increase clearance of magnesium from the extracellular fluid. The use of magnesium-free cathartics or enemas to accelerate clearance of ingested magnesium from the gastrointestinal tract, together with vigorous intravenous hydration, is generally successful in reversing hypermagnesemia. Refractory cases, especially those with advanced renal insufficiency, may require hemodialysis.[649] Infusions of intravenous calcium have been advocated as an effective antidote to hypermagnesemia.[648, 658, 665]

Hypomagnesemia

Hypomagnesemia may occur because of impaired intestinal absorption of magnesium, defective renal tubular reabsorption of magnesium, or a combination of these (Table 24–11). Because only 1% of the body's magnesium content is present in extracellular fluid, measurements of serum magnesium concentration may not reflect total-body magnesium or the magnesium status of the intracellular compartment in critical tissues such as muscle.[1, 666] Thus patients with deficiency of tissue magnesium may fail to manifest overt hypomagnesemia[667] but have enhanced retention (i.e., >50% in 24 h) of infused magnesium, a maneuver that may be employed to assess magnesium status.[668, 669]

INTESTINAL CAUSES OF HYPOMAGNESEMIA

Selective dietary magnesium deficiency does not occur, and it is difficult to induce magnesium depletion by feeding magnesium-deficient diets, probably because renal magnesium conservation is so efficient. Large amounts of magnesium may be lost in chronic diarrheal states (this fluid may contain more than 5 mmol/L [12 mg/dL] of magnesium) or via intestinal fistulae or prolonged gastrointestinal drainage.[670] More commonly magnesium becomes trapped within fatty acid soaps in disorders associated with chronic malabsorption.[671–674] In a rare syndrome termed *primary hypomagnesemia* a defect in the saturable component of intestinal magnesium absorption causes hypomagnesemia that can be partially overcome by administering large amounts of oral magnesium.[675, 676]

RENAL CAUSES OF HYPOMAGNESEMIA

Renal magnesium wasting can occur from a primary tubular transport defect, as in Bartter's syndrome and other rare

TABLE 24–11. Causes of Hypomagnesemia

Impaired Intestinal Magnesium Absorption

Primary infantile hypomagnesemia
Malabsorption syndromes

Increased Intestinal Magnesium Losses

Protracted vomiting or diarrhea
Intestinal drainage
Intestinal fistulae

Impaired Renal Tubular Magnesium Reabsorption

Congenital Magnesium-Wasting Syndromes

Bartter's syndrome
Gitelman's syndrome
Magnesuria with nephrocalcinosis

Acquired Renal Disease

Tubulointerstitial disease
After obstruction, acute tubular necrosis (diuretic phase)
Renal transplantation

Drugs and Toxins

Ethanol
Diuretics (loop, thiazide, osmotic)
Cisplatin
Pentamidine
Cyclosporine
Aminoglycosides
Foscarnet
Amphotericin B

Endocrine and Metabolic Abnormalities

Extracellular fluid volume expansion
Hyperaldosteronism (primary, secondary)
Syndrome of inappropriate antidiuretic hormone
   secretion
Diabetes mellitus
Hypercalcemia
Phosphate depletion
Metabolic acidosis
Hyperthyroidism

Rapid Shifts of Magnesium Out of Extracellular Fluid

Intracellular Redistribution

Recovery from diabetic ketoacidosis
Refeeding syndrome
Correction of respiratory acidosis
Catecholamines

Accelerated Net Bone Formation

After parathyroidectomy
Osteoblastic metastases
Intensive erythropoietin, G-CSF therapy
Treatment of vitamin D deficiency
Calcitonin therapy

G-CSF, granulocyte colony-stimulating factor.

inherited magnesium-wasting renal tubular disorders (see Table 24–11).[677–681] Most often, however, it is due to an acquired defect in tubular magnesium reabsorption. In normal subjects magnesium conservation is virtually complete within several days of instituting a magnesium-deficient diet, even before serum magnesium has declined substantially.[682] Thus the finding of more than 2 mmol/d of urinary magnesium in a hypomagnesemic patient indicates a defect in renal tubular magnesium reabsorption. The causes of acquired primary tubular magnesium wasting include various tubulointerstitial disorders, recovery from acute tubular necrosis or obstruction, renal transplantation, various endocrinopathies, alcoholism, and exposure to certain drugs (see Table 24–11).

Hypomagnesemia or magnesium depletion due to subnormal renal reabsorption may complicate hyperaldosteronism, hyperthyroidism, and disorders associated with hypercalcemia, hypercalciuria, or phosphate depletion.[699] In primary hyperparathyroidism PTH stimulates increased tubular magnesium reabsorption, but this stimulation is opposed by a direct tubular effect of hypercalcemia. As a result serum magnesium

in primary hyperparathyroidism is usually normal or only slightly reduced.[683] In hypoparathyroidism serum and urinary magnesium levels are low. The magnesium depletion in hypoparathyroidism may reflect both impaired renal reabsorption due to PTH deficiency and subnormal intestinal absorption due to low $1,25(OH)_2D$.[684]

Diabetes mellitus is among the most common diagnoses associated with hypomagnesemia.[685, 686] The severity of the hypomagnesemia in diabetes correlates with indices of glycosuria and poor glycemic control,[687] suggesting that urinary losses of magnesium on the basis of glycosuria may partly explain the magnesium depletion. Rapid correction of hyperglycemia with insulin therapy causes magnesium to enter cells and may further lower the extracellular magnesium level during treatment.

Alcoholism is another common cause of hypomagnesemia.[688] Magnesium depletion in alcoholism may result in part from deficient intake of magnesium, overall caloric deprivation and ketosis, and gastrointestinal losses due to vomiting or diarrhea,[2, 687, 689] but the magnesuric effect of alcohol probably plays the major role.[688, 690–692] This effect of alcohol is most evident during the rising phase of blood ethanol and may be related to transient suppression of PTH secretion.[690, 692] Other factors that may contribute to hypomagnesemia in alcoholism include pancreatitis, malabsorption, secondary hyperaldosteronism, respiratory alkalosis, and elevated plasma catecholamines, which increase intracellular sequestration of magnesium.[669]

Several drugs can impair renal tubular magnesium reabsorption and cause hypomagnesemia.[669] These include diuretics of all classes (especially loop diuretics), cisplatin, pentamidine, cyclosporine, aminoglycosides, foscarnet, and amphotericin. Drug-induced hypomagnesemia is usually mild and reversible, particularly that associated with diuretic therapy; however, in over half of patients who develop hypomagnesemia with cisplatin therapy the hypomagnesemia persists for many months or even years. The median duration of hypomagnesemia in cisplatin-treated patients is about 2 mo, but recovery may not occur for up to 2 y after treatment.[693] Cisplatin may induce a more global nephropathy and azotemic renal failure, but the magnesium wasting is usually an isolated functional abnormality. The renal magnesium-wasting syndrome may be prevented by intravenous magnesium administration (12 to 20 mmol) before or during cisplatin infusion.[694] Such findings suggest that cisplatin may selectively impair magnesium reabsorption by binding competitively to sites or cells involved in the binding and transport of magnesium.

A syndrome similar to that with cisplatin occurs in transplant recipients who receive cyclosporin A.[695–697] In these patients exposure to other drugs that may impair magnesium reabsorption, including aminoglycosides and amphotericin B, may compound the hypomagnesemia induced by cyclosporine.

OTHER CAUSES OF HYPOMAGNESEMIA

Magnesium, like phosphate, is a major intracellular ion, and significant shifts of magnesium from the extracellular compartment can occur during recovery from chronic respiratory acidosis or acute ketoacidosis, during refeeding, with hyperalimentation, and in response to elevations of circulating catecholamines.[669] Rapid loss of extracellular magnesium may also occur during periods of greatly accelerated net bone formation (after parathyroidectomy, during recovery from vitamin D deficiency, with osteoblastic metastases)[688] or with losses due to pancreatitis,[698] cardiopulmonary bypass surgery,[699] massive transfusion,[700] extensive burns,[701] excessive sweating,[702] pregnancy, or lactation.[703]

CONSEQUENCES OF HYPOMAGNESEMIA

Most of the signs and symptoms of hypomagnesemia reflect alterations in neuromuscular function: tetany, hyperreflexia, positive Chvostek's and Trousseau's signs, tremors, fasciculations, seizures, ataxia, nystagmus, vertigo, choreoathetosis, muscle weakness, apathy, depression, irritability, delirium, and psychosis.[2, 669, 682] Patients usually are not symptomatic unless serum magnesium falls below 0.5 mmol/L (1.2 mg/dL), although symptoms, like intracellular magnesium levels, may not correlate well with serum magnesium levels. Atrial or ventricular arrhythmias may occur, as may various electrocardiographic abnormalities: prolonged PR or QT intervals, T-wave flattening or inversion, and ST straightening.[669, 704] Hypomagnesemia also increases myocardial sensitivity to digitalis intoxication.[705, 706]

Hypomagnesemia causes alterations in mineral ion and potassium homeostasis that frequently aggravate the clinical syndrome. Magnesium deprivation causes hypocalcemia, hypocalciuria, hypokalemia (due to impaired tubular reabsorption of potassium), and positive calcium and sodium balance.[682, 707] Sustained correction of hypocalcemia or hypokalemia cannot be achieved with administration of calcium or potassium alone, respectively, whereas both abnormalities respond to administration of magnesium.[674, 708]

The etiology of hypocalcemia in this setting may be multifactorial. Inappropriately normal or low serum PTH, despite hypocalcemia, indicates a defect in PTH secretion.[503, 709, 710] Hypomagnesemia may also impair PTH action on bone and kidney, although the issue remains controversial.[502–504, 708–711]

Vitamin D resistance is also a feature of hypomagnesemia,[673, 712] owing mainly to impaired renal 1α-hydroxylation of 25(OH)D, although tissue resistance to 1,25(OH)$_2$D may play a role.[684, 713] The serum 1,25(OH)$_2$D level is usually low with hypomagnesemia, possibly owing to magnesium depletion itself, to parathyroid insufficiency, or to coexistent vitamin D deficiency.[714–716] Deficiency of 1,25(OH)$_2$D probably is not the main cause of hypocalcemia in these patients, however, because the hypocalcemia can be rapidly corrected (within hours to days) by magnesium therapy alone, prior to a measurable increase in the serum 1,25(OH)$_2$D level.[714, 715]

THERAPY FOR HYPOMAGNESEMIA

Patients with mild, asymptomatic hypomagnesemia can be treated with oral magnesium salts, i.e., MgCl$_2$, MgO, Mg(OH)$_2$, usually given in divided doses totaling 40 to 60 mEq/d (480 to 720 mg/d) (see Table 24–6). Diarrhea sometimes occurs with larger doses but generally is not a problem. The gluconate preparation (58 mg of magnesium/g) is said to cause less diarrhea.[669] Patients with malabsorption or ongoing urinary magnesium losses may require chronic oral therapy to avoid recurrent magnesium depletion. Although intestinal magnesium absorption is severely impaired in renal failure,[717] oral magnesium must be administered with great caution in this setting, especially in patients receiving concomitant therapy with calcitriol.

Symptomatic or severe (<0.5 mmol/L [<1.2 mg/dL]) hypomagnesemia, especially if complicated by hypocalcemia, usually signifies magnesium deficits of at least 0.5 to 1 mmol/kg body weight and is best treated promptly with parenteral magnesium salts. The use of intramuscular MgSO$_4$ is to be discouraged, as the injections are painful and provide relatively little magnesium (2 mL of 50% MgSO$_4$ supplies only 4 mmol of magnesium, compared with typical magnesium deficits in excess of 50 mmol). Moreover because unretained sulfate ions also may increase urinary calcium excretion, intravenous magnesium chloride or gluconate probably is the most logical approach to initial parenteral therapy for patients who

may also be hypocalcemic. In adult hypomagnesemic patients with normal renal function, infusion of 1 to 2 mmol/h (i.e., 25 to 50 mmol/d) is generally required to maintain serum magnesium in the range of 1 to 1.5 mmol/L (2.4 to 3.6 mg/dL).[674, 714, 718] Up to 50 mmol/d for 2 d can be safely administered without elevating serum magnesium above 2 mmol/L (5 mg/dL), whereas doses of 100 mmol/d may increase serum magnesium to 2.2 to 2.8 mmol/L (5.3 to 6.8 mg/dL) and thus are excessive.[718] In patients with active seizures or other urgent indications, the infusion may be preceded by a slowly administered bolus of 5 to 10 mmol, followed by a higher rate of infusion (i.e. 5 to 7.5 mmol/h) for the first 1 to 2 h only. Patients with normal renal function can readily excrete over 200 mmol/d of magnesium in the urine without becoming hypermagnesemic, but even mild renal failure may limit magnesium excretion. Therefore doses of magnesium supplements should be reduced two- to three-fold, and serum magnesium should be monitored carefully in patients with compromised renal function.

A large fraction of parenterally administered magnesium may be excreted in the urine, even in patients with profound magnesium deficiency. Many patients excrete as much as 50 to 75% of infused magnesium, whereas in normal subjects this rate approaches 100%.[674] Moreover, because equilibration of the intracellular and extracellular magnesium pools is relatively slow, it is usually necessary to continue magnesium therapy for 3 to 5 d to achieve adequate repletion of the typical deficit of 0.5 to 1 mmol/kg body weight. Because serum magnesium may become normal before tissue stores are repleted, monitoring of urinary magnesium excretion is a more reliable measure of full repletion, especially after patients are switched to oral therapy.

The need for calcium, potassium, and phosphate supplementation should be considered in the usual clinical setting of hypomagnesemia. Vitamin D deficiency also frequently coexists and should be treated with oral or parenteral vitamin D or calcifediol. Use of calcitriol is not necessary, does not hasten recovery, and may actually worsen hypomagnesemia by suppressing PTH secretion and thereby promoting renal magnesium excretion.[719] Initial parenteral magnesium therapy in hypocalcemic patients may cause hypophosphatemia via the rapid stimulation of PTH secretion. This is most likely to be significant in those with underlying phosphate depletion (malabsorption, alcoholism, diabetes mellitus), in whom magnesium therapy may provoke acute neuromuscular dysfunction; the latter may be avoided by concomitant intravenous calcium therapy.

REFERENCES

1. Elin RJ, Armstrong WD, Singer L. Body fluid electrolyte composition of chronically magnesium-deficient and control rats. Am J Physiol 1971; 220:543–548.
2. Wacker WEC, Parisi AF. Magnesium metabolism. N Engl J Med 1968; 278:712–717.
3. de Rouffignac C, Quamme G. Renal magnesium handling and its hormonal control. Physiol Rev 1994; 74:305–322.
4. Hendy GN, Kronenberg HM, Potts JT, Jr, et al. Nucleotide sequence of cloned cDNAs encoding human preproparathyroid hormone. Proc Natl Acad Sci USA 1981; 78:7365–7369.
5. Kronenberg HM, McDevitt BE, Majzoub JA, et al. Cloning and nucleotide sequence of DNA coding for bovine preproparathyroid hormone. Proc Natl Acad Sci USA 1979; 76:4981–4985.
6. Heinrich G, Kronenberg HM, Potts JT Jr, et al. Gene encoding parathyroid hormone: nucleotide sequence of the rat gene and deduced amino acid sequence of rat preproparathyroid hormone. J Biol Chem 1984; 259:3320–3329.
7. Schmelzer H-J, Gross G, Widera G, et al. Nucleotide sequence of a full-length cDNA clone encoding preproparathyroid hormone from pig and rat. Nucleic Acids Res 1987; 15:6740.
8. Khosla S, Demay M, Pines M, et al. Nucleotide sequence of cloned cDNAs encoding chicken preproparathyroid hormone. J Bone Miner Res 1988; 3:689–698.

9. Russell J, Sherwood LM. Nucleotide sequence of the DNA complementary to avian (chicken) preproparathyroid hormone mRNA and the deduced sequence of the hormone precursor. Mol Endocrinol 1989; 3:325–331.

10. Rosol TJ, Steinmeyer CL, McCauley LK, et al. Sequences of the cDNAs encoding canine parathyroid hormone–related protein and parathyroid hormone. Gene 1995; 160:241–243.

11. Karaplis AC, Hiou-Tim FF-T, Al-Akad B, et al. Genomic organization and nucleotide sequence of the mouse gene encoding parathyroid hormone (in preparation).

12. Arnold A, Horst SA, Gardella RJ, et al. Mutation of the signal peptide-encoding region of the preproparathyroid hormone gene in familial isolated hypoparathyroidism. J Clin Invest 1990; 86:1084–1087.

13. Karaplis AC, Lim S-K, Baba H, et al. Inefficient membrane targeting, translocation, and proteolytic processing by signal peptidase of a mutant preproparathyroid hormone protein. J Biol Chem 1995; 270:1629–1635.

14. Wiren KM, Potts JT Jr, Kronenberg HM. Importance of the propeptide sequence of human preproparathyroid hormone for signal sequence function. J Biol Chem 1988; 263:19771–19777.

15. Hashizume Y, Waguri S, Watanabe T, et al. Cysteine proteinases in rat parathyroid cells with special reference to their correlation with parathyroid hormone (PTH) in storage granules. J Histochem Cytochem 1993; 41:273–282.

16. MacGregor RR, Hamilton JW, Shofstall RE, et al. Isolation and characterization of porcine parathyroid cathepsin B. J Biol Chem 1979; 254:4423–4427.

17. Flueck JA, DiBella FP, Edis AJ, et al. Immunoheterogeneity of parathyroid hormone in venous effluent serum of hyperfunctioning parathyroid glands. J Clin Invest 1977; 69:1367–1375.

18. Mayer GP, Keaton JA, Hurst JG, et al. Effects of plasma calcium concentration on the relative proportion of hormone and carboxyl fragments in parathyroid venous blood. Endocrinology 1979; 104:1778–1784.

19. D'Amour P, Palardy J, Bahsali G, et al. The modulation of circulating parathyroid hormone immunoheterogeneity in man by ionized calcium concentration. J Clin Endocrinol Metab 1992; 74:525–532.

20. Habener JF, Kemper B, Potts JT Jr. Calcium-dependent intracellular degradation of parathyroid hormone: a possible mechanism for the regulation of hormone stores. Endocrinology 1975; 97:431–441.

21. Chu LLH, MacGregor RR, Anast CS, et al. Studies on the biosynthesis of rat parathyroid hormone and proparathyroid hormone: adaptation of the parathyroid gland to dietary restriction of calcium. Endocrinology 1973; 93:915–924.

22. Brown EM. PTH secretion in vivo and in vitro. Miner Electrolyte Metab 1982; 8:130–150.

23. Brown EM. Four-parameter model of the sigmoidal relationship between parathyroid hormone release and extracellular calcium concentration in normal and abnormal parathyroid tissue. J Clin Endocrinol Metab 1983; 56:572–581.

24. Parfitt AM: Calcium homeostasis. In: Mundy GR, Martin TJ, eds. Physiology and Pharmacology of Bone. Berlin: Springer-Verlag, 1993:1–65.

25. Grant FD, Conlin PR, Brown EM. Rate and concentration dependence of parathyroid hormone dynamics during stepwise changes in serum ionized calcium in normal humans. J Clin Endocrinol Metab 1990; 71:370–378.

26. Brown EM, Gamba G, Riccardi D, et al. Cloning and characterization of an extracellular Ca^{2+}-sensing receptor from bovine parathyroid. Nature 1993; 366:575–580.

27. Garrett JE, Capuano IV, Hammerland LG, et al. Molecular cloning and functional expression of human parathyroid calcium receptor cDNAs. J Biol Chem 1995; 270:12919–12925.

28. Rogers KV, Dunn CK, Hebert SC, et al. Pharmacological comparison of bovine parathyroid, human parathyroid, and rat kidney calcium receptors expressed in HEK 293 cells. J Bone Miner Res 1995; 10(Suppl 1):S483.

29. Pollak MR, Brown EM, Chou YHW, et al. Mutations in the human Ca^{2+}-sensing receptor gene cause familial hypocalciuric hypercalcemia and neonatal severe hyperparathyroidism. Cell 1993; 75:1297–1303.

30. Ho C, Conner DA, Pollack MR, et al. A mouse model of human familial hypocalciuric hypercalcemia and neonatal severe hyperparathyroidism. Nat Genet 1995; 11:389–394.

31. Heath H, III, Sanguinetti EL, Oglesby S, et al. Inhibition of human parathyroid hormone secretion in vivo by NPS R-568, a calcimimetic drug that targets the parathyroid cell-surface calcium receptor. Bone 1995; 16:85S.

32. Vasicek T, McDevitt BE, Freeman MW, et al. Nucleotide sequence of genomic DNA encoding human parathyroid hormone. Proc Natl Acad Sci USA 1983; 80:2127–2131.

33. Reis A, Hecht W, Groger R, et al. Cloning and sequence analysis of the human parathyroid hormone gene region. Hum Genet 1990; 84:119–124.

34. Weaver CA, Gordon DF, Kissil MS, et al. Isolation and complete nucleotide sequence of the gene for bovine parathyroid hormone. Gene 1984; 28:319–329.

35. Silver J, Russell J, Sherwood LM. Regulation by vitamin D metabolites of messenger ribonucleic acid for preproparathyroid hormone in isolated bovine parathyroid cells. Proc Natl Acad Sci USA 1985; 82:4270–4273.

36. Russell J, Lettieri D, Sherwood LM. Suppression by 1,25(OH)$_2$D$_3$ of transcription of the pre-proparathyroid hormone gene. Endocrinology 1986; 119:2864–2866.

37. Silver J, Naveh-Many T, Mayer H, et al. Regulation by vitamin D metabolites of parathyroid hormone gene transcription in vivo in the rat. J Clin Invest 1986; 78:1296–1301.

38. Hawa NS, O'Riordan JLH, Farrow SM. Binding of 1,25-dihydroxyvitamin D$_3$ receptors to the 5′-flanking region of the bovine parathyroid hormone gene. Endocrinology 1994; 142:53–60.

39. Demay MB, Kiernan MS, DeLuca HF, et al. Sequences in the human parathyroid hormone gene that bind the 1,25-dihydroxyvitamin D$_3$ receptor and mediate transcriptional repression in response to 1,25-dihydroxyvitamin D$_3$. Proc Natl Acad Sci USA 1992; 89:8097–8101.

40. Russell J, Sherwood LM. The effects of 1,25(OH)$_2$D$_3$ and high calcium on transcription of the pre-proparathyroid hormone gene are direct. Trans Assoc Am Physicians 1987; 100:256–262.

41. Brown AJ, Zhong M, Finch J, et al. The roles of calcium and 1,25-dihydroxyvitamin D$_3$ in the regulation of vitamin D receptor expression by rat parathyroid glands. Endocrinology 1995; 136:1419–1425.

42. Russell J, Bar A, Sherwood LM, et al. Interaction between calcium and 1,25-dihydroxyvitamin D$_3$ in the regulation of pre-proparathyroid hormone and vitamin D receptor mRNA in avian parathyroids. Endocrinology 1993; 132:2639–2643.

43. Naveh-Many T, Friedlaender MM, Mayer H, et al. Calcium regulates parathyroid hormone messenger ribonucleic acid (mRNA), but not calcitonin mRNA in vivo in the rat: dominant role of 1,25-dihydroxyvitamin D. Endocrinology 1989; 125:275–280.

44. Yamamoto M, Igarashi T, Muramatsu M, et al. Hypocalcemia increases and hypercalcemia decreases the steady-state level of parathyroid hormone messenger ribonucleic acid in the rat. J Clin Invest 1989; 83:1053–1058.

45. Moallem E, Silver J, Naveh-Many T. Post-transcriptional regulation of PTH gene expression by hypocalcemia due to protein binding to the PTH mRNA 3′ UTR. J Bone Miner Res 1995; 10(Suppl 1):S142.

46. Hawa NS, O'Riordan JLH, Farrow SM. Post-transcriptional regulation of bovine parathyroid hormone synthesis. Mol Endocrinol 1993; 10:43–49.

47. Parfitt AM. Parathyroid growth: normal and abnormal. In: Bilezikian JP, ed. The Parathyroids. New York: Raven Press, 1994: 373–405.

48. Szabo A, Merke J, Beier E, et al. 1,25-(OH)$_2$-vitamin D$_3$ inhibits parathyroid cell proliferation in experimental uremia. Kidney Int 1989; 35:1049–1056.

49. Wernerson A, Widholm SM, Svensson O, et al. Parathyroid cell number and size in hypocalcemic young rats. Acta Pathol Microbiol Immunol Scand 1991; 99:1096–1102.

50. Naveh-Many T, Rahamimov R, Livni N, et al. Parathyroid cell proliferation in normal and chronic renal failure rats: the effects of calcium, phosphate and vitamin D. J Clin Invest 1995; 96:1786–1793.

51. Raisz LG. Regulation by calcium of parathyroid growth and secretion in vitro. Nature 1963; 197:1115–1117.

52. Lee MJ, Roth SI. Effect of calcium and magnesium on deoxyribonucleic acid synthesis in rat parathyroid glands in vitro. Lab Invest 1975; 1:72–79.

53. Kremer R, Bolivar I, Goltzman D, et al. Influence of calcium and 1,25-dihydroxycholecalciferol on proliferation and proto-oncogene expression in primary cultures of bovine parathyroid cells. Endocrinology 1989; 125:935–941.

54. Henry HL, Taylor AN, Normal AW. Response of chick parathyroid glands to the vitamin D metabolites, 1,25-dihydroxycholecalciferol and 24,25-dihydroxycholecalciferol. J Nutr 1977; 107:1918–1926.

55. Nygren P, Larsson R, Johansson H, et al. 1,25(OH)$_2$D$_3$ inhibits hormone secretion and proliferation but not functional dedifferentiation of cultured bovine parathyroid cells. Calcif Tissue Int 1988; 43:213–218.

56. Berson SA, Yallow RS. Immunochemical heterogeneity of parathyroid hormone in plasma. J Clin Endocrinol Metab 1968; 28:1037–1047.

57. Bringhurst FR, Stern AM, Yotts M, et al. Peripheral metabolism of [^{35}S]parathyroid hormone in vivo: influence of alterations in calcium availability and parathyroid status. J Endocrinol 1989; 122:237–245.

58. Rouleau MF, Warshawsky H, Goltzman D. Parathyroid hormone binding in vivo to renal, hepatic, and skeletal tissues of the rat using a radioautographic approach. Endocrinology 1986; 118:919–931.

59. Segre GV, D'Amour P, Potts JT, Jr. Metabolism of radioiodinated bovine parathyroid hormone in the rat. Endocrinology 1976; 99:1645–1652.

60. Martin KJ, Hruska KA, Freitag JJ, et al. The peripheral metabolism of parathyroid hormone. N Engl J Med 1979; 302:1092–1098.

61. Friedman PA, Gesek FA. Calcium transport in renal epithelial cells. Am J Physiol 1993; 264:F181–F198.

62. Bourdeau JE. Mechanisms and regulation of calcium transport in the nephron. Semin Nephrol 1993; 13:191–201.

63. Gesek FA, Friedman PA. On the mechanisms of parathyroid hormone stimulation of calcium uptake by mouse distal convoluted tubule cells. J Clin Invest 1992; 90:749–758.

64. Shimizu T, Yoshitomi K, Nakamura M, et al. Effect of parathyroid hormone on the connecting tubule from the rabbit kidney: biphasic response of transmural voltage. Pflugers Arch 1990; 416:254–261.

65. Bouhtiauy I, LaJeunesse D, Brunette MG. The mechanism of parathyroid hormone action on calcium reabsorption by the distal tubule. Endocrinology 1991; 128:251–258.

66. Bijvoet OLM. Relation of plasma phosphate concentration to renal tubular reabsorption of phosphate. Clin Sci 1969; 37:23–36.

67. Murer H. Cellular mechanisms in proximal tubular Pi reabsorption: some answers and more questions. J Am Soc Nephrol 1992; 2:1649–1665.

68. Sorribas V, Markovich D, Hayes G, et al. Cloning of a NaPi cotransporter from opossum kidney cells. J Biol Chem 1994; 269:6615–6621.

69. Kempson SA, Lotscher M, Kaissling B, et al. Parathyroid hormone action on phosphate transporter mRNA and protein in rat renal proximal tubules. Am J Physiol 1995; 268:F784–F791.

70. Kempson SA, Helmle C, Abraham MI, et al. Parathyroid hormone action on phosphate transport is inhibited by high osmolality. Am J Physiol 1990; 268:F1336–F1344.

71. Fraser DR, Kodicek E. Regulation of 25-hydroxycholecalciferol-1-hydroxylase activity in kidney by parathyroid hormone. Nature 1973; 241:163–166.

72. Garabedian M, Holick MF, DeLuca HF, et al. Control of 25-hydroxycholecalciferol metabolism by parathyroid glands. Proc Natl Acad Sci USA 1972; 69:1673–1676.

73. Shigematsu T, Horiuchi N, Ogura Y, et al. Human parathyroid hormone inhibits renal 24-hydroxylase activity of 25-hydroxyvitamin D_3 by a mechanism involving adenosine 3',5'-monophosphate in rats. Endocrinology 1986; 118:1583–1589.

74. Alpern RJ. Cell mechanisms of proximal tubule acidification. Physiol Rev 1990; 70:79–114.

75. Humes HD, Ichikawa I, Troy JL, et al. Evidence for a parathyroid hormone–dependent influence of calcium on the glomerular ultrafiltration coefficient. J Clin Invest 1978; 61:32–40.

76. McSheehy PMGJ, Chambers TJ. Osteoblastic cells mediate osteoclastic responsiveness to parathyroid hormone. Endocrinology 1986; 118:824–828.

77. McSheehy PMJ, Chambers TJ. Osteoblast-like cells in the presence of parathyroid hormone release soluble factor that stimulates osteoclastic bone resorption. Endocrinology 1986; 119:1654–1659.

78. Chambers TJ, Athanasou NA, Fuller K. Effect of parathyroid hormone and calcitonin on the cytoplasmic spreading of isolated osteoclasts. J Endocrinol 1984; 102:281–286.

79. Vaes G. Cellular biology and biochemical mechanism of bone resorption. Clin Orthop 1988; 231:239–271.

80. Uy HL, Guise TA, De La Mata J, et al. Effects of parathyroid hormone (PTH)–related protein and PTH on osteoclasts and osteoclast precursors in vivo. Endocrinology 1995; 136:3207–3212.

81. Hakeda Y, Hiura K, Sato T, et al. Existence of parathyroid hormone-binding sites on murine hemopoietic blast cells. Biochem Biophys Res Commun 1989; 163:1481–1486.

82. Takahashi N, Yamana H, Yoshiki S. Osteoclast-like cell formation and its regulation by osteotropic hormones in mouse marrow cultures. Endocrinology 1988; 122:1373–1377.

83. Takashashi N, Akatsu T, Udagawa N. Osteoblastic cells are involved in osteoclast formation. Endocrinology 1988; 123:2600–2603.

84. Rouleau MF, Mitchell L, Goltzman D. In vivo distribution of parathyroid hormone receptors in bone: evidence that a predominant osseous target cell is not the mature osteoblast. Endocrinology 1988; 123:187–191.

85. Dietrich JW, Canalis EM, Maina DM, et al. Hormonal control of bone collagen synthesis in vitro: effects of parathyroid hormone and calcitonin. Endocrinology 1976; 98:943–949.

86. Bellows CG, Ishida H, Aubin JE, et al. Parathyroid hormone reversibly suppresses the differentiation of osteoprogenitor cells into functional osteoblasts. Endocrinology 1990; 127:3111–3116.

87. Canalis E, Centrella M, Burch W, et al. Insulin-like growth factor I mediates selective anabolic effects of parathyroid hormone in bone cultures. J Clin Invest 1989; 83:60–65.

88. Chase LR, Aurbach GD. Parathyroid function and the renal secretion of 3',5'-adenylic acid. Proc Natl Acad Sci USA 1967; 58:518–525.

89. Jüppner H, Abou-Samra A-B, Freeman M, et al. A G protein–linked receptor for parathyroid hormone and parathyroid hormone–related peptide. Science 1991; 254:1024–1026.

90. Abou-Samra AB, Jüppner H, Force T, et al. Expression cloning of a common receptor for parathyroid hormone and parathyroid hormone–related peptide from rat osteoblast-like cells: a single receptor stimulates intracellular accumulation of both cAMP and inositol triphosphates and increases intracellular free calcium. Proc Natl Acad Sci USA 1992; 89:2732–2736.

91. Schipani E, Karga H, Karaplis AC, et al. Identical complementary deoxyribonucleic acids encode a human renal and bone parathyroid hormone (PTH)/PTH-related peptide receptor. Endocrinology 1993; 132:2157–2165.

92. Karperien M, van Dijk TB, Hoeijmakers T, et al. Expression pattern of parathyroid hormone/parathyroid hormone–related peptide receptor mRNA in mouse postimplantation embryos indicates involvement in multiple developmental processes. Mech Dev 1994; 47:29–42.

93. Smith DP, Zhang X-Y, Frolik CA, et al. Structure and functional expression of a complementary DNA for porcine parathyroid hormone/parathyroid hormone–related peptide receptor. Biochem Biophys Acta 1996; 1307:339–347.

94. Bergwitz C, unpublished.

95. Schneider H, Feyen JHM, Seuwen K, et al. Cloning and functional expression of a human parathyroid hormone receptor. Eur J Pharm (Mol Pharmacol Sect) 1993; 246:149–155.

96. Kronenberg HM, Abou-Samra A-B, Bringhurst FR, et al. The PTH/PTHrP receptor: one receptor for two ligands. In: Thakker RV, ed. Molecular Genetics of Endocrine and Metabolic Disorders. London: Chapman & Hall, 1997: 389–420.

97. Kronenberg HM, Bringhurst FR, Nussbaum SR, et al. Parathyroid hormone: biosynthesis, secretion, chemistry and action. In: Mundy GR, Martin TJ, eds. Handbook of Experimental Pharmacology. Heidelberg: Springer-Verlag, 1993:185–201.

98. Segre GV. Receptors for parathyroid hormone and parathyroid hormone–related protein. In: Bilezikian JP, ed. The Parathyroids. New York: Raven Press, 1994:213–229.

99. Kong XF, Schipani E, Lanske B, et al. The rat, mouse and human genes encoding the receptor for parathyroid hormone and parathyroid hormone–related peptide are highly homologous [published erratum appears in Biochem Biophys Res Commun 1994 June 15; 201(2):1058]. Biochem Biophys Res Commun 1994; 200:1290–1299.

100. McCuaig KA, Lee HS, Clarke JC, et al. Parathyroid hormone/parathyroid hormone–related peptide receptor gene transcripts are expressed from tissue-specific and ubiquitous promoters. Nucleic Acids Res 1995; 23:1948–1955.

101. Joun H, Lanske B, Karperien M, et al. Tissue-specific transcription start sites and alternative splicing of the parathyroid hormone (PTH)/PTH-related peptide (PTHrP) receptor gene: a new PTH/PTHrP receptor splice variant that lacks the signal peptide. Endocrinology 1997; 138:1742–1749.

102. Urena P, Kong XF, Abou-Samra A-B. Parathyroid hormone (PTH)–related peptide (PTHrP) receptor mRNA is widely distributed in rat tissues. Endocrinology 1993; 133:617–623.

103. Lee K, Deeds JD, Segre GV. Expression of parathyroid hormone–related peptide and its receptor messenger ribonucleic acids during fetal development of rats. Endocrinology 1995; 136:453–463.

104. Schwindinger WF, Watkins L, Pines M, et al. Direct demonstration that the PTH/PTHrP receptor activates G-proteins G_s and $G_{Q/11}$. The Endocrine Society 77th Annual Meeting, Washington, DC, 1995: Abstract #OR41–6.

105. Offermanns S, Iida-Klein A, Segre GV, et al. Gαq family members couple PTH/PTHrP and calcitonin receptors to phospholipase C in COS-7 cells. Mol Endocrinol 1996; 10:566–574.

106. Mitchell J, Mayeenuddin L, Sargeant J. Dual, G protein–mediated regulation of phospholipase C activity in osteosarcoma cells. J Bone Miner Res 1995; 10(Suppl 1):S321.

107. Murray TM, Rao LG, Muzaffar SA, et al. Human parathyroid hormone carboxyterminal peptide (53–84) stimulates alkaline phosphatase activity in dexamethasone-treated rat osteosarcoma cells in vitro. Endocrinology 1989; 124:1097–1099.

108. Kaji H, Sugimoto T, Kanatani M, et al. Carboxyl-terminal parathyroid hormone fragments stimulate osteoclast-like cell formation and osteoclastic activity. Endocrinology 1994; 134:1897–1904.

109. Schlüter K-D, Hellstern H, Wingender E, et al. The central part of parathyroid hormone stimulates thymidine incorporation of chondrocytes. J Biol Chem 1989; 264:11087–11092.

110. Orloff JJ, Ganz MB, Ribaudo AE, et al. Analysis of PTHrP binding and signal transduction mechanisms in benign and malignant squamous cells. Am J Physiol 1992; 262:E599–E607.

111. Whitfield JF, Chakravarthy BR, Durkin JP, et al. Parathyroid hormone stimulates protein kinase C but not adenylate cyclase in mouse epidermal keratinocytes. J Cell Physiol 1992; 150:299–303.

112. Gaich G, Orloff JJ, Atillasoy EJ, et al. Amino-terminal parathyroid hormone–related protein: specific binding and cytosolic calcium responses in rat insulinoma cells. Endocrinology 1993; 132:1402–1409.

113. Orloff JJ, Kats Y, Urena P, et al. Further evidence for a novel receptor for amino-terminal parathyroid hormone–related protein on keratinocytes and squamous carcinoma cell lines. Endocrinology 1995; 136:3016–3023.

114. Inomata N, Akiyama M, Kubota N, et al. Characterization of a novel parathyroid hormone (PTH) receptor with specificity for the carboxyl-terminal region of PTH-(1–84). Endocrinology 1995; 136:4732–4740.

115. Usdin TB, Gruber C, Bonner TI. Identification and functional expression of a receptor selectively recognizing parathyroid hormone, the PTH2 receptor. J Biol Chem 1995; 270:15455–15458.

116. Chorev M, Rosenblatt M: Structure-function analysis of parathyroid hormone and parathyroid hormone–related peptide. In: Bilezikian JP, ed. The Parathyroids. New York, Raven Press, 1994, pp 139–156.

117. Pines M, Adams AE, Stueckle S, Bessalle R, Rashti-Behar V, Chorev M, Rosenblatt M, Suva LJ. Generation and characterization of human kidney cell lines stably expressing recombinant human PTH/PTHrP receptor: Lack of interaction with a C-terminal human PTH peptide. Endocrinology 1994; 135:1713–1716.

118. Nussbaum SR, Rosenblatt M, Potts JT Jr. Parathyroid hormone/renal receptor interactions: demonstration of two receptors-binding domains. J Biol Chem 1980; 255:10183–10187.

119. Rosenblatt M, Callahan EN, Mahaffey JE, et al. Parathyroid hormone inhibitors: design, synthesis, and biologic evaluation of hormone analogues. J Biol Chem 1977; 252:5847–5851.

120. Horiuchi N, Holick MF, Potts JT Jr, et al. A parathyroid hormone inhibitor in vivo: design and biologic evaluation of a hormone analog. Science 1983; 220:1053–1055.

121. McKee RL, Caulfield MP, Rosenblatt M. Treatment of bone-derived ROS 17/2.8 cells with dexamethasone and pertussis toxin enables detection of partial agonist activity for parathyroid hormone antagonists. Endocrinology 1990; 127:76–82.

122. Nutt RF, Caulfield MP, Levy JJ, et al. Removal of partial agonism from parathyroid hormone (PTH)–related protein-(7–34)NH_2 by substitution of PTH amino acids at positions 10 and 11. Endocrinology 1990; 127:491–493.

123. Gardella TJ, Jüppner H, Wilson AK, et al. Determinants of [Arg2]PTH-(1–34) binding and signaling in the transmembrane region of the parathyroid hormone receptor. Endocrinology 1994; 135:1186–1194.

124. Lee CW, Luck MD, Jüppner H, et al. Homolog scanning mutagenesis of the parathyroid hormone (PTH) receptor reveals PTH(1–34) binding

determinants in the third extracellular loop. Mol Endocrinol 1995; 9:1269–1278.

125. Gardella TJ, Luck MD, Fan MH, et al. Mutations in the transmembrane domains of the PTH receptor impair binding of PTH-(1–34) but not PTH-(3–34). J Biol Chem 1996; 271:12820–12825.

126. Jüppner H, Schipani E, Bringhurst FR, et al. The extracellular, amino-terminal region of the PTH/PTHrP receptor determines the binding affinity for carboxyl-terminal fragments of PTH(1–34). Endocrinology 1994; 134:879–884.

127. Marx UC, Austermann S, Bayer P, et al. Structure of human parathyroid hormone 1–37 in solution. J Biol Chem 1995; 270:15194–15202.

128. Schertler GFX, Villa C, Henderson R. Projection structure of rhodopsin. Nature 1993; 362:770–772.

129. Suryanarayana S, von Zastrow M, Kobilka BK. Identification of intramolecular interactions in adrenergic receptors. J Biol Chem 1992; 267:21991–21994.

130. Lee CW, Gardella TJ, Abou-Samra A-B, et al. Role of the extracellular regions of the parathyroid hormone (PTH)/PTH-related peptide receptor in hormone binding. Endocrinology 1994; 135:1488–1495.

131. Schipani E, Kruse K, Jüppner H. A constitutively active mutant PTH-PTHrP receptor in Jansen-type metaphyseal chondrodysplasia. Science 1995; 268:98–100.

132. Schipani E, Jensen G, Parfitt AM, et al. Constitutively active PTH/PTHrP receptors in Jansen metaphyseal chondrodysplasia: identification of a novel T410P mutation and further characterization of position 223. N Engl J Med 1996; 335:708–714.

133. DeHaas WHD, DeBoer W, Griffioen F. Metaphysial dysostosis. J Bone Joint Surg 1969; 51B:290–299.

134. Kruse K, Schütz C. Calcium metabolism in the Jansen type of metaphyseal dysplasia. Eur J Pediatr 1993; 152:912–915.

135. Wells H, Lloyd W. Hypercalcemic and hypophosphatemic effects of dibutyryl cyclic AMP in rats after parathyroidectomy. Endocrinology 1969; 84:861–867.

136. Agus ZS, Puschett JB, Senesky D, et al. Mode of action of parathyroid hormone and adenosine 3′,5′-cyclic monophosphate on renal tubular phosphate reabsorption in the dog. J Clin Invest 1971; 50:617–626.

137. Sugimoto T, Fukase M, Tsutsumi M, et al. Additive effects of parathyroid hormone and calcitonin on adenosine 3′,5′-monophosphate release in newly established perfusion system of rat femur. Endocrinology 1985; 117:1901–1905.

138. Caverzasio J, Rizzoli R, Bonjour JV. Sodium-dependent phosphate transport inhibited by parathyroid hormone and cyclic AMP stimulation in an opossum kidney cell line. J Biol Chem 1986; 261:3233–3237.

139. Civitelli R, Hruska KA, Jeffrey JJ, et al. Second messenger signaling in the regulation of collagenase production by osteogenic osteosarcoma cells. Endocrinology 1989; 124:2928–2934.

140. Bringhurst FR, Zajac JD, Daggett AS, et al. Inhibition of parathyroid hormone responsiveness in clonal osteoblastic cells expressing a mutant form of 3′,5′-cyclic adenosine monophosphate–dependent protein kinase. Mol Endocrinol 1989; 3:60–67.

141. Segal J, Pollock AS. Transfection-mediated expression of a dominant cAMP-resistant phenotype in the opossum-kidney (OK) cell line prevents parathyroid hormone–induced inhibition of Na-phosphate cotransport. J Clin Invest 1990; 86:1442–1450.

142. Dunlay R, Hruska K. PTH receptor coupling to phospholipase C is an alternate pathway of signal transduction in bone and kidney. Am J Physiol 1990; 258:F223–F231.

143. Malstrom K, Stange G, Murer H. Intracellular cascades in the parathyroid-hormone–dependent regulation of Na⁺/phosphate cotransport in OK cells. Biochem J 1988; 251:207–213.

144. Janulis M, Tembe V, Favus MJ. Role of protein kinase C in parathyroid hormone stimulation of renal 1,25-dihydroxyvitamin D₃ secretion. J Clin Invest 1992; 90:2278–2283.

145. Fukayama S, Tashjian AH Jr, Davis JN, et al. Signaling by N- and C-terminal sequences of parathyroid hormone–related protein in hippocampal neurons. Proc Natl Acad Sci USA 1995; 92:10182–10186.

146. Gonzalez EA, Zhong M, Brown AJ, et al. Effects of dietary calcium and calcitriol administration on the levels of parathyroid hormone, serum calcium and PTH receptor mRNA in vitamin D–deficient rats. J Bone Miner Res 1995; 10(Suppl 1):S483.

147. Turner G, Coureau C, Rabin MR, et al. Parathyroid hormone (PTH)/PTH-related protein receptor messenger ribonucleic acid expression and PTH response in a rat model of secondary hyperparathyroidism associated with vitamin D deficiency. Endocrinology 1995; 136:3751–3758.

148. Xie LY, Leung A, Segre GV, et al. Dramatic downregulation of the PTH/PTHrP receptor protein and transcript by 1,25(OH)₂ vitamin D₃ in the osteoblast-like ROS 17/2.8 cells. Am J Physiol 1996; 270:E654–E660.

149. Urena P, Iida-Klein A, Kong XF, et al. Regulation of parathyroid hormone (PTH)/PTH-related peptide receptor messenger ribonucleic acid by glucocorticoids and PTH in ROS 17/2.8 and OK cells. Endocrinology 1994; 134:451–456.

150. Abou-Samra AB, Goldsmith PK, Xie LY, et al. Down-regulation of parathyroid (PTH)/PTH-related peptide receptor immunoreactivity and PTH binding in opossum kidney cells by PTH and dexamethasone. Endocrinology 1994; 135:2588–2594.

151. Huang Z, Bambino T, Chen Y, et al. Biochemical and confocal microscopic studies of constitutive and agonist-stimulated endocytosis of the PTH-PTHrP receptor. J Bone Miner Res 1995; 10:S94.

152. Huang Z, Chen Y, Nissenson RA. The cytoplasmic tail of the G-protein–coupled receptor for parathyroid hormone and parathyroid hormone–related protein contains positive and negative signals for endocytosis. J Biol Chem 1995; 270:151–156.

153. Suva LJ, Winslow GA, Wettenhall RE, et al. A parathyroid hormone–related protein implicated in malignant hypercalcemia: cloning and expression. Science 1987; 237:893–896.

154. Mangin M, Webb AC, Dreyer BE, et al. Identification of a cDNA encoding a parathyroid hormone–like peptide from a human tumor associated with humoral hypercalcemia of malignancy. Proc Natl Acad Sci USA 1988; 85:597–601.

155. Thiede MA, Strewler GJ, Nissenson RA, et al. Human renal carcinoma expresses two messages encoding a parathyroid hormone–like peptide: evidence for the alternative splicing of a single-copy gene. Proc Natl Acad Sci USA 1988; 85:4605–4609.

156. Karaplis AC, Yasuda T, Hendy GN, et al. Gene-encoding parathyroid hormone–like peptide: nucleotide sequence of the rat gene and comparison with the human homologue. Mol Endocrinol 1990; 4:441–446.

157. Thiede MA, Rutledge SJ. Nucleotide sequence of a parathyroid hormone–related peptide expressed by the 10-day chicken embryo. Nucleic Acids Res 1990; 18:3062.

158. Mangin M, Ikeda K, Broadus AE. Structure of the mouse gene encoding parathyroid hormone–related peptide. Gene 1990; 95:195–202.

159. Gardella TJ, Luck MD, Jensen GS, et al. Converting parathyroid hormone–related peptide (PTHrP) into a potent PTH-2 receptor agonist. J Biol Chem 1996; 271:18888–19893.

160. Abou-Samra A-B, Uneno S, Jüppner H, et al. Non-homologous sequences of parathyroid hormone and the parathyroid hormone–related peptide bind to a common receptor on ROS 17/2.8 cells. Endocrinology 1989; 125:2215–2217.

161. Caulfield MP, McKee RL, Goldman ME, et al. The bovine renal parathyroid hormone (PTH) receptor has equal affinity for two different amino acid sequences: the receptor binding domains of PTH and PTH-related protein are located within the 14–34 region. Endocrinology 1990; 127:83–87.

162. Barden JA, Kemp BE. NMR study of a 34-residue N-terminal fragment of the parathyroid-hormone–related protein secreted during humoral hypercalcemia of malignancy. Eur J Biochem 1989; 184:379–394.

163. Orloff JJ, Reddy D, DePapp AE, et al. Parathyroid hormone–related protein as a prohormone: posttranslational processing and receptor interactions. Endocr Rev 1994; 15:40–59.

164. Soifer NE, Dee KE, Insogna KL, et al. Parathyroid hormone–related protein. J Biol Chem 1992; 267:18236–18243.

165. Wu TL, Vasavada RC, Yang KH, et al. Structural and physiological characterization of the mid-region secretory species of parathyroid hormone–related protein. J Biol Chem 1996; 271:24371–24381.

166. Henderson JE, Shustik C, Kremer R, et al. Circulating concentrations of parathyroid hormone–like peptide in malignancy and in hyperparathyroidism. J Bone Miner Res 1990; 5:105–113.

167. Ratcliffe WA, Norbury S, Stott RA, et al. Immunoreactivity of plasma parathyrin-related peptide: three region-specific radioimmunoassays and a two-site immunoradiometric assay compared. Clin Chem 1991; 37:1781–1787.

168. Burtis WJ, Brady TG, Orloff JJ, et al. Immunochemical characterization of circulating parathyroid hormone–related protein in patients with humoral hypercalcemia of cancer. N Engl J Med 1990; 322:1106–1112.

169. Martin TJ. Parathyroid hormone–related protein: molecular biology, chemistry, and actions. In: Mundy GR, Martin TJ, eds. Physiology and Pharmacology of Bone. Berlin: Springer-Verlag, 1993:617–639.

170. Orloff JJ, Wu TL, Stewart AF. PTH-like protein, biochemical responses, and receptor interactions. Endocr Rev 1989; 10:476–495.

171. Strewler GJ, Nissenson RA. Peptide mediators of hypercalcemia in malignancy. Annu Rev Med 1990; 41:35–44.

172. Rodda CP, Kubota M, Heath JA, et al. Evidence for a novel parathyroid hormone–related protein in fetal lamb parathyroid glands and sheep placenta: comparisons with a similar protein implicated in humoral hypercalcaemia of malignancy. J Endocrinol 1988; 117:261–271.

173. Abbas SK, Pickard DW, Rodda CP, et al. Stimulation of ovine placental calcium transport by purified natural and recombinant parathyroid hormone–related protein (PTHrP) preparations. Q J Exp Physiol 1989; 74:549–552.

174. Kovacs CS, Lanske B, Hunzelman JL, et al. Parathyroid hormone–related protein (PTHrP) regulates fetal-placental calcium transport through a receptor distinct from the PTH/PTHrP receptor. Proc Natl Acad Sci USA 1996; 93:15233–15238.

175. Halloran BP, DeLuca HF. Skeletal changes during pregnancy and lactation: the role of vitamin D. Endocrinology 1980; 107:1923–1929.

176. Hodnett DW, DeLuca HF, Jorgensen NA. Bone mineral loss during lactation occurs in absence of parathyroid tissue. Am J Physiol 1992; 262:E230–E233.

177. Ratcliffe WA, Hutchesson ACJ, Bundred NJ, et al. Role of assays for parathyroid-hormone–related protein in investigation of hypercalcaemia. Lancet 1992; 339:164–167.

178. Yamamoto M, Duong LT, Fisher JE, et al. Suckling-mediated increases in urinary phosphate and 3′,5′-cyclic adenosine monophosphate excretion in

lactating rats: possible systemic effect of parathyroid hormone–related protein. Endocrinology 1991; 129:2614–2622.

179. Grill V, Hillary J, Ho PMW, et al. Parathyroid hormone–related protein: a possible endocrine function in lactation. Clin Endocrinol 1992; 37:405–410.

180. Bucht E, Rong H, Bremme K, et al. Midmolecular parathyroid hormone–related peptide in serum during pregnancy, lactation and in umbilical cord blood. Eur J Endocrinol 1995; 132:438–443.

181. Khosla S, van Heerden JA, Gharib H, et al. Parathyroid hormone–related protein and hypercalcemia secondary to massive mammary hyperplasia. N Engl J Med 1990; 322:1157.

182. Lepre F, Grill V, Ho PWM, et al. Hypercalcemia in pregnancy and lactation associated with parathyroid hormone–related protein. N Engl J Med 1993; 328:666–667.

183. Sato K, Taira M, Yoshiwara I, et al. A case of humoral hypercalcemia of pregnancy: hypercalcemic crisis at the postpartum period due to markedly elevated plasma PTHrP levels without malignancy. J Bone Miner Res 1995; 10(Suppl 1):S401.

184. Philbrick WM, Wysolmerski JJ, Galbraith S, et al. Defining the roles of parathyroid hormone–related protein in normal physiology. Physiol Rev 1996; 76:127–173.

185. Karaplis AC, Luz A, Glowacki J, et al. Lethal skeletal dysplasia from targeted disruption of the parathyroid hormone–related peptide gene. Genes Dev 1994; 8:277–289.

186. Holick MF, Ray S, Chen TC, et al. A parathyroid hormone antagonist stimulates epidermal proliferation and hair growth in mice. Proc Natl Acad Sci USA 1994; 91:8014–8016.

187. Wysolmerski JJ, Broadus AE, Zhou J, et al. Overexpression of parathyroid hormone–related protein in the skin of transgenic mice interferes with hair follicle development. Proc Natl Acad Sci USA 1994; 91:1133–1137.

188. Copp DH, Cameron EC, Cheney B, et al. Evidence for calcitonin: a new hormone from the parathyroid that lowers blood calcium. Endocrinology 1962; 70:638–649.

189. Hirsch PF, Voelkel EF, Munson PL. Thyrocalcitonin hypocalcemic hypophosphatemic principle of the thyroid gland. Science 1964; 146:412–413.

190. Pearse AGE. The cytochemistry of the thyroid C cells and their relationship to calcitonin. Proc R Soc Lond 1966; 170:71–80.

191. Pearse AGE, Cavalheira AF. Cytochemical evidence for an ultimobranchial origin of rodent thyroid C cells. Nature 1967; 214:929–930.

192. Copp DH, Cockcroft DW, Kueh Y. B Calcitonin from ultimobranchial glands from dogfish and chickens. Science 1967; 158:924–926.

193. Niall HD, Keutmann HT, Copp DH, et al. Amino acid sequence of salmon ultimobranchial calcitonin. Proc Natl Acad Sci USA 1969; 63:771–778.

194. Neher R, Riniker B, Rittel W, et al. Mensehliches calcitonin III. Struktur von calcitonin M and D. Helv Chim Acta 1968; 51:1900–1905.

195. Potts JT, Niall HD, Keutmann HT, et al. The amino acid sequence of porcine thyrocalcitonin. Proc Natl Acad Sci USA 1968; 59:1321–1328.

196. Potts JT Jr. Chemistry of the calcitonins. Bone Miner 1992; 16:169–173.

197. Jacobs JW, Goodman RH, Chin WW, et al. Calcitonin messenger RNA encodes multiple polypeptides in a single precursor. Science 1981; 213:457–459.

198. Hoppener JWM, Steenbergh PH, Zandberg J, et al. The second human calcitonin/CGRP gene is located on chromosome 11. Hum Genet 1985; 70:259–263.

199. Amara SG, Jones V, Rosenfeld MG, et al. Alternative RNA processing in calcitonin gene expression generates mRNAs encoding different polypeptide products. Nature 1982; 298:240–244.

200. Care AD, Cooper CW, Duncan T, et al. A study of thyrocalcitonin secretion by direct measurement of in vivo secretion rates in pigs. Endocrinology 1968; 83:161–169.

201. Cooper CW, Borosky SA, Farrell PE, et al. Effects of the calcium channel activator BAY-K-8644 on in vitro secretion of calcitonin and parathyroid hormone. Endocrinology 1986; 118:545–549.

202. Pento JT. Influence of the calcium ionophores A123187 and X537A on calcitonin secretion from the isolated perfused porcine thyroid. Mol Cell Endocrinol 1986; 45:71–75.

203. Garrett JE, Tamir H, Kifor O, et al. Calcitonin-secreting cells of the thyroid express an extracellular calcium receptor gene. Endocrinology 1995; 136:5202–5211.

204. Care AD. The regulation of the secretion of calcitonin. Bone Miner 1992; 16:182–185.

205. Cote GJ, Gagel RF. Dexamethasone differentially affects the levels of calcitonin and calcitonin gene–related peptide mRNAs expressed in a human medullary thyroid carcinoma cell line. J Biol Chem 1986; 261:15524–15528.

206. Aron DC, Muszynski M, Birnbaum RS, et al. Somatostatin elaboration by monolayer cell cultures derived from transplantable rat medullary thyroid carcinoma: synergistic stimulatory effects of glucagon and calcium. Endocrinology 1981; 109:1830–1834.

207. Bean BP. Neurotransmitter inhibition of neuronal calcium currents by changes in channel voltage dependence. Nature 1989; 340:153–155.

208. Naveh-Many T, Raue F, Grauer A, et al. Regulation of calcitonin gene expression by hypocalcemia, hypercalcemia, and vitamin D in the rat. J Bone Miner Res 1992; 7:1233–1237.

209. Peleg S, Abruzzese RV, Cooper CW, et al. Down-regulation of calcitonin gene transcription by vitamin D requires two widely separated enhancer sequences. Mol Endocrinol 1993; 7:999–1008.

210. Cote GJ, Rodgers DG, Huang ESC, et al. The effect of 1,25-dihydroxyvitamin D_3 treatment on calcitonin and calcitonin gene–related peptide mRNA levels in cultured human thyroid C-cells. Biochem Biophys Res Commun 1987; 149:239–243.

211. Friedman PA, Gesek FA. Cellular calcium transport in renal epithelial: measurement, mechanisms and regulation. Physiol Rev 1995; 75:429–471.

212. Chambers TJ, McSheehy PM, Thomson BM, et al. The effect of calcium-regulating hormones and prostaglandins on bone resorption by osteoclasts disaggregated from neonatal rabbit bones. Endocrinology 1985; 116:234–239.

213. Talmage RV, Vanderwiel CJ, Decker SA, et al. Changes produced in postprandial urinary calcium excretion by thyroidectomy and calcitonin administration in rats on different calcium regimes. Endocrinology 1979; 105:459–464.

214. Hurley DL, Tiegs RD, Wahner HW, et al. Axial and appendicular bone mineral density in patients with long-term deficiency or excess of calcitonin. N Engl J Med 1987; 317:537–541.

215. Wimalawansa SJ. Long- and short-term side effects and safety of calcitonin in man: a prospective study. Calcif Tissue Int 1993; 52:90–93.

216. Lin HY, Harris TL, Flannery MS, et al. Expression cloning of an adenylate cyclase–coupled calcitonin receptor. Science 1991; 254:1022–1024.

217. Chakraborty M, Chatterjee D, Kellokumpu S, et al. Cell cycle–dependent coupling of the calcitonin receptor to different G proteins. Science 1991; 251:1078–1082.

218. Houssami S, Findley DM, Brady CL, et al. Isoforms of the rat calcitonin receptor: consequences for ligand binding and signal transduction. Endocrinology 1994; 135:183–190.

219. Ikegame M, Rakopoulos M, Zhou H, et al. Calcitonin receptor isoforms in mouse and rat osteoclasts. J Bone Miner Res 1995; 10:59–65.

220. Nakamura M, Hashimoto T, Nakajima T, et al. A new type of human calcitonin receptor isoform generated by alternative splicing. Biochem Biophys Res Commun 1995; 209:744–751.

221. Nussenzveig DR, Mathew S, Gershengorn MC. Alternative splicing of a 48-nucleotide exon generates two isoforms of the human calcitonin receptor. Endocrinology 1995; 136:2047–2051.

222. Yamin M, Gorn AH, Flannery MR, et al. Cloning and characterization of a mouse brain calcitonin receptor complementary deoxyribonucleic acid and mapping of the calcitonin receptor gene. Endocrinology 1994; 135:2635–2643.

223. Albrandt K, Brady EMG, Moore CX, et al. Molecular cloning and functional expression of a third isoform of the human calcitonin receptor and partial characterization of the calcitonin receptor gene. Endocrinology 1995; 136:5377–5384.

224. Goldring SR, Gorn AH, Yamin M, et al. Characterization of the structural and functional properties of cloned calcitonin receptor cDNAS. Horm Metab Res 1993; 25:477–480.

225. Rosenfeld MG, Mermod JJ, Amara SG, et al. Production of a novel neuropeptide encoded by the calcitonin gene via tissue-specific RNA processing. Nature 1983; 304:129–135.

226. Goltzman D, Mitchell J. Interaction of calcitonin and calcitonin gene–related peptide at receptor sites in target tissues. Science 1985; 227:1343–1345.

227. Kapas S, Clark AJ. Identification of an orphan receptor gene as a type 1 calcitonin gene–related peptide receptor. Biochem Biophys Res Commun 1995; 217:832–838.

228. Sexton PM, Houssami S, Brady CL, et al. Amylin is an agonist of the renal porcine calcitonin receptor. Endocrinology 1994; 134:2103–2107.

229. Wilding JPH, Khandan-Nia N, Bennet WM, et al. Lack of acute effect of amylin (islet-associated polypeptide) on insulin sensitivity during hyperinsulinaemic euglycaemic clamp in humans. Diabetologia 1994; 37:166–169.

230. Lorenzo A, Razzaboni B, Weir GC, et al. Pancreatic islet cell toxicity of amylin associated with type-2 diabetes mellitus. Nature 1994; 368:756–757.

231. Poyner D. Pharmacology of receptors for calcitonin gene–related peptide and amylin. Trends Pharmacol Sci 1995; 16:424–428.

232. Niccoli P, Brunet P, Roubicek C, et al. Abnormal calcitonin basal levels and pentagastrin response in patients with chronic renal failure on maintenance hemodialysis. Eur J Endocrinol 1995; 132:75–81.

233. Bugalho MJGM, Roque L, Sobrinho LG, et al. Calcitonin-producing insulinoma: clinical, immunocytochemical and cytogenetical study. Clin Endocrinol 1994; 41:257–260.

234. Rambaud JC, Nisard A, Modigliani R, et al. Hypercalcitoninaemia in vipomas. Lancet 1978; 1:220.

235. Roos BA, Lindall AW, Baylin SB, et al. Plasma immunoreactive calcitonin in lung cancer. Endocr Res Commun 1979; 6:169–190.

236. O'Neill WJ, Jordan MH, Lewis MS, et al. Serum calcitonin may be a marker for inhalation injury in burns. J Burn Care Rehabil 1992; 13:605–616.

237. Sperber SJ, Blevins DD, Francis JB. Hypercalcitoninemia, hypocalcemia, and toxic shock syndrome. Rev Infect Dis 1990; 12:736–739.

238. Canale DD, Donabedian RK. Hypercalcitoninemia in acute pancreatitis. J Clin Endocrinol Metab 1975; 40:738–741.

239. Szanto J, Ady N, Jozsef S. Pain killing with calcitonin nasal spray in patients with malignant tumors. Oncology 1992; 49:180–182.

240. Jaeger H, Maier C. Calcitonin in phantom limb pain: a double-blind study. Pain 1992; 48:21–27.

241. Holick MF, MacLaughlin JA, Clark MB, et al. Photosynthesis of previtamin D_3 in human skin and the physiologic consequences. Science 1980; 210:203–205.

242. Holick MF, Shao Q, Liu WW, et al. The vitamin D content of fortified milk and infant formula. N Engl J Med 1992; 326:1178–1181.

243. Bikle DD, Gee E, Halloran B, et al. Assessment of the free fraction of 25-hydroxyvitamin D in serum and its regulation by albumin and the vitamin D–binding protein. J Clin Endocrinol Metab 1986; 63:954–959.

244. Bikle DD, Siiteri PK, Ryzen E, et al. Serum protein binding of 1,25-dihydroxyvitamin D: a reevaluation by direct measurement of free metabolite levels. J Clin Endocrinol Metab 1985; 61:969–975.

245. Tanaka Y, DeLuca HF. The control of 25-hydroxyvitamin D metabolism by inorganic phosphorus. Arch Biochem Biophys 1973; 154:566–574.

246. Glass AR, Eil C. Ketoconazole-induced reduction in serum 1,25-dihydroxyvitamin D and total serum calcium in hypercalcemic patients. J Clin Endocrinol Metab 1988; 66:934–938.

247. Tanaka Y, Halloran B, Schnoes HK, et al. In vitro production of 1,25-dihydroxyvitamin D_3 by rat placental tissue. Proc Natl Acad Sci USA 1979; 76:5033–5035.

248. Breslau NA, McGuire JL, Zerwekh JE, et al. Hypercalcemia associated with increased serum calcitriol levels in three patients with lymphoma. Ann Intern Med 1984; 100:1–7.

249. Barbour GL, Coburn JW, Slatopolsky E, et al. Hypercalcemia in an anephric patient with sarcoidosis: evidence for extrarenal generation of 1,25-dihydroxyvitamin D. N Engl J Med 1981; 305:440–443.

250. Adams JS, Sharma OP, Diz MM, et al. Ketoconazole decreases the serum 1,25-dihydroxyvitamin D and calcium concentration in sarcoidosis-associated hypercalcemia. J Clin Endocrinol Metab 1990; 70:1090–1095.

251. Adams JS, Diz MM, Sharma OP. Effective reduction in the serum 1,25-dihydroxyvitamin D and calcium concentration in sarcoidosis-associated hypercalcemia with short-course chloroquine therapy. Ann Intern Med 1989; 111:437–438.

252. Ohyama Y, Noshiro M, Okuda K. Cloning and expression of cDNA encoding 25-hydroxyvitamin D_3 24-hydroxylase. FEBS Lett 1991; 278:195–198.

253. DeLuca HF. The vitamin D story: a collaborative effort of basic science and clinical medicine. FASEB J 1988; 2:224–236.

254. Canterbury JM, Gavellas G, Bourgoignie JJ, et al. Metabolic consequences of oral administration of 24,25-dihydroxycholecalciferol to uremic dogs. J Clin Invest 1980; 65:571–576.

255. Schwartz Z, Brooks B, Swain L, et al. Production of 1,25-dihydroxyvitamin D_3 and 24,25-dihydroxyvitamin D_3 by growth zone and resting zone chondrocytes is dependent on cell maturation and is regulated by hormones and growth factors. Endocrinology 1992; 130:2495–2504.

256. Kumar R. Metabolism of 1,25-dihydroxyvitamin D. Physiol Rev 1984; 64:478–504.

257. Baker AR, McDonnell DP, Hughes M, et al. Cloning and expression of full-length cDNA encoding human vitamin D receptor. Proc Natl Acad Sci USA 1988; 85:3294–3298.

258. Pettifor JM, Bikle DD, Cavaleros M, et al. Serum levels of free 1,25-dihydroxyvitamin D in vitamin D toxicity. Ann Intern Med 1995; 122:511–513.

259. Kliewer SA, Umesono K, Mangelsdorf DJ, et al. Retinoid X receptor interacts with nuclear receptors in retinoic acid, thyroid hormone and vitamin D_3 signalling. Nature 1992; 355:446–449.

260. Demay MB, Kiernan MS, DeLuca HF, et al. Characterization of 1,25-dihydroxyvitamin D_3 receptor interactions with target sequences in the rat osteocalcin gene. Mol Endocrinol 1992; 6:557–562.

261. Noda M, Vogel RL, Craig AM, et al. Identification of a DNA sequence responsible for binding of the 1,25-dihydroxyvitamin D_3 receptor and 1,25-dihydroxyvitamin D_3 enhancement of mouse secreted phosphoprotein 1 (Spp-1 or osteopontin) gene expression. Proc Natl Acad Sci USA 1990; 87:9995–9999.

262. Gill RK, Christakos S. Identification of sequence elements in mouse calbindin-D28k gene that confer 1,25-dihydroxyvitamin D_3– and butyrate-inducible responses. Proc Natl Acad Sci USA 1993; 90:2984–2988.

263. Cao X, Ross FP, Zhang L, et al. Cloning of the promoter for the avian integrin β_3 subunit and its regulation by 1,25-dihydroxyvitamin D_3. J Biol Chem 1993; 268:27371–27380.

264. Chen K-S, DeLuca HF. Cloning of the human 1-alpha,25-dihydroxyvitamin D_3 24-hydroxylase gene promoter and identification of two vitamin D–responsive elements. Biochem Biophys Acta Gene Struct Expression 1995; 1263:1–9.

265. Jurutka PW, Terpening CM, Haussler MR. The 1,25-dihydroxy-vitamin D_3 receptor is phosphorylated in response to 1,25-dihydroxy-vitamin D_3 and 22-oxacalcitriol in rat osteoblasts, and by casein kinase II, in vitro. Biochemistry 1993; 32:8184–8192.

266. MacDonald PN, Sherman DR, Dowo DR Jr, et al. The vitamin D receptor interacts with general transcription factor IIB. J Biol Chem 1995; 270:4748–4752.

267. Godschalk M, Levy JR, Downs RW Jr. Glucocorticoids decrease vitamin D receptor number and gene expression in human osteosarcoma cells. J Bone Miner Res 1992; 7:21–27.

268. Iida K, Shinki T, Yamaguchi A, et al. A possible role of vitamin D receptors in regulating vitamin D activation in the kidney. Proc Natl Acad Sci USA 1995; 92:6112–6116.

269. Caffrey JM, Farach-Carson MC. Vitamin D_3 metabolites modulate dihydropyridine-sensitive calcium currents in clonal rat osteosarcoma cells. J Biol Chem 1989; 264:20265–20274.

270. Nemere I, Dormanen MC, Hammond MW, et al. Identification of a specific binding protein for 1α,25-dihydroxyvitamin D_3 in basal-lateral membranes of chick intestinal epithelium and relationship to transcaltachia. J Biol Chem 1994; 269:23750–23756.

271. Norman AW, Okamura WH, Farach-Carson MC, et al. Structure-function studies of 1,25-dihydroxyvitamin D_3 and the vitamin D endocrine system. J Biol Chem 1993; 268:13811–13819.

272. Barsony J, Marx SJ. Rapid accumulation of cyclic GMP near activated vitamin D receptors. Proc Natl Acad Sci USA 1991; 88:1436–1440.

273. Hughes MR, Malloy PJ, Kieback DG, et al. Point mutations in the human vitamin D receptor gene associated with hypocalcemic rickets. Science 1988; 242:1702–1705.

274. van Os CH. Transcellular calcium transport in intestinal and renal epithelial cells. Biochim Biophys Acta 1987; 906:195–222.

275. Wasserman RH, Fullmer CS. Calcium transport proteins, calcium absorption, and vitamin D. Annu Rev Physiol 1983; 45:375–390.

276. Karbach U. Paracellular calcium transport across the small intestine. J Nutr 1992; 122:672–677.

277. de Boland AR, Nemere I, Norman AW. Ca^{2+}-channel agonist BAY K8644 mimics 1,25(OH)$_2$-vitamin D_3 rapid enhancement of Ca^{2+} transport in chick perfused duodenum. Biochem Biophys Res Commun 1990; 166:217–222.

278. Nemere I, Norman AW. 1,25-dihydroxyvitamin D_3–mediated vesicular transport of calcium in intestine: time-course studies. Endocrinology 1988; 122:2962–2969.

279. Fullmer CS. Intestinal calcium absorption: calcium entry. J Nutr 1992; 122:644–650.

280. Wasserman RH, Chandler JS, Meyer SA, et al. Intestinal calcium transport and calcium extrusion processes at the basolateral membrane. J Nutr 1992; 122:662–671.

281. Kaune R, Munson S, Bikle DD. Regulation of calmodulin binding to the ATP extractable 110-kDa protein (myosin I) from chicken duodenal brush border by 1,25(OH)$_2$D$_3$. Biochim Biophys Acta 1994; 1190:329–336.

282. Kretsinger RH. Structure and evolution of calcium-regulated proteins. CRC Crit Rev Biochem 1980; 8:119–174.

283. Cai Q, Chandler JS, Wasserman RH, et al. Vitamin D and adaptation to dietary calcium and phosphate deficiencies increase intestinal plasma membrane calcium pump gene expression. Proc Natl Acad Sci USA 1993; 90:1345–1349.

284. Ghijsen WEJM, DeJong MD, van Os CH. Kinetic properties of Na^+/Ca^{2+} exchange in basolateral plasma membranes of rat small intestine. Biochim Biophys Acta 1983; 730:85–94.

285. Harrison JR, Petersen DN, Lichtler AC, et al. 1,25-Dihydroxyvitamin D_3 inhibits transcription of type I collagen genes in the rat osteosarcoma line ROS 17/2.8. Endocrinology 1989; 125:327–333.

286. Price PA. Vitamin K–dependent bone proteins. In: Cohn DV, Martin TJ, Meunier PJ, eds. Calcium Regulation and Bone Metabolism: Basic and Clinical Aspects. Vol 9. Amsterdam: Exerpta Medica, 1987:419–426.

287. Raisz LG, Trummel CL, Holick MF, et al. 1,25-Dihydroxycholecalciferol: a potent stimulator of bone resorption in tissue culture. Science 1972; 175:768–769.

288. Holtrop ME, Cox KA, Clark MB, et al. 1,25-Dihydroxycholecalciferol stimulates osteoclasts in rat bones in the absence of parathyroid hormone. Endocrinology 1981; 108:2293–2301.

289. Medhora MM, Teitelbaum S, Chappel J, et al. 1α,25-Dihydroxyvitamin D_3 up-regulates expression of the osteoclast integrin $\alpha_v\beta_3$. J Biol Chem 1993; 268:1456–1461.

290. Underwood JL, DeLuca HF. Vitamin D is not directly necessary for bone growth and mineralization. Am J Physiol 1984; 246:E493–E498.

291. Weinstein RS, Underwood JL, Hutson MS, et al. Bone histomorphometry in vitamin D–deficient rats infused with calcium and phosphorus. Am J Physiol 1984; 246:E499–E506.

292. Balsan S, Garabedian M, Larchet M, et al. Long-term nocturnal calcium infusions can cure rickets and promote normal mineralization in hereditary resistance to 1,25-dihydroxyvitamin D. J Clin Invest 1986; 77:1661–1667.

293. Walling MW. Intestinal Ca and phosphate transport: differential responses to vitamin D_3 metabolites. Am J Physiol 1977; 2:E488–E494.

294. Kumar R. Vitamin D and calcium transport. Kidney Int 1991; 40:1177–1189.

295. Massheimer V, Fernandez LM, Boland R, et al. Regulation of Ca^{2+} uptake in skeletal muscle by 1,25-dihydroxyvitamin D_3: role of phosphorylation and calmodulin. Mol Cell Endocrinol 1992; 84:15–22.

296. Pointon JJ, Francis MJO, Smith R. Effect of vitamin D deficiency on sarcoplasmic reticulum function and troponin C concentration of rabbit skeletal muscle. Clin Sci 1979; 57:257–263.

297. Zhou JY, Norman AW, Chen DL, et al. 1,25-Dihydroxy-16-ene-23-yne-vitamin D prolongs survival time of leukemic mice. Proc Natl Acad Sci USA 1990; 87:3929–3932.

298. Shabahang M, Buras RR, Davoodi F, et al. Growth inhibition of HT-29 human colon cancer cells by analogues of 1,25-dihydroxyvitamin D_3. Cancer Res 1994; 54:4057–4064.

299. Halline AG, Davidson NO, Skarosi SF, et al. Effects of 1,25-dihydroxyvitamin D_3 on proliferation and differentiation of Caco-2 cells. Endocrinology 1994; 134:1710–1717.

300. Colston KW, Mackay AG, James SY, et al. EB 1089: a new vitamin D analogue that inhibits the growth of breast cancer cells in vivo and in vitro. Biochem Pharmacol 1992; 44:2273–2280.

301. Mathieu C, Laureys J, Waer M, et al. Prevention of autoimmune destruction of transplanted islets in spontaneously diabetic NOD mice by KH1060, a 20-epi analog of vitamin D: synergy with cyclosporine. Transplant Proc 1994; 26:3128–3129.

302. Brown AJ, Ritter CR, Finch JL, et al. The noncalcemic analogue of vitamin D, 22-oxacalcitriol, suppresses parathyroid hormone synthesis and secretion. J Clin Invest 1989; 84:728–732.

303. Holick MF, Smith E, Pincus S. Skin as the site of vitamin D synthesis and target tissue for 1,25-dihydroxyvitamin D_3: use of calcitriol (1,25-dihydroxyvitamin D_3) for treatment of psoriasis. Arch Dermatol 1987; 123:1677–1683.

304. Hoeck HC, Laurberg G, Laurberg P. Hypercalcemia crisis after excessive topical use of a vitamin D derivative. J Intern Med 1994; 235:281–282.

305. Kamimura S, Gallieni M, Kubodera N, et al. Differential catabolism of 22-oxacalcitriol and 1,25-dihydroxyvitamin D_3 by normal human peripheral monocytes. Endocrinology 1993; 133:2719–2722.

306. Gill HS, Londowski JM, Corradino RA, et al. The synthesis and biological activity of 25-hydroxy-26,27-dimethylvitamin D_3 and 1,25-dihydroxy-26,27-dimethylvitamin D_3: highly potent novel analogs of vitamin D_3. J Steroid Biochem 1988; 31:147–160.

307. Peleg S, Sastry M, Collins ED, et al. Distinct conformational changes induced by 20-epi analogues of 1α,25-dihydroxyvitamin D_3 are associated with enhanced activation of the vitamin D receptor. J Biol Chem 1995; 270:10551–10558.

308. Norman AW, Sergeev IN, Bishop JE, et al. Selective biological response by target organs (intestine, kidney, and bone) to 1,25-dihydroxyvitamin D_3 and two analogues. Cancer Res 1993; 53:3935–3942.

309. Nussbaum SR, Zahradnik RJ, Lavigne JR, et al. Highly sensitive two-site immunoradiometric assay of parathyrin and its clinical utility in evaluating patients with hypercalcemia. Clin Chem 1987; 33:1364–1367.

310. Bilezikian JP. Clinical utility of assays for parathyroid hormone–related protein. Clin Chem 1992; 38:179–181.

311. Grill V, Ho P, Body JJ, et al. Parathyroid hormone–related protein: elevated levels in both humoral hypercalcemia of malignancy and hypercalcemia complicating metastatic breast cancer. J Clin Endocrinol Metab 1991; 73:1309–1315.

312. Henderson J, Bernier S, D'Amour P, et al. Effects of passive immunization against PTH-like peptide in hypercalcemic tumor–bearing rats and normocalcemic controls. Endocrinology 1990; 127:1310–1316.

313. Pandian MR, Morgan CH, Carlton E, et al. Modified immunoradiometric assay of parathyroid hormone–related protein: clinical application in the differential diagnosis of hypercalcemia. Clin Chem 1992; 38:282–288.

314. Weissel M, Kainz H, Tyl E, et al. Clinical evaluation of new assays for determination of serum calcitonin concentrations. Acta Endocrinol 1991; 124:540–544.

315. Kao PC, Gharib H. Clinical performance of an extraction calcitonin radioimmunoassay. Mayo Clin Proc 1993; 68:1165–1170.

316. Wimalawansa SJ, Bailey F. Validation, role in perioperative assessment, and clinical applications of an immunoradiometric assay for human calcitonin. Peptides 1995; 16:307–312.

317. Weber CJ, Sewell CW, McGarity WC. Persistent and recurrent sporadic primary hyperparathyroidism: histopathology, complications, and results of reoperation. Surgery 1994; 116:991–998.

318. LiVolsi VA: Embryology, anatomy, and pathology of the parathyroids. In: Bilezikian JP, ed. The Parathyroids. New York: Raven Press, 1994:1–14.

319. Rosen IB, Young JEM, Archibald SD, et al. Parathyroid cancer: clinical variations and relationships to autotransplantation. Can J Cancer 1994; 37:465–469.

320. Shane E, Bilezikian JP. Parathyroid carcinoma: a review of 62 patients. Endocr Rev 1982; 3:218–226.

321. Albright F, Aub J, Bauer W. Hyperparathyroidism: a common and polymorphic condition as illustrated by seventeen proved cases from one clinic. JAMA 1934; 102:1276–1287.

322. Cope O. The study of hyperparathyroidism at the Massachusetts General Hospital. N Engl J Med 1966; 274:1174–1182.

323. Keating FR, Jr, Cook EN. Recognition of primary hyperparathyroidism: analysis of 24 cases. JAMA 1945; 129:994–1002.

324. Pyrah LN. Primary hyperparathyroidism. Br J Surg 1966; 53:245–316.

325. Patten BM, Bilezikian JP, Mallette LE, et al. Neuromuscular disease in hyperparathyroidism. Ann Intern Med 1974; 80:182–193.

326. Grey AB, Evans MC, Stapleton JP, et al. Body weight and bone mineral density in postmenopausal women with primary hyperparathyroidism [see comments]. Ann Intern Med 1994; 121:745–749.

327. Rubinoff H. Hypercalcemia: long-term follow-up with matched controls. J Chron Dis 1983; 36:859–868.

328. Palmer M, Adami HO, Bergstrom R, et al. Mortality after surgery for primary hyperparathyroidism: a followup of 441 patients operated on from 1956–1979. Surgery 1987; 102:1–7.

329. Palmer M, Adami HO, Krusemo UB, et al. Increased risk of malignant diseases after surgery for primary hyperparathyroidism: a nationwide cohort study. Am J Epidemiol 1988; 127:1031–1040.

330. Parisien M, Silverberg SJ, Shane E, et al. The histomorphometry of bone in primary hyperparathyroidism: preservation of cancellous bone structure. J Clin Endocrinol Metab 1990; 70:930–938.

331. Silverberg S, Shane E, de la Cruz L, et al. Skeletal disease in primary hyperparathyroidism [see comments]. J Bone Miner Res 1989; 4:283–291.

332. Alhava EM. Bone mineral density and surgical treatment of primary hyperparathyroidism. Acta Chir Scand 1988; 154:345–347.

333. Rao DS, Wilson RJ, Kleerekoper M, et al. Lack of biochemical progression or continuation of accelerated bone loss in mild asymptomatic primary hyperparathyroidism: evidence for biphasic disease course. J Clin Endocrinol Metab 1988; 67:1294–1298.

334. Martin P. Long-term irreversibility of bone loss after surgery. Arch Intern Med 1990; 150:1495–1497.

335. Silverberg SJ, Gartenberg F, Jacobs TP, et al. Longitudinal measurements of bone density and biochemical indices in untreated primary hyperparathyroidism. J Clin Endocrinol Metab 1995; 80:723–728.

336. Melton LI, Atkinson E, O'Fallon W, et al. Long-term fracture prediction by bone mineral assessed at different skeletal sites. J Bone Miner Res 1993; 8:1227–1233.

337. Mitlak B, Daly M, Potts JJ, et al. Asymptomatic primary hyperparathyroidism. J Bone Miner Res 1991; 6:S103–S110.

338. Parfitt AM, Rao DS, Kleerekoper M. Asymptomatic primary hyperparathyroidism discovered by multichannel biochemical screening: clinical course and considerations bearing on the need for surgical intervention. J Bone Miner Res 1991; 6(Suppl):S97–S101.

339. Silverberg SJ, Shane E, Jacobs TP, et al. Nephrolithiasis and bone involvement in primary hyperparathyroidism. Am J Med 1990; 89:327–334.

340. Arnold A, Staunton CE, Kim HG, et al. Monoclonality and abnormal parathyroid hormone genes in parathyroid adenomas. N Engl J Med 1988; 318:658–662.

341. Arnold A. Molecular basis of hyperparathyroidism. In: Bilezikian JP, ed. The Parathyroids. New York: Raven Press, 1994:407–421.

342. Cryns VL, Yi SM, Tahara H, et al. Frequent loss of chromosome arm 1p DNA in parathyroid adenomas. Genes Chromosomes Cancer 1995; 13:9–17.

343. Tahara H, Smith AP, Gas RD, et al. Genomic localization of novel candidate tumor suppressor gene loci in human parathyroid adenomas. Cancer Res 1996; 56:599–605.

344. Friedman E, Sakaguchi K, Bale AE, et al. Clonality of parathyroid tumors in familial multiple endocrine neoplasia type I. N Engl J Med 1989; 321:213–218.

345. Bystrom C, Larsson C, Blomberg C, et al. Localization of the MEN 1 gene to a small region within chromosome 11q13 by deletion mapping in tumors. Proc Natl Acad Sci USA 1990; 87:1968–1972.

346. Motokura T, Bloom T, Kim HG, et al. A BCL1-linked candidate oncogene which is rearranged in parathyroid tumors encodes a novel cyclin. Nature 1991; 350:512–515.

347. Hsi E, Zukerberg LR, Yang WI, et al. Cyclin D1/PRAD1 expression in parathyroid adenomas: an immunohistochemical study. J Clin Endocrinol Metab 1996; 81:1736–1739.

348. Schneider AB, Gierlowski TC, Shore-Freedman E, et al. Dose-response relationships for radiation-induced hyperparathyroidism. J Clin Endocrinol Metab 1995; 80:254–257.

349. Carling T, Kindmark A, Hellman P, et al. Vitamin D receptor genotypes in primary hyperparathyroidism. Nat Med 1995; 1:1309–1311.

350. Falchetti A, Bale AE, Amorosi A, et al. Progression of uremic hyperparathyroidism involves allelic loss on chromosome 11. J Clin Endocrinol Metab 1993; 76:139–144.

351. Arnold A, Brown MF, Urena P, et al. Monoclonality of parathyroid tumors in chronic renal failure and in primary parathyroid hyperplasia. J Clin Invest 1995; 95:2047–2053.

352. Davies M. Hyperparathyroidism in X-linked hypophosphataemic osteomalacia. Clin Endocrinol 1995; 42:205–206.

353. Mallette LE, Khouri K, Zengotita H, et al. Lithium treatment increases intact and midregion parathyroid hormone and parathyroid volume. J Clin Endocrinol Metab 1989; 68:654–660.

354. Stancer HC, Forbath N. Hyperparathyroidism, hypothyroidism and impaired renal function after 10 to 20 years of lithium treatment. Arch Intern Med 1989; 149:1042–1045.

355. Thakker RV, Bouloux P, Wooding C, et al. Association of parathyroid tumors in multiple endocrine neoplasia type 1 with loss of alleles on chromosome 11. N Engl J Med 1989; 321:218–224.

356. Brown EM, Gardner DG, Brennan MF, et al. Calcium-regulated parathyroid hormone release in primary hyperparathyroidism. Am J Med 1979; 66:923–931.

357. LeBoff MS, Shoback D, Brown EM, et al. Regulation of parathyroid hormone release and cytosolic calcium by extracellular calcium in dispersed and cultured bovine and pathological human parathyroid cells. J Clin Invest 1985; 75:49–57.

358. Kifor O, Moore FD, Wang P, et al. Reduced immunostaining for the extracellular Ca^{2+}-sensing receptor in primary and uremic secondary hyperparathyroidism. J Clin Endocrinol Metab 1996; 81:1598–1606.

359. Rizzoli R, Green J, Marx SJ. Primary hyperparathyroidism in familial multiple endocrine neoplasia type 1. Am J Med 1985; 78:467–474.

360. Hellman P, Skogseid B, Juhlin C, et al. Findings and long-term results of parathyroid surgery in multiple endocrine neoplasia type 1. World J Surg 1992; 16:718–723.

361. Hofstra RMW, Landsvater RM, Ceccherini I, et al. A mutation in the RET proto-oncogene associated with multiple endocrine neoplasia type 2B and sporadic medullary thyroid carcinoma. Nature 1994; 367:375–383.

362. Santoro M, Carlomagno F, Romano A, et al. Activation of RET as a

dominant transforming gene by germline mutations of MEN2A and MEN2B. Science 1995; 267:381–383.

363. Pausova Z, Soliman E, Amizuka N, et al. Role of the RET proto-oncogene in sporadic hyperparathyroidism and in hyperparathyroidism of multiple endocrine neoplasia type 2. J Clin Endocrinol Metab 1996; 81:2711–2718.

364. Wassif WS, Moniz CF, Friedman E, et al. Familial isolated hyperparathyroidism: a distinct genetic entity with an increased risk of parathyroid cancer. J Clin Endocrinol Metab 1993; 77:1485–1489.

365. Szabo J, Heath B, Hill VM, et al. Heredity hyperparathyroidism–jaw tumor syndrome: the endocrine tumor gene HRPT2 maps to chromosome 1q21-q31. Am J Hum Genet 1995; 56:944–950.

366. Potts JT Jr, ed. Proceedings of the NIH Consensus Development Conference on Diagnosis and Management of Asymptomatic Primary Hyperparathyroidism. J Bone Miner Res 1991; 6:S9–S13.

367. Ohrvall U, Akerstrom G, Ljunghall S, et al. Surgery for sporadic primary hyperparathyroidism in the elderly. World J Surg 1994; 18:612–618.

368. Chigot JP, Menegaux F, Achrafi H. Should primary hyperparathyroidism be treated surgically in elderly patients older than 75 years? Surgery 1995; 117:397–401.

369. Scholz DA, Purnell DC. Asymptomatic primary hyperparathyroidism: 10-year prospective study. Mayo Clin Proc 1981; 56:473–478.

370. Kleerekoper M, Bilezkian JP. A cure in search of a disease: parathyroidectomy for nontraditional features of primary hyperparathyroidism [editorial; comment]. Am J Med 1994; 96:99–100.

371. Insogna KL, Mitnick ME, Stewart AF, et al. Sensitivity of the parathyroid hormone–1,25-dihydroxyvitamin D axis to variations in calcium intake in patients with primary hyperparathyroidism. N Engl J Med 1985; 313:1126–1130.

372. Gallagher JC, Wilkinson R. The effect of ethinyloestradiol on calcium and phosphorus metabolism of post-menopausal women with primary hyperparathyroidism. Clin Sci Mol Med 1973; 45:782–785.

373. Marcus R. Estrogens and progestins in the management of primary hyperparathyroidism. J Bone Miner Res 1991; 6(Suppl):S125–S129.

374. Selby PL, Peacock M. Ethinyl estradiol and norethindrone in the treatment of primary hyperparathyroidism in postmenopausal women. N Engl J Med 1986; 314:1481–1485.

375. Broadus AE, Magee JS. A detailed evaluation of oral phosphate therapy in selected patients with primary hyperparathyroidism. J Clin Endocrinol Metab 1983; 56:953–961.

376. Reasner CA, Stone MD, Hosking DJ, et al. Acute changes in calcium homeostasis during treatment of primary hyperparathyroidism with risedronate. J Clin Endocrinol Metab 1993; 77:1067–1071.

377. Russell CF, Edis AJ. Surgery for primary hyperparathyroidism: experience with 500 consecutive cases and evaluation of the role of surgery in the asymptomatic patient. Br J Surg 1982; 69:244–247.

378. Thompson NW. Localization studies in patients with primary hyperparathyroidism. Br J Surg 1988; 75:97–98.

379. Doppman JL, Miller DL. Localization of parathyroid tumors in patients with asymptomatic hyperparathyroidism and no previous surgery. J Bone Miner Res 1991; 6(Suppl):S153–S158.

380. Akerstrom G, Rundberg C, Grimelius L, et al. Causes of failed primary exploration and technical aspects of reoperation in primary hyperparathyroidism. World J Surg 1992; 16:562–569.

381. Mitchell BK, Merrell RC, Kinder BK. Localization studies in patients with hyperparathyroidism. Surg Clin North Am 1995; 75:483–498.

382. Levin KE, Clark OH. The reasons for failure in parathyroid operations. Arch Surg 1989; 124:911–915.

383. Proye CAG, Carnaille B, Bizard JP, et al. Multiglandular disease in seemingly sporadic primary hyperparathyroidism revisited: where are we in the early 1990's? A plea against unilateral parathyroid exploration. Surgery 1992; 112:1118–1122.

384. Heller KS, Attie JN, Dubner S. Parathyroid localization: inability to predict multiple gland involvement. Am J Surg 1993; 166:357–359.

385. Oertli D, Richter M, Kraenzlin M, et al. Parathyroidectomy in primary hyperparathyroidism: preoperative localization and routine biopsy of unaltered glands are not necessary. Surgery 1995; 117:392–396.

386. Duh QY, Uden P, Clark OH. Unilateral neck exploration for primary hyperparathyroidism: analysis of a controversy using a mathematical model. World J Surg 1992; 16:654–662.

387. LiVolsi VA, Hamilton R. Intraoperative assessment of parathyroid gland pathology: a common view from the surgeon and the pathologist. Am J Clin Pathol 1994; 102:365–373.

388. Billingsley KG, Fraker DL, Doppman JL, et al. Localization and operative management of undescended parathyroid adenomas in patients with persistent primary hyperparathyroidism. Surgery 1994; 116:982–989.

389. Sandelin K, Auer G, Bondeson L, et al. Prognostic factors in parathyroid carcinoma: a review of 95 cases. World J Surg 1992; 16:724–731.

390. Sandelin K, Thompson NW, Bondeson L. Metastatic parathyroid carcinoma: dilemmas in management. Surgery 1991; 110:978–988.

391. Gaz R, Doubler PB, Wang C. The management of 50 unusual hyperfunctioning parathyroid glands. Surgery 1987; 102:949–957.

392. Kollmorgen CF, Aust MR, Ferreiro JA, et al. Parathyromatosis: a rare yet important cause of persistent or recurrent hyperparathyroidism. Surgery 1994; 116:111–115.

393. Brennan MF, Norton JA. Reoperation for persistent and recurrent hyperparathyroidism. Ann Surg 1985; 201:40–44.

394. Bergenfelz A, Valdermarsson S, Ahren B. Functional recovery of the parathyroid glands after surgery for primary hyperparathyroidism. Surgery 1994; 116:827–836.

395. Brasier AR, Wang CA, Nussbaum SR. Recovery of parathyroid hormone secretion after parathyroid adenomectomy. J Clin Endocrinol Metab 1988; 66:495–500.

396. Thule P, Thakore K, Vansant J, et al. Preoperative localization of parathyroid tissue with technetium-99m sestamibi ^{123}I subtraction scanning. J Clin Endocrinol Metab 1994; 78:77–82.

397. Hindie E, Melliere D, Simon D, et al. Primary hyperparathyroidism: is technetium 99m-sestamibi/iodine-123 subtraction scanning the best procedure to locate enlarged glands before surgery? Clin Endocrinol 1995; 80:302–307.

398. Mitchell BK, Kinder BK, Cornelius E, et al. Primary hyperparathyroidism: preoperative localization using technetium-sestamibi scanning [editorial]. J Clin Endocrinol Metab 1995; 80:7–10.

399. Prinz RA, Barbato AL, Braithwaite SS, et al. Simultaneous primary hyperparathyroidism and nodular thyroid disease. Surgery 1982; 92:454–458.

400. Laing VO, Frame B, Block MA. Associated primary hyperparathyroidism and thyroid lesions. Arch Surg 1969; 98:709–712.

401. McIntyre RJ, Kumpe DA, Liechty RD. Reexploration and angiographic ablation for hyperparathyroidism. Arch Surg 1994; 129:499–503.

402. Doherty GM, Doppman JL, Miller DL, et al. Results of a multidisciplinary strategy for management of mediastinal parathyroid adenoma as a cause of persistent primary hyperparathyroidism. Ann Surg 1992; 215:101–106.

403. MacFarlane MP, Fraker DL, Shawker TH, et al. Use of preoperative fine-needle aspiration in patients undergoing reoperation for primary hyperparathyroidism. Surgery 1994; 116:959–964.

404. Smythe WR, Bavaria JE, Hall RA, et al. Thoracoscopic removal of mediastinal parathyroid adenoma. Ann Thorac Surg 1995; 59:236–238.

405. Prinz RA, Lonchyna V, Carnaille B, et al. Thoracoscopic excision of enlarged mediastinal parathyroid glands. Surgery 1994; 116:999–1004.

406. Mautalen C, Reyes HR, Ghiringhelli G, et al. Cortical bone mineral content in primary hyperparathyroidism: changes after parathyroidectomy. Acta Endocrinol 1986; 111:494–497.

407. Wells S Jr. Surgical therapy of patients with primary hyperparathyroidism: long-term benefits. J Bone Miner Res 1991; 6(Suppl):S143–S149.

408. Siminovitch JM, Esselstyn CB, Jr, Straffon RA. Renal lithiasis and hyperparathyroidism: diagnosis, management and prognosis. J Urol 1981; 126:720–722.

409. Deaconson TF, Wilson SD, Lemann J Jr. The effect of parathyroidectomy on the recurrence of nephrolithiasis. Surgery 1987; 102:910–913.

410. Hedback G, Tisell LE, Bengtsson BA, et al. Premature death in patients operated on for primary hyperparathyroidism. World J Surg 1990; 14:829–836.

411. Khosla S, Ebeling PR, Firek AF, et al. Calcium infusion suggests a "set-point" abnormality of parathyroid gland function in familial benign hypercalcemia and more complex disturbances in primary hyperparathyroidism. J Clin Endocrinol Metab 1993; 76:715–720.

412. Marx SJ, Attie MF, Levine M, et al. The hypocalciuric or benign variant of familial hypercalcemia: clinical and biochemical features in fifteen kindreds. Medicine 1981; 60:397–412.

413. Nordenstrom J, Strigard K, Perbeck L, et al. Hyperparathyroidism associated with treatment of manic-depressive disorders by lithium. Eur J Surg 1992; 158:207–211.

414. Brown EM. Lithium induces abnormal calcium-regulated PTH release in dispersed bovine parathyroid cells. J Clin Endocrinol Metab 1981; 52:1046–1048.

415. McHenry CR, Racke F, Meister M, et al. Lithium effects on dispersed bovine parathyroid cells grown in tissue culture. Surgery 1991; 110:1061–1066.

416. Ralston SH, Gallacher SJ, Patel U, et al. Cancer-associated hypercalcemia: morbidity and mortality. Ann Intern Med 1990; 112:499–504.

417. Mundy GR, Martin TJ. Pathophysiology of skeletal complications of cancer. In: Mundy GR, Martin TJ, eds. Physiology and Pharmacology of Bone. Berlin: Springer-Verlag, 1993: 641–671.

418. Garrett IR, Durie BGM, Nedwin GE, et al. Production of the bone-resorbing cytokine lymphotoxin by cultured human myeloma cells. N Engl J Med 1987; 317:526–532.

419. Mundy GR: Cytokines of bone. In: Mundy GR, Martin TJ, eds. Physiology and Pharmacology of Bone. Berlin: Springer-Verlag, 1993:186–214.

420. Berenson JR, Lichtenstein A, Porter L, et al. Efficacy of pamidronate in reducing skeletal events in patients with advanced multiple myeloma. N Engl J Med 1996; 334:488–493.

421. Bundred NJ, Ratcliffe WA, Walker RA, et al. Parathyroid hormone–related protein and hypercalcaemia in breast cancer. Br Med J 1991; 303:1506–1509.

422. Guise TA, Yin JJ, Taylor SD, et al. Evidence for a causal role of parathyroid hormone–related protein in the pathogenesis of human breast cancer–mediated osteolysis. J Clin Invest 1996; 98:1544–1549.

423. Stewart AF, Horst R, Deftos LJ, et al. Biochemical evaluation of patients with cancer-associated hypercalcemia. N Engl J Med 1980; 303:1377–1383.

424. Thiede MA, Smock SL, Petersen DN, et al. Presence of messenger ribonucleic acid encoding osteocalcin, a marker of bone turnover, in bone marrow megakaryocytes and peripheral blood platelets. Endocrinology 1994; 135:927–937.

425. Kukreja SC, Shevrin DH, Wimbiscus SA, et al. Antibodies to parathyroid hormone–related protein lower serum calcium in athymic mouse models of malignancy-associated hypercalcemia due to human tumors. J Clin Invest 1988; 82:1798–1802.

426. Strewler GJ, Wronski TJ, Halloran BP. Pathogenesis of hypercalcemia in nude mice bearing a human renal carcinoma. Endocrinology 1986; 119:303–309.

427. Bushinsky DA, Riera GS, Favus MJ, et al. Evidence that blood ionized calcium can regulate serum 1,25(OH)$_2$D$_3$ independently of parathyroid hormone and phosphorus in the rat. J Clin Invest 1985; 76:1599–1604.

428. Ikeda K, Ogata E. Humoral hypercalcemia of malignancy: some enigmas on the clinical features. J Cell Biochem 1995; 57:384–391.

429. DeLaMata J, Uy HL, Guise TA, et al. Interleukin-6 enhances hypercalcemia and bone resorption mediated by parathyroid hormone–related protein in vivo. J Clin Invest 1995; 95:2846–2852.

430. Seymour JF, Gagel RF, Hagemeister FB, et al. Calcitriol production in hypercalcemic and normocalcemic patients with non-Hodgkin lymphoma. Ann Intern Med 1994; 121:633–640.

431. Yoshimoto K, Yamasaki R, Sakai H, et al. Ectopic production of parathyroid hormone by small cell lung cancer in a patient with hypercalcemia. J Clin Endocrinol Metab 1989; 68:976–981.

432. Nussbaum S, Gaz R, Arnold A. Hypercalcemia and ectopic secretion of parathyroid hormone by an ovarian carcinoma with rearrangement of the gene for parathyroid hormone. N Engl J Med 1990; 323:1324–1326.

433. Strewler GJ, Budayr AA, Clark OH, et al. Production of parathyroid hormone by a malignant nonparathyroid tumor in a hypercalcemic patient. J Clin Endocrinol Metab 1993; 76:1373–1375.

434. Rizzoli R, Pache J-C, Didierjean L, et al. A thymoma as a cause of true ectopic hyperparathyroidism. J Clin Endocrinol Metab 1994; 79:912–915.

435. Jacobus CH, Holick MF, Shao Q, et al. Hypervitaminosis D associated with drinking milk. N Engl J Med 1992; 326:1173–1177.

436. Streck WF, Waterhouse CW, Haddad JG. Glucocorticoid effects in vitamin D intoxication. Arch Intern Med 1979; 139:974–977.

437. Bell NH, Stern PH, Pantzer E, et al. Evidence that increased circulating 1-alpha, 25-dihydroxyvitamin D is the probable cause for abnormal calcium metabolism in sarcoidosis. J Clin Invest 1979; 66:852–855.

438. Kruithoff KL, Gyetko MR, Scheiman JM. Giant splenomegaly and refractory hypercalcemia due to extrapulmonary sarcoidosis. Arch Intern Med 1993; 153:2793–2796.

439. Adams JS, Sharma OP, Gacad MA, et al. Metabolism of 25-hydroxyvitamin D$_3$ by cultured pulmonary alveolar macrophages in sarcoidosis. J Clin Invest 1983; 72:1856–1860.

440. Reichel H, Koeffler HP, Barbers R, et al. Regulation of 1,25-dihydroxyvitamin D$_3$ production by cultured alveolar macrophages from normal human donors and from patients with pulmonary sarcoidosis. J Clin Endocrinol Metab 1987; 65:1201–1209.

441. Bell NH, Gill JF, Bartter FC. On the abnormal calcium absorption in sarcoidosis: evidence for increased sensitivity to vitamin D. Am J Med 1964; 36:500–513.

442. Basile JN, Leil Y, Shary J, et al. Increased calcium intake does not suppress circulating 1,25-dihydroxyvitamin D in normocalcemic patients with sarcoidosis. J Clin Invest 1993; 91:1396–1398.

443. Shaker JL, Redlin KC, Warren GV, et al. Case report: hypercalcemia with inappropriate 1,25-dihydroxyvitamin D in Wegener's granulomatosis. Am J Med Sci 1994; 308:115–118.

444. Ahmed B, Jaspan JB. Case report: hypercalcemia in a patient with AIDS and *Pneumocystis carinii* pneumonia. Am J Med Sci 1993; 306:313–316.

445. Auwerx J, Bouillon R. Mineral and bone metabolism in thyroid disease: a review. Q J Med 1986; 60:737–752.

446. Daly JG, Greenwood RM, Himsworth RL. Serum calcium concentration in hyperthyroidism at diagnosis and after treatment. Clin Endocrinol 1983; 19:397–404.

447. Mosekilde L, Melsen F, Bagger JP, et al. Bone changes in hyperthyroidism: interrelationships between bone morphometry, thyroid function, and calcium-phosphorus metabolism. Acta Endocrinol (Copenh) 1977; 85:515–525.

448. Mallette LE, Rubenfeld S, Silverman V. A controlled study of the effects of thyrotoxicosis and propranolol treatment on mineral metabolism and parathyroid hormone immunoreactivity. Metabolism 1985; 34:999–1006.

449. Valentic JP, Elias AN, Weinstein GD. Hypercalcemia associated with oral isotretinoin in the treatment of severe acne. JAMA 1986; 250:1899–1900.

450. Frame B, Jackson CE, Reynolds WA, et al. Hypercalcemia and skeletal effects in chronic hypervitaminosis A. Ann Intern Med 1974; 80:44–48.

451. Walser M, Robinson BH, Duckett JW. The hypercalcemia of adrenal insufficiency. J Clin Invest 1963; 42:456–464.

452. Muls E, Bouillon R, Boelaert J, et al. Etiology of hypercalcemia in a patient with Addison's disease. Calcif Tissue Int 1982; 34:523–526.

453. Christensson T, Hellstrom K, Wengle B. Hypercalcemia and primary hyperparathyroidism: prevalence in patients receiving thiazides as detected in a health screen. Arch Intern Med 1977; 137:1138–1142.

454. Porter RH, Cox BG, Heaney P, et al. Treatment of hypoparathyroid patients with chlorthalidone. N Engl J Med 1978; 298:577–581.

455. McMillan DE, Freeman RB. The milk alkali syndrome: a study of the acute disorder with comments on the development of the chronic condition. Medicine 1965; 44:485–501.

456. Abreo K, Adlakha A, Kilpatrick S, et al. The milk-alkali syndrome. Arch Intern Med 1993; 153:1005–1010.

457. Beall DP, Scofield RH. Milk-alkali syndrome associated with calcium carbonate consumption. Medicine 1995; 74:89–96.

458. Naftchi NE, Viaa AT, Sell GH, et al. Mineral metabolism in spinal cord injury. Arch Phys Med Rehabil 1980; 61:139–142.

459. Stewart AF, Alder M, Byers CM. Calcium homeostasis in immobilization: an example of resorptive hypercalciuria. N Engl J Med 1982; 306:1136–1140.

460. Minaire P, Meunier P, Edouard C, et al. Quantitative histological data on disuse osteoporosis: comparison with biological data. Calcif Tissue Res 1974; 17:57–73.

461. Meythaler JM, Tuel SM, Cross LL. Successful treatment of immobilization hypercalcemia using calcitonin and etidronate. Arch Phys Med Rehabil 1993; 74:316–319.

462. Llach F, Felsenfeld AJ, Haussler MR. The pathophysiology of altered calcium metabolism in rhabdomyolysis-induced acute renal failure. N Engl J Med 1981; 305:117–123.

463. Akmal M, Bishop JE, Telfer N, et al. Hypocalcemia and hypercalcemia in patients with rhabdomyolysis with and without acute renal failure. J Clin Endocrinol Metab 1986; 63:137–142.

464. Hadjis T, Grieff M, Lockhat D, et al. Calcium metabolism in acute renal failure due to rhabdomyolysis. Clin Nephrol 1993; 39:22–27.

465. Coburn JW, Salusky IB. Hyperparathyroidism in renal failure. In: Bilezikian JP, ed. The Parathyroids. New York: Raven Press, 1994: 721–745.

466. Williams JCP, Barratt-Boyes BG, Lowe JB. Supravalvular aortic stenosis. Circulation 1961; 24:1311–1318.

467. Jones KL. Williams syndrome: an historical perspective of its evolution, natural history, and etiology. Am J Med Genet 1990; 6:89–96.

468. Garabedian M, Jacqz E, Guillozo H, et al. Elevated plasma 1,25-dihydroxyvitamin D concentrations in infants with hypercalcemia and an elfin facies. N Engl J Med 1985; 312:948–952.

469. Ewart AK, Morris CA, Atkinson D, et al. Hemizygosity at the elastin locus in a developmental disorder, Williams syndrome. Nature 1993; 5:11–16.

470. Ewart AK, Jin W, Atkinson D, et al. Supravalvular aortic stenosis associated with a deletion disrupting the elastin gene. J Clin Invest 1994; 93:1071–1077.

471. Frangiskakis JM, Ewart AK, Morris CA, et al. LIM-kinase 1 hemizygosity implicated in impaired visuospacial constructive cognition. Cell 1996; 86:59–69.

472. Kruse K, Pankau R, Gosch A, et al. Calcium metabolism in Williams-Beuren syndrome. J Pediatr 1992; 121:902–907.

473. Weir E, Philbrick WM, Amling M, et al. Targeted overexpression of parathyroid hormone–related peptide in chondrocytes causes chondrodysplasia and delayed endochondral bone formation. Proc Natl Acad Sci USA 1996; 93:10240–10245.

474. Bilezikian JP. Management of acute hypercalcemia. N Engl J Med 1992; 326:1196.

475. Suki WN, Yiumm JJ, vonMinden M, et al. Acute treatment of hypercalcemia with furosemide. N Engl J Med 1970; 283:836–840.

476. Wimalawansa SJ. Optimal frequency of administration of pamidronate in patients with hypercalcemia of malignancy. Clin Endocrinol 1994; 41:591–595.

477. Hosking DJ, Gilson D. Comparison of the renal and skeletal actions of calcitonin in the treatment of severe hypercalcemia of malignancy. Q J Med 1984; 53:359–368.

478. Ralston SH, Alzaid AA, Gardner MD, et al. Treatment of cancer-associated hypercalcaemia with combined aminohydroxypropylidene diphosphonate and calcitonin. Br Med J 1986; 292:1549–1550.

479. Warrell RP, Israel R, Frisone M, et al. Gallium nitrate for acute treatment of cancer-related hypercalcemia: a randomized, double-blind comparison to calcitonin. Ann Intern Med 1988; 108:669–674.

480. Shackney S, Hasson J. Precipitous fall in serum calcium, hypotension, and acute renal failure after intravenous phosphate therapy for hypercalcemia: report of two cases. Ann Intern Med 1967; 66:906–916.

481. Doroghazi RM, Childers R. Time-related changes in the Q-T interval in acute myocardial infarction: possible relation to local hypocalcemia. Am J Cardiol 1978; 41:684–688.

482. Reddy CVR, Gould L, Gomprecht RF. Unusual electrocardiographic manifestations of hypocalcemia. Angiology 1974; 25:764–768.

483. Connor TB, Rosen BL, Blaustein MP, et al. Hypocalcemia precipitating congestive heart failure. N Engl J Med 1982; 307:869–872.

484. Tambyah PA, Ong BKC, Lee KO. Reversible parkinsonism and asymptomatic hypocalcemia with basal ganglia calcification from hypoparathyroidism 26 years after thyroid surgery. Am J Med 1993; 94:444.

485. Zaloga GP, Willey S, Tomasic P, et al. Free fatty acids alter calcium binding: a cause for misinterpretation of serum calcium values and hypocalcemia in critical illness. J Clin Endocrinol Metab 1987; 64:1010–1014.

486. Karayiorgou M, Morris MA, Morrow B, et al. Schizophrenia susceptibility associated with interstitial deletions of chromosome 22q11. Proc Natl Acad Sci USA 1995; 92:7612–7616.

487. Budarf ML, Collins J, Gong W, et al. Cloning a balanced translocation associated with DiGeorge syndrome and identification of a disrupted candidate gene. Nat Genet 1995; 10:269–278.

488. Scire G, Dallapiccola B, Iannetti P, et al. Hypoparathyroidism as the major manifestation in two patients with 22q11 deletions. Am J Med Genet 1994; 52:478–482.

489. Bockman DE, Kriby ML. Dependence of thymus development on derivatives of the neural crest. Science 1984; 223:498–500.

490. Chisaka O, Capecchi MR. Regionally restricted developmental defects resulting from targeted disruption of the mouse homeobox gene hox-1.5. Nature 1991; 350:473–479.

491. Thakker RV, Davies KE, Whyte MP, et al. Mapping the gene causing X-linked recessive idiopathic hypoparathyroidism to Xq26-Xq27 by linkage studies. J Clin Invest 1990; 86:40–45.

492. Ahn TG, Antonarakis SE, Kronenberg HM, et al. Familial isolated hypoparathyroidism: a molecular genetic analysis of 8 families with 23 affected persons. Medicine 1986; 65:73–81.

493. Baldellou A, Bone J, Tamparillas M, et al. Congenital hypoparathyroidism, ocular colobomata, unilateral renal agenesis and dysmorphic features. Genet Couns 1991; 2:245–247.

494. Dahlberg PJ, Borer WZ, Newcomer KL, et al. Autosomal or X-linked recessive syndrome of congenital lymphedema, hypoparathyroidism, nephropathy, prolapsing mitral valve, and brachytelephalangy. Am J Med Genet 1983; 16:99–104.

495. Bilous RW, Murty G, Parkinson DB, et al. Brief report: autosomal dominant familial hypoparathyroidism, sensorineural deafness, and renal dysplasia. N Engl J Med 1992; 327:1069–1074.

496. Parkinson DB, Thakker RV. A donor splice site mutation in the parathyroid hormone gene is associated with autosomal recessive hypoparathyroidism. Nat Genet 1992; 2:149–152.

497. Northcutt RC, Levinson JD, Earnest JB. Hypocalcemia resulting from infarction of a parathyroid adenoma. Ann Intern Med 1969; 70:353–356.

498. Hammes M, DeMory A, Sprague SM. Hypocalcemia in end-stage renal disease: a consequence of spontaneous parathyroid gland infarction. Am J Kidney Dis 1994; 24:519–522.

499. Burch WM, Posillico JT. Hypoparathyroidism after I-131 therapy with subsequent return of parathyroid function. J Clin Endocrinol Metab 1983; 57:398–401.

500. Gertner JM, Broadus AE, Anast CS, et al. Impaired parathyroid response to induced hypocalcemia in thalassemia major. J Pediatr 1979; 95:210–213.

501. Carpenter TO, Carnes DL, Anast CS. Hypoparathyroidism in Wilson's disease. N Engl J Med 1983; 309:873–877.

502. Suh SM, Tashjian AH, Matsuo N, et al. Pathogenesis of hypocalcemia in primary hypomagnesemia: normal end-organ responsiveness to parathyroid hormone, impaired parathyroid gland function. J Clin Invest 1973; 52:153–160.

503. Rude RK, Oldham SB, Singer FR. Functional hypoparathyroidism and parathyroid hormone end-organ resistance in human magnesium deficiency. Clin Endocrinol 1976; 5:209–224.

504. Estep H, Shaw WA, Watlington C, et al. Hypocalcemia due to hypomagnesemia and reversible parathyroid hormone unresponsiveness. J Clin Endocrinol Metab 1969; 29:842–848.

505. Krapf R, Jaeger P, Hulter HN, et al. Chronic respiratory alkalosis induces renal PTH-resistance, hyperphosphatemia and hypocalcemia in humans. Kidney Int 1992; 42:727–734.

506. Pollak MR, Brown EM, Estep HL, et al. Autosomal dominant hypocalcemia caused by a Ca^{2+}-sensing receptor gene mutation. Nat Genet 1994; 8:303–307.

507. Pearce SH, Williamson C, Kifor O, et al. A familial syndrome of hypocalcemia and hypocalciuria due to mutations in the calcium-sensing receptor. N Engl J Med 1996; 335:1115–1122.

508. Albright F, Burnett CH, Smith PH, et al. Pseudo-hypoparathyroidism: an example of "Seabright-Bantam syndrome." Endocrinology 1942; 30:922–932.

509. Mallette LE, Kirkland JL, Gagel RF, et al. Synthetic human parathyroid hormone-(1–34) for the study of pseudohypoparathyroidism. J Clin Endocrinol Metab 1988; 67:964–972.

510. Chase LR, Melson GL, Aurbach GD. Pseudohypoparathyroidism: defective excretion of 3',5'-AMP in response to parathyroid hormone. J Clin Invest 1969; 48:1832–1844.

511. Farfel Z, Brickman AS, Kaslow HR, et al. Defect of receptor-cyclase coupling protein in pseudohypoparathyroidism. N Engl J Med 1980; 303:237–242.

512. Carter A, Bardin C, Collins R, et al. Reduced expression of multiple forms of the a subunit of the stimulatory GTP-binding protein in pseudohypoparathyroidism type 1a. Proc Natl Acad Sci USA 1987; 84:7266–7269.

513. Levine MA, Ahn TG, Klupt SF, et al. Genetic deficiency of the α subunit of the guanine nucleotide-binding protein Gs as the molecular basis for Albright hereditary osteodystrophy. Proc Natl Acad Sci USA 1988; 85:617–621.

514. Patten JL, Johns DR, Valle D, et al. Mutation in the gene encoding the stimulatory G protein of adenylate cyclase in Albright's hereditary osteodystrophy. N Engl J Med 1990; 322:1412–1419.

515. Weinstein LS, Gejman PV, de Mazancourt P, et al. A heterozygous 4-bp deletion mutation in the Gsa gene (GNAS1) in a patient with Albright hereditary osteodystrophy. Genomics 1992; 13:1319–1321.

516. Farfel Z, Friedman E. Mental deficiency in pseudohypoparathyroidism Type I is associated with Ns-protein deficiency. Ann Intern Med 1986; 105:197–199.

517. Iiri T, Herzmark P, Nakamoto JM, et al. Rapid GDP release from Gsα in patients with gain and loss of endocrine function. Nature 1994; 371:164–168.

518. Levine MA, Jap TS, Mauseth RS, et al. Activity of the stimulatory guanine nucleotide-biding protein is reduced in erythrocytes from patients with pseudohypoparathyroidism and pseudopseudohypoparathyroidism: biochemical, endocrine and genetic analysis of Albright's hereditary osteodystrophy in six kindreds. J Clin Endocrinol Metab 1986; 62:497–502.

519. Davies SJ, Hughes HE. Imprinting in Albright's hereditary osteodystrophy. J Med Genet 1993; 30:101–103.

520. Wilson LC, Oude Luttikhuis ME, Clayton PT, et al. Parental origin of Gs alpha gene mutations in Albright's hereditary osteodystrophy. J Med Genet 1994; 31:835–839.

521. Barrett D, Breslau NA, Wax MB, et al. New form of pseudohypoparathyroidism with abnormal catalytic adenylate cyclase. Am J Physiol 1989; 257:E277–E283.

522. Schipani E, Weinstein LS, Bergwitz C, et al. Pseudohypoparathyroidism Type Ib is not caused by mutations in the coding exons of the human parathyroid hormone (PTH)/PTH-related peptide receptor gene. J Clin Endocrinol Metab 1995; 80:1611–1621.

523. Murray TM, Rao LG, Wong MM, et al. Pseudohypoparathyroidism with osteitis fibrosa cystica: direct demonstration of skeletal responsiveness to parathyroid hormone in cells cultured from bone. J Bone Miner Res 1993; 8:83–91.

524. Silve C, Suarez F, El Hessni A, et al. The resistance to parathyroid hormone of fibroblasts from some patients with Type Ib pseudohypoparathyroidism is reversible with dexamethasone. J Clin Endocrinol Metab 1990; 71:631–638.

525. Suarez F, Lebrun JJ, Lecossier D, et al. Expression and modulation of the parathyroid hormone (PTH)/PTH-related peptide receptor messenger ribonucleic acid in skin fibroblasts from patients with Type Ib pseudohypoparathyroidism. J Clin Endocrinol Metab 1995; 80:965–970.

526. Drezner M, Neelon FA, Lebovitz HE. Pseudohypoparathyroidism Type II: a possible defect in the reception of the cyclic AMP signal. N Engl J Med 1973; 289:1056–1060.

527. Koo BB, Schwindinger WF, Levine MA. Characterization of Albright hereditary osteodystrophy and related disorders. Acta Paediatr Sin 1995; 36:3–13.

528. Minagawa M, Yasuda T, Kobayashi Y, et al. Transient pseudohypoparathyroidism of the neonate. Eur J Endocrinol 1995; 133:151–155.

529. Silve C. Pseudohypoparathyroidism syndromes: the many faces of parathyroid hormone resistance. Eur J Endocrinol 1995; 133:145–146.

530. Kidd GS, Schaaf M, Adler RA, et al. Skeletal responsiveness in pseudohypoparathyroidism. Am J Med 1980; 68:772–781.

531. Kolb FO, Steinbach HL. Pseudohypoparathyroidism with secondary hyperparathyroidism and osteitis fibrosa. J Clin Endocrinol Metab 1962; 22:59–70.

532. Kruse K, Kracht U, Wohlfart K, et al. Biochemical markers of bone turnover, intact serum parathyroid hormone and renal calcium excretion in patients with pseudohypoparathyroidism and hypoparathyroidism before and during vitamin D treatment. Eur J Pediatr 1989; 148:535–539.

533. Frame B, Hanson CA, Frost HM, et al. Renal resistance to parathyroid hormone with osteitis fibrosa. Am J Med 1972; 52:311–321.

534. Breslau NA, Moses AM, Pak CYC. Evidence for bone remodeling but lack of calcium mobilization response to parathyroid hormone in pseudohypoparathyroidism. J Clin Endocrinol Metab 1983; 57:638–644.

535. Ish-Shalom S, Rao LG, Levine MA, et al. Normal parathyroid hormone responsiveness of bone-derived cells from a patient with pseudohypoparathyroidism. J Bone Miner Res 1996; 11:8–14.

536. Rao DS, Parfitt AM, Kleerekoper M, et al. Dissociation between the effects of endogenous parathyroid hormone on adenosine 3',5'-monophosphate generation and phosphate reabsorption in hypocalcemia due to vitamin D depletion: an acquired disorder resembling pseudohypoparathyroidism Type II. J Clin Endocrinol Metab 1985; 61:285–290.

537. Holick MF. The use and interpretation of assays for vitamin D and its metabolites. J Nutr 1990; 120:1464–1469.

538. Gloth FM, Gundberg CM, Hollis BW, et al. Vitamin D deficiency in homebound elderly persons. JAMA 1995; 274:1683–1686.

539. Chapuy MC, Arlot ME, Duboeuf F, et al. Vitmain D_3 and calcium to prevent hip fractures in elderly women. N Engl J Med 1992; 327:1637–1642.

540. Arnaud C, Maijer R, Reade T, et al. Vitamin D dependency: an inherited postnatal syndrome with secondary hyperparathyroidism. Pediatrics 1970; 46:871–880.

541. Hahn TJ, Hendin BA, Scharp CR, et al. Effect of chronic anticonvulsant therapy on serum 25-hydroxycalciferol levels in adults. N Engl J Med 1972; 287:900–904.

542. Greenwood RH, Pruntz FTG, Silver J. Osteomalacia after prolonged glutethimide administration. Br Med J 1973; 1:643–645.

543. Brodie MJ, Boobis AR, Hillyard CJ, et al. Effect of rifampicin and isoniazid on vitamin D metabolism. Clin Pharmacol Ther 1982; 32:525–530.

544. Casella SJ, Reiner BJ, Chen TC, et al. A possible genetic defect in 25-hydroxylation as a cause of rickets. J Pediatr 1994; 124:929–932.

545. Andress DL, Norris KC, Coburn JW, et al. Intravenous calcitriol in the treatment of refractory osteitis fibrosa of chronic renal failure. N Engl J Med 1989; 321:274–279.

546. Mazzaferro S, Pasquali M, Ballanti P, et al. Intravenous versus oral calcitriol therapy in renal osteodystrophy: results of a prospective, pulsed and dose-comparable study. Miner Electrolyte Metab 1994; 20:122–129.

547. Martin KJ, Ballal HS, Domoto DT, et al. Pulse oral calcitriol for the treatment of hyperparathyroidism in patients on continuous ambulatory peritoneal dialysis: preliminary observations. Am J Kidney Dis 1992; 19:540–545.

548. Liou HH, Chiang SS, Huang TP, et al. Comparative effect of oral or intravenous calcitriol on secondary hyperparathyroidism in chronic hemodialysis patients. Miner Electrolyte Metab 1994; 20:97–102.

549. Shigematsu T, Kawaguchi Y, Unemura S, et al. Suppression of secondary hyperparathyroidism in chronic dialysis patients by single oral weekly dose of 1,25-dihydroxycholecalciferol. Intern Med 1993; 32:695–701.

550. Drezner MK, Feinglos MN. Osteomalacia due to 1α,25-dihydroxycholecalciferol deficiency. J Clin Invest 1977; 60:1046–1053.

551. Delvin EE, Glorieux FH, Marie PJ, et al. Vitamin D dependency: replacement therapy with calcitriol. Pediatrics 1981; 99:26–34.

552. Scriver CR, Reade TM, DeLuca HF, et al. Serum 1,25-dihydroxyvitamin D levels in normal subjects and in patients with hereditary rickets or bone disease. N Engl J Med 1978; 299:976–979.

553. Fraser D, Kooh SW, Kind HP, et al. Pathogenesis of hereditary vitamin-D–dependent rickets: an inborn error of vitamin D metabolism involving defective conversion of 25-hydroxyvitamin D to 1α,25-dihydroxyvitamin D. N Engl J Med 1973; 289:817–822.

554. Glorieux FH. Calcitriol treatment in vitamin D–dependent and vitamin D–resistant rickets. Metabolism 1990; 39:10–12.

555. Reade TM, Scriver CR, Glorieux FH, et al. Response to crystalline 1α-hydroxyvitamin D₃ in vitamin D dependency. Pediatr Res 1975; 9:593–599.

556. Hughes M, Malloy P, Kieback D, et al. Human vitamin D receptor mutations: identification of molecular defects in hypocalcemic vitamin D–resistant rickets. Adv Exp Med Biol 1989; 255:491–503.

557. Hughes MR, Malloy PJ, O'Malley BW, et al. Genetic defects of the 1,25-dihydroxyvitamin D₃ receptor. J Recept Res 1991; 11:699–716.

558. Saijo T, Ito M, Takeda E, et al. A unique mutation in the vitamin D receptor gene in three Japanese patients with vitamin D–dependent rickets type II: utility of single-strand conformation polymorphism analysis for heterozygous carrier detection. Am J Hum Genet 1991; 49:668–673.

559. Sone T, Scott RA, Hughes MR, et al. Mutant vitamin D receptors which confer hereditary resistance to 1,25-dihydroxyvitamin D₃ in humans are transcriptionally inactive in vitro. J Biol Chem 1989; 264:20230–20234.

560. Sone T, Marx SJ, Liberman UA, et al. A unique mutation in the human vitamin D receptor chromosomal gene confers hereditary resistance to 1,25-dihydroxyvitamin D₃. Mol Endocrinol 1990; 4:623–631.

561. Yagi H, Ozono K, Miyake H, et al. A new point mutation in the deoxyribonucleic acid–binding domain of the vitamin D receptor in a kindred with hereditary 1,25-dihydroxyvitamin D–resistant rickets. J Clin Endocrinol Metab 1993; 76:509–512.

562. Ritchie HH, Hughes MR, Thompson ET, et al. An ochre mutation in the vitamin D receptor gene causes hereditary 1,25-dihydroxyvitamin D₃–resistant rickets in three families. Proc Natl Acad Sci USA 1989; 86:9783–9787.

563. Brooks MH, Bell NH, Love L, et al. Vitamin D–dependent rickets Type II: resistance of target organs to 1,25-dihydroxyvitamin D. N Engl J Med 1978; 298:996–999.

564. Fraher LJ, Karmali R, Hinde FRJ, et al. Vitamin D–dependent rickets type II: extreme end-organ resistance to 1,25-dihydroxyvitamin D₃ in a patient without alopecia. Eur J Pediatr 1986; 145:389–395.

565. Liberman UA, Halabe A, Samuel R, et al. End-organ resistance to 1,25-dihydroxycholecalciferol. Lancet 1980; 1:504–506.

566. Bell NH. Vitamin D–dependent rickets type II. Calcif Tissue Int 1980; 31:89–91.

567. Chen TL, Hirst MA, Cone CM, et al. 1,25-Dihydroxyvitamin D resistance, rickets, and alopecia: analysis of receptors and bioresponse in cultured fibroblasts from patients and parents. J Clin Endocrinol Metab 1984; 59:383–388.

568. Eil C, Liberman UA, Marx SJ. The molecular basis for resistance to 1,25-dihydroxyvitamin D: studies in cells cultured from patients with hereditary hypocalcemic 1,25(OH)₂D₃-resistant rickets. Adv Exp Med Biol 1986; 196:407–422.

569. Takeda E, Yokota I, Kawakami I, et al. Two siblings with vitamin-D–dependent rickets type II: no recurrence of rickets for 14 years after cessation of therapy. Eur J Pediatr 1989; 149:54–57.

570. Marx SJ, Liberman UA, Eil C, et al. Hereditary resistance to 1,25-dihydroxyvitamin D. Recent Prog Horm Res 1984; 40:589–615.

571. Harrison HC, Harrison HE. Inhibition of vitamin D–stimulated active transport of calcium of rat intestine by diphenylhydantoin-phenobarbital treatment. Proc Soc Exp Biol Med 1976; 153:220–224.

572. Relkin R. Hypocalcemia resulting from calcium accretion by a chondrosarcoma. Cancer 1974; 34:1834–1837.

573. Dembinski TC, Yatscoff RW, Blandford DE. Thyrotoxicosis and hungry bone syndrome: a cause of posttreatment hypocalcemia. Clin Biochem 1994; 27:69–74.

574. Jacobson MA, Gambertoglio JG, Aweeka FT, et al. Foscarnet-induced hypocalcemia and effects of foscarnet on calcium metabolism. J Clin Endocrinol Metab 1991; 72:1130–1135.

575. Aggeler PM, Perkins HA, Watkins HB. Hypocalcemia and defective hemostasis after massive blood transfusion: report of a case. Transfusion 1967; 7:35–39.

576. Greco RJ, Hartford CE, Haith LR, et al. Hydrofluoroic acid–induced hypocalcemia. J Trauma 1988; 28:1593–1596.

577. Tsang RC, Kleinman LI, Sutherland JM, et al. Hypocalcemia in infants of diabetic mothers. J Pediatr 1972; 80:384–395.

578. Tsang RC, Light IJ, Sutherland JM, et al. Possible pathogenetic factors in neonatal hypocalcemia of prematurity. J Pediatr 1973; 82:423–429.

579. Kaplan EL, Burrington JD, Klementschitsch P, et al. Primary hyperparathyroidism, pregnancy and neonatal hypocalcemia. Surgery 1984; 96:717–722.

580. Stewart AF, Longo W, Kreutter D, et al. Hypocalcemia associated with calcium-soap formation in a patient with a pancreatic fistula. N Engl J Med 1986; 315:496–498.

581. Dettelbach MA, Deftos LJ, Stewart AF. Intraperitoneal free fatty acids induce severe hypocalcemia in rats: a model for the hypocalcemia of pancreatitis. J Bone Miner Res 1990; 5:1249–1255.

582. Norberg HP, DeRoos J, Kaplan EL. Increased parathyroid hormone secretion and hypocalcemia in experimental pancreatitis: necessity for an intact thyroid gland. Surgery 1975; 77:773–779.

583. Weir GC, Lesser PB, Drop LJ, et al. The hypocalcemia of acute pancreatitis. Ann Intern Med 1975; 83:185–189.

584. Desai TK, Carlson RW, Geheb MA. Prevalence and clinical implications of hypocalcemia in acutely ill patients in a medical intensive care setting. Am J Med 1988; 84:209–214.

585. Slatopolsky E, Robson AM, Elkan I, et al. Control of phosphate excretion in uremic man. J Clin Invest 1968; 47:1865–1874.

586. Okano K, Furukawa Y, Hirotoshi M, et al. Comparative efficacy of various vitamin D metabolites in the treatment of various types of hypoparathyroidism. J Clin Endocrinol Metab 1982; 55:238–242.

587. Howard JE, Hopkins TR, Connor TB. On certain physiologic responses to intravenous injection of calcium salts into normal, hyperparathyroid and hypoparathyroid persons. J Clin Endocrinol 1953; 13:1–19.

588. Corvilain J, Abramow M. Growth and renal control of plasma phosphate. J Clin Endocrinol Metab 1972; 34:452–459.

589. Hammerman MR, Karl IE, Hruska KA. Regulation of canine renal vesicle Pi transport by growth hormone and parathyroid hormone. Biochim Biophys Acta 1980; 603:322–335.

590. Schwartz E, Wiedman E, Simon S, et al. Estrogenic antagonism of metabolic effects of administered growth hormone. J Clin Endocrinol Metab 1969; 29:1176.

591. Recker RR, Hassing GS, Lau JR, et al. The hyperphosphatemic effect of disodium ethane-1-hydroxy-1, 1-diphosphonate (EHDP): renal handling of phosphorus and the renal response to parathyroid hormone. J Lab Clin Med 1973; 81:258–260.

592. Lyles KW, Halsey DL, Friedman NE, et al. Correlations of serum concentrations of 1,25-dihydroxyvitamin D, phosphorus, and parathyroid hormone in tumoral calcinosis. J Clin Endocrinol Metab 1985; 67:88–92.

593. Lufkin EG, Kumar R, Heath H, III. Hyperphosphatemic tumoral calcinosis: effects of phosphate depletion on vitamin D metabolism, and of acute hypocalcemia on parathyroid hormone secretion and action. J Clin Endocrinol Metab 1983; 56:1319–1322.

594. Prince MG, Schaefer PC, Goldsmith RS, et al. Hyperphosphatemic tumoral calcinosis: association with elevation of serum 1,25-dihydroxycholecalciferol concentration. Ann Intern Med 1982; 96:586–591.

595. Chernow B, Rainey TG, Georges LP, et al. Iatrogenic hyperphosphatemia: a metabolic consideration in critical care medicine. Crit Care Med 1981; 9:772–774.

596. McConnell TH. Fatal hypocalcemia from phosphate absorption from laxative preparation. JAMA 1971; 216:147–148.

597. Chesney RW, Houghton PB. Tetany following phosphate enemas in chronic renal disease. Am J Dis Child 1974; 127:584–586.

598. Biberstein M, Parker BA. Enema-induced hyperphosphatemia. Am J Med 1985; 79:645–646.

599. Jimenez RAH, Larson EB. Tumoral calcinosis: an unusual complication of the laxative abuse syndrome. Am J Med Sci 1981; 282:141–147.

600. Oxnard SA, O'Bell J, Grupe WE. Severe tetany in an azotemic child related to a sodium phosphate enema. Pediatrics 1974; 53:105–106.

601. Tsokos GL, Balow JE, Spiegel RJ, et al. Renal and metabolic complications of undifferentiated and lymphoblastic lymphomas. Medicine 1981; 60:218–229.

602. Zusman J, Brown DM, Nesbit ME. Hyperphosphatemia, hyperphosphaturia and hypocalcemia in acute lymphoblastic leukemia. N Engl J Med 1973; 289:1335–1340.

603. Brereton HD, Anderson T, Johnston RE, et al. Hyperphosphatemia and hypocalcemia in Burkitt lymphoma. Arch Intern Med 1975; 135:307–309.

604. Armata J, Depowska T. Hyperphosphatemia and hypocalcemia in neoplastic disorders. N Engl J Med 1974; 290:858.

605. O'Connor LR, Klein KL, Bethune JE. Hyperphosphatemia in lactic acidosis. N Engl J Med 1977; 297:707–709.

606. Miller PD, Heinig RE, Waterhouse C. Treatment of alcoholic ketoacidosis. Arch Intern Med 1978; 138:57–72.

607. Oster JR, Perez GO, Vaamode CA. Relationship between blood pH and potassium and phosphorus during acute metabolic acidosis. Am J Physiol 1978; 235:345–351.

608. Tranquada RE, Grant WJ, Peterson CR. Lactic acidosis. Arch Intern Med 1982; 117:192–202.

609. Spencer H, Lewin I, Samachson J, et al. Changes in metabolism in obese persons during starvation. Am J Med 1966; 40:27–37.

610. Silvis SE, Paragas PU Jr. Paresthesias, weakness, seizures and hypophosphatemia in patients receiving hyperalimentation. Gastroenterology 1972; 62:513–520.

611. Eisenberg E. Effects of serum calcium level and parathyroid extracts on phosphate and calcium excretion in hypoparathyroid patients. J Clin Invest 1965; 44:942–946.

612. Amiel C, Kuntziger H, Couette S, et al. Evidence for a parathyroid hormone–independent calcium modulation of phosphate transport along the nephron. J Clin Invest 1976; 57:256–263.

613. Reid IR, Hardy DC, Murphy WA, et al. X-linked hypophosphatemia: a clinical, biochemical and histopathologic assessment of morbidity in adults. Medicine 1989; 68:336–352.

614. Hruska KA, Rifas L, Cheng SL, et al. X-linked hyposphosphatemic rickets and the murine Hyp homologue. Am J Phys 1995; 268:F357–362.

615. Ryan EA, Reiss E. Oncogenous osteomalacia: a review of the world literature of 42 cases and report of two new cases. Am J Med 1984; 77:501–512.

616. Cai Q, Hodgson SF, Kao PC, et al. Inhibition of renal phosphate transport by a tumor product in a patient with oncogenic osteomalacia. N Engl J Med 1994; 330:1645–1649.

617. Larsson L, Rebel K, Sorbo B. Severe hypophosphatemia: a hospital survey. Acta Med Scand 1983; 214:221–223.

618. Daily WH, Tonnesen AS, Allen SJ. Hypophosphatemia: incidence, etiology and prevention in the trauma patient. Crit Care Med 1990; 18:1210–1214.

619. Betro MG, Pain RW. Hypophosphatemia and hyperphosphatemia in a hospital population. Br Med J 1972; 1:273–276.

620. Fiaccadori E, Coffrini E, Ronda N, et al. Hypophosphatemia in course of chronic obstructive pulmonary disease: prevalence, mechanisms, and relationships with skeletal muscle phosphorus content. Chest 1990; 97:857–868.

621. Vanneste J, Hage J. Acute severe hypophosphatemia mimicking Wernicke's encephalopathy. Lancet 1986; 1:44.

622. Weintraub MI, Chakravorty HP. Nutrient deficiencies after intensive parenteral alimentation. N Engl J Med 1974; 291:799.

623. Silvis SE, DiBartolomeo AG, Aaker HM. Hypophosphatemia and neurological changes secondary to oral caloric intake. Am J Gastroenterol 1980; 73:215–222.

624. Furlan AJ, Hanson M, Cooperman A, et al. Acute areflexic paralysis: association with hyperalimentation and hypophosphatemia. Arch Neurol 1975; 32:706–707.

625. Singhal PC, Kumar A, Desroches L, et al. Prevalence and predictors of rhabdomyolysis in patients with hypophosphatemia. Am J Med 1992; 92:458–464.

626. Gabow PA, Kaehny WD, Kelleher SP. The spectrum of rhabdomyolysis. Medicine 1982; 61:141–152.

627. Knochel JR, Bilbrey GL, Fuller TJ, et al. The muscle cell in chronic alcoholism: the possible role of phosphate depletion in alcoholic myopathy. Ann NY Acad Sci 1975; 252:274–286.

628. Agusti AG, Torres A, Estopa R, et al. Hypophosphatemia as a cause of failed weaning: the importance of metabolic factors. Crit Care Med 1984; 12:142–143.

629. Aubier M, Murciano D, Lecocguic Y, et al. Effect of hypophosphatemia on diaphragmatic contractility in patients with acute respiratory failure. N Engl J Med 1985; 3131:420–424.

630. Newman JH, Neff TA, Ziporin P. Acute respiratory failure associated with hypophosphatemia. N Engl J Med 1977; 296:1101–1103.

631. Davis SV, Olichwier KK, Chakko SC. Reversible depression of myocardial performance in hypophosphatemia. Am J Med Sci 1988; 295:183–187.

632. Bollaert PE, Levy B, Nace L, et al. Hemodynamic and metabolic effects of rapid correction of hypophosphatemia in patients with septic shock. Chest 1995; 107:1698–1701.

633. Rasmussen A, Buus S, Hessov I. Postoperative myocardial performance during glucose-induced hypophosphatemia. Acta Chir Scand 1985; 151:13–15.

634. Vered Z, Battler A, Motro M, et al. Left ventricular function in patients with chronic hypophosphatemia. Am Heart J 1984; 107:796–798.

635. Lichtman MA, Miller DR, Cohen J, et al. Reduced red cell glycolysis, 2,3-diphosphoglycerate and adenosine triphosphate concentration and increased hemoglobin oxygen affinity caused by hypophosphatemia. Ann Intern Med 1971; 74:562–568.

636. Craddock PR, Yawata Y, VanSanten L, et al. Acquired phagocyte dysfunction: a complication of the hypophosphatemia of parenteral hyperalimentation. N Engl J Med 1974; 290:1403–1407.

637. Yawata Y, Hebbel RP, Silvis S, et al. Blood cell abnormalities complicating the hypophosphatemia of hyperalimentation: erythrocyte and platelet ATP deficiency associated with hemolytic anemia and bleeding in hyperalimented dogs. J Lab Clin Med 1974; 84:643–653.

638. Travis SF, Sugerman HJ. Alterations in red-cell glycolytic intermediates and oxygen transport as a consequence of hypophosphatemia in patients receiving intravenous hyperalimentation. N Engl J Med 1971; 285:763–768.

639. DeFronzo RA, Lang R. Hypophosphatemia and glucose intolerance: evidence for tissue insensitivity to insulin. N Engl J Med 1980; 303:1259–1263.

640. Franks M, Berris RF, Kaplan NO, et al. Metabolic studies in diabetic acidosis. II. The effect of the administration of sodium phosphate. Arch Intern Med 1948; 81:42–55.

641. Wilson HK, Keuer SP, Lea AS, et al. Phosphate therapy in diabetic ketoacidosis. Arch Intern Med 1982; 142:517–520.

642. Keller U, Berger W. Prevention of hypophosphatemia by phosphate infusion during treatment of diabetic ketoacidosis and hyperosmolar coma. Diabetes 1980; 29:87–95.

643. Rosen GH, Boullata JI, O'Rangers EA, et al. Intravenous phosphate repletion regimen for critically ill patients with moderate hypophosphatemia. Crit Care Med 1995; 23:1204–1210.

644. Clark CL, Sacks GS, Dickerson RN, et al. Treatment of hypophosphatemia in patients receiving specialized nutrition support using a graduated dosing scheme: results from a prospective clinical trial. Crit Care Med 1995; 23:1504–1511.

645. Kingston M, Al-Siba'i MB. Treatment of severe hypophosphatemia. Crit Care Med 1985; 13:16–18.

646. Reinhart RA, Desbiens NA. Hypomagnesemia in patients entering the ICU. Crit Care Med 1985; 13:506–507.

647. Broner CW, Stidham GL, Westenkirchner DF, et al. Hypermagnesemia and hypocalcemia as predictors of high mortality in critically ill pediatric patients. Crit Care Med 1990; 18:921–928.

648. Mordes JP, Wacker WE. Excess magnesium. Pharmacol Rev 1978; 29:273–300.

649. Alfrey AC, Terman DS, Brettschneider L, et al. Hypermagnesemia after renal homotransplantation. Ann Intern Med 1970; 73:367–371.

650. Cruikshank DP, Pitkin RM, Reynolds WA, et al. Effects of magnesium sulfate treatment on perinatal calcium metabolism. I. Maternal and fetal responses. Am J Obstet Gynecol 1979; 134:243–249.

651. Green KW, Key TC, Coen R, et al. The effects of maternally administered magnesium sulfate on the neonate. Am J Obstet Gynecol 1983; 146:29–33.

652. Rasch DK, Huber PA, Richardson CJ, et al. Neurobehavioral effects of neonatal hypermagnesemia. J Pediatr 1982; 100:272–276.

653. Donovan EF, Tsang RC, Steichen JJ, et al. Neonatal hypermagnesemia: effect on parathyroid hormone and calcium homeostasis. J Pediatr 1980; 96:305–310.

654. Brand JM, Greer FR. Hypermagnesemia and intestinal perforation following antacid administration in a premature infant [see comments]. Pediatrics 1990; 85:121–124.

655. Zwanger ML. Hypermagnesemia and perforated viscus. Ann Emerg Med 1986; 15:1219–1220.

656. Engbaek L. The pharmacological actions of magnesium ions with particular reference to the neuromuscular and the cardiovascular system. Pharmacol Rev 1952; 4:396–414.

657. Randall RE, Cohen MD, Spray CC, et al. Hypermagnesemia and renal failure: etiology and toxic manifestations. Ann Intern Med 1964; 61:73–88.

658. Mordes JP, Swartz R, Arky RA. Extreme hypermagnesemia as a cause of refractory hypotension. Ann Intern Med 1975; 83:657–658.

659. Ferdinandus J, Pederson JA, Whang R. Hypermagnesemia as a cause of refractory hypotension, respiratory depression, and coma. Arch Intern Med 1981; 141:669–670.

660. Suzuki K, Nonaka K, Kono N, et al. Effects of the intravenous administration of magnesium sulfate on corrected serum calcium level and nephrogenous cyclic AMP excretion in normal human subjects. Calcif Tissue Int 1986; 39:304–309.

661. Cholst IN, Steinberg SF, Tropper PJ, et al. The influence of hypermagnesemia on serum calcium and parathyroid hormone levels in human subjects. N Engl J Med 1984; 310:1221–1225.

662. Carney SL, Wong NLM, Quamme GA, et al. Effect of magnesium deficiency on renal magnesium and calcium transport in the rat. J Clin Invest 1980; 65:180–188.

663. Cruikshank DP, Pitkin RM, Donnelly E, et al. Urinary magnesium, calcium, and phosphate excretion during the magnesium sulfate infusion. Obstet Gynecol 1981; 58:430–434.

664. Buckle RM, Care AD, Cooper CW, et al. The influence of plasma magnesium concentration on parathyroid hormone secretion. J Endocrinol 1968; 42:529–534.

665. Fassler CA, Rodriguez RM, Badesch DB, et al. Magnesium toxicity as a cause of hypotension and hypoventilation: occurrence in patients with normal renal function. Arch Intern Med 1985; 145:1604–1606.

666. Alfrey AC, Miller NL, Butkus D. Evaluation of body magnesium stores. J Lab Clin Med 1974; 84:153–162.

667. Lim P, Jacob E. Magnesium status of alcoholic patients. Metabolism 1972; 21:1045–1051.

668. Ryzen E, Elbaum N, Singer FR, et al. Parenteral magnesium tolerance testing in the evaluation of magnesium deficiency. Magnesium 1985; 4:137–147.

669. Al-Ghamdi SMG, Cameron EC, Sutton RAL. Magnesium deficiency: pathophysiologic and clinical overview. Am J Kidney Dis 1994; 24:737–752 (review).

670. Barnes BA. Magnesium conservation: a study of surgical patients. Ann NY Acad Sci 1969; 162:786–801.

671. Goldman AS, Van Fossan DD, Baird EE. Magnesium deficiency in celiac disease. Pediatrics 1962; 29:948–952.

672. Booth CC, Hanna S, Babouris N, et al. Incidence of hypomagnesaemia in intestinal malabsorption. Br Med J 1963; 2:141–144.

673. Heaton FW, Fourman P. Magnesium deficiency and hypocalcaemia in intestinal malabsorption. Lancet 1965; 2:50–52.

674. Rude RK, Singer FR. Magnesium deficiency and excess. Annu Rev Med 1981; 32:245–259.

675. Milla PJ, Aggett PJ, Wolff OH, et al. Studies in primary hypomagnesemia: evidence for defective carrier-mediated small intestinal transport of magnesium. Gut 1979; 20:1028–1033.

676. Pronicka E, Gruszczynska B. Familial hypomagnesemia with secondary hypocalcemia: autosomal or X-linked inheritance? J Inherit Metab Dis 1991; 14:397–399.

677. Bettinelli A, Bianchetti MG, Borella P, et al. Genetic heterogeneity in

25

METABOLIC BONE DISEASE

Lawrence G. Raisz, Barbara E. Kream, and Joseph A. Lorenzo

STRUCTURE AND FUNCTION OF THE SKELETON

The skeleton is one of the largest organ systems in the body. It consists of a large mineralized matrix and a small but highly active cellular fraction. The skeleton serves the dual functions of maintaining the structure of the body and providing a storehouse of minerals and protein. Imbalance between the structural and the storage functions of the skeleton can be important in the pathogenesis of metabolic bone disease.[1]

Embryology and Anatomy

In the embryo, skeletal development begins with the condensation of mesenchyme into cartilage. The cartilage template is then converted into bone through one of two distinct pathways.[2] The growth of long bones and the vertebrae involves *endochondral bone formation* (Fig. 25–1). The cartilage growth plate cells proliferate and then undergo hypertrophy; this is followed by partial degradation of the matrix, which then mineralizes. The cartilage is invaded by vessels, and the spicules of mineralized cartilage are covered by osteoblasts to

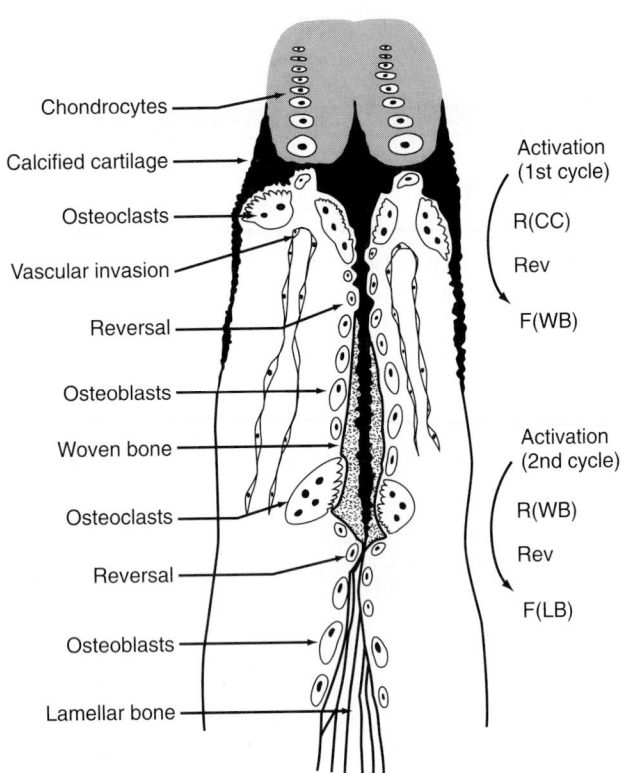

Figure 25–1. The steps in endochondral bone formation. R, resorption; Rev, reversal; F, formation; CC, calcified cartilage; WB, woven bone; LB, lamellar bone. (Redrawn from Baron R. Anatomy and ultrastructure of bone. In: Favus MJ, ed. Primer on the Metabolic Bone Diseases and Disorders of Mineral Metabolism. 2nd ed. New York: Lippincott-Raven, 1993: 3–9. Copyright 1993, American Society for Bone and Mineral Research.)

form a cancellous or trabecular bone mass called the primary spongiosa. These structures are then resorbed and replaced by trabecular plates made up entirely of bone, termed the secondary spongiosa. This bone undergoes rapid remodeling. In the adult, it is most abundant at the ends of the long bones and in the bodies of the vertebrae.

Intramembranous bone formation occurs typically in flat bones, such as the skull, scapula, and ileum, and on the outer surfaces of long bones. Initially, relatively disorganized woven bone is formed, but this rapidly converts to more organized lamellar bone produced by oriented layers of osteoblasts. The main difference between endochondral and intramembranous bone formation is that the latter does not use calcified cartilage as a direct template for osteoblasts.

Cortical bone is the dense bone that is found, for example, in the shafts of long bones. It makes up 80% of the mass of the skeleton, determines its shape, and provides much of its strength. Modeling of cortical bone involves not only new bone formation but also resorption to alter skeletal shape (see Fig. 25–1). The wide cortex at the epiphyseal plate of long bones must be resorbed, because these bones elongate to maintain the narrow tubular structure of the diaphysis. Although remodeling begins early in cancellous bone, remodeling of cortical bone begins only after the cortex reaches a critical thickness. In smaller animals such as rodents, cortical bone can remain lamellar. In large animals and humans, lamellar cortical bone is gradually replaced through haversian remodeling to form cylindrical osteons.

Chemistry of Matrix and Mineral

Bone matrix consists of fibers of type I collagen laid down in layers that have various orientations, which may add to the strength of the matrix. The matrix contains many additional proteins, including small amounts of other collagen types on the fibrillar surface that may be important in the interaction of type I collagen with noncollagen proteins.[3] The noncollagen proteins represent about 10% of the total protein in bone and may serve to direct the formation of fibers, enhance mineralization, strengthen the attachment between cells and matrix, and provide signals for bone remodeling (Table 25–1). These proteins range from the large cell-attachment proteins, such as thrombospondin and fibronectin, with molecular weights higher than 400 kd, to the small, vitamin K–dependent gamma-carboxylated proteins, matrix Gla protein and osteocalcin, which are 6-kd calcium-binding proteins. Osteocalcin may regulate both mineralization and resorption of bone. A number of the noncollagen proteins, such as biglycan, decorin, bone sialoprotein, and osteopontin, are highly acidic. In addition to cell-attachment sequences, these proteins contain varying amounts of carbohydrate and may be termed glycoproteins or proteoglycans. Noncollagen proteins of bone are often highly phosphorylated, which enables them to bind calcium, and may regulate mineralization. The matrix is also a storehouse for growth factors and their binding proteins (see later discussion).

COLLAGEN SYNTHESIS. Type I collagen, a rigid, rod-like, insoluble molecule composed of two $\alpha1$ and one $\alpha2$ chains, consists of repeating triplets of amino acids with glycine in every third position and a high content of proline and lysine (Fig. 25–2). These chains form a triple helix that is stabilized by the hydroxylation of proline and lysine residues, which requires ascorbic acid. Collagen is initially synthesized as a soluble propeptide with large nonhelical extensions at both the COOH and NH_2 termini. Procollagen also contains COOH-terminal interchain disulfide bonds that help initiate triple helix formation. Procollagen is released into the cisternae of the rough endoplasmic reticulum, packaged in the Golgi vesicles, and secreted extracellularly. The procollagen peptides are then removed by specific peptidases to produce mature insoluble collagen molecules, which are further stabilized by intramolecular and intermolecular cross-links. The major cross-links are formed by lysine and hydroxylysine residues that ultimately form pyridinium ring structures (see later discussion).

MINERALIZATION. Bone mineral is made up of small, imperfect hydroxyapatite crystals, which contain carbonate, magnesium, sodium, and potassium. When bone forms in the presence of fluoride ions, the fluorapatite crystal is larger and less soluble than hydroxyapatite and may increase bone fragility.[4]

Mineralization occurs by two distinct mechanisms. The initial mineralization of calcified cartilage and woven bone probably occurs by means of matrix vesicles.[5] These membrane-bound bodies are released from chondrocytes and osteoblasts, contain alkaline phosphatase, and can form a nidus

TABLE 25–1. Principal Noncollagen Proteins of the Bone Matrix

Name	Approximate Size (kd)	Potential Function
Thrombospondin	450 (trimer)	Cell attachment
Fibronectin	440 (dimer)	Cell attachment, spreading
Biglycan (proteoglycan I)	170 (monomer)	Unknown
Decorin (proteoglycan II)	120 (monomer)	Collagen fibrillogenesis
Bone sialoprotein	75 (monomer)	Cell attachment
Osteopontin	50 (monomer)	Cell attachment, spreading
Osteonectin	35 (monomer)	Ca^{2+}, mineral binding
Matrix gla protein	9 (monomer)	Ca^{2+} binding
Osteocalcin	6 (monomer)	Ca^{2+} binding

Adapted from Termine JD. Bone matrix proteins and the mineralization process. In: Primer on the Metabolic Bone Diseases. Favus MJ, ed. New York: Lippincott-Raven, 1993: 21–25. Copyright 1993, American Society for Bone and Mineral Research.

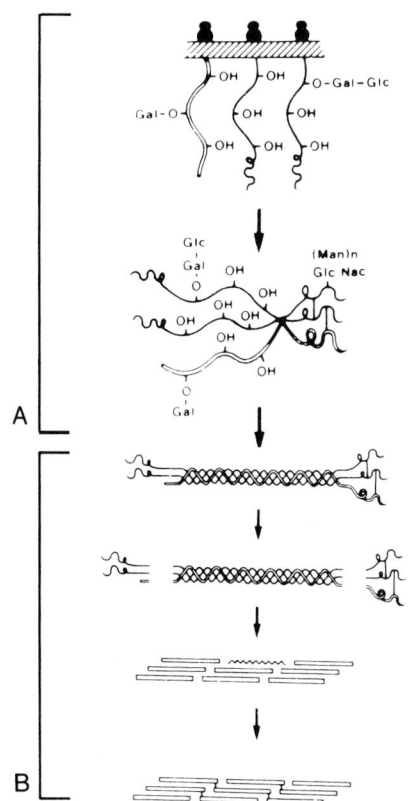

Figure 25–2. Synthesis and assembly of collagen fibrils. *A,* Intracellular post-translational modifications of pro alpha chains, association of propeptide domains, and folding into triple-helical conformation. Gal, galactose; Glc, glucose; Glc Nac, *N*-acetylglucosamine; (Man)n, mannose. *B,* Enzymatic cleavage of procollagen to collagen, self-assembly of collagen monomers into fibrils, and cross-linking of fibrils. (Modified from Prockop DJ, Kivirikko K. Heritable diseases of collagen. Reprinted with permission from The New England Journal of Medicine, 1984; 311:376–386.)

for crystallization. In lamellar bone, the collagen fibers are tightly packed, and matrix vesicles are rarely seen. Mineralization does not occur immediately after collagen deposition, and there is a layer of 10 to 100 μm of unmineralized osteoid between the mineralization front and the osteoblast. Presumably, changes in the packing of the fibrils and in the composition of the noncollagen proteins are required for mineralization. Mineralization of collagen fibrils begins in the "hole zones," where there is more room for inorganic ions to accumulate (Fig. 25–3). Mineralization requires calcium, phosphate, and alkaline phosphatase. This process is impaired in vitamin D deficiency and hypophosphatasia.

Osteoblast Differentiation and Function

Bone is formed by osteoblasts,[6] which are highly differentiated cells that have many unique features (Fig. 25–4). They are initially derived from mesenchymal stem cells, which were termed "inducible" osteoprogenitors by Friedenstein.[7] Adult bone also contains less pluripotent bone cell precursors, termed "committed" osteoprogenitors.

Osteoprogenitor cells (or preosteoblasts) replicate and differentiate into active osteoblasts that may not all have the same phenotypic characteristics. For example, osteoblasts in early development and during repair produce woven bone, whereas more mature osteoblasts produce lamellar bone. The distribution of noncollagen proteins in cortical and trabecular bone may also be different. The activity of osteoblasts can vary during bone formation. Some cells are tall and closely packed

and produce a large amount of matrix in a small area; others are flatter and produce matrix at a slower rate over a larger area. Nevertheless, all differentiated osteoblasts share certain features. They are connected by gap junctions and contain a dense network of rough endoplasmic reticulum and a large Golgi complex. They secrete collagen and noncollagen proteins in an oriented fashion and produce more type I collagen and alkaline phosphatase than other mesenchymal cells. Some products, such as osteocalcin, are produced almost uniquely by osteoblasts; others, such as osteopontin, are produced by a limited number of cell types. Mature osteoblasts have a finite capacity to produce matrix, and bone formation is sustained by the arrival of new populations of cells at the bone surface. After osteoblasts have completed their matrix formation, they may become embedded in the matrix as osteocytes, undergo apoptotic cell death, or be converted to flattened lining cells, which cover a large percentage of the surface of bone with a thin cytoplasmic layer.

The conversion of osteoblasts to osteocytes involves a reduction but not a complete loss of metabolic activity.[8] A critical feature is the development of an extensive network of cytoplasmic connections. The osteoblasts have multiple cell processes that are connected to underlying osteocytes through small canaliculi. After mineralization is complete, the processes persist as connections between osteocytes (Fig. 25–5). This extended syncytium is probably important in maintaining

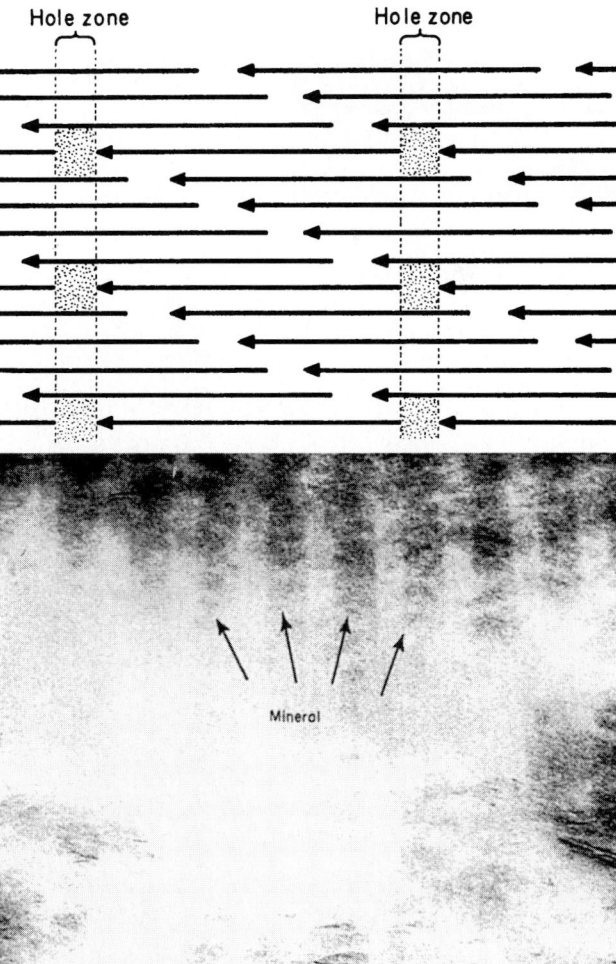

Figure 25–3. The staggered arrangement of individual molecules in collagen fibers results in hole zones between the head of one molecule and the tail of the next. Mineral deposition *(bottom)* begins within the hole zones. (From Glimcher MJ, Krane SM. Treatise on Collagen 2: Part B. New York: Academic, 1968: 67–251.)

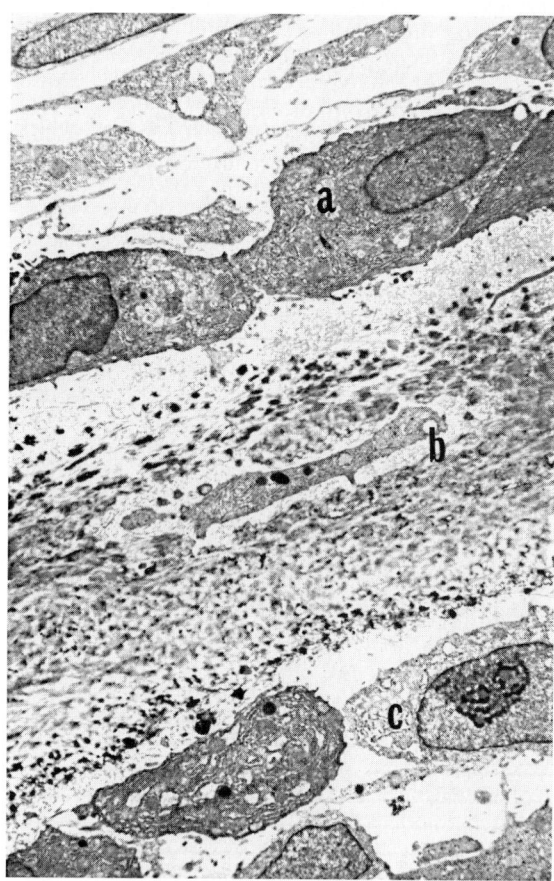

Figure 25–4. Electron micrograph of rat calvarial bone showing (a) mature osteoblasts with their dense, rough endoplasmic reticulum and large Golgi apparatus, (b) an osteocyte embedded in the bone, and (c) a less differentiated cell which may represent a preosteoblast. (Courtesy of Dr. Marijke E. Holtrop.)

Figure 25–5. *A*, Cross-section of an osteon. *B*, Cultured cells from avian bone, showing osteocytes and their cytoplasmic connections. (From Aarden EM, et al. Function of osteocytes and bone. J Cell Biochem 1994; 55:287–299. Reprinted by permission of Wiley-Liss, Inc., a subsidiary of John Wiley & Sons, Inc.)

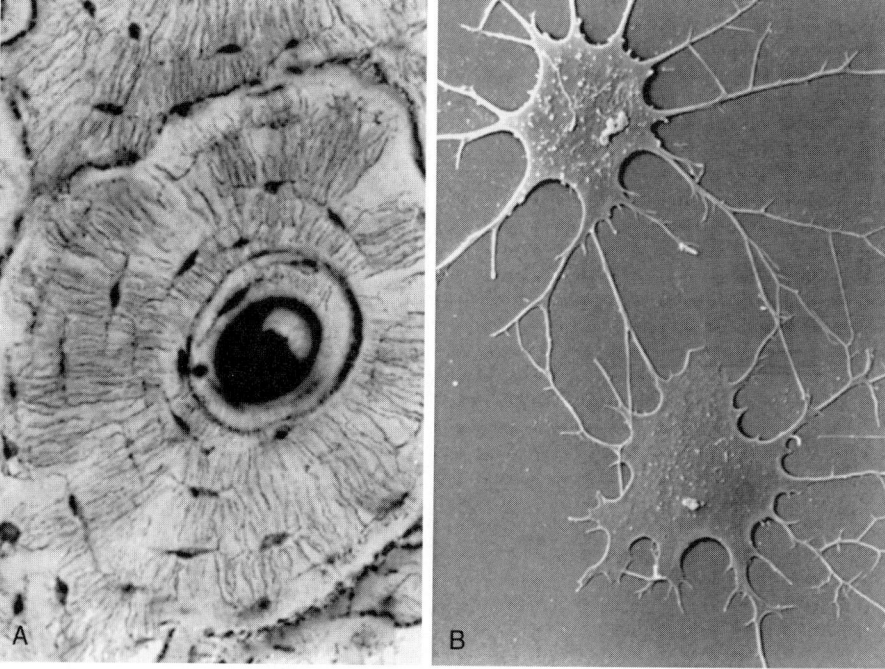

the viability of the osteocytes, which otherwise would be separated from the extracellular fluid. Initially, osteocytes may continue to synthesize collagen and play a role in mineralization. Later, the major role of the osteocyte-osteoblast syncytium may be to sense mechanical forces.[9] One hypothesis is that small strains produce fluid shear stress in the canaliculi between osteocytes. This could result in intracellular signaling through changes in ion channels or the production of biologically active molecules (e.g., prostaglandins) from the phospholipid membrane.

Cells of the osteoblastic lineage are important not only in forming bone but also in initiating resorption.[10] It is still not clear which cells of the osteoblast lineage activate resorption or how they interact with the hematopoietic cells that form osteoclasts. Nevertheless, all of the factors that stimulate bone resorption act on osteoblasts. Osteoblasts also produce local factors that can influence resorption, including cytokines, prostaglandins, and growth factors. In cell culture, contact between osteoblastic cells and hematopoietic cells appears to be necessary for osteoclast formation (see Fig. 25–6). Osteoblasts may also play a role in initiating bone resorption by releasing enzymes that prepare the bone surface. Hormones and local factors that stimulate bone resorption increase the production of collagenase, other metalloproteinases, and plasminogen activator by osteoblasts. These enzymes may remove the surface proteins of bone, which block the access of osteoclasts to the mineralized matrix. Osteoblasts may also influence the development and maintenance of the marrow, because they are sources of growth factors and cytokines that could act on hematopoietic cells.

Osteoclast Differentiation and Function

Although osteoclasts are derived from hematopoietic progenitors, their relation to other hematopoietic lineages is not fully defined. Hematopoietic stem cells under the direction of granulocyte-macrophage colony-stimulating factor (GM-CSF) and colony-stimulating factor-1 (macrophage colony-stimulating factor, M-CSF) may differentiate into either monocyte-macrophages or preosteoclasts.[11] The latter fuse to form highly differentiated multinucleated osteoclasts that resorb bone (Fig. 25–6). Progression through the osteoclast pathway probably involves multiple local and systemic hormones that may include 1,25-dihydroxyvitamin D [1,25-(OH)$_2$D], prostaglandins, and the cytokines interleukin-1 (IL-1), IL-6, and tumor necrosis factor (TNF). A specific osteoclast trophic factor may be produced by osteoblasts, but it has not yet been identified.

The formation of multinucleated osteoclast-like cells in vitro requires both hematopoietic precursors and cells of the osteoblastic lineage. In vivo or in cultures with devitalized bone, mononuclear preosteoclasts attach to the bone surface and form multinucleated osteoclasts by fusion. The accumulation of additional nuclei into osteoclasts by fusion probably continues while the cell is actively resorbing. The life span of the osteoclast is limited. As osteoclasts become inactive, the nuclei become apoptotic. Hormones that enhance bone resorption may delay apoptosis, and inhibitors of resorption can accelerate it. The mechanisms that limit the extent of osteoclastic resorption are incompletely understood and may involve inhibition by calcium ions, which accumulate under the osteoclast resorbing surface, or by local inhibitory factors (e.g., transforming growth factor β [TGF β]), which are released and activated during resorption.

The mature osteoclast is a unique and highly specialized cell (Fig. 25–7). It usually contains 10 to 20 nuclei, but giant osteoclasts with up to 100 nuclei can be seen in Paget's disease or giant cell tumors of bone. The large size of osteoclasts is probably essential for their resorptive function, which depends on their ability to isolate a region of the bone surface from the extracellular fluid and produce a local environment that can dissolve bone mineral and degrade matrix. The resorbing apparatus consists of a central ruffled border area, which secretes hydrogen ions and proteolytic enzymes, surrounded by a clear or sealing zone that anchors the cell to the bone surface by a ring of contractile proteins linked to integrin receptors. The osteoclast may secrete adhesion proteins, such as osteopontin and bone sialoprotein, that anchor the cell to bone by binding both to mineral and to cell-surface integrins.

Acidification of the ruffled border area requires that osteoclasts have proton pumps. These pumps are similar to the vacuolar proton pumps that acidify intracellular organelles, but in the osteoclast they are exteriorized to increase extracellular hydrogen ion concentration.[12] The hydrogen ions dissociate from carbonic acid, which is synthesized by carbonic anhydrase; the bicarbonate generated by this dissociation is removed from the cell by chloride-bicarbonate exchange. Ion pumps can transport the dissolved calcium from the bone surface through the cell to the extracellular fluid. However,

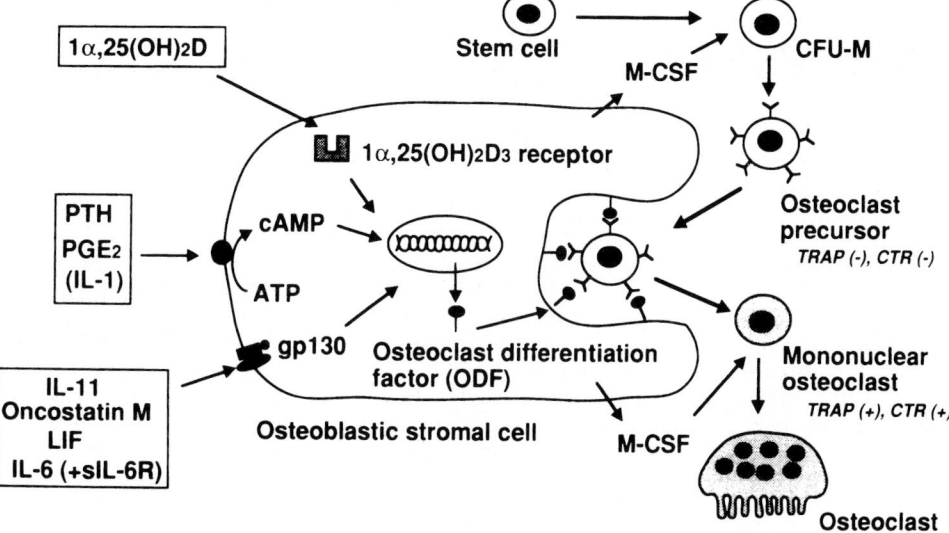

Figure 25–6. Possible regulation of osteoclast differentiation by factors acting on stromal cells. (From Suda P, et al. Modulation of osteoclast differentiation: Update 1995. Endocr Rev 1995; 4:266–270. Copyright © 1995, by The Endocrine Society.)

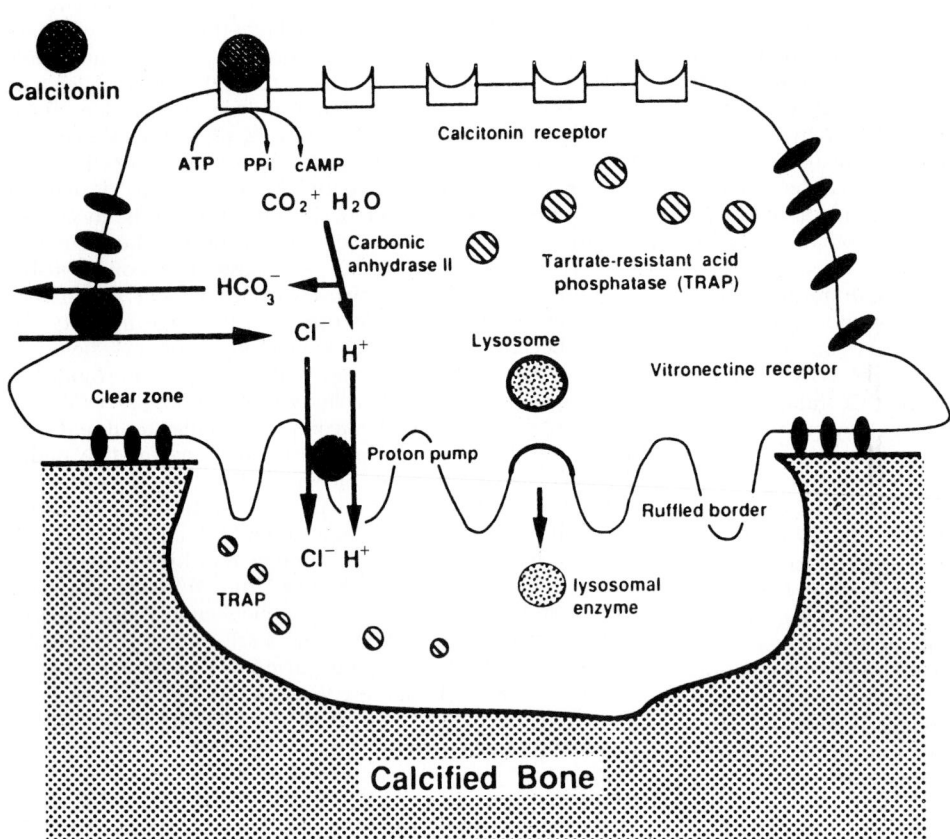

Figure 25–7. Functional elements of the fully differentiated osteoclast. (From Suda T, et al. Modulation of osteoclast differentiation. Endocr Rev 1992; 13:66–80. Copyright © 1992, by The Endocrine Society.)

calcium can also reach the extracellular fluid directly if the sealing zone is disrupted. The proteolytic enzymes produced by the osteoclast include lysosomal enzymes and metalloproteinases. Lysosomal proteases can degrade collagen at the low pH present in the ruffled border area; metalloproteinases, which are active at neutral pH, have also been detected at the resorption site.[13] In trabecular bone, osteoclasts characteristically resorb to a limited depth and then move laterally to produce irregular, plate-like resorption areas that are termed Howship lacunae. In cortical remodeling, the path of directed resorption is longer, possibly because of renewal of osteoclasts from hematopoietic cells brought to the site through the haversian canal.

BONE REMODELING AND ITS REGULATION[14, 15]

After peak bone mass has been achieved, the cellular activity in the skeleton is largely devoted to an orderly sequence of bone resorption and formation termed *remodeling.* This process produces plate-like structures on trabecular surfaces and cylindrical structures (osteons) in cortical bone that are termed *basic multicellular* or *basic structural units.* The remodeling cycle can be divided into four steps: activation, resorption, reversal, and formation (Figs. 25–8 and 25–9). Similar sequences are seen in trabecular and cortical remodeling. In young adults, this cycle is tightly coupled, and the amount of new bone formed by osteoblasts is equal to the amount that is resorbed by osteoclasts. Postmenopausal and age-related bone loss begins when resorption increases and formation no longer keeps pace. The activation of new remodeling sites may also increase with age. Although 80% of skele-

tal mass is cortical bone, the surface area of cortical bone is only about one fifth that of cancellous bone. Moreover, more osteoclast precursor cells are available in cancellous bone and on the endosteal surfaces of cortical bone. Turnover is greater on these surfaces than on periosteal bone, which normally undergoes little remodeling. However, subperiosteal resorption can be activated in hyperparathyroidism, and the periosteal surface contains preosteoblasts that may become active late in life and cause an age-related increase in the periosteal diameter of long bones. This periosteal expansion may maintain bone strength and compensate for losses at the endosteal surfaces and in cancellous bone.

Remodeling can be activated by both systemic and local factors and probably serves several physiological functions. Changes in mechanical force can activate remodeling to improve the skeletal strength. Remodeling may serve to repair microdamage, particularly in cortical bone, and this could explain the fact that remodeling is sustained in the aging skeleton.[16] Systemic hormones influence bone remodeling to regulate the movement of mineral from bone to extracellular fluid and as part of their overall effects on growth. Local factors mediate the response to mechanical forces and may also modulate the effects of systemic hormones.

Calcium-Regulating Hormones

PARATHYROID HORMONE. Parathyroid hormone (PTH) acts on bone to stimulate resorption.[17] PTH does not act on osteoclasts in the absence of cells of the osteoblastic lineage; moreover, PTH receptors are abundant on osteoblasts, but not on osteoclasts. PTH acts on osteoblasts to cause cell contraction; to induce immediate-early response genes, including c-*fos* and the inducible form of prostaglandin G/H synthase (cyclooxygenase); and to increase the synthesis of

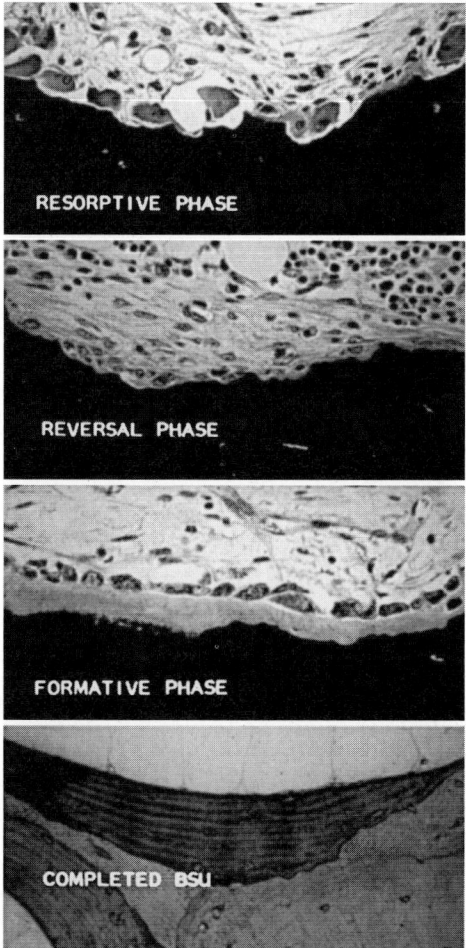

Figure 25–8. Stages of bone remodeling. This figure illustrates the resorptive, reversal, and formative phases of bone remodeling and a completed bone structural unit (BSU) on a trabecular surface. The morphologic features of the activation step have not been defined. (Courtesy of Dr. Robert E. Schenk, University of Berne, Switzerland.)

local mediators, including insulin-like growth factor I (IGF-I) and IL-6.[18] High concentrations of PTH in vitro inhibit expression of type I collagen, but intermittent administration of PTH can stimulate bone formation. High amounts of PTH increase bone turnover, which is low in hypoparathyroidism.

VITAMIN D. The hormonal form of vitamin D, 1,25-$(OH)_2D$, is necessary for intestinal calcium and phosphorus absorption and therefore for mineralization. 1,25-$(OH)_2D$ also has effects on the skeleton,[19] but its physiological role in bone remodeling is not clear. It is a potent stimulator of osteoclast growth in cell culture,[10] and high concentrations increase osteocalcin synthesis by osteoblasts and inhibit collagen synthesis. Lower concentrations may increase bone formation but not to the extent seen with intermittent administration of PTH.

CALCITONIN. Calcitonin inhibits bone resorption by acting directly on the osteoclast[20] but appears to play a small role in the regulation of bone turnover in adults. Bone mass is not greatly altered in patients with medullary thyroid carcinoma (MTC), who have an excess of calcitonin production, or in athyreotic patients on adequate thyroid hormone replacement, who have low calcitonin levels.[21] In fact, bone turnover is increased in MTC patients.[22] Nevertheless, subtle alterations in calcitonin production or response may play a role in metabolic bone disease.

Other Systemic Hormones

GROWTH HORMONE. Deficiency and excess of growth hormone have marked effects on skeletal growth.[23] Growth hormone increases both circulating and local levels of IGF-I, which mediates the skeletal effects of growth hormone. Both exogenous growth hormone and IGF-I increase bone remodeling. Growth hormone also stimulates cartilage growth, probably through an increase in local IGF production and direct stimulation of cartilage cell proliferation. Whether systemic IGF plays a role in skeletal growth is not known, but low levels of growth hormone receptors are present in bone cells, and administration of IGF-I together with its major binding protein, IGFBP-3, can increase skeletal growth.

GLUCOCORTICOIDS. Glucocorticoids exert biphasic effects on bone formation and resorption.[24] In vivo, glucocorticoids may increase bone resorption indirectly by diminishing calcium absorption and producing secondary hyperparathyroidism. Low levels of glucocorticoids increase osteoclastic activity in organ culture, whereas high levels inhibit it, perhaps by decreasing the production of cytokines and prostaglandins. Glucocorticoids enhance differentiation of osteoblast precursors in cell culture and cause a transient increase in collagen synthesis in bones in organ culture, possibly as a result of increased sensitivity to endogenous IGF-I. However, glucocorticoids act in the long term in vitro and in vivo to inhibit bone formation, decrease osteoblast replication and differentiation, and decrease IGF-I synthesis.

THYROID HORMONES.[25] In children, hyperthyroidism is associated with increased skeletal growth, and hypothyroidism results in decreased growth. Thyroid hormones are critical for cartilage growth and differentiation, enhance the response to growth hormone, and stimulate bone resorption. However, their effects on bone formation are less clear. Increased resorption as a result of hyperthyroidism could result in a coupled increase in bone formation, but thyroid hormone may also directly stimulate bone cell replication.

INSULIN.[26] Normal skeletal growth depends on an adequate amount of insulin. Excess insulin production by the fetuses of mothers with uncontrolled diabetes results in excessive growth of the skeleton and other tissues, and undertreated diabetes mellitus impairs skeletal growth and mineralization. In vitro, insulin at physiological concentrations selectively stimulates osteoblastic collagen synthesis by a pretranslational mechanism. Insulin can mimic the effects of IGF-I but only at supraphysiological levels. Insulin does not appear to affect bone resorption.

GONADAL HORMONES. Both estrogens and androgens are critical for skeletal development and maintenance. Bone cells contain estrogen and androgen receptors, but it is difficult to demonstrate direct effects of gonadal steroids on bone formation or resorption in cell and organ culture.[27] Gonadal hormones are critical for the pubertal growth spurt, and estrogen is necessary for epiphyseal closure.[28] Deficiency of estrogen or androgen increases bone resorption in vivo, possibly by increasing local synthesis or sensitivity to cytokines, such as IL-1, TNF, or IL-6, and to prostaglandins.[29–31] Androgens can increase bone formation in vivo.[32] The effect of estrogens on bone formation is less clear. The absolute rate of bone formation is increased in estrogen deficiency states, possibly because of an increase in the activation frequency and the number of remodeling sites in bone. However, the fact that estrogen deficiency causes bone loss implies a relative deficiency in bone formation. Estrogens may also stimulate osteoblasts directly.

Local Regulators

Characterization of local regulators produced within the bone itself represents a major advance in bone biology.[33]

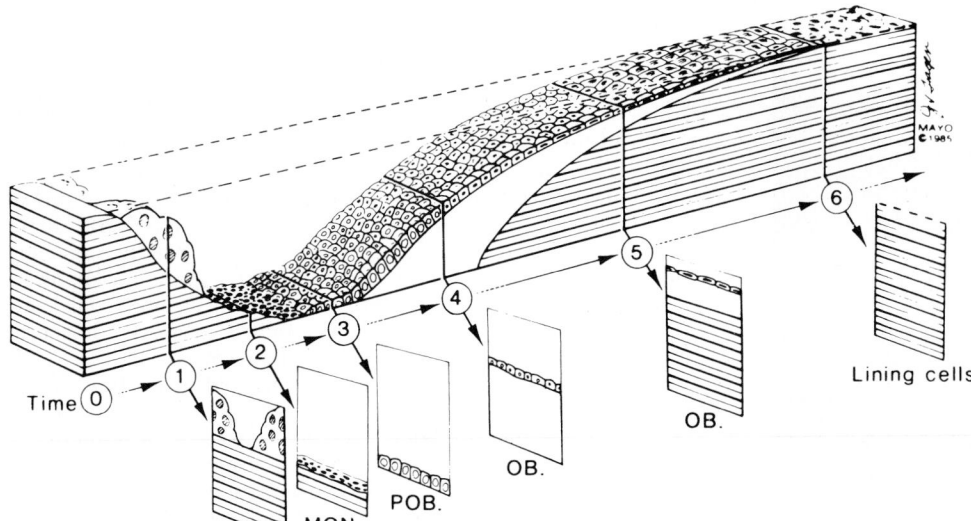

Figure 25–9. Three-dimensional reconstruction of the remodeling sequence in human trabecular bone. 1, Early bone resorption with osteoclasts (OCL); 2, late bone resorption with mononuclear cells (MON); 3, reversal phase with preosteoblasts (POB); 4, early matrix formation by osteoblasts (OB); 5, late bone formation with mineralization; 6, completed remodeling cycle with reversion to lining cells. (From Eriksen, EF. Normal and pathological remodeling of human trabecular bone: three-dimensional reconstruction of the remodeling sequence in normals and in metabolic bone disease. Endocr Rev 1986; 7:379–408. Copyright © 1986, by The Endocrine Society.)

These local factors can be synthesized by bone cells or by adjacent hematopoietic cells and can interact both with each other and with systemic hormones. They are critical in the repair of skeletal damage and in the response to mechanical forces.

CYTOKINES. IL-1α, IL-1β, TNF α, and TNF β are potent stimulators of bone resorption and inhibitors of bone formation[34] and may mediate bone loss after estrogen withdrawal.[35] IL-6 is not very effective in stimulating bone resorption but increases osteoclastogenesis in cell cultures.[31] IL-6 is produced by osteoblasts, and its production is stimulated by PTH, by prostaglandin E_2 (PGE$_2$), and by other factors that increase resorption. As noted previously, colony-stimulating factors are probably important in the early stages of osteoclast formation. IL-4 inhibits resorption and prostaglandin synthesis in bone cells,[36] and leukemia inhibitory factor has biphasic effects on bone formation.[37] Interferon γ can inhibit resorption, probably by inhibiting osteoclast differentiation. The responses to cytokines can be blocked by inhibitors, such as the IL-1 receptor antagonist and the soluble TNF receptor, and they can be enhanced by activators such as the soluble IL-6 receptor.

TRANSFORMING GROWTH FACTOR α (TGF α) AND EPIDERMAL GROWTH FACTOR (EGF). These peptides stimulate bone resorption through the same receptor and act by both prostaglandin-dependent and prostaglandin-independent pathways. TGF α and EGF are potent mitogens in bone that probably act on both mesenchymal and hematopoietic precursors.[38] TGF α is produced by neoplasms and may play a role in the increased bone resorption that occurs in certain malignancies.

PROSTAGLANDINS. Prostaglandins are potent regulators of bone cell metabolism and are synthesized by many cell types in the skeleton.[39] Prostaglandin production in bone is regulated by local and systemic hormones and by mechanical forces. Increased prostaglandin production may contribute to the increase in bone resorption with immobilization, the increase in bone formation with impact loading, and the changes after estrogen withdrawal. Many of the hormones, cytokines, and growth factors that stimulate bone resorption also increase prostaglandin production. Prostaglandins have biphasic effects on bone formation. Stimulation of bone formation is seen in vivo, and inhibition of collagen synthesis occurs in osteoblast cultures. Bone cells produce PGE$_2$, PGF$_{2α}$, prostacyclin, and lipoxygenase products (e.g., leukotriene B$_4$), which may also stimulate bone resorption.

Growth Factors

A large number of growth factors have been identified in bone, and their production by bone cells has been established by measurements of mRNA and protein.[40] Bone cells also produce binding proteins for growth factors, which may regulate storage in bone.

INSULIN-LIKE GROWTH FACTORS.[41] IGFs increase bone cell replication, matrix synthesis, and bone formation. Both IGF-I and IGF-II are synthesized by bone cells and stored in bone matrix. More IGF-II is stored in human bone, but IGF-I is a more potent stimulator of osteoblasts. Binding of IGF-I and IGF-II to matrix may be mediated by specific IGF-binding proteins. Five of the six known binding proteins have been identified in bone, and these both inhibit and enhance IGF responses. Because PTH and PGE$_2$ increase and glucocorticoids decrease skeletal IGF-I synthesis, IGFs may mediate the effects of these hormones on bone growth. IGF-I may also stimulate osteoclast formation.[42]

TRANSFORMING GROWTH FACTOR β AND BONE MORPHOGENETIC PROTEINS (BMP). This family of peptides has many complex actions on bone metabolism. TGF β acts to stimulate bone formation and to inhibit bone resorption.[43, 44] Because it is stored in bone matrix and released in an active form by bone-resorbing hormones, it may play a role in the reversal phase of bone remodeling when resorption stops and formation starts. The BMPs, like TGF β, stimulate mitosis and growth of bone cells and have similar effects on other mesenchymal cells, particularly cartilage. TGF β and BMPs accelerate the healing of bony defects in vivo.

FIBROBLAST GROWTH FACTORS (FGFs). Acidic and basic fibroblast growth factors (FGF-1 and FGF-2, respectively) are critical for cartilage growth and differentiation.[45] FGFs inhibit collagen synthesis in cell culture but increase bone formation in vivo. The in vivo effect may be caused in part by stimulation of prostaglandin synthesis.[46] FGF can stimulate bone resorption by both prostaglandin-dependent and prostaglandin-independent pathways. FGFs are heparin-binding growth factors, and this binding can influence their cellular activity and their sequestration in extracellular matrix.

PLATELET-DERIVED GROWTH FACTOR (PDGF).[47] PDGF was originally isolated from blood platelets, and it is also present in bone. The two gene products, PDGF-A and PDGF-B, form dimers. PDGF-AA is the major product of bone cells, but PDGF-BB is a more active stimulator of osteoblast replication. PDGF also stimulates bone resorption by a prostaglandin-dependent mechanism but inhibits osteoclast formation in cell cultures.

CLINICAL EVALUATION OF METABOLIC BONE DISEASE

Bone Densitometry

The most widely used procedure for measuring bone mass is dual-energy x-ray absorptiometry (DXA).[48] Other methods include quantitative computed tomography (QCT), quantitative radiography, single-energy x-ray absorptiometry (SXA), and ultrasound.[49, 50]

DUAL-ENERGY X-RAY ABSORPTIOMETRY. DXA can provide accurate and reproducible values for bone mineral content (BMC) and density (BMD) in the lumbar spine, the proximal femur, the distal radius, and the whole body. BMD is calculated from the BMC and the area of bone scanned (g/cm²). DXA has many advantages. Radiation exposure is minimal (<10 mrem), and scanning time is short (5 to 20 min). Variability of repeat readings is less than 1% for phantom standards; less than 2% for lumbar spine, total body, and radius; and less than 3% for proximal femur. The major disadvantages are (1) changes with disease progression or therapy are small in relation to the variability of the measurement, (2) the test is moderately expensive, and (3) anteroposterior measurements of the lumbar spine in older patients are subject to errors caused by aortic calcification and osteoarthritic changes. The last disadvantage can be overcome by performing lateral densitometry of the lumbar spine. Newer DXA systems can accomplish this accurately and may have sufficient resolution to measure changes in vertebral body height (Fig. 25–10).

QUANTITATIVE COMPUTED TOMOGRAPHY. QCT, which employs instruments available in most radiology departments, can assess true bone density (g/cm³) and separate cancellous and cortical bone in the vertebral body. It has also been used to measure cortical and trabecular bone density in the appendicular skeleton. The radiation exposure (100 to 300 mrem) is larger than for DXA, and the precision and accuracy are lower, but within the acceptable range. A major disadvantage is its cost.

OTHER METHODS. SXA, single-energy photon absorptiometry (SPA), or ultrasound can be used to assess bone mass in the appendicular skeleton with readily available instruments. Ultrasound, particularly of the calcaneus, may also provide information on the microarchitecture of bone[55] and may predict fractures. These instruments are useful for population studies and large-scale prevention programs.

Biochemical Measurements

Biochemical measurements can be used to assess bone formation and resorption.[51] One application is in the assessment of therapeutic response. High bone turnover correlates inversely with bone mass and may predict a high rate of bone loss. For this reason, the combined measurement of bone

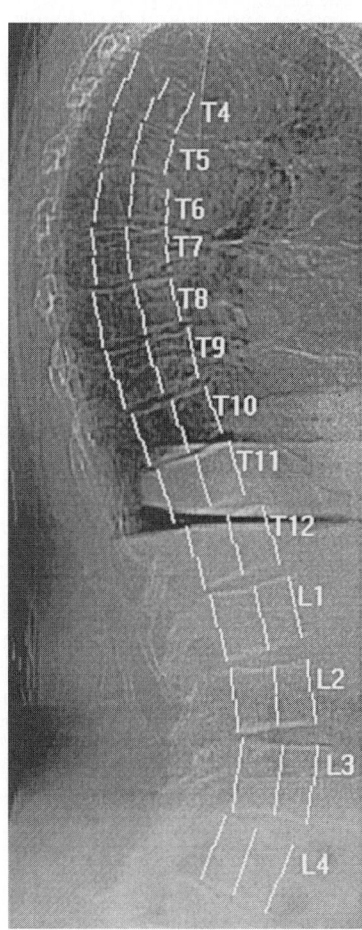

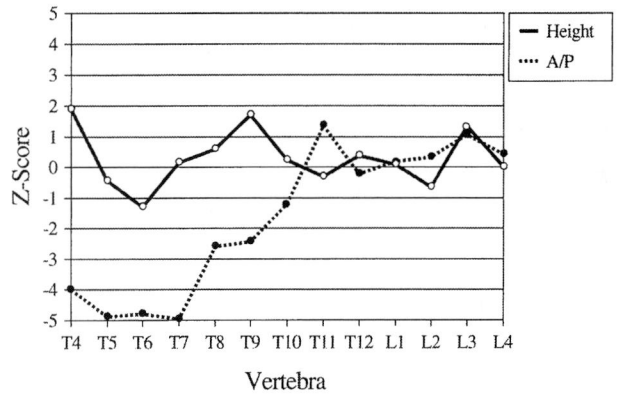

Region		HEIGHT (mm)	Z	A/P Ratio	Z
T4	>	18.6	+1.9	0.74	-4.0
T5	>	16.2	-0.5	0.69	-4.9
T6	>	15.6	-1.4	0.66	-4.8
T7	>	17.6	+0.2	0.64	-5.0
T8		18.7	+0.7	0.77	-2.6
T9		20.7	+1.8	0.81	-2.5
T10		20.0	+0.2	0.88	-1.2
T11		20.5	-0.3	1.00	+1.4
T12		23.5	+0.4	0.93	-0.2
L1		24.4	+0.1	0.96	+0.2
L2		23.9	-0.7	1.01	+0.4
L3		28.3	+1.5	1.07	+1.1
L4		25.7	+0.1	1.07	+0.5

Figure 25–10. Use of dual-energy X-ray absorptiometry for vertebral body morphometry. Posterior vertebral body heights and the ratio of anterior to posterior height (A/P) are presented in terms of standard deviation scores. Note that minor anterior wedging alone may not indicate an osteoporotic fracture. (Courtesy of Dr. Richard B. Mazess.)

markers and bone mass may improve the assessment of fracture risk. However, most of the markers show a wide normal range, so their usefulness in individual patients may be limited. Moreover, the variability in successive samples from the same patient may be as high as 20 to 40%.

Markers of Bone Formation

ALKALINE PHOSPHATASE. Total serum alkaline phosphatase is measured to assess osteoblastic activity in Paget's disease, primary hyperparathyroidism, osteomalacia, and rickets. An immunoassay that selectively measures the bone isoenzyme may increase the usefulness of this test in osteoporosis, in which changes in osteoblastic activity are small.

OSTEOCALCIN. The bone γ-carboxyglutamic acid–containing protein, osteocalcin, is one of the few proteins that are relatively specific for skeletal tissue. A fraction of the osteocalcin synthesized by osteoblasts is released into the circulation. Carboxy-terminal cleavage of the molecule may occur after release, but both the intact and amino terminal portions can be measured by specific immunoassays. Serum osteocalcin correlates with skeletal growth rates in childhood and puberty and is increased when bone turnover is accelerated (e.g., hyperparathyroidism, hyperthyroidism). In Paget's disease, osteocalcin is elevated to a lesser degree than alkaline phosphatase. Because osteocalcin production is increased by 1,25-$(OH)_2D$, the levels may be low in osteomalacia and rickets even when alkaline phosphatase is elevated.

PROCOLLAGEN PEPTIDES. The amino- and carboxy-terminal extension peptides of procollagen (see Fig. 25–2), which are removed during processing of collagen, are released into the circulation. Their measurement is an index of total body collagen synthesis, the bulk of which is derived from bone. The carboxy-terminal procollagen peptide correlates with histologic measures of bone formation. Levels of procollagen peptides are high in infants and may provide a clinically useful index of growth.

Markers of Bone Resorption

CALCIUM. Measurement of fasting urinary calcium excretion is convenient but shows wide variation, reflecting the net result of intestinal absorption, bone resorption, and mineralization. The assay is most useful for detecting a marked increase in osteoclastic activity with little change in formation, for example, in patients with osteolytic bone metastases.

HYDROXYPROLINE. Collagen degradation releases hydroxyproline into the circulation in both free and peptide-bound forms. Because bone resorption is by far the largest contributor to collagen breakdown, urinary hydroxyproline excretion has been used as a measure of bone resorption. However, 80 to 90% of the released hydroxyproline is metabolized, and hydroxyproline from collagen or gelatin in the diet is excreted in urine. Therefore, the sample should be obtained after a 12-hour fast or while the patient is on a gelatin-free diet. The hydroxyproline assay has been most useful in conditions in which resorption is markedly increased, such as Paget's disease, hyperparathyroidism, and malignancy.

COLLAGEN CROSS-LINKS.[58] Unlike hydroxyproline, the pyridinoline and deoxypyridinoline cross-links that stabilize collagen in the extracellular matrix (Fig. 25–11) are not metabolized but are excreted in the urine in either a free or peptide-bound form. The deoxypyridinoline cross-link is almost entirely derived from skeletal tissue and therefore is a more sensitive indicator of bone resorption than pyridinoline, which is also found in skin and other connective tissues. Measurement of total urinary pyridinoline or deoxypyridinoline by high-performance liquid chromatography is expensive and time-consuming, and immunoassays have been developed for free pyridinoline and deoxypyridinoline as well as for the amino- and carboxy-terminal peptides that contain these cross-links and are released during resorption. These measurements correlate with bone turnover and change in response to agents that affect resorption and should be useful in assessing changes in resorption in the course of disease or in response to therapy. They may also be useful in identifying patients with high bone turnover, who have low bone mass, lose bone rapidly, and are more likely to develop osteoporosis.

OTHER ASSAYS. Immunoassays for collagen degradation products in serum are being evaluated. Tartrate-resistant acid phosphatase is secreted by osteoclasts into serum and may be useful as a measure of bone resorption. Other collagen

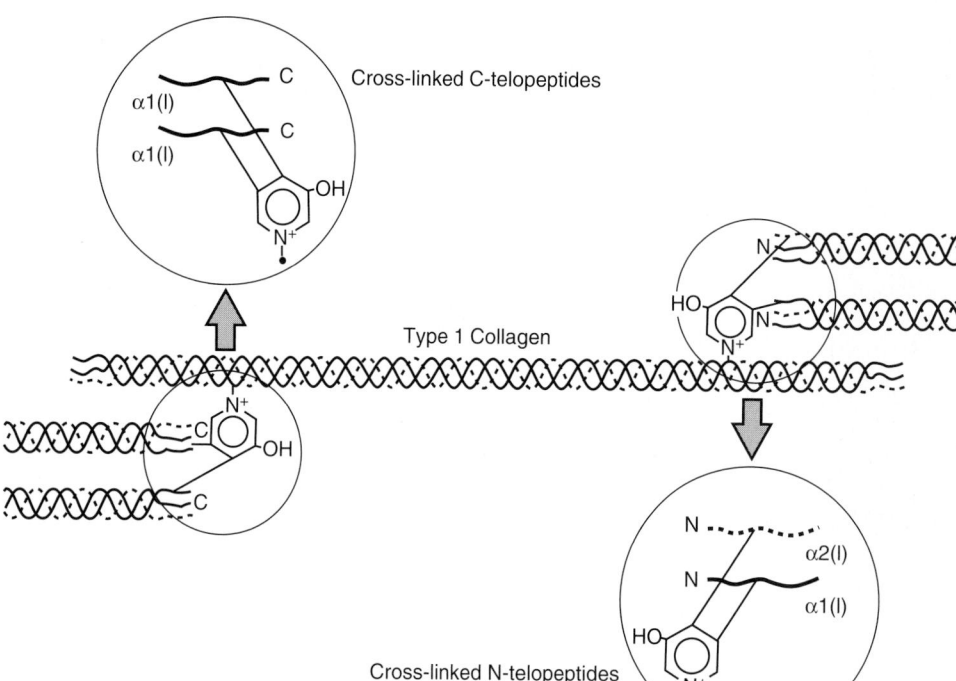

Figure 25–11. Collagen cross-links. Cross-links are formed between the COOH- and NH_2-terminal nonhelical portions of collagen and adjacent helical molecules. Immunoassays are available for the pyridinoline and deoxypyridinoline molecules themselves and for the adjacent nonhelical peptides. (Redrawn from Eyre DR. The specificity of collagen cross-links as markers of bone and connective tissue degradation. Acta Orthop Scand 1995; 266:166–170 [review].)

breakdown products such as glycosylated hydroxylysines may be measured to assess resorption.

Bone Biopsy

Transiliac bone biopsy can provide direct information about cancellous bone volume, the density of connections between trabecular plates (connectivity), and the function of bone cells.[52] The rate of bone formation and mineralization can be measured by this technique with the use of dynamic histomorphometry after tetracycline labeling (Fig. 25–12), but bone resorption is more difficult to assess by bone biopsy. Bone biopsy requires the use of a large needle with a 7- to 9-mm internal bore and the technical skill to obtain a sample that is not crushed or distorted. The sample must be processed without decalcification and stained appropriately. Unstained sections are needed to see fluorescent tetracycline labels. Special stains may be used to identify mast cells in mastocytosis or aluminum in renal osteodystrophy.[53] Biopsies may be useful in patients with atypical skeletal lesions or in men and premenopausal women who have osteoporotic fractures with no apparent cause.

Radiographs and Bone Scans

The use of radiographs and bone scans in diagnosis is covered under the discussions of specific disorders. Radiographs are most important in detecting fractures.[54] The trabec-

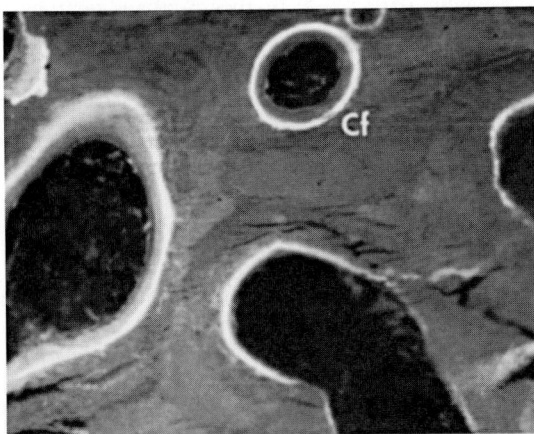

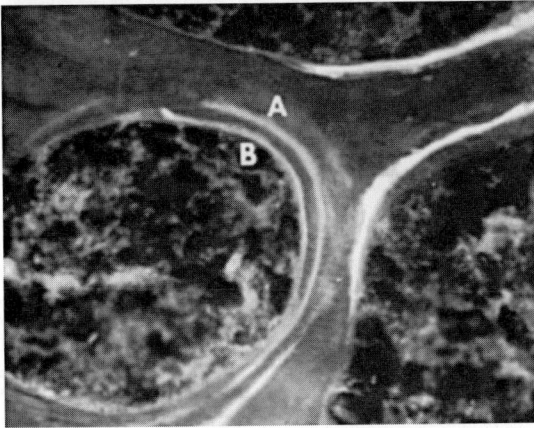

Figure 25–12. Tetracycline labels sites of active mineralization and is deposited at the calcification front (Cf) *(top)*. A double-label technique can be used to measure the rate of mineralization; label A was administered about 10 d before label B *(bottom)*. Undecalcified iliac crest, ultraviolet light, magnification × 113. (From Aaron J. Histology and microanatomy of bone. In: Nordin BEC, ed. Calcium, Phosphate and Magnesium Metabolism. Edinburgh: Churchill Livingstone, 1976: 298–356.)

ular pattern in the proximal femur (the Singh index) correlates with bone density and may predict the risk of fracture. High-resolution radiographs have also been used to assess cortical porosity.

Bone scans using technetium 99m linked to a bisphosphonate are useful in localization of bone lesions.[55] Uptake is a function of blood flow to the region and the amount of mineralizing bone. The test does not give information about the nature of the lesion but serves as a guide for further studies.

PRIMARY OSTEOPOROSIS

Definition

Although osteoporosis is by far the most common metabolic bone disease, there is variability in the use of this term among clinicians. In the past, osteoporosis was not diagnosed until fractures occurred, but the disorder has been better defined by the Consensus Development Conference[56] as "a disease characterized by low bone mass and microarchitectural deterioration of bone tissue, leading to enhanced bone fragility and a consequent increase in fracture risk."

Diagnostic categories for postmenopausal women are based on measurements of bone mass or density[57] (Table 25–2). These categories can aid in treatment and follow-up of patients but are applicable only to those who have had bone density measured but have not yet experienced fractures. The use of bone mass measurements to diagnose osteoporosis may not be widely applicable because it is expensive and not always available. If the diagnosis is based on low bone density at any site, the validity of the diagnosis may depend on the site measured; site-specific measurements may best predict fractures at those sites, particularly in the proximal femur. The frequency of osteoporosis is high in older persons (Fig. 25–13). As many as 70% of women more than 80 years old who have not been treated with estrogen have sufficiently low bone mass to warrant the diagnosis, and the incidence of fractures in such women is also high.

Epidemiology[59]

Osteoporosis is frequently considered a disorder of postmenopausal women of Northern European descent, primarily because they have high rates of fractures. However, the frequency of hip fractures is also high in other populations and is likely to increase further as life expectancy increases. Moreover, there appears to be an increase in the age-adjusted incidence of hip fractures around the world, possibly related to increasing industrialization and decreasing physical activity.

TABLE 25–2. Diagnostic Categories for Osteoporosis Based on Measurements of Bone Mineral Density (BMD) and Bone Mineral Content (BMC)

Category	Definition
Normal	A value for BMD or BMC ± 1 SD of the young adult reference mean.
Low bone mass (osteopenia)	A value for BMD or BMC >1 SD and <2.5 SD lower than the young adult mean.
Osteoporosis	A value for BMD or BMC >2.5 SD lower than the young adult mean.
Severe osteoporosis (established osteoporosis)	A value for BMD or BMC >2.5 SD lower than the young adult mean in the presence of one or more fragility fractures.

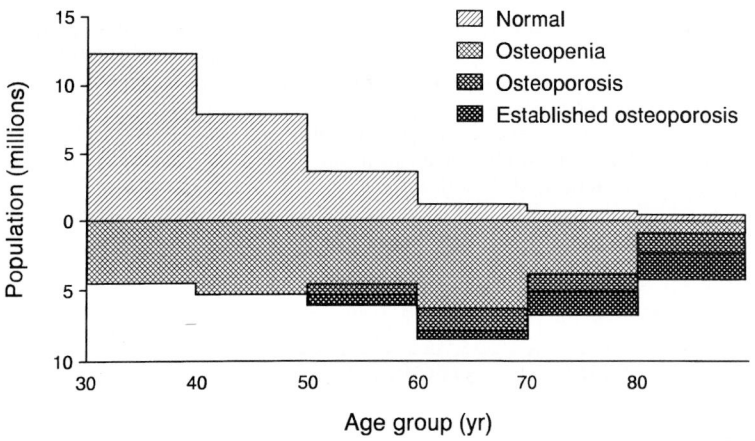

Figure 25–13. Estimation of the current prevalence of osteoporosis in the United States. Based on World Health Organization criteria, there are more than 9 million women in the United States with osteoporosis, of whom more than half have established osteoporosis with fractures. In addition, 17 million postmenopausal women have osteopenia or low bone mass and are at risk for developing osteoporosis. (Melton LJ. How many women have osteoporosis now? J Bone Miner Res 1995; 10:175–177.)

Most of the epidemiologic data are for hip fractures, but vertebral fractures are also common. In one study, the lifetime risk of osteoporotic fractures after the age of 50 years was about 40% in women and 13% in men (Table 25–3). The temporal pattern for the increase in fracture incidence differs for the hip, spine, and wrist (Fig. 25–14).

The incidence of osteoporotic fractures varies in different populations, possibly because of variations in skeletal architecture and turnover and in bone mass. For example, in South Africa the incidence of hip fracture in Bantus is only a fraction of that in whites, who have lower bone densities.[60]

Pathogenesis

Understanding of the pathogenesis of primary osteoporosis remains largely descriptive.[1, 61] Decreased bone mass and increased fragility can occur because of (1) failure to achieve optimal peak bone mass, (2) bone loss caused by increased bone resorption, or (3) inadequate replacement of lost bone as a result of decreased bone formation. Moreover, an analysis of the pathogenesis of osteoporosis must take into account the heterogeneity of clinical expression.

INADEQUATE PEAK BONE MASS. Studies of twins suggest that 70 to 80% of the variation in peak bone mass can be accounted for by genetic determinants.[62] Different alleles of the gene for the vitamin D receptor may be associated with differences in bone mass and in remodeling rates.[63–65] Additional genetic factors undoubtedly influence peak bone mass and strength. Furthermore, structural features of the skeleton, such as the length of the femoral neck, are genetically determined and can influence fracture incidence.[66] High levels of physical activity and a good calcium intake during childhood and puberty can help achieve maximal peak bone mass.[67]

Skeletal development involves a number of systemic hormones, including glucocorticoids, growth hormone, thyroid hormones, and, most particularly, gonadal steroids. Gonadal hormones are responsible for the initiation of the pubertal growth spurt, and a delay in puberty is associated with a decrease in peak bone mass.[68] Estrogen probably plays the primary role in epiphyseal closure and decreased bone remodeling after puberty; a man with defective estrogen receptors showed continued linear growth, low bone mass, and high bone turnover.[28]

INCREASED BONE RESORPTION. After peak bone mass is achieved, bone mass remains stable for a period of years because resorption and formation are equal. However, bone loss in women, particularly in the distal radius, may begin well before menopause.[69] The incidence of Colles' fractures increases in women in their forties. In contrast, the increase in vertebral crush fractures is greatest 5 to 15 y after the menopause, and hip fractures show a logarithmic increase (see Fig. 25–14). These differences indicate that rates of bone loss, although menopause- and age-related, differ in different sites.

Excessive bone resorption probably reflects increased activation frequency more than an increase in the amount of bone resorbed at each site. However, trabecular perforation can occur when the mechanisms for stopping osteoclast activity fail. The finding that markers of bone turnover are increased in postmenopausal women, even in the elderly, suggests that excessive bone resorption is the predominant cause of osteoporosis. However, morphologic studies do not always support this concept.[70–72]

DECREASED BONE FORMATION. Skeletal bone mass can

TABLE 25–3. Estimated Lifetime Fracture Risk in Women and Men from Rochester, Minnesota, at the Age of 50 Years

Fracture Site	Women (% [95% Confidence Interval])	Men (% [95% Confidence Interval])
Proximal femur	17.5 (16.8–18.2)	6.0 (5.6–6.5)
Vertebra*	15.6 (14.8–16.3)	5.0 (4.6–5.4)
Distal forearm	16.0 (15.7–16.7)	2.5 (2.2–3.1)
Any of the above	39.7 (38.7–40.6)	13.1 (12.4–13.7)

*Clinically diagnosed fractures.
From Melton LJ III, Chrischilles EA, Cooper C, et al. How many women have osteoporosis? J Bone Miner Res 1992; 7:1005–1010.

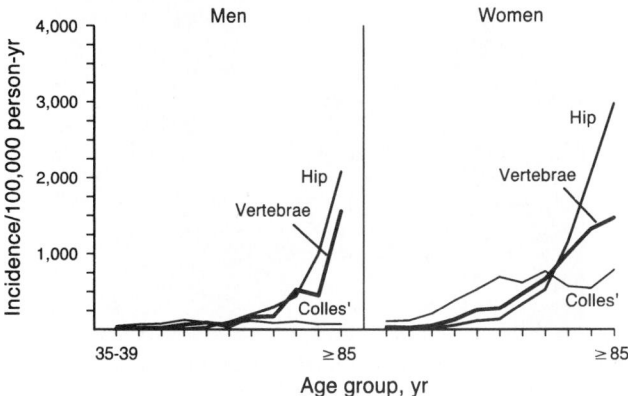

Figure 25–14. Age-specific incidence rates for hip, vertebral, and Colles' fractures in Rochester, Minnesota. (From Cooper C, Melton LJ. Epidemiology of osteoporosis. Trends Endocrinol Metab 1992; 3:224. Copyright © 1992, by Elsevier Science Inc.)

be maintained or even increased during puberty and young adult life, when the rate of resorption is high. Menopausal and age-related bone loss involve relative impairment of bone formation. With age, the amount of bone formed decreases with each bone structural unit, as evidenced by a decrease in mean wall thickness. Histomorphometric studies show a decrease in mean wall thickness and in the area of osteoblastic surfaces in osteoporosis.[70] As yet, no biochemical abnormality of matrix or mineral has been identified.[73, 74]

Pathogenetic Factors

SYSTEMIC HORMONES. The search for pathogenetic factors in osteoporosis has focused primarily on systemic hormones. A critical role for gonadal hormone deficiency is supported by the fact that postmenopausal women have the highest incidence of osteoporosis and by the occurrence of osteoporosis in hypogonadal men and in younger women with estrogen deficiency.[75, 76] Nevertheless, osteoporosis can occur, albeit rarely, in the absence of gonadal hormone deficiency, and there is no difference in estrogen production in postmenopausal women with or without osteoporosis. However, androgen production may be decreased in osteoporotic women compared with age-matched controls.[77, 78]

Other systemic hormones may play a role in age-related bone loss. PTH levels increase with age, probably because of decreased dietary intake and impaired intestinal absorption of calcium and decreased synthesis of 1,25-$(OH)_2D$ in the kidney.[79] Increased PTH could accelerate cortical bone loss. However, PTH levels in patients with vertebral fractures are not different from those in age-matched controls, and the PTH response to phosphate loading is actually blunted.[80] Levels of 1,25-$(OH)_2D$ are not consistently altered, although some older patients with hip fractures do have low levels.[81] Calcitonin deficiency does not appear to play a role in osteoporosis,[82] although pharmacologic doses of calcitonin can prevent bone loss or increase bone mass in patients with high bone turnover.[83] Glucocorticoid excess can produce secondary osteoporosis but does not appear to play a major role in primary osteoporosis. Growth hormone secretion and circulating IGF-I decrease with age, but the changes are similar in osteoporotic patients and in controls.[84] Thyroid hormone excess may aggravate osteoporosis.[85, 86]

LOCAL FACTORS. Several features of osteoporosis suggest a role for local factors in pathogenesis: (1) no systemic hormone plays an essential role; (2) differential bone loss occurs in different parts of the skeleton; (3) levels of cytokines, prostaglandins, and local growth factors may be altered in osteoporosis.

Production of IL-1, TNF α, and IL-6 may be increased in estrogen-deficient and osteoporotic patients.[87, 88] The loss of bone after ovariectomy in rats can be blocked by inhibiting the activity of IL-1 and TNF α.[35] PGE_2 production is increased in bones from oophorectomized animals and decreased by estrogen administration.[89] Nonsteroidal anti-inflammatory drugs that inhibit prostaglandin synthesis can slow bone loss in ovariectomized animals and postmenopausal women, although the effect is limited.[90, 91] IL-6 levels increase with age in humans,[92] and estrogens and androgens can decrease IL-6 production.[31, 93] However, there are also negative studies on the role of cytokines in osteoporosis.[94, 95]

Levels of IGF-I decrease with age, but no consistent difference has been observed in osteoporotic patients. It is more likely that skeletal production of IGF or IGF-binding proteins plays a role.[96] TGF β and BMPs may regulate bone remodeling, and TGF β levels are decreased in bones from oophorectomized animals.[97] Decreased TGF β levels may not only impair bone formation but also increase bone resorption.

NUTRITION AND LIFESTYLE. Calcium deficiency and de-creased physical activity in early life can lead to a lower peak bone mass[98] and may accelerate bone loss later in life. Calcium loading, particularly when given with vitamin D, can slow bone loss.[99] There are also correlations between body fat, lean body mass, and bone density. One mechanism for protection of bone density in overweight people may be conversion of adrenal androgens to estrogens in fat. Another pathway may be the decrease in testosterone-binding globulin associated with increased body mass index.[100]

Clinical Features

VERTEBRAL CRUSH FRACTURES. Compression fractures of the vertebrae, which occur spontaneously or with minimal trauma, are the most common manifestation of osteoporosis. The terms *postmenopausal osteoporosis* and *type I osteoporosis* have been applied to vertebral crush fracture at a younger age and mainly in women, whereas *senile osteoporosis* and *type II osteoporosis* have been used for hip fractures in older women and men.[101] These distinctions may not be helpful clinically. The disorders certainly are not separate, because patients with any type of osteoporotic fracture are more likely to have subsequent fractures of either the spine or the hip. Moreover, the difference in incidence between women and men is the same for vertebral and hip fractures (see Table 25–3).

The clinical course of the vertebral crush fracture syndrome varies. Some patients have compression of one vertebra, and others develop collapse of multiple vertebrae. Vertebrae may show extensive loss of trabecular structure before they collapse (Fig. 25–15). Radiologically, fractures can vary from mild end-plate deformities or anterior wedging to complete vertebral collapse (Fig. 25–16). The most frequent fractures are in the thoracic vertebrae below T6 and in the lumbar vertebrae.

Patients with vertebral crush fractures usually develop back pain that leads to radiologic assessment. Pain in the lumbar or sacral area is less likely to be associated with vertebral compression than is pain in the thoracic area. Height loss is a sensitive indicator of compression, but height loss can occur without fractures as a result of narrowing of vertebral disks and postural changes. Many patients are asymptomatic,

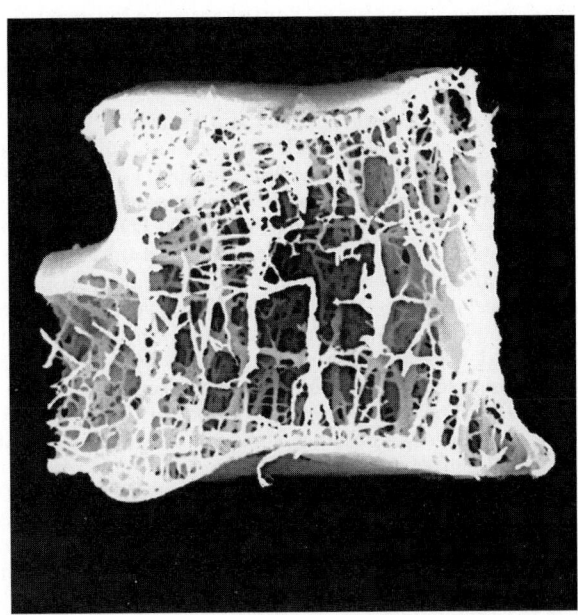

Figure 25–15. Cross-section of an osteoporotic vertebra showing extensive loss of trabecular bone architecture. (Courtesy of Dr. Anders Odgaard, Aarhus, Denmark.)

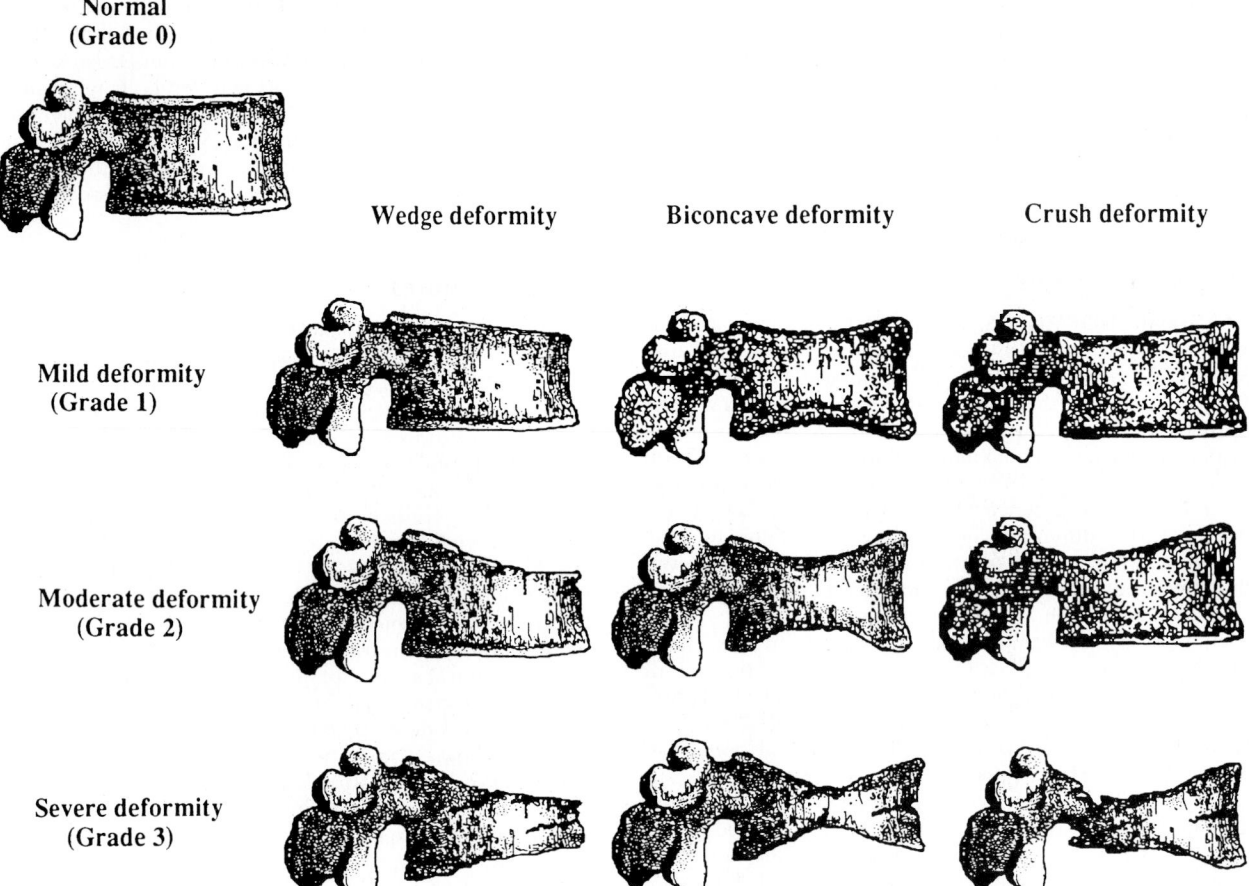

**Normal
(Grade 0)**

Wedge deformity   Biconcave deformity   Crush deformity

**Mild deformity
(Grade 1)**

**Moderate deformity
(Grade 2)**

**Severe deformity
(Grade 3)**

Figure 25–16. Types of vertebral compression fractures. Changes in vertebral height can be quantitated by measuring percent change or standard deviations from expected normal heights. (From Genant HK, et al. Vertebral fracture assessment using a semiquantitative technique. J Bone Miner Res 1993; 8:1137–1148, with permission.)

particularly those who have only anterior wedging. Anterior wedging in the upper thoracic vertebrae (T5 to T8) is common in older women and is not necessarily associated with severe compression fractures. Bone density measurements can help predict fracture risk in these patients. Anterior wedging may also develop early in life, probably during pubertal growth. This is termed Scheuermann's disease, and it may be transmitted as an autosomal dominant disorder.[102]

Multiple vertebral crush fractures cause severe impairment. Kyphosis and the loss of the lumbar lordosis are deforming and can aggravate back pain. Impairment of chest wall function may reduce the vital capacity.[103] The compression of abdominal contents may be disfiguring and uncomfortable. Ultimately, impingement of the ribs on the iliac crest is another source of pain. Many patients have additional spinal abnormalities, including spondylolisthesis, intervertebral disk disease, and osteoarthritis, particularly in the spinal facets. Osteoporosis itself rarely compresses nerve roots or the spinal cord. Although patients with severe osteoarthritis are less likely to have osteoporosis, these two common disorders frequently occur in the same patient.[104]

HIP FRACTURE. Fractures of the proximal femur are a major cause of morbidity and mortality in the elderly. Most fractures are in the femoral neck or at the base of the greater trochanter and are associated with trauma, which may be minimal. The risk is influenced by factors that increase the risk of falling and by the type of fall.[105] The increased incidence of hip fractures with age is caused both by increased falls and by continued bone loss.[106] Hip fracture is usually treated surgi-

cally, and the costs are substantial. In addition, perioperative and postoperative complications are associated with a 5 to 20% mortality rate. Many elderly patients cannot return to their previous level of activity after hip fracture and require long-term nursing home care. It is important to perform a diagnostic evaluation and develop a prevention plan in these patients, because a second hip fracture or a fragility fracture at another site is likely to occur.

COLLES' FRACTURE. Colles' fractures of the distal radius, which is composed largely of trabecular bone, are caused by falling on the outstretched hand.[107] The incidence in women begins to increase after 40 years of age. Unlike vertebral and hip fractures, the incidence of Colles' fractures in men does not increase with age. Colles' fractures usually heal well and result in little long-term morbidity. Women older than age 40 with a Colles' fracture should be assessed for osteoporosis so that an appropriate treatment plan can be provided.

OTHER FRACTURES. Fractures at any site, with the possible exception of the face and skull, can be associated with osteoporosis. Measurements of bone mass and further diagnostic work-up are indicated for all fractures that occur with minimal trauma.

Osteoporosis in Men

The incidence of hip and spine fractures in men increases with age and is about one third that in women. In men the increase in frequency tends to occur later in life, and a higher proportion of men have definable secondary causes.[108] Bone histomorphometry shows increased resorption in most patients.[109] A diagnostic work-up and therapeutic plan should be provided for men with fragility fractures, but this is rarely carried out in practice. Screening for osteoporosis in older men has not yet been evaluated but may be justified after preventive therapy becomes available.

Juvenile Osteoporosis

Juvenile osteoporosis[110] is a rare, self-limiting disease that can begin between the ages of 8 and 14 years with back pain and vertebral compression. Bone turnover is high, and antiresorptive or anti-inflammatory agents may be beneficial.[111] However, spontaneous remission usually occurs, and the disorder usually does not lead to permanent deformity.

Idiopathic Osteoporosis

Osteoporosis with no obvious secondary cause in premenopausal women or younger men is termed *idiopathic osteoporosis*. The term is not used consistently, and the patients so defined include individuals with both high and low bone turnover.[112] Some patients have a transient, self-limited condition, whereas others develop a progressive and disabling disease. Idiopathic osteoporosis can be associated with nonspecific inflammatory changes, and these cases may be caused by abnormal cytokine activity. Careful evaluation should be made for secondary causes.[113–115]

Osteoporosis in Pregnancy[116]

Osteoporosis in pregnancy occurs rarely and may be related to the fact that a large amount of calcium must be provided to the fetus during pregnancy. Ordinarily, maternal bone mass is well maintained during pregnancy, presumably because the high levels of estrogen protect the skeleton and because high levels of $1,25\text{-}(OH)_2D$ stimulate calcium absorption. Prolonged lactation is also associated with bone loss.[117]

Localized Osteoporosis

Immobilization is the most common cause of localized osteoporosis (see later discussion). However, regional migratory osteoporosis can occur without immobilization, particularly in the lower extremities.[118] This phenomenon may be associated with local inflammation or autonomic dysfunction with vasomotor changes and hyperesthesia, a syndrome termed *reflex sympathetic dystrophy*.[119]

SECONDARY OSTEOPOROSIS

The division of osteoporosis into primary and secondary forms is somewhat arbitrary. For example, patients with diseases that lead to hypogonadism early in life are considered to have secondary osteoporosis, whereas osteoporosis in women with natural menopause is termed primary. Moreover, many patients have a combination of primary and secondary causes. Although most postmenopausal women and older men do not have a definable secondary cause, the few that do can be treated more effectively. Therefore, this possibility should be considered in every patient. There are many causes of secondary osteoporosis (Table 25–4), only a few of which are discussed here.

Glucocorticoid-Induced Osteoporosis

The most common form of secondary osteoporosis is that induced by exogenous glucocorticoids.[24] Cushing's syndrome,

TABLE 25–4. Causes of Secondary Osteoporosis

A. Endocrine disorders
  1. Hyperparathyroidism
  2. Cushing's syndrome
  3. Hypogonadism
  4. Hyperthyroidism
  5. Prolactinoma
  6. Diabetes mellitus
  7. Acromegaly
  8. Pregnancy and lactation
B. Hematopoietic disorders
  1. Plasma cell dyscrasias: multiple myeloma and macroglobulinemia
  2. Systemic mastocytosis
  3. Leukemias and lymphomas
  4. Sickle cell disease and thalassemia minor
  5. Lipidoses: Gaucher's disease
  6. Myeloproliferative disorders: polycythemia
C. Connective tissue disorders
  1. Osteogenesis imperfecta
  2. Ehlers-Danlos syndrome
  3. Marfan syndrome
  4. Homocystinuria and lysinuria
  5. Menkes' syndrome
  6. Scurvy
D. Drug-induced disorders
  1. Glucocorticoids
  2. Heparin
  3. Anticonvulsants
  4. Methotrexate, cyclosporin A
  5. Leuteinizing hormone–releasing hormone (LHRH) agonist or antagonist therapy
  6. Aluminum-containing antacids
E. Immobilization
F. Renal disease
  1. Chronic renal failure
  2. Renal tubular acidosis
G. Nutritional and gastrointestinal disorders
  1. Malabsorption
  2. Total parenteral nutrition
  3. Gastrectomy
  4. Hepatobiliary disease
  5. Chronic hypophosphatemia
H. Miscellaneous
  1. Familial dysautonomia (Riley-Day syndrome)
  2. Reflex sympathetic dystrophy

caused by excess of endogenous glucocorticoids, is less common but can also involve osteoporosis at presentation. Patients with rheumatoid arthritis, chronic pulmonary disease, or gastrointestinal disease who receive exogenous glucocorticoids are at additional risk, because disease-associated inflammation, poor nutrition, and immobilization can aggravate bone loss. Glucocorticoid-induced osteoporosis is particularly common in postmenopausal women, presumably because they also have primary osteoporosis. However, fragility fractures can occur in any patient treated with glucocorticoids at moderate to high doses for a long period. Glucocorticoid-induced osteoporosis is a result of both increased bone resorption and decreased bone formation. Increased resorption may be caused by decreased calcium absorption and the resulting secondary hyperparathyroidism. Decreased bone formation is probably caused by direct inhibition of osteoblasts, which are highly sensitive to glucocorticoids; for example, as little as 2.5 mg of prednisone given at bedtime can block the normal nocturnal rise in osteocalcin.[120] Glucocorticoids also increase urinary calcium and phosphate and can inhibit gonadal hormone production by blocking gonadotrophin release. Levels of testosterone are low in men receiving 20 mg or more of prednisone per day.[121] In postmenopausal women exogenous glucocorticoids decrease secretion of corticotropin, thereby decreasing the production of adrenal androgens, which are the major precursors for estrone formation.

Glucocorticoid-induced osteoporosis is similar clinically to primary osteoporosis. Initial bone loss is predominantly trabecular and best assessed in the spine or distal radius.

However, rib fractures and aseptic necrosis of the femoral or humeral heads or of the vertebrae are common in glucocorticoid-induced osteoporosis, although they are rare in primary osteoporosis. Glucocorticoid-induced osteoporosis can be reversible, particularly in young patients who are cured of Cushing's syndrome.[122] In patients who cannot discontinue glucocorticoid therapy, early preventive therapy may be effective.[123, 124]

Hypogonadism

Hypogonadism can occur in either sex and from multiple causes. Patients with primary hypogonadism due to ovarian or testicular failure or secondary hypogonadism due to hypothalamic or pituitary disease lose bone rapidly and often develop fragility fractures. The hypogonadotrophic group includes patients with anorexia nervosa, athletic amenorrhea, prolactinoma, or lesions of the pituitary or hypothalamus, including tumors and hypogonadotropis hypogonadism. Loss of growth hormone may also play a role in the osteoporosis of pituitary tumors. Patients with prolactinomas can secrete parathyroid hormone–related peptide (PTHrP), which may cause bone loss.[125]

Other Endocrine Causes

Hyperthyroidism can produce bone loss; however, the increase in formation in young individuals is usually adequate, and, if the disease is treated early, changes in bone mass are small.[25, 126] In individuals at risk for osteoporosis, primary hyperthyroidism may be missed, or excessive amounts of exogenous thyroid hormone may be administered for many years. Osteoporosis is seen both in growth hormone deficiency and in acromegaly, but the latter may be caused by gonadotropin deficiency and the loss of gonadal hormones with large pituitary tumors.[127–129] Patients with insulin-dependent diabetes mellitus often have low bone mass and diminished bone formation,[26] particularly at the onset of the disease, but osteoporotic fractures are not a major problem. The role of non–insulin-dependent diabetes mellitus in the pathogenesis of osteoporosis is unclear.[130, 131] Bone loss may occur, particularly in patients who are not obese, but the data on fracture incidence are inconsistent.

Malignancy

Multiple myeloma and other lymphoproliferative malignancies can produce a clinical picture that resembles primary osteoporosis.[132, 133] It is particularly important to exclude myeloma in patients with rapidly progressive vertebral crush fracture syndrome. Metastases to the spine may also cause vertebral compression and should be considered in the differential diagnosis, particularly in patients with normal bone density.

Other Diseases

The incidence and severity of osteoporosis are increased in chronic hepatic and intestinal disorders, probably both on a nutritional basis and because these patients often receive glucocorticoids or other drugs that affect the skeleton.[134, 135] Although it was initially thought that impairment of vitamin D function in hepatic and intestinal disease would cause osteomalacia, the most common lesion in such patients is osteoporosis. Severe alcoholics also can develop osteoporosis; however, low intakes of ethanol may be associated with increased bone mass and a decreased fracture risk.[136] Mastocytosis causes both osteoporosis and osteosclerosis, and the number of mast cells may be increased in the marrow of patients with primary osteoporosis.[115, 137] The functional significance of the mast cells

is not known, although mast cells produce heparin, which can cause bone loss (see later discussion). Hyperplastic anemias such as thalassemia can also cause bone loss,[138] partly because of bone erosion by the marrow and partly because of hypogonadism consequent to transfusion-induced hemochromatosis.[139] Osteoporosis after organ transplantation results both from the underlying disease and from the drugs used to prevent graft rejection.[134, 140–143]

Drugs

A number of drugs can produce osteoporosis. Heparin stimulates bone resorption and inhibits bone formation and can cause osteoporosis.[144, 145] Patients on anticonvulsants, including phenytoin, barbiturates, and carbamazepine, often show low bone mass.[146] Impairment of vitamin D metabolism has been described, but most patients develop osteoporosis with normal mineralization. Immunosuppressive agents such as cyclosporin A and FK-506 are associated with bone loss.[143] Gonadotropin-releasing hormone antagonists, which decrease production of gonadal hormones, can lead to osteoporosis.[147] Some agents used in cancer chemotherapy probably act both by inhibiting osteoblasts and by suppressing gonadal hormones.[148, 149]

DIAGNOSIS OF OSTEOPOROSIS

Based on the definition of the World Health Organization, osteoporosis can be diagnosed before fracture by measuring bone density.[56, 57] The incidence of diagnosis therefore depends on the frequency, site, and timing of bone density measurements. There is no general agreement as to who should be screened or when screening should be done. Screening at the menopause is recommended for those women in whom bone density results may affect the decision for or against hormone replacement therapy. Screening is also recommended for high-risk groups such as persons with multiple risk factors or a strong family history of osteoporosis. Nevertheless, most patients are not diagnosed until after their first fracture. Bone density measurements establish the severity of bone loss and provide a baseline to follow the patient's therapeutic response. The subsequent work-up should be the same whether osteoporosis is diagnosed on the basis of screening or after the finding of a fragility fracture.[150]

The history should include a detailed analysis of calcium intake and nutrition, physical activity and lifestyle, smoking history, menstrual and reproductive history, and family history of osteoporosis or other metabolic or endocrine disorders that may affect the skeleton. Physical examination should include a careful height measurement, assessment of the spine, and evaluation for thyroid or adrenal disease.

In addition to routine radiologic assessment of fractures, magnetic resonance imaging (MRI) or computed tomography (CT) imaging may be indicated if there are neurologic changes or if fractures are associated with normal bone density, raising the possibility of malignancy.

A minimal laboratory screen should include measurement of serum calcium, preferably as an ionized calcium, fasting calcium excretion (most easily measured as the calcium/creatinine ratio in the second-voided morning specimen), and appropriate tests to exclude secondary causes of osteoporosis. Serum phosphorus and alkaline phosphatase are useful in ruling out hyperparathyroidism and osteomalacia. Measurements of vitamin D metabolites, urine phosphorus, and PTH are indicated if the screening test results are abnormal. Serum electrophoresis, blood count, and sedimentation rate can help to rule out myeloma, and thyroid function should be assessed. Laboratory studies for Cushing's syndrome are indicated in patients with suggestive clinical features.

PREVENTION OF AND THERAPY FOR OSTEOPOROSIS

Although it is important to relieve pain and limit the impact of deformities in established osteoporosis, the primary goal of treatment is to prevent further fractures. Therefore, prevention and therapy are considered together.

Nutrition and Calcium Supplementation

The calcium intakes recommended for prevention and treatment of osteoporosis range from 1 to 2 g/day.[151] Most studies indicate that calcium supplementation slows but does not stop bone loss. These high calcium intakes are generally safe, although it may be worthwhile to check urine calcium levels. There is no advantage for any particular calcium formulation. Calcium carbonate is inexpensive and, when taken with meals, is usually well absorbed, even in patients with achlorhydria.[152] Calcium citrate and other salts may be absorbed better than calcium carbonate in the fasting state. It is also worthwhile to include foods high in calcium in the diet. Patients should be informed as to the calcium content of the major food sources, such as dairy products. Vitamin D intake should be at least 400 U/day, and up to 2000 U/day is probably safe; higher levels may produce hypercalciuria or hypercalcemia. Calcium and vitamin D increase bone mass and decrease the incidence of fractures, particularly in populations likely to have deficient intakes or limited sun exposure.[153-155] Other forms of vitamin D have been used, including calcidiol (25-(OH)D), calcitriol (1,25-(OH)$_2$D), and 1α-(OH)D, but there is no direct evidence that these are superior to ordinary vitamin D, which is less expensive.[156] Dietary intakes of other minerals and of vitamins C and K, which are important for bone matrix synthesis, should be adequate.

Exercise and Lifestyle

Although immobilization decreases bone mass and muscle strength, the role of exercise in treatment of osteoporosis has not been defined.[157] Based on limited data, one-half hour of weight-bearing exercise per day is recommended for patients who can tolerate it.[158] Epidemiologic data suggest that lifetime leisure exercise is associated with higher bone mineral density at the hip but has no effect on fracture incidence.[159] Patients often are better able to develop and maintain a suitable exercise program under the supervision of a physical therapist. Patients should also be instructed in body mechanics and posture, so as to minimize musculoskeletal damage and the likelihood of falls. They should stop smoking and limit their intake of alcohol. Pain relief for patients with vertebral crush fractures can usually be achieved with mild analgesics and local physical therapy. Calcitonin has analgesic effects and may be useful in patients with severe pain.[160] Help should be provided for coping with osteoporosis and for designing a lifestyle that maintains function and minimizes fracture risk.[161]

Hormone Replacement Therapy

Unless there are specific contraindications, postmenopausal women with or without osteoporosis should be offered hormone replacement therapy. Many different regimens and forms of estrogen slow bone loss and decrease the incidence of fractures,[162, 163] including several oral preparations and transdermal estrogen, and the choice is based on tolerance and convenience. Estrogen induces a detectable decrease in bone resorption,[164] and bone formation also decreases. However, bone mass usually increases, perhaps primarily by filling in of the "remodeling space," because the rate of increase in bone mass tends to decrease with time, unlike the continuous responses with anabolic agents such as fluoride.[165] Patients with an intact uterus should be given progestagens to prevent endometrial hyperplasia and an increased risk of endometrial cancer. Intermittent progestagen usually causes the return of menses. Low-dose, continuous progestagen may be more acceptable in older patients, because it usually causes only transient breakthrough bleeding. All patients on estrogen should have annual mammograms and undergo appropriate evaluation if atypical uterine bleeding occurs (see Chapter 15).

The most important contraindication to the use of estrogen is breast cancer, and a strong family history of breast cancer is a relative contraindication. Tamoxifen may slow bone loss in patients with breast cancer, but it is not as effective as estrogen in reducing bone turnover.[166, 167] The presence of hypertension, thromboembolic disease, or migraine headaches may make management with hormones more difficult.

Despite the effectiveness of estrogen in osteoporosis and the likelihood that hormone replacement therapy reduces cardiovascular disease, patient compliance often is poor because of side effects or fear of cancer. The most common side effects are breast tenderness and recurrence of menstrual bleeding.

Bisphosphonates

Bisphosphonates are pyrophosphate analogues that bind to bone mineral and inhibit resorption. The first compound available for clinical use, etidronate, inhibits bone mineralization at high doses but increases bone mass without impairing mineralization when given intermittently at low doses.[168] Second-generation bisphosphonates such as alendronate, risedronate, and tiludronate do not impair mineralization at therapeutic doses and can be given continuously.[169] Alendronate is approved for use in the United States, based on evidence that it decreases bone resorption, increases bone mass in the spine and hip, and decreases the incidence of vertebral fractures in patients with osteoporosis.[170, 171] The bisphosphonates are useful in treating established osteoporosis, particularly in patients who cannot or will not take estrogen. Moreover, because they act by a different mechanism, they can be added to estrogen in patients who are responding poorly or have severe disease. However, data for the efficacy of combined therapy are limited.

Calcitonin

Calcitonin, an inhibitor of bone resorption, can increase bone mass, particularly in patients with high turnover.[83] Calcitonin also has some analgesic properties and may be particularly useful in patients with recent painful vertebral fractures. It is available either as a subcutaneous injection or as a nasal spray.[172] The former is probably more effective but is less well tolerated, often producing gastrointestinal side effects. Calcitonin is usually given three times a week or daily for 3 to 12 mo, followed by a rest period. Although the ability of calcitonin to prevent bone loss in postmenopausal women is well documented, the evidence that it can decrease the incidence of osteoporotic fractures is limited.[162]

Other Therapeutic Approaches

Fluoride increases bone formation and is used in the treatment of vertebral crush fractures. The incidence of vertebral fractures was not decreased in a prospective controlled trial of high-dose sodium fluoride,[173] but one study of slow-release fluoride reported a decrease in fractures in a small number of osteoporotic patients.[174]

PTH given intermittently in low doses increases bone mass in animals and can increase trabecular bone mass in humans.[175] The loss of cortical bone caused by PTH is a concern, but addition of an antiresorptive drug may prevent this problem.

Anabolic steroids such as nandrolone may increase bone as well as muscle mass. However, they have unacceptable androgenic side effects in many women[176] and are not documented to be effective in men who are not hypogonadal.

Thiazides can decrease urinary calcium excretion and may cause a positive calcium balance and increased bone mass.[177] The incidence of hip fractures may be lower in patients on thiazides, but the data are inconsistent.[178] Thiazides can be combined with amiloride to minimize potassium loss. This therapy may be appropriate in patients with hypercalciuria and osteoporosis.

Estrogen analogues such as raloxifene and droloxifene, which are agonists in bone but antagonists for the breast, prevent bone loss in experimental animals but are not approved for human use.[179, 180]

Many other therapeutic approaches are being explored. The use of growth hormone or IGF-I to stimulate bone formation is attractive but may be limited by side effects.[181]

Future Challenges in Osteoporosis

Major advances have been made in prevention, diagnosis, and treatment of osteoporosis. However, the pathogenesis of this disease is not sufficiently understood to develop a specific therapy. It is not possible to assess noninvasively the architectural abnormalities in osteoporosis that undoubtedly contribute to fragility. Laboratory and clinical studies clearly show that bone formation can be stimulated, but documentation of the efficacy of inducers of bone formation is limited. Finally, widespread application of current knowledge is limited by cost, and less expensive approaches are needed.

RICKETS AND OSTEOMALACIA

Rickets and osteomalacia are disorders of the mineralization of newly synthesized organic matrix. In adults, this involves only bone, but in children defects also occur in the growth plate and in the mineralization of cartilage, leading to characteristic deformities.

Pathogenesis

To understand the pathogenesis of rickets and osteomalacia, it is important to recognize that vitamin D is a prohormone that can be synthesized in the skin or supplied in the diet.[182] Vitamin D deficiency is usually the combined result of deficient sun exposure and decreased dietary intake. Rickets and osteomalacia can also be caused by metabolic defects in the vitamin D hormone system, including inadequate activation in the liver and kidney and abnormalities of the vitamin D receptor (see Chapter 24). Mineralization can also be impaired when the supply or transport of mineral is inadequate in renal, intestinal, or bone cell disorders.

NUTRITIONAL AND GASTROINTESTINAL DISORDERS. Inadequate vitamin D intake is relatively uncommon in the United States because many foods are supplemented with vitamin D. However, the combination of inadequate sunlight or lack of the appropriate ultraviolet wavelengths, which oc-

curs during the winter in the northern half of the United States, and failure to provide vitamin D supplements in the diet can cause rickets in infants and osteomalacia in older persons. Individuals with darker pigmentation of the skin are more prone to vitamin D deficiency because they are less efficient in converting 7-dehydrocholesterol to vitamin D. Intestinal malabsorption of fat can also cause deficiency of vitamin D and of other fat-soluble vitamins. Inability to produce adequate amounts of 25-(OH)D can occur in advanced liver disease and with use of antiepileptic drugs.

Calcium-deficiency rickets may differ from other forms of rickets and osteomalacia, particularly in adolescents, who may develop genu valgum without end-plate deformities.[183] In contrast, phosphate deficiency causes typical rickets. Because most foods contain phosphate, this form of rickets requires markedly unbalanced nutrition, such as can occur with prolonged intravenous feeding, removal of phosphate by dialysis with a low-phosphate solution, or use of aluminum-containing antacids, which bind phosphate in the intestine.[184]

RENAL DEFECTS. Impairment of 1α-hydroxylase can occur because of loss of renal mass or in renal tubular disorders such as the Fanconi syndrome. A hereditary deficiency of 1α-hydroxylase, termed *vitamin D–dependent rickets type 1* or *pseudo–vitamin D deficiency*, is a rare autosomal recessive disorder in which rickets develops during the first year of life; it responds to physiological doses of calcitriol.[185]

HEREDITARY RESISTANCE TO VITAMIN D. Families with severe rickets who have defects in the vitamin D receptor sometimes have alopecia. They may respond to high doses of calcium and phosphorus.[186]

FAMILIAL X-LINKED HYPOPHOSPHATEMIA. Originally termed vitamin D–resistant rickets, this syndrome is caused by a defect in phosphate transport. Although the most apparent abnormality is decreased renal tubular reabsorption of phosphate, phosphate transport may be impaired in other cells, particularly osteoblasts. Mutations in a gene (PEX) that shares sequence homology with endopeptidases have been found in this disorder.[187] These patients may also have some impairment in 1α-hydroxylase, and treatment involves a combination of calcitriol and phosphate.[188] However, it is difficult to achieve normal growth rates in this disorder. The condition exhibits genetic and phenotypic heterogeneity.[189] Autosomal dominant, autosomal recessive, and X-linked transmission have been described. Although most cases are familial, some severe, sporadic cases have their onset at puberty.

ONCOGENIC OSTEOMALACIA. This severe form of osteomalacia may be caused by production of an inhibitor of 1α-hydroxylase or of a phosphaturic factor[190] by fibrous and mesenchymal tumors that are often small and difficult to identify. Removal of the tumor causes rapid reversal of the osteomalacia.

HYPOPHOSPHATASIA. This rare autosomal recessive disorder is characterized by decreased production of the tissue-nonspecific (liver-bone-kidney) isoenzyme of alkaline phosphatase.[191] The clinical manifestations vary from death in utero due to severe deformities through infantile and childhood rickets to adult-onset osteomalacia. Premature loss of deciduous teeth and impaired dentition in adults are common. Levels of organic phosphate compounds such as pyridoxal 5'-phosphate in the plasma are decreased.

FLUORIDE AND BISPHOSPHONATE. High doses of sodium fluoride or of first-generation bisphosphonates such as etidronate can produce osteomalacia.[192] However, high calcium and high vitamin D intake can overcome the fluoride effect. Anticonvulsant therapy in patients with a marginal vitamin D supply can cause osteomalacia by decreasing 25-hydroxylation of vitamin D in the liver.

Clinical Features

Rickets differs from osteomalacia in that it occurs before closure of the epiphyses. Enlargement of cartilage at the

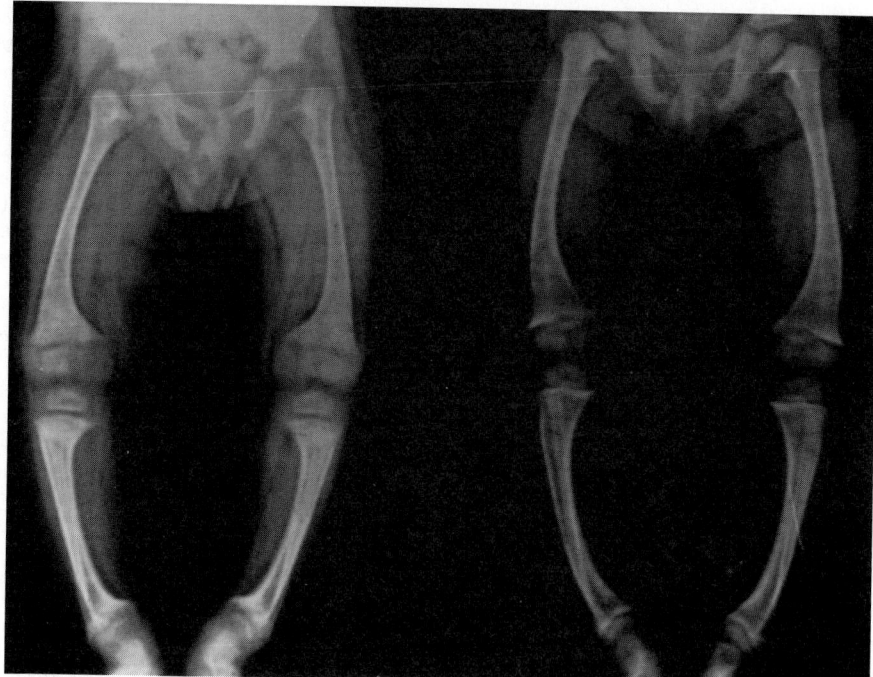

Figure 25–17. *Left,* Active rickets in a patient with tissue resistance to 1,25-(OH)₂D at age 21 mo with genu varum, irregular metaphyses, and widened growth plates. *Right,* Inactive rickets in the same patient at age 27 mo after treatment with massive doses of ergocalciferol. (From Marx SJ, Spiegel AM, Brown EM, et al. Familial syndrome of decrease in sensitivity to 1,25-hydroxyvitamin D. J Clin Endocrinol Metab 1978; 47:1303–1310. Copyright © 1978, by The Endocrine Society.)

growth plate causes the "rachitic rosary" at the costochondral junctions of the ribs and widening of the cartilaginous ends of the long bones. Impaired mineralization results in bowing of long bones. Radiologically, there is widening, cupping, and fraying of the metaphyses (Fig. 25–17). Severe vitamin D deficiency causes muscle weakness, and this weakness, combined with the deformity of the chest wall, causes an increased incidence of pneumonia. The clinical expression of osteomalacia in adults varies widely. The most common deformity is bowing of the legs, and in severe cases bone pain and weakness may cause the patient to be bedridden.

Radiographic changes include subperiosteal erosions caused by marked secondary hyperparathyroidism and a virtually pathognomonic but relatively uncommon lesion, the so-called pseudofracture (Looser zones or Milkman's syndrome) of the long bones, ribs, scapulae, or pubic rami (Fig. 25–18). Coarsening of the trabecular pattern in the spine may be present, but it is also seen in osteoporosis.

Diagnosis

Although clinical features may point to rickets or osteomalacia, the diagnosis depends on laboratory studies. The biochemical picture can vary with different pathogenic mechanisms and with different stages of disease. In infants with vitamin D deficiency, serum calcium may be low and serum phosphorus concentration may be normal initially, but as secondary hyperparathyroidism develops the calcium concentration usually returns to the low-normal range and the serum phosphorus falls further. In advanced stages, serum calcium concentration may fall again. This has been attributed to the inability of secondary hyperparathyroidism to maintain the serum calcium level when the bone surface is covered by osteoid and is resistant to attack by osteoclasts. In adults, the characteristic picture is a low-normal or slightly decreased serum calcium level, a decreased urinary calcium level, and a low serum phosphate level. Increased alkaline phosphatase levels reflect the activity of the osteoblasts, which form unmineralized matrix. PTH levels may be markedly increased. The key diagnostic test in vitamin D deficiency is demonstration of an increased serum 25-(OH)D value. 25-(OH)D levels may

also be decreased in hepatic disease or with drugs that impair 25-hydroxylase. The 1,25-(OH)₂D levels may be normal in vitamin D deficiency, presumably because of a maximal stimulation of 1α-hydroxylase by the low serum phosphorus and high PTH levels. Nevertheless, the amount of this hormone is inadequate to activate the receptors in intestine and bone. Because of the high activity of 1α-hydroxylase, administration of vitamin D to these patients causes a further increase in 1,25-(OH)₂D to supernormal levels.

Other forms of rickets and osteomalacia can be diagnosed by measuring vitamin D metabolite levels. For example, low values for 1,25-(OH)₂D and normal levels of 25-(OH)D suggest a defect in 1α-hydroxylase that may be genetic or acquired as a result of loss of renal function or tumor-induced osteomalacia. High levels of 1,25-(OH)₂D and normal levels of 25-(OH)D are seen in patients with vitamin D receptor defects. In X-linked hypophosphatemia the serum phosphorus is low and the levels of serum calcium and vitamin D metabolites are normal. If alkaline phosphatase is low, a definitive diagnosis of hypophosphatasia should be sought by measuring pyridoxal 5′-phosphate; elevated levels are relatively specific for hypophosphatasia and correlate with clinical severity.

Although the diagnosis of osteomalacia usually can be made on the basis of clinical findings and laboratory studies, a bone biopsy is sometimes needed for a definitive diagnosis. The characteristic finding is markedly widened osteoid seams and impaired mineralization with diffuse or absent tetracycline labeling. The bone also shows great variation in trabecular width and resorption lacunae from secondary hyperparathyroidism. A modest increase in osteoid width can occur in a high turnover state, such as hyperparathyroidism, thyrotoxicosis, or Paget's disease; however, tetracycline labeling shows a normal mineralization front in these conditions.

Therapy

Vitamin D is effective in the treatment of nutritional and malabsorptive rickets and osteomalacia.[193] High doses (50,000 to 100,000 U/day) may be given for a few days, but it is important not to overtreat patients, because vitamin D is stored in the fat and excessive amounts can cause hypercalce-

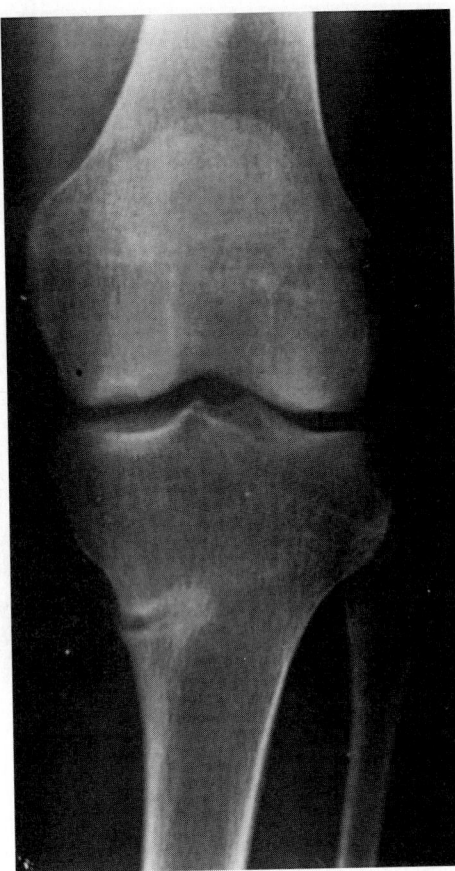

Figure 25–18. Active osteomalacia in a patient (a sibling of the patient in Fig. 25–17) with hereditary tissue resistance to 1,25-(OH)₂D at age 18 with pseudofracture of the left tibia. (From Marx SJ, Spiegel AM, Brown EM, et al. Familial syndrome of decrease in sensitivity to 1,25-hydroxyvitamin D. J Clin Endocrinol Metab 1978; 47:1303–1310. Copyright © 1978, by The Endocrine Society.)

mia and hypercalciuria. Monitoring of urinary calcium excretion is useful to determine when the vitamin D dose should be decreased. Patients with malabsorption may require large doses, parenteral vitamin D, or calcidiol, which is absorbed even by patients with impaired fat absorption. Patients with defects in 1α-hydroxylase can be treated with calcitriol. If the cause is tumor-induced osteomalacia, the treatment is to find and remove the lesion. Severe defects in the vitamin D receptor are most difficult to treat. Massive does of calcium and phosphorus have been given to these patients, but normal growth is rarely achieved. Similarly, normal growth may not occur despite repletion of phosphorus and administration of calcitriol in patients with X-linked hypophosphatemia, although bone mineralization can be restored.[188] Careful monitoring of levels of calcium, phosphorus, and vitamin D metabolites is important to prevent impairment of renal function. At present, there is no effective therapy for hypophosphatasia.[191]

HYPERPARATHYROID BONE DISEASE

Early severe cases of primary hyperparathyroidism showed "osteitis fibrosa cystica generalisata," manifested by generalized bone loss with increased bone resorption, including both subperiosteal and endosteal surfaces.[194] The formation of fibrotic cystic lesions in the long bones and jaw (called brown tumors) caused swelling, pathologic fractures, and bone pain. This bone disease is now rarely seen in primary hyperparathy-

roidism but may occur in poorly managed secondary hyperparathyroidism. With the common forms of hyperparathyroidism,[195] the major finding is an increased rate of remodeling in bone. Bone mass is decreased in the cortex, largely because of endosteal resorption, but trabecular bone is preserved.[196] Bone density is low in the cortical bone of the radius, but bone density in the metaphyses and vertebrae, which represent largely trabecular bone, is normal or only moderately decreased.[197, 198] Patients with mild to moderate disease do not have progressive bone loss,[198] but when these patients are cured surgically, bone density in the spine can increase by as much as 15%,[199] even in postmenopausal women who are at the highest risk for fracture. Bone density also increases in the radius and hip. Moreover, bone loss is attenuated in postmenopausal women with hypoparathyroidism.[200] Based on these results, patients with primary hyperparathyroidism and low levels of bone density who are at risk for fractures are candidates for parathyroid surgery.

RENAL OSTEODYSTROPHY

In view of the central role of the kidney in regulating mineral metabolism, it is not surprising that patients with chronic renal failure frequently develop skeletal abnormalities.[201] In renal failure, the decreased capacity to synthesize 1,25-(OH)₂D and to excrete phosphate causes secondary hyperparathyroidism. This results from the lowering of serum calcium by phosphate, the impairment of calcium absorption in the intestine, and the loss of the feedback inhibitory effect of 1,25-(OH)₂D on PTH production. The increased secretion of PTH ultimately leads to osteitis fibrosis cystica. Development of bone disease can be slowed or prevented by phosphate restriction or by treatment with phosphate binders and calcitriol. In the past, aluminum hydroxide was used to bind phosphate, a therapy that sometimes caused aluminum-induced adynamic bone disease.[202] This condition is less common with the use of calcium salts to decrease phosphate absorption, but low-turnover bone disease still occurs, particularly in patients in whom secondary hyperparathyroidism has been reversed. Osteomalacia can occur in patients on dialysis if they have an inadequate supply of vitamin D and calcium, but this is unusual.

Renal osteodystrophy causes growth retardation and skeletal deformities in children, and both children and adults have bone pain and muscle weakness. Soft-tissue calcifications are particularly dangerous when they occur in blood vessels and lead to ischemia and gangrene. Calcification may be the result of a high calcium-phosphorus product and of vessel wall changes secondary to renal failure or direct effects of PTH. To prevent calcification, it is important to avoid a high serum calcium-phosphorus ion product and to minimize secondary hyperparathyroidism.

The diagnosis of a specific form of renal osteodystrophy can often be made on biochemical grounds. Levels of PTH are very high in patients with severe secondary hyperparathyroidism. Plasma aluminum levels may be elevated in patients with aluminum-induced osteodystrophy but do not necessarily reflect the stores in bone. Deferoxamine chelates aluminum, and this agent can be used to measure the body burden and to treat aluminum overload. The interpretation of biochemical markers of bone turnover is difficult in renal disease because their clearance may be altered.

A bone biopsy may clarify the pathogenesis of renal osteodystrophy.[203] Using double tetracycline labeling, it is possible to determine whether mineralization is impaired. Sections that have not been decalcified show the extent of osteoid seams and resorption surfaces. Aluminum can be identified by special stains. Amyloid deposits, which consist largely of B_2-microglobulin, may be seen in the bone. Amyloidosis of the bone is associated with cystic lesions but not necessarily with bone pain.

The treatment of renal osteodystrophy can be highly successful if it is correctly focused on specific pathogenetic mechanisms. The goal should be to maintain normal serum calcium and phosphorus levels and minimize exposure to aluminum. Phosphate restriction should be instituted relatively early in renal failure, but diets low in phosphorus are difficult to achieve. Therefore, after the filtration rate is reduced below 25% of normal, it is usually necessary to administer phosphate-binding salts such as calcium carbonate, calcium acetate, or calcium citrate.[204] The ability of citrate to increase aluminum absorption is a concern. Correction of acidosis is also important in preventing bone disease.[205]

Early in renal failure, modest supplementation with vitamin D may be sufficient to maintain 1,25-$(OH)_2$D levels, but eventually calcitriol itself should be administered.[206] Low doses (0.25 to 0.5 μg/day) are well tolerated, but higher doses can lead to hypercalcemia. In severe secondary hyperparathyroidism, low doses are often not sufficient to suppress PTH secretion, and intravenous calcitriol may be used.[206] In some, parathyroidectomy may be required. Persistent hypercalcemia in patients with renal failure, intractable pruritus, extracellular calcifications, and severe skeletal lesions are all indications for surgery. However, parathyroidectomy should be avoided in patients with aluminum-induced bone disease, because symptoms may be worsened.

Renal transplantation corrects many of the biochemical disturbances that lead to renal osteodystrophy, but bone disease may persist.[207] Usually secondary hyperparathyroidism slowly resolves, but patients with persistent hypercalcemia or autonomy of the parathyroid glands (tertiary hyperparathyroidism) may require surgery. A major concern, particularly in older patients, is progressive osteoporosis; glucocorticoids and immunosuppressants aggravate bone loss in these patients. Finally, osteonecrosis or avascular necrosis, particularly of the proximal femur, is common after renal transplantation.

PAGET'S DISEASE

Paget's disease may affect as many as 3% of adults older than 40 years of age; it is often asymptomatic and usually progresses slowly.[208]

Pathogenesis

The primary abnormality in Paget's disease is the localized, uncontrolled formation of large, highly active osteoclasts. The initial lesion is an increase in bone resorption. The response to this resorption, particularly in bones that are subject to mechanical force, is an intense but chaotic increase in osteoblastic activity. The characteristic histologic appearance is of focal lesions with many giant osteoclasts and active osteoblasts. The bone that forms in the lesions is disorganized and has a mosaic pattern with loss of the usual lamellar structure. The marrow shows a pattern of fibrosis and increased vascularity.[209]

The concept of a viral origin for Paget's disease is based on the finding of nuclear inclusion bodies in osteoclasts (Fig. 25–19) and the detection of viral transcripts in hematopoietic cells from patients with the disease. Several paramyxoviruses have been suggested, including measles and canine distemper virus.[210] However, further work is needed to establish pathogenetic links between viral sequences and production of abnormal osteoclasts. Pagetic osteoclasts differ from normal osteo-

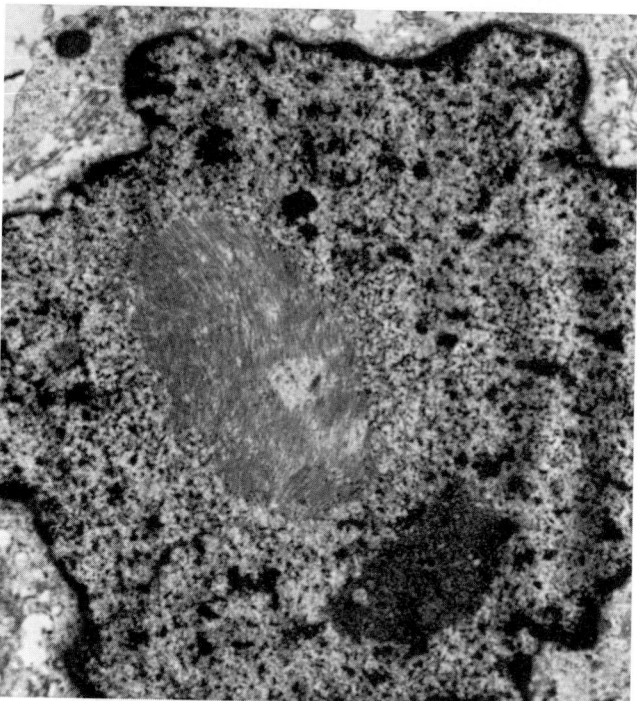

Figure 25–19. Electron micrograph of an osteoclast nucleus from a patient with Paget's disease showing characteristic intranuclear inclusion (consisting of 125-Å diameter microfilaments). Decalcified bone magnified × 32,400. (Courtesy of Dr. Barbara G. Mills and Dr. Frederick R. Singer.)

clasts not only by their greater size and the presence of viral inclusions but also because they express IL-6, which may play a role in pathogenesis.[211]

There may also be a genetic component to Paget's disease.[212] As many as 15 to 30% of patients have a positive family history, and the first-degree relatives of patients with Paget's disease have a sevenfold greater relative risk of having the disorder than individuals with no affected relatives. There is also an ethnic and geographic clustering. The incidence is high in some areas of northern Europe, particularly in northern England, but low in Norway and Sweden.

Clinical Features

Paget's disease affects men and women almost equally, but men tend to be more symptomatic. The disease usually is not clinically apparent until age 50 to 60. It usually progresses slowly and does not develop in new sites. Many different bones can be affected, and the lesions can vary from single, monostotic lesions to involvement of almost the entire skeleton. The pelvis, femur, spine, skull, and tibia are most commonly involved, whereas hands and feet are rarely affected.

Paget's disease is often discovered in asymptomatic patients because of an elevated serum alkaline phosphatase measurement obtained on routine screening or because of a radiograph taken for an unrelated problem. The most common symptom is bone pain at the site of pagetic involvement. Pain also commonly occurs in adjacent joints as a result of secondary degenerative arthritis. Bowing of the legs is common (Fig. 25–20), and pathologic fractures can occur. Vertebral involvement can cause kyphosis and compression of the spinal cord. Neural changes can also result from vascular steal because of the high blood flow to the lesion. The most common consequence of Paget's disease of the skull is hearing loss, which can be both conductive and neurosensory. Extensive involvement of the base of the skull can produce basilar impression

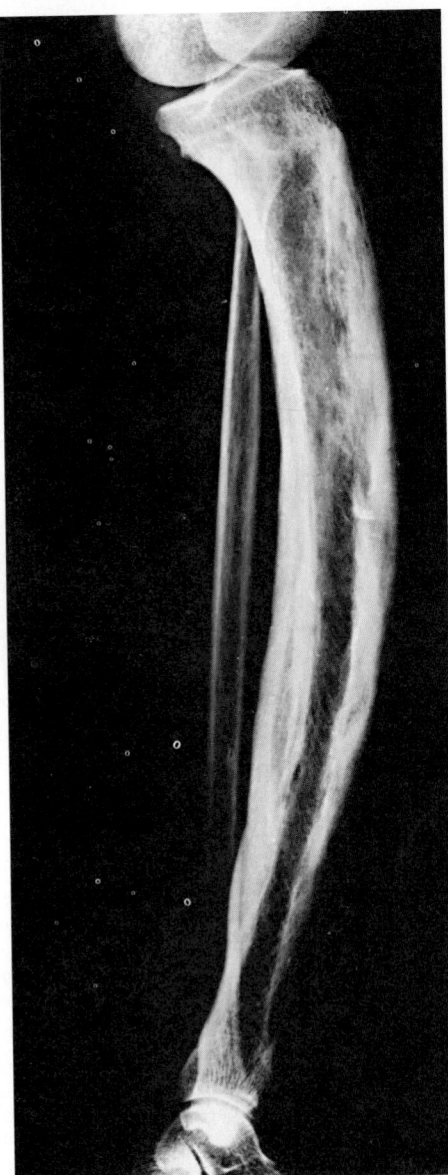

Figure 25–20. Paget's disease of the tibia. Note the bowing, marked irregularity of the anterior cortex, and "flame-shaped" lytic lesion of the posterior cortex. (Courtesy of Dr. Ethel S. Siris.)

and, rarely, brain stem compression (Fig. 25–21). Facial and skull deformities and dental problems are common.

The incidence of osteosarcoma is increased but is less than 1%. When it does occur, it is highly malignant, and most patients do not live longer than 1 to 3 years. Fibrosarcomas, chondrosarcomas and benign giant cell tumors are also occasionally seen. The giant cell tumors, termed *reparative granulomas,* may represent an extension of pagetic tissue outside the skeleton. These tumors are sensitive to antipagetic therapy and may also respond to glucocorticoids.

Patients with Paget's disease may have an increased incidence of primary hyperparathyroidism. Angioid streaks are often seen in the fundus. Pseudogout, gout, and osteoarthritis occur. Patients with heart disease may show worsening of heart failure, which has been attributed to the increase in blood flow in pagetic lesions.

Diagnosis

As noted previously, the diagnosis of Paget's disease may be made by the finding of an elevated alkaline phosphatase

concentration or after a routine radiograph. In older persons with deformities or bone pain, the diagnosis should be considered, and a careful family history and review of the musculoskeletal system by both history and physical examination should be obtained. A bone scan should be carried out to localize possible pagetic sites. Positive scans do not necessarily indicate Paget's disease, and radiographs should be obtained to confirm that Paget's disease is the cause of the increased uptake. Rarely, pagetic sites in bone are not evident by bone scan because there is a minimal formation response in the lesion. Pagetic lesions in the skull are termed *osteoporosis circumscripta.* An audiogram should be obtained in patients with involvement of the petrous bone or complaints of hearing loss. Because of the high incidence of hyperparathyroidism, ionized calcium levels should be measured in the initial workup. Monostotic Paget's disease, particularly in the vertebrae, may be difficult to distinguish from metastatic disease. In addition, some patients with vertebral disease may have impingement on the spinal canal. In these individuals, the area should be examined by CT or MRI. Bone biopsies can be useful in atypical cases. An ordinary aspiration biopsy sometimes yields the giant osteoclasts that are pathognomonic of Paget's disease. Samples of bone that show the irregular "marble bone" pattern can also be diagnostic.

After the initial work-up has been completed, the patient can usually be monitored biochemically by serial measurements of total alkaline phosphatase and urinary hydroxyproline. Although 24-h urine measurements of hydroxyproline are often recommended, a morning fasting measurement avoids the dual problems of collecting a 24-h sample and maintaining a diet free from gelatin products. The newer markers, including bone-specific alkaline phosphatase and collagen cross-links in the urine, offer no advantage in Paget's disease.[213]

Therapy

In the past, patients with Paget's disease were often simply observed until symptoms were clear-cut or there was evidence of progression in critical areas of the skeleton. With the newer bisphosphonates, treatment is instituted earlier. Pamidronate is available for intravenous use, and a single infusion of 60 mg

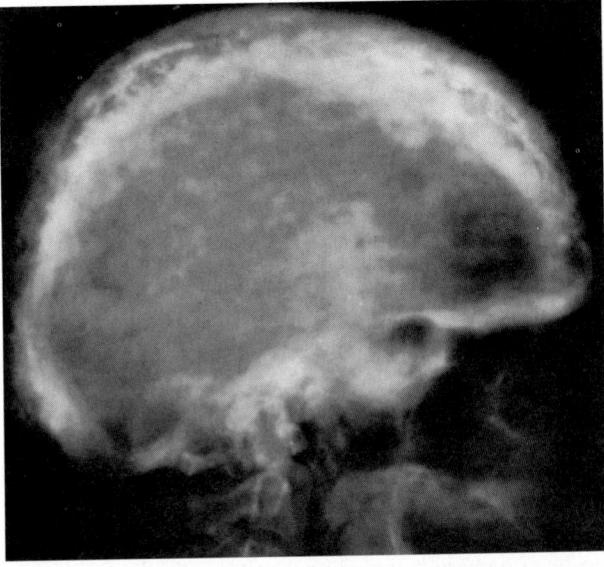

Figure 25–21. Radiograph of the skull in a patient with advanced Paget's disease showing thickening, disordered new bone formation (cotton-wool patches), and basilar impression. (From Singer FR. Paget's Disease of Bone. New York: Plenum, 1977.)

of pamidronate can produce remission for 6 mo or longer in mild or limited Paget's disease. Patients with more extensive disease require multiple doses. Intravenous pamidronate is generally safe, although transient fever and a transient increase in bone pain may occur. Rare idiosyncratic reactions include uveitis. Other bisphosphonates are given orally. Alendronate (40 mg/day) is approved in the United States, and risedronate and tiludronate are undergoing clinical trials. These treatments may replace therapy with calcitonin, etidronate, or plicamycin. All of these agents act by inhibiting osteoclastic activity, so the earliest indication of therapeutic response is a drop in resorption markers, followed by a decrease in alkaline phosphatase levels.

The indications for treatment are pain that can be attributed to Paget's disease and deformities that might produce neurologic changes or are likely to lead to fracture, such as the osteolytic "flame" or "blade of grass" lesions in weight-bearing bones (see Fig. 25–20). Hearing loss may be an indication for therapy, although most patients do not show major improvement. Patients with heart disease and extensive Paget's disease should be treated in the hope that decreased pagetic activity will improve management. With the advent of safe and effective therapy, patients with mild to moderate disease, particularly those with the potential for complications (i.e., those with lesions in weight-bearing bone, the vertebral bodies, or the base of the skull), are being treated before symptoms develop. Early treatment is logical in young patients with Paget's disease to prevent progression if possible.

Many patients with Paget's disease have pain from joint damage that does not respond to antipagetic therapy. These patients may respond to anti-inflammatory drugs. If osteoarthritis is advanced, knee and hip replacement may be appropriate, but biochemical remission should be obtained before surgery. A high calcium intake may be useful in Paget's disease. Bisphosphonate therapy can lower the serum calcium level and cause secondary hyperparathyroidism, which is probably not advantageous; increased calcium intake may prevent this development. Moreover, calcium loading can produce an increase in endogenous calcitonin secretion that may have beneficial effects. However, the urine calcium should be checked before calcium supplementation is given, because an increase in the incidence of renal stones has been reported in pagetic patients.

Hereditary Hyperphosphatasia

Although hereditary hyperphosphatasia has been termed juvenile Paget's disease, it involves all of the skeleton and develops in infants.[214] The serum alkaline phosphatase levels are very high. There are severe bony deformities, and the histologic appearance resembles that of Paget's disease with high bone turnover, although the osteoclasts are not enlarged. Treatment with bisphosphonates or calcitonin may be effective in reducing bone turnover and improving bone lesions.

OSTEOGENESIS IMPERFECTA

Osteogenesis imperfecta, or brittle bone disease, is a heterogenous, congenital disorder in which increased bone fragility leads to fractures and deformity.[215] It ranges in severity from a lethal perinatal form to a mild disorder that results only in increased fractures.

Pathogenesis

Most patients with osteogenesis imperfecta have defects in the genes for type I collagen. Bones, ligaments, skin, sclerae, and teeth are affected. The incidence of osteogenesis imperfecta is estimated at 1 in 200,000 to 500,000. The heterogeneity of the features is caused by the variety of genetic defects, although phenotypic variation occurs even with the same genetic abnormality (Table 25–5). The more severe forms, types II and III, involve mutations in the helical portion of the collagen molecule that prevent normal assembly and produce unstable triple helices. Point mutations in this portion of the collagen gene can be associated with mild disease (type IV). Type I osteogenesis imperfecta differs from the other forms in that there is usually a deletion of one allele of the α1(I) procollagen gene, resulting in decreased collagen production but a normal molecular structure.[216] This disorder is of particular interest because familial osteoporosis may also exhibit such defects.[217]

Classification and Clinical Features

The classification devised by Sillence and modified by Byers[215] is summarized in Table 25–5. In addition to the bone involvement, there may also be ligament laxity, joint hypermobility, and easy bruising. Dentin formation is often abnormal, and the teeth are fragile and discolored. Blue sclerae are a variable manifestation and do not correlate with severity. Because of the thoracic deformities, patients with severe manifestations are predisposed to pulmonary infections and usually have a shortened life span. Intelligence is not affected, and individuals with marked deformities can be highly productive if appropriate conditions are provided.

TABLE 25–5. Classification of Osteogenesis Imperfecta

Type	Clinical Features	Inheritance	Common Biochemical Abnormality
I	Normal stature, little or no deformity, blue sclerae, hearing loss in 50% of families. Dentinogenesis imperfecta may distingush a subset.	AD	Nonfunctional allele of the α1(I) procollagen gene (COL1A1)
II	Lethal in the perinatal period; minimal calvarial mineralization, beaded ribs, compressed femurs, marked long bone deformity, platyspondyly	AD (new mutations) AR (rare)	Substitution of glycine in triple helix of COL1A1 or COL1A2
III	Progressively deforming bones, usually with moderate deformity at birth. Scleral hue varies, often lightening with age. Dentinogenesis imperfecta common, hearing loss common. Stature very short.	AD AR (uncommon)	Substitution of glycine in triple helix of COL1A1 or COL1A2
IV	Normal sclerae, mild to moderate bone deformity and variable short stature; dentinogenesis imperfecta is common and hearing loss occurs in some families.	AD	Substitution of glycine in triple helix of COL1A1 or COL1A2. Exon-skipping in COL1A2

AD, autosomal dominant; AR autosomal recessive.
Classification from Sillence et al. as modified from Byers PH. Osteogenesis imperfecta. In: Royce PM, Steinman B, eds. Connective Tissue and Its Heritable Disorders: Molecular, Genetic and Medical Aspects. New York: Wiley-Liss, 1993: 317–350. Reprinted by permission of Wiley-Liss, Inc., a subsidiary of John Wiley & Sons, Inc.

Diagnosis

The clinical features make the diagnosis relatively straightforward in patients with moderate to severe disease, but in the milder forms the diagnosis may be missed. In children without deformities, multiple fractures are usually attributed to trauma, and in infants this may lead to an accusation of parental abuse. In the absence of typical clinical features, the diagnosis can be made only biochemically. Culture of fibroblasts from skin biopsies and analysis of the collagen by gel electrophoresis can point to a defect, and the techniques of molecular biology can identify the mutation more specifically. This analysis is useful for families, because specific DNA polymorphisms may allow for prenatal diagnosis if the mutation has already been identified in other affected family members.

In children and adolescents with multiple fractures but no deformity, measurements of bone density and turnover may point toward the diagnosis. In the type I disorder both bone density and serum type I procollagen peptide levels are likely to be decreased.[218] However, because excretion of collagen cross-links is increased in all types of osteogenesis imperfecta, increased bone resorption may play a role in pathogenesis.[219]

Therapy

There is no established therapy for osteogenesis imperfecta. Supportive treatment is important. The Osteogenesis Imperfecta Foundation works with patients and families to improve the quality of life. Orthopedic and rehabilitation services can be helpful in dealing with deformities. Genetic counseling and prenatal diagnosis, including ultrasound examination and testing for informative DNA polymorphisms, are important for the family. Antiresorptive treatment with calcitonin and bisphosphonates has been used, but there are no controlled trials. Gene therapy is now being explored.[220]

Other Connective Tissue Disorders Affecting the Skeleton

Other inherited disorders of connective tissue with impairment of skeletal development or increased bone fragility include Ehlers-Danlos syndrome, Menkes' disease, lysinuric protein intolerance, and homocystinuria.[221–224] In these disorders abnormalities of collagen cross-linking can affect bone and other connective tissues. In Ehlers-Danlos syndrome the cross-linking enzyme lysyl oxidase is deficient, and in Menkes' disease copper deficiency impairs the function of the enzyme. Lysinuric protein intolerance and homocystinuria probably also impair cross-linking of collagen.

OSTEOPETROSIS

Osteopetrosis, also termed Albers-Schönberg or marble bone disease is a heterogeneous group of disorders characterized by an increase in bone density.[226, 227] Most cases are inherited and involve a defect in bone resorption. Acquired osteopetrosis occurs in fluorosis,[228] and a localized form is seen in certain metastatic malignancies, particularly cancers of the prostate and breast. Osteopetrotic rats and mice with specific defects in osteoclasts have been found as a result of spontaneous mutations and developed using gene knock-out techniques. The *op/op* mouse has a genetic defect in the production of M-CSF that results in failure of osteoclast formation[229] and that can be corrected by treatment with M-CSF. Knockouts of the proto-oncogenes *c-src* and *c-fos* also cause osteopetrosis.[230, 231] In *c-src* deficiency, osteoclasts are present but

nonfunctional, and in *c-fos* deficiency osteoclasts are not formed. Similar mutations may cause human osteopetrosis, but the only specific genetic cause identified in humans is carbonic anhydrase type II deficiency.[232]

Infantile Osteopetrosis

Infantile osteopetrosis is a rare, autosomal recessive disorder in which failure to resorb bone and calcified metaphyseal cartilage causes near-obliteration of the marrow spaces. Extramedullary hematopoiesis occurs in the liver and spleen. The cranial nerve foramina do not form normally, causing optic atrophy and other cranial nerve defects. The bones, although dense, are brittle, and pathologic fractures can occur. The impaired function of the hematopoietic system causes death in the first decade from hemorrhage or infection. Based on studies in animal models in which transfer of hematopoietic tissue resulted in cure, patients have been treated with total body radiation and grafting of marrow from HLA-identical donors (Fig. 25–22). When suitable donors cannot be found, therapy with high doses of calcitriol or interferon γ has improved bone resorption.[233]

Carbonic Anhydrase II Deficiency

Carbonic anhydrase II deficiency, a nonlethal autosomal recessive disorder, is associated with a complete deficiency of the type II carbonic anhydrase that provides carbonic acid for hydrogen ion secretion by osteoclasts and by the distal tubules. Hence, osteopetrosis is accompanied by renal tubular acidosis that may involve both distal and proximal lesions.[232] Affected individuals are shorter than their siblings and may develop calcification of the basal ganglia.

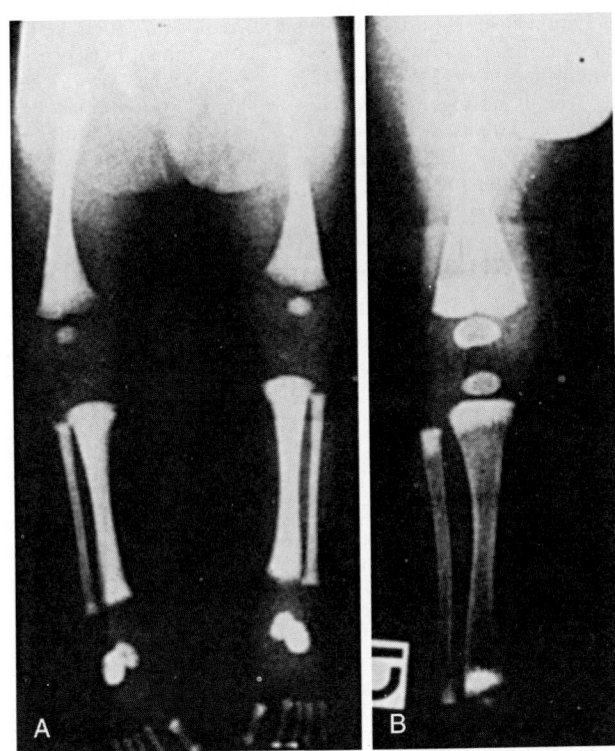

Figure 25–22. Radiographs of the lower limb in a patient with osteopetrosis (A) at age 2 mo before a bone marrow transplant and (B) at age 9 mo, after transplantation, showing formation of normal medullary bone. (From Ballet JJ, Griscelli C. Lymphoid cell transplantation in human osteopetrosis. In: Horton JE, Tarpley TM, Davis WF, eds. Mechanisms of localized bone loss. [A Special Supplement of Calcified Tissue Abstracts]. J London: IRI., 1978: 399–414, by permission of Oxford University Press.)

Other Forms of Osteopetrosis

Mild to moderate osteopetrosis has been described in familial and isolated cases. Two familial autosomal dominant forms have different defects in osteoclast function.[234] In one type, there is diffuse osteosclerosis and a decrease in the number and size of osteoclasts. In the other type, generalized osteosclerosis is also present, but there is an increased number of large osteoclasts that appear to be functionally defective.

FIBROUS DYSPLASIA

Fibrous dysplasia is characterized by expanding lesions within the bone that contain both fibroblastic and osteoblastic elements.[235] The disorder can occur as a monostotic lesion without any associated abnormalities or in a polyostotic form as part of the McCune-Albright syndrome, which is associated with functional abnormalities of one or more endocrine glands and irregular hyperpigmented macules called café au lait spots. The most common endocrine manifestation is precocious puberty, particularly in girls (see Chapter 31). The molecular defect in the McCune-Albright syndrome is somatic mosaicism for an activating mutation of the $G_{\alpha s}$ subunit of the nucleotide-binding regulatory protein that couples receptors to adenylyl cyclase.[236] The bone lesions may show increased expression of the c-*fos* oncogene.[237]

Monostotic fibrous dysplasia is usually diagnosed in the second or third decade of life as an expanding bone lesion that can cause fracture, deformity, or nerve entrapment. Sarcomatous degeneration can occur. In polyostotic fibrous dysplasia any skeletal site can be affected, but the femur, tibia, ribs, and face are most often involved. Histologically, the lesions contain many spindle-shaped fibroblasts and islands of woven bone. Bone lesions can worsen during pregnancy, and estrogen receptors have been identified in the bone lesions of patients with McCune-Albright syndrome.[238]

The course of both monostotic and polyostotic fibrous dysplasia is variable. Patients who show progression, nerve compression, or pathologic fractures may require surgery. Careful assessment of the endocrine system is critical in the McCune-Albright syndrome, because early intervention can prevent irreversible changes resulting from precocious puberty. The bone lesions may respond to bisphosphonate.[239]

SCLEROSING BONE DYSPLASIAS

A number of rare, congenital skeletal disorders cause irregular bone structure and varying degrees of sclerosis.[226, 240]

Pycnodysostosis

Pycnodysostosis is an autosomal recessive disorder characterized by short stature, a large cranium, and small facies.[241] Unlike patients with osteopetrosis, these patients do not have loss of the marrow cavity and are not anemic. Histologically, trabecular bone volume is increased despite an increase in the number of osteoclasts, suggesting a defect in osteoclast function.

Progressive Diaphyseal Dysplasia[242]

This disorder, known as Camurati-Engelmann disease, consists of patchy thickening of the bone on both periosteal and endosteal surfaces and is associated with gait abnormalities and muscle wasting. The histologic picture is one of in-

creased bone formation rather than decreased resorption. Glucocorticoid therapy relieves bone pain and reverses the histologic abnormalities in some cases.

Endosteal Hyperostosis

The term van Buchem's disease is applied to both severe and mild forms of hyperostosis.[240] The disorder begins in infancy, and progressive enlargement of the jaw commences at puberty. Some subjects have cranial nerve deficits caused by impingement of the foramina. This disorder may be related to sclerosteosis, in which there is also syndactyly. Subjects with both disorders are usually tall and heavy.

Other Disorders[226]

Unusual disorders that affect bone structure include osteopoikilosis, which is characterized by many small foci of sclerosis in cancellous bone; osteopathia striata, in which there are linear striations of the ends of the long bones; and melorheostosis, in which patchy areas of hyperostosis affect both the cortex and the medullary canal, sometimes associated with thickening of the overlying skin. Mixed pictures involving several different forms of sclerosis have been described.

Axial osteomalacia and fibrogenesis imperfecta ossium[226] are rare disorders characterized by a coarse and dense appearance of trabecular bone. These disorders may be forms of osteomalacia because they show defective mineralization, presumably because of a defect in the matrix produced by osteoblasts.

Pachydermoperiostosis is a disorder characterized by periostitis, sclerosis of the distal portions of the tubular bones, and thickening of the skin.[243] It is also termed primary hypertrophic osteoarthropathy and must be distinguished from the secondary hypertrophic osteoarthropathy that occurs in patients with chronic pulmonary disease.

Infantile cortical hyperostosis is characterized by overgrowth of cortical bone. The similarity of this disorder to the changes seen after prolonged infusion of PGE_1 in neonates has suggested a possible cause, and the disorder has been treated with glucocorticoids and nonsteroidal anti-inflammatory drugs.[244, 245]

EXTRASKELETAL CALCIFICATION AND OSSIFICATION

Mineral deposition in soft tissues is a common consequence of tissue damage and of a local elevation in extracellular calcium-phosphate product. Ectopic bone formation can occur at sites of injury or surgical trauma and may be related to the presence of an inductive protein matrix. This form of bone induction stimulated the search for bone morphogenetic proteins. The frequency of ossification after hip replacement can be decreased by treatment with nonsteroidal anti-inflammatory drugs that inhibit prostaglandin synthesis or by local irradiation. Extensive subcutaneous calcium deposition may be crippling in inflammatory disorders such as dermatomyositis. The term *myositis ossificans* is used when bone formation occurs in traumatized muscle, but similar masses can be formed in tendon, ligaments, joint capsules, and fascia without trauma.[246]

Tumoral Calcinosis

Tumoral calcinosis is an inherited disorder characterized by periarticular calcification and hyperphosphatemia.[247] It is associated with defective phosphate transport and sometimes with excessive activity of renal 1α-hydroxylase. The primary disorder must be differentiated from secondary tumoral calcinosis, which occurs in association with renal failure and with hypercalcemic disorders. Treatment by phosphate depletion using phosphate-binding antacids or diuretics[248] and with calcitonin to reduce serum calcium and phosphorus has been attempted.

Fibrodysplasia Ossificans Progressiva

This rare congenital disorder is most often sporadic but can be transmitted as an autosomal dominant disorder.[249] Characteristic short phalanges and soft tissue swelling can be detected at birth. Painful, tender lesions caused by true ectopic bone can develop in connective tissues. Progressive deformities may include scoliosis and ankylosis of the spine and rib cage. This disorder may be caused by ectopic expression of a bone morphogenetic protein. There is no known therapy.

REFERENCES

1. Raisz LG, Shoukri KC. Pathogenesis of osteoporosis. In: Mundy GR, Martin TJ, eds. Physiology and Pharmacology of Bone. New York: Springer-Verlag, 1993: 299–323.
2. Baron R. Anatomy and ultrastructure of bone. In: Favus MJ, ed. Primer on the Metabolic Bone Diseases and Disorders of Mineral Metabolism. 2nd ed. New York: Lippincott, Raven, 1993: 3–9.
3. Termine JD. Bone matrix proteins and the mineralization process. In: Favus MJ, ed. Primer on the Metabolic Bone Diseases and Disorders of Mineral Metabolism. 2nd ed. New York: Lippincott, Raven, 1993: 21–25.
4. Boivin G, Grousson B, Meunier PJ. X-ray microanalysis of fluoride distribution in microfracture calluses in cancellous iliac bone from osteoporosis patients treated with fluoride and untreated. J Bone Miner Res 1991; 6:1183–1190.
5. Anderson HC. Molecular biology of matrix vesicles. Clin Orthop 1995; 314:266–280.
6. Raisz LG, Kream BE. Regulation of bone formation, part 2. N Engl J Med 1983; 309:83–89.
7. Friedenstein AJ. Marrow stromal fibroblasts. Calcif Tissue Int 1995; 56(Suppl 1):S17.
8. Aarden EM, Burger EH, Nijweide PJ. Function of osteocytes in bone. J Cell Biochem 1994; 55:287–299.
9. Klein-Nulend J, van der Plas A, Semeins CM, et al. Sensitivity of osteocytes to biomechanical stress in vitro. FASEB J 1995; 9:441–445.
10. Suda T, Takahashi N, Martin TJ. Modulation of osteoclast differentiation: update 1995. Endocr Rev 1995; 4:266–270.
11. Grooth RD, Mieremet RHP, Haas EWKD, et al. Murine macrophage precursor cell lines are unable to differentiate into osteoclasts: a possible implication for osteoclast ontogeny. Int J Exp Pathol 1994; 75:265–275.
12. Ravesloot JH, Eisen T, Baron R, et al. Role of Na-H exchangers and vacuolar H+ pumps in intracellular pH regulation in neonatal rat osteoclasts. J Gen Physiol 1995; 105:177–208.
13. Delaisse JM, Eeckhout Y, Neff L, et al. (Pro)collagenase (matrix metalloproteinase-1) is present in rodent osteoclasts and in the underlying bone-resorbing compartment. J Cell Sci 1993; 106:1071–1082.
14. Parfitt AM. Osteonal and hemi-osteonal remodeling: the spatial and temporal framework for signal traffic in adult human bone. J Cell Biochem 1994; 55:273–286.
15. Eriksen EF. Normal and pathological remodeling of human trabecular bone: three-dimensional reconstruction of the remodeling sequence in normals and in metabolic bone disease. Endocr Rev 1986; 7:379–408.
16. Burr DB. Remodeling and the repair of fatigue damage. Calcif Tissue Int 1993; 53(Suppl 1):S75–S80.
17. Raisz LG. Bone resorption in tissue culture: factors influencing the response to parathyroid hormone. J Clin Invest 1965; 44:103–116.
18. Dempster DW, Cosman F, Parisien M, et al. Anabolic actions of parathyroid hormone on bone. Endocr Rev 1994; 15:261.
19. Raisz LG. Recent advances in bone cell biology: interactions of vitamin D with other local and systemic factors. Bone Miner 1990; 9:191–197.
20. Martin TJ, Findlay DM, Houssami S, et al. Heterogeneity of the calcitonin receptor: functional aspects in osteoclasts and other sites. J Nutr 1995; 125(Suppl 7):2009S–2014S.
21. Hurley DL, Tiegs RD, Wahner HW, et al. Axial and appendicular bone mineral density in patients with long-term deficiency or excess of calcitonin. N Engl J Med 1987; 317:537–541.
22. Eriksen EF, Kudsk H, Emmertsen K, et al. Bone remodeling during calcitonin excess: reconstruction of the remodeling sequence in medullary thyroid carcinoma. Bone 1993; 14:399–401.
23. Beshyah SA, Kyd P, Thomas E, et al. The effects of prolonged growth hormone replacement on bone metabolism and bone mineral density in hypopituitary adults. Clin Endocrinol 1995; 42:249–254.
24. Lukert BP, Raisz LG. Glucocorticoid-induced osteoporosis. Rheum Dis Clin North Am 1994; 20:629–650.
25. Baran DT, Braverman LE. Thyroid hormones and bone mass. J Clin Endocrinol Metab 1991; 72:1182–1183.
26. Bouillon R, Bex M, Van Herck E, et al. Influence of age, sex, and insulin on osteoblast function: osteoblast dysfunction in diabetes mellitus. J Clin Endocrinol Metab 1995; 80:1194–1202.
27. Benz DJ, Haussler MR, Komm BS. Estrogen binding and estrogenic responses in normal human osteoblast-like cells. J Bone Miner Res 1991; 6:531–541.
28. Smith EP, Boyd J, Frank GR, et al. Estrogen resistence caused by a mutation in the estrogen-receptor gene in a man. N Engl J Med 1994; 331:1056–1061.
29. Horowitz MC. Cytokines and estrogen in bone: anti-osteoporotic effects. Science 1993; 260:626–627.
30. Bellido T, Jilka RL, Boyce BF, et al. Regulation of interleukin-6, osteoclastogenesis, and bone mass by androgens: the role of the androgen receptor. J Clin Invest 1995; 95:2886–2895.
31. Manolagas SC, Jilka RL. Bone marrow, cytokines, and bone remodeling: emerging insights into the pathophysiology of osteoporosis. N Engl J Med 1995; 332:305–311.
32. Vanderschueren D, Bouillon R. Androgens and bone. Calcif Tissue Int 1995; 56:341–346.
33. Raisz LG. Local and systemic factors in the pathogenesis of osteoporosis. N Engl J Med 1988; 318:818–827.
34. Lorenzo JA. The role of cytokines in the regulation of local bone resorption. Crit Rev Immunol 1991; 11:195–213.
35. Kimble RB, Matayoshi AB, Vannice JL, et al. Simultaneous block of interleukin-1 and tumor necrosis factor is required to completely prevent bone loss in the early postovariectomy period. Endocrinology 1995; 136:3054–3061.
36. Lacey DL, Erdmann JM, Teitelbaum SL, et al. Interleukin 4, interferon-gamma, and prostaglandin E impact the osteoclastic cell-forming potential of murine bone marrow macrophages. Endocrinology 1995; 136:2367–2376.
37. Malaval L, Gupta AK, Aubin JE. Leukemia inhibitory factor inhibits osteogenic differentiation in rat calvaria cell cultures. Endocrinology 1995; 136:1411–1418.
38. Lorenzo JA, Quinton J, Sousa S, et al. Effects of DNA and prostaglandin synthesis inhibitors on the stimulation of bone resorption by epidermal growth factor in fetal rat long-bone cultures. J Clin Invest 1986; 77:1897–1902.
39. Kawaguchi H, Pilbeam CC, Harrison JR, et al. The role of prostaglandins in the regulation of bone metabolism. Clin Orthop 1995; 313:36–46.
40. Canalis E. Skeletal growth factors and aging. J Clin Endocrinol Metab 1994; 78:1009–1010.
41. Jones JI, Clemmons DR. Insulin-like growth factors and their binding proteins: biological actions. Endocr Rev 1995; 16:3–34.
42. Hill PA, Reynolds JJ, Meikle MC. Osteoblasts mediate insulin-like growth factor-I and -II stimulation of osteoclast formation and function. Endocrinology 1995; 136:124–131.
43. Bonewald LF, Dallas SL. Role of active and latent transforming growth factor β in bone formation. J Cell Biochem 1994; 55:350–357.
44. Centrella M, Horowitz MC, Wozney JM, et al. Transforming growth factor-beta gene family members and bone. Endocr Rev 1994; 15:27–39.
45. Muenke M, Schell U. Fibroblast-growth-factor receptor mutations in human skeletal disorders. Trends Genet 1995; 11:308–313.
46. Kawaguchi H, Pilbeam CC, Gronowicz G, et al. Transcriptional induction of prostaglandin G/H synthase-2 by basic fibroblast growth factor. J Clin Invest 1995; 96:923–930.
47. Canalis E, Varghese S, McCarthy TL, et al. Role of platelet-derived growth factor in bone cell function. Growth Regul 1992; 2:151–155.
48. Mazess RB. Dual-energy x-ray absorptiometry for the management of bone disease. Phys Med Rehabil Clin North Am 1995; 6:507–537.
49. Engelke K, Grampp S, Gluer CC, et al. Significance of QCT bone mineral density and its standard deviation as parameters to evaluate osteoporosis. J Comput Assist Tomogr 1995; 19:111–116.
50. Bauer DC, Gluer CC, Genant HK, et al. Quantitative ultrasound and vertebral fracture in postmenopausal women: Fracture Intervention Trial Research Group. J Bone Miner Res 1995; 10:353–358.
51. Delmas PD. Biochemical markers of bone turnover. J Bone Miner Res 1993; 8(Suppl 2):S549–S555.
52. Recker RR. Bone biopsy and histomorphometry in clinical practice. Rheum Dis Clin North Am 1994; 20:609–627.
53. McCarthy JT, Dayton JM, Fitzpatrick LA, et al. The importance of bone biopsy in managing renal osteodystrophy. Advan Renal Replac Ther 1995; 2:148–159.
54. Cummings SR, Melton LJ, Felsenberg D, et al. Assessing vertebral fractures. J Bone Miner Res 1995; 10:518–523.
55. Ryan PJ, Fogelman I. The bone scan: where are we now? Semin Nucl Med 1995; 25:76–91.
56. Consensus Development Conference: Diagnosis, prophylaxis and treatment of osteoporosis. Am J Med 1993; 94:636–638.
57. Kanis JA, Melton LJ, Christiansen C, et al. Perspective: the diagnosis of osteoporosis. J Bone Miner Res 1994; 9:1137–1142.

58. Cummings SR, Black DM, Nevitt MC, et al. Bone density at various sites for prediction of hip fractures. Lancet 1993; 341:72–75.
59. Cooper C, Melton LJ. Epidemiology of osteoporosis. Trends Endocrinol Metab 1992; 3:224–228.
60. Schnitzler CM. Bone quality: a determinant for certain risk factors for bone fragility. Calcif Tissue Int 1993; 53(Suppl 1):S27–S31.
61. Dempster DW, Lindsay R. Pathogenesis of osteoporosis. Lancet 1993; 341:797–801.
62. Young D, Hopper JL, Nowson CA, et al. Determinants of bone mass in 10- to 26-year-old females: a twin study. J Bone Miner Res 1995; 10:558–567.
63. Eisman JA. Vitamin D receptor gene alleles and osteoporosis: an affirmative view. J Bone Miner Res 1995; 10:1289–1293.
64. Peacock M. Vitamin D receptor gene alleles and osteoporosis: a contrasting view. J Bone Miner Res 1995; 10:1294–1297.
65. Tokita A, Kelly PJ, Nguyen TV, et al. Genetic influences on type I collagen synthesis and degradation: further evidence for genetic regulation of bone turnover. J Clin Endocrinol Metab 1994; 78:1461–1466.
66. Faulkner KG. Hip axis length and osteoporotic fractures. J Bone Miner Res 1995; 10:506–509.
67. Johnston CC, Miller JZ, Slemenda CW, et al. Calcium supplementation and increases in bone mineral density in children. N Engl J Med 1992; 327:82–87.
68. Finkelstein JS, Neer RM, Biller BM, et al. Osteopenia in men with a history of delayed puberty. N Engl J Med 1992; 326:600–604.
69. Rannevik G, Jeppsson S, Johnell O, et al. A longitudinal study of the perimenopausal transition: altered profiles of steroid and pituitary hormones, SHBG and bone mineral density. Maturitas 1995; 21:103–113.
70. Parfitt AM, Villanueva AR, Foldes J, et al. Relations between histologic indices of bone formation: implications for the pathogenesis of spinal osteoporosis. J Bone Miner Res 1995; 10:466–473.
71. Rehman MTA, Hoyland JA, Denton J, et al. Histomorphometric classification of postmenopausal osteoporosis: implications for the management of osteoporosis. J Clin Pathol 1995; 48:229–235.
72. Khosla S, Lufkin EG, Hodgson SF, et al. Epidemiology and clinical features of osteoporosis in young individuals. Bone 1994; 15:551–556.
73. Bailey AJ, Wotton SF, Sims TJ, et al. Biochemical changes in the collagen of human osteoporotic bone matrix. Connect Tissue Res 1993; 29:119–132.
74. Pocock AE, Francis MJO, Smith R. Type I collagen biosynthesis by skin fibroblasts from patients with idiopathic juvenile osteoporosis. Clin Sci 1995; 89:69–74.
75. Young N, Formica C, Szmukler G, et al. Bone density at weight-bearing and nonweight-bearing sites in ballet dancers: the effects of exercise, hypogonadism, and body weight. J Clin Endocrinol Metab 1994; 78:449–454.
76. Arisaka O, Arisaka M, Nakayama Y, et al. Effect of testosterone on bone density and bone metabolism in adolescent male hypogonadism. Metabolism 1995; 44:419–423.
77. Longcope C, Baker RS, Hui SL, et al. Androgen and estrogen dynamics in women with vertebral crush fractures. Maturitas 1985; 6:308–318.
78. Jassel SK, Barrettconnor E, Edelstein SL. Low bioavailable testosterone levels predict future height loss in postmenopausal women. J Bone Miner Res 1995; 10:650–654.
79. Young G, Marcus R, Minkoff JR, et al. Age-related rise in parathyroid hormone in man: the use of intact and midmolecule antisera to distinguish hormone secretion from retention. J Bone Miner Res 1987; 2:367–374.
80. Silverberg SJ, Shane E, de la Cruz L, et al. Abnormalities in parathyroid hormone secretion and 1,25-dihydroxyvitamin D₃ formation in women with osteoporosis. N Engl J Med 1989; 320:277–281.
81. Lips P, Van Ginkel FC, Jongen MJM, et al. Determinants of vitamin D status in patients with hip fracture and in elderly control subjects. Am J Clin Nutr 1987; 46:1005–1010.
82. Tiegs RD, Body JJ, Wahner HW, et al. Calcitonin secretion in postmenopausal osteoporosis. N Engl J Med 1985; 312:1097–1100.
83. Civitelli R, Gonnelli S, Zacchei F, et al. Bone turnover in postmenopausal osteoporosis: effect of calcitonin treatment. J Clin Invest 1988; 82:1268–1274.
84. Rosen CJ, Donahue LR, Hunter SJ. Insulin-like growth factors and bone: the osteoporosis connection. Proc Soc Exp Biol Med 1994; 206:83–102.
85. Cummings SR, Nevitt MC, Browner WS, et al. Risk factors for hip fracture in white women. N Engl J Med 1995; 332:767–773.
86. Baran DT. Thyroid hormone and bone mass: the clinician's dilemma. Thyroid 1994; 4:143–144.
87. Pacifici R, Brown C, Puscheck E, et al. Effect of surgical menopause and estrogen replacement on cytokine release from human blood mononuclear cells. Proc Natl Acad Sci USA 1991; 88:5134–5138.
88. Bismar H, Diel I, Ziegler R, et al. Increased cytokine secretion by human bone marrow cells after menopause or discontinuation of estrogen replacement. J Clin Endocrinol Metab 1995; 80:3351–3355.
89. Kawaguchi H, Pilbeam CC, Vargas SJ, et al. Ovariectomy enhances and estrogen replacement inhibits the activity of bone marrow factors that stimulate prostaglandin production in cultured mouse calvariae. J Clin Invest 1995; 96:539–548.
90. Lane N, Coble T, Kimmel DB. Effect of naproxen on cancellous bone in ovariectomized rats. J Bone Miner Res 1990; 5:1029–1036.
91. Bell NH, Hollis BW, Shary JR, et al. Diclofenac sodium inhibits bone resorption in postmenopausal women. Am J Med 1994; 96:349–353.
92. McKane WR, Khosia S, Peterson JM, et al. Circulating levels of cytokines that modulate bone resorption: effects of age and menopause in women. J Bone Miner Res 1994; 9:1313–1318.
93. Bellido T, Jilka RL, Boyce BF, et al. Regulation of interleukin-6, osteoclastogenesis, and bone mass by androgens: the role of the androgen receptor. J Clin Invest 1995; 95:2886–2895.
94. Khosla S, Peterson JM, Egan K, et al. Circulating cytokine levels in osteoporotic and normal women. J Clin Endocrinol Metab 1994; 79:707–711.
95. Kassem M, Khosla S, Spelsberg TC, et al. Cytokine production in the bone marrow microenvironment: failure to demonstrate estrogen regulation in early postmenopausal women. J Clin Endocrinol Metab 1996; 81:513–518.
96. Nicolas V, Mohan S, Honda Y, et al. An age-related decrease in the concentration of insulin-like growth factor binding protein-5 in human cortical bone. Calcif Tissue Int 1995; 57:206–212.
97. Finkelman RD, Bell NH, Strong DD, et al. Ovariectomy selectively reduces the concentration of transforming growth factor beta in rat bone: implications for estrogen deficiency–associated bone loss. Proc Natl Acad Sci USA 1992; 89:12190–12193.
98. Matkovic V, Kostial K, Simonovic I, et al. Bone status and fracture rates in two regions of Yugoslavia. Am J Clin Nutr 1979; 32:540–549.
99. Heaney RP. Skeletal development and maintenance: the role of calcium and vitamin D. Adv Endocrinol Metab 1995; 6:17–38.
100. Heiss CJ, Sanborn CF, Nichols DL, et al. Associations of body fat distribution, circulating sex hormones, and bone density in postmenopausal women. J Clin Endocrinol Metab 1995; 80:1591–1596.
101. Riggs BL, Melton LJ III. Involutional osteoporosis. N Engl J Med 1986; 314:1676–1686.
102. McKenzie L, Sillence D. Familial Scheuermann disease: a genetic and linkage study. J Med Genet 1992; 29:41–45.
103. Culham EG, Jimenez HA, King CE. Thoracic kyphosis, rib mobility, and lung volumes in normal women and women with osteoporosis. Spine 1994; 19:1250–1255.
104. Osman AAH, Bassiouni H, Koutri R, et al. Aging of the thoracic spine: distinction between wedging in osteoarthritis and fracture in osteoporosis—a cross-sectional and longitudinal study. Bone 1994; 15:437–442.
105. Greenspan SL, Myers ER, Maitland LA, et al. Fall severity and bone mineral density as risk factors for hip fracture in ambulatory elderly. JAMA 1994; 271:128–133.
106. Greenspan SL, Maitland LA, Myers ER, et al. Femoral bone loss progresses with age: a longitudinal study in women over age 65. J Bone Miner Res 1994; 9:1959–1966.
107. Mallmin H, Ljunghall S. Incidence of Colles' fracture in Uppsala: a prospective study of a quarter-million population. Acta Orthop Scand 1992; 63:213–215.
108. Orwoll ES, Klein RF. Osteoporosis in men. Endocr Rev 1995; 16:87–116.
109. Delichatsios HK, Lane JM, Rivlin RS. Bone histomorphometry in men with spinal osteoporosis. Calcif Tissue Int 1995; 56:359–363.
110. Smith R. Idiopathic juvenile osteoporosis: experience of twenty-one patients. Br J Rheumatol 1995; 34:68–77.
111. Wright NM, Metzger DL, Key LL. Estrogen and diclofenac sodium therapy in a prepubertal female with idiopathic juvenile osteoporosis. J Pediatr Endocrinol Metab 1995; 8:135–140.
112. Khosla S, Lufkin EG, Hodgson SF, et al. Epidemiology and clinical features of osteoporosis in young individuals. Bone 1994; 15:551–555.
113. Ljunghall S, Johansson AG, Burman P, et al. Low plasma levels of insulin-like growth factor I (IGF-1) in male patients with idiopathic osteoporosis. J Intern Med 1992; 232:59–64.
114. Zerwekh JE, Sakhaee K, Breslau NA, et al. Impaired bone formation in male idiopathic osteoporosis: further reduction in the presence of concomitant hypercalciuria. Osteoporos Int 1992; 2:128–134.
115. Chines A, Pacifici R, Avioli LV, et al. Systemic mastocytosis presenting as osteoporosis: a clinical and histomorphometric study. J Clin Endocrinol Metab 1991; 72:140–144.
116. Dunne F, Walters B, Marshall T, et al. Pregnancy-associated osteoporosis. Clin Endocrinol 1993; 39:487–490.
117. Sowers M, Eyre D, Hollis BW, et al. Biochemical markers of bone turnover in lactating and nonlactating postpartum women. J Clin Endocrinol Metab 1995; 80:2210–2216.
118. Banas MP, Kaplan FS, Fallon MD, et al. Regional migratory osteoporosis: a case report and review of the literature. Clin Orthop 1990; 250:303–309.
119. Inhofe PD, Garcia-Moral CA. Reflex sympathetic dystrophy: a review of the literature and a long-term outcome study. Orthop Rev 1994; 23:655–661.
120. Nielsen HK, Charles P, Moskilde L. The effect of single oral doses of prednisone on the circadian rhythm of serum osteocalcin in normal subjects. J Clin Endocrinol Metab 1988; 67:1025–1030.
121. Reid IR, Heap SW. Determinants of vertebral mineral density in patients receiving long-term glucocorticoid therapy. Arch Intern Med 1990; 150:2545–2548.
122. Hermus AR, Smals AG, Swinkels LM, et al. Bone mineral density and bone turnover before and after surgical cure of Cushing's syndrome. J Clin Endocrinol Metab 1995; 80:2859–2865.
123. Sambrook P, Birmingham J, Kelly P, et al. Prevention of corticosteroid bone loss. Osteoporos Int 1993; 3(Suppl 1):141–143.
124. Lukert BP, Johnson BE, Robinson RG. Estrogen and progesterone replacement therapy reduces glucocorticoid-induced bone loss. J Bone Miner Res 1992; 7:1063–1069.

125. Stiegler C, Leb G, Kleinert R, et al. Plasma levels of parathyroid hormone–related peptide are elevated in hyperprolactinemia and correlated to bone density status. J Bone Miner Res 1995; 10:751–759.

126. Ross DS. Hyperthyroidism, thyroid hormone therapy, and bone. Thyroid 1994; 4:319–326.

127. Beshyah SA, Freemantle C, Thomas E, et al. Abnormal body composition and reduced bone mass in growth hormone–deficient hypopituitary adults. Clin Endocrinol 1995; 42:179–190.

128. Kotzmann H, Bernecker P, Hubsch P, et al. Bone mineral density and parameters of bone metabolism in patients with acromegaly. J Bone Miner Res 1993; 8:459–465.

129. Ezzat S, Melmed S, Endres D, et al. Biochemical assessment of bone formation and resorption in acromegaly. J Clin Endocrinol Metab 1993; 76:1452–1457.

130. Barrett-Connor E, Holbrook TL. Sex differences in osteoporosis in older adults with non–insulin-dependent diabetes mellitus. JAMA 1992; 268:3333–3337.

131. Melchior TM, Sorensen H, Torp-Pedersen C. Hip and distal arm fracture rates in peri- and postmenopausal insulin-treated diabetic females. J Intern Med 1994; 236:203–208.

132. Mundy GR, Bertolini DR. Bone destruction and hypercalcemia in plasma cell myeloma. Semin Oncol 1986; 13:291–299.

133. Cohn SL, Morgan ER, Mallette LE. The spectrum of metabolic bone diseases in lymphoblastic leukemia. Cancer 1987; 59:346–350.

134. Hawkins FG, Leon M, Lopez MB, et al. Bone loss and turnover in patients with liver transplantation. Hepatogastroenterology 1994; 41:158–161.

135. Bernstein CN, Seeger LL, Sayre JW, et al. Decreased bone density in inflammatory bowel disease is related to corticosteroid use and not disease diagnosis. J Bone Miner Res 1995; 10:250–256.

136. Bikle DD. Alcohol-induced bone disease. World Rev Nutr Diet 1993; 73:53–79.

137. de Gennes C, Kuntz D, de Vernejoul MC. Bone mastocytosis: a report of nine cases with a bone histomorphometric study. Clin Orthop 1992; 279:281–291.

138. Katz K, Horev G, Goshen J, et al. The pattern of bone disease in transfusion-dependent thalassemia major patients. Isr J Med Sci 1994; 30:577–580.

139. Diamond T, Stiel D, Posen S. Effects of testosterone and venesection on spinal and peripheral bone mineral in six hypogonadal men with hemochromatosis. J Bone Miner Res 1991; 6:39–43.

140. Epstein S, Shane E, Bilezikian JP. Organ transplantation and osteoporosis. Curr Opin Rheumatol 1995; 7:255–261.

141. Wolpaw T, Deal CL, Fleming-Brooks S, et al. Factors influencing vertebral bone density after renal transplantation. Transplantation 1994; 58:1186–1189.

142. Berguer DG, Krieg MA, Thiebaud D, et al. Osteoporosis in heart transplant recipients: a longitudinal study. Transplant Proc 1994; 26:2649–2651.

143. Cvetkovic M, Mann GN, Romero DF, et al. The deleterious effects of long-term cyclosporine A, cyclosporine G, and FK506 on bone mineral metabolism in vivo. Transplantation 1994; 57:1231–1237.

144. Barbour LA, Kick SD, Steiner JF, et al. A prospective study of heparin-induced osteoporosis in pregnancy using bone densitometry. Am J Obstet Gynecol 1994; 170:862–869.

145. van der Wiel HE, Lips P, Huijgens PC, et al. Effects of short-term low-dose heparin administration on biochemical parameters of bone turnover. Bone Miner 1993; 22:27–32.

146. Gotfredsen A, Borg J, Nilas L, et al. Representativity of regional to total bone mineral in healthy subjects and "anticonvulsive treated" epileptic patients: measurements by single and dual photon absorptiometry. Eur J Clin Invest 1986; 16:198–203.

147. Orwoll ES, Yuzpe AA, Burry KA, et al. Nafarelin therapy in endometriosis: long-term effects on bone mineral density. Am J Obstet Gynecol 1994; 171:1221–1224.

148. Ratcliffe MA, Lanham SA, Reid DM, et al. Bone mineral density (BMD) in patients with lymphoma: the effects of chemotherapy, intermittent corticosteroids and premature menopause. Hematol Oncol 1992; 10:181–187.

149. Kother M, Schindler J, Oette K, et al. Abnormalities in serum osteocalcin values in children receiving chemotherapy including ifosfamide. In Vivo 1992; 6:219–221.

150. Kleerekoper M. Extensive personal experience: the clinical evaluation and management of osteoporosis. J Clin Endocrinol Metab 1995; 80:757–763.

151. Bilezikian JP, Bailey L, Elmer PJ, et al. Optimal calcium intake. JAMA 1994; 272:1942–1948.

152. Recker RR. Calcium absorption and achlorhydria. N Engl J Med 1985; 313:70–73.

153. Chapuy MC, Arlot ME, Delmas PD, et al. Effect of calcium and cholecalciferol treatment for three years on hip fractures in elderly women. BMJ 1994; 308:1081–1082.

154. Reid IR, Ames RW, Evans MC, et al. Long-term effects of calcium supplementation on bone loss and fractures in postmenopausal women: a randomized controlled trial. Am J Med 1995; 98:331–335.

155. Ooms ME, Roos JC, Bezemer PD, et al. Prevention of bone loss by vitamin D supplementation in elderly women: a randomized double-blind trial. J Clin Endocrinol Metab 1995; 80:1052–1058.

156. Bikle DD. Role of vitamin D, its metabolites, and analogs in the management of osteoporosis. Rheum Dis Clin North Am 1994; 759–775.

157. Anonymous. ACSM position stand on osteoporosis and exercise. American College of Sports Medicine. Med Sci Sports Exerc 1995; 27:i–vii.

158. Dalsky GP, Stock KS, Ehsani AA, et al. Weight-bearing exercise training and lumbar bone mineral content in postmenopausal women. Ann Intern Med 1988; 108:824–828.

159. Greendale GA, Barrett-Connor E, Edelstein S, et al. Lifetime leisure exercise and osteoporosis: the Rancho Bernardo study. Am J Epidemiol 1995; 141:951–959.

160. Overgaard K, Riis BJ. Nasal salmon calcitonin in osteoporosis. Calcif Tissue Int 1994; 55:79–81.

161. Gold DT, Lyles KW, Bales CW, et al. Teaching patients coping behaviors: an essential part of successful management of osteoporosis. J Bone Miner Res 1990; 4:799–802.

162. Kanis JA, Johnell O, Gullberg B, et al. Evidence for efficacy of drugs affecting bone metabolism in preventing hip fracture. BMJ 1992; 305:1124–1128.

163. Lafferty FW, Fiske ME. Postmenopausal estrogen replacement: a long-term cohort study. Am J Med 1994; 97:66–77.

164. Prestwood KM, Pilbeam CC, Burleson JA, et al. The short-term effects of conjugated estrogen on bone turnover in older women. J Clin Endocrinol Metab 1994; 79:366–371.

165. Heaney RP. The bone-remodeling transient: implications for the interpretation of clinical studies of bone mass change. J Bone Miner Res 1994; 9:1515–1524.

166. Love RR, Bardon HS, Mazess RB, et al. Effect of tamoxifen on lumbar spine bone mineral density in postmenopausal women after 5 years. Arch Intern Med 1994; 154:2585–2588.

167. Kenny AM, Prestwood KM, Pilbeam CC, et al. The short-term effects of tamoxifen on bone turnover in older women. J Clin Endocrinol Metab 1995; 80:3287–3291.

168. Harris ST, Watts NB, Jackson RD, et al. Four-year study of intermittent cyclic etidronate treatment of postmenopausal osteoporosis: three years of blinded therapy followed by one year of open therapy. Am J Med 1993; 95:557–567.

169. Kanis JA, Gertz BJ, Singer F, et al. Rationale for the use of alendronate in osteoporosis. Osteoporos Int 1995; 5:1–13.

170. Liberman UA, Weiss SR, Broll J, et al. Effect of oral alendronate on bone mineral density and the incidence of fractures in postmenopausal osteoporosis. N Engl J Med 1995; 333:1437–1443.

171. Chestnut CH, McClung MR, Ensrud KE. Alendronate treatment of the postmenopausal osteoporotic woman: effect of multiple dosages on bone mass and bone remodeling. Am J Med 1995; 99:144–152.

172. Reginster JY, Deroisy R, Lecart MP, et al. A double-blind, placebo-controlled dose-finding trial of intermittent nasal salmon calcitonin for prevention of postmenopausal lumbar spine bone loss. Am J Med 1995; 98:452–458.

173. Riggs BL, Hodgson SF, O'Fallon WM, et al. Effect of fluoride treatment on fracture rate in postmenopausal women with osteoporosis. N Engl J Med 1990; 322:802–809.

174. Pak CY, Sakhaee K, Adams-Huet B, et al. Treatment of postmenopausal osteoporosis with slow-release sodium fluoride: final report of a randomized controlled trial. Ann Intern Med 1995; 123:401–408.

175. Finkelstein JS, Klibanski A, Schaefer EH, et al. Parathyroid hormone for the prevention of bone loss induced by estrogen deficiency. N Engl J Med 1994; 331:1618–1623.

176. Lyritis GP, Androulakis C, Magiasis B, et al. Effect of nandrolone decanoate and 1-alpha-hydroxy-calciferol on patients with vertebral osteoporotic collapse: a double-blind clinical trial. Bone Miner 1994; 27:209–217.

177. Morton DJ, Barrett-Connor EL, Edelstein SL. Thiazides and bone mineral density in elderly men and women. Am J Epidemiol 1994; 139:1107–1115.

178. Cauley JA, Cummings SR, Seeley DG, et al. Effects of thiazide diuretic therapy on bone mass, fractures, and falls: the Study of Osteoporotic Fractures Research Group. Ann Intern Med 1993; 118:666–673.

179. Black LJ, Sato M, Rowley ER, et al. Raloxifene (LY139481 HCl) prevents bone loss and reduces serum cholesterol without causing uterine hypertrophy in ovariectomized rats. J Clin Invest 1994; 93:63–69.

180. Ke HZ, Simmons HA, Pirie CM, et al. Droloxifene, a new estrogen antagonist agonist, prevents bone loss in ovariectomized rats. Endocrinology 1995; 136:2435–2441.

181. Holloway L, Butterfield G, Hintz RL, et al. Effects of recombinant human growth hormone on metabolic indices, body composition, and bone turnover in healthy elderly women. J Clin Endocrinol Metab 1994; 79:470–479.

182. Holick MF. The photobiology of vitamin D and its consequences for humans. Ann NY Acad Sci 1985; 453:1–13.

183. Schnitzler CM, Pettifor JM, Patel D, et al. Metabolic bone disease in black teenagers with genu valgum or varum without radiologic rickets: a bone histomorphometric study. J Bone Miner Res 1994; 9:479–486.

184. Godsall JW, Baron R, Insogna KL. Vitamin D metabolism and bone histomorphometry in a patient with antacid-induced osteomalacia. Am J Med 1984; 77:747–750.

185. Glorieux FH, Arabian A, Delvin EE. Pseudo-vitamin D deficiency: absence of 25-hydroxyvitamin D 1α-hydroxylase activity in human placenta decidual cells. J Clin Endocrinol Metab 1995; 80:2255–2258.

186. Kruse K, Feldmann E. Healing of rickets during vitamin D therapy despite defective vitamin D receptors in two siblings with vitamin D–dependent rickets type II. J Pediatr 1995; 126:145–148.

187. The HYP Consortium. A gene (PEX) with homologies to endopeptidases is mutated in patients with X-linked hypophosphatemic rickets. Nature Genet 1995; 11:130–136.

188. Petersen DJ, Boniface AM, Schranck FW, et al. X-Linked hypophosphatemic rickets: a study (with literature review) of linear growth response to calcitriol and phosphate therapy. J Bone Miner Res 1992; 7:583–597.

189. Hanna JD, Niimi K, Chan JC. X-linked hypophosphatemia: genetic and clinical correlates. Am J Dis Child 1991; 145:865–870.

190. Wilkins GE, Granlesse S, Hegele RG, et al. Oncogenic osteomalacia: evidence for a humoral phosphaturic factor. J Clin Endocrinol Metab 1995; 80:1628–1663.

191. Whyte MP. Hypophosphatasia and the role of alkaline phosphatase in skeletal mineralization. Endocr Rev 1994; 15:439–461.

192. Jones G, Sambrook PN. Drug-induced disorders of bone metabolism: incidence, management and avoidance. Drug Saf 1994; 10:480–489.

193. Gallagher JC. Vitamin D metabolism and therapy in elderly subjects. South Med J 1992; 85:2S43–2S47.

194. Albright F, Reifenstein EC Jr. The Parathyroid Glands and Metabolic Bone Disease: Selected Studies. Baltimore, Williams & Wilkins, 1948.

195. Bilezikian JP, Silverberg SJ, Shane E, et al. Characterization and evaluation of asymptomatic primary hyperparathyroidism. J Bone Miner Res 1991; 6(Suppl 2):S85–S89.

196. Parisien M, Mellish RW, Silverberg SJ, et al. Maintenance of cancellous bone connectivity in primary hyperparathyroidism: trabecular strut analysis. J Bone Miner Res 1992; 7:913–919.

197. Casez JP, Troendle A, Lippuner K, et al. Bone mineral density at distal tibia using dual-energy X-ray absorptiometry in normal women and in patients with vertebral osteoporosis or primary hyperparathyroidism. J Bone Miner Res 1994; 9:1851–1858.

198. Silverberg SJ, Gartenberg F, Jacobs TP, et al. Longitudinal measurements of bone density and biochemical indices in untreated primary hyperparathyroidism. J Clin Endocrinol Metab 1995; 80:723–728.

199. Silverberg SJ, Gartenberg F, Jacobs TP, et al. Increased bone mineral density after parathyroidectomy in primary hyperparathyroidism. J Clin Endocrinol Metab 1995; 80:729–734.

200. Fujiyama K, Kiriyama T, Ito M, et al. Attenuation of postmenopausal high turnover bone loss in patients with hypoparathyroidism. J Clin Endocrinol Metab 1995; 80:2135–2138.

201. Hruska KA, Teitelbaum SL. Renal osteodystrophy. N Engl J Med 1995; 333:166–174.

202. Goodman WG, Ramirez JA, Belin TR, et al. Development of adynamic bone in patients with secondary hyperparathyroidism after intermittent calcitriol therapy. Kidney Int 1994; 46:1160–1166.

203. Malluche HH, Monier-Faugere MC. The role of bone biopsy in the management of patients with renal osteodystrophy. J Am Soc Nephrol 1994; 4:1631–1642.

204. Pflanz S, Henderson IS, McElduff N, et al. Calcium acetate versus calcium carbonate as phosphate-binding agents in chronic haemodialysis. 1994; 9:1121–1124.

205. Bushinsky DA. The contribution of acidosis to renal osteodystrophy. Kidney Int 1995; 47:1816–1832.

206. Mazzaferro S, Pasquali M, Ballanti P, et al. Intravenous versus oral calcitriol therapy in renal osteodystrophy: results of a prospective, pulsed and dose-comparable study. Miner Electrolyte Metab 1994; 20:122–129.

207. Boot AM, Nauta J, Hokkenkoelega ACS, et al. Renal transplantation and osteoporosis. Arch Dis Child 1995; 72:502–506.

208. Siris ES. Paget's disease of bone. J Clin Endocrinol Metab 1995; 80:335–338.

209. Singer FR. Paget's disease of bone: classical pathology and electron microscopy. Semin Arthritis Rheum 1994; 23:217–218.

210. Reddy SV, Singer FR, Roodman GD. Bone marrow mononuclear cells from patients with Paget's disease contain measles virus nucleocapsid messenger ribonucleic acid that has mutations in a specific region of the sequence. J Clin Endocrinol Metab 1995; 80:2108–2111.

211. Roodman GD, Kurihara N, Ohsaki Y, et al. Interleukin 6: a potential autocrine/paracrine factor in Paget's disease of bone. J Clin Invest 1992; 89:46–52.

212. Siris ES. Epidemiological aspects of Paget's disease: family history and relationship to other medical conditions. Semin Arthritis Rheum 1994; 23:222–225.

213. Alvarez L, Guanabens N, Peris P, et al. Discriminative value of biochemical markers of bone turnover in assessing the activity of Paget's disease. J Bone Miner Res 1995; 10:458–465.

214. Chosich N, Long F, Wong R, et al. Post-partum hypercalcemia in hereditary hyperphosphatasia (juvenile Paget's disease). J Endocrinol Invest 1991; 14:591–597.

215. Byers PH. Osteogenesis imperfecta. In: Royce PM, Steinmann B, eds. Connective Tissue and Its Heritable Disorders: Molecular, Genetic, and Medical Aspects. New York: Wiley-Liss, 1993, 317–350.

216. Willing MC, Deschenes SP, Scott DA, et al. Osteogenesis imperfecta type I: molecular heterogeneity for COL1A1 null alleles of type I collagen. Am J Hum Genet 1994; 55:638–647.

217. Spotila LD, Constantinou CD, Sereda L, et al. Mutation in a gene for type I procollagen (COL1A2) in a woman with postmenopausal osteoporosis:

218. Davie MWJ, Haddaway MJ. Bone mineral content and density in healthy subjects and in osteogenesis imperfecta. Arch Dis Child 1994; 70:331–334.

219. Brenner RE, Vetter U, Bollen AM, et al. Bone resorption assessed by immunoassay of urinary cross-linked collagen peptides in patients with osteogenesis imperfecta. J Bone Miner Res 1994; 9:993–997.

220. Khillan JS, Li SW, Prockop DJ. Partial rescue of a lethal phenotype of fragile bones in transgenic mice with a chimeric antisense gene directed against a mutated collagen gene. Proc Natl Acad Sci USA 1994; 91:6298–6328.

221. Deodhar AA, Woolf AD. Ehlers-Danlos syndrome and osteoporosis. Ann Rheum Dis 1994; 53:841–842.

222. Bankier A. Menkes' disease. J Med Genet 1995; 32:213–215.

223. Kraus JP. Molecular basis of phenotype expression in homocystinuria. J Inherit Metab Dis 1994; 17:383–390.

224. Parto K, Penttinen R, Paronen I, et al. Osteoporosis in lysinuric protein intolerance. J Inherit Metab Dis 1993; 16:441–450.

225. Gray JR, Bridges AB, Mole PA, et al. Osteoporosis and the Marfan syndrome. Postgrad Med J 1993; 69:373–375.

226. Whyte MP. Osteopetrosis and the heritable forms of rickets. In: Royce PM, Steinmann B, eds. Connective Tissue and Its Heritable Disorders: Molecular, Genetic, and Medical Aspects. New York: Wiley-Liss, 1993, 563–589.

227. Shapiro F. Osteopetrosis: current clinical considerations. Clin Orthop 1993; 294:34–44.

228. Wang YZ, Yin YM, Gilula LA, et al. Endemic fluorosis of the skeleton: radiographic features in 127 patients. Am J Roentgenol 1994; 162:93–98.

229. Felix R, Hofstetter W, Wetterwald A, et al. Role of colony-stimulating factor-1 in bone metabolism. J Cell Biochem 1994; 55:340–349.

230. Lowe C, Yoneda T, Boyce BF, et al. Osteopetrosis in Src-deficient mice is due to an autonomous defect of osteoclasts. Proc Natl Acad Sci USA 1993; 90:4485–4490.

231. Grigoriadis AE, Wang ZQ, Cecchini MG, et al. c-Fos: a key regulator of osteoclast-macrophage lineage determination and bone remodeling. Science 1994; 266:443–448.

232. Whyte MP. Carbonic anhydrase II deficiency. Clin Orthop 1993; 294:52–63.

233. Key LL Jr, Rodriguiz RM, Willi SM, et al. Long-term treatment of osteopetrosis with recombinant human interferon gamma. N Engl J Med 1995; 332:1594–1599.

234. Bollerslev J, Mosekilde L. Autosomal dominant osteopetrosis. Clin Orthop 1993; 294:45–51.

235. Park YK, Unni KK, McLeod RA, et al. Osteofibrous dysplasia: clinicopathologic study of 80 cases. Hum Pathol 1993; 24:1339–1347.

236. Malchoff CD, Reardon G, MacGillivray DC, et al. An unusual presentation of McCune-Albright syndrome confirmed by an activating mutation of the Gs alpha-subunit from a bone lesion. J Clin Endocrinol Metab 1994; 78:803–806.

237. Candeliere GA, Glorieux FH, Prud'homme J, et al. Increased expression of the c-fos proto-oncogene in bone from patients with fibrous dysplasia. N Engl J Med 1995; 332:1546–1551.

238. Kaplan FS, Fallon MD, Boden SC, et al. Estrogen receptors in bone in a patient with polyostotic fibrous dysplasia (McCune-Albright syndrome). N Engl J Med 1988; 319:421–425.

239. Liens D, Delmas PD, Meunier PJ. Long-term effects of intravenous pamidronate in fibrous dysplasia of bone. Lancet 1994; 343:953–954.

240. Greenspan A. Sclerosing bone dysplasias: a target-site approach. Skeletal Radiol 1991; 20:561–583.

241. Edelson JG, Obad S, Geiger R, et al. Pycnodysostosis: orthopedic aspects with a description of 14 new cases. Clin Orthop 1992; 280:263–276.

242. DeVits A, Keymeulen B, Bossuyt A, et al. Progressive diaphyseal dysplasia (Camurati-Engelmann's disease): improvement of clinical signs and of bone scintigraphy during pregnancy. Clin Nucl Med 1994; 19:104–107.

243. Matucci-Cerinic M, Lotti T, Jajic I, et al. The clinical spectrum of pachydermoperiostosis (primary hypertrophic osteoarthropathy). Medicine 1991; 70:208–214.

244. Barr DG, Belton NR. Mineral balance in infantile cortical hyperostosis: effects of corticosteroids. Arch Dis Child 1991; 66:140–142.

245. Gardiner JS, Zauk AM, Donchey SS, et al. Prostaglandin-induced cortical hyperostosis: case report and review of the literature. J Bone Joint Surg Am 1995; 77:932–936.

246. Cushner FD, Morwessel RM. Myositis ossificans in children. Orthopedics 1995; 18:287–291.

247. Slavin RE, Wen J, Kumar D, et al. Familial tumoral calcinosis: a clinical, histopathologic, and ultrastructural study with an analysis of its calcifying process and pathogenesis. Am J Surg Pathol 1993; 17:788–802.

248. Yamaguchi T, Sugimoto T, Imai Y, et al. Successful treatment of hyperphosphatemic tumoral calcinosis with long-term acetazolamide. Bone 1995; 16:S247–S250.

249. Cohen RB, Hahn GV, Tabas JA, et al. The natural history of heterotopic ossification in patients who have fibrodysplasia ossificans progressiva: a study of forty-four patients. J Bone Joint Surg Am 1993; 75:215–219.

stones (5%) are principally hydroxyapatite or brushite (CaH-PO$_4$·2H$_2$O).

The most common noncalcareous stones, 15 to 20% of the total, are composed of struvite (MgNH$_4$PO$_4$·6H$_2$O). Often called "infection" stones, they typically occur as mixtures with carbonate apatite, tricalcium diphosphate, or calcium oxalate. Pure struvite stones are rare. Stones of uric acid (approximately 5%) or cystine (1 to 3%) usually occur alone but may be found as mixtures with calcium oxalate or calcium phosphate. Rarely stones are composed of sodium urate, xanthine, 2,8-dihydroxyadenine,[7] or triamterene.

Calcium oxalate stones are more common in men than in women, and middle-aged white men are particularly susceptible. Struvite and calcium phosphate stones are more common in women. The chemical composition of the stone may sometimes provide the diagnosis (e.g., cystine stones for cystinuria, struvite stones for urinary tract infection with urea-splitting organisms, and uric acid stones for gout). The finding of calcium phosphate as the predominant component suggests the diagnosis of distal renal tubular acidosis or primary hyperparathyroidism. However the identification of the most common stones—calcium oxalate stones—has limited diagnostic value because they can result from a wide variety of metabolic and environmental disturbances.

Physical Chemistry of Stone Formation

A current scheme for stone formation, based on physicochemical principles, considers the process to begin by nucleation of a crystal nidus, followed by transformation of the nidus into a stone through crystal growth, crystal aggregations, and crystal-cell interaction.[8, 9, 9a] Nucleation, the mechanism by which a crystal nidus is formed, is influenced by the degree of saturation of the urine with the chemical constituents of the crystal nidus and by the limit of metastability.

STATE OF SATURATION. The concentration products or the concentrations of individual ions such as calcium or oxalate generally provide a poor measure of urinary saturation. Urinary activity products of the ions making up stones provide the best estimates of the state of saturation. The activity of an ion is the product of ionic concentration and activity coefficient, where activity coefficient is an inverse function of ionic strength. Although several techniques have been described for estimating the state of saturation from activity products, the different methods have yielded varying results.

Two general approaches have been used for this purpose. In one the activity product is calculated from an estimate of ionic activities and compared with the thermodynamic solubility product.[10, 11] The ratio of the activity product to the thermodynamic solubility product yields the relative saturation ratio. This technique for calcium oxalate may overestimate the true state of saturation by as much as a factor of 3, mainly because of errors in calculating ionic concentrations.[12]

In another approach (activity product ratio method)[13] the activity product is calculated for a urine sample before and after incubation of that urine to "equilibrium" with a synthetic solid phase against which the state of saturation is being measured. The ratio of activity products before and after incubation represents the state of saturation; the ratio of 1 indicates saturation, greater than 1 supersaturation, and less than 1 undersaturation. The activity product ratio has physicochemical validity because it indicates the extent to which the synthetic solid phase undergoes growth or dissolution in urine. When the urine is supersaturated there is growth of the solid phase, as indicated by a decrease in concentration of constituent ions in the ambient fluid. When the urine sample is undersaturated there is dissolution of the solid phase, with an increase in concentration of constituent ions in the ambient fluid. A simpler approach yielding a close approximation

of urinary saturation is the concentration product ratio (or the ratio of concentration products before and after incubation).[12]

The urinary environment of patients with stones is typically supersaturated with respect to stone constituents. The urine of individuals without stones may also be supersaturated, but it is generally less supersaturated than the urine of stone-forming patients.[13]

METASTABILITY. Metastability is the condition in which spontaneous nucleation or precipitation of stone-forming salts does not occur during the period of observation, even though urine may be supersaturated with respect to those salts.[8] Urine supports varying degrees of metastable supersaturation with respect to stone-forming salts because of the presence of inhibitors that increase and promoters that reduce metastability. The limit of metastability indicates the point at which nucleation (or formation of a crystal nidus) occurs; it may be defined by the formation product ratio.

The formation product ratio[13] represents the lowest supersaturated state at which nucleation is initiated. At greater than this value nucleation proceeds. It is measured in urine samples free from crystalline constituents as follows. For brushite the urine sample is rendered increasingly supersaturated with respect to calcium phosphate by adding a solution of calcium chloride. The lowest calcium concentration that elicits spontaneous precipitation of calcium phosphate at the prescribed time is then noted. The corresponding activity of Ca^{2+} and HPO$_4$$^{2-}$ represents the formation product. The ratio of the formation product and the activity product at saturation is the formation product ratio. Thus the formation product ratio is a direct measure of the degree to which urine must be supersaturated for spontaneous precipitation to occur. The formation product ratio of calcium oxalate is obtained similarly by adding increasing amounts of oxalate (as oxalic acid or sodium oxalate) to urine. Because of the particle "impurities" in urine, the nucleation that proceeds in urine may be nonhomogeneous. The formation product ratios of brushite and calcium oxalate are sensitive to both low- and high-molecular-weight inhibitors. Thus they are augmented by pyrophosphate, citrate, and glycopeptide.

The urine of patients with calcium stones not only is supersaturated with calcium oxalate and calcium phosphate but also has a reduced formation product ratio.[13] Thus the nucleation process is facilitated in the "stone-forming" urinary environment. This increased propensity for nucleation is reflected by the reduced amount of soluble oxalate or calcium required to elicit spontaneous precipitation of calcium oxalate and calcium phosphate in the urine of stone-forming patients.[14]

HETEROGENEOUS NUCLEATION. Nucleation from a metastably supersaturated solution can be induced by a heterologous "seed." This process of heterogeneous nucleation may be the basis for the formation of stones of mixed crystalline composition. Because the solution is metastable, spontaneous precipitation would not occur without seeding. To be biologically meaningful the heterogeneous nucleation should have some degree of specificity.

Several forms of heterogeneous nucleation have been described. An example is nucleation of calcium oxalate by seeds of calcium phosphate or monosodium urate.[15, 16] For some systems epitaxial fit or crystalline spatial conformity has been demonstrated between the seed crystal and the induced phase.[17]

CRYSTAL GROWTH. The growth of crystals of the same chemical composition as the nidus may be measured by adding to solution a small amount of a synthetic solid phase (representing stone) and determining its rate of growth.[8] Because the rate of growth is a function of the amount of solid phase added, the duration of growth, and the extent of metastable supersaturation, these variables must be controlled.

TABLE 26–1. Classification of Nephrolithiasis

Type of Nephrolithiasis	Occurring Alone* (%)	Occurring with Multiple Diagnosis* (%)
Calcium nephrolithiasis		
Hypercalciuric nephrolithiasis		
Absorptive	15	45
Renal	1	2
Resorptive	1	2
Hyperuricosuric calcium nephrolithiasis	8	30
Hyperoxaluric calcium nephrolithiasis	1	10
Enteric hyperoxaluria		
Primary hyperoxaluria		
Dietary hyperoxaluria		
Hypocitraturic calcium nephrolithiasis	5	30
Distal renal tubular acidosis		
Chronic diarrheal syndrome		
Hypomagnesiuric calcium nephrolithiasis	1	7
Gouty diathesis	3	7
Cystinuria	1	1
Infection stones	2	4
Low urine volume	2	14
No disturbance and miscellaneous causes	3	0

*The percentage for each diagnosis is an approximate estimate based on experience in Dallas. Some patients present with more than one abnormality.

This technique is difficult to apply to whole urine because large amounts of inhibitors are normally present. Therefore crystal growth is typically measured in a standard synthetic metastable solution to which a small amount of urine (1 to 5%) has been added.[18] Unfortunately such assessments with diluted urine samples may have limited biologic significance.

The inhibition of crystal growth of calcium phosphate in urine is due largely to low-molecular-weight substances (e.g., citrate and pyrophosphate),[19, 20] whereas the inhibition of crystal growth of calcium oxalate is due largely to high-molecular-weight substances (glycopeptides and glycosaminoglycans).[18, 20–22] The rate of crystal growth of calcium oxalate and calcium phosphate may be increased in urine of patients with calcium stones.[13]

CRYSTAL AGGREGATION. Crystal aggregation is the process by which preformed crystals (25 to 50 μm in diameter individually) aggregate into large clusters.[23] Crystal aggregates of calcium oxalate 100 to 200 μm in diameter have been found in stone-forming urine. Normal urine may contain substances that inhibit the aggregation of calcium oxalate crystals, thereby allowing passage of the crystals through the urinary tract. These inhibitors may be deficient or absent in stone-forming urine. For example rapid aggregation of calcium oxalate crystals has been reported in the urine of patients with hypocitraturic nephrolithiasis.[24] Moreover some substances (e.g. Tamm-Horsfall protein) may be inhibitors in dilute urine but promoters in concentrated urine.[25]

CRYSTAL-CELL INTERACTION. For crystal nidus to grow into a stone in the kidney, the rate of crystallization should be rapid enough to allow crystals to attain a sufficient size to be lodged in the renal tubule. Alternatively, stone-forming crystals may be toxic to tubular cells and become adherent to cells and degradation products.

CLASSIFICATION OF NEPHROLITHIASIS

One method of diagnostic differentiation of nephrolithiasis is based on the categorization of underlying metabolic or environmental abnormalities, assuming that these disturbances are important in stone formation (Table 26–1). Although complete validation is lacking, excessive renal excretion of calcium, uric acid, oxalate, or cystine, or defective excretion of citrate (hypocitraturia) or magnesium, may contribute to stone formation. This classification is based on the presumed principal abnormality. Several disturbances may in fact coexist in a given disorder. The pathogenetic significance of the metabolic disturbances in stone formation is presented in Table 26–2.

Role of Hypercalciuria

Hypercalciuria plays a major role in calcium stone formation. First, it increases the saturation of urine with respect to stone-forming calcium salts. There is a direct correlation between urinary saturation of calcium oxalate or brushite and urinary calcium concentration.[13] Although a rise in urinary calcium concentration may reduce the ionic oxalate concentration through increased formation of oxalate complexes, this effect is generally less prominent than is the increase in ionic calcium concentration. Calcium in the diet can form a complex with oxalate in the intestine as well and modestly decrease its absorption. Nevertheless the net effect of a high-calcium diet, despite suggestions to the contrary,[25a] is to cause hypercalciuria and to increase the saturation of calcium salts in the urine.[26] Second, hypercalciuria reduces the urinary inhibitor activity against the crystallization of calcium salts through binding and inactivation of negatively charged inhibitors.[27]

Persistent hypercalciuria is one of the most important determinants of continued stone formation during therapy.[28] Correction of hypercalciuria by the administration of thiazide or sodium cellulose phosphate restores the normal urinary physicochemical environment[29] and retards the formation of new stones.[30]

Hypercalciuria is not uniformly a consequence of a high calcium intake. In stone-forming patients with normal intestinal calcium transport, a high-calcium diet may produce only a modest and transient hypercalciuria because of intestinal adaptation (a fall in calcium absorption from suppressed parathyroid hormone [PTH] and 1,25-$(OH)_2$D secretion).[31] In

TABLE 26–2. Pathogenetic Significance of Various Derangements in Stone Formation

Derangement	Physicochemical Effect in Urine
Hypercalciuria	Increased saturation of calcium oxalate and calcium phosphate
	Attenuation of inhibitor activity of citrate and chondroitin sulfate
Hyperuricosuria	Increased saturation of monosodium urate
	Facilitated urate-induced crystallization of calcium oxalate
Hyperoxaluria	Increased saturation of calcium oxalate
Hypocitraturia	Increased saturation of calcium salts via reduced formation of calcium-citrate complexes
	Reduced inhibitor activity against crystallization of calcium salts resulting from loss of inhibitor activity of citrate
Hypomagnesiuria	Increased saturation of calcium oxalate because of reduced binding of oxalate
Low urinary pH	Low uric acid solubility
Cystinuria	Increased saturation of cystine
High urinary pH	Increased phosphate dissociation
	Increased saturation of calcium phosphate and struvite (if ammonium ion concentration is high)
Low urine volume	Increased saturation of stone-forming salts (because of the rise in concentration of stone-forming constituents)

patients with absorptive hypercalciuria, however, a sustained, marked hypercalciuria may ensue from the loss of intestinal adaptation.[32]

Role of Hyperuricosuria

Recurrent calcium nephrolithiasis (stones of calcium oxalate or calcium phosphate, or both) can occur in patients with hyperuricosuria and no other discernible cause for nephrolithiasis provided that the urinary pH is greater than the dissociation constant (pK_a) of 5.47 for the first proton of uric acid.[33] The association of hyperuricosuria with calcium nephrolithiasis has led to the suggestion that hyperuricosuria is pathogenetically important in calcium stone formation.[34] The following scheme has been proposed: the urine may be supersaturated with respect to monosodium urate because it has a high content of uric acid and a pH (>5.5) in which monosodium urate is stable.[35] Either a colloidal or a crystalline monosodium urate can form in such a supersaturated environment[36] and initiate the formation of calcium stones by (1) direct induction of heterogeneous nucleation of calcium oxalate[23] or (2) absorption of glycosaminoglycans (which are inhibitors of crystal aggregation or spontaneous nucleation of calcium oxalate).[37]

The scheme is supported by the demonstration of supersaturation of urine with monosodium urate,[23] by the ability of monosodium urate to induce heterogeneous nucleation of calcium oxalate,[23] and by the capacity of monosodium urate to attenuate the inhibitory activity of heparin (model mucopolysaccharide)[37] or naturally occurring urinary macromolecules.[38] Moreover the induction of hyperuricosuria by oral purine loading facilitates spontaneous precipitation of calcium oxalate in urine, commensurate with a rise in urinary saturation of monosodium urate.[36] Unfortunately the presence of crystalline monosodium urate in urine has not yet been documented.

Role of Hyperoxaluria

A role for hyperoxaluria in stone formation is suggested by its identification as a risk factor for stone formation and by its frequent association with calcium nephrolithiasis. Hyperoxaluria facilitates stone formation by increasing urinary saturation of calcium oxalate.

Role of Hypocitraturia

Hypocitraturia may be a risk factor for the formation of calcium stones because citrate is known to inhibit stone formation. Citrate reduces urinary saturation of calcium oxalate or calcium phosphate by forming a soluble complex with calcium and thereby reducing calcium ion activity.[39] The spontaneous nucleation of calcium oxalate is retarded by the ensuing decline in the urinary saturation of calcium oxalate as well as by a direct inhibitor action of citrate.[40] Citrate is an effective inhibitor of calcium phosphate crystal growth and a modest inhibitor of calcium oxalate crystal growth.[18] Citrate may also be a potent inhibitor of the agglomeration or aggregation of preformed calcium oxalate crystals.[24]

Other simple (low-molecular-weight) and complex (macromolecular) inhibitors of the crystallization of calcium salts in urine include pyrophosphate, glycopeptides,[41] glycosaminoglycans,[19] ribonucleic acids, nephrocalcin,[9a, 21] and uropontin.[21a] Renal excretion of these substances may be disturbed in certain patients with nephrolithiasis, but this has never been fully substantiated. However the finding that a specific urinary glycoprotein in patients with calcium nephrolithiasis may be abnormal structurally and functionally is intriguing and could be important pathogenetically.[21] Measurement of these inhibitors may have diagnostic or predictive utility if simple and reliable assays can be developed. Furthermore therapeutic approaches to augmenting the activity of these inhibitors in urine may be developed.

Role of Hypomagnesiuria

Magnesium is a weak direct inhibitor of the crystallization of stone-forming calcium salts. It attenuates the crystallization of calcium oxalate indirectly by forming a complex with oxalate,[42] thereby reducing the ionic oxalate concentration and the urinary saturation of calcium oxalate. Thus calcium oxalate crystallization could be enhanced in the setting of hypomagnesiuria.

Role of Altered Urinary pH

Persistent passage of unusually acidic urine (pH <5.5) may cause both uric acid and calcium stones. When urinary pH is close to or less than the dissociation constant of uric acid,[33] the concentration of undissociated uric acid is high, promoting uric acid crystallization. The uric acid crystals in turn may promote the crystallization of calcium oxalate by the mechanism described for monosodium urate. Although uric acid is less efficient than monosodium urate in inducing heterogeneous nucleation of calcium oxalate (on a weight basis), its crystalline dimensions are more compatible with induction of ordered crystalline overgrowth of calcium oxalate.[25] Moreover uric acid can bind naturally occurring urinary macromolecular inhibitors of stone formation, thereby attenuating their activity.[38]

In contrast a high urinary pH (neutral or alkaline) favors formation of calcium phosphate stones. It increases urinary saturation of calcium phosphate by enhancing the dissociation of hydrogen phosphate and raising the concentration of trivalent phosphate ion. If a high concentration of ammonium ion is also present (e.g., as a result of infection with urea-splitting organisms), struvite (magnesium ammonium phosphate) saturation could increase, promoting formation of infection stones.[43]

Role of Urinary Cystine

Cystine is sparingly soluble in urine. Its solubility is greater at higher pH and is enhanced by electrolytes and macromolecules[44]; however it rarely exceeds 1.7 mmol/L (400 mg/L). Cystine stones may form when the urinary cystine concentration exceeds the solubility of cystine.

Role of Low Urine Volume

Low urine volume contributes to stone formation by increasing the concentration of stone-forming constituents and raising the saturation of stone-forming salts.[45] Volume changes affect both cationic and anionic components of the stone-forming salt (e.g., calcium and oxalate in calcium oxalate). For instance a reduction in urine output by one half generally increases urinary saturation by up to fourfold. Therefore marked urinary supersaturation may result from reduced urine output even when the total renal excretion of stone-forming constituents is normal.

PATHOPHYSIOLOGICAL DERANGEMENTS

Hypercalciuria

The association of hypercalciuria with calcium nephrolithiasis has long been recognized. The term *idiopathic hypercalci-*

uria has been used to denote this entity.[46] Progress in pathophysiological elucidation mandates that this term be discarded because hypercalciuria of nephrolithiasis is composed of several entities of different origin (Fig. 26–1).[47] In the original description[48] hypercalciuria of nephrolithiasis was categorized into absorptive, renal, and resorptive variants. Subsequently additional presentations have been suggested. They may be categorized as subvariants of the three main categories.

ABSORPTIVE HYPERCALCIURIA. The primary abnormality in absorptive hypercalciuria is intestinal hyperabsorption of calcium. The consequent increase in the circulating concentration of calcium increases the renal filtered load and suppresses parathyroid function. Hypercalciuria ensues from the increased filtered load and the reduced tubular reabsorption of calcium associated with suppression of PTH secretion. The excessive renal loss of calcium compensates for the high calcium absorption from the intestinal tract and helps maintain serum calcium concentration in the normal range.

Absorptive hypercalciuria is heterogeneous and may be broadly categorized into vitamin D–independent and vitamin D–dependent subvariants. The former may be a primary jejunal abnormality[49, 50] because the high calcium absorption has been observed only in the jejunum, and the absorption of magnesium and phosphate is normal. Moreover the restoration of normal serum 1,25-(OH)$_2$D by ketoconazole does not correct the exaggerated intestinal absorption or renal excretion of calcium.[51]

In vitamin D–dependent absorptive hypercalciuria there may be 1,25-(OH)$_2$D overproduction or hypersensitivity. Ketoconazole therapy completely or partially corrects the hyperabsorption of calcium and hypercalciuria.[51] 1,25-(OH)$_2$D overproduction is supported by the finding of high serum 1,25-(OH)$_2$D concentration in about one fourth of patients[52, 53] and of accelerated 1,25-(OH)$_2$D synthesis in vivo in some of them.[54, 55] This subvariant may include hypophosphatemic absorptive hypercalciuria. Hypophosphatemia ensuing from renal phosphate leak is thought to cause intestinal hyperabsorption of calcium by stimulating the renal synthesis of 1,25-(OH)$_2$D.[56, 57] However hypophosphatemia is found uncommonly and the full spectrum of this entity is rarely encountered in stone-forming patients.[58]

Hypersensitivity to vitamin D is supported by the state of intestinal hyperabsorption of calcium in patients with normal circulating concentrations of 1,25-(OH)$_2$D, in which ketoconazole challenge restores normal calcium absorption.[51] It resembles the state of up-regulation of the vitamin D receptor produced by long-term treatment with calcitriol in normal subjects.[59]

Fasting urinary calcium levels may be high in some patients with absorptive hypercalciuria. In most it is probably due to the incomplete renal clearance of calcium that is excessively absorbed[60] and, perhaps, stimulation of bone resorption by 1,25-(OH)$_2$D.[61] Suppressed parathyroid function may contribute to fasting hypercalciuria by impairing renal tubular reabsorption of calcium. In some patients fasting hypercalciuria may reflect the resorptive action on bone of vitamin D excess or hypersensitivity.[62]

Some patients with absorptive hypercalciuria may show evidence of excessive bone loss. Spinal bone density may be depressed, although radial shaft density is generally normal.[63] Calcium balance may be negative.[64] The exact cause for bone loss is not known. It may be related to vitamin D excess or hypersensitivity.[62]

RENAL HYPERCALCIURIA. The primary abnormality in renal hypercalciuria is thought to be impairment of renal tubular reabsorption of calcium.[65] The consequent reduction in the circulating concentration of calcium stimulates parathyroid function. There may be excessive mobilization of calcium from bone and enhanced intestinal absorption of calcium because of excess PTH and ensuing stimulation of the renal synthesis of 1,25-(OH)$_2$D.[52] These compensatory mechanisms restore the serum calcium level toward normal. Unlike the situation in primary hyperparathyroidism, the serum calcium concentration is normal and the state of hyperparathyroidism is secondary.

Some patients with hypercalciuric nephrolithiasis, albeit a minority in most series, have a biochemical presentation in keeping with the foregoing scheme. The combination of high serum PTH or urinary cAMP concentration, elevated serum 1,25-(OH)$_2$D concentration, and enhanced intestinal calcium absorption has been shown in such patients in the setting of a normal serum calcium level and fasting hypercalciuria (indicative of renal calcium leak).[52] Correction of the renal calcium leak by thiazide restores the normal serum 1,25-(OH)$_2$D level and fractional calcium absorption commensurate with the correction of hyperparathyroidism.[66] These findings support the contention that 1,25-(OH)$_2$D synthesis is enhanced by secondary parathyroid stimulation and that intestinal calcium absorption is high because of 1,25-(OH)$_2$D excess.

The occurrence of a primary renal calcium leak is supported by three lines of evidence. First, fasting hypercalciuria is associated with parathyroid stimulation and is poorly corrected by inhibition of intestinal calcium absorption (and removal of any effect of absorbed calcium) with sodium cellulose phosphate.[60] Second, there is a unique natriuretic response to thiazide. When thiazide is given to block reabsorption of calcium and sodium in the distal (renal) tubule, impaired proximal tubular function causes an exaggerated renal excretion of these cations. The enhanced natriuretic and calciuric responses to thiazides are encountered only in patients with renal hypercalciuria with secondary hyperpara-

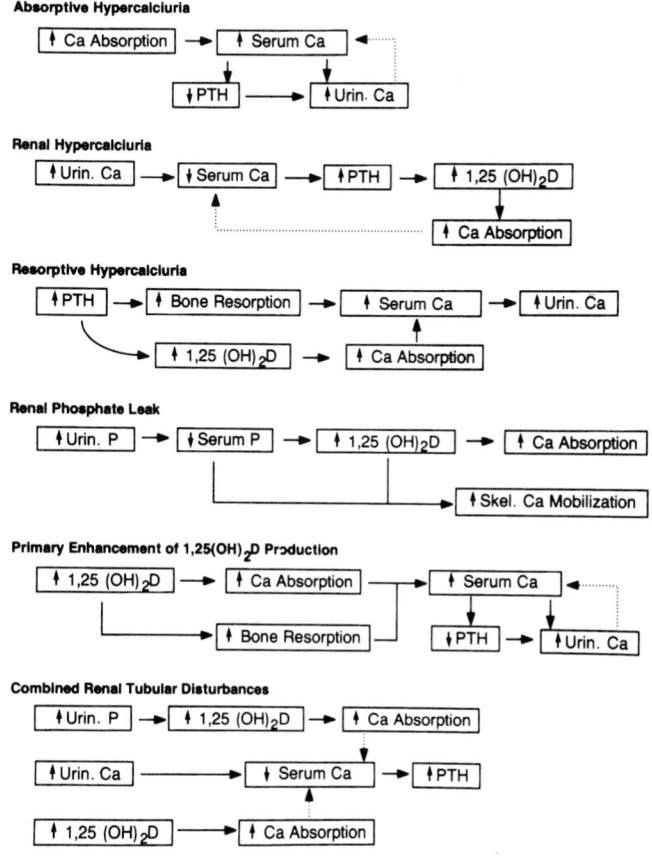

Figure 26–1. Pathophysiological schemes for the various forms of hypercalciuria associated with nephrolithiasis.

thyroidism.[67] Third, an exaggerated calciuric response to a glucose load occurs in patients with renal hypercalciuria but not in those with absorptive hypercalciuria.[68] Ingestion of readily metabolizable carbohydrate (without calcium) normally augments renal calcium excretion, probably through an alteration in renal proximal tubular function.[69]

It has been suggested that renal calcium leak might be secondary to an excessive dietary intake of sodium.[70] However institution of a low sodium intake (9 mmol/d) does not eliminate fasting hypercalciuria in patients with renal hypercalciuria.

The fact that renal calcium leak (and secondary hyperparathyroidism) can be long-standing is shown by changes in bone density. Although clinical bone disease is rare, mean bone density as measured by photon absorptiometry in the distal third of the radius is reduced in subjects with renal hypercalciuria (compared with age- and sex-matched controls).[71] These results indicate that secondary hyperparathyroidism has deleterious effects on the skeleton. The lack of more serious involvement is probably due to the compensatory intestinal hyperabsorption of calcium that results from the PTH-induced renal synthesis of 1,25-(OH)$_2$D. This compensation is often inadequate, and negative calcium balance can occur when the urinary calcium level exceeds calcium absorption. Fasting hypercalciuria with normal parathyroid function occurring in absorptive hypercalciuria should not be confused with renal hypercalciuria.[60] Recently three uncommon disorders of X-linked hypercalciuric nephrolithiasis have been associated with mutations in the gene encoding a renal chloride channel.[71a] How these mutations cause hypercalciuria is unknown. Specific features distinguishing absorptive hypercalciuria and renal hypercalciuria are presented in Table 26–3.

RESORPTIVE HYPERCALCIURIA. Resorptive hypercalciuria resulting in kidney stones is generally due to primary hyperparathyroidism (also see Chapter 24). The initial event is excessive resorption of bone resulting from hypersecretion of PTH. Intestinal absorption of calcium is frequently elevated because of PTH-mediated stimulation of the renal synthesis of 1,25-(OH)$_2$D.[72] These effects increase the circulating concentration and the filtered load of calcium in urine. Development of hypercalciuria in primary hyperparathyroidism seems paradoxical because the primary effect of PTH in the kidney is to stimulate tubular reabsorption of calcium. However hypercalciuria occurs in primary hyperparathyroidism when the PTH-dependent augmentation of renal tubular reabsorption of calcium is "overcome" by an increase in the renal filtered load

and by a suppressive effect of hypercalcemia on the renal reabsorption of calcium.

Stone formation has become less common in primary hyperparathyroidism, probably because of earlier diagnosis. Hypercalciuria is characteristic of stone-forming patients with primary hyperparathyroidism and may be one of the causes of renal stone formation. The hypercalciuria may result from excessive PTH-dependent bone resorption or enhanced intestinal absorption of calcium resulting from PTH-dependent synthesis of 1,25-(OH)$_2$D, or both. The component of the hypercalciuria that results from enhanced intestinal absorption may be of particular importance for the formation of kidney stones.[55] Thus a predilection for nephrolithiasis has been reported in patients with primary hyperparathyroidism who have a high circulating concentration of 1,25-(OH)$_2$D and increased intestinal absorption of calcium. Conversely patients presenting with bone disease are reported to have lower glomerular filtration, lower levels of 25-hydroxycholecalciferol (25-OHD), and higher values of serum PTH than those without bone disease. Impairment of renal function or decreased levels of vitamin D prohormones, or both, might lead to impaired synthesis of 1,25-(OH)$_2$D. From the resulting loss of a normal inhibitory action of 1,25-(OH)$_2$D, PTH synthesis is increased, worsening bone disease.[73]

Many patients with primary hyperparathyroidism who present with renal stones cannot be distinguished from those without stones on the basis of biochemical or physicochemical features.[74] First, there is no unique histologic pattern in the parathyroid glands characteristic of stone formation. The prevalence of nephrolithiasis is similar in patients with parathyroid hyperplasia and those with parathyroid adenoma. Second, mean bone density as assayed by photon absorptiometry is reduced in both the stone-forming and the non–stone-forming groups. The mean value for the fractional change in bone density is actually lower in patients with stones than in those without stones, although the difference is not significant. It thus seems clear that skeletal involvement is a characteristic feature of PTH excess. Third, biochemical findings for patients with stones cannot be distinguished from those for patients without stones, at least in a group with surgically proven primary hyperparathyroidism.[74] Patients with stones and those without stones have similar degrees of elevation of serum calcium, serum PTH, and serum 1,25-(OH)$_2$D levels; fractional calcium absorption; and urinary calcium levels. Most patients without stones have high fractional calcium absorption, and some patients with stones have normal absorption.

Finally, the urine of patients with stones cannot be distinguished from that of non–stone-forming patients by measurements of urinary composition or saturation with stone-forming salts.[74] It is not known why certain patients with primary hyperparathyroidism form stones, whereas others do not.

Although the overall scheme for resorptive hypercalciuria in primary hyperparathyroidism is generally accepted, the mechanisms by which intestinal calcium absorption is controlled are not entirely clear. The high intestinal calcium absorption is customarily ascribed to the enhanced PTH-mediated synthesis of 1,25-(OH)$_2$D. Thus the fractional calcium absorption is directly related to serum 1,25-(OH)$_2$D levels.[53] However in some patients with primary hyperparathyroidism, the intestinal hyperabsorption of calcium persists after parathyroidectomy and after restoration of normal serum 1,25-(OH)$_2$D levels.[75] Therefore factors other than 1,25-(OH)$_2$D may contribute to the maintenance of high intestinal calcium absorption in hyperparathyroid patients in the postoperative state.

There are other causes of resorptive hypercalciuria associated with nephrolithiasis. Other sources of excessive bone resorption, such as oncogenic hypercalcemia, thyrotoxicosis, and sarcoidosis, occasionally result in stone formation. En-

TABLE 26–3. Distinction Between Absorptive and Renal Hypercalciurias

	Absorptive Hypercalciuria		Renal Hypercalciuria
Physiological parameter	Vitamin D–dependent	Vitamin D–independent	
Primary derangement	Vitamin D excess, hypersensitivity	Unknown	Renal calcium leak
Parathyroid function	Normal, suppressed	Normal, suppressed	Stimulated
Fasting hypercalciuria	Secondary	Secondary	Primary
Serum 1,25(OH)$_2$D	Primary increased synthesis or hypersensitivity	Normal	Secondary increase (PTH-dependent)
Intestinal calcium absorption	Secondary increase (vitamin D–dependent)	Primary increase	Secondary increase (vitamin D–dependent)
Bone loss	Increased (vitamin D–dependent)	Normal	Increased (PTH-dependent)

PTH, parathyroid hormone.

hanced renal excretion of prostaglandin E_2 has been reported in patients with hypercalciuric nephrolithiasis.[76] Treatment with inhibitors of prostaglandin synthesis corrected the hypercalciuria in such patients and reduced urinary calcium in normocalciuric patients with nephrolithiasis but not in normal individuals.

Hyperuricosuria

Uric acid is an end product of purine metabolism and cannot be degraded in humans because they lack uricase, which is present in other mammalian species. A major site of disposal of uric acid is the kidney, where filtration, reabsorption, and secretion all occur.

Hyperuricosuria may ensue when the serum concentration and the renal filtered load of uric acid are increased as a result of (1) the availability of an excessive amount of substrate, e.g., from a diet high in purine-rich foods[77] or from accelerated degradation and turnover of nucleic acids or (2) a disturbance in purine biosynthesis that causes overproduction of purine substrates for uric acid synthesis (Table 26–4). A high urinary uric acid level can occur transiently when renal tubular reabsorption of uric acid is impaired, as during early stages of extracellular volume expansion or after administration of uricosuric agents such as probenecid. In the steady state, however, normal urinary uric aid concentration is restored in the latter conditions because of the secondary decline in the serum concentration and renal filtered load of uric acid, even though renal tubular reabsorption of uric acid remains impaired.[78]

Hyperuricosuria may be the only observed physiological abnormality in patients with calcium nephrolithiasis. Such a defect (hyperuricosuric calcium urolithiasis) exists alone in approximately 10% of patients with renal calculi.[79, 80] Although hyperuricosuria may coexist with the various forms of hypercalciuria, only the pure disorder is considered in this section.

The most common cause of hyperuricosuria in patients with hyperuricosuric calcium oxalate nephrolithiasis is probably dietary overindulgence in purine-rich foods.[77] Such individuals have a history of a liberal intake of meat, poultry, and fish, and their estimated purine intake is higher than that of control groups. Hyperuricosuria in such patients can be ameliorated by dietary purine deprivation.[36, 77, 81]

However about 30% of patients with hyperuricosuric calcium oxalate nephrolithiasis have hyperuricosuria as the result of uric acid overproduction. Hyperuricosuria persists despite long-term purine deprivation. No further studies have been performed to elucidate the nature of this apparent urate overproduction.

During long-term thiazide therapy hyperuricosuria and hyperuricemia may be encountered.[82] Besides its customary action of augmenting renal tubular reabsorption of urate, thiazide may stimulate urate production or decrease the extrarenal disposal of urate.

Hyperoxaluria

Oxalate is derived from both in vivo synthesis and intestinal absorption. Once synthesized or absorbed it is not further degraded, and the principal route of excretion is the kidney. Data on renal handling of oxalate are limited and conflicting. Of the 30 mg of oxalate excreted normally each day, 80% is derived from in vivo synthesis and the remainder is derived from the diet.

No primary derangement in renal handling of oxalate has been recognized. Rather hyperoxaluria is due to increased serum concentrations and increased renal filtered loads resulting from (1) high substrate availability, as caused by administration of methoxyflurane or ascorbic acid; (2) enzymatic disturbances in the oxalate biosynthetic pathway that cause overproduction, as in primary hyperoxaluria (rare); or (3) increased intestinal absorption of oxalate (see Table 26–4), as in the hyperoxaluria of ileal disease.[83, 84]

Two factors probably act in concert to cause intestinal hyperabsorption of oxalate: (1) intestinal transport of oxalate may be primarily increased because of the action of bile salts and fatty acids on the permeability of intestinal mucosa to oxalate and (2) the total amount of oxalate absorbed may be increased because of an enlarged intraluminal pool of oxalate available for absorption. The intestinal fat malabsorption characteristic of ileal disease may exaggerate soap formation with divalent cations, limit the amount of "free" divalent cations available to form complexes with oxalate, and thereby enlarge the available oxalate pool.

The formation of calcium oxalate stones has multifactorial causes in the setting of intestinal disease. In addition to the disturbance in oxalate metabolism, the intestinal absorption and renal excretion of calcium are often decreased in enteric hyperoxaluria, probably because of the loss of the intestinal site of calcium absorption as a result of disease or resection, intraluminal binding of calcium by nonabsorbed fatty acids, and vitamin D deficiency associated with fat malabsorption. Urine volume may be reduced because of fluid loss from the intestinal tract. Urinary citrate concentration may be depressed because of hypokalemia and metabolic acidosis,[85, 86] and urinary magnesium concentration may be low because of impaired intestinal magnesium absorption. Saturation of urine with calcium oxalate may be increased because of the high oxalate concentration, even though the urinary calcium level may be low, and low urine volume exaggerates urinary supersaturation. Urinary saturation of calcium oxalate is further increased because the intestinal loss of electrolytes reduces urinary ionic strength, thereby increasing the activity coefficient and the fraction of ionic calcium and oxalate. Moreover inhibitor activity against crystallization of calcium salts is reduced because of low renal excretion of citrate and magnesium.

Hypocitraturia

Urinary citrate excretion is a function of filtration, reabsorption, peritubular transport, and synthesis by the renal tubular cell. Approximately 80 to 90% of filtered citrate is

TABLE 26–4. Derangements Other Than Hypercalciuria That Can Cause Nephrolithiasis

Derangement	Physicochemical Effect in Urine
Hyperuricosuria	Primary overproduction
	Dietary purine overindulgence or increased cellular degradation
Hyperoxaluria	High substrate availability (e.g., vitamin C or oxalate intake)
	Primary overproduction
	Intestinal hyperabsorption of oxalate (enteric hyperoxaluria)
Hypocitraturia	Renal tubular acidosis
	Enteric hyperoxaluria
	Hypokalemia (e.g., thiazide therapy)
	Diet high in animal protein
	Urinary tract infection
	Other
Hypomagnesiuria	Insufficient dietary intake of magnesium
Low urinary pH (uric acid stones)	Gout and chronic diarrheal syndrome
	Diet high in animal protein
Cystinuria	Impaired renal tubular reabsorption of cystine
High urinary pH and ammonium (struvite stones)	Infection with urea-splitting organisms

normally reabsorbed, and citrate secretion is usually negligible.

Although the exact physiology of renal handling of citrate has not been elucidated, several factors influence citrate excretion: it is enhanced by alkalosis,[86] PTH, vitamin D, growth hormone, and estrogen and is decreased by acidosis,[87] hypokalemia,[88] androgen, and urinary tract infection (probably because of bacterial degradation of citrate). Acid-base status probably plays the most important role in citrate excretion. Acidosis reduces the urinary citrate concentration by enhancing both the renal tubular reabsorption and the metabolism of citrate by stimulating citrate lyase activity.[88a] The mechanism accounts for the occurrence of hypocitraturia in distal renal tubular acidosis (complete or incomplete),[89] chronic diarrheal states (resulting from intestinal alkali loss),[90, 91] hypokalemia (from intracellular acidosis), thiazide therapy (from hypokalemia),[88] and a diet high in animal protein (from elevated acid-ash content) (see Table 26–4).[92] Urinary citrate concentration may also be low after strenuous physical exercise (because of lactic acidosis)[93] and after high sodium intake (probably because of sodium-induced potassium loss).[94]

Distal acidification defect (type I) is the only form of renal tubular acidosis associated with nephrolithiasis. The stone formation is the result of high urinary pH and calcium levels and low urinary citrate levels. Calcium phosphate crystallization is promoted by increased urine saturation (resulting from increased dissociation of phosphate and hypercalciuria) and reduced inhibitor activity (from hypocitraturia). Crystallization of calcium oxalate may also be enhanced because of increased saturation (resulting from hypercalciuria and reduced citrate complexation of calcium) and impaired inhibitor activity (from hypocitraturia). The predominant stone constituent is hydroxyapatite (a form of calcium phosphate), but calcium oxalate is also typically present as a minor constituent. Nephrocalcinosis commonly coexists with nephrolithiasis.

Nephrolithiasis is not associated with proximal renal tubular acidosis (type II) or hyporeninemic hypoaldosteronism (type IV). In these disorders the urinary citrate and calcium levels may be low.[95] Moreover urinary pH is normal in type IV nephrolithiasis.

Distal renal tubular acidosis should not be confused with calcium oxalate nephrolithiasis of the chronic diarrheal syndrome. In the latter disorder metabolic acidosis is secondary to intestinal alkali loss in the stool. Stone (calcium) formation is due to low urinary citrate concentration and low urine volume. Gastrointestinal disorders that cause this syndrome include the postgastrectomy state, inflammatory disease of the small bowel, bowel resection or bypass, and colitis. States of malabsorption of fat, hyperoxaluria, and low urinary magnesium level may contribute to calcium oxalate stone formation. Uric acid lithiasis may develop as a result of low urinary pH.

In many patients with hypocitraturic calcium nephrolithiasis, the cause of low urinary citrate concentration is unknown. It is not due to a primary defect in citrate absorption from the gastrointestinal tract.[96] Dietary habits that lead to a low gastrointestinal absorption of net alkali may be an important factor.[97]

Hypomagnesiuria

Urinary magnesium concentrations may be low in chronic diarrheal states, especially in the setting of fat malabsorption, because of impaired intestinal absorption of magnesium.[90] Hypomagnesiuria may also occur in the absence of gastrointestinal disease in a minority of patients with calcium nephrolithiasis.[98, 99] It is probably due to a diet insufficient in magnesium content.

Gouty Diathesis

Gouty diathesis is exemplified by primary gout, which is usually associated with a low urinary pH, hyperuricosuria, and stones. More commonly hyperuricosuria represents a forme fruste or early phase of primary gout before the onset of arthritic manifestations.[100, 101] It is noteworthy that stone disease often precedes the onset of articular symptoms in patients with primary gout.[102]

Gouty diathesis[100, 101] is characterized by a low urinary pH (<5.5) of unknown cause, occurring independently of excessive alkali loss or consumption of a diet rich in acid-ash content. Stones may be composed of uric acid alone, calcium alone, or both calcium and uric acid. Finally, some patients present with hyperuricemia, hypertriglyceridemia, frank gouty arthritis, and a family history of gout.

The stone formation in gouty diathesis is probably due to the increased amount of undissociated uric acid in the acidic urinary environment, which leads to the development of uric acid stones.[100] Calcium stones could form by heterogeneous nucleation or binding of inhibitors by uric acid itself or its salt (monosodium urate).

Noncalcareous Stones

URIC ACID LITHIASIS. Critical determinants for uric acid lithiasis are a urinary pH lower than the dissociation constant for uric acid (5.47) or hyperuricosuria, or both.[33] Besides primary gout other causes of uric acid nephrolithiasis include certain inborn errors of uric acid metabolism, secondary causes of urate overproduction, chronic diarrheal states, and use of uricosuric agents. Three well-studied enzymatic disorders of uric acid metabolism are hypoxanthine-guanine phosphoribosyltransferase deficiency (Lesch-Nyhan syndrome), phosphoribosyl pyrophosphate synthetase overactivity, and glucose-6-phosphatase deficiency (type I glycogen storage disease). Affected patients have marked overproduction of uric acid. In myeloproliferative disorders, leukemia, neoplasia, and hemolytic anemia, hyperuricemia and hyperuricosuria occur because of an increased rate of nucleic acid turnover. As many as half of patients with myeloproliferative disorders may form uric acid stones, which may be the initial clinical manifestation.

Certain drugs such as probenecid, high-dose salicylates, and x-ray contrast agents may produce an acute uricosuria by inhibiting net uric acid reabsorption and increasing the fractional excretion of uric acid. Chronic administration of these agents, however, results in a new steady state in which the rate of uric acid excretion should be no greater than the pretreatment rate. Thus the risk of stone formation occurs early. A high incidence of uric acid lithiasis is associated with gastrointestinal disorders, including ulcerative colitis and regional enteritis, and with the presence of ileostomy.[103] Uric acid stones in these cases are related to variable degrees of dehydration and bicarbonate loss, resulting in an unusually acidic and concentrated urine. The excretion rate of uric acid is usually normal. Uric acid stones may form after strenuous exercise because of concentrated urine (from sweat loss) and low urinary pH (from lactic acidosis).[93]

CYSTINURIA. Normally cystine is filtered and almost completely reabsorbed in the proximal nephron so that less than 20 mg is excreted in urine each day. In cystinuria the serum concentration, and hence the renal filtered load of cystine, is reduced. Exaggerated cystine excretion under this circumstance suggests a disturbance in renal handling of cystine. More than one defect can impair tubular reabsorption and back-diffusion of cystine.[104]

Similar defects in the transport of other dibasic amino acids are present. However, exaggerated renal excretion of these amino acids and cystine may not be due to a single transport defect.[105] Increasing the filtered load of one of these amino acids does not necessarily augment the excretion of others.[106]

The intestinal transport of dibasic amino acids may also be defective in cystinuria. The disorder has been classified into three types based on varying intestinal transport disturbances for these amino acids.[107] The intestinal transport has been assessed by the in vitro uptake of radiolabeled amino acid by specimens of jejunal mucosa obtained through peroral biopsy and by studies of plasma cystine levels after oral cystine administration. In type I cystinuria there is no uptake of cystine, lysine, or arginine by jejunal mucosa, and the plasma cystine concentration is not elevated after an oral cystine load. Thus there is defective intestinal transport of all three dibasic amino acids. In cystinuria types II and III the intestinal transport of dibasic amino acids is disturbed but less severely than in the type I presentation. In type II cystinuria some cystine is taken up by jejunal mucosa but at a reduced rate, and oral cystine loading does not increase the plasma cystine level. In type III cystinuria cystine and lysine uptake by jejunal mucosa is variably reduced and the increment in plasma cystine after oral cystine loading is blunted but present. In the homozygous state all three types of cystinuria involve excessive renal excretion of all four dibasic amino acids.[107] In the heterozygous state type I cystinuria is characterized by normal cystine excretion, whereas type II and type III cystinuria have elevated cystine and lysine excretion (although not quite up to the level encountered in the homozygous state), probably because of a prevailing (although reduced) intestinal uptake of these amino acids. Discrete mutations in the dibasic amino acid transporter gene have been found in certain cystinuric patients.[108]

INFECTION STONES. Infection of the urinary tract with urea-splitting organisms may be associated with renal stones of struvite and calcium carbonate apatite.[43] The critical determinant is the formation of ammonia in urine because of enzymatic degradation of urea by bacterial urease. The ammonia is hydrated to form ammonium and hydroxyl ions. The resulting alkalinity of the urine augments dissociation of phosphate to form triphosphate ions and reduces the solubility of struvite. Thus the urinary environment becomes supersaturated with struvite. Although struvite stones may form de novo from infection alone, they more commonly occur from infection resulting from other causes of renal calculi, such as hypercalciuria.

DIAGNOSTIC CONSIDERATIONS

Most diagnostic protocols are based on underlying metabolic-environmental derangements or on stone composition.

Such protocols differ in the exactness of diagnostic separation, especially of the hypercalciurias. Most protocols include analysis of urine for certain stone-forming risk factors (calcium, uric acid, oxalate, citrate, sodium, magnesium, pH, and volume) and screening of blood for calcium, phosphorus, electrolytes, and uric acid.[1, 109] Urinary risk factors are typically assessed in urine collected from patients with a random diet and fluid intake. Some measurements are repeated after imposition of a restricted diet (e.g., with limited calcium and sodium content) to assess the contribution of dietary factors.[1] The assay of urinary risk factors on a single urine sample is now available commercially. Differentiation of the different hypercalciurias requires determination of the fasting urinary calcium level (to obtain a measure of renal calcium leak),[110] the calciuric response to oral calcium load (for an indirect measure of intestinal calcium absorption),[110] and the serum PTH level. A qualitative cystine determination, stone analysis, urine culture, and appropriate radiologic examination of stones are necessary for a full examination.

The following simplified approach to diagnosis has gained wide acceptance.[111] In patients presenting with their first stone episode (single stone-formers) who are not at risk for further stone formation, the evaluation may comprise simply stone analysis, urinalysis, and culture; an abdominal roentgenogram; systematic multichannel analysis of serum; and a careful history for dietary aberrations and fluid loss. In single stone-formers who are at risk for further stone formation (family history of stones, bone or gastrointestinal disease, gout, and nephrocalcinosis), as well as patients with recurrent stone formation, a more thorough evaluation is warranted. It would include a collection of two 24-h urine samples, one on a random diet and the other following a dietary modification, for a full analysis of risk factors for stone formation. Thus both environmental and metabolic risk factors could be discerned.

Diagnostic criteria for the major forms of nephrolithiasis are summarized in Table 26-5. Absorptive hypercalciuria type I[1] is characterized by normal serum calcium and phosphorus levels; a slightly high or normal fasting urinary calcium (<0.03 mmol/L [<0.11 mg/100 mL] glomerular filtrate), increased ratio of urinary calcium to creatinine after an oral calcium load (>5 mmol/mg [>0.2 mg/dL]), normal or suppressed parathyroid function (normal serum immunoreactive PTH level), and urinary calcium level for a restricted diet (10 mmol [400 mg] calcium and 100 mmol sodium/d) of more than 5 mmol/d (200 mg/d). These values reflect increased intestinal calcium absorption, resultant parathyroid suppression, and hypercalciuria. Spinal bone density may be low in some patients,[63] although radial shaft bone density is generally normal.[71]

TABLE 26–5. Diagnostic Criteria for Major Forms of Nephrolithiasis*

Form	Serum				Urine								Bone Density†
	Calcium	Phosphorus	Immunoreactive Parathyroid Hormone	1,25-(OH)₂D	Calcium (Fasting)	Calcium (Calcium Load)	Calcium (24 h)	Uric Acid	Oxalate	Citrate	pH	Fractional Calcium Absorption	
AH-I	N	N	N	N/↑	N/↑	↑	↑	N	N	N	N	↑	N/↓
AH-II	N	N	N	N	N	↑	N	N	N	N	N	↑/N	N
RH	N	N	↑	↑	↑	N/↑	↑	N	N	N	N	↑	↓
HUCU	N	N	N	N	N	N	N	↑	N	N	N	N	N
EH	N/↓	N/↓	N/↑	N	↓	↓	↓	↓	↑	↓	↓	↓	↓
Hypocrit	N	N	N	N	N	N	N	N	N	↓	N	N	N
RTA	N	N	N/↑	N	↑	N	N/↑	N	N	↓	N/↑	↓	↓
Gouty diathesis	N	N	N	N	N	N	N	N	N	N	↓	N	N

*Fasting samples represent 2-h collections obtained in the morning after an overnight fast. Calcium load samples were obtained over a 4-h period after oral ingestion of 1 g calcium; they provide an indirect measure of intestinal calcium absorption. Fractional calcium absorption was estimated from fecal recovery of radioactivity after oral administration of radiocalcium with 100 mg calcium.

†Measured in the distal third of the radius by photon absorptiometry.

↑, high; ↓, low; N, normal; AH-I, absorptive hypercalciuria type I; AH-II, absorptive hypercalciuria type II; RH, renal hypercalciuria; HUCU, hyperuricosuric calcium nephrolithiasis; EH, enteric hyperoxaluria; Hypocrit, idiopathic hypocitraturic calcium nephrolithiasis; RTA, incomplete renal tubular acidosis. Data reflect criteria for sole presentations.

Absorptive hypercalciuria type II[1] is characterized by the same biochemical features as type I except for a normal urine calcium level (<5 mmol/d [<200 mg/d]) for a restricted diet of 10 mmol (400 mg) calcium and 100 mmol sodium/d. If these patients are placed on a diet of 25 mmol/d (1000 mg/d) calcium and 100 mmol/d sodium, the urinary calcium level exceeds 0.1 mmol/kg body weight/d (4 mg/kg/d) or 6 mmol/d (250 mg/d).

Renal hypercalciuria[1] has the following features: a normal serum calcium level, a fasting urinary calcium level greater than 0.03 mmol/L glomerular filtrate (>0.11 mg/100 mL glomerular filtrate), and enhanced parathyroid activity (high serum immunoreactive PTH level). These results indicate a renal leak of calcium with compensatory parathyroid stimulation. Evidence of parathyroid stimulation (high serum PTH level) is critical for the diagnosis of renal hypercalciuria. Radial shaft bone density may be low in patients with renal hypercalciuria.[71]

Primary hyperparathyroidism is characterized by hypercalcemia, hypophosphatemia, hypercalciuria, and an increased or inappropriately high serum PTH level. Bone density in the radial diaphysis is often low.[71] Hypercalcemic symptoms, peptic ulcer, or bone disease (osteitis, pathologic fractures, osteoporosis) may be present. A decline in femoral neck and spinal bone density occurs less commonly.[112]

Hyperuricosuric calcium oxalate nephrolithiasis[113] is characterized by hyperuricosuria (urinary uric acid level >3.6 mmol/d [>600 mg/d] in at least two of three urine samples), normal serum calcium levels, a normal fasting and calcium load response, normal urinary calcium levels, normal urinary oxalate levels (<500 μmol/d [<45 mg/d]), and calcium nephrolithiasis. Hyperuricosuria, defined functionally here by the upper normal limit of 3.6 mmol/d (600 mg/d), correlates with the urinary supersaturation with monosodium urate associated with the increased propensity for calcium stone formation.[35] (Other laboratories employ a higher upper limit for urinary uric acid, e.g., 4.5 mmol/d [750 mg/d] for women and 4.8 mmol/d [800 mg/d] for men.) Urinary pH is typically greater than 5.5. Hyperuricosuria may be the only abnormality in patients with calcium stones, or it may coexist with various forms of hypercalciuria.

Hypocitraturic calcium nephrolithiasis in the pure presentation is the condition in which hypocitraturia (urinary citrate <1.7 mmol/d [<320 mg/d]) is present alone without other physiological derangements (e.g., hypercalciuria or hyperuricosuria).[85] Hypocitraturia may be caused by distal renal tubular acidosis, metabolic acidosis of chronic diarrheal states, or thiazide-induced hypokalemia. Complete distal renal tubular acidosis is characterized by hyperchloremic metabolic acidosis (high serum chloride and low serum potassium and carbon dioxide levels) and high urinary pH (>6.8) in the absence of infection of the urinary tract. A more common presentation of renal tubular acidosis in stone disease is the incomplete form, which is characterized by normal serum electrolyte levels but an impaired ability to acidify the urine after an ammonium chloride load. Both complete and incomplete forms may be associated with hypercalciuria, hypocitraturia, calcium nephrolithiasis, and nephrocalcinosis. Stone analysis typically shows a preponderance of hydroxyapatite with calcium oxalate as a minor constituent.

Chronic diarrheal states[90] capable of producing hypocitraturia and calcium nephrolithiasis include ileal disease or ileal resection, gastrectomy, ulcerative colitis, and colectomy. The degree of hypocitraturia is generally proportional to the severity of intestinal fluid loss. In severe diarrheal states urinary citrate concentration may be very low (<0.3 mmol/d [<50 mg/d]); serum electrolyte abnormalities of acquired metabolic acidosis (caused by intestinal fluid loss) and low urinary

pH may also be present. Some patients show full features of enteric hyperoxaluria.

In thiazide-induced hypocitraturia[88] the serum potassium level is low or low normal and the urinary citrate level is low (<1.7 mmol/d [<320 mg/d]). Thiazide action may also cause a high serum bicarbonate and a low serum chloride concentration.

The invariant feature in gouty diathesis is the persistent passage of an acidic urine (pH <5.5).[100, 101] The cause of low urinary pH is not always evident. Some patients may give a personal or family history of gouty arthritis. Others may present with hyperuricemia or hypertriglyceridemia. The stones may be composed of uric acid alone or calcium oxalate-phosphate alone, or a mixture of the two. Some patients may form pure uric acid stones on one occasion and calcium stones on another occasion. Uric acid stones are radiolucent.

In cystinuria the cyanide-nitroprusside test provides a qualitative measure of the cystine content of urine. If positive results are obtained, a quantitative test should be performed. In patients with cystine stones the urinary cystine concentration is greater than 1 mmol/g creatinine (>250 mg/g creatinine).

Lithiasis resulting from infection is diagnosed by showing that the stones are composed of magnesium ammonium phosphate. Such struvite stones are often associated with pyuria, a positive urine culture for urea-splitting organisms (*Proteus*, certain species of *Staphylococcus*, *Pseudomonas*, or *Klebsiella*), and high urinary pH (>7.5). Struvite stones are radiopaque and sometimes may attain a large (staghorn) size; they usually occur as mixtures with calcium carbonate apatite or less commonly with calcium oxalate.

RATIONAL THERAPY FOR NEPHROLITHIASIS

Urolithiasis is characterized by a high recurrence rate. Moreover the removal of stones, e.g., by lithotripsy, does not modify the propensity for further stone formation. Thus a medical prophylactic program is essential.

All patients should be offered a conservative treatment program of increased fluid intake, sodium and oxalate restriction, avoidance of excessive meat intake, and increased citrus fruit intake. This program alone may be sufficient in controlling stone recurrence, especially in single stone-formers without risk. However in patients with active recurrent disease presenting with metabolic derangements (e.g., hypercalciuria or hypocitraturia), specific drug treatment is generally necessary.

Elucidation of the pathophysiology and formulation of diagnostic criteria for different causes of nephrolithiasis make it possible to devise individual and specific treatment programs.[2, 79, 114] Such regimens ideally should (1) reverse the underlying physicochemical and physiological derangements, (2) inhibit new stone formation, (3) prevent nonrenal complications of the disease process, and (4) be free from serious side effects.[114] The underlying assumption is that the physicochemical and physiological aberrations identified are etiologically important in the formation of renal stones (as previously discussed) and that the correction of such disturbances will prevent new stone formation. Moreover such a selected treatment program is assumed to be more effective and safer than a "random" treatment. Considerable information is available about the physicochemical and physiological effects for many of these treatment programs (Table 26–6).

The selective approach has been supported by two placebo-controlled randomized trials. Compared with placebo, allopurinol[114a] and potassium citrate[114b] have been shown to

TABLE 26–6. Optimal Treatment Programs for Nephrolithiasis

Indication	Treatment	Physiological Action*	Physicochemical Action*
Absorptive hypercalciuria type I	Sodium cellulose phosphate	↓ Intestinal calcium absorption ↓ Urinary calcium	↓ Urinary saturation of calcium ↓ Calcium phosphate saturation
	Thiazide	= Intestinal calcium absorption ↓ Urinary calcium (transient) ↓ Urinary citrate	↓ Urinary saturation of calcium salts
Absorptive hypercalciuria type II	Low-calcium diet	↓ Intestinal calcium absorption ↓ Urinary calcium ↓ Urinary calcium (sustained)	↓ Urinary saturation of calcium oxalate and calcium phosphate ↓ Urinary saturation of calcium salts
Renal hypercalciuria	Thiazide	↓ Intestinal calcium absorption	↓ Urate-induced crystallization of calcium salts
Hyperuricosuric calcium nephrolithiasis	Allpurinol	↓ Urinary uric acid	↓ Urinary saturation of calcium oxalate
	Potassium citrate	↑ Urinary citrate	↓ Urate-induced crystallization of calcium salts
Enteric hyperoxaluria	↓ Oxalate intake	↓ Urinary oxalate	↓ Urinary saturation of calcium oxalate
	Potassium citrate	↑ Urinary citrate ↑ Urinary pH	↓ Urinary saturation of calcium oxalate ↑ Inhibitor activity
	Magnesium gluconate	↑ Urinary magnesium	↓ Urinary saturation of calcium oxalate
	Calcium citrate	↑ Urinary citrate ↑ Urinary pH	↑ Inhibitor activity
Hypocitraturic calcium nephrolithiasis	Potassium citrate	↑ Urinary citrate ↑ Urinary pH ↓/= Urinary calcium	↓ Urinary saturation of calcium oxalate ↑ Inhibitor activity
Gouty diathesis	Potassium citrate	↑ Urinary pH ↓ Undissociated uric acid ↑ Urinary citrate	↓ Urinary saturation of uric acid ↓ Calcium oxalate crystallization
Cystinuria	Penicillamine or tiopronin†	Mixed disulfide with cysteine ↓ Urinary cystine	↓ Urinary saturation of cystine
Infection stones	Acetohydroxamic acid	↓ Urease activity ↓ NH₄⁺ ↓ pH	Urinary saturation of struvite

* ↓, decrease; ↑, increase; =, no change.
†α-Mercaptopropionylglycine.

be more effective in controlling stone formation due to hyperuricosuria and hypocitraturia, respectively.

Primary Hyperparathyroidism

Parathyroidectomy is the optimal treatment for nephrolithiasis of primary hyperparathyroidism (also see Chapter 24). After successful surgery urinary calcium excretion, serum concentration of calcium, and intestinal calcium absorption are restored to normal.[115] The urine becomes less saturated with calcium oxalate and brushite, and the limit of metastability (formation product ratio) for these calcium salts increases.[116] The rate of new stone formation is reduced unless urinary tract infection is present. Parathyroidectomy is contraindicated in secondary hyperparathyroidism of renal hypercalciuria and in absorptive hypercalciuria.

There is no established medical treatment for the nephrolithiasis of primary hyperparathyroidism. Although orthophosphates have been recommended for disease of mild to moderate severity, their safety and efficacy have not yet been proved.[117] The use of estrogen in postmenopausal women with this condition has shown some promise.[118] A medical approach should be applied only when parathyroid surgery cannot be undertaken.

Absorptive Hypercalciuria Type I

No treatment program is capable of correcting the basic abnormality of absorptive hypercalciuria, although several drugs restore normal calcium excretion. Sodium cellulose phosphate administration is not an optimal therapy.[119] When given orally this nonabsorbable ion-exchange resin binds calcium and inhibits calcium absorption.[47, 119] However, decreased calcium absorption is due to limitation of the amount of intraluminal calcium available for absorption and not to correction of the disturbance in calcium transport.

There are two potential complications of sodium cellulose phosphate therapy.[114, 120] First, the agent may cause magnesium depletion by binding dietary magnesium. Second, sodium cellulose phosphate may produce secondary hyperoxaluria[121] by binding divalent cations in the intestinal tract, reducing the formation of divalent cation-oxalate complexes, and making more oxalate available for absorption. These complications may be prevented by oral magnesium supplementation (magnesium citrate, 10 mEq given twice a day separately from sodium cellulose phosphate) and moderate dietary restriction of oxalate. Under such circumstances sodium cellulose phosphate (10 to 15 g/d, given with meals) lowers urinary calcium levels, reduces urinary saturation of calcium salts, and retards new stone formation without significantly altering urinary oxalate or magnesium levels.[2] This drug is contraindicated in other forms of hypercalciuria because it may further stimulate parathyroid function and worsen negative calcium balance. Because of this potential complication, sodium cellulose phosphate should be given only in severe cases of absorptive hypercalciuria type I and in thiazide-resistant hypercalciuria in which there is normal bone density.

Thiazide does not decrease intestinal calcium absorption[52] but it is widely used to treat this disorder because of its hypocalciuric action. However thiazide may have limited long-term effectiveness in absorptive hypercalciuria type I.[122] It is usually effective in reducing the urinary calcium level during the first 2 y of treatment, but thereafter urinary calcium levels generally return to the pretreatment range (Fig. 26–2). Intestinal calcium absorption persistently remains elevated throughout thiazide treatment. Thiazide may cause accretion of calcium in bone during the early years of therapy; eventually a low turnover state of bone interferes with continued calcium accretion in the skeleton.[39] The "rejected" calcium would then be excreted in urine. In contrast calcium retention does not occur in renal hypercalciuria because thiazide causes a decrease in intestinal calcium absorption commensurate with the reduction in urinary calcium level.[66, 122]

The following guidelines for the use of these two agents are recommended until more selective therapies are found. Sodium cellulose phosphate is appropriate for patients with

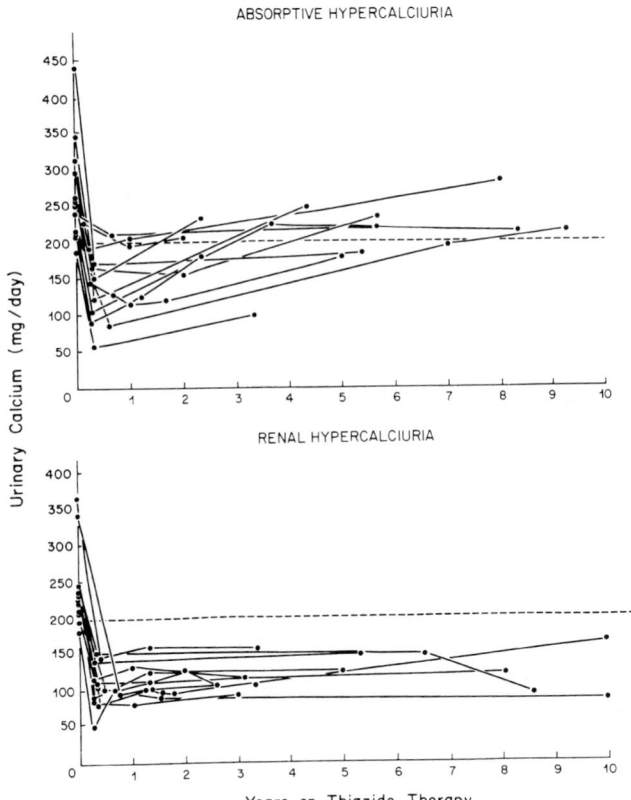

Figure 26-2. Contrasting effect of thiazide on urinary calcium in absorptive hypercalciuria versus renal hypercalciuria. (From CYC Pak, Medical management of nephrolithiasis in Dallas: update 1987, J Urol, 140, 461-467, © by Williams & Wilkins, 1988.)

severe absorptive hypercalciuria type I (urinary calcium >8.75 mmol/d [>350 mg/d]) and for patients without osteopenia who are resistant to or intolerant of thiazide therapy. In patients at risk for bone disease (growing children, postmenopausal women, or elderly men), thiazide is the first choice. When thiazide becomes ineffective in lowering the urinary calcium level, this treatment may be temporarily replaced by sodium cellulose phosphate or orthophosphate treatment (for approximately 6 mo). Restoration of the hypocalciuric response to thiazide may then ensue, permitting resumption of thiazide therapy. Potassium citrate (e.g., 15 to 20 mEq twice a day) should be given along with thiazide (e.g., trichlormethiazide 4 mg/d) to prevent hypokalemia and to augment citrate excretion.[123]

Recent studies suggest a promising treatment approach with slow-release neutral potassium phosphate.[124] It reduces intestinal absorption of calcium by direct binding of calcium in the intestinal tract and by impairing renal 1,25-(OH)$_2$D synthesis. A sustained reduction in urinary calcium is accompanied by a rise in urinary inhibitors (citrate and pyrophosphate).

In absorptive hypercalciuria type II a low-calcium diet (10 to 15 mmol/d [400 to 600 mg/d]) and a high fluid intake (sufficient to maintain urine output greater than 2 L/d) are appropriate[2] because normocalciuria can be restored by dietary calcium restriction alone and because increased urine volume reduces urinary saturation of calcium oxalate, brushite, and monosodium urate and inhibits spontaneous nucleation of calcium oxalate.

Renal Hypercalciuria

Thiazide is the treatment of choice for renal hypercalciuria.[52, 66] This agent corrects the renal leak of calcium directly by augmenting calcium absorption in the distal tubule and by causing extracellular volume depletion, which stimulates proximal tubular reabsorption of calcium. The ensuing correction of secondary hyperparathyroidism restores normal serum 1,25-(OH)$_2$D levels and intestinal calcium absorption. Physicochemically the urine becomes less saturated with calcium oxalate and brushite, largely because of the reduced calcium excretion.[125] Moreover urinary inhibitor activity, as reflected by an increase in the limit of metastability, occurs by an unknown mechanism. These effects are shared by hydrochlorothiazide (50 mg twice a day), chlorthalidone (25 mg/d), and trichlormethiazide (4 mg/d). Potassium supplementation (15 to 20 mEq twice a day) may be required to prevent hypokalemia and attendant hypocitraturia. Concurrent use of triamterene, a potassium-sparing agent, should be undertaken with caution because of the possibility of triamterene stone formation.[126] Amiloride may be used with thiazide (because it may also exert a hypocalciuric action) to exaggerate the hypocalciuric action of thiazide and to prevent hypokalemia.[127] However amiloride does not augment citrate excretion. Thus in patients with hypercalciuric nephrolithiasis and hypocitraturia, in whom the use of potassium citrate is contemplated, it is probably wise to use thiazide alone without a potassium-sparing diuretic. Thiazide is contraindicated in primary hyperparathyroidism because of potential aggravation of hypercalcemia.

Hyperuricosuric Calcium Oxalate Nephrolithiasis

Allopurinol (300 mg/d) is the drug of choice in hyperuricosuric calcium oxalate nephrolithiasis resulting from uric acid overproduction because of its ability to reduce uric acid synthesis and to lower urinary uric acid concentration.[34] Its use in hyperuricosuria associated with dietary purine overindulgence is also reasonable because dietary purine restriction may be impractical. Physicochemical changes ensuing from restoration of a normal urinary uric acid level include an increase in the urinary limit of metastability of calcium oxalate.[36] Thus the spontaneous nucleation of calcium oxalate is retarded by treatment, probably by inhibition of monosodium urate–induced stimulation of calcium oxalate crystallization.[37] Because of the potential exaggeration involved in the latter process, a moderate sodium restriction (<150 mmol/d) may be advisable.

Potassium citrate is an effective alternative to allopurinol for the treatment of this condition.[128] Citrate can inhibit the heterogeneous nucleation of calcium oxalate by monosodium urate. When potassium citrate is given to patients with hyperuricosuric calcium oxalate nephrolithiasis, the urinary citrate concentration rises. Not only does the induced hypercitraturia reduce urinary saturation of calcium oxalate (by forming a complex with calcium) but it also inhibits urate-induced crystallization of calcium oxalate.

Enteric Hyperoxaluria

Stone formation in enteric hyperoxaluria is multifactorial. The treatment should therefore be directed at correcting the various disturbances, including hyperoxaluria, hypocitraturia and low urinary pH, hypomagnesiuria, and low urine volume.

Oral administration of large amounts of calcium (0.25 to 1.0 g four times a day) or magnesium has been recommended for the control of calcium nephrolithiasis of ileal disease. Although the urinary oxalate concentration may decrease (probably because of binding of oxalate by divalent cations), the concurrent rise in urinary calcium concentration may obviate the beneficial effect of this therapy, at least in some patients.[129] Cholestyramine does not cause a sustained reduction in oxalate excretion, but limitation of dietary oxalate intake and partial replacement of dietary fat with medium chain fatty acids may be helpful in patients with malabsorption.

The treatment of low urinary citrate and pH levels with potassium citrate is considered in the section on chronic diarrheal syndrome. Hypomagnesiuria results from impaired intestinal absorption of magnesium. It contributes to calcium oxalate stone formation because of reduced formation of oxalate and magnesium complexes and a consequent rise in the urinary saturation of calcium oxalate. Oral magnesium supplementation can partially correct hypomagnesiuria, although it may worsen diarrhea. Magnesium citrate (10 mEq two to four times a day) is better tolerated and absorbed than is magnesium oxide or hydroxide. Magnesium chloride is contraindicated because it exaggerates metabolic acidosis.

A high fluid intake is recommended to ensure adequate urine volume. Control of excessive intestinal fluid loss with an antidiarrheal agent may be necessary before sufficient urine output can be achieved.

Calcium citrate may theoretically have a role in the management of enteric hyperoxaluria. This treatment may lower the urinary oxalate level by binding oxalate in the intestinal tract and increase urinary citrate and pH levels by providing an alkali load.[130] Finally, it may correct the malabsorption of calcium and reverse demineralization of the skeleton by enhancing calcium absorption. If hypercalciuria develops, thiazide may be added.

Hypocitraturic Calcium Nephrolithiasis

RENAL TUBULAR ACIDOSIS (DISTAL). Potassium citrate therapy is capable of correcting both metabolic acidosis and hypokalemia.[89] Moreover it may restore normal urinary citrate concentration, although large doses (up to 120 mEq/d) may be required in severe acidotic states. Urinary calcium concentration typically decreases with the correction of acidosis. The overall rise in urinary pH is small because the urinary pH is high to begin with; urinary pH is generally less than 7.5 during treatment unless a urinary tract infection is present.

Thus potassium citrate treatment produces a sustained decline in the urinary saturation of calcium oxalate (through a reduction in the urinary calcium level and a rise in the formation of a citrate-calcium complex). The urinary saturation of calcium phosphate does not increase because the rise in phosphate dissociation is relatively small (as a result of the modest rise in pH) and is adequately compensated by a decrease in ionic calcium concentration. Moreover inhibitor activity against the crystallization of calcium oxalate and calcium phosphate is augmented by the direct action of citrate. Treatment with potassium citrate improves calcium balance by increasing intestinal calcium absorption (through an unknown mechanism) and by reducing urinary calcium levels.[131]

If renal sodium leak is significant, alkali might be provided as a mixed sodium-potassium salt. However, renal sodium wasting is not prominent in most patients with renal tubular acidosis presenting with stones.

CHRONIC DIARRHEAL SYNDROME. In patients with mild to moderate severity of intestinal fluid loss in whom hypocitraturia is not severe (urinary citrate in the range of 0.5 to 1.5 mmol/d [100 to 300 mg/d]), potassium citrate (40 to 60 mEq in three or four divided doses in a liquid form) is generally effective in restoring normal urinary citrate and pH levels.[91] Urinary calcium concentration generally remains low. In those with severe hypocitraturia (urinary citrate <0.5 mmol/d [<100 mg/d]), even high doses of potassium citrate (up to 120 mEq/d) may be ineffective in restoring a normal urinary citrate level.

A liquid preparation of potassium citrate is preferable to a slow-release tablet preparation in these states because some of the patients may have abnormal intestinal motility and may be more prone to obstruction caused by a tablet preparation. Furthermore a slow-release tablet medication may be poorly absorbed because of rapid intestinal transit.

A frequent dose schedule (three or four times a day) is recommended for the liquid preparation because of the relatively short duration of biologic action. In other hypocitraturic conditions the solid slow-release preparation is preferable or is better tolerated. A less frequent dose schedule (twice a day) is acceptable for the solid preparation because of its slow-release characteristic.

THIAZIDE-INDUCED HYPOKALEMIA. Hypokalemia resulting from thiazide may cause hypocitraturia, probably by causing intracellular acidosis and may thereby attenuate the beneficial hypocalciuric effect of therapy on renal stone formation.[122]

It has been suggested that potassium citrate may be less effective than potassium chloride in correcting the thiazide-induced hypokalemia because of the poor reabsorbability of citrate from the renal tubules.[132] However, severe chloride depletion is uncommon in patients with thiazide-induced hypocitraturia. Potassium citrate (15 to 20 mEq twice a day) is usually effective in preventing hypokalemia and maintaining normal urinary citrate levels.

IDIOPATHIC HYPOCITRATURIC CALCIUM NEPHROLITHIASIS. Idiopathic hypocitraturic calcium oxalate nephrolithiasis can be the result of isolated hypocitraturia with calcium stones or of hypocitraturia occurring in conjunction with absorptive and renal hypercalciurias or with hyperuricosuric calcium oxalate nephrolithiasis.[133] The stones formed are composed predominantly of calcium oxalate.

Potassium citrate treatment (15 to 30 mEq twice a day) produces a sustained increase in urinary citrate excretion.[133] Urinary pH can be maintained at 6.5 to 7. Along with these changes the urinary saturation of calcium oxalate declines to normal limits.

Gouty Diathesis

Potassium citrate is the treatment of choice for gouty diathesis. A dosage of 30 to 60 mEq/d in divided doses increases the low urinary pH (<5.5) to the desired range (>6).[100] Because of the resulting enhanced dissociation of uric acid, the amount of undissociated uric acid decreases to levels found in normal controls (<0.9 mmol/d [<150 mg/d]). Thus potassium citrate therapy increases the solubility of uric acid, preventing uric acid stone formation. Moreover this treatment inhibits the formation of calcium stones by reducing urinary saturation of calcium oxalate and retarding the crystallization of calcium oxalate.

Sodium alkali is as effective as potassium citrate in preventing uric acid nephrolithiasis because it has a similar capacity for raising urinary pH. However calcium stones may sometimes occur with sodium alkali therapy.[100] In patients with hyperuricemia or moderate to marked hyperuricosuria, allopurinol (e.g., 300 mg/d) is recommended as well.

Cystine Stones

A low-methionine diet has often been recommended for the control of cystine nephrolithiasis because methionine is a precursor of cystine. Although such a dietary maneuver may reduce cystine excretion, rigid methionine restriction is impractical. Dietary sodium restriction may also reduce cystine excretion,[134] but this beneficial effect may be neutralized by reduced solubility of cystine resulting from loss of the "solubilizing" action of sodium.[44]

In patients with cystine calculi and moderate cystinuria (1 to 2 mmol/d [250 to 500 mg/d]), conservative measures of high fluid intake and alkali administration should be attempted. The aim of fluid therapy is to increase urine volume sufficiently to reduce the cystine concentration to less than the solubility limit. At least 3 L of fluid should be provided, including two 8-oz servings with each meal and at bedtime. Patients should be directed to wake up at night to urinate and drink water. Additional fluids should be consumed when excessive sweating or intestinal fluid loss is present. A minimal urine output of 2 L/d on a consistent basis is attainable by most patients with proper and persistent instruction.

In theory alkali therapy would enhance cystine solubility by raising urinary pH. However, substantial increases in cystine solubility do not occur until the urinary pH exceeds 7.5. The provision of alkali, no matter how much, rarely raises the urinary pH to greater than 7.5. When the urinary pH increases to greater than 7 with alkali therapy, calcium phosphate nephrolithiasis may be enhanced because of the enhanced urinary supersaturation of hydroxyapatite in an alkaline environment. Excessive alkali therapy therefore is not indicated.[105]

Thus a modest amount of alkali is recommended to maintain urinary pH in a high normal range (6.5 to 7). Potassium citrate has an advantage over sodium citrate in that it does not cause hypercalciuria, is less likely to promote the development of calcium stones,[100, 135] and does not induce increased cystine excretion.[134]

The object of treatment with penicillamine or tiopronin (α-mercaptopropionylglycine) is to reduce total cystine excretion of complexing cysteine, the monomeric form of cystine. Penicillamine or tiopronin may be added to the conservative treatment program in patients with moderate cystinuria when the conservative treatment is ineffective in controlling stone formation. In patients with severe cystinuria (>2 mmol/d [>500 mg/d]), in whom conservative management alone is not likely to be effective, penicillamine or tiopronin therapy (together with conservative measures) may be started.

Penicillamine and tiopronin share with cysteine a free sulfhydryl group.[136] Thus they undergo thiol-disulfide exchange with cystine to form penicillamine-cysteine or tiopronin–cysteine disulfide, which is much more soluble than cystine. After oral administration a sufficient amount of penicillamine or tiopronin can be excreted in urine to form a complex with cysteine and thereby lower cystine excretion. Unfortunately penicillamine therapy is associated with frequent and sometimes severe side effects, including nephrotic syndrome, dermatitis, and pancytopenia.[137] Tiopronin has biochemical and clinical actions similar to those of penicillamine.[138] However it has a lower toxicity profile than that of penicillamine.

Infection Stones

If long-standing control of infection with urea-splitting organisms can be achieved, new stone formation may be averted and some existing stones may be dissolved. Unfortunately such control is difficult to obtain with antibiotic therapy. If a struvite stone is present, it is difficult to eradicate infection completely because the stone may harbor the organisms within its interstices. Even if "sterilization" of urine can be achieved with antibiotic therapy, reinfection by organisms harbored by the stones can occur. For this reason surgical removal of the struvite stones is usually recommended.

Acetohydroxamic acid, a urease inhibitor, reduces urinary saturation of struvite by preventing the formation of ammonium and hydroxyl ions.[139] It may prevent stone growth and sometimes cause dissolution of existing stones. However, it

may cause hemolytic anemia, thrombophlebitis, and nonspecific neurologic symptoms (disorientation, tremulousness, and headache).[140]

Conservative Management

The conservative measures of high fluid intake and avoidance of dietary excess should be applied in all patients with nephrolithiasis.[141] They may be applied alone in patients with a single stone episode and inactive stone disease but should be instituted together with a specific medical treatment program in patients with recurrent stone disease, particularly if extrarenal manifestations are present. Some conservative programs are applicable to all forms of stone disease, whereas others are useful for particular causes.

High fluid intake is the only nutritional modification that is useful in all forms of nephrolithiasis.[45] By increasing urine output, urinary concentration of constituent ions and saturation of stone-forming salts are lowered. Increased intake of water alone has been shown to reduce stone formation in a randomized trial.[142] Although dietary restriction of oxalate may be beneficial in all types of nephrolithiasis, it is particularly indicated when intestinal absorption of oxalate is increased, as in ileal disease and when calcium absorption is increased. Rigid calcium restriction (<10 mmol/d [<400 mg/d]) is ill advised, even in patients who have high intestinal calcium absorption, because it is difficult to adhere to, may adversely affect general nutrition, and may cause negative calcium balance. However, moderate calcium restriction (10 to 15 mmol/d [400 to 600 mg/d]) may be useful in absorptive hypercalciuria because it alone may control hypercalciuria in the less severe (type II) presentation and permit reduction of the dosage of medication necessary to restore normal urinary calcium concentration in the more severe (type I) presentation. Calcium restriction is neither necessary nor indicated in patients with nephrolithiasis and normal intestinal absorption of calcium.

Moderate sodium restriction (100 mmol/d) may be helpful in all forms of nephrolithiasis. Sodium excess raises urinary calcium and lowers urinary citrate.[94] Moreover it attenuates the hypocalciuric action of thiazide and increases urinary saturation of monosodium urate.[135]

REFERENCES

1. Pak CYC, Britton F, Peterson R, et al. Ambulatory evaluation of nephrolithiasis: classification, clinical presentation and diagnostic criteria. Am J Med 1980; 69:19–30.
2. Pak CYC, Peters P, Hurt G, et al. Is selective therapy of recurrent nephrolithiasis possible? Am J Med 1981; 71:615–622.
3. Frangos DN, Rous SN. Incidence and economic factors in urolithiasis. In: Rous SN, ed. Stone Disease: Diagnosis and Management. Orlando, FL: Grune & Stratton, 1987: 3–10.
4. Chulkaranta S, Van Reen R, Valyasevi A. Studies of bladder stone disease in Thailand. XV: Factors affecting the solubility of calcium oxalate. Invest Urol 1971; 9:246–250.
5. Fine JK, Pak CYC, Preminger GM. Effect of medical management and residual fragments on recurrent stone formation following shock wave lithotripsy. J Urol 1995; 153:27–33.
6. Prien EL, Prien EL Jr. Composition and structure of urinary stone. Am J Med 1968; 45:654–672.
7. Simmonds HA, Van Acker KJ, Cameron JS, et al. The identification of 2,8-dihydroxyadenine, a new component of urinary stones. Biochem J 1976; 157:485–487.
8. Nancollas G. The kinetics of crystal growth and renal stone formation. In: Fleisch H, Robertson WG, Smith LH, et al, eds. Urolithiasis Research. New York: Plenum, 1976: 5–23.
9. Meyer JL. Physicochemistry of stone formation. In: Resnick MI, Pak CYC, eds. Urolithiasis. Philadelphia: WB Saunders, 1990: 11–34.
9a. Coe FL, Parks JH, Asplin JR. The pathogenesis and treatment of kidney stones. N Engl J Med 1992; 327:1141–1152.
10. Robertson WG, Peacock M, Nordin BEC. Activity products in stone-forming and non–stone-forming urine. Clin Sci 1968; 34:579–594.
11. Finlayson B. Calcium stones: some physical and clinical aspects. In: David

D, ed. Calcium Metabolism in Renal Failure and Nephrolithiasis. New York: John Wiley & Sons, 1979: 337.

12. Pak CYC, Hayashi Y, Finlayson B, et al. Estimation of the state of saturation of brushite and calcium oxalate in urine: a comparison of three methods. J Lab Clin Med 1977; 89:891–901.

13. Pak CYC, Holt K. Nucleation and growth of brushite and calcium oxalate in urine of stone-formers. Metabolism 1976; 25:665–673.

14. Nicar MJ, Hill K, Pak CYC. A simple technique for assessing the propensity for crystallization of calcium oxalate and brushite in urine from the increment in oxalate or calcium necessary to elicit precipitation. Metabolism 1983; 32:906–910.

15. Pak CYC, Holt K, Britton F, et al. Assessment of pathogenetic roles in uric acid, monopotassium urate, monoammonium urate and monosodium urate in hyperuricosuric calcium oxalate nephrolithiasis. Miner Electrolyte Metab 1980; 4:130–136.

16. Meyer JL, Bergert JH, Smith LH. Epitaxial relationship in urolithiasis: the calcium oxalate monohydrate-hydroxyapatite system. Clin Sci Mol Med 1975; 49:369–374.

17. Lonsdale K. Epitaxy as a growth factor in urinary calculi and gallstones. Nature 1968; 217:56–58.

18. Meyer JL, Smith LH. Growth of calcium oxalate crystals. II: Inhibition by natural urinary crystal growth inhibitors. Invest Urol 1975; 13:36–39.

19. Bisaz S, Felix R, Neiman W, et al. Quantitative determination of inhibitors of calcium phosphate precipitation in whole urine. Miner Electrolyte Metab 1978; 1:74.

20. Smith LH, Meyer JL, McCall JT. Chemical nature of crystal inhibitors isolated from human urine. In: Cifuentes L, Rapado A, Hodgkinson A, eds. Urinary Calculi: International Symposium on Renal Stone Research. Basel: S. Karger, 1973: 318.

21. Nakagawa Y, Kaiser ET, Coe FL. Isolation and characterization of calcium oxalate crystal growth inhibitors from human urine. Biochem Biophys Res Commun 1978; 84:1038–1044.

21a. Worcester EM, Blumenthal SS, Beshensky AM, et al. The calcium oxalate crystal growth inhibitor protein produced by mouse kidney cortical cells in culture is osteopontin. J Bone Miner Res 1992; 7:1029–1036.

22. Bowyer RC, Brockis JG, McCulloch RK. Glycosaminoglycans as inhibitors of calcium oxalate crystal growth and aggregation. Clin Chim Acta 1979; 95:23–28.

23. Robertson WG, Peacock M, Nordin BEC. Inhibitors of the growth and aggregation of calcium oxalate crystals in vitro. Clin Chim Acta 1973; 43:31–37.

24. Kok DJ, Papapoulos SE, Bijvoet OLM. Excessive crystal agglomeration with low citrate excretion in recurrent stone-formers. Lancet 1986; 1:1056–1058.

25. Hess B. Tamm-Horsfall glycoprotein and calcium nephrolithiasis. Miner Electrolyte Metab 1996; 20:393–398.

25a. Jaeger P, Portmann L, Jacquet A, et al. Influence of the calcium content of the diet on the incidence of mild hyperoxaluria in idiopathic renal stone formers. Am J Nephrol 1985;5:40–44.

26. Pak CYC. Idiopathic renal lithiasis: new developments in evaluation and treatment. In: Fleisch H, Robertson WG, Smith LH, et al, eds. Urolithiasis Research. New York: Plenum, 1976: 213–244.

27. Zerwekh JE, Hwang TIS, Poindexter J, et al. Modulation by calcium of the inhibitor activity of citrate, chondroitin sulfate and urinary glycoprotein against calcium oxalate crystallization. Kidney Int 1988; 33:1005–1008.

28. Strauss AL, Coe FL, Deutsch L, et al. Factors that predict relapse of calcium nephrolithiasis during treatment. Am J Med 1982; 71:17–24.

29. Pak CYC, Galosy RA. Propensity for spontaneous nucleation of calcium oxalate. Quantitative assessment by urinary FPR-APR discriminant score. Am J Med 1980; 69:681–689.

30. Yendt ER, Cohanim M. Prevention of calcium stones with thiazides. Kidney Int 1978; 13:397–409.

31. Sakhaee K, Baker S, Zerwekh J, et al. Limited risk of kidney stone formation during long-term calcium citrate supplementation in non–stone forming subjects. J Urol 1994; 152:324–327.

32. Pak CYC. Calcium metabolism. J Am Coll Nutr 1989; 8:465–535.

33. Finlayson B, Smith A. Stability of first dissociable proton of uric acid. J Chem Eng Data 1974; 19:94.

34. Coe FL. Hyperuricosuric calcium oxalate nephrolithiasis. Kidney Int 1978; 13:418–426.

35. Pak CYC, Waters O, Arnold L, et al. Mechanism for calcium nephrolithiasis among patients with hyperuricosuria: supersaturation of urine with respect to monosodium urate. J Clin Invest 1977; 59:426–431.

36. Pak CYC, Barilla DE, Holt K, et al. Effect of oral purine load and allopurinol on the crystallization of calcium salts in urine of patients with hyperuricosuric calcium urolithiasis. Am J Med 1978; 65:593–599.

37. Pak CYC, Holt K, Zerwekh JE. Attenuation by monosodium urate of the inhibitory effect of glycosaminoglycans on calcium oxalate nucleation. Invest Urol 1979; 17:138–140.

38. Zerwekh JE, Holt K, Pak CYC. Natural urinary macromolecular inhibitors: Attenuation of inhibitory activity by urate salts. Kidney Int 1983; 23:838–841.

39. Pak CYC, Nicar MJ, Northcutt C. The definition of the mechanism of hypercalciuria is necessary for the treatment of recurrent stone formers. Contrib Nephrol 1982; 33:136–151.

40. Nicar MJ, Hill K, Pak CYC. Inhibition by citrate of spontaneous precipitation of calcium oxalate, in vitro. J Bone Miner Res 1987; 2:215–220.

41. Kitamura T, Zerwekh JE, Pak CYC. Partial biochemical and physicochemical characterization of organic macromolecules in urine from patients with renal stones and control subjects. Kidney Int 1981; 21:379–386.

42. Lindberg JS, Zobitz MM, Poindexter JR, et al. Magnesium bioavailability from magnesium citrate and magnesium oxide. Am J Coll Nutr 1990; 9:48–55.

43. Griffith DP, Musher DM. Prevention of infected urinary stones by urease inhibition. Invest Urol 1973; 11:228–233.

44. Pak CYC, Fuller CJ. Assessment of cystine solubility in urine and of heterogeneous nucleation between cystine and calcium salts. Invest Urol 1983; 129:1066–1070.

45. Pak CYC, Sakhaee K, Crowther C, et al. Evidence justifying a high fluid intake in treatment of nephrolithiasis. Ann Intern Med 1980; 93:36–39.

46. Henneman PH, Benedict PH, Forbes AP. Idiopathic hypercalciuria. N Engl J Med 1958; 259:801–807.

47. Pak CYC. Pathogenesis of hypercalciuria. In: Peck WA, ed. Bone and Mineral Research. Vol 4. New York: Elsevier, 1986: 303–334.

48. Pak CYC, Ohata M, Lawrence EC, et al. The hypercalciurias: causes, parathyroid functions and diagnostic criteria. J Clin Invest 1974; 54:387–400.

49. Brannan PG, Morawski S, Pak CYC. Selective jejunal hyperabsorption of calcium in absorptive hypercalciuria. Am J Med 1979; 66:425–428.

50. Pak CYC, Nicar MJ, Krejs GJ. Intestinal absorption of calcium, magnesium, phosphate and oxalate: deviation from normal in idiopathic urolithiasis. In: Schwille PO, Smith LH, Robertson WG, et al, eds. Urolithiasis and Related Clinical Research. New York: Plenum, 1985: 127–133.

51. Breslau NA, Preminger GM, Adams BV, et al. Use of ketoconazole to probe the pathogenetic importance of 1,25-$(OH)_2$D in absorptive hypercalciuria. J Clin Endocrinol Metab 1992; 75:1446–1452.

52. Pak CYC. Physiological basis for absorptive and renal hypercalciurias. Am J Physiol 1979; 237:F415–F423.

53. Kaplan RA, Haussler MR, Deftos LJ, et al. The role of 1α,25-dihydroxyvitamin D in the mediation of intestinal hyperabsorption of calcium in primary hyperparathyroidism and absorptive hypercalciuria. J Clin Invest 1977; 59:756–760.

54. Insogna KL, Broadus AE, Dreyer BE, et al. Elevated production rate of 1,25-dihydroxyvitamin D in patients with absorptive hypercalciuria. J Clin Endocrinol Metab 1985; 61:490–495.

55. Broadus AE, Horst RL, Lang R, et al. The importance of circulating 1,25-dihydroxyvitamin D in the pathogenesis of hypercalciuria and renal-stone formation in primary hyperparathyroidism. N Engl J Med 1980; 302:421–426.

56. Shen FH, Baylink DJ, Nielson RL, et al. Increased serum 1,25-dihydroxyvitamin D in idiopathic hypercalciuria. J Lab Clin Med 1977; 90:955–962.

57. Gray RW, Wilz DR, Caldas AE, et al. The importance of phosphate in regulating plasma 1,25-$(OH)_2$vitamin D levels in humans: studies in healthy subjects, in calcium-stone formers and in patients with primary hyperparathyroidism. J Clin Endocrinol Metab 1977; 45:299–306.

58. Barilla DE, Zerwekh JE, Pak CYC. A critical evaluation of the role of phosphate in the pathogenesis of absorptive hypercalciuria. Miner Electrolyte Metab 1979; 2:302–309.

59. Broadus AE, Erickson SB, Gertner JM, et al. An experimental human model of 1,25-dihydroxyvitamin D–mediated hypercalciuria. J Clin Endocrin Metabol 1984; 59:202–206.

60. Pak CYC, Galosy RA. Fasting urinary calcium and adenosine $3'$-$5'$-monophosphonate: a discriminant analysis for the identification of renal and absorptive hypercalciuria. J Clin Endocrinol Metab 1979; 48:260–265.

61. Raisz LG, Trummel CL, Holick MF, et al. 1,25-Dihydroxycholecalciferol: a potent stimulator of bone resorption in tissue culture. Science 1972; 175:768–769.

62. Reynolds JJ, Holick MF, DuLuca HF. The role of vitamin D metabolites on bone resorption. Calcif Tissue Res 1973; 12:295–301.

63. Pietschmann F, Breslau NA, Pak CYC. Reduced vertebral bone density in hypercalciuric nephrolithiasis. J Bone Miner Res 1992; 7:1383–1388.

64. Coe FL, Favus MJ, Crockett T, et al. Effects of low-calcium diet on urine calcium excretion, parathyroid function and serum 1,25-$(OH)_2D_3$ levels in patients with idiopathic hypercalciuria and in normal subjects. Am J Med 1982; 72:25–32.

65. Coe FL, Canterbury JM, Firpo JJ, et al. Evidence for secondary hyperparathyroidism in idiopathic hypercalciuria. J Clin Invest 1973; 52:134–142.

66. Zerwekh JE, Pak CYC. Selective effects of thiazide therapy on serum 1,25-dihydroxyvitamin D and intestinal calcium absorption in renal and absorptive hypercalciurias. Metabolism 1980; 29:13–17.

67. Sakhaee K, Nicar MJ, Brater DC, et al. Exaggerated natriuretic and calciuric responses to hydrochlorothiazide in renal hypercalciuria but not in absorptive hypercalciuria. J Clin Endocrinol Metab 1985; 61:825–829.

68. Barilla DE, Townsend J, Pak CYC. An exaggerated augmentation of renal calcium excretion following oral glucose ingestion in patients with renal hypercalciuria. Invest Urol 1978; 15:486–488.

69. Lemann J, Piering WF, Lennon EJ. Possible role of carbohydrate-induced calciuria in calcium oxalate kidney-stone formation. N Engl J Med 1969; 280:232–237.

70. Muldowney FP, Freaney R, Moloney MF. Importance of dietary sodium in the hypercalciuria syndrome. Kidney Int 1982; 22:292–296.

71. Lawoyin S, Sismilich S, Browne R, et al. Bone mineral content in patients with primary hyperparathyroidism, osteoporosis, and calcium urolithiasis. Metabolism 1979; 28:1250–1254.

71a. Lloyd SE, Pearce SHS, Fisher SE, et al. A common molecular basis for three inherited kidney stone diseases. Nature 1996; 379:445–449.

72. Garabedian M, Holick MF, DeLuca HF, et al. Control of 25-hydroxycholec-alciferol metabolism by parathyroid glands. Proc Natl Acad Sci USA 1972; 69:1673.

73. Patron P, Gardin J-P, Paillard M. Renal mass and reserve of vitamin D: determinants of plasma 1,25-(OH)₂D₃ in primary hyperparathyroidism. Kidney Int 1987; 31:1174–1180.

74. Pak CYC, Nicar MJ, Peterson R, et al. A lack of unique pathophysiologic background for nephrolithiasis of primary hyperparathyroidism. J Clin Endocrinol Metab 1981; 53:536–542.

75. Bone HG III, Zerwekh JE, Haussler MR, et al. Effect of parathyroidectomy on serum 1,25-dihydroxyvitamin D and on intestinal calcium absorption in primary hyperparathyroidism. J Clin Endocrinol Metab 1979; 48:877–879.

76. Buck AC, Lote CJ, Sampson WF. The influence of renal prostaglandins on urinary calcium excretion in idiopathic urolithiasis. J Urol 1983; 129:421–426.

77. Coe FL, Kavalach AG. Hypercalciuria and hyperuricosuria in patients with calcium nephrolithiasis. N Engl J Med 1974; 291:1344–1350.

78. Breslau NA, Pak CYC. Lack of effect of salt intake on urinary uric acid excretions. J Urol 1983; 129:531–532.

79. Pak CYC. Medical management of nephrolithiasis in Dallas: update 1987. J Urol 1988; 140:461–467.

80. Levy FL, Huet-Adams B, Pak CYC. Ambulatory evaluation of nephrolithiasis: an update from 1980. Am J Med 1995; 98:50–59.

81. Loffler W, Grobner W, Medina R, et al. Influence of dietary purines on pool size, turnover, and excretion of uric acid during balance condition. Res Exp Med (Berl) 1982; 181:113–123.

82. Pak CYC, Tolentino R, Stewart A, et al. Enhancement of renal excretion of uric acid during long-term thiazide therapy. Invest Urol 1978; 3:191–193.

83. Earnest DL, Williams HE, Admirand WH. A physicochemical basis for treatment of enteric hyperoxaluria. Trans Assoc Am Phys 1975; 88:224–234.

84. Smith LH, Fromm H, Hofmann AF. Acquired hyperoxaluria, nephrolithiasis and intestinal disease: description of a syndrome. N Engl J Med 1972; 286; 1371–1374.

85. Nicar MJ, Skurla C, Sakhaee K, et al. Low urinary citrate excretion in nephrolithiasis. Urology 1983; 21:8–14.

86. Simpson DP. Regulation of renal citrate metabolism by bicarbonate ion and pH: observations in tissue slices and mitochondria. J Clin Invest 1967; 16:225–238.

87. Morrissey JF, Ocha M, Lotspeich WD, et al. Citrate excretion in renal tubular acidosis. Ann Intern Med 1963; 55:159–166.

88. Nicar MJ, Peterson R, Pak CYC. Use of potassium citrate as potassium supplement during thiazide therapy of calcium nephrolithiasis. J Urol 1984; 131:430–433.

88a. Melnick JZ, Srere PA, Elshourbagy NA, et al. ATP citrate lyase mediates hypocitraturia of chronic metabolic acidosis in rats. J Clin Invest 1996; 98:2381–2387.

89. Preminger GM, Sakhaee K, Skurla C, et al. Prevention of recurrent calcium stone formation with potassium citrate therapy in patients with distal renal tubular acidosis. J Urol 1985; 134:20–23.

90. Rudman D, Dedonis JL, Fountain MT, et al. Hypocitraturia in patients with gastrointestinal malabsorption. N Engl J Med 1980; 303:657–661.

91. Pak CYC, Fuller C, Sakhaee K, et al. Long-term treatment of calcium nephrolithiasis with potassium citrate. Therapy in patients with distal renal tubular acidosis. J Urol 1985; 134:11–19.

92. Breslau NA, Brinkley L, Hill KD, et al. Relationship role of animal protein-rich diet to kidney stone formation and calcium metabolism. J Clin Endocrinol Metab 1988; 66:140–146.

93. Sakhaee K, Nigam S, Snell P, et al. Assessment of the pathogenetic role of physical exercise in renal stone formation. J Clin Endocrinol Metab 1987; 65:974–979.

94. Sakhaee K, Harvey JA, Padalino PK, et al. Potential role of salt abuse on the risk for kidney stone formation. J Urol 1991; 150:310–312.

95. Uribarri J, Oh MS, Pak CYC. Renal stone risk factors in patients with type IV renal tubular acidosis. Am J Kidney Dis 1994; 23:784–787.

96. Fegan J, Khan R, Poindexter J, et al. Gastrointestinal citrate absorption in nephrolithiasis. J Urol 1992; 147:1212–1214.

97. Sakhaee K, Williams RH, Oh MS, et al. Alkali absorption and citrate excretion in calcium nephrolithiasis. J Bone Miner Res 1993; 8:787–792.

98. Drach GW, Gaines J, Donovan J. Is magnesium metabolism related to calcium urolithiasis? In: Schwille PO, Smith LH, Robertson WG, et al, eds. Urolithiasis and Related Clinical Research. New York: Plenum, 1985: 241–244.

99. Preminger GM, Baker S, Peterson R, et al. Hypomagnesiuric hypocitraturia: an apparent new entity for calcium nephrolithiasis. J Lith Stone Dis 1989; 1:22–25.

100. Pak CYC, Sakhaee K, Fuller C. Successful management of uric acid nephrolithiasis with potassium citrate. Kidney Int 1986; 30:422–428.

101. Khatchadourian J, Preminger GM, Whitson PM, et al. Clinical and biochemical presentation of gouty diathesis: comparison of uric acid versus pure calcium stone formation. J Urol 1995; 154:1665–1669.

102. Yu TF. Uric acid nephrolithiasis. In: Kelly WN, Weiner IM, eds. Handbook of Experimental Pharmacology. Vol 51. New York: Springer-Verlag, 1978: 397–422.

103. Deren JJ, Porush JG, Levitt MF, et al. Nephrolithiasis as complication of ulcerative colitis and regional ileitis. Ann Intern Med 1962; 56:843–853.

104. Broadus A, Thier S. Metabolic basis of renal stone disease. N Engl J Med 1979; 300:839–845.

105. Dent CE, Rose GA. Amino acid metabolism in cystinuria. Q J Med 1951; 20:205–219.

106. Thier SO, Segal S. Cystinuria. In: Stanbury JB, Wyngaarden JB, Fredrickson DS, eds. The Metabolic Basis of Inherited Disease. New York: McGraw-Hill, 1972: 1504–1519.

107. Rosenberg LE, Downing S, Durant JL, et al. Cystinuria: biochemical evidence for three genetically distinct diseases. J Clin Invest 1966; 45:365–371.

108. Calonge MJ, Gasparini P, Chillarón J, et al. Cystinuria caused by mutations in rBAT, a gene involved in the transport of cystine. Nat Genet 1994; 6:420–425.

109. Pak CYC, Skurla C, Harvey J. Graphic display of urinary risk factors for renal stone formation. J Urol 1985; 134:867–870.

110. Pak CYC, Kaplan RA, Bone H, et al. A simple test for the diagnosis of absorptive, resorptive and renal hypercalciurias. N Engl J Med 1975; 292:497–500.

111. Pak CYC, Griffith DP, Menon M, et al. Urolithiasis. In: Current Practice of Medicine. Series Ed. Bone RC; Volume Ed. Glassock R. Current Medicine, Inc. Philadelphia, 1996: Vol 4. pp 13.3–13.4.

112. Silverberg SJ, Shane E, Cruz L, et al. Skeletal disease in primary hyperparathyroidism. J Bone Miner Res 1989; 4:283–291.

113. Coe FL, Boro ES. Hypercalciuria and hyperuricosuria in patients with calcium nephrolithiasis. N Engl J Med 1974; 291:1344–1350.

114. Pak CYC. Medical management of nephrolithiasis. J Urol 1982; 128:1157–1164.

114a. Ettinger B, Tang A, Citron JT, et al. Randomized trial of allopurinol in the prevention of calcium oxalate calculi. N Engl J Med 1986; 315:1386–1389.

114b. Barcelo P, Wuhl O, Servitge E, et al. Randomized double-blind study of potassium citrate in idiopathic hypocitraturic calcium nephrolithiasis. J Urol 1993; 150:1761–1764.

115. Kaplan RA, Snyder WH, Stewart A, et al. Metabolic effects of parathyroidectomy on asymptomatic primary hyperparathyroidism. J Clin Endocrinol Metab 1976; 42:415–426.

116. Pak CYC. Effect of parathyroidectomy on crystallization of calcium salts in urine of patients with primary hyperparathyroidism. Invest Urol 1979; 17:146–148.

117. Broadus AE, Magee JS, Mallette LE, et al. A detailed evaluation of oral phosphate therapy in selected patients with primary hyperparathyroidism. J Clin Endocrinol Metab 1983; 56:953–961.

118. Selby PL, Peacock M. Ethinyl estradiol and norethindrone in the treatment of primary hyperparathyroidism in postmenopausal women. N Engl J Med 1986; 314:1481–1485.

119. Pak CYC. Sodium cellulose phosphate: mechanism of action and effect on mineral metabolism. J Clin Pharmacol 1973; 13:15–27.

120. Pak CYC. A cautious use of sodium cellulose phosphate in the management of calcium nephrolithiasis. Invest Urol 1981; 19:187–190.

121. Hayashi Y, Kaplan RA, Pak CYC. Effect of sodium cellulose phosphate therapy on crystallization of calcium oxalate in urine. Metabolism 1975; 24:1273–1278.

122. Preminger GM, Pak CYC. Eventual attenuation of hypocalciuric response to hydrochlorothiazide in absorptive hypercalciuria. J Urol 1987; 137:1104–1109.

123. Pak CYC, Peterson R, Sakhaee K, et al. Correction of hypocitraturia and prevention of stone formation by combined thiazide and potassium citrate therapy in thiazide-unresponsive hypercalciuric nephrolithiasis. Am J Med 1985; 79:284–288.

124. Breslau NA, Padalino P, Kok DJ, et al. Physicochemical effects of a new slow-release potassium phosphate preparation (UroPhos-K) in absorptive hypercalciuria. J Bone Miner Res 1993; 10:394–400.

125. Woelfel A, Kaplan RA, Pak CYC. Effect of hydrochlorothiazide therapy on crystallization of calcium oxalate in urine. Metabolism 1977; 26:201–205.

126. Ettinger B, Oldroyd NO, Sorge F. Triamterene nephrolithiasis. JAMA 1980; 244:2443–2445.

127. Leppla D, Browne R, Hill K, et al. Effect of amiloride with or without hydrochlorothiazide on urinary calcium and saturation of calcium salts. J Clin Endocrinol Metab 1983; 57:920–924.

128. Pak CYC, Peterson R. Successful treatment of hyperuricosuric calcium oxalate nephrolithiasis with potassium citrate. Arch Intern Med 1986; 146:863–868.

129. Barilla DE, Notz C, Kennedy D, et al. Renal oxalate excretion following oral oxalate loads in patients with ileal disease and with renal and absorptive hypercalciurias: Effect of calcium and magnesium. Am J Med 1978; 64:576–585.

130. Harvey JA, Zobitz MM, Pak CYC. Calcium citrate: reduced propensity for the crystallization of calcium oxalate in urine resulting from induced hypercalciuria of calcium supplementation. J Clin Endocrinol Metab 1985; 61:1223–1225.

131. Preminger GM, Sakhaee K, Pak CYC. Hypercalciuria and altered intestinal calcium absorption occurring independently of vitamin D in incomplete distal renal tubular acidosis. Metabolism 1987; 36:176–179.

132. Kassirer JP, Berkman PM, Lawrenz DR, et al. The critical role of chloride in the correction of hypokalemic alkalosis in man. Am J Med 1965; 38:172–189.

133. Pak CYC, Fuller C. Idiopathic hypocitraturic calcium oxalate nephrolithiasis successfully treated with potassium citrate. Ann Intern Med 1986; 104:33–37.

134. Jaeger P, Portmann L, Saunders A, et al. Anticystinuric effects of glutamine and of dietary sodium restriction. N Engl J Med 1986; 315:1120–1123.

135. Sakhaee K, Nicar M, Hill K, et al. Contrasting effects of potassium citrate and sodium citrate therapies on urinary chemistries and crystallization of stone-forming salt. Kidney Int 1983; 24:348–352.

136. Perrett D. The metabolism and pharmacology of D-penicillamine in man. J Rheumatol 1981; 8(S7):41–50.

137. Halperin EC, Thier SO, Rosenberg LE. The use of D-penicillamine in cystinuria: efficacy and untoward reactions. Yale J Biol Med 1981; 54:439–446.

138. Pak CYC, Fuller C, Sakhaee K, et al. Management of cystine nephrolithiasis with alpha-mercaptopropionylglycine (Thiola). J Urol 1986; 136:1003–1008.

139. Griffith DP. Struvite stones. Kidney Int 1978; 13:372–382.

140. Williams JJ, Rodman JS, Peterson CM. A randomized double-blind study of acetohydroxamic acid in struvite nephrolithiasis. N Engl J Med 1984; 311:760–764.

141. Pak CYC, Smith LH, Resnick MI, et al. Dietary management of idiopathic calcium urolithiasis. J Urol 1984; 131:850–852.

142. Borghi L, Meschi T, Amato F, et al. Urinary volume, water and recurrences in idiopathic calcium nephrolithiasis: a 5-year randomized prospective study. J Urol 1996; 155:839–843.

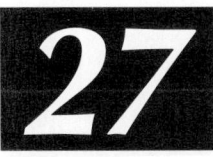

ENDOCRINE CHANGES OF PREGNANCY

M. Linette Casey and Paul C. MacDonald†

During the past 75 years, the endocrinologic and physiological changes that accompany human pregnancy have been defined in appreciable detail.[1] Although it is commonly believed that the endocrinology/physiology of human pregnancy is similar to that of other mammalian species, this is not the case. That misconception probably exists because of our greater understanding of the hormonal changes of human pregnancy and therefore our greater familiarity with the endocrine milieu of human gestation than with those of other mammalian species. In most mammals the corpus luteum is the site of steroid hormone formation during pregnancy (mouse, rat, rabbit, hamster, cat, dog, goat, and cow). The placenta is a steroid hormone–producing organ in only a few species, such as primates (including humans), sheep, horses, and guinea pigs. More importantly, the amounts of steroid and protein hormones produced during human pregnancy are orders of magnitude greater than those produced during gestation in most other mammals, including subhuman primates. At or near term, the daily production rate of estradiol in women is about 70 μmol (20 mg) and that of estriol is about 300 μmol (80 mg). By comparison, the plasma levels of estrogen in the pregnant cow are comparable to those in postmenopausal women. Progesterone production in preg-

nant women during the third trimester is about 1 mmol (300 mg), and in multifetal pregnancies much more is produced. In the elephant, progesterone cannot be detected in plasma at any time during pregnancy, and the level of plasma progesterone in pregnant rhesus monkeys is only 2% of that in women.

The rate of aldosterone secretion in human pregnancy is about 3 μmol (1 mg) per day, and the daily production rate of deoxycorticosterone is approximately 30 μmol (10 mg). The levels of plasma renin, angiotensinogen, and angiotensin II increase strikingly. The daily rate of secretion of human placental lactogen (hPL, also called human chorionic somatomammotropin [hCS]) near term is about 1 g, and large quantities of human chorionic gonadotropin (hCG) are formed. In addition, the placenta produces human growth hormone variant (hGH-V) and hypothalamic-like releasing factors, including luteinizing hormone–releasing hormone (LHRH), growth hormone–releasing hormone (GHRH), thyrotropin-releasing hormone (TRH), and corticotropin-releasing hormone (CRH). Consequently, a remarkable aspect of human pregnancy is the establishment of mechanisms whereby the gravid woman and the fetus are able to adapt to this unusual endocrine milieu.[1] What is the physiological purpose of these massive endocrine changes in human pregnancy? We can only speculate. The pregnant human uterus is a thick muscular

†Deceased.

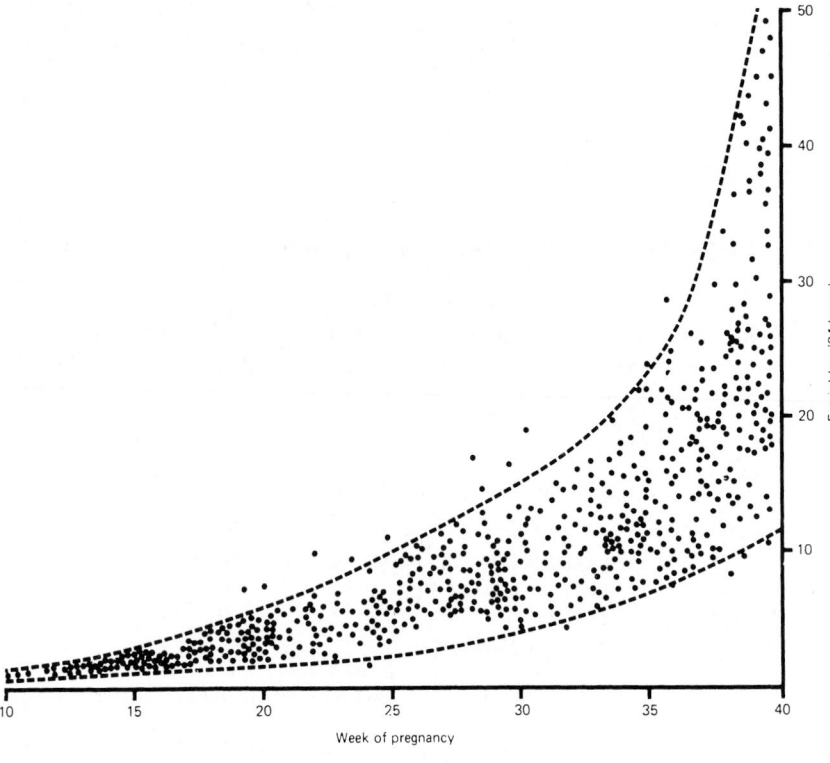

Figure 27–1. Urinary excretion of estriol-16-glucuronoside in 31 healthy pregnant women followed throughout pregnancy. Upper and lower dashed lines are the 95% confidence limits. (From Beling C. Estrogens. In: Fuchs F, Klopper A, eds. Endocrinology of Pregnancy. 2nd ed. New York: Harper & Row, 1977: 86, with permission.)

structure that undergoes violent contractions during the time of labor and delivery of the fetus. Immediately after delivery, women experience appreciable blood loss, which is not the case with the delivery of young in other species. One function of the endocrine milieu of pregnancy is to increase blood volume. On average, the blood volume expands by about 1500 mL during normal human gestation, which protects against the effects of blood loss that varies from 500 to 1500 mL in most spontaneous vaginal deliveries. Other endocrine changes of human pregnancy may represent vestiges of evolutionary development. For example, hPL and hGH-V may have played a critical physiological role in pregnancy thousands of years ago when our ancestors were hunter-gatherers and were obliged to experience frequent periods of near-starvation. Placental lactogen and hGH-V act to mobilize free fatty acids and to antagonize insulin action, thereby serving to ensure a continuing source of nutrients to the fetus, even at the expense of maternal well-being. Whatever the reasons for the endocrine changes of pregnancy, most women successfully adapt to the alterations during pregnancy.

ESTROGEN FORMATION DURING PREGNANCY

Large quantities of estrogens are produced during normal human pregnancy (Fig. 27–1), and after the first 3 to 4 wk of gestation nearly all of the estrogen (estradiol and estriol) is produced in the syncytiotrophoblast of the placenta. The mechanism by which estrogen is produced in the human trophoblast, however, is unique. Steroid 17α-hydroxylase (CYP17) is not expressed in the human placenta; consequently, C_{21}-steroids cannot be converted to C_{19}-steroids in trophoblast. Thus, progesterone is not metabolized further within the placenta, except by C-6-hydroxylation (in limited amounts). Therefore, estrogens cannot be produced de novo, that is, from acetate or cholesterol, in the human trophoblast. Nonetheless the human placenta is endowed with a remark-

able capacity for the aromatization of C_{19}-steroids, and androstenedione, testosterone, and dehydroepiandrosterone are efficiently converted to estrone and estradiol by minces of placental tissue and placental tissue microsomes.[2] As an important corollary, Frandsen and Stakeman[3] found that the levels of urinary estrogens are low in women pregnant with an anencephalic fetus; the fetal adrenal is usually atrophic in anencephalic fetuses, and they suggested that the fetal adrenal may participate in estrogen formation in the human placenta.

Placental Aromatization of Circulating C_{19}-Steroids

In the early 1960s three groups of investigators demonstrated that the human placenta synthesizes estrogen from circulating C_{19}-steroid precursors, principally dehydroepiandrosterone sulfate (Fig. 27–2).[4–6] Dehydroepiandrosterone sulfate is desulfurylated in placenta by steroid sulfatase and then converted to androstenedione. The product of the aromatization of androstenedione is estrone, which is converted by

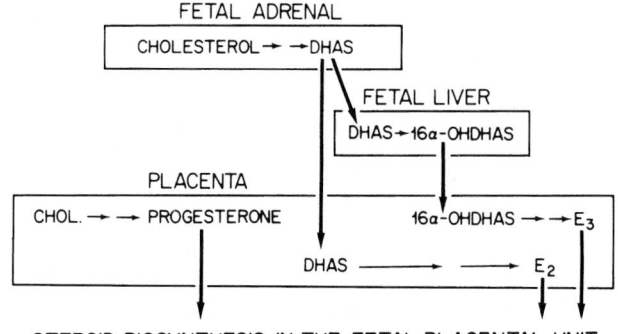

STEROID BIOSYNTHESIS IN THE FETAL-PLACENTAL UNIT

Figure 27–2. Schematic representation of steroid hormone biosynthesis in the fetal-placental unit. DHAS, dehydroepiandrosterone sulfate; E2, estradiol; E3, estriol; CHOL, cholesterol.

17β-hydroxysteroid dehydrogenase (17β-HSD) type I in the trophoblast to estradiol, which then enters the maternal circulation.[7] It is not clear whether 17β-HSD type II is expressed in trophoblast. The 17β-HSD type II isoform of the enzyme preferentially catalyzes the oxidation of the 17β-hydroxyl group of estradiol and the 20α-hydroxyl group of 20α-dihydroprogesterone. This enzyme activity is readily demonstrable in microsome-enriched fractions of whole placental tissue but has not been demonstrated specifically in trophoblast. The 17β-HSD type II enzyme activity in placental tissue might be localized in nontrophoblastic tissue of the placenta, namely, fetal blood vessels. The contribution of trophoblast to the total mass of the placenta is small compared with the contribution of fetal vascular tissue. If 17β-HSD type II were present only in vascular tissue of placenta, it would explain the finding that estradiol is secreted from trophoblast into the maternal compartment, whereas estrone appears to be secreted into the fetal compartment. It is possible that estradiol is the secretory product of the syncytiotrophoblast but is converted to estrone in the fetal blood vessels of the placenta before reaching the umbilical venous blood.[8]

A second feature of estrogen formation in human pregnancy is that the amount of estriol in the blood and urine of pregnant women is elevated disproportionately, as compared with the amount of estrone and estradiol in the blood and urine of nonpregnant women. In nonpregnant women, estriol is totally accounted for by the metabolism of estrone and estradiol, whereas estriol in pregnant women is secreted directly by the syncytiotrophoblast by a pathway involving desulfurylation of plasma 16α-hydroxydehydroepiandrosterone sulfate[9, 10] and aromatization of the 16α-hydroxyandrostenedione formed by the action of 3β-hydroxysteroid dehydrogenase.

Near term, approximately half of the estradiol synthesized in the placenta is derived from precursors in the fetal circulation and half from precursors in the maternal circulation.[10] By contrast, approximately 90% of estriol in the near-term pregnant woman is produced from 16α-hydroxydehydroepiandrosterone sulfate in the fetal plasma. Dehydroepiandrosterone sulfate is synthesized in the fetal adrenal cortex and is converted to 16α-hydroxydehydroepiandrosterone sulfate in the fetal adrenal and liver. Steroid sulfatase activity in the placenta is high.[11, 12]

Role of Fetal Adrenal in Placental Estrogen Biosynthesis

The adrenals of the human fetus at term are as large as those of adults, weighing 8 to 10 g or more (Fig. 27–3).[13]

Morphologically the fetal adrenals are composed principally of an inner fetal zone that accounts for 85% of the volume of the fetal glands. The outer zone (i.e., the neocortex), which ultimately develops into the mature adrenal cortex, makes up 15% or less of the total volume. The capacity of the fetal adrenals for steroidogenesis is remarkable. Near term, the fetal adrenals secrete 100 to 200 mg/d of steroid, compared with the total daily steroid production of only about 35 mg/d by the adrenals of nonstressed adults. The principal products of the fetal adrenal are dehydroepiandrosterone sulfate and pregnenolone sulfate.

In addition to its role in providing precursors for placental estrogen formation, the fetal adrenal cortex may participate in the biochemical processes that lead to maturation of the fetal lung and the initiation of parturition.[14, 15] Therefore the regulation of steroidogenesis in the human fetal adrenal is important to human pregnancy. Corticotropin levels in human fetal blood decline as gestation advances,[16] whereas the adrenals continue to grow in late gestation when corticotropin levels are falling. The pattern of steroids secreted by the fetal adrenals also is different from that of the adult. For these reasons a trophic role has been proposed for other hormones including growth hormone, hCG, prolactin, hPL, and α-melanocyte–stimulating hormone. There is little convincing evidence, however, that any of these hormones serve an important role in controlling growth or steroidogenesis in the fetal adrenals. It is likely that one or more unidentified growth factors (possibly of placental origin) regulate growth of the adrenal without directly enhancing the rate of synthesis of adrenal steroidogenic enzymes and that the increase in the rate of steroid secretion as gestation progresses is caused primarily by the growth of the adrenals rather than by a specific increase in the rate of adrenal steroid synthesis per cell.

The principal precursor for fetal adrenal steroid biosynthesis is cholesterol, which can arise from two sources: de novo synthesis from two-carbon precursors or assimilation from plasma low-density lipoprotein (LDL),[17] but the LDL cholesterol level in cord blood of newborns is only about 0.8 mmol/L (30 mg/dL), approximately one fourth to one fifth of that in the plasma of normal adults.[18] The total LDL cholesterol in the entire plasma volume of the human fetus near term is only 0.08 mmol (30 mg). Thus if LDL is the principal source of cholesterol for fetal adrenal steroidogenesis, its turnover in fetal plasma must be rapid compared with that in the adult; indeed, LDL cholesterol is the form of cholesterol preferentially utilized for steroidogenesis in human fetal adre-

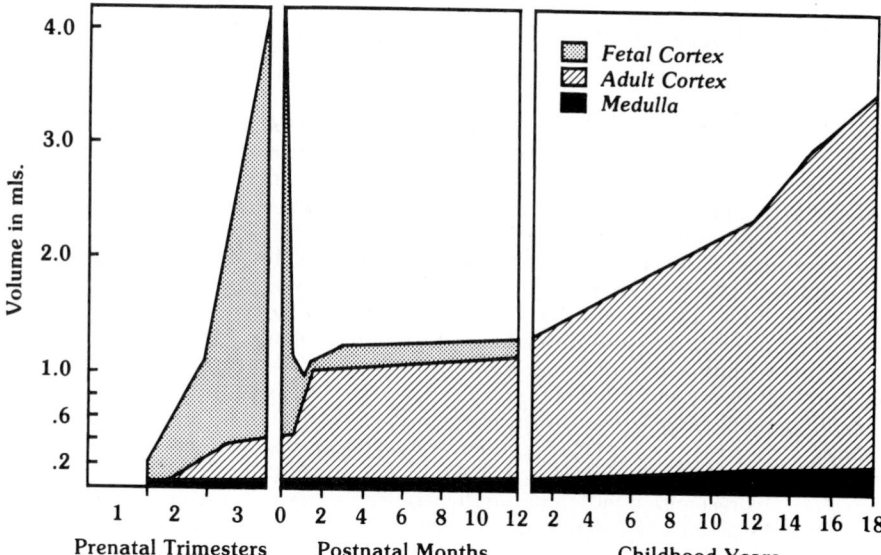

Figure 27–3. Size of adrenal gland and its component parts in utero, during infancy, and during childhood. (Adapted from Bethune JE, ed. The Adrenal Cortex, A Scope Monograph. Kalamazoo, MI: Upjohn, 1974: 11, with permission.)

nal tissue fragments maintained in organ culture.[19] In these studies it was estimated that 50 to 70% of the pregnenolone sulfate, dehydroepiandrosterone sulfate, and cortisol secreted by the fetal adrenal are derived from LDL cholesterol and that the remainder is derived from the de novo synthesis of cholesterol in the adrenal gland.[19] LDL is the preferred lipoprotein, high-density lipoprotein (HDL) is less effective, and very-low-density lipoprotein (VLDL) is not used.[20] The rate of fetal adrenal steroidogenesis may be regulated, in part, by the levels of LDL in the fetal plasma and hence by the rate of synthesis of lipoproteins in the fetus. Only about 20% of fetal cholesterol is derived from the maternal circulation.[21]

LDL is ultimately derived from VLDL through the hydrolysis of the triacylglycerol portion of VLDL by lipoprotein lipase. Because there is little adipose tissue in the human fetus before the 36th wk of gestation, lipoprotein lipase in the fetal rat lung may be important in LDL formation. Prolactin stimulates lipoprotein lipase in other tissues[22] and may facilitate adrenal steroidogenesis by enhancing the conversion of VLDL to LDL in fetal tissues. In keeping with this possibility, the levels of prolactin in fetal plasma increase in parallel to the rate of increase in the size of the fetal adrenal cortex. Therefore prolactin may be an indirect trophic agent for the fetal adrenal, even though the hormone does not seem to stimulate fetal adrenal steroidogenesis directly.

Secretion of Placental Steroids into Maternal and Fetal Compartments

More than 90% of the estradiol and estriol and 85% or more of the progesterone formed in the trophoblast are secreted into the maternal compartment,[23] and little of the progesterone in the maternal circulation enters the fetus.[24] The distribution of steroids from trophoblast to maternal and fetal compartments is dictated by the nature of placentation (hemochorioendothelial) in human pregnancy. The syncytiotrophoblast is bathed directly by maternal blood in the intervillous space but is separated from the fetal blood by several layers of tissue. Steroids secreted from syncytiotrophoblast into the fetal compartment must enter the intravillous space and cross the fetal capillary and the fetal capillary endothelial cells before entering the fetal blood. In consequence, the net transfer of steroids to maternal blood is approximately ten times that of the net transfer to fetal blood. The same anatomic considerations are involved in the limited transfer of steroids from maternal blood across the placenta to fetal blood.

Placental Sulfatase Deficiency

With fetal sulfatase deficiency there is failure of hydrolysis of dehydroepiandrosterone sulfate or 16α-hydroxydehydroepiandrosterone sulfate in the placenta, and the formation of estrogen by the placenta is consequently impaired.[25] In such instances the levels of estradiol and estriol in the plasma and urine of pregnant women are quite low, indeed similar to the low levels associated with death of the fetus. Infants with placental sulfatase deficiency are male, are usually normal at birth, and develop ichthyosis later in life. In some pregnancies associated with fetal sulfatase deficiency, there is a delay in the onset of parturition, or refractoriness to the induction of labor by the intravenous administration of oxytocin, or both. In the past, pregnancies in which there was fetal sulfatase deficiency were thought to be associated with hypertension. Placental sulfatase deficiency per se, however, does not predispose to pregnancy-associated hypertension; it is likely that sulfatase deficiency was recognized more often in hypertensive women because of the practice of monitoring of estriol levels in hypertensive pregnant women.

Aromatase Deficiency

Fetal aromatase deficiency was previously believed to be incompatible with the establishment of pregnancy, based on evidence in several animal species of estrogen formation for implantation of the blastocyst. Clearly, this view is not entirely correct. Aromatase deficiency in a pregnant woman was reported by Shozu and co-workers in 1991.[26] In this instance fetal aromatase enzyme deficiency was severe, the levels of estrogens in maternal blood were extremely low, and there was no significant increase in the maternal plasma levels of estriol and estradiol after the intravenous infusion of dehydroepiandrosterone sulfate into the mother. Because of the aromatase deficiency in placenta, the normal (large) amounts of dehydroepiandrosterone sulfate in fetal blood were converted in trophoblast to dehydroepiandrosterone and thence to androstenedione and testosterone. The androgenic C_{19}-steroids produced in trophoblast entered the fetal and maternal compartments, causing virilization of both the pregnant woman and her female fetus. The deficiency in aromatase enzyme activity was due to a mutation of the aromatase (*CYP19*) gene, namely, a homozygous mutation caused by the insertion of 87 base pairs "in frame," giving rise to an abnormal protein containing 29 additional amino acids and possessing only 6% of normal enzyme activity. Additional cases of aromatase deficiency have subsequently been reported.[27]

PROGESTERONE FORMATION

During the last 8 to 10 wk of pregnancy the placenta secretes about 1 mmol (300 mg) or more of progesterone per day (Fig. 27–4). Indeed, in pregnancies with multiple fetuses, 2 mmol (600 mg) of progesterone or more may be formed per day. Progesterone in the human placenta is derived from circulating maternal cholesterol.[28, 29] Normally, the fetus does not contribute precursors for placental progesterone formation; indeed, ligation of the umbilical cord with the placenta

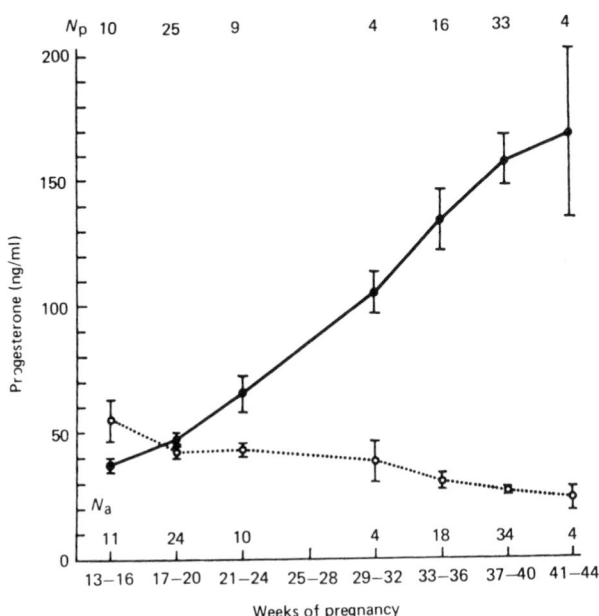

Figure 27–4. Progesterone levels in maternal plasma *(solid line)* and amniotic fluid *(dotted line)* from the same subjects. Values were grouped in 4-wk periods. Np, number of plasma samples; Na, number of amniotic fluid samples in each period. (From Johansson ED, Johansson LE. Progesterone levels in amniotic fluid and plasma from women: I. Levels during normal pregnancy. Acta Obstet Gynecol Scand 1971; 50:339–343, with permission.)

remaining in situ does not cause an immediate reduction in the level of progesterone in plasma or in the level of pregnanediol in maternal urine.[30] Furthermore, in a study of women pregnant with an anencephalic and who were given radiolabeled cholesterol under conditions that approximated an isotopic steady state, Hellig and co-workers showed that the specific activities of plasma progesterone and urinary pregnanediol are similar to those of maternal plasma cholesterol.[29]

Mechanism of Placental Progesterone Formation

In near-term pregnant women the amount of progesterone formed per day is equivalent to one fourth to one third of the daily rate of LDL cholesterol turnover in nonpregnant adults. Nonetheless, the incorporation of [^{14}C]acetate into cholesterol by placental tissue in the human is low, as is the activity of the rate-limiting step in cholesterol biosynthesis, namely, 3-hydroxy-3-methylglutaryl coenzyme A reductase, in human placental microsomes. Therefore, it is likely that de novo synthesis of cholesterol in the placenta is low. In cultured choriocarcinoma cells and human trophoblasts, maternal plasma lipoproteins are the principal source of cholesterol for progesterone synthesis and LDL is the preferred lipoprotein.[31] LDL binds to a saturable population of plasma membrane receptors on syncytiotrophoblast with high affinity for LDL (also see Chapter 23) and is internalized through a process of endocytosis. The endocytotic vesicles fuse with lysosomes, and lysosomal enzymes hydrolyze the lipoprotein. The protein moiety of LDL is broken down to amino acids, and the hydrolysis of the cholesterol esters gives fatty acids and cholesterol. Amino acids derived from hydrolysis of the protein component are one source of amino acids for the fetus; linoleic acid derived from hydrolysis of the cholesterol esters of LDL can fill the essential fatty acid requirement for the fetus. The liberated cholesterol is a precursor for pregnenolone formation in mitochondria, and pregnenolone is converted to progesterone in the endoplasmic reticulum. The mechanism by which progesterone is synthesized from circulating LDL cholesterol is illustrated in Figure 27–5.

Although the mechanism of progesterone biosynthesis in normal pregnancy is well established, other mechanisms may be operative under certain circumstances. In a full-term pregnancy in a woman with familial homozygous hypobetalipoproteinemia, the plasma level of progesterone was low but not absent.[32] The rate of production of progesterone by the corpus luteum during an ovulatory cycle in this woman was negligible.[33] Estrogen levels in this pregnancy were reduced modestly, probably because of some attenuation in fetal adrenal dehydroepiandrosterone sulfate production caused by reduced levels of circulating LDL in the fetus, who was a heterozygous carrier of the mutant gene.

Ordinarily, the uptake of LDL by a tissue is associated with an increase in cholesterol ester synthesis through LDL stimulation of acyl-CoA:cholesterol acyltransferase (ACAT) activity.[34] In contrast, there are few or no cholesterol esters in trophoblastic tissue progesterone that inhibit ACAT activity in placenta.[35, 36] Indeed, by inhibiting ACAT activity almost completely, progesterone prevents the sequestration of cholesterol in ester storage form, ensuring a continuing supply of cholesterol for progesterone biosynthesis.

Progesterone Metabolism to Bioactive Products

No class of steroid hormones other than estrogens and progesterone appears to be formed or secreted by the placenta. For example, there is no evidence for the placental synthesis of glucocorticosteroids or mineralocorticoids. All of the effects of progesterone, however, cannot be accounted for solely by processes mediated by the progesterone receptor. Progesterone also acts through a nongenomic plasma membrane mechanism, and plasma progesterone is metabolized to bioactive products that act through progesterone receptor-independent mechanisms. Plasma progesterone is converted to the mineralocorticoid deoxycorticosterone in extra-adrenal, extrahepatic tissues in a reaction catalyzed by a steroid 21-hydroxylase distinct from the steroid 21-hydroxylase (CYP21B) in the adrenal cortex.[37] In addition, plasma progesterone is 5α-reduced to 5α-dihydroprogesterone, the immediate precursor of 5α-pregnan-3α-ol-20-one, a potent anesthetic/antianxiety agent.[38] This steroid acts by binding to the gamma-aminobutyric acid (GABA)$_A$ receptor-chloride channel complex to increase the binding affinity for GABA,[39] a neuroinhibitory amino acid. Therefore, this acts to mitigate anxiety in a manner similar to that of barbiturates and the benzodiazepines.[40] The blood production rate of 5α-dihydroprogesterone during the third trimester of human pregnancy may exceed 100 mg/d,[41] and, consequently, a large supply of precursor for 5α-pregnan-3α-ol-20-one formation is available during pregnancy. The abrupt removal of this steroid after delivery may be involved in the development of puerperal depression in some women.[42]

Transfer of Steroid Hormones from Maternal to Fetal Compartments

Little of the steroids in the maternal circulation reaches the fetal compartment. The rapid clearance of steroids from maternal plasma minimizes the availability of maternal plasma steroids to the trophoblast, and steroids that enter the trophoblast re-enter the maternal compartment preferentially rather than the fetal compartment. For example, little cortisol in maternal plasma crosses the placenta, both because the re-entry pathway dominates and because cortisol within the trophoblast is converted largely to cortisone through the action of 11β-hydroxysteroid dehydrogenase.[43]

Circulating C$_{19}$-steroids in the maternal compartment, namely, dehydroepiandrosterone sulfate, dehydroepiandrosterone, androstenedione, and testosterone, do not reach the fetal compartment in significant quantities because of the large capacity of the 3β-hydroxysteroid dehydrogenase and aromatase enzymes of the syncytiotrophoblast for the conversion of C$_{19}$-steroids to estrogens. In most circumstances the aromatase activity of the human trophoblast is not rate limiting in the conversion of C$_{19}$-steroids to estrogens, as evidenced by the fact that the fractional conversion of circulating C$_{19}$-steroids to estradiol is not altered by wide fluctuations in

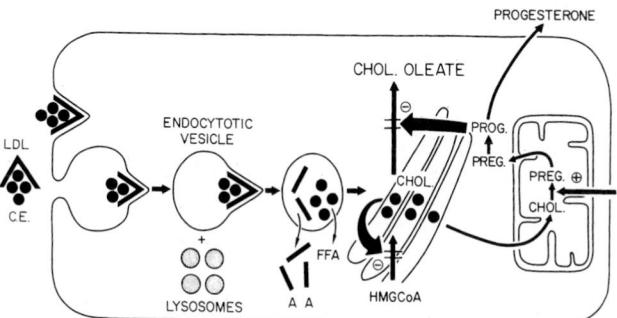

Figure 27–5. Pathways of cholesterol metabolism and its regulation in human placenta. PREG., pregnenolone; PROG., progesterone; LDL, low-density lipoprotein; C.E., cholesteryl esters; FFA, free fatty acids; AA, amino acids; CHOL., cholesterol; HMGCoA, 3-hydroxy-3-methylglutaryl CoA.

the levels of these precursors in the maternal circulation.[44] This mechanism prevents virilization of the female fetus in women who develop androgen-secreting tumors of the ovary during pregnancy. When virilization of the female fetus does occur as a result of excessive androgen formation in the maternal compartment, it is probably caused by C_{19}-steroids that are not estrogen prehormones, such as 5α-dihydrotestosterone or 5α-androstanedione; alternatively, such fetuses may become virilized early in pregnancy before the placenta can clear testosterone efficiently by aromatization.

PROTEIN HORMONES OF THE PLACENTA

Human Chorionic Gonadotropin

Human chorionic gonadotropin, the "pregnancy hormone" is a glycoprotein (molecular weight of about 36,700) that is composed of an α- and a β-subunit and is secreted by the syncytiotrophoblast. hCG is sometimes referred to as a "surrogate" luteinizing hormone (LH) because it binds to the LH/hCG receptor and mimics the action of LH. hCG is produced almost exclusively in the placenta, although small amounts may be formed by a number of tissues, including the anterior pituitary. In addition, malignant tumors may produce hCG, sometimes in reasonably large amounts. Nonetheless, using commercial assays commonly available, the detection of immunoreactive hCG in blood or urine of reproductive age women is almost always diagnostic of pregnancy. hCG is produced in the syncytiotrophoblast and not in the cytotrophoblast, although the maximal rate of hCG secretion coincides in time with the greatest abundance of cytotrophoblasts in placenta (Fig. 27–6). Because the cytotrophoblast is the progenitor of the syncytiotrophoblast, the correlation between formation and secretion of hCG with numbers of cytotrophoblasts may simply reflect increased conversion of cytotrophoblast to syncytiotrophoblasts. Alternatively, the cytotrophoblast is the site of synthesis of LHRH; thus a paracrine mechanism may exist in which LHRH of cytotrophoblast origin acts on syncytiotrophoblast to stimulate the production of hCG.

The rate of secretion of hCG increases rapidly in the first few weeks of pregnancy, and maximal levels are attained in maternal blood and urine at approximately 10 wk gestation. When the maximal levels of hCG are attained, the mean

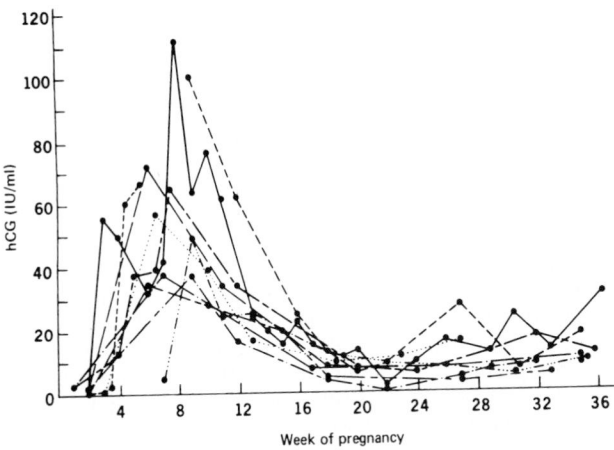

Figure 27–6. Plasma hCG levels of eight women followed longitudinally throughout gestation. Week of pregnancy is indicated, relative to time of ovulation. (From Vaitukaitis J. Human chorionic gonadotropin. In: Fuchs F, Klopper A, eds. Endocrinology of Pregnancy. 2nd ed. New York: Harper & Row, 1977: 67, with permission.)

concentration in the plasma of most pregnant women is of the order of 100,000 IU/L. Thereafter hCG levels in both maternal serum and urine slowly decline, reaching a nadir of approximately 20,000 IU/L at approximately 120 d gestation that persists until delivery.

Levels of hCG are elevated in women with multiple fetuses and in women with hydatidiform mole or choriocarcinoma. Late in pregnancy, the plasma levels of hCG also may increase in women with Rh isoimmunization and an affected fetus and in some women with diabetes mellitus. In these latter two circumstances, cytotrophoblasts reappear in the placenta late in gestation. If hCG concentrations rise above 500,000 IU/L of plasma, the diagnosis of hydatidiform mole is virtually ensured, but serum hCG levels below 500,000 IU/L do not exclude the possibility of trophoblastic disease. Interestingly, levels of hPL do not increase in women with hydatidiform mole. Rather, the finding of high levels of hCG together with low levels of hPL is characteristic of this abnormality. Development of theca lutein cysts of the ovary during pregnancy usually indicates high levels of hCG. These lesions are found most often in women with hydatidiform mole and also occur in women with multiple fetuses, diabetes mellitus, or Rh isoimmunization.

The physiological role of hCG in human pregnancy is not fully defined. hCG acts as a luteotropin to maintain the corpus luteum and serves to convert the corpus luteum of menstruation to the corpus luteum of pregnancy through its capacity to stimulate the secretion of progesterone and relaxin. hCG induces the secretion of testosterone by the fetal testes before the onset of LH secretion by the fetal pituitary. LH/hCG receptors are in myometrium and myometrial blood vessels, and hCG may promote myometrial smooth muscle relaxation or myometrial vasodilation.[45]

hCG Stimulation of the Thyroid

In many women with neoplastic trophoblast disease (e.g., hydatidiform mole or choriocarcinoma), clinical and biochemical evidence of hyperthyroidism sometimes develops. At one time it was believed that chorionic thyrotropin produced by the neoplastic trophoblast was the cause of the hyperthyroid-like condition that develops in these women; however, some forms of hCG itself bind to the thyroid receptors of thyroid cells, and treatment of normal men with hCG increases thyroid activity.[46] Thyroid-stimulatory activity in plasma of first-trimester pregnant women, however, varies widely because modifications of the oligosaccharides of hCG determine the thyroid stimulatory activity of the hCG molecule. In addition, the LH/hCG receptor is expressed in the thyroid, and it is possible that hCG stimulates thyroid activity through the LH/hCG receptor and through the thyroid-stimulating hormone (TSH) receptor as well.[47]

Placental Lactogen

The secretion of hPL by the syncytiotrophoblast commences soon after implantation; the pattern of hPL secretion, however, differs from that of hCG (Fig. 27–7). Levels of hPL in maternal blood increase slowly in parallel with placental mass, and maximal levels are attained after the 32nd wk of gestation and remain relatively constant thereafter. The rate of hPL secretion in pregnant women is higher than that of any other protein hormone in women or men, with daily production rates reaching 1 g or more late in pregnancy. Little hPL enters the fetal circulation. The hormone has both lactogenic and somatotrophic properties, but its capacity to promote growth is only about 1/100 that of growth hormone. hPL is an insulin antagonist and may be responsible in part for the development of gestational diabetes mellitus in women

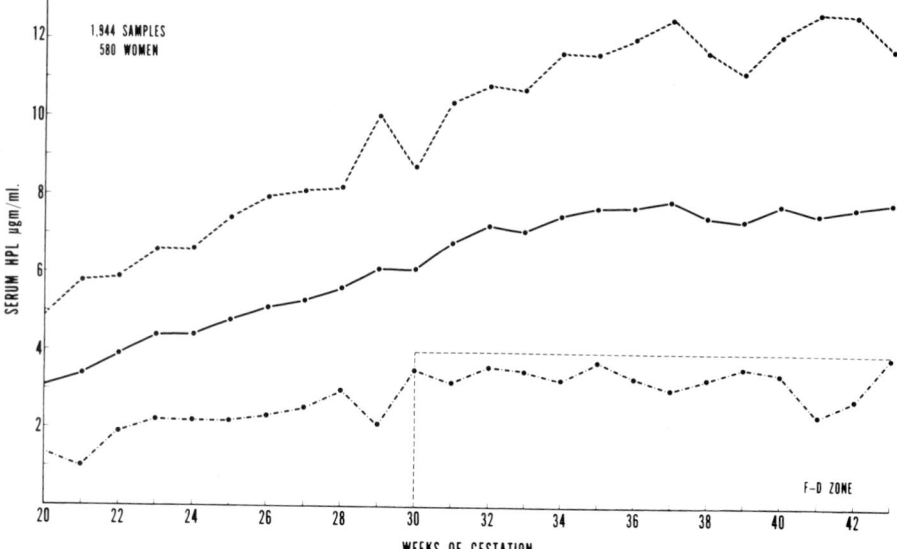

Figure 27–7. Plasma levels of hPL as a function of gestational age (±2 SD). If, after 30-wk gestation, the level of hPL is less than 4 µg/mL, the fetus is considered to be in danger (F-D zone). (From Spellacy WN. Human placental lactogen in high-risk pregnancy. Clin Obstet Gynecol 1973; 16:298–312, with permission.)

who did not have the disease before they became pregnant and who may not require insulin after pregnancy is terminated. Apparently normal pregnancies have been described in which hPL could not be detected in maternal blood or in placenta.[48]

Human Growth Hormone Variant

The hGH-V gene encodes a growth hormone variant that is expressed in syncytiotrophoblast but not in the pituitary. hGH-V, also referred to as placental growth hormone, is a 191-amino-acid protein that differs in 15 amino acid residues from hGH. hGH-V is synthesized in placenta, but the pattern of synthesis of hGH-V has not been characterized in detail.[49] It is believed that hGH-V appears in maternal plasma during the second trimester and that the concentrations increase until about 36 wk gestation. The biologic action of hGH-V is similar to that of hPL. Apparently normal pregnancies are known in which there were complete deletions of both the hGH-V and hPL genes.

Hypothalamic-Like Releasing Hormones

For each of the known hypothalamic-releasing or -inhibiting hormones (e.g., LHRH, thyroid-releasing hormone [TRH], corticotropin-releasing hormone [CRH], GHRH, and somatostatin), a similar peptide is produced in the placenta. The role of these placental factors is not well understood, but they may act as paracrine factors in the placenta in a manner analogous to that of hypothalamic factors in the pituitary, namely, to regulate the synthesis/release of their respective protein hormones. In addition, some are secreted into the maternal and fetal compartments. For example, placental CRH enters the maternal circulation. In nonpregnant women, the plasma level of CRH is about 15 ng/L. During pregnancy the maternal plasma levels of CRH increase to about 250 ng/L in the early third trimester and up to 1 to 2 µg/L at term, having increased abruptly during the last 5 to 6 wk of pregnancy.[50] CRH in plasma is bound to the CRH-binding protein, plasma levels of which remain constant until the final weeks of pregnancy when the levels decrease as the levels of CRH increase.[51] The physiologic role of placental CRH is not established, but CRH in the fetal circulation may stimulate release of ACTH by the fetal pituitary and, thereby, contribute to the growth and enhanced steroidogenesis of the fetal adrenal late in pregnancy. Nevertheless, the levels of CRH in fetal

plasma are quite low, and the levels of ACTH in fetal plasma do not increase appreciably late in gestation. The increase in the levels of CRH in maternal plasma late in pregnancy might be involved in the initiation of parturition. However, although CRH receptors are present in human myometrium, a role for CRH in the initiation of parturition is not yet easily envisioned because CRH normally acts to increase intracellular cyclic adenosine monophosphate and promote uterine relaxation.[52] Possibly, a change in the CRH receptor isoform[53] or a change in the G-protein phenotype in the myometrium could favor the stimulation of phospholipase C by CRH and thereby increase intracellular levels of calcium.

MEASUREMENT OF PLACENTAL HORMONES AS AN INDEX OF FETAL WELL-BEING

For decades physicians have sought to monitor the levels of various placental or fetal hormones as a means of evaluating the well-being of the fetus. If alterations in hormone concentrations reflect changes in the health of the fetus, that information would allow intervention in high-risk pregnancies to effect preterm delivery when the intrauterine environment of the fetus is deteriorating.

In most cases fetal *stress* is due to fetal hypoxia from decreased uteroplacental blood flow, such as in pregnancies complicated by chronic hypertension, pregnancy-induced hypertension (preeclampsia-eclampsia), placental insufficiency (from unknown causes), impaired fetal growth (for unknown reasons), or severe diabetes mellitus. Fetal stress is commonly equated with stress in the adult, which is associated with increased corticotropin secretion. If pituitary corticotropin secretion were increased in the stressed fetus, increased estriol levels in the maternal plasma or urine would be expected because the principal precursor of placental estriol is fetal 16α-hydroxydehydroepiandrosterone sulfate formed from dehydroepiandrosterone sulfate secreted by the fetal adrenal. Thus, if fetal pituitary secretion of corticotropin were increased with stress, increased secretion of fetal adrenal dehydroepiandrosterone sulfate should cause an increase in the secretion of 16α-hydroxydehydroepiandrosterone sulfate and estriol. This is not the case. During fetal hypoxia the secretion of fetal pituitary corticotropin decreases, the rate of secretion of fetal adrenal dehydroepiandrosterone sulfate declines, and the rate of estriol secretion decreases.[54, 55]

During fetal hypoxia there is a decrease in body[56] and thoracic[57] movements, suggesting that hypoxia induces longer sleep periods for the fetus; and the levels of plasma LDL in the cord blood of newborns of mothers with chronic and pregnancy-induced hypertension are higher than in the newborns of normotensive mothers.[58] These data, together with the finding that the fetal adrenal preferentially uses LDL cholesterol for steroidogenesis in vitro, support the view that fetal hypoxia is associated with a decrease in the utilization of circulating LDL for steroidogenesis by the fetal adrenal.

Estriol

After fetal death the levels of estriol in maternal plasma and urine are reduced. Indeed, the diagnosis of fetal death can be established with some reliability by the determination of estriol levels in the maternal compartment. Furthermore, in pregnancies in which the fetus is believed to be at risk, marked reductions in estriol levels or persistently low levels of estriol are predictive of impending fetal demise. Consequently, it was reasoned that the measurement of estriol in the maternal compartment would provide a reliable index of fetal well-being. Unfortunately, in some pregnancies in which the fetus is undoubtedly at risk, estriol levels are not decreased. For example, in pregnancies associated with Rh isoimmunization that affects the fetus and pregnancies complicated by maternal diabetes mellitus, the levels of estriol in maternal plasma and urine may be higher than in normal pregnant women at the same stage of gestation.

Consequently, the question is whether the measurement of estriol in maternal plasma or urine provides a sufficiently sensitive index of fetal well-being to allow the physician to choose the ideal timing of delivery of a fetus when the intrauterine environment is compromised. The choice is usually between preterm delivery on the one hand and a deteriorating intrauterine environment of the fetus on the other hand. Measurements of estriol in maternal blood or urine do not provide meaningful information over and above that available from the clinical assessment of the pregnancy unit.[59] Clinical assessment is accomplished by measurement of the rate of fetal growth by clinical and ultrasonographic criteria, by systematic evaluation of maternal blood pressure, and by monitoring renal function or the status of carbohydrate metabolism in pregnant women. It is not difficult to conclude that the fetus is at risk when maternal hypertension is worsening or when carbohydrate metabolism is not controlled in a pregnant diabetic woman. It is also easy to recognize that the fetus is at risk when the biparietal diameter of the fetal head fails to increase at a proper rate. These considerations, together with the fact that estriol levels fluctuate widely in the same pregnant woman and from woman to woman, have led us to the view that more harm than good can come from the timing of delivery solely on the basis of estriol levels in the maternal compartment. Most investigators now share this view. There has been only one controlled, prospective study of the utility of estriol measurements, and in this investigation measurement of estriol levels was not helpful in decreasing perinatal mortality or morbidity.[59]

Placental Lactogen

Because hPL is secreted by the trophoblast and because the rate of its secretion generally is proportional to the placental mass, measurements of hPL in maternal plasma are obtained to evaluate placental function and, indirectly, fetal well-being. Again, the objective of such measurements is to predict the optimal time of delivery for a potentially adversely affected fetus in complicated pregnancies. In some high-risk pregnancies, especially those complicated by hypertension, there is a reasonable correlation between the level of hPL and the outcome for the newborn.[60] Unfortunately, however, this correlation is no better than, and probably not as good as, that between the level of estriol and fetal outcome.

Placental Clearance of Maternal Plasma Dehydroepiandrosterone Sulfate and the Dehydroepiandrosterone Sulfate Loading Test

A convenient test for placental sulfatase deficiency or aromatase deficiency involves the intravenous administration of dehydroepiandrosterone sulfate. Because of extensive clearance of dehydroepiandrosterone sulfate from the maternal circulation by way of its conversion to estradiol in the placenta, the failure of an increase in the levels of estrogens in maternal plasma after dehydroepiandrosterone sulfate administration is indicative of a profound deficiency in estrogen synthesis by the trophoblast.

OVARIAN FUNCTION DURING PREGNANCY

In most mammalian species, the corpus luteum of the ovary is the site of estrogen and progesterone synthesis throughout pregnancy. In human pregnancy, however, the ovarian contribution to the maintenance of pregnancy appears to be limited to the first 8 wk of gestation. Bilateral oophorectomy as early as the 78th day of pregnancy is not associated with a reduction in the levels of urinary estrogens or with abortion.[61] By the 7th wk of pregnancy more than 50% of estrogen entering the maternal circulation is produced in the placenta. Progesterone secretion by the human corpus luteum begins to decline by 6 wk of gestation, and the maximum secretion of relaxin by the corpus luteum corresponds in time with the maximum levels of hCG in plasma (i.e., about 10 wk of pregnancy). Thereafter, the levels of relaxin in plasma also decline abruptly. Therefore, the endocrine milieu of human pregnancy is primarily dependent on placental, not ovarian, function.

MATERNAL ADAPTATIONS TO PREGNANCY

As stated earlier, a remarkable feature of pregnancy is the successful adaptation of the gravid woman to the enormous endocrine changes effected by steroid and protein hormones produced by the placenta. Women experience considerable blood loss at delivery. On average, 500 mL of blood is lost at the time of vaginal delivery, 1000 mL is lost with cesarean section, and 1500 ml is lost with cesarean section-hysterectomy.[62] This loss is usually well tolerated because the maternal blood volume increases from 3.5 L before pregnancy to 5 L by the latter part of pregnancy. In spite of the increase in blood volume, levels of plasma renin activity and angiotensin II are elevated, and the rate of aldosterone secretion in late pregnancy is 10 to 40 times that of nonpregnant women. Yet systolic and diastolic blood pressures are usually lower during pregnancy than before or after. This process of adaptation is not fully understood, but some of the individual components of the adaptation have been clarified.

Estrogen stimulates the hepatic synthesis of angiotensinogen, the precursor of angiotensin I and, in turn, of angiotensin II. Estrogen and progesterone, alone or together, stimulate the secretion of renin, the enzyme that catalyzes the conversion of angiotensinogen to angiotensin I. The net consequence is an enhancement in the synthesis of angiotensin II. The zona glomerulosa of the maternal adrenal remains responsive to the trophic action of angiotensin II as aldosterone secretion increases during pregnancy whereas the maternal vasculature becomes refractory to the pressor effects of angiotensin II. These two phenomena, acting in concert, are probably important for the expansion of blood volume during pregnancy. Refractoriness to the pressor effect of angiotensin II develops early in pregnancy and persists throughout gestation in women who do not develop pregnancy-induced hypertension (preeclampsia and eclampsia). In normal men and nonpregnant women, on average, the intravenous infusion of angiotensin II at a rate of 7 ng/kg body weight/min causes a rise of 20 mm Hg in diastolic pressure. By contrast, infusion of more than 16 ng/kg body weight/min of angiotensin II is required, on average, to effect a similar pressor response in pregnant women; and in some there is little pressor response even to 40 ng/kg body weight/min of angiotensin II. A prostaglandin or a prostaglandin-like substance is believed to mediate this process, because prostaglandin synthase inhibitors such as indomethacin and aspirin abolish the refractoriness of pregnant women to the pressor effects of angiotensin II.[63]

Failure of the normal physiological adaptations of pregnancy may be catastrophic. In a prospective study of young primigravid women who were at risk of developing pregnancy-induced hypertension, those who ultimately developed preeclampsia became refractory to the pressor effects of angiotensin II early in pregnancy and thereafter began to lose refractoriness to angiotensin II—some as early as 22 wk of gestation—long before hypertension developed.[64] This failure in the adaptive process of pregnancy is believed to be important in the pathophysiology of pregnancy-induced hypertension. After the development of hypertension, the levels of renin, angiotensin II, and aldosterone in the plasma of affected pregnant women decline, sometimes to values only slightly greater than those in nonpregnant women.

The plasma levels of the mineralocorticoid deoxycorticosterone (DOC) increase strikingly during pregnancy,[65, 66] principally in the last trimester, and the rate of DOC production in pregnant women is not controlled by the same mechanisms that modulate the secretion of aldosterone or cortisol. The administration of corticotropin or dexamethasone to near-term pregnant women does not change the level of DOC in plasma,[66] and DOC secretion from the adrenal is not regulated by the action of angiotensin II. Although the levels of DOC and DOC sulfate in umbilical cord plasma are greater than that in the maternal plasma, maternal plasma DOC levels cannot be accounted for by transfer from the fetus.[67] In adults plasma progesterone is converted to DOC in nonadrenal tissues,[68] and the fractional conversion of plasma progesterone to DOC is similar in men and in nonpregnant and pregnant women. Thus, the rate of extra-adrenal DOC formation is proportional to the plasma level of progesterone. Interestingly, the fractional conversion of circulating progesterone to DOC varies widely among normal persons (i.e., 0.002 to 0.03).[68] When progesterone secretion is high, as at the midluteal phase of the ovarian cycle (0.1 mmol/d [40 mg/d]) or during pregnancy (0.8 to 2.0 mmol/d [250 to 600 mg/d]), extraglandular formation of DOC from plasma progesterone is the principal source of DOC in plasma. The amount of DOC formation from plasma progesterone varies, depending on the fractional conversion of plasma progesterone to DOC in a given woman. In some pregnant women, 20 μmol (7.5 mg) or more of DOC is produced each day from plasma progesterone.

The level of plasma cortisol is increased in pregnant women, partly because of a three- to fourfold increase in the level of corticosteroid-binding globulin.[69] The rate of secretion of cortisol by the maternal adrenal is not increased in pregnancy, but the rate of clearance is decreased so that the half-life of the hormone in plasma is prolonged. The corticotropin level is suppressed in women during pregnancy,[70] presumably because of the action of estrogen and progesterone.[71] The lowest level of corticotropin is found early in pregnancy, rising to a maximum between 26 wk and term.[70]

The rate of secretion of dehydroepiandrosterone sulfate by the maternal adrenal has not been studied systematically in pregnant women, but dehydroepiandrosterone sulfate levels in plasma decline appreciably[72] during pregnancy because of increased metabolic clearance due to utilization for estradiol formation in the placenta and extensive 16α-hydroxylation in the maternal liver.

Prolactin secretion increases steadily during pregnancy; in near-term pregnant women, the level of prolactin (of pituitary origin) in plasma ranges from 150 to 250 μg/L. The role of prolactin in adrenal function, if any, however, is not defined. Prolactin also is produced in the decidua of pregnant women, which is believed to be the source of the high levels of this hormone in amniotic fluid. Decidual prolactin secretion does not account for that present in maternal or fetal blood. The synthesis of decidual prolactin during pregnancy is not inhibited by dopamine or dopamine agonists.[73]

The physiological adaptation of the pregnant woman assures the fetus of adequate placental transfer of the nutrients required for growth and development and protects the mother from the trauma and blood loss of delivery by an expansion of blood volume without a concomitant increase in arterial blood pressure.

ENDOCRINOLOGY OF PARTURITION

Phases of Parturition

Human parturition is divisible into four distinct but overlapping phases.[74, 75] *Phase 0* of parturition is defined as the period of uterine tranquillity and refractoriness to contraction, which exists in all mammalian species for approximately the first 95% of pregnancy. Despite the expansion of the uterine cavity by 1000-fold or more, the myometrium remains remarkably relaxed during this phase of uterine tranquillity. This phenomenon is even more curious considering the fact that the myometrium is a tissue with an inherent propensity to contract. Factors believed to operate in human pregnancy to guarantee contractile refractoriness of the myometrium during phase 0 of parturition include estrogen, progesterone, and unidentified agents. Several seven-transmembrane-spanning domain receptors that are linked to G-proteins are expressed in human myometrium, including receptors for β-adrenergic agents, hCG,[76–79] parathyroid hormone–related protein,[80] CRH,[52, 53, 81] vasoactive intestinal peptide, and several prostaglandins. Most of these receptors are linked to the $G_{\alpha s}$-protein, which activates adenylate cyclase and increases the intracellular level of cyclic adenosine monophosphate. In addition, relaxin and calcitonin gene-related peptide increase myometrial cyclic adenosine monophosphate, which in turn is believed to promote myometrial relaxation,[82] and the $G_{\alpha s}$-protein directly activates calcium-dependent potassium channels.

Phase 1 of parturition is the time of uterine awakening. The transition from phase 0 to phase 1 is defined as the initiation of parturition. During phase 1 changes in the uterus include an increase in the number of gap junctions between myometrial cells,[83] an increase in the number of oxytocin receptors in myometrium,[84] an increase in uterine contractile responsiveness, and changes in the cervix.[1] Whereas the return of contractile responsiveness can be induced in most pregnant mammals by progesterone withdrawal, phase 1 of parturition in human pregnancy occurs in the absence of progesterone withdrawal. Phase 2 of parturition encompasses the stages of active labor—from the onset of labor to the delivery of the placenta. Phase 3 of human parturition involves the expulsion of the placenta and the final uterine contraction.

Progesterone and Parturition

It was long presumed that progesterone is primarily responsible for uterine quiescence during phase 0 of parturition. This view was based on the finding that progesterone withdrawal by physiological, pharmacologic, or surgical means brings about the onset of labor in most mammalian species. Indeed, spontaneous progesterone withdrawal heralds the onset of parturition in the mouse, rat, hamster, dog, cat, cow, sheep, and goat. In some mammalian species such as the sheep the mechanism by which progesterone withdrawal occurs is well defined. A parturition signal, likely CRH,[85] is formed in the fetal sheep brain and is transported by means of the hypophyseal-portal vessels to the fetal pituitary. In consequence, there is an increase in ACTH secretion from the anterior pituitary and, thence, an increase in the production of cortisol by the fetal sheep adrenal.[86] Cortisol acts in some way to increase the activity of steroid CYP17 (17α-hydroxylase) activity in the trophoblast. In consequence, progesterone production declines and the formation of estrogen increases.[87] Other mechanisms are operative in the mouse, rat, hamster, dog, cat, and cow to effect progesterone withdrawal. Progesterone withdrawal, however, does not precede the onset of labor in primates, including humans, and in some other species such as the guinea pig. In fact, in women, the levels of progesterone in plasma are maintained after labor begins and only decline after delivery of the placenta, a finding that raised doubts as to the obligatory nature of progesterone in the maintenance of primate pregnancy.[1] In addition, the administration of progesterone receptor antagonists to primates late in the course of pregnancy does not bring about labor and delivery. Investigators have searched for another mechanism by which progesterone action might be blocked during human parturition, such as a decline in the production rate of progesterone or an increase in its metabolic clearance, a decrease in the number of progesterone receptors in the myometrium, an increase in the metabolism (inactivation) of progesterone in the uterus, or the binding or sequestering of progesterone to prevent interaction with uterine progesterone receptors. None of these mechanisms appears to be operative.[1] Another possibility is that progesterone action may be attenuated or blocked in a gene-specific manner. For example, transforming growth factor-β inhibits the ability of progesterone to induce specific genes.[88] Accordingly, the local production of active transforming growth factor-β or some agent may prevent the action of progesterone at the level of gene expression in a gene- and cell-specific manner and, thereby, promote the transition from phase 0 to phase 1 of parturition.

Estrogen and Parturition

The role of estrogen, produced in very high amounts during human pregnancy, in modulating myometrial quiescence and contractility is not defined precisely. Whereas it is believed that progesterone attenuates contractile responsiveness, it is also commonly believed that estrogen causes myometrial contractions. Reference is made frequently to the "estrogen:progesterone ratio" as being a critical factor in determining the effects of these two steroids on myometrial function and uterine contractility. It is unlikely that this is a correct interpretation. The plasma levels of both estrogen and progesterone in normal human pregnancy are so great that there must be an excess of both in terms of the classic estrogen and progesterone receptors. It is not likely, therefore, that subtle changes in the estrogen:progesterone ratio modulate uterine function in human pregnancy. It is possible, however, that estrogen and progesterone function by nongenomic mechanisms or via nonclassic receptors. For example, estrogen acts in some cells by an estrogen receptor–independent (nongenomic) mechanism to stimulate adenylyl cyclase[89]; such an action in myometrial cells would promote myometrial quiescence.

On the other hand, there is evidence that estrogen promotes myometrial changes that facilitate myometrial contractility. In pregnancies with placental sulfatase deficiency, fetal anencephaly, or fetal adrenal hypoplasia, estrogen production is decreased.[1] In placental sulfatase deficiency the hydrolysis of dehydroepiandrosterone sulfate in placenta is limited and, thence, the availability of dehydroepiandrosterone for placental aromatization to estrogen is decreased. In fetal anencephaly and fetal adrenal hypoplasia, the production of dehydroepiandrosterone sulfate is reduced markedly, leading to decreased estrogen production. In some of these pregnancies with decreased estrogen formation, parturition is delayed. Estrogen, acting directly or indirectly, effects a number of changes in myometrium that enhance the capacity of the myometrium to generate powerful contractile force. These include myometrial cell hypertrophy, myometrial cell contractile potential,[90] uterotonin receptors, and cell-to-cell communicability (by increasing the synthesis of the myometrial smooth muscle gap junction protein, connexin43).[91, 92] A clearer definition of the effects of estrogen and progesterone that are mediated by classic and nonclassic steroid receptors and by nongenomic mechanisms is of the utmost importance in defining the roles of these steroids in modulating uterine quiescence and contractility. It is highly likely that redundant (i.e., fail-safe) mechanisms are operative in human pregnancy to ensure the maintenance of pregnancy and the timely initiation of parturition.

Uterotonins

In the absence of progesterone withdrawal in the initiation of labor in humans, agents that have been considered as potential uterotonins include oxytocin, prostaglandins, endothelin, and others. Each of these agents acts on the myometrium to increase the levels of intracellular calcium and, subsequently, to cause contraction.

Although *oxytocin* is a potent uterotonin, it does not appear to be involved in the initiation of human parturition. The plasma levels of oxytocin increase after the initiation of parturition and the onset of labor, but the fact that the number of oxytocin receptors increases during phase 1 of parturition suggests that oxytocin is involved somehow in the parturitional process, probably in phases 2 and 3 of parturition. During phase 2 of parturition, oxytocin may act to promote uterine contraction and facilitate the expulsive stage of labor. Oxytocin acts during phase 3 of parturition, together with other uterotonins, to facilitate myometrial contraction and uterine retraction after delivery of the placenta to limit uterine blood loss.[1]

Oxytocin may be produced in decidua, in the placenta, and in the amnion (a fetal membrane), and this locally produced oxytocin may be important in modulating the function of the uterus and the placental/fetal membrane system.[93–95] It is not known whether oxytocin produced in these sites can reach the myometrium in an active form, and the levels of the oxytocin-inactivating enzyme oxytocinase are high in the chorion laeve (a fetal membrane)[96] and other uterine tissues.

Prostaglandins were also considered as candidate uterotonins for the initiation of parturition and the onset of labor in women. Prostaglandins are produced during labor by uterine decidua and possibly the myometrium, and the levels of selected prostaglandins increase in amniotic fluid and maternal and fetal blood during labor. However, there is no evidence that the production of prostaglandins increases before the onset of labor, and instead the enhancement of prostaglandin production during labor appears to be the consequence of the normal processes of labor.[75, 97, 98] For example, the levels of prostaglandins E_2 and $F_{2\alpha}$ in amniotic fluid increase after labor begins as a result of cervical dilatation and the consequent inflammation of the exposed tissues of the presenting fetal membranes and uterine decidual fragments.[97, 98] These tissues are traumatized during the process of cervical dilatation, are exposed to inflammatory cytokines in vaginal fluid and normal bacterial flora in the vagina, and synthesize prostaglandins in large amounts as a part of this inflammatory process.[97] Moreover, the amniotic fluid becomes separated into two compartments during labor, and the accumulation of prostaglandins is limited to one of these compartments, namely, the forebag compartment, which is the presenting portion of the fetal membranes. The levels of prostaglandins in the upper compartment do not increase as labor progresses. Thus, although the administration of prostaglandins to pregnant women will cause the onset of uterine contractions (as is likely the case for any uterotonin for which receptors are present), there is no convincing evidence for a role for these agents in the initiation of parturition.

Endothelin-1 is a potent uterotonin and is produced in uterine tissues and fetal membranes.[99] Like prostaglandins, the levels of endothelin-1 in amniotic fluid increase during labor, but not before, probably as a consequence of the labor process.[100] The findings concerning *platelet-activating factor* are similar; namely, whereas the levels of this uterotonin increase in amniotic fluid during labor, there is evidence that this agent is produced as a consequence of the inflammatory process after cervical dilatation during labor. *Histamine* and other agents that increase intracellular calcium in myometrium have also been considered, but there is no evidence for a role for these agents in the initiation of parturition.

Human Parturition

The understanding of human parturition is incomplete. The profound uterine quiescence of phase 0 of parturition is central to the successful maintenance of pregnancy. The mechanisms that alleviate this state of pregnancy and facilitate a return to the usual state of myometrial contractile responsiveness must be key in the definition of the initiation of parturition, and the profound changes in the endocrine milieu with pregnancy must be involved in the maintenance of quiescence during pregnancy and in the initiation of parturition at its termination. It is likely that many bioactive agents, including hormones, growth factors, cytokines, and others acting in endocrine, paracrine, and autocrine fashions, likely are involved in the modifications of myometrial function that accommodate each phase of pregnancy.

REFERENCES

1. Cunningham FG, MacDonald PC, Gant NF, et al. Williams Obstetrics. 20th ed. Stamford, CT: Appleton & Lange, 1997.
2. Ryan KJ. Aromatization of steroids. J Biol Chem 1959; 234:268–272.
3. Frandsen VA, Stakeman G. The site of production of oestrogenic hormones in human pregnancy: hormone excretion in pregnancy with anencephalic fetus. Acta Endocrinol 1961; 38:383–391.
4. Siiteri PK, MacDonald PC. The utilization of circulating dehydroisoandros-
terone sulfate for estrogen synthesis during human pregnancy. Steroids 1963; 2:713–730.
5. Baulieu EE, Dray F. Conversion of ³H-dehydroisoandrosterone (3β-hydroxy-Δ⁵-androsten-17-one) sulfate to ³H-estrogens in normal pregnant women. J Clin Endocrinol Metab 1963; 23:1298–1301.
6. Bolte E, Mancuso S, Eriksson G, et al. Studies on the aromatization of neutral steroids in pregnant women: I. Aromatization of C-19 steroids by placentas perfused in situ. Acta Endocrinol 1964; 45:535–559.
7. Wu L, Einstein M, Geissler WM, et al. Expression cloning and characterization of human 17β-hydroxysteroid dehydrogenase type 2, a microsomal enzyme possessing 20α-hydroxysteroid dehydrogenase activity. J Biol Chem 1993; 168:12964–12969.
8. Gurpide E, Marks C, deZiegler D, et al. Asymmetric release of estrone and estradiol derived from labeled precursors in perfused human placentas. Am J Obstet Gynecol 1982; 144:551–555.
9. Magendantz HG, Ryan KJ. Isolation of an estriol precursor, 16α-hydroxydehydroepiandrosterone, from human umbilical sera. J Clin Endocrinol Metab 1964; 24:1155–1162.
10. Siiteri PK, MacDonald PC. Placental estrogen biosynthesis during human pregnancy. J Clin Endocrinol Metab 1966; 26:751–761.
11. Pulkkinen MO. Arylsulphatase and the hydrolysis of some steroid sulphates in developing organism and placenta. Acta Physiol Scand 1961; 52(Suppl 180):90–92.
12. Warren JC, Timberlake CE. Steroid sulfatase in the human placenta. J Clin Endocrinol Metab 1962; 22:1148–1151.
13. Spector WS, ed. Handbook of Biological Data. Philadelphia: WB Saunders, 1956: 353.
14. MacDonald PC, Porter JC, Schwarz BE, et al. Initiation of parturition in the human female. Semin Perinatol 1978; 2:273–286.
15. Liggins GC. Premature delivery of foetal lambs infused with glucocorticoids. J Endocrinol 1969; 45:515–523.
16. Winters AJ, Oliver C, Colston C, et al. Plasma ACTH levels in the human fetus and neonate as related to age and parturition. J Clin Endocrinol Metab 1974; 39:269–273.
17. Goldstein JL, Brown MS. Binding and degradation of low density lipoproteins by cultured human fibroblasts. J Biol Chem 1974; 249:5153–5162.
18. Glueck CJ, Mellies MJ, Tsang RC, et al. Low and high density lipoprotein cholesterol interrelationships in neonates with low density lipoprotein cholesterol above the 10th percentile and in neonates with high density lipoprotein cholesterol below the 90th percentile. Pediatr Res 1977; 11:957–959.
19. Simpson ER, Carr BR, Parker CR, et al. The role of serum lipoproteins in steroidogenesis by the human fetal adrenal cortex. J Clin Endocrinol Metab 1979; 49:146–148.
20. Carr BR, Parker CR, Milewich L, et al. The role of low density, high density, and very low density lipoprotein in steroidogenesis by the human fetal adrenal gland. Endocrinology 1980; 106:1854–1860.
21. Lin DS, Pitkin RM, Connor WE. Placental transfer of cholesterol into the human fetus. Am J Obstet Gynecol 1977; 128:735–739.
22. Zinder O, Hamosh M, Fleck TRC, et al. Effect of prolactin on lipoprotein lipase in mammary gland and adipose tissue of rats. Am J Physiol 1974; 226:744–748.
23. Gurpide E, Schwers J, Welch MT, et al. Fetal and maternal metabolism of estradiol during pregnancy. J Clin Endocrinol Metab 1966; 26:1355–1365.
24. Gurpide E, Tseng J, Escarcena L, et al. Fetomaternal production and transfer of progesterone and uridine in sheep. Am J Obstet Gynecol 1972; 113:21–32.
25. Tabei T, Heinrichs WL. Diagnosis of placental sulfatase deficiency. Am J Obstet Gynecol 1976; 124:409–414.
26. Shozu M, Akasofu K, Harada T, Kubota Y. A new cause of female pseudohermaphroditism: placental aromatase deficiency. J Clin Endocrinol Metab 1991; 72:560–566.
27. Simpson ER, Zhao Y, Agarwal V, et al. Aromatase expression in health and disease. Recent Prog Horm Res 1997; 52:185–214.
28. Bloch K. Biological conversion of cholesterol to pregnanediol. J Biol Chem 1945; 157:661–666.
29. Hellig H, Gattereau D, Lefebvre Y, et al. Steroid metabolism from plasma cholesterol. I. Conversion of plasma cholesterol to placental progesterone in humans. J Clin Endocrinol Metab 1970; 30:624–631.
30. Cassmer O. Hormone production of the isolated human placenta. Acta Endocrinol 1959; 45(Suppl):3–82.
31. Simpson ER, Bilheimer DW, MacDonald PC, et al. Uptake and degradation of plasma lipoproteins by human choriocarcinoma cells in culture. Endocrinology 1979; 104:8–16.
32. Parker CR Jr, Illingworth DR, Bissonnette J, et al. Endocrine changes during pregnancy in a patient with homozygous familial hypobetalipoproteinemia. N Engl J Med 1986; 314:557–560.
33. Illingworth DR, Corbin DK, Kemp ED, et al. Hormone changes during the menstrual cycle in abetalipoproteinemia: reduced luteal phase progesterone in a patient with homozygous hypobetalipoproteinemia. Proc Natl Acad Sci USA 1982; 79:6685–6689.
34. Brown MS, Dana SE, Goldstein JL. Cholesterol ester formation in cultured human fibroblasts. J Biol Chem 1975; 250:4025–4027.
35. Simpson ER, Burkhart MF. AcylCoA:cholesterol acyltransferase activity in human placental microsomes: inhibition by progesterone. Arch Biochem Biophys 1980; 200:79–85.

36. Simpson ER, Burkhart MF. Regulation of cholesterol metabolism by human choriocarcinoma cells in culture: effect of lipoproteins and progesterone on cholesteryl ester synthesis. Arch Biochem Biophys 1980; 200:86–92.

37. Mellon SH, Miller WL. Extraadrenal steroid 21-hydroxylation is not mediated by P450c21. J Clin Invest 1989; 84:1497–1502.

38. Gee KW, Bolger MB, Brinton RE, et al. Steroid modulation of the chloride ionophore in rat brain: structure-activity requirements, regional dependence and mechanism of action. J Pharmacol Exp Ther 1988; 246:803–812.

39. Paul SM, Purdy RH. Neuroactive steroids. FASEB J 1992;6;2311–2322.

40. Majewska MD, Harrison NL, Schwartz RD, et al. Steroid hormone metabolites are barbiturate-like modulators of the GABA receptor. Science 1986; 232:1004–1007.

41. Dombroski RA, Casey ML, MacDonald PC. The metabolic disposition of 5α-dihydroprogesterone [5α-pregnane-3,20-dione (5α-DHP)] in women and men. J Clin Endocrinol Metab 1993; 77:944–948.

42. Majewska MD, Ford-Rice F, Falkay G. Pregnancy-induced alterations of GABA$_A$ receptor sensitivity in maternal brain: An antecedent of postpartum blues? Brain Res 1989; 482:397–401.

43. Murphy BEP, Clark SJ, Donald IR, et al. Conversion of maternal cortisol to cortisone during placental transfer to the human fetus. Am J Obstet Gynecol 1974; 118:538–541.

44. MacDonald PC, Siiteri PK. Origin of estrogen in women pregnant with an anencephalic fetus. J Clin Invest 1965; 44:465–474.

45. Kornyei JL, Lei ZM, Rao CV. Human myometrial smooth muscle cells are novel targets of direct regulation by human chorionic gonadotropin. Biol Reprod 1993; 49:1149–1157.

46. Kenimer JG, Hershman JM, Higgins P. The thyrotropin in hydatidiform moles is human chorionic gonadotropin. J Clin Endocrinol Metab 1975; 40:482–491.

47. Tomer Y, Huber GK, Davies TF. Human chorionic gonadotropin (hCG) interacts directly with recombinant human TSH receptors. J Clin Endocrinol Metab 1992; 74:1477–1479.

48. Nielsen PV, Pedersen J, Kampmann EM. Absence of human placental lactogen in an otherwise uneventful pregnancy. Am J Obstet Gynecol 1979; 135:322–326

49. Ogren L, Talamantes F. The placenta as an endocrine organ: polypeptides. In: Knobil E, Neill JD, eds. The Physiology of Reproduction. New York: Raven Press, 1994: 875–969.

50. Goland RS, Wardlaw SL, Blum M, et al. Biologically active corticotropin-releasing hormone in maternal and fetal plasma during pregnancy. Am J Obstet Gynecol 1988; 159:884–890.

51. Linton EA, Perkins AV, Woods RJ, et al. Corticotropin releasing hormone-binding protein (CRH-BP): plasma levels decrease during the third trimester of normal human pregnancy. J Clin Endocrinol Metab 1993; 76:260–262.

52. Grammatopoulos D, Milton NGN, Hillhouse EW. The human myometrial CRH receptor: G proteins and second messengers. Mol Cell Endocrinol 1994; 99:245–250.

53. Hillhouse EW, Grammatopooulos D, Milton NGN, et al. The identification of a human myometrial corticotropin-releasing hormone receptor that increases in affinity during pregnancy. J Clin Endocrinol Metab 1993; 76:736–741.

54. Parker CR, Simpson ER, Bilheimer DW, et al. Inverse relationships between the plasma concentrations of LDL-cholesterol and the placental estrogen precursor, dehydroisoandrosterone sulfate, in the human fetus. Science 1980; 208:512–514.

55. Parker CR, Leveno K, Carr BR, et al. Umbilical cord plasma levels of dehydroisoandrosterone sulfate (DS) during human gestation. J Clin Endocrinol Metab 1982; 54:1216–1220.

56. Pearson JF, Weaver JB. Fetal activity and fetal well-being: an evaluation. BMJ 1976; 1:1305–1307.

57. Boddy K, Mantell CD. Observations of fetal breathing movements transmitted through maternal abdominal wall. Lancet 1972; 2:1219–1220.

58. Parker CR, Hankins GDV, Carr BR, et al. The effect of hypertension in pregnant women on fetal adrenal function and plasma lipoprotein-cholesterol metabolism. Am J Obstet Gynecol 1984; 150:263–269.

59. Duenhoelter JH, Whalley PJ, MacDonald PC. An analysis of the utility of plasma immunoreactive estrogen measurements in determining delivery time of gravidas with a fetus considered at high risk. Am J Obstet Gynecol 1976; 125:889–898.

60. Spellacy WN, Buhi WC, Birk SA, et al. Distribution of human placental lactogen in the last half of normal and complicated pregnancies. Am J Obstet Gynecol 1974; 120:214–223.

61. Diczfalusy E, Borell U. Influence of oophorectomy on steroid excretion in early pregnancy. J Clin Endocrinol 1961; 21:1119–1127.

62. Pritchard JA, MacDonald PC. Obstetric hemorrhage. In: Williams Obstetrics. 16th ed. New York: Appleton-Century-Crofts, 1980: 487–489.

63. Everett RB, Worley RJ, MacDonald PC, et al. Effect of prostaglandin synthetase inhibitors on pressor response to angiotensin II in human pregnancy. J Clin Endocrinol Metab 1978; 46:1007–1010.

64. Gant NF, Daley GL, Chand S, et al. A study of angiotensin II pressor response throughout primigravid pregnancy. J Clin Invest 1973; 52:2682–2689.

65. Brown RD, Strott CA, Liddle GW. Plasma deoxycorticosterone in normal and abnormal human pregnancy. J Clin Endocrinol Metab 1972; 35:736–742.

66. Nolten WE, Lindheimer MD, Oparil S, et al. Deoxycorticosterone in pregnancy. I. Sequential studies of the secretory patterns of desoxycorticosterone, aldosterone, and cortisol. Am J Obstet Gynecol 1978; 132:414–420.

67. Parker CR, Cutrer S, Casey ML, et al. Concentrations of deoxycorticosterone, deoxycorticosterone sulfate, and progesterone in maternal venous and umbilical arterial and venous sera. Am J Obstet Gynecol 1983; 145:427–432.

68. Winkel CA, Milewich L, Parker CR, et al. Conversion of plasma progesterone to deoxycorticosterone in men, nonpregnant and pregnant women, and adrenalectomized subjects: evidence for steroid 21-hydroxylase activity in non-adrenal tissues. J Clin Invest 1980; 66:803–812.

69. Doe RP, Fernandez R, Seal US. Measurement of corticosteroid-binding globulin in man. J Clin Endocrinol Metab 1964; 24:1029–1039.

70. Carr BR, Parker CR, Madden JD, et al. Maternal plasma adrenocorticotropin (ACTH) and cortisol relationships throughout human pregnancy. Am J Obstet Gynecol 1981; 139:416–422.

71. Vale W, Rivier C, Yang L, et al. Effects of purified hypothalamic corticotropin-releasing factor and other substances on the secretion of adrenocorticotropin and β-endorphin-like immunoreactivities in vitro. Endocrinology 1978; 103:1910–1915.

72. Milewich L, Gomez-Sanchez CE, Madden JD, et al. Dehydroisoandrosterone sulphate in peripheral blood of premenopausal, pregnant and postmenopausal women and men. J Steroid Biochem 1978; 9:1159–1164.

73. Friesen H, Forsbach G. Prolactin secretion during pregnancy. In: Jaffe RB, ed. Prolactin. New York: Elsevier, 1981: 167–180.

74. Cunningham FG, MacDonald PC, Gant NF, et al. Williams Obstetrics, Norwalk, CT: Appleton & Lange, 1993.

75. MacDonald PC, Casey ML. Preterm Birth. In: Scientific American Science and Medicine. Vol 3. Scientific American, 1996: 42–51.

76. Zuo J, Lei ZM, Rao CV. Human myometrial chorionic gonadotropin/luteinizing hormone receptors in preterm and term deliveries. J Clin Endocrinol Metab 1994; 79:907–911.

77. Flowers B, Ziecik AJ, Caruolo EV. Effects of human chorionic gonadotrophin on contractile activity of steroid-primed pig myometrium in vitro. J Reprod Fertil 1991; 92:425.

78. Ziecik AJ, Derecka-Reszka K, Rzucidlo SJ. Extragonadal gonadotropin receptors, their distribution and function. J Physiol Pharmacol 1992; 43:33–49.

79. Lei ZM, Reshef E, Rao V. The expression of human chorionic gonadotropin/luteinizing hormone receptors in human endometrial and myometrial blood vessels. J Clin Endocrinol Metab 1992; 75:651–659.

80. Casey ML, Mibe M, Erk A, et al. Transforming growth factor-1 stimulation of parathyroid hormone-related protein expression in human uterine cells in culture: mRNA levels and protein secretion. J Clin Endocrinol Metab 1992; 74:950–952.

81. Grammatopoulos D, Thompson S, Hillhouse EW. The human myometrium expresses multiple isoforms of the corticotropin-releasing hormone receptor. J Clin Endocrinol Metab 1995; 80:2388–2393.

82. Kotlikoff MI, Kamm KE. Molecular mechanisms of β-adrenergic relaxation of airway smooth muscle. Annu Rev Physiol 1996; 58:115–141.

83. Garfield RE, Sims SM, Daniel EE. Gap junctions: their presence and necessity in myometrium during parturition. Science 1977; 198:958–960.

84. Soloff MS, Alexandrova M, Fernström MJ. Oxytocin receptors: triggers for parturition and lactation? Science 1979; 204:1313–1315.

85. Myers DA, McDonald TJ, Nathanielsz PW. Effect of bilateral lesions of the ovine fetal hypothalamic paraventricular nuclei at 118–122 days of gestation on subsequent adrenocortical steroidogenic enzyme gene expression. Endocrinology 1992; 131:305–314.

86. McDonald TJ, Nathanielsz PW. Bilateral destruction of the fetal paraventricular nuclei prolongs gestation in sheep. Am J Obstet Gynecol 1991; 165:764–770.

87. Challis JRG, Lye SJ. Parturition. In: Knobil E, Neill JD, eds. The Physiology of Reproduction. 2nd ed. Vol II. New York, Raven Press, 1994: 985.

88. Casey ML, MacDonald PC. Transforming growth factor-β inhibits progesterone-induced enkephalinase expression in human endometrial stromal cells. J Clin Endocrinol Metab 1996; 81:4022–4027.

89. Aronica SM, Kraus WL, Katzenellenbogen BS. Estrogen action via the cAMP signaling pathway: stimulation of adenylate cyclase and cAMP-regulated gene transcription. Proc Natl Acad Sci USA 1994; 19:8517–8521.

90. Pepe GJ, Albrecht ED. Actions of placental and fetal steroid hormones in primate pregnancy. Endocr Rev 1995; 16:608–648.

91. Burghardt RC, Mitchell PA, Kurten RC. Gap junction modulation in rat uterus. II. Effects of antiestrogens on myometrial and serosal cells. Biol Reprod 1984; 30:249–255.

92. Petrocelli T, Lye SJ. Regulation of transcripts encoding the myometrial gap junction protein, connexin-43, by estrogen and progesterone. Endocrinology 1993; 133:284–290.

93. Chibbar R, Miller FD, Mitchell BF. Synthesis of oxytocin in amnion, chorion, and decidua may influence the timing of human parturition. J Clin Invest 1993; 91:185–192.

94. Zingg HH, Rozen F, Chu K, et al. Oxytocin and oxytocin receptor gene expression in the uterus. Recent Prog Horm Res 1995; 50:255–273.

95. Lefebvre DL, Giaid A, Zingg HH. Expression of the oxytocin gene in rat placenta. Endocrinology 1992; 130:1185–1192.

96. Germain A, Smith J, MacDonald PC, et al. Human fetal membrane contribution to the prevention of parturition: uterotonin degradation. J Clin Endocrinol Metab 1994; 78:463–470.

97. Cox SM, King MR, Casey ML, et al. Interleukins-1βα, -6, and prostaglandins in vaginal/cervical fluids of pregnant women before and during labor. J Clin Endocrinol Metab 1993; 77: 805–815.

98. MacDonald PC, Casey ML. The accumulation of prostaglandins (PG) in amniotic fluid is an aftereffect of labor and not indicative of a role for PGE_2 and $PGE_{2\alpha}$ in the initiation of human parturition. J Clin Endocrinol Metab 1993; 76:1332–1339.

99. Casey ML, Word RA, MacDonald PC. Endothelin-1 gene expression and regulation of endothelin mRNA and protein biosynthesis in avascular human amnion: potential source of amniotic fluid endothelin. J Biol Chem 1991; 266:5762–5768.

100. Casey ML, Brown CEL, Peters M, et al. Endothelin levels in human amniotic fluid at midtrimester and at term before and during spontaneous labor. J Clin Endocrinol Metab 1993; 76:1647–1650.

TABLE 28–1. Features of the Fetal Endocrine Environment

Placental hormone production
  Estrogens
  Progesterone
  Polypeptide hormones
  Neuropeptides
  Growth factors
Unique fetal endocrine systems
  Fetal adrenal cortex
  Para-aortic chromaffin system
  Intermediate lobe of the pituitary
Prominent fetal hormones or metabolites
  Vasotocin
  Calcitonin
  Cortisone
  Reverse triiodothyronine (rT$_3$)
  Sulfated iodothyronines
  Ectopic neuropeptides
Fetal endocrine system adaptations
  Adrenal-placental interactions
  Testicular control of male phenotypic differentiation
  Neuropeptides and fetal water metabolism
  Parathyroid glands and placental calcium transport
  Catecholamine and vasopressin responses to hypoxia
  Catecholamine and cortisol control of extrauterine adaptation
  Developmentally regulated growth factor control of fetal growth
  Perinatal hormonal imprinting
  Cortisol programming for extrauterine exposure

MATERNAL INTERVILLOUS SPACE

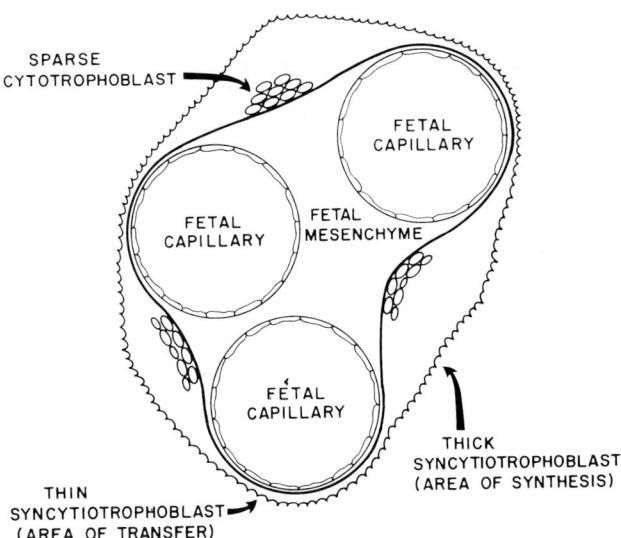

Figure 28–1. Diagrammatic representation of a cross-section of chorionic villus extending into the maternal blood lake and showing fetal capillaries in the fetal mesenchyme. The villus is sheathed by the syncytiotrophoblast. The residual sparse areas of cytotrophoblast probably provide cells to renew and maintain the syncytiotrophoblast layer. The syncytiotrophoblast surface membrane is microvillous, which massively increases the effective surface area. The villus is surrounded by maternal blood in the maternal intervillous space. (Modified from Chard T. Proteins of the human placenta: some general concepts. In: Grudzinskas JG, Seppala M, eds. Pregnancy Proteins. North Ryde, Australia: Academic, 1982: 6, with permission.)

ous cytoplasm, the syncytiotrophoblast, which forms the early fetal-maternal interface. Pockets of cytotrophoblast cells in the mature placenta serve as a reservoir of stem cells for continuing syncytiotrophoblast development. The predominantly syncytiotrophoblastic placenta grows progressively throughout gestation. As the placenta develops, the chorionic villi containing the fetal capillaries extend into the maternal lakes of blood within the maternal decidua. Within the villi three layers of fetal tissue separate the fetal circulation from the maternal circulation: the cytotrophoblast-syncytiotrophoblast layer, the fetal mesenchyme layer of extraembryonic connective tissue, and the fetal capillary endothelium. The syncytiotrophoblast is the major site of diffusion between the maternal lakes of blood in the placenta and the fetal capillaries (Fig. 28–1). The syncytiotrophoblast also manufactures steroid and protein hormones, and after the eighth week of pregnancy it is the most active fetal or maternal endocrine organ. The steroid hormones are produced from both fetal and maternal substrates. The protein hormones are synthesized in the rough endoplasmic reticulum of the syncytiotrophoblast from amino acids of maternal origin. Secretion is predominantly into the maternal circulation, but significant amounts reach the fetal compartment.

Placental Hormone Transfer

The placenta regulates maternal-fetal molecular exchange, and "thin" areas of the syncytiotrophoblast adjacent to the fetal capillaries seem to be specialized for this function (see Fig. 28–1).[1] However, the fetal endocrine milieu is largely autonomous of maternal hormones because the placenta is impermeable to most peptide hormones. There are two major routes for the transfer of molecules across the placenta: an extracellular route via fluid-filled intercellular channels and a transcellular route. The rate of extracellular diffusion relates to the luminal diameter of the intercellular or paracellular channels and to the molecular weight (molecular radius or size) and lipid solubility or hydrophilicity of the transferred molecule. The placenta is more permeable to lipid-soluble molecules, and the permeability of both lipid-soluble and lipid-insoluble molecules decreases with increasing molecular weight.[3, 4] The transfer or diffusion of L-glucose is believed to be accomplished by extracellular diffusion.

The placental transfer of a number of hormones is summarized in Table 28–2.[5–29] The differences in placental structure among species have a limited influence on placental hormone transfer, and data derived from some animal and primate species are included. Hormones larger than 0.7 to 1.2 kd have little or no access to the fetal compartment.

Placental cell membranes contain a variety of receptors for polypeptide hormones and growth factors, including insulin, the IGFs, and epidermal growth factor (EGF).[30, 31] These receptors bind and in some instances degrade their respective ligands but do not facilitate placental transfer.

Hormones that traverse the placenta via the transcellular

TABLE 28–2. Placental Transfer of Hormones

Hormone	Approximate Molecular Size (Daltons)	Placental Transfer
Catecholamine	180	Yes
Melatonin	230	Yes
Steroid hormones	350	Yes
Vitamin D	350	Yes
Thyrotropin-releasing hormone (TRH)	360	Yes
Thyroid hormones	800	Limited
Oxytocin (OT)	1,000	No
Vasopressin	1,100	No
Luteinizing hormone–releasing hormone (LHRH)	1,200	Yes
Atrial natriuretic hormone	3,080	No
Calcitonin (CT)	3,400	No
Glucagon	3,600	No
Corticotropin	4,500	No
Corticotropin-releasing hormone (CRH)	4,800	No
Insulin	6,000	No
Parathyroid hormone (PTH)	9,000	No
Growth hormone (GH)	22,000	No
Thyrotropin	27,000	No
Luteinizing hormone (LH)	30,000	No
Erythropoietin	30,400	No
Renin	40,000	No

route and are metabolized en route[5, 11, 14, 32, 33] include glucocorticoids, thyroid hormones, and catecholamines. The placental cells contain an active 11β-hydroxysteroid dehydrogenase (11β-HSD) that catalyzes the conversion of most of the cortisol to inactive cortisone; cortisol/cortisone ratios in human placental tissue are less than a factor of 1 near term.[11, 33] Placental tissue also contains an iodothyronine inner ring monodeiodinase, which deiodinates most of the T_4 to inactive reverse triiodothyronine (rT_3) and converts active 3,5,3'-triiodothyronine (T_3) to inactive diiodothyronine.[14] In addition catecholamine-degrading enzymes in placental tissue include both monoamine oxidase and catechol O-methyltransferase,[14, 32] and both metanephrine and dihydroxymandelic acid metabolites of catecholamines are present in placental homogenates.

Placental Hormone Production

Placental Estrogen Production

The human placenta near term secretes large amounts of estrogens, including estrone, estradiol, and estriol (see also Chapter 27).[34–37] Daily excretion rates of these steroids during the latter third of pregnancy approximate 2, 1, and 30 to 40 mg, respectively, whereas total estrogen production in nonpregnant women is less than 1 mg/d. This production is due to the combined effects of the fetal adrenal gland and the placenta, first characterized by Diczfalusy as the human fetoplacental unit.[37a] Most of the estrogen is secreted into the maternal circulation, but fetal concentrations and levels in amniotic fluid are high. The major substrates for placental estrogen synthesis are dehydroepiandrosterone (DHEA) and androstenedione. These inactive adrenal steroids are derived from both fetal and maternal adrenals.[33–35] The fetal zone of the adrenal cortex is deficient in an enzyme with 3β-hydroxysteroid dehydrogenase (3β-HSD) and $\Delta^{4,5}$-isomerase activities but has high steroid sulfokinase activity.[34, 35] Thus the conversion of pregnenolone to progesterone is limited, and the major product of fetal adrenal steroidogenesis is DHEA sulfate (DHEAS), which is transported to the liver for 16-hydroxylation. DHEAS and 16-hydroxy-DHEAS are hydrolyzed in the placenta by the steroid sulfatase and converted to androstenedione and 16-hydroxyandrostenedione. Androstenedione in turn is a substrate for placental estrone biosynthesis; 16-hydroxyandrostenedione is the major substrate for placental estriol synthesis. The features of the fetoplacental unit are summarized in Figure 28–2. The rate of placental estrogen biosynthesis is a function of placental mass and the amount of C_{19}-steroid production by the fetal adrenal gland.[33–35]

Estrogens have important roles in the maintenance of pregnancy. They support placental progesterone synthesis by stimulating placental low-density lipoprotein (LDL) cholesterol uptake and cholesterol side chain cleavage enzyme (CYP11A1) activity, increasing and maintaining maternal blood volume and uteroplacental blood flow, promoting uterine growth and placental neovascularization, stimulating production of albumin and globulins in the maternal liver, and augmenting mammary growth.[36] In conditions associated with decreased placental estrogen production (placental sulfatase deficiency, placental aromatase deficiency, fetal anencephaly), both estrogen production and estrogen levels may be reduced 80 to 90%, but placental progesterone production and fetal development are normal.[36] Thus in normal pregnancy there is a considerable excess of estrogen production relative to the levels necessary for estrogen receptor–mediated effects.[36]

Placental Progesterone Production

During normal pregnancy there is a marked and progressive increase in progesterone production. The maternal cor-

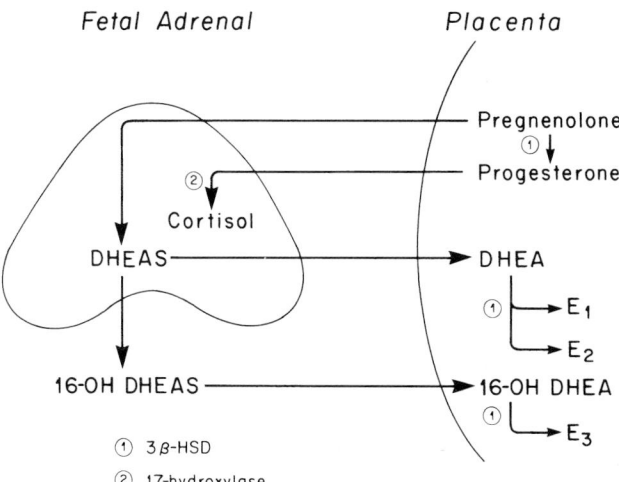

Figure 28–2. Diagrammatic representation of the fetoplacental unit composed of the fetal adrenal cortex and the placenta. The placenta is deficient in 17-hydroxylase activity and cannot synthesize estrogens from progesterone. The fetal adrenal has low β-hydroxysteroid dehydrogenase (β-HSD) and D[4,5]-isomerase activity and cannot synthesize progesterone. Sulfokinase activity is high in fetal adrenal tissue, and steroid sulfatase activity is high in placental tissue. Thus the placenta produces progesterone, which is predominantly converted to dehydroepiandrosterone (DHEA) by the fetal adrenal; the DHEA can be sulfated to form DHEA sulfate (DHEAS). Part of this is 16-hydroxylated by the fetal liver, and both DHEA and DHEAS are used by the placenta as substrates for estrogen synthesis. Placental sulfatase converts DHEAS and 16-hydroxy-DHEAS to DHEA and 16-hydroxy-DHEA. DHEA serves as a substrate for estrone (E_1) and estradiol (E_2) synthesis; 16-hydroxy-DHEA is utilized for estriol (E_3) synthesis. See text and references for further details.

pus luteum is the major source of plasma progesterone during the first 5 to 6 wk of gestation; after 12 wk the placenta is the major source.[34, 35, 38] The principal substrate for placental progesterone synthesis is circulating maternal LDL and very-low-density lipoprotein (VLDL) cholesterol; de novo placental synthesis of cholesterol from acetate is limited. Placental progesterone production is largely independent of the maternal pituitary or adrenal glands, and fetal death in utero has little acute effect on maternal progesterone levels.[35, 38] Progesterone production is regulated by the number of LDL receptors and thus placental mass. The major factor in control of placental progesterone production appears to be the expression of steroidogenic enzymes, including CYP11A1 and 3β-HSD, in cytotrophoblast cells.[38] The type I 3β-HSD enzyme is expressed in placenta, whereas type II activity is expressed in adrenal and gonadal tissues. mRNA expression for all the placental steroidogenic enzymes is stimulated by cAMP, which appears to be produced constitutively in mature cytotrophoblast cells. There is some evidence that endogenous steroids may modulate placental progesterone production.[38]

The production of progesterone approximates 200 mg daily during the third trimester, a value some 10-fold higher than that during the midluteal phase of the normal menstrual cycle; 90% of this amount is secreted into the maternal circulation.[35, 38] Progesterone acts on the uterine musculature to maintain a state of quiescence and inhibits maternal cell-mediated immune responses to foreign (fetal) antigens. Despite the predominant secretion of progesterone into the maternal circulation, fetal blood progesterone levels are two- to threefold higher than maternal values because of a lower metabolic clearance of progesterone by the fetus.[35] The significance of this progesterone to the fetus is not clear.

Placental Polypeptide Hormone Production

The placenta produces several pituitary-like hormones. The most abundant are human chorionic gonadotropin (hCG) and human placental lactogen (hPL, also called human chorionic somatomammotropin [hCS]).[2, 38] hCG is a glycoprotein of 36 to 40 kd with structural, biologic, and immunologic similarities to the pituitary gonadotropins and thyrotropin (also called thyroid-stimulating hormone [TSH]); hCG also has weak thyrotropic hormone–like activity. hPL is a 191-amino-acid protein with 96% homology to human growth hormone (hGH). It has 3% or less of the growth-promoting bioactivity of hGH and equivalent prolactin (PRL)-like effects. hCG is secreted predominantly during the first half of gestation, and hPL is secreted mainly during the second half. The control of synthesis and secretion of these placental hormones is not well understood,[38] but hormone secretion is related to placental mass and continues in the absence of the fetus. Luteinizing hormone–releasing hormone (LHRH; also called chorionic gonadotropin-releasing hormone [GnRH]), EGF, activin, and hCG increase hCG synthesis in placental tissue in vitro, whereas inhibin and progesterone suppress synthesis.[38, 39]

hCG probably plays a role in the maintenance of the corpus luteum early in pregnancy as well as stimulation of the fetal testes and stimulation of placental progesterone production.[38, 39] hCG has weak thyrotropin-like activity; there is less than 0.5 mU of thyrotropin per unit of hCG; and hCG produces minimal changes in maternal thyroid function during normal pregnancy.[40, 41] hPL has weak hGH-like and PRL-like bioactivities and may exert an anti-insulin effect on maternal carbohydrate and lipid metabolism,[38] thereby increasing maternal glucose and amino acid levels and augmenting maternal-to-fetal substrate flow. In addition hPL appears to be an important stimulus of fetal growth.

The same gene is responsible for the β subunit expressed in the placenta for hCG and in the pituitary for production of luteinizing hormone (LH), follicle-stimulating hormone, and thyrotropin.[42] Also there is a single gene for the β subunit of LH, whereas there are seven genes or pseudogenes, or both, for the hCG β subunit. These hCG and LH beta genes have similar structures, and it appears that the hCG gene arose from the LH beta and that the hCG beta gene family is early in the process of evolution of pseudogenes.[42, 43] The PRL, hGH, and hPL genes are also closely related.[38, 44, 45] The PRL gene is presumed to be the ancestral gene; hGH evolved nearly 400 million years ago, whereas hPL evolved within the last 10 million years. The hGH gene cluster includes five similar gene loci, two for hGH and three for hPL; these loci have 93% sequence homology in mRNA and probably evolved by repeated duplication over time.[38, 45] Only two of the hPL sequences are expressed in the placenta and produce identical hPL molecules. Placental tissue also expresses pituitary PRL and one of the hGH genes (hGH-V), and placental hGH may contribute to the maternal hGH-like effects mediated by somatomedins during pregnancy.[38, 46, 47]

The human placenta synthesizes a pro-opiomelanocortin (POMC) and contains the POMC-derived peptides corticotropin (also called adrenocorticotropic hormone [ACTH], adrenocorticotropin), α- and β-lipotropin, β-endorphin, α-melanocyte–stimulating hormone (α-MSH), and three forms of endorphin.[37, 38] Corticotropin-releasing hormone (CRH) is also produced by the placenta, and CRH stimulates corticotropin production from perfused human placental fragments, suggesting a possible paracrine role for placental CRH in modulating corticotropin production in the placenta.[48] Glucocorticoids, however, have no effect on placental CRH or corticotropin release, and oxytocin (OT) stimulates placental POMC release but has no effect on pituitary release of corticotropin.[49] Also β-endorphin and α-MSH are released from placenta in larger amounts than is corticotropin. Thus control and processing of placental POMC are different than in the anterior pituitary.[49] The increased plasma levels of POMC-derived peptides in pregnant women and the resistance of

maternal plasma corticotropin to glucocorticoid suppression in pregnancy suggest that the placenta may be involved in regulation of the maternal pituitary-adrenal axis during pregnancy.[37, 49, 50]

Inhibin and activin are produced by placental tissue.[51] mRNAs for inhibin subunits (α, $β_A$, and $β_B$) are present in the placenta, and inhibin A ($αβ_A$) and activin A ($β_A$-$β_A$) are produced throughout pregnancy. Inhibin and activin A levels in maternal serum increase progressively during pregnancy and decrease rapidly after delivery.[51] Immunoreactive and bioactive inhibins also are present in umbilical cord serum and amniotic fluid; umbilical artery and vein concentrations are similar and lower than maternal values.[51] Activin A is present in cord serum only at term, whereas activin B is present in fetal blood and amniotic fluid before birth; activin B is largely absent from maternal serum.[51] The role of these hormones during pregnancy is not clear. Inhibin production in placenta is stimulated by hCG, follicle-stimulating hormone, EGF, and prostaglandins; inhibin suppresses hCG production, whereas activin can stimulate growth hormone–releasing hormone (GHRH), LHRH, progesterone, and prostaglandin by placental cells in culture.[51, 52] A paracrine role for these hormones in the placenta is suggested.

Renin activity is present in homogenates and in cultured explants of placenta and has been localized in chorionic tissue by immunohistochemical assay.[53, 54] The amino acid composition and NH_2-terminal sequence of chorionic renin are identical to kidney renin.[55] Renin mRNA is present in the chorion throughout pregnancy; no mRNA has been detected in decidua, amnion, or myometrium.[54] Placental renin mRNA concentrations at term are about 10% of kidney levels, and the total placental renin mRNA level approximates 20% of kidney content. Angiotensinogen mRNA has not been detected in placenta.

Functional angiotensin II receptors (AT_2) are present in skeletal muscle and connective tissue of the late-gestation rat embryo.[55] In fetal skin fibroblasts these receptors are coupled to membrane phospholipid turnover and mediate increases in cellular inositol phosphate and cytosolic calcium concentrations. Moreover injection of angiotensin II into 18-d-old rat fetuses increases amino acid incorporation into skin protein.[55] These observations suggest a role for angiotensin II in fetal growth, and placental renin may play a role in the production of fetal angiotensin II.

The placenta produces a parathyroid hormone (PTH)–like bioactivity that is similar in composition to the PTHrP produced by tumors associated with hypercalcemia.[56, 57] Bioactivity of sheep placental PTH-like protein is inhibited by an antiserum against synthetic human PTHrP, whereas antiserum that neutralizes bovine PTH bioactivity has no effect on the ovine placental PTH-like bioactivity.[56] In the sheep, placental PTH-like bioactivity is highest in midgestation placentas. PTHrP is also present in fetal ovine parathyroid glands. Calcitonin mRNA and a calcitonin-like immunoreactivity are also present in the rat placenta.[58] The significance of these proteins is discussed later in the section describing the fetal PTH-calcitonin system.

Placental Neuropeptide Production

The human placenta contains and produces LHRH, thyrotropin-releasing hormone (TRH), somatostatin (also called somatotropin release-inhibiting factor [SRIF]), CRH, and GHRH.[59–76] LHRH is produced in the cytotrophoblast and can bind to receptors in the syncytiotrophoblast. Because synthetic LHRH increases in vitro production of hCG and perhaps of progesterone, estrone, estradiol, and estriol from placental explants, endogenous chorionic LHRH may have a paracrine role in the regulation of placental hCG and steroid hormone production.[38, 39]

Placental TRH immunoreactivity and chromatographic characteristics are similar to those of synthetic TRH, and bioactivity has been demonstrated.[62–64] Sheep placental TRH levels vary with the thyroid status of the fetus, increasing with hypothyroidism and decreasing after administration of T_3 to the fetus.[65] These data suggest that regulation of placental *TRH* gene transcription resembles that of hypothalamic TRH.

Immunoreactive chorionic somatostatin, like LHRH, is localized in the cytotrophoblast.[66, 67] The finding that the somatostatin-containing cells in the placenta disappear as pregnancy progresses and that hPL production increases progressively during the second half of gestation led to the speculation that chorionic somatostatin may exert negative paracrine control on the production of hPL by the syncytiotrophoblast.[67]

Immunoreactive CRH has been identified in human and sheep placental extracts and in third-trimester pregnancy plasma.[37, 71, 72] It is not detected in plasma of pregnant women during the first or second trimesters, and it disappears postpartum.[70–72] CRH mRNA is present in full-term human placental tissue, and immunoreactive CRH, with chromatographic characteristics similar to those of synthetic CRH, is produced by placental fragments in vitro.[48, 73, 74] The lack of correlation of maternal plasma corticotropin or cortisol and CRH levels has suggested that placental CRH is not primarily involved in maternal pituitary corticotropin regulation.[71, 72] However maternal plasma CRH levels correlate with gestational age, which suggests a relationship to placental function.[72] Moreover studies in the baboon, which resembles the human with regard to CRH metabolism during pregnancy, have shown a blunted maternal pituitary corticotropin response to CRH after CRH infusion.[75] These studies support a role of placental CRH in modulating maternal pituitary and adrenal function during pregnancy. In contrast to the negative-feedback effect of glucocorticoid on hypothalamic CRH production, glucocorticoid stimulates placental CRH mRNA and CRH production.[73, 74] This observation and the parallel increases in placental CRH and CRH mRNA concentrations during the last 5 wk of pregnancy suggest that the increase in fetal glucocorticoid production near term may stimulate placental CRH and POMC production and may further augment prenatal fetal cortisol production.

Immunoreactive GHRH and biologically active GHRH are present in rat placenta.[76] Two forms of GHRH activity were identified by high-performance liquid chromatography, one eluting identically with synthetic GHRH and one similar to the methionine sulfoxide analogue. By analogy with other placental releasing factors, chorionic GHRH may be involved in paracrine control of hPL or placental hGH production. Plasma GHRH levels, like CRH concentrations, are elevated during the third trimester of human gestation, correlate with gestational age and hPL concentrations, and become undetectable 3 d postpartum.[72] A relationship to placental function seems likely.

The placenta also produces a variety of neurotransmitter and transcription factor molecules that may have roles in the regulation of placental neuropeptide and polypeptide hormone secretion. These include catecholamines, prostaglandins, pituitary factor-1 (Pit-1), and neuropeptide Y.[39, 77, 78] Neuropeptide Y stimulates CRH production, and Pit-1 stimulates hPL and hGH gene transcription in placental tissue in vitro.[77, 78] Prostaglandins and catecholamines stimulate CRH and LHRH secretion in vitro.[78, 79]

Placental Growth Factor Production

Human placental tissue contains both IGF-I (also called somatomedin-C) and IGF-II mRNA species,[80, 81] and translation of placental RNA in vitro results in the production of a 14-kd protein that is immunoprecipitable with IGF-I antiserum.[80] Term placental explants also produce a 24-kd immunoprecipitable IGF-I–like protein.[80] The IGF-II cDNA isolated from human placenta has a 5′-untranslated region different from that produced in human liver, and IGF-II mRNA in placenta may differ from that in liver or kidney.[81] Only one IGF-II gene is present in the human genome, so there may be unique tissue-specific and developmental alteration of somatomedins by human placental tissue. The role of placental somatomedins and control of their production remain to be characterized. Placental cells possess IGF-I receptors by the sixth week of gestation, and placental IGF-I may have an autocrine or a paracrine role in placental growth.[80]

Nerve growth factor β (NGF-β) from human placenta has similar molecular weight, chromatographic properties, and biologic (neurite-promoting) activity as mouse salivary gland NGF-β.[82, 83] Human placental NGF does not cross-react, however, with antisera to mouse NGF-β. The significance of placental NGF with regard to fetal development is not clear.

EGF and TGF α mRNAs and proteins have been demonstrated in pools of placental tissue from early, middle, and late gestation.[84, 85] Placental levels of TGF α protein are relatively high throughout gestation (90 to 180 ng/mg protein), whereas EGF values are low (3 to 9 ng/mg protein).[84] The placenta is richly endowed with receptors that bind both EGF and TGF α.[30, 85, 86] TGF α mRNA is localized in the maternal decidua early in gestation in the mouse and is present in fetal tissues.[87, 88] Moreover EGF induces differentiation of human trophoblast to syncytiotrophoblast, and this differentiation is associated with increased production of hCG and hPL.[89] These studies have suggested that TGF α or EGF, or both, may influence placental maturation and function.

Transforming growth factor β has been purified from human placenta, and precursor mRNA is present in placental tissue.[90] PTHrP, platelet-derived growth factor, vascular endothelial growth factor, endothelin-1, tumor necrosis factor α, and several colony-stimulating factors and receptors also have been demonstrated in placental tissue and conditioned media.[91–95] These factors also are postulated to have autocrine-paracrine roles in placental growth and function.

ECTOPIC FETAL HORMONE PRODUCTION

Ectopic Fetal Polypeptide Hormone Production

Kidney, liver, and testes from 16- to 20-week-old human fetuses produce immunoreactive and bioactive hCG in vitro.[96] Kidney tissue produces nearly half as much hCG (per milligram of protein) as placenta, and liver activity is lower. Corticotropin-like immunoreactivity is present in relatively high concentrations in neonatal rat pancreas and kidney.[97] This material is presumably derived from a POMC parent molecule.

Extraneural Fetal Neuropeptide Production

Hypothalamic neuropeptides are present in a variety of adult tissues, particularly in the pancreas and gut.[98–104] In the fetus, hypothalamic neuropeptides are also present in the gut and tissues derived from it. High concentrations of TRH and somatostatin immunoreactivity have been reported in neonatal rat pancreas and gastrointestinal tract tissues, whereas hypothalamic concentrations of these immunoreactive substances are low.[105–108] These neuropeptides have immunoreactive and chromatographic properties similar to those of the synthetic hypothalamic peptides. Other peptides cleaved from pre-proTRH are present in perinatal rat pancreas.[109] In addition, encephalectomy does not alter the circulating TRH levels in the neonatal rat, whereas significant reductions are produced by pancreatectomy.[109] TRH production by monolayer cultures of fetal rat pancreatic cells is stimulated by serotonin and is inhibited by carbachol; catecholamines, γ-aminobutyric acid, and histamine have no effect.[110] Specific neurotransmitter control has been postulated. In the sheep fetus, thyroid hormones modulate pancreatic and gut TRH concentrations, which suggests thyroid hormone control of extrahypothalamic TRH gene transcription or translation in the fetus.[65]

TRH and somatostatin are present in the human neonatal pancreas[111, 112] and in blood of the human newborn.[113-115] It seems likely that both hormones are derived mostly from extrahypothalamic sources.[70, 110, 114] The presence of TRH at high concentrations in fetal ovine blood and the control of fetal pancreatic, placental, and blood TRH levels by thyroid hormones suggest a role for extrahypothalamic TRH in the control of fetal pituitary thyrotropin secretion before the near-term maturation of hypothalamic TRH.[65] Infusion of TRH into the fetal sheep also evokes behavioral arousal, causes increased body and eye movements, and stimulates fetal breathing.[116] The role of extraneural somatostatin in the fetus is undefined.

There is a general tendency toward hypersecretion of fetal pituitary hormones during the last half of gestation, and pituitary hormones found at high levels in cord blood from aborted human fetuses and premature human infants include hGH, thyrotropin, corticotropin, β-endorphin, β-lipotropin, LH, and follicle-stimulating hormone.[117, 118] Maturation of hypothalamic-pituitary control is complex, involving maturational events in the cortex and midbrain, the hypothalamus and hypothalamic-pituitary portal vascular system, peripheral endocrine systems, and the placenta itself, including hormone, growth factor, and neuropeptide production. The fetal pituitary hyperfunction appears to relate more to relatively delayed maturation of the central nervous system and hypothalamic control with unrestrained secretion of stimulating hypothalamic hormones than to the action of placental neuropeptides, but details of fetal-placental interactions during endocrine systems ontogenesis remain to be defined.[118]

FETAL ENDOCRINE SYSTEMS

Anterior Pituitary and Target Organs

Development

The human fetal forebrain is identifiable by 3 wk of gestation; the diencephalon and telencephalon are distinguishable by 5 wk. Rathke's pouch, the buccal precursor of the anterior pituitary gland, separates from the primitive pharyngeal stomodeum by 5 wk of gestation.[118-120] The neural components of the transducer system—the hypothalamus, the pituitary stalk, and the posterior pituitary—are largely developed by 7 wk of gestation, and the bony floor of the sella turcica is present by this time and separates the adenohypophysis from the primitive gut. Capillaries develop within the proliferating anterior pituitary mesenchymal tissue around Rathke's pouch and the diencephalon by 8 wk of gestation, and intact hypothalamic-pituitary portal vessels are present by 12 to 17 wk.[121] Maturation of the pituitary portal vascular system continues, and the system becomes functionally intact during the period of histologic differentiation of the hypothalamus and development of the portal vascular extension into

hypothalamic tissue; this maturation process extends to 30 to 35 wk of gestation.

The median eminence of the hypothalamus is evident by 9 to 10 wk of gestation, and the hypothalamic cell condensations, which represent the hypothalamic nuclei, and the interconnecting fiber tracts are demonstrable histologically by 15 to 18 wk of gestation.[118, 122] Hypothalamic cells and diencephalic fiber tracts for the hypothalamic neuropeptides somatostatin, CRH, GHRH, and LHRH are also visible by this time.[123-127] Concentrations of dopamine, TRH, LHRH, and somatostatin are significant in hypothalamic tissue by 10 to 14 wk of gestation.[118, 128, 129] Specialized anterior pituitary cell types, including lactotropes, somatotropes, corticotropes, thyrotropes, and gonadotropes, can be recognized in the anterior pituitary between 7 and 16 wk of gestation.[130, 131] Anterior pituitary hormones—including hGH, PRL, thyrotropin, LH, follicle-stimulating hormone, and corticotropin—are detectable by radioimmunoassay between 10 and 17 wk of gestation.[118] Thus the anatomy and biosynthetic mechanisms that make up the hypothalamic-pituitary neuroendocrine transducer appear to be functional by 12 to 17 wk of gestation in the human.

Human Fetal Pituitary Growth Hormone and Prolactin

The human fetal pituitary can synthesize and secrete hGH by 8 to 10 wk of gestation.[117, 118] Pituitary hGH content increases from about 1 nmol (20 ng) at 10 wk to 45 nmol (1000 ng) at 16 wk of gestation. Fetal plasma hGH levels in cord blood samples are in the 1 to 4 nmol/L range during the first trimester and increase to a mean peak of approximately 6 nmol/L at midgestation (Fig. 28-3). Plasma hGH levels fall progressively during the second half of gestation to a mean value of 1.5 nmol/L at term.[118] Pituitary hGH mRNA and hGH content generally parallel the increase in plasma hGH concentration between 16 and 24 wk of gestation.[132] This pattern of ontogenesis of plasma hGH reflects a progressive maturation of hypothalamic-pituitary and forebrain function. The responses of plasma hGH to somatostatin and GHRH and to insulin and arginine are mature at term in human infants.[117, 118] Plasma hGH levels are low in anencephalic infants.[118]

The high plasma hGH concentrations at midgestation after the development of the pituitary portal vascular system may reflect unrestrained secretion.[118] Studies of 9- to 16-week-old human fetal pituitary cells in culture have shown a predominant response to GHRH and a limited effect of somatostatin, which suggests that the inhibitory action of somatostatin develops later in gestation.[133] This interpretation has been substantiated by in vivo studies in the sheep fetus, which have shown a failure of somatostatin to inhibit GHRH-stimulated GH release early in the third trimester and maturation of the inhibitory effect of somatostatin near term.[134] Thus a predominant GHRH enhancement and limited somatostatin inhibition of hGH secretion at midgestation are presumably associated with a limited capacity for inhibition of hGH release by somatomedin feedback. In addition there may be unrestrained hGH secretion at the pituitary cell level and/or immaturity of limbic and forebrain inhibitory circuitry that modulates hypothalamic function.[118] Whatever the mechanisms, control of hGH secretion matures progressively during the last half of gestation and the early weeks of postnatal life so that mature responses to sleep, glucose, and L-dopa are present by 3 months of age.

The ontogenesis of fetal plasma PRL differs significantly from that of hGH (see Fig. 28-3); levels are low until 25 to 30 wk of gestation and increase to a mean peak value of approximately 11 nmol/L at term.[118] Pituitary PRL content

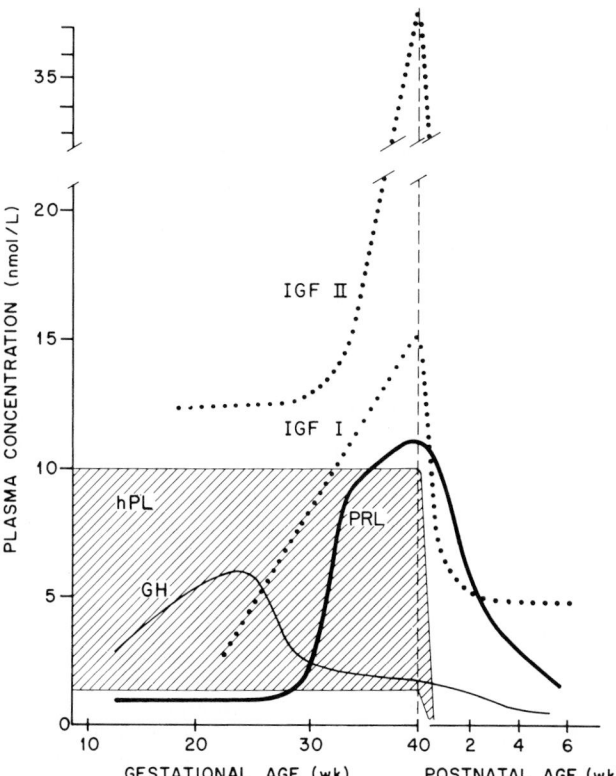

Figure 28–3. Patterns of change of average fetal plasma human placental lactogen (hPL), growth hormone (GH), prolactin (PRL), insulin-like growth factor I (IGF-I), and insulin-like growth factor II (IGF-II) during gestation and in the neonatal period. The range of fetal plasma hPL concentrations is shown as the hatched area. (Data from Bennett A, Wilson DM, Liu R, et al. Levels of insulin like growth factors I and II in human cord blood. J Clin Endocrinol Metab 1983; 57:609–612; Kaplan SL, Grumbach MM, Aubert ML. The ontogenesis of pituitary hormones and hypothalamic factors in the human fetus: maturation of central nervous system regulation of anterior pituitary function. Recent Prog Horm Res 1976; 32:161–243; and Bala RM, Lopatka J, Leung A, et al. Serum immunoreactive somatomedin levels in normal adults, pregnant women at term, children at various ages, and children with constitutionally delayed growth. J Clin Endocrinol Metab 1981; 52:508–512, with permission.)

increases progressively from 12 to 15 wk, and in vitro fetal pituitary cells from midgestation fetuses show limited autonomous PRL secretion, although PRL release increases in response to TRH and decreases in response to dopamine.[117] Brain and hypothalamic control of PRL matures late in gestation and during the first months of extrauterine life.[117, 118] Estrogen stimulates PRL synthesis and release by pituitary cells, and the marked increase in fetal plasma PRL concentration in the last trimester parallels the increase in fetal plasma estrogen levels, although lagging by several weeks.[117, 118] Anencephalic fetuses have plasma PRL concentrations in the normal or low-normal range.[118] These data support a role for estrogen in stimulating fetal PRL release. The fetal sheep exhibits a similar pattern of fetal plasma PRL levels, indicating that maturation and integration of brain and hypothalamic mechanisms modulating PRL release develop late in gestation and in the postnatal period, accounting for the delayed postnatal fall in plasma PRL level in the neonate of this species.[118]

The somatomedins IGF-I and IGF-II are important factors in fetal growth. mRNA and protein for both factors are present early in gestation in essentially all fetal tissues.[118, 135] IGF-II transcripts are more abundant than those of IGF-I and are predominant in fibroblasts and mesenchymal tissues.[135] Receptors for the IGFs also are widespread in fetal tissues. Studies of transgenic mice with null mutations of the genes encoding IGF-I, IGF-II, and IGF-I receptor have defined the role of the

somatomedins; the birth weight of the embryos lacking IGF-I or IGF-II is 60% of the control mice.[136] When both genes are inactive birth weight is reduced another 30%, and mice lacking IGF-I receptor have birth weights averaging 45% of controls.[136]

Postnatally GH acts via receptors in liver and other tissues to stimulate production of IGF-I and, to a lesser degree, IGF-II. Prenatally, in contrast, GH receptor mRNA levels and receptor binding are low in fetal liver, although receptor mRNA is present in other fetal tissues.[118] The growth of anencephalic fetuses is near normal, however, suggesting that factors other than GH stimulate fetal somatomedin production. hPL may play a role[136, 137]; ovine placental lactogen stimulates glycogen synthesis in fetal ovine liver, and hPL stimulates amino acid transport, DNA synthesis, and IGF-I production in human fetal fibroblasts and muscle cells. GH and PRL have little activity in these tissues.[137, 138] Nutritional factors also play a role in modulating fetal somatomedin production.[139]

Fetal Pituitary-Adrenal System

The primordium of the fetal adrenal gland can be recognized just cephalad to the developing mesonephros at 3 to 4 wk of gestation. By 6 to 8 wk an inner fetal zone of cells is surrounded by a subcapsular rim of immature cells referred to as the outer or definitive zone. The fetal adrenal gland grows rapidly and progressively in mass; the combined glandular weight approximates 8 g at term, when the fetal zone makes up about 80% of the mass of the gland.[140, 141] The large eosinophilic cells of the fetal zone are well differentiated by 9 to 12 wk of gestation and are capable of active steroidogenesis. The regulation of fetal adrenal growth is complex and involves fetal pituitary and placental factors and growth factors acting via paracrine and endocrine routes at different times.[142]

The fetal adrenal can produce the same five steroidogenic apoenzymes as the adult gland, including the mitochondrial cytochrome P450 (CYP) enzymes for cholesterol side-chain cleavage (CYP11A1) and hydroxylation of C-11 and C-18 of the steroid nucleus (CYP11/18), and CYP enzymes with 17-hydroxylase and 17,20-desmolase (CYP17) and 21-hydroxylase (CYP21) activities.[140–142] The fifth enzyme, also in the microsomes, has both 3β-HSD and Δ4,5-isomerase activities. Expression of these genes appears to be independent of fetal pituitary stimulation because specific mRNA levels are similar in the adrenal tissue of normal and anencephalic fetuses.[142, 143] However, quantitative differences in relative enzymatic activities in the zones of the fetal adrenal influence the pattern of steroids produced; e.g., there is a paucity of 3β-HSD activity in the fetal zone.[34–36, 140, 141]

The fetal adrenal gland also has relatively high steroid sulfotransferase activity,[144] and because of the low 3β-HSD and high sulfotransferase activities, the major steroid products of the fetal adrenal are DHEA, DHEAS, pregnenolone sulfate, several Δ5-3β-hydroxysteroids, and limited amounts of Δ5-3-ketosteroids, including cortisol and aldosterone.[140, 141, 145] The definitive zone contributes only a small fraction of total fetal adrenal steroid output compared with the fetal zone but may produce more cortisol per cell.[140, 141] Cholesterol, the major substrate for fetal adrenal steroidogenesis, is derived from circulating LDL and from de novo adrenal synthesis[140, 141, 146, 147]; LDL cholesterol, largely of fetal liver and testicular origin, contributes 70% of the total. The fetal zone contains more LDL binding sites and manifests a greater rate of de novo cholesterol synthesis than does the definitive zone, in keeping with its greater steroidogenic activity.[148]

The major control of fetal adrenal function is mediated by fetal pituitary corticotropin. In the anencephalic fetus the fetal adrenal involutes between 14 and 20 wk of gestation, and in the rhesus monkey hCG, PRL, and α-MSH have little effect on fetal adrenal activity, suggesting that any role of placental factors in control of fetal corticotropin is limited.[140, 141, 149, 150] Other pituitary peptides—including β-endorphin, β-lipotropin, α-MSH, and corticotropin-like intermediate peptide—also have little adrenotropic effect.[140] Maternal levels of CRH are elevated during the last trimester of gestation and reach values of 0.5 to 1 nmol/L at term; normal nonpregnant values are less than 0.01 nmol/L.[151] This CRH is bioactive, and levels correlate with maternal cortisol concentrations, suggesting that CRH plays a role in stimulating maternal corticotropin release.[151] Fetal plasma CRH levels at term, however, approximate 0.03 nmol/L and, relative to the presumably high levels in pituitary portal blood, probably have little role in modulating fetal corticotropin release.[151] Midgestation fetal plasma corticotropin concentrations average about 55 pmol/L (250 pg/mL), levels that maximally stimulate fetal adrenal steroidogenesis, and concentrations are higher throughout gestation than in postnatal life, although they fall near term (Fig. 28–4).[140, 152] Fetal corticotropin secretion in the sheep fetus during the third trimester is approximately 1 pmol/min/kg body weight (5 ng/min/kg), compared with the adult rate of about 0.3 pmol/min/kg body weight.[153]

Thus the fetal adrenal cortex is maximally stimulated by pituitary corticotropin and produces large quantities of DHEA and pregnenolone and their sulfate conjugates. Much of the DHEA is converted to 16-hydroxy-DHEAS by the fetal adrenal and fetal liver. As already discussed, DHEA serves as a substrate for placental estrone and estradiol production; 16-hydroxy-DHEA undergoes metabolism to estriol in the placenta. In the

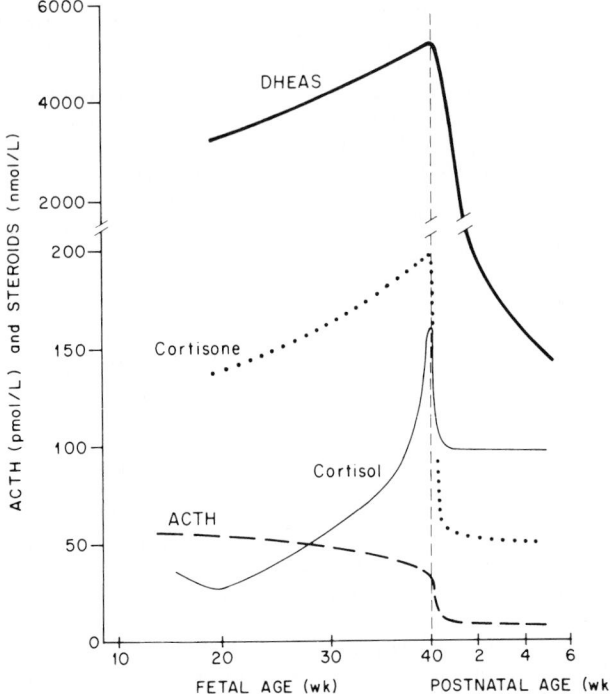

Figure 28–4. Patterns of change of fetal plasma corticotropin (ACTH), cortisol, cortisone, and DHEAS during gestation and in the neonatal period. The trend of average values is shown for each hormone in nanomoles per liter. Note the broken scale for DHEAS. (Data from Winters AJ, Oliver C, Colston C, et al. Plasma ACTH levels in the human fetus and neonate as related to age and parturition. J Clin Endocrinol Metab 1974; 39:269–273; Murphy BEP. Human fetal serum cortisol levels related to gestational age: evidence of a midgestational fall and a steep late gestational rise, independent of sex or mode of delivery. Am J Obstet Gynecol 1982; 144:276–282; Beitins IZ, Bayard F, Ances FIG, et al. The metabolic clearance rate, blood production, interconversion and transplacental passage of cortisol and cortisone in pregnancy near term. Pediatr Res 1973; 7:509–513; and Winter JSD. Fetal and neonatal adrenocortical physiology. In: Polin RA, Fox WW, eds. Neonatal and Fetal Medicine. Philadelphia: WB Saunders, 1992: 1829–1841, with permission.)

anencephalic fetus placental estrogen production is reduced to about 10% of normal.[34] An important factor in fetal adrenal function appears to be substrate inhibition of 3β-HSD activity by placental estrogens and intracellular adrenal steroids.[140, 154] The fetus also produces significant amounts of cortisol; indeed the fetal cortisol production rate in blood, per unit body weight, is similar to that in the adult.[155] About two thirds of fetal cortisol is derived from the fetal adrenal glands, and one third is derived via placental transfer.[141] Both fetal adrenal cortisol and placental estradiol regulate hepatic synthesis of cholestrol in the fetus.[141]

The corticotropin feedback control system matures progressively during the second half of gestation and the early neonatal period. Dexamethasone can suppress the human fetal pituitary-adrenal axis at term but not at 18 to 20 wk of gestation.[140, 141, 156, 157] In the fetal sheep hypothalamic and pituitary glucocorticoid receptors are present at midgestation, and corticotropin suppressibility can be demonstrated by the midpoint of the third trimester of gestation.[158, 159] The number of glucocorticoid receptors in the pituitary gland increases at term at the time of increasing glucocorticoid levels, suggesting that some process in the fetus allows the normal autoregulation of glucocorticoid receptors to be overriden at term.[159]

Fetal cortisol is converted to cortisone via an 11β-HSD in fetal tissues, and levels of circulating cortisone in the midgestation fetus are four- to fivefold higher than cortisol concentrations (see Fig. 28–4). Cortisone is a relatively inactive glucocorticoid, so this metabolism protects the anabolic milieu of the fetus because cortisol can retard both placental and fetal growth.[160] Glucocorticoid receptors are present at birth and probably are present at midgestation in most tissues, including placenta, lung, brain, liver, and gut.[159, 161, 162] As term approaches, selected fetal tissues including liver and lung express 11-ketosteroid reductase activity that promotes local conversion of cortisone to cortisol.[11, 140] Cortisol serves as an important stimulus to prepare the fetus for extrauterine survival. The increase in fetal cortisol concentration occurs during the last 10 wk of gestation and is the result of increased cortisol secretion and decreased conversion of cortisol to cortisone (see Fig. 28–3).[140] This fetal cortisol increase has an important role in the maturation of several fetal systems or functions that are critical to extrauterine survival[140, 161, 163, 164] (see the section on extrauterine adaptation).

The human fetal adrenal is capable of aldosterone secretion near term, and fetal plasma aldosterone concentrations in infants who are born by cesarean section are three- to fourfold higher than are maternal levels.[140, 165] Vaginal delivery and maternal salt restriction increase levels in both mother and infant.[165] The increased aldosterone levels in the fetus are due to increased secretion and persist during the first year of extrauterine life.[166] However, there is a poor correlation between plasma renin activity (PRA) and aldosterone levels in cord blood.[167] Aldosterone secretion is low in the midgestation human fetal adrenal and is unresponsive to the secretagogues that are known to modulate aldosterone production in the adult.[145] In sheep, fetal aldosterone becomes responsive to PRA and angiotensin II in the neonatal period.[168] In this species, in which late fetal aldosterone levels are also high relative to the adult, furosemide stimulates PRA but not aldosterone during the third trimester; the aldosterone response to furosemide (and PRA) is delayed until the neonatal period.[168, 169] This situation appears to be the case also in the human fetus and neonate.[145]

Angiotensin II levels in the sheep fetus are similar to maternal values, and blockade of fetal production with angiotensin-converting enzyme inhibitors decreases the fetal glomerular filtration rate.[169] Two subtypes of angiotensin receptors, AT_1 and AT_2, are detectable in various tissues early in fetal development.[170] AT_1 receptor mRNA expression in the fetal sheep kidney is low early in gestation, increases in the latter third of pregnancy, and decreases postnatally; AT_2 mRNA levels, in contrast, are high at midgestation and decrease during the third trimester.[170] These changes are believed to reflect growth factor–mediated changes in cells that contain AT in various tissues. Hormonal factors modulate fetal renal AT gene expression in sheep; angiotensin II suppresses both AT_1 and AT_2, and cortisol increases AT_1 gene expression.[170] The role of the fetal renin-angiotensin system is not clear; the fetal renin-angiotensin system, rather than modulating renal sodium excretion via aldosterone, may maintain renal excretion of salt and water into amniotic fluid to prevent oligohydramnios.[169] This renal effect presumably is mediated via modulation of arterial pressure. The mechanism for the high aldosterone levels in the fetal and neonatal periods remains unclear. Plasma atrial natriuretic factor concentrations are high in the fetus, so the increased PRA and aldosterone levels are not due to relative atrial natriuretic factor deficiency.[171]

Aldosterone affects renal sodium excretion in the fetal sheep and in premature infants.[140, 165, 168] Despite the fact that the newborn human kidney is relatively unresponsive to exogenous aldosterone, manifestations of mineralocorticoid deficiency in the newborn term infant can occur as a result of aldosterone deficiency or because of competition for binding to renal mineralocorticoid receptors by other steroids such as 17-hydroxyprogesterone.[140] Relatively reduced glomerular filtration in the newborn limits sodium loss initially, but by 1 wk of age aldosterone deficiency produces the characteristic manifestations of hyponatremia, hyperkalemia, and volume depletion.

Fetal Pituitary-Thyroid System

The thyroid gland is a derivative of the primitive buccopharyngeal cavity and develops from contributions of two anlagen, a midline thickening of the pharyngeal floor (median anlage) and paired caudal extensions of the fourth pharyngobranchial pouches (lateral anlagen).[172, 173] These structures are discernible by 16 to 17 d of gestation, and by 24 d the median anlage develops a thin, flask-like diverticulum extending from the floor of the buccal cavity to the fourth branchial arch. By 50 d of gestation the median and lateral anlagen have fused and the buccal stalk has ruptured. During this period the thyroid gland migrates caudally to its definitive location in the anterior neck. By 70 d of gestation colloid is visible histologically and thyroglobulin synthesis and iodide accumulation can be demonstrated within the gland. During the final follicular phase of development colloid spaces increase in size and there is progressive cell growth and accumulation of thyroid hormones. At 12 wk of gestation the fetal thyroid gland weighs about 80 mg and at term it weighs 1 to 2 g.

The parathyroid glands develop between 5 and 12 wk of gestation from the third and fourth pharyngeal pouches. The third pouches encounter the migrating thyroid anlage, and the parathyroid anlagen are carried caudally with the thyroid gland and finally come to rest at the lower poles of the thyroid lobes as the inferior parathyroid glands. The fourth pouches encounter the thyroid anlage later and come to rest at the upper poles of the thyroid lobes as the superior parathyroid glands. The individual parathyroid glands increase in diameter from less than 0.1 mm at 14 wk of gestation to 1 to 2 mm at birth. The fifth pouches contribute paired ultimobranchial bodies that are incorporated into the developing thyroid gland as the parafollicular or C cells that secrete calcitonin.[174]

As indicated earlier, maternal-fetal transfer of T_4 and T_3 occurs. T_4 is detectable in human coelomic fluid at levels of 0.5 to 2 nmol/L between 6 and 11 wk of gestation, before the onset of fetal thyroid function.[175] At term serum T_4 levels in the athyroid fetus range from 30 to 70 nmol/L (2.3 to 5.4 µg/dL).[176] Isotopic equilibrium studies with pregnant rats at term suggest that 15 to 20% of the T_4 in fetal tissues is of maternal origin.[177] Fetal serum T_4 and T_3 concentrations are low before midgestation and can be largely accounted for by maternal transfer, if similar maternal-fetal hormone kinetics early and late in gestation are assumed.

Pituitary and plasma thyrotropin concentrations begin to increase during the second trimester in the human fetus, about the time that pituitary portal vascular continuity develops (Fig. 28–5).[178–183] Plasma thyrotropin levels increase progressively during the last half of gestation (see Fig. 28–5). Plasma thyroxine-binding globulin and total T_4 concentrations increase progressively from low levels at 16 to 18 wk of gestation to maximal levels at 35 to 40 wk. Free T_4 levels also increase as a consequence of the increase in T_4 production.

The increases in plasma thyrotropin and T_4 levels during the third trimester reflect a progressive maturation of hypothalamic-pituitary control of thyrotropin and of thyroid gland responsiveness to thyrotropin (see Fig. 28–5). Thyrotropin is responsive to TRH early in the third trimester. Premature infants born at 26 to 28 wk of gestation respond to exogenous TRH with an increase in plasma thyrotropin concentration comparable to that in adults.[183] Moreover injection of T_4 into the amniotic fluid 24 h before elective cesarean section increases fetal plasma T_4 and decreases thyrotropin levels, which indicates negative-feedback control of thyrotropin.[179, 183] The ratios of free T_4 to thyrotropin and free T_3 to thyrotropin mature progressively after birth and approach adult values by 2 mo of age.[173, 180]

The adult thyroid follicular cell can modify iodine transport or uptake with changes in dietary iodine intake, independent of variations in serum thyrotropin levels.[184] Before 36 to 40 wk of gestation the thyroid lacks this autoregulatory mechanism and is susceptible to iodine-induced inhibition of thyroid hormone synthesis.[185, 186] The fetal thyroid follicular cell, when exposed to high circulating levels of iodide, is

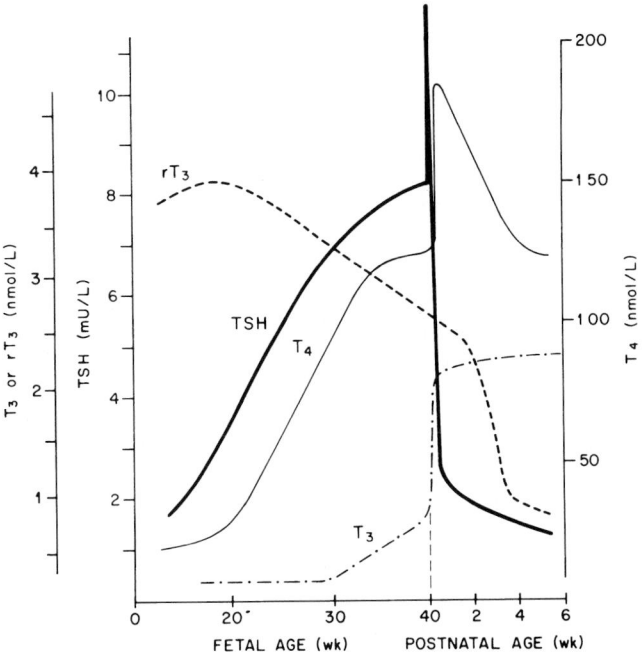

Figure 28–5. Patterns of change of average fetal plasma thyrotropin (also called thyroid-stimulating hormone [TSH]), thyroxine (T_4), triiodothyronine (T_3), and reverse T_3 (rT_3) levels during gestation and in the neonatal period. (Data from Fisher DA, Klein AH. Thyroid development and disorders of thyroid function in the newborn. N Engl J Med 1981; 304:702–712, with permission.)

unable to reduce iodide trapping and prevent the high intracellular iodide concentrations that produce the blockade of hormone synthesis referred to as the Wolff-Chaikoff effect.[185] The membrane autoregulatory mechanism is not well characterized, but the failure of the immature thyroid to exhibit autoregulation may relate to the absence or reduced iodination of an 8- to 10-kd protein in the thyroid follicular cell.[185] In addition to maturation of autoregulation, thyroidal responsiveness to thyrotropin increases during the last trimester.[179, 180]

These data and studies in rats, sheep, and nonhuman primates indicate that hypothalamic-pituitary-thyroid control matures during an interval corresponding to the third trimester and early neonatal period of human development.[173, 180, 183] This maturation includes coordinate maturation of hypothalamic TRH secretion, pituitary TRH sensitivity, thyrotropin negative-feedback control, and thyroid follicular cell responsiveness to thyrotropin. The fetus progresses from a state of both primary (thyroidal) and tertiary (hypothalamic) hypothyroidism at midgestation through a state of mild tertiary hypothyroidism during the final weeks in utero to a fully mature hypothalamic-pituitary-thyroid axis by 2 mo postnatally (see Fig. 28–5).

The catabolism of thyroid hormones proceeds through a progressive series of monodeiodinations[178, 187] (see also Chapter 11). Several enzymes act on the iodines in the outer (phenolic) ring or the inner (tyrosyl) iodothyronine ring. Most of the circulating, biologically active T_3 in adults is derived via outer ring monodeiodination of T_4 to T_3 in liver and other nonthyroidal tissues; biologically inactive reverse T_3 (rT_3) derives from inner ring deiodination of T_4 in peripheral tissues. Several iodothyronine monodeiodinase subtypes have been characterized. Type I outer ring monodeiodinase in liver and kidney is a high–Michaelis constant (K_m) enzyme inhibited by propylthiouracil and stimulated by thyroid hormone. This enzyme also has inner ring deiodinative activity and catalyzes the conversion of rT_3 to 3,3′-diiodothyronine. Type II outer ring monodeiodinase in brain, pituitary, and brown adipose tissue is a low-K_m enzyme insensitive to propylthiouracil and inhibited by thyroid hormone.[178] Type III monodeiodinase in liver, heart, skin, and placenta is responsible for inner ring deiodination of T_4 to rT_3. The type I monodeiodinase is believed to be responsible for production of T_3 that escapes from the cells into the circulation, whereas the type II enzyme is responsible for production of local T_3 in brain, pituitary, and brown adipose tissue. rT_3 apparently diffuses out of most tissues to appear in plasma.

The type III enzyme that catalyzes conversion of T_4 to rT_3 and T_3 to diiodothyronine (T_2) is expressed in most fetal tissues and in the placenta early in gestation and is responsible for production of the high levels of fetal plasma rT_3, which peak at midgestation in the range of 3 to 4 nmol/L (200 to 300 ng/dL).[179, 180] The persistence of the high plasma levels of rT_3 in the neonate for several weeks after birth indicates that most circulating rT_3 is produced by fetal tissues rather than by the placenta (see Fig. 28–5).[179]

There is little conversion of T_4 to circulating T_3 in the midgestation human fetus; plasma T_3 levels are low (<0.2 nmol/L [<15 ng/dL]) until 30 wk of gestation, after which the mean value increases to 0.7 nmol/L (50 ng/dL) at term (see Fig. 28–5).[178–182] Sulfation is active in fetal tissues, and the predominant thyroid hormone metabolites in the fetus are iodothyronine sulfates.[178] In the last third of gestation in fetal sheep the plasma production rates for T_4 and metabolites average the following: T_4 = 40 μg/kg/body weight/d, T_4 sulfate (T_4S) = 10 μg/kg/body weight/d, rT_3 = 5 μg/kg/body weight/d, rT_3S = 12 μg/kg/body weight/d, T_3 = 2 μg/kg/body weight/d, and T_3S = 2 μg/kg/body weight/d. All are biologically inactive except for T_3 and perhaps T_3S so that 90% of the T_4 metabolites in the fetus are biologically inac-

tive.[187] The sulfated metabolites accumulate in fetal serum as a result of the low type I monodeiodinase activity in fetal tissues and because the sulfated iodothyronines are not substrates for type III monodeiodinase.[178, 187] The production rate of T_3 increases progressively until term because of maturation of type I monodeiodinase activity in the liver and other tissues. In the fetal sheep, hepatic type I monodeiodinase activity increases progressively during the last trimester.[188] Type II monodeiodinase activity is present in the brain at midgestation and helps guarantee adequate brain T_3 in the sheep, a species in which brain maturation depends on thyroid hormone during the second half of gestation.[188] Both enzyme activities are T_4-responsive during the third trimester.[188]

Relatively high levels of nuclear T_3 receptors are present in brain tissue of the fetal sheep at midgestation; liver binding matures during the third trimester to reach adult levels at term.[189, 190] The sheep is relatively mature at birth, and the sensitivity of brain maturation to thyroid hormones begins about midgestation. The effects of thyroid hormone on skin and bone are evident during the third trimester, whereas thyroid hormone effects on heart, lung, kidney, and liver appear to be delayed until the early weeks of postnatal life.[180, 190]

There is limited information on maturation of thyroid hormone receptors and responses to thyroid hormones in the human fetus and neonate. In the human fetus, thyroid receptors are present in lung, brain, heart, and liver at 13 to 19 wk of gestation.[191, 192] However, there are few manifestations of thyroid hormone deficiency in the infant born without thyroid tissue and with very low plasma T_4 and high thyrotropin concentrations.[179, 180] Size, weight, appearance, behavior, biochemical parameters, extrauterine adaptation, and neonatal course are usually normal. However, the occurrence of marked fetal hypothyroidism in the Pit-1–deficient infant of a Pit-1–deficient mother and with undetectable serum T_4 levels in mother and infant at term argues for an important role for maternal thyroid hormone in the developing fetus.[193]

Fetal Pituitary-Gonadal Axis (also see Chapter 29)

The mammalian gonad is derived from two tissue anlagen, the primordial germ cells of the yolk sac wall and somatic, stromal cells that migrate from the primitive mesonephros.[194–196] By 4 to 5 wk of gestation the germ cells have begun their migration from the yolk sac, and the gonadal ridge has appeared as a derivative of the mesonephros. The germ cells are incorporated into the developing gonadal ridge during the sixth week, when the primitive gonad is composed of a surface epithelium, primitive gonadal cords continuous with the epithelium, and a dense cellular mass referred to as the gonadal blastema.[196] Development of the undifferentiated gonads into testes or ovaries after 6 wk of gestation is regulated by genetic determinants. The first gene to be characterized in the testis-determining pathway is the *SRY* gene on the Y chromosome, which functions to initiate the process of testicular differentiation.[197] The product of this gene is a DNA-binding zinc finger protein that acts as a transcriptional modulator.[197] Other sex-determining genes on the X and Y chromosomes remain to be identified.

Male gonadal differentiation begins at 7 wk of gestation, with organization of the gonadal blastema into interstitium and germ cell–containing testicular cords. The primitive cords lose their connections with the epithelium; primitive Sertoli cells and spermatogonia become visible within the cords; and the epithelium differentiates to form the tunica albuginea.[196] Leydig cells derived from the undifferentiated interstitium are visible by the end of the eighth week of gestation and are capable of androgen synthesis at this time. By 14 wk of gestation these cells make up as much as 50% of the cell mass, but as the tubules develop they account for a smaller percentage of the tissue. The fetal testes grow from approximately 20 mg at 14 wk of gestation to 800 mg at birth; at 5 to 6 mo they descend into the inguinal canal in association with the epididymis and the ductus deferens.[196]

In females differentiation of ovaries begins during the seventh week of gestation. The gonadal blastema differentiates into interstitium and medullary cords containing the primitive germ cells now referred to as oogonia. The cords degenerate and cortical layers of surface epithelium, containing individual small oogonia, appear. By 11 to 12 wk of gestation clusters of dividing oogonia are surrounded by cord cells within the cortex; the medulla at this time consists largely of connective tissue.[196] At 12 wk of gestation primitive granulosa cells begin to replicate, and many of the large oogonia in the deepest layers of the cortex enter their first meiotic division; other oogonia degenerate. Maturation continues toward the superficial layers through the ninth month, by which time all the surviving oogonia have undergone the first meiotic division to become primary oocytes. Primordial follicles are present by 5 mo of gestation, and during the seventh month stroma-derived thecal cells develop around the primordial follicles as they mature to primary follicles. This process continues after birth, again progressing toward the superficial layers. Each fetal ovary weighs about 15 mg at 14 wk of gestation and 300 to 350 mg at birth.[196]

In the male the development of Leydig cells leads to an increase in fetal testosterone production between gestational weeks 10 and 20 (Fig. 28–6). In vitro studies in the rat have shown that hCG binding to fetal testis cells does not down-regulate LH receptors.[198] If this is true in vivo, continuous exposure of the Leydig cell to hCG would not desensitize the fetal testis and would allow the maintenance of augmented testosterone production during development. Fetal LH may contribute to fetal Leydig cell function, but quantitatively hCG is the predominant gonadotropin (see Fig. 28–6). Testoste-

rone itself, acting via the androgen receptor, stimulates differentiation of the primitive mesonephric ducts into bilateral ductus deferens, epididymides, seminal vesicles, and ejaculatory ducts. Dihydrotestosterone stimulates male differentiation of the urogenital sinus and external genitalia, including differentiation of the prostate, growth of the genital tubercle to form a phallus, and fusion of the urogenital folds to form the penile urethra. Dihydrotestosterone is formed from testosterone via the 5α-reductase enzyme within the urogenital sinus and urogenital tubercle and acts via the same androgen receptor that mediates the action of testosterone in the wolffian ducts.

The fetal testis also produces antimüllerian hormone (AMH), which causes dedifferentiation of the müllerian duct system in the male fetus.[198, 199] AMH is a glycoprotein with a monomer molecular size of approximately 72 kd and multimer sizes ranging from 145 to 235 kd.[198, 199] It is produced by testicular Sertoli cells and reaches the müllerian ducts largely by diffusion; duct regression in vitro requires a 24- to 36-h exposure to AMH, which is synthesized early in gestation, production peaking at the time of müllerian duct regression. Biosynthesis continues throughout gestation and decreases after birth.[198, 199] *AMH* gene expression is activated by the *SRY* gene.[200] AMH may have a role in testicular descent and is present in adult granulosa cells.[198, 201]

Male phenotypic differentiation is mediated by testicular testosterone and AMH and occurs between 8 and 14 wk of gestation. In the female fetus the müllerian duct system differentiates in the absence of AMH, the mesonephric ducts fail to develop in the absence of testosterone, and the undifferentiated urogenital sinus and external genitalia mature into female structures.

Gonadal hormones also control gonadotropin production in the brain that results in cyclic ovarian function and normal function of the testes. Testosterone administration to neonatal female rats produces permanent inhibition of cyclic hypothalamic control via local aromatization to estradiol and estrogen receptor binding.[202, 203] In primates and humans estrogens per se seem to be more effective in this regard.[203–205] However, there is no evidence for permanent programming in the primate, and there appear to be no major tissue biochemical differences between the sexes in utero to account for sexual dimorphic behavioral or gonadotropic programming.[205] Thus the mechanisms for these effects are not yet clear in the primate and human fetus.

Intermediate Lobe of the Pituitary

The intermediate lobe of the pituitary gland is prominent in both the human and the sheep fetus.[206, 207] Intermediate lobe cells begin to disappear near term and are virtually absent in the adult human pituitary, although the intermediate lobe in the adult of some lower species is anatomically and functionally distinct.[206] The major secretory products of the intermediate lobe are α-MSH and β-endorphin derived from cleavage of the POMC molecule. Cleavage of POMC in the anterior lobe results predominantly in corticotropin and β-lipotropin formation.

In rhesus monkeys and humans the fetal pituitary contains high concentrations of compounds resembling α-MSH and corticotropin-like intermediate lobe peptide[141,208]; α-MSH levels in the human fetus decrease with increasing fetal age.[118, 209] The circulating levels of both β-endorphin and β-lipotropin are high in the fetal lamb, and the ratio of β-endorphin to β-lipotropin increases during hypoxic stimulation of the anterior pituitary.[118] Because hypoxia provokes corticotropin release and β-lipotropin production from the anterior pituitary, these data have been interpreted to suggest that basal β-endorphin levels in the fetus originate in the

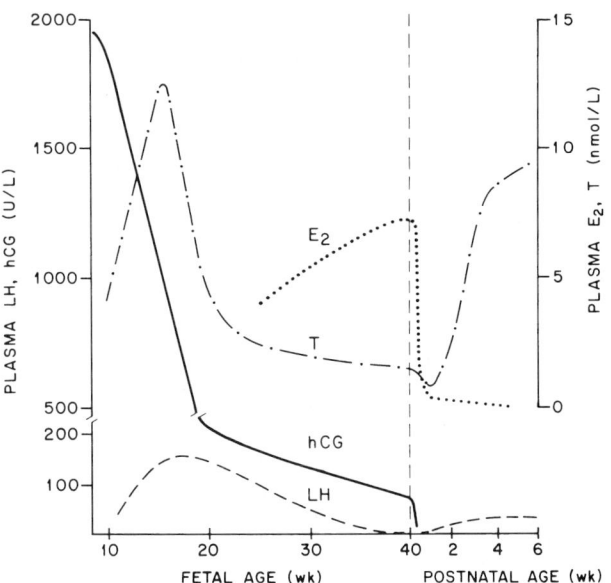

Figure 28–6. Patterns of change of average plasma levels of human growth hormone (hCG), luteinizing hormone (LH), testosterone (T), and estradiol (E₂) in a male fetus during gestation and in the neonatal period. (Data from Reyes FI, Boroditsky RS, Winter JS, et al. J Clin Endocrinol Metab 1974; 38:612–617; Kaplan SL, Grumbach MM, Aubert ML. Recent Prog Horm Res 1976; 32:161–243; Winter JS, Faiman C, Hobson WC, et al. J Clin Endocrinol Metab 1975; 40:545–551; Forest MG, Cathiard AM. J Clin Endocrinol Metab 1975; 41:977–980; and Penny R, Parlow AF, Frasier SD. Pediatrics 1979; 64:604–608, with permission.)

intermediate lobe.[114] α-MSH and corticotropin-like intermediate lobe peptide may play a role in fetal adrenal activation, and α-MSH may play a role in fetal growth.[141, 210, 211] However, these effects are probably minor; the processing of pituitary POMC in the human fetus by the end of the second trimester is similar to that in the adult,[212] but the role of these intermediate lobe peptides in the fetus remains obscure.[140, 141]

Posterior Pituitary

The fetal neurohypophysis is well developed by 10 to 12 wk of gestation and contains both arginine vasopressin (AVP, also called antidiuretic hormone [ADH]) and oxytocin (OT).[213–215] In addition, arginine vasotocin (AVT), the parent neurohypophyseal hormone in submammalian vertebrates, is present in the fetal pituitary and pineal glands and in adult pineal glands from several mammalian species, including humans.[215–218] AVT is present in the pituitary during fetal life and disappears in the neonatal period.[216] In adult mammals the instillation of AVT into cerebrospinal fluid inhibits gonadotropin and corticotropin release and stimulates PRL release by the anterior pituitary and induces sleep; however, its physiological importance in these regards remains unclear.[217] The role of AVT in the fetal pineal gland is unknown.

In the fetal sheep the baseline fetal plasma AVP concentrations are similar to maternal levels after midgestation. During the last trimester of gestation fetal hypothalamic and pituitary responsiveness to both volume and osmolar stimuli for AVP secretion are well developed, and AVP exerts antidiuretic effects on the fetal kidney.[213, 219, 220] Baseline plasma levels of AVT in fetal sheep during the last trimester approximate values for AVP and OT.[218] Presumably this AVT is derived from the posterior pituitary, but the stimuli for AVT secretion in the fetus is not defined. The neurohypophyseal peptides are synthesized as large precursor molecules (neurophysins) and processed to bioactive amidated peptides.[221] Enzymatic processing involves progressive cleavage of carboxy terminal–extended peptides producing sequentially (for OT) OT-glycine-lysine-arginine (OT-GKR), OT-GK, OT-G, and OT. Similar progressive processing yields AVP-G and AVP from the AVP neurophysin. Enzymatic processing of neurophysins matures progressively in the fetus so that early in gestation fetal plasma contains relatively large concentrations of the extended peptides. For OT the ratio of OT extended peptides to OT in fetal sheep serum approximates 35:1 early in gestation and 3:1 late in gestation.[221]

In the fetus AVP appears to function as a stress-responsive hormone. Perhaps the major potential stress for the fetus is hypoxia, and the response of AVP to hypoxia is increased relative to the maternal response and relative to the fetal AVP responses to osmolar stimuli.[222–226] Plasma AVP concentrations in human cord blood are elevated with intrauterine bradycardia and meconium passage.[225] The vasopressor action of AVP may be important in the maintenance of fetal circulatory homeostasis during hemorrhage and hypoxia; AVP has a limited effect on fetoplacental blood flow.[227, 228] Fetal hypoxia is also a major stimulus for catecholamine release.[229] There is little information on interaction between AVP and catecholamines during fetal hypoxia, but both fetal hypoxia and AVP stimulate anterior pituitary function.[226, 229] A role for AVP as a CRH is established in the adult, and the ovine fetal pituitary responds separately and synergistically to AVP and CRH early in the third trimester.[230–232] The role of AVP in controlling fetal corticotropin release seems to decrease with gestational age.[231] It is not known whether AVT functions as a fetal CRH.

There is little information on maturation of neurohypophyseal hormone receptors and their physiological effects in the fetus. OT receptors have been demonstrated in neonatal rat brain and in human fetal membranes at term; AVP

receptors have been found in renal medullary membranes of newborn sheep.[233–235] Both AVP and AVT have antidiuretic actions in the sheep fetus during the last third of gestation.[236, 237] In vitro AVP stimulates contracture of aortic rings from neonatal rats and may have an effect on water transport via the amniotic membranes.[238, 239] Thus both hormones act to conserve water for the fetus by inhibiting fluid loss into amniotic fluid via the lungs and kidneys (Fig. 28–7). Whether AVT exerts its effects via AVP receptors or separate fetal AVT receptors is not clear. The ability of the newborn human infant to respond to isotonic dextran or hypertonic saline with appropriate alterations in kidney free water clearance indicates that both volume and osmolar control systems for modulation of AVP secretion are mature at birth.[240] Maximal concentrating capacity by the fetal kidney is limited to about 600 mmol/L. This limitation is not due to inadequate AVP stimulation but rather to inherent immaturity of the renal tubules.[240]

Fetal Autonomic Nervous System

The primordia of the sympathetic trunk ganglia are visible in the human fetus by 6 to 7 wk of gestation. The preaortic sympathetic primordia at this time are composed of primitive sympathetic neurons and chromaffin cells, which condense into chains of cell masses along the abdominal aorta. By 10 to 12 wk of gestation the paired adrenal masses are well developed. In addition, numerous extramedullary paraganglia (derived from preaortic condensations of sympathetic neurons and chromaffin cells) are scattered throughout the abdominal and pelvic sympathetic plexuses (Fig. 28–8).[241] Each of these extramedullary paraganglia may reach a maximal diameter of 2 to 3 mm by 28 to 30 wk of gestation. The largest of the paraganglia, the organs of Zuckerkandl near the origin of the inferior mesenteric arteries, enlarge to 10 to 15 mm in length at term. After birth the paraganglia gradually atrophy and disappear by 2 to 3 y of age. Progressive growth of the adrenal medullae, increasing catecholamine content of the adrenal medullae with increasing gestational age, and a progressive maturation of medullary functional capacity occur (see Fig. 28–8).[241, 242] Histologically the adrenal medullae are somewhat immature at birth, but by the age of 1 they resemble the adult glands.[241]

Both chromaffin and sympathetic nerve cells are derived from common neuroectodermal stem cells, and both respond to NGF.[243, 244] Sympathetic nervous system development is NGF dependent, and injections of NGF antiserum into neonatal rats lead to degeneration of immature chromaffin cells, sympa-

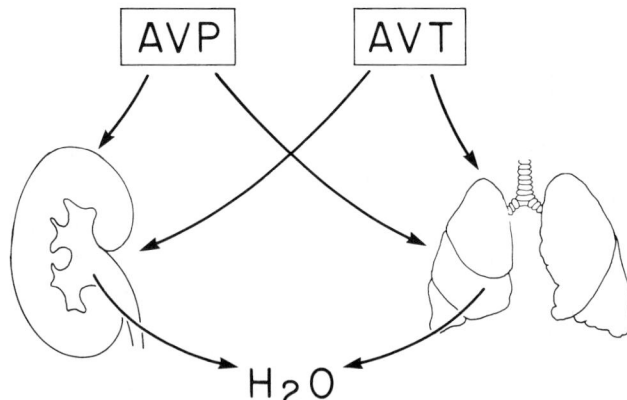

Figure 28–7. Effect of arginine vasopressin (AVP) and arginine vasotocin (AVT) on fetal water metabolism. Both peptides act to decrease output of urine and to decrease tracheal fluid outflow in the fetus. Thus both act to decrease production of amniotic fluid. See text for details.

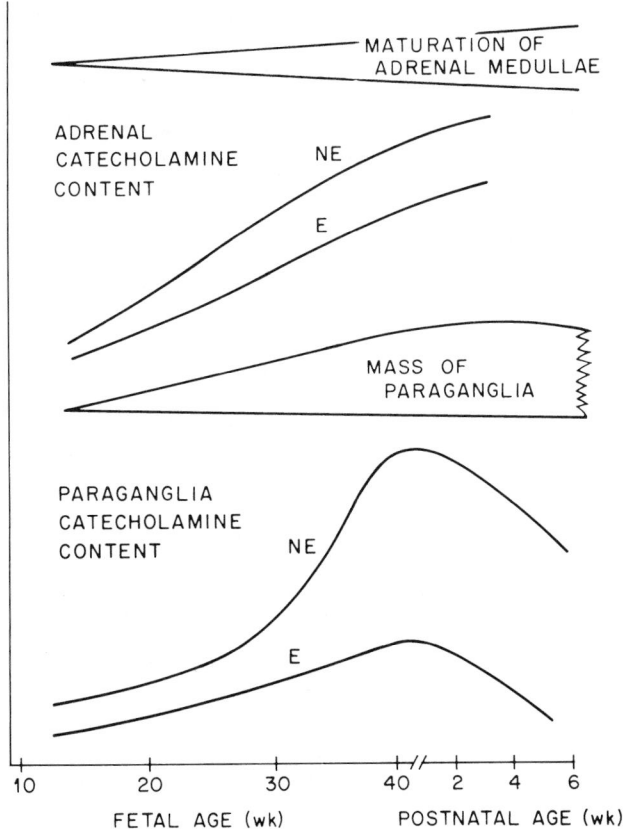

Figure 28–8. Patterns of maturation of chromaffin tissue and chromaffin tissue catecholamine concentrations in the human fetus during gestation and infancy. The general patterns of change in norepinephrine (NE) and epinephrine (E) levels in adrenomedullary and aortic paraganglial tissue are shown. (Modified from Fisher DA. Fetal endocrinology: endocrine disease and pregnancy. In: DeGroot LJ, Besser GM, Cahill GF Jr, et al, eds. Endocrinology. 2nd ed. Philadelphia: WB Saunders, 1989: 2102–2120, with permission.)

thetic cells, and pheochromoblasts.[244] Whether NGF and other growth factors are involved in the transient life span and function of the paraganglia in the human fetus and neonate remains to be clarified. The role of placental NGF in maturation of the fetal autonomic nervous system is also unclear.[82, 83]

Catecholamines are present in the para-aortic chromaffin tissue by 10 to 15 wk of gestation, and concentrations increase until term.[242] The predominant catecholamine is norepinephrine (NE), presumably because of low activity of phenylethanolamine N-methyltransferase in para-aortic chromaffin tissue. This enzyme, which catalyzes the methylation of NE to epinephrine, appears to be activated by the high levels of cortisol that diffuse into the adrenal medulla from the adrenal cortex; in contrast, cortisol levels in extramedullary chromaffin tissue are low.[245] Fetal hypophysectomy reduces adrenomedullary epinephrine content in rats, and corticotropin restores this content.[246] In fetal mammals the chromaffin cells of the adrenal medulla can respond directly to asphyxia, long before splanchnic innervation develops, by secreting NE; it is likely that the noninnervated para-aortic tissue responds similarly.[246, 247] In the developing rat splanchnic innervation of the adrenal medulla develops by day 10 postnatally, and in neonatal rats acute hypoxia increases adrenal catecholamine synthesis and plasma epinephrine and NE levels.[248] In the fetal sheep a similar developmental transition occurs between days 120 and 135 of the 150-d gestation.[247–250] The central nervous system responds to stimuli that evoke sympathetic nervous system responses before the adrenomedullary splanchnic innervation, but the adrenal medulla is relatively unresponsive

to such stimuli. The transition is heralded by an adrenomedullary response to hypoglycemia mediated by the central nervous system.[249] This response is present in developing sheep, monkeys, and human fetuses during the third trimester of gestation.[251–253] Central and adrenal enkephalins are also involved in fetal autonomic nervous system function.[249, 250] Pretreatment with naloxone potentiates, and methadone inhibits, the catecholamine response to hypoxia.[249, 250]

There is limited information about the source of catecholamines in the human fetus. Basal plasma epinephrine, NE, and dopamine levels during the last third of gestation decrease as term approaches.[254] The metabolic clearance rate of epinephrine increases with gestational age, whereas the production rate remains unchanged,[255] indicating that the decreasing basal catecholamine levels that occur with fetal age are due to maturation of clearance mechanisms. The fetal sheep responds to maternal exercise or hypoxia with increased catecholamine levels.[256] The human neonate responds to parturition with an increase in plasma epinephrine and NE concentrations, and these responses are augmented by hypoxia and acidosis.[249, 257, 258] In the newborn infant catecholamine secretion also increases after cold exposure and hypoglycemia.[249, 253]

Catecholamines are critical for fetal cardiovascular function and fetal survival. Gene knockout studies in mice targeting either tyrosine hydroxylase or dopamine β-hydroxylase produce fetal catecholamine deficiency and midgestation fetal death in 90% of the mutant embryos.[259, 260] Additionally fetal catecholamines are the major stress hormones in the fetus.[249, 251, 252] The fetal adrenal and the para-aortic chromaffin masses discharge large amounts of catecholamines directly into the circulation in response to fetal hypoxia.[249] Moreover the defense against fetal hypoxia involves catecholamine actions mediated through cardiac α-receptors that are unique to immature animals.[249, 261] α-Adrenergic receptors predominate in immature cardiac tissue and gradually decline in number as β-adrenergic receptors increase with maturation. Chromaffin tissue in the fetus is also innervated by opiate receptors and contains relatively large amounts of opiate peptides that appear to be cosecreted with the catecholamines.[249, 250] The extent to which these peptides or pituitary endorphins are involved in modulating fetal catecholamine secretion remains unclear.

Parathyroid Hormone–Calcitonin System

As indicated earlier, the fetal parathyroid glands and the thyroid parafollicular C cells (the calcitonin-secreting cells) are identifiable at the end of the first trimester, and both endocrine systems are functional during the second and third trimesters. Studies in fetal sheep and monkey and measurements in human preterm and term infants indicate that high concentrations of fetal calcium (averaging 2.75 to 3 mmol/L in the last trimester) are maintained by active placental transport from maternal blood.[262, 263] The transport of calcium probably occurs across the syncytiotrophoblast. This tissue contains a calcium-binding protein that buffers intracellular calcium ions as they are transported across the syncytial cell to the basement membrane. An adenosine triphosphate–dependent calcium pump transports the calcium across the cell membrane to the fetal circulation.[263] PTH levels in human cord blood during the last trimester are relatively low and calcitonin concentrations are high.[262–265] 25-Hydroxycholecalciferol and 1,25-dihydroxycholecalciferol (1,25(OH)$_2$D) are transported across the placenta, and free vitamin D concentrations in the fetal circulation are similar to or higher than maternal values.[264, 266, 267] The high prevailing levels of total and ionized calcium maintained in fetal blood by active maternal-fetal transport are believed to suppress fetal PTH and stimulate fetal calcitonin secretion.

Thyroparathyroidectomy in the fetal sheep causes a rapid decrease in fetal plasma calcium concentration and a loss of the placental calcium gradient.[268, 269] Thyroparathyroidectomy produces a deficiency of PTH, but ovine fetal parathyroid glands also contain relatively high concentrations of a PTHrP with chemical and immunologic characteristics of the PTHrP synthesized by tumors that cause hypercalcemia.[56, 269–271] PTHrP gene expression and protein also are present in placenta and a variety of fetal tissues.[95] PTHrP has a major role in fetal bone development and metabolism as well as fetal calcium homeostasis. PTHrP(1–34) has structural homology to PTH(1–34) and binds to and activates the PTH receptor.[269–271] Carboxy terminus fragments may have other actions, including inhibition of osteoclast activity [PTHrP(107–111)] and stimulation of placental calcium transport [PTHrP(1–84) or PRHrP(1-141)].[263, 271, 272] PTHrP knockout mice die immediately after birth with a multitude of skeletal anomalies.[272] PTH and PTHrP act on the fetal kidney to decrease calcium and increase cAMP excretion.[269] PTH receptors are localized in the brush border and apical plasma membranes of human placental cells, and PTH stimulates adenylate cyclase activity in these membranes.[273, 274] Placental receptors for carboxy terminus PTHrP have not been described. Human cord blood contains higher concentrations of PTHrP than do paired maternal samples (1.5 vs. 0.8 pmol/L), and maternal blood PTH levels are higher than cord values, supporting the postulated role of fetal PTHrP in human fetal calcium metabolism.[275]

Fetal nephrectomy also reduces fetal calcium concentrations, and the hypocalcemia can be prevented by administration of 1,25(OH)$_2$D.[266, 268] Moreover infusion into the sheep fetus of antibody to 1,25(OH)$_2$D reduces the placental calcium gradient.[266] Thus fetal PTHrP and PTH appear to stimulate fetal renal 1,25(OH)$_2$D production, which acts to enhance maternal-fetal transport of calcium by the placenta. The fetal kidney can synthesize 1,25(OH)$_2$D, and the placenta contains both 1,25(OH)$_2$D receptors and a vitamin D–dependent calcium-binding protein.[264, 266] In the sheep fetus the endogenous production rate of 1,25(OH)$_2$D during the last third of gestation is six times greater than that in the mother.[276] The metabolic clearance of 1,25(OH)$_2$D is also higher in the fetus than in the mother.[276]

The fetal parathyroid-placental axis promotes maternal-fetal transfer of bone mineral and accretion of fetal bone mineral. The high blood levels of calcitonin in the fetus, probably due to the chronic stimulation by fetal hypercalcemia, are thought to contribute to the fetal bone mineral accretion.[262, 263, 265] A prominent effect of calcitonin is to inhibit bone resorption, and the high fetal serum calcium concentrations coupled with high circulating calcitonin promote bone mineral anabolism.[277] Calcitonin has been called a vestigial hormone because of its limited role in postnatal calcium regulation,[277] but it may have an important role in the fetus. Placental calcitonin production may contribute to the calcitonin in fetal plasma, but the persistence of high plasma levels in neonatal plasma argues for predominant fetal production.[262] 1,25(OH)$_2$D or 24,25(OH)$_2$D may play a role in fetal cartilage growth and bone mineral accretion.[278] These concepts are summarized in Figure 28–9.

Endocrine Pancreas: Insulin and Glucagon

The fetal pancreas is identifiable by 4 wk of gestation, and alpha and beta cells can be recognized by 8 to 9 wk. Insulin, glucagon, somatostatin, and pancreatic polypeptide are measurable by 8 to 10 wk of gestation.[279–283] Alpha cells are more numerous than are beta cells in the early fetal pancreas

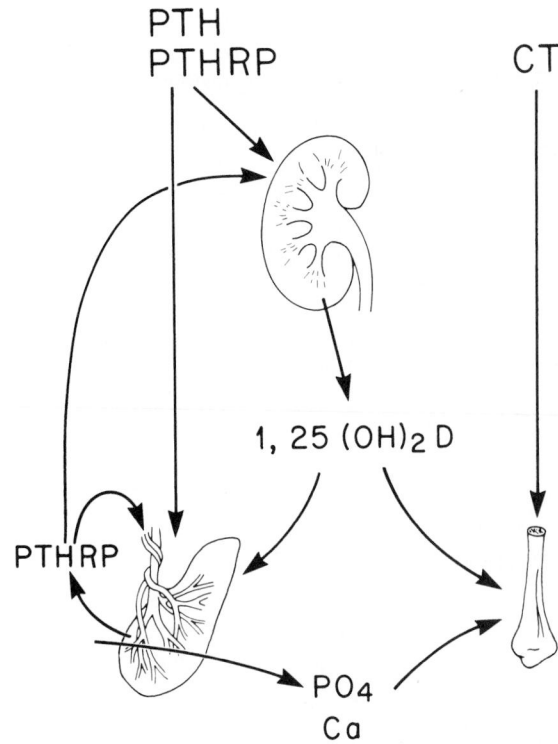

Figure 28–9. Proposed actions of parathyroid hormone (PTH), PTH-related protein (PTHRP), and calcitonin (CT) in the fetus. PTHrP and perhaps PTH from the parathyroid glands and PTHrP from the placenta act on the placenta to promote calcium (Ca) and phosphate (PO$_4$) transport from the maternal to the fetal circulation to maintain the relative fetal hypercalcemia and the high rate of fetal bone formation during the last half of gestation. PTHrP also acts on the kidney to promote 1-hydroxylation of 25-hydroxycholecalciferol to 1,25(OH)$_2$D, which augments placental calcium transport and promotes fetal bone growth. High fetal CT levels tend to promote bone accretion. See text for details.

and reach a relative peak at midgestation; beta cells increase throughout the second half of gestation so that by term the ratio of alpha cells to beta cells approximates 1:1.[282, 283] The insulin content of the pancreas increases from less than 3.6 pmol/g (0.5 U/g) at 7 to 10 wk to 30 pmol/g (4 U/g) at 16 to 25 wk of gestation and 93 pmol/g (13 U/g) near term; the concentration in the adult pancreas approximates 14 pmol/g (2 U/g).[280, 282]

Although the fetal beta cell is functional by 14 to 24 wk of gestation and although fetal pancreatic hormone concentrations are high, secretion of insulin by the fetal pancreas is low. Insulin release from the fetal rat pancreas in vitro in response to glucose or pyruvate is minimal but can be stimulated by leucine, arginine, tolbutamide, or potassium chloride so that parts of the secretory mechanism are functional in the fetus.[282, 284] Insulin secretion in adult islets is mediated by two or more mechanisms, including stimulation of the adenylate cyclase system with production of cAMP and inhibition of potassium efflux, which leads to depolarization of the cell membrane and opening of voltage-dependent calcium channels.[284] The former mechanism, although suppressed in the fetal islets, can be augmented by theophylline, but calcium channel activation does not occur in fetal islets in response to initiators of insulin release that cause depolarization of adult islet cells.[284] The infusion of glucose or arginine to pregnant women prior to hysterotomy fails to provoke fetal insulin secretion at midgestation or near term, and plasma insulin levels in the late human fetus are relatively unresponsive to high glucose concentrations before the onset of labor.

Similar observations have been made in the monkey. In this species neither glucose nor arginine stimulates fetal insulin release near term, whereas glucagon evokes prompt insulin secretion.[282] Late in gestation in the ovine fetus, epinephrine inhibits insulin release via a receptor pathway.[282] In the anencephalic human fetus, the endocrine pancreas develops normally if maternal carbohydrate metabolism is not impaired, but beta cell hypertrophy and hyperplasia do not occur in the anencephalic fetus or in decapitated fetal rabbits exposed to chronic hyperglycemia. This lack of beta cell response to hyperglycemia may be the result of GH deficiency because GH stimulates insulin gene expression and may exert a permissive role in beta cell hyperplasia and hypertrophy.[285]

Pancreatic glucagon concentrations are also relatively high in fetal plasma and increase progressively with fetal age. The fetal pancreatic glucagon content at midgestation is approximately 6 μg/g compared with an adult level of 2 μg/g.[281–283] As is true for insulin, the capacity for glucagon secretion is blunted in the fetus. Hyperglycemia does not suppress fetal plasma glucagon levels in rats, monkeys, or sheep and acute hypoglycemia does not evoke glucagon secretion in the rat fetus. Amino acids, which are important secretagogues for insulin and glucagon in the adult, probably have little role in modulating insulin and glucagon secretion in the preterm fetus.[283] However, infusion of alanine into women at term increases both maternal and cord blood glucagon levels, indicating a fetal glucagon reponse to amino acids in the term fetus. Catecholamines also evoke glucagon release in the near-term ovine fetus.[282]

Thus the fetal pancreatic islet cells, although histologically mature and capable of hormone synthesis and hyperplasia, are functionally immature at birth in regard to the capacity to secrete both insulin and glucagon. The relatively rapid maturation of responsiveness to glucose in the neonatal period in both premature and mature infants suggests that this blunted state may be a secondary result of the relatively stable fetal serum glucose levels maintained by placental transfer of maternal glucose, rather than a primary, temporally fixed maturation process. The blunted capacity for insulin and glucagon secretion has been related to a deficient capacity of the fetal pancreatic islet cells to generate cAMP or to a rapid destruction of cAMP by phosphodiesterase, or both. A two- to threefold increase in islet cell cAMP concentration occurs in newborn rats during the first 72 h after birth, in keeping with this hypothesis.[286] The metabolism of nutrient secretagogues (such as glucose) in the fetal islets fails to couple with the potassium channel to depolarize the cell membrane.[287]

Insulin and glucagon normally are not necessary for substrate metabolism in the fetus.[283, 288] Glucose is obtained by placental transfer via facilitated diffusion. The fetal respiratory quotient approximates 1, which suggests that glucose is the primary energy substrate for the fetus. Other substrates such as amino acids and lactate may also be utilized in the human as in the sheep fetus.[288] However, at least early in gestation, hepatic metabolism and substrate utilization appear to be independent of insulin and to be modulated in an autoregulatory fashion by glucose.[282] In addition, the constant supply of glucose normally precludes the necessity for endogenous gluconeogenesis, and gluconeogenic enzyme activities are low in the fetal liver.[282, 289, 290]

Glycogen storage in the fetus is modulated by fetal glucocorticoids and probably by placental hPL. Fetal insulin plays a role near term, when insulin also has the capacity to increase fetal glucose uptake and lipogenesis.[282, 283, 291] Insulin receptors are present on most fetal cells in higher numbers than on adult cells; moreover hyperinsulinemia fails to down-regulate fetal insulin receptors.[282, 292] Fetal hepatic glucagon receptors, in contrast, are reduced in number, and fetal liver is relatively resistant to the glycemic effect of glucagon.[293] These conditions tend to potentiate the fetal anabolic milieu during the period of rapid growth in the last trimester of gestation.

NEUTRALIZATION OF HORMONE ACTIONS IN THE FETUS

Production of Inactive Metabolites

Throughout the latter part of gestation, cortisol is metabolized in fetal tissues to inactive cortisone via an 11β-HSD. The placenta is permeable to steroid hormones including cortisol. During midgestation placental 11β-HSD activity is low, and cortisol is transferred to the fetus. Placental 11β-HSD activity increases during the second half of pregnancy under the control of placental estrogens, and enzyme activity near term is high.[36, 141] Thus maternal-fetal cortisol transfer decreases progressively. In addition, although many adult tissues can convert cortisone to cortisol, conversion is reduced during most of fetal life. Consequently most of the cortisol that crosses the placenta or is produced by the fetus is inactivated to cortisone by the placenta or by fetal tissues. Levels of cortisone in fetal plasma exceed those of cortisol by three- to fourfold until after 30 wk of gestation (see Fig. 28–4). Teleologically this would help preserve the anabolic and growth-promoting milieu of the fetus and minimize premature maturational and parturitional effects of cortisol. After 30 wk the ratio of cortisol to cortisone in fetal tissues and plasma increases as a result of increased fetal secretion and decreased conversion of cortisol to cortisone within the placenta and fetal tissues.[11, 36, 140, 141] Cortisol has important maturational action on several fetal tissues (see later in the section on the transition to extrauterine life).

Fetal thyroid hormone metabolism is characterized by conversion of T_4 to inactive rT_3 and to inactive sulfated iodothyronines and by limited receptor and postreceptor responsiveness to thyroid hormone in selected tissues.[178, 187] The placenta contains an iodothyronine inner ring monodeiodinase that catalyzes conversion of maternal T_4 to rT_3.[178, 179, 188] In addition, the fetal sheep liver and kidney, in contrast to the adult liver and kidney, manifest little or no iodothyronine outer ring monodeiodinase activity so that there is limited conversion of T_4 to active T_3 and accumulation of large amounts of inactive iodothyronine sulfoconjugates.[178, 179, 188] As a consequence, plasma T_3 levels in the fetus remain low until the last few weeks of gestation (see Fig. 28–5). Selected fetal tissues (brain, brown adipose tissue) have active iodothyronine outer ring monodeiodinase activities that contribute to local tissue T_3 concentrations; local T_3 is important in development, particularly in the hypothyroid fetus.[178, 193, 294, 295] Near term and in the neonatal period in the human fetus, the dramatic increase in plasma T_3 levels and presumably in T_3 production heralds the onset of thyroid hormone actions on growth and development and on metabolism.

Receptor or Postreceptor Immaturity

Selected human fetal tissues seem relatively unresponsive to thyroid hormones. Fetal ovine liver and kidney thermogenesis (as evidenced by oxygen consumption, Na^+,K^+-ATPase activity, and mitochondrial α-glycerophosphate activity) is also unresponsive to exogenous T_3 during the third trimester.[189, 190] Moreover thyroid hormone responsiveness in a number of tissues (cardiac, hepatic, renal, and skin) develops only during the perinatal period; β-adrenergic–receptor binding in heart and lung of the ovine fetus is unresponsive to T_3 late in the third trimester but increases in response to T_3 in the neonatal period.[296] Rat pituitary GH concentrations become responsive to thyroid hormone only during the first weeks of extrauterine life.[297] Mouse submandibular gland EGF and NGF levels become responsive to thyroid hormone during the second week of life,[298, 299] as do urine and kidney EGF concentrations[299] and hepatic EGF receptor levels.[300] Mouse skin EGF levels and EGF receptors are responsive during the first neonatal week.[301, 302] Thus despite the presence of nuclear T_3 receptors in significant concentrations in developing rat and sheep, many thyroid hormone actions in these species are delayed.[190, 303] The mechanism of this delayed thyroid hormone responsiveness is not clear; suppressor nuclear proteins may block gene expression in response to thyroid hormones during fetal development, and the levels of these suppressor proteins may determine the onset and degree of action of thyroid hormones during development.[303a]

The effect of the high circulating concentrations of GH in the fetus is also limited. Fetal somatic growth is only partially GH dependent; indeed the GH-deficient fetus has little or no growth retardation.[118] The paucity of fetal GH effects is likely due to delayed maturation of GH receptors or postreceptor mechanisms. In animals such as sheep, hepatic GH receptor binding appears only during the neonatal period.[118, 137, 138] Receptor deficiency may also be a factor in the limited PRL bioactivity in the fetus near term.[137, 138]

There is less information on fetal hormone responsiveness in other systems. β-Adrenergic–receptor binding in heart and lung of the sheep fetus is relatively low near term and, as indicated earlier, increases in the neonatal period in response to thyroid hormones.[296] Moreover premature lambs have an augmented plasma catecholamine surge at birth but have a relatively mild increase in plasma free fatty acid levels, which suggests reduced catecholamine responsiveness.[304] The high levels of progesterone and estrogens in fetal blood also seem to have limited effects in the fetus. Progesterone receptors are present in low concentration in fetal guinea pig kidney, lung, and uterus at midgestation and increase progressively until term.[305] Immunohistochemically, estrogen receptors appear in neonatal rat uterus, oviduct, cervix, and vagina during the first 10 d of extrauterine life.[306] The human neonate often manifests mild breast enlargement at birth, and vaginal estrogenation may be evident in female infants at birth. Estrogen effects otherwise appear limited.

FETAL GROWTH

Somatomedins

During the first decade of postnatal life, growth and development are largely programmed by pituitary hGH and thyroid hormones. Somatic growth is mediated by the somatomedins (IGF-I and IGF-II), molecules of approximately 7 kd and 43 and 41% homologies, respectively, with insulin. Unlike most hormones the somatomedins are synthesized in many tissues and act via ubiquitous (types I and II) receptors.[135, 136] The somatomedins are active via autocrine and paracrine as well as endocrine routes. The liver is a major source of circulating IGF-I, but other tissues contribute to circulating somatomedin levels as well.

The somatomedins circulate bound to high-molecular-weight carrier proteins, which prolong the plasma half-life and provide a reservoir of circulating peptide available for target tissues.[135, 136] The carrier proteins also may be essential for somatomedin actions by facilitating delivery to receptors.[136] The type I receptor for IGF is a 300-kd heterotetramer composed of two 135-kd α subunits and two 90-kd β subunits. The β subunit is a tyrosine kinase that is autophosphorylated subsequent to IGF-I binding. The type II receptor is a single chain 250-kd protein without tyrosine kinase activity. The type I receptor binds IGF-II and, with lower affinity, insulin, and it probably mediates the mitogenic responses to these molecules. Insulin-like actions of the somatomedins are mediated by insulin receptors. Amino acid uptake is stimulated by IGF-I or

insulin acting via both somatomedin type I and insulin receptors. The postnatal function of type II receptors is not clear.[135]

GH and nutritional status are the primary regulators of postnatal somatomedin production. GH receptors in liver and in most tissues can modulate IGF-I mRNA levels. In adult rats GH has little effect on hepatic or pancreatic IGF-II mRNA levels but important effects on brain tissue. The negative-feedback effect of IGF-I on GH production is mediated by a direct action on pituitary GH mRNA synthesis and by increased hypothalamic somatostatin release.[135, 136] Food deprivation decreases tissue IGF-I mRNA levels; both dietary energy and protein appear to be involved. Thyroid hormones increase circulating somatomedin levels, predominantly via enhancement of pituitary GH production. Actions of estrogens and androgens on somatomedin levels also appear to be mediated via effects on GH production. Glucocorticoids inhibit the growth-promoting actions of somatomedins at the postreceptor tissue level.[135]

The somatomedins probably play an important role in the regulation of uterine and placental growth during pregnancy and in early embryonic and fetal development. IGF-I, EGF, and estrogens are mitogens for endometrial stromal cells, and the endometrial contents of IGF-I and IGF-I mRNA are high at implantation and during early embryogenesis in the sow.[307] Uterine IGF-I and IGF-I mRNA levels decrease progressively with advancing gestation.[307] Placental tissue also contains IGF-I and IGF-II mRNAs, significant concentrations of the respective proteins, and IGF-I receptors.[80, 81] Autocrine and paracrine roles for the IGFs in uterine and placental tissues are postulated. IGF-I and insulin are produced by embryonic tissues during the prepancreatic stage of mouse development, and both factors stimulate growth of embryonic mouse cells.[308]

Immunoreactive IGF-I is present in most fetal tissues, and fetal growth is regulated by the somatomedins.[311–315] Transgenic mice with null mutations of IGF-I, IGF-II, and IGF-I receptor have reduced birth weights, organ hypoplasia, and delayed bone development.[313–315] Animals deficient in IGF-I receptor and some mice deficient in IGF-I die at birth; mice deficient in IGF-II survive and have near-normal postnatal growth, whereas surviving IGF-I–deficient animals have deficient postnatal growth.[313, 315] IGF-II deficiency impairs placental growth, whereas IGF-I deficiency does not.[315]

IGF-I and IGF-II mRNAs are localized in mesenchymal and fibroblast-like cells in interstitial and perivascular connective tissues and surrounding capsular tissues.[311] In addition, immunoreactive IGF-I is produced by in vitro explant cultures of fetal mouse tissues, and fibroblasts cultured from fetal rat lung and skin synthesize both IGFs.[312, 316] These findings are consistent with a predominantly paracrine mode of action for these growth factors in the fetus.[309]

Somatomedin-binding proteins are present as early as 5 wk of gestation, and prenatally, as postnatally, somatomedins circulate associated with binding proteins.[136, 309] Thus during fetal and postnatal life, plasma concentrations of somatomedins are relatively high compared with tissue concentrations. In the fetus, IGF-II levels are higher than those of IGF-I, in contrast to these levels in children and adults (see Fig. 28–3). Fetal levels of both peptides at term are 30 to 50% of adult levels. In most studies cord blood IGF-I concentrations correlate with birth size.[309, 317] In the rat IGF-II concentrations are elevated in fetal plasma relative to maternal serum, and levels fall to adult values during the early weeks of postnatal life; IGF-I levels are low and increase postnatally.[318] Somatomedin receptors have been identified as early as 5 wk of gestation and are widespread in fetal tissues.[309, 319, 320] IGF-I stimulates glycogenesis in cultured fetal rat hepatocytes and induces formation of myotubes in cultured myoblasts.[309, 321] IGF-II is active in cultured muscle and neonatal rat astroglial cells.[309, 320] Insulin receptors are increased in fetal cells and are resistant to down-regulation[292]; there are no similar data available for the IGF-I receptor.

As discussed earlier GH receptors are relatively deficient, and receptors for hPL predominate in fetal tissues.[137, 138] Moreover hPL stimulates IGF-I production and augments amino acid transport and DNA synthesis in human fetal fibroblasts and muscle cells.[137, 138] In addition, nutrition influences somatomedins in developing mammals. IGF-I levels fall in suckling rats deprived of milk,[309] and IGF-I and IGF-II levels are reduced in fetuses of protein-starved pregnant rats and placentally restricted sheep.[139, 322] hPL reverses the low IGF-II levels in the protein-starved rats.[322] There is no evidence that thyroid hormones modulate GH or somatomedin levels in the mammalian fetus but, as mentioned earlier, glucocorticoids can inhibit fetal growth, presumably by inhibiting somatomedin action.[160]

These data support the view that the somatomedins are important in embryonic and fetal growth and that they are regulated, at least in part, in the fetus by hPL and by nutritional substrate derived transplacentally. The high levels of IGF-II in fetal rat serum, the high levels of IGF-II mRNA in fetal tissues, and the presence of a truncated form of IGF-I in human fetal brain tissue suggest unique developmental actions of these peptides.[309, 318, 323]

Insulin

Insulin has been proposed to act as a fetal growth factor. Infants born to women with diabetes mellitus may have hyperinsulinemia associated with increased birth weight.[324] Most of this increased weight is accounted for by body fat; there is little increase in body length, but some organomegaly may occur. Infants with hyperinsulinemia caused by nesidioblastosis or the Beckwith-Wiedemann syndrome may also have increased somatic growth in utero. Conversely the human fetus with pancreatic agenesis is small and has decreased muscle bulk and little or no adipose tissue.[324] Homozygosity for a null mutation of the insulin receptor gene in fetal mice leads to early neonatal death with hyperglycemia and ketonemia; the pups, however, manifest normal birth weight.[325] Similar homozygosity in the human fetus results in leprechaunism associated with intrauterine growth retardation, lack of subcutaneous fat, decreased muscle mass, hirsutism, and death during infancy.[326] These and other studies suggest that insulin may act as a fetal growth factor by promoting growth or hypertrophy of selected tissues. In clinical conditions associated with fetal hyperinsulinemia, insulin may act via insulin receptors (in adipose and liver tissues) or via type I IGF-I receptors. Insulin may also have a role in regulating IGF-I release.[324]

Epidermal Growth Factor–Transforming Growth Factor α System

The EGF–TGF α system has been characterized in considerable detail.[327–330] EGF is a 6-kd peptide product of a large 1207-amino-acid precursor molecule and acts via a 170-kd membrane receptor glycoprotein.[329] This receptor, like the somatomedin receptor, has intrinsic tyrosine kinase activity, and tyrosine kinase–mediated autophosphorylation is a critical event in EGF signal transduction. TGF α, which has 35% amino acid homology with murine EGF and 44% homology with human EGF, also acts via the EGF receptor system.[327, 328] Several additional family members have been characterized, including amphiregulin, heparin-binding EGF, cripto, betacellulin and neuregulins.[328, 329] Three additional receptors are referred to as human EGF receptors (HER) 2, 3, and 4.[328, 330] All were characterized in malignant tissues, where they function as oncogenes, and all are widely distributed in normal mammalian tissues.

EGF is a potent mitogen for ectodermal and mesodermal cells in tissue and organ culture.[327, 330] These cells include keratinocytes derived from skin and conjunctival and pharyngeal tissues, corneal endothelial cells, vascular smooth muscle cells, chondrocytes, fibroblasts, liver cells, thyroid follicular cells, granulosa cells, and mammary gland cells. In adult humans EGF is present in highest concentrations in sweat glands, salivary glands, Brunner's (duodenal) glands, stomach, pancreas, bone marrow, prostate, kidney, and endocrine glands (pituitary, adrenal, and thyroid). High concentrations of EGF are also present in urine.[327]

The roles of EGF and TGF α in humans are incompletely understood. In rodents and sheep, EGF provokes precocious eyelid opening and tooth eruption in neonatal animals; stimulates lung maturation; promotes palatal development in organ culture; stimulates gastrointestinal maturation; evokes secretion of pituitary hormones, including GH, PRL, and corticotropin; and stimulates secretion of chorionic gonadotropin and placental lactogen by the placenta.[243, 327] Both EGF and TGF α compete for binding to the EGF receptor, and both factors accelerate eye opening and tooth eruption in the neonatal rodent, presumably via interaction with the same "EGF" receptor.[327] Moreover either TGF α or EGF in combination with TGF β stimulates proliferation of rat kidney cells in agar.[331]

EGF and pre-pro-EGF mRNA are present in most tissues in the postnatal rodent.[332] EGF and EGF mRNA are present in most adult mouse tissues, but mRNA levels are highest in salivary glands and kidneys.[332] EGF and pre-pro-EGF mRNA levels are absent or low in the fetal rodent, and levels remain low in mouse tissues during the early neonatal period.[327] Tissue concentrations of both EGF and EGF mRNA increase in the mouse during the first 2 mo of postnatal life; indeed levels of EGF in the salivary glands increase several thousand–fold between 3 wk and 3 mo of age. Mouse urine levels increase 200-fold, and kidney concentrations increase 10-fold between 1 wk and 2 mo of age. EGF concentrations in mouse ocular tissues increase 100-fold during the first week of life.[327] Liver EGF concentrations increase more slowly, as do serum levels, and there is a high degree of correlation between serum and liver EGF levels in the developing mouse.[327, 333] Thus the production of EGF in the rodent is accelerated during the early neonatal period, and it is during this time that most hormone-stimulated growth and development occur.

There are few data on tissue TGF α concentrations in developing mammals.[327, 334] Immunoreactive TGF α concentrations are measurable at relatively high levels in lung and brain tissues at 20 d of gestation in the rat and show minimal changes through day 50 postnatally.[334] Liver, which also has high TGF α levels at 20 d of gestation, shows a progressive reduction in TGF α concentrations postnatally to nadir values in the young adult. Kidney tissue has low concentrations of TGF α in late gestation, and levels increase progressively during the first 2 mo of postnatal life. Thus the ontogenic pattern of TGF α is tissue specific; most late fetal tissues studied contain TGF α, and levels persist or increase in most tissues through the period of growth and development.[334]

EGF plays an important role in pregnancy and fetal development. Maternal salivary gland and plasma EGF concentrations in the mouse increase four- to fivefold during pregnancy.[335] Removal of the salivary glands prevents the increase in plasma EGF; moreover salivary gland removal reduces the number of mice completing term pregnancy (by 50%), decreases the percent of live pups, and decreases the crown-rump length of fetuses delivered.[335] Administration of EGF antiserum to pregnant mice without salivary glands further increases the abortion rate, whereas administration of EGF improves pregnancy outcome.[335] These observations suggest an important role of EGF in pregnancy in the mouse. Maternal EGF is too large a molecule to traverse the placental barrier so that an effect on maternal metabolism and an effect on the placenta are likely.[335] The placenta is richly endowed with EGF receptors, and placental tissue binds and degrades EGF to constituent amino acids.[243, 327]

EGF receptors are present in embryonal and fetal tissues, and EGF stimulates protein synthesis during the morula-blastocyst transition and in postimplantation mouse embryo tissue.[243, 327] In vitro EGF stimulates differentiation of the inner cell mass during early embryonic development.[336] However, EGF and EGF precursor mRNA levels are absent or present at low levels in selected fetal mouse tissues.[327] Low levels are also present in submandibular gland and kidney during the early neonatal period.[327] Fetal mouse and human tissues have high levels of TGF α, suggesting that this factor may be the ligand for the fetal EGF receptor.[87, 337] TGF α is produced by the maternal decidua during the first half of gestation in rodents, and pro-TGF α mRNA is present in decidua.[87] Decidual pro-TGF α mRNA levels peak at 8 d of gestation (term = 21 d) and decline through day 15, when the decidua is being absorbed. EGF receptors are present in decidua, and TGF α may stimulate proliferation of decidual tissue and enhance decidual PRL production.[87]

Inactivation of the gene encoding the EGF receptor in mice leads to fetal or neonatal death of homozygous fetuses.[338] The receptor-deficient animals manifest impaired epithelial development in several organs, including skin, lungs, and gastrointestinal tract.[338] Thorburn and co-workers[339] observed that the intravenous infusion of recombinant human EGF to the ovine fetus for 3 to 14 d produced skin hypertrophy and increased liver, kidney, adrenal, and thyroid weights; thymus gland weight was decreased. As indicated earlier, EGF receptors are present in a variety of fetal tissues, but it is not clear whether EGF or TGF α, or both, are produced by the ovine fetus. Freemark and Comer[88] reported the presence of TGF α–like transforming bioactivity in ovine fetal kidney and high-affinity EGF receptors in ovine fetal liver. These authors were unable to identify EGF in fetal kidney extracts and suggested that TGF α may play a role in ovine fetal development. Further evidence for a role of EGF in early mammalian development comes from studies of the effect of the administration of EGF antiserum to neonatal mice—namely to delayed eye and ear opening, delayed tooth eruption, accelerated hair growth, and reduced weight gain during the first 30 d of life.[340]

The factors that control EGF and TGF α production are incompletely understood. The increases in EGF concentration in tissues, blood, and urine of the neonatal rodent correlate with and may be conditioned by the increases in thyroid and gonadal hormone levels.[327] EGF concentrations in the mouse submandibular gland are increased by thyroid hormones and testosterone. Thyroid hormones increase EGF concentrations in skin, ocular tissue, kidney, and urine in the developing mouse and up-regulate EGF gene expression and the production of pro-EGF in rat kidney; thyroid hormones also increase EGF receptor levels in developing mouse skin and liver.[300, 302, 327, 341] GH increases urine EGF concentrations in the neonatal mouse, and estrogens increase EGF and EGF mRNA levels in mouse uterus.[327, 342] Testosterone stimulates EGF and EGF mRNA levels in submandibular gland and increases EGF receptor levels in prostatic tissue.[343, 344] Thus EGF may mediate growth and developmental actions of a variety of hormones in selected tissues. There is little information about the regulation of TGF α production postnatally or prenatally. Amphiregulin binds to and stimulates EGF receptor and HER2 in human epithelial cells and has been localized to breast and colonic epithelium.[345] Transgenic mice with a deficiency of neuregulin, HER2, or HER4 die in midgestation with aborted development of myocardial trabecular and nervous system anomalies.[330]

Considerable evidence suggests a role for the EGF family of growth factors in mammalian central nervous system development.[327, 346–350] EGF, TGF α, neuregulins, EGF receptor, HER2, and HER4 are widely distributed in the nervous system.[327, 345–349] EGF promotes cell proliferation of astroglial cells, acts as an astroglial differentiation factor, and enhances survival and outgrowth of selected neuronal cells.[346, 347] Mice lacking neuregulin, HER2, or HER4 die in utero with cardiac anomalies and developmental anomalies of the hindbrain, midbrain, and ventral forebrain.[330, 348, 349] The HER3 receptor also is widely distributed, but its role remains unclear.

Nerve Growth Factor

NGF is a 13-kd protein that is present at high concentrations in mouse salivary gland and at low concentrations in many adult tissues.[328, 351] It also is produced by human placental tissue.[81, 82] NGF is the original member of an expanding family of neurotropic growth factors now including brain-derived neurotropic factor, neurotropin 3, and two less well characterized factors and involving two receptors, NGF and NGF2 (or Trk).[328, 351–354] NGF binds to high-affinity plasma membrane receptors and is internalized and transported to subcellular organelles, including the nucleus, in neurons of the peripheral nervous system.[328, 351] It promotes neurite outgrowth and enhances tryosine hydroxylase and dopamine β-hydroxylase activities in developing sympathetic neurons. It acts on undifferentiated sympathetic cell precursors to evoke both hyperplastic and hypertrophic effects[243, 328, 351] and plays a permissive role to stimulate development of immature autonomic neurons along either a sympathetic or a cholinergic pathway.[243]

The injection of neonatal mice with NGF causes a marked increase in the volume of the superior cervical ganglia and increases in RNA polymerase, ornithine decarboxylase, and tyrosine hydroxylase activities. This growth factor also increases the nerve supply of body organs. Likewise, injection of NGF antiserum during early neonatal life results in a decrease in the size of the superior cervical ganglia, reduction in tyrosine hydroxylase activity, and permanent sympathectomy.[243] Maternal NGF autoantibodies in rats and rabbits impair autonomic nervous system development in utero.[352, 355] This impairment affects sympathetic and dorsal root ganglia and autonomic innervation of peripheral organs. NGF is produced by neonatal mouse astroglial cells in tissue culture, is present in developing mouse brain tissue and, with brain-derived neurotropic factor and neurotropin 3, plays an important role in brain development.[353, 354, 356, 357] Thyroid hormones and testosterone modulate postnatal NGF levels in the submandibular gland of the mouse. Thyroid hormones increase NGF, neurotropin 3, and brain-derived neurotropic factor mRNA levels in adult rat brain.[358]

Other Factors

Additional growth factors are involved in fetal growth and development, including hematopoietic growth factors, fibroblast growth factors, platelet-derived growth factors, and members of the TGF β family.[328] Hematopoietic growth factors are also active in the fetus during development[359]; erythropoietin (EP) in the fetal sheep is produced by the liver rather than the kidney; a switch to kidney production occurs after parturition.[360] Postnatally thyroid hormones, testosterone, and hypoxia modulate EP production. Although thyroid hormones have little effect on fetal hepatic EP production, their administration to the fetus accelerates the switch to kidney EP production.[360] It is not known whether factors other than hypoxia modulate fetal EP production.

Basic fibroblast growth factor may play a role in the

growth and differentiation of endodermal and mesodermal tissues of mammalian embryos. Infusion of recombinant fibroblast growth factor into the renal artery of kidneys containing a subcapsular transplant of a 10-day-old rat embryo stimulated growth of the embryo.[361] Antiserum to fibroblast growth factor retards the growth of all tissues of endodermal origin and some of mesodermal origin.[361] Fibroblast growth factor, like EGF, stimulates the production of hCG from a choriocarcinoma cell line.[361] These observations and the fact that the placenta contains fibroblast growth factor, NGF, TGF α and β, IGF-I, and IGF-II suggest that the placenta may play a critical role in modulating fetal growth.[80-95]

TRANSITION TO EXTRAUTERINE LIFE

The transition to extrauterine life involves abrupt delivery from the protected intrauterine environment and succor by the placenta to the relatively hostile extrauterine environment. The neonate must initiate air breathing and defend against hypothermia, hypoglycemia, and hypocalcemia as the placental supply of energy and nutritional substrate is removed. Both the adrenal cortex and the autonomic nervous system, including the para-aortic chromaffin system, are essential for extrauterine adaptation. Longer term transition requires adaptation to an environment of intermittent nutrient supply and transient substrate deficiency and requires maturation of the secretory control mechanisms for the PTH-calcitonin system and the endocrine pancreas.

Cortisol Surge

In most mammals a cortisol surge occurs near term and is mediated by increased cortisol production by the fetal adrenal and a decreased rate of conversion of cortisol to cortisone (see Fig. 28–4). Pepe and Albrecht have proposed that the preterm fetal cortisol surge is due to the progressive stimulation by estrogens of placental 11β-HSD activity and the subsequent increase in placental conversion of cortisol to cortisone.[36] The resulting decrease in maternal-to-fetal cortisol transfer results in stimulation of fetal CRH and corticotropin secretion via the negative-feedback control loop. The concomitant estrogen-stimulated increase in 11β-HSD activity in fetal tissues potentiates the relative fetal cortisol deficiency and the CRH-corticotropin response.[36] Placental CRH also may potentiate the fetal adrenal activation.[36]

The cortisol surge augments surfactant synthesis in lung tissue; increases lung liquid reabsorption; increases adrenomedullary phenylethanolamine N-methyltransferase activity, which in turn increases methylation of NE to epinephrine; increases hepatic iodothyronine outer ring monodeiodinase activity and hence increases conversion of T_4 to T_3; decreases sensitivity of the ductus arteriosus to prostaglandins, which facilitates ductus closure; induces maturation of several enzymes and transport processes of the small intestine; and stimulates maturation of hepatic enzymes.[140, 161, 163, 164, 362] In some cases these events involve increased synthesis of specific proteins or enzymes. In other instances, such as the action on the ductus arteriosus, the mechanism remains obscure. These effects are summarized in Figure 28–10. Secondary effects of cortisol also promote extrauterine adaptations. The increased

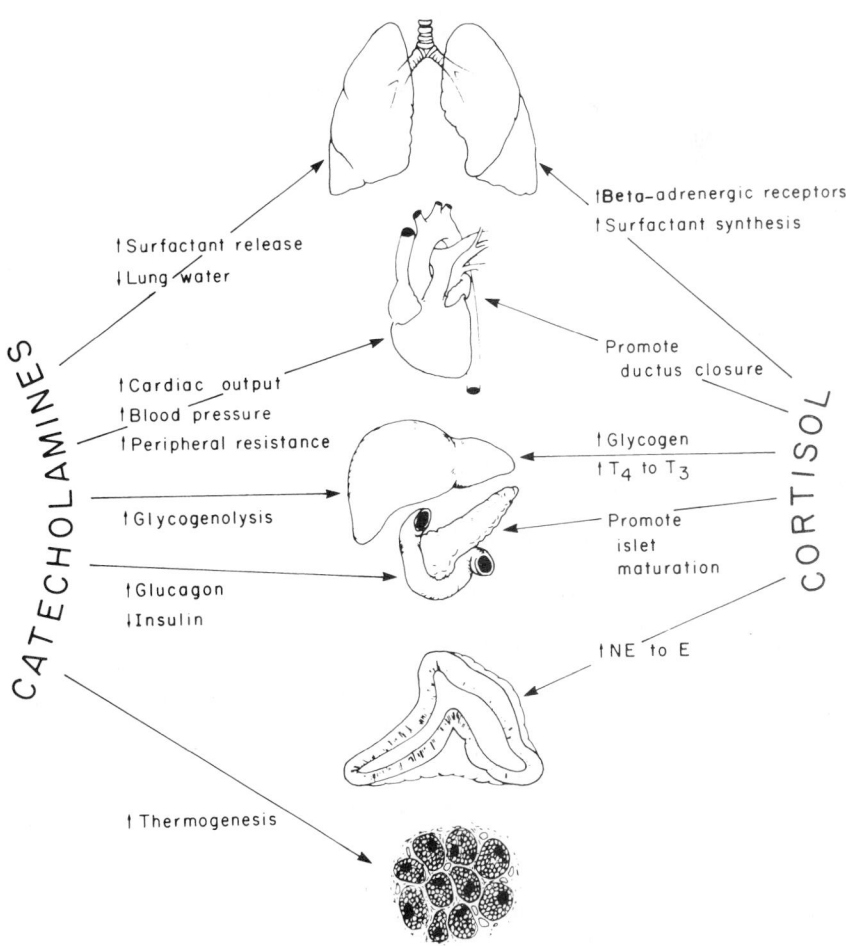

Figure 28–10. Actions of cortisol and catecholamines during fetal adaptation to the extrauterine environment. The prenatal cortisol surge acts to promote functional maturation of several organ systems as indicated. The neonatal catecholamine surge triggers or potentiates a number of the extrauterine cardiopulmonary and metabolic functional adaptations that are critical to extrauterine survival. See text for details.

T_3 levels stimulate β-adrenergic–receptor binding and potentiate surfactant synthesis in lung tissue and increase the sensitivity of brown adipose tissue to NE. The significance of prenatal cortisol is demonstrated by the effects of gene-targeted CRH or glucocorticoid receptor deficiency in mice; the progeny of homozygous CRH or glucocorticoid receptor–deficient animals die in the first 12 h with lung dysplasia and surfactant deficiency.[363, 364]

Catecholamine Surge

Parturition also evokes a dramatic catecholamine surge in the newborn, resulting in extraordinarily high levels of NE, epinephrine, and dopamine in cord blood.[365] As indicated earlier, plasma NE concentrations exceed epinephrine levels because of peripheral and adrenomedullary and para-aortic catecholamine release. Cord blood NE levels of 15 nmol/L (2500 pg/mL) and epinephrine levels of 2 nmol/L (370 pg/mL) are common after spontaneous delivery of term infants.[365] Levels of 25 nmol/L (4200 pg/mL) of NE and 35 nmol/L (640 pg/mL) of epinephrine are common in cord blood of premature infants.[258] These changes evoke critical cardiovascular adaptations, including increased blood pressure and increased cardiac inotropic effects; increased glucagon secretion; decreased insulin secretion; increased thermogenesis in brown adipose tissue and increased plasma free fatty acid levels; and pulmonary adaptation, including mobilization of pulmonary fluid and increased surfactant release.[249, 250, 362, 365] These events are summarized in Figure 28–10.

Thermogenesis in Neonatal Brown Adipose Tissue

Brown adipose tissue is the major site for thermogenesis in the newborn and is especially prominent in the mammalian fetus. The largest accumulations of brown adipose tissue envelop the kidneys and adrenal glands, and smaller amounts surround the blood vessels of the mediastinum and neck.[366] The mass of brown adipose tissue peaks at the time of birth and gradually decreases during the early weeks of life. Surgical removal of this tissue leads to neonatal hypothermia. NE, via β-adrenergic receptors, stimulates thermogenesis by brown adipose tissue, and optimal responsiveness of this tissue to NE is thyroid hormone dependent.[367] Brown adipose tissue is rich in mitochondria containing a unique 32-kd uncoupling protein (thermogenin) that uncouples oxidation and phosphorylation of adenosine diphosphate to adenosine triphosphate and consequently enhances thermogenesis.[366] Thermogenin is T_3 dependent, and brown adipose tissue contains a 5′-monoiodothyronine deiodinase that synthesizes T_3 locally from T_4.[368] Full maturation of catecholamine-stimulated cellular respiration in brown adipose tissue occurs before delivery in the ovine fetus and requires thyroid hormone.[369–371] Fetal thyroidectomy in this species leads to marked hypothermia, with low plasma free fatty acid levels and increased plasma epinephrine concentrations.[370] In vitro basal brown adipose tissue thermogenesis and NE and dibutyryl cAMP-stimulated thermogenesis are decreased by fetal thyroidectomy.[370] The rapid onset of thermogenesis in brown adipose tissue is essential for survival in newborn infants. Catecholamine release is the stimulus for brown adipose tissue thermogenesis in the early neonatal period, and responsiveness to catecholamines is markedly increased by cutting of the umbilical cord.[367] Fetal hypoxia and placental inhibitors, including prostaglandin E_2 and adenosine, appear to inhibit brown adipose tissue thermogenesis in utero.[367] Cord cutting, neonatal cooling, catecholamine stimulation, and augmented T_4 to T_3 conversion in brown adipose tissue in the neonatal period are the essential features that mediate and condition newborn thermogenesis.

Calcium Homeostasis

The neonate must adjust rapidly from a high-calcium environment regulated by PTHrP and calcitonin to a low-calcium environment that requires regulation by PTH and vitamin D. With removal of the placenta in term infants, plasma total calcium concentration falls and reaches a nadir of approximately 2.3 mmol/L (9 mg/dL),[262, 263, 364] and the ionized calcium concentration reaches a low level of about 1.2 mmol/L (4.8 mg/dL) by 24 h of life.[372] Plasma PTH levels are relatively low in the neonatal period and are minimally responsive to hypocalcemia during the first 2 to 3 d of life.[373] Calcitonin concentrations are high in cord blood (about 2000 ng/L), increase further during the early neonatal period, and remain high for several days after birth.[262, 263, 374] The relatively obtunded PTH response and the high calcitonin levels lead to a 2- to 3-d period of transient neonatal hypocalcemia.[374, 375] Inhibition of calcitonin secretion and stimulation of PTH secretion gradually result in increased serum calcium levels in the neonate. The disappearance of PTHrP in the neonatal lamb is approximately coincident with the time of restoration of calcium levels to the adult range.[263] The mechanism for the transition from PTHrP to PTH secretion by the neonatal parathyroid glands is not clear.

Calcium homeostasis is also affected in the human newborn period by the low level of glomerular filtration that persists for several days.[262] In addition, renal responsiveness to PTH is reduced in the first few days of life.[262] These factors limit phosphate excretion and predispose the neonate to hyperphosphatemia, particularly if the diet includes high-phosphate milk such as unmodified cow's milk. Premature infants tend to have lower PTH and higher calcitonin levels and more immature kidney function; in these infants neonatal hypocalcemia may be more marked and prolonged, and the incidence of symptomatic hypocalcemia is higher. Birth asphyxia also predisposes the neonate to hypocalcemia.[262, 375] Infants born to mothers with hypercalcemia due to hyperparathyroidism have a high incidence of sympatomatic hypocalcemia. These infants have a more marked suppression of parathyroid function and a longer period of transient hypoparathyroidism in the neonatal period. PTH secretion and calcium homeostasis usually return to normal in 1 to 2 wk in full-term infants and within 2 to 3 wk in the small premature infant.

Glucose Homeostasis

The abrupt withdrawal of the placental glucose supply leads to a prompt fall in plasma glucose in the term neonate.[282, 283, 376] The low glucose and high catecholamine levels stimulate glucagon secretion, and the plasma glucagon level peaks within 2 h after birth.[282, 283, 362, 376] Plasma insulin levels are low at birth and tend to fall further with hypoglycemia. The early glucagon response is short-lived; however, levels remain in the 100 ng/L range for the first 12 to 24 h, and the glucagon/insulin ratio is high enough to stabilize glucose levels in the 2.8 to 4 mmol/L (50 to 70 mg/dL) range during this period. The early glucagon and catecholamine surges deplete hepatic glycogen stores so that return of plasma glucose levels to normal after 12 to 18 h requires maturation of hepatic gluconeogenesis under the stimulus of a high plasma glucagon/insulin ratio.[283, 376] Glucagon secretion gradually increases during the early hours after birth, especially with protein feeding, which stimulates gut glucagon release and pancreatic glucagon secretion.[282, 283, 376] Premature infants have more severe and prolonged hypoglycemia because of reduced glycogen stores and impaired hepatic gluconeogenesis. Infants born to diabetic mothers have more severe neonatal hypoglycemia because of relative hyperinsulinism. In the healthy term infant, glucose homeostasis is achieved within 5 to 7 d of life; in premature infants 1 to 2 wk may be required.

Other Hormonal Adaptations

Changes in other hormone systems are summarized in Figures 28–3 to 28–6. Delivery of the placenta results in decreases in fetal blood levels of estrogens, progesterone, hCG, and hPL. The fall in estrogen levels (see Fig. 28–6) presumably removes the major stimulus to fetal PRL release, and PRL levels decrease within several weeks (see Fig. 28–3). The relatively delayed rate of fall may be due to lactotrope hyperplasia in the fetal pituitary or to delayed maturation of hypothalamic dopamine secretion. The gradual fall of hGH levels during the early weeks of life is due to delayed maturation of hypothalamic-pituitary and feedback control of hGH release.[118, 134] In the neonatal primate there are concomitant decreases in plasma GH levels and GH responsiveness to exogenous GHRH.[377] The mechanisms remain unclear. Changes in secretion or in pituitary sensitivity to GHRH or somatostatin, or both, may be involved. Somatomedin levels fall to infantile values within a few days, presumably because of the removal of placental hPL and placental somatomedin production (see Fig. 28–3).

In male infants (see Fig. 28–6) after a transient fall in testosterone levels as the hCG stimulus abates, pituitary LH secretion rebounds and there is a secondary surge of plasma testosterone that persists at significant levels for several weeks.[378] This surge is mediated by hypothalamic LHRH, and blockade of neonatal activation of the pituitary-testicular axis with an LHRH agonist in neonatal monkeys ablates the neonatal increments in LH and testosterone.[379] Such a blockade also results in subnormal increments in plasma LH and testosterone levels and subnormal testicular enlargement at puberty in these animals, which suggests that neonatal LHRH release with pituitary-testicular activation may be critical for normal sexual maturation of male primates.[379] In females a transient, secondary surge in follicle-stimulating hormone may transiently elevate estrogen levels.

Delivery results in a reversal of the high fetal cortisone/cortisol ratio, and plasma cortisol concentrations are higher in the neonate despite relatively lower plasma corticotropin concentrations (see Fig. 28–4). Presumably this increase is due to decreased inhibition of adrenal 3β-HSD by estrogen[140, 144] and perhaps to removal of a placental CRH action on fetal pituitary corticotropin release. Plasma DHEAS and DHEA levels fall as the fetal adrenal atrophies (see Fig. 28–4).

The increase in serum thyrotropin levels during the early minutes after birth is due to cooling of the neonate in the extrauterine environment.[179, 180] The thyrotropin surge peaks at 30 min at concentrations approximating 70 mU/L (see Fig. 28–5). This peak evokes increased secretion of T_4 and T_3 by the thyroid. In addition, increased conversion of T_4 to T_3 by liver and other tissues maintains the T_3 level in the extrauterine range of 1.6 to 3.4 nmol/L (105 to 220 ng/dL) (see Fig. 28–5).[179, 180] The re-equilibration of thyrotropin levels to the normal extrauterine range is probably due to the readjustment of prevailing serum T_3 levels and to maturation of feedback control of thyrotropin by thyroid hormones during the early weeks of life. rT_3 production by fetal and neonatal tissues abates by 3 to 4 wk of age at which time serum rT_3 reaches adult levels.

IMPRINTING OF DEVELOPING ENDOCRINE SYSTEMS

Data in several mammalian species indicate that hormonal imprinting occurs during a critical, usually perinatal, period of development. In the female rodent, transient neonatal androgen administration masculinizes the pattern of hypothalamic control of LHRH secretion and pituitary gonadotropin secretion, masculinizes adult behavior and adult sexual activity, permanently alters the pattern of GH secretion, increases longitudinal bone growth and body weight, and masculinizes the pattern of hepatic steroid metabolism.[380-383] Estrogen administration to pregnant rats during the last third of gestation produces cryptorchid male offspring and may permanently suppress spermatogenesis in adult males.[384] Perinatal estrogen administration to the developing female rodent produces long-term effects, including persistent vaginal cornification, hyperplastic vaginal lesions, and cervicovaginal cancer; synthetic nonsteroidal estrogen (diethylstilbestrol) has similar effects.[385] Chronic hyperprolactinemia also occurs, presumably secondary to the low-level continuous estrogen secretion in these anovulatory animals.[385] Female rats given a single neonatal dose of estradiol or diethylstilbestrol manifest decreased uterine estradiol receptor binding as adults, and neonatal administration of dexamethasone causes decreased glucocorticoid binding in adult thymus tissue.[386, 387]

Transient levothyroxine administration to neonatal rodents leads to growth retardation, delayed puberty, decreased adult pituitary weight, decreased pituitary TRH concentrations, low serum thyrotropin levels, and decreased thyrotropin responsiveness to propylthiouracil challenge.[388-390] Adult adrenal function and EGF metabolism are also altered.[389, 391] Neonatal administration of insulin or alloxan to rats produces permanent alteration of glucose tolerance,[392, 393] and a single neonatal dose of vasopressin to the neonatal rat permanently enhances adult response to vasopressin.[394] Neonatal catecholamine administration alters the response of adult rat vascular tissue to NE.[386] Fetal exposure to high maternal glucocorticoid levels in the rat inhibits fetal growth and leads to subsequent hypertension in the offspring.[395]

There is much less information about hormonal imprinting in primates and humans. Blockade of LHRH in neonatal monkeys with an LHRH agonist results in obtundation of plasma LH and testosterone levels and decreased testicular size at puberty.[379] Diethylstilbestrol administration to pregnant women increases the prevalence of vaginal adenocarcinoma in female offspring during the second and third decades of life.[396, 397] Congenital hypothyroidism in human infants may be associated with alteration of the set point for feedback control of thyrotropin release such that serum thyrotropin levels remain inappropriately elevated after return of serum T_4 levels to normal by treatment.[398, 399]

The mechanisms for imprinting remain obscure. Neonatal administration of testosterone can cause permanent effects on brain structure.[382] The effect in some instances may be transmitted to subsequent generations.[388, 392] A functional overlap of hormone-mediated imprinting may also occur; the administration of both thyrotropin and follicle-stimulating hormone to the neonate alters the adult response to thyrotropin, and neonatal OT or vasopressin exposure can alter the adult response to vasopressin.[386, 394] Hormonal imprinting is also demonstrable in cell lines and in unicellular organisms in which a single exposure to a hormone can produce persistent alteration of the hormonal response characteristics.[386] These observations suggest that hormone imprinting is due to hormone receptor plasticity during a critical period of receptor maturation and that exposure to abnormal amounts of ligand during this period somehow alters the adult pattern of hormone receptor expression. Nuclear receptors and plasma membrane receptors may be involved. Plasticity of prohormone processing may also be involved; in newborn rat intermediate pituitary lobe cells, in vitro treatment with dexamethasone decreases production of α-MSH and increases production of corticotropin-related peptides.[400] Whatever the mechanisms, the developing endocrine systems have significant plasticity, and the maturation of endocrine control systems can be influenced by alterations in the prevailing hormone concentrations.

CONCLUSION

The foregoing review summarizes current understanding of the intrauterine endocrine milieu and highlights progress in this challenging frontier of medicine. This progress has set the stage for advances in the management of the infant of the diabetic mother, the infant with disordered sexual differentiation, and neonates with congenital thyroid, parathyroid, or pituitary disease. In addition, important advances in the management of premature labor and abnormalities of fetal growth have resulted. Most therapeutic approaches to intrauterine abnormalities to date have been indirect.

We are now entering a new era of direct access and management of the intrauterine environment, entailing both potential advantages and risks.[401–404] With expansion of the application and scope of amniotic fluid and fetal cell sampling and the advent of fetal visualization and intrauterine fetal blood sampling, direct access to the fetus and diagnosis are now possible.[181, 182, 401] Manipulation of the menstrual cycle, artificial insemination, and in vitro fertilization are routine procedures. Selective embryocide has been used to control induced multiple embryo pregnancy.[405] Women are treated with glucocorticoids or glucocorticoids plus TRH to stimulate fetal lung maturation.[406] There are now many instances of intrauterine diagnosis and treatment of human fetal adrenal and thyroid disorders.[407–410] Intravenous nutritional supplementation of fetal sheep can prevent some forms of growth retardation,[411] and chronic fetal therapy via indwelling pumps is feasible in animal fetuses.[188] These approaches, coupled with increasing availability of synthetic hormones and growth factor agonists and antagonists, will facilitate direct fetal endocrine therapy.

In addition, transplantation of fetal neuroendocrine tissues in rodents can alter neuroendocrine, cognitive, and motor functions of the host. Transplantation of fetal preoptic area tissue restores mating and pregnancy in genetically hypogonadal mice,[412] transplantation of fetal hypothalamic vasopressin-containing neurons corrects diabetes insipidus in adult hosts,[413] and fetal brain grafts improve motor function in adults with Parkinson's disease.[414] Fetal neuroendocrine tissue appears to survive after transplantation to adult rodent hosts, and preliminary studies demonstrate that cryopreserved human fetal brain tissue can be transplanted successfully to primate hosts.[415] The use of fetal tissues for transplantation involves difficult moral and ethical issues, but continuing progress in both technical and ethical areas is inevitable.[416, 417] The next decades will witness continuing expansion of our understanding of the endocrinology and metabolism of the fetus and increasing effectiveness of efforts to diagnose and manage abnormal pregnancies, including direct fetal diagnosis and therapy and the use of fetal tissues in the treatment of adult disease.

REFERENCES

1. Chard T. Proteins of the human placenta: some general concepts. In: Grudzinskas JG, Seppala M (eds): Pregnancy Proteins. New York: Academic Press, 1982: 3–21.
2. Ogren L, Talamantes F. The placenta as an endocrine organ; polypeptides. In: Knobil E, Neill JD (eds): The Physiology of Reproduction. 2nd ed. New York: Raven, 1994: 875–945.
3. Faber JJ, Thornburg KL, Binder ND. Physiology of placental transfer in mammals. Am Zool 1992; 32:343–354.
4. Sibley CP, Boyd RDH. Mechanisms of transfer across the human placenta. In: Polin RA, Fox WW (eds): Fetal and Neonatal Physiology. Philadelphia: WB Saunders, 1992: 62–74.
5. Sodha RJ, Proegler M, Schneider H. Transfer and metabolism of norepinephrine studied from maternal to fetal and fetal to maternal sides in the in vitro perfused human placental life. Am J Obstet Gynecol 1984; 148:474–481.
6. Sandler M, Ruthven CRJ, Contractor SF. Transmission of noradrenaline across the human placenta. Nature 1963; 197:598.
7. Weaver DR, Namboodiri A, Reppert SM. Iodinated melatonin mimics melatonin action and reveals discrete binding sites in fetal brain. FEBS Lett 1988; 228:123–127.
8. Solomon S, Friesen HG. Endocrine relations between mother and fetus. Annu Rev Med 1968; 19:399–430.
9. Smith W, Adams W. Transplacental influence of androgens upon ovulatory mechanisms in the rat. J Endocrinol 1970; 48:477–478.
10. Pepe GJ, Albrecht ED. Transutero placental metabolism of cortisol and cortisone during mid and late gestation in the baboon. Endocrinology 1984; 115:1946–1951.
11. Murphy BEP. Cortisol and cortisone in human fetal development. J Steroid Biochem 1979; 11:509–513.
12. Boyard F, Ances IG, Tapper AJ, et al. Transplacental passage and fetal secretion of aldosterone. J Clin Invest 1970; 49:1389–1392.
13. Ron M, Levitz M, Chuba J, et al. Transfer of 25-hydroxyvitamin D_3 and 1,25-dihydroxyvitamin D_3 across the perfused human placenta. Am J Obstet Gynecol 1984; 148:370–374.
14. Roti E, Gnudi A, Braverman LE. The placental transport, synthesis and metabolism of hormones and drugs which affect thyroid function. Endocr Rev 1983; 4:131–149.
15. Glatz TH, Weitzman RE, Nathanielsz PW, et al. Metabolic clearance rate and transplacental passage of oxytocin in the pregnant ewe and fetus. Endocrinology 1980; 106:1006–1011.
16. Stegner H, Leake RD, Palmer SM, et al. Permeability of the sheep placenta to ^{125}I-arginine vasopressin. Dev Pharmacol Ther 1984; 7:140–144.
17. Sopelak VM, Hodgen GD. Infusion of gonadotropin releasing hormone agonist during pregnancy: maternal and fetal responses in primates. Am J Obstet Gynecol 1987; 156:755–760.
18. Garel JM, Milhaud G, Sizonenko PC. Inactivation de la calcitonine porcine par differents organes foetaux et maternels du rat. C R Acad Sci Paris 1970; 270:2469–2471.
19. Adam PAJ, King KC, Schwartz R, et al. Human placental barrier to ^{125}I-glucagon early in gestation. J Clin Endocrinol Metab 1972; 34:772–782.
20. Sperling MA, Erenberg A, Fiser RH, et al. Placental transfer of glucagon in sheep. Endocrinology 1973; 93:1435–1438.
21. Miyakawa I, Ikeda I, Maeyama M. Transport of ACTH across human placenta. J Clin Endocrinol Metab 1974; 39:440–442.
22. Campbell EA, Linton EA, Wolfe CDA, et al. Plasma corticotropin releasing hormone concentrations during pregnancy and parturition. J Clin Endocrinol Metab 1987; 64:1054–1059.
23. Wolf H, Sabata V, Frerichs H, et al. Evidence for impermeability of the human placenta for insulin. Horm Metab Res 1969; 1:224–227.
24. Balabanova S, Lang T, Wolf AS, et al. Placental transfer of parathyroid hormone. J Perinat Med 1986; 14:243–250.
25. King KC, Adam PAJ, Schwartz R, et al. Human placental transfer of human growth hormone. Pediatrics 1971; 48:534–539.
26. Foster DL, Karsch FJ, Nalbandov AV. Regulation of luteinizing hormone (LH) in the fetal and neonatal lamb. II: Study of placental transfer of LH in the sheep. Endocrinology 1972; 90:589–592.
27. Symonds EM, Furler I. Plasma renin levels in the normal and anephric fetus at birth. Biol Neonate 1973; 23:133–138.
28. Deloot S, VanCamp G, Chatelain A. Absence of placental transfer of atrial natriuretic peptide in the rat: direct experimental evidence. Med Sci Res 1995; 23:347–349.
29. Zanjani ED, Pixley JS, Slotnik N, et al. Erythropoietin does not cross the placenta. Am J Reprod Immunol 1993; 30:136–145.
30. Blay J, Hollenberg MD. The nature and function of the polypeptide growth factor receptors in the human placenta. J Dev Physiol 1989; 12:237–248.
31. Jones CJP, Hartmann M, Desoye G. Ultrastructural localization of insulin receptors in human placenta. Am J Reprod Immunol 1993; 30:136–145.
32. Iisalo E, Castren O. The enzymatic inactivation of noradrenaline in human placental tissue. Ann Med Exp Biol Fenn 1967; 45:253–257.
33. Murphy BEP, Branchaud CL. The fetal adrenal. In: Tulchinsky D, Little AB (eds): Maternal-Fetal Endocrinology. 2nd ed. Philadelphia: WB Saunders, 1994: 276–295.
34. Falcone T, Little AB. Placental synthesis of steroid hormones. In: Tulchinsky D, Little AB (eds): Maternal-Fetal Endocrinology. 2nd ed. Philadelphia: WB Saunders, 1994: 2–14.
35. Albrecht ED, Pepe GJ. Placental steroid hormone biosynthesis in primate pregnancy. Endocr Rev 1990; 11:124–150.
36. Pepe GJ, Albrecht ED. Actions of placental and fetal adrenal steroid hormones in primate pregnancy. Endocr Rev 1995; 16:608–648.
37. Waddell BJ. The placenta as hypothalamus and pituitary: possible impact on maternal and fetal adrenal function. Reprod Fertil Dev 1993; 5:479–497.
37a. Diczfalusy E. Endocrine functions of the human fetoplacental unit. Fed Proc 1964; 23:791–798.

38. Strauss JF III, Gafvels M, King BF. Placental hormones. In: DeGroot LJ, Besser M, Burger HG, et al (eds): Endocrinology. 3rd ed. Philadelphia: WB Saunders, 1995: 2171–2206.

39. Falcone T, Little AB. Placental polypeptides. In: Tulchinsky D, Little AB (eds): Maternal-Fetal Endocrinology. 2nd ed. Philadelphia: WB Saunders, 1994: 15–32.

40. Glinoer D, DeNayer P, Robyn C, et al. Serum levels of intact human chorionic gonadotropin (HCG) and its free αβ subunits in relation to maternal thyroid stimulation during normal pregnancy. J Endocrinol Invest 1993; 16:881–888.

41. Yoshimura M, Hershman JM. Thyrotropic action of human chorionic gonadotropin. Thyroid 1995; 5:425–434.

42. Miller WL, Eberhardt NL. Structure and evolution of the growth hormone gene family. Endocr Rev 1983; 4:97–130.

43. Barsh GS, Seeburg PH, Gelinas RE. The human growth hormone gene family: structure and evolution of the chromosomal locus. Nucleic Acids Res 1983; 11:3939–3985.

44. Walker WH, Fitzpatrick AL, Barrera-Saldana HA, et al. The human placental lactogen genes: structure, function, evolution, and transcriptional regulation. Endocr Rev 1991; 12:316–328.

45. MacLeod JN, Lee AK, Liebhaber A, et al. Developmental control and alternative splicing of the placentally expressed transcripts from the human growth hormone gene cluster. J Biol Chem 1992; 267:14219–14226.

46. Golander A, Hurley T, Barrett J, et al. Prolactin synthesis by human chorion-decidual tissue. A possible source of prolactin in the amniotic fluid. Science 1978; 202:311–313.

47. Jara CS, Salud AT, Bryant-Greenwood GD, et al. Immunocytochemical localization of the human growth hormone variant in the human placenta. J Clin Endocrinol Metab 1989; 69:1069–1072.

48. Grino M, Chrousos GP, Margioris AN. The corticotropin releasing hormone gene is expressed in human placenta. Biochem Biophys Res Commun 1987; 148:1208–1214.

49. Margioris AN, Grino M, Protos P, et al. Corticotropin releasing hormone and oxytocin stimulate the release of placental proopiomelanocortin peptides. J Clin Endocrinol Metab 1988; 66:922–926.

50. Abboud TK. Maternal and fetal β-endorphin: effects of pregnancy and labor. Arch Dis Child 1988; 63:707–709.

51. Qu J, Thomas K. Inhibin and activin production in human placenta. Endocr Rev 1995; 16:485–507.

52. Yamaguchi M, Endo H, Tasaka K, et al. Mouse growth hormone releasing factor secretion is activated by inhibin and inhibited by activin in placenta. Biol Reprod 1995; 16:368–372.

53. Egan DA, Grzegorczyk V, Tricarico KA, et al. Placental chorionic renin: production, purification and characterization. Biochim Biophys Acta 1988; 965:68–75.

54. Ihara Y, Taii S, Mori T. Expression of renin and angiotensinogen genes in the human placental tissues. Endocrinol Jpn 1987; 34:887–896.

55. Millan MA, Carvallo P, Izumi SI, et al. Novel sites of expression of functional angiotensin II receptors in the late gestation fetus. Science 1989; 244:1340–1342.

56. Rodda CP, Kubota M, Heath JA, et al. Evidence for a novel parathyroid hormone–related protein in fetal lamb, parathyroid glands and sheep placenta: comparisons with a similar protein implicated in humoral hypercalcemia of malignancy. J Endocrinol 1988; 117:261–271.

57. Ferguson JE, Gorman JV, Bruns DE, et al. Abundant expression of parathyroid hormone related protein in human amnion and its association with labor. Proc Natl Acad Sci USA 1992; 89:8384–8388.

58. Jousset V, Legendre B, Besnard P, et al. Calcitonin-like immunoreactivity and calcitonin gene expression in the placenta and in the mammary gland of the rat. Acta Endocrinol 1988; 119:443–451.

59. Radovick S, Wondiford FE, Nakayama Y, et al. Isolation and characterization of the human gonadotropin releasing hormone gene in the hypothalamus and placenta. Mol Endocrinol 1990; 4:476–480.

60. Iwashita M, Evans MI, Catt KJ. Characterization of a gonadotropin releasing hormone receptor site in term placenta and chorionic villi. J Clin Endocrinol Metab 1986; 62:127–133.

61. Lin LS, Roberts VJ, Yen SS. Expression of human gonadotropin-releasing hormone receptor gene in the placenta and its functional relationship to human chorionic gonadotropin secretion. J Clin Endocrinol Metab 1995; 80:580–585.

62. Gibbons JM Jr, Mitnick M, Chieffo V. In vitro biosynthesis of TSH and LH releasing factors by the human placenta. Am J Obstet Gynecol 1975; 121:127–131.

63. Shambaugh GD, Kubek M, Wilber JF. Thyrotropin releasing hormone activity in the human placenta. J Clin Endocrinol Metab 1979; 48:483–486.

64. Youngblood WW, Humm J, Lipton MA, et al. Thyrotropin releasing hormone bioactivity in placenta: evidence for the existence of substances other than pyroglu-his-pro-NH$_2$ (TRH) capable of stimulating pituitary thyrotropin release. Endocrinology 1980; 106:541–546.

65. Polk DH, Reviczky AL, Lam RW, et al. Thyrotropin releasing hormone. Effect of thyroid status on tissue concentrations in fetal sheep. Clin Res 1988; 36:203A.

66. Kumasaka T, Nishi N, Yaoi Y, et al. Demonstration of immunoreactive somatostatin-like substance in villi and decidua in early pregnancy. Am J Obstet Gynecol 1979; 134:39–44.

67. Watkins WB, Yen SSC. Somatostatin in cytotrophoblast of the immature human placenta: localization by immunoperoxidase cytochemistry. J Clin Endocrinol Metab 1980; 50:969–971.

68. Shibasaki T, Dagiri E, Shizume K, et al. Corticotropin-releasing factor–like activity in human placental extracts. J Clin Endocrinol Metab 1982; 55:384–386.

69. Jones CT, Gu W, Parer JT. Production of corticotrophin releasing hormone by sheep placenta in vivo. J Dev Physiol 1989; 11:97–101.

70. Sasaki A, Liotta AS, Luckey MM, et al. Immunoreactive corticotropin releasing factor is present in human plasma during the third trimester of pregnancy. J Clin Endocrinol Metab 1984; 59:812–814.

71. Campbell EA, Linton EA, Wolfe CDA, et al. Plasma corticotropin-releasing hormone concentrations during pregnancy and parturition. J Clin Endocrinol Metab 1987; 64:1054–1059.

72. Jeske W, Soszyński P, Rogoziński W, et al. Plasma GHRH, CRH, ACTH, β-endorphin, human placental lactogen, GH, and cortisol concentrations at the third trimester of pregnancy. Acta Endocrinol 1989; 120:785–789.

73. Robinson BG, Emanuel RL, Frim DM, et al. Glucocorticoid stimulates expression of corticotropin-releasing hormone gene in human placenta. Proc Natl Acad Sci USA 1988; 85:5244–5248.

74. Frim DM, Emanuel RL, Robinson BG, et al. Characterization and gestational regulation of corticotropin releasing hormone messenger RNA in human placenta. J Clin Invest 1988; 82:287–292.

75. Goland RS, Stark RI, Wardlaw SL. Response to corticotropin-releasing hormone during pregnancy in the baboon. J Clin Endocrinol Metab 1990; 70:925–929.

76. Baird A, Wehrenberg WB, Bohlen P, et al. Immunoreactive and biologically active growth hormone releasing factor in rat placenta. Endocrinology 1985; 117:1598–1601.

77. Bamberger AM, Bamberger CM, Pu LP, et al. Expression of pit-1 messenger RNA and protein in the human placenta. J Clin Endocrinol Metab 1995; 80:2021–2026.

78. Petraglia F, Calza L, Giardino L, et al. Identification of neuropeptide Y in human placenta: localization, secretion and binding sites. Endocrinology 1989; 124:2016–2022.

79. Petraglia F, Lim ATW, Vale W. Adenosine 3′,5′ monophosphate, prostaglandins, and epinephrine stimulate the secretion of immunoreactive gonadotropin releasing hormone from cultured human placental tissue. J Clin Endocrinol Metab 1987; 65:1020–1025.

80. Mills NC, D'Ercole AJ, Underwood LE, et al. Synthesis of somatomedin C/insulin-like growth factor I by human placenta. Mol Biol Rep 1986; 11:231–236.

81. Shen SJ, Daimon M, Wang CY, et al. Isolation of an insulin-like growth factor II cDNA with a unique 5′ untranslated region from human placenta. Proc Natl Acad Sci USA 1988; 85:1947–1951.

82. Goldstein LD, Reynolds CP, Perez Polo JR. Isolation of human nerve growth factor from placental tissue. Neurochem Res 1978; 3:185–193.

83. Walker P, Weichsel ME Jr, Fisher DA. Human nerve growth factor: lack of immunoreactivity with mouse nerve growth factor. Life Sci 1980; 26:195–200.

84. Bissonnette F, Cook C, Geoghegan T, et al. Transforming growth factor and epidermal growth factor messenger ribonucleic acid and protein levels in human placentas from early, mid and late gestation. Am J Obstet Gynecol 1992; 166:192–199.

85. Hofmann GEJ, Drews MR, Scott RT Jr, et al. Epidermal growth factor and its receptor in human implantation trophoblast: immunohistochemical evidence for autocrine/paracrine function. J Clin Endocrinol Metab 1992; 74:981–988.

86. Hock RA, Hollenberg MD. Characterization of the receptor for epidermal growth factor—urogastrone in human placental membranes. J Biol Chem 1980; 255:10731–10736.

87. Han VKM, Hunter ES III, Pratt RM, et al. Expression of rat transforming growth factor alpha mRNA during development occurs predominantly in the maternal decidua. Mol Cell Biol 1987; 7:2335–2343.

88. Freemark M, Comer M. Epidermal growth factor (EGF)-like transforming growth factor (TGF) activity and EGF receptors in ovine fetal tissues: possible role for TGF in ovine fetal development. Pediatr Res 1987; 22:609–615.

89. Morrish DW, Bhardwaj D, Dabbagh LK, et al. Epidermal growth factor induces differentiation and secretion of human chorionic gonadotropin and placental lactogen in normal human placenta. J Clin Endocrinol Metab 1987; 65:1282–1290.

90. Frolick CA, Dart LL, Meyers CA, et al. Purification and initial characterization of a type B transforming growth factor from human placenta. Proc Natl Acad Sci USA 1983; 80:3676–3680.

91. Cheung CY, Singh M, Ebaugh E, et al. Vascular endothelial growth factor gene expression in ovine placenta and fetal membranes. Am J Obstet Gynecol 1995; 173:753–759.

92. Horwitz MJ, Clarke MR, Kanbour-Shakir A, et al. Developmental expression and anatomical localization of endothelin-1 messenger ribonucleic acid and immunoreactivity in the rat placenta: a Northern analysis and immunohistochemical study. J Lab Clin Med 1995; 125:713–718.

93. Yang Y, Yelavarthi KK, Chen HL, et al. Molecular, biochemical and functional characteristics of tumor necrosis factor-α produced by human placental cytotrophoblastic cells. J Immunol 1993; 150:5614–5624.

94. Saito S, Fukunaga R, Ichijo M, et al. Expression of granulocyte colony-stimulating factor and its receptor at the fetomaternal interface in murine and human pregnancy. Growth Factors 1994; 10:135–143.

95. Dunne FP, Ratcliffe WA, Mansour P, et al. Parathyroid hormone related protein (PTHrP) gene expression in fetal and extra-embryonic tissues of early pregnancy. Hum Reprod 1994; 9:149–156.

96. Goldsmith PC, McGregor WG, Raymoure WJ, et al. Cellular localization of chorionic gonadotropin in human fetal liver and kidney. J Clin Endocrinol Metab 1983; 57:654–661.

97. Kapcala LP. Immunoassayable adrenocorticotropin in peripheral organs: concentrations during early development. Life Sci 1985; 37:2283–2290.

98. Martino E, Lernmark A, Seo H, et al. High concentration of thyrotropin releasing hormone in pancreatic islets. Proc Natl Acad Sci USA 1978; 75:4265–4267.

99. Pekary AE, Meyer NV, Vaillant C, et al. Thyrotropin releasing hormone and a homologous peptide in the male rat reproductive system. Biochem Biophys Res Commun 1980; 95:993–1000.

100. Suda T, Tomori N, Tozawa J, et al. Distribution and characterization of immunoreactive corticotropin-releasing factor in human tissues. J Clin Endocrinol Metab 1984; 59:861–866.

101. Petrusz P, Merchenthaler I, Maderdrut JL, et al. Corticotropin releasing factor (CRF)-like immunoreactivity in the vertebrate endocrine pancreas. Proc Natl Acad Sci USA 1983; 80:1721–1725.

102. Nieuwenhuyzen Kruseman AC, Linton EA, Ackland J, et al. Heterogeneous immunocytochemical reactivities of oCRF-41-like material in the human hypothalamus, pituitary and gastrointestinal tract. Neuroendocrinology 1984; 38:212–216.

103. Thompson RC, Seasholtz AF, Herbert E. Rat corticotropin releasing hormone gene: sequence and tissue specific expression. Mol Endocrinol 1987; 1:363–370.

104. Shibaski T, Kiyosawa Y, Masuda A, et al. Distribution of growth hormone releasing hormone–like immunoreactivity in human tissue extracts. J Clin Endocrinol Metab 1984; 59:263–268.

105. Koivusalo F, Leppaluoto J. High TRH immunoreactivity in purified pancreatic extracts of fetal and newborn rats. Life Sci 1979; 24:1655–1658.

106. Engler P, Scanlon MF, Jackson IMD. Thyrotropin releasing hormone in the systemic circulation of the neonatal rat is derived from the pancreas and other extraneural tissues. J Clin Invest 1981; 67:800–808.

107. McIntosh N, Pictet RL, Kaplan SL, et al. The developmental pattern of somatostatin in the embryonic and fetal rat pancreas. Endocrinology 1977; 101:825–829.

108. Koshimizu T. The development of pancreatic and gastrointestinal somatostatin-like immunoreactivity and its relationship to feeding in neonatal rats. Endocrinology 1983; 112:911–916.

109. Wu P, Jackson IMD. Identification, characterization and localization of thyrotropin releasing hormone precursor peptides in perinatal rat pancreas. Regul Pept 1988; 22:347–360.

110. Lamberton P, Wu P, Jackson IMD. Thyrotropin releasing hormone release from rat pancreas is stimulated by serotonin but inhibited by carbachol. Endocrinology 1985; 117:1834–1838.

111. Rahier J, Wallon J, Henquin JC. Abundance of somatostatin cells in the human neonatal pancreas. Diabetologia 1980; 18:251–254.

112. Leduque P, Aratan-Spire S, Czernichow P, et al. Ontogenesis of thyrotropin-releasing hormone in the human fetal pancreas. J Clin Invest 1986; 78:1028–1034.

113. Saito H, Saito S, Sano T, et al. Fetal and maternal plasma levels of immunoreactive somatostatin at delivery: evidence for its increase in the umbilical artery and its arterio-venous gradient in the feto-placental circulation. J Clin Endocrinol Metab 1983; 56:567–571.

114. Koshimizu T, Ohyama Y, Yokota Y, et al. Peripheral plasma concentrations of somatostatin-like immunoreactivity in newborns and infants. J Clin Endocrinol Metab 1985; 61:78–82.

115. Perelman AH, Klein AH, Fisher DA. Cord blood thyrotropin releasing hormone (TRH). Clin Res 1981; 29:111A.

116. Umans JG, Umans HR, Szeto HH. Effects of thyrotropin releasing hormone in the fetal lamb. Am J Obstet Gynecol 1986; 155:1266–1271.

117. Mulchahey JJ, DiBlasio AM, Martin MC, et al. Hormone production and peptide regulation of the human fetal pituitary gland. Endocr Rev 1987; 8:406–425.

118. Grumbach MM, Gluckman PD. The human fetal hypothalamus and pituitary gland: the maturation of neuroendocrine mechanisms controlling secretion of fetal pituitary growth hormone, prolactin, gonadotropins, adrenocorticotropin-related peptides and thyrotropin. In: Tulchinsky D, Little AB (eds): Maternal-Fetal Endocrinology. 2nd ed. Philadelphia: WB Saunders, 1994: 193–261.

119. Falin LI. The development of human hypophysis and differentiation of cells of the anterior lobe during embryonic life. Acta Anat (Basel) 1961; 44:188–205.

120. Conklin JL. The development of the human fetal adenohypophysis. Anat Rec 1968; 160:79–91.

121. Thiveris JA, Currie RW. Observations in the hypothalamo-hypophyseal portal vasculature in the developing human fetus. Am J Anat 1980; 157:441–444.

122. Hyyppa M. Hypothalamic monoamines in human fetus. Neuroendocrinology 1972; 9:257–266.

123. Bresson JL, Clavequin MC, Fellman D, et al. Ontogeny of the neuroglandular system revealed with HPGRF-44 antibodies in human hypothalamus. Neuroendocrinology 1984; 39:68–73.

124. Bugnon C, Fellman D, Gouget A, et al. Corticolibrin neurons: cytophysiology, phylogeny and ontogeny. J Steroid Biochem 1984; 20:183–195.

125. Bresson JL, Clavequin MC, Fellman D, et al. Human corticolibrin hypothalamic neuroglandular system: comparative immunocytochemical study with anti-rat and anti-ovine corticotropin-releasing factor sera in the early stages of development. Dev Brain Res 1987; 32:241–246.

126. Bugnon C, Fellmann D, Block B. Immunocytochemical study of the ontogenesis of hypothalamic somatostatin-containing neurons in the human fetus. Cell Tissue Res 1977; 183:319–328.

127. Bugnon C, Block B, Lenys D, et al. Cytoimmunological study of the LH-RH neurons in humans during fetal life. In: Scott DE, Koslowski GP, Weindl A (eds): Brain Endocrine Interactions. III: Neural Hormones and Reproduction. Basel: S. Karger, 1978: 183–196.

128. Winters AJ, Eskay RL, Porter JC. Concentration and distribution of TRH and LRH in the human fetal brain. J Clin Endocrinol Metab 1974; 39:269–273.

129. McNeilly S, Gilmore D, Dobbie G, et al. Prolactin releasing activity in the early foetal hypothalamus. J Endocrinol 1977; 73:533–534.

130. Baker BL, Jaffe RB. The genesis of cell types in the adenohypophysis of the human fetus as observed by immunohistochemistry. Am J Anat 1975; 143:137–161.

131. Begeot M, Dubois MP, Dubois PM. Immunologic localization of α and β-endorphins and β-lipotropin in corticotrophic cells of the normal and anencephalic fetal pituitaries. Cell Tissue Res 1978; 193:413–422.

132. Suganuma N, Seo H, Yamamoto N, et al. The ontogeny of growth hormone in the human fetal pituitary. Am J Obstet Gynecol 1989; 160:729–733.

133. Goodyear CG, Sellen JM, Fuks M, et al. Regulation of growth hormone secretion from human fetal pituitaries, interactions between growth hormone releasing factor and somatostatin. Reprod Nutr Dev 1987; 27:461–470.

134. de Zegher F, Daaboul J, Grumbach MM, et al. Hormone ontogeny in the ovine fetus and neonate. XXII: The effect of somatostatin on the growth hormone (GH) response to GH-releasing factor. Endocrinology 1989; 124:1114–1117.

135. D'Ercole AJ. Growth factors and development. In: Polin RA, Fox WW (eds): Fetal and Neonatal Physiology. Philadelphia: WB Saunders, 1992: 1820–1828.

136. Jones JI, Clemmons DR. Insulin like growth factors and their binding proteins: biological actions. Endocr Rev 1995; 16:3–34.

137. Freemark M, Comer M. Purification of a distinct placental lactogen receptor, a new member of the growth hormone/prolactin receptor family. J Clin Invest 1989; 83:883–889.

138. Hill DJ, Freemark M, Strain AH, et al. Placental lactogen and growth hormone receptors in human fetal tissues: relationship to fetal plasma hPL concentrations and fetal growth. J Clin Endocrinol Metab 1988; 66:1283–1290.

139. Kind KL, Owens JA, Robinson JS, et al. Effect of restriction of placental growth on expression of IGFs in fetal sheep: relationship to fetal growth, circulating IGFs and binding proteins. J Endocrinol 1995; 146:23–34.

140. Winter JSD. Fetal and neonatal adrenocortical physiology. In: Polin RA, Fox WW (eds): Maternal-Fetal Endocrinology. Philadelphia: WB Saunders, 1992: 1829–1841.

141. Pepe GJ, Albrecht ED. Regulation of the primate fetal adrenal cortex. Endocr Rev 1990; 11:151–176.

142. Voutilainen R, Miller WL. Developmental expression of genes for the steroidogenic enzymes P450scc (20,20-desmolase), P450c17 (17 α-hydroxylase/17,20-lyase), and P450c21 (21-hydroxylase) in the human fetus. J Clin Endocrinol Metab 1986; 63:1145–1150.

143. John ME, Simpson ER, Carr BR, et al. Ontogeny of adrenal steroid hydroxylase: evidence for cAMP independent gene expression. Mol Cell Endocrinol 1987; 50:263–268.

144. Korte K, Hemsell PG, Mason JI. Sterol sulfate metabolism in the adrenals of the human fetus, anencephalic newborn and adult. J Clin Endocrinol Metab 1982; 55:671–675.

145. Nelson HP, Kuhn RW, Deyman ME, et al. Human fetal adrenal definitive and fetal zone metabolism of pregnenolone and corticosterone: alternative biosynthetic pathways and absence of detectable aldosterone synthesis. J Clin Endocrinol Metab 1990; 70:693–698.

146. Carr BR, Porter JC, MacDonald PC, et al. Metabolism of low density lipoprotein by human fetal adrenal tissue. Endocrinology 1980; 107:1034–1040.

147. Carr BR, Simpson ER. De novo synthesis of cholesterol by human fetal adrenal gland. Endocrinology 1981; 108:2154–2162.

148. Carr BR, Ohashi M, Simpson ER. Low density lipoprotein binding and de novo synthesis of cholesterol in the neocortex and fetal zones of the human fetal adrenal gland. Endocrinology 1982; 110:1994–1998.

149. Gray ES, Abramovitch DR. Morphologic features of the anencephalic adrenal gland in early pregnancy. Am J Obstet Gynecol 1980; 137:491–495.

150. Walsh SW, Norman RL, Novy MJ. In utero regulation of rhesus monkey fetal adrenals: effects of dexamethasone, adrenocorticotropin, thyrotropin-releasing hormone, prolactin, human chorionic gonadotropin, and α-melanocyte-stimulating hormone on fetal and maternal plasma steroids. Endocrinology 1979; 104:1805–1813.

151. Goland RS, Wardlow SL, Blum M, et al. Biologically active corticotropin-releasing hormone in maternal and fetal plasma during pregnancy. Am J Obstet Gynecol 1988; 159:884–890.

152. Winters AJ, Oliver C, Colston C, et al. Plasma ACTH levels in the human fetus and neonate as related to age and parturition. J Clin Endocrinol Metab 1974; 39:269–273.

153. Jones CT, Luther E, Ritchie JWK, et al. The clearance of ACTH from the adult and fetal sheep. Endocrinology 1975; 96:231–234.

154. Byrne GC, Perry YS, Winter JSD. Steroid inhibitory effects upon human adrenal 3β-hydroxysteroid dehydrogenase activity. J Clin Endocrinol Metab 1986; 62:413–418.

155. Beitins IZ, Bayard F, Ances FIG, et al. The metabolic clearance rate, blood production, interconversion and transplacental passage of cortisol and cortisone in pregnancy near term. Pediatr Res 1973; 7:509–519.

156. Dorr HG, Versmold HT, Sippell WG, et al. Antenatal betamethasone therapy: effects on maternal, fetal, and neonatal mineralocorticoids, glucocorticoids and progestins. J Pediatr 1986; 108:990–993.

157. Charnvises S, Fencl MD, Osathanondh R, et al. Adrenal steroids in maternal and cord blood after dexamethasone administration at midterm. J Clin Endocrinol Metab 1985; 61:1220–1222.

158. Rose JC, Turner CS, Ray DeW, et al. Evidence that cortisol inhibits basal adrenocorticotropin secretion in the sheep fetus by 0.70 gestation. Endocrinology 1988; 123:1307–1313.

159. Yang K, Jones SA, Challis JRG. Changes in glucocorticoid receptor number in the hypothalamus of the sheep fetus with gestational age and after adrenocorticotropin treatment. Endocrinology 1990; 126:11–17.

160. Johnson JW, Mitzner W, Beck JC, et al. Long term effects of betamethasone in fetal development. Am J Obstet Gynecol 1981; 141:1053–1064.

161. Ballard PL. Glucocorticoids and differentiation. In: Baxter JD, Rousseau GG (eds): Monographs on Endocrinology. Vol 12: Glucocorticoid Action. Berlin: Springer-Verlag, 1979: 493–575.

162. Pavlik A, Buresova M. The neonatal cerebellum: the highest level of glucocorticoid receptors in the brain. Dev Brain Res 1984; 12:13–20.

163. Liggins GC. The role of cortisol in preparing the fetus for birth. Reprod Fertil Dev 1994; 6:141–150.

164. Fisher DA. The unique endocrine milieu of the fetus. J Clin Invest 1986; 78:603–611.

165. Beitins IZ, Bayard F, Levitsky L, et al. Plasma aldosterone concentrations at delivery and during the newborn period. J Clin Invest 1972; 51:386–394.

166. Beitins IZ, Graham GG, Kowarski A, et al. Adrenal function in normal infants and in marasmus and kwashiorkor: plasma aldosterone concentration and aldosterone secretion rate. J Pediatr 1974; 84:444–451.

167. Katz FH, Beck P, Makowski EL. The renin-aldosterone system in mother and fetus at term. Am J Obstet Gynecol 1974; 118:51–55.

168. Siegel SR, Fisher DA. Ontogeny of the renin-angiotensin-aldosterone system in the fetal and newborn lamb. Pediatr Res 1980; 14:99–102.

169. Lumbers ER. Functions of the renin-angiotensin system during development. Clin Exp Pharmacol Physiol 1995; 22:499–505.

170. Robillard JE, Page WV, Matthews MS, et al. Differential gene expression and regulation of renal angiotensin II receptor subtypes (AT1 and AT2) during fetal life in sheep. Pediatr Res 1995; 38:896–904.

171. Ito Y, Matsumoto T, Ohbu K, et al. Concentrations of human atrial natriuretic peptide in the cord blood and the plasma of the newborn. Acta Paediatr Scand 1988; 77:76–78.

172. Pintar JE, Toran-Alerand CO. Normal development of the hypothalamic-pituitary-thyroid axis. In: Braverman LE, Utiger Rd (eds): The Thyroid. 6th ed. Philadelphia: LB Lippincott, 1991: 7–21.

173. Fisher DA, Dussault JH, Sack J, et al. Ontogenesis of hypothalamic-pituitary-thyroid function and metabolism in man, sheep and rat. Recent Prog Horm Res 1977; 33:59–116.

174. Moseley JM, Matthews EW, Breed RH, et al. The ultimobranchial origin of calcitonin. Lancet 1968; 1:108–110.

175. Contempre B, Jauniaux E, Calvo R, et al. Detection of thyroid hormones in human embryonic cavities during the first trimester of pregnancy. J Clin Endocrinol Metab 1993; 77:1719–1722.

176. Vulsma T, Gons MH, de Vijlder JJ. Maternal-fetal transfer of thyroxine in congenital hypothyroidism due to a total organification defect or thyroid agenesis. N Engl J Med 1989; 321:13–16.

177. Morreale De Escobar G, Calvo R, Obregon MJ, et al. Contribution of maternal thyroxine to fetal thyroxine pools in normal rats near term. Endocrinology 1990; 126:2765–2767.

178. Burrow GN, Fisher DA, Larsen PR. Maternal and fetal thyroid function. N Engl J Med 1994; 331:1072–1078.

179. Fisher DA, Klein AH. Thyroid development and disorders of thyroid function in the newborn. N Engl J Med 1981; 304:702–712.

180. Fisher DA, Polk DA. Development of the thyroid. Baillieres Clin Endocrinol Metab 1989; 3:627–657.

181. Ballabio M, Nicolini V, Jowett T, et al. Maturation of thyroid function in the normal human fetus. Clin Endocrinol 1989; 31:565–571.

182. Thorpe Beeston JG, Nicolaides KH, McGregor AM. Fetal thyroid function. Thyroid 1992; 2:207–217.

183. Roti E. Regulation of thyroid stimulating hormone (TSH) secretion in the fetus and neonate. J Endocrinol Invest 1988; 11:145–158.

184. Ingbar SH. Autoregulation of the thyroid: response to iodide excess and depletion. Mayo Clin Proc 1972; 47:814–823.

185. Sherwin JR. Development of regulatory mechanisms in the thyroid: failure of iodide to suppress iodide transport activity. Proc Soc Exp Biol Med 1982; 169:458–462.

186. Castaign H, Fournet JP, Leger FA, et al. Thyroid of the newborn and postnatal iodine overload. Arch Fr Pediatr 1979; 36:356–368.

187. Polk DH, Reviczky A, Wu SY, et al. Metabolism of sulfoconjugated thyroid hormone derivatives in developing sheep. Am J Physiol 1994; 266:E892–E896.

188. Polk DH, Wu WY, Wright C, et al. Ontogeny of thyroid hormone effect on tissue 5'-monodeiodinase activity in fetal sheep. Am J Physiol 1988; 254:E337–E341.

189. Polk DH, Cheromcha D, Reviczky A, et al. Nuclear thyroid hormone receptors: ontogeny and thyroid hormone effects in sheep. Am J Physiol 1989; 256:E543–E549.

190. Fisher DA, Polk DH. Maturation of thyroid hormone actions. In: Delange F, Fisher DA, Glinoer D (eds): Research in Congenital Hypothyroidism. New York: Plenum, 1989: 61–77.

191. Bernal J, Pekonen F. Ontogeny of nuclear 3,5,3'-triiodothyronine receptors in human fetal brain. Endocrinology 1984; 114:677–679.

192. Gonzales LW, Ballard PL. Identification and characterization of nuclear 3,5,3'-triiodothyronine-binding sites in fetal human lung. J Clin Endocrinol Metab 1981; 53:21–28.

193. DeZegher F, Pernasetti F, Vanhole C, et al. The prenatal role of thyroid hormone evidenced by fetomaternal pit-1 deficiency. J Clin Endocrinol Metab 1995; 80:3127–3130.

194. Jost A. A new look at the mechanisms controlling sexual differentiation in mammals. Johns Hopkins Med J 1972; 130:38–53.

195. Wilson JD. Sexual differentiation. Annu Rev Physiol 1978; 40:279–306.

196. Pelliniemi LJ, Dym M. The fetal gonad and sexual differentiation. In: Tulchinsky D, Little AB (eds): Maternal-Fetal Endocrinology. 2nd ed. Philadelphia: WB Saunders, 1994: 298–320.

197. Dubin RA, Ostrer H. Sry is a transcriptional activator. Mol Endocrinol 1994; 8:1182–1192.

198. Josso N. Antimullerian hormone: new perspectives for a sexist molecule. Endocr Rev 1986; 7:421–433.

199. Donahoe PK, Budzik GP, Trelstad M, et al. Müllerian inhibiting substance: an update. Recent Prog Horm Res 1982; 38:279–326.

200. Haqq CM, King CY, Ukiyama E, et al. Molecular basis of mammalian sexual determination: activation of müllerian inhibiting substance gene expression by SRY. Science 1994; 266:1494–1500.

201. Voutilainen R, Miller WL. Human müllerian inhibitory factor messenger ribonucleic acid is hormonally regulated in the fetal testis and in adult granulosa cells. Mol Endocrinol 1987; 1:604–608.

202. Barraclough CA, Gorski RA. Evidence that the hypothalamus is responsible for androgen-induced sterility in the female rat. Endocrinology 1961; 68:68–79.

203. Naftolin F, Brawer JB. The effect of estrogens on hypothalamic structure and function. Am J Obstet Gynecol 1978; 132:758–765.

204. Ryan KJ, Naftolin F, Reddy V, et al. Estrogen formation in the brain. Am J Obstet Gynecol 1972; 114:454–460.

205. Sholl SA, Goy RW, Kim KL. 5α-Reductase, aromatase, and androgen receptor levels in the monkey brain during fetal development. Endocrinology 1989; 124:627–634.

206. Visser M, Swaab DF. Life span changes in the presence of melanocyte-stimulating-hormone-containing cells in the human pituitary. J Dev Physiol 1979; 1:161–178.

207. Perry RA, Mulvogue HM, McMillen IC, et al. Immunohistochemical localization of ACTH in the adult and fetal sheep pituitary. J Dev Physiol 1985; 7:397–404.

208. Silman RE, Holland T, Chard T, et al. The ACTH family tree of the rhesus monkey changes with development. Nature 1978; 276:526–528.

209. Osamura RY, Tsutsumi Y, Watanabe K. Light and electron microscopic localization of ACTH and proopiomelanocortin-derived peptides in human developmental and neoplastic cells. J Histochem Cytochem 1984; 32:885–893.

210. Glickman JA, Carson GD, Challis JRG. Differential effects of synthetic adrenocorticotropin and melanocyte stimulating hormone on adrenal formation in human and sheep fetus. Endocrinology 1979; 104:34–39.

211. Swaab DF, Martin JT. Functions of alpha melanotropin and other opiomelanocortin peptides in labour, intrauterine growth and brain development. Ciba Found Symp 1981; 81:196–221.

212. Facchinetti F, Storchi AR, Petraglia F, et al. Ontogeny of pituitary β-endorphin and related peptides in the human embryo and fetus. Am J Obstet Gynecol 1987; 156:735–739.

213. Fisher DA. Maternal-fetal neurohypophyseal system. Clin Perinatol 1983; 10:695–708.

214. Leake RD, Fisher DA. Ontogeny of vasopressin in man. In: Czernichow P, Robinson AG (eds): Diabetes Insipidus in Man. Frontiers in Hormone Research. Vol 13. Basel: S. Karger, 1985: 42–51.

215. Leake RD. The fetal-maternal neurohypophysial system. In: Tulchinsky D, Little AB (eds): Maternal-Fetal Endocrinology. 2nd ed. Philadelphia: WB Saunders, 1994: 264–274.

216. Perks AM. Developmental and evolutionary aspects of the neurohypophysis. Am Zool 1977; 17:833–849.

217. Pavel S. Arginine vasotocin as a pineal hormone. J Neural Transm Suppl 1978; 13:135–155.

218. Ervin MG, Leake RD, Ross MG, et al. Arginine vasotocin in ovine maternal and fetal blood, fetal urine, and amniotic fluid. J Clin Invest 1985; 75:1696–1701.

219. Bell RJ, Congiu M, Hardy KJ, et al. Gestation-dependent aspects of the response of the ovine fetus to osmotic stress induced by maternal water deprivation. Q J Exp Physiol 1984; 69:187–195.

220. Daniel SS, Stark RI, Husain MK, et al. Role of vasopressin in fetal homeostasis. Am J Physiol 1982; 242:F740–F744.

221. Morris M, Castro M, Rose JC. Alterations in prohormone processing during early development in the fetal sheep. Am J Physiol 1992; 263:R738–R740.

222. DeVane GW, Naden RP, Porter JC, et al. Mechanism of arginine vasopressin release in the sheep fetus. Pediatr Res 1982; 16:504–507.

223. Stark RI, Daniel SS, Hussain MK, et al. Vasopressin concentration in amniotic fluid as an index of fetal hypoxia: mechanisms of release in sheep. Pediatr Res 1984; 18:552–558.

224. Stegner H, Leake RD, Palmer SM, et al. The effect of hypoxia on neurohypophyseal hormone release in fetal and maternal sheep. Pediatr Res 1984; 18:188–191.

225. DeVane GW, Porter JC. An apparent stress-induced release of arginine vasopressin by human neonates. J Clin Endocrinol Metab 1980; 51:1412–1416.

226. Matthews SG, Challis JRG. Regulation of CRH and AVP mRNA in the developing ovine hypothalamus: effects of stress and glucocorticoids. Am J Physiol 1995; 268:E1096–E1107.

227. Kelly RT, Rose JC, Meis PJ, et al. Vasopressin is important for restoring cardiovascular homeostasis in fetal lambs subjected to hemorrhage. Am J Obstet Gynecol 1983; 146:807–812.

228. Irion GL, Mack CE, Clark KE. Fetal hemodynamic and fetoplacental vascular response to exogenous arginine vasopressin. Am J Obstet Gynecol 1990; 162:1115–1120.

229. Jones CT, Ritchie JW. The effects of adrenergic blockade on fetal response to hypoxia. J Dev Physiol 1983; 5:211–222.

230. Norman LJ, Challis JRG. Dose dependent effects of arginine vasopressin on endocrine and blood gas responses of fetal sheep during the last third of pregnancy. Can J Physiol Pharmacol 1987; 65:2291–2296.

231. Norman LJ, Challis JRG. Synergism between systemic corticotropin-releasing factor and arginine vasopressin on adrenocorticotropin release in vivo varies as a function of gestational age in the ovine fetus. Endocrinology 1987; 120:1052–1058.

232. Brooks AN, White A. Activation of pituitary adrenal function in fetal sheep by corticotrophin-releasing factor and arginine vasopressin. J Endocrinol 1990; 124:27–35.

233. Benedetto MT, DeCicco F, Rossiello F, et al. Oxytocin receptor in human fetal membranes at term and during labor. J Steroid Biochem 1990; 35:205–208.

234. Tribollet E, Charpak S, Schmidt A, et al. Appearance and transient expression of oxytocin receptors in fetal, infant and peripubertal rat brain studied by autoradiography and electrophysiology. J Neurosci 1989; 9:1764–1773.

235. Ervin MG, Miller SJ, Ramseyer LJ, et al. Renal arginine vasopressin receptors in newborn and adult sheep. Clin Res 1990; 38:170A.

236. Robillard JE, Weitzman RE. Developmental aspects of the fetal renal response to exogenous arginine vasopressin. Am J Physiol 1980; 238:F407–F414.

237. Ervin MG, Ross MG, Leake RD, et al. Changes in steady state plasma arginine vasotocin levels affect ovine fetal renal and cardiovascular function. Endocrinology 1986; 118:759–765.

238. Kullama LK, Balaraman V, Claybaugh JR, et al. Ontogeny of vasoconstrictor neurohypophysial hormone function in rats. Am J Physiol 1990; 258:R263–R268.

239. Manku MS, Mtabaji JB, Horrobin DF. Effect of cortisol, prolactin and ADH on the amniotic membrane. Nature 1975; 258:78–80.

240. Fisher DA, Pyle HR Jr, Porter JC, et al. Control of water balance in the newborn. Am J Dis Child 1963; 106:137–146.

241. Coupland RS. The prenatal development of the abdominal paraaortic bodies in man. J Anat 1952; 86:357–372.

242. Niemineva R, Pekkarinen A. The noradrenaline and adrenaline content of human fetal adrenal glands and aortic bodies. Ann Med Exp Biol Fenn 1952; 30:274–286.

243. Gospodarowicz D. Epidermal and nerve growth factors in mammalian development. Annu Rev Physiol 1981; 43:251–263.

244. Aloe L, Levi-Montalcini R. Nerve growth factor–induced transformation of immature chromaffin cells in vivo into sympathetic neurons: effect of antiserum to nerve growth factor. Proc Natl Acad Sci USA 1979; 76:1246–1250.

245. Wurtman RJ. Control of epinephrine synthesis in the adrenal medulla by the adrenal cortex: hormonal specificity and dose-response characteristics. Endocrinology 1966; 79:608–614.

246. Margolis EL, Rotti J, Jost A. Norepinephrine methylation in fetal rat adrenals. Science 1966; 154:275–276.

247. Comline RS, Silver M. Development of activity in the adrenal medulla of the foetus and newborn animal. Br Med Bull 1966; 22:16–20.

248. Shaul PW, Cha CJM, Oh W. Neonatal sympathoadrenal response to acute hypoxia: impairment after experimental intrauterine growth retardation. Pediatr Res 1989; 25:466–472.

249. Slotkin TA, Seidler FJ. Adrenomedullary catecholamine release in the fetus and newborn: secretory mechanisms and their role in stress and survival. J Dev Physiol 1988; 10:1–16.

250. Padbury JF, Agata Y, Polk DH, et al. Neonatal adaptation: naloxone increases the catecholamine surge at birth. Pediatr Res 1987; 21:590–593.

251. Stonestreet BS, Piasecki GJ, Susa JB, et al. Effects of insulin infusion on catecholamine concentration in fetal sheep. Am J Obstet Gynecol 1989; 160:740–745.

252. Cohen WR, Piasecki GJ, Cohn HE, et al. Plasma catecholamines in the hypoxaemic fetal rhesus monkey. J Dev Physiol 1987; 9:507–515.

253. Pryds O, Christensen NJ, Friis-Hansen B. Increased cerebral blood flow and plasma epinephrine in hypoglycemic, preterm neonates. Pediatrics 1990; 85:172–176.

254. Palmer SM, Oakes GK, Lam RW, et al. Catecholamine physiology in the ovine fetus. I: Gestational age variation in basal plasma concentrations. Am J Obstet Gynecol 1984; 149:420–425.

255. Palmer SM, Oakes GK, Lam RW, et al. Catecholamine physiology in the ovine fetus. II: Metabolic clearance rate of epinephrine. Am J Physiol 1984; 246:E350–E355.

256. Palmer SM, Oakes GK, Champion JA, et al. Catecholamine physiology in the ovine fetus. III: Maternal and fetal response to acute maternal exercise. Am J Obstet Gynecol 1984; 149:426–434.

257. Padbury JF, Roberman B, Oddie TH, et al. Fetal catecholamine release in response to labor and delivery: the role of fetal acid-base status, sex, and heart rate patterns at term. Obstet Gynecol 1982; 60:607–611.

258. Newnham JP, Marshall JC, Padbury JF, et al. Fetal catecholamine release with preterm delivery. Am J Obstet Gynecol 1984; 149:888–893.

259. Zhou QY, Ouaife CJ, Palmiter RD. Targeted disruption of the tyrosine hydroxylase gene reveals that catecholamines are required for mouse fetal development. Nature 1995; 374:640–643.

260. Thomas SA, Matsumoto AM, Palmiter RD. Noradrenaline is essential for mouse fetal development. Nature 1995; 374:643–646.

261. Seidler FJ, Brown KK, Smith PG, et al. Toxic effects of hypoxia on neonatal cardiac function in the rat: alpha-adrenergic mechanisms. Toxicol Lett 1987; 37:79–84.

262. Schedewie HK, Fisher DA. Perinatal mineral homeostasis. In: Tulchinsky D, Ryan KJ, eds. Maternal-Fetal Endocrinology. Philadelphia: WB Saunders, 1980: 355–386.

263. Care AD. Development of endocrine pathways in the regulation of calcium homeostasis. Baillieres Clin Endocrinol Metab 1989; 3:671–688.

264. Bouillon R, Van Assche FA. Perinatal vitamin D metabolism. Dev Pharmacol Ther 1982; 4(Suppl 1):38–44.

265. Stevenson JC. Mineral needs of the fetus. Curr Top Exp Endocrinol 1983; 5:177–196.

266. Moore ES, Langman CB, Favus MJ, et al. Role of fetal 1,25-dihydroxyvitamin D production in intrauterine phosphorus and calcium homeostasis. Pediatr Res 1985; 19:566–569.

267. Abbas SK, Care AD, Van Baelen H, et al. Plasma vitamin D-binding protein and free 1,25-dihydroxyvitamin D_3 index in pregnant ewes and their fetuses in the last month of gestation. J Endocrinol 1987; 115:7–12.

268. Care AD, Caple IW, Abbas SK, et al. The effect of fetal thyroparathyroidectomy on the transport of calcium across the ovine placenta to the fetus. Placenta 1986; 7:417–424.

269. MacIsaac RJ, Horne RSC, Caple IW, et al. Effects of thyroparathyroidectomy, parathyroid hormone, and PTHrP on kidneys of ovine fetuses. Am J Physiol 1993; 264:E37–E44.

270. MacIsaac RJ, Caple IW, Danks JA, et al. Ontogeny of parathyroid hormone–related protein in the ovine parathyroid gland. Endocrinology 1991; 129:757–764.

271. Rouffet J, Barlet JP. Peptide apparente a la hormone parathyroidienne (PTHrP) et metabolisme osseux. Arch Physiol Biochem 1995; 103:3–13.

272. MacIsaac RJ, Heath JA, Rodda CP, et al. Role of the fetal parathyroid glands and parathyroid hormone–related protein in the regulation of placental transport of calcium, magnesium, and inorganic phosphate. Reprod Fertil Dev 1991; 3:337–457.

273. Brunette MG, Anger D, Lafond J. Effect of parathyroid hormone on PO_4 transport through the human placenta microvilli. Pediatr Res 1989; 25:15–18.

274. Lafond J, Auger D, Fortier J, et al. Parathyroid hormone receptor in human placental syncytiotrophoblast brush border and basal plasma membranes. Endocrinology 1988; 123:2834–2840.

275. Thiebaud D, Janisch S, Koelbl H, et al. Direct evidence of a parathyroid related protein gradient between the mother and newborn in humans. Bone Miner 1993; 23:213–221.

276. Ross R, Halbert K, Tsang RC. Determination of the production and metabolic clearance rates of 1,25-dihydroxyvitamin D_3 in the pregnant sheep and its chronically catheterized fetus by primed infusion technique. Pediatr Res 1989; 26:633–638.

277. Austin LA, Heath N. Calcitonin, physiology and pathophysiology. N Engl J Med 1981; 304:269–278.

278. Takigawa M, Enomoto M, Shirai E, et al. Differential effects of 1α,25-dihydroxycholecalciferol and 24,25-dihydroxycholecalciferol on proliferation and the differentiated phenotype of rabbit costal chondrocytes in culture. Endocrinology 1988; 122:831–839.

279. Liu HM, Potter EL. Development of the human pancreas. Arch Pathol 1962; 74:439–452.

280. Steinke J, Driscoll S. The extractable insulin content of pancreas from fetuses and infants of diabetic and control mothers. Diabetes 1965; 14:573–578.

281. Assan R, Boillot J. Pancreatic glucagon and glucagon-like material in tissues and plasmas from human fetuses 6–26 weeks old. Pathol Biol 1973; 21:149–157.

282. Sperling MA. Carbohydrate metabolism: insulin and glucagon. In: Tulchinsky D, Little AB (eds): Maternal-Fetal Endocrinology. 2nd ed. Philadelphia: WB Saunders, 1994: 380–400.

283. Girard J. Control of fetal and neonatal glucose metabolism by pancreatic hormones. Baillieres Clin Endocrinol Metab 1989; 3:817–836.

284. Ammon HP, Glocker C, Waldner RG, et al. Insulin release from pancreatic islets of fetal rats mediated by leucine, b-BCH, tolbutamide, glibenclamide, arginine, potassium chloride, and theophylline does not require stimulation of Ca^{2+} net uptake. Cell Calcium 1989; 10:441–450.

285. Formby B, Ullrich A, Coussens L, et al. Growth hormone stimulates insulin gene expression in cultured human fetal pancreatic islets. J Clin Endocrinol Metab 1988; 66:1075–1079.

286. Muntz DH, Levey GS, Schenk A. Adenosine 3'5'-cyclic monophosphate and phosphodiesterase activities in isolated fetal and neonatal rat pancreatic islets. Endocrinology 1973; 92:614–617.

287. Hole RL, Pian-Smith MCM, Sharp GWG. Development of the biphasic response to glucose in fetal and neonatal rat pancreas. Am J Physiol 1988; 254:E167–E174.

288. Hay WW Jr, Sparks JW, Wilkening RB, et al. Fetal glucose uptake and utilization as functions of maternal glucose concentration. Am J Physiol 1984; 246:E237–E242.

289. Duee PH, Pegorier JP, El Manoubi L, et al. Development of gluconeogenesis from different substrates in newborn rabbit hepatocytes. J Dev Physiol 1986; 8:387–394.

290. Herbin C, Duee PH, Pegorier JP, et al. Premature appearance of gluconeogenesis and fatty acid oxidation in the liver of the post term rabbit fetus. Pediatr Res 1988; 23:224–228.

291. Bloch CA, Menon RK, Sperling MA. Effects of somatostatin and glucose infusion on glucose kinetics in fetal sheep. Am J Physiol 1988; 255:E87–E93.

292. Kaplan SA. The insulin receptor. J Pediatr 1984; 104:327–336.

293. Devaskar SU, Ganguli S, Styer D, et al. Glucagon and glucose dynamics in sheep: evidence for glucagon resistance in the fetus. Am J Physiol 1984; 246:E256–E265.

294. Kaplan MM, Yakoski KA. Maturational patterns of iodothyronine phenolic and tyrosyl ring deiodinase activities in rat cerebrum, cerebellum and hypothalamus. J Clin Invest 1981; 67:1208–1214.

295. Ruiz de Ona C, Jesus Obregon M, Escobar del Rey F, et al. Developmental changes in rat brain 5'-deiodinase and thyroid hormones during the fetal period. The effects of fetal hypothyroidism and maternal thyroid hormones. Pediatr Res 1988; 24:588–594.

296. Padbury JF, Klein AH, Polk DH, et al. The effect of thyroid status in lung and heart beta adrenergic receptors in fetal and newborn sheep. Dev Pharmacol Ther 1986; 9:44–53.

297. Coulombe P, Ruel J, Dussault JH. Effects of neonatal hypo- and hyperthyroidism on pituitary growth hormone content in the rat. Endocrinology 1980; 107:2027–2033.

298. Lakshmanan J, Beri U, Perheentupa J, et al. Acquisition of submandibular gland nerve growth factor (SMG-NGF) responsiveness to thyroxine in neonatal mice. J Neurosci Res 1984; 12:71–85.

299. Lakshmanan J, Perheentupa J, Macaso T, et al. Acquisition of urine, kidney and submandibular gland epidermal growth factor responsiveness to thyroxine administration in neonatal mice. Acta Endocrinol 1985; 109:511–516.

300. Alm J, Scott SM, Fisher DA. Epidermal growth factor receptor ontogeny in mice with congenital hypothyroidism. J Dev Physiol 1986; 8:377–385.

301. Hoath SB, Lakshmanan J, Fisher DA. Thyroid hormone effects on skin and hepatic epidermal growth factor concentrations in neonatal and adult mice. Biol Neonate 1984; 45:49–52.

302. Hoath SB, Lakshmanan J, Fisher DA. Epidermal growth factor binding to neonatal mouse skin explants and membrane preparations—effect of triiodothyronine. Pediatr Res 1985; 19:277–280.

303. Perez-Castillo A, Bernal J, Ferriero B, et al. The early ontogenesis of thyroid hormone receptor in the rat fetus. Endocrinology 1985; 117:2457–2461.

303a. Anderson GW, Larson RJ, Strait KA, et al. Developmentally regulated nucleoproteins may regulate brain gene responsivity to transcriptional control by triiodothyronine. Tenth International Congress of Endocrinology, San Francisco, 1996, 728 (OR55–5).

304. Padbury JF, Lam RW, Newnham JP, et al. Neonatal adaptation: greater neurosympathetic system activity in preterm than full term sheep at birth. Am J Physiol 1985; 248:E443–E449.

305. Pasqualini JR, Sumida C, Gelly C, et al. Progesterone receptors in the fetal uterus and ovary of the guinea pig: evolution during fetal development and induction and stimulation in estradiol-primed animals. J Steroid Biochem 1976; 7:1031–1038.

306. Yamashita S, Newbold RR, McLachlan JA, et al. Developmental pattern of estrogen receptor expression in female mouse genital tracts. Endocrinology 1989; 125:2888–2896.

307. Simmen FA, Simmon RCM, Letcher LR, et al. IGFs in pregnancy: developmental expression in uterus and mammary gland and paracrine actions during embryonic and neonatal growth. In: LeRoith D, Raizada MK (eds): Molecular and Cellular Biology of Insulin-Like Growth Factors and Their Receptors. New York: Plenum, 1989: 195–208.

308. Spaventi R, Antica M, Pavelic K. Insulin and insulin-like growth factor I (IGF I) in early mouse embryogenesis. Development 1990; 108:491–495.

309. D'Ercole AJ. Somatomedins/insulin-like growth factors and fetal growth. J Dev Physiol 1987; 9:481–495.

310. Han VKM, Hill DJ, Strain AJ, et al. Identification of somatomedin/insulin-like growth factor immunoreactive cells in the human fetus. Pediatr Res 1987; 22:245–249.

311. Han VKM, D'Ercole AJ, Lund PK. Cellular localization of synthesis of somatomedin (insulin-like growth factor) messenger RNA in the human fetus. Science 1987; 236:193–197.

312. D'Ercole AJ, Applewhite GT, Underwood LE. Evidence that somatomedins are synthesized by multiple tissues in the fetus. Dev Biol 1980; 75:315–328.

313. De Chiara TM, Efstradiadis A, Robertson EJ. A growth deficiency phenotype in heterozygous mice carrying an insulin like growth factor II gene disrupted by targeting. Nature 1990; 345:78–80.

314. Liu JKP, Baker J, Perkins AS, et al. Mice carrying null mutations of the genes encoding insulin-like growth factor I and type I IGF receptor. Cell 1993; 75:59–72.

315. Baker J, Liu JP, Robertson EJ, et al. Role of insulin-like growth factors in embryonic and postnatal growth. Cell 1993; 75:73–82.

316. Adams SO, Nissley SP, Handwerger S, et al. Developmental patterns of insulin-like growth factor I and II synthesis and regulation in rat fibroblasts. Nature 1983; 302:150–153.

317. Bennett A, Wilson DM, Liu R, et al. Levels of insulin like growth factors I and II in human cord blood. J Clin Endocrinol Metab 1983; 57:609–612.

318. Moses AC, Nissley SP, Short PA. Elevated levels of multiplication-stimulating activity, an insulin-like growth factor, in fetal rat serum. Proc Natl Acad Sci USA 1980; 77:3649–3653.

319. Sara VR, Hall K, Misaki M, et al. Ontogenesis of somatomedin and insulin receptors in the human fetus. J Clin Invest 1983; 71:1084–1094.

320. Han VKM, Lauder IM, D'Ercole AJ. Characterization of somatomedin–insulin like growth factor receptors and correlation with biological activity in cultured neonatal rat astroglial cells. J Neurosci 1987; 7:501–511.

321. Freemark M, D'Ercole AJ, Handwerger S. Somatomedin C stimulates glycogen synthesis in fetal rat hepatocytes. Endocrinology 1985; 116:2578–2582.

322. Pilistine SJ, Moses AC, Munro HN. Placental lactogen administration reverses the effect of low protein diet on maternal and fetal somatomedin levels in the pregnant rat. Proc Natl Acad Sci USA 1984; 81:5853–5857.

323. Sara VR, Carlsson-Skwirut C, Andersson C, et al. Characterization of somatomedins from human fetal brain: identification of a variant form of insulin-like growth factor I. Proc Natl Acad Sci USA 1986; 83:4904–4907.

324. Hill DJ, Milner RDG. Insulin as a growth factor. Pediatr Res 1985; 19:879–886.

325. Accili D, Drago J, Lee EJ, et al. Early neonatal death in mice homozygous for a null allele of the insulin receptor gene. Nat Genet 1996; 12:106–109.

326. Krook A, Brueton L, O'Rahilly S. Homozygous nonsense mutation in the insulin receptor gene in infant with leprechaunism. Lancet 1993; 342:277–278.

327. Fisher DA, Lakshmanan J. Metabolism and effects of EGF and related growth factors in mammals. Endocr Rev 1990; 11:418–442.

328. Russell WE, Van Wyk JJ. Peptide growth factors. In: DeGroot LJ, Besser M, Burger HC, et al (eds): Endocrinology. 3rd ed. Philadelphia: WB Saunders, 1995: 2590–2623.

329. Meyer D, Birchmeier C. Multiple essential functions of neuregulin in development. Nature 1995; 378:386–390.

330. Gassmann M, Casagranda F, Orioli D, et al. Aberrant neural and cardiac development in mice lacking the Erb B4 neuregulin receptor. Nature 1995; 378:390–394.

331. Anzano MA, Roberts AB, Meyers CA, et al. Synergistic interaction of two classes of transforming growth factors from murine sarcoma cells. Cancer Res 1982; 19:4776–4778.

332. Rall LB, Scott J, Bell GI, et al. Mouse prepro-epidermal growth factor synthesis by the kidney and other tissues. Nature 1985; 313:228–231.

333. Laborde NP, Grodin M, Buenaflor G, et al. Ontogenesis of epidermal growth factor in liver of BALB mice. Am J Physiol 1988; 255:E28–E32.

334. Brown PI, Lam R, Lakshmanan J, et al. Transforming growth factor alpha (TGFα) in the developing rat. Am J Physiol 1990; 259:E256–E260.

335. Kamei Y, Tsutsumi O, Kuwabara Y, et al. Intrauterine growth retardation and fetal losses are caused by epidermal growth factor deficiency in mice. Am J Physiol 1993; 264:R597–R600.

336. Goldman S, Dirnfeld M, Koifman M, et al. The effect of epidermal growth factor on growth and differentiation of mouse preimplantation embryos in vitro. Hum Reprod 1993; 9:1459–1462.

337. Hemmings R, Langlais J, Falcone T, et al. Human embryos produce transforming growth factor α activity and insulin-like growth factor II. Fertil Steril 1992; 58:101–104.

338. Meittinen PJ, Berger JE, Menesses J, et al. Epithelial immaturity and multiorgan failure in mice lacking epidermal growth factor receptor. Nature 1995; 376:337–341.

339. Thorburn GD, Waters MJ, Young IR, et al. Epidermal growth factor: a critical factor in fetal maturation? Ciba Found Symp 1981; 86:172–198.

340. Zschiesche W. Retardation of growth and epithelial differentiation in suckling mice by anti-EGF antisera. Biomed Biochim Acta 1989; 48:103–109.

341. Tang MJ, Lin YJ, Huang JJ. Thyroid hormone upregulates gene expression, synthesis and release of pro-epidermal growth factor in adult rat kidney. Life Sci 1995; 57:1477–1485.

342. Korach KS, McLachlan JA, Teng CT. Influence of estrogens on mouse uterine epidermal growth factor precursor protein and messenger ribonucleic acid. Endocrinology 1988; 122:2355–2363.

343. Walker P, Weichsel ME Jr, Hoath SB, et al. Effect of T₄, testosterone and corticosterone on NGF and EGF concentrations in adult female mouse SMG: dissociation of EGF and NGF responses. Endocrinology 1981; 109:582–587.

344. Abdulmaged MT, Notiz HH. Prostatic epidermal growth factor receptors and their regulation by androgens. Endocrinology 1987; 121:1461–1467.

345. Johnson GR, Kannan B, Shoyab M, et al. Amphiregulin induces tyrosine phosphorylation of the epidermal growth factor receptor and p185 erbB2. J Biol Chem 1993; 268:2924–2931.

346. Mazzoni IE, Kenigsberg RL. Effects of epidermal growth factor in the mammalian central nervous system. Drug Dev Res 1992; 26:111–128.

347. Kitchens DL, Snyder EY, Gottlieb DI. FGF and EGF are mitogens for immortilized neural progenitors. J Neurobiol 1990; 21:356–375.

348. Santa-Olalla J, Covarrubias L. Epidermal growth factor, transforming growth factor-α, and fibroblast growth factor differentially influence neural precursor cells of mouse embryonic mesencephalon. J Neurosci Res 1995; 42:172–183.

349. Lee KF, Simon H, Chen C, et al. Requirement for neuregulin receptor erbB2 in neural and cardiac development. Nature 1995; 378:394–398.

350. Kaser MR, Lakslmanan J, Fisher DA. Comparison between epidermal growth factor, transforming growth factor alpha, and EGF receptor levels in regions of adult rat brain. Mol Brain Res 1992; 16:316–322.

351. Bradshaw RA. Nerve growth factor. Annu Rev Biochem 1978; 47:191–216.

352. Gorin PD, Johnson EM. Effects of exposure to nerve growth factor antibodies on the developing nervous system of the rat, an experimental autoimmune approach. Dev Biol 1980; 80:313–323.

353. Sendtner M, Holtmann B, Kolbeck R, et al. Brain derived neurotrophic factor prevents the death of motoneurons in newborn rats after nerve section. Nature 1992; 360:757–759.

354. Yan Q, Elliott J, Snider WD. Brain derived neurotrophic factor reserves spinal motor neurons from axotomy-induced cell death. Nature 1992; 360:753–755.

355. Padbury JF, Lam RW, Polk DH, et al. Autoimmune sympathectomy in fetal rabbits. J Dev Physiol 1986; 8:369–376.

356. Tarris RH, Weichsel ME Jr, Fisher DA. Synthesis and secretion of a nerve growth stimulating factor by neonatal mouse astrocyte cells in vitro. Pediatr Res 1986; 20:367–372.

357. Lakshmanan J, Weichsel ME Jr, Tarris R, et al. Nerve growth factor in developing mouse cerebral cortical synaptosomes: measurement by competitive radioimmunoassay and bioassay. Pediatr Res 1986; 20:391–397.

358. Giordano T, Pan JB, Casuto D, et al. Thyroid hormone regulation of NGF, NT3 and BDNF RNA in the adult rat brain. Mol Brain Res 1992; 16:239–245.

359. Sieff CA. Hematopoietic growth factors. J Clin Invest 1987; 79:1549–1557.

360. Zanjani ED, Ascensau JL, McGlave PB. Studies on the liver to kidney switch of erythropoietin production. J Clin Invest 1981; 67:1183–1188.

361. Oberbauer AM, Linkhart TA, Mohan S, et al. Fibroblast growth factor enhances human chorionic gonadotropin synthesis independent of mitogenic stimulation in Jar choriocarcinoma cells. Endocrinology 1988; 123:2696–2700.

362. Wallace MJ, Hooper SB, Harding R. Effects of elevated fetal cortisol concentrations on the volume, secretion, and reabsorption of lung liquid. Am J Physiol 1995; 269:R881–R887.

363. Muglia L, Jacobson L, Dikkes P, et al. Corticotropin-releasing hormone deficiency reveals major fetal but not adult glucocorticoid need. Nature 1995; 373:427–432.

364. Cole TJ, Blendy JA, Monaghan P, et al. Targeted disruption of the glucocorticoid receptor gene blocks adrenergic chromaffin cell development and severely retards lung maturation. Genes Dev 1995; 9:1608–1621.

365. Padbury JF. Functional maturation of the adrenal medulla and peripheral sympathetic nervous system. Baillieres Clin Endocrinol Metab 1989; 3:689–705.

366. Polk DH. Thyroid hormone effects on neonatal thermogenesis. Semin Perinatol 1988; 12:151–156.

367. Gunn TR, Gluckman PD. Perinatal thermogenesis. Early Hum Dev 1995; 42:169–183.

368. Obregon MJ, Pitamber R, Jacobsson A, et al. Euthyroid status is essential for the perinatal increase in thermogenin mRNA in brown adipose tissue of rat pups. Biochem Biophys Res Commun 1987; 148:9–14.

369. Klein AH, Reviczky A, Chou P, et al. Development of brown adipose tissue thermogenesis in the ovine fetus and newborn. Endocrinology 1983; 112:1662–1666.

370. Polk DH, Padbury JF, Callegari CC, et al. Effect of fetal thyroidectomy on newborn thermogenesis in lambs. Pediatr Res 1987; 21:453–457.

371. Fisher DA, Polk DH, Wu SY. Fetal thyroid metabolism: a pluralistic system. Thyroid 1994; 4:367–371.

372. Longhead JL, Minouni F, Tsang RC. Serum ionized calcium concentrations in normal neonates. Am J Dis Child 1988; 142:516–518.

373. Dincsoy MY, Tsang RC, Laskarzewski P, et al. The role of postnatal age and magnesium on parathyroid hormone responses during exchange blood transfusion in the newborn period. J Pediatr 1982; 100:277–283.

374. Venkataraman PS, Tsang RC, Chen IW, et al. Pathogenesis of early neonatal hypocalcemia: studies of serum calcitonin, gastrin and plasma glucagon. J Pediatr 1987; 110:599–603.

375. Mimoumi F, Tsang RC. Perinatal mineral metabolism. In: Tulchinsky D, Little AB (eds): Maternal-Fetal Endocrinology. 2nd ed. Philadelphia: WB Saunders, 1994: 402–417.

376. Menon RK, Sperling MA. Carbohydrate metabolism. Semin Perinatol 1988; 12:157–162.

377. Wheeler MD, Styne DM. Longitudinal changes in growth hormone response to growth hormone–releasing hormone in neonatal rhesus monkeys. Pediatr Res 1990; 28:15–18.

378. Penny R, Parlow AF, Frasier O. Testosterone and estradiol concentrations in paired maternal and cord sera and their correlation with the concentration of chorionic gonadotropin. Pediatrics 1979; 64:604–608.

379. Mann DR, Gould KG, Collins DC, et al. Blockade of neonatal activation of the pituitary-testicular axis: effect on peripubertal luteinizing hormone and testosterone secretion and on testicular development in male monkeys. J Clin Endocrinol Metab 1989; 68:600–607.

380. Barraclough CA. Production of anovulatory sterile rats by single injection of testosterone propionate. Endocrinology 1961; 68:62–67.

381. Janson JD, Ekberg S, Isacksson D, et al. Imprinting of growth hormone secretion, body growth, and hepatic steroid metabolism by neonatal testosterone. Endocrinology 1985; 117:1881–1889.

382. Gorski RA. Sexual differentiation of brain structure in rodents. In: Serio M, Zanisi M, Martini L (eds): Sexual Differentiation: Basic and Clinical Concepts. New York: Raven, 1984: 65–77.

383. Dohler KD. The special case of hormonal imprinting. The neonatal influence on sex. Experientia 1986; 42:759–769.

384. Grocock CA, Charlton HM, Pike MC. Role of fetal pituitary in cryptorchidism induced by exogenous maternal oestrogen during pregnancy in mice. J Reprod Fertil 1988; 83:295–300.

385. Bern HA, Talamentes FJ Jr. Neonatal mouse models and their relation to disease in the human female. In: Herbst AL, Bern HA (eds): Developmental Effects of Diethylstilbestrol (DES) in Pregnancy. New York: Thieme-Stratton, 1981: 129–147.

386. Csaba G. Receptor ontogeny and hormonal imprinting. Experientia 1986; 42:750–759.

387. Csaba G, Inczefi-Gonda A. Lifelong effect of a single neonatal treatment with estradiol or progesterone on rat uterine estrogen receptor binding capacity. Horm Metab Res 1992; 24:167–171.

388. Bakke JL, Lawrence NL, Bennet J, et al. Endocrine syndromes produced by neonatal hyperthyroidism, hypothyroidism, or altered nutrition and effects seen in untreated progeny. In: Fisher DA, Burrow GN (eds): Perinatal Thyroid Physiology and Disease. New York: Raven, 1975: 79–112.

389. Martin SM, Moberg GP. Effects of early neonatal thyroxine treatment on development of the thyroid and adrenal axes in rats. Life Sci 1981; 29:1683–1688.

390. Walker P, Courtin F. Transient neonatal hyperthyroidism results in hypothyroidism in the adult rat. Endocrinology 1985; 116:2246–2250.

391. Alm J, Lakshmanan J, Hoath S, et al. Neonatal hyperthyroidism alters hepatic epidermal growth factor receptor ontogeny in mice. Pediatr Res 1988; 23:557–560.

392. Spiegel G, Levy LJ, Goldner MG. Glucose intolerance in the progeny of rats treated with single subdiabetogenic dose of alloxan. Metabolism 1971; 20:401–413.

393. Csaba G, Inczefi Gonda A, Dobozy O. Hereditary transmission in the F₁ generation of hormonal imprinting (receptor memory) induced in rats by neonatal exposure to insulin. Acta Physiol Hung 1984; 63:93–99.

394. Csaba G, Ronai A, Laszlo V, et al. Amplification of hormone receptors by neonatal oxytocin and vasopressin treatment. Horm Metab Res 1980; 12:28–31.

395. Benediktsson R, Lindsay RD, Noble J, et al. Glucocorticoid exposure in utero: new model for adult hypertension. Lancet 1993; 341:339–341.

396. Herbst AL, Ulfelder H, Poskjanzer DC. Adenocarcinoma of the vagina: association of maternal stilbestrol therapy with tumor appearance in young women. N Engl J Med 1971; 284:878–881.

397. Herbst AL. The epidemiology of vaginal and cervical clear cell adenocarcinoma. In: Herbst AL, Bern HA (eds): Developmental Effects of Diethylstilbestrol (DES) in Pregnancy. New York: Thieme-Stratton, 1981: 63–70.

398. Sato T, Suzuki Y, Taketani T, et al. Age related change in pituitary threshold for TSH release during thyroxine replacement therapy for cretinism. J Clin Endocrinol Metab 1977; 44:553–559.

399. McCrossin RB, Sheffield LJ, Robertson EF. Persisting abnormality in the pituitary-thyroid axis in congenital hypothyroidism. In: Stockigt JR, Nagataki S (eds): Thyroid Research. VIII. Canberra: Australian Academy of Science, 1980: 37–40.

400. Sato SM, Mains RE. Plasticity in the adrenocorticotropin-related peptides produced by primary cultures of neonatal rat pituitary. Endocrinology 1988; 122:68–77.

401. Evans MI, Adzick MS, Johnson MP, et al. Fetal therapy 1994. Curr Opin Obstet Gynecol 1994; 6:58–64.

402. Donner C, Vermeylen D, Kirkpatrick C, et al. Management of the growth-restricted fetus: the role of noninvasive tests and fetal blood sampling. Obstet Gynecol 1995; 85:965–970.

403. Garmel SH, D'Alton ME. Fetal ultrasonography. West J Med 1993; 159:273–285.

404. Harrison MR. Fetal surgery. West J Med 1993; 159:341–349.

405. O'Keane JA, Yuen BH, Farquharson DF, et al. Endocrine response to selective embryocide in a gonadotropin-induced quintuplet pregnancy. Am J Obstet Gynecol 1988; 158:364–367.

406. Morales WJ, O'Brien WF, Angel JL, et al. Fetal lung maturation: the combined use of corticosteroids and thyrotropin releasing hormone. Obstet Gynecol 1989; 73:111–116.

407. Forest MG, David M, Morel Y. Prenatal diagnosis and treatment of 21 hydroxylase deficiency. J Steroid Biochem Mol Biol 1993; 45:75–82.

408. Lightner ES, Fisher DA, Giles H, et al. Intraamniotic injection of thyroxine to a human fetus: evidence for conversion of T₄ to reverse T₃. Am J Obstet Gynecol 1977; 127:487–490.

409. Wallace C, Couch R, Ginsberg J. Fetal thyrotoxicosis: a case report and recommedations for prediction, diagnosis, and treatment. Thyroid 1995; 5:125–128.

410. Check JH, Rezvani I, Goodner D, et al. Prenatal treatment of thyrotoxicosis to prevent intrauterine growth retardation. Obstet Gynecol 1982; 60:122–124.

411. Charlton V, Johengen M. Fetal intravenous nutritional supplementation ameliorates the development of embolization-induced growth retardation in sheep. Pediatr Res 1987; 22:55–61.

412. Gibson MJ, Krieger DT, Charlton HM, et al. Mating and pregnancy can occur in genetically hypogonadal mice with preoptic area brain grafts. Science 1984; 225:949–951.

413. Gash D, Sladek JR Jr, Sladek CD. Functional development of grafted vasopressin neurons. Science 1980; 210:1367–1369.

414. Freed CR, Breeze RE, Rosenberg NL, et al. Survival of implanted fetal dopamine cells and neurologic improvement 12 to 46 months after transplantation for Parkinson's disease. N Engl J Med 1992; 327:1549–1555.

415. Redmond DE Jr, Naftolin F, Collier TJ, et al. Cryopreservation, culture and transplantation of human fetal mesencephalic tissue into monkeys. Science 1988; 242:768–771.

416. Annas GJ, Elias S. The politics of transplantation of human fetal tissue. N Engl J Med 1982; 320:1079–1082.

417. Sanders LM, Giudice L, Raffin TA. Ethics of fetal tissue transplantation. West J Med 1993; 159:400–407.

29

DISORDERS OF SEX DIFFERENTIATION

Melvin M. Grumbach and Felix A. Conte

Under most circumstances the distinction between male and female is considered absolute, and these terms are often used to epitomize opposites. Usually, the components of an individual's sexual make-up are indeed dominantly of one gender and conform to the chromosomal pattern established in the zygote at the time of fertilization. Most sexual characteristics, however, emerge from identical bipotential precursors in the embryo, and a spectrum of differentiation is possible at each level of sexual organization.

The remarkable accumulation of knowledge over the past four decades and new and continuing insights in the field of sex determination and differentiation represent major landmarks in biomedical science. No aspect of prenatal development is better understood. Advances in embryology, steroid biochemistry, molecular and cell biology, cytogenetics and genetics, endocrinology, immunology and transplantation biology, and the behavioral sciences all have contributed to the understanding of sexual anomalies in humans and to the improved clinical management of these disorders. Major contributions to this understanding have stemmed from studies of patients with abnormalities of sex differentiation. Of special note are the advances that have resulted from application of the techniques of molecular genetics.

Failure at any of the sequential stages of sexual development, whether the cause is genetic or environmental, can have a profound effect on the phenotype and lead to complete sex reversal, various degrees of ambisexual development, or less overt abnormalities in sexual function that first become apparent after sexual maturity. For general works on sex determination and differentiation see references 1 through 17. The diversity of sex-determining mechanisms in multicellular organisms is extraordinary and varies from a repertoire of genetic sex-determining models, including the X chromosome/autosome ratio in fruit flies and worms and the evolution of the highly conserved, dominant, testis-determining, Y-linked gene SRY in mammals, to the temperature-dependent sex determination model in many egg-laying reptiles.[18–21]

NORMAL SEX DETERMINATION AND SEX DIFFERENTIATION

Sex determination and differentiation are sequential processes that involve successive establishment of chromosomal (and genetic) sex in the zygote at the moment of conception, determination of gonadal (primary) sex by the genetic sex, and regulation by the gonadal sex of the differentiation of the genital apparatus and, hence, the phenotypic sex. At puberty the development of sex-specific secondary sexual characteristics reinforces and provides more visible phenotypic manifestations of this sexual dimorphism. Sex determination is concerned with control of the development of the primary or gonadal sex, and sex differentiation encompasses the events subsequent to gonadal organogenesis. These processes are regulated by at least 50 different genes located on sex chromosomes and autosomes that act through a variety of mechanisms, including organizing factors, gonadal steroid and peptide hormones, and tissue receptors. Early embryos of both sexes possess indifferent, common primordia that have an inherent tendency to feminize unless there is active interference by masculinizing factors. The indifferent embryonic gonad develops into an ovary unless it is diverted by a testis-organizing factor regulated by the Y chromosome; female differentiation of the somatic sex structures (the internal and external genital tract) is probably independent of gonadal hormones and takes place in the absence of fetal testes whether ovaries are present or not. Thus, the sexual dimorphism in phenotype in placental mammals is mediated by the fetal testis and its dual hormonal secretions and not by the ovary (Table 29–1). When testicular secretions are present, male differentiation takes place despite an environment in which the concentration of circulating estrogens and progestogens is high.

Abnormalities of sexual development can be classified into two broad categories: (1) disorders of sex determination, which most often are caused by sex chromosome or gene abnormalities that affect gonadogenesis, and (2) disorders of sex differentiation, which usually are caused by a genetic defect, less often by adverse factors in the intrauterine environ-

TABLE 29–1. Ontogeny of Sexual Characteristics

Characteristic	How Identified	Origin	Factors Determining Differentiation

Chromosomal sex	Karyotype analysis	Sex chromosomes of parental germ cell	Normal: chromosomal composition of sperm
			Abnormal:
			  Nondisjunction during meiotic divisions of parental germ cells
			  Nondisjunction or anaphase lag in early mitotic divisions of zygote
			  Structural errors caused by chromosome breakage

X chromatin	Buccal smear; neutrophil spreads; smears or sections of other peripheral tissues	Late-replicating (heterochromatinized) X chromosome	Partial inactivation and heterochromatin formation of all X chromosomes in excess of one
Y body	Same as for X chromatin; also seen in sperm	Y chromosome	Distal heterochromatic segment of long arm of Y
Gonadal sex	Histologic appearance	Testis	Testis: SRY gene on the Y chromosome just proximal to the pseudoautosomal boundary; upstream and downstream autosomal genes
		Ovary	Ovary: ovary-determining genes on two X chromosomes [DSS(?DAX1)]
Genital ducts	Pelvic examination and imaging; pelvic exploration	Müllerian and wolffian ducts	Intrinsic tendency to feminize; müllerian involution requires AMH from fetal Sertoli cells and the AMH receptor testosterone stimulates male duct development
External genitalia	Inspection; investigation of urogenital sinus by urethroscopy and/or radiographic contrast study	Genital tubercle, urethral folds, labioscrotal folds, and urogenital sinus	Intrinsic tendency to feminize; masculinization requires androgenic stimulation before 12th fetal week Normal male: testosterone from fetal testes converted to dihydrotestosterone at end organ Virilized female: adrenal hyperplasia (21- and 11-hydroxylase deficiency); maternal androgen; aromatase deficiency Incompletely differentiated male: insufficient testosterone secretion by fetal testes; 5α-reductase deficiency; end-organ androgen resistance

Hormonal sex	*Secondary sexual characteristics*
	  Male: sexual hair pattern; voice; muscularity; phallus size
	  Female: breast development; rounding of contours; growth of reproductive tract; menstruation; ovulation
	Hormonal patterns
	  Male: testosterone secretion from testes; gonadotropin release
	  Female: cyclic secretion of gonadotropins, estrogen, and progesterone
		Hypothalamus and other neural centers; LHRH
		Pituitary gonadotropin
		Secretory cells of testes, ovaries, and adrenals
			Hypothalamus and neural centers: LHRH
			
			Pituitary: gonadotropin release governed by pulsatile secretion of hypothalamic LHRH and circulating levels of gonadal steroids and inhibin
			
			Gonads: differentiation of secretory cells and biosynthetic enzymes; stimulation by pituitary gonadotropins
			Hormone expression may be modified by end-organ sensitivity

Gender identity	Identification of self as either male or female	Appearance of external genitalia, environmental factors, sex hormones, genes, pubertal sex characteristics	Psychological environment during early years of paramount importance in establishing gender identity:
			  Attitudes of parents
			  Interactions of both sexes
			  Conformity of genitalia and secondary sexual characteristics at puberty to assigned sex
			Hormonal factors: adult sexual postures in lower species conditioned by hormonal factors in fetal and perinatal periods
			Unidentified genes on Y

ment. Before the genetic control of sex determination and gonadogenesis are discussed, a description of aspects of cytogenetics that are important to understanding abnormalities of sex determination is presented.

Chromosomal Sex and X and Y Chromatin

A systematized array of metaphase chromosomes from a single cell is known as a karyotype.[22] The meaning of this term is usually extended to imply that the chromosomal pattern in that cell typifies all the diploid cells of that individual or even of that species, although this is by no means always true. The 22 autosomes and two sex chromosomes (i.e., two X chromosomes or an X and a Y) are arranged and serially numbered according to size. The X chromosomes resemble the larger autosomes in the medium-sized group with submedian centromeres (group 6 to 12). The Y chromosome resembles the short acrocentric autosomes in chromosomes 21 and 22[22] (Fig. 29–1).

Each of the pairs of chromosomes can be identified with chromosome banding techniques.[22] The pattern of DNA replication in human chromosomes can be studied by pulse-labeling cell cultures with tritiated thymidine and preparing autoradiographs of the chromosomal spreads[23, 24] or by using the bromodeoxyuridine dye technique.[22] One of the two X chromosomes in the female replicates late during DNA synthesis in the cell cycle,[23, 24] and this X chromosome gives rise to the distinctive X chromatin or Barr body seen in female somatic cells (see later discussion).

Chromosome banding techniques differentially stain chromosome segments. Caspersson and associates[25, 26] introduced a fluorescent staining method referred to as the Q-staining method, in which substances such as quinacrine mustard or quinacrine hydrochloride are used to give a distinctive banding pattern (Q bands) for each chromosome (Fig. 29–2). The distal portion of the Y chromosome flouresces intensely. Pardue and Gall[27] subsequently reported a Giemsa staining technique that preferentially stains the centromeric regions of the chromosome; the areas of constitutive (centromeric) heterochromatin are known as C bands.[22] The Giemsa staining

technique[28] has been modified by use of a multitude of pretreatment procedures on fixed metaphase chromosomes (e.g., hypertonic saline, sodium hydroxide, variation of pH, temperature, cation concentration, proteolytic enzymes), which produce Giemsa-stained bands that are identical (with minor exceptions) to the Q bands described by Caspersson[25]; this method yields permanent preparations for conventional light microscopy (see Fig. 29–2), and the resulting bands are designated G bands.[22] Reverse (R) banding is a Giemsa staining method that produces a pattern of chromosome banding that is the reverse of either the Q or G bands. The structural components of the chromosome that give rise to the banding patterns are uncertain, but the differential distribution of base composition and the state of condensation of the chromatin appear to be involved. The Q bands result from binding of quinacrine stains to adenine- and thymine-rich (A-T–rich) regions of DNA, whereas guanine- and cytosine-rich (G-C–rich) regions of the chromosome quench the fluorescence. The G bands appear to be a consequence of differential binding of dye to nonhistone protein overlying the A-T–rich regions.

High-resolution chromosome banding procedures provide precise methods for identification of each chromosome and analysis of chromosome abnormalities, including chromosome rearrangements (see Fig. 29–2). A standard nomenclature for identification and designation of individual chromosomes, chromosome regions and bands, and structurally altered chromosomes is embodied in the report of the 1995 International System for Human Cytogenetics Nomenclature.[22] Table 29–2 summarizes the nomenclature applied to sex chromosome anomalies.

The identification of normal and structurally abnormal chromosomes, of supernumary chromosomes, and of specific DNA sequences and genes (chromosome microdissection) has been revolutionized by the development of fluorescence in situ hybridization (FISH), the labeling of normal or abnormal DNA with fluorescent dyes,[29–32] so-called chromosome painting.[30] With the use of special cameras (multiplex FISH) or Fourier spectroscopy (spectral karyotyping), a variety of fluorophores, and computer programs, the karyotype of normal and complex chromosome spreads can be determined rapidly.[31]

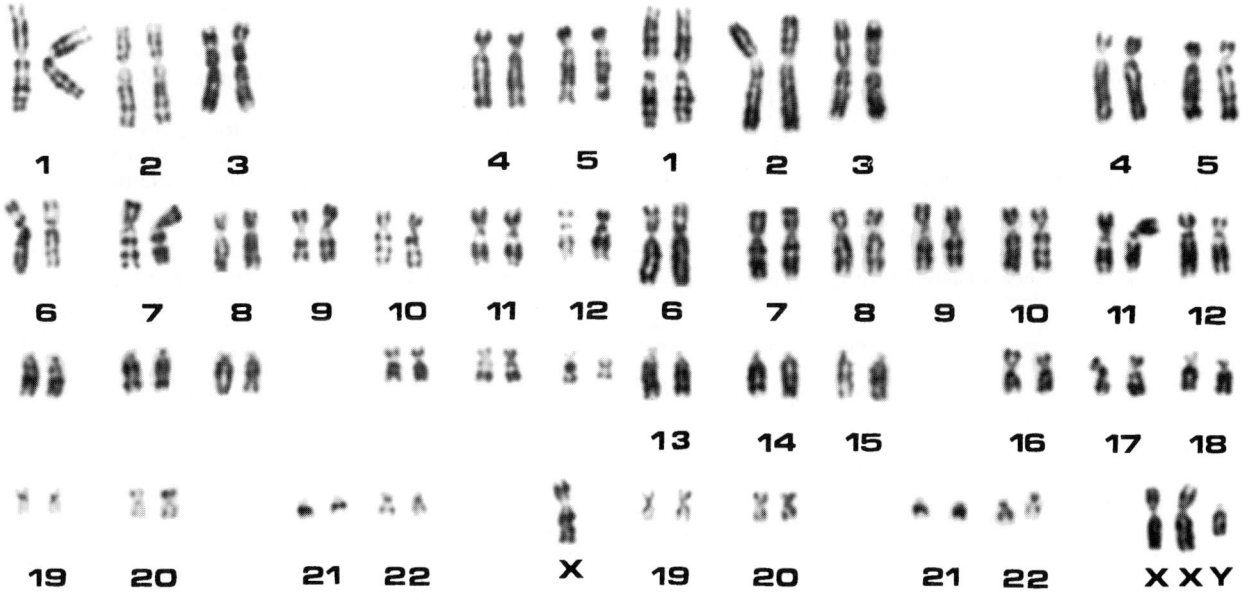

Figure 29–1. Typical G-banded karyotypes of patients with abnormal gonadal differentiation. *Left,* The 45,X karyotype of a patient with streak gonads, short stature, and physical stigmata of Turner syndrome. *Right,* The 47,XXY karyotype of a phenotypic male with seminiferous tubule dysgenesis (chromatin-positive Klinefelter's syndrome).

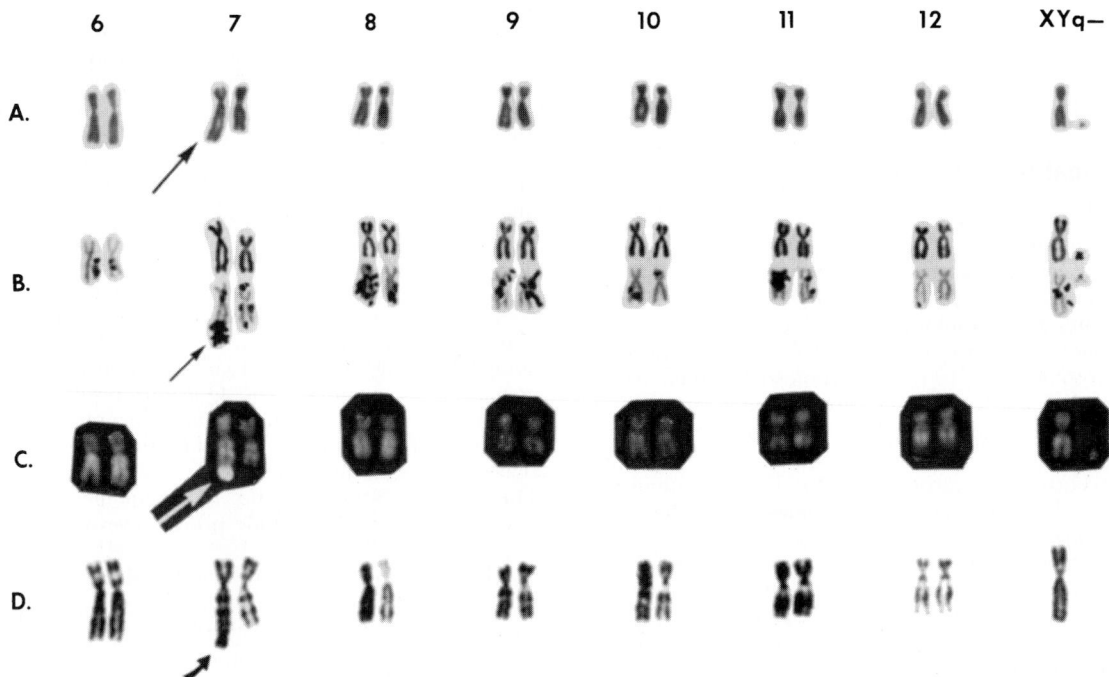

Figure 29–2. A partial karyotype of C group (chromosome numbers 6 to 12) and X and Y in a patient with a 46,X,t(Y;7) (q11;q36) karyotype. Standard Giemsa staining, autoradiography, fluorescent (Q), and Giemsa (G) banding techniques were used to identify the chromosome anomaly. *A,* The standard staining technique for karyotype analysis revealed an enlarged C group chromosome and a deleted G group chromosome. *B,* Autoradiography after incubation of lymphocyte culture with tritiated thymidine showed a late-labeling segment on the distal arms of the C chromosome and absence of a late-labeling segment on the deleted long arm of the presumptive Y. *C,* Quinacrine hydrochloride staining and fluorescence microscopy demonstrated a translocation of the brightly fluorescent segment of the long arm of the Y chromosome to the long arm of chromosome 7. *D,* Giemsa banding confirmed that the C group chromosome involved in the translocation was chromosome 7.

Mechanisms of Chromosome Anomalies

Chromosome errors can arise from faulty replication of the germ cells during spermatogenesis or oogenesis or from faulty mitotic division of cells in the zygote after fertilization.

ANEUPLOIDY. Aneuploid cells contain a total number of chromosomes different from that characteristic of the species. One mechanism producing aneuploidy is nondisjunction, which can occur during either mitotic or meiotic division. Nondisjunction is characterized by failure of either of a pair of sister chromatids or members of a pair of homologous chromosomes to separate during anaphase. As a result, one daughter cell receives an extra chromosome and the other is one short (Fig. 29–3). Aneuploidy can also be caused by anaphase lag, in which there is a simple loss of a chromosome from one or both of the two daughter cells, presumably because of failure of one chromosome to become properly oriented at the equatorial plate during metaphase. If both chromatids are lost, both daughter cell lines lack this chromosome.

If only one member of the chromatid pair is lost, the descendants of one daughter cell are normal, and those of the other are one chromosome short (see Fig. 29–3). Nondisjunction in the oocyte increases with advanced maternal age[33]; an abnormality in reciprocal recombination in the fetus manifested as a compromised exchange configuration predisposes to missegration during the completion of meiosis I (less frequently of meiosis II) immediately before ovulation 10 to 40 years later.[34, 35]

MOSAICISM. Mosaicism is the presence in an individual of two or more cell lines that differ in chromosomal constitution but originate from a single zygote. This condition can arise only from errors in mitosis after fertilization has occurred, but embryos with abnormal chromosomal make-up are prone to further errors of replication.[29] Mosaicism is more common than first supposed, and many of the seeming paradoxes between genotype and phenotype are attributable to studies in which mosaicism was not rigorously excluded.[36] The difficulty in detecting or, especially, in excluding sex chromo-

TABLE 29–2. Nomenclature for Describing Human Karyotypes Pertinent to Designating Sex Chromosome Abnormalities

ISCN 1995 (22)	Description	Standard Nomenclature
46,XX	Normal female karyotype	XX
46,XY	Normal male karyotype	XY
47,XXY	Karyotype with 47 chromosomes including an extra X chromosome	XXY
45,X	Monosomy X	XO
45,X/46,XY	Mosaic karyotype composed of 45,X and 46,XY cell lines	XO/XY
p	Short arm	p
q	Long arm	q
46,X,del(X)(p21)	Deletion of short arm of X distal to band Xp21	Xp−
46,X,del(X)(q21)	Deletion of long arm of X distal to band Xq21	Xq−
46,X,i(Xq)(q10)	Isochromosome of long arm of X	Xqi
46,X,r(X)(q22;q25)	Ring X chromosome	Xr
46,XY,del(7)t(Y;7)(q11;q13)	Translocation of distal fluorescent portion of Y chromosome to long arm of chromosome 7	46,XYt(Yq−,7q+)

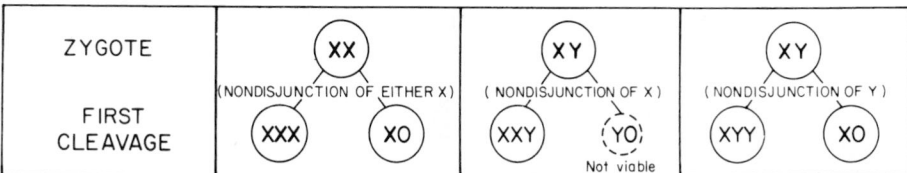

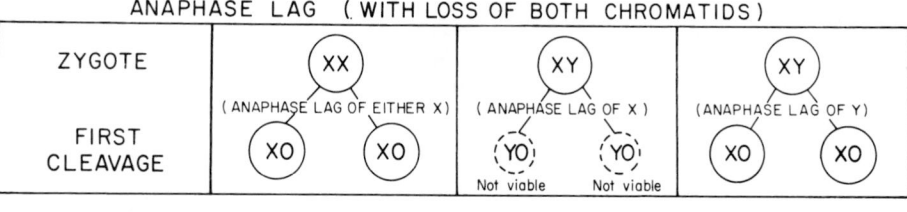

Figure 29–3. Daughter cell lines can arise from mitotic nondisjunction or anaphase lag during first mitotic division in the zygote. More complex mosaicism can result if the zygote is aneuploid or if replication errors arise beyond the one-cell stage. In females, nondisjunction or anaphase lag may involve either the maternal or paternal X chromosome. Deductions regarding the origin of X chromosomes in aneuploid patients can be made by correlating sex-linked traits with those in parents and by using specific DNA probes for analysis.

some mosaicism cytogenetically was formidable in the past, but recombinant DNA techniques provide more specific and more accurate detection.[37] The use of X and Y DNA probes together with the polymerase chain reaction (PCR) makes it possible to detect the presence and quantity of both X- and Y-specific chromosome material in tissues not amenable to routine cytogenetic analyses. For example, direct visualization of PCR products can detect 0.01% mosaicism for Y chromosome material in putative 45,X or 46,XX patients.[37] Therefore, more accurate phenotype-genotype correlations can be made in patients with sex chromosome mosaicism and/or structural abnormalities of the X or Y chromosome.

CHIMERISM. Chimerism is the existence in an individual of two or more cell lines, each of which has a different genetic origin. In the freemartin, a common form of intersex in cattle, chimerism is derived by admixture of hemopoietic and primordial germ cells between biovular twins of opposite sex through anastomotic placental channels. Although in humans it may be difficult to recognize the presence of chimerism if the separate cell lines have the same sex, the presence of cell lines of different sex is marked by a 46,XX/46,XY karyotype. Ford[38] discussed mechanisms by which chimerism can occur: (1) double fertilization (dispermy) of a binucleate ovum, (2) fusion of two complete zygotes or morulae before implantation, and (3) fertilization by separate sperm of an ovum and its polar body. The difference between mosaicism and chimerism depends solely on whether the lineage of the different cell lines are of the same or different genetic origin.

STRUCTURAL ERRORS. With the increased ability to characterize the morphology of human chromosomes by banding, FISH, and molecular biologic techniques, subtle as well as more obvious abnormalities of structure can be recognized. Structural errors result from chromosome breakage or partial deletion, often followed by improper reunion of the fragments (Fig. 29–4). Most structural abnormalities that are of sufficient size to be visible by light microscopy are characterized by an abnormally long or short chromosome. Chromosome fragments lacking a centromere or containing an additional functional centromere are usually eliminated from the cell. The following are the more common structural abnormalities (see Table 29–2).[22]

Isochromosomes are chromosomes with almost identical arms. They were thought to arise by transverse rather than longitudinal division of the chromosome (termed *centric fission*) (Fig. 29–5). This error involves primarily the X and Y chromosomes and usually results in a chromosome consisting of two long arms (e.g., Xqi or Yqi). Isochromosomes may have either one or two centromeric bands, and some isochromosomes have subtle differences in banding patterns and size of the two arms. These features and the limited evidence that centric fission can occur in human cells led to the hypothesis that most Xq isochromosomes arise from breaks in the short arm close to the centromere (not by centromeric misdivision), with fusion of the sister chromatids, followed by normal division of the centromere and duplication of the entire chromatid to form an isochromosome; this view was supported by detailed molecular studies[39, 40] (see Fig. 29–5).

PRODUCTION OF SOME STRUCTURAL ABNORMALITIES OF A CHROMOSOME

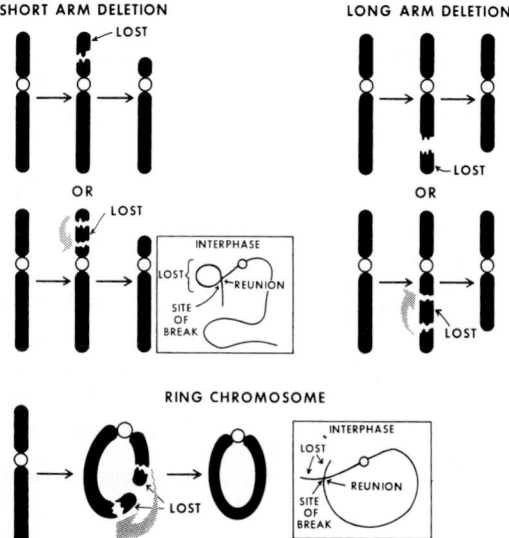

Figure 29–4. A diagram of chromosome breakage and recombination to form long and short arm deletions and ring chromosomes. Deleted segments may also be transposed to terminal portions of other chromosomes as additions, or there may be reciprocal translocations of deleted segments with those from another chromosome.

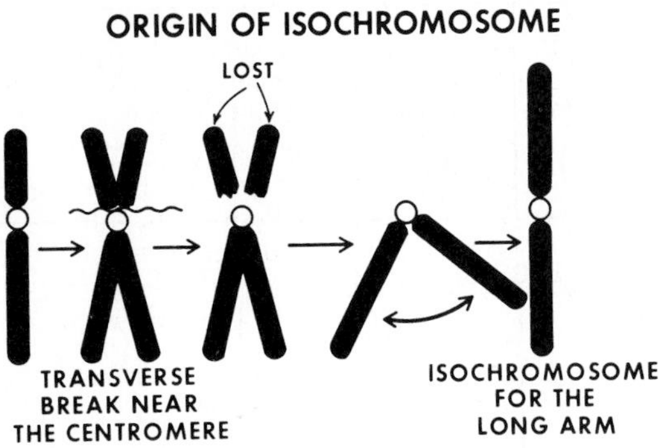

ORIGIN OF ISOCHROMOSOME

Figure 29–5. Long arm isochromosomes of the X, Xqi, were postulated to result from centric fission, that is, transverse rather than longitudinal division of the centromere. A more likely mechanism is shown. A deletion occurs above the centromere on the short arm. Fusion of chromatids followed by division of the centromere and duplication of entire chromatid results in an isochromosome with either one or two centromeres. The acentric fragment is lost.

Deletion is characterized by detachment and loss of a portion of a chromosome. The notation q− refers to deletion of a portion of the long arm, and p− refers to deletion of a portion of the short arm.

Duplication occurs when a deleted segment is incorporated into another chromosome, usually the other member of a homologous pair.

Translocations are characterized by exchanges of chromosome segments between two chromosomes.

Ring chromosomes—for example, a ring X (Xr)—arise by deletions from the ends (telomeres) of a chromosome, with reunion of the new distal portions to form a ring (see Fig. 29–4).

Biologic Functions of the Y Chromosome

Until the advent of human chromosome analysis, it was widely believed that the Y chromosome (Fig. 29–6) was inert and that male determinants were carried on the autosomes. The finding of a 47,XXY sex chromosome constitution in men with Klinefelter's syndrome and only a single X chromosome in women with the syndrome of gonadal dysgenesis (Turner syndrome) provided convincing evidence that the Y chromosome carries male-determining genes that can induce testicular development even in the presence of two or more X chromosomes. The presence of a Y chromosome causes testicular differentiation even in individuals with a 49,XXXXY sex chromosome constitution, whereas testicular differentiation

does not occur in 45,X individuals. In addition, the Y is essential to spermatogenesis. In subsequent work the testis-determining function was localized to the short arm of the Y chromosome.

The Y chromosome contains putative genes that influence stature in addition to the gene affecting growth located in the pseudoautosomal region of the Y and X chromosomes. For example, XYY boys have a mean final height of about 188 cm, more than 13 cm taller than their fathers.[641a] Whether the increased stature is related solely to the extra dose of the pseudoautosomal *PHOG/SHOX* gene (see below) or to other Y-borne genes is not known.

The length of the human Y chromosome varies as much as threefold in normal men. The length and morphology of the Y are heritable, are relatively constant in first-degree male relatives, and exhibit ethnic variation. Most of this variation is in the length of the long arm and in particular in the length of its distal, heterochromatic, brilliantly fluorescent segment in Q-stained preparations (see Fig. 29–6). This polymorphism in the size of the fluorescent portion and even loss of part of the distal nonfluorescent portion of the long arm are consistent with normal male sex differentiation and are not associated with known phenotypic effects; consequently, it is likely that a large segment of the long arm of the Y is not engaged in gene transcription. The long arm of the Y contains highly repetitious Y chromosome–specific and non-Y–specific sequences of DNA. The euchromatic short arm and the proximal portion of the long arm of the human Y chromosome make up about 0.5% of the diploid genome (XY + 44 autosomes).

The euchromatic portion of the Y chromosome[41] contains two regions, a Y-specific segment and regions at the distal ends of the short and long arms—the so-called pseudoautosomal regions (PARs)—that are homologous to the distal ends of the short and the long arms, respectively, of the X chromosome. The X and Y chromosomes pair and recombine obligately only along these small segments at the distal ends during meiosis. They form chiasmata primarily in the PARs of the short arms, thereby maintaining sequence homology and allowing for the proper distribution of sex chromosomes to the daughter cells. This process is critical to sex determination.[42–44] One gene identified in the PAR of the long arm of the X and Y chromosomes is the interleukin-9 receptor (*IL9R*).[45] Genes on the distal short and long arms of the X and Y are paired and are not subject to dosage compensation (i.e., gene inactivation); hence, they are expressed like autosomal genes rather than sex-linked genes, leading to the PAR designation (see Fig. 29–6).

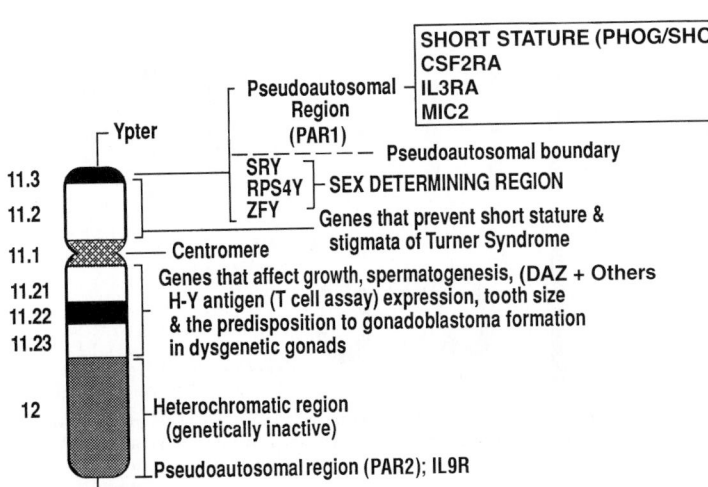

Figure 29–6. Diagrammatic representation of a G-banded Y chromosome. Y-linked genes are shown. *PHOG*, pseudoautosomal homeobox-containing osteogenic gene; *CSF2RA*, colony-stimulating factor-2α receptor; *IL3RA*, interleukin-3α receptor; *MIC2*, a cell-surface antigen recognized by monoclonal antibody 12E7; *SRY*, sex-determining region Y; *ZFY*, zinc finger Y; *RPS4Y*, ribosomal protein S4 Y; *DAZ*, deleted in azoospermia; *IL9R*, interleukin-9 receptor.

At least eight genes are located on the PAR of the short arm of the X and Y chromosomes.[46–48] The short arm PAR (PAR1) is about 2500 kb in length, the boundaries being demarcated distally by the telomeres of the X and Y chromosomes and proximally by the Alu repeat sequence on the Y chromosome.[49] The PARs of the X and Y chromosomes are 99% homologous distal to the Alu sequence.[49] Distally on the short arm PAR is CSF2RA, which encodes the α subunit of the granulocyte colony-stimulating factor receptor.[46, 47] Proximal to CSF2RA is IL3RA (encoding the α subunit for the IL-3A receptor), followed by ANT3 (adenine nucleotide translocase), ASMT (acetyl serotonin methyl transferase), XE7 (function unknown), MIC2, and, at the PAR boundary, PBDY (a gene that is not transcribed by the Y chromosome but whose homologue is PBDX on the X chromosome, a candidate for the XG locus).[46, 47]

The association between short stature and deletions of either Xp or Yp[50] suggests that a gene for stature is present in the distal 700 kb of the PAR1, since patients with only a single copy of this region have short stature. A gene from this 700-kb distal PAR region of Xp and Yp (PAR1), called PHOG (pseudoautosomal homeobox-containing osteogenic gene), is expressed mainly in osteogenic cells and bone marrow stromal fibroblasts[48] and encodes a transcription regulatory factor. Its location in the distal PAR, the nature of its predicted protein, and its expression in bone make deletions of this gene a strong candidate for the gene responsible for the short stature in patients with gonadal dysgenesis.[48] An identical gene was cloned from a 170-kb critical segment of PAR1 and termed SHOX (short stature homeobox-containing gene).[48a] This gene (SHOX or PHOG), which is alternatively spliced, encodes proteins of 292 and 225 amino acids and was deleted in 36 patients with short stature and rearrangements on Xp22 or Yp11.3. Of 91 patients with uncomplicated idiopathic short stature, 1 had a nonsense mutation in the gene that produces a truncated SHOX protein,[48a] and the same mutation was detected in 4 other short family members in three generations.

The second region of the euchromatic portion of the Y chromosome is the so-called sex-specific region, which extends from the proximal boundary of the PAR to the heterochromatic portion of the long arm. Deletion analyses of the Y chromosome in 46,XX males and 46,XY females indicate that the segment just proximal to the PAR on the short arm of the Y chromosome carries a gene or genes critical to testicular organogenesis and subsequent male sex differentiation. A 35-kb region immediately adjacent to the PAR boundary contains a gene termed SRY (sex-determining region Y).[51, 52] This gene encodes a testis-specific transcript that exhibits structural homology to two DNA-binding proteins: Mc, a mating-type protein of the fission yeast Schizosaccharomyces pombe, and HMG-1 and HMG-2, so-called nuclear high-mobility-group proteins.[52] Proximal to SRY is a gene for ribosomal protein subunit-4 (RPS4Y), which has a homologue on the long arm of the X chromosome and whose exact function is not yet determined.[47] On the short arm of the Y chromosome proximal to RPS4Y is a gene that encodes for a protein that has 13 Cys-Cys/His-His zinc fingers and both an acidic and a basic domain and that has been termed ZFY (zinc finger Y).[53, 54] By analogy to similar zinc finger proteins, such as Xenopus transcription factor IIIA, the protein is thought to bind to DNA in a sequence-specific manner and to regulate transcription.[55] Two other genes on the proximal short arm of the Y chromosome are TSPY (testis-specific protein, Y encoded) and AMELY (amelogenin), the gene that encodes the major extracellular matrix enamel protein in the developing tooth bud.[47]

The genes localized to the euchromatic region of the long arm of the Y chromosome include a pseudogene for steroid sulfatase (STS),[56–58] a gene (SMCY) that controls the expression of histocompatibility Y (H-Y) antigen,[59] and a gene family, the Y-located RNA binding motif (YRBM), that may include a gene with a role in spermatogenesis, the azoospermic factor (AZF).[60] Another gene in this region, termed DAZ (deleted in azoospermia), encodes an RNA-binding protein and is expressed in the testes.[61] Both DAZ and one or more members of the YRBM genes have been found to be absent in a small proportion of men with azoospermia or severe oligospermia.[61–63] However, further studies are needed to define the precise roles of DAZ and the YRBM family of genes in spermatogenesis.

Other genes postulated to reside on the Y chromosome but not yet cloned include genes affecting height[64] other than SHOX (or PHOG) and genes that prevent the stigmata of gonadal dysgenesis.[65] A gene that predisposes to the formation of gonadoblastoma (GBY, gonadoblastoma locus on Y) in patients with an XY karyotype and dysgenetic testes[66, 67] has been sublocalized to a 1- to 2-Mb region (regions 3 and 4) near the centromere.

Y CHROMATIN (Y BODY). The fluorescent end of the human Y chromosome in metaphase, when stained with the fluorochrome quinacrine hydrochloride or its mustard derivative, is visualized as a small, brightly fluorescent body (Y body) in a high proportion of diploid interphase nuclei of cells from male buccal mucosal smears, lymphocytes and polymorphonuclear leukocytes in peripheral blood cells, hair root sheath cells, and cells grown in culture.[28] In 46,XY males a single Y body, sometimes bipartite in structure, is present in interphase nuclei (Fig. 29–7), whereas two Y bodies are detectable in more than 15% of nuclei in 47,XYY and 48,XXYY males (Table 29–3). In a small percentage of normal males (<0.05%), a small Y chromosome is present that lacks all or most of the distal fluorescent segment, and a Y body is absent in somatic nuclei. Q-stained X chromatin bodies have been observed in cultured female fibroblasts and certain other female tissues, but the intensity of fluorescence of the X body is less, and the size is three to five times larger than that of the Y body (see Fig. 29–7).

Biologic Functions of the X Chromosome

The biologic functions of the X chromosome are more complex than those of the Y chromosome. The X chromosome consists of about 160 Mb; as of 1997, landmark DNA sequences (sequence-tagged sites) have been determined at about every 75 kb over the entire X chromosome. Genes on the X have a critical influence on sex determination in both the female and the male and on the differentiation of the somatic sex structures in the male. More than 200 gene loci unrelated to sex development are known to be X linked.[8]

The organization of the X chromosome resembles that of the Y chromosome in that it has both a PAR on its distal short arm, homologous to that on the Y (Xp22.3→pter)[46] and an X-specific region (Fig. 29–8). The PAR of the X chromosome is the locus for at least eight genes (CSF2RA, PHOG, IL3RA, ANT3, ASMT, XE7, MIC2, and PBDX).[46, 47] The locus of the PBDX gene (the Xg blood group gene) is unusual in that it appears to span the PAR boundary on the X chromosome.[46, 68] Immediately proximal to the boundary of the PAR are the loci for many genes, including chondrodysplasia punctata, steroid sulfatase (STS),[56, 57] the gene encoding the amelogenin enamel protein in the developing tooth bud,[69] and the locus for the zinc finger X gene (ZFX),[70] which cross-hybridizes with DNA probes with the ZFY gene. Because the ZFX protein has 13 zinc fingers with 97% amino acid sequence homology to ZFY, it appears that both these zinc finger proteins may bind to the same nucleic acid sequences. Furthermore, ZFX is transcribed in 46,XX cell lines.[70] Genes in the area of the X chromosome immediately proximal to the PAR (i.e., XG [also

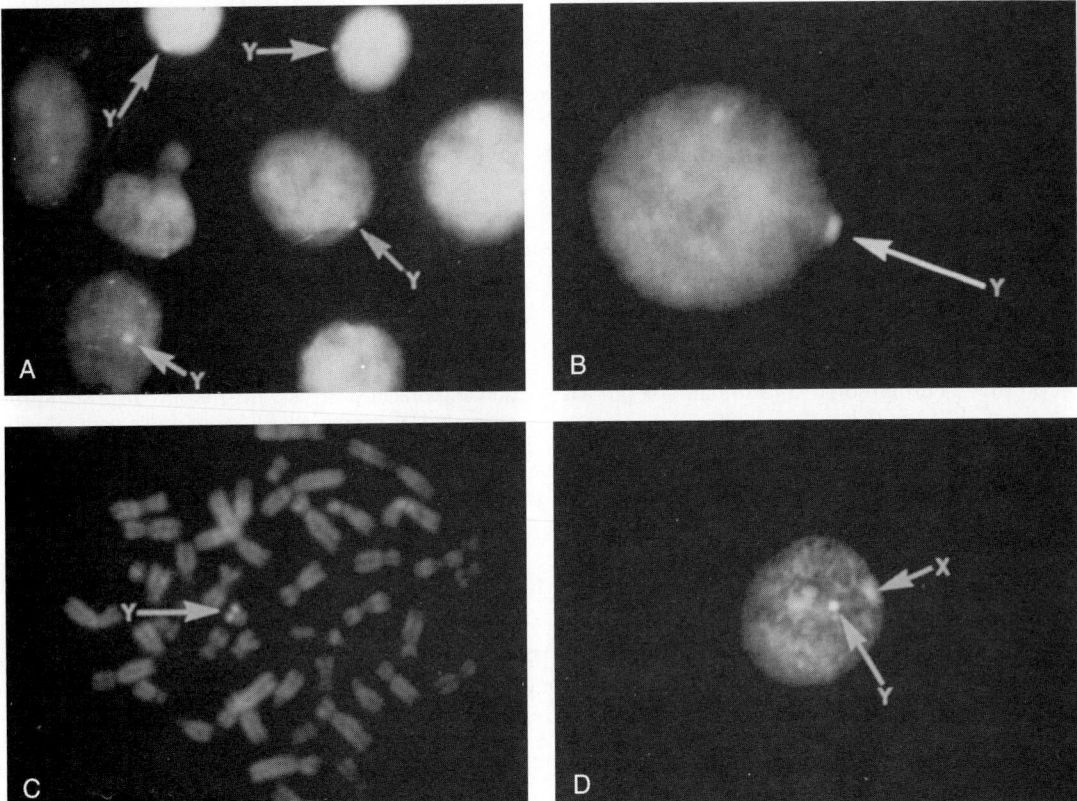

Figure 29–7. A, Q staining and fluorescence microscopy of interphase cells from a normal male, illustrating typical Y bodies. B, An enlarged photograph of one cell, showing a fluorescent Y body at the periphery of the nucleus. C, Metaphase chromosomes from a normal male, illustrating the brightly fluorescent distal segment of the long arm of the Y chromosome. D, An interphase nucleus in a buccal smear of a patient with a 47,XXY karyotype. A brightly fluorescent Y body and an X chromatin body (which exhibits much weaker fluorescence) were identified by Q staining and fluorescence microscopy.

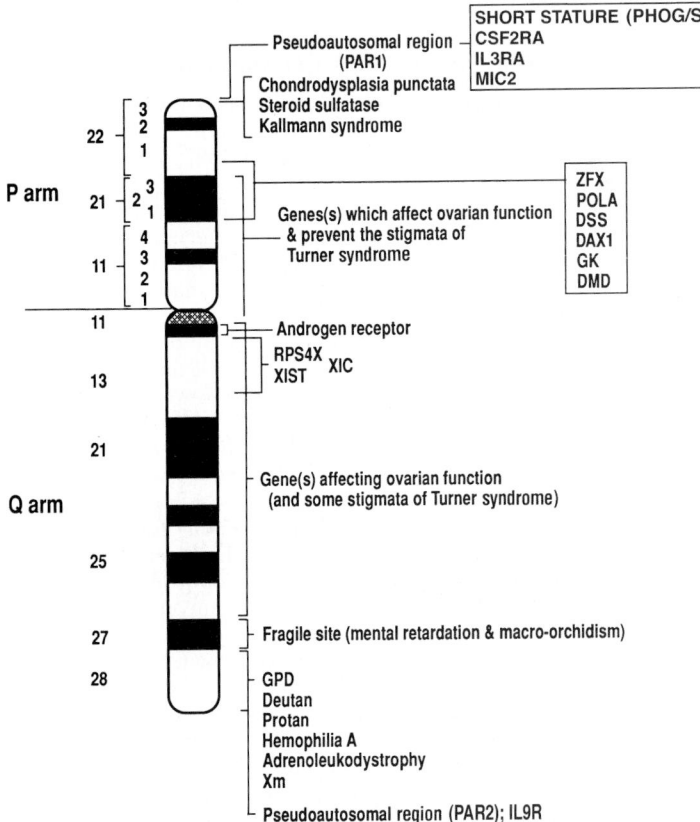

Figure 29–8. Diagrammatic representation of a G-banded X chromosome. Selected X-linked genes are shown. *PHOG*, pseudoautosomal homeobox-containing osteogenic gene; *CSF2RA*, colony-stimulating factor-2α receptor; *IL3RA*, interleukin-3α receptor; *MIC2*, a cell-surface antigen recognized by monoclonal antibody 12E7; *ZFX*, zinc finger X; *POLA*, RNA polymerase; *DSS*, dosage-sensitive sex reversal; *DAX1*, Dosage-sensitive sex reversal congenital adrenal hypoplasia critical region on the X chromosome-1; *GK*, glycerol kinase; *DMD*, Duchenne's muscular dystrophy; *RPS4X*, ribosomal protein S4X; *XIST*, Xi-specific transcripts; XIC, X inactivation center; *IL9R*, interleukin-9 receptor.

TABLE 29–3. Sex Chromosome Complement Correlated with X Chromatin and Y Bodies in Somatic Interphase Nuclei*

Sex Chromosomes	Maximal Number in Diploid Somatic Nuclei	
	X Bodies	Y Bodies
45,X	0	0
46,XX	1	0
46,XY	0	1
47,XXX	2	0
47,XXY	1	1
47,XYY	0	2
48,XXXX	3	0
48,XXXY	2	1
48,XXYY	1	2
49,XXXXX	4	0
49,XXXXY	3	1
49,XXXYY	2	2

*Maximal number of X chromatin bodies in diploid somatic nuclei is one less than the number of Xs, whereas maximal number of Y fluorescent bodies is equivalent to the number of Ys in the chromosome constitution.

termed the *PBDX* gene[68]], *STS, KAL1, ZFX*) escape X inactivation.[56] Other genes are postulated to reside in this region, including a gene or genes that prevent many of the somatic abnormalities found in the syndrome of gonadal dysgenesis.[65, 71, 72] Proximal to this region are genes that are not homologous to sequences on the Y chromosome and are subject to dosage compensation by X inactivation on all X chromosomes in excess of one.

Several genes that play a role in sex determination and differentiation are present on the short arm of the X chromosome. These include the Kallmann's syndrome gene, *KAL1*, deletion or mutation of which results in anosmia and hypogonadotropic hypogonadism.[73] *KAL1* maps about 1.5 Mb proximal to *STS* on Xp22.3[74] and encodes a neural factor that is critical for the migration of the neurosecretory neurons that secrete luteinizing hormone–releasing hormone (LHRH) from the olfactory placode to the hypothalamus.[73] A closely related homologue to *KAL1* is found on Yq11.2; however, it is nonfunctional.[75] Proximal to the genes for Duchenne's muscular dystrophy *(DMD)* and glycerol kinase *(GK)* in the Xp21 region is a locus that contains two overlapping genes, *AHC* (congenital adrenal hypoplasia) and *DSS* (dosage-sensitive sex reversal). A gene, *DAX1* (*DSS*-*AHC* critical region on the X chromosome)[76] has been cloned from this region. Deletions and mutations in the *DAX1* gene are associated in the male with adrenal hypoplasia and hypogonadotropic hypogonadism.[77] Duplication of the *DSS* locus, a 160-kb region adjacent to and overlapping the *DAX1* gene on Xp21, results in testicular dysgenesis and lack of masculization or incomplete masculinization in 46,XY patients.[78] In contrast, deletions of this locus have no effect on testicular determination and differentiation and subsequent in utero masculinization of 46,XY individuals; duplications in 46,XX females do not affect ovarian function.[78] *DSS* may have a role in ovarian development and function as a link between ovary and testis formation.[78]

Two X chromosomes are required in the human for normal ovarian differentiation and follicular maturation: 45,X individuals have bilateral streak gonads. Studies of patients with deletions of the X chromosome indicate that loci on both the short and long arms of the X chromosome are involved in ovarian differentiation and maturation.[65, 71, 72, 79]

The long arm of the X chromosome contains a large number of genes that are subject to X inactivation and are responsible for a wide variety of X-linked traits. The gene for the androgen receptor protein is located in the paracentromeric region of the long arm of the X.[80, 81] The *RPS4X* gene is also located in this region and is subject to X inactivation.[47]

This region also contains the putative X inactivation center, XIC, the site around which the X chromosome condenses to form the sex chromatin body and from which X inactivation spreads.[82]

X CHROMATIN (X OR BARR BODY). Whereas the Y chromosome is one of the smallest human chromosomes and is mainly concerned with testis organogenesis, the X chromosome is the eighth longest and contains about 5% of the total DNA content of the haploid genome (X + 22 autosomes). Furthermore, the X chromosome contains genes that encode functions involving every system in the body. Because females have twice as much of this genetic material in their cells as males, the biologic differences between the sexes should be far greater than is the case. Theories proposed to explain this paradox are an outgrowth of Barr's pioneering observations of the X chromatin body in somatic cells of females.

In 1949 Barr and Bertram[83] described the presence of a stainable chromatin mass at the periphery of the nucleus in resting ganglion cells of female but not of male cats. This distinguishing characteristic of the female sex is present in most mammalian cells and can be used as a cytologic means of assessing the number of X chromosomes in humans (Fig. 29–9; see Table 29–3).

The X chromatin body is usually planoconvex, with the flattened side in apposition to the inner surface of the nuclear membrane; in some nuclei it has a bipartite structure. It is about 1 μm in diameter and stains positively for DNA. In certain tissues, such as amniotic membrane, almost every interphase nucleus is chromatin positive. In buccal mucosal smears (the most commonly used preparation for determining the X chromatin pattern), the proportion of X chromatin–positive nuclei in females may be lower than in other somatic tissues, but in most studies they are detected in no less than 20% of nuclei.

In polymorphonuclear leukocytes in females, 1 to 15% of neutrophils (mean, 2.5%) have a drumstick-shaped, dense chromatin accessory nuclear appendage not found in normal

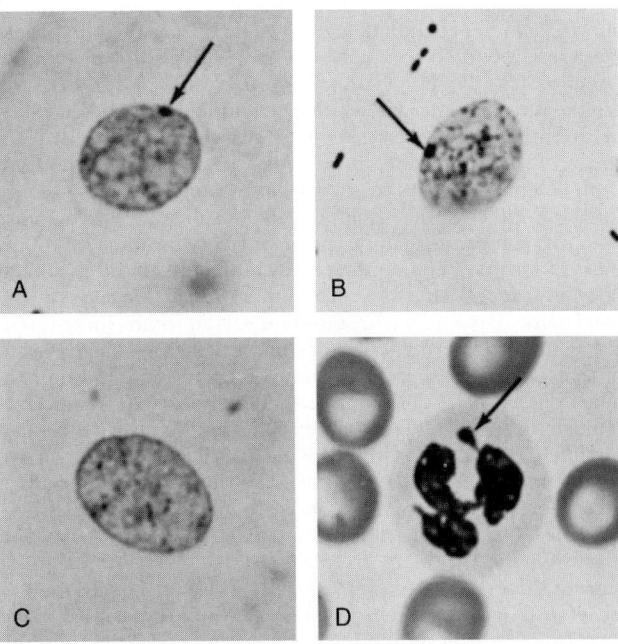

Figure 29–9. *A* and *B*, Photomicrographs showing the X chromatin body (Barr body, *arrow*) in the nucleus of buccal mucosal cells from a normal female (thionine stain, ×2000). Such cells are found in about 25% of well-preserved nuclei. *C*, A buccal mucosal cell from a normal male, illustrating absence of this body (thionine stain ×2000). *D*, A typical "drumstick" nuclear appendage *(arrow)* found in a variable proportion of leukocytes of female subjects.

males (see Fig. 29–9*D*). These appendages have the same significance as X chromatin in other somatic tissues.

In patients with more than one X chromosome, the maximal number of X chromatin bodies in any diploid nucleus is one less than the total number of X chromosomes. In 47,XXX females or 48,XXXY males, for example, at most two Barr bodies are present in diploid nuclei, whereas 46,XY and 45,X individuals are X chromatin negative (see Table 29–3). Abnormalities in shape and size of the X chromatin body can often be correlated with structural abnormalities of the X chromosome. The X chromatin body is small in females with one normal X and one deleted X chromosome (46,XXp −) and in those with one ring X chromosome (46,XXr). A large X body is associated with a long arm isochromosome (Xqi). When an X is structurally abnormal, the aberrant X chromosome replicates late and gives rise to the X chromatin (except when the structurally abnormal X is an X-autosome translocation).

X CHROMATIN AND GENE EXPRESSION. In 1959 Ohno and co-workers[84] reported the first evidence that X chromatin arises from only one of the two X chromosomes in the interphase nuclei of female somatic cells. The staining characteristics of such nuclei arise from the fact that a portion of one X chromosome is highly condensed (heteropyknotic); the other X, like the autosomes, is extended and filamentous.[85] This difference in staining quality betokens a striking difference in the functional roles of the two X chromosomes. By studying the sequence of incorporation of tritiated thymidine into replicating chromosomes, Grumbach and colleagues[23, 24] showed that the X chromosome that gives rise to X chromatin completes DNA synthesis later than any other chromosome and that the maximal number of X chromatin bodies in a single diploid nucleus is equal to the number of late-replicating X chromosomes (Fig. 29–10). These observations and the incisive genetic studies of Lyon, Beutler, and others led to the concept that only one X chromosome in each cell is genetically active during interphase, the other X chromosome being heterochromatinized and genetically inactive for most functions.[23, 24, 86–88]

The change in state (heterochromatinization) of one X chromosome in each female cell occurs during the late blastocyst stage, between the 12th and the 18th day in the human embryo. The female germ cells beyond the stage of oogonia are the only cell lines known to be exempted from heterochromatinization, a finding in keeping with the requirement for a second X chromosome for normal ovarian differentiation. Both X chromosomes in mouse oocytes are active and code for the X-linked genes for glucose-6-phosphate dehydrogenase and hypoxanthine-guanine phosphoribosyltransferase.[89] This observation has been confirmed in human fetal and postnatal oocytes.[90] In all somatic cells, either the maternally or the paternally derived X chromosome is randomly inactivated. Once this transformation is accomplished, the inactive state of that particular X chromosome is transmitted to all descendants of that cell. This control system appears to function as a mechanism of dosage compensation by which each female somatic cell functions virtually as if it had only one active X chromosome.[87, 88, 88a] The female, in effect, has only a little more active genetic material than does the male. This hypothesis is variously referred to as the Lyon hypothesis, the inactive-X theory, or the fixed differentiation hypothesis of X chromosome behavior (Fig. 29–11). Although inactivation of structurally normal X chromosomes in individuals with more than one X chromosome in their genome is usually random, instances of apparent nonrandom inactivation are well documented.[90] XX individuals heterozygous for X-linked immunodeficiencies, Lesch-Nyhan syndrome, or adrenoleukodystrophy may appear to have nonrandom activation of their X chromosomes due to postinactivation selection (i.e., in vivo selection

against those cells in which the normal allele is inactivated in tissues where the gene product is required).[90, 91] Nonrandom inactivation of the X chromosome has been reported in families with X-linked diseases and in monozygotic twins discordant for an X-linked disease.[90] If inactivation occurs normally as a random event in a small number of cells, 10% of "normal females" may show an 80:20 proportion of inactivated X chromosomes from one parent and even manifest symptoms of an X-linked mutant allele.[90] Nonrandom inactivation also occurs in patients with a structurally abnormal X chromosome: the structurally abnormal X chromosome is inactivated, unless it is a part of an X-autosome translocation. A skewed pattern of X inactivation also has been described in a multigenerational study suggesting that this character is controlled in some families by one or more X-linked genes.[92]

The fact that normal females function as genetic mosaics insofar as X-linked traits are concerned has been documented in the mouse and in humans. For example, Davidson and associates[93] demonstrated two populations of cells in females heterozygous for a mutant form of the X-linked gene for glucose-6-phosphate dehydrogenase (see Fig. 29–11). Heterochromatinization of all X chromosomes in excess of one also explains the relatively minor phenotypic changes in women with more than two X chromosomes, because the supernumerary X chromosomes are also heterochromatinized and therefore relatively inactive (Fig. 29–12). By contrast, trisomy for an autosome as small as chromosome 21, as in Down's syndrome, is usually associated with profound effects. Biochemical analysis of DNA methylation of active and inactive X chromosomes and studies with 5-azacytidine (which impairs methylation of cytosine) suggest that DNA methylation plays an important role in the maintenance of X chromosome inactivation, late replication, and sex chromatin formation.[94] DNA methylation differs in the two X chromosomes. The double-stranded palindromic cytosine-guanine dinucleotide clusters, the so-called CpG islands, commonly found at the 5′ end of genes, are methylated mainly in genes on the inactive X chromosome. The methylated cytosine residues serve to maintain the suppressed transcriptional activity and relative resistance to nuclease. The chromatin of the inactive X contains more unacetylated histones (histones H3 and H4) than the chromatin of the active X chromosome does.[95] Underacetylated histones bind more tightly to nearby DNA and inhibit transcription of DNA to RNA; in short, transcriptional silencing and down-regulation of gene expression. Acetylation, a common requisite for the activation of gene expression, is mediated by histone acetyl transferase A, encoded by the *HATA* gene.[96] The mechanism of the initiation and termination of X inactivation during the meiotic cycle is not known.

In contrast to the mouse, human X chromosome inactivation does not involve the entire chromosome. The heteropyknotic X in the human female is only segmentally inactive in terms of transcriptional activity. Genes on the PAR of the short arm as well as genes scattered along the short and long arms of the heteropyknotic X escape inactivation.[88, 97] Individuals with a 45,X or 47,XXY constitution, for example, have abnormalities in sexual development and in somatic features unrelated to sex. Further, as noted previously, the gene for the red blood cell antigen Xg (*PBDX* gene), the *STS* gene, and the *ZFX* genes escape inactivation and are active on both X chromosomes in the female; these genes have been mapped to the distal part of the short arm of the X,[56, 70] outside the PAR. Two genes, *XIST* (*Xi*-specific *t*ranscripts)[98] and *RPS4*,[99] which are located on the proximal long arm of the X chromosome, escape inactivation on the heteropyknotic X chromosome. Inactivation of the X chromosome is mediated by a *cis*-acting region of the X chromosome, the XIC, from which inactivation spreads along the X. The *XIST* gene is an essential component of the XIC, at Xq13.[88, 100–103]

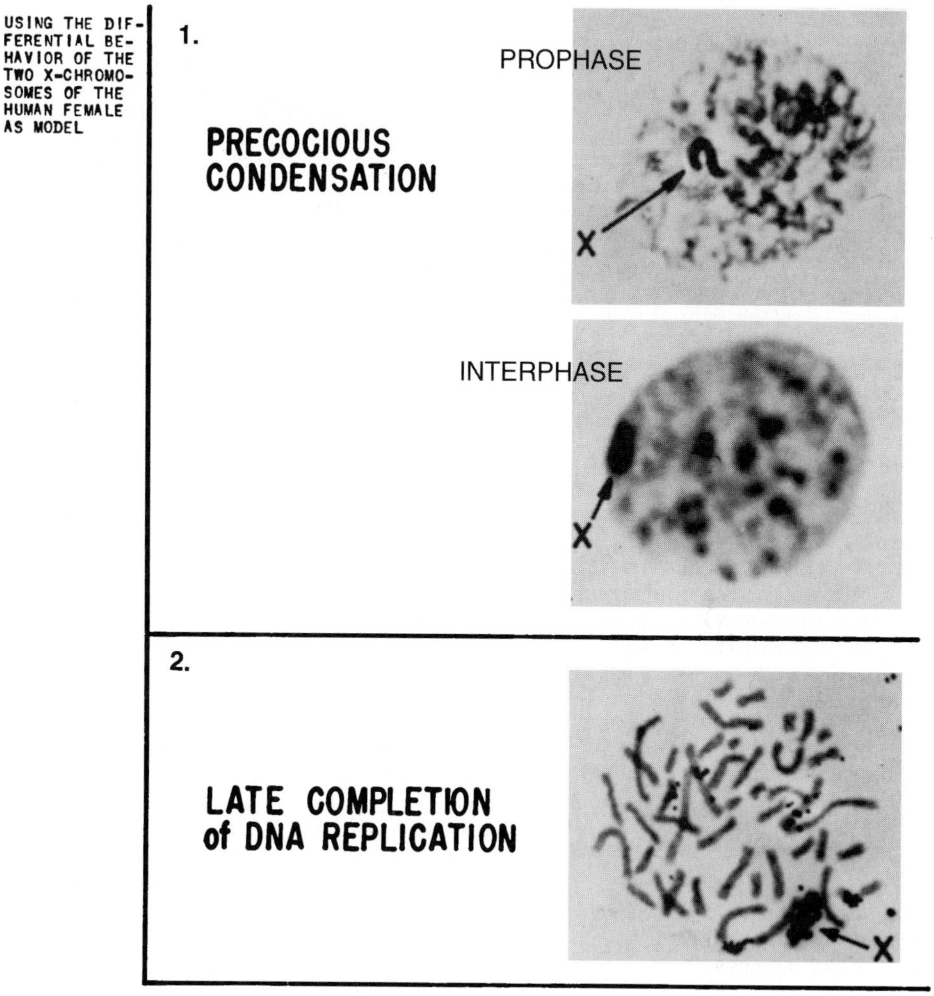

USING THE DIF-
FERENTIAL BE-
HAVIOR OF THE
TWO X-CHROMO-
SOMES OF THE
HUMAN FEMALE
AS MODEL

1.

PROPHASE

**PRECOCIOUS
CONDENSATION**

X

INTERPHASE

X

Figure 29–10. Characteristics of heterochromatin formation as exemplified by differential behavior of the two X chromosomes of the female in somatic cells. *1,* Precocious condensation of a large part of one of the two X chromosomes in prophase and formation of the X chromatin body in interphase nuclei. *2,* Delayed replication of DNA in one of the X chromosomes (*arrow* indicates silver grains overlying one X chromosome in the autoradiogram of metaphase chromosomes from a normal female exposed to tritiated thymidine late in the synthetic period). With some exceptions (PAR region, etc.) gene activity on the heterochromatic late-replicating X chromosome is silenced or modified. (From Grumbach MM. On the significance of sex chromatin. In: Second International Conference on Congenital Malformations. New York: International Medical Congress, 1964: 62–67.)

2.

**LATE COMPLETION
of DNA REPLICATION**

X

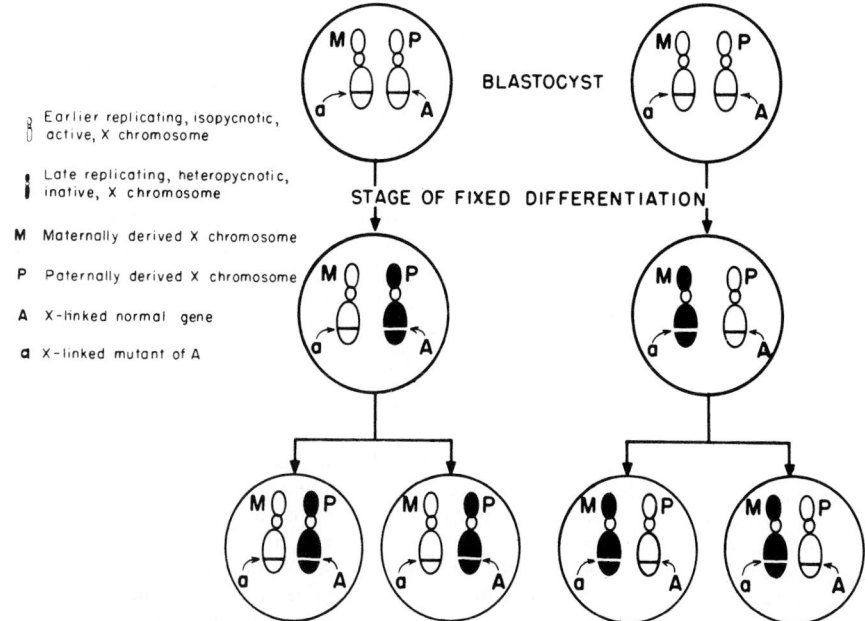

BLASTOCYST

○ Earlier replicating, isopycnotic,
   active, X chromosome

▌ Late replicating, heteropycnotic,
   inactive, X chromosome

M   Maternally derived X chromosome

P   Paternally derived X chromosome

A   X-linked normal gene

a   X-linked mutant of A

STAGE OF FIXED DIFFERENTIATION

Figure 29–11. A diagrammatic representation of the fixed differentiation or Lyon hypothesis of X chromosome behavior in somatic cells of the human female. At the late blastocyst stage (the time when X chromatin can first be identified), one of the two X chromosomes becomes heterochromatinized in each cell and gives rise to an X chromatin body; it is by chance in each cell whether this differentiation involves a maternally derived X (M) or a paternally derived X (P). Once differentiation has occurred, this characteristic is fixed in succeeding generations of somatic cells. Most of the genes on the heterochromatic portion of an X chromosome are suppressed or inactivated, thus serving as a means of "dosage compensation" for the greater number of X-linked genes in the female than in the male. This mechanism has an important bearing on expressivity and penetrance of an X-linked mutant gene in a heterozygous female. In the diagram, the maternally derived X carries a mutant gene (a) that is expressed only in cells in which this X is the isopyknotic, euchromatic active X (white X^M). Although the heterochromatinized X (black X) in this diagram is represented as wholly inactive, some loci on the heterochromatinized X do remain active and exert genetic effects. The female germ cell line beyond the oogonia stage is exempted from heterochromatinization.

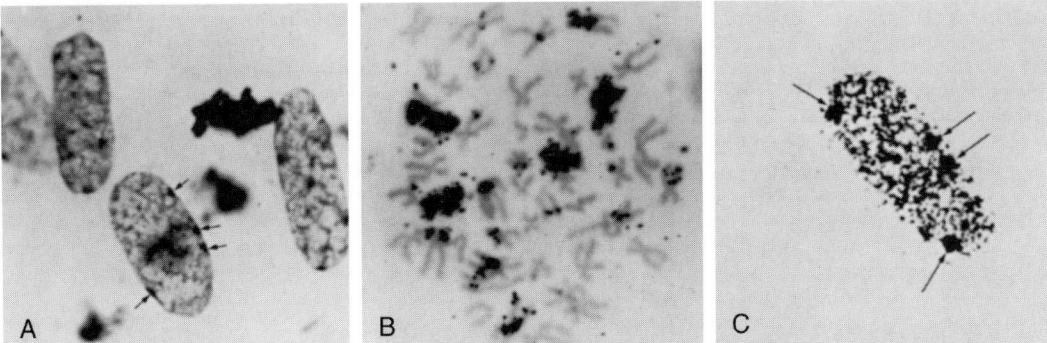

Figure 29–12. Diploid somatic cells from a girl with a 49,XXXX karyotype. *A,* Four X chromatin bodies *(arrows)* in an interphase nucleus from a culture of skin fibroblasts. *B,* Autoradiogram of metaphase chromosomes, illustrating four areas of high grain density overlying four of the five X chromosomes. *C,* An autoradiogram of an interphase nucleus in a culture of skin fibroblasts; four peripheral "hot" areas *(arrows)* of high grain density overlie four X chromatin bodies and provide direct evidence that each X chromatin body is derived from one late-labeling X chromosome. (Modified from Grumbach MM, Morishima A, Taylor JA. Human sex chromosome abnormalities in relation to DNA replication and heterochromatization. Proc Natl Acad Sci USA 1963; 49:581–589; and Grumbach MM. On the significance of sex chromatin. In: Second International Congress on Congenital Malformations. New York: International Medical Congress, 1964: 62–67.)

XIST is a unique gene in that it is expressed only on the inactive X chromosome.[90, 104] Its expression correlates with the inactivation of the X chromosome in female somatic cells and with meiosis in spermatogonia.[90, 106] Hence, its lack of expression suggests that the genes encoded by the X chromosome are transcriptionally active. Human and mouse *XIST* genes encode a long messenger RNA transcript that does not code for a protein and is retained in the nucleus associated with the inactive X chromosome.[90, 104] Knockout of the *XIST* gene in embryonic stem cells prevents X inactivation in *cis*.[102] Further, the insertion of ectopic copies of *XIST* into autosomes of murine stem cells results in the molecular and heterochromatic features of X inactivation, including XIST RNA association in *cis*, gene inactivation, late replication, and a decrease in histone H4 acetylation.[106a–106c] *XIST* apparently is not required for maintenance of X inactivation.[98, 105] The silent *XIST* gene on the active X chromosome is fully methylated at its 5′ end.[106] More studies are needed to clarify the relationship of XIST to the XIC[104, 106c] and to the mechanism of X chromosome counting[107] by which all but one X is inactivated.[107]

Some patients with a 45,X/46,X, "tiny" ring X chromosome karyotype differ in phenotype from other patients with gonadal dysgenesis with a ring X chromosome in their genome.[108] These tiny ring X chromosomes do not express *XIST,* have histone H4 acetylation at a level consistent with that found on an active X chromosome, and contain genes that are active.[108] These tiny ring X chromosomes that lack the *XIST* gene do not undergo X inactivation; as a consequence, the phenotype in these patients results from functional disomy caused by lack of dosage compensation.[108] In one instance, a deleted X and a large ring X that originated from the same maternal X chromosome (maternal isodisomy) escaped inactivation despite the presence of the XIC locus, suggesting that the X chromosomes were imprinted before X inactivation took place.[103]

Genes and Testicular Organogenesis

The genetic sex of the zygote is established by fertilization of a normal ovum by an X- or Y-bearing sperm, and the mechanisms involved in the translation of genetic sex into a testis or an ovary are understood in broad terms. From the early days of human chromosome analysis, compelling evidence was obtained for the regulation of testicular gonadogenesis by a gene (or genes) on the Y chromosome. Indeed, sex determination is essentially testis differentiation. The short arm of the Y chromosome contains a gene that controls testis determination and, hence, maleness. The gene acts in a domi-

nant fashion and leads to differentiation of the bipotential gonad as a testis. Several hypotheses have been proposed to explain testicular morphogenesis (Fig. 29–13). H-Y antigen and *ZFY* were proposed as the sex-determining genes and later discarded. More recent studies provide compelling evidence that the *SRY* gene is the master gene that controls male sex determination.

H-Y ANTIGEN. In 1955 Eichwald and Silmser[109] discovered in males of a highly inbred strain of mice the H-Y antigen, a male-specific cell membrane component encoded by the Y chromosome that causes rejection by female mice of skin grafts from male donors of the same strain. Antibodies to H-Y antigen were identified serologically in male-grafted female mice by Goldberg and associates in 1971 and were utilized for measurement of H-Y antigen. Initial reports suggested that H-Y antigen was a good candidate for the testicular determining factor (TDF) on the Y chromosome, but the lack of reproducibility of the H-Y antigen assay led to increasing skepticism about its role in testicular determination.[110] Finally, it was demonstrated that the gene for H-Y antigen is located on the long arm of the Y chromosome, separate and distinct from the gene for male sex determination.[59, 111]

ZFY GENE. In 1987 Page and co-workers[53] proposed that the sex-determining function of the Y chromosome is located within a 140-kb segment of the short arm of the Y chromosome. A gene in this region encodes a protein with 13 Cys-Cys/His-His zinc fingers at the COOH terminus (and a basic and acidic region at the NH_2 terminus).[112] By analogy to *Xenopus* transcription factor IIIA, it was suggested that this protein binds to DNA and/or RNA in a sequence-specific manner and regulates transcription[53] and that this zinc finger protein, ZFY, is the primary sex-determining signal on the Y chromosome. A sequence homologous to *ZFY* is present on the X chromosome *(ZFX)* in the Xp21.2-p22.1 region.[53] The latter finding initially suggested that X inactivation (dosage compensation) might play a role in sex determination,[113–115] but *ZFX* escapes inactivation, so X chromosome inactivation cannot play a role in this process.[70] Convincing evidence has shown that *ZFY* is not the testis-determining gene. Further, in metatherian species (marsupials), sex determination is Y dependent even though ZFY-related sequences are not located on the X and Y chromosomes of these animals but rather on autosomes.[116]

SRY GENE. The long quest for the TDF finally met with success with the identification of the *SRY* gene. In 1989, Palmer and co-workers[51] described three 46,XX males and one true hermaphrodite, the sibling of one of the 46,XX males. They were all ZFY negative, in spite of evidence for a Y-to-X

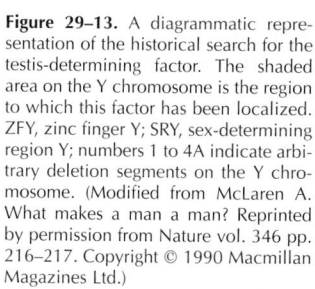
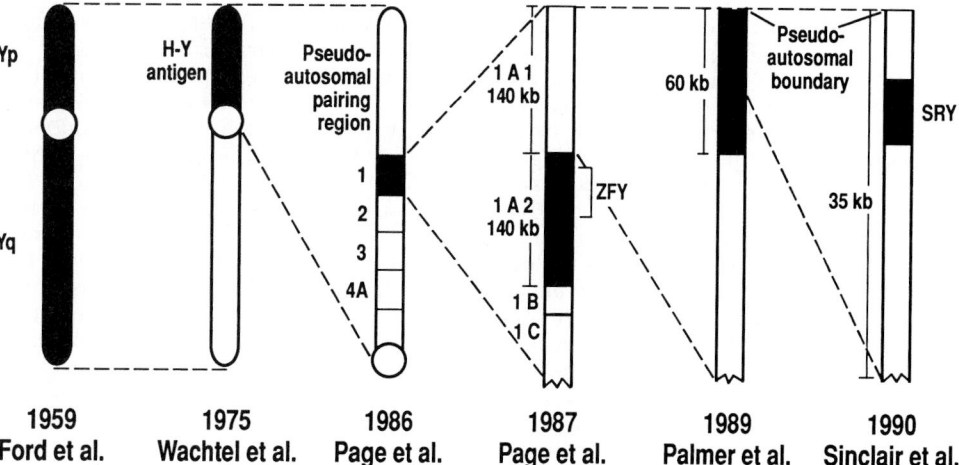

Figure 29–13. A diagrammatic representation of the historical search for the testis-determining factor. The shaded area on the Y chromosome is the region to which this factor has been localized. ZFY, zinc finger Y; SRY, sex-determining region Y; numbers 1 to 4A indicate arbitrary deletion segments on the Y chromosome. (Modified from McLaren A. What makes a man a man? Reprinted by permission from Nature vol. 346 pp. 216–217. Copyright © 1990 Macmillan Magazines Ltd.)

chromosome exchange as the mechanism of their XX karyotype in the presence of testes with male sex differentiation.[51] The fragment of Y chromosome translocated to the X chromosome in these patients involved sequences that were distal to the ZFY locus on the short arm of the Y chromosome. This demonstration of testes in patients with a Y fragment but no ZFY sequences, along with studies in marsupials[116, 117] and mice,[118] doomed the hypothesis that ZFY is the TDF on the Y chromosome. The Y-to-X exchange in these four patients involved Y-specific sequences located within 35 kb of the boundary of the PAR on the short arm of the Y chromosome (Fig. 29–14).[51] A 2.1-kb clone, pY53.3, was identified in this region within 8 kb of the PAR boundary.[119] This probe detected male sequences in a wide variety of eutherian mammals.[119]

Studies in mice established that Sry (the mouse homologue of the human SRY gene) is the TDF. Sry is present in the Sxr' mouse, a male mouse that has the smallest piece of Y chromosome known to code for testicular determination and differentiation.[119] Sry is absent in the XY fertile "female"

mouse,[121, 122] which has an 11-kb deletion involving the testes-determining region.[122] Further studies in the mouse model demonstrated that Sry is expressed in the embryonic genital ridge for only a brief period, from 10.5 to 12.5 days after coitus—a time when the genital ridge differentiates into a testes.[123] Sry expression is limited to pre-Sertoli cells in the genital ridge; in contrast, Sry in the adult testes is expressed in the germ cells.[124] The function of Sry transcripts in the adult mouse testes is unknown, since the transcripts are circular and are not associated with polyribosomes; they appear not to be translated into a protein.[124] Definitive proof that Sry was the TDF came from the demonstration that 46,XX mice with a transgene that contains a 14-kb piece of the Y chromosome including Sry differentiate as males with testes.[125] In the first series of animals, one 46,XX progeny that expressed the transfected Sry gene[2] was a well-differentiated 46,XX male that exhibited appropriate male sexual mating behavior.[125] Histologic examination of the testes revealed normal somatic elements, absent spermatogenesis, and degenerating germ

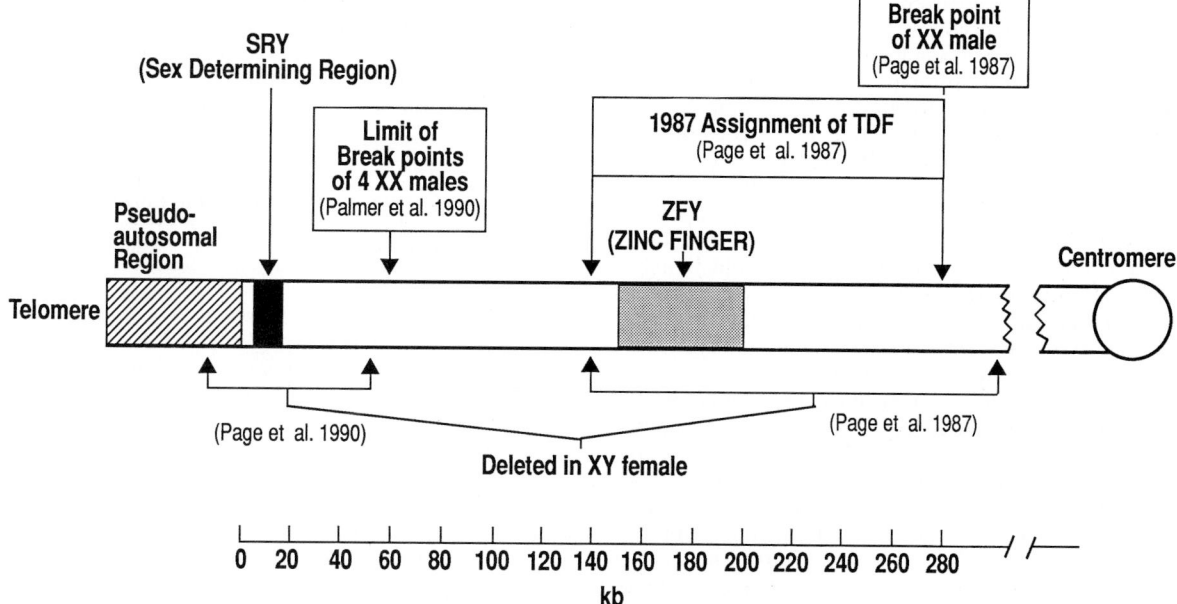

Figure 29–14. Localization of the putative sex-determining region, SRY, on the short arm of the Y chromosome. The zinc finger locus ZFY (the suggested site of the testis-determining factor in 1987) is shown, as well as the break points observed in four 46,XX males described by Palmer and co-workers.[51] The break points of one 46,XX male and one 46,XY female studied by Page and colleagues[53] are also indicated. Note that the 46,XY female has a noncontinuous deletion that involves both ZFY and SRY. (From Page DC, Fisher EMC, McGillivray B, et al: Additional deletion in the sex-determining region of the human Y chromosome resolves the paradox of Xt(y;22) female. Nature 1990; 346:279–281.)

cells.[2] The two other mice were 46,XX females; one was able to transmit the *Sry* transgene to her progeny, resulting in the generation of 46,XX males; 46,XX hemaphrodites; and 46,XX females.[2] That the *Sry* transgene produced sex reversal in only 25% of transfected embryos may be attributable to the incorporation of the transgene into a region of the genome where it is either not expressed, expressed at a low level, or expressed late in relation to gonadal determination and differentiation.[2] Nevertheless, this critical transgene experiment proved conclusively that *Sry* is the only gene on the Y chromosome necessary for testes determination and differentiation and that *Sry* is the testes-determining gene. Further, these studies indicated that Y-borne genes other than *Sry* are involved in the regulation of spermatogenesis.

Evidence in the human from sex-reversed 46,XX males and 46,XY females confirms the conclusion that *SRY* is the TDF. In humans, an aberrant Y-to-X interchange during paternal spermatogenesis can transfer Y-specific loci to the X chromosome,[126, 127] and 80% of 46,XX males have a variable amount of the Y chromosome translocated to the X.[127] All these patients are *SRY* positive.[127] In general, the *SRY*-negative 46,XX males have an increased prevalence of ambiguity of the external genitalia and siblings with true hermaphroditism.[127] The familial occurrence of 46,XX males and 46,XX true hermaphrodites who are *SRY* negative suggests the constitutional activation or inactivation of an X-linked or autosomal downstream gene (or genes) in the sex determination and differentiation cascade that is normally regulated by *SRY*.[128]

Approximately 15 to 20% of females with the complete form of 46,XY gonadal dysgenesis have inactivating mutations in the *SRY* gene.[127, 129] With two exceptions, all the mutations have occurred in the DNA-binding domain of the SRY protein, the high-mobility-group (HMG) box.[127, 129] Therefore, the data in the mouse and in humans with sex reversal support the critical role of *SRY* in the sex determination and differentiation cascade.

The human *SRY* gene contains no introns and produces a 900-base-pair transcript[130] that encodes a protein of 204 residues with three domains: an NH$_2$-terminal domain, a central DNA-binding domain consisting of a single HMG box, and a COOH-terminal domain.[4, 52] Comparison of nucleotide sequences of the *SRY* gene from different species indicates that only the HMG box is conserved.[131] The HMG box is an 80-residue domain that is homologous to the DNA-binding domain of a number of transcription factors, including lymphoid enhancer–binding factor-1 (LEF1), T cell factor-1 (TCF1), and a family of genes referred to as *SOX* (*SRY*-like HMG box) genes, in which the HMG region exhibits more than 60% sequence homology with that of *SRY*.[132, 133] The SRY protein binds specifically to the linear consensus DNA sequence A/TAACAAT/A and nonspecifically to cruciform (four-way junction) DNA.[134] The SRY-HMG protein is made up of three helices and NH$_2$- and COOH-terminal domains.[135] The HMG box has an L or boomerang shape and presents a concave surface to the DNA for sequence-specific binding.[135–137] DNA binding occurs in the minor groove of the DNA and results in a bend of approximately 85 degrees in the DNA, conforming to the shape of the HMG box.[135–137] Additional conformational changes in the DNA include helix unwinding and minor groove expansion.[135–137]

SRY has no recognizable transactivation domain.[2, 4] The control of gene expression by SRY may be mediated by the conformational changes in DNA that result in the approximation of distant regulatory elements of the transcriptional apparatus, thereby allowing them to interact with one another.[135, 136, 137] Analysis of mutations in the HMG box in women with 46,XY gonadal dysgenesis suggests that the spatial rearrangements (bending) in DNA produced by the HMG-domain protein are critical to its activity, as is its binding.[134] Mutations

in the SRY-HMG box that affect either binding or bending activity can result in the loss of transcriptional activity.[138] The transcriptional activity of *SRY* has been demonstrated in vitro with the use of FOS-related antigen-1 promoter constructs.[139] However, neither the upstream regulatory genes nor the downstream targets of *SRY* have been ascertained. Both the antimüllerian hormone (AMH) and the aromatase genes are candidate target genes for regulation by *SRY*, because their promoters contain putative specific consensus binding sequences for SRY-HMG. However, as Goodfellow and associates[2] noted, the consensus sequence A/TAACAAT/A is rather ubiquitous in the human genome, occurring at more than 10^5 sites, which makes it difficult to ascribe specificity to the interaction of *SRY* with a gene based solely on the presence of the consensus sequence in its promoter. Furthermore, the temporal sequence of *Amh* and *Sry* expression in the mouse genital ridge does not indicate a proximate sequential relation between these two genes.[140] In addition, humans with AMH gene or AMH receptor mutations develop testes.[140] To demonstrate that a specific gene is a target gene for SRY, one must establish that SRY both binds and bends the DNA specifically and that it directly initiates transactivation of the gene. Because of the lack of an apparent strict relation between the absence of *SRY* and testicular development in some 46,XX males and 46,XX true hermaphrodites, McElreavey and associates[141] proposed that the main function of SRY is to repress a putative gene termed "Z" which itself represses male development. At present, there are little data to either support or refute the repressor hypothesis.

Autosomal and X Chromosomal Genes. Several other genes on autosomes and the X chromosome participate in the testis determination cascade (Table 29–4). 46,XY individuals with duplication of the Xp21 region of the short arm of the X chromosome have dysgenetic gonads and consequent male-to-female sex reversal.[78] The presence of two active copies of a gene at this *DSS* locus impairs testicular differentiation in spite of a normal *SRY* gene.[78] The *DSS* locus maps to a 160-kb region of Xp21 and overlaps the gene for congenital adrenal hypoplasia and hypogonadotropic hypogonadism *(DAX1)*.[77, 78] Duplication of the *DSS* locus on one X in 46,XX females has no effect on ovarian differentiation (possibly related to X inactivation), and deletion of the *DSS* locus in 46,XY males does not affect normal testicular differentiation. These observations taken together suggest a putative role for the *DSS* gene locus in ovarian differentiation.[78]

The association of male pseudohermaphroditism with

TABLE 29–4. Genes Implicated in Gonadogenesis

Stage of Development	Chromosomal Locus
Primitive Genital Ridge	
Autosomal genes	
WT1	11p13
SF1	9q33
Gonads	
Testis	
Sex chromosomal genes	
Y chromosome: SRY	Yp11.3
Autosomal genes	
SOX9	17q24.3-q25.1
Unidentified	9p24-pter
Unidentified	10q26-qter
Ovary	
Sex chromosomal genes	
X chromosome: DSS (?DAX1)	Xp21-p22
Unidentified	Xq13-qter
Autosomal genes	
Unidentified	?

Wilms' tumor led to the identification of the Wilms' tumor suppressor gene *(WT1)*[142] and its important role in urogenital development.[143] The gene, located on 11p13, contains 10 exons, including two alternative splice sites in exons 5 and 7; therefore it can produce four different mRNA transcripts.[142–144] The full-length WT1 protein has four zinc fingers, is localized in the nucleus, and has an NH_2 terminus rich in proline and glutamine, all characteristics compatible with a role as a transcriptional factor.[142–144] *WT1* is expressed in fetal renal mesenchyme, in the primordial gonads (i.e., genital ridge), and in adult Sertoli and granulosa cells.[142, 143] Constitutive heterozygous mutations, most of which affect base pairs on one allele involved in the expression of amino acids in or near the third zinc finger, or heterozygous deletion can result in Wilms' tumor and dysgenetic gonads in both sexes as well as ambiguous genitalia in 46,XY males.[144] Conclusive evidence for the role of *WT1* in early renal and gonadal development has come from the mouse *WT1* gene knockout model.[145] Homozygous mutation of the *WT1* repressor gene prevents development of kidneys and gonads.[145] Gonadal development is arrested at a very early stage, and the gonads are streak-like.[145]

Steroidogenic factor 1 (SF1), an orphan (ligand unknown) nuclear receptor that shows sequence homology with receptors of the thyroid-steroid-retinoid family, is critical to the tissue-specific expression of cytochrome P450 (CYP) genes involved in steroid hormone synthesis,[146, 147] AMH synthesis,[148] and pituitary differentiation.[149] It is expressed in the mouse genital ridge at 9 to 9.5 days after coitus, in steroidogenic cells, in the hypothalamus, and in the pituitary gonadotrope.[147, 149] *Sf1* colocalizes with *Dax1* in many cell types, and its expression precedes or is concurrent with *Dax1* expression in the urogenital ridge and brain of mouse embryos.[150] However, *Dax1* expression is not compromised in the *Sf1* knockout mouse, indicating that *Dax1* expression is not dependent on *Sf1*.[150] The gene encoding for human SF1 is on chromosome 9.[149] It is the human homologue of the *Drosophila* gene FTZ-F1 receptor, which regulates the expression of the fushi tarazu *(FTZ)* homeobox gene during early blastoderm development in the fly.[151] Knockout of the *Sf1* gene in mice results in female phenotype sex differentiation in both sexes and the absence of both the adrenals and gonads.[152] SF1 deficiency has not been described in humans. On the basis of the mouse knockout experiments, a severely affected 46,XY individual would be expected to lack gonads and adrenals and to have a female phenotype. Müllerian duct development would be normal. Adrenal crisis would ensue in infancy because of the lack of adrenals, and at puberty sexual infantilism with low gonadotropins would be present. *SF1* has a very low level of expression in the placenta and appears not to be essential for placental progesterone synthesis. Accordingly, it is possible that *SF1* mutations in the human may not be lethal in utero.

SOX9. Campomelic dysplasia, a skeletal malfunction syndrome, is associated with an increased prevalence of 46,XY gonadal dysgenesis and sex reversal.[153] The campomelic dysplasia locus and a sex reversal locus have been mapped to 17q24.3-q25.1,[153] and a gene designated *SOX9* has been cloned from this locus.[154] Mutations in one allele of this gene are causes of both campomelic dysplasia and gonadal dysgenesis in 46,XY patients.[154, 155] 46,XX females with mutations in this gene have normal ovaries.[154–156] *SOX9* is expressed in the developing testes[156, 157] and in mesenchymal condensations, precursors of cartilage and bone.[158, 159] *SOX9* expression is apparently specific to the Sertoli cell linkage in the developing gonad.[156] Its expression during gonadal development suggests that it plays a critical role in the sex determination cascade, possibly downstream of *SRY*.[157]

46,XY individuals with deletions of the short arm of chromosome 9 (9p−) or deletions of the long arm of chromosome 10 (10q−) can have gonadal dysgenesis and sexual ambiguity.[160, 161] The postulated genes that affect testis organogenesis on chromosome 9p24 and 10q26.1-qter have not been identified.

A hypothetical scheme of genes on the sex chromosomes and autosomes that are implicated in sex determination and differentiation is shown in Figure 29–15. The upstream regulatory genes for *SRY* and its downstream target genes in the sex determination cascade remain to be determined.[162]

Genes and Ovarian Organogenesis

As early as 1958[163] it was suggested that two intact X chromosomes are required in the human for differentiation of the indifferent gonad into a normal ovary, in contrast to the mouse and some other mammals, in which an XO sex

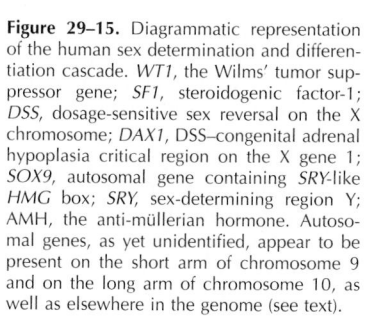

Figure 29–15. Diagrammatic representation of the human sex determination and differentiation cascade. *WT1,* the Wilms' tumor suppressor gene; *SF1,* steroidogenic factor-1; *DSS,* dosage-sensitive sex reversal on the X chromosome; *DAX1,* DSS–congenital adrenal hypoplasia critical region on the X gene 1; *SOX9,* autosomal gene containing *SRY*-like *HMG* box; *SRY,* sex-determining region Y; *AMH,* the anti-müllerian hormone. Autosomal genes, as yet unidentified, appear to be present on the short arm of chromosome 9 and on the long arm of chromosome 10, as well as elsewhere in the genome (see text).

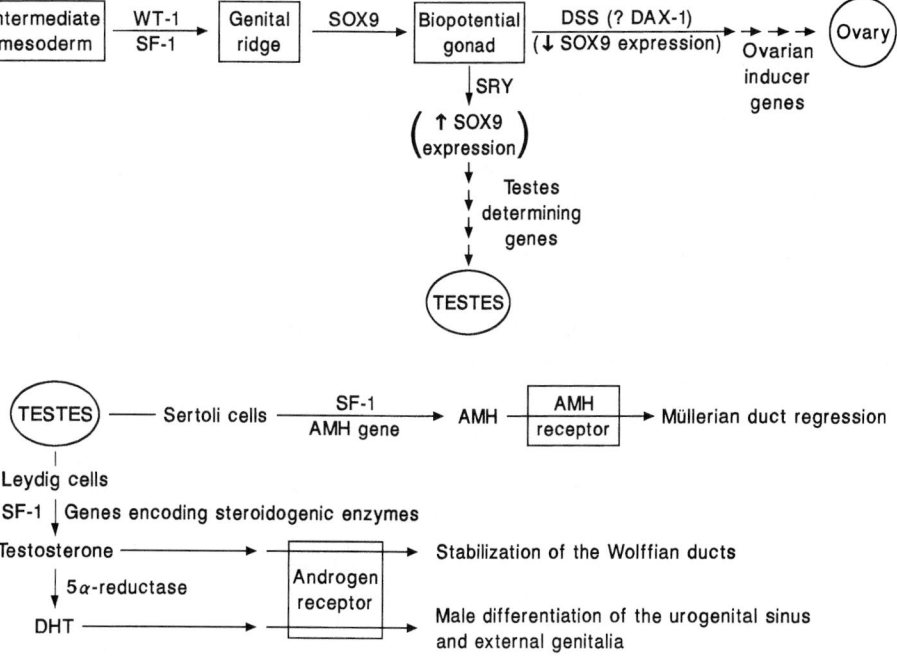

chromosome constitution does not prevent the development of a fertile ovary (although it leads to accelerated atresia of ovarian follicles). In 45,X individuals and in those with deletions of the short (Xp) or long (Xq) arm of the X chromosome, ovarian development commences in utero; however, oocytes usually do not survive meiosis, and folliculogenesis fails to occur or is defective. This results in loss of germ cells, oocyte degeneration, and, secondarily, gonadal dysgenesis (streak gonads). Both X chromosomes appear to be active in the germ cell and oocyte from the onset of meiosis to ovulation,[164] suggesting that genes controlling ovarian differentiation and function are located on both arms of the X chromosome and that viability of the germ cells and oocytes depends on the genetic contribution of both X chromosomes. The occurrence of familial 46,XX gonadal dysgenesis, which is transmitted as an autosomal recessive trait, suggests that autosomal genes, expressed through direct or indirect actions on the germ cell, are essential for ovarian organogenesis. A homozygous inactivating mutation in the gene encoding the follicle-stimulating hormone (FSH) receptor leads to ovarian dysgenesis and hypergonadotropic hypogonadism in family cohorts, as reported in Finland.[165] Other possible causes of familial 46,XX gonadal dysgenesis include a mutant autosomal gene that leads to a defect in development of the rete ovarii or in the synthesis or action of the putative meiosis-stimulating factor.

Gametogenesis

ORIGIN OF PRIMORDIAL GERM CELLS. Primordial germ cells of both sexes migrate to the undifferentiated gonads. In the 24-d embryo, germ cells are located in the dorsal endoderm of the yolk sac close to the allantoic evagination. From this site, the cells, increasing in number by mitosis, migrate during the fourth and fifth weeks to the hindgut and then through the dorsal mesentery to the primordial gonad in the urogenital ridge.[166–168] In the absence of primordial germ cells, the gonadal ridges in the female remain undeveloped, but germ cells are not essential for differentiation of testes.[71] Germ cells that fail to reach the gonads by the time of sex differentiation usually disappear, although they may persist outside the gonads and give rise to germ cell neoplasms.[168]

SPERMATOGENESIS. During early testicular differentiation the primordial germ cells become distributed throughout the primitive seminiferous tubules as progenitors of spermatogonia. A series of mitotic divisions occurs, and the prespermatogonia then enter a long quiescent phase during childhood, followed by an increase in mitotic activity late in the prepubescent period. With the onset of puberty, the basement membrane of the spermatogenic tubule becomes lined by proliferating spermatogonia that arise by the mitotic division of prespermatogonia.[169, 170] The spermatogonia in turn give rise by mitotic division to primary spermatocytes, which enter meiosis at puberty.

The formation of haploid secondary spermatocytes from the euploid primary spermatocytes is accomplished by the special form of cell division termed *meiosis*. Whereas in mitotic division both daughter cells receive duplicates of each of the 46 parental chromosomes, in the first meiotic division each daughter cell receives only 23 chromosomes, one from each of the homologous pairs (Fig. 29–16). Thus, half of the secondary spermatocytes contain 22 autosomes and an X chromosome, and the other half contain 22 autosomes and a Y chromosome. Each haploid daughter cell receives by random chance either the maternally or the paternally derived chromosomes of each homologous pair, but not both. This process ensures great diversity in the genetic composition of the gametes, because by independent assortment and recombination

of the 23 pairs of paternal and maternal chromosomes it is possible to obtain 2^{23} different kinds of gametes. This is not the only mechanism for ensuring genetic variation, however, because the special nature of the prophase during this reduction division facilitates exchanges of DNA (crossover) between homologous chromosomes. The details of this complex process are described in standard genetics texts. Secondary spermatocytes give rise to spermatids by a second meiotic division, but this division is more analogous to mitosis than to the first meiotic division, because daughter cells are again produced by a longitudinal split of the two chromatid filaments constituting each of the unpaired chromosomes (see Fig. 29–16); the haploid number is not altered.

Spermatids do not undergo further division but rather develop into spermatozoa by metamorphosis. Germ cells in the adult male are continually being renewed and undergoing maturation. Heller and Clermont[171] estimated that the complete cycle in adult males from spermatogonium to mature sperm requires about 74 ± 5 d.

The X chromosome undergoes inactivation in pachytene spermatocytes during meiosis.[170] The condensed sex chromosomes form a sex vesicle or XY body. X-Y pairing must occur during normal meiosis,[172] and X inactivation may be involved in the heterochromatinization of those regions of the X chromosome that are similar to but not homologous to regions on the Y chromosome.

OOGENESIS. Female germ cells pursue a different course. During ovarian differentiation, the primary germ cells undergo vigorous mitotic replication and successive differentiation into oogonia. When mitotic division ceases and the cells enter meiosis, they are then termed oocytes. Meiosis is influenced by the mesonephric tissue by means of a meiosis-stimulating factor. The period of oogonial proliferation results in a peak population of about 6 million to 7 million germ cells in the two ovaries at 5 mo gestational age, including oogonia, oocytes in various stages of prophase, and degenerating oocytes.[173, 174] Oocytes degenerate at different stages of meiosis. Only 5% of the peak number of germ cells in the fetal ovary reach the diplotene stage.[173] Formation of oogonia from primary germ cells ceases by the seventh month of gestation. Some oocytes remain in undifferentiated nests, whereas others form primordial follicles.[166] A follicle is formed when presumptive granulosa cells surround the diplotene oocyte and an intact basal lamina encloses this unit. If the oocyte is not enclosed in a follicle, it degenerates.[168] The number of primordial follicles in the ovary is maximal at birth, and the number thereafter diminishes. In the germ cells that survive, the oocyte is arrested at late prophase of the first meiotic division (diplotene state) and remains in this state from before birth until ovulation occurs many years later. The arrest of the oocyte in late prophase of meiosis is thought to be caused by a meiosis-preventing factor. The long life span of female germ cells, in contrast to those of the male, may explain the increased prevalence of certain chromosomal anomalies with advanced maternal age (see section on aneuploidy).

Before ovulation, the first polar body is extruded, thus completing the first meiotic division. The haploid secondary oocyte immediately begins a second meiotic division but remains in metaphase and does not extrude the second polar body until the ovum is penetrated by a sperm. The triploidy that is common in spontaneously aborted fetuses may be caused either by failure of extrusion of the second polar body (polygyny) or by double fertilization (polyspermy).

Differentiation of the Testis and the Ovary

The gonads of both sexes develop from anlagen located on the medioventral border of the urogenital ridge, adjacent

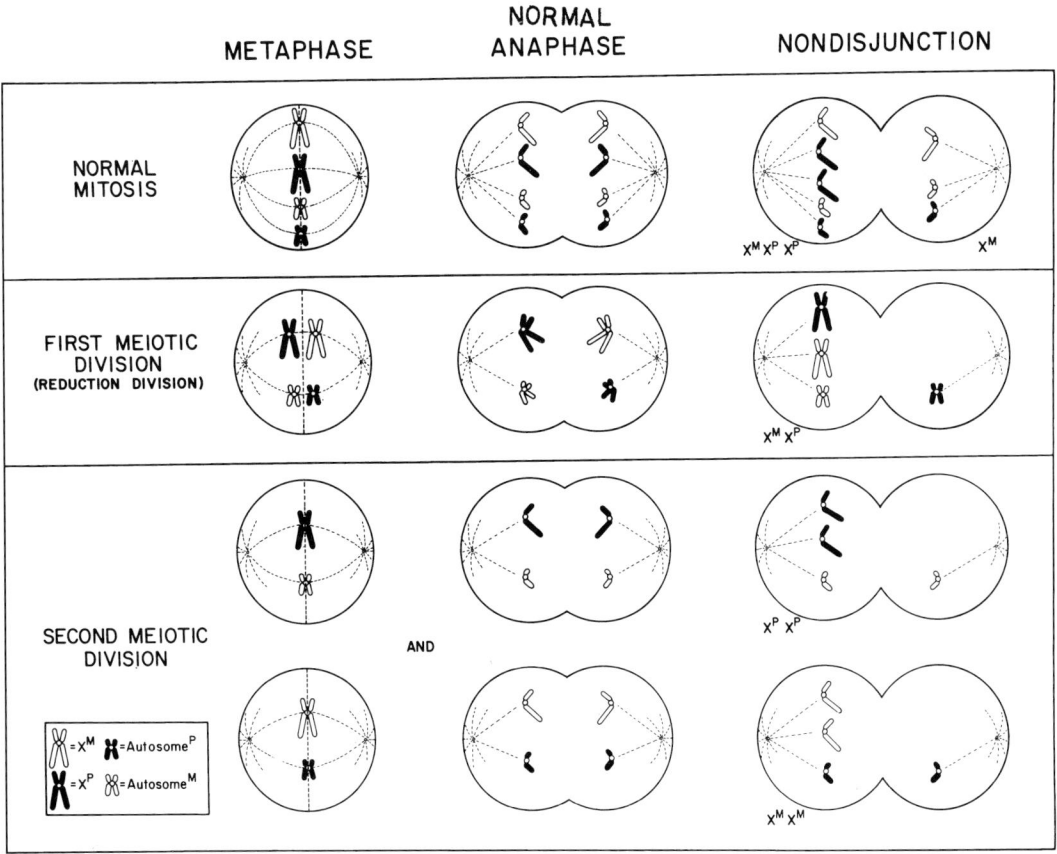

METAPHASE | NORMAL ANAPHASE | NONDISJUNCTION

NORMAL MITOSIS

FIRST MEIOTIC DIVISION (REDUCTION DIVISION)

SECOND MEIOTIC DIVISION

Figure 29–16. Types of cell division. A female somatic cell undergoing mitosis is represented. At the metaphase plate are two X chromosomes and two homologous autosomes of group 21 to 22. Division occurs through the centromere, giving rise to two daughter cells of identical chromosomal composition. Replication of each arm into two chromatids takes place while the chromosomes are extended and before the next metaphase. The first meiotic division involves pairing of homologous chromosomes. The centromere does not divide in this cell division. It is by chance whether the maternal (X^M) or paternal (X^P) member of each pair goes to the respective daughter cells. During the complex prophase of first meiotic division (not shown), multiple chiasmata are formed between the chromosomes of each pair, facilitating exchanges of chromosomal segments (crossing over) between them. During the second meiotic division, the centromere again divides, giving rise to daughter cells identical to the parent cell. This division more nearly resembles mitosis than the first meiotic division. Nondisjunction can take place in mitosis or in the first or second meiotic division; representative examples are illustrated.

to the kidney and the primitive adrenal (Fig. 29–17).[5, 168, 175] Until the 12-mm stage (approximately 42 d of gestation), the gonads of the male and female are indistinguishable on morphologic grounds and could potentially differentiate either as testes or as ovaries. The close ontogenic and anatomic relation between gonadal and adrenal cells at this early stage is noteworthy, because as differentiation proceeds nests of adrenal cells frequently separate with the gonad and are found as adrenal rests in the hilum of the mature ovary or testis. Such rests may become a problem in patients with long-standing untreated adrenal hyperplasia. Adrenal cell rests in testes, for example, may enlarge under persistent corticotropin (ACTH, adrenocorticotropin) stimulation and be mistaken for testicular tumors or true testicular enlargement.

The primitive undifferentiated gonad is derived from proliferation of the mesodermal coelomic epithelium, the mesenchymal cell mass in the urogenital ridge, mesonephric elements,[176, 177] and the large alkaline phosphatase–containing primordial germ cells that have migrated from the posterior endoderm of the yolk sac through the mesenchyme of the mesentery to the gonad.[167, 178] Little is known about the factors that regulate migration and proliferation.[178] According to Witschi,[166] the number of migrating germ cells in the human embryo is about 700 to 1300, and by the eighth week of embryogenesis about 600,000 germ cells are present, which later become either oogonia or spermatogonia. Lack of germ cells is incompatible with ovarian differentiation but does not prevent testicular morphogenesis. However, in the mouse,

genes such as the steel *(S1)* gene, which encodes a peptide growth factor (SCF, stem cell factor), and the proto-oncogene *c-kit* (also known as white spotting *[W]*), which encodes a tyrosine kinase receptor in the plasma cell membrane (a receptor for Sl), affect the proliferation, mobility, and migration of primordial germ cells to the urogenital ridge.[167, 179, 180] SCF, in its transmembrane second form, is expressed in Sertoli cells and acts as an adhesion protein, binding germ cells.[179] The precursor of the Sertoli cell of the testis and its counterpart in the ovary, the granulosa cell, are not established. Byskov and Høyer[16] and Wartenberg and co-workers[181] suggested a dual origin from both the germinal epithelium and cells of mesonephric origin. In the mouse the rete ovarii, derived from the mesonephric tubules, appear to give rise to the first granulosa cells.[16, 182]

There is a striking sexual dimorphism in the timing of gonadal differentiation. Under the influence of the testis-determining genes, testis organization begins at about 45 d of gestation (6 to 7 wk); the testis develops more rapidly than the ovary.[183] The ovary does not emerge from the indifferent stage until 3 mo of gestation, when the earliest sign appears: the beginning of meiosis, as evidenced by the maturation of oogonia into oocytes.[5, 184]

TESTIS. In the past it was believed that the testis is derived primarily from the medullary portion of the primitive gonad and the ovary from the cortical portion. According to this concept, the testis and ovary are not strictly homologous. Witschi and co-workers[185] suggested that in genetic males the

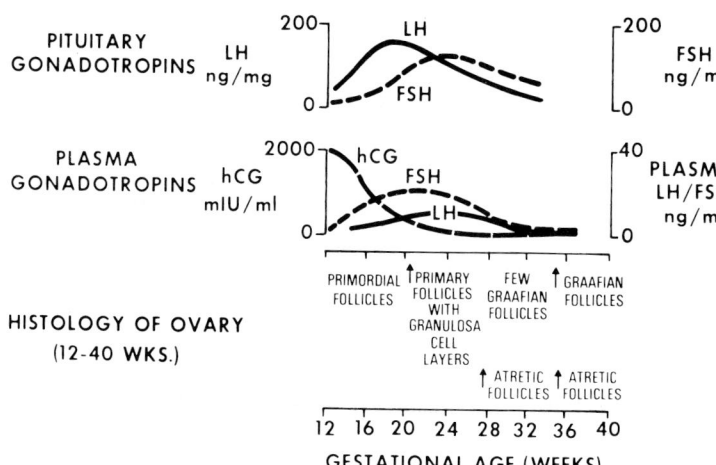

Figure 29–19. Comparison of the pattern of serum FSH, LH, and hCG and pituitary FSH and LH in the human female fetus during gestation with the developmental histology of the fetal ovary. (Adapted from Kaplan SL, Grumbach MM. Pituitary and placental gonadotropins and sex steroids in the human and sub-human primate fetus. Clin Endocrinol Metab 1978; 7:487–511.)

mary follicles are formed (Fig. 29–19). By the 20th to the 25th week the gonad has the morphologic characteristics of a definitive ovary. As discussed earlier, the maximal number of germ cells decreases from a peak of 6 to 7 million to 2 million at term. The last oogonia enter meiosis at 7 mo of gestation. In the late anencephalic female fetus, the ovaries are small and have a decreased number and hypoplasia of primary follicles, whereas the hilar cells seem to be similar in anencephalic and normal fetuses, suggesting that the hilar cells differentiate independently of the effect of pituitary gonadotropins.[168, 197, 201] Whereas the meiosis-inducing factor of the rete may be essential for meiosis and the formation of primordial follicles, the growth, development, and maintenance of follicles appear to be regulated in late gestation by fetal pituitary gonadotropins, mainly FSH.

The sequence and timing of events in gonadal organogenesis and their relation to the differentiation of male and female somatic sexual characteristics are shown in Figure 29–20.

Differentiation of the Genital Ducts

At the seventh week of intrauterine life, the fetus is equipped with both male and female genital ducts derived from the mesonephros. The müllerian ducts serve as the anlagen of the uterus and fallopian tubes, whereas the mesonephric or wolffian ducts have the potential to differentiate further into the epididymis, vas deferens (ejaculatory ducts of the male), and seminal vesicles. During the third fetal month, either the müllerian or wolffian ducts complete their development, and involution occurs simultaneously in the opposite structures (Fig. 29–21).

Jost[207, 208] demonstrated that secretions from the fetal testis play a decisive role in determining the direction of genital duct development. In the presence of functional testes, the müllerian structures involute and undergo programmed cell death and the wolffian ducts complete their development; in the absence of testes, the wolffian ducts do not develop and the müllerian structures differentiate (Fig. 29–22). The regres-

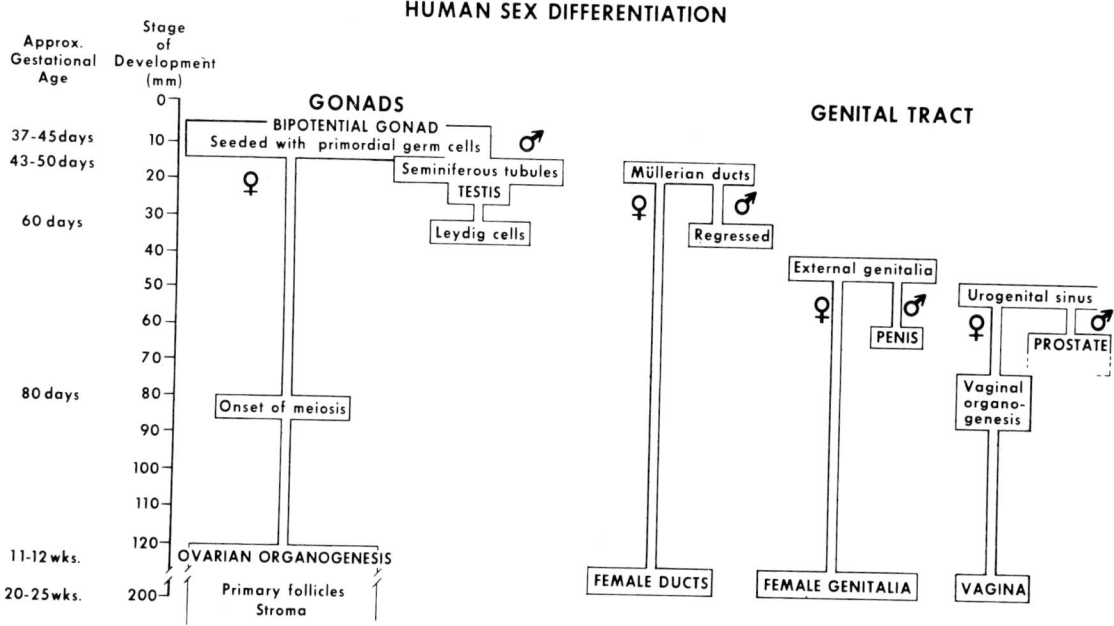

Figure 29–20. The sequence of sexual differentiation in the human fetus. The sequence as schematically depicted here emphasizes that testicular development in the male fetus precedes all other forms of sexual dimorphism. There is an inherent propensity of the gonads, genital ducts, and external genitalia to feminize, whereas masculinization requires Y chromosome–mediated (SRY) differentiation of the fetal testes. (Modified from Jost A. Hormonal factors in the sex differentiation of the mammalian foetus. Philos Trans R Soc Lond [Biol] 1970; 259:119–130.)

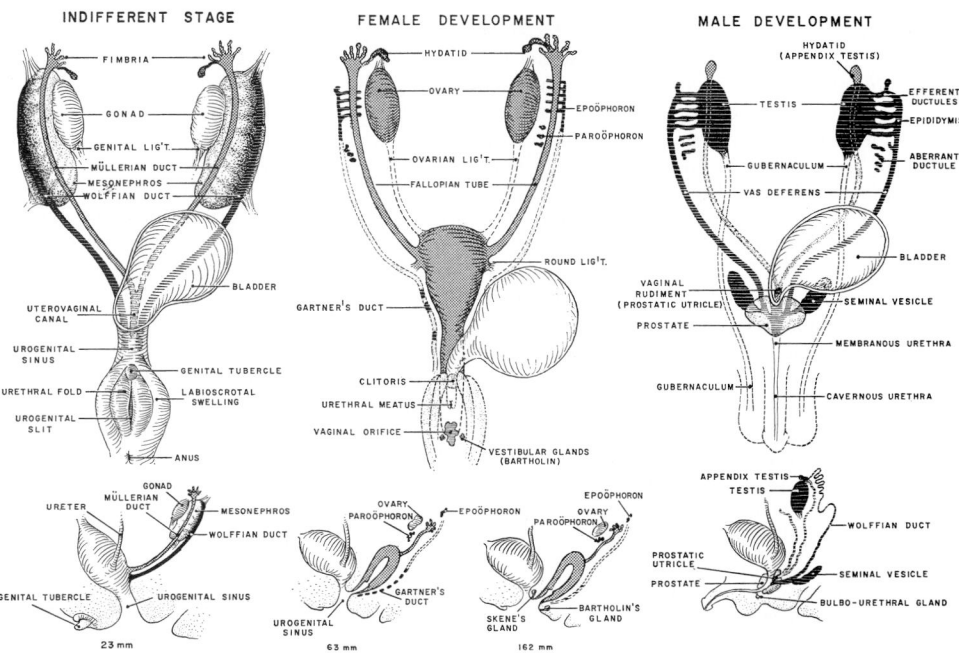

Figure 29–21. Embryonic differentiation of male and female genital ducts from wolffian and müllerian primordia. *Left,* An indifferent stage showing large mesonephric body. *Middle,* Female ducts. Remnants of mesonephros and wolffian ducts are now termed the epoophoron, paroöphoron, and Gartner duct. *Right,* Male ducts before descent into scrotum. The only müllerian remnant is the testicular appendix. Prostatic utricle (vagina masculina) is derived from urogenital sinus. (Modified from Corning HK. Lehrbuch der Entwicklungsgeschichte des Menschen. Munich: JF Bergmann, 1921; and Wilkins L. The Diagnosis and Treatment of Endocrine Disorders in Childhood and Adolescence. 3rd ed. 1965. Courtesy of Charles C Thomas, Publisher, Springfield, IL.)

sion of the müllerian ducts and the stabilization and differentiation of the wolffian ducts are mediated by different secretions of the fetal testes: the glycoprotein AMH secreted by the fetal Sertoli cells[191] and the steroid testosterone synthesized by the fetal Leydig cells.

Female development is not contingent on the presence of an ovary, because development of the uterus and tubes occurs if no gonad is present. However, the müllerian duct (paramesonephric duct) fails to differentiate in the absence of the mesonephric ducts, which serve as the anlage for both the male urogenital tract and the metanephros (primordial kidney); and therefore renal aplasia is commonly associated with hypoplasia of the fallopian tubes and uterus and vaginal agenesis.

The influence of the fetal testis on duct development is

exerted locally and unilaterally; if one testis is removed at an early stage of development, the oviduct develops normally on that side but müllerian regression occurs on the side of the intact testis.[208]

Systemic administration of androgen to an early embryo does not cause regression of müllerian structures. Even when large amounts of androgen are implanted locally in the gonadal region of female fetuses, the müllerian ducts do not atrophy, although the differentiation of the wolffian ducts is stimulated.[207, 208] On the other hand, if a testis is grafted onto an ovary, müllerian regression and wolffian stimulation occur on that side (see Fig. 29–22). For these reasons, Jost proposed that the fetal testis secretes a müllerian duct–inhibiting substance that is distinct from ordinary androgens.

Jost and co-workers[7] and Josso and associates[191] studied

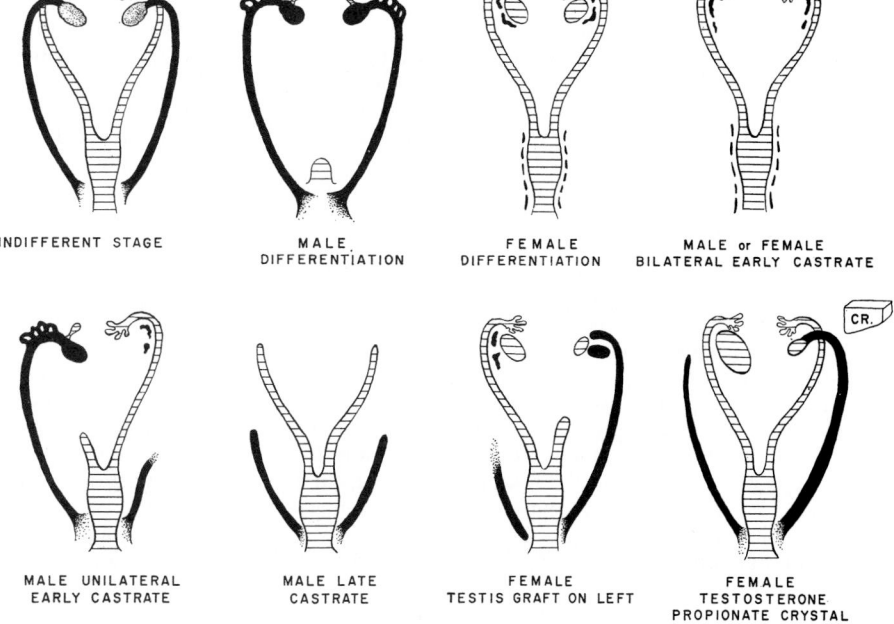

Figure 29–22. A schematic summary of Jost's experiments with rabbit embryos. The fetal testis plays a decisive role in determining the differentiation of the genital ducts. Testosterone stimulates wolffian development but fails to effect involution of müllerian structures. (Data from Jost A. Embryonic sexual differentiation [morphology, physiology, abnormalities]. In: Jones HW, Scott WW, eds. Hermaphroditism, Genital Anomalies and Related Endocrine Disorders. 2nd ed. Baltimore: Williams & Wilkins, 1971: 16.)

the influence of the fetal testis on müllerian duct inhibition in organ culture. Direct contact between the testis and the müllerian anlage was not necessary to bring about this inhibition. By separating the testis from the müllerian ducts with dialysis membranes, they concluded that the material secreted from the testis was a protein and not a steroid. They also demonstrated that the human fetal testis, regardless of age, inhibits the müllerian ducts of 14.5-day-old fetal rats in similar organ culture studies and that AMH activity is present in human testes until 8 to 10 years of age.[209-213] Using bovine fetal testes in which tubules and interstitial tissue were isolated and assayed separately, they showed that AMH activity is derived from the Sertoli cell, with peak levels occurring at the time of müllerian duct regression.[191, 211] Thereafter, the levels remain high until birth, after which a steady decline occurs until the prepubertal period.[191, 211] AMH is present in the ovarian follicle and is synthesized and secreted by the granulosa cells, but only after birth.[210-212] Elevated serum levels of AMH have been detected in patients with granulosa cell tumors.[214] Hence, AMH secretion by the postnatal ovary does not affect the fallopian tubes and the uterus, because they are apparently insensitive to AMH after the fetal period.

In the freemartin the fetal ovary and the müllerian structures are exposed to AMH before the refractory period. AMH secreted by the fetal Sertoli cells of the male twin passes by means of placental vascular anastomoses to the female twin and results in müllerian regression, ovarian inhibition, tunica albuginea formation, and development of seminiferous tubule–like cords.[215, 216] Studies show that transgenic female mice that persistently express the human AMH gene resemble the bovine freemartin.[217, 218] The transgenic female mice lack müllerian derivatives, and at birth the ovaries have fewer germ cells than normal. During the first 2 weeks of life germ cells are lost, and the somatic cells become organized into seminiferous tubule–like structures that do not persist to adulthood.[217] The "virilized" ovaries are not found in adult female mice transgenic for *AMH*.[217, 218] In the transgenic male mice, sex differentiation is usually normal, although some males have incomplete virilization of the external genitalia, incomplete wolffian duct development, and undescended testes.[217, 218] The relevance of these studies to normal sex differentiation is unclear, because the levels of AMH and its continuous secretion are different from those in the normal mouse fetus. Gene knockout of Amh (murine antimüllerian hormone) produced normal female mice with normal müllerian duct derivatives that were fertile, indicating that AMH is not required for normal ovarian function, at least in mice.[218, 219] The AMH-deficient males, as expected, had persistence of the müllerian derivatives.[218, 219] Ninety percent of the AMH-deficient mice were infertile because of interference by the müllerian duct derivatives with the passage of sperm from the epididymis and vas deferens to the urethra.[218, 219] The testes showed normal spermatogenesis but marked Leydig cell hypoplasia and tumor function, suggesting that AMH may affect Leydig cell proliferation.[218, 219] The mechanism of action of AMH is still to be defined; it acts on the müllerian duct mesenchyme where AMH receptors are located and not directly on the duct epithelium.[220] Donahoe and co-workers[221] suggested that AMH acts by blocking tyrosine phosphorylation. Physiological roles for AMH in males after regression of the müllerian ducts and in adult females are yet to be defined.

AMH is a dimeric glycoprotein composed of identical subunits linked by disulfide bonds.[191, 210] The monomer has a molecular mass of 72 kd, and the multimer ranges from 145 to 235 kd.[191, 210] The COOH-terminal domain exhibits marked homology with transforming growth factor β and the beta chain of inhibin and activin.[221] The gene for AMH, located on the short arm of chromosome 19,[221,222] is expressed only in the gonad. AMH is cleaved from its prohormone by specific protein convertases to its bioactive form within the fetal testis and at its target site.[223]

Studies of humans with various forms of intersex have confirmed that regression of the müllerian ducts is the only documented effect of AMH in the human male.[210] In patients with rudimentary gonads, the uterus and fallopian tubes develop normally regardless of the chromosomal sex. In true hermaphrodites who have a testis on one side and an ovary on the other, regression of the müllerian ducts is most marked on the side of the testis. Similarly, müllerian derivatives are absent in 46,XY women with the androgen resistance syndrome, a condition characterized by unresponsiveness of tissues to the action of androgens. Conversely, early intrauterine exposure of human female fetuses to high levels of androgens (as in congenital adrenal hyperplasia) fails to hinder normal development of the uterus and fallopian tubes.

Although müllerian involution is not androgen dependent, the differentiation of primitive wolffian ducts into the epididymides, vas deferens, and seminal vesicles requires testosterone and the androgen receptor.[224, 225] Mice, rats, and dogs treated with cyproterone acetate (an agent that blocks androgen action) and androgen-resistant XY humans and animals show the expected regression of the müllerian ducts, but structures derived from wolffian ducts remain vestigial.[226] Jost showed that the implantation of a crystal of testosterone adjacent to the fetal rabbit ovary stimulates differentiation of male ducts on that side and to a lesser extent on the contralateral side; similar results were obtained by grafting a fetal testis adjacent to the ovary (see Fig. 29–22).

The lateralization of these effects suggests that higher local concentrations of androgen are required for male duct stimulation than for masculinization of the external genitalia and derivatives of the urogenital sinus. Unlike the masculinization of the urogenital sinus and external genitalia, in which testosterone reaches these target tissues systemically through the circulation (a classic endocrine effect), local diffusion of testosterone from the testis may be involved in stabilization and differentiation of wolffian duct derivatives. The local effect of a hormone from one cell on neighboring cells resulting from local dissemination is referred to as a *paracrine* action.

During differentiation of the wolffian ducts to form the epididymides, vasa deferentia, and seminal vesicles, the wolffian ducts lack the enzyme 5α-reductase, which converts testosterone to dihydrotestosterone (DHT).[227] Experimental data and studies in humans with steroid 5α-reductase type 2 deficiency provide additional evidence that testosterone (not DHT) mediates the differentiation of the wolffian ducts. This is in striking contrast to the urogenital sinus and genital tubercle, which express steroid 5α-reductase-2 even before the testis has developed the capacity to synthesize testosterone.[228] DHT mediates the masculinization of the urogenital sinus and external genitalia. Despite this difference in the action of testosterone and DHT on the primordia of the genital tract, the androgen receptor, at least in the rabbit fetus, is the same in the wolffian duct and in the anlage of the urogenital sinus and external genitalia.[229]

In patients with ambiguous genitalia, male genital ducts are well differentiated only in those who have testes. Females with congenital adrenal hyperplasia (CAH) do not display wolffian duct differentiation even though their external genitalia may be highly virilized in utero. Patients with asymmetrical gonadal differentiation likewise have asymmetrical male duct development that correlates with the degree of testicular differentiation on that side.

If the critical role of the testis in male duct development is to provide a high local concentration of testosterone, male duct development would be expected to be deficient, even though testes are present, in patients with severe defects in steroid biosynthesis (e.g., deficiency of steroidogenic acute regulatory protein [StAR]) and in XY patients whose tissues are unresponsive to testosterone (complete syndrome of androgen resistance). The epididymides and vasa deferentia of these patients are indeed hypoplastic or rudimentary. During sex differentiation testosterone and AMH seem to effect their morphogenetic actions on the underlying mesenchymal cells rather than directly affecting the epithelial cells.[220, 230] Action of the hormone-stimulated mesenchyme on the epithelial cells mediates the morphogenesis of the male ducts and retrogression of the müllerian ducts[220, 230]; keratinocyte growth factor (FGF7), a member of the fibroblast growth factor family produced by mesenchymal cells, may be an important mediator of mesenchymal-epithelial interactions by androgen.[231]

Differentiation of the External Genitalia and Urogenital Sinus

Origin of the External Genitalia

At the eighth fetal week the external genitalia of both sexes are identical and have the capacity to differentiate in either direction.[232] They consist of a urogenital slit bounded by paired urethral folds and, more laterally, by labioscrotal swellings. The urogenital slit is surmounted by a genital tubercle consisting of corpora cavernosa and glans (Fig. 29–23). The mucosa-lined urethral folds may remain separate, in

which case they are called labia minora, or they may fuse to form a corpus spongiosum enclosing a phallic urethra. The fleshy labioscrotal swellings may remain separate to form labia majora or fuse in the midline to form a scrotum and the ventral epidermal covering of the penis. The distinction between a clitoris and a penis is based primarily on size and whether or not the labia minora fuse to form a corpus spongiosum.

By the 50-mm crown-rump stage, male and female fetuses can be distinguished by inspection of the external genitalia; in the male, the urethral folds have fused completely in the midline to form the cavernous urethra and corpus spongiosum by 12 to 14 wk of gestation. Penile length in the male increases linearly, at about 0.7 mm/wk, from 10 wk to normal term; a 12-fold increase occurs from 0.3 cm at 10 wk to 3.5 cm at term, a rate of growth about 3.5 times that of the clitoris.[233]

Origin of the Vagina

The urogenital sinus separates from a common cloaca in early fetal life.[234] There is disagreement about the relative contribution of the müllerian duct and the urogenital sinus to the vagina, but the contact and interaction of the fused müllerian ducts with the urogenital sinus is essential for normal development of the vagina.[235, 236] In normal female devel-

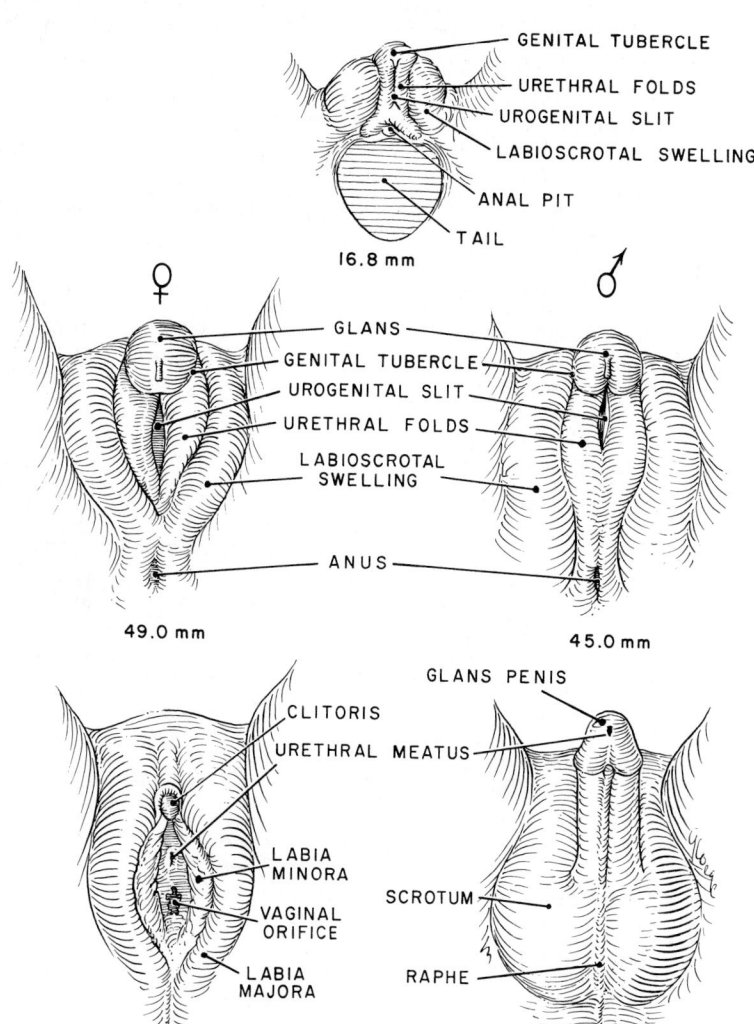

Figure 29–23. Differentiation of male and female external genitalia from indifferent primordia. Male development occurs only in the presence of androgenic stimulation during the first 12 fetal weeks. (Adapted from Spaulding MH. The development of the external genitalia in the human embryo. Contrib Embryol Carnegie Inst 1921; 13:69–88.)

TABLE 29–5. Homologies Between Male and Female Sexual Structures

Male Derivative	Primordial Structure	Female Derivative
	Gonad	
	Indifferent gonad derived from	
Seminiferous tubules	Coelomic epithelium	Graafian follicles
Sertoli cells	Mesenchymal cell mass	Granulosa cells
Leydig cells	Mesonephric elements	Theca cells
		Interstitial cells
Rete testes		Rete ovarii
Septa and tunica albuginea		
Tunica vaginalis		
Spermatogonia → sperm	Primordial germ cells	Oogonia → ova
	Genital Ducts	
	Mesonephric tubules	Epoöphoron
Ductuli efferentes		Paroöphoron
Aberrant ductules	Mesonephric (wolffian) ducts	Gartner ducts
Epididymis		
Vas deferens		
Seminal vesicles		
Ejaculatory ducts	Müllerian ducts	Fallopian tubes
Appendix testis (hydatid)		Uterus
		Upper vagina
	External Genitalia	
	Genital tubercle	Clitoris
Penis		Corpora cavernosa
Corpora cavernosa		Glans clitoris
Glans penis	Urethral folds	Labia minora
Corpus spongiosum (enclosing penile urethra)	Labioscrotal swellings	Labia majora
Scrotum and ventral epidermis of penis	Urogenital sinus	Paraurethral glands (of Skene)
Prostrate		Bartholin glands
Bulbourethral glands (of Cowper)		Vagina (lower)
Prostatic utricle (vagina masculina)		

opment, proliferation of the vesicovaginal septum pushes the vaginal orifice posteriorly so that it acquires a separate external opening; thus no urogenital sinus, as such, is preserved. In male development, the vaginal pouch is usually obliterated when the müllerian ducts are resorbed, although a vestigial blind vaginal pouch known as the prostatic utricle can sometimes be demonstrated.

The prostate gland and bulbourethral glands of Cowper in the male are outgrowths of the urogenital sinus; their differentiation is mediated by DHT and requires the presence of androgen receptors. In the female, the paraurethral glands of Skene and the vestibular glands of Bartholin have homologous origins (Table 29–5).

Mechanism of Androgen Action

The effects of testosterone are varied and tissue specific and reflect the sum of its action and the actions of its conversion products, DHT and estradiol (Fig. 29–24).[237, 238] Testosterone enters the cell by diffusion. It can be 5α-reduced to DHT or aromatized to estradiol. Subsequently, testosterone and DHT bind to a high-affinity androgen receptor; this receptor

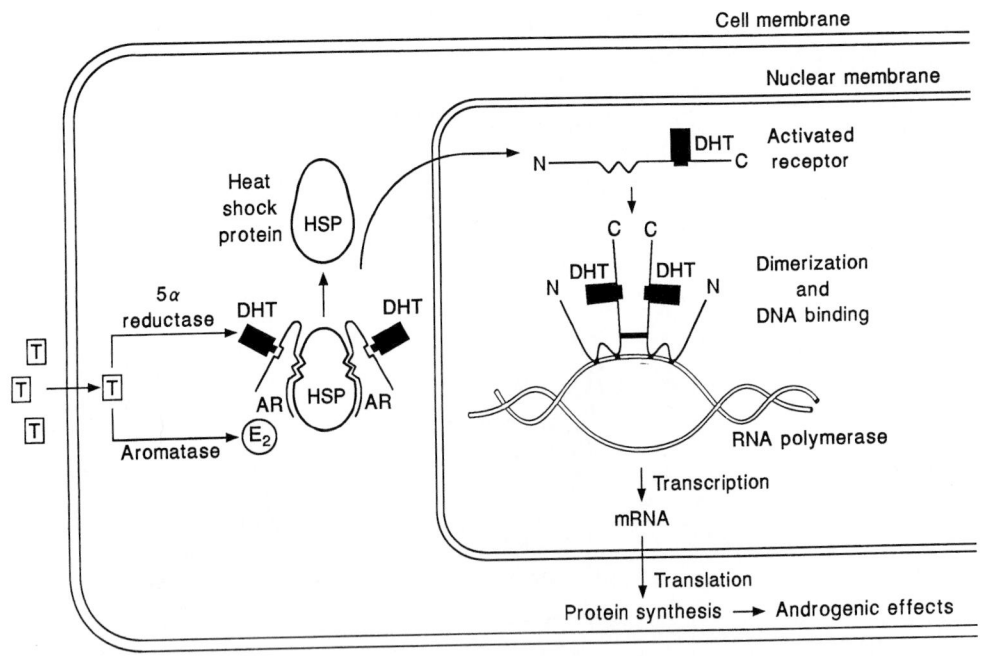

Figure 29–24. A diagrammatic representation of the putative mechanism of action of testosterone on target cells. Testosterone (T) enters the cell, where it is either 5α-reduced to dihydrotestosterone (DHT) or aromatized to estradiol (E₂). DHT binds to the androgen receptor (AR) in the nucleus and "activates" it with the release of heat shock proteins (HSP). The activated AR complex then binds as a dimer (not shown) to specific hormone response elements of the DNA and initiates transcription, translation, and protein synthesis, with consequent androgenic effects. N, NH₂ terminus; C, COOH terminus.

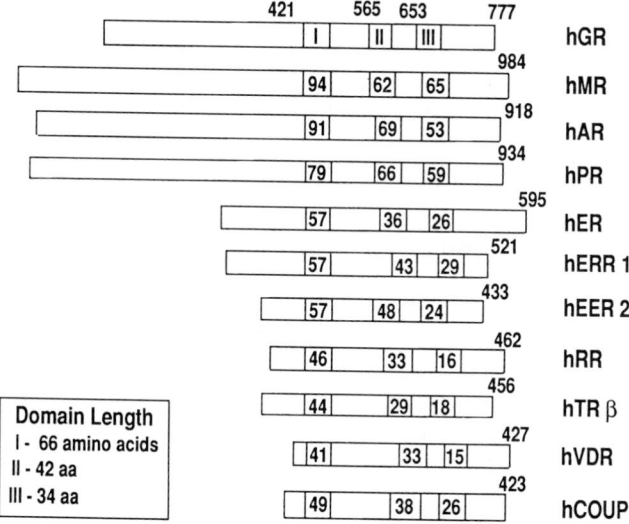

Figure 29–25. Linear representations of the steroid/thyroid hormone receptor superfamily are shown to illustrate sequence homology. hGR is the glucocorticoid receptor; hMR, the mineralocorticoid receptor; hAR, the androgen receptor; hPR, the progesterone receptor; hER, the estrogen receptor; hERR 1 and hERR 2, estrogen-related receptors; hRR, the retinoic acid receptor; hTRβ, the thyroid hormone receptor; hVDR, the vitamin D receptor; and hCOUP, the chicken ovalbumin upstream promotor. The DNA binding site (region I) and the hormone binding regions (II and III) are shown. (From B O'Malley. The steroid receptor superfamily: more excitement predicted in the future. Mol Endocrinol 1990; 4:363–369. © by The Endocrine Society.)

has a greater binding affinity for DHT than for testosterone, and the DHT-receptor complex also is more stable. The androgen receptor is encoded by a gene located between the centromere and Xq13 on the X chromosome[81] and is present in androgen-sensitive target tissues of both males and females. The androgen receptor, a ligand-activated transcriptional factor, is a phosphoprotein and a member of a family of regulatory proteins that includes the nuclear receptors for other steroid hormones and for vitamin D, thyroid hormone, retinoic acid and 9-*cis*-retinoic acid, ecdysone, and a group of orphan receptors, the ligands for which are unknown[237, 239] (Fig. 29–25; also see Chapter 4). These nuclear receptors have in common three domains: (1) an NH$_2$-terminal domain thought to be involved in gene transcription; (2) a central DNA-binding domain that contains two zinc fingers (see Fig. 29–25), of which one has information for sequence-specific binding to DNA and the other is thought to stabilize binding of the receptor to DNA (Fig. 29–26); and (3) a COOH-terminal signal-receiving domain that binds the ligand (androgen).[237–240] Between the DNA- and androgen-binding domains is a hinge domain. The degree of homology among the recep-

tors in this family is highest in the DNA-binding domain and second highest in the ligand-binding domain.[237, 239] The NH$_2$-terminal domains of these receptors show little homology.

In the absence of ligand, steroid hormone receptors (but not the thyroid hormone receptor) are complexed to chaperone proteins that are heat shock proteins and form large receptor complexes.[239] Ligand binding causes a conformational change in the receptor, additional phosphorylation of serine residues located in the NH$_2$-terminal transactivation domain,[240a] dissociation of the receptor from heat shock proteins, and "activation" of the receptor.[237, 239] The monomeric activated steroid-receptor complex is smaller (≤4S) than the unactivated complex (≥8S).[237, 239] The steroid-receptor complex dimerizes and binds to palindromic steroid-responsive elements in genomic DNA that are upstream from CAAT and TATA boxes.[237, 239] RNA polymerase and other transcription factors and co-activators (e.g., androgen receptor–associated protein, ARA70[241]) are recruited to initiate transcription of the steroid response gene at a point 19 to 27 kb downstream of the TATA box. Despite intense study, the mechanism of transactivational transcription is incompletely understood.[237] After transcription and processing of the mRNA, the RNA moves to the cytoplasm, where it is translated by cytoplasmic ribosomes and results in synthesis of new proteins and hence androgenic effects.

It is thought that testosterone and DHT have different roles. The testosterone-receptor complex modulates the secretion of LH by the hypothalamic-pituitary unit and affects the stabilization of the wolffian ducts, whereas the DHT-receptor complex acts in the fetus to promote masculinization of the urogenital sinus and external genitalia of the fetus and acts at puberty to induce maturation.[238] A defect in any of the essential steps in the action of androgen in a male fetus impairs masculinization of the urogenital sinus and external genitalia (Fig. 29–27).

Role of Androgens in the Differentiation of The External Genitalia and Urogenital Sinus

The induction of male differentiation of the external genitalia and urogenital sinus is affected by DHT, the 5α-reduced metabolite of testosterone. Testosterone is the prohormone that is delivered through the bloodstream to these

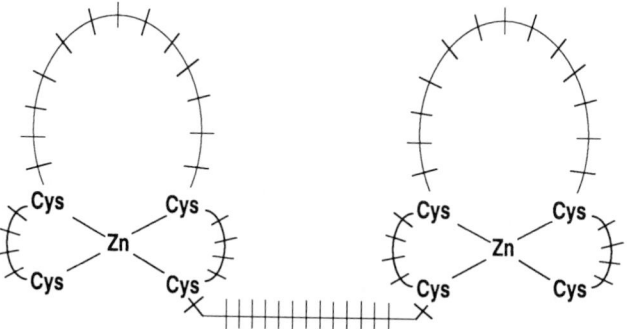

Figure 29–26. Type II zinc fingers. ╫╫╫ indicates the amino acid skeleton of the zinc fingers, which specifies DNA binding in a sequence-specific manner.

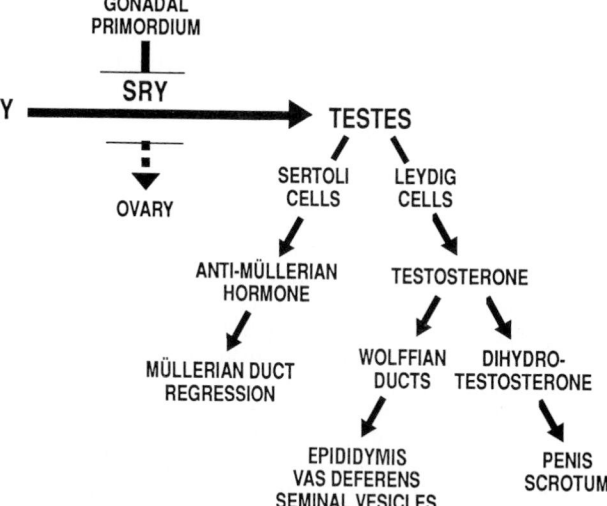

Figure 29–27. A scheme of male sex differentiation. (Modified from Grumbach MM. Genetic mechanisms of sex development. In: Vallet HL, Porter IH, eds. Genetic Mechanisms of Sexual Development. New York: Academic, 1979: 33–73.)

target tissues, which are rich in the enzyme 5α-reductase and can readily convert testosterone to DHT, even before the fetal testis acquires the capacity to secrete testosterone.[228] DHT binds to the androgen receptor and initiates the events that lead to androgen action. As in the case of the genital ducts, there is an inherent tendency for the external genitalia and urogenital sinus to feminize in the absence of fetal gonadal secretions. Complete male differentiation of the external genitalia and urogenital sinus occurs only if the androgenic stimulus is received during the critical period of development (8 to 12 wk) in fetal life. DHT stimulates growth of the genital tubercle and induces fusion of the urethral folds and labioscrotal swellings. It also induces differentiation of the prostate[242] and inhibits growth of the vesicovaginal septum, thereby preventing the development of the vagina. These morphogenetic effects of androgen seem to be mediated by the mesenchyme of these tissues and not by the overlying epithelium.[230] After about the 12th week, when the vagina has separated from the urogenital sinus, fusion of the labioscrotal folds and urethral groove cannot occur, even with an intense androgenic stimulus.[243] However, androgenic stimulation can cause clitoral hypertrophy at any time during fetal life or after birth. The male fetus with steroid 5α-reductase deficiency and impaired conversion of testosterone to DHT has defective masculinization of the external genitalia and urogenital sinus, including absence or hypoplasia of the prostate. The failure of testosterone to masculinize the fetal external genitalia has been ascribed primarily to inability of the target tissues to form DHT. The growth of the external genitalia at puberty in patients with steroid 5α-reductase-2 deficiency has been attributed to the postnatal expression of the isozyme 5α-reductase-1.

Whereas in some species fetal pituitary gonadotropins are required to sustain the secretion of testosterone by the fetal testes, in humans placental hCG stimulates fetal Leydig cell development and function; human fetal pituitary gonadotropin plays a role only after differentiation of the external genitalia is already advanced. This probably explains why the external genitalia of male infants with anencephaly or hypopituitarism and pituitary gonadotropin deficiency usually differentiate normally but remain small. Incomplete fusion of the labial folds and retention of the vaginal pouch in male infants may therefore be caused by deficient androgen secretion or by failure of the target tissues to respond to androgenic stimulation. Conversely, if female infants are subjected in utero to androgenic stimulation from some extragonadal source, the external genitalia can masculinize, ranging from clitoral hypertrophy to the formation of a normal-appearing penis. Thus, similar external abnormalities can be produced in the male by androgen deficiency (or failure of the target tissues to respond) and in the female by exposure to androgen from some pathologic source in the fetus or mother.

Endocrine and Paracrine Control Mechanisms in Sex Differentiation

The regulation of sex differentiation by chemical messengers involves two types of control mechanisms. One is the classic endocrine mechanism: a cell, usually in a discrete endocrine gland, secretes a hormone into the bloodstream, where it is transported to a distant target tissue to regulate or induce differentiation. Testosterone is a striking example of an endocrine secretion; testosterone secreted by the fetal Leydig cell is delivered through the circulation to the anlagen of the external genitalia and urogenital sinus. Similarly, hCG synthesized by the syncytiotrophoblast acts on the Leydig cell to stimulate testosterone secretion.

The second type of regulation in sex differentiation is paracrine control. This local and more primitive regulatory mechanism involves the dissemination of a hormone from its

site of synthesis to its target cells by local diffusion through the extracellular space. Examples of this delivery system for chemical messengers are the action of AMH on the müllerian duct and the action of testosterone on the wolffian duct (in this instance testosterone is a paracrine secretion).

Hormonal Sex Differentiation

Sex differentiation is not complete until the secondary sexual characteristics have matured, fertility is attained, and the ultimate goal, reproduction, becomes possible (Fig. 29–28). These developments occur during puberty. In the past, puberty was regarded as a de novo event because of the dramatic changes brought about by the maturation of the gonads and the increased secretion of gonadal steroids. However, the development of gonadal function is actually a continuum extending from the differentiation of the gonad and the ontogeny of the hypothalamic-pituitary-gonadal system in the fetus, through puberty, to the attainment of full sexual maturation and fertility. Puberty is not an isolated event but rather a critical stage in a sequence of complex maturational changes. The hypothalamic-pituitary unit (including the pulsatile secretion of hypothalamic LHRH and of FSH and LH) functions in the fetus, is suppressed to a low level of activity for about a decade during childhood, and is reactivated at the onset of puberty.[244] The hormonal changes and the neuroendocrinology of puberty, including adrenarche and gonadarche, are reviewed in Chapter 31.

Sex Differentiation in the Hypothalamus

Although the control of gonadal function in both sexes is mediated by both FSH and LH, the secretory patterns of the gonadotropins differ in males and females. The male pituitary characteristically secretes both FSH and LH in a pulsatile but relatively constant and sustained manner, whereas in the mature female the pulsatile secretion of FSH and LH is cyclic and is characterized by a preovulatory gonadotropin surge that leads to ovulation.

In 1936 Pfeiffer[245] reported that the rat pituitary becomes differentiated during the early postnatal period according to the nature of the gonads, but the cyclic secretory pattern characteristic of the female pituitary is not an innate property of the pituitary itself. The pituitary of a male animal, when grafted under the hypothalamus of an adult female, is fully able to sustain the rhythm of repeated estrous cycles. When the male pituitary is grafted elsewhere in the recipient, ovulation fails to occur. Therefore the hypothalamus or higher neural centers function differently in the two sexes.[246–248] In the rat, mouse, hamster, guinea pig, and sheep there is an inherent tendency to a female hypothalamic-hypophyseal pattern of gonadotropin release, and this pattern is converted to a male pattern if the newborn animal is exposed to androgens or estrogens during the neonatal period[247–249]; in the guinea pig and sheep the androgen must be administered prenatally. Once the male pattern is imprinted on "sex centers" in the hypothalamus (usually by testicular androgens), the potential for cyclic activity on the part of the hypophysis is irrevocably lost. In the rat, the critical period is the first 10 d of life; the administration of as little as 1 μg of testosterone to female rats during this period causes structural changes in the hypothalamus,[249, 250] permanent infertility because gonadotropin secretion at maturity is sustained rather than cyclic, and failure of ovulation. The ovaries of these rats develop multiple follicular cysts and no corpora lutea. Similarly, if male rats are castrated during the first few days of life, later ovarian implants form corpora lutea in a normal female manner.

In contrast, sex differentiation of the central nervous system mechanisms mediating gonadotropin secretion in the

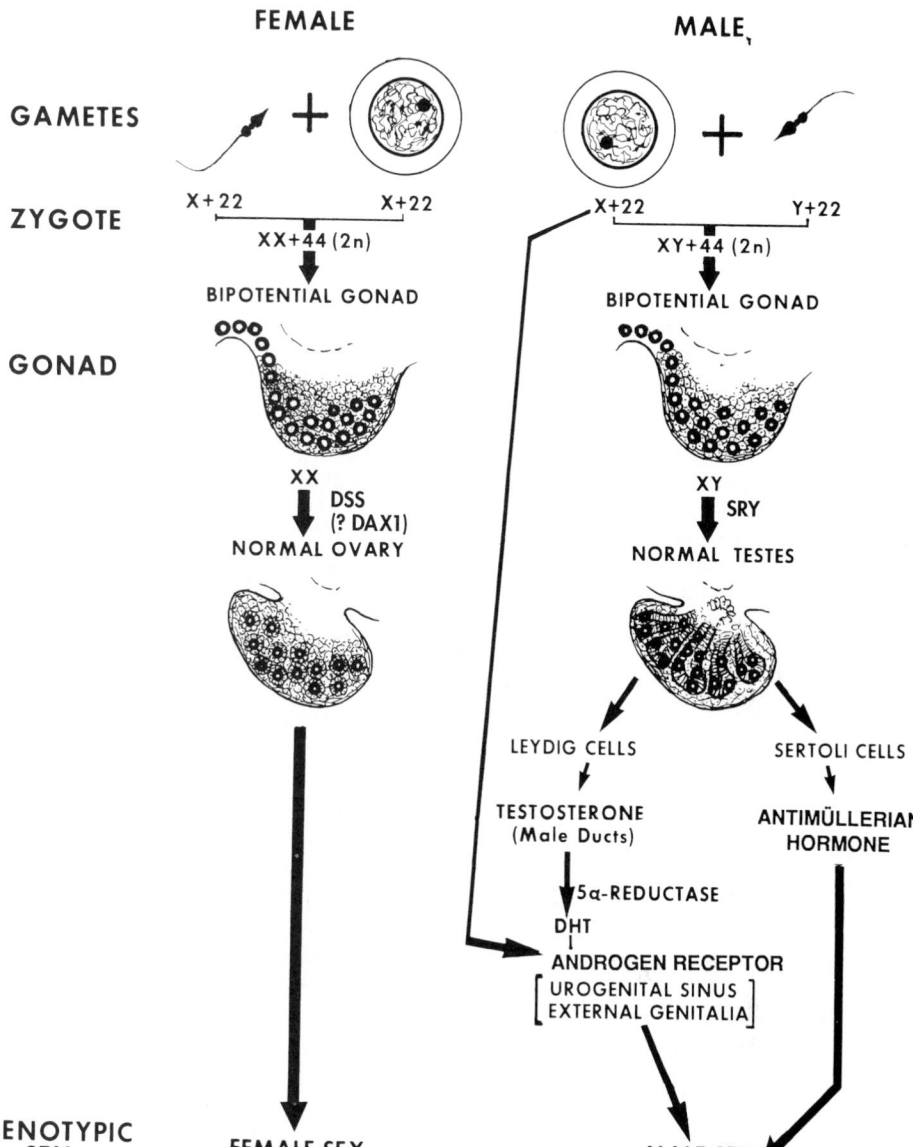

FEMALE   MALE

GAMETES

ZYGOTE

GONAD

PHENOTYPIC
SEX

Figure 29–28. A diagrammatic representation of human sex determination and differentiation. Intrinsic or extrinsic factors adversely affecting any stage of these processes can lead to anomalies of sex (see text).

primate does not occur even when testosterone is administered to pregnant monkeys beginning early in gestation. Furthermore, girls with virilizing CAH and girls who have been exposed to androgens in utero later develop a female-type FSH response to the administration of LHRH[251] and normal ovulatory cycles, although cystic ovaries may be present.[252] Moreover, in both castrate men and male monkeys,[253, 254] an acute rise in concentration of serum estradiol after estrogen administration can elicit a surge in LH secretion; this suggests that in primates the potential for cyclic gonadotropin secretion is intact and that androgen-induced differentiation of the gonadotropin regulatory mechanism described in rodents and sheep does not occur in humans. Anatomic differences between human male and female brains can be detected in the hypothalamus and adjacent brain; the functional implications of these sex differences are unclear.[255–257]

Psychosexual Differentiation

Sexually dimorphic human behavior may be classified into four broad categories (Table 29–6)[12, 258, 259]: (1) *gender identity*, which is defined as the identification of self as either male or female; (2) *gender role*, which means the aspects of behavior in which males and females differ from one another in our culture at this time; (3) *gender orientation*, which is the choice of erotic partner, whether homosexual, heterosexual, or bisexual; and (4) *cognitive differences*.[260–263]

Studies in lower species suggest that the sexual role adopted at maturity is determined by the hormonal environment in early life.[260–263] As with other aspects of sex differentia-

TABLE 29–6. Gender-Related Behavior

Gender identity	Identification of self as male or female
Gender role	Sexually dimorphic behavior
	Energy expenditure
	Aggression
	Parenting rehearsal
	Peer and group interaction—preference of playmates by sex
	Labeling ("tomboy," "sissy")
	Grooming behavior (e.g., clothes, hair)
Gender orientation	Choice of sexual partner
Cognition	Sexually dimorphic cognitive abilities

tion, there appears to be an innate tendency to develop female sexual postures. Development of male patterns of sexual behavior in lower species is influenced to a large extent by exposure to androgens, in particular testosterone, during the prenatal and perinatal period.[263, 264] This organizing capacity of testosterone administered at a critical stage of development has been localized to specific areas of the brain.[247, 257, 263, 264] There is a difference between the sexes in the volume of the sexually dimorphic nucleus in the preoptic area of the rat brain, and structural differences of the brains of the two sexes are now recognized in many species including humans[255, 256, 265]; however, in the human brain the morphologic sex differences are not apparent before about 2 to 5 years of age.[256] Moreover, sexually dimorphic organization of target cell nuclei and behavior-related events in lower species are the result of aromatization of testosterone to estradiol in the central nervous system of these species.[263, 264, 266] The so-called protection hypothesis holds that physiological levels of estradiol cannot enter the brain and masculinize the central nervous system of the female rodent fetus because the estrogen is bound to α-fetoprotein.[264] However, in humans, α-fetoprotein does not retard the transport of estradiol to the central nervous system, and testosterone-binding globulin (TeBG), also called sex hormone–binding globulin (SHBG), has a greater affinity for testosterone than for estradiol. Therefore, the protection hypothesis does not appear to be applicable to humans. Human males are more frequently left-handed than are females, a difference that has been ascribed, at least in part, to the prenatal effect of testosterone on the brain.[267] Females with virilizing CAH are more commonly left biased, as assessed by an index of cerebral lateralization, than their normal sisters, whereas affected males do not differ in handedness from their normal brothers.[268]

Gender identity—the identification of self as either male or female—is a complex, poorly understood, sexually dimorphic phenomenon applicable only to humans. The behavioral changes attributed to prenatal exposure to androgens and progestogens in girls with CAH or to estrogens and progestogens in boys are subtle, do not appear to affect gender identity, and are within the range of normal for sexually dimorphic behavior.[259, 260, 269, 270] Individuals who have been reared in a sex opposite to their chromosomal and/or gonadal sex, as well as prenatally androgenized females with CAH, provide evidence that gender identity cannot be attributed solely to sex chromosome constitution or to prenatal exposure to testosterone.[12, 260, 271] Gender identity is evident early in the postnatal years, and both experience and learning have a profound effect.[12, 260, 271, 271a]

For the past 30 years, the dogma has prevailed that gender identity is concordant with the assigned sex in the intersex patient, provided that the child is raised unambiguously, free from doubt about his or her phenotypic sex, and that appropriate surgical correction and hormone therapy are instituted to ensure as far as possible that the child has an unambiguously male or female phenotype.[12] This generally accepted hypothesis is based on the notion of psychosexual neutrality at birth.[12] However, this hypothesis is now being rigorously challenged (reviewed by Diamond and Sigmundson[271b]) by those who favor a varying degree of inherent prenatal psychosexual differentiation, precipitated by the reassessment of a critical study of a sex-reversed patient. The prismatic case involved a 46,XY phenotypic male identical twin who sustained an accidental phallic ablation at circumcision. He was castrated, the external genitalia were anatomically modified to a female phenotype, and he was assigned a female gender role. In spite of continuing medical and psychological support and early claims to the contrary, follow-up study indicated that the patient was unable to accept the female gender assignment.[271b] He subsequently made a successful adaptation as a male.[271b]

The authors encountered a similar case in an adolescent 46,XY identical twin with ambiguous genitalia in contrast to the normal male phenotype of the twin. A female sex assignment was made at another institution and surgery was performed to modify the external genitalia. This sex assignment was not accepted by the patient despite counseling. These cases, confounded by monozygotic twinning, call into question the concept of the neutrality of gender identity at birth in the human and raise the question of the magnitude of the effect of prenatal hormone exposure and genotype on gender identity.

Sexual identity is usually established by 18 to 30 months of age.[12] Thereafter, even the development of secondary sexual characteristics of the opposite sex at puberty may not shake the conviction of gender identity if it has been firmly established in early life and if any discordant genital anatomy is corrected.[260] On the other hand, if at puberty discordant secondary sexual characteristics are allowed to mature, some individuals may develop doubts about their true gender identity. This has been described in some patients with 5α-reductase-2 deficiency, 17β-hydroxysteroid dehydrogenase 3 (17β-HSD 3) deficiency, or 45,X/46,XY mosaicism. Invariably the change has been from assigned female sex to male consequent to virilization by the retained gonads at puberty in 46,XY patients. Imperato-McGinley and associates[272] reported on a geographic and cultural isolate of male pseudohermaphrodites with 5α-reductase deficiency who masculinized at puberty. In these patients, a change in gender behavior was common but not invariable.[272] More recent evidence supports the effect of gonadal hormones on neuronal plasticity of the adult brain in rats.[273] Furthermore, differentiation of the sexually dimorphic nucleus of the preoptic area of the human hypothalamus is detectable between about 5 years of age and puberty,[256] although its role in gender identity is unknown. These studies have cast doubt on the hypothesis that gender identity is irreversibly fixed by environmental factors by 2 to 3 years of age.[274] They also emphasize the effect of gonadal steroids at puberty on gender identity and behavior and attest to the plasticity of gender identity in the cultural-genetic isolates studied.[272] In another genetic isolate of patients with 5α-reductase deficiency in New Guinea, gender role appeared to be affected primarily by social-experiential and cultural factors rather than by hormonal mechanisms.[275]

Stronger credence is now given to the role of early hormonal influences on sexually dimorphic behavior in humans. As noted, studies of women and girls with prenatal virilization caused by virilizing CAH or maternal ingestion of progestagens demonstrate no effect on gender identity in well-managed patients.[269, 276] However, gender-related behavior can be affected. Prenatally androgenized girls have more interest in outdoor play and competitive sports and are more "tomboyish" than are unaffected girls.[260] As a group, they are more career oriented and tend to lack a strong interest in doll play and mothering.[260] The pattern is persistent and is not abnormal for female behavior in our culture. According to some studies,[277, 278] a higher proportion of young women with virilizing CAH rated themselves as bisexual or homosexual; another study did not support this contention.[279]

The eventual outcome of this "nature versus nurture" controversy is of practical importance. The evidence related to hypogonadal males, patients with the complete form of androgen resistance, and prenatally virilized girls supports the thesis that exposure to androgens before birth can contribute to the programming of sexually dimorphic behavior. However, these hormonal factors are rarely decisive in patients with abnormalities of sex differentiation, and more important elements in the development of gender identity are the assigned sex of rearing, the reinforcement that this assignment receives during infancy and early childhood, and reinforcement by appropriate gonadal steroid secretion or replacement therapy at the normal age of puberty. If this reinforcement is weak because of ambiguous attitudes of the parents and the community setting, the outlook for attaining a normal gender identity in adult life is diminished.

These interpretations are supported by experience gained from a pragmatic approach to the assignment of sex in patients with ambiguous genitalia (see later).

CLASSIFICATION OF ERRORS IN SEX DIFFERENTIATION

In the past, individuals with hermaphroditism were classified according to their gonadal morphology. In the terminology of Klebs, a *true hermaphrodite* is a person who possesses both ovarian and testicular tissue. A *male pseudohermaphrodite* is one whose gonads are exclusively testes but whose genital ducts or external genitalia, or both, exhibit the phenotype of a female or incompletely differentiated male. A *female pseudohermaphrodite* is a person with ovaries whose external genitalia exhibit some masculine characteristics. The authors have classified errors in sex differentiation by a modification and expansion of this broad framework and have attempted to blend etiologic mechanisms and clinical entities into a simplified rational classification (Table 29–7). The clinical and etiologic heterogeneity of syndromes with similar anatomic findings merits emphasis.

Disorders of Gonadal Differentiation and Sex Chromosome Anomalies

Not all patients with anomalies of sex chromosomes have abnormal gonads; conversely, congenital defects in gonadal differentiation are not always caused by chromosomal errors. The association is so frequent, however, that these topics are inseparable. Exceptions to this association are of special importance in defining the genetic and chromosomal determinants of gonadogenesis (see Table 29–4).

Seminiferous Tubule Dysgenesis: Klinefelter's Syndrome and Its Variants

47,XXY SEMINIFEROUS TUBULE DYSGENESIS (TYPICAL KLINEFELTER'S SYNDROME). Seminiferous tubule dysgenesis is a common cause of primary hypogonadism and male infertility (Table 29–8). This syndrome, as defined by Klinefelter and associates,[280] usually becomes manifest first during adolescence as gynecomastia, a variable degree of androgen deficiency, small atrophic testes with hyalinization of the seminiferous tubules, aggregation of Leydig cells, aspermatogenesis, and increased plasma gonadotropins, especially plasma FSH.

In 1956 several groups found that a high proportion of patients with this syndrome are X chromatin positive despite their phenotypic male appearance. In 1959 Jacobs and Strong[281] and Ford and co-workers[282] first reported a 47,XXY sex chromosome constitution in patients with this disorder, explaining the positive sex chromatin pattern. Various other sex chromosome compositions, including mosaicism, were described subsequently. Virtually all these variants have in common the presence of at least two X chromosomes and a Y chromosome, except for the rare group that has a 46,XX sex chromosome complement by karyotype analysis of multiple tissues.

The differentiation of testes and lack of ovarian differentiation in patients with 47,XXY and, more strikingly, in those with 49,XXXXY complements indicate that a single Y chromo-

TABLE 29–7. Classification of Anomalous Sexual Development

I. Disorders of gonadal differentiation
  A. Seminiferous tubule dysgenesis (Klinefelter's syndrome)
  B. Syndrome of gonadal dysgenesis and its variants (Turner syndrome)
  C. Complete and incomplete forms of XX and XY gonadal dysgenesis
  D. True hermaphroditism
II. Female pseudohermaphroditism
  A. Androgen-induced
    1. Congenital virilizing adrenal hyperplasia
    2. CYP19 (P45$_{arom}$) aromatase deficiency
    3. Androgens and synthetic progestagens transferred from maternal circulation
  B. Other teratologic factors (non–androgen-induced) associated with malformations of intestine and urinary tract
III. Male pseudohermaphroditism
  A. Testicular unresponsiveness to hCG and LH (Leydig cell agenesis or hypoplasia due to hCG/LH receptor defect)
  B. Inborn errors of testosterone biosynthesis
    1. Enzyme deficits affecting synthesis of both corticosteroids and testosterone (variants of congenital adrenal hyperplasia)
      a. StAR deficiency (congenital lipoid adrenal hyperplasia)
      b. 3β-Hydroxysteroid dehydrogenase/Δ^5 isomerase type II (3β-HSD II) deficiency
      c. CYP17 (P450$_{c17}$ [17α-hydroxylase/17,20 lyase]) deficiency
    2. Enzyme defects primarily affecting testosterone biosynthesis by the testes
      a. CYP17 (P450$_{c17}$ [17,20 lyase]) deficiency
      b. 17β-Hydroxysteroid dehydrogenase type 3 (17β-HSD 3) deficiency
  C. Defects in androgen-dependent target tissues
    1. End-organ resistance to androgenic hormones
      a. Syndrome of complete androgen resistance and its variants (testicular feminization and its variant forms)
      b. Syndrome of incomplete androgen resistance and its variants (Reifenstein's syndrome)
      c. Androgen resistance in phenotypically normal males
    2. Defects in testosterone metabolism by peripheral tissues; 5α-reductase-2 (SRD5A2) deficiency (pseudovaginal perineoscrotal hypospadias)
  D. Dysgenetic male pseudohermaphroditism
    1. XY gonadal dysgenesis (incomplete)
    2. XO/XY mosaicism, structurally abnormal Y chromosome, Xp+, 9p−, 10q−
    3. Denys-Drash syndrome (*WT1* mutation)
    4. WAGR syndrome (*WT1* deletion)
    5. Campomelic dysplasia (*SOX9* mutation)
    6. ? *SF1* mutation
    7. Testicular regression syndrome
  E. Defects in synthesis, secretion, or response to antimüllerian hormone: persistent müllerian duct syndrome (female genital ducts in otherwise normal men; herniae uteri inguinale)
  F. Maternal ingestion of progestagens and estrogens
  G. ?Environmental chemicals
IV. Unclassified forms of abnormal sexual development
  A. In males
    1. Hypospadias
    2. Ambiguous external genitalia in XY males with multiple congenital anomalies
  B. In females, absence or anomalous development of the vagina, uterus, and uterine tubes (Rokitansky-Küster syndrome)

some and the expression of the testis-determining gene *(SRY)* are sufficient to bring about testis organogenesis and male sex differentiation in the presence of as many as four X chromosomes.

Clinical Features.[283–285] In the postpubertal patient, the only constant clinical features are a male phenotype, small testes (<3 cm in length, and often <1.5 cm), and azoospermia (Fig. 29–29). Gynecomastia is common. Prepubertal studies indicate that children with a 47,XXY karyotype, as a group, have lower birth weights; smaller mean head circumference; a slightly increased incidence of congenital anomalies, especially clinodactyly; height percentiles that increase with age; a lower verbal I.Q. than normal boys; and delayed emotional development and poor motor control.[285–287] Impairment in verbal I.Q. is slight (10 to 20 points), and the mean I.Q. falls between 85 and 90, with a wide range of variation.[288–291] Most boys with

TABLE 29–8. Clinical Features of Klinefelter's Syndrome

Karyotype:	47,XXY
Inheritance:	Sporadic; associated with advanced maternal age; nondisjunction during first or second meiotic division in either parent (67% maternal, 33% paternal); mitotic nondisjunction
Genitalia:	Male
Wolffian duct derivatives:	Normal
Müllerian duct derivatives:	Absent
Gonads:	Small, firm testes; seminiferous tubule dysgenesis; azoospermia; Leydig cell hyperplasia
Habitus:	Poor to normal virilization at puberty: gynecomastia; disproportionately long legs
Hormone profile:	Testosterone levels variable but usually decreased; increased levels of plasma LH and FSH postpubertally

Klinefelter's syndrome require help in reading and spelling.[292] Severe retardation is uncommon.[293] One study of 13 47,XXY males monitored from birth through adolescence noted a mean I.Q. 21 points lower than that of a matched control group.[292] Despite difficulties with reading and writing, 12 of 13 graduated from high school, and 4 attended college. In general, lack of motor skills hindered participation in competitive sports; 3 of 13 were successful in achieving personal goals and in their family relationships.[292] The families of these 3 boys were among the most stable and supportive of the study group.[292] Most patients with Klinefelter's syndrome do not have behavioral disorders,[290] and, in spite of verbal deficits, adult men with Klinefelter's syndrome are not significantly different as a group from other hypogonadal males or even normal controls as far as education, employment, socioeconomic status,[290] social adjustment, and criminal behavior are concerned.[294]

Patients with a 47,XXY karyotype tend to be taller than average because of disproportionate length of the legs.[289, 295] This finding is present before clinical signs of puberty are evident and may not be accompanied by a proportional increase in arm span. The prepubertal onset suggests that disproportionate leg length is not related to androgen deficiency or delayed epiphyseal closure. Androgen deficiency after the age of puberty augments the prepubertal deviation in skeletal proportions.[295]

Prepubertally, the basal plasma concentration of FSH and LH and the response to LHRH are within the normal range for age.[296–298] The timing and onset of secondary sexual characteristics and puberty were reported as normal in one study[298] and as delayed in another.[299] With the onset of puberty, testicular histology becomes abnormal and testosterone synthesis is impaired. In postpubertal patients the plasma concentrations of testosterone[298] tend to be low, the levels of plasma estradiol are normal or increased, and the gonadotropin levels are elevated. Testosterone responses to hCG appear to be normal in childhood and early adolescence and blunted in adulthood.[298] Potency is usually diminished in the adult, and Leydig cell reserve is impaired, as reflected by a subnormal increase in the concentration of serum testosterone after administration of hCG and an increased concentration of LH in plasma.[300] The testosterone production rate, levels of total and free testosterone, and rates of metabolic clearance of testosterone and estradiol tend to be low, whereas plasma estradiol levels are normal or elevated.[283, 301] Gynecomastia and signs of androgen deficiency, such as diminished facial and body hair, a female escutcheon, a small phallus, poor muscular development, and a further increase in the disproportion between leg and body length, usually become evident during or after puberty. The testicular failure in Klinefelter's syndrome appears to progress with age. Gynecomastia, which occurs in about 90% of patients, is considered to be secondary to an increased ratio of serum estradiol to testosterone[298] (also see Chapter 17).

Associated Abnormalities. Abnormalities in thyroid function include a diminished thyroid response to thyrotropin, decreased uptake of radioactive iodine, and a subnormal increase in serum thyrotropin concentration after administration of thyrotropin-releasing hormone.[302] Clinically significant

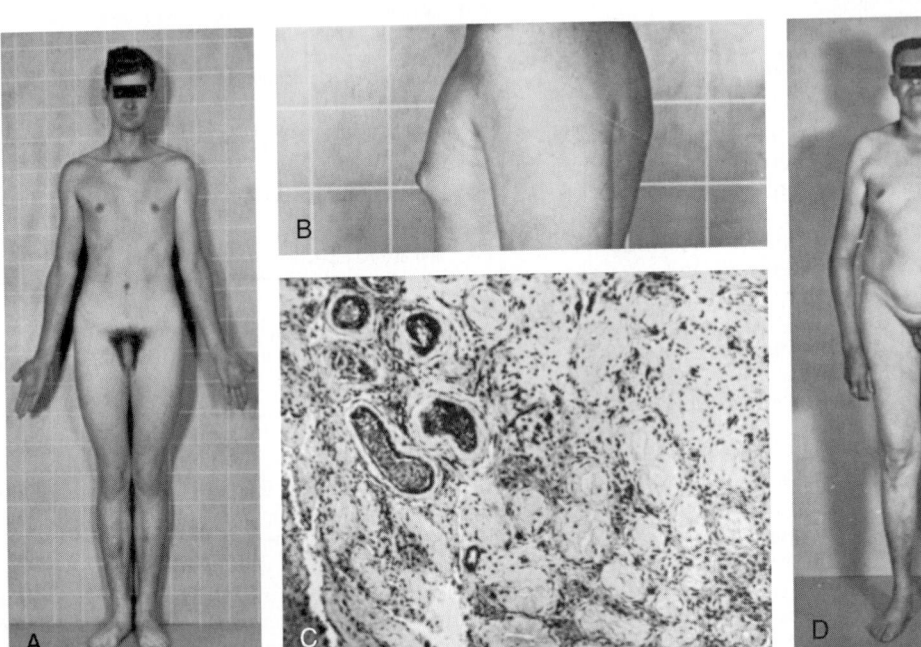

Figure 29–29. *A,* A 19-year-old phenotypic male with chromatin-positive seminiferous tubule dysgenesis (Klinefelter's syndrome). The karyotype was 47,XXY, gonadotropin levels were elevated, and testosterone levels were low normal. Note normal virilization with long legs and gynecomastia *(B).* The testes were small and firm and measured 1.8 × 0.9 cm. Testicular biopsy *(C)* revealed a severe degree of hyalinization of the seminiferous tubules and clumping of Leydig cells. *D,* A 48-year-old male with 47,XXY Klinefelter's syndrome with severe leg varicosities.

thyroid disease is uncommon. Approximately 10% of men with Klinefelter's syndrome have antibodies to thyroglobulin.[286]

The frequency of diabetes mellitus is increased. Nielsen[303] reported that 19% had impaired glucose tolerance and that 8% had overt diabetes. The prevalence of diabetes mellitus was also increased in the parents. The patients with diabetes mellitus were usually younger than 50 years of age, and the type II diabetes was usually mild. Insulin resistance with secondary hyperinsulinemia may be the cause of glucose intolerance.[304]

47,XXY patients with gynecomastia have an increased predisposition to cancer of the breast. In a survey of 187 males with breast cancer, 8 patients with chromatin-positive seminiferous tubule dysgenesis were detected, about 18 times the expected prevalence.[305] Whether this increased incidence is solely the consequence of the gynecomastia is unclear (see Chapter 17). Infiltrating ductal carcinoma is the most common histologic type.[306] Even though a study of 696 men with Klinefelter's syndrome did not report an overall increase in cancer incidence,[307] the prevalence of germ cell tumors (particularly in the mediastinum) that secrete hCG and cause LHRH-independent sexual precocity is increased.[308-310] About 20% of patients with primary mediastinal germ cell tumors have Klinefelter's syndrome.[310] The latter diagnosis is suggested by the association of prepubertal-size testes with sexual precocity. Routine screening is not indicated, given an estimated incidence of germ cell tumors of 1.5 per 1000 persons with Klinefelter's syndrome.[310]

About 25% of adults with Klinefelter's syndrome have osteoporosis.[311] Chronic pulmonary disease and varicose veins with stasis ulcers may also be more prevalent in adults. Patients with both androgen resistance and a 47,XXY karyotype have been reported.[312] These patients had female or ambiguous male genitalia and some clinical features of the 47,XXY karyotype. This combined defect is probably caused by fertilization of an oocyte containing two X chromosomes, each bearing a defect in the X-linked gene coding for the androgen receptor, by a normal sperm containing a Y chromosome. Several males with 46,XY plus a marker chromosome have been reported. In these patients, the marker found was a small ring X chromosome that did not express *XIST* and hence was not inactivated. The abnormal dosage of X-active chromosome genes caused developmental delay and dysmorphic features.[313]

Frequency. Surveys of the prevalence of 47,XXY fetuses by karyotype analysis of unselected newborn infants indicate an incidence of about 1 per 1000 males. No racial or geographic predilection has been observed.[314]

Testicular Lesions. Changes in the histologic structure of the testis become more marked with age in 47,XXY individuals.[315] A limited number of studies of fetal testes have been reported, and the findings are variable. Grumbach and associates[316] reported normal histology for the testes of a 1700-g chromatin-positive premature infant, as was similarly reported in a 49,XXXXY 21-week fetus,[317] but examination of several other affected fetuses suggested that the germinal epithelium was deficient and that germ cells were heterotopic[318]; these observations indicate that the histology of the fetal testes varies. In three infants aged 3 to 12 months with a 47,XXY karyotype, spermatogonia were decreased.[319] In later childhood, testicular biopsies have revealed small tubules with progressive reduction in spermatogonia.[320] In considering the testicular lesion, it seems that a normal or near-normal complement of germ cells is present early in fetal life. During late gestation and early infancy, a drastic loss of spermatogonia ensues, possibly because of an exaggeration of the normal degeneration of spermatogonia in the neonatal period. Excessive germ cell loss could result from either defective maturation[321] or failure of the germ cells to migrate to the periphery

of the tubule and align in opposition to the basement membrane.

With the approach of adolescence, even before pubertal signs are well advanced, the actions of pituitary gonadotropins on the intrinsically defective testis induce progressive hyalinization of the seminiferous tubules and pseudoadenomatous clumping of Leydig cells. Despite this clumping, the mean volume of Leydig cells usually is normal.[322] After pubescence, the testes are characterized by small dysgenetic tubules with arrested development, fibrosis, and hyalinization. The result is testes that are small in size and firm in consistency. Peritubular elastic tissue is usually absent or diminished.[315, 320] That gonadotropin secretion plays a direct or indirect role in the progressive degeneration of the testes was suggested in a 7-year-old 48,XXXY boy with true precocious puberty and elevated urinary gonadotropin levels. Unlike the relatively normal testicular architecture in most boys of this age with Klinefelter's syndrome, the testes of this boy exhibited extensive hyalinization and fibrosis of the tubules and clumping of Leydig cells (Fig. 29–30). Conversely, 47,XXY patients with gonadotropin deficiency do not exhibit changes in testicular histology.

Hyalinization of the tubules is usually extensive but varies in degree from patient to patient and even between the testes of the same patient. The fibrosis tends to progress with age, and in some older patients few tubules can be identified. Conversely, in some patients the tubules are lined by Sertoli cells, tubular fibrosis is relatively slight, and the histologic appearance resembles that of germinal cell aplasia. Rarely, spermatogenesis is found in isolated tubules. This finding could represent hidden mosaicism in the gonad or possibly mitotic nondisjunction or anaphase lag in germ cells giving rise to 46,XY cells that would then go on to spermatogenesis. There have been sporadic reports of paternity; most fertile individuals proved to have sex chromosome mosaicism, and in others acceptable documentation of paternity was not provided. Fertile patients with 46,XY/47,XXY mosaicism often lack features that distinguish them from patients with typical Klinefelter's syndrome. Analyses of sperm chromosomes from a 46,XY/47,XXY male showed that 1% of sperm had a 24,XY haplotype, which suggests that some 47,XXY cells can undergo meiosis and form XY-bearing spermatozoa.[323]

Origin of 47,XXY Constitution. 47,XXY males may develop through nondisjunction of the sex chromosomes during either the first or second meiotic division in either parent or, less commonly, through mitotic nondisjunction in the zygote at the time of or after fertilization[33] (see Figs. 29–3 and 29–16). Fertilization of a 46,XX ovum by a Y-bearing sperm or of an X ovum by a 46,XY-bearing sperm would create a 47,XXY zygote. Mitotic nondisjunction of the sex chromosomes in a 46,XY zygote could yield a 47,XXY and a 45,Y daughter cell (Fig. 29–31). Because the 45,Y cell line is nonviable, only the 47,XXY cell line would survive.

These abnormalities of meiosis almost always occur in parents with normal sex chromosome constitution. However, Rosenkranz[324] described two 47,XXY patients whose mothers were, respectively, 47,XXX and 46,XX/47,XXX mosaic. Whether a 47,XXY karyotype is derived more frequently than previously suspected from a polysomic X constitution in the mother remains to be determined.

In a study of 47,XXY males, Jacobs and colleagues[325] found that the XXY constitution resulted from paternal nondisjunction in the first meiotic division in 53% of the patients, from maternal nondisjunction during the first meiotic division in 34%, and from maternal nondisjunction during the second meiotic division in 9%. Three percent of cases appeared to be related to postzygotic mitotic nondisjunction. Ferguson-Smith and colleagues[326] and others reported a positive association with advanced maternal age in 47,XXY patients, although this association is less marked than in trisomy-

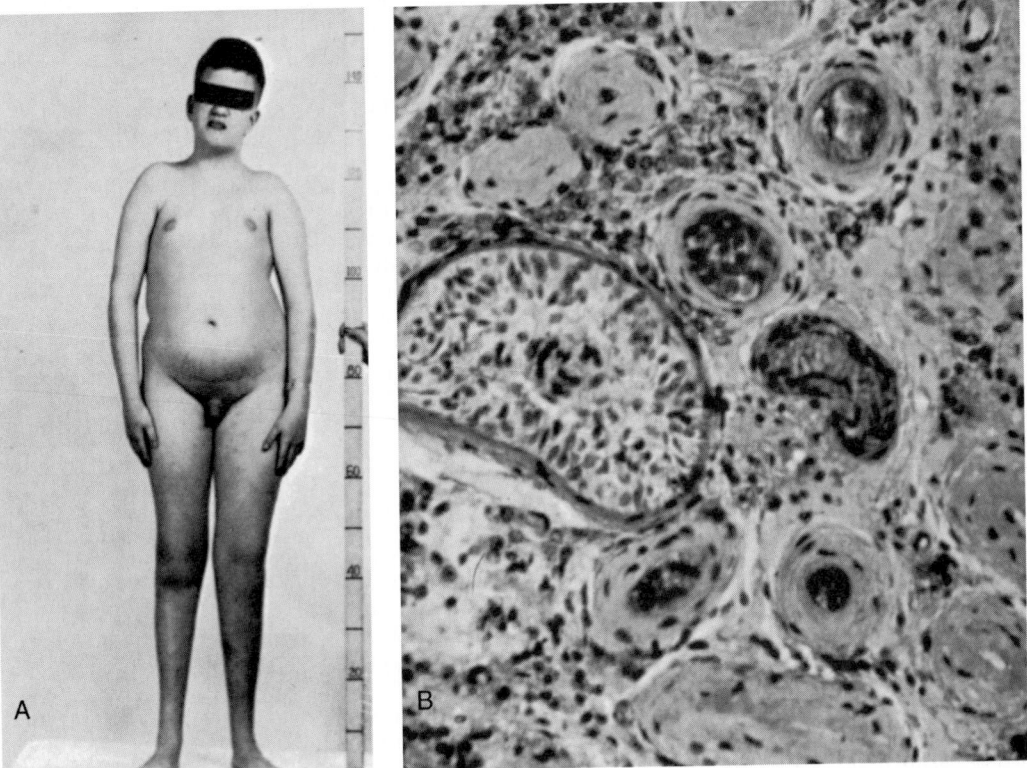

Figure 29–30. *A,* An 8½-year-old boy with a 48,XXXY chromosome constitution, mental retardation, precocious sexual development, and accelerated growth. The appearance of pubic hair was noted at age 6. By 8 years, acne, a deep voice, tall stature, and axillary hair were present. Height was 148 ± 2.9 cm, weight 47.7 ± 3.9 kg, span 140 cm, and upper segment/lower segment ratio 0.87. Testes measured 2.1 × 1.3 cm. Note the long legs, prognathism, small hands and feet, gynecomastia, and secondary sexual characteristics. The I.Q. was 62. The urinary 17-ketosteroid level was 3.2 mg/d and urinary gonadotropin levels were between 10 and 50 mouse units/d. Bone age was 13½ years. Roentgenogram of chest was normal. The buccal smear contained diploid nuclei with a maximum of two X chromatin bodies. Karyotype of cells derived from skin and blood was 48,XXXY. *B,* Testicular biopsy showed hyalinized tubules and clumping of Leydig cells; germ cells were absent. The findings suggest that true precocious puberty, with stimulation of juvenile testes by pituitary gonadotropin, led to premature appearance of typical histologic changes of seminiferous tubule dysgenesis. (M.M. Grumbach and A. Morishima, unpublished data.)

21. The association with advanced maternal age correlates with first meiotic division errors.[34, 35, 325] Studies in $X^M X^P Y$ individuals indicate that paternal nondisjunction does not depend on age,[325–327] a finding reminiscent of that in patients with autosomal trisomy. Nevertheless, the prevalence of XY, YY, and XX disomy in human sperm appears to be increased in older men.[328]

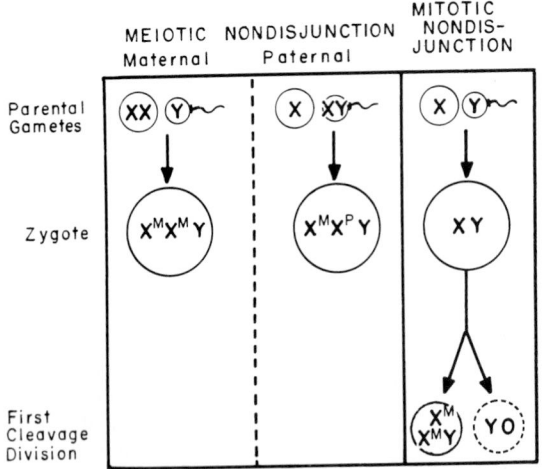

Figure 29–31. Origin of the 47,XXY karyotype. Superscripts M and P designate, respectively, maternal and paternal X chromosomes. The interrupted circle indicates a nonviable cell line. (From Grumbach MM. The testes. In: Beeson PB, McDermott W, eds. Cecil-Loeb Textbook of Medicine. 13th ed. Philadelphia: WB Saunders, 1971: 1804–1818.)

Rarely, Klinefelter's syndrome is associated with a supernumerary X chromosome that is structurally abnormal; for example, an X-autosome translocation or an isochromosome for the long arm of the X.

Etiologic Factors. An important factor in the origin of the 47,XXY chromosome constitution is advanced maternal age and maternal nondisjunction.[33, 325–327] As discussed previously, the maternal age effect in chromosome abnormalities may be a consequence of the long diplotene stage of human ova. Oocytes remain suspended in prophase of the first meiotic division from birth to ovulation, which may not occur for many years. The defective segregation of the two X chromosomes could be caused, at least in part, by reduction of the length of the chiasma as the length of the diplotene stage increases (see section on aneuploidy). As in the syndrome of gonadal dysgenesis, the prevalence of twinning in sibships of 47,XXY individuals may be increased.

Genetic factors that predispose to nondisjunction have been demonstrated in lower species. Although chromosome abnormalities are usually sporadic, families have been reported in which leukemia and various chromosome abnormalities have occurred in siblings and relatives. In addition, patients with more than one form of trisomy seem to occur more frequently than expected by chance alone. A role for radiation, viruses, environmental toxins, or autoimmunity as a predisposing factor has not been established.

Diagnosis and Treatment. The diagnosis of Klinefelter's syndrome in the postpubertal male is suggested by the typical phenotype and hormonal changes and confirmed by the finding of a 47,XXY karyotype or a variant sex chromosome complement in blood, skin, or gonads. Treatment should be directed toward androgen replacement therapy when there is evidence of androgen deficiency. In general, parenteral androgens are more effective in inducing virilization and are safer than oral preparations (also see Chapters 16 and 31). Hepatic tumors and abnormalities in liver function have been associated with chronic administration of oral androgens that have substitutions at the 17α position (e.g., a methyl group), but such abnormalities are not a problem with testosterone ester preparations such as propionate or enanthate. Testosterone enanthate in oil, 200 mg IM every 2 to 3 wk, is recommended for full replacement therapy, but it is wise to begin therapy at a lower dose (e.g., 50 mg IM every 4 wk) to avoid rapid virilization and bone maturation, especially in adolescent males. In general, conspicuous and long-standing gynecomastia does not diminish as a result of androgen replacement. However, in some patients, especially those with less striking gynecomastia, regression can occur with androgen replacement therapy. Severe or psychologically disturbing gynecomastia is corrected by reduction mammoplasty.

The diagnosis of Klinefelter's syndrome should be suspected in prepubertal patients with one or more of the following: (1) long legs, (2) smaller than normal prepubertal testes and/or penis, (3) learning disorders, and (4) developmental delay in speech and language. Many of these features are amenable to therapy, so early detection and intervention may be beneficial. Nielsen and Pelsen[294] suggested that prepubertally diagnosed patients with Klinefelter's syndrome should be offered therapy with testosterone at 11 to 12 years of age to initiate puberty and to prevent the physical and psychological complications of hypogonadism. The authors have employed, primarily for patients with hypogonadotropic hypogonadism, a regimen that begins replacement therapy with 50 mg of testosterone enanthate in oil intramuscularly each month at a bone age of 12 years.[329] When the bone age has advanced to 14 years, the dose may be increased to 100 mg IM monthly. After several years of treatment at these doses, a height is usually attained that is appropriate for genetic height potential of the individual and pubertal progression is usually adequate. If full virilization is desired, an adult replacement dose of 200 mg every 2 wk or 300 mg every 3 wk may be given.

VARIANT FORMS OF KLINEFELTER'S SYNDROME

46,XY/47,XXY Mosaicism.
46,XY/47,XXY mosaicism is the second most common karyotype in chromatin-positive men. The presence of a normal XY cell line in these patients can modify the clinical expression of the 47,XXY cell line. In general, these patients manifest a lesser degree of gynecomastia, androgen deficiency, and testicular pathology. As a group they are older (mean age, 45 years) at the time of diagnosis than 47,XXY patients. Decreased libido and potency may not appear until the fourth or fifth decade. At the time of diagnosis, serum FSH levels are elevated and serum testosterone concentrations often are in the normal male range. Secondary sexual characteristics are more normal than those of patients with 47,XXY karyotypes, and seminiferous tubules exhibit spermatogenesis more commonly than in 47,XXY patients.[284] Some patients with 46,XY/47,XXY mosaicism are fertile.[284]

The diagnosis of 46,XY/47,XXY mosaicism is established by the finding of at least 5% XY cells in blood, skin, or gonads in which the second cell line is 47,XXY. 46,XY/47,XXY mosaicism may result from nondisjunction or anaphase lag in a 47,XXY zygote.

48,XXYY.
Individuals with a 48,XXYY karyotype have the typical findings of Klinefelter's syndrome and often exhibit additional features. They constitute about 3% of chromatin-positive males and most are mentally retarded, although this may in part relate to ascertainment bias, because a significant proportion of cases are detected in screening mental and psychiatric hospitals. The 48,XXYY karyotype is usually associated with tall stature (the mean height of 26 patients was 181

cm, compared with 172 cm for 47,XXY males), disproportionately long lower extremities, gynecomastia, delinquent behavior, and unusual dermatoglyphic patterns. Peripheral vascular disease, especially varicose veins and stasis dermatitis, has been observed. Secondary sexual characteristics are poorly developed, and testicular histology is similar to that of 47,XXY patients. The sex chromatin pattern is indistinguishable from that of the 47,XXY groups; however, two fluorescent Y bodies are present in a high proportion of somatic nuclei.

To have two Y chromosomes, nondisjunction must occur in paternal meiosis. In two informative matings the Xg blood groups indicated that the father contributed an X as well as two Y chromosomes, suggesting that an X ovum was fertilized by an XYY sperm (arising from successive nondisjunction in the first and second meiotic divisions). The 48,XXYY karyotype in a patient whose mother was 47,XXX[330] could have arisen by the fertilization of an XX ovum by a YY sperm.

48,XXXY and 49,XXXYY.
All reported patients with a 48,XXXY karyotype have moderate to severe mental retardation, normal to tall stature, facial dysmorphology, small testes, and signs of androgen deficiency.[331] With the increase in the number of X chromosomes, the severity and frequency of somatic anomalies such as short neck, epicanthal folds, radioulnar synostosis, and clinodactyly increase. Mental retardation, somatic anomalies, and small testes also occur in 49,XXXYY patients.[332]

49,XXXXY.
The 49,XXXXY karyotype has been reported in more than 100 patients since the first report by Fraccaro and colleagues in 1960.[333] The diagnosis may be suspected from the clinical features. Mental deficiency can vary from moderate to profound. Phenotypic features include (1) skeletal abnormalities, especially radioulnar synostosis, genu valgum, pes cavus, and clinodactyly, and (2) hypoplastic external genitalia with a small penis, underdeveloped scrotum, and very small and frequently undescended testes; external genitalia may be ambiguous because of hypospadias, bifid scrotum, hypoplastic phallus, and cryptorchidism.[332, 334, 335] Fifteen to 20% of patients have cardiac defects, the most common of which is patent ductus arteriosus.[332] In adults, androgen deficiency is severe and gynecomastia is absent. In contrast to other males with multiple X chromosomes in their constitution, most affected patients are short.[332] Before puberty, the testes often contain hypoplastic seminiferous tubules. Other anomalies include congenital heart disease, cleft palate, strabismus, and microcephaly. The face may have a characteristic appearance, with a Down's syndrome–like slant of the eyes, epicanthal folds, hypertelorism, strabismus, and a wide nose.[334, 335] Sarto and co-workers[336] suggested that the phenotypic abnormalities noted in patients with aneuploidy involving supernumerary X chromosomes result from an effect of nonactivated genes on the X chromosomes and/or asynchronous replication of the supernumerary X chromosomes, so that more than one X chromosome is active in cells. Analyses of the parental origin of sex chromosome polysomies indicate that the extra sex chromosomes are always derived from one parent, probably by successive nondisjunction during the first and second meiotic divisions of either paternal or maternal gametogenesis.[337]

46,XX Males.
A 46,XX karyotype is present in about 1 of every 20,000 phenotypic males.[127, 338] These patients have a male phenotype and psychosocial orientation and are similar clinically and endocrinologically to individuals with classic Klinefelter's syndrome except for minor differences. Postpubertally, as in Klinefelter's syndrome, they have varying degrees of testosterone deficiency, gynecomastia, and small testes with azoospermia.[339, 340] Testosterone production is usually decreased, as is the response to hCG.[339] Both basal and LHRH-induced FSH and LH levels are increased.[339, 340] There is a 10% incidence of hypospadias that is attributed to a deficiency

of testosterone formation by the fetal Leydig cells. 46,XX males with genital abnormalities tend to lack evidence for Y chromosomal DNA in their genome and to manifest a greater prevalence and degree of gynecomastia than 46,XX men in whom a Y-to-X translocation is present.[340, 341] Compared with males with a 47,XXY karyotype, 46,XX males have a lower frequency of intellectual and psychosocial problems; they are shorter (mean height, 168 cm) than 47,XXY or normal males; they have smaller tooth crowns (Y-linked gene) than normal males; and, in contrast to 47,XXY individuals, they usually have normal skeletal proportions.[115, 127, 340, 341]

The histology of the testes is similar to that in 47,XXY males; seminiferous tubules are decreased in size and number, germinal cells usually are absent, and peritubular and interstitial fibrosis occurs. The Leydig cells appear hyperplastic. In some patients the morphology of the testes is similar to that in germinal cell aplasia or intermediate between it and the morphology in Klinefelter's syndrome. In contrast to 47,XXY patients, maternal age is not increased.

The paradoxical finding of males with a 46,XX karyotype has fascinated investigators and led to an expansion of the understanding of the genes that control sex determination. Several theories have been advanced to explain this type of sex reversal: (1) loss of a Y chromosome early in embryogenesis, (2) cryptic sex chromosome mosaicism in a 46,XX male with an undetected and/or circumscribed cell line containing a Y chromosome,[342] (3) translocation between a Y chromosome and an X chromosome or autosome resulting in the presence of the testis-determining gene (or genes) on an X chromosome or autosome,[343] and (4) a mutation involving either an autosomal or X-linked gene in the pathway to testis differentiation.[341, 344] Studies involving X- and Y-linked marker genes,[345] cytogenetic observations,[346, 347] and direct molecular genetic analyses[51, 127, 348–358] suggest that 80 to 90% of 46,XX males result from an anomalous Y-to-X translocation during meiosis.

As discussed earlier, the X and Y chromosomes have a homologous region on the distal short arms, the PAR1. The homology of this region and the proper segregation of sex chromosomes are maintained by an obligate crossover within the region at meiotic pairing. The *SRY* gene is located just proximal to the boundary of the PAR.[52] 46,XX males can arise from a balanced aberrant nonhomologous interchange between Yp and Xp that includes the sex-determining locus[127, 354] (Fig. 29–32) or from aberrant unequal nonhomologous exchange resulting in an X chromosome that has part of its PAR as well as the sex-determining region of the Y and its PAR[355, 359] (see Fig. 29–32B). Such 46,XX patients have had three copies of the pseudoautosomal gene *MIC2*. The resulting Y chromosome in both the anomalous balanced and unbalanced exchanges lacks the testes-determining region of the Y chromosome and hence could give rise to a 46,XY phenotypic female with XY gonadal dysgenesis.[127, 360, 361] The Y-to-X translocation in *SRY*-positive 46,XX males is heterogeneous, involving most of the short arm in approximately 40% of cases but as little as the *SRY* sequence and the PAR.[127, 362] In general, the greater amount of Y material present, the more virilized the phenotype.[127, 362] Anomalous Y-to-X recombinations can also occur in homologous segments of the X and Y chromosome that are outside the PAR[362] (see Fig. 29–32). Three patients with 47,XXX karyotypes and male sex differentiation have been reported.[358, 363] All three were Y chromosome positive. Two of the three had two maternal X chromosomes, and the third had two paternal X chromosomes. These findings suggest that both anomalous Y-to-X exchange and maternal or paternal nondisjunction occurred in these patients.[362]

Approximately 20% of 46,XX males are *SRY* negative.[127, 362] These males have a higher prevalence of sexual ambiguity than those who are *SRY* positive.[127, 362, 364] *SRY*-negative (Y DNA–negative) 46,XX males have been reported in several familial cohorts associated with true hermaphroditism.[51, 354, 356, 364–367] These observations are consistent with the origin of a small proportion of 46,XX males as a consequence of a mutation in a downstream autosomal or X-linked gene

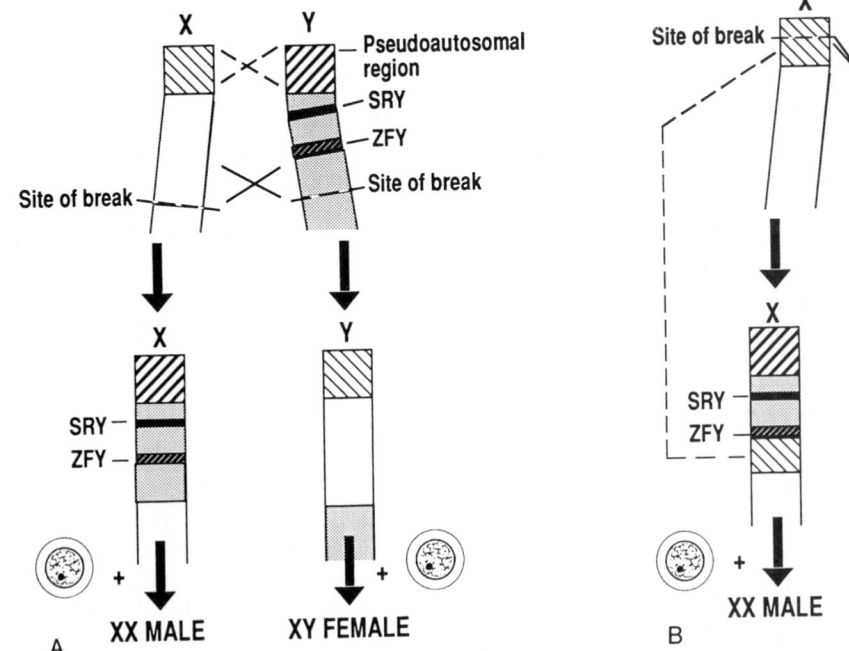

Figure 29–32. A diagrammatic representation of the short arms of the X and Y chromosomes during meiotic pairing. *A,* A crossover *(interrupted lines)* usually occurs between the pseudoautosomal regions of the X and Y chromosomes. Anomalous but equal crossovers *(solid lines)* can occur that result in an X chromosome with the sex-determining region (SRY) and a Y chromosome deficient in the SRY. Zygotes with these sex chromosomes will become XX males or XY females as indicated. *B,* Anomalous unequal crossovers *(solid lines)* during male meiosis can result in an X chromosome with an SRY gene as well as the pseudoautosomal regions of both the X and Y chromosomes. *SRY,* sex-determining region Y; *ZFY,* zinc finger Y.

(or genes) involved in the testes-determining cascade (see Fig. 29–15). They also suggest that 46,XX males and 46,XX true hermaphrodites may arise by similar pathogenetic mechanisms. In sum, the 46,XX male syndrome arises mainly as a result of a Y-to-X translocation; other possible mechanisms include mutation in an X chromosomal or autosomal gene and cryptic mosaicism that involves a Y-bearing cell line in at least the Sertoli cells.

Syndrome of Gonadal Dysgenesis: Turner Syndrome and Its Variants

In 1938 Turner described seven phenotypic women with short stature, sexual infantilism, webbing of the neck, and cubitus valgus. Studies of this syndrome and its variants have made a major contribution to the evolution of current concepts of sex differentiation. (For reviews, see references 13, 36, and 368 through 374).

In the early 1940s Albright and colleagues and Varney and associates found that the excretion of urinary gonadotropin was increased in affected adolescents and adults. Wilkins and Fleischmann soon thereafter described the gonads as bilateral, pale "streaks" of connective tissue situated in the mesosalpinges and devoid of any germ cells. Wilkins proposed, in light of Jost's fetal castration experiments in the rabbit, that some of these functionally agonadal patients might be genetic males, because fetal castration of either sex invariably leads to a female phenotype. The discovery in 1954 that many of these patients, contrary to their phenotype, were X chromatin negative seemed initially to confirm that hypothesis, but after techniques became available for analysis of the chromosome constitution Ford and co-workers[375] reported that the sex chromosome constitution in a 14-year-old phenotypic female with this syndrome was 45,X rather than 46,XY. Work in many laboratories thereafter defined more precisely the chromosomal basis of this and related disorders.

The absence of a second sex chromosome (X chromosome monosomy with haploinsufficiency) is associated with five cardinal features: female phenotype, short stature, sexual infantilism owing to rudimentary gonads, a variety of associ-

TABLE 29–9. Clinical Features of 45,X Gonadal Dysgenesis: Turner Syndrome

Karyotype:	45,X
Inheritance:	Sporadic; meiotic or mitotic nondisjunction
Genitalia:	Female
Wolffian duct derivatives:	Absent
Müllerian duct derivatives:	Normal female
Gonads:	Streak
Habitus:	Short stature; sexual infantilism at puberty; somatic stigmata
Hormone profile:	Increased plasma LH and FSH concentrations; decreased plasma estradiol levels

ated somatic abnormalities, and embryonic lethality. These features may be modified by the presence of lesser degrees of sex chromosome deficiency. It is therefore useful to consider the syndrome of gonadal dysgenesis and its variants as a continuum of features ranging from those of the typical 45,X phenotype to that of a normal female or male. The functional importance of chromosomal additions to the basic 45,X pattern can be deduced from the extent to which they modify toward normal, in at least some cases, the short stature, sexual infantilism, and somatic anomalies that typify the 45,X patient.

Partial sex chromosome monosomy (haploinsufficiency) may be attributed to a structurally abnormal second sex chromosome (X or Y), sex chromosome mosaicism involving a 45,X cell line, or both. Even though the modified clinical forms are almost invariably associated with partial sex chromosome monosomy, the contrary is not necessarily true; partial sex chromosome monosomies can cause the typical clinical picture found in 45,X patients.

TYPICAL 45,X GONADAL DYSGENESIS (TURNER SYNDROME).[13, 72, 368–373] In patients with the cardinal features of sex chromosome monosomy, the X chromatin pattern is negative in about 60%; most of these patients have a 45,X sex chromosome constitution (Table 29–9). Significant variability occurs in expression of the somatic anomalies associated with sex chromosome monosomy (Fig. 29–33).

Clinical Aspects. The typical patient (see Fig. 29–33) is

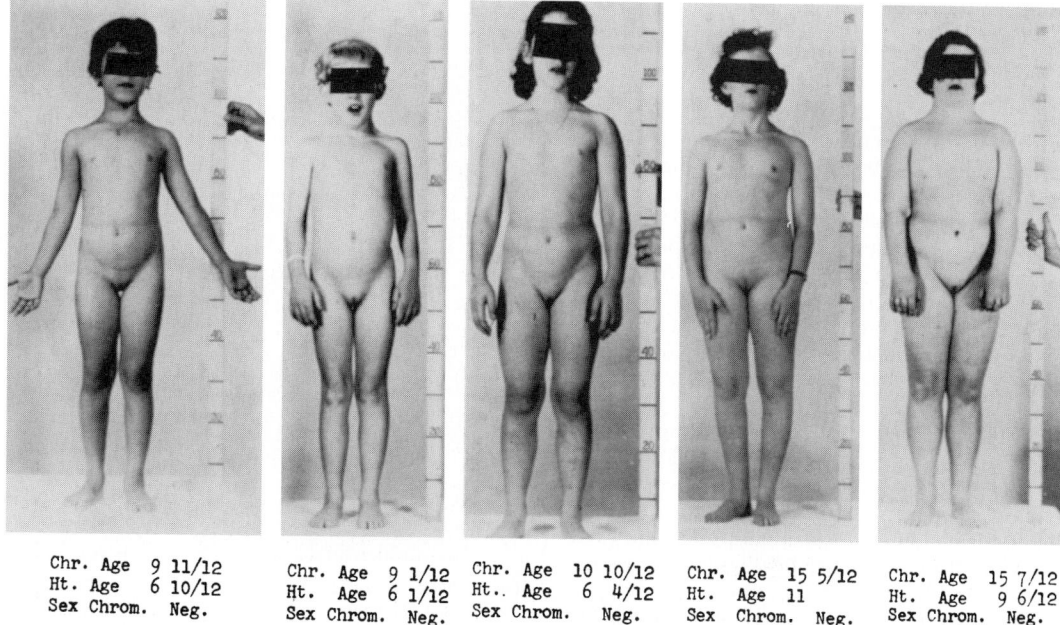

Chr. Age	9 11/12	Chr. Age	9 1/12	Chr. Age	10 10/12	Chr. Age	15 5/12	Chr. Age	15 7/12
Ht. Age	6 10/12	Ht. Age	6 1/12	Ht. Age	6 4/12	Ht. Age	11	Ht. Age	9 6/12
Sex Chrom.	Neg.	Sex Chrom.	Neg.	Sex Chrom.	Neg.	Sex Chrom.	Neg.	Sex Chrom.	Neg.

Figure 29–33. Variation in physical appearance in five patients with the typical form of the syndrome of gonadal dysgenesis. All of these patients had a 45,X karyotype, and all had differences between height age and chronological age of 3 y or more. (Modified from Grumbach MM. Some considerations of the pathogenesis and classification of anomalies of sex in man. In: Astwood EB, ed. Clinical Endocrinology. New York: Grune & Stratton, 1960: 407–436.)

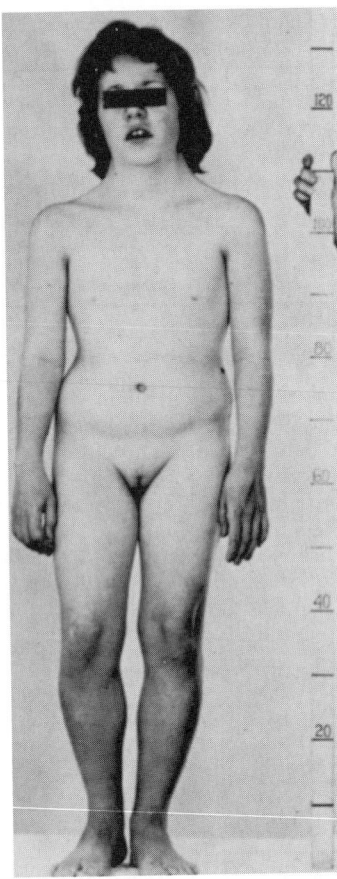

Figure 29–34. A 14 10/12-year-old patient with the typical form of the syndrome of gonadal dysgenesis. The X chromatin pattern was negative and karyotype was 45,X. She was short (height 134.5 cm, height age 9⁵/₁₂ years), was sexually infantile except for the appearance of sparse pubic hair, and exhibited characteristic stigmata of the syndrome: a short webbed neck, shield-like chest with widely separated nipples, bilateral short fourth metacarpals, puffiness over dorsum of fingers, cubitus valgus, and an increased number of pigmented nevi. The facies were characteristic and the ears low set. The bone age was 13½ years. The urinary 17-ketosteroid level was 5.1 mg/d; plasma and urinary gonadotropin levels were elevated. Vaginal smears and urocytogram showed an immature pattern in which cornified squamous cells were absent. With estrogen therapy, female secondary sexual characteristics were induced; cyclic administration resulted in periodic estrogen-withdrawal bleeding.

often recognizable by the distinctive facies, in which micrognathia; epicanthal folds; prominent, low-set, rotated and/or deformed ears; a fish-like mouth with a narrow, high-arched palate; ptosis; and strabismus are present with varying degrees of frequency. The chest is usually square and shield-like with microthelia and inverted nipples. The areolae appear to be widely spaced. The neck is short and broad, and the hairline in back is low. Webbing of the neck is present in 25 to 40%, and coarctation of the aorta occurs in 10 to 20%. Those with coarctation usually also have webbing of the neck. Additional anomalies include congenital lymphedema of the feet and hands (30%) (Fig. 29–34) or puffiness of the dorsum of the fingers; short fourth metacarpals (50%); renal abnormalities (40%); high-arched palate; various skeletal anomalies, including cubitus valgus, Madelung's deformity of the wrist, genu valgum, and scoliosis[373]; increased number of pigmented nevi; tendency to keloid formation; abnormal nails; recurrent otitis media, which may result in conductive hearing loss (as well as progressive sensorineural loss of hearing); unexplained hypertension[376]; and, rarely, gastrointestinal bleeding secondary to intestinal telangiectasia, hemangiomatoses, or dilated veins.[373] Money and others have reported that impairments of directional sense and space-form recognition, visual-motor coordi-

nation, and motor learning are common; this perceptual disability results in a lower mean performance I.Q. than in the general population and is evidence of diffuse or multifocal cerebral dysfunction,[377, 378] whereas verbal ability (including comprehension and vocabulary) is normal. In general, patients with gonadal dysgenesis do not tend to differ from siblings in overall intelligence[379, 380]; however, two studies suggest that mental retardation (I.Q. <70) may be more common than the 1 to 3% incidence reported in the general population.[381, 382] Gender identity and sexual attitudes are feminine. Girls with gonadal dysgenesis are generally more immature and distractable and have less self-esteem, poorer peer relations, and more difficulty at school than peers.[383, 384] Skuse and associates described poorer adjustment and "social cognition" in 45,Xᴹ (Xᴹ, maternally derived X chromosome) than in 45,Xᴾ (Xᴾ, paternally derived X chromosome) individuals with Turner syndrome. This difference was attributed to genomic imprinting, the silencing of some gene on the maternal X chromosome located in the pericentric region of the short arm or on the long arm of the X chromosome.[384a] This putative gene, which apparently escapes inactivation, is the first imprinted gene proposed for the human X chromosome.

As adults, women with gonadal dysgenesis exhibit more conservative sexual attitudes and a more negative body image.[385] Lack of ovarian function (including infertility), rather than height, was the major concern of adult women with gonadal dysgenesis in one study.[386] Severe psychopathic manifestations are uncommon. In general, most women with gonadal dysgenesis are independent, self-sufficient, and sexually active.[381] The risk of anorexia nervosa and inflammatory bowel disease may be increased.[374]

The eponym Bonnevie-Ullrich syndrome has been applied to phenotypic female infants with lymphedema of the distal extremities and loose folds of skin over the back of the neck in addition to the typical features of gonadal dysgenesis (Fig. 29–35). In the neonate, pleural effusions and ascites that clear spontaneously are not uncommon,[387] and pericardial effusion has been reported. The serous effusions and the lymphedema are attributable to hypoplasia and other defects

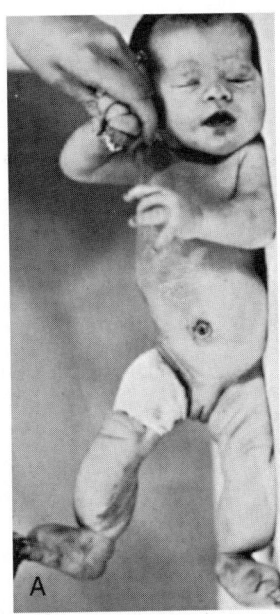
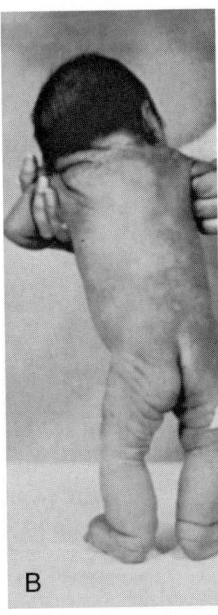

Figure 29–35. A and B, An infant with the syndrome of gonadal dysgenesis (karyotype 45,X) and associated lymphedema of extremities. The term Bonnevie-Ullrich syndrome is applied when this characteristic swelling of the feet or hands or both is associated with other features of gonadal dysgenesis. (From Grumbach MM. Chromosomal sex and the prepubertal diagnosis of gonadal dysgenesis. Reproduced by permission of Pediatrics 20:740. Copyright 1957.)

of the lymphatic system.[388] 45,X abortuses commonly exhibit generalized edema and a large hygroma of the neck.[389, 390] Postnatally, the latter abnormality results in webbing of the neck. These findings can be detected by prenatal ultrasonography.[389] Shephard and Fantel[391] suggested that the severe edema that occurs secondary to hypoalbuminemia and lymphatic duct hypoplasia in 45,X fetuses is responsible for many of the malformations involving the ears, hairline, neck, nipples, nails, and kidneys. The increased incidence of congenital heart disease associated with webbed neck has led to the suggestion that lymphatic obstruction is involved in the pathogenesis of both types of deformation.[392, 393]

The prevalence of cardiovascular abnormalities has varied from 20 to 50%. In a Danish study of 179 patients, 26% had cardiovascular malformations.[394] Coarctation of the aorta was the most common, occurring in 10% of patients, primarily those with a 45,X karyotype.[394] The prevalence of bicuspid aortic valves in gonadal dysgenesis determined by echocardiography has ranged from 9 to 34%.[373, 394, 395] Bicuspid aortic valves carry an increased risk for subacute bacterial endocarditis and tend to evolve with age into stenotic and/or insufficient aortic valves.[373, 394] An increased incidence of mitral valve prolapse has been reported in patients with gonadal dysgenesis.[373] Other studies have reported an increased incidence of partial anomalous venous drainage[395] and hypoplastic left heart syndrome.[396] On echocardiography, 8 to 29% of patients with gonadal dysgenesis have aortic root dilatation,[397, 398] and rupture from aortic dilatation has been reported in more than 20 patients.[398] Therefore, all patients with gonadal dysgenesis should have a thorough baseline cardiac evaluation, including an echocardiogram and/or magnetic resonance imaging (MRI) study in infancy and again at adolescence.[399-401] Patients with increased risk factors for dissection and rupture (e.g., those with coarctation, hypertension, and aortic root dilatation) require yearly follow-up and therapeutic measures to decrease the risk of dissection. Patients with bicuspid aortic valves should be given prophylactic antibiotic therapy before surgery or dental procedures, to prevent subacute bacterial endocarditis.

The most common renal abnormalities are rotation of the kidney, horseshoe kidney, duplication of the renal pelvis and ureter, and hydronephrosis secondary to ureteropelvic obstruction. Complete absence of the kidney and gross renal ectopia in 7 of 141 patients was reported by Lippe and associates.[402] Malformation of the kidneys and upper collecting system are so common that intravenous urography or a renal sonogram should be obtained routinely at the time of diagnosis.

Skeletal maturation is normal or slightly delayed in childhood and lags further in adolescence as a result of gonadal steroid deficiency. In most cases, the skeleton exhibits localized areas of rarefaction (fishnet appearance), especially of the hands, feet, elbows, and upper femurs.[403-405] Prepubertal girls with gonadal dysgenesis have normal bone density for height and age but decreased density at the wrist for bone age and body mass index.[406] The risk of wrist fractures is increased.[406] Patients not treated with estrogen often develop a severe form of the postmenopausal type of osteoporosis and may develop fractures and vertebral collapse. Osteochondrosis-like changes of the spine, vertebral hypoplasia, and scoliosis are common.[403, 404] In addition to the metacarpal sign (shortening of the fourth metacarpal), Kosowicz described a carpal sign characterized by a more acute angular configuration of the proximal row of carpal bones. The Madelung's or "bayonet" deformity of the wrist is present in about 10% of patients. Cubitus valgus (an increased carrying angle) occurs in half and is a consequence of a developmental abnormality of the trochlear head. The knee may show deformities of the medial tibial and femoral condyles with obliquely tipped tibial

epiphyses and medial projections of the tibial metaphyses that can result in genu valgum.[373] The pelvis tends to have a male-type inlet. Midface hypoplasia is common. The growth of the temporal bone, condylar cartilage, and spheno-occipital synchondrosis are abnormal.[373] Scoliosis is present in approximately 10% of patients, secondary either to hemivertebrae, leg length inequality, or idiopathic causes, and requires monitoring.[373] Gonadotrope hyperplasia may cause enlargement of the sella turcica, especially in untreated adults with hypergonadotropic hypogonadism. An "empty sella" was noted on computed tomographic (CT) scan in two of the authors' patients.

Short Stature. Short stature is an invariant feature in 45,X individuals and may be evident in utero. Intrauterine growth retardation is common, and the average birth weight $(2.83 \pm 0.57 \text{ kg})$ and length $(48.2 \pm 3.2 \text{ cm})$ are 1 standard deviation (SD) below the mean value for normal infants of comparable gestational age[407, 408]; the growth retardation is evident by the middle of the second trimester of gestation and affects all long bones.[409] The mean final height of patients in different series ranged from 142 to 147 cm.[407, 408, 410-412] In a survey of 12 European countries, a total of 661 patients were found, 51% of whom were 45,X and had a mean final height of 144.3 ± 6.7 cm; none had received estrogen therapy before the age of 14 years.[413] The ratio of sitting to standing height is frequently increased by late childhood and reflects the greater retardation in growth of the legs.[373, 414]

For the first 3 years of life, growth velocity is usually within the normal range.[408] Subsequently velocity decelerates, so that by a bone age of 9 years the difference in mean height between patients and normal individuals (16 cm) is close to the difference at maturity (20 cm).[408] Hence, there is little additional loss of height relative to normal individuals after a bone age of 9 years despite the lack of a pubertal growth spurt (Fig. 29–36). This may be a result of prolongation of growth as a consequence of the effect of estrogen deficiency on bone maturation. Although final height in untreated patients may not be achieved until late in the second decade of life, there is no major gain in height after the age of 16 years.[413] Final height correlates with birth weight and target height.[407, 410, 411, 413]

The short stature is not attributable to a deficiency of growth hormone, insulin-like growth factor I (IGF-I, also called somatomedin-C), IGF-II,[415] or adrenal or gonadal steroids[416] (see Chapter 30). Decreased amplitude and frequency of growth hormone pulses have been reported after 8 years of age.[417] Likewise, IGF-I levels that are normal up to 10 years of age are low thereafter[417]; however, administration of either estrogen[415] or growth hormone induces a rise in the concentration of plasma IGF-I. The changes in growth hormone secretory dynamics and IGF-I concentrations after 8 to 10 years of age are probably secondary to the lack of the estrogen-induced rise in plasma growth hormone concentration and IGF-I levels at puberty. The cause of the progressive growth failure is attributable, at least in part, to the missing *PAR1* gene, *PHOG* or *SHOX*, on the absent or structurally abnormal second sex chromosome.

Sexual Infantilism. The genital tract and external genitalia in this syndrome are female in character but immature. Located in the mesosalpinges parallel to the fallopian tubes are long, attenuated, pale, fibrous streaks of connective tissue. Typically, these streak-like or spindle-shaped structures consist of fibrous stroma arranged in whorls similar to those in ovarian stroma, but they lack primordial follicles. Vestigial medullary elements and rudimentary mesonephric tubules like those found in the primitive genital ridge are common at the hilus. After puberty, aggregates of epithelioid cells resembling Leydig or hilus cells are present in variable quantity.

Singh and Carr[388] studied the gonadal ridges of eight spontaneously aborted embryos and fetuses ranging in gesta-

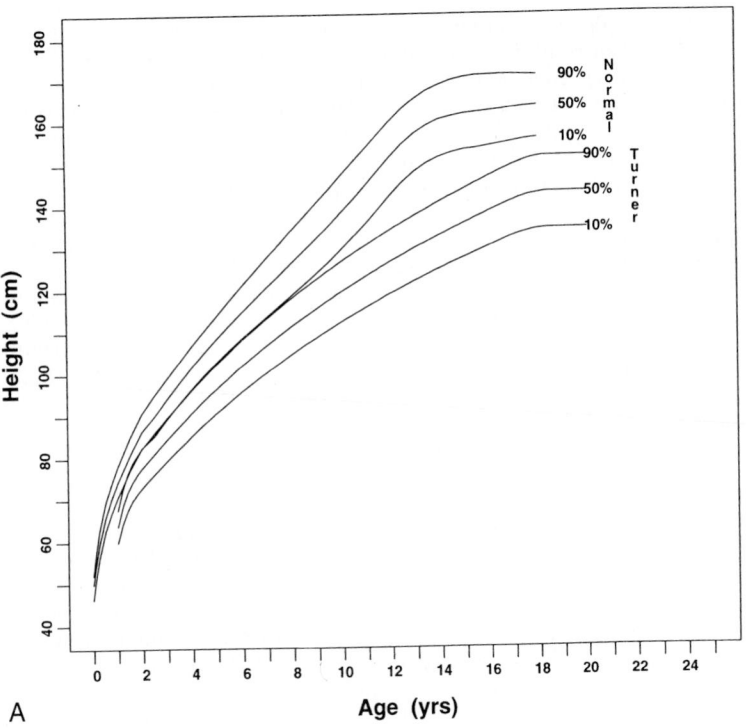

A

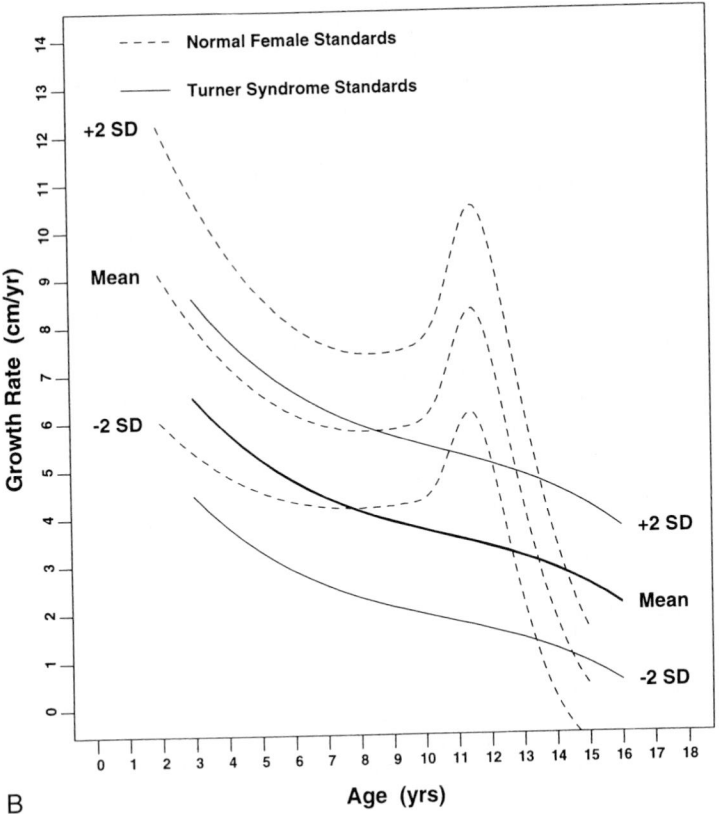

B

Figure 29–36. *A*, The mean height (50th percentile) in untreated patients with gonadal dysgenesis (mainly 45,X karyotype), compared with the growth curve of normal females. *B*, The mean height velocity in patients with gonadal dysgenesis and in normal females. Data derived from various sources. Note the lack of a pubertal growth spurt. (*B*, Courtesy of J. Frame and K. Attie, Genentech, Inc.)

tional age from 5 wk to 4 mo. Primordial germ cells were observed in all eight specimens. Until the third month of gestation, no appreciable differences were noted between these gonads and those from 46,XX fetuses; after that, connective tissue stroma increased and formation of follicles was impaired, suggesting that primordial germ cells seed the 45,X gonad, that many degenerate during oocyte formation and

folliculogenesis, and that surviving oocytes undergo accelerated atresia.[418] Jirasek[419] reported that oocytes in patients with a 45,X karyotype degenerate shortly after formation of the primary follicle, possibly because the surrounding follicular cell layer is incomplete. Two active X chromosomes appear to be required for the normal development of human oogonia and oocytes. Follicles are common in the gonadal streaks of

45,X infants at birth but are uncommon by late childhood and adolescence. Nevertheless, spontaneous puberty, menses, and fertility can occur in putative 45,X patients.

Longitudinal studies of both basal and LHRH-evoked gonadotropin secretion demonstrate a lack of feedback inhibition of the hypothalamic-pituitary axis by the dysgenetic gonads in infants and young children with gonadal dysgenesis.[420, 421] In 58 patients aged 2 days to 20 years, plasma FSH levels were elevated in those aged 2 days to 4 years and decreased to high-normal values between 5 and 10 years of age (Fig. 29–37). After 10 years, the plasma FSH level rose again into the castrate range.[420] Therefore, the pattern of plasma FSH concentration followed a diphasic curve similar to but higher than that in normal infants and children. The pattern of change in LH levels was similar, but the concentrations were one third to one tenth those of FSH. LHRH-induced LH and FSH responses exhibited a diphasic pattern with age, similar to those of basal levels.[421] In patients younger than 5 years of age, both the mean basal levels and the rise in gonadotropin levels induced by administration of LHRH were increased. Between ages 5 and 10 years, basal levels of FSH and LH and LHRH-evoked responses were less than those of younger patients with gonadal dysgenesis (see Fig. 29–37). In some patients between ages 6 and 10 years, both FSH and LH concentrations and the LHRH-induced gonadotropin responses were comparable to those in normal children. After age 11 years a striking rise in basal and readily releasable LH and FSH levels was observed. Therefore, between the ages of 5 and 10 years, basal and LHRH-elicited gonadotropin responses may not reflect the functional status of the gonads in all patients with gonadal dysgenesis.

Although streak gonads are the rule in 45,X gonadal dysgenesis, exceptions have been documented. Primary follicles have been described in the gonadal ridges of some 45,X individuals at adolescence, and this correlates with the rare occurrence of menarche and a variable but attenuated period of regular menses. By means of sonography, 30% of a series of 32 45,X females were found to have nonstreak gonads.[422] In this study, 3 of the 32 patients had breast development but had not menstruated.[422] This number correlates with previous data suggesting that 5 to 10% of patients with gonadal dysgenesis have a sufficient number of ovarian follicles ($>10^4$) at adolescence to initiate breast development.[423] Conceptions have been documented despite extensive karyotypic studies revealing only a 45,X cell line in multiple tissues.[424–426] In addition to variability in the rate of follicular atresia, another possible explanation for the presence of oogonia in 45,X

individuals is that a certain number of 45,X germ cells may undergo mitotic nondisjunction with the formation of 46,XX oogonia.[427] This process normally occurs in the female creeping vole and serves as a sex-determining mechanism in this species. Alternatively, some fertile 45,X patients may be unrecognized sex chromosome mosaics. Women with a 45,X cell line have increased fetal wastage and an increased number of chromosomally abnormal liveborn infants, including those with gonadal dysgenesis and Down syndrome.[426, 428–430]

Adrenarche in patients with gonadal dysgenesis is associated with a normal rise in adrenal androgen production in childhood but sparse pubic and axillary hair. Before the age of 10 years, the plasma concentration of adrenal androgens is normal,[431] but levels of dehydroepiandrosterone (DHEA), testosterone, and androstenedione are lower than normal after age 15, reflecting absence of the gonadal contribution.[432]

Rarely, enlargement of the clitoris may be present at birth or develop at puberty. Secretion of androgens by "Leydig cells" in the gonadal streak is a possible cause, as is the presence of a cryptic Y cell line.

Males with a 45,X karyotype have a Y-autosome translocation involving variable segments of the euchromatic (sex-determining) region of the Y chromosome.[433–437] Translocations have been reported involving the short arm of chromosomes 5, 14, 15, and 18 and the X chromosome.[438] Most patients have had either minor or major anomalies not usually associated with the syndrome of gonadal dysgenesis, such as the cri du chat syndrome. These additional anomalies are no doubt related to the autosome involved in the translocation and to the degree of deletion involved.

Incidence in Abortuses, Newborns, and Twins. The incidence of gonadal dysgenesis is approximately 1 per 2000 live female births,[439, 440] and approximately 50% of the patients have a 45,X karyotype. There is, in addition, a considerable loss of 45,X embryos and fetuses.[441] About 7% of spontaneous abortuses have a 45,X constitution.[441] It is estimated that frequency of 45,X zygotes is 2%, probably the most common chromosome anomaly in humans, but fewer than 1% of 45,X conceptuses survive to term.[442] Hook and Warburton[443] have analyzed chromosome karyotypes in embryonic and fetal deaths and demonstrated a significant disparity between the 45,X karyotype and those with mosaicism and/or an isochromosome for the long arm of the X chromosome (Xqi). They postulated a "fetoprotective" effect of more than one dose of some locus or loci on the long arm of the X chromosome.[443]

Associated Disorders. The incidence of autoimmune disorders is increased; the most prevalent is autoimmune thyroiditis and Grave's disease, which occurs in 15 to 20%. The prevalence of thyroid antibodies and hypothyroidism (or hyperthyroidism) increases during childhood and adolescence[444, 445] and in adulthood may approach 50% of patients. Early diagnosis may be facilitated by monitoring levels of thyroid antibody and basal thyroid-stimulating hormone with the use of new, sensitive assays. Basal and thyrotropin-releasing hormone–induced concentrations of prolactin may be elevated in euthyroid patients with gonadal dysgenesis. Prevalences of rheumatoid arthritis and inflammatory bowel disease are increased in patients with a 45,X karyotype.[446]

Carbohydrate intolerance with mild insulin resistance is common, especially after age 16 years, and may become worse with obesity or during treatment with growth hormone or oxandrolone.[447, 448] Mean cholesterol levels may be elevated after 11 years of age, independent of age and body mass index.[449]

During childhood, problematic otitis media is common and may result in conductive hearing loss.[450] Abnormalities in the growth of the temporal bone, condylar cartilage, and spheno-occipital synchondrosis result in an abnormality in the positioning of the external auditory meatus and the relation

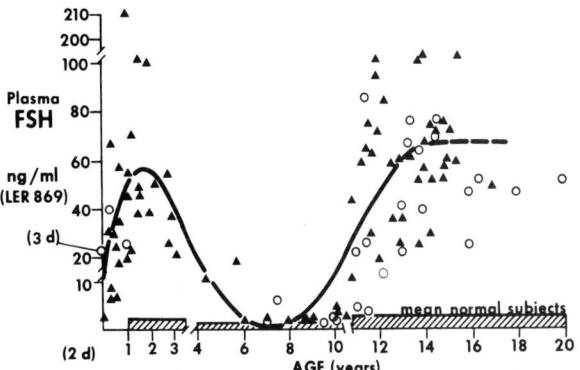

Figure 29–37. The pattern of plasma FSH concentration in relation to age in 58 patients with the syndrome of gonadal dysgenesis. ▲, patients with 45,X karyotype; ○, patients with structural abnormalities of the X chromosome and mosaics. The hatched area shows the range of FSH values in normal females. (From Conte FA, Grumbach MM, Kaplan SL. A diphasic pattern of gonadotropin secretion in patients with the syndrome of gonadal dysgenesis. J Clin Endocrinol Metab 40:670–674, 1975. © The Endocrine Society.)

of the middle ear to the eustachian tube in patients with gonadal dysgenesis.[450] These changes, along with abnormalities in the shape of the palate, are thought to be responsible for the increased incidence of otitis media. Sensorineural deafness has also been reported in two thirds of adult patients.[451] The frequent episodes of otitis media and the sensorineural hearing loss are independent variables in gonadal dysgenesis; the sensorineural hearing loss may be related to loss of genes on the X chromosome responsible for the gonadal dysgenesis phenotype.[452]

In a survey of 289 patients with gonadal dysgenesis stigmata, Wertelecki and co-workers[453] found eight patients with nongonadal tumors, suggesting a possible increased risk of malignancy. As noted previously, the prevalence of anorexia nervosa is increased.

Origin of 45,X Constitution and Phenotype. A 45,X chromosome constitution (see Figs. 29–3 and 29–13) may be a consequence of nondisjunction or chromosome loss during gametogenesis in either parent which results in a sperm or ovum lacking a sex chromosome. Although errors of mitosis in a normal zygote often lead to mosaicism, a purely 45,X constitution may arise at the first cleavage division from anaphase lag with loss of a sex chromosome or, less likely, from mitotic nondisjunction with failure of the complementary 47,XXX or 47,XYY cell line to survive (see Fig. 29–3). Loss of one X or Y chromosome between fertilization and the first cleavage division may be a frequent but not the only cause of a 45,X embryo.[36]

Several lines of evidence support the hypothesis of a mitotic error in this syndrome: (1) the lack of association with advanced maternal age, in contrast to XXY Klinefelter's syndrome (indeed the incidence of 45,X conceptuses is increased in teenage pregnancies)[454, 455]; (2) the prevalence of sex chromosome mosaicism; (3) the increased frequency of twinning in sibships with a 45,X individual[456]; and (4) the occurrence of a 46,XY monozygotic co-twin of a 45,X individual.[457]

Family studies of X-linked traits (e.g., color blindness, Xg blood group) indicate that loss of the paternally derived X chromosome is more common than would be expected with random loss of either the maternally or the paternally derived X chromosome; in informative pedigrees, 77% of 45,X individuals have loss of the paternal sex chromosome (45,X^M), and 23% have loss of the maternal X chromosome (45,X^P). Similar findings have been obtained with the use of DNA analysis.[458, 459]

The deviation in parental origin of the retained X chromosome raised the possibility that retention of the maternal X chromosome might play a role in survival in addition to affecting the phenotype through "imprinting." However, the percentage of aborted fetuses with a 45,X^M karyotype is the same as in liveborn infants.[460, 461] Therefore, imprinting does not appear to affect fetal survival in 45,X individuals. Although some studies showed no effect of imprinting on phenotype,[462] 45,X^M patients appear to have an increased prevalence of cardiovascular anomalies and webbed neck; furthermore, the height in 45,X^M correlates more strongly with maternal height than with midparental height.[463] An imprinted gene on the maternal X chromosome,[384a] which affects social cognition, is discussed above in the section on clinical aspects.

The very high embryonic and fetal mortality of 45,X conceptuses as opposed to those with 45,X/46,XX or 45,X/46,XY mosaicism or a structurally abnormal X chromosome, raised the possibility that all liveborn individuals with the gonadal dysgenesis syndrome are mosaics.[443] This hypothesis has not been supported by cytogenetic data[464] or by molecular analysis with X chromosome probes.[465, 466] However, the possibility of prenatal mosaicism and in vivo loss of structurally abnormal sex chromosomes postnatally has not been ruled out. Molecular analysis with the use of Y-specific probes has

been inconclusive.[37] From 0 to 33% of patients with gonadal dysgenesis whose karyotype is other than 45,X/46,XY have a low percentage of Y chromosome material.[37, 467] Chu and colleagues[37] studied 87 patients with the use of multiple Y chromosome probes and found 3.4% to be positive for low-percentage mosaicism for all or part of the Y chromosome. The similar results obtained by Binder and colleagues[468] indicate a low level of Y chromosome mosaicism in 45,X and chromatin-positive individuals with gonadal dysgenesis. The significance of low-percentage mosaicism for Y chromosome material and its relation to gonadal differentiation and the risk of malignancy are still to be determined.

The classic gonadal dysgenesis phenotype is usually associated with absence of all or a proximal portion of the short arm of the X or Y chromosome. The haploinsufficiency of genes in these loci that are not inactivated is postulated to cause the phenotype. Page and co-workers suggested that the genes that encode ribosome protein S4X (*RPS4X*), and its homologue on the Y chromosome (*RPS4Y*), are candidate genes.[469] However, the location of this gene on the long arm of the X chromosme and the fact that it is expressed in patients with 46,XXp− and 46,X,Xqi karyotypes make it an unlikely candidate.[470] Other candidate genes are being sought.

Ogata and Matsuo[471] postulated that the gonadal dysgenesis phenotype is multifactoral in origin. According to their construct, the phenotype is related to (1) quantitative loss or alteration of euchromatic or noninactivated genes (haploinsufficiency), leading to global nonspecific developmental defects; (2) haploinsufficiency of pseudoautosomal and/or Y-specific growth genes and lymphogenic genes, resulting in short stature and the "deformative" stigmata; (3) oocyte loss and gonadal dysgenesis due to impaired or failed chromosome pairing during meiotic prophase.[471]

The underlying cause of this sex chromosome abnormality is not known. An increased frequency of thyroid autoimmunity in patients with the syndrome of gonadal dysgenesis and in their parents suggests that the genetic predisposition to develop autoantibodies in one or both parents is associated with an increased prevalence of the 45,X constitution and other chromosome abnormalities in the offspring. Infants with the syndrome of gonadal dysgenesis have been born after artificial insemination.[472] Familial occurrence of 45,X gonadal dysgenesis is rare.

Diagnosis and Treatment. Phenotypic females with the following features should have a karyotype analysis: (1) short stature (>2.5 SD below the mean height value for age), (2) somatic stigmata associated with gonadal dysgenesis, and (3) delayed adolescence with increased plasma or urinary gonadotropin levels. In the past, X chromatin was assessed to screen for gonadal dysgenesis. Normal females have 20 to 30% sex chromatin–positive cells at all ages, including the neonatal period. 45,X patients lack an X chromatin body in interphase nuclei, and 45,X/46,XX mosaics usually have between 3 and 19% chromatin-positive cells. Although determination of the X chromatin pattern is a rapid method of screening, karyotype analysis is the definitive procedure. The concentration of plasma FSH is useful in assessing the functional status of the gonads.

The following studies should be done in women when the diagnosis of gonadal dysgenesis is made: an intravenous pyelogram or ultrasonographic examination to exclude a renal anomaly; an echocardiogram or MRI study to assess cardiovascular function; periodic hearing examination and evaluation of thyroid function and thyroid antibodies; regular measurements of plasma glucose levels after adolescence; and monitoring for scoliosis and bone density in late adolescence and adulthood for evidence of osteopenia.[473]

Therapy is directed toward augmenting stature, correcting somatic anomalies, and inducing secondary sexual characteristics and menses. As noted, the short stature in gonadal dysgenesis is not related to a deficiency of growth hormone, insulin-like growth factors, thyroid hormone, or adrenal or gonadal steroids. However, administration of pharmacologic doses of biosynthetic human growth hormone increases growth rate and augments final height by a mean of 5 to 10 cm.[474–478] The heterogeneity in response appears to be related to the chronologic age at the start of therapy, the duration of therapy, the dose and frequency of growth hormone administration, the use of oxandrolone and/or estrogen, the growth standards used, the height of the parents, and the growth hormone peak elicited by pharmacologic stimuli.[474–481] Rosenfeld and co-workers have the longest and most extensive study.[474] Starting in 1983, 70 patients between the ages of 4.7 and 12.4 years with normal growth hormone responses to provocative stimuli were studied.[474] They were randomly assigned to (1) a control group for 1 year; (2) the anabolic steroid oxandrolone at a dose of 0.125 mg/kg by mouth daily; (3) growth hormone 0.125 mg/kg subcutaneously three times per week; or (4) a combination of oxandrolone and growth hormone.[474] After 12 to 24 mo, all groups except the growth hormone alone group were placed on combination therapy; however, the oxandrolone dose was lowered to 0.0625 mg/kg because of signs of virilization.[474] After 3 y, most patients received daily growth hormone rather than thrice weekly; however, the dose of 0.375 mg/kg/wk was unchanged. The mean height in patients who completed therapy was 151.7 cm, for a net mean gain of 9 cm over projected height and historical controls.[474]

Uncertainty exists as to the magnitude of the increase in final height that can be attributed to ethnic differences,[476, 477] the possibility of a secular trend in growth since the baseline standard was derived, and the methods of evaluation of growth and prediction of final height in gonadal dysgenesis.[412, 482] For this reason, two trials using concurrent randomized controls are in progress to evaluate the effect of growth hormone treatment on final height, its safety, and the psychosocial effects of years of injections.[483] Growth hormone therapy is now approved by the U.S. Food and Drug Administration for the treatment of patients with gonadal dysgenesis, and it was approved previously in Japan and many Western European countries. It is prudent to discuss growth hormone therapy with the parents and patients, including its efficacy and side effects, in all patients with gonadal dysgenesis whose height is more than 2.5 SD below the mean value for age, especially those whose growth rate is less than 5 cm/y. Studies are in progress to evaluate the effects of initiating growth hormone therapy at 5 to 6 years of age before the growth deficit is severe. In general, the authors recommend the guidelines proposed by Rosenfeld and co-workers.[484] Growth hormone therapy is usually continued until the growth rate falls to less than 2 cm/y or the bone age exceeds 15 years.

Estrogen therapy has commonly been deferred until age 15 or later on the assumption that treatment at an earlier age leads to rapid skeletal maturation and diminished height. This premise was based largely on the fact that pharmacologic doses of estrogens can accelerate bone maturation and lead to premature epiphyseal fusion without a proportionate increase in height. Studies in patients with aromatase deficiency and in a patient with a mutation in the estrogen receptor indicate that estrogen rather than androgen is the principal gonadal hormone involved in bone maturation and fusion and bone mineral accretion.[485–487] The authors examined the effect of early low-dose, conjugated estrogen therapy on linear growth, bone age, and the development of secondary sexual characteristics in a group of patients with gonadal dysgenesis.[410] Low-dose conjugated estrogens (9 μg/kg body weight/d) or ethinyl estradiol (141 ng/kg body weight/d) was given to 21 patients with gonadal dysgenesis who had a mean age of

13 years and mean bone age of 10.7 years. Growth rate was transiently accelerated but declined to below the pretherapy rate after 12 mo of therapy. The final height of the patients treated with low-dose estrogen was not different from that of control nontreated patients or that of a group of six girls with the syndrome of gonadal dysgenesis in whom normal ovarian function was present and spontaneous puberty ensued. Hence, no increase or decrease in mean final height was noted in the authors' study. However, girls who received estrogen with a bone age of less than 11 years were shorter than the girls who began low-dose estrogen therapy after a bone age of 11 years.[410] Similar results have been obtained subsequently in other studies.[488–493]

Serious psychological effects are frequently associated with a prolonged delay in the treatment of sexual infantilism.[494] The institution of low-dose, conjugated estrogen or synthetic estrogen therapy alone at approximately 13 years of age (bone age >11 years) elicits a growth spurt without inordinate advancement of skeletal maturation or reduction in final height and induces the development of secondary sexual characteristics at an age comparable to that of normal peers, thereby obviating the undesirable psychological consequences of a prolonged delay in sexual maturation. Studies in which growth hormone treatment was combined with early estrogen therapy (i.e., in patients younger than 12 years of age) indicate a shorter final height than in patients who received growth hormone treatment and "late" estrogen substitution therapy.[490, 492] Therefore, in the treatment of girls with gonadal dysgenesis, the goal of increased adult stature must be balanced against the desire for sexual maturation in each individual patient.

A number of instances of endometrial carcinoma have been reported in patients with gonadal dysgenesis.[495] The evidence suggests that estrogens, especially when unopposed by progesterone, can produce a progression of histologic changes from endometrial hyperplasia to invasive carcinoma (also see Chapter 15). To clarify the relation between estrogen therapy and endometrial pathology in gonadal dysgenesis, Rosenwaks and colleagues[496] studied 41 patients receiving estrogen replacement therapy. Increased risk of abnormal endometrial histology correlated with (1) a lifetime dosage of conjugated estrogens of more than 2500 mg, (2) more than 7 y of estrogen therapy, and (3) a daily dose of conjugated estrogens greater than 1.25 mg. Progestagens can modify the effect of estrogens on endometrial histology. It is therefore prudent to treat patients with gonadal dysgenesis with low-dose cyclic estrogen replacement therapy, with progestagen added at the end of each cycle. Further studies are necessary to assess the optimal dose of estrogen that reduces the risk of endometrial carcinoma while concurrently preventing osteoporosis. Rarely, patients with a 45,X karyotype and no cytogenetic evidence of Y chromosome material develop gonadoblastomas.[497] However, studies employing multiple Y-specific DNA probes indicate that 3.4% of apparent 45,X patients have Y chromosomal material present.[37] These 45,X patients may be at risk for gonadoblastoma formation. Most patients with a 45,X karyotype have little or no risk of neoplastic transformation of the streak gonads.

Replacement Therapy. The authors routinely initiate therapy (depending on the height) at about 13 years of age with 0.3 mg of conjugated estrogen or 5 μg of ethinyl estradiol by mouth. The dose is gradually increased over the next 2 to 3 y to 0.6 to 1.25 mg of conjugated estrogens or 10 μg of ethinyl estradiol daily for the first 21 d of the month. The patient is maintained on the minimal dose of estrogen needed to maintain secondary sexual characteristics, permit withdrawal bleeding, and prevent osteopenia. Medroxyprogesterone acetate, 5 to 10 mg/d, is given from the 10th through the 21st day of

have an X chromosome that consists primarily of two long arms (Xq) and lacks a short arm (Xp); it arises mainly as a consequence of a break in sequence in the proximal short arm and not by centromere misdivision[40] (Fig. 29–40). The Xqi chromosomes may be either monocentric or dicentric X.[505] In a review of 89 cases, 29 were monocentric. Of these, only 5 of 17 were associated with mosaicism for a 45,X cell line.[506] In contrast, 49 of 60 patients with a dicentric isochromosome had a 45,X cell line. Dicentric X isochromosomes are more unstable than monocentric forms and probably result more frequently in sex chromosome mosaicism through loss of the heteromorphic dicentric X chromosome. In 14 patients studied with molecular biologic techniques, Xp markers were found in 3 dicentric Xqi chromosomes and in 3 monocentric Xqi chromosomes.[507] In 5 instances the Xqi was paternally derived.[507] Isochromosome for the long arm of the X is the most common form of structural rearrangement of the X chromosome, occurring in approximately 15% of patients with the syndrome of gonadal dysgenesis.

Patients with a long arm X isochromosome are invariably short and have streak gonads,[36, 72, 471] although some menstruate spontaneously.[423, 508] In general, the somatic stigmata of gonadal dysgenesis are less severe than in 45,X patients. Coarctation of the aorta and severe lymphedema of the hands and feet are less common in 46,XXqi patients. Webbing of the neck, if present, is usually slight. The findings indicate that absence of the short arm on the second X, even in the presence of an X chromosome composed of two long arms, leads to short stature, failure of ovarian development, and some somatic stigmata of gonadal dysgenesis. The prevalence of autoimmune thyroiditis,[509] decreased glucose tolerance, and inflammatory bowel disease may be higher in patients with structural abnormalities of the X chromosome, especially 46,XXqi, than in 45,X individuals.

Structurally abnormal X chromosomes are usually late replicating (except in balanced X-autosome translocations), and they give rise to the X chromatin body. Therefore X chromatin bodies are larger than normal in patients with a 46,XXqi constitution, but their increased size may be less evident in buccal smears than in other tissues. Karyotype analysis reveals a metacentric X chromosome with two arms of equal length whose banding pattern is similar to that of the long arm of the normal X chromosome.

46,XXpi. There is controversy about the existence of an isochromosome for the short arm of the X chromosome. Of the 11 reported cases, 3 have been revised to long arm deletions, 4 were reported as presumptive, and 2 have been questioned on cytogenetic grounds.[510] The controversy revolves around the difficulty in distinguishing Xpi from deletions of the long arm of the X chromosome, because the banding pattern of Xp is quite similar to that of Xq from the centromere to Xq24. There have been no reports of either high-resolution chromosome banding or molecular genetic analysis in a patient with 46,XXpi.

46,XXr or 45,X/46,XXr. A ring X chromosome usually occurs as part of 45,X/46,XXr mosaicism or a more complex karyotype (see Fig. 29–40).[13, 511] Short stature is present in most patients, and most have minor stigmata of gonadal dysgenesis; none have a webbed neck or coarctation of the aorta. Approximately one third have spontaneous menses and develop secondary sexual characteristics. A mother and daughter with 45,X/46,XXr have been described.[512] Although most patients with 45,X/46,XXr have the gonadal dysgenesis phenotype, patients with severe mental retardation, syndactly, and abnormal facies have been reported. *XIST*, a gene that is transcribed only by the inactive X chromosome, is not expressed in these patients.[108, 513, 514] All genes analyzed on the proximal short and long arms of the ring X were expressed,[108] suggesting that the abnormal phenotype in these patients is caused by disomy for these genes on the X chromosome resulting from lack of dosage compensation.[108]

The proportion of X chromatin–positive cells is decreased in patients with a ring X chromosome, and the X chromatin bodies tend to be small. The ring X chromosome, with rare exceptions, exhibits late DNA replication.[36]

The ring X chromosome arises by loss of both ends (telomeres) of the chromosome and union of the proximal breaks; as a consequence, a variable amount of chromatin material is lost from each arm (see Fig. 29–4). Ring chromosomes are unstable, and the size of the ring varies in different cells of the same subject. In relation to gonadal dysgenesis, studies of patients with a ring X chromosome have established that loss of both telomeres of an X chromosome need not lead to the development of streak gonads.

It is sometimes difficult to be sure of the cytogenetic origin of the ring chromosome, a distinction that is critical in view of the increased risk of gonadal tumors associated with dysgenetic gonads and Y cell lines. DNA analysis with specific X and Y chromosome probes have made identification easier.[515, 516]

46,XXp– and 45,X/46,XXp–. Deletions of the short arm of the X chromosome (Xp–) are rare and are frequently associated with 45,X mosaicism. Phenotypic-karyotypic analysis of 40 nonmosaic patients indicated considerable variation in somatic stigmata and gonadal function.[13, 517–521] Patients with a terminal deletion of the short arm of the X (distal to Xp21)

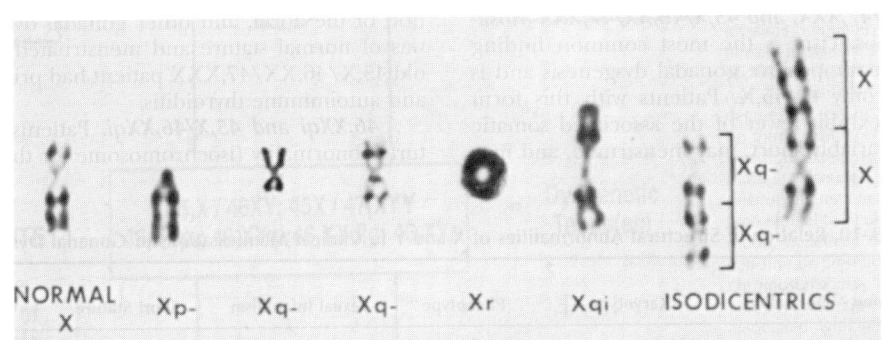

Figure 29–40. Structural anomalies of the X chromosome. The normal X at the left is G banded. A dark band on the short arm and two major dark bands on the long arm are visible. The first Xq– and the ring X chromosome (Xr) are not banded. They show late replication with tritiated thymidine. Note symmetry of the arms of the second Xq–. Even with G banding, it is difficult to distinguish this chromosome from a possible short arm isochromosome. The long arm isochromosome (Xqi) appears to be dicentric. The two chromosomes to the far right are apparent isodicentric X chromosomes. Both have two C bands but only one functional centromere. There is a mirror-like band pattern on both sides of a point between the two C bands. The first isodicentric presumably represents a break in the long arm of X at q22 with fusion of chromatids and duplication of entire chromatid. The second isodicentric appears to represent a terminal break in the short arm so that reduplication of the chromatids has produced what appears to be almost two X chromosomes.

can have normal ovarian function and no somatic stigmata of gonadal dysgenesis with the possible exception of a modest degree of short stature.[108, 502] Patients with deletions proximal to Xp21 usually have short stature, variable stigmata of gonadal dysgenesis, and gonadal dysfunction (Fig. 29–41).

The abnormal X chromosome is usually the late DNA-replicating X and is responsible for the small X chromatin body in interphase nuclei in these patients. Of interest is the report of a familial group of seven patients with the syndrome of gonadal dysgenesis secondary to a deletion of the short arm of an X chromosome in which the disorder was transmitted by carriers of a balanced translocation between the X and chromosome 1.[522]

46,XXq− and 45,X/46,XXq− . Patients have been re-

ported with a deletion of the long arm of the X chromosome (Xq−). In general, patients with only a 46,XXq− cell line are normal in stature or have moderately short stature and exhibit few manifestations of gonadal dysgenesis but have primary amenorrhea, sexual infantilism, and streak gonads. The authors have studied two patients with 46,XXq− karyotypes, and the findings in one are summarized in Figure 29–42. Exceptions to the rule that 46,XXq− patients lack stigmata of gonadal dysgenesis and are of normal height were reported before chromosome banding techniques became available. Such cases may represent either hidden mosaicism or complex structural rearrangements of the X chromosome, including inversions and interstitial rather than terminal deletions. Studies with FISH and Southern blotting suggest that

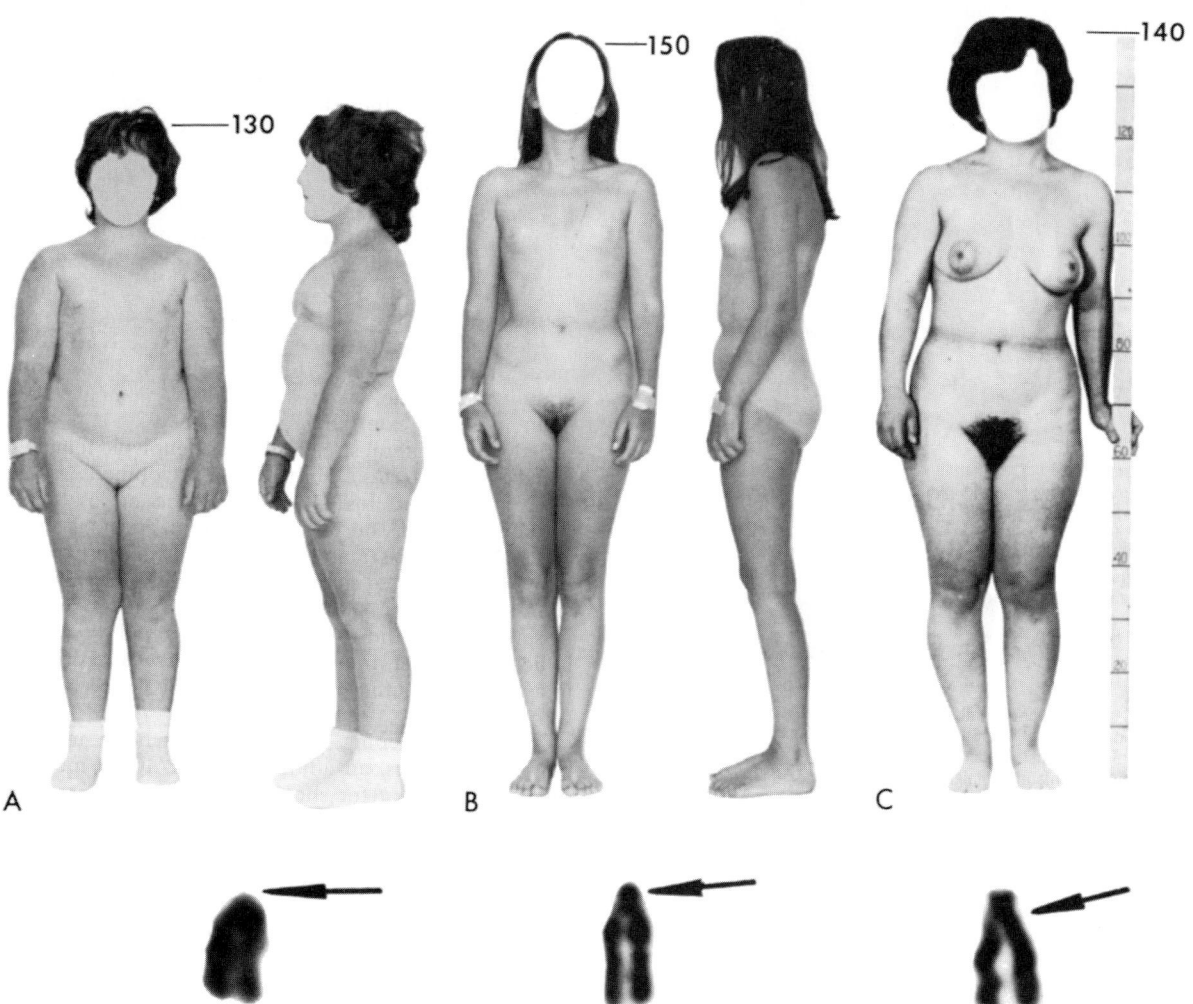

Figure 29–41. Variable gonadal function and phenotypic stigmata in three patients with a deletion of the short arm of the X chromosome (Xp−) of different degrees. *A*, A 13-year-old phenotypic female of short stature (−3.5 SD) with low-set ears, high-arched palate, low hairline, broad chest with wide-spaced areolae, cubitus valgus, puffy hands and feet, and short fourth metacarpals. There was no evidence of secondary sexual characteristics. The plasma FSH level was elevated at 26 μg/L (LER-869); the plasma estradiol level was less than 22 pmol/L (6 pg/mL). The buccal smear contained a normal proportion of X chromatin bodies in interphase nuclei, which were conspicuously small. Karyotype analysis and autoradiography revealed a 46,XXp− karyotype. The abnormal X chromosome appeared to lack the entire short arm. *B*, A 17⁴/₁₂-year-old phenotypic female with the stigmata of the syndrome of gonadal dysgenesis. Her height was 151 cm (−3 SD), and she had multiple nevi, cubitus valgus, and a short fourth metacarpal on the right hand. At age 13 the patient noted spontaneous onset of breast development, which did not progress. Plasma gonadotropin levels were elevated: LH 7.3 μg/L (LER-960) and FSH 53 μg/L (LER-869). The concentration of plasma estradiol was 70 pmol/L (19 pg/mL). On buccal smear, the cells had a normal proportion of X chromatin bodies, which appeared small. Karyotype analysis and autoradiography indicated an Xp− chromosome that had been deleted close to the centromere, but a small segment of the short arm was visible distal to the centromere. *C*, A 20-year-old phenotypic female with a chief complaint of dysfunctional uterine bleeding. She had short stature, slight puffiness of hands and feet, and short fourth metacarpals. Female secondary sexual characteristics appeared at age 11, and menarche at age 13 was followed by regular menses, which later became irregular. The buccal smear contained nuclei with a normal proportion, but small sex chromatin bodies. Bilateral ovaries were identified grossly and histologically during an appendectomy. Karyotype was 46,XXp−. The extent of deletion of the short arms of the abnormal X chromosome in this patient is less than that seen in patients in *A* and *B*. A segment of the short arm is readily discernible above the centromere. It appears that, in these three patients with XXp− karyotypes, somatic and gonadal manifestations of the syndrome of gonadal dysgenesis correlated with the magnitude of deletion of the short arm of the X chromosome.

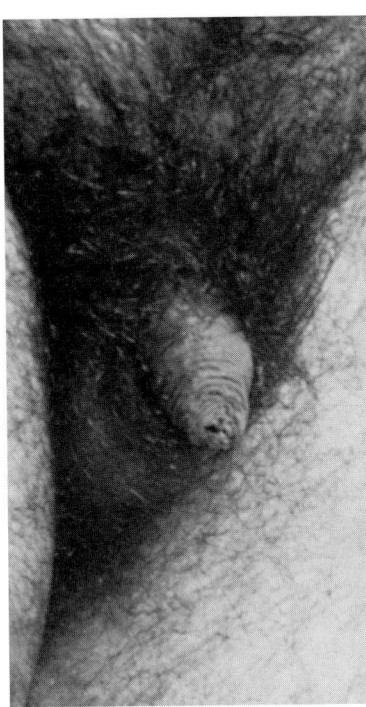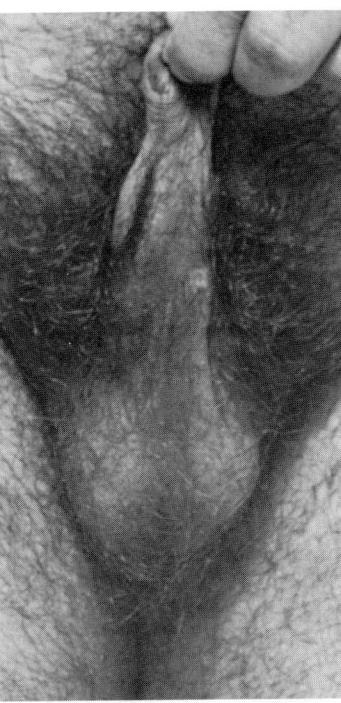

Figure 29–44. The external genitalia of a normally differentiated male with 45,X/46,XY mosaicism. Karyotype analyses revealed 16 and 68% mosaicism for a 45,X cell line in blood and skin, respectively. Gonadotropin levels, both basal and LHRH stimulated, were normal. Fertility was documented in vitro and by the conception of a normal male fetus.

testosterone levels, both basally and in response to LHRH, were within the normal range for adult men. On pelvic ultrasonography, müllerian duct derivatives were absent, and the testes appeared normal and homogeneous. The sperm count was 17,000,000/mL, and the patient demonstrated fertility as evidenced by the fathering of a "normal" 46,XY fetus. The finding of a short, otherwise normal fertile male with 45,X/46,XY mosaicism extends the phenotypic spectrum of this disorder.

Ascertainment bias may be responsible for the lack of well-differentiated males in reports of this disorder.[532] A review of the chromosome analyses of 58 patients in the literature who were ascertained because of ambiguous genitalia shows a preponderance of 45,X cells,[500] suggesting that only individuals whose abnormality occurred in the first few cell divisions are represented in this group of patients. However, 90% of the fetuses diagnosed by amniocentesis and confirmed postnatally as 45,X/46,XY mosaics have normal male genitalia.[532–534] Follow-up of these patients is limited, and hypothalamic-pituitary-gonadal function has not been characterized. However, their lack of presentation at a later date with either gonadal tumors or gonadal dysfunction suggests that most (at least 75%), like the authors' patient, have normal hypothalamic-pituitary-gonadal function and are at low risk for testicular tumors.

The restricted local or paracrine action of the testes on the differentiation of genital ducts is well demonstrated in patients with asymmetrical gonadal development. In such patients, development of male ducts and involution of the müllerian structures are also asymmetrical and parallel the degree of testicular development on each side. As discussed previously, local action of the testis on müllerian duct regression is mediated through AMH, whereas unilateral differentiation of male ducts is mediated by high local levels of testosterone in the wolffian ducts and their derivatives. The presence of Sertoli cells in the ipsilateral gonad correlates with the absence of müllerian structures on the same side in patients with 45,X/46,XY mosaicism.[535] This observation is consistent with the local secretion of AMH by embryonic and fetal Sertoli cells. Male differentiation of the external genitalia is, however, brought about by the systemic effects of testosterone secreted by a fetal testis. Hence, the external phenotype may range from a simulant female to a completely male configuration. Although the secretion of androgenic hormones at adolescence is usually predictable from the degree of masculinization of the external genitalia in utero, virilization may occur at puberty in patients with a female phenotype. Breast development at or after the age of puberty occurs in about one fourth of cases and is usually associated with a gonadal neoplasm. The authors studied two adolescent 45,X/46,XY subjects who had breast development and had pubertal levels of plasma estradiol; at laparotomy a gonadoblastoma that secreted estradiol was found (Fig. 29–45).

The propensity of patients with 45,X/46,XY mosaicism to develop gonadal tumors is high, and prophylactic removal of the streak gonads or dysgenetic undescended testes is indicated. Gonadoblastoma, a complex tumor composed of large germ cells, Sertoli cells, and stromal derivatives, is the neoplasm most often found, and it can give rise to a malignant germinoma. Therefore, after the removal of the gonads, serial sections should be examined for evidence of a tumor. The risk of tumor is about 20%[536] and is age related. Four 45,X/46,XY patients with incomplete virilization have been described in whom carcinoma in situ (CiS) was present in biopsies of the gonads.[537] CiS is thought to be a premalignant lesion leading to germ cell tumors.[537] Because 45,X/46,XY mosaics not only may harbor gonadoblastomas, roughly 30% of which are associated with germ cell tumors, but also have an increased prevalence of CiS, gonadal biopsy is indicated in all individuals with a male phenotype and 45,X/46,XY mosaicism. If the testis is histologically normal and is in the scrotum or can be placed in the scrotum, it can be retained. However, careful, close follow-up is mandatory. Müller, Skakkeback, and associates recommend sonography of the gonads and biopsy of the retained testis at the start of puberty. If biopsy and sonography show lack of evidence of CiS, they suggest an annual sonographic examination and a second biopsy at 20 years of age.[537a] The absence of CiS at age 20 suggests that the risk of a gonadal germ cell tumor is minimal. The risk of gonadal germ cell tumors in phenotypically normal males ascertained by chance to be 45,X/46,XY mosaics has not been defined and must await further studies. Modalities

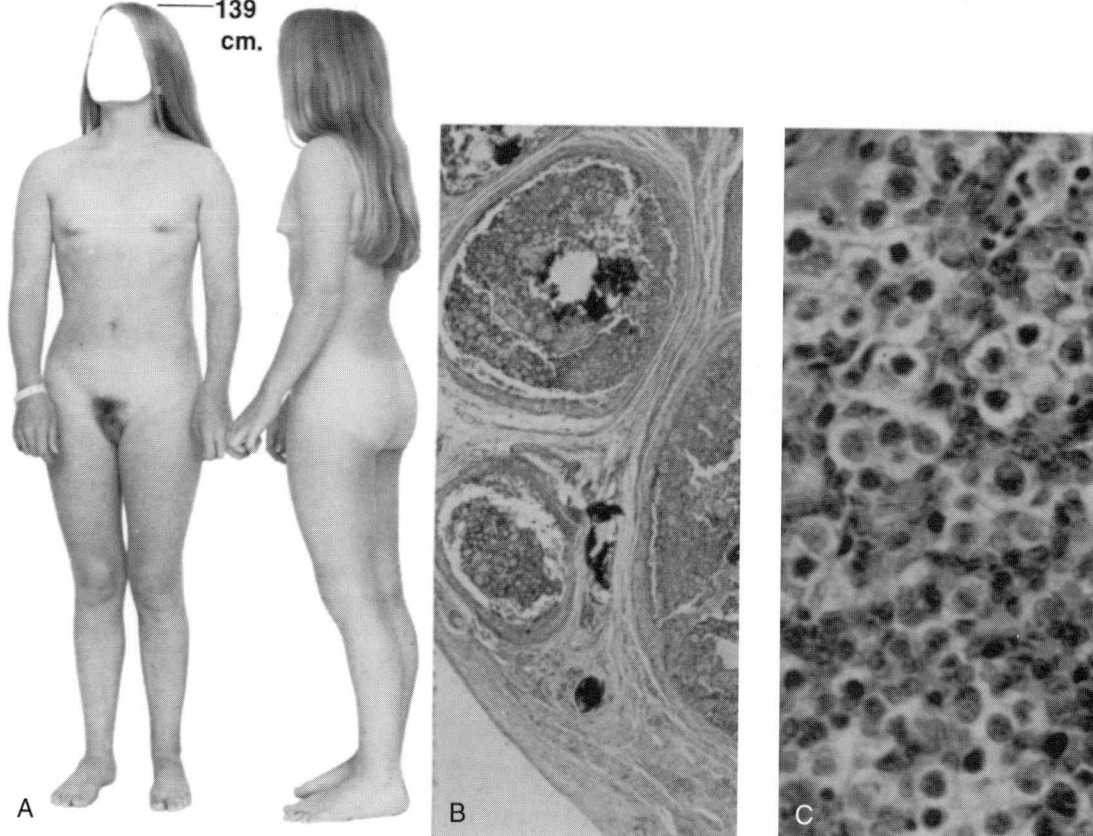

Figure 29–45. 45,X/46,XY mosaicism with a feminizing gonadoblastoma. *A,* A 20-year-old female with many stigmata of the syndrome of gonadal dysgenesis, including short stature, multiple nevi, cubitus valgus, and hyperconvex, small nails. The buccal smear was X chromatin negative; on fluorescence microscopy, 30% of interphase nuclei had a single Y body. Karyotype was 45,X/46,XY. The patient had spontaneous development of pubic and axillary hair at age 12. At age 18, breast development was noted. Her height was 139 cm (-5.1 SD) and weight 39 kg (-2.5 SD). Bone age was 17 years; an intravenous pyelogram was normal. The concentration of plasma gonadotropins at 20 years of age was elevated; plasma LH 8 μg/L (LER-960) and FSH 50 μg/L (LER-869). A urocystogram showed a moderate estrogen effect. The concentration of plasma estradiol was 95 pmol/L (26 pg/mL) and of estrone was 117 pmol/L (32 pg/mL); plasma testosterone level was less than 0.7 nmol/L (0.2 ng/mL). On exploratory laparotomy, normal-appearing fallopian tubes and a uterus were found. The right gonad was a typical "streak," with whorls of fibrous connective tissue. *B,* The left gonad was replaced by a 1.3 × 1 × 1 cm tumor mass, which, on histologic section, revealed well-defined nests and islands of Sertoli-Leydig–like cells and germ cells, as well as calcification consistent with diagnosis of gonadoblastoma. *C,* Higher magnification illustrates aggregates of germ cells and small epithelial cells resembling immature Sertoli cells, as well as cells indistinguishable from Leydig cells. After gonadectomy the concentration of plasma estradiol was prepubertal (<18 pmol/L [<5 pg/mL]).

such as sonography, CT, or MRI of the testes are useful noninvasive approaches to screening for gonadal neoplasms.

The presence of functional testicular elements can be detected before puberty by the rise in the concentration of serum testosterone above prepubertal values after a course of hCG.

In some patients with 45,X/46,XY or 45,X/47,XXY mosaicism, the brightly fluorescent portion of the Y chromosome is absent. Caspersson and colleagues[538] noted the absence of bright fluorescence of the Y chromosome in four of seven patients. In one patient, a Y–to–chromosome 2 translocation during gametogenesis was suspected. In other such patients[539, 540] no evidence of translocation or deletion of the Y chromosome was found. Fluorescence, C banding, and replication of the Y chromosome were altered compared with normal.

Magenis and Donlon[541] studied 12 structurally altered Y chromosomes with a panel of banding techniques. They concluded that the nonfluorescent Y chromosome is an isodicentric chromosome that most likely arises from a chromatid break at the heterochromatic-euchromatic junction on the long arm of the Y chromosome with sister chromatid fusion and duplication of the Y. Subsequent studies with Y-specific DNA probes verified their interpretation but revealed variability in the break point on the Y. Isodicentric chromosomes are more prone to mitotic errors that result in a 45,X cell

line.[542, 543] In patients bearing a Y cell line who have "dysgenetic gonads," gonadal extirpation is prudent. Some patients have mosaicism with a cell line containing a minute nonfluorescent chromosome fragment whose exact nature (i.e., either X or Y) is not apparent by standard chromosome banding techniques. Molecular DNA analyses or FISH should be performed in these cases to ascertain the origin of the fragment.

Mixed, asymmetrical, or atypical gonadal dysgenesis is a term that has sometimes been used to describe patients with a streak gonad on one side and a testis on the other. Although this association is common in 45,X/46,XY mosaicism, these gonadal findings are not specific for this mosaicism and also occur with a 46,XY karyotype (e.g., in familial 46,XY gonadal dysgenesis).[544]

45,X/46,XY mosaicism probably arises mainly through anaphase lag and is frequently associated with structurally abnormal Y chromosomes.[542, 543] Interchromosomal rearrangements with loss of the structurally abnormal Y may be a common mechanism for the production of 45,X/46,XY mosaicism.

Diagnosis and Treatment. The diagnosis is established by demonstration of 45,X/46,XY mosaicism in blood, skin, or gonadal tissue. A Y chromosome, even one lacking the distal fluorescent portion of its long arm, can be recognized by its size and morphologic appearance (parallel long arms and short, fuzzy short arms) and the presence of a segment of Giemsa 11-positive heterochromatin; it can also be identified by use of Y-specific DNA probes for the centromeric region as well as for the long and short arms.[515] The decision as to the sex of rearing should be based on the potential for normal function of the external genitalia. In patients assigned a female gender role, the gonads should be removed, and the external genitalia should be repaired by clitoral recession, vaginoplasty, and labioscrotal reduction. Estrogen therapy should be initiated at the age of normal puberty to induce female secondary sexual characteristics. In affected infants for whom a male gender assignment is selected, all gonadal tissue except that which appears functionally and histologically normal and is in the scrotum should be removed, and prosthetic testes should be placed in the reconstructed scrotal sac if appropriate. In these patients, removal of the müllerian duct remnants is indicated, as is repair of any hypospadias.

As discussed previously, most 45,X/46,XY mosaic males detected by amniocentesis are born with normal male genitalia.[532–534] In these infants, it is prudent to obtain an MRI scan of the pelvis and testes to detect any müllerian structures and any inhomogeneity of the testes suggestive of dysgenesis or neoplasm. Hypothalamic-pituitary-gonadal integrity can be assessed by serial determinations of plasma gonadotropin and testosterone levels. Plasma AMH and inhibin levels are markers of the functional integrity of the Sertoli cells. If there is hormonal or imaging evidence of testicular dysgenesis, testicular biopsy or gonadectomy (or both) is indicated in infancy. Even in the absence of evidence for testicular dysgenesis, close follow-up is indicated, including a testicular biopsy at puberty and at age 20 to ascertain malignant potential (e.g., CiS).[537, 537a, 545] The need for androgen replacement therapy at adolescence depends on the capacity of the testis to secrete testosterone.

Structural Abnormalities of the Y Chromosome.[534, 546] Structural abnormalities of the Y chromosome that are of clinical significance are rarer than those of the X chromosome. This may be because the abnormal Y chromosome, being smaller than most structurally abnormal X chromosomes, is more readily lost from the cell during mitosis. The 45,X composition may therefore occur as a consequence of a structural abnormality of the Y that is lost at an early cleavage division. Deletions of both the long and short arms of the Y chromosome, as well as rings, isochromosomes of both arms, and dicentric chromosomes, have been described, and the PARs of the Y chromosome have been defined.[46, 47, 534] Proximal to the PAR on the short arm of the Y chromosome are the sex-determining region and the sex-determining gene *SRY*.[51, 52] In general, males with deletions of the short arm of the Y do not differentiate as males and may manifest gonadal dysgenesis stigmata, especially lymphedema.[534] They are not short.[534] The findings in these patients support earlier evidence that genes responsible for the stigmata of gonadal dysgenesis are primarily on the short arms of the X and Y chromosomes, whereas a gene for stature (*PHOG/SHOX* on PAR1) and certain skeletal abnormalities resides on the proximal long arm of the Y chromosome.[64, 471] Deletions of the long arm of the Y chromosome and, to a lesser extent, the long arm of the X chromosome do not result in gonadal dysgenesis somatic stigmata.

The genes mapped to the long arm of the Y chromosome include a locus for H-Y antigen (*SMCY*) as assessed by the cytotoxic T cell assay, the pseudogene for STS, the *YRBM* family of genes,[60] and a putative locus that affects spermatogenesis.[61, 62, 63, 547] A gene (*GBY*) that has a role in gonadoblastoma formation in patients with dysgenetic gonads is colocalized to a 1- to 2-Mb region (regions 3 and 4) near the centromere of the Y chromosome.[66] A small number of patients with putative isochromosomes for the short and long arms of the Y chromosome are not mosaics.[534] Three fourths of the patients reported with short arm isochromosomes, Ypi,

were phenotypic males[534]; the others had ambiguous genitalia.[534] Seven patients with long arm isochromosomes, Yqi, were phenotypic females with gonadal dysgenesis.[534] Gonadal dysgenesis stigmata and short stature were present in half the patients. In other words, the phenotype in 46,XYqi individuals was that expected with the loss of Yp and thus *SRY* and the genes that prevent gonadal dysgenesis stigmata, whereas patients with Ypi invariably had male differentiation.[534] Patients with ring Y chromosomes usually have an associated 45,X cell line and hence are mosaics. The phenotypes vary from that of a normal male (depending on the presence of the *SRY* gene) through individuals with ambiguous genitalia and male pseudohermaphroditism to women with infantile female external genitalia and bilateral streak gonads. The variation in phenotype is best explained by the effect of the 45,X cell line as well as the loss of genes on the Y chromosome.[534] Instances of apparently balanced Y-autosome translocations are known[534]; usually the distal heterochromatic region of the long arm of the Y chromosome is translocated to either a D or G autosome. Other reciprocal balanced and unbalanced Y-autosome translocations have been reported[534] in which male sex differentiation is normal (see Fig. 29–2).

As noted previously, Y-to-X translocations involving the sex-determining portion of the Y chromosome and a variable portion of the short arm of the X chromosome (usually the PAR) are found in more than 90% of XX males. There have also been reports of males with a 46,Yt(Xp22:Yq11) karyotype who inherited the t(X:Y) from their mothers.[534, 548] These males have an intact Y chromosome and a variable deletion of the short arm of the X chromosome. The phenotypic features are variable and correlate with the extent of the deletion of the short arm of the X chromosome. Hence, short stature, mild mental retardation, chondrodysplasia punctata, STS deficiency with ichthyosis, anosmia, and hypogonadotropic hypogonadism (Kallmann's syndrome) are variable features of this contiguous gene deletion syndrome.[56, 534, 548] Phenotypically normal females with a 46,Xt(X:Y) karyotype have been reported.[534, 548] All females with Xp22:Yq11 translocations have been normal except for short stature and increased fetal wastage. In patients with Y-to-X translocation, careful cytogenetic and molecular DNA studies should be performed to define the exact break points on the X and Y chromosomes. One can assess the functional integrity of the gonads by measuring the concentration of basal and LHRH-evoked plasma gonadotropins and gonadal steroids. Pelvic MRI is helpful in defining the pelvic contents and gonads.

Y-autosome translocations have been reported in 45,X males.[534] In general there appear to be two preferential locations, on chromosomes 5p and 18p, resulting in monosomy for 5p and 18p and multiple congenital anomalies.[534] Three unrelated phenotypic males with an XYq− karyotype had severe mental retardation, generalized hypotonia, and microcephaly with evidence of partial X chromosome disomy.[549] Aberrant X-Y exchange involving the distal long arm of the X and the distal euchromatic region of the long arm of the Y chromosome results in functional disomy for X-linked genes, and the phenotype has been designated the XYxq syndrome.[549]

Pure Gonadal Dysgenesis

This term has been applied to phenotypic females with a 46,XX or 46,XY karotype who have rudimentary streak gonads and remain sexually infantile but are of normal or tall stature and lack the somatic stigmata of gonadal dysgenesis. At puberty, they exhibit the usual effects of prepubertal castration, and plasma and urinary gonadotropin values are increased. The X chromatin pattern may be either positive or negative. Some X chromatin–negative patients have clitoral enlargement, which may be present at birth or first become manifest at puberty; clitoral enlargement is rarely present in X chromatin–positive patients. The designation *pure gonadal dysgenesis* was introduced by Harnden and Stewart in 1959 in their report of a 19-year-old phenotypic female with the described phenotype and 46,XY karyotype.[550] It is now known that a variety of etiologic factors may lead to the development of this clinical picture. The authors have chosen to restrict the term pure gonadal dysgenesis to patients with XX or XY gonadal dysgenesis (see later discussion).

FAMILIAL AND SPORADIC 46,XX GONADAL DYSGENESIS AND ITS INCOMPLETE FORMS. 46,XX gonadal dysgenesis is characterized by normal stature, sexual infantilism, bilateral streak gonads (similar in structure to those of 45,X gonadal dysgenesis), normal female internal and external genitalia, primary or secondary amenorrhea, elevated gonadotropin levels, absence of the somatic stigmata of the syndrome of gonadal dysgenesis, and a 46,XX karyotype[13, 551] (Table 29–13).

The habitus is often eunuchoid. Rare patients have had a few somatic abnormalities including cubitus valgus, but none have the typical gonadal dysgenesis phenotype. McDonough and associates[552] reviewed the phenotypic and cytogenetic findings in 82 phenotypic female patients with primary gonadal failure. Sex chromosome anomalies were found in association with ovarian failure in 52 of 82 patients, all of whom were less than 160 cm tall. Conversely, all patients taller than 160 cm with ovarian failure had either a 46,XX or a 46,XY karyotype.[552]

Occasionally, women with clitoral enlargement, hirsutism, and other signs of virilization have serum testosterone levels above the range for normal women.[553] The streak gonads secrete testosterone, presumably from nests of hilus cells. The high concentration of gonadotropins apparently leads to hilus cell hyperplasia and a modest increase in circulating androgen levels, which, in the presence of meager estrogen production, have potent biologic action.

Families may have multiple siblings affected,[13, 551] and within families the expression of the disease may vary in affected siblings. The gonads may range from bilateral streak gonads to hypoplastic ovaries with varying degrees of ovarian function resulting in secondary rather than primary amenorrhea. In the familial cases transmission is consistent with an autosomal recessive trait.[554] A locus for XX gonadal dysgenesis was mapped to the short arm of chromosome 2 in a large group of Finnish women.[165, 554, 555] A homozygous missense mutation in the gene encoding the FSH receptor was detected[165]; it resulted in a substitution of valine for alanine at residue 189 of the FSH receptor protein, and receptor activity was decreased but not absent in transfected cells.[165] The affected women with XX gonadal dysgenesis had either primary or secondary amenorrhea, variable development of secondary sexual characteristics, and elevated gonadotropins.[556] However, women with the FSH receptor mutation had primary follicles present in their ovaries, whereas women with primary ovarian failure of other causes had no or few ovarian follicles.[556] Males

homozygous for the same mutation of the FSH receptor had variable degrees of spermatogenic failure but not azoospermia.[557] Abnormal folliculogenesis in patients without the FSH receptor mutation may result from the effect of a mutant gene on germ cell migration, the gonadal blastema, or the rate of germ cell attrition; a defect in the putative ovary-organizing factor or its receptor; or accelerated atresia.

Familial 46,XX gonadal dysgenesis has been associated with sensorineural deafness.[558, 559] Genetic heterogeneity is suggested by concordance of the gonadal defect with deaf-mutism in these families and by other families in which short stature, 46,XX gonadal dysgenesis, microcephaly, and arachnodactyly occurred in affected siblings. Hamet and colleagues[560] described three sisters with renal failure, adrenal hyperplasia, hypertension, sensorineural deafness, and primary hypogonadism. A kindred with cerebellar ataxia and hypergonadotropic hypogonadism and a family with mental retardation, streak gonads, myopathy, and various neurologic abnormalities have been described.[561] The association of XX gonadal dysgenesis and blepharophimosis can occur in families.[562, 563] The gene locus for this syndrome, blepharophimosis-ptosis-epicanthus inversus syndrome (BPES type 1), maps to chromosome 3q22-q23.[563]

Sporadic cases of 46,XX gonadal dysgenesis are heterogenous. For example, ovarian hypoplasia has been associated with aneuploidy, especially trisomy-13 and trisomy-18. Patients with 46,XX gonadal dysgenesis should be distinguished from those with ovarian failure caused by infection (e.g., mumps in childhood, autoimmune oophoritis) and from patients with antibodies to gonadotropin receptors, biologically inactive FSH, galactosemia, or biosynthetic errors that affect estrogen formation (e.g., deficiency of steroid 17α-hydroxylase and/or 17,20-lyase [CYP17]).

Rare 46,XX patients with absent gonads, hypoplastic müllerian duct derivatives, and other congenital anomalies have been described in sibships with similarly affected 46,XY phenotypic females.[564, 565] The term *46,XX gonadal agenesis or agonadism* has been applied to these patients because of the complete absence of gonads, even gonadal streaks, and the occurrence of müllerian duct abnormalities.[564, 565]

In contrast to 46,XY gonadal dysgenesis, gonadal neoplasms are rare in 46,XX gonadal dysgenesis. The diagnosis of 46,XX gonadal dysgenesis is based on finding a normal karyotype in a sexually infantile phenotypic female with hypergonadotropic hypogonadism. In sporadic cases, it is important to confirm the presence of streak or hypoplastic gonads by sonography, pelvic MRI, or laparoscopy. Replacement therapy with estrogen is similar to that for patients with 45,X gonadal dysgenesis.

FAMILIAL AND SPORADIC 46,XY GONADAL DYSGENESIS AND ITS INCOMPLETE FORMS. 46,XY gonadal dysgenesis was first described by Swyer.[566] This syndrome in its complete form is characterized by a female phenotype, normal to tall stature, bilateral dysgenetic gonads, sexual infantilism with

TABLE 29–13. 46,XX Gonadal Dysgenesis and Variant Form

Parameter	Complete Syndrome	Incomplete Form
Karyotype:	46,XX	Same
Inheritance:	Autosomal recessive in familial cases (sensorineural deafness in about 10%); FSH receptor mutation in some cases	Same
Genitalia:	Normal female	Same
Wolffian duct derivatives:	Absent	Same
Müllerian duct derivatives:	Normal female	Same
Gonads:	Bilateral streak gonads	Hypoplastic ovary and streak or bilateral hypoplastic ovaries
Habitus:	Normal stature, no somatic stigmata of gonadal dysgenesis	Same
	Sexual infantilism	Incomplete puberty, premature ovarian failure
Hormone profile:	Increased plasma FSH and LH concentration	Plasma estradiol variable: decreased or normal

primary amenorrhea, eunuchoid habitus, and a 46,XY karyotype (Table 29–14). Somatic features of gonadal dysgenesis are usually absent. The internal structures are female with bilateral fallopian tubes, a uterus, and a vagina. Clitoral enlargement is not uncommon, and gonadal neoplasms, especially gonadoblastoma and germinoma (seminoma, dysgerminoma), occur 10 to 30%. In individuals with the incomplete or variant form, both the internal and external genitalia may be ambiguous.[567] Breast development after the normal age of puberty suggests the presence of an estrogen-secreting gonadal tumor, especially a gonadoblastoma.[568] Plasma and urinary gonadotropin levels are increased. In some patients the concentration of serum testosterone is higher than in adult women, presumably because of the secretion of androgens from the hilus cells of the streak gonads. A male proportion of single fluorescent Y bodies is present in interphase nuclei. Excluded from this syndrome are patients with variants of the syndrome of gonadal dysgenesis (e.g., 45,X/46,XY mosaicism) and those with microscopically visible structural abnormalities of the Y chromosome.

XY gonadal dysgenesis is a heterogenous condition that can result from deletions of the short arm of the Y chromosome,[534, 568] mutations in the *SRY* gene,[127, 129, 569] mutations in autosomal genes,[141, 143, 145, 154, 160, 161] or duplications of the *DSS* locus on the X chromosome.[78] As noted previously, patients with extensive contiguous deletions of the short arm of the Y chromosome can manifest gonadal dysgenesis stigmata as well as XY gonadal dysgenesis.[534] Point mutations in the *SRY* gene have been found in 10 to 20% of patients with complete XY gonadal dysgenesis.[127, 129, 570] Presumably, most patients with XY gonadal dysgenesis who do not have a mutation in the *SRY* gene have mutations either in upstream or downstream genes in the testes determination and differentiation cascade. Almost all the mutations in the *SRY* gene in patients with the complete form of XY gonadal dysgenesis,[571] except for one in the 3′ region[572] and a deletion in the 5′ region of the gene, are in the DNA-binding (HMG) box domain of the SRY protein.[573] These mutations are usually nonsense or missense single-amino-acid substitutions (15 of 23 mutations) and affect DNA binding or bending.[129, 574-578]

Familial aggregates of 46,XY gonadal dysgenesis have been reported.[13, 574, 577, 579, 580] The presence of complete 46,XY dysgenesis in "daughters" of fathers who have the same mutation in the SRY HMG box is perplexing. Possible explanations for this phenomenon include (1) another mutation in the father which allows for normal testicular determination and differentiation; (2) segregation of another polymorphic locus that interacts with *SRY;* and (3) variations in the timing and the critical level of *SRY* expression achieved[129]; and (4) mosaicism. Two novel *SRY* missense mutations causing reduced

DNA binding have been identified in XY females and their fathers.[574] Analyses of DNA from the fathers indicated that they were mosaics for both the wild-type and mutant *SRY* genes and quite likely are mosaic for the *SRY* mutation in their testes.[574]

Familial 46,XY gonadal dysgenesis without an apparent mutation in the *SRY* may be transmitted as an X-linked, sex-limited autosomal dominant or possibly as an autosomal recessive trait.[579] Within a family, affected individuals may vary in the appearance of the external genitalia and the development of secondary sexual characteristics. Usually, the external genitalia and internal genital ducts are female, and the patient is sexually infantile (complete form). However, affected siblings may have ambiguous external genitalia, ambiguous genital ducts, and a urogenital sinus (incomplete or variant form). The spectrum of findings suggests heterogeneity in transmission or variable expression of the mutant gene in the same cohort. In a family reported by Chemke and colleagues,[579] two siblings had 46,XY gonadal dysgenesis with bilateral streak gonads and another had the incomplete form with genital ambiguity, bilateral dysgenetic testes, and müllerian derivatives. An infant born to the "normal" 46,XX sister in this family had a 46,XY karyotype, ambiguous external genitalia, bilateral dysgenetic testes, and müllerian duct derivatives; inheritance in this family is consistent with an X-linked recessive or male-limited autosomal dominant trait.

46,XY gonadal dysgenesis can be caused by a duplication of the *DSS* locus on the short arm of the X chromosome.[78, 581, 582] This locus overlaps with the gene *(DAX1)* encoding congenital adrenal hypoplasia, which is located in the Xp21 region of the X chromosome. Duplication of the locus in 46,XY individual leads to sex reversal; deletion of the *DAX1* gene and the *DSS* locus has no effect on testicular development. *DSS* (?*DAX1*) is postulated to be an ovary-determining gene, but its role in both testicular and ovarian gonadogenesis is uncertain.

46,XY gonadal dysgenesis occurs in association with campomelic dysplasia,[154, 155, 583] which is caused by a mutation in the *SOX9* gene on 17q21. Mutations in a single allele for this gene in males can result in both XY gonadal dysgenesis and campomelic dysplasia.[154, 155] 46,XX affected females have normal ovarian development. Homozygous mutations are probably lethal owing to the critical function of *SOX9* in chondrogenesis.[159]

9p− and 10q− deletions also can cause 46,XY gonadal dysgenesis.[160, 161] As yet undefined genes in the testis determination cascade are probably localized in these regions. Mutations of *WT1* result in the Denys-Drash and WAGR syndromes (see later discussions).[142-145] 46,XY gonadal dysgenesis has also been associated with multiple congenital anomalies (genito-

TABLE 29–14. Salient Features of 46,XY Gonadal Dysgenesis and Variant Form

Parameter	Complete Syndrome*	Incomplete Form
Karyotype:	46,XY	Same
Inheritance:	Familial cases consistent with X linked (or male-limited autosomal dominant); *SRY* mutation or deletion in 15%	Same: No *SRY* mutation detected
Genitalia:	Female	Ambiguous
Wolffian duct derivatives:	Absent	Rudimentary → hypoplastic
Müllerian duct derivatives:	Normal	Variable, rudimentary → hypoplastic
Gonads:	Bilateral streak gonads	Bilateral dysgenetic testes or streak gonad + dysgenetic testes (mixed gonadal dysgenesis)
	Increased risk of gonadal tumor, gonadoblastoma	Same
Habitus:	Sexual infantilism at puberty	Variable degree of virilization at puberty
	Breast development suggests presence of gonadal tumor	Same
Hormone profile:	Increased plasma FSH and LH and decreased testosterone concentrations postpubertally	Same

palato-cardiac syndrome)[567] and with the Smith-Lemli-Opitz syndrome.[584] The latter disorder is associated with low serum cholesterol concentrations and a marked elevation of the cholesterol derivative 7-dehydrocholesterol; it is apparently caused by deficient 7-dehydrocholesterol C-7 reductase.[585]

Like some 45,X individuals, some patients with 46,XY gonadal dysgenesis have ovarian follicles in the dysgenetic gonads. Cussen and MacMahon[586] described germ cells and follicles in the underdeveloped gonads of a 3-month-old 46,XY female. Subsequent examination at age 3 years 10 months revealed bilateral streak gonads and a gonadoblastoma in one gonad.[586] Some ovarian follicles persisted and functioned at puberty in 46,XY phenotypic females who underwent spontaneous puberty and experienced menarche.[587] Examination of the gonads after development of secondary amenorrhea revealed only gonadal streaks with a few hilus cells.

There is a high prevalence of gonadal tumors, especially gonadoblastoma and germinoma, in 46,XY gonadal dysgenesis, and they can occur bilaterally in childhood. Bilateral prophylactic gonadectomy is indicated in all patients with 46,XY gonadal dysgenesis, even those who have deletions or mutations involving the *SRY* gene.[588]

The sex of rearing of patients with the incomplete form of 46,XY gonadal dysgenesis is determined by the extent of genital ambiguity and the age at diagnosis. Patients raised as females should be placed on estrogen replacement therapy at age 12 to 13 years and should eventually be cycled monthly with estrogen and progestagen. In patients raised as males, testosterone replacement therapy should begin at the age of puberty.

"MALE TURNER SYNDROME." Many phenotypic males have been reported with short stature, webbed neck, and other somatic abnormalities associated with the syndrome of gonadal dysgenesis in whom the testes were hypoplastic and frequently undescended. The resemblance of these males to females with 45,X gonadal dysgenesis suggested a pathogenetic parallelism or gonadal dysgenesis in the male. However, with rare exceptions, this relation is no longer tenable. A few patients with the phenotypic features of gonadal dysgenesis syndrome have a sex chromosome abnormality (e.g., 45,X/46,XY mosaicism) and represent a variant form of gonadal dysgenesis. The other patients have a 46,XY sex chromosome constitution. The 46,XY cases form a heterogeneous clinical group; unless partial sex chromosome monosomy can be demonstrated, these patients ought not to be considered as the clinical parallel in the male of gonadal dysgenesis. Many of the cases previously categorized under this term are examples of the syndrome of webbed neck, ptosis, hypogonadism, and short stature usually associated with congenital heart disease and mental retardation (Noonan's syndrome).[331]

Noonan's Syndrome

Among the group of phenotypic males previously classified as having male gonadal dysgenesis syndrome, a distinctive clinical entity was identified that led to the identification of its counterpart in the female and its distinction from the syndrome of gonadal dysgenesis.[331, 589-592] Various names have been applied to this now well established syndrome (Noonan's syndrome, 46,XX and 46,XY Turner phenotype, pseudo-Turner syndrome, Ullrich's syndrome), but the authors prefer to exclude "Turner" from the designation. Table 29–15 lists the clinical features of 2 phenotypic males and 12 phenotypic females with this entity studied by us. These patients have a characteristic facies that includes hypertelorism, downslanting palpebral tissues, epicanthal folds, ptosis, low-set anteriorly rotated ears, and, frequently, a webbed neck and short stature (Fig. 29–46); in 12 of the 14 cases, congenital heart disease was present. The most common cardiac malformation is pulmonary valvular stenosis (50 to 60%). Hypertrophic cardiomyopathy occurs in 20% of patients and can manifest in the neonatal period[593]; the electrocardiogram is frequently abnormal. Atrial septal defects are found in 10% of patients.[593] Coarctation of the aorta and aortic stenosis, the most common cardiovascular anomalies in the syndrome of gonadal dysgenesis, are infrequent (10%). Pectus carinatum superiorly, pectus excavatum inferiorly, and cubitus valgus are often present. Mental development is impaired in about 15% of patients. There are few reports of cognition and intelligence in individuals with Noonan's syndrome.[594, 595] In a study of 8 patients

TABLE 29–15. Summary of Clinical Findings in 14 Patients with the Syndrome of Webbed Neck, Ptosis, Hypogonadism, Congenital Heart Disease, and Short Stature

Clinical Characteristics	No. Males	No. Females	Clinical Characteristics	No. Males	No. Females
Short stature (>2 SD below mean)	2/2	8/12	ECD + patent ductus arteriosus and mitral insufficiency	0/2	1/10
Typical facies	2/2	12/12	Both PS and ASD	2/2	3/10
Triangular shape of face	2/2	7/12	Patent ductus arteriosus (PDA)	0/2	2/10
Prominent brow	2/2	12/12	Undiagnosed heart disease	0/2	2/10
Hypertelorism	2/2	12/12	Incompletely evaluated	0/2	2/12
Epicanthus	2/2	9/12	Extremities		
Antimongoloid palpebral slant	2/2	10/12	Cubitus valgus	2/2	9/12
Ptosis	2/2	12/12	Gracile fingers	1/2	8/12
Depressed nasal bridge	1/2	2/12	Short stubby fingers	1/2	2/12
Broad apex nasi	2/2	11/12	Lymphedema	0/2	3/12
Low-set and/or malformed ears	2/2	8/12	Dystrophic nails	2/2	2/12
High-arched palate	2/2	8/12	Shortened fourth metacarpal(s)	0/2	3/12
Neck			Clinodactyly of fifth finger(s)	1/2	2/12
Short	2/2	10/12	Palmar simian crease	1/2	1/12
Webbing	2/2	10/12	Undescended testes	2/2	—
Low hairline	2/2	10/12	Delayed puberty	1/1	3/3
Chest			Skeletal retardation	2/2	8/10
Shield-like	1/2	11/12	Mental development		
Wide-spaced nipples	2/2	11/11	Retarded	2/2	4/12
Pectus exacavatum	2/2	5/12	Borderline	0/2	5/12
Cardiac abnormalities	2/2	11/12	Normal	0/2	3/12
Pulmonic stenosis (PS)	2/2	5/10	Intrauterine growth retardation	1/2	4/12
PS and ventricular septal defect	0/2	1/10	Renal collecting system		
Atrial septal defect (ASD)	2/2	6/10	Normal	2/2	7/8
ASD with anomalous pulmonary venous return	0/2	1/10	Abnormal	0/2	1/8
Endocardial cushion defect (ECD)	0/2	2/10	Normal karyotype	2/2	12/12

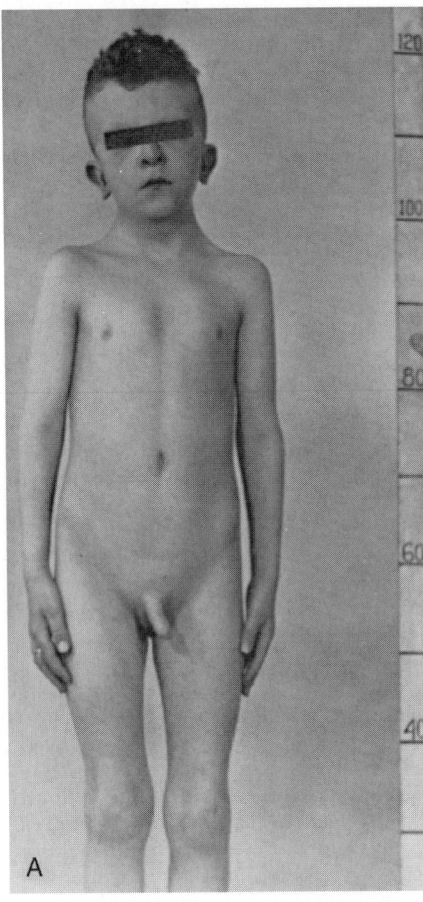 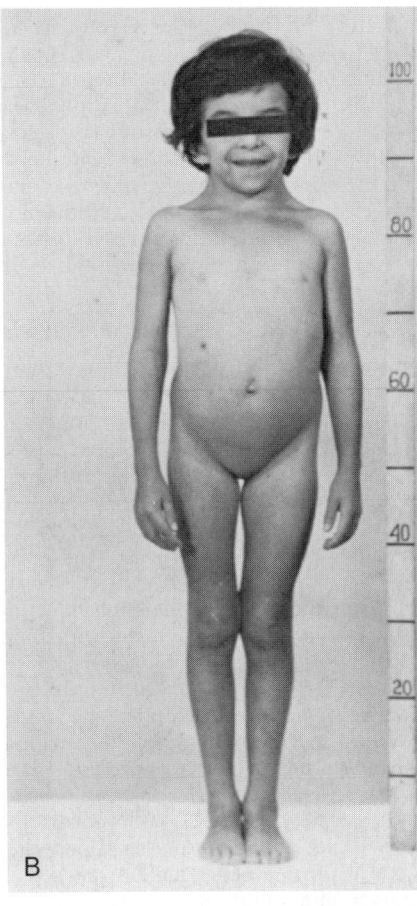

Figure 29–46. Phenotypic male and female with syndrome of webbed neck, ptosis, congenital heart disease, short stature, and hypogonadism (pseudo-Turner syndrome, Noonan syndrome). *A,* A 9⁷/₁₂-year-old boy who exhibited characteristic abnormalities: triangular facies, prominent brow, hypertelorism, ptosis, antimongoloid slant of palpebral fissures, broad apex nasi, low-set ears, webbed neck, pectus excavatum, pulmonic stenosis and atrial septal defect, short stature (−3.5 SD), bilateral undescended testes, and high-grade mental retardation. At age 18, he was 154.0 cm in height (height age 12⁵/₁₂ years); the boy had Leydig cell hypofunction. Biopsy of testes showed germinal aplasia. (From Grumbach MM, Barr ML. Cytologic tests of chromosomal sex in relation to sexual anomalies in man. Recent Prog Horm Res 1958; 14:255–334.) *B,* An 8-year-old girl with similar features. Height was 106.2 cm (height age 4⁴/₁₂ years). Pulmonic stenosis was present, and the karyotype was 46,XX.

aged 13 to 36 years, the I.Q. ranged from 64 to 127, with a median of 102.[595] Refractive errors and strabismus are common. Lymphedema occurs in 15% of patients.[596] Sixty-five percent of patients have easy bruising or excessive postoperative bleeding as a result of a variety of coagulation defects.[597] The chromosome constitution is normal, and gonadal differentiation is appropriate for the phenotypic and chromosomal sex. Cryptorchidism is common in males, and the testes may be hypoplastic and exhibit germinal aplasia. Puberty is delayed, and androgen deficiency is not uncommon. However, 50% of affected males have normal testicular function, including fertility in the absence of cryptorchidism. Affected females have functioning ovaries and, although the onset of puberty may be delayed, female secondary sexual characteristics eventually emerge.

Most cases are sporadic. Familial clusters are consistent with autosomal dominant inheritance.[598] Linkage analysis in a large Dutch kindred suggested location of a gene for Noonan's syndrome on the long arm of chromosome 12 (12q22-qter).[598] The abnormality of gonadal function and the higher incidence of congenital heart disease in males may play a part in the apparently higher maternal transmission of the mutant gene. However, the authors and others have seen familial cases transmitted through an affected male.

The diagnosis is based on the constellation of stigmata, the most prominent of which are short stature, webbed neck, pectus excavatum, ptosis, and right-sided congenital heart disease in a patient with a normal sex chromosome constitution. The differential diagnosis of this syndrome is extensive and includes structural abnormalities of the Y chromosome (especially those involving the short arm), 45,X/46,XY mosaicism, and dysmorphic syndromes secondary to hydantoin, primidone, or alcohol exposure during gestation.[331] At puberty, affected males may require testosterone replacement therapy.

True Hermaphroditism

The diagnosis of true hermaphroditism requires the presence of both ovarian and testicular tissue in either the same or opposite gonads.[599–601] Failure to adhere to this definition has led to considerable confusion. Gonadal stroma arranged in whorls, similar to those found in the ovary but lacking oocytes, should not be considered sufficient evidence to designate the rudimentary gonad as an ovary. Similarly, if testicular tissue is present in the contralateral gonad, the authors do not consider the presence of a few oocytes in a streak gonad to be adequate evidence for the diagnosis of true hermaphroditism. Because rare female-type germ cells may be found in patients with 45,X gonadal dysgenesis, it is of little value from the clinical, cytogenetic, embryologic, or nosologic standpoint to classify as true hermaphrodites the 45,X/46,XY mosaics in whom a dysgenetic gonad contains rare oocytes.[530] Similarly, the status of the internal and external genitalia, which invariably exhibit some degree of ambisexual development, should not be used as a criterion for classification of an individual as a true hermaphrodite.

CLASSIFICATION. True hermaphroditism is uncommon but has been reported in more than 400 individuals.[601–604a] Patients with this syndrome may be subclassified according to the type and location of the gonads.

Lateral. A testis is present on one side and an ovary is present on the other in about 20% of patients.[601–604] The ovary is frequently found on the left side.

Bilateral. Both testicular and ovarian tissue are present bilaterally, usually as ovotestes, in about 30% of patients.[601–604a]

Unilateral. Testicular and ovarian tissue is present on one side and a testis or ovary is found on the other side in slightly less than one half of cases.[601–604a] A testis or ovotestis may be situated along the normal pathway of descent of a testis, but an ovary is almost invariably in its normal position.

TABLE 29–16. Clinical Features of True Hermaphroditism

Karyotype:	46,XX (most common), 46,XX/46,XY, or 46,XY (rare)
Inheritance:	Familial cases (autosomal recessive, autosomal dominant transmission) rare
Genitalia:	Ambiguous; cryptorchidism frequent; ovotestis possibly located in labioscrotal fold
Wolffian duct derivatives: ⎱ Müllerian duct derivatives: ⎰	Duct differentiation after that of the homolateral gonad
Gonad:	Testis, ovary, or ovotestis
Habitus:	Breast development and virilization common at puberty
Molecular studies:	Approximately 10% of 46,XX true hermaphrodites are *SRY* positive

CLINICAL FEATURES. The differentiation of the genital tract and the development of secondary sexual characteristics are variable (Table 29–16; Fig. 29–47). The external genitalia may simulate those of either a male or a female, or they may be ambiguous; most of the patients are reared as males because of the size of the phallus and because of social factors.[601, 602] Almost all have hypospadias, which varies in extent from perineal to penile, and incomplete fusion of the labioscrotal folds. The labioscrotal folds are asymmetrical in half of the patients, with the right side more predominant.[602] In rare cases a penile urethra is present. Cryptorchidism is common, but at least one gonad is usually palpable in the labioscrotal fold or in the inguinal region.[603] An inguinal hernia, which may contain a gonad or uterus, is present in about one half of the cases, and a vagina and a uterus are present in most patients; the uterus may be underdeveloped (hemiuterus), rudimentary, or absent.[602, 603] The differentiation of the genital ducts usually follows that of the gonads. The ovotestis is the

most common gonad in true hermaphrodites, followed by the ovary and, least commonly, the testis.[602–609] In patients with a testis on one side and an ovary on the other, the development of the homolateral duct is usually consistent with that of the gonad, despite the varied appearance of the external genitalia. Most patients with an ovotestis have predominantly female development of the genital ducts. The relation between gonadal structure and differentiation of the genital tract in true hermaphroditism provides additional evidence for the local action of AMH secreted by the Sertoli cells of the embryonic and fetal testes.

Breast development is common during puberty in true hermaphrodites, and menses occur in more than half of the patients. Periodic hematuria associated with menstruation is a late clue to the diagnosis. Spermatogenesis is rare; seminiferous tubules in an ovotestis or testes are abnormal in most cases, and interstitial fibrosis of the testes is common.[603, 604] Ovulation is not uncommon, and pregnancy and childbirth can occur in patients with a 46,XX karyotype,[607, 610, 611] whereas only one 46,XY true hermaphrodite has been reported to have fathered a child.[613]

Few studies of hypothalamic-pituitary-gonadal function have been carried out in true hermaphrodites. Whereas an ovary or ovarian portion of an ovotestis may function normally, the testis or testicular component of the ovotestis is usually abnormal.[603, 612] The cyclic pattern of FSH and LH secretion can be similar to that in normal women.[613] As in other men with gynecomastia, a low ratio of testosterone to estradiol, caused by enhanced secretion of estradiol by the ovotestis and/or testes, plays a role in the breast development that is seen frequently in postpubertal true hermaphrodites.[614]

CHROMOSOMAL FINDINGS. By far the most common karyotype found in true hermaphrodites is 46,XX, followed

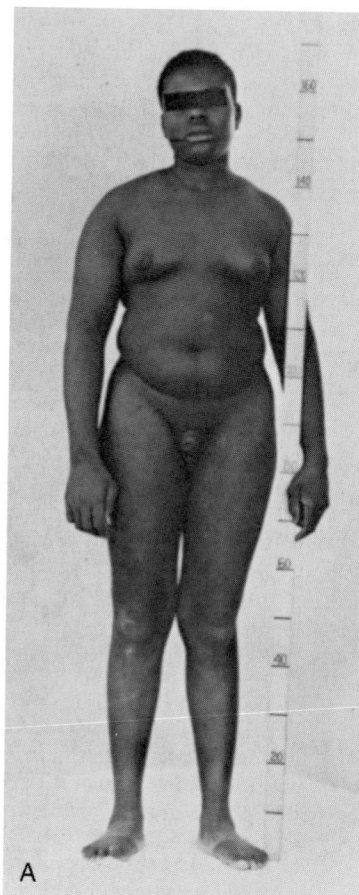

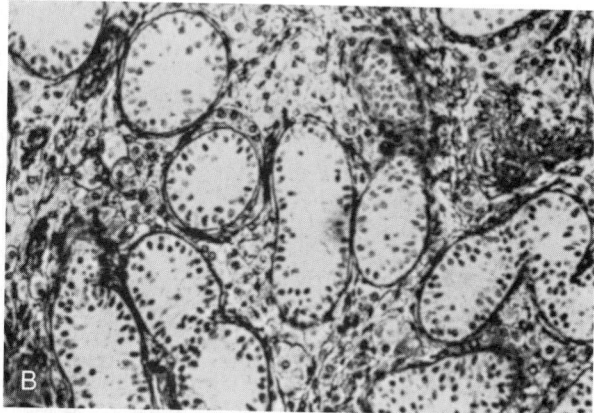

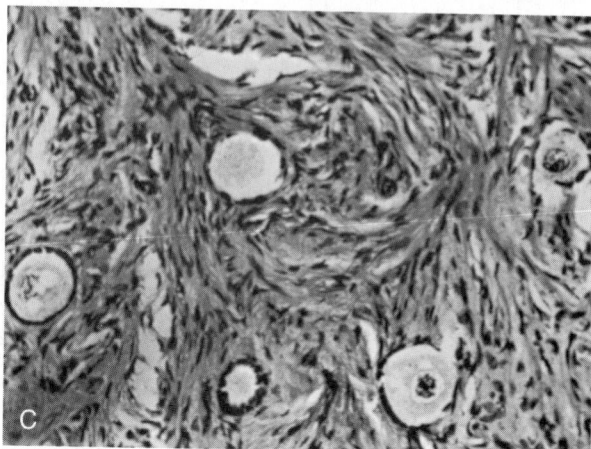

Figure 29–47. *A*, A 17-year-old true hermaphrodite with bilateral scrotal ovotestes and a 46,XX sex chromosome constitution in cultures of peripheral blood and skin, perineal hypospadias (partially repaired in photograph), moderate bilateral gynecomastia and pubic hair (recently shaved in picture), sparse axillary hair, a high-pitched voice, and absent facial hair. Height was 168 cm. Urinary 17-ketosteroid level was 1.3 mg/d; urinary gonadotropin levels were between 10 and 80 mouse units/d. A male type of urethra, bilateral scrotal fallopian tubes and ovotestes, and rudimentary bicornuate uterus and vagina attached to the posterior urethra were seen at operation. The photomicrographs show histopathology of demarcated ovarian and testicular portion of one ovotestis: *B*, immature seminiferous tubules lined with Sertoli cells and spermatogonia and Leydig cells; *C*, ova and follicles. (From Grumbach MM, Barr ML. Cytologic tests of chromosomal sex in relation to sexual anomalies in man. Recent Prog Horm Res 1958; 14:255–334.)

by 46,XX/46,XY chimerism, mosaicism, and, rarely, 46,XY (7%).[602-606]

ORIGINS OF TRUE HERMAPHRODITISM. True hermaphroditism could result from sex chromosome mosaicism (apparent or cryptic), chimerism, Y-to-autosome or Y-to-X chromosome translocation,[365, 366, 615, 616] or mutation of either X-linked or autosomal genes involved in sex determination.[367] Most 46,XX true hermaphrodites are *SRY* negative.[617-619] The gene (or genes) responsible for true hermaphroditism in these patients has not yet been identified; however, it is probably a downstream gene in the sex determination pathway which, when mutated, allows for testicular differentiation. That Y sequence–negative 46,XX males and 46,XX true hermaphrodites can occur in the same pedigree is well documented.[367, 619, 620] Kuhnle and associates[367] studied a pedigree with two 46,XX true hemaphrodites and a 46,XX male who were first cousins. The three patients were negative for Y sequences, including *PABY* (*pseudoautosomal boundary Y*), *SRY*, and *ZFY*. The pattern of inheritance of 46,XX true hermaphroditism and 46,XX maleness was compatible with an autosomal dominant or an X-linked dominant mode of transmission with variable expression.[367] In the case of a putative X-linked gene mutation, it has been postulated that random inactivation would result in true hermaphroditism and nonrandom inactivation would lead to an XX male.[621] However, no evidence for nonrandom X inactivation in *SRY*-negative 46,XX males has been reported. Because of the postulated role of a gene on the X chromosome as a cause of true hermaphroditism, Spurdle and colleagues carried out a detailed DNA analysis of the X chromosome in a study of sixteen 46,XX *SRY*-negative true hermaphrodites and found no evidence of uniparental disomy of the X chromosome.[622]

A small number of "Y-positive" 46,XX true hermaphrodites have been reported in kindreds with 46,XX males.[619, 623] It has been postulated that inactivation of the X chromosome bearing the Y chromosome translocation could lead to inactivation of the *SRY* gene by the spread of inactivation into the translocated segment. However, in one *SRY*-positive 46,XX true hermaphrodite, the translocated X was randomly inactivated; on the other hand, nonrandom inactivation of the X chromosome bearing the Y translocation was found in another *SRY*-positive 46,XX male.[623] Accordingly, in some instances X inactivation may play a role in the gonadal phenotype of 46,XX *SRY*-positive males.

Sex chromosome mosaicism arises from mitotic or meiotic errors. In contrast, 46,XX/46,XY chimerism is usually a consequence of double fertilization or, possibly, fusion of two normally fertilized ova.[38, 624] Chimeric individuals have two distinct populations of cells, each of which has a different genetic origin (in contrast to mosaicism). Study of 46,XX/46,XY chimeras provides evidence for the fertilization of a binucleate ovum by two sperms, one bearing an X and the other a Y.[625, 626] Not all patients with whole body chimerism have true hermaphroditism. One 46,XX/46,XY patient was a phenotypic male without true hermaphroditism; a likely mechanism for the chimerism in this case, based on the blood group studies and other findings, is fusion of two zygotes or fertilization of an ovum and its polar body. The experiments of Tarkowski[627] with XX and XY mouse blastocytes demonstrated that random fusion of two blastocytes seldom produces 46,XX/46,XY true hermaphroditism; fused mouse blastocysts usually develop testes rather than ovaries or ovotestes. A 46,XY true hermaphrodite, the least common form,[615] had an apparently normal Y chromosome and *SRY* gene. However, DNA analysis of the "ovotestes" uncovered mosaicism for a normal *SRY* gene and a mutated *SRY* gene with a nonconservative amino acid substitution.[615] This suggested that a postzygotic gonadal mutation in *SRY* resulted in ovotestes and, thus, true hermaphroditism.[615] It may be that all 46,XY true hermaphro-

dites are cryptic gonadal mosaics for an *SRY* mutation or another gene mutation in the gonadal differentiation cascade, or they may harbor a 46,XX cell line. Rare familial cases of putative XY true hermaphroditism have been reported in the past; however, these have not been studied with newer cytogenetic or molecular biologic techniques.[628]

DIAGNOSIS AND THERAPY. The diagnosis of true hermaphroditism should be considered in all patients with ambiguous genitalia. A 46,XX/46,XY karyotype in a patient with ambiguous external genitalia strongly suggests the diagnosis, and a 46,XX or 46,XY karyotype does not exclude the diagnosis. The finding of a gonad in the labioscrotal fold (especially on the right side) with a lobulated bipolar consistency compatible with an ovotestis is suggestive. In one study, 11 of 12 46,XX true hermaphrodites examined before 6 months of age had basal plasma testosterone levels greater than 40 ng/dL (upper range of normal in females of this age, 15 ng/dL), suggesting the presence of Leydig cells.[603] All children examined after 6 months of age in the same study had basal testosterone levels lower than 15 ng/dL; however, administration of hCG induced testosterone responses that were greater than 40 ng/dL.[603] Therefore, both basal testosterone values in infants younger than 6 months of age and hCG-induced testosterone responses are useful for ascertaining the presence of Leydig cells. Plasma AMH levels are detectable in true hermaphrodites with functional Sertoli cells.[211] If all other forms of pseudohermaphrodism have been ruled out, the diagnosis of true hermaphroditism should be confirmed by the demonstration of both ovarian and testicular tissues histologically.

The management is contingent on the age at diagnosis and assessment of the functional capacity of the internal and external genitalia. In infants in whom gender identity has not already been established, either a male or female assignment of sex can be made. However, in 46,XX true hermaphrodites the authors are of the view that, except for patients who have a well-developed phallic structure and who lack a uterus or possess a vestigial one, a female sex assignment is prudent because ovarian tissue is usually functional, pregnancy has been documented, and surgical reconstruction of the external genitalia is generally easier and the results more functional.[603, 607] The risk of malignant transformation in the ovarian tissue of 46,XX true hermaphrodites is unknown.[629] If a male gender role is assigned, all müllerian and ovarian structures should be removed. The testis or testicular component of an ovotestis is usually dysgenetic, and the risk of neoplasm is increased. The prevalence of gonadoblastoma and/or germinoma arising in the testicular tissue of 46,XX true hermaphrodites has been estimated at 3 to 4%.[601, 603] Accordingly, in 46,XX true hermaphrodites raised as males the authors recommend gonadectomy, the insertion of prosthetic testes, and hormone replacement at puberty. In 46,XX/46,XY chimeras and 46,XY true hermaphrodites, especially when a testis is present on one side and an ovary on the contralateral side and the size of the phallus is adequate, one should weigh the alternative of retaining a histologically normal-appearing testis in the scrotum and raising the patient as a male, even though the risk of gonadal malignancy may be increased. In true hermaphrodites reared as females, all testicular tissue should be removed. Postoperative assessment of the plasma testosterone response to hCG is useful to ascertain the persistence of Leydig cells as well as plasma AMH, markers of retained testicular tissue. In older patients, gender identity is the major consideration; usually it conforms to the sex of rearing. The discordant gonad and dysgenetic gonadal tissue should be removed, and plastic repair of the external genitalia should be carried out. Appropriate gonadal hormone replacement therapy is recommended at the age of puberty.

Sex Chromosome Abnormalities Unassociated with Gonadal Defects

The addition of one or more sex chromosomes to the genome has a deleterious effect on cognitive function. The following five sex chromosome abnormalities are not accompanied by a typical gonadal defect but are frequently associated with mental retardation.

47,XXX. This common chromosome abnormality has the frequency of about 1 per 1000 newborn female infants. The prevalence of 47,XXX individuals in institutions for the mentally retarded is 4.3 per 1000,[630] suggesting an increased risk for severe mental retardation. 47,XXX females have reduced general intelligence and low scores on tests of attention, concept formation, spatial thinking, verbal fluency, and academic skills.[292, 631, 632] XXX individuals demonstrated less overall psychosocial adaptation and a greater degree of psychological disturbance, compared with patients with Klinefelter's syndrome or gonadal dysgenesis.[292] Although some have delayed menarche or premature ovarian failure, most 47,XXX females have normal ovarian function. 47,XXX females can rarely give birth to 47,XXY sons,[330] and the prevalence of congenital malformations is increased in the progeny of 47,XXX women.[633] Subtle clinical features in infants ascertained by karyotype analysis include the following: a tendency to low birth weight, decreased head circumference, advanced mean parental age, an increased incidence of clinodactyly, normal postnatal growth patterns, an increased risk of speech and language problems, and a lower mean I.Q. than the siblings or a control group.[292, 632] The extra X chromosome is of maternal origin in most instances, arising mainly from nondisjunction during the first or second meiotic divisions.[634]

The diagnosis of 47,XXX can be confirmed by the finding of two sex chromatin bodies in interphase cells and by the demonstration of a 47,XXX karyotype through the use of appropriate banding techniques. Because of the increased risk in the offspring of a sex chromosome abnormality (47,XXY and 47,XXX) and congenital malformations, prenatal counseling and amniocentesis should be considered in 47,XXX females who become pregnant.

48,XXXX. This rare anomaly[332, 635, 636] is associated with considerable phenotype heterogeneity, making identification by clinical means difficult. The most constant feature is a variable degree of mental retardation affecting speech.[636] Ovarian function is usually normal.[636] Average adult height is 169 cm; the prevalence of skeletal anomalies, such as clinodactyly and radioulnar synostosis, is increased.[332] The diagnosis is suggested by finding three sex chromatin bodies in 6 to 9% of somatic nuclei and is confirmed by karyotype analysis.

49,XXXXX.[13, 332, 637] The rare penta-X syndrome is invariably associated with severe prenatal and postnatal growth delay and mental retardation. Other stigmata include microcephaly, hypertelorism, epicanthal folds, upslanted palpebral fissures, depressed nasal bridge, abnormal dentition, a short neck, congenital heart disease, clinodactyly, overlapping toes, and joint laxity. The external genitalia and gonadal function are usually normal; however, fertility is still to be documented.[332] A proportion of interphase nuclei contain four X chromatin bodies.

47,XYY. The first subject reported by Sandberg and associates[638] was an essentially normal fertile man of average intelligence who was detected only because he had a daughter with Down syndrome. However, surveys in penal institutions suggested an increase in prevalence of this anomaly, especially in tall prisoners, and gave rise to an undeserved stereotype that has been modified by later studies.[639–641] Among 43 47,XYY boys 1 to 12 years of age, ascertained by routine karyotype analysis in the newborn period, no clearcut 47,XYY syndrome emerged in childhood.[285] No major deviations could be attributed to an extra Y chromosome, with the possible exception of a skew to the left in I.Q. scores, although full-scale I.Q. scores ranged from 80 to 140.[290] In general, 47,XYY patients tend to be easily distractible and hyperactive and to have low tolerance of frustration.[290] The prevalence of antisocial and other behavioral difficulties is increased.[641a] 47,XYY is a common sex chromosome abnormality, occurring in 1 per 1000 male births. Among the features are tall stature,[641a] nodulocystic acne, and skeletal anomalies such as radioulnar synostosis. Sexual development is usually normal, and the rare reports of hypospadias in 47,XYY patients may be coincidental. The diagnosis should be suspected in hyperactive tall men with nodulocystic acne and can be confirmed by demonstration of two fluorescent Y bodies in somatic interphase nuclei or by karyotype analysis.

48,XYYY. The variable phenotypes associated with this rare karyotype include multiple somatic abnormalities and mental retardation.[642] The diagnosis is confirmed by finding three fluorescent Y bodies in interphase nuclei or by karyotype analysis.

Gonadal Neoplasms in Dysgenetic Gonads

The prevalence of gonadal neoplasms is increased in patients with certain types of dysgenetic gonads, in particular all those with a Y-bearing cell line.[643–649] Germinoma (dysgerminoma, seminoma), teratoma, and gonadoblastoma have been found. Cryptorchid testes, even when not associated with intersexuality, are also associated with an increased risk of malignancy. The probability that cryptorchid testes will undergo malignant degeneration is difficult to assess, but it is at least 10 times greater than the probability for normally descended testes.[647, 648] Approximately 7% of males with testicular neoplasms have been or are cryptorchid at the time of diagnosis.[648] In addition, in one third of patients with cryptorchidism who develop carcinoma of the testis, the neoplasm occurs after orchiopexy; in patients with unilateral cryptorchidism, 25% of tumors were located in the contralateral descended testes.[647, 648] CiS is a premalignant lesion of the testes.[537, 650, 651] It is characterized by germ cells that are larger than normal spermatogonia, have clumped chromatin, are highly aneuploid, and are positive for placental alkaline phosphatase.[650, 651] CiS, also called intratubular germ cell neoplasm (IGCN), is commonly seen adjacent to germ cell tumors in adults.[650] However, CiS is not found adjacent to tumors before puberty, and the cells differ morphologically from those in postpubertal males. The natural history of CiS in prepubertal patients remains to be determined.[650] About 50% of postpubertal patients with CiS develop germ cell tumors within 5 y of diagnosis; it has been suggested that, with time, the incidence may approach 100%.[650] CiS is thought to originate from primordial germ cells.[650] It occurs in 2 to 3% of males with cryptorchidism, in a higher proportion of individuals with dysgenetic testes and an XY cell line (XY gonadal dysgenesis, XO/XY mosaicism), and in the syndrome of androgen resistance.[650]

Gonadal neoplasms are uncommon in patients with 47,XXY seminiferous tubule dysgenesis, but a small number of patients have gonadal or extragonadal germ cell tumors.[307, 308, 648, 651a] Similarly, gonadal tumors are rare in the streak gonads of 45,X patients and in 45,X mosaics with a normal or structurally abnormal X chromosome in the second cell line. Gonadoblastoma and dysgerminoma,[648, 652–654] mucinous cystadenoma,[655] and a hilus cell tumor with signs of virilization have been reported in gonadal dysgenesis.[656, 657] However, these patients have not been studied for a low percentage of Y chromosome mosaicism by molecular analyses.[37]

Gonadoblastomas are usually composed of three elements—large germ cells, sex cord derivatives (Sertoli-granulosa cells), and stromal elements (theca cells, Leydig cells). They are found almost exclusively in patients who have a 46,XY cell line. They may be microscopic or large, especially if overgrown by other germ cell elements, and often are calcified. A comprehensive review of gonadoblastoma was published by Scully[646] (see Fig. 29–45). In 27 of 74 patients, a tumor was present in both gonads. Thirty patients were younger than 15 years of age when the tumor was diagnosed, and 10 were younger than 10 years. A third of these tumors were detected incidentally on histologic examination of dysgenetic gonads removed for other indications. In patients in whom chromosomal studies were carried out, the predominant karyotypes were 45,X/46,XY and 46,XY. Although 80% of 46,XY patients are reared as females, most display some degree of clitoromegaly or hirsutism; rarely, the tumors secrete enough estrogen to induce breast development (see Fig. 29–45). Pure gonadoblastomas can be regarded as germ cell tumors in situ and as such do not metastasize.[647, 648] In half the cases, however, the germ cells infiltrate the stroma of the tumor to form a seminoma.[658, 660] Gonadoblastomas are also associated with more highly malignant germ cell tumors such as endodermal sinus tumors, embryonal carcinoma, and choriocarcinoma (10%).[647, 659] There is an increased risk of gonadal tumors (gonadoblastoma and/or germinoma) in patients with 46,XY gonadal dysgenesis and particularly in familial cases.[659] The strikingly disparate propensity for neoplastic transformation in the streak or dysgenetic gonads of patients with 46,XY gonadal dysgenesis in contrast to 46,XX gonadal dysgenesis must be emphasized.

In view of the well-documented malignant potential of dysgenetic gonads, the question of prophylactic gonadectomy merits serious attention. The neoplasms are infrequent in childhood,[645, 660] but the risk rises appreciably in young adults.[645–648] High gonadotropin levels may play a role in their growth, and substitution therapy with gonadal steroids may afford some protection. A prudent course is to advise laparotomy and removal of the dysgenetic gonads of all patients with 46,XY gonadal dysgenesis (complete and incomplete forms) and of all patients with the syndrome of gonadal dysgenesis who have a cell line with a normal or a structurally abnormal Y chromosome or who have Y chromosomal material as determined by molecular biologic studies. Exceptions to this rule occur in patients who are 45,X/46,XY mosaics with normal male genitalia, histologically normal testes, and normal gonadotropin levels and in patients with 45,X/46,XY mosaicism with ambiguous genitalia who have been assigned a male gender role and in whom a histologically normal gonad is located in the scrotum. However, the fact that a gonad is located in the scrotum or labial folds and is palpable does not guarantee against a disastrous result, because seminomas can metastasize at an early stage, before a local mass is obvious. Hence, it is prudent to biopsy these testes postpubertally to ascertain the presence of CiS (a premalignant lesion).[537] Patients with 45,X gonadal dysgenesis who have no suggestion of clitoromegaly are not at risk. The incidence of gonadal tumors in patients with other X chromosome abnormalities, such as 45,X/46,XX, 46,XXr, 46,XXp−, and 46,XXq−, is low; however, these patients should be examined at regular intervals and, if indicated, monitored by sonography of the pelvis for signs of gonadal or uterine neoplasm.

Female Pseudohermaphroditism

Female pseudohermaphroditism (Table 29–17) is the easiest of the sexual anomalies to comprehend, because the ovaries and müllerian derivatives are normal and anatomic abnormality is limited to the external genitalia. Because in the absence of testes there is an inherent tendency for the external genitalia to feminize, a female fetus is masculinized only

TABLE 29–17. Classification of Female Pseudohermaphroditism

I. Androgen-induced
  A. Fetal source
    1. Congenital adrenal hyperplasia
      a. Virilism only, defective adrenal 21-hydroxylation (CYP21)
      b. Virilism with salt-losing syndrome, defective adrenal 21-hydroxylation (CYP21)
      c. Virilism with hypertension, defective adrenal 11β-hydroxylation (CYP11B1)
      d. Virilism with adrenal insufficiency, deficient 3β-HSD II (HSD3B II)
    2. P450 aromatase (CYP19) deficiency
  B. Maternal source
    1. Iatrogenic
      a. Testosterone and related steroids
      b. Certain synthetic oral progestagens and rarely diethylstilbestrol
    2. Virilizing ovarian or adrenal tumor
    3. Virilizing luteoma of pregnancy
    4. Congenital virilizing adrenal hyperplasia in mother
  C. Undetermined source
    1. ? Virilizing luteoma of pregnancy
II. Non–androgen-induced disturbances in differentiation of urogenital structures

if exposed to androgens. The degree of fetal masculinization is determined by the stage of differentiation at the time of exposure. Once the vagina has separated from the urogenital sinus (at about the 12th fetal week), androgens cause only clitoral hypertrophy (Fig. 29–48). Even with severe masculinization of the external genitalia, the uterus and fallopian tubes are normal, because regression of the primordia for these structures, the müllerian ducts, requires secretion of AMH by fetal testes, and this action cannot be mimicked by androgens. Although the presence of virilized genitalia usually provides prima facie evidence of an androgenic influence during gestation, ambiguous genitalia, superficially resembling those produced by androgen, are an occasional feature of other, more generalized teratologic malformations. The genes involved in sex differentiation are listed in Table 29–18.

Congenital Adrenal Hyperplasia

CAH[661–663] accounts for most of the cases of female pseudohermaphroditism and approximately half of all patients with ambiguous external genitalia.

BIOCHEMICAL VARIANTS OF CONGENITAL ADRENAL HYPERPLASIA. Mutations in five genes, four that encode biosynthetic enzymes for steroid hormone synthesis (CYP21, CYP17, CYP11A1, and HSD3B2) and one that encodes the intracellular cholesterol transport protein (StAR), can cause CAH, each resulting in distinctive biochemical consequences and clinical features[661–663] (Fig. 29–49; see Chapter 12). All are transmitted as autosomal recessive traits. The common denominator in all six biochemical defects is impaired cortisol secretion, which results in hypersecretion of corticotropin and consequent hyperplasia of the adrenal cortex. Only deficiencies of 21-hydroxylase (CYP21) and 11β-hydroxylase (CYP11B1), however, are predominantly virilizing disorders. In patients with "classic" forms of these defects, the most striking abnormality of the sexual phenotype is masculinization of the female fetus because of overproduction of adrenal androgens and androgen precursors. Affected males have no abnormalities of the genitalia. These inborn errors of steroid biosynthesis are discussed in this section as causes of female pseudohermaphroditism.

Patients with 3β-HSD, CYP17, and StAR deficiencies have defects that not only block cortisol synthesis but also impair the production of gonadal steroids by the gonads and by the adrenal glands. Affected males have varying degrees of male pseudohermaphroditism because of deficient testosterone production by the fetal Leydig cells, whereas affected females may or may not exhibit virilization. If present, virilization in

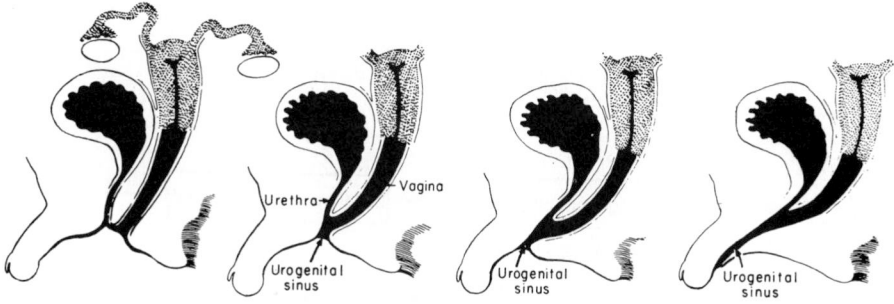

Figure 29–48. Female pseudohermaphroditism induced by prenatal exposure to androgens. Exposure after 12th fetal week leads only to clitoral hypertrophy (diagram on left). Exposure at progressively earlier stages of differentiation (depicted from left to right in drawings) leads to retention of the urogenital sinus and labioscrotal fusion. If exposure occurs sufficiently early, the labia fuse to form a penile urethra. (From Grumbach MM, Ducharme JR. The effects of androgens on fetal sexual development: androgen-induced female pseudohermaphroditism. Fertil Steril 1960; 11:157–180. Reproduced with permission of the publisher. The American Fertility Society.)

females is usually less severe than in CYP21 and CYP11B1 deficiencies. These forms of CAH in the male are discussed in the section on male pseudohermaphroditism. Administration to the pregnant rat of selective synthetic inhibitors of the enzymes involved in adrenal and testicular steroid biogenesis produced abnormalities of sex differentiation in the offspring that are the counterparts of CAH in humans and served to clarify the role of steroidogenic enzymes in the control of fetal sex differentiation.[664]

CYP21 (21-HYDROXYLASE) DEFICIENCY

Simple Virilizing Form of CYP21 Deficiency. Deficiency of CYP21 (cytochrome P450$_{c21}$), the most common cause of ambiguous genitalia in infants, is inherited (as are the other forms) as an autosomal recessive trait. The simple virilizing form of CYP21 deficiency has an incidence of about 1 per 50,000 persons and accounts for approximately 25% of subjects with CYP21 deficiency[665] (Table 29–19).

The abnormality in adrenal biosynthesis in patients with the simple virilizing form of CYP21 deficiency is primarily defective hydroxylation at C-21 of progesterone and 17-hydroxyprogesterone in the adrenal gland, which results in increased production of progesterone and 17-hydroxyprogesterone and impaired synthesis of cortisol.[661–663, 666] As a consequence of defective cortisol synthesis, hypersecretion of corticotropin causes hyperpigmentation and stimulation of the adrenals to produce excessive amounts of cortisol precursors, including androgen precursors, proximal to the block

in the biosynthetic pathway. Hence, in affected patients the concentrations of plasma 17-hydroxyprogesterone and 21-deoxycortisol are increased, as are the plasma levels of androstenedione, testosterone, and, to a lesser extent, progesterone and 17α-hydroxypregnenolone. Postnatally, metabolites of these steroids are excreted as urinary 17-ketosteroids, pregnanetriol, and 11-ketopregnanetriol. Prenatally, excess adrenal androgen synthesis in the fetus, which exceeds in the first trimester the capacity of placental aromatase to convert C$_{19}$-steroids to estrogens,[667] results in elevated circulating testosterone levels. Before the 12th week of gestation, high fetal androgen levels lead to a varying degree of labioscrotal fusion and clitoral enlargement in the affected female fetus; exposure to androgen after week 12 causes isolated clitorimegaly.[243] Exposure to excess androgens in the male during gestation can result in phallic enlargement (e.g., testotoxicosis, virilizing adrenal hyperplasia).

The genitalia of females with the virilizing forms of CAH (CYP21, CYP11B1, and 3β-HSD deficiencies) may exhibit a spectrum of masculinization from simple enlargement of the clitoris to complete labioscrotal fusion with a penile urethra (see Fig. 29–48). In severe cases the urogenital sinus is usually preserved and serves as a common outlet for both the urethra and vagina. The hypersecretion of androgens and androgen precursors begins before the 12th week of gestation, especially in patients who manifest more than simple clitorimegaly. The uterus and fallopian tubes (müllerian structures) and the

TABLE 29–18. Genes Involved in Sex Differentiation

Gene	Chromosomal Locus	Function
AMH (antimüllerian hormone)	19p13.3	Regression (apoptosis) of müllerian ducts
AMH type II receptor	12q13	Receptor for AMH
hCG (β subunit)*	19	Stimulates testosterone synthesis by fetal testis
hCG/LH receptor	2p21	Receptor for hCG/LH
StAR (steroid acute regulatory protein)	8p11.2	Labile protein that stimulates transport of cholesterol from outer to inner mitochondrial membrane; not expressed in placenta
CYP11A1 (P450$_{scc}$)†	15q23-q24	Enzyme that converts cholesterol to pregnenolone located on inner mitochondrial membrane
3β-HSD2	1p13.1	Catalyzes in adrenal and gonad conversion of C21 and C19 Δ^5 steroids to Δ^4 steroids
3β-HSD1†	1p13	Catalyzes conversion of Δ^5 steroids to Δ^4 steroids in extra-adrenal and extragonadal tissues; expressed in placenta
CYP17 (P450$_{c17}$)	10q24-q25	Has both 17α-hydroxylase and C-17,20 lyase (mainly Δ^5 17,20 lyase) activities
CYP21 (P450$_{c21}$)	6p21.3	21α-Hydroxylase activity
CYP11B1 (P450$_{c11}$)	8q21-q22	11β-Hydroxylase activity
17β-HSD type 3	9q22	Converts androstenedione to testosterone by the testis
AR	Xq11-q12	Androgen receptor
5α-reductase-2 (*SRD5A2*)	2p23	Converts testosterone to dihydrotestosterone
CYP19 (P450$_{arom}$)	15q21	Placental aromatase; aromatizes C19 androgens and androgen precursors to C18 estrogens and serves to protect the female fetus from masculinization by C19 steroids produced by the normal fetal and maternal adrenal

*No naturally occurring α-subunit mutations have been described; mutations in hCG would be expected to be lethal in utero because of involution of maternal corpus luteum.
†Expressed in placenta; essential for placental progesterone synthesis; severe mutations probably lethal in utero.

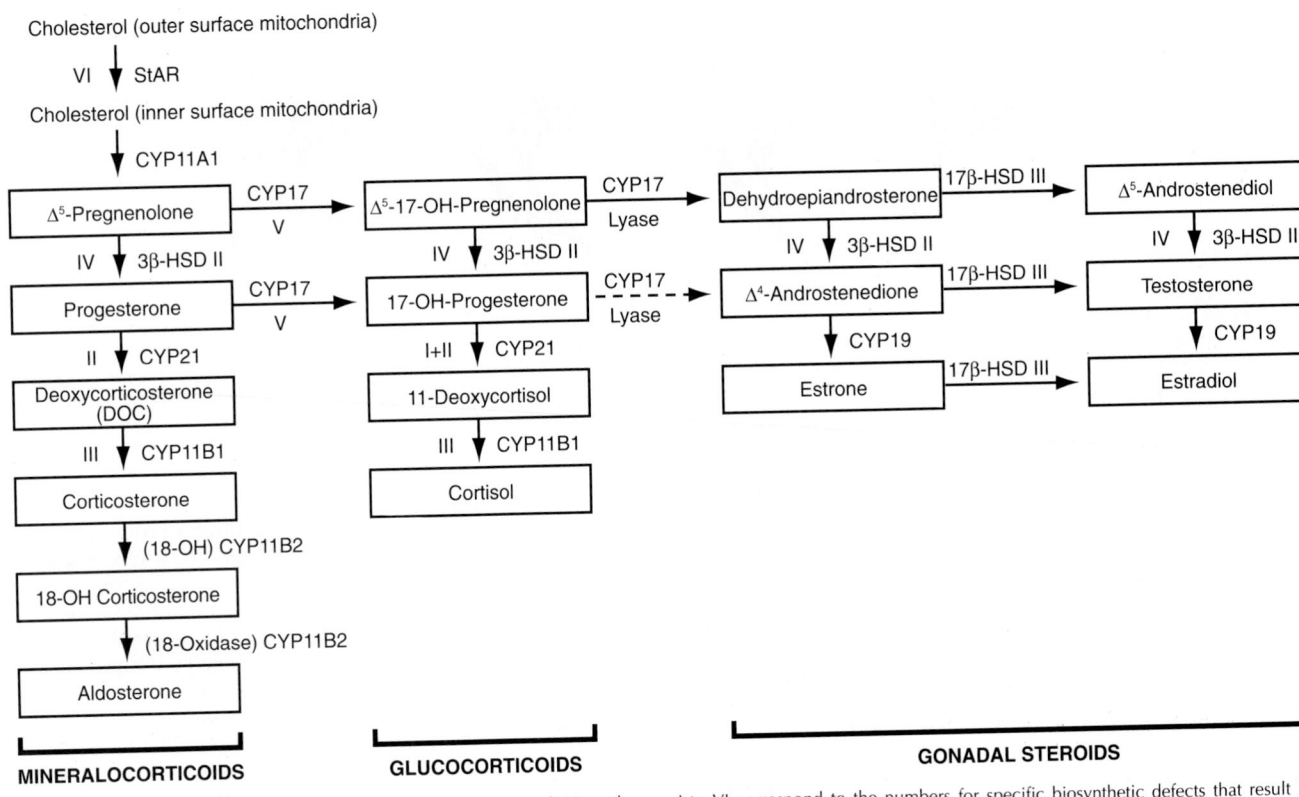

Figure 29–49. A diagrammatic representation of the steroid biosynthetic pathways. I to VI correspond to the numbers for specific biosynthetic defects that result in congenital adrenal hyperplasia. The defect in patients with lipoid adrenal hyperplasia is not in the CYP11A1 (cholesterol side-chain cleavage) enzyme but in StAR, the steroidogenic acute regulatory protein. This protein is involved in the transport of cholesterol from the outer mitochondrial membrane to the inner membrane where the CYP11A1 enzyme is located. CYP11B1 (11β-hydroxylase) catalyzes 11-hydroxylation of deoxycorticosterone and 11-deoxycortisol primarily. CYP17 (17α-hydroxylase/17,20-lyase) catalyzes both 17-hydroxylation and splitting of the 17,20 bond, but for the latter it has preferential Δ5-17,20-lyase activity (see text). CYP19 (aromatase) catalyzes the conversion of androstenedione to estrone and testosterone to estradiol. CYP11B2 (aldosterone synthetase) catalyzes the conversion of corticosterone to aldosterone. 3β-HSD I and 3β-HSD II, 3β-hydroxysteroid dehydrogenase/Δ4, 5-isomerase types I and II; CYP21 (P450-c21), 21-hydroxylase; 17β-HSD 3, 17β-hydroxysteroid dehydrogenase type 3. In the human, deletion of or a homozygous null mutation of CYP11A1 is probably lethal in utero (see text).

ovaries are normally formed, except in rare cases. Wolffian duct development is consistently absent regardless of the degree of virilization of the external genitalia in affected females. Thus, internal genital morphogenesis corresponds to gonadal sex in females and males.

Postnatally, secretion of testosterone by the adrenal gland and conversion of androstenedione to testosterone in periph-

TABLE 29–19. Incidence of Classic Congenital Virilizing Adrenal Hyperplasia (CYP21 Deficiency) After Screening

Population	Number of Newborns Screened	Newborns Affected/ Live Births	Incidence by Case Survey
Alaska	1,131	1/282	1/490
La Réunion, France	31,472	1/3,147	
Rome, Italy	22,400	1/5,600	
Lille (Lyon), France	199,624	1/11,090	1/23,000
Illinois	357,825	1/11,928	1/15,000 Wisconsin 1/40,000 USA
Sweden	370,000	1/12,758	
Portugal	100,000	1/14,285	
Emilia-Romagna, Italy	73,000	1/14,600	
Scotland	119,960	1/17,137	1/20,907
Washington	255,527	1/18,251	1/15,000 Wisconsin
New Zealand	168,965	1/18,773	
Japan	585,000	1/20,892	1/43,674

Reprinted by permission of the publisher from Pang S, Clark A. Newborn screening, prenatal diagnosis, and prenatal treatment of congenital adrenal hyperplasia due to 21-hydroxylase deficiency. Trends Endocrinol Metab 1990; 1:302. Copyright 1990 by Elsevier Science Publishing Co., Inc.

eral tissues result in continued virilization of the untreated patient. In the simple virilizing form of CYP21 deficiency, the 21-hydroxylation of C_{21} 17-hydroxysteroids and 17-deoxysteroids is primarily impaired.[666, 668] However, even in patients with "mild," late-onset CYP21 deficiency the 21-hydroxylation of mineralocorticoids is defective, as evidenced by elevated plasma 21-deoxycorticosterone levels after corticotropin stimulation.[668] Untreated patients with simple virilizing CYP21 deficiency usually, but not always, have normal plasma renin levels and normal aldosterone secretion rates.[669] In untreated patients, increased androgen production leads to the early appearance of pubic hair, acne, clitorimegaly (or phallic enlargement in the male), increased muscular development, other signs of virilization, rapid growth during childhood, and disproportionate increase in the rate of skeletal maturation, which results in premature closure of the epiphyses and short stature in adolescence and adulthood.[670]

CYP21 Deficiency with Salt Loss. In patients with severe CYP21 deficiency, both virilization and salt loss can occur. This variant, which occurs in about 75% of patients with classic CYP21 deficiency (1 in 16,000 persons),[665] is caused by a severe or complete defect in adrenal 21-hydroxylation that leads to impaired cortisol (adrenal fasciculata) and aldosterone (adrenal glomerulosa) secretion[661–663] and increased plasma renin activity. Electrolyte and fluid losses cause hyponatremia, hyperkalemia, acidosis, dehydration, vascular collapse, and, if untreated, death. About 50% of patients have the first salt-losing adrenal crisis at between 6 and 14 days of age; it is infrequent before that time. However, plasma potassium concentrations may be elevated before 6 d. Rarely, the "crisis" may occur as late as 6 to 12 weeks, usually in association with a concomitant stress. Masculinization of the external genitalia and urogenital sinus in affected females tends to be more severe in complete CYP21 deficiency than in simple CYP21 or CYP11B1 deficiency. Without specific therapy, death can result from hyperkalemia, dehydration, and shock. In the affected male whose genitalia are normal, the differential diagnosis includes sepsis, pyloric stenosis, gastroenteritis, congenital heart disease, and congenital adrenal hypoplasia.

Nonclassic CYP21 Deficiency. Studies of families affected with 21-hydroxylase deficiency have revealed heterogeneity in the biochemical and clinical manifestations of this condition, including asymptomatic as well as symptomatic "late-onset" disease.[661-663, 671-674] Affected females have no genital ambiguity at birth, in contrast to those with classic CYP21 deficiency, but can manifest symptoms of androgen excess, such as premature development of pubic hair in early childhood,[675] accelerated linear growth and bone maturation with resulting short stature, cystic acne, male-pattern baldness, hirsutism, and menstrual abnormalities. Symptoms and findings in women may be similar to those in women with polycystic ovary disease.[661, 662]

In affected males, premature development of pubic hair, beard growth, growth spurt, and phallic maturation can occur prepubertally as a result of the increased adrenal androgen production. Oligospermia and decreased fertility have also been attributed to late-onset CYP21 deficiency.[676]

In studies of families with classic CYP21 deficiency, some individuals have hormonal criteria of this disease (i.e., elevated basal and/or corticotropin-stimulated 17-hydroxyprogesterone, androstenedione, and testosterone levels) but no clinical signs of androgen excess.[661] These patients have been designated as having "cryptic" CYP21 deficiency. Symptoms of hyperandrogenism may wax and wane in these patients, who therefore may not be truly asymptomatic over a period of time.[661]

New and co-workers,[677] using corticotropin-induced rises in 17-hydroxyprogesterone, have defined hormone reference data in the form of a nomogram. Their studies provide a means of distinguishing patients with classic CYP21 deficiency from those with milder variant forms, heterozygotes, and normal individuals. These hormonal data in conjunction with linkage studies with human leukocyte antigen (HLA) typing, and in some instances genotyping, indicated that all three variants—classic CYP21 deficiency and the cryptic and late-onset variants—resulted from a defect in the same gene. The features of the cryptic and late-onset forms can occur in families with the classic disease and can be present in the same patient at different times of life. The cryptic and late-onset forms arise from allelic variants of the gene that causes classic CYP21 deficiency. Genotypically, patients may be compound heterozygotes with a classic mutation and a variant allele, or they may have two variant alleles.[671] Using hormonal data and linkage studies, Speiser and co-workers[671, 678, 681] estimated that nonclassic CYP21 deficiency is the most common autosomal recessive disorder in humans, the frequency being 0.01 in all ethnic groups. The gene frequency is higher in Ashkenazi Jews, Hispanics, and Yugoslavs.[678, 679]

Molecular Genetics of CYP21 Deficiency.[680, 681] CYP21, a member of the cytochrome P450 superfamily of monooxygenases, is a heme-containing enzyme that is bound to endoplasmic reticulum and receives electrons from NADPH by way of a flavoprotein, P450 reductase. The gene for this enzyme is located within the major HLA locus on the short arm of chromosome 6 (6p21.3)[661] (Fig. 29–50). HLA types are codominantly inherited and can be used in informative families (those containing an affected child and the parents) to distinguish homozygotes, heterozygotes, and unaffected individuals (Fig. 29–51). Although a wide variety of HLA antigens and haplotypes is found in affected patients, genetic disequilibrium has been found for certain specific types and haplotypes. In particular, HLA-Bw47 has a high degree of association with the salt-losing form of CYP21 deficiency, and HLA-DR1,B14 occurs more frequently in patients with the nonclassic form of the disease.[671]

Two *CYP21* genes are located on each chromosome 6 between HLA-B and HLA-DR[682] (Fig. 29–52), a functional *CYP21B* gene and a nonfunctional *CYP21A* pseudogene. The *CYP21* gene, the gene for the fourth component of complement (C4)[692] and a gene for a large extracellular matrix protein called tenascin X[683] are duplicated in tandem in the sequence C4A, CYP21A, XA, C4B, CYP21B, and XB; this locus is one of the most complex in the human genome. The *CYP21* genes and X genes overlap one another on opposite strands of DNA.[690, 693] The *CYP21A* and *CYP21B* genes are about 3.3 kb long, have 10 exons each, and are 98% homologous; *CYP21A* is a pseudogene that is transcribed,[683a] but it has nine deleterious mutations that impair translation of the mRNA, including an eight-base pair deletion in exon 3, insertion of a thymidine residue in exon 7, and a cytosine-to-thymidine substitution in exon 8.[684-686] Each of these changes results in stop codons, and, as a consequence, the gene is nonfunctional (a pseudogene).

The molecular genetics of 21-hydroxylase deficiency are unique (Fig. 29–53). The tandem organization of the *CYP21* and *C4* genes, as well as their sequence homology, may lead to unequal pairing during meiosis of the *CYP21-C4* genes on one chromosome 6 with the *CYP21-C4* genes on its homologue and result in duplication/deficiency products (see Fig. 29–52). Approximately 95% of mutations that cause 21-hydroxylase deficiency are a consequence of recombination between the *CYP21B* gene and the highly homologous *CYP21A* pseudogene. Approximately 15% of severely affected *CYP21B* genes

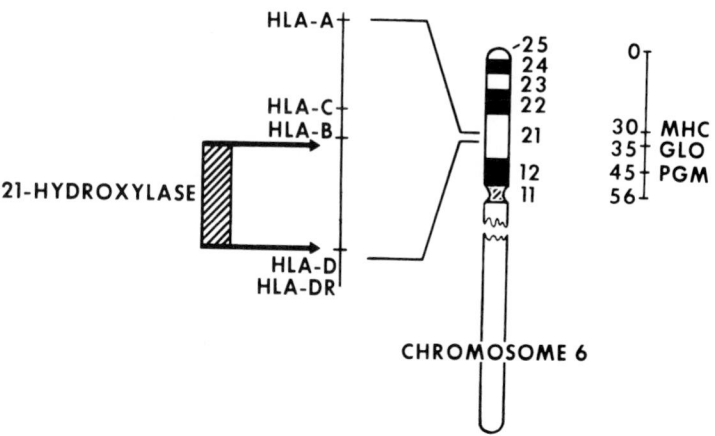

Figure 29–50. A diagrammatic representation of chromosome 6. Only the banding pattern of the short arm is shown. Numbers 11 to 25 delineate bands according to the Paris nomenclature. To right of the centromere, the sites of genes for the major histocompatibility complex (MHC), glyoxalase I (GLO), and phosphoglucomutase (PGM) are indicated on a recombinant unit scale. To left is a scheme of genes in the MHC complex. The gene for 21-hydroxylase is closely linked to HLA-B and resides between the HLA-B and HLA-D loci.

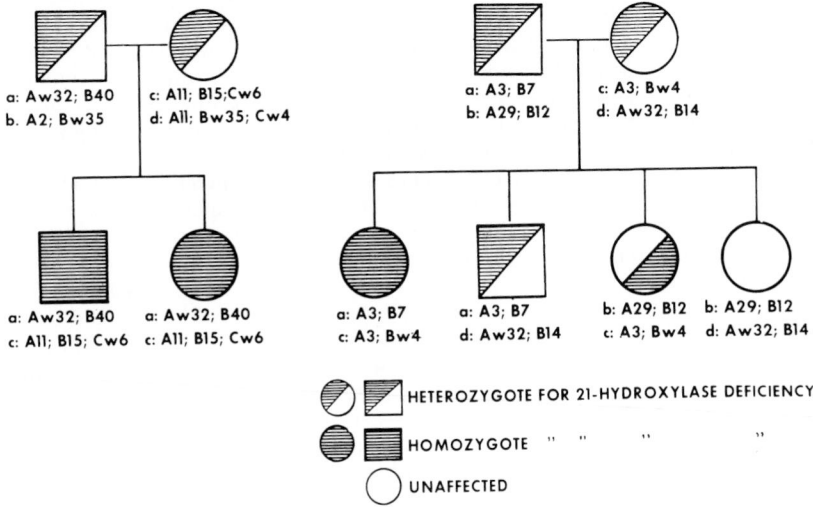

Figure 29–51. Pedigrees of two families with children with 21-hydroxylase deficiency. HLA haplotypes for HLA-A, HLA-B, and HLA-C are indicated for each individual. a, b indicate paternal haplotypes and c, d maternal haplotypes. Parents are heterozygotes for 21-hydroxylase deficiency. Patients with haplotype a, c are homozygous for 21-hydroxylase deficiency. Haplotype b, d indicates a child who has two normal genes for 21-hydroxylase activity. (Redrawn from Levine LS, Zachmann M, New MI, et al. Genetic mapping of the 21-hydroxylase deficiency gene within the HLA linkage group. Reprinted, by permission of the New England Journal of Medicine, 1978; 299:911–915.)

have a deletion that extends from exon 3 to exon 8 of the *CYP21A* pseudogene to a similar region of the *CYP21B* gene. This results in a fusion *CYP21A/CYP21B* gene that is nonfunctional because of the presence of the eight-base-pair deletion in exon 3 of *CYP21A*.[661, 680, 681] The remaining 80% of patients have gene "conversions" (i.e., transfer of sequences usually found on *CYP21A*, the pseudogene, to *CYP21B*), which result in a variable decrease in 21-hydroxylase activity.[661, 680, 681] The conversions most commonly involve the transfer of any of the nine deleterious mutations on the pseudogene to the *CYP21B* gene. Approximately 10% of severely deficient alleles have macroconversions (the entire gene is converted), and the rest have microconversions that resemble point mutations and correspond to the nine expressed noncorrespondences between the pseudogene and the functional *CYP21B* gene.[681]

The most common mutation in classic CAH is the gene conversion mutation, guanine for adenine (or cytosine) near the 3' end of intron 2, which causes a premature splice of the intron and a frameshift (see Fig. 29–53). This mutation results in minimal 21-hydroxylase activity; however, a small amount of normally spliced mRNA has been detected in transfected cultured cells with this mutation.[661, 680, 681] Hence, this mutation can be associated with both the salt-losing and the simple virilizing forms of the disease. An Ile172Asn mutation in patients with simple virilizing adrenal hyperplasia[680, 681] causes the formation of an enzyme with 3 to 7% of the activity of the normal enzyme but allows for enough aldosterone production to prevent clinical salt wasting.[681, 684] Mutations associated with nonclassic CAH, such as Val281Leu and Pro30Leu, have 20 to 50% of normal activity in transfected cultured cells.[681, 684, 685] Several mutations have been identified that appear to be true point mutations and not gene conversions.[686]

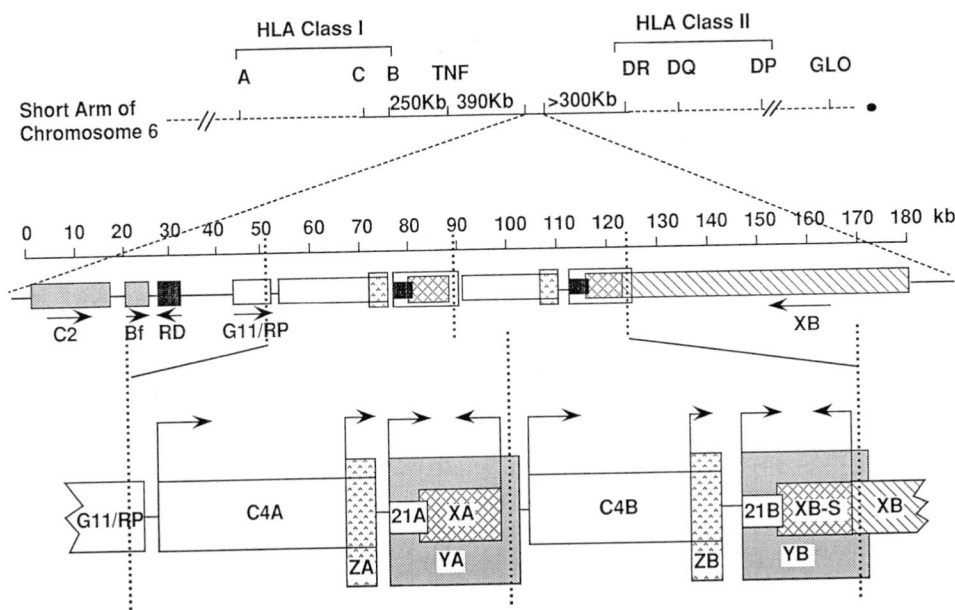

Figure 29–52. Genetic anatomy of the 21-hydroxylase locus. The upper line shows the large-scale organization of the short arm of chromosome 6, with the telomere at the left and the centromere at the right. A 180-kb segment (note scale) of the class III region of the HLA locus is shown in the middle. The genes include C2, second component of complement; Bf, properdin factor Bf; RD and G11/RP—widely expressed genes of unknown function. The C4/CYP21/TNX locus is enlarged below. C4A and C4B, fourth component of complement; 21A, CYP21 pseudogene; 21B, functional CYP21 gene; ZA and ZB, adrenal-specific transcripts corresponding to the C-termini of C4A and C4B; YA and YB, alternate transcripts arising from the CYP21 promoters; XA, truncated tenascin-X pseudogene expressed in the adrenal; XB-S, short, adrenal-specific tenascin-X–like protein; XB, gene for the extracellular matrix protein, tenascin-X. Arrows indicate transcriptional orientation. Vertical dotted lines designate the duplication boundaries of the A and B regions. (Redrawn from Tee MK, Babalola GO, Aza-Blanc P, et al. A promoter within intron 35 of the human C4A gene initiates abundant adrenal-specific transcription of a 1 kb RNA: location of a cryptic CYP21 promoter element? Hum Mol Genet 1995; 4:2109–2116.)

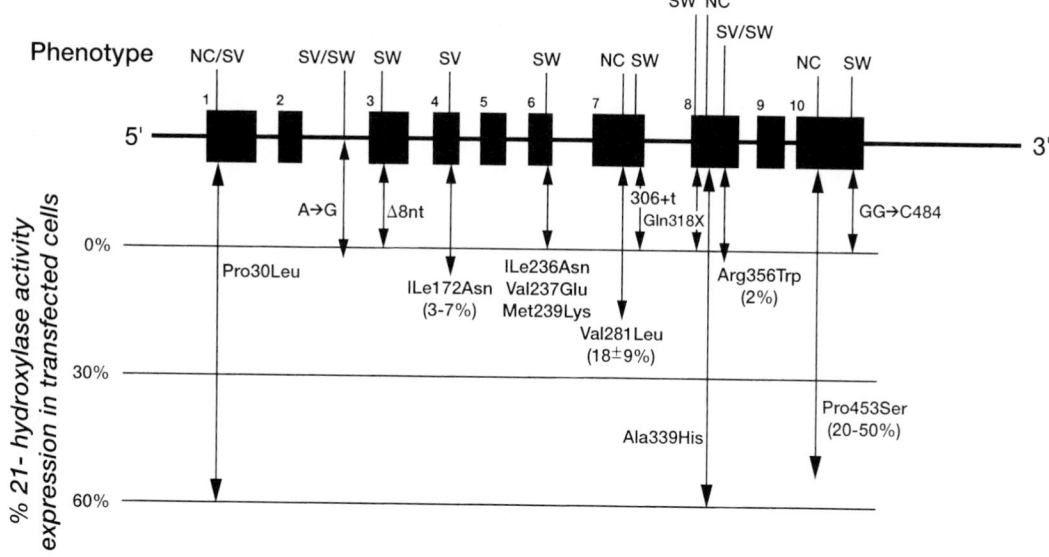

Figure 29–53. Diagrammatic representation of the *CYP21B* gene and the site of microconversions which cause 21-hydroxylase deficiency. The numbered black boxes are the exons. SW, salt wasting; SV, simple virilizing; NC, nonclassic form. A→G indicates an adenine to guanine transition near the end of intron 2, which causes premature splicing resulting in an aberrant 11-amino-acid string and a stop codon. Δ8nt indicates an eight-nucleotide deletion in exon 3. 306+t indicates a thymidine insertion at codon 306, which causes a frameshift and stop. GG→C is a guanine-to-cytosine transition at codon 484. As noted in the text, all of these deleterious mutations which inactivate or diminish 21-hydroxylase activity are normally present in the *CYP21A* pseudogene. The lengths of the arrows and the percentages in parentheses designate the magnitude of activity of the 21-hydroxylase enzyme in transfected cells.

Classic salt-wasting CYP21 deficiency is commonly associated with gene deletions or conversions that abolish or severely reduce 21-hydroxylase activity; functionally less severe mutations cause the nonclassic form of the disease.[680, 681, 685] Most patients are compound heterozygotes harboring, for example, a deletion on one chromosome 6 and a gene conversion (less commonly, a point mutation) on the other. The functionally less severe genetic defect is the major determinant of the severity of the enzyme deficiency and thus the phenotype (e.g., classic salt-wasting or cryptic form). However, the difference between the simple salt-wasting and nonclassic variants of CYP21 deficiency may be both quantitative and qualitative. Not only the amount of enzyme produced but also its specificity may be determined by the specific combination of deletions, point mutations, and gene conversions. Indeed, individuals who are either homozygous for a *CYP21B* gene deletion or heterozygous for a deletion and a large gene conversion of *CYP21B* to *CYP21A* (null mutations) are classic salt wasters. Simple virilizing phenotypes result from dysfunctional mutations or compound heterozygosity in which the less severe mutation dictates the phenotype. Some mutations can cause more than one phenotype. These variations in phenotype may be mediated, in part, by extra-adrenal 21-hydroxylase activity coded for by genes other than *CYP21B*.[680, 687, 688]

Screening for CYP21 Deficiency. Newborn screening programs for CYP21 deficiency have been instituted in a number of regions and countries by measurement of heel-blot 17-hydroxyprogesterone levels.[665, 689, 690] A blood heel-blot specimen is obtained at 3 to 5 days of life in conjunction with screening for hypothyroidism and a variety of other inborn metabolic diseases. The 17-hydroxyprogesterone level is determined either by direct radioimmunoassay or after organic solvent extraction.[675] Variability in the "normal" levels reported from one study to another reflects differences in assay technique, antibody specificity, and thickness of the blood spot. Each screening program must establish its own diagnostic standards and take into account confounding variables such as illness and prematurity.[690]

In results from screening studies worldwide, an average of 1 in 14,500 infants is homozygous for the classic (simple or salt-wasting) forms of CYP21 deficiency, and 1 in 60 is a heterozygote.[665] However, the prevalence of homozygosity varies from 1 in 282 among the Yupik Eskimos of southwest Alaska to 1 in 17,942 infants in the state of Washington.[665] Seventy-five percent of individuals identified in such screens have the salt-losing form. Screening for CYP21 deficiency is reliable and cost-effective, reduces morbidity and unexpected mortality in newborn males with severe CYP21 deficiency, and prevents erroneous assignment of male sex to affected female infants.[665]

Diagnosis. The diagnosis of CYP21 deficiency should be considered in (1) subjects with ambiguous genitalia and the features of female pseudohermaphroditism, (2) phenotypic males with bilateral cryptorchidism, (3) infants who present in shock or in a severely dehydrated condition, and (4) boys and girls who virilize before puberty. The family history may reveal a previously affected sibling, an unexpected death in infancy, or a male sibling with sexual precocity. The initial evaluation of patients with suspected CYP21 deficiency includes measurement of plasma electrolytes, 17-hydroxyprogesterone, androstenedione, and testosterone levels. A karyotype should be obtained. Pelvic ultrasonography is useful to determine the nature of internal genital structures. Increased excretion of urinary 17-ketosteroids and pregnanetriol and an elevated concentration of plasma 17-hydroxyprogesterone and androstenedione establish the diagnosis in affected infants and children. The level of plasma 17-hydroxyprogesterone is normally elevated in umbilical cord blood (mean 50 nmol/L [1640 ng/dL]) but rapidly decreases to 3 to 6 nmol/L (100 to 200 ng/dL) by 24 h after birth[691] (Fig. 29–54). After 24 h, infants with CYP21 deficiency can usually be distinguished from normal infants by measurement of 17-hydroxyprogesterone and androstenedione levels. However, "sick" unaffected infants and premature infants may have elevated androstenedione and 17-hydroxyprogesterone levels that can confound the diagnosis.[692–694]

In affected patients, plasma 17-hydroxyprogesterone values usually range from 90 to 1200 nmol/L (3000 to 40,000 ng/dL), depending on age and the severity of the enzyme defect. Rarely, salt losers have a borderline 17-hydroxyproges-

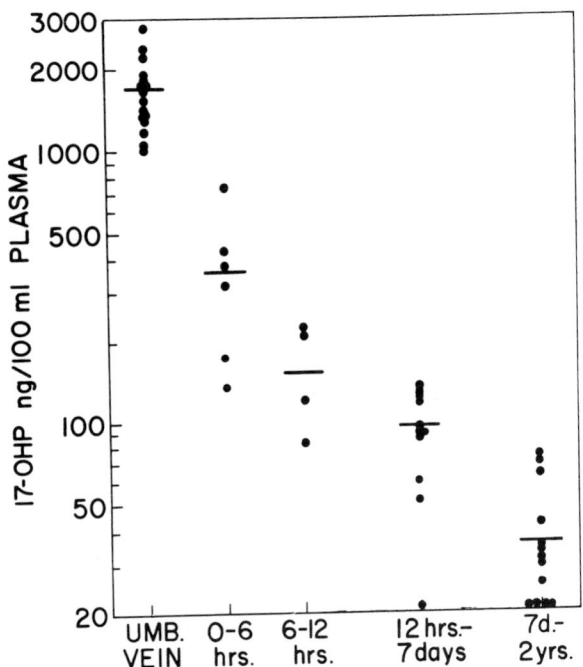

Figure 29–54. Normal plasma 17-hydroxyprogesterone levels in nonstressed infants from birth to 2 years of age. To convert 17-hydroxyprogesterone values to nanomoles per liter, multiply by 0.03026. (From Jenner MR, Grumbach MM, Kaplan SL. Plasma 17-OH progesterone in maternal and umbilical cord plasma in children, and in congenital adrenal hyperplasia [CAH]: application to neonatal diagnosis of CAH. Pediatr Res 1970; 4:380 [abstract].)

terone concentration early in the neonatal period. Patients with nonclassic CYP21 deficiency and heterozygotes may have borderline or nondiagnostic levels of 17-hydroxyprogesterone. In these instances, the corticotropin-induced increase of 17-hydroxyprogesterone, androstenedione, and 21-deoxycortisol levels identifies affected infants.[677, 695] In a kinship with an affected infant, HLA genotyping often can be used to distinguish between heterozygosity and a mild homozygous form of the disorder.

In the past, diagnosis of CYP21 deficiency was based on assessment of the excretion of urinary 17-ketosteroids and pregnanetriol. The excretion of 17-ketosteroids varies with age, and in the first few days of life in unaffected infants it can be as high as 7 to 14 μmol/d (2 to 4 mg/24 h). After 1 month of age, urinary 17-ketosteroid levels decrease to an upper limit of approximately 1.6 μmol/d (0.5 mg per year of age) until the onset of adrenarche. An elevated level of pregnanetriol, the metabolite of 17-hydroxyprogesterone, is a hallmark of 21-hydroxylase deficiency. However, in the neonatal period the urinary pregnanetriol level may be within the normal range in affected infants. Thereafter, the levels rise and are useful diagnostically.

Infants with salt wasting usually have clinical evidence of frank or incipient adrenal insufficiency or crisis after the sixth day of life and especially during the second week. Early diagnosis of the salt-losing form of CAH is usually based on the clinical findings of poor appetite, weight loss, vomiting, hyponatremia, hyperkalemia, and often renal acidosis. The plasma concentration and excretion of aldosterone are low, and plasma renin activity is high. Mild salt losers may have normal electrolytes under basal conditions but exhibit elevated plasma renin activity and hyponatremia, hyperkalemia, and inappropriate natriuresis with salt restriction.

Prenatal Diagnosis and Therapy. The striking elevation in the level of plasma 17-hydroxyprogesterone is such a distinctive marker of 21-hydroxylase deficiency that prenatal diagno-

sis has been attempted by determining its concentration in amniotic fluid in pregnancies at risk.[661, 662, 696, 697] HLA typing of cells obtained from amniotic fluid of mothers who had a previously affected offspring has also been used to identify fetuses homozygous or heterozygous for CYP21 deficiency.[698] Advances in prenatal diagnosis using amniotic fluid cells at 15 to 18 weeks, or chorionic villus biopsy samples and application of allele-specific hybridization and Southern blot analyses at about 12 weeks, have provided methods for more accurate identification of female fetuses affected with CYP21 deficiency.[699, 700]

The success of prenatal diagnosis has led to attempts at prenatal treatment.[701] Dexamethasone crosses the placenta and suppresses the fetal adrenal gland if given in sufficient doses[699, 701]; unlike cortisol or prednisolone, the placenta does not convert the 11β-hydroxy group of dexamethasone to the inactive 11-keto group. Dexamethasone administration to pregnant women early in gestation (starting at 4 to 6 weeks) can decrease the virilization of the external genitalia in approximately 75% of affected female infants,[661, 699–702] particularly if fetal adrenal suppression is monitored by regular determination of maternal serum or urine estriol. The use of prenatal dexamethasone therapy in pregnancies with a fetus at risk for CYP21 deficiency has engendered much discussion and debate, since only one in eight pregnancies in a family with an index case results in an affected female fetus. If all were treated, seven (out of eight) fetuses not at risk for ambiguous genitalia would be exposed to supraphysiological doses (20 μg/kg of maternal body weight per day) of dexamethasone for up to 13 weeks during the first trimester of gestation; in an affected female, fetal treatment is continued for the duration of pregnancy. An increase in morbidity or mortality has not been reported as yet in fetuses treated to term and monitored through infancy and early childhood.[699–702] Dexamethasone therapy, however, can result in weight gain, hypertension, striae, and glucose intolerance in the mothers. The potential risks and benefits of long-term prenatal dexamethasone therapy and the importance of long-term follow-up of all infants, affected and unaffected, who have been subjected to prenatal dexamethasone therapy have been reviewed.[703]

Treatment. Therapy for CAH resulting from CYP21 deficiency can be divided into two phases, acute and chronic. In acute adrenal crises in infants and children with the salt-losing form of the disorder, deficiency of cortisol and aldosterone rapidly leads to dehydration, hypoglycemia, electrolyte imbalance, hypotension, and, consequently, vascular collapse and cardiac arrest. An intravenous infusion of normal saline should be started immediately, and fluid and electrolyte intakes should be adequate to ensure correction of the electrolyte disorder and maintenance of normal plasma electrolyte levels and body water. In the first hour, restoration of intravascular volume is imperative.

Hypoglycemia should be treated with a bolus of 0.25 g of glucose per kilogram of body weight (maximum dose, 25 g). If the patient is hypotensive, isotonic saline (20 mL/kg) may be administered by rapid infusion. (Note that, if 5% glucose in isotonic saline is used, 1 g of glucose per kilogram of body weight will be given, and this may result in hyperglycemia.) Hydrocortisone sodium succinate (50 mg/m²) should be administered as a bolus intravenously, and another 50 to 100 mg/m² should be added to the infusion fluid over the first 24 h. When hyponatremia and hyperkalemia are present, fludrocortisone 0.1 mg should be given. These tablets can be crushed and given in a small volume of liquid by nasogastric tube. Alternatively if the child cannot take oral medication, hydrocortisone and saline therapy may suffice, since 25 mg of hydrocortisone has the equivalent mineralocorticoid action of 0.1 mg of fludrocortisone. The frequency and amount of mineralocorticoid and the amount and type of intravenous fluids are adjusted according to the serum electrolyte levels, state of hydration, body weight, and blood pressure. Excess mineralocorticoid and salt can cause hypertension, congestive heart failure, and hypertensive encephalopathy, and insufficient salt and mineralocorticoid will not correct the electrolyte imbalance and hypovolemia. Severe hyperkalemia may result in life-threatening cardiac arrhythmias. Under these circumstances, intravenous sodium bicarbonate and calcium and rectal cation-exchange resins are useful adjuvants for rapid correction of the serum potassium level.

After diagnosis and stabilization, maintenance therapy is begun. During the first 2 years of life, the authors prefer to treat infants with intramuscular cortisone acetate, avoiding the problems of regurgitation and variable absorption of oral medication. The initial suppressive dose in infants is 20 to 25 mg of intramuscular cortisone acetate daily for 5 d. This initial depot is used to "suppress" the increased secretion of androgen precursors and androgens. Thereafter, intramuscular cortisone acetate is given every 3 d in a dose of 15 to 20 mg. The cortisol secretory rate in children is about 8 ± 1 mg/m^2/d,[704, 705] but the dose of cortisol necessary to suppress corticotropin and the adrenal and achieve normal growth and development varies from individual to individual and is larger than that required to correct the glucocorticoid deficiency. With stress, febrile episodes, acute gastrointestinal disorders, and surgery, the dose is increased by giving the injection daily rather than every 3 d. This regimen of glucocorticoid replacement is usually continued until 18 to 24 months of age.

The dose of glucocorticoid (Table 29–20) is empirical and must be adjusted for each patient by assessing bone age, linear growth, 24-h excretion of 17-ketosteroids, and clinical evidence of glucocorticoid deficiency or excess. Plasma levels of testosterone, 17-hydroxyprogesterone, and androstenedione fluctuate with the time of day and the length of time from the previous dose of glucocorticoid. Therefore, random plasma steroid measurements are difficult to interpret in relation to the adequacy of therapy in infants and children. The estimation of circadian rhythms of plasma 17-hydroxyprogesterone by measurement of salivary or heel-stick blood levels may be useful but is costly and often is not practical.[706]

After 18 to 24 mo of intramuscular therapy, oral glucocorticoids are substituted. The oral dose of cortisone acetate is approximately 22 mg/m^2/d (for hydrocortisone, 18 mg/m^2/d) and is divided into three equal doses. These doses of cortisone acetate or hydrocortisone usually permit normal growth and development[670]; the dose must be readjusted on an individual basis, depending on the clinical findings, pattern of growth, skeletal maturation, and hormone findings. Adjustment of the oral dose of the more potent and longer-acting glucocorticoids (e.g., methylprednisolone, dexamethasone) is more difficult in infants and children, and their use can result

in overtreatment, manifested by suppression of growth and development of cushingoid features. Therefore the authors tend to avoid these long-acting glucocorticoid analogues in the treatment of infants and young children. On the other hand, such analogues are useful in postpubertal girls because their long action leads to less fluctuation in adrenal suppression and may facilitate normal hypothalamic-pituitary-gonadal function and menses.[707] Many affected women with the simple virilizing form of CAH, when treated appropriately, give birth to normal children. Polycystic ovaries and infertility can occur in women with undertreated CAH, although the prevalence is not known.

Patients with salt wasting require long-term therapy with mineralocorticoids and salt as well as glucocorticoids. After the infant has been diagnosed and stabilized, fludrocortisone (0.05 to 0.3 mg/d) and sodium chloride supplements (1 to 3 g/d by mouth) are given to maintain normal electrolyte levels, blood pressure, and plasma renin activity.

Plasma renin activity measurements are a useful index of the adequacy of mineralocorticoid replacement therapy. Insufficient mineralocorticoid and sodium chloride therapy not only results in hypovolemia, hyperkalemia, and hyponatremia but can lead to increased secretion of glucocorticoid precursors and adrenal androgens.[708] For optimal therapy and to ensure normal growth and development, it is recommended that all salt losers and all patients with elevated plasma renin activity be maintained on mineralocorticoid; the dosage should be assessed periodically, especially before an increase in the maintenance dose of glucocorticoid therapy is instituted. By the age of 2 to 3 years, patients with salt wasting can regulate their own dietary salt intake ad libitum.

Long-term follow-up studies on the effects of glucocorticoid and mineralocorticoid replacement in patients with CAH indicate that the mean adult height of both males and females is less than that of unaffected siblings and less than the normal mean adult height.[709–711] In addition, in a retrospective study the prevalence of learning disorders was increased in children with the salt-losing form, probably related to unrecognized hypoglycemia and to electrolyte derangements.[712] Retrospective studies in adult women have described a high prevalence of an inadequate introitus, lack of or decreased interest in sexual activity, and a below-average proportion who were married or had sexual partners.[713, 714] The fertility rate among the heterosexual sexually active women, especially those with the salt-losing form, was low.[713] An apparent increase in the frequency of homosexual and bisexual fantasies[278] and an increased propensity for homosexual and bisexual behavior has been reported,[277] but this finding was not confirmed in another study of 45 adult patients.[279] Puberty and even fertility have been reported in untreated adult males with CAH. However, men who discontinue therapy or are noncompliant are at risk for (1) hyperplasia of adrenal rests in the testes that produce bilateral, less commonly unilateral, testicular tumor-like masses that may respond to glucocorticoid suppression[715–718]; (2) pituitary hyperplasia; (3) adrenal adenoma or carcinoma[719] and adrenal incidentalomas, which may occur in more than 70% of affected adults including those with the nonclassic form and heterozygotes[720]; and (4) adrenal crises with stress. It is recommended that all patients receive treatment throughout life with a glucocorticoid and, if indicated, a mineralocorticoid (Fig. 29–55).

Surgical repair of the external genitalia of female infants with ambiguous external genitalia should be inititated after the adrenal insufficiency is stabilized and before 6 months of age. Clitoroplasty is the procedure of choice, not clitoridectomy.[721, 722] Vaginoplasty is usually deferred until later childhood or adolescence,[723] although early, one-stage reconstructions have been recommended.[724] The parents must be reassured that with appropriate treatment and compliance the

TABLE 29–20. Mean Estimated Optimal Dose of Glucocorticoids for Growth in Patients with Congenital Adrenal Hyperplasia, Compared with Anti-inflammatory Potencies

Glucocorticoid	Actual Dose in mg/m^2/24 h	Equivalent Dose	Reported Potency Based on Anti-inflammatory Effect
Dexamethasone	0.23	1	1
Methylprednisolone	2.4	10	5
Prednisone	3.7	16	7
Hydrocortisone	18.4	80	27
Cortisone acetate (IM)	13.9	60	17
Cortisone acetate (PO)	22.0	96	33

From Styne DM, Richards GE, Bell JJ, et al. Growth patterns in congenital adrenal hyperplasia. Correlation of glucocorticoid therapy with stature. In: Lee PA, Plotnick LP, Kowarski AA, et al., eds. Congenital Adrenal Hyperplasia. Baltimore: University Park Press, 1977: 247–261.

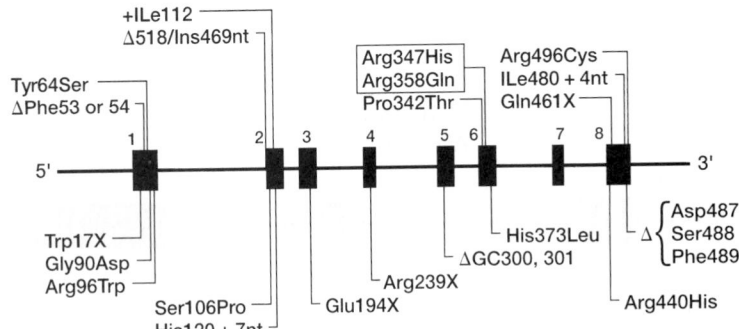

Figure 29–58. Diagrammatic representation of mutations in the CYP17 gene (17α-hydroxylase/17,20-lyase deficiency). The exons are the numbered black boxes. Missense mutations causing amino acid substitutions in the enzyme are indicated by the three-letter abbreviation for the wild-type amino acid, followed by the amino acid number in the enzyme and the three-letter abbreviation for the substituted amino acid. X indicates a nonsense (stop) mutation. ΔPhe53 or 54 is a deletion of phenylalanine at codon 53 or 54. Δ518/Ins469nt is a deletion of 518 nucleotides and an insertion of 469 nucleotides. His 120 + 7nt is a seven-nucleotide duplication at codon 120 (histidine). +ILe112 is a duplication of isoleucine at codon 112. ΔGC300,301 is a deletion of two nucleotides, guanine and cytosine, at codon 300 and 301. ILe480 + 4nt is a four-nucleotide duplication (cytosine-adenine-thymidine-cytosine) at codon 480. ΔAsp487, Ser488, Phe489 indicates a deletion of aspartic acid (codon 487), serine (codon 488), and phenylalanine (codon 489). All of these mutations cause 17α-hydroxylase deficiency. Missense mutations at codons 347 and 358, indicated by the box, have been associated with "isolated" 17,20-lyase deficiency.

46,XY male with this same mutation had only hypospadius and cryptorchidism.[794] Another 46,XY male with ambiguous genitalia was a compound heterozygote with a stop codon (TGA) at amino acid position 239 in exon 4 (a null mutation) on one allele and a missense mutation on the other allele that changes a proline to threonine at amino acid 342 (Pro342Thr) in exon 6.[790] This patient had 20% of normal 17α-hydroxylase activity in transfected cells.[790, 793] Analysis of these patients suggests that 5% of normal activity in a 46,XX female is sufficient to allow estrogen production with normal secondary sexual characteristics and irregular menses,[790, 793] whereas more than 25% of normal activity appears to be necessary to achieve normal virilization of the external genitalia of affected 46,XY males.[790, 793]

Diagnosis. 17α-Hydroxylase/17,20-lyase deficiency should be considered in all patients with ambiguous genitalia and hypergonadotrophic hypogonadism and in all phenotypic females with or without sexual infantilism, including absent adrenarche, who have hypertension and hypokalemic alkalosis. Elevated levels of 17-deoxy-C_{21}-steroids such as progesterone, pregnenolone, DOC, and corticosterone in plasma and increased urinary excretion of their metabolites establish the diagnosis. The basal plasma concentrations of DOC, corticosterone, 18-hydroxycorticosterone, and 18-hydroxy-DOC, and their response to a corticotropin challenge can be used to discriminate among homozygous, heterozygous, and unaffected individuals.[795, 796]

Glucocorticoid therapy for 21-hydroxylase deficiency suppresses DOC and corticosterone secretion. With suppression of the excess circulating mineralocorticoids, the blood pressure and serum potassium level return to normal. At puberty, both affected males and affected females usually require gonadal steroid replacement.

StAR DEFICIENCY (CONGENITAL LIPOID ADRENAL HYPERPLASIA): MALE PSEUDOHERMAPHRODITISM, SEXUAL INFANTILISM, AND ADRENAL INSUFFICIENCY. This autosomal recessive form of CAH is associated with severe glucocorticoid and mineralocorticoid deficiency, in which no C_{18^-}, C_{19^-}, or C_{21}-steroids are elaborated by the adrenal glands or gonads because of failure to convert cholesterol to pregnenolone. This disorder is the most severe genetic defect in steroidogenesis.[797–799] Affected males have female external genitalia with a blind vaginal pouch and absent müllerian derivatives. Females with this disorder have normal internal and external genital differentiation. Clinical manifestations of adrenal insufficiency, including hyponatremia, hypokalemia, acidosis, dehydration, and hypoglycemia, usually become apparent in the

first few weeks of life, but survival for months without therapy has been described.[798–800] Hyperpigmentation is common, and respiratory distress occurs in about one fourth of neonates. On ultrasound, CT, or MRI scans, markedly enlarged, lipid-laden adrenals displace the kidneys downward.

Most of the more than 80 patients with StAR deficiency are of Japanese and Korean origin[798–814]; it is second to CYP21 deficiency in prevalence in Japan and Korea. There is an unexplained 3:1 male/female sex ratio.[803] Many affected individuals die in infancy (approximately one third survive with replacement therapy); the authors have cared for one patient for more than 30 y.[802]

In contrast to the severe fetal and postnatal testosterone deficiency in affected 46,XY individuals, surviving affected 46,XX females can enter puberty and menstruate; they later develop polycystic ovaries and progressive ovarian failure.[800, 804] The prolonged survival described in a few patients before the onset of adrenal insufficiency, and the puberty and menses described in females, have been perplexing.[800] As proposed by Bose, two separate events seem responsible for these phenomena.[800] The first event is the loss of steroid hormone synthesis, which is dependent on StAR in steroid-producing cells.[800] The second event is the accumulation of cholesterol which cannot be converted to pregnenolone by the cell. Eventually this accumulation engorges the cell and results in disruption of the structural and functional integrity of the cell.[800] It is assumed that the functional activity of the cell in question mediates the time course to functional and structural disruption. Hence, postnatal survival for a period of time may reflect the relatively low level of activity of the definitive adrenal glands prenatally.[800] Postnatally, the zona glomerula and fasciculata can make a limited amount of steroids independent of StAR until they become engorged and dysfunctional.[800] The ovaries, in contrast to the testes, remain relatively quiescent through fetal life and childhood. At puberty, estrogen synthesis independent of StAR can occur, leading to feminization and menses.[800, 812, 812a] Progressive gonadal failure due to cholesterol engorgement of steroidogenic cells then results (Fig. 29–59; see color section between pages 875 and 877).[800, 812, 812a] In support of the two-hit hypothesis, no surviving XY patient has had evidence of testicular function at the expected age of puberty. All patients are markedly pigmented.

Initially it was thought that the disorder was caused by a mutation in *CYP11A1*, the gene for the side-chain cleavage enzyme. As opposed to the homozygous *CYP11A1* gene deletion discovered in the rabbit, which causes congenital lipoid adrenal hyperplasia in this species,[815] analyses in affected hu-

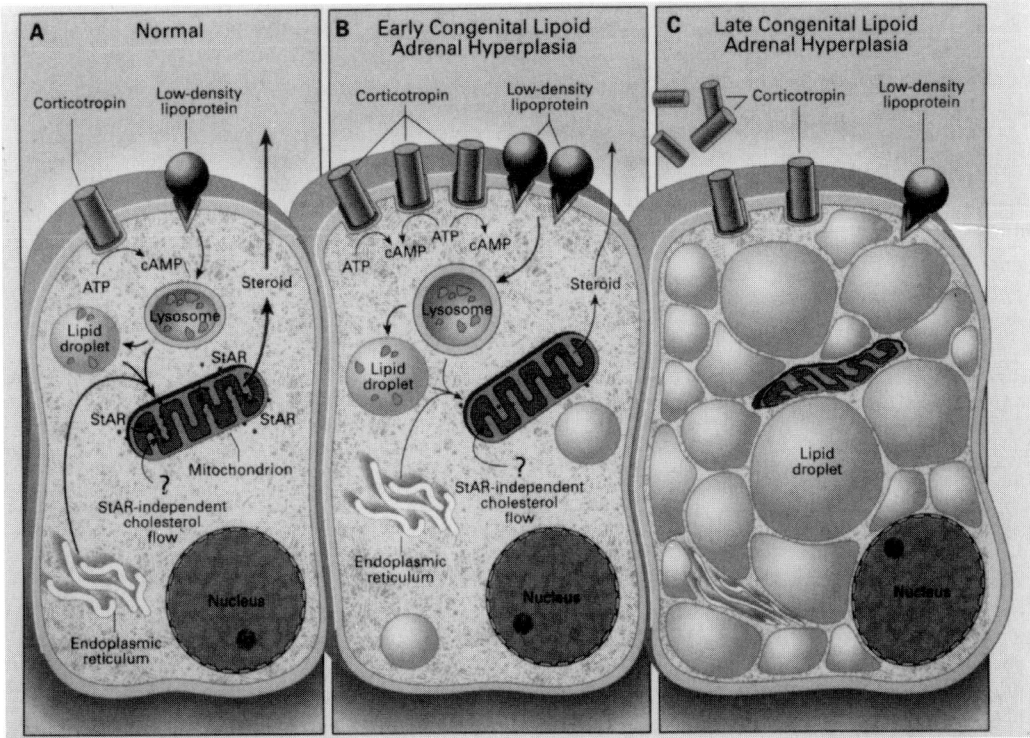

Figure 29–59. Model of the steroid-synthesizing cell (adrenal/gonadal) showing conversion of cholesterol to steroids (see color section between pages 875 and 877). *A,* Cholesterol from low-density lipoprotein, from cholesterol esters stored in lipid droplets, and from endogenous synthesis in the endoplasmic reticulum is transported from the outer mitochondrial membrane to the inner membrane. This transport, which is a rate-limiting step in steroid synthesis, is facilitated by StAR (steroidogenic acute regulatory protein) as well as by other, StAR-independent mechanisms. In the mitochondria, steroid synthesis then ensues as a result of the conversion of cholesterol to Δ^5-pregnenolone by the enzyme CYP11A1 (P450$_{scc}$). *B,* In patients with congenital lipoid adrenal hyperplasia, a mutation in the gene encoding StAR results in little or no activity of the mutant StAR, causing greatly diminished cholesterol transport into the mitochondria. Low levels of steroidogenesis via mechanisms independent of StAR can occur; however, increased ACTH (LH/FSH) secretion results in cholesterol accumulation in the cells as lipid droplets. *C,* Continued stimulation and resultant accumulation of cholesterol causes engorgement of these cells, with both mechanical and chemical perturbation of the cell function. Females with congenital lipoid adrenal hyperplasia feminize at puberty and menstruate but have progressive hypergonadotropic hypogonadism. It has been hypothesized by Bose and co-workers that this occurs because the follicular cells are relatively quiescent in utero and before puberty; hence, they are undamaged. At the beginning of each cycle, they are recruited, and a small amount of estradiol can be produced as a result of StAR-independent mechanisms. This can occur until the follicular cells are engorged and rendered nonfunctional. (From Bose HS, Sujiwara T, Strauss III JF, Miller WL. The pathophysiology and genetics of congenital lipoid adrenal hyperplasia. N Engl J Med 1996; 335:1870–1878. Copyright 1996, Massachusetts Medical Society. All rights reserved.) (See text.)

mans have failed to detect a derangement of the CYP11A1, adrenodoxin reductase, or adrenodoxin genes.[806, 807, 809] Because side-chain cleavage of cholesterol in the primate is essential for the placental synthesis of progesterone and therefore the maintenance of pregnancy, mutations in the gene encoding the CYP11A1 enzyme may be incompatible with sustained human pregnancy.

The transfer of cholesterol from the outer to the inner mitochondrial membrane is the rate-limiting step in acute or rapid steroid synthesis.[816, 817] A 30-kd mitochondrial protein in adrenal cells rapidly increases in response to corticotropin stimulation and is inhibited by cyclohexamide; it is also present in the gonads.[818–821] The cDNA for this factor has been cloned, and the protein transcript for this gene was named the *st*eroidogenic *a*cute *r*egulatory (StAR) protein.[818, 819] As with other steroid hormone hydroxylases, the StAR gene is transcriptionally regulated by SF1.[821] The stimulation of StAR by corticotropin and by LH is mediated through a cAMP/protein kinase A–dependent pathway and involves the phosphorylation of the StAR protein.[821] The stimulation of cholesterol transport by StAR from the outer to the inner mitochondrial membrane, the site of the cholesterol side-chain cleavage complex, apparently does not require the import of StAR across the mitochondrial membrane.[822] Human StAR is encoded by a gene on chromosome 8p11.2 and is expressed in the adrenal gland and gonad, but not in the placenta or the central nervous system.[811, 819, 820, 821, 823, 824] Fifteen patients with congenital lipoid adrenal hyperplasia (studied from 10 coun-

tries) have been found to have mutations in the gene encoding StAR (Fig. 29–60).[800] In 80% of affected alleles from affected Japanese and Korean individuals, a Gln258Stop mutation was detected, whereas an Arg182Leu mutation was present in 78% of alleles from affected Arabs.[800] Study of congenital lipoid adrenal hyperplasia provided the decisive evidence of the critical role of StAR in steroid hormone biosynthesis in humans. Unlike *CYP11A1,* the gene encoding the StAR protein is not expressed in the human placenta, and mutations in StAR do not impair progesterone synthesis by the placenta.

In patients with StAR deficiency, little or no C_{18}-, C_{19}-, and C_{21}-steroids are detectable in plasma or urine, even after corticotropin stimulation. In 46,XX females the differential diagnosis includes congenital adrenal hypoplasia. Demonstration of greatly enlarged adrenals in StAR deficiency by imaging techniques readily differentiates these two entities. Affected males are raised as females, and their functionless testes are removed to reduce the risk of malignant transformation and for cosmetic reasons. Therapy requires replacement with glucocorticoids and mineralocorticoids and the addition of estrogen when gonadal failure ensues.

In obligate heterozygotes with a StAR mutation, unlike heterozygotes with other forms of CAH, steroid responses to corticotropin are normal.[810] Prenatal diagnosis of StAR deficiency was successfully demonstrated in a family with two previously affected children.[810] Amniotic fluid levels of progesterone and pregnenolone were 30% and 50% of normal, respectively, but the concentrations of steroids such as 17-

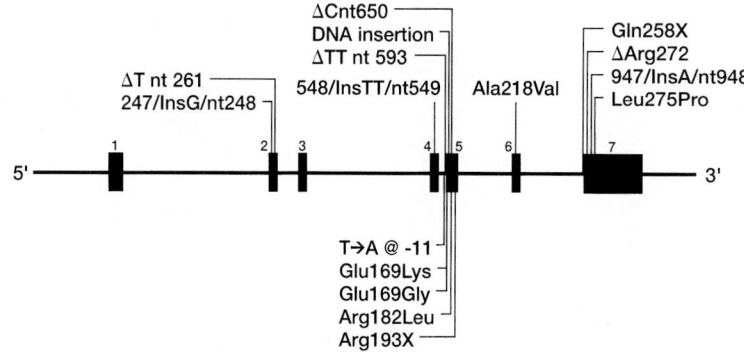

Figure 29–60. Diagrammatic representation of the mutations identified in the StAR gene associated with congenital lipoid adrenal hyperplasia. Nucleotide (nt) and amino acid numbers are given according to the cDNA sequence. Missense mutations causing amino acid substitutions are indicated by the three-letter abbreviation for the wild-type amino acid, followed by the amino acid number in the protein and the three-letter abbreviation for the substituted amino acid. X indicates a nonsense (stop) mutation. 247/InsG/nt248 is an insertion of a guanine causing a frameshift between nucleotides 247 and 248. ΔT nt261 is a deletion of a thymidine at nucleotide 261. 548/InsTT/nt549 is an insertion of two thymidines in exon 4 between nucleotides 548 and 549, causing a frameshift. ΔTT nt 593 is a deletion of two thymidines at nucleotide 593, causing a frameshift. ΔCnt650 is a deletion of a cytosine at nucleotide 650, causing a frameshift. T→A @ −11 is a thymidine-to-adenine transition minus 11 nucleotides (5′) from the intron 4/exon 5 junction. 947/InsA/nt948 is the insertion of an adenine between nucleotides 947 and 948, which results in a frameshift. (Data from Bose H, Sugawara T, Stauss JF, Miller WL. The pathophysiology and genetics of congenital lipoid adrenal hyperplasia. N Engl J Med 1996; 335:1870–1878.)

hydroxyprogesterone, cortisol, DHEA, androstenedione, and estradiol were low or undetectable.[810] Absent fetal steroidogenesis and subsequent failure to synthesize fetal adrenal precursors for transformation to estrogens by the placenta result in low maternal plasma and urine estriol values.

The clinical manifestations of each form of CAH are summarized in Table 29–21.

Placental Aromatase Deficiency

Aromatase (CYP19, cytochrome P450$_{arom}$, formerly estrogen synthetase) catalyzes the conversion of testosterone to estradiol and androstenedione to estrone in many tissues, including the gonads, placenta, brain, liver, and adipose tissue.[825] Placental aromatase deficiency causes female pseudohermaphroditism. Only one CYP19 gene has been isolated; its tissue-specific expression is mediated by tissue-specific promoters using alternative promoter choice, but the protein translated is the same in all tissues.[825]

Description of female pseudohermaphroditism occurring in five 46,XX females as a result of autosomal recessive inheritance of mutations in the CYP19 gene illustrates the critical role that this enzyme plays in protecting the fetus from excess androgen exposure in utero.[728, 729, 826–830] The placenta lacks CYP17 enzymatic activity and thus cannot convert C$_{21}$-steroids such as progesterone to C$_{19}$-steroids and thereafter to estrogens.[831] During gestation, large quantities of DHEAS are produced in the fetal adrenal gland and by the maternal adrenal.

DHEAS is 16α-hydroxylated in the fetal adrenal and liver. 16α-Hydroxy-DHEAS from the fetus and DHEAS from the fetus and mother are transferred to the placental unit, where the sulfate moiety is cleaved by placental sulfatase. These steroids can then be converted to androstenedione and 16α-hydroxyandrostenedione by 3β-HSD/Δ$^{4, 5}$-isomerase, to testosterone and 16α-hydroxytestosterone by 17β-HSD and to estrogens (mainly estriol from 16α-hydroxy-DHEA) by placental aromatase (Fig. 29–61). Androstenedione and 16α-hydroxyandrostenedione may be directly aromatized to estrogens.[832] In the absence of aromatase, estrogen cannot be synthesized by the placenta, and large quantities of placental testosterone and androstenedione are transferred to the fetal and maternal circulation, resulting in masculinization of the urogenital sinus and of the genital tubercle of the female fetus and virilization of the mother during pregnancy. Putative CYP19 deficiency has been described in the spotted hyena, which provides an explanation for the strikingly masculinized external genitalia and aggressive behavior of the female spotted hyena.[729, 833]

Affected females are born with clitoromegaly, varying degrees of posterior fusion, scrotalization of the labioscrotal folds, and, in some infants with a urogenital sinus, a single perineal orifice (Table 29–22). Müllerian structures are normal.[728, 729, 828, 829, 830] During infancy, basal and LHRH-induced FSH and LH are elevated.[824] The histology of the ovaries in infancy is normal, but under increased FSH stimulation in the absence of ovarian CYP19, multiple enlarged follicular cysts develop. At puberty affected females have hypergonadotropic

TABLE 29–21. Clinical Manifestations of Various Types of Congenital Adrenal Hyperplasia

Type	Type VI		Type IV		Type V		Type III		Types II and I	
Gene	StAR‡		HSD3B2		CYP17		CYP11B1		CYP21	
Enzymatic defect			3β-HSD II		P-450$_{c17}$		P-450$_{c11}$		P-450$_{c21}$	
	(no defect)				(17α-Hydroxylase)		(11β-Hydroxylase)		(21α-Hydroxylase)	
Chromosomal sex	XX	XY	XX	XY	XX	XY	XX	XY	XX	XY
External genitalia	Female	Female	Female (clitorimegaly)	Ambiguous	Female	Female or ambiguous	Ambiguous	Male	Ambiguous	Male
Postnatal virilization	−*	−†	±	Mild to moderate	−	+	+		+	
Addisonian crises	+		±		−		−		+ in 80% (type II)	
Hypertension	−		−		+		±		−	

*At puberty, female secondary sex characteristics develop, followed by ovarian failure.
†Sexual infantilism at puberty.
‡StAR mutations impair transport of cholesterol to the inner mitochondrial membrane and thus by substrate deprivation impair steroid biogenesis; the disorder leads as well to storage of lipid in the cells of the adrenal and gonad—congenital lipoid adrenal hyperplasia.

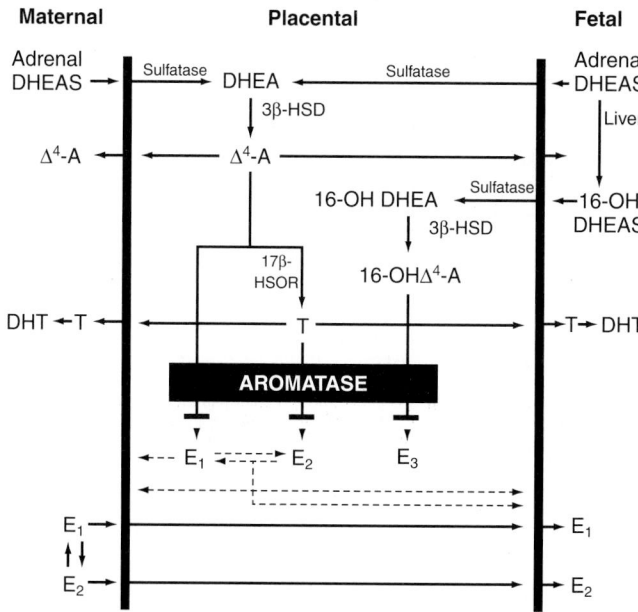

Figure 29–61. The biosynthetic defects in converting C_{19}-steroids (androgens, androgen precursors) to C_{18}-steroids (estrogens) in the CYP19 (P450$_{arom}$)–deficient fetal placental unit. 3β-HSD, 3β-hydroxysteroid dehydrogenase/$\Delta^{4, 5}$ isomerase; 17β-HSD, 17β-hydroxysteroid dehydrogenase; DHEA, dehydroepiandrosterone; DHEAS, DHEA sulfate; DHT, dihydrotestosterone; T, testosterone; Δ^4-A, androstenedione; E_1, estrone; E_2, estradiol; E_3, estriol. (Modified and redrawn from Conte FA, Grumbach MM, Ito Y, Fisher CR, Simpson ER. A syndrome of female pseudohermaphrodism, hypergonadotropic hypogonadism, and multicystic ovaries associated with missense mutations in the gene encoding aromatase (P450$_{arom}$). J Clin Endocrinol Metab 1994; 78:1287–1292. © 1994, The Endocrine Society.)

hypogonadism, fail to develop female secondary sexual characteristics, and exhibit progressive virilization.[728, 729, 828] Plasma androstenedione and testosterone are elevated, and estrone and estradiol levels are low or unmeasurable.[728, 729, 828] The ovaries enlarge and develop multiple cysts at puberty; in one affected female, polycystic ovaries were detected in infancy. The hypergonadotropism and the multiple ovarian cysts respond to estrogen replacement therapy.

All three postpubertal patients had tall stature, delayed bone maturation and epiphyseal fusion, and osteopenia, suggesting that estrogens are essential for the prevention of osteoporosis in males and females and for normal skeletal maturation and proportion (but not for linear growth in men).[728, 729, 828]

TABLE 29–22. Clinical Features of CYP19 Deficiency in the Female

Karyotype:	46,XX
Inheritance:	Autosomal recessive
Maternal history:	Virilization of mother during pregnancy (usually)
Genitalia:	Ambiguous or female with clitorimegaly
Wolffian duct derivatives:	Absent
Müllerian duct derivatives:	Present
Gonads:	Ovaries: multicystic in infancy and postpubertally
Habitus:	Tall stature and virilization at puberty
	Severe estrogen deficiency with increased plasma gonadotropins in infancy and at puberty
	Polycystic ovaries
	Increased plasma androstenedione and testosterone
	Delayed bone age; osteoporosis
	Normal psychosocial orientation
	Response to estrogen therapy

The affected adult man had normal sex differentiation and pubertal maturation with macro-orchidism and elevated concentrations of FSH, LH, and testosterone in plasma.[728] He also had osteoporosis, hyperinsulinemia, and abnormal plasma lipids, similar to the findings in a tall man with a null mutation in the estrogen receptor.[727] These observations suggest that estrogens as well as testosterone and inhibin play a role in the regulation of gonadotropin secretion in males and females and that estrogen deficiency in males can be associated with insulin resistance and hyperinsulinemia and an abnormal plasma lipid profile.[728, 729]

The finding of apparently normal psychosexual development in the three aromatase-deficient adolescent or adult patients and in the man with an estrogen receptor defect suggests that estrogen does not play a critical role in sex differentiation of the human brain, as has been reported in nonprimate mammals.[728, 834, 835] The detection of severe defects in critical regions of the gene encoding CYP19 that lead to generalized aromatase deficiency is strong evidence that survival of the conceptus can occur in the absence of estrogen synthesis by the implanting blastocyst, the fetus, and the fetal compartment of the placenta.[728, 828]

Analysis of the CYP19 gene in the six affected individuals has revealed seven different mutations (Fig. 29–62). The patient of Shozu and colleagues was homozygous for a point mutation (GT→GC) in the consensus 5′-splice acceptor sequence in the gene.[836] This mutation resulted in a CYP19 protein with a 29-amino-acid insert and less than 0.3% of normal enzyme activity.[836] A second patient was a compound heterozygote with two missense mutations.[827] Assay of the expressed mutated proteins showed that one allele had 1.1% of the activity of the wild-type CYP19, whereas the other had no activity.[827] The male and female siblings reported by Morishima and associates were both homozygous for a single base change that resulted in an amino acid substitution.[728] Expression of this mutant cDNA showed that it had 0.2% of the wild-type aromatase activity. The patient of Mullis and co-workers had a cytosine deletion in one allele (codon 408, proline) which corresponds to the consensus aromatic region of the enzyme.[829] This mutation results in a frameshift causing a stop codon 37 amino acids downstream.[829] The other allele, inherited from the father, had a guanine-to-thymidine (G→T) transversion at the splice junction between exon 3 and intron 3.[829] Both mutations resulted in a complete lack of enzymatic activity.[829] Another patient described from France had a homozygous mutation that resulted in a stop codon (Arg457X) in exon 10 of the CYP19 gene.[830] As in other patients, this mutation occurs in the critical heme-binding region of the aromatase enzyme.[728, 729, 825]

The diagnosis of CYP19 deficiency should be suspected in female pseudohermaphrodites in whom CAH has been excluded. The presence of elevated concentrations of androstenedione and testosterone of gonadal origin and elevated plasma gonadotropin levels can be observed even in infancy. Prenatal diagnosis of CYP19 deficiency is possible. Signs of an affected fetus include unexplained maternal virilization during pregnancy, which was observed in four of the five pregnancies with affected infants, and the detection of increased maternal levels of Δ^4-androstenedione, testosterone, and DHT and low levels of plasma estriol and urinary estriol. The absence of maternal virilization in the patient reported by the authors may result from the fact that this patient, unlike the others reported, had 1.1% activity of Arg435Cys mutation, which may have allowed for some degree of aromatization in the placenta during gestation and therefore lower levels of maternal androgens.[829] Amniotic fluid concentrations of androstenedione and testosterone are high, and those of estrone, estradiol, and estriol are low.

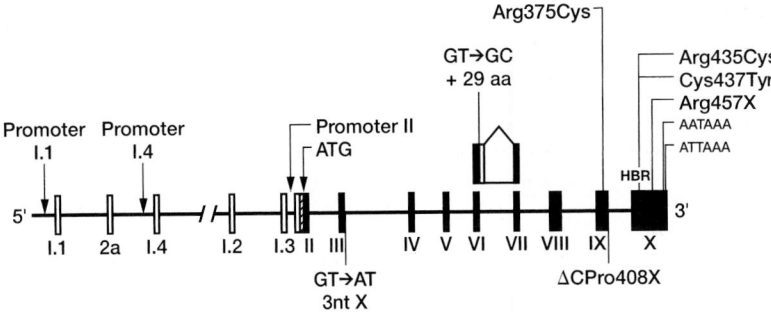

Figure 29–62. Diagrammatic representation of the *CYP19* (P450$_{arom}$) gene and the mutations causing aromatase deficiency. The numbered black boxes represent translated exons. The septum in the open box in exon II represents the 3' acceptor splice junction for the untranslated exons. The multiple alternate promotors and the untranslated exons (open boxes) are indicated. Missense mutations causing amino acid substitutions in the enzyme are indicated by the three-letter abbreviation for the wild-type amino acid, followed by the amino acid number in the enzyme and the three-letter abbreviation for the substituted amino acid. X indicates a nonsense (stop) mutation. GT→AT 3nt X is a guanine-to-adenine transition at the splice junction between exon 3 and intron 3, resulting in a stop codon (X) three nucleotides downstream (3'). GT→GC +29 aa is a thymidine-to-cytosine transition at the splice junction between exon 6 and intron 6, giving rise to a 29-amino-acid insert in the protein. ΔCPro408X, a deletion of a cytosine occurring in codon 408 (proline), results in a frameshift and a stop codon 111 nucleotides (37 amino acids) downstream (3'). HBR, heme-binding region. (Modified from Morishima A, Grumbach MM, Simpson ER, Fisher C, Qin K. Aromatase deficiency in male and female siblings caused by a novel mutation and the physiological role of estrogens. J Clin Endocrinol Metab 1995; 80:3689–3698. © 1995, The Endocrine Society.)

Maternal Androgens and Progestagens

Masculinization of the external genitalia of female infants has been observed after maternal ingestion of testosterone or synthetic progestational agents during the first trimester of pregnancy[837–841] (see Fig. 29–55). If the exposure occurs after the 12th week of gestation, the labioscrotal folds do not fuse, although the clitoris may enlarge.[843] Severe masculinization of the external genitalia of a female fetus may be caused, for example, by methyltestosterone in dosages as low as 3 mg daily, even though androgenic effects are not noticeable in the mother.[243]

Because progesterone itself is only slightly active when administered orally, various synthetic derivatives that may be taken by mouth were prescribed in the past for women with habitual or threatened abortion. Most of these progestagens are 19-nortestosterone derivatives; they are intrinsically androgenic to some degree and can cause virilization of female fetuses in experimental animals. Principal among the offenders have been norethindrone and ethisterone and, less commonly, norethynodrel and the C$_{21}$-steroid medroxyprogesterone acetate.[839] Ishizuka and co-workers[841] reported some degree of masculinization of the external genitalia in 2.75% of female infants whose mothers received synthetic progestagens of various types during pregnancy. This consequence of synthetic progestagen administration to the pregnant female is dose and time dependent.

Danazol, the 2,3-D-isoxazole derivative of 17α-ethinyltestosterone, a progestagen, is used for the treatment of endometriosis. Danazol crosses the placenta and can cause virilization of the external genitalia of the fetus in a manner similar to other androgenic compounds.[842] Several instances of female pseudohermaphroditism are believed to be the consequence of maternal ingestion of danazol.[842–844]

In four cases of female pseudohermaphroditism, the mothers received only stilbestrol in large doses.[845] The mechanism of masculinization is unknown but may be related to inhibition of 3β-HSD by stilbestrol or its metabolites.

Masculinization of the female fetus occurs on occasion if the mother has a virilizing ovarian tumor (usually arrhenoblastoma or Krukenberg's tumor) or adrenal tumor, a virilizing form of CAH, or virilization of some other cause during pregnancy.[838, 840, 843–849] Luteoma of pregnancy, an ovarian pseudotumor composed of hyperplastic luteinized thecal cells that regress after delivery, has been associated with masculinization of the external genitalia of female infants, especially in the presence of maternal virilization.[850, 851] Ovarian lutein cysts in pregnancy (hyperreactio luteinalis), considered by some to be

a cystic form of luteoma, are less frequently associated with maternal virilization and only rarely with fetal masculinization.[852, 853] Placental aromatization of androgens such as testosterone and androstenedione protects the mother and the female fetus from virilization[729, 828, 852, 853] unless the placental CYP19 activity is insufficient for the androgen steroid load or unless the androgen is not a substrate for CYP19.

Some of the rare cases of female pseudohermaphroditism of undetermined origin may have resulted from a luteoma of pregnancy that regressed spontaneously after delivery or an undiagnosed placental aromatase deficiency.[728, 828] In these patients a history of maternal ingestion of androgenic steroids is lacking and the postpartum course of the mother is inconsistent with a virilizing neoplasm, but the clinical features are most compatible with fetal exposure to androgens. The absence of virilism in the mother does not exclude a maternal source of androgen in these children, because the amounts of androgen required to masculinize the external genitalia of a female fetus may be less than those required to cause overt manifestations in the mother.

Female pseudohermaphroditism caused by the transfer of androgenic steroids from the mother to the fetus is the most easily treated of all types of ambisexual development. No hormone therapy is necessary, postnatal virilism does not occur, and female secondary sexual characteristics can be expected to emerge at the usual age of adolescence. Surgical correction of the external genitalia, if deemed necessary for cosmetic and psychological indications, restores feminine appearance and permits normal sexual function.

Malformations of the Intestine and the Urinary Tract (Non–Androgen-Induced Female Pseudohermaphroditism)

Genital abnormalities are frequently associated with imperforate anus, renal agenesis or dysplasia, and other congenital malformations of the lower intestine and urinary tract.[854–857] Carpentier and Potter reviewed the findings in such infants and suggested the term "nonspecific female pseudohermaphroditism."[856] Some, but not all, of these anomalies are incompatible with life. Renal failure, often accompanied by pyelonephritis, is common and may confuse the clinical picture with that of adrenal insufficiency. In contrast to other forms of female pseudohermaphroditism, the female müllerian derivatives may also be malformed. The findings in these patients may be bizarre; persistence of a primitive cloaca, imperforate anus, and fistulae are not infrequent. The pathogenesis of these anomalies is different from that of other types of ambisexual development and should be considered in the context of other forms of developmental field defects. Familial occurrence of nonadrenal female pseudohermaphroditism with multiple anomalies has been reported.[840]

Male Pseudohermaphroditism

Male pseudohermaphroditism is a heterogeneous condition in which the gonads are exclusively testes but the genital ducts and/or external genitalia are incompletely masculinized. The clinical spectrum varies from individuals with female external genitalia to those with mild impairment of masculinization of the external genitalia, as represented by hypospadias, cryptorchidism, and minimal ambiguity of the external genitalia.

With the advances in the knowledge of pathogenesis, systems of nomenclature based on phenotype have become less important. There are at least six major etiologic categories of male pseudohermaphroditism, with many subtypes, all of which are associated with incomplete masculinization of the fetal genital tract and/or incomplete regression of the müllerian ducts.

In this section, forms of male pseudohermaphroditism in 46,XY individuals with relatively normal embryonic differentiation of the testes are discussed. In such patients, defective male development must be ascribed to a more specific failure of the fetal testes to overcome the inherent tendency toward feminization of the somatic sex structures. This failure may stem either from a secretory failure of the testes during the critical period of sex differentiation or from a failure of target tissues to respond normally to androgen stimulation or to AMH. Table 29–23 reflects an attempt to classify the many forms of male pseudohermaphroditism on the basis of cause, insofar as that is known.

The ability of the testes to virilize at adolescence is in many ways a recapitulation of their capacity to masculinize the external genitalia in utero. The greater the development of the phallus in an infant, the greater likelihood that male secondary sexual characteristics will emerge at the time of expected puberty. Individuals with ambiguous genitalia may remain eunuchoid, exhibit mild virilism, or develop breast enlargement and other female secondary sexual characteristics. Those with an external female phenotype usually either feminize or remain sexually infantile. These are only approximate guides, however, and the development of male sexual characteristics at adolescence may occur, especially in patients with partial androgen resistance, 17β-hydroxysteroid dehydrogenase-3 deficiency, or 5α-reductase-2 deficiency.

Male pseudohermaphroditism can result from (1) testicular unresponsiveness to hCG and LH and consequent Leydig cell aplasia or hypoplasia; (2) a specific enzyme defect in testosterone biosynthesis; (3) familial end-organ resistance to androgen caused by abnormalities in the cytosolic receptor for testosterone and DHT or by an enzyme defect in the intracellular metabolism of testosterone; (4) aberrations in testicular organogenesis (dysgenetic male pseudohermaphroditism); (5) defective synthesis, secretion, or response to AMH; (6) administration of progestagens during pregnancy; and (7) environmental exposures. Apart from dysgenetic male pseudohermaphroditism and the persistent müllerian duct syndrome, all other forms of male pseudohermaphroditism are characterized by the absence of müllerian duct derivatives. Except for some variants of dysgenetic male pseudohermaphroditism and the maternal ingestion of progestagens, all forms of male pseudohermaphroditism are familial and characterized by genetic heterogeneity. No doubt many subtypes will be defined and characterized by molecular, genetic, and biochemical techniques. Although dysgenetic male pseudohermaphrodit-

TABLE 29–23. Male Pseudohermaphroditism

A. Testicular unresponsiveness to hCG and LH (Leydig cell agenesis or hypoplasia due to hCG/LH receptor defect)
B. Inborn errors of testosterone biosynthesis
   1. Enzyme deficits affecting synthesis of both corticosteroids and testosterone (variants of congenital adrenal hyperplasia)
      a. StAR deficiency (congenital lipoid adrenal hyperplasia)
      b. 3β-Hydroxysteroid dehydrogenase/Δ⁵-isomerase type II (3β-HSD II) deficiency
      c. P450$_{c17}$ (CYP17[17α-hydroxylase/17,20 lyase]) deficiency
   2. Enzyme defects primarily affecting testosterone biosynthesis by the testes
      a. P450$_{c17}$ (CYP17[17,20 lyase]) deficiency
      b. 17β-hydroxysteroid dehydrogenase type 3 (17-HSD 3) deficiency
C. Defects in androgen-dependent target tissues
   1. End-organ resistance to androgenic hormones
      a. Syndrome of complete androgen resistance and its variants (testicular feminization and its variant forms)
      b. Syndrome of incomplete androgen resistance and its variants (Reifenstein's syndrome)
      c. Androgen resistance in phenotypically normal males
   2. Defects in testosterone metabolism by peripheral tissues; steroid 5α-reductase-2 deficiency (pseudovaginal perineoscrotal hypospadias) (SRD5A2)
D. Dysgenetic male pseudohermaphroditism
   1. XY gonadal dysgenesis (incomplete)
   2. XO/XY mosaicism, structurally abnormal Y chromosome, Xp+, 9p−, 10q−
   3. Denys-Drash syndrome (WT1 mutation)
   4. WAGR syndrome (WT1 deletion)
   5. Campomelic dysplasia (SOX9 mutation)
   6. ? SF1 mutation
   7. Testicular regression syndrome
E. Defects in synthesis, secretion, or response to antimüllerian hormone duct inhibitory factor: persistent müllerian duct syndrome (female genital ducts in otherwise normal men; herniae uteri inguinale)
F. Maternal ingestion of progestagens and estrogens
G. ? Environmental chemicals

Unclassified Forms of Abnormal Sexual Development

A. In males
   1. Hypospadias
   2. Ambiguous external genitalia in XY males with multiple congenital anomalies
B. In females, absence or anomalous development of the vagina, uterus, and uterine tubes (Rokitansky-Küster syndrome)

---

ism—the group of disorders associated with defective organogenesis of the testes—has already been discussed, it is included under male pseudohermaphroditism because this category of intersexuality must be considered by the clinician in the differential diagnosis of male pseudohermaphroditism. In Table 29–4 and Fig. 29–15 genes implicated in sex determination (gonadogenesis) are shown; Table 29–18 lists genes involved in sex differentiation.

Testicular Unresponsiveness to hCG and LH, LH/hCG Resistance (Leydig Cell Agenesis or Hypoplasia)

The production of testosterone by fetal Leydig cells is critical to male sexual differentiation of the wolffian ducts and the external genitalia. Leydig cell unresponsiveness to hCG-LH can result in male pseudohermaphroditism (Fig. 29–63) with Leydig cell agenesis or hypoplasia[858–870] (Table 29–24).

Phenotypically, the external genitalia vary, from those of a normal-appearing female to those of a male with microphallus and hypoplastic external genitalia.[867, 869] Müllerian derivatives are absent in all patients; wolffian derivatives have been present in some of the most severely affected patients despite the presence of female external genitalia.[859, 860] Basal FSH and LH concentrations and LHRH-evoked responses are elevated in postpubertal patients.[867] Plasma levels of 17-hydroxyprogesterone, androstenedione, and testosterone are low, and stimulation with hCG elicits little or no increase. Plasma LH levels decrease after testosterone administration.[861]

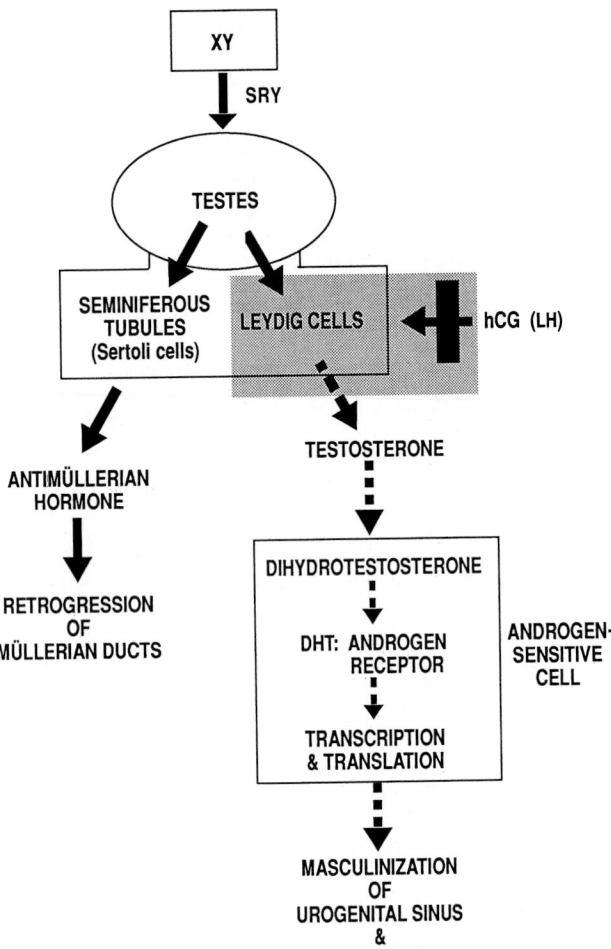

Figure 29–63. hCG/LH resistance. A diagrammatic scheme of male sex determination and differentiation showing a defect in the hCG/LH receptor that causes Leydig cell unresponsiveness to hCG (LH) and results in male pseudohermaphroditism. Solid bar delineates defect, and stippled area designates general site of defect. Interrupted lines indicate that subsequent processes may be completely or partially affected.

On histologic examination, the testes lack distinct Leydig cells in prepubertal patients. Postpubertal patients have absent or decreased numbers of Leydig cells without Reinke's crystalloids, normal-appearing Sertoli cells, and seminiferous tubules with spermatogenic arrest.[859–861, 868] In five patients in whom the LH receptor was studied, there was absent or diminished binding of labeled hCG and LH to Leydig cells.[862, 863] Familial studies are consistent with autosomal recessive trans-

TABLE 29–24. Clinical Features of Testicular Unresponsiveness to hCG/LH (Leydig Cell Aplasia or Hypoplasia)

Karyotype:	46,XY
Inheritance:	Familial; mutations in the LH/hCG receptor gene
Genitalia:	Female → ambiguous male → hypoplastic male
Wolffian duct derivatives:	Absent → hypoplastic
Müllerian duct derivatives:	Absent
Gonads:	Small undescended testes with absent or decreased number of Leydig cells
Habitus:	Lack of or poor virilization at puberty
Hormone profile:	Increased gonadotropins postpubertally, decreased testosterone levels with decreased or absent response to hCG stimulation, decreased or normal binding of hCG/LH by Leydig cell depending on mutation

mission.[868] The counterpart to this disorder described in the rat is termed the vestigial testis syndrome and is apparently caused by an LH-receptor defect.[871]

Kremer and associates studied two 46,XY siblings who had female external genitalia and hypergonadotropic hypogonadism.[872] Plasma levels of testosterone and its precursors were low, and hCG elicited no response.[872] Leydig cells were sparse in the testes. Both siblings had a homozygous missense mutation, Ala593Pro, in the sixth transmembrane domain of the gene encoding the LH receptor (Fig. 29–64). In vitro, this mutated receptor binds hCG normally but does not evoke an increase in cAMP or testosterone synthesis.[872] A sibship reported by Latronico and colleagues contained four affected individuals, three 46,XY females with Leydig cell hypoplasia and hypergonadotropic hypogonadism and a sexually mature 46,XX female with elevated plasma LH levels and amenorrhea.[873] All four siblings were homozygous for an Arg554Stop (null) mutation within the third cytosolic loop of the LH receptor, which resulted in a truncated receptor protein incapable of transducing the LH signal.[873] A 6-year-old 46,XY male with a micropenis, descended testes, and no testosterone response to the administration of hCG had a homozygous mutation (Ser616Tyr) in the seventh transmembrane domain of the LH receptor gene.[873] The mutant receptor did not bind hCG.[873] Homozygous mutations in eight 46,XY males analyzed resulted in fetal and postnatal testosterone deficiency, in female external genitalia or a micropenis, and in hypergonadotropic hypogonadism.[873] Laue and colleagues described a nonsense mutation in exon 11 of the LH receptor in one allele in two 46,XY females with Leydig cell hypoplasia and LH/hCG resistance.[874] This mutation, Cys545X, truncated the LH receptor in the fifth transmembrane loop, which led to decreased LH-binding activity. Since the father of the 46,XY female was found to have the mutation, it was presumed that these patients were compound heterozygotes and that another as yet unidentified mutation existed in the second allele.[874] Null mutations of the LH receptor in 46,XX females do not prevent normal development of female secondary sexual characteristics at puberty, but affected women have high plasma concentrations of LH, normal FSH levels, and amenorrhea.[873]

In patients with testicular unresponsiveness to hCG-LH, fetal testosterone deficiency impairs masculinization of the external genitalia, but müllerian duct regression is complete because the secretion of AMH by the fetal Sertoli cells is intact. Of interest is the paradoxical finding of wolffian derivatives, which are testosterone dependent, in some patients with minimal masculinization of the external genitalia (only posterior labial fusion). One explanation, supported by the variation in masculinization of the external genitalia, is that the defect in the hCG-LH receptor is of variable severity. A second possibility is that during the early fetal period, sufficient testosterone may have been secreted locally, possibly autonomously,[199] and independently of circulating hCG, to induce male duct development, but the concentration of testosterone in the fetal circulation was too low to evoke normal male differentiation of the external genitalia and urogenital sinus. hCG is necessary to sustain Leydig cell differentiation and growth and testosterone secretion by the fetal testes, at least by about the 10th week of gestation, but, as discussed previously, it may not be essential for initiation of these functions at week 8. Variation in the magnitude of hCG-LH resistance of the undifferentiated embryonic and fetal Leydig cells would result in variable degrees of fetal testosterone deficiency and thus a variable degree of failure to develop normal male external genitalia.

Therapy depends on the age at diagnosis and the degree of virilization. In the severe form of testicular unresponsiveness to hCG/LH with female external genitalia, sex assignment is usually female. The gonads are removed, and estrogen

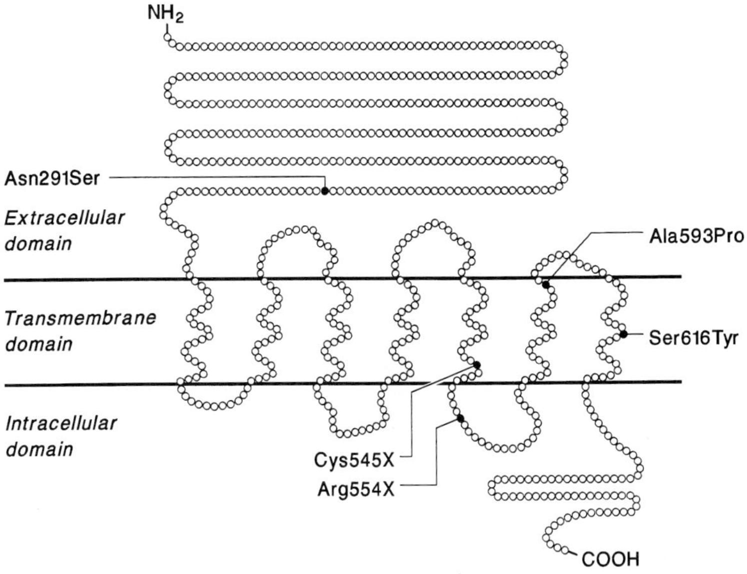

NH$_2$

Asn291Ser

Extracellular domain

Ala593Pro

Transmembrane domain

Ser616Tyr

Intracellular domain

Cys545X

Arg554X

COOH

Figure 29–64. Diagrammatic representation of the LH/hCG receptor with its seven transmembrane alpha helices and the mutations that can cause male pseudohermaphroditism. The open circles represent the amino acid residues on the LH/hCG receptor protein. The solid circles indicate the amino acid substitutions in patients with male pseudohermaphroditism. The mutations are indicated by the three-letter abbreviation of the wild-type amino acid, followed by the position number of the amino acid in the protein and the three-letter abbreviation for the substituted amino acid or the letter X, which indicates a nonsense (stop) mutation leading to an inactive, truncated receptor.

replacement therapy is instituted at the time of expected puberty. In the less extreme forms with predominantly male external genitalia, testosterone therapy augments phallic development and virilizes the patient at puberty.

In the human male fetus, deficient fetal pituitary gonadotropin secretion associated with anencephaly, hypothalamic hypopituitarism, and isolated gonadotropin deficiency (including Kallmann's syndrome) is not associated with ambiguous external genitalia (with one possible exception[875]), although undescended testes, hypoplasia of the scrotum, and microphallus are common. These clinical observations are consistent with the important role of hCG in testosterone secretion by the human fetal testis during the critical period of male sex differentiation; fetal pituitary FSH and LH are not required for normal differentiation of testes or male external genitalia but do play a role in their growth during the last half of gestation.

Enzyme Defects of Testosterone Biosynthesis Affecting Both Adrenal Steroid and Testosterone Biosynthesis (Variants of Congenital Adrenal Hyperplasia)

Defects in testosterone biosynthesis (Fig. 29–65) have been described, one at each of the enzymatic steps required for the conversion of cholesterol to testosterone[661–663] (Fig. 29–66). Two of the defects (3β-HSD and CYP17) involve enzymes, and the third, StAR, a protein that affects both glucocorticoid and gonadal steroid biosynthesis; these errors in steroid biosynthesis are discussed, in part, in the section on CAH.

StAR DEFICIENCY (CONGENITAL LIPOID ADRENAL HYPERPLASIA). Infants with this defect (Table 29–25; see previous discussion in the section on CAH) present with severe adrenal insufficiency and accumulation of lipid in the cells of both the adrenal cortex and the gonads. Affected males have female external genitalia with a blind vaginal pouch and hypoplastic male genital ducts but no uterus or fallopian tubes; the genitalia of affected females are normal. In males, the testes may be abdominal, inguinal, or in the labia. All reported patients are diffusely pigmented; glucocorticoid and mineralocorticoid insufficiency is severe; and adrenal crises in infancy can lead to death if untreated. However, three male pseudohermaphrodites survived the perinatal period without therapy and presented at 6 weeks, 12 weeks, and 8 months of age[801–803]

(see discussion of StAR and its mutations in the section on female pseudohermaphroditism). The patient reported by Hauffa and co-workers[802] (and in the previous editions of this chapter) is more than 30 years old and well maintained on glucocorticoid and mineralocorticoid replacement therapy. Sexual hair is absent unless small doses of testosterone are given; female secondary sexual characteristics are induced by estrogen replacement. As described in the section on CAH, no secondary sexual characteristics (either male or female) develop at the age of puberty in affected males, in contrast to females with this disorder.[800, 804] Pedigree analysis of families and DNA analysis of affected patients and parents indicate autosomal recessive transmission.[800] The male/female ratio in this disorder appears to be 3:1.[800, 803] The unusual ratio of affected patients is yet to be explained and may represent, at least in part, ascertainment bias. The molecular genetics of StAR deficiency is illustrated in Figure 29–60.

The diagnosis of StAR deficiency should be suspected in patients with male pseudohermaphroditism, including all phenotypic female infants with evidence of adrenal insufficiency. The diagnosis can be confirmed by documentation of low or absent mineralocorticoids, glucocorticoids, and gonadal steroids and their metabolites in plasma and urine and an absent steroid response to corticotropin and hCG administration. The adrenals are large and lipid laden and displace the kidneys caudad on CT or MRI scans. Therapy requires replacement doses of glucocorticoid and mineralocorticoid from the time of diagnosis. All affected 46,XY males have been reared as females. Estrogen replacement therapy to induce female sexual characteristics at puberty and low-dose testosterone treatment to elicit development of sexual hair are indicated; prophylactic orchidectomy is appropriate.

3β-HYDROXYSTEROID DEHYDROGENASE/Δ⁴,⁵-ISOMERASE TYPE II DEFICIENCY. This autosomal recessive disorder is a consequence of mutations in *HSD3B2*, the gene encoding the 3β-HSD/Δ^{4,5}-isomerase type II isozyme, which is expressed mainly in the adrenals and gonads. This enzyme catalyzes a crucial step in the biosynthesis of all steroid hormones, the conversion of Δ^5- to Δ^4-steroids. The type I isozyme is expressed predominantly in the placenta and in peripheral tissues (e.g., skin, breast), has 93% homology in structure with the type II isozyme, is about five times as active, and is closely linked to the type II isozyme (both are encoded by genes on chromosome 1p13).[757–763] The type I isozyme is not associated with CAH, and mutations in the coding region of type I are

TABLE 29–27. Clinical Features of CYP17 Mutations with Both 17α-Hydroxylase and 17,20-Lyase Deficiencies in 46,XY Males

Karyotype:	46,XY
Inheritance:	Autosomal recessive; CYP17 (P450$_{c17}$) gene mutations
Genitalia:	Female → ambiguous → hypospadiac male; blind vaginal pouch
Wolffian duct derivatives:	Absent → hypoplastic
Müllerian duct derivatives:	Absent
Gonads:	Testes
Habitus:	Absent or poor virilization at puberty, gynecomastia
Hormone and metabolic profile:	Decreased plasma testosterone; increased plasma LH and FSH levels; increased plasma deoxycorticosterone, corticosterone, and progesterone concentrations; decreased plasma renin activity Low renin hypertension with hypokalemic alkalosis

CYP17 (17α-HYDROXYLASE/17,20-LYASE) DEFICIENCY.
17α-Hydroxylase/17,20 lyase deficiency (due to mutations in a single gene, CYP17) is a defect that impairs both adrenal and gonadal steroidogenesis (Table 29–27; see previous discussion in the section on CAH). The phenotype of 46,XY males with 17α-hydroxylase deficiency varies from that of an individual with normal-appearing female external genitalia and a blind vaginal pouch to (rarely) that of a male with hypospadias and a small phallus.[775, 781, 784–787, 790, 793, 885, 886] The magnitude of the impaired masculinization in the male fetus correlates with the severity of the block in 17α-hydroxylation and the magnitude of the consequent impairment in fetal testosterone synthesis.[775, 787, 790, 793] A male with a homozygous deletion of the phenylalanine codon (TTC) at amino acids 53 or 54 of exon 1 of the CYP17 gene had mild hypospadias and cryptorchidism.[793] Analysis of the 17α-hydroxylase and 17,20-lyase activity of this mutant protein showed less than 23% and 5% activity, respectively, compared with the wild-type enzyme.[793] Hence, it appears that more than 25% of normal enzymatic activity is necessary for normal fetal masculinization of the external genitalia.[790, 793] The testes may be intra-abdominal, in the inguinal canal, or in the labioscrotal folds. Inguinal hernias are commonly present. In one affected 46,XY patient, no gonads were found at laparotomy.[887] Müllerian structures are absent, and wolffian derivatives are usually hypoplastic. Excessive secretion of DOC and corticosterone, the consequence of the failure of 17α-hydroxylation of the C$_{21}$-steroids, usually leads to hypertension, hypokalemia, and alkalosis. The adrenal zona fasciculata is the source of the increased plasma concentration of DOC, corticosterone, 18-hydroxy-DOC, and 18-hydroxycorticosterone.[795] Salt and water retention, volume expansion, and hypertension suppress renin and consequently aldosterone secretion in the classic form (although aldosterone concentrations are normal or elevated in some patients).[886] This process is reversible with cortisol therapy. Because gonadal steroid secretion is low, severely affected patients fail to develop secondary sexual characteristics, including pubic and axillary hair. Plasma and urinary FSH and LH levels are increased. One patient with a partial deficiency of 17α-hydroxylase activity developed prominent gynecomastia and incomplete male secondary sexual characteristics at the expected time of puberty.[888] As previously discussed in the section on CAH, mutations in the CYP17 gene (see Fig. 29–58) that are associated with less than 25% of normal 17α-hydroxylase activity in intact transfected cells result in female (complete deficiency) or ambiguous genitalia in affected 46,XY males, whereas activity equal to at least 25% of that of the normal enzyme is associated with normal male genitalia.[790, 793, 888]

The diagnosis of 17α-hydroxylase deficiency should be suspected in male pseudohermaphrodites, including 46,XY phenotypic females, who have hyporeninemic hypertension and hypokalemic alkalosis. Plasma concentrations of corticotropin, DOC, corticosterone, and progesterone are high, and those of aldosterone, 17-hydroxyprogesterone, cortisol, and gonadal steroids are low. Replacement therapy with physiological doses of glucocorticoids suppresses DOC and corticosterone secretion and causes return of serum potassium levels, blood pressure, and plasma renin and aldosterone levels to normal. At puberty, appropriate gonadal steroid replacement therapy is indicated, and gonadectomy should be performed in 46,XY patients who have been assigned a female sex of rearing.

Enzyme Defects Primarily Affecting Testosterone Biosynthesis by the Testes

CYP17 (ISOLATED 17,20-LYASE) DEFICIENCY (Table 29–28). The 17α-hydroxylation of pregnenolone and progesterone and the conversion of the C$_{21}$-steroids 17-hydroxypregnenolone and 17-hydroxyprogesterone to the C$_{19}$-steroids DHEA and androstenedione are mediated by a single microsomal enzyme encoded by the CYP17 gene located on chromosome 10q24-25.[773–778] In the adrenal gland, CYP17 catalyzes 17α-hydroxylation in the biosynthesis of glucocorticoids, and in both the adrenal and the gonad it catalyzes the 17α-hydroxylation of C$_{21}$-steroids and the subsequent conversion of 17-hydroxypregnenolone and 17-hydroxyprogesterone to the C$_{19}$-steroids DHEA and androstenedione (17,20-lyase activity). The Δ^5-17,20-lyase activity of CYP17 is much greater in the human than its Δ^4-17,20-lyase activity.[776] Little or no Δ^4-17,20-lyase activity can be demonstrated in the human testis or in cultured human theca cells.[776] The control of 17,20-lyase activity in the adrenal appears to be independent of that in the gonad; adrenal 17,20-lyase activity is age dependent, as illustrated by adrenarche. Data suggest that the ratio of 17α-hydroxylase to 17,20-lyase activity of the CYP17 enzyme is a function of the molar ratio of electron transfer (redox) partners.[889, 890] Increasing the amount of either NADPH–P450 reductase or cytochrome b$_5$ increases the activity of 17,20-lyase several fold.[889–891] Furthermore, the CYP17 enzyme undergoes post-translational modification through phosphorylation of serine and threonine residues by cAMP-dependent protein kinase A.[892] Phosphorylation of the enzyme increases 17,20-lyase activity, and dephosphorylation reduces or eliminates it.[890, 892] Both these mechanisms appear to play a role in control of 17,20-lyase activity in the adrenal and gonads.

There have been 14 case reports of putative isolated 17,20-lyase deficiency,[775, 790] despite the fact that one gene

TABLE 29–28. Clinical Features of CYP17 Mutations with Only 17,20-Lyase Deficiency in 46,XY Males

Karyotype:	46,XY
Inheritance:	Autosomal recessive—certain mutations in CYP17 (P450$_{c17}$) gene (Arg347His; Arg358Gln)
Genitalia:	Female → male with perineal hypospadias → hypoplastic male; blind vaginal pouch
Wolffian duct derivatives:	Rudimentary → normal
Müllerian duct derivatives:	Absent
Gonads:	Testes
Habitus:	Normal stature; sexual infantilism
Hormone profile:	Decreased plasma testosterone, androstenedione, dehydroepiandrosterone (DHEA), and estradiol concentrations; abnormal increase in plasma 17-hydroxyprogesterone and 17-hydroxypregnenolone and increased ratio of 17-hydroxy C$_{21}$-deoxysteroids to C$_{19}$-steroids (DHEA, Δ^4-androstenedione) after hCG stimulation test; plasma LH and FSH elevated

encodes a single enzyme with both 17α-hydroxylase and 17,20-lyase activities. Zachmann and colleagues[893] initially reported two first cousins with a familial form of male pseudohermaphroditism ascribed to a partial deficiency of 17,20-lyase in both the adrenals and testes. The patients had ambiguous genitalia, inguinal or intra-abdominal testes, and a 46,XY sex chromosome constitution. Both cousins had severe hypospadias with a male-type urethra and male duct development. Only urinary steroids were examined. A sample of testicular tissue from one cousin studied in vitro exhibited a defect in the conversion of C_{21}-steroids to testosterone (C_{19}-steroids). Subsequent studies of the cousins at ages 12 and 13 years disclosed a putative partial defect in the conversion of Δ^5- and Δ^4-C_{21}-steroids to C_{19}-steroids.[894] Analysis of the CYP gene in one cousin detected compound heterozygosity with two different mutant alleles. Transfection studies indicated combined 17α-hydroxylase and 17,20-lyase deficiencies despite the clinical findings.[895] Further study of the steroid pattern in this patient revealed that although 17α-hydroxylase activity had been normal in childhood and adolescence, it was decreased in adulthood.[894] Mendonca and coworkers described two male pseudohermaphrodites from consanguineous marriages with presumed isolated 17,20-lyase deficiency.[896] Both had 46,XY karyotypes, microphallus, perineal hypospadias, bifid scrotum, a blind vaginal pouch, and cryptorchidism.[896] Basal LH and FSH concentrations were elevated in the postpubertal case, and testosterone levels were low. The administration of hCG resulted in a marked rise in plasma 17-hydroxyprogesterone with a paucity of response in DHEA, androstenedione, and testosterone, consistent with isolated 17,20-lyase deficiency. Molecular modeling and site-directed mutagenesis indicated that the Arg347Ala mutation selectively ablates 17,20-lyase activity in the rat or human enzyme while leaving 17α-hydroxylase activation intact.[890, 897, 898] Analyses of CYP17 in these patients showed one to be homozygous for an Arg347His mutation and the other to have an Arg358Gln mutation (see Fig. 29–58).[899] These two mutations are located in the redox partner binding site of the CYP17 enzyme and therefore cause a decrease in 17,20-lyase activity by reducing electron transfer.[890] These are the first patients with "isolated" 17,20-lyase deficiency defined by molecular analyses and the first example of prediction of the specific location for a mutation by site-directed mutagenesis and modeling.[890, 899]

Depending on the degree of impairment in 17,20-lyase activity and its effect on fetal testosterone production during gestation, the external appearance may vary from female to ambiguous to hypoplastic male. The testes may be intra-abdominal, in the inguinal region, or in the scrotum. As with other defects in testosterone synthesis, wolffian duct derivatives are either hypoplastic or normal, depending on the severity of the testosterone deficiency, and müllerian duct derivatives are absent. In the 46,XX females, putative isolated 17,20-lyase deficiency leads to failure of pubertal development and elevated gonadotropin levels.[900]

The diagnosis of 17,20-lyase deficiency should be considered in male pseudohermaphrodites with absent müllerian derivatives and in 46,XX females who have no abnormality in glucocorticoid or mineralocorticoid synthesis but fail to develop secondary sexual characteristics at the expected time of puberty and have elevated concentrations of FSH and LH. In prepubertal male pseudohermaphrodites, 17,20-lyase deficiency must be distinguished from the partial form of androgen resistance, 5α-reductase-2 deficiency, and 17β-HSD type 3 deficiency.

In the prepubertal patient, both corticotropin and hCG stimulation may be useful in unmasking the defect. Prenatal diagnosis is possible by the measurement of amniotic fluid C_{21}- and C_{19}-steroids[901] and by DNA analysis. The age at diagnosis and the degree of masculinization of the external genitalia

are important determinants of the sex of rearing. Gonadal steroid replacement therapy usually is necessary in both sexes at puberty. Gonadectomy is recommended in 46,XY patients raised as females.

17β-HYDROXYSTEROID DEHYDROGENASE TYPE 3 DEFICIENCY. The 17β-HSD reaction is mediated by five known isozymes[902, 903] that catalyze the reduction of androstenedione, DHEA, and estrone to testosterone, Δ^5-androstenediol, and estradiol, respectively, as well as the reverse reaction. The type 1 (17β-HSD 1) isozyme is cytosolic, is expressed at highest levels in the ovary and placenta, and primarily interconverts estrone and estradiol[903, 904]; its gene is located on chromosome 17q21.[903, 905] A second gene, located on chromosome 16q24, encodes the 17β-HSD 2 isozyme,[903, 906] which is expressed in placental liver and endometrial microsomes and oxidizes (inactivates) both androgens and estrogens.[903, 907] The 17β-HSD 3 isozyme is a microsomal enzyme that utilizes NADPH as a cofactor[902, 903]; it is encoded by a gene on chromosome 9q22 that is 23% homologous to the genes for 17β-HSD 1 and 17β-HSD 2 and is expressed primarily in the testes, where it favors the reduction of androstenedione to testosterone.[902, 903] 17β-HSD 4 encodes a 17β-estradiol dehydrogenase and is expressed in multiple tissues.[902, 903, 908] 17β-HSD 5 is encoded by a gene on chromosome 10p14,15 and catalyzes the reduction reaction.[909]

Male pseudohermaphroditism caused by 17β-HSD deficiency (also called 17β-HYDROXYSTEROID OXIDOREDUCTASE or 17-KETOSTEROID REDUCTASE) was first reported by Saez and colleagues[910, 911] (Table 29–29). Many patients have been described, including a cohort of 68 subjects from a highly inbred population in the Gaza Strip.[912, 913] Except for a few 46,XY individuals with ambiguous genitalia at birth,[914–916] most affected 46,XY males have predominantly female external genitalia, testes (usually located in the inguinal canal), male wolffian duct derivatives (epididymes, vas deferens, seminal vesicles, and ejaculatory ducts), and a blind vaginal pouch.[902, 903, 916] Because of unambiguous female genitalia at birth, such individuals are usually assigned a female sex and raised as females. However, at the age of puberty, gonadotropin levels and plasma concentrations of androstenedione, estrone, and testosterone increase. The levels of testosterone in some cases approach the normal male range, and some virilization invariably ensues.[903, 916–919] In the patients described by Rösler from the Gaza Strip, the phallus, although bound down in chordee, reached lengths of 4 to 8 cm.[912, 913] Deepening of the voice, male body hair distribution, and increased muscle mass ensue. Gynecomastia is a variable most likely related to the severity of the enzymatic defect and the ratio of androgens to estrogens.[920] The latter are derived from the conversion of androstenedione by aromatase in extraglandular tissue and the action of the 17β-HSD 1 or 17β-HSD 2 isoen-

---

TABLE 29–29. Clinical Features of 17β-Hydroxysteroid Dehydrogenase Type 3 Deficiency in 46,XY Males

Karyotype:	46,XY
Inheritance:	Autosomal recessive; mutations in 17β-HSD 3 gene
Genitalia:	Female → ambiguous; blind vaginal pouch
Wolffian duct derivatives:	Hypoplastic
Müllerian duct derivatives:	Absent
Gonads:	Testes
Habitus:	Virilization at puberty (phallus enlargement, deepening of voice, and development of facial and body hair); gynecomastia variable
Hormone profile:	Increased plasma estrone and androstenedione; decreased ratio of plasma testosterone/androstenedione and estradiol/estrone after hCG stimulation test; increased plasma FSH and LH levels

zymes. The striking virilization at puberty is in sharp contrast to the impaired masculinization of the external genitalia in utero. Like patients with 5α-reductase-2 deficiency, some patients, especially those from the Gaza Strip, have changed their gender role from female to male at puberty.[912, 913, 919] Studies in the authors' patients and in others indicate that the principal source of plasma testosterone in patients with a severe defect in 17β-HSD 3 is extraglandular conversion rather than direct testicular secretion.[903, 921] In two patients studied in San Francisco, testicular vein sampling indicated that androstenedione levels were markedly increased, whereas testosterone secretion was estimated at 0.05 and 0.2 mg/day, as opposed to about 4 mg/day in adult males. Although 17β-HSD 3 activity appears to be completely deficient in infancy, a progressive rise occurs in plasma testosterone from puberty to adulthood.[922–924] This apparent "recovery" of 17β-HSD enzymatic activity is undoubtedly a result of the increase with puberty in gonadotropin and androstenedione secretion as well as the extragonadal activity of the other 17β-HSD isozymes in converting androstenedione to testosterone.[903, 924] However, the patients described from the Gaza Strip had a less severe enzyme block, with 15 to 20% of normal 17β-HSD 3 activity and evidence of synthesis of testosterone by the testes at the expected time of puberty.

Analyses of 17 patients with classic 17β-HSD deficiency, including 4 from San Francisco, revealed 14 mutations in the *HSD17B3* gene.[902, 903, 916] Twelve patients had homozygous mutations, four were compound heterozygotes, and one was a presumed heterozygote[902, 903, 916] (Fig. 29–68). The mutations included a frameshift, 3 splice site abnormalities, and 10 missense mutations.[902, 903, 916] Expression of eight of the nine missense mutations revealed complete absence of 17β-HSD 3 enzymatic activity.[916] The Arg80Gln missense mutation in the Gaza Strip Arab patients resulted in an enzyme with partial (15 to 20%) activity.[902, 916] Of note, 46,XX females homozygous for the Gaza Strip mutation are completely asymptomatic and fertile; the expression of the 17β-HSD 3 isozyme is limited to the testes.[924]

The presence of wolffian duct derivatives in these patients with homozygous mutations of the 17β-HSD 3 isoenzyme that result in complete absence of enzymatc activity is unexplained.[916] Andersson and colleagues[903] suggested that because the androgen receptor in the wolffian duct appears to be identical to the mature androgen receptor,[925] there must be an alternate pathway for testosterone synthesis by a 17β-HSD in utero to induce wolffian duct stabilization.

The diagnosis of 17β-HSD 3 deficiency should be considered in (1) male pseudohermaphrodites who have no abnor-mality in adrenal steroid biosynthesis, absent müllerian ducts, and normal wolffian duct structures and (2) male pseudohermaphrodites who virilize at puberty either with or without gynecomastia. The absence of müllerian duct derivatives distinguishes patients with defective testosterone biosynthesis or androgen resistance from those with dysgenetic male pseudohermaphroditism. In the prepubertal or young adolescent patient, basal androstenedione and estrone levels may not be elevated for age. However, at any age the defect in testosterone biosynthesis can be demonstrated by a prolonged hCG stimulation test.[912] In response to hCG, there is a disproportionate rise in plasma androstenedione and estrone levels, compared with testosterone and estradiol concentrations.[912, 923, 926–928]

In a previous edition of this chapter, the authors postulated that severely affected females would feminize spontaneously at puberty but not menstruate regularly and that the biochemical hallmark of the defect, elevated androstenedione, estrone, and gonadotropin concentrations, would be present. Putative affected females have been reported.[929, 930] Because little or no 17β-HSD 3 is expressed in the ovary, further molecular studies are necessary to determine whether these patients have a mutation in one of the other 17β-HSD isozyme genes.[903] Likewise, a putative late-onset form of 17β-HSD deficiency causing gynecomastia and hypogonadism in males has been reported[931] but has not been confirmed by DNA analyses of the coding sequence of the HSD17β3 gene.[903]

In patients reared as females (the usual case), the treatment involves castration followed by estrogen substitution therapy at puberty, but this approach needs to be re-examined, especially in view of the dramatic advances in neonatal diagnosis and DNA analysis. In the patient with ambiguous genitalia reared as a male, testosterone therapy to augment phallic size and genitoplasty are indicated in infancy. As noted previously, male pseudohermaphroditism caused by 17β-HSD 3 deficiency is relatively common among Arabs of the Gaza Strip.[913, 924] The natural history in this isolate is virilization at puberty; furthermore, a change in gender role behavior from female to male is the rule. Because of this, Gross and colleagues[927] proposed that these patients should be given male gender assignment at diagnosis. They described seven young affected 46,XY males with female external genitalia who after biochemical confirmation were treated with testosterone enanthate, 25 to 50 mg each month for 3 mo. Most patients received two or three courses of testosterone therapy, which resulted in an increase in phallic length into the normal range for age.[927] First-stage genitoplasty was then undertaken when the patients were between 2 and 3 years of age. Ten of the 11 children treated in this way were reported to have a "pleasing

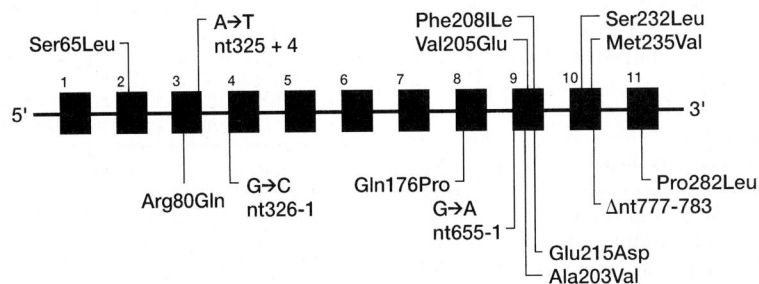

Figure 29–68. Diagrammatic representation of the gene encoding 17β-hydroxysteroid dehydrogenase type 3 with the mutations reported to cause 17β-HSD deficiency. The exons are the numbered black boxes. Missense mutations causing amino acid substitutions in the enzyme are indicated by the three-letter abbreviation for the wild-type amino acid, followed by the amino acid number in the enzyme and the three-letter abbreviation for the substituted amino acid. nt325+4 is a splice junction mutation, a transition of adenine (A) to thymidine (T), located four nucleotides downstream (3') of the boundary between exon 3 and intron 3; nucleotide 325 is the closest base pair in the exon to the mutation. nt326−1 is a splice junction mutation, a transition of guanine (G) to cytosine (C), located one nucleotide upstream (5') of the boundary between intron 3 and exon 4. nt665−1 is a splice junction mutation, a transition of guanine (G) to adenine (A), located one nucleotide upstream (5') of the splice junction between intron 8 and exon 9. Δnt777-783 indicates a deletion of nucleotides 777 to 783 in the gene. (Redrawn from Andersson S, Geissler WM, Wu L, David DL, Grumbach MM, New MI, Schwarz HP, Blethen SL, Mendonca BB, Bloise W, et al. Molecular genetics and pathophysiology of 17β-hydroxysteroid dehydrogenase 3 deficiency. J Clin Endocrinol Metab 1996; 81:130–136. © 1996, The Endocrine Society.)

TABLE 29–30. Clinical Features of Complete Androgen Resistance

Karyotype:	46,XY
Inheritance:	X-linked recessive; mutations in *AR* gene
Genitalia:	Female with blind vaginal pouch
Wolffian duct derivatives:	Usually absent; less commonly, rudimentary or hypoplastic
Müllerian duct derivatives:	Absent or vestigial
Gonads:	Testes
Habitus:	Scant or absent pubic and axillary hair; breast development and female habitus at puberty; primary amenorrhea ("hairless woman")
Hormone and metabolic profile:	Increased plasma LH and testosterone concentration; increased estradiol (for men); FSH levels often normal or slightly increased Resistance to androgenic and metabolic effects of testosterone
Androgen receptor studies:	Genetic heterogeneity; mutations can lead to low or undetectable amount of normal receptor (receptor-negative), unstable receptor (thermolabile, partial receptor deficiency), or the receptor-positive form

appearance" of their external genitalia with phallic length within 1 SD of the normal mean value.[932] Cosmetic and functional results in adolescents were also reported to be "encouraging"; however, the results of this treatment in adults were "poor."[932]

When the patient is reared as a male, testosterone replacement therapy at the age of puberty is necessary to achieve full masculinization and to prevent, at least in some, the appearance of gynecomastia. A plausible explanation for the absence of spermatogenesis in these patients, aside from cryptorchidism, is the low concentration of testosterone in the testis. In patients raised as males with retained gonads, cryptorchidism and elevated gonadotropin levels (postpubertally) may increase the risk for testicular neoplasm.

Defects in Androgen-Dependent Target Tissues

A defect at any step in the mechanism of action of androgens on their target cells (see Fig. 29–24)—5α-reduction of

testosterone, binding of DHT to the receptor, nuclear localization of the steroid receptor complex to hormone response elements on DNA and subsequent transcription, or translation—can lead to impaired androgen action and result in male pseudohermaphroditism. Two major forms have been identified: end-organ resistance to androgenic hormones (androgen receptor defects) and errors in testosterone metabolism in target tissues (5α-reductase deficiency).

END-ORGAN RESISTANCE TO ANDROGENS (ANDROGEN RECEPTOR DEFECTS).[238, 933–935] The spectrum of phenotypes in 46,XY individuals with androgen resistance syndromes varies from patients with normal female external genitalia, the so-called "complete" form, through those with genital ambiguity to those with a normal male phenotype who have a small phallus and are fertile.

Complete Androgen Resistance and Its Variants (Androgen Insensitivity Syndrome, Testicular Feminization, Feminizing Testes). The term "testicular feminization," coined by Morris and Mahesh,[936] but no longer used, was applied to a highly distinctive X-linked disorder in which affected males are phenotypic females and develop female secondary sexual characteristics at puberty but fail to menstruate (Table 29–30). That affected individuals are genetic males is shown by the 46,XY karyotype and the presence of testes. The prevalence of this disorder is estimated at 1 in 20,000 live male births.[937] Phenotypically, these patients have unambiguous female external genitalia; hypoplastic labia majora[938]; a blind vaginal pouch; absent or, rarely, vestigial müllerian structures (uterus and tubes)[939, 940]; testes located in the labia, the inguinal canal, or the abdomen; and absent or vestigal wolffian derivatives[940] (Fig. 29–69). Histologically, the testes are difficult to distinguish from normal before puberty. After puberty, seminiferous tubules are small, spermatogonia are sparse, and spermatogenesis is absent.[941, 942] The Leydig cells are hyperplastic and tend to form adenomatous clumps. The testes are predisposed to malignant transformation.[937, 939] CiS and seminoma have been reported, especially in patients with the incomplete form of androgen resistance.[651, 933] The overall risk of a testicular neoplasm in the affected adult has been estimated at 4%[648] to

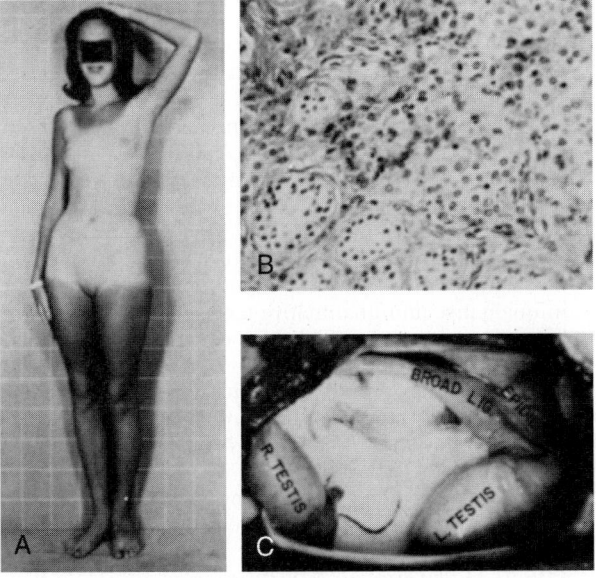

COMPLETE FORM OF SYNDROME

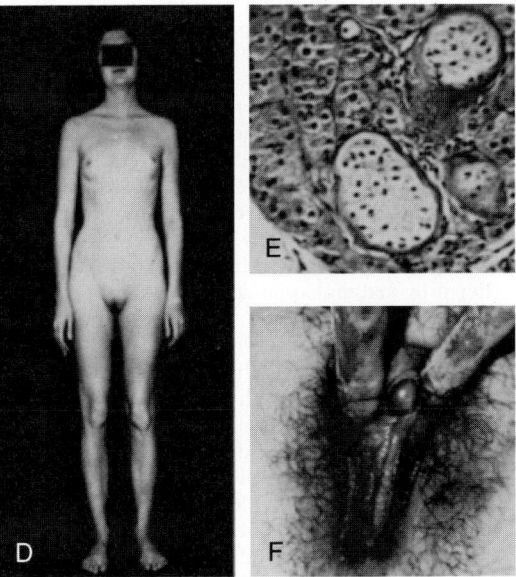

VARIANT FORM OF SYNDROME

Figure 29–69. The syndrome of complete androgen resistance and its variant form. *A*, A 17-year-old patient with the complete syndrome. This phenotypic female was chromatin-negative, had a 46,XY karyotype, and had total absence of sexual hair with female secondary sexual characteristics. A small vagina ended blindly. *B*, The testes exhibited Leydig cell hyperplasia and seminiferous tubules that lacked germinal elements. *C*, At laparotomy, abdominal testes, rudimentary wolffian structures, and no müllerian structures were found. *D*, The variant form of syndrome in a 25-year-old female. Sexual hair was present, although sparse. *E*, The testes exhibited Leydig cell hyperplasia. *F*, The clitoris was hypertrophied, but there was no labial fusion. A shallow vagina ended blindly. At laparotomy, hypoplastic wolffian structures and absent müllerian structures were noted.

9%[939]; however, the risk appears to be significantly less in those younger than 20 years of age.[648]

At birth and in childhood the diagnosis should be suspected in phenotypic females with an inguinal hernia and a testis-like mass in the inguinal region or in the labia. It has been estimated that 1 to 2% of phenotypic females with inguinal hernias have androgen resistance.[943] At adolescence, female secondary sexual characteristics develop and include normal breasts and female body habitus but no menses. Pubic and axillary hair is usually sparse and is completely lacking in about one third of patients. A small amount of vulval hair is usually present. The clitoris is normal or small, the vagina is shallow and ends in a blind pouch, and the labia minora tend to be underdeveloped. Wolffian duct derivatives are absent, rudimentary, or hypoplastic; vestigial müllerian structures are present in about one third of patients.[939] Approximately 10% of patients have slight ambiguity of the external genitalia at birth, with partial fusion of the labioscrotal folds and modest clitorimegaly (the *incomplete form* of androgen resistance). In these patients, in whom wolffian duct derivatives are hypoplastic, slight clitorimegaly and virilization often occur at puberty, as do pubic and axillary hair and feminization (breast development and a female habitus).[238, 944] The authors prefer to classify this condition as the incomplete variant of complete androgen resistance. Intelligence is normal, as are thyroid and adrenal function; there are no associated clinical anomalies. Gender identity is that of a normal female with strong maternal instincts.

Pathophysiology and Hormone Profile

The Androgen Receptor. Understanding of the pathogenesis of this syndrome has advanced rapidly over the past few years. In 1950 Wilkins first suggested that failure of androgenization of the male fetus and the development of female rather than male secondary sexual characteristics at puberty could be explained by end-organ unresponsiveness to androgen (Fig. 29–70). Studies by subsequent workers supported this contention by failing to demonstrate a clinical or metabolic response to testosterone administration in patients with the complete form of this syndrome.[945] This X-linked disorder has been described in several mammalian species, including mouse, rat, bull, and chimpanzee.[946]

Studies in two animal models, the tfm mouse and rat, by Bardin and co-workers,[871] Stanley and associates,[946] Gehring and colleagues,[947] and Goldstein and Wilson[948] suggested that the primary defect is a deficient number of androgen receptors for DHT and testosterone. Soon thereafter, Keenan and colleagues[949] reported an undetectable or low amount of androgen receptor activity in cultured fibroblasts from the genital skin of karyotypic males with the syndrome. Their observations were amply confirmed by others.[950, 951] The lack of androgen binding in genital skin fibroblasts from patients with this disorder provided an explanation for the observed failure of androgen action.

Subsequent studies, mainly from the laboratories of Migeon and of Wilson, indicated that genetic heterogeneity in the defect exists in patients with androgen resistance.[238, 933, 952–954] Initial studies of patients with complete androgen resistance revealed two groups: those with absent DHT binding and those with apparently normal cytosolic and nuclear binding. Additional observations of the receptor-positive patients showed that the receptor was thermolabile[955, 956] and/or unstable in the presence of molybdate.[957] Other qualitative abnormalities in androgen binding or kinetics have been described in some receptor-positive patients, including (1) an increase in the rate of dissociation of the steroid-receptor complex,[956, 958] (2) defective up-regulation of the androgen receptor,[959] (3) decreased affinity of ligand binding,[960] (4) impaired nuclear retention of the ligand,[961, 962] and (5) lability of the androgen receptor under transforming conditions.[963]

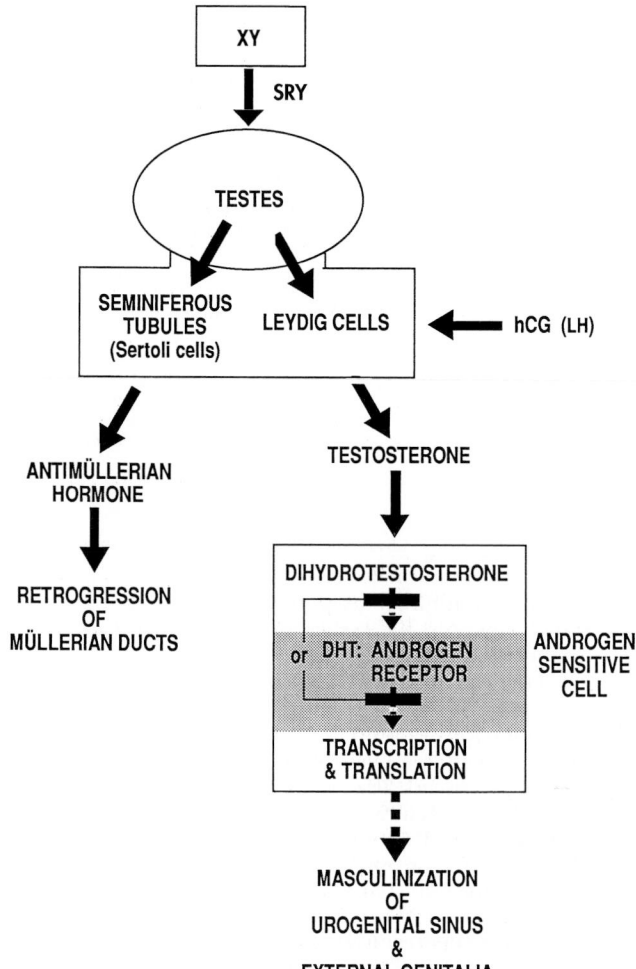

Figure 29–70. A diagrammatic scheme of male pseudohermaphroditism caused by complete or partial androgen resistance illustrating defects in the androgen receptor that result in absent or reduced binding of DHT or impaired function of the ligand-bound receptor.

In general, the severity of the defect in androgen receptor quantity or quality correlates with the phenotype.[238] Patients with complete androgen resistance usually have absent binding or severe qualitative abnormalities, whereas those with more masculinized phenotypes (i.e., Reifenstein's syndrome or infertile males) have lesser qualititative and quantitative deficits in androgen receptor activity.[238] Individuals varying in phenotype from complete testicular feminization to the infertile male syndrome have had an apparently normal receptor in qualitative and quantitative terms when assessed by steroid-binding properties.[238] The lack of strict correlation between phenotype and receptor binding, as well as the apparently normal binding found in patients with androgen resistance, was clarified by studies of the molecular biology of the androgen receptor and of mutations in the gene encoding the receptor.[238]

Molecular Biology of the Androgen Receptor. The androgen receptor is encoded by a gene (*AR*) that maps to Xq11-q12.[964, 965] The gene has eight exons (1 to 8) and encodes a 110- to 114-kd protein that varies in length from 910 to 919 amino acids[964–966] (Fig. 29–71). The androgen receptor, a typical member of the nuclear receptor superfamily of transcription factors, is structurally and functionally similar to other steroid hormone receptors and is related to receptors for thyroid hormone, Vitamin D, and retinoic acid in that it has three major functional domains.[967, 968]

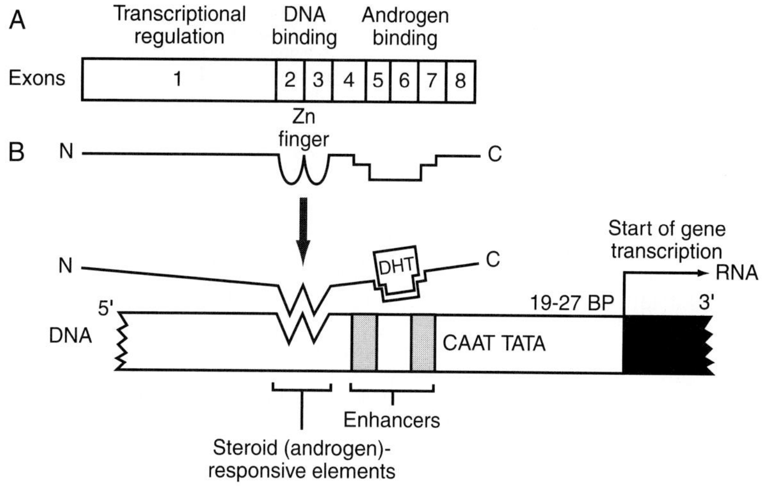

Figure 29–71. *A,* A diagrammatic representation of the androgen receptor gene divided into its eight exons. Exon 1 codes for the NH$_2$-terminal domain and regulates transcription. Exons 2 and 3 code for two zinc fingers. Exons 4 through 8 code for the androgen binding domain of the receptor. *B,* The organization of a steroid-responsive gene. Ligand binding activates the receptor, and it binds to the steroid response elements of the gene (as a dimer; not shown). Enhancers as well as a CAAT and a TATA box are present. Gene transcription begins 19 to 27 base pairs downstream of the TATA box (see also Fig. 29–24).

The NH$_2$-terminal domain is encoded by exon 1. This large domain is critical for the regulation of target gene transcription.[969] The NH$_2$-terminal domain contains two repeat sequences in the coding region that are polymorphic and composed of 16 to 27 trinucleotide repeats of a GGN (polyglycine) and 11 to 31 repeats of a CAG (polyglutamine).[966] The function of these two repetitive domains is unknown, although expansion of repeated glutamine residues is found in spinal and bulbar muscular atrophy[970, 971] and Kennedy's disease, an adult-onset motor neuron disease characterized by degeneration of spinal cord and bulbar motor neurons.[971] The latter disease usually becomes manifest in the third or fourth decade of life, and affected males have subtle signs of androgen resistance (i.e., gynecomastia, testicular atrophy, and reduced fertility).[971] The polymorphic glutamine repeats in the NH$_2$-terminal position of the androgen receptor are expanded to 45 to 68 repeats in affected males.[970–972] The relation between the number of glutamine repeats in the androgen receptor and the neuronal degeneration is still to be defined.

Although complete deletion of the *AR* gene has been reported in two families and is associated with the complete androgen resistance phenotype (the null phenotype),[938, 973] few mutations causing either a stop codon or frameshift have been reported in exon 1, which encodes the NH$_2$-terminal portion of the androgen receptor.[974, 975] In two patients, a deletion of the X chromosome affected both *AR* and gene loci more proximal and distal.[976] Both patients had mental retardation as well as complete androgen resistance, suggesting that a gene for mental retardation is located on the X chromosome in immediate proximity to the gene encoding the androgen receptor.[976, 977]

The highly conserved DNA-binding domain of the androgen receptor is encoded by exons 2 and 3 (see Fig. 29–70). It has about 80% homology with other steroid hormone receptors. Exons 2 and 3 encode two zinc fingers, which bind to hormone response elements (transcriptional enhancer nucleotide sequences) of DNA.[967, 968] Sequences in the second zinc finger mediate dimerization of the androgen-receptor complex.[966] Mutations in the DNA-binding region of the androgen receptor can result in a receptor that binds the androgen substrate normally but is unable to induce transactivation because of faulty binding to DNA, destabilization of the protein structure, or lack of dimerization of the receptor.[934, 935, 966, 978] As with mutations or deletions in other areas of the androgen receptor, the degree of impairment of transactivation correlates with the phenotype (i.e., complete versus partial androgen resistance). Specific mutations in the second zinc finger have been reported in patients with partial androgen resistance and infiltrating carcinoma of the breast.[979, 980] In two studies, the mutation involved a glycine and lysine substitution of the arginine at residues 607 and 608, respectively. The similarity of the mutations and the occurrence of breast cancer in all three patients raises the possibility of a causal relation.[979, 980]

Between the DNA-binding region and the ligand-binding region of the androgen receptor is the hinge region, encoded by the 5′ portion of exon 4. This region contains a nuclear localization signal necessary for the transfer of the ligand receptor complex from the cytoplasm to the nucleus.[981, 982] As yet, no mutations in the nuclear localization signal region have been reported in patients with androgen resistance.[966]

The steroid-binding region is located in the COOH-terminal third of the androgen receptor; it is encoded by the 3′ portion of exon 4 and by exons 5 through 8. Binding of androgen to its high-affinity binding site induces a conformational change in the receptor, further phosphorylation, dimerization, nuclear localization, and consequently transactivation. This region apparently interacts in its ligand-free conformation with the chaperone heat shock proteins which inhibit binding to DNA.[969] The majority of mutations in the androgen receptor affect the steroid-binding domain (see Fig. 29–71). These mutations influence androgen binding, the specificity of androgen binding, and the kinetics of association and dissociation of androgen with its receptor and can result in receptors that cannot bind androgens or that bind androgens but exhibit qualitative abnormalities such as thermolability or accelerated dissociation of androgen from the receptor.

The distribution of point mutations in the androgen receptor is similar for patients with complete androgen resistance and those with partial androgen resistance (Fig. 29–72). Most mutations involve exons 5 and 7 of the *AR* gene.[983] Arginine constitutes 4% of the amino acid residues of the androgen receptor, whereas 40% of reported mutations involve an arginine residue.[983] Four arginine residues, at positions 774, 831, 840, and 855, and a valine residue at 866 are mutated in many cases.[933, 966, 984] The replacement of arginine 855 by a cystine or leucine results in complete androgen resistance, whereas a substitution of histidine for arginine at position 855 results in partial androgen resistance. The difference in phenotype is the result of the effect of the substitution on the ability of the receptor to induce transactivation. In general, patients with similar mutations in the androgen receptor have the same phenotype; however, patients with androgen resistance are described who have different phenotypes despite apparently harboring an identical mutation[983, 984a] (see Fig. 29–71). The latter observation suggests

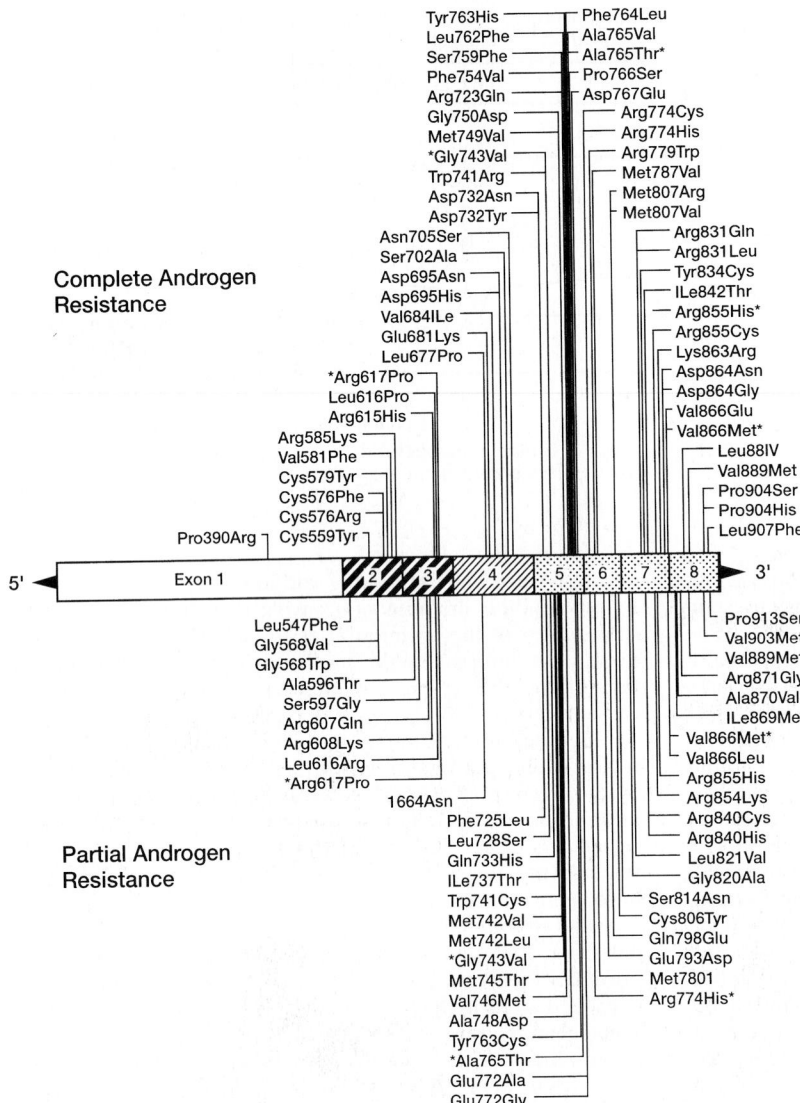

Figure 29–72. Diagrammatic representation of the androgen receptor gene (AR) with missense mutations that cause complete androgen resistance (CAR) and partial androgen resistance (PAR). Asterisks indicate mutations that have been found to cause both complete and partial androgen resistance. Each mutation is indicated by the three-letter abbreviation for the wild-type amino acid, followed by the position number of the amino acid in the protein and the three-letter abbreviation for the substituted amino acid. Exon 1, indicated by the open box, regulates transcription. Exons 2 and 3, indicated by heavy diagonal lines, encode the DNA-binding region of the androgen receptor. Part of exon 4 (thin diagonal lines) encodes the "hinge region" of the androgen receptor, which contains a nuclear localization signal. The 3' end of exon 4 through exon 8 (stippled) encodes the ligand (androgen)–binding region. A mutational hot spot is located in exon 5 and can cause both CAR and PAR. Not shown are nonsense, frameshift, and splice junction mutations and deletions that can cause either CAR or PAR. (Redrawn from Quigley CA, De Bellis A, Marschke KB, el-Awad MK, Wilson EM, French FS. Androgen receptor defects: historical, clinical and molecular perspectives. Endocr Rev 1995; 16:271–321. © 1995, The Endocrine Society.)

that there are other factors in the androgenization cascade, as yet unidentified, that influence the relation of genotype to phenotype.

In summary, impaired androgen-induced transactivation leads to androgen resistance.[238, 933, 934, 935] A wide variety of defects affecting the androgen transactivation pathway have been found. These include complete or partial deletion of the receptor, nonsense and missense mutations, and expansion of the trinucleotide repeats of exon 1.[238, 933–935] Complete androgen resistance has been associated with all these defects, whereas partial androgen resistance is in general associated with amino acid substitutions in the DNA- and androgen-binding domains of the receptor protein. Usually these amino acid substitutions produce a quantitative or qualitative change in the transactivation activity of the androgen receptor complex and result in partial androgen resistance.[238, 933–935]

Hormone Profile. In the complete form of androgen resistance, lack of effect of testosterone and DHT during embryogenesis blocks stabilization of the wolffian ducts and masculinization of the external genitalia. Secretion of AMH by the fetal Sertoli cells leads to complete regression of the müllerian ducts in two thirds of the patients. The hormone profile is similar in all variants of androgen resistance but has been characterized best in those with the complete form. The hallmark is an elevated concentration of plasma LH and

testosterone in the absence of virilization (or in the presence of a minimal degree of virilization). However, plasma LH and testosterone levels were normal in the first 4 months of life in four patients with the complete form of androgen resistance (personal communication, J. L. Chaussain),[933] in contrast to the elevated plasma levels of LH and testosterone found during the same period in two patients with partial androgen resistance.[985, 986] Furthermore, a lack of the neonatal surge in LH and testosterone has been reported in infants with complete androgen resistance.[933] The authors have observed elevated basal plasma LH and testosterone after 6 months of age in patients with the complete form, in contrast to the reports of others,[987, 988] which suggest that patients with complete androgen resistance differ from those with partial androgen resistance with respect to the function of the hypothalamic-pituitary-gonadal axis during the first 6 months of life. At puberty, androgen resistance at the hypothalamic-pituitary level leads to an increase in LH pulse frequency and amplitude in these patients, compared with normal individuals.[989] This results in augmented LH secretion, which in turn stimulates an increase in testosterone secretion, but the conversion of testosterone to DHT is reduced.[987, 990, 991] Increased testicular secretion of estradiol and, to a lesser degree, peripheral conversion of androstenedione and testosterone to estradiol result in elevated plasma estradiol concentrations, which, in the presence of end-organ resistance to androgens, cause feminization.[992, 993] At puberty, these patients exhibit the type of growth spurt induced by estrogen, with a peak height velocity of 7.4 cm/y at a mean chronologic age of 12.7 years.[994] Mean final height in five adult patients was 172 ± 4.1 cm, which is +1.4 SD of the mean value for women and −.6 SD of that for men.[994] The growth of sexual hair, normally mediated by androgens, is either absent, sparse, or diminished, depending on the degree of androgen resistance. Concentrations of adrenal androgens, including DHEAS, are normal. The elevated estradiol evokes an increase in the concentration of plasma TeBG, which, along with the increased secretion of testosterone by the testes, results in an increase in the mean plasma testosterone level.[991, 993] On the other hand, the concentration of plasma DHT tends to be lower than normal because of a decrease in peripheral 5α-reduction of C_{19}-steroids.[991] Plasma FSH levels are variable, either normal or slightly elevated. Castration results in a further elevation of plasma LH concentration and a rise in FSH concentration, which suggests that both estradiol and inhibin play a role in the negative feedback of gonadotropins in patients with androgen resistance.[995]

Diagnosis. The diagnosis of complete androgen resistance (testicular feminization) can be established by clinical criteria alone after puberty and can be strongly suspected before puberty. The patients may present with an inguinal hernia or labial mass, primary amenorrhea despite female secondary sexual characteristics, and a history of an affected sister, aunt, or cousin. A phenotypic female with primary amenorrhea, breast development, scant or absent pubic and axillary hair, a shallow vagina and absent cervix on gynecological examination, and a 46,XY karyotype has the complete form of androgen resistance. Similarly, the detection of a 46,XY karyotype in a female infant or child with an inguinal hernia and/or labial mass suggests the diagnosis. A presumptive diagnosis of androgen resistance can be made in infants in whom the concentration of plasma LH and/or testosterone is elevated despite lack of virilization[985, 986]; however, as noted previously, this may not hold true in the neonatal period for patients with the complete form of androgen resistance. Absence of the uterus can be confirmed by sonography or pelvic MRI. Before puberty, the differential diagnosis includes defects in testosterone biosynthesis and 5α-reductase deficiency. In the prepubertal patient, the family history, phenotype, endocrine evaluation including C_{19}- and C_{21}-steroid responses to hCG and corticotropin, determination of androgen receptor activity, and, if necessary, metabolic response to testosterone are used to establish the diagnosis. In addition, the poor suppression of TeBG by the nonaromatizable anabolic steroid stanozolol and the determination of plasma AMH levels have been used as clues to the diagnosis of androgen resistance, but these tests have not yet been extensively evaluated and confirmed.[996, 997] The combination of a smaller decrease in the concentration of TeBG and a rise in the level of testosterone 2 days after a 3-day course of hCG has been proposed as a screening test for both the complete and partial forms of androgen resistance.[998] Although the preliminary results are promising, more patients must be assessed before this relatively simple screen can be validated, especially in the newborn period. DNA analysis of the *AR* gene is definitive (although laborious and expensive) and is becoming more readily available.

46,XX females heterozygous for an androgen receptor mutation can manifest delayed puberty[999] and/or reduced or asymmetrical development of pubic and axillary hair,[960] and the carrier status in a female suspected of having androgen resistance can be confirmed by molecular analysis of the *AR* gene by a number of techniques, such as PCR/SSCP (polymerase chain reaction/single strand conformation polymorphism), allele-specific PCR, and analysis of the length of CAG

repeats in exon 1.[933] The segregation of the two X chromosomes in a carrier female can be followed by examination of polymorphic markers such as CAG repeat sequences in exon 1 and the intronic *Hind* III restriction site.[1000]

These molecular genetic techniques have been used in prenatal diagnosis of infants affected with androgen receptor defects.[1000, 1001] Prenatal diagnosis in the complete form of androgen resistance may not routinely be necessary, because this condition is associated with a normal female phenotype and a normal life span.[1000] It is, however, associated with infertility and the possible psychological stress of being an 46,XY female. Parents must decide whether they wish a prenatal diagnosis. In families with partial androgen insensitivity, carrier detection and prenatal diagnosis are more appropriate,[1002] but even in these patients, phenotypic variability with the same mutation makes prenatal diagnosis and counseling problematic. Repeated ultrasonic examination of the fetus is useful in evaluating the external genitalia.

Treatment. Therapy includes affirmation and reinforcement of the female phenotype and gender identity. Prepubertal orchidectomy is indicated when the testes of patients with complete androgen resistance are located in the labia majora or when an inguinal hernia is present. Otherwise, castration can be deferred until late adolescence to allow the patient to undergo spontaneous feminization at puberty; the status of the intra-abdominal testes can be monitored by periodic sonography or MRI scans of the pelvis. Girls with the incomplete variant of complete androgen resistance (with clitorimegaly and slight posterior labial fusion) may exhibit mild virilization as well as feminization at puberty; in these patients, it is prudent to remove the testes before puberty or soon after puberty begins. When the testes are removed, estrogen substitution is necessary to promote development of secondary sexual characteristics at the expected age of puberty. The vagina may be adequate in length for sexual intercourse; in patients with a short vaginal pouch, the initiation during adolescence of manual dilatation with a prosthesis is effective in increasing the size of the vagina.

The question of when, if ever, to inform the patient about the discordance in genetic and phenotype sex is controversial.[238, 1003–1005] In the era of informed consent and the Freedom of Information Act, it has become increasingly difficult and inappropriate to withhold information in order to "protect" the patient. In fact, the worst scenario is that in which the patient learns of her diagnosis inadvertently. The authors recommend that, with the consent of the parents and the establishment of an appropriate psychological support system, the pathophysiology of the disorder be disclosed to the patient carefully, stage by stage, in an age-appropriate manner. The patient must be counseled and reassured of her ability to lead a functional, normal life, except for fertility, including marriage and adoptive parenthood. With proper therapy and reassurance and support, these patients can become "normal" adult females. A national androgen resistance support group has been formed and is active in educating physicians as well as affected females about the special concerns and problems of women with androgen resistance.

Partial Form of Androgen Resistance and Its Variants (Reifenstein's Syndrome). A heterogenous group of 46,XY individuals have partial androgen resistance[238, 933] (Table 29–31). The external genitalia range from perineoscrotal hypospadias with cryptorchidism and micropenis to clitorimegaly with partial labial fusion. The patients described in the past by Lubs, Gilbert-Dreyfus, Reifenstein, Rosewater, Walker, and their associates quite likely had partial androgen resistance.[238, 933, 1006, 1007] The variable degree of masculinization of affected males within and between kinships is well illustrated by one family studied by Wilson and colleagues.[1008] Eleven males were affected; two had a relatively mild defect in masculinization of

TABLE 29–31. Clinical Features of Partial Androgen Resistance

Karyotype:	46,XY
Inheritance:	X-linked recessive; mutations in *AR* gene
External genitalia:	Ambiguous with blind vaginal pouch → hypoplastic male → normal male with infertility
Wolffian duct derivatives:	Rudimentary → hypoplastic → normal
Müllerian duct derivatives:	Absent
Gonads:	Testes
Habitus:	Decreased to normal axillary and pubic hair, beard growth, and body hair; gynecomastia common at puberty
Hormone and metabolic profile:	Increased plasma LH and testosterone concentrations; increased estradiol (for men); FSH levels may be normal or slightly increased
	Partial resistance to androgenic and metabolic effects of testosterone
Androgen receptor studies:	Genetic heterogeneity; partial deficiency of normal receptor; mutations lead to qualitatively abnormal receptor

the external genitalia (small penis and bifid scrotum), eight had perineal hypospadias, and one had hypospadias, a urogenital sinus with a blind vaginal pouch, and an absent vas deferens. All lacked müllerian structures. In contrast, families with the complete form of androgen resistance exhibit little variability in expression of the mutant gene. The most common presentation in infancy is that of an apparent male with third-degree hypospadias (the urethral orifice located at the base of the phallus), a small penis, and, often, cryptorchidism. Müllerian duct derivatives are absent; wolffian duct derivatives are usually present but hypoplastic. At puberty, pubic and axillary hair and gynecomastia usually develop, male secondary sexual characteristics are incompletely developed, and the testes remain small and exhibit azoospermia because of germinal cell arrest beyond the primary spermatocyte stage. Less severely affected men may exhibit a bifid scrotum, infertility, and poor virilization at puberty. More severely affected males may have ambiguous genitalia, a blind vaginal pouch, and poorly developed wolffian structures. As in other patients with androgen insensitivity, the concentrations of plasma LH and testosterone are elevated, and the high LH levels are resistant to suppression by exogenous androgens. Estradiol and testosterone production rates are increased. However, the degree of feminization at puberty, despite elevated estradiol secretion, is less than in the complete form of androgen resistance (Fig. 29–73).

Molecular biologic studies in patients with androgen resistance indicate that partial androgen resistance is associated with amino acid substitutions in the DNA- and androgen-binding domains of the androgen receptor. These substitutions are distributed throughout these domains and are similar to those causing complete androgen resistance. They tend to be more conservative than those causing complete androgen resistance (for example, substitution of a basic amino acid such as arginine for another basic amino acid such as histidine, or substitution of methionine for valine, both of which are hydrophobic amino acids).[238, 933] These conservative amino acid mutations disrupt the function of the androgen receptor less than those found in complete androgen resistance and produce the less severe phenotypic manifestations observed in patients with partial androgen resistance. However, phenotypic variability is common in families with affected males with partial androgen resistance and the same mutation in the *AR* gene, a finding that is consistent with the influence of epistatic factors, other than a derangement of the gene, that affect the phenotypic manifestations in these families.[983, 985, 1009]

Androgen Resistance in Infertile Men. Analysis of a large kindred with Reifenstein's syndrome led to the detection of two phenotypically normal males who were infertile and lacked the clinical features of androgen resistance. These infertile males could not be distinguished endocrinologically or by androgen receptor studies from their more severely affected relatives.[238, 1010] Subsequently, Aiman and co-workers[1011] reported infertility in three unrelated men with uninformative family histories and a quantitative deficiency of the androgen receptor. Two of the men had a normal adult male phenotype; one had slight gynecomastia, decreased body hair, and a modest reduction in testicular size. All were infertile and had severe oligospermia or azoospermia. The significant hormonal findings were normal or elevated serum concentrations of testosterone in the presence of high plasma concentrations of LH. Two of the three men had increased blood production rates for testosterone, androstenedione, and estradiol. The decreased amount of androgen receptor in genital skin fibroblasts was consistent with a quantitative deficiency of the androgen receptor. Further studies suggested the existence of both quantitative and qualitative abnormalities in the androgen receptor in infertile males.[1011] To estimate the frequency of androgen receptor abnormalities in men with idiopathic infertility, Aiman and Griffin[1012] studied 28 unrelated, phenotypically normal men with idiopathic azoospermia or oligospermia. Using genital skin fibroblasts, they observed a partial deficiency of the receptor in 9 (40%) of 22 of the azoospermic or oligospermic subjects.[1012] In contrast to previously studied patients with androgen resistance, six of nine infertile men had normal levels of plasma LH and testosterone, and the plasma production rate of testosterone was elevated in only two of six.[1012] Other studies have detected subtle defects in the androgen receptor in some subfertile men.[1013]

Androgen Resistance in Fertile Men. It was postulated that infertility in otherwise normal men was the most consistent and most subtle clinical manifestation of quantitative and qualitative defects in the androgen receptor.[1012, 1013] However, families have now been described which include men with normal male genitalia, postpubertal gynecomastia, and poor virilization in spite of elevated plasma testosterone levels.[1014, 1015] Studies of the androgen receptor in affected individuals detected several qualitative abnormalities, including receptor instability, failure of up-regulation, increased dissociation of receptor–synthetic androgen complexes, and thermal instability.[1014, 1015] Molecular analysis of the *AR* gene in one cohort revealed a single nucleotide substitution in the androgen-binding domain, a leucine-to-phenylalanine change at amino acid 789 (Leu789Phe).[1015] Expression of the mutant gene in transfected cells demonstrated a decrease in transactivational activity with this substitution compatible to that seen in this mild form of androgen resistance. Hence, subtle undervirilization (phallus length, 5 to 6 cm in two patients) with or without gynecomastia, rather than infertility, may represent the extreme of the phenotypic spectrum of subtle defects in androgen receptor function.[1014, 1015]

Diagnosis. Partial androgen resistance must be differentiated from other forms of male pseudohermaphroditism caused by androgen deficiency or 5α-reductase deficiency. There is no readily available in vivo or in vitro assay of the transactivational capacity of the androgen receptor.[1016] However, the pattern of inheritance and measurement of the levels of plasma LH and testosterone and its precursors, as well as TeBG levels, before and after the administration of hCG may distinguish patients with partial androgen resistance from those with other forms of male pseudohermaphroditism.[998] As with complete androgen resistance, a lesser decrease in TeBG levels after a short course of the synthetic anabolic androgen, stanozolol, has been suggested as a biologic test of androgen resistance.[997] However, this bioassay is not useful in newborn infants because of the normal decrease in the concentration of TeBG in the neonate. Few confirmatory data have been

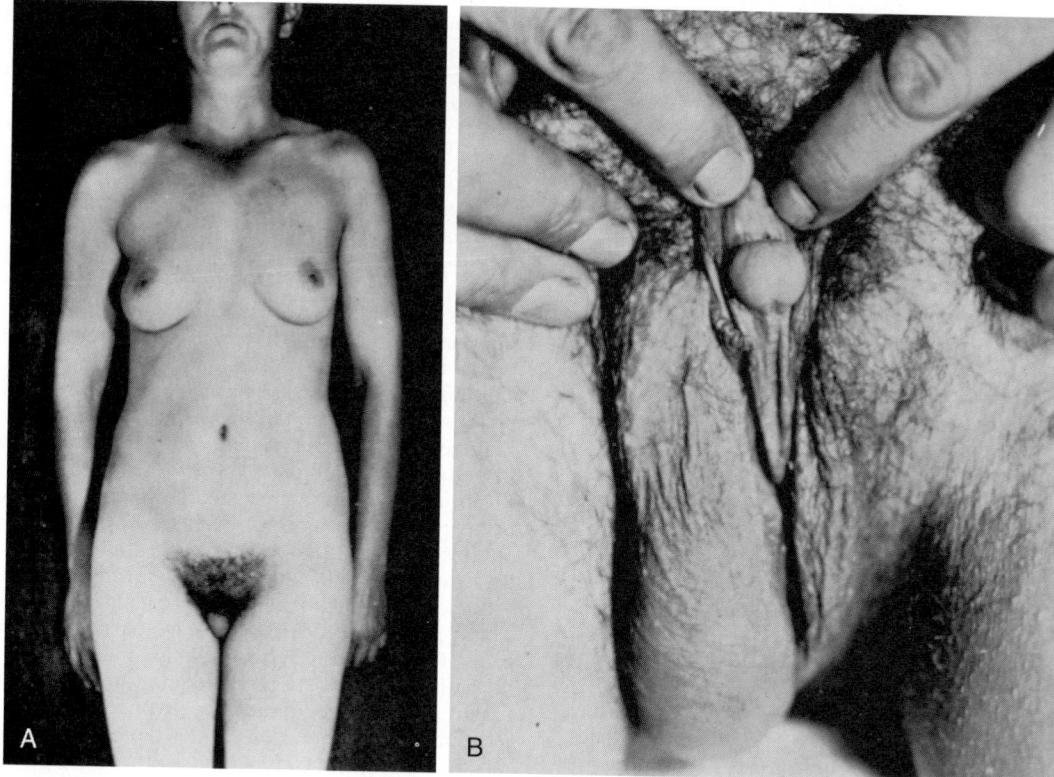

Figure 29–73. A patient with partial androgen resistance (Reifenstein's syndrome). Both the patient and his brother had hypospadias, poor masculinization, and marked gynecomastia. Both had a normal 46,XY karyotype, normal wolffian duct derivatives, and no müllerian structures. (Reproduced, with permission, from Bowen P, Lee CSN, Migeon CJ, et al. Hereditary male pseudohermaphroditism with hypogonadism, hypospadias, and gynecomastia [Reifenstein's syndrome]. Ann Intern Med 1965; 62:252–270. Courtesy of Dr. E. C. Reifenstein, Jr.)

published in older patients. An increased plasma level of AMH may be a useful marker of androgen resistance during the first year of life and after the onset of puberty.[996, 1017] The phallic response to a course of testosterone has been used as a predictive test of androgen responsiveness and future phallic growth, but in some cases the results have been equivocal and a neonatal response has not been invariably followed by a response at puberty.[1018] Studies of the binding of DHT in fibroblasts cultured from genital skin may show quantitative and/or qualitative deficits in the androgen receptor, and molecular analysis of the *AR* gene (e.g., by exon-specific amplification using PCR, SSCP, and nucleotide sequence analysis) has been used for the definitive diagnosis of androgen receptor defects.[1019] However, these studies are labor intensive and require specialized laboratories that are not universally available. A promising new approach, currently undergoing evaluation, is the delivery of an androgen-responsive reporter gene into a culture of genital skin fibroblasts from affected individuals to assess the function of the androgen receptor.[1016]

There is no specific therapy for partial androgen resistance. However, some patients respond at least partially to high-dose androgen therapy.[1020, 1021] The sex of rearing depends on the age at diagnosis and the degree of genital ambiguity. In view of the limited response to testosterone in patients with this condition and the appearance of gynecomastia at puberty, it may be prudent to raise many of the patients with partial androgen resistance who have ambiguous genitalia as females. In patients assigned a female gender identity, surgical repair of the genitalia and gonadectomy are indicated before 6 months of age. At the age of puberty, estrogen replacement therapy should be initiated.

DEFECTS IN TESTOSTERONE METABOLISM BY PERIPHERAL TISSUES: STEROID 5α-REDUCTASE TYPE 2 DEFICIENCY (MALE PSEUDOHERMAPHRODITISM WITH VIRILIZATION AT PUBERTY).

In 1961 Nowakowski and Lenz[1022] described a familial type of male pseudohermaphroditism, which they termed "pseudovaginal perineoscrotal hypospadias," that was transmitted as an autosomal recessive trait.[1023] The patients resemble those with other forms of male pseudohermaphroditism by having a 46,XY karyotype, normally differentiated testes, male internal ducts, and ambiguous external genitalia. At puberty, striking but selective signs of masculinization appear.

In 1974 Walsh and associates[1024] and Imperato-McGinley and colleagues[1025–1028] reported a defect in the conversion of testosterone to its 5α-reduced metabolite DHT in patients with this syndrome (Fig. 29–74). Imperato-McGinley described a genetic isolate from villages in the southwestern part of the Dominican Republic. In 24 families, 38 male pseudohermaphrodites were identified, 24 of whom were postpubertal[1026] (Table 29–32). The classic features of this form of male pseudohermaphroditism in infancy include a clitoris-like, hypospadiac phallus bound in chordee of variable degree, a bifid scrotum, and a urogenital sinus that opens on the perineum. A blind vaginal pouch opens either into the urogenital sinus or onto the perineum behind the urethral orifice. The testes are well differentiated and are located in the inguinal canal or the labioscrotal folds. No müllerian structures are present. The wolffian structures (epididymis, vas deferens, and seminal vesicle) are well differentiated; the ejaculatory ducts usually terminate in the blind vaginal pouch. If a vaginal pouch is not present, the wolffian ducts terminate on the perineum next to the urethra. The prostate is hypoplastic. At puberty, plasma testosterone levels increase into the adult male range, whereas DHT levels remain disproportionately low but measurable. Affected males virilize to a variable degree without gynecomastia: the voice deepens; muscle mass increases; the phallus, although bound in chordee of variable severity, enlarges to 4

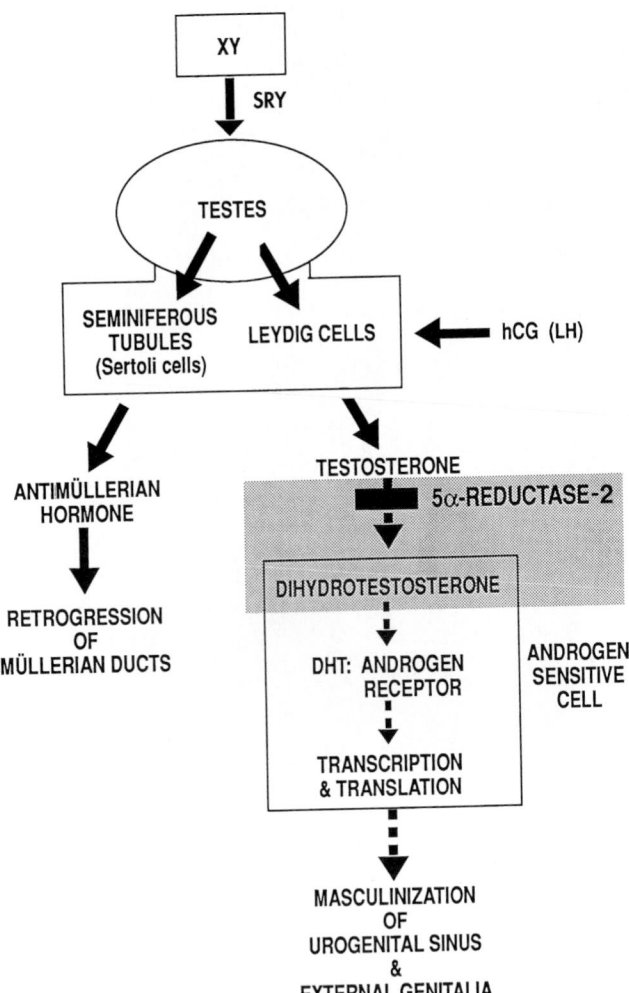

Figure 29–74. A diagrammatic scheme of male pseudohermaphroditism resulting from 5α-reductase deficiency.

to 8 cm in length; libido ensues; and penile erections occur.[238, 1029] The bifid scrotum becomes rugated and pigmented, and the testes enlarge and descend into the labioscrotal folds. However, none of the postpubertal affected males have acne, more than sparse facial or body hair, temporal hair recession, or enlargement of the prostate. Histologic examination of the adult testes in affected males shows Leydig cell hyperplasia

TABLE 29–32. Clinical Features of 5α-Reductase-2 Deficiency

Karyotype:	46,XY
Inheritance:	Autosomal recessive; mutations in *SRD5A2* gene
Genitalia:	Usually ambiguous with small, hypospadiac phallus; blind vaginal pouch
Wolffian duct derivatives:	Normal
Müllerian duct derivatives:	Absent
Gonads:	Normal testes
Habitus:	Partial virilization at puberty without gynecomastia; decreased facial and body hair, no temporal hair recession; prostate not palpable
Hormone profile:	Decreased ratio of 5α/5β C_{21}- and C_{19}-steroids in urine; increased plasma testosterone/dihydrotestosterone (T/DHT) ratio before and after hCG stimulation; modest increase in plasma LH and decreased conversion of T to DHT in vivo

and decreased spermatogenesis.[1030, 1031] In general, spermatogenesis is either absent or profoundly impaired.[1030, 1031] Semen analyses of nine patients with 5α-reductase-2 deficiency from the Dominican cohort revealed normal sperm concentration, total count, and mobility in one patient with hypospadias and bilaterally descended testes and in a second patient after hypospadias repair.[1031] Semen volume and viscosity were abnormal in all nine patients. The finding of a normal sperm count and concentration in a male with 5α-reductase-2 deficiency suggests that DHT, in contrast to testosterone, does not play a major role in spermatogenesis.[1031, 1031a]

As with other forms of male pseudohermaphroditism, phenotypic variability has been described both within and between cohorts.[237] Approximately 55% of patients have had a pseudovagina; the rest have a urogenital sinus, a hypospadiac phallus, or even a microphallus with a penile urethra.[1032–1035] Eighteen of 19 46,XY patients with 5α-reductase-2 deficiency from the Dominican cohort who were raised "unambiguously" as females changed their gender identity and gender role behavior to male after the onset of puberty (Fig. 29–75).[272] Similar observations were reported in 19 of 40 families with 5α-reductase-2 deficiency, as well as in male pseudohermaphrodites with 17β-HSD deficiency or XO/XY mosaicism.[238, 1036] This phenomenon appears to be particularly prevalent, although not exclusively so, in 46,XY male pseudohermaphrodites whose gonads are retained and who produce testosterone that results in masculinization at puberty.[1037] These patients raise provocative questions about the effect of sex of rearing, social and cultural factors, and learning on psychosexual development. Another genetic isolate of individuals deficient in 5α-reductase-2 was described from New Guinea by Herdt and Davidson.[275] As in the Dominican cohort, a third category of sex was identified in this cultural isolate, the so-called "Turnim man." However, sex reversal at puberty has not been as com-

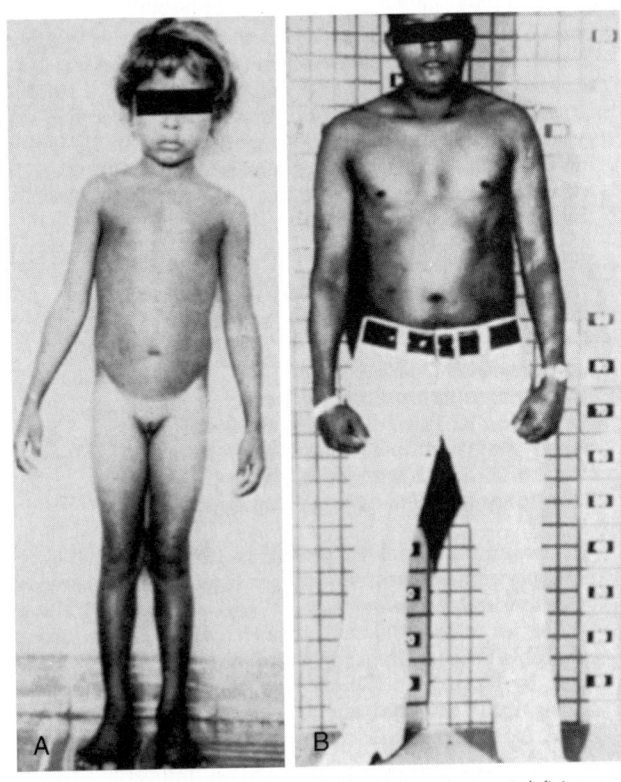

Figure 29–75. *A,* A prepubertal 46,XY child with 5α-reductase-2 deficiency who was raised as a female. *B,* A postpubertal male with 5α-reductase-2 deficiency who has virilized and changed gender role behavior. (From Peterson RE, Imperato-McGinley J, Gautier T, et al. Male pseudohermaphroditism due to 5α-steroid deficiency. Am J Med 1977; 62:170–191.)

mon in this cultural isolate as in others, where the sex reversal appears to be in part a consequence of social and cultural pressure rather than solely a sex hormone effect on behavior.[275]

Females homozygous for 5α-reductase-2 deficiency are phenotypically normal and undergo normal pubertal maturation except for delayed menarche.[1036, 1038, 1039] They have an absence of hair on the arms and legs and decreased axillary and pubic hair, which suggests an important effect of DHT on the growth of body hair.[1039] Fertility is normal, and two of the three homozygous females studied in the Dominican kindred gave birth to nonidentical twins, which suggests a role for DHT in the regulation of ovarian follicular maturation[1039]; the human ovary has 5α-reductase-2 activity.

In infancy and childhood, patients with 5α-reductase-2 deficiency have normal to elevated plasma concentrations of testosterone and decreased levels of DHT after the administration of hCG.[238, 1024, 1040] In affected postpubertal patients, the testosterone/DHT ratio in peripheral blood is increased from 12 ± 31 (mean $\pm$ SD) to 35 to 84.[1040] Postpubertally, plasma LH levels are either normal or slightly elevated; plasma FSH levels are elevated in about 50% of patients.[238] Studies of estrogen and androgen synthesis demonstrate normal male androgen and estrogen production; this explains the lack of gynecomastia postpubertally in these patients, compared with patients with partial androgen resistance.[238, 1028] Additional biochemical features of 5α-reductase-2 deficiency are a diminished ratio of urinary 5α- to 5β-reduced C_{19}- and C_{21}-steroids and deficient or abnormal 5α-reductase-2 activity in fibroblasts cultured from genital skin.[238, 1028] Heterozygotes for 5α-reductase-2 deficiency have no clinical manifestations and have intermediate ratios of urinary 5α-reduced to 5β-reduced C_{19}-steroids (e.g., androsterone/etiocholanolone).[238]

Genetics. The disorder is transmitted as an autosomal recessive trait. There are two steroid 5α-reductase enzymes.[1041-1043] Both isozymes, which share 50% homology, are located in microsomes and catalyze the NADPH-dependent conversion of testosterone to the more androgenic DHT.[1043] Steroid 5α-reductase-1 is encoded by a gene located on chromosome 5p15[1042]; the gene, *SRD5A1*, has 5 exons and 4 introns and encodes a protein with a neutral to basic pH optimum.[1043] It is expressed at birth in the liver and nongenital skin.[1043, 1044] Although the expression of the type 1 enzyme persists in the liver throughout postnatal life,[1043] its expression decreases in skin to unmeasurable levels after 2 to 3 years of age and remains low until puberty, when it is again present in nongenital skin, especially the sebaceous glands of the scalp.[1043] No mutations in the type 1 gene have as yet been described.

Steroid 5α-reductase-2 is encoded by the *SRD5A2* gene on chromosome 2 in band p23[1042] which, like the type 1 gene, contains 5 exons and 4 introns. The type 2 isozyme has a lower Michaelis constant (K_m) for testosterone than the type 1 does; 5α-reductase-2 has an acidic pH optimum and is more sensitive to inhibition by finasteride.[238, 1043] Most of the 5α-reductase activity in the early fetus is caused by the type 2 enzyme.[1044] It is expressed in the primordia of the prostate and external genitalia before their differentiation,[1044] but it is not expressed in the embryonic wolffian duct until after the differentiation of the epididymides, vas deferens, and seminal vesicles, which are induced by testosterone and not by DHT.[227] Type 2 expression increases in liver and nongenital skin at birth.[1044] It persists in the liver throughout life but diminishes to unmeasurable levels in nongenital skin after 3 years of age. A pseudogene has been mapped to the long arm of the X chromosome at band q24-qter.[1045]

Steroid 5α-reductase-2 deficiency is inherited as an autosomal recessive trait and is genetically heterogenous. More than 40 mutations have been detected in the gene (Fig. 29–76).[238, 1029, 1034-1036, 1046] In most patients, missense mutations cause amino acid substitutions.[238, 1029, 1034-1036, 1046] Less commonly, deletions, splice junction, and nonsense mutations are described. The mutations are distributed throughout the coding region of the gene. In general, mutations involving the 3′ end of the gene and the COOH terminus of the enzyme are associated with a decrease in the affinity for the cofactor NADPH, whereas mutations that affect the binding of testosterone involve exons that encode either the NH_2- or COOH-terminal ends of the enzyme.[238, 1043] DNA analysis indicates that approximately 75% of patients are homozygous for a mutation and 25% are compound heterozygotes. Consanguinity has been described in approximately 40% of patients.[1042] The occurrence of the disorder in three genetic isolates in the Dominican Republic (Arg246Trp), the Sambia tribe of the New Guinea highlands (deletion of the *SRD5A2* gene),[1047] and cohorts in Turkey is probably the result of a "founder effect."[238] However, the detection of similar mutations in patients from all over the world suggests the presence of mutational "hot spots" in the type 2 gene.

The finding of two 5α-reductase genes with different tissue distributions and different temporal expressions has clarified the nature of the pubertal masculinization in this disorder, which contrasts with the failure of masculinization of the external genitalia during embryogenesis. Even patients with a deletion of the *SRD5A2* gene (null genotypes) have measurable levels of DHT at puberty, which is attributed to the conversion of testosterone to DHT in peripheral tissues by the expression of the type 1 enzyme in nongenital skin and liver at puberty. The masculinization at puberty can result from the increased plasma DHT levels as well as the chronic effect of adult levels of testosterone on the androgen receptor.

Diagnosis. The diagnosis of 5α-reductase-2 deficiency can be difficult, especially before the age of puberty. It should

Figure 29–76. Diagrammatic scheme of the gene encoding 5α-reductase-2 with representative mutations causing 5α-reductase-2 deficiency. The exons are the numbered black boxes. Missense mutations causing amino acid substitutions in the enzyme are indicated by the three-letter abbreviation for the wild-type amino acid, followed by the position number of the amino acid in the enzyme and the three-letter abbreviation for the substituted amino acid. X indicates a nonsense (stop) mutation. G→T nt725 + 1 is a splice junction mutation of guanine (G) to thymidine (T) one nucleotide downstream of the boundary between exon 4 and intron 4. Nucleotide 725 is the closest nucleotide in the exon to the mutation. A cohort of patients from New Guinea has been described with complete deletion of the 5α-reductase-2 gene. (Redrawn from Wilson JD, Griffin JE, Russell DW. Steroid 5α-reductase deficiency. Endocr Rev 1993; 14:577–593. © 1993, The Endocrine Society.)

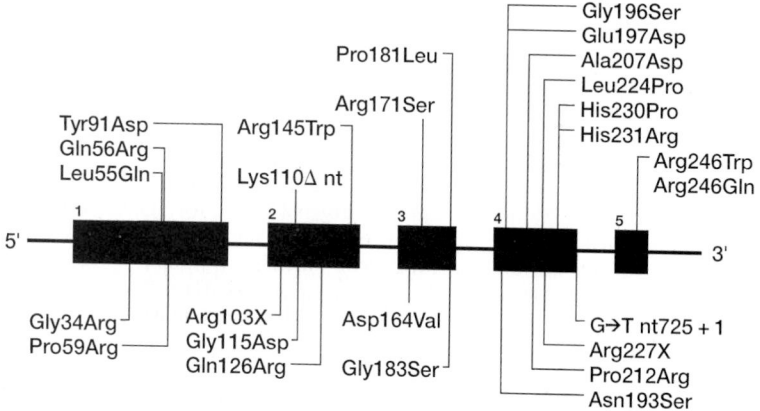

be suspected in all prepubertal male pseudohermaphrodites, especially those with perineoscrotal hypospadias with or without a blind vaginal pouch, in males with hypospadias and microphallus, and in male pseudohermaphrodites who virilize at puberty without evidence of gynecomastia. Virilization at puberty and the absence of gynecomastia in male pseudohermaphrodites are not unique to 5α-reductase-2 deficiency. For example, patients with 17β-HSD III deficiency or partial androgen resistance may present in this manner, but they can be distinguished biochemically or by DNA analysis from patients with 5α-reductase-2 deficiency. The diagnosis of 5α-reductase-2 deficiency can be confirmed prepubertally and postpubertally by demonstration of an abnormally high testosterone/DHT ratio in peripheral blood before and/or after hCG administration.[1032, 1033, 1040, 1048–1050] The testosterone/DHT ratio under basal conditions in postpubertal affected males is 35 to 84, whereas the ratio in normal men is 12 ± 3.1. In normal male infants, when plasma testosterone and DHT are detectable, the testosterone/DHT ratio ranges from 1.7 to 17 (mean ± SD, 4.9 ± 2.9).[1040] In view of the low levels of testosterone and DHT in prepubertal males, it is usually necessary to administer hCG (1500 U/m² IM every 24 h × 3) to demonstrate the defect. Patients with 5α-reductase-2 deficiency have high testosterone/DHT ratios after hCG administration. After a course of hCG, the ratio is 5.2 ± 1.5 SD in normal male infants (17 days to 6 months) and 11 ± 4.4 SD in normal prepubertal males (6 months to 14 years).[1040] Similarly, the ratio of 5α- to 5β-metabolites of testosterone in urine is a marker both prepubertally and postpubertally of 5α-reductase-2 deficiency.[1032, 1033, 1050] Using both basal and hCG-induced increases in testosterone level and urinary analyses of 5α- and 5β-steroid metabolites, Imperato-McGinley and co-workers detected 5α-reductase-2 deficiency in three infants between the ages of 1 and 3 months.[1051] Less readily available but more direct studies that can be used to confirm the diagnosis of 5α-reductase-2 deficiency include determination of the in vitro conversion of testosterone to DHT by genital skin fibroblasts[1028, 1052] and measurement of the blood production rate of DHT.[1028] 5α-Reductase-2 activity can be diminished in patients with other disorders, including the receptor-negative form of androgen resistance, porphyria, hypothyroidism, the low-triiodothyronine syndrome (e.g., anorexia nervosa, chronic illness), and Cushing's syndrome.[1028] DNA analyses of the SRD5A2 gene are both confirmatory and diagnostic.[1029]

Early diagnosis of 5α-reductase-2 deficiency is important because of its bearing on the assignment of sex in the affected infant. Although the majority of missense mutations in the SRD5A2 gene are associated with less than 0.4% of normal activity, mutations with 3 to 15% residual activity have been reported in 46,XY individuals with sufficient masculinization of the external genitalia at birth to be assigned a male gender.[1049, 1050] Masculinization in utero and the plasma testosterone/DHT ratio in early infancy correlate with the degree of residual 5α-reductase-2 activity.[1049] The natural history of patients with this deficiency—that is, the propensity in some patients for change to male gender role behavior and for virilization at puberty—makes male assignment of neonatally diagnosed patients appealing, especially in affected individuals with ambiguous or hypoplastic male genitalia.[1032, 1033, 1049] On the other hand, this decision usually necessitates extensive surgical repair as well as hormone therapy. Therapy with DHT should increase phallic length into the normal range for age and enable repair of hypospadias. However, DHT has not been generally available,[1053] and its long-term efficacy and safety have not been established.[1054] Carpenter and co-workers[1055] described a 9-month-old infant with 5α-reductase-2 deficiency who had been assigned a male gender at birth. The genitalia exhibited penoscrotal hypospadias with a phallus 1.9 cm in length and bound down in chordee. The testes were normal

and in the scrotum. No müllerian structures were present on pelvic sonography. Therapy was instituted with DHT, 25 mg/d (2% by weight in a cold cream base), applied to the patient's abdomen. The plasma DHT level 12 h after application was 2.0 nmol/L (58 ng/dL), which is within the normal adult male range.[1055] Four months of therapy resulted in an increase of stretched phallus length from 1.8 to 3.8 cm. No advancement in bone maturation was noted. Hypospadias repair was undertaken, and a second course of DHT was given without consequence.[1055] The authors' experience with males with microphallus suggests that it would be prudent to maintain the phallic length at or above the 50% range for age by using additional short courses of DHT until the onset of puberty and spontaneous phallus development. In adults with 5α-reductase-2 deficiency, supraphysiological doses of testosterone have resulted in normal DHT levels and partial masculinization[1020]; the conversion to DHT is mediated by the type 1 5α-reductase isozyme. In patients reared as females, gonadectomy before puberty, plastic repair of genitalia, and estrogen replacement at an age appropriate for puberty are indicated.

Dysgenetic Male Pseudohermaphroditism (Ambiguous Genitalia Resulting from Dysgenetic Gonads)

Ambiguous development of the genital ducts, urogenital sinus, and external genitalia occurs in patients with dysgenetic gonads. They usually present with evidence of AMH deficiency as well as androgen deficiency and therefore have müllerian duct derivatives and ambiguous external genitalia. Mutations and deletions of any and all of the genes involved in the testes determination and differentiation cascade (see Fig. 29–15 and Table 29–4) have been implicated in the etiology of dysgenetic male pseudohermaphroditism. The differential diagnosis encompasses a spectrum of abnormalities of the Y chromosome as well as mosaicism involving a 45,X chromosome cell line and a cell line with Y-chromosome DNA which the authors have classified as "abnormalities of gonadal differentiation" (see sections on X-chromatin–negative variants of the syndrome of gonadal dysgenesis and familial and sporadic XY gonadal dysgenesis). These patients, all of whom have in common a defect in testes differentiation, can present with the clinical syndrome of "dysgenetic male pseudohermaphroditism"[1056, 1057] (Fig. 29–77).

Certain abnormalities of the X chromosome or an autosome are associated with dysgenetic male pseudohermaphroditism (see Fig. 29–15 and Table 29–4). Duplication of a locus in the Xp21 region can cause dysgenetic male pseudohermaphroditism as well as other extragenital anomalies and mental retardation[78, 1058] in 46,XY males with a functionally intact SRY gene.[581, 582] This locus, termed DSS (dosage-sensitive sex reversal), has been mapped to a 160-kb region of Xp21 and contains a gene DAX1 (DSS-AHC critical region on the X, gene 1) that is a putative candidate for DSS[3, 76, 77, 1059]; mutations in DAX1 cause X-linked congenital adrenal hypoplasia and hypogonadotropic hypogonadism. DAX1 encodes a protein with three and one half repeats of a motif that may be a DNA-binding domain.[76] The gene is expressed in the ovaries, testes, hypothalamus, and pituitary gland[1060] and has a steroidogenic factor (SF1) response element in its promoter.[1061] Mutations in DAX1 in XY males have no apparent effect on either the differentiation of the testes or male differentiation of the external genitalia; DNA analysis of 46,XY phenotypic females has failed to detect an abnormality in the DAX1 gene.[76] Duplication of DAX1 in transgenic XY or XX mouse embryos has not been studied as yet, so that the postulated identity of DAX1 and DSS is still to be demonstrated. Irrespective of the function of DAX1, deletion of the DSS region does not impair testicular determination and differentiation, but

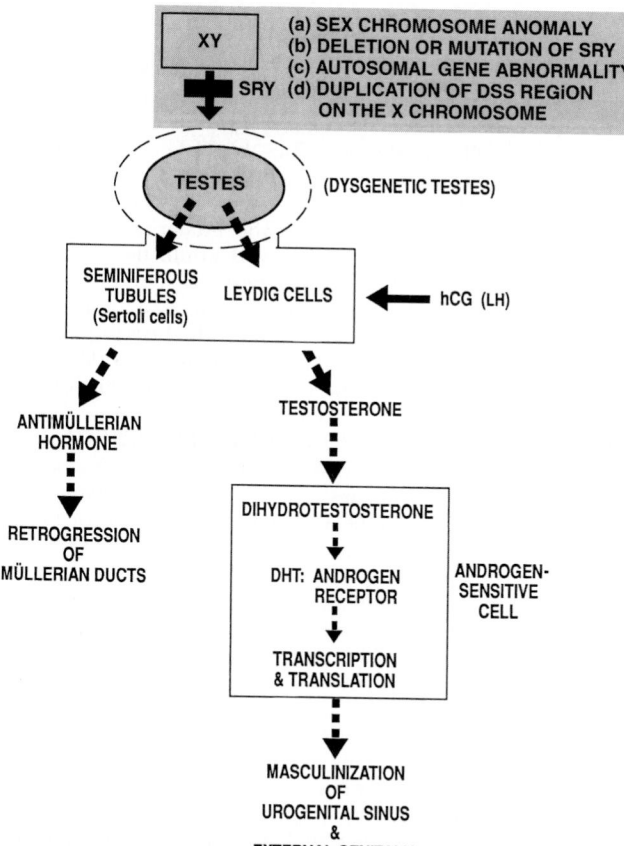

Figure 29–77. A diagrammatic representation of the pathogenesis of dysgenetic male pseudohermaphroditism. This condition can result from a sex chromosome anomaly or from a mutant gene in the male sex determination or differentiation cascade. The degree of masculinization is dependent on the functional ability of the dysgenetic gonads to produce antimüllerian hormone and testosterone.

duplications of *DSS* impair testicular differentiation and ovarian differentiation in 46,XY individuals. This observation has led to the suggestion that *DSS* is required for ovarian organogenesis and that it may function as a repressor of male differentiation.[78, 1059, 1062] Furthermore, it has been proposed that *SRY* may act as a repressor of DSS in the testis differentiation cascade (hence, *DSS* is a candidate for the putative testis repressor gene *Z*).[141, 1059]

46,XY dysgenetic male pseudohermaphroditism has been associated with mental retardation and α-thalassemia, the "ATR-X syndrome."[1063] Mutations in a gene called *XH2*, located at Xq13.3, that encodes a DNA helicase are described in patients with an atypical form of this syndrome.[1064] Terminal deletions at chromosome 10q (10q26-qter) and at 9p24-pter are associated with dysgenetic male pseudohermaphroditism and dysmorphic features.[160, 161, 1064a] The putative genes on these autosomes involved in testes development have not been ascertained.

Anomalies of the urinary tract are common in patients with abnormalities of genital differentiation.[1065] Less common is the association of dysgenetic male pseudohermaphroditism with congenital or early-onset renal disease (diffuse mesangial sclerosis) and Wilms' tumor (i.e., the Denys-Drash syndrome)[144, 1066] or with the childhood onset of renal disease and gonadal tumors (the Frasier syndrome).[1067, 1068]

Patients with Denys-Drash syndrome usually present in the newborn period with ambiguous genitalia, although both normal male and normal female genitalia have been reported.[1066] The karyotype is 46,XY, albeit affected 46,XX females with renal disease and normal genitalia have been re-

ported. Gonadal development in males varies from streak gonads to dysgenetic testes. The differentiation of the genital ducts varies depending on the functional status of the Sertoli cells of the gonads. Diffuse mesangial sclerosis, leading to renal failure, is seen on renal biopsy.[1066] Wilms' tumor occurs in the first decade of life, and 4% of patients with Denys-Drash syndrome develop a gonadoblastoma.[1066] Frasier and associates described a pair of 46,XY monozygotic twins with streak gonads and gonadoblastoma, one of whom developed renal failure[1067]; these patients may represent an entity separate from Denys-Drash syndrome.[1068] DNA analysis of patients with Denys-Drash syndrome has revealed heterozygous mutations of the Wilms' tumor suppressor gene (*WT1*) located on 11p13.[142–144, 1069, 1070] The *WT1* gene in patients with Frasier's syndrome appears to be normal.[1071] The *WT1* gene encodes a transcription factor with four Cys-Cys/His-His zinc fingers[143] which is expressed in the fetal kidney, gonad, and genital ridge.[142] Heterozygous mutations, mostly missense mutations, are most common in exon 9 of the *WT1* gene with Arg394Trp being the most frequent.[143, 170] Phenotypic variation is common with this mutation; some affected males exhibit ambiguous genitalia and others female external genitalia.[1071a] The majority of *WT1* mutations in Denys-Drash syndrome are de novo and appear to act as dominant negative mutations.[1072]

Heterozygous deletions of *WT1* and contiguous genes produce the WAGR syndrome (*W*ilms' tumor, *a*niridia [absence or malformation of the iris], *g*enitourinary abnormalities, and mental *r*etardation).[1073] The genitourinary anomalies in the WAGR syndrome include renal agenesis, horseshoe kidney, urethral atresia, hypospadias, and cryptorchidism,[1073] and they are usually less severe than those observed in the Denys-Drash syndrome. (A mutation or deletion of *WT1* has not been found in SRY-positive patients with dysgenetic gonads who do not have evidence of renal disease.[1074])

Heterozygous mutations of the autosomal *SOX9* gene cause campomelic dysplasia, often a lethal skeletal malformation, in which three fourths of affected 46,XY patients have dysgenetic male pseudohermaphroditism.[1075, 1076] The disorder has an incidence of 0.05 to 1.6 per 10,000 live births.[1076–1078] Manifestations include bowed long bones, hypoplastic scapula, a deformed pelvis, 11 pairs of ribs, a small thoracic cage, cleft palate, macrocephaly, micrognothia, hypertelorism, and a variety of cardiac and renal defects.[1076] Death from respiratory distress usually occurs in the neonatal period, but long-term survival has been reported.[1075, 1076] The external genitalia of affected 46,XY males varies from that of normal males with descended testes through ambiguous genitalia to female external genitalia, depending on the functional status of the fetal gonads.[1075, 1076, 1079] Affected 46,XX females have normal external genitalia and apparently normal ovarian function.[1076] Histologic examination of the gonads from 46,XY patients with ambiguous or female external genitalia showed varying degrees of testicular dysgenesis extending to streak gonads with primordial follicles.[1075, 1076, 1079]

Tommerup and co-workers[153] mapped the sex-reversal locus associated with campomelic dysplasia to 17q24.3-q25.1 from studies of three patients with balanced de novo reciprocal translocations. The break point in these patients was distal to the growth hormone locus and proximal to the thymidine locus on 17q.[153, 1080] Because the murine gene *Sox9* had been localized to a region in the murine genome that is homologous to 17q and this gene is expressed in skeletal tissue, the corresponding human gene *SOX9* was considered to be a candidate for campomelic dysplasia.[1081] Subsequently, missense, nonsense, frameshift, and splice junction mutations were detected in the *SOX9* gene in patients with campomelic dysplasia with or without gonadal dysgenesis.[154, 155] However, no correlation between the mutations and the gonadal phenotype (sex reversal) has been found.[1082] In one family, the same

SOX9 mutation resulted in siblings with campomelic dysplasia as a result of a germ-line mosaicism for a *SOX9* mutation in the father.[1083] However, the gonadal phenotype varied in the two 46,XY males from dysgenetic gonads to "normal" ovaries, and the affected 46,XX female had "normal" ovaries.[1083] In all patients studied, the mutation has been identified in only one *SOX9* allele (heterozygous), which suggests that both the campomelic dysplasia and sex reversal are caused by haploinsufficiency of the *SOX9* gene.[154, 1079] The absence of sex reversal in approximately one quarter of 46,XY individuals with campomelic dysplasia and in patients with translocations that involve break points in 17q more than 130 kilobases from the *SOX9* gene in which no mutations have been found is unexplained.

The *SOX9* gene has three exons and two introns,[154] the first of the *SOX* genes to have introns,[154] and encodes a 509-residue protein that localizes to the nucleus and contains an HMG box with 71% homology to that of the SRY protein.[2, 1084] The HMG box binds to the same DNA motif—AACAAAG—as other HMG transcription factors and transactivates transcription of a downstream target gene or genes.[1084] The transactivation function of *SOX9* appears to reside in the COOH-terminal domain of the protein.[1084] *SOX9* is expressed in the developing gonad, rete testis, and seminiferous tubule and in the mesenchyme that gives rise to skeletal tissue.[155, 156, 159] During chondrogenesis *SOX9* is coexpressed with *COL2A1*, the gene that encodes type II collagen[1084a]; the SOX9 protein binds to regulatory gene sequences in the *COL2A1* gene and regulates its expression.[1084b] It is apparent from the study of patients with campomelic dysplasia that *SOX9* is an integral part of testicular development cascade.

SF1. Steroidogenic factor-1 (SF1, or Ad4BP, adrenal 4 binding protein), a zinc-finger "orphan" nuclear receptor,[146, 1085, 1086] is a member of the steroid hormone/thyroid hormone receptor superfamily of transcription regulatory factors. SF1 is encoded by a gene on chromosome 9q33[1087] and binds to a DNA motif consisting of an estrogen receptor half-site, AGGTCA, and to nucleotides 5′ to this half-site.[1088] The presence of this motif in the promoters of CYP steroid hydroxylase genes, as well as in in vivo expression studies, suggests that SF1 is a key regulator of CYP steroidogenic enzymes in the adrenals and gonads.[146, 1085, 1086, 1089] However, in the placenta the expression of *CYP11A1* and other CYP steroidogenic genes occurs in the absence of expression of the *SF1* gene,[1090] as is the case in the central nervous system where neurosteroids are produced locally.[1091] The *SF1* gene is critical to the in vivo expression of AMH and the β-subunit of LH.[148, 1086, 1092]

Sf1 and the embryonal long terminal repeat binding protein (ELP, a protein that suppresses expression of Moloney murine leukemia virus in mouse undifferentiated embryonal carcinoma cells) are isoforms transcribed from the same gene by alternative promoter usage and splicing.[1086, 1092] Sf1/ELP is the mouse homologue of Drosophila FTZ-F1, a transcription factor that regulates the fushi-tarazu gene.[151, 1093, 1094] "Knockout" of the *Sf1* gene in mice causes complete absence of the adrenals and gonads.[152] All male and female knockout mice die of presumed adrenal insufficiency in the neonatal period.[152] The external genitalia are female in both XX and XY mice, müllerian duct derivatives are normally developed, and the ventromedial nucleus of the hypothalamus is aplastic or hypoplastic.[1095] The expression of *Sf1* in the developing gonad is sexually dimorphic. At 12.5 days of embryonic development, when the bipotential gonad develops into an ovary or testis in the mouse and before expression of the CYP steroidogenic genes, *Sf1* expression persists in the Leydig and Sertoli cells of the testes but is extinguished in the primordial ovary.[152]

In Sf1 knockout mice the genital ridges developed normally until 10.5 d after coitus and thereafter underwent apoptosis.[152] Therefore, Sf1 appears to play a critical role in the development of the adrenals, ovaries, testes, hypothala-

mus, and gonadotropes and in modulation of AMH and CYP steroidogenic enzymes. SF1 deficiency has not been described in humans as yet. As adduced from the "knockout" experiment in mice, one would expect the human without SF1 to manifest severe adrenal insufficiency in the neonatal period (Table 29–33). Plasma steroid values would be unmeasurable and corticotropin levels elevated, owing to absence of the adrenal glands. The external genitalia would be female in both XX and XY individuals, and the müllerian derivatives would be intact. Gonadal steroid levels would be unmeasurable in infancy and at the age of puberty because of gonadal absence. A key finding would be the absence of elevated gonadotropin levels in an agonadal individual during infancy and at puberty. The phenotype of mutations in the *SF1* gene would undoubtedly reflect the degree of impairment of SF1 function resulting from the mutation.

VANISHING TESTES SYNDROME (EMBRYONIC TESTICULAR REGRESSION SYNDROME). Various terms (XY gonadal dysgenesis, XY gonadal agenesis, rudimentary testis syndrome, congenital anorchia) have been used to describe the spectrum of genital anomalies resulting from cessation of testicular function during the middle phase of male sex differentiation, between 8 and 14 weeks of gestation. The authors first used the term *vanishing testes syndrome* for this form of male pseudohermaphroditism in 1957 because the genitalia in these cases suggested that the testes functioned initially and then "vanished" (for obscure reasons) at some time during the process of male sex differentiation.[163] These patients have a 46,XY karyotype. Gonadal elements are absent, and differentiation of the genital ducts, urogenital sinus, and external genitalia is variable. At one end of the spectrum is the group of 46,XY individuals with female external and internal genitalia in whom the deficiency of embryonic testicular function presumably occurred before 8 weeks of gestation.[1096] These individuals have either no gonads (46,XY agonadism) or streak gonads.[1096] Loss of function of the fetal testes at 8 to 10 weeks of gestation would lead to ambiguous genitalia and variable development of the genital ducts, from complete absence of both müllerian and wolffian ducts to partial development of either, a constellation referred to by some as the *XY gonadal agenesis syndrome*.[1097-1099] Loss of testicular function after the critical phase of male differentiation (about 12 to 14 weeks) results in anorchia, a syndrome characterized by normal male differentiation both internally and externally but no gonadal tissue. The presence of normal male genitalia and absence of müllerian duct derivatives implies that fetal testicular function was normal before its loss. Sporadic and familial forms of unilateral and bilateral anorchia, including monozygotic twins concordant and discordant for anorchia, have been described.[1100-1102] Fetal testicular insufficiency and incomplete regression of the fetal testes after 12 to 14 weeks would be expected to produce a syndrome similar to that described by Bergada and col-

TABLE 29–33. Features of Hypothetical Severe SF1 Deficiency in the Human*

Karyotype:	46,XY
Inheritance:	Autosomal recessive
Genitalia:	Female
Wolffian duct derivatives:	Absent
Müllerian duct derivatives:	Present
Gonads:	Absent
Habitus:	Severe adrenal insufficiency with "crisis" in early infancy
Hormonal profile:	Absent or low plasma glucocorticoids, mineralocorticoids and sex steroids; low gonadotropins despite absent gonads in infancy and at puberty

*Postulated from observations in mice with interrupted *Sf1* gene.

leagues,[1103–1105] that is, small, rudimentary testes with microphallus and male ejaculatory ducts.

The nature of the underlying defect, which in some cases leads to absence or regression of genital ducts as well as testes and in some cases other congenital anomalies, is not known.[1106, 1107] Several sibships with multiple affected individuals have been described. Josso and Briard[1108] reported on two siblings, one of whom was a normally differentiated male with microphallus and anorchia. The other sibling had a 46,XY karyotype but was raised as a female. She had a normal clitoris, fused labioscrotal folds, a single perineal opening that led into a urogenital sinus, and a vagina. At laparotomy, absent gonads with coexistent müllerian and wolffian structures were found. This patient's phenotype was compatible with a diagnosis of XY gonadal agenesis. Despite the absent gonads, the patients had distinct phenotypic differences in the internal and external genitalia. The coexistence of so-called XY gonadal agenesis and anorchia in the same sibship suggests that the disorders are related and are caused by embryonic testicular regression occurring at different stages of male development in utero; the familial cases support the operation of a rare, mutant gene in at least some patients with this syndrome.

The diagnosis of "true" anorchia (in contrast to the testicular regression syndrome with ambiguous external genitalia) can be suspected in normally differentiated males with bilateral cryptorchidism and elevated gonadotropin levels. It is infrequently familial. The authors have demonstrated a diphasic childhood pattern of gonadotropin levels in anorchic males similar to that seen in females with gonadal dysgenesis.[1109] In particular, plasma FSH levels are elevated in infancy, decrease into the normal range in middle childhood, and rise into the agonadal range after age 9 to 10 years. LHRH-induced increases in plasma FSH and LH concentrations are elevated throughout infancy and childhood. Hence, the LHRH test may be helpful diagnostically in middle childhood, when basal gonadotropin levels are normal. It has been proposed that the finding of elevated plasma FSH levels in conjunction with lack of a plasma testosterone response to hCG (1500 U/m² IM every 48 h × 7) establishes the diagnosis of anorchia and obviates the need for laparotomy.[1110] This approach has been called into question by the finding of testes at laparotomy in two prepubertal males in whom no testosterone response to hCG was elicited.[1111] Immunoassay of plasma AMH in infancy and childhood is a useful additional test to assess for the presence of a testis; the concentration of plasma AMH in anorchia is very low.[210, 211] Furthermore, CT or MRI, sonography, and laparoscopy are useful procedures for evaluation of the patient with suspected anorchia. The authors have cautiously deferred laparoscopic exploration of males with presumed "true" anorchia (phenotypic males with nonpalpable testes, elevated gonadotropin levels, and no rise in the plasma concentration of testosterone in response to hCG) until the time of insertion of prosthetic testes.

Defects in Synthesis, Secretion, or Response to Antimüllerian Hormone

PERSISTENT MÜLLERIAN DUCT SYNDROME (FEMALE DUCTS IN OTHERWISE NORMAL MEN; HERNIAE UTERI INGUINALE). AMH, a 148-kd glycoprotein homodimer, is secreted by the Sertoli cells of the testes beginning with differentiation of the fetal seminiferous tubules and continuing until pubertal maturation. AMH is not secreted by the fetal ovary,[210] but postnatally it is expressed in the granulosa cells of antral and preantral ovarian follicles.[210] AMH, a member of the transforming growth factor β (TGF-β) superfamily of growth and differentiation factors,[210, 1112] is processed intracellularly and secreted in its mature, bioactive form.[1113, 1114] It binds to a type II serine/threonine kinase receptor located in the mesen-

chyme surrounding the müllerian ducts before 8 weeks of gestation (when the müllerian ducts respond to AMH), causing epithelial-mesenchymal interaction, apoptosis of the müllerian duct epithelium, and regression of the müllerian duct.[210, 1115, 1116, 1116a] Studies in the bovine freemartin and in transgenic mice overexpressing AMH indicate that AMH can cause regression of germ cells in the ovary and reorganization of the ovary into cord-like seminiferous tubules and can inhibit CYP19 activity.[210, 217, 218] Five of 21 transgenic male mice that chronically expressed human AMH exhibited mammary gland development, arrested wolffian duct differentiation, and undescended testes.[217, 218] These observations suggest that high levels of AMH can impair Leydig cell function and steroidogenesis in the testes.[218] AMH levels are measurable in the normal male in plasma until pubertal maturation.[210]

AMH is encoded by a 2.75-kb gene containing five exons in the region of chromosome 19p13.3.[222] The gene has an upstream regulatory element, the estrogen response element, half-site AGGTCA type, to which SF1 binds to regulate AMH secretion.[1092, 1117]

The AMH receptor, a serine/threonine kinase with a single transmembrane domain, is a member of the family of type II receptors for TGF-β–related proteins.[1015, 1116a, 1118] The type II receptor binds ligand but requires the type I receptor for signal transduction.[1119] The AMH-II receptor is encoded by a gene that contains 11 exons.[1112, 1118] Exons 1 to 3 code for the signal sequence and the extracellular domain of the AMH receptor, exon 4 codes for the transmembrane domain, and exons 5 through 11 code for the intracellular serine/threonine domain.[1112, 1118] In addition to the mesenchyme surrounding the fetal müllerian ducts (but not the epithelial cells), this receptor is expressed in adult granulosa and Sertoli cells, which suggests a possible autocrine action of AMH in these cells.[1118]

A distinctive disorder, persistent müllerian duct syndrome (PMDS), has been described in which 46,XY men and boys have well-developed testes, normal male ducts and external genitalia, and müllerian duct derivatives[210, 1120–1123] (Fig. 29–78). The diagnosis often is not made until a Fallopian tube and uterus are encountered in patients undergoing inguinal hernia repair, orchiopexy, or abdominal surgery. Because of the trend for early surgical repair of an inguinal hernia or undescended testis, more cases are detected in infancy.[1124] There are two anatomic forms.[1123] In the more prevalent form, there is a hernia containing a partially descended or scrotal testis, and the ipsilateral tube and uterus are in the hernia.[1123] In some instances the contralateral testis and tube are present in the hernial sac as well. The presence of transverse testicular ectopia should suggest PMDS.[1123] In the second form, the uterus, tubes, and testes are in the pelvis.

PMDS is a heterogenous condition that is inherited in a sex-limited autosomal recessive manner. Females homozygous for null mutations in the *AMH* gene have normal müllerian ducts, external genitalia, and ovarian function, including fertility.[1125] Therefore *AMH* does not appear to play a critical role in ovarian differentiation or formation.

The retention of müllerian structures in normally differentiated males can result from failure of the testes to synthesize or secrete AMH or from a defect in the response of the duct to AMH—because of an AMH receptor defect or possibly an abnormality in the timing or secretion of the hormone.[1126, 1127] Mutations in the *AMH* gene can lead to absence of AMH as a cause of PMDS (Fig. 29–79).[210, 218, 1125, 1128] *AMH* mutations are most common in Mediterranean and Arab countries with high rates of consanguinity, and most familial mutations are homozygous; on the other hand, AMH type II receptor mutations are more common in France and Northern Europe and are often heterozygous mutations.[1129, 1130]

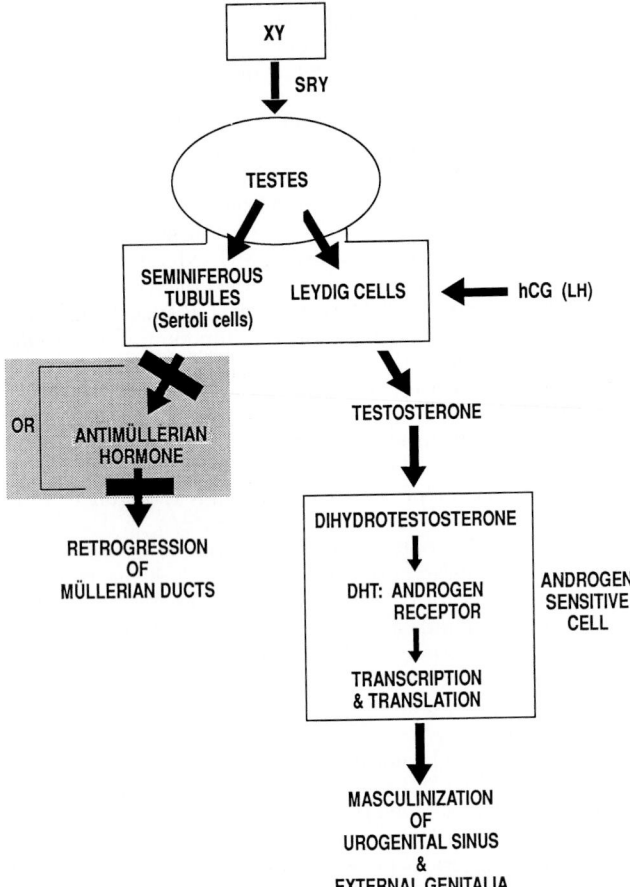

Figure 29–78. A diagrammatic representation of the pathogenesis of the persistent müllerian duct syndrome.

In an extensive study of 38 families, mutations in the *AMH* gene were detected in 16 families (see Fig. 29–79).[1125, 1129] Both homozygous and compound heterozygous mutations were found in affected families,[1125] including splicing, missense, nonsense, and deletion mutations affecting the whole gene but mainly exon 1 and the 3′ half of exon 5.[1125, 1129] In 16 families, deleterious mutations in the type II AMH receptor were detected, including deletion, missense, and nonsense mutations[1129] (Fig. 29–80). The most common mutation was a 27-base-pair deletion in exon 10, which was found on at least one allele in 10 out of 16 families and stands in contrast to the diverse mutations in the AMH gene.[1129] In the remaining six families, no abnormality in AMH or AMH receptor genes was detected. Patients with PMDS caused by mutations of the AMH gene have low or undetectable levels of serum AMH; in contrast, AMH concentrations are high normal or elevated in patients with mutations of the AMH receptor.[1131]

Treatment of PMDS is directed toward an attempt to ensure fertility in males, a difficult issue because of the anatomic findings. Testicular differentiation and function are normal in these patients, but an increased prevalence of testicular degeneration has been described, which is probably secondary to torsion of the testes.[1132] Anatomic abnormalities of the epididymis and the vas deferens are common. Infertility may result from late orchiopexy or from mechanical problems associated with entrapment of the vas deferens in the müllerian derivatives, which is usually present.[210, 1124] Early orchiopexy, proximal salpingectomy (leaving the epididymis attached to the fibrae of the fallopian tube), dissection of the vas deferens from the lateral walls of the uterus, and a complete hysterectomy are recommended as a useful surgical approach.[1123, 1124] Despite these recommendations, men with high pelvic testes rarely have successful orchiopexy, and many of these individuals are androgen deficient.[1133]

Maternal Ingestion of Progestagens and Estrogens

Progestagens and synthetic estrogens, alone or in combination, have been implicated as rare causes of male pseudohermaphroditism. Courrier and Jost[1134] in 1942 demonstrated an antiandrogen effect on the male fetus induced by a synthetic progestagen, ethisterone. Neumann and colleagues[226] observed that relatively high doses of progesterone or of synthetic progestagens impaired urethral groove fusion in fetal male rats. Aarskog[1135] reported on 130 patients with hypospadias who were studied retrospectively. A history of maternal ingestion of oral progestagens in early pregnancy was obtained in 11 cases. In six, the agent was administered for threatened abortion, and in five progestagen in combination with estrogens was given as a pregnancy test. Hypospadias occurred anywhere from the glans to the base of the penile shaft; the location correlated with the week of gestation in which therapy was initiated. Other studies have also suggested an association between progestagens and hypospadias,[1136, 1137] although this relation has been questioned.[1138]

Aarskog postulated that maternal progestagens may inhibit testosterone synthesis by the fetal testes or impair the reduction of testosterone to DHT at the target tissue and thereby lead to failure of urethral groove fusion and hypospadias. Some progestagens can inhibit 5α-reductase activity in vitro.[1139] Inhibition of this enzymatic activity at an early fetal stage (e.g., through placental transfer of drugs given to the mother), could impair masculinization of the male external genitalia. Alternatively, progestagens may bind to androgen receptors and impair androgen action.

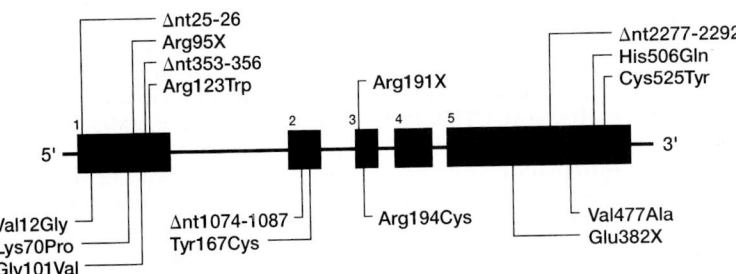

Figure 29–79. Diagrammatic representation of the mutations in the antimüllerian hormone gene that cause the persistent müllerian duct syndrome. Exons are the black numbered boxes. Mutations are indicated by the three-letter abbreviation for the wild-type amino acid in the protein and the three-letter abbreviation for the substituted amino acid or X for a nonsense (stop) mutation. Δnt25-26 is a deletion of nucleotides 25 and 26; Δnt353-356, Δnt1074-1087, and Δnt2277-2292 indicate similar deletions of the respective nucleotides. (Redrawn from Imbeaud S, Carré Eusebe D, Rey R, Belville C, Josso N. Molecular genetics of the persistent müllerian duct syndrome: a study of 19 families. Hum Mol Genet 1994; 3:125–131. By permission of Oxford University Press.)

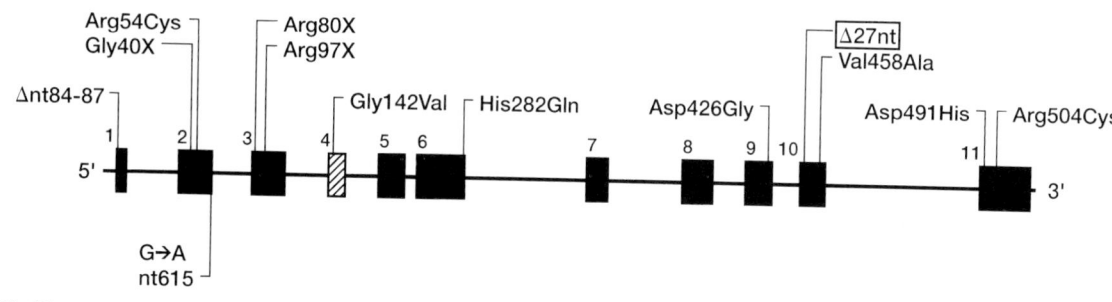

Figure 29–80. Diagrammatic representation of the mutations in the gene for the AMH receptor type II. Black numbered boxes are exons. Exons 1 to 3 encode the extracellular domain of the receptor. Exon 4 (diagonal lines) encodes the transmembrane domain, and exons 5 through 11 encode the intracytoplasmic domain. Mutations are indicated by the three-letter abbreviation for the wild-type amino acid, followed by the position number of the amino acid in the receptor protein and the three-letter abbreviation for the substituted amino acid or X for a nonsense (stop) mutation. Δnt84-87 designates a deletion/insertion at nucleotides 84-87. G→A nt615 is a guanine-to-adenine transition at nucleotide 615, which is at the splice site between exon 2 and intron 2. Δ27nt (open box) is a 27-nucleotide deletion, the most common mutation causing the AMH-positive form of the persistent müllerian duct syndrome, a mutation present in 25% of the patients studied with this form. (Redrawn from Imbeaud S, Belville C, Messike-Zeitoun L, Rey R, di Clemente N, Josso N, Picard J-Y. A 27 base-pair deletion of the anti-müllerian type II receptor gene is the most common cause of the persistent müllerian duct syndrome. Hum Mol Genet 1996; 5:1269–1277. By permission of Oxford University Press.)

Kaplan[1140] described male pseudohermaphroditism in a boy whose mother received large doses of diethylstilbestrol during early pregnancy. However, no additional reports of this association have appeared. Because of the report of Herbst linking maternal diethylstilbestrol therapy during pregnancy with vaginal and cervical adenocarcinoma in daughters, abnormalities in the genital tract have been sought in males.[1141] Increased incidences of meatal stenosis, epididymal cysts, hypoplastic testes, and abnormal semen have been observed, but hypospadias has not been reported.[1142, 1143]

Environmental Chemicals

An increase in the prevalence of disorders of the development and function of the male reproductive system, especially hypospadias and cryptorchidism, and in some European countries a fall in the sperm count and a rise in cancer of the testis, has occurred during the past 50 years.[1144, 1145] Some investigators have speculated that the increase in reproductive abnormalities observed in human males is related to an increase in the exposure in utero to exogenous estrogenic chemicals, so-called environmental estrogens, in the maternal diet, either as a natural occurrence or as a result of chemical contamination.[1144] Administration of diethylstilbestrol or the putative environmental estrogen, 4-octylphenol, to pregnant rats resulted in decreased expression of CYP17 mRNA and protein in Leydig cells of XY male offspring.[1146] Suppression of CYP17 may play a role in the putative adverse effect of environmental estrogens on fetal masculinization. The dichlorodiphenyltrichloroethane (DDT) metabolite p,p'-DDE (1,1-dicloro-2,2-bis (p-chlorophenyl) ethylene), unlike DDT itself, has little ability to bind to the estrogen receptor,[1147] but it binds to the androgen receptor and inhibits androgen action in the developing urogenital tract of rodents.[1147] In addition, the combination of four weakly estrogenic pesticides in a yeast model elicited an enormous increase in in vitro estrogenic activity, but this finding has not been confirmed.[1148–1150] Further studies on the levels and risks of natural and environmental estrogens and antiandrogens in humans are necessary before the putative increased prevalence of certain abnormalities of the reproductive tract can be attributed to these agents.

Unclassified Forms of Abnormal Sexual Development

Extraordinary advances in the understanding of male pseudohermaphroditism and its heterogeneity have been made since the first edition of this textbook. The major subgroups are now defined, and genetic defects in testosterone

biosynthesis, androgen action, and testis organogenesis are recognized. Nonetheless, some forms of male pseudohermaphroditism are not readily categorized, and their pathogenesis is obscure.

Sexual Abnormalities of Unknown Cause in Males

HYPOSPADIAS. Hypospadias, which may be defined as incomplete fusion of the penile urethra, is one of the common congenital anomalies. It has an estimated incidence of 4 to 8 per 1000 male births.[1024, 1145, 1151, 1152] As noted previously, the rate appears to have doubled in some countries in the 1970s and 1980s.[1144] Analysis of the family histories of patients with hypospadias revealed an increase in the occurrence of hypospadias in males in the pedigrees.[1153, 1154] This finding suggested a multifactorial mode of inheritance in some cases; the cause in most instances is unknown.[1151, 1154]

On theoretical grounds, incomplete masculinization of the external genitalia implies either subnormal Leydig cell function in utero, a mild degree of androgen resistance or of 5α-reductase-2 deficiency, or a transient, functional, timing-related abnormality in the availability or action of DHT on the primordia of the external genitalia.

Aarskog carried out a careful prospective study of 100 consecutive patients with hypospadias without other somatic anomalies, most of which were referred from a surgery clinic.[1155] One patient was a genetic female with virilizing CAH, five had sex chromosome abnormalities, one had the incomplete form of 46,XY gonadal dysgenesis, and nine were from pregnancies in which the mother had taken synthetic progestational agents during the first trimester.[1155] Thus, in 15% of the patients a pathogenetic mechanism was found or suspected. Both maternal cocaine use and environmental estrogens and antiandrogens have also been implicated in the development of hypospadias.[1144, 1145, 1156] Even though androgen receptor defects have been suggested to play a significant role in the origin of hypospadias,[1157–1159] androgen receptor defects are a rare cause of isolated hypospadias.[1160, 1161]

Hypospadias is a feature of many malformation syndromes, such as the Opitz syndrome.[1162] The cardinal manifestations of this syndrome are widely spaced eyes and hypospadias. This disorder is genetically heterogenous; an X-linked form involves a locus at Xp22, and an autosomal form involves a locus at 22q11.2.[1162] Hypospadias is also a feature of the hand-foot-genital syndrome in males.[1163] Limb anomalies include short first metacarpals, short distal phalanges of the thumbs, and a short great toe.[1163] A mutation in the *HOXA13* gene was detected in a pedigree with this syndrome.[1163]

270. Meyer-Bahlburg HFL. Hormones and psychosexual differentiation: implications for the management of intersexuality, homosexuality and transsexuality. Clin Endocrinol Metab 1982; 11:681–701.

271. Money J, Higham E. Sexual behavior and endocrinology (normal and abnormal). In: DeGroot LJ, Besser GM, Cahill GF Jr, et al., eds. Endocrinology. 2nd ed. Philadelphia: WB Saunders, 1989: 1848–1859.

271a. Money J. Hormones, hormonal anomalies and psychologic health care. In: Kappy MS, Blizzard RM, Migeon CJ, eds. Wilkins, The Diagnosis and Treatment of Endocrine Disorders in Childhood and Adolescence. Springfield, Illinois: Charles C Thomas, 1994: 1141–1178.

271b. Diamond M, Sigmundson K. Sex reassignment at birth. Arch Pediatr Adol Med 1997; 151:248–304.

272. Imperato-McGinley JL, Peterson MD, Gautier T, et al. Androgens and the evolution of male-gender identity among male pseudohermaphrodites with 5α-reductase deficiency. N Engl J Med 1979; 300:1233–1237.

273. García-Segura LM, Chowen JA, Párducz A, et al. Gonadal hormones as promoters of structural synaptic plasticity: cellular mechanisms. Prog Neurobiol 1994; 44:279–307.

274. Money J, Hampson JG, Hampson JL. An examination of some basic sexual concepts: the evidence of human hermaphroditism. Johns Hopkins Med J 1955; 97:301–319.

275. Herdt GH, Davidson J. The Sambia "Turnim-man": sociocultural and clinical aspects of gender formation in male pseudohermaphrodites with 5-alpha-reductase deficiency in Papua, New Guinea. Arch Sex Behav 1988; 17:33–55.

276. Ehrhardt AA, Epstein R, Money J. Fetal androgens and female gender identity in the early-treated adrenogenital syndrome. Johns Hopkins Med J 1968; 122:160–167.

277. Money J, Schwartz M, Lewis VG. Adult erotosexual status and fetal hormonal masculinization and demasculinization: 46,XX congenital virilizing adrenal hyperplasia and 46,XY androgen-insensitivity compared. Psychoneuroendocrinology 1984; 9:405–414.

278. Dittmann RW, Kappes ME, Kappes MH. Sexual behavior in adolescent and adult females with congenital adrenal hyperplasia. Psychoneuroendocrinology 1992; 17:153–170.

279. Kuhnle U, Bullinger M, Schwarz HP. The quality of life in adult female patients with congenital adrenal hyperplasia: a comprehensive study of the impact of genital malformations and chronic disease on female patients life. Eur J Pediatr 1995; 154:708–716.

280. Klinefelter HF Jr, Reifenstein EC Jr, Albright F. Syndrome characterized by gynecomastia, aspermatogenesis without a Leydigism and increased excretion of follicle-stimulating hormone. J Clin Endocrinol 1942; 2:615–627.

281. Jacobs PA, Strong JA. A case of human intersexuality having a possible XXY sex-determining mechanism. Nature 1959; 83:302–303.

282. Ford CE, Jones KW, Miller OH, et al. The chromosomes in a patient showing both mongolism and the Klinefelter syndrome. Lancet 1959; 1:709–710.

283. Hsueh WA, Hsu TH, Federman DD. Endocrine features of Klinefelter's syndrome. Medicine (Baltimore) 1978; 57:447–461.

284. Leonard JM, Paulsen CA, Ospina LF, et al. The classification of Klinefelter's syndrome. In: Vallet HL, Porter IH, eds. Genetic Mechanisms of Sexual Development. New York: Academic Press, 1978: 407–423.

285. Robinson A, Lubs HA, Bergsma D. Summary of clinical findings: profiles of children with 47,XXY, 47,XXX and 47,XYY karyotypes. Birth Defects 1979; 15:261–281.

286. Schwartz ID, Root AW. The Klinefelter syndrome of testicular dysgenesis. Endocrinol Metab Clin North Am 1991; 20:153–163.

287. Mandokim W, Gavla SS, Hofman RP, et al. A review of Klinefelter syndrome in children and adolescents. J Am Acad Child Adolesc Psychiatry 1991; 30:167–172.

288. Ratcliffe SG, Bancroft J, Axworthy D, et al. Klinefelter's syndrome in adolescence. Arch Dis Child 1982; 57:6–12.

289. Stewart DA, Netley CT, Park E. Summary of clinical findings of children with 47,XXY, 47,XYY and 47,XXX karyotypes. Birth Defects 1982; 18:1–5.

290. Robinson A, Bender BG, Linden MG. Summary of clinical findings in children and young adults with sex chromosome anomalies. In: Evans JA, Hamerton JL, Robinson A, eds. Birth Defect Original Article Series. Vol 26. New York: Wiley-Liss, 1991; 26:225–228.

291. Graham JM Jr, Bashir AS, Stark RE, et al. Oral and written language abilities of XXY boys: implications for anticipatory guidance. Pediatrics 1988; 81:795–806.

292. Bender B, Harmon RJ, Linden MG, Robinson A. Psychosocial adaptation of 39 adolescents with sex chromosome abnormalities. Pediatrics 1995; 96:302–308.

293. Klinefelter syndrome. Lancet 1988; 2:1316–1317 (editorial).

294. Nielsen J, Pelsen B. Followup 20 years later of 34 Klinefelter males with karyotype 47,XXY and 16 hypogonadal males with karyotype 46,XY. Hum Genet 1987; 77:188–192.

295. Schibler D, Brook CGD, Kind HP, et al. Growth and body proportions in 54 boys and men with Klinefelter's syndrome. Helv Paediatr Acta 1974; 29:325–333.

296. Illig R, Tolkdorf M, Murset G, et al. LH and FSH responses to synthetic LH-RH in children and adolescents with Turner's and Klinefelter's syndrome. Helv Paediatr Acta 1975; 30:221–231.

297. Ratcliffe SG. The sexual development of boys with the chromosome constitution 47,XXY (Klinefelter's syndrome). Clin Endocrinol Metab 1982; 11:703–716.

298. Salenblatt JA, Bender BG, Puck MH, et al. Pituitary-gonadal function in Klinefelter syndrome before and during puberty. Pediatr Res 1985; 19:82–86.

299. Sorenson K. Klinefelter's Syndrome in Childhood, Adolescence and Youth: A Genetic, Clinical, Developmental, Psychiatric and Psychological Study. Lancaster, UK: Parthenon, 1988.

300. Smals AHG, Kloppenberg WC, Bernard TJ. Effect of short and long term human chorionic gonadotropin (hCG) administration on plasma testosterone levels in Klinefelter's syndrome. Acta Endocrinol 1974; 77:753–764.

301. Wang C, Baker HWG, Burger HG, et al. Hormonal studies in Klinefelter syndrome. Clin Endocrinol 1975; 4:399–411.

302. Smals AHG, Kloppenborg PWC, Lequin RL, et al. The pituitary-thyroid axis in Klinefelter's syndrome. Acta Endocrinol 1977; 84:72–79.

303. Nielsen J. Diabetes mellitus in patients with aneuploid chromosome aberrations and in their parents. Humangenetik 1972; 16:165–170.

304. Geffner ME, Kaplan SA, Bersche N, et al. Insulin resistance in Klinefelter syndrome. J Pediatr Endocrinol 1987; 2:173–177.

305. Harnden DG, Maclean N, Langlands AO. Carcinoma of the breast and Klinefelter's syndrome. J Med Genet 1971; 8:460–461.

306. Sanchez AG, Villanueva AG, Redoudo C. Lobular carcinoma of the breast in a patient with Klinefelter syndrome: a case with bilateral, synchronous, histologically different breast tumors. Cancer 1986; 57:1180–1183.

307. Hasle H, Mellemgaard A, Nielsen J, et al. Cancer incidence in men with Klinefelter syndrome. Br J Cancer 1995; 71:416–420.

308. Chaussain J-L, Lemerle J, Roger M, et al. Klinefelter syndrome, tumor and sexual precocity. J Pediatr 1980; 97:607–609.

309. Nichols CR, Heerema NA, Palmer C, et al. Klinefelter syndrome associated with mediastinal germ cell neoplasms. J Clin Oncol 1987; 5:1290–1294.

310. Derenoncourt AN, Castro-Magana M, Jones KL. Mediastinal teratoma and precocious puberty in a boy with mosaic Klinefelter syndrome. Am J Med Genet 1995; 55:38–42.

311. Horowitz M, Wishart JM, O'Loughlin PD, et al. Osteoporosis and Klinefelter's syndrome. Clin Endocrinol 1992; 36:113–118.

312. Eil C. Case 13-1990: case records of the Massachusetts General Hospital. N Engl J Med 1990; 322:917–925.

313. Rauch A, Pfeiffer RA, Trautmann U, et al. A study of ten small supernumerary (marker) chromosomes identified by fluorescence in situ hybridization (FISH). Clin Genet 1992; 42:84–90.

314. Hook EB, Hamerton JG. The frequency of chromosome abnormalities detected in consecutive newborn studies: difference between studies. Results by sex and severity of phenotypic involvement. In: Hook EB, Porter IH, eds. Population Cytogenetics Studies in Humans. New York: Academic Press 1977: 63–79.

315. Rutgers JL, Scully RE. Pathology of the testis in intersex syndromes. Semin Diagn Pathol 1987; 4:275–291.

316. Grumbach MM, Blanc WA, Engle ET. Sex chromatin pattern in seminiferous tubule dysgenesis and other testicular disorders: relationship to true hermaphrodism and to Klinefelter's syndrome. J Clin Endocrinol Metab 1957; 17:703–736.

317. Fryns JP, Moerman PL, Kleczkowska A. Normal testicular histology in a mid-trimester 49,XXXXY fetus. Clin Genet 1995; 47:331 (letter).

318. Citoler P, Aechter J. Histology of testis in XXY-fetuses. In: Murken J-D, Stengel-Rutkowski S, Schwinger E, eds. Prenatal Diagnosis: Proceedings of the 3rd European Conference on Prenatal Diagnosis of Genetic Disorders. Stuttgart: Ferdinand Enke, 1979: 336–337.

319. Mikano K, Aguercif M, Hazeghi P, et al. Chromatin-positive Klinefelter syndrome. Fertil Steril 1968; 19:731–739.

320. Ferguson-Smith MA. The prepubertal testicular lesions in chromatin positive Klinefelter's syndrome (primarily micro-orchidism) as seen in mentally handicapped children. Lancet 1959; 1:219–222.

321. Ohno S. Control of meiotic processes. In: Troen P, Nankin HR, eds. The Testis in Normal and Infertile Men. New York: Raven Press, 1977: 1–33.

322. Ahmad KN, Dykes JRW, Ferguson-Smith MA, et al. Leydig cell volume in chromatin-positive Klinefelter's syndrome. J Clin Endocrinol Metab 1971; 33:517–520.

323. Cozzi J, Chevret S, Rousseaux S, et al. Achievement of meiosis in XXY germ cells: study of 543 sperm karyotypes from an XY/XXY mosaic patient. Hum Genet 1994; 93:32–34.

324. Rosenkranz VW. Klinefelter Syndrom bei Kindern von Frauen mit Geschlechtschromosomen-Anomalien. Helv Paediatr Acta 1965; 20:359–368.

325. Jacobs PA, Hassold TJ, Whittington E, et al. Klinefelter's syndrome: an analysis of the origin of the additional sex chromosome using molecular probes. Ann Hum Genet 1988; 52:147–151.

326. Ferguson-Smith MA, Mack WS, Ellis PM, et al. Parental age and the source of the X chromosomes in XXY Klinefelter's syndrome. Lancet 1964; 1:46.

327. Carothers AD, Filippi G. Klinefelter's syndrome in Sardinia and Scotland: comparative studies of parenteral age and other aetiological factors in 47,XXY. Hum Genet 1988; 81:71–75.

328. Griffin DK, Abruzzo MA, Millie EA, et al. Non-disjunction in human sperm: evidence for an effect of increasing paternal age. Hum Mol Genet 1995; 4:2227–2232.

329. Van Dop C, Burstein S, Conte FA, et al. Isolated gonadotropin deficiency in boys: clinical characteristics and growth. J Pediatr 1987; 111:684–692.

330. Zizka J, Balicek P. XXYY son of a triple-X mother. Humangenetik 1975; 26:159–160.

331. Jones KL, ed. Smith's Recognizable Patterns of Human Malformation: Genetic, Embryologic and Clinical Aspects. 4th ed. Philadelphia: WB Saunders, 1996.

332. Linden MG, Bender BG, Robinson A. Sex chromosome tetrasomy and pentasomy. Pediatrics 1995; 96:672–682.

333. Fraccaro M, Kaljser K, Lindsten J. A child with 49 chromosomes. Lancet 1960; 2:899–902.

334. Curts LM, Scheppers-Tijdink G, Wiegers A, et al. The 49,XXXXY syndrome: clinical and psychological findings in five patients. J Intellect Disabil Res 1990; 34:277–282.

335. Borghgraeff M, Fryns JP, Smeets E, et al. The 49,XXXXY syndrome: clinical and psychologic follow-up data. Clin Genet 1988; 33:429–434.

336. Sarto GE, Otto PG, Kuhn EM, et al. What causes the abnormal phenotype in a 49,XXXXY male? Hum Genet 1987; 76:1–4.

337. Leal CA, Belmont JW, Nachtman R, et al. Parental origin of the extra chromosomes in polysomy X. Hum Genet 1994; 94:423–426.

338. de la Chapelle A. The etiology of maleness in XX men. Hum Genet 1981; 58:105–116.

339. Perez-Palacios G, Medina M, Ullao-Aguirre, et al. Gonadotropin dynamics in XX males. J Clin Endocrinol Metab 1981; 53:254–257.

340. Boucekkine C, Toublanc JE, Abbas N, et al. Clinical and anatomical spectrum in XX sex reversed patients: relationship to the presence of Y specific DNA-sequences. Clin Endocrinol 1994; 40:733–742.

341. Ferguson-Smith MA, Cooke A, Affara NA, et al. Genotype-phenotype correlations in XX males and their bearing on current theories of sex determination. Hum Genet 1990; 84:198–202.

342. Miro R, Cabellin MR, Marsini S, et al. Mosaicism in XX males. Hum Genet 1978; 45:103–106.

343. Ferguson-Smith MA. X-Y chromosomal interchange in the aetiology of true hermaphroditism and XX Klinefelter's syndrome. Lancet 1966; 2:475–476.

344. de la Chapelle A, Koo GC, Wachtel SS. Recessive sex-determining genes in human XX male syndrome. Cell 1978; 15:837–842.

345. de la Chapelle A, Tippett PA, Wetterstrand G, et al. Genetic evidence of X-Y interchange in a human XX male. Nature 1984; 307:170–171.

346. Evans HJ, Buckton KE, Spowart G, et al. Heteromorphic X chromosomes in 46,XX males: evidence for the involvement of X-Y interchange. Hum Genet 1979; 49:11–31.

347. Magenis RE, Webb MJ, McKeon RS, et al. Translocation (X:Y) (p22:33; p11.2) in XX males: etiology of male phenotype. Hum Genet 1982; 62:271–276.

348. Guellaen G, Casanova M, Bishop C, et al. Human XX males with Y single-copy DNA fragments. Nature 1984; 307:172–173.

349. Muller U, La Lande M, Donlon T, et al. Moderately repeated sequences for the short arm of the human Y chromosome are present in XX males and reduced in copy number in an XY female. Nucleic Acids Res 1986; 14:1325–1340.

350. Affara NA, Ferguson-Smith MA, Tolmie J, et al. Variable transfer of Y specific sequences in XX males. Nucleic Acids Res 1986; 14:5375–5387.

351. Andersson M, Page DC, de la Chapelle A. Chromosome Y-specific DNA is transferred to the short arm of X chromosome in human XX males. Science 1986; 223:786–788.

352. Buckle VJ, Boyd Y, Fraser N, et al. Localization of Y chromosome sequences in normal and XX males. J Med Genet 1987; 24:197–203.

353. Kalaitzidakis M, Therialt A, Boyd E, et al. The destination of Y specific sequences in X-Y interchange males. Development 1987; 101(Suppl):195 (abstract).

354. Petit C, de la Chapelle A, Levilliers J, et al. An abnormal X-Y interchange accounts for most but not all cases of human XX maleness. Cell 1987; 49:595–602.

355. Rouyer F, Simmler MC, Page DC, et al. A sex chromosome rearrangement in a human XX male caused by Alu-Alu recombination. Cell 1987; 51:417–425.

356. de la Chapelle A. The Y chromosome and autosomal testes-determining genes. Development 1987; 101(Suppl):33–38.

357. Magenis RE, Casanova M, Fellous M, et al. Further cytologic evidence of Xp-Yp translocation in XX males using in situ hybridization with Y-derived probe. Hum Genet 1987; 75:228–233.

358. Muller U, Latt SA, Donlon T. Y specific DNA sequences in male patients with 46,XX and 47,XXX karyotypes. Am J Med Genet 1987; 28:393–401.

359. Stalvey JRD, Durbin EJ, Erickson RP. Sex vesicle "entrapment": translocation or nonhomologous recombination of misaligned Yp and Xp as alternative mechanisms for abnormal inheritance of the sex-determining region. Am J Med Genet 1989; 32:564–572.

360. Disteche CM, Casanova M, Saal M, et al. Small deletions of the short arm of the Y chromosome in 46,XY females. Proc Natl Acad Sci U S A 1986; 83:7841–7844.

361. Page DC, Fisher EMC, McGillivray B, et al. Additional deletion in sex determining region of human Y chromosome resolves paradox of X,t(Y:22) female. Nature 1990; 346:279–281.

362. Weil D, Wang I, Dietrich A, et al. Highly homologous loci on the X and Y chromosomes are hot-spots for ectopic recombinations leading to XX maleness. Nat Genet 1994; 7:414–419.

363. Sherer G, Schempp W, Baccichetti C, et al. Analysis of two 47,XXX males reveals X-Y interchange and maternal and paternal nondisjunction. Hum Genet 1989; 81:247–251.

364. Turner B, Fechner PY, Fuqua JS, et al. Combined Leydig cell and Sertoli cell dysfunction in 46,XX males lacking the sex determining region Y gene. Am J Med Genet 1995; 57:440–443.

365. Skordis NA, Stetka DG, MacGillivray MH, et al. Familial 46,XX males coexisting with familial 46,XX true hermaphrodites in same pedigree. J Pediatr 1987; 110:224–248.

366. Pereira ET, Cabral de Almeida JC, Gunha A, et al. Use of probes for ZFY, SRY, and the Y pseudoautosomal boundary in XX males, XX true hermaphrodites and an XY female. J Med Genet 1991; 28:591–595.

367. Kuhnle U, Schwarz HP, Löhrs U, et al. Familial true hermaphroditism: paternal and maternal transmission of true hermaphroditism (46,XX) and XX maleness in the absence of Y-chromosomal sequences. Hum Genet 1993; 92:571–576.

368. Engel E, Forbes AP. Cytogenetic and clinical findings in 48 patients with congenitally defective or absent ovaries. Medicine (Baltimore) 1965; 44:135–165.

369. Palmer CG, Reichman A. Chromosomal and clinical findings in 110 females with Turner syndrome. Hum Genet 1976; 35:35–49.

370. Hall JG, Sybert VP, Williamson RA, et al. Turner's syndrome. West J Med 1982; 137:32–44.

371. Rosenfeld R, Grumbach MM, eds. Turner Syndrome. New York: Marcel Dekker, 1990.

372. Hibi I, Takano K. Basic and Clinical Approach to Turner Syndrome. Amsterdam: Elsevier Science Publishers BV, 1993.

373. Lippe BM. Turner syndrome. In: Sperling M, ed. Pediatric Endocrinology. Philadelphia: WB Saunders, 1996: 384–421.

374. Albertsson-Wikland K, Ranke MB. Turner syndrome in a life span perspective: research and clinical aspects. Amsterdam: Elsevier Science BV, 1995.

375. Ford CE, Jones KW, Polani PE, et al. A sex chromosome anomaly in a case of gonadal dysgenesis (Turner's syndrome). Lancet 1979; 1:711–713.

376. Virdis R, Cantu MC, Ghizzoni L, et al. Blood pressure behavior and control in Turner syndrome. Clin Exp Hypertens 1986; 8:787–791.

377. Money J, Alexander D, Ehrhardt A. Visual constructional deficit in Turner's syndrome. J Pediatr 1966; 69:126–127.

378. Bender B, Puck M, Sallenblatt J, et al. Cognitive development of unselected girls with complete and partial X monosomy. Pediatrics 1984; 73:175–182.

379. Garron DC. Intelligence among persons with Turner's syndrome. Behav Genet 1977; 7:105–127.

380. Downey JI, Ehrhardt AA. The long-term behavior of patients with Turner syndrome—an update. In: Rosenfeld RG, Grumbach MM, eds. Turner Syndrome. New York: Marcel Dekker, 1990: 483–490.

381. Sybert VP. The adult patient with Turner syndrome. In: Albertsson-Wikland K, Ranke M, eds. Turner Syndrome in a Life Span Perspective: Research and Clinical Aspects. Amsterdam: Elsevier Science BV, 1995, pp 205–218.

382. Swillen A, Fryns JP, Kleczkowska A, et al. Intelligence, behavior and psychosocial development in Turner syndrome: A cross sectioned study of 50 pre-adolescent and adolescent girls (4–20 years). Genet Couns 1993; 4:7–18.

383. Rovet J, Ireland L. Behavioral phenotype in children with Turner syndrome. J Pediatr Psychology 1994; 19:779–790.

384. McCauley E, Ross JL, Kushner H, Cutler G Jr. Self-esteem and behavior in girls with Turner syndrome. J Dev Behav Pediatr 1995; 16:82–88.

384a. Skuse DH, James RS, Bishop DVM, et al. Evidence from Turner's syndrome of an unprinted X-linked locus affecting cognitive function. Nature 1997; 387:705–708.

385. Pavlidis K, McCauley E, Sybert VP. Psychosocial and sexual functioning in women with Turner syndrome. Clin Genet 1995; 47:85–89.

386. Sylven L, Magnusson C, Hagenfeldt K, von Schoultz B. Life with Turner's syndrome: a psychosocial report from 22 middle-aged women. Acta Endocrinol 1993; 129:188–194.

387. Gordon RR, O'Neill EM. Turner's infantile phenotype. Br Med J 1969; 1:483–485.

388. Singh RF, Carr DH. The anatomy and histology of XO human embryos and fetuses. Anat Rec 1966; 155:369–384.

389. van der Putte SCJ. Lymphatic malformation in human fetuses: a study of fetuses with Turner's syndrome or status Bonnevie-Ullrich. Virchows Arch [A] 1977; 376:233–246.

390. Boyd PA, Anthony M, Mannning N, et al. Antenatal diagnosis of cystic hygroma or nuchal pad: Report of 92 cases with follow up survivors. Arch Dis Child Fetal Neonatal Ed 1996; 74:F38–F42.

391. Shephard TH, Fantel AG. Pathogenesis of congenital defects associated with Turner's syndrome: the role of hypoalbuminemia and edema. Acta Endocrinol 1986; 113(Suppl 279):440–447.

392. Clark EB. Web neck and congenital heart defects: a pathogenic association in 45XO Turner syndrome? Teratology 1984; 29:355–361.

393. Lacro RV, Jones KL, Benirschke K. Coarctation of the aorta in Turner syndrome: a pathologic study of fetuses with nuchal cystic hygromas, hydrops fetalis, and female genitalia. Pediatrics 1988; 81:445–451.

394. Gøtzsche CO, Krag-Olsen B, Nielsen J, et al. Prevalence of cardiovascular malformations and association with karyotypes in Turner's syndrome. Arch Dis Child 1994; 71:433–436.

a Life Span Perspective: Research and Clinical Aspects. New York: Marcel Dekker, 1990: 37–54.

517. Hoo JJ. A note on the Xp−. Hum Genet 1979; 50:339–40.

518. Herva R, Kaluzewski B, de la Chapelle A. Inherited interstitial del(Xp) with minimal consequences: with a note on the location of genes controlling phenotypic features. Am J Med Genet 1979; 3:43–58.

519. Kalousek D, Schiffrin A, Berguer A-M, et al. Partial short arm deletions of the X chromosome and spontaneous pubertal development in girls with short stature. J Pediatr 1979; 94:891–894.

520. Fryns JP, Petit P, Van den Berghe H. The various phenotypes in Xp deletion: observation in eleven patients. Hum Genet 1981; 57:385–387.

521. Wilson MG, Modebe O, Towner JW, et al. Ullrich-Turner syndrome associated with interstitial deletion of Xp11.4p22.31. Am J Med Genet 1983; 14:567–576.

522. Leichtman DA, Schmickel RD, Gelehrter TD, et al. Familial Turner syndrome. Ann Intern Med 1978; 89:473–476.

523. Geerkens C, Just W, Vogel W. Deletions of Xq and growth deficit: a review. Am J Med Genet 1994; 50:105–113.

524. Maraschio P, Tupler R, Barbierato L, et al. An analysis of Xq deletions. Hum Genet 1996; 97:375–381.

525. Mirzayants GG, Baranovskaya LI. X-X translocation in a patient with gonadal dysgenesis and the problem of phenotypic-karyotypic correlations. Hum Genet 1978; 40:249–257.

526. Madan K. Balanced structural changes involving the human X: effect on sexual phenotype. Hum Genet 1983; 63:216–221.

527. Schmidt M, Du Sart D. Functional disomies of the X chromosome influence the cell selection and hence X inactivation pattern in females with balanced X-autosome translocation: a review of 122 cases. Am J Med Genet 1992; 42:161–169.

528. Zah W, Kalderon HE, Tucci JR. Mixed gonadal dysgenesis. Acta Endocrinol report 1975; 79(Suppl 197):3–39.

529. Donahoe PK, Crawford JD, Hendren WH. Mixed gonadal dysgenesis, pathogenesis and management. J Pediatr Surg 1979; 14:287–300.

530. Akin JW, Tho SPT, McDonough PG. Reconsidering the difference between mixed gonadal dysgenesis and true hermaphroditism. Adolesc Pediatr Gynecol 1993; 6:102–104.

531. Robboy SJ, Miller T, Donahoe PK, et al. Dysgenesis of testicular and streak gonads in the syndrome of mixed gonadal dysgenesis: perspective derived from clinicopathologic analysis of 21 cases. Hum Pathol 1982; 13:700–716.

532. Wheeler M, Peakman D, Robinson A, et al. 45X/46XY mosaicism: contrast of prenatal and postnatal diagnosis. Am J Med Genet 1988; 29:565–571.

533. Chang HJ, Clark RD, Bachman H. The phenotype of 45,X/46,XY mosaicism: an analysis of 92 prenatally diagnosed cases. Am J Med Genet 1990; 46:156–168.

534. Hsu LYF. Phenotype/karyotype correlations of Y chromosome aneuploidy with emphasis on structural aberrations in postnatally diagnosed cases. Am J Med Genet 1994; 53:108–140.

535. Bonaventura L, Roth LM, Cleary RE. The Sertoli cell in mixed gonadal dysgenesis. Obstet Gynecol 1979; 53:324–329.

536. Simpson JL. Male pseudohermaphroditism: genetics and clinical delineation. Hum Genet 1978; 44:1–49.

537. Müller J, Skakkeback NE, Ritzen M, et al. Carcinoma in situ of the testis in children with 45,X/46,XY gonadal dysgenesis. J Pediatr 1985; 106:431–436.

537a. Müller J, Ritzen M, Rujpert-De Meyts E, et al. Management of males with 45,X/46,XY gonadal dysgenesis. 5th Joint Meeting of the European Society for Pediatric Endocrinology/Lawson Wilkins Pediatric Endocrine Society. Horm Res 1997; 48(Suppl 2):28 (abstr. 109).

538. Caspersson TA, Hulten M, Jonasson J, et al. Translocation causing non-fluorescent Y chromosomes in human XO/XY mosaicism. Hereditas 1971; 68:317–324.

539. Kluzewski B, Jokineu A, Hortling H, et al. A theory explaining the abnormality in 45,X/46,XY mosaicism with non-fluorescent Y chromosome: presentation of 3 cases. Ann Genet 1978; 21:5–11.

540. Madan K, Gooren L, Shoemaker J. Three cases of sex chromosome mosaicism with a nonfluorescent Y. Hum Genet 1979; 46:295–304.

541. Magenis E, Donlon T. Non-fluorescent Y chromosomes: cytologic evidence of origin. Hum Genet 1982; 60:133–138.

542. Weckworth PF, Johnson HW, Pantzer JT, et al. Dicentric Y chromosome and mixed dysgenesis. J Urol 1988; 139:91–94.

543. Sugarman ID, Crolla JA, Malone PS. Mixed gonadal dysgenesis and cell line differentiation: case presentation and literature review. Clin Genet 1994; 46:313–315.

544. Mendez JP, Ulloa-Aguirre A, Kofman-Alfaro S, et al. Mixed gonadal dysgenesis: clinical, cytogenetic, endocrinological, and histopathological findings in 16 patients. Am J Med Genet 1993; 46:263–267.

545. Borer JG, Ntti VW, Glassberg KI. Mixed gonadal dysgenesis and dysgenetic male pseudohermaphroditism. J Urol 1995; 153:1267–1273.

546. Yanagisawa S. Structural abnormalities of the Y chromosome and abnormal external genitalia. Hum Genet 1980; 53:183–188.

547. Cooke HJ, Elliott DJ. RNA-binding proteins and human male infertility. Trends Genet 1997; 13:87–89.

548. Bernstein R. X:Y chromosome translocations and their manifestations. In: Sandberg AA, ed. Progress and Topics in Cytogenetics, the Y Chromosome. New York: Alan R Liss, 1985: 171–206.

549. Lahn BT, Ma N, Breg WR et al. Xq-Yq interchange resulting in supernormal X-linked gene expression in severely retarded males with 46,XYq-karyotype. Nat Genet 1994; 8:243–250.

550. Harnden DG, Stewart JSS. The chromosomes in a case of pure gonadal dysgenesis. Br Med J 1959; 2:1285–1287.

551. Granat M, Amar A, Mor-Yosef S, et al. Pure gonadal dysgenesis (type XX): report on a family with four affected sibs. Hum Genet 1977; 37:117–120.

552. McDonough PG, Byrd JR, Tho PT, et al. Phenotypic and cytogenetic findings in eighty-two patients with ovarian failure: changing trends. Fertil Steril 1977; 28:638–641.

553. Judd HL, Scully RE, Atkins L, et al. Pure gonadal dysgenesis with progressive hirsutism: demonstration of testosterone production by gonadal streaks. N Engl J Med 1970; 282:881–885.

554. Aittomäki K. The genetics of XX gonadal dysgenesis. Am J Hum Genet 1994; 54:844–851.

555. Heufelder AE. Gonads in trouble: follicle-stimulating hormone receptor gene mutation as a cause of inherited streak ovaries. Eur J Endocrinol 1996; 134:296–297.

556. Aittomaki K, Herva R, Stenman U-H, et al. Clinical features of primary ovarian failure caused by a point mutation in the follicle-stimulating hormone receptor gene. J Clin Endocrinol Metab 1995; 81:3722–3726.

557. Tapanainen JS, Aittomaki K, Min J, et al. Men homozygous for an inactivating mutation of the follicle-stimulating hormone (FSH) receptor gene present variable suppression of spermatogenesis and fertility. Nat Genet 1997; 15:205–206.

558. Pallister PD, Opitz JM. The Perrault syndrome: autosomal recessive ovarian dysgenesis with facultative, non-sex-limited sensorineural deafness. Am J Med Genet 1979; 4:239–246.

559. Nishi Y, Hamamoto K, Kajiyama M, et al. The Perrault syndrome: clinical report and review. Am J Med Genet 1988; 31:623–629.

560. Hamet P, Kuchel O, Nowaczynski W, et al. Hypertension with adrenal, genital, renal defects, and deafness. Arch Intern Med 1973; 131:563–569.

561. Skre H, Bassoe HH, Berg K, et al. Cerebellar ataxia and hypergonadotropic hypogonadism in two kindreds: chance occurrence, pleiotropism or linkage? Clin Genet 1976; 9:234–244.

562. Nicolino M, Bost M, David M, et al. Familial blepharophenosis: an uncommon marker of ovarian dysgenesis. J Pediatr Endocrinol Metab 1995; 8:127–133.

563. Amati P, Gasparini P, Zlotogora J, et al. A gene for premature ovarian failure associated with eyelid malformation maps to chromosome 3q22-q23. Am J Hum Genet 1996; 58:1089–1092.

564. Kennerknecht I, Sorgo W, Oberhoffer R, et al. Familial occurrence of agonadism and multiple internal malformations in phenotypically normal girls with 46,XY and 46,XX karyotypes, respectively: a new autosomal recessive syndrome. Am J Med Genet 1993; 47:1166–1170.

565. Mendonca BB, Barbosa AS, Arnhold IJP, et al. Gonadal dysgenesis in XX and XY sisters: evidence for the involvement of an autosomal gene. Am J Med Genet 1994; 52:39–43.

566. Swyer GIM. Male pseudohermaphrodism: a hitherto undescribed form. Br Med J 1955; 2:709–712.

567. Simpson JL. Genetic heterogeneity in XY sex reversal: potential pitfalls. In: Wachtel S, ed. Isolating the Testes-Determining Factor (TDF) in Evolutionary Mechanism in Sex Determination. Boca Raton, Florida: CRC Press, 1989: 266–276.

568. Warner BA, Monsaert RP, Stumpf PG, et al. 46,XY gonadal dysgenesis: is oncogenesis related to H-Y antigen phenotype or breast development? Hum Genet 1985; 69:79–85.

569. Blagowidow N, Page DC, Huff D, et al. Ullrich-Turner syndrome in an XY female fetus with deletion of the sex determining portion of the Y chromosome. Am J Med Genet 1989; 34:159–162.

570. Affara NA, Chalmers IJ, Ferguson-Smith MA. Analysis of the SRY gene in 22 sex-reversed XY females identifies four new point mutations in the conserved DNA binding domain. Hum Mol Genet 1993; 2:785–789.

571. Hawkins JR, Taylor A, Goodfellow PN, et al. Evidence for increased prevalence of SRY mutations in XY females with complete rather than partial gonadal dysgenesis. Am J Hum Genet 1992; 51:979–984.

572. Tajima T, Nakae J, Shinohara N, et al. A novel mutation localized in the 3′ non-HMG box region of the SRY gene in 46,XY gonadal dysgenesis. Hum Mol Genet 1994; 3:1187–1189.

573. McElreavy K, Vilain E, Abbas N, et al. XY sex reversal associated with a deletion 5′ to the SRY "HMG box" in the testis-determining region. Proc Natl Acad Sci U S A 1992; 89:11016–11020.

574. Schmitt-Ney M, Thiele H, Kaltwasser P, et al. Two novel SRY missense mutations reducing DNA binding identified in XY females and their mosaic fathers. Am J Hum Genet 1995; 56:862–869.

575. Nasrin N, Buggs C, Kong XF, et al. DNA-binding properties of the product of the testes-determining gene and related protein. Nature 1991; 354:317–320.

576. Harley VR, Jackson DI, Hextall PJ, et al. DNA binding activity of recombinant SRY from normal males and XY females. Science 1992; 255:453–456.

577. Jäger RJ, Harley VR, Pfeifter RA, et al. A familial mutation in the testis-determining gene SRY shared by both sexes. Hum Genet 1992; 90:350–355.

578. Poulat F, Soullier S, Goze C, et al. Description and functional implications of a novel mutation in the sex-determining gene SRY. Hum Mutat 1994; 3:200–204.

579. Chemke J, Carmichael R, Stewart JM, et al. Familial XY gonadal dysgenesis. J Med Genet 1970; 7:105–111.

580. Vilain E, McElreavy K, Jaubert F, et al. Familial case with sequence variant in the testis-determining region associated with two sex phenotypes. Am J Hum Genet 1992; 50:1008–1011.

581. Bernstein R, Koo GC, Wachtel SS. Abnormality of the X chromosome in human 46,XY female siblings with dysgenetic ovaries. Science 1980; 207:768–769.

582. Scherer G, Shempp W, Baccichetti C, et al. Duplication of an Xp segment that includes the ZFX locus causes sex inversion in man. Hum Genet 1989; 81:291–294.

583. Hofnagel D, Wurster-Hill DH, Dupree WB, et al. Camptomelic dwarfism associated with XY-gonadal dysgenesis and chromosome anomalies. Clin Genet 1978; 13:489–499.

584. Bialer MG, Penchaszadeh VB, Kahn E, et al. Female external genitalia and müllerian duct derivatives in a 46,XY infant with the Smith-Lemli-Opitz syndrome. Am J Med Genet 1987; 28:723–731.

585. Tint GS, Salen G, Batta AK, et al. Correlation of severity and outcome with plasma sterol levels in variants of the Smith-Lemli-Opitz syndrome. J Pediatr 1995; 127:82–87.

586. Cussen LJ, MacMahon RA. Germ cells and ova in dysgenetic gonads of a 46,XY female dizygotic twin. Am J Dis Child 1979; 133:373–375.

587. Russel MH, Wachtel SS, Davis BW, et al. Ovarian development in 46,XY gonadal dysgenesis. Hum Genet 1982; 60:196–199.

588. Barbosa AS, Ferraz-Costa T, Semer M, et al. XY gonadal dysgenesis with gonadoblastoma: a study of two sisters with a cryptic deletion of the Y chromosome involving the SRY gene. Hum Genet 1995; 95:63–66.

589. Grumbach MM, Morishima A, Liu N. A distinctive clinical entity simulating Turner's syndrome in boys and girls associated with congenital heart disease, appropriate gonadal differentiation, and a normal sex chromosome constitution. J Pediatr 1965; 67:966 (abstract).

590. Noonan J. Hypertelorism with Turner phenotype: a new syndrome with associated congenital heart disease. Am J Dis Child 1968; 116:373–380.

591. Sharland M, Burch M, McKenna WM, Paton MA. A clinical study of Noonan syndrome. Arch Dis Child 1992; 67:178–183.

592. Noonan JA. Noonan syndrome: an update and review for the primary pediatrician. Clin Pediatr 1994; 33:548–555.

593. Sharland M, Morgan M, Smith G, et al. Genetic counselling in Noonan syndrome. Am J Med Genet 1993; 45:437–440.

594. Wood A, Massarano A, Super M, et al. Behavioral aspects and psychiatric findings in Noonan's syndrome. Arch Dis Child 1995; 72:153–155.

595. Money J, Kolus ME. Noonan syndrome: IQ and specific disabilities. Am J Dis Child 1979; 133:846–850.

596. Miller M, Motulsky AC. Noonan syndrome in an adult family presenting with chronic lymphedema. Am J Med 1978; 65:379–383.

597. Sharland M, Patton MA, Talbot S, et al. Coagulation-factor deficiencies and abnormal bleeding in Noonan's syndrome. Lancet 1992; 339:19–21.

598. Jamieson CR, van der Burgt I, Brady AF, et al. Mapping a gene for Noonan syndrome to the long arm of chromosome 12. Nat Genet 1994; 8:357–360.

599. Jones HW, Scott WW. Hermaphroditism, Genital Anomalies, and Related Endocrine Disorders. 2nd ed. Baltimore: Williams & Wilkins, 1971.

600. van Niekerk WA. True hermaphroditism: an analytic review with a report of 3 new cases. Am J Obstet Gynecol 1976; 126:890–907.

601. van Niekerk WA. True hermaphrodism. In: Josso N, ed. The Intersex Child: Pediatric and Adolescent Endocrinology. Vol 8. Basel: S Karger, 1981: 80–99.

602. Aaronson IA. True hermaphroditism: a review of 41 cases with observations in testicular histology and function. Brit J Urol 1985; 57:775–779.

603. Hadjiathanasiou CG, Brauner R, Lortat-Jacob S, et al. True hermaphroditism: genetic variants and clinical management. J Pediatr 1994; 125:738–744.

604. Krob G, Braun A, Kuhnle U. True hermaphroditism: geographical distribution, clinical findings, chromosomes and gonadal histology. Eur J Pediatr 1994; 153:2–10.

604a. Damiani D, Fellows M, McElreavey K, et al. True hermaphroditism: clinical aspects and molecular studies in 16 cases. Eur J Endocrinol 1997; 136:201–204.

605. Torres L, Lopez M, Mendez JP, et al. Molecular analysis in true hermaphrodites with different karyotypes and similar phenotypes. Am J Med Genet 1996; 63:348–355.

606. Van Niekerk WA, Retief AE. The gonads of human true hermaphrodites. Hum Genet 1981; 58:117–122.

607. McKelvie J, Jaubert F, Nezelof C. True hermaphroditism: a primary germ cell disorder. Pediatr Pathol 1987; 7:31–41.

608. Nihoul-Fekete C, Lortat-Jacob S, Cahin O, Josso N. Preservation of gonadal function in true hermaphroditism. J Pediatr Surg 1984; 19:50–55.

609. Ramsay M, Bernstein R, Zwane W, et al. XX true hermaphroditism in southern African blacks: an enigma of primary sexual differentiation. Am J Hum Genet 1988; 43:4–13.

610. Williamson HO, Phansey SA, Mathur RS. True hermaphroditism with term vaginal delivery and a review. Am J Obstet Gynecol 1981; 141:262–265.

611. Starceski PJ, Sieber WK, Lee PA. Fertility in true hermaphroditism. Adolesc Pediatr Gynecol 1988; 1:55–156.

612. Shannon R, Nicolaides NJ. True hermaphrodism with oogenesis and spermatogenesis. Aust N Z J Obstet Gynaecol 1973; 13:184–187.

613. Armendares S, Salamanca F, Cantu JM, et al. Familial true hermaphrodism in three siblings: clinical, cytogenetic, histologic and hormonal studies. Humangenetik 1975; 29:99–109.

614. Aiman J, Hemsell DJ, MacDonald PC. Production and origin of estrogen in two true hermaphrodites. Am J Obstet Gynecol 1978; 132:401–409.

615. Braun A, Kammerer S, Cleve A, et al. True hermaphroditism in a 46,XY individual, caused by a postzygotic somatic point mutation in the male gonadal sex-determining locus (SRY): molecular genetics and histological findings in a sporadic case. Am J Hum Genet 1993; 52:578–585.

616. Jüger RJ, Ebensperger C, Fraccaro M, et al. A ZFY-negative 46,XX true hermaphrodite is positive for the Y pseudoautosomal boundary. Hum Genet 1990; 85:666–668.

617. McElreavy K, Rappaport R, Vilain E, et al. A minority of 46,XX true hermaphrodites are positive for the Y-DNA sequence including SRY. Hum Genet 1992; 90:121–125.

618. Ramos ES, Moreira-Filho CA, Vincente YA, et al. SRY-negative true hermaphrodites and XX males in two generations of the same family. Hum Genet 1996; 97:596–598.

619. Abbas NE, Toublanc JE, Boucekkine C, et al. A possible common origin of "Y-negative" human XX males and XX true hermaphrodites. Hum Genet 1990; 84:356–360.

620. Pereira ET, Cabal de Almeida JC, Gunha A, et al. Use of probes for ZFY, SRY, and the Y pseudoautosomal boundary in XX males, XX true hermaphrodites and an XY female. J Med Genet 1991; 28:591–595.

621. Affara NA. Sex and the single Y. Bioessays 1991; 13:475–478.

622. Spurdle AB, Shankman S, Ramsay M. XX true hermaphroditism in southern African blacks: exclusion of SRY sequences and uniparental disomy of the X chromosome. Am J Med Genet 1995; 55:53–56.

623. Fechner PY, Rosenberg C, Stetten G, et al. Nonrandom inactivation of the Y-bearing X chromosome in a 46,XX individual: evidence for the etiology of 46,XX true hermaphroditism. Cytogenet Cell Genet 1994; 66:22–26.

624. Benirschke K, Naftolin F, Gittes R, et al. True hermaphroditism and chimerism. Am J Obstet Gynecol 1972; 113:449–458.

625. Gartler SM, Waxman SH, Giblett E. An XX/XY human hermaphrodite resulting from double fertilization. Proc Natl Acad Sci U S A 1962; 48:332–335.

626. Josso N, de Grouchy J, Auvert J, et al. True hermaphroditism with XX/XY mosaicism, probably due to double fertilization of the ovum. J Clin Endocrinol Metab 1965; 25:114–126.

627. Tarkowski AK. Mouse chimaera developed from fused eggs. Nature 1961; 190:857–860.

628. Lowry RB, Honore LH, Arnold WJD, et al. Familial true hermaphroditism. In: Bergsma D, ed. Genetic Forms of Hypogonadism. New York: National Foundation of March of Dimes, 1975: 105–113.

629. Schwartz IS, Cohen CJ, Deligdisch L. Dysgerminoma of the ovary associated with true hermaphroditism. Obstet Gynecol 1980; 56:102–106.

630. Barr ML, Sergovich FR, Carr DH, et al. The triplo-X female: an appraisal based on a study of 12 cases and a review of the literature. Can Med Assoc J 1969; 101:247–258.

631. Bender BG, Linden MG, Robinson A. Neuropsychological impairment in 42 adolescents with sex chromosome abnormalities. Am J Med Genet 1993; 48:169–173.

632. Linden M, Bender BG, Harmin RJ, et al. 47,XXX: what is the prognosis? Pediatrics 1988; 82:619–630.

633. Fryns JP, Kleczkowska A, Petit P, et al. X-chromosome polysomy in the female: personal experience and review of the literature. Clin Genet 1983; 23:341–349.

634. MacDonald M, Hassold T, Harvey J, et al. The origin of 47,XXY and 47,XXX aneuploidy: heterogeneous mechanisms and role of aberrant recombination. Hum Mol Genet 1994; 3:1365–1371.

635. Nielsen J, Homma A, Christiansen F, et al. Women with tetra-X (48XXXX). Hereditas 1977; 85:151–156.

636. Collen RJ, Falk RE, Lippe BM, et al. A 48,XXXX female with absent ovaries. Am J Med Genet 1980; 6:275–278.

637. Kassai R, Hamada I, Furuta K, et al. Penta X syndrome: a case report with review of the literature. Am J Med Genet 1991; 40:51–56.

638. Sandberg AA, Koepf GF, Ishihara T, et al. An XYY human male. Lancet 1961; 2:488–489.

639. Hook EB. Extra sex chromosomes and human behavior: the nature of the evidence regarding XYY, XXY, XXYY, and XXX genotypes. In: Vallet HL, Porter IH, eds. Genetic Mechanisms of Sexual Development. New York: Academic Press, 1979: 437–463.

640. Owen DR. Psychological studies in XYY men. In: Vallet HL, Porter IH, eds. Genetic Mechanisms of Sexual Development. New York: Academic Press, 1979: 465–471.

641. Fryns JP, Kleczkowska A, Kubien E, et al. XYY syndrome and other Y chromosome polysomies: mental status and psychosocial functioning. Genet Couns 1995; 6:197–206.

641a. Ratcliffe SG. The psychological and psychiatric consequences of sex chromosome abnormalities in children, based on population studies. In: Poustka F, ed. Basic Approaches to Genetic and Molecular-Biological, Developmental Psychiatry. Berlin: Quintessenz, 1994: 99–122.

642. Mazauric-Stuber M, Kordt G, Brodersen D. Y aneuploidy: a further case of a male patient with a 48,XYYY karyotype and literature review. Ann Genet 1992; 35:237–240.

643. Schellhas F. Malignant potential of the dysgenetic gonad. Obstet Gynecol 1974; 44:298–309 (Part I) and 455–562 (Part II).

644. Simpson JL, Photopulos G. The relationship of neoplasia to disorders of abnormal sexual differentiation. Birth Defects 1976; 12:15–50.

645. Manuel M, Katayama K, Jones HW Jr. The age of occurrence of gonadal tumors in intersex patients with a Y chromosome. Am J Obstet Gynecol 1976; 124:293–300.

646. Scully RE. Gonadoblastoma: a review of 74 cases. Cancer 1970; 25:1340–1356.

647. Scully RE. Neoplasia associated with anomalous sexual development and abnormal sex chromosomes. In: Josso N, ed. The Intersex Child: Pediatric and Adolescent Endocrinology. Vol 8. Basel: S Karger, 1981: 203–217.

648. Verp MS, Simpson JL. Abnormal sexual differentiation and neoplasia. Cancer Genet Cytogenet 1987; 25:191–218.

649. Savage MO, Lowe DG. Gonadal neoplasia and abnormal sexual differentiation. Clin Endocrinol 1990; 32:519–533.

650. Jørgensen N, Müller J, Giwercman A, et al. Clinical and biologic significance of carcinoma in situ of the testis. Cancer Surv 1990; 9:288–302.

651. Ramani P, Yeung CK, Habeebu SM. Testicular intratubular germ cell neoplasia in children and adolescents with intersex. Am J Surg Pathol 1993; 17:1124–1133.

651a. Sogge MR, McDonald SD, Cofold PB. The malignant potential of the dysgenetic germ cell in Klinefelter's syndrome. Am J Med 1979; 66:515–518.

652. Greenblatt RB, Byrd JR, McDonough PG, et al. The spectrum of gonadal dysgenesis: a clinical, cytogenetic and pathologic study. Am J Obstet Gynecol 1967; 98:151–172.

653. Lindsay AN, Sills IN, MacGillivray MH, et al. Dysgerminoma in a patient with the syndrome of gonadal dysgenesis with a 45,X karyotype. Am J Med Genet 1981; 10:21–24.

654. Patel SK, Prentice SA. Gonadoblastoma, distinctive ovarian tumor. Arch Pathol 1972; 94:165–170.

655. Goldberg MB, Scully AL, Solomon IL, et al. Gonadal dysgenesis in phenotypic female subjects: a review of 87 cases, with cytogenetic studies in 53. Am J Med 1968; 45:529–543.

656. Warren JC, Erkman B, Cheatum S, et al. Hilus cell adenoma in a dysgenetic gonad with XX/XO mosaicism. Lancet 1964; 1:141–143.

657. Müller J, Skakkebaek NE. Gonadal malignancy in individuals with sex chromosome anomalies in children and young adults with sex chromosome aneuploidy. In: Evans JA, Haverton JL, Robinson A, eds. Birth Defects Original Article Series. Vol 26. New York: Wiley-Liss, 1991; 247–255.

658. Hart WR, Burkons DM. Germ cell neoplasms arising in gonadoblastomas. Cancer 1979; 43:669–678.

659. Boczkowski K, Teter J, Sternandel Z. Sibship occurrence of XY gonadal dysgenesis with dysgerminoma. Am J Obstet Gynecol 1972; 113:952–955.

660. Gourlay WA, McGillivray B, Johnson HW, et al. Gonadal tumors in disorders of sexual differentiation. Urology 1994; 43:537–540.

661. New MI. Congenital adrenal hyperplasia. In: De Groot L, ed. Endocrinology, 3rd ed. Philadelphia: WB Saunders, 1995: 1813–1835.

662. Donohoue PA, Parker K, Migeon CJ. Congenital adrenal hyperplasia. In: Scriver CR, Beaudet AL, Sly WS, Valle D, eds. The Metabolic and Molecular Basis of Inherited Disease. 7th ed. New York: McGraw-Hill, 1995: 2929–2966.

663. Miller WL, Tyrell JB. The adrenal cortex. In: Felig P, Baxter JD, Frohmer LA, eds. Endocrinology and Metabolism. 3rd ed. New York: McGraw-Hill 1995; 555–711.

664. Goldman AS. Animal models of inborn errors of steroidogenesis and steroid action. Colloq Ges Biol Chem 1970; 21:389–436.

665. Pang S, Wallace MA, Hofman L, et al. Worldwide experience in newborn screening for congenital adrenal hyperplasia due to 21 hydroxylase deficiency. Pediatrics 1988; 81:866–874.

666. Biglieri EG, Wajchenberg BL, Malerbi DA, et al. The zonal origins of the mineralocorticoid hormones in the 21-hydroxylation deficiency of congenital adrenal hyperplasia. J Clin Endocrinol Metab 1981; 53:964–969.

667. Kitawaki J, Inoue S, Tamara T, et al. Increasing aromatase cytochrome P450 level in human placenta during pregnancy studied by immunohistochemistry and enzyme linked immunoabsorbent assay. Endocrinology 1992; 130:2751–2757.

668. Fiet J, Gueux B, Raux-Demay M-C, et al. Increased plasma 21-deoxycorticosterone (21-DB) levels in late onset adrenal 21-hydroxylase deficiency suggest a mild defect of the mineralocorticoid pathway. J Clin Endocrinol Metab 1989; 68:542–547.

669. Kowarski A, Finkelstein JW, Spaulding JS, et al. Aldosterone secretion rate in congenital adrenal hyperplasia: a discussion of the theories on the pathogenesis of the salt-losing form of the syndrome. J Clin Invest 1965; 44:1505–1513.

670. Styne DM, Richards GE, Bell JJ, et al. Growth pattern in congenital adrenal hyperplasia: correlation of glucocorticoid therapy with stature. In: Lee PA, Plotnick LP, Kowarski AA, et al., eds. Congenital Adrenal Hyperplasia. Baltimore: University Park Press, 1977: 247–263.

671. Speiser PW, New MI. Genotype and hormonal phenotype in nonclassical 21-hydroxylase deficiency. J Clin Endocrinol Metab 1987; 64:86–91.

672. Levine LS, Dupont B, Lorenzen F, et al. Cryptic 21-hydroxylase deficiency in families of patients with classical congenital adrenal hyperplasia. J Clin Endocrinol Metab 1980; 51:1316–1324.

673. Kohn B, Levine LS, Pollack MS, et al. Late-onset steroid 21-hydroxylase deficiency: a variant of classical congenital adrenal hyperplasia. J Clin Endocrinol Metab 1982; 55:817–827.

674. Rosenwaks Z, Lee PA, Jones GS. An attenuated form of congenital virilizing adrenal hyperplasia. J Clin Endocrinol Metab 1979; 49:335–339.

675. Temeck JW, Pang S, Nelson C, et al. Genetic defects of steroidogenesis in premature pubarche. J Clin Endocrinol Metab 1987; 64:609–617.

676. Wischusen J, Bakker HWG, Hudson B. Reversible male infertility due to congenital adrenal hyperplasia. Clin Endocrinol 1981; 14:571–577.

677. New MI, Lorenzen F, Lerner AJ, et al. Genotyping steroid 21-hydroxylase deficiency: hormonal reference data. J Clin Endocrinol Metab 1983; 57:320–326.

678. New MI, Speiser PW. Genetics of adrenal steroid 21-hydroxylase deficiency. Endocr Rev 1986; 7:331–349.

679. Speiser PW, Dupont B, Rubinstein P, et al. High frequency of nonclassical steroid 21-hydroxylase deficiency. Am J Hum Genet 1985; 37:650–667.

680. Miller WL. Genetics, diagnosis and management of 21-hydroxylase deficiency. J Clin Endocrinol Metab 1994; 78:241–246.

681. New MI, White PC. Genetic disorders of steroid hormone synthesis and metabolism. Baillieres Clin Endocrinol Metab 1995; 9:525–554.

682. White PC, Grossberger D, Onufer BJ, et al. Two genes encoding steroid 21-hydroxylase are located near the genes encoding the fourth component of complement in man. Proc Natl Acad Sci U S A 1985; 82:1089–1093.

683. Bristow J, Tee MK, Gitelman SE, et al. Tenascin-X: a novel extracellular matrix protein encoded by the human XB gene overlapping P450c21B. J Cell Biol 1993; 122:265–278.

683a. Bristow J, Gitelman SE, Tee MK, et al. Abundant adrenal-specific transcription of the human P450c21A "Pseudogene." J Biol Chem 1993; 268:1219–1224.

684. Tusie-Luna M-T, Traktmon P, White PC. Determination of functional effects of mutations in the steroid 21-hydroxylase gene (CYP21) using recombinant vaccinia virus. J Biol Chem 1990; 265: 20916–20922.

685. Speiser PW, Dupont J, Zhu D, et al. Disease expression and molecular genotype in congenital adrenal hyperplasia due to 21-hydroxylase deficiency. J Clin Invest 1992; 90:584–595.

686. Helmberg A. Twin genes and endocrine disease: CYP21 and CYP11B genes. Acta Endocrinol 1993; 129:97–108.

687. Speiser PW, Agdere L, Ueshiba H, et al. Aldosterone synthesis in salt-wasting congenital adrenal hyperplasia with complete absence of adrenal 21-hydroxylase. N Engl J Med 1991; 324:145–149.

688. Wilson RC, Mercado AB, Cheng KC, New MI. Steroid 21-hydroxylase deficiency: genotype may not predict phenotype. J Clin Endocrinol Metab 1995; 80:2322–2329.

689. Pang S, Clark A. Congenital adrenal hyperplasia due to 21-hydroxylase deficiency: newborn screening and its relationship to the diagnosis and treatment of the disorder. Screening 1993; 2:105–139.

690. Thompson R, Seargeant L, Winter JSD. Screening for congenital adrenal hyperplasia: distribution of 17α-hydroxyprogesterone concentrations in neonatal blood spot specimens. J Pediatr 1989; 114:400–404.

691. Jenner MR, Grumbach MM, Kaplan SL. Plasma 17OH-progesterone in maternal and umbilical cord plasma in children, and in congenital adrenal hyperplasia (CAH): application to neonatal diagnosis of CAH. Pediatr Res 1970; 4:380 (abstract).

692. Pang S, Levine LS, Chow DM, et al. Serum androgen concentration in neonates and young infants with congenital adrenal hyperplasia due to 21 hydroxylase deficiency. Clin Endocrinol 1979; 11:575–584.

693. Godo B, Visser HKA, Degenhart JH. Plasma 17OH-progesterone in full-term and preterm infants at birth and during the early neonatal period. Horm Res 1981; 15:65–71.

694. de Peretti E, Forest M. Pitfalls in the etiologic diagnosis of congenital adrenal hyperplasia in the early neonatal period. Horm Res 1982; 16:10–22.

695. Fiet J, Gueux B, Gourmelen M, et al. Comparison of basal and adrenocorticotropin-stimulated plasma 21-deoxycortisol and 17-hydroxyprogesterone values as biological markers of late-onset adrenal hyperplasia. J Clin Endocrinol Metab 1988; 66:659–667.

696. Frasier SD, Thorneycroft IH, Weiss BA, et al. Elevated amniotic fluid concentration of 17α-hydroxyprogesterone in congenital adrenal hyperplasia. J Pediatr 1975; 86:310–311 (letter).

697. Gueux B, Fiet J, Couillin P, et al. Prenatal diagnosis of 21-hydroxylase deficiency congenital adrenal hyperplasia by simultaneous radioimmunoassay of 21-deoxycortisol and 17-hydroxyprogesterone in amniotic fluid. J Clin Endocrinol Metab 1988; 66:534–537.

698. Pollack M, Levine LS, Duchon M, et al. Prenatal diagnosis of CAH due to 21 hydroxylase deficiency by HLA typing of cultured amniotic fluid cells. Pediatr Res 1979; 13:384 (abstract).

699. Speiser PW, Laforgia N, Kato K, et al. First trimester prenatal treatment and molecular genetic diagnosis of congenital adrenal hyperplasia (21-hydroxylase deficiency). J Clin Endocrinol Metab 1990; 70:838–848.

700. Speiser PW, White PC, Dupont J, et al. Prenatal diagnosis of congenital adrenal hyperplasia due to 21-hydroxylase deficiency by allele-specific hybridization and Southern blot. Hum Genet 1994; 93:424–428.

701. Forest MG, David M, Morel Y. Prenatal diagnosis and treatment of 21-hydroxylase deficiency. J Steroid Biochem Mol Biol 1993; 45:75–82.

702. Mercado AB, Wilson RC, Cheng KC, et al. Extensive personal experience:

prenatal treatment and diagnosis of congenital adrenal hyperplasia owing to steroid 21-hydroxylase deficiency. J Clin Endocrinol Metab 1995; 80:2014–2020.

703. Seckl JR, Miller WL. How safe is long term prenatal glucocorticoid treatment? JAMA 1997; 277:1077–1079.

704. Linder BL, Esteban NV, Yergey AL, et al. Cortisol production rate in children. J Pediatr 1990; 117:892–896.

705. Kerrigan JR, Veldhuis JD, Leyo SA, et al. Estimation of daily cortisol production and clearance rates in normal prepubertal males by deconvolution analysis. J Clin Endocrinol Metab 1993; 76:1505–1510.

706. Young MC, Robinson JA, Read GF. 17OH-Progesterone rhythms in congenital adrenal hyperplasia. Arch Dis Child 1988; 63:617–623.

707. Richards GE, Grumbach MM, Kaplan SL, et al. The effect of long acting glucocorticoids in menstrual abnormalities in patients with virilizing congenital adrenal hyperplasia. J Clin Endocrinol Metab 1978; 47:1208–1215.

708. Horner JM, Hintz RL, Leutscher JA. The role of renin and angiotensin in salt-losing, 21-hydroxylase-deficient congenital adrenal hyperplasia. J Clin Endocrinol Metab 1979; 48:776–783.

709. Urban MD, Lee PA, Migeon CJ. Adult height and fertility in men with congenital virilizing adrenal hyperplasia. N Engl J Med 1978; 299:1392–1396.

710. Brook CGD, Zachmann M, Prader A, et al. Experience with long-term therapy in congenital adrenal hyperplasia. J Pediatr 1974; 85:12–19.

711. Klingensmith GJ, Garcia SC, Jones HW Jr, et al. Glucocorticoid treatment of girls with congenital adrenal hyperplasia: effects on height, sexual maturation, and fertility. J Pediatr 1977; 90:996–1004.

712. Donaldson MDC, Thomas PH, Love JG, et al. Presentation, acute illness, and learning difficulties in salt wasting 21-hydroxylase deficiency. Arch Dis Child 1994; 70:214–218.

713. Mulaikal RM, Migeon CJ, Rock JA. Fertility rates in female patients with congenital adrenal hyperplasia due to 21-hydroxylase deficiency. N Engl J Med 1987; 316:178–182.

714. Kuhnle U, Bullinger M, Schwarz HP, Knorr D. Partnership and sexuality in adult female patients with congenital adrenal hyperplasia: first results of a cross-sectional quality-of-life evaluation. J Steroid Biochem Mol Biol 1993; 45:123–126.

715. Cunnah D, Perry L, Dacie JA, et al. Bilateral testicular tumors in congenital adrenal hyperplasia: a continuing diagnostic and therapeutic dilemma. Clin Endocrinol 1989; 30; 141–147.

716. Srikanth MS, West BR, Ishitani M, et al. Benign testicular tumors in children with congenital adrenal hyperplasia. J Pediatr Surg 1992; 27:639–641.

717. Combes-Moukhovsky ME, Kottler ML, Valensi P, et al. Gonadal and adrenal catheterization during adrenal suppression and gonadal stimulation in a patient with bilateral testicular tumors and congenital adrenal hyperplasia. J Clin Endocrinol Metab 1994; 79:1390–1394.

718. Avila NA, Premkumar A, Shawker TH, et al. Testicular adrenal rest tissue in congenital adrenal hyperplasia: findings at gray-scale and color Doppler US. Radiology 1996; 198:99–104.

719. Bhatia V, Shukla R, Mishra SK, Gupta RK. Adrenal tumor complicating untreated 21-hydroxylase deficiency in a 5½-year-old boy. Am J Dis Child 1993; 147:1321–1323.

720. Ravichandran R, Lafferty F, McGinniss MJ, Taylor HC. Congenital adrenal hyperplasia presenting as massive adrenal incidentalomas in the sixth decade of life: report of two patients with 21-hydroxylase deficiency. J Clin Endocrinol Metab 1996; 81:1776–1779.

721. Sotiropoulos A, Morishima A, Homsy Y, et al. Long-term assessment of genital reconstruction in female pseudohermaphrodites. J Urol 1976; 115:599–601.

722. Gearhart JP, Burnett A, Owen JH. Measurement of pudendal evoked potentials during feminizing genitoplasty: technique and applications. J Urol 1995; 153:486–487.

723. Hendren WH, Donahoe PK. Correction of congenital abnormalities of the vagina and perineum. J Pediatr Surg 1980; 16:751–763.

724. Donahoe PK, Gustafson ML. Early one-stage surgical reconstitution of the extremely high vagina in patients with congenital adrenal hyperplasia. J Pediatr Surg 1994; 29:352–358.

725. Van Wyk JJ, Gunter DF, Ritzén EM, et al. The use of adrenalectomy as a treatment for congenital adrenal hyperplasia. J Clin Endocrinol Metab 1996; 81:3180–3190.

726. Laue L, Mecke DP, Jones JV, et al. A preliminary study of flutamide, testolactone, and reduced hydrocortisone dose in the treatment of congenital adrenal hyperplasa. J Clin Endocrinol Metab 1996; 3535–3539.

727. Smith EP, Boyd J, Frank GR, et al. Estrogen resistance caused by a mutation in the estrogen receptor gene in a man. N Engl J Med 1994; 331:1056–1061.

728. Morishima A, Grumbach MM, Simpson ER, et al. Aromatase deficiency in male and female siblings caused by a novel mutation and the physiological role of estrogens. J Clin Endocrinol Metab 1995; 80:3689–3698.

729. Grumbach MM. Mutations in the human gene encoding cytochrome P450 aromatase: female pseudohermaphrodism, polycystic ovaries, macroorchidism, tall stature, osteopenia, and the female spotted hyena. In: Hibi I, Tanaka T, eds. Sexual Differentiation and Maturation: Frontiers in Endocrinology. Ares-Serono Symposia 1996; 17:175–188.

730. Eberlein WR, Bongiovanni AM. Congenital adrenal hyperplasia with hypertension: unusual steroid pattern in blood and urine. J Clin Endocrinol Metab 1955; 15:1531–1534.

731. Zachmann M, Tassinari D, Prader A. Clinical and biochemical variability of congenital adrenal hyperplasia due to 11β-hydroxylase deficiency: a study of 25 patients. J Clin Endocrinol Metab 1983; 56:222–229.

732. White PC, Curnow KM, Pascoe L. Disorders of steroid 11β-hydroxylase isozymes. Endocr Rev 1994; 15:421–438.

733. White PC, Speiser PW. Steroid 11β-hydroxylase deficiency and related disorders. Endocrinol Metab Clin North Am 1994; 23:325–339.

734. Mornet E, Dupont J, Vitek A, et al. Characterization of two genes encoding human steroid 11β-hydroxylase (P45011B). J Biol Chem 1989; 264:20961–20967.

735. Chua SC, Szabo P, Vitek A, et al. Cloning of cDNA encoding steroid 11β-hydroxylase (P450c11). Proc Natl Acad Sci U S A 1987; 84:7193–7197.

736. Rösler A, Leiberman E, Cohen T. High frequency of congenital adrenal hyperplasia (classic 11β-hydroxylase deficiency) among Jews from Morocco. Am J Med Genet 1992; 42:827–834.

737. Levine LS, Rauh W, Gottesdiener K, et al. New studies of the 11β-hydroxylase and 18-hydroxylase enzymes in the hypertensive form of congenital adrenal hyperplasia. J Clin Endocrinol Metab 1980; 50:258–263.

738. Rodriguez Portales JA, Arteaga E, Lopez Moreno JM, et al. Zona glomerulosa function after life-long suppression in two siblings with the hypertensive virilizing form of congenital adrenal hyperplasia. J Clin Endocrinol Metab 1988; 66:349–354.

739. Holcombe JH, Keenan BS, Nichols BL, et al. Neonatal salt loss in the hypertensive form of congenital adrenal hyperplasia. Pediatrics 1980; 65:777–781.

740. Hochberg Z, Benderly A, Kahana L, et al. Requirement of mineralocorticoid in congenital adrenal hyperplasia due to 11β-hydroxylase deficiency. J Clin Endocrinol Metab 1986; 63:36–40.

741. Rosler A, Leiberman E. Enzymatic defects of steroidogenesis: 11β-hydroxylase deficiency congenital adrenal hyperplasia. In: New MI, Levine LS, eds. Adrenal Diseases in Childhood: Pediatric Adolescent Endocrinology. Vol 13. Basel: S Karger, 1984: 47–71.

742. Birnbaum MD, Rose LI. Late onset adrenocortical 11β-hydroxylase deficiency associated with menstrual dysfunction. Obstet Gynecol 1984; 63:445–451.

743. Reboul P, Merceron RE, Cordray JP, et al. Blocs enzymatiques surrénaliens à révélation tardive par déficit de la 11-hydroxylase: a propos de 29 observations. [Adrenal enzymatic block with late-onset caused by 11-hydroxylase deficiency: apropos of 29 cases.] Ann Endocrinol (Paris) 1992; 53:187–195.

744. Nakagawa Y, Yamada M, Ogawa H, et al. Missense mutation in CYP11B1 (CGA [Arg384]→GGA[Gly]) causes steroid 11β-hydroxylase deficiency. Eur J Endocrinol 1995; 132:286–289.

745. Geley S, Kapelaari K, Jöherer K, wr L. CYP11B1 mutations causing congenital adrenal hyperplasia due to 11β-hydroxylase deficiency. J Clin Endocrinol Metab 1996; 81:2896–2901.

746. Charnow KM, Slutsker L, Vitek J, et al. Mutations in the CYP11B1 gene causing adrenal hyperplasia and hypertension cluster in exons 6, 7, and 8. Proc Natl Acad Sci U S A 1993; 90:4552–4556.

747. White PC, Dupont J, New MI, et al. A mutation in CYP11β1 (Arg-448→His) associated with steroid 11β-hydroxylase deficiency in Jews of Moroccan origin. J Clin Invest 1991; 87:1664–1667.

748. Ulick S, Wang JZ, Morton DH. The biochemical phenotypes of two inborn errors in the biosynthesis of aldosterone. J Clin Endocrinol Metab 1992; 74:1415–1420.

749. Mitsuuchi Y, Kawamoto T, Miyahara K, et al. Congenitally defective aldosterone biosynthesis in humans: inactivation of the P450c18 gene (CYP11B2) due to nucleotide deletion in CMO 1 deficient patients. Biochem Biophys Res Commun 1993; 190:864–869.

750. Pascoe L, Curnow KM, Slutsker L, et al. Mutations in the human CYP11B2 (aldosterone synthase) gene causing corticosterone methyloxidase II deficiency. Proc Natl Acad Sci U S A 1992; 89:4996–5000.

751. Lee PDK, Patterson BD, Hintz RL, et al. Biochemical diagnosis and management of corticosterone methyl oxidase type II deficiency. J Clin Endocrinol Metab 1986; 62:225–229.

752. Ulick S, Chan CK, Gill JR Jr, et al. Defective fasciculata zone function as the mechanism of glucocorticoid-remediable aldosteronism. J Clin Endocrinol Metab 1990; 71:1151–1157.

753. Lashansky G, Saenger P, Fishman K, et al. Normative data for adrenal steroidogenesis in a healthy pediatric population: age- and sex-related changes after adrenocorticotropin stimulation. J Clin Endocrinol Metab 1991; 73:674–686.

754. Pang S, Levine LS, Lorenzen F, et al. Hormonal studies in obligate heterozygotes and siblings of siblings with 11β-hydroxylase deficiency congenital adrenal hyperplasia. J Clin Endocrinol Metab 1980; 50:586–589.

755. Schumert Z, Rosenmann A, Landau H, et al. 11-Deoxycortisol in amniotic fluid: prenatal diagnosis of congenital adrenal hyperplasia due to 11β-hydroxylase deficiency. Clin Endocrinol 1980; 12:257–260.

756. Rosler A, Lieberman E, Rosenmann A, et al. Prenatal diagnosis of 11β-hydroxylase deficiency congenital adrenal hyperplasia. J Clin Endocrinol Metab 1979; 49:546–551.

757. Labrie F, Simard J, Pelletier G, et al. Structure, regulation and role of 3β-hydroxysteroid dehydrogenase, 17β-hydroxysteroid dehydrogenase and aromatase enzymes in the formation of sex steroids in classical and

peripheral intracrine tissues. Ballieres Clin Endocrinol Metab 1994; 8:451–474.

758. Simard J, Rheaume E, Mebarki F, et al. Molecular basis of human 3β-hydroxysteroid dehydrogenase deficiency. J Steroid Biochem Mol Biol 1995; 53:127–138.

759. Mason JI. The 3β-hydroxysteroid dehydrogenase gene family of enzymes. Trends Endocrinol Metab 1993; 4:199–203.

760. Martel C, Melner MA, Gagné D, et al. Widespread tissue distribution of steroid sulfatase, 3β-hydroxysteroid dehydrogenase/Δ^5-Δ^4 isomerase (3β-HSD), 17β-HSD, 5α-reductase and aromatase activities in the rhesus monkey. Mol Cell Endocrinol 1994; 104:103–111.

761. Bérube D, Luu-The V, La Chance Y, et al. Assignment of the human 3β-hydroxysteroid dehydrogenase gene (HSDβ3) to the p13 band of chromosome 1. Cytogenet Cell Genet 1989; 52:199–200.

762. La Chance Y, Luu-The V, Verrault H, et al. Characterization of the human 3β-hydroxysteroid dehydrogenase/Δ^5-Δ^4 isomerase gene and its expression in mammalian cells. J Biol Chem 1990; 265:469–475.

763. Rhéaume E, Lachance Y, Zhao H-F, et al. Structure and expression of a new complementary DNA encoding the almost exclusive 3β-hydroxysteroid dehydrogenase/Δ^5-Δ^4 isomerase gene in human adrenals and gonads. Mol Endocrinol 1991; 5:1147–1157.

764. Rhéaume E, Simard J, Morel Y, et al. Congenital adrenal hyperplasia due to point mutations in the type II 3β-hydroxysteroid dehydrogenase gene. Nat Genet 1992; 1:239–245.

765. Bongiovanni AM. The adrenogenital syndrome with deficiency of 3β-hydroxysteroid dehydrogenase. J Clin Invest 1962; 41:2086–2092.

766. Pang S, Levine LS, Stoner E, et al. Nonsalt-losing congenital adrenal hyperplasia due to 3β-hydroxysteroid dehydrogenase deficiency with normal glomerulosa function. J Clin Endocrinol Metab 1983; 56:808–818.

767. Rosenfield RL, Rich BH, Wolfsdorf JL, et al. Pubertal presentation of congenital Δ^5-3β-hydroxysteroid dehydrogenase deficiency. J Clin Endocrinol Metab 1980; 51:345–353.

768. Mendonca BB, Russell AJ, Vasconcelos-Leite M, et al. Mutation in 3β-hydroxysteroid dehydrogenase type II associated with pseudohermaphroditism in males and premature pubarche or cryptic expression in females. J Mol Endocrinol 1994; 12:119–122.

769. Chang YT, Zhang L, Aikaddour HS, et al. Absence of molecular defect in the type II 3β-hydroxysteroid dehydrogenase (3β-HSD) gene in premature pubarche children and hirsute female patients with moderately decreased adrenal 3β-HSD activity. Pediatr Res 1995; 37:820–824.

770. Luu-The V, Lachance Y, Le Blanc G, et al. Human 3β-hydroxysteroid dehydrogenase/Δ^5-Δ^4 isomerase: characterization of three additional related genes. Abstract 1499. In: Proceedings of the 74th Annual Meeting of the Endocrine Society, 1994: 426.

771. Pang S, Lerner AJ, Stoner E, et al. Late onset adrenal steroid 3β-hydroxysteroid dehydrogenase: a cause of hirsutism in pubertal and postpubertal women. J Clin Endocrinol Metab 1985; 60:428–438.

772. Bongiovanni AM. Urinary steroidal pattern of infants with congenital hyperplasia due to 3β-hydroxysteroid dehydrogenase deficiency. J Steroid Biochem 1980; 13:809–811.

773. Nakajin S, Shively JE, Yuan P-M, Hall PF. Microsomal cytochrome P-450 from neonatal pig testis: two enzymatic activities (17α-hydroxylase and $C_{17,20}$-lyase) associated with one protein. Biochemistry 20:4037–4042, 1981.

774. Chung B-C, Picardo-Leonard J, Haniu M, et al. Cytochrome P450c17 (steroid 17α-hydroxylase/17,20-lyase) cloning of the human adrenal and testes cDNAs indicate the same gene is expressed in both tissues. Proc Natl Acad Sci U S A 1987; 84:407–411.

775. Yanase T, Simpson ER, Waterman MR. 17α-Hydroxylase/17,20-lyase deficiency: from clinical investigation to molecular definition. Endocr Rev 1991; 12:91–108.

776. Lin D, Black SM, Nagahama Y, Miller WL. Steroid 17α-hydroxylase and 17,20-lyase activities of P450c17: contributions of serine[106] and P450 reductase. Endocrinology 1993; 132:2498–2506.

777. Sparkes RS, Klisak I, Miller WL. Regional mapping of genes encoding human steroidogenic enzymes: P450scc to 15q23-q24; adrenodoxin to 11q22; adrenodoxin reductase to 17q24-q25; and P450c17 to 10q24-q25. DNA Cell Biol 1991; 10:359–365.

778. Matteson KJ, Picardo-Leonard J, Chung B, et al. Assignment of the gene for adrenal P450c17 (17α-hydroxylase/17,20-lyase) to human chromosome 10. J Clin Endocrinol Metab 1986; 63:789–791.

779. Oei SG, Derksen J, Weusten JJAM, et al. A case of 16-ene-synthetase deficiency in male pseudohermaphroditism due to combined 17α-hydroxylase/17,20-lyase deficiency. Eur J Endocrinol 1995; 132:281–285.

780. Biglieri EG, Herron MA, Brust N. 17-Hydroxylation deficiency in man. J Clin Invest 1966; 45:1946–1954.

781. New MI. Male pseudohermaphrodism due to a 17α-hydroxylase deficiency. J Clin Invest 1970; 49:1930–1941.

782. Dean HJ, Shackelton CHL, Winter JSD. Diagnosis and natural history of 17-hydroxylase deficiency in a newborn male. J Clin Endocrinol Metab 1984; 59:513–520.

783. Winter JSD, Couch RM, Muller J, et al. Combined 17-hydroxylase and 17/20 desmolase deficiencies: evidence for synthesis of a defective cytochrome P450c17. J Clin Endocrinol Metab 1989; 68:309–316.

784. Lin D, Harikrishna JA, Moore CCD, et al. Missense mutation serine 106 → proline causes 17α-hydroxylase deficiency. J Biol Chem 1991; 266:15992–15998.

785. Fardella CE, Zhang L-H, Mahachoklertwattana P, et al. Deletion of amino acids Asp487-Ser488-Phe489 in human cytochrome P450c17 causes severe 17α-hydroxylase deficiency. J Clin Endocrinol Metab 1993; 77:489–493.

786. Fardella CE, Hum DW, Homoki J, et al. Point mutation of Arg 440 to His in cytochrome P450c17 causes severe 17α-hydroxylase deficiency. J Clin Endocrinol Metab 1994; 79:160–164.

787. Kater CE, Biglieri EG. Disorders of steroid 17α-hydroxylase deficiency. Endocrinol Metab Clin North Am 1994; 23:341–357.

788. Moreira AC, Leal AMO, Castro M. Characterization of adrenocorticotropin secretion in a patient with 17α-hydroxylase deficiency. J Clin Endocrinol Metab 1990; 71:86–91.

789. Fardella CE, Hum DW, Homoki J, et al. Point mutation of Arg 440 to His in cytochrome P450c17 causes severe 17α-hydroxylase deficiency. J Clin Endocrinol Metab 1994; 79:160–164.

790. Yanase T. 17α-hydroxylase/17,20-lyase defects. J Steroid Biochem Mol Biol 1995; 53:153–157.

791. Oshiro C, Takasu N, Wakugami T, et al. Seventeen α-hydroxylase deficiency with one base pair deletion of the cytochrome P450c17 (CYP17) gene. J Clin Endocrinol Metab 1995; 80:2526–2529.

792. Imai T, Yanasi T, Waterman M, et al. Canadian Mennonites and individuals residing in the Friesland region of The Netherlands share the same molecular basis of 17α-hydroxylase deficiency. Hum Genet 1992; 89:95–96.

793. Miura K, Yasuda K, Yanase T, et al. Mutation of cytochrome P-45017α gene (CYP17) in a Japanese patient previously reported as having glucocorticoid-responsive hyperaldosteronism: with a review of Japanese patients with mutations of CYP17. J Clin Endocrinol Metab 1996; 81:3797–3801.

794. Kaneko E, Kobayashi Y, Yasukochi Y, et al. Genomic analysis of two siblings with 17α-hydroxylase deficiency and hypertension. Hypertens Res 1994; 17:143–147.

795. Kater CE, Biglieri EG, Brust N, et al. The unique patterns of plasma aldosterone and 18-hydroxycorticosterone concentrations in the 17α-hydroxylase deficiency syndrome. J Clin Endocrinol Metab 1982; 55:295–302.

796. D'Armiento M, Reda G, Kater C, et al. 17α-Hydroxylase deficiency: mineralocorticoid hormone profiles in an affected family. J Clin Endocrinol Metab 1983; 56:697–701.

797. Miller WL. Molecular biology of steroid hormone synthesis. Endocr Rev 1988; 9:295–318.

798. Prader A, Gurtner HP. Das Syndrom des Pseudohermaphroditismus masculinus bei kongenitaler Nebennierenrinden-Hyperplasie ohne Androgenuberproduktion (adrenaler Pseudohermaphrotidismus masculinus). Helv Paediatr Acta 1955; 10:397–412.

799. Koizumi S, Kyoya S, Miyawaki T, et al. Cholesterol side-chain cleavage enzyme activity and cytochrome P-450 content in adrenal mitochondria of a patient with congenital lipoid adrenal hyperplasia (Prader disease). Clin Chim Acta 1977; 77:301–306.

800. Bose HS, Sugawara T, Strauss III JF, et al. The pathophysiology and genetics of congenital lipoid adrenal hyperplasia. N Engl J Med 1996; 335:1870–1878.

801. Kirkland RT, Kirkland JL, Johnson CM, et al. Congenital lipoid adrenal hyperplasia in an eight-year old phenotypic female. J Clin Endocrinol Metab 1973; 56:488–496.

802. Hauffa BP, Miller WL, Grumbach MM, et al. Congenital adrenal hyperplasia due to deficient cholesterol side-chain cleavage activity (20,22 desmolase) in a patient treated for 18 years. Clin Endocrinol 1985; 23:481–493.

803. Matsuo N, Tsuzaki S, Anzo M, et al. The phenotypic definition of congenital lipoid adrenal hyperplasia: analysis of the 67 Japanese patients. Abstract 200. 33rd Annual European Society of Pediatric Endocrinology Meeting. Horm Res 1994; 41:106.

804. Matsuo N, Ogata T, Sato S, et al. Polycystic ovaries in congenital lipoid adrenal hyperplasia: a characteristic pubertal manifestation. Abstract 204. 34th Annual European Society of Pediatric Endocrinology Meeting. Horm Res 1995; 44(Suppl):52.

805. Müller J, Torsson A, Damkjaer Nielsen M, et al. Gonadal development and growth in 46,XX and 46,XY individuals with P450scc deficiency (congenital lipoid adrenal hyperplasia). Horm Res 1991; 36:203–208.

806. Lin D, Gitelman SE, Saenger P, Miller WL. Normal genes for the cholesterol side chain cleavage enzyme, P450scc, in congenital adrenal hyperplasia. J Clin Invest 1991; 88:1955–1962.

807. Saenger P, Lin D, Gitelman SE, Miller WL. Congenital lipoid adrenal hyperplasia: genes for P450scc, side chain cleavage enzyme, are normal. J Steroid Biochem Mol Biol 1993; 45:87–97.

808. Izumi H, Saito N, Ichiki S, et al. Prenatal diagnosis of congenital lipoid adrenal hyperplasia. Obstet Gynecol 1993; 81:839–841.

809. Sakai Y, Yanase T, Okabe Y, et al. No mutation in cytochrome P450 side chain cleavage in a patient with congenital adrenal hyperplasia. J Clin Endocrinol Metab 1994; 79:1198–1201.

810. Saenger P, Klonari Z, Black SM, et al. Prenatal diagnosis of congenital lipoid adrenal hyperplasia. J Clin Endocrinol Metab 1995; 80:200–205.

811. Lin D, Sugawara T, Strauss JF III, et al. Role of steroidogenic acute regulatory protein in adrenal and gonadal steroidogenesis. Science 1995; 267:1828–1831.

812. Bose HS, Pescouitz OH, Miller WL. Spontaneous feminization in a 46,XX female patient with adrenal hyperplasia due to a homozygous frame shift

mutation in the steroidogenic reactive protein. J Clin Endocrinol Metab 1997; 82:1511–1515.

812a. Fujieda K, Tajima T, Nakae J, et al. Spontaneous puberty in a 46,XX subject with congenital lipoid adrenal hyperplasia. J Clin Invest 1997; 99:1265–1271.

813. Tee M-K, Lin D, Sugawara T, et al. T → A transversion 11 bp from a splice acceptor site in the human gene for steroidogenic acute regulatory protein causes congenital lipoid adrenal hyperplasia. Hum Mol Genet 1995; 4:2299–2305.

814. Portat-Doven S, Leheup B, Chaussain J-L, et al. Three new mutations of the steroidogenic acute regulatory gene (StAR) in 2 families with congenital lipoid adrenal hyperplasia. Abstract P2-726. 10th Intl Cong of Endocrinology, 1996: 586.

815. Yang X, Iwamoto K, Wang M, et al. Inherited congenital adrenal hyperplasia in the rabbit is caused by a deletion in the gene encoding cytochrome P450 cholesterol side-chain cleavage enzyme. Endocrinology 1993; 132:1977–1982.

816. Lambeth JD, Xu XX, Glover M. Cholesterol sulfate inhibits adrenal mitochondrial cholesterol side chain cleavage at a site distinct from cytochrome P-450$_{scc}$. J Biol Chem 1987; 262:9181–9188.

817. Jefcoate CR, Di Bartolomeas MJ, Williams CA, et al. ACTH regulation of cholesterol movement in isolated adrenal cells. J Steroid Biochem 1987; 27:721–729.

818. Stocco DM, Sodeman TC. The 30 kDA mitochondrial proteins induced by hormone stimulation in MA-10 mouse Leydig tumor cells are processed from larger precursors. J Biol Chem 1991; 266:19731–19738.

819. Clark BJ, Wells J, King SR, et al. The purification, cloning and expression of a novel luteinizing hormone-induced mitochondrial protein in MA-10 mouse Leydig tumor cells: characterization of the steroidogenic acute regulatory protein (StAR). J Biol Chem 1994; 269:28314–28322.

820. Stocco DM, Clark BJ. Regulation of the acute production of steroids in steroidogenic cells. Endocr Rev 1996; 17:221–244.

821. Stocco DM, Clark BJ. The role of the steroidogenic acute regulatory protein in steroidogenesis. Steroids 1997; 62:29–36.

822. Arakane F, Sugawara T, Nishino H, et al. Steroidogenic acute regulatory protein (StAR) retains activity in the absence of its mitochondrial import sequence: implications for the mechanism of StAR action. Proc Natl Acad Sci U S A 1996; 93:13731–13736.

823. Sugawara T, Holt JA, Driscoll D, et al. Human steroidogenic acute regulatory protein: functional activity in COS-1 cells, tissue-specific expression, and mapping of the structural gene to 8p11.2 and a pseudogene to chromosome 13. Proc Natl Acad Sci U S A 1995; 92:4778–4782.

824. Miller WL. Mitochondrial specificity of the early steps in steroidogenesis. J Steroid Biochem Mol Biol 1995; 55:607–616.

825. Simpson ER, Mahendroo MS, Means GD, et al. Aromatase cytochrome P450, the enzyme responsible for estogen biosynthesis. Endocr Rev 1994; 15:342–355.

826. Shozu M, Akasofu K, Takenori H, Kubota Y. A new cause of female pseudohermaphroditism: placental aromatase deficiency. J Clin Endocrinol Metab 1991; 72:560–566.

827. Ito Y, Fisher CR, Conte FA, et al. Molecular basis of aromatase deficiency in an adult female with sexual infantilism and polycystic ovaries. Proc Natl Acad Sci U S A 1993; 90:11673–11677.

828. Conte FA, Grumbach MM, Ito Y, et al. A syndrome of female pseudohermaphrodism, hypergonadotropic hypogonadism, and multicystic ovaries associated with missense mutations in the gene encoding aromatase (P450arom). J Clin Endocrinol Metab 1994; 78:1287–1292.

829. Mullis PE, Yoshimura N, Kuhlmann B, et al. Aromatase deficiency in a girl compound heterozygote for two point mutations in the P450arom gene: impact of estrogens in hypergonadotrophic hypogonadism, multicystic ovaries, body composition and bone density in childhood. J Clin Endocrinol Metab 1997; 82:1739–1745.

830. Portat-Doyen S, Forrest MG, Nicolino M, et al. Female pseudohermaphroditism (FPH) resulting from aromatase (P450arom) deficiency associated with a novel mutation in the CYP19 gene. Abstract 14. Horm Res 1996; 46(Suppl):4.

831. Casey ML, MacDonald PC. Alterations in steroid production by the human placenta. In: Pasqualini JR, Sholler R, eds. Hormones and Fetal Pathophysiology. New York: Marcel Dekker, 1992: 251–270.

832. Yoshida N, Osawa Y. Purification of human placental aromatase cytochrome P-450 with monoclonal antibody and its characterization. Biochemistry 1991; 30:3003–3010.

833. Yalcinkaya TM, Siiteri PK, Vigne J-L, et al. A mechanism for virilization of female spotted hyenas in utero. Science 1993; 260:1929–1931.

834. Hodgkin J. Sex determination and the generation of sexually dimorphic nervous systems. Neuron 1991; 6:177–185.

835. Pilgrim C, Reisert I. Differences between male and female brains: developmental mechanisms and implications. Horm Metab Res 1992; 24:353–359.

836. Harada N, Ogawa H, Shozu M, et al. Biochemical and molecular genetic analyses on placental aromatase (P-450$_{arom}$) deficiency. J Biol Chem 1992; 267:4781–4785.

837. Grumbach MM, Ducharme JR, Moloshok RE. On the fetal masculinizing action of certain oral progestins. J Clin Endocrinol Metab 1959; 19:1369–1380.

838. Kirk JM, Perry LA, Shard WS. Female pseudohermaphroditism due to a maternal adrenocortical tumor. J Clin Endocrinol Metab 1990; 70:1280–1284.

839. Wilkens L. Masculinization of female fetus due to use of orally given progestins. JAMA 1960; 172:1028–1032.

840. Jones HW Jr. Nonadrenal female pseudohermaphroditism. In: Josso N, ed. The Intersex Child: Pediatric and Adolescent Endocrinology. Vol 8. Basel: S Karger, 1981: 65–79.

841. Ishizuka N, Kawashima Y, Nakanishi T, et al. Statistical observations on genital anomalies of newborns following the administration of progestins to their mothers. Obstet Gynecol Surv 1964; 19:496–497.

842. Duck SC, Katayama KP. Danazol may cause female pseudohermaphrodism. Fertil Steril 1981; 35:230–231.

843. Brunskill J. The effects of fetal exposure to Danazol. Br J Obstet Gynaecol 1992; 99:212–214.

844. Picco P, Garibaldi LR, Di Rocco M, et al. In utero virilization by Danazol: effects on adrenal steroidogenesis. Adolesc Pediatr Gynecol 1995; 8:97–100.

845. Bongiovanni AM, Di George AM, Grumbach MM. Masculinization of the female infant associated with estrogenic therapy alone during gestation: four cases. J Clin Endocrinol Metab 1959; 19:1104–1110.

846. Krik JM, Perry LA, Shard WS. Female pseudohermaphroditism due to a maternal adrenocortical tumor. J Clin Endocrinol Metab 1990; 70:1280–1284.

847. Novak DJ, Lauchlan SC, McCawley JC, et al. Virilization during pregnancy. Am J Med 1970; 49:281–290.

848. Verhoeven ATM, Mastboom JL, Van Leusden HAIM, et al. Virilization in pregnancy coexisting with an (ovarian) mucinous cystadenoma: a case report and review of virilizing ovarian tumors in pregnancy. Obstet Gynecol Surv 1973; 28:597–622.

849. Kai H, Nose O, Iida Y, et al. Female pseudohermaphrodism caused by maternal congenital adrenal hyperplasia. J Pediatr 1979; 95:418–420.

850. Manganiello PD, Adams LV, Harris RD, Ornvold K. Virilization during pregnancy with spontaneous resolution postpartum: a case report and review of the English literature. Obst Gynec Surv 1995; 50:404–410.

851. Joshi R, Dunaif A. Ovarian disorders of pregnancy. Endocrinol Metab Clin North Am 1995; 24:153–169.

852. Hensleigh PA, Carter RP, Grotjan HE Jr. Fetal protection against masculinization with hyperreactio luteinalis and virilization. J Clin Endocrinol Metab 1975; 40:816–823.

853. Hensleigh PA, Woodruff JD. Differential maternal-fetal response to androgenizing luteoma or hyperreactio luteinalis. Obstet Gynecol Surv 1978; 33:262–271.

854. Park IJ, Johanson A, Jones HW, et al. Special female hermaphroditism associated with multiple disorders. Obstet Gynecol 1972; 39:100–106.

855. Gearhart JP, Rock JD. Female pseudohermaphroditism: unusual variants and their management. Adolesc Pediatr Gynecol 1989; 2:3–9.

856. Carpentier PJ, Potter EL. Nuclear sex and genital malformation in 48 cases of renal agenesis, with especial reference to nonspecific female pseudohermaphroditism. Am J Obstet Gynecol 1959; 78:235–258.

857. Wenstrup RJ, Pagon RA. Female pseudohermaphroditism with anorectal, müllerian duct, and urinary tract malformations: report of four cases. J Pediatr 1985; 107:751–754.

858. Perez-Palacios G, Scaglia H, Kofman-Alfaro S, et al. Inherited deficiency of gonadotropin receptor in Leydig cells: a new form of male pseudohermaphroditism. Am J Hum Genet 1975; 27:71a (abstract).

859. Berthezene F, Forest MG, Grimaud JA, et al. Leydig cell agenesis: a cause of male pseudohermaphroditism. N Engl J Med 1976; 295:969–972.

860. Brown DM, Markland C, Dehner LP. Leydig cell hypoplasia: a cause of male pseudohermaphroditism. J Clin Endocrinol Metab 1978; 46:1–7.

861. Perez-Palacios G, Scaglia H, Kofman-Alfaro S, et al. Inherited male pseudohermaphrodism due to gonadotropin unresponsiveness. Acta Endocrinol 1981; 98:148–156.

862. Schwartz M, Imperato-McGinley J, Peterson RE, et al. Male pseudohermaphroditism secondary to an abnormality in Leydig cell differentiation. J Clin Endocrinol Metab 1981; 53:123–127.

863. Perez-Palacios G, Ulloa-Aguirre A, Kofman-Alfaro S. Inherited male pseudohermaphroditism: analogies between human and rodent models. In: Serio M, Motta M, Zanisi M, et al., eds. Sexual Differentiation: Basic and Clinical Aspects. New York: Raven Press, 1984: 287–299.

864. Lee PA, Rock JA, Brown TR, et al. Leydig cell hypofunction resulting in male pseudohermaphroditism. Fertil Steril 1982; 37:675–679.

865. David R, Yoon D, Landin L, et al. A syndrome of gonadotropin resistance possibly due to an LH receptor defect. Endocr Soc Abstr 1983; 468:197.

866. Eil C, Austin RM, Sesterhenn I, et al. Leydig cell hypoplasia causing male pseudohermaphroditism: diagnosis 13 years after prepubertal castration. J Clin Endocrinol Metab 1984; 58:441–448.

867. Toledo SPA, Arnhold IJP, Luthold W, et al. Leydig cell hypoplasia determining familial hypergonadotrophic hypogonadism. Prog Clin Biol Res 1985; 200:311–314.

868. Saldanha PH, Arnhold IJP, Mendonca BB, et al. A clinico-genetic investigation of Leydig cell hypoplasia. Am J Med Genet 1987; 26:337–344.

869. Toledo SPA. Leydig cell hypoplasia leading to two different phenotypes: male pseudohermaphroditism and primary hypogonadism not associated with this. Clin Endocrinol 1992; 36:521–522 (Letter).

870. Themmen APN, Brunner HG. Luteinizing hormone receptor mutations and sex differentiation. Eur J Endocrinol 1996; 134:533–540.

871. Bardin CW, Bullock LP, Sherins RJ, et al. Androgen metabolism and mechanism of action in male pseudohermaphroditism: a study of testicular feminization. Recent Prog Horm Res 1973; 29:65–109.

872. Kremer H, Kraaij R, Toledo SPA, et al. Male pseudohermaphroditism due to a homozygous missense mutation of the luteinizing hormone receptor gene. Nat Genet 1995; 9:160–164.

873. Latronico AC, Anasti J, Arnhold IJP, et al. Brief report: testicular and ovarian resistance to luteinizing hormone caused by homozygous inactivating mutations of the luteinizing hormone receptor gene. N Engl J Med 1996; 334:507–512

874. Laue L, Wu S-M, Kudo M, et al. A nonsense mutation of the human luteinizing hormone receptor gene in Leydig cell hypoplasia. Hum Mol Genet 1995; 4:1429–1433.

875. Burgner DP, Kinmond S, Wallace AM, et al. Male pseudohermaphroditism secondary to panhypopituitarism. Arch Dis Child 1996; 75:153–155.

876. Mendonca BB, Bloise W, Arnhold IJP, et al. Male pseudohermaphroditism due to non-salt losing 3β-hydroxysteroid dehydrogenase deficiency: gender role change and absence of gynecomastia at puberty. J Steroid Biochem 1987; 28:669–675.

877. Parks GA, Bermudez JA, Anast CS, et al. Pubertal boy with the 3β-hydroxysteroid dehydrogenase defect. J Clin Endocrinol Metab 1971; 33:269–278.

878. Schneider G, Genel M, Bongiovanni AM, et al. Persistent testicular Δ⁵-isomerase-3β-hydroxysteroid dehydrogenase (Δ⁵-3β-HSD) deficiency in the Δ⁵-3β-HSD form of congenital adrenal hyperplasia. J Clin Invest 1975; 55:681–690.

879. Simard J, Rhéaume E, Sanchez R, et al. Molecular basis of congenital adrenal hyperplasia due to 3β-hydroxysteroid dehydrogenase deficiency. Mol Endocrinol 1993; 7:716–728.

880. Sanchez R, Mebarki F, Rhéaume E, et al. Functional characterization of the novel L108W and P186L mutations detected in the type II 3β-hydroxysteroid dehydrogenase gene of a male pseudohermaphrodite with congenital adrenal hyperplasia. Hum Mol Genet 1994; 3:1639–1645.

881. Morel Y, Mebarki F, Rheáume E, et al. Structure-function relationship of 3β-hydroxysteroid dehydrogenase: contribution made by molecular genetics of 3β-hydroxysteroid dehydrogenase deficiency. Steroids 1997; 62:176–184.

882. Russel AJ, Wallace AM, Forest MG, et al. Mutation in the human gene for 3β-hydroxysteroid dehydrogenase type II leading to male pseudohermaphroditism without salt loss. J Mol Endocrinol 1994; 12:225–237.

883. Zerah M, Rhéaume E, Mani P, et al. No evidence of mutations in the genes for type I and type II 3β-hydroxysteroid dehydrogenase (3β-HSD) in nonclassical 3β-HSD deficiency. J Clin Endocrinol Metab 1994; 79: 1811–1817.

884. Cara JF, Moshang T Jr, Bongiovanni AM, et al. Elevated 17-hydroxy-progesterone and testosterone in a newborn with 3-beta-hydroxysteroid dehydrogenase deficiency. N Engl J Med 1985; 313:618–621.

885. Jones HW Jr, Lee PA, Rock JA, et al. A genetic male patient with 17α-hydroxylase deficiency. Obstet Gynecol 1982; 59:254–259.

886. Peter M, Sippell WG, Wernze H. Diagnosis and treatment of 17-hydroxylase deficiency. J Steroid Biochem Mol Biol 1993; 45:107–116.

887. Tvedegaard M, Frederiksen V, Olgaard K, et al. Two cases of 17α-hydroxylase deficiency: one combined with complete gonadal agenesis. Acta Endocrinol 1981; 98:267–273.

888. Ahlgren R, Yanase T, Simpson ER, et al. Compound heterozygous mutations (Arg 239 → stop, Pro 342 → Thr) in the CYP17 (P450 17α) gene lead to ambiguous external genitalia in a male with partial combined 17α-hydroxylase/17,20-lyase deficiency. J Clin Endocrinol Metab 1992; 74:667–672.

889. Yanagibashi K, Hall PF. Role of electron transport in the regulation of the lyase activity of C21 side-chain cleavage P450 from porcine adrenal and testicular microsomes. J Biol Chem 1986; 261:8429–8433.

890. Miller WL, Auchus RJ, Geller DH. The regulation of 17,20-lyase activity. Steorids 1997; 62:133–142.

891. Katagiri M, Kagawa N, Waterman MR. The role of cytochrome b_5 in the biosynthesis of androgens by human P450$_{c17}$. Arch Biochem Biophys 1995; 317:343–347.

892. Zhang L-H, Rodriguez H, Ohno S, Miller WL. Serine phosphorylation of human P450c17 increases 17,20-lyase activity: implications for adrenarche and the polycystic ovary syndrome. Proc Natl Acad Sci U S A 1995; 92:10619–10623.

893. Zachmann M, Vollmin JA, Hamilton W, et al. Steroid 17,20-desmolase deficiency: a new cause of male pseudohermaphroditism. Clin Endocrinol 1972; 1:369–385.

894. Zachmann M, Kempkin B, Manella B, Navarro E. Conversion from pure 17,20-desmolase to combined 17,20-desmolase/17α-hydroxylase deficiency with age. Acta Endocrinol 1992; 127:97–99.

895. Yanase T, Waterman MR, Zachmann M, et al. Molecular basis of apparent isolated 17,20-lyase deficiency: compound heterozygous mutations in the C-terminal region (Arg(496)→Cys, Gln(461)→Stop) actually cause combined 17α-hydroxylase/17,20-lyase deficiency. Biochim Biophys Acta 1992; 1139:275–279.

896. Mendonca BB, Arnhold IJP, Pelegrinelli AC, et al. Male pseudohermaphroditism due to isolated 17,20-lyase deficiency. Abstract P3-617. Proceedings of the 77th Annual Meeting of the Endocrine Society, Washington, DC, 1995.

897. Kitamura M, Buczbo E, Dufau ML. Dissociation of hydroxylase and lyase activities by site-directed mutagenesis of the rat P450$_{17α}$. Mol Endocrinol 1991; 5:1373–1380.

898. Lin D, Zhang L-H, Chiao E, Miller WL. Modeling and mutagenesis of the active site of human P450c17. Mol Endocrinol 1994; 8:392–402.

899. Geller DH, Auchus RJ, Mendonca BB, et al. The genetic and functional basis of isolated 17,20-lyase deficiency. Nat Genet 1997; 17:201–205.

900. Larrea F, Lisker R, Banuelos R, et al. Hypergonadotropic hypogonadism in an XX female subject due to 17,20-desmolase deficiency. Acta Endocrinol 1983; 103:400–405.

901. Forest MG. Familial male pseudohermaphroditism due to 17-20 desmolase deficiency. I. In vivo endocrine studies. J Clin Endocrinol Metab 1980; 50:826–833.

902. Geissler WM, Davis DL, Wu L, et al. Male pseudohermaphroditism caused by mutations of testicular 17β-hydroxysteroid dehydrogenase 3. Nat Genet 1994; 7:34–39.

903. Andersson S, Russell DW, Wilson J. 17β-hydroxysteroid dehydrogenase 3 deficiency. Trends Endocrinol 1996; 7:121–125.

904. Luu-The V, Labrie C, Simard J, et al. Structure of two in tandem human 17β-hydroxysteroid dehydrogenase genes. Mol Endocrinol 1990; 4:268–275.

905. Luu-The V, Labrie C, Zhao HF, et al. Characterization of cDNAs for human estradiol 17β-dehydrogenase and assignment of one gene to chromosome 17: evidence for two mRNA species with distinct 5′-termini in human placenta. Mol Endocrinol 1989; 3:1301–1309.

906. Wu L, Einstein M, Geissler WM, et al. Expression cloning and characterization of human 17β-hydroxysteroid dehydrogenase type 2, a microsomal enzyme possessing 20 α-hydroxysteroid dehydrogenase activity. J Biol Chem 1993; 268:12964–12969.

907. Casey ML, MacDonald PC, Andersson S. 17β-hydroxysteroid dehydrogenase type 2: chromosomal assignment and progestin regulation of gene expression in human endometrium. J Clin Invest 1994; 94:2135–2141.

908. Adamski J, Normand T, Leenders F, et al. Molecular cloning of a novel widely expressed 80 kDA 17β-hydroxysteroid dehydrogenase IV. Biochem J 1995; 311(Part 2):437–443.

909. Zhang Y, Dufort I, Soucy P, et al. Cloning and expression of human type V 17β-hydroxysteroid dehydrogenase. Abstract P3-614. Proceedings, 77th Annual Meeting of the Endocrine Society, Washington, DC. Bethesda, MD, The Endocrine Society, 1995, p 622.

910. Saez JM, de Peretti E, Morera AM, et al. Familial male pseudohermaphroditism with gynecomastia due to a testicular 17-ketosteroid reductase defect. I. In vivo studies. J Clin Endocrinol Metab 1971; 32:604–601.

911. Saez JM, Morera AM, de Peretti E, Bertand J. Further in vivo studies in male pseudohermaphroditism with gynecomastia due to a testicular 17-ketosteroid reductase defect (compared to a case of testicular feminization). J Clin Endocrinol Metab 1972; 34:598–600.

912. Rösler A, Kohn G. Male pseudohermaphroditism due to 17β-hydroxysteroid dehydrogenase deficiency: studies on the natural history of the defect and effect of androgens on gender role. J Steroid Biochem 1983; 19:663–674.

913. Rösler A. Steroid 17β-hydroxysteroid dehydrogenase deficiency in man: an inherited form of male pseudohermaphroditism. J Steroid Biochem Mol Biol 1992; 43:989–1002.

914. Dumic M, Plavsic V, Fattorini I, et al. Absent spermatogenesis despite early bilateral orchiopexy in 17-ketoreductase deficiency. Horm Res 1985; 22:100–106.

915. Ulloa-Aguirre A, Bassol S, Poo J, et al. Endrocine and biochemical studies in a 46,XY phenotypically male infant with 17-ketosteroid reductase deficiency. J Clin Endocrinol Metab 1985; 60:639–643.

916. Andersson S, Geissler WM, Wu L, et al. Molecular genetics and pathophysiology of 17β-hydroxysteroid dehydrogenase 3 deficiency. J Clin Endocrinol Metab 1996; 81:130–136.

917. Givens JR, Wiser WL, Summitt RL, et al. Familial male pseudohermaphroditism without gynecomastia due to deficient testicular 17-ketosteroid reductase activity. N Engl J Med 1974; 291:938–944.

918. Pittaway DE, Andersen RN, Givens JR. Deficient 17β-hydroxysteroid oxidoreductase activity in testes from a male pseudohermaphrodite. J Clin Endocrinol Metab 1976; 43:457–461.

919. Imperato-McGinley J, Peterson RE, Stoller R, et al. Male pseudohermaphroditism secondary to 17β-hydroxysteroid dehydrogenase deficiency: gender role change with puberty. J Clin Endocrinol Metab 1979; 49:391–395.

920. Millan M, Audi L, Martinez-Mora J, et al. 17-Ketosteroid reductase deficiency in an adult patient without gynecomastia but with female psychosocial orientation. Acta Endocrinol 1983; 102:633–640.

921. Akesode FA, Meyer WJ, Migeon CJ. Male pseudohermaphroditism with gynecomastia due to testicular 17-ketosteroid reductase deficiency. Clin Endocrinol 1977; 7:443–452.

922. Rösler A, Belanger A, Labrie F. Mechanisms of androgen production in male pseudohermaphroditism due to 17β-hydroxysteroid dehydrogenase deficiency. J Clin Endocrinol Metab 1992; 75:773–778.

923. Eckstein B, Cohen S, Farkas S, Rösler A. The nature of the defect in familial male pseudohermaphroditism in Arabs of the Gaza. J Clin Endocrinol Metab 1994; 64:477–485.

924. Rösler A, Silverstein S, Abeliovich D. A (R80Q) mutation in 17β-hydroxysteroid dehydrogenase type 3 gene among Arabs of Israel is associated with pseudohermaphroditism in males and normal asymptomatic females. J Clin Endocrinol Metab 1996; 81:1827–1831.

925. Bentvelsen FM, McPhaul MJ, Wilson JD, George FW. The androgen receptor of the urogenital tract of the fetal rat is regulated by androgen. Mol Cell Endocrinol 1994; 105:21–26.

926. Harkness RA, Thistlethwaite D, Darling JAB, et al. 17β-Hydroxysteroid oxidoreductase deficiency causing male pseudohermaphroditism in a child. J Endocrinol 1975; 67:16P–17P.

927. Gross DJ, Landau H, Kohn G, et al. Male pseudohermaphroditism due to 17β-hydroxysteroid dehydrogenase deficiency: gender assignment in early infancy. Acta Endocrinol 1986; 112:238–246.

928. Gregory JW, Aynsley-Green A, Evans BAJ, et al. Deficiency of 17-ketoreductase presenting before puberty. Horm Res 1993; 40:145–148.

929. Pang S, Softness B, Sweeney WJ III, et al. Hirsutism, polycystic ovarian disease and ovarian 17-ketosteroid reductase deficiency. N Engl J Med 1987; 316:1295–1301.

930. Toscano V, Balducci R, Bianchi P, et al. Ovarian 17-ketosteroid reductase deficiency as a possible cause of polyceptic ovarian disease. J Clin Endocrinol Metab 1990; 71:288–292.

931. Castro-Magana M, Angulo M, Uy J. Male hypogonadism with gynecomastia caused by late onset deficiency of testicular 17-ketosteroid reductase. N Engl J Med 1993; 328:1297–1301.

932. Farkas A, Rösler A, et al. Ten years experience with masculinizing genitoplasty in male pseudohermaphroditism due to 17β-hydroxysteroid dehydrogenase deficiency. Eur J Pediatr 1993; 152(Suppl 2):S88–S90.

933. Quigley C, De Bellis A, Marschke KB, et al. Androgen receptor defects: historical, clinical, and molecular perspectives. Endocr Rev 1995; 16:271–321.

934. Patterson MN, McPhaul MJ, Hughes IA. Androgen insensitivity syndrome. Baillieres Clin Endocrinol Metab 1994; 8:379–404.

935. MacLean HE, Warne GL, Zajac JD. Defects of androgen receptor function: from sex reversal to motor neurone disease. Mol Cell Endocrinol 1995; 112:133–141.

936. Morris JM, Mahesh VB. Further observations on the syndrome, "testicular feminization." Am J Obstet Gynecol 1963; 87:731–734.

937. Bangsbøll S, Qvist I, Lebech PE, Lewinsky M. Testicular feminization syndrome and associated gonadal tumors in Denmark. Acta Obstet Gynecol Scand 1992; 71:63–66.

938. Quigley CA, Friedman KJ, Johnson A, et al. Complete deletion of the androgen receptor gene: definition of the null phenotype of the androgen insensitivity syndrome and determination of carrier status. J Clin Endocrinol Metab 1992; 74:927–933.

939. Rutgers JL, Scully RE. The androgen insensitivity syndrome (testicular feminization): a clinicopathologic study of 43 cases. Int J Gynaecol Pathol 1991; 10:126–144.

940. Bale PM, Howard NJ, Wright JE. Male pseudohermaphroditism in XY children with female phenotype. Pediatr Pathol 1992; 12:29–49.

941. O'Leary JA. Comparative studies of the gonad in testicular feminization and cryptorchidism. Fertil Steril 1965; 16:813–819.

942. Ferenczy A, Richart RM. The fine structures of the gonads in the complete form of testicular feminization syndrome. Am J Obstet Gynecol 1972; 113:399–409.

943. German J, Simpson JL, Morillo-Cucci G, et al. Testicular feminization and inguinal hernias. Lancet 1978; 1:891.

944. Madden JD, Walsh PC, MacDonald PC, et al. Clinical and endocrinologic characterization of a patient with the syndrome of incomplete testicular feminization. J Clin Endocrinol Metab 1973; 41:751–760.

945. French FS, Van Wyk JJ, Baggett B, et al. Further evidence of a target organ defect in the syndrome of testicular feminization. J Clin Endocrinol Metab 1966; 26:493–503.

946. Stanley AJ, Gumbreck LG, Allison JE. Male pseudohermaphroditism in the laboratory Norway rat. Recent Prog Horm Res 1973; 29:43–64.

947. Gehring U, Tomkins GM, Ohno S. Effect of the androgen-insensitivity mutation on a cytoplasmic receptor for dihydrotestosterone. Nat New Biol 1971; 232:106–107.

948. Goldstein JL, Wilson JD. Studies on the pathogenesis of the pseudohermaphroditism in the mouse with testicular feminization. J Clin Invest 1972; 51:1647–1658.

949. Keenan BS, Meyer WJ III, Hadjian AJ, et al. Syndrome of androgen insensitivity in man: absence of 5α-dihydrotestosterone binding protein in skin fibroblasts. J Clin Endocrinol Metab 1974; 38:1143–1146.

950. Griffin JE, Punyashthiti K, Wilson JD. Dihydrotestosterone binding by cultured fibroblasts: comparison of cells from control subjects and from patients with hereditary male pseudohermaphroditism due to androgen resistance. J Clin Invest 1976; 57:1342–1351.

951. Kaufman M, Straidfeld C, Pinsky L. Male pseudohermaphroditism presumably due to target organ unresponsiveness to androgens: deficient 5α-dihydrotestosterone binding in cultured skin fibroblasts. J Clin Invest 1976; 58:345–350.

952. Amrhein JA, Meyer WJ III, Jones HW Jr, et al. Androgen insensitivity in man: evidence for genetic heterogeneity. Proc Natl Acad Sci U S A 1976; 73:891–894.

953. Kaufman M, Pinsky L, Baird PH, et al. Complete androgen insensitivity with a normal amount of 5α-dihydrotestosterone–binding activity in labium majus skin fibroblasts. Am J Med Genet 1979; 4:401–411.

954. Berkovitz GD, Brown TR, Migeon CJ. Androgen receptors. Clin Endocrinol Metab 1983; 12:155–173.

955. Griffin JE. Testicular feminization associated with a thermolabile androgen receptor in cultured fibroblasts. J Clin Invest 1979; 64:1624–1631.

956. Pinsky L, Kaufman M, Summitt RL. Congenital androgen insensitivity due to a qualitatively abnormal androgen receptor. Am J Med Genet 1981; 10:91–99.

957. Griffin JE, Durrant JL. Qualitative receptor defects in families with androgen resistance: failure of stabilization of the fibroblast cytosol androgen receptor. J Clin Endocrinol Metab 1982; 55:465–474.

958. Brown TR, Maes M, Rothwell SW, et al. Human complete androgen insensitivity with normal dihydrotestosterone receptor binding capacity in cultured genital skin fibroblasts: evidence for a qualitative abnormality of the receptor. J Clin Endocrinol Metab 1982; 55:61–69.

959. Kaufman M, Pinsky L, Feder-Hollander R. Defective up-regulation of the androgen receptor in human androgen insensitivity. Nature 1981; 293:735–737.

960. Pinsky L, Kaufman M, Chudley AE. Reduced affinity of the androgen receptor for 5α-dihydrotestosterone but not methyltrienolone in a form of partial androgen resistance. J Clin Invest 1985; 75:1291–1296.

961. Eil C. Familial incomplete male pseudohermaphroditism associated with impaired nuclear androgen retention. J Clin Invest 1983; 71:850–858.

962. Brown TR, Migeon CJ. Androgen binding in nuclear matrix of human genital skin fibroblasts from patients with androgen insensitivity syndrome. J Clin Endocrinol Metab 1986; 62:542–550.

963. Kovacs WJ, Griffen JE, Weaver DD, et al. A mutation that causes lability of the androgen receptor under conditions that normally promote transformation to the DNA-binding state. J Clin Invest 1984; 73:1095–1104.

964. Lubahn DR, Joseph DR, Sar M, et al. The human androgen receptor: complementary deoxyribonucleic acid cloning, sequence analysis, and gene expression in prostate. Mol Endocrinol 1988; 2:1265–1275.

965. Kupier GGJM, Faber PW, von Rooij HCJ, et al. Structural organization of the human androgen receptor gene. J Mol Endocrinol 1989; 2:R1–4

966. Brown TR. Human androgen insensitivity syndrome. J Androl 1995; 16:299–303.

967. O'Malley B. The steroid receptor superfamily: more excitement predicted for the future. Mol Endocrinol 1990; 4:363–369.

968. Ribeiro RCJ, Kushner PJ, Baxter JD. The nuclear hormone receptor gene superfamily. Annu Rev Med 1995; 46:443–453.

969. Zhou Z-X, Wong C-I, Sar M, et al. The androgen receptor: an overview. Recent Prog Horm Res 1994; 49:249–274.

970. La Spada AR, Wilson EM, Lubahn DB, et al. Androgen receptor gene mutations in X-linked spinal and bulbar muscular atrophy. Nature 1991; 352:77–79.

971. Trifiro MA, Kazemi-Esfarjani P, Pinsky L. X-linked muscular atrophy and the androgen receptor. Trends Endocrinol Metab 1994; 5:416–421.

972. Lumbroso S, Lobaccaro J-M, Vial C, et al. Molecular analysis of the androgen receptor gene in Kennedy's disease. Horm Res 1997; 47:23–29.

973. Trifiro M, Gottlieb B, Pinsky L, et al. The 56/58 kDa androgen-binding protein in male genital skin fibroblasts with a deleted androgen receptor gene. Mol Cell Endocrinol 1991; 75:37–47.

974. Batch JA, Williams DM, Davies HR, et al. Androgen receptor gene mutations identified by SSCP in fourteen subjects with androgen insensitivity syndrome. Hum Mol Genet 1992; 1:497–503.

975. McPhaul MJ, Marcelli M, Zoppi S, et al. Genetic basis of endocrine disease 4: the spectrum of mutations in the androgen receptor gene that causes androgen resistance. J Clin Endocrinol Metab 1993; 76:17–23.

976. Davies HR, Hughes IA, Savage MO, et al. Androgen insensitivity with mental retardation: a continuous gene syndrome? J Med Genet 1997; 34:158–160.

977. Gedeon AK, Donnelly AJ, Mulley JC, et al. How many X-linked genes for non-specific mental retardation (MRX) are there? Am J Med Genet 1996; 64:158–162.

978. Lobaccaro J-M, Poujol N, Chiche L, et al. Molecular modeling and in vitro investigations of the human androgen receptor DNA-binding domain: applications for the study of two mutations. Mol Cell Endocrinol 1996; 116:137–147.

979. Wooster R, Magion J, Eeles R, et al. A germline mutation in the androgen receptor gene in two brothers with breast cancer and Reifenstein syndrome. Nat Genet 1992; 2:132–134.

980. Lobaccaro J-M, Lumbroso S, Belon C, et al. Androgen receptor gene mutation in male breast cancer. Hum Mol Genet 1993; 2:1799–1802.

981. Jenster G, Trapman J, Brinkmann AO. Nuclear import of the human androgen receptor. Biochem J 1993; 293:761–768.

982. Zhou Z-X, Sar M, Simental JA, et al. A ligand-dependent bipartite nuclear targeting signal in the human androgen receptor: requirement for the DNA-binding modulation by NH2-terminal and carboxyl-terminal sequences. J Biol Chem 1994; 269:13115–13123.

983. McPhaul MJ, Marcelli M, Zoppi S, et al. Mutations in the ligand-binding domain of the androgen receptor cluster in two regions of the gene. J Clin Invest 1992; 90:2097–2101.

984. Murono K, Mendonca BB, Arnhold IJP, et al. Human androgen insensitivity due to point mutations encoding amino acid substitutions in the androgen receptor steroid-binding domain. Hum Mutat 1995; 6:152–162.

984a. Balducci R, Ghirri P, Brown TR, et al. A clinician looks at androgen resistance. Steroids 1996; 61:205–211.

985. Lee PA, Brown TR, LaTorre HA. Diagnosis of partial androgen insensitivity syndrome during infancy. JAMA 1986; 25:2207–2209.

986. Nagel BA, Lippe BM, Griffen JE. Androgen resistance in the neonate: use of hormones of hypothalamic-pituitary-gonadal axis for diagnosis. J Pediatr 1986; 109:486–488.

987. Tremblay RR, Foley TP Jr, Corvol P, et al. Plasma concentration of testosterone, dihydrotestosterone, testosterone-oestradiol binding globulin, and pituitary gonadotropins in the syndrome of male pseudohermaphroditism with testicular feminization. Acta Endocrinol 1972; 70:331–341.

988. Cicognani A, Cacciari E, Tacconi M, et al. Effect of gonadectomy on growth hormone, IGF-I, and sex steroids in children with complete and incomplete androgen insensitivity. Acta Endocrinol (Copenh) 1989; 121:777–783.

989. Boyar RM, Moore RJ, Rosner W, et al. Studies on gonadotropin-gonadal dynamics in patients with androgen insensitivity. J Clin Endocrinol Metab 1978; 47:1116–1117.

990. Faiman C, Winter JSD. The control of gonadotropin secretion in complete testicular feminization. J Clin Endocrinol Metab 1974; 39:631–638.

991. Imperato-McGinley J, Peterson RE, Gautier T, et al. Hormonal evaluation of a large kindred with complete androgen insensitivity: evidence for secondary 5α-reductase. J Clin Endocrinol Metab 1982; 54:931–941.

992. MacDonald PC, Madden JD, Brenner PF, et al. Origin of estrogen in normal men and in women with testicular feminization. J Clin Endocrinol Metab 1979; 49:905–916.

993. Kelch RP, Jenner MR, Weinstein R, et al. Estradiol and testosterone secretion by human, simian, and canine testes, in males with hypogonadism and in male pseudohermaphrodites with the feminizing testes syndrome. J Clin Invest 1972; 51:824–830.

994. Zachmann M, Prader A, Sobel E, et al. Pubertal growth in patients with androgen insensitivity: indirect evidence for the importance of estrogens in pubertal growth of girls. J Pediatr 1986; 108:694–697.

995. Conte FA, Grumbach MM. Bearing of abnormalities of sex differentiation on the hypothalamic-pituitary-gonadal axis at puberty. In: Serio M, Motta M, Zanisi M, et al., eds. Sexual Differentiation: Basic and Clinical Aspects. New York: Raven Press, 1984: 275–285.

996. Rey R, Mebarki F, Forest MG, et al. Anti-müllerian hormone in children with androgen insensitivity. J Clin Endocrinol Metab 1994; 79:960–964.

997. Sinnecker G, Dohler S. Sex hormone binding globulin response to the anabolic steroid stanozolol: evidence for its suitability as a biologic androgen sensitivity test. J Clin Endocrinol Metab 1989; 68:1195–1200.

998. Bertelloni S, Federico G, Baroncelli GI, Cavallo L, et al. Biochemical selection of prepubertal patients with androgen insensitivity syndrome by sex hormone-binding globulin response to the human chorionic gonadotropin test. Pediatr Res 1997; 41:266–271.

999. Sai T, Seino S, Chang C, et al. An exonic point mutation of the androgen receptor gene in a family with complete androgen insensitivity. Am J Hum Genet 1990; 46:1095–1100.

1000. Hughes IA, Patterson MN. Prenatal diagnosis of androgen insensitivity. Clin Endocrinol 1994; 40:295–296.

1001. Lobaccaro J-M, Belon C, Lumbroso S, et al. Molecular prenatal diagnosis of partial androgen insensitivity syndrome based on the Hind III polymorphism of the androgen receptor gene. Clin Endocrinol 1994; 40:297–302.

1002. Morel Y, Mebarki F, Forest MG. What are the indications for prenatal diagnosis in the androgen insensitivity syndrome? Facing clinical heterogeneity of phenotypes for the same genotype. Eur J Endocrinol 1994; 130:325–326.

1003. Goodall J. Helping a child to understand her own testicular feminisation. Lancet 1991; 337:33–35.

1004. Minoque BP, Taraszewski R. The whole truth and nothing but the truth? Hastings Cent Rep 1988; 18:34–35.

1005. Money J. Hormones, hormonal anomalies and psychologic health care. In: Kappy MS, Blizzard RM, Migeon CJ, eds. Wilkins Diagnosis and Treatment of Endocrine Disorders in Childhood and Adolescence. 4th ed. Springfield, Illinois: Charles C Thomas, 1994: 1141–1178.

1006. Reifenstein EC Jr. Hereditary familial hypogonadism. Clin Res 1947; 3:86.

1007. Bowen P, Lee CSN, Migeon CJ, et al. Hereditary male pseudohermaphroditism with hypogonadism, hypospadias, and gynecomastia (Reifenstein's syndrome). Ann Intern Med 1965; 62:252–270.

1008. Wilson JD, Harrod MJ, Goldstein JL, et al. Familial incomplete male pseudohermaphrodism, type I. N Engl J Med 1974; 290:1097–1103.

1009. Batch JA, Davies HR, Evans BA, et al. Phenotypic variation and detection of carrier status in the partial androgen insensitivity syndrome. Arch Dis Child 1993; 68:453–457.

1010. Amrhein JA, Jones Klingensmith G, Walsh PC, et al. Partial androgen insensitivity: the Reifenstein syndrome revisited. N Engl J Med 1977; 297:350–356.

1011. Aiman J, Griffin JE, Gazak JM, et al. Androgen insensitivity as a cause of infertility in otherwise normal men. N Engl J Med 1979; 300:223–227.

1012. Aiman J, Griffin JE. The frequency of androgen receptor deficiency in infertile men. J Clin Endocrinol Metab 1982; 54:725–732.

1013. Morrow AF, Gyorki S, Warne GL, et al. Variable androgen receptor levels in infertile men. J Clin Endocrinol Metab 1987; 64:1115–1121.

1014. Grino PB, Griffin JE, Cushard WG Jr, et al. A mutation of the androgen receptor associated with partial androgen resistance, familial gynecomastia and fertility. J Clin Endocrinol Metab 1988; 66:754–761.

1015. Tsukada T, Inoue M, Tachibana S, et al. An androgen receptor mutation causing androgen resistance in undervirilized male syndrome. J Clin Endocrinol Metab 1994; 79:1202–1207.

1016. McPhaul MJ, Deslypere JP, Allman DR, Gerard RD. The adenovirus-mediated delivery of a receptor gene permits the assessment of androgen receptor function in genital skin fibroblast cultures. J Biol Chem 1993; 268:26063–26066.

1017. Rey R, Josso N. Regulation of testicular anti-Müllerian hormone secretion. Eur J Endocrinol 1996; 135:144–152.

1018. Forest MG, Mollard P, David M, et al. Syndrome d'insensibilite incomplete aux androgenes. Arch Fr Pediatr 1990; 47:107–113.

1019. Hiort O, Wodtke A, Struve D, et al. Detection of point mutations in the androgen receptor gene using non-isotopic single strand confirmation polymorphism analysis. German Collaborative Intersex Group. Hum Mol Genet 1994; 3:1163–1166.

1020. Price P, Wass JAH, Griffin JE, et al. High dose androgen therapy in male pseudohermaphroditism due to 5α-reductase deficiency and disorders of the androgen receptor. J Clin Invest 1984; 74:1496–1508.

1021. Grino PB, Isidro-Gutierrez F, Griffin JE, et al. Androgen resistance associated with a qualitative abnormality of the androgen receptor and responsive to high dose androgen therapy. J Clin Endocrinol Metab 1989; 68:578–584.

1022. Nowakowski H, Lenz W. Genetic aspects in male hypogonadism. Recent Prog Horm Res 1961; 17:53–95.

1023. Opitz JM, Simpson JL, Sarto GE, et al. Pseudovaginal perineoscrotal hypospadias. Clin Genet 1972; 3:1–26.

1024. Walsh PC, Madden JD, Harrod MJ, et al. Familial incomplete male pseudohermaphroditism, type 2: decreased dihydrotestosterone formation in pseudovaginal perineoscrotal hypospadias. N Engl J Med 1974; 291:944–949.

1025. Imperato-McGinley JL, Guerrero L, Gautier T, et al. Steroid 5α-reductase deficiency in man: an inherited form of male pseudohermaphrodism. Science 1974; 186:1213–1215.

1026. Imperato-McGinley JL, Peterson RE. Male pseudohermaphroditism: the complexities of male phenotypic development. Am J Med 1976; 61:251–272.

1027. Peterson RE, Imperato-McGinley J, Gautier T, et al. Male psuedohermaphroditism due to steroid 5α-reductase deficiency. Am J Med 1977; 62:170–191.

1028. Imperato-McGinley JL, Peterson RE, Gautier T. Primary and secondary 5α-reductase deficiency. In: Serio M, Motta M, Zanisi M, et al., eds. Sexual Differentiation: Basic and Clinical Aspects. New York: Raven Press, 1984: 233–245.

1029. Wilson JD, Griffin JE, Russell DW. Steroid 5α-reductase 2 deficiency. Endocr Rev 1993; 14:577–593.

1030. Johnson L, George FW, Neaves WB, et al. Characterization of the testicular abnormality in 5α-reductase deficiency. J Clin Endocrinol Metab 1986; 63:1091–1099.

1031. Cai L-Q, Fratianni CM, Gautier T, Imperato-McGinley J. Dihydrotestosterone regulation of semen in male pseudohermaphrodites with 5α-reductase-2 deficiency. J Clin Endocrinol Metab 1994; 79:409–414.

1031a. Katz MD, Kligman I, Cai L-Q, et al. Paternity by intrauterine insemination with sperm from a man with 5α-reductase-2 deficiency. N Engl J Med 1997; 336:994–997.

1032. Odame I, Donaldson MCD, Wallace AM, et al. Early diagnosis and management of 5α-reductase deficiency. Arch Dis Child 1992; 67:720–723.

1033. Ng WK, Taylor NF, Hughes IA, et al. 5α-reductase deficiency without hypospadias. Arch Dis Child 1990; 65:1166–1167.

1034. Mendonca BB, Inacio M, Costa EMF, et al. Male pseudohermaphroditism due to steroid 5α-reductase 2 deficiency. Medicine (Baltimore) 1996; 75:64–76.

1035. Sinnecker GHG, Hiort O, Dibbelt L, et al. Phenotypic classification of male pseudohermaphroditism due to steroid 5α-reductase 2 deficiency. Am J Med Genet 1996; 63:223–230.

1036. Hochberg Z, Chayen R, Reiss N, et al. Clinical, biochemical and genetic findings in a large pedigree of male and female patients with 5α-reductase 2 deficiency. J Clin Endocrinol Metab 1966; 81:2821–2823.

1037. Boudon C, Lumbroso S, Lobaccaro JM. Molecular study of the 5α-reductase type 2 gene in three European families with 5α-reductase deficiency. J Clin Endocrinol Metab 1995; 80:2149–2153.

1038. Milewich L, Mendonca BB, Arnhold I, et al. Women with steroid 5α-reductase 2 deficiency have normal concentrations of plasma 5α-dihydroprogesterone during the luteal phase. J Clin Endocrinol Metab 1995; 80:3136–3139.

1039. Katz MD, Cai L-Q, Zhu Y-S, et al. The biochemical and phenotypic characterization of females homozygous for 5α-reductase 2 deficiency. J Clin Endocrinol Metab 1995; 80:3160–3167.

1040. Pang S, Levine LS, Chow D, et al. Dihydrotestosterone and its relationship to testosterone in infancy and childhood. J Clin Endocrinol Metab 1979; 48:821–826.

1041. Andersson S, Berman DM, Jenkins EP, et al. Deletion of steroid 5α-reductase 2 gene in male pseudohermaphroditism. Nature 1991; 354:159–161.

1042. Thigpen AE, Davis DL, Milatovich A, et al. Molecular genetics of steroid 5α-reductase 2 deficiency. J Clin Invest 1992; 90:799–809.

1043. Russell DW, Wilson JD. Steroid 5α-reductase: two genes/two enzymes. Ann Rev Biochem 1994; 63:25–61.

1044. Thigpen AE, Silver RI, Guileyardo JM, et al. Tissue distribution and ontogeny of steroid 5α-reductase isozyme expression. J Clin Invest 1993; 92:903–910.

1045. Jenkins EP, Hsieh C-L, Milatovich A, et al. Characterization and chromosomal mapping of a human steroid 5α-reductase gene and pseudogene and mapping of the mouse homologue. Genomics 1991; 11:1102–1112.

1046. Boudon C, Lobaccaro JM, Lumbroso S, et al. A new deletion of 5α-reductase type 2 gene in a Turkish family with 5α-reductase deficiency. Clin Endocrinol 1995; 43:183–188.

1047. Imperato-McGinley J, Miller M, Wilson JD, et al. A cluster of male pseudo-hermaphrodites with 5α-reductase deficiency in Papua New Guinea. Clin Endocrinol (Oxf) 1991; 34: 293–298.

1048. Saenger P, Goldman AS, Levine LS, et al. Prepubertal diagnosis of steroid 5α-reductase deficiency. J Clin Endocrinol Metab 1978; 46:627–634.

1049. Forti G, Falchetti A, Santoro S, et al. Steroid 5α-reductase 2 deficiency: virilization in early infancy may be due to partial function of a mutant enzyme. Clin Endocrinol 1996; 44:447–482.

1050. Greene S, Zachmann M, Manella B, et al. Comparison of two tests to recognize or exclude 5α-reductase deficiency in prepubertal children. Acta Endocrinol 1987; 114:113–117.

1051. Imperato-McGinley J, Gautier T, Pichardo M, et al. The diagnosis of 5α-reductase deficiency in infancy. J Clin Endocrinol Metab 1986; 63:1313–1318.

1052. Pinsky L, Kaufman M, Straidfeld C, et al. 5α-Reductase activity of genital and nongenital skin fibroblasts from patients with 5α-reductase deficiency, androgen insensitivity, or unknown forms of male pseudohermaphroditism. Am J Med Genet 1978; 1:407–416.

1053. Keenan BS, Eberle AJ, Sparrow JT, et al. Dihydrotestosterone heptanoate: synthesis, pharmacokinetics, and effects on hypothalamic-pituitary-testicular function. J Clin Endocrinol Metab 1987; 64:557–563.

1054. Kuhn JM, Rieu M, Laudat MH, et al. Effects of 10 days of pericutaneous dihydrotestosterone on the pituitary-testicular axis of normal men. J Clin Endocrinol Metab 1982; 58:231–235.

1055. Carpenter TO, Imperato-McGinley J, Boulware SD, et al. Variable expression of 5α-reductase deficiency: presentation with male phenotype in a child of Greek origin. J Clin Endocrinol Metab 1990; 71:318–322.

1056. Rajfer J, Mendelsohn G, Arnheim J, et al. Dysgenetic male pseudohermaphrodism. J Urol 1978; 119:525–527.

1057. Rajfer J, Walsh PC. Mixed gonadal dysgenesis: dysgenetic male pseudohermaphroditism. In: Josso N, ed. The Intersex Child: Pediatric and Adolescent Endocrinology. Basel: S. Karger, 1981; 8:105–115.

1058. Baumstark A, Barbi G, Djalali M, et al. Xp-duplications with and without sex reversal. Hum Genet 1996; 97:79–86.

1059. Jiminez R, Sanchez A, Burgos M, Diaz de la Guardia R. Puzzling out the genetics of mammalian sex determination. Trends Genet 1996; 12:164–166.

1060. Burris TP, Guo W, McCabe ERB. The gene responsible for adrenal hypoplasia congenita, DAX-1, encodes a nuclear hormone receptor that defines a new class within the superfamily. Recent Prog Horm Res 1996; 51:241–259.

1061. Burris TP, Guo W, Le T, McCabe ER. Identification of a putative steroidogenic factor-1 response element in the DAX-1 promoter. Biochem Biophys Res Commun 1995; 214:576–581.

1062. Swain A, Zanaria E, Hacker A, et al. Mouse Dax1 expression is consistent with a role in sex determination as well as adrenal and hypothalamus function. Nat Genet 1996; 12:404–409.

1063. McPherson EW, Clemens MM, Gibbons RJ, et al. X-linked α-thalassemia/mental retardation (ATR-X) syndrome: a new kindred with severe genital anomalies and mild hematologic expression. Am J Med Genet 1995; 55:302–306.

1064. Ion A, Telvi L, Chaussain JL, et al. A novel mutation in the putative DNA helicase XH2 is responsible for male to female sex reversal associated with an atypical form of ATR-X syndrome. Am J Hum Genet 1996; 58:1185–1191.

1064a. Ogata T, Muroya K, Matsus N, et al. Impaired male sex development in an infant with molecular defined partial 9p monosomy: implication for a testis forming gene(s) on 9p. J Med Genet 1997; 34:331–334.

1065. Curry CJR, Jensen K, Holland J, et al. The Potter sequence: a clinical analysis of 80 cases. Am J Med Genet 1984; 19:679–702.

1066. Drash A, Sherman F, Hartmann WH, et al. A syndrome of pseudohermaphroditism, Wilms' tumor, hypertension and degenerative renal disease. J Pediatr 1970; 76:585–593.

1067. Frasier SD, Bashne RA, Mosler HD. Gonadoblastoma associated with pure gonadal dysgenesis in monozygous twins. J Pediatr 1964; 64:740–745.

1068. Moorthy AV, Chesney RW, Lubinsky M. Chronic renal failure and XY gonadal dysgenesis: Frasier syndrome. A commentary on reported cases. Am J Med Genet 1987; 3(Suppl):297–302.

1069. Call KM, Glaser T, Ito CY, et al. Isolation and characterization of a zinc finger polypeptide gene at the human chromosome 11 Wilms tumor locus. Cell 1990; 60:509–520.

1070. Baird PN, Santos A, Groves N, et al. Constitutional mutations in the WT1 gene in patients with Denys-Drash syndrome. Hum Mol Genet 1992; 1:301–305.

1071. Poulat F, Morin D, Konig A, et al. Distinct molecular origins for Denys-Drash and Frasier syndromes. Hum Genet 1993; 91:285–286.

1071a. Little M, Wells C. A clinical overview of WT1 gene mutations. Hum Mutat 1997; 9:209–225.

1072. Pelletier J, Bruening W, Kashtan CE, et al. Germline mutations in the Wilms tumor suppressor gene are associated with abnormal urogenital development in Denys-Drash syndrome. Cell 1991; 67:437–447.

1073. Von Heyninger V, Boyd PA, Seawright A, et al. Molecular analysis of chromosome 11 deletions in aniridia: Wilms tumor syndrome. Proc Natl Acad Sci U S A 1985; 82:8592–8596.

1074. Nordenskjöld A, Fricke G, Anvret M. Absence of mutations in the WT1 gene in patients with XY gonadal dysgenesis. Hum Genet 1995; 96:102–104.

1075. Houston CS, Opitz JM, Spranger JW, et al. The campomelic syndrome: review, report of 17 cases, and follow-up on the currently 17-year-old boy first reported by Maioteaux et al. in 1971. Am J Med Genet 1983; 15:3–28.

1076. Mansour S, Hall CM, Pembrey ME, Young ID. A clinical and genetic study of campomelic dysplasia. J Med Genet 1995; 32:415–420.

1077. Camera G, Mastroiacovo P. Birth prevalence of skeletal dysplasias in the Italian Multicultural Monitoring System for Birth Defects. In: Papadatos CJ, Bartosocca CS, eds. Skeletal Dysplasias. New York: Alan R. Liss, 1982: 441–449.

1078. Normann EK, Pederson JC, Stiris G, van der Hagen CB. Campomelic dysplasia: an underdiagnosed condition? Eur J Pediatr 1993; 152:331–333.

1079. Kwok C, Weller P, Guioli S, et al. Mutations in SOX9, the gene responsible for campomelic dysplasia and autosomal sex reversal. Am J Hum Genet 1995; 57:1028–1036.

1080. Wirth J, Wagner T, Meyer J, et al. Translocation breakpoints in three patients with campomelic dysplasia and autosomal sex reversal map more than 130 kb from Sox9. Hum Genet 1996; 97:186–193.

1081. Ballabio A. The rise and fall of positional cloning? Nature Genet 1993; 3:277–279.

1082. Meyer J, Sudbeck P, Held M, et al. Mutational analysis of SOX9 gene in campomelic dysplasia and autosomal sex reversal: lack of genotype/phenotype correlations. Hum Mol Genet 1997; 6:91–98.

1083. Cameron FJ, Hageman RM, Cooke-Yarborough C, et al. A novel germ line mutation in SOX9 causes familial campomelic dysplasia and sex reversal. Hum Mol Genet 1996; 5:1625–1630.

1084. Sudbeck P, Schmitz M, Baeuerle PA, Scherer G. Sex reversal by loss of the C-terminal transactivation domain of human SOX9. Nat Genet 1996; 13:230–232.

1084a. Ng LJ, Wheatley S, Muscat GE, et al. SOX9 binds DNA, activates transcription and co-expresses with type II collagen during chondrogenesis in the mouse. Devel Biol 1997; 183:108–121.

1084b. Bell DM, Leung KKH, Wheatley SC, et al. SOX9 directly regulates the type-II collagen gene. Nat Genet 1997; 16:174–178.

1085. Honda S, Morohashi K, Nomura M, et al. Ad4BP regulating steroidogenic P-450 gene is a member of steroid hormone receptor superfamily. J Biol Chem 1993; 268:7494–7502.

1086. Parker KL, Ikeda Y, Luo X. The role of steroidogenic factor-1 in reproductive function. Steroids 1996; 61:161–165.

1087. Taketo M, Parker KL, Howard TA, et al. Homologs of Drosophila fushi-tarazu factor 1 map to mouse chromosome 2 and human chromosome 9q33. Genomics 1995; 25:565–567.

1088. Wilson TE, Fahrner TJ, Millbrandt J. The orphan receptors NGFI-B and steroidogenic factor 1 establish monomer binding as a third paradigm of nuclear receptor-DNA interaction. Mol Cell Biol 1993; 13:5794–5804.

1089. Lala DS, Rice DA, Parker KL. Steroidogenic factor 1, a key regulator of steroidogenic enzyme expression, is the mouse homolog of fushi-tarazu factor 1. Mol Endocrinol 1992; 6:1249–1258.

1090. Sadovsky Y, Crawford PA, Woodson KG, et al. Mice deficient in the orphan receptor steroidogenic factor 1 lack adrenal glands and gonads but express P450 side-chain cleavage enzyme in the placenta and have normal embryonic serum levels of corticosteroids. Proc Natl Acad Sci U S A 1995; 92:10939–10943.

1091. Compagnone NA, Bulfone A, Rubenstein JL, Mellon SH. Steroidogenic enzyme P450c17 is expressed in the embryonic central nervous system. Endocrinology 1995; 136:5212–5223.

1092. Giuili G, Shen W-H, Ingraham HA. The nuclear receptor SF-1 mediates sexually dimorphic expression of müllerian inhibiting substance in vivo. Development 1997; 124:1799–1807.

1093. Ikeda Y, Lala DS, Luo X, et al. Characterization of the mouse FTZ-F1 gene, which encodes a key regulator of steroid hydroxylase gene expression. Mol Endocrinol 1993; 7:852–860.

1094. Tsukiyama T, Ueda H, Hirose S, Niwa O. Embryonal long terminal repeat binding protein is a murine homolog of FTZ-F1, a member of the steroid receptor superfamily. Mol Cell Biol 1992; 12:1286–1291.

1095. Ikeda Y, Luo X, Abbud R, et al. The nuclear receptor steroidogenic factor 1 is essential for the formation of the ventromedial hypothalamic nucleus. Mol Endocrinol 1995; 9:478–486.

1096. Cleary RE, Caras J, Rosenfield R, et al. Endocrine and metabolic studies in a patient with male pseudohermaphrodism and true agonadism. Am J Obstet Gynecol 1977; 128:862–867.

1097. Sarto GE, Opitz JM. The XY gonadal agenesis syndrome. J Med Genet 1973; 10:288–293.

1098. Edman CD, Winters A, Porter J, et al. Embryonic testicular regression. A clinical spectrum of XY agonadal individuals. Obstet Gynecol 1977; 49:208–217.

1099. Coulam CB. Testicular regression syndrome. Obstet Gynecol 1979; 53:44–49.

1100. Goldberg LM, Skaist LB, Morrow JM. Congenital absence of testes: anorchism and monorchism. J Urol 1974; 111:840–845.

1101. Hall JG, Morgan A, Blizzard RM. Familial congenital anorchia. Birth Defects 1975; 11:115–119.

1102. Aynsley-Green AA, Zachmann M, Illig R, et al. Congenital bilateral anorchia in childhood: a clinical, endocrine and therapeutic evaluation of 21 cases. Clin Endocrinol 1976; 5:381–391.

1103. Bergada C, Cleveland WW, Jones HW Jr, et al. Variants of embryonic testicular dysgenesis: bilateral anorchia and the syndrome of rudimentary testes. Acta Endocrinol 1962; 40:521–536.

1104. Najjar SS, Takla RJ, Nassar VH. The syndrome of rudimentary testes: occurrence in five siblings. J Pediatr 1974; 84:119–122.

1105. Marcantonio SM, Fechner PY, Migeon CJ, et al. Embryonic testicular regression sequence: a part of the clinical spectrum of 46,XY gonadal dysgenesis. Am J Med Genet 1994; 49:1–5.

1106. Kushnick T, Wiley JE, Palmer SM. Agonadism in a 46,XY patient with CHARGE association. Am J Med Genet 1992; 42:96–99.

1107. Maaswinkel-Mooij, PD, Stokvis-Brantsma WH. Phenotypically normal girl with male pseudohermaphroditism, hypoplastic left ventricle, lung aplasia, horsehoe kidney, and diaphragmatic hernia. Am J Med Genet 1992; 42:647–648.

1108. Josso N, Briard M-L. Embryonic testicular regression syndrome: variable phenotypic expression in siblings. J Pediatr 1980; 97:200–204.

1109. Lustig RH, Conte FA, Grumbach MM, et al. Ontogeny of gonadotropin secretion in congenital anorchia: sexual dimorphism versus syndrome of gonadal dysgenesis and diagnostic considerations. J Urol 1987; 138:587–591.

1110. Levitt SB, Kogan SJ, Engel RM, et al. The impalpable testis: a rational approach to management. J Urol 1978; 120:515–520.

1111. Bartone FF, Huseman CA, Maizels M, et al. Pitfalls in using human chorionic gonadotropin (hCG) stimulation test to diagnose anorchia. J Urol 1984; 132:563–567.

1112. Cate RL, Mattaliano RJ, Hession C, et al. Isolation of the bovine and human genes for müllerian inhibiting substance and expression of the human gene in animal cells. Cell 1986; 45:685–689.

1113. MacLaughlin DT, Epstein J, Donahoe PK. Bioassay, purification, cloning, and expression of müllerian inhibiting substance. Methods in Enzymology 1991; 198:358–369.

1114. Nachtigal MW, Ingraham HA. Bioactivation of müllerian inhibiting substance during gonadal development by a kex2/subtilisin-like endoprotease. Proc Am Acad Sci U S A 1996; 93:7711–7716.

1115. Baarends WM, van Helmond MJ, Post M, et al. A novel member of the transmembrane serine/threonine kinase receptor family is specifically expressed in the gonads and in mesenchymal cells adjacent to the müllerian duct. Development 1994; 120:189–197.

1116. Tsuji M, Shima H, Yonemura CY, et al. Effect of human recombinant müllerian inhibiting substance on isolated epithelial and mesenchymal cells during müllerian duct regression in the rat. Endocrinology 1992; 131:1481–1488.

1116a. Josso N, diClemente N. Serine/threonine kinase receptors and ligands. Curr Opin Genet Dev 1997; 7:371–377.

1117. Shen W-H, Moore CCD, Ikeda Y, et al. Nuclear receptor steroidogenic factor 1 regulates the müllerian inhibiting substance gene: a link to the sex determination cascade. Cell 1994; 77:651–661.

1118. di Clemente N, Wilson C, Faure E, et al. Cloning, expression, and alternative splicing of the receptor for anti-Müllerian hormone. Mol Endocrinol 1994; 8:1006–1020.

1119. Massagué J. Receptors for the TGF-β family. Cell 1992; 69:1067–1070.

1120. Brook CGD, Wagner H, Zachmann M, et al. Familial occurrence of persistent müllerian structures in otherwise normal males. Br Med J 1973; 1:771–773.

1121. Brook CGD. Persistent müllerian duct syndrome. In: Josso N, ed. The Intersex Child: Pediatric and Adolescent Endocrinology. Vol 8. Basel: S. Karger, 1981: 100–104.

1122. Josso N, Fekete C, Cachin O, et al. Persistence of müllerian ducts in male pseudohermaphroditism, and its relationship to cryptorchidism. Clin Endocrinol 1983; 19:247–258.

1123. Guerrier D, Tran D, Vanderwinden JM, et al. The persistent müllerian duct syndrome: a molecular approach. J Clin Endocrinol Metab 1989; 68:46–52.

1124. Loeff D, Imbeaud S, Reyes HM, et al. Surgical and genetic aspects of persistent müllerian duct syndrome. J Pediatr Surg 1994; 29:61–65.

1125. Imbeaud S, Carré-Eusebe D, Rey R, et al. Molecular genetics of the persistent müllerian duct syndrome: a study of 19 families. Hum Mol Genet 1994; 3:125–131.

1126. Taguchi O, Cunha GR, Lawrence WD, et al. Timing and irreversibility of müllerian duct inhibition in the embryonic reproductive tract of the human male. Dev Biol 1984; 106:394–398.

1127. Fuqua JS, Sher ES, Perlman EJ, et al. Abnormal gonadal differentiation in two subjects with ambiguous genitalia, Müllerian structures, and normally developed testes: evidence for a defect in gonadal ridge development. Hum Genet 1996; 97:506–511.

1128. Knebelmann B, Boussin L, Guerrier D, et al. Anti-Müllerian hormone Bruxelles: a nonsense mutation associated with the persistent Müllerian duct syndrome. Proc Natl Acad Sci U S A 1991; 88:3767–3771.

1129. Imbeaud S, Belville C, Messika-Zeitoun L, et al. A 27 base-pair deletion of the anti-müllerian type II receptor gene is the most common cause of the persistent müllerian duct syndrome. Hum Mol Genet 1996; 5:1269–1277.

1130. Carré-Eusebe D, Imbeaud S, Harbison M, et al. Variants of the anti-müllerian hormone gene in a compound heterozygote with the persistent Müllerian duct syndrome and his family. Hum Genet 1992; 90:389–394.

1131. Imbeaud S, Faure E, Lamarre I, et al. Insensitivity to anti-müllerian hormone due to a mutation in the human anti-müllerian hormone receptor. Nat Genet 1995; 11:382–388.

1132. Imbeaud S, Rey R, Berta P, et al. Testicular degeneration in three patients with the persistent müllerian duct syndrome. Eur J Pediatr 1995; 154:187–190.

1133. Personal communication, J. D. Wilson, M.D.

1134. Courrier R, Jost A. Intersexualité totale provoqué par la pregneninolone au cours de la grossesse. C R Soc Biol (Paris) 1942; 136:395–396.

1135. Aarskog D. Maternal progestins as a possible cause of hypospadias. N Engl J Med 1979; 300:75–78.

1136. Sweet RA, Schrott HG, Kurland R, et al. Study of the incidence of hypospadias in Rochester, Minnesota, 1940–1970, and a case control comparison of possible etiologic factors. Mayo Clin Proc 1974; 49:52–58.

1137. Lorber CA, Cassidy SB, Engel E. Is there an embryo-fetal exogenous sex steroid exposure syndrome (EFESSES)? Fertil Steril 1979; 31:21–24.

1138. Czezel A, Toth J. Correlation between the birth prevalence of hypospadias and parental subfertility. Teratology 1990; 41:167–172.

1139. Voight W, Hsia SL. Further studies on testosterone 5α-reductase of human skin: structural features of steroid inhibitors. J Biol Chem 1973; 248:4280–4285.

1140. Kaplan NM. Male pseudohermaphrodism: report of a case, with observations on pathogenesis. N Engl J Med 1959; 261:641–644.

1141. Henderson BE, Benton B, Cosgrove M, et al. Urogenital tract abnormalities in sons of women treated with diethylstilbestrol. Pediatrics 1976; 58:505–507.

1142. Driscoll SG, Taylor SH. Effects of prenatal maternal estrogen on the male urogenital system. Obstet Gynecol 1980; 56:537–542.

1143. Penny R. The effect of DES on male offspring. West J Med 1982; 136:329–330.

1144. Sharpe RM, Skakkebaek NE. Are oestrogens involved in falling sperm counts and disorders of the male reproductive tract? Lancet 1993; 341:1392–1395.

1145. Paulozzi LJ, Erickson JD, Jackson RJ. Hypospadias trends in two US surveillance systems. Pediatrics 1997; 100:831–834.

1146. Majdic G, Sharpe RM, O'Shaughnessy, et al. Expression of cytochrome P450 17α-hydroxylase/c17-20 lyase in fetal rat testes is reduced by maternal exposure to exogenous estrogens. Endocrinology 1996; 137:1063–1070.

1147. Kelce WR, Stone CR, Laws SC, et al. Persistent DDT metabolite p,p'-DDE is a potent androgen receptor antagonist. Nature 1995; 375:581–585.

1148. Arnold SF, Klotz DM, Collins BM, et al. Synergistic activation of estrogen receptor with combinations of environmental chemicals. Science 1996; 272:1489–1492.

1149. Simons SS Jr. Environmental estrogens: can two "alrights" make a wrong? Science 1996; 272:1451.

1150. Heufelder AE, Hofbauer LC. Environmental endocrinology: hidden but potent ways of activating the estrogen receptor. Eur J Endocrinol 1996; 135:653–655.

1151. Carter CO. Multifactorial genetic disease. In: McKusick VA, Claiborne R, eds. Medical Genetics. New York: HP Publishing, 1973.

1152. Belman AB. Hypospadias and other urethral abnormalities. In: Kelalis PP, King LR, Belman AB, eds. Clinical Pediatric Urology. 3rd ed, Vol 1. Philadelphia: WB Saunders, 1992: 619–663.

1153. Bauer SB, Relik AB, Colodny AA. Genetic aspects of hypospadias. Urol Clin North Am 1981; 8:559.

1154. Harris EL, Beaty TH. Segregation analysis of hypospadias: a reanalysis of published pedigree data. Am J Med Genet 1993; 45:420–425.

1155. Aarskog D. Clinical and cytogenetic studies in hypospadias. Acta Paediatr Scand 1970; 203(Suppl):1–62.

1156. Battin M, Albersheim S, Newman D. Congenital genitourinary tract abnormalities following cocaine exposure in utero. Am J Perinatol 1995; 12:425–428.

1157. Svensson J, Snochowski M. Androgen receptor levels in preputial skin from boys with hypospadias. J Clin Endocrinol Metab 1979; 49:340–345.

1158. Warne GL, Gyorski S, Risibridger GP, et al. Fibroblast studies on clinical androgen insensitivity. J Steroid Biochem 1983; 18:583–586.

1159. Keenan BS, McNeel RL, Gonzales ET. Abnormality of intracellular 5α-dihydrotestosterone binding in simple hypospadias: studies on equilibrium steroid binding in sonicates of genital skin fibroblasts. Pediatr Res 1984; 18:216–220.

1160. Allera A, Herbst MA, Griffin JE, et al. Mutations of the androgen receptor coding sequence are infrequent in patients with isolated hypospadius. J Clin Endocrinol Metab 1995; 80:2697–2699.

1161. Sutherland RW, Wiener JS, Hicks JP, et al. Androgen receptor gene mutations are rarely associated with isolated penile hypospadias. J Urol 1996; 156:828–831.

1162. Robin NH, Feldman GJ, Aronson AL, et al. Opitz syndrome is genetically heterogenous with one locus on Xp22, and a second locus on 22q11.2. Nat Genet 1995; 11:459–461.

1163. Mortlock DP, Innis JW. Mutation of HOXA13 in hand-foot-genital syndrome. Nat Genet 1997; 15:179–180.

1164. Sandberg DE, Meyer-Bahlburg HFL, Yager TJ, et al. Gender development in boys born with hypospadias. Psychoneuroendocrinology 1995; 20:693–709.

1165. Walsh PC, Wilson JD, Allen TD, et al. Clinical and endocrinological evaluation of patients with congenital microphallus. J Urol 1978; 120:90–95.

1166. Burstein S, Grumbach MM, Kaplan SL. Early determination of androgen-responsiveness is important in the management of microphallus. Lancet 1979; 2:983–986.

1167. Lovinger RD, Kaplan SL, Grumbach MM. Congenital hypopituitarism associated with neonatal hypoglycemia and microphallus: four cases secondary to hypothalamic hormone deficiencies. J Pediatr 1975; 87:1171–1181.

1168. Rozanski TA, Bloom DA. The undescended testis: theory and management. Urol Clin North Am 1995; 22:107–118.

1169. Hadziselimovic F. Cryptorchidism: the disease and its management. Acta Urol Belg 1995; 63:83–88.

1170. Lee PA. Consequence of cryptorchidism: relationship to etiology and treatment. Curr Probl Pediatr 1995; 25:232–236.

1171. Cortes D, Thorup JM, Beck BL. Quantitative histology of germ cells in the undescended testes of human fetuses, neonates and infants. J Urol 1995; 154:1188–1192.

1172. Jones KL. Smith's Recognizable Patterns of Human Malformation. 5th ed. Philadelphia: WB Saunders, 1997.

1173. Park IJ, Burnett LS, Jones HW Jr, et al. A case of male pseudohermaphrodism associated with elevated LH, normal FSH and low testosterone possibly due to the secretion of an abnormal LH molecule. Acta Endocrinol 1976; 83:173–181.

1174. Meyer WJ III, Keenan BS, De Lacerda L, et al. Familial male pseudohermaphroditism with normal Leydig cell function at puberty. J Clin Endocrinol Metab 1978; 46:593–603.

1175. Griffin JE, Edwards C, Madden JD, et al. Congenital absence of the vagina: the Mayer-Rokitansky-Küster-Hauser syndrome. Ann Intern Med 1976; 85:224–236.

1176. Neinstein LS, Castle G. Congenital absence of the vagina. Am J Dis Child 1983; 137:671.

1177. Ross GT, van de Wiele RL. The ovaries. In: Williams RH, ed. Textbook of Endocrinology. 5th ed. Philadelphia: WB Saunders, 1974: 368–422.

1178. Fraser ID, Baird DT, Hobson BM, et al. Cyclical ovarian function in women with congenital absence of the uterus and vagina. J Clin Endocrinol Metab 1973; 36:634–637.

1179. Strubbe EH, Cremers CW, Dikkers FG, Willemsen WN. Hearing loss and the Mayer-Rokitansky-Küster-Hauser syndrome. Am J Otol 1994; 15:431–436.

1180. Strubbe EH, Cremers CW, Willemsen WN, et al. The Mayer-Rokitansky-Küster-Hauser (MRKH) syndrome without and with associated features: two separate entities? Clin Dysmorphol 1994; 3:192–199.

1181. Strubbe EH, Lemmens JA, Thijn CJ, et al. Spinal abnormalities and the atypical form of the Mayer-Rokitansky-Küster-Hauser syndrome. Skeletal Radiol 1992; 21:459–462.

1182. Pinsky L. A community of human malformation syndromes involving the müllerian ducts, distal extremities, urinary tract and ears. Teratology 1974; 9:65–79.

1183. Michels VV, Caskey TC. Müllerian aplasia with hypoplastic thumbs: two case reports. Int J Gynaecol Obstet 1979; 17:6–10.

1184. Duncan PA, Shapiro LR, Stangel JJ, et al. The MURCS association: müllerian duct aplasia, renal aplasia, and cervicothoracic somite dysplasia. J Pediatr 1979; 95:399–402.

1185. Haskins JL, Gysler M, Cowell CA. Anatomical amenorrhea: the problems of congenital vaginal agenesis and its surgical correction. Pediatr Clin North Am 1981; 28:345–354.

1186. Fliegner JR, Pepperell RJ. Management of vaginal agenesis with a functioning uterus: is hysterectomy advisable? Aust N Z J Obstet Gynecol 1994; 34:467–470.

1187. Hendren WH, Atala A. Use of bowel for vaginal reconstruction. J Urol 1994; 152:752–755.

1188. Hecker BR, McGuire LS. Psychosocial function in women treated for vaginal agenesis. Am J Obstet Gynecol 1977; 129:543–547.

1189. Taha SA. Male pseudohermaphroditism: factors determining the gender of rearing in Saudi Arabia. Urology 1994; 43:370–374.

1190. Money J, Hampson JC, Hampson JL. Hermaphroditism: recommendations concerning assignment of sex, change of sex, and psychologic management. Johns Hopkins Med J 1955; 97:284.

1191. Forest MG. Pattern of the response of testosterone and its precursors to human chorionic gonadotropin stimulation in relation to age in infants and children. J Clin Endocrinol Metab 1979; 49:132–137.

1192. Aaronson IA. Micropenis: medical and surgical implications. J Urol 1994; 152:4–14.

1193. McMahon DR, Kramer SA, Husmann DA. Micropenis: does early treatment with testosterone do more harm than good? J Urol 1995; 154:825–829.

1194. Sutherland RS, Kogan BA, Baskin LS, et al. The effect of pre-pubertal androgen exposure on adult penile length. J Urol 1996; 156(Pt 2):783–787.

1195. Choi SK, Han SW, Kim DH, et al. Transdermal dihydrotestosterone therapy and its effects on patients with microphallus. J Urol 1993; 150(Pt 2):657–660.

1196. Money J. Sex Errors of the Body and Related Syndromes: A Guide to Counseling Children, Adolescents and Their Families. 2nd ed. Baltimore: Paul H Brookes, 1994.

1197. Caron AM, D'Avino R. Legal implications of intersexuality. In: Josso N, ed. The Intersex Child: Pediatric and Adolescent Endocrinology. Vol 8. Basel: S Karger, 1981: 218–227.

1198. Gross RE, Randolph J, Crigler JF Jr. Clitorectomy for sexual abnormalities: indications and technique. Surgery 1966; 59:300–308.

1199. Lattimer JK. Relocation and recession of the enlarged clitoris with preservation of the glans: an alternative to amputation. J Urol 1961; 86:113–116.

1200. Spense HM, Allen TD. Genital reconstruction in the female with the adrenogenital syndrome. Br J Urol 1973; 45:126–130.

1201. Shaw A. Subcutaneous reduction clitoroplasty. J Pediatr Surg 1977; 12:331–338.

1201a. Hutson JM, Voight RW, Kelly JM, et al. Girth reduction clitoroplasty: a new technique with 15 years experience in 38 patients. Pediatr Surg Intl 1991; 6:336–340.

1202. Masters HW, Johnson VE. Human Sexual Response. Boston: Little, Brown, 1966.

1203. Jones HW Jr, Garcia SC, Klingensmith GJ. Necessity for and the technique of secondary surgical treatment of masculinized external genitalia of patients with virilizing adrenal hyperplasia. In: Lee PA, Plotnick LP, Kowarski AA, et al., eds. Congenital Adrenal Hyperplasia. Baltimore: University Park Press, 1977: 347–353.

1204. Wabrek AJ, Millard R, Wilson WB Jr, et al. Creation of a neovagina by the Frank nonoperative method. Obstet Gynecol 1971; 37:408–413.

1205. Thomsen C, Jensen KE, Giwercman A, et al. Magnetic resonance: in vivo tissue characterization of the testes in patients with carcinoma in situ of the testis and healthy subjects. Int J Androl 1987; 10:191–198.

1206. Baker SW. Psychological management of intersex children. In: Josso N, ed. The Intersex Child: Pediatric and Adolescent Endocrinology. Vol 8. Basel: S Karger, 1981: 261–269.

1207. Meyer-Bahlburg HFL. Gender identity development in intersex patients. Child Adolesc Clin North America 1993; 2:501–512.

30

NORMAL AND ABERRANT GROWTH

Edward O. Reiter and Ron G. Rosenfeld

NORMAL GROWTH

Childhood is a time of growth; it is a process that is complex and involves the interaction of multiple, diverse factors; it is the "cumulative sum of millions of unsynchronized cell replications."[1-3] Growth is common to all multicellular organisms and occurs by cell replication and enlargement along with the nonhomogeneous processes of cell and organ differentiation. The overall morphologic development, the rates of cellular division in different organ systems at different times, and the ultimate outcome are determined by the genetic composition of the individual interacting with external factors, including nutrition and psychosocial and economic factors.

The very nature of linear height growth, whether occurring as a continuous process or with periodic bursts of growth and arrest,[3-5] has been hard to characterize definitively. Nonetheless despite the fact that the process of growth is multifactorial and complex, children normally grow in a remarkably predictable manner. Deviation from a normal pat-

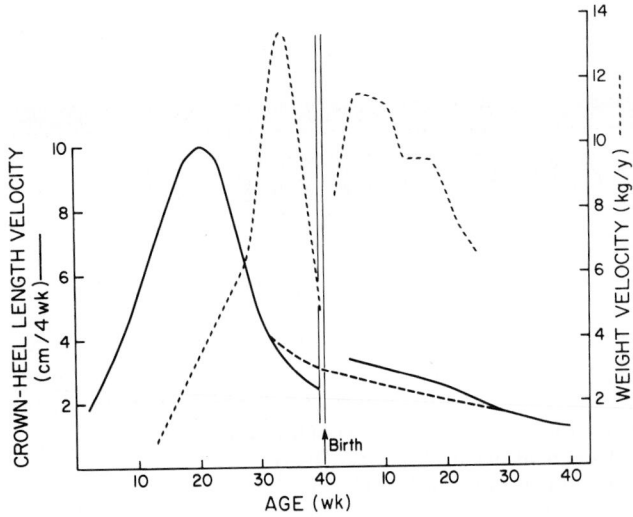

Figure 30–1. The rate of linear growth and weight gain in utero and during the first 40 wk after birth. Note that length velocity is expressed in centimeters per week. The solid line depicts the actual linear growth rate; the dashed line connecting the prenatal and postnatal length velocity lines depicts the theoretical curve for no uterine restriction late in gestation. The lighter dashed line depicts weight velocity. (From data in Tanner JM. Foetus into Man. Cambridge, MA: Harvard University Press, 1978, with permission.)

tern of growth can be the first manifestation of a wide variety of disease processes, including both endocrine and nonendocrine disorders and involving virtually any organ system of the body. Frequent and accurate assessment of growth is therefore of primary importance in the care of children.

Phases of Normal Growth

Growth occurs at differing rates during intrauterine life, early and middle childhood, and adolescence prior to its cessation after the fusion of long bone and vertebral epiphyseal growth plates. Prenatal growth averages 1.2 to 1.5 cm/wk but varies dramatically (Fig. 30–1); a midgestational length growth velocity of 2.5 cm/wk falls to almost 0.5 cm/wk immediately before birth. Growth velocity (Figs. 30–2 and 30–3) during the first 2 y of life averages about 15 cm/y and slows

to approximately 6 cm/y during middle childhood. Pubertal growth begins earlier in girls than in boys but is 3 to 5 cm greater in magnitude in boys than in girls. The peak height velocity during the pubertal growth spurt is comparable to the rate of growth during the second year of life. The time of onset of the pubertal growth spurt varies in normal children, reflecting the concept of a "tempo of growth" or rate of maturation, as emphasized by Tanner.[2, 6–10] In most normal children the final height is not influenced by the chronologic time of onset of the pubertal growth spurt, although the sex-related differences in adult height of approximately 13 cm are due to an earlier cessation of growth in females.[9] Growth ceases when the skeleton achieves adult maturity.

Karlberg and colleagues have resolved the normal linear growth curve into three additive, partially superimposable phases.[11, 12] The components of this model include an

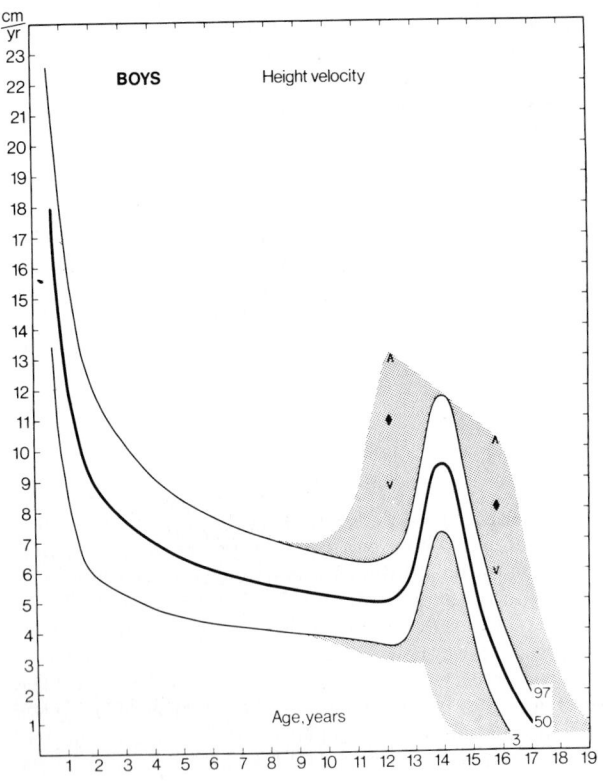

Figure 30–2. Height velocity chart for boys constructed from longitudinal observations of British children. The 97th, 50th, and 3rd percentile curves define the general pattern of growth during puberty. Shaded areas define velocities of children who have peak velocities at ages up to 2 SD before or after the average age depicted by the percentile lines. Arrows and diamonds mark the 97th, 50th, and 3rd percentiles of peak velocity when the peak occurs at these early or late limits. (Modified from charts prepared by Tanner JM, Whitehouse RH, from data published in Tanner JM, Whitehouse RH, Takaishi M. Arch Dis Child 1966; 41:613–635; Iranmanesh A, Lizarralde G, Veldhuis JD. J Clin Endocrinol Metab 1991; 73:1081–1088; and Tanner JM, Whitehouse RH. Arch Dis Child 1976; 51:170–179. Reproduced with permission of Tanner JM and Castlemead Publications, Ward's Publishing Services, Herts, UK.)

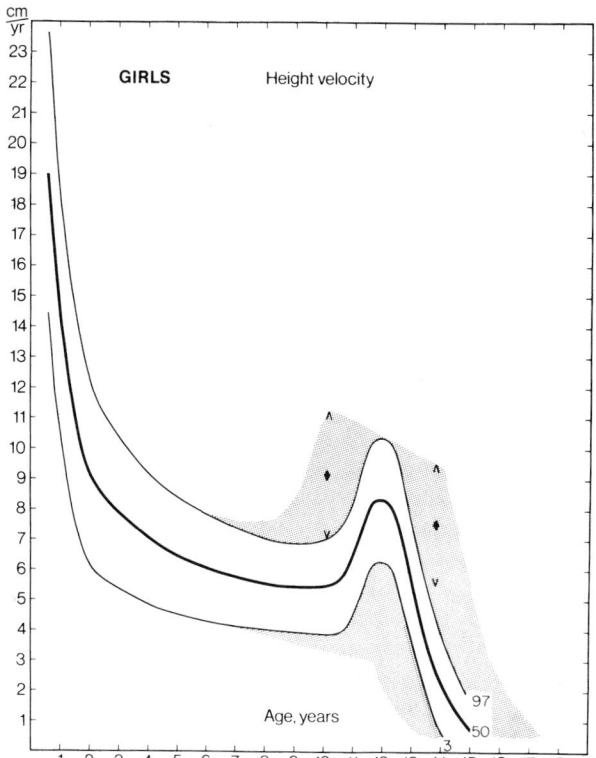

Figure 30–3. Height velocity chart for girls. (See legend for Fig. 30–2.) (Modified and reproduced with permission of Tanner JM and Castlemead Publications, Ward's Publishing Services, Herts, UK.)

"infancy" phase, starting in midgestation and then rapidly decelerating to about 3 to 4 y of age; a "childhood" phase, slowly decelerating during early adolescence; and a sigmoid-shaped "puberty" phase that involves the adolescent growth spurt. Hormonal concomitants of these phases have been suggested but, as seen in this chapter, the interplay of the growth hormone (GH)–insulin-like growth factor (IGF) axis, gonadal steroids, and thyroxine is complex, and attempts to define individual predominance of one hormone at any time of life is likely an oversimplification.

Measurement

Assessment of growth requires accurate and reproducible determinations of height.[13–15] Supine length is routinely measured in children less than 2 y of age, and erect height is assessed in older children. The inherent inaccuracies involved in measuring length in infants are often obscured by the rapid skeletal growth during this period. For measurement of supine length (Fig. 30–4) it is best to use a firm box with an inflexible board against which the head lies, with a movable footboard on which the feet are placed perpendicular to the plane of the supine length of the infant. Optimally the child should be

relaxed, the legs should be fully extended, and the head should be positioned in the "Frankfort plane," with the line connecting the outer canthus of the eyes and the external auditory meatus perpendicular to the long axis of the trunk.

When children are old enough (and physically able) to stand erect, it is best to employ a wall-mounted "Harpenden" stadiometer, similar to that designed by Tanner and Whitehouse for the British Harpenden Growth Study. Free-standing stadiometers are also available but require frequent recalibration. The traditional measuring device of a flexible arm mounted to a weight balance is notoriously unreliable and does not provide accurate serial measurements.

As with length measurements in infants, positioning of the child in the stadiometer is critical (Fig. 30–5). The child should be fully erect, with the head in the Frankfort plane; the back of the head, thoracic spine, buttocks, and heels should touch the vertical axis of the stadiometer, and the heels should be together. Every effort should be made to correct discrepancies related to lordosis or scoliosis and, ideally, serial measurements should be made at the same time of day because standing height may undergo diurnal variation.[16]

Height determinations should be performed by a trained individual rather than by an inexperienced member of the staff. We recommend that lengths and heights be measured in triplicate, that variation be no more than 0.3 cm, and that the mean height be recorded. For determination of height velocity when several measurements are being made within a short period, the same individual should perform the determinations to eliminate interobserver variability. Even when every effort is made to obtain accurate height measurements, a minimum interval of 6 mo is necessary for meaningful height velocity computation. Data gathered over 9 to 12 mo are preferable so that errors of measurement are minimized and the seasonal variation in height velocity[17] is assimilated into the data.

Growth Charts

Evaluation of a child's height must be performed in the context of normal standards. Such standards can be either *cross-sectional* or *longitudinal.* Most American pediatric endocrine clinics continue to use the cross-sectional data provided by the National Center for Health Statistics (NCHS) (Figs. 30–6 and 30–7).[18–20] These charts compare individual children with the 3rd, 10th, 25th, 50th, 75th, 90th, and 97% percentiles of normal American children. There are, however, two major limitations of these charts when applied to the individual child. First, they do not satisfactorily define children below the 3rd or above the 97th percentile, the very children in whom it is most critical to define the degree to which deviation from the normal growth percentiles occurs. The NCHS data are useful in computing standard deviation (SD) scores, which are more helpful because a short child can be described as, e.g., −4.2 or −2.5 SD scores from normal. A height SD score for age is calculated as follows: SD scores equal height minus mean height for normal children at this age and sex divided by the SD of height for normal children at this age and sex.

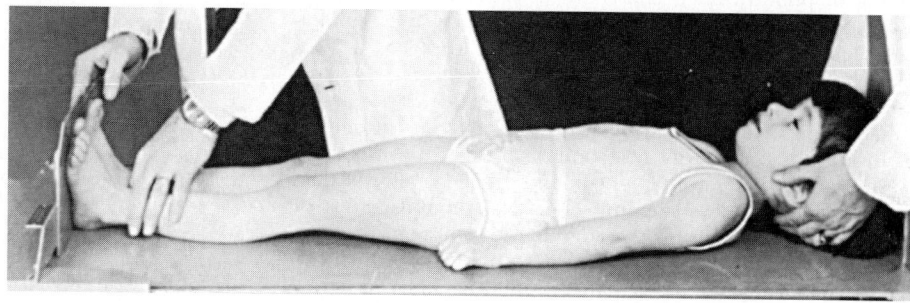

Figure 30–4. Technique for measuring recumbent length. (Courtesy of Noel Cameron. A device suitable for measurement of length of infants can be purchased from Raven Equipment Limited, Unit 4, Ford Farm Industrial Complex, Braintree Rd, Dunmow Essex CMG 1 HU, UK.)

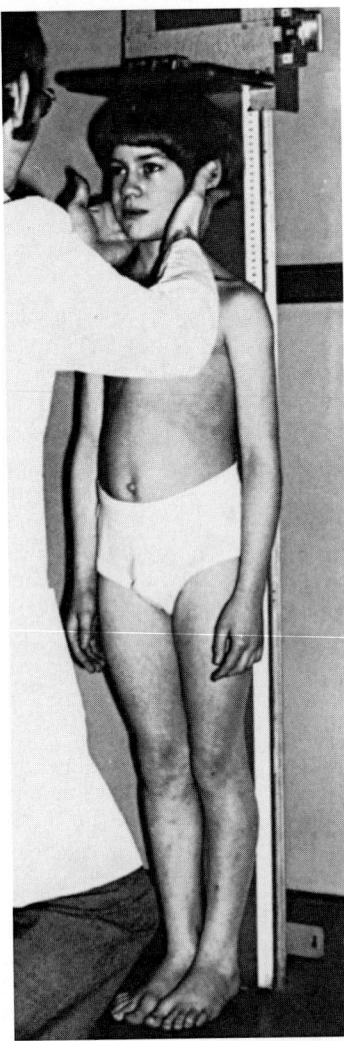

Figure 30–5. Technique for measuring erect height using the Harpenden stadiometer with direct digital display of height. (Devices of this type are available from Holtain Ltd, Crosswell, Crymych, Dyfed SA41, 3UF, Wales, UK. In the United States, they may be obtained from Seritex Inc, 450 Barell Avenue, Carlstadt, NM, 07072.)

Because these are defined by cross-sectional data, however, childhood SD scores are not directly comparable with SD scores during adolescence, when variation in growth rate and maturational tempo can be large. Second, cross-sectional data are of greater value during infancy and childhood than in adolescence because differences in the timing of pubertal onset can considerably influence normal growth rates. To address this issue Tanner and colleagues[6] developed longitudinal growth charts, combining longitudinal data to construct the curve shapes with percentile widths obtained from a large cross-sectional survey, thus accounting for variability in the timing of puberty. Such charts are of particular value in assessing growth during adolescence and puberty and for plotting sequential growth data on any given child.

The data from cross-sectional and longitudinal growth studies have been employed to develop *height velocity* standards, enhancing the value of linear growth velocity measurements in an individual (see Figs. 30–2 and 30–3). [6, 21] It is important to emphasize that carefully documented height velocity data are invaluable in assessing the child with abnormalities of growth. Although there is considerable variability in the normal height velocity in children of different ages, between the age of 2 y and the onset of puberty children normally grow

with remarkable fidelity relative to the normal growth curves. Any "crossing" of height percentiles during this age period should be noted by the physician, and abnormal height velocities always warrant further evaluation.

Syndrome-specific growth curves have been developed for a number of clinical conditions associated with growth failure, such as gonadal dysgenesis (Turner's syndrome),[22] achondroplasia,[23] and Down's syndrome.[24] Such growth profiles are invaluable for tracking the growth of children with these clinical conditions. Deviation of growth from the appropriate disease-related growth curve suggests the possibility of a second underlying cause.

Body Proportions

Many abnormal growth states, including both short stature and excessive stature, are characterized by *disproportionate* growth. The following determinations should be made as part of the evaluation of short stature:

Occipitofrontal head circumference
Lower body segment: distance from the top of the pubic symphysis to the floor
Upper body segment: sitting height (height of stool should be subtracted from standing height)
Arm span

Published standards exist for these body proportion mea-

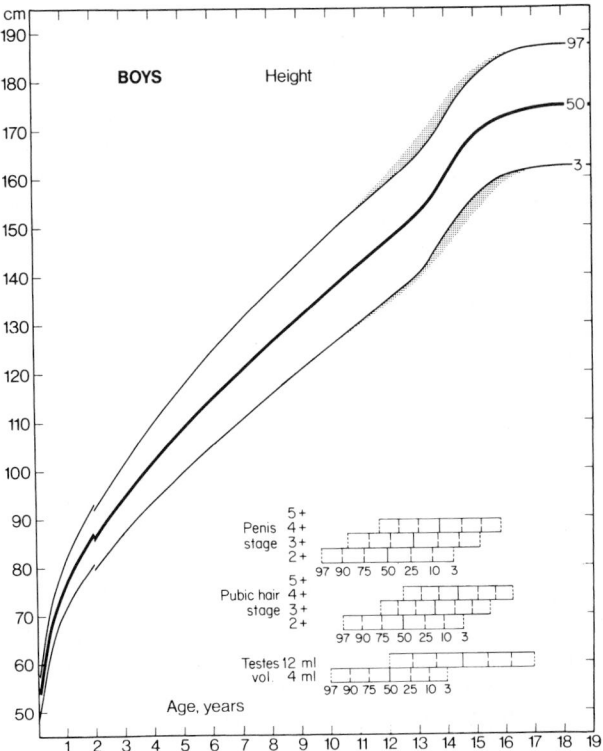

Figure 30–6. Cumulative (height-attained) growth chart for boys. The 97th, 50th, and 3rd percentile curves depict the normal growth pattern from data collected by longitudinal as well as cross-sectional observations of British children. Outer (*upper and lower*) margins of shaded areas represent 97th and 3rd percentile standards collected by cross-sectional observations. The ages of attainment of stages of pubertal development (Tanner) are plotted by percentiles, the 97th percentile being the early limit of occurrence of a given pubertal stage and the 3rd being the late limit. (Modified from charts prepared by Tanner JM, Whitehouse RH, from data published in Tanner JM, Whitehouse RH, Takaishi M. Arch Dis Child 1966; 41:613–635; Tanner JM, Whitehouse RH. Arch Dis Child 1976; 51:170–179; and Tanner JM, Whitehouse RH, Takaishi M. Arch Dis Child 1966; 41:454–471. Original charts also contain 10th, 25th, 75th, and 90th percentile lines. Reproduced with permission of Tanner JM and Castlemead Publications, Ward's Publishing Services, Herts, UK.)

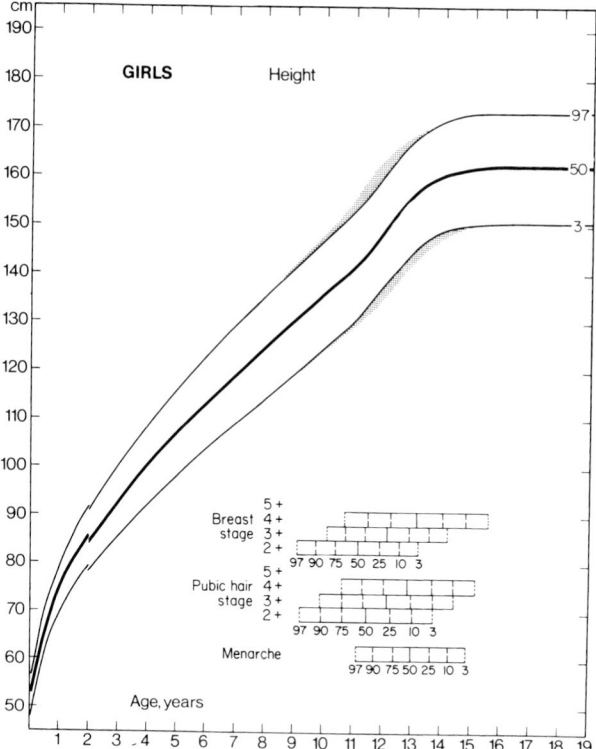

Figure 30–7. Cumulative growth chart for girls. (See legend for Fig. 30–6.) (Adapted and reproduced with permission of Tanner JM and Castlemead Publications, Ward's Publishing Service, Herts, UK.)

surements, which must be evaluated relative to the patient's age.[25] The upper segment/lower segment ratio, e.g., ranges from 1.7 in the neonate to slightly less than 1 in the adult.

Skeletal Maturation (Bone Age)

The growth potential in the tubular bones can be assessed by evaluation of the progression of ossification within the epiphyses. The ossification centers of the skeleton appear and progress in a predictable sequence in normal children, and skeletal maturation can be compared with normal age-related standards. This forms the basis of "bone age" or "skeletal age," which is the only readily available quantitative determination of net somatic maturation and thus is a mirror of the tempo of growth and maturation. It is not clear what factors determine this normal maturational pattern, but it is certain that genetic factors and multiple hormones, including thyroxine, GH, and gonadal steroids, are involved. After the neonatal period a radiograph of the left hand and wrist is commonly used for comparison with the published standards of Greulich and Pyle.[26] An alternative method for assessing bone age from radiographs of the left hand involves a scoring system for developmentally identified stages of each of 20 individual bones,[27] a technique that has been adapted for computerized assessment.[28, 29] The left hand is used because radiographs of the entire skeleton would be tedious and expensive and would involve additional radiation exposure. However, the hand does not contribute to height, and accurate evaluation of growth potential might require radiographs of the legs and spine.

A number of important caveats concerning bone age must be considered. Experience in determination of bone age is essential to minimize intraobserver variance, and clinical studies involving bone age generally benefit from having a single reader perform all interpretations. The normal rate of skeletal maturation differs between boys and girls and among

different ethnic groups. The standards of Greulich and Pyle are separable by sex but were developed in American white children between 1931 and 1942. Finally, both the Greulich and Pyle and the Tanner and Whitehouse standards involved *normal* children[30] and may not be applicable to children with skeletal dysplasias, endocrine abnormalities, or other forms of growth retardation.

Prediction of Adult Height

The extent of skeletal maturation observed in an individual can be employed to predict the ultimate height potential. Such predictions are based on the observation that the more delayed the bone age (relative to the chronologic age), the longer the time before epiphyseal fusion prevents further growth. The most commonly used method for height prediction, based on Greulich and Pyle's *Radiographic Atlas of Skeletal Development*,[26] was developed by Bayley and Pinneau,[31] and relies on bone age, height, and a semiquantitative allowance for chronologic age (Table 30–1). The system of Tanner and colleagues[27, 32] employs height, bone age, chronologic age and, during puberty, height and bone age increments during the previous year and menarchal status. Roche and co-workers[33] employ the combination of height, bone age, chronologic age, and midparental height and weight. Furthermore, attempts have been made to calculate final height predictions without requiring the use of skeletal age[34, 35] by using multiple regression analyses with available data such as height, weight, birth measurements, and midparental stature. All of these systems are, by nature, empirical and are not absolute predictors. The more advanced the bone age, the greater the accuracy of the adult height prediction because a more advanced bone age places a patient closer to final height.

All methods of predicting adult height are based on data from normal children, and none has been documented to be accurate in children with growth abnormalities. For this kind of precision it would be necessary to develop disease-specific (e.g., achondroplasia, gonadal dysgenesis) atlases of skeletal maturation.

Parental Target Height

Since genetic factors are important determinants of growth and height potential, it is useful to assess a patient's stature relative to that of siblings and parents. Tanner and associates developed a growth chart modifying the heights of children, aged 2 to 9 y, by the midparental height.[36] Furthermore, the child's predicted adult height (see earlier) may be related to a "parental target height," namely the mean parental height with the addition or subtraction of 6.5 cm for boys and girls, respectively. The 2 SD range for this calculated parental target height is about ±10 cm so that calculated target heights, like predicted adult heights, are approximations. Nevertheless when a child's growth pattern clearly deviates from that of parents or siblings, the possibility of an underlying pathologic condition should be considered.

ENDOCRINE REGULATION OF GROWTH

Pituitary

The concept of the pituitary as a "master gland" controlling the endocrine activities of the body has been replaced by recognition of the importance of the brain and, particularly, the hypothalamus in regulating hormonal production and

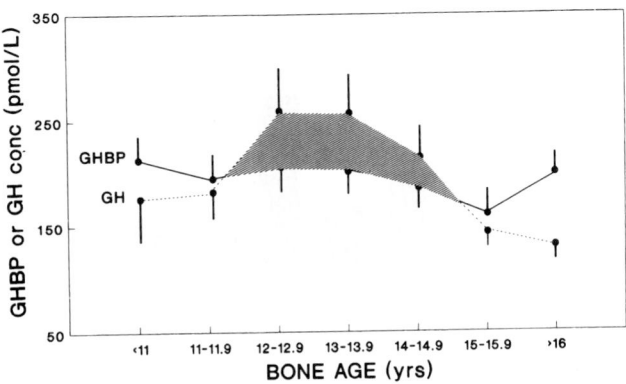

Figure 30–12. Levels of hGH and GHBP measured in normal pubertal boys throughout adolescence. The GHBP levels do not significantly change during puberty, but there is a significant increment of hGH production and, therefore, of hGH levels during this same time. These data suggest that there may be greater amounts of "free hGH" during this period, leading to greater production of IGF-I. (Based on data from Martha PM, Rogol AD, Veldhuis JD, et al. J Clin Endocrinol Metab 1989; 69:563–570; and Martha PM Jr, Rogol AD, Blizzard RM, et al. J Clin Endocrinol Metab 1991; 73:175–181, with permission.)

production.[131] The age-dependent decrements in sleep-related GH secretion may play an important role in the somatopause.[132] Ho and colleagues[67] reported that serum estradiol levels are the major factor affecting GH secretion. Neither age nor sex influenced the integrated serum levels of GH when the effects of estradiol were removed from analysis. When testosterone was administered to boys with delayed puberty, spontaneous GH release was enhanced, but such a change was not duplicated by administration of oxandrolone, a nonaromatizable androgen, again emphasizing the possible unique importance of estrogen on GH secretion.[71a, 108, 133–136] The effects of testosterone on serum IGF-I levels may be independent of GH, at least in part, because individuals with mutations of the GH receptor still experience a rise in serum IGF-I during puberty.[137]

Obesity is characterized by markedly decreased GH production, reflected by a decrease of nearly 70% in number of GH secretory bursts and of 25% in half-life duration.[128] Obesity in childhood and adolescence, similarly, is characterized by decreased GH production but normal IGF levels and often increased linear growth. Endogenous GH secretion and levels achieved during provocative tests in these obese subjects[135] are in the diagnostic range of GH deficiency. Fasting increases both the number and amplitude of GH secretory bursts, presumably reflecting decreased somatostatin secretion and enhanced GHRH release. Veldhuis and colleagues[99] suggested that rapid changes in levels of IGF-binding proteins (IGFBPs) in response to altered nutrition and changes of insulin levels may modify the effect of IGF-I on its negative feedback sites. Body mass also influences GH production in normal prepubertal and pubertal children and adults.[103, 110, 138]

Growth Hormone Receptor–Growth Hormone–Binding Protein

Leung and colleagues[139] cloned both rabbit and human cDNAs for the GH receptor. Each contains an open reading frame of 638 amino acids and encodes a mature receptor of 620 amino acids and a predicted molecular weight of 70 kd before glycosylation. There are three domains—an extracellular, hormone-binding domain; a single membrane-spanning domain; and a cytoplasmic domain. In humans the most important circulating GHBP appears to be derived from proteolytic cleavage of the extracellular domain of the receptor.[140] Conversely in the mouse[141, 142] and rat[143] there are multiple transcripts for the GH receptor: the larger 3.4- to 4.8-kb tran-

script codes for the intact receptor and the 1.2- to 1.9-kb transcript codes for the soluble GHBP.

The coding and 3'-untranslated regions of the human GH receptor are encoded by nine exons, numbered 2 to 10.[144, 145] The gene for the human GH receptor is located on chromosome 5p13.1-p12, where it spans more than 87 kb.[146] The GH receptor shows sequence homology with the prolactin receptor and with receptors for interleukin-2, 3, 4, 6, and 7, as well as receptors for erythropoietin, granulocyte-macrophage colony stimulating factor, and interferon.[144]

After binding to its receptor GH stimulates phosphorylation of a protein with an apparent molecular weight of 120 kd.[147] JAK2 has recently been identified as a major GH receptor–associated tyrosine kinase.[148] The presumed sequence of steps in GH action involves (1) binding of GH to the membrane-associated GH receptor, (2) dimerization of the GH receptor, (3) interaction of the GH receptor with JAK2, (4) tyrosine phosphorylation of both JAK2 and the GH receptor, (5) changes in cytoplasmic and nuclear protein phosphorylation and dephosphorylation, and (6) stimulation of target gene transcription. Although GH stimulates *IGF-I* gene transcription, it is likely that additional genes are also regulated by GH.

The major GHBP in human plasma binds GH with high specificity and affinity but with relatively low capacity, as about 45% of circulating GH is bound.[122, 149–152] The GHBP is, in essence, the extracellular domain of the GH receptor and has an apparent molecular weight of approximately 55 kd. An additional GHBP, not related to the GH receptor, binds approximately 5 to 10% of circulating GH with lower affinity.[122, 152] GHBP prolongs the half-life of GH, presumably by impairing its glomerular filtration, and modulates its binding to the GH receptor. In general, GHBP levels reflect GH receptor levels and activity; i.e., low levels are associated with states of GH resistance.[122, 152] However, in the rapidly growing child levels of GHBP are low.[153, 154] Initial assays for GHBP involved incubation of serum with [125I]-GH and separation of bound from free radioligand.[122] Carlsson and colleagues[155] have developed a ligand-mediated immunofunctional assay (LIFA) for measurement of GHBP.

Levels of GHBP are low in early life, rise through childhood, and plateau during puberty and adulthood.[121, 152–154] Levels are usually constant for a given individual once puberty is reached.[121] Impaired nutrition, diabetes mellitus, hypothyroidism, chronic liver disease, and a spectrum of inherited abnormalities of the GH receptor are associated with low levels of GHBP, whereas obesity, refeeding, early pregnancy, and estrogen treatment can cause elevated levels of GHBP.[122, 152] A direct correlation exists between GHBP levels and body mass index.[156] Serum GHBP levels correlate inversely with 24-h GH production[121]; this reciprocal relationship between GH production and GHBP in normal individuals (and in persons with idiopathic short stature) [157, 158] may result from adjustments of GH secretion to accommodate GH receptor levels, which may be genetically determined or modulated by environmental factors such as nutritional status.[156, 159]

Assays of serum levels of GHBP are useful in identifying persons with GH resistance caused by genetic abnormalities of the GH receptor.[160, 161] Patients with GH resistance due to nonreceptor abnormalities, defects of the intracellular domain of the GH receptor, or inability of the receptor to dimerize may, however, have normal serum levels of GHBP.[950, 954]

Growth Hormone Actions

According to the somatomedin hypothesis (see later), the anabolic actions of GH are mediated through the IGF peptides.[163, 164] Although this theory is largely true, GH is also capable of inducing effects that are independent of IGF activity. Indeed the actions of GH and IGF are, on occasion, contradictory, as evident in the "diabetogenic" actions of GH[165, 166] and the glucose-lowering activity of IGFs. Green and colleagues[167] have attempted to resolve some of these differences in a "dual effector" model, in which GH stimulates precursor cells, such as prechondrocytes, to differentiate. When differentiated cells or neighboring cells then secrete IGFs, these peptides act as mitogens and stimulate clonal expansion. This hypothesis is based on the ability of IGF peptides to work not only as hormones that are transported through the blood but also as paracrine or autocrine growth factors.

GH has a variety of metabolic actions, some of which appear to be independent of IGF production, such as enhancement of lipolysis,[168] stimulation of amino acid transport in diaphragm[169] and heart,[170] and enhancement of hepatic protein synthesis. The concept of IGF-independent actions of GH is supported by in vivo studies in which IGF-I cannot duplicate all of the effects of GH, such as nitrogen retention and insulin resistance.[171] The administration of GH for 1 to 3 wk to calorically restricted normal or obese men results in significant nitrogen retention, although this effect does not persist with prolonged therapy.[172] The effects of GH in normal human aging[173] and in catabolic states[174] are subjects under active investigation.

Insulin-Like Growth Factors

Historical Background

The IGFs (also called somatomedins) are a family of peptides that are, in part, GH-dependent and that mediate many of the anabolic and mitogenic actions of GH. Originally identified in 1957 by their ability to stimulate [^{35}S]sulfate incorporation into rat cartilage and termed *sulfation factor,*[163] concurrent investigations indicated that only a component of the insulin-like activity of normal serum could be blocked by the addition of anti-insulin antibodies. The remaining activity, termed *nonsuppressible insulin-like activity* (NSILA), was subsequently demonstrated to contain two soluble, low-molecular-weight (7-kd) forms, named NSILA-I and II.[175, 176] A third line of investigation arose from studies by Dulak and Temin[177] of the mitogenic nature of bovine serum; the mitogenic factor was termed *multiplication stimulating activity* and shares metabolic and mitogenic activities with both sulfation factor and NSILA.

In 1972 the restrictive labels of sulfation factor and NSILA were replaced by the term *somatomedin.*[178] The following criteria for a somatomedin were established: (1) the concentration in serum must be GH-dependent; (2) the factor must possess insulin-like activity in extraskeletal tissues; (3) the factor must promote the incorporation of sulfate into cartilage; and (4) the factor must stimulate DNA synthesis and cell multiplication. Purification yielded two somatomedin peptides, a basic peptide (SM-C) and a neutral peptide (SM-A).[179, 180] In 1978 Rinderknecht and Humbel[181, 182] isolated two active somatomedins from human plasma and demonstrated a striking structural resemblance to proinsulin. Accordingly these two peptides were renamed *insulin-like growth factors.*

Insulin-Like Growth Factor Structure and Molecular Biology

IGF-I is a basic peptide of 70 amino acids that is also called SM-C, and IGF-II is a slightly acidic peptide of 67 amino acids. The two peptides share 45 of 73 possible amino acid positions and have approximately 50% amino acid homology to insulin.[164, 181, 182] Like insulin both IGFs have A and B chains connected by disulfide bonds. The connecting C-peptide re-

gion is 12 amino acids long for IGF-I and 8 amino acids for IGF-II and bears no homology with the C-peptide region of proinsulin. IGF-I and IGF-II also differ from proinsulin in possessing carboxyl terminal extensions, or D-peptides, of eight and six amino acids, respectively. This structural similarity explains the ability of both IGFs to bind to the insulin receptor and of insulin to bind to the type 1 IGF receptor (see later). Conversely, structural differences also explain the failure of insulin to bind to the IGFBPs (see later).

INSULIN-LIKE GROWTH FACTOR VARIANTS

There are several variants of the two IGF peptides. Rinderknecht and Humbel[182] reported that up to a quarter of the IGF-II isolated from human plasma lacked the NH$_2$-terminal alanine. Jansen and co-workers[183] demonstrated that an IGF-II cDNA isolated from a human liver library predicted an IGF-II variant in which Ser[29] was replaced by Arg-Leu-Pro-Gly, and Zumstein and colleagues[184] identified this variant peptide in human plasma. Zumstein and colleagues isolated a 10-kd IGF-II variant from human plasma that contains a 21-residue carboxyl extension, representing a portion of the E domain of pro-IGF-II (see later). In one peptide fragment isolated, Ser[33] was replaced by Cys-Gly-Asp. A 25-kd IGF-II variant was isolated by Gowan and colleagues, presumably representing a carboxyl terminal extension.[185]

The significance of "big" IGF-II forms is still uncertain. In general these variants appear capable of binding to IGF and insulin receptors and to IGFPBs and can participate in formation of the 150-kd IGF/IGFBP-3/acid-labile subunit ternary complex. Big IGF-II can be produced by mesenchymal tumors and can cause non–islet-cell tumor hypoglycemia. Daughaday and co-workers[186] described a patient with a leiomyosarcoma and recurrent hypoglycemia, in whom 70% of serum IGF-II was in higher molecular weight forms. Removal of the tumor eliminated big IGF-II from the serum and corrected the hypoglycemia. The presence of big IGF-II in non–islet-cell tumor hypoglycemia has been confirmed in multiple laboratories, but it is unclear why hypoglycemia occurs in the face of normal *total* serum IGF-II levels. Zapf[187] has proposed that non–islet-cell tumor hypoglycemia occurs when secretion of big IGF-II results in suppression of GH, insulin, and 7-kd IGF-II, leading to decreased production of IGF-I, IGFBP-3, and the acid-labile subunit and increased production of IGFBP-2. This leads to a shift in the distribution of IGF-II from the 150-kd ternary complex to the 40- to 50-kd molecular weight complex, composed of IGFBP-3, IGFBP-2, and a number of other low-molecular-weight IGFBPs. It is presumed that this results in increased bioavailability of IGF-II to target tissues, enhances glucose consumption, and decreases hepatic glucose production.

Big forms of IGF-I have not been as thoroughly documented as IGF-II. Powell and co-workers,[188] however, have reported that IGF-I forms with an apparent molecular weight as high as 19 kd may be found in uremic serum. Large molecular forms of IGF-I have also been identified in conditioned media of human fibroblast cell lines.

Two IGF-I precursor molecules have been identified.[164] The first 134 amino acids of each are identical, comprising the signal peptide (48 amino acids), the mature IGF-I molecule (70 amino acids), and the first 16 amino acids of the E domain of the precursor. IGF-IA has an additional 19 amino acids and IGF-IB has an additional 61 amino acids (total 195 residues). Alternative splicing of the *IGF-I* gene presumably generates the two mRNAs. The primary IGF-II translation product in human, rat, and mouse contains 180 amino acids, including a 24-residue signal peptide, the 67-amino-acid mature IGF-II sequence, and a carboxyl-terminal E peptide of 89 amino acids.

INSULIN-LIKE GROWTH FACTOR GENES

The IGF genes (Fig. 30–13) are expressed differently in the embryo, fetus, child, and adult.[164, 189–191] Both IGF-I and IGF-II are encoded by single large genes. The human *IGF-I* gene is located on the long arm of chromosome 12.[192, 193] The human *IGF-I* gene contains at least five or six exons. Exons 1 and 2 encode alternative signal peptides, probably each containing several transcription start sites. Exons 3 and 4 encode the remaining signal peptide, the remainder of the mature IGF-I molecule, and part of the trailer peptide (E peptide). Exons 5 and 6 encode alternatively used segments of the trailer peptide (resulting in the IGF-IA and IGF-IB forms) and 3'-untranslated sequences with multiple different polyadenylation sites. The wide diversity of IGF-I mRNAs thus reflects (1) multiple leader exons and transcription start sites, (2) alternative splicing of exons 5 or 6, and (3) multiple polyadenylation sites in exon 6.

The human *IGF-II* gene (Fig. 30–14) is located on the short arm of chromosome 11[192–194] adjacent to the insulin gene and spans 35 kb of genomic DNA, containing nine exons. Exons 1 to 6 encode 5'-untranslated RNA, exon 7 encodes the signal peptide and most of the mature protein, and exon 8 encodes the carboxyl terminal portion of the protein and part of the trailer peptide, whose coding is completed in exon 9.

Thus multiple mRNA species exist for both IGF-I and IGF-II, allowing for tissue-specific expression of specific transcripts and for developmental and hormonal regulation. The mechanisms involved in the regulation of IGF gene expression include the existence of multiple promoters, heterogeneous transcription initiation within each of the promoters, alternative splicing of various exons, differential RNA polyadenylation, and variable mRNA stability. Translation of *IGF-I* genes may also be under complex control.

REGULATION OF EXPRESSION OF INSULIN-LIKE GROWTH FACTOR GENES

GH appears to be the primary regulator of *IGF-I* gene transcription, which begins as early as 30 min after intraperitoneal injection of GH into hypophysectomized rats.[195] Transcriptional activation by GH affects both IGF-I promoters equivalently, resulting in a 20-fold rise in IGF-I mRNA. This coordinated, rapid induction of all IGF-I mRNA species coincides with induction of *Spi 2.1* gene by GH, although the relationship between these two processes is still not clear.[195] Furthermore there may be tissue-to-tissue variability in GH-induced expression of IGF-I mRNA.[196] Other factors that influence *IGF-I* gene expression include estrogen, which stimulates IGF-I mRNA expression in the uterus but inhibits GH-stimulated *IGF-I* transcription in the liver.[197] The pubertal rise in serum IGF-I levels reflects the effect of gonadal steroids on *IGF-I* transcription, some of which results from the pubertal rise in GH secretion and some of which is due to a direct effect of gonadal steroids on IGF synthesis or secretion, since a pubertal rise in serum IGF levels is also observed in patients with GH resistance.

The factors involved in the regulation of *IGF-II* gene expression are less clear.[198] In humans and rats, *IGF-II* gene

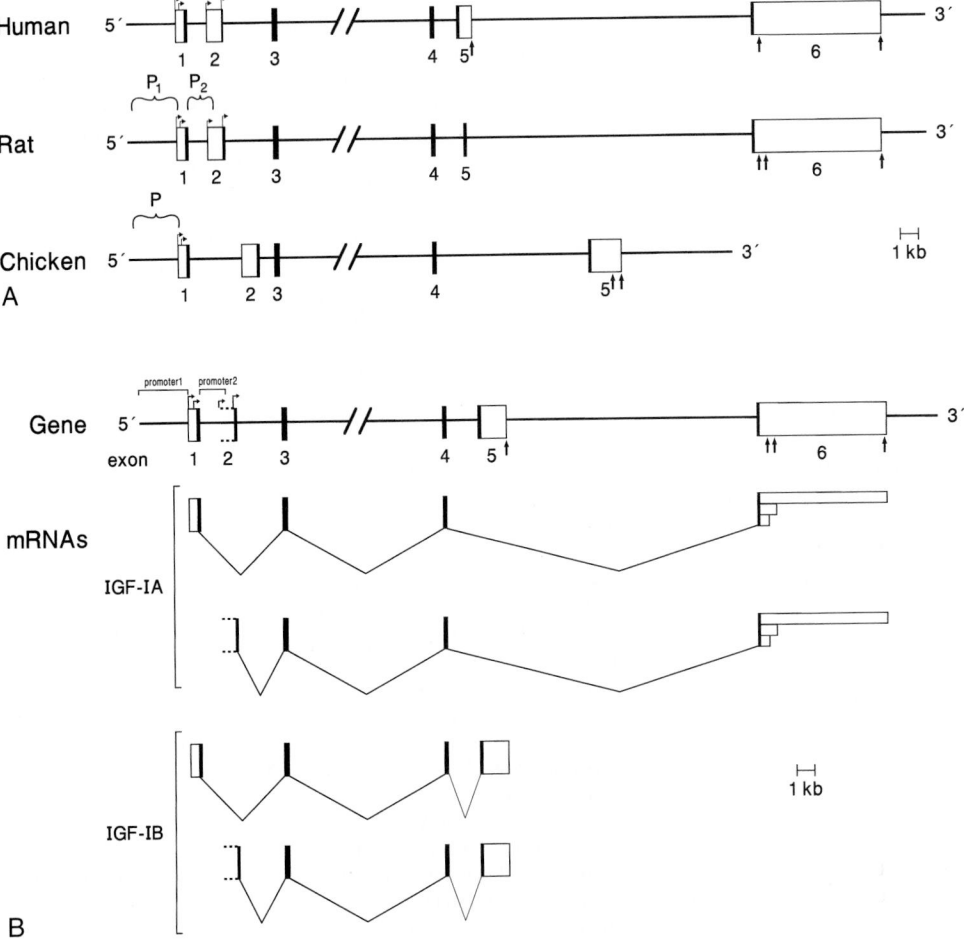

Figure 30–13. Structure of the *IGF-I* gene. *A,* The organization of the genes encoding human, rat, and chicken IGF-I is depicted. Exons are represented by boxes (coding regions are in black, noncoding regions in white), polyadenylation sites are represented by arrows, and promoter regions are represented by a bracket and the letter P. The full extent of the second and last human exons and the second rat exon has not been determined, as indicated by the dotted lines. *B,* Structure and expression of the human *IGF-I* gene. The structure of the different human IGF-I mRNAs is displayed below the map of the gene. Sites of pre-mRNA processing are indicated by the thin lines. Sites of differential polyadenylation are marked at the 3' end of the gene by vertical arrows and in the mRNAs by horizontal boxes of varying length. (From Rotwein P. Structure, evolution, expression and regulation of insulin-like growth factors I and II. Growth Factors 1991; 5:3–18, with permission.)

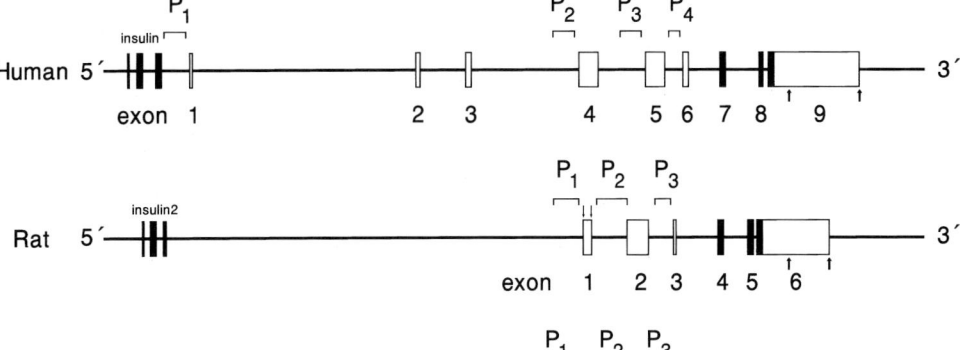

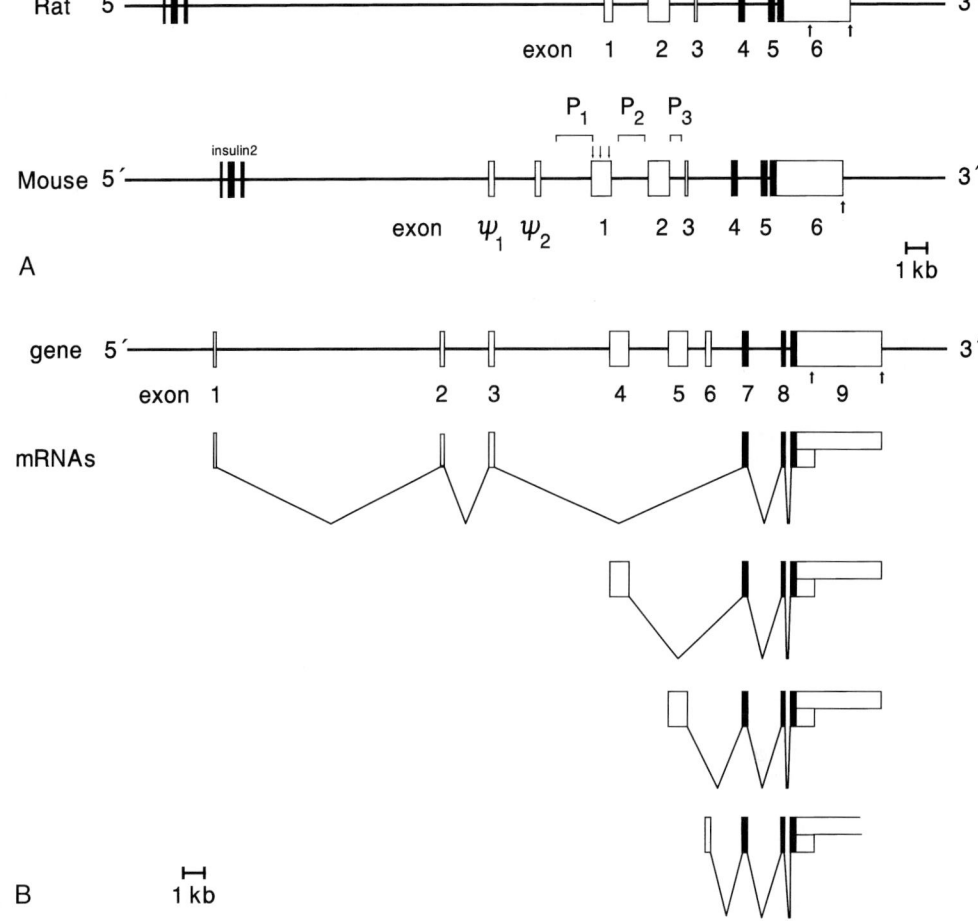

Figure 30–14. Structure of the *IGF-II* gene. *A,* The organization of human, rat, and mouse *Igf-II* genes is shown. Exons are represented by boxes (coding regions are in black, and noncoding regions in white), polyadenylation sites are represented by thick vertical arrows, and promoter regions are represented by a bracket and the letter P. The multiple transcription initiation sites for mouse and rat exon 1 are marked by the thin vertical arrows. The locations of mouse pseudoexons 1 and 2 are indicated. *B,* Structure and expression of the human *IGF-II* gene. The structure of different human IGF-II mRNAs is displayed below the map of the gene. The patterns of mRNA processing are indicated by the thin lines. Sites of differential polyadenylation are marked at the 3' end of the gene by vertical arrows and in the mRNAs by horizontal boxes of varying length. (From Rotwein P. Structure, evolution, expression and regulation of insulin-like growth factors I and II. Growth Factors 1991; 5:3–18, with permission.)

expression is high in fetal life and has been detected as early as the blastocyst stage in mice.[199] Serum levels of IGF-II are high in midgestation in pregnant rabbits.[200] Fetal tissues generally have high IGF-II mRNA levels that decline postnatally, although brain IGF-II mRNA remains high in the adult rat.[201] IGF-II mRNA is expressed constitutively in a number of mesenchymal and embryonic tumors, including Wilms' tumor,[202, 203] rhabdomyosarcoma, neuroblastoma, pheochromocytoma, hepatoblastoma, leiomyoma and leiomyosarcoma, liposarcoma, and colon carcinoma.[204–208] Production of "big" IGF-II by these tumors may cause non–islet-cell tumor hypoglycemia (see earlier).[186] A tumor suppressor gene associated with Wilms' tumor *(WT-1)* has been mapped to chromosome 11p13, close to the *IGF-II* locus (chromosome 11p15.5), consistent with the possibility of a direct effect of *WT-1* on *IGF-II* gene transcription and suggesting an autocrine role for IGF-II in some tumors.[209] This may be relevant in the embryonal tumors of Beckwith-Wiedemann syndrome, where there may be loss of heterozygosity in the 11p15 maternally derived chromosome and paternal isodisomy, consistent with parental imprinting and a twofold increase in gene dosage of the active *IGF-II* allele.[210]

INSULIN-LIKE GROWTH FACTOR IMPRINTING

Gene regulation for the IGF system may also be subject to genomic imprinting, a process that influences the expression of specific genes. Namely, certain autosomal genes are expressed from only one of the two theoretically available alleles in a manner that is specific for the parent of origin. The result is a heritable difference in gene expression depending on whether a specific allele is inherited from the mother or from the father. Allele-specific imprinting is exemplified by abnormalities of chromosome 15q11-13, where deletions of the paternal chromosome result in the Prader-Willi syndrome, and deletions of the maternal locus are associated with Angelman syndrome, two phenotypically distinct conditions. The molecular mechanisms responsible for genomic imprinting are still unclear but may involve variable DNA methylation.

The first evidence for imprinting in the IGF axis emerged from studies of targeted gene disruption of *Igf-II* in the mouse[211] that caused fetal growth retardation only when the disrupted allele was inherited from the father (i.e., maternally imprinted).[212] The human *IGF-II* gene is similarly imprinted.[210,]

[213, 214] In tissues in which only maternal chromosomes are present, such as ovarian teratomas, no *IGF-II* expression is observed, whereas gene expression is observed in tissues in which only paternal chromosomes are present (complete hydatidiform mole).[215] Loss of imprinting (or "relaxation" of imprinting) of the *IGF-II* gene has been observed in rhabdomyosarcomas, lung cancers, Wilms' tumor, and choriocarcinoma.[203, 204, 207] In such situations, IGF-II may act as an autocrine or paracrine growth factor for neoplastic tissue. Furthermore in Wilms' tumor, loss of imprinting of the *IGF-II* gene is associated with reduced expression of the putative tumor suppressor gene *H19*.[216] The *H19* gene appears to be imprinted in a reciprocal manner to *Igf-II/IGF-II*, and the two genes may be coordinately regulated, since the genes are located near each other on the same chromosome.

The genes for the type 2 IGF receptor, which is the same as the cation-independent mannose-6-phosphate receptor, are also imprinted, although in a different manner.[217] Thus the mouse Igf-II receptor gene and the human IGF type 2 receptor gene are both expressed by the maternal allele (i.e., paternally imprinted). If IGF-II functions as a fetal growth factor, there is potential for both maternal and paternal regulation of fetal size.

TARGETED DISRUPTION OF INSULIN-LIKE GROWTH FACTOR GENES

The role of the IGF axis in fetal growth has been firmly established by a series of studies involving IGF and IGF receptor null mutations. Mice with knockouts of the gene for either IGF-I *or* IGF-II have birth weights approximately 60% of normal.[212, 218] These observations indicate that both IGF-I and IGF-II are important embryonic and fetal growth factors. Although fetal size was proportionately reduced in both situations and morphogenesis was grossly normal, a higher neonatal death rate was observed after disruption of the gene for IGF-I. Growth delay began on day 11 for *IGF-II* knockouts and on day 13.5 for *IGF-I* knockouts. Those mice with *IGF-I* gene disruptions who survived the immediate neonatal period continued to have growth failure postnatally, with weights 30% of normal by 2 mo of age. Indeed postnatal growth was poorer than that observed in mice with GHRH receptor mutations or *Pit-1* mutations, indicating that both GH-dependent and GH-independent factors are necessary for normal growth. When the genes for both IGF-I and IGF-II were disrupted, weight at birth was only 30% of normal, and all animals died shortly after birth, apparently from respiratory insufficiency secondary to muscular hypoplasia.

Knockout of the gene for the type 1 IGF receptor resulted in birth weights 45% of normal and in 100% neonatal lethality. Concurrent knockout of genes for IGF-I and the type 1 IGF receptor resulted in no further reduction in birth size (45% of normal), which is consistent with the concept that all IGF-I actions in fetal life are mediated through this receptor. Conversely, simultaneous knockout of the genes for IGF-II and the type 1 IGF receptor resulted in further reduction of birth size to 30% of normal (as with simultaneous knockouts of *IGF-I* and *IGF-II*), suggesting that some of the fetal anabolic actions of IGF-II are mediated by a secondary mechanism. This pathway does not appear to involve the type 2 IGF receptor, since knockout of this gene results in an *increased* birth weight but death in late gestation or at birth. Knockout of the genes for the type 2 IGF receptor plus IGF-II causes a birth weight 60% of normal (as is the case with knockout of IGF-II alone) but allows fetal survival.[219]

Several conclusions can be drawn from these studies:

1. IGF-I is important for both fetal and postnatal growth.
2. IGF-I is more important than GH for postnatal growth.

3. IGF-II is a major fetal growth factor.
4. The type 1 IGF receptor mediates anabolic actions of both IGF-I and IGF-II.
5. The type 2 IGF receptor is bifunctional, serving both to target lysosomal enzymes and to enhance IGF-II turnover.
6. IGF-I production is involved in normal fertility.
7. Placental growth is impaired only with *IGF-II* knockouts.

Whether these studies in mice are applicable to humans is of course unknown.

INSULIN-LIKE GROWTH FACTOR PEPTIDE ASSAYS

Bioassay methods for IGF activity included stimulation of [35S]sulfate incorporation, using various modifications of the original method described by Salmon and Daughaday.[163, 220, 221] A wide variety of other bioassays used stimulation of the synthesis of DNA,[222] RNA,[223] or protein[224] or of glucose uptake.[224] Such assays are cumbersome, subject to interference by IGFBPs, and incapable of distinguishing between IGF-I and IGF-II. When SM-C (and later IGF-I and IGF-II) were purified, it became possible to develop radioreceptor[225, 226] and competitive protein-binding assays,[227, 228] and development of specific antibodies made possible the development of accurate and specific measurement of IGF-I and IGF-II.[229–233]

Nevertheless the issue of IGFBPs must be dealt with in any IGF assay.[234] For example, the discrepant results found in uremic sera assayed for IGF by bioassay, radioreceptor assay, and immunoassay are due to the interference of IGFBPs[235]; such interference is a particular problem in conditions with a relatively high IGFBP/IGF peptide ratio and at the extremes of the assay (i.e., GH deficiency or acromegaly). The most effective way of dealing with IGFBPs is to separate them from IGF peptides by chromatography under acidic conditions.[236] This is, however, a labor-intensive procedure and has occasionally been replaced by an acid ethanol extraction procedure.[237] Although this latter method may be reasonably effective for most serum samples, it is problematic in conditions of high IGFBP/IGF peptide ratios, such as conditioned media from cell lines and sera from newborns and from individuals with GH deficiency or uremia.

Alternative methods include the use of antibodies generated against synthetic peptides, such as the C peptide region of IGF-I or IGF-II, which does not bind to IGFBPs. In general such antibodies have high specificity but relatively low affinity. An alternative approach, developed by Blum and co-workers,[238] involves the use of an antibody with high specificity for IGF-II, which permits the addition of excess unlabeled IGF-I to saturate endogenous IGFBPs. Bang and colleagues[239] have bypassed the interference of IGFBPs by employing a truncated IGF-I radioligand, which has decreased affinity for IGFBPs.

Serum Levels of Insulin-Like Growth Factor Peptides

In human fetal serum IGF-I levels are relatively low and are positively correlated with gestational age.[240, 241] A correlation between fetal cord serum IGF-I levels with birth weight has been reported by some[240–242] but not all groups.[243] IGF-I levels in human newborn serum are generally 30 to 50% of adult levels. Serum levels rise during childhood and attain adult levels at the onset of sexual maturation[244] (Fig. 30–15*A* and *B*). During puberty IGF-I levels rise to two to three times the adult range.[245] Thus levels during adolescence correlate better with Tanner stage (or bone age) than with chronologic age. Girls with gonadal dysgenesis show no adolescent increase in serum IGF-I, clearly establishing the association of the pubertal rise in IGF-I with the production of gonadal steroids.[246–248] The pubertal rise in gonadal steroids may stimulate IGF-I

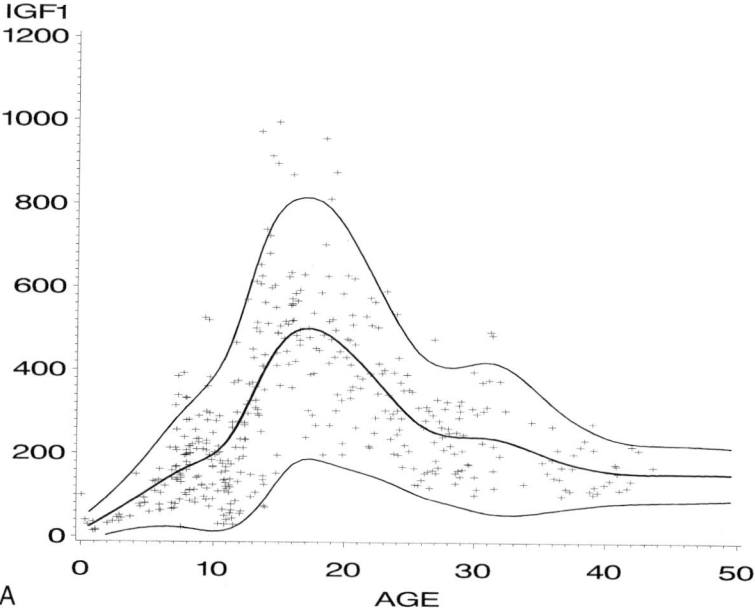

A

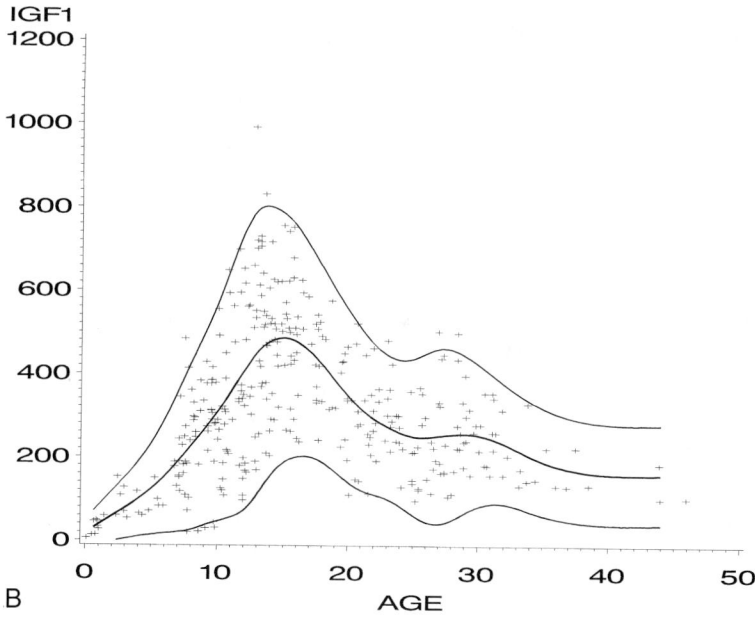

B

Figure 30–15. Normal serum levels of IGF-I (µg/L) for males *(A)* and females *(B)*. Lines represent the 3rd, 50th, and 97th percentiles. (Data courtesy of Diagnostic Systems Laboratories, Inc., Webster, Texas; and Drs. Phillip Lee and Darrell Wilson.)

production indirectly by first leading to a rise in GH secretion, but patients with GH resistance due to GH receptor mutations show a pubertal rise in serum IGF-I despite a *decline* in GH levels, thereby suggesting a direct effect of gonadal steroids on IGF-I.[96]

After adolescence, or at least after age 20 to 30, serum IGF-I levels demonstrate a gradual and progressive age-associated decline,[173, 249] a decline that is possibly responsible for the negative nitrogen balance, decrease in muscle mass, and osteoporosis of aging.[173] This provocative hypothesis is unproved but has generated interest in the potential use of GH or IGF-I therapy, or both, in normal aging (see later).

Human newborn levels of IGF-II are generally 50% of adult levels. By age 1, however, adult levels are attained, with little if any subsequent decline, even up to the seventh or eighth decade of life. This pattern of IGF-II levels in humans is different from that in the rat or mouse, in which serum IGF-II levels are also high in the fetus but rapidly decline postnatally to undetectable levels in the adult.[250, 251]

Measurement of Insulin-Like Growth Factor Levels in Growth Disorders

The GH dependency of the IGFs was established in the initial report from Salmon and Daughaday[163] and further clarified with the development of sensitive and specific immunoassays that distinguish between IGF-I and IGF-II.[232] IGF-I levels are more GH-dependent than are IGF-II levels and are more likely to reflect subtle differences in GH secretory patterns. However, serum IGF-I levels, as stated earlier, are influenced by age, degree of sexual maturation, and nutritional status. As a result, construction of age-defined normative values may be misleading. IGF-I levels in normal children less than 5 y of age are low and there is overlap between the normal range and values in GH-deficient children. Assessment of serum IGF-II levels is less age-dependent, especially after 1 y of age, but IGF-II is less GH-dependent than is IGF-I.

Moore and colleagues[252] performed GH stimulation tests in 78 children with heights below the 5th percentile and serum IGF-I levels less than 0.5 U/mL. Although 19 of these children were subsequently diagnosed as GH-deficient on the basis of standard provocative tests, there was overlap of serum IGF-I levels between GH-deficient children and children with other forms of short stature and normal provocative GH levels. It was only in children with bone ages greater than 12 y that serum IGF-I levels permitted discrimination between GH deficiency and normal short children. Similarly Reiter and Lovinger[253] found that 4 of 16 children with low provocative GH levels had normal serum IGF-I levels, whereas 7 of 25 children with normal provocative GH levels had low serum IGF-I levels.

Rosenfeld and co-workers[233] evaluated the efficacy of IGF-I and IGF-II measurements in 68 GH-deficient patients, 197 normal children with normal stature, and 44 normal children with short stature (Figs. 30–16 and 30–17). Eighteen percent of the GH-deficient children had serum IGF-I levels within the normal range for age, and 32% of normal short children had low IGF-I levels. Low IGF-II levels were found in 52% of GH-deficient children and in 35% of normal short children. However, the use of combined IGF-I–IGF-II assays provided better discrimination. Only 4% of GH-deficient children had normal plasma levels of both IGF-I and IGF-II. Furthermore only 0.5% of normal children and 11% of normal short children had low serum levels of both IGF-I and IGF-II.

The observation that many "normal short" children have low serum levels of IGF-I or IGF-II, or both, calls into question the criteria by which the diagnosis of GH deficiency is made. Given that provocative GH testing is both arbitrary and non-physiological and given the inherent variability in GH assays, it is not surprising that the correlation between IGF-I levels and provocative GH levels is imperfect. These points are further supported by recent observations with immunoassays for IGFBP-3 (see later).

Insulin-Like Growth Factor Receptors

The binding of IGFs to the insulin receptor provided an explanation for their insulin-like activity.[254] Shortly thereafter Megyesi and colleagues[255] identified distinct receptors for insulin and IGF in rat hepatic membranes. At least two classes of IGF receptors exist; insulin, at high levels, competes for occupancy of one form of IGF receptor but has essentially no affinity for the second form of receptor.

Structural characterization of these receptors documented the differences in the two forms of receptor (Fig. 30–18).[256–261] The type 1 IGF receptor is closely related to the insulin receptor; both are heterotetramers composed of two membrane-spanning α subunits and two intracellular β subunits. The α subunits contain the binding sites for IGF-I and are linked by disulfide bonds. The β subunits contain a transmembrane domain and an adenosine triphosphate–binding site and a tyrosine kinase domain that constitute the presumed signal transduction mechanism for the receptor. One mole of the full heterotetrameric receptor appears to bind 1 mole of ligand.

Although the type 1 IGF receptor has been commonly termed the *IGF-I receptor,* the receptor binds both IGF-I and IGF-II with high affinity, and both IGF peptides appear capable of activating tyrosine kinase by binding to this receptor. In studies involving transfection and overexpression of the type 1 IGF receptor cDNA, the K_D for IGF-I is typically in the 0.2 to 1 nM range; affinity for IGF-II is usually slightly less but varies from study to study. The affinity of the type 1 receptor for insulin is generally 100-fold less, thereby explaining the relatively weak mitogenic effect of insulin.

Ullrich and colleagues[262] deduced the structure of the human type 1 IGF receptor from cDNA; the mature peptide constitutes 1337 amino acids with a predicted molecular mass

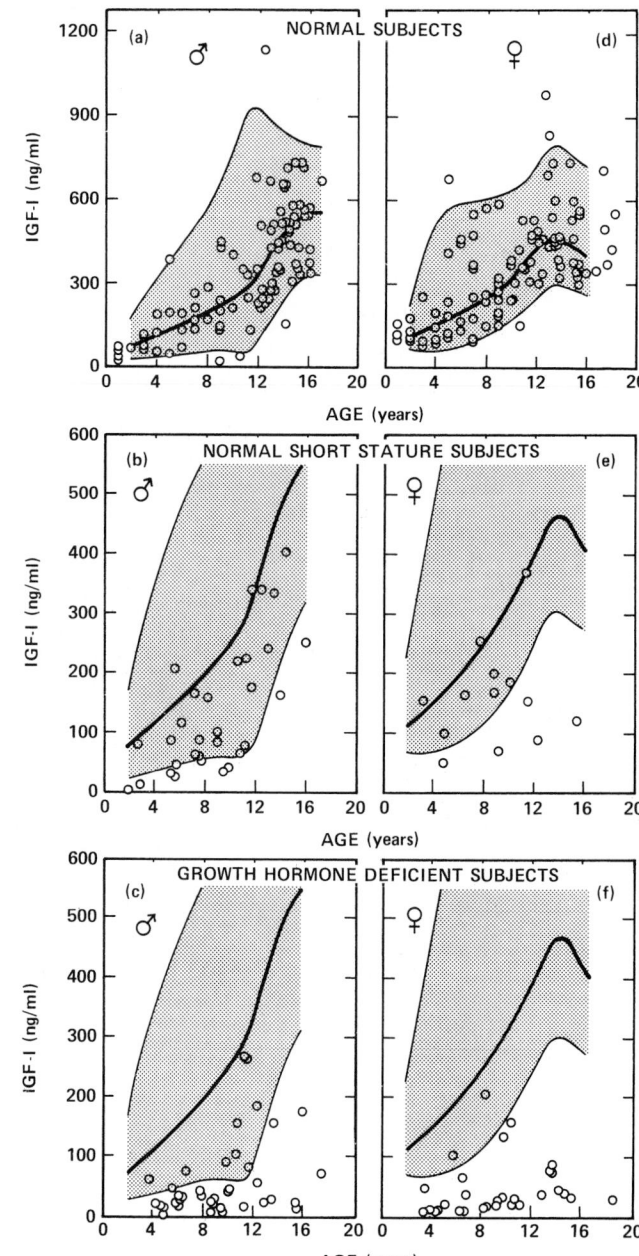

Figure 30–16. Serum IGF-I levels in the evaluation of growth disorders. (From Rosenfeld RG, Wilson DM, Lee PDK, et al. Insulin-like growth factors I and II in the evaluation of growth retardation. J Pediatr 1986; 109:428–433, with permission.)

of 151,869 kd (Fig. 30–19). The translated $\alpha\beta$ heterodimer is subsequently cleaved at an Arg-Lys-Arg-Arg sequence at positions 707 to 710, and the released α- and β-subunits are linked by disulfide bonds to form the mature $(\alpha\beta)_2$-receptor in which two α chains are joined by secondary disulfide bonds. The α-subunits are extracellular and contain a cysteine-rich domain, which is critical for IGF binding. As is the case with the insulin receptor, the β subunit has a short extracellular domain, a hydrophobic transmembrane domain, and the intracellular tyrosine kinase domain and adenosine triphosphate–binding site. Like the insulin receptor the type 1 IGF receptor undergoes ligand-induced autophosphorylation, principally on tyrosines 1131, 1135, and 1136.[263–266] Both receptors are believed to have evolved from a common ancestor protein but are encoded by genes on separate chromosomes (chromosome 15

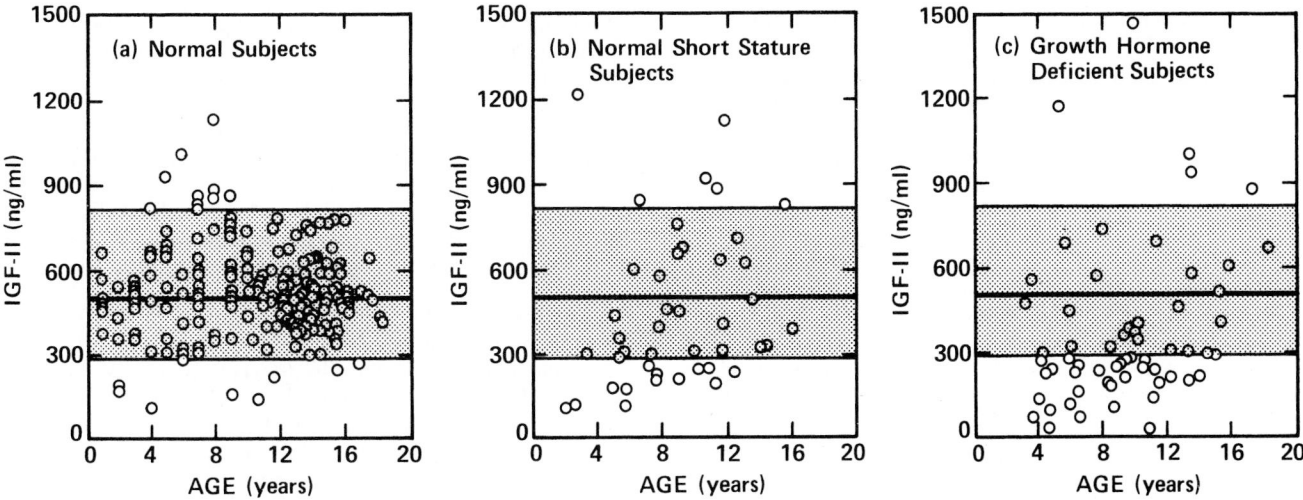

Figure 30–17. Serum IGF-II levels in the evaluation of growth disorders. (From Rosenfeld RG, Wilson DM, Lee PDK, et al. Insulin-like growth factors I and II in the evaluation of growth retardation. J Pediatr 1986; 109:428–433, with permission.)

for the type 1 IGF receptor[267] and chromosome 19 for the insulin receptor).

The type 1 IGF receptor gene spans greater than 100 kb of genomic DNA, with 21 exons; the genomic organization resembles that of the insulin receptor gene.[262, 268] Figure 30–19 depicts the structure of the type 1 IGF receptor precursor. Exons 1 to 3 code for the 5′-untranslated region, the signal peptide, the NH$_2$-terminal region, and the cysteine-rich domain of the α subunit involved in ligand binding. The remainder of the α subunit is encoded by exons 4 to 10. The peptide cleavage site involved in generation of the α- and β-subunits is encoded by exon 11, and the tyrosine kinase domain of the β subunit is encoded by exons 16 to 20. It is in the latter region that the type 1 IGF receptor and insulin receptor share the greatest sequence homology, ranging from 80 to 95%; interspecies homology in this region of the receptors is also high. Exon 21 encodes 3′-untranslated sequences.

Type 1 IGF receptor mRNA has been identified in virtually every tissue except liver.[269, 270] By Northern blot hybridization, human mRNA reveals two bands of 11 and 7 kb; rat tissues contain only the 11-kb band.[271] Type 1 IGF receptor mRNA is most abundant in embryonic tissues and appears to decrease with age. The type 1 IGF receptor is present at the embryonic eight-cell stage (the type 2 IGF receptor is first demonstrable at the two-cell stage) and becomes widely expressed after implantation, consistent with the observation that this receptor is essential for normal fetal growth.

As with other growth factor receptor tyrosine kinases, binding of ligand (IGF-I or IGF-II) induces receptor autophosphorylation of critical tyrosine residues in the type 1 receptor.[263–266] Mutations of the adenosine triphosphate–binding site or of critical tyrosine residues in the β subunit result in loss of IGF-stimulated thymidine incorporation and glucose uptake. Autophosphorylation appears to occur by transphosphorylation of sites on the opposite β subunit.[272, 273] The activated type 1 IGF receptor is capable of phosphorylating other tyrosine-containing substrates, such as IRS-1 (insulin receptor substrate 1), a 185-kd protein that is the predominant substrate of the insulin receptor kinase (Fig. 30–20).[274] IRS-1 contains specific phosphotyrosine motifs that can associate with proteins con-

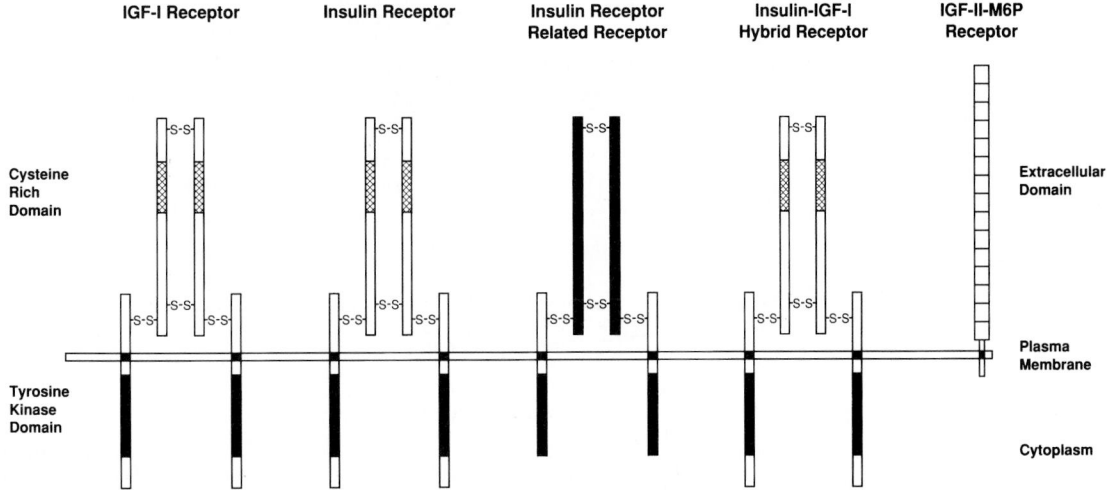

Figure 30–18. Structure of the IGF receptors. The insulin and IGF-I receptors are both heterotetrameric complexes composed of extracellular α subunits that bind the ligands and β subunits that anchor the receptor in the membrane and that contain tyrosine kinase activity in their cytoplasmic domains. The tyrosine kinase domain of the insulin receptor–related receptor is homologous to the tyrosine kinase domains of the insulin and IGF-I receptors. The C-terminal domain is deleted in the insulin receptor–related receptor. Hybrids consist of a hemireceptor from both insulin and IGF-I receptors. The IGF-II/mannose-6-phosphate receptor is not structurally related to the IGF-I and insulin receptors or the insulin receptor–related receptor, having a short cytoplasmic tail and no tyrosine kinase activity. (From LeRoith D, Werner H, Geitner-Johnson D, et al. Molecular and cellular aspects of the insulin-like growth factor I receptor. Endocr Rev 1995; 16:143–163. © The Endocrine Society)

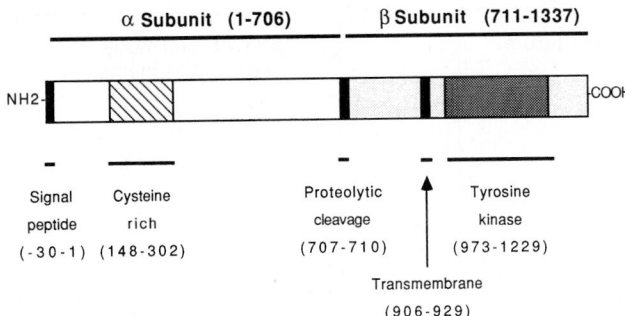

α Subunit (1-706)

Figure 30–19. Structure of the human IGF-I receptor precursor. Molecular cloning of human IGF-I receptor cDNAs isolated from a placental library revealed the presence of an open reading frame of 4101 nucleotides. The 1337-amino-acid polypeptide contains, at its N terminus, a 30-amino-acid hydrophobic signal peptide, which is responsible for the transfer of the nascent protein chain into the endoplasmic reticulum. After digestion by endopeptidases at a proteolytic cleavage site (Arg-Lys-Arg-Arg) located at residues 707 to 710, α and β subunits are released and linked by disulfide bonds to give the configuration of the mature heterotetrameric receptor. Shown in this diagrammatic representation are, in addition, the cysteine-rich domain of the α subunit and the transmembrane and tyrosine kinase domains of the β subunit. (From LeRoith D, Werner H, Beitner-Johnson D, et al. Molecular and cellular aspects of the insulin-like growth factor I receptor. Endocr Rev 1995; 16:143–164. © The Endocrine Society)

either the type 1 IGF or insulin receptor activates multiple signaling cascades that ultimately influence nuclear transcription and gene expression. It is presumably at this level that the IGF peptides exert their mitogenic and anabolic actions. Given that insulin and IGF peptides activate similar, if not identical, signaling pathways through their own specific receptors, it is unclear how the cell distinguishes between these overlapping ligands. Whether this merely reflects the relative levels of receptors or whether divergent downstream pathways exist for insulin and IGF action remain issues for future investigation.[281]

Interestingly, although targeted disruption of the gene for the type 1 IGF receptor causes fetal growth retardation, a clear role for this receptor in the cell cycle has not been established. Fibroblast cell lines derived from mouse embryos homozygous for the knockout gene still undergo cell cycle–dependent division, although at a slower rate.[282–284] Conversely, the transformed phenotype of some cells may be critically dependent on expression of the type 1 IGF receptor. The SV40TAg is capable of inducing a transformed phenotype in a cell only in the presence of intact type 1 IGF receptors.[284] NIH 3T3 cells and Rat-1 fibroblasts that are made to overexpress the type 1 IGF receptor develop IGF-I–dependent neoplastic transformation, with colony formation in soft agar and tumor formation in nude rats.[285] Prager and colleagues[286] have shown that truncation of the type 1 IGF receptor at the amino terminus increases transforming potential, suggesting that the α subunit normally restricts this function and that the binding of IGF to the receptor releases constraints on mitogenic stimulation.

Variants of both the α- and β-subunits are present in placenta,[287] muscle,[287, 288] and brain.[289] These variants may explain seemingly anomalous competitive binding studies.[290–292] The molecular mechanisms for the formation of such receptor

taining SH2 (src homology 2) domains, such as PI3-kinase (phosphatidylinositol-3 kinase),[275] Grb2 (growth factor receptor–bound protein 2),[276] Syp (a phosphotyrosine phosphatase),[275] and Nck (an oncogenic protein).[277] Activation of the type 1 IGF receptor also leads to tyrosine phosphorylation of Shc (src homology domain–containing protein),[278] which then associates with Grb2 and activates Ras, leading to a cascade of protein kinases, including Raf, MAP kinase kinases, MAP kinases, and S6 kinase.[279, 280] Thus phosphorylation of IRS-1 by

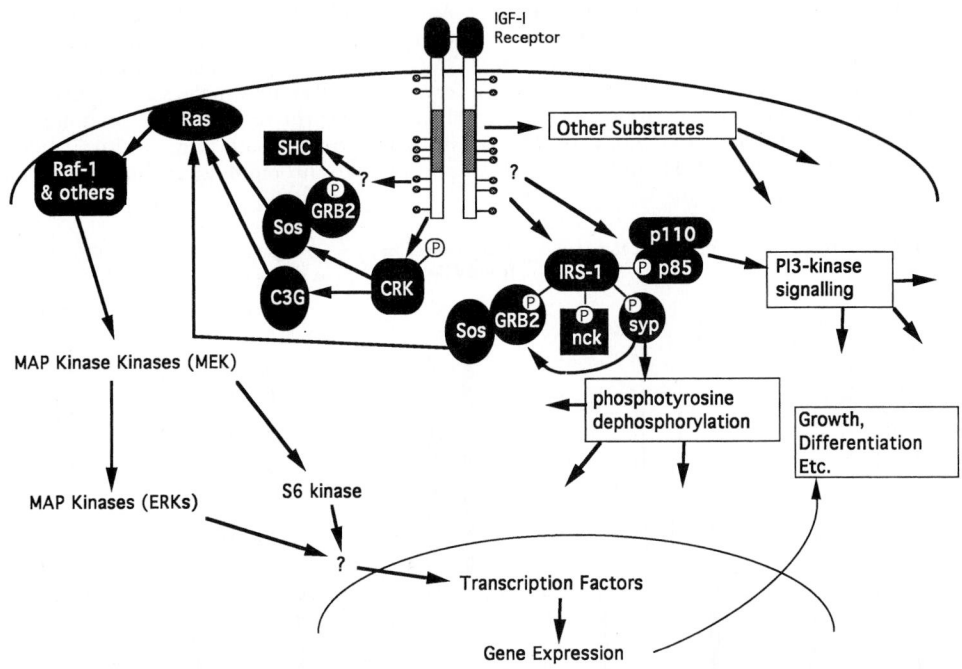

Figure 30–20. Schematic representation of intracellular signaling pathways of the IGF-I receptor. On binding IGF-I the IGF receptor undergoes autophosphorylation at multiple tyrosine residues. The intrinsic kinase activity of the receptor also phosphorylates IRS-1 at multiple tyrosine residues. Various SH domain–containing proteins, including PI3-kinase, Grb2, Syp, and Nck, associate with specific phosphotyrosine-containing motifs within IRS-1, as shown. Activation of the IGF-I receptors also results in tyrosine phosphorylation of the Shc, which then forms a complex with Grb2. Grb2 is tightly associated with the mammalian guanine nucleotide exchange factor Sos, which activates Ras. IGF-I can apparently activate Ras via both the IRS-1–Grb2-Sos or the Shc-Grb-Sos pathways. This leads to the activation of a cascade of protein kinases including Raf-1 and one or more related kinases, MAP kinase kinases (or MEKs), the MAP kinases (or ERKs), and S6 kinase. These protein kinases in turn activate various other elements, including nuclear transcription factors. Alterations in expression of various IGF-I–responsive genes results in longer term effects of IGF-I, including growth and differentiation. (From LeRoith D, Werner H, Beitner-Johnson D, et al. Molecular and cellular aspects of the insulin-like growth factor I receptor. Endocr Rev 1995; 16:143–163. © The Endocrine Society)

variants have not been identified, nor is it clear if they differentially bind IGF-I, IGF-II, or insulin. The formation of IGF-insulin receptor hybrids that contain an α-IGF hemireceptor disulfide linked to an α-insulin hemireceptor (see Fig. 30–18)[293–295] appears to be ligand-dependent,[296] and studies with monoclonal antibodies specific for the insulin or type 1 IGF receptor suggest that such receptors develop in cells with abundant native receptors, such as muscle and placenta.[297, 298] Such hybrids have near-normal affinity for IGF-I but decreased affinity for insulin. The physiological significance of such hybrid receptors is unknown.

The type 2 IGF receptor bears no structural homology to either the insulin or type 1 IGF receptors. It has an apparent molecular weight of 220,000 kd under nonreducing conditions and 250,000 kd after reduction, indicating that it is a monomeric protein. The cloned human type 2 receptor cDNA predicts a molecular mass of 270,294 kd and a lengthy extracellular domain containing 15 repeat sequences of 147 residues each, a 23-residue transmembrane domain, and a small cytoplasmic domain consisting of only 164 residues.[299] The receptor does not contain an intrinsic tyrosine kinase domain or any other recognized signal transduction mechanism. The type 2 IGF receptor is identical to the cation-independent mannose-6-phosphate receptor, a protein involved in the intracellular lysosomal targeting of acid hydrolases and other mannosylated proteins.[300, 301] Most of these receptors are located on intracellular membranes, in equilibrium with receptors on the plasma membrane.[302]

Why this receptor binds both IGF-II and mannose-6-phosphate–containing lysosomal enzymes is unknown. Unlike the type 1 IGF receptor, which binds both IGF peptides with high affinity and insulin with 100-fold lower affinity, the type 2 receptor binds only IGF-II with high affinity, the K_D ranging from 0.017 to 0.7 nM; IGF-I binds with lower affinity, and insulin does not bind at all.[302] One mole of IGF-II binds one mole of receptor. IGF-II and mannose-6-phosphate bind to different portions of the receptor, but the two ligands do show some reciprocal inhibitory effects on receptor binding, suggesting that IGF-II may affect the sorting of lysosomal enzymes. Alternatively this receptor may be important to the degradation of IGF-II. Knockout of the gene for the type 2 IGF receptor in mice causes macrosomia and fetal death.

The mitogenic and metabolic actions of both IGF-I and IGF-II appear to be mediated through the type 1 IGF receptor because monoclonal antibodies directed against the IGF-I–binding site on the type 1 IGF receptor inhibit the ability of both IGF-I and IGF-II to stimulate thymidine incorporation and cell replication.[303, 304] Similarly polyclonal antibodies that block IGF-II binding to the type 2 IGF/mannose-6-phosphate receptor do not block IGF-II actions.[305–307] In addition, IGF-II analogues with decreased affinity for the type 1 receptor but preserved affinity for the type 2 receptor are less potent than IGF-II in stimulating DNA synthesis,[181] and the mannose-6-phosphate receptor in hepatic tissues from chicken[308] or frog[309] does not bind IGF-II. Presumably the mitogenic actions of IGF-II in these species are mediated solely through the type 1 IGF receptor.

Nevertheless some IGF-II actions may be mediated via the type 2 IGF receptor. Rogers and Hammerman[310] have suggested that the type 2 receptor is involved in production of inositol triphosphate and diacylglycerol in proximal tubules and canine kidney membranes. Tally and co-workers[290] have reported that IGF-II stimulates the growth of a K562 human erythroleukemia cell line, an action not duplicated by either IGF-I or insulin. Minniti and colleagues[291] reported that IGF-II appears capable of acting as an autocrine growth factor and cell motility factor for human rhabdomyosarcoma cells, actions apparently mediated through the type 2 receptor, and IGF-II may activate a calcium-permeable cation channel via the

type 2 IGF receptor, perhaps through coupling to a pertussis toxin–sensitive guanine nucleotide–binding protein (G_i protein).[292, 296, 311–314] In cells transfected with the human type 2 IGF receptor cDNA, IGF-II decreased cAMP accumulation promoted by cholera toxin or forskolin. Mutations or truncation of the small cytoplasmic domain of the receptor prevented these IGF-II actions.

Insulin-Like Growth Factor–Binding Proteins

In contrast to insulin the IGFs circulate in plasma in complex with a family of binding proteins (Fig. 30–21) that extend the serum half-life of the IGF peptides, transport the IGFs to target cells, and modulate the interaction of the IGFs with surface membrane receptors.[315–318] The identification and characterization of IGFBPs in body fluids[319] and in conditioned media from cultured cells has been facilitated by the development of a number of biochemical and assay techniques, including gel chromatography, radioreceptor assays, affinity cross-linking, Western ligand blotting,[320] immunoblotting, and specific radioimmunoassays. However, study of the molecular biologic characteristics of the IGFBPs has provided the most information concerning their structural interrelationship.

INSULIN-LIKE GROWTH FACTOR–BINDING PROTEIN STRUCTURE

To date, the cDNAs for six distinct human and rat IGFBPs have been cloned and sequenced[316, 317, 321]; another potential member of the IGFBP family is mac25, a protein whose cDNA was cloned from human meningioma cells and that has 40 to 45% homology with IGFBPs 1 to 6 at the amino acid level.[322] The ability of a mac25 protein to bind IGF has not, however, been demonstrated. Their structural characteristics are summarized in Table 30–2 and Figure 30–22. The amino acid sequences of the six cloned mammalian IGFBPs (and mac25) are highly conserved. Within a species the IGFBPs share an overall amino acid sequence homology on the order of 50%, and between species there is more than 80% sequence homology for individual IGFBPs. Perhaps the most impressive similarity in structure is the conservation of the number and placement of the cysteine residues. The total number of cysteines varies from 16 to 20 (18 cysteines are conserved in human IGFBPs 1 to 5; IGFBP-6 conserves 16 of the 18, and IGFBP-4 has 2 additional cysteines in the middle region of the protein), and each of the IGFBPs has cysteine-rich regions at the amino and carboxyl termini. Conservation of the spatial order of the

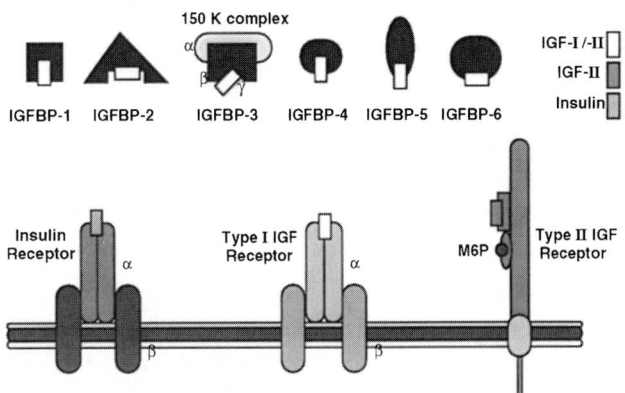

Figure 30–21. Schematic representation of the IGF axis, including IGF ligands, receptors, and binding proteins. (From Cohen P, Fielder PJ, Hasegawa Y, et al. Clinical aspects of insulin-like growth factor binding proteins. Acta Endocrinol 1991; 124[Suppl 2]:74–85, with permission.)

TABLE 30–2. Insulin-Like Growth Factor–Binding Proteins

Insulin-Like Growth Factor Binding Protein (IGFBP)	Molecular Weight (kd)	No. of Amino Acids	No. of Cysteines	RGD Sequence	Glycosyl Sites	mRNA Size (kb)
IGFPB-1	29,600	234	18	+	0	1.6
IGFBP-2	31,300	289	18	+	0	1.5
IGFBP-3	28,500	264	18	−	3	2.4
IGFBP-4	25,974	237	20	−	1	1.7
IGFBP-5	28,572	252	18	−	0	?
IGFBP-6	22,862	216	16	−	0	1.1

cysteines presumably indicates that the secondary structure of the IGFBPs, which is dependent on disulfide bonding, must also be conserved. Disulfide bonding is essential for formation of the IGF-binding site of each IGFBP; reduction of the disulfide proteins results in loss of IGF binding. Conversely, the middle region of the IGFBPs is not well conserved, containing N-glycosylation sites for IGFBP-3 and IGFBP-4, and two additional cysteine residues in IGFBP-4. Some of the more specialized properties of the IGFBPs, such as cell association, IGF enhancement, and IGF-independent actions (see later) may be dependent on specific sequences in these midregions.

An RGD (arginine-glycine-aspartic acid) sequence near the carboxyl terminus of IGFBP-1 and IGFBP-2[323] is the minimal sequence required for the binding of many extracellular matrix proteins to membrane receptors of the integrin protein family, and IGFBPs may associate with the cell surface through such amino acid sequences.[324] However, IGFBP-3, which lacks an RGD sequence, also binds to cell membranes,[325, 326] possibly to specific receptors[327] (see later).

Under most conditions the IGFBPs appear to inhibit IGF action, presumably by competing with IGF receptors for binding IGF peptides.[328] For example, IGF analogues with decreased affinity for IGFBPs have increased biologic potency.[329–331] In studies involving transfection of the human *IGFBP-3* gene into fibroblasts, increased expression of *IGFBP-3* inhibited cell growth, even in the absence of added IGF, suggesting a direct inhibitory role of the binding protein.[332] Under some conditions, however, the IGFBPs appear to enhance IGF action, perhaps by facilitating the delivery of IGF to target receptors[333] (see later).

Analysis of IGFBPs is further complicated by the presence of IGFBP proteases, which degrade IGFBP.[334, 335] Initially reported in the serum of pregnant women,[334, 335] proteases for

IGFBP-2, 3, 4, and 5 are present in serum, seminal plasma,[336] cerebrospinal fluid,[337] and urine.[338] It is likely that multiple IGFBP proteases exist, including calcium-dependent serine proteases, kallikreins, cathepsins,[339] and matrix metalloproteases.[340] Proteolysis of IGFBPs complicates their assay and must be taken into consideration when measuring the various IGFBPs in biologic fluids.[341] The physiological significance of limited proteolysis of IGFBPs remains to be determined, although protease activity usually decreases the affinity of the IGFBP for IGF peptides (Fig. 30–23) and may enhance the mitogenic and anabolic effects of IGF peptides in this way. In prostate epithelial cells[342–344] prostate specific antigen acts as a potent IGFBP-3 protease (Figs. 30–24 and 30–25), and in rat granulosa cells[345] follicle-stimulating hormone induces an IGFBP-5 protease.

INSULIN-LIKE GROWTH FACTOR–BINDING PROTEINS AS CARRIER PROTEINS

Given the high affinity of the IGFBPs for IGF-I and IGF-II (K_d 10 to 100 fM), virtually all IGF-I and IGF-II in serum are in complex with IGFBPs.[346] In normal adult serum 75 to 80% of the IGF peptides is carried in a ternary complex consisting of one molecule of IGF plus one molecule of IGFBP-3 plus one molecule of an 88-kd protein termed the acid-labile subunit (ALS).[347, 348] Binding of the ALS to form the full ternary complex occurs after the binding of IGF by IGFBP-3, although the ALS may bind to IGFBP-3 even in the absence of IGF.[349] The 150-kd ternary complex is too large to leave the vascular compartment and extends the half-life of IGF peptides from approximately 10 min for IGF alone to 1 to 2 h for IGF in the IGF-I–IGFBP-3 binary complex to 12 to 15 h for IGF in the ternary complex.[350] The fact that both

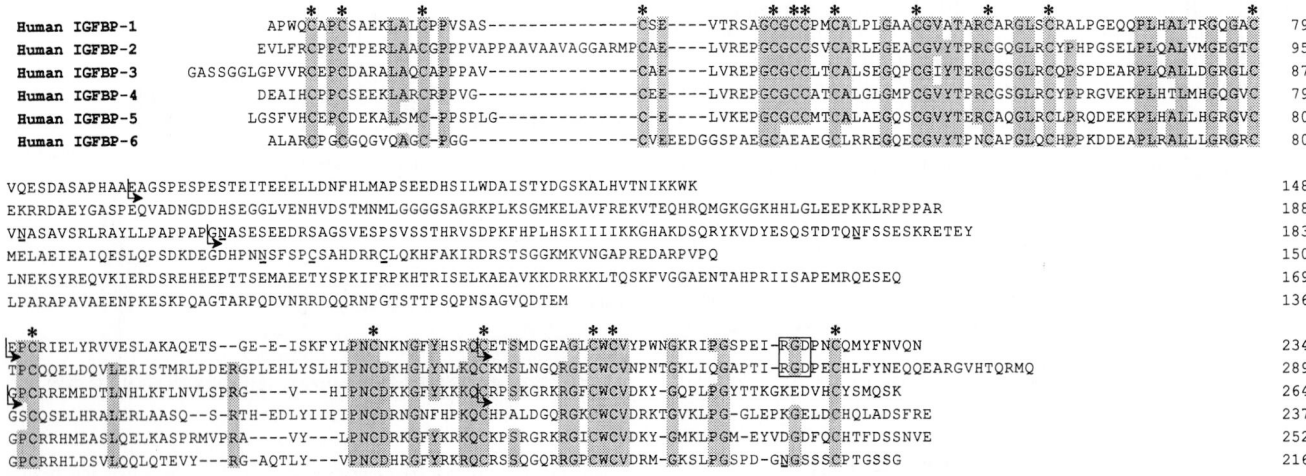

Figure 30–22. Amino acid sequences of human IGFBP-1 to -6, deduced from nucleotide sequences. Sequences in the amino terminal and carboxy terminal residues are aligned to show maximal homologies. Dashes indicate gaps. Residues that are identical in five or six of the six IGFBPs are shaded. (From Rechler MM. Insulin-like growth factor binding proteins. Vitam Horm 1993; 47:114, with permission.)

Theoretical mechanism of the actions of IGFBP proteases

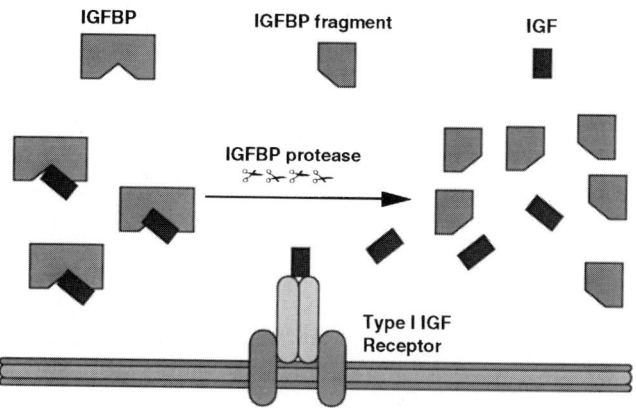

Figure 30–23. Schematic representation of the effect of IGFBP proteases on IGF action. In this model proteolysis of IGFBPs results in a reduction in their affinity for IGF ligands, resulting in enhanced binding of IGF peptides by IGF receptor. (Adapted from Shiverick K, Rosenbloom A, eds. Human Growth Hormone Pharmacology: Basic and Clinical Aspects. Boca Raton, FL: CRC Press, 1995:48.)

GH administration to GH-deficient patients shifts IGF from the 40- to 50-kd low-molecular-weight peak to the 150-kd high-molecular-weight peak,[356, 357] a similar phenomenon is not observed following IGF-I treatment.[356]

IGF peptides in the 40- to 50-kd molecular weight peak may not be restricted to the vascular compartment. IGFBP-1, 2, and 4, at least, can probably cross endothelial barriers.[358] In the fetus and neonate, in whom IGFBP-3 levels are relatively low, and in GH deficiency and GH resistance, binding of IGFs by IGFBP-1, -2, -4, and -5 may predominate over binding to IGFBP-3.[250, 356, 359] Similarly, in tumor-induced hypoglycemia associated with increased serum levels of IGF-II, ternary complex formation may be decreased, and most IGF peptides are found in the low-molecular-weight peak.

INSULIN-LIKE GROWTH FACTOR–BINDING PROTEINS AS MODULATORS OF INSULIN-LIKE GROWTH FACTOR ACTION

In general the binding affinity of IGFBPs for IGF peptides is higher than that of IGF receptors, implying that IGFBPs can modulate IGF binding to its receptors, thereby modulating IGF biologic actions (Fig. 30–26).[346] Coincubation of cells with IGF-I and a molar excess of IGFBP-3 results in an inhibition of IGF-I–stimulated thymidine incorporation in human fibroblasts, lipogenesis in rat epididymal adipocytes,[360] and glucose consumption in mouse fibroblasts.[361] Termination of inhibition apparently requires dissociation of IGFs from the IGF-I–IGFBP complex by mass action, proteolysis, or other mechanisms. IGFBP proteases have been identified in a wide variety of body fluids and cell culture media[339, 340, 342, 343, 345] and are postulated to play a role in altering IGF availability by lowering the affinities of IGFBPs for their ligand, thereby increasing the availability of IGFs to cell membrane receptors[344, 362] (see earlier).

Under certain conditions the IGFBPs potentiate IGF ac-

IGFBP-3 and ALS are GH-dependent provides an additional mechanism for GH regulation of the IGF axis. Although IGF-I administration to hypophysectomized rats increases serum levels of IGFBP-3,[351–353] no sustained increase in serum levels of IGFBP-3 occurs in humans following administration of IGF-I.[96, 354] ALS levels may even decline after IGF-I administration, presumably reflecting IGF feedback inhibition of pituitary GH secretion.[354, 355] Thus in serum of patients with GH deficiency or GH resistance, little IGF is present in the 150-kd ternary complex, most being found in the lower molecular weight IGF-I–IGFBP-3 complex or bound by other IGFBPs. Although

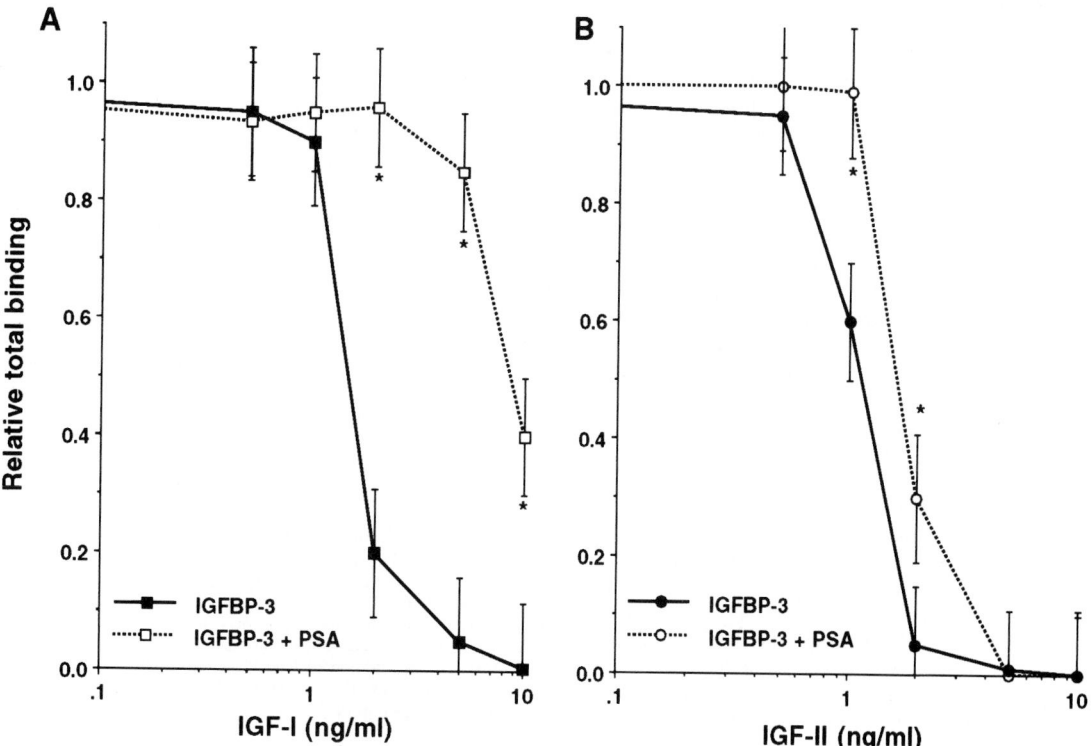

Figure 30–24. The effect of IGFBP-3 proteolysis by prostate-specific antigen (PSA) on IGFBP-3 affinity for IGF-I (A) and IGF-II (B). (From Cohen P, Peehl DM, Graves HC, et al. Biological effects of prostate-specific antigen as an insulin-like growth factor binding protein-3 protease. J Endocrinol 1994; 142:407–415, with permission.)

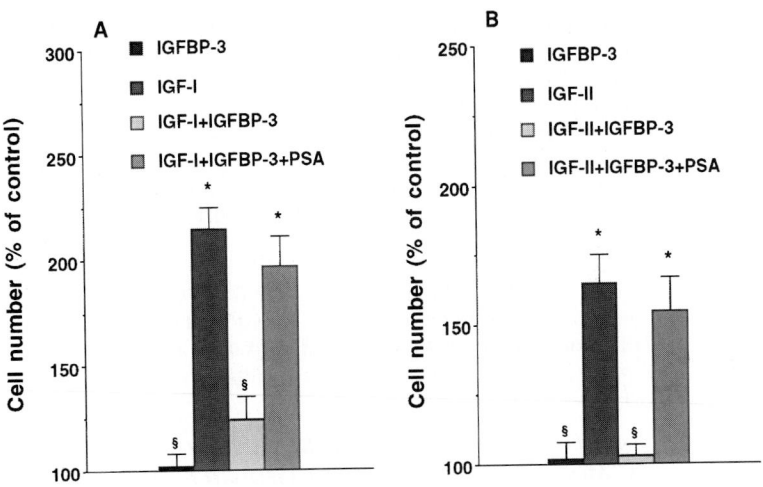

Figure 30–25. The effect of IGFBP-3 proteolysis by prostate-specific antigen (PSA) on the ability of IGFBP-3 to inhibit IGF-I *(A)* and IGF-II *(B)* action. (From Cohen P, Peehl DM, Graves HC, et al. Biological effects of prostate-specific antigen as an insulin-like growth factor binding protein-3 protease. J Endocrinol 1994; 142:407–415, with permission.)

tion. In human and bovine fibroblasts, DNA synthesis and α-aminoisobutyric acid transport are potentiated when cells are preincubated with IGFBP-3, whereas IGFBP-3 is inhibitory if added at the same time as IGF-I.[363, 364] These observations have suggested that cell association of IGFBP-3 during preincubation is essential for its IGF-potentiating effect, perhaps allowing IGFBP-3 to serve as a reservoir for IGFs and bringing the ligand into closer proximity to the type 1 IGF receptors. This cell surface association of IGFBP-3 may involve interaction with heparin and heparin sulfate proteoglycans on the cell membrane or specific IGFBP-3 receptors.[327]

INSULIN-LIKE GROWTH FACTOR–INDEPENDENT ACTIONS OF INSULIN-LIKE GROWTH FACTOR–BINDING PROTEINS

IGFBP-3 itself appears to have intrinsic inhibitory effects on cells, independent of its interaction with IGF. Villaudy and co-workers[365] found that the stimulation of DNA synthesis by basic IGF is inhibited by simultaneous treatment with IGFBP-3, even in the presence of levels of insulin, suggesting that sequestration of IGF peptides from type 1 IGF receptors is not the only means whereby IGFBP-3 inhibits cell growth. IGFBP-3 is also more effective than immunoneutralization of IGF-I in inhibiting serum-stimulated DNA synthesis, and IGFBP-3 inhibits follicle-stimulating hormone–stimulated DNA synthesis in cultured ovarian granulosa cells, with or without added IGF.[366] Under the same conditions IGFBP-2 is less inhibitory, despite its higher affinity for IGF peptides. Expression of a transfected human IGFBP-3 cDNA in mouse fibroblasts inhibits both IGF-stimulated and insulin-stimulated cell proliferation (Fig. 30–27).[332] Similar studies in fibroblasts derived from mouse embryos homozygous for a targeted disruption of the type 1 IGF receptor again demonstrated inhibition with overexpression of IGFBP-3.[367] These studies strongly support an IGF-independent action for IGFBP-3 (Fig. 30–28).

IGFBP-3 binds with high affinity to the surface of various cell types, including human breast cancer cells, and inhibits monolayer growth of these cells in an IGF-independent manner (Fig. 30–29).[327, 368] Furthermore transcriptional regulation of *IGFBP-3* expression may be the mechanism for the inhibition of breast cancer cell growth by both TGF-β₂ and retinoic acid (Fig. 30–30).[369–372] Reduction of IGFBP-3 production through the use of IGFBP-3 antisense oligodeoxynucleotides decreases the inhibitory effects of both TGF-β₂ and retinoic acid, suggesting that IGFBP-3 production may be a common pathway for multiple hormones and growth factors involved in the modulation of cell growth.[369] For example, estrogen inhibits expression and secretion of IGFBP-3, whereas anties-

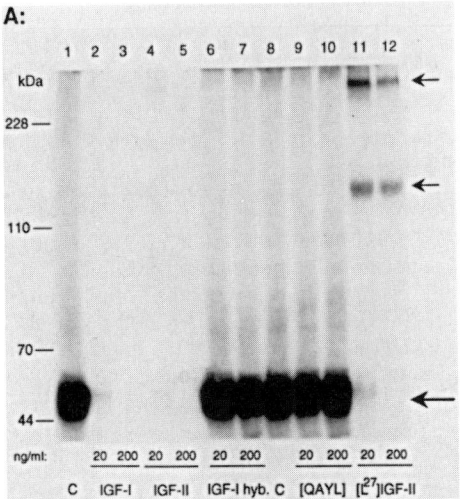

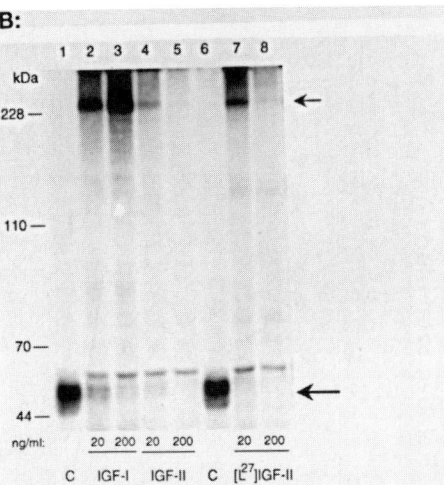

Figure 30–26. Affinity cross-linking of [125I]IGF-I *(A)* and [125I]IGF-II *(B)* to membranes from Hs578T breast cancer cells. In the absence of unlabeled IGF peptide (1), IGF was predominantly bound to 40- to 45-kd IGFBP-3; no type 1 or type 2 IGF receptors were observed. Iodinated IGF was readily displaceable by unlabeled IGF-I or IGF-II (2 to 5), but not by unlabeled IGF-I/insulin hybrid molecule (6 to 7) or by an IGF analogue with decreased affinity for IGFBPs (QAYL; 9 to 10 in *A*). However addition of [Leu²⁷] IGF-II, which has decreased affinity for the type 1 IGF receptor (11 to 12 in *A* and 7 to 8 in *B*, resulted in "unmasking" of the 130-kd α subunit of the type 1 IGF receptor *(A)* and the 250-kd type 2 IGF receptor. (From Oh Y, Muller HL, Lamson G, et al. Insulin-like growth factor (IGF)-independent action of IGF-binding protein-3 in hs578T human breast cancer cells: cell surface binding and growth inhibition. J Biol Chem 1993; 268:14964–14971, with permission.)

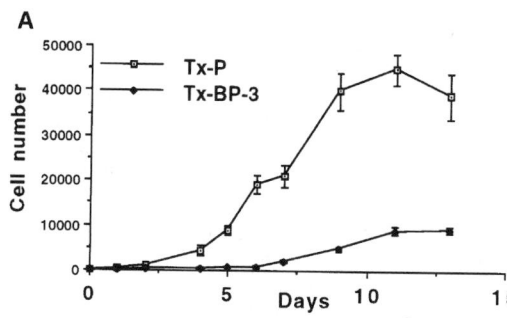 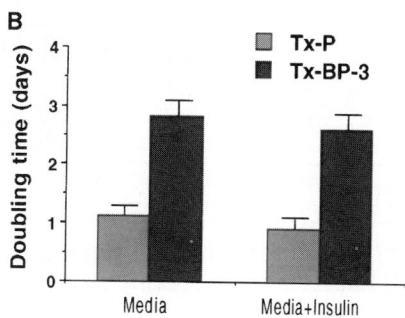

Figure 30–27. Effect of transfection of Balb/c fibroblasts with a human IGFBP-3 cDNA (Tx-BP-3) or with the control plasmid (Tx-P) on cell growth. Transfection with the IGFBP-3 cDNA resulted in a decreased cell proliferation *(A)* and increased cell doubling time *(B)*. The latter effect could not be overcome with insulin, supporting the concept that the inhibitory effects of IGFBP-3 are IGF-independent. (From Cohen P, Lamson G, Okajima T, et al. Transfection of the human insulin-like growth factor binding protein-3 gene into Balb/c fibroblasts inhibits cellular growth. Mol Endocrinol 1993; 7:380–386. © The Endocrine Society.)

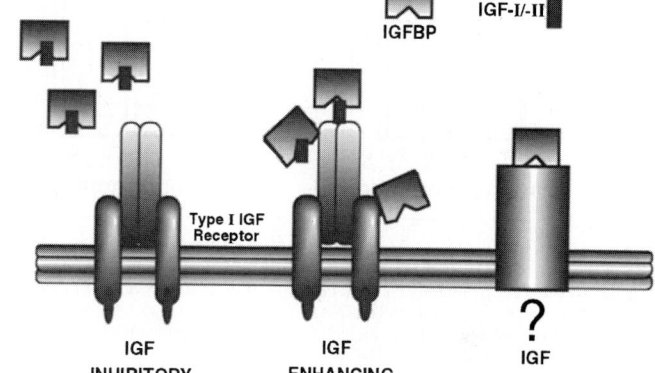

Figure 30–28. Theoretical mechanisms of cellular IGFBP actions.

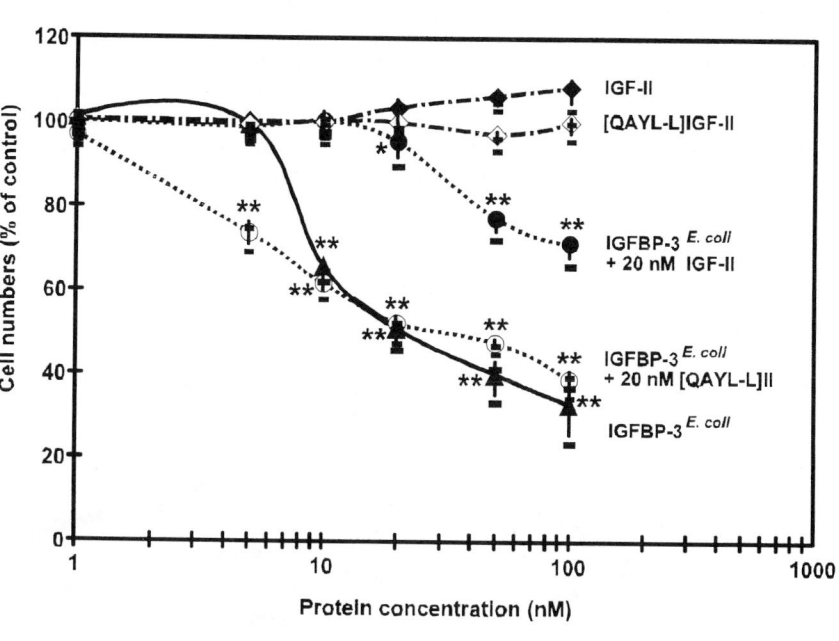

Figure 30–29. Inhibition of Hs578T breast cancer cell growth by IGFBP-3 is IGF-independent. Recombinant IGFBP-3 from *Escherichia coli* results in decreased cell number and cannot be overcome by the addition of an IGF analogue with normal affinity for IGF receptors but decreased affinity for IGFBP-3 (QUAY-L-Leu-IGF-II). Conversely IGF-II, which itself does not stimulate cell proliferation in Hs578T cells, partially releases cells from the growth inhibitory effects of IGFBP-3, presumably by causing dissociation of IGFBP-3 from the cell membrane. (From Oh Y, Muller HL, Lamson G, et al. Insulin-like growth factor (IGF)-independent action of IGF binding protein-3 in Hs578T human breast cancer cells. J Biol Chem 1993; 268:14964–14971, with permission.)

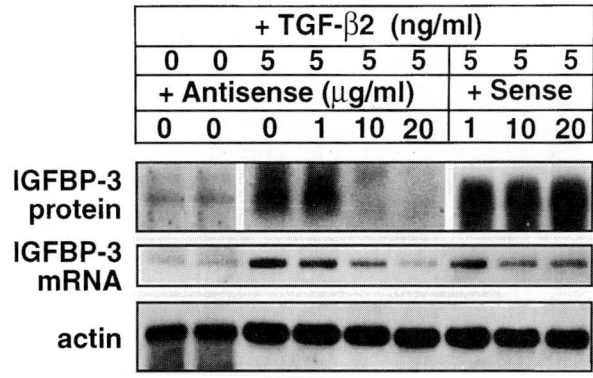

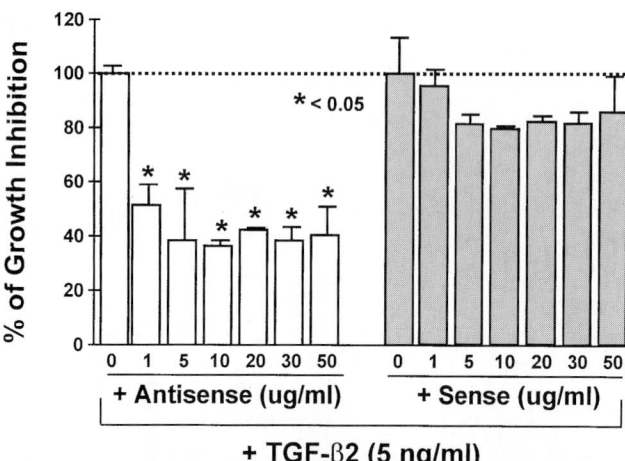

Figure 30–30. TGF β_2 inhibits Hs578T cell growth by transcriptional regulation of IGFBP-3. Reduction in IGFBP-3 mRNA and protein levels through the use of an IGFBP-3 antisense oligodeoxynucleotide resulted in significant reduction in the growth inhibitory actions of TGF β_2. (From Oh Y, Muller HL, Ng L, et al. TGF-β_2–induced cell growth inhibition in human breast cancer cells is mediated through IGFBP-3 action. J Biol Chem 1995; 270:13589–13592, with permission.)

trogens stimulate production of IGFBP-3 in estrogen receptor–positive human breast cancer cells.[373] Similarly the mitogenic action of epidermal growth factor in human cervical epithelial cells is associated with inhibition of *IGFBP-3* expression, and the inhibitory effect of retinoic acid is accompanied by increased *IGFBP-3* expression.[374] Regulation of *IGFBP-3* gene expression plays a role in signaling by p53, a potent tumor suppressor protein.[375]

The presence of cell membrane proteins or receptors that specifically bind IGFBP-3 provides a potential mechanism for IGF-independent growth inhibitory actions of IGFBP-3 (Fig. 30–31).[327] IGFBP-3 may inhibit cell growth both by sequestering IGF ligands (IGF-dependent action of IGFBP-3) and also by binding to the cell surface (IGF-independent action of IGFBP-3). IGFBP-3 proteases not only may degrade intact IGFBP-3 to forms with lower affinities for IGFs but also may generate IGFBP-3 fragments with enhanced affinity for cell surface IGFBP-3–interacting proteins or receptors. A proteolytic fragment of IGFBP-3 that fails to bind IGFs still retains its ability to inhibit cell proliferation.[376]

CHARACTERISTICS OF INSULIN-LIKE GROWTH FACTOR–BINDING PROTEINS 1 TO 6

Insulin-Like Growth Factor–Binding Protein-1

IGFBP-1 was the first of the IGFBPs to be purified and to have its cDNA cloned.[377] The protein was actually identified

and purified from several different tissues, including amniotic fluid[378] and Hep G2–conditioned media,[379] placental membranes (placental protein 12),[380] and endometrium (pregnancy-associated α_1-globulin).[381] Its gene is 5.2 kb long, located on the short arm of chromosome 7, and composed of four exons.[382] The mature protein is 30 kd and is nonglycosylated. mRNA for IGFBP-1 is strongly expressed in decidua (although not in placental trophoblasts), liver, and kidney.

IGFBP-1 may be involved in reproductive functions, including endometrial cycling,[383] oocyte maturation,[384] and fetal growth.[359, 385] It is the major IGFBP in fetal serum in early gestation, reaching levels as high as 3000 $\mu g/L$ by the second trimester. Levels of IGFBP-1 in newborn serum are inversely correlated with birth weight, which is consistent with an inhibitory role on fetal IGF action.

IGFBP-1 also appears to have an important metabolic role because its gene expression is enhanced in catabolic states,[250, 386, 387] and serum levels undergo diurnal variation.[388] Insulin suppresses and glucocorticoids enhance IGFBP-1 mRNA levels.[386, 389] The acute modulation of serum IGFBP-1 levels may regulate the free fraction of circulating IGF peptides.[386, 388] For example, administration of IGFBP-1 transiently reduces the glucose-lowering capability of IGF-I in rats.[390]

Although most in vitro studies are consistent with an inhibitory effect of IGFBP-1 on IGF actions, presumably reflecting interference with IGF ligand receptor interactions,[318] IGFBP-1 potentiates IGF effects in certain cell systems,[391] possibly as the result of the binding of IGFBP-1 to cell membranes through its Arg-Gly-Asp (RGD) sequence; RGD is an integrin receptor recognition sequence that presumably allows IGFBP-1 to associate with the $\alpha_5\beta_1$ integrin (fibronectin) receptor.[324] The ability of IGFBP-1 to inhibit or potentiate IGF action may depend on post-translational modifications of IGFBP-1, such as phosphorylation, which appears to enhance IGFBP-1 affinity for IGF-I and thereby inhibit IGF action.[392]

Insulin-Like Growth Factor–Binding Protein-2

The *IGFBP-2* gene is located on the long arm of chromosome 2.[393, 394] A single 1.6-kb mRNA yields a mature protein of approximately 34 kd. Like *IGFBP-1*, *IGFBP-2* is highly expressed in fetal tissues, particularly in the CNS.[395] IGFBP-2 is also similar to IGFBP-1 in its lack of *N*-glycosylation and in the presence of an RGD sequence, perhaps allowing cell association and potentiation of IGF action.[396] Nevertheless knockout of the *IGFBP-2* gene[397] or overexpression of *IGFBP-1* in transgenic mice[398] appears to have little effect on phenotype, possibly reflecting "redundancy" in the IGFBP system, in which one IGFBP can compensate for loss of another.

The existence of a low-molecular-weight IGFBP in cere-

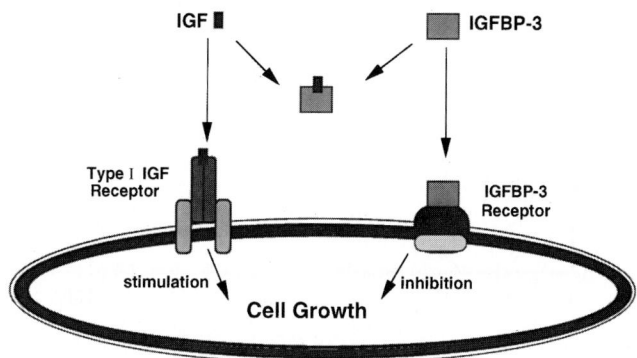

Figure 30–31. Schematic diagram of IGF-dependent and IGF-independent actions of IGFBP-3, the latter being mediated through a putative membrane-associated IGFBP-3 receptor.

brospinal fluid was inferred from studies demonstrating a 34-kd IGFBP that did not react with antibodies to IGFBP-1 (or IGFBP-3).[399] This IGFBP appeared to be consistent with a previous observation of CSF IGFBPs with preferential affinity for IGF-II.[400]

IGFBP-2 is expressed in secretory endometrium and endometrial tumors[383] and is the major IGFBP in seminal fluid and in the conditioned media of prostatic epithelial cells.[401] Interestingly *IGFBP-2* gene expression is markedly reduced in prostatic stromal cells from patients with benign prostatic hyperplasia, suggesting that IGFBP-2 may inhibit stromal growth.[402] Serum levels of IGFBP-2 are frequently elevated in patients with prostatic carcinoma.[403]

Insulin-Like Growth Factor–Binding Protein-3

The *IGFBP-3* gene is located on chromosome 7 in proximity to the gene for IGFBP-1.[404] It contains four exons homologous to those of IGFBP-1 and 2 and a fifth exon, consisting of 3'-untranslated sequences. In all human tissues studied to date, a single 2.6-kb mRNA has been observed, whereas an additional 1.7-kb mRNA species suggests alternative splicing in baboons.[405] mRNA levels are high in liver, but IGFBP-3 appears to be synthesized in hepatic endothelia (portal venous and sinusoidal) and Kupffer's cells, whereas ALS is synthesized in hepatocytes.[406, 407]

IGFBP-3 is GH-dependent because of either a direct GH effect or regulation by IGF. IGF-I administration to hypophysectomized rats increases serum levels of IGFBP-3.[351–353] Conversely, IGF-I treatment of patients with GH resistance does not alter serum IGFBP-3 levels,[96, 324, 339] whereas GH treatment of GH-deficient patients does increase serum levels. Whether these observations mean that GH has a direct effect on IGFBP-3 or reflect GH regulation of ALS and ternary complex formation is unclear.

The mature IGFBP-3 protein has a molecular weight of approximately 29 kd, but because it is *N*-glycosylated, it normally migrates as a doublet-triplet of 40 to 46 kd. Glycosylation does not appear to alter its affinity for IGF-I or IGF-II.[408] IGFBP-3 also undergoes serine phosphorylation, although its physiological significance is uncertain.[409] Perhaps the most significant post-translational modification of IGFBP-3 is proteolysis (see earlier). Discrepancies between immunoblot analyses and radioimmunoassays for IGFBP-3 reflect the altered affinity of IGFBP-3 fragments for IGF ligands, although some proteolytic fragments of IGFBP-3 are capable of ternary complex formation.[341] In pregnancy serum the predominant form of IGFBP-3 is a glycosylated 29-kd fragment. A similar-sized IGFBP-3 fragment is present in serum from postsurgical patients or those who are catabolic[410] and from patients with non–insulin-dependent diabetes mellitus.[411]

IGFBP-3 is the predominant IGFBP in adult serum, in which it carries approximately 75% of the total IGF, primarily as part of the 150-kd ternary complex. Serum levels are reduced in patients with GH deficiency or GH resistance, conditions in which assays for serum IGFBP-3 have important diagnostic value (see later).

IGFBP-3 associates with cell membranes. Affinity cross-linking studies employing [^{125}I]IGF-I and a human breast cancer cell line have demonstrated no binding to the type 1 IGF receptor but rather to membrane-associated 45-kd IGFBP-3 (see Fig. 30–26). When IGF analogues with selective affinity for IGFBPs were added, a typical 135-kd α subunit of the type 1 IGF receptor was uncovered, demonstrating that membrane-associated IGFBP-3, with its high affinity for IGF peptides, normally "masks" the IGF receptors. Oh and colleagues[369] demonstrated that the binding of IGFBP-3 to cell membrane proteins was specific, cation-dependent, and of high affinity. Whether these proteins constitute genuine "IGFBP-3 recep-

tors" remains to be demonstrated, although they may mediate IGF-independent actions of IGFBP-3. Alternatively IGFBP-3 may associate with heparin-containing proteoglycans both in the extracellular matrix and in the cell membrane, since both IGFBP-3 and IGFBP-5 contain heparin-binding consensus sequences in their COOH termini.[412] However, treatment of cell monolayers with heparinase or chondroitinase has only minor effect on IGFBP-3 binding.

Like other IGFBPs, IGFBP-3 inhibits IGF action, especially when the binding protein is present in excess. Presumably inhibition of IGF action by IGFBP-3 reflects a sequestering of IGF peptides away from the type 1 receptor. Proteolysis of IGFBP-3, resulting in a decrease in affinity for IGF ligands, decreases the inhibitory effects of the binding protein.

Insulin-Like Growth Factor–Binding Protein-4

The *IGFBP-4* gene, located on chromosome 17, contains four exons.[413] A single 2.6-kb mRNA has been identified with high expression in liver. The protein is the smallest of the IGFBPs, with 237 amino acids in humans including 20 cysteines and one *N*-linked glycosylation site. In immunoblots of most biologic fluids, IGFBP-4 is a 24/28-kd doublet; deglycosylation eliminates the 28-kd band.[414] IGFBP-4 appears to interact with connective tissues,[415] but there is no evidence of membrane association, which is consistent with a primary role for IGFBP-4 as a soluble extracellular IGFBP.

IGFBP-4 was initially isolated on the basis of its ability to inhibit IGF-stimulated cell proliferation in bone,[416] and there is no evidence for any IGF-potentiating effects. The inhibitory effects of IGFBP-4 are reduced by proteolysis of the protein, much as has been observed with IGFBP-3 degradation. IGFBP-4 proteases are produced by a wide variety of cells, including neuroblastoma,[417] smooth muscle,[418] fibroblasts,[419] osteoblasts[420] and prostatic epithelium.[421] Activation of IGFBP-4 proteolysis occurs in the presence of IGF-I or IGF-II, presumably reflecting a conformational change in IGFBP-4 resulting from IGF occupancy.[422, 423]

Insulin-Like Growth Factor–Binding Protein-5

cDNAs for IGFBP-5 have been isolated and sequenced from rat ovary and human placenta and from a human osteosarcoma.[321, 424] The gene is located on chromosome 5 and contains four exons. A single 6-kb mRNA is expressed in a wide variety of tissues, particularly in kidney. Mature IGFBP-5 is produced as a 252-amino-acid protein with no *N*-linked glycosylation sites but with one *O*-linked glycosylation site.[425]

The addition of excess IGFBP-5 to human osteosarcoma cells inhibits IGF-I-stimulated DNA and glycogen synthesis.[426] However, when IGFBP-5 adheres to fibroblast extracellular matrix, it potentiates the growth stimulatory effects of IGF on DNA synthesis.[427] The affinity of IGFBP-5 for IGF-I is reduced approximately sevenfold when the binding protein is associated with extracellular matrix, providing a potential mechanism for release of IGFs to cell surface receptors. Association of IGFBP-5 with extracellular matrix also appears to protect it from proteolysis.[428] Addition of IGFBP-5 to conditioned medium from fibroblasts results in proteolysis to a 21-kd fragment that does not potentiate IGF action, whereas the deposition of IGFBP-5 in extracellular matrix of fibroblasts makes it relatively resistant to degradation. Andress and Birnbaum[429] have purified a 23-kd IGFBP-5 fragment from U-2 osteosarcoma cells that has reduced affinity for IGFs but enhances IGF-I-stimulated mitogenesis. The 23-kd IGFBP-5 fragment stimulates mitogenesis in an IGF-independent manner, presumably by binding to a specific "receptor" on the cell membrane.

Unlike proteolysis of IGFBP-4, which is enhanced by addition of IGFs, degradation of IGFBP-5 is inhibited by the binding of IGF peptides.[35, 345, 425] Proteolysis of IGFBP-5 results in the formation of 16- to 23-kd fragments demonstrated on immunoblots. Degradation of IGFBP-5 may have particular importance in the regulation of granulosa cell activity. In healthy ovarian follicles neither IGFBP-4 nor IGFBP-5 is expressed, whereas both binding proteins are expressed in atretic follicles, thereby providing a mechanism for intrafollicular regulation of IGF action.[430, 431] Furthermore follicle-stimulating hormone enhances IGF action in the ovary and stimulates IGFBP-5 proteolysis.[345]

IGFBP-5 and IGFBP-4 also appear to be major IGFBPs in bone where, in addition to inhibiting IGF actions, IGFBP-5 may promote IGF-receptor interactions. Thus depending on the conditions, IGFBP-5 can either inhibit or potentiate IGF actions.

Insulin-Like Growth Factor–Binding Protein-6

The human *IGFBP-6* gene is located on chromosome 12 and contains four exons. *IGFBP-6* transcripts include a major 1.3-kb mRNA and a minor 2.2-kb transcript.[432] The mature peptide contains 216 amino acids and has a molecular weight of approximately 23 kd, although it may migrate at a higher molecular weight on sodium dodecyl sulfate gels, presumably reflecting *O*-glycosylation.[433] Although IGFBP-6 binds both IGF-I and IGF-II, it has a significantly greater affinity for IGF-II.[434] IGFBP-6 is found in relatively high levels in cerebrospinal fluid, as is also the case for IGFBP-2, which also binds IGF-II with selectively high affinity. IGFBP-6 may also have a role in regulating ovarian activity, perhaps by functioning as an antigonadotropin.[435]

RADIOIMMUNOASSAYS FOR THE INSULIN-LIKE GROWTH FACTOR–BINDING PROTEINS

Specific radioimmunoassays have been developed for IGFBP-1,[436–438] IGFBP-2,[403] IGFBP-3,[341, 439, 440] IGFBP-4,[441] IGFBP-5, and IGFBP-6. Measurement of IGFBP-3 appears to have the greatest clinical value because it is GH-dependent (Fig. 30–32).

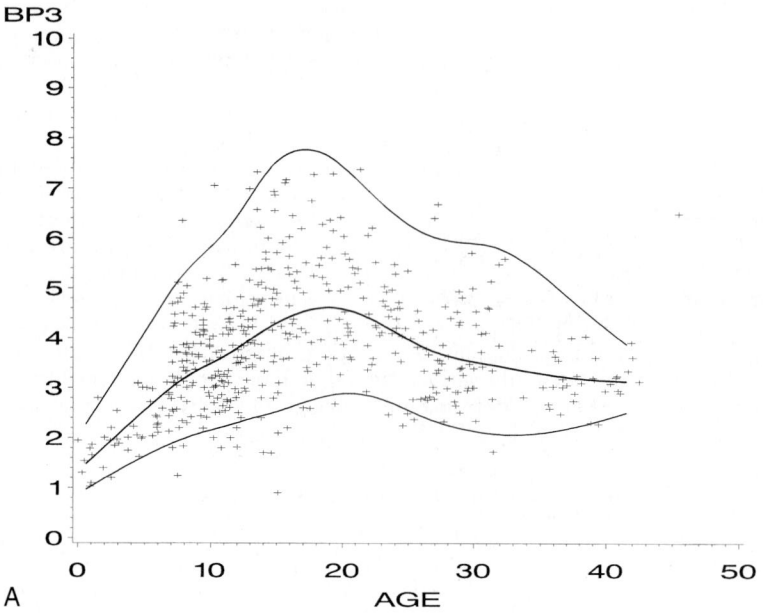

Figure 30–32. Normal serum levels of IGFBP-3 (μg/mL) for males *(A)* and females *(B)*. Lines represent the 3rd, 50th, and 97th percentiles. (Data courtesy of Diagnostic Systems Laboratories, Inc., Webster, Texas; and Phillip Lee, M.D. and Darrell Wilson, M.D.)

Blum and colleagues[440] have suggested that immunoassay of serum levels of IGFBP-3 may be superior to IGF-I assays in the diagnosis of GH deficiency because normal levels of IGF-I are so low in young children and because many "normal" short children have low levels of IGF-I. Because IGFBP-3 determinations reflect the levels of both IGF-I and IGF-II, their age dependency is not nearly as striking as that of IGF-I; even in young children normal levels are greater than 500 μg/L. The use of IGFBP assays in the evaluation of IGF deficiency and GH deficiency is discussed later. Measurement of IGFBP levels in biologic fluids may be useful for evaluation of malignancies or other pathologic states in which the IGFBP levels may be altered.

Gonadal Steroids

Although androgens and estrogens do not contribute substantially to normal growth before puberty, the adolescent rise in serum gonadal steroid levels is an important part of the pubertal growth spurt. States of androgen or estrogen excess prior to epiphyseal fusion cause rapid linear growth and skeletal maturation. Thus just as growth deceleration requires evaluation, growth acceleration can be just as abnormal and may be a sign of precocious puberty or virilizing congenital adrenal hyperplasia.

A GH-replete state is obligatory for a normal growth response to gonadal steroids, and children with GH deficiency do not have a normal growth response to either endogenous or exogenous androgens. Androgens work in part by enhancing GH secretion and also stimulate IGF-I production directly, as evidenced by the rise in serum IGF-I levels and a pubertal growth spurt in children with mutations of the GH receptor.[137]

Both androgens and estrogens increase skeletal maturation, and it is likely that androgens act in this regard after conversion to estrogens by aromatase in extraglandular tissues. Indeed mutation of the estrogen receptor in a man was associated with tall stature and open epiphyses,[442] and similar findings occur in patients with mutations of the gene encoding the aromatase enzyme.[443, 444] In addition women with an estrogen receptor variant have increased height.[445]

Skeletal development, in terms of bone mass accretion, is an important pubertal phenomenon and is largely mediated by estrogen action.[446-449] More than 90% of skeletal mass is present by age 18[450, 451] and estrogens appear to regulate the timing of the growth spurt, stabilization of bone modeling, and endosteal mineral apposition.[446] Independent and synergistic effects of gonadal steroids, GH, and IGF-I contribute to the attainment of peak bone mass in adults.[448]

Thyroid Hormone

Thyroid hormone is a major contributor to postnatal growth, although like GH it is of relatively little importance to growth of the fetus. Hypothyroidism postnatally can cause profound growth failure and virtual arrest of skeletal maturation. In addition to a direct effect on epiphyseal cartilage, thyroid hormones appear to have a permissive effect on GH secretion. Patients with hypothyroidism have decreased spontaneous GH secretion and blunted responses to GH provocative tests. Treatment with thyroid hormone results in rapid "catch-up" growth, which is typically accompanied by marked skeletal maturation, potentially causing overly rapid epiphyseal fusion and compromise of adult height (see later).

GROWTH RETARDATION

A classification of growth retardation is shown in Table 30–3. Growth disorders are subdivided into (1) *primary growth*

TABLE 30–3. Classification of Growth Retardation

Primary Growth Abnormalities

Osteochondrodysplasias
Chromosomal abnormalities
Intrauterine growth retardation (IUGR)

Secondary Growth Disorders

Malnutrition
Chronic disease
Endocrine disorders
  Hypothyroidism
  Cushing's syndrome
  Pseudohypoparathyroidism
  Rickets
    Vitamin D-resistant rickets
  IGF deficiency
    Hypothalamic dysfunction
    Pituitary GH deficiency
    GH resistance
      Primary GH resistance
      Secondary GH resistance

Idiopathic Short Stature

Genetic short stature
Constitutional delay of growth and maturation
Heterozygous defects of the GH receptor

IGF, insulin-like growth factor; hGH, human growth hormone.

abnormalities, in which the defect or defects appear to be intrinsic to the growth plate; (2) *secondary growth disorders*, i.e., growth failure resulting from chronic disease or endocrine disorders—the category of *IGF deficiency* can result from GHRH deficiency, GH deficiency, or GH resistance; and (3) *idiopathic short stature*, including variants of normal (constitutional delay of growth and maturation and genetic short stature) and heterozygous mutations of the GH receptor gene, a variant of GH resistance.

Primary Growth Abnormalities

Osteochondrodysplasias

The osteochondrodysplasias encompass a heterogeneous group of disorders characterized by intrinsic abnormalities of cartilage or bone, or both.[452, 453] These conditions share the following features: (1) genetic transmission; (2) abnormalities in the size or shape, or both, of bones of the limbs, spine, or skull; and (3) radiologic abnormalities of the bones (generally). More than 100 osteochondrodysplastic conditions have been identified to date on the basis of physical features and radiologic characteristics, and biochemical, molecular, and genetic studies of these conditions will undoubtedly lead to the recognition of additional types. An international classification for the osteochondrodysplasias developed in 1970[454] and revised in 1978[455] and 1992[452] is summarized in Table 30–4. It is of note that the category of dysostoses has been dropped from the classification, which now focuses on developmental disorders of bone and cartilage.

Diagnosis of osteochondrodysplasias can be difficult. Although the underlying molecular and biochemical defects have been identified in many of these conditions, clinical and radiologic evaluation remains central to the diagnosis. Frequently the clinical features are characteristic, and the diagnosis can be made at birth or even prenatally by ultrasound. The family history is critical, although many cases are due to fresh mutations, as is generally the case in the classic autosomal dominant achondroplasia and hypochondroplasia. Measurement of body proportions should include arm span, sitting height, upper and lower body segments, and head circumference. Clinical and radiologic evaluation should be used to determine whether involvement is of the long bones,

TABLE 30–4. Classification of Osteochondrodysplasias

Defects of the Tubular (and Flat) Bones or Axial Skeleton, or Both

Achondroplasia group
Achondrogenesis
Spondylodysplastic group (perinatally lethal)
Metatropic dysplasia group
Short rib dysplasia group (with or without polydactyly)
Atelosteogenesis/diastrophic dysplasia group
Kniest-Stickler dysplasia group
Spondyloepiphyseal dysplasia congenita group
Other spondyloepi-(meta)-physeal dysplasias
Dysostosis multiplex group
Spondylometaphyseal dysplasias
Epiphyseal dysplasias
Chondrodysplasia punctata (stippled epiphyses) group
Metaphyseal dysplasias
Brachrachia (short spine dysplasia)
Mesomelic dysplasias
Acro/acromesomelic dysplasias
Dysplasias with significant (but not exclusive) membranous bone involvement
Bent bone dysplasia group
Multiple dislocations with dysplasias
Osteodysplastic primordial dwarfism group
Dysplasias with increased bone density
Dysplasias with defective mineralization

Disorganized Development of Cartilaginous and Fibrous Components of the Skeleton

Idiopathic Osteolyses

skull, or vertebrae, or a combination of these structures, and whether abnormalities are primarily at the epiphyses, metaphyses, or diaphyses.

Two of the more common osteochondrodysplasias are achondroplasia and hypochondroplasia.

ACHONDROPLASIA

Achondroplasia is the most common of the osteochondrodysplasias, with a frequency of approximately 1 in 26,000 individuals. Although transmitted as an autosomal dominant disorder, 90% of cases appear to be due to new mutations. Achondroplasia results from a mutation in a transmembranous domain of the gene for fibroblast growth factor receptor 3 (FGFR3)[456, 457] located on the short arm of chromosome 4(4p16.3).[456, 458–460] Most cases identified to date are due to mutations at a "hot spot" at nucleotide 1138 of the FGFR3 gene,[456, 457, 461, 462] and because these mutations create new recognition sites for restriction enzymes they can be easily diagnosed. To date the mutation rate reported at this site indicates that it may be the most mutable gene in the human genome.[461, 462] The homogeneity of mutation in achondroplasia probably explains the minimal heterogeneity in its phenotype. Infants homozygous for this condition have severe disease, typically dying in infancy from respiratory insufficiency resulting from the small thorax. Diminished growth velocity is present from infancy, although short stature may not be evident until after 2 y of age. Mean adult heights in males and females are 130 and 120 cm, respectively.[463] Growth curves for achondroplasia have been developed and are of value in following patients.[23]

With increasing age the diagnosis of achondroplasia becomes easier, as these patients have characteristic abnormalities of the skeleton, including megalocephaly, a low nasal bridge, lumbar lordosis, a short trident hand, and rhizomelia (shortness of the proximal legs and arms) with skin redundancy. Radiologic findings include small, cuboid-shaped vertebral bodies with short pedicles and progressive narrowing of the lumbar interpedicular distance. The iliac wings are small, with narrow sciatic notches. The small foramen magnum may lead to hydrocephalus, and spinal cord or root compression

(or both) may result from kyphosis, stenosis of the spinal canal, or disc lesions.[464, 465] The relationship of the mutation of the FGFR3 gene to the clinical and skeletal structural and biochemical abnormalities for achondroplasia is not apparent. GH secretion in these children is comparable to that in normal children.[466]

HYPOCHONDROPLASIA

Hypochondroplasia is an autosomal dominant disorder that was described as a "mild form" of achondroplasia, but the two disorders do not occur in the same family and are not the result of mutations of the same gene.[467] Mullis and co-workers, using restriction enzyme analysis, suggested that the IGF-I gene may be a candidate gene for hypochondroplasia.[468] The facial features of achondroplasia are absent, and both the short stature and rhizomelia are less pronounced. Adult heights typically are in the 120- to 150-cm range. In contrast to achondroplasia, poor growth may not be evident until after 2 y of age, but stature then deviates progressively from normal. Occasionally the disproportionate short stature is not apparent until adulthood. Outward bowing of the legs may be accompanied by genu varum. Lumbar interpedicular distances diminish between L1 and L5 and, as with achondroplasia, there may be flaring of the pelvis and narrow sciatic notches. Mild variants of the syndrome may not be clinically distinguishable from normal, and radiologic studies should be performed if a question arises.

Chromosomal Abnormalities

Abnormalities of autosomes or sex chromosomes may cause growth retardation frequently associated with somatic abnormalities and mental retardation, as in deletion of chromosome 5 or trisomy 18 or 13. Such abnormalities, however, may be subtle, and the diagnosis of gonadal dysgenesis must be considered in any girl with unexplained short stature.

Down's Syndrome

Trisomy 21, or Down's syndrome, is probably the most common chromosomal disorder associated with growth retardation, affecting approximately 1 in 600 live births. On average, newborns with Down's syndrome have birthweights 500 g less than normal and are 2 to 3 cm shorter. Growth failure continues postnatally and is typically associated with delayed skeletal maturation and a delayed and incomplete pubertal growth spurt. Adult heights range from 135 to 170 cm in men and 127 to 158 cm in women.[24] The cause of growth failure in Down's syndrome and in other autosomal defects is unknown. Attempts to find underlying hormonal explanations for growth retardation have been unsuccessful, even though hypothyroidism due to Hashimoto's thyroiditis is more common than normal in Down's syndrome and should be sought. Marginal levels of GH secretion and low serum levels of IGF-I have been reported in Down's syndrome,[469–472] and exogenous GH may be efficacious in the short term.[473–477] It is more likely, however, that the growth failure reflects a generalized biochemical abnormality of the epiphyseal growth plate.

Gonadal Dysgenesis

In girls with gonadal dysgenesis short stature is the single most common feature, occurring more frequently than delayed puberty, cubitus valgus, or webbing of the neck.[478–480] In large series of such individuals short stature occurs in 95 to 100% of girls with a 45,X karyotype (see Chapter 29).[481–483] Several distinct phases of growth have been identified in girls with gonadal dysgenesis[484]: (1) mild intrauterine growth retardation (IUGR), with mean birth weights and length of 2800 g and 48.3 cm, respectively; (2) normal height gain between birth and 3 y of age; (3) progressive decline in height velocity from age 3 y until approximately 14 y of age, resulting in progressive deviation from normal height percentiles; and (4) a prolonged adolescent growth phase, characterized by a partial return toward normal height, followed by delayed epiphyseal fusion. Mean adult heights in the United States and Europe range from 142 to 146.8 cm (lower in Asia). There are important genetic and ethnic influences on growth in these girls. Parental height correlates well with final patient height[485, 486] and a cross-cultural study in 15 countries demonstrated a strong correlation $(r = 0.91)$ between final height in gonadal dysgenesis and in the normal population.[481]

The cause of growth failure in gonadal dysgenesis remains unclear. Most patients have normal GH and IGF levels during childhood; reports of low GH or IGF levels in adolescents with gonadal dysgenesis are likely due to low serum levels of gonadal steroids.[487] Growth impairment is evident prior to the period when activity of the GH-IGF axis is decreased. Nevertheless GH therapy is capable of both accelerating short-term growth and increasing adult height.[247, 488, 489] Gonadal dysgenesis is described in greater detail in Chapter 29. Its diagnosis should be considered in all girls with unexplained growth failure.

Intrauterine Growth Retardation

Infants with IUGR are a heterogeneous group with birth weight or length, or both, below the 10th percentile for gestational age.[490, 491] They may also be referred to as small-for-gestational age infants, in contrast to those who are appropriate for gestational age. The importance of this distinction, in addition to a number of issues influencing neonatal morbidity, is in the prediction of later growth: most appropriate-for-gestational age, low–birth weight infants experience catch-up growth during the first 2 y of life, in contrast to the slower, attenuated growth of small-for-gestational age infants who may have persistent height deficits throughout childhood and adolescence.[492–495] The earlier in gestation that fetal growth is impaired, the less likely that complete recapture of lost growth will occur.

IUGR can arise from abnormalities in the fetus, the placenta, or the mother (Table 30–5). Factors affecting fetal

TABLE 30–5. Causes of Intrauterine Growth Retardation

Intrinsic Fetal Abnormalities	Maternal Disorders
Chromosomal disorders	Malnutrition
Syndromes associated with primary growth failure	Constraints on uterine growth
IGF-I gene deletion	Vascular disorders
Russell-Silver syndrome	Hypertension
Seckel's syndrome	Toxemia
Noonan's syndrome	Severe diabetes mellitus
Progeria	Uterine malformations
Cockayne's syndrome	Drug ingestion
Bloom syndrome	Tobacco
Prader-Willi syndrome	Alcohol
Rubenstein-Taybi syndrome	Narcotics
Congenital infections	
Congenital anomalies	
Placental Abnormalities	
Abnormal implantation of the placenta	
Placental vascular insufficiency; infarction	
Vascular malformations	

Modified from Underwood LE, Van Wyk JJ: Normal and aberrant growth. In: Wilson JD, Foster DW (eds): Williams Textbook of Endocrinology. 8th ed. Philadelphia: WB Saunders, 1992: 1110, with permission.

growth include nutrition provided by the maternal-placental system, alterations of fetal IGF production, and as yet unclarified genes. Although it is understandable why uterine constraint or twin pregnancies might result in limited fetal growth, the reason for abnormal fetal growth in most cases of IUGR is unclear.

The implications of IUGR may extend beyond fetal life. In a retrospective study of 47 individuals who had IUGR, 23 men had an adult height of 162 cm, and 24 women had an adult height of 148 cm.[496] Furthermore small-for-gestational age infants have an increased risk of hypertension, maturity-onset diabetes, and cardiovascular disease later in life.[497, 498] Whether IUGR is *causally* related to these disorders or is a symptom of an underlying inborn metabolic disorder is not known.

Intrinsic Fetal Factors

In contrast to the role of the endocrine system in postnatal growth, intrauterine growth is less dependent on fetal pituitary hormones.[499, 500] Athyreotic and agonadal infants are of normal length and weight at birth. The ontogeny of GH production is discussed later; in summary, pituitary GH is synthesized and secreted by the latter half of the first trimester, with midgestational levels peaking at 150 μg/L and then falling to around 30 μg/L at term.[112] Since the anencephalic fetus is normal in size, the pituitary was thought to be unnecessary for fetal growth.[501, 502] However, documentation of birth size of rats and humans with congenital GH deficiency[503–506] and of human newborns with mutations of the GH or GH receptor genes[137] indicate that GH from the fetal pituitary makes a small contribution to birth size. Infants with neonatal GH deficiency are around -0.5 to -1.5 SD below the mean in length and are heavy for this length.[504–506]

These observations should not be interpreted to mean that the IGF axis is unimportant in fetal growth. Gene knockout studies causing elimination of paracrine-autocrine production of IGF-I and IGF-II, as well as of the type 1 IGF receptor, impair fetal growth.[507, 508] Circulating IGF-I levels in fetal and cord blood correlate with fetal size and are reduced in IUGR, especially in situations associated with decreased growth velocity.[120, 242, 509–512] The initial case of a deletion of the *IGF-I* gene showed profound IUGR.[513] The implication of that report is that local tissue production of IGF-I is critical for intrauterine growth and that its regulation is largely GH-independent. Human umbilical cord lymphocytes have increased numbers of IGF receptors,[514] and mRNAs for both IGF-I and IGF-II are abundant in fetal tissues.[515, 516] Hepatic levels of GH receptor mRNA and of GH receptor are low,[112, 517, 518] perhaps explaining the modest impact of GH on IGF production and linear growth. In neonates with IUGR, GH levels are elevated[519] and exogenous GH treatment has little or no effect on growth, body composition, or energy expenditure,[520, 521] further supporting a state of relative resistance to GH at this developmental stage. With defects of the GH receptor neonatal IGF levels are low,[112] suggesting a role for GH in regulating IGF production. Similarly the IGFBPs are identifiable in serum and other biologic fluids in the fetus and newborn.[359] However, serum levels of IGFBP-3 and ALS, the major serum carriers of IGF peptides in the adult, are low in the fetus and newborn. Thus the components of the IGF system are apparently regulated directly by glucose levels or indirectly by fetal insulin secretion, with less impact on GH levels.[509, 522, 523] The role of insulin production in fetal growth is demonstrated by somatic overgrowth of the hyperinsulinemic infants of diabetic mothers and of infants with the syndrome of persistent neonatal hyperinsulinemic hypoglycemia (nesidioblastosis).[490, 524, 525] In contrast, infants with pancreatic agenesis or with abnormalities of the insulin receptor in the "leprechaun" syndrome are small for gestational age.[490] Furthermore, the inverse relationship of insulin and IGFBP-1 levels and the finding that fetal IGFBP-1 levels are elevated in IUGR[523] support an important role for insulin in fetal growth regulation.

Infants with IUGR frequently exhibit poor postnatal growth, particularly when the abnormalities are intrinsic to the fetus. Such conditions have frequently been categorized as *primordial growth failure*. Several syndromes are briefly noted below.

RUSSELL-SILVER SYNDROME

The Russell-Silver syndrome was independently described by Russell[526] and by Silver.[527] Although this syndrome is probably due to a heterogeneous group of disorders, the common findings include IUGR, postnatal growth failure, congenital hemihypertrophy, and small triangular facies.[528–531] Nonspecific findings include clinodactyly, precocious puberty, delayed closure of the fontanelles, and delayed bone age.[528–530] Adults are short, with final heights about −4 SD below the mean.[529, 531] Endogenous GH secretion in prepubertal children with the Russell-Silver syndrome is similar to that in other short children with IUGR and less than in appropriate-for-gestational age short children.[532] Because no genetic or biochemical basis for this disorder has been identified, the Russell-Silver syndrome is often used incorrectly as a designation for IUGR of unknown cause.

SECKEL'S SYNDROME

Although originally described by Mann and Russell in 1959,[533] this autosomal recessive disorder characterized by IUGR and severe postnatal growth failure, combined with microcephaly, prominent nose, and micrognathia, is most commonly termed *Seckel's syndrome* or *Seckel's birdheaded dwarfism*.[534] Final height is typically 90 to 110 cm, with moderate to severe mental retardation. The nature of the underlying defect is unknown.

NOONAN'S SYNDROME

Although Noonan's syndrome shares certain phenotypic features with gonadal dysgenesis, the two disorders are clearly distinct.[535] In Noonan's syndrome the sex chromosomes are normal, and transmission is apparently autosomal dominant; neither the gene locus nor product are identified. Both males and females may be affected, explaining the misleading terms *Turner-like syndrome* and *male gonadal dysgenesis*. Affected individuals typically have webbing of the neck, a low posterior hairline, ptosis, cubitus valgus, and malformed ears. Cardiac abnormalities are primarily right-sided (pulmonary valve) rather than the left-sided (aorta, aortic valve) lesions characteristic of gonadal dysgenesis. Although birth weight is generally within the normal range, mean growth in length and weight is below the 3rd percentile through much of childhood, with a falling height velocity not dissimilar to that seen in gonadal dysgenesis, except for the late and attenuated pubertal increment.[536, 537] GH secretory abnormalities do not account for the short stature, although endogenous GH production may be reduced somewhat.[538, 539] Microphallus and cryptorchidism are common, and puberty may be delayed or incomplete. Mental retardation of variable degrees is present in approximately 25 to 50% of patients.

PROGERIA

The senile appearance characteristic of progeria (Hutchinson-Gilford syndrome) is typically apparent by 2 y of age.[540] There is a progressive loss of subcutaneous fat, accompanied by alopecia, hypoplasia of the nails, joint limitation, and early onset of atherosclerosis, typically followed by angina, myocardial infarction, hypertension, and congestive heart failure. Skeletal hypoplasia results in severe growth retardation, which typically becomes evident by 6 to 18 mo of age.

COCKAYNE'S SYNDROME

Cockayne's syndrome, like progeria, is characterized by a premature senile appearance.[541] Retinal degeneration, photosensitivity of the skin, and impaired hearing may also be present. Growth failure typically appears at 2 to 4 y of age. Transmission is in an autosomal recessive manner.

PRADER-WILLI SYNDROME

Growth failure may be evident at birth and is more impressive postnatally in Prader-Willi syndrome.[542] The neonatal period is characterized by hypotonia and, in the male, cryptorchidism and microphallus. Hypogonadotropic hypogonadism may persist into adult life. With advancing age hyperphagia and obesity become prominent. The cause of growth failure is unclear. Low mean serum GH levels or inadequate responses after provocative testing[543–545] may reflect the impact of obesity and are not necessarily causal. Many patients with Prader-Willi syndrome have deletions of the short arm of the paternally derived chromosome 15, and in the absence of structural abnormalities of chromosome 15 both copies may be maternally derived, so-called uniparental disomy.[546]

Other syndromes associated with moderate to profound growth failure include Bloom syndrome, de Lange's syndrome, leprechaunism (mutations of the insulin receptor gene), Ellis-van Creveld syndrome, Aarskog syndrome, Rubenstein-Taybi syndrome, mulibrey nanism (Perheentupa syndrome), Dubovitz syndrome, and Johanson-Blizzard syndrome.[547]

Maternal and Placental Factors

Maternal factors and placental insufficiency can impair fetal growth. Although such affected infants have better growth potential than do those with "primordial growth failure," postnatal growth is not always normal. Maternal nutrition is an important contributor to fetal growth and to growth during the first year of life.[548] Fetal growth retardation may also result from alcohol consumption during pregnancy[549–551] and from the use of cocaine,[552, 553] marijuana,[553] and tobacco.[554] The mechanisms for such drug-induced fetal growth retardation are unclear but probably include uterine vasoconstriction and vascular insufficiency, placental abruption, and premature rupture of membranes. Although maternal tobacco use is statistically a major contributor to reduced fetal size, it is unlikely by itself to result in severe IUGR. The maternal hormonal milieu is affected by placental steroids and peptides, especially placental GH and human placental lactogen, which influence the production of maternal IGF-I.[509] Maternal IGF affects placental function and may facilitate transport of nutrients to the fetus, and maternal IGF-I levels correlate with fetal growth.[555, 556] Hasegawa and colleagues[556a] have found increased levels of free (non–IGFBP-bound) IGF-I levels during normal human pregnancy, possibly due to accelerated proteolysis of IGFBP-3.

The placenta has multiple functions, including transporting of nutrients, oxygen, and waste and production of hormones, and it consumes oxygen and glucose brought to it by the uterine circulation. Placental GH affects maternal IGF production, which in turn affects placental function. Human placental lactogen is a major regulator of glucose, amino acid, and lipid metabolism in the mother, aiding in the mobilization of nutrients for transport into the fetus. Damage to the placenta by vascular disease, infection, or intrinsic abnormalities of the syncytiotrophoblasts can impair these important functions. Sometimes, but not always, examination of the placenta will yield diagnostic information as to the cause of IUGR.

Secondary Growth Disorders

Malnutrition

Given the worldwide presence of undernutrition, it is not surprising that inadequate caloric or protein intake, or both, is the most common cause of growth failure.[557] Marasmus refers to an overall deficiency of calories including protein malnutrition. Subcutaneous fat is minimal and protein wasting is marked. Kwashiorkor, in contrast, refers to inadequate protein intake, although it may also be characterized by some caloric undernutrition. In both conditions multiple deficiencies of vitamins and minerals are apparent.[558] Frequently the two conditions overlap. Decreased weight growth generally precedes the failure of linear growth by a short time in the neonatal period and by several years at older ages.

Both acute and chronic malnutrition affect the GH-IGF system.[559, 560] The impaired growth is usually associated with elevated basal or stimulated serum GH levels, or both,[561] but in generalized malnutrition (marasmus) GH levels may be normal or low.[562] In both conditions serum IGF-I levels are reduced.[563, 564] Malnutrition may consequently be considered a form of GH resistance (see later), with serum IGF-I levels reduced despite normal or elevated GH levels. GHBP levels, as a reflection of GH receptor content, are decreased.[559, 560] GH resistance may be an adaptive response, whereby protein is spared by the lipolytic and anti-insulin actions of GH.[565, 566] Reduced serum IGF-I levels would serve to shift calories from anabolic to survival requirements. These adaptive mechanisms are accompanied by changes in serum IGFBPs to further limit IGF action during periods of malnutrition.[560, 567]

Inadequate calorie-protein intake complicates many chronic diseases that are characterized by growth failure. Anorexia is a common feature of renal failure and inflammatory bowel disease and occurs with cyanotic heart disease, congestive heart failure, CNS disease, and other illnesses. Some of these conditions may furthermore be characterized by deficiencies of specific dietary components such as zinc, iron, and vitamins necessary for normal growth and development.

Undernutrition may also be voluntary, as with dieting and food fads (Fig. 30–33).[568] Caloric restriction is especially common in girls during adolescence, when it may be associated with anxiety concerning obesity, and in gymnasts and ballet dancers. Anorexia nervosa and bulimia are extremes of "voluntary" caloric deprivation and are commonly associated with impaired growth prior to epiphyseal fusion that may result in diminished final adult height.[569–573] Later in adolescence malnutrition may cause delayed puberty or menarche, or both, and a variety of metabolic alterations. In anorexia nervosa hormonal profiles are similar to those in protein-energy malnutrition,[569–575] with high basal levels of GH but low levels of IGF-I, IGFBP-3, and GHPB. GHBP and IGFBP-3 levels correlate with body mass index, as in normal children.[121, 569, 576] The hormones of the GH-IGF axis return to normal levels with refeeding.[560, 569, 576]

Chronic Diseases[577]

MALABSORPTION AND GASTROINTESTINAL DISEASES

Intestinal disorders that impair absorption of calories or protein cause growth failure, for many of the reasons cited earlier.[565, 578–580] Growth retardation may predate other manifestations of malabsorption or chronic inflammatory bowel dis-

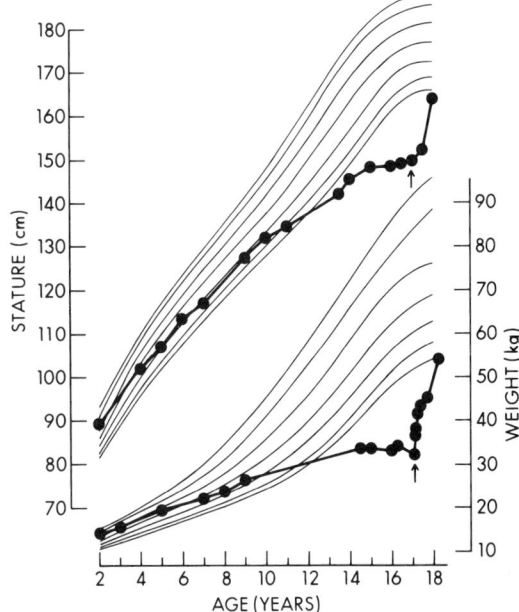

Figure 30–33. Curves of weight and height in a child who had growth failure resulting from prolonged self-imposed caloric restriction because of a fear of becoming obese. Note that crossing of percentiles on the weight curve preceded that for the height curve, and when the caloric intake was normalized *(arrow)*, the gain in weight occurred before the improvement in linear growth. Also note that at the end of the prolonged period of caloric restriction, weight age (10.2 y) was less than height age (12 y). (From Pugliese MT, Lifshitz F, Grad G, et al. Fear of obesity: a cause of short stature and delayed puberty. N Engl J Med 1983; 309:513–518. Reprinted by permission of the New England Journal of Medicine.)

ease, or both. Accordingly, celiac disease (gluten-induced enteropathy) and regional enteritis (Crohn's disease) should be considered in the differential diagnosis of unexplained growth failure. Serum levels of IGF-I may be reduced,[565, 581, 582] reflecting the malnutrition, and it is critical to discriminate between these conditions and GH deficiency or related disorders causing IGF-I deficiency. Documentation of malabsorption requires demonstration of fecal wasting of calories, especially fecal fat, along with other measures of gut dysfunction such as the D-xylose or breath hydrogen studies.

In celiac disease (Fig. 30–34) impaired linear growth may be the first manifestation of disease,[565, 583–588] although the degree of growth impairment may be similar in patients with and those without gastrointestinal symptoms.[565] In European studies celiac disease is the cause of unexplained growth impairment in 5 to 20% of unselected patients.[585–588] The onset and progression of puberty may be delayed and menarche may be late.[578, 583] Accordingly a screening test for celiac disease is needed to obviate the standard diagnostic tests involving multiple intestinal biopsies[589] when assessing asymptomatic patients. Both IgG and IgA antigliadin, antiendomysial, and antijejunal antibodies have relatively high sensitivity and specificity[583, 590, 591] and improve screening efficacy. Nonetheless demonstration of the characteristic mucosal flattening in small bowel biopsy, return of jejunal mucosa to normal after gluten withdrawal, and reappearance of abnormalities on gluten challenge are necessary to *confirm* the diagnosis. Although some have recommended jejunal biopsy to rule out celiac disease in all cases of unexplained growth failure during the first 5 y of life,[578, 583] this aggressive approach usually is not necessary.[581] An alternative is to reserve biopsies for children with a history of diarrhea or steatorrhea, or both, in the first 2 y of life; abnormal D-xylose absorption tests; and IgG or IgA antigliadin antibodies. Gluten withdrawal is a highly effective treatment for celiac disease and results in rapid catch-up growth and decreased

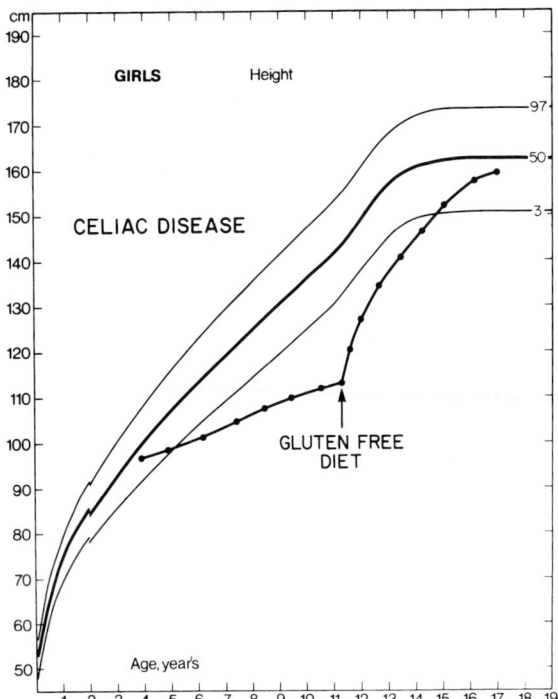

Figure 30–34. Catch-up growth in a girl with gluten-induced enteropathy (celiac disease). After 8 y of growth impairment the patient was placed on a gluten-free diet and demonstrated substantial catch-up growth. Note the return to the previous growth percentiles. (Courtesy of JM Tanner.)

clinical symptoms during the first 6 to 12 mo of treatment.[565, 583] Low IGF-I and IGFBP-3 levels return to normal during this period.[585, 592] Most children who receive appropriate dietary management ultimately achieve a normal final height.[593, 594]

The growth failure in Crohn's disease is probably due to a combination of malnutrition from malabsorption and anorexia, chronic inflammation,[595] inadequacy of trace minerals in the diet, and the use of glucocorticoids.[596–598] IGF-I levels are low, especially with impaired growth.[565, 582] One third to two thirds or more of children with Crohn's disease have impaired growth at diagnosis,[565, 599–601] and occasional patients have significant growth failure as the first evidence of Crohn's disease.[565, 597, 601] For this reason a screening test would be valuable. An elevated erythrocyte sedimentation rate is a useful clue, but diagnosis ultimately requires endoscopy and biopsy. Long-term treatment includes enteral and parenteral nutrition, alternate-day steroid therapy, and judicious operative intervention.[565, 597] Permanent impairment of linear growth and deficits of final height may occur in 30% of patients.[597, 602]

CHRONIC LIVER DISEASE

Impaired linear growth and short stature with chronic liver disease in childhood[603–608] are caused by decreased food intake, fat and fat-soluble vitamin malabsorption, trace element deficiencies, and abnormalities of the GH-IGF system.[606–608] Decreased levels of IGF-I, IGF-II, and IGFBP-3, and increased GH secretion define the acquired GH resistance syndrome.[609–614] A close correlation between GH-dependent peptides and liver function indicates the dominant regulatory role of the damaged hepatocyte in end-stage liver failure.[609] Diminished levels of GHBP substantiate the GH resistance.[612] Despite the provision of adequate calories, resistance to the action of GH persists.[608, 611] Liver transplantation prolongs life expectancy,[615–617] but in the early post-transplantation years, linear growth is

often inadequate.[614, 618–620] The administration of exogenous glucocorticoids and immunosuppressive agents presumably plays a major role in the continued growth retardation; GH and IGF-I production are normal, but the amount of "free IGF" may be decreased as IGFBP-3 levels are relatively high.[614, 619] Long-term growth improvement has been reported with the use of alternate-day glucocorticoids in children who undergo transplantation after 2 y of age.[620] Exogenous GH treatment, for a period of 18 mo, enhances growth rates in such patients and increases median height SD scores from -3.9 to -2.6.[621]

CARDIOVASCULAR DISEASE

Congenital heart disease with cyanosis or chronic congestive failure can cause growth failure.[622–624] As many as 27% of children with varied cardiac lesions were below the 3rd percentile for height and weight in one survey,[625] and 70% were lower than the 50th percentile in another.[626] As cardiac defects are usually congenital, many infants have dysmorphic features and IUGR.[627] Inadequate caloric intake is the most common cause of growth impairment in children with congenital heart disease,[624, 626, 628] frequently associated with anorexia and vomiting. Chronic congestive heart failure is associated with malabsorption that includes protein-losing enteropathy, intestinal lymphangiectasia, and steatorrhea.[624, 629, 630] Greater cardiac and respiratory work and the relatively higher ratio of metabolically active, energy-utilizing brain and heart to the growth-retarded body mass (cardiac cachexia[631]) causes an increased basal metabolic rate in these children.[632, 633] Food intake that appears adequate for the child's weight thus is inadequate for normal growth. The degree of cyanosis or hypoxia does correlate with the degree of growth impairment.[624, 626, 634] Decreased levels of IGF-I and IGFBP-3,[635, 636] normal levels of GH, and hepatic GH receptors in chronically hypoxemic newborn sheep[636] suggest GH resistance distal to the GH receptor.

Corrective surgery may restore normal growth, frequently after a phase of "catch-up" growth. Surgery must, on occasion, be delayed until the infant reaches an appropriate size, resulting in the conundrum that surgery corrects growth failure but cannot be performed because the infant is too small. In these situations meticulous attention to caloric support and alleviation of hypoxia and heart failure is necessary to promote growth prior to surgery. Fortunately this problem has diminished because of operative successes in the neonatal period. The nutritional management of these infants includes calorie-dense feedings because of the need to restrict fluids, calcium supplementation because of the use of diuretics that may cause calcium loss in the urine, and iron to maintain an enhanced rate of erythropoiesis.[633]

RENAL DISEASE

All conditions that impair renal function can impair growth.[637–643] Uremia and renal tubular acidosis can cause growth failure before other clinical manifestations become evident. The growth impairment results from multiple mechanisms—including inadequate formation of 1,25-dihydroxy-cholecaliferol $(1,25(OH)_2D)$ with resultant osteopenia, decreased caloric intake, loss of electrolytes necessary for normal growth, metabolic acidosis, protein wasting, insulin resistance, chronic anemia, and compromised cardiac function—as well as from impairment of GH and IGF production and action. In nephropathic cystinosis, acquired hypothyroidism contributes to the inadequate growth.[644] Sixty to 75% of patients with chronic renal failure treated prior to the GH therapeutic era had final adult heights more than -2 SD below the mean.[642]

Children and adolescents have normal or elevated circulating levels of GH, depending on the degree of renal failure.[639–641, 645–648] In children with end-stage renal disease (ESRD) who are receiving dialysis or in children with preterminal chronic renal failure, the half-life of GH is prolonged twofold.[609] The number of secretory bursts was increased in patients with ESRD by two- to threefold over that in patients with chronic renal failure and in controls, and mean levels of GH were 2.5-fold higher in patients with ESRD than in patients with chronic renal failure or in controls. Overall, children with ESRD had a substantially higher GH production than did either chronic renal failure patients or controls. Early reports of decreases in serum IGF levels in uremia were an artifact due to inadequate separation of IGF from IGFBPs prior to assay.[235] Decreased hepatic IGF production[649] is possibly due to low hepatic GH receptor gene expression.[650] Serum IGF-I and IGF-II levels are, however, usually normal,[639, 640, 645, 651] but increases in serum IGFBPs, especially IGFBP-1,[639–641, 651, 652] may inhibit IGF action.[653–656] In nephrotic syndrome serum levels of IGF-I and IGFBP-3 are low because of urinary loss of IGF–I–IGFBP complexes.[643] Chronic glucocorticoid therapy for a variety of renal disorders can exacerbate growth retardation by diminishing GH release and blunting IGF-I action at growth plates.[655, 657–659] Chronic renal disease, especially ESRD, with increased GH levels and production, low levels of IGF-I, and poor growth is thus a state of relative resistance to GH and, in some instances, to IGF-I.[642, 653–656, 660]

Even after successful renal transplantation growth may not be normal.[644, 659, 661–663] In the large cohort of patients in the North American Pediatric Renal Transplant Cooperative Study,[217, 663] mean height increased after transplantation by only 0.11 SD in the first 4.5 y. The youngest age group (<2 y) had the largest deficit and the most catch-up (0.94 SD); children between 6 and 17 y had no improvement in SD score. Unfortunately the younger age group had a 16% mortality, suggesting that transplantation may have an unacceptably high risk in such patients.[663] In another study only 30% of prepubertal patients experienced appreciable catch-up during the first 2 y after transplantation,[661] with none having significant improvement in height SD scores for age if undergoing transplantation after age 5. Growth-retarded children, whether receiving daily or alternate-day glucocorticoid treatment after transplantation, have decreased GH secretion, normal levels of IGF-I and IGFBP-1, and elevated levels of IGFBP-3. They differ from patients with ESRD in that IGFBP-1 levels are not strikingly elevated, perhaps because of altered glucose tolerance due to chronic glucocorticoid therapy.[655] Overall, height SD scores at the time of transplantation and use of alternate-day glucocorticoid therapy after transplantation correlate positively with final height, and a longer duration of reduced glomerular filtration rate and a higher cumulative dose of prednisone have a negative impact; other factors such as gender, age at transplantation, diagnosis, and number of transplants do not seem to have significant impact on adult height.[661] The importance of height at the time of transplantation in determining final adult height, despite the complex post-transplantation health issues, confirms the value of improving growth velocity and absolute height prior to transplantation.

Although the growth failure of renal disease in the pretransplantation period is not specifically due to either GH or IGF deficiency, GH therapy accelerates skeletal growth (see later) and is approved by the Food and Drug Administration for use. Such treatment probably increases the molar ratio of IGF peptides to IGFBPs and may override the inhibitory actions of IGFBPs. GH administration may also be useful for the treatment of post-transplantation growth failure.[664–668]

HEMATOLOGIC DISORDERS

Chronic anemias, such as sickle cell disease, are characterized by growth failure.[669–673] In general the decrease in height and weight is greater in adolescent years than it is earlier, as the onset of the adolescent growth spurt is delayed and menarche is late.[672–675] The adolescent growth and final adult height in sickle cell disease, however, may be normal.[674] The causes of growth retardation probably include impaired oxygen delivery to tissues, increased work of the cardiovascular system, energy demands of increased hematopoiesis, and impaired nutrition. The GH-IGF system probably does not have an important role in the growth impairment of sickle cell anemia.

In thalassemia, in addition to the consequences of chronic anemia, endocrine deficiencies can result from chronic transfusions and accompanying hemosiderosis.[676–678] Despite vigorous efforts to maintain hemoglobin levels near normal and to avoid iron overload, growth failure is still a common feature of thalassemia, especially in adolescents. It is likely that anemia, impaired IGF-I synthesis,[679, 680] hypothyroidism, gonadal failure, and hypogonadotropic hypogonadism all contribute to growth failure in this disorder. GH resistance is suggested by generally adequate GH production with low IGF-I levels.[681, 682] In most patients GH treatment increases growth at least initially.[681, 683]

DIABETES MELLITUS

Although weight loss may occur immediately before the onset of clinically apparent insulin-dependent diabetes mellitus (IDDM), children with new-onset diabetes are frequently taller than their peer group, possibly because GH and insulin levels are increased during the preclinical evolution of the disease.[684–686] Most children with IDDM grow normally, even those with marginal control,[687] especially in prepubertal years, although growth velocity may decrease during puberty.[688, 689] Growth failure, however, can occur in diabetic children with long-standing poor glycemic control.[690, 691] The Mauriac syndrome[692] describes children with poorly regulated IDDM, severe growth failure, and hepatosplenomegaly due to excess hepatic glycogen deposition. This type of growth retardation has become increasingly rare.[693]

Many pathophysiologic processes, including malnutrition, chronic intermittent acidosis, increased glucocorticoid production, hypothyroidism, impaired calcium balance, and "end organ unresponsiveness" to either GH or IGF, may contribute to growth failure in IDDM.[685, 694–696] IGF-I and IGFBP-3 levels are diminished in the face of enhanced GH production[6, 55, 691, 697–704] reflecting acquired GH resistance; GHBP levels are decreased,[694, 704] supporting the concept of impaired GH receptor number or function. Further IGFBP-1 is normally suppressed by insulin, and hypoinsulinemia results in elevated serum IGFBP-1 levels, which may inhibit IGF action.[703–709] In contrast to the situation in adolescents and adults IGFBP-1 levels are not elevated in well-growing prepubertal children.[703, 706–708] On the contrary, increased IGFBP-3 proteolysis may enhance the bioactivity of the available IGF-I.[710] Most children with IDDM, however, attain normal cellular nutrition and growth factor action despite intermittent hypoinsulinemia and derangements of peripheral indices of the GH-IGF system.

Although glycemic control is inversely correlated with IGF-I levels,[695, 697–699, 701, 703–705] the correlation between glycemic control and growth is weak, with conflicting reports as to the influence of glycemic regulation on growth.[685, 686, 699, 711–717] A longitudinal study[715] of 46 children whose diabetes began before age 10 indicated that initial heights at diagnosis were normal and that the final height SD scores were minimally reduced from those at the onset. Despite a delay of about 2.5 y in the onset of puberty in boys, total pubertal height gain was normal. In girls with diabetes, however, total pubertal height gain was diminished and the age of menarche was delayed; the effects of altered insulin and IGF-I levels on ovarian function have not been assessed in such patients.

Chronic metabolic control did not correlate with the pubertal height gain nor with the normal final heights. Nevertheless good glycemic control at certain maturational periods, such as puberty, may improve growth during those intervals.[685, 702, 718]

INBORN ERRORS OF METABOLISM

Inborn errors of metabolism are often accompanied by growth failure, which may be pronounced. Glycogen storage disease, the mucopolysaccharidoses, glycoproteinoses, and mucolipidoses are characterized by poor growth. Many inborn metabolic disorders are also associated with significant skeletal dysplasia. In a small number of patients with organic acidoses, such as methylmalonic and propionic acidurias, IGF-I levels are low and GH levels are normal, suggesting a possible state of GH resistance related to nutritional status.[719] Preliminary data suggest that exogenous GH treatment may improve the metabolic status of such children.[719, 720]

PULMONARY DISEASE

Growth can be retarded in children with asthma who have not received glucocorticoid therapy.[721, 722] Mean height and growth velocity and the degree of growth failure are related to the severity of the asthma.[721, 722] Delayed pubertal maturation in such patients is also associated with growth deceleration in the early teenage years.[721, 723] Impaired nutrition and increased energy requirements along with chronic stress, especially with nocturnal asthma and enhanced endogenous glucocorticoid production, cause poor linear growth. Glucocorticoid therapy, generally given to more severely affected patients, further impairs growth throughout childhood.[724–726] Synthetic glucocorticoids, such as prednisone or dexamethasone, may have a greater growth-suppressive effect than equivalent therapeutic doses of cortisol, presumably because the biopotency of the synthetic agents may be underestimated. Alternate-day or aerosolized glucocorticoid therapy often ameliorates growth retardation and can be associated with an accelerated catch-up phase.[721, 725] The use of spacer devices and effective nebulizer solutions may permit the use of inhaled glucocorticoids in young children without growth impairment.[727, 728] Clearly, however, sufficient glucocorticoid delivered by any route can diminish growth and impede the function of the adrenal gland.[729] The impaired growth in asthmatic children does not appear to be associated with abnormalities of the GH-IGF axis.[730] Normal adult height is usually achieved.[731, 732]

Bronchopulmonary dysplasia, a sequela of hyaline membrane disease and prematurity, has an incidence as high as 35% in very low birth weight infants (<1500 g).[733] The use of dexamethasone in the neonatal treatment of bronchopulmonary dysplasia causes a transient cessation of growth.[734] Growth in surviving infants is poor through early childhood,[735–737] but the defect disappears by 8 y of age.[738–740] Long-term hypoxemia, poor nutrition, chronic pulmonary infections, and reactive airway disease are responsible for the poor early growth.

Cystic fibrosis (CF), chronic pulmonary infection with bronchiectasis, pancreatic insufficiency with exocrine and endocrine inadequacy, malabsorption, and malnutrition[577, 741–746] all contribute to decreased growth and late sexual maturation. In 17,857 patients with CF, mean height was at the 21st percentile and mean weight was at the 9th perecentile.[747] Early impairment of height and weight growth and retardation of skeletal maturation may progress or plateau during the middle childhood years but may become most marked in the preadolescent period when growth and maturational changes are delayed.[741, 747–750] The degree of growth retardation is related most closely to the severity and variability of the pulmonary disease rather than to pancreatic dysfunction.[577, 743, 744] The degree of steatorrhea does not correlate well with growth impairment, although improved nutrition programs enhance the overall clinical picture.[745, 746] Adult heights of surviving patients with CF approach the normal range.[577] Endocrine abnormalities, such as failure of both alpha and beta islet cells with decreased glucagon and insulin production, do not seem to influence prepubertal growth patterns in children with CF. The incidence of diabetes mellitus increases as patients live past the second decade of life.[747] Alterations of vitamin D metabolism, although potentially affecting skeletal mineralization, do not diminish growth.[751] In delayed sexual maturation in which LHRH administration evokes a prepubertal pattern of pituitary gonadotropin secretion similar to that in constitutional delay of growth and maturation (CDGM),[749, 750] the GH-IGF axis shows evidence for acquired GH resistance with lowered mean IGF-I and elevated GH levels.[752] Treatment of nine prepubertal children with CF using GH for 1 y resulted in an anabolic effect with increased growth velocity, increased nitrogen retention, and increased protein and decreased fat stores.[753] Systematic longitudinal studies of nutritional status and the function of the GH-IGF axis have not been performed.

CHRONIC INFECTION

Exposure to human immunodeficiency virus in children and adolescents occurs through perinatal transmission, blood transfusions, drug usage, and sexual contact, but most commonly via perinatal transmission from human immunodeficiency virus–infected mothers. Growth failure is a cardinal feature of childhood acquired immunodeficiency syndrome.[754–759] Mean length and weight measurements during early childhood years are at or less than 1 SD below the mean, but weight-for-height data may be normal,[757, 759] in contrast to the "wasting" syndrome described in adult patients with acquired immunodeficiency syndrome.[760, 761] In a drug treatment study of 88 human immunodeficiency virus–infected children with the mean age being 3.1 y, more than 90% were below the 50th percentile for both height and weight; only 44% of this group survived 4 y after initiation of the study. Height and growth velocity are not useful predictive indicators for survival.[757] In hemophiliac boys with human immunodeficiency virus growth impairment, delayed pubertal onset and progression and younger skeletal age were common.[758] Despite the delayed pubertal maturation, serum testosterone levels were not significantly decreased.

In many developing countries chronic infestation with parasites, such as schistosomiasis, hookworm, and roundworm, contribute to nutritional debilitation and growth failure.[762] A complex cascade of cytokines, acting as part of the inflammatory response to acute and chronic infection, can affect the endocrine system at many levels,[763, 764] impairing mineral and nutrient metabolism and the growth and remodeling of bone.[765]

Endocrine Disorders

HYPOTHYROIDISM

Growth may be retarded in children with hypothyroidism, but the development of newborn screening programs for congenital hypothyroidism has resulted in more prompt diagnosis and treatment of such newborns (approximately 1 in 4100 live births). Growth in appropriately treated infants and children with congenital hypothyroidism is normal for age[766, 767] so that skeletal maturation approximates chronologic age.[767] Many features of adult myxedema are not present in children with hypothyroidism. The most prominent manifestation of acquired hypothyroidism is growth failure, which may be profound.[768] In acquired hypothyroidism growth retardation may take several years to become clinically evident but, once present, is typically severe and progressive. The poor growth is more apparent in height than in weight gain so that children tend to be overweight in relation to their height. Rivkees and co-workers[768] have reported a mean 4.2-y delay between slowing of growth and the diagnosis of hypothyroidism. At diagnosis girls were 4.04 SD below and boys 3.15 SD below the mean heights for age. (This is one of several situations in which the diagnosis of short stature is made later in girls than in boys.) Body proportion is immature, with an increased upper/lower body segment ratio. Skeletal age is usually markedly delayed. Although chronic hypothyroidism is usually associated with delayed puberty, precocious puberty and premature menarche can occur in hypothyroid children (see Chapter 31).

The diagnosis of primary hypothyroidism is usually straightforward. Serum levels of T_4 are reduced, and thyrotropin levels are elevated. The presence of antithyroid antibodies (usually thyroperoxidase antibodies) is consistent with a diagnosis of Hashimoto's thyroiditis, the most common cause of acquired childhood hypothyroidism in the United States. Isolated secondary or tertiary hypothyroidism, caused by thyrotropin or thyrotropin-releasing hormone deficiency, respectively, are rare causes of hypothyroidism.

Replacement therapy results in rapid catch-up growth. Nevertheless accelerated growth may not restore full growth potential because rapid skeletal maturation is rapid during the first 18 mo of treatment. In one study of profoundly hypothyroid children, those treated at a mean chronologic age of 11 y had adult heights approximately 2 SD below the mean—final heights that were lower than midparental and predicted adult heights.[768] The deficit in adult stature correlated with the duration of hypothyroidism before initiation of treatment. In a study of hypothyroid children treated at a mean age of 9 y and with a 3-y delay of bone age,[769] mean height SD scores for bone age fell from +0.59 to −0.55 in girls and from +1.6 to −0.87 in boys. Catch-up growth may be particularly compromised when therapy is initiated near puberty.[770] Based on these studies it may be appropriate to use lower than usual replacement dosages of levothyroxine or to consider a pharmacologic delay of puberty and epiphyseal fusion, or both.

CUSHING'S SYNDROME

Glucocorticoid excess impairs skeletal growth,[771, 772] interferes with normal bone metabolism by inhibiting osteoblastic activity, and enhances bone resorption,[773–775] effects related to the duration of steroid excess,[776] regardless of whether Cushing's syndrome is due to corticotropin (also called adrenocorticotropic hormone [ACTH]) hypersecretion, adrenal tumor, or glucocorticoid administration. The effects of glucocorticoids are probably at the level of the epiphysis[655, 657, 658, 777] because GH secretion and serum concentrations of IGF peptides and IGFBPs are usually normal.[775, 778] GH treatment cannot completely overcome the growth-inhibiting effects of excess glucocorticoids, although short-term GH or IGF-I administration can diminish many of the catabolic effects.[174, 774, 779] Linear growth in children receiving glucocorticoids falls during GH therapy if the exogenous prednisone dose is less than 0.35 mg/kg/d.[775, 780] The "toxic" effects of glucocorticoids on the epiphysis may persist, in part, after correction of chronic glucocorticoid excess, and patients frequently do not attain target heights.[781, 782] The longer the duration and the greater the intensity of glucocorticoid excess, the less likely catch-up growth will be completed. Therefore exposure to excess glucocorticoids should be limited as much as the underlying condition allows, frequently by the use of alternate-day therapy.[721, 725, 780, 783]

Adrenal tumors secreting large amounts of glucocorticoids can produce excess androgens, which may mask the growth-inhibiting effects of glucocorticoids. In addition Cushing's syndrome in children may not cause all the clinical signs and symptoms associated with the disorder in adults and may present with growth arrest. However, Cushing's syndrome is an unlikely diagnosis in children with obesity because exogenous obesity is associated with normal or even accelerated skeletal growth and because growth deceleration is generally evident by the time other signs of Cushing's syndrome appear (Fig. 30–35).

PSEUDOHYPOPARATHYROIDISM

Pseudohypoparathyroidism is discussed in detail in Chapter 24 but is included here because growth failure is a common feature.[784] This condition typically combines growth failure, characteristic dysmorphic features, and hypocalcemia and hyperphosphatemia secondary to end organ resistance to parathyroid hormone. Children with pseudohypoparathyroidism are short and exhibit truncal obesity with short metacarpals, subcutaneous calcifications, round facies, and mental retardation.

RICKETS

In the past, hypovitaminosis D was a major cause of short stature, often associated with other causes of growth failure such as malnutrition, prematurity, malabsorption, hepatic disease, or chronic renal failure (see Chapters 24 and 25.). In

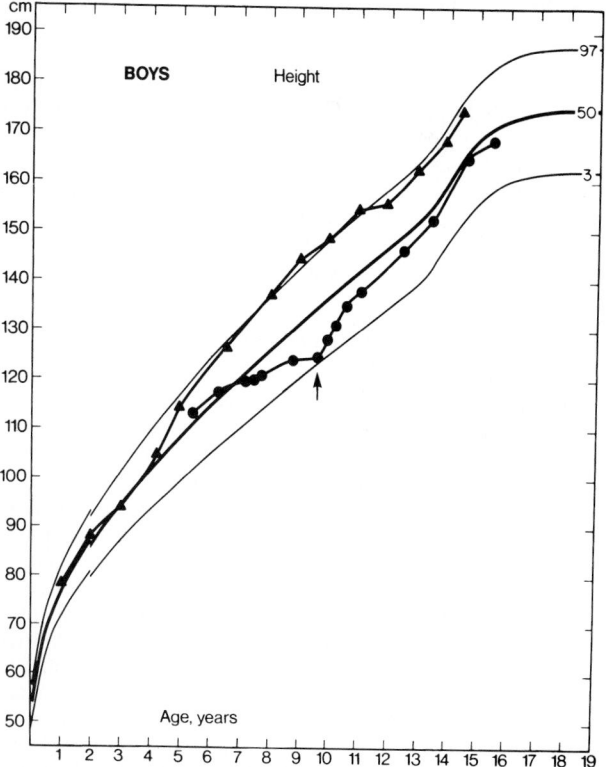

Figure 30–35. Growth curves of two boys with obesity. The boy depicted by the circles had cortisol excess related to Cushing's disease. He had an onset of rapid weight gain associated with a decrease in linear growth velocity at age 7. Diagnosis was made and an adrenalectomy *(arrow)* was performed at age 9½ with an almost immediate increase in growth rate and striking catch-up growth. The boy whose growth is depicted by triangles had exogenous obesity. At age 9½, his weight was approximately the same as that of the patient with Cushing's disease, but his height was at the 97th percentile, reflecting the enhancement of linear growth in this individual with exogenous obesity.

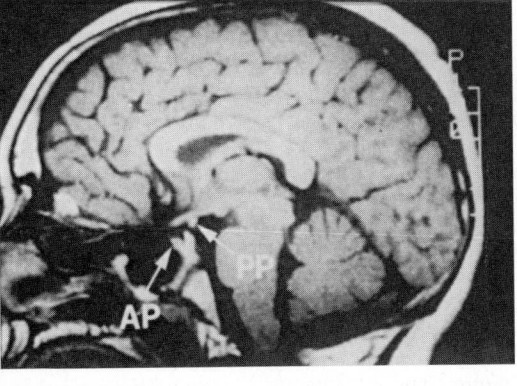

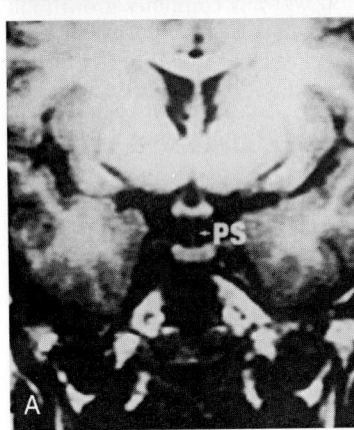

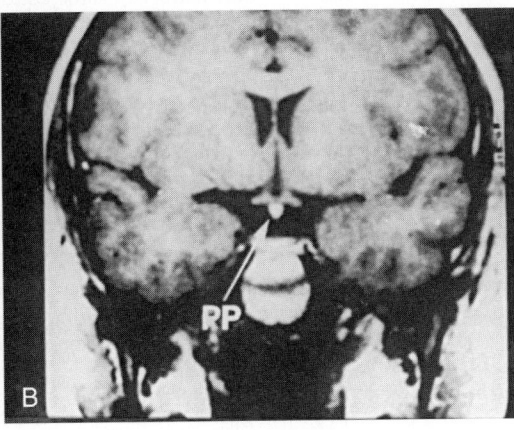

Figure 30–36. Magnetic resonance images of infundibular dysgenesis. *A,* T1-weighted sagittal and coronal images of the hypothalamic-pituitary area in a normal 8-year-old girl. The anterior (AP) and posterior pituitary (PP) lobes and the pituitary stalk (PS) are marked. *B,* T1-weighted sagittal and coronal images of the hypothalamic-pituitary area of a 17-year-old boy with isolated hGH deficiency. The anterior pituitary lobe (AP) is hypoplastic, the posterior pituitary (PP) is ectopic, and the pituitary stalk (PS) is absent. (From Root AW, Martinez CR. Magnetic resonance imaging in patients with hypopituitarism. Trends Endocrinol Metab 1992; 3:283–287, with permission.)

isolated vitamin D deficiency infants typically have poor exposure to sunlight and are not nutritionally supplemented with vitamin D. Characteristic skeletal manifestations of rickets include frontal bossing, craniotabes, rachitic rosary, and bowing of the legs. Such children usually begin to synthesize $1,25(OH)_2D$ as they become older, broaden their diet, and have increased exposure to sunlight with amelioration of the transient early decrease of linear growth velocity.

Vitamin D–Resistant (Hypophosphatemic) Rickets

Vitamin D–resistant rickets is an X-linked disorder due to decreased renal tubular reabsorption of phosphate (see Chapter 25). The features are usually more severe in boys and include short stature, prominent bowing of the legs, and (sometimes) rachitic signs.[785] The metabolic and skeletal abnormalities cannot be overcome by vitamin D therapy alone, hence the name vitamin D–resistant rickets. Treatment of hypophosphatemic rickets requires oral phosphate replacement, but such therapy may result in poor calcium absorption from the intestine. The addition of calcitriol to oral phosphate increases intestinal phosphate absorption and prevents hypocalcemia and secondary hyperparathyroidism. Such combined therapy does improve the rickets but does not necessarily correct growth.[786–791] There is no clear association between endogenous GH secretion, IGF-I, or phosphate levels and height in this disorder.[792–794] Nevertheless GH therapy, at least to age 3, has resulted in an enhancement of skeletal growth and improvement in bone mineral density.[795–798]

INSULIN-LIKE GROWTH FACTOR I DEFICIENCY

Because IGF-I is a major mediator of skeletal growth, its deficiency can result in severe growth failure. Causes of IGF-I

deficiency include (1) central hypothalamic-pituitary dysfunction with failure of pituitary GH production, i.e., hypopituitarism or GH deficiency (it may be impossible to discriminate between hypothalamic and pituitary dysfunction if both organs have the same pathologic process) and (2) primary or secondary GH resistance. This chapter uses the term IGF-I deficiency syndrome to describe the generic condition—whether caused by GH deficiency, dysfunction, or resistance—to illustrate this unifying concept.

Clinical Features of Insulin-Like Growth Factor Deficiency

Patients with IGF-I deficiency due to hypothalamic dysfunction with abnormalities of GHRH or somatostatin synthesis or secretion, primary or secondary decreased pituitary GH production, or GH resistance share a common phenotype. The similarity among these patients emphasizes the role of IGF-I in mediating most of, if not all, the anabolic and growth-promoting actions of GH. This point is further supported by the ability of IGF-I therapy to correct growth in children with mutations of the GH receptor gene (see later). Accordingly the typical clinical features of severe IGF deficiency are shared by all these conditions. If GH or IGF deficiency is acquired, clinical signs and symptoms will appear at a later age.

Birth size is normal or nearly normal in most children with IGF-I deficiency but is low in severe congenital GH deficiency, GH resistance, and in the single case of a deletion of the *IGF-I* gene.[513] Birth length and weight are typically within 10% of normal, and severe IUGR is *not* part of typical IGF deficiency but is present in infants with profound IGF deficiency, confirming the critical role of IGF-I in intrauterine growth. Infants with early-onset GH deficiency have a birth length about 2 SD below the mean.[504–506] Although at least half of infants diagnosed before age 2 y have a birth length more than 2 SD below the mean (both in isolated GH and in multiple pituitary hormone deficiencies), mean birth weight is about −1 SD, lending an appearance of relative adiposity, even in the neonatal period.[505] These data further support an intrauterine role of the GH-IGF system in growth regulation, along with the high frequency of abnormalities of the hypothalamic-pituitary area defined by magnetic resonance imaging (MRI).[112, 799] The anatomic abnormalities include dysgenesis of the pituitary stalk, ectopic placement of the posterior pituitary inferior to the median eminence, and diminished volume of the anterior pituitary (Fig. 30–36).[800–808] There is a high frequency of breech deliveries and perinatal asphyxia.[112, 504–506, 809–811] Neonatal morbidity can include hypoglycemia and prolonged jaundice with direct hyperbilirubinemia due to cholestasis and giant cell hepatitis.[812, 813] When GH deficiency is combined with deficiency of corticotropin and thyrotropin, hypoglycemia may be severe. The combination of GH deficiency with gonadotropin deficiency can cause microphallus, cryptorchidism, and hypoplasia of the scrotum.[814] GH deficiency (or GH resistance) should therefore be considered in the differential diagnosis of neonatal hypoglycemia and of microphallus-cryptorchidism.

Postnatal growth is abnormal in severe congenital IGF deficiency (Fig. 30–37). Most surveys of GH deficiency and GH resistance indicate that growth failure can occur during the first months of life.[504–506, 809] By age 6 to 12 mo the growth rate is definitely slow and deviates from the normal growth curve, with length measurements 3 to 4 SD below the mean. This stresses the importance of normal IGF-I production and action in the neonatal period and early childhood. We emphasize that the single most important clinical manifestation of IGF deficiency of all causes is growth failure, and careful documentation of growth rates is critical to making the correct diagnosis. Deviation from the normal growth curve should always be a cause of concern; growth deceleration (or acceleration) between age 2 y and the onset of puberty is *always* pathologic.

Skeletal proportions tend to be relatively normal but may correlate better with bone age than with chronologic age. Skeletal age may be delayed to less than 60% of chronologic age but in the absence of hypothyroidism is similar to the height age.[809] In acquired GH deficiency, as from a CNS tumor that causes increased intracranial pressure, bone age may approximate the chronologic age; delayed skeletal maturation should not therefore be required for the diagnosis of GH deficiency. Weight/height ratios tend to be increased, and fat distribution is often "infantile" or "doll-like" in pattern. Musculature is poor, especially in infancy, and can cause a delay in gross motor development and lead to the erroneous

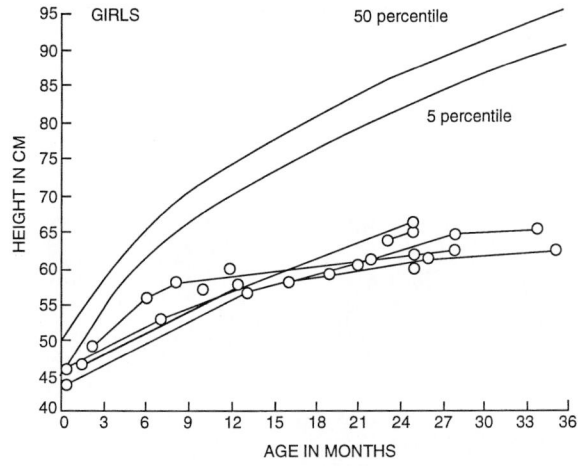

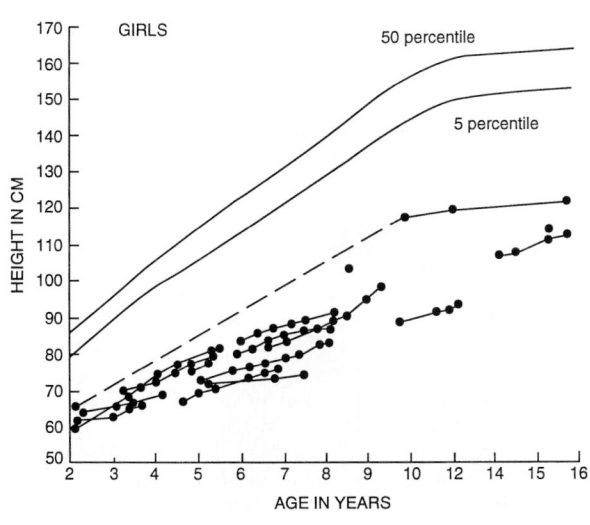

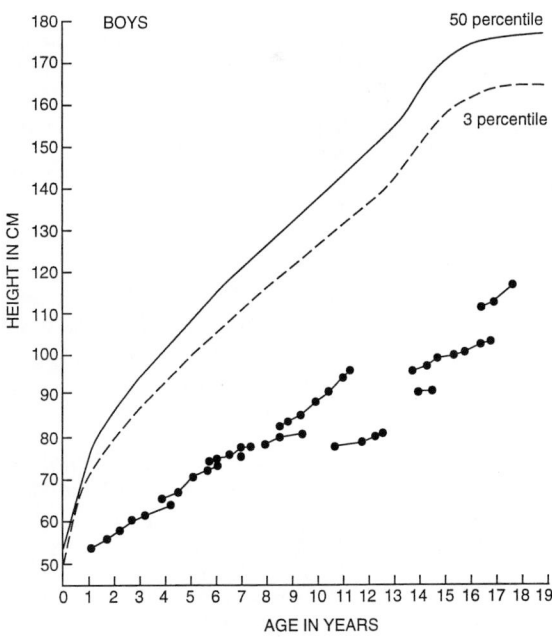

Figure 30–37. Height measurements for Ecuadorian children with IGF deficiency resulting from hGH resistance. (From Rosenfeld RG, Rosenbloom AL, Guevara-Aguirre J. Growth hormone (GH) resistance due to primary GH receptor deficiency. Endocr Rev 1994; 15:369–390. © The Endocrine Society.)

impression of mental retardation in an immature-appearing child. Facial bone growth may be particularly retarded, with an underdeveloped nasal bridge and frontal bossing (Fig. 30–38). Fontanelle closure is often delayed but the overall growth of the skull is normal, leading to cephalofacial disproportion and the appearance of hydrocephalus. The voice is infantile because of hypoplasia of the larynx. Hair growth is sparse and thin, especially during early life; nail growth is also slow. Even with normal gonadotropin production, the penis is small and puberty is usually delayed.

Final height data in patients with untreated GH deficiency are not plentiful. Wit and colleagues[1085] summarized data[815–817] from 22 untreated men and 14 untreated women with severe isolated GH deficiency who had a mean final height SD score of −4.7. In 19 patients with multiple pituitary hormone deficiencies, thus lacking in gonadal steroids, the mean final height SD score was −3.1.[817]

Causes of Insulin-Like Growth Factor I Deficiency

Two surveys of more than 22,000 GH-treated patients, in databases managed by Pharmacia (KIGS) and Genentech (National Cooperative Growth Study), cared for by pediatric endocrinologists throughout the world include more than half of the internationally treated patients.[818, 819] The patients are diverse and include individuals with GH deficiency and with gonadal dysgenesis and miscellaneous other disorders. Nonetheless about 55% of the total group, or approximately 12,000 patients, had GH deficiency (as defined by a stimulated GH level of <10 μg/L) of whom 76% had "idiopathic" GH deficiency and 24% had "acquired" or "organic" causes of GH deficiency (neoplasms, trauma, inflammation, miscellaneous). The latter group includes patients with congenital (develop-

mental) GH deficiency–associated syndromes (described later). The organic-acquired group is probably underestimated because many of the patients classified as having idiopathic GH deficiency had not had definitive assessments of the hypothalamic-pituitary region.

With the availability of synthetic IGF-I for the treatment of patients with inherited abnormalities of the GH receptor, about 200 patients with primary GH resistance have been identified. This is an exceedingly small number of individuals, even with the addition of the potentially larger group of individuals with heterozygous abnormalities of the GH receptor[820, 821] (see earlier). In contrast, patients with secondary GH resistance, including those with malnutrition or chronic systemic disease, must be considered as a potentially huge number on a worldwide basis.

An incidence of GH deficiency of 1 in 60,000 live births has been reported from the United Kingdom,[822] and a survey of Scottish schoolchildren indicated a prevalence as high as 1 in 4000 live births.[823] The best estimate in the United States population is approximately 1 in 3480 live births.[824]

CENTRAL: HYPOTHALAMIC-PITUITARY ABNORMALITIES. Many of the disorders that affect hypothalamic regulation of GH synthesis and secretion also have a direct impact on pituitary function. Consequently it is not always possible to establish definitively the primacy of hypothalamic or pituitary dysfunction, hence the term *idiopathic*. Nevertheless congenital (developmental) or functional abnormalities of the hypothalamus account for most idiopathic cases of hypopituitarism, and many such cases of GH deficiency will prove to have a molecular basis. Acquired structural damage to this area (neoplastic, traumatic, and so on) causes a quarter of GH deficiency cases.

Hypothalamic Dysfunction: Genetic Abnormalities. Hypothalamic factors involved in regulating GH synthesis and secre-

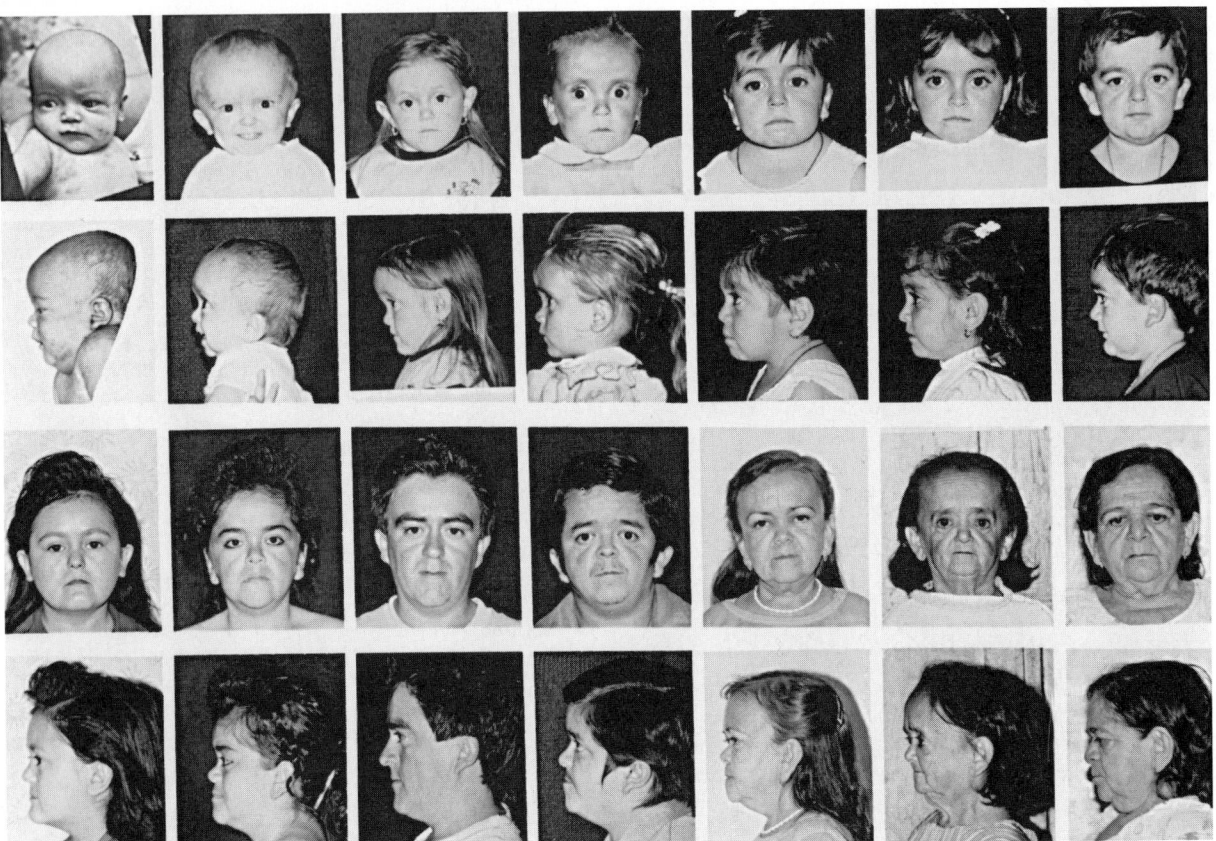

Figure 30–38. Facial appearance of Ecuadorian patients with IGF deficiency due to hGH resistance. (From Rosenfeld RG, Rosenbloom AL, Guevara-Aguirre J. Growth hormone (GH) resistance due to primary GH receptor deficiency. Endocr Rev 1994; 15:369–390. © The Endocrine Society; photography by A.L. Rosenbloom, M.D.)

tion include, but may not be limited to, GHRH,[52, 53] PACAP,[82, 83] galanin,[63] and somatostatin,[54] and mutations of the genes encoding these or other hypothalamic peptides may explain some cases of IGF deficiency due to hypothalamic dysfunction. To date, however, mutations of the genes encoding GHRH have not been identified.[825-827] A Gsh-1 homeobox gene, expressed in varied parts of the developing murine CNS,[59] plays an important role in pituitary development, as mutant strains have impaired production of GHRH with anterior pituitary hypoplasia and GH deficiency.[60] The broad impact of defects of this gene on hypothalamic releasing factors may be similar to mutations of the *Pit-1* gene, since deficiencies of prolactin and LH also occur.[60]

Congenital Malformations Involving the Hypothalamus. Hypothalamic dysfunction from congenital malformations of the brain or hypothalamus is a common cause of hypopituitarism. As noted earlier, patients with early diagnosed congenital GH deficiency frequently have an abnormal pituitary stalk, ectopia of the posterior pituitary, and hypoplasia of the anterior pituitary. Anencephaly results in a pituitary gland that is small or abnormally formed and frequently ectopic.[112, 828, 829] During intrauterine life serum GH and IGF-I levels are 30 to 50% of the normal range,[120] and pituitary GH content at birth is about 15 to 20% of normal,[112, 120] with similarly low neonatal plasma GH levels.[113, 830, 831] Holoprosencephaly, due to abnormal midline development of the embryonic forebrain, is typically associated with hypothalamic insufficiency.[832, 833] Facial dysmorphism of holoprosencephaly ranges from cyclopia to hypertelorism, accompanied by an absence of the nasal septum, midline clefts of the palate or lip, and sometimes a single central incisor. GH deficiency may be accompanied by other pituitary hormone insufficiencies. The incidence of GH deficiency is increased in cases of simple clefts of both the lip and the palate or the palate alone,[834, 835] and children with cleft palates who grow abnormally require further evaluation.

In its complete form the syndrome of septo-optic dysplasia combines hypoplasia or absence of the optic chiasm or optic nerves, or both; agenesis or hypoplasia of the septum pellucidum or corpus callosum, or both; and hypothalamic insufficiency.[835-837] The extent of the anatomic and functional abnormalities can vary.[836, 837] GH deficiency can occur by itself or in combination with deficiencies of thyrotropin, corticotropin, or gonadotropins. About 50% of children with severe anatomic defects have hypopituitarism,[112, 838] and the diagnosis should be considered in any child with growth failure associated with pendular or rotatory nystagmus or impaired vision and a small optic nerve disc. In some patients hypoplastic or interrupted pituitary stalks and ectopic posterior pituitary placement have been identified by MRI.[112] It is not clear whether this disorder is inherited but there is an increased incidence in offspring of young mothers and in first-born children.

In most patients, so-called idiopathic hypopituitarism or GH deficiency is due to abnormalities of synthesis or secretion of the hypothalamic hypophysiotropic factors.[76-78] In a number of reports idiopathic GH deficiency is associated with MRI findings of an ectopic neurohypophysis, pituitary stalk dysgenesis, and hypoplasia or aplasia of the anterior pituitary.[800-808] In series involving 341 children with isolated GH deficiency or with multiple pituitary hormone deficiencies, 54% had the characteristic MRI findings; 93% of patients with multiple pituitary hormone deficiencies were abnormal in contrast to 32% of patients with isolated GH deficiency.[803-808] Abrahams and colleagues[801] studied 35 patients with idiopathic GH deficiency and found that those with MRI abnormalities could be divided into two groups: (1) 43% had an ectopic neurohypophysis (neurohypophysis located near the median eminence), absent infundibulum, and absence of the normal posterior pituitary bright spot; (2) 43% had a small anterior pituitary,

either as an isolated finding or combined with an ectopic neurohypophysis. Overall those patients with the most striking abnormalities of the hypothalamic-pituitary region, largely those with multiple pituitary hormone deficiencies, had the smallest anterior pituitary glands.[807, 808]

Although the increased incidence of breech presentation and birth trauma with neonatal asphyxia in congenital idiopathic hypopituitarism has led some to suggest a causative role for these occurrences,[802, 804] the syndrome of pituitary stalk dysgenesis with congenital hypopituitarism is probably due to abnormal development, and the perinatal difficulties are likely to be the consequence rather than the cause of the abnormalities. Findings of a similar MRI appearance in patients with septo-optic dysplasia[112] in association with type I Arnold-Chiari syndrome and syringomyelia,[112, 807, 809] and possibly in holoprosencephaly,[112] and the occurrence of micropenis with this syndrome[112, 504-506, 814] all support the concept that congenital hypopituitarism is a malformation, not a birth injury. Further indirect evidence in studies[839] of isolated complete anterior pituitary aplasia indicates that hypothalamic hypopituitarism and breech delivery are consequences of congenital midline brain defects, although perinatal residua of breech delivery may exacerbate ischemic damage to the hypothalamic-pituitary unit.

The MRI findings described previously for patients diagnosed early with hypopituitarism are also found in children diagnosed at a later age. Most of these children have hypothalamic dysfunction as the cause of diminished pituitary hormone secretion. In the older group, as in the infants, structural, acquired hypothalamic, stalk, or pituitary abnormalities must be considered.

Trauma of the Brain and Hypothalamus. Head trauma may cause isolated GH deficiency or multiple anterior pituitary deficiencies,[840] and some series of patients with GH deficiency indicate an increased incidence of birth trauma, such as breech deliveries, extensive use of forceps, prolonged labor, or abrupt delivery.[802, 804, 810, 811] Although GH deficiency *may* be a consequence of a difficult delivery or hypoxemic perinatal period, it is more commonly an associated developmental abnormality (as discussed earlier) or due to head trauma later in life.

Inflammation of the Brain and Hypothalamus. Bacterial, viral, or fungal infections may result in hypothalamic-pituitary insufficiency,[841, 842] and the hypothalamus or pituitary, or both, may also be involved in sarcoidosis.[843]

Tumors of the Brain and Hypothalamus. Brain tumors are a major cause of hypothalamic insufficiency,[844] especially midline brain tumors, such as germinomas, meningiomas, gliomas, colloid cysts of the third ventricle, ependymomas, and gliomas of the optic nerve. Although metastasis from extracranial carcinomas is rare in children, hypothalamic insufficiency can result from local extension of craniopharyngeal carcinoma or Hodgkin's disease of the nasopharynx. Craniopharyngiomas and histiocytosis can cause hypothalamic dysfunction but are discussed in the section on pituitary GH deficiency.

Radiation of the Brain and Hypothalamus. Cranial radiation appears to be an increasing cause of hypothalamic-pituitary dysfunction.[21, 845-850] Radiation may impair both hypothalamic and pituitary function and it is often not easy to discriminate between damage at the two levels. The hypothalamus is more radiosensitive than is the pituitary and is more often the site of damage, especially in the dose range usually given to children with malignancy.[848] Thyroidal and gonadal function may also be directly impaired by certain radiation therapies. The degree of pituitary dysfunction is a function of the dose of radiation received. Low doses typically cause isolated GH deficiency and higher doses cause multiple pituitary deficiencies. Within 5 y of radiation, nearly 100% of children receiving greater than or equal to 3000 Gy over 3 wk to the hypothalamic-pituitary axis had subnormal GH responses to provocative tests.[844, 849, 850] The degree of pituitary deficiency is also a function of the length of time after radiation[851]; children who test normally 1 y after therapy may acquire pituitary deficiencies later. Prior to the development of GH secretory deficiency, GH resistance with low levels of IGF-I, IGFBP-3, and GHBP (presumably caused by the malignancy and the intensive chemotherapy and radiotherapy regimens) may decrease growth velocity.[852, 853] Chemotherapy regimens by themselves may impair final adult height, although not nearly to the extent seen after radiation.[853, 854] Even when serum GH responses to provocative testing are normal, spontaneous GH secretion may be blunted at x-ray doses as low as 1800 to 2400 Gy.[855] Although acquired GH deficiency impairs final height,[854, 856] the relation of diminished GH production to levels of the GH-dependent peptides IGF-I and IGFBP-3 is variable.[857, 858] With long-term follow-up, however, correlations were found among nocturnal GH secretion, levels of IGF-I and IGFBP-3, and pituitary size.[857]

Poor linear growth from decreased GH secretion may be exacerbated by impact radiation itself and by an inadequate pubertal acceleration of spinal growth.[848, 850, 859–861] Surprisingly, cranial radiation can result in precocious puberty, especially in children undergoing radiation at a young age,[862–864] causing early epiphyseal fusion. Sexual precocity appears to occur more frequently with low doses of radiation,[862, 865] and gonadotropin deficiency is likely at high doses.[866] The rate of pubertal progression, however, does not appear to be accelerated.[863] Treatment with LHRH analogues may be necessary to suppress the hypothalamic-pituitary gonadal axis in an attempt to attain normal final height.[867]

Three possibilities must be considered in following children after craniospinal radiation: evolving hypopituitarism, decreased spinal growth potential, and early puberty with premature epiphyseal fusion. Children with documented GH deficiency and growth failure are candidates for exogenous GH treatment[848, 863, 868]; there is no evidence for enhanced relapses of the primary neoplasm in patients treated with GH,[869, 870] but there appears to be a variable growth response to GH[863, 871, 872]; spinal growth impairment, inadequate or delayed treatment, and sexual precocity may limit linear growth.

Bone marrow transplantation (BMT) for patients with inborn errors of metabolism, aplastic anemias, and malignancies requires preparative regimens that include total lymphoid or total body radiation, often with chemotherapy and sometimes including cranial radiation.[868, 873] Children in whom the clinical condition requires modest treatment programs before BMT have minimal loss of growth after BMT.[868, 873–875] In children who had cranial radiation followed by high-dose chemotherapy and total body radiation (especially in a single dose) as preparative regimens, growth failure is almost inevitable 2 to 5 y after BMT.[875–880] Pubertal growth is most affected.[875] If the total body radiation is fractionated and if cranial radiation was not previously needed, growth velocity and height 3 y after BMT are not compromised.[57, 873, 879, 880] In the absence of cranial radiation, there is a poor correlation between GH production and levels of IGF-I or IGFBP-3 and growth in children after BMT,[868, 880, 881] suggesting the importance of factors such as nutrition and radiation-induced vertebral dysplasia or hypothyroidism.[882] Mean final height data in 28 long-term survivors of BMT were about 1 SD lower than those at the time of transplantation but still within the normal range in all except one patient[883]; such data suggest a conservative approach with regard to exogenous hormonal treatment.

Psychosocial Dwarfism. An extreme form of "failure to thrive" is termed *psychosocial dwarfism* or *emotional deprivation dwarfism.*[884–886] Most cases of failure to thrive can be traced back to a poor home environment and inadequate parenting, with improved weight gain and growth on removal of the infant from the dysfunctional home. Some children have dramatic behavioral manifestations beyond those in the typical infant with failure to thrive, namely bizarre eating and drinking habits, such as drinking from toilets, social withdrawal, and primitive speech.[885] Hyperphagia and abnormalities of GH production are associated.[887] Studies have shown that GH secretion was low in response to pharmacologic stimuli but returned to normal on removal from the home. Concomitantly, eating and behavioral habits returned to normal, and a period of catch-up growth ensued. Careful assessment of endogenous GH secretion showed reversal of the GH insufficiency within 3 wk, including enhancement of GH pulse amplitude and a variable increase in pulse frequency.[887–889] The reversibility of GH secretion and the later growth increment in the context of the clinical findings described earlier confirm the diagnosis of psychosocial dwarfism.[886, 889–891]

The neuroendocrinologic mechanisms involved in psychosocial dwarfism remain to be elucidated. GH secretion is abnormal and corticotropin and thyrotropin levels may also be low, although some patients have high plasma cortisol levels.[886] Even when GH secretion is reduced, treatment with GH is not usually of benefit until the psychosocial situation is improved.[886] Management of the environmental causes of the growth failure is imperative and often associated with substantial growth. In our experience although psychosocial dysfunction is a common cause of failure to thrive in infancy, the constellation of bizarre behaviors described in psychosocial dwarfism is rare.

The fact that GH production is impaired in adults with varied psychiatric disorders,[892, 893] as well as the growth aberrations of functional GH deficiency with psychosocial dwarfism, suggests that children with emotional problems may have impaired GH secretion and growth.[894] Indeed depression in children, as in adults, can lower GH production,[895] and in girls anxiety disorders predict a modest height loss in adults.[894]

Growth Hormone Neurosecretory Dysfunction. Because tests of GH secretion after pharmacologic provocation may not accurately reflect normal GH secretion, it has been argued that a subset of children with "GH neurosecretory dysfunction" may be identified by frequent or continuous serum sampling over a 12- to 24-h period.[896, 897] This condition is characterized by short stature and poor growth, normal serum GH response to provocative testing, and reduced IGF-I and 24-h serum GH levels. Prior cranial radiation may be the most common cause of these findings. Patients with *idiopathic short stature* (see later) do not appear to have diminished 24-h GH production rates, especially when the broad range of data in normal and short normal children is considered.[71, 103, 898–900] There appears to be little doubt that some children with "GH neurosecretory dysfunction" secrete insufficient amounts of GH, even if they pass provocative GH testing; whether they should be identified by 24-h GH sampling or by determination of the GH-dependent peptides is unclear.

Pituitary Growth Hormone Deficiency. As discussed earlier, many of the disease processes that impair hypothalamic regulation of GH secretion also impair pituitary function. Another group of abnormalities specifically affect pituitary somatotrope development and function.

Genetic Abnormalities of Growth Hormone Production and Secretion. As many as 3 to 30% of children with GH deficiency have an affected parent, sibling, or child,[825, 826, 901–903] and several genetic causes of GH deficiency have been described.[902, 904] We discuss inborn errors of the *Pit-1,* GHRH receptor, and *GH* genes, each of which can cause GH deficiency and IGF deficiency.

The *Pit-1* (GHF-1) gene (chromosome 3) is a member of a large family of transcription factors, referred to as POU-domain proteins, and is responsible for pituitary-specific transcription of genes for GH, prolactin, thyrotropin, and the GHRH receptor.[84, 86, 87] Additionally Pit-1 activates transcription of genes that regulate differentiation, proliferation, and survival of somatotropes, lactotropes, and thyrotropes.[826, 902, 905, 906] At least seven point mutations of the *Pit-1* gene have been found in Dutch, American, Japanese, and Tunisian families with GH deficiency and prolactin deficiency and variable defects in thyrotropin secretion.[827, 902, 907–911] These mutations of the *Pit-1* gene are transmitted as autosomal recessive or co-dominant traits and cause variable peptide hormone deficiencies with or without anterior pituitary hypoplasia.[827, 902, 908–913] Phenotypic variability can occur among patients with apparently similar genotypes.[913] The mutations involve sites affecting Pit-1 DNA-binding, dimerization, or target gene *trans*-activation. Both Snell (dw/dw) and Jackson (dw/dwJ) dwarf mice have GH, prolactin, and thyrotropin deficiency and mutations or rearrangements of the *Pit-1* gene.[914, 915]

Wajnrajch and co-workers[916] reported the first human cases of a mutation in the GHRH receptor gene (chromosome 7) in two cousins with IGF deficiency. The gene defect resulted in a truncated GHRH receptor protein that lacked the membrane-spanning regions and the G-protein–binding site. The affected children had undetectable GH release during standard provocative tests and after exogenous GHRH administration but responded to GH treatment. Another series of 18 patients with the same point mutation was found in Pakistan ("dwarfism of Sindh").[917] Mutation of the gene for the GHRH receptor in its ligand-binding domain has also been identified in the *little* mouse (lit/lit), leading to dwarfism and decreased numbers of somatotropes,[905, 918, 919] but in this model the fetal somatotrope mass is normal, and hypoplasia, but not absence of the somatotropes, is evident postnatally only.[905, 906, 918, 919] These data suggest that GHRH is not an essential factor for fetal differentiation of the somatotropes and that GHRH-independent cells persist or that mutation does not cause total loss of GHRH function.

Four forms of isolated GH deficiency due to errors of the GH gene have been reported (Table 30–6).[825, 826, 901, 920, 921] The gene encoding GH *(GH-1)* is located on chromosome 17 in a cluster that includes two genes for placental lactogen, a pseudogene for human placental lactogen, and the *GH-2* gene that encodes placental GH.[825, 901] Isolated GH deficiency IA results from deletions or mutations of the *GH-1* gene that prevent synthesis or secretion of the hormone.[922] Isolated GH deficiency IA is inherited as an autosomal recessive trait and affected individuals have profound congenital GH deficiency. Since GH is not produced even in fetal life, patients are immunologically intolerant of GH and typically acquire anti-GH antibodies when treated with either pituitary-derived or recombinant DNA-derived GH. When antibodies prevent patients from responding to GH, isolated GH deficiency IA can be viewed as a form of GH resistance, and such patients are candidates for IGF-I therapy (see later). The less severe form of autosomal recessive GH deficiency (isolated GH deficiency IB) also results from mutations or rearrangements of the *GH-1* gene, which cause production of a GH molecule that retains some function. These patients usually respond to exogenous GH therapy. In a group of 65 children with isolated GH deficiency IB, the GHRH receptor gene was normal.[923]

Isolated GH deficiency II is inherited as an autosomal dominant trait. If such patients also prove to have abnormalities of the *GH-1* gene, it is likely that they function in a dominant-negative manner. Isolated GH deficiency III is transmitted as an X-linked trait. Despite extensive assessment mutations of the gene encoding GHRH, which causes a similar phenotype, have not been identified.[825–827] Mutations causing constitutive or enhanced ligand-mediated activation of the G-protein–related somatostatin receptor to yield chronic inhibition of GH also have not yet been reported.

Trauma. See earlier discussion.

Inflammation. See earlier discussion.

Tumors Involving the Pituitary. Many tumors that impair hypothalamic function also impair pituitary secretion of GH.[844] In addition, *craniopharyngiomas* are a major cause of pituitary insufficiency.[924, 925] These tumors arise from remnants of Rathke's pouch, which is the diverticulum of the roof of the embryonic oral cavity that normally gives rise to the anterior pituitary. This tumor is a congenital malformation present at birth and gradually grows over the ensuing years. The tumor arises from rests of squamous cells at the junction of the adenohypophysis and neurohypophysis and it forms a cyst as it enlarges, which contains degenerated cells and may calcify but does not undergo malignant degeneration. The cyst fluid ranges from a "machinery oil" to a shimmering cholesterol-laden liquid, and the calcifications may be microscopic or gross.[926] About 75% of craniopharyngiomas arise in the su-

TABLE 30–6. Classification of Familial Human Growth Hormone Deficiency

	Genetics	Endogenous Growth Hormone	Response to Growth Hormone	Associated Deficiencies	Molecular Basis
Isolated Human Growth Hormone Deficiency					
1A	AR	Absent	Transient	—	GH1 deletion or mutation
1B	AR	Reduced	+	—	? hGH1 mutation
II	AD	Reduced	+	—	? Dominant negative
III	X-Linked	Reduced	+	—	?
Multiple Pituitary Deficiencies					
I	AR	Reduced	+	LH, FSH, thyrotropin, ± corticotropin	?
IB	AR	Absent or severely reduced	+	Prolactin, thyrotropin	*Pit-1* mutation or deletion
II	X-Linked	Reduced	+	LH, FSH, thyrotropin	?

LH, luteinizing hormone; FSH, follicle-stimulating hormone.

prasellar region, the remainder resembling pituitary adenomas.[926–931]

Craniopharyngiomas can cause manifestations at any age from infancy to adulthood, but they usually occur in middle childhood. The most common presentation is due to increased intracranial pressure, including headaches, vomiting, and oculomotor abnormalities. Visual field defects may result from compression of the optic chiasm, and papilledema or optic atrophy may be present. Visual and olfactory hallucinations have been reported, as have seizures and dementia. Most children with craniopharyngiomas have evidence of growth failure at the time of presentation. GH and the gonadotropins are the most commonly affected pituitary hormones in children and adults, but deficiency of thyrotropin or corticotropin, or both, may also occur; diabetes insipidus is present in 25 to 50% of these patients.[926–928, 932] Fifty to 80% of patients have abnormalities of at least one anterior pituitary hormone at diagnosis.[927, 932] Although lateral skull films may demonstrate enlargement or distortion of the sella turcica, frequently accompanied by suprasellar calcifications, some children have normal plain films. Magnetic resonance imaging is the most sensitive diagnostic technique, allowing identification of cystic and solid components and delineation of anatomic relationships necessary for a rational operative approach. Operative intervention may result in partial or almost complete removal of the lesion. In some patients, especially those who become obese, a syndrome of normal linear growth without GH may occur. The circulating growth-promoting substance or substances in this condition include insulin and other poorly characterized mitogens.[933]

Pituitary adenomas are infrequent during childhood and adolescence, accounting for less than 5% of patients operated on at large centers[930, 931, 934] (see Chapter 9). Nearly two thirds of tumors stain immunochemically for prolactin, and a small number stain positive for GH. GH-secreting pituitary adenomas are exceedingly unusual in youth. There is a variable experience as to the invasive nature of pituitary adenomas, although the prevailing opinion is that they are less aggressive in children than in adults.[930, 934] In 56 patients at the Mayo Clinic with non–corticotropin-secreting adenomas removed transsphenoidally, macroadenomas were about one-third more frequent than microadenomas, girls outnumbering boys 3.3:1.[930] The macroadenoma patients had about a 50% incidence of hypopituitarism, compared with none in patients with microadenomas; long-term cure rates were 55 to 65% for both tumor sizes.

The localized or generalized proliferation of mononuclear macrophages (histiocytes) characterizes Langerhans cell histiocytosis, a diverse disorder occurring at all ages, with a peak incidence at ages 1 to 4.[935] Endocrinologists are more familiar with the term histiocytosis X, which includes three related disorders: solitary bony disease (eosinophilic granuloma), Hand-Schüller-Christian disease (chronic disease with diabetes insipidus, exophthalmos, and multiple calvarial lesions), and disseminated histiocytosis X (Letterer-Siwe disease, with widespread visceral involvement). These syndromes are characterized by an infiltration and accumulation of Langerhans cells in the involved areas, such as skull, hypothalamic-pituitary stalk, CNS, and viscera. Although these disorders, especially Hand-Schüller-Christian disease, are classically associated with diabetes insipidus, approximately 50 to 60% of patients in selected series have growth failure and GH deficiency at the time of presentation,[936, 937] in contrast to only 1% of children with Langerhans cell histiocytosis living in Canada during a 15-y period.[938] GH deficiency may be isolated or may be associated with deficiencies of other pituitary hormones.

Bioinactive Growth Hormone. Serum GH exists in multiple molecular forms, the consequences of alternative post-transcriptional or post-translational processing of the mRNA or protein, respectively (see earlier). Some of these forms are presumed to have defects in the amino acid sequences required for binding of GH to its receptor, and different molecular forms of GH may have varying potencies for stimulating skeletal growth, although this remains to be rigorously proved. It has been suggested that some cases of short stature may be characterized by serum GH forms with normal immunoreactivity but reduced biopotency.[939, 940] The molecular abnormalities in such situations have not been characterized. Takahashi and colleagues[941] described a child with extreme short stature (−6.1 SD scores) with a mutant GH caused by a single missense mutation (cys to arg, codon 77 of *GH-1* gene) that bound with greater affinity than normal to GHBP and the GH receptor and inhibited the action of normal GH. The child grew appreciably during a period of exogenous GH administration in moderate dosage. Strangely the father had the same genetic abnormality but did not express the mutant hormone.

PERIPHERAL: INHERITED AND ACQUIRED SYNDROMES OF RESISTANCE TO GROWTH HORMONE ACTION (Table 30–7)

Growth Hormone Resistance. GH resistance describes a condition in which patients have the phenotype of GH deficiency but normal or elevated serum GH levels and diminished production of IGF-I (Fig. 30–39; Table 30–8).[137, 942] These individuals clearly have IGF-I deficiency. *Primary* GH resistance denotes (1) abnormalities of the GH receptor, including the extracellular GH-binding domain, the extracellular GH receptor dimerization domain, or the intracellular domain; (2) postreceptor abnormalities of GH signal transduction; and (3) primary defects of IGF-I biosynthesis. *Secondary* GH resistance is an acquired and relatively common condition that can be due to (1) malnutrition; (2) hepatic, renal, and other chronic diseases; (3) circulating antibodies to GH; and (4) antibodies to the GH receptor. Illness-related GH resistance is discussed in the specific text sections.

The initial report by Laron and colleagues of primary GH resistance described "...three siblings with hypoglycemia and other clinical and laboratory signs of growth hormone deficiency, but with abnormally high levels of immunoreactive serum growth hormone."[943] To date approximately 200 cases have been identified worldwide,[137] most from the Mediterranean region or from Ecuador (presumed Spanish conversos, that is, Jews who converted to Christianity).[944] These individuals do not respond to exogenous GH in terms of growth, metabolic changes, or increases in serum levels of IGF-I and IGFBP-3.[96] Cellular unresponsiveness to GH was demonstrated in vitro by the failure of GH to stimulate erythroid progenitor cells from the peripheral blood of patients,[945] and direct evidence of receptor dysfunction was provided by the demonstration that microsomes obtained by liver biopsy do not bind radiolabeled GH.[946]

TABLE 30–7. Classification of Growth Hormone Resistance Syndromes

Primary GH resistance syndromes (Laron syndrome; hereditary-congenital defects)
    GH receptor deficiency (encompassing quantitative and qualitative defects in the GH receptor)
    Abnormalities of GH signal transduction (postreceptor defects)
    Primary defects of synthesis of IGF-I
Secondary GH resistance syndromes (acquired conditions; sometimes transitory)
    Circulating antibodies to GH that inhibit GH action
    Antibodies to the GH receptor
    GH resistance caused by malnutrition
    GH resistance caused by liver disease
    Other conditions that cause GH resistance

GH, growth hormone; IGF-I, insulin-like growth factor I.
From Laron Z, Blum W, Chatelain P, et al. Classification of growth hormone insensitivity syndrome. J Pediatr 122:241, 1993, with permission.

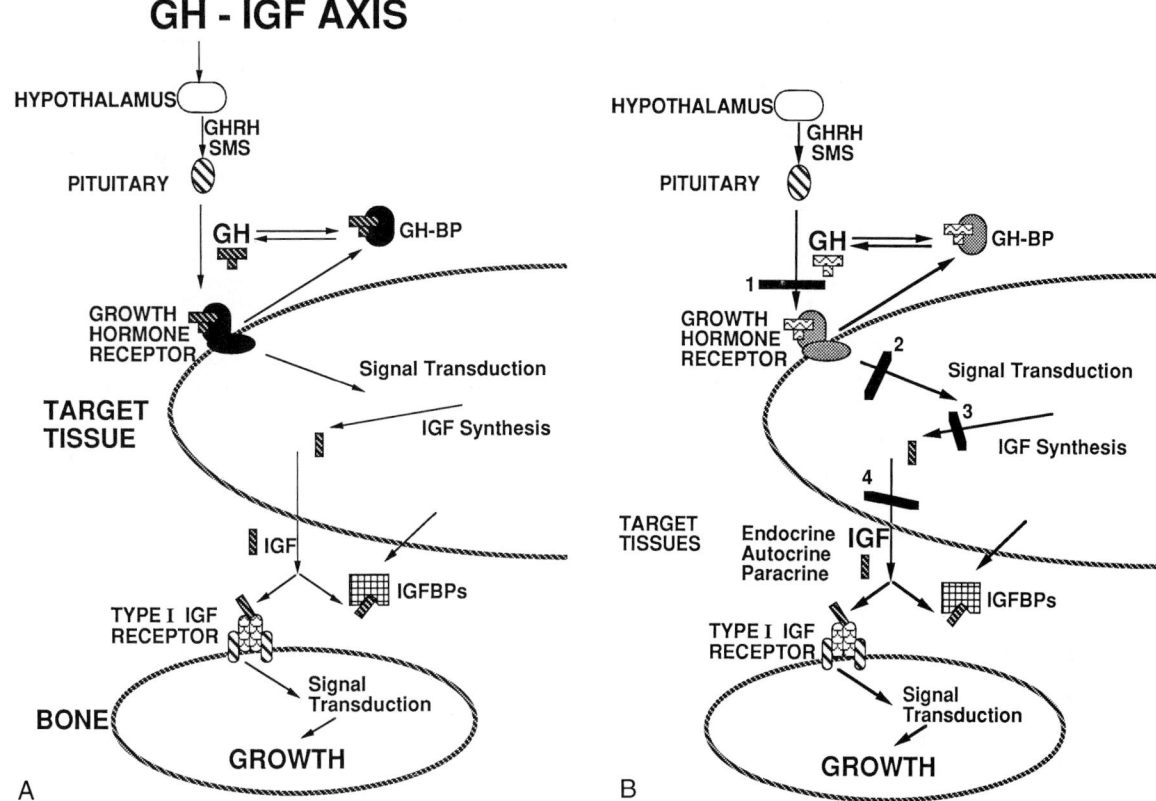

Figure 30–39. The normal hGH-IGF axis (A) and the hGH-IGF axis showing four potential biochemical defects capable of causing hGH resistance (B): abnormalities of the GH receptor or binding protein, or both (1); abnormal signal transduction, resulting from a defect in the intracellular domain of the GH receptor or postreceptor (2); defect of IGF synthesis (3); defect of IGF secretion (4). (From Rosenfeld RG, Rosenbloom AL, Guevara-Aguirre J. Growth hormone (GH) resistance due to primary GH receptor deficiency. Endocr Rev 1994; 15:369–390. © The Endocrine Society.)

GHBP activity is undetectable in the sera of patients with this disorder.[160, 161] When GHBP was purified and the cDNA was cloned and sequenced, it was found to be virtually identical to the extracellular domain of the GH receptor.[139] Studies of the GH receptor gene in Israeli patients indicated that some, but not most, contained gene deletions,[947] and a wide

TABLE 30–8. Clinical Features of Growth Hormone Resistance

Growth and Development

Birth weight: near normal
Birth length: may be slightly decreased
Postnatal growth: severe growth failure
Bone age: delayed, but may be advanced relative to height age
Genitalia: micropenis in childhood; normal for body size in adults
Puberty: delayed 3–7 y
Sexual function and fertility: normal

Craniofacies

Hair: sparse before age 7
Forehead: prominent; frontal bossing
Skull: normal head circumference; craniofacial disproportion due to small facies
Facies: small
Nasal bridge: hypoplastic
Orbits: shallow
Dentition: delayed eruption
Sclerae: blue
Voice: high-pitched

Musculoskeletal, Metabolic, Miscellaneous

Hypoglycemia: in infants and children; fasting symptoms in some adults
Walking and motor milestones: delayed
Hips: dysplasia; avascular necrosis of femoral head
Elbow: limited extensibility
Skin: thin, prematurely aged osteopenia

variety of point mutations in this gene (missense, nonsense, and abnormal splicing) have subsequently been identified (Table 30–9).[137, 948, 949] Most of the mutations are in the extracellular (GH-binding) domain of the GH receptor, and one mutation of the extracellular domain does not affect GH binding but prevents dimerization of the receptor.[950] In these situations the genotype does not uniformly characterize the phenotype. There is one report of a patient with two separate amino acid substitutions in the intracellular domain, but because both mutations are on the same allele, which comes from the unaffected mother, the diagnosis of GH resistance in this patient is in doubt.[951] Chujo and colleagues[952] additionally found that a specific heterozygous missense exon 10 (which codes for most of the GH receptor intracellular domain) mutation[951] was present in 14 of 96 volunteers; there was no significant impact on stature, suggesting that this mutation represents a normal polymorphism. Another individual with compound heterozygous mutations in exon 10 was extremely short (−4 SD scores) but grew in response to a very high dose of GH.[953] At this time inadequate data exist to determine whether these intracellular domain substitutions represent genuine mutations or innocent polymorphisms. Woods and co-workers[954] described two cousins with severe GH resistance and homozygous mutations at the splice site of exon 8, resulting in a mutant GH receptor without functional transmembrane or intracellular domains. Serum levels of GHBP were elevated as the mutant receptor protein apparently becomes detached from the cell receptor surface. Heterozygosity for defects of the GH receptor may cause relative GH resistance,[820, 821, 955] with modest growth occurring only in response to high doses of GH. Such observations raise the important issue of whether heterozygosity for GH resistance can result in

TABLE 30–9. Mutations of the Growth Hormone Receptor Gene

Category	Ethnicity	Nucleotides	Exon (Intron)	Amino Acids	Extra/Intra	Growth Hormone–Binding Protein	Physiology
Missense	United States	184: G-A	4	E44K	Extra	Negative	Double heterozygous
Missense	Mediterranean	266: G-A	4	R71K	Extra	Negative	
Missense	Mediterranean	341: T-C	5	F96S	Extra	Negative	
Missense	European	428: T-C	5	V125A	Extra	Negative	
Missense	Mediterranean	485: T-A	6	V144D	Extra	Negative	
Missense	Asian	508: G-C	6	D152H	Extra	Positive	
Missense	Middle East	535: C-T	6	R161C	Extra	Negative	
Missense	United States	535: C-T	6	R161C	Extra	Negative	Double heterozygous
Missense	Mediterranean	685: C-G	7	R211G	Extra	Negative	
Missense	United States	686: G-A	7	R211H	Extra	Negative	Heterozygous
Missense	United States	726: G-A	7	E224D	Extra	Negative	Heterozygous
Missense	United States	1362: G-T	10	C422F	Intra (exon 10)	Positive	
Missense	United States	1778: C-A	10	P561T	Intra (exon 10)	Positive	
Nonsense	Europe	168: C-A	4	C38X	Extra	Negative	
Nonsense	Mediterranean	168: C-A	4	C38X	Extra	Negative	
Nonsense	Mediterranean	181: C-T	4	R43X	Extra	Negative	
Nonsense	Ecuador	181: C-T	4	R43X	Extra	Negative	
Nonsense	United States	418: T-A	5	C122X	Extra	Negative	Heterozygous
Nonsense	Mexico		6	E183X	Extra	Negative	
Nonsense	Middle East	703: C-T	7	R217X	Extra	Negative	
Nonsense	United States	703: C-T	7	R217X	Extra	Negative	
Splice	Europe	266 + 1: G-A	exon 4/intron 4	Splice 71 + 1	Extra	Negative	Splice 5' intron 4
Splice	Mediterranean	266 + 1: G-A	exon 4/intron 4	Splice 71 + 1	Extra	Negative	Splice 5' intron 4
Splice	Mediterranean	440 − 1: G-C	intron 5/exon 6	Splice 130 − 1	Extra	Negative	
Splice	Ecuador	594: A-G	6	Splice E180	Extra	Negative	
Splice	Israel	594: A-G	6	Splice E180	Extra	Negative	
Splice	Brazil	610 − 1: G-T	intron 6/exon 7	Splice 189 − 1	Extra	Negative	Splice 3' intron 6
Splice	United Kingdom		8	Splice: R274T	Trans/Intra	Positive	Lose exons 8–10
Frameshift	Mediterranean	192–193 del TT	4	46 del TT	Extra	Negative	
Frameshift	South Africa	743–744 del TA or AT	7	230 del TA or AT	Extra	Negative	

a clinically important phenotype and whether some children labeled as having "idiopathic short stature" may harbor such mutations (see later). Given the requirement for dimerization of the GH receptor, there is the potential for an abnormal protein to have a dominant negative effect.

The clinical features of GH resistance due to GH receptor deficiency are identical to those of other forms of severe IGF deficiency, such as congenital GH deficiency (see Table 30–8). Basal serum GH levels are typically elevated in children but may be normal in adults (Fig. 30–40). Most patients have decreased serum GHBP levels, but a normal serum GHBP concentration does not exclude the diagnosis of GH receptor deficiency, since mutations of the GH receptor dimerization domain and of the intracellular domain have been identified. Serum IGF-I, IGF-II, and IGFBP-3 levels are profoundly reduced (Fig. 30–41).

Woods and colleagues[513] described a 15-year-old boy with a partial deletion of the *IGF-I* gene yielding a truncated IGF-I molecule. Severe prenatal and postnatal (−6.7 SD scores) growth retardation and resistance to exogenous GH were consistent with the expectations of the phenotype of IGF-I deficiency. Sensorineural deafness, mental retardation, and microcephaly suggest a role for prenatal IGF-I in CNS development. Although IGF-I levels were exceedingly low, IGFBP-3 and GHBP levels were normal.

Diagnosis of Insulin-Like Growth Factor Deficiency Syndrome: Growth Hormone Deficiency

Since the proper means of diagnosing GH deficiency is controversial,[956] the concept of the IGF deficiency syndrome becomes even more relevant. With the availability of highly specific assays for the IGF peptides and binding proteins and

with increasing understanding of the GH-IGF axis, evaluation of patients with growth failure should include a combination of careful auxologic assessment and appropriate measures of the GH-IGF system. Documenting a deficiency of IGF levels and concomitant alterations in serum concentrations of IGFBPs suggests an abnormality of GH secretion or activity and makes a thorough evaluation of hypothalamic-pituitary-IGF function necessary.

The foundation for the diagnosis of IGF deficiency is the careful documentation of serial heights and determination of height velocity. In the absence of other evidence of pituitary GH secretory dysfunction it is usually unnecessary to perform tests of GH secretion. Thus even in children below the 5th percentile in height (which obviously applies to 5% of the normal population), documentation of a normal height velocity (above the 25th percentile for several years) makes the diagnosis of IGF deficiency and GH deficiency highly unlikely.

Assessment of pituitary GH production is difficult because GH secretion is pulsatile, with the most consistent surges occurring at times of slow-wave electroencephalographic rhythms during phases 3 and 4 of sleep. The regulation of GH secretion involves at least two hypothalamic factors, GHRH and somatostatin, and multiple other peptides and neurotransmitters. Spontaneous GH secretion varies with gender, age, pubertal stage, and nutritional status, all of which must be factored into the evaluation of GH production.

Between normal pulses of GH secretion, serum GH levels are low (often <0.1 μg/L), below the limits of sensitivity of most conventional assays (usually <1 μg/L). Accordingly measurement of a random serum GH concentration is virtually useless in diagnosing GH deficiency but may be useful in the diagnosis of GH resistance and GH excess. Measurement of GH "secretory reserve" therefore relies on the use of physiologic or pharmacologic stimuli, and such "provocative

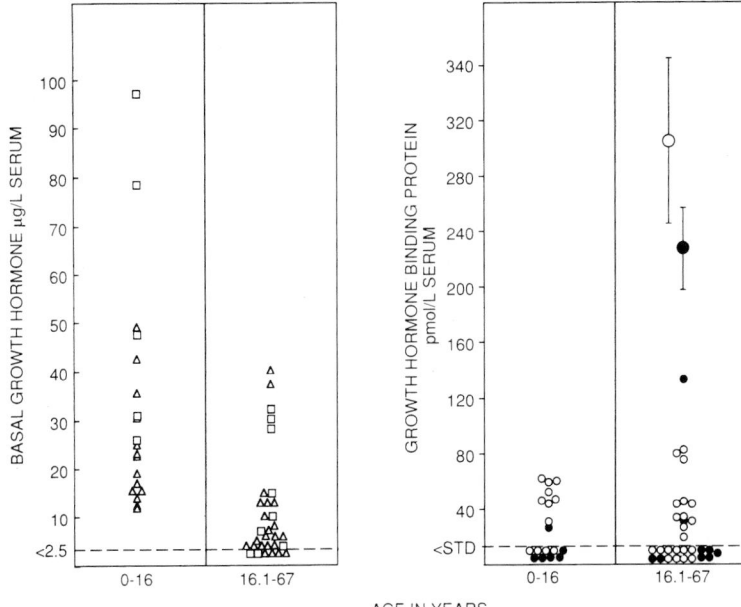

Figure 30–40. Serum hGH and GHBP levels in the sera of patients with GH receptor deficiency from Ecuador. (From Rosenfeld RG, Rosenbloom AL, Guevara-Aguirre J. Growth hormone (GH) resistance due to primary GH receptor deficiency. Endocr Rev 1994; 15:369–390. © The Endocrine Society.)

tests" have been the basis for the diagnosis of GH deficiency for more than 30 y.[956, 957] "Physiological" stimuli include fasting, sleep,[958] and exercise,[959, 960] and pharmacologic stimuli include levodopa,[961] clonidine,[962] glucagon,[963] propranolol, arginine,[964] and insulin.[965, 966] Stimulation tests have often been divided into "screening tests" (exercise, fasting, levodopa, clonidine), which are characterized by ease of administration, low toxicity, low risk, and low specificity, and "definitive tests" (arginine, insulin, glucagon). To improve specificity, provocative tests are customarily combined or given sequentially.[967–969] We have, e.g., often used fasting plus oral clonidine as a "screening test," to be followed by fasting plus intravenous sequential arginine or levodopa and insulin as a "definitive test." It is generally accepted that a child must "fail" provoca-

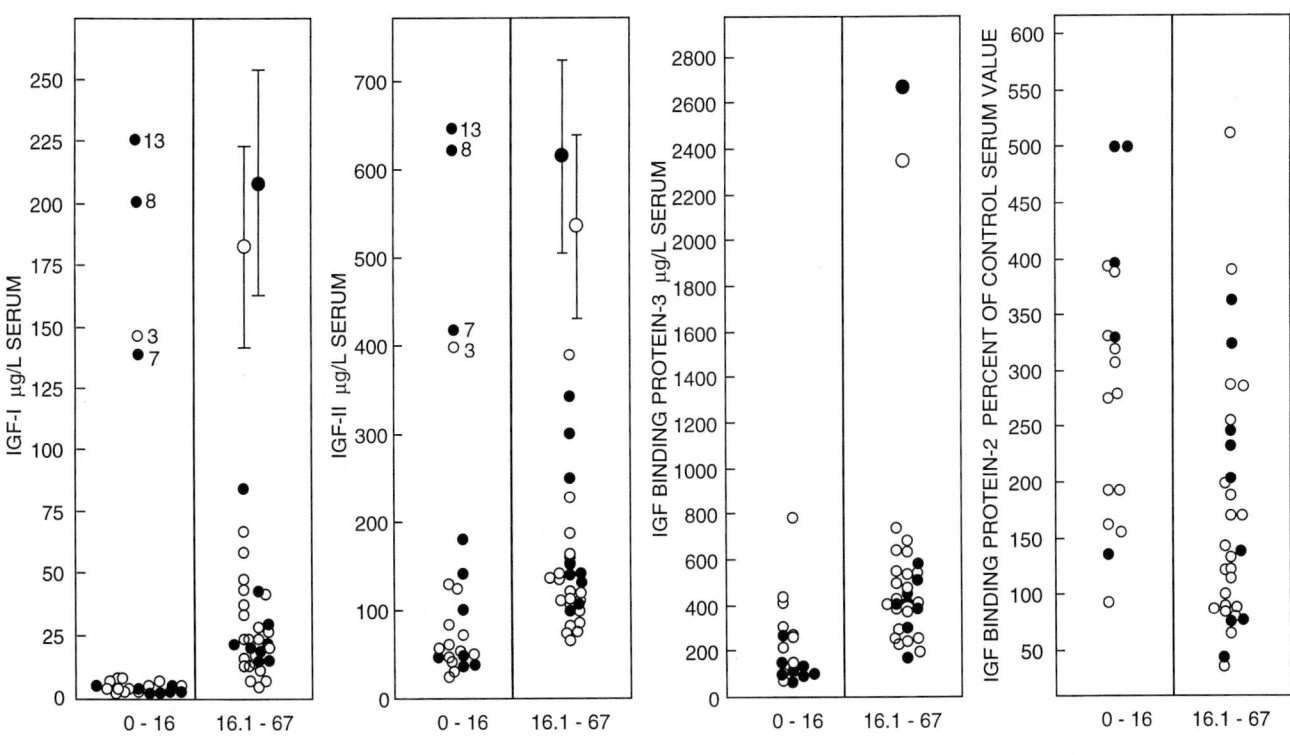

AGE IN YEARS

Figure 30–41. Serum levels of IGF-I, IGF-II, IGFBP-2, and IGFBP-3 in patients with GH receptor deficiency from Ecuador. (From Rosenfeld RG, Rosenbloom AL, Guevara-Aguirre J. Growth hormone (GH) resistance due to GH receptor deficiency. Endocr Rev 1994; 15:369–390. © The Endocrine Society.)

tive tests with at least two separate stimuli to be considered GH deficient. Standard provocative GH tests are summarized in Table 30–10.

Although provocative GH testing has been the foundation for the diagnosis of GH deficiency since GH assays first became available, it has been criticized for a number of reasons, which are discussed in the following sections.[956, 970]

Provocative Growth Hormone Testing is Nonphysiological. None of the standard pharmacologic provocative tests satisfactorily mimic the normal secretory pattern of pituitary GH. Even when naturally occurring regulatory peptides are used for stimulation, their dosage, route of administration, and interactions with other regulatory factors are artificial. Furthermore since most endocrine centers use several different stimulation tests, there is no validated means of resolving conflicting data from two or more provocative tests.[971]

Arbitrary Definitions of "Subnormal" Response to Provocative Tests. Different centers vary in the definition of a "normal" response to stimulation tests. Although early reports generally employed a cutoff level of 2.5 μg/L, this cutoff was gradually increased to 7 μg/L and with the availability of recombinant DNA–derived GH, this level was increased to 10 μg/L, although there are no data for validating higher arbitrary cutoff values. The initial levels of GH that were used to define GH deficiency were based on the study of patients with profound "classic" findings or organic destruction of the adenohypophysis. The lack of documentation of defined normal responses can be seen in the use of vague terminology such as "lack of adequate endogenous GH secretion"[972] and "inadequate secretion of normal endogenous GH."[973]

Age Dependence and Use of Gonadal Steroids. Serum GH levels generally rise during puberty, typically because of an increase in pulse amplitude rather than an increase in pulse frequency.[103, 133, 974] Prior to puberty and during the early phases of puberty, GH secretion may normally be so low as to blur the discrimination between GH deficiency and constitutional delay of growth and maturation.[71, 975] Many children who "fail" provocative testing before the onset of puberty prove to have "normal" GH secretion after puberty or after administration of exogenous gonadal steroids.[976–979] A study of provocative GH testing in children of normal stature documented the inherent problems with provocative GH testing and the need for standardization of gonadal steroid administration during stimulation tests in peripubertal children.[980] When exercise and arginine-insulin stimulation tests were administered to these normal children, the lower limit of normal (−2 SD) for peak serum GH concentration in prepubertal children was only 1.9 μg/L, whereas in children of Tanner stage 5 puberty this level was 9.3 μg/L. When estrogen was administered before provocative testing, the lower 95% confidence limit for the normal serum GH range rose to 7.2 μg/L. When estrogen was not administered the serum GH level did not rise to greater than 7 μg/L during three provocative tests in 61% of normal prepubertal children. These normally growing children could, potentially, have been erroneously labeled as GH deficient. Furthermore the finding of similar GH values in slow-growing, short children emphasizes the difficulty of basing this important diagnosis on provocative test data that use a "magic" number as an arbitrary cutoff for normal.

Variability of Growth Hormone Assays Limit Discriminatory Power. Several studies have demonstrated as much as a threefold variability in the measurement of serum GH levels among established laboratories.[981–983] This is explained, at least in part, by the presence of several molecular forms of GH in serum and by the use of different monoclonal antibodies, in contrast to older polyclonal antibodies and variations in the choice of standards, labeling techniques, and assay buffers (matrix). The consequence is that children labeled as GH deficient by one assay are considered normal by another. This is an unacceptable situation for clinicians, who may be unaware of the type and source of GH assay being used by a given laboratory.[984]

Expense, Discomfort, and Risks of Provocative Growth Hormone Testing. Provocative testing typically requires multiple, timed blood samples and the parenteral administration of drugs. The resulting discomfort to the patient and the expense are self-evident. In addition, tests involving insulin administration carry the risk of hypoglycemia and seizures and should be performed only by experienced medical personnel under appropriate supervision. Deaths have been reported from insulin-induced hypoglycemia and from its overly vigorous correction with parenteral glucose.[985]

Poor Reproducibility of Provocative Tests. The reproducibility of provocative GH tests has never been adequately documented, even when GH levels are measured with the same assay.[986]

ALTERNATIVE MEANS OF DIAGNOSING GH DEFICIENCY. Another diagnostic approach involves measurement of spontaneous GH secretion. This can be performed either by multiple sampling (every 5 to 30 min) over a 12- to 24-h period or by continuous blood withdrawal over 12 to 24 h.[896, 897, 987–989] The former method allows one to evaluate and characterize GH pulsatility, whereas the latter permits determination of mean GH concentration only. Both approaches are subject to many of the same limitations as provocative GH

TABLE 30–10. Tests to Provoke Growth Hormone Secretion

Stimulus	Dosage	Times Samples are Taken (min)	Comments
Exercise	Step climbing; exercise cycle for 10 min	0, 10, 20	Observe child closely when on the steps
Levodopa	<15 kg: 125 mg 10–30 kg: 250 mg >30 kg: 500 mg	0, 60, 90	Nausea, rarely emesis
Clonidine	0.15 mg/m²	0, 30, 60, 90	Tiredness, postural hypotension
Arginine HCl (IV)	0.5 g/kg (max 30 g) 10% arginine HCl in 0.9% NaCl over 30 min	0, 15, 30, 45, 60	
Insulin (IV)	0.05–0.1 unit/kg	0, 15, 30, 60, 75, 90, 120	Hypoglycemia, requires close supervision
Glucagon (IM)	0.03 mg/kg (maximum 1 mg)	0, 30, 60, 90, 120, 150, 180	Nausea, occasional emesis
GHRH (IV)	1 μg/kg	0, 15, 30, 45, 60, 90, 120	Flushing, metallic taste

Tests should be performed after an overnight fast. Many investigators suggest that prepubertal children should be "primed" with gonadal steroids, e.g., 5 mg Premarin (conjugated estrogens) orally the night before and the morning of the test or with 50 to 100 μg/d ethinyl estradiol for 3 consecutive d before testing or 100 mg depot testosterone 3 d before testing. This, of course, alters the patient's steady state and performs the provocative test in a steroid-rich environment. Patients must be euthyroid at the time of testing.

* Insulin-induced hypoglycemia is a potential risk of this procedure, which is designed to lower the blood glucose by at least 50%. Documentation of appropriate lowering of blood glucose is recommended. If GH deficiency is suspected, the lower dosage of insulin is usually administered, especially in infants. D₁₀W and glucagon should be available.

IV, intravenous; IM, intramuscular; GHRH, growth hormone–releasing hormone.

testing. The expense and discomfort of such testing is obvious, and although it was thought that this approach is more reproducible than provocative GH tests, variability is a problem.[990–992] The ability of such tests to discriminate between GH deficiency and normal short children is also an issue. Rose and colleagues[898] reported that measurement of spontaneous GH secretion identified only 57% of children with GH deficiency as defined by provocative testing. Similarly Lanes[899] reported that one fourth of normally growing children have low overnight GH levels, and a longitudinal study of normal boys through puberty demonstrated a wide intersubject variance, including many "low" 24-h GH production rates, despite fully normal growth.[71, 103]

Given the problems with GH testing it is not surprising that provocative tests and 24-h GH profiles do not always correlate. It is likely that the 12- to 24-h GH profile can identify most children with GH deficiency and is superior, both in sensitivity and specificity, to provocative GH testing. "Neurosecretory dysfunction" probably does exist in children after cranial radiation and likely does characterize a subgroup of children with GH deficiency and IGF deficiency. The expense and discomfort of such GH profiles and the problems in GH determinations preclude them from being the test of choice in establishing the diagnosis of GH deficiency.

The measurement of GH levels in urine is an alternative means of estimating "integrated" GH secretion (or at least excretion).[993–995] This technique requires timed urine collections and anti-GH antibodies of high affinity, since urinary GH levels are normally low. Adequate age- and gender-related standards have not been developed, and the diagnostic use of urinary GH determinations remains to be defined.[994, 996–998]

Still another way of diagnosing GH deficiency is the assessment of IGF-I and IGF-II and their binding proteins.[229, 230, 232, 253] GH deficiency then becomes part of the differential diagnosis of IGF deficiency, which includes hypothalamic dysfunction, pituitary insufficiency, and GH resistance. With the development of sensitive and specific assays for IGF-I, IGF-II, and the IGFBPs, it is clear that these peptides accurately reflect integrated GH status. Furthermore IGF-I and IGF-II normally circulate in serum in sufficiently high levels that assay sensitivity is not an issue. Serum levels of both peptides are relatively constant during the day so that provocative testing or multiple sampling is not necessary. However, IGF-I assays do have potential limitations:

1. IGFBPs potentially interfere with radioimmunoassays, radioreceptor assays, and bioassays.[235–237] These binding proteins must either be removed by acid gel chromatography (which is labor intensive)[235–237] or blocked by the addition of excess IGF-II (which requires a high-affinity, high-specificity antibody for IGF-I).[241] An alternative approach is to employ a radiolabeled IGF-I analogue with reduced affinity for IGFBPs.[239]

2. Serum IGF-I levels are age-dependent,[231, 244, 245] being lowest in young children (<5 y), a period during which one most wishes to have an accurate diagnostic test.

3. Serum IGF-I levels may be low in conditions other than GH deficiency, such as primary GH resistance (Laron syndrome) and secondary GH resistance (malnutrition, liver disease, and so on).

Even when these caveats are considered the correlation between serum IGF-I levels and provocative or spontaneous GH measurements is imperfect, possibly because of limitations of GH testing rather than inadequacies of IGF measurements. However, when serum levels of both IGF-I and IGF-II are determined, the correlation with GH testing improves because serum IGF-II levels are low in GH deficiency and normally do not increase with age after 1 y.[232] In one study 18% of patients with low provocative GH levels had IGF-I concentrations in the normal range, but only 4% of "GH deficiency" patients had normal serum levels of both IGF-I and IGF-II.[232] Serum levels of IGF-I and IGF-II were both reduced in only 0.5% of normal children and in 11% of normal short children.

The assay of GH-dependent IGFBP-3, normally the major serum carrier of IGF peptides, is an additional means of diagnosing IGF deficiency due to GH deficiency[341, 439, 440] because the concentrations of IGFBP-3 correlate with the sum of the levels of IGF-I and IGF-II:

1. The immunoassay of IGFBP-3 is technically simple and does not require separation of the binding protein from IGF peptides.

2. Normal serum levels of IGFBP-3 are high, typically in the 1- to 5-mg/L range so that assay sensitivity is not an issue.

3. Serum IGFBP-3 levels vary with age to a lesser degree than is the case for IGF-I. Even in infants serum IGFBP-3 levels are sufficiently high to allow discrimination of low values from the normal range.

4. Serum IGFBP-3 levels are less dependent on nutrition than are IGF-I levels, reflecting the "stabilizing" effect of IGF-II levels.

5. IGFBP-3 levels are GH-dependent.

The utility of IGFBP-3 assays in the diagnosis of GH deficiency was evaluated by Blum and colleagues,[440] who found that serum IGFBP-3 levels were below the 5th percentile for age in 128 of 132 children (97%) diagnosed as GH deficient by conventional criteria (height <3rd percentile, height velocity <10th percentile, and peak serum GH <10 μg/L). At the same time, 124 of 130 (95%) non–GH-deficient, short children had normal IGFBP-3 levels; it is likely that this group of patients consisted largely of children with severe GH deficiency, since such a clear correlation between provocative GH testing and serum IGFBP-3 levels has not been consistently observed. For example, in one study the sensitivity of the IGFBP-3 assay in complete GH deficiency (peak GH <5 μg/ L) was 93% but was only 43% in partial GH deficiency (peak GH 5 to 10 μg/L).[999] In another study 100% of children with severe GH deficiency (peak GH ≤1 μg/L) and low serum IGF-I also had decreased serum IGFBP-3, 4 of 8 children with GH deficiency and normal serum IGF-I levels had reduced IGFBP-3 levels, and 10 of 23 normal short children (43%) had decreased serum IGFBP-3.[1000] In the latter study 18% of patients had discordance between IGFBP-3 levels and provocative GH testing. The addition of a radioimmunoassay for IGFBP-2 further enhanced the ability of IGF axis measures to identify children who were GH deficient by conventional criteria.[1000]

The correlation between IGF and IGFBP-3 levels and assessments of spontaneous GH secretion is also imperfect. Even in normal children the correlation between 24-h GH secretion and serum IGF-I and IGFBP-3 levels is modest ($r = 0.78$ and $r = 0.62$, respectively).[995]

It is not possible to resolve fully conflicts between assays of the IGF axis and measurements of GH secretion, as there is no definitive way of diagnosing GH deficiency, but studies of patients with GH receptor deficiency support the utility of IGF-related determinations.[137, 999, 1001] Although such patients may have normal or elevated serum GH levels, mutations or deletions of the GH receptor gene render them unresponsive to GH, making them "functionally GH-deficient." In approximately 70 instances of GH receptor gene mutations, there were markedly reduced serum levels of both IGF-I and IGFBP-3.[1001] Even so, both IGF-I and IGFBP-3 correlated significantly with height. Measurements of IGF-I and IGFBP-3 levels have been used in other studies to establish the diagnosis of GH resistance.[1002, 1003]

Ultimately the diagnosis of GH deficiency (or IGF deficiency) should be made on the basis of combined clinical and laboratory criteria. Short children who have well-documented normal height velocities do not generally require evaluation of GH secretion, and the finding of normal serum levels of IGF-I or IGFBP-3, or both, is confirmatory. Children with gonadal dysgenesis and short stature should not be required to undergo GH testing to qualify for GH therapy, since such treatment is not predicated on abnormal GH secretion. Conversely the child with documented growth deceleration requires further evaluation, even if tests of GH secretion appear normal. Documentation of decreased serum IGF-I and IGFBP-3 levels would then substantiate the diagnosis of IGF deficiency, and the differential diagnosis of GH deficiency and GH resistance would need to be considered. The child with a history of cranial radiation, decreased height velocity, and reduced serum levels of IGF-I and IGFBP-3 should be considered to have GH deficiency (or GH resistance), even in the face of normal provocative tests.[855]

This approach still leaves a place for measurements of GH secretion. Such determinations are critical for distinguishing between GH deficiency and GH resistance as causes of IGF deficiency. Documentation of abnormal pituitary GH secretion raises the possibility of intracranial tumors and the potential for deficiency of other pituitary hormones. Evaluation of

GH deficiency permits concomitant assessment of corticotropin-cortisol secretion during insulin-induced hypoglycemia.

Ultimately the most important parameter in assessing children with growth failure is careful clinical evaluation, including accurate serial measurements of height and height velocity. The possibility of hypothalamic-pituitary dysfunction should always be considered in children with documented growth deceleration, particularly in the face of a known or suspected CNS pathologic condition (tumors, radiation, malformations, infection, trauma, blindness, nystagmus, and so on). Similarly the neonate with hypoglycemia or microphallus, or both, warrants evaluation of pituitary function (including MRI), and children with documented thyrotropin, corticotropin, arginine vasopressin (ADH), or gonadotropin deficiency are candidates for GH deficiency. For children with proportional short stature and documented growth deceleration, assessment of serum IGF-I and IGFBP-3 is warranted and, based on the results, the possibilities of hypothalamic dysfunction, pituitary insufficiency, and GH resistance can be investigated.

Figure 30–42 provides an algorithm for the biochemical evaluation of growth failure.

BIOCHEMICAL EVALUATION OF GROWTH FAILURE

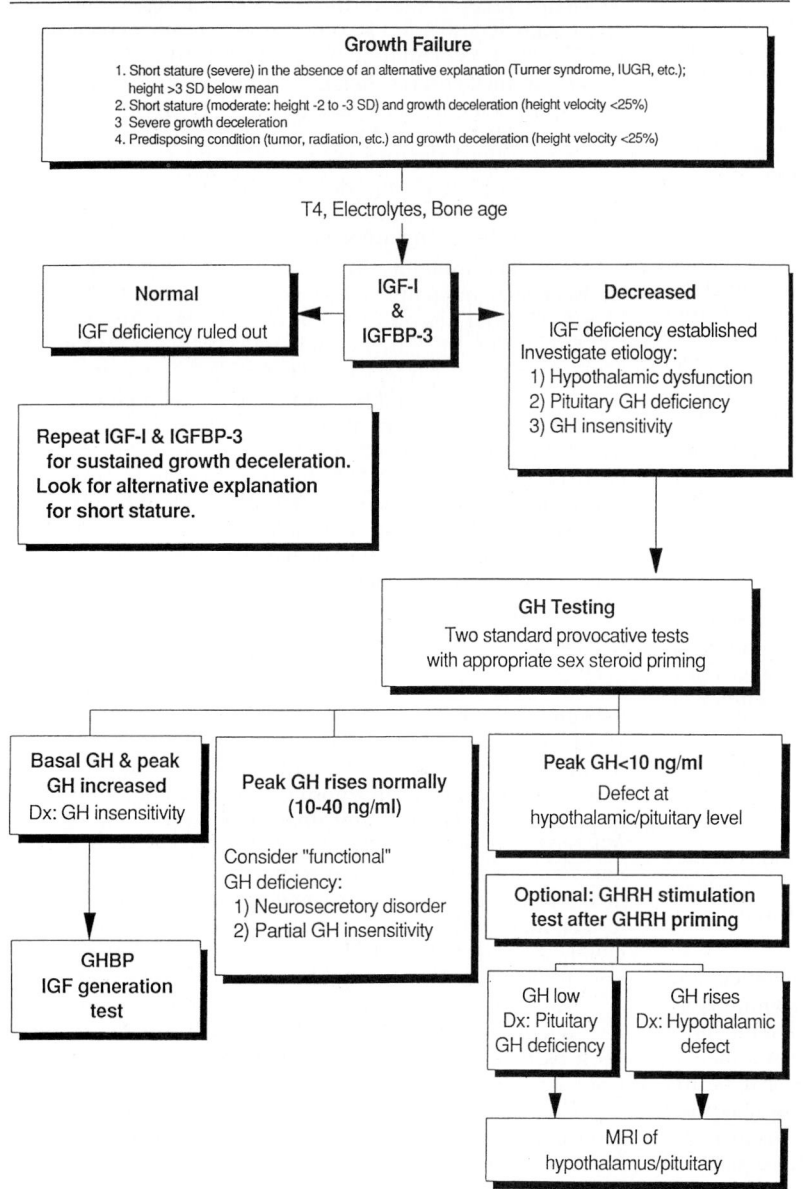

Figure 30–42. Biochemical evaluation of growth failure. Primary evaluation is for "IGF deficiency," with studies designed to delineate hypothalamic abnormalities, pituitary abnormalities, or GH resistance.

Diagnosis of Insulin-Like Growth Factor Deficiency Syndrome: Growth Hormone Resistance

The combination of decreased serum levels of IGF-I, IGF-II, and IGFBP-3, plus increased serum levels of GH, is highly suggestive of a diagnosis of GH resistance.[137] The possibility of GH receptor deficiency is supported by a family history consistent with autosomal recessive transmission. Savage and colleagues[999] devised a scoring system for evaluating short children for the diagnosis of GH receptor deficiency based on five parameters: (1) basal serum GH greater than 10 mU/L (approximately 5 μg/L), (2) serum IGF-I less than or equal to 50 μg/L, (3) height SD scores less than −3 SD, (4) serum GHBP levels less than 10% (based on binding of [^{125}I]hGH), and (5) a rise in serum IGF-I levels after GH administration of less than twofold the intra-assay variation (approximately 10%). Blum and co-workers[1004] proposed that these criteria could be strengthened by (1) evaluating GH secretory profiles, rather than isolated basal levels; (2) employing an age-dependent range and the 0.1 percentile as the cutoff level for evaluation of serum IGF-I concentrations; (3) employing highly sensitive IGF-I immunoassays and defining a failed GH response as the inability to increase serum IGF-I levels by at least 15 μg/L; and (4) measuring both basal and GH-stimulated IGFBP-3 levels. These criteria fit well with the population of GH receptor deficiency patients in Ecuador, but that is a homogeneous population with severe GH resistance.[137, 1001] The applicability of these criteria elsewhere remains to be evaluated. An important biochemical marker is the response of IGF-I (and possibly IGFBP-3) to GH stimulation. Normal ranges and age-defined responses of serum IGF-I levels have not been established.[1005, 1006]

Decreased serum levels of GHBP suggest the diagnosis of GH receptor deficiency, but some individuals with GH receptor deficiency have normal serum concentrations of GHBP.[137, 954] Such cases may represent mutations in the dimerization site or in the intracellular domain of the receptor or abnormalities of postreceptor signal transduction mechanisms. Conversely, polymorphisms of the GH receptor gene, without associated reductions in levels of IGF-I or IGFBP-3, should not be considered examples of GH resistance. At this point definitive diagnosis of GH resistance requires (1) the classic phenotype, (2) decreased serum levels of IGF-I and IGFBP-3, and (3) identification of an abnormality of the GH receptor gene.

IDIOPATHIC SHORT STATURE

Many children and early adolescents are short (<3rd percentile); have slowed impairment of linear growth velocity (<25 percentile); may have delayed skeletal maturation and an impaired or attenuated pubertal growth spurt, with or without a family history manifesting some or all of these clinical features; and have no chronic illnesses or apparent endocrinopathies. Such children usually have normal GH secretory dynamics, although provocative test results may be blunted under some circumstances; GH-dependent peptides are lower than expected on a chronologic, although usually not skeletal, age basis; treatment with exogenous GH usually augments linear growth. Such children are usually considered variants of normal and achieve a final adult height within the range considered acceptable for the family. The cause of the slowed childhood growth and frequently delayed pubertal spurt has not been established in most of these children. As this is the largest group of short children, continuing efforts are under way to develop a rational categorization and to develop the means of separating these children from those with an abnormality of the GH-IGF axis. Several groups of patients, including those with constitutional delay of growth

and maturation, genetic or familial short stature, and heterozygous abnormalities of the GH receptor are described later. Additional causes of idiopathic short stature will likely be identified at each level of the hypothalamic-pituitary-IGF axis.[821]

Constitutional Delay of Growth and Maturation

The term *constitutional delay*[1007–1010] describes children with a normal variant of maturational tempo characterized by short stature but relatively normal growth rates during childhood, delayed puberty with a late and attenuated pubertal growth spurt, and attainment of normal adult height. Most children with constitutional delay begin to deviate from the normal growth curve during the early years of life and by age 2 are at or slightly below the 5th percentile for height.[1011] Final height, although usually within the normal population range, is often in the lower part of the parental height target zone,[1012–1014] with few patients exceeding that target height. The predicted final height, especially when the skeletal age is extremely delayed, is greater than that usually achieved.[1015–1017] The delayed growth spurt may adversely affect growth of the spine and mineralization of the vertebrae, which is not overcome when the pubertal growth acceleration finally occurs, thus limiting the final height.[1016, 1018]

GH secretion may be decreased with transient partial GH deficiency at the time of the delayed pubertal growth spurt, which is apparently the consequence of inadequate production of gonadal steroids.[108, 978, 1019, 1020] Such children would be expected to have delayed skeletal ages, normal or slightly low serum IGF-I and IGFBP-3 levels for skeletal age, and normal GH provocative test results (if pretreated with gonadal steroids). Overnight GH secretion is generally normal in these children when control groups are carefully matched.[900] By definition children with pure CDGM should have bone ages sufficiently delayed to result in normal predicted adult heights (>163 cm in males and >150 cm in females) (Table 30–11), although the correlation between predicted and final height is imperfect and must be viewed with caution.[1015–1017] When CDGM occurs in the context of familial short stature (see later), however, children may experience both a delayed adolescent growth spurt *and* a short final height.

As stated earlier, some have attributed the diminished growth in the peripubertal period in CDGM to a transient GH deficiency or to a "lazy" pituitary, a concept that is probably due to the inadequacies of GH testing, especially to the failure to pretreat patients with a brief course of gonadal steroids.[108, 980] Low serum levels of IGF-I and IGFBP-3 or a poor GH response to provocative testing (after priming with gonadal steroids), or both, should mandate an investigation for an underlying pathologic condition, such as intracranial tumors.

TABLE 30–11. Criteria for Presumptive Diagnosis of Constitutional Delay of Growth and Maturation

No history of systemic illness
Normal nutrition
Normal physical examination, including body proportions
Normal thyroid and GH levels
Normal CBC, sedimentation rate, electrolytes, BUN
Height at or below the 3rd percentile, but with annual growth rate >5th percentile for age
Delayed puberty:
  Males: failure to achieve Tanner G2 stage by age 13.8 y or P2 by 15.6 y
  Females: failure to achieve Tanner B2 stage by age 13.3 y
Delayed bone age
Normal predicted adult height:
  Males: >163 cm (64 inches)
  Females: >150 cm (59 inches)

GH, growth hormone; CBC, complete blood count; BUN, blood urea nitrogen.

Genetic (Familial) Short Stature

The control of growth in childhood and the final height attained are polygenic in nature. For this reason familial height has an impact on the growth of an individual, and evaluation of a specific growth pattern must be placed in the context of familial growth and stature. Formulas have been developed for determination of parental target height, and growth curves that relate a child's height to parental height are available.[36] As a general rule a child who is growing at a rate that is inconsistent with that of siblings or parents warrants further evaluation.

Furthermore many organic diseases characterized by growth retardation are genetically transmitted. This list includes many conditions such as GH resistance due to mutations of the GH receptor gene, GH gene deletions, mutations of the *Pit-1* gene, pseudohypoparathyroidism, diabetes mellitus, and some forms of hypothyroidism. Inherited nonendocrine diseases characterized by short stature include osteochondrodysplasias (see earlier), dysmorphic syndromes associated with IUGR (see earlier), inborn errors of metabolism, renal disease, and thalassemia (see later). Identifying short stature as inherited thus does not, by itself, relieve the physician of responsibility for determining the underlying cause of growth failure.

Nonetheless a constellation of clinical findings describes a normal variant referred to as genetic short stature (or familial short stature) that differs from the syndrome of constitutional delay of growth and maturation discussed earlier. In genetic short stature childhood growth is at or below the 5th percentile, but the velocity is generally normal. The onset and progression is normal or even slightly early and more rapid than normal so that skeletal age is concordant with chronologic age. Parental height is short (both parents are often below the 10th percentile) and pubertal maturation is normal. Final heights in these individuals are short and in the target zone for the family.[1014] The GH-IGF system is normal but exogenous GH therapy during middle childhood years increases linear growth velocity substantially without disproportionate augmentation of skeletal maturation.[1157] Whether long-term GH treatment enhances final height outcome is not clear.

Heterozygous Mutations of the Growth Hormone Receptor

The level of the GH receptor may be genetically determined, although modulated by factors such as nutritional status; GH production appears to be inversely related to GH receptor–GHBP levels.[156, 159] Accordingly GHBP levels have been assessed in individuals with idiopathic short stature.[157, 158, 1021] Serum levels of GHBP in 90% of children with idiopathic short stature are lower than the normal mean, 20% being less than the normal range, especially a subgroup with low IGF-I and higher mean 12-h levels of GH.[157, 158] Such data raise the possibility that an abnormality in the GH receptor content or structure could impair GH action. The inverse relationship of GHBP levels to GH production is normal.[121] Heterozygous GH receptor mutations were present in 28% of a small group of patients with growth failure, low levels of IGF-I, and poor response to exogenous GH.[820] In contrast to the rarity of homozygous GH receptor mutations in GH resistance, heterozygosity is more common and may be a frequent cause of short stature.[821, 955] In heterozygotes protein from the mutant allele may disrupt the normal dimerization that occurs when GH interacts with its receptor, leading to diminished GH action and growth impairment.

TREATMENT OF GROWTH DISORDERS

When growth failure is the result of a chronic underlying disease such as renal failure, cystic fibrosis, or malabsorption, therapy must be directed at treatment of the underlying condition.[577] Although growth acceleration may occur in such children with GH or IGF-I therapy, complete catch-up requires correction of the primary medical problem. If treatment of the underlying condition involves glucocorticoids, growth failure may be profound and is unlikely to be correctable until steroids are reduced or discontinued.

Correction of growth failure associated with chronic hypothyroidism requires appropriate thyroid replacement. As discussed earlier, thyroid therapy causes dramatic catch-up growth but also markedly accelerates skeletal maturation, potentially limiting adult height. More gradual thyroid replacement or the use of gonadotropin inhibitors to delay puberty may be necessary to obtain maximal final height.

Treatment of Constitutional Delay

CDGM is a normal variant, with (by definition) potential for a normal (although delayed) pubertal maturation and a normal (albeit diminished for target zone) adult height. Most patients can be managed by careful evaluation to rule out other causes of abnormal growth or delayed puberty, or both, combined with appropriate explanation and counseling. The skeletal age and Bayley-Pinneau table are often helpful in explaining the potential for normal growth to the patient and parents. A family history of constitutional delay is also frequently a source of reassurance. On occasion, however, the stigmata of short stature and delayed maturation may be psychologically disabling for the preadolescent or teenager. Some adolescents with delayed puberty have poor self-images and limited social involvement.[1022] In such patients, and in some in whom pubertal delay is predicted based on the overall clinical picture, there is a role for the judicious use of short-term gonadal steroids.

Two aspects of this syndrome are addressed by androgen treatment: *short stature,* especially in boys between ages 10 and 14, and *delayed puberty* after age 14. In the younger group, in whom CDGM is apparent, the orally administered synthetic androgen oxandrolone has been used extensively.[1023] In several controlled studies,[1024–1029] oxandrolone therapy for 3 mo to 4 y resulted in increased linear growth velocity of 3 to 5 cm/y without adverse affects or decreasing either actual[1029–1031] or predicted[1026, 1030, 1032] final height. The growth-promoting effects of oxandrolone appear related to its androgenic and anabolic effects rather than to augmentation of the GH-IGF axis.[1033, 1034] Currently recommended treatment, through an available research IND (investigational new drug) protocol, is 0.1 mg/kg/d oxandrolone orally. In older boys in whom delayed pubertal maturation is unbearable testosterone enanthate has been administered intramuscularly with success.[1023, 1024, 1035] Criteria for therapy of such adolescents should include (1) a minimal age of 14 y, (2) height below the 3rd percentile, (3) prepubertal or early Tanner G2 stage with an early morning serum testosterone level less than 3.5 nmol/L (<1 ng/mL), and (4) a poor self-image that does not respond to reassurance alone. Therapy consists of intramuscular testosterone enanthate, 50 to 200 mg every 3 to 4 wk for a total of four to six injections.[1022, 1036] Patients typically show evidence of beginning virilization by the fourth injection and grow an average of 10 cm in the ensuing year. Despite attempts to choose subjects carefully for treatment programs in CDGM, a spectrum of activation of the reproductive system is inevitable; growth responses to short courses of therapy are best in boys who have early pubertal gonadotropin secretory patterns.[1037]

Testosterone enhances growth velocity by direct actions and increases GH production.[71a, 108, 133–136] Brief testosterone regimens do not cause overly rapid skeletal maturation, compromise adult height, or suppress pubertal maturation.[1038] It is important to emphasize to the patient that he is normal, that therapy is short-term and designed to provide some pubertal development earlier than he would on his own, and that treatment will not increase adult height. In such situations the combination of short-term androgen therapy, reassurance, and counseling helps boys with constitutional delay cope with a difficult adolescence.

Patients must be re-evaluated to ensure that they enter "true" puberty. One year after testosterone treatment boys should exhibit testicular enlargement and a serum testosterone level in the pubertal range. If this is not the case the diagnosis of hypothalamic-pituitary insufficiency or hypogonadotropic hypogonadism should be considered. Although the diagnosis of constitutional growth delay remains most likely in such patients, some eventually prove to be gonadotropin deficient especially if still prepubertal late in the teenage years.

Referrals for constitutional delay are more common in boys than in girls, undoubtedly reflecting our cultural values. Nonetheless, an increased number of girls are being assessed. When constitutional delay is a problem in girls, short-term estrogen therapy can be employed. The use of GH in patients with constitutional delay is discussed later.

Treatment of Growth Hormone Deficiency

Nomenclature and Potency Estimation

The nomenclature for the various biosynthetic GH preparations reflects the source and the chemical composition of the product. Somatropin refers to GH of the same amino acid sequence as that in naturally occurring GH. Somatropin from human pituitary glands is abbreviated hGH or pit-hGH; recombinant origin somatropin is termed recombinant GH or rGH. Somatrem refers to the methionine derivative of recombinant GH, and is abbreviated met-rGH. Although the latter preparation is a more antigenic preparation, that propensity is not clinically relevant; despite the presence of anti-GH antibodies, growth responses to met-rGH are similar to those seen in patients treated with rGH.[1039, 1040] We will refer to these biosynthetic preparations as GH in the subsequent discussions.

The biopotency of commercially available biosynthetic GH preparations, expressed as international units per milligram of the new WHO rhGH reference reagent for somatropin (88/624), is 3 IU/mg.[1041] It was necessary to standardize the early GH preparations by bioassay because of variable production techniques (extraction, column purification, and so on). The most common bioassays have been the hypophysectomized rat weight gain assay and the tibial width assay.[1041–1043] With the availability of purified and essentially equivalent recombinant GH products, the requirement for bioassays has become a Food and Drug Administration requisite to substantiate biologic activity rather than to assess potential differences among preparations. The bioassays are likely to be replaced by in vitro binding assays using GH receptors or GHBP derived from molecular techniques.[1041]

Historical Perspective

The action of GH is highly species-specific and humans do not respond to animal-derived GH.[1044–1049] Unlike most other hormones the only GH that is biologically active in humans is primate GH. Human cadaver pituitary glands were for many years the only practical source of primate GH for treatment of GH deficiency, and more than 27,000 children with GH deficiency worldwide were treated with pit-hGH.[1050] The limited supplies of pit-hGH, low doses, and interrupted treatment regimens resulted in incomplete growth increments; usually therapy was discontinued in boys who reached 5 feet 5 inches and in girls who reached 5 feet. Nonetheless this treatment did increase linear growth and in many patients enhanced final adult height. The dose-response relationship and the relation of age to GH response was recognized during this period.[1051]

Distribution of pit-hGH was halted in the United States and most of Europe in 1985 because of concern about a causal relationship with Creutzfeldt-Jakob disease, a rare and fatal spongiform encephalopathy that had been previously reported to be capable of iatrogenic transmission through human tissue.[1052, 1053] In North America and Europe this disorder has an incidence of approximately 1 case per million in the general population; it is exceedingly rare before age 50. To date more than 30 young adults who had received human cadaver pituitary products have died from Creutzfeldt-Jakob disease and at least 60 to 70 cases of Creutzfeldt-Jakob disease have been identified in such recipients.[1054, 1055]

Fortunately by the time the risks of pituitary-derived hGH were discovered, rGH was being tested for safety and efficacy.[1039, 1056, 1057] The original rGH included an NH_2-terminal methionine, added as a start signal for transcription (met-rGH). This preparation mimicked pit-hGH in regard to both anabolic and metabolic actions. Subsequent recombinant hGH preparations do not contain the additional methionine. rGH has replaced pit-GH as the treatment for children with GH deficiency.

Treatment Regimens

The recommended starting dose of hGH in GH deficiency is 0.175 to 0.35 mg/kg body weight/wk, administered in seven daily doses. Alternative regimens include a 6 d/wk or 3 d/wk schedule, with the same weekly dosage. In general the growth response to GH is a function of the log-dose given so that increasing dosages further enhance growth velocities,[1050, 1051] but daily dosing may be the most important treatment parameter.[1058] Either subcutaneous or intramuscular administration has equivalent growth-promoting activity[1059]; the former is now used almost exclusively. A sustained-release form of injectable GH is under evaluation for once monthly hormone treatment.[1060] Treatment may be continued after growth ceases because GH has other important metabolic effects, including support of normal gonadal function[1061] and attainment of normal adult bone mineral density.[1062, 1063] A report from the Drug and Therapeutics Committee of the Lawson Wilkins Pediatric Endocrine Society summarized that society's views on the use of GH in children with diverse syndromes of short stature.[1064]

Growth responses to exogenous GH vary, depending on the frequency of administration, dosage, age (greater absolute gain in a younger child, although not necessarily of growth velocity SD scores), weight, and GH receptor amount, as assessed by serum GHBP levels.[156, 159, 1065] On this general regimen, nonetheless, growth in the typical GH-deficient child accelerates from a pretreatment rate of 3 to 4 cm/y to 10 to 12 cm/y in year 1 of therapy and 7 to 9 cm/y in years 2 and 3. Progressive waning of GH efficacy occurs and is poorly understood. The importance of dosage frequency is illustrated (Figs. 30–43 and 30–44) by data from a carefully performed assessment of growth responses of prepubertal GH-deficient children randomly assigned to receive thrice-weekly or daily GH at the same total weekly dose (0.30 mg/kg/wk).[1058] The mean total height gain during this period was 9.7 cm greater in the daily-treated patients (38.4 vs 28.7 cm, $p < .0002$) with

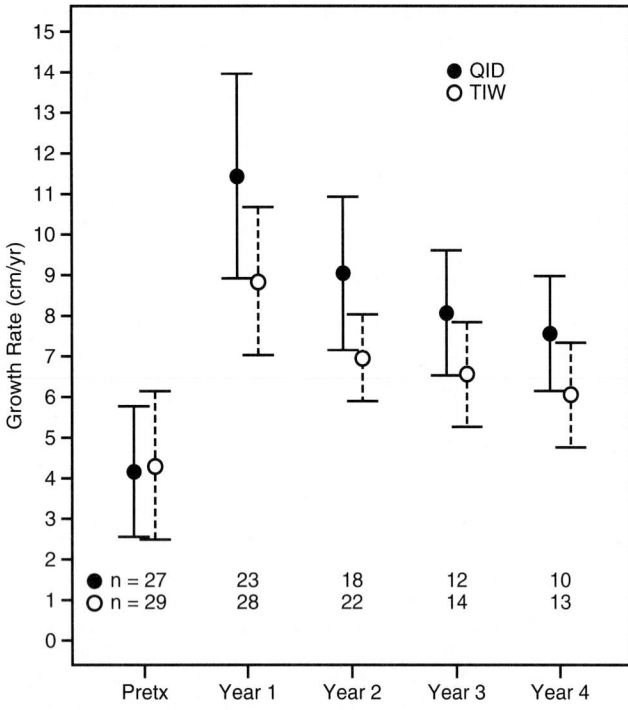

Figure 30–43. Annual growth velocity (mean ±SD) for prepubertal hGH deficiency patients prior to and during 4 y of GH treatment, contrasting results with daily (QID) and thrice-weekly (TIW) injections. The mean annual growth velocity in the QID group was significantly greater than that of the TIW group during each year, although significance diminished from year 1 to year 4. (From MacGillivray MH, Baptista J, Johanson A, et al. Outcome of a four year randomized study of daily versus three times weekly somatropin treatment in prepubertal naive growth hormone deficient children. J Clin Endocrinol Metab 1996; 81:1806–1809, with permission.)

similar increments in skeletal maturation and no acceleration of the onset of puberty. Mean height SD scores at the end of 4 y were +0.2, or at the midpoint of normal for age. At a dosage of 0.30 mg/kg/wk, the approximate current cost of GH therapy for a 20-kg child is $15,000/y.

Longer Term Results

Much information on growth has been reported about children given pit-hGH, generally thrice-weekly and intramuscularly administered. Bundak and colleagues[1066] have provided 5-y data on a group of 58 prepubertal and 20 pubertal children with GH deficiency. The younger group increased its height from −3.6 SD scores to −2 SD scores, whereas the pubertal children grew to −2.3 SD scores. The height SD scores for bone age, however, did not increase; thus further loss of adult height was prevented but there was no increase in the adult height prediction. The importance of early initiation of treatment is stressed by such data. Similarly Libber and co-workers[1067] found that GH therapy increased mean height from about −4.2 SD scores to −2.3 SD scores. Bierich reviewed nine trials of pit-hGH to determine the effect on final height.[1068] Overall a dose-response relationship was noted between doses of 0.11 and 0.25 mg/kg/wk. The greatest SD score increment of 2.7 occurred with the highest dosage of pit-hGH. The pretreatment heights ranged from −5.6 to −3.6 SD scores, with adult heights achieving −3.6 to −1.6 SD scores.

Patients treated largely with biosynthetic GH[1039, 1065, 1069–1073] have improved actual or near-final adult height SD scores, with average final height in more than 350 patients approximating −1.3 SD below the mean. The use of higher doses of

GH, the ability to treat until growth, early initiation of treatment,[1074–1076] progressive weight-related dose increments,[1075] attention to compliance with daily administration, and appropriate thyroid hormone and glucocorticoid replacement therapy are important factors in this improved adult height outcome. Indeed, a report on 121 children treated for 8 y with 0.3 mg/kg/wk showed an adult height outcome of −0.7 SD.[1242] As final height correlates with height at the onset of puberty in GH-deficient patients,[1065, 1072, 1073, 1077, 1078] every effort must be made to enhance growth velocity during prepuberty. When normal or precocious puberty limits the response to GH, it may be appropriate to delay puberty by the use of an LHRH analogue.[1079, 1080] Use of this strategy in pubertal patient groups, however, is not yet documented to enhance final height.[1081–1084] Nevertheless the earlier the age of pubertal onset, the lower the final height outcome and GH-deficient patients with delayed puberty or hypogonadotropic hypogonadism have a taller adult height.[1065, 1085, 1086]

Multiple Pituitary Hormone Deficiencies

If GH deficiency is part of a multiple pituitary insufficiency, it is necessary to address each endocrine deficiency both for general medical reasons and to ensure a maximal effect from GH therapy. Thyrotropin deficiency is often "unmasked" during the initial phase of therapy, and thyroid function should be assessed both before the onset of therapy and during the first 3 mo of GH treatment[1087] and at least on an annual basis thereafter. The pituitary-adrenal axis is customarily evaluated during the insulin stimulation test in the work-up for GH deficiency. If corticotropin secretion is impaired, patients should receive the lowest safe maintenance dose of glucocorticoids, certainly no more than 10 mg/m²/d

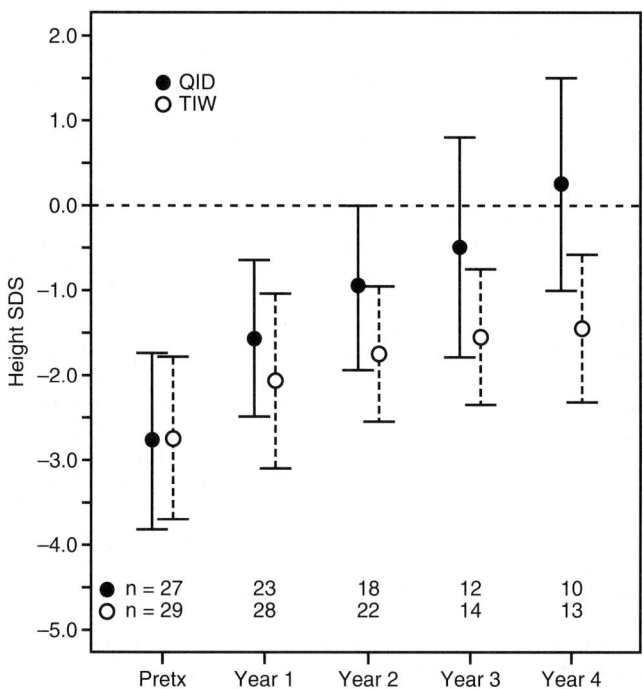

Figure 30–44. Height SD scores (mean ±SD) for prepubertal hGH-deficient patients prior to and during 4 y of GH treatment, contrasting results with daily (QID) and thrice-weekly (TIW) injections. The mean SD score in the QID group was significantly greater throughout the treatment period. Younger patients had the greatest increase in height SD scores and the effect of age was more marked in the QID group. (From MacGillivray MH, Baptista J, Johanson A, et al. Outcome of a four-year randomized study of daily versus three times weekly somatropin treatment in prepubertal naive growth hormone deficient children. J Clin Endocrinol Metab 1996; 81:1806–1809, with permission.)

of hydrocortisone and less if possible. Higher doses impair the growth response to GH therapy but may be necessary during times of stress.

Gonadotropin deficiency may be evident in the infant with microphallus. This can usually be treated with three to four monthly injections of 25 mg of testosterone enanthate.[1088] Management at puberty can be more complicated because the physical and psychological benefits of promoting sexual maturation must be balanced against the effects of epiphyseal fusion. When GH therapy is initiated in childhood and growth is normal prior to adolescence, it is appropriate to begin gonadal steroid replacement at a normal age (e.g., age 11 to 12 in girls and 12 to 13 in boys). In boys this can be accomplished by beginning with monthly injections of 50 to 100 mg of testosterone enanthate, gradually increasing to 200 mg/mo, and eventually moving to the appropriate adult replacement regimen as determined by the monitoring of plasma testosterone levels (see Chapter 16). In girls therapy involves the use of conjugated estrogens or ethinyl estradiol and eventual cycling with estrogen and progesterone, as described in Chapter 15.

Poor Growth Responses

As stated earlier the growth response to GH typically attenuates after the first year but should continue to be equal to or greater than the normal height velocity for age throughout treatment. A suboptimal response to GH can be due to several causes: (1) poor compliance, (2) improper preparation of GH for administration or incorrect injection techniques, (3) subclinical hypothyroidism, (4) coexisting systemic disease, (5) excessive glucocorticoid therapy, (6) prior radiation of the spine, (7) epiphyseal fusion, (8) anti-GH antibodies,[1040, 1089] or (9) incorrect diagnosis of GH deficiency as an explanation for growth retardation. Although 10 to 20% of recipients of rGH acquire anti-GH antibodies, growth failure is rarely due to such antibodies.[498, 1039, 1040, 1090] Maximal growth response to GH can usually be obtained by early diagnosis and initiation of therapy and by careful attention to compliance and psychological support. Although in some old studies as many as 50% of boys and 85% of girls with idiopathic GH deficiency do not achieve adult heights above the 3rd percentile,[1077] it is our belief that normal height (i.e., reaching the family-specific target height) is presently achievable in most cases.[1039, 1065, 1069–1073, 1242]

Despite the efficacy of GH in accelerating growth in GH-deficient children and to bring adult height into the normal range if treatment is begun sufficiently early, several studies have indicated that the long-term prognosis for such patients is guarded.[1091, 1092] The educational, vocational, and social outlook for adults who had childhood GH deficiency is frequently suboptimal. Whether this reflects subtle intellectual deficits or the consequences of lower expectations of patients, families, or teachers remains to be determined. In any case GH deficiency should be followed carefully throughout life.

The clinical consequences of GH deficiency in adults and the potential benefits of GH therapy in this population is a subject of intense interest.[1092, 1093] Signs and symptoms of adult GH deficiency include reduced lean body mass and musculature, increased body fat, reduced bone mineral density, reduced exercise tolerance, and increased plasma cholesterol levels. Adults with GH deficiency have an increased risk of death from cardiovascular causes, possibly due to the increase in adiposity and serum cholesterol levels.[1094] GH-deficient adults have been found to have "impaired psychological well-being and quality of life"[1095] characterized by depression, anxiety, reduced energy and vitality, and social isolation.[1096, 1097] In several placebo-controlled studies, GH therapy of adult GH-deficient patients resulted in marked improvement in lean body mass, fat distribution, bone density, and sense of well-

being.[1096–1099] Whether these effects of GH therapy will be sustained and, if so, what the optimal GH regimen will be remain to be determined.

Growth Hormone Treatment of Other Forms of Short Stature

The availability of GH has made it possible to use the hormone for treatment of other forms of short stature. Theoretically it should be possible to accelerate growth in any child to achieve height greater than that indicated by genetic potential. Whether such therapy is safe and whether it justifies the cost and potential risks is more complicated. Additionally questions have been raised about the appropriateness of "cosmetic" hormonal therapy.

A survey of 251 pediatric endocrinologists suggested that 30 to 50% would consider treating short children with a wide array of diagnoses, including Russell-Silver and Noonan's syndromes, IUGR, steroid-induced growth suppression, and Prader-Willi syndrome.[984] Such a wide range of potential treatment conditions far exceeds those that have received or are likely to receive Food and Drug Administration approval or that have been shown to respond to GH treatment. Guidelines have been developed by the Lawson Wilkins Pediatric Endocrine Society to provide a rational framework in this area.[1064] Another set of criteria based on an auxology system is used in Australia; when carefully monitored and rationally modified, this program uses GH doses in the middle range of doses used in other countries.[1100]

Chronic Renal Failure

GH accelerates growth in children with chronic renal failure (Figs. 30–45 and 30–46) at least over several years of therapy.[664, 1099, 1101–1105] Using a GH dosage of 0.05 mg/kg/d Fine and colleagues[1106] reported a mean first-year growth rate of 10.7 cm in GH recipients and 6.5 cm in the placebo group;

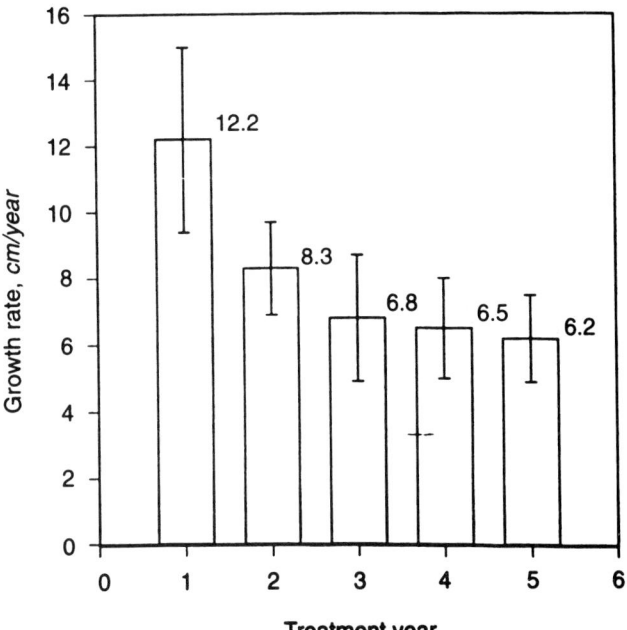

Figure 30–45. Annual growth velocity in 20 growth-retarded prepubertal patients with chronic renal insufficiency who were treated with GH. (From Fine RN, Kohaut E, Brown D, et al. Long-term treatment of growth-retarded children with chronic renal insufficiency with recombinant human growth hormone. Kidney Int 1996; 49:781–785, with permission.)

heterozygous mutations of the GH receptor gene. Even though they are grouped in one category, this group includes some children who have normal provocative GH responses but are, nevertheless, relatively IGF deficient, reflecting the inadequacies of GH testing. This group will also contain children with unidentified syndromes and unidentified chronic illnesses or endocrine disorders. For example, children with heterozygous mutations of the GH receptor have subnormal growth, diminished IGF and GHBP levels, and impaired responsiveness to exogenous GH administration.

Such issues make it difficult to evaluate clinical trials in this group. The failure to report levels of IGF-I, IGFBP-3, and GHBP in many studies, and differing interpretations of endogenous GH secretion studies (assay variance, control group size, and so on) confound data assessment. Furthermore published clinical trials have not contained long-term control groups and have reported variable growth responses.[1150–1154] Most normal short children treated with GH have growth acceleration (catch-up) that, generally, is sustained over the first several years of therapy (although attenuation of the response occurs as in all other instances of GH treatment). It appears that slower pretreatment growth velocity and higher weight/height ratio, factors suggesting GH deficiency, and less degree of bone age retardation are associated with better early growth responses.[1155] Longer term data are inadequate, however, to determine the impact of therapy on adult height. Zadik and co-workers[1153] report a mean increase of 5.4 ± 5.5 cm (SD) increase of final height predictions over 4 y of GH treatment of 43 prepubertal boys with low endogenous GH secretion. To the contrary, other investigators found that long-term GH treatment did not generally increase final target height and that height SD scores for bone age did not improve longitudinally.[1150, 1154, 1156] Concern had been raised that GH therapy of normal short children may result in an earlier onset of puberty and, as a result, earlier fusion of the epiphyses, thereby offsetting the positive response observed during the early years of GH treatment.[1157] Overall the available evidence does not clearly affirm the value of GH therapy in children who do not have evidence of IGF deficiency, but more precise patient selection, differing dosage levels, and frequency of administration may yet alter that conclusion.

Important questions have also been raised about the financial, ethical, and psychosocial impact of GH therapy in normal short children.[1158, 1159] Given the cost of GH, the financial implications of treating normal short children (whether at the bottom 5, 3, 1, or 0.1%) is considerable. The point is well taken that 5% of the population will always be below the 5th percentile, whether we treat with GH or not, and focusing on short stature potentially handicaps an otherwise normal child, psychologically or socially. No convincing data have been presented to date that GH treatment of normal short children improves psychological, social, or educational function. Furthermore the final adult height in children with CDGM (probably the most frequent diagnosis) will be adequate without any treatment.[1012–1014] Finally the treatment risks of GH therapy, both known and unknown, must be considered when treatment of otherwise normal children is an issue.

Conversely, given (1) the current limitations in the definitive discrimination between GH deficiency and normal short stature, (2) the inadequate understanding of neurosecretory defects of GH secretion, (3) the inadequate recognition of "partial" GH deficiency or GH resistance, and (4) the need to move to a more global concept of "IGF deficiency," it seems unfair to prevent GH therapy of short children who do not meet a narrow definition of GH deficiency (i.e., provocative testing), which we recognize as inadequate. Many of these children behave clinically and biochemically and respond to

GH treatment, as in classic GH deficiency. Accordingly we recommend the following approach:

1. Controlled therapeutic trials of "normal short stature" must be carried out to adult height.

2. Appropriate evaluation should include extensive analysis of the GH-IGF axis (with GHBP levels, IGF responses to GH treatment, and possibly GH releasing peptide–GHRH testing) before labeling a short child as "normal."

3. Proper assessment of pretreatment growth velocity should be over a minimum of a 6-mo period and preferably for 12 mo.

4. In the otherwise normal child with severe short stature (at least 2.5 SD below the mean for age) *and* a poor height velocity (e.g., <25th percentile for age: <6 cm/y before age 4; <5 cm/y at age 4 to 8; <4 cm/y anytime before puberty), the possibility of a *trial* of GH therapy should be discussed with the patient and family. This discussion should include an assessment of normal growth patterns, familial growth patterns, and the predicted pubertal and statural development. The inconveniences, discomforts, and potential risks of GH treatment should be fully described. It is the physician's responsibility to ensure that expectations of the child and the parents are realistic in regard to short-term growth and ultimate height. When appropriate, counseling and psychological support should be provided.

5. If a trial of GH therapy is desired, treatment should be for a minimum of 6 mo. There are no good guidelines for dosage; we recommend 0.05 mg/kg/d.

6. Therapy with GH should be continued beyond 6 mo only if growth is accelerated (defined as an increase in the height velocity of at least 2 cm/y). Efficacy of treatment requires continuous monitoring, especially in patients with partial GH resistance when the possibility of IGF-I therapy is a future alternative.

7. Growth acceleration with GH treatment does not relieve the physician of the need to investigate the cause of the child's growth failure. Appropriate studies should be repeated when indicated.

8. Treatment must be carefully monitored for side effects of GH treatment.

9. Continued psychological support should be provided for the child and family. This includes guiding the patient through puberty and providing post-treatment follow-up.

The evaluation and treatment of a "normal short child" with GH should be conducted by physicians trained in the management of growth disorders.

Miscellaneous Causes of Growth Failure

In addition to the clinical conditions described earlier, GH has been employed in the treatment of short stature associated with Prader-Willi syndrome,[1160] Noonan's syndrome,[1161, 1162] neurofibromatosis, and a variety of other conditions associated with postnatal growth failure. In general such trials have been uncontrolled and have not included sufficient numbers of individuals for efficacy to be evaluated.

Normal Aging and Other Catabolic States

Detailed consideration of the potential use of GH in normal aging is beyond the scope of this chapter.[173] The rationale for such therapy is based on the concept of the "somatopause," referring to the fact that GH secretion normally declines progressively after age 30, as reflected in decreasing IGF-I levels. Aging can be viewed as a catabolic state, with the potential that GH therapy must reverse or retard the loss of muscle mass and strength and the decrease in bone density with aging. Clinical studies are in progress.

As noted earlier, growth failure, often with impaired final adult height, is a characteristic clinical finding in endogenous or exogenous Cushing's syndrome. Excess glucocorticoids cause a catabolic state characterized by increased proteolysis, decreased protein synthesis, lowered osteoblastic and increased osteolytic activity, and insulin resistance.[1163] GH treatment blunts some of these catabolic actions but increases the insulin resistance.[789] Mauras and Beaufrere[779] showed that IGF-I therapy similarly induces an anabolic response despite excess glucocorticoids but does not cause insulin resistance. GH treatment in the post-transplantation period[1108–1110] and in other glucocorticoid-treated children[775] causes some height increments but not as good a response as in individuals not receiving glucocorticoids. GH does enhance bone formation and increases osteoblastic activity in such children.[1164] The marked increase in IGF-I levels during GH treatment may be sufficient to overcome the local resistance to IGF action.[657, 658, 777]

GH therapy is also being investigated in catabolic states,[174] such as burns, tumor cachexia, major abdominal surgery, acquired immunodeficiency syndrome, sepsis, metabolic acidosis, and situations requiring total parenteral alimentation.

Side Effects of Growth Hormone

As stated earlier pituitary-derived hGH had an enviable safety record for a quarter of a century but proved to be the agent for transmission of the fatal spongiform encephalopathy Creutzfeldt-Jakob disease.[1052, 1053] Although pit-hGH was removed from use in the United States in 1985, and later throughout the world, approximately 70 more patients with pit-GH–derived Creutzfeldt-Jakob disease have been identified and cases are likely to continue to be found over the next several decades.[1054, 1055] Although this risk does not exist with recombinant DNA–derived hGH, the experience with pit-hGH serves as a grim reminder of the potential toxicity that can reside in "normal" products and "physiological replacement."

Extensive experience with rGH over 15 y has been encouraging.[1165–1168] Every attempt has been made to seek physiological replacement rather than pharmacologic therapy, but often this is not possible. Concerns have been raised about a number of potential complications, which clearly require continued follow-up and assessment. This evaluation has been greatly facilitated by the extensive data bases established by GH manufacturers, in particular Genentech (National Cooperative Growth Study, NCGS)[1165] and Pharmacia-Upjohn (Kabi International Growth Study, KIGS).[1167]

Development of Leukemia

The development of leukemia as a complication of GH therapy was first reported in five patients from Japan in 1988,[1169] and to date more than 50 cases of leukemia have been reported in GH-treated patients. Many of the cases are from Japan[1170] but some are from the United States.[1165, 1171] One difficulty in assessing the role of GH treatment in this disorder is that many GH-deficient children have conditions that may predispose them to the development of leukemia, such as histories of prior malignancies, radiation, or syndromes associated with the development of leukemia (Bloom's syndrome, Down's syndrome, Fanconi's anemia). GH-treated patients who acquire leukemia do so at a later age than occurs in the normal population. Patients have included recipients of both pit-hGH and rGH, and leukemia has occurred both during treatment and after termination of therapy. Calculations of relative risk are imprecise but vary from sevenfold in Japan to two- to fourfold in the United States. Leukemia has been reported in GH-deficient individuals *without any history*

of GH therapy, raising the possibility that the GH-deficient state, by itself, might be a predisposing factor.[1166, 1167]

It is not possible to be certain whether GH is a causative agent in the development of leukemia. If it is, the increase in risk appears modest and may arise from the underlying state rather than from GH therapy. The number of cases of new leukemia in non-Japanese children treated with GH but in whom there are no known risk factors is approximately what would be expected on a patient-year basis.[1165] This issue should be discussed with all potential recipients of GH, but it appears that the risk is limited to those children with high-risk factors. Particular care should be used in prescribing GH therapy for children with past histories of leukemia or lymphoma or other disorders conveying an increased risk of leukemia. In a study of more than 200 children with prior leukemia who were treated with GH, the relapse rate was within the expected range, which was consistent with no effect of GH replacement therapy on recurrence of leukemia.[1165, 1172] In addition, data from 12,209 GH-treated patients with more than 51,000 patient-years at risk did not reveal an increased risk of nonleukemic extracranial neoplasms.[1173]

Recurrence of Central Nervous System Tumors

Since many recipients of GH have acquired GH deficiency from CNS tumors or from their treatment, the possibility of tumor recurrence with therapy is of obvious importance. Estimates of CNS tumor recurrence rates in non–GH-treated children and adolescents are difficult to obtain, bearing in mind the vast array of treatment programs used in the past three decades. In a total of 1083 patients not treated with GH compiled in 11 reports, 209 or 19.3% had recurrences.[1172, 1174–1183] Such data in a heterogeneous group, whose conditions included craniopharyngiomas, gliomas, ependymomas, medulloblastomas, and germ cell tumors, provide a background for assessing recurrence rates in GH-treated youth. Reports from six centers, encompassing 210 patients, indicate recurrence in 29 patients, or 13.8%, at the time of publication,[1172, 1174, 1183–1186] which is not much different from the larger number of untreated patients. Extensive analysis of the approximately 1262 patients with brain tumor histories prior to GH therapy in the National Cooperative Growth Study at Genentech showed a similar lack of increased tumor recurrence, as had been reported by the European Society of Pediatric Endocrinology.[1165, 1187, 1188] In the National Cooperative Growth Study series recurrence rates of the most common CNS neoplasms, craniopharyngioma (6.4%), primary neuroectodermal tumors (medulloblastoma, ependymoma) (7.2%), and low-grade glioma (18.1%) were lower or similar to those reported in non–GH-treated children.[1172, 1189, 1190]

Pseudotumor Cerebri

Pseudotumor cerebri (idiopathic intracranial hypertension) has been reported in about 30 GH-treated patients.[1165, 1191] The disorder may develop within months of starting treatment or as long as 5 y into the course; it appears to be more frequent in patients with renal failure than in those with GH deficiency.[1165] The mechanism for the effect is unclear but may reflect changes in fluid dynamics within the CNS. Pseudotumor has also been described following thyroid hormone replacement in hypothyroidism. In any case physicians should be alert to complaints of headache, nausea, dizziness, ataxia, or visual changes. Significant fluid retention with edema or hypertension is rare.[1192] Because of the possible association of pseudopapilledema with GH deficiency, perhaps representing a variant of optic nerve hypoplasia,[1193] careful ophthalmologic evaluation should be undertaken in patients with suspected

GH therapy–associated pseudotumor cerebri to avoid overdiagnosis and invasive treatments.

Slipped Capital Femoral Epiphysis

Slipped capital femoral epiphysis is associated with both hypothyroidism and GH deficiency.[1194–1196] Whether GH therapy plays a role in slipped capital femoral epiphysis has been difficult to determine, in part because the incidence of slipped capital femoral epiphysis varies with age, sex, race, and geographic locale, being reported in between 2 and 142 cases per 100,000 population. Accordingly, although slipped capital femoral epiphysis cannot be attributed to GH therapy per se, complaints of hip and knee pain, or limp, or both, should be evaluated carefully.

Miscellaneous Side Effects

Other potential side effects[1167] of GH therapy include prepubertal gynecomastia,[1197] pancreatitis,[1198] growth[1199, 1200] but not malignant degeneration of nevi,[1165] behavioral changes, scoliosis and kyphosis, worsening of neurofibromatosis, hypertrophy of tonsils and adenoids, and sleep apnea. This list is obviously only partial. It is best for the clinician to remember that GH and the peptide growth factors it regulates are potent mitogens with diverse metabolic and anabolic actions. All patients receiving GH treatment, even as replacement therapy, must be carefully monitored for side effects.

Treatment of Growth Hormone Resistance Syndrome: Use of Insulin-Like Growth Factor I

The production of IGF peptides by recombinant DNA technology has permitted clinical trials of IGF therapy. IGF-I administration to normal adult male volunteers as a single intravenous injection of 100 µg/kg caused hypoglycemia within 15 min.[1201] On a molar basis IGF-I has approximately 6% of the hypoglycemic potency of insulin, presumably reflecting increases in "free" IGF-I. In contrast, intravenous infusions of IGF-I to normal men at a rate of 20 µg/kg/h resulted in serum IGF-I levels within the normal range and did not produce hypoglycemia but did suppress GH levels, increase creatinine clearance, and decrease plasma urea nitrogen.[95]

The most obvious clinical use of IGF-I therapy is in patients with GH resistance. In patients with GH receptor deficiency, intravenous bolus administration of IGF-I caused acute symptomatic hypoglycemia, presumably because of low serum levels of IGFBP-3.[1202] The subcutaneous administration of IGF-I to eight GH receptor deficiency patients, at a dosage of 150 µg/kg/d for 7 d, did not cause symptomatic hypoglycemia.[1203]

Vaccarello and colleagues[96] treated six adults with GH receptor deficiency for 7 d with subcutaneous IGF-I at a dosage of 40 µg/kg every 12 h. Normal serum IGF-I levels were maintained for 2 to 6 h after injection, followed by a rapid decline because of low serum levels of IGFBP-3. Hypoglycemia did not occur, mean 24-h GH levels were suppressed, and urinary calcium was increased. In longer studies Laron and co-workers[1204] reported growth acceleration to rates of 8.8 to 13.6 cm/y in five children treated with a single daily dose of 150 µg IGF-I/kg for 3 to 10 mo. Similarly Walker and colleagues[1205] reported an increase in growth rate from 6.5 to 11.4 cm/y in a GH receptor deficiency patient treated with twice-daily subcutaneous injections of 120 µg IGF-I/kg. Wilton[1206] reported preliminary data on the treatment of 30 individuals, ages 3 to 23 y, with GH resistance from GH receptor deficiency or GH deficiency IA with anti-GH antibodies; the

TABLE 30–12. Therapeutic Potential of Insulin-Like Growth Factor Peptides

Growth-related indications
  Syndromes of GH resistance (see Table 30–8)
  Chronic renal failure–related growth failure
  Glucocorticoid-related growth failure
  Intrauterine growth retardation (IUGR)
    Administration to mother (stimulate placental growth)
    Administration to fetus
Catabolic states
  Malnutrition
  After surgery
  Burns
  Sepsis
  Cancer cachexia
  Acquired immunodeficiency syndrome (AIDS)-related cachexia
  Hyperalimentation
Aging
Insulin-resistant diabetes mellitus
Insulin-dependent diabetes mellitus

GH, growth hormone.

dosage of IGF-I varied from 40 to 120 µg/kg given twice daily. With the exception of the two oldest individuals, growth rates increased in all individuals by at least 2 cm/y, and the good growth response has continued in most patients.[1207] Side effects included hypoglycemia, headache, convulsions, urolithiasis, and papilledema; the latter suggests the possibility of pseudotumor cerebri.

A randomized, double-blind, placebo-controlled trial of IGF-I therapy in GH receptor deficiency has been performed in Ecuador, probably the only place where the patient population is sufficiently large and homogeneous to permit such investigation.[1208, 1208a] Growth rates in subjects receiving IGF-I increased from 2.9 to 8.6 cm/y over the first year of therapy and then 6.4 cm/y in year 2. The placebo group grew 4.4 cm/y during the same time, and then their growth rate increased to 8.4 cm/y during IGF-I treatment. The incidence of hypoglycemia was equal in the two groups. One recipient of IGF-I acquired papilledema, which resolved spontaneously while the patient was receiving treatment.

Although these early studies are promising, little is known about the long-term effects of IGF-I or about the optimal dose or frequency of administration. The failure of IGFBP-3 serum levels to increase with IGF-I administration underscores the relevance of the IGFBPs to IGF pharmacokinetics.[96, 1209] Nevertheless these data indicate that the IGF peptides, long considered to function as autocrine or paracrine growth factors, can act as classic hormones.

These studies provide the basis for studies of IGF therapy in a wide variety of growth-related catabolic and metabolic disorders. These are summarized in Table 30–12.

EXCESS GROWTH AND TALL STATURE

Although as many children have heights greater than 2 SD above the mean as have heights greater than 2 SD below the mean, referral for tall stature is less common than it is for short stature. This pattern speaks eloquently to the psychosocial pressures to which children with "growth disorders" are subjected. Nevertheless it is critical to identify those situations in which tall stature or an accelerated growth rate provides a clue for the diagnosis of an underlying disorder (see Table 30–12).

Statural Overgrowth in the Fetus

Maternal diabetes mellitus is the most common cause of large-for-gestational age infants (height or weight greater than the 90th percentile for gestational age). Even in the absence of clinical symptoms or a family history the birth of an excessively large infant should lead to evaluation for maternal (or gestational) diabetes.

Two relatively rare syndromes can also cause large-for-gestational age infants. Children with cerebral gigantism (also known as Sotos' syndrome)[1209, 1210] are typically above the 90th percentile for both length and weight at birth. Additional clinical features include a prominent forehead; dolichocephaly; macrocephaly; high arched palate; hypertelorism with an unusual slant to the eyes; prominent ears, jaw, and chin; mental retardation; and motor incoordination. Although such children continue to grow rapidly during the early years of childhood, puberty is usually early and causes premature epiphyseal fusion. GH secretion and serum IGF levels are normal, and no cause of the overgrowth in cerebral giantism has been identified.

Beckwith-Wiedemann syndrome is characterized by fetal macrosomia with omphalocele.[1211] Many of the clinical features of this syndrome are due to selective organomegaly, including macroglossia, renal medullary hyperplasia, and neonatal hypoglycemia due to islet cell hyperplasia.[1212] As with cerebral gigantism excessive fetal, neonatal, and childhood growth ultimately leads to early epiphyseal fusion, without an increase in adult height.[1213] An association between Beckwith-Wiedemann syndrome and disordered regulation of *IGF-II* gene transcription has been reported, but no consistent abnormality of the GH-IGF axis has been identified to date.[1214, 1215] The paternally derived gene for IGF-II is overexpressed and the maternally transmitted gene is not active.[1216] Four children with somatic overgrowth but not the diagnostic features of Beckwith-Wiedemann syndrome had *IGF-II* gene overexpression.[1217]

Postnatal Statural Overgrowth

As stated earlier, both cerebral gigantism and the Beckwith-Wiedemann syndrome are associated with rapid perinatal growth, but rapid growth usually ends by early to middle childhood. Nevertheless these conditions should be considered when tall stature in childhood is accompanied by the characteristic phenotypic features or with a history of unexplained fetal overgrowth. As in the case of the child with growth failure, crossing height percentiles between infancy and the onset of puberty is an indication for further evaluation. Although such growth patterns are frequently not of concern to parents, such overly rapid statural growth can indicate a serious underlying pathologic condition. Furthermore as with short stature, children with tall stature must be evaluated in the context of familial growth and pubertal patterns.

Familial (Constitutional) Tall Stature

GH secretion and levels of IGF-I and IGFBP-3 in familial tall stature are often in the upper range of normal.[1218] Tauber and colleagues[1219] divided 65 children with familial tall stature into a subset with high GH secretion rates (5.4 ± 2.3 mg/L/mm) and frequent secretory bursts (5.1 ± 1.6/d) and another subset with lower GH secretion (2.1 ± 0.5 mg/L/mm) and fewer episodic spikes (3.3 ± 1.3/d). IGF-I levels were higher in the group producing more GH and were normal in the low-GH group. They postulated that both enhanced secretion of GH and greater efficiency of GH-mediated IGF-I production might be potential causes of familial tall stature.

As with short stature, children with tall stature must be evaluated relative to familial growth patterns and parental target height (see earlier).[1220] When a family history of tall stature is available, support and reassurance are frequently all

that is required. A careful assessment of pubertal status and bone age facilitates prediction of adult height and usually obviates the need for hormonal therapy. Standard height prediction using Bayley-Pinneau tables, especially in children younger than age 12, tends to overestimate final height with large confidence limits,[1221–1223] particularly in boys. We discourage therapy for boys with predicted adult heights less than or equal to 198 cm (6 feet 6 inches) and girls with predicted adult heights less than or equal to 183 cm (6 feet). Indeed societal changes in attitudes toward tall individuals appear to discourage treatment except in extreme circumstances. Therapy, when necessary, is aimed at the acceleration of puberty in order to cause premature epiphyseal fusion.[1224, 1225] Accordingly the optimal time for treatment is before the onset of puberty. The earlier the intervention, the more likely that adult height can be decreased, although patients are not usually referred until late childhood or early puberty. Although some success with lower dosages had been reported, administration of ethinyl estradiol at a dose of 0.15 to 0.30 mg/d is a reasonable starting level in girls and can be increased, if necessary and well tolerated, to 0.50 mg/d. Conjugated estrogens, 7.5 to 10 mg/d have also been successful. If breakthrough bleeding occurs, cyclic progestagens may be added to the estrogen therapy. Treatment should be continued until the epiphyses fuse, as post-treatment growth may be substantial if treatment is stopped early.[1223]

The mechanism of estrogen action is probably complex, since estrogen can affect both GH secretion and serum IGF levels and, more importantly, act directly on the epiphysis. Estrogen mediates epiphyseal fusion in both girls and boys.[442–444] In prepubertal girls estrogen therapy reduces adult height by as much as 5 to 6 cm, relative to predictions. When therapy is initiated after the onset of puberty the decrement in adult height is not likely to be as large.

The use of high-dose estrogen in otherwise normal children must be weighed against the known (and unknown) toxicity of such therapy,[1226] including nausea, weight gain, edema, and hypertension. During the initial phases of therapy growth is paradoxically accelerated as the child rapidly progresses through puberty. Other potential problems, such as thromboembolism, cystic hyperplasia of the breast, endometrial hyperplasia, and cancer, have not been definitively related to estrogen therapy in children but should be discussed with the patient and family.

Therapy in boys with tall stature is even more problematic. For the reasons discussed earlier, estrogen is likely to be most efficacious in accelerating epiphyseal fusion but is obviously undesirable in males. Androgens will also accelerate skeletal maturation, presumably via aromatization to estrogen but at the price of rapid virilization.

Obesity

Obesity is frequently associated with rapid skeletal growth and an early onset of puberty.[1227] This association is so characteristic that the child with obesity and *short stature* should always be evaluated for an underlying pathologic condition such as hypothyroidism, GH deficiency, Cushing's syndrome, and disorders such as the Prader-Willi syndrome. Patients with obesity tend to have diminished overall GH production but normal high GHBP and IGF-I levels maintaining adequate or enhanced linear growth velocity. Early activation of adrenal androgenesis and premature pubarche are common. Bone age is usually modestly accelerated so that both puberty and epiphyseal fusion occur early and adult height is normal.

Excess Growth Hormone Secretion

Pituitary gigantism is a rare condition analogous to acromegaly in the adult[1228–1230] (see Chapter 9). GH-secreting tumors of the pituitary are typically eosinophilic or chromophobe adenomas. Their cause is uncertain, although many result from somatic mutations that generate constitutively activated G proteins with reduced guanosine triphosphatase activity[1231] (see Chapter 6). The resulting increase in intracellular cAMP in the pituitary leads to increased GH secretion. The McCune-Albright syndrome, which is also caused by mutations resulting in constitutive activation of G proteins, may also be characterized by somatotropic tumors and excess GH secretion.[1232, 1233] GH-secreting tumors have also been reported in multiple endocrine neoplasia and in association with neurofibromatosis and tuberous sclerosis[1234] (see Chapter 32.)

GH excess that occurs prior to epiphyseal fusion results in rapid growth and attainment of adult heights to greater than the expected genetic potential. When GH hypersecretion is accompanied by gonadotropin deficiency, accelerated linear growth may persist for decades, as in the case of the Alton giant, who reached a height of 280 cm by the time of his death in his 20s.[1235] Manifestations typical of acromegaly may also appear, such as soft tissue swelling; enlargement of the nose, ears, and jaw, with coarsening of the facial features; pronounced increases in hand and foot size; diaphoresis; galactorrhea; and menstrual irregularity.

Serum IGF-I levels are elevated, although high IGF-I levels may also be a normal manifestation of puberty. Basal serum GH levels may be normal or increased, but serum GH is not suppressed by the administration of glucose (1.75 g/kg body weight, up to a maximum of 100 g).

Although abnormalities of the sella turcica are often evident on lateral skull films, the demonstration of increased GH-IGF secretion should lead to radiologic evaluation of the hypothalamus and pituitary by MRI or computed tomography. Definitive therapy requires surgical ablation of the tumor. Fortunately this can usually be accomplished by transsphenoidal pituitary surgery, although macroadenomas may require a more aggressive surgical approach. As described in Chapter 9, the use of somatostatin analogues is an important part of treatment for GH excess.

Precocious Puberty

Precocious puberty, whether centrally mediated (increased gonadotropin secretion, LHRH dependent) or peripherally mediated (increased androgen or estrogen secretion, or both, LHRH dependent) results in accelerated linear growth in childhood, mimicking the pubertal growth spurt. Since skeletal maturation is also accelerated, adult height is frequently compromised. The diagnostic evaluation and management of precocious puberty is discussed in Chapter 31.

Miscellaneous Causes of Tall Stature

Marfan syndrome, an autosomal dominant disorder of collagen metabolism, is characterized by hyperextensible joints, dislocation of the lens, kyphoscoliosis, and dissecting aortic aneurysm and often leads to long, thin bones that result in arachnodactyly and moderately tall stature. Homocystinuria, an autosomal recessive disorder, phenotypically resembles Marfan syndrome, although patients are usually mentally retarded. Males with an XYY karyotype may also have moderate tall stature. Of note, however, men with Klinefelter's syndrome (XXY karyotype) usually have normal adult stature. The rate of linear growth may increase modestly in hyperthyroidism.

It is worth commenting that although delayed puberty may be associated with short stature in childhood, as with constitutional delay, failure to enter puberty and complete sexual maturation may result in sustained growth during adult life with ultimate tall stature and a characteristic eunuchoid habitus. The description of tall stature with open epiphyses

resulting from mutation of the estrogen receptor or from aromatase deficiency underscores the fundamental role of estrogen in promoting epiphyseal fusion and termination of normal skeletal growth.[442-444]

REFERENCES

1. Kaplan SL. Normal and abnormal growth. In: Rudolph AM, ed. Pediatrics. New York: Appleton-Century Crofts, 1977: 95–120
2. Reiter EO, Witt MR. Physical growth and development. In: Braham RL, Morris, ME, eds. Textbook of Pediatric Dentistry. Baltimore: Williams & Wilkins, 1985: 2–23.
3. Heinrich C, Munson PJ, Counts DRG, et al. Patterns of human growth. Science 1995; 268:442–444.
4. Lampl M, Veldhuis JD, Johnson ML. Saltation and stasis: a model of human growth. Science 1992; 258:801–803.
5. Lampl M, Cameron N, Veldhuis JD, et al. Patterns of human growth: response. Science 1995; 268:445–447.
6. Tanner JM, Davies SWD. Clinical longitudinal standards for height and height velocity for North American children. J Pediatr 1985; 107:317.
7. Tanner JM, Whitehouse RH, Takaishi M. Standards from birth to maturity for height, weight, height velocity, and weight velocity: British children, 1965. Part II. Arch Dis Child 1966; 41:613–635.
8. Tanner JM, Whitehouse RH, Hughes PCR, et al. Relative importance of growth hormone and sex steroids for growth at puberty of trunk length, limb length, and muscle width in growth hormone–deficient children. J Pediatr 1976; 89:1000–1010.
9. Tanner JM. Auxology. In: Kappy MS, Blizzard RM, Migeon CJ, eds. The Diagnosis and Treatment of Endocrine Disorders. Springfield, IL, Charles C Thomas, 1994: 137–192.
10. Tanner JM. Foetus into Man. Cambridge: Harvard University Press, 1990.
11. Karlberg J, Engstrom I, Karlberg P, et al. Analysis of linear growth using a mathematical model. 1: From birth to three years. Acta Paediatr Scand 1987; 76:478–488.
12. Karlberg J, Fryer JG, Engstrom I, et al. Analysis of linear growth using a mathematical model. II: From 3 to 21 years. Acta Paediatr Scand 1987; 337(Suppl):12–29.
13. Cameron N. The methods of auxological anthropometry. In: Falkner F, Tanner JM, eds. Human Growth: A Comprehensive Treatise. New York: Plenum, 1986: 35–90.
14. Tanner JM. Normal growth and techniques of growth assessment. Clin Endocrinol Metab 1986; 15:411.
15. Underwood LE, Van Wyk JJ. Normal and aberrant growth. In: Wilson JD, Foster DW, eds. Williams Textbook of Endocrinology. Philadelphia: WB Saunders, 1991: 1079–1138.
16. Whitehouse RH, Tanner JM, Healy MJR. Diurnal variation in stature of sitting height in 12–14 year old boys. Ann Hum Biol 1974; 1:103–106.
17. Marshall WA. Evaluation of growth rate in height over periods of less than one year. Arch Dis Child 1971; 46:414–420.
18. Hamill PVV, Drizd TA, Johnson CL, et al. Physical growth: National Center for Health Statistics percentiles. Am J Clin Nutr 1979; 32:607–629.
19. Anonymous. National Center for Health Statistics: NCH Growth Charts, 1976. Monthly Vital Statistics Report. Rockville, MD. Health Resources Administration. 1976; 3(Suppl):76–1120.
20. Anonymous. National Center for Health Statistics: NCH Growth Curves for Children 0–18 years. United States, Vital and Health Statistics, Series 11, No 165. Washington, DC: Health Resources Administration, US Government Printing Office, 1977.
21. Albertsson-Wikland K, Lannering B, Marky I, et al. A longitudinal study on growth and spontaneous growth hormone (GH) secretion in children with irradiated brain tumors. Acta Paediatr Scand 1987; 76:966–973.
22. Lyon AL, Preece MA, Grant DB. Growth curve for girls with Turner syndrome. Arch Dis Child 1985; 60:932–935.
23. Horton WA, Rotter JI, Rimoin DL, et al. Standard growth curves for achondroplasia. J Pediatr 1978; 93:435–438.
24. Cronk C, Crocker AC, Pueschel SM, et al. Growth charts for children with Down syndrome: 1 month to 18 y of age. Pediatrics 1988; 81:102–110.
25. Bayer LM, Bayley L. Growth Diagnosis. Chicago: University of Chicago Press, 1959: 226 pp.
26. Greulich WW, Pyle SI. Radiographic Atlas of Skeletal Development of the Hand and Wrist. Stanford: Stanford University Press, 1959.
27. Tanner JM, Whitehouse RH, Cameron, N, et al. Assessment of Skeletal Maturity and Prediction of Adult Height (TW2 Method). New York: Academic, 1983.
28. Tanner JM, Oshman D, Lindgren G, et al. Reliability of computer-assisted estimates of Tanner-Whitehouse skeletal maturity [CASAS]: comparison with manual method. Horm Res 1994; 42:288–294.
29. Van Teunenbroek A, De Waal W, Roks A, et al. Computer-aided skeletal age scores in healthy children, girls with Turner syndrome, and in children with constitutionally tall stature. Pediatr Res 1996; 39:360–367.
30. Roche AF, Davila GH, Eyman SL. A comparison between Greulich-Pyle and Tanner-Whitehouse assessments of skeletal maturity. Radiology 1971; 98:273–280.
31. Bayley N, Pinneau SR. Tables for predicting adult height from skeletal

age: revised for use with the Greulich-Pyle hand standards. J Pediatr 1952; 40:423–441.

32. Tanner JM, Whitehouse RH, Marshall WA, et al. Prediction of adult height from height, bone age, and occurrence of menarche at ages 4–16 with allowance for midparent height. Arch Dis Child 1975; 50:14–26.

33. Roche AF, Wainer H, Thissen D. The RWT method for the prediction of adult stature. Pediatrics 1975; 56:1026–1033.

34. Karlberg J, Lawrence C, Albertsson-Wikland K. Prediction of final height in short, normal and tall children. Acta Paediatr 1994; 406(Suppl):3–9.

35. Khamis HJ, Roche AF. Predicting adult stature without using skeletal age: The Khamis-Roche method. Pediatrics 1994; 94:504–507.

36. Tanner JM, Goldstein H, Whitehouse RH. Standards for children's height at ages 2–9 years allowing for height of parents. Arch Dis Child 1970; 45:755–762.

37. Ikeda H, Suzuki J, Sasano N, et al. The development and morphogenesis of the human pituitary gland. Anat Embryol (Berl) 1988; 178:327–336.

38. Goodyer CG. Ontogeny of pituitary hormone secretion. In: Collu R, Ducharme JR, Guyda HJ, eds. Pediatric Endocrinology. New York: Raven, 1989: 125–169.

39. Stanfield JP. The blood supply of the human pituitary gland. J Anat 1960; 94:257–273.

40. Gorcyzca W, Hardy J. Arterial supply of the human anterior pituitary gland. Neurosurgery 1987; 20:369–378.

41. Thorner MO, Vance ML, Horvath E, et al. The anterior pituitary. In: Wilson JD, Foster DW, eds. Williams Textbook of Endocrinology. 8th ed. Philadelphia: WB Saunders, 1992: 210–221.

42. Scheithauer BW, Sano T, Kovacs K, et al. The pituitary gland in pregnancy: a clinicopathologic and immunohistochemical study of 69 cases. Mayo Clin Proc 1990; 65:461–474.

43. Boyd JD. Observations on human pharyngeal hypophysis. J Endocrinol 1956; 14:66–77.

44. Underwood LE, Radcliffe WB, Guinto FC. New standards for the assessment of sella turcica volume in children. Radiology 1976; 119:651–854.

45. Hoyt WF, Kaplan SL, Grumbach MM, et al. Septo-optic dysplasia and pituitary dwarfism. Lancet 1970; 1:893–894.

46. Lewis UJ, Singh RNP, Tutwiler GH, et al. Human growth hormone: a complex of proteins. Recent Prog Horm Res 1980; 36:477–508.

47. Baumann G. Heterogeneity of growth hormone. In: Bercu B, ed. Basic and Clinical Aspects of Growth Hormone. New York: Plenum, 1988: 13–31.

48. Frankenne F, Closset J, Gomez F, et al. The physiology of growth hormones (GH) in pregnant women and partial characterization of the placental GH variant. J Clin Endocrinol Metab 1988; 66:1171–1180.

49. Cooke NE, Ray J, Watson MA, et al. Human growth hormone gene and the highly homologous growth hormone variant gene display different splicing patterns. J Clin Invest 1988; 82:270–275.

50. Miller WL, Eberhardt NL. Structure and evaluation of the growth hormone gene family. Annu Rev Med 1983; 34:519.

51. DeNoto FM, Moore DD, Goodman HM. Human growth hormone DNA sequence and mRNA structure: possible alternative splicing. Nucleic Acids Res 1981; 9:3719–3730.

52. Barinaga M, Yamonoto G, Rivier C, et al. Transcriptional regulation of growth hormone gene expression by growth hormone–releasing factor. Nature 1983; 306:84–85.

53. Esch FS, Bohlen P, Ling NC, et al. Guillemin. Primary structure of three human pancreas peptides with growth hormone releasing activity. J Biol Chem 1983; 258:1806.

54. Holl RW, Thorner MO, Leong DA. Intracellular calcium concentration and growth hormone secretion in individual somatotropes: effects of growth hormone–releasing factor and somatostatin. Endocrinology 1988; 122:2927–2932.

55. Ahmad I, Finkelstein JA, Downs TR, et al. Obesity-associated decrease in growth hormone–releasing hormone gene expression: a mechanism for reduced growth hormone mRNA levels in genetically obese Zucker rats. Neuroendocrinology 1993; 58:332–337.

56. Szabo M, Butz MR, Banerjee SA, et al. Autofeedback suppression of growth hormone (GH) secretion in transgenic mice expressing a human GH reported targeted by tyrosine hydroxylase 5′-flanking sequences to the hypothalamus. Endocrinology 1995; 136:4044–4048.

57. Horikawa R, Hellmann P, Cella SG, et al. Growth hormone–releasing factor (GRF) regulates expression of its own receptor. Endocrinology 1996; 137:2642–2645.

58. Kineman RD, Aleppo G, Frohman LA. The tyrosine hydroxylase–human growth hormone (GH) transgenic mouse as a model of hypothalamic GH deficiency: growth retardation is the result of a selective reduction in somatotrope numbers despite normal somatotrope function. Endocrinology 1996; 137:4630–4636.

59. Valerius MT, Li H, Stock JL, et al. Gsh-1: a novel murine homeobox gene expressed in the central nervous system. Dev Dynamics 1995; 203:337–351.

60. Li H, Zeitler PS, Valerius MT, et al. Gsh-1, an orphan Hox gene, is required for normal pituitary development. EMBO J 1996; 15:714–724.

61. Hartman ML, Faria ACS, Vance ML, et al. Temporal sequence of in vivo growth hormone secretory events in man. Am J Physiol 1991; 260:E101–E110.

62. Frohman LA. Neurotransmitters as regulators of endocrine function. In: Krieger DT, Hughes JC, eds. Neuroendocrinology. Sunderland, MA: Sinauer Associates, 1980: 44–58.

63. Melander T, Hokfelt T, Rokaeus A. Distribution of galaninlike immunoreactivity in the rat central nervous system. J Comp Neurol 1986; 218:175–217.

64. Phelps CJ. Pituitary hormones as neurotrophic signals: anomalous hypophysiotrophic neuron differentiation in hypopituitary dwarf mice. Proc Soc Exp Biol Med 1994; 206:6–23.

65. Deller JJ, Plunket DC, Forsham PH. Growth hormone studies in growth retardation: therapeutic response to administration of androgen. Calif Med 1966; 104:359.

66. Zeitler P, Argente J, Chowen-Breede JA, et al. Growth hormone releasing hormone messenger ribonucleic acid in the hypothalamus of the adult male rat is increased by testosterone. Endocrinology 1990; 127:362–368.

67. Ho KY, Evans WS, Bilzzard RM, et al. Effects of sex and age on the 24-h profile of growth hormone secretion in man: importance of endogenous estradiol concentrations. J Clin Endocrinol Metab 1987; 64:51–58.

68. Katz HP, Youlton R, Kaplan SL, et al. Growth and growth hormone. III: Growth hormone release in children with primary hypothyroidism and thyrotoxicosis. J Clin Endocrinol Metab 1969; 29:346.

69. Frantz AG, Rabkin MT. Human growth hormone. Clinical measurement, response to hypoglycemia and suppression by corticosteroids. N Engl J Med 1964; 271:1375–1381.

70. Thompson RG, Rodriguez A, Kowarski A, et al. Growth hormone: metabolic clearance rates in normal adults and effect of prednisone. J Clin Invest 1972; 51:3193–3199.

71. Martha PM, Rogol AD, Veldhuis JD, et al. Alterations in the pulsatile properties of circulating growth hormone concentrations during puberty in boys. J Clin Endocrinol Metab 1989; 69:563–570.

71a. Link K, Blizzard RM, Evans WS, et al. The effect of androgens on the pulsatile release and twenty-four-hr mean concentration of growth hormone in peripubertal males. J Clin Endocrinol Metab 1986; 62:159–164.

72. Bowers CY, Momany F, Reynolds GA, et al. On the in vitro and in vivo activity of a new synthetic hexapeptide that acts on the pituitary to specifically release growth hormone. Endocrinology 1984; 114:1537–1545.

73. Sartor O, Bowers CY, Reynolds GA, et al. Variables determining the GH response of His-D-Trp-Ala-Trp-D-Phe-Lys-NH (GHRP-6) in the rat. Endocrinology 117:1441–1447.

74. Malozowski S, Hao EH, Ren SG, et al. Growth hormone (GH) responses to hexapeptide GH-releasing peptide and GH-releasing hormone (GHRH) in the cynomologus Macaque: evidence for non–GHRH-mediated responses. J Clin Endocrinol Metab 1991; 73:314–317.

75. Bellone G, Aimaretti G, Bartolotta E, et al. Growth hormone–releasing activity of hexarelin, a new synthetic hexapeptide, before and during puberty. J Clin Endocrinol Metab 1995; 80:1090–1094.

76. Tuilipakov AN, Bulatov AA, Peterkova AV, et al. Growth hormone (GH)-releasing effects of synthetic peptide GH-releasing peptide-2 and GH-releasing hormone (1-29NH2) in children with GH insufficiency and idiopathic short stature. Metabolism 1995; 44:1199–1204.

77. Pombo M, Barreiro J, Penalva A, et al. Absence of growth hormone (GH) secretion after administration of GH-releasing hormone (GHRH), GH-releasing peptide (GHRP-6), or GHRH plus GHRP-6 in children with neonatal pituitary stalk transection. J Clin Endocrinol Metab 1995; 80:3180–3184.

78. Korbonits M, Grossman AB. Growth hormone–releasing peptide and its analogues. Trends Endocrinol Metab 1995; 6:43–49.

79. Howard AD, Feighner SD, Cully DF, et al. A receptor in pituitary and hypothalamus that functions in growth hormone release. Science 1996; 273:974–977.

80. Smith RG, Cheng K, Schoen WR, et al. A non peptidyl growth hormone secretagogue. Science 1993; 260:1640–1643.

81. Bowers CY. On a peptidomimetric growth hormone–releasing peptide. J Clin Endocrinol Metab 1994; 79:940–942 (editorial).

82. Goth MI, Lyons CE, Canny BJ, et al. Pituitary adenylate cyclase activating polypeptides, growth hormone (GH) releasing peptide and GH releasing hormone stimulate GH release through distinct pituitary receptors. Endocrinology 1992; 130:939–944.

83. Cauvin A, Robberecht P, De Neef P, et al.Properties and distribution of receptors for pituitary adenylate cyclase activating peptide (PACAP) in rat brain and spinal cord. Regul Peptides 1991; 35:161–173.

84. Nelson C, Albert VR, Elsholtz HP, et al. Activation of cell-specific expression of rat growth hormone and prolactin genes by a common transcription factor. Science 1988; 239:1400–1405.

85. Puy LA, Asa SL. The ontogeny of Pit-1 expression in the human fetal pituitary gland. Neuroendocrinology 1996; 63:349–355.

86. Mangalam HJ, Albert VR, Ingraham HA, et al. A pituitary POU domain protein, pit-1, activates both growth hormone and prolactin promoters transcriptionally. Genes Dev 1989; 3:946–958.

87. Li S, Crenshaw EB III, Rawson EJ, et al. Dwarf locus mutants lacking three pituitary cell types result from mutations in the POU-domain gene pit-1. Nature 1990; 347:528–532.

88. Berelowitz M, Szabo M, Frohman LA, et al. Somatomedin-C mediates growth hormone negative feedback by effects on both the hypothalamus and pituitary. Science 1981; 212:1279–1281.

89. Yamashita S, Melmed S. Insulin-like growth factor I action on rat anterior

pituitary cells: suppression of growth hormone secretion and messenger ribonucleic acid levels. Endocrinology 1986; 118:176–182.

90. Abe H, Molitch M, Van Wyk JJ, et al. Human growth hormone and somatomedin-C suppress the spontaneous release of growth hormone in unanesthetized rats. Endocrinology 1983; 113:1319–1324.

91. Rosenfeld RG, Ceda G, Cutler CW, et al. Insulin and insulin-like growth factor (somatomedin) receptors on cloned rat pituitary tumor cells. Endocrinology 1985; 117:2008–2016.

92. Rosenfeld RG, Ceda G, Wilson DM, et al. Characterization of high-affinity receptors for insulin-like growth factors-I and -II on rat anterior pituitary cells. Endocrinology 1984; 114:1571–1575.

93. Ceda GP, Hoffman AR, Silverberg GD, et al. Regulation of growth hormone release from cultured human pituitary adenomas of somatomedins and insulin. J Clin Endocrinol Metab 1985; 60:1204–1209.

94. Ceda GP, Davis RG, Rosenfeld RG, et al. The growth hormone (GH) releasing hormone (GHRH)-GH-somatomedin axis: evidence for rapid inhibition of GHRH-elicited GH release by insulin-like growth factors I and II. Endocrinology 1987; 120:1658–1662.

95. Guler HP, Zapf J, Froesch ER. Short-term metabolic effects and half-lives of intravenously administered insulin-like growth factor I in healthy adults. N Engl J Med 1987; 317:137–140.

96. Vaccarello MA, Diamond FB Jr, Guevara-Aguirre J, et al. Hormonal and metabolic effects and pharmacokinetics of recombinant insulin-like growth factor-I in growth hormone receptor deficiency (GH receptor deficiency)/Laron syndrome. J Clin Endocrinol Metab 1993; 77:273–280.

97. Hartman ML, Veldhuis JD, Thorner MO. Normal control of growth hormone secretion. Horm Res 1993; 40:37–47.

98. Hartman ML, Faria ACS, Vance ML, et al. Temporal structure of in vivo growth hormone secretory events in humans. Am J Physiol 1991; 260:E101–E110.

99. Veldhuis JD, Liem AY, South S, et al. Differential impact of age, sex steroid hormones, and obesity on basal versus pulsatile growth hormone secretion in men as assessed in an ultrasensitivie chemiluminescence assay. J Clin Endocrinol Metab 1995; 80:3209–3222.

100. Veldhuis JD, Carlson ML, Johnson ML. The pituitary gland secretes in bursts: appraising the nature of glandular secretory impulses by simultaneous multiple-parameter deconvolution of plasma hormone concentrations. Proc Natl Acad Sci USA 1987; 84:7686–7690.

101. Iranmanesh A, Grisso B, Veldhuis JD. Low basal and persistent pulsatile growth hormone secretion are revealed in normal and hyposomatotropic men studied with a new ultrasensitive chemiluminescence assay. J Clin Endocrinol Metab 1994; 78:526–535.

102. Chapman IM, Hartman ML, Straume M, et al. Enhanced sensitivity growth hormone chemiluminescence assay reveals lower-post-glucose nadir GH concentrations in men than women. J Clin Endocrinol Metab 1994; 78:1312–1319.

103. Martha PM Jr, Gorman KM, Blizzard RM, et al. Endogenous growth hormone secretion and clearance rates in normal boys, as determined by deconvolution analysis: relationship to age, pubertal status and body mass. J Clin Endocrinol Metab 1992; 74:336–344.

104. Faria ACS, Bekenstein LW, Booth RA, et al. Pulsatile growth hormone release in normal women during the menstrual cycle. Clin Endocrinol (Oxf) 1992; 36:591–596.

105. Mauras D, Rogol AD, Veldhuis JD. Increased hGH production rate after low-dose estrogen therapy in prepubertal girls with Turner's syndrome. Pediatr Res 1990; 28:626–630.

106. Ho KY, Veldhuis JD, Johnson ML, et al. Fasting enhances growth hormone secretion and amplifies the complex rhythms of growth hormone secretion in man. J Clin Invest 1988; 81:968–975.

107. Hartman ML, Veldhuis JD, Johnson ML, et al. Augmented growth hormone (GH) secretory burst frequency and amplitude mediate enhanced GH secretion during a two day fast in normal men. J Clin Endocrinol Metab 1992; 74:757–765.

108. Martha PM Jr, Reiter EO. Pubertal growth and growth hormone secretion. Endocrinol Metab Clin North Am 1991; 20:165–182.

109. Albertsson-Wikland K, Rosberg L, Libre E, et al. Growth hormone secretory rates in children as estimated by deconvulution analysis of 24-hr plasma concentration profiles. Am J Physiol 1989; 257:E804–E814.

110. Martin-Hernandez T, Diaz Galvez M, Torres Cuadro A, et al. Growth hormone secretion in normal prepubertal children; importance of relations between endogenous secretion, pulsatility and body mass. Clin Endocrinol 1996; 44:327–334.

111. Veldhuis JD, Johnson ML. Deconvolution analysis of hormone data. Methods Enzymol 1992; 210:539–575.

112. Grumbach MM, Gluckman PD. The human fetal hypothalamic and pituitary gland: the maturation of neuroendocrine mechanisms controlling secretion of fetal pituitary growth hormone, prolactin, gonadotropin, adrenocorticotropin-related peptides and thyrotropin. In: Tulchinsky D, Little AB, eds. Maternal and Fetal Endocrinology. Philadelphia: WB Saunders, 1994: 193–261.

113. Kaplan SL, Grumbach MM, Aubert ML. The ontogenesis of pituitary hormones and hypothalamic factors in the human fetus: maturation of central nervous system regulation of anterior pituitary function. Recent Prog Horm Res 1976; 32:161–243.

114. Siler-Khodr TM, Morgenstern IL, Greenwood FC. Hormone synthesis and release from human fetal adenohypophysis in vitro. J Clin Endocrinol Metab 1974; 39:891–905.

115. Atwell WJ. The development of the hypophysis cerebri in man, with special reference to the pars tuberalis. Am J Anat 1926; 37:159–193.

116. Falin LI. The development of the human hypophysis and differentiation of cells of its anterior lobe during embryonic life. Acta Anat 1961; 44:188–205.

117. Thliveris JA, Currie RW. Observations of the hypothalamophypophyseal portal vasculature in the developing human fetus. Am J Anat 1980; 157:441–444.

118. Hindmarsh P, Brook C, Radeck C, et al. Hormonal levels in the human fetus between 14 and 22 weeks gestation. Early Hum Dev 1987; 15:253–254.

119. Gluckman PD, Grumbach MM, Kaplan SL. The neuroendocrine regulation and function of growth hormone and prolactin in the mammalian fetus. Endocr Rev 1981; 2:363–395.

120. Arosio M, Cortelazzi D, Persani L, et al. Circulating levels of growth hormone, insulin-like growth factor-I and prolactin in normal, growth-retarded and anencephalic human fetuses. J Endocrinol Invest 1995; 18:346–353.

121. Martha PM Jr, Rogol AD, Blizzard RM, et al. Growth hormone–binding protein activity is inversely related to 24-h growth hormone release in normal boys. J Clin Endocrinol Metab 1991; 73:175–181.

122. Baumann G, Shaw MA, Amburn K. Circulating growth hormone binding proteins. J Endocrinol Invest 1994; 17:67–81.

123. MacGillivray MH, Frohman LA, Doe J. Metabolic clearance and production rates of human growth hormone in subjects with normal and abnormal growth. J Clin Endocrinol Metab 1970; 30:632–638.

124. Dudl RJ, Ensinck JW, Palmer HE, et al. Effect of age on growth hormone secretion in man. J Clin Endocrinol Metab 1973; 37:11–16.

125. Rudman D, Kutner MH, Rogers CM, et al. Impaired growth hormone secretion in the adult population: relation to age and adiposity. J Clin Invest 1981; 67:1361–1369.

126. Sassin JF, Parker DC, Mace JW, et al. Human growth hormone release. Relation to slow-wave sleep and sleep-waking cycles. Science 1969; 165:513.

127. Van Cauter E, Kerkhofs M, Van Onderbergen A, et al. Modulation of spontaneous and GHRH-stimulated growth hormone secretion by sleep. Endocr Soc Proc 1989; 220 (abstract 792).

128. Veldhuis JD, Iranmanesh A, Ho KK, et al. Dual defects in pulsatile growth hormone secretion and clearance subserve the hyposomatotropism of obesity in man. J Clin Endocrinol Metab 1991; 72:51–59.

129. Schalch DS. The influence of physical stress and exercise on growth hormone and insulin secretion in man. J Lab Clin Med 1967; 69:256.

130. Holl RW, Hartman ML, Veldhuis JD, et al. Thirty second sampling of plasma growth hormone in man: correlation with sleep stages. J Clin Endocrinol Metab 1991; 72:854–861.

131. Jaffe CA, Turgeon DK, Friberg RD, et al. Nocturnal augmentation of growth hormone (GH) secretion is preserved during repetitive bolus administration of GH–releasing hormone: Potential involvement of endogenous somatostatin-A clinical research center study. J Clin Endocrinol Metab 1995; 80:3321–3326.

132. Van Cauter E, Plat L. Physiology of growth hormone secretion during sleep. J Pediatr 1996; 128:532–537.

133. Mauras N, Blizzard RM, Link K, et al. Augmentation of growth hormone secretion during puberty: evidence for a pulse amplitude–modulated phenomenon. J Clin Endocrinol Metab 1987; 64:596–601.

134. Metzger DL, Kerrigan JR. Androgen receptor blockade with flutamide enhances growth hormone secretion in late pubertal males: evidence for independent actions of estrogen and androgen. J Clin Endocrinol Metab 1993; 76:1147–1152.

135. Metzger DL, Kerrigan JR. Estrogen blockade with tamoxifen diminishes growth hormone secretion in boys: evidence for a stimulatory role of endogenous estrogens during male adolescence. J Clin Endocrinol Metab 1994; 79:513–518.

136. Keenan BS, Richards GE, Ponder SW, et al. Androgen-stimulated pubertal growth: the effects of testosterone and dihydrotestosterone on growth hormone and insulin-like growth factor-I in the treatment of short stature and delayed puberty. J Clin Endocrinol Metab 1993; 76:996–1001.

137. Rosenfeld RG, Rosenbloom AL, Guevara-Aguirre J. Growth hormone (GH) insensitivity due to primary GH receptor deficiency. Endocr Rev 1994; 15:369–390.

138. Iranmanesh A, Lizarralde G, Veldhuis JD. Age and relative adiposity are specific negative determinants of the frequency and amplitude of growth hormone (GH) secretory bursts and the half-life of endogenous GH in healthy men. J Clin Endocrinol Metab 1991; 73:1081–1088.

139. Leung DW, Spencer SA, Cachianes G, et al. Growth hormone receptor and serum binding protein: purification, cloning and expression. Nature 1987; 330:537–543.

140. Trivedi B, Daughaday WH. Release of growth hormone binding protein from IM-9 lymphocytes by endopeptidase is dependent on sulfhydryl group inactivation. Endocrinology 1988; 123:2201–2206.

141. Smith WC, Linzer DH, Talamantes F. Detection of two growth hormone receptor mRNAs and primary translation products in the mouse. Proc Natl Acad Sci USA 1988; 85:9576–9579.

142. Smith WC, Kuniyoshi J, Talamantes F. Mouse serum growth hormone (GH) binding protein has GH receptor extracellular and substituted transmembrane domains. Mol Endocrinol 1989; 3:984–990.

143. Sadeghi H, Wang BS, Lumunglas AL, et al. Identification of the origin of the growth hormone-binding protein in rat serum. Mol Endocrinol 1990; 4:1799–1805.

144. Kelly PA, Djiane J, Postel-Vinay M, et al. The prolactin/growth hormone receptor family. Endocr Rev 1991; 12:235–251.

145. Mathews L. Molecular biology of growth hormone receptors. Trends Endocrinol Metab 1991; 2:176–180.

146. Barton DE, Foellmer BE, Wood WI, et al. Chromosome mapping of the growth hormone receptor gene in man and mouse. Cytogenet Cell Genet 1989; 50:137–141.

147. Carter-Su C, Stubbart JR, Wang XY, et al. Phosphorylation of highly purified growth hormone receptors by a growth hormone receptor–associated tyrosine kinase. J Biol Chem 1989; 264:18654–18661.

148. Argetsinger LS, Campbell GS, Yang X, et al. Identification of JAK2 as a growth hormone receptor–associated tyrosine kinase. Cell 1993; 74:237–244.

149. Baumann G, Stolar MW, Amburn K, et al. A specific growth hormone–binding protein in human plasma: initial characterization. J Clin Endocrinol Metab 1986; 62:134–141.

150. Herington AC, Ymer S, Stevenson J. Identification and characterization of specific binding proteins for growth hormone in normal human sera. J Clin Invest 1986; 77:1817–1823.

151. Herington AC, Ymer SI, Stevenson JL. Affinity purification and structural characterization of a specific binding protein for human growth hormone in human serum. Biochem Biophys Res Commun 1986; 138:150–155.

152. Baumann G. Growth hormone binding to a circulating receptor fragment: the concept of receptor shedding and receptor splicing. Exp Clin Endocrinol 1995; 103:2–6.

153. Holl RW, Snehotta R, Siegler B, et al. Binding protein for human growth hormone: effects of weight and age. Horm Res 1991; 35:190–197.

154. Massa G, deZegher F, Vanderschueren-Lodeweyckx M. Serum growth hormone binding proteins in the human fetus and infant. Pediatr Res 1992; 32:69–72.

155. Carlsson LMS, Rowland AM, Clark RG, et al. Ligand-mediated immuno-functional assay for quantitation of growth hormone–binding protein in human blood. J Clin Endocrinol Metab 1991; 73:1216–1223.

156. Martha PM, Reiter EO, Davila N, et al. The role of body mass in the response to growth hormone therapy. J Clin Endocrinol Metab 1992; 75:1470–1473.

157. Attie KM, Carlsson LMS, Rundle AC, et al. Evidence for partial growth hormone insensitivity among patients with idiopathic short stature. J Pediatr 1995; 127:244–250.

158. Carlsson LMS, Attie KM, Compton PG, et al. Reduced concentration of serum growth hormone–binding protein in children with idiopathic short stature. J Clin Endocrinol Metab 1994; 78:1325–1330.

159. Martha PM, Reiter EO, Davila N, et al. Serum growth hormone (GH)-binding protein/receptor: an important determinant of GH responsiveness. J Clin Endocrinol Metab 1992; 75:1464–1469.

160. Daughaday WH, Trivedi B. Absence of serum growth hormone binding protein in patients with growth hormone receptor (Laron dwarfism). Proc Natl Acad Sci USA 1987; 84:4636–4640.

161. Baumann G, Shaw MA. Absence of plasma growth hormone–binding protein in Laron-type dwarfism. J Clin Endocrinol Metab 1987; 65:814–816.

162. Buchanan CR, Maheshwari HG, Norman MR, et al. Laron-type dwarfism with apparently normal high affinity serum growth hormone–binding protein. Clin Endocrinol (Oxf) 1991; 35:179–185.

163. Salmon WD Jr, Daughaday WH. A hormonally controlled serum factor which stimulates sulfate incorporation by cartilage in vitro. J Lab Clin Med 1957; 49:825–836.

164. Daughaday WH, Rotwein P. Insulin-like growth factors I and II. Peptide, messenger ribonucleic acid and gene structures, serum and tissue concentrations. Endocr Rev 1989; 10:68–91.

165. Sherwin RS, Schulman GA, Hendler R, et al. Effect of growth hormone on oral glucose tolerance and circulating metabolic rules in man. Diabetologia 1983; 24:155–161.

166. Rosenfeld RG, Wilson DM, Dollar LA, et al. Both human pituitary growth hormone and recombinant DNA–derived human growth hormone cause insulin resistance at a postreceptor level. J Clin Endocrinol Metab 1982; 54:1033–1038.

167. Green H, Morikawa M, Nixon T. A dual effector theory of growth hormone action. Differentiation 1985; 29:195–198.

168. Gerich JE, Lorenzi M, Bier DM, et al. Effects of physiologic levels of glucagon and growth hormone on human carbohydrate and lipid metabolism. Studies involving administration of exogenous hormone during suppression of endogenous hormone secretion with somatostatin. J Clin Invest 1976; 57:875–884.

169. Kostyo JL, Hotchkiss J, Knobil E. Stimulation of amino acid transport in isolated diaphragm by growth hormone added in vitro. Science 1959; 130:1653–1656.

170. Hjalmarson A, Isaksson O, Ahmen K. Effects of growth hormone and insulin on amino acid transport in perfused rat heart. Am J Physiol 1969; 217:1795–1802.

171. Griffin EE, Miller LL. Effects of hypophysectomy of liver donor on net synthesis of specific plasma proteins by the isolated perfused rat liver: modulation of synthesis of albumin, fibrinogen, alpha 1-acid glycoprotein, alpha 2-(acute phase)-globulin, and haptoglobin by insulin, cortisol, triio-dothyronine, and growth hormone. J Biol Chem 1974; 249:5062–5069.

172. Snyder DK, Clemmons DR, Underwood LE. Treatment of obese, diet-restricted subjects with growth hormone for 11 weeks: effects on anabolism, lipolysis, and body composition. J Clin Endocrinol Metab 1988; 67:54–61.

173. Rudman D, Feller AG, Nagraj H, et al. Effects of human growth hormone in men over 60 years old. N Engl J Med 1990; 323:1–6.

174. Horber FF, MV Haymond. Human growth hormone prevents the protein catabolic side effects of prednisone in humans. J Clin Invest 1990; 86:265–272.

175. Burgi H, Muller WA, Humbel RE, et al. Non-suppressible insulin-like activity of human serum. I: Physicochemical properties, extraction and partial purification. Biochim Biophys Acta 1966; 121:349–359.

176. Froesch ER, Zapf J, Meuli C, et al. Biologic properties of NSILA-S. Adv Metab Disord 1975; 8:211–235.

177. Dulak NC, Temin HM. A partially purified polypeptide fraction from rat liver cell conditioned medium with multiplication-stimulating activity for embryo fibroblasts. J Cell Physiol 1973; 81:153–160.

178. Daughaday WH, Hall K, Raben MS, et al. Somatomedin: proposed designation for sulphation factor. Nature 1972; 235:107.

179. Hall K, Takano K, Fryklund L, et al. Somatomedins. Adv Metab Disord 1975; 8:19–46.

180. Van Wyk JJ, Underwood LE, Hintz RL, et al. The somatomedins: a family of insulin like hormones under growth hormone control. Recent Prog Horm Res 1974; 30:259–318.

181. Rinderknecht E, Humbel RE. The amino acid sequence of human insulin-like growth factor I and its structural homology with proinsulin. J Biol Chem 1978; 253:2769–2776.

182. Rinderknecht E, Humbel RE. Primary structure of human insulin-like growth factor II. FEBS Lett 1978; 89:283–286.

183. Jansen M, Van Schaik SM, Van Tol H, et al. Nucleotide sequence of cDNAs encoding precursors of human insulin-like growth factor II (IGF2) and an IGF2 variant. FEBS Lett 1985; 179:243.

184. Zumstein PP, Luthi C, Humbel RE. Amino acid sequence of a variant pro-form of insulin-like growth factor II. Proc Natl Acad Sci USA 1985; 82:3169.

185. Gowan LK, Hampton B, Hill DJ, et al. Purification and characterization of a unique high molecular weight form of insulin-like growth factor II. Endocrinology 1987; 121:449–458.

186. Daughaday WH, Emanuele MA, Brooks MH, et al. Insulin-like growth factor II synthesis and secretion by a leiomyosarcoma with associated hypoglycemia. N Engl J Med 1988; 319:1434–1440.

187. Zapf J. Insulin-like growth factor binding proteins and tumor hypoglycemia. Trends Endocrinol Metab 1995; 6:37–42.

188. Powell DR, Lee PDK, Chang D, et al. Antiserum developed for the E-peptide region of insulin-like growth factor IA prohormone recognizes a serum protein by both immunoblot and radioimmunoassay. J Clin Endocrinol Metab 1987; 65:868.

189. Sussenbach JS. The gene structure of the insulin-like growth factor family. Prog Growth Factor Res 1989; 1:33–48.

190. Lund PK, Moats-Staats BM, Hynes MA, et al. Somatomedin-C/insulin-like growth factor-I and insulin-like growth factor-II mRNAs in rat fetal and adult tissues. J Biol Chem 1986; 261:14539–14544.

191. Brown AL, Graham DE, Nissley SP, et al. Developmental regulation of insulin-like growth factor II mRNA in different rat tissues. J Biol Chem 1986; 261:13144–13150.

192. Brissenden JE, Ullrich A, Francke U. Human chromosomal mapping of genes for insulin-like growth factors I and II and epidermal growth factor. Nature 1984; 310:781–784.

193. Tricoli JV, Rall LB, Scott J, et al. Localization of insulin-like growth factor genes to human chromosomes 11 and 12. Nature 1984; 310:784–785.

194. Bell GI, Gerhard DS, Fong NM, et al. Isolation of the human insulin-like growth factor genes. Insulin-like growth factor II and insulin genes are contiguous. Proc Natl Acad Sci USA 1985; 82:6450–6454.

195. Yoon, JB, Berry SA, Seelig S, et al. An inducible nuclear factor binds to a growth hormone–regulated gene. J Biol Chem 1990; 265:19947–19954.

196. Lowe WL Jr, Roberts CT Jr, Lasky SR, et al. Differential expression of alternative 5' untranslated regions in mRNAs encoding rat insulin-like growth factor I. Proc Natl Acad Sci USA 1987; 84:8946–8950.

197. Murphy LJ, Friesen HG. Differential effects of estrogen and growth hormone on uterine and hepatic insulin-like growth factor I gene expression in the ovariectomized hypophysectomized rat. Endocrinology 1988; 122:325–332.

198. Holthuizen PE, Rodenburg RJT, Scheper W, et al. Regulation of IGF2 gene expression and posttranscriptional processing of IGF2 mRNAs. In: Baxter RC, Gluckman PD, Rosenfeld RG, eds. The Insulin-like Growth Factors and Their Regulatory Proteins. Amsterdam: Elsevier Science, 1994: 43–53.

199. Rappolee DA, Sturm KS, Behrendtsen O, et al. Insulin-like growth factor II acts through an endogenous growth pathway regulated by imprinting in early mouse embryos. Genes Dev 1992; 6:939–952.

200. Nason KS, Binder ND, Labarta JI, et al. IGF2 and IGF-binding proteins increase dramatically during rabbit pregnancy. J Endocrinol 1996; 148:121–130.

201. Stylianopoulou F, Herbert J, Soares MB, et al. Expression of the insulin-

like growth factor II gene in the choroid plexus and the leptomeninges of the adult rat central nervous system. Cell Biol 1988; 85:141–145.

202. Reeve AE, Eccles MR, Wilkins RJ, et al. Expression of insulin-like growth factor-II transcripts in Wilms tumour. Nature 1985; 317:258–260.

203. Ogawa O, Eccles MR, Szeto J, et al. Relaxation of insulin-like growth factor II gene imprinting implicated in Wilms' tumor. Nature 1993; 362:749–751.

204. Zhan S, Shapiro D, Zhang L, Hirschfeld S, et al. Concordant loss of imprinting of the human insulin-like growth factor II gene promoters in cancer. J Biol Chem 1995; 270:27983–27986.

205. El-Badry OM, Helman LJ, Chatten J, et al. Insulin-like growth factor II–mediated proliferation of human neuroblastoma. J Clin Invest 1991; 87:648–657.

206. Haselbacher GK, Irminger JC, Zapf J, et al. Insulin-like growth factor in human adrenal pheochromocytomas and Wilms tumors: expression of the mRNA and protein level. Proc Natl Acad Sci USA 1987; 84:1104–1106.

207. Rainier S, Johnson LA, Dobry CJ, et al. Relaxation of imprinted genes in human cancer. Nature 1993; 362:747–749.

208. Tricoli JV, Rall LB, Karakousis CP, et al. Enhanced levels of insulin-like growth factor messenger RNA in human colon carcinomas and liposarcomas. Cancer Res 1986; 46:6169–6173.

209. Werner H, Roberts CT Jr, LeRoith D. Transcriptional repression of the IGF2 and IGF1 receptor genes by tumor suppressor WT1: implications for normal kidney development and Wilms' tumor. In: Baxter RC, Gluckman PD, Rosenfeld RG, eds. The Insulin-like Growth Factors and Their Regulatory Proteins. Amsterdam: Elsevier Science, 1994: 107–115.

210. Ohlsson R, Nystrom A, Pfeifer-Ohlsson S, et al. IGF2 is parentally imprinted during human embryogenesis and in the Beckwith-Wiedemann syndrome. Nature Genet 1993; 4:94–97.

211. DeChiara TM, Efstratiadis A, Robertson EJ. A growth-deficiency phenotype in heterozygous mice carrying an insulin-like growth factor II gene disrupted by targeting. Nature 1990; 345:78–80.

212. Baker J, Liu JP, Robertson EJ, et al. Role of insulin-like growth factors in embryonic and postnatal growth. Cell 1993; 75:73–82.

213. Giannoukakis N, Deal C, Paquette J, et al. Parental genomic imprinting of the human IGF2 gene. Nature Genet 1993; 4:98–100.

214. Deal CL. Parental genomic imprinting. Curr Opin Pediatr 1995; 7:445–458.

215. Mutter GL, Stewart CL, Chaponot ML, et al. Oppositely imprinted genes H19 and insulin-like growth factor 2 are coexpressed in human androgenetic trophoblast. Am J Hum Genet 1993; 53:1096–1102.

216. Steenman MJC, Rainier S, Dobry CJ, et al. Loss of imprinting of IGF2 is linked to reduced expression and abnormal methylation of H19 in Wilms' tumor patients. Nat Genet 1994; 7:433–438.

217. Barlow DP, Stoger R, Hermann BG, et al. The mouse insulin-like growth factor type-2 receptor is imprinted and closely linked to the Tme locus. Nature 1991; 349:84–87.

218. Liu JP, Baker J, Perkins AS, et al. Mice carrying null mutations of the genes encoding insulin-like growth factor I (Igf-1) and type 1 IGF receptor (Igf1r). Cell 1993; 75:73–82.

219. Filson AJ, Louvi A, Efstratiadis A, et al. Rescue of the T-associated maternal effect in mice carrying null mutations in Igf-2 and Igf-2r, two reciprocally imprinted genes. Development 1993; 118:731–736.

220. Hall K. Quantitative determination of the sulphation factor activity in human serum. Acta Endocrinol (Kbh) 1970; 63:338–350.

221. Phillips LS, Herington AC, Daughaday WH. Somatomedin stimulation of sulfate incorporation in porcine costal cartilage discs. Endocrinology 1974; 94:856–863.

222. Garland JT, Lottes ME, Kozak S, et al. Stimulation of DNA synthesis in isolated chondrocytes by sulfation factor. Endocrinology 1972; 90:1086–1090.

223. Garland JT, Buchanan F. Stimulation of RNA and protein synthesis in isolated chondrocytes by human serum. J Clin Endocrinol Metab 1976; 43:842–846.

224. Meuli C, Froesch ER. Effects of insulin and of NSILA-S on the perfused rat heart: glucose uptake, lactate production and efflux of 3-O-methyl glucose. Eur J Clin Invest 1975; 5:93–99.

225. Hall K, Takano K, Fryklund L. Radioreceptor assay for somatomedin A. J Clin Endocrinol Metab 1974; 39:973–976.

226. Van Wyk JJ, Underwood LE, Baseman JB, et al. Explorations of the insulin-like and growth-promoting properties of somatomedin C by membrane receptor assays. Adv Metab Disord 1975; 8:128–150.

227. Zapf J, Kaufmann U, Eigenmann EJ, et al. Determination of nonsuppressible insulin-like activity in human serum by a sensitive protein-binding assay. Clin Chem 1977; 23:677–682.

228. Schalch DS, Heinrich UE, Koch JG, et al. Nonsuppressible insulin-like activity (NSILA). Development of a new sensitive competitive protein-binding assay for determination of serum levels. J Clin Endocrinol 1978; Metabolism 46:664–671.

229. Furlanetto RW, Underwood LE, Van Wyk JJ, et al. Estimation of somatomedin-C levels in normals and patients with pituitary disease by radioimmunoassay. J Clin Invest 1977; 60:646–756.

230. Zapf J, Walter H, Froesch ER. Radioimmunological determination of insulin-like growth factors I and II in normal subjects and in patients with growth disorders and extrapancreatic tumor hypoglycemia. J Clin Invest 1981; 68:1321–1330.

231. Bala RM, Bhaumick B. Radioimmunoassay of a basic somatomedin: comparison of various assay techniques and somatomedin levels in various sera. J Clin Endocrinol Metab 1979; 49:770–777.

232. Baxter RC, Axiak S, Raison RL. Monoclonal antibody against human somatomedin-C/insulin-like growth factor I. J Clin Endocrinol Metab 1982; 54:474–476.

233. Rosenfeld RG, Wilson DM, Lee PDK, et al. Insulin-like growth factors I and II in the evaluation of growth retardation. J Pediatr 1986; 109:428–433.

234. Daughaday WH, Kapadia M, Mariz I. Serum somatomedin binding proteins: physiologic significance and interference in radioligand assay. J Lab Clin Med 1986; 109:355–363.

235. Powell DR, Rosenfeld RG, Baker BK, et al. Serum somatomedin levels in adults with chronic renal failure: the importance of measuring insulin-like growth factor (IGF)-1 and -2 in acid chromatographed uremic serum. J Clin Endocrinol Metab 1986; 63:1186–1192.

236. Horner JM, Liu F, Hintz RL. Comparison of [125I] somatomedin-A and [125I] somatomedin C radioreceptor assays for somatomedin peptide content in whole and acid-chromatographed plasma. J Clin Endocrinol Metab 1978; 47:1287–1295.

237. Daughaday WH, Mariz IK, Blethen SL. Inhibition of access of bound somatomedin to membrane receptor and immunobinding sites: a comparison of radioreceptor and radioimmunoassay of somatomedin in native and acid-ethanol-extracted serum. J Clin Endocrinol Metab 1980; 51:781–788.

238. Blum WF, Ranke MB, Bierich JR. A specific radioimmunoassay for IGF2: the interference of IGF binding proteins can be blocked by excess IGF1. Acta Endocrinol 1988; 118:374–380.

239. Bang P, Ericksson U, Sara V, et al. Comparison of acid ethanol extraction and acid gel filtration prior to IGF1 and IGF2 radioimmunoassays: improvement of determinations in acid ethanol extracts by the use of a truncated IGF1 as radioligand. Acta Endocrinol (Copenh) 1991; 124:620–629.

240. Bennett A, Wilson DM, Liu F, et al. Levels of insulin-like growth factor-I and -II in human cord blood. J Clin Endocrinol Metab 1983; 57:609–612.

241. Gluckman PD, Barrett-Johnson JJ, Butler JH, et al. Studies of insulin-like growth factor I and II by specific radioligand assays in umbilical cord blood. Clin Endocrinol 1983; 19:405–413.

242. Lassare C, Hardouin S, Daffos F, et al. Serum insulin-like growth factors and their binding proteins in the human fetus. Relationships with growth in normal subjects and in subjects with intrauterine growth retardation. Pediatr Res 1991; 29:219–225.

243. Hall K, Hansson U, Lundin G, et al. Serum levels of somatomedins and somatomedin-binding protein in pregnant women with type I or gestational diabetes and their infants. J Clin Endocrinol Metab 1986; 63:1300–1305.

244. Luna AM, Wilson DM, Wibbelsman CJ, et al. Somatomedins in adolescence: a cross-sectional study of the effect of puberty on plasma insulin-like growth factor I and II levels. J Clin Endocrinol Metab 1983; 57:258–271.

245. Cara JF, Rosenfield RL, Furlanetto RW. A longitudinal study of the relationship of plasma somatomedin-C concentration to the pubertal growth spurt. Am J Dis Child 1987; 141:562–564.

246. Cuttler L, Van Vliet G, Conte FA, et al. Somatomedin-C levels in children and adolescents with gonadal dysgenesis: differences from age-matched normal females and effect of chronic estrogen replacement therapy. J Clin Endocrinol Metab 1985; 60:1087–1091.

247. Rosenfeld RG, Hintz RL, Johanson AJ, et al. Methionyl human growth hormone and oxandrolone in Turner syndrome: preliminary results of a prospective randomized trial. J Pediatr 1986; 109:936–940.

248. Copeland KC. Effects of acute high dose and chronic low dose estrogen on plasma somatomedin-C and growth in patients with Turner's syndrome. J Clin Endocrinol Metab 1988; 66:1278–1282.

249. Johanson AJ, Blizzard RM. Low somatomedin-C levels in older men rise in response to growth hormone administration. Johns Hopkins Med J 1981; 149:115–117.

250. Donovan SM, Oh Y, Pham H, et al. Ontogeny of serum insulin-like growth factor binding proteins in the rat. Endocrinology 1989; 125:2621–2627.

251. Glasscock GF, Gelber SE, Lamson G, et al. Pituitary control of growth in the neonatal rat: effects of neonatal hypophysectomy on somatic and organ growth, serum insulin-like growth factors (IGF)-I and -II levels, and expression of IGF binding proteins. Endocrinology 1990; 127:1792–1803.

252. Moore DC, Ruvalcaba RHA, Smith EK, et al. Plasma somatomedin-C as a screening test for growth hormone deficiency in children and adolescents. Horm Res 1982; 16:49–55.

253. Reiter EO, Lovinger RD. The use of a commercially available somatomedin-C radioimmunoassay in patients with disorders of growth. J Pediatr 1981; 99:720–724.

254. Hintz RL, Clemmons DR, Underwood LE, et al. Competitive binding of somatomedin to the insulin receptors of adipocytes, chondrocytes and liver membranes. Proc Natl Acad Sci USA 1972; 69:2351–2353.

255. Megyesi K, Kahn CR, Roth J, et al. Insulin and non-suppressible insulin-like activity (NSILA-s): evidence for separate plasma membrane receptor sites. Biochem Biophys Res Commun 1974; 57:307–315.

256. Massague J, Czech MP. The subunit structures of two distinct receptors for insulin-like growth factors I and II and their relationship to the insulin receptor. J Biol Chem 1982; 257:5038–5045.

257. Kasuga M, Van Obberghen E, Nissley SP, et al. Demonstration of two subtypes of insulin-like growth factor receptors by affinity crosslinking. J Biol Chem 1981; 256:5305–5308.

258. Chernausek SD, Jacobs S, Van Wyk JJ. Structural similarities between receptors for somatomedin C and insulin: analysis by affinity labeling. Biochemistry 1981; 20:7345–7350.

259. Rosenfeld RG, Hintz RL. Somatomedin receptors: structure, function and regulation. In: Conn M, ed. The Receptors. New York: Academic Press, 1986: 281–329.

260. Oh Y, Muller H, Neely EK, et al. New concepts in insulin-like growth factor receptor physiology. Growth Reg 1993; 3:113–123.

261. LeRoith D, Werner H, Beitner-Johnson D, et al. Molecular and cellular aspects of the insulin-like growth factor I receptor. Endocr Rev 1995; 16:143–163.

262. Ullrich A, Gray A, Tam AW, et al. Insulin-like growth factor I receptor primary structure: comparison with insulin receptor suggests structural determinants that define functional specificity. EMBO J 1986; 5:2503–2512.

263. Kato H, Faria TN, Stannard B, et al. Role of tyrosine kinase activity in signal transduction by the insulin-like growth factor-I (IGF1) receptor. J Biol Chem 1993; 265:2655–2661.

264. Kato H, Faria TN, Stannard B, et al. Essential role of tyrosine residues 1131, 1135, and 1136 of the insulin-like growth factor-I (IGF1) receptor in IGF1 action. Mol Endocrinol 1994; 8:40–50.

265. Yamaski H, Prager D, Gebremedhin S, et al. Human insulin-like growth factor I receptor 950 tyrosine is required for somatotroph growth factor signal transduction. J Biol Chem 1992; 267:20953–20958.

266. Gronborg M, Wulff BS, Rasmussen JS, et al. Structure-function relationship of the insulin-like growth factor-I receptor tyrosine kinase. J Biol Chem 1993; 258:23435–23440.

267. Abbott AM, Bueno R, Pedrini MT, et al. Insulin-like growth factor I receptor gene structure. J Biol Chem 1992; 267:10759–10763.

268. Ullrich A, Bell JR, Chen EY, et al. Human insulin receptor and its relationship to the tyrosine kinase family of oncogenes. Nature 1985; 313:756–761.

269. Bondy CA, Werner H, Roberts CT Jr, et al. Cellular pattern of insulin-like growth factor-I (IGF1) and type I IGF receptor gene expression in early organogenesis: comparison with IGF2 gene expression. Mol Endocrinol 1990; 4:1386–1398.

270. Werner H, Woloschak M, Adamo M, et al. Developmental regulation of the rat insulin-like growth factor I receptor gene. Proc Natl Acad Sci USA 1989; 86:7451–7455.

271. Lowe WL Jr, Adamo M, Werner H, et al. Regulation by fasting of rat insulin-like growth factor I and its receptor. Effects on gene expression and binding. J Clin Invest 1989; 84:619–626.

272. Frattali AL, Pessin JE. Relationship between alpha subunit ligand occupancy and beta subunit autophosphorylation in insulin/insulin-like growth factor-1 hybrid receptors. J Biol Chem 1993; 268:7393–7400.

273. Treadway JL, Morrison BD, Soos MA, et al. Transdominant inhibition of tyrosine kinase activity in mutant insulin/insulin-like growth factor I hybrid receptors. Proc Natl Acad Sci USA 1991; 88:214–218.

274. Shemer J, Adamo M, Wilson GL, et al. Insulin and insulin-like growth factor-I stimulate a common endogenous phosphoprotein substrate (pp185) in intact neuroblastoma cells. J Biol Chem 1987; 262:15476–15482.

275. Kuhne MR, Pawson T, Lienhard GE, et al. The insulin receptor substrate-1 associates with the SH2-containing phosphotyrosine phosphatase Syp. J Biol Chem 1993; 268:11479–11481.

276. Skolnik EY, Batzer A, Li N, et al. The function of GRB2 in linking the insulin receptor to ras signaling pathways. Science 1993; 260:1953–1955.

277. Lee CH, Li W, Nishimura R, et al. Nck associates with the SH2 domain-docking protein IRS-1 in insulin-stimulated cells. Proc Natl Acad Sci USA 1993; 90:11713–11717.

278. Sasaoka T, Rose DW, Juhn BH, et al. Evidence for a functional role of Shc proteins in mitogenic signaling induced by insulin, insulin-like growth factor-I, and epidermal growth factor. J Biol Chem 1994; 269:13689–13694.

279. Lamphere L, Leinhard GE. Components of signaling pathways for insulin and insulin-like growth factor-I in muscle myoblasts and myotubes. Endocrinology 1992; 131:2196–2202.

280. Oemar BS, Law NM, Rosenweig SA. Insulin-like growth factor-I induces tyrosyl phosphorylation of nuclear proteins. J Biol Chem 1991; 266:27241–27244.

281. Chao MV. Growth factor signaling: where is the specificity? Cell 1992; 68:995–997.

282. Porcu P, Ferber A, Pietrzkowski Z, et al. The growth-stimulatory effect of simian virus 40 T antigen requires the interaction of insulin-like growth factor I with its receptor. Mol Cell Biol 1992; 12:5069–5077.

283. Baserga R. The double life of the IGF1 receptor. Receptor 1992; 2:261–266.

284. Sell C, Rubini M, Rubin R, et al. Simian virus 40 large tumor antigen is unable to transform mouse embryonic fibroblasts lacking type I insulin-like growth factor receptor. Proc Natl Acad Sci USA 1993; 90:11217–11221.

285. Kaleko M, Rutter WJ, Miller AD. Overexpression of the human insulin-like growth factor I receptor promotes ligand-dependent neoplastic transformation. Mol Cell Biol 1990; 10:464–473.

286. Prager D, Li HL, Asa S, et al. Dominant negative inhibition of tumorigenesis in vivo by human insulin-like growth factor I receptor mutant. Proc Natl Acad Sci USA 1994; 91:2181–2185.

287. Alexandrides TK, Chen JH, Bueno R, et al. Evidence for two insulin-like growth factor I receptors with distinct primary structure that are differentially expressed during development. Regul Pept 1993; 48:279–290.

288. Alexandrides TK, Smith RJ. A novel fetal insulin-like growth factor (IGF) I receptor. Mechanism for increased IGF1 and insulin-stimulated tyrosine kinase activity in fetal muscle. J Biol Chem 1989; 264:12922–12930.

289. Garofalo RS, Rosen OM. Insulin and insulin-like growth factor I (IGF1) receptors during central nervous system development: expression of two immunologically distinct IGF1 receptor b subunits. Mol Cell Biol 1989; 9:2806–2817.

290. Tally M, Li CH, Hall K. IGF-2 stimulated growth mediated by the somatomedin type 2 receptor. Biochem Biophys Res Commun 1987; 148:811–816.

291. Minniti CP, Kohn EC, Grubb JH, et al. The insulin-like growth factor II (IGF2)/mannose 6-phosphate receptor mediates IGF2-induced motility in human rhabdomyosarcoma cells. J Biol Chem 1992; 267:9000–9004.

292. Nishimoto I, Murayama Y, Katada T, et al. Possible direct linkage of insulin-like growth factor-II receptor with guanine nucleotide-binding proteins. J Biol Chem 1989; 264:14029–14038.

293. Moxham CP, Duronio V, Jacobs S. Insulin-like growth factor I receptor beta subunit heterogeneity. Evidence for hybrid tetramers composed of insulin-like growth factor I and insulin receptor heterodimers. J Biol Chem 1989; 264:13238–13244.

294. Soos MA, Siddle K. Immunological relationships between receptors for insulin and insulin-like growth factor I. Evidence for structural heterogeneity of insulin-like growth factor I receptors involving hybrids with insulin receptors. Biochem J 1989; 263:553–563.

295. Moxham CP, Jacobs S. Insulin/IGF1 receptor hybrids: a mechanism for increasing receptor diversity. J Cell Biochem 1992; 48:136–140.

296. Misra P, Hintz RL, Rosenfeld RG. Structural and immunological characterization of insulin-like growth factor II binding to IM-9 cells. J Clin Endocrinol Metab 1986; 63:1400–1405.

297. Soos MA, Field CE, Siddle K. Purified hybrid insulin/insulin-like growth factor-I, but not insulin, binds with high affinity. Biochem J 1993; 290:419–425.

298. Kasuya J, Paz B, Madduz BA, et al. Characterization of human placental insulin-like growth factor-I/insulin hybrid receptors by protein microsequencing and purification. Biochemistry 1993; 32:13531–13536.

299. Morgan DO, Edman JC, Strandring DN, et al. Insulin-like growth factor II receptor as a multifunctional binding protein. Nature 1987; 329:301–307.

300. MacDonald RG, Pfeffer SR, Coussens L, et al. A single receptor binds both insulin-like growth factor II and mannose-6-phosphate. Science 1988; 239:1134–1137.

301. Kornfeld S. Trafficking of lysosomal enzymes. FASEB J 1987; 1:462–468.

302. Rosenfeld RG, Conover CA, Hodges D, et al. Heterogeneity of insulin-like growth factor-I affinity for the insulin-like growth factor-II receptor: comparison of natural, synthetic and recombinant DNA-derived insulin-like growth factor-I. Biochem Biophys Res Commun 1987; 143:195–205.

303. Beukers M, Oh Y, Zhang H, et al. [Leu27] Insulin-like growth factor II is highly selective for the type II IGF receptor in binding, cross-linking and thymidine incorporation. Endocrinology 1991; 128:1201–1203.

304. Furlanetto RW, DiCarlo JN, Wisehart C. The type II insulin-like growth factor receptor does not mediate deoxyribonucleic acid synthesis in human fibroblasts. J Clin Endocrinol Metab 1987; 64:1142–1149.

305. Mottola C, Czech MP. The type II insulin-like growth factor receptor does not mediate DNA synthesis in H-35 hepatoma cells. J Biol Chem 1984; 259:12705–12713.

306. Kiess W, Haskell JF, Lee L, et al. An antibody that blocks insulin-like growth factor (IGF) binding to the type II IGF receptor is neither an agonist nor an inhibitor of IGF-stimulated biologic response in L6 myoblasts. J Biol Chem 1987; 162:12756–12761.

307. Adashi EY, Resnick CE, Rosenfeld RG. Insulin-like growth factor-I (IGF1) hormonal action in cultured rat granulosa cells: mediation via type I but not type II IGF receptors. Endocrinology 1989; 126:216–222.

308. Canfield WM, Kornfeld S. The chicken liver cation-independent mannose-6-phosphate receptor lacks the high affinity binding site for insulin-like growth factor II. J Biol Chem 1989; 264:7100–7103.

309. Clairmont KB, Czech MP. Chicken and *Xenopus* mannose 6-phosphate receptors fail to bind insulin-like growth factor II. J Biol Chem 1989; 264:16390–16392.

310. Rogers SA, Hammerman MR. Insulin-like growth factor II stimulates production of inositol triphosphate in proximal tubular basolateral membranes from canine kidney. Proc Natl Acad Sci USA 1988; 85:4037–4041.

311. Jonas HA, Cox AJ. Insulin-like growth factor binding to the atypical insulin receptors of a human lymphoid-derived cell line (IM-9). Biochem J 1990; 266:737–742.

312. Feltz SM, Swanson SM, Wemmie JA, et al. Functional properties of an isolated heterodimeric human placenta insulin-like growth factor I complex. Biochemistry 1988; 27:3234–3242.

313. Treadway JL, Morrison BD, Goldfine ID, et al. Assembly of insulin/insulin-like growth factor-1 hybrid receptors in vitro. J Biol Chem 1989; 264:21450–21453.

314. Soos MA, Siddle K. Immunological relationships between receptors for insulin and insulin-like growth factor I. Biochemistry 1989; 263:553–563.

315. Rosenfeld RG, Lamson G, Pham H, et al. Insulin-like growth factor binding proteins. Recent Prog Horm Res 1990; 46:99–163.

316. Lamson G, Giudice L, Rosenfeld RG. The insulin-like growth factor binding proteins: structural and molecular relationships. Growth Factors 1991; 5:19–28.

317. Rechler MM. Insulin-like growth factor binding proteins. Vitamins Hormones 1993; 47:1–114.

318. Jones JI, Clemmons DR. Insulin-like growth factors and their binding proteins: biologic actions. Endocr Rev 1995; 16:3–34.

319. Hintz RL, Liu F. Demonstration of specific plasma protein binding sites for somatomedin. J Clin Endocrinol Metab 1977; 45:988–995.

320. Hossenlopp P, Surin D, Segovia-Quinson B, et al. Analysis of serum insulin-like growth factor binding proteins using western blotting: use of the method for titration of the binding proteins and competitive binding studies. Anal Biochem 1986; 154:138–143.

321. Shimasaki S, Shimonaka J, Zhang HP, et al. Identification of five different insulin-like growth factor binding proteins (IGFBPs) from adult rat serum and molecular cloning of a novel IGFBP-5 in rat and human. J Biol Chem 1991; 266:10646–10653.

322. Swisshelm K, Ryan K, Tsuchiya K, et al. Enhanced expression of an insulin growth factor-like binding protein (mac25) in senescent human mammary epithelial cells and induced expression with retinoic acid. Proc Natl Acad Sci USA 1995; 92:4472–4476.

323. Brewer MT, Stetler GL, Squires CH, et al. Cloning, characterization, and expression of a human insulin-like growth factor binding protein. Biochem Biophys Res Commun 1988; 152:1289–1297.

324. Jones JI, Gockerman A, Busby WH, et al. Insulin-like growth factor binding protein 1 stimulates cell migration and binds to the a5b1 integrin by means of its Arg-Gly-Asp sequence. Proc Natl Acad Sci USA 1993; 90:10553–10557.

325. Oh Y, Muller H, Pham H, et al. Non–receptor mediated, post-transcriptional regulation of insulin-like growth factor binding protein (IGFBP)-3 in H578T human breast cancer cells. Endocrinology 1992; 131:3123–3125.

326. Oh Y, Muller H, Lamson G, et al. Insulin-like growth factor (IGF)-independent action of IGF binding protein (BP)-3 in H578T human breast cancer cells. Cell surface binding and growth inhibition. J Biol Chem 1993; 268:14964–14971.

327. Oh Y, Muller HL, Pham H, et al. Demonstration of receptors for insulin-like growth factor binding protein-3 (IGFBP-3) on H578T human breast cancer cells. J Biol Chem 1993; 268:26045–26048.

328. Ritvos O, Ranta T, Julkanen J, et al. Insulin-like growth factor (IGF) binding protein from human decidua inhibits the binding and biologic action of IGF1 in cultured choriocarcinoma cells. Endocrinology 1988; 122:2150–2157.

329. Ross M, Francis GL, Szabo L, et al. Insulin-like growth factor (IGF)-binding proteins inhibit the biologic activities of IGF1 and IGF2 but not des-(1-3)-IGF1. Biochem J 1989; 258:267–272.

330. Clemmons DR, Cascieri MA, Camacho-Hubner C, et al. Discrete alterations of the insulin-like growth factor I molecule which alter its affinity for insulin-like growth factor-binding proteins result in changes in bioactivity. J Biol Chem 1990; 265:12210–12216.

331. Okajima T, Nakamura K, Zhang H, et al. Sensitive colorimetric bioassays for insulin-like growth factor (IGF) stimulation of cell proliferation and glucose consumption: use in studies of IGF analogues. Endocrinology 1992; 130:2201–2212.

332. Cohen P, Lamson G, Okajima T, et al. Transfection of the human insulin-like growth factor binding protein-3 gene into Balb/c fibroblasts inhibits cellular growth. Mol Endocrinol 1993; 7:380–386.

333. Elgin RC, Busby WH, Clemmons DR. An insulin-like growth factor (IGF) binding protein enhances the biologic response to IGF1. Proc Natl Acad Sci USA 1987; 84:3254–3258.

334. Giudice LC, Farrell EM, Pham H, et al. Insulin-like growth factor binding proteins in the maternal serum throughout gestation and in the puerperium: effects of a pregnancy-associated protease activity. J Clin Endocrinol Metab 1990; 71:1330–1338.

335. Hossenlopp P, Segovia B, Lassaree C, et al. Evidence of enzymatic degradation of insulin-like growth factor binding proteins in the 150K complex during pregnancy. J Clin Endocrinol Metab 1990; 71:797–805.

336. Cohen P, Graves HCB, Peehl DM, et al. Prostate-specific antigen (PSA) is an insulin-like growth factor binding protein-3 protease found in seminal plasma. J Clin Endocrinol 1992; 75:1046–1053.

337. Muller H, Oh Y, Gargosky SE, et al. Concentrations of insulin-like growth factor binding protein-3, insulin-like growth factors and IGFBP-3 protease activity in cerebrospinal fluid (CSF) of children with leukemia, brain tumors, or meningitis. J Clin Endocrinol Metab 1993; 77:1113–1119.

338. Lee D, Park S, Yorgin P, et al. Alteration in insulin-like growth factor binding proteins (IGFBPs) and IGFBP-3 protease activity in serum and urine from acute and chronic renal failure. J Clin Endocrinol Metab 1994; 79:1376–1382.

339. Conover CA, De Leon DD. Acid-activated insulin-like growth factor-binding protein-3 proteolysis in normal and transformed cells. Role of cathepsin. J Biol Chem 1994; 269:7076–7080.

340. Fowlkes JL, Enghild JJ, Suzuki K, et al. Matrix metalloproteinases degrade insulin-like growth factor-binding protein-3 in dermal fibroblast cultures. J Biol Chem 1994; 269:16766–16773.

341. Gargosky SE, Pham H, Wilson KF, et al. Measurement and characterization of insulin-like growth factor binding protein-3 in human biologic fluids: discrepancies between radioimmunoassay and ligand blotting. Endocrinology 1992; 131:3051–3060.

342. Cohen P, Graves HC, Peehl DM, et al. Prostate-specific antigen (PSA) is an insulin-like growth factor binding protein-3 protease found in seminal plasma. J Clin Endocrinol Metab 1992; 75:1046–1053.

343. Angelloz-Nicoud P, Binoux M. Autocrine regulation of cell proliferation by the insulin-like growth factor (IGF) and IGF binding protein-3 protease system in a human prostate carcinoma cell line (PC-3). Endocrinology 1995; 136:5485–5492.

344. Cohen P, Peehl DM, Graves HC, et al. Biologic effects of prostate specific antigen as an insulin-like growth factor binding protein-3 protease. J Endocrinol 1994; 142:407–415.

345. Fielder PJ, Pham H, Adashi EY, et al. Insulin-like growth factors (IGFs) block follicle-stimulating hormone-induced proteolysis of IGF-binding protein-5 (BP-5) in cultured rat granulosa cells. Endocrinology 1993; 133:415–418.

346. Oh Y, Muller HL, Lee DY, et al. Characterization of the affinities of insulin-like growth factor (IGF)-binding proteins 1–4 for IGF1, IGF2, IGF1/insulin hybrid, and IGF1 analogues. Endocrinology 1993; 132:1337–1344.

347. Leong SR, Baxter RC, Camerato T, et al. Structure and functional expression of acid labile subunit of the insulin-like growth factor binding protein complex. Mol Endocrinol 1992; 6:870–876.

348. Baxter RC, Martin JL. Structure of the Mr 140,000 growth hormone-dependent insulin-like growth factor binding protein complex: demonstration by reconstitution and affinity labeling. Proc Natl Acad Sci USA 1989; 86:6898–6902.

349. Barreca A, Ponzani P, Arvigo M, et al. Effect of the acid-labile subunit on the binding of insulin-like growth factor (IGF)-binding protein-3 to [125I]IGF1. Endocrinol Metab 1995; 80:1318–1324.

350. Guler HP, Zapf J, Schmid C, et al. Insulin-like growth factors I and II in healthy man. Estimations of half-lives and production rates. Acta Endocrinol 1989; 121:753–758.

351. Zapf J, Hauri C, Waldvogel M, et al. Recombinant human insulin-like growth factor I induces its own specific carrier protein in hypophysectomized and diabetic rats. Proc Natl Acad Sci USA 1989; 86:3813–3817.

352. Clemmons DR, Thissen JP, Maes M, et al. Insulin-like growth factor-I (IGF1) infusion into hypophysectomized or protein-deprived rats induces specific IGF binding proteins in serum. Endocrinology 1989; 125:2967–2972.

353. Glasscock GF, Hein AN, Miller JA, et al. Effects of continous infusion of insulin-like growth factor I and II, alone and in combination with thyroxine or growth hormone, on the neonatal hypophysectomized rat. Endocrinology 1992; 130:203–210.

354. Wilson KF, Fielder PJ, Guevara-Aguirre J, et al. Long-term effects of insulin-like growth factor (IGF)-I treatment on serum IGFs and IGF binding proteins in adolescent patients with growth hormone receptor deficiency. Clin Endocrinol 1995; 42:399–407.

355. Walker JL, Baxter RC, Young S, et al. Effects of recombinant insulin-like growth factor I on IGF binding proteins and the acid-labile subunit in growth hormone insensitivity syndrome. Growth Regul 1993; 3:109–112.

356. Gargosky SE, Wilson KF, Fielder PJ, et al. The composition and distribution of insulin-like growth factors (IGFs) and IGF-binding proteins (IGFBPs) in the serum of growth hormone receptor-deficient patients: effects of IGF1 therapy on IGFBP-3. J Clin Endocrinol Metab 1993; 77:1683–1689.

357. Gargosky SE, Tapanainen P, Rosenfeld RG. Administration of growth hormone (GH), but not insulin-like growth factor-I (IGF1), by continous infusion can induce the formation of the 150-kilodalton IGF-binding protein-3 complex in GH-deficient rats. Endocrinology 1994; 134:2267–2276.

358. Bar RS, Boes M, Clemmons DR, et al. Insulin differentially alters transcapillary movement of intravascular IGFBP-1, IGFBP-2 and endothelial cell IGF binding proteins in rat heart. Endocrinology 1990; 127:497–499.

359. Giudice LC, de Zegher F, Gargosky SE, et al. Insulin-like growth factors and their binding proteins in the term and pre-term human fetus with normal and extremes of intrauterine growth and in the neonatal period. J Clin Endocrinol Metab 1995; 80:1548–1555.

360. Rechler MM, Nissley SP. Insulin-like growth factors. In: Sporn MB, Roberts AB, eds. Peptide Growth Factors and Their Receptors. Berlin: Springer-Verlag, 1990: 263–367.

361. Okajima T, Iwashita M, Takeda Y, et al. Inhibitory effects of insulin-like growth factor (IGF)-binding proteins-1 and -3 on IGF-activated glucose consumption in mouse Balb/c 3T3 fibroblasts. J Endocrinol 1993; 136:457–470.

362. Lamson G, Giudice LC, Cohen P, et al. Proteolysis of IGFBP-3 may be a common regulatory mechanism of IGF action in vivo. Growth Regul 1993; 3:91–95.

363. De Mellow JSM, Baxter RC. Growth hormone–dependent insulin-like growth factor (IGF) binding protein both inhibits and potentiates IGF1-stimulated DNA synthesis in human skin fibroblasts. Biochem Biophys Res Commun 1988; 156:199–204.

364. Conover CA, Ronk M, Lombana F, et al. Structural and biologic characterization of bovine insulin-like growth factor binding protein-3. Endocrinology 1990; 127:2795–2803.

365. Villaudy J, Delbe J, Blat C, et al. An IGF binding protein is an inhibitor of FGF stimulation. J Cell Physiol 1991; 149:492–496.

366. Bicsak TA, Simonaka M, Malkowski M, et al. Insulin-like growth factor binding protein (IGFBP) inhibition of granulosa cell function: effect of cyclic adenosine 3′,5′-monophosphate, deoxyribonucleic acid synthesis, and comparison with the effect of an IGF1 antibody. Endocrinology 1990; 126:2184–2189.

367. Valentis B, Bhala A, DeAngelis T, et al. The human insulin-like growth factor (IGF) binding protein-3 inhibits the growth of fibroblasts with a targeted disruption of the IGF1 receptor gene. Mol Endocrinol 1995; 9:361–367.

368. Oh Y, Muller HL, Lamson G, et al. Insulin-like growth factor (IGF)-independent action of IGF binding protein-3 in H578T human breast cancer cells. J Biol Chem 1993; 268:14964–14971.

369. Oh Y, Muller HL, Ng L, et al. TGF-β₂-induced cell growth inhibition in human breast cancer cells is mediated through IGFBP-3 action. J Biol Chem 1995; 270:13589–13592.

370. Martin JL, Coverley JA, Pathon ST, et al. Insulin-like growth factor binding protein-3 production by MCF-7 breast cancer cells: stimulation by retinoic acid and cyclic adenosine monophosphate and differential effects of estradiol. Endocrinology 1995; 136:1219–1226.

371. Fontana JA, Burrows-Meszu A, Clemmons DR, et al. Retinoid modulation of insulin-like growth factor binding proteins and inhibition of breast carcinoma proliferation. Endocrinology 1991; 128:1115–1122.

372. Sheikh MS, Shao ZM, Hussain A, et al. Regulation of insulin-like growth factor binding protein-1,2,3,4,5, and 6: synthesis, secretion, and gene expression in estrogen receptor-negative human breast cancer cells. J Cell Physiol 1993; 155:556–567.

373. Huynh H, Yang X, Pollak M. Estradiol and antiestrogens regulate a growth inhibitory insulin-like growth factor binding protein-3 autocrine loop in human breast cancer cells. J Biol Chem 1996; 271:1016–1021.

374. Leyen SA, Hembree JR, Eckert RL. Regulation of insulin-like growth factor-I binding protein-3 levels by epidermal growth factor and retinoic acid in cervical epithelial cells. J Cell Physiol 1994; 160:265–274.

375. Buckbinder L, Talbott R, Velasco-Miguel S, et al. Induction of the growth inhibitor IGF-binding protein-3 by p53. Nature 1995; 377:646–649.

376. Lalou C, Lassarre C, Binoux M. A proteolytic fragment of insulin-like growth factor binding protein-3 (IGFBP-3) that fails to bind IGFs is a growth inhibitor. Tuebingen, Germany: 3rd International Symposium of IGFBPs, 1995.

377. Lee YL, Hintz RL, James PM, et al. Insulin-like growth factor (IGF) binding protein complementary deoxyribonucleic acid from human HEP G2 hepatoma cells: predicted protein sequence suggests an IGF binding domain different from those of the IGF1 and IGF2 receptors. Mol Endocrinol 1988; 2:404–411.

378. Drop SLS, Valiquette G, Guyda HJ, et al. Partial purification and characterization of a binding protein for insulin-like activity (ILAs) in human amniotic fluid: a possible inhibitor of insulin-like activity. Acta Endocrinol (Copenh) 1979; 90:505–518.

379. Moses AC, Freinkel AJ, Knowles BB, et al. Demonstration that a human hepatoma cell line produces a specific insulin-like growth factor carrier protein. J Clin Endocrinol Metab 1983; 56:1003–1008.

380. Rutanen EM, Koistinen R, Wahlstrom T, et al. Synthesis of placental protein 12 by human decidua. Endocrinology 1985; 116:1304–1309.

381. Koistinen R, Kalkkinen N, Huhtala M, et al. Placental protein 12 is a decidual protein that binds somatomedin and has an identical N-terminal amino acid sequence with somatomedin-binding protein from human amniotic fluid. Endocrinology 1986; 118:1375–1378.

382. Brinkman A, Groffen CAH, Kortleve DJ, et al. Organization of the gene encoding the insulin-like growth factor binding protein IBP-1. Biochem Biophys Res Commun 1988; 157:898–907.

383. Giudice LC, Irwin JC, Dsupin BA, et al. Insulin-like growth factors (IGFs), IGF binding proteins (IGFBPs) and IGFBP protease in human uterine endometrium. Their potential relevance to endometrial cyclic function and maternal-embryonic interactions. In: Baxter RC, Gluckman PD, Rosenfeld RG, eds. The Insulin-like Growth Factors and Their Regulatory Proteins. Amsterdam: Elsevier, 1994: 351–361.

384. Adashi EY. Regulation of intrafollicular IGFBPs: possible relevance to ovarian follicular selection. In: Baxter RC, Gluckman PD, Rosenfeld RG, eds. The Insulin-like Growth Factors and Their Regulatory Proteins. Amsterdam: Elsevier, 1994: 341–350.

385. Unterman TG, Simmons RA, Glick RP, et al. Circulating levels of insulin, insulin-like growth factor-I (IGF1), IGF2, and IGF-binding proteins in the small for gestational age fetal rat. Endocrinology 1993; 132:327–336.

386. Lee PDK, Conover CA, Powell DA. Regulation and function of insulin-like growth factor binding protein-1. Proc Soc Expl Biol Med 1993; 204:4–29.

387. Thissen JP, Ketelslegers JM, Underwood LE. Nutritional regulation of the insulin-like growth factors. Endocr Rev 1994; 15:80–101.

388. Cotterill AM, Cowell CT, Baxter RC, et al. Regulation of the growth hormone-independent growth factor–binding protein in children. J Clin Endocrinol Metab 1988; 67:882–887.

389. Powell DR, Suwanichkul A, Cubbage ML, et al. Insulin inhibits transcription of the human gene for insulin-like growth factor binding protein-1. J Biol Chem 1991; 266:18868–18876.

390. Lewitt MS, Saunders H, Cooney GJ, et al. Effect of human insulin-like growth factor–binding protein-1 on the half-life and action of administered insulin-like growth factor-I in rats. J Endocrinol 1993; 136:253–260.

391. Koistinen R, Itkonen O, Selenius P, et al. Insulin-like growth factor binding protein-1 inhibits binding of IGF1 on fetal skin fibroblasts but stimulates their DNA synthesis. Biochem Biophys Res Commun 1990; 173:408–415.

392. Jones JI, D′Ercole AJ, Camacho-Hubner C, et al. Phosphorylation of insulin-like growth factor binding protein in cell culture and in vivo. Effects on affinity for IGF1. Proc Natl Acad Sci USA 1991; 88:7481–7485.

393. Binkert C, Margot JB, Landwehr J, et al. Structure of the human insulin-like growth factor binding protein-2 gene. Mol Endocrinol 1992; 6:826–836.

394. Agarwal N, Hieh CL, Sills D, et al. Sequence analysis, expression and chromosomal localization of a gene, isolated from a subtracted human retina cDNA library, that encodes an insulin-like growth factor binding protein (IGFBP2). Exp Eye Res 1991; 52:549–561.

395. Lamson G, Pham H, Oh Y, et al. Expression of the BRL-3A insulin-like growth factor binding protein (rBP-30) in the rat central nervous system. Endocrinology 1989; 123:1100–1102.

396. Bourner MJ, Busby WH, Seigel NR, et al. Cloning and sequence determination of bovine insulin-like growth factor binding protein-2 (IGFBP-2). Comparison of its structural and functional properties with IGFBP-1. J Cell Biochem 1992; 48:215–226.

397. Wood TL, Rogler L, Streck RD, et al. Targeted disruption of IGFBP-2 gene. Growth Regul 1993; 3:5–8.

398. Dai Z, Xing Y, Borney CM, et al. Human insulin-like growth factor binding protein-1 (hIGFBP-1) in transgenic mice. Characterization and insights into the regulation of IGFBP-1 expression. Endocrinology 1994; 135:1316–1327.

399. Rosenfeld RG, Pham H, Conover CA, et al. Structural and immunological comparison of insulin-like growth factor (IGF) binding proteins of cerbrospinal and amniotic fluids. J Clin Endocrinol Metab 1989; 68:638–646.

400. Binoux M, Hardouin S, Lassarre C, et al. Evidence for production by the liver of two IGF binding proteins with similar molecular weights but different affinities for IGF1 and IGF2. Their relationship with serum and cerebrospinal fluid IGF binding proteins. J Clin Endocrinol Metab 1982; 55:600–602.

401. Rosenfeld RG, Pham H, Oh Y, et al. Identification of insulin-like growth factor binding protein-2 (IGFBP-2) and a low molecular weight IGFBP in human seminal plasma. J Clin Endocrinol Metab 1990; 70:551–553.

402. Cohen P, Peehl DM, Baker B, et al. Insulin-like growth factor axis abnormalities in prostatic stromal cells from patients with benign prostatic hyperplasia. J Clin Endocrinol Metab 1994; 79:1410–1415.

403. Cohen P, Peehl DM, Stamey TA, et al. Elevated levels of insulin-like growth factor binding protein-2 in the serum of prostate cancer patients. J Clin Endocrinol Metab 1993; 76:1031–1035.

404. Cubbage ML, Suwanichkal A, Powell DR. Insulin-like growth factor binding protein-3. Organization of the human chromosomal gene and demonstration of promoter activity. J Biol Chem 1990; 265:12642–12649.

405. Gargosky SE, Giudice LC, Rosenfeld RG, et al. Different molecular and messenger ribonucleic acid forms of insulin-like growth factor binding protein-3 in the pregnant baboon. J Endocrinol 1995; 147:449–461.

406. Arany E, Afford S, Strain AJ, et al. Different cellular synthesis of insulin-like growth factor binding protein-1 (IGFBP-1) and IGFBP-3 within human liver. J Clin Endocrinol Metab 1994; 79:1871–1976.

407. Chin E, Zhou J, Dai J, et al. Cellular localization and regulation of gene expression for components of the insulin-like growth factor ternary binding complex. Endocrinology 1994; 134:2498–2504.

408. Baxter RC. Insulin-like growth factor binding proteins in the human circulation. A review. Horm Res 1994; 42:140–144.

409. Hoech WG, Mukku VR. Identification of the major sites of phosphorylation in IGF binding protein-3. J Cell Biochem 1994; 56:262–273.

410. Holly J, Claffey DCP, Cwyfan-Hughes SC, et al. Proteases acting on IGFBPs. Their occurrence and physiological significance. Growth Regul 1992; 3:88–91.

411. Bang P, Brismar K, Rosenfeld RG. Increased proteolysis of insulin-like growth factor-binding protein-3 (IGFBP-3) in noninsulin-dependent diabetes mellitus serum, with elevation of a 29-kilodalton (kd) glycosylated IGFBP-3 fragment contained in the approximately 130- to 150-kd ternary complex. J Clin Endocrinol Metab 1994; 78:1119–1127.

412. Booth BA, Boes M, Andress DL, et al. IGFBP-3 and IGFBP-5 association with endothelial cells: role of C-terminal heparin binding domain. Growth Regul 1995; 5:1–17.

413. Gao L, Ling N, Shimasaki S. Structure of the rat insulin-like growth factor binding protein-4 gene. Biochem Biophys Res Commun 1993; 190:1053–1059.

414. Ceda GP, Fielder PJ, Henzel WJ, et al. Differential effects of insulin-like growth factor (IGF)-I and IGF-II on the expression of IGF binding proteins (IGFBPs) in a rat neuroblastoma cell line. Isolation and characterization of two forms of IGFBP-4. Endocrinology 1991; 128:2815–2824.

415. Boes M, Booth BA, Sandra A, et al. Insulin-like growth factor binding protein (IGFBP)-4 accounts for the connective tissue distribution of endothelial cell IGFBPs perfused through the isolated heart. Endocrinology 1992; 133:327–330.

416. Mohan S, Bautista CM, Wergedal J, et al. Isolation of an inhibitory insulin-like growth factor (IGF) binding protein from bone cell–conditioned medium. A potential local regulator of IGF action. Proc Natl Acad Sci USA 1989; 88:8338–8342.

417. Cheung PT, Wu J, Banach W, et al. Glucocorticoid regulation of an insulin-like growth factor binding protein-4 protease produced by a rat neuronal cell line. Endocrinology 1994; 135:1328–1335.

418. Cohick WS, Gockerman A, Clemmons DR. Vascular smooth muscle cells synthesize two forms of insulin-like growth factor binding proteins which are regulated differently by the insulin-like growth factors. J Cell Physiol 1993; 157:52–60.

419. Conover CA, Kiefer MC, Zapf J. Postranslational regulation of insulin-like growth factor binding protein-4 in normal and transformed human fibroblasts. J Clin Invest 1993; 91:1129–1137.

420. Durham SK, Kiefer MC, Roggs BL, et al. Regulation of insulin-like growth factor binding protein-4 by a specific insulin-like growth factor binding protein-4 proteinase in normal osteoblast-like cells. Implications in bone cell physiology. J Bone Miner Res 1994; 9:111–117.

421. Lee KO, Oh Y, Giudice LC, et al. Identification of insulin-like growth factor binding protein-3 (IGFBP-3) fragments and IGFBP-5 proteolytic activity in human seminal plasma. A comparison of normal and vasectomized men. J Clin Endocrinol Metab 1994; 79:1367–1372.

422. Neely EK, Rosenfeld RG. Insulin-like growth factors (IGFs) reduce IGF-binding protein-4 (IGFBP-4) concentration and stimulate IGFBP-3 independently of IGF receptors in human fibroblasts and epidermal cells. Endocrinology 1992; 130:985–993.

423. Fowlkes J, Freemark M. Evidence for a novel insulin-like growth factor (IGF)-dependent protease regulating IGF binding protein-4 in dermal fibroblasts. Endocrinology 1992; 131:2071–2076.

424. Kiefer MC, Ioh RS, Bauer DM, et al. Molecular cloning of a new human insulin-like growth factor binding protein. Biochem Biophys Res Commun 1991; 176:219–225.

425. Conover CA, Kiefer MC. Regulation and biologic effect of endogenous insulin-like growth factor binding protein-5 in human osteoblast cells. J Clin Endocrinol Metab 1993; 76:1153–1159.

426. Kiefer MC, Schmid C, Waldvogel M, et al. Characterization of recombinant human insulin-like growth factor binding proteins 4, 5 and 6 produced in yeast. J Biol Chem 1992; 267:12692–12699.

427. Jones JL, Gockerman A, Busby WH, et al. Extracellular matrix contains insulin-like growth factor binding protein-5: potentiation of the effects of IGF1. J Cell Biol 1993; 121:679–687.

428. Clemmons DR, Nam TJ, Busby WH, et al. Modification of IGF action by insulin-like growth factor binding protein-5. In: Baxter RC, Gluckman PD, Rosenfeld RG, eds. The Insulin-like Growth Factors and Their Regulatory Proteins. Amsterdam: Elsevier, 1994; 183–191.

429. Andress DL, Birnbaum RS. Human osteoblast-derived insulin-like growth factor (IGF) binding protein-5 stimulates osteoblast mitogenesis and potentiates IGF action. J Biol Chem 1992; 267:22467–22372.

430. Adashi EY, Resnick CE, Hurwitz A, et al. The intra-ovarian IGF system. Growth Regul 1992; 2:10–15.

431. Shimasaki S, Tanahashi H, Onoda N, et al. Transcriptional and posttranscriptional regulation of IGFBP-4 and -5 in cultured rat granulosa cells. In: Baxter RC, Gluckman PD, Rosenfeld RG, eds. The Insulin-like Growth Factors and Their Regulatory Proteins. Amsterdam: Elsevier, 1994; 193–204.

432. Kiefer MC, Masiarz FR, Bauer DM, et al. Identification and molecular cloning of two new 30 kd insulin-like growth factor binding proteins isolated from adult human serum. J Biol Chem 1991; 266:9043–9049.

433. Bach LA, Thotakura NR, Rechler MM. Human insulin-like growth factor binding protein-6 is O-glycosylated. Growth Reg 1993; 3:59–62.

434. Roghani M, Lassarre C, Zapf J, et al. Two insulin-like growth factor (IGF) binding proteins are responsible for the selective affinity for IGF2 of cerebrospinal fluid binding proteins. J Clin Endocrinol Metab 1991; 73:658–666.

435. Rohan RM, Ricciarelli E, Kiefer MC, et al. Rat ovarian insulin-like growth factor binding protein-6, a hormonally regulated theca-interstitial-selective species with limited antigonadotropic activity. Endocrinology 1993; 132:2507–2512.

436. Drop SLS, Valiquette G, Guyda HJ, et al. Partial purification and characterization of a binding protein for insulin-like activity (ILAs) in human amniotic fluid: a possible inhibitor of insulin-like activity. Acta Endocrinol 1979; 90:505–518.

437. Povoa G, Roovete A, Hall K. Cross-reaction of a serum somatomedin-binding protein in a radioimmunoassay developed for somatomedin-binding protein isolated from human amniotic fluid. Acta Endocrinol 1984; 107:563–570.

438. Baxter RC, Cowell CT. Diurnal variation of growth hormone–independent binding protein for insulin-like growth factors in humans. Clin Endocrinol Metab 1987; 65:432–440.

439. Baxter RC, Martin JL. Radioimmunoassay of growth hormone dependent insulin-like growth factor binding protein in human plasma. J Clin Invest 1986; 78:1504–1512.

440. Blum WF, Ranke MB, Kietzmann K, et al. A specific radioimmunoassay for the growth hormone–dependent somatomedin-binding protein: its use for diagnosis of GH deficiency. J Clin Endocrinol Metab 1990; 70:1292–1298.

441. Honda Y, Landale EC, Strong DD, et al. Recombinant synthesis of insulin-like growth factor-binding protein-4 (IGFBP-4): development, validation and application of a radioimmunoassay for IGFBP-4 in human serum and other biologic fluids. J Clin Endocrinol Metab 1996; 81:1389–1396.

442. Smith EP, Boyd J, Frank GR, et al. Estrogen resistance caused by a mutation in the estrogen-receptor gene in a man. N Engl J Med 1994; 331:1056–1061.

443. Conte FA, Grumbach MM, Ito Y, et al. A syndrome of female pseudohermaphroditism, hypergonadotropic hypogonadism, and multicystic ovaries associated with missense mutations in the gene encoding aromatase (P450arom). J Clin Endocrinol Metab 1994; 78:1287–1292.

444. Morishima A, Grumbach MM, Simpson ER, et al. Aromatase deficiency in male and female siblings caused by a novel mutation and the physiological role of estrogens. J Clin Endocrinol Metab 1995; 80:3689–3698.

445. Lehrer S, Rabin J, Stone J, et al. Association of an estrogen receptor variant with increased height in women. Horm Metab Res 1994; 26:486–488.

446. Matkovic V. Skeletal development and bone turnover revisited (editorial). J Clin Endocrinol Metab 1996; 81:2013–2016.

447. Abrams SA, O'Brien KO, Stuff JE. Changes in calcium kinetics associated with menarche. J Clin Endocrinol Metab 1996; 81:2017–2020.

448. Mauras N, Doi SQ, Shapiro JR. Recombinant human insulin-like growth factor-I, recombinant human growth hormone, and sex steroids: effects on markers of bone turnover in humans. J Clin Endocrinol Metab 1996; 81:2222–2226.

449. Slemenda CW, Reister TK, Hui SL, et al. Influences on skeletal mineralization in children and adolescents: evidence for varying effects of sexual maturation and physical activity. J Pediatr 1996; 125:201–207.

450. Matkovic V, Fontana D, Tominac C, et al. Factors which influence peak bone mass formation: a study of calcium balance and the inheritance of bone mass in adolescent females. Am J Clin Nutr 1990; 52:878–888.

451. Theintz G, Buch B, Rizzoli R, et al. Longitudinal monitoring of bone mass accumulation in healthy adolescents: evidence for a marked reduction after 16 years of age at the levels of lumbar spine and femoral neck in female subjects. J Clin Endocrinol Metab 1992; 75:1060–1065.

452. Spranger J. International classification of osteochondrodysplasias. Eur J Pediatr 1992; 151:407–415.

453. Pauli RM. Osteochondrodysplasia with mild clinical manifestations: a guide for endocrinologists and others. Growth Genetics Hormone 1995; 11:1–5.

454. Maroteaux P. Nomenclature internationale des maladies osseuses constitutionnelles. Ann Radiol 1970; 13:455–464.

455. Rimoin DL. International nomenclature of constitutional diseases of bone: revision—May 1977. J Pediatr 1978; 93:614–616.

456. Shiang R, Thompson LM, Zhu Y, et al. Mutation in the transmembrane domain of FGFR3 causes the most common genetic form of dwarfism, achondroplasia. Cell 1994; 78:335–342.

457. Rousseau F, Bonaventure J, Legeai-Mallet L, et al. Mutations in the gene encoding fibroblast growth factor receptor-3 in achondroplasia. Nature 1994; 371:252–254.

458. Velinov M, Slaughenhaupt SA, Stoilov I, et al. The gene for achondroplasia maps to the telomeric region of chromosome 4p. Nat Genet 1994; 6:314–317.

459. Le Merrer M, Rousseau F, Legeai-Mallet L, et al. A gene for achondroplasia-hypochondroplasia maps to chromosome 4p. Nat Genet 1994; 3:18–21.

460. Francomano CA, Ortiz de Luna RI, Hefferon TW, et al. Localization of the achondroplasia gene to the distal 25 Mb of human chromosome 4p. Hum Mol Genet 1994; 3:787–792.

461. Francomano CA. The genetic basis of dwarfism. N Engl J Med 1995; 332:58–59.

462. Bellus GA, Hefferon TW, Ortiz de Luna RI, et al. Achondroplasia is defined by recurrent G380R mutations of FGFR3. Am J Human Genet 1995; 56:368–373.

463. Yamate T, Kanzaki S, Tanaka H, et al. Growth hormone (GH) treatment in achondroplasia. J Pediatr Endocrinol 1993; 6:45–52.

464. Hecht JT, Butler IJ. Neurologic morbidity associated with achondroplasia. J Child Neurol 1990; 5:84–97.

465. Hahn YS, Engelhard HH, Naidish T, et al. Paraplegia resulting from thoracolumbar stenosis in a seven-month-old achondroplastic dwarf. Pediatr Neurosci 1989; 15:39–43.

466. Waters KA, Kirjavainen T, Jimenez M, et al. Overnight growth hormone secretion in achondroplasia: deconvolution analysis, correlation with sleep state, and changes after treatment of obstructive sleep apnea. Pediatr Res 1996; 39:547–553.

467. Stollov I, Kilpatrick M, Tsipouras P. A common FGFR3 gene mutation is present in achondroplasia but not in hypochondroplasia. Am J Med Genet 1995; 55:127–133.

468. Mullis PE, Patel MS, Brickell PM, et al. Growth characteristics and response to growth hormone therapy in patients with hypochondroplasia: genetic linkage of the insulin-like growth factor I gene at chromosome 12q23 to the disease in a subgroup of these patients. Clin Endocrinol 1991; 34:265–274.

469. Castells S, Torrado C, Bastian W, et al. Growth hormone deficiency in Down's syndrome children. J Intellect Disabil Res 1992; 36:29–43.

470. Pueschel SM. Growth hormone response after administration of L-dopa, clonidine, and growth hormone releasing hormone in children with Down syndrome. Res Dev Disabil 1993; 14:291–298.

471. Barreca A, Quartino AR, Acutis MS, et al. Assessment of growth hormone insulin like growth factor-I axis in Down's syndrome. J Endocrinol Invest 1994; 17:431–436.

472. Sara VR, Gustavson KH, Anneren G, et al. Somatomedins in Down's syndrome. Biol Psychiatry 1983; 18:803–811.

473. Anneren G, Sara VR, Hall K, et al. Growth and somatomedin responses to growth hormone in Down's syndrome. Arch Dis Child 1986; 61:48–52.

474. Anneren G, Gustavson KH, Sara VR, et al. Normalized growth velocity in children with Down's syndrome during growth hormone therapy. J Intellect Disabil Res 1993; 37:381–387.

475. Neyzi O, Darendeliler F. Growth hormone treatment in syndromes with short stature including Down syndrome, Prader-Labhardt-Willi syndrome, von Recklinghausen syndrome, Williams syndrome and others. In: Ranke B, Gunnarsson R, eds. Progress in Growth Hormone Therapy—5 Years of KIGSM. Mannheim: J&J Verlag, 1994: 240–245.

476. Torrado C, Bastian W, Wisniewski KE, et al. Treatment of children with Down syndrome and growth retardation with recombinant human growth hormone. J Pediatr 1991; 119:478–483.

477. Allen DB, Frasier SD, Foley TP, et al. Growth hormone for children with Down syndrome. J Pediatr 1993; 123:742–743.

478. Rosenfeld RG, Grumbach MM, eds. Turner Syndrome. New York: Marcel Dekker, 1990.

479. Ranke MB, Rosenfeld RG, eds. Turner Syndrome: Growth Promoting Therapies. New York: Elsevier, 1991.

480. Hibi I, Takano K, eds. Basic and Clinical Approach to Turner Syndrome. Amsterdam: Excerpta Medica, 1993.

481. Rochiccioli P, David M, Malpuech G, et al. Study of final height in Turner's syndrome: ethnic and genetic influences. Acta Paediatr 1994; 83:305–308.

482. Nilsson KO, Wikland KA, Alm J, et al. Improved final height in girls with Turner's syndrome treated with growth hormone and oxandrolone. J Clin Endocrinol Metab 1996; 81:635–640.

483. Rosenfeld RG, Chernausek S, Frane J, et al. Growth hormone treatment of Turner syndrome: effect on final height. Pediatr Res 1996; 39:97(A).

484. Ranke MB, Pfluger H, Rosendahl W, et al. Turner syndrome: spontaneous growth in 150 cases and review of the literature. Eur J Pediatr 1983; 141:81–88.

485. Brook CGD, Gasser T, Werder EA, et al. Height correlations between parents and mature offspring in normal subjects and in subjects with Turner's and Klinefelter's and other syndromes. Ann Hum Biol 1977; 4:17–22.

486. Massa G, Vanderschueren-Lodeweyckx M, Malvaux P. Linear growth in patients with Turner syndrome: influence of spontaneous puberty and parental height. Eur J Pediatr 1990; 149:246–150.

487. Ross JL, Long LM, Loriaux DL, et al. Growth hormone secretory dynamics in Turner syndrome. J Pediatr 1985; 106:202–206.

488. Rosenfeld RG, Hintz RL, Johanson AJ, et al. Three-year results of a randomized prospective trial of methionyl human growth hormone and oxandrolone in Turner syndrome. J Pediatr 1988; 113:393–400.

489. Rosenfeld RG, Frane J, Attie KM, et al. Six-year results of a randomized, prospective trial of human growth hormone and oxandrolone in Turner syndrome. J Pediatr 1992; 121:49–55.

490. Warshaw JB. Intrauterine growth restriction revisited. Growth Genetics Hormones 1992; 8:5–8.

491. Kitchen WH, Ford GW, Doyle LW. Growth and very low birthweight. Arch Dis Child 1989; 64:379–382.

492. Fitzhardinge PM, Stevens EM. The small for date infant: later growth patterns. Pediatrics 1972; 49:671–681.

493. Westwood DM, Kramer MS. Growth and development of full term nonasphyxiated small for gestational age newborns: follow-up through adolescence. Pediatrics 1983; 376–382.

494. Hack M, Merkatz IR, McGrath SK, et al. Catch-up growth in very low birthweight infants. Am J Dis Child 1984; 138:370–375.

495. Fitzhardinge PM, Inwood S. Long term growth in small for date children. Acta Paediatr Scand 1989; 349:27–33.

496. Chaussain JL, Colle M, Ducret JP. Adult height in children with prepubertal short stature secondary to intrauterine growth retardation. Acta Paediatr 1994; 399(Suppl):72–73.

497. Barker DJP, Gluckman PD, Dodrey KM, et al. Fetal nutrition and cardiovascular disease in adult life. Lancet 1993; 341:938–941.

498. Barker DJP. Growth in utero and coronary heart disease. Nutr Rev 1996; 54:S1–S7.

499. D'Ercole AJ, Underwood LE. Regulation of fetal growth by hormones and growth factors. In: Falkner F, Tanner JM, eds. Human Growth: A Comprehensive Treatise. Vol I: Developmental Biology, Prenatal Growth. New York: Plenum, 1986: 327–338.

500. Sizonenko PC, Aubert ML. Pre- and perinatal endocrinology. In: Falkner F, Tanner JM, eds. Human Growth: A Comprehensive Treatise. Vol I: Developmental Biology Prenatal Growth. New York: Plenum, 1986: 339–376.

501. Gluckman P, Harding J. The regulation of fetal growth. In: Hernandez M, Argente J, eds. Human Growth: Basic and Clinical Aspects. Amsterdam: Elsevier, 1992: 253–276.

502. Cooke PS, Nicoll CS. Hormonal control of fetal growth. Physiologist 1983; 26:317–323.

503. Kim JD, Nanto-Salonen K, Szcepankiewicz JR, et al. Evidence of pituitary regulation of somatic growth, insulin-like growth factors-I and -II and their binding proteins in the fetal rat. Pediatr Res 1993; 33:144–151.

504. Wit JM, van Unen H. Growth of infants with neonatal growth hormone deficiency. Arch Dis Child 1992; 67:920–924.

505. Gluckman PD, Gunn AJ, Wray A, et al. Congenital idiopathic growth hormone deficiency associated with prenatal and early postnatal growth failure. J Pediatr 1992; 121:920–923.

506. DeLuca F, Bernasconi S, Blandino A, et al. Auxological, clinical, and neuroradiological findings in infants with early onset growth hormone deficiency. Acta Paediatr Scand 1995; 84:561–565.

507. Liu JP, Baker J, Perkins AS, et al. Mice carrying null mutations of the genes encoding insulin-like growth factor I (Igf-1) and type 1 IGF receptor (Igf1r). Cell 1993; 75:73–82.

508. Jones JI, Clemmons. Insulin-like growth factors and their binding proteins: biologic actions. Endocr Rev 1995; 16:3–34.

509. Evain-Brion D. Hormonal regulation of fetal growth. Horm Res 1994; 42:207–214.

510. Ashton IK, Zapf J, Einschenk I, et al. Insulin-like growth factors IGF 1 and 2 in human fetal plasma and relationship to gestational age and fetal size during mid pregnancy. Acta Endocrinol 1985; 110:558–563.

511. Spencer JAD, Chang TC, Jones J, et al. Third trimester fetal growth and umbilical venous blood concentrations of IGF1, IGFBP-1, and growth hormone at term. Arch Dis Child 1995; 73:F87–F90.

512. Leger J, Oury JF, Noel M, et al. Growth factors and intrauterine growth retardation. I: Serum growth hormone, insulin-like growth factor (IGF)-I, IGF2, and IGF binding protein 3 levels in normally grown and growth-retarded human fetuses during the second half of gestation. Pediatr Res 1996; 40:94–100.

513. Woods KA, Camacho-Hubner C, Savage MO, et al. Intrauterine growth retardation and postnatal growth failure associated with deletion of the insulin-like growth factor I gene. N Engl J Med 1996; 335:1342–1349.

514. Rosenfeld RG, Thorsson AV, Hintz RL. Increased somatomedin receptor sites in newborn circulating mononuclear cells. J Clin Endocrinol Metab 1979; 48:456–461.

515. D'Ercole AJ. Somatomedins/insulin-like growth factors and fetal development. J Dev Physiol 1987; 9:481–495.

516. Han VK, D'Ercole AJ, Lund PK. Cellular localization of somatomedin (insulin-like growth factor) messenger RNA in the human fetus. Science 1987; 236:193–197.

517. Klempt M, Bingham B, Breier BH, et al. Tissue distribution and ontogeny of growth hormone receptor mRNA and ligand binding to hepatic tissue in the midgestation fetus. Endocrinology 1993; 132:1071–1077.

518. Gluckman PD, Butler JH, Elliott TB. The ontogeny of somatotropic binding sites in ovine hepatic membranes. Endocrinology 1983; 112:1607–1612.

519. de Zegher FJ, Kimpen J, Raus J, et al. Hypersomatotropism in the dysmature infant at term and preterm birth. Biol Neonate 1990; 58:188–191.

520. Wollmann HA, Ranke MB. GH treatment in neonates. Acta Paediatr 1996; 85:398–400.

521. van Toledo-Eppinga LEC, Houdijk AM, Cranendonk A, et al. Effects of recombinant human growth hormone treatment in intrauterine growth-retarded preterm newborn infants on growth, body composition and energy expenditure. Acta Paediatr 1996; 85:476–481.

522. Oliver MH, Harding JE, Breier BH, et al. Glucose but not a mixed amino acid infusion regulates insulin-like growth factor I concentrations in fetal sheep. Pediatr Res 1993; 34:62–65.

523. Chard T. Insulin-like growth factors and their binding proteins in normal and abnormal fetal growth. Growth Regul 1994; 4:91–100.

524. Milner RDG. Nesidioblastosis unravelled. Arch Dis Child 1996; 74:369–372.

525. Soliman AT, Alsalmi I, Darwish A, et al. Growth and endocrine function after near total pancreatectomy for hyperinsulinemic hypoglycemia. Arch Dis Child 1996; 74:379–385.

526. Russell AA. A syndrome of "intrauterine" dwarfism recognizable at birth with craniofacial dysostosis, disproportionately short arms and other anomalies (5 examples). Proc R Soc Med 1954; 47:1040–1044.

527. Silver HK. Asymmetry, short stature and variations in sexual development: syndrome of congenital malformations. Am J Dis Child 1964; 107:495–515.

528. Angehrn V, Zachmann M, Prader A. Silver-Russell syndrome. Observations in 20 patients. Helv Paediatr Acta 1979; 34:297–308.

529. Davies PSW, Valley R, Preece MA. Adolescent growth and pubertal progression in the Silver-Russell syndrome. Arch Dis Child 1988; 63:130–135.

530. Saal HM, Pagon RA, Pepin MG. Re-evaluation of Russell-Silver syndrome. J Pediatr 1985; 107:733–737.

531. Wollman HA, Kirchner T, Enders H, et al. Growth and symptoms in Silver-Russell syndrome: review on the basis of 386 patients. Eur J Pediatr 1995; 154:958–968.

532. Boguszewski M, Rosberg S, Albertsson-Wikland K. Spontaneous 24-h growth hormone profiles in prepubertal small for gestational age children. J Clin Endocrinol Metab 1995; 80:2599–2602.

533. Mann TP, Russell A. Study of a microcephalic midget of extreme type. Proc R Soc Med 1959; 52:1024–1027.

534. Harper RG, Orti E, Baker RK. Birdheaded dwarfs (Seckel's syndrome). A familial pattern of developmental, dental, skeletal, genital, and central nervous system anomalies. J Pediatr 1967; 70:799–804.

535. Collins E, Turner G. The Noonan syndrome—a review of the clinical and genetic features of 27 cases. J Pediatr 1973; 83:941–950.

536. Patton MA. Noonan syndrome: a review. Growth Genetics Hormones 1994; 10:1–3.

537. Ranke MB, Heidemann P, Knupfer C, et al. Noonan syndrome: growth and clinical manifestations in 144 cases. Eur J Pediatr 1988; 148:22–27.

538. Witt DR, Keena BA, Hall JG, et al. Growth curves for height in Noonan syndrome. Clin Genet 1986; 30:150–153.

539. Bernardini S, Spadoni GL, Cianfarani S, et al. Growth hormone secretion in Noonan's syndrome. J Pediatr Endocrinol 1991; 4:217–221.

540. Rosenbloom AL, DeBusk FL. Progeria of Hutchinson-Gilford: a caricature of aging. Am Heart J 1971; 82:287–289.

541. MacDonald WB, Fitch KD, Lewis IC. Cockayne's syndrome. An heredo-familial disorder of growth and development. Pediatrics 1960; 25:997–1007.

542. Bray GA, Dahms WT, Swerdloff RS, et al. The Prader-Willi syndrome. A study of 40 patients and review of the literature. Medicine 1983; 62:59–80.

543. Costeff H, Holm VA, Ruvalcaba R, et al. Growth hormone secretion in Prader Willi syndrome. Acta Paediatr Scand 1990; 79:1059–1062.

544. Cappa M, Grossi A, Borrelli P, et al. Growth hormone (GH) response to combined pyridostigmine and GH-releasing hormone administration in patients with Prader-Labhard-Willi syndrome. Horm Res 1993; 39:51–55.

545. Angulo M, Castro-Magana M, Uy J. Pituitary evaluation and growth hormone treatment in Prader-Willi syndrome. J Pediatr Endocrinol 1991; 4:167–173.

546. Francke U. Prader-Willi syndrome: chromosomal and gene aberrations. Growth Genetics Hormones 1994; 10:4–7.

547. Jones KL. Smith's Recognizable Patterns of Human Malformation. 5th ed. Philadelphia: WB Saunders, 1997.

548. Edwards LE, Alton IR, Barrada MI, et al. Pregnancy in the underweight woman: course, outcome and growth patterns of the infant. Am J Obstet Gynecol 1979; 135:297–302.

549. Ouellette EM, Rosett HL, Rosman NP, et al. Adverse effects on offspring of maternal alcohol abuse during pregnancy. N Engl J Med 1977; 297:528–530.

550. Jones KL, Smith DW, Streissguth AP. Outcome in offspring of chronic alcoholic women. Lancet 1974; 1:1076–1078.

551. Abel EL. Consumption of alcohol during pregnancy: a review of effects on growth and development of offspring. Hum Biol 1982; 54:421–453.

552. Chasnoff IJ, Griffith DR, MacGregor S, et al. Temporal patterns of cocaine use in pregnancy: perinatal outcome. JAMA 1989; 261:1741–1744.

553. Zuckerman B, Frank DA, Hingson R, et al. Effects of maternal marijuana and cocaine use on fetal growth. N Engl J Med 1989; 320:762–768.

554. Abel EL. Smoking during pregnancy: a review of effects on growth and development of offspring. Hum Biol 1980; 52:593–625.

555. Hall K, Enberg G, Hellem D, et al. Somatomedin levels in pregnancy: longitudinal study in healthy subjects and in pregnancies with intrauterine growth retardation. J Clin Endocrinol Metab 1984; 59:587–594.

556. Mirlesse V, Frankenne F, Alsat E, et al. Placental growth hormone levels in normal pregnancy and in pregnancies with intrauterine growth retardation. Pediatr Res 1993; 34:439–442.

556a. Hasegawa T, Hasegawa Y, Takada M, et al. The free form of insulin-like growth factor increases in circulation during normal human pregnancy. J Clin Endocrinol Metab 1995; 80:3284–3286.

557. Graham GC, Adrianzen T, Rabold J, et al. Later growth of malnourished children. Am J Dis Child 1982; 136:348–352.

558. Allen LH. Nutritional influences on linear growth: a general review. Eur J Clin Nutr 1994; 48(Suppl):S75–S89.

559. Thissen J, Ketelslegers J, Underwood LE. Nutritional regulation of the insulin-like growth factors. Endocr Rev 1994; 15:80–101.

560. Zamboni G, Dufillot D, Antoniazzi F, et al. Growth hormone–binding proteins and insulin-like growth factor–binding proteins in protein-energy malnutrition, before and after nutritional rehabilitation. Pediatr Res 1996; 39:410–414.

561. Pimstone B, Berbezat G, Hansen JD, et al. Growth hormone and protein-calorie malnutrition. Impaired suppression during induced hyperglycemia. Lancet 1967; 2:1333–1334.

562. Beas F, Contreras I, Maccioni A, et al. Growth hormone in infant malnutrition: the arginine test in marasmus and kwashiorkor. Br J Nutr 1971; 26:169–175.

563. Grant DB, Hambley J, Becker D, et al. Reduced sulphation factor in undernourished children. Arch Dis Child 1973; 48:596–600.

564. Soliman AT, Hassan AEHI, Aref MK, et al. Serum insulin-like growth factors I and II concentrations and growth hormone and insulin responses to arginine infusion in children with protein-energy malnutrition before and after nutritional rehabilitation. Pediatr Res 1986; 20:1122–1130.

565. Mayer E, Stern M. Growth failure in gastrointestinal diseases. Baillieres Clin Endocrinol Metab 1992; 6:645–663.

566. Phillips LS. Nutrition, somatomedins, and the brain. Metabolism 1986; 35:78–87.

567. Donovan SM, Atilano LC, Hintz RL, et al. Differential regulation of the insulin-like growth factors (IGF1 and IGF2) and IGF binding proteins during malnutrition in the neonatal rat. Endocrinology 1991; 129:149–157.

568. Pugliese MT, Lifshitz F, Grad G, et al. 1983; Fear of obesity: a cause of short stature and delayed puberty. N Engl J Med 309:513–518.

569. Golden NH, Kreitzer P, Jacobson MS, et al. Disturbances in growth hormone secretion and action in adolescents with anorexia nervosa. J Pediatr 1994; 125:655–660.

570. Root AW, Powers PS. Anorexia nervosa presenting as growth retardation in adolescents. J Adolesc Health Care 1983; 4:25–30.

571. Nussbaum M, Baird D, Sonnenblick M, et al. Short stature in anorexia nervosa patients. J Adolesc Health Care 1985; 6:453–455.

572. Russell GFM. Premenarchal anorexia nervosa and its sequelae. J Psychiatry Res 1985; 19:363–369.

573. Huseman C, Johanson A. Growth hormone deficiency in anorexia nervosa. J Pediatr 1975; 87:946–948.

574. Hochberg Z, Barkley RJ, Even L, et al. The effects of growth hormone therapy on GH binding protein in GH-deficient children. Acta Endocrinol 1991; 125:23–27.

575. Postel-Vinay C, Saab C, Gourmelen M. Nutritional status and growth hormone-binding protein. Horm Res 1995; 44:177–181.

576. Counts DR, Gwirtsman H, Carlsson LMS, et al. The effects of anorexia nervosa and refeeding on growth hormone-binding protein, the insulin-like growth factors (IGFs), and the IGF-binding proteins. J Clin Endocrinol Metab 1992; 75:762–767.

577. Preece MA, Law CM, Davies PSW. The growth of children with chronic paediatric disease. Clin Endocrinol Metab 1986; 15:453–477.

578. Groll A, Candy D, Preece M, et al. Short stature as the primary manifestation of coeliac disease. Lancet 1980; 2:1097–1099.

579. Mock DM. Growth retardation in chronic inflammatory bowel disease. Gastroenterology 1986; 91:1019–1023.

580. Rosenthal SR, Snyder JD, Hendricks KM, et al. Growth failure and inflammatory bowel disease: approach to treatment of a complicated adolescent problem. Pediatrics 1983; 72:481–490.

581. Lecornu M, David L, Francois R. Low serum somatomedin activity in celiac disease. Helv Paediatr Acta 1978; 33:509–516.

582. Kirschner BS, Sutton MM. Somatomedin-C levels in growth-impaired children and adolescents with chronic inflammatory bowel disease. Gastroenterology 1986; 91:830–836.

583. Auricchio S, Greco L, Troncone R. Gluten-sensitive enteropathy in childhood. Pediatr Clin North Am 1988; 35:157–187.

584. Young WF, Pringle EM. 110 children with coeliac disease, 1950–1969. Arch Dis Child 1971; 46:421–436.

585. Verkasalo M, Kuitunen P, Leisti S, et al. Growth failure from symptomless celiac disease. Helv Paediatr Acta 1978; 33:489–495.

586. DeLuca F, Astori M, Pandullo E, et al. Effects of a gluten-free diet on catch-up growth and height prognosis in coeliac children with growth retardation recognized after the age of 5 years. Eur J Pediatr 1988; 47:188–191.

587. Stenhammar L, Fallstrom SP, Jansson G, et al. Coeliac disease in children of short stature without gastrointestinal symptoms. Eur J Pediatr 1986; 145:185–186.

588. Radzikowski T, Zalewski TK, Kapuscinska A, et al. Short stature due to unrecognized coeliac disease. Eur J Pediatr 1988; 147:334–335.

589. Meuwisse GW. Diagnostic criteria for celiac disease. Acta Paediatr Scand 1970; 59:461–463.

590. Chan KN, Phillips AD, Mirakian R, et al. Endomysial antibody screening in children. J Pediatr Gastroenterol Nutr 1994; 18:316–320.

591. Volta U, Molinaro N, Fratangelo D, et al. IgA antibodies to jejunem. Specific immunity directed against target organ of gluten-sensitive enteropathy. Dig Dis Sci 1994; 39:1924–1929.

592. Hernandez M, Argente J, Navarro A, et al. Growth in malnutrition related to gastrointestinal diseases: coeliac disease. Horm Res 1992; 38(Suppl): 79–84.

593. Bode SH, Bachmann EH, Gudmand-Hoyer E, et al. Stature of adult coeliac patients: no evidence for decreased attained height. Eur J Clin Nutr 1991; 45:145–149.

594. Cacciari E, Corazza GR, Salardi S, et al. What will be the adult height of coeliac patients? Eur J Pediatr 1991; 150:407–409.

595. Murch SH, Lamkin V, Savage MO, et al. Serum concentrations of tumor necrosis factor alpha in childhood chronic inflammatory bowel disease. Gut 1991; 32:913–917.

596. Booth IW, Harries JT. Inflammatory bowel disease in childhood. Gut 1984; 25:188–202.

597. Kirschner BS. Growth and development in chronic inflammatory bowel disease. Acta Paediar Scand 1990; 366(Suppl):98–104.

598. Kelts DG, Grand RJ, Shen G, et al. Nutritional basis of growth failure in children and adolescents with Crohn's disease. Gastroenterology 1979; 76:720–727.

599. Gryboski JD, Spiro HM. Prognosis in children with Crohn's disease. Gastroenterology 1978; 74:807–817.

600. Kanof ME, Lake AM, Bayless TM. Decreased height velocity in children and adolescents before the diagnosis of Crohn's disease. Gastroenterology 1988; 95:1523–1527.

601. McCaffery TD, Nast K, Lawrence AM, et al. Severe growth retardation in children with inflammatory bowel disease. Pediatrics 1970; 45:386–393.

602. Markowitz J, Grancher K, Rosa J, et al. Growth failure in inflammatory bowel disease. J Pediatr Gastroenterol Nutr 1993; 16:373–380.

603. Alagille D, Estrada A, Hadchouel M, et al. Syndromic paucity of interlobular bile ducts (Alagille syndrome or arteriohepatic dysplasia): review of 80 cases. J Pediatr 1987; 110:195–200.

604. Kobayashi A, Itabashi F, Ohbe Y. Long-term prognosis in biliary atresia after hepatic portoenterostomy; analysis of 35 patients who survived beyond 5 years of age. J Pediatr 1984; 105:243–246.

605. Urbach AH, Gartner JC, JJ Malatack, et al. Linear growth following pediatric liver transplantation. Am J Dis Child 1987; 141:547–549.

606. Kaufman SS, Murray ND, Wood RP, et al. Nutritional support for the infant with extrahepatic biliary atresia. J Pediatr 1987; 110:679–686.

607. Russell WE. Growth hormone, somatomedins, and the liver. Semin Liver Dis 1985; 5:46–58.

608. Bucuvalas JC, Cutfield W, Horn J, et al. Resistance to the growth promoting and metabolic effects of growth hormone in children with chronic liver disease. J Pediatr 1990; 117:397–402.

609. Donaghy A, Ross R, Gimson A, et al. Growth hormone, insulin-like growth factor binding proteins 1 and 3 in chronic liver disease. Hepatology 1995; 21:680–688.

610. Moller S, Becker U. Insulin-like growth factor I and growth hormone in chronic liver disease. Digest Dis 1992; 10:239–248.

611. Quirk P, Owens P, Moyse K, et al. Insulin-like growth factors I and II are reduced in plasma from growth-retarded children with chronic liver disease. Growth Reg 1994; 4:35–38.

612. Hattori N, Kurahachi H, Ikekubo K, et al. Serum growth hormone–binding protein, insulin-like growth factor I, and growth hormone in patients with liver cirrhosis. Metabolism 1992; 41:377–381.

613. Cuneo RC, Hickman PE, Wallace JD, et al. Altered endogenous growth hormone secretory kinetics and diurnal GH-binding protein profiles in adults with chronic liver disease. Clin Endocrinol 1995; 43:265–275.

614. Holt GRI, Jones JS, Stone NM, et al. Sequential changes in insulin-like growth factor I (IGF1) and IGF-binding proteins in children with end stage liver disease before and after successful orthotopic liver transplantation. J Clin Endocrinol Metab 1996; 81:160–168.

615. Chin SE, Shepherd RW, Cleghorn GJ, et al. Survival, growth and quality of life in children after orthotopic liver transplantation. J Paediatr Child Health 1991; 27:380–385.

616. Stewart SM, Uauy R, Waller DA, et al. Mental and motor development, social competence and growth one year after successful pediatric liver transplantation. J Pediatr 1989; 114:574–581.

617. Paradis GKJ, Freese DK, Sharp HL. A pediatric perspective on liver transplantation. Pediatr Clin North Am 1988; 35:409–433.

618. Sarna S, Sipila I, Jalanko H, et al. Factors affecting growth after pediatric liver transplantation. Transplant Proc 1994; 26:161–164.

619. Sarna S, Sipila I, Vihervuori E, et al. Growth delay after liver transplantation in childhood: studies of underlying mechanisms. Pediatr Res 1995; 38:366–372.

620. Codoner-French P, Bernard O, Alvarez F. Long-term follow-up of growth in height after successful liver transplantation. J Pediatr 1994; 124:368–373.

621. Sarna S, Sipila I, Ronnholm K, et al. Recombinant human growth hormone improves growth in children receiving glucocorticoid treatment after liver transplantation. J Clin Endocrinol Metab 1996; 81:1476–1482.

622. Bayer LM, Robinson SJ. Growth history of children with congenital heart defects. Am J Dis Child 1969; 117:564–572.

623. Feldt RH, Strickler GB, Weidman WH. Growth of children with congenital heart disease. Am J Dis Child 1969; 117:573–579.

624. Gilger M, Mensen C, Kessler B, et al. Nutrition, growth and the gastrointestinal system: basic knowledge for the pediatric cardiologist. In: Garson A Jr, Bricker JT, McNamara DG, eds. The Science and Practice of Pediatric Cardiology. Philadelphia: Lea & Febiger, 1990: 2354–2370.

625. Mehrizi A, Drash A. Growth disturbances in congenital heart disease. J Pediatr 1962; 61:418–429.

626. Nadas AS, Rosenthal A, Crigler JF. Nutritional considerations in the prognosis and treatment of children with congenital heart disease. In: Suskind RM, ed. Textbook of Pediatric Nutrition. New York: Raven, 1987: 537–544.

627. Noonan JA. Association of congenital heart disease with syndromes of other defects. Pediatr Clin North Am 1978; 25:797–816.

628. McLean WC. Protein energy malnutrition. In: Grand RJ, Sutphen JL, Dietz WH, eds. Pediatric Nutrition: Theory and Practice. Stoneham, MA: Butterworth's, 1987: 421–431.

629. Nelson DL, Blaese RM, Strober W. Constrictive pericarditis, intestinal lymphangiectasia and reversible immunologic deficiency. J Pediatr 1975; 86:548–554.

630. Sondheimer JM, Hamilton JR. Intestinal function in infants with severe congenital heart disease. J Pediatr 1978; 92:572–578.

631. Naeye RL. Anatomic features of growth failure in congenital heart disease. Pediatrics 1967; 39:433–440.

632. Heymsfield SB, Andrews JS, Hood R, et al. Nutrition and the heart. In: Grand RJ, Sutphen JL, Dietz WH, eds. Pediatric Nutrition: Theory and Practice. Stoneham, MA: Butterworth's, 1987: 597–613.

633. Wahlig TM, Georgieff MK. The effects of illness on neonatal metabolism and nutritional management. Clin Prenatal 1995; 22:77–79.

634. Linde LM, Dunn OJ, Schireson R, et al. Growth in children with congenital heart disease. J Pediatr 1967; 70:413–419.

635. Barton JS, Hindmarsh PC, Preece MA. Serum insulin-like growth factor I in congenital heart disease. Arch Dis Child 1996; 75:162–163.

636. Bernstein D, Jasper JR, Rosenfeld RG, et al. Decreased serum insulin-like growth factor-I associated with growth failure in newborn lambs with experimental cyanotic heart disease. J Clin Invest 1992; 89:1128–1132.

637. Holliday MA. Symposium on metabolism and growth in children with kidney disease. Kidney Int 1978; 14:299–382.

638. Rizzoni G, Broyer M, Guest G, et al. Growth retardation in childhood renal disease: scope of the problem. Am J Kidney 1986; 7:256–261.

639. Kohaut EC. Chronic renal disease and growth in childhood. Curr Opin Pediatr 1995; 7:171–175.

640. Tonshoff B, Mehls O. Growth retardation in children with chronic renal insufficiency: current aspects of pathophysiology and treatment. J Nephrol 1955; 8:133–142.

641. Mehls O, Blum WF, Schaefer F, et al. Growth failure in renal disease. Bailieres Clin Endocrinol Metab 1992; 6:665–685.

642. Warady BA, Jabs K. New hormones in the therapeutic arsenal of chronic renal failure. Pediatr Clin North Am 1995; 42:1551–1577.

643. Lee D-Y, Park SK, Kim J-S. Insulin-like growth factor-I (IGF1) and IGF-binding proteins in children with nephrotic syndrome. J Clin Endocrinol Metab 1996; 81:1856–1860.

644. Kimonis VE, Troendle J, Rose SR, et al. Effects of early cysteamine therapy on thyroid function and growth in nephropathic cystinosis. J Clin Endocrinol Metab 1995; 80:3257–3261.

645. Tonshoff B, Veldhuis JD, Heinrich U, et al. Deconvolution analysis of spontaneous nocturnal growth hormone secretion in prepubertal children with preterminal chronic renal failure and with end-stage renal disease. Pediatr Res 1995; 37:86–93.

646. Ramirez G, O'Neill WM Jr, Bloomer A, et al. Abnormalities in the regulation of growth hormone in chronic renal failure. Arch Intern Med 1978; 138:267–271.

647. Hokken-Koelega SAC, Hackeng WHL, Stijen T, et al. Twenty-four-hour plasma growth hormone (GH) profiles, urinary GH excretion, and plasma insulin-like growth factor-I and -II levels in prepubertal children with chronic renal insufficiency and severe growth retardation. J Clin Endocrinol Metab 1990; 71:688–695.

648. Schaefer F, Hamill G, Stanhope R, et al. Cooperative Study Group on Pubertal Development in Chronic Renal Failure 1991. Pulsatile growth hormone secretion in peri-pubertal patients with chronic renal failure. J Pediatr 1991; 119:568–577.

649. Blum WF. Insulin-like growth factors (IGFs) and IGF binding proteins in chronic renal failure: evidence for reduced secretion of IGFs. Acta Paediatr Scand 1991; 379(Suppl):24–31.

650. Tonshoff B, Eden S, Weiser E, et al. Reduced hepatic growth hormone (GH) receptor gene expression and increased plasma GH binding protein in experimental uremia. Kidney Int 1994; 45:1085–1092.

651. Hokken-Koelega SAC, Stijnen T, De Muinck Keizer-Schrama SMPF, et al. Placebo-controlled, double-blind, cross-over trial of growth hormone treatment in prepubertal children with chronic renal failure. Lancet 1991; 338:585–590.

652. Rees L, Maxwell H. The hypothalamo-pituitary-growth hormone insulin-like growth factor 1 axis in children with chronic renal failure. Kidney Int 1996; 47(Suppl):S109–S114.

653. Blum WF, Ranke MB, Kietzmann K, et al. Growth hormone resistance and inhibition of somatomedin activity by excess of insulin-like growth factor binding protein in uremia. Pediatr Nephrol 1991; 5:539–545.

654. Saenger P, Wiedemann E, Schwartz E, et al. Somatomedin and growth after renal transplantation. Pediatr Res 1974; 8:162–169.

655. Hokken-Koelega ACS, Stijnen T, De Muinck Keizer-Schrama SMPF, et al. Levels of growth hormone, insulin-like growth factor-I (IGF-I) and -II, IGF-binding protein-1 and -3, and cortisol in prednisone-treated children with growth retardation after renal transplantation. J Clin Endocrinol Metab 1993; 77:932–938.

656. Hanna JD, Santos F, Foreman JW, et al. Insulin-like growth factor-I gene expression in the tibial epiphyseal growth plate of growth hormone–treated uremic rats. Kidney Int 1995; 17:1374–1382.

657. Unterman TG, Phillips LS. Glucocorticoid effects on somatomedins and somatomedin inhibitors. J Clin Endocrinol Metab 1985; 61:618–626.

658. Allen DB. Growth suppression by glucocorticoid therapy. Pediatr Rounds 1995; 4:1–5.

659. Fine RN, Tejani A. Renal transplantation in children. Nephron 1987; 47:81–896.

660. Ding H, Gao X-L, Hirschberg R, et al. Impaired actions of insulin-like growth factor I on protein synthesis and degradation in skeletal muscle of rats with chronic renal failure: evidence for a postreceptor defect. J Clin Invest 1996; 97:1064–1075.

661. Hokken-Koelega ACS, Van Zaal MAE, de Ridder MAJ, et al. Growth after renal transplantation in prepubertal children: impact of various treatment modalities. Pediatr Res 1994; 35:367–371.

662. Hokken-Koelega ACS, Van Zaal MAE, Van Bergen W, et al. Final height and its predictive factors after renal transplantation in childhood. Pediatr Res 1994; 36:323–328.

663. Tejani A, Fine R, Alexander S, et al. Factors predictive of sustained growth in children after renal transplantation. J Pediatr 1993; 122:397–402.

664. Van Es A. Growth hormone treatment in short children with chronic renal failure and after renal transplantation: combined data from European clinical trials. Acta Paediatr Scand 1991; 379(Suppl):42–48.

665. Hokken-Koelega ACS, de Ridder MAJ, De Muinck Keizer-Schrama SMPF, et al. Growth hormone treatment in growth-retarded adolescents after renal transplant. Lancet 1994; 343:1313–1317.

666. Van Dop C, Jabs KL, Donohoue PA, et al. Accelerated growth rates in children treated with growth hormone after renal transplantation. J Pediatr 1992; 120:244–250.

667. Fine RN. Recombinant human growth hormone in children with chronic renal insufficiency—clinical update: 1995. Kidney Int 1996; 49(Suppl): S115–S116.

668. Ingulli E, Tejani A. An analytical review of growth hormone studies in children after renal transplantation. Pediatr Nephrol 1995; 9:S61–S65.

669. Platt OS, Rosenstock W, Espeland MA. Influence of sickle hemoglobinopathies on growth and development. N Engl J Med 1984; 311:7–12.

670. Stevens MCG, Maude GH, Cupidore L. Prepubertal growth and sexual maturation in children with sickle cell disease. Pediatrics 1986; 78:124–132.

671. Phebus CK, Gloninger MF, Maciak BJ. Growth patterns in children with sickle cell disease. J Pediatr 1984; 105:28–33.

672. Henderson RA, Saavedra JM, Dover GJ. Prevalence of impaired growth in children with homozygous sickle cell anemia. Am J Med Sci 1994; 307:405–407.

673. Modebe O, Ifenu SA. Growth retardation in homozygous sickle cell disease: role of calorie intake and possible gender-related differences. Am J Hematol 1994; 44:149–154.

674. Singhal A, Thomas P, Cook R, et al. Delayed adolescent growth in homozygous sickle cell disease. Arch Dis Child 1994; 71:404–408.

675. Zago MA, Kerbauy J, Souza HM, et al. Growth and sexual maturation of Brazilian patients with sickle cell disease. Trop Geogr Med 1992; 44:317–321.

676. Borgna-Pignatti C, De Stefano P, Zonta L, et al. Growth and sexual maturation in thalassemia major. J Pediatr 1985; 106:150–155.

677. Deluca F, Simone E, Corona G, et al. Adult height in thalassemia major without hormonal treatment. Eur J Pediatr 1987; 146:494–496.

678. Saka N, Sukur M, Bundak R, et al. Growth and puberty in thalassemia major. J Pediatr Endocrinol Metab 1995; 8:181–186.

679. Saenger P, Schwartz E, Markenson AL, et al. Depressed serum somatomedin activity in beta-thalassemia. J Pediatr 1980; 96:214–218.

680. Werther GA, Matthews RN, Burger HG, et al. Lack of response of nonsuppressible insulin-like activity to short-term administration of human growth hormone in thalassemia major. J Clin Endocrinol Metab 1981; 53:806–809.

681. Low LCK, Kwan EYW, Lim YJ, et al. Growth hormone treatment of short Chinese children with β-thalassemia major without GH deficiency. Clin Endocrinol 1995; 42:359–363.

682. Deluca G, Maggioline M, Bria M, et al. GH secretion in thalassemic patients with short stature. Horm Res 1995; 44:158–163.

683. Scacchi M, Danesi L, DeMartin M, et al. Treatment with biosynthetic growth hormone of short thalassemic patients with impaired growth hormone secretion. Clin Endocrinol 1991; 35:335–339.

684. Herber SM, Dunsmore IR. Does control affect growth in diabetes mellitus? Acta Paediatr Scand 1988; 77:303–305.

685. Malone JI. Growth and sexual maturation in children with insulin-dependent diabetes mellitus. Curr Opin Pediatr 1993; 5:494–498.

686. Thon A, Heinze E, Feilen KD, et al. Development of height and weight in children with diabetes mellitus: report on two prospective multicentre studies, one cross-sectional, one longitudinal. Eur J Pediatr 1992; 151:258–262.

687. Hjelt K, Braendholt V, Kamper J, et al. Growth in children with diabetes mellitus. Dan Med Bull 1983; 30:28–33.

688. White P, Marble A, Bogan IK, et al. Enlargement of the liver in diabetic children. II: Effect of raw pancrease, betaine hydrochloride and protamine insulin. Arch Intern Med 1938; 62:751–764.

689. Jackson RL, Holland E, Chatman ID, et al. Growth and maturation of children with insulin-dependent diabetes mellitus. Diabetes Care 1978; 1:96–107.

690. Vanelli M, DeFanti J, Adinolfi B, et al. Clinical data regarding the growth of diabetic children. Horm Res 1992; 37:65–69.

691. Rogers DG, Sherman LD, Gabbay KH. Effect of puberty on insulin-like growth factor I and HbA1 in type I diabetes. Diabetes Care 1991; 14:1031–1035.

692. Mandell F, Berenberg W. The Mauriac syndrome. Am J Dis Child 1974; 127:900–902.

693. White P. Childhood diabetes: its course, and influence on the second and third generation. Diabetes 1960; 9:345–355.

694. Menon RK, Arslaninan S, May B, et al. Diminished growth hormone binding protein in children with insulin-dependent diabetes mellitus. J Clin Endocrinol Metab 1992; 74:934–938.

695. Froesch ER, Hussain M. Metabolic effects of insulin-like growth factor I with special reference to diabetes. Acta Paediatr Scand 1994; 399:165–170.

696. Malone JI, Lowitt S, Duncan JA, et al. Hypercalciuria, hyperphosphaturia and growth retardation in children with diabetes mellitus. Pediatrics 1986; 78:298–304.

697. Clayton KL, Holly JMP, Carlsson LMS. Loss of the normal relationship between growth hormone, growth hormone binding protein and insulin like growth factor in adolescents with insulin dependent diabetes mellitus. Clin Endocrinol 1994; 41:517–524.

698. Amiel SA, Sherwin RS, Hintz RL, et al. Effect of diabetes and its control on insulin-like growth factors in the young subject with type I diabetes. Diabetes 1984; 33:1175–1179.

699. Dills DG, Allen C, Palta M, et al. Insulin-like growth factor-I is related to glycemic control in children and adolescents with newly diagnosed insulin-dependent diabetes mellitus. J Clin Endocrinol Metab 1995; 80:2139–2143.

700. Bereket A, Lang CH, Blethen SL, et al. Effect of insulin on IGF system in children with new onset insulin dependent diabetes mellitus. J Clin Endocrinol Metab 1995; 80:1312–1317.

701. Winter RJ, Phillips LS, Klein MN, et al. Somatomedin activity and diabetic control in children with insulin-dependent diabetes. Diabetes 1979; 28:952–954.

702. Rudolf MCJ, Sherwin RS, Markowitz R, et al. Effect of intensive insulin treatment on linear growth in the young diabetic patient. J Pediatr 1982; 101:333–339.

703. Knip M, Tapanainen P, Pekonen F, et al. Insulin-like growth factor binding proteins in prepubertal children with insulin dependent diabetes mellitus. Eur J Endocrinol 1995; 133:440–444.

704. Munoz MT, Barrios V, Pozo J, et al. Insulin-like growth factor I, its binding proteins 1 and 3, and growth hormone–binding protein in children and adolescents with insulin-dependent diabetes mellitus: clinical implications. Pediatr Res 1996; 39:992–998.

705. Dunger DB. Insulin and insulin-like growth factors in diabetes mellitus. Arch Dis Child 1995; 72:469–471.

706. Suikkari AM, Koivisto VA, Rutanen EM, et al. Insulin regulates the serum levels of low molecular weight insulin-like growth factor binding protein. J Clin Endocrinol Metab 1988; 66:266–272.

707. Holly JMP, Biddlecomb RA, Dunger DB, et al. Circadian variation of GH-dependent IGF-binding protein in diabetes mellitus and its relation to insulin. A new role for insulin? Clin Endocrinol 1988; 29:667–677.

708. Batch JA, Baxter RC, Werther G. Abnormal regulation of insulin-like growth factor binding proteins in adolescents with insulin-dependent diabetes mellitus. J Clin Endocrinol Metab 1991; 73:964–968.

709. Taylor AM, Dunger DB, Preece MA, et al. The growth hormone independent insulin-like growth factor-I binding protein BP-28 is associated with serum insulin-like growth factor I inhibitory bioactivity in adolescent insulin-dependent diabetes mellitus. Clin Endocrinol 1990; 32:229–239.

710. Bereket A, Lang CH, Blethen SL, et al. Insulin-like growth factor binding protein-3 proteolysis in children with insulin dependent diabetes mellitus: a possible role for insulin in the regulation of IGFBP-3 protease activity. J Clin Endocrinol Metab 1995; 80:2282–2288.

711. Jivani SKM, Rayner PHW. Does control influence the growth of diabetic children? Arch Dis Child 1973; 48:109–115.

712. Tattersall RB, Pyke DA. Growth in diabetic children. Studies in identical twins. Lancet 1973; 2:1105–1109.

713. Clarson D, Daneman D, Ehrlich RM. The relation of metabolic control to growth and pubertal development in children with insulin-dependent diabetes. Diabetes Res 1985; 2:237–241.

714. Dunger DB, Brown M. Diabetes and growth in puberty. Growth Matters 1990; 5:10–14.

715. Du Caju MVL, Rooman RP, Op De Beeck L. Longitudinal data on growth and final height in diabetic children. Pediatr Res 1995; 38:607–611.

716. Pitukcheewanont P, Alemzadeh R, Jacobs WR, et al. Does glycemic control affect growth velocity in children with insulin-dependent diabetes mellitus? Acta Diabetol 1995; 32:148–152.

717. Jackson RL. Growth and maturation of children with insulin-dependent diabetes mellitus. Pediatr Clin North Am 1984; 31:545–567.

718. Tamborlane WV, Hintz RL, Bergman M, et al. Insulin-infusion-pump treatment of diabetes: influence of improved metabolic control on plasma somatomedin levels. N Engl J Med 1981; 305:303–307.

719. Marsden D, Barshop BA, Capistrano-Estrada S, et al. Anabolic effect of human growth hormone: management of inherited disorders of catabolic pathways. Biochem Med Metab Biol 1994; 52:145–154.

720. Bain MD, Nussey SS, Jones M, et al. Use of human somatotropin in the treatment of a patient with methylmalonic aciduria. Eur J Pediatr 1995; 154:850–852.

721. Russell G. Asthma and growth. Arch Dis Child 1993; 69:695–698.

722. Cohen MB, Abram LE. Growth patterns of allergic children. J Allergy 1948; 19:165–171.

723. Balfour-Lynn L. Growth and childhood asthma. Arch Dis Child 1986; 61:1049–1055.

724. Ninan TK, Russell G. Asthma, inhaled corticosteroid treatment and growth. Arch Dis Child 1992; 67:703–705.

725. Nassif E, Weinberger M, Sherman B, et al. Extrapulmonary effects of maintenance corticosteroid therapy with alternate-day prednisolone and inhaled beclomethasone in children with chronic asthma. J Allergy Clin Immunol 1987; 80:518–528.

726. Falliers CJ, Tan LS, Szentivanyi J, et al. Childhood asthma and steroid therapy as influences on growth. Am J Dis Child 1963; 105:127–137.

727. Versano I, Volovitz B, Malik H, et al. Safety of 1 year of treatment with budesonide in young children with asthma. J Allergy Clin Immunol 1990; 85:914–920.

728. Volovitz B, Amir J, Malik H, et al. Growth and pituitary-adrenal function in children with severe asthma treated with inhaled budesonide. N Engl J Med 1996; 329:1703–1708.

729. Todd G, Dunlop K, McNaboe J, et al. Growth and adrenal suppression in asthmatic children treated with high-dose fluticasone propionate. Lancet 1996; 348:27–29.

730. Crowley S, Hindmarsh PC, Matthews DR, et al. Growth and the growth hormone axis in prepubertal children with asthma. J Pediatr 1995; 126:297–303.

731. Martin AJ, McLennan LA, Landau LI, et al. The natural history of childhood asthma to adult life. BMJ 1980; 280:1397–1400.

732. Shohat M, Shohat T, Kedem R, et al. Childhood asthma and growth outcome. Arch Dis Child 1987; 62:63–65.

733. Avery ME, Tooley W, Keller J, et al. Is chronic lung disease in low birth weight infants preventable? A survey of eight centers. Pediatrics 1987; 79:26–30.

734. Gibson AT, Pearse RG, Wales JKH. Growth retardation after dexamethasone administration: assessment by knemometry. Arch Dis Child 1993; 69:505–509.

735. Kurzner SI, Garg M, Bautista D, et al. Growth failure in infants with bronchopulmonary dysplasia: nutrition and elevated resting metabolic expenditure. Pediatrics 1988; 81:379–384.

736. Yu V, Orgill A, Lim S, et al. Growth and development of very low-birth-weight infants recovering from bronchopulmonary dysplasia. Arch Dis Child 1983; 58:791–794.

737. Meisels S, Plunkett J, Roloff D, et al. Growth and development of preterm infants with respiratory distress syndrome and bronchopulmonary dysplasia. Pediatrics 1986; 77:345–352.

738. Vrlenich LA, Bozynski MEA, Shyr Y, et al. The effect of bronchopulmonary dysplasia on growth at school age. Pediatrics 1995; 95:855–859.

739. Ross G, Lipper E, Auld P. Growth achievement of very low-birthweight premature children at school age. J Pediatr 1990; 117:307–309.

740. Robertson M, Etches P, Goldson E, et al. Eight year school performance, neurodevelopmental, and growth outcome of neonates with bronchopulmonary dysplasia: a comparative study. Pediatrics 1992; 89:365–372.

741. Landon C, Rosenfeld RG. Short stature and pubertal delay in male adolescents with cystic fibrosis. Am J Dis Child 1984; 138:388–391.

742. Sproul A, Huang N. Growth patterns in children with cystic fibrosis. J Pediatr 1964; 65:664–676.

743. Lapey A, Kattwinkel J, DiSant'Agnese PA, et al. Steatorrhea and azotorrhea and their relation to growth and nutrition in adolescents and young adults with cystic fibrosis. J Pediatr 1974; 84:328–334.

744. Mearns M. Growth and development. In: Hodson E, Norman A, Batten J, eds. Cystic Fibrosis. London: Bailliere Tindall, 1983: 183–196.

745. Shepherd RW, Holt TL, Thomas BJ, et al. Nutritional rehabilitation in cystic fibrosis: controlled studies of effects on nutritional growth retardation, body protein turnover, and course of pulmonary disease. J Pediatr 1986; 109:788–794.

746. Reiter EO, Gerstle RS. Cystic fibrosis in puberty and adolescence. In: Lerner RM, Petersen AC, Brooks-Gunn J, eds. Encyclopedia of Adolescence. New York: Garland, 1991: 187–195.

747. FitzSimmons SC. The changing epidemiology of cystic fibrosis. J Pediatr 1993; 122:1–9.

748. Karlberg J, Kjellmer I, Kristiansson B. Linear growth in children wth cystic fibrosis. I: Birth to 8 years of age. Acta Paediatr Scand 1991; 80:508–514.

749. Reiter EO, Stern RC, Root AW. The reproductive system in cystic fibrosis. I: Basal gonadotropin and sex steroid levels. Am J Dis Child 1981; 135:422–426.

750. Reiter EO, Stern RC, Root AW. The reproductive system in cystic fibrosis. II: Changes in gonadotrophins and sex steroids following LHRH. Clin Endocrinol 1982; 16:127–137.

751. Reiter EO, Brugman SM, Pike JW, et al. Vitamin D metabolites in adolescents and young adults with cystic fibrosis: effects of sun and season. J Pediatr 1985; 106:21–26.

752. Laursen EM, Juul A, Lanng S, et al. Diminished concentrations of insulin-like growth factor I in cystic fibrosis. Arch Dis Child 1995; 72:494–497.

753. Huseman CA, Columbo JL, Brooks MA, et al. Anabolic effect of biosynthetic growth hormone in cystic fibrosis. Pediatr Pulmonol 1996; 22:90–95.

754. Abrams EJ, Rogers MF. Pediatric HIV infection. Baillieres Clin Haematol 1991; 4:333–339.

755. McKinney RE, Robertson JWR, the Duke Pediatric AIDS Clinical Trials Unit. Effect of human immunodeficiency virus infection on the growth of young children. J Pediatr 1993; 123:579–582.

756. Saavedra JM, Henderson RA, Perman JA, et al. Longitudinal assessment of growth in children born to mothers with human immunodeficiency virus infection. Arch Pediatr Adolesc Med 1995; 149:497–502.

757. McKinney RE, Wilfert C, the AIDS Clinical Trials Group Protocol 043 Study Group. Growth as a prognostic indicator in children with immunodeficiency virus infection treated with zidovudine. J Pediatr 1994; 125:728–733.

758. Gertner JM, Kaufman FR, Donfield SM, et al. Delayed somatic growth and pubertal development in human immunodeficiency virus-infected hemophiliac boys: hemophilia growth and development study. J Pediatr 1994; 124:896–902.

759. Moye J, Rich KC, Kalish LA, et al. Natural history of somatic growth in infants born to women infected by human immunodeficiency virus. J Pediatr 1996; 128:58–69.

760. Grunfeld C. What causes wasting in AIDS? N Engl J Med 1995; 333:123–124.

761. Grunfeld C, Feingold KR. Metabolic disturbances and wasting in the acquired immunodeficiency syndrome. N Engl J Med 1992; 327:329–337.

762. Anonymous. Infections as deterrants of growth. Nutr Rev 1981; 39:328.

763. Mccann SM, Lyson K, Karanth S, et al. Role of cytokines in the endocrine system. Ann NY Acad Sci 1994; 50–63.

764. Vassilopoulou-Sellin R. Endocrine effects of cytokines. Oncology 1994; 8:43–50.

765. Skerry TM. The effects of the inflammatory response on bone growth. Eur J Clin Nutr 1994; 48(Suppl):S190–S198.

766. Chiesa A, de Papendieck G, Keselman A, et al. Growth follow-up in 100 children with congenital hypothyroidism before and during treatment. J Pediatr Endocrinol 1994; 7:211–217.

767. Grant DB. Growth in early treated congenital hypothyroidism. Arch Dis Child 1994; 70:464–468.

768. Rivkees SA, Bode HH, Crawford JD. Long-term growth in juvenile acquired hypothyroidism. N Engl J Med 1988; 318:599–602.

769. Pantsiouou S, Stanhope R, Urena M, et al. Growth prognosis and growth after menarche in primary hypothyroidism. Arch Dis Child 1991; 66:838–840.

770. Boersma B, Otten BJ, Stoelings GBA, et al. Catch-up growth after prolonged hypothyroidism. Eur J Pediatr 1996; 155:362–367.

771. Magiakou MA, Mastorakos G, Oldfield EH, et al. Cushing's syndrome in children and adolescents. Presentation, diagnosis, and therapy. N Engl J Med 1994; 331:629–636.

772. Lee PA, Weldon VV, Migeon CJ. Short stature as the only clinical sign of Cushing's syndrome. J Pediatr 1975; 86:89–91.

773. Reid IR. Pathogenesis and treatment of steroid osteoporosis. Clin Endocrinol 1989; 30:83–103.

774. Giustina A, Bussi AR, Jacobello C, et al. Effects of recombinant human growth hormone (GH) on bone and intermediary metabolism in patients receiving chronic glucocorticoid treatment with suppressed endogenous GH response to GH-releasing hormone. J Clin Endocrinol Metab 1995; 80:122–129.

775. Allen DB, Goldberg BD. Stimulation of a collagen synthesis and linear growth by growth hormone in glucocorticoid-treated children. Pediatrics 1992; 89:416–421.

776. Schatz M, Dudl J, Zeiger RS, et al. Osteoporosis in corticosteroid-treated asthmatic patients: clinical correlates. Allergy Proc 1993; 14:341–345.

777. Luo J, Murphy LJ. Dexamethasone inhibits growth hormone induction of insulin-like growth factor-I (IGF-I) messenger ribonucleic acid (mRNA) in hypophysectomized rats and reduces IGF-I mRNA abundance in the intact rat. Endocrinology 1989; 125:165–171.

778. Magiakou MA, Mastorakos G, Gomez MT, et al. Suppressed spontaneous and stimulated growth hormone secretion in patients with Cushing's disease before and after surgical cure. J Clin Endocrinol Metab 1994; 78:131–137.

779. Mauras N, Beaufrere B. rhIGF-I enhances whole body protein anabolism and significantly diminishes the protein-catabolic effects of prednisone in humans without a diabetogenic effect. J Clin Endocrinol Metab 1995; 80:869–874.

780. Rivkees SA, Danon M, Herrin J. Prednisone dose limitation of growth hormone treatment of steroid-induced growth failure. J Pediatr 1994; 125:322–325.

781. Mosier HD, Smith FG, Schultz MA. Failure of catch-up growth after Cushing's syndrome in childhood. Am J Dis Child 1972; 124:251–253.

782. Leong GM, Mercado-Asis LB, Reynolds JC, et al. The effect of Cushing's disease on bone mineral density, body composition, growth and puberty; a report of identical adolescent twin pair. J Clin Endorinol Metab 1996; 81:1905–1911.

783. Reimer LG, Morris HG, Ellis FE. Growth of asthmatic children during treatment with alternate day steroids. J Allergy Clin Immunol 1975; 55:224–231.

784. Schwindinger WF, Levine MA. Albright hereditary osteodystrophy. Endocrinologist 1994; 4:17–27.

785. Chan JCM. Renal hypophosphatemic rickets—a review. Int J Pediatr Nephrol 1982; 3:305–310.

786. Glorieux FH, Marie PJ, Pettifor JM, et al. Bone response to phosphate salts, ergocalciferol and calcitriol in hypophosphatemic vitamin D resistant rickets. N Engl J Med 1980; 303:1023–1031.

787. Petersen DJ, Boniface AM, Schranck FW, et al. X-linked hypophosphatemic rickets: a study (with literature review) of linear growth response to calcitriol and phosphate therapy. J Bone Miner Res 1992; 7:583–597.

788. Balsan S, Tieder M. Linear growth in patients with hypophosphatemic vitamin D-resistant rickets: influence of treatment regimen and parental height. J Pediatr 1990; 116:365–371.

789. Reusz GS, Hoyer PF, Lucas M, et al. X linked hypophosphatemia: treatment, height gain, and nephrocalcinosis. Arch Dis Child 1990; 65:1125–1128.

790. Herweijer TJ, Steendijk R. The relation between attained adult height and the methaphyseal lesions in hypophosphatemic vitamin D–resistant rickets. Acta Paediatr Scand 1985; 74:196–200.

791. Stickler GB, Morgenstern BZ. Hypophosphatemic rickets: final height and clinical symptoms in adults. Lancet 1989; 2:902–905.

792. Bistritzer T, Chalew SA, Hanukoglu A, et al. Does growth hormone influence the severity of phosphopenic rickets? Eur J Pediatr 1990; 150:26–29.

793. Jasper H, Cassinelli H. Growth hormone and insulin-like growth factor I plasma levels in patients with hypophosphatemic rickets. J Pediatr Endocrinol 1993; 6:179–184.

794. Saggese G, Barancelli GI, Vertelloni S, et al. Growth hormone secretion in poorly growing children with renal hypophosphatemic rickets. Eur J Pediatr 1994; 153:548–555.

795. Wilson DM, Olney RC, Tyerman G, et al. Preliminary results of multicenter, controlled study of growth hormone treatment in children with X-linked hypophosphatemic rickets (XLHR). Endocrinol Metab 1994; 1(Suppl):16.

796. Wilson DM, Lee PD, Morris AH, et al. Growth hormone therapy in hypophosphatemic rickets. Am J Dis Child 1991; 145:1165–1170.

797. Saggese G, Barancelli GI, Bertelloni S, et al. Long-term growth hormone treatment in children with renal hypophosphatemic rickets: effects on growth, mineral metabolism and bone density. J Pediatr 1995; 127:395–402.

798. Wilson DM, Olney RC, Tyerman GPD, et al. A trial of growth hormone treatment of X-linked hypophosphatemic rickets—results of the second year 10th International Congress of Endocrinology. San Francisco, 1996 P1-136 (abstract).

799. Maghnie M, Genovese E, Villa A, et al. Dynamic MRI in the congenital agenesis of the neural pituitary stalk syndrome: the role of the vascular pituitary stalk in predicting residual anterior pituitary function. Clin Endocrinol 1996; 45:281–290.

800. Fujisawa I, Kikuchi K, Nishimura K, et al. Transection of the pituitary stalk: development of anectopic posterior lobe assessed with MR imaging. Radiology 1987; 165:487–489.

801. Abrahams JJ, Trefelner E, Boulware SD. Idiopathic growth hormone deficiency: MR findings in 35 patients. Am J Neuroradiol 1991; 12:155–160.

802. Kuroiwa T, Okabe Y, Hasuo K, et al. MR imaging of pituitary dwarfism. Am J Neuroradiol 1991; 12:161–164.

803. Cacciari E, Zucchini S, Carla G, et al. Endocrine function and morphological findings in patients with disorders of the hypothalamo-pituitary area: a study with magnetic resonance. Arch Dis Child 1990; 65:1199–1202.

804. Maghnie M, Larizza D, Triulzi F, et al. Hypopituitarism and stalk agenesis: a congenital syndrome worsened by breech delivery? Horm Res 1991; 35:104–108.

805. Brown RS, Bhatia V, Hayes E. An apparent cluster of congenital hypopituitarism in central Massachusetts: magnetic resonance imaging and hormonal studies. J Clin Endocrinol Metab 1991; 72:12–18.

806. Root AW, Martinez CR. Magnetic resonance imaging in patients with hypopituitarism. Trends Endocrinol Metab 1992; 3:283–287.

807. Argyopoulou M, Perignon F, Brauner R, et al. Magnetic resonance imaging in the diagnosis of growth hormone deficiency. J Pediatr 1992; 120:886–891.

808. Triulzi F, Scotti G, diNatale B, et al. Evidence of a congenital midline brain anomaly in pituitary dwarfs: a magnetic resonance imaging study in 101 patients. Pediatrics 1994; 93:409–416.

809. Goodman HG, Grumbach MM, Kaplan SL. Growth and growth hormone II. A comparison of isolated growth hormone deficiency and multiple pituitary hormone deficiency in 35 patients with idiopathic hypopituitary disease. N Engl J Med 1968; 278:57–68.

810. Albertsson-Wikland K, Niklasson A, Karlberg P. Birth data for patients who later develop growth hormone deficiency: preliminary analysis of a national register. Acta Paediatr Scand 1990; 370(Suppl):115–120.

811. Craft WH, Underwood LE, Van Wyk JJ. High incidence of perinatal insult in children with idiopathic hypopituitarism. J Pediatr 1980; 96:397–402.

812. Copeland KC, Franks RC, Ramamurthy R. Neonatal hyperbilirubinemia and hypoglycemia in congenital hypopituitarism. Clin Pediatr 1981; 20:523–526.

813. Choo-Kang LR, Sun C-CJ, Counts DR. Cholestasis and hypoglycemia: manifestations of congenital anterior hypopituitarism. J Clin Endocrinol Metab 1996; 81:2786–2789.

814. Lovinger RD, Kaplan SL, Grumbach MM. Congenital hypopituitarism associated with neonatal hypoglycemia and microphallus: four cases secondary to hypothalamic hormone deficiences. J Pediatr 1975; 87:1171–1181.

815. Rimoin DL, Merimee TJ, Rabinowitz D, et al. Genetic aspects of clinical endocrinology. Recent Prog Horm Res 1968; 24:365–437.

816. Ranke MB. A note on adults with growth hormone deficiency. Acta Paediatr Scand 1987; 331(Suppl):80–82.

817. van der Werff ten Bosch JJ, Bot A. Growth of males with idiopathic hypopituitarism without growth hormone treatment. Clin Endocrinol 1990; 32:707–717.

818. Wilson P. Panorama of the diagnoses in the Kabi International Growth Study. In: Ranke B, Gunnarsson R, eds. Progress in Growth Hormone Therapy—5 Years of KIGSM. Mannheim: J&J Verlag, 1994: 62–66.

819. Cumulative Data Review. Genentech National Cooperative Growth Study Summary Report. San Francisco: Genentech, 1994; 18:6–13.

820. Goddard AD, Covello R, Shiuh ML, et al. Mutation of the growth hormone receptor in children with idiopathic short stature. N Engl J Med 1995; 333:1093–1098.

821. Rosenfeld RG. Broadening the growth hormone insensitivity syndrome. N Engl J Med 1995; 333:1145–1146.

822. Parkin JM. Incidence of growth hormone deficiency. Arch Dis Child 1974; 49:904–905.

823. Vimpani GV, Vimpani AF, Lidgard GP, et al. Prevalence of severe growth hormone deficiency. Br Med J 1977; 2:427–430.

824. Lindsay R, Feldkamp M, Harris D, et al. Utah Growth Study: growth standards and the prevalence of growth hormone deficiency. J Pediatr 1994; 125:29–35.

825. Perez Juarado LA, Argente J. Molecular basis of familial growth hormone deficiency. Horm Res 1994; 42:189–197.

826. Parks JS, Pfaffle RW, Brown MR, et al. Growth hormone deficiency. In: Weintraub BD, ed. Molecular Endocrinology: Basic Concepts and Clinical Correlations. New York: Raven, 1995: 473–490.

827. Cogan JD, Phillips JA, Sakati N, et al. Heterogeneous growth hormone (GH) gene mutations in familial GH deficiency. J Clin Endocrinol Metab 1993; 76:1224–1228.

828. Chin KY. The endocrine glands of anencephalic foetuses. Chinese Med J 1938; 2(Suppl):63–90.

829. Lemire RJ, Beckwith JB, Warkany J. Anencephaly. New York: Raven, 1978.

830. Grumbach MM, Kaplan SL. Ontogenesis of growth hormone, insulin, prolactin and gonadotropin secretion in the human foetus. In: Cross DW, Nathanielsz P, eds. Foetal and Neonatal Physiology: Proceedings of Sir Joseph Barcroft Centenary Symposium. Cambridge: Cambridge University Press, 1973: 462.

831. Grumbach MM, Kaplan SL. Fetal pituitary hormones and the maturation of central nervous system regulation of anterior pituitary function. In: Gluck L, ed. Modern Perinatal Medicine. Chicago: Year Book Medical, 1974: 247.

832. Hintz RL, Menking M, Sotos JF. Familial holoprosencephaly with endocrine dysgenesis. J Pediatr 1968; 72:81–87.

833. Lieblich JM, Rosen SW, Guyda H, et al. The syndrome of basal encephalocele and hypothalamic pituitary dysfunction. Ann Intern Med 1978; 89:910–916.

834. Rudman D, Davis GT, Priest JH, et al. Prevalence of growth hormone deficiency in children with cleft lip or palate. J Pediatr 1978; 93:378–382.

835. Izenberg N, Rosenblum M, Parks JS. The endocrine spectrum of septo-optic dysplasia. Clin Pediatr 1984; 23:632–636.

836. Wilson DM, Enzmann DR, Hintz RL, et al. Cranial computed tomography in septo-optic dysplasia: discordance of clinical and radiological features. Neuroradiology 1984; 26:279–283.

837. Willnow S, Kiess W, Butenandt O, et al. Endocrine disorders in septo-optic dysplasia (De Morsier syndrome)—evaluation and follow-up of 18 patients. Eur J Pediatr 1996; 155:179–184.

838. Kaplan SL, Grumbach MM. Pathophysiology of GH deficiency and other disorders of GH metabolism. In: LaCauza C, Root AW, eds. Problems in Pediatric Endocrinology, Serono Symposia, Vol 32. London: Academic, 1980: 45.

839. de Zegher F, Kaplan SL, Grumbach MM, et al. The foetal pituitary, postmaturity and breech presentation. Acta Paediatr 1995; 83:1100–1102.

840. Miller WL, Kaplan SL, Grumbach MM. Child abuse as a cause of post-traumatic hypopituitarism. N Engl J Med 1980; 302:724–728.

841. Mayfield RK, Levine JH, Gordon L, et al. Lymphadenoid hypophysitis presenting as a pituitary tumor. Am J Med 1980; 69:619–623.

842. Bartsocas CS, Pantelakis SN. Human growth hormone therapy in hypopituitarism due to tuberculous meningitis. Acta Paediatr Scand 1973; 62:304–306.

843. Stuart CA, Neelon FA, Lebovitz HE. Hypothalamic insufficiency: the cause of hypopituitarism in sarcoidosis. Ann Intern Med 1978; 88:589–594.

844. Costin G. Endocrine disorders associated with tumors of the pituitary and hypothalamus. Pediatr Clin North Am 1979; 26:15–31.

845. Brauner R, Rappaport R, Prevot C, et al. A prospective study of the development of growth hormone deficiency in children given cranial irradiation, and its relation to statural growth. J Clin Endocrinol Metab 1989; 68:346–351.

846. Shalet SM. Irradiation-induced growth failure. Pediatr Clin North Am 1986; 15:591–606.

847. Blatt J, Bercu BB, Gillin JC, et al. Reduced pulsatile growth hormone secretion in children after therapy for acute lymphoblastic leukemia. J Pediatr 1984; 104:182–186.

848. Sklar CA, Constine LS. Chronic neuroendocrinological sequelae of radiation therapy. Int J Radiat Oncol Biol Phys 1995; 31:1113–1121.

849. Clayton PE, Shalet SM. Dose dependency of time of onset of radiation-induced growth hormone deficiency. J Pediatr 1991; 118:226–228.

850. Rappaport R, Brauner R. Growth and endocrine disorders secondary to cranial irradiation. Pediatr Res 1989; 25:561–567.

851. Littley MD, Shalet SM, Beardwell CG, et al. Radiation-induced hypopituitarism is dose-dependent. Clin Endocrinol 1989; 31:361–373.

852. Nivot S, Benelli C, Clot JP, et al. Nonparallel changes of growth hormone (GH) and insulin-like growth factor-I, insulin-like growth factor binding protein-3, and GH-binding protein, after craniospinal irradiation and chemotherapy. J Clin Endocrinol Metab 1995; 78:597–601.

853. Ogilvy-Stuart AL, Shalet SM. Effect of chemotherapy on growth. Acta Paediatr 1995; 411(Suppl):52–56.

854. Sklar C, Mertens A, Walter A, et al. Final height after treatment for childhood acute lymphoblastic leukemia: comparison of no cranial irradiation with 1800 and 2400 centigrays of cranial irradiation. J Pediatr 1993; 123:56–64.

855. Stubberfield TG, Byrne GC, Jones TW. Growth and growth hormone secretion after treatment for acute lymphoblastic leukemia in childhood. J Pediatr Hematol Oncol 1995; 17:167–171.

856. Katz JA, Pollack BH, Jacaruso D, et al. Finally attained height in patients successfully treated for childhood acute lymphoblastic leukemia. J Pediatr 1993; 123:546–552.

857. Talvensaari KK, Lanning M, Paako E, et al. Pituitary size assessed with

magnetic resonance imaging as a measure of growth hormone in long term survivors of childhood cancer. J Clin Endocrinol Metab 1994; 79:1122–112.

858. Sklar CA, Sarafoglou K, Whittam E. Effects of insulin-like growth factor binding protein 3 in predicting the growth hormone response to provacative testing in children treated with cranial irradiation. Acta Endocrinol 1993; 129:511–515.

859. Donaldson SS, Kaplan H. Complications of treatment of Hodgkin's disease in children. Cancer Treat Rep 1982; 66:977–989.

860. Wallace WHB, Shalet SM, Morris-Jones PH, et al. Effect of abdominal irradiation on growth in boys treated for a Wilms' tumor. Med Pediatr Oncol 1990; 18:441–446.

861. Davies HA, Didcock E, Didi A, et al. Growth, puberty obesity after treatment for leukemia. Acta Paediatr 1995; 411:45–50.

862. Leiper AD, Stanhope R, Kitching P, et al. Precocious and premature puberty associated with treatment of acute lymphoblastic leukemia. Arch Dis Child 1987; 62:1107–1112.

863. Ogilvy-Stuart AL, Shalet SM. Growth and puberty after growth hormone treatment after irradiation for brain tumors. Arch Dis Child 1995; 73:141–146.

864. Oberfield SE, Soranno D, Nirenberg A, et al. Age at onset of puberty following high dose central nervous system radiation. Arch Pediatr Adolesc Med 1996; 150:589–592.

865. Quigley C, Cowell C, Jimenez M, et al. Normal or early development of puberty despite gonadal damage in children treated for acute lymphoblastic leukemia. N Engl J Med 1989; 321:143–151.

866. Constine LS, Woolf PD, Cann D, et al. Hypothalamic-pituitary dysfunction after radiation for brain tumors. N Engl Med 1993; 328:87–94.

867. Cara JF, Kreiter ML, Rosenfield RL. Height prognosis of children with true precocious puberty and growth hormone deficiency: effect of combination therapy with gonadotropin releasing hormone agonist and growth hormone. J Pediatr 1992; 120:709–715.

868. Sklar CA. Growth following therapy for childhood cancer. Cancer Invest 1995; 13:511–516.

869. Ogilvy-Stuart AL, Ryder WDJ, Gattamanemi HR, et al. Growth hormone and tumor recurrence. Br Med J 1992; 304:1601–1605.

870. Moshang T. Is brain tumor recurrence increased following growth hormone treatment? Trends Endocrinol Metab 1995; 6:205–209.

871. Sulmont V, Brauner R, Fontoura M, et al. Response to growth hormone treatment and final height after cranial or craniospinal irradiation. Acta Paediatr Scand 1990; 79:542–549.

872. Lannering B, Marky I, Mellander L, et al. Growth hormone secretion and response to growth hormone therapy after treatment for brain tumor. Acta Pediatr Scand 1988; 343:146–151.

873. Sklar C. Growth and endocrine disturbances after bone marrow transplantation in childhood. Acta Paediatr 1995; 411(Suppl):57–61.

874. Bushhouse S, Ramsay NKC, Pescovitz OH, et al. Growth in children following irradiation for bone marrow transplantation. Am J Pediatr Hematol Oncol 1989; 11:134–140.

875. Clement-De Boers A, Oostdijk W, Van Weel-Sipman MH, et al. Final height and hormonal function after bone marrow transplantation in children. J Pediatr 1996; 129:544–550.

876. Giri N, Davis EAC, Vowels MR. Long-term complications following BMT in children. J Pediatr Child Health 1993; 29:201–205.

877. Sanders JE. Endocrine problems in children after bone marrow transplant for hematologic malignancies. Bone Marrow Transplant 1991; 8(Suppl): 2–4.

878. Bozzola M, Giorgiani G, Locatelli F, et al. Growth in children after bone marrow transplantation. Horm Res 1993; 39:122–6.

879. Brauner R, Fontoura M, Zucker JM, et al. Growth and growth hormone secretion after bone marrow transplantation. Arch Dis Child 1993; 68:458–463.

880. Thomas BC, Stanhope R, Plowman PN, et al. Endocrine function following single fraction and fractionated total body irradiation for bone marrow transplantation in childhood. Acta Endocrinol 1993; 128:508–512.

881. Ogilvy-Stuart AL, Clark DJ, Wallace WHB, et al. Endocrine deficit after fractionated total body irradiation. Arch Dis Child 1992; 67:1107–1110.

882. Sklar CA, Kim TH, Ramsay NKC. Thyroid function among long-term survivors of bone marrow transplantation. Am J Med 1982; 73:688–694.

883. Cohen A, Rovelli A, Van-Lint MT, et al. Final height of patients who underwent bone marrow transplantation during childhood. Arch Dis Child 1996; 74:437–440.

884. Blizzard RM. Psychosocial short stature. In: Lifshitz F, ed. Pediatric Endocrinology. New York: Marcel Dekker, 1985: 87–107.

885. Powell GF, Brasel JA, Blizzard RM. Emotional deprivation and growth retardation simulating idiopathic hypopituitarism. I: Clinical evaluation of the syndrome. N Engl J Med 1967; 276:1271–1278.

886. Blizzard RM, Bulatovic A. Psychosocial short stature: a syndrome with many variables. Clin Endocrinol Metab 1992; 6:687–712.

887. Skuse D, Albanese A, Stanhope R, et al. A new stress-related syndrome of growth failure and hyperphagia in children, associated with reversibility of growth-hormone insufficiency. Lancet 1996; 348:353–358.

888. Stanhope R, Adlard P, Hamill G, et al. Physiological growth hormone (GH) secretion during the recovery from psychosocial dwarfism; a case report. Clin Endocrinol 1988; 28:335–339.

889. Albanese A, Hamill G, Jones J, et al. Reversibility of physiological growth

hormone secretion in children with psychosocial dwarfism. Clin Endocrinol 1994; 40:687–692.

890. Skuse D. Emotional abuse and delay in growth. Br Med J 1989; 299:113–115.

891. Miller JD, Tannenbaum GS, Colle E, et al. Daytime pulsatile growth hormone secretion in short prepubertal children. Clin Endocrinol 1982; 27:581–591.

892. Brambilla F, Perna G, Garberi A, et al. Alpha-2 adrenergic receptor sensitivity in panic disorder. I: GH response to GHRH and clonidine stimulation in panic disorder. Psychoneuroendocrinology 1995; 20:1–9.

893. Charney DS, Heninger GR, Sternberg DE, et al. Adrenergic receptor sensitivity in depression. Effects of clonidine in depressed patients and healthy subjects. Arch Gen Psychiatry 1982; 39:290–294.

894. Pine DS, Cohen P, Brook J. Emotional problems during youth as predictors of stature during early adulthood: results from a prospective epidemiologic study. Pediatrics 1996; 97:856–863.

895. Jensen JB, Garfinkel BD. Growth hormone dysregulation in children with major depressive disorder. J Am Acad Child Adolesc Psychiatry 1990; 29:295–301.

896. Spiliotis BE, August GP, Hung W, et al. Growth hormone neurosecretory dysfunction: a treatable cause of short stature. JAMA 1984; 252:2223–2230.

897. Bercu BB, Shulman D, Root AW, et al. Growth hormone (GH) provocative testing frequently does not reflect endogenous GH secretion. J Clin Endocrinol Metab 1986; 63:709–716.

898. Rose SR, Ross JL, Uriarte M, et al. The advantage of measuring stimulated as compared with spontaneous growth hormone levels in the diagnosis of growth hormone deficiency. N Engl J Med 1988; 319:201–207.

899. Lanes R. Diagnostic limitations of spontaneous growth hormone measurements in normally growing prepubertal children. Am J Dis Child 1989; 143:1284–1286.

900. Rose SR, Municchi G, Barnes K, et al. Overnight growth hormone concentrations are usually normal in pubertal children with idiopathic short stature—a clinical research center study. J Clin Endocrinol Metab 1996; 81:1063–1068.

901. Phillips JA, Cogan JD. Molecular basis of familial human growth hormone deficiency. J Clin Endocrinol Metab 1994; 76:11–16.

902. Parks JS, Kinoshita EI, Pfaffle RW. Pit-1 and hypopituitarism. Trends Endocrinol Metab 1993; 4:81–85.

903. Phillips JA III, Prince MA, Kostalova L, et al. Molecular analysis of growth hormone genes in GH deficient subjects. 10th International Congress of Endocrinology. San Francisco, 1996; P3-807 (abstract).

904. Woods KA, Weber A, Clark AJL. The molecular pathology of pituitary hormone deficiency and resistance. Baillieres Clin Endocrinol Metab 1995; 9:453–487.

905. Lin S, Lin CR, Gukovsky I, et al. Molecular basis of the little mouse phenotype and implications for cell type-specific growth. Nature 1993; 364:208–213.

906. Montminy M. The road not taken. Nature 1993; 364:190–191.

907. Wit JM, Drayer NM, Jansen M, et al. Total deficiency of growth hormone and prolactin and partial deficiency of thryoid stimulating hormone in two Dutch families: a new variant of hereditary pituitary deficiency. Horm Res 1989; 32:170–177.

908. Cogan JD, Phillips JA, Schenkman SS, et al. Familial growth hormone deficiency: a model of dominant and recessive mutations affecting a monomeric protein. J Clin Endocrinol Metab 1994; 79:1261–1265.

909. Cohen LE, Wondisford PE, Salvatoni A, et al. A "hot spot" in the Pit-1 gene responsible for combined pituitary hormone deficiency: clinical and molecular correlates. J Clin Endocrinol Metab 1995; 80:679–684.

910. Tatsumi KI, Miyai K, Notomi T, et al. Cretinism with combined hormone deficiency caused by a mutation in the Pit-1 gene. Nat Genet 1992; 1:56–58.

911. Pellegrini-Bouiller I, Belicar P, Barlier A, et al. A new mutation of the gene encoding the transcription factor Pit-1 is responsible for combined pituitary hormone deficiency. J Clin Endocrinol Metab 1996; 81:2790–2796.

912. Radovick S, Nations M, Du Y, et al. A mutation in the POU-homeodomain of pit-1 responsible for combined pituitary hormone deficiency. Science 1992; 257:1115–1118.

913. Pfaffle R, Kim C, Otten B, et al. Pit 1: clinical aspects. Horm Res 1996; 45(Suppl):25–28.

914. Pfaffle RW, DiMattia GE, Parks JS, et al. Mutation of the POU-specific domain of Pit-1 and hypopituitarism without pituitary hypoplasia. Science 1992; 257:1118–1121.

915. Buckwalter MS, Katz RW, Camper SA. Localization of the panhypopituitary dwarf mutation (df) on mouse chromosome 11 in an intersubspecific backcross. Genomics 1991; 10:515–526.

916. Wajnrajch MP, Gertner JM, Harbison MD, et al. Nonsense mutations of the human growth hormone releasing hormone receptor (GHRHR) causes growth failure analogous to that of the little (lit) mouse. Nat Genet 1996; 12:88–90.

917. Maheshwari H, Silverman BL, Dupois J, et al. Dwarfism of Sindh: a novel form of familial isolated GH deficiency linked to the locus for the GH releasing hormone receptor. 10th International Congress of Endocrinology. San Francisco, 1996; OR46-2 (abstract).

918. Godfrey P, Rahal JO, Beamer WG, et al. GHRH receptor of little mouse

contains missense mutation in the extracellular domain that disrupts receptor function. Nat Genet 1993; 4:227–232.

919. Mayo KE, Godfrey PA, Suhr ST, et al. Growth hormone–releasing hormone: synthesis and signaling. Recent Prog Horm Res 1995; 50:35–73.

920. Phillips JA, Hjell BL, Seeburg PH, et al. Molecular basis for familial isolated growth hormone deficiency. Proc Natl Acad Sci USA 1981; 78:6372.

921. Phillips JA. Genetic defects in processing growth hormone. In: Bercu BB, ed. Basic and Clinical Aspects of Growth Hormone. New York: Plenum, 1988: 57–67.

922. Illig R, Prader A, Ferrandez A, et al. Hereditary prenatal growth hormone deficiency with increased tendency to growth hormone antibody formation ("A-type" of isolated growth hormone deficiency). Acta Paediatr Scand 1971; 60:607.

923. Cao Y, Wagner JK, Hindmarsh PC, et al. Isolated growth hormone deficiency: testing the little mouse hypothesis in man and exclusion of mutations within the extracellular domain of the growth hormone releasing hormone receptor. Pediatr Res 1995; 38:962–966.

924. Jenkins JS, Gilberg CJ, Ang V. Hypothalamic-pituitary function in patients with craniopharyngiomas. J Clin Endocrinol Metab 1976; 43:394–399.

925. Thomsett MJ, Conte FA, Kaplan SL, et al. Endocrine and neurologic outcome in childhood craniopharyngioma. Review of effect of treatment in 42 patients. J Pediatr 1980; 97:728–735.

926. Laws ER, Thapar K. The diagnosis and management of craniopharyngioma. Growth Genetics Hormones 1994; 10:6–10.

927. Paja M, Lucas T, Garcia-Uria J, et al. Hypothalamic-pituitary dysfunction in patients with craniopharyngioma. Clin Endocrinol 1995; 42:467–473.

928. Rivarola M, Mendilaharzu H, Warman M, et al. Endocrine disorders in 66 suprasellar and pineal tumors of patients with prepubertal and pubertal ages. Horm Res 1992; 37:1–6.

929. Kane LA, Leinung MC, Scheithauer BW, et al. Pituitary adenomas in childhood and adolescence. J Clin Endocrinol Metab 1994; 79:1135–1140.

930. Frailioli B, Ferrante L, Celli P. Pituitary adenomas with onset during puberty: features and treatment. J Neurosurg 1983; 59:590–595.

931. Maira G, Anile C. Pituitary tumors in childhood and adolescence. Can J Neurol Sci 1990; 65:733–744.

932. Devile CJ, Grant DB, Hayward RD, et al. Growth and endocrine sequelae of craniopharyngioma. Arch Dis Child 1996; 75:108–114.

933. Geffner ME. The growth without growth hormone syndrome. Endocrinol Metab Clin North Am 1996; 25:649–663.

934. Richmond IL, Wilson CB. Pituitary adenomas in childhood and adolescence. J Neurosurg 1978; 49:163–168.

935. Egeler RM, D'Angio GJ. Langerhans' cell histiocytosis. J Pediatr 1996; 127:1–11.

936. Braunstein GD, Kohler PO. Pituitary function in Hand-Schüller-Christian disease. Evidence for deficient growth hormone release in patients with short stature. N Engl J Med 1972; 286:1225–1229.

937. Broadbent V, Dunger DN, Yeomans E, et al. Anterior pituitary function and computed tomography/magnetic resonance imaging in patients with Langerhans cell histiocytosis and diabetes insipidus. Med Pediatr Oncol 1993; 21:649–654.

938. Dean HJ, Bishop A, Winter JSD. Growth hormone deficiency in patients with histiocytosis X. J Pediatr 1996; 109:615–618.

939. Valenta LJ, Sigel MB, Lesniak MA, et al. Pituitary dwarfism in a patient with circulating abnormal growth hormone polymers. N Engl J Med 1985; 312:214–217.

940. Kowarski AA, Schneider J, Ben-Galim E, et al. Growth failure with normal serum RIA-GH and low somatomedin activity: somatomedin restoration and growth acceleration after exogenous GH. J Clin Endocrinol Metab 1978; 47:461–464.

941. Takahashi Y, Kaji H, Okimura Y, et al. Short stature caused by a mutant growth hormone. N Engl J Med 1996; 334:432–436.

942. Laron Z, Blum W, Chatelain P, et al. Classification of growth hormone insensitivity syndrome. J Pediatr 1993; 122:241.

943. Laron Z, Pertzelan A, Mannheimer S. Genetic pituitary dwarfism with high serum concentration of growth hormone—a new inborn error of metabolism? Isr J Med Sci 1966; 2:152–155.

944. Rosenbloom AL, Guevara-Aguirre J, Rosenfeld RG, et al. The little women of Loja: growth hormone receptor deficiency in an inbred population of southern Ecuador. N Engl J Med 1990; 323:1367–1374.

945. Golde DW, Bersch N, Kaplan SA, et al. Peripheral unresponsiveness to human growth hormone in Laron dwarfism. N Engl J Med 1980; 303:1156–1159.

946. Eshet R, Laron Z, Pertzelan A, et al. Defect of human growth hormone receptors in the liver of two patients with Laron-type dwarfism. Isr J Med Sci 1984; 20:8–11.

947. Godowski PJ, Leung DW, Meacham LR, et al. Characterization of the human growth hormone receptor gene and demonstration of a partial gene deletion in two patients with Laron-type dwarfism. Proc Natl Acad Sci USA 1989; 86:8083–8087.

948. Amselem S, Duquesnoy P, Attree O, et al. Laron dwarfism and mutations of the growth hormone–receptor gene. N Engl J Med 1989; 321:989–995.

949. Berg MA, Guevara-Aguirre J, Rosenbloom AL, et al. Mutuation creating a new splice site in the growth hormone receptor genes of 37 Ecuadorean patients with Laron syndrome. Hum Mutat 1992; 1:24–34.

950. Douquesnoy P, Sobrier ML, Duriez B. A single amino acid substitution in the exoplasmic domain of the human growth hormone (GH) receptor confers familial GH resistance (Laron syndrome) with positive GH-binding activity by abolishing receptor homodimerization. EMBO J 1994; 13:1386–1395.

951. Kou K, Lajara R, Rotwein P. Amino acid substitutions in the intracellular part of the growth hormone receptor in a patient with Laron syndrome. J Clin Endocrinol Metab 1993; 76:54–59.

952. Chujo S, Kaji H, Takahashi Y, et al. No correlation of growth hormone receptor gene mutation P561t with body height. Eur J Endocrinol 1996; 134:560–562.

953. Goddard AM, Dowd P, Covello R, et al. Association of mutations in the intracellular domain of the growth hormone receptor with IGF1 deficiency and growth failure. 10th International Congress of Endocrinology. San Francisco, 1996; P3-69 (abstract).

954. Woods KA, Fraser NC, Postel-Vinay MC, et al. A homozygous splice site mutation affecting the intracellular domain of the growth hormone (GH) receptor resulting in Laron syndrome with elevated GH-binding protein. J Clin Endocrinol Metab 1996; 81:1686–1690.

955. Attie KM. Mutations of the growth hormone receptor—widening the search. J Clin Endocrinol Metab 1996; 81:1683–1685 (editorial).

956. Rosenfeld RG, Albertsson-Wikland K, Cassorla F, et al. The diagnosis of childhood growth hormone deficiency revisited. J Clin Endocrinol Metab 1995; 80:1532–1540.

957. Frasier SD. A review of growth hormone stimulation tests in children. Pediatrics 1974; 53:929–937.

958. Underwood LE, Azumi K, Voina SJ, et al. Growth hormone levels during sleep in normal and growth hormone deficient children. Pediatrics 1971; 48:946–954.

959. Buckler JMH. Plasma growth hormone response to exercise as a diagnostic aid. Arch Dis Child 1973; 48:565–567.

960. Lacey KA, Hewison A, Parkin JM. Exercise as a screening test for growth hormone deficiency in children. Arch Dis Child 1973; 48:508–512.

961. Coller R, Leboeuf G, Letarte J. Stimulation of growth hormone secretion by levodopa propranolol in children and adolescents. Pediatrics 1975; 56:262–266.

962. Lanes R, Hurtado E. Oral clonidine—an effective growth hormone–releasing agent in prepubertal subjects. J Pediatr 1982; 100:710–714.

963. Mitchell ML, Bryne MJ, Sanchez Y, et al. Detection of growth hormone deficiency. The glucagon stimulation test. N Engl J Med 1970; 282:539–541.

964. Merimee TJ, Rabinowitz D, Fineberg SE. Arginine-initiated release of human growth hormone. N Engl J Med 1969; 280:1434–1438.

965. Kaplan SL, Abrams CAL, Bell JJ. Growth and growth hormone. I: Changes in serum levels of growth hormone following hypoglycemia in 134 children with growth retardation. Pediatr Res 1968; 2:43–63.

966. Root AW, Rosenfield RL, Bongiovanni AM, et al. The plasma growth hormone response to insulin-induced hypoglycemia in children with retardation of growth. Pediatrics 1967; 39:844–852.

967. Penny R, Blizzard RM, Davis WT. Sequential arginine and insulin tolerance tests on the same day. J Clin Endocrinol Metab 1969; 29:1499–1501.

968. Fass B, Lippe BM, Kaplan SA. Relative usefulness of three growth hormone stimulation screening tests. Am J Dis Child 1979; 133:931–933.

969. Weldon VV, Gupta SK, Klingensmith G. Evaluation of growth hormone release in children using arginine and L-dopa in combination. J Pediatr 1975; 87:540–544.

970. Reiter EO, Martha PM Jr. Pharmacological testing of growth hormone secretion. Horm Res 1990; 33:121–127.

971. Raiti S, Davis WT, Blizzard RM. A comparison of the effects of insulin hypoglycemia and arginine infusion on release of human growth hormone. Lancet 1967; 2:1182–1183.

972. Physicians' Desk Reference. Montvale, NJ: Medical Economics Data Production, 1994: 1004.

973. Physicians' Desk Reference. Montvale, NJ: Medical Economics Data Production, 1994: 1228.

974. Finkelstein JW, Roffwarg HP, Boyar RM, et al. Age-related change in twenty-four-hour spontaneous secretion of growth hormone. J Clin Endocrinol Metab 1972; 35:665–670.

975. Rosenfeld RG. Evaluation of growth and maturation in adolescence. Pediatr Rev 1982; 4:175–183.

976. Lippe B, Wong S, Kaplan SA. Simultaneous assessment of growth hormone and ACTH reserve in children pretreated with diethylstilbesterol. J Clin Endocrinol 1971; 33:949–956.

977. Chernausek SD. Laboratory diagnosis of growth disorders. In: Hintz RL, Rosenfeld RG, eds. Growth Abnormalities. Contemporary Issues in Endocrinology and Metabolism. New York: Churchill Livingstone, 1987: 231–254.

978. Gourmelen M, Pham-Huu-Trung MT, Girard F. Transient partial GH deficiency in prepubertal children with delay of growth. Pediatr Res 1979; 13:221–224.

979. Cacciari E, Tassoni P, Parisi G, et al. Pitfalls in diagnosing impaired growth hormone (GH) secretion: retesting after replacement therapy of 63 children defined as GH deficient. J Clin Endocrinol Metab 1992; 74:1284–1289.

980. Marin G, Domene HM, Barnes KM, et al. The effects of estrogen priming and puberty on the growth hormone response to standardized treadmill exercise and arginine-insulin in normal girls and boys. J Clin Endocrinol Metab 1994; 79:537–541.

981. Blethen SL, Chaslow FI. Use of a two-site radioimmunometric assay for growth hormone (GH). J Endocrinol Metab 1983; 57:1031–1035.

982. Reiter EO, Morris AH, MacGillivray MH, et al. Variable estimates of serum growth hormone concentrations by difference radioassay systems. J Clin Endocrinol Metab 1988; 66:68–71.

983. Celniker AC, Chem AB, Wert RM Jr, et al. Variability in the quantitation of circulating growth hormone using commercial immunoassays. J Clin Endocrinol Metab 1989; 68:469–476.

984. Wyatt DT, Mark D, Slyper A. Survey of growth hormone treatment practices by 251 pediatric endocrinologists. J Clin Endocrinol Metab 1995; 80:3292–3297.

985. Shah A, Stanhope R, Matthews D. Hazards of pharmacological tests of growth hormone secretion in childhood. Br Med J 1992; 304:173–174.

986. Eddy RL, Gilliland PF, Ibarra JD Jr, et al. Human growth hormone release. Comparison of provocative test procedures. Am J Med 1974; 56:179–185.

987. Zadik Z, Chalew SA, Raiti S, et al. Do short children secrete insuffcent growth hormone? Pediatrics 1985; 76:355–360.

988. Thompson RG, Rodriguez A, Kowarski AA, et al. Growth hormone: metabolic clearance rates, integrated concentrations and production rates in normal adults and the effects of prednisone. J Clin Invest 1972; 51:3193–3199.

989. Zadik Z, Chalew SA, McCarter RJ, et al. The influence of age on the 24-hour integrated concentrations of growth hormone in normal individuals. J Clin Endocrinol Metab 1985; 60:153.

990. Zadik Z, Chalew SA, Gilula Z, et al. Reproducibility of growth hormone testing procedures: a comparison between 24-hour integrated concentration and pharmacological stimulation. J Clin Endocrinol Metab 1990; 71:1127–1130.

991. Tassoni P, Cacciari E, Cau M, et al. Variability of growth hormone response to pharmacological and sleep tests performed twice in short children. J Clin Endocrinol Metab 1990; 71:230–234.

992. Donaldson DL, Hollowell JG, Pan F, et al. Growth hormone secretory profiles: variation on consecutive nights. J Pediatr 1989; 115:51–56.

993. Hourd P, Edwards R. Current methods for the measurement of growth hormone in urine. Clin Endocrinol 1994; 40:155–170.

994. Albini CH, Quattrin T, Vandlen RL, et al. Quantitation of urinary growth hormone in children with normal and subnormal growth. Pediatr Res 1988; 23:89–92.

995. Granada ML, Sanmarti A, Lucas A, et al. Clinical usefulness of urinary growth hormone measurements in normal and short growth hormone data. Pediatr Res 1992; 32:73–76.

996. Girard J, Celniker A, Price A, et al. Urinary measurement of growth hormone secretion. Acta Paediatr Scand 1990; 366(Suppl):149–154.

997. Phillip M, Chalew SA, Stene MA, et al. The value of urinary growth hormone determination for assessment of growth hormone deficiency and compliance with growth hormone therapy. Am J Dis Child 1993; 147:553–557.

998. Skinner AM, Clayton PE, Price DA, et al. Urinary growth hormone excretion in the assessment of children with disorders of growth. Clin Endocrinol 1993; 39:201–206.

999. Savage MO, Blu WF, Ranke MB, et al. Clinical features and endocrine status in patients with growth hormone insensitivity (Laron syndrome). J Clin Endocrinol Metab 1993; 77:1465–1471.

1000. Smith WJ, Nam TJ, Underwood LE, et al. Use of insulin-like growth factor binding protein-2 (IGFBP-2), IGFBP-3, and IGF1 for assessing growth hormone status in short children. J Clin Endocrinol Metab 1993; 77:1294–1299.

1001. Guevara-Aguirre J, Rosenbloom AL, Fielder PJ, et al. Growth hormone receptor deficiency in Ecuador: clinical and biochemical phenotype in two populations. J Clin Endocrinol Metab 1993; 76:417–423.

1002. Thalange NKS, Price DA, Gill MS, et al. Insulin-like growth factor binding protein-3 generation: an index of growth hormone insensitivity. Pediatr Res 1996; 39:849–855.

1003. Blum WF, Cotterill AM, Postel-Vinay MC, et al. Improvement in the diagnostic criteria in growth hormone insensitivity syndrome: solutions and pitfalls. Acta Paediatr Scand 1994; 399(Suppl):117–124.

1004. Blum WF, Ranke MB, Savage MO. Insulin-like growth factors and their binding proteins in patients with growth hormone receptor deficiency: suggestions for new diagnostic criteria. Acta Paediatr Scand 1992; 383(Suppl):125–126.

1005. Rosenfeld RG, Kemp SF, Hintz RL. Constancy of somatomedin response to growth hormone treatment of hypopituitary dwarfism and lack of correlation with growth rate. J Clin Endocrinol Metab 1981; 53:611–617.

1006. Albertsson-Wikland K, Hall K. Growth hormone treatment in short children: relationship between growth and serum insulin-like growth factor I and II levels. J Clin Endocrinol Metab 1987; 65:671–678.

1007. Bierich JR. Constitutional delay of growth and adolescent development. Eur J Pediatr 1982; 139:221–224.

1008. Clayton PE, Shalet SM, Price DA. Endocrine manipulation of constitutional delay in growth and puberty. J Endocrinol 1988; 116:321–323.

1009. Styne DM. 1987; Delayed puberty. In: Hintz RL, Rosenfeld RG, eds. Growth Abnormalities. New York: Churchill Livingstone, 141–161.

1010. Burstein S, Rosenfield RL. Constitutional delay in growth and development. In: Hintz RL, Rosenfeld RG, eds. Growth Abnormalities. New York: Churchill Livingstone, 1987: 167–186.

1011. Horner JM, Thorsson AV, Hintz RL. Growth deceleration pattern in children with constitutional short stature: an aid to diagnosis. Pediatrics 1978; 62:529–534.

1012. Crowne EC, Shalet SM, Wallace WHB, et al. Final height in boys with untreated constitutional delay in growth and puberty. Arch Dis Child 1990; 65:1109–1112.

1013. LaFranchi S, Hanna CE, Mandel SH. Constitutional delay of growth: expected versus final adult height. Pediatrics 1991; 87:82–87.

1014. Ranke MB, Grauer ML, Kistner K, et al. Spontaneous adult height in idiopathic short stature. Horm Res 1995; 44:152–157.

1015. Blethen SL, Gaines S, Weldon V. Comparison of predicted and adult heights in short boys: effect of androgen therapy. Pediatr Res 1984; 18:467–469.

1016. Albanese A, Stanhope R. Predictive factors in the determination of final height in boys with constitutional delay of growth and puberty. J Pediatr 1995; 126:545–550.

1017. Volta C, Ghizzoni L, Buono T, et al. Final height in a group of untreated children with constitutional growth delay. Helv Paediat Acta 1988; 43:171–176.

1018. Finkelstein JS, Neer RM, Biller BMK, et al. Osteopenia in men with a history of delayed puberty. N Engl J Med 1992; 326:600–604.

1019. Eastman CJ, Lazarus L, Stuart MC, et al. The effect of puberty on growth hormone secretion in boys with short stature and delayed adolescence. Aust NZ J Med 1971; 1:154–159.

1020. Deller JJ Jr, Boulis MW, Harriss WE, et al. Growth hormone response patterns to sex hormone administration in growth retardation. Am J Med Sci 1970; 259:292–297.

1021. Davila N, Moreira-Andres M, Alcanez J, et al. Serum growth hormone–binding protein is decreased in prepubertal children with idiopathic short stature. J Endocrinol Invest 1996; 19:348–352.

1022. Rosenfeld RG, Northcraft GB, Hintz RL. A prospective, randomized trial of testosterone treatment of constitutional short stature in adolescent males. Pediatrics 1982; 69:681–687.

1023. Blizzard RM, Hindmarsh PC, Stanhope R. Oxandrolone therapy: 25 years experience. Growth Genetics Hormones 1991; 7:1–6.

1024. Buyukgebiz A, Hindmarsh C, Brook CDG. Treatment of constitutional delay of growth and puberty with oxandrolone compared with growth hormone. Arch Dis Child 1990; 65:448–449.

1025. Clayton PE, Shalet SM, Price DA, et al. Growth and growth hormone responses to exandrolone in boys with constitutional delay of growth and puberty (CDGP). Clin Endocrinol 1988; 23:123–130.

1026. Joss EE, Schmidt JA, Zuppinger KA. Oxandrolone in constitutionally delayed growth, a longitudinal study up to final height. J Clin Endocrinol Metab 1989; 69:1109–1115.

1027. Marti-Henneberg C, Niirianen A, Rappaport MD. Oxandrolone treatment of constitutional short stature in boys during adolescence: effect on linear growth, bone age, pubic hair and testicular development. J Pediatr 1975; 86:783–788.

1028. Stanhope R, Buchanan CR, Fenn GC, et al. Double-blinded placebo controlled trial of low dose oxandrolone in the treatment of boys with constitutional delay of growth and puberty. Arch Dis Child 1988; 63:501–505.

1029. Wilson DM, McCauley E, Brown DR, et al. Oxandrolone treatment in constitutionally delayed growth and puberty. Pediatrics 1995; 96:1095–1100.

1030. Tse WY, Buyukgebiz A, Hindmarsh PC, et al. Long-term outcome of oxandrolone treatment in boys with constitutional delay of growth and puberty. J Pediatr 1990; 117:588–591.

1031. Papadimitriou S, Wacharasindhu S, Preece MA, et al. Treatment of constitutional growth delay in prepubertal boys with a prolonged course of low dose oxandrolone. Arch Dis Child 1991; 66:841–843.

1032. Hochberg Z, Korman S. Oxandrolone therapy for short stature. J Pediatr Endocrinol (Isr) 1987; 2:115–120.

1033. Link K, Blizzard RM, Evans WS, et al. The effect of androgens on growth hormone response in children with constitutional growth delay. J Clin Endocrinol Metab 1986; 52:159–164.

1034. Malhotra A, Poon E, Tse WY, et al. The effects of oxandrolone on the growth hormone and gonadal axes in boys with constitutional delay of growth and puberty. Clin Endocrinol 1993; 38:393–398.

1035. Kulin HE, Reiter EO. Managing the patient with delay in puberty development. Endocrinologist 1992; 2:231–239.

1036. Richman RA, Kirsch LR. Testosterone treatment in adolescent boys with constitutional delay in growth and development. N Engl J Med 1988; 319:1563–1567.

1037. Crowne EC, Wallace WH, Moore C, et al. Degree of activation of the pituitary-testicular axis in early pubertal boys with constitutional delay of growth and puberty determines the growth response to treatment with testosterone or oxandrolone. J Clin Endocrinol Metab 1995; 80:1869–1875.

1038. Wilson DM, Kei J, Hintz RL, et al. Effects of testosterone enanthate therapy for pubertal delay. Am J Dis Child 1988; 142:96–99.

1039. Kaplan SL, Underwood LE, August GP, et al. Clinical studies with recombinant-DNA-derived methionyl human growth hormone in growth hormone deficient children. Lancet 1986; 1:697–700.

1040. Underwood LE, Moore WV. Antibodies to growth hormone: measurement and meaning. Growth Genetics Hormones 1987; 3:1–3.

1041. MacGillivray MH, Blizzard RM. Rationale for dosing recombinant human growth hormone by weight rather than units. Growth Genetics Hormones 1994; 10:7–9.

1042. Marx W, Simpson ME, Evans HM. Bioassay of growth hormone of anterior pituitary. Endocrinology 1942; 30:1–10.

1043. Wilhelmi AE. Measurement: Bioassay. In: Berson SA, Yalow RS, eds. Peptide Hormones: Methods in Investigative and Diagnostic Endocrinology. New York: North-Holland, 1973: 296–302.

1044. Bennett LL. Failure of hypophyseal growth hormone to produce nitrogen storage in a girl with hypophyseal dwarfism. J Clin Endocrinol 1950; 10:492–495.

1045. Shelton EK, Cavanaugh RA, Evans HM. Hypophyseal infantilism; treatment with anterior hypophyseal extract; final report. Am J Dis Child 1936; 52:100–113.

1046. Shelton EK, Cavanaugh RA, Long ML. Studies on effects of human blood serum on growth of rat. Endocrinology 1936; 19:543–548.

1047. Wilhelmi AE. Comparative biochemistry of growth hormone from ox, sheep, pig, horse and fish pituitaries. In: Smith RW Jr, Gaebler OH, Long CNH, eds. The Hypophyseal Growth Hormone: Nature and Actions. New York: McGraw-Hill, 1955: 59–69.

1048. Knobil E, Greep RO. Physiological effects of growth hormone of primate origin in the hypophysectomized monkey. Fed Proc 1956; 15:111–112.

1049. Knobil E, Wolf RC, Greep RO. Some physiologic effects of primate pituitary growth-hormone preparations in the hypophysectomzed rhesus monkey. J Clin Endocrinol 1956; 16:916.

1050. Frasier SD. Human pituitary growth hormone (hGH) therapy in growth hormone deficiency. Endocr Rev 1983; 4:155–170.

1051. Frasier SD, Costin G, Lippe BM, et al. A dose-response curve for human growth hormone. J Clin Endocrinol Metab 1981; 53:1213–1217.

1052. Fradkin JE. Creutzfeldt-Jakob disease in pituitary growth hormone recipients. Endocrinologist 1993; 3:108–114.

1053. Buchanan CR, Preece MA, Milner RDG. Mortality, neoplasia, and Creutzfeldt-Jakob disease in patients treated with human pituitary growth hormone in the United States. Br Med J 1991; 302:824–828.

1054. Tintner R, Brown P, Hedley-Whyte ET, et al. Neuropathologic verification of Creutzfeldt-Jakob disease in the exhumed American recipient of human growth hormone: epidemiologic and pathogenetic implications. Neurology 1986; 36:932–936.

1055. Hintz RL. The prismatic case of Creutzfeldt-Jakob disease associated with pituitary growth hormone treatment. J Clin Endocrinol Metab 1995; 80:2298–2301.

1056. Rosenfeld RG, Aggarwal BB, Hintz RL, et al. Recombinant DNA–derived methionyl growth hormone is similar in membrane binding properties to human pituitary growth hormone. Biochem Biophys Res Commun 1982; 106:202–209.

1057. Hintz RL, Rosenfeld RG, Wilson DM, et al. Biosynthetic methionyl–human growth hormone is biologically active in adult humans. Lancet 1982; 1:1276–1279.

1058. MacGillivray MH, Baptista J, Johanson A, et al. Outcome of a four year randomized study of daily versus three times weekly somatropin treatment in prepubertal naive growth hormone deficient children. J Clin Endocrinol Metab 1996; 81:1806–1809.

1059. Wilson DM, Baker B, Hintz RL, et al. Subcutaneous versus intramuscular growth hormone therapy: growth and acute somatomedin response. Pediatrics 1985; 76:361–364.

1060. Johnson OL, Cleeand JL, Lee HJ, et al. A month-long effect from a single injection of microencapsulated human growth hormone. Nat Med 1996; 2:795–799.

1061. Ranke MB. Growth hormone therapy in children: when to stop? Horm Res 1995; 43:122–125.

1062. Inzucchi SE, Robbins RJ. Effects of growth hormone on human bone biology. J Clin Endocrinol Metab 1994; 79:691–694.

1063. De Boer H, Blok GJ, Van Lingen A, et al. Consequences of childhood-onset growth hormone deficiency for adult bone mass. J Bone Miner Res 1994; 9:1319–1326.

1064. Drug and Therapeutics Committee of the Lawson Wilkins Pediatric Endocrine Society. Guidelines for the use of growth hormone in children with short stature. J Pediatr 1995; 127:857–867.

1065. Price DA, Ranke MB. Final height following growth hormone treatment. In: Ranke B, Gunnarsson R, eds. Progress in Growth Hormone Therapy—5 Years of KIGSM. Mannheim: J&J Verlag, 1994: 129–144.

1066. Bundak R, Hindmarsh PC, Brook CGD. Long-term auxologic effects of human growth hormone. J Pediatr 1988; 127:875–879.

1067. Libber SM, Plotnick LP, Johanson AJ, et al. Long-term follow-up of hypopituitary patients treated with human growth hormone. Medicine 1990; 69:46–55.

1068. Bierich JR. Final height in hypopituitary patients after treatment with HGH. In: Bierch JR, Cacciari E, Raiti S, eds. Growth Abnormalities. New York: Raven, 1989: 161–174.

1069. Bramswig JH, Schlosser H, Kiese K. Final height in children with growth hormone deficiency. Horm Res 1995; 43:126–128.

1070. Blethen SL, Foley T, LaFranchi S, et al. Adult height (AH) in growth hormone (GH) deficient (GHD) children treated with recombinant GH (rhGH). Pediatr Res 1995; 27:85A.

1071. Chipman JJ, Hicks JR, Holcombe JH, et al. Approaching final height in children treated for growth hormone deficiency. Horm Res 1995; 43:129–131.

1072. Frisch H, Birnbacher R. Final height and pubertal development in children with growth hormone deficiency after long-term treatment. Horm Res 1995; 43:132–134.

1073. Severi F. Final height in children with growth hormone deficiency. Horm Res 1995; 43:138–140.

1074. Josefsberg Z, Bauman B, Pertzelan A, et al. Greater efficiency of human growth hormone therapy in children below five years of age with growth hormone deficiency: a 5-year follow-up study. Horm Res 1987; 27:126–133.

1075. Blethen SL, Compton P, Lippe BM, et al. Factors predicting the response to growth hormone (GH) therapy in prepubertal children with GH deficiency. J Clin Endocrinol Metab 1993; 74:574–579.

1076. Arrigo T, DeLuca F, Bernasconi S, et al. Catch-up growth and height prognosis in early treated children with congenital hypopituitarism. Horm Res 1996; 44(Suppl):26–31.

1077. Burns EC, Tanner JM, Preece MA, et al. Final height and pubertal development in 55 children with idiopathic growth hormone deficiency, treated for between 2 and 15 years with human growth hormone. Eur J Pediatr 1981; 137:155–164.

1078. Bourguignon JP, Vandeweghe M, Vanderschuren-Lodeweyckx M, et al. Pubertal growth and final height in hypopituitary boys: a minor role of bone age at onset of puberty. J Clin Endocrinol Metab 1986; 63:376–382.

1079. Saggese G, Cesaretti G, Andreani G, et al. Combined treatment with growth hormone and gonadotropin-releasing hormone analogues in children with isolated growth hormone deficiency. Acta Endocrinol 1992; 127:307–312.

1080. Toublanc JE, Couptrie C, Garnier P, et al. The effects of treatment combining an agonist of gonadotropin-releasing hormone with growth hormone in pubertal patients with isolated growth hormone deficiency. Acta Endocrinol 1989; 120:795–799.

1081. Balducci R, Toscano V, Mangiantini A, et al. Adult height in short normal adolescent girls treated with gonadotropin-releasing hormone analog and growth hormone. J Clin Endocrinol Metab 1995; 80:3596–3600.

1082. Saggese G, Pasquino AM, Bertelloni S, et al. Effect of combined treatment with gonadotropin releasing hormone analogue and growth hormone in patients with central precocious puberty who had subnormal growth velocity and impaired height prognosis. Acta Paediatr 1995; 84:299–304.

1083. Pasquino AM, Municchi G, Pucarelli I, et al. Combined treatment with gonadotropin-releasing hormone analog and growth hormone in central precocious puberty. J Clin Endocrinol Metab 1996; 81:948–951.

1084. Job JC, Toublanc JE, Landier F. Growth of short normal children in puberty treated for three years with growth hormone alone or in association with gonadotropin-releasing hormone agonist. Horm Res 1994; 41:177–184.

1085. Wit JM, Kamp G, Rikken B. Spontaneous growth and response to growth hormone treatment in children with growth hormone deficiency and idiopathic short stature. Pediatr Res 1996; 39:295–302.

1086. Hibi I, Tanaka T, Tanae A, et al. The influence of gonadal function and the effect of gonadal suppression treatment on final height in growth hormone (GH)-treated GH-deficient children. J Clin Endocrinol Metab 1989; 69:221–226.

1087. Lippe BM, Van Herle AJ, Lafranchi SH, et al. Reversible hypothyroidism in growth-hormone deficient children treated with human growth hormone. J Clin Endocrinol Metab 1975; 40:612–618.

1088. Guthrie RD, Smith SW, Graham CB. Testosterone treatment for micropenis during early childhood. J Pediatr 1973; 83:247–252.

1089. Retegui LA, Masson PL, Paladini AC. Specificities of antibodies to human growth hormone (hGH) in patients treated with hGH: longitudinal study and comparison with the specificities of animal antisera. J Clin Endocrinol Metab 1985; 60:184–190.

1090. Pirazzoli P, Cacciari E, Mandini M, et al. Follow-up of antibodies to growth hormone in 210 growth hormone–deficient children treated with different commercial preparations. Acta Paediatr 1995; 84:1223–1226.

1091. Dean HJ, McTaggart TL, Fish DG, et al. The educational vocational, and marital status of growth hormone–deficient adults treated with growth hormone during childhood. Am J Dis Child 1985; 139:1105–1110.

1092. Salomon F, Cuneo RC, Hesp R, et al. The effects of treatment with recombinant human growth hormone on body composition and metabolism in adults with growth hormone deficiency. N Engl J Med 1989; 321:1797–1803.

1093. Bengtsson B, Eden S, Lonn L, et al. Treatment of adults with growth hormone deficiency with recombinant human growth hormone. J Clin Endocrinol Metab 1993; 76:309–317.

1094. Rosen T, Bengtsson B. Premature mortality due to cardiovascular disease in hypopituitarism. Lancet 1990; 336:285–288.

1095. McGauley GA, Cuneo RC, Salomon F, et al. Psychological well-being before and after growth hormone treatment in adults with growth hormone deficiency. Horm Res 1990; 33(Suppl):52–54.

1096. Shalet SM, Rahim A, Toogood AA. Growth hormone therapy for adult growth hormone deficiency. Trends Endocrinol Metab 1996; 7:287–290.

1097. Rosen T, Wiren L, Wilhelmsen L, et al. Decreased psychological well-being in adult patients with growth hormone deficiency. Clin Endocrinol (Oxf) 1994; 40:111–116.

1098. Sonksen PH, Cuneo RC, Salomon F, et al. Growth hormone therapy in adults with growth hormone deficiency. Acta Paediatr Scand 1991; 379(Suppl):139–146.

1099. Mardh G, Lundin K, Borg B, et al. Growth hormone replacement therapy in adult hypopituitary patients with growth hormone deficiency: combined data from 12 European placebo-controlled clinical trials. Endocrinol Metab 1994; 1(Suppl):43–49.

1100. Werther GA. Growth hormone measurements versus auxology in treatment decisions: the Australian experience. J Pediatr 1996; 128:S47–S51.

1101. Tonshoff B, Mehls O, Heinrich U, et al. Growth-stimulating effects of recombinant human growth hormone in children with end-stage renal disease. J Pediatr 1990; 116:561–566.

1102. Fine RN, Attie KM, Kuntze J, et al. The use of recombinant human growth hormone (rhGH) in infants and children with chronic renal insufficiency. Pediatr Res 1994; 35:364A.

1103. Hokken-Koelega ACS, Stijnen T, de John MCJW, et al. Double blind trial comparing the effects of two doses of growth hormone in prepubertal patients with chronic renal insufficiency. J Clin Endocrinol Metab 1994; 79:1185–1190.

1104. Mehls O, Broyer M, European/Australian Study Group. Growth response to recombinant human growth hormone in short prepubertal children with chronic renal failure with or without dialysis. Acta Paediatr 1994; 399(Suppl):1–7.

1105. Fine RN, Kohaut E, Brown D, et al. Long-term treatment of growth retarded children with chronic renal insufficiency with recombinant human growth hormone. Kidney Int 1996; 49:781–785.

1106. Fine RN, Kohaut EC, Brown D, et al. Growth after recombinant human growth hormone treatment in children with chronic renal failure: report of a multicenter randomized double-blind placebo-controlled study. J Pediatr 1994; 124:374–382.

1107. Watkins SL. Bone disease in patients receiving growth hormone. Kidney Int 1996; 49(Suppl):S126–S127.

1108. Fine RN. Allograft rejection in growth hormone and non–growth hormone treated children. J Pediatr Endocrinol 1994; 7:127–133.

1109. Chavers BM, Doherty L, Nevins TE, et al. Effects of growth hormone on kidney function in pediatric transplant recipients. Pediatr Nephrol 1995; 9:176–181.

1110. Benfield MR, Parker KL, Waldo FB, et al. Growth hormone in the treatment of growth failure in children after renal transplantation. Kidney Int 1993; 44(Suppl):S62–S64.

1111. Laine J, Krogerus L, Sarna S, et al. Recombinant human growth hormone treatment; its effect on renal allograft function and histology. Transplantation 1996; 61:898–903.

1112. Crock P, Werther GA, Wettenhall HN. Oxandrolone increases final height in Turner syndrome. J Pediatr Child Health 1990; 26:221–224.

1113. Joss E, Zuppinger K. Oxandrolone in girls with Turner's syndrome: a pair-matched controlled study up to final height. Acta Paediatr Scand 1984; 73:674–679.

1114. Lenko HL, Soderholm A, Perheentupa J. Turner syndrome: effect of hormone therapies on height velocity and adult height. Acta Paediatr Scand 1988; 77:699–704.

1115. Lev-Ran A. Androgens, estrogens, and the ultimate height in XO gonadal dysgenesis. Am J Dis Child 1977; 131:648–649.

1116. Moore DC, Tattoni DS, Ruvalcaba RHA, et al. Studies of anabolic steroids. J Pediatr 1977; 90:462–466.

1117. Muritano MR, Job JC. Effects of weakly androgenic anabolic steroids on growth in Turner's syndrome. Arch Fr Pediatr 1985; 42:265–271.

1118. Naeraa RW, Nielsen J, Pediatrersen IL, et al. Effect of oxandrolone on growth and final height in Turner's syndrome. Acta Paediatr Scand 1990; 9:784–749.

1119. Stanke N, Lingstaedt K, Willig RP. Oxandrolone increased final height in Turner's syndrome. Pediatr Res 1985; 19:620.

1120. Sybert VP. Adult height in Turner syndrome with and without androgen therapy. J Pediatr 1984; 104:365–369.

1121. Urban MD, Lee PA, Dorst JP, et al. Oxandrolone therapy in patients with Turner syndrome. J Pediatr 1979; 94:823–827.

1122. Bohnet HG. New aspects of oestrogen/gestation-induced growth and endocrine changes in individuals with Turner syndrome. Eur J Pediatr 1986; 145:275–279.

1123. Demetriou E, Emans SJ, Crigler JF Jr. Final height in estrogen-treated patients with Turner syndrome. J Obstet Gynecol 1984; 64:459–464.

1124. Job JC. How sex steroids can modify the effect of growth hormone on growth in Turner syndrome. In: Hibi I, Takano K, eds. Basic and Clinical Approach to Turner Syndrome. Amsterdam: Elsevier Science Publishers, 1993: 279–286.

1125. Kastrup KW: Oestrogen therapy in Turner syndrome. Acta Paediatr Scand 1988; 343(Suppl):43–46.

1126. Kastrup KW: Growth and development in girls with Turner's syndrome during early therapy with low doses of estradiol. Acta Endocrinol (Copenh) 1986; 279(Suppl):157–163.

1127. Knudtzon J, Aarskog D. Results of two years of growth hormone treatment followed by combined growth hormone and oestradiol in Turner syndrome. The Norwegian Turner Study Group. Horm Res 1993; 39(Suppl): 7–17.

1128. Martinez A, Heinrich JJ, Domene H, et al. Growth in Turner's syndrome: long-term treatment with low dose ethinyl estradiol. J Clin Endocrinol Metab 1987; 65:253–257.

1129. Naeraa RW, Nielsen J, Kastrup KW. Growth hormone and 17B-oestradiol treatment of Turner girls—2 year results. Eur J Pediatr 1994; 153:72–77.

1130. Pasquino AM, Boscherini B. Effect of low-dose estrogen on growth in Turner syndrome. In: Ranke MB, Rosenfeld RG, eds. Turner syndrome: Growth Promoting Therapies. Amsterdam: Elsevier Science, 1991: 181–185.

1131. Ranke MB, Haug F, Blum WF, et al. Effect on growth of patients with Turner's syndrome treated with low estrogen doses. Acta Endocrinol (Copenh) 1986; 279(Suppl):153–156.

1132. Ross JL, Cassorla FG, Skerda MC, et al. A preliminary study of the effect of estrogen dose on growth Turner's syndrome. N Engl J Med 1983; 309:1104–1106.

1133. Schwartzberg M, Senior B, Sadeghi-Nejad AB. Final height in girls with Turner syndrome treated with low-dose ethinyl estradiol (EE2). Pediatr Res 1992; 31:84A.

1134. Rudman D, Goldsmith M, Kutner M, et al. Effect of growth hormone and oxandrolone singly and together on growth rate in girls with X chromosome abnormalities. J Pediatr 1980; 96:132–135.

1135. Forbes AP, Jacobsen JG, Carroll EL, et al. Studies of growth arrest in gonadal dysgenesis: response to exogenous human growth hormone. Metabolism 1962; 11:56–75.

1136. Takano K, Hizuka N, Shizume K. Treatment of Turner's syndrome with methionyl human growth hormone for six months. Acta Endocrinol (Copenh) 1986; 112:130–137.

1137. Rongen-Westerlaken C, Wit JM, Drop SLS, et al. Methionyl human growth hormone in Turner's syndrome. Arch Dis Child 1988; 63:1211–1217.

1138. Massa G, Otten BJ, De Muinck Keizer-Schrama SMPF, et al. Treatment with two growth hormone regimens in girls with Turner's syndrome: final height results. Horm Res 1995; 43:144–146.

1139. Rocchiccioli P, Battin J, Bertrand AM, et al. Final stature in cases of Turner's syndrome treated with growth hormone. Arch Pediatr 1994; 1:359–362.

1140. Chatelain PG. Auxology and response to growth hormone treatment of patients with intrauterine growth retardation or Silver-Russell syndrome: analysis of data from the Kabi Pharmacia International Growth Study. Acta Paediatr 1993; 391(Suppl):79–81.

1141. de Zegher F, Maes M, Heinrich C, et al. High-dose growth hormone therapy for short children born small for gestational age. Acta Paediatr 1994; 399(Suppl):77–78.

1142. Seino Y, Yamate T, Kanzaki S, et al. Achondroplasia: effect of growth hormone in 40 patients. Clin Pediatr Endocrinol 1994; 3(Suppl):41–45.

1143. Leger J, Noel M, Limal JM, et al. Growth factors and intrauterine growth retardation. II: Growth hormone, insulin-like growth factor (IGF) I, and IGF-binding protein 3 levels in children with intrauterine growth retardation compared with normal control subjects: prospective study from birth to two years of age. Pediatr Res 1996; 40:101–107.

1144. Chatelain P, Job JC, Blanchard J, et al. Dose-dependent catch-up growth after 2 years of growth hormone treatment in intrauterine growth retarded children. J Clin Endocrinol Metab 1994; 78:1454–1460.

1145. Job JC, Chaussain JL, Job B, et al. Follow-up of three years of treatment with growth hormone and of one post-treatment year, in children with severe growth retardation of intrauterine onset. Pediatr Res 1996; 39:354–359.

1146. Chaussain JL, Colle M, Landier F. Effects of growth hormone therapy in prepubertal children with short stature secondary to intrauterine growth retardation. Acta Paediatr 1994; 399:74–75.

1147. de Zegher F, Maes M, Gargosky SE, et al. High-dose growth hormone treatment of short children born small for gestational age. J Clin Endocrinol Metab 1996; 81:1887–1892.

1148. Albanese A, Stanhope R. Growth and metabolic data following growth hormone treatment of children with intrauterine growth retardation. Horm Res 1993; 39:8–13.

1149. Bridges NA, Brook CGD. Progress report: growth hormone in skeletal dysplasia. Horm Res 1994; 42:231–234.

1150. Van Vliet G, Styne DM, Kaplan SL, et al. Growth hormone treatment for short stature. N Engl J Med 1983; 309:1016–1022.

1151. Gertner JM, Genel M, Gianfredi SP, et al. Prospective clinical trial of human growth hormone in short children without growth hormone deficiency. J Pediatr 1984; 104:172–176.

1152. Hopwood NJ, Hintz RL, Gertner JM, et al. Growth response of children with non–growth hormone deficiency and marked short stature during three years of growth hormone therapy. J Pediatr 1993; 123:215–222.

1153. Zadik Z, Chalew S, Zung A, et al. Effect of long-term growth hormone therapy on bone age and pubertal maturation in boys with and without classical growth hormone deficiency. J Pediatr 1994; 125:189–195.

1154. Loche S, Cambiaso P, Setzu S, et al. Final height after growth hormone therapy in non-growth-hormone-deficient children with short stature. J Pediatr 1994; 125:196–200.

1155. Spagnoli A, Spadoni GL, Cianfarani S, et al. Prediction of the outcome of growth hormone therapy in children with idiopathic short stature. J Pediatr 1995; 126:905–909.

1156. Kaplan SL, Grumbach MM. Long-term treatment with growth hormone of children with non–growth hormone deficient short stature. In: Isaksson O, Binder G, Hall K, eds. Growth Hormone: Basic and Clinical Aspects. Amsterdam: Excerpta Medica, 1987: 197–204.

1157. Cowell CT. Growth hormone therapy in idiopathic short stature in the Kabi International Growth Study. In: Ranke B, Gunnarsson R, eds. Progress in Growth Hormone Therapy—5 Years of KIGSM. Mannheim: J&J Verlag, 1994: 216–229.

1158. Underwood LE, Rieser PA. Is it ethical to treat healthy short children with growth hormone? Acta Paediatr Scand 1989; 362(Suppl):18–23.

1159. Allen DB, Brook CGD, Bridges NA, et al. Therapeutic controversies: growth hormone (GH) treatment of non–GH deficient subjects. J Clin Endocrinol 1994; 79:1239–1248.

1160. Lee PDK, Wilson DM, Rountree L, et al. Growth hormone treatment of short stature in Prader-Willi syndrome. J Pediatr Endocrinol 1987; 2:31–34.

1161. Cotterill AM, McKenna WJ, Brady AF, et al. The short-term effects of growth hormone therapy on height velocity and cardiac ventricular wall thickness in children with Noonan's syndrome. J Clin Endocrinol Metab 1996; 81:2291–2297.

1162. Romano AA, Blethen SL, Dana K, et al. Growth hormone treatment in Noonan syndrome: the National Cooperative Growth Study experience. J Pediatr 1996; 128:S18–S21.

1163. Robinson ICAF, Gabrielsson B, Klaus G, et al. Glucocorticoids and growth problems. Acta Paediatr 1995; 411(Suppl):81–86.

1164. Sanchez CP, Goodman WG, Brandli D, et al. Skeletal response to recombinant human growth hormone (rhGH) in children treated with long-term glucocorticoids. J Bone Miner Res 1995; 10:2–6.

1165. Blethen SL, Allen DB, Graves D, et al. Safety of recombinant DNA–derived growth hormone (rhGH): The National Cooperative Growth Study experience. J Clin Endocrinol Metab 1996; 81:1704–1710.

1166. Wilton P. Adverse events during growth hormone treatment: 5 years' experience. In: Ranke B, Gunnarsson R, eds. Progress in Growth Hormone Therapy—5 Years of KIGSM. Mannheim: J&J Verlag, 1994: 291–307.

1167. Blethen SL. Complications of growth hormone therapy in children. Curr Opin Pediatr 1995; 7:466–471.

1168. Cowell CT, Dietsch S. Adverse events during growth hormone therapy. J Pediatr Endocrinol Metab 1995; 8:243–252.

1169. Watanabe S, Yamaguchi N, Tsunematsu Y, et al. Risk factors for leukemia occurrence among growth hormone users. Jpn J Cancer 1989; 80:822–825.

1170. Fisher DA, Job J, Preece M, et al. Leukemia in patients treated with growth hormone. Lancet 1988; 1:1159–1160.

1171. Fradkin JE, Mills JL, Schonberger LB, et al. Risk of leukemia after treatment with pituitary growth hormone. JAMA 1993; 270:2829–2832.

1172. Ogilvy-Stuart AL, Ryder WD, Gattamaneni HR, et al. Growth hormone and tumor recurrence. Br Med J 1992; 304:1601–1605.

1173. Tuffli GA, Johanson A, Rundle AC, et al. Lack of increased risk for extracranial, nonleukemic neoplasms in recipients of recombinant deoxyribonucleic acid growth hormone. J Clin Endocrinol Metab 1995; 80:1416–1422.

1174. Arslanian SA, Becker DJ, Lee PA, et al. Growth hormone therapy and tumor recurrence: findings in children with brain neoplasms and hypopituitarism. Am J Dis Child 1985; 139:347–350.

1175. Bloom HJG, Glees J, Bell J. The treatment and long-term prognosis of children with intracranial tumors: a study of 610. cases, 1950–1981. Int J Radiat Oncol Biol Phys 1990; 18:723–745.

1176. Davis CH, Joglekar VM. Cerebellar astrocytomas in children and young adults. J Neurol Neurosurg Psychiatry 1981; 44:820–828.

1177. Halperin EC. Pediatric brain stem tumors: patterns of treatment failure and their implications for radiotherapy. Int J Radiat Oncol Biol Phys 1985; 11:1293–1298.

1178. Hoffman HJ, De Silva M, Humphreys RP, et al. Aggressive surgical management of craniopharyngiomas in children. J Neurosurg 1992; 76:47–52.

1179. Lapras C, Patet JD, Mottolese C, et al. Craniopharyngiomas in childhood: analysis of 42 cases. Prog Exp Tumor Res 1987; 30:350–358.

1180. Nishio S, Fukui M, Takeshita I, et al. Recurrent medulloblastoma in children. Neurol Med Chir 1986; 26:19–25.

1181. Schuler D, Somolo P, Borsi J, et al. New drug combination for the treatment of relapsed brain tumors in children. Pediatr Hematol Oncol 1988; 5:153–156.

1182. Torres CF, Rebsamen S, Silber JH, et al. Surveillance scanning of children with medulloblastoma. N Engl J Med 1994; 330:892–895.

1183. Uematsu Y, Tsuura Y, Miyamoto K, et al. The recurrence of primary intracranial germinomas. J Neurooncol 1992; 13:247–256.

1184. Clayton PE, Shalet SM, Gattamaneni HR, et al. Does growth hormone cause relapse of brain tumors? Lancet 1987; 1:711–713.

1185. Rodens KP, Kaplan SL, Grumbach MM, et al. Does growth hormone therapy increase the frequency of tumor recurrence in children with brain tumors? Acta Endocrinol 1987; 28(Suppl):188–189.

1186. Moshang T Jr. Is brain tumor recurrence increased following growth hormone treatment? Trends Endocrinol Metab 1995; 6:205–209.

1187. Mancilla EE, Orlando S, Albright AL, et al. Leukemia and craniopharyngioma: coexistence in the absence of human growth hormone therapy or irradiation. Pediatr Res 1994; 35:103A.

1188. Moshang T, Rundle AC, Graves DA, et al. Brain tumor recurrence in children treated with growth hormone: the National Cooperative Growth Study experience. J Pediatr 1996; 128:S4–S7.

1189. Weiss M, Sutton L, Marcial V, et al. The role of radiation therapy in the management of childhood craniopharyngioma. J Radiat Oncol Biol Phys 1989; 17:1313–1321.

1190. Packer RJ, Sutton LN, Elterman R, et al. Outcome for children with medulloblastoma treated with radiation and cisplatin, CCNU, and vincristine chemotherapy. J Neurosurg 1994; 81:690–698.

1191. Malozowski S, Tanner LA, Wysoluski D, et al. Growth hormone, insulin-like growth factor-I, and benign intracranial hypertension. N Engl J Med 1993; 329:665–666.

1192. Ranke MB. Effects of growth hormone on the metabolism of lipids and water and their potential causing adverse events during growth hormone treatment. Horm Res 1993; 39:104–106.

1193. Collett-Solberg P, Liu GT, Satin-Smith M, et al. Pseudopapilledema and congenital disc anomalies in patients with growth hormone deficiency (GHD). 10th International Congress of Endocrinology. San Francisco, 1996; P2-301 (abstract).

1194. Harris WR. The endocrine basis for slipping of the upper femoral epiphysis: an experimental study. J Bone Joint Surg 1950; 32B:5–11.

1195. Kelsey JL. Epidemiology of slipped capital femoral epiphysis: a review of the literature. Pediatrics 1973; 51:1042–1050.

1196. Rappaport EB, Fife D. Slipped capital femoral epiphysis in growth hormone–deficient patients. Am J Dis Child 1985; 139:396–399.

1197. Malozowski S, Stadel BV. Prepubertal gynecomastia during growth hormone therapy. J Pediatr 1995; 126:659–661.

1198. Malozowski S, Hung W, Scott DC. Acute pancreatitis associated with growth hormone therapy for short stature. N Engl J Med 1995; 332:401–402.

1199. Bourguignon JP, Pierard GE, Ernould C, et al. Effects of human growth hormone therapy on melanocytic naevi. Lancet 1993; 341:1505–1506.

1200. Pierard GE, Pierard-Franchimont C. Morphometric evaluation of the growth of nevi. Ann Dermatol Venereol 1993; 120:605–609.

1201. Guler HP, Schmid C, Zapf J, et al. Effects of recombinant insulin-like growth factor-I on insulin secretion and renal function in normal human subjects. Proc Natl Acad Sci USA 1989; 86:2868–2872.

1202. Laron Z, Klinger B, Erster B, et al. Effects of acute administration of insulin-like growth factor-I in patients with Laron-type dwarfism. Lancet 1988; 2:1170–1172.

1203. Laron Z, Klinger B, Jensen JT, et al. Biochemical and hormonal changes induced by one week of administration of rIGF-I to patients with Laron type dwarfism. Clin Endocrinol (Oxf) 1991; 35:145–150.

1204. Laron Z, Anin S, Klipper-Auerbach Y, et al. Effects of insulin-like growth factor-I on linear growth, head circumference, and body fat in patients with Laron-type dwarfism. Lancet 1992; 339:1258–1261.

1205. Walker J, Van Wyk JJ, Underwood LE. Stimulation of statural growth by recombinant insulin-like growth factor-I in a child with growth hormone insensitivity syndrome (Laron type). J Pediatr 1992; 121:641–646.

1206. Wilton P. Treatment with recombinant insulin-like growth factor-I of children with growth hormone receptor deficiency (Laron syndrome). Acta Paediatr 1992; 282(Suppl):137–141.

1207. Savage MO, Wilton P, Ranke MB, et al. Therapeutic response to recombinant IGF-I in thirty-two patients with growth hormone insensitivity (abstract). Pediatr Res 1993; 33:S5.

1208. Guevara-Aguirre J, Vasconez O, Martinez V, et al. A randomized, double-blind, placebo-controlled trial on safety and efficacy of recombinant human insulin-like growth factor-I in children with growth hormone receptor deficiency. J Clin Endocrinol Metab 1995; 80:1393–1398.

1208a. Guevara-Aguirre J, Rosenbloom AL, Vascomez O, et al. Two-year treatment of growth hormone (GH) receptor deficiency with insulin-like growth factor I in 22 children: comparison of two-dosage levels and two GH-treated GH deficiency. J Clin Endocrinol Metab 1997; 82:629–633.

1209. Sotos JF, Cutler EA, Dodge P. Cerebral gigantism. Am J Dis Child 1977; 131:625–627.

1210. Wit JM, Beemer FA, Barth PG, et al. Cerebral gigantism (Sotos syndrome). Compiled data of 22 cases. Eur J Pediatr 1985; 144:131–140.

1211. Sotelo-Avila C, Gonzalez-Crussi F, Fowler JW. Complete and incomplete forms of Beckwith-Wiedemann syndrome: their oncogenic potential. J Pediatr 1980; 96:47–50.

1212. Elliott M, Bayly R, Cole T, et al. Clinical features and natural history of Beckwith-Wiedemann syndrome: presentation of 74 new cases. Clin Genet 1994; 46:168–174.

1213. Weng EY, Moeschler JB, Graham JM Jr. Longitudinal observations on 15 children with Wiedemann-Beckwith syndrome. Am J Med Genet 1995; 56:366–373.

1214. Drummond IA, Madden Rohwer-Nutter SL, Bell GI, et al. Repression of the insulin-like growth factor II gene by the Wilm's tumor suppressor WT1. Science 1992; 257:674–678.

1215. Schofield PN, Nystrom A, Smith J, et al. Expression of a high molecular weight form of insulin-like growth factor II in a Beckwith-Wiedemann syndrome associated adrenocortical adenoma. Cancer Lett 1995; 94:71–77.

1216. Kubota T, Saitoh S, Matsumoto T, et al. Excess functional copy of allele at chromosomal region 11p15 may cause Wiedemann-Beckwith syndrome. Am J Med Genet 1994; 49:378–383.

1217. Morison IM, Becroft DM, Taniguchi T, et al. Somatic overgrowth associated with overexpression of insulin-like growth factor II. Nat Med 1996; 2:311–316.

1218. Blum WF, Albertsson-Wikland K, Rosberg S, et al. Serum levels of insulin-like growth factor I (IGF1) and IGF binding protein 3 reflect spontaneous growth hormone secretion. J Clin Endocrinol Metab 1993; 76:1610–1616.

1219. Tauber M, Pienkowski C, Rochiccioli P. Growth hormone secretion in children and adolescents with familial tall stature. Eur J Pediatr 1994; 153:311–316.

1220. Dickerman Z, Loewinger J, Laron Z. The pattern of growth in children with constitutional tall stature from birth to age 9 years: a longitudinal study. Acta Paediatr Scand 1984; 73:530–536.

1221. Josse EE, Temperli R, Mullis PE. Adult height in constitutionally tall stature: accuracy of five different height prediction methods. Arch Dis Child 1992; 67:1357–1362.

1222. Ignatius A, Lenko HL, Perheentupa J. Oestrogen treatment of tall girls: effect decreases with age. Acta Paediatr Scand 1991; 80:712–717.

1223. De Waal WJ, Greyn-Fokker MH, Stijnen TH, et al. Accuracy of final height prediction and effect of growth reductive therapy in 362 constitutionally tall children. J Clin Endocrinol Metab 1996; 81:1206–1216.

1224. Bierich JR. Estrogen treatment of girls with constitutional tall stature. Pediatrics 1978; 62(Suppl):1196–1201.

1225. Sorgo W, Scholler K, Heinze F, et al. Critical analysis of height reduction in oestrogen-treated tall girls. Eur J Pediatr 1984; 142:260–265.

1226. Trygstad O. Oestrogen treatment of adolescent tall girls; short term side effects. Acta Endocrinol 1986; 113(Suppl):170–173.

1227. Forbes GB. Nutrition and growth. J Pediatr 1977; 91:40.

1228. Spence HJ, Trias EP, Raiti S. Acromegaly in a 9½-year-old boy. Am J Dis Child 1972; 123:504–506.

1229. AvRuskin TW, Sau K, Tang S, et al. Childhood acromegaly: successful therapy with conventional radiation and effects of chlorpromazine on growth hormone and prolactin secretion. J Clin Endocrinol Metab 1973; 37:380.

1230. DeMajo SF, Onativia A. Acromegaly and gigantism in a boy: comparison with three overgrown non-acromegalic children. Pediatrics 1960; 57:382.

1231. Lefkowitz RJ. G proteins in medicine. N Engl J Med 1995; 332:186–187.

1232. Lightner ES, Winter JSD. Treatment of juvenile acromegaly with bromocriptine. J Pediatr 1981; 98:494–496.

1233. Geffner ME, Nagel RA, Dietrich RB, et al. Treatment of acromegaly with a somatostatin analog in a patient with McCune-Albright syndrome. J Pediatr 1987; 3:740–743.

1234. Hoffman WH, Perrin JS, Halac E, et al. Acromegalic gigantism and tuberous sclerosis. J Pediatr 1978; 93:478.

1235. Daughaday WH. Extreme gigantism. Analysis of growth velocity and occurrence of severe peripheral neuropathy and neuropathic arthropathy (Charcot joints). N Engl J Med 1977; 297:1267–1269.

1236. Post EM, Richman RA. A condensed table for predicting adult stature. J Pediatr 1981; 98:440–442.

1237. Tanner JM, Whitehouse RH. Clinical longitudinal standards for height, weight, height velocity, weight velocity and the stages of puberty. Arch Dis Child 1976; 51:170–179.

1238. Tanner JM, Whitehouse RH, Takaishi M. Standards from birth to maturity for height, weight, height velocity and weight velocity. British children, 1965. Arch Dis Child 1966; 41:454–471.

1239. Cohen P, Rosenfeld RG. The IGF axis. In: Rosenbloom AL, ed. Human Growth Hormone, Basic and Scientific Aspects. Boca Raton, FL: CRC Press, 1995: 279–285.

1240. Rotwein P. Structure, evolution, expression and regulation of insulin-like growth factors I and II. Growth Factors 1991; 5:3–18.

1241. Cohen P, Fielder PJ, Hasegawa Y, et al. Clinical aspects of insulin-like growth factor binding proteins. Acta Endocrinol 1991; 124:74–85.

1242. Blethen SL, Baptista J, Kuntze J, et al. Adult height in growth hormone (GH)–deficient children treated with biosynthetic GH. J Clin Endocrinol Metab 1997; 82:418–420.

31

PUBERTY: ONTOGENY, NEUROENDOCRINOLOGY, PHYSIOLOGY, AND DISORDERS

Melvin M. Grumbach and Dennis M. Styne

INTRODUCTION

Puberty is not a de novo event but rather a phase in the continuum of development of hypothalamic-pituitary-gonadal function from fetal life, through puberty, to the attainment of full sexual maturation and fertility. By puberty, secondary sexual characteristics and the adolescent growth spurt result in the striking sexual dimorphism of mature individuals, fertility is achieved, and profound psychological effects ensue.[1] These changes are a consequence of stimulation of the gonads by pituitary gonadotropins and the increase in gonadal steroid output. Adolescence is accompanied by the onset of adult patterns of sociosexual and economic behavior.[2]

The human is, reproductively, the most successful of mammals, and many anthropologists attribute this success to the prolonged pattern of human growth and development and to the delay in attaining full sexual maturity.[2, 3] Human growth involves the development of two phases: a childhood stage and an adolescent stage that includes an adolescent or pubertal growth spurt (Fig. 31–1). Our closest biologic relative, the chimpanzee, which matures twice as rapidly as the human, does not exhibit these two stages, including the adolescent spurt in height. (The estimated date for divergence of the chimpanzee and human lineages is 4 to 5 million years ago.) Theorists have proposed that a portion of human success and many biosocial characteristics emanate from learning and practicing adult behaviors related to sex and childrearing, particularly providing children, not just infants, with food.[2] These behaviors include learning skills related to the production of food, cooperative hunting, division of labor according to sex, sharing food, tool making, and adjustment to the social organization and cultural environment. On the other hand, Bogin, noting that tool making preceded the evolutionary development of adolescence, suggested that the evolution and value of human childhood and adolescence and this unique pattern of growth and development contribute to the reproductive advantage and success of the human.[2–5] Mayr has called this process "selection for reproductive success."[6]

Historical evidence suggests that puberty occurs at an earlier age today than in the past.[7–11] The average age of menarche in industrialized European countries has decreased 2 to 3 mo per decade over the past 150 y, and in the United States the decrease averaged 2 to 3 mo per decade in the last century[8–10] (Fig. 31–2). However, this trend ceased in developed countries, such as the United States and the Netherlands, beginning approximately in 1940, presumably owing to improved socioeconomic status and health and the benefits of urbanization.[12] Remarkably, a reverse trend in Northern Italy

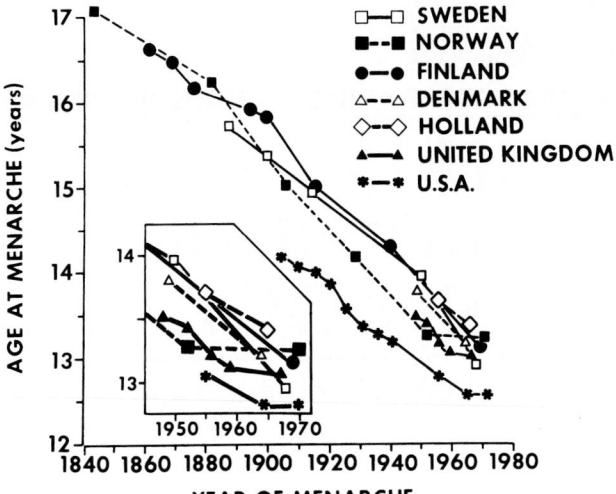

Figure 31–2. Changes in age at menarche, 1840 to 1978, illustrating the advance in the age at menarche in Western Europe and the United States since 1840 and the slowing of this trend over the last 30 y. (Modified from Tanner M, Eveleth PB. Variability between populations in growth and development at puberty. In: Berenberg SR, ed. Puberty, Biologic and Psychosocial Components. Leiden: H. E. Stenfert Kroese, 1975: 256–273. Reprinted by permission of Kluwer Academic Publishers.)

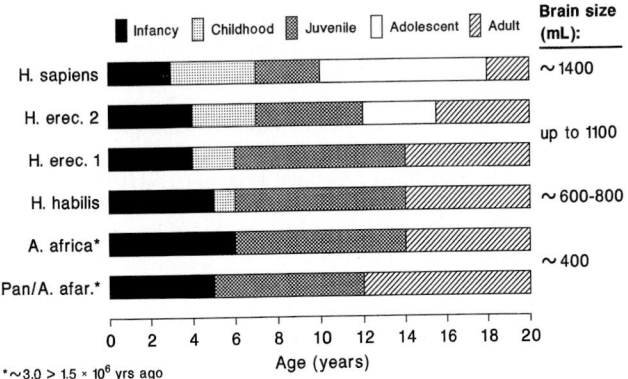

Figure 31–1. A summary and proposed scheme of the evolution of the human pattern of postnatal growth and development during the first 20 years of life. A. afar, *Australopithecus afarensis*, a "bipedal chimpanzee"; A. africa, *Australopithecus africanus*; H. habilis, *Homo habilis* (the toolmaker); H. erec 1, early *Homo erectus*; H. erec 2, late *Homo erectus*; H. sapiens, *Homo sapiens*. The early hominid australopithecine specimens from South Africa date back about 3.0 to 1.5 million years ago. *H. afarensis*, while a hominid (the family of all human species), retained many anatomic features of nonhominid species, e.g., an adult brain size of about 400 mL compared with *H. habilis* (650 to 800 mL), early *H. erectus* (850 to 900 mL), late *H. erectus* (up to 1100 mL), and modern *H. sapiens* (about 1400 mL). Infancy is defined as the period when the mother's breast milk is the sole or most important source of nutrition, and in preindustrialized societies ends at about 36 months. Childhood is the period after weaning, when the child is dependent on others for food and protection; this period ends when the growth of the brain in weight is almost complete, at about age 7 years. The juvenile stage is defined as prepubertal individuals who are no longer dependent on their parents for survival. The adolescent stage that begins with the onset of puberty, ends when adult height is attained.[2, 3] The pattern in *A. afarensis* is no different than that in the chimpanzee (*Pan troglodytes*). Note the first appearance of the childhood stage, *H. habilis* (arising about 2 million years ago) and the first appearance of the adolescent stage in *H. erectus* 2 (about 500,000 years ago); *H. sapiens* arose about 120,000 to 150,000 years ago. (Modified from Bogin B. Growth and development: recent evolutionary and biocultural research. In: Boaz NT, Wolfe LD, eds. Biological Anthropology: The State of the Science. Bend, OR: International Institute for Human Evolutionary Research, 1995: 49–70, with permission.)

(in women born between 1950 and 1959) leading to a later age at menarche has been attributed to a resurgence of physical and psychological stress.[13] In South America and Africa a different type of reversal has occurred in which rural children fare better and have earlier puberty and taller stature than do urban children, the opposite of the expected pattern.[14] Thus socioeconomic conditions, nutritional status, and states of health influence the age at onset of puberty and the progression of pubertal development.[15–18] The interaction of nutrition, energy expenditure, and puberty is of particular importance when nutrition is suboptimal.

If the age at onset of puberty was later in past centuries, the age of attaining adult height was also later. Records of army recruits, schoolchildren, workers in Europe and America, and slaves indicate that large portions of the population in the past two centuries continued to grow a considerable amount into their early 20s, whereas modern adolescents cease to grow and reach stable heights by about 17 years of age.[8, 9] The final heights attained during the 18th and 19th centuries were often at modern 25th percentiles or less.

The progressive decline in the age at onset of puberty is probably a result of improvements in socioeconomic conditions, nutrition, and general health. In nomadic Lapps, for whom the standard of living changed little between 1870 and 1930, there has been no trend toward earlier puberty.[17] The tendency for earlier menarche in Western Europe and the United States (see Fig. 31–1) has slowed or ceased over the past 40 y,[8–11, 18–21] and the social class difference in menarcheal age has narrowed or disappeared in most countries. According to one survey by the U.S. National Center for Health Statistics, the age at onset of menarche in the United States is 12.8 years,[22, 23] and this age remains true for white girls, although the age at menarche is about 6 mo earlier in black girls.[24]

Moderate obesity (up to 30% above normal weight for age) is associated with earlier menarche, whereas menarche is delayed with pathologic obesity.[25] Delayed puberty is a feature of chronic disease and malnutrition; strenuous physical activity in girls, especially when associated with low body weight, can delay or arrest puberty.[26] On the contrary, inactive, bedridden children with mental retardation reach menarche at an earlier age and with a lower proportion of body fat value than do similarly retarded children who are more active.[27] Early studies suggesting that blindness may advance the age at onset of puberty[28] have not been confirmed. Puberty starts at a later age, and the duration of pubertal development is longer at high altitudes than at low ones, even when nutritional status is similar.[29]

Genetic factors play an important role in the onset of puberty, as illustrated by the similar age at onset of menarche in members of ethnic groups and in mother-daughter, monozygotic twin, and sibling pairs. Secondary sexual development occurs earlier in black girls than in white girls in the United States, and there is no apparent effect of social or economic factors on this relationship (see later). Thus when nutrition, health, and infant care are good, the age at onset of puberty is determined largely by genetic factors.[8, 18, 30]

PHYSICAL CHANGES OF PUBERTY

Secondary Sexual Characteristics

Characterization of the physical changes in individuals and in populations requires objective and reproducible methods of describing the features under study. Tanner[8, 10] developed standards for assessing sexual maturation that have been widely used throughout the world (see Figs. 31–3 to 31–5). Self-assessment scales of adolescent sexual maturation are used in some studies to avoid the embarrassment of physical examination in normal children and adolescents.[31, 32]

Girls

Two distinct phenomena occur in the female. The development of the breast[33, 34] is under the control primarily of estrogens secreted by the ovaries (Fig. 31–3); the growth of pubic and axillary hair (Fig. 31–4) is under the influence mainly of androgens secreted by the adrenal cortex and the ovary. The glandular and connective tissues of the mammary gland begin to develop at the onset of pubertal maturation. Thus lobules, composed of small ductules and cellular connective tissue, develop to a more pronounced degree in the female. Proliferation of fatty and connective tissue accounts for 80% of the volume of the adult nonlactating female breast.[33]

The classification of female breast development[35] depends

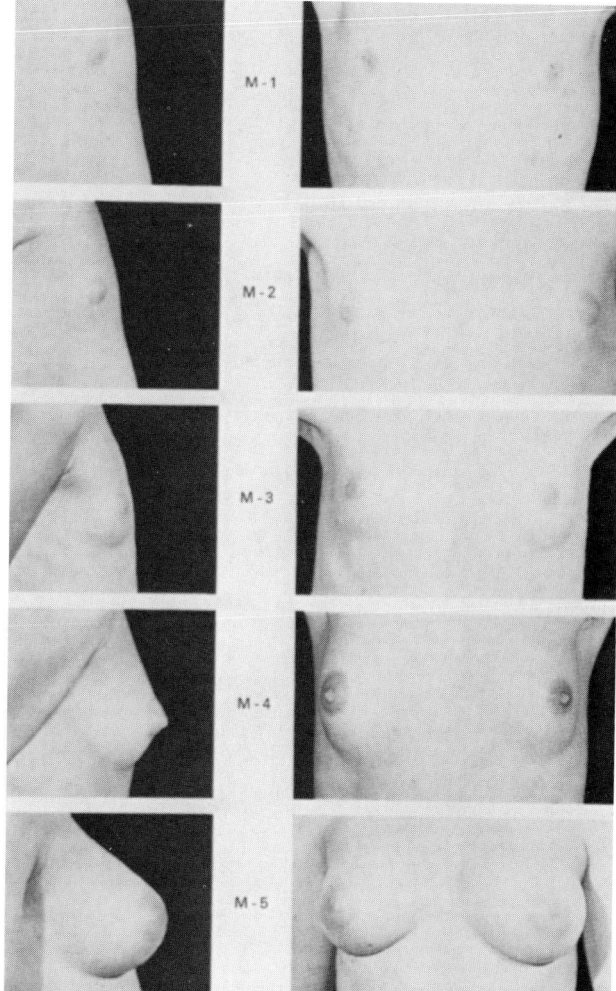

Figure 31–3. Stages of breast development according to Marshall and Tanner[75] and Reynolds and Wines.[36] Stage 1: preadolescent; elevation of papilla only. Stage 2: breast bud stage; elevation of breast and papilla as a small mound, enlargement of areolar diameter. Stage 3: further enlargement of breast and areola with no separation of their contours. Stage 4: projection of areola and papilla to form a secondary mound above the level of the breast. Stage 5: mature stage; projection of papilla only, resulting from recession of the areola to the general contour of the breast. (Photographs from Van Wieringen JD, Wafelbakker F, Verbrugge HP, et al. Growth Diagrams 1965 Netherlands: Second National Survey on 0–24 Year Olds. Netherlands Institute for Preventative Medicine TNO. Groningen: Wolters-Noordhoff, 1971. © Wolters-Noordhoff, Groningen.[1428])

on specific characteristics common to the breast but does not include size or inherent shape, which are determined by genetic and nutritional factors (see Fig. 31–3). Four stages were described by Stratz;[35] a fifth was added by Reynolds and Wines;[36] and modifications were made to the schema by Tanner,[10] in the most widely utilized staging. The initial breast development may be unilateral for several months and may be cause for unfounded concern by girls or parents. Indeed, surgical biopsies have been performed inappropriately when it was not appreciated that asymmetrical development is normal. In unusual cases of agenesis of the breast, no glandular or fat enlargement occurs regardless of the level of estrogen stimulation.

Changes in the diameter of the papilla of the nipple are sequential and linked to the stages of pubertal development. Nipple papilla diameter does not increase much during pubic hair stages 1 to 3 or breast stages 1 to 3 (diameter is 3 to 4 mm) but increases after breast stage 3, providing an objective method of differentiating stage 4 from 5 (the final diameter of the papilla is approximately 9 mm)[37] (Table 31–1).

TABLE 31–1. Nipple Diameter Compared with Breast and Pubic Hair Stages: Comparison of Longitudinal and Cross-Sectional Data

Stage	Nipple Size (mm)*	
	Cross-Sectional Data	Longitudinal Data
Breast		
1	2.89 (0.81)	3.0 (0.77)
2	3.28 (0.89)	3.37 (0.96)
3	4.07 (1.32)	4.72 (1.40)†
4	7.74 (1.64)†	7.25 (1.46)†
5	9.94 (1.38)†	9.41 (1.45)†
Pubic hair		
1	2.95 (1.02)	3.14 (1.31)
2	3.32 (0.91)	3.69 (1.34)
3	4.11 (1.54)	4.44 (1.17)†
4	7.15 (1.81)†	6.54 (1.47)†
5	9.66 (1.59)†	8.98 (1.56)†

*Results are means ± standard deviation (SD; in parentheses).
†Significantly different from previous stage, P <.05.
Reprinted by permission of Elsevier Science Publishing Co., Inc. from Papilla (nipple) development during female puberty, by Rohn RD. Journal of Adolescent Health Care, Vol. 2, pp. 217–220. Copyright 1982 by The Society for Adolescent Medicine.[37]

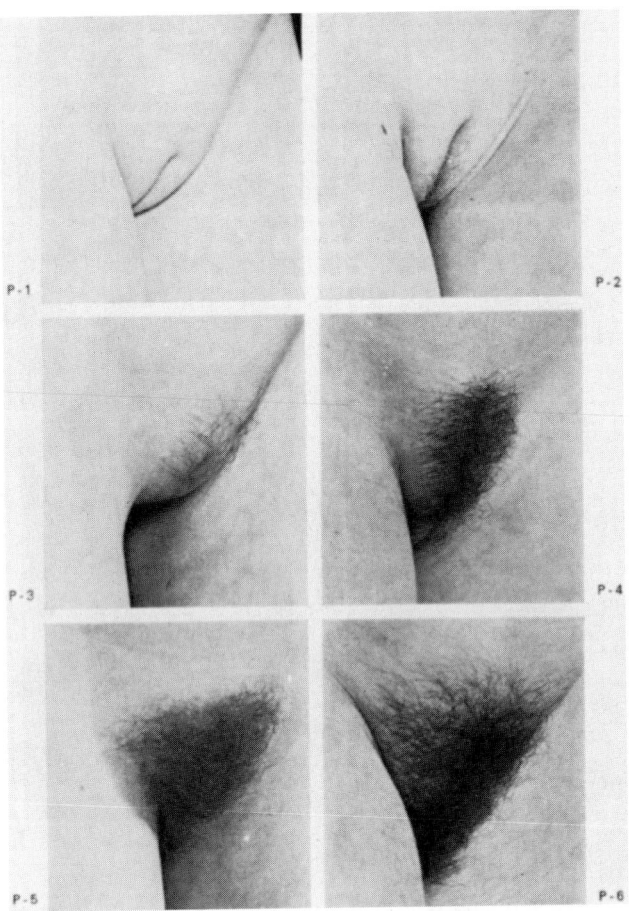

Figure 31–4. Stages of female pubic hair development, according to Marshall and Tanner,[75] Reynolds and Wines,[36] and Dupertuis et al.[1429] Stage 1: preadolescent; the vellus over the pubes is not further developed than that over the anterior abdominal wall; i.e., there is no pubic hair. Stage 2: sparse growth of long, slightly pigmented, downy hair, straight or only slightly curled, appearing chiefly along the labia. This stage is difficult to see on photographs. Stage 3: hair is considerably darker, coarser, and curlier. The hair spreads sparsely over the junction of the pubes. Stage 4: hair is now adult in type, but the area covered by it is still considerably smaller than in most adults. There is no spread to the medial surface of the thighs. Stage 5: hair is adult in quantity and type, distributed as an inverse triangle of the classic feminine pattern. The spread is to the medial surface of the thighs but not up the linea alba or elsewhere above the base of the inverse triangle. (Photographs from Van Wieringen JD, Wafelbakker F, Verbrugge HP, et al. Growth Diagrams 1965 Netherlands: Second National Survey on 0–24 Year Olds. Netherlands Institute for Preventative Medicine TNO. Groningen. Wolters-Noordhoff, 1971. © Wolters-Noordhoff, Groningen.)

The stage of breast development is usually equal to the pubic hair stage in normal girls, but as different endocrine organs control these two processes, breast and pubic hair stages should be assessed separately (Tables 31–2 and 31–3).

Areolar diameter also increases in boys at puberty, and many boys have palpable glandular enlargement of the breast at some time during adolescence (see Chapter 17).

Although rarely evident, an increase in height velocity, rather than breast development, is actually the first sign of puberty in girls.

TABLE 31–2. Reported Mean Ages (Years) at Onset of Sexual Maturity Stages in Females

Study	No. of Subjects	Age Range	Breast Stages				Pubic Hair Stages			
			B2	B3	B4	B5	PH2	PH3	PH4	PH5
Marshall and Tanner (1969) United Kingdom	192	8–18	11.1	12.1	13.1	15.3	—	12.4	12.9	14.4
Billewicz et al. (1981) United Kingdom			10.8	12.0	13.1	14.0	—	—	—	—
Roy et al. (1972) France			11.4	12.5	13.4	—	11.3	12.4	13.2	—
Taranger (1976) Sweden			11.0	11.8	13.1	15.6	11.5	12.0	12.9	15.2
Largo and Prader (1983) Switzerland			10.9	12.2	13.2	14.0	10.4	12.2	13.0	14.0
Roede and Van Wieringen (1985) Holland			11.0	12.1	13.4	15.2	11.3	12.2	13.3	14.9
Neyzi et al. (1975) Turkey			10.0	11.6	12.8	15.2	10.8	11.6	12.3	13.6
Villarreal et al. (1989) Mexican-American	699	10–17	10.9	12.2	13.9	15.1	11.2	12.4	14.1	15.5
Roche et al. (1995) USA (Ohio)	67	9.5–16	11.2	12.0	12.4	—	11.0	11.8	12.4	13.1
Herman-Giddens (1997) USA	17,077	3–12								
African-American	1,638		8.9	10.2	—	—	8.8	10.4		
White	15,439		10.0	11.3	—	—	10.5	11.5		

Modified from Roche AF, Wellens R, Attie KM, et al. The timing of sexual maturation in a group of U.S. white youths. J Pediatr Endocrinol Metab 1995; 8:11–18, with permission.[43]

The pattern of development and growth of pubic hair in girls is illustrated in Figure 31–4. The vaginal mucosa changes from the prepubertal glistening, reddish hue to a thicker, duller appearance because of the cornification of the lining cells, and the secretion of clear or whitish discharge increases in the months before menarche as a result of estrogen action. The vaginal pH decreases as menarche approaches because of the increased lactic acid production by lactobacilli in the vaginal flora. The length of the vagina increases from about 8 cm at onset of puberty to 11 cm at menarche. Thickening, protrusion, and rugation of the labia majora and minora occur. Fat is deposited in the area of the mons pubis, and the labia majora become wrinkled in appearance. The clitoris enlarges slightly, and the urethral opening becomes more prominent. Photographic atlases of normal female prepubertal genitalia include standards for variation in appearance of the hymenal opening; this information is invaluable in the examination of a victim of suspected child abuse.[38]

TABLE 31–3. Descriptive Statistics for the Timing of Sexual Maturity Stages in Females

Breast Stages

	Onset of Stage		Mean Age for Stage	
STAGE	MEAN	SD	MEAN	SD
Stage 2				
Roche et al. (Ohio)	11.2	0.7	11.3	1.1
Herman-Giddens et al. (USA)				
African-American	8.9	1.9		
White	10.0	1.8		
Stage 3				
Roche et al. (Ohio)	12.0	1.0	12.5	1.5
Herman-Giddens et al. (USA)				
African-American	10.2	1.4		
White	11.3	1.4		
Stage 4				
Roche et al. (Ohio)	12.4	0.9		

Tanner Pubic Hair

	MEAN	SD		
Tanner Stage 2				
Roche et al. (Ohio)	11.0	0.5		
Herman-Giddens et al. (USA)				
African-American	8.8	2.0		
White	10.5	1.7		
Tanner Stage 3				
Roche et al. (Ohio)	11.8	1.0		
Herman-Giddens et al. (USA)				
African-American	10.4	1.6		
White	11.5	1.2		
Tanner Stage 4				
Roche et al. (Ohio)	12.4	0.8		

Menarche

Herman-Giddens et al. (USA)				
African-American	12.2	1.2		
White	12.9	1.2		
	At Age 11		At Age 12	
African-American	27.9%*		62.1%	
White	13.4%*		35.2%	
Onset Axillary Hair (Stage 2)				
African-American	10.1 ± 2.0			
White	11.8 ± 1.9			

*African-American girls enter puberty approximately 1 to 1½ years earlier than white girls and begin menses 8½ months earlier.

From Herman-Giddens ME, Slora EJ, Wasserman RC, et al. Secondary sexual characteristics and menses in young girls seen in office practice: a study from the Pediatric Research in Office Settings Network. Pediatrics 1997; 99:505–512, with permission.[44]

Boys

The growth and maturation of the penis usually correlate with pubic hair development, because both processes are under the control of androgen. However, the stages of the pubic hair and genital development should be determined independently and recorded separately; in this way, discordant stages will indicate potential disorders of the adrenal gland or testes (Fig. 31–5 and Tables 31–4 and 31–5).

Growth of the testes is usually the first sign of puberty in the male, and it begins approximately 6 mo after the initiation of breast development in girls. In general, pubertal testicular enlargement has begun when the longitudinal measurement of a testis is greater than 2.5 cm (excluding the epididymis). The testicular volume index—(length × width of right testis + length × width of left testis/2) and testicular volume, measured by comparing the testes with ellipsoids of known volume, correlate with the stages of puberty[39, 40] (Table 31–6). A useful sign of the onset of puberty is a testicular length of more than 2.5 cm or volume of 4 mL or greater. Stage 2a refers to a testicular volume of 3 mL; further pubertal progression occurs within 6 mo in 82% of boys whose testes reach this 3 mL size[40a] (Table 31–7). The right testis is usually larger than the left, and the left testis is located lower in the scrotum than the right.

The phallus is most accurately measured in the stretched, flaccid state. The length of the erectile tissue (excluding the foreskin) increases from an average of 6.2 cm in the prepubertal state to 12.4 ± 2.7 cm in the white adult; in black men the mean length is 14.6 cm, and in Asians it is 10.6 cm.[41]

Limits of Normal Pubertal Development

Data on the normal variation in pubertal development in the United States are becoming more plentiful but are still incomplete. A United States survey of the age of attainment of the various stages of puberty that began with subjects of 12 years of age was useful in defining the upper limits of normal pubertal development but uninformative about the lower limits of the age at onset of puberty.[23, 24, 42] A longitudinal study (see Table 31–5 for males) of white boys and girls started at 9.5 years of age and provided information about the mean age of stages of puberty[43] but started too late to include those normal children entering puberty at the earlier limits (see Table 31–3 for females). A cross-sectional study sponsored by the American Academy of Pediatrics of 17,070 girls visiting the offices of pediatricians across the United States and examined by trained observers started at 3 years of age but ended at 12 years of age and so excluded a proportion of children who enter puberty at a later age.[44] The standard deviation of the longitudinal study[43] was low, 1.0 year or less in most cases, while the cross-sectional study had a larger standard deviation of approximately 2 years.[44]

A comprehensive, large, preferably longitudinal study that would include the youngest normal pubertal subjects and the oldest is needed in the United States. For example, the longitudinal study by Roche and colleagues[43] of 78 white boys and 67 white girls used self-assessment beginning at age 9.5 years and lasting to age 16 or 17 years. In the absence of such a study, the authors define the normal onset of puberty as occurring between 2.5 standard deviations (SD) above and below the mean (including 99.4% of the population) as determined by a combination of studies discussed above; regrettably, this is an arbitrary rather than a statistical definition, but it serves the purpose of defining the children in need of medical evaluation. The mean age for a boy to reach genital stage 2 or pubic hair stage 2 in the longitudinal study was 11.2 years (±0.7 SD), and the mean age of the population in stage 2 was 11.3 years (±1 SD).[43] For simplicity, the authors

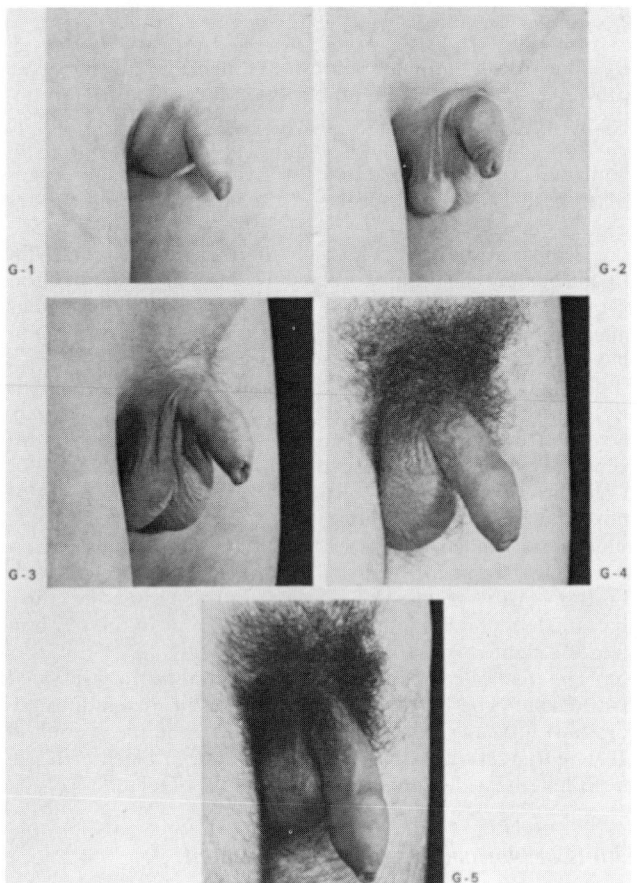

Figure 31–5. Stages of male genital development and pubic hair development, according to Marshall and Tanner,[75] Reynolds and Wines,[36] and Dupertuis et al.[1429] *Genital Development:* Stage 1: preadolescent. Testes, scrotum, and penis are about the same size and proportion as in early childhood. Stage 2: the scrotum and testes have enlarged; the scrotal skin shows a change in texture and also some reddening. Stage 3: growth of the penis has occurred, at first mainly in length but with some increase in breadth; there is further growth of the testes and scrotum. Stage 4: the penis is further enlarged in length and breadth with development of the glans. The testes and scrotum are further enlarged. The scrotal skin has further darkened. Stage 5: genitalia are adult in size and shape. No further enlargement takes place after stage 5 is reached. *Pubic Hair Development:* Stage 1: preadolescent; the vellus over the pubes is not further developed than that over the abdominal wall; i.e., there is no pubic hair. Stage 2: sparse growth of long, slightly pigmented, downy hair, straight or slightly curled, appearing chiefly at the base of the penis. Stage 3: hair is considerably darker, coarser, and curlier and spreads sparsely over the junction of the pubes. Stage 4: hair is now adult in type, but the area it covers is still considerably smaller than in most adults. There is no spread to the medial surface of the thighs. Stage 5: hair is adult in quantity and type, distributed as an inverse triangle. The spread is to the medial surface of the thighs but not up the linea alba or elsewhere above the base of the inverse triangle. Most men will have further spread of the pubic hair. (Photographs from Van Wieringen JD, Wafelbakker F, Verbrugge HP, et al. Growth Diagrams 1965 Netherlands: Second National Survey on 0–24 Year Olds. Netherlands Institute for Preventative Medicine TNO. Groningen: Wolters-Noordhoff, 1971. © Wolters-Noordhoff, Groningen.[1428])

combined the data from Roche and colleagues[43] to set the mean age of onset of puberty in boys as 11 years, with the normal limits between 9 and 13.5 years (these limits are similar to those of a prior United States national study).[45]

The evaluation of girls is more complicated because it may be difficult even for a trained observer to detect the onset of stage 2 breast development during an office visit, whereas ascertainment of stage 3 is generally straightforward. Using the longitudinal study of Roche,[43] which found a mean age of onset of stage 2 breast development of 11.2 years (±0.7 SD) and a mean age of girls in stage 2 as 11.3 years (±1.1 SD),

the authors simplified these data so that the mean age of onset of puberty is 11 years, with limits between 9 and 13 years. If we collate the information from the large cross-sectional study of 17,000 girls by Herman-Giddens et al[44] and average the age of onset of stage 2 and stage 3 breast development, to allow for the difficulty in assessment of the start of stage 2, with the data from the smaller longitudinal study, we consider the mean age at onset of breast development as 10.6 years for white girls with limits between 7 and 13 years, and 9.5 years for black girls with limits between 6 and 13 years.

Thus, apparently normal boys who develop secondary

TABLE 31–4. Reported Mean Ages (Years) at Onset of Sexual Maturity Stages in Males

Study	Genital Stages				Pubic Hair Stages			
	G2	G3	G4	G5	PH2	PH3	PH4	PH5
Marshall and Tanner (1970) United Kingdom	11.6	12.9	13.8	14.9	—	13.9	14.4	15.2
Roy (1972) France	12.0	13.1	14.3	—	12.4	13.4	14.3	—
Taranger (1976) Sweden	12.2	13.1	13.9	15.1	12.5	13.4	14.1	15.5
Largo and Prader (1983) Switzerland	11.2	12.9	13.8	14.7	12.2	13.5	14.2	14.9
Roede and Van Wieringen (1985) Holland	11.3	13.1	14.0	15.3	11.7	13.1	14.0	15.0
Neyzi et al. (1975) Turkey	—	—	—	—	12.3	13.8	16.1	—
Villarreal et al. (1989) Mexican-American	12.4	13.5	14.6	16.3	12.8	13.6	14.6	16.1
Roche et al. (1995) USA (Ohio)	11.2	12.1	13.5	14.3	11.2	12.1	13.4	14.3

Modified from Roche AF, Wellens R, Attie KM, et al. The timing of sexual maturation in a group of U.S. white youths. J Pediatr Endocrinol Metab 1995; 8:11–18, with permission.[37]

TABLE 31–5. Descriptive Statistics for the Timing of Sexual Maturity Stages in White Males (Ohio)

Genital Stages

	Onset of Stage		Mean Age for Stage	
STAGE	MEAN	S.D.	MEAN	S.D.
2	11.2	0.7	11.3	1.0
3	12.1	0.8	12.6	1.0
4	13.5	0.7	14.5	1.1
5	14.3	1.1	—	—

Pubic Hair Stages

	Onset of Stage		Mean Age for Stage	
STAGE	MEAN	S.D.	MEAN	S.D.
2	11.2	0.8	11.3	0.9
3	12.1	1.0	12.4	1.0
4	13.4	0.9	13.7	0.9
5	14.3	0.8	14.8	1.0
6	15.3	0.8	—	—

TABLE 31–6. Correlation of Testicular Volume with Stage of Pubertal Development

	Pubertal Stage				
Parameter	1	2	3	4	5
TV*	1.8	4.5	8.2	10.5	—
Volume (cm³)†	2.5	3.4	9.1	11.8	14
Volume (cm³)‡	1.8	4.2	10	11	15
Volume (cm³)§	1.8	5.0	9.5	12.5	17

*Testicular volume index calculated by (length × width of right testis + length × width of left testis) ÷ 2. Data from Burr et al.[275] and August et al.[277]
†Volume estimated by comparison with ellipsoid of known volume (orchidometer) that is equal to or smaller than the testes. Data from Zachmann et al.[39]
‡Volume by comparison with orchidometer. Data from Waaler et al.[1433]
§Measurement with calipers and average volume of both testes calculated by 0.52 × longitudinal axis × transverse axis. Data from Waaler et al.[1433]

sexual characteristics before 9 years of age and those who do not develop these characteristics by 13.5 years of age are out of the range of normal. White girls younger than 7 years and black girls younger than 6 years who develop breasts and girls who do not develop breasts by 13 years of age are out of the range of normal.

Black girls have about a 1-year earlier onset of breast development, even though the average age at menarche in the cross-sectional study was only 0.7 year different (12.2 years for blacks and 12.9 for whites). However, in the cross-sectional study, 3.0% of white girls had stage 2 breast development by 6 years, and 5.0% by 7 years, whereas 6.4 of blacks had stage 2 breast development by 6 years, and 15.4% by 7 years. This must make us careful in choosing candidates for expensive diagnostic tests and long-term therapy, as many of the children who appear to have mild sexual precocity represent normal variation. It would be inappropriate to study extensively all girls found in these lower limits of normal. Family history, the rapidity of development, the presence or absence of central nervous system (CNS) symptoms and signs, and the concern of the parents must enter into the decision of whether to evaluate a child at the lower limits of the age range for normal children.

International cross-sectional and longitudinal studies are available for the age at onset of pubertal stages. The results show similarities to United States data for boys (Fig. 31–6), but the data differ for girls (Fig. 31–7).

There are no differences between black and white boys in the ages of attainment of pubertal stages. Black girls are advanced in secondary sexual development compared with white girls of the same age during the first three stages of puberty, a difference that may be related, in part, to the higher prevalence in black girls of obesity, which can advance the age at onset of puberty.[24, 45] Growth patterns for black and white children are usually plotted on the standard North American growth charts, but ethnic-specific growth charts are available for some groups.[46]

Other Sexually Dimorphic Physical Changes

In boys the membranous and cartilaginous components of the vocal cords lengthen during puberty. The length of the prepubertal vocal cords in both boys and girls is about 12 to 15 mm, of which the membranous portion is 7 to 8 mm. In adult men the vocal cords attain a length of 18 to 23 mm (membranous portion 12 to 16 mm), whereas in women the cords enlarge only slightly (13 to 18 mm). In men who are castrated prepubertally, the membranous component of the vocal cords is the same length as that in prepubertal boys and is even shorter than that in women.[47] During puberty the male larynx, cricothyroid cartilage, and laryngeal muscles enlarge; the voice breaks at approximately 13.9 years, and the adult voice is achieved by about 15 years.[48]

Facial hair in boys first appears on the corners of the upper lip and the upper cheeks and then spreads to the

TABLE 31–7. Mean Values of Age, Height, Weight, Body Mass Index, and Serum Hormone Levels by Pubertal Stage, in 515 (Ohio) Boys (237 African-American, 278 White; Age 10–15 y at Intake) Followed Every 6 Months for 3 Years ANOVA, with Duncan Post-Hoc Analysis, by Pubertal Stage

	Pubertal Stage					
Variable	PS1†	PS2a	PS2b	PS3	PS4	PS5
Age (y)	11.44*	12.18*	12.79*	13.74*	14.63*	15.19*
Height (cm)	144.2*	149.8*	154.6*	162.3*	169.9*	173.3*
Weight (kg)	38.18*	41.65*	47.27*	54.67*	61.11*	66.88*
Body mass index (kg/m²)	18.1*	18.4*	19.5*	20.6*	21.0*	22.2*
Testosterone: nmol/L (ng/dL)						
Black subjects	0.8 (23)*	3.0 (86)*	4.9 (141)*	11.5 (331)*	13.4 (338)*	15.5 (449)*
White subjects	0.6 (16)*	2.9 (83)*	4.6 (132)*	9.7 (281)*	13.3 (383)*	14.6 (422)*
Free testosterone: pmol/L (ng/dL)	11 (0.33)*	60 (1.74)*	114 (3.28)*	294 (8.49)*	413 (11.9)*	504 (14.5)*
DHEAS: μmol/L (μg/dL)	2.71 (99.7)*	3.31 (121.8)*	4.04 (148.7)*	4.75 (175.0)*	5.08 (187.0)*	5.89 (217.0)*
TEBG (nmol/L)	34.6	33.3	28.4*	21.5*	14.4*	10.7*

*Duncan post-hoc analysis significant at P < 0.01.
†PS1: absence of pubic hair, testicular volume < 3 mL. PS2a: absence of pubic hair, testicular volume ≥ 3 mL. PS2b: Tanner stage 2 pubic hair. PS3-5: Tanner pubic hair stages. Modified from Biro FM, Lucky AW, Hoster GA, et al. Pubertal staging in boys. J Pediatr 1995; 127:40–46, with permission.[40a]

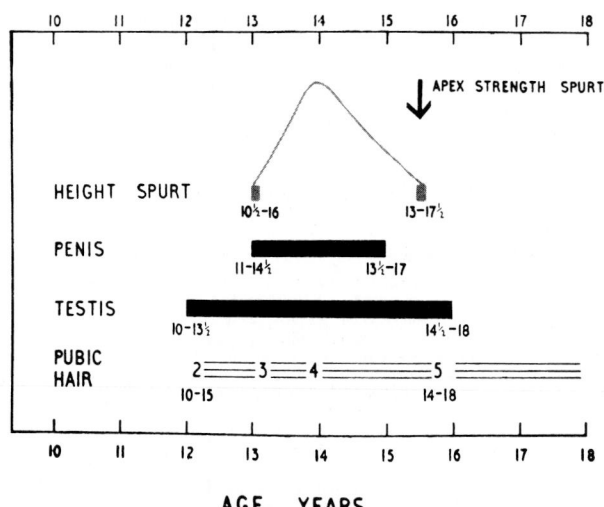

Figure 31–6. Diagram of the sequence of events at puberty in males. An average is represented in relation to the scale of ages; the range of ages within which some of the changes occur is indicated by the figures below. (From Marshall WA, Tanner JM. Variations in the pattern of pubertal changes in boys. Arch Dis Child 1970; 45:13–23.)

midline of the lower lip and, finally, to the sides and the lower border of the chin. The first stage of facial hair development usually occurs during pubic hair stage 3 (average age of 14.9 years in the United States), and the last stage occurs after pubic hair stage 5 and genital stage 5.

Axillary hair appears at approximately 14 years in boys. A total of 93% of black girls and 68% of white girls have axillary hair by age 12.[44] Axillary sweat glands begin to function as the hair appears. Circumanal hair usually appears prior to axillary hair in boys.

Comedones, acne, and seborrhea of the scalp are a consequence of the increased secretion of gonadal and adrenal steroids.[51] Early-onset acne correlates with the development of severe acne later in puberty. The most serious variety, acne fulminans, occurs mainly in pubertal males.[52] Acne vulgaris, the most prevalent skin disorder in adolescence, occurs at a mean age of 12.2 years ± 1.4 SD (range 9 to 15 years) in boys and progresses with advancement through puberty. Acne vulgaris can be the first notable sign of puberty in a girl, preceding pubic hair and breast development.[51] At late prepuberty comedones are present in many boys, and all boys have comedones by genital stage 5.

Dental hygiene is often worse in boys than girls after the onset of puberty; this is also the age when gingivitis begins and pockets form at the gum line.[49] There is a positive correlation between gonadal steroid levels in blood and the presence of the bacteria most responsible for the inflammation of gingivitis in boys and girls.[50]

Gonadal Development and Function

Female

OVARIAN DEVELOPMENT IN PUBERTY. (See Chapters 15 and 29.)[53, 53a, 54, 778] The peak number of germ cells is attained at 16 to 20 weeks of gestation. Primordial follicles appear beginning at 20 weeks of fetal life, and primary follicles develop soon thereafter. Follicle-stimulating hormone (FSH) receptors have not been detected in midtrimester human fetal ovaries, and fetal pituitary FSH is not required for proliferation of oogonia, oocyte differentiation, or formation of primordial follicles.[53] During fetal life and childhood, follicles grow to the large antral stage, but follicles that develop prior

to puberty are destined to undergo atresia[54, 55] (Fig. 31–8). During follicular growth, the oocyte enlarges, and granulosa cells are transformed from spindle-shaped to cuboidal cells that, along with the ovum, secrete the zona pellucida.[778] The granulosa cells multiply with a substantial increase in volume of the follicle, and ultimately a plasma transudate, the follicular fluid, forms in response to FSH and fills the antrum. The theca develops during the time of antrum formation. During reproductive life, the follicle undergoes luteinization or terminal differentiation into a corpus luteum, which is the major source of gonadal steroids after ovulation. After 8 d of gonadal steroid secretion in the absence of fertilization, the corpus luteum undergoes programmed cell death,[55a, 886] and cytolysis results in an avascular scar. If fertilization occurs, fetal tissue, through the secretion of human chorionic gonadotropin (hCG), inhibits apoptosis and supports the maternal corpus luteum throughout pregnancy.[54, 55, 55a]

Ultrasonographic studies (Fig. 31–9) indicate that the corpus of the uterus increases during pubertal progression from an initial tubular shape to a bulbous structure, that the length of the uterus increases from 2 to 3 cm to 5 to 8 cm,[56] and that the uterine volume increases from 0.4 to 1.6 mL to 3 to 15 mL.[57] During prepuberty the ovarian volume is 0.2 to 1.6 mL on ultrasound scans, and after the onset of puberty ovarian volume increases to 2.8 to 15 mL.[57, 58, 59] Tall girls have larger ovarian volume than average-sized girls. The multicystic appearance of the ovaries on ultrasound increases with the progression through puberty and should not be considered a sign of disease.[59]

MENARCHE. (See Chapter 15.) Menarche usually occurs during the 6 mo preceding or following the fusion of the second and first distal phalanges and the appearance of the sesamoid bone.[60] Anovulatory cycles are common in the first years after menarche. Apter and Vihko[61] reported a prevalence of 55% anovulation in the first 2 y after menarche that decreased to 20% anovulatory cycles by the fifth year; others have observed a lower number of ovulatory events shortly after menarche.[62, 63] While most pubertal females are infertile in terms of the risk of pregnancy, some are fertile, as evidenced by early teenage pregnancy.

Male

TESTICULAR DEVELOPMENT IN PUBERTY. (See Chapters 16 and 29.) During puberty the testes increase in size,

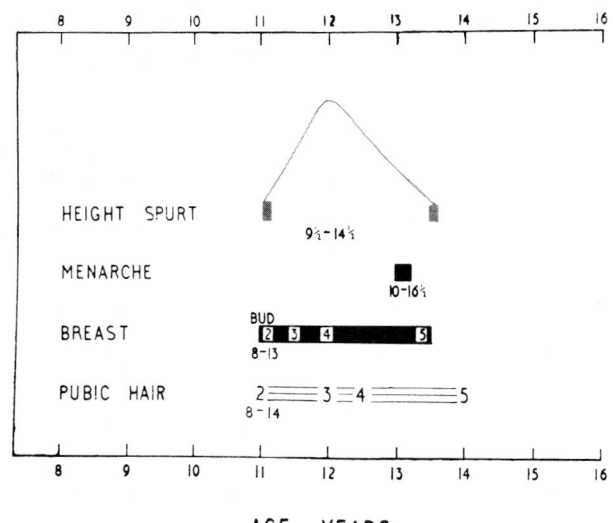

Figure 31–7. The sequence of events at puberty in females. The design of the figure is described in the legend of Figure 31–6. (From Marshall WA, Tanner JM. Variations in pattern of pubertal changes in girls. Arch Dis Child 1969; 44:291–303.)

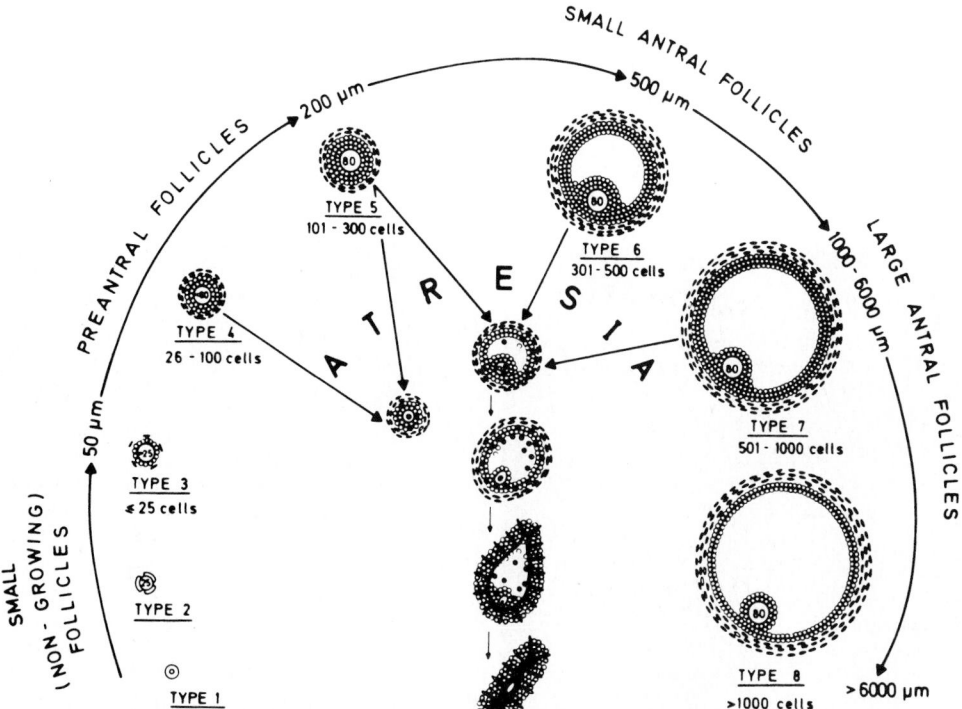

Figure 31–8. Schematic representation of the growth of ovarian follicles during infancy and childhood. Type 1 (primordial follicle) and type 2 (primary follicle) are composed of a small oocyte and a few to a ring of flat granulosa cells. In the diplotene (nesting) stage of prophase, primary follicles are the predominant form of oocyte and constitute the reservoir of cells from which follicular growth occurs. Types 3 to 5 (preantral follicles) are follicles that have entered the growth phase; the oocyte is enlarging and is surrounded by a zona pellucida, and granulosa cells increase in number and differentiate. The growth of the oocyte is complete by the end of the preantral stage, and the increased follicular size is due to follicular growth and fluid accumulation. Types 6 to 8 represent antral follicles (graafian follicles) and contain a fully grown oocyte, a large number of granulosa cells, a fluid-filled cavity, and a well-developed theca external to the basement membrane. Large preovulatory follicles are absent (10,000 to 15,000 μm). Follicular growth and atresia take place throughout childhood; all follicles that enter the growth phase become atretic, and this can occur at any stage in their development but mainly involves large antral follicles. (From Peters H, Byskov AG, Grinsted J. Follicular growth in fetal and prepubertal ovaries of humans and other primates. Clin Endocrinol Metab 1978; 7:469–485.[55])

principally because growth of the seminiferous tubules is associated with the onset of spermatogenetic activity, and because of mitoses of Sertoli cells[64] (Fig. 31–10 and Table 31–8). Testosterone production increases. The Sertoli cells are the major cell type in the seminiferous cords in prepuberty and early puberty, but germ cells predominate in the adult.[65] During puberty the Sertoli cells cease to undergo mitosis, differentiate into adult-type Sertoli cells, and form occlusive junctions that are the anatomic basis of the blood-testicular barrier. Although Leydig cells can be detected in early gestation and during the neonatal period of testosterone secretion, in childhood the interstitial tissue is composed principally of undifferentiated mesenchymal cells. With pubertal development and rising levels of serum luteinizing hormone (LH), adult-type Leydig cells appear. The seminal vesicle enlarges through childhood to puberty and eventually holds 3.4 to 4.5 mL, or 70% of the seminal fluid.[66] The mean blood flow in the testes increases to adult values in boys with a testicular volume greater than 4 mL.[67]

SPERMATOGENESIS. Spermatogenesis becomes histologically apparent between ages 11 and 15 years. Sperm can be detected in the first morning urine specimen at a mean age of 13.3 years, a phenomenon that probably reflects the maturation of spermatogenesis,[68, 69] but sperm concentration, morphology, and motility do not reach adult levels until a bone age of 17 years.[70, 71] Hence, the onset of spermatogenesis (spermarche) is a relatively early pubertal event that occurs at a mean pubic hair stage of 2.5, before the adult plasma testosterone level and peak height velocity (PHV) are attained.[68] The first conscious ejaculation occurs at a mean chronologic age of 13.5 years in normal boys and at a mean bone age of 13.5 years in boys with delayed puberty.[72] There

is a higher incidence of sperm in urine in early puberty than in late puberty, suggesting that sperm may flow continuously through the urethra in early puberty but that ejaculation is necessary for sperm to appear in the urine in late puberty.[73] The potential for fertility is reached before the adult phenotype is attained; spermaturia was present in 2 of 28 normal boys with bilateral testicular volumes of 3 mL and no other signs of puberty.[74]

Adolescent Growth

Pubertal Growth Spurt

Prepubertal height and growth velocity are similar in boys and girls. Maximal growth occurs in infancy and decreases to the nadir termed the *minimal prespurt velocity* just before the pubertal growth spurt. The pubertal growth spurt can be divided, for purposes of comparison, into three stages: the stage of minimal growth velocity in peripuberty just before the spurt (takeoff velocity); the stage of most rapid growth, or PHV; and the stage of decreased velocity and cessation of growth at epiphyseal fusion. Boys reach PHV approximately 2 y later than girls and are taller at takeoff (Fig. 31–11); PHV occurs during stages 3 to 4 of puberty in most boys (see Tables 31–3 and 31–4 and Fig. 31–5) and is completed by stage 5 in more than 95% of boys.[8, 77, 78] The pubertal growth spurt in girls occurs between stages 2 and 3 (see Table 31–2 and Fig. 31–7).[75, 76] Boys grew a mean of 28 cm and girls grew 25 cm between takeoff and cessation of growth in one study.[77] The mean height difference of 12.5 cm between adult men and women results partly from the greater prespurt growth of boys (+1.5 cm); partly from the height difference at age of takeoff,

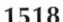

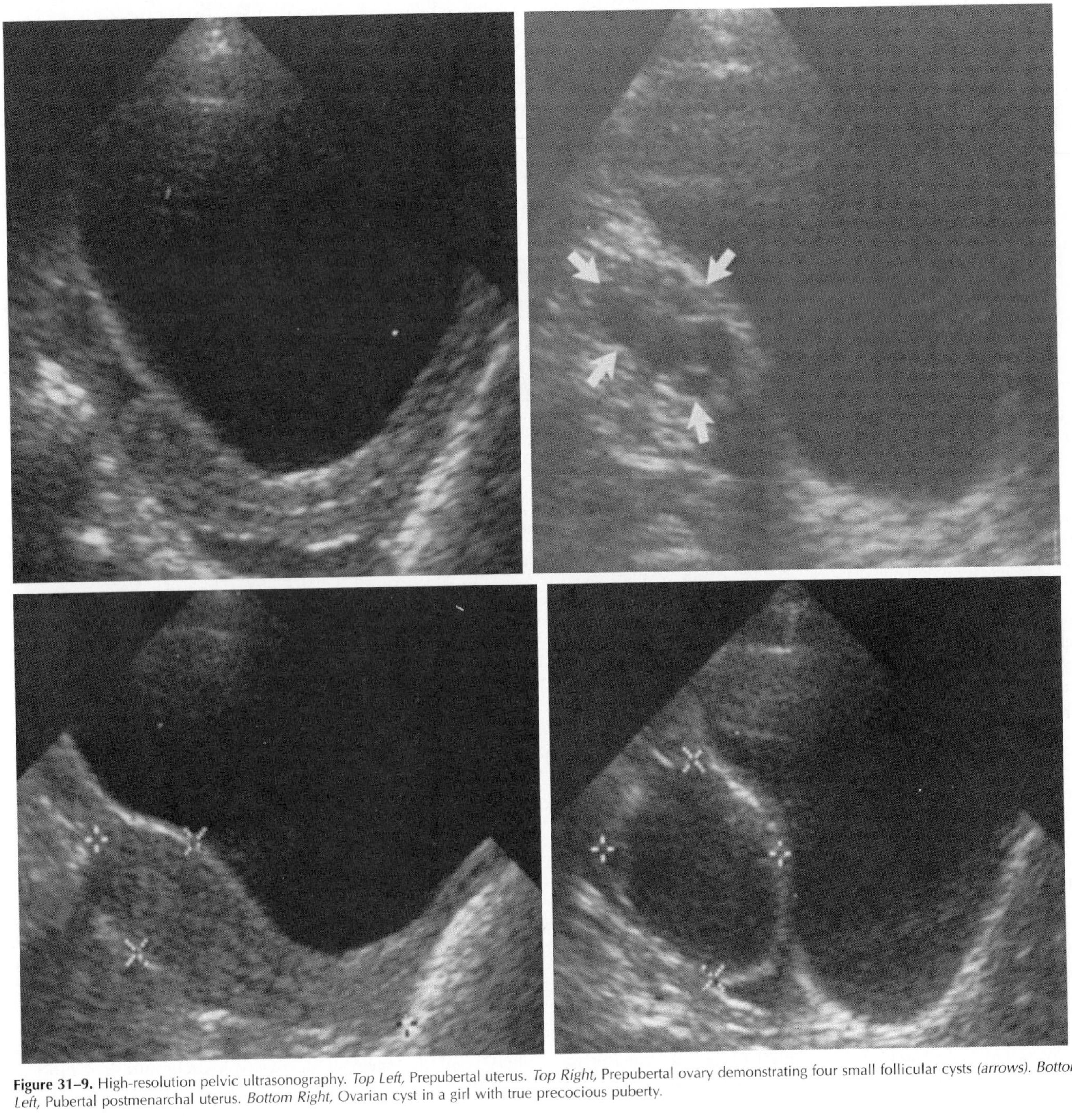

Figure 31–9. High-resolution pelvic ultrasonography. *Top Left,* Prepubertal uterus. *Top Right,* Prepubertal ovary demonstrating four small follicular cysts *(arrows). Bottom Left,* Pubertal postmenarchal uterus. *Bottom Right,* Ovarian cyst in a girl with true precocious puberty.

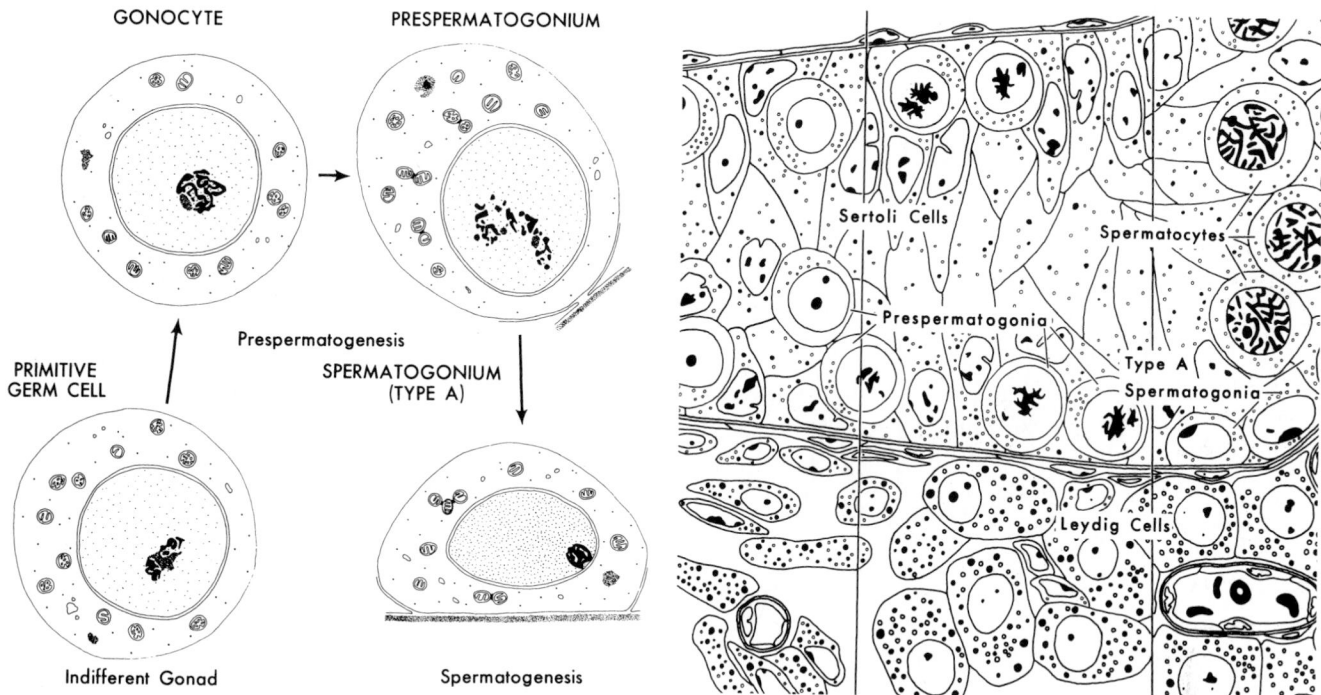

Figure 31–10. *Left,* Diagram illustrating developmental stages of testicular germ cells based on electron microscopic findings in the rabbit. Note differences between prespermatogonium and spermatogonium. *Right,* Diagram showing maturation of testicular cell types in the rabbit from prepubertal appearance at left to onset of spermatogenesis at right. Interstitial cells undergo changes in shape, size, and arrangement in the process of Leydig cell differentiation. (From Gondos B. Testicular development. In: Johnson AD, Gomes WR, eds. The Testis. Vol 4. New York: Academic, 1977: 1–37.)

with boys being taller at their later age of takeoff (+6.5 cm); partly from the greater gain in height of boys during the pubertal growth spurt (+6 cm); and partly from the greater postspurt growth in girls (−1.5 cm).[78]

A mathematical model of growth separates the infancy, childhood, and pubertal phases of growth and allows evaluation of growth despite the variation in age at onset of puberty. A slowly decelerating childhood component is the base, with a sigmoidal pubertal component added during secondary sexual development (Fig. 31–12). This model provides a new means of predicting adult height, the height adjusted for pubertal onset (HAPO) method.[79] Variations on this technique of height prediction use the ICP (infancy-childhood-puberty) growth curve either (1) without bone age (IPP) or (2) without bone age but with the use of parental height information (ICPN) when available.[80] Tanner and Davies[81] have constructed growth curves for American children (using longitudinal data from the National Center for Health Statistics and calculated data from theoretical growth curves thereafter; see Chapter 30); these curves can be adjusted for time of PHV and appear to be more useful for evaluation of the growth of individual children during adolescence than are the standard cross-sectional charts.

Many other physiological and biochemical parameters change with the onset of puberty and must be interpreted in terms of the stage of pubertal development. The mean heart

rate and maximal oxygen uptake do not change in boys with the passage of PHV, but the respiratory quotient increases at the time of PHV.[82] Levels of serum inorganic phosphate, alkaline phosphatase, and osteocalcin (Gla-protein level) and of urinary pyridinoline, deoxypyridinoline, and galactosylhydroxylysine reflect the increased osteoblastic activity and growth rate in both sexes.[83–87] Serum urate levels rise at the end of pubertal development in average boys, but obese boys experience an increase earlier in puberty.[88]

Because girls reach PHV about 1.3 y before menarche, growth potential is limited after menarche. Most girls have attained all but an average of 2.5% of their adult height by the time of menarche,[75] usually adding no more than 5 to 7.5 cm after menarche, although there is a variation from 1 to as much as 11 cm. Boys have no event comparable to menarche during pubertal development to mark the amount of remaining growth; however, boys in early puberty are likely to have significant subsequent growth, whereas in late puberty growth is limited. The ages at menarche, takeoff, and PHV are not good predictors of adult height because the duration of pubertal growth is a more important determinant of final height; later onset of puberty and the consequent increase in height at takeoff of the pubertal growth spurt can be balanced by a decrease in actual height achieved during PHV and result in no net change in adult height. However, the early onset of puberty usually diminishes ultimate adult stature,[89] whereas

TABLE 31–8. Cellular Activity in Human Testis at Different Stages of Development

Stage	Germ Cells	Sertoli Cells	Leydig Cells
Prepubertal	Prespermatogenic cells present	Predominant cells in seminiferous cords	Scattered, partially differentiated cells present
Pubertal	Initiation of spermatogenesis	Increased complexity, formation of occlusive junctions	Fully differentiated cells appear
Adult	Active spermatogenesis, predominant cells	Individual cells associated with groups of germ cells	Groups of fully differentiated cells present

From Gondos B, Kogan S. Testicular development during puberty. In: Grumbach MM, Sizonenko PC, Aubert ML, eds. Control of the Onset of Puberty, Baltimore: Williams & Wilkins, 1990: 387–398. © 1990, the Williams & Wilkins Co., Baltimore.[65]

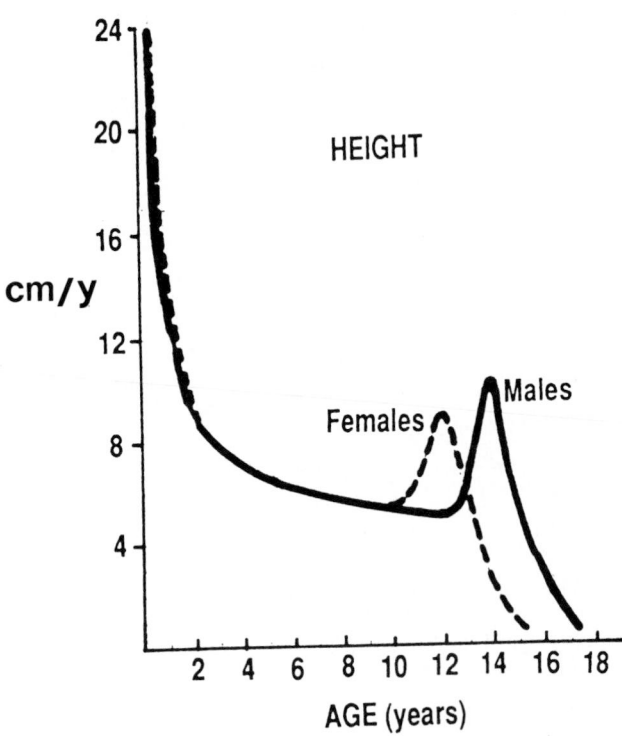

Figure 31–11. The adolescent growth spurt in boys and girls (growth velocity curves). Note the later onset and the greater peak height velocity in boys.

as the length from the top of the pubic ramus to the top of the head divided by the distance from the top of the pubic ramus to the sole of the foot, change during the peripubertal and early pubertal periods because of the elongation of the extremities.[91] The legs begin to grow before the trunk, although later in puberty, growth of the legs is similar to that of the upper torso.[92] The mean upper/lower segment ratio of white adults is 0.92, and that of black adults is 0.85. There are no differences in upper/lower segment ratio between the sexes, but the ratio of sitting height to standing height is higher in pubertal and adult females than in males.[8, 10] In general, hypogonadal individuals have delayed epiphyseal fusion and do not undergo a pubertal growth spurt; therefore, the extremities grow for a prolonged period, leading to a decreased upper/lower segment ratio and an increased span for height (eunuchoid body proportions). The distal parts of the extremities, the hands and feet, grow before the proximal parts; a rapid increase in shoe size heralds the pubertal growth spurt.

The shoulders widen in boys, whereas the hips enlarge more in girls; the ratio of biacromial (shoulder) breadth to bicristal (hip) breadth remains constant in boys at about 1.37 but decreases in girls from 1.35 to 1.27.[8, 10] The female pelvic inlet widens, mainly because of the growth of the os acetabuli.

The brain reaches 95% of adult size by the onset of puberty.[10] The head approaches the adult size by age 10, but changes in the relationships of the parts of the face are apparent during puberty. Although the mandible and nose enlarge more in boys, these bones and the maxilla, brow, frontal sinuses, and middle and posterior fossae enlarge in both sexes, mainly during the pubertal growth spurt. Children with isosexual precocity have the facial appearance of older children, and individuals with delayed puberty have the facial features of younger children. The pituitary gland enlarges more in the female during puberty. In a magnetic resonance imaging (MRI) study, the height of the pituitary gland was no greater

prolonged delay of puberty[90] can increase stature. The age at PHV and the age at initiation of puberty correlate with the rate of passage through the stages of pubertal development.[78]

Both stature and the upper/lower segment ratio, defined

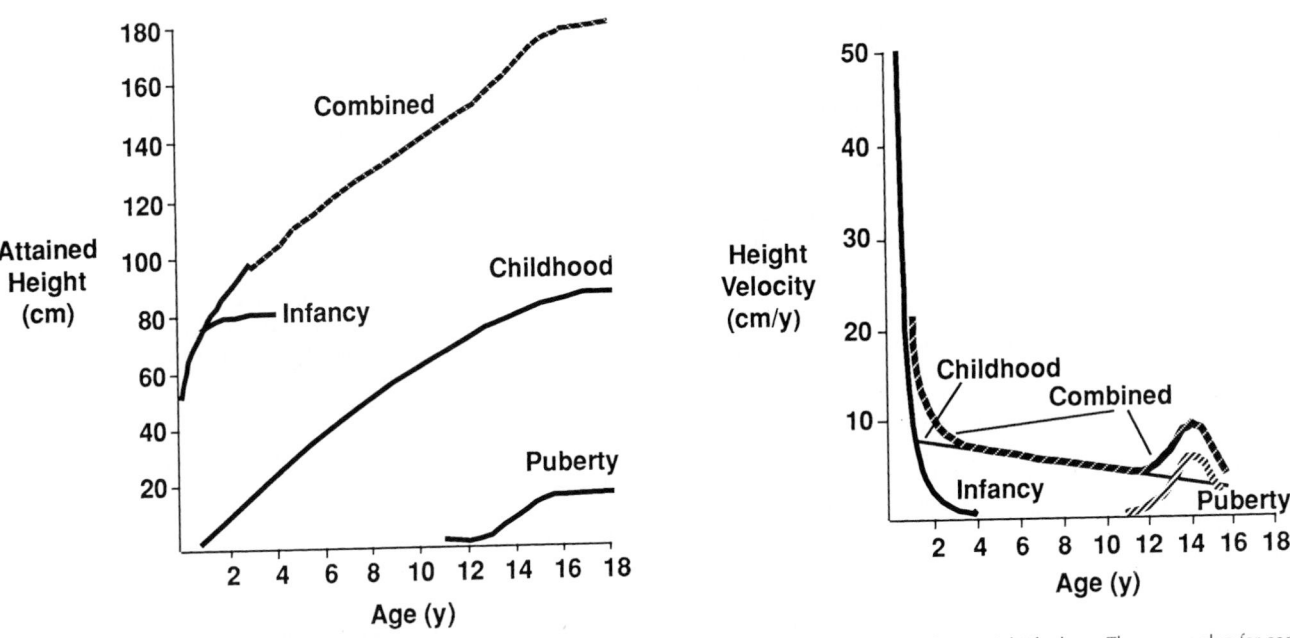

Figure 31–12. The infancy, childhood, and puberty (ICP) model of Karlberg for mean attained height (*left*) and height velocity (*right*) for boys. The mean value for each component (infancy, childhood, puberty) and their sums (combined growth, right; combined velocity, left) are plotted. The growth curve for an individual represents the additive effect of the three biologic phases of the growth process (ICP). Karlberg has provided mathematical functions for each component of his model. *Infancy:* This component starts before birth and falls off by age 3 to 4 years. It can be described by the exponential function $y = a + b[1 - \exp(-ct)]$. Average total gain in height for Swedish boys is 79.0 cm (44.0% of final height) and for girls is 76.8 cm (46.2%). *Childhood:* This phase begins at the end of the first year of life and continues to mature height. A second-degree polynomial function describes this component: $y = a + bt + ct^2$. Average total gain in height for boys is 85.2 cm (47.4%) and for girls is 78.4 cm (47.3%). *Puberty:* The model for the pubertal growth spurt is a logistic function: $y = a/[1 + \exp(-b(t - t_v))]$. Average total gain in height for boys is 15.4 cm (8.6%) and for girls is 10.9 cm (6.5%); y designates attained height at time t in years from birth; a, b, and c are constants; t_v is the age at peak height velocity. (Adapted from Karlberg J. On the construction of the infancy-childhood-puberty growth standard. Acta Paediatr Scand [Suppl] 1989; 356:26–37.)

than 6 mm before puberty, was 8 to 10 mm in teen-age females, was no greater than 7 mm in teen-age males, and was decreased in young adults of both sexes.[93]

Growth of lymphoid tissue reaches a maximum at about age 12 and thereafter decreases with pubertal progression.

Hormonal Control of the Pubertal Growth Spurt

Hormonal control of the pubertal growth spurt is complex (Figs. 31–13 and 31–14). Growth hormone (GH) increases growth at puberty through the stimulation of production of insulin-like growth factor I (IGF-I, also called somatomedin-C). Gonadal steroids have two effects on pubertal growth: (1) enhancement of GH secretion and thus enhancement of IGF-I production, and (2) a direct effect on cartilage and bone by stimulating production of local factors such as IGF-I (reviewed in references 94 and in 95). Gonadal steroids have both growth-promoting and maturational effects on chondrocytes and osteoblasts; the latter action, eventually leading to epiphyseal fusion and the cessation of longitudinal growth in both boys and girls, is mediated mainly by estrogen either secreted directly (in girls) or arising from the extraglandular conversion of testosterone and androstenedione to estrogen.[96–98] Thyroid hormone also plays an important permissive role in pubertal growth.

GROWTH HORMONE. The secretion of GH increases with pubertal development in boys and girls.[99–107] Increased GH pulse amplitude and the amount of GH secreted per pulse

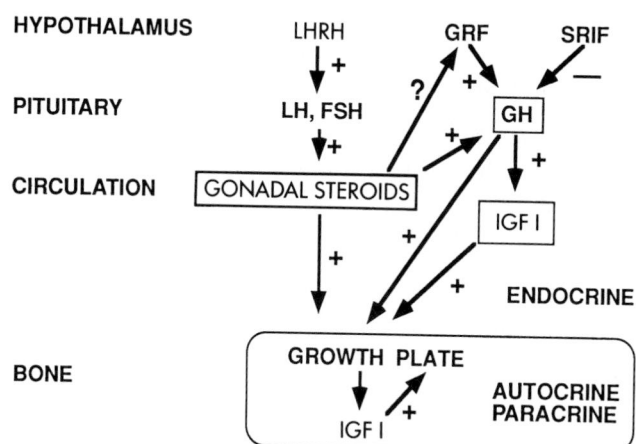

Figure 31–14. Interactions of the major growth-promoting hormones during puberty. Plus (+) indicates stimulatory action, minus (−) inhibitory action. Gonadal steroids in the circulation refer primarily to gonadal estrogens and androgens. Circulating IGF-I arises mainly from liver, but other tissues also contribute (endocrine action). Growth hormone and gonadal steroids have a direct stimulatory effect on the generation of IGF-I (paracrine action) locally in bone and cartilage cells. For simplification, the feedback loops for IGF-I and gonadal steroids on the hypothalamic-pituitary unit are omitted.

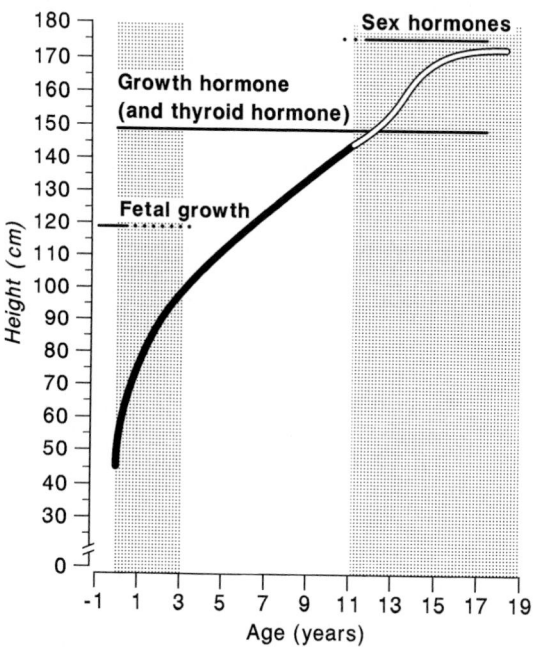

Figure 31–13. A schematic male growth chart with the features of the ICP (infancy, childhood, puberty) pattern overlaid and illustrating the predominant endocrine mechanisms controlling each phase of growth. The first shaded area emphasizes the decreasing velocity of infantile growth as the individual leaves the rapid growth phase of fetal life. The clear area is the childhood phase, which continues and magnifies the decreased velocity of growth into a plateau of rather constant growth during childhood. These two phases depend, in large part, on the effects of GH and thyroid hormone with no or little effect derived from gonadal steroids. Finally, the period of the pubertal growth spurt in which gonadal steroids exert their direct and indirect effects. Gonadal steroids exert direct effects on the bone by stimulating the generation of IGF-I and other growth factors locally, and exert indirect effects by stimulating increased GH secretion which, in turn, exerts its own effects on bone and stimulates the production of IGF-I. In the female, the major gonadal steroid involved in the pubertal growth spurt is estradiol, whereas in the male, testosterone and estradiol (arising mainly from the aromatization of testosterone) are the major gonadal steroids.

are mainly responsible for the augmented GH levels in the basal state.[105, 108] The increase in GH secretion occurs earlier in girls coincident with the onset of breast development (Tanner stage 2) and is maximal at Tanner stage 3 to 4 breast development; in boys the increase occurs later and peaks at stage 4 genital development. Levels of GH and IGF-I decrease from the higher pubertal values to adult values after late puberty in both sexes. Stimulated GH secretion also increases at puberty[109, 110]; indeed, a study of 88 subjects of normal height found that in 61% of prepubertal children GH peak levels did not increase above 7 ng/mL after exercise, arginine, or levodopa, only 56% met the 7 ng/mL level by stage 2, 89% met the level by stage 3, and 100% did so at stages 4 and 5.[109] Remarkably, hexarelin, a six-amino-acid GH-releasing peptide, stimulates as much GH release during prepuberty as it does in puberty, in contrast to the changes in response to other secretagogues with puberty.[111] The increase in serum gonadal steroid levels is the major cause of the higher GH secretion during puberty, as pubertal serum levels of both estrogen and testosterone promote GH release. The effect, however, is mediated mainly through estrogen, as evidenced by the facts that estrogen receptor blockade with tamoxifen decreases GH secretion in boys and that the administration of androgens that cannot be aromatized to estrogen (e.g., oxandrolone and dihydrotestosterone) has less effect on GH secretion than the administration of testosterone, which is aromatized to estrogen. Contrariwise, administration of the androgen receptor inhibitor flutamide increases GH secretion.[112–114] Dihydrotestosterone, which is not aromatized to estrogen, does not increase GH secretion or the plasma concentration of IGF-I, may even inhibit the integrated GH secretion, but stimulates growth, suggesting a direct effect of androgen on growth independent of GH[94, 114] or estradiol. GH secretion is increased in sexual precocity and decreases with the fall in gonadal steroid levels after treatment of children with true precocious puberty with luteinizing hormone–releasing hormone (LHRH) agonists.[100, 115, 116]

Patients with isolated GH deficiency[117] or GH resistance[118] have an attenuated pubertal growth spurt, indicating the importance of GH and IGF-I in this form of rapid growth. Individuals with severe primary or secondary hypogonadism have a minimal or no pubertal growth spurt, demonstrating the critical role of gonadal steroids in pubertal growth. Patients deficient in both GH and gonadotropins do not have an adolescent growth spurt when GH alone is replaced; gonadal steroids must also be given, substantiating the interaction of GH and gonadal steroids in the pubertal growth spurt.[92, 119] However, in normal puberty neither the magnitude of the increase in GH secretion nor the level of plasma IGF-I correlates with the PHV of the pubertal growth spurt. Thus although a threshold level of GH secretion is necessary, the extent of the growth spurt correlates with gonadal steroid secretion. Individuals with both true precocious puberty and GH deficiency (usually a consequence of cranial irradiation for a brain tumor) can exhibit a growth spurt almost as great as that of children with true precocious puberty and normal GH secretion.[94] After treatment with an LHRH agonist for sexual precocity, children with GH deficiency and true precocious puberty have a slowing of growth velocity along with suppression of pubertal progression,[94] illustrating the direct effects of gonadal steroids on the pubertal growth spurt.

Plasma IGF-I levels increase during puberty and reach an earlier peak in girls than in boys[116, 120] and then decrease to adult levels (Fig. 31–15). Increased GH secretion at puberty induces the increase in IGF-I level, and the increase in both hormones is temporally associated with the pubertal growth spurt. The rise in both GH and IGF-I secretion at the onset of puberty suggests transient relative resistance of the hypothalamic-pituitary GH feedback mechanism to IGF-I, a suppressor of GH release, possibly related to the effect of estrogen. The plasma level of IGF-I is high for chronologic age in sexual precocity and low in delayed puberty. Although the precise role of gonadal steroids in the pubertal increase in IGF-I levels is uncertain, the major effect appears to be mediated through increased secretion of GH and IGF-I,[116] and through enhanced local generation of IGF-I in cartilage and bone.[94] Bone contains receptors for both estrogen and androgen as well as the enzyme aromatase. Studies of patients with true precocious puberty show elevated serum GH levels in the untreated state and suppressed GH levels for age and a decrease of plasma IGF-I concentration, but not to prepubertal values, after treatment with an LHRH agonist, further indicating that GH is the major factor that increases IGF-I levels in puberty.[115, 116]

GONADAL STEROIDS. The adolescent growth spurt in normal girls and boys depends on both estradiol and GH.[96–98] A pubertal growth spurt, which leads to a final height that is close to that of normal men, occurs in 46,XY women with the complete form of androgen resistance,[121] a finding that

supports the critical role of estrogen in the adolescent growth spurt. The detection of estrogen resistance due to a null mutation in the gene encoding the estrogen receptor and of derangements in the aromatase (CYP19) gene leading to severe aromatase deficiency also indicates a major role of estradiol, but not testosterone, in epiphyseal maturation, and normal skeletal proportions and mineralization in both sexes.[96–98] Further, plasma estradiol levels in prepubertal boys correlate with the pubertal growth rate.[122] The serum estrogen level also correlates with the serum testosterone level, but not with that of serum GH, again implicating estrogen in the pubertal growth spurt and skeletal maturation of boys and girls.

Children with chronic adrenal insufficiency who are given appropriate replacement therapy have a normal pubertal growth spurt despite deficient adrenal androgen secretion, indicating a minimal impact of adrenal androgens on growth at puberty.[123]

Thyroid hormone is a requisite for normal growth. Children with primary hypothyroidism may not have a growth spurt even when the disorder is accompanied by sexual precocity[124] (see the section on juvenile hypothyroidism).

Bone Age

Skeletal maturation is assessed by comparing radiographs of the hand, the knee, or the elbow with standards of maturation in a normal population.[125, 126] Ossification centers appear in early life, the bones mature in shape and size and develop articulation of surfaces, and ultimately the epiphyses or growth plates fuse with the shafts. In normal children, bone age, an index of physiological maturation, does not have a well-defined relationship to the onset of puberty and is as variable as chronologic age. However, bone age is useful for predicting age at menarche and correlates in delayed puberty better with the onset of secondary sexual development than does chronologic age. The relation between the initiation of the pubertal growth spurt and the rate of maturation of bone age is uncertain. Some studies suggest a strong relationship between the timing of the pubertal growth spurt and the rate of skeletal maturation,[127] and that the timing and rate of growth in stature and the rate of skeletal maturation are tightly integrated genetic processes.[128] Another view is that while the PHV occurs during a limited range of bone ages, the takeoff of the pubertal spurt occurs during a wider range of bone ages.[129] In addition, bone age, height, and chronologic age can be used to predict final adult height from the Bayley-Pinneau tables[130] or with the Roche-Wainer-Thissen (RWT),[131] Tanner-Whitehouse,[126] or Walker[132] techniques. Separate standards are used for boys and girls; skeletal maturation is more advanced in girls than in boys of the same age. For example, the bone ages of 11 years in girls and 13 in boys (bone ages of early puberty in each sex) are equivalent stages of bone maturation. Although there are no separate standards of bone age, black children have slightly more advanced bone ages than do white children of the same chronologic age.[133] A difference between bone age and chronologic age must exceed 2 SD (according to tables available in the respective bone age atlases) to be of biologic significance. As commonly estimated, bone age is an imprecise, qualitative measure. Development of techniques for scanning radiographs and computer analysis should increase the precision of the procedure.[134–136]

The estimation of skeletal age may be confounded by asymmetrical conditions. For example, children with hemiplegia due to cerebral palsy have a less advanced bone age on the affected side than on the normal side.[137] This difference (mean of 7.3 months) is greater than the differences between the left and the right sides in normal children (less than 6 months).

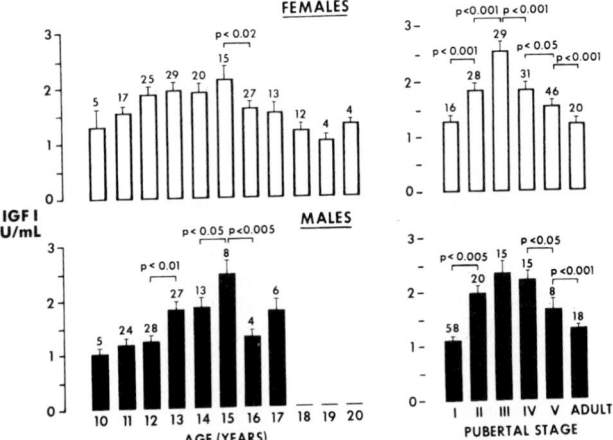

Figure 31–15. Serum IGF-I (also called somatomedin-C, SM-C) in females and males stratified by age (left) and by pubertal stage (right). Males attain peak IGF-I levels at 15 years (2.5 ± 0.2 U/mL) at pubertal (genital) stage 3 (2.3 ± 0.2 U/mL). IGF-I concentrations reach a plateau between ages 12 and 15 in females (about 2 U/mL) and peak at pubertal (breast) stage 3 (2.5 ± 0.2 U/mL). The mean concentrations during puberty are higher than both adult and prepubertal values.

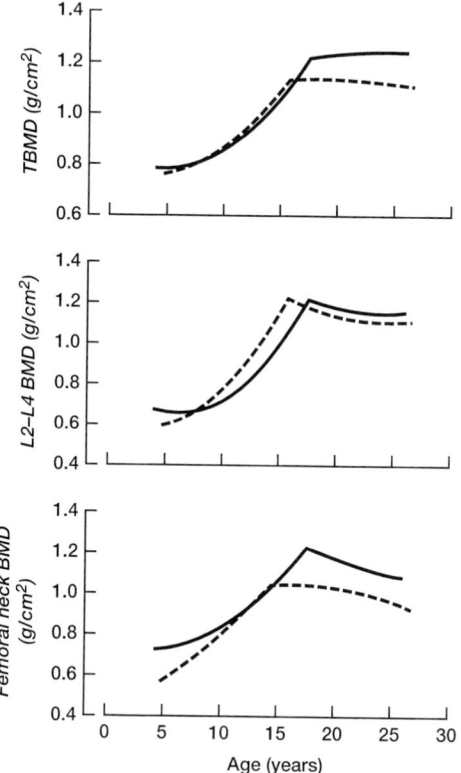

Figure 31–16. Mean predictions for bone mineral density are plotted to show sex differences. Males, *solid lines;* females, *dotted lines.* There was no sex difference in total bone mineral density (TBMD) until the late teen years, when TBMD became higher in males. Girls had an earlier increase in age related L2-L4 BMD, but no sex differences occurred in peak L2-4 BMD nor was there a sex difference in femoral neck BMD. (From Lu PW, Briody JN, Ogle GD, et al. Bone mineral density of total body, spine, and femoral neck in children and young adults: a cross-sectional and longitudinal study. J Bone Miner Res 1994; 9:1451–1458, with permission.[155])

Skeletal Density

Bone mineral density (BMD) increases throughout childhood, but the major increases occur during the first 3 years of life and during pubertal growth, a plateau being reached at or after the end of puberty.[138–147] Bone mineral density of the total body, lumbar spine, and femoral neck increases at a mean annual rate of 0.047 g/cm² for boys and 0.039 g/cm²

for girls. A peak is reached at 17.5 years for boys and 15.8 years for girls (although femoral neck BMD peaks at 14.1 years); the difference in the timing of the peak is related to the difference in the time of PHV.[144–148] The peak bone mass is reached after the PHV of puberty, a factor that may result in a period of increased fragility and susceptibility to trauma.[148] While cortical bone density of the lumbar spine increases predictably with age, cancellous bone density does not correlate with age until the later stages of puberty.[149] The increase in BMD correlates with height, weight, age, pubertal development, and body mass index (BMI) but has less relationship with serum IGF-I.[150, 151] Weight is a main determinant of bone density in postpubertal girls.[152] The strength of the femoral head increases markedly during puberty, and the femoral neck increases in density more with impact loading sports such as running than with active loading sports such as swimming (Fig. 31–16 and Table 31–9).[153] The latter table contains bone volumetric density, BMD (g/cm³), which corrects, in part, for variations in bone size.[154, 155]

Bone density accrual is related to calcium intake.[156, 157] The calcium intake of girls during puberty is commonly below recommended levels, and recommended levels may be too low for optimal bone mineralization.[140, 158] Black children retain more calcium than white children, and the bone structure is thicker in black children.[159] The difference in vertebral bone density appears to develop by late puberty, as there is no prepubertal difference between the two ethnic groups.[160] Extra calcium administration may increase bone accretion and may be accomplished with increased intake of dairy products,[161–164] but the effect of increased ingestion of calcium may last only as long as the calcium is actually administered.[165] Increased calcium intake does not disturb magnesium balance. Administration of testosterone to normal prepubertal boys and hypogonadal men increases calcium retention and bone growth,[166, 167] an effect mediated mainly by conversion of testosterone to estradiol in peripheral tissues, including bone. Increased thickness of bone in boys is the cause of increased bone mineral content, rather than an increase in actual bone density.[168]

Absence or delay of puberty impairs bone accretion in both sexes and is mainly a consequence of estrogen deficiency due either to decreased estrogen secretion or to impaired peripheral aromatization of androgens. Boys with constitutional delay in puberty are reported to have decreased bone density as adults.[169, 170] Treatment of hypogonadotropic hypogonadism in boys with testosterone raises serum osteocalcin levels and increases bone density.[171] Individuals with Kline-

TABLE 31–9. Bone Mineral Density (BMD) and Bone Volumetric Density (BMDᵥₒₗ) at the Spine and Femoral Neck in Study Subjects*

Age (y)	Spine (L2-4)		Femoral Neck	
	BMD (g/cm²)	BMD_{vol} (g/cm³)	BMD (g/cm²)	BMD_{vol} (g/cm³)
Females	(n = 37)		(n = 32)	
7–9	0.712±0.124	0.282±0.053	0.692±0.079	0.345±0.023
10–11	0.808±0.093	0.304±0.033	0.810±0.061	0.388±0.029
12–13	0.957±0.097	0.330±0.039	0.924±0.101	0.402±0.065
14–15	1.091±0.179	0.355±0.046	1.056±0.207	0.456±0.070
16–17	1.115±0.162	0.355±0.045	0.981±0.122	0.406±0.047
18–20	1.118±0.116	0.356±0.032	0.962±0.072	0.390±0.018
Males	(n = 28)		(n = 20)	
7–9	0.708±0.058	0.260±0.012	0.824	0.446
10–11	0.740±0.097	0.282±0.042	0.965±0.072	0.451±0.055
12–13	0.800±0.041	0.300±0.023	0.910±0.119	0.377±0.048
14–15	1.055±0.093	0.329±0.027	1.169±0.132	0.447±0.040
16–17	1.100±0.088	0.333±0.034	1.044±0.096	0.391±0.044
18–20	1.217±0.129	0.341±0.028	1.258±0.109	0.440±0.026

*Values are means ± SD.

From Kröger H, Kotaniemi A, Kröger L, et al. Development of bone mass and bone density of the spine and femoral neck—a prospective study of 65 children and adolescents. Bone Miner 1993; 23:171–182.[143]

felter's syndrome and decreased testosterone concentrations have decreased bone density; full testosterone replacement is recommended at puberty to avoid this outcome.[172] Loss of bone density also occurs in girls with anorexia nervosa, hypothalamic amenorrhea, or ovarian failure.[173, 174] Children with true precocious puberty have increased bone density, but treatment with LHRH agonists decreases bone density again.[175–179] Bone density is increased in women with excess androgens.[180, 180a, 181] Bone density is decreased in GH-deficient children and becomes more severe in the absence of GH replacement during puberty.[182]

The bone density of children of parents with osteoporosis is decreased, demonstrating the importance of genetic factors in bone accretion during adolescence. Indeed, there is a relationship of bone density between generations when the effects of age and puberty are eliminated.[183, 184]

Bone turnover is reflected by changes in biochemical markers,[83] such as bone-specific alkaline phosphatase, osteocalcin, and urinary deoxpyridinoline, which peak at midpuberty and decrease thereafter. Lesser changes in bone density are reflected in levels of plasma carboxyterminal pyridinoline cross-linked telopeptide, immunoreactive urinary pyridinolines, and urinary galactosylhydroxylysine. Estrogen levels correlate negatively with bone turnover.[185]

Body Composition

Body composition and energy requirements change during puberty.[186, 187] Lean body mass, skeletal mass, and body fat are equal in prepubertal boys and girls, but mature men have 1.5 times the lean body mass and almost 1.5 times the skeletal mass of women, whereas women have twice as much body fat.[187–193]

The increase in lean body mass starts at 6 years in girls and 9.5 years in boys. Weight is not necessarily a reflection of body fat: BMI, calculated as weight/height^2 is useful in assessing the shape of the body in age-adjusted terms,[194] and the use of weight/height$^{2.88}$ is used as an index of obesity unrelated to age or height; the mean values are 12.74 in boys and 12.45 in girls prior to stage 4 pubertal development.[195] Other easily performed measurements of body fat, such as triceps skinfold, are also used but require training. MRI can be employed to quantify abdominal (visceral) fat.[196] Fat oxidation increases in prepubertal obese children compared with nonobese children, apparently limiting the tendency to become more obese.[197]

Hips enlarge with pubertal development in girls and there is no change in waist circumference, so that the waist/hip ratio drops; the waist/hip ratios of various ethnic groups develop differently.[198] The usual distribution of fat in males (central fat or apple-shaped; android) is different from that in females (lower body fat predominance or pear-shaped; gynoid).[199, 200] Furthermore, girls at breast stage 2 with predominant fat on the hips have higher estrogen and gonadotropin levels, and girls with predominant fat in the abdomen have lower androgen/estrogen ratios, probably because of increased aromatization of androgens to estrogens in adipose tissue.[200] Fat distribution and testosterone-binding globulin (TeBG; sex hormone–binding globulin) levels may be related.[201]

A "strength spurt" occurs during puberty after the pubertal growth spurt.[8, 10, 186] The discrepancy in adult strength between men and women is due partly to the fact that men have more muscle cells and partly to the greater size of individual muscle cells; the muscle mass is 54% of body weight in adolescent boys and 42% of body weight in adolescent girls. With the change in fat composition, body water increases by 5% in men and decreases by 5% in women. Whereas extracellular water is about 25% of body weight in boys and girls, intracellular water increases at puberty in boys from 36 to 39% and decreases in girls from 36 to 29%. Frisch and Revelle[202] pointed out the relation between menarche and the maintenance of menstrual function and the percentage and absolute amount of body fat.

By 9 to 10 years of age, black girls have a higher caloric intake, ingest more fat, and engage in less physical activity than white girls: by 9 to 10 years the incidence of obesity is higher in black girls than in white girls.[203] Black and white girls have an equal prevalence of dieting, but black girls more frequently attempt to gain weight, usually by parental influence, possibly related to the average 20-pound greater weight of their mothers.[45, 204]

At 10 years of age there is increased concern about eating and weight gain in girls compared to boys.[205] Excessive weight in childhood correlates with adult mortality.[205, 206]

Blood Pressure

Basal systolic and diastolic blood pressures increase with age, weight, height, surface area, and pubertal stage[207–210] at the time of puberty, as does the rise in systolic blood pressure induced by exercise. Postmenarcheal girls have higher blood pressure than premenarcheal girls.[206] In sexual precocity, blood pressure increases above prepubertal levels in proportion to body size.[211] A circadian rhythm of blood pressure, with values lowest at 2300 to 0530 h, is more common in midpubertal individuals (80 to 90%) than in early or prepubertal subjects (50%), suggesting development of a circadian pacemaker.[212] Blood pressure in adolescence is responsive to stress, making it difficult to measure resting blood pressure in a brief clinic visit.[207] Blood pressure in childhood and adolescence is predictive of adult blood pressure. While blood pressure is higher at certain chronologic ages in black adolescents than in white adolescents, this difference appears to be due to the earlier pubertal maturation in black children.[210]

HEMATOPOIETIC SYSTEM. Testosterone induces an increase in the concentration of hemoglobin and in the red blood cell mass at puberty.

BEHAVIORAL CHANGES OF PUBERTY

The prolongation of adolescence, from the ages of 11 years to 20 years in America, dates to no more than the last 100 y in Western society. In the "less-developed, simpler societies,"[213] the acquisition of an adult role in society occurs within a few years of achievement of reproductive maturity. In general, the more technologically advanced the society, the more protracted the time society relegates to adolescent psychosocial development.[214]

The most important psychological and psychosocial changes in adolescence are the emergence of abstract thinking, the growing ability of absorbing the perspectives or viewpoints of others, an increased ability of introspection, the development of personal and sexual identity, the establishment of a system of values, increasing autonomy from family and personal independence, greater importance of peer relationships of sometimes subcultural quality, and the emergence of skills and coping strategies to overcome problems and crises.[201]

The process may be divided into early, middle, and late adolescence.[213] Ages 11 to 15 years, early adolescence, is the time of most of the biologic changes of puberty outlined in this chapter, the profound social change from the sheltered, single-classroom environment of elementary school to the multiple-classroom and multiple-teacher experience of junior high school, the wide exposure to new peers often with different life experiences and behavior patterns, and maturing, but not mature, abstract thought and decision-making processes developing out of the concrete reasoning of childhood. Middle adolescence, ages 15 to 17 years, the high school years, is a calmer period, as the school experience is not a wrenching change from the past and most of the biologic changes of puberty are past. Partial independence becomes an issue, as some increased autonomy is accepted by societies in the form of driver's licenses while the individual still lives at home. The adolescent emotionally moves away from the family and is less influenced by the peer group than are early adolescents; friendships are increasingly important. Late adolescence may be considered to start at the senior year of high school and is the time of assuming adult roles in work and in relation to the family and community. Individuals who attend a college have a more prolonged time to achieve these changes than do those who do not.

Early and middle adolescence is the period of introduction to sexuality for some, but not for most, teen-agers. The incidence of sexual intercourse in urban teen-age girls increased between 1971 and 1981 more than 50% in white girls, with 17.3% of white girls and 23.2% of black girls reporting sexual intercourse at 15 years, and 39.5% of white girls and 46.7% of black girls reporting sexual intercourse by 17 years of age.[221] The mean age at first intercourse is 17.5 years for white boys, 15.5 years for black boys, 17 years for Latino boys, 18.5 years for white girls, 17.5 years for black girls, and 18.5 years for Latino girls.[222]

Fertility is attained before adult phenotype is acquired, and the lack of forethought and planning in early and middle adolescence contributes to the remarkable rate of teen-age pregnancy in the United States[218, 219]; one million adolescents become pregnant in the United States each year, a rate of 110 per 100,000. However, the number of pregnancies has decreased during the last 20 years in adolescents; namely, a 27% decrease in pregnancies in black 15- to 17-year-olds (99.5 to 72.9 per 1000), and a 6% decrease in whites (25.7 to 24.1 per 1000). At the same time, abortions increased among teen-agers.[223]

At the beginning of the century, Hall[224] characterized the maturing child restrained by cultural influences as experiencing "Sturm und Drang" (storm and stress), and many depictions of adolescent turmoil followed. Contrary to this view, which is prominent in the popular mind and press, most empirical studies describe adolescent development as a continuous, adaptive phase of emotional growth characterized by stability, rather than disorder, and harmonious relationships between generations, rather than conflict.[214, 215] In a longitudinal study of 320 first-year high school students in the United States followed for 4 y, and of 64 followed for 8 y, 25% experienced "continuous growth" characterized by smooth, well-adjusted function despite stressful situations; 34% experienced "surgent growth" demonstrating good adaptation in general but short periods of difficulty and distress after some stressful situations; and 21% were judged to be in "turmoil (the tumultuous group) characterized by mood swings, anxiety, and depression. Thus 79% had successful adaptive development, and the tumultuous 21% came mainly from homes characterized by conflict, familial mental illness, and socioeconomic distress.[225] Furthermore, many individuals with adolescent turmoil "do not grow out of it" when studied 5 y later and are eventually diagnosed with unipolar and bipolar depressive disorders.[226] On balance, about 80 to 90% of adolescents do well during puberty and are happy individuals, and 10 to 20% have significant difficulties.[228] The normal fluctuation of mood over the period of hours or days due to the adolescent developmental process should be differentiated from long-standing mood and behavior changes of serious psychopathology, the "turmoil" that reflects actual psychopathology and will require diagnosis and treatment.[213]

A variety of psychopathologic states increase in prevalence during adolescence. Panic attack first appears during pu-

berty.[229] Migraine headaches are rare before puberty but begin to appear at this stage.[230] The frequency of attempted suicide increases abruptly, and suicide is fourth as a cause of death among 15- to 19-year-olds.[214, 215] Adolescents who commit suicide have the onset of depression in childhood or early puberty, but the act occurs later in puberty.[231] An estimated 1.7 to 5.5% of adolescents have seasonal affective disorders,[232] and the frequency of depression is equal in pubertal boys and girls.[233] Schizophrenia usually starts no earlier than puberty. Some psychiatric conditions in children and adolescents do not readily fit the categories in the *Diagnostic and Statistical Manual of Mental Disorders*, Fourth Edition (DSM-IV).[234] A longitudinal study of childhood-onset schizophrenia described changes in affected children on brain MRI and positron-emission tomography (PET) scans.[235]

Adolescents who remain at lower levels of cognitive complexity or concrete thinking and have an early onset of puberty have an increased incidence of risk-taking behavior.[236] The age at which an adolescent starts smoking cigarettes and using alcohol is proportional to the age at onset of puberty; earlier maturing girls and boys partake earlier.[220, 237] The changes in behavior in adolescents are related to the changes in gonadal steroid levels.[217, 227, 238, 239] Aggressive behavior appears to decrease through puberty, although some adolescents retain such tendencies throughout development; there is, however, no relationship between the actual serum concentrations of testosterone, TeBG, or adrenal androgens and violent, unmanageable behavior (conduct disorders).[240–247]

Sexuality correlates with testosterone production in boys in some studies, but in others it appears more related to social effects of pubertal maturation.[243] The hormonal influences on female sexual behavior may follow the same pattern.[244] Nonetheless, the earlier onset of puberty today compared with previous centuries has had a profound effect on societal norms of sexual behavior.[245, 246]

A negative self-image is common in girls at the beginning of puberty, but body image improves with breast development.[216] The onset of eating disorders is earlier in the affected girls with an earlier onset of puberty; it appears that prevention of eating disorders must start before puberty.[247, 248]

Sleep patterns change in puberty; left to their own devices adolescents would stay up later and awaken hours later than a normal weekday schedule would allow.[249] Daytime sleepiness is prevalent. This change to eveningness from morningness appears to be biologic in origin.[250] Changes in electroencephalographic patterns during puberty indicate an increasing complexity of brain function during this period.[251]

The timing of the onset of puberty affects psychosocial development. In general, early-developing boys are perceived to be more mature and are given more leadership roles and are accepted as smarter and more attractive by their peers. Late-developing boys are more insecure and more vulnerable to peer pressure, especially in working class and minority groups. On the other hand, early-maturing girls tend to experience more difficulty, especially in junior high school, where they may attract the attention of older, more mature boys. Late-maturing girls are usually more comfortable, remaining within the support structure of their families longer, and are less often brought to medical attention than late-maturing boys.[217]

HORMONAL AND METABOLIC CHANGES IN PUBERTY (Table 31–10)

Puberty is a stage in a continuum extending from sexual differentiation and the ontogeny of the hypothalamic-pituitary–gonadotropin-gonadal apparatus in the fetus to the com-

TABLE 31–10. Cardinal Hormonal Characteristics of Puberty

Increased amplitude and frequency of LH pulses (initially at night)
Increased LH response to intravenous LHRH
Increased estradiol secretion in girls and testosterone secretion in boys
Increased GH secretion
Increased serum IGF–I concentration
Increased prolactin secretion in girls

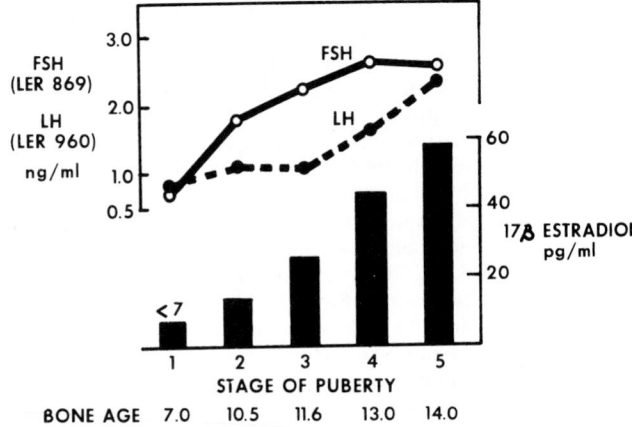

Figure 31–17. Mean plasma estradiol, FSH, and LH concentrations in prepubertal and pubertal females by pubertal stage of maturation (1 = prepubertal; 5 = menstruating adolescents) and the mean bone age for each stage. Single daytime values of gonadotropins have limited usefulness because of pulsatility of gonadotropin release and the increased amplitude of LH pulses during sleep through puberty. The gonadal steroid values, however, are useful in determining the stage of pubertal development. To convert FSH values (LER-869) to international units per liter, multiply by 8.4. To convert LH values (LER-960) to international units per liter, multiply by 3.8. To convert estradiol values to picomoles per liter, multiply by 3.671. (From Grumbach MM. Onset of puberty. In: Berenberg SR, ed. Puberty, Biologic and Social Components. Leiden: H. E. Stenfert Kroese, 1975: 1–21. Reprinted by permission of Kluwer Academic Publishers.[1])

pletion of sexual maturation.[252, 253] Changes in the CNS and increased frequency and amplitude of LHRH secretion at puberty initiate and regulate increases in the secretion of pituitary gonadotropins and gonadal steroids, which culminate in sexual maturity and fertility.

Gonadotropins

The pulsatile secretion of LHRH causes pulsatile secretion of gonadotropins. Plasma levels of LH and FSH in the fetus rise after the establishment of the hypothalamic-pituitary portal system until midgestation and then decrease toward term as inhibitory control begins to function; mean levels of fetal plasma FSH are higher in females than in males.[53, 253, 254] During the first 2 y after birth, plasma levels of LH and FSH rise intermittently to adult values and occasionally higher. Then, from middle childhood, plasma levels of FSH and LH remain low until puberty. Ultrasensitive assays for LH and FSH[255–259] document that pulsatile secretion of the gonadotropins occurs during prepuberty[260–263] and that the basal immunoreactive levels of LH are lower than initially reported.[255–257] Amplitude of LH secretion increases approximately 2 y before the onset of secondary sexual development and has been detected in boys with a testicular volume of 3 mL, but not at 1 to 2 mL; amplitude increases about 28-fold, whereas the frequency of LH pulses through the onset of puberty increases only 1.8-fold.[258] The serum FSH level is higher than the LH level in prepubertal boys and girls.[254] The temporal concordance of LH and FSH pulses is about 43%. Primary testicular failure causes enhanced amplitude and frequency of both FSH and LH pulses.[252, 261]

In the prepubertal period, measurements of LH provide indirect evidence of a diurnal variation of LHRH secretion, with a preponderance at night; the frequency is very similar to that of the early pubertal period, although the amplitude of LH pulses does not increase until the peripubertal period.[257, 259, 264–266] During this stage, enhanced release of LH can first be shown in response to intravenous LHRH, and pulsatile LH secretion is augmented during sleep.[262, 265, 267–272] During puberty, the episodic secretion of FSH and LH becomes more clear-cut as the amplitude and frequency of the gonadotropin pulses increase.[270–272] The amplitude and frequency of such peaks increase, and daytime secretion becomes apparent with the progression of pubertal development.[255, 256, 261, 263, 265, 266, 270, 272, 273] Single daytime serum measurements do not reliably indicate the stage of puberty. Nonetheless, studies of a large number of individuals using single daytime samples indicate that changes in the mean serum gonadotropin levels increase between prepuberty and puberty.[274–278] In girls, FSH levels rise during the early stages, and LH levels tend to rise in the later stages; from beginning to late puberty, the LH concentration rises over 100-fold. In boys, FSH levels rise progressively through puberty, and LH levels rise and reach an early plateau (Figs. 31–17 and 31–18).[257, 275–280]

Improved, more sensitive assays indicate that basal levels of serum LH and FSH in early pubertal subjects are lower than previous assays indicated. The basal values of serum LH and FSH with such assays are thought to predict the onset of pubertal development as well as the results of LHRH test-

ing.[274, 279, 281, 1092] For example, a random value of serum LH greater than 0.3 IU/mL measured by immunochemiluminometric assay is consistent with the onset of puberty.[1092] Serum LH amplitude increases strikingly in early puberty and in later male prepuberty, and FSH rises through male puberty owing to increased amplitude, but not frequency.[257, 282, 283] Moreover, measurement of LH and FSH with ultrasensitive assays reveals a pattern of a 5-fold increase in urinary FSH in boys and girls, a 50-fold increase in urinary LH in boys, and a 100-fold increase in urinary LH in girls during puberty.[284] An increase in LH in the first morning void precedes the physical signs of the onset of puberty. Doses of exogenous LHRH that are ineffective in stimulating gonadotropin or gonadal steroid secretion before puberty become effective with the onset of puberty[252]; thus an amplification occurs in the hypothalamic-pituitary–gonadal axis with progression of puberty.[252, 267, 282]

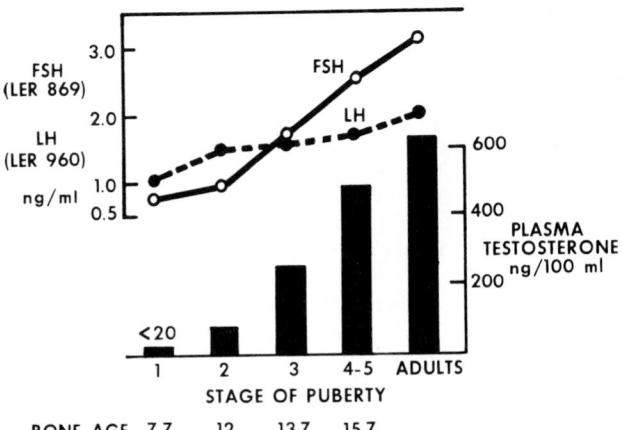

Figure 31–18. Mean plasma testosterone and gonadotropin levels in normal boys by stage of maturation (1 = prepubertal) and mean bone age for each stage. (See legend for Fig. 31–17.) To convert testosterone values to nanomoles per liter, multiply by 0.03467. (From Grumbach MM. Onset of puberty. In: Berenberg SR, ed. Puberty, Biologic and Social Components. Leiden: H. E. Stenfert Kroese, 1975: 1–21. Reprinted by permission of Kluwer Academic Publishers.[1])

While the LHRH test usually requires multiple samplings after the administration of LHRH, a single determination at 30, 45, or 60 min may suffice with the new, ultrasensitive assay, but only if a positive result is obtained.[285, 1092] Furthermore, the use of an LHRH agonist (e.g., nafarelin) in a single dose followed by measurement of serum gonadotropins and gonadal steroids can help differentiate the pubertal from the prepubertal state.[286, 287]

Levels of biologically active LH, as determined by rat or mouse interstitial cell assays, and of biologically active FSH, as assessed by rat Sertoli or granulosa cell assays, have been compared with immunoreactive LH and FSH levels estimated by radioimmunoassay.[283, 288–292] Measurement of biologically active LH may provide a more accurate indication of the state of pubertal development than measurement of immunoreactive LH[283] (Fig. 31–19). This discordance may be related to changes in the glycosylation of the LH molecule or to technical factors, such as the purity of LH standards, the quality of the radiolabeled LH, and the specificity of the antiserum.[289] Bioactive LH peaks do not always correspond to immunoactive LH pulses, further emphasizing the discrepancies between the two moieties. Levels of biologically active LH in serum increase more than those of immunoreactive LH during male pubertal development,[292–294] but this observation has not been confirmed with other sensitive immuno- (IFMA) and bioassays.[291]

Qualitative changes also occur in FSH and LH in the pituitary gland, serum, and urine during development. The pattern of glycosylation of the α and the β subunits of the gonadotropins is influenced by maturation, LHRH secretion, and the action of gonadal steroids on the pituitary gonadotropes. Variation in glycosylation affects the size and charge of the hormone and is the principal cause of the heterogeneity of FSH and LH and the large number of isoforms that vary

according to the more acidic or more basic charge.[295, 296] This pleomorphism affects the turnover rate and biologic activity of the gonadotropins.[283, 292–298]

Although it has been difficult to characterize a diurnal variation of immunoreactive FSH secretion, secretion of bioactive FSH increases at night during sleep and is more resistant to testosterone-induced suppression than is immunoreactive LH.[283, 290]

Gonadal Steroids

Estrogen exerts effects different from those of testosterone, and many actions of testosterone on growth, skeletal maturation, and accretion of bone mass are the result of its aromatization to estrogen.

Testosterone

The Leydig cells of the testes produce testosterone and, in lesser amounts, androstenedione, Δ^5-androstenediol, dihydrotestosterone, and estradiol. In addition to direct secretion, a small amount of testosterone is derived from extraglandular conversion of androstenedione secreted by the testes and the adrenal.[299] Although testosterone induces development of a male body habitus and voice change, dihydrotestosterone formed from the 5α-reduction of testosterone in the target cell is the major mediator of growth of the phallus and the prostate, temporal hair recession, and beard growth.[300] In the female, extraglandular conversion of ovarian and adrenal androstenedione accounts for almost all of the circulating testosterone.

Prepubertal boys and girls have plasma testosterone concentrations of less than 0.3 nmol/L (0.1 ng/mL),[257, 277, 301] except during the first 3 to 5 mo of infancy in the male, when pubertal levels are found. Nighttime elevations of serum testosterone levels are detectable in the male before the onset of physical signs of puberty and during early puberty after development of sleep-entrained secretion of LH[257, 270, 302] and increased pituitary sensitivity to LHRH; there is a lag of about 60 min between the peak of LH and the increase in testosterone secretion.[257, 303] In the daytime, testosterone levels begin to increase at approximately 11 y in boys after the testis volume is at least 4 mL, and continue to increase throughout puberty.[277, 301] The steepest increment in testosterone levels in boys occurs between pubertal stages 2 and 3 (see Fig. 31–14); mean testosterone levels can rise from 0.7 to 8 nmol/L (from 0.2 to 2.4 ng/mL) within 10 mo.[301] Although the measurement of the ratio of testosterone to its metabolites has been advocated as a means of detecting the use of illicit androgen preparations by athletes,[304] the ratio of testosterone to epitestosterone in the urine may be elevated normally during the progression through puberty, casting doubts on the validity of this procedure during puberty.[304, 305]

Testosterone can be measured in saliva (as can other types of steroids) for screening purposes and for monitoring therapy.[306, 307]

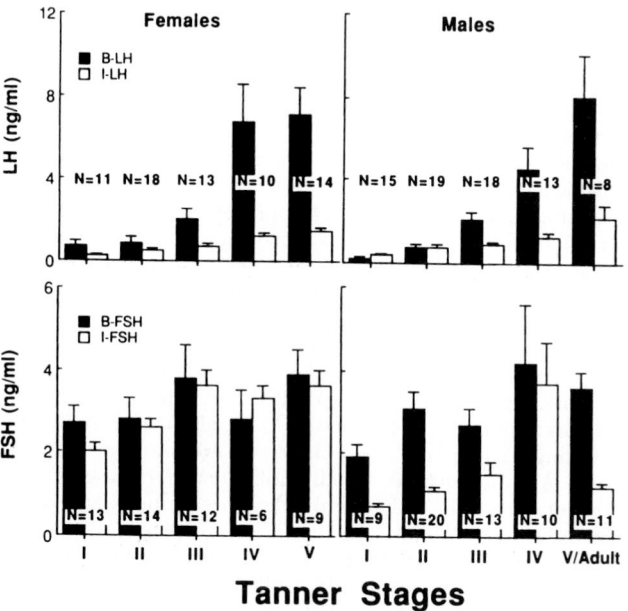

Figure 31–19. Bioactive and immunoreactive plasma LH and FSH levels in prepubertal and pubertal girls and boys. Filled bars designate bioactive LH and FSH, and open bars immunoreactive LH and FSH. The concentration of LH is expressed as nanograms per milliliter (LER-960) and that of FSH as nanograms per liter (hFSH-I-3). For conversion to SI units, see the legend of Figure 31–17. (Data from Reiter EO, Beitins IZ, Ostrea TR, et al. Bioassayable luteinizing hormone during childhood and adolescence and in patients with delayed pubertal development. J Clin Endocrinol Metab 1982; 54:155–161; and from Beitins IZ, Padmanabhan V, Kasa-Vubu J, et al. Serum bioactive follicle-stimulating hormone concentrations from prepuberty to adulthood: a cross-sectional study. J Clin Endocrinol Metab 1990; 71:1022–1027. Figure courtesy of I.Z. Beitins.)

Estrogens

In the female, most of the major estrogen, estradiol, is secreted principally (90%) by the ovary, a small fraction arising from the extraglandular conversion of testosterone and androstenedione. In the male, approximately 75% or more of estradiol is derived from extraglandular aromatization of testosterone and (indirectly) androstenedione, and the remainder is secreted by the testes.[299] Aromatase is absent or barely detectable in prepubertal testes but is easily measurable in late puberty; in normal testes aromatase is predominantly present in Leydig cells, but tumors of either Sertoli or Leydig cells can have increased aromatase activity.[308, 309]

In the fetus and at term, levels of estrogen are high because of the conversion of fetal and maternal C_{19}-steroids such as dehydroepiandrosterone (DHEA) and its sulfate (DHEAS) to estrogen by the placenta. Plasma levels of estrogen drop precipitously in the first few days of life, and estrogen levels are so low in prepuberty that detection requires a highly sensitive bioassay.[122] Estradiol is present in serum in both boys and girls before puberty, with higher levels in girls than boys.[122] The mean level of serum estradiol equivalents in 21 prepubertal girls (7.7 ± 1.9 years) was 2.2 ± 2.2 pmol/L (0.6 ± 0.6 [SD] pg/mL) higher than the levels, 0.3 ± 0.7 pmol/L (0.08 ± 0.2 pg/mL), in 23 boys (9.4 ± 2.0 years). The higher estrogen levels in girls may explain in part the more advanced skeletal maturation and earlier onset of sexual maturation in girls than in boys. Plasma estradiol levels rise steadily through puberty until maturity[278] (see Fig. 31–15), Estrone levels rise early and reach a plateau by midpuberty.[278] The daily peak of estradiol in early pubertal girls occurs about 6 to 9 h after the peak of serum LH detected during the night,[310] probably reflecting the time necessary for synthesis and release of estradiol. In all stages of puberty, boys have higher concentrations of estrone than estradiol, and levels of both estrogens are lower than those in girls at comparable stages.[257, 311] In boys levels of estradiol rise throughout puberty until the pubertal growth spurt occurs, and decrease thereafter.[312]

Adrenal Androgens

There is a progressive increase in plasma levels of DHEA and DHEAS in both boys and girls beginning before age 8 (skeletal age of 6 to 8) and continuing throughout early adulthood (Table 31–11). The increase in the secretion of adrenal androgen and its precursors is known as adrenarche. Plasma DHEA has a diurnal rhythm similar to that of cortisol, but levels of plasma DHEAS show less variation and serve as a useful biochemical marker of adrenarche. The role of adrenarche in puberty is discussed in the section on adrenal androgens and adrenarche.

Testosterone-Binding Globulin (TeBG)

Between 97 and 99% of circulating testosterone and estradiol is reversibly bound to TeBG, and only the free steroid is physiologically active.[313] TeBG is a glycoprotein of 90 to 100 kd, consists of heterogeneous monomers, and has one steroid-binding site per dimeric molecule.[314] Prepubertal levels of TeBG are approximately equal in boys and girls, and TeBG levels decrease with advancing prepubertal age and the con-

comitant increase in the plasma gonadal steroid levels; the decrease in TeBG levels is small in girls and, as a consequence of testosterone, more pronounced in boys. The rise in adrenal androgen levels at adrenarche may cause the early drop in TeBG levels, which allows more circulating free hormone at a given concentration of testosterone.[315] The plasma level of testosterone is 20 times higher and the level of free testosterone is 40 times greater in men than women.[313, 316–318] Levels of TeBG in boys with hypogonadotropic hypogonadism and individuals with androgen resistance syndrome fall at puberty to values that are intermediate between those of normal men and women.[319, 320] TeBG production is down-regulated by GH administration to prepubertal children, perhaps by the action of IGF-I,[321] and is decreased in prepubertal children with diabetes mellitus.[322]

Prolactin

Prolactin levels rise in girls during puberty. Prepubertal mean (± standard error) plasma prolactin levels are 4.0 ± 0.5 μg/L in boys and 4.5 ± 0.6 μg/L in girls. Late pubertal girls and adult women have higher concentrations of prolactin (7.5 ± 0.7 and 8.3 ± 0.7 μg/L), whereas the mean concentration in adult men is 5.2 ± 0.4 μg/L.[323] This sex difference seems to be the consequence of the higher estradiol levels in girls and in women.

Inhibin, Activin, and Folliculostatin

Inhibin, activin, and folliculostatin were characterized on the basis of their effects on FSH secretion: inhibin and folliculostatin inhibit and activin stimulates expression of the FSH β subunit and, hence, biosynthesis and secretion of FSH. These hormones are synthesized in a variety of tissues in addition to the gonads and have diverse activities apart from those on the reproductive apparatus.[324] Distinct binding proteins for inhibin and activin are present in the circulation, the gonads, and other tissues: α_2-macroglobulin, a high-capacity, low-affinity binding protein; and folliculostatin, a glycosylated single peptide chain that functions both as a high-affinity binding protein and a regulator of activin bioactivity (e.g., in the pituitary gland, a site of synthesis of both activin and folliculostatin).[324, 325]

Inhibin, a heterodimeric glycoprotein product of the Sertoli cell of the testes and the ovarian granulosa cells (as well as the placenta and other tissues), exerts a negative-feedback action on the secretion of FSH from the pituitary. Inhibin is composed of an α subunit and one of two β subunits, β_A or β_B, which form inhibin A or inhibin B, respectively, dimers with apparently identical function. Inhibin is a member of the transforming growth factor β (TGF β) superfamily, which includes antimüllerian hormone (AMH, also called müllerian-inhibiting factor) and the dimers of two inhibin subunits, activin A and activin B, which stimulate the release of FSH from pituitary cells.[324] FSH enhances the synthesis and secretion of gonadal inhibin, which appears to play a role in the feedback regulation of FSH secretion during puberty in boys and girls.[324, 325] Thus, while LH remains predominantly under the control of LHRH, the regulation of FSH secretion is more complex.[324]

The assay for plasma "inhibin" is confounded by the fact that the dimeric inhibins occur in multiple molecular weights, including combinations of precursor forms of each of the subunits. One radioimmunoassay detects the dimeric inhibins, inhibin A and B, a precursor of the α subunit, and related peptides and is thus a nondiscriminatory total inhibin assay.[326] More specific enzyme-linked immunoabsorbent assays that detect the mature 31-kd inhibin A and inhibin B dimers have

TABLE 31–11. Mean Serum Concentrations of DHEAS During Childhood

	Concentration, μmol/L (ng/mL), at Chronologic Age					
	6–8 y	8–10 y	10–12 y	12–14 y	14–16 y	16–20 y
Boys	0.5 (188)	1.6 (586)	3.4 (1260)	3.6 (1330)	7.2 (2640)	7.2 (2640)
Girls	0.8 (306)	3.2 (1170)	3.1 (1130)	4.6 (1690)	6.9 (2540)	6.3 (2320)

	Concentration, μmol/L (ng/mL), at Bone Age				
	6–8 y	8–10 y	10–12 y	12–14 y	14–16 y
Boys	0.98 (360)	1.6 (574)	3.4 (1250)	5.8 (2150)	10.9 (4030)
Girls	0.73 (276)	3.1 (1130)	4.33 (1560)	7.1 (2610)	3.9 (1450)

Modified from Reiter EO, Fuldauer VG, Root AW. Secretion of the adrenal androgen, dehydroepiandrosterone sulfate, during normal infancy, childhood, and adolescence, in sick infants, and in children with endocrinologic abnormalities. J Pediatr 1977; 90:766–770, with permission.[641]

advanced our knowledge of the biologic and clinical roles of inhibin.[327, 328]

During pregnancy the placenta secretes inhibin A, and the fetal membranes secrete both inhibins A and B,[329] whereas during the first 20 weeks of gestation, only inhibin A is detected in maternal serum. In umbilical cord serum from term female newborn infants, no inhibin dimer was detected, whereas cord serum from male newborns contained inhibin B, the inhibin of adult males; the median value was 167 ng/L.[329] In the human fetal testis α and β_B (but not β_A) subunits are present in both Sertoli and Leydig cells at 16 weeks of gestation; by 24 weeks levels of both subunits were greater in the Sertoli cells. Postnatally, the expression of both subunits decreased by 4 months of age. Inhibin subunits were not detected in the fetal ovary, nor was immunoreactive folliculostatin present in fetal or neonatal gonads.[330]

Immunoreactive "inhibin-like" activity increases in both boys and girls during puberty, with mean plasma levels increasing in boys from 161 to 442 U/L and in girls from 97 to 231 U/L between stage 1 and stage 5.[331] In boys, serum immunoreactive "inhibin" increases 1.5-fold between a testis volume of 1 mL and 10 mL.[332] However, in a large cross-sectional study,[333] using a highly specific inhibin B immunoassay that correlates with the bioactivity of inhibin and distinguishes inhibin B from inhibin A, the mean level of serum inhibin B increased between prepuberty (a stage when it is higher than the undetectable levels in castrate men[334]) and the first stage of puberty; when the strong correlation with chronologic age was taken into account, a correlation with LH and testosterone values remained. From stage II puberty on, inhibin B levels are relatively constant, despite an increase in the mean level of serum FSH between stages II and III. By stage III a negative correlation was found between inhibin B and FSH levels and persisted as puberty advanced.[333]

Serum inhibin A and B levels increase early in puberty in girls; inhibin B is predominant in the follicular phase, and inhibin A predominates during the luteal phase.[327, 328]

Serum inhibin and FSH levels are elevated in chronic renal failure and decline after renal transplantation.[335] Early pubertal boys with testicular defects have high FSH and low inhibin levels.[336] In adult men the serum inhibin B level is an indicator of Sertoli cell function.[334]

Antimüllerian Hormone (AMH) and Prostate-Specific Antigen

AMH (or MIS, müllerian inhibitory substance), a 145-kd glycoprotein dimer structurally related to the subunit of inhibin and TGF β, is produced by the Sertoli cell of the fetal testis and, later in gestation, by granulosa cells of the fetal ovary.[337, 338] Plasma levels of AMH rise from birth in newborn boys to relatively high levels by the end of the first year, decrease by age 10, and decrease further during puberty.[339] Serum levels of AMH are low or undetectable in newborn girls and are nondetectable in most girls just before puberty.[337, 338, 340] There is an inverse relationship between serum AMH and androgen levels in pubertal boys and in boys with true precocious puberty, in which values are appropriate for pubertal stage rather than chronologic age; in addition, subjects with androgen resistance have elevated serum AMH levels in the newborn period and again at puberty and thereafter.[341–343] Values are elevated in men with primitive Sertoli-like tumors and in girls and women with granulosa cell tumors, so AMH is a useful marker for these tumors.[339] Levels of AMH are slightly higher in individuals with delayed puberty and lower in boys with testicular dysgenesis associated with impaired virilization. However, boys with isolated cryptorchidism have normal values of AMH. Measurements of serum AMH are useful in determining the presence of testicular tissue to dif-

ferentiate anorchia from bilateral cryptorchidism in prepubertal boys; in the former, AMH is absent, while in the latter AMH is in the normal range.[343, 344] Patients with dysgenetic testes often have low serum levels of AMH.[344]

Prostate-specific antigen (PSA) is detectable in cord blood in both sexes and in the serum of infants but becomes undetectable during childhood. PSA levels in males increase to the measurable range with the onset of puberty and correlate with pubertal stage, the size of the testes, and presumably the size of the prostate, and serum LH and testosterone levels.[345, 346]

Growth Hormone

Serum GH levels rise during pubertal development in both boys and girls as a result of increased gonadal steroid secretion.[347] In individuals with delayed puberty GH secretion can be increased by the adminstration of exogenous androgens. The increased secretion in girls starts at an earlier chronologic age than in boys, owing to the earlier onset of puberty.[8, 9] In adolescents of normal height, there is an inverse relationship between weight and GH levels.[348] The amplitude and amount of GH secretion, but not secretory episodes, are increased by puberty or androgen administration. Following pubertal development, GH secretion decreases with advancing age.

The aromatization of testosterone to estradiol mainly accounts for the effect of testosterone on GH secretion.[112, 114, 349] Treatment of late pubertal boys with the estrogen antagonist tamoxifen leads to smaller GH secretory peaks and, to a lesser degree, fewer GH secretory episodes, supporting the critical role of estrogen.[112] Furthermore, the administration of exogenous estrogen increases the peak GH levels reached after insulin-induced hypoglycemia, exercise, and arginine.[109] Growth hormone release is stimulated by hypothalamic growth hormone–releasing hormone (GHRH), but another class of peptides (growth hormone–releasing peptide [GHRP]) also stimulate GH release independently and in a manner additive to GHRH. GHRH stimulates the release of GH in the absence of GHRH as well as in its presence. Growth hormone secretion is increased in puberty, both in the basal state and after GHRH or GHRP stimulation.[350, 351] Urinary GH excretion reflects serum levels and changes with pubertal development;[352–354] urinary GH content is higher in boys than in girls.[354] Urinary GH levels after intravenous administration of arginine correlate inversely with BMI, and GH excretion in pubertal, but not in prepubertal, short normal children or in patients with gonadal dysgenesis.[355]

Growth hormone–binding protein (GHBP) has the same amino acid sequence as the extracellular component of the GH receptor (GHR) and is directly related to the amount of cellular GHR; in normal children, plasma GHBP is inversely related to 24-h GH secretion.[356] Serum GHBP levels rise early in childhood and throughout puberty in some,[357–359] but not in other studies.[352, 360]

Insulin-Like Growth Factor I

Serum free IGF-I levels slowly increase in prepuberty, followed by a steeper rise during puberty.[361, 367] The concentration of IGF-I during puberty is higher than in prepubertal or adult subjects, remains elevated past the time of PHV with a peak attained 1 or 2 y after the pubertal growth spurt (thus later in boys than in girls), and then falls to adult levels[116, 362–367] (see Fig. 31–13).

The pubertal pattern of the GH-dependent serum insulin-like growth factor–binding protein-3 (IGFBP-3) is similar to that of serum IGF-I. However, serum IGFBP-3 concentrations correlate with BMI even when IGF-I does not.[365, 367] Free IGF-I levels show the same development pattern as total IGF-I, but the magnitude of the change differs.[361] Free IGF-I levels decrease in the later stages of puberty.[366] The increase in the serum ratio of IGF-I to IGFBP-3 at the time of the pubertal growth spurt appears to be due to differences in production of these moieties.[365, 367, 368] However, IGFBP-3 proteolysis increases in children with poorly controlled diabetes mellitus.[367] The urinary excretion of IGF-I changes with pubertal stage. The rise in testosterone level in boys and the estradiol level in girls correlates with the rise in IGF-I concentration.

The major effects of estrogen and testosterone on IGF-I generation are mediated indirectly via augmented release of GH (see earlier). Children with true precocious puberty have the plasma IGF-I values of normal children in the same pubertal stage, rather than of children of the same chronologic age.[116] After treatment of true precocious puberty with LHRH agonists to lower plasma gonadotropin and gonadal steroid levels, IGF-I values slowly decrease, along with the secretion of GH.

Serum IGF-II levels show no pubertal peak and fall during adulthood in boys.

Insulin

Serum fasting insulin concentration increases two- to threefold at PHV, and increased insulin secretion after glucose administration suggests a degree of insulin resistance during puberty.[369-376] This impairment of insulin-stimulated glucose metabolism can be demonstrated by the euglycemic insulin clamp technique[371] and is more marked in adolescents with diabetes mellitus. Pubertal children compensate for this defect by increasing insulin secretion. In contrast, the insulin resistance does not impair the effect of insulin on amino acid metabolism.[369, 375] Thus the enhanced insulin response to glucose in puberty due to the relative resistance may increase the anabolic effects of insulin with regard to protein synthesis.[369]

The response of insulin to oral glucose is greater in black subjects than in white subjects at all stages of pubertal development; this ethnic difference in insulin resistance may contribute to the increased incidence of non–insulin-dependent diabetes mellitus (NIDDM) in black adults.[377]

Children with insulin-dependent diabetes mellitus (IDDM) usually require an increase in the dose of insulin for glucose control at puberty.[369, 373, 374] The cause of insulin resistance is attributed, at least in part, to increased fat oxidation at puberty.[378] Insulin sensitivity is related both to pubertal stage and to BMI; in a longitudinal study insulin sensitivity inversely correlated with BMI, decreased with pubertal progression from pubertal stage 2 to stage 3, and was lower in girls than boys at either stage 2 or stage 3.[379] Insulin resistance is present early in the course of gonadal dysgenesis and thalassemia.[380]

In well-managed children with IDDM the growth rate may decrease slightly and transiently in the 10 y after diagnosis; slowing of bone age advancement during this period leads to a transient slowing of development, but the effect of diabetes mellitus on growth is less than the influence of parental height. While growth velocity in diabetic children increases again during puberty, weight gain increases even more during puberty, leading to a high incidence of obesity in children with IDDM.[381] One study reported a decrease in final height if the diagnosis of IDDM was made prior to 5 years of age, but not if the diagnosis of IDDM was made later; the pubertal growth rate was reduced in all patients, particularly in girls.[382]

Adolescents with IDDM have lower serum levels of IGF-I than control subjects.[383] Elevated GH levels in IDDM are associated with low serum IGF-I and low serum GHBP concentrations, and the usual reciprocal relationship between serum GH and GHBP does not exist.[383-385]

Obese teen-age girls with prominent abdominal adiposity

have insulin resistance and are at higher risk for breast cancer; abdominal adiposity in the prepubertal state is associated with early puberty, early menarche, and a longer exposure to hormones that predispose to breast cancer.[386-390] Plasma insulin in obese adolescent boys correlates with fasting plasma glucose, plasma triglycerides, uric acid, and systolic blood pressure and in obese adolescent girls correlates with plasma triglycerides and systolic and diastolic blood pressure. Plasma insulin correlates inversely with HDL cholesterol in both boys and girls.[391]

Retinopathy in IDDM characteristically appears in the teen-age years or later, but the duration and degree of diabetes control in the prepubertal years are contributing factors; retinopathy can occur in the prepubertal years.[392-398] An increase in the vitreous fluorophotometry penetration ratio at the time of puberty indicates that the blood-retinal barrier decreases during this period.[399]

The American Diabetes Association recommends screening for microalbuminuria as an index of the development of diabetic nephropathy; microalbuminuria can develop quite early in puberty.[400]

While NIDDM has been recognized in children and adolescents in the past, the incidence is increasing, probably owing to the increase in obesity in these age groups. NIDDM appears most often among children and adolescents of ethnic minority populations and should be considered in subjects with acanthosis nigricans (a marker for insulin resistance); girls with hyperandrogenism not otherwise explained are also of concern. NIDDM in the young is a heterogeneous disorder, and obesity, while common, is variable (reviewed in references 401 to 403; see Chapter 21).

Early-onset NIDDM is prevalent among the Native American and Mexican American populations. Several variations of maturity-onset diabetes of the young (MODY) have been defined,[403] all with progressive loss of pancreatic beta cell function and inherited as autosomal dominant traits in individuals who need not be obese; type 2 MODY is linked to a defect in mitochondrial glucokinase. MODY patients may require insulin therapy.

Several syndromes of insulin resistance combine hyperglycemia and virilization.[401, 402] The type A disorder features include a lean, muscular adolescent female with acanthosis nigricans, hirsutism, oligomenorrhea or amenorrhea, and ovarian hyperthecosis and stromal hyperplasia associated with abnormalities of the insulin receptor gene. A less severe combination of hyperandrogenism, insulin resistance, and acanthosis nigricans (HAIR-AN) syndrome and the polycystic ovary syndrome can also be manifested in adolescent females. Rabson-Mendenhall syndrome is associated with severe insulin resistance (sometimes leading to diabetic ketoacidosis), dysmorphic facies, acanthosis nigricans, thickened nails, hirsutism, dental dysplasia, abdominal distention, and phallic or clitoral enlargement. Rabson-Mendenhall syndrome shares features with leprechaunism and is due to homozygous or compound heterozygous defects in the insulin receptor gene. The type B syndrome is due to inhibitory or stimulatory antibodies to the insulin receptor, sometimes with acanthosis nigricans and ovarian hyperandrogenism; this disorder can occur with ataxia-telangiectasia or as an isolated defect in otherwise normal adolescents. Individuals with Berardinelli-Seip syndrome have severe insulin resistance, lipodystrophy with complete or partial absence of subcutaneous fat, increased growth and skeletal maturation, muscle hypertrophy, acanthosis nigricans, hypertrichosis, organomegaly, and mild hypertrophy of the external genitalia. Most of these NIDDM syndromes can be treated with oral hypoglycemic agents initially but may require insulin.

Serum Lipids

Testosterone increases serum low-density lipoprotein (LDL) cholesterol and decreases high-density lipoprotein

(HDL) cholesterol levels and thereby accounts for the adverse LDL/HDL ratio in adult males.[404, 405] Postheparin hepatic lipase activity is increased by exogenous androgens (and decreased by estrogens), possibly explaining the decrease in HDL after androgen treatment or after an increase in endogenous androgen secretion.[406] Serum lipoprotein A is not related to pubertal stage in normal subjects but is determined by genetic factors.[407] Even though there is an increased risk of coronary heart disease in patients with IDDM, and lipoprotein A is related to coronary heart disease, lipoprotein A levels in children with IDDM are not different from those of control subjects.[408] In a longitudinal study, 9-year-old girls with high LDL cholesterol retained high LDL concentrations 12 y later, while those starting with lower LDL levels remained so,[409] and in another study obesity was related to elevation of apolipoprotein B and the ratio of apolipoprotein B/apolipoprotein AI; these measures correlate with the development of atherosclerosis.[410] Waist circumference and the waist-to-hip ratio inversely correlate with serum HDL and correlate directly with serum triglycerides, while the BMI correlates with serum triglycerides and diastolic blood pressure; waist circumference correlates with apolipoprotein B and the apolipoprotein B/apolipoprotein AI ratio.[411]

Patients with familial hypercholesterolemia have carotid intimal atherosclerotic plaques demonstrable by B-mode ultrasonography by the age of puberty.[412] Further, intra-abdominal adipose tissue assessed by MRI correlates with serum total and LDL cholesterol and triglycerides in obese adolescents 10 to 15 years of age, indicating cardiovascular risk at these early ages.[413]

A 40-y longitudinal study found that obese children and adolescents continue to be obese as adults; the heaviest subjects and those that gained the most weight during the study had a greater risk of death, cardiovascular disease, and diabetes mellitus.[414]

Cortisol

Although the secretory rate of cortisol does not change at puberty, salivary cortisol values increase slightly and correlate with pubertal stage in both sexes.[415]

CENTRAL NERVOUS SYSTEM AND PUBERTY

The onset of puberty is a consequence of maturational changes that are incompletely understood.[252, 253, 416] The development of secondary sexual characteristics, the adolescent growth spurt, the attainment of fertility, and the psychosocial changes proceed from the maturation of the gonads and the increase in gonadal steroid secretion. The development of gonadal function is a continuum extending from sexual differentiation and the ontogenesis of the hypothalamic-pituitary-gonadotropin-gonadal system[53, 254, 417] through a juvenile pause (in which the system is largely quiescent)[253, 418] to the attainment of full sexual maturation and fertility during puberty. The end point of this process is the capacity for procreation. Two independent, but associated, processes (controlled by different mechanisms but temporally linked) are involved in the increased secretion of gonadal steroids during puberty. The first, adrenarche, the increase in adrenal androgen secretion,[123] precedes by 2 y or so the second, gonadarche, which is the consequence of the pubertal reactivation of the hypothalamic-pituitary-gonadotropin-gonadal apparatus.[253, 418] These two processes and their role in puberty are considered separately.

Puberty is not an isolated de novo event but rather a stage in development that involves the reactivation or augmentation of the hypothalamic LHRH pulse generator and gonadotropin secretion. This system, which is functional during fetal life and infancy,[53, 253, 254, 417, 419] is suppressed to a low level of activity in childhood.

Understanding the mechanisms involved in the restraint of gonadotropin secretion during childhood is essential for understanding the onset of puberty. Certain CNS lesions involving the hypothalamus and nearby structures can advance or delay the onset of puberty.[252, 253, 419–422] For example, true precocious puberty (including cyclic ovulation in girls and spermatogenesis in boys) can occur secondary to CNS tumors, developmental defects, or inflammatory lesions that involve the hypothalamus and activate the hypothalamic-pituitary-gonadal complex prematurely (Table 31–12).

Several regulatory systems are involved in the control of human sexual maturation (Fig. 31–20):

1. In humans and nonhuman primates the neural component that controls gonadotropin secretion resides in the medial basal hypothalamus and includes the arcuate region[423] and its transducer LHRH neurosecretory neurons, which are few in number (about 1500 to 2500 neurons), and are dispersed—and not segregated into a specific nucleus—but are functionally interconnected. These LHRH neurons act in a

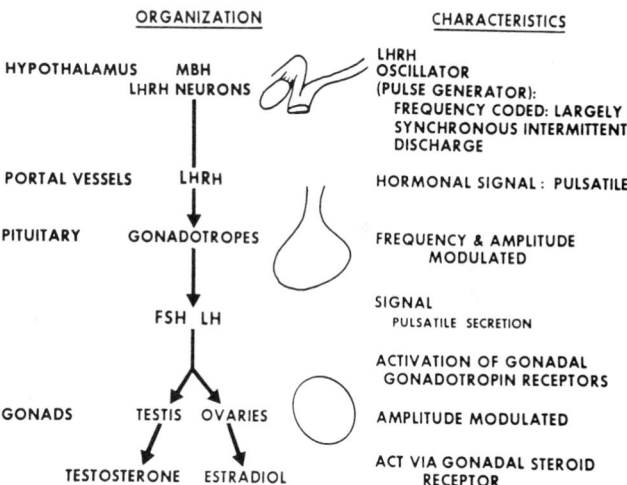

Figure 31–20. Organization and characteristics of the hypothalamic–pituitary gonadotrope–gonadal system. The medial basal hypothalamus (MBH) contains the transducer LHRH neurosecretory neurons. These neurons translate neural signals into a periodic, oscillatory chemical signal, LHRH. This MBH complex functions as an LHRH pulse generator (oscillator), which is frequency coded and releases LHRH from its axon terminals at the median eminence as a largely synchronous intermittent discharge into the primary capillary plexus of the hypothalamic-hypophyseal portal circulation. The LHRH pulse generator is influenced by biogenic amine neurotransmitters, peptidergic neuromodulators, neuroexcitatory amino acids, and neural pathways. During the follicular phase in the adult female and the adult male, an LHRH pulse (estimated indirectly by monitoring LH pulses in peripheral blood) occurs approximately every 90 to 120 min throughout the day. Changes in the frequency and probably in the amplitude of the LHRH-secretory episodes modulate the pattern of LH and FSH. The major site of action of testosterone and progesterone is on the LHRH pulse generator, as these two classes of steroids decrease LH pulse frequency, but a pituitary site of action has also been described. Estrogens have major direct inhibitory and stimulatory effects on the LHRH-primed pituitary gonadotrope; the inhibitory, or negative, feedback action is associated with a decrease in both the frequency and the amplitude of pituitary LH secretion. On the other hand, evidence also supports a negative- and positive-feedback action of estrogen on the LHRH pulse generator. Inhibin has a direct inhibitory effect on the pituitary gland and the secretion of FSH. The secretion of gonadal steroids by the gonads is controlled mainly by the amplitude of the gonadotropin signal. (Adapted from Grumbach MM, Kaplan SL. The neuroendocrinology of human puberty: an ontogenetic perspective. In: Grumbach MM, Sizonenko PC, Aubert ML, eds. Control of the Onset of Puberty. Baltimore: Williams & Wilkins, 1990: pp. 1–68. © 1990, the Williams & Wilkins Co., Baltimore.)

TABLE 31–12. Hypothesis of the Control of the Onset of Human Puberty

1. *Central Dogma:* The CNS exercises the only major restraint on the onset of puberty. The neuroendocrine control of puberty is mediated by the hypothalamic LHRH-secreting neurosecretory neurons in the medial basal hypothalamus, which act as an endogenous pulse generator (oscillator).
2. The development of reproductive function is a continuum extending from sexual differentiation and the ontogeny of the hypothalamic-pituitary-gonadal system in the fetus to the attainment of full sexual maturation and fertility.
3. In the prepubertal child the LHRH pulse generator, operative in the fetus and infant, functions at a low level of activity (the juvenile pause) because of steroid-independent and steroid-dependent inhibitory mechanisms.
4. Puberty represents the *reactivation* (disinhibition) of the CNS suppressed LHRH pulse generator characteristic of late infancy and childhood, leading to increased amplitude and frequency of LHRH pulsatile discharges, to increased stimulation of the pituitary gonadotropes, and finally to gonadal maturation. Hormonally, puberty is initiated by the recrudescence of augmented pulsatile LHRH and gonadotropin secretion, mainly at night.

From Grumbach MM, Kaplan SL. The neuroendocrinology of human puberty: an ontogenetic perspective. In: Grumbach MM, Sizonenko PC, Aubert ML, eds. Control of the Onset of Puberty. Baltimore: Williams & Wilkins, 1990: 1–68. © 1990, the Williams & Wilkins Co., Baltimore.[253]

coordinated manner to translate neural signals into a periodic, oscillatory release of a chemical signal, LHRH associated with episodic electrical activity in the hypothalamus of the same frequency.[424–426] LHRH, a decapeptide, is synthesized as part of a larger precursor protein; the encoding gene is located on the short arm of chromosome 8.[427] The LHRH-secreting neurons of the hypothalamic LHRH pulse generator exhibit spontaneous authorhythmicity[425, 426, 428, 429] and function intrinsically as an oscillator for entrainment of the repetitive release of LHRH (Fig. 31–21). The mechanism for pulse generation, the coordinated synchronous discharge of LHRH from neighboring but dispersed cells, is unknown but may involve synaptic connections among LHRH neurons and electronic coupling of cells through gap junctions[424, 430, 431] and through autocrine factors such as LHRH itself[432] and nitric oxide.[433, 434] LHRH is synthesized in these neurons and released episodically from axon terminals at the median eminence into the primary plexus of the hypothalamic-hypophyseal portal circulation. The hormone is then transported by the portal vessels to the anterior pituitary gland (see Chapter 8). LHRH is essential for the release of both FSH and LH. In some species, notably rodents, extrahypothalamic CNS structures, including the limbic system (hippocampus and amygdala),[436, 437] influ-

ence gonadotropin secretion. The amplitude and frequency of the pulsatile LHRH signal are modified by catecholaminergic and serotoninergic neurons, through their effect on hypothalamic norepinephrine, dopamine, and serotonin, by opioid peptide, by neuropeptide Y (NPY), galanin, and corticotropin-releasing hormone (CRH), and by γ-aminobutyric acid and excitatory amino acid neuronal networks.[435–440, 440a] In humans and nonhuman primates, the inhibitory effects of γ-aminobutyric acid, opioid peptides, and CRH on the LHRH pulse generator and the stimulatory effects of excitatory amino acids and adrenergic pathways are the most firmly established. The hypothalamic-pituitary-gonadotropin unit is influenced by gonadal steroids, inhibin, activin, and folliculostatin[441, 442] and by neural influences that integrate intrinsic stimuli and environmental factors and cues. In vitro studies suggest that the generation of the LHRH pulse is an intrinsic property of the LHRH neurosecretory neuronal network, and that a variety of factors modulate the autorhythmicity of these neurons.[443–445]

2. The pituitary gonadotropes, in response to the LHRH rhythmic signal, release LH and FSH in a pulsatile manner. Each LH (and FSH) pulse is induced by a pulse of LHRH.

3. The gonads, which are modulated primarily by the amplitude of the gonadotropin pulse, transmit the episodic gonadotropin signal into pulsatile secretion of gonadal steroids.

This system and its three components (medial basal hypothalamic LHRH neurosecretory neurons, pituitary gonadotropes, and gonadotropin-responsive elements of the gonad) are common to all mammals (see Fig. 31–20). In the pituitary gland and the gonad, target cells contain receptors for the peptide hormones that mediate the cellular response to the signal.[446, 447]

Although the hypothalamic LHRH pulse generator–pituitary-gonadal complex is similar in all mammalian species, diverse adaptive mechanisms and strategies have evolved among species and between the sexes that influence the biology and timing of puberty.[448, 449] Photoperiodicity and seasonal breeding, biologic clocks, and pheromones are integral parts of the pubertal process in some species, but not in the control of human puberty. Many well-established CNS regulatory mechanisms that affect the LHRH pulse generator and the onset of puberty in nonprimates are of minor or of no documented significance in primates. Other environmental factors and cues that play a role in the human and nonhuman primate are less critical in most mammals.

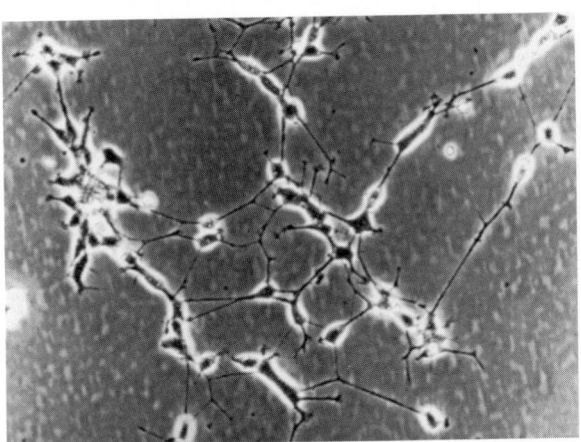 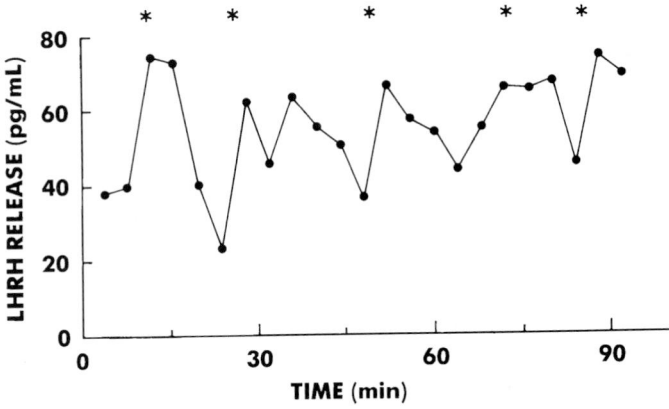

Figure 31–21. The immortalized hypothalamic LHRH neuronal cell line. *Left,* Phase contrast micrograph illustrating the neuronal phenotype (GT1–3 cell line) including the extension of multiple long neurites, cell-cell contacts, and growth cones. The neuroendocrine function of GT cells is limited to expression of LHRH and GAP. Magnification × 175. *Right,* Demonstration of autonomous LHRH (GnRH) pulses at about 20-min intervals by the LHRH neurons in culture. This is the same frequency as that for LH pulses in vivo, in castrated adult mice and rats. To convert LHRH values to picomoles per liter, multiply by 0.8460 (Micrograph from Mellon PL, Windle JJ, Goldsmith PC, et al. Immortalization of hypothalamic GnRH neurons by genetically targeted tumorigenesis. Neuron 1990; 5:1–10. Copyright by Cell Press. Graph courtesy of G. Martinez de la Escalera and R. I. Weiner.[424])

The human hypothalamic LHRH pulse generator–pituitary system functions during fetal life and early infancy.[53, 253, 254, 418] The system is suppressed to a low level of activity during childhood (the juvenile pause) and is derepressed or reactivated during puberty.[253, 254, 416, 418] In this light, puberty does not represent the initiation or first occurrence of pulsatile secretion of LHRH or pituitary gonadotropins but the reactivation or disinhibition of LHRH neurosecretory neurons and maintenance of the self-sustaining oscillatory secretion of LHRH thereafter.

A large body of evidence indicates that the CNS—and not the hypothalamic LHRH pulse generator itself, the pituitary gland, the gonads, or gonadal steroid target tissues—restrains the hypothalamic-pituitary-gonadal system during the prepubertal years.[252, 253, 420, 421, 451, 452] The inhibitory effect of the CNS appears to be mediated through the hypothalamus acting on the neurosecretory neurons that synthesize and secrete LHRH.

Pattern of Gonadotropin Secretion

There are two pulsatile secretory patterns of gonadotropins: tonic and cyclic. Tonic, or basal, secretion is regulated by a negative, or inhibitory, feedback mechanism in which changes in the concentration of circulating gonadal steroids and inhibin cause reciprocal changes in the secretion of pituitary gonadotropins. This is the pattern of secretion in the male and one of the control mechanisms in the female. Cyclic secretion involves a positive, or stimulatory, control mechanism in which an increase in circulating estrogens, to a critical level and of sufficient duration, initiates the synchronous release of LH and FSH (the preovulatory LH surge) that is characteristic of the normal ovulatory woman before menopause. The secretion of FSH and LH is probably always pulsatile or episodic, regardless of whether the pattern is tonic or cyclic and regardless of age (i.e., in the fetus, infant, or child, during puberty, or in the adult). However, it is difficult to detect small pulses when the plasma gonadotropin levels are low (as in prepubertal individuals) because of methodologic limitations.

In men, the pulsatile release of LH has a periodicity of about 90 to 120 min and precedes testosterone secretion by about 40 min.[435] In women LH pulse frequency and amplitude vary during the menstrual cycle from about 1 pulse/h in the midfollicular phase to 1 pulse/5 h in the late luteal phase.[453]

Changes in the pattern of the gonadotropin spikes and their circadian rhythm occur in the peripubertal period and during puberty. Even though LHRH stimulates the release of both FSH and LH, the pulsatile secretion of immunoreactive FSH in normal adults is less prominent; this discordance in FSH and LH pulses is due largely to the longer half-life of FSH than LH, to differences in the factors that modulate the action of LHRH on FSH and LH release by the gonadotropes (especially gonadal steroids, inhibin, and possibly activin and folliculostatin), and to intrinsic differences in the secretory pattern of the two gonadotropins. For example, a change in the frequency of LHRH pulses can modify the ratio of release of FSH to LH; midfollicular phase levels of estradiol and adult male concentrations of plasma testosterone inhibit the response of FSH more than that of LH to pulsatile injections of LHRH.[454–456]

The inherent oscillatory characteristic of gonadotropin secretion is a consequence of the pulsatile release of LHRH. However, the physiological significance of the episodic, rhythmic pattern of gonadotropin secretion was unclear until Knobil and Belchetz and associates[425, 457, 458] demonstrated the essential nature of a periodic, oscillatory LHRH signal for the regulation of gonadotropin secretion. Gonadotropin secretion is inhibited by the continuous infusion of LHRH because of desensitization of LHRH receptors on the gonadotrope.[446, 447, 459] Intermittent or pulsatile administration (e.g., LHRH, 1 μg/min for 6 min every hour) restores pulsatile release of LH and FSH in adult monkeys in which destruction of the LHRH pulse generator abolishes endogenous LHRH secretion.[457, 458] Pulsatile LHRH administration also re-establishes gonadotropin secretion in animals in which gonadotropin secretion is suppressed by the continuous infusion of LHRH (Fig. 31–22). These studies indicate that the LHRH signal to the pituitary gonadotropes is frequency coded. Pulsatile administration of natural LHRH has made it possible to induce ovarian and testicular maturation, including fertility, in patients with hypothalamic hypogonadism, and gonadotropin secretion can be suppressed in boys and girls with true precocious puberty by long-acting potent LHRH analogues (see section on sexual precocity).

Ontogeny

In the mouse,[460–462] rhesus monkey,[463] human,[464, 465] and all vertebrates examined,[466] LHRH neurons do not originate in

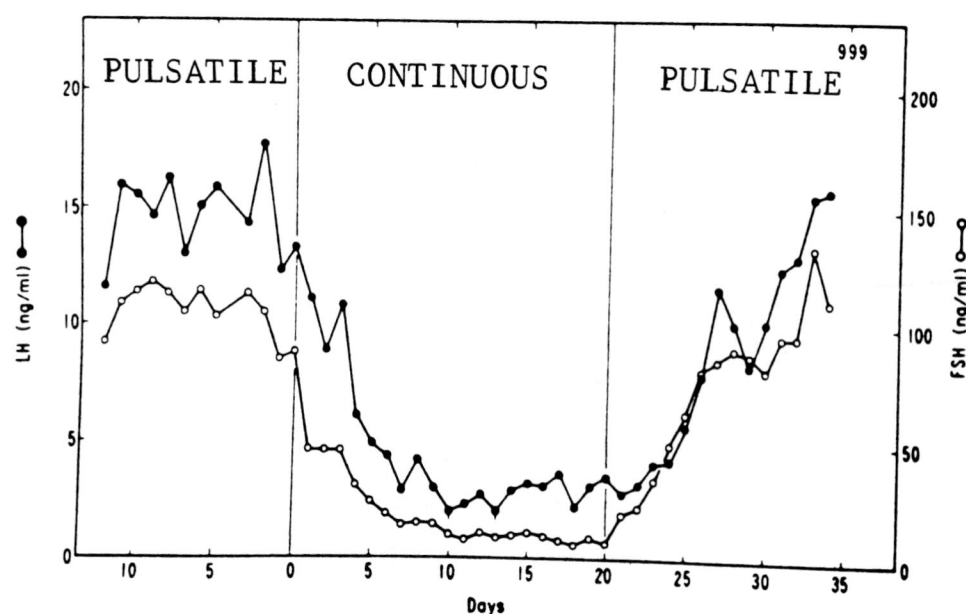

Figure 31–22. Effect of pulsatile administration of LHRH in contrast to continuous infusion of LHRH in adult oophorectomized rhesus monkeys in which gonadotropin secretion has been abolished by lesions that ablated the medial basal hypothalamic LHRH pulse generator. Note the high concentrations of plasma LH and FSH in monkeys given one LHRH pulse per hour, the suppression of gonadotropin secretion by continuous infusion of LHRH even though the total dose of LHRH was the same, and the restoration of FSH and LH secretion when the pulsatile mode of LHRH administration was reinitiated. (From Belchetz PE, Plant TM, Nakai Y, et al. Hypophysial responses to continuous and intermittent delivery of hypothalamic gonadotropin releasing hormone. Science 1978; 202:631–633. Copyright 1978 by the AAAS.[458])

the CNS but arise in the embryo from the epithelium of the olfactory placode and migrate to the forebrain by an ordered course along the pathway of the nervus terminalis–vermonasal complex, which also originates in the olfactory placode and forms a connection between the nasal septum and the forebrain (Fig. 31–23). In the mouse embryo,[460–462] the LHRH cells can be identified by embryonic day 9.5, undergo mitosis between days 10 and 11, and express LHRH messenger RNA and immunoreactive LHRH by day 10.5. By day 12.5, all cells that make up the mature population of LHRH neurosecretory neurons are present. The cells migrate in a rostrocaudal direction through the nasal septum into the forebrain from days 12.5 to 15.5 along with the terminalis nerve. By embryonic day 16.5 the LHRH neurosecretory neurons have a postnatal distribution in the hypothalamus (see Fig. 31–23). LHRH cells are limited to the nasal region in the 36-day-old monkey embryo, are present in the basal hypothalamus by day 47, and after day 50 are in the same area of the medial basal hypothalamus as in the adult (Fig. 31–24).[463]

The Human Fetus

Schwanzel-Fukuda and co-workers[464] studied a male human fetus of 19 weeks of gestation with Kallmann's syndrome (see later). No LHRH neurosecretory neurons were detected in the brain, including the hypothalamus. However, dense clusters of LHRH cells and fibers were present in the nose, including the nasal septum and cribriform plate, and within the dural layers of the meninges under the forebrain. The olfactory bulbs were absent. In contrast, normal male fetuses at 19 weeks of gestation had the expected distribution of

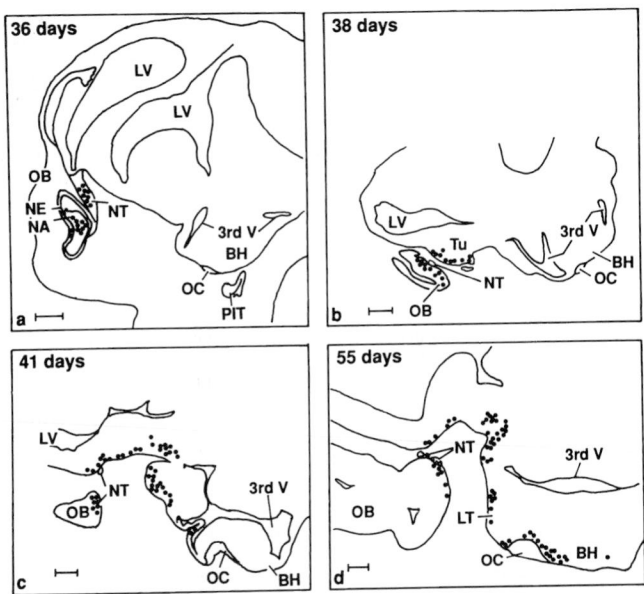

Figure 31–24. Ontogeny of the LHRH neurons in the rhesus monkey. In the 36-day embryo the LHRH cells *(black dots)* are located deep in the nasal septum along the path of the nervus terminals but not within the brain. By day 38 LHRH cells are clustered along the dorsal region of the olfactory bulbs and nervus terminalis with a few cells arching back along the ventral surface of the forebrain. By 55 days the LHRH neurons are in the process of migration, but clusters of LHRH cells have entered the CNS and reached the basal hypothalamus. BH, basal hypothalamus; LT, lamina terminalis; LV, lateral ventricle; NA, nasal area; NE, nasal epithelium; NT, nervus terminalis; OB, olfactory bulb; OC, optic chiasm; Tu, olfactory tubercle. (Adapted from Ronnekiev OK, Resko JA. Ontogeny of gonadotropin-releasing hormone-containing neurons in early development of rhesus macaques, Endocrinology, 126, 498–511, 1990, © by The Endocrine Society.[463])

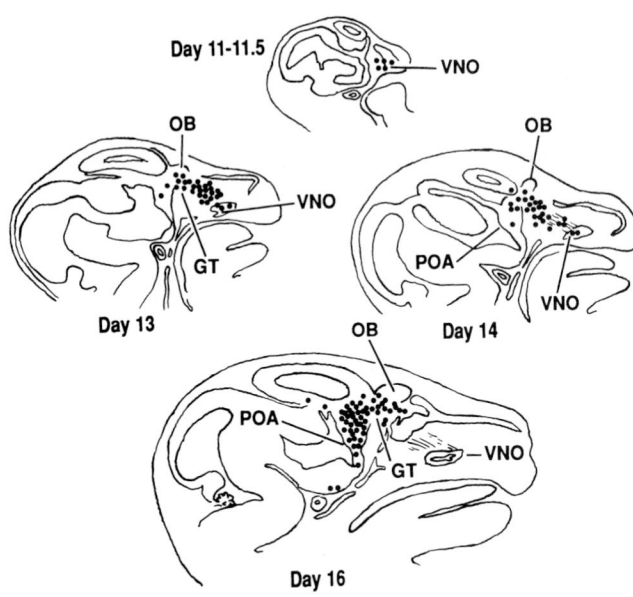

Figure 31–23. Ontogeny of LHRH neurons in the mouse. The route of migration of the LHRH neurosecretory neurons *(black dots)* in the mouse embryo is shown from their origin in the medial olfactory placode (a plate-like thickening of embryonic ectoderm) in the nasal region through the forebrain into the hypothalamus and preoptic areas. At embryonic (E) day 11 to 11.5 LHRH cells are in the anlage of the vomeronasal organ and medial wall of the olfactory placode. By E day 13 the number of LHRH neurons has increased, and most are in the nasal septum with the nervus terminalis and the vomeronasal nerves; only a few cells are in the brain. By E day 14 the majority of LHRH cells are in the ganglion terminale and the central root of the nervus terminalis and arch through the forebrain to the hypothalamus. By E day 16 most of the LHRH neurons are in the hypothalamus and preoptic areas, and the migration is almost complete. GT, ganglion terminale; OB, olfactory bulb; POA, preoptic area, VNO, vomeronasal organ. (Adapted from Schwanzel-Fukuda M, Pfaff DW. Origin of luteinizing hormone-releasing hormone neurons. Nature 1989; 338:161–164. Reprinted by permission from Nature, Vol. 338, pp. 161–164. Copyright © 1989 Macmillan Magazines Ltd.[460])

LHRH neurons in the hypothalamus. In subsequent studies, LHRH immunoreactivity was present in the epithelium of the medial aspect of the olfactory placode by 42 days of gestation, but not at 28 to 32 days.[465] These findings in the human are consistent with the migration of LHRH neurosecretory neurons from the olfactory placode to the hypothalamus in other mammals. Adults have about 1500 hypothalamic LHRH neurons.

LHRH has been detected in human embryonic brain extracts by 4.5 weeks and in the early fetal hypothalamus (Table 31–13), and fetal pituitary gonadotropes are responsive to LHRH.[53, 254] The hypothalamic-hypophyseal portal system is functional by 11.5 weeks of gestation.[467, 468] By 9 weeks, LHRH neurons are detectable in the fetal hypothalamus, and by 16 weeks axons that contain LHRH are present in the median eminence and terminate in contact with capillaries of the portal system (reviewed in references 53, 253, and 254). Thus the human fetal hypothalamic LHRH pulse generator develops by at least the end of the first trimester. In fetal sheep the hypothalamus secretes LHRH in a pulsatile manner.[469, 470]

The human fetal gonad is affected by chorionic gonadotropin and by fetal pituitary FSH and LH (reviewed in reference 53). Early in gestation, the placental gonadotropin hCG might play an important role in the secretion of testosterone by the Leydig cells of the fetal testes during the masculinization of the wolffian ducts and the external genitalia. However, it is uncertain whether functional hCG/LH and FSH receptors are present in the fetal testis before 12 weeks of gestation[471–473] and whether the early fetal testis responds to hCG at the time of onset of testosterone biosynthesis. Fetal Leydig cells are unique to the fetus and infant and regress, to be followed by the differentiation of adult-type Leydig cells in the peripubertal period (reviewed in references 53 and 474 to 476). In

TABLE 31–13. The Early Development of the Human Fetal Pituitary and Hypothalamus

Gestational Age (wk)	Hypothalamus	Pituitary	Portal Circulation
3	Forebrain appears		
4		Rathke's pouch in contact with stomodeum	
5	Diencephalon differentiated	Rathke's pouch separated from stomodeum and in contact with infundibulum; pituitary in culture can secrete corticotropin, prolactin, GH, FSH	
6	Premamillary preoptic nucleus; LHRH detected	Intermediate-lobe primordia; cell cords penetrate mesenchyme around Rathke's pouch	
7	Arcuate, supraoptic nucleus	Sphenoidal plate forms	
8	Median eminence differentiated: TRH detected*	Basophils appear	Capillaries in mesenchyme
9	Paraventricular nucleus; dorsal medial nucleus	Pars tuberalis formed: β-endorphin detected*	
10	Serotonin and norepinephrine detected*	Acidophils appear	
11	Mamillary nucleus; primary (hypothalamic) portal plexus present; β-endorphin and opioidergic neurons detected*	Secondary (pituitary) portal plexus present catecholamines (IF)†	Functional hypothalamic-hypophyseal portal system
12	Dopamine present		
13	Corticotropin-releasing hormone detected*	α-Melanocyte–stimulating hormone detected	
14	Fully differentiated hypothalamus	Adult form of hypophysis developed	

*Hormone detected at this gestational age but may be present earlier.
†IF, detected by immunofluorescence.
Modified from Gluckman P, Grumbach MM, Kaplan SL. The human fetal hypothalamus and pituitary gland. In: Tulchinsky D, Ryan KJ, eds. Maternal-Fetal Endocrinology. Philadelphia: WB Saunders, 1980: 196–232, with permission.

comparison with the adult cells, fetal Leydig cells form tightly opposed clusters joined by gap junctions and lack Reinke crystals, are resistant to hCG/LH-induced desensitization—indeed, hCG/LH up-regulate fetal LH/hCG receptors—and contain little aromatase activity and few estradiol receptors.

FSH receptors have not been detected in the fetal ovary early in gestation,[473] but later in gestation, after completion of male phenotypic differentiation, fetal FSH and LH affect the growth and maturation of both fetal testis and ovary. The stage of gestation at which fetal pituitary gonadotropins are important for development of the fetal gonad differs in the two sexes. In the anencephalic fetus (which is deficient in hypothalamic LHRH and pituitary gonadotropins), the testes are hypoplastic early in the third trimester, but the ovaries in this disorder are normal until at least 32 weeks of gestation.[53, 419, 477]

FSH and LH are detectable in the human fetal pituitary gland by 10 weeks of gestation, and the content increases until approximately 25 to 29 weeks of gestation[53, 254, 417, 419] (Figs. 31–25 and 31–26). The fetal pituitary not only synthesizes and stores FSH and LH but also secretes these hormones by 11 to 12 weeks. The fetal serum LH and FSH levels increase to peak levels by midgestation and then decrease; levels in umbilical venous blood at term are low (see Figs. 31–25 and 31–26). Studies of fetal blood obtained by cordocentesis and using highly sensitive gonadotropin immunoassays provided new information on the pattern of change in both immunoreactive and bioactive gonadotropins and gonadal steroids between 17 weeks and term. The serum levels of FSH and LH and of bioactive FSH at 17 to 24 weeks of gestation were higher in female than male fetuses and in both sexes decreased between 25 and 40 weeks of gestation.[478] Similarly, mean FSH and LH

Figure 31–25. Comparison of the pattern of change of serum testosterone, hCG, and serum and pituitary LH (LER-960) and FSH (LER-869) levels in the human male fetus during gestation in relation to the morphologic changes in fetal testis. The top graph illustrates the regression curve for the increment (Δ) between a baseline plasma LH and FSH level and the 15-min response to administration of LHRH to the male fetus plotted as a function of gestational age. The scale masks the slight increase in plasma FSH. Data were recalculated from Takagi et al.[483] The evidence supports the hypothesis that the hypothalamic LHRH pulse generator is functional early in gestation and mediates the rise in serum concentration of fetal pituitary gonadotropes. To convert plasma hCG values to international units per liter, multiply by 1.0. Other conversions are in the legends of Figures 31–17 and 31–18. (Modified from Kaplan SL, Grumbach MM. Pituitary and placental gonadotrophins and sex steroids in the human and sub-human primate fetus. Clin Endocrinol Metab 1978[419]; 7:487–511; and Gluckman PD, Grumbach MM, Kaplan SL. The human fetal hypothalamus and pituitary gland. In: Tulchinsky D, Ryan KJ, eds. Maternal-Fetal Endocrinology. Philadelphia: W. B. Saunders, 1980: 196–232.)

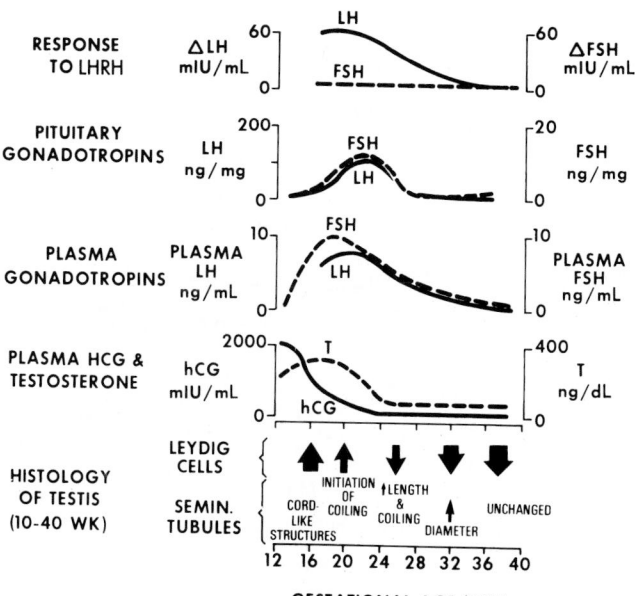

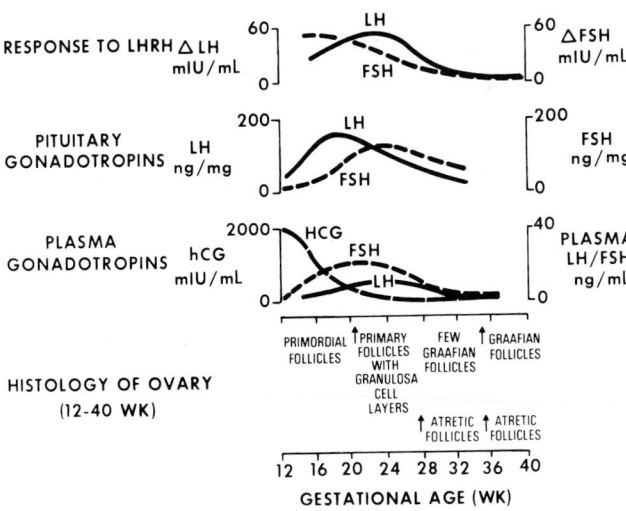

Figure 31–26. Pattern of change of serum FSH, LH, and hCG levels; concentration of pituitary FSH and LH; and increment (Δ) between baseline FSH and LH and the 15-min response to administration of LHRH in human female fetus during gestation with the development of the fetal ovary. See legends of Figures 31–17, 31–18, and 31–25 for conversions to SI units. (Modified from Kaplan SL, Grumbach MM. Pituitary and placental gonadotrophins and sex steroids in the human and subhuman primate fetus. Clin Endocrinol Metab 1978; 7:487–511.[419])

levels were elevated at the beginning of the third trimester and decreased with advancing gestational age to become undetectable in term fetuses.[478] The mean FSH value was higher in female fetuses between 26 and 36 weeks, and the mean LH level was higher in males.[479] Thus FSH and LH secretion continues during late gestation but at decreasing rates. In the ovine fetus LH and FSH are secreted in a pulsatile manner in response to the episodic secretion of fetal hypothalamic LHRH (Fig. 31–27); human fetal pituitary gonadotropins are probably also secreted in pulses. The mean FSH and LH content of fetal pituitary glands and the level of fetal serum FSH are greater in female than in male fetuses at midgestation. This difference has been ascribed to the higher concentration of plasma testosterone between 11 and 24 weeks in the male fetus (the only major difference in circulating gonadal steroids between the male and the female fetus) and higher levels of fetal testicular inhibin.[53] The decrease in both serum FSH and LH levels during late gestation is attributed to the

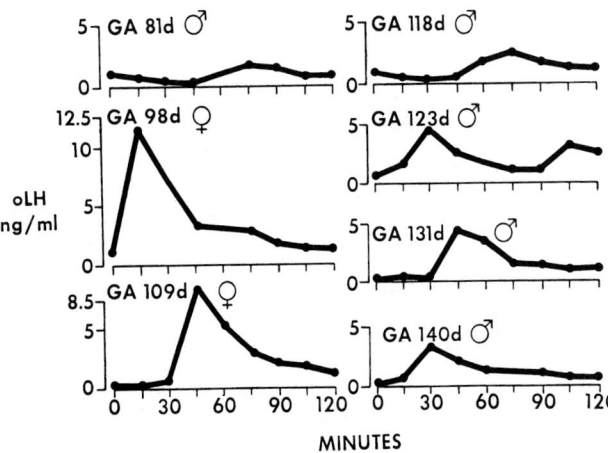

Figure 31–27. Pulsatile LH secretion in the ovine fetus. GA, gestational age. The length of gestation is 145 days in the sheep. (From Clark SJ, Ellis N, Styne DM, et al. Hormone ontogeny in the ovine fetus. XVII. Demonstration of pulsatile luteinizing hormone secretion by the fetal pituitary gland. Endocrinology, 115:1774–1779, 1984, © by The Endocrine Society.[469])

maturation of the negative-feedback mechanism, the development of gonadal steroid receptors in the hypothalamic-pituitary unit,[254, 417, 480] and the effects of inhibin.[53]

The human fetal pituitary gland is responsive in vitro to LHRH as early as 10 weeks of gestation,[481] and the LHRH-stimulated release of LH is greater in second-trimester fetal pituitary cells cultured from females and is augmented by estradiol in both sexes.[482] In vivo studies[483] during middle and late gestation demonstrate that exogenous LHRH stimulates fetal FSH and LH release by 16 weeks of gestation, with a fall in responsivity to LHRH in late gestation (see Figs. 31–25 and 31–26). The anencephalic infant and some neonatal infants with hypothalamic hypopituitarism[53] have an absent or a diminished gonadotropin response to LHRH.[53, 254]

The changes in FSH and LH levels in the fetal pituitary glands and serum are consistent with a sequence of increasing synthesis and secretion in which peak serum gonadotropin levels reach castrate levels, followed by a decline after midgestation that persists to term.[254] The high serum concentrations of FSH and LH in the female and of LH in the male in early and midgestation are probably the result of relatively autonomous, unrestrained activity of the fetal hypothalamic LHRH pulse generator and the consequent stimulation of the fetal gonadotropes by LHRH.[254] As a consequence of the pulsatile secretion of LHRH, the release of fetal LH and FSH is pulsatile (Fig. 31–28; see Fig. 31–27). As fetal development advances, the negative-feedback mechanism matures, and the hypothalamus secretes less LHRH, which in turn leads to decreased secretion of FSH and LH.[480] This inhibition of hypothalamic LHRH release and pituitary gonadotropin secretion appears to be a consequence of the development of sensitivity of the hypothalamus and its LHRH pulse generator to the inhibitory effects of gonadal steroids in the fetal circulation[253, 254] and in the male fetus to a contributory effect by testicular inhibin in late gestation on the decrease in FSH.[53] The increasing CNS control of gonadotropin secretion seems to require maturation of gonadal steroid receptors in the fetal hypothalamus and in the pituitary gonadotropes.[484]

The Sheep Fetus

Studies in the human fetus did not provide insight into the mechanisms of maturation or regulation of the hypothalamic LHRH-pituitary–gonadotropin-gonadal apparatus. The fetal sheep model in which indwelling vascular catheters are placed in the fetus and mother makes it possible to do mechanistic studies.[467] The length of gestation in sheep is about 145 d. The ontogeny of fetal gonadotropins, hypothalamic LHRH, and gonadal steroids is similar to that in the human fetus.[53, 253, 254] Secretion of FSH and LH is not autonomous in the ovine fetus.[253, 469, 470, 480, 485] By midgestation the secretion of fetal LH and FSH is pulsatile[469] and is mediated by the hypothalamic LHRH pulse generator.[470] The ovine fetal hypothalamic-pituitary-gonadotropin unit can respond to gonadal steroid negative feedback by the middle of gestation.[253, 480] A sex difference in gonadotropin secretion[253] is demonstrated by the fact that orchiectomy (but not oophorectomy) leads to an increase in pulsatile secretion of LH (and, to a lesser degree, FSH) in the ovine fetus.[486] Opioidergic neurons have a tonic suppressive effect on the pulsatile release of LHRH in the fetus.[253, 485] The excitatory amino acid analogue N-methyl-D-aspartate (NMDA) evokes an LH pulse mediated by LHRH,[487] providing additional evidence for the function of the fetal LHRH neurosecretory neurons and the capacity of the excitatory amino acids glutamate and aspartate to stimulate[450] the LHRH pulse generator.[443, 601, 602, 605]

Furthermore, FSH stimulates inhibin synthesis by the ovine fetal testis and ovary, and administration of inhibin inhibits secretion of fetal FSH, but not LH, indicating the

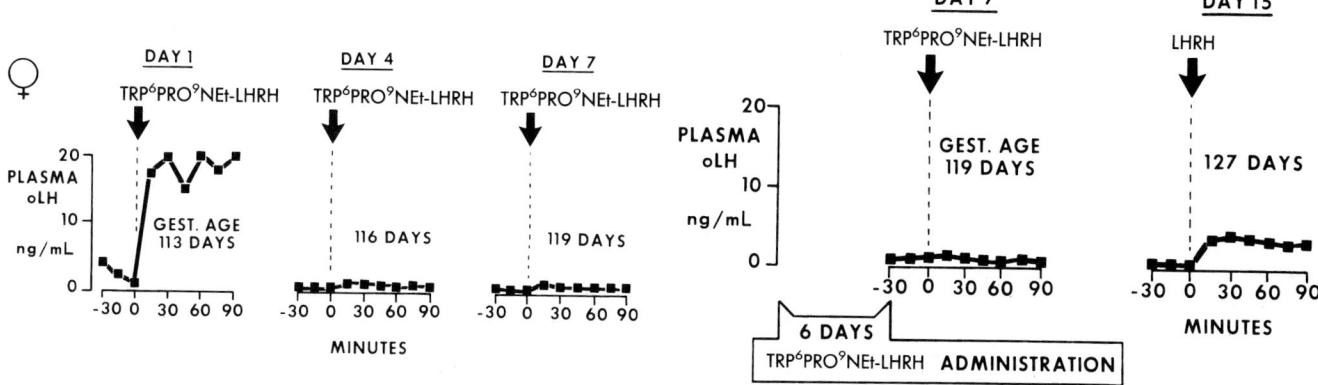

Figure 31–28. *Left,* The effect in the ovine fetus of administration for 7 d of LHRH agonist (10 μg intravenously daily) on the acute LH response to LHRH agonist. *Right,* Recovery of the LH response was impaired 8 d after discontinuing LHRH agonist administration to the ovine fetus. (From Grumbach MM, Kaplan SL. The neuroendocrinology of human puberty: an ontogenetic perspective. In: Grumbach MM, Sizonenko PC, Aubert ML, eds. Control of the Onset of Puberty. Baltimore: Williams & Wilkins, 1990.1–68. © 1990, the Williams & Wilkins Co., Baltimore.[253])

functional capacity of the fetal FSH inhibin feedback system.[488, 489] These observations in the human and ovine fetus, including the pattern of change of fetal FSH and LH, suggest that the hypothalamic LHRH-pituitary-gonadotropin unit is operative by at least the end of the first third of gestation in the human fetus and slightly later in the ovine fetus.

The Human Neonate

Hypothalamic regulatory control of pituitary gonadotropins, as for other pituitary hormones, is not fully mature at birth.[253] Within a few minutes after birth the concentration of LH increases abruptly in peripheral blood (about 10-fold) in the male neonate. This short-lived surge in LH release is followed by an increase in serum testosterone level during the first 3 h that persists for 12 h or more.[490] In the female neonate LH levels do not increase, and FSH levels in both sexes are low during the first days of neonatal life. After the fall in circulating levels of placental steroids (especially estrogens) during the first few days after birth, levels of serum FSH and LH increase and exhibit a pulsatile pattern, with wide perturbations for several months. FSH pulse amplitude is greater in the female infant, and FSH response to LHRH is higher in females throughout childhood; LH pulses are higher in the male (Fig. 31–29). This sex difference is also present in agonadal male and female infants[253, 491] and in the infant rhesus monkey.[492] The high gonadotropin concentrations are associated with a transient second wave of differentiation of fetal-type Leydig cells and increased serum testosterone levels in male infants and with elevated estradiol levels intermittently during the first 1 to 2 years of life in females.[493, 494] The mean FSH level is higher in females than in males during the first few years of life. By approximately 6 months of age in the male and 2 to 3 years of age in the female, the levels of plasma gonadotropins decrease to low values until the onset of puberty. Thus the restraint of the hypothalamic LHRH pulse generator and the suppression of pulsatile LHRH secretion (and thus LH release) attain the prepubertal level of quiescence in late infancy or early childhood and earlier in boys than girls.[253, 495]

Neural Control

The neural regulation of puberty involves two major components: the timing and the control of sexual maturation.

Timing and Onset of Puberty

The onset of puberty and its course are influenced by genetic factors and by environmental forces operating through the CNS. The latter include socioeconomic factors, nutrition, general health, geography, and altitude. Although multiple genes (quantitative or polygenic inheritance) are involved in the time of onset of puberty, little is known about the actual genes involved in this complex trait or the effects of gene interactions (epistasis) on the process.[496–499]

Frisch and Revelle[202] suggested that in healthy girls, despite different ages, there is an "invariant mean weight" (48 kg) for the initiation of the pubertal spurt in weight, the maximal rate of weight gain, and the timing of menarche and that this association is related primarily to fatness.[500–502] The Frisch hypothesis has generated controversy[503–507] in part because the empirical estimations and the equations used to determine fat mass have been challenged. However, the role of nutritional factors and body composition in the onset of menarche[501, 502, 508] is supported by the earlier age of menarche in moderately obese girls;[25] delayed menarche in states of

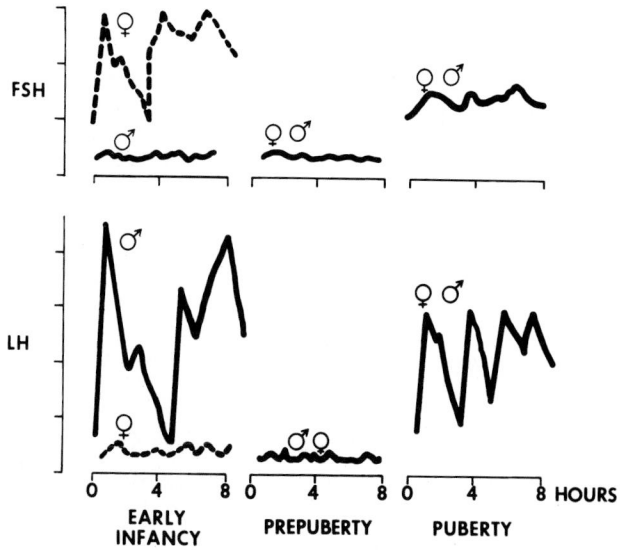

Figure 31–29. Change in the pattern of pulsatile FSH and LH secretion in early infancy, childhood, and puberty. The data for early infancy are derived from Waldhauser et al.[610] Note the pulsatile secretion in the infant and the striking difference in the amplitude of FSH and LH pulses between male and female infants. After infancy the amplitude and frequency of gonadotropin pulses decrease greatly for almost a decade (juvenile pause) until the onset of puberty. (From Grumbach MM, Kaplan SL. The neuroendocrinology of human puberty: an ontogenetic perspective. In: Grumbach MM, Sizonenko PC, Aubert ML, eds. Control of the Onset of Puberty. Baltimore: Williams & Wilkins, 1990: 1–68. © 1990, the Williams & Wilkins Co., Baltimore.[253])

malnutrition and chronic disease, in twins, and after early rigorous athletic or ballet training; and the relationship of weight and diminished body fat to changes in gonadotropin secretion and amenorrhea in girls with anorexia nervosa,[509] voluntary weight loss, and strenuous physical conditioning.[510–513] Long-term studies of girls who had had malnutrition in infancy suggest that no permanent delay in puberty persists if they are treated early.[514]

The proposed causal relationship of "critical body weight," "critical metabolic rate," and body fat to *onset* of puberty in girls has not been substantiated by direct measurements.[515–517] When increments in the excretion of urinary gonadotropins were correlated with changes in body composition at puberty, both developmental events occurred simultaneously rather than sequentially.[518] Moreover, menarche is a late event in the pubertal process and is remote from the factors that control the initial hormonal and physical signs of sexual maturation. Nevertheless, it has long been postulated that some alteration of body/energy metabolism may affect the CNS restraints on pubertal onset and progression.[449, 508, 519] The cloning of the *ob* gene and its product, leptin[520–523]—a 16-kd cytokine-like protein that is expressed and secreted by fat cells (and the placenta)—provides challenging new leads for research.

Leptin, the adipocyte hormone, reflects body fat and hence adipose energy stores.[522, 524] It appears to function as a "lipostat" in the hypothalamus,[525–527] decreasing appetite as a satiety factor and increasing energy expenditure and sympathetic activity. Thus it has an important role in the control of body weight and the regulation of metabolism. The leptin receptor is expressed in the hypothalamus and other tissues including the ovary.[528, 529] In the human, leptin is secreted in a pulsatile fashion[530] and circulates in a bound form.[524, 524a] Serum leptin is increased in rodents with a mutation in the *ob* gene or its receptor,[531] and levels correlate with adipose tissue mass and body fat distribution.[522, 524, 530, 532]

Leptin is also thought to play a role in the neuroendocrine regulation of reproduction. In leptin-deficient mice homozygous for a mutation in the *ob* gene (the Lep^ob^/Lep^ob^ mouse), the administration of leptin repaired the infertility;[533–535] leptin advanced puberty in normal female mice[536, 537] (despite the lower body weight of the treatment group) and repaired the delayed puberty of the food-restricted female rat.[538] Further, leptin at low concentrations stimulates LHRH release from hypothalamic explants from adult rats, LH secretion in intact rats, and LH and FSH release from rat pituitary glands.[539] It is unclear whether the effects of leptin on the hypothalamus are direct or indirect. In the human, anorexia nervosa and athletic amenorrhea are associated with low serum levels of leptin.[524]

These studies suggest that leptin may be a factor in the onset of human puberty. Does leptin provide a peripheral, somatic trigger for the onset of puberty to the central neural neurons, or does it have a permissive role, signaling the hypothalamus and the LHRH pulse generator that a critical energy store for puberty has been attained?[501, 508, 540] In one study leptin levels rose before the initial rise in testosterone in eight boys.[541] But this observation was not confirmed in the male rhesus monkey[542] or in other studies of normal children.[543, 544, 544a, 545] Further, in a large cross-sectional study of prepubertal and pubertal children, leptin levels correlated best with BMI, percent body fat, and age, less with early pubertal maturation[544, 544a, 545] (Fig. 31–30). The rise in leptin levels over the prepubertal and early pubertal years was similar in both sexes, but the rise occurred 1 y earlier in girls. The level in boys peaked at Tanner genital stage 2 and decreased by stage 5; in girls leptin levels increased in breast stage 2 and peaked at stage 5. In addition, a major quantitative locus on human chromosome 2 influenced serum leptin levels and fat mass[546] (the leptin gene is located on chromosome 7.[520]) Further, a group of 9- to 10-year-old boys, followed during the months leading up to an increase in morning salivary testosterone

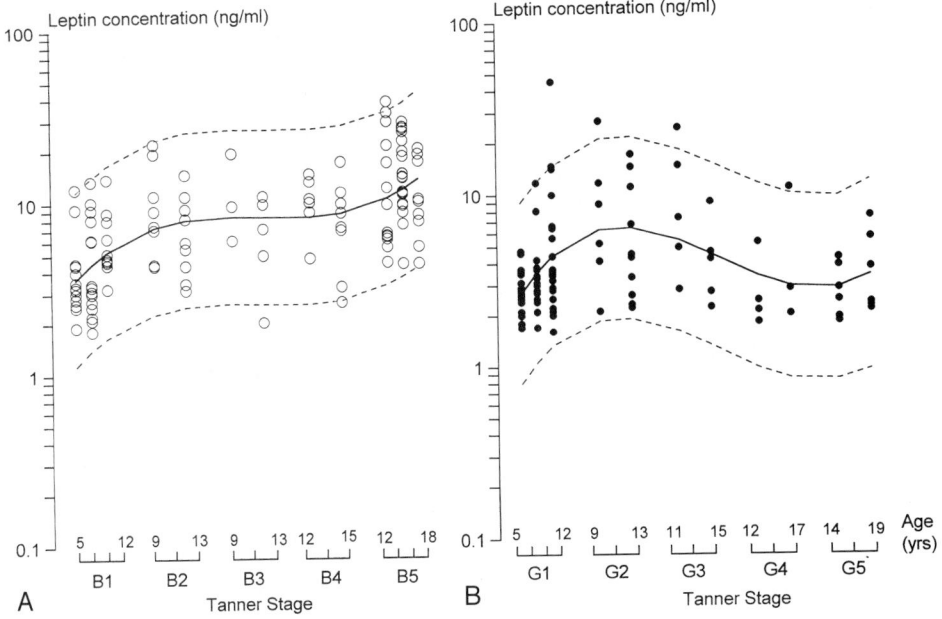

Figure 31–30. Serum leptin concentration (ng/mL) (on a log$_{10}$ scale) versus pubertal stage (females: breast stage; males: genital stage), and age in girls *(A)* and boys *(B)*. The best fit line (shown in bold) for the girls was log$_{10}$[leptin] = $0.029x^3 - 0.275x^2 + 0.858x + 0.036$ (r = 0.6, P < .001) and for the boys was log$_{10}$[leptin] = $0.047x^3 - 0.47x^2 + 1.337x - 0.364$ (r = 0.44, P < .001) where x = pubertal stage, ranked by age. The dashed line represents 95% prediction intervals around the best fit line. Throughout the prepubertal and pubertal years, BMI has a significant effect on leptin in both males and females. The concentration of leptin was similar in prepubertal girls and boys.

Note the decline in serum leptin levels in boys in G4 and G5, whereas leptin concentration rose to a peak in girls in B5. In boys and girls, leptin was positively correlated with BMI standard deviation scores (38 to 41% in girls; 31 to 35% in boys). In B1 and B2 and G1 and G2, leptin also correlated positively with age. In boys in G3 to G5, leptin correlated negatively with testicular volume. Girls reached a leptin level of more than 5 ng/mL more than 1 y earlier than boys (mean 8.6 years vs. 10.4 years). (From Clayton PE, Gill MS, Hall CM, et al. Serum leptin through childhood and adolescence. Clin Endocrinol 1997; 46:727–733.[545])

levels, had a relatively constant basal metabolic rate (BMR)/lean body mass (LBM) ratio but an increase in the ratio of BMR/total daily energy expenditure, suggesting that a subtle energy-dependent process is in play.[547]

The present data seem to be more consistent with the concept that leptin, especially in girls, serves a permissive role in the timing of human puberty by signaling the central nervous system that energy stores, as reflected in the level of serum leptin, are adequate for pubertal development, than that it is a critical trigger for pubertal onset (Fig. 31–31). Leptin may play a more critical role in the onset of puberty in some animals.[542]

The timing of puberty has been linked to the vague concept of "maturation" of the CNS; maturation in this sense is the outcome or consequence of all environmental and genetic factors that retard or accelerate the onset of puberty. A provocative but unproven hypothesis is that a metabolic signal related to body composition is a critical factor in the reactivation of the hypothalamic LHRH pulse generator, and that this activation is not just the consequence of the early changes in hormones and body composition in human puberty. In either event, the factors that influence the timing of puberty are expressed through CNS regulation of its onset.[252, 253, 420, 421, 548–550] In the human, the pineal gland and melatonin do not appear to have a major effect on this control system.[253, 551–560]

Mechanisms of Control

In some species, the neural control mechanism[448, 449] is exquisitely sensitive to the environment. In the rat and the mouse, exteroceptive factors and cues, including light, olfaction, and pheromones, influence gonadotropin secretion by way of the CNS.[448, 449] In seasonal breeding species, such as sheep, the length of the light-dark cycle is critical, and the pattern of gonadotropin secretion is different.[561] In contrast, both male and female primates exhibit an estrogen-provoked LH surge. In brief, diverse strategies and adaptive mechanisms have evolved to control puberty in different species.[253, 451, 452, 561–563]

In both the human and the subhuman primate, the increase in LH and FSH secretion in early infancy is followed

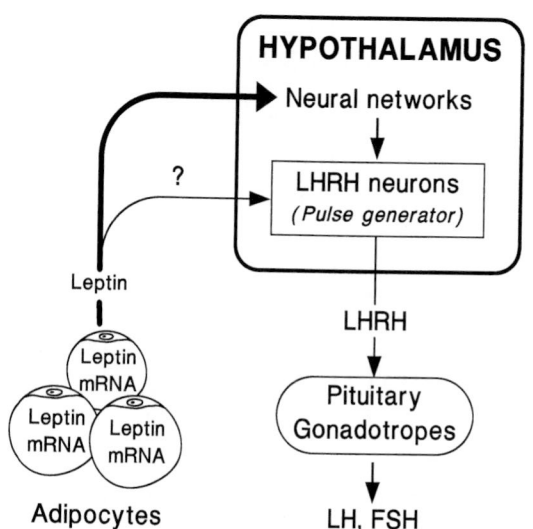

Figure 31–31. The postulated action of leptin secreted by adipocytes on the hypothalamic LHRH pulse generator. Its indirect action through hypothalamic neural networks is illustrated. A direct action, indicated by the thin arrow and ?, on the LHRH pulse generator has not been established. Although leptin is reported to advance puberty in rodents, its role in "triggering" puberty in humans has not been established and is speculative. (*See text.*)

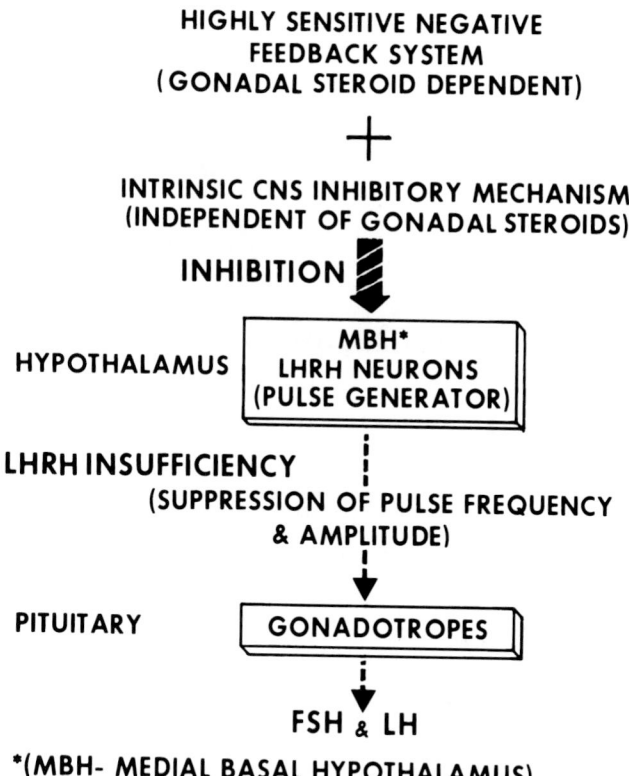

Figure 31–32. Postulated dual mechanism of restraint of puberty involves both gonadal steroid–dependent and gonadal steroid–independent (intrinsic CNS inhibitory mechanism) processes. (Modified from Grumbach MM, Kaplan SL. The neuroendocrinology of human puberty: an ontogenetic perspective. In: Grumbach MM, Sizonenko PC, Aubert ML, eds. Control of the Onset of Puberty. Baltimore: Williams & Wilkins, 1990. 1–68. © 1990, the Williams & Wilkins Co., Baltimore.[253])

by a long period in which the hypothalamic LHRH pulse generator is suppressed and the pituitary gonadotropin-gonadal axis is quiescent (see Table 31–15).[253, 452] In humans this juvenile pause lasts approximately one decade. Two interacting mechanisms have been proposed to explain the pause.[253, 564] One is a hypothalamic-pituitary-gonadal negative-feedback system in infancy and early childhood that is exquisitely sensitive to small amounts of gonadal steroids. The other is a steroid-independent mechanism that involves "intrinsic" CNS inhibition of the LHRH pulse generator in the medial basal hypothalamus[253, 416, 418, 564] throughout childhood (Fig. 31–32).

NEGATIVE-FEEDBACK MECHANISM (GONADAL STEROID–DEPENDENT). The principal evidence for an operative negative-feedback mechanism in prepubertal children is as follows:[252, 253]

1. The pituitary of the prepubertal child secretes small amounts of FSH and LH, suggesting that the hypothalamic-pituitary-gonadal complex is operative in childhood, but at a low level of activity.

2. In the absence of functional gonads prepubertally, as in infants and children with gonadal dysgenesis or other forms of gonadal deficiency, secretion of FSH and, to a lesser degree, LH is increased. The elevated gonadotropin levels in infancy and early childhood in patients with gonadal dysgenesis suggest that even low levels of hormones secreted by the normal prepubertal gonad inhibit gonadotropin secretion[253, 494, 564, 565] (Fig. 31–33).

3. The low level of gonadotropin secretion in childhood is shut off by administration of small amounts of gonadal

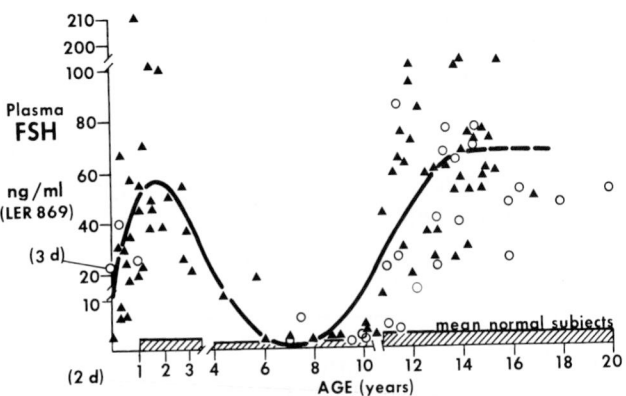

Figure 31–33. Change in pattern of the plasma concentration of FSH with age in 58 patients with the syndrome of gonadal dysgenesis. Mixed longitudinal (n = 23) and cross-sectional (n = 35) data. Triangles designate patients with 45,X karyotype. Circles indicate Turner's syndrome patients with X chromosome mosaicism and/or structural abnormalities of the X chromosome. Note the values in the 2- and 3-day-old infants. The solid line represents a regression line of best fit. The hatched area indicates the mean plasma values in normal females. To convert FSH values to international units per liter, multiply by 8.4. (From Conte FA, Grumbach MM, Kaplan SL. A diphasic pattern of gonadotropin secretion in patients with the syndrome of gonadal dysgenesis. J Clin Endocrinol Metab, 40, 670–675, 1975, © by The Endocrine Society.[565])

steroids, further supporting the idea that the hypothalamic-pituitary unit is highly sensitive to the feedback effect of gonadal steroids.[253, 566] Figure 31–34 shows the striking sensitivity of the hypothalamic-pituitary-gonadotropin complex to the administration of small amounts of ethinyl estradiol. The prepubertal hypothalamic-pituitary unit appears to be approximately 6 to 15 times more sensitive than the adult system.[252] However, as discussed later, this is not the predominant mechanism of LHRH and gonadotropin suppression during the juvenile phase.

The negative feedback becomes operative in the fetus during middle to late gestation[252, 253] (see Figs. 31–25 and 31–26). The lower pituitary content of FSH and LH, the lower serum concentration of FSH in the male fetus, and the decrease in serum FSH and LH levels in late gestation in both female and male fetuses can be explained by the maturation of the gonadal steroid–dependent negative-feedback mechanism. The sex differences in FSH and LH levels during midgestation appear to be a consequence of the high plasma testosterone level in the male fetus and, possibly, inhibin.[53] Estrogen levels increase to a similar extent with advancing gestation in both sexes, presumably arising from placental aromatization of fetal and maternal androgens. However, in the newborn infant there is a sharp decrease in circulating levels of estrogen and other gonadal steroids during the first week of life. Consequently, the plasma levels of FSH and LH increase from the low levels at birth in response to the diminished feedback suppression of the hypothalamic-pituitary-gonadotropin unit.[253, 493] The increased amplitude and frequency of pulsatile gonadotropin secretion in the second week of life evoke an increase in the plasma concentrations of testosterone and inhibin B in male infants and of estradiol in female infants. The gonadal steroid values fall to prepubertal levels by approximately 6 months of age, and by about 6 months of age in the male and 2 to 3 years in the female gonadotropin levels have fallen to values characteristic of the prepubertal child.[493, 494]

"INTRINSIC" CNS INHIBITORY MECHANISM (GONADAL STEROID–INDEPENDENT). The diphasic pattern of basal and LHRH-induced FSH and LH secretion from infancy to adulthood is similar in normal individuals and in agonadal patients, but in the latter gonadotropin levels are higher, except during the middle childhood nadir.[564, 565] The high

concentration of plasma FSH and LH in agonadal children between infancy and age 4 years and the increased gonadotropin reserve reflect the absence of gonadal steroid inhibition (see Fig. 31–35) of the hypothalamic-pituitary unit.[253] However, the striking fall in gonadotropin secretion between ages 4 and 11 suggests the presence of a CNS inhibitory mechanism that, independent of gonadal steroid secretion, restrains the hypothalamic LHRH pulse generator during this pause. This mechanism suppresses LHRH and gonadotropin synthesis and pulsatile secretion and prevents the onset of puberty. The fall in gonadotropin secretion in agonadal children cannot be explained by gonadal steroid feedback (because functional gonads are lacking) or by increased secretion of adrenal steroids (because concentrations are low, and glucocorticoid suppression of the adrenal does not augment the concentration of circulating gonadotropins).[253] Thus a steroid-independent mechanism for suppression of the hypothalamic LHRH pulse generator in the CNS seems to be the dominant factor in restraint of puberty between ages 4 and 11.[253, 567] Gradual loss of this intrinsic CNS inhibitory mechanism leads to disinhibition or reactivation of the LHRH pulse generator at puberty.

INTERACTION OF NEGATIVE FEEDBACK AND INTRINSIC CNS INHIBITORY MECHANISMS (Fig. 31–35). During the first 2 to 3 years of life the gonadal steroid negative-feedback mechanism seems dominant, as evidenced by the striking difference in gonadotropin secretion between the agonadal and the intact infant and young child. Extrapolating from the changing pattern of plasma FSH and LH levels in agonadal infants and children, beginning at about 3 years of age the intrinsic CNS inhibitory mechanism is dominant during the rest of the juvenile pause, as evidenced by the fall in FSH and LH levels between ages 3 and 10 despite the lack of functional gonads. During this segment of the juvenile pause, the negative-feedback mechanism is also operative; agonadal patients in this age group have higher mean plasma FSH levels than normal prepubertal children and a greater FSH and LH response to the acute administration of LHRH.[564, 565] However, the negative-feedback mechanism probably plays a secondary role. As puberty approaches, the CNS inhibitory mechanism

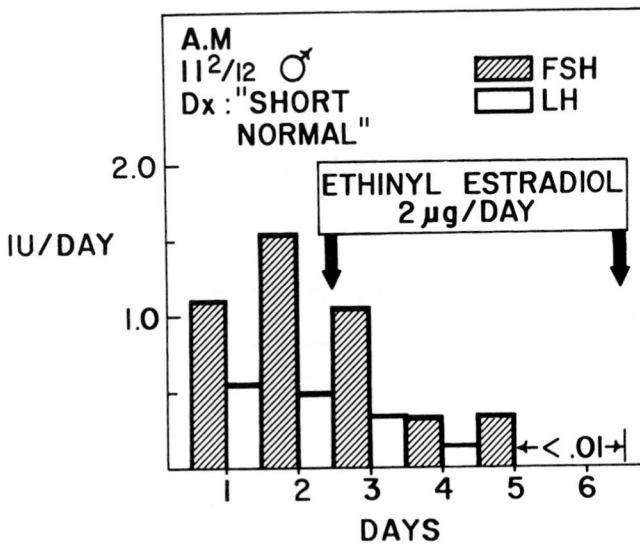

Figure 31–34. Effect of administration of ethinyl estradiol (2 μg/d) on the urinary excretion of LH and FSH in a prepubertal normal male aged 11 years, 2 months. Note the rapid and significant decrease in LH and FSH levels by day 3 after treatment with estradiol; by day 4 the excretion of FSH and LH is less than 0.01 IU. (From Kelch RP, Kaplan SL, Grumbach MM. Suppression of urinary and plasma follicle-stimulating hormone by exogenous estrogens in prepubertal and pubertal children. Reproduced from the Journal of Clinical Investigation, 1973, vol. 52, pp. 1122–1128 by copyright permission of the American Society for Clinical Investigation.[566])

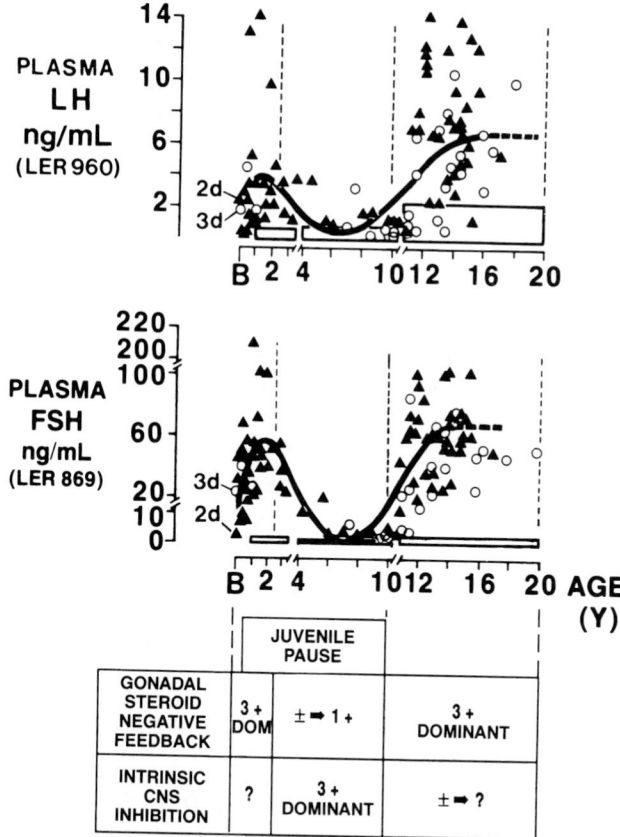

		JUVENILE PAUSE		
GONADAL STEROID NEGATIVE FEEDBACK	3 + DOM	± ➡ 1 +	3 + DOMINANT	
INTRINSIC CNS INHIBITION	?	3 + DOMINANT	± ➡ ?	

Figure 31–35. Interaction of the negative-feedback mechanism and the putative intrinsic CNS inhibitory mechanism in restraining puberty as extrapolated from the pattern of change in the concentrations of FSH and LH in agonadal infants, children, and adolescents. (See Fig. 31–33 for key to symbols; the solid line is the regression curve of best fit; the solid bars connote the mean normal concentrations + 1 SD of FSH and LH.) For about the first 3 years of life the sensitive gonadal steroid, negative-feedback mechanism has a dominant role in restraining gonadotropin secretion, as exemplified by the high gonadotropin concentrations in this age group in the absence of gonads (and gonadal steroid feedback). A major role of the intrinsic CNS inhibitory mechanism in this age group is unlikely in light of the rise in gonadotropins to castrate levels in the absence of functional gonads. From 4 to 6 years of age the postulated intrinsic CNS inhibitory mechanism is dominant, as indicated by the fall in FSH and LH concentrations in the absence of gonads. Even in this age group the augmented gonadotropin response evoked by LHRH and the slightly higher mean basal gonadotropin concentrations in agonadal individuals support a role, although a subsidiary one, for gonadal steroid negative feedback in the suppression of gonadotropin secretion during this period of the juvenile pause. The authors suggest that the intrinsic CNS inhibitory mechanism suppresses the functional LHRH pulse generator. Finally, after about 10 years of age the CNS inhibition gradually wanes, resulting in disinhibition of the LHRH pulse generator. The gonadal steroid negative-feedback mechanism with an adult-type set point and inhibin play a dominant role in regulating the LHRH pulse generator–pituitary gonadotropin system. For conversion to SI units, see the legend of Figure 31–17. (Modified from Grumbach MM, Kaplan SL. The neuroendocrinology of human puberty: an ontogenetic perspective. In: Grumbach MM, Sizonenko PC, Aubert ML, eds. Control of the Onset of Puberty. Baltimore: Williams & Wilkins, 1990: 1–68. © 1990, the Williams & Wilkins Co., Baltimore.[253])

gradually wanes, initially during nighttime sleep, and the hypothalamic LHRH pulse generator becomes less sensitive to gonadal steroid negative feedback (see Fig. 31–35).[253] After the onset of puberty gonadal steroid negative feedback attains the set point characteristic of the adult and is again the dominant mechanism in controlling gonadotropin secretion (along with inhibin), as reflected in the increased gonadotropin levels in the adolescent with primary hypogonadism (see Fig. 31–35). A similar phenomenon has been described in the infant monkey.[492] The postulated ontogeny of this dual mechanism of restraint of puberty is illustrated in Figure 31–36.

Many neural, neurotransmitter/neuromodulator, hor-

monal, growth, and metabolic factors[568–574] and exteroceptive stimuli and cues can influence the activity of the LHRH pulse generator, but the nature of the intrinsic inhibitory mechanism remains speculative. In the rhesus monkey, despite the damping of the LHRH pulse generator during the juvenile pause,[575] the contents of hypothalamic LHRH and LHRH messenger RNA during this phase are similar to those in the infant and adult monkey.[452, 575a] Quiescence of the LHRH pulse generator during the juvenile pause is not absolute. Infrequent LH and FSH pulses are detectable by sensitive and specific immunoradiometric assays.[257–259, 264] The end of the juvenile pause is marked by an increase in both LH pulse amplitude and frequency first evident during the early hours of sleep.

POTENTIAL COMPONENTS OF THE INTRINSIC CNS INHIBITORY MECHANISM. Indirect evidence of an inhibitory neural network that arises or projects through the posterior hypothalamus and suppresses the LHRH pulse generator has been derived from studies of children with true (or central) precocious puberty (reviewed in reference 253) and studies in the female and male monkey.[452, 576–578]

Children with true precocious puberty due to posterior hypothalamic neoplasms (usually a pilocytic astrocytoma), radiation of the CNS, midline CNS developmental abnormalities such as septo-optic dysplasia with deficiency of one or more pituitary hormones, or other CNS lesions provide indirect evidence of an inhibitory neural component located in or projecting through the posterior hypothalamus. As a consequence of these lesions, the neural pathway inhibiting the hypothalamic LHRH pulse generator is compromised, resulting in its disinhibition and reactivation.[253] For example, a suprasellar arachnoid cyst can cause true precocious puberty by compressing and distorting the hypothalamus.[253] In some children with such cysts, the puberty is reversed after decompression of the cyst (Fig. 31–37), suggesting that the disinhibition of the CNS inhibitory mechanism was reversed by treatment of the cyst.

The LHRH-secreting hypothalamic hamartoma, a heterotypic mass of nervous tissue that contains LHRH neurosecretory neurons attached to the tuber cinereum or the floor of the third ventricle[579, 580] can also cause true precocious puberty. The LHRH neurons within the hamartoma secrete LHRH in pulsatile fashion, acting as an "ectopic LHRH generator" that functions independently of the CNS inhibitory mechanisms that normally restrain the hypothalamic LHRH pulse generator (Fig. 31–38).[253] An analogy is the rescue of fertility in the LHRH-deficient hypogonadal mouse *(hpg/hpg)* by transplantation of fetal or neonatal hypothalamic tissue into the third ventricle.[581, 582]

The ontogeny of the fetal LHRH pulse generator suggests that its initial function is unrestrained,[253] similar to the spontaneous, synchronized autorhythmicity in the release of LHRH by the immortalized LHRH neurosecretory neuronal cell line.[424, 426, 428] Taken together, these observations suggest that in the human[253] and nonhuman primate[425, 451, 623] stimulatory input is not required for pulsatile LHRH secretion. In addition, precocious sexual maturation can be induced in the female rhesus monkey by posterior hypothalamic lesions,[576] which advance the age at onset of a pubertal increase in LH secretion and the first positive-feedback effects of estrogen.[577]

Factors that may play a role in the restraint of the LHRH pulse generator during the juvenile pause include noradrenergic, dopaminergic, serotoninergic, and opioidergic pathways; inhibitory neurotransmitters (e.g., γ-aminobutyric acid); excitatory amino acids (e.g., glutamic and aspartic acids); nitrergic (nitric oxide) transmitters; other brain peptides, including neurotrophic and growth factors; and CRH[440, 451, 487, 562, 568–574, 583–588] (Table 31–14). However, the precise mechanism of the CNS restraint is uncertain. Studies in the monkey[452] and

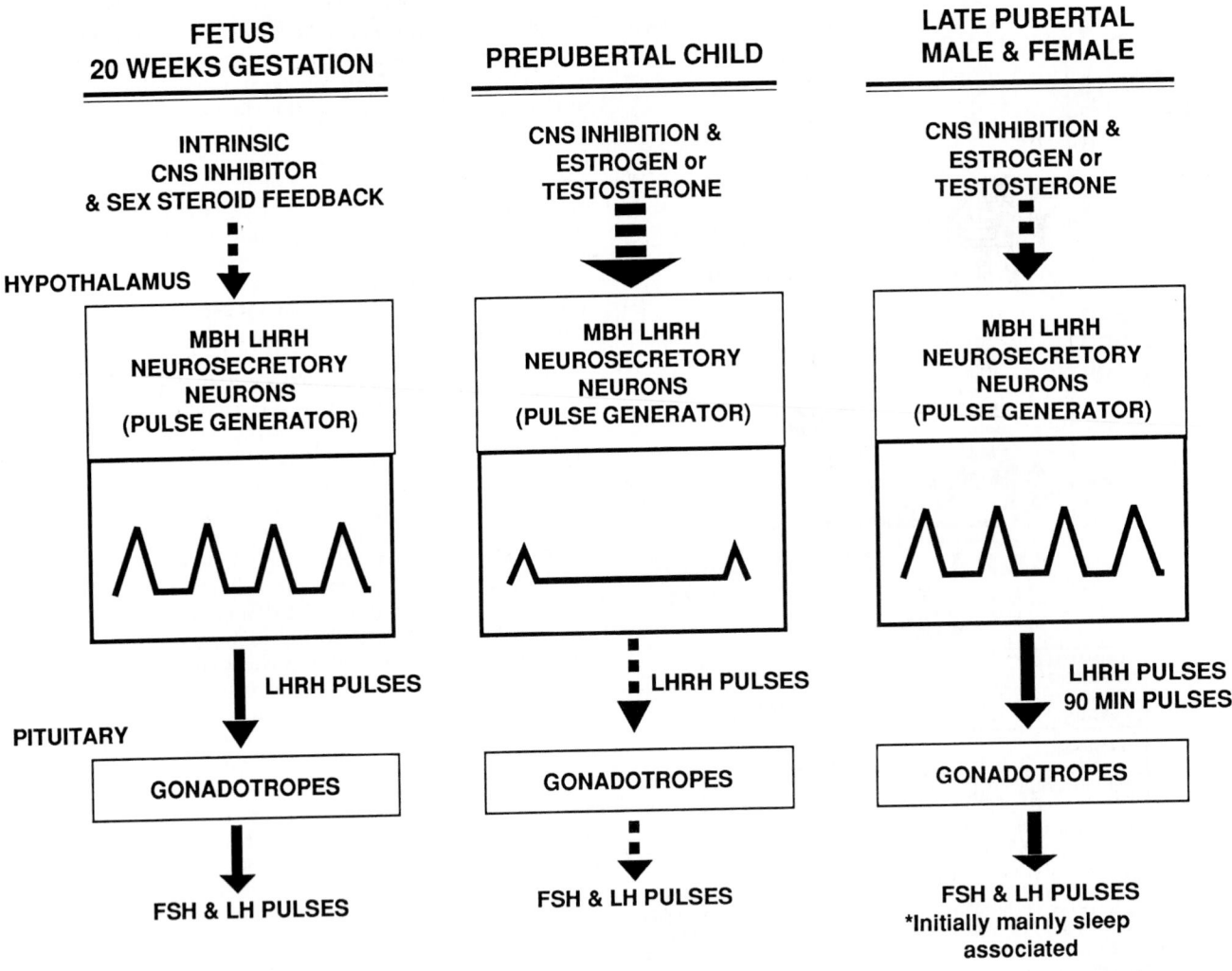

Figure 31–36. Postulated ontogeny of the dual mechanism for the inhibition of puberty. Interrupted arrows indicate inhibition. Note the action of both components during the juvenile pause (prepuberty). See Figure 31–35 for the relative role of these two mechanisms during development. LHRH is given as LRF in the figure; MBH, medial basal hypothalamus. (Modified from Grumbach MM, Kaplan SL. The neuroendocrinology of human puberty: an ontogenetic perspective. In: Grumbach MM, Sizonenko PC, Aubert ML, eds. Control of the Onset of Puberty. Baltimore: Williams & Wilkins, 1990: 1–68. © 1990, the Williams & Wilkins Co., Baltimore.[253])

the human exclude melatonin as a critical restraining factor in primates (see review in references 253, 552 to 554, and 589). Furthermore, there is no evidence of an important role for endogenous opioid peptide in the juvenile pause.[590–594]

γ-Aminobutyric acid (GABA) is the most important known inhibitory neurotransmitter in the primate brain, including the hypothalamus.[595–597] In vivo studies of the median eminence of prepubertal, early pubertal, and midpubertal monkeys, the direct infusion of bicuculline, a GABA$_A$ receptor blocker, evoked a rapid and large increase in LHRH release in prepubertal, but not pubertal, monkeys. In contrast, infusion of GABA itself suppressed LHRH release in pubertal, but not in prepubertal, monkeys. Furthermore, endogenous GABA release is higher and LHRH release much lower in prepubertal monkeys than in pubertal monkeys (Fig. 31–39). These findings suggest that GABA is a potent inhibitor of the LHRH pulse generator in prepuberty and that exogenous administration of GABA in prepuberty is ineffective because of the high local endogenous levels.[595] Glutamic acid decarboxylase (GAD) is the enzyme that catalyzes the conversion of glutamate to GABA. Two classes of GAD, GAD65 and GAD67, are present in mammalian brain. Both GAD mRNAs are detectable in the medial basal hypothalamus, the site of the LHRH pulse generator. Infusion of antisense oligodeoxynucleotides for GAD67 and GAD65 mRNAs into the median

eminence of prepubertal monkeys inhibited GABA synthesis and induced a striking increase in LHRH release.[596] These studies provide additional support for the role of GABA in the juvenile pause.[597] GABA probably has a direct effect on the LHRH pulse generator neuron because it affects LHRH secretion in an LHRH-releasing mouse neuronal cell line, as well as indirect effects.[598]

Among the facilitatory neurotransmitters that affect the release of LHRH, norepinephrine, NPY, and galanin do not appear to have a critical role in the control of the onset of puberty in primates,[452, 599] even though they may play roles as facilitators once the LHRH pulse generator is reactivated. The potential role of leptin in the onset of puberty, controversial in the human but established in the rodent, was discussed earlier.

Excitatory NMDA amino acid neurotransmitter receptors are widely distributed throughout the CNS, including the hypothalamus.[450] NMDA stimulates LH release in neonatal[600] and adult[601] rats, fetal sheep,[487] and prepubertal[602] and adult[603] monkeys. NMDA evokes LHRH secretion from rat hypothalamic explants[604] and from an LHRH neuronal cell line but does not have a direct effect on pituitary gonadotropes.[487]

Chronic intermittent administration of NMDA to prepubertal monkeys induces true precocious puberty and activation of the hypothalamic LHRH-pituitary-gonadal system,[253] and the effect of NMDA on LHRH and LH release can be blocked

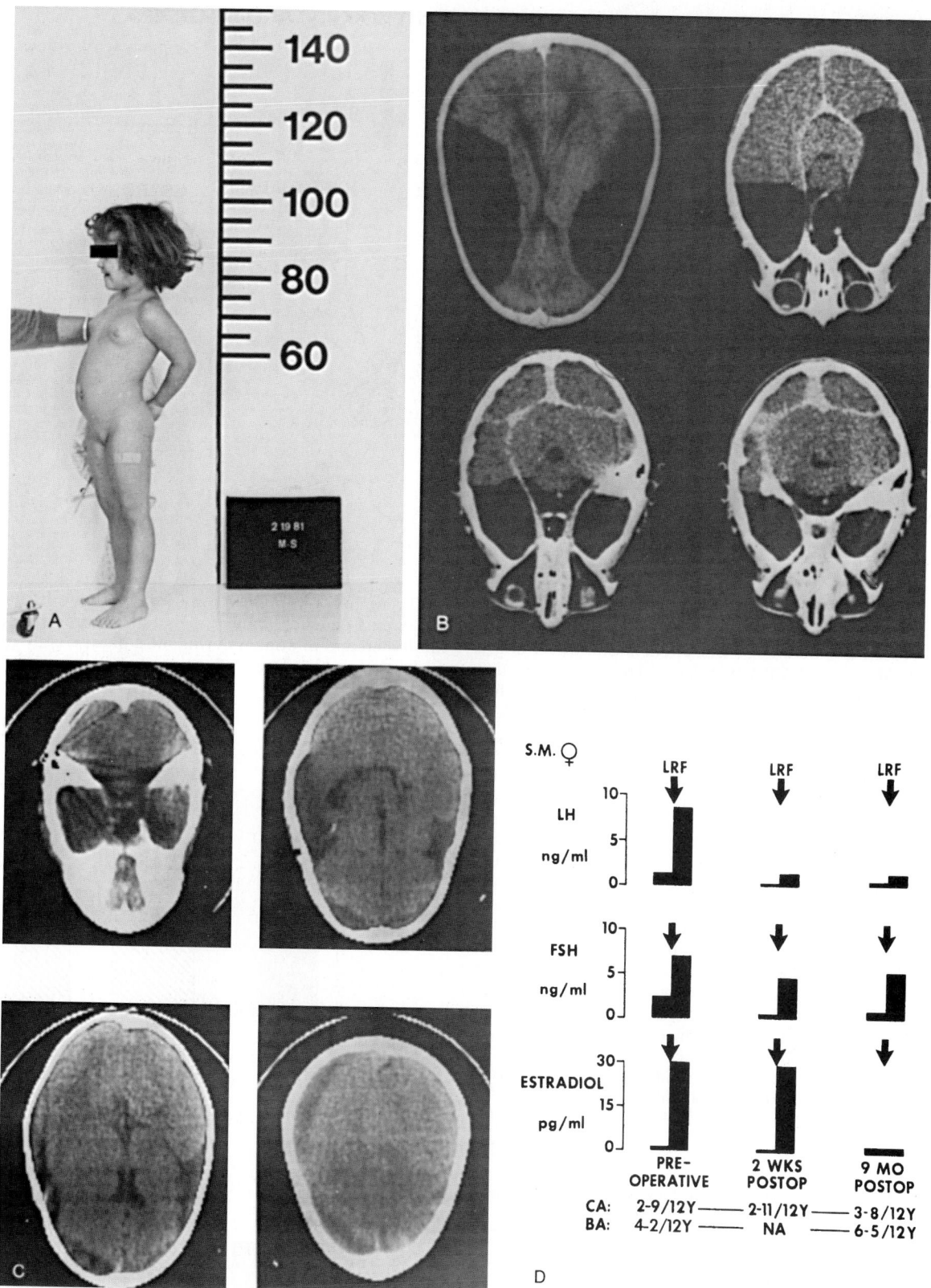

Figure 31–37. *A,* True precocious puberty in a 2 9/12-year-old girl (SM) secondary to a large bilateral congenital suprasellar arachnoid cyst. Signs of sexual precocity were noted during the preceding year. The head circumference was + 5 SD above the mean value for age, and frontal bossing was present. Breasts were Tanner stage 3. Serum estradiol, 26 pg/mL; estrone, 38 pg/mL; DHEAS, < 3 μg/dL. The serum LH concentration rose from 1.4 to 8.7 ng/mL (LER-960) after intravenous administration of LHRH, a pubertal response. Bone age, 3 6/12 years. Pelvic ultrasonography showed pubertal-size uterus and ovaries. To convert estrone values to picomoles per liter, multiply by 3.699. To convert DHEAS values to micromoles per liter, multiply by 0.02714. For other conversions see legend of Figure 31–17. *B,* Cranial CT scans for SM showing low-density fluid collection in the middle cranial fossa, thinning of the cortex, and striking compression of the lateral and third ventricles. *C,* Cranial CT scans 8 mo later, after decompression of the arachnoid cyst and creation of a communication between the cyst and the basal cerebrospinal fluid cisterns and a cystoperitoneal shunt. Note the striking decrease in size of the fluid collections and expansion of the cerebral cortex. *D,* Basal and peak LH and FSH concentrations after LHRH administration in SM and serum estradiol values before and 2 wk and 9 mo after surgical decompression of the arachnoid cyst. Note prepubertal LH response to LHRH and fall in serum estradiol level by 9 mo after surgery. The bone age had increased by 3 y over an 11-mo period, but the velocity has now returned to normal. The patient remained prepubertal during follow-up. (From Grumbach MM, Kaplan SL. The neuroendocrinology of human puberty: an ontogenetic perspective. In: Grumbach MM, Sizonenko PC, Aubert ML, eds. Control of the Onset of Puberty. Baltimore: Williams & Wilkins, 1990: 1–68. © 1990, the Williams & Wilkins Co., Baltimore.[251])

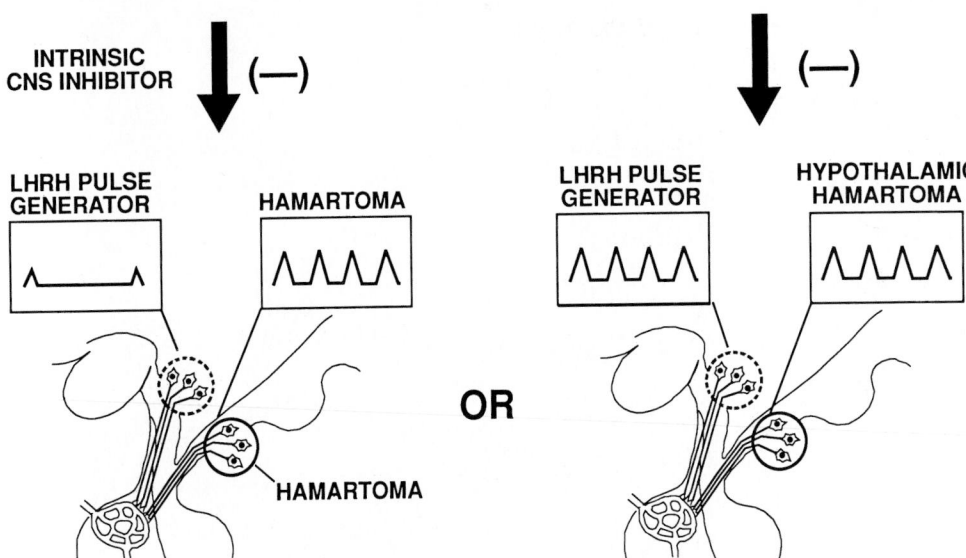

Figure 31–38. Hypothalamic hamartoma as an ectopic LHRH pulse generator that escapes the intrinsic CNS inhibitory mechanism and results in true precocious puberty. Two possible mechanisms are proposed. *Left,* The LHRH neurosecretory neurons in the hamartoma functioning as an LHRH pulse generator without activation of the suppressed normally located LHRH pulse generator. *Right,* The hamartoma acting as an ectopic LHRH pulse generator but communicating with and activating (possibly through axonic connections or by LHRH itself) the normally located hypothalamic LHRH pulse generator, which then functions synchronously with the hamartoma.

by the NMDA receptor antagonist DL-2-amino-5-phosphonopentanoic acid.[583] Furthermore, NMDA receptors are present on LHRH-secreting neurons,[605] consistent with a direct effect of NMDA. Moreover, NMDA stimulates LHRH release in the ovine fetus.[487] These observations establish that the hypothalamic LHRH neurosecretory neuron is not a limiting factor in puberty. The pulse generator, the pituitary, gonads, and gonadal steroid end-organs all are functionally intact prepubertally and in the fetus and can be activated before puberty by the appropriate stimulus. Hence, the restraint of puberty occurs above the level of the LHRH neurosecretory neurons in the hypothalamus. Figure 31–40 contrasts the effects of the GABA inhibitory and the excitatory amino acid (as represented by NMDA and other glutamate receptors) stimulatory neurotransmitters on LHRH release. Hence, in the primate the GABA network seems to be a major component of the intrinsic CNS inhibition during the juvenile pause.

SLEEP-ASSOCIATED LH RELEASE AND ONSET OF PUBERTY. Episodic, or pulsatile, secretion of pituitary LH and FSH is evoked by the pulsatile LHRH signal originating from the hypothalamic LHRH oscillator. Discrete episodic bursts of LH release occur approximately once every 120 min (about 12 episodes over a 24-h period) in adult men[258, 606] and about once every hour during the midfollicular phase in women.[453] Secretory pulses of LH can also be detected in prepubertal

children;[590, 607] the pulses are of lower amplitude and usually of lower frequency than in pubertal children or adults. In adult men and in women during most phases of the menstrual cycle, the amplitude and frequency of these episodic pulses

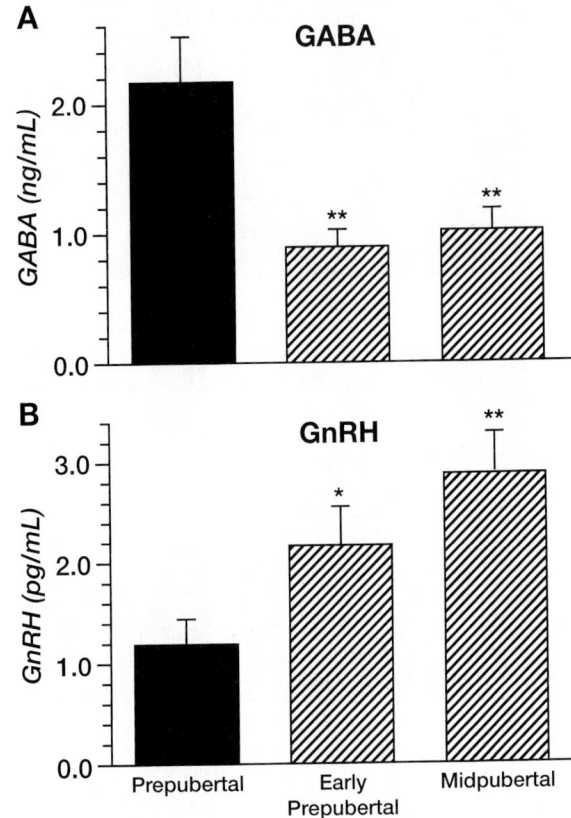

Figure 31–39. The striking developmental changes in γ-aminobutyric acid (GABA) and GnRH (LHRH) release between the prepubertal and the pubertal rhesus monkey as measured in 10-min perfusate samples from the stalk-median eminence. In each animal, multiple samples were obtained. Mean ± SEM; **P < .01; *P < .05 versus prepubertal monkeys. (From Mitsushima D, Hei DL, Terasawa E. γ-Aminobutyric acid is an inhibitory neurotransmitter restricting the release of luteinizing hormone–releasing hormone before the onset of puberty. Proc Natl Acad Sci USA 1994; 91:395–399, with permission.[596])

TABLE 31–14. Potential Components of the Intrinsic CNS Inhibitory Mechanism ("Juvenile Pause")

I. Inhibitory
  A. Inhibitory central neurotransmitter–neuromodulatory pathways
    1. γ-Aminobutyric acid (the main inhibitory factor)
    2. Endogenous opioid peptides
II. Stimulatory
  A. Stimulatory central neurotransmitter-neuromodulatory pathways
    1. Excitatory amino acids
    2. Noradrenergic
    3. Dopaminergic
    4. Neuropeptide Y (NPY)
    5. Nitric oxide
    6. Prostaglandins, PGE_2
    7. Calcium-mobilizing agonists
  B. Other brain peptides
    1. Neurotrophic and growth peptides
    2. Activin A
    3. Endothelin-1, -2, -3

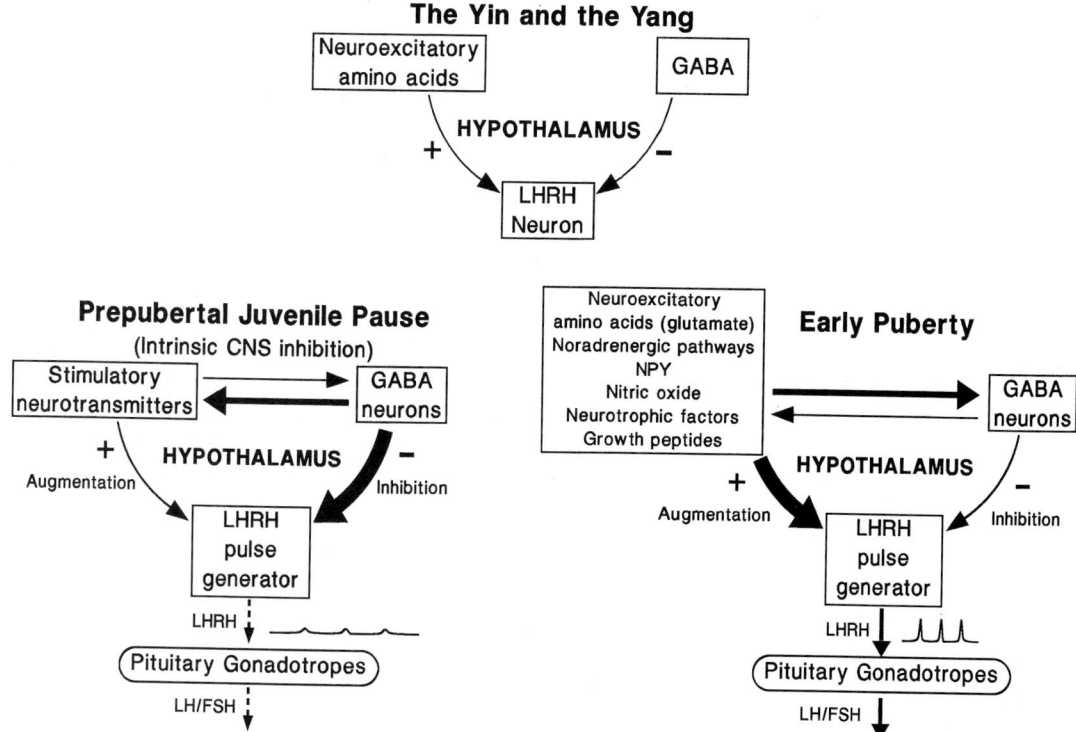

Figure 31–40. The yin and the yang of the neuroendocrinology of the prepubertal juvenile pause and its intrinsic central inhibition of the LHRH pulse generator and the reversal of this inhibition and termination of the juvenile pause, which leads to the onset of puberty. The GABAergic neuronal network and its neurotransmitter GABA is the most ubiquitous inhibitory transmitter in the hypothalamus as well as the brain. During the prepubertal juvenile pause, this neurotransmitter system appears to play the major neural role in inhibiting the LHRH pulse generator. (Suppression of GABA inhibition during this period promptly results in reactivation of the suppressed LHRH pulse generator in the rhesus monkey.) With the approach of puberty GABA inhibition of the LHRH pulse generator wanes, and its reactivation gradually occurs. This reactivation is quite likely augmented by stimulatory neurotransmitters (e.g., excitatory amino acids), some of which are dependent on increased gonadal steroids for their activation, and by neurotrophic factors and growth peptides. As a consequence, the amplitude and, to a lesser extent, the frequency of LHRH pulses increase, which, in turn, leads to increased pulsatile secretion of FSH and LH and the activation of the ovary and testis. As shown experimentally in the monkey, the LHRH pulse generator can function in the absence of hypothalamic stimulatory factors. The nature of and factor or factors responsible for this transition from central inhibition and the postulated dominance of GABA to the release of inhibition and reactivation of the LHRH pulse generator are unknown.

are similar at all times of the day. In pubertal children, however, pulsatile release of LH in early and midpuberty is mainly sleep-associated (see Fig. 31–41),[608] and prominent LH-secretory episodes are detected during the day only in late puberty. Urinary LH in prepubertal children is also excreted mainly at night, although the absolute differences are small.[609]

Gonadotropin secretion in infants is episodic, with a striking sex difference[610] (see Fig. 31–29); the amplitude of the pulses is large and correlates with the increased plasma gonadotropin levels during the first 6 months in boys and the first 1 to 2 years in girls. After this age, pulsatile secretion is demonstrable at low amplitude and frequency mainly at night[253, 555, 606–612] (see Fig. 31–29). In peripubertal boys, augmented LH release during sleep leads to increased testosterone secretion and a rise in the plasma testosterone level at night (Fig. 31–41).[270] This pattern of sleep-associated LH secretion occurs in agonadal patients during the pubertal age period,[608] suggesting that it is not dependent on gonadal function. Furthermore, sleep-related gonadotropin release occurs in children with idiopathic true precocious puberty[612] and in glucocorticoid-treated children with congenital adrenal hyperplasia who have an advanced bone age and an early onset of true puberty.

Sleep-enhanced LH secretion is a phenomenon of maturation of the CNS and the hypothalamic control of LHRH release. However, the factors involved in the initiation of this circadian rhythm are unclear. Episodic release of gonadotropins is suppressed by anti-LHRH antibodies and by the administration of gonadal steroids or of certain catecholaminergic agonists and antagonists and is augmented by the opioid an-

tagonist naloxone. Naloxone does not alter the testosterone-mediated suppression of LH or the effects of testosterone on LH pulsatility in boys in early to middle puberty.[613]

The authors have suggested that an increase in LHRH secretion at puberty has a priming effect on the gonadotrope[252, 267] and leads to increased sensitivity of the pituitary to LHRH (either endogenous or exogenous). In the monkey, the pulse amplitude (and to a lesser degree, pulse frequency) increases between prepuberty and puberty.[452, 614] Sleep-associated LH release in the peripubertal period correlates with the increased sensitivity of the pituitary gonadotropes to administration of LHRH in the peripubertal period.

The increased pulsatile secretion of gonadotropins that is entrained during sleep is the neuroendocrine hallmark of the onset of puberty.

PITUITARY AND GONADAL SENSITIVITY TO TROPIC STIMULI. Maturational changes with puberty involve, sequentially, the extra–medial basal hypothalamus, the hypothalamic LHRH pulse generator, the pituitary, the gonads, and the gonadal hormone target organs.[252, 253] If the increased secretion of gonadotropins at the onset of puberty is due to changes in both neural and hormonal restraints on the pulsatile secretion of LHRH, disinhibition of the LHRH pulse generator should lead to increased amplitude and frequency of pulses initially, increased pulsatile gonadotropin secretion from the pituitary, and finally augmented output of hormones by the gonads. LHRH release is not directly measurable in the human, but it can be estimated indirectly and qualitatively by determining the pulsatile pattern of LH and by the gonadotropin response to exogenous LHRH. The pituitary sensitivity to

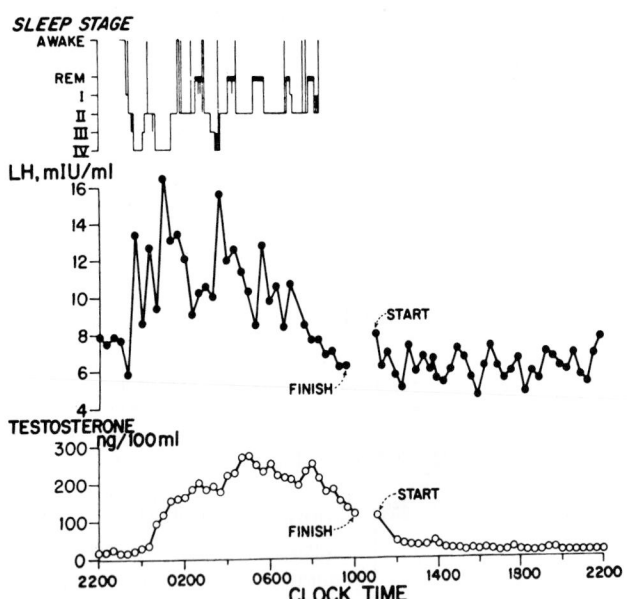

Figure 31–41. Plasma LH and testosterone sampled every 20 min in a 14-year-old boy in pubertal stage 2. The histogram displaying sleep stage sequence is depicted above the period of nocturnal sleep. Sleep stages are REM with stages I to IV shown by depth of line graph. Plasma LH is expressed as mIU/mL. Plasma testosterone is expressed as nanograms per 100 mL. To convert LH values to international units per liter, multiply by 1.0. To convert testosterone values to nanomoles per liter, multiply by 0.03467. (From Boyar RM, Rosenfeld RS, Kapen S, et al. Human puberty. Simultaneous augmented secretion of luteinizing hormone and testosterone during sleep. Reproduced from the Journal of Clinical Investigation, 1974, vol. 54, pp. 609–618 by copyright permission of the American Society for Clinical Investigation.[270])

synthetic LHRH and the reserve of pituitary gonadotropins have been studied at different stages[268, 269] and in disorders of the hypothalamic-pituitary-gonadal system. The results support the concept that the prepubertal state is characterized by functional LHRH deficiency.[252, 253, 416, 418, 614]

The release of LH after administration of LHRH is minimal in prepubertal children beyond infancy, increases during the peripubertal period and puberty,[252, 253] (Fig. 31–42), and is still greater in adults (depending on the phase of the menstrual cycle in women).[615, 616] The change in the pattern of FSH release with maturation is different from that of LH and results in a striking reversal of the FSH/LH ratio after the administration of LHRH to both males and females between prepuberty and puberty.[252] FSH release after the administration of LHRH is comparable in prepubertal, pubertal, and adult males (see Fig. 31–42), but there is a sex difference in the FSH response: prepubertal and pubertal females release more FSH than do males at all stages of sexual maturation.[252, 268] Prepubertal girls also have a larger readily releasable pool of pituitary FSH than do prepubertal or pubertal males, possibly related in part to the higher concentration of inhibin B in prepubertal boys (see Fig. 31–42). The sex difference in sensitivity to LHRH and releasable FSH and the low inhibin levels in the prepubertal female may be factors in the higher frequency of idiopathic true precocious puberty in girls and in the occurrence of premature thelarche.[617] The available data suggest that less LHRH is required for FSH than for LH release.

The responses to LHRH in peripubertal children prior to the onset of sexual maturation suggest that endogenous LHRH augments or primes pituitary responsiveness to exogenous LHRH and that this process is an important factor in the increased gonadotropin secretion at puberty;[252, 253] the increased LH response to synthetic LHRH is one of the earliest hormonal markers of the onset of puberty.

Studies of the effects of acute and chronic administration of synthetic LHRH in hypergonadotropic hypogonadism, hypogonadotropic hypogonadism, constitutional delayed growth and adolescence, and idiopathic precocious puberty support this concept of "self-priming."[252, 267, 269, 282, 453, 618–622] The prepubertal pituitary gland has a smaller pool of releasable LH and decreased responsiveness to the acute administration of synthetic LHRH. With the approach of puberty, the derepression of the hypothalamic LHRH pulse generator and the increased pulsatile secretion of LHRH augment pituitary sensitivity to LHRH and enlarge the reserve of LH. The reason for the discordance in FSH and LH release prepubertally is not clear, but the frequency of LHRH pulses may be a factor[451, 454, 455, 457, 623] as well as the effect of inhibin secreted by the prepubertal testis on FSH release. In rhesus monkeys with ablative hypothalamic lesions that eliminate endogenous LHRH secretion, reduction in the frequency of exogenous LHRH pulses from 1/h to 1/3 h increases the FSH/LH ratio.[454] Inhibin and endogenous gonadal steroids may also affect this ratio.

These observations and the previously discussed role of the pulsatility of the LHRH signal in the control of gonadotro-

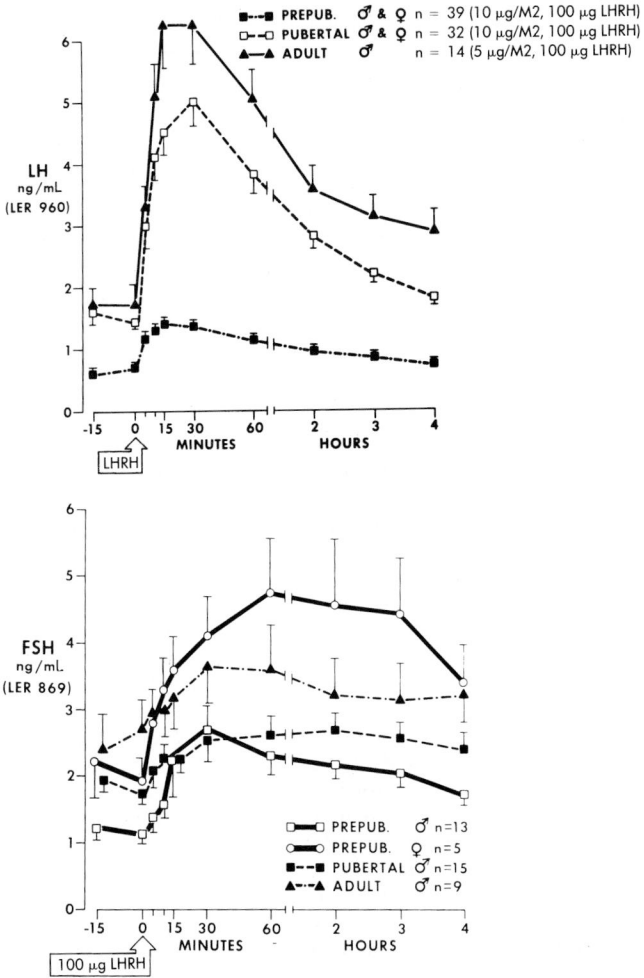

Figure 31–42. Changes in plasma LH *(top)* and FSH *(bottom)* levels in prepubertal, pubertal, and adult individuals. Note the limited LH response in prepubertal children compared with that of pubertal and adult subjects. The FSH response to LHRH is similar in prepubertal, pubertal, or adult males. In females, the FSH response is significantly greater than that of prepubertal, pubertal, or adult males. For conversion to 51 units, see the legend of Figure 31–17. (Modified from Grumbach MM, Roth JC, Kaplan SL, et al. Hypothalamic-pituitary regulation of puberty in man: evidence and concepts derived from clinical research. In: Grumbach MM, Grave GD, Mayer FE, eds. Control of the Onset of Puberty. New York: John Wiley & Sons, 1974: 115–166.[252])

pin secretion have important implications for the induction of puberty. Pulsatile administration of LHRH to prepubertal monkeys promptly initiates puberty (and, in females, ovulatory menstrual cycles) and restores complete gonadal function in adult monkeys with hypothalamic lesions.[451, 452, 623–625] Studies in prepubertal children and in adults with hypothalamic hypogonadotropic hypogonadism are similar.[455, 590, 607, 618–622, 626] Responsiveness of the gonads to gonadotropins also increases during puberty. For example, the augmented response in testosterone secretion to administration of hCG in boys at puberty[627] is probably a consequence of the priming effect of the endogenous LH (in the presence of FSH)[628] on the Leydig cell.

MATURATION OF POSITIVE-FEEDBACK MECHANISM. Estradiol has both negative- and positive-feedback effects on the hypothalamic-pituitary system. The midcycle surge of LH and FSH secretion in women is due to the positive feedback of increased plasma estradiol during the latter part of the follicular phase.[457, 615, 629] Although the suppressive effect is probably operative from late fetal life on, the positive feedback of endogenous (or exogenous) estradiol on gonadotropin release does not occur in prepubertal and early pubertal children.[252, 253, 630] Hence, acquisition of positive feedback, a requisite for ovulation, is a late maturational event in puberty.[252, 253, 630, 631]

A positive-feedback action of estradiol on gonadotropin release at puberty[252] requires (1) ovarian follicles primed by FSH to secrete sufficient estradiol to reach and maintain a critical level in the circulation, (2) a pituitary gland that is sensitized to LHRH and contains a large enough pool of releasable LH to engender an LH surge, and (3) possibly, sufficient LHRH stores for the LHRH neurosecretory neurons to respond with an acute increase in LHRH release above the usual adult pattern of pulsatile LHRH secretion.

Estradiol acts to induce positive feedback at the level of the anterior pituitary. Indeed, positive as well as negative feedback can occur in adult ovariectomized female rhesus monkeys in whom the medial basal hypothalamus has been surgically disconnected from the CNS.[425, 451, 623, 632] In monkeys with hypothalamic lesions, unvarying, pulsatile LHRH administration leads to sufficient estradiol release from the ovary to induce an ovulatory LH surge in the absence of an increase in the LHRH pulses.[457, 625] Estradiol also exerts a positive-feedback effect directly on the pituitary gland in women, and prolonged administration of estradiol causes an augmented LH response to LHRH administration in women.[616] The fact that the major positive-feedback action of estradiol on the pituitary gland is demonstrable in the absence of an increase in pulsatile LHRH secretion suggests that the failure to elicit a positive-feedback action of estradiol in prepubertal girls could be related to the functional immaturity of either the CNS or the pituitary; the consequence is inadequate LHRH pulses or insufficient LH reserve, respectively, or both.

The fact that gonadotropin cyclicity[633, 634] and estradiol-induced positive feedback can be demonstrated by midpuberty and before menarche does not imply that the positive-feedback loop is complete.[1, 252, 495, 630, 631] Indeed, the output of estradiol by the pubertal ovary may be insufficient to induce an ovulatory LH surge even when the pituitary store of readily releasable LH and FSH is adequate. Inadequate production of estradiol by the immature ovary could be due to lack of sufficient gonadotropin stimulation, decreased responsiveness, or other local factors. We visualize the process leading to ovulation as a gradual one in which the ovary[457] and the hypothalamic-pituitary-gonadotropin complex become progressively more integrated and synchronous until, finally, an ovary primed for ovulation secretes sufficient estradiol to induce an ovulatory LH surge.[495]

Studies of basal body temperature[633] and of plasma pro-

gesterone levels[61, 635] indicate that as many as 55 to 90% of cycles are anovulatory during the first 2 y after menarche and that the proportion decreases to less than 20% of cycles by 5 y after menarche[61] (see Chapter 15). A cyclic surge of LH occurs during some anovulatory cycles in adolescence, but the mechanism of ovulation seems unstable and immature and does not appear to have attained the fine-tuning and synchronization requisite for maintenance of regular ovulatory cycles.

Summary of Present Concept

Our present view of the role of the onset of puberty is illustrated in Table 31–15. Clearly, the understanding of this complex process is incomplete.

Puberty is not immutable; it can be arrested or even reversed. Environmental factors and disorders that impair puberty mediate their effects by direct or indirect suppression of the hypothalamic LHRH pulse generator. For example, strenuous physical conditioning in girls (but not boys) and anorexia nervosa can delay or arrest puberty or cause the reversion of the hypothalamic-pituitary unit to a prepubertal state, depending on the magnitude of the functional LHRH insufficiency. With a decrease in physical activity in the former disorder and with resumption of weight gain and attainment of sufficient body mass in the latter, puberty is reactivated. In

---

TABLE 31–15. Postulated Ontogeny of the Hypothalamic-Pituitary-Gonadal Circuit

Fetus
Medial basal hypothalamic LHRH neurosecretory neurons (pulse generator) operative by 80 d of gestation
Pulsatile secretion of FSH and LH by 80 d of gestation
Initially unrestrained secretion of LHRH (100 to 150 d)
Maturation of negative gonadal steroid feedback mechanisms by 150 d of gestation—sex difference
Low level of LHRH secretion at term

Early Infancy
Hypothalamic LHRH pulse generator functional after 12 d of age
Prominent FSH and LH episodic discharges until approximately 6 mo of age in males and 12 mo of age in females with transient increase in plasma levels of testosterone and estradiol in males and females, respectively

Late Infancy and Childhood
Intrinsic CNS inhibition of hypothalamic LHRH pulse generator operative; predominant mechanism in childhood; maximal sensitivity by approximately 4 y of age
Negative-feedback control of FSH and LH secretion highly sensitive to gonadal steroids (low set point)
LHRH pulse generator inhibited; low amplitude and frequency of LHRH discharges
Low secretion of FSH, LH, and gonadal steroids

Late Prepubertal Period
Decreasing effectiveness of intrinsic CNS inhibitory influences and decreasing sensitivity of hypothalamic-pituitary unit to gonadal steroids (increased set point)
Increased amplitude and frequency of LHRH pulses, initially most prominent with sleep (nocturnal)
Increased sensitivity of gonadotropes to LHRH
Increased secretion of FSH and LH
Increased responsiveness of gonad to FSH and LH
Increased secretion of gonadal hormones

Puberty
Further decrease in CNS restraint of hypothalamic LHRH pulse generator and of the sensitivity of negative-feedback mechanism to gonadal steroids
Prominent sleep-associated increase in episodic secretion of LHRH gradually changes to adult pattern of pulses about every 90 min
Pulsatile secretion of LH follows pattern of LHRH pulses
Progressive development of secondary sexual characteristics
Spermatogenesis in males
Middle to late puberty—operative positive-feedback mechanism and capacity to exhibit an estrogen-induced LH surge
Ovulation in females

Modified from Grumbach MM, Roth JC, Kaplan SL, et al. Hypothalamic-pituitary regulation of puberty in man: evidence and concepts derived from clinical research. In: Grumbach MM, Grave GD, Mayer FE, eds. Control of the Onset of Puberty. New York: John Wiley & Sons, 1974: 115–166.[252]

rare instances, true precocious puberty caused by an extrinsic mass lesion that impinges on the hypothalamus can be reversed by decompression or removal of the mass (e.g., a subarachnoid cyst).[253, 636]

ADRENAL ANDROGENS AND ADRENARCHE

The adrenal contribution to puberty (adrenarche) and the interactions between adrenal and gonadal hormones are poorly understood.[123, 637, 638]

Nature and Regulation of Adrenal Androgens

The major androgens secreted by the adrenal cortex are DHEA, DHEAS, and androstenedione. The adrenal androgens can be converted to physiologically active testosterone and

estradiol by extraglandular metabolism. In normal women, only androstenedione is an important precursor; androstenedione is the major androgen secreted by the ovary during and after puberty. DHEA and DHEAS contribute little to circulating testosterone and estradiol but can be converted locally to these steroids in some tissues; the metabolism and kinetics of DHEA and DHEAS in prepubertal children are poorly characterized. However, DHEA and especially DHEAS are useful biochemical markers of adrenal androgen secretion and the onset of adrenarche.

The plasma concentrations of DHEA and DHEAS in boys and girls begin to increase by the age of 7 or 8 (6 to 8 years of skeletal age) about 2 years before the increase in gonadotropin and gonadal steroid levels,[638, 642] and continue to rise through puberty (ages 13 to 15),[123, 639–641] reaching a peak at ages 20 to 30 and then gradually decreasing thereafter (Fig. 31–43). The 20-fold increase in the concentration of DHEAS between the onset of adrenarche and midpuberty is accompanied by increased excretion of urinary 17-ketosteroids, especially 11-deoxy C_{19}-steroids. The increase is not asso-

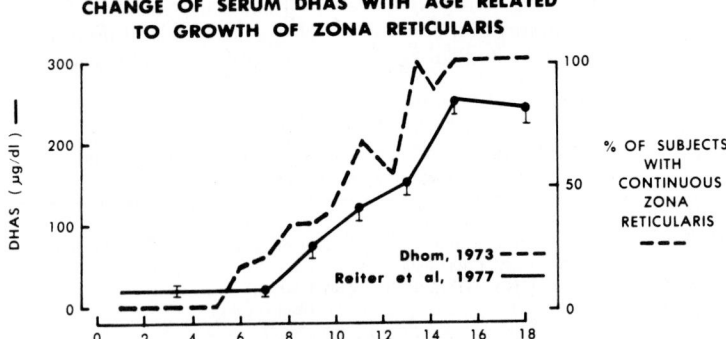

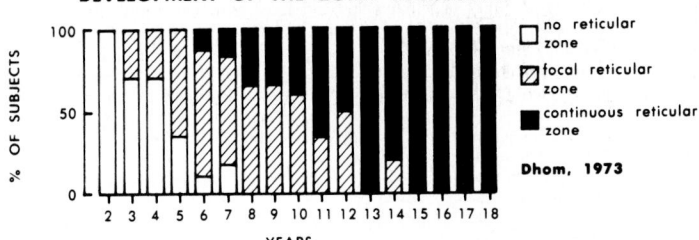

Figure 31–43. Relation of plasma DHEAS (DHAS) to growth of the zona reticularis and increase in adrenal volume with age. *Top,* The close correlation between the development of the zona reticularis and the increase in plasma DHEAS level. *Middle,* The age at which either focal islands of reticular tissue or a continuous reticular zone was found in a series of patients with sudden death who had not had an antecedent illness. *Bottom,* The increase in adrenal volume at the time of puberty. For conversion to SI units, see the legend of Figure 31–37. (From Grumbach MM, Richards HE, Conte FA, et al. Clinical disorders of adrenal function and puberty: assessment of the role of the adrenal cortex and abnormal puberty in man and evidence for an ACTH-like pituitary adrenal androgen stimulating hormone. In: James VHT, Serio M, Giusti G, et al., eds. The Endocrine Function of the Human Adrenal Cortex. New York: Academic, 1978: 583–612.[123])

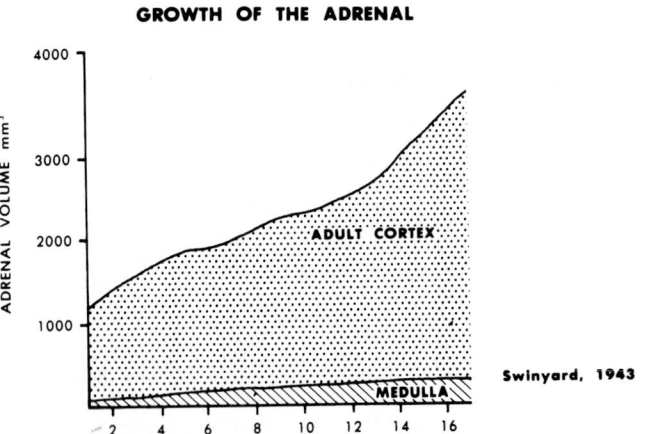

ciated with enhanced sensitivity of the pituitary gonadotropes to LHRH[617] or with sleep-associated LH secretion and occurs at an age when the hypothalamic-pituitary-gonadal complex functions at a low level.[123]

The increase in the adrenal secretion of DHEA and DHEAS at adrenarche (independent of a change in the secretion of cortisol or aldosterone) is accompanied by growth of the zona reticularis (see Fig. 31–43)[642] (see Chapter 12). The zona reticularis, the innermost zone of the adrenal cortex, is the last zone to develop in the adrenal cortex and the principal source of DHEA and DHEAS. Four features distinguish the zona reticularis from the zona glomerulosa and zona fasciculata:

1. A low level of expression of 3β-hydroxysteroid/$\Delta^{4, 5}$-isomerase type 2 and steroid 21-hydroxylase (CYP21) mRNA and enzyme activities.[643–645]

2. Abundant dehydroepiandrosterone (hydroxysteroid) sulfotransferase activity.[643, 644]

3. A relative increase in 17,20-lyase to 17α-hydroxylase activity of CYP17, the enzyme that catalyzes both activities.[643, 644] The above characteristics are shared by the fetal zone of the adrenal cortex.[643, 646, 647]

4. Expression of major histocompatibility complex (MHC) class II (HLA-DR) antigens[648, 649] (antigens not expressed in the fetal zone of the adrenal cortex[649]).

The CYP17 enzyme catalyzes both adrenal 17α-hydroxylase and 17,20-lyase activities. In contrast to the zona fasciculata, the zona reticularis has an increased ratio of 17,20-lyase/17α-hydroxylase activity. Tissue-specific regulation of the 17,20-lyase activity is well described. In the human Leydig cell (and quite likely the zona reticularis) pregnenolone is 17α-hydroxylated, and the 17α-hydroxypregnenolone is oxidized to DHEA, whereas in the zona fasciculata, the 17α-hydroxypregnenolone is converted to 17α-hydroxyprogesterone and 21-hydroxylated and oxidation to DHEA is inhibited. In the rat, site-directed mutagenesis of arginine 346 to alanine in CYP17 led to retention of 80% of 17α-hydroxylase activity but reduced 17,20-lyase activity by 93%.[650] Similarly, mutation of the corresponding residue in human CYP17 (arginine 347 to

alanine) decreased 17,20-lyase activity but had no effect on 17α-hydroxylase activity.[651, 653] Two 46,XY phenotypic females with hypergonadotropic hypogonadism and normal mineralocorticoid and glucocorticoid function had isolated 17,20-lyase deficiency owing to homozygous mutations at either the arginine 347 residue or arginine 350 in CYP17.[651, 653]

In contrast, Miller and colleagues[651, 652] showed that the ratio of human 17,20-lyase/17α-hydroxylase activities is increased by phosphorylation of serine and threonine residues on the CYP17 enzyme and by increased abundance of redox partners such as P450 reductase and b_5.[653] These latter studies may provide insight into the relatively increased 17,20-lyase activity of the zona reticularis, but not into its regulation (Fig. 31–44).

The control of adrenal androgen secretion is poorly understood.[123, 637, 653] Regulation of adrenal androgen secretion in the zona reticularis may involve a dual control mechanism: (1) corticotropin (ACTH, adrenocorticotropin) which appears to be obligatory, as evidenced, for example, by the findings in ACTH deficiency or resistance, and (2) an unidentified adrenal androgen–stimulating factor, possibly from the pituitary or from an adrenal or nonadrenal source[123] (Fig. 31–45). Rejected alternatives to a unique adrenal androgen–stimulating factor are the known hormones, including endorphin, pro-opiomelanocortin (residues 79–96; the hinge peptide), prolactin, FSH, LH, GH, melatonin,[556] and estrogen. Despite much effort, a distinct hormone or factor that stimulates the zona reticularis and adrenal androgen secretion in addition to corticotropin has not been isolated.

A distinct adrenal androgen–stimulating factor, whether of pituitary, intra-adrenal, or other origin, could explain the following observations:[123]

1. The spurt in adrenal growth and the growth of the zona reticularis at adrenarche occur independent of an increase in corticotropin or cortisol secretion but correlate with the increase in plasma DHEAS (see Fig. 31–43).

2. The secretion of cortisol and adrenal androgen varies independently with age, during normal as well as premature adrenarche, and in Cushing's disease, starvation, malnutrition, anorexia nervosa, and chronic disease.

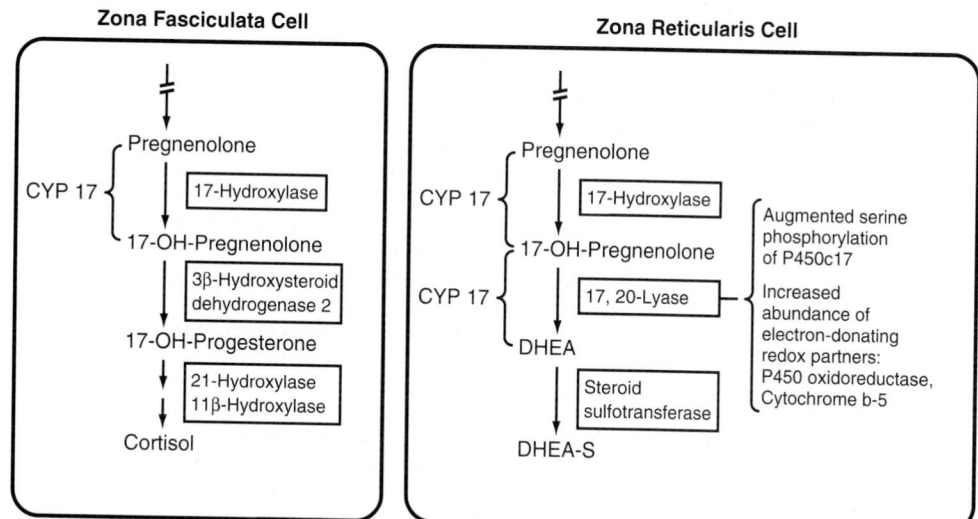

Figure 31–44. Adrenarche and the zona reticularis. The rise in circulating dehydroepiandrosterone sulfate is the biochemical hallmark of adrenarche. The diagram compares and contrasts the major steroidogenic pathway in the zona fasciculata with that in the zona reticularis. In contrast to the zona fasciculata, the expression of 3β-hydroxysteroid, $\Delta^{4,5}$-isomerase type 2 mRNA and its activity (the enzyme that irreversibly traps Δ^5 precursors into Δ^4 steroids) is very low in the zona reticularis, whereas the expression of and activity of steroid sulfotransferase is high. A single gene, CYP17, encodes a single enzyme that has both 17α-hydroxylase and 17,20-lyase activity, but the ratio of 17,20-lyase/17α-hydroxylase activity is relatively high in the zona reticularis compared with that in the zona fasciculata. Some of the factors that seem to augment the increased 17,20-lyase activity of CYP17 are the augmented serine phosphorylation of the enzyme and the apparent increased abundance of electron-donating redox partners, including P450 reductase and cytochrome b-5. *(See text.)*

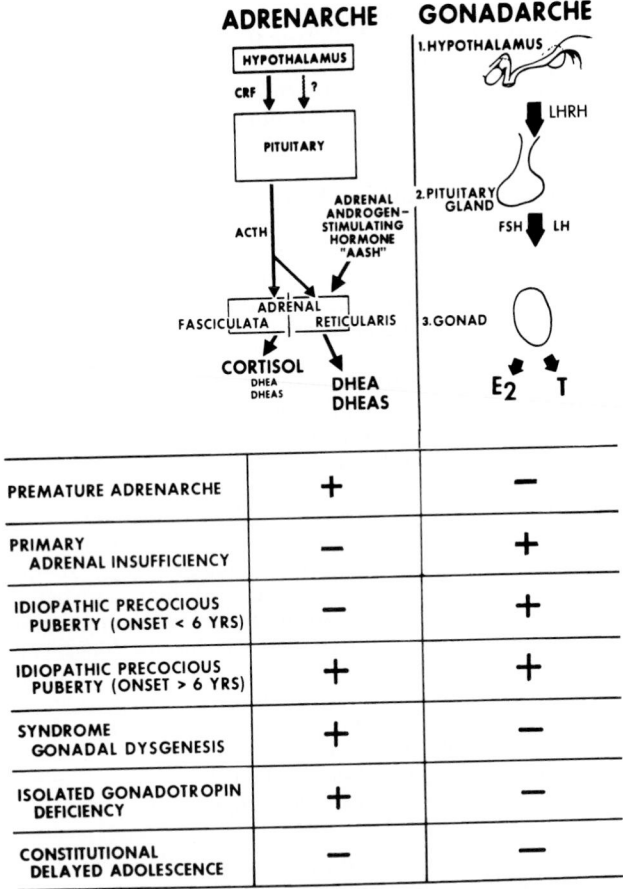

	ADRENARCHE	GONADARCHE
PREMATURE ADRENARCHE	+	−
PRIMARY ADRENAL INSUFFICIENCY	−	+
IDIOPATHIC PRECOCIOUS PUBERTY (ONSET < 6 YRS)	−	+
IDIOPATHIC PRECOCIOUS PUBERTY (ONSET > 6 YRS)	+	+
SYNDROME GONADAL DYSGENESIS	+	−
ISOLATED GONADOTROPIN DEFICIENCY	+	−
CONSTITUTIONAL DELAYED ADOLESCENCE	−	−

Figure 31–45. Hypothesis of the control of pituitary adrenal androgen secretion by a putative separate adrenal androgen–stimulating hormone acting on an corticotropin (ACTH)-primed adrenal cortex. Although this diagram suggests that "AASH" arises from the pituitary gland, a distinct pituitary factor with "AASH" activity has not been isolated; an extrapituitary factor is not excluded. The lower part of the diagram shows the relationship of adrenarche to gonadarche, including dissociation in various clinical disorders of sexual development (+, present; −, absent). (Modified from Sklar CA, Kaplan SL, Grumbach MM. Evidence for dissociation between adrenarche and gonadarche: studies in patients with idiopathic precocious puberty, gonadal dysgenesis, isolated gonadotropin deficiency, and constitutionally delayed puberty, J Clin Endocrinol Metab, 51, 548–556, 1980, © by The Endocrine Society.[638])

3. Unlike cortisol secretion, the secretion of DHEA and DHEAS in response to corticotropin administration varies with age.

4. Dissociation of adrenarche and gonadarche occurs in several disorders of sexual maturation (see Fig. 31–45), including premature adrenarche (onset of pubic or axillary hair before age 8), chronic adrenal insufficiency, true precocious puberty (when the onset is before age 6), primary hypogonadism, isolated gonadotropin deficiency, and anorexia nervosa.[638]

Adrenal Androgens and Puberty

Although true precocious puberty may occur when the prepubertal child has previously been exposed to excessive levels of endogenous or exogenous androgens (e.g., after the initiation of glucocorticoid therapy in congenital virilizing adrenal hyperplasia),[123, 654] there is little evidence that adrenal androgens play an important or rate-limiting role in the normal onset of puberty.[123]

Most patients with premature adrenarche, who secrete excessive amounts of adrenal androgens for their age, enter puberty and experience menarche within the normal age

range.[123] Moreover, prepubertal children with adrenal insufficiency and, consequently, deficient or absent adrenal androgen secretion usually have a normal onset and progression of puberty when given appropriate glucocorticoid and mineralocorticoid replacement therapy.[123] Furthermore, growth studies in children with chronic adrenal insufficiency, isolated gonadotropin deficiency, hypergonadotropic hypogonadism, and androgen resistance suggest that adrenal androgens are not essential for the adolescent growth spurt in girls and boys, whereas steroids secreted by the testis and ovary are important in the process in concert with GH.[123] A transient increase in height velocity (about 1.5 cm/y in both sexes) that occurs in middle childhood (6 to 7 y) and lasts about 2 y has been attributed by some to adrenarche. However, this middle childhood spurt, which terminates while serum DHEAS levels continue to increase, is related to the cyclic pattern of prepubertal growth and to genetic factors rather than to an increase in secretion of adrenal androgen or GH.[652, 655]

DISORDERS OF PUBERTY

Delayed Puberty and Sexual Infantilism
(Table 31–16)

A useful definition of delayed puberty is absence of physical manifestations of sexual maturation in boys and girls at a chronologic age that is 2.5 SD above the mean age at onset of puberty. As discussed in the section on limits of normal pubertal development, it seems prudent to combine several sources of data, as no single study has established the range of normal puberty. In the United States, the ages of 13 years in girls and 13.5 years in boys serve as practical guidelines for determining the need for evaluation. It is important to separate children destined to undergo spontaneous but delayed puberty from those with disorders of permanent sexual infantilism that require treatment. Diagnosis is aimed at determining whether a given individual has constitutional (idiopathic) delay, hypogonadotropic hypogonadism, or primary gonadal failure with hypergonadotropic hypogonadism. Functionally, delayed puberty can be divided into disorders that affect the LHRH pulse generator, the pituitary gland, or the gonad.

Idiopathic (Constitutional) Delay in Growth and Puberty[422, 656]

Healthy individuals who spontaneously enter puberty after the age of 13 for girls and 13.5 for boys have constitutional delay in growth and adolescence. They usually are short (2 SD below the mean value for height for age) at evaluation and have been shorter than their classmates for years, although growth velocity and height are usually appropriate for bone age (Fig. 31–46 and Table 31–17). Family history often reveals that the mothers had delayed menarche and that the fathers and siblings entered puberty late (ages 14 to 18). Such individuals have a constitutional delay at all stages of physical development and may be considered physiologically immature; as a result of the delay in the reactivation of the LHRH pulse generator, LHRH secretion is deficient for chronologic age but not for the stage of physiological development. Adrenarche and gonadarche occur later in these individuals, whereas adrenarche is usually at a normal age in patients with isolated gonadotropin deficiency.[638, 657]

In patients with constitutional delay in growth and puberty, bone age correlates better with the time at onset and the stage of puberty than with chronologic age. These patients have a retarded bone age at presentation, but, on achieving a bone age of approximately 12 to 14 years for boys and 11 to

TABLE 31–16. Classification of Delayed Puberty and Sexual Infantilism

Idiopathic (Constitutional) Delay in Growth and Puberty (Delayed Activation
  of Hypothalamic LRF Pulse Generator)
Hypogonadotropic Hypogonadism: Sexual Infantilism Related to
  Gonadotropin Deficiency
  CNS Disorders
    Tumors
      Craniopharyngiomas
      Germinomas
      Other germ cell tumors
      Hypothalamic and optic gliomas
      Astrocytomas
      Pituitary tumors
    Other causes
      Langerhans' histiocytosis
      Postinfectious lesions of the CNS
      Vascular abnormalities of the CNS
      Radiation therapy
      Congenital malformations especially associated with craniofacial
        anomalies
      Head trauma
  Isolated Gonadotropin Deficiency
    Kallmann's syndrome
      With hyposmia or anosmia
      Without anosmia
    Congenital adrenal hypoplasia (DAX1 mutation)
    Isolated LH deficiency
    Isolated FSH deficiency
  Idiopathic and Genetic Forms of Multiple Pituitary Hormone Deficiencies
  Miscellaneous Disorders
    Prader-Willi syndrome
    Laurence-Moon and Bardet-Biedl syndromes
    Functional gonadotropin deficiency
      Chronic systemic disease and malnutrition
        Sickle-cell disease
        Cystic fibrosis
        Acquired immunodeficiency syndrome (AIDS)
        Chronic gastroenteric disease
        Chronic renal disease
    Malnutrition
    Anorexia nervosa
    Bulimia
    Psychogenic amenorrhea

    Impaired puberty and delayed menarche in female
      athletes and ballet dancers (exercise amenorrhea)
    Hypothyroidism
    Diabetes mellitus
    Cushing's disease
    Hyperprolactinemia
    Marijuana use
    Gaucher's disease

Hypergonadotropic Hypogonadism
  Males
    The syndrome of seminiferous tubular dysgenesis and its
      variants (Klinefelter's syndrome)
    Other forms of primary testicular failure
      Chemotherapy
      Radiation therapy
      Testicular biosynthetic defects
      Sertoli only syndrome
      LH resistance
      Anorchism and cryptorchidism
  Females
    The syndrome of gonadal dysgenesis (Turner's syndrome)
      and its variants
    XX and XY gonadal dysgenesis
      Familial and sporadic XX gonadal dysgenesis and its
        variants
      Familial and sporadic XY gonadal dysgenesis and its
        variants
    Other forms of primary ovarian failure
      Premature menopause
      Radiation therapy
      Chemotherapy
      Autoimmune oophoritis
      Resistant ovary
      Galactosemia
      Glycoprotein syndrome type 1
      FSH receptor gene mutations
      LH/hCG resistance
      Polycystic ovarian disease
      Noonan's or Pseudo-Turner's syndrome

13 years for girls, early stages of sexual maturation become
evident. In the U.S. Health Examination Survey 5.7% of boys
with a bone age of 14 years lacked pubic hair (stage 1) and
4% were in genital stage 1, whereas at age 15 years only 0.2%
were in pubic hair stage 1 and 0.8% were in genital stage 1.[42]
(Unfortunately, the same descriptive information could not be
determined for girls[24].) In contrast to isolated gonadotropin
deficiency due to Kallmann's syndrome, olfaction is normal,
and undescended testes are uncommon in this disorder.
Plasma gonadal hormone levels may be low at the time of
presentation (adrenarche as well as gonadarche is usually delayed), but as bone age advances, gonadotropin levels and
pulsatile LH secretion increase (initially at night), and both
the basal serum gonadotropin levels measured by third-generation assays and the LH response to LHRH increase to reflect
maturation of the hypothalamic-pituitary system.

In most cases, the first signs of sexual maturation occur
within 1 y after LH rises more than 2.0 IU/L in third-genera-

tion assays after administration of 100 μg of synthetic LHRH
intravenously or within 1 y after gonadotropin and testosterone or estradiol concentrations begin to increase spontaneously.[252, 253]

In its pure form, constitutional delay in growth and adolescence is an extreme physiological variant of the normal
velocity of development, a counterpart for constitutional true
precocious puberty. Affected children attain full sexual maturity, but the process takes longer. Patients with isolated familial
short stature do not have delayed puberty. Thus, familial short
stature is a physiological variant in which the velocity of development and bone age are normal, whereas constitutional delay in growth and adolescence is a disorder of tempo that
secondarily impairs growth distance. Of course, some children
may have both genetic short stature and constitutional delay,
and such patients most often seek medical advice. The combination of delayed pubertal maturation and decreased stature
during adolescence, superimposed on a familial tendency toward short stature, leads to more conspicuous shortness, especially in the peripubertal period, than with either condition
alone. Growth rate before the actual onset of puberty in these
patients is often suboptimal for chronologic age, and GH
secretion after provocative stimuli or after the administration
of GHRH may be decreased. Growth velocity and GH secretion in subjects with constitutional delay in growth and adolescence return to normal after the onset of puberty. The amplitude of GH secretion and the GH response to GHRH also
increase after the administration of exogenous androgens or
estrogens.[104, 658–661] Thus, constitutional delay in puberty may result from

TABLE 31–17. Constitutional Delay in Growth and Adolescence

A variation of normal
Males more often seek assistance
Family history of delayed menarche or delayed secondary sexual characteristics
Height is often below the fifth percentile, but growth rate is normal for skeletal
  age
Onset of adrenarche is delayed
The combination of genetic short stature and constitutional delay leads to more
  profound short stature
Final height is less than predicted

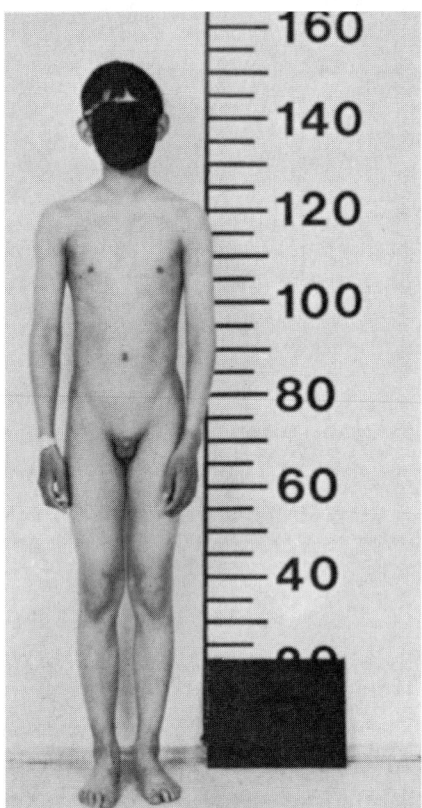

Figure 31–46. A boy 16 years, 2 months of age, with constitutional delay in growth and puberty. Height, 149.5 cm (4 SD below the mean value for age); upper/lower body ratio, 1.1 (retarded for age); phallus, 6.0 × 1.6 cm; testes, 2.5 × 1.4 cm; the scrotum showed early thinning. At a chronologic age of 15 years, 4 months the bone age was 11 years and the sella turcica was normal. The plasma concentration of LH was 0.7 ng/mL (LER-960); FSH, 0.5 ng/mL (LER-869). On LHRH testing the plasma concentration of LH increased to 2.2 ng/mL (an increment of 1.5 ng/mL), and the testosterone level rose from 52 to 77 ng/dL. The testes subsequently spontaneously enlarged, and the patient progressed through puberty. For conversion to SI units, see the legends of Figures 31–17 and 31–18. (From Styne DM, Grumbach MM. Puberty in the male and female: its physiology and disorders. In: Yen SCC, Jaffe RB, eds. Reproductive Endocrinology. 2nd ed. Philadelphia. W. B. Saunders, 1986: 313–384.[1430])

temporary functional GH insufficiency for chronologic age but not for bone age; there is no rationale for treatment of constitutional delay with GH. IGF-I and gonadotropins interact in the ovary and testis, and the relatively low secretion of GH (and presumably low intragonadal IGF-I) in subjects with constitutional delayed puberty may impair the gonadal response to gonadotropins.[662] Affected boys seem to be more distressed by short stature than by delay in sexual development.[663–666]

Occasionally, individuals with constitutional delayed puberty are of normal stature. In such instances the genetic tendency for tall stature is greater than in cases with short stature. In these patients diagnostic and therapeutic decisions should focus on the pubertal status.

Patients with constitutional delay in adolescence and growth often do not reach the predicted height.[666–668] This has been attributed in a retrospective study to a lack of growth of the spine in relation to leg length and is said to result in eunuchoid body proportions when the subject reaches adulthood (associated with a decreased upper/lower segment ratio); the greater the segmental disproportion, the closer the patient is to reaching target height.[669, 670] An alternative explanation for reduced adult stature is that the patients most likely to be evaluated are those that have both genetic short stature and constitutional delay in growth and puberty.[668] While the

use of exogenous androgens may improve self-image and start the secondary sexual changes of puberty, these agents do not improve final height or prevent the eunuchoid body proportions.[671] Furthermore, GH therapy has not been shown to increase the final height in patients with constitutional delay even if growth velocity does transiently increase.[672] The use of GH to increase the height of short normal children is similarly disappointing,[673] although the issue as to the use of pharmacologic doses of GH in short children remains unresolved.

Girls with constitutional delay in growth and puberty seek evaluation less commonly than boys, but they also reach suboptimal heights; since they may present at an older age than boys and their predicted height is calculated at a later age, they may reach their predicted adult height but not their target height, in contrast to some affected boys who may reach neither.[667]

Some studies have combined LHRH agonist therapy with GH treatment to increase final height, but the results are inconclusive.[674, 675] However, in some studies, LHRH agonist therapy administered to delay the normal onset of puberty in short normal children increased predicted or near-final height; again, this treatment is experimental.[676–678]

Men with a history of constitutional delay in puberty had a mean femoral neck bone mineral density about −1 SD below normal values, which increases the risk of sustaining osteoporotic fracture, including hip fracture.[169, 170]

Hypogonadotropic Hypogonadism: Sexual Infantilism Related to Gonadotropin Deficiency

Insufficient pulsatile secretion of LHRH and the resulting FSH and LH deficiency lead to sexual infantilism. The magnitude of the LHRH deficiency and hence the phenotype can vary from severe sexual infantilism to instances in which the separation from constitutional delay of puberty is difficult. LHRH deficiency may be secondary to a genetic or developmental defect not detected until the age of expected puberty, or it may be due to a tumor, an inflammatory process, a vascular lesion, or trauma. The deficiency of pulsatile LHRH can be quantitative—either absolute or relative—or qualitative, especially in females; it may involve abnormalities in the amplitude or frequency of LHRH pulses or in both components[453, 679, 680] (Fig. 31–47). Similarly, gonadotropin deficiency may arise from lesions or defects that involve the pituitary gland directly. When GH is affected as well as gonadotropins, growth velocity decreases, and eventual stature is short. Patients with isolated deficiencies of FSH and LH usually are of normal height for age in the early or middle adolescent years, whereas patients with constitutional, or idiopathic, delay in growth and puberty usually have a normal growth rate for bone age but are short for chronologic age. In contrast to subjects with constitutional delay in growth and puberty, gonadotropin-deficient patients usually do not have a normal LH response to LHRH stimulation or a pulsatile LH profile commensurate with bone age, and the levels of plasma FSH and LH and of urinary gonadotropins are frequently low.[826]

CNS DISORDERS: TUMORS. CNS tumors that delay puberty are usually extrasellar masses that interfere with LHRH synthesis, secretion, or stimulation of pituitary gonadotropes. Virtually all gonadotropin-deficient patients with hypothalamic-pituitary tumors also have deficiency of one or more additional pituitary hormones (or, in the case of prolactin-secreting adenomas, an increased level of plasma prolactin). GH deficiency due to neoplasms often is associated with relatively late onset of growth failure as contrasted to idiopathic and familial hypopituitary dwarfs, who usually have growth failure early in life. Similarly, the development of both anterior and posterior pituitary deficiencies after infancy suggests an

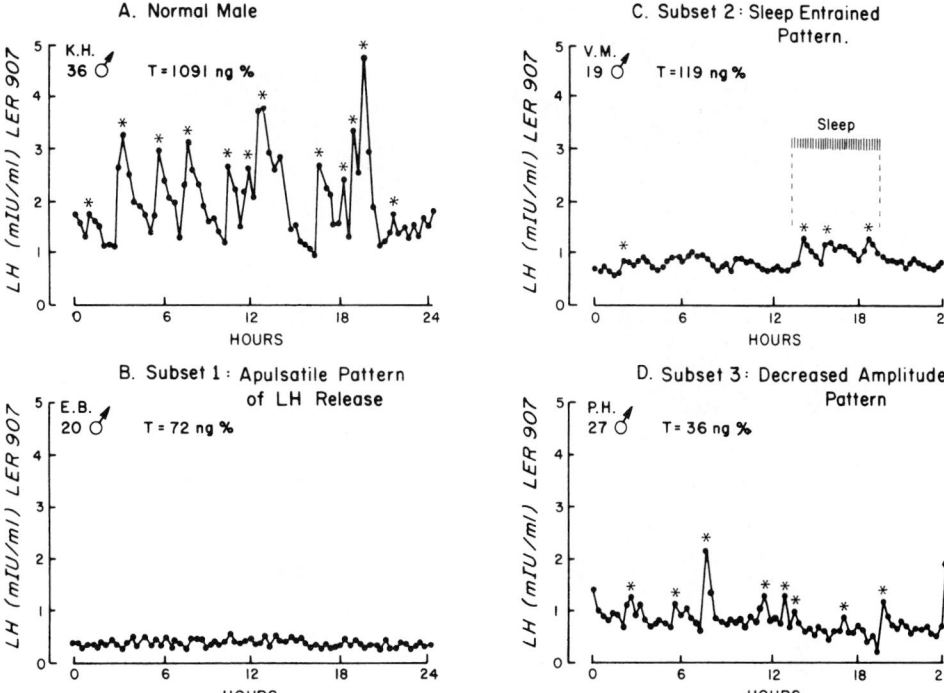

Figure 31–47. The various patterns of pulsatile LH secretion that can occur in isolated hypogonadotropic hypogonadism (*B* to *D*) compared with LH secretion in a normal man *(A)*. *A*, The discrete LH pulses occurring about every 2 h in a normal 36-year-old man. *B*, Typical apulsatile LH pattern associated with a low testosterone concentration usually found in isolated hypogonadotropic hypogonadism. *C*, Pattern of developmental arrest with low-amplitude nocturnal LH pulses apparent only during sleep. *D*, Low-amplitude LH pulse pattern during sleep and wake periods. To convert LH values to international units per liter, multiply by 1.0. (From Spratt DI, Crowley WF. Hypogonadotropic hypogonadism: GnRH therapy. In: Krieger DT, Bardin CW, eds. Current Therapy in Endocrinology and Metabolism, 1985–1986. Toronto: B. C. Decker, 1985: 155–159.[1431])

expanding lesion; this combination in infancy suggests a midline developmental defect.

Craniopharyngioma. This is the most common brain neoplasm of nonglial origin and the most common brain tumor associated with hypothalamic-pituitary dysfunction and sexual infantilism (see Chapters 8 and 9). This Rathke's pouch tumor, which is usually suprasellar, originates from epithelial rests along the pituitary stalk that extend superiorly to the hypothalamus; craniopharyngiomas may reside within the sella turcica or, more rarely, may be found in the nasopharynx[681] or the third ventricle.[682] Craniopharyngiomas are usually symptomatic before age 20; the peak incidence is between ages 6 and 14.[683–685] CNS signs are the consequence of encroachment of the tumor on surrounding structures.

Clinical manifestations include headache, visual disturbances, short stature, symptoms of diabetes insipidus, and weakness of one or more limbs.[684, 685] Physical findings include visual defects (including bilateral temporal field deficits), optic atrophy or papilledema, and signs of GH deficiency, delayed puberty, and hypothyroidism.[684, 685] Although only a few patients seek evaluation because of short stature, most are below the mean in height and height velocity at the time of diagnosis.[685] Laboratory evaluation often indicates deficiencies in one or more pituitary hormones, including gonadotropins, GH, thyrotropin (thyroid-stimulating hormone [TSH]), corticotropin, and vasopressin (AVP). The plasma level of prolactin may be normal or increased. Radiographic examination often shows retarded bone age.

Suprasellar or intrasellar calcification occurs in approximately 70% of patients with craniopharyngioma but fewer than 1% of normal individuals, and an abnormal sella is present in 70% of patients.[685] Some asymptomatic patients have been diagnosed by the demonstration of calcification or abnormalities of the sella on skull radiographs taken for other indications.[683–686] Computed tomography (CT) scans (but not MRI scans) can reveal fine calcifications that are not apparent on routine radiographs, and CT or MRI scans with contrast (the latter is the diagnostic procedure of choice) can determine whether the tumor is cystic or solid and whether hydrocephalus is present (Fig. 31–48).[687]

Smaller craniopharyngiomas, primarily intrasellar, can be resected or decompressed with transsphenoidal microsurgery, but larger or suprasellar masses usually require craniotomy. Because of the wide variation in the size and behavior of the tumor, the therapeutic approach must be determined on an individual basis. Complete surgical removal is often attempted, but the recurrence rate is high; a survey of 40 patients in whom complete removal was attempted without radiation therapy revealed a recurrence rate of 42%.[688] The combination of limited tumor removal and radiation therapy of large craniopharyngiomas leads to at least as satisfactory a neurologic prognosis and better cognitive outcome and to a better endocrinologic outcome than attempts at complete surgical extirpation.[685, 689–692] Attempts at radical removal of craniopharyngioma frequently result in hypopituitarism; virtually all require replacement with gonadal steroids and GH; 91% required glucocorticoids; half of the patients developed severe obesity postoperatively.[688] Postoperative hyperphagia and obesity, which can be striking (BMI > 5 SD), correlate with the magnitude of the hypothalamic damage as evidenced by cranial MRI[693] and are probably manifestations of injury to the hypothalamic ventromedial nuclei (associated with increased parasympathetic activity and hyperinsulinemia) and/or the paraventricular nuclei.[694] Aberrant sleep patterns can follow treatment for craniopharyngioma with awakenings at night and, in some cases, daytime somnolence.[695]

Other Extrasellar Tumors. Sexual infantilism can be caused by other extrasellar tumors that arise in or encroach on the hypothalamus. Germinomas (previously termed pinealomas, ectopic pinealomas, atypical teratomas, or dysgerminomas)[696] or other germ cell tumors of the CNS are the extrasellar tumors that most commonly cause sexual infantilism, although, when all primary CNS tumors are considered, germinomas are rare. The diagnosis is usually made during the second decade of life. Polydipsia and polyuria are among the most common symptoms,[697] followed by visual difficulties and abnormalities of growth and puberty.[698] The most common endocrine abnormalities are deficiencies of vasopressin and GH, but other anterior pituitary hormone deficiencies (including gonadotropin deficiency) and elevated serum prolac-

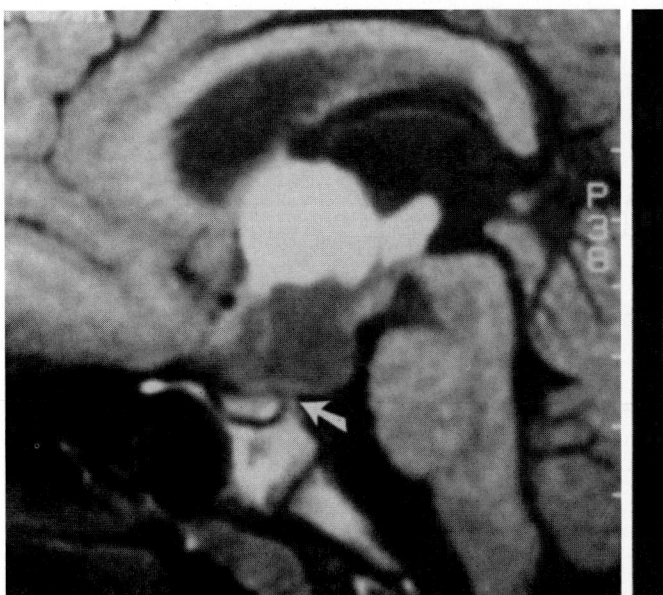 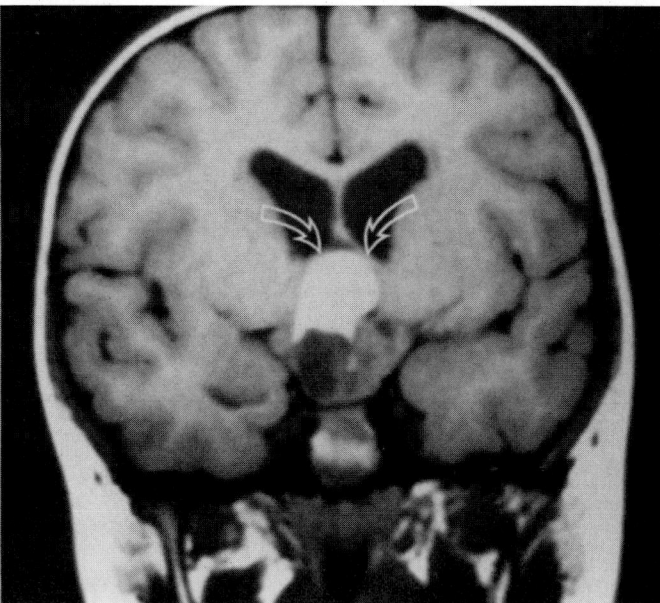

Figure 31–48. Craniopharyngioma in a short 5-year-old girl with a history of frontal headaches, impaired vision, and poor growth. *Left,* Midline sagittal T1-weighted image that shows a hyperintense region superiorly and an inferior hypointense region. The combination of hyper- and hypointense areas in a non–contrast-enhanced examination is the most characteristic finding in craniopharyngioma. Note erosion of dorsum sellae (*solid white arrow*) and posterior pituitary bright spot. *Right,* Coronal-weighted T1 image shows tumor extending upward to the inferior frontal horns, narrowing the foramen of Monro and causing mild hydrocephalus. The open white arrows indicate the upper border of the hyperintense area of the tumor.

tin levels are frequent. Germ cell tumors in boys occasionally cause isosexual precocity as the result of secretion of hCG. The level of hCG in spinal fluid especially, and levels of serum hCG and α-fetoprotein, are useful tumor markers in children and adolescents with CNS germ cell tumors. The tumor may be located in the suprasellar hypothalamic region, in the pineal region, or in another area of the CNS. A single case is reported of an hCG-secreting suprasellar teratoma that produced mild isosexual precocity in a 6-year-old girl with nondetectable serum concentrations of LH and FSH possibly related to aromatase activity of the teratoma; with therapy and regression of the tumor, the breast budding disappeared.[699] Subependymal spread can occur along the lining of the third ventricle, and seeding can lead to involvement of the lower spinal cord and corda equina. MRI scans with contrast enhancement are useful in the diagnosis of tumors more than 0.5 cm in diameter and for the detection of isolated enlargement of the pituitary stalk, an early finding on MRI scans.[697] Hypothalamic-pituitary abnormalities on MRI are related to functional defects, such as diabetes insipidus.[697, 698, 700, 701] Unlike the pituitary, which increases in size 100% between years 1 and 15, the size of the pineal gland does not change after age 1.[702] Pure germinomas are radiosensitive, and radiation is the preferred treatment; the clinical features and the response to radiation therapy are so characteristic that surgery is rarely indicated except for biopsy to establish a tissue diagnosis.[697, 703] When a mixed germ cell tumor is found, both radiation therapy and chemotherapy may be required.

Hypothalamic and optic gliomas or astrocytomas, occurring either as part of neurofibromatosis (von Recklinghausen's disease) or independently, can also cause sexual infantilism.[704–706]

Pituitary Tumors. Chromophobe adenomas are uncommon in children. Hyperprolactinemia due to micro- or macroprolactinomas (>10 mm in diameter) of the pituitary is uncommon in childhood and adolescence and a rare cause of delayed puberty.[707–710] In our series only 2 of 29 children with prolactinomas had delayed onset of puberty,[710] although primary amenorrhea was the presenting symptom in 13 of 20 pubertal females. Galactorrhea may be absent by history but is often demonstrable by manual manipulation of the nipples.

Transsphenoidal resection of microprolactinomas in children and adolescents has an 89% cure rate.[710] The dopamine agonist bromocriptine is also useful for decreasing serum prolactin concentrations and decreasing the size of the tumors;[711] the authors use this approach in children and adolescents in whom resection of the adenoma is incomplete and to reduce the size of the tumor in macroprolactinomas before attempted surgical removal. Puberty progresses in affected boys and girls and menstrual function becomes normal in girls after serum prolactin levels are reduced.

OTHER CNS DISORDERS LEADING TO DELAYED PUBERTY

Langerhans Cell Histiocytosis (Hand-Schüller-Christian Disease, or Histiocytosis X). This disorder, now thought to be a clonal proliferative disorder of Langerhans histiocytes or their precursors,[712] is characterized by the infiltration of lipid-laden histiocytic cells or foam cells in the skin, viscera, and bone.[713–715] Diabetes insipidus, usually resulting from infiltration of the hypothalamus and/or the pituitary stalk, is the most common endocrine manifestation, and GH deficiency and delayed puberty may occur. The lungs, liver, and spleen may or may not be involved. Other findings include cyst-like areas in flat bones of the skull, ribs, pelvis, and scapula; in the long bones of the arms and legs; and in the dorsolumbar spine. Lesions of the mandible lead to the radiographic impression of "floating teeth" within rarefied bone and the clinical finding of absent or loose teeth. Infiltration of the orbit may lead to exophthalmos, and mastoid or temporal bone involvement may cause chronic otitis media. Treatment with glucocorticoids, antineoplastic agents, and radiation is promising in terms of survival, but more than 50% of patients have late sequelae or progression.[715–717] The natural waxing and waning course of this disease makes evaluation of therapy difficult.[716, 717]

Postinfectious Inflammatory Lesions of the CNS, Vascular Abnormalities, and Head Trauma. These are unusual causes of hypogonadotropic hypogonadism. Rarely, tuberculous or sarcoid granulomas of the CNS are associated with delayed puberty.[718] Hydrocephalus may cause delayed puberty, which can be reversed with decompression.[719]

Radiation of the Head. Radiation of the head for treatment of CNS tumors, leukemia, or neoplasms may cause the gradual onset of hypothalamic-pituitary failure.[720] GH deficiency is the most common hormone disorder resulting from radiation, followed by gonadotropin deficiency. The final height of children with acute lymphocytic leukemia treated with CNS radiation is decreased, the consequence of decreased growth and early onset of puberty.[721] The advance in the age at onset of puberty correlates positively with the age at diagnosis of the condition for which the radiation was given and with BMI at diagnosis.[722] Newer treatment regimens that use 18 Gy, instead of 24 Gy, may have less influence on advancing the age at menarche and may lead to less long-term morbidity.[723] One study found that girls receiving 25 Gy of CNS irradiation after 7 years of age are more likely to have delayed puberty, while those treated earlier had normal onset of puberty but ultimately had diminished height;[724] the latter part of this study contrasts with the advance of puberty, noted earlier.

Developmental Defects. Midline malformations of the head and the CNS are associated with a variety of endocrine deficiencies.[53] Septo-optic or optic dysplasia is caused by abnormal development of the prosencephalon. The optic nerve is usually affected, leading to small, dysplastic, pale optic discs, and pendular (evenly moving side to side) nystagmus; severely affected patients may be blind. The midline hypothalamic defect can lead to GH deficiency and diabetes insipidus and can be associated with deficient secretion of corticotropin, TSH, and gonadotropin; short stature and delayed puberty are common, although true precocious puberty may alternatively occur (see later).[725] The septum pellucidum is often absent in association with optic hypoplasia or dysplasia, which is readily demonstrable by imaging techniques.[53, 726] The pituitary may be hypoplastic, presumably owing to the lack of hypothalamic stimulatory factors, and the neurohypophysis may have an ectopic location.[727] In the authors' series, the syndrome is associated with decreased maternal age. Other congenital midline defects range from complete dysraphism and holoprosencephaly to cleft palate or lip and can be associated with hypothalamic-pituitary dysfunction.[53] Twenty cases of duplication of the hypophysis are reported with delayed puberty in at least one.[728] Patients with myelomeningocele (myelodysplasia) may have endocrine abnormalities, including hypothalamic hypothyroidism, hyperprolactinemia, and elevated gonadotropin levels; and true precocious puberty may occur.[729, 730]

ISOLATED GONADOTROPIN DEFICIENCY (Table 31–18).[622, 626, 680, 707, 731]

Isolated gonadotropin deficiency may occur in families or sporadically. In contrast to patients with CNS tumors, which are usually associated with GH deficiency and growth failure, and to patients with constitutional delay in growth and adolescence, who are short for chronologic age, patients with isolated gonadotropin deficiency are usually of appropriate height for age (Fig. 31–49). Because levels of gonadal steroids are too low to fuse the epiphyses, these patients develop increased arm span for height and decreased upper/lower ratios (eunuchoid body proportions) and, if untreated, become tall adults.[732] An autosomal recessive form has been described in the mouse (*hpg/hpg*) in which part of the LHRH gene is deleted.[733]

Kallmann's Syndrome. (Table 31–19.) This genetically heterogeneous syndrome is the most common form of isolated hypogonadotropic hypogonadism with delayed puberty; anosmia or hyposmia due to agenesis or hypoplasia of the olfactory lobes and/or sulci is associated with LHRH deficiency.[734] The prevalence in boys is about four times that in girls (Fig. 31–50). While the extent of the defect in olfaction usually correlates with the degree of LHRH deficiency, even in patients with complete anosmia, LHRH deficiency may be partial (the fertile eunuch syndrome).[735] The magnitude of the LHRH deficiency correlates with the size of the testes[736] (Fig. 31–51). Affected individuals often do not notice impaired olfaction, particularly partial impairment; testing with graded dilutions of pure scents is necessary.[737] Undescended testes and gynecomastia are common in all types of hypogonadotropic hypogonadism in boys.[736] About one half of males with Kallmann's syndrome have a micropenis.[738]

Inconstant defects include cleft lip, cleft palate, imperfect facial fusion, seizure disorders, short metacarpals, pes cavus, neurosensory hearing loss, cerebellar ataxia, ocular motor

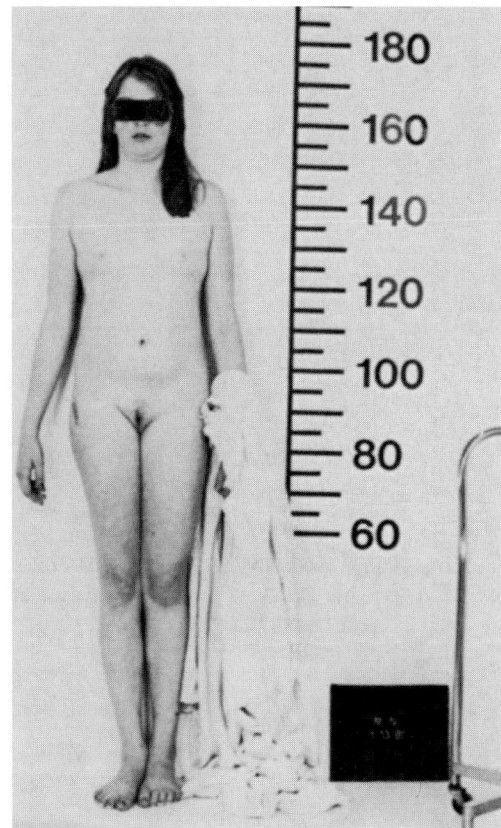

Figure 31–49. A girl 18 years, 8 months of age, with isolated gonadotropin deficiency (sexual infantilism and primary amenorrhea). Height was 173 cm (+1 SD), weight was 66.5 kg (+1 SD), and skeletal age was 13 years. Adrenarche with pubic hair development occurred at age 13 1/2 years. At the time of the photograph, pubic hair was in stage 3 and there was slight breast and nipple development resulting from a previous short course of estrogen therapy. Immature labia minora and majora were noted, and no estrogen effect was present on the vaginal mucosa. Olfactory testing was normal. The plasma LH (LER-960) level after LHRH administration rose from 0.5 to 1.8 ng/mL (a prepubertal response). Serum estradiol was undetectable. DHEAS level was 92 µg/dL (appropriate for pubic hair stage 2). Note the discrepancy between adrenarche and gonadarche. For conversion to SI units, see the legends of Figures 31–17 and 31–37. (From Styne DM, Grumbach MM. Puberty in the male and female: its physiology and disorders. In: Yen SCC, Jaffe RB, eds. Reproductive Endocrinology. 2nd ed. Philadelphia: W. B. Saunders, 1986: 313–384.[1430])

TABLE 31–18. Isolated Gonadotropin Deficiency

Males more commonly affected
Familial or sporadic
Height normal for age; tall adult height if untreated
Eunuchoid skeletal proportions
Delayed bone age
Small, often cryptorchid testes: Diameter <2.5 cm prepubertal size; phallus may be small
Normal adrenarche
Examine for anosmia or hyposmia (Kallmann's syndrome)
Look for associated malformations (facial, CNS, skeletal, renal)

TABLE 31–19. Features of Kallmann's Syndrome

Clinical
  LHRH deficiency: absent or arrested puberty
  Anosmia or hyposmia
  In infancy: microphallus; cryptorchidism
  Normal stature and growth in childhood
  Normal adrenarche
  Eunuchoid proportions
  Associated midline defects (e.g., cleft lip, cleft palate, midline cranial
    anomalies)
  MRI: aplasia or hypoplasia of olfactory bulbs and/or sulci
Prevalence: approximately 1 in 7500 males, 1 in 50,000 females; one tenth
  prevalence of Klinefelter's syndrome
Inheritance: sporadic and familial cases; genetic heterogeneity
  X linked
    X-linked recessive (Kallmann et al.[734])
    X chromosome deletion: Xp22.3 (Ballabio et al.[746])
  Autosomal
    Dominant (sex limitation) (Santen and Paulsen;[750] Merriam et al.[751])
    Recessive (White et al.[752])
Anatomy: developmental field defect
  Aplasia or hypoplasia of olfactory bulb and sulcus
  Arrested migration of LHRH neurosecretory neurons from olfactory placode to
    medial basal hypothalamus

abnormalities,[739] and, limited to the X-linked form, unilateral (or rarely bilateral) renal aplasia or dysplasia[740] and mirror movements of the upper extremities[734, 741] (Table 31–20).

Coronal and axial cranial MRI scans of the olfactory bulbs and sulci are useful as an ancillary approach to diagnosis,[742, 743] especially in affected infants and prepubertal-age children.[743] In a review of MRI findings in 64 individuals with Kallmann's syndrome, 56% had bilateral agenesis of the olfactory bulbs (in 2% the agenesis was unilateral); 56% had absent or abnormal olfactory sulci bilaterally (in 17% the abnormality was unilateral).[744] Hence, in this study fewer than 10% had a normal cranial MRI.

Serum LH and FSH levels are indistinguishable from those of prepubertal children except for absent or impaired nocturnal pulses of gonadotropin in Kallmann's syndrome.[745]

This syndrome is genetically heterogeneous and can be inherited as an X-linked, autosomal dominant or autosomal recessive trait. Reports of affected men who were infertile suggested an X-linked mode of inheritance,[734] and X linkage has been substantiated by gene-mapping techniques at Xp22.3, the locus of the *KAL1* gene, an X-linked gene that escapes X-inactivation and maps 1.5 megabases proximal to the steroid sulfatase gene in the same region. The *KAL1* gene encodes a 680-amino-acid glycoprotein with characteristics of an extracellular neural adhesion molecule and that may function as a pathfinder in guiding the migration of LHRH neurons to the medial basal hypothalamus (see earlier discussion).

The molecular genetics of the X-linked form is well established. A variety of deletions and mutations of the *KAL* gene have been described, including large and small deletions,[746–748] point mutations, and a variety of nonsense mutations that lead to frameshift and premature stop codons.[744, 747] A small number of familial cases in which X-linked inheritance is likely do not have a mutation in the coding region of the *KAL* gene; the defect in some of these patients may be located in the promoter region of the *KAL* gene.[749] Contiguous gene dele-

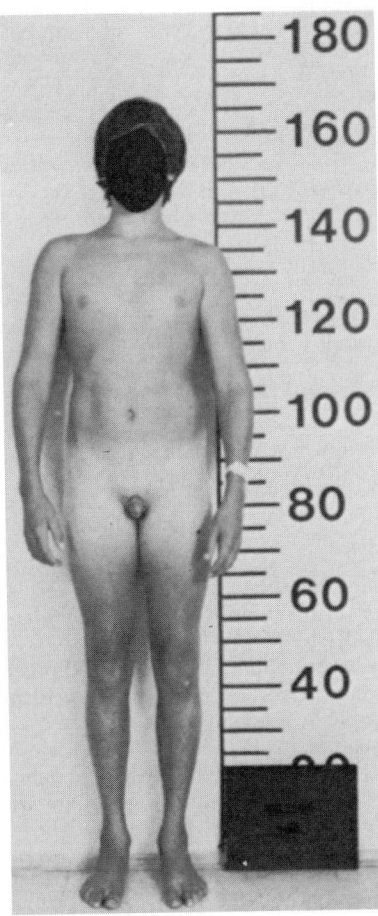

Figure 31–50. A boy of 15 years, 10 months, with isolated gonadotropin deficiency and anosmia (Kallmann's syndrome). He had undescended testes, but after administration of 10,000 U of hCG the testes descended and were palpable in the scrotum. Height, 163.9 cm (−1.5 SD); the upper/lower body ratio was 0.86, which is eunuchoid. The phallus measured 6.3 × 1.8 cm, and the testes were 1.2 × 0.8 cm. The concentration of plasma LH was less than 0.3 ng/mL; of FSH, 1.2 ng/mL; of testosterone, 16 ng/dL. After 100 μg of LHRH the plasma LH (LER-960) was 0.7 ng/mL and FSH (LER-869) 2.4 ng/mL. For conversion to SI units, see the legends of Figures 31–17 and 31–18. (From Styne DM, Grumbach MM. Puberty in the male and female: its physiology and disorders. In: Yen SCC, Jaffe RB, eds. Reproductive Endocrinology. 2nd ed. Philadelphia: W. B. Saunders, 1986: 313–384.[1430])

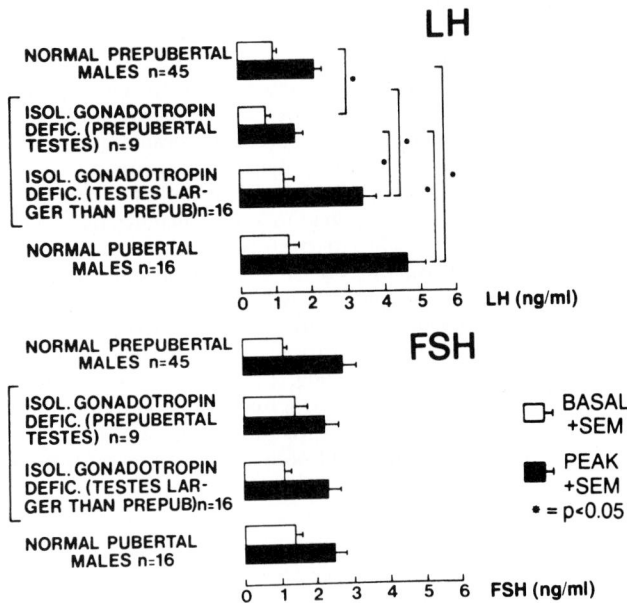

Figure 31–51. Serum LH and FSH responses to the administration of LHRH in 25 males with an isolated gonadotropin deficiency with or without anosmia, segregated according to whether the volume of the testes was prepubertal or >2.5 cm³; testicular volume in those with testes >2.5 cm³ were as large as 4 cm³. Basal and LHRH-stimulated gonadotropin levels after the intravenous injection of 100 μg LHRH (peak value) are shown.* $P < .05$. For conversion to SI units, see the legend of Figure 31–17. (From Van Dop C, Burstein S, Conte FA, et al. Isolated gonadotropin deficiency in boys: clinical characteristics and growth. J Pediatr 1987; 111:684–692.[736])

TABLE 31-20. Isolated Gonadotropin Deficiency: Clinical Features in 20 Adolescent Boys

Classification	Age and Range* (y)	Testicular Enlargement	Undescended Testes	Gynecomastia	Ocular Anomalies	Other Anomalies
Euosmic	$3^{5}/_{12}-20^{6}/_{12}$	3/10	3/10	2/10	3/10	6/10†
Anosmic or hyposmic	7–18	2/10	8/10	6/10	7/10	7/10‡
Total		5/20	11/20	8/20	10/20	13/20

*First evaluated at University of California, San Francisco, Pediatric Endocrine Clinic. All of the patients had delayed puberty; mean height was normal for age.
†Cohen syndrome (1); congenital adrenal hypoplasia (1).
‡Absent kidney (1); talipes, camptodactyly (1).

tions in this region of the X chromosome can lead to an association of Kallmann's syndrome with X-linked ichthyosis (due to steroid sulfatase deficiency), mental retardation, and chondroplasia punctata.[746, 747]

The phenotype in some families appears to be inherited as an autosomal dominant trait,[738, 750] and this possibility is supported by a report of an affected man who fathered an affected son after treatment with hCG.[751] In other kindreds, the disorder appears to be inherited by an autosomal recessive mechanism.[752] Thus the various forms of Kallmann's syndrome are due to heterogeneous mutations,[738, 750, 752] and the phenotype can be variable in each type. For example, a 20-year-old man with the complete picture of Kallmann's syndrome had an identical twin brother (proved by genetic fingerprinting) with anosmia but with a normal adult phenotype and normal male plasma testosterone and gonadotropin levels.[753]

In Kallmann's syndrome fetal LHRH neurosecretory neurons fail to migrate from the olfactory placode, where they arise, to the medial basal hypothalamus, where they form the LHRH pulse generator (see earlier discussion). The defect may be absolute or relative. The fetal LHRH-containing cells and neurites are arrested in their migration to the brain and end in a tangle around the cribriform plate and in the dural layers adjacent to the meninges beneath the forebrain;[464] in some patients this abnormality can be seen in cranial MRI scans[743] (Fig. 31–52).

Other Forms of Isolated Hypogonadotropic Hypogonadism. Hypogonadotropic hypogonadism can be transmitted by autosomal recessive inheritance with none of the other features of Kallmann's syndrome. In the mouse, a genetic form of isolated gonadotropin deficiency secondary to absent or low levels of hypothalamic LHRH is transmitted as an autosomal trait[733] (see earlier). Males with cerebellar ataxia and deficient gonadotropin production have been reported in kindreds with X-linked inheritance (possibly a variant form of Kallmann's syndrome), and hypogonadotropic hypogonadism may be associated with the multiple lentigines and basal cell nevus syndromes.

In all types of congenital gonadotropin deficiency, male patients are likely to manifest micropenis (phallic length in infancy less than 2 cm at birth or 2.5 SD below the mean) owing to lack of gonadotropin stimulation of fetal testes during the last half of gestation. Occasionally, patients with congenital GH deficiency have micropenis. Infants and children with micropenis due to hypothalamic deficiencies should be treated with one or two 3-mo courses of testosterone enanthate, 25 mg/mo IM to enlarge the size of the penis.[754] While concern was raised that this therapy might not allow the attainment of a normal adult penile size, experience has proved otherwise. Furthermore, the concern that the penis might not respond to androgens later in life if exposed to testosterone in childhood, a pattern noted in the rat, proved incorrect.[41] Thus it is appropriate to treat male infants and children with micropenis due to gonadotropin or GH deficiency with short courses of androgens to enlarge the penis into the normal childhood range.

X-Linked Congenital Adrenal Hypoplasia and Hypogona-dotropic Hypogonadism. This uncommon X-linked recessive disorder of adrenocortical organogenesis is due to a deletion or mutation in the *DAX1* gene, (*d*osage-sensitive sex reversal-*a*drenal hypoplasia congenita gene on the X chromosome gene *1*)[755–758] and is characterized by severe glucocorticoid, mineralocorticoid, and, at puberty, androgen deficiency.[759–763] A mature adrenal cortex is lacking, and the adrenal cortex resembles that of the fetal zone made up of disorganized vacuolated cytomegalic cells.[761, 763–765] In the majority of affected boys, the severe primary adrenal insufficiency is lethal if untreated.[761, 763] Less commonly, the onset of symptomatic adrenal insufficiency is delayed into later childhood, an early sign of which is increased skin pigmentation. In some instances, glucocorticoid deficiency precedes the electrolyte abnormalities, but they are usually congruent and include deficient secretion of the zona reticularis steroids dehydroepiandrosterone and its sulfoconjugate. The testes are undescended in many of the patients; micropenis is rare, but urogenital abnormalities and hearing loss may be present. At the age of expected puberty, signs of sexual maturation do not develop, including the lack of development of pubic and axillary hair and testicular enlargement, and persistent low levels of serum FSH, LH, and testosterone.[759–763] Two advances clarified the pathogenesis. First, as discussed later, intragenic mutations in the *DAX1* gene[756, 757, 766, 767] indicate that the hypogonadotropic hypogonadism is an intrinsic characteristic of the single gene mutation and is not due to the involvement of a contiguous gene. Second, the *DAX1* gene is expressed in the adrenal cortex, testes, ovary (weakly),[755, 766] hypothalamus, and pituitary.[758, 768] There is evidence of both LHRH deficiency and an abnormality in the gonadotropes, giving a mixed picture of both hypothalamic and gonadotrope defects, but in some instances one or the other defect is predominant, usually the pituitary deficit (reviewed in reference 763). The pulsatile secretion of LH is absent or erratic; basal immunoreactive LH and FSH levels may be normal, but the gonadotropins seem to lack bioactivity.[769] In the only infant male in which hypothalamic-pituitary–gonadotropin-testicular function was assessed at birth and in early infancy, the serum testosterone level was normal (i.e., elevated to pubertal levels), as were the levels of FSH and LH, and an LHRH test at 98 days induced a positive but modest LH and FSH response. In addition to the glucocorticoid and mineralocorticoid deficiencies, the serum DHEAS levels were low.[770] Furthermore, one boy with this disorder had true precocious puberty in early childhood. Both observations suggest that, at least in some affected boys, the LHRH pulse generator–pituitary gonadotropin apparatus is intact and functional in infancy and early childhood and that the LHRH-gonadotrope defects are not manifested until later in childhood or the peripubertal period.

In addition to deletions most mutations of DAX-1 result in nonsense mutations and frameshifts; missense mutations that change a single amino acid are relatively uncommon.[755, 756, 766–769]

Contiguous gene syndromes are not uncommon in association with X-linked congenital adrenal hypoplasia; the gene for this disorder maps to Xp21, distal to the glycerol kinase

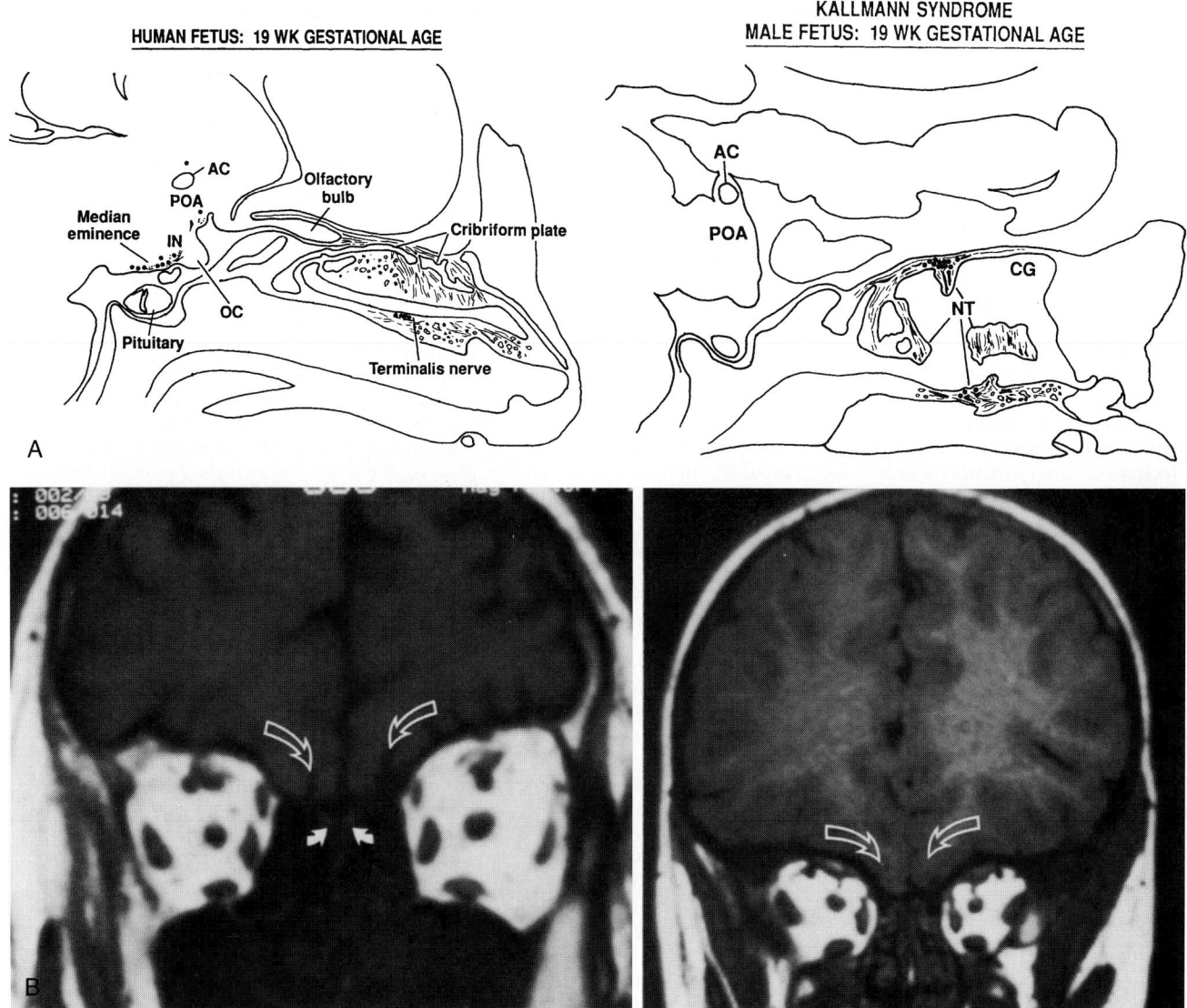

Figure 31–52. Comparison of the brain and nasal cavities of a normal 19-week-old male fetus *(upper left)* and those of a male fetus of similar age with Kallmann's syndrome caused by an X chromosome deletion at Xp22.3 *(upper right).* In the normal fetal brain the LHRH neurosecretory neurons *(black dots)* are located in the hypothalamic area including the medial basal hypothalamus; the anterior hypothalamic area; and, of interest regarding hypothalamic hamartoma as an ectopic LHRH pulse generator, the premamillary and retromamillary areas. A small cluster of LHRH neurons is present among the fibers of the terminalis nerve on the floor of the nasal septum. In the male fetus with Kallmann's syndrome, no LHRH neurons were detected in the hypothalamic region including the basal hypothalamus, median eminence, and preoptic area. The LHRH cells fail to migrate to and enter the brain from their origin in the nose; these cells end in a tangle beneath the forebrain on the dorsal surface of the cribriform plate and in the nasal cavity. AC, anterior commissure; CG, crista galli; IN, infundibular nucleus; NT, terminalis nerve; OC, optic chiasm; POA, preoptic area. Lower panels show MRI scans of brain (coronal section, TI-weighted image). *Lower left,* Normal olfactory sulci *(open white arrows)* and bulbs *(small solid white arrows)* in a 15-year-old boy. *Lower Right,* Absent olfactory sulci *(open white arrows)* and bulbs in a 17-year-old anosmic, sexually infantile boy with Kallmann's syndrome. (Adapted from Schwanzel-Fukuda M, Bick D, Pfaff DW. Luteinizing hormone–releasing hormone [LHRH]–expressing cells do not migrate normally in an inherited hypogonadal [Kallman] mouse. Mol Brain Res 1989; 6:311–326.[464])

(GK) gene and the Duchenne's muscular dystrophy (DMD) gene and proximal to the gene associated with mental retardation.[771] Hence a deletion of the congenital adrenal hypoplasia locus can include the GK and DMD genes if it extends toward the centromere or mental retardation if it extends toward the telomere.

The *DAX1* gene, a member of the nuclear receptor superfamily, encodes an orphan receptor that is a putative transcription factor. *DAX1* locus undergoes X-inactivation. The gene overlaps with the DSS (*d*osage-*s*ensitive *s*ex reversal) locus; a double dose of the DAX1 is associated with a female phenotype or ambiguous genitalia in XY males (see Chapter 29). It remains to be firmly established whether DSS and DAX1 are the same gene.[771a] DAX1 protein has a novel domain in the amino terminus that contains two putative unique zinc finger

motifs, and the carboxyl terminus contains a ligand-binding domain;[756, 758] the gene product binds DNA, localizes to the nucleus, and appears to have a steroidogenic factor-1 (SF-1) response element in the 5′ promoter region.[772] SF-1 is another orphan member of the nuclear hormone receptor superfamily; both DAX1 and SF-1 are expressed in the adrenals, gonads, pituitary, and hypothalamus,[773] raising the possibility of interaction between the products of these two genes.

Isolated LH Deficiency. Isolated LH deficiency (the fertile eunuch syndrome) is associated with deficient testosterone production (which responds to administration of hCG) and variable degrees of spermatogenesis; in most instances the isolated gonadotropin deficiency is incomplete;[774] the disorder may be idiopathic or secondary to a hypothalamic neoplasm. Rarely it is due to a mutation in the gene that encodes the

LH β subunit. A man with a history of delayed puberty and infertility, increased immunoreactive levels of serum LH that lacked bioactivity, and normal serum FSH concentrations, had a homozygous mutation in exon 3 of the LH β subunit gene (glutamine 54–arginine). Biopsy of the testis showed absent Leydig cells and arrested spermatogenesis. Treatment with hCG increased testosterone secretion and spermatogenesis. The serum LH of the heterozygous mother exhibited only 50% of normal binding to the LH receptor.[775]

Isolated FSH Deficiency. Isolated FSH deficiency can be caused by deficient production of the β subunit of FSH.[776] A homozygous nonsense mutation in the FSH β subunit gene (arginine 554 stop) was detected in a woman with primary amenorrhea and infertility, normal pubertal feminization, and isolated FSH deficiency.[777] The fact that pubertal feminization was not delayed (see later) is a surprising finding in view of current concepts of the action of FSH on folliculogenesis.[778] Low levels of FSH and of FSH receptor activity may be sufficient to sustain sufficient estradiol secretion to induce puberty. In an adolescent girl with isolated FSH deficiency who had adrenarche but sexual infantilism, compound heterozygous mutations of the gene encoding the FSH β subunit were detected; these mutations led to undetectable immuno- and bio-FSH levels and pubertal failure.[778a]

IDIOPATHIC HYPOPITUITARY DWARFISM. (Fig. 31–53.) Idiopathic hypopituitarism is usually caused by a deficiency of hypothalamic releasing factors. In the untreated state, patients usually have delayed puberty. However, patients with isolated GH deficiency ultimately undergo spontaneous pubertal development, without exogenous gonadal steroids, when the bone age reaches the pubertal stage of 11 to 13 y.[117, 779, 780] Patients with associated gonadotropin deficiency do not undergo spontaneous puberty, even when the bone age advances to the pubertal stage with GH therapy. Common to many patients with idiopathic hypopituitary dwarfism is early onset of growth failure; late onset of diminished growth suggests the presence of a CNS tumor. There is an association between breech delivery (especially in males), perinatal distress, and idiopathic hypopituitarism,[53, 779] and malformations of the pituitary stalk demonstrable by MRI are common in such patients.[53] The familial forms of multiple pituitary hormone deficiencies with either autosomal recessive or X-linked inheritance are less common.[117, 118] The absence of GH and gonadotropins may allow slow, long-term growth to increase final height; the height at the onset of puberty and the height in relation to bone age determine the final height. One patient was reported to be taller than expected for family after the diagnosis of panhypopituitarism was made at 25 years of age and after treatment was given.[781] In the authors' experience, treatment with GH in prepubertal children with isolated GH deficiency can increase the rate of pubertal development, thereby limiting the amount of growth attained with GH treatment; in these instances the use of LHRH agonists to suppress pubertal development is useful. The judicious use of low-dose testosterone in affected boys of pubertal age with associated gonadotropin deficiency does not seem to impair the final height attained with GH replacement.[782]

MISCELLANEOUS CONDITIONS

Prader-Willi Syndrome. This syndrome of early-onset childhood hyperphagia, massive obesity and carbohydrate intolerance, infantile central hypotonia and lethargy, poor fetal activity, short stature by 15 years of age, small hands and feet, mild to moderate mental retardation, emotional instability (including perseveration, obsessions and compulsions), and characteristic facies with almond-shaped eyes, triangular mouth, and narrow bifrontal cranial diameter is associated with delayed puberty and hypogonadism caused by hypothalamic dysfunction despite a tendency to early adrenarche.[783–788] Affected boys often have micropenis and cryptorchidism. Se-

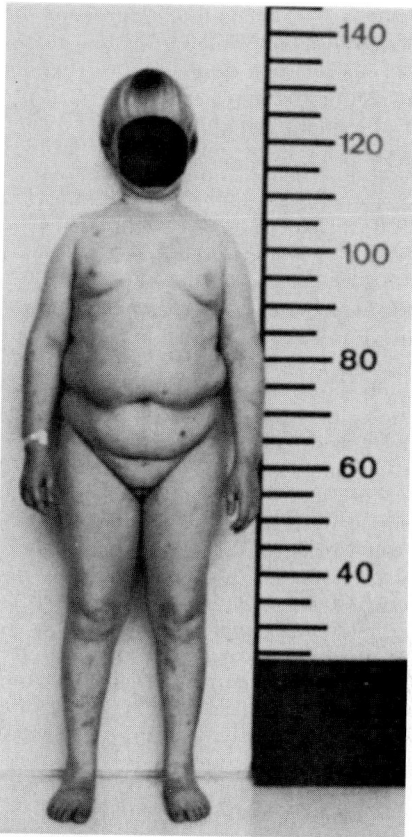

Figure 31–53. A 20-year-old male with idiopathic hypopituitary dwarfism and deficiencies of gonadotropins, thyrotropin, corticotropin, and GH, who had a history of arrested hydrocephalus. Height, 129 cm (−8 SD); the phallus was 2 cm in length, and the testes measured 1.5 × 1 cm. He had received thyroid and glucocorticoid replacement. Basal LH was less than 0.2 ng/mL (LER-960), FSH was 0.5 ng/mL (LER-869), and testosterone was less than 0.1 ng/mL. In response to 100 μg of LHRH, the plasma LH concentration increased slightly to 0.6 ng/mL, and there was no increase in plasma testosterone. The excretion of urinary 17-ketosteroids was 1.1 mg/24 h. The bone age was 10 years, and the volume of the sella turcica was small on skull radiographs. For conversion to SI units, see the legends of Figures 31–17 and 31–18. (From Styne DM, Grumbach MM. Puberty in the male and female: its physiology and disorders. In: Yen SCC, Jaffe RB, eds. Reproductive Endocrinology. 2nd ed. Philadelphia: W. B. Saunders, 1986: 313–384.[1430])

vere obesity may play a role in the impaired puberty, and weight reduction has been associated with menarche in some females. The assessment of GH secretion is confounded by the obesity and is difficult to interpret. In a controlled, short-term study in 13 affected individuals, GH therapy increased the mean rate of growth, decreased free fat mass, increased lean body mass (decreasing the BMI), and increased serum IGF-I levels,[789] but the long-term benefits on height, body composition, and behavior are unknown. Further, if the daily dose of GH is based on the actual rather than ideal body weight, there is an increased risk of untoward reactions.[790]

This genetic disorder has a frequency of about 1 in 20,000, is rarely familial (the estimated recurrence risk is 1.6%), and is caused by abnormalities of the long arm of chromosome 15 in the region q11-q13. Approximately 70% of Prader-Willi patients have a paternal deletion of 15q11-q13 (commonly about 3 to 5 mega-base pairs in size). A total of 20 to 25% of cases have maternal uniparental disomy (either isodisomy or heterodisomy) in which both chromosomes 15 are derived from the mother, possibly by nondisjunction during maternal meiosis, and represent a striking example of genomic imprinting. In 2 to 5%, a defect in the imprinting center is detected;[787, 788, 791–794] The lack of a functional paternal

15q11-q13 region is the common feature of these various forms. One candidate imprinted gene that maps to this region, snRPN (small nuclear ribonucleoprotein-associated polypeptide SmN), which is implicated in splicing pre-mRNA, is expressed in the brain, including the hypothalamus, and has been suggested as a critical gene in the syndrome.[795, 796] Little is known about the fine structure of the brain in this disorder, but a decrease in the number of immunoreactive oxytocin-containing cells—"putative satiety" neurosecretory neurons—has been described in the paraventricular nucleus of the hypothalamus.[797]

Laurence-Moon and Bardet-Biedl Syndromes.[798, 799] Laurence-Moon syndrome and Bardet-Biedl syndrome are now regarded as distinct entities. Both are autosomal recessive traits, and both have retinitis pigmentosa and hypogonadism of various etiologies: many of Bardet-Biedl patients have developmental delay, as do all Laurence-Moon patients. Laurence-Moon syndrome, however, is associated with spastic paraplegia, whereas Bardet-Biedl syndrome involves polydactyly and obesity. Biemond syndrome II is associated with iris coloboma, hypogenitalism (hypogonadism), obesity, polydactyly, and developmental delay.

Functional Gonadotropin Deficiencies. Chronic systemic disorders and malnutrition are associated with delayed puberty or failure to progress through the stages of puberty. It is necessary to distinguish the effects of malnutrition, which can lead to functional hypogonadotropic hypogonadism, from the primary effects of the disease. For example, a group of malnourished rural children from Kenya had chronologic delay in pubertal development and excreted less urinary FSH and LH than did well-nourished urban children of the same age. However, when the two groups were matched by pubertal stage rather than chronologic age, differences in gonadotropin excretion disappeared.[800, 801] Another study of girls who had previously had kwashiorkor demonstrated no delay in breast development or PHV but a delay in pubic hair development and menarche.[514] In general, weight loss of any cause to less than 80% of ideal weight for height can lead to gonadotropin deficiency[501, 802] and low serum leptin levels; weight regain usually restores hypothalamic-pituitary gonadal function over a variable period.[803] If adequate nutrition and body weight are maintained in patients with regional enteritis or chronic pulmonary disease,[804, 805] gonadotropin secretion is usually adequate.

Cystic fibrosis also delays puberty, in large part through malnutrition.[806, 807] However, even with normal pubertal progression, boys with cystic fibrosis almost universally have oligospermia caused by obstruction of the spermatic ducts unrelated to their nutritional status.[808] The greater prevalence of reproductive difficulties in male patients with cystic fibrosis compared with female patients[811] may be due to the more important role of the cystic fibrosis transmembrane regulator (CFTR) in the male reproductive tract, such as the epididymis and vas deferens, and a consequent viscoid luminal secretion which ultimately blocks sperm transport.[809] Normal ovaries do not express the CFTR, and endometrial tissue expresses it only after puberty to various degrees in cervical epithelium and fallopian tubes. Further, boys with cystic fibrosis have an autoimmunity to sperm that is detectable at the time of the appearance of spermatogenesis.[810] Boys with cystic fibrosis have antisperm IgM antibodies prepubertally and IgA, IgM, and IgG antibodies during puberty, and men with congenital absence of the vas deferens had predominantly IgM and IgG antisperm antibodies.[810]

Jamaican boys and girls with sickle-cell disease have a mean 1.4-y delay in the pubertal growth spurt and a 1.6-y delay in PHV, although final height is comparable to normal adults; girls have a 2.3-y mean delay in the onset of menstruation.[811] There is a similar delay in Brazilian children with sickle-cell disease.[812] Boys with sickle cell anemia often have impaired Leydig cell function, due to ischemia of the testes or gonadotropin deficiency, or both.[813]

Thalassemia carries the risk of hemochromatosis, which causes multiple endocrine abnormalities; delayed puberty with decreased gonadotropin secretion is most common, and GH deficiency is second in prevalence.[843]

Thalassemia major impairs sexual maturation in 65 to 80% of boys and in 75% of girls, and similar percentages of patients experience growth failure.[814] The primary hypothyroidism in this condition contributes to growth failure, but hypogonadotropic hypogonadism is also present in many.[815] The alkylating agents used to prepare thalassemia patients for bone marrow transplant may contribute to growth failure as well.[816] Further, iron deposition in the pituitary causes hypogonadotropic hypogonadism and complete absence of pubertal development in 40% of patients with thalassemia;[817] the gonads can be stimulated by exogenous gonadotropins, and satisfactory sexual development including fertility can be promoted by the use of hCG and hFSH.[818-820]

The Hemophilia Growth and Development Study followed more than 180 boys affected with acquired immunodeficiency syndrome (AIDS). Growth in stature was delayed, but weight for height was equal to normal boys. Remarkably, serum testosterone concentrations were not affected, but bone age and the progression through puberty were delayed. As GH secretion is usually not affected by AIDS, the poor growth appeared to be related to the delay in pubertal development.[821]

Chronic gastrointestinal disorders such as Crohn's disease are often accompanied by delayed puberty; therapy to restore nutrition, if successful, enables puberty to progress. The delayed puberty may allow a longer period of prepubertal growth that compensates, to some degree, for the poor rate of growth in this disorder. The pubertal growth in patients with active inflammatory bowel disease is further compromised if glucocorticoid therapy is necessary.[822] Celiac disease decreases the growth rate in childhood and adolescence, but with appropriate dietary therapy final adult height appears to be normal.[823]

Chronic renal disease is associated with delayed pubertal development[824, 825] and decreased pulsatile gonadotropin secretion due to a decrease in the amount of bioactive and immunoactive LH secreted, rather than an alteration of pulse frequency; successful renal transplantation usually restores gonadotropin secretion.[825] Patients with nephrotic syndrome have poor pubertal growth, poor secondary sexual development, and deficient gonadotropin secretion in a pattern resembling constitutional delay in puberty.[827] Treatment of glomerulonephritis with alternate-day glucocorticoid therapy leads to a late, diminished but prolonged pubertal growth spurt that can lead to a normal final height.[828] Children with end-stage renal disease receiving renal or peritoneal dialysis often are delayed in reaching sequential pubertal stages and deficient in linear growth, resulting in decreased final height, even despite the improved growth experienced after renal transplantation.[829, 830] Immunoreactive gonadotropin levels may be elevated, presumably because of impaired renal clearance, but the response to LHRH is blunted by severe renal impairment.[831, 832] TeBG levels are elevated in chronic renal failure, and free testosterone is low.[833] While growth and pubertal development usually improve after renal transplantation, glucocorticoid treatment after transplantation presents its own problems. Survivors of renal transplantation who receive immune suppression and alternate-day steroid treatment often have delayed onset of puberty and decreased pulsatile secretion of GH and gonadotropins at night.[827]

Advances in the treatment have improved the prognosis of leukemia. Children with early-onset and long-term remission undergo puberty at an appropriate age or with only slight delay, whereas patients who present with leukemia in late childhood may have profound delay of pubertal development.[834]

The type of therapy for malignancy also influences the age of puberty; radiation to the head may cause hypogonadotropic hypogonadism and/or GH deficiency, and radiation to the abdomen or pelvis and certain types of chemotherapy, especially if administered during puberty, can impair gonadal function and cause primary hypogonadism.[835]

Total body irradiation for bone marrow transplant may impair growth despite normal secretion of GH. Girls treated with CNS irradiation for leukemia have a diminished pubertal growth spurt and low final height, regardless of whether 24 Gy or 18 Gy is used, but the final height in similarly treated boys was reduced only with the higher dose.[836, 837] Treatment with 24 Gy before the age of 6 years carries a high risk of short stature.[838] Interestingly, the risk of short stature in children treated with chemotherapy and radiation to the CNS is due mainly to decreased growth of the spine.[839] However, patients who have undergone chemotherapy treatment without irradiation have normal final height after a period of catch-up growth following chemotherapy.[840] Secondary malignancies, such as papillary thyroid carcinoma and pulmonary fibrosis, are additional risks to total body irradiation.[841] In more than 100 patients treated for acute lymphocytic leukemia before puberty, the incidence of obesity was over 45%, indicating the need for dietary counseling in such cases.[842]

Hypothyroidism may delay the onset of puberty or menarche; treatment with levothyroxine reverses this pattern. Loss of height may be permanent if diagnosis is delayed, even though growth may continue for a longer period after menarche with levothyroxine therapy.[844]

Poorly controlled diabetes mellitus can lead to poor growth, fatty infiltration of the liver, and sexual infantilism (Mauriac syndrome),[845, 846] probably related to poor nutritional status; prepubertal children are most vulnerable to poor glycemic control, while pubertal subjects exhibit normal growth unless severe hyperglycemia occurs.[847] The degree of control necessary to avoid these complications cannot be quantified exactly, but adolescents with even moderately poor control may have some growth impairment and delayed puberty or irregular menses.[848] Serum IGF-I is decreased in children with diabetes mellitus regardless of pubertal stage.[849]

Cushing's disease can cause delayed onset or arrest of gonadarche, which usually is corrected by surgical removal of a pituitary adenoma.[850] The ACTH-secreting pituitary adenoma is the most common prepubertal pituitary tumor.[851]

Anorexia nervosa, a common cause of gonadotropin deficiency in adolescence, is a functional disorder, apparently increasing in prevalence in girls but rare in boys, and is characterized by a distorted body image, obsessive fear of obesity, and food avoidance that can cause severe weight loss, primary or secondary amenorrhea in affected females, and even death (see Chapter 22).[852] Other features include onset in middle adolescence, hyperactivity, defective thermoregulation with hypothermia and sensitivity to cold, constipation, bradycardia and hypotension, decreased basal metabolic rate, dry skin, fine downy hypertrichosis, peripheral edema, and parotid enlargement.[853–855] The clinician should be aware of the existence of subclinical forms. The pathogenesis is multifactorial and includes a genetic risk factor and a psychological component. Anorexia nervosa may rarely occur in association with a primary psychiatric disorder. It is important to exclude organic disease before the diagnosis of anorexia nervosa is made; one girl with a macroprolactinoma had manifestations consistent with anorexia nervosa.[708] The prevalence of anorexia nervosa is increased in gonadal dysgenesis. Hypogonadotropic hypogonadism is present in many patients with anorexia nervosa and, at least in part, is related to weight loss.[853, 854, 855] However, unidentified factors, including a low plasma level of leptin, may contribute to the amenorrhea of anorexia nervosa, especially when the onset of amenorrhea precedes the onset of severe weight loss (see Chapter 22).

It is not uncommon for patients with anorexia nervosa to be referred months after the onset; growth failure may be the first sign, and this condition must be considered in the differential diagnosis of growth failure.[856]

In anorexia nervosa the levels of plasma FSH, LH, leptin, and estradiol and of urinary gonadotropins are low. In adult women, there may be a reversion to a circadian rhythm of LH secretion with the sleep-associated episodic LH secretion characteristic of puberty; in severe cases, the amplitude of pulsatile secretion is diminished and resembles the pattern in prepubertal children.[621] Similarly, the LH response to LHRH correlates with the severity of the weight loss.[858, 859] In patients who weigh less than 75% of the appropriate weight and have major reductions in BMI and percent body fat, the LH response to the administration of synthetic LHRH is absent or blunted. Long-term administration of intravenous LHRH at 90- to 120-min intervals stimulates the pituitary to produce LH pulses indistinguishable from the normal pubertal pattern.[857] This response further supports the important role of functional LHRH deficiency in the amenorrhea of anorexia nervosa. Serum leptin levels are low, remarkably so with severe malnutrition, consistent with the strikingly decreased mass of adipose tissue, and increase with regaining of weight.[860–862] Other hormonal changes include increased levels of plasma GH and cortisol; low levels of plasma IGF-I, DHEAS, and plasma triiodothyronine with normal levels of thyroxine (unless associated with the "low thyroxine syndrome") and TSH; a decreased rise in serum prolactin after the administration of thyrotropin-releasing hormone (TRH) or insulin-induced hypoglycemia;[863] and a diminished capacity to concentrate urine.

The restoration of normal endocrine and metabolic function after weight gain indicates that many of these changes are secondary to starvation and severe weight loss; nevertheless, the amenorrhea may persist for months after weight gain, suggesting persistent hypothalamic dysfunction[864] (see Chapter 22). Treatment of this disorder requires skillful management, understanding, patience, and psychiatric consultation. Various approaches have been used to increase the food intake. In view of the mortality, parenteral alimentation may be useful in resistant patients with severe weight loss, especially in the presence of infection or an electrolyte imbalance.

Functional amenorrhea can also occur in women of normal weight and is characterized by normal levels of gonadotropin and normal gonadotropin response to LHRH stimulation but an absent or inadequate midcycle LH surge and a decrease in normal pulsatile secretion (amplitude and/or frequency) of gonadotropins.[865] The consequences range in severity from severe estrogen deficiency to anovulation to a short luteal phase.

Bulimia nervosa is a variant of anorexia nervosa;[867] it occurs in about 1.5% of young women. In this disorder, the individual consumes large amounts of food, but food gorging is followed by induced vomiting.[864, 867] A hand lesion from the induced vomiting (Russell's sign) and abnormal serum electrolytes are useful clinical markers. Abuse of laxatives, diet pills, and diuretics is common. Although weight loss is not frequent, amenorrhea is common.[867] Bulimia is especially prevalent in women in high school and college. A history of childhood sexual abuse is more frequent than in unaffected adolescents.

Cessation of growth can occur in infants and young children with psychosocial dwarfism. Stressful social situations can also inhibit growth and physical pubertal development at adolescence.[868]

Exercise, Hypo-ovarianism, and Amenorrhea. In the late

1970s amenorrhea in female long-distance runners and delayed menarche in other female athletes, including ballet dancers, figure skaters, and gymnasts, were reported.[869] A link between increased physical activity and abnormalities of puberty in the female is now established (reviewed in references 869 and 870). Bulimia, anorexia nervosa, or anorexia athletica occurred in 15% of 603 Norwegian girl athletes, particularly those engaged in sports that emphasize low weight.[871] In healthy ballet dancers and female athletes, factors other than decreased body weight can delay menarche and impair pubertal progression by inhibition of the hypothalamic LHRH pulse generator.[506, 510–513, 864, 869, 872] Teenage ballet dancers weigh less, have less body fat, and have a high incidence of delayed puberty and amenorrhea. When the strenuous physical activity is interrupted (e.g., by injury), puberty advances, and menarche often occurs within a few months, in some cases before body composition or weight has changed.[864] Female athletes of normal weight who have less fat and more muscle than nonathletic girls (e.g., ice skaters or swimmers) are also at risk for delayed puberty and for primary and secondary amenorrhea.[26, 513] However, the mechanism in the latter group is different from that of the hypothalamic amenorrhea in runners and ballet dancers.[873] Thinness and strenuous physical activity appear to act synergistically, but strenuous exercise training by itself may inhibit the LHRH pulse generator. The effect on pulsatile LHRH secretion may be mediated in part by endogenous opioidergic pathways involving β-endorphin. Even though gonadarche is retarded, adrenarche is normal.[26, 510] Athletes who began strenuous training before menarche have a delay in menarche,[506] and osteopenia can result from chronic hypoestrogenism.

A prospective study of 22 gymnasts demonstrated decreased growth velocity, stunting in leg length growth, and decreased height prediction, suggesting that heavy training starting before and continuing through puberty impairs ultimate height.[874] Gymnasts have a delayed age of menarche and less body fat, are shorter, and weigh less. The gymnasts had a decreased growth spurt, and the final height in 6 of 21 studied was 3.5 to 7.5 cm shorter than expected.[875] These studies suggest that extensive training (10 to 12 h/wk) may be excessive for prepubertal girls. On the contrary, a study of 222 intensively trained adolescent girls and their mothers showed a positive correlation between the delayed menarche in the girls and the age of menarche of their mothers, again illustrating the role of genetic factors in the onset of menarche.[876] Despite the endocrine effects of excessive athletic training in girls, elite prepubertal and pubertal athletes suffer relatively few physical injuries.[877]

Although less common than in women, men may also be affected by rigorous physical training; LH response to LHRH and spontaneous LH pulse frequency and amplitude are decreased; the serum testosterone is normal or low.

Ballet dancers have a higher incidence of scoliosis and delayed puberty than that of the general population; idiopathic scoliosis in the general population is associated with an earlier age at menarche (0.4 y earlier) and an early adolescent growth spurt.[878] An even stronger association is tall stature at the time of the early pubertal growth spurt; with scoliosis this combination leads to a slight increase in final height.[879] Scoliosis usually develops during the pubertal growth spurt and more often occurs in girls with a more rapid growth spurt.[879] Final height in familial scoliosis does not vary from the family norm.[880]

Prolactin levels may be elevated in women athletes and contribute to the delayed menarche found in this group.[710, 881] Marijuana use is associated with gynecomastia[882] and is a putative cause of pubertal delay.[883] Gaucher's disease caused delay in pubertal development in two thirds of patients in one study.[884]

Hypergonadotropic Hypogonadism: Sexual Infantilism with Primary Gonadal Disorders

Impaired secretion of gonadal steroids in primary gonadal failure results in decreased negative feedback and elevated LH and FSH levels. The most common forms of primary gonadal failure are associated with sex chromosome abnormalities.[885] Isolated testicular or ovarian dysfunction is less common.[886]

KLINEFELTER'S SYNDROME (SYNDROME OF SEMINIFEROUS TUBULAR DYSGENESIS) AND ITS VARIANTS. (See Chapter 29.) Klinefelter's syndrome, or seminiferous tubular dysgenesis, and its variants occur in approximately 1 in 1000 males and are the most common forms of male hypogonadism.[885, 887] Invariable features include small, firm testes (less than 3.5 cm in length), impaired spermatogenesis, and a male phenotype, usually with gynecomastia and eunuchoid body proportions[885] (Fig. 31–54). Gonadotropin levels are elevated postpubertally, but before age 12 gonadotropin concentrations are in the prepubertal range. Rarely, gonadotropin concentrations are low when hypogonadotropic hypogonadism is associated with 47,XXY Klinefelter's syndrome.[888] Hyalinization and fibrosis of the seminiferous tubules and pseudoadenomatous changes of Leydig cells develop after puberty; prepubertal testes show only subtle histologic changes, although the testes are small and the germ cell content is reduced. Prepubertally, patients can be detected by the disproportionate length of the extremities: decreased upper/lower body ratio without an increase in arm span.[889] The plasma testosterone level tends to be normal until about age 14, after which age it may fail to rise to normal adult levels.[890, 891] The onset of puberty usually is not delayed, but impaired Leydig cell reserve and low testosterone levels may slow or arrest pubertal changes. Testosterone replacement should be considered when the LH level rises above the normal range of values. Ratios of serum estradiol/testosterone and TeBG levels are higher than normal, indicating increased estrogen and decreased testosterone effects. These factors probably account, at least in part, for the characteristic gynecomastia[891–893] (see Chapter 17). Testosterone administration does not appear to reduce the gynecomastia.[894] If gynecomastia worsens, a reduction mammoplasty may be required. Tall stature in this disorder is due to the disproportionate growth of the legs.

Affected individuals detected by karyotype analysis at birth and in screening studies have minimal impairment (10 to 20 points) in verbal I.Q. but normal full-scale I.Q. Severe retardation is uncommon, although speech, learning disorders, and adjustment problems may be apparent in adolescence. Psychopathology is rare, and a 20-y follow-up of 47,XXY individuals showed little or no difference from control subjects in employment, social status, mental or physical health, or criminality.[895–897]

Conditions associated with Klinefelter's syndrome include aortic valvular disease and ruptured berry aneurysms (six times the normal rate);[898] breast cancer—20 times the rate in normal men (but no different from that in other types of gynecomastia) and one fifth that of women[899]—acute leukemia, lymphoma, and germ cell tumors at any midline site;[895] systemic lupus erythematosus;[900, 901] and osteoporosis.[172, 902] About 25% of men with Klinefelter's syndrome have osteoporosis. The prevalence of diabetes mellitus and thyroid disease is increased.

About 20% of mediastinal germ cell tumors are associated with Klinefelter's syndrome. These germ cell tumors may secrete hCG and induce sexual precocity, and the diagnosis should be considered in boys with hCG-secreting germ cell tumors, especially if the tumor is located in the mediastinum or CNS.[903–905] The incidence of fatigue, varicose veins, and essential tremor is increased.

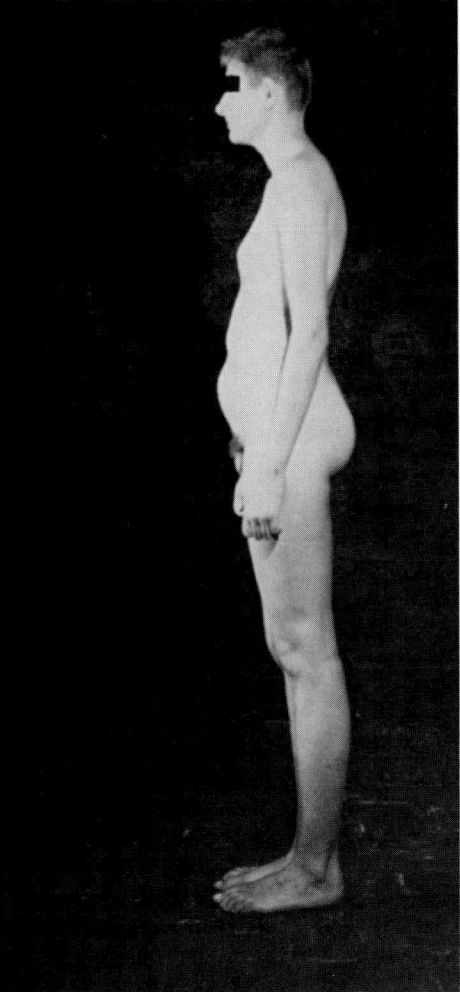 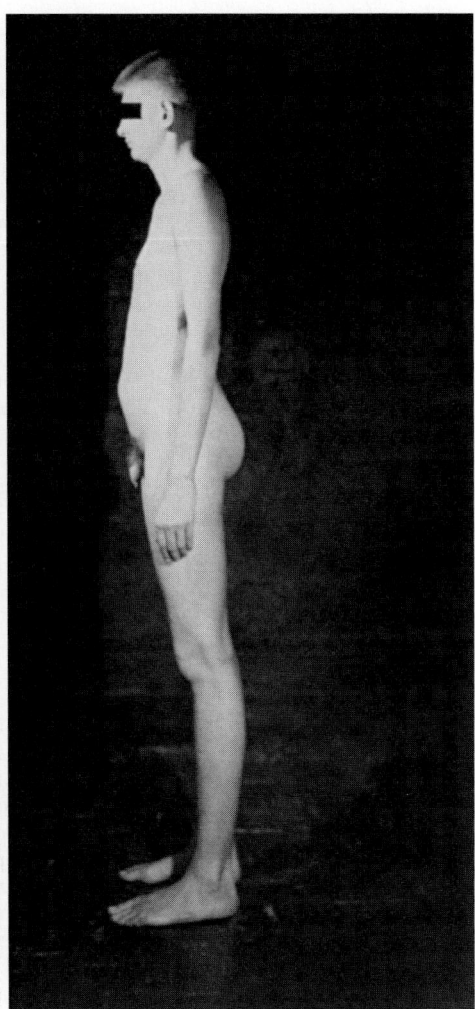

Figure 31–54. 47,XXY Klinefelter's syndrome in 17-year-old identical twins. At age 15 gynecomastia was noted. The twins had a eunuchoid habitus and poorly developed male secondary sexual characteristics. Both were 187 cm in height; armspans were 187 cm and 189.5 cm; the voices were high-pitched; the testes measured 1.8 × 1.5 cm; penis length was 7.5 cm. Gynecomastia and signs of androgen deficiency were more evident in the twin on the left. Urinary gonadotropins, >50 mU/24 h. The testes exhibited extensive tubular fibrosis, small dysgenetic tubules, and clumping or pseudoadenomatous formation of Leydig cells; germ cells were rare. The microscopic appearance was typical of seminiferous tubule dysgenesis. Patients are described in Grumbach MM, Barr ML. Cytologic tests of chromosome sex in relation to sexual anomalies in man. Recent Prog Horm Res 1958; 14:255–324.[1432]

Most patients have a 47,XXY chromosomal karyotype. The next most common variant is 46,XY/47,XXY; 48,XXYY and 48,XXXY karyotypes also occur and are associated with a higher incidence of mental retardation and somatic anomalies. The rare 46,XX male has some features of Klinefelter's syndrome[885] (see Chapter 29). The 49,XXXXY karyotype causes a syndrome characterized by severe mental deficiency, skeletal abnormalities (e.g., radioulnar synostosis), and hypoplastic external genitalia with a small penis and undescended testes.[885]

OTHER FORMS OF PRIMARY TESTICULAR FAILURE

Chemotherapeutic Agents. Chemotherapeutic agents used in the treatment of nephrotic syndrome or leukemia, such as cyclophosphamide and chlorambucil, can cause Sertoli cell and germ cell damage in prepubertal patients; these effects are sometimes reversible. Chemotherapy for childhood Hodgkin's disease, including chlorambucil, vinblastine, Mustargen (mechlorethamine), Oncovin (vincristine), procarbazine, and prednisone, may allow spontaneous progression through puberty, but both FSH and LH concentrations may be elevated in later life, indicative of persistent gonadal damage.[906] The basal serum FSH level and the rise in LH and FSH after LHRH correlate with the dose of cyclophosphamide.[907–909] COPP/MOPP therapy* for Hodgkin's disease can cause severe damage to germinal cells without much effect on

*COPP = cyclophosphamide, Oncovin (vincristine), procarbazine, prednisone; MOPP = Mustargen hydrochloride (mechlorethamine hydrochloride), Oncovin, procarbazine, prednisone.

Sertoli cells or Leydig cells, even with therapy in the prepubertal period.[910] Serum FSH is often elevated in patients treated with chemotherapy; basal LH levels are normal, although the response of serum LH to LHRH stimulation is elevated; thus germinal cell damage is evident, but Leydig cell function appears relatively normal.[911] Adriamycin (doxorubicin), bleomycin, vinblastine, and dacarbazine (ABVD) also can cause germ cell depletion. Although some degree of gonadal maturation is generally considered necessary before these drugs cause gonadal damage, in fact gonadal damage in the prepubertal period may not be demonstrable until the age of puberty.[912]

Radiation of the gonads can cause primary testicular damage, manifested by azoospermia, although testosterone levels may be normal in association with elevated LH and FSH values (compensated Leydig cell failure).[913] The gonads should be excluded from radiation therapy fields, if possible. While doses of 0.35 Gy to the testes may lead to temporary aspermia, more than 2 Gy leads to permanent aspermia, and more than 15 Gy can cause Leydig cell dysfunction.[914]

Testicular Biosynthetic Defects. (See Chapter 29.) Male pseudohermaphroditism caused by 17α-hydroxylase/17,20-lyase (CYP17) deficiency is associated with sexual infantilism and a female phenotype; the defect blocks the synthesis of testosterone and adrenal androgens and impairs masculinization at all stages of development. Associated cortisol deficiency and increased mineralocorticoid lead to hypertension, decreased serum potassium levels, and metabolic alkalosis. Glucocorticoid replacement suppresses corticotropin and mineralocorticoid excess and corrects the electrolyte abnormalities, but sexual development does not occur until exogenous gonadal steroids are administered. Less severe deficiencies are associated with ambiguous genitalia; one case of delayed puberty in a phenotypic male was attributed to partial deficiency of 17,20-lyase and 17α-hydroxylase.[915] CYP17 mutations leading to isolated 17,20-lyase deficiency occur rarely.

Deficiency of *s*teroidogenic *a*cute *r*egulatory protein (StAR) results in a defect in the movement of cholesterol into mitochondria; as a consequence little or no substrate is available for steroidogenesis.[916] Severely affected patients have lipid-laden adrenal glands (congenital lipoid adrenal hyperplasia), which can be visualized on ultrasonographic, CT, or MRI scans. Death often occurs in infancy because of unrecognized adrenal insufficiency. Affected XY individuals appear to be sexually infantile females; because of the absence of gonadal and adrenal androgens affected 46,XY phenotypic females do not develop secondary sexual characteristics, including pubic hair.[885] However, 46,XX females even with null mutations[917, 918] of StAR develop female sex characteristics at puberty, including pubic hair and multicystic ovaries, despite having either primary or secondary amenorrhea. Apparently, in contrast to the fetal testis, the fetal ovary, which is insensitive to FSH and steroidogenically inactive, is undamaged in fetal life and remains so until the onset of puberty when, under FSH stimulation and the recruitment of ovarian follicles, the ovaries undergo progressive damage and cyst formation.

Luteinizing Hormone Resistance. Presumptive evidence of LH resistance caused by an LH receptor abnormality on the Leydig cell was reported in an 18-year-old boy with a male phenotype, no male secondary sexual development, gynecomastia, elevated plasma LH levels, and early pubertal plasma testosterone concentrations that did not increase after hCG administration; levels of testosterone precursors were normal.[919] The testes were prepubertal in size and had the microscopic appearance of normal prepubertal testes. Plasma membrane receptor preparations from the testes bound only one half as much radiolabeled hCG as control testes. This autosomal recessive disorder is due to a mutation in the gene encoding the G protein–coupled seven transmembrane LH/CG cell receptor in 46,XY individuals (see Chapter 29) and is usually associated with severe male pseudohermaphroditism.

Nephropathic cystinosis in boys leads to hypergonadotropic hypogonadism.[920]

Anorchism and Cryptorchidism.[921, 922] In the 46,XY male without palpable testes, it is important to determine whether any testicular tissue is present. The finding may be due to intra-abdominal testes, which carry an increased risk of malignant degeneration; anorchia (the "vanishing testes syndrome"), in which no testes are found at laparotomy; or retractile testes, a variant of normal.[491, 885] The presence of a male phenotype and male internal ducts indicates that functioning fetal testes capable of secreting testosterone and AMH were present early during fetal life but degenerated thereafter. When functional Leydig cells are present, administration of 2000 U of hCG intramuscularly usually evokes an increased concentration of plasma testosterone after 72 h;[923] the lack of a rise in testosterone concentration, in conjunction with an increased plasma concentration of FSH and LH or an augmented gonadotropin response to LHRH, suggests the diagnosis of bilateral anorchia. Alternatively, measurement of male levels of AMH documents the presence of testicular tissue in a variety of disorders, from presumed anorchia to male pseudohermaphroditism and true hermaphroditism.[340, 343]

Cryptorchid testes may descend into the scrotum during more prolonged treatment with hCG (3000 U/m² surface area intramuscularly every other day for six doses) or intranasal LHRH,[924] although such descent occurs only in retractile,

rather than true cryptorchid, testes (see Chapter 16). Testicular descent normally occurs by 1 year of age, although later descent is described (see reviews in references 921 and 922). Orchiopexy should be performed by 2 years of age in testes not expected to descend spontaneously; postpubertal orchiopexy is associated with a high (>85%) prevalence of azoospermia or oligospermia.[925–927] It has been surmised that cryptorchid testes, even if replaced in the scrotum, may never have normal spermatogenic function as a consequence of an early abnormality in germ cell maturation, vascular damage to the testicular circulation during orchiopexy, or an intrinsic testicular defect.[921, 922, 927] However, results are improving with the move to ever earlier orchiopexy, and the phenomenon may have been based on a sample of boys who underwent orchiopexy later than is optimal.

Early orchiopexy may reduce the risk of carcinoma of the testes,[922, 928] although dysgenetic testes, even if located in the scrotum, carry an increased risk of malignant transformation.[885] Undescended testes remain at a higher temperature than descended testes, and undescended testes have a maturation arrest at the conversion of the gonocyte to the spermatogonium, and this appears to direct the testes toward malignant degeneration.[922] The incidence of testicular carcinoma is about 0.5 in 100,000 in boys and higher in adolescents.[929] However, in one study of 794 men with testicular cancer, orchiopexy before 10 years of age appeared to reduce the increased risk of testicular carcinoma associated with undescended testes.[930] The risk of carcinoma of the testes in prepuberty is small, but the absence of carcinoma in situ in prepuberty is not an assurance that carcinoma will not develop in adult life. Men who have had orchiopexy should be followed carefully because of the lifelong risk of cancer development. Annual ultrasonography of the testis is recommended in addition to periodic physical examination after the onset of puberty.[931, 932] At present, the earlier the orchiopexy is carried out, the better for ultimate function and the greater the decrease in the risk of malignant degeneration.[922, 927] One year is a useful age to consider orchiopexy for undescended testes, as it is the age at which the likelihood of spontaneous descent lessens but the benefits to the testes of orchiopexy remain.

The risk of breast cancer is increased in men with a history of undescended testes, orchiopexy, orchitis, testicular injury, infertility, or any cause of delayed puberty; this risk is principally due to the gynecomastia associated with these conditions (see Chapter 17).[933]

SYNDROME OF GONADAL DYSGENESIS AND ITS VARIANTS (TURNER'S SYNDROME) (see Chapter 29).[885, 934] The most common form of hypergonadotropic hypogonadism in the female is the syndrome of gonadal dysgenesis (Turner's syndrome) and its variants, a sporadic disorder with an incidence of 1 in 2500 to 10,000 liveborn girls[934–936] in which all or part of the second sex chromosome is absent. About 99% of 45,X conceptuses abort spontaneously, and 1 in 15 spontaneous abortions has a 45,X karyotype.[937, 938] The 45,X karyotype is associated with a female phenotype, short stature, sexual infantilism, various somatic abnormalities, and frequent fetal demise. Sex chromosome mosaicism or structural abnormalities of an X or a Y chromosome may modify the features, although about 40% of the individuals with the full complement of features noted above have mosaicism or structural abnormalities of the X chromosome. Thus the syndrome of gonadal dysgenesis and its variants is a continuum ranging from the typical 45,X phenotype to a normal male or female phenotype.[885]

45,X Gonadal Dysgenesis (Fig. 31–55) (see Chapter 29). Short stature and sexual infantilism are invariable features of 45,X gonadal dysgenesis. This karyotype is found in about 60% of women with the full syndrome.[885, 938] Short stature is thought to be due to loss of a homeobox-containing gene in

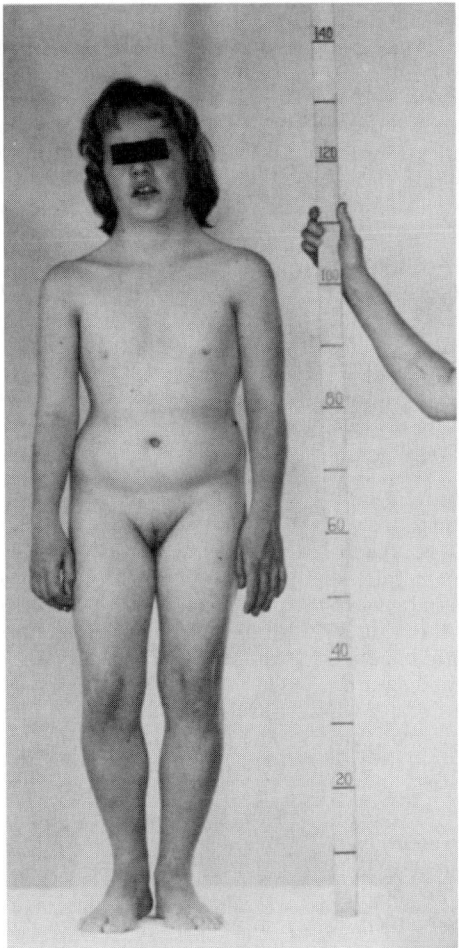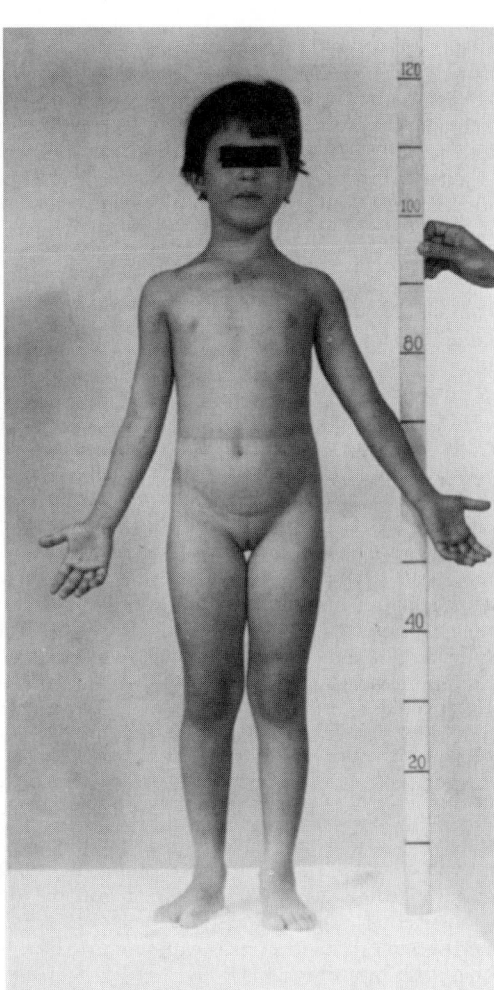

Figure 31-55. *Left,* A 14 10/12-year-old patient with the typical form of the syndrome of gonadal dysgenesis (Turner's syndrome). The X chromatin pattern was negative, and the karyotype was 45,X. She was short (height 134.5 cm; height age 9 5/12 years) and sexually infantile except for the appearance of sparse pubic hair, and exhibited characteristic stigmata of the syndrome: a short webbed neck, shield-like chest with widely separated nipples, bilateral metacarpal signs, puffiness over the dorsum of the fingers, cubitus valgus, increased number of pigmented nevi, characteristic facies, and low-set ears. The bone age was 13 6/12 y; urinary 17-ketosteroids 5.1 mg/d; urinary gonadotropin >100 mU/d. Vaginal smears and the urocytogram showed an immature pattern in which cornified squamous cells were absent. With estrogen therapy, female secondary sexual characteristics were induced; the cyclic administration resulted in periodic estrogen-withdrawal bleeding. *Right,* A 45,X, 9 11/12-year-old patient with Turner's syndrome. Apart from short stature (height 118 cm; age 6 10/12 years), increased pigmented nevi, and subtle changes in the fingers and toes, she had few somatic anomalies. In contrast to the patient in the left panel, the main clinical feature was short stature.

the pseudoautosomal region (PAR 1) of the short arms of the X (Xp22) and Y (Yp11.3) chromosomes.[939, 940] The gene that encodes an osteogenic factor[940] is called SHOX (short *s*tature *homeobox*-containing gene[939] or PHOG (*p*seudoautosomal *ho*meobox *o*steogenic *gene*).[940]

The syndrome may be recognized in the newborn period. 45,X abortuses have edema and large hygromas of the neck, which may be recognized on prenatal ultrasound studies; this lymphatic defect is the basis for the loose skin folds that may scar down to form the webbed neck (pterygium colli). Affected newborn infants may also have lymphedema of the extremities; the term *Bonnevie-Ullrich syndrome* has been applied to newborn infants with these features. It is important to determine whether coarctation of the aorta and/or a bicuspid aortic valve is present because of the risk of hypertension and aortic rupture (see Chapter 29).

Frequent features include distinct facies with micrognathia, "fishmouth" appearance, dysplastic nails, high-arched palate with dental abnormalities, epicanthal folds, ptosis, low-set or deformed ears, short neck with low hairline and webbing (pterygium colli), and recurrent otitis media (often leading to impaired hearing).[885, 941] A broad shield-like chest causes the nipples to appear to be wide-spaced; the areolae are often hypoplastic. Skeletal defects include short fourth metacarpals and cubitus valgus (which may develop after birth), Madelung's deformity of the wrist, genu valgum, and scoliosis. Extensive pigmented nevi, tendency to keloid formation, and hypoplastic nails may be present.[885, 942] Lymphatic obstruction causes infantile puffiness of extremities, pterygium colli, and a distinctive shape of the ears. Cardiovascular

anomalies include coarctation of the aorta (40% of whom also have webbing of the neck), aortic stenosis, and bicuspid aortic valves; the latter individuals are at risk for dissecting aortic aneurysm.[943] An echocardiogram of the cardiovascular system must be performed. Abnormal pelvicaliceal collecting systems, malposition or misalignment of the kidneys, abnormal vascular supply to the kidney, and recurrent urinary tract infections occur with increased frequency.[944] Defects of the gastrointestinal system include intestinal telangiectasias and hemangiomatoses that can rarely lead to massive gastrointestinal bleeding; the prevalence of inflammatory bowel disease is increased.[945-947] The uterus and fallopian tubes are infantile but can be detected with pelvic ultrasonography or MRI. Hashimoto's thyroiditis and Graves' disease are common. Insulin resistance and diabetes mellitus may develop after the age of puberty, in some made worse by the associated obesity.[948] Serum cholesterol levels are elevated prior to treatment with GH and/or estrogen.[949]

Intelligence is normal when verbal ability, comprehension, and vocabulary are considered, but spatiotemporal processing, visuomotor coordination,[950, 951] and mathematical ability (particularly in geometry) may be impaired, leading to a decrease in the overall performance of IQ;[948, 952] difficulties associated with social adjustment and cognition are common.[953] 45,X individuals in whom the X is of paternal origin (X^P) are better adjusted and have better "social cognition" as a group than X^m individuals.[954, 955] This difference has been attributed to the imprinting of a gene inherited from the mother located on X^m (but which is not imprinted on X^P).[954] In the first example of an imprinted gene on the X chromosome, the locus resides in the pericentric region of the short arm or on the long arm of the X chromosome. Skuse and colleagues[954] postulate that this maternally imprinted gene may play a role in male-female differences in social behavior and in developmental disorders. It is useful to monitor the progress of these patients in high school mathematics. Gender identity and sexual orientation are female.[948] While it has been generally accepted that these patients do well in their psychological development,[954] a study of 103 children with the disorder demonstrated a significant decrease in social competence scores; an increase in behavior problems; difficulty in schooling, peer relationships and concentration; and immaturity, hyperactivity, and nervousness. The origin of the X chromosome was not determined in that study. Structural abnormalities of the X chromosome were associated with more behavior problems than X chromosome absence or mosaicism.[956] Hyperactive behavior usually improves after puberty.[951] The risk of anorexia nervosa is increased.[953]

Patients are usually small at birth, owing to intrauterine growth retardation, and exhibit a relatively normal growth rate until a bone age of about 3 years and then an impaired growth pattern, a profound reduction in growth rate at the time of expected puberty, and failure of the pubertal growth spurt.[957-959] Women with gonadal dysgenesis in the United Kingdom and United States have a mean final height of about 142 to 143 cm;[958] adult stature correlates with midparental height.[960] The pattern of growth is due to the loss of a gene (SHOX or PHOG) in the pseudoautosomal region on the short arm of the X and Y (see earlier). hGH in pharmacologic doses is now approved for use in this disorder and increases the mean final height variably (discussed below).[958, 959] Specific growth curves are available for plotting the growth of affected children. In a group of girls with gonadal dysgenesis and spontaneous puberty, height velocity was transiently higher during puberty than in girls with amenorrhea, but final adult height was not different.[885]

As discussed earlier, the biphasic pattern of gonadotropin secretion in infancy and childhood (see Fig. 31–33) is exaggerated in gonadal dysgenesis. Thus baseline gonadotropin concentrations and peak LH and FSH values after LHRH administration are above normal between birth and 4 years of age and again after age 10. Baseline values of FSH are 3 to 10 times higher than LH values. However, between ages 4 and 10, mean gonadotropin levels are similar to the mean values in normal girls (see Figs. 31–33 and 31–35).[564, 565]

The appearance of pubic hair is often delayed in girls with gonadal dysgenesis, even though adrenarche, as assessed by the increase in plasma DHEAS, occurs at the normal age.[638] The pubic hair of affected women is sparse, and estrogen therapy increases the growth of pubic hair despite a lack of increase in adrenal androgen secretion.[961] The streak gonads are the cause of the sexual infantilism; in about 10% of cases, puberty, menarche, and, rarely, pregnancy may occur.[885]

Girls with gonadal dysgenesis have a tendency toward impaired glucose tolerance.[962] This feature may be of importance in view of the tendency to treat with GH, which at pharmacologic doses can be a diabetogenic.

Decreased bone density, due at least in part to hypogonadism, becomes more severe with age in patients who do not receive estrogen or discontinue replacement therapy.

Sex Chromatin–Positive Variants of Gonadal Dysgenesis.
Mosaicism of 45,X/46,XX, 45,X/47,XXX, or 45,X/46,XX/47,XXX chromosomes is associated with a chromatin-positive buccal smear and usually fewer manifestations. Structural abnormalities of the X chromosome can also be associated with fewer phenotypic features. Lack of genetic material on the long or the short arm of the second X chromosome can impair gonadal function; loss of all or part of the short arm of the X chromosome leads to the physical findings of gonadal

dysgenesis (see Chapter 29).[885] Depending on the location and extent of the deletion on the short arm of the X chromosome, these patients are more likely to have modest pubertal growth and some pubertal development.[963]

Sex Chromatin–Negative Variants of Gonadal Dysgenesis.
These variants include 45,X/46,XY mosaicism and structural abnormalities of the Y chromosome. Affected individuals vary in phenotype from that of typical gonadal dysgenesis to ambiguous genitalia to phenotypic males.[885] Patients may present with short stature, delayed puberty, and a history of hypospadias repair.[964] Testicular differentiation can range from a streak gonad to functioning testes. Patients with mosaicism involving a Y cell line or structural abnormalities of the Y chromosome are at risk for neoplastic transformation of the dysgenetic testes. Gonadoblastomas, benign nonmetastasizing tumors, can arise within the gonad and produce either testosterone or estrogens and may be calcified sufficiently to be detected on an abdominal radiograph. Thus the appearance of feminization or virilization in a patient with dysgenetic gonads and a Y cell line suggests gonadoblastoma formation. Of greater significance is the development of malignant germ cell tumors in the dysgenetic gonad or in a gonadoblastoma.[965] Such tumors usually occur in postpubertal subjects and rarely in children.[966] The management of the dysgenetic gonads in patients with a Y cell line is discussed in Chapter 29 and reference 885.

46,XX AND 46,XY GONADAL DYSGENESIS. Women with pure gonadal dysgenesis have sexual infantilism and a 46,XX or 46,XY karyotype without identifiable chromosomal abnormalities.[885]

Familial and Sporadic 46,XX Gonadal Dysgenesis and Its Variants.
The usual phenotype of 46,XX gonadal dysgenesis includes normal stature, sexual infantilism, bilateral streak gonads, normal female internal and external genitalia, and primary amenorrhea. The streak gonad occasionally produces estrogens or androgens, but malignant transformation is rare. Incomplete forms result in hypoplastic ovaries that produce enough estrogen to cause some breast development and a few menstrual periods followed by secondary amenorrhea. This heterogeneous syndrome[866] occurs sporadically or with autosomal recessive inheritance and may be associated with other congenital malformations such as sensorineural deafness (Perrault syndrome)[885] (see later).

Familial and Sporadic 46,XY Gonadal Dysgenesis and Its Variants.
Women with 46,XY gonadal dysgenesis have female genitalia with or without clitoral enlargement, normal or tall stature, bilateral streak gonads, normal müllerian structures, sexual infantilism, and a eunuchoid habitus. About 15% have a deletion or mutation in the SRY gene. If the dysgenetic testes produce significant amounts of testosterone, clitoral enlargement may be present at birth, and virilization can ensue at puberty. The incomplete form of 46,XY gonadal dysgenesis may involve any degree of ambiguity of the external genitalia and internal ducts. The risk of neoplastic transformation of the streak gonads or dysgenetic testes is increased, and gonadectomy is indicated.[885] The disorder is usually transmitted as an X-linked or sex-limited autosomal dominant trait, less commonly as an autosomal recessive trait[885] (see Chapter 29).

OTHER CAUSES OF PRIMARY OVARIAN FAILURE. Primary ovarian failure secondary to cytotoxic chemotherapy and radiation is increasing in prevalence as these agents prolong life in children and adolescents with cancer.

Radiation Therapy.
Radiation therapy that includes the ovaries can cause primary ovarian failure;[913] a dose of 4 Gy to the ovaries leads to sterility in 30% of young women and 100% of older women.[914] It may be useful to move the ovaries surgically out of the radiation field; such a procedure before radiation therapy is compatible with normal menses, pubertal development, and pregnancy in most cases.[968] The uterus may

also be affected by radiation and may not expand normally during pregnancy.

Chemotherapy. In a study by Quigley and colleagues,[969] after cytotoxic chemotherapy for acute lymphoblastic leukemia, boys and girls had extensive germ cell damage as evidenced by increased FSH secretion, and boys had decreased testicular size for the stage of puberty. The concentration of plasma inhibin was usually decreased. At puberty many of the girls had a compensated decrease in ovarian follicular function. Probably because of cranial irradiation, the mean age at menarche was advanced about 12 mo despite the ovarian damage; puberty was not advanced in boys. The type of chemotherapy determines the effects on the gonads. Use of nitroso compounds (carmustine and lomustine) or procarbazine for treatment of brain tumors in particular is linked to primary gonadal failure.[912, 970, 971] It was previously thought that cancer therapy in prepubertal individuals does not cause gonadal damage, but prepubertal boys and girls treated with abdominal radiation for Wilms' tumor plus chemotherapy (dactinomycin, vincristine with Adriamycin, or cyclophosphamide) may experience gonadal damage, whereas those given chemotherapy alone usually do not.[971–973] Attempts to protect the gonads by suppressing the pituitary-gonadal axis with gonadal steroids or LHRH agonists are ineffective.

Autoimmune Oophoritis. Premature menopause may occur at any age before the normal climacteric, including in adolescent girls; cessation of ovarian function presents as secondary amenorrhea. Autoimmune oophoritis can cause ovarian failure, leading to primary amenorrhea, oligomenorrhea, arrest of puberty, and, occasionally, cystic enlargement of the ovaries,[974–978] most often associated with other autoimmune endocrinopathies, especially autoimmune adrenal insufficiency[974, 978, 979] (see Chapter 33). Furthermore, autoimmune oophoritis is present in more than 20% of patients with autoimmune adrenal insufficiency. Thirty-six percent of women with type I polyglandular autoimmune syndrome (hypoparathyroidism, adrenal insufficiency, gonadal failure, diabetes mellitus, pernicious anemia, hypothyroidism, chronic hepatitis, mucocutaneous candidiasis, dystrophic nail hypoplasia, vitiligo, alopecia, keratinopathy, and intestinal malabsorption) exhibited ovarian failure before age 20, whereas only 4% of affected men had testicular failure by this age.[976] Various autoantibodies have been detected in autoimmune oophoritis, including autoantibodies to cytochrome P450 steroidogenic enzymes;[974, 978–980] some are organ specific, and others react with more than one tissue and cell type.[975, 981] Glucocorticoid therapy may improve ovarian function at least temporarily.[981]

Resistant Ovary. Resistant ovary is a rare heterogeneous cause of primary hypogonadism, a syndrome associated with elevated concentrations of plasma FSH and LH and ovaries that contain primordial follicles.[982, 983]

Galactosemia. Galactosemia is commonly associated with primary ovarian failure (either failure to develop puberty or primary or secondary amenorrhea and premature menopause), but puberty and testicular function are usually normal in galactosemic males.[984, 985] Dietary restriction programs do not prevent the ovarian failure.[986]

Carbohydrate-Deficient Glycoprotein Syndrome Type I. This syndrome is an autosomal recessive neurologic disorder associated with circulating glycoproteins deficient in carbohydrate moieties, including glycoprotein enzymes, binding proteins, and coagulation factors. A typical isoform pattern of serum transferrin by isoelectric focusing is used as a diagnostic test. The dominant clinical feature is the neurologic manifestations of involvement of the central and peripheral nervous system. Among the other organ systems affected is the pituitary-gonadal system.[987, 988]

The principal endocrine manifestation, hypergonadotropic-hypogonadism, is more severe in females than males.

Both the ovary and the pituitary gland are affected. Affected girls have sexual infantilism; the ovaries are hypoplastic or atrophic. High serum FSH and LH levels appear to have decreased but not absent FSH bioactivity in an FSH bioassay, and the administration of human menopausal gonadotropin causes an increase in serum estradiol and, occasionally, ovarian follicular growth.

FSH Receptor Gene Mutations and Hypergonadotropic Hypogonadism. The FSH receptor is a member of the seven transmembrane G protein–linked superfamily of receptors.[989] An autosomal recessive disorder due to a mutation in the extracellular ligand-binding domain of the FSH receptor in girls[990] results in delayed (40%) or normal puberty, primary amenorrhea, elevated plasma gonadotropin levels, and arrest of ovarian follicular development at the primary follicle stage.[990, 991] This disorder is probably responsible for most cases of the "resistant" ovary syndrome; a similar phenotype has been produced by targeted disruption of the gene encoding the FSH β subunit in mice.[992] The receptor disorder was described in six Finnish families who have an alanine-189–valine substitution in the extracellular domain.[993] Expression of the mutation in transfected cells indicated impairment of the FSH effect on cAMP production, a striking reduction in FSH-binding capacity, and normal FSH binding affinity.[993]

Affected males in these families are normally masculinized at puberty but tend to have small testes, a variable degree of spermatogenic insufficiency—but not azoospermia—increased plasma levels of FSH and LH, decreased inhibin B levels, and normal plasma testosterone levels.[994]

These patients illustrate the striking sex difference in the role of FSH in the ovary and testis.

LH/hCG resistance due to mutations in the gene encoding the LH/hCG receptor is discussed in Chapter 29. In affected 46,XY individuals this disorder leads to varying degrees of male pseudohermaphroditism. In the affected female, other LH/hCG resistance does not affect pubertal maturation but leads to amenorrhea with high serum LH levels but normal FSH and estradiol levels.[995]

Polycystic Ovary Disease. Polycystic ovary disease does not delay the onset of puberty but often delays menarche or causes menstrual abnormalities[996, 997] (see Chapter 15).

Noonan's Syndrome (Pseudo-Turner's Syndrome, Ullrich's Syndrome) (see Chapter 29). Individuals with Noonan's syndrome have webbed neck, ptosis, down-slanting palpebral fissures, low-set ears, short stature, cubitus valgus, and lymphedema, and hence this phenotype has been called pseudo-Turner's syndrome.[885] Features that differentiate this disorder from gonadal dysgenesis (Turner's syndrome) include triangular facies, pectus excavatum, right-sided heart disease (e.g., pulmonic stenosis or atrial septal defect), hypertrophic cardiomyopathy, and an increased incidence of developmental delay. Women with Noonan's syndrome have normal ovarian function. Males may have undescended testes, germinal aplasia or hypoplasia, and impaired Leydig cell function.[998] Noonan's syndrome is inherited as an autosomal dominant mutation[885] of a gene on the long arm of chromosome 12.[967] The incidence is estimated at 1 in 1000 to 1 in 5000. About half of patients are thought to be the result of new mutations.

The diagnosis of *Frasier syndrome* (chronic renal failure combined with gonadal dysgenesis)[981] should be considered in any phenotypic female with end-stage renal disease and sexual infantilism; the karyotype may be 46,XY or 46,XX.[999]

Diagnosis of Delayed Puberty and Sexual Infantilism (Figs. 31–56 and 31–57; Table 31–21)

When prepubertal girls present at age 13 or prepubertal boys present at age 13.5, the physician must make a clinical judgment as to which are variants of normal and which require

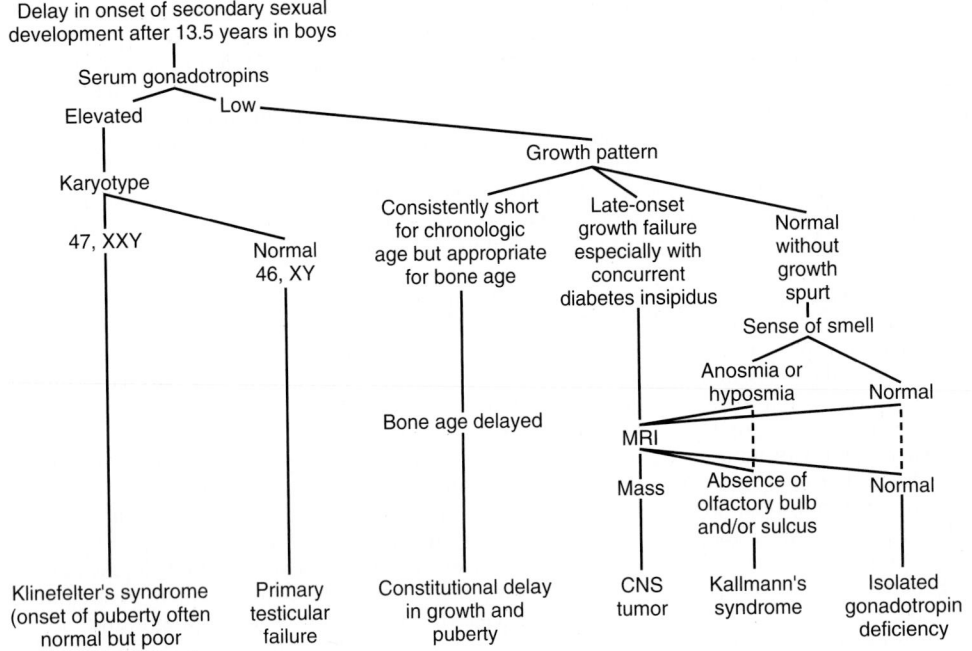

Figure 31–56. The evaluation of delayed puberty in boys.

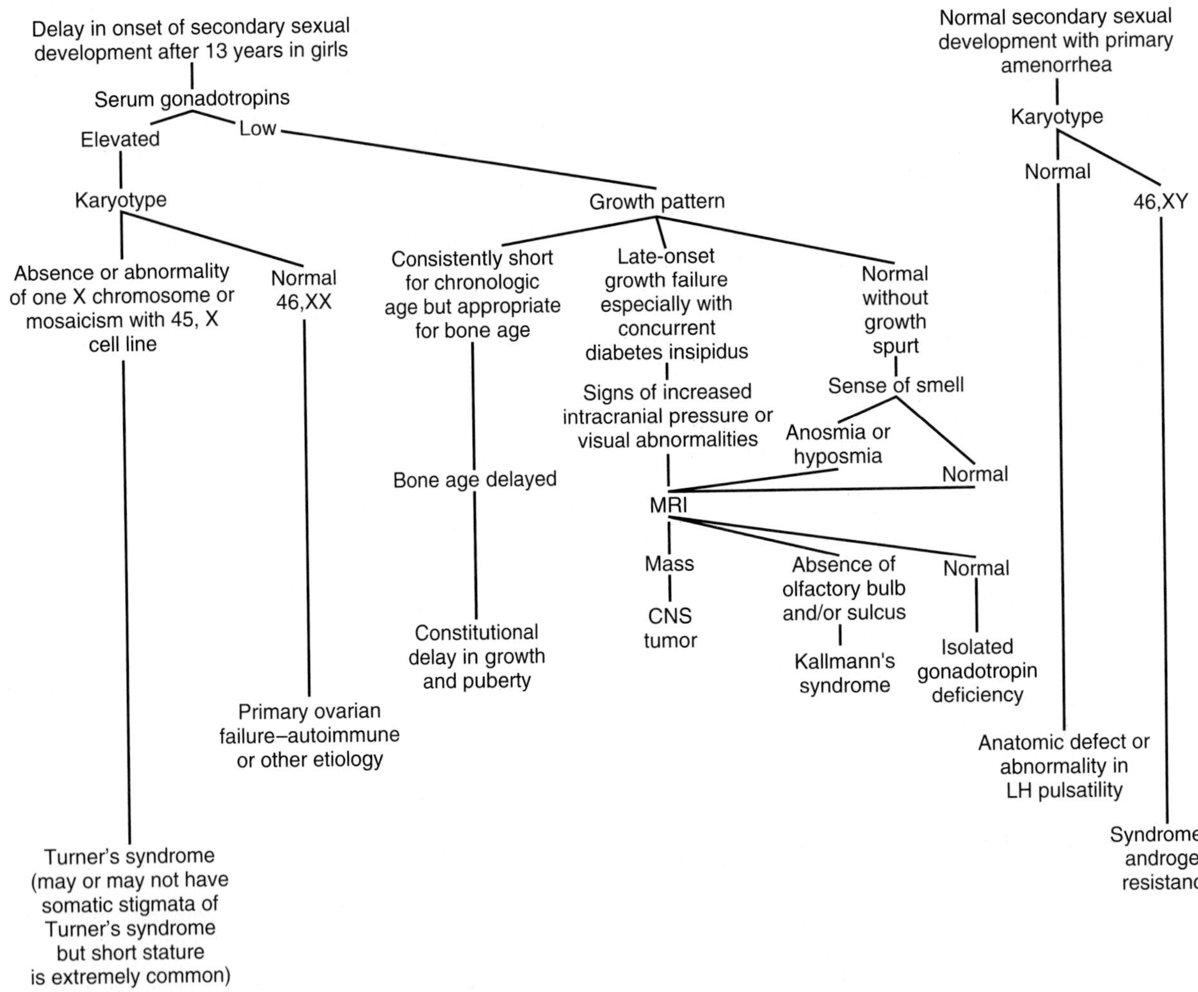

Figure 31–57. The evaluation of delayed puberty in girls.

TABLE 31–21. Differential Diagnostic Features of Delayed Puberty and Sexual Infantilism

	Stature	Plasma Gonadotropins	LRF Test LH Response	Plasma Gonadal Steroids	Plasma DHEAS	Karyotype	Olfaction
Constitutional delay in growth and adolescence	Short for chronologic age, usually appropriate for bone age	Prepubertal, later pubertal	Prepubertal, later pubertal	Low, later normal	Low for chronologic age, appropriate for bone age	Normal	Normal
Hypogonadotropic Hypogonadism							
Isolated gonadotropin deficiency	Normal, absent pubertal growth spurt	Low	Prepubertal or no response	Low	Appropriate for chronologic age	Normal	Normal
Kallmann's syndrome	Normal, absent pubertal growth spurt	Low	Prepubertal or no response	Low	Appropriate for chronologic age	Normal	Anosmia or hyposmia
Idiopathic multiple pituitary hormone deficiencies	Short stature and poor growth since early childhood	Low	Prepubertal or no response	Low	Usually low	Normal	Normal
Hypothalamic-pituitary tumors	Late onset decrease in growth velocity	Low	Prepubertal or no response	Low	Normal or low for chronologic age	Normal	Normal
Primary Gonadal Failure							
Syndrome of gonadal dysgenesis (Turner's syndrome) and variants	Short stature since childhood	High	Hyper-response for age	Low	Normal for chronologic age	45,X or variant	Normal
Klinefelter's syndrome and variants	Normal to tall	High	Hyper-response at puberty	Low or normal	Normal for chronologic age	47,XXY or variant	Normal
Familial XX or XY gonadal dysgenesis	Normal	High	Hyper-response for age	Low	Normal for chronologic age	46,XX or 46,XY	Normal

evaluation and treatment.[24, 42, 43] Lack of progression through the stages of puberty, even if the age at onset is normal, may also require evaluation; a boy who has not completed secondary sexual maturation within 4.5 y after onset of puberty or a girl who does not menstruate within 5 y after onset may have a hypothalamic, pituitary, or gonadal disorder.

The diagnosis of hypergonadotropic hypogonadism is readily established by documenting elevation of basal plasma LH and FSH levels. However, the differential diagnosis of hypogonadotropic hypogonadism versus constitutional delay in growth and adolescence is more difficult because of the overlap in findings in the two conditions, including inability to separate normal from low levels of serum gonadotropins (Table 31–22).

A presumptive diagnosis can usually be formed during the initial evaluation on the basis of the history and physical examination. The history should address all manifestations of chronic or intermittent illnesses, the details of growth and development, and the sense of smell. Disorders of pregnancy, abnormalities of labor and delivery, and birth trauma, if present, suggest that a congenital or neonatal event may be related to the delay in puberty. Poor linear growth and poor nutritional status during the neonatal period and childhood may reflect abnormalities of development. A growth chart is plotted to characterize the increase in stature and assess growth velocity from birth (see Chapter 30). The family history may reveal disorders of fertility, anosmia or hyposmia, or delay in the age at onset of puberty in parents or siblings. Recalled age at pubertal onset is relatively reliable, especially in women.[1000] A history of consanguinity is important in the identification of autosomal recessive disorders.

The physical examination starts with determining height and weight; the upper/lower segment ratio or sitting height is calculated, and the arm span is measured and compared with the height. The height velocity should be documented over a period of at least 6 mo, preferably 12 mo. The signs of puberty are noted, and the stage of secondary sexual development is determined (see Figs. 31–3 to 31–5) Assessment questionnaires utilizing pictures to allow children to determine their own stages of puberty are commonly used in survey studies but do not replace the physical examination because there is a tendency to overestimate development early in puberty and underestimate development late in puberty.[31, 32, 1001, 1002] The sizes of the testes and penis are measured in boys, and the diameter of glandular breast tissue and areolar size are noted in girls. The presence or absence of galactorrhea is defined. Obese boys may appear to have a small penis because of excessive adipose tissue surrounding the phallus; only when the fat is retracted can the full extent of phallic development be assessed. Cryptorchidism, or retractile testes, should be noted if no testes are palpated in the scrotum. Neurologic examination, including examination of the optic discs, assessment of visual fields by frontal confrontation perimetry, and evaluation of olfaction may reveal findings suggesting the presence of a CNS neoplasm or Kallmann's syndrome. The stigmata of gonadal dysgenesis or the small testes and gynecomastia of Klinefelter's syndrome may suggest one of these diagnoses. The lungs, heart, kidneys, and gastrointestinal tract should also be examined.

Laboratory studies (Table 31–23) include measurement of plasma LH and FSH, measurement of the rise in LH level after LHRH administration, determination of testosterone levels in boys and estradiol levels in girls, and measurements of thyroxine and prolactin concentrations in both sexes if the clinical features warrant. Levels of estradiol below 15 pg/mL can be measured with confidence in only a few available clinical estradiol assays. Radiographic examination includes bone age determination and, if the diagnosis seems to lead to the CNS, an MRI with contrast of the brain with specific attention to the pituitary and hypothalamic area; only advanced pituitary tumors or calcified craniopharyngiomas will appear on lateral skull films, and a negative radiograph does not exclude a CNS condition.[1003] Ultrasound evaluation of the uterus and ovaries is usually not indicated initially in work-up

TABLE 31–22. Endocrine Diagnosis of Constitutional Delayed Adolescence and Hypogonadotropic Hypogonadism

No single test reliably discriminates between the two diagnoses.
Onset of puberty in boys is indicated by
  Testes > 2.5 cm in diameter
  Serum testosterone concentration > 50 ng/dL
  Pubertal LH response to LHRH bolus
  Pubertal pattern of LH pulsatility

TABLE 31–23. Endocrine and Imaging Studies in Delayed Adolescence

Initial assessment
  Plasma testosterone or estradiol
  Plasma FSH and LH
  Plasma thyroxine (and prolactin)
  Bone age and lateral skull roentgenograph
  Test of olfaction
Follow-up studies
  Karyotype (short, phenotypic females)
  MRI with contrast enhancement
  Pelvic ultrasonography (females)
  LHRH test
  hCG test (males)
  Pattern of pulsatile LH secretion
  Visual acuity and visual fields

of delayed puberty but provides information about the state of development of these structures;[56] one study demonstrated streak gonads in 50% of patients with gonadal dysgenesis.[1004] Assessment of the chromosomal karyotype should be considered in all short girls without a diagnosis, even in the absence of signs of gonadal dysgenesis, and in all boys with suspected Klinefelter stigmata.

A presumptive diagnosis of constitutional delay in growth and adolescence can be made if the history and growth chart reveal a history of short stature but a growth rate consistent with skeletal age (and no signs or symptoms of hypothalamic lesions), if the family history includes parents or siblings with delayed puberty, if the physical examination (including the olfactory threshold) is normal, if optic discs and visual fields are normal, and if the bone age is significantly delayed. In classic cases of constitutional delay in growth and puberty an MRI of the hypothalamic-pituitary region may not be necessary. The rate of growth in these patients is appropriate for bone age; a decrease in growth velocity occurs in some normal children just before the appearance of secondary sexual characteristics and may awaken concerns when it occurs in these subjects. Furthermore, in these children the onset of puberty correlates better with bone age than with chronologic age. Levels of gonadotropins determined by supersensitive third-generation immunoassays and gonadal steroids become elevated months prior to pubertal development; thus measurements of serum LH, FSH, estradiol, or testosterone may aid in predicting future development. The third-generation LH assays are sufficiently sensitive to allow the determination of the onset of endocrine puberty from a morning blood sample in most boys, but an LHRH test is still characteristically performed. An increase in the concentration of LH of more than 7.5 IU/L (2 ng/mL LER-960) determined by conventional polyclonal RIA after intravenous administration of 100 μg of LHRH usually precedes the first physical sign of sexual maturation by less than 1 y.

Clomiphene citrate, an antiestrogen with weak estrogenic effects, decreases secretion of gonadotropins in prepubertal patients but increases gonadotropin secretion in pubertal patients and in adults. However, the authors have not found administration of clomiphene citrate to be useful in the diagnosis of constitutional delay in growth and adolescence.

Various diagnostic schemes for differentiating hypogonadotropic hypogonadism from constitutional delay in puberty, including assessment of the prolactin response to TRH,[1005, 1006] chlorpromazine,[1007] metoclopramide,[1008] or domperidone,[1009] either failed or gave inconsistent results.[1008, 1009] The combination of the prolactin response to metoclopramide and the gonadotropin response to LHRH[1010] and the use of priming doses of LHRH with subsequent evaluation of gonadotropin response to a subsequent dose of LHRH[1011–1013] or of a superactive LHRH agonist[1014, 1015] have been suggested. The FSH re-

sponse is higher in patients with hypothalamic-pituitary disorders who will undergo pubertal development.[1016] A sensitive immunofluorometric or immunochemiluminometric[1092] assay for LH may help differentiate between constitutional delay in growth and adolescence and hypogonadotropic hypogonadism.[1017] Urinary gonadotropin excretion is lower in hypogonadotropic patients than in delayed puberty, but this approach may require years of observation before the difference is apparent.[826] Although these latter methods are promising, their efficacy must be established. Hypogonadotropic patients usually undergo adrenarche at a normal age and may have higher DHEAS levels than those with constitutional delay in growth and puberty, and this pattern may be helpful in the differential diagnosis.[638, 1018, 1019]

Measurement of 8 AM serum testosterone is an indicator of impending pubertal development; a value greater than 0.7 nmol/L (20 ng/dL) predicts enlargement of testes to greater than 4 mL within 12 mo in 77% of cases and within 15 mo in 100% of cases; in boys with a value less than 0.7 nmol/L only 12% entered puberty in 12 mo, and only 25% entered puberty within 15 mo. This technique may help predict spontaneous pubertal development but requires watching and waiting.[1020] At present there does not appear to be a practical and reliable endocrine test for differentiating indisputably between constitutional delay in growth and adolescence and hypogonadotropic hypogonadism.

A typical patient with isolated gonadotropin deficiency is of average height for age and has eunuchoid proportions; low plasma levels of gonadal steroids, LH, and FSH; and no increase in or a blunted response of LH after LHRH administration. The amplitude and usually the frequency of LH pulses are decreased when blood is serially sampled over a 24-h period. In Kallmann's syndrome, the sense of smell is frequently absent or impaired. However, differentiation of isolated gonadotropin deficiency, in the absence of hyposmia or anosmia, from constitutional delay in puberty may be difficult. Gonadotropin-deficient patients may be as short as those with constitutional delay in growth and adolescence, and concentrations of LH and FSH in hypogonadotropic hypogonadism may be indistinguishable from those of normal prepubertal children or children with constitutional delay. Sometimes years of observation are necessary to detect signs of secondary sexual development or to document rising levels of gonadotropins and gonadal steroids before the diagnosis is clear. In general, absence of signs of sexual maturation or failure of a rise in gonadotropins or gonadal steroid levels by age 18 in the presence of normal levels of serum DHEAS for chronologic age supports the diagnosis of isolated gonadotropin deficiency.

Patients with combined deficiency of gonadotropins and other pituitary hormones require careful evaluation for CNS neoplasms. Visual field or optic disc abnormalities support the diagnosis of CNS tumor; even if these tests are normal, CT scans and especially MRI with contrast of the head are valuable in detecting mass lesions and developmental abnormalities of the hypothalamic-pituitary region.[1003, 1021]

Treatment of Delayed Puberty and Sexual Infantilism

Treatment of delayed puberty (Table 31–24) depends on the diagnosis. Patients with constitutional delay in growth and adolescence ultimately have spontaneous onset and progression through puberty. However, if puberty is inordinately delayed, bone mineral accretion may not be optimal, which can increase the risk of osteoporotic fracture in adult life.[169, 170] Reassurance and continued observation to ensure that the expected sexual maturation occurs may be sufficient. However, the stigma of appearing less mature than one's peers can

TABLE 31–24. Management and Treatment of Delayed Puberty

Objectives
Determine site and etiology of abnormality
Induce and maintain secondary sexual characteristics
Induce pubertal growth spurt
Prevent the potential short-term and long-term psychological, personality, and social handicaps of delayed puberty
Ensure normal libido and potency
Attain fertility

Therapy
Concerned but not anxious or socially handicapped adolescent:
  Reassurance and follow-up (tincture of time)
  Repeat evaluation (including serum testosterone or estradiol) in 6 mo
Psychosocial handicaps, anxiety, highly concerned:
  Therapy for 4 mo with
  Boys: testosterone enanthate 100 mg intramuscularly every 4 wk at 14–14.5 y of age
  Girls: ethinyl estradiol 5–10 μg daily by mouth or conjugated estrogens 0.3 mg daily by mouth at 13 y of age
  No therapy for 4–6 mo; re-evaluate status including serum testosterone or estradiol; if indicated repeat treatment regimen

cause psychological stress; such individuals may be unable to participate in social and athletic activities, immature appearance may lead to ridicule especially in the locker room, and school work may suffer because of poor self-image.[1022, 1023] Some children feel such intense peer pressure and low self-esteem that only the appearance of signs of puberty will reassure them and enable them to function with their peers, and poor self-image in late-maturing boys may carry over into adulthood even after normal puberty ensues (reviewed in references 1022 and 1023). The growth retardation may be more responsible for stress than delay in pubertal development itself.[1024]

For psychological reasons, a 4 to 6-mo course of low-dose testosterone enanthate (50 to 100 mg intramuscularly every 4 wk) may be helpful in boys of age 14 or older who show no signs of puberty[1025–1027] (Table 31–25). The low dose and short course of testosterone enanthate does not compromise final height.[1037] Oral treatment with 2.5 mg of fluoxymesterone for 6 to 60 mo will allow increased pubertal development without adverse effect on final height; compliance may be a problem.[1028] Low-dose oxandrolone (2.5 mg/d orally)[1029] has also been used as an oral alternative to intramuscular testosterone enanthate; this androgen increases growth through androgenic effects as reflected by suppression of LH and FSH but does not stimulate GH secretion because it is not aromatized to estrogen.[1030] The temporary increase in growth velocity with oxandrolone does not affect final height.[1031–1033] Increased growth response to 50 mg of intramuscular testosterone enanthate per mouth or 2.5 mg/d of oxandrolone by mouth is greatest in patients in whom puberty advances most rapidly after the termination of treatment. Short-term treatment with fluoxymesterone (2.5 mg/d orally) also does not compromise adult height.[1028] Oral testosterone undecanoate at 40 mg/d is an alternative treatment available in some countries.[1034–1036]

TABLE 31–25. Hormonal Substitution Therapy in Boys with Hypogonadism

Goal: to approximate normal adolescent development *when diagnosis is established*
Initial therapy: at 13 y of age, testosterone enanthate (or other long-acting testosterone ester) 50 mg intramuscularly every month for about 9 mo (6–12 mo)
Over the next 3 to 4 y: gradually increase dose to adult replacement dose of 200 mg every 2–3 wk
Begin *replacement therapy in boys with suspected hypogonadotropic hypogonadism* by bone age ≤14 y
To induce fertility at appropriate time: pulsatile LHRH or FSH and hCG therapy

For girls of age 13 or older, a 3- to 4-mo course of ethinyl estradiol (5 μg/d orally) or of conjugated estrogens (0.3 mg/d orally) may initiate maturation of the secondary sexual characteristics without unduly advancing bone age or limiting final height[1038] (Table 31–26).

If, during the 3 to 6 mo after discontinuing gonadal steroid therapy in either boys or girls, spontaneous puberty does not ensue or the concentrations of plasma gonadotropins and plasma testosterone in boys or plasma estradiol in girls do not increase, the treatment may be repeated. Usually, only one or two courses of therapy are necessary. When treatment is discontinued after bone age has advanced, for example, at ages 12 to 13 years in girls or 13 or 14 years in boys, patients with constitutional delay usually continue pubertal development, whereas those with gonadotropin deficiency do not progress and may in fact regress.

Functional hypogonadotropic hypogonadism associated with chronic disease is treated by alleviating the underlying problem. In this situation delayed puberty is usually the result of inadequate nutrition and low weight; when weight returns to normal, puberty usually occurs spontaneously.

Treatment with thyroxine promotes normal pubertal development in hypothyroid patients with delayed puberty.

Congenital or acquired gonadotropin deficiency due to CNS lesions requires replacement therapy with gonadal steroids at the normal age at onset of puberty (see Tables 31–25 and 31–26). An exception may occur when GH deficiency coexists with gonadotropin deficiency; if bone age advancement and epiphyseal fusion are brought about by testosterone or estradiol replacement before therapy with GH causes adequate linear growth, adult height will be compromised. However, if puberty is not initiated early enough, the patient may suffer psychological damage. It is generally advisable to initiate puberty in such patients with low-dose gonadal steroids by age 14 in boys and age 13 in girls regardless of the definitive diagnosis of gonadotropin deficiency; thus children with GH deficiency are treated as if they had isolated delayed puberty. Patients with isolated growth hormone deficiency have a delayed onset of puberty; with hGH administration puberty usually occurs at an appropriate age but may progress faster than normal.[1039, 1040] In more than 200 children with growth hormone deficiency treated with hGH the age at onset of induced puberty in subjects who were also gonadotropin deficient correlated with final height, while those who underwent spontaneous puberty, which occurred earlier than the age at hormone-induced puberty in the gonadotropin-deficient children, had a lower final height; it is thus advisable to wait to initiate puberty in subjects deficient in both GH and gonadotropin.[1041] Height at the onset of puberty also correlates with final height in GH-deficient children.[1042] Trials have not met with success in artificially delaying puberty with an

TABLE 31–26. Hormonal Substitution Therapy in Girls with Hypogonadism

When diagnosis of hypogonadism is firmly established (e.g., girls with 45,X gonadal dysgenesis), begin hormonal substitution therapy at 12–13 y of age
Goal: to approximate normal adolescent development
Initial therapy: ethinyl estradiol 5 μg by mouth or conjugated estrogen 0.3 mg (or less) by mouth daily for 4–6 mo
After 6 mo of therapy (or sooner if "breakthrough" bleeding occurs) begin cyclic therapy:
  Estrogen: first 21 d of month
  Progestagen: (e.g., medroxyprogesterone acetate 5 mg by mouth) 12th to 21st day of month
  Gradually increase dose of estrogen *over next 2–3 y* to conjugated estrogen 0.6–1.25 mg or ethinyl estradiol 10–20 μg daily for first 21 d of month
In hypogonadotropic hypogonadism: to induce ovulation at appropriate time: pulsatile LHRH or FSH and hCG therapy

LHRH analogue to achieve a greater final height in patients with isolated GH deficiency treated with hGH.[675, 1043]

Micropenis due to fetal androgen deficiency caused either by a primary testicular defect or by gonadotropin deficiency[1044] can be successfully treated with small doses of testosterone enanthate (25 to 50 mg/mo IM), administered for short periods during infancy[754, 1044] (see Chapter 29). Patients with isolated congenital GH deficiency occasionally have micropenis, which is successfully treated with hGH replacement alone.[1045]

As discussed earlier, episodic administration of LHRH can elicit pulsatile LH and FSH release and gonadal stimulation in normal prepubertal children and in hypogonadotropic patients.[618–622] Administration of LHRH in episodic fashion over prolonged periods with portable pumps or frequent injections (see Chapters 15 and 16)[620] can induce puberty and promote the development of secondary sexual characteristics and spermatogenesis in men[1046–1050] and ovulation in women;[1051, 1052] with this regimen women with hypogonadotropic hypogonadism have become pregnant. A lower frequency of LHRH administration favors FSH secretion; more frequent injections favor LH secretion and have been associated with ovarian changes similar to polycystic ovary syndrome.[1053] A comparison of two different regimens did not reveal a difference between an LHRH pulse given subcutaneously every 3 h and one given every 45 min in the time of onset of pubertal development or in serum LH, FSH, or gonadal steroid levels; this indicates that the pituitary-gonadal axis is sufficiently robust to accommodate various frequencies of LHRH secretion.[1054]

The use of pulsatile LHRH administration is not practical for the routine induction of puberty in adolescent boys and girls with gonadotropin deficiency. Human menopausal gonadotropin and hCG can be used as effective substitutes for human FSH and LH to produce full gonadal maturation, but this regimen is cumbersome and expensive.[1055, 1056] Consequently, long-term gonadal steroid replacement is the treatment of choice for hypothalamic or pituitary gonadotropin deficiency until fertility is desired.

Hypergonadotropic hypogonadism is treated with replacement of testosterone in boys and estradiol in girls. For treatment of gonadal dysgenesis, estrogen therapy should be initiated when the patient is age 13 (bone age ≥ 11 years) to allow secondary sexual development at an appropriate chronological age and to sustain bone mineral accretion. Klinefelter's syndrome is compatible with varying degrees of masculinization at puberty, but the levels of plasma testosterone and LH in such boys should be monitored every 6 months during puberty and yearly thereafter. If the LH level rises more than 2.5 SD above the mean value or if the testosterone level decreases below the normal range for age, testosterone replacement therapy is indicated.

Gonadal steroid treatment regimens are the same in both hypogonadotropic hypogonadism and hypergonadotropic hypogonadism (see Tables 31–25 and 31–26). Boys are given testosterone enanthate, 50 to 100 mg every 4 wk intramuscularly at the start; later, when the pubertal growth spurt is well underway, the dosage is gradually increased to 200 to 300 mg every 2 to 3 wk[89] (see Chapter 16). Skin patches of testosterone that are applied to the scrotum or nonsexual skin have been successful in adults and maintain a more constant level of serum testosterone than injections of testosterone esters, but teenage boys may be less likely to comply with daily applications; nonetheless, 2.5-mg and 5-mg patches may be useful in motivated teenagers.

Girls age 12 to 13 are initially given ethinyl estradiol, 5 μg/d orally, or conjugated estrogens, 0.3 mg/d by mouth, daily for the first 6 months and then for the first 21 d of the month. The dose is gradually increased over the next 2 to 3 y to 10 μg of ethinyl estradiol or 0.6 to 1.25 mg of conjugated estrogen for the first 21 d of the month. The maintenance dose should be the minimal amount to maintain secondary sexual characteristics, sustain withdrawal bleeding, and prevent osteoporosis. After breakthrough bleeding occurs, or no later than 6 mo after the start of cyclic therapy, a progestagen (e.g., medroxyprogesterone acetate, 5 to 10 mg/d) is added on days 12 through 21 of the month. Undesirable effects are uncommon but may include weight gain, headache, nausea, peripheral edema, and mild hypertension (see Chapter 15). There is a concern about the increased risk of endometrial and breast carcinoma in patients receiving chronic estrogen replacement therapy, including patients with gonadal dysgenesis. The use of progestational agents to antagonize the effect of estrogens reduces the risk (see Chapter 15).

Patients with hypopituitarism may complain of sparse pubic hair growth or, in girls, total absence of pubic hair. Pubic hair thickens in affected males after testosterone treatment. Growth hormone therapy in boys who are deficient in both GH and gonadotropin enhances the steroidogenic response of the testes to hCG administration.[1057] Furthermore, adolescent or young adult women have been given a low dose (25 mg) of long-acting intramuscular testosterone, every 4 wk to stimulate the growth of pubic hair without virilization.[1058]

Testosterone treatment in boys with radiation-induced testicular failure results in normal final height, although the upper/lower segment ratio may be much reduced because of impaired spinal growth if concurrent spinal irradiation is given.[1059]

Human GH therapy in gonadal dysgenesis causes an increase in growth rate and final height but the magnitude of the increase in final height and hence the cost-benefit relationship remains uncertain.[1060, 1061] The addition of estrogen therapy in replacement doses can reduce the final height obtained with GH therapy alone[1062–1066] (see Chapter 30). Counseling and a peer support group are important components of the long-term management.[1040]

Sexual Precocity

Sexual precocity (Table 31–27) is defined as the appearance of any sign of secondary sexual maturation at an age more than 2.5 SD below the mean age (see Tables 31–3 and 31–5). There are few data in the United States to establish this limit, so the ages of 8 in girls and 9 in boys were defined as the lower limits of the normal onset of puberty based on longitudinal data available from European studies, such as those from Switzerland, that appeared most compatible with American children.[76, 1067] However, as noted earlier (see section on physical changes of puberty), the fact that breast development and pubic hair development may occur in normal American girls as young as 6 years, especially in black girls, makes it mandatory to evaluate carefully and conservatively girls with minimal, relatively nonprogressive signs of sexual precocity. The lower limit of "normal" age at onset of puberty, as evidenced by breast development, can be set at 7 years for white girls and 6 years for black girls. For both black and white American boys, the lower limit of "normal" age at onset of puberty as marked by Tanner genitalia stage 2 is about 9 years, an age similar to some European studies (see Table 31–4). If the sexual precocity results from premature reactivation of the hypothalamic LHRH pulse generator–pituitary–gonadotropin-gonadal axis, the condition is called complete isosexual precocity, or true or central precocious puberty, and is LHRH dependent. Pulsatile LH release has a pubertal pattern, and the rise in the level of LH after LHRH administration is indistinguishable from the normal pubertal pattern. If extrapituitary secretion of gonadotropins or secretion of gonadal steroids independent of pulsatile LHRH stimulation leads to virilization in boys or feminization in girls, the condition is termed incomplete isosexual precocity, pseudoprecocious puberty, or LHRH-independent sexual precocity. The production

TABLE 31–27. Classification of Sexual Precocity

TRUE PRECOCIOUS PUBERTY OR COMPLETE ISOSEXUAL PRECOCITY
(LHRH-DEPENDENT SEXUAL PRECOCITY OR PREMATURE ACTIVATION OF
THE HYPOTHALAMIC LHRH PULSE GENERATOR)

Idiopathic true precocious puberty
CNS tumors
    Optic glioma associated with neurofibromatosis type I
    Hypothalamic astrocytoma
Other CNS disorders:
    Developmental abnormalities including hypothalamic hamartoma of the tuber
        cinereum
    Encephalitis
    Static encephalopathy
    Brain abscess
    Sarcoid or tubercular granuloma
    Head trauma
    Hydrocephalus
    Arachnoid cyst
    Myelomeningocele
    Vascular lesion
    Cranial irradiation
True precocious puberty after late treatment of congenital virilizing adrenal
    hyperplasia or other previous chronic exposure to sex steroids

INCOMPLETE ISOSEXUAL PRECOCITY (HYPOTHALAMIC
LHRH-INDEPENDENT)

Males
    Gonadotropin-secreting tumors
        hCG-secreting CNS tumors (e.g., chorioepitheliomas, germinoma, teratoma)
        hCG-secreting tumors located outside the CNS (hepatoma, teratoma,
            choriocarcinoma)
    Increased androgen secretion by adrenal or testis
        Congenital adrenal hyperplasia (CYP21 and CYP11B1 deficiencies)
        Virilizing adrenal neoplasm
        Leydig cell adenoma
        Familial testotoxicosis (sex-limited autosomal dominant pituitary
            gonadotropin-independent precocious Leydig cell and germ cell
            maturation)
        Cortisol resistance syndrome

Females
    Ovarian cyst
    Estrogen-secreting ovarian or adrenal neoplasm
    Peutz-Jeghers syndrome
In Both Sexes
    McCune-Albright syndrome
    Hypothyroidism
    Iatrogenic or exogenous sexual precocity (including inadvertent exposure to
        estrogens in food, drugs, or cosmetics)

VARIATIONS OF PUBERTAL DEVELOPMENT

Premature thelarche
Premature isolated menarche
Premature adrenarche
Adolescent gynecomastia in boys
Macro-orchidism

CONTRASEXUAL PRECOCITY

Feminization in Males
    Adrenal neoplasm
    Chorionepithelioma
    CYP11B1 deficiency
    Late-onset adrenal hyperplasia
    Testicular neoplasm (Peutz-Jeghers syndrome)
    Increased extraglandular conversion of circulating adrenal androgens to
        estrogen
    Iatrogenic (exposure to estrogens)
Virilization in Females
    Congenital adrenal hyperplasia
        CYP21 deficiency
        CYP11B1 deficiency
        3β-HSD deficiency
    Virilizing adrenal neoplasm (Cushing's syndrome)
    Virilizing ovarian neoplasm (e.g., arrhenoblastoma)
    Iatrogenic (exposure to androgens)
    Cortisol resistance syndrome

LHRH, luteinizing hormone–releasing factor (GnRH); CYP21, 21-hydroxylase; CYP11B1, 11-hydroxylase; 3β-HSD, 3β-hydroxysteroid dehydrogenase 4,5-isomerase.
Modified from Grumbach MM. True or central percocious puberty. In: Kreiger DT, Bordin CW, eds. Current Therapy in Endocrinology and Metabolism, 1985–1986. Toronto: BC Decker, 1985: 4–8.[1121]

of excessive estrogens in boys causes inappropriate feminization, and the production of increased androgens in girls causes virilization; these conditions are termed contrasexual precocity (also termed heterosexual precocity). The various disorders that cause sexual precocity can be separated into those in which the increased secretion of gonadal steroids depends on LHRH stimulation of pituitary gonadotropins and those in which the precocity is unrelated to activation of the LHRH pulse generator.

In all forms of sexual precocity, increased gonadal steroid levels increase height velocity, somatic development, and the rate of skeletal maturation and, because of premature epiphyseal fusion, can lead to the paradox of tall stature in childhood but short adult height. Data on the final height in true precocious puberty are scarce (Table 31–28), but several studies of untreated females with idiopathic central precocious puberty demonstrated a mean final height of 151 to 155 cm.[636, 1068–1075] There are a few reports of final height in boys (see Table 31–28). In one study[1069] the mean height was 155.4 cm ± 8.3 SD and all boys were well below midparent height and below the father's height.

Blood pressure is that of height- and weight-related normal subjects rather than of age-matched normal people; thus elevated blood pressure for age in patients with sexual precocity may not indicate hypertension.[211] Serum alkaline phosphatase and IGF-I levels reflect sexual development rather than chronologic age.[85]

True, or Central, Precocious Puberty: Complete Isosexual Precocity (LHRH-Dependent Sexual Precocity)

In our series of more than 200 patients with true precocious puberty,[636] precocious puberty was five times more com-

mon in girls than boys, and the idiopathic form was eight times more common in girls (Table 31–29). Neurologic causes were as common as idiopathic true precocious puberty in boys, whereas neurologic lesions were only a fifth as common as idiopathic disorders in girls. Thus it is especially important to search for a neurologic etiology for true precocious puberty, especially in boys[567, 636] (Table 31–30).

LONG-TERM FOLLOW-UP OF TRUE PRECOCIOUS PUBERTY. Pregnancy has occurred in patients with true precocious puberty as early as 5 y of age.[1076] Of course, such pregnancies are in fact the result of childhood sexual abuse of a child regardless of the cause of the precocious puberty. Fertility in later life is less well documented, but normal pregnancies have occurred in women who had idiopathic true preco-

TABLE 31–28. Historical Controls of Untreated Children with True Precocious Puberty

Reference	No. of Patients (Women/Men)	Final Ht (cm)* Women	Final Ht (cm)* Men
Thamdrup[1070]			
Sigurjonsdottir and	26/8	151.3 ± 8.8	155.4 ± 8.3
Hayles[1073]	40/11	152.7 ± 8.0	156.0 ± 7.3
Werder[1074]	4/0	150.9 ± 5.0	
Lee[1072]	15/0	155.3 ± 9.6	
UCSF	8/4	153.8 ± 6.8	159.6 ± 8.7
Total	93/23	152.7 ± 8.6	155.6 ± 7.7

*Mean ± 1SD.
From Paul D, Conte FA, Grumbach MM, Kaplan SL. Long-term effect of gonadotropin-releasing hormone agonist therapy on final and near-final height in 26 children with true precocious puberty treated at a median age of less than 5 years. J Clin Endocrinol Metab 1995; 80:546–551, with permission.[1068]

TABLE 31–29. Distribution by Sex of Children with Idiopathic and Neurogenic Precocious Puberty

| | Idiopathic | | Neurogenic | |
Series	Male	Female	Male	Female
Thamdrup (1961)[1070]	4	34	7	11
Wilkins (1965)[422]	13	67	10	5
Sigurjonsdottir and Hayles (1968)[1073]	8	54	16	16
University of California, San Francisco (1981)*	13	121	26	45

*Unpublished.

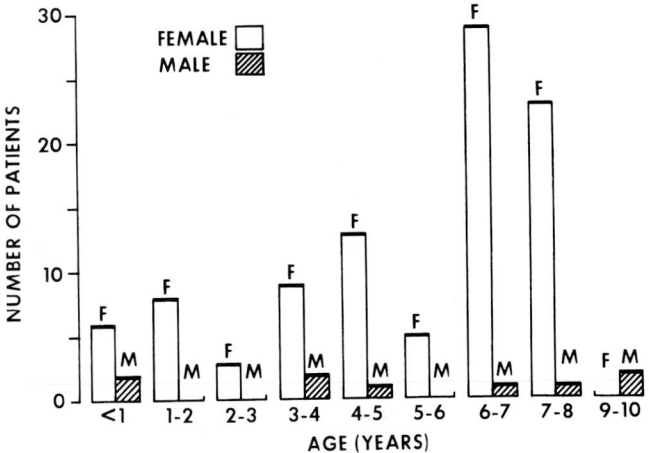

Figure 31–58. Age at onset of idiopathic true precocious puberty in 106 children. Open bars, female; hatched bars, male. At all ages, the frequency is greater in females than in males. The peak prevalence in girls is between ages 6 and 8 years. (From Kaplan SL, Grumbach MM. The neuroendocrinology of human puberty: an ontogenetic perspective. In: Grumbach MM, Sizonenko PC, Aubert ML, eds. Control of the Onset of Puberty. Baltimore: Williams & Wilkins, 1990: 1–68. © 1990, the Williams & Wilkins Co., Baltimore.[253])

cious puberty,[1076, 1077] a CNS abnormality triggering true precocious puberty,[636, 1073] or premature menarche. There are also reports of adult fertility in the isosexual precocity of McCune-Albright syndrome.[422, 1078, 1079]

IDIOPATHIC TRUE PRECOCIOUS PUBERTY. Many girls age 6 to 8 with idiopathic precocious puberty represent the left-hand end of the bell-shaped curve for the onset of normal puberty and are examples of early normal puberty. There may be a history of early maturation in the family; rarely, true precocious puberty is inherited as an autosomal recessive trait in boys and girls.[636, 1080] Most children with true precocious puberty, however, have the idiopathic disorder with no familial tendency toward early maturation and no signs of organic disease. This condition, which can be manifested in infancy, is more common in girls than in boys and is usually associated with electroencephalographic abnormalities.[1081] The age at onset in girls in about 50% of cases is 6 to 7 y, in about 25% it is 2 to 6 y, and in 18% it is in infancy[636] (Fig. 31–58).

In boys (Fig. 31–59) the testes usually enlarge under gonadotropin stimulation before other signs of puberty are seen; in girls (see Fig. 31–59) an increase in the rate of growth, breast development, enlargement of the labia minora, and maturational changes in the vaginal mucosa are the usual presenting signs, with variable manifestations of pubic hair. Progression of sexual maturation is often more rapid than normal. A waxing and waning course of development may be encountered. The rapid growth is associated with increased GH secretion and elevation of serum IGF-I levels because of stimulation by gonadal steroids.[100, 116] The ratio of bone age to chronologic age and the rise of IGF-I above normal values for age are predictive of outcome: children with modest clinical signs progress less rapidly and maintain their target heights.[1082] Furthermore, in girls slowly progressing cases may have little or no loss of predicted final height and have normal or

only slightly elevated estrogen and IGF-I levels.[1082] If height prediction is normal at the time of diagnosis, the patients may not require therapy.[1082] Spermatogenesis in males and ovulation in females make fertility possible.

The uterus and ovaries increase in size. The ovaries also may develop a polycystic appearance that persists even after successful treatment with an LHRH agonist.[1083] True precocious puberty does not lead to premature menopause, but there is an increased risk of the development of carcinoma of the breast in women. Psychosexual development[1084, 1085] is advanced only modestly (about 1.5 y in girls with idiopathic true precocious puberty).[1086]

The pituitary gland increases in size on MRI scans in patients with central precocious puberty.[93, 1087, 1088] T1-weighted images indicate a convex upper border of the pituitary in true precocious puberty, indicating its similarity to normal puberty. Two sisters had pituitary gland hyperplasia (height greater than 1 cm) with central precocious puberty.[1089] Although the empty-sella syndrome (see Chapter 9) may be associated with central precocious puberty, the empty-sella syndrome is more common in patients with pituitary hypofunction. Empty sella was found in 10% of children imaged for suspected hypothalamic-pituitary disorders, including hypogonadotropic hypogonadism, but the incidence in the general population is not known.[1090, 1091, 1094]

The plasma gonadotropin and gonadal steroid levels, the LH response to LHRH administration, and the amplitude and frequency of LH pulses are in the normal pubertal range[278, 612, 617] (Figs. 31–60 and 31–61). Third-generation gonadotropin assays may allow the diagnosis of true precocious puberty by random LH analyses in the basal state or after administration of a single subcutaneous dose of LHRH.[1092, 1093] Adrenarche usually does not accompany gonadarche in girls below age 5 or 6 with true precocious puberty; pubic hair is sparse or initially absent in girls of this age.[636, 638] When true precocious puberty begins after age 6, adrenarche is usually early for chronologic age, but not for bone age.[638]

A small number of patients with central precocious puberty revert spontaneously to a more immature pubertal state, persist without further progression, or fluctuate between progression and regression.[636, 1095] Thus the course may not be inexorably progressive.

CNS TUMORS CAUSING TRUE PRECOCIOUS PUBERTY.

TABLE 31–30. Etiology of True Precocious Puberty*

Etiology	Number and Sex
Idiopathic	121F, 13M
Other causes	
CNS-hypothalamic tumors including hamartomas	11F, 15M
Arachnoid cyst	2F, 1M
Hydrocephalus	6F, 1M
Head trauma (child abuse)	1F
Perinatal asphyxia, cerebral palsy	3F, 1M
Encephalitis or meningitis	3F, 1M
Sex chromosome abnormalities (47,XXY; 48,XXXY)	2M
Nonspecific seizure disorder or mental retardation	26F, 16M
Degenerative CNS disease	3M
Congenital virilizing adrenal hyperplasia with secondary true precocious puberty	3M

*Data from University of California, San Francisco, Pediatric Endocrine Clinic.
From Kaplan SL, Grumbach MM. Pathogenesis of sexual precocity. In: Grumbach MM, Sizonenko PC, Aubert ML, eds. Control of the Onset of Puberty. Baltimore: Williams & Wilkins, 1990: 620–660. © 1990, the Williams & Wilkins Co., Baltimore.[636]

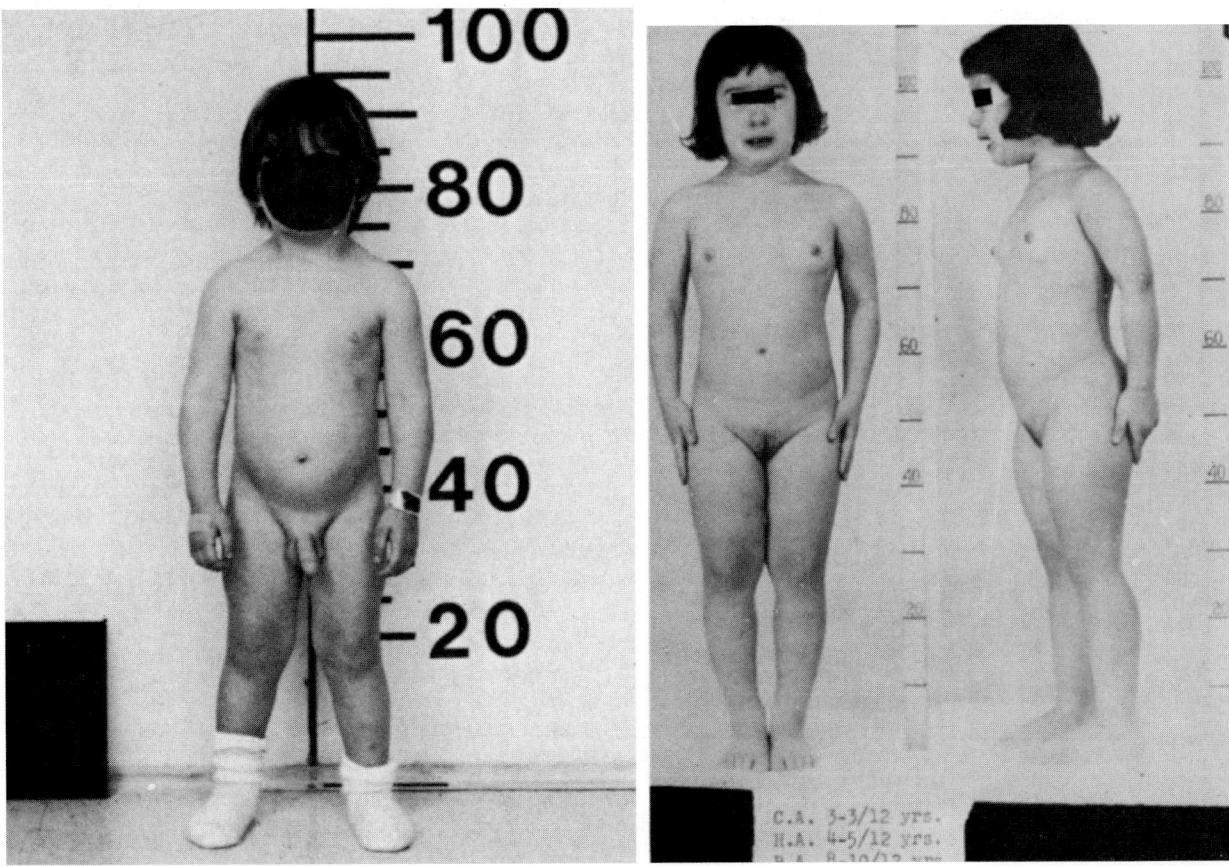

Figure 31–59. *Left,* A boy 2 years, 5 months of age with idiopathic precocious puberty. He had pubic hair and phallic and testicular enlargement by 10 months of age. At 1 year of age, his height was 86 cm (+4 SD); the phallus measured 10 × 3.5 cm, and the testes measured 2.5 × 1.5 cm. Plasma LH was 1.9 ng/mL (LER-960); FSH 1.2 ng/mL (LER-869); and testosterone 416 ng/dL. After 100 μg of LHRH, the plasma LH increased to 8.4 ng/mL, and FSH to 1.8 ng/mL, a pubertal response. When photographed, the patient had been treated with medroxyprogesterone acetate for 1.5 y. His height was 95.2 cm (+ 1 SD), the phallus was 6 × 3 cm, and the testes were 2.4 × 1.3 cm. Basal concentrations of LH (LER-960) were 0.9 ng/mL; FSH (LER-869) 0.8 ng/mL; and testosterone 7 ng/dL. After 100 μg of LHRH, LH concentrations rose to 2.3 ng/mL, whereas FSH concentrations did not change when he was on treatment with medroxyprogesterone acetate. For conversion to SI units, see the legends of Figures 31–17 and 31–18. (*Left Panel,* From Styne DM, Grumbach MM. Puberty in the male and female: its physiology and disorders. In: Yen SCC, Jaffe RB, eds. Reproductive Endocrinology. 2nd ed. Philadelphia: W. B Saunders, 1986: 313–384.[1430]) *Right,* A 3 3/12-y-old girl with idiopathic true precocious puberty who had recurrent vaginal bleeding since 9 mo of age. Height age, 4 5/12 years; bone age, 8 10/12 y.

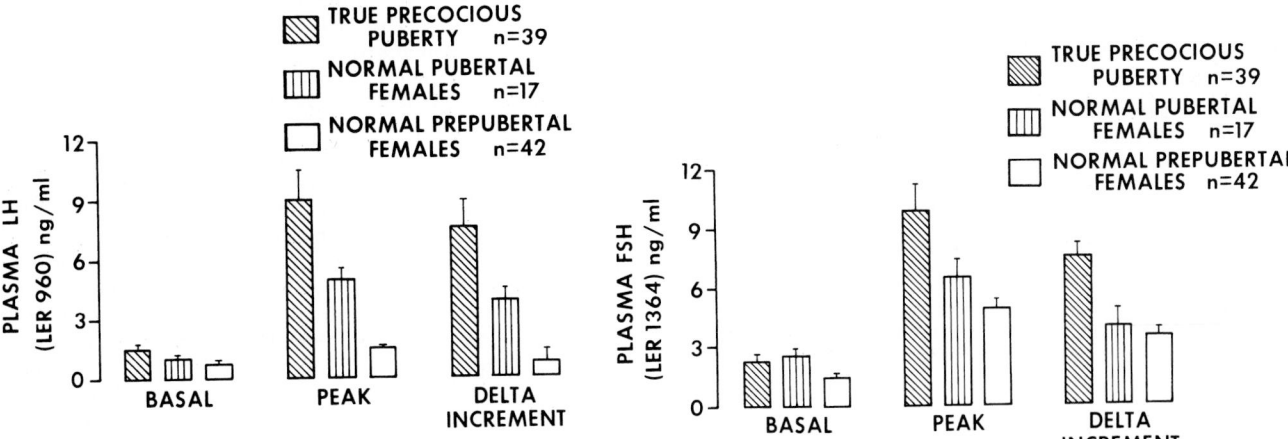

Figure 31–60. *Left,* Mean basal plasma LH level (LER-960) and mean peak and increment after intravenous LHRH (100 μg) in normal prepubertal and pubertal females and in females with idiopathic true precocious puberty. The mean peak and increments of plasma LH are higher in true precocious puberty than in normal puberty. *Right,* Basal FSH level (LER-1364) and mean peak and increment after intravenous LHRH (100 μg) in normal prepubertal and pubertal females with true precocious puberty. The concentration of FSH and the response to LHRH were greater in females with true precocious puberty and normal puberty than in prepubertal females. (From Kaplan SL, Grumbach MM. Pathogenesis of sexual precocity. In: Grumbach MM, Sizonenko PC, Aubert ML, eds. Control of the Onset of Puberty. Baltimore: Williams & Wilkins, 1990: 620–660. © 1990, the Williams & Wilkins Co., Baltimore.[636])

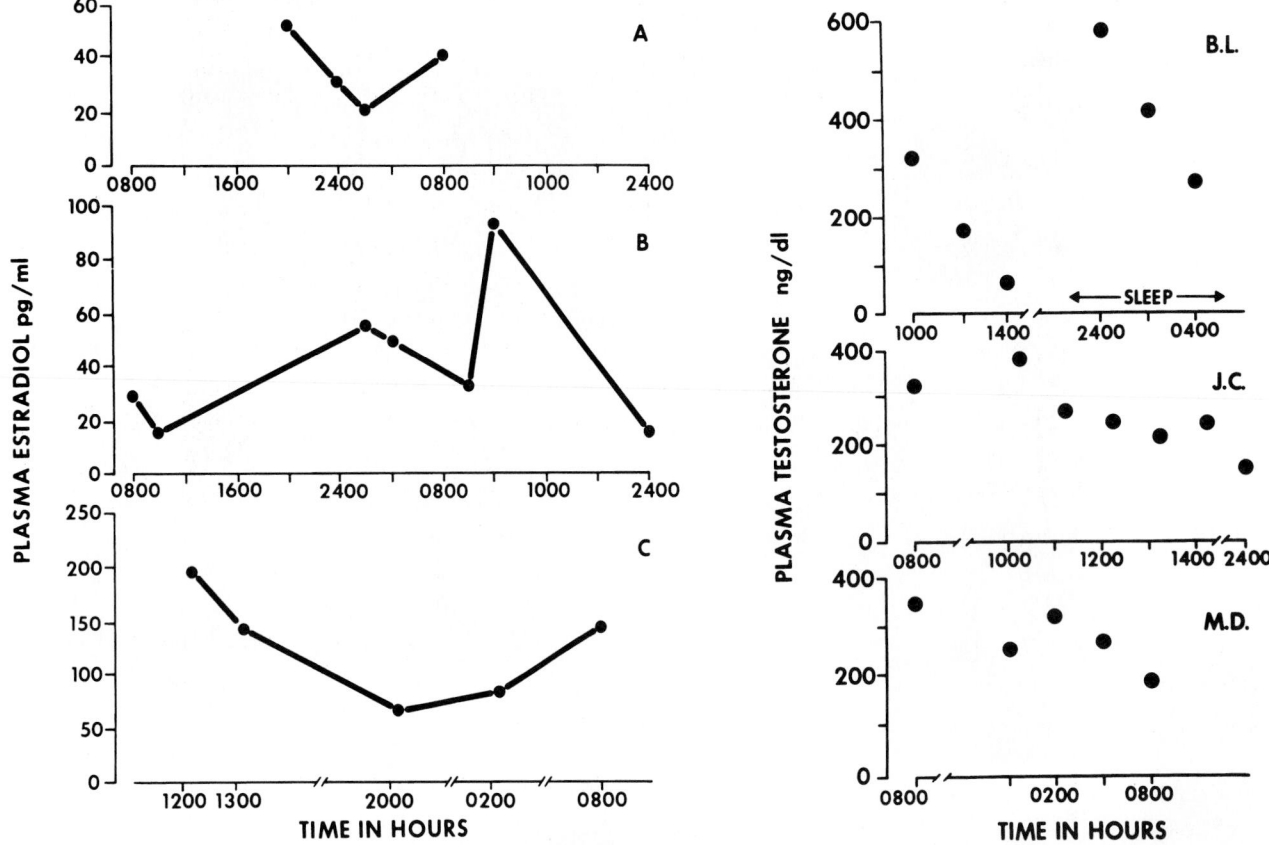

Figure 31–61. *Left,* Serial determinations of plasma estradiol in three girls with idiopathic true precocious puberty. Note the striking fluctuations in values. *Right,* Serial determinations of plasma testosterone in three boys with true precocious puberty (B.L. and J.C. have a hypothalamic hamartoma; M.D. has the idiopathic form). For conversion to SI units, see the legends of Figures 31–17 and 31–18. (From Kaplan SL, Grumbach MM. Pathogenesis of sexual precocity. In: Grumbach MM, Sizonenko PC, Aubert ML, eds. Control of the Onset of Puberty. Baltimore: Williams & Wilkins, 1990: 620–660. © 1990, the Williams & Wilkins Co., Baltimore.[636])

True precocious puberty from CNS tumors (Table 31–31; see Tables 31–29 and 31–30) has a similar prevalence in boys and girls; however, in boys, neurologic abnormalities account for two thirds of instances of true precocious puberty, and in the authors' experience a CNS tumor was present in at least half of this group.[636] A CNS neoplasm must be considered in the differential diagnosis of true precocious puberty.[422, 567, 705, 1073, 1096] Optic and hypothalamic glioma (often associated with neurofibromatosis),[704, 705, 1097] astrocytoma, ependymoma, and, rarely, craniopharyngioma can cause true precocious puberty, either by impinging on the pathways that inhibit the LHRH pulse generator in childhood or as a consequence of cranial radiation of a brain tumor. The prevalence of true precocious puberty is increased after cranial radiation for local tumors or

leukemia.[94, 722, 1098, 1099] Even radiotherapy targeting the pituitary can cause true precocious puberty.[1100]

The unusual combination of GH deficiency and central precocious puberty can occur in children who have received CNS radiation for neoplasms or in children with a variety of CNS abnormalities, including developmental malformations and head trauma.[94] The lack of GH may not be apparent because of accelerated growth from the elevated gonadal steroid levels. Nonetheless, GH-deficient children with central precocious puberty grow slower than GH-sufficient children with central precocious puberty but faster than GH-deficient children without sexual precocity. Furthermore, in GH-deficient children with central precocious puberty the IGF-I levels are intermediate between the higher levels in GH-sufficient children with sexual precocity and the lower levels in the prepubertal GH-deficient children.[94] GH deficiency and true precocious puberty can occur with CNS radiation doses of only 18 Gy, while gonadotropin deficiency, thyrotropin deficiency, corticotropin deficiency, and hyperprolactinemia occur with doses greater than 40 Gy.[1101] Both boys and girls are subject to an earlier onset of puberty in combination with GH deficiency and CNS irradiation of 25 to 47 Gy for tumors outside of the hypothalamic-pituitary area.[94] Treatment with both hGH and an LHRH agonist is indicated and results in better growth and improved height prognosis over the use of LHRH agonist alone.[94, 1063, 1102] Since GH secretion is related to BMI, it is important to exclude a decrease in GH secretion due to increased BMI in true precocious puberty before one interprets the decrease as evidence of GH deficiency.[1103]

Hamartomas of the tuber cinereum, congenital malformations composed of a heterotopic mass of neurosecretory neurons,

TABLE 31–31. Classification of CNS Tumors Associated with Isosexual Sexual Precocity at University of Caifornia, San Francisco

10% of all true precocious puberty patients: CNS tumors, hypothalamic (n = 26)

Males—IPP*/organic precocious puberty = 13/15 = 0.9/1	
Females—IPP/organic precocious puberty = 121/11 = 12/1	
LHRH-dependent true precocious puberty	
Astrocytoma	3M, 5F
Hamartomas	3M, 3F
Neurofibromatosis	5M, 1F
Craniopharyngioma	2F
LHRH-independent incomplete sexual precocity	
hCG-secreting tumor†	4M

*IPP, idiopathic precocious puberty.
†CNS and extra-CNS neoplasms.

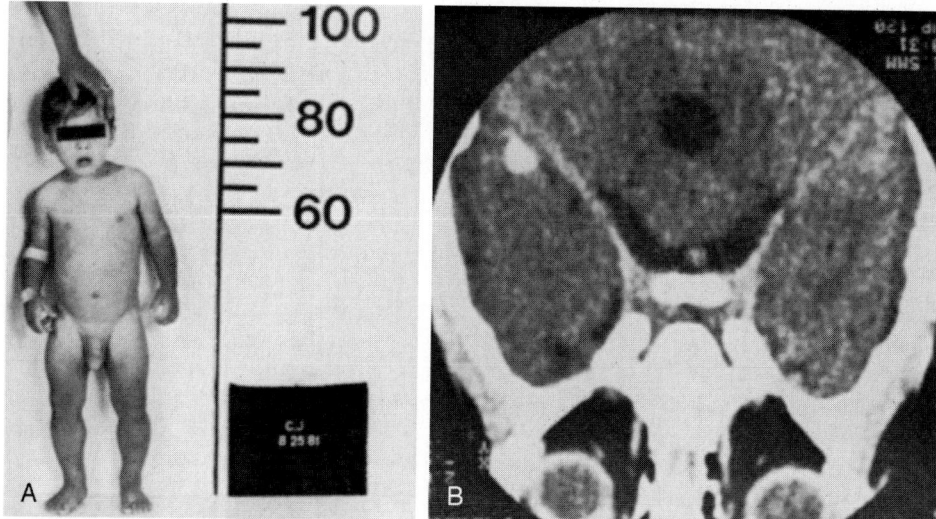

Figure 31–62. *A,* A 17-month-old male infant with hamartoma of the tuber cinereum and true precocious puberty. At 8 months of age, secondary sexual development was noted, and the patient was misdiagnosed as having congenital virilizing adrenal hyperplasia. He was treated with glucocorticoids, which slowed his growth but did not affect his sexual development and bone age advancement. When he was first seen at 17 months, height was 84.2 cm; weight was 14.8 kg; the pubic hair stage was stage II; the penis was 10.4 × 2.2 cm; the testes were 1.5 × 2.8 cm; and the scrotum was thinned and rugated. The bone age was 4 3/12 years. After LHRH administration, the LH level rose from 0.5 to 3.1 ng/dL (LER-960), the FSH level from 0.5 to 1.2 ng/mL (LER-869), and the testosterone level from 409 to 450 ng/dL. DHEAS was 17 µg/dL (preadrenarchal value). The patient was treated with a potent long-acting LHRH-agonist deslorelin (D-Trp⁶Pro⁹NEt-LHRH), which resulted in arrest of his pubertal advancement and a striking decrease in the plasma concentration of testosterone, LH pulses, and the response to exogenous LHRH. *B,* CT scan of the patient, demonstrating a 1.5-cm mass posterior and rostral to the dorsum sella, which depresses the flow of the third ventricle. For conversion to SI units, see the legends of Figures 31–17, 31–18, and 31–37. (From Styne DM, Grumbach MM. Puberty in the male and female: its physiology and disorders. In: Yen SCC, Jaffe RB, eds. Reproductive Endocrinology. 2nd ed. Philadelphia W. B. Saunders, 1986: 313–384.[1430])

fiber bundles, and glial cells, can cause true precocious puberty (Fig. 31–62), usually before the age of 3 years (Table 31–32).[579, 580, 636, 1104] Such hypothalamic hamartomas can be associated with laughing (gelastic) seizures, petit mal, or generalized tonic-clonic seizures; developmental delay; behavioral disturbances; and dysmorphic syndromes.[1104–1106] Seizures are unusual when the mass diameter of the hamartoma is less than 10 mm, whereas larger masses are associated with a high risk.[1106] With CT and MRI brain scans, hamartomas of the tuber cinereum are now detected in many boys and girls previously thought to have idiopathic true precocious puberty and are now the most common known cause of true precocious puberty (Fig. 31–63); before 1980 37 patients had been described with hamartomas of the tuber cinereum, and more than 80 additional patients have subsequently been reported[1104, 1106–1108] (see Table 31–32), an increase attributable to the use of CT and MRI brain scans.[1109] For example, Pescovitz and colleagues,[1110] in reviewing the experience at the National Institutes of Health, reported that of 87 girls with true precocious puberty, 16% had a hypothalamic hamartoma, 40% had other CNS abnormalities, and 60% had idiopathic true

precocious puberty. Among 20 boys with true precocious puberty, 2 had idiopathic true precocious puberty, 10 had a hypothalamic hamartoma, and 8 had other CNS abnormalities, including hypothalamic neoplasms.

The LHRH-secreting hypothalamic hamartoma contains a heterotopic mass of nervous tissue, including LHRH neurosecretory neurons; the tumors may be sessile or pedunculated and are usually attached to the posterior hypothalamus between the tuber cinereum and the mammillary bodies. The pedunculated hamartoma has a distinct stalk; hamartomas have a characteristic appearance that does not change with time. On CT or MRI scan they cause an isodense fullness of the interpeduncular, prepontine, and posterior suprasellar cisterns, occasionally with distortion of the anterior third ventricle.[1111, 1112] There is no enhancement with contrast material.[1113] MRI gives the best visualization of the lesion[1106, 1114, 1115] (see Fig. 31–63).

The etiology of the hypothalamic hamartoma may be the opposite of the failure of migration of LHRH neurons in Kallmann's syndrome; in the hypothalamic hamartoma, LHRH neurons may have enhanced migration to the site of the hamartoma or alternatively there may be a stimulus to progenitor cells to develop the capacity to synthesize LHRH in the hamartoma.

Hamartomas of the tuber cinereum are not true neoplasms and do not progress or enlarge.[579, 580, 1106, 1108, 1116, 1117] Hamartomas associated with true precocious puberty contain LHRH neurosecretory cells similar to the LHRH-containing neurons in the medial basal hypothalamus. Such hamartomas exert their endocrine effects by the pulsatile release of LHRH.[567, 636] Indeed, LHRH-containing fibers may extend from the hamartoma toward the median eminence.[636, 1116] The LHRH-containing neurosecretory neurons in the malformation appear to be unrestrained by the intrinsic CNS mechanisms that inhibit the normal LHRH pulse generator and consequently act as ectopic LHRH pulse generators,[253, 421] either independently or in synchrony with the LHRH neurosecretory neurons in the medial basal hypothalamus to produce

TABLE 31–32. Clinical and Laboratory Characteristics of Children with True Precocious Puberty Caused by Hypothalamic Hamartoma

Characteristic	University of California, San Francisco (n = 12: 6M, 6F)	Hochman et al.,[579]* (n = 27: 18M, 9F)
Age at onset of pubertal signs		
Birth to 1 y	4	6
1 to 2 y	4	17
2 to 4 y	3	6
7 y	1	1
Neurological signs		
Seizures including gelastic type	3/12	11/24
Headache and visual symptoms	1/12	5/24
None	7/12	7/24

*Literature review.

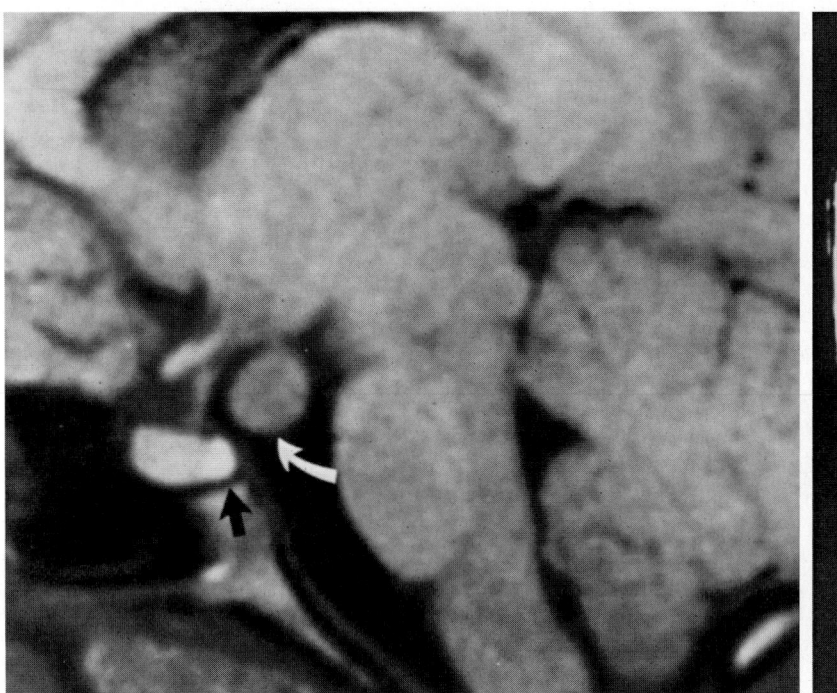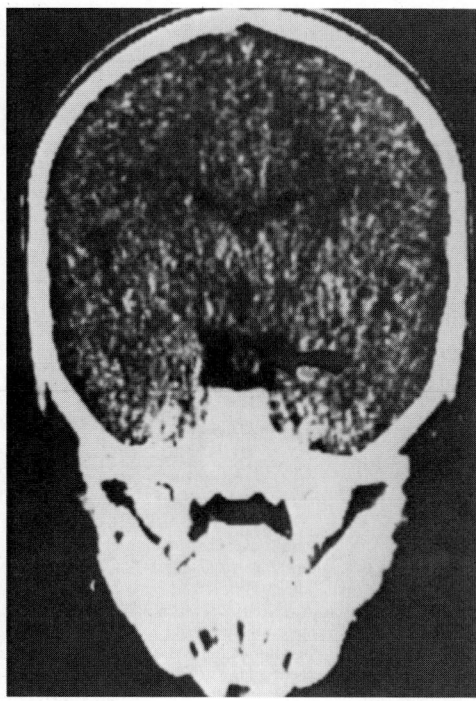

Figure 31–63. *Left,* MRI scan demonstrating a hypothalamic hamartoma *(solid white arrow)* in a 4-year-old boy with true precocious puberty; sagittal T1-weighted image. The posterior pituitary hot spot is designated by the solid black arrow. *Right,* CT brain scan (coronal section) showing an isodense, pedunculated, collar button–shaped hypothalamic hamartoma *(arrow)* in a 2-year-old girl with true precocious puberty.

intermittent secretory bursts of LHRH[253] (see Fig. 31–38). The LHRH acts like endogenous LHRH to elicit pulsatile release of LH (Fig. 31–64). If the hamartoma secreted LHRH in a continuous fashion, true precocious puberty should not occur, as the LHRH receptors would be desensitized. (About 10% of hypothalamic hamartomas are not associated with true precocious puberty.)

Hamartomas of the tuber cinereum should not be approached surgically except in unusual circumstances. Although removal of a hypothalamic hamartoma has led to reversal of the pubertal process,[579, 1107, 1116, 1117] operative removal has also caused death.[579] Hamartomas associated with true precocious puberty are congenital malformations that do not grow, as evidenced by periodic CT or MRI scans,[1106, 1118] and the precocious puberty can be controlled by LHRH agonist therapy.[1119] Accordingly, although some advocate neurosurgical removal of these hamartomas[1120] the authors do not recommend surgery in the absence of strong evidence of growth of the mass or of a complication such as intractable seizures or hydrocephalus.[567, 636, 1106, 1121, 1122]

CNS NEOPLASMS. Sexual precocity may be the first manifestation of a hypothalamic tumor of any cell type when it arises in or impinges on the posterior hypothalamus. In addition, headaches and visual disturbances may develop, and children may have diabetes insipidus, hydrocephalus, or optic atrophy due to enlarging tumors.[636, 1073]

The locations of CNS tumors that cause true precocious puberty make surgical removal difficult. A conservative approach calls for biopsy of the neoplasm and radiation, chemotherapy or both, depending on the pathologic findings.

OTHER CNS CONDITIONS. True precocious puberty may occur secondary to encephalitis, static cerebral encephalopathy, brain abscess, or sarcoid or tuberculous granulomas of the hypothalamus.[636, 1124] Central precocious puberty can occur after severe head trauma[1125] (usually in girls), and it has been associated with cerebral atrophy or focal encephalomalacia or following cerebral edema complicating the treatment of severe diabetic ketoacidosis.[1126] Children with hydrocephalus, even if shunted, may have early pubertal development, and those who are not adequately treated can develop true precocious puberty.[251, 636, 1123, 1127] Children with severe hydrocephalus often have poor prepubertal growth, an early pubertal growth spurt, and decreased final height.[1128]

Arachnoid cysts arising de novo, after infection, or after

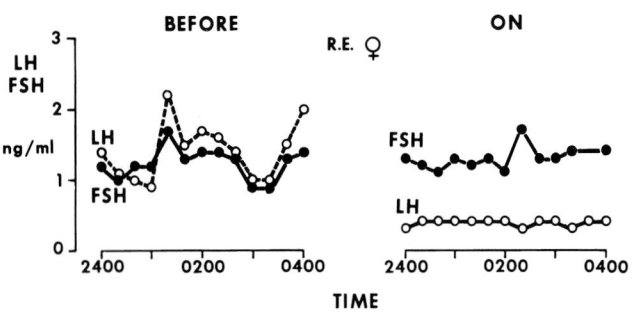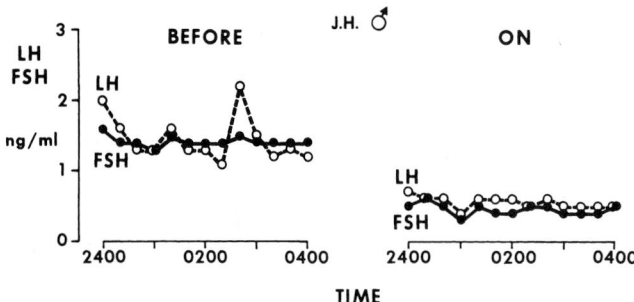

Figure 31–64. Pulsatile LH secretion before and during LHRH agonist therapy in a boy *(right)* and a girl *(left)* with true precocious puberty secondary to a hypothalamic hamartoma. For conversion to SI units, see the legend of Figure 31–17.

surgery can cause premature sexual development, sometimes with associated GH deficiency.[253, 636, 1129] Head nodding, abnormal gait, and abnormalities of visual fields occur commonly. The sella turcica can be eroded or enlarged. Decompression and extirpation of a suprasellar arachnoid cyst may reverse the sexual precocity[253, 1130, 1131] (see Fig. 31–37).

Neurofibromatosis type 1 (von Recklinghausen's disease) is associated with a propensity to develop the optic chiasmal tumors that are the most common[1132] but not the only[1133] cause of true precocious puberty in the disorder. Most optic gliomas appear in the first decade; these tumors rarely progress after diagnosis.[506, 1132, 1134, 1135, 1140] The tumor suppressor *NFI* gene is widely expressed, even though neurofibromatosis 1 involves mainly tissues derived from the neural crest.[1136–1138] A wide variety of mutations in neurofibromatosis type 1 have been reported, including especially deletions, nonsense, and truncating mutations.[1135, 1139] In sporadic cases, the new mutations usually originate in the paternal NF1 allele, suggesting a role for genomic imprinting.[1139]

Neurofibromatosis type 1 is characterized by multiple pigmented areas including café au lait spots and overgrowth of nerve sheaths and fibrous tissue elements (Fig. 31–65).[704, 705, 1140, 1141] Diagnosis requires two or more of the following: (1) six or more café au lait macules, the greatest diameter of which is more than 5 mm in prepubertal and more than 12.5 mm in postpubertal subjects; (2) two or more neurofibromas of any type or one plexiform neurofibroma; (3) freckling in the axilla or inguinal region; (4) optic glioma; (5) two or more iris Lisch nodules (ophthalmic hamartomas); (6) a distinctive osseous lesion, such as sphenoid dysplasia or pseudoarthrosis; and (7) a first-degree relative with neurofibromatosis type 1 according to the preceding criteria (reviewed in references 1135, 1140, 1141, and 1142).

Neurofibromas of the skin in neurofibromatosis may be subcutaneous sessile or deep plexiform masses in children; pedunculated lesions develop in later childhood. Bone abnormalities include cysts and pseudarthrosis, hemihypertrophy, bowing, scoliosis, and skull and facial defects (20%); dumbbell-shaped tumors of spinal nerve roots can cause pain, sensory and motor dysfunction, and bone erosions; gliomas or neurofibromas of any part of the CNS, including the optic nerves and hypothalamus, may calcify. Lisch nodules of the iris are frequent.[1140, 1142] Sarcomas develop in 5 to 15% of patients. Other neoplasms include CNS astrocytomas often involving the visual pathways, ependymomas, meningiomas, neurofibrosarcomas, rhabdomyosarcomas, nonlymphocytic leukemias, and pheochromocytomas.[1143]

Manifestations include seizures, visual defects, and either delayed or true precocious puberty.[1140] Developmental delay occurs but is usually mild;[1144] there is also an increased incidence of psychiatric disease.[1145] Most affected children have some manifestations of the disease by 1 year of age.[704, 705, 1138, 1140, 1141] CNS tumors can be diagnosed with screening MRI scans.

Other CNS abnormalities associated with true precocious puberty include epilepsy,[1081] laughing seizures,[1146] developmental delay, and the post-traumatic state.[1147] Septo-optic dysplasia (described earlier) is associated not only with multiple pituitary hormone deficiencies and delayed puberty but also rarely with true precocious puberty.[1148, 1149] Thus there may be coexisting deficiencies of some pituitary hormones and excessive secretion of others, including prolactin.[1149] Patients with myelomeningocele (myelodysplasia) have an increased prevalence of endocrine abnormalities, including hypothalamic hypothyroidism, hyperprolactinemia, and elevated gonadotropin levels, which may cause true precocious puberty.[730]

TRUE PRECOCIOUS PUBERTY IN CHILDREN ADOPTED FROM DEVELOPING COUNTRIES. An increased prevalence of true precocious puberty occurred in children (who had documented birth dates) from developing countries adopted after 3 years of age into families in Sweden and in children re-fed after kwashiorkor prior to 3 years of age.[1150, 1151] The etiology is not established but may relate to the effects of undernutrition or its rapid repair during a sensitive time in development. In Sweden, the adopted children had pubertal growth spurts similar to those of Swedish children, but the loss of height in childhood and the early puberty appeared to decrease adult height.[1151]

TRUE PRECOCIOUS PUBERTY AFTER VIRILIZING DISORDERS. If a virilizing condition has been long-standing, correction of the virilization may be followed by development of true precocious puberty with activation of the hypothalamic-

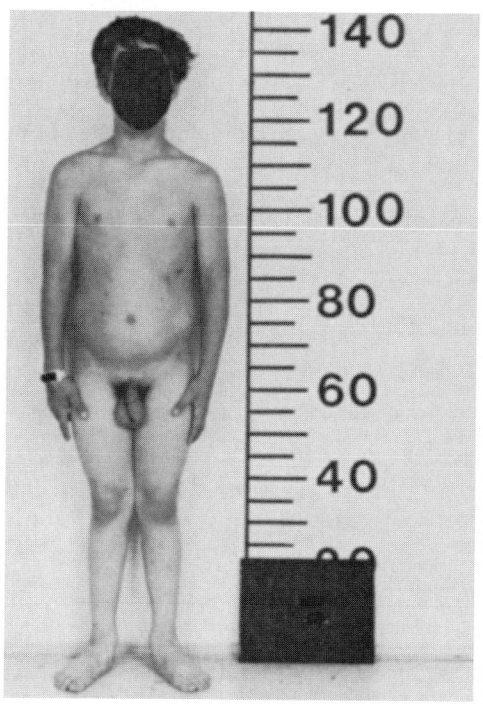
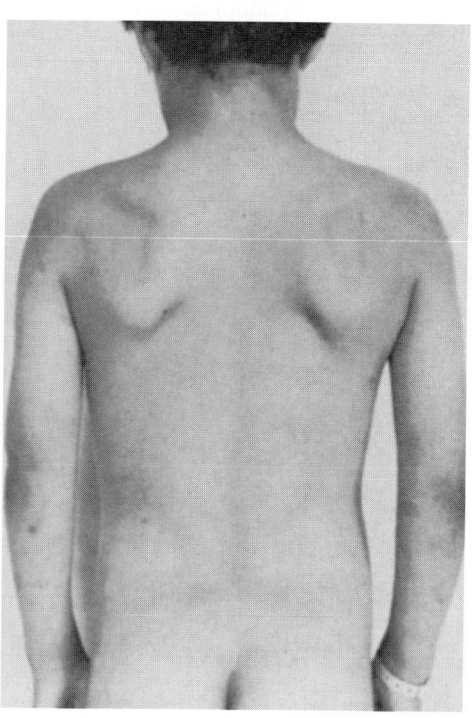

Figure 31–65. A boy of 8 years, 8 months with neurofibromatosis and precocious puberty, secondary to a hypothalamic glioma. He had tonic-clonic seizures at 2 1/2 years and rapid growth starting at 4 years; an enlarged penis and testes and the presence of pubic hair were first noted at 7 1/2 years. At this time, his height was 139.9 cm (+ 1.4 SD); the phallus was 9 × 3 cm; the right testis measured 5.5 × 3.2 cm and the left measured 5.4 × 2.9 cm. He had stage 3 pubic hair and 24 large café au lait spots. CT scans and pneumoencephalography revealed a 1.5 × 2.5 cm hypothalamic mass, which was treated with radiation. The plasma concentration of LH was 0.5 ng/mL (LER-960); FSH 0.4 ng/mL (LER-869); testosterone 221 ng/dL. After 100 µg of intravenous LHRH the peak concentration of LH was 4.9 ng/mL, and that of FSH 1.4 ng/mL, a pubertal response. For conversion to SI units, see the legends of Figures 31–17 and 31–18. (From Styne DM, Grumbach MM. Puberty in the male and female: its physiology and disorders. In: Yen SCC, Jaffe RB, eds. Reproductive Endocrinology. 2nd ed. Philadelphia: W. B. Saunders, 1986: 313–384.[1430])

TABLE 31–33. Objectives of the Management and Treatment of True Precocious Puberty

Detection and treatment of an expanding intracranial lesion
Arrest of premature sexual maturation until the normal age at onset of puberty
Regression of secondary sexual characteristics already present
Attainment of normal mature height; suppression of the rapid rate of skeletal maturation
Prevention of emotional disorders and handicaps and alleviation of parental anxiety; promotion of understanding by counseling, early sex education, and acceleration of social age
Reduction of risk of sexual abuse and early sexual debut
Prevention of pregnancy in girls
Preservation of future fertility
Diminish the increased risk of breast cancer associated with early menarche

From Grumbach MM. True or central precocious puberty. In: Krieger DT, Bardin CW, eds. Current Therapy in Endocrinology and Metabolism, 1985–1986. Toronto: B. C. Decker, 1985: 4–8.[1121]

TABLE 31–34. Action of LHRH Agonists in True Precocious Puberty

A selective, highly specific pharmacologic clamp on the secretion of gonadotropin that produces a "medical gonadectomy"
Chronic administration induces desensitization of the pituitary gonadotrope to the action of endogenous LHRH
As a consequence:
    Inhibition of pulsatile secretion of LH and FSH
    Inhibition of gonadotropin secretion results in a striking decrease in gonadal steroid output by testes or ovaries and reduction in gonadal size

pituitary–gonadotropin-gonadal system. This phenomenon, secondary true precocious puberty, occurs in boys and girls with congenital virilizing adrenal hyperplasia who began to receive glucocorticoid replacement therapy after ages 4 to 8 and who had an advanced bone age.[123, 422, 617, 1152] True precocious puberty may also occur in children who received androgens or estrogens for long periods during early childhood.

MANAGEMENT OF TRUE PRECOCIOUS PUBERTY. The management and treatment of true precocious puberty are summarized in Table 31–33.[1121] Psychosocial issues must be dealt with to provide optimal management of affected children.[1086]

Three principal agents have been used in the treatment of true precocious puberty whether idiopathic or neurologic: medroxyprogesterone acetate, cyproterone acetate, and LHRH agonists. Medroxyprogesterone and cyproterone reverse or arrest the progression of secondary sexual characteristics but have at best a minor effect on final height, especially in girls.[1072, 1074, 1075] In none of the early studies with medroxyprogesterone or cyproterone was the concentration of plasma estradiol in girls and of testosterone in boys systematically monitored and the dosage of these agents adjusted accordingly. More encouraging results from long-term treatment with medroxyprogesterone acetate on final height are reported in a later study.[1154] In addition, both medroxyprogesterone acetate and cyproterone acetate have undesirable effects in high doses.[1121, 1153]

Medroxyprogesterone Acetate and Cyproterone Acetate.
The dose of medroxyprogesterone acetate is 5 to 10 mg twice a day orally or 100 to 200 mg/m² surface area intramuscularly

every 1 or 2 wk. The authors prefer the oral route.[567, 1153] This agent inhibits gonadotropin secretion by its action on the hypothalamic LHRH pulse generator–pituitary gonadotropin unit and suppresses gonadal steroidogenesis directly. Medroxyprogesterone acetate has glucocorticoid-like actions and can suppress corticotropin and cortisol secretion, increase appetite and cause excessive weight gain, and induce hypertension and a cushingoid facies and appearance.[567, 636, 1153]

Cyproterone acetate, which has antiandrogenic, antigonadotropic, and progestational properties, is used outside the United States for the treatment of true precocious puberty.[1074, 1075, 1155] Its advantages and disadvantages are similar to those of medroxyprogesterone acetate.[567] The usual oral dose is 70 to 100 mg/m² surface area daily, given in two doses; the intramuscular dose is 100 to 200 mg/m² every 14 to 28 d. Cyproterone acetate suppresses the secretion of corticotropin and the plasma concentration of cortisol. Fatigue and weakness are common side effects, probably as a consequence of secondary adrenal insufficiency. This agent lacks gluconeogenic activity and does not appear to produce cushingoid features. The long-term effects of either of these agents on fertility are not known.

Medroxyprogesterone and cyproterone acetate have been replaced in the treatment of true precocious puberty by LHRH agonists; at present they are useful as back-up agents for occasional patients who develop untoward effects from LHRH agonist therapy.

LHRH Agonists. The LHRH agonists, synthetic analogues of the natural LHRH decapeptide, are the treatment of choice for true precocious puberty of all types (reviewed in reference 1156; Tables 31–34 and 31–35). Chronic administration of these agents suppresses pulsatile LH and FSH release, gonadal steroid output, and gametogenesis[457, 458, 632, 1157] after an initial, brief stimulation of gonadotropin release. Suppression is due to binding of the agonist to the LHRH receptor on gonadotropes and desensitization of the gonadotrope to LHRH. Initially, down-regulation and loss of receptors occur. When re-

TABLE 31–35. LHRH Agonists: Pharmacologic Treatment of True Precocious Puberty

Structure of Natural LHRH and Substitutions in LHRH Agonist Analogues		Relative Potency	Formula	Dosage Form	Dose	References
<Glu-His-Pro-Ser-Trp-Gly-Leu-Arg-Pro-Gly-NH₂ 1 2 3 4 5 6 7 8 9 10		1	LHRH			
Deslorelin	D-Trp⁶ −NEt	150	[D-Trp⁶Pro⁹NEt]LHRH	Subcutaneous Depot-intramuscular	4–8 µg/kg/d	567, 1110, 1119, 1162–1165, 1168, 1435
Nafarelin	D-Nal(2)⁶	150	[D-Nal(2)⁶Pro⁹NEt]LHRH	Subcutaneous Intranasal	4 µg/kg/d 800–1600 µg/d	567, 1168 567, 1168, 1436
Leuprolide	D-Leu⁶ −NEt	20	[D-Leu⁶-Pro⁹NEt]LHRH	Subcutaneous Depot-intramuscular	20–50 µg/kg/d 140–300 µg/kg/mo	1437 1183, Kaplan and Grumbach 1991*
Buserelin	D-Ser(tBu)⁶ −NEt	20	[D-Ser(tBu)⁶Pro⁹NEt]LHRH	Subcutaneous Intranasal	20–40 µg/kg/d 1200–1800 µg/d	1166, 1438, 1439, 1440 1166, 1167, 1438, 1440, 1441, 1442, 1443
Tryptorelin	D-Trp⁶	35	[D-Trp⁶]LHRH	Subcutaneous Depot-intramuscular	20–40 µg/kg/d 60 µg/kg/mo	1444 1184, 1434
Histerelin	D-His(Bzt)⁶ −NEt	150	[D-His(Bzt)⁶NEt]LHRH	Subcutaneous	8–10 µg/kg/d	Boepple and Crowley 1991*

*Not published.
Modified from Grumbach MM, Kaplan SL. Recent advances in the diagnosis and management of sexual precocity. Acta Paediatr Jpn 1988; 30(Suppl):155–175.[567]

ceptor levels return to normal, desensitization persists owing to uncoupling of the receptors from the intracellular signaling effector pathway.[446, 447, 1158] Administration of a potent LHRH agonist subcutaneously once a day desensitizes the gonadotropes to LHRH within a few days. In children with true precocious puberty this regimen blocks the action of endogenous LHRH and acts as a selective, highly specific pharmacologic clamp on the secretion of gonadotropins without interfering directly with the release of the other pituitary hormones. In essence, the regimen induces a reversible medical gonadectomy (see Table 31–34). The superactive agonist analogues of LHRH are about 15 to 200 times as potent as the natural LHRH decapeptide, have prolonged action, and are of low toxicity (see Table 31–35).

These agonist are more resistant to enzymatic degradation, have increased binding affinity for the receptor on the pituitary gonadotrope, have increased hydrophobicity, and, with some analogues, have increased binding to plasma proteins.[446, 447, 567, 1159–1161]

The suppressive effects of the agonists on gonadotropin secretion are the basis for their usefulness in the treatment of true precocious puberty.[567, 1156, 1162–1168] Various agonists are available (see Table 31–35). A comparison of intranasal buserelin to every-month intramuscular triptorelin demonstrated the superiority of the latter in regard to final height, although intranasal preparations can also improve final height in affected children.[1156, 1169–1173] The depot formulation of leuprorelin (leuprolide acetate), the only once-a-month depot preparation approved by the U.S. Food and Drug Administration as of 1997, is effective and safe.[1156, 1174–1176] The bioavailability of intranasal agonists is reduced,[567, 1177] as reflected in the need to use a high dose at frequent intervals. The effectiveness of LHRH agonists in the treatment of true precocious puberty is a function of the potency of the analogue, dose, route of administration, and compliance.[567, 1156, 1168]

In both the idiopathic and the organic forms of true precocious puberty, treatment with a potent LHRH agonist initially enhances FSH and LH release and causes a rise in circulating gonadal steroid levels; chronic therapy suppresses the pulsatile secretion of LH and FSH and blocks the pubertal LH response to the administration of native LHRH (Figs. 31–66 and 31–67). The isoforms of gonadotropins with a more basic charge increase, suggesting that the LHRH agonist also has effects on metabolism of gonadotropins in the pituitary.[297] Within 2 to 4 wk in girls and 6 wk in boys, gonadal steroid secretion is reduced to prepubertal levels and maintained in the prepubertal state by chronic treatment (Fig. 31–68; see Figs. 31–66 and 31–67). A plasma estradiol concentration of less than 18 pmol/L (5 pg/mL) in girls and a plasma testosterone level of less than 0.7 nmol/L (20 ng/dL) in boys indicate adequate gonadal suppression. LHRH agonist therapy does not affect the secretion of adrenal androgens.[567, 1119, 1164] Careful monitoring of serum gonadotropins and gonadal steroids is necessary for the evaluation of the effectiveness of LHRH agonist treatment.

Changes in secondary sexual characteristics occur within the first 6 mo of therapy (see Fig. 31–68). In girls, these effects include reduction in breast size and decrease in pubic hair, cessation of menses if present before treatment, and decreased size of the uterus and ovaries as assessed by pelvic ultrasonography. Occasional girls have recurrent episodes of hot flushes and moodiness. In boys, pubic hair thins, the testes decrease in size, acne and seborrhea regress, penile erections and masturbation become much less frequent, the high energy level and aggressive behavior diminish, and self-esteem improves.

Height velocity decreases about 60% during the first year of therapy. Skeletal maturation slows dramatically during the first 3 y, to a rate often less than the progression in chronologic age. From the second year on, height velocity for bone

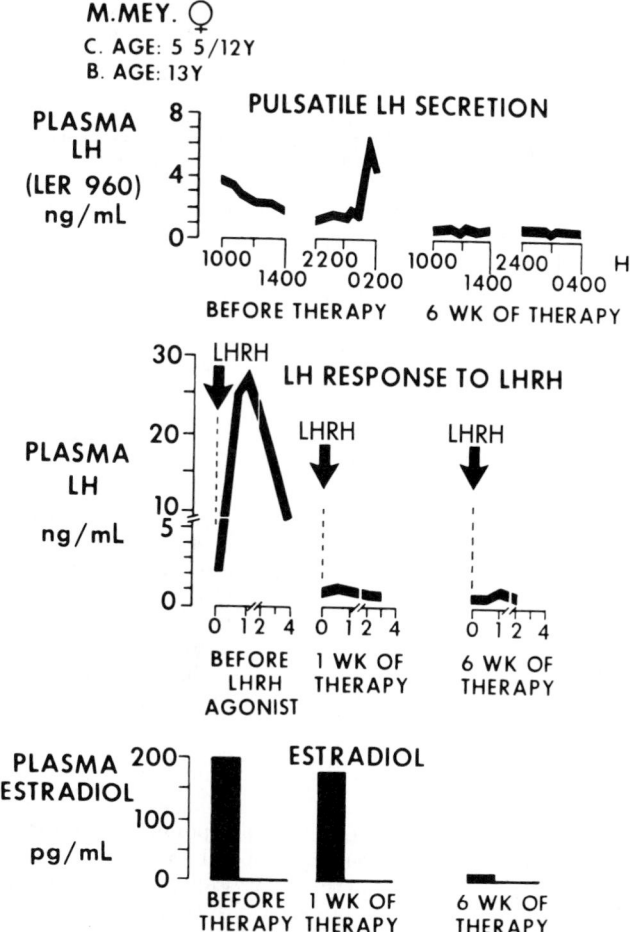

Figure 31–66. Effect of administration of the LHRH agonist deslorelin (4 μg/kg/d subcutaneously) on pulsatile secretion of LH (top), LH response to LHRH (middle), and plasma concentration of estradiol (bottom) in a 5 1/12-year-old girl with idiopathic true precocious puberty. This patient, who had a bone age of 13 years when treatment was begun, has been administered deslorelin for 7 y. During this period, the estimated predicted final height increased by 15 cm. Surprisingly, the bone age advanced by only about 6 mo on serial examinations for several years. For conversion to SI units, see the legend of Figure 31–17. (Modified from Grumbach MM, Kaplan SL. Recent advances in the diagnosis and management of sexual precocity. Acta Paediatr Jpn 1988; 30[Suppl]:155–175.[567])

age is usually appropriate (Fig. 31–69). The available growth data for compliant patients suggest that adult height is improved in young children with true precocious puberty, especially when treatment is begun soon after the onset of precocity and when the bone age is advanced only a few years.[1068, 1156] Effective therapy improves final height predictions or maintains the normal target height in young children.[1068, 1156, 1178–1180] In 26 children (Table 31–36)[1068] there was a striking benefit if children were treated before 5 years of age (girls' adult height 164.3±7.7 cm) compared to those treated after age 5 years (157.6±6.6 cm) or to untreated patients (152.7±8.6 cm).[1068]

Children with true precocious puberty have higher mean circulating IGF-I levels for chronologic age, comparable to levels in normal puberty. The IGF-I concentration correlates best with the stage of puberty and with the plasma level of testosterone or estradiol.[116] The fact that treatment with LHRH agonists reduces the level of IGF-I to the normal range for bone age but not for chronologic age[116] indicates that gonadal steroids increase plasma IGF-I levels in true precocious puberty and in normal puberty. Secretion of GH is increased in true precocious puberty to levels comparable to those in normal puberty.[100, 101] Treatment with LHRH agonists usually results in a decrease in GH secretion, most strikingly

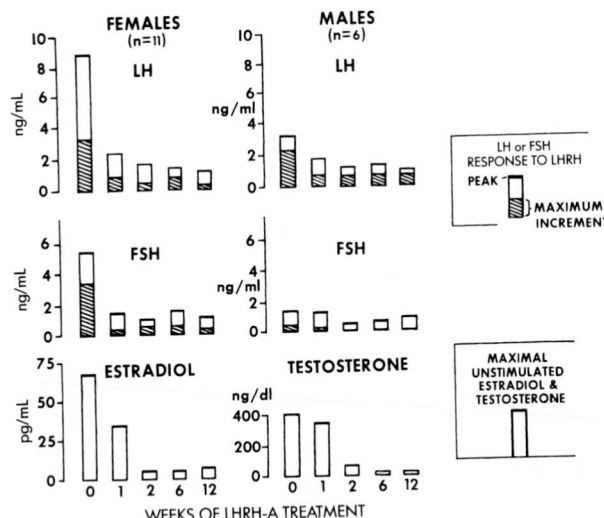

Figure 31–67. Deslorelin treatment (4 μg/kg/d subcutaneously) of girls and boys with true precocious puberty: effect during the first 12 wk of treatment on the LH and FSH response to a challenge with LHRH (mean peak response and maximum increment) and on the maximal unstimulated concentration of plasma estradiol in the girls and of plasma testosterone in the boys. Note the relatively rapid change from pubertal values to prepubertal values. For conversion to SI units, see the legends of Figures 31–17 and 31–18. (From Styne DM, Harris DA, Egli CA, et al. Treatment of true precocious puberty with a potent luteinizing-hormone releasing factor agonist: effect on growth, sexual maturation, pelvic sonography, and the hypothalamic-pituitary gonadal axis, J Clin Endocrinol Metab, 61, 142–181, 1985, © by The Endocrine Society.[1119])

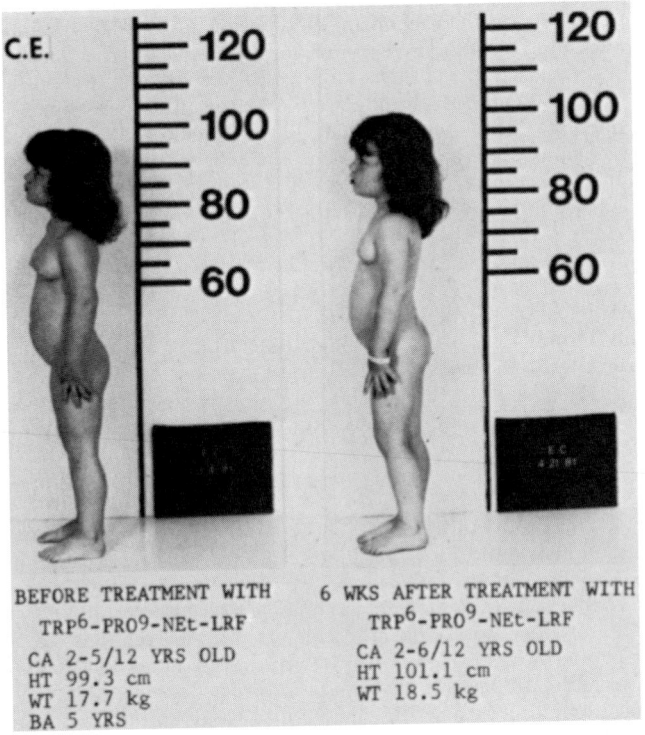

Figure 31–68. A 2 5/12-year-old girl with true precocious puberty after 6 wk of deslorelin therapy (4 μg/d subcutaneously). Note the regression in the size of the breasts; however, the rapid rate of growth had not decreased. At the end of 1 y of therapy, growth rate was suppressed to 4 cm/y, and bone age advanced only 1 y. CA, chronologic age; HT, height; WT, weight; BA, bone age. (From Styne DM, Grumbach MM. Puberty in the male and female: its physiology and disorders. In: Yen SCC, Jaffe RB. Reproductive Endocrinology. 2nd ed. Philadelphia: W. B. Saunders, 1986: 313–384.[1430])

during sleep, and in a decrease in GH response to provocative stimuli. The serum concentrations of GH and GHBP activity may be a better reflection of the suppression of growth velocity with LHRH agonist than serum IGF-I and IGFBP-3 levels.[1181, 1182] The reason for the fall in GH secretion is unclear but may involve both a decrease in plasma gonadal steroid levels and an increase in BMI.

The serum levels of the propeptide of type III procollagen (P-III-NP) in normal puberty and in true precocious puberty parallel the normal pubertal growth curve and the changes in growth rate in children treated with LHRH agonists.

Chronic administration of LHRH agonists induces a pharmacologic gonadectomy with reversion to a prepubertal level of gonadal steroid output. The use of depot formulations of LHRH agonists with a single intramuscular injection every 4

wk minimizes the problem of compliance.[805, 967, 1068, 1183, 1184] Regular assessment, initially at intervals of 1 to 3 mo, requires periodic measurements of plasma testosterone levels in boys and estradiol levels in girls; basal levels of LH and FSH with third-generation assays or the LH and FSH response to exogenous LHRH; measurement of growth, bone age, and secondary sexual characteristics; and in girls serial evaluations of ovarian morphology and uterine size by pelvic ultrasonography. Urinary gonadotropin determinations are not sufficiently sensitive to be used for monitoring purposes. The size of

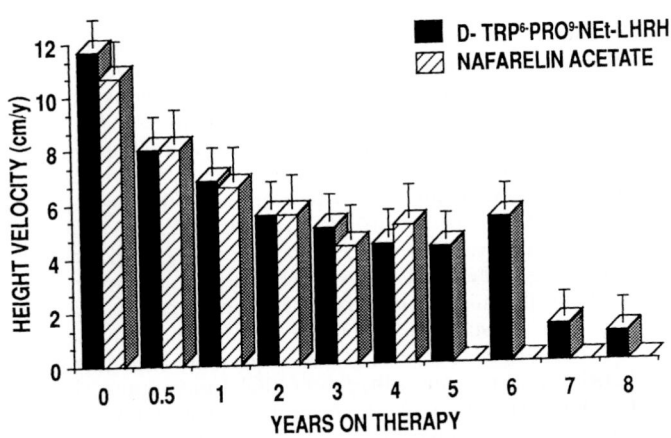

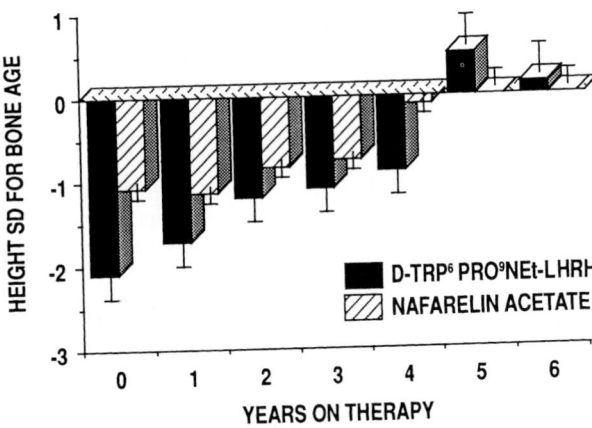

Figure 31–69. Effect of LHRH agonist therapy in true precocious puberty on growth. *Left,* Changes in mean height velocity (cm/y ± 1 SE) after the initiation of LHRH agonist therapy with D-Trp⁶Pro⁹Net[LHRH] (deslorelin) *(filled bars)* or with nafarelin *(hatched bars).* A sharp decrease in height velocity occurred within 1 y. *Right,* Mean (±1 SE) height for bone age before and during LHRH agonist treatment. The discrepancy between height and the more advanced bone age decreases (reverts to normal) with chronic LHRH agonist treatment. (From Kaplan SL, Grumbach MM. True precocious puberty: treatment with GnRH-agonists. In: Delemarre-Van de Waal H, Plant TM, van Rees GP, et al., eds. Control of the Onset of Puberty III. Amsterdam: Elsevier, 1989: 357–373.[1168])

TABLE 31–36. Comparison of Current Height (Final or Near Final) and Height Gain of LHRH Agonist-Treated Patients

| | No. of Patients | Mean Current Ht (cm) | | Mean Ht Gain (cm)[a] |
		Female	Male	
Untreated[b]				
Total	116	152.7 ± 8.6	155.6 ± 7.7	
<5 yr	41	150.2 ± 7.6	153.3 ± 7.1	
>5 yr	75	153.4 ± 8.4	161.3 ± 6.0	
LHRH-treated[d]				
UCSF	26	160.5 ± 6.6	166.3 ± 12.2	
<5 yr[c]	11	164.3 ± 7.7	172.1	10.0 (female); 11.1 (male)
>5 yr[c]	15	157.6 ± 6.6	163.3 ± 13.0	4.0 (female); 6.0 (male)
Ref.				
Oerter[1435]	40	157.8 ± 5.9	168.8 ± 8.3	5.2 (female), 6.7 (male)
Kauli[1436]	8	151.2 ± 5.9		5.8 (female)
Boepple[1437]	26	154.4		4.1 (female)

[a]Final predicted height − initial predicted height (Bayley-Pinneau method).
[b]Final height.
[c]CA at start of therapy.
[d]Final or nearly final height.
From Paul D, Conte FA, Grumbach MM, Kaplan SL. Long-term effect of gonadotropin-releasing hormone agonist therapy on final and near-final height in 26 children with true precocious puberty treated at a median age of less than 5 years. J Clin Endocrinol Metab 1995; 80:546–551, with permission.[1068]

ovaries and uterus on pelvic ultrasonography decreases with successful treatment with LHRH agonists.[1119, 1185]

A large number of patients have been taken off treatment after years of therapy. In 46 girls who were treated for at least 2 y and were taken off therapy at a mean age of 11 years, menarche occurred at a mean age of 12.1 years, an average of 1.2 years after discontinuing therapy. Ovulation occurred in 50% of girls 1 y after menarche and in 90% within 2 y or more after menarche.[1186] This pattern is similar to normal pubertal maturation. Development of the hypothalamic-pituitary axis is not delayed in girls with true precocious puberty treated with LHRH agonist therapy.[1187]

Treatment of true precocious puberty is not indicated if the pattern of pulsatile LH secretion is not pubertal during sleep or if the LH response to exogenous LHRH is not pubertal (Table 31–37). Before beginning treatment it is essential to establish the progressive nature of the sexual precocity.[1188, 1189] Girls who do not have a reduced height potential do not require LHRH agonist therapy to ensure an appropriate final height outcome; these girls tend to have lower serum IGF-I and estradiol levels and may have lesser signs of estrogenization.[1190, 1191] The most severely affected girls respond best to LHRH agonist therapy.[1188, 1192] In a subset of girls with precocious puberty the tempo is relatively slow, and sexual precocity may not be sustained.[636, 1168] The growth rate slows to normal for age, skeletal maturation progresses in

accordance with chronologic age, and there is little or no risk of impairment of final height. In some girls over a 1- to 2-mo period the pattern of LH pulsatility during sleep, the LH response to LHRH, and the levels of plasma estradiol return to a pubertal state; unlike the typical patient, such girls do not exhibit the initial hyperresponse of plasma estradiol and LH to the LHRH agonist. Many girls in this subset have clinical and hormonal features between those of premature thelarche and true precocious puberty and are typical of neither condition,[1193] so-called exaggerated thelarche. In contrast, some girls with typical premature thelarche progress to true precocious puberty with no signs at the time of first presentation to separate them from girls with isolated premature thelarche.[1194]

Psychosocial factors and parental anxiety that adversely affect the well-being of the child need to be assessed in the decision to initiate LHRH agonist treatment.

Adverse Effects. Untoward reactions to LHRH agonists include local and systemic allergic reactions in a few patients, including asthmatic episodes when the agent is given intranasally. Sterile abscesses can occur at the sites of intramuscular injection of leuprorelin and triptorelin (5 to 10%), believed to be due to the polylactic and polyglycotic polymer, and not to the LHRH agonist itself.[1175, 1195] When treatment is discontinued, even after 8 y, the gonadal suppression is reversed within a few weeks to months with a rise in plasma gonadal steroid levels, progression of sexual maturation, and return of menses.[1196] Serum prolactin levels may be increased in girls following treatment with LHRH agonist unassociated with galactorrhea.[1197] Bone density is increased in central precocious puberty, but the use of LHRH agonists reverses this trend.[175–179] Despite these encouraging results, one must be alert to the possible emergence of unforeseen long-term side effects.

Psychosocial Aspects. Psychological management is a critical aspect of the therapy for true precocious puberty.[567, 1023, 1121, 1198] With the advanced physical maturation for chronologic age, such children tend to seek friends close to their size, strength, and physical development but tend to lack the social skills of older children. Sex education of the child and the family is essential and must be given in a skillful, sensitive, and explicit manner; the risks of sexual abuse in both sexes and of pregnancy in girls need to be discussed. The parents need to be informed about the management of menses. The onset of sexual activity may be earlier than average but is usually within the normal range.[1084] It is imperative to provide

TABLE 31–37. Indications for Therapy with LHRH Agonists in True or Central Precocious Puberty

In children with clinical and unequivocal endocrine features of idiopathic true precocious puberty:
  Rapid advancement over a period of 6 mo to 1 y of secondary sex characteristics, height, height velocity, and bone age (increased >2.5 SD for chronologic age) in affected boys and girls
  A plasma testosterone concentration sustained >2.5 nmol/L (>75 ng/dL) in boys younger than 8 y of age determined by sensitive, specific immunoassay
  A plasma estradiol, recurrently ≥36 pmol/L (≥10 pg/ml) determined by a sensitive, specific assay capable of quantifying low concentrations of estradiol
  Onset of menarche (and recurrent menses) in girls younger than 9 y of age
  Psychosocial factors and parental anxiety, including evidence that the child's psychosocial well-being is adversely affected
In children with neurogenic or organic true precocious puberty, especially those with associated GH deficiency, the course is almost invariably progressive and LHRH treatment should not be delayed

support in handling the increased height, the advanced sexual maturation, and the effects of gonadal steroids on behavior, activity, and emotional stability. The unrealistic demands and expectations that arise from the discrepancy between the physique and the chronologic, mental, and psychosexual age require wise counseling, including the reaction to ridicule by peers and the concern about being different from age mates. Some of these problems have been mitigated by school acceleration, advancing the child one or two grades, if consistent with the mental and emotional development. These problems are similar in children with all forms of sexual precocity. The effectiveness of LHRH agonists has reduced but not eliminated many of the management problems in true precocious puberty.[1121]

LHRH agonists are effective in both boys and girls with idiopathic true precocious puberty, the androgen-induced form of secondary true precocious puberty following therapy for virilizing congenital adrenal hyperplasia with glucocorticoids, and the true precocious puberty associated with hamartomas of the tuber cinereum, hypothalamic neoplasms, and other CNS lesions.[1119, 1164, 1199] Although hamartomas of the tuber cinereum have been treated surgically,[580, 1107, 1117, 1200–1203] the ease of medical treatment of this form of sexual precocity, the fact that the mass does not enlarge with time on MRI or CT brain scans, and the risks of adverse outcome in surgical intervention in this disorder[580] support the choice of LHRH agonists over surgical intervention.

LHRH agonists are useful in conjunction with GH in the management of patients with true precocious puberty associated with GH deficiency (usually as a result of radiation of the brain).[1102] Such a regimen allows a longer period of GH treatment before epiphyseal fusion.[1043] A few, mostly short-term studies utilized GH and/or LHRH agonist in short normal children to increase final height; two studies suggest that an increase may occur, but this regimen is experimental.[678, 1204]

Incomplete Form of Isosexual Precocity: LHRH-Independent Sexual Precocity (Precocious Pseudopuberty)

In this disorder the secretion of testosterone in boys and of estrogen in girls is independent of the hypothalamic LHRH pulse generator (see Table 31–38). Affected individuals do not have a pubertal-type LH response to the administration of LHRH or a pubertal pattern of pulsatile LH secretion, nor do they respond to chronic administration of an LHRH agonist with suppression of gonadal steroid output. Incomplete isosexual precocity or precocious pseudopuberty is a consequence of the secretion of gonadal or adrenal steroids independent of LHRH, of iatrogenic exposure to gonadal steroids, or, in boys, of rare hCG- or LH-secreting tumors.

BOYS

Chorionic Gonadotropin–Secreting Tumors. Several types of germ cell tumors can secrete a glycoprotein hormone that has the bioactivity of LH or hCG and can cross-react with LH in some radioimmunoassay systems. Studies with specific antisera to the β subunit of hCG, however, established that the gonadotropin is hCG. Boys with these hCG-secreting neoplasms may have slightly enlarged testes and may be difficult to differentiate from boys with true precocious puberty on the basis of physical examination.[636, 1205, 1206] Plasma hCG levels are elevated without an increase in the concentration of FSH or LH.[1205] In addition to germ cell tumors, hepatomas and hepatoblastomas can also secrete hCG (Fig. 31–70); in one case α-fetoprotein was found in the embryonal-type tumor cells spread throughout the hepatoblastoma.[1207] The average survival is only 10.7 mo after diagnosis; the mean age at onset is 2 years, 8 months.[1206, 1208, 1209]

Some teratomas, chorioepitheliomas, or mixed germ cell tumors in the hypothalamus, mediastinum, lungs, gonads, or retroperitoneum and certain hypothalamic pineal tumors

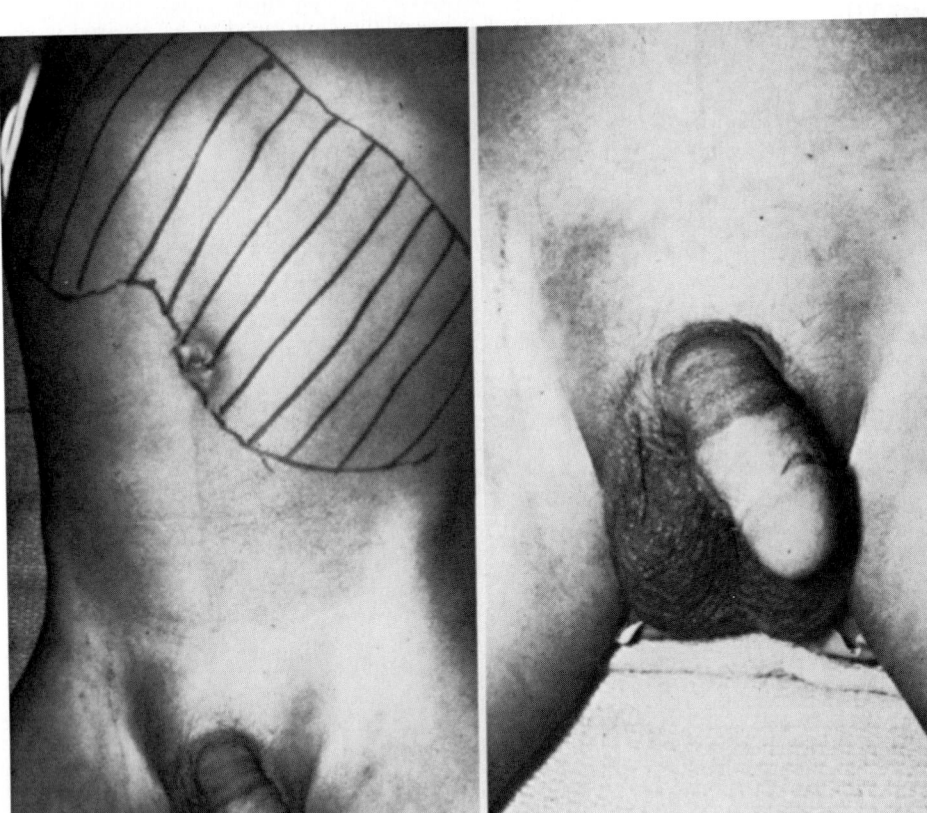

Figure 31–70. A 1 5/12-year-old boy with an hCG-secreting hepatoblastoma. Note the outline of the large liver (*left*) and the penile enlargement (*right*). The testes were 2 × 1 cm, and pubic hair was stage 2. The plasma hCG level was 50 mIU/mL; plasma testosterone 168 ng/dL; and plasma α-fetoprotein 160,000 ng/mL. Metastatic lesions in both lungs were seen on the roentgenogram of the chest. To convert testosterone values to SI units, see the legend of Figure 31–17. To convert hCG values to international units per liter, multiply by 1.0. To convert α-fetoprotein values to micrograms per liter, multiply by 1.0. (From Kaplan SL, Grumbach MM. Pathogenesis of sexual precocity. In: Grumbach MM, Sizonenko PC, Aubert ML, eds. Control of the Onset of Puberty. Baltimore: Williams & Wilkins, 1990: 620–660. © 1990, the Williams & Wilkins Co., Baltimore.[636])

(usually a germ cell tumor or mixed germ cell tumor)[1205, 1210, 1211]—less commonly a chorioepithelioma or its variants—cause sexual precocity in boys by secreting hCG rather than by activating the hypothalamic LHRH pulse generator.[1205] The prevalence of hCG-secreting embryonal neoplasms, especially of the mediastinum, is increased in boys with Klinefelter's syndrome. About 20% of mediastinal germ cell tumors occur in boys with Klinefelter's syndrome, a prevalence 30 to 50 times more common than in 46,XY boys.[903, 905, 1212, 1213] Plasma α-fetoprotein is a useful marker for yolk sac (endodermal sinus) or mixed germ cell tumors.[1214]

Such tumors are rare in girls and, if they occur, rarely cause isosexual precocity. In prepubertal girls, hCG has few effects. However, hCG-secreting tumors of the CNS can rarely cause true precocious puberty by disinhibition of the hypothalamic LHRH pulse generator by a local effect; rarely, germ cell tumors contain sufficient aromatase activity to convert circulating C_{19}-steroids of adrenal origin to estradiol, which in some instances is sufficient to induce breast development.

Germinomas limited to the CNS secrete insufficient hCG to be readily detectable in the circulation, but in some patients hCG can be detected in the cerebrospinal fluid.[697] In mixed germ cell tumors, on the other hand, hCG is commonly present in blood and cerebrospinal fluid.

In children germ cell tumors in the suprasellar-hypothalamic region do not exhibit a sex predominance and are frequently associated with pituitary hormone deficiencies including diabetes insipidus.[697] Germ cell tumors that secrete hCG occasionally arise in the thalamus and basal ganglia. Germ cell tumors of the hypothalamus or pineal region constitute fewer than 1% of primary CNS tumors in Western countries but account for 4.5% of such tumors in Japan. Mixed germ cell tumors and especially "pure" germinomas may respond to chemotherapy and/or radiotherapy, and regression of sexual precocity may occur if the bone age is less than 11 years, to be followed later by normal puberty.[1205] The pineal is calcified in 8 to 11% of 8- to 11-year-old children, and by itself calcification is not indicative of a tumor.

An LH- and prolactin-secreting pituitary adenoma in a boy caused sexual precocity.[1215] The concentration of serum LH was elevated (900 IU/L) and did not increase further after the administration of LHRH. The elevated levels of serum testosterone 7 nmol/L (200 ng/dL), prolactin (215 μg/L), and LH fell to prepubertal values after removal of a "chromophobe" adenoma.

Precocious Androgen Secretion Caused by Congenital Adrenal Hyperplasia, Virilizing Adrenal Tumor, or Leydig Cell Tumor.
Virilizing congenital adrenal hyperplasia caused by a defect in steroid 21-hydroxylase (CYP21, cytochrome P450-c21) leads to elevated androgen concentrations and masculinization and is a common cause of LHRH-independent sexual precocity in boys[885] (see Chapter 29). Approximately 75% of patients with CYP21 deficiency have salt loss resulting from impaired aldosterone secretion, and low serum sodium and high serum potassium levels. Increased plasma concentrations of 17-hydroxyprogesterone, increased urinary excretion of 17-ketosteroids and pregnanetriol, and advanced bone age and rapid growth are characteristic. Treatment with glucocorticoids and mineralocorticoids (when appropriate) suppresses the abnormal androgen secretion and arrests virilization and corrects electrolyte imbalance. A rarer form of virilizing adrenal hyperplasia is usually accompanied by hypertension and is caused by steroid 11β-hydroxylase deficiency (CYP11); the progressive virilization ceases and the blood pressure falls to normal with glucocorticoid therapy. All forms of congenital adrenal hyperplasia are inherited as autosomal recessive traits.[885] Virilizing congenital adrenal hyperplasia, if untreated, can cause anovulatory amenorrhea in females and oligospermia in males; with treatment, the infertility is usually corrected

(see Chapter 29). Treatment of virilizing congenital adrenal hyperplasia (CAH) may unmask LHRH-dependent sexual precocity (secondary true precocious puberty) as a consequence of the advanced somatic and hypothalamic maturation caused by exposure to androgen before initiation of glucocorticoid therapy.

Virilizing adrenal carcinomas and adenomas secrete large amounts of DHEA, DHEAS, and on occasion testosterone. Glucocorticoids do not suppress the increased secretion of adrenal androgens or the urinary excretion of 17-ketosteroids in adrenal carcinoma, but they readily decrease plasma 17-hydroxyprogesterone or 11-deoxycortisol levels and 17-ketosteroid excretion in congenital adrenal hyperplasia. Adrenal carcinoma can cause isosexual precocity and growth failure in boys. Rare adrenal adenomas produce both testosterone and aldosterone, leading to sexual precocity and hypertension with hypokalemia.[1216]

Adrenal rests, or heterotopic adrenal tissue in the testes, may enlarge with endogenous corticotropin stimulation in boys with untreated or inadequately treated congenital adrenal hyperplasia and may mimic bilateral or unilateral interstitial cell tumors, occasionally leading to massive enlargement of the testes (see Chapter 29).

Leydig cell tumors in boys occasionally cause sexual precocity; this neoplasm causes unilateral enlargement (often nodular) of the testis, in contrast to the normal size of both testes for chronologic age in most boys with congenital adrenal hyperplasia or a virilizing adrenal tumor.[422]

Women with a previous history of congenital adrenal hyperplasia or a virilizing tumor may develop ovarian hyperandrogenism with persistent elevation of LH despite successful treatment of childhood virilization; such an outcome does not occur in women with late-onset congenital adrenal hyperplasia.[1217]

Familial and Sporadic Testotoxicosis (Familial Male-Limited Gonadotropin-Independent Sexual Precocity with Premature Leydig Cell and Germ Cell Maturation).
Pituitary gonadotropin-independent familial premature Leydig cell and germ cell maturation, or testotoxicosis,[1215, 1218–1223] has been recognized as an LHRH-independent form of male isosexual precocity since 1981, although the phenotype was described earlier.[1224] Affected boys have penile enlargement, which may be present at birth,[1219] and bilateral enlargement of the testes to the early or midpubertal range (Fig. 31–71). The testes exhibit premature Leydig and Sertoli cell maturation and spermatogenesis; Leydig cell hyperplasia may be present.[1218, 1219, 1221] Linear growth and skeletal maturation are accelerated, and muscular development is prominent. Basal and LHRH-stimulated gonadotropin concentrations are prepubertal and there is no evidence of LH pulsatility, whether measured by immunologic or bioassay techniques[1219] (Table 31–38). Plasma testosterone values are in the normal pubertal or adult range. The onset of adrenarche and its biochemical marker, serum DHEAS, correlate with bone age rather than chronologic age. Treatment with LHRH agonists does not suppress the testicu-

---

TABLE 31–38. Testotoxicosis: Clinical and Laboratory Characteristics

Sex-limited autosomal dominant inheritance; activating mutation in the gene encoding the LH receptor
Early-onset of sexual precocity in boys with bilateral testicular enlargement
Prepubertal immunologic and biologic LH response to LHRH, prepubertal LH pulse secretory pattern
Concentration of plasma testosterone in pubertal range
Premature Leydig cell and seminiferous tubule maturation
No CNS, adrenal, or testicular abnormalities demonstrable by radiologic or hormonal studies
Lack of suppression of plasma testosterone or physical signs of puberty by LHRH agonist

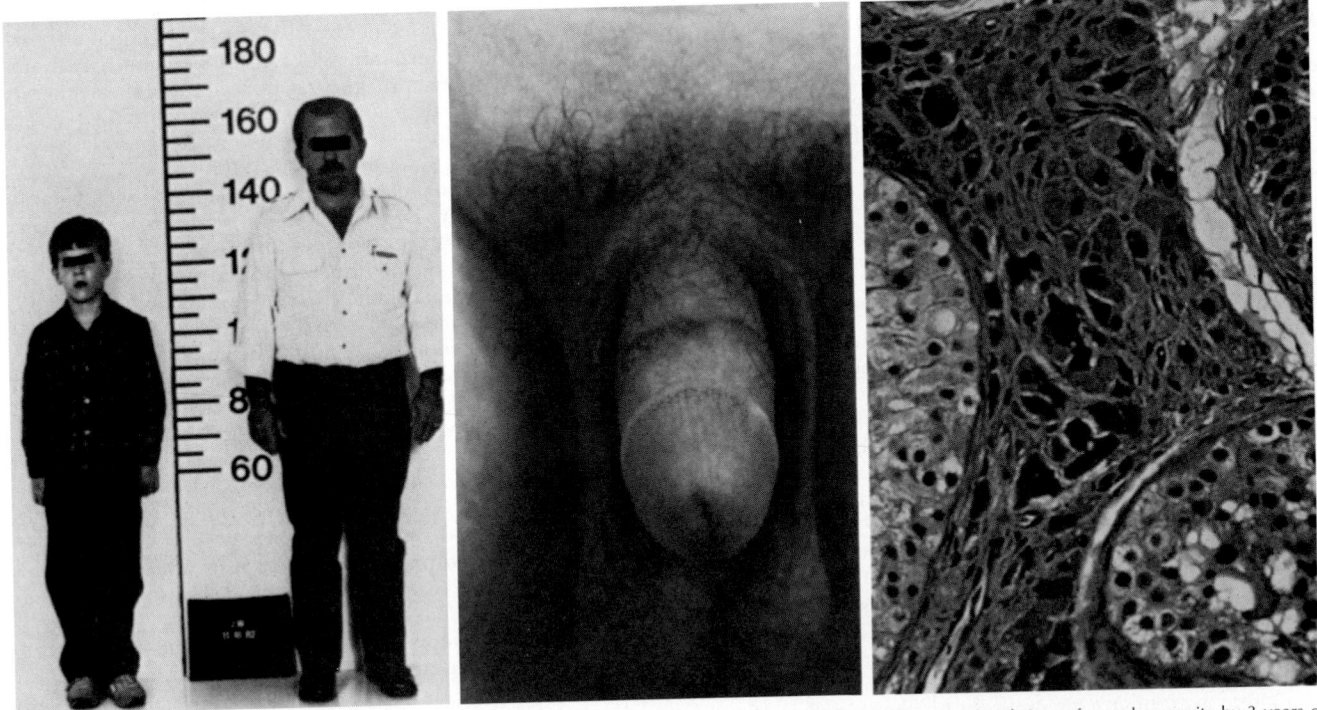

Figure 31–71. Familial testotoxicosis *Left,* A 5 1/2-year-old boy and his 28-year-old father with the disorder. The boy exhibited signs of sexual precocity by 3 years of age. Height was 130.6 cm (+4.8 SD); bone age 12 1/2 years. The plasma testosterone level was 267 ng/dL; dihydrotestosterone 46 ng/dL; DHEAS 23 µg/dL. The plasma LH and FSH levels were low, and neither rose after treatment. Pulsatile LH secretion was not demonstrable. Treatment with deslorelin, an LHRH agonist, was without effect. The father had begun sexual maturation by 3 years of age and had reached a final height of 162.6 cm in his early teens. The plasma testosterone level was 294 ng/dL; LH 0.5 ng/mL (LER-960); and FSH 0.5 ng/mL (LER-869). The father had an adult-type LH and FSH response to LHRH; the LH level increased to 7.5 ng/mL, and the FSH level to 2 ng/mL. At least 28 male family members over nine generations are affected. To convert dihydrotestosterone values to nanomoles per liter, multiply by 0.03467. For other conversions to SI units, see the legends of Figures 31–17 and 31–18. *Center,* External genitalia of the 5 1/2-year-old boy. The penis measured 12 × 2.8 cm; the right testis was 4 × 2 cm, and the left testis 3.5 × 2.5 cm. *Right,* Testis of the boy showed Leydig cell maturation without Reinke crystalloids and spermatogenesis Mallory trichome.

lar function or maturation.[1219, 1223] When untreated affected individuals reach late childhood or early adolescence, fertility is achieved, and the pattern of LH secretion and response to LHRH is adult in character;[1220] secondary LHRH-dependent true precocious puberty is superimposed on the substrate of testotoxicosis.[1220, 1221, 1225] In some adults, spermatogenic function is impaired, and levels of plasma FSH are elevated.[1220] This disorder occasionally occurs sporadically but is commonly inherited as a male-limited autosomal dominant trait.[1220] Nine generations of males were affected in one kindred;[1220] female carriers of the trait are unaffected.[1220, 1225]

In 1993 Shenker and colleagues[1226] and Kremer and co-workers[1227] described the nature of the disorder, namely heterozygous activating mutations of the heterotrimeric Gs protein-coupled LH/hCG receptor which, in concert, transduce the LH/hCG signal to the main effector, adenylate cyclase (Fig. 31–72). The LH receptor[1228–1231] is a glycoprotein of 80 to 90kd encoded by a gene localized to chromosome 2p21. A single exon, the large exon 11, encodes the entire G protein–linked seven transmembrane domain, almost two thirds of the receptor[1232–1234] (Fig. 31–72A). More than 11 constitutively activating heterozygous missense mutations have been described in exon 11 (see Fig. 31–72B); six involve the transmembrane helix VI, two the flanking third cytoplasmic loop, and one each in helix V and helix II.[1226, 1227, 1235, 1236, 1241] Thus nine mutations are between amino acid residues 542 and 581. A model of the transmembrane domain of the receptor provides novel suggestions on the structural and functional effects of these activating mutations.[1236a] Inactivating mutations of the LH/hCG receptor and their clinical consequences are discussed in Chapter 29.

Boys with LHRH and pituitary gonadotropin-independent maturation of the testes do not respond to chronic administra-

tion of LHRH agonists with suppression of testosterone secretion, in contrast to the characteristic response in patients with true precocious puberty.[1219] However, testosterone secretion, height velocity and rate of bone maturation, and aggressive and hyperactive behavior have been decreased by treatment with oral medroxyprogesterone acetate.[567, 1219]

Two other therapies have been used (Table 31–39). Ketoconazole, an orally active substituted imidazole derivative, suppresses gonadal and adrenal biosynthesis at several steps.[1237] In the dosage used in testotoxicosis (200 mg every 8 to 12 h orally)[1222, 1238] ketoconazole inhibits mainly the enzyme CYP17, which is responsible for the 17α-hydroxylation and scission of 17α-hydroxypregnenolone to dehydroepiandrosterone (see adrenarche and Chapter 29). However, the agent produces a mild transient decrease in cortisol secretion and interferes with binding of testosterone to TeBG. Secondary true precocious puberty often occurs when the bone age advances to or has already reached the pubertal range (usually >11.5 years), at which time addition of an LHRH agonist is appropriate.[1222] Ketoconazole can cause hepatic injury, which is usually mild and reversible but may be severe.[1237] Some side effects may be dose related.[1239]

Another approach is the use of the antiandrogen (and antimineralocorticoid) spironolactone combined with testolactone, an inhibitor of cytochrome P450 aromatase (CYP19), the key enzyme in the conversion of androgens to estrogens.[1240] Because these boys often develop secondary central precocious puberty after control with spironolactone and testolactone, the addition of an LHRH agonist may be required to suppress pituitary gonadotropin secretion.[1240] More potent antiandrogens such as flutamide and nilutamide[1242] and aromatase inhibitors such as letrozole[1243, 1243a] have greater therapeutic potential.

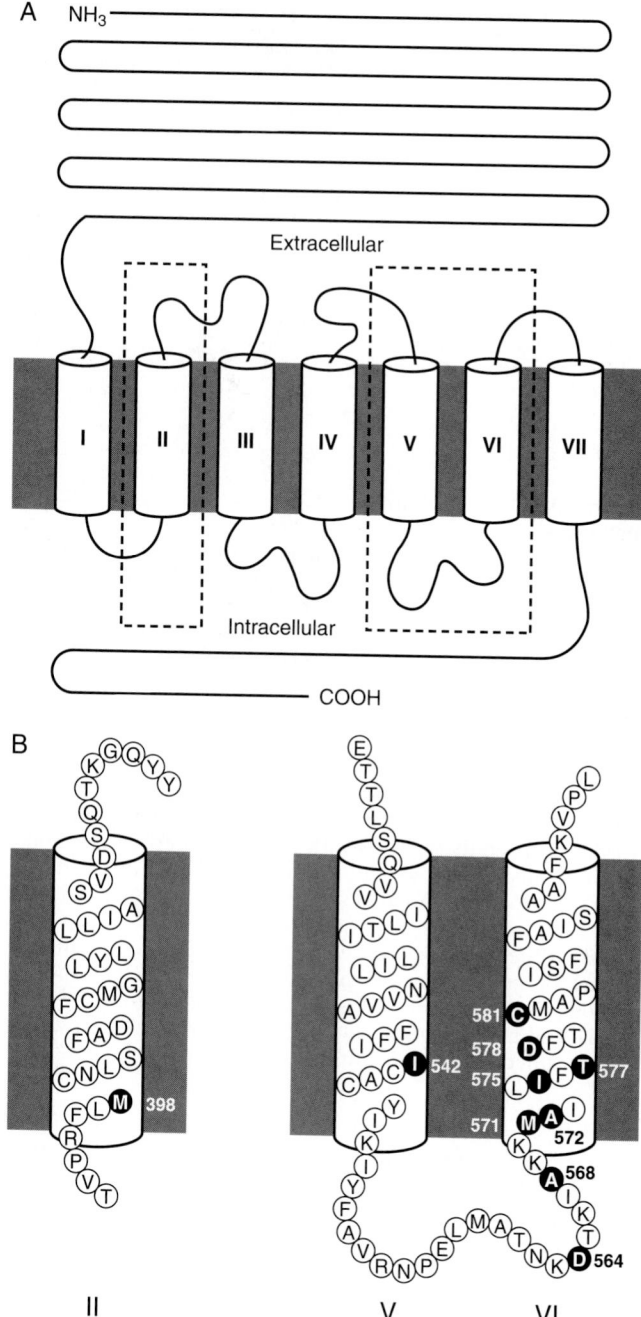

Figure 31–72. *A*, The serpentine seven transmembrane G$_s$ protein coupled hLH/hCG receptor with its large extracellular domain and the intracellular domain. The seven helical transmembrane domains are indicated by Roman numerals. *B*, The two-dimensional seven transmembrane topology of the hLH/hCG receptor with positions of constitutively activating mutations causing testotoxicosis (male-limited autosomal dominant sexual precocity). The mutations are indicated by solid circles and the residue number. Note the cluster of mutations in the VI transmembrane helix and third cytoplasmic loop. The aspartine 578–glycine mutation is the most common. (Redrawn from Yano K, Kohn LD, Saji M, et al. A case of male-limited precocious puberty caused by a point mutation in the second transmembrane domain of the luteinizing hormone choriogonadotropin receptor gene. Biochem Biophys Res Comm 1996; 220:1036–1042, with permission.[1236])

Table 31–39 lists the various agents used in the treatment of testotoxicosis.

GIRLS. Incomplete isosexual precocity in girls (see Table 31–27) is caused by estrogen secretion by ovarian cysts or tumors or adrenal neoplasms or by inadvertent exposure to estrogen. In a pure hCG-secreting tumor in girls, signs of isosexual precocity are absent; teratomas or teratocarcinomas (or a CNS germ cell tumor) that secrete hCG have caused sexual precocity in girls due to the concurrent estrogen secretion by the tumor.

Autonomous Ovarian Follicular Cysts. The most common estrogen-secreting ovarian mass of childhood is the follicular cyst.[1244] Antral follicles up to about 8 mm in diameter are common in normal prepubertal ovaries[55, 1245–1247] and may be present in third-trimester fetuses and newborn infants.[1248–1250, 1252] They can appear and regress spontaneously. Large follicular cysts may be discovered because of the presence of an abdominal mass or abdominal pain or as an unexpected finding on pelvic ultrasonography performed for other reasons. Occasionally, the antral follicles secrete estrogen and cause sexual precocity and recurrent acyclic vaginal bleeding. Enlarged antral follicles or cysts also occur in girls with premature thelarche, true precocious puberty, and transient or incomplete sexual precocity.[636, 1253–1256] In some girls with ovarian follicular cysts the transient or recurrent sexual precocity is LHRH independent (Fig. 31–73). The concentration of estradiol fluctuates, usually correlating with changes in the size of the follicular cyst or cysts[1257] and may increase to levels found with granulosa cell tumors.[278, 636, 1256] The level of LH is suppressed, and the pattern of pulsatile LH and the LH rise induced by LHRH are prepubertal.[636, 1254–1256]

It is curious that a constitutive activating mutation of the FSH receptor has not been described in women, since a heterozygous mutation, asparagine 567 to glycine, has been detected in the third intracellular loop of the FSH receptor in a hypophysectomized man who, despite gonadotropin deficiency, was fertile and had normal-sized testes.[1258] Accordingly, it is possible that some girls with recurrent ovarian cysts may harbor an activating mutation of the FSH receptor.

An unusual syndrome of estradiol-secreting ovarian cysts occurs in preterm infants born before 30 weeks of gestation and is associated with edema of the labia majora and, in some instances, of the lower abdominal wall.[1250] In four preterm neonates the syndrome appeared weeks after birth and 1 to 4 weeks before the putative date of a full-term gestation. The follicular cysts, which may be unilateral or bilateral, were detected by abdominal and pelvic ultrasonography. The LH and FSH response to LHRH suggested that the cysts were LHRH dependent. Treatment with medroxyprogesterone acetate was associated with regression of the cysts.

LHRH agonists are useful in the treatment of ovarian follicular cysts associated with true precocious puberty (LHRH dependent) but not so-called autonomous cysts.[1259] However, girls with "autonomously" functioning ovarian follicular cysts may respond to treatment with oral medroxyprogesterone acetate. Medroxyprogesterone acetate seems to prevent recurrence and to accelerate involution of the follicular cysts[636, 1256] and reduce the risk of torsion. The use of potent aromatase inhibitors, such as letrozole, to reduce estradiol secretion is another potential treatment.[1243, 1243a] Surgical intervention is rarely indicated; a large or persistent cyst can be reduced with percutaneous aspiration guided by ultrasonography.

Plasma estradiol concentrations in girls with recurrent cysts (>7 cm) may be as high as in girls with granulosa cell tumors of the ovary.[636, 1256] Alternatively, the levels of estrogen in blood and urine may be in the early pubertal range. A characteristic feature with recurrent cysts is waxing and waning of estrogen levels in accord with changes in the appearance of the ovary on pelvic ultrasonography.[1257, 1260] Luteinization of follicular cysts may be due to subtle elevations of plasma FSH. A cyst that secretes estrogen autonomously differs from the follicular cysts that may occur in girls with true precocious puberty. In the latter case, removal or reduction of the cyst does not correct sexual precocity.[1256, 1261] Further-

TABLE 31–39. Pharmacologic Therapy for Sexual Precocity

Disorder	Treatment	Action and Rationale
LHRH dependent True or central precocious puberty	LHRH agonists	Desensitization of gonadotropes; blocks action of endogenous LHRH
LHRH independent Incomplete sexual precocity		
Girls		
Autonomous ovarian cysts	Medroxyprogesterone acetate	Inhibition of ovarian steroidogenesis; regression of cyst (inhibition of FSH release)
McCune-Albright syndrome	Medroxyprogesterone acetate* Testolactone* or letrozole	Inhibition of ovarian steroidogenesis; regression of cyst (inhibition of FSH release) Inhibition of P-450 aromatase; blocks estrogen synthesis
Boys		
Familial testotoxicosis	Ketoconazole* Spironolactone* or flutamide *and* testolactone or letrozole Medroxyprogesterone acetate*	Inhibition of P-450-c17 (CYP17) (mainly 17,20-lyase activity) Antiandrogen Inhibition of aromatase; blocks estrogen synthesis Inhibition of testicular steroidogenesis

*If true precocious puberty develops, an LHRH agonist can be added.
Modified from Grumbach MM, Kaplan SL. Recent advances in the diagnosis and management of sexual precocity. Acta Paediatr Jpn 1988; 30(Suppl):155–175, with permission.[567]

more, the autonomously secreting cysts are not associated with augmented pulsatile LH secretion or with a pubertal LH response to LHRH administration. Ovarian cysts and sexual precocity have been associated with the fragile X syndrome in girls.[1262]

Granulosa Cell Tumor of the Ovary. This tumor is rare in childhood, and theca cell tumors are even less common.[1261, 1263] Juvenile granulosa cell tumors have distinctive histologic features that include nodular architecture, follicle formation, abundant interstitial and intrafollicular acid mucopolysaccharide-rich fluid, irregular microcysts, individual cell necrosis, and high mitotic activity. The size can vary from 2.5 to 25 cm with a mean diameter of 12 cm. The interstitial mucinous fluid contains hyaluronic acid.[1264] The vast majority of granulosa cell tumors can be palpated on bimanual examination. Fewer than 5% are bilateral or clinically malignant, and only about 3% of patients die of the disease. The concentration of plasma estradiol may increase to high levels;[278] FSH and LH concentrations are usually suppressed. The tumors secrete AMH and inhibin, which are sensitive tumor markers.[1265–1269] Sonograms of the ovary facilitate diagnosis. If the patient is younger than age 9, an elevated estradiol, and an elevation in concentration of

plasma AMH or inhibin at any age, suggest recurrence or metastasis.

Occasionally, gonadoblastomas in streak gonads, rare lipoid tumors, cystadenomas, and ovarian carcinomas secrete estrogens or androgens, or both hormones. Even with successful resection of a gonadal steroid-secreting neoplasm, the child is at risk for development of secondary central precocious puberty in the future. Gonadal tumors composed of a mixture of germ cells and sex cord stromal cells that are distinct from gonadoblastoma are usually benign when discovered in 46,XY female infants or children,[1270, 1271] although neoplastic transformation can occur.[1272, 1273] Two cases of metastasizing malignant mixed germ cell–sex cord–stromal tumors have been described in prepubertal girls with isosexual precocity.[1273] Some of these neoplasms secrete α-fetoprotein and other tumor markers. Most childhood ovarian tumors are benign,[1274] and early diagnosis allows successful cure.[1275]

Peutz-Jeghers Syndrome. This autosomal dominant syndrome of mucocutaneous pigmentation of the lips, buccal mucosa, fingers, and toes; gastrointestinal hamartomatous polyposis; and a predisposition to malignancy is associated with a rare, distinctive sex cord tumor with annular tubules in both

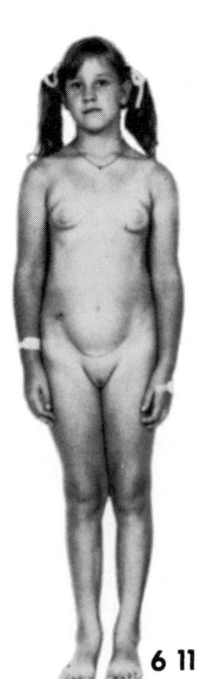

FOLLICULAR CYST OF OVARY   **(Pt. G.B.)**

<u>**AGE OF ONSET:**</u> 2 10/12 Y

<u>**P.E. AT AGE**</u> 4 10/12 Y

　HT: 122.8 cm (+3.2 SD)

　BREASTS: III, PH: 2

<u>**LAB:**</u> LRF: LH: 0.4 to 0.7 ng/ml, FSH: 0.4 to 0.8 ng/ml

　E₂: 180 pg/ml

　BA: 6 Y, CA: 4 10/12

Rx: 5 3/12: REMOVAL OF OVARIAN CYST

　CYST FLUID: 25,000 pg/ml E₁

　　　　　>34,000 pg/ml E₂

<u>**MPA:**</u> AGE 5 5/12 to 9 0/12 Y

　LRF: PREPUBERTAL LH RESPONSE

　E₂:<10 pg/ml

　REMISSION WITH NO PROGRESSION OF

　PUBERTAL SIGNS

6 11/12 Y, ON MPA

Figure 31–73. A 4 10/12-year-old girl with recurrent "autonomous" follicular cysts of the ovary. MPA, medroxyprogesterone acetate (oral). For conversion to SI units, see the legend of Figure 31–17. (From Kaplan SL, Grumbach MM. Pathogenesis of sexual precocity. In: Grumbach MM, Sizonenko PC, Aubert ML, eds. Control of the Onset of Puberty. Baltimore: Williams & Wilkins, 1990: 620–660. © 1990, the Williams & Wilkins Co., Baltimore.[636])

boys and girls.[1276-1278] Estrogen secretion by the tumor can lead to feminization and incomplete sexual precocity in boys as well as girls. Less frequently, an epithelial tumor of the ovary, dysgerminoma, or a feminizing Sertoli-Leydig cell tumor has been found in patients with Peutz-Jeghers syndrome.[1279, 1280] Children with this disorder should be examined at regular intervals for the presence of gonadal tumors by pelvic ultrasonography. The putative tumor suppressor gene is located on the distal short arm of chromosome 19.[1281]

INCOMPLETE SEXUAL PRECOCITY: BOYS AND GIRLS

McCune-Albright Syndrome. This syndrome,[1079, 1282, 1283] which occurs about twice as often in girls as in boys, is due to somatic activating mutations in the gene (GNAS1) that encodes the α subunit of the trimeric guanosine triphosphate (GTP)–binding protein ($G_{\alpha s}$) that stimulates adenylate cyclase. The disorder is characterized by the triad of irregularly edged hyperpigmented macules (café au lait spots); a slowly progressive bone disorder, polyostotic fibrous dysplasia, that can involve any bone and is frequently associated with facial asymmetry and hyperostosis of the base of the skull; and, more common in girls, LHRH-independent sexual precocity[1079, 1284, 1285] (Fig. 31–74; Table 31–40). Autonomous hyperfunction most commonly involves the ovary, but other endocrine involvement includes the thyroid (nodular hyperplasia with thyrotoxicosis or euthyroid status[906]), adrenal (multiple hyperplastic nodules with Cushing's syndrome[1285]), pituitary (somatotrope adenoma or hyperplasia with gigantism and acromegaly and hyperprolactinemia[1286]), and parathyroids (adenoma or hyperplasia with hyperparathyroidism[1079]). In addition, hypophosphatemic vitamin D–resistant rickets or osteomalacia can occur either because of secretion of a putative phosphaturic factor, phosphatonin,[1287] by the bone lesions or because of an intrinsic renal abnormality leading to the excess generation of nephrogenous cyclic AMP and, as a result, decreased reabsorption of phosphate.[1288] At least two of the features must be present to consider the diagnosis. This sporadic condition can be discordant in monozygotic twins.[1289]

The skin manifestations may not be conspicuous in infancy. The café au lait macules usually do not cross the midline, are usually located on the same side as the main bone lesions, and have a segmental distribution.[1282]

The skeletal lesions are dysplastic and are filled with spindle cells with poorly organized collagen support; they take the form of scattered cystic areas of rarefaction on radiography and often result in pathologic fractures and progressive deformities[1079, 1290] (Fig. 31–75). Bone lesions can be detected by technetium bone scan before they are visible radiographically. If the skull is involved, the optic or auditory nerve foramina may be compressed and lead to blindness, deafness, facial asymmetry, and ptosis.

The sexual precocity in girls, the onset of which is often in the first 2 years of life and is frequently heralded by menstrual bleeding, is due to autonomously functioning luteinized follicular cysts of the ovary (Table 31–41).[636, 1079] The ovaries contain multiple follicular cysts, but not corpora lutea, and commonly exhibit asymmetrical enlargement as a result of a large solitary cyst, which characteristically enlarges and regresses only to recur (Fig. 31–76).[636, 1223, 1079, 1285, 1291, 1292] Serum estradiol is elevated; in contrast, the LH response to LHRH is prepubertal, and the pubertal pattern of nighttime LH pulses is absent at the onset and during the initial years.[636, 1293, 1294] When the bone age approaches 12 years, the LHRH pulse generator becomes operative, and ovulatory cycles ensue. Thus, an affected girl may progress from LHRH-independent puberty to LHRH-dependent puberty[636, 1293, 1295] (see Table 31–39). LHRH agonists are not effective for treatment in the LHRH-independent stage. Testolactone (40 mg/kg/d orally),[1296] a relatively weak aromatase inhibitor, is of equivocal usefulness;[1297, 1298]

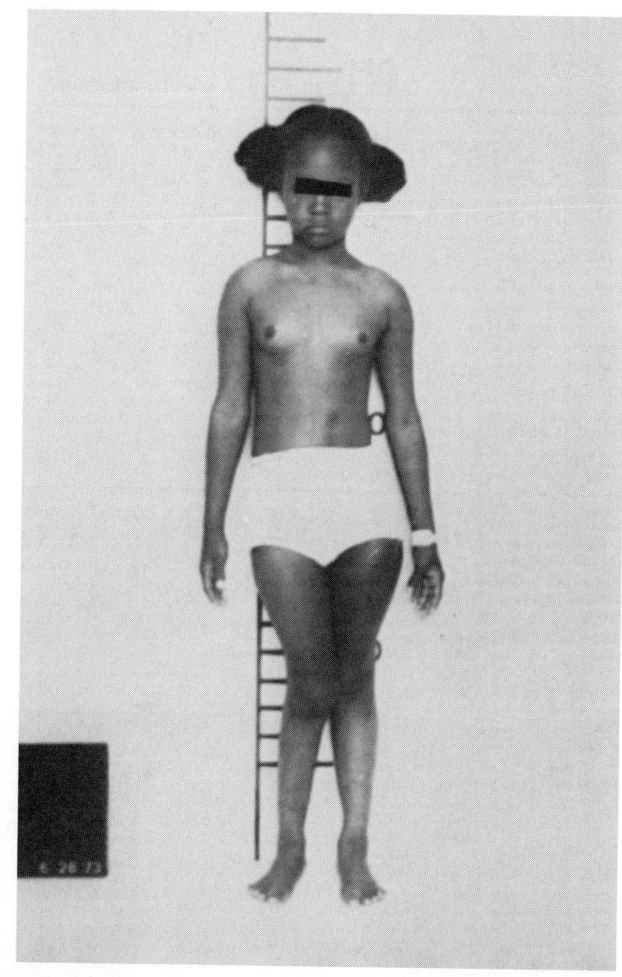

Figure 31–74. A 7 4/12-year-old girl with LHRH-independent sexual precocity associated with McCune-Albright syndrome. She had breast development since infancy, and it increased noticeably at about 3 years of age; 6 mo later episodes of recurrent vaginal bleeding began. Growth of pubic hair was noted at about 4 to 5 years of age. At age 5 1/12 years the bone age was 6 11/12 years; height was +1 SD above the mean value for age. By 6 1/2 years of age, when she was seen at the University of California, San Francisco, the bone age had advanced to 9 years, and height was +1 SD. Breasts were at Tanner stage 4; pubic hair at stage 3. Extensive irregular café au lait macules cover the right side of the face, left lower abdomen and thigh, and both buttocks. A bone survey showed widespread involvement of the long bones with typical polyostotic fibrous dysplasia, and the floor of the anterior fossa of the skull was sclerotic and the diploetic space widened. She has had two pathologic fractures through bone cysts in the right upper femur. Note the osseous deformities. Plasma estradiol concentrations were consistently in the pubertal range; LH response to LHRH was prepubertal. Results of thyroid function studies were normal, including the TSH response to TRH administration and antithyroid antibodies were not detected. Treatment with oral medroxyprogesterone acetate suppressed menses and arrested pubertal development but did not slow skeletal maturation. Her final height is 142 cm (−2.5 SD). Menstrual cycles are regular.

more potent aromatase inhibitors, for example, letrozole, may be more effective.[1243a]

Sexual precocity is rare in boys with McCune-Albright syndrome,[1079, 1299] but affected boys may have asymmetrical enlargement of the testes in addition to signs of sexual precocity. The seminiferous tubules are enlarged and exhibit spermatogenesis; Leydig cells may be hyperplastic.[1299] The LH response to LHRH was prepubertal in two cases. The hormonal data (although scanty) and the testicular findings appear similar to those in boys with familial testotoxicosis (for review see reference 1079).

The pathogenesis was uncertain for many years. The disorder may occur concordantly or discordantly in monozygotic twins; familial cases have not been described. In 1986, Hap-

TABLE 31–40. Clinical Manifestations of McCune-Albright Syndrome in 158 Reported Patients*

Manifestation	Patients (%) (n = 158)	Male (n = 53)	Female (n = 105)	Age at Diagnosis (yr)	(range)	Comments
Fibrous dysplasia	97	51	103	7.7	(0–52)	Polyostotic more common than monostotic
Café au lait lesion	85	49	86	7.7	(0–52)	Variable size and number of lesions, irregular border ("coast of Maine")
Sexual precocity	52	8	74	4.9	(0.3–9)	Common initial manifestation
Acromegaly/gigantism	27	20	22	14.8	(0.2–42)	17/26 with adenoma on MRI/CT
Hyperprolactinemia	15	9	14	16.0	(0.2–42)	23/42 of acromegalic with ↑ PRL
Hyperthyroidism	19	7	23	14.4	(0.5–37)	Euthyroid goiter is common
Hypercortisolism	5	4	5	4.4	(0.2–17)	All primary adrenal
Myxomas	5	3	5	34	(17–50)	Extremity myxomas
Osteosarcoma	2	1	2	36	(34–37)	At site of fibrous dysplasia, not related to prior radiation therapy
Rickets/osteomalacia	3	1	3	27.3	(8–52)	Responsive to phosphorus plus calcitriol
Cardiac abnormalities	11	8	9		(0.1–66)	Arrhythymias and CHF reported
Hepatic abnormalities	10	6	10	1.9	(0.3–4)	Neonatal icterus is most common

Abbreviations: MRI = magnetic resonance imaging; CT = computed tomography; PRL = prolactin; CHF = congestive heart failure.

*Evaluations include clinical and biochemical data; other rarely described manifestations include metabolic acidosis, nephrocalcinosis, developmental delay, thymic and splenic hyperplasia, and colonic polyps.

Modified from Ringel MD, Schwindinger MD, Levine MA. Clinical implication of genetic defects in G proteins: the molecular basis of McCune-Albright syndrome and Albright hereditary osteodystrophy. Medicine 1996; 75:171–184, with permission.[1284]

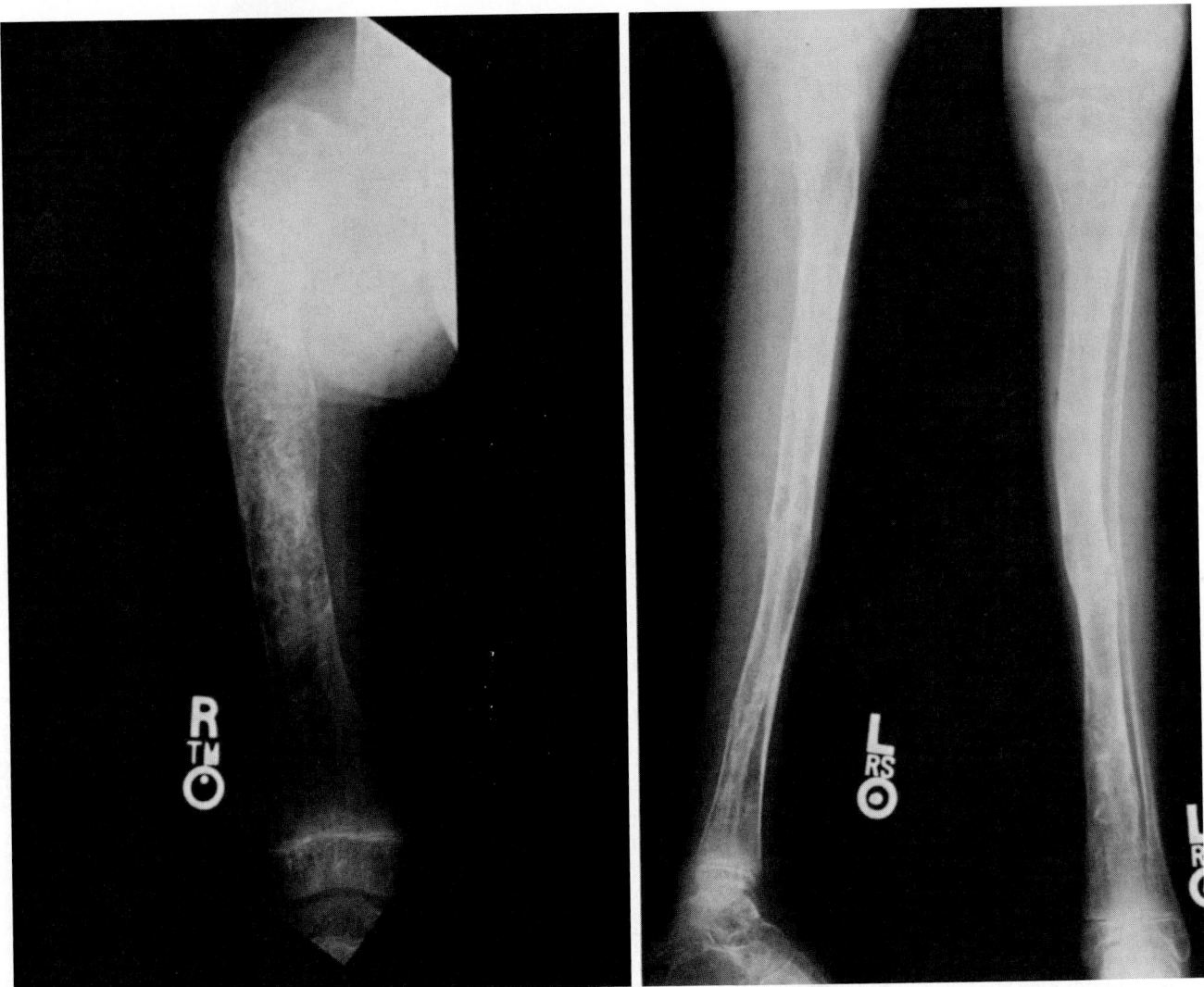

Figure 31–75. Bone lesions in McCune-Albright syndrome (see text for description).

TABLE 31–41. A Patient with McCune-Albright Syndrome and Recurrent Ovarian Cysts

Chronologic Age (y)	Bone Age (y)	Height (cm)	Physical Signs*	Basal and Post-LHRH‡	Plasma Estradiol, pmol/L (pg/mL)	Radiograph, Long Bones
$1^{4/12}$	$1^{3/12}$	81.1	Café au lait pigmentation, B2, PH1 Vaginal bleeding (× 2 mo)	LH 0.6–1.3† (LER-960) FSH 1.9–3.2† (LER-869) (DHEAS <0.14 μmol/L [<50 ng/mL])	40 (11)	Normal
$1^{8/12}$			B1, PH1			
$2^{6/12}$	$2^{6/12}$	92.4	B2, PH2 Vaginal bleeding	LH 0.6–1.1 FSH 1.9–3.2 (DHEAS <0.14 μmol/L [<50 ng/mL])	55–66 (15–18)	Normal
$3^{3/12}$		98.3	B1, PH1			
$3^{10/12}$	$3^{10/12}$		B2, PH1	LH 1.1–2.0 FSH 1–1.7	51–95 (14–26)	Normal
$4^{3/12}$			B1, PH1		7.3–7.3 (20–20)	Polyostotic fibrous dysplasia of femurs
$5^{11/12}$	6	123.4	B3, PH2 Vaginal bleeding (× 2 mo)	LH 1.1–4.3 FSH 1.0–2.0		
$6^{6/12}$	$7^{10/12}$	128.5	B3, PH2 Oral medroxyprogesterone acetate, 10 mg bid started		<5	
$7^{10/12}$	$8^{10/12}$	136.8				
$8^{7/12}$		142.2				

*B2, breast stage 2; PH1, pubic hair stage 1.
†ng/mL. To convert ng/mL to IU/L, multiply LH value by 3.8 and FSH value by 8.4.
‡Note the prepubertal LH response to LHRH consistent with LHRH-independent sexual precocity until age $5^{11/12}$ y, and the pubertal LH response at $5^{11/12}$ y consistent with the development of secondary true precocious puberty (LHRH-dependent). Note discrepancy between gonadarche and adrenarche as evidenced by preadrenarchal concentration of DHEAS.

ple[1300] posited that the disorder is caused by an autosomal "dominant" lethal gene that results in loss of the zygote in utero and that cells bearing this mutation survive only in embryos mosaic for the lethal gene. The early somatic mutation would lead to a mosaic cell pattern of the distribution of cells containing the mutation. The severity would depend on the proportion of mutant cells in various embryonic tissues. The description of somatic mutations in human endocrine tumors that convert the peptide chain of the G_s protein into a putative oncogene (referred to as a *gsp* mutation)[1301] raised the possibility of a similar defect in McCune-Albright syndrome. These hypotheses have now been established. Mutations in the gene encoding the α subunit of the stimulatory G protein for adenylate cyclase have been identified in the tissues of children with McCune-Albright syndrome (see later).

The heterotrimeric guanine nucleotide–binding proteins (G proteins) are reviewed in Chapter 5.[1302–1304] The heterotrimer is composed of (1) an α subunit (39 to 45 kd) that binds GTP and has intrinsic GTPase activity that converts GTP to GDP; (2) a β subunit (35 to 36 kd) and a smaller α subunit (7 to 8 kd) that are tightly but noncovalently associated with each other. Each of the subunits is encoded by a distinct gene. The G proteins function as "conformational switches." The GDP-liganded α subunit is bound to the βγ subunits and is in an inactivated state. When the cell surface receptor is activated by its ligand or agonists, the GDP is catalytically released

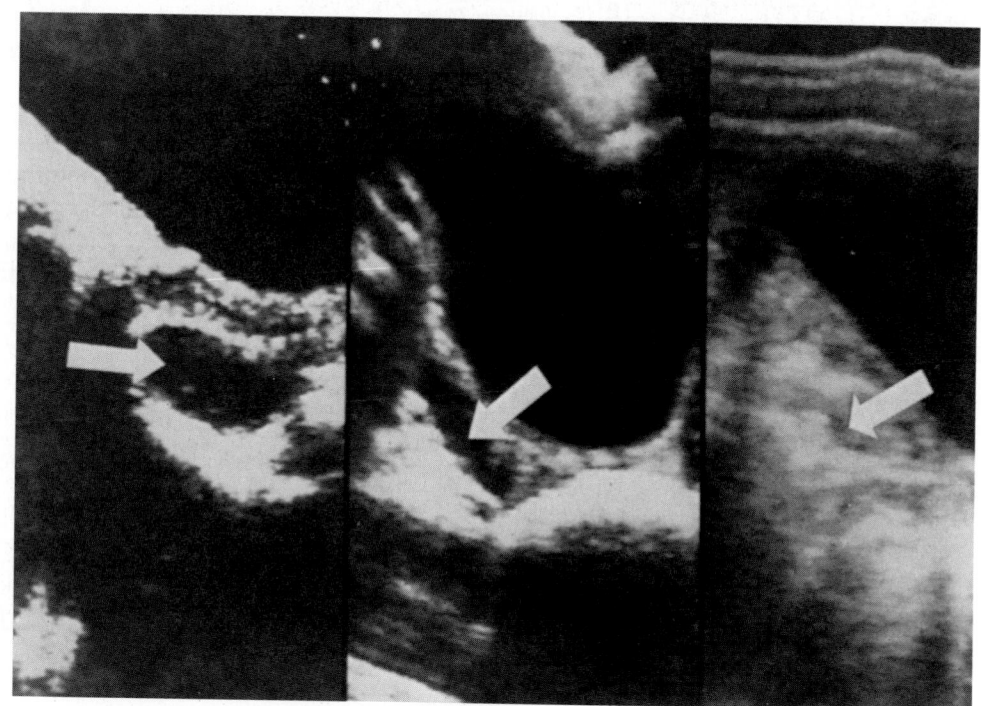

Figure 31–76. Serial pelvic ultrasonograms at 2-wk intervals in a 6-year-old girl with McCune-Albright syndrome. Breast development and vaginal bleeding coincided with the enlargement of the ovarian cyst. With the spontaneous regression of the large ovarian cyst, the breasts regressed in size and vaginal bleeding ceased. (From Kaplan SL, Grumbach MM. Pathogenesis of sexual precocity. In: Grumbach MM, Sizonenko PC, Aubert ML, eds. Control of the Onset of Puberty. Baltimore: Williams & Wilkins, 1990:620–660. © 1990, the Williams & Wilkins Co., Baltimore.[636])

from the α subunit and enables GTP to bind. This leads to dissociation of the GTP-activated α subunit, its dissociation from the bound βγ subunits, and activation of the effector, adenylate cyclase. When GTP is hydrolyzed by the intrinsic GTPase activity of $G_{\alpha s}$, the α and βγ subunits reassociate and the α subunit is now in the off, or inactive, conformation. The three-dimensional structure of the heterotrimeric G proteins has been determined.[1305–1309]

Activating heterozygous somatic mutations in the α subunit of the G_s protein in McCune-Albright syndrome lead to excess cAMP production and in some tissues cAMP-induced hyperplasia.[1308] The somatic constitutive activating mutations are expressed in a mosaic fashion, and the fact that the proportion of mutant to normal cells varies in different tissues is a cause of the variability in clinical findings and severity, even in monozygotic twins. A germ line mutation is presumed to be lethal to the embryo. Two gain-of-function somatic missense mutations have been described in this order, arginine 201 with either a cysteine or histidine substitution (Fig. 31–77).[1284, 1302, 1310–1312] The arginine 201 residue is critical for α subunit GTPase activity, and each of the described mutations decreases the GTPase activity of the $G_{\alpha s}$ subunit and leads to constitutive activation. These activating mutations have been found in all tissues affected in the syndrome,[1313, 1314] including bone lesions. Manifestations of McCune-Albright syndrome in infancy include Cushing's syndrome due to macronodular adrenal cortical hyperplasia, hyperthyroidism caused by thyroid adenomas, jaundice associated with hepatobiliary disease, and pancreati-

tis.[1315] Another nonendocrine manifestation is cardiac disease, which carries the risk of arrhythmia and sudden death.

Gonadotropin-Independent Sexual Precocity and Pseudo-hypoparathyroidism Type Ia Due to a $G_{\alpha s}$ Mutation. Mutations in $G_{\alpha s}$, can either constitutively activate or inactivate adenylate cyclase.[1302] Two boys who presented in infancy with classic pseudohypoparathyroidism type Ia (PHPIa), a disorder characterized by resistance to hormones whose action is mediated by cyclic AMP, developed signs of sexual precocity with features suggesting testotoxicosis (gonadotropin-independent sexual precocity) at about 24 months of age.[1316] Each had an alanine 366-to–serine mutation[1316] in one allele of the $G_{\alpha s}$ gene; PHPIa is due to a wide variety of inactivating mutations in $G_{\alpha s}$ that lead to about a 50% reduction in $G_{\alpha s}$ activity in functional assays.[1284]

The paradox of a $G_{\alpha s}$ mutation causing both inactivation (pseudohypoparathyroidism) and constitutive activation (testotoxicosis) was resolved by in vitro studies.[1317] In cultured cells, the $G_{\alpha s}$ alanine 366-to–serine mutant protein is rapidly degraded at 37°C but constitutively activates adenylate cyclase at 33°C.[1317] Unlike other activating mutations of $G_{\alpha s}$, which impair its intrinsic GTPase activity and decrease the hydrolysis of GTP to GDP, the mutation in the two boys accelerated dissociation of GDP at 33°C but was rapidly degraded at 37°C.[1316, 1317] These observations provide a theoretical explanation for increased $G_{\alpha s}$ activity in the testes which are 3 to 5°C cooler than the body, and low activity in other tissues.[1317] The mother of one patient appeared to be a mosaic for the $G_{\alpha s}$

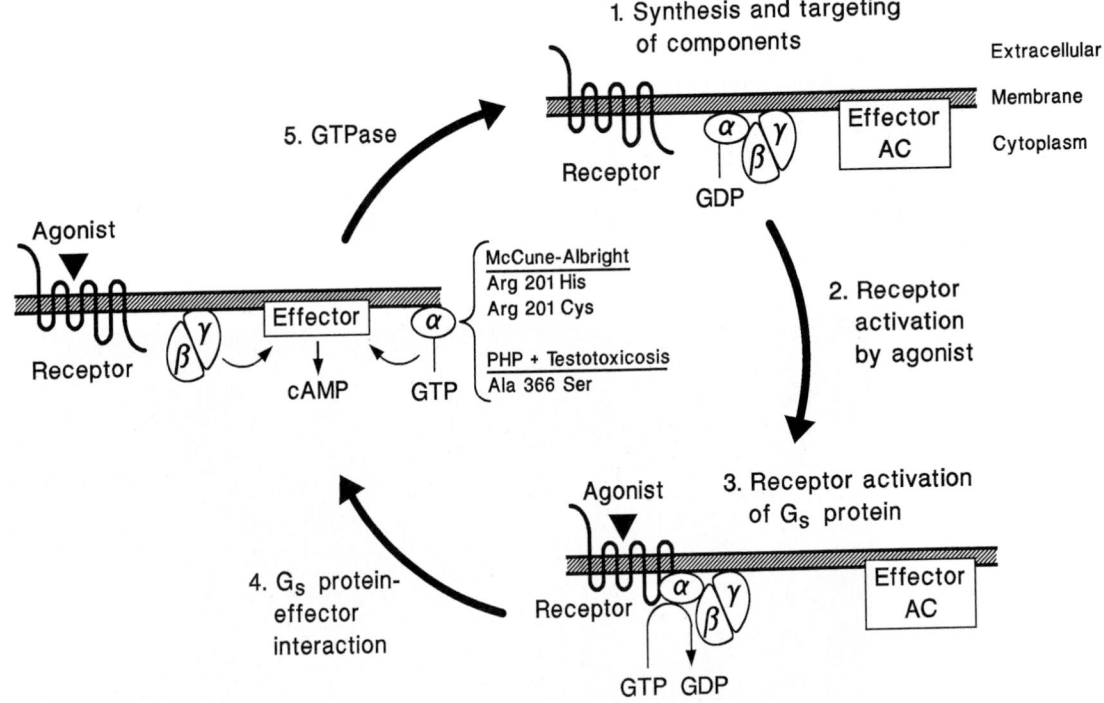

Figure 31–77. The G protein GTPase cycle. The heterotrimeric guanine nucleotide-binding proteins (G protein) composed of three subunits (α, β, γ) couple cell surface receptors consisting of a single serpentine polypeptide having seven helical membrane-spanning domains with an effector, in this instance, adenylate cyclase (AC) that catalyzes the transformation of ATP to cAMP. The G protein stimulation subunit α, $G_{\alpha s}$, mediates the stimulation of cAMP generation. In the inactive, unstimulated state, the G protein is a heterotrimer and GDP is tightly bound to the α subunit. When the cell surface receptor is activated by its cognate agonist, the receptor catalyzes the release of the tightly bound GDP, which enables GTP to bind to the α subunit. The GTP-bound α subunit (α-GTP) dissociates from the tightly bound βγ dimer, and both play a role in the G protein activation of the effector, adenylate cyclase. The intrinsic GTPase activity of the α subunit ends the stimulation of the effector by converting the bound α-GTP to α-GDP; as a consequence the α subunit again returns to its inactive state and reassociates with high affinity with the βγ subunit, yielding the α, β, γ heterotrimer. Disorders of signal transduction can arise from germ cell or somatic mutations at any of the five stages of the cycle.

The gain-of-function, activating somatic mutations in the *GNAS1* gene that encodes the $G_{\alpha s}$ subunit and leads to McCune-Albright syndrome (shown in the bracket) involve the highly conserved arginine 201 residue. These mutations inhibit the intrinsic GTPase activity of the α subunit, and hence the conversion of the bound GTP to GDP. *(See text)*. Alanine 366-to–serine mutation (shown in the bracket) was detected in two boys, both of whom had pseudohypoparathyroidism Ia (PHP) and testotoxicosis. The mutant protein was constitutively activated in the Leydig cells at the scrotal temperature (32–33°C), leading to testotoxicosis, but was rapidly degraded at body temperature, 37°C, which led to PHP1a. *(See text)*. (Modified from Spiegel AM. Mutations in G proteins and G protein–coupled receptors in endocrine disease. J Clin Endocrinol Metab 1996; 81:2434–2442, with permission.[1312])

mutation, whereas a germ line mutation is likely in the other boy.[1316]

Juvenile Hypothyroidism. Long-standing untreated primary hypothyroidism, usually a consequence of Hashimoto's thyroiditis, can cause incomplete isosexual precocity[124, 1318, 1319] in both girls and boys and occurs in association with impaired growth and delayed skeletal maturation. If the level of plasma prolactin is elevated, galactorrhea may be demonstrable, more commonly in girls (Fig. 31–78). The signs of sexual maturation are not accompanied by a pubertal growth spurt; rather, growth is impaired[124] (Fig. 31–79). Girls have breast development, enlarged labia minora, and estrogenic changes in the vaginal smear, usually without the appearance of pubic hair;[124, 1320–1323] some girls have irregular vaginal bleeding,[124, 1324] and solitary or multiple ovarian cysts may be demonstrable with pelvic ultrasonography or by physical examination.[124] In most boys with juvenile hypothyroidism, the testes are enlarged because of an increase in the size of the seminiferous tubules, but signs of virilization and Leydig cell maturation are absent[1322, 1325] and the plasma concentration of testosterone is prepubertal. Enlargement of the sella turcica and the pituitary gland (see Fig. 31–79) has led to the misdiagnosis of a pituitary neoplasm. The hypothyroidism, incomplete sexual maturation, galactorrhea, and pituitary enlargement are reversed or corrected by levothyroxine therapy within a few months.[124]

In 1960, Van Wyk and Grumbach[124] suggested that the syndrome resulted from hormonal "overlap" in negative-feedback regulation with increased secretion of gonadotropins, prolactin, and TSH as a consequence of the chronic hypothyroidism. With the advent of radioimmunoassays for pituitary hormones, increased prolactin secretion was documented in children[1318, 1319] and adults with primary hypothyroidism and in affected girls with the syndrome.[1320] Hyperprolactinemia correlates with the increased production of TSH.[1318] GH release is usually decreased, as in uncomplicated primary hypothyroidism.[1326, 1327] Hypothalamic TRH stimulates the release of both prolactin and TSH, and the increased TRH production in children with primary hypothyroidism seems to account for the rise in serum prolactin and TSH levels.[1318]

However, the explanation for the sexual maturation remains uncertain. Pubertal development in primary hypothyroidism is usually delayed and is only rarely advanced for chronologic age. With radioimmunoassays for FSH and LH, in which the cross-reaction with TSH is negligible, an increased (pubertal) concentration of plasma immunoreactive and bioactive FSH, but not LH, has been detected.[1326–1328] Bioactive LH activity is also low. In addition, pulsatile release of FSH, mainly at night, but not of LH, was demonstrated in patients with the syndrome and in some children with primary hypothyroidism who do not exhibit premature sexual maturation.[1326–1328] The increased FSH release and the high FSH/LH ratio (in contrast to that in normal puberty) seem to account for the increased ovarian estrogen secretion in girls and for the enlarged testes without signs of virilization in affected boys; FSH-induced Sertoli cell proliferation may be a determinant of mature testis size.[64, 1329, 1330] An LHRH-independent mechanism is likely because an LHRH agonist does not suppress the pubertal LH levels.[1328] Pulsatile TSH release is increased at night; administration of TRH increases FSH release in normal children (but not adults); moreover, the FSH response to TRH, but not LHRH, is augmented in primary hypothyroidism.[1327] Thus, incomplete sexual precocity and the increased prolactin secretion and galactorrhea may be a consequence of the increased release of TRH, the increased sensitivity of the mammotropes and gonadotropes to TRH, or both.

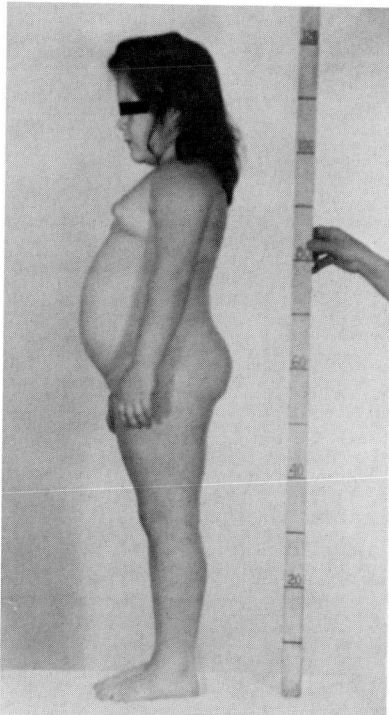 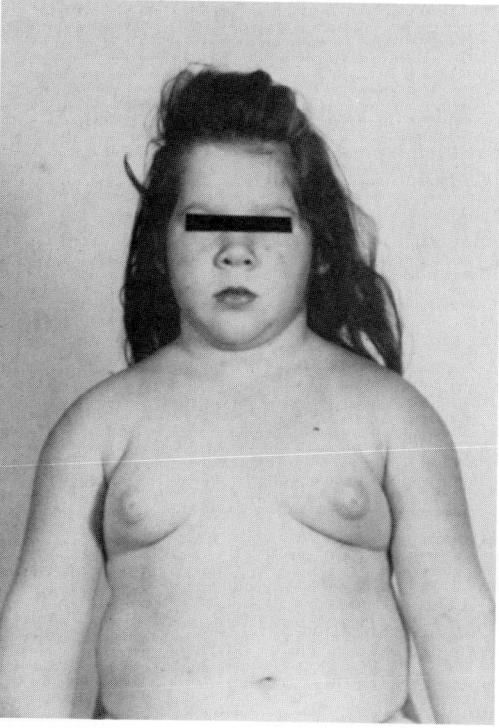 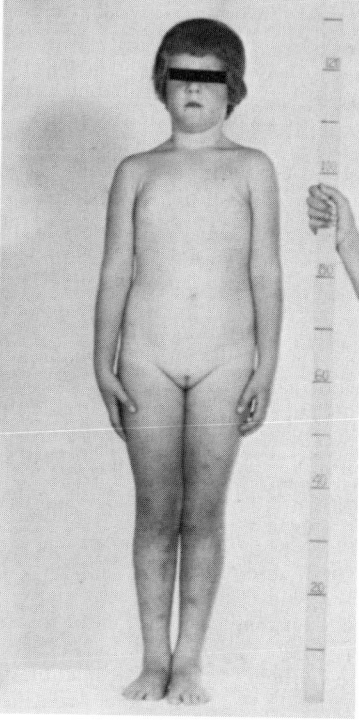

Figure 31–78. *Left and center,* Severe, chronic hypothyroidism of Hashimoto's thyroiditis in a 7 1/12-year-old girl with sexual precocity (without pubic or axillary hair), episodic vaginal bleeding, and galactorrhea. She had symptoms of hypothyroidism and a sharply decreased rate of growth over the previous 2 y (height, −1 SD; bone age, 5 3/12 years). Breast development was Tanner stage 3; the labia minora were enlarged, and the vaginal mucosa was dull pink, thickened, and rugated with evidence of an estrogenic effect. No acne, seborrhea, or hirsutism was present. The uterus was of adolescent size, and the endometrial mucosa was in a proliferative phase. Urinary gonadotropins were barely detectable by bioassay. *Right,* Striking change in appearance after 8 mo of thyroid hormone treatment. She had grown 7 cm in height and lost 8.1 kg in weight; the breasts had decreased in size, galactorrhea was no longer demonstrable, the labia minora had regressed, and the vaginal mucosa was pink and glistening (no estrogen effect). Ten weeks after the initiation of thyroid hormone replacement therapy, she developed a right slipped capital femoral epiphysis that was repaired surgically; recovery was uneventful.

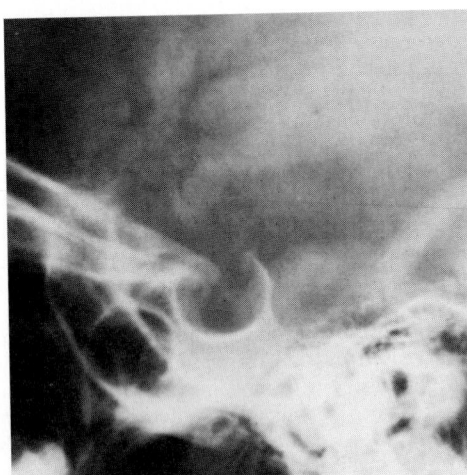 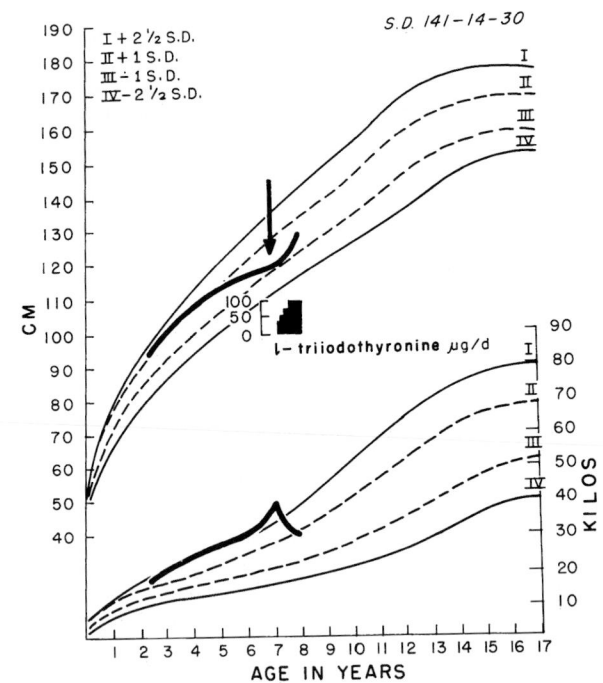

Figure 31–79. *Left,* Radiograph of the skull of a patient with hypothyroidism illustrating an enlarged pituitary fossa in the lateral view. The dorsum sellae was thin and demineralized, and the floor had a double contour line. The area of the sella turcica was 150 mm². Pneumoencephalography showed a suprasellar mass impinging on the cisterna chiasmatica. After thyroid hormone treatment for 8 mo, the area of the sella had decreased 30% in volume to 100 mm², the dorsum sellae had remineralized, and the double floor was no longer evident. *Right,* Growth curve illustrating the decrease in growth rate despite the sexual precocity and the catch-up growth induced by thyroid hormone therapy. (From Van Wyk JJ, Grumbach MM. Syndrome of precocious menstruation and galactorrhea in juvenile hypothyroidism: an example of hormonal overlap in pituitary feedback. J Pediatr 1960; 57:416–435.)

This mechanism,[124] which has gained support,[1328] would explain the relatively rapid and complete reversal of the syndrome by levothyroxine treatment. Human recombinant TSH in a very high dose evoked a dose-dependent cAMP response in COS-7 cells transfected with the human FSH receptor, suggesting another possible mechanism for the FSH (or FSH-like)-dependent, LHRH-independent sexual precocity.[1331] A direct effect of hypothyroidism on the prepubertal testis leading to overproliferation of Sertoli cells also has been advanced as an explication of the enlarged testes.[1325]

Diagnosis of Sexual Precocity (Table 31–42; Figs. 31–80 to 31–82)

The separation of patients with self-limited benign disorders, such as premature adrenarche or premature thelarche, or normal but early puberty, from those with serious or potentially fatal disorders is the first step in evaluation. The history may reveal symptoms suggesting perinatal abnormalities or injuries, previous infections, adventitious ingestion of or exposure to gonadal steroids, or the presence of similar conditions in family members. In addition, previous measurements should be plotted on a growth chart to determine height velocity and the age at onset of any increase in the rate of growth.

Important aspects of the physical examination include description of the secondary sexual development according to the Tanner stages; measurement of the penis and the testes in boys and breast tissue in girls; and examination for acne, oily skin, facial and body hair, pubic and axillary hair development, apocrine gland odor, muscular development, and galactorrhea. A careful examination of the external genitalia should be done with a nonrelated chaperone present, as the performance of such an examination has been interpreted by patients as sexual abuse in several cases.[1332] A thorough neurologic examination is indicated, with emphasis on assess-

ment of the visual fields and optic discs and search for signs of increased intracranial pressure; evaluation for skin lesions of McCune-Albright syndrome or neurofibromatosis; and examination for abdominal, gonadal, or adnexal masses and for coexisting endocrine disease.

Radiographs should be obtained for determination of bone age, and an MRI with contrast enhancement should be obtained in all boys with evidence of LHRH-dependent sexual precocity and in selected girls. Ultrasonography of the ovary and uterus is useful in evaluation of affected girls.[50, 57–59, 1260, 1333–1335] The largest measurements of uterine size by ultrasonography in infants and children are found at puberty and in the neonatal period.[1335] The upper limit of uterine length in the prepubertal state is 3.5 cm.[1333] Furthermore, a uterine volume of more than 1.8 mL is specific for the onset of puberty, whereas increased ovarian size is less specific; patients with premature thelarche are indistinguishable from age-matched control subjects when this ultrasonographic standard was used.[57] Microcysts and macrocysts of the ovary can be detected on ultrasound as well.[1260] Cysts may be found in the ovaries in true precocious puberty or LHRH-independent isosexual precocity, but the cysts usually are less than 9 mm in the former and greater than 9 mm in the latter.[1336]

Measurements of plasma gonadotropin levels using third-generation assays, the plasma concentration of testosterone in boys and of estradiol in girls, and the LH response to administration of LHRH (or the amplitude and frequency of LH pulses, especially at night) are useful. Girls early in the course of true precocious puberty have elevation of estradiol levels associated with increasing LH levels, but not necessarily an increase in the concentration of FSH.[1337] Thyroxine concentration should be measured when hypothyroidism is suspected.

True precocious puberty in boys usually begins with enlargement of the testes, followed by other signs of secondary sexual maturation. Leydig cell tumors usually cause asymmetri-

TABLE 31–42. Differential Diagnosis of Sexual Precocity

	Plasma Gonadotropins	LH Response to LHRH	Serum Sex Steroid Concentrations	Gonadal Size	Miscellaneous
True Precocious Puberty (premature reactivation of LHRH pulse generator)	Prominent LH pulses, initially during sleep	Pubertal LH response	Pubertal values of testosterone or estradiol	Normal pubertal testicular enlargement or ovarian and uterine enlargement (by ultrasonography)	MRI of brain to rule out CNS tumor or other abnormality; skeletal survey for McCune-Albright syndrome
Incomplete Sexual Precocity (pituitary gonadotropin-independent) *Males*					
Chorionic gonadotropin–secreting tumor in males	High hCG, low LH	Prepubertal LH response	Pubertal value of testosterone	Slight to moderate uniform enlargement of testes	Hepatomegaly suggests hepatoblastoma; CT scan of brain if chorionic gonadotropin–secreting CNS tumor suspected
Leydig cell tumor in males	Suppressed	No LH response	Very high testosterone	Irregular asymmetrical enlargement of testes	
Familial testotoxicosis	Suppressed	No LH response	Pubertal values of testosterone	Testes symmetrical and larger than 2.5 cm but smaller than expected for pubertal development; spermatogenesis occurs	Familial; probably sex-limited, autosomal dominant trait
Virilizing congenital adrenal hyperplasia	Prepubertal	Prepubertal LH response	Elevated 17-OHP in CYP21 deficiency or elevated 11-deoxycortisol in CYP11B1 deficiency	Testes prepubertal	Autosomal recessive, may be congenital or late-onset form, may have salt loss in CYP21 deficiency or hypertension in CYP11B1 deficiency
Virilizing adrenal tumor	Prepubertal	Prepubertal LH response	High DHEAS and androstenedione values	Testes prepubertal	CT, MRI, or ultrasonography of abdomen
Premature adrenarche	Prepubertal	Prepubertal LH response	Prepubertal testosterone, DHEAS, or urinary 17-ketosteroid values appropriate for pubic hair stage II	Testes prepubertal	Onset usually after 6 years of age; more frequent in CNS-injured children
Females					
Granulosa cell tumor (follicular cysts may present similarly)	Suppressed	Prepubertal LH response	Very high estradiol	Ovarian enlargement on physical examination, CT, or ultrasonography	Tumor often palpable on abdominal examination
Follicular cyst	Suppressed	Prepubertal LH response	Prepubertal to very high estradiol	Ovarian enlargement on physical examination, CT, or ultrasonography	Single or recurrent episodes of menses and/ or breast development; exclude McCune-Albright syndrome
Feminizing adrenal tumor	Suppressed	Prepubertal LH response	High estradiol and DHAS values	Ovaries prepubertal	Unilateral adrenal mass
Premature thelarche	Prepubertal	Prepubertal LH, pubertal estradiol response	Prepubertal or early	Ovaries prepubertal	Onset usually before 3 years of age
Premature adrenarche	Prepubertal	Prepubertal LH response	Prepubertal estradiol; DHAS or urinary 17-ketosteroid values appropriate for pubic hair stage II	Ovaries prepubertal	Onset usually after 6 years of age; more frequent in brain-injured children
Late-onset virilizing congenital adrenal hyperplasia	Prepubertal	Prepubertal LH response	Elevated 17-OHP in basal or corticotropin stimulated state	Ovaries prepubertal	Autosomal recessive
In Both Sexes McCune-Albright syndrome	Suppressed	Suppressed	Sex steroids pubertal or higher	Ovarian (on ultrasound); slight testicular enlargement	Skeletal survey for polyostotic fibrous dysplasia and skin examination for café au lait spots
Primary hypothyroidism	LH prepubertal; FSH may be slightly elevated	Prepubertal FSH may be increased	Estradiol may be pubertal	Testicular enlargement; ovaries cystic	TSH and prolactin elevated; T$_4$ low

cal enlargement of the testes, whereas extragonadal hCG-secreting tumors are associated with less marked testicular enlargement than occurs at the same stage of masculinization in true precocious puberty. Adrenal rests in the testes may enlarge under chronic stimulation from corticotropin in inadequately treated congenital adrenal hyperplasia and may be bilateral, although they are unlikely to mimic normal pubertal testicular development.[1338] An elevated hCG level with a prepu-

bertal LHRH test is diagnostic of gonadotropin-secreting tumor. If this tumor is in the CNS, abnormalities are present on MRI or CT brain scans. Enlargement of the liver or a mediastinal or retroperitoneal mass in boys suggests an hCG-producing hepatic or germ cell tumor; the possibility of Klinefelter's syndrome should be considered with the latter. Pubertal concentrations of LH and FSH, a pubertal mode of pulsatile LH secretion (initially during sleep), and/or pubertal LH re-

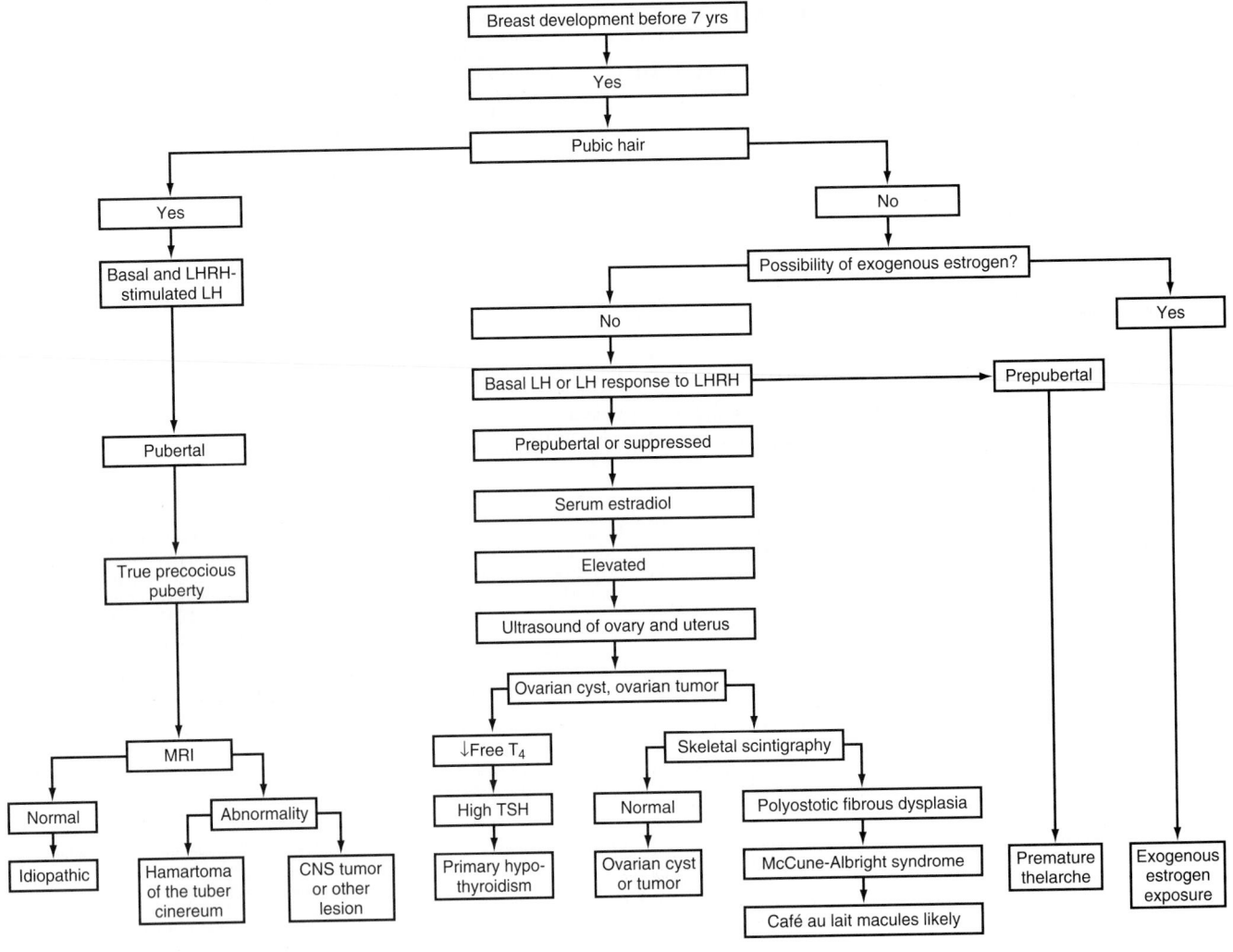

Figure 31–80. The diagnosis of sexual precocity in girls.

sponse in the LHRH test confirms the diagnosis of true precocious puberty (and in boys differentiates true precocity from familial testotoxicosis).

A CNS tumor must be considered as a potential cause of this premature activation of the hypothalamic LHRH pulse generator. The evaluation for a CNS tumor as a cause of true precocious puberty is similar to the investigation of an hCG-secreting tumor of the CNS. Although CT scanning is useful for identifying CNS abnormalities,[1339] MRI with contrast enhancement is more sensitive for the detection of small masses in the hypothalamus, such as hamartomas of the tuber cinereum[1106, 1115, 1340] and germ cell tumors (see Fig. 31–53). The use of contrast enhancement adds to diagnostic certainty and is recommended for MRI of the CNS.[1341] The height of the pituitary gland on MRI correlates with age and pubertal development;[1087, 1342] patients with true precocious puberty and higher peak LH/FSH ratios had pituitary heights exceeding 6 mm on the average, while those with a lower LH/FSH ratio or precocious thelarche had lower heights of approximately 5 mm.[1343] The shape of the pituitary gland is also of importance; a convex rather than a flat top is associated with true precocious puberty of all etiologies.[1088]

The premature appearance of pubic hair, phallic enlargement, and other signs of virilization in a male who does not have enlargement of the testes or the liver suggests the diagnosis of congenital virilizing adrenal hyperplasia, virilizing adrenal tumor, or, rarely, Cushing's syndrome.

If growth rate is suppressed, the possibility of primary hypothyroidism or of Cushing's syndrome is raised; elevated plasma levels of cortisol and urinary free cortisol and 17-hydroxycorticosteroid values establish the latter diagnosis. The development in a girl of pubic hair and other signs of virilization, such as clitoral enlargement, acne, deepening voice, muscular development, and growth spurt, is caused by congenital virilizing adrenal hyperplasia, virilizing adrenal tumor, or virilizing ovarian tumor; Cushing's syndrome caused by an adrenocortical carcinoma can cause virilization associated with growth failure. Virilizing ovarian tumors can be detected with pelvic ultrasound.

The appearance of pubic hair without other signs of puberty in boys or girls is usually a result of premature adrenarche but may be the first sign of sexual precocity or of adrenal virilism from other causes.

In a girl, breast development associated with dulling and thickening of the vaginal mucosa and enlargement of the labia minora indicates significant estrogen secretion or iatrogenic exposure to estrogen. The differential diagnosis includes true precocious puberty, an estrogen-secreting neoplasm, and a cyst of the ovary. If the plasma levels of gonadotropins are in the pubertal range, if LH pulses of pubertal amplitude are

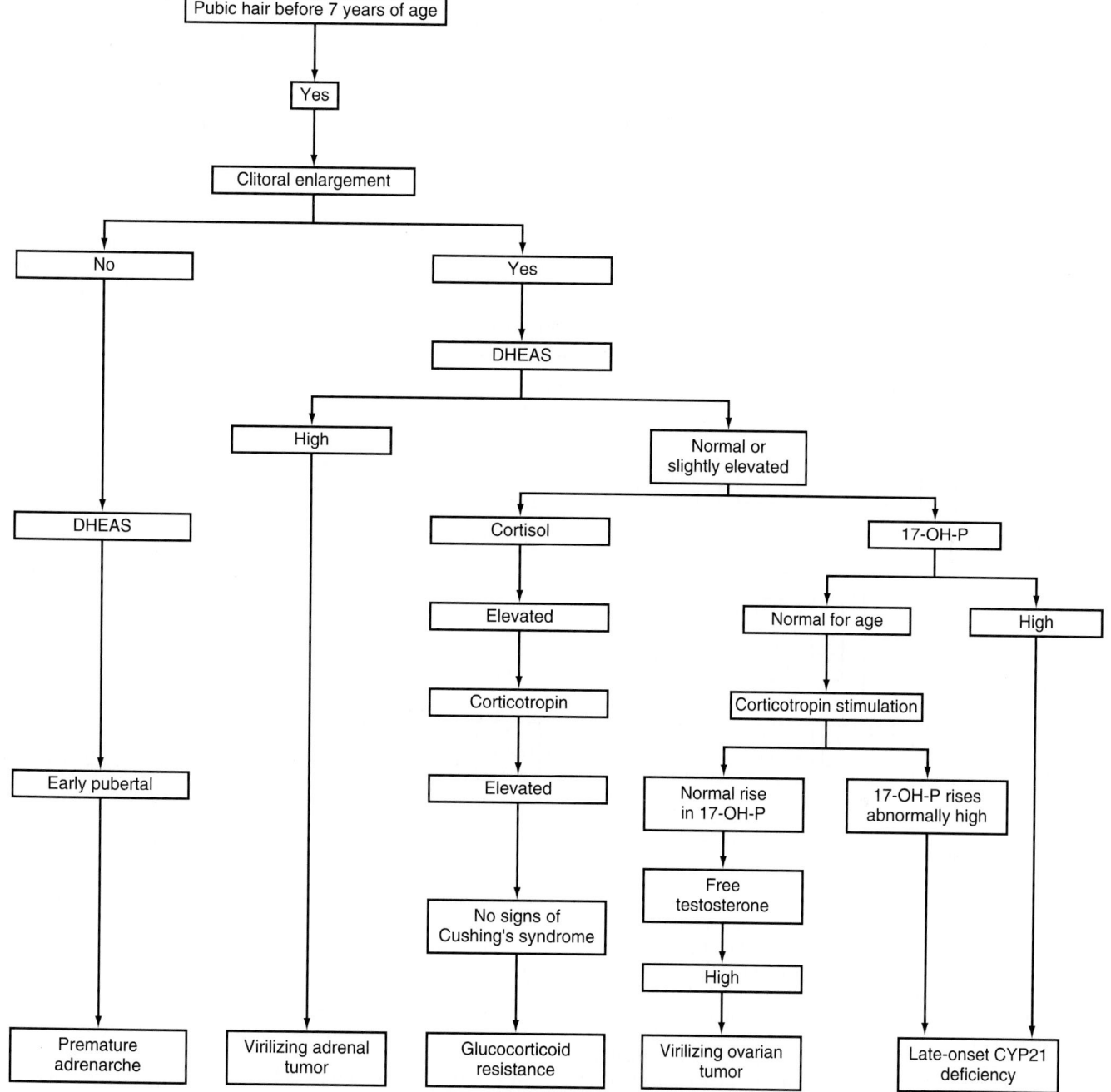

Figure 31–81. The evaluation of pubic hair in normal phenotypic girls before 7 years.

detected, or if the LH response to LHRH is pubertal, true precocious puberty is present. Estrogen levels in girls early in normal or true precocious puberty are in the prepubertal range much of the day, and a single determination may be inadequate to reflect ovarian function[636] (see Fig. 31–61).

A CNS tumor is less likely in girls than in boys to be the cause of this premature reactivation of the hypothalamic LHRH pulse generator–pituitary gonadal system. However, hypothalamic hamartomas are more prevalent in both boys and girls with "idiopathic" true precocious puberty than was previously suspected.

If the level of plasma estradiol is elevated but gonadotropin levels are low, an estrogen-secreting cyst or neoplasm is present. Ovarian tumors of moderate size can be palpated with bimanual examination. Pelvic ultrasonography allows the delineation of ovarian cysts or tumors and determination of

uterine size, and this procedure is an essential component of the diagnostic evaluation.[56] An estrogen-secreting neoplasm of the ovary is usually accompanied by high estradiol concentrations. However, some ovarian cysts are associated with equally high levels of estradiol; the differential diagnosis between such cysts and ovarian neoplasms rarely requires exploratory laparotomy or laparoscopy and usually can be resolved with pelvic ultrasonography and with the use of tumor markers. Breast development in the absence of other estrogen effects is almost always a result of premature thelarche.

Iatrogenic Sexual Precocity

Prepubertal children are remarkably sensitive to exogenous gonadal steroids and may show signs of sexual maturation resulting from overlooked sources of androgens or estro-

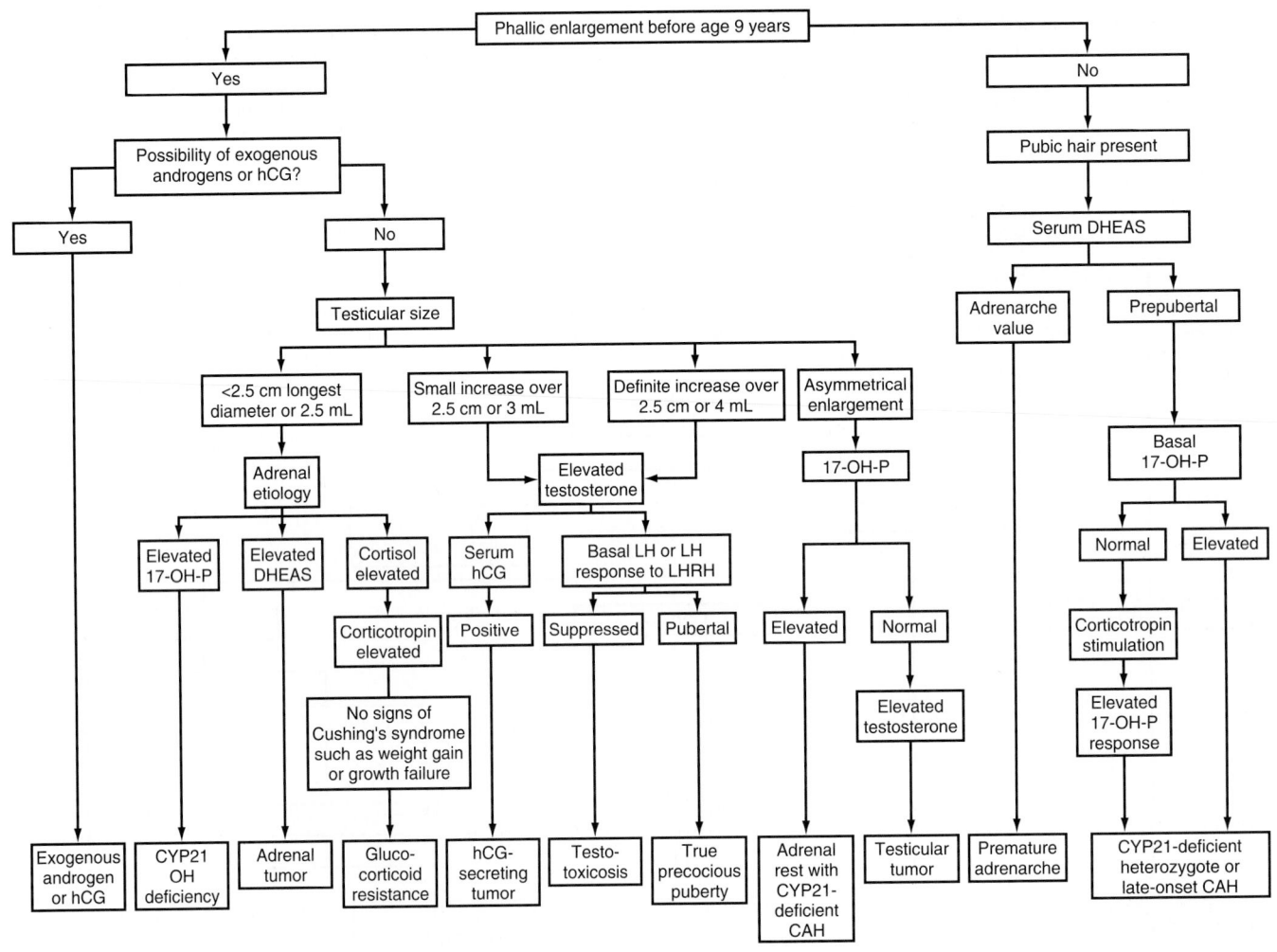

Figure 31–82. The diagnosis of sexual precocity in a phenotypic male.

gens, such as ingested or absorbed tonics, lotions, or creams that contain or are inadvertently contaminated with estrogen.[1344] Children who inhaled estrogen dust have developed sexual precocity. Likewise, estrogens can be absorbed from cosmetics. A short course of estrogen cream may be successful in treating labial adhesions, but long courses can cause breast development or even withdrawal bleeding. In addition to breast development, pigmentation of the areolae and the linea alba and the appearance of pubic hair may be seen in children exposed to estrogen. Epidemics of gynecomastia in boys and thelarche in girls have occurred in schoolchildren in Italy and Puerto Rico.[1345, 1346] During a 10-y period more than 600 cases of gynecomastia in boys and premature thelarche or incomplete sexual precocity in girls were discovered in Puerto Rico. Ovarian cysts were present in two thirds of affected girls.[1347, 1348] The possibility was raised that the food supply had been contaminated by the clandestine use of estrogens as growth-promoting agents for meat production. This contention has not been confirmed by selected analyses of meat, poultry, and milk in Puerto Rico by the U.S. Department of Agriculture, but it has also not been excluded.[1348] Careful investigation of sources of possible exposure to exogenous hormones is mandatory in every case of sexual precocity.

Feminization in Boys and Virilization in Girls (Contrasexual Precocity)

BOYS. Feminization in a boy before the age of puberty is on rare occasions due to an estrogen-secreting adrenal adenoma[1349] or a germ cell tumor including chorionepithelioma (choriocarcinoma). Gynecomastia has been reported in a 1-year-old boy with CYP11B1 deficiency[1350] and in boys with late-onset congenital adrenal hyperplasia. Gynecomastia in prepubertal boys can also be caused by increased extraglandular aromatization of C_{19}-steroids of adrenal origin, such as androstenedione, and hence increased extraglandular estrogen production.[1351, 1352, 1371] Feminizing testicular tumors may cause gynecomastia in boys below age 6 with the Peutz-Jeghers syndrome.[1276–1278] Both testes may be enlarged, and the histology indicates sex cord or Sertoli cell tumors that form annular tubules and often have areas of calcification; estradiol secretion is increased in the basal state and increases further after hCG administration. Otherwise, feminizing Sertoli cell and Leydig cell tumors are very rare in boys.[1280] Ultrasonography or MRI scans of the testes may be useful in the diagnosis.[1280, 1353]

GIRLS. Except for premature adrenarche, virilization in a girl indicates organic disease. Congenital adrenal hyperplasia resulting from CYP21 or CYP11B1 deficiency and androgen-producing tumors of the adrenal can cause virilization, and were discussed earlier as occurring in males. 3β-Hydroxydehydrogenase/$\Delta^{4,5}$-isomerase deficiency is a rare type of congenital adrenal hyperplasia characterized by elevated 17-hydroxypregnenolone, DHEA, and DHEAS levels. Severely affected patients also have mineralocorticoid and glucocorticoid deficiency and may die in infancy. Excess adrenal androgens lead to virilization in utero and to ambiguous external genitalia, including clitoral enlargement in girls with continued virilization after birth[885] (see Chapter 29). Mild forms of this disorder can cause hirsutism in women. 46,XY phenotypic women with incomplete forms of androgen resistance syndrome or with 17β-hydroxysteroid dehydrogenase type 3 deficiency may have virilization as well as breast development at the time of expected puberty. Mutations in the CYP19 gene that encodes aromatase are associated not only with intrauterine masculinization of the external genitalia in affected XX individuals, but also with progressive virilization, lack of female secondary sex characteristics, multicystic ovaries at the age of puberty, tall stature, and osteopenia[96,98] (see Chapter 29).

Cushing's syndrome resulting from adrenal carcinoma usually manifests as growth failure with or without virilization, obesity, moon facies, and hypertension; striae may not appear for months to years later.

The *syndrome of glucocorticoid resistance* causes variable manifestations. Some children have evidence of virilization, including acne, hirsutism, male type baldness, menstrual irregularities, and oligo- or anovulation and infertility.[1354] Dexamethasone decreased the excessive adrenal androgen secretion, virilization, and advancing bone age in a prepubertal body with generalized glucocorticiod resistance.[1355]

Arrhenoblastoma (androblastoma), the most common virilizing ovarian tumor, is rare in children, and lipoid cell tumors and gonadoblastomas are even more unusual sources of androgens.[1356,1357]

Variations of Pubertal Development

PREMATURE THELARCHE. Unilateral or bilateral breast enlargement without other signs of sexual maturation (e.g., sexual hair and growth of the labia minora and the uterus) is common in infancy and childhood and is referred to as premature thelarche. The disorder occurs usually by age 2 and rarely after age 4.[1358] In a study in Minnesota, premature thelarche occurred with an incidence of 21.2 per 100,000 patient-years, 60% of instances occurred between 6 months and 2 years of age, and most regressed within 6 mo to 6 y following diagnosis, although a few persisted until puberty. A 10- to 35-y follow-up was available in 25 cases, and no untoward effects on later health, growth, or fertility were evident.[1359] The breast enlargement is characteristically cyclical and usually regresses after a few months[1360] but occasionally persists for years or lasts until the onset of normal puberty; in about half of affected girls the breast development lasts 3 to 5 y. Significant nipple and areolae development is usually absent, and estrogen-induced thickening and dulling of the vaginal mucosa is uncommon. The uterus on ultrasonography is usually normal (<1.8 mL volume and length <36 mm). Measurement of the ellipsoid volume of the uterus (V = longitudinal diameter × anteroposterior diameter × transverse diameter × 0.523) is the most sensitive and specific discriminator between premature thelarche and early true precocious puberty[57] and provides better early discrimination than the LH response to LHRH. Growth in stature is normal.[422, 1358, 1361–1363]

This common, benign self-limited disorder is compatible with normal pubertal development at an appropriate age; only reassurance and follow-up are usually necessary. In occasional cases as discussed earlier, the appearance of premature thelarche can be the harbinger of further sexual maturation.[422, 1361, 1364, 1371] Because the development may be unilateral, it is important to consider the diagnosis in girls with unilateral breast development so that needless worry about a breast neoplasm does not lead to unnecessary surgery. Indeed, the removal of tissue in premature thelarche may leave the child with no possibility of future breast development. In selected instances, ultrasonography of the breast is useful in distinguishing unilateral premature thelarche from less benign conditions.

The most common cause of breast mass in the pubertal girl is fibroadenoma; while metastatic disease may locate in the pubertal breast, breast carcinoma is rare in children.[1365]

Plasma estradiol levels may be slightly elevated for age in premature thelarche, but some patients have nondetectable levels when studied, possibly because samples are obtained after the transient episode of estrogen secretion or because of the insensitivity of the radioimmunoassay for estradiol, increased aromatase activity in the breast, or end-organ sensitivity. One report described a slight elevation of free estrogen levels.[1366] However, there is usually no increase in plasma levels of thyroxine-binding globulin, as an indicator of estrogen action on circulating plasma proteins,[1367] but TeBG levels for age may be moderately increased.[1035] The urocytogram often reveals an estrogen effect on squamous epithelial cells in the urine.[278, 1368]

The concentration of serum FSH may be in the pubertal range, nocturnal FSH pulsatility has been detected, and the rise in FSH elicited by the administration of LHRH may be augmented for chronologic age, with an FSH/LH ratio higher in precocious thelarche than in normal girls or girls with true precocious puberty.[617, 1358, 1369, 1370] However, these results overlap those in normal prepubertal girls. Ultrasonograms of the ovary often show one or several cysts larger than 0.5 cm that disappear and reappear, usually correlating with changes in the size of the breasts,[1260, 1370] but the volume of the ovary and uterus is prepubertal.[57, 1335] As noted, there is evidence for intermittent secretion of small amounts of estrogen from the ovary. Thus, as postulated for some recurrent ovarian cysts, premature thelarche appears to result from the ovarian response to transient increases in FSH levels and possible variations in ovarian sensitivity to FSH.[617, 1368] The LH response to LHRH is prepubertal in all cases.[617, 1372] Plasma inhibin and activin concentrations have not been reported.

"Exaggerated thelarche" is described as premature thelarche with the added findings of advanced bone age and increased growth rate, and estrogen effects in addition to thelarche. The endocrine measurements in the basal state are in the normal prepubertal range, and after LHRH agonist stimulation, the levels of FSH, but not of LH, rose higher than in control subjects or true precocious puberty.[1373]

PREMATURE ISOLATED MENARCHE. Rarely, girls begin periodic vaginal bleeding at ages 1 to 9 without other signs of secondary sexual development.[1374, 1375] The bleeding can recur for 1 to 6 y and then cease. At the normal age of puberty (3 to 11 y later), secondary sexual development and menses ensue and follow a normal pattern, as does stature. After a normal onset of puberty, women with this variant of pubertal development are fertile. The etiology is uncertain, but it may be a counterpart of premature thelarche. Isolated menarche may appear before other manifestations of sexual precocity in McCune-Albright syndrome and in the premature sexual maturation that can occur in juvenile hypothyroidism.

Before the diagnosis of premature menarche is accepted, all other causes of vaginal bleeding and precocious estrogen secretion and of exposure to exogenous estrogens should be excluded, including neoplasms, granulomas, infection of the vagina or cervix, and foreign bodies.[1376] In a series of 50 girls who had vaginal bleeding before age 10, a local lesion was found in about 50%; half of the latter had a malignant neoplasm (usually a rhabdomyosarcoma).[1377] In another report, a foreign body was responsible for 25% of vaginal bleeding in prepubertal girls.[1378] A careful examination for trauma, such as that caused by sexual abuse, is indicated. Urethral prolapse may be misdiagnosed as vaginal bleeding.

PREMATURE ADRENARCHE (PUBARCHE). Premature adrenarche[1379–1381] is the precocious appearance of pubic hair and/or axillary hair and, less commonly, an apocrine odor, comedones, and acne, without other signs of puberty or virilization; it is characterized by premature, mild hyperandrogenism. In the past, this designation was assigned to the appearance of these clinical features before age 8 in girls or age 9 in boys. While in boys the age of 9 still seems appropriate, the age of 8 can no longer be used for American girls. In a cross-sectional study, involving physical examination in 17,077 girls, striking differences were detected in pubic hair (and breast) development between black and white girls.[44] At 6 years of age, 9.5% (range 5.7 to 16.4%) and, at 8 years of age, 34.3% of black girls had at least Tanner stage 2 pubic hair, whereas 1.4% (range 0.9 to 2.2%) and 7.7% of white girls, at these ages, respectively, had pubic hair (mean ages are shown in Table 31–3). Accordingly, the authors recommend that the diagnosis of premature pubarche be limited to black girls up to 5 years of age and to white American girls younger than age 7, which affects the age at which laboratory studies are initiated unless other signs of virilization such as clitoromegaly or rapid growth are present.

Premature adrenarche is more common in girls than in boys, and the prevalence is increased in children with CNS abnormalities. The electroencephalogram may be abnormal[435, 1081] in the absence of other neurologic findings. Familial occurrence is uncommon.[1382] Premature adrenarche is a nonprogressive disorder compatible with progression of the usual secondary sexual maturation at the normal age of puberty.[123]

Plasma levels of DHEA, DHEAS, androstenedione, testosterone, 17-hydroxyprogesterone, and 17-hydroxypregnenolone are comparable to values normally found in pubic hair stage 2.[640, 1379, 1383–1385] Corticotropin stimulation increases serum DHEA and DHEAS levels and urinary 17-ketosteroid excretion, but the levels of plasma 17-hydroxyprogesterone and 17-hydroxypregnenolone do not increase to the same extent as in virilizing forms of congenital adrenal hyperplasia.[651, 1384, 1386] As in congenital adrenal hyperplasia, dexamethasone suppresses secretion of adrenal androgens and androgen precursors.[1384, 1385] Serum gonadotropin levels in the basal state and after LHRH are in the prepubertal range.[617, 1387] Premature adrenarche occurs independently of gonadarche and is due to some factor other than increased secretion of LHRH or corticotropin (see section on adrenarche).[638] Bone age and height are slightly advanced for chronologic age, but adult height is normal,[1388, 1389] with the rare exception of some individuals with unusually high values of adrenal androgens, hirsutism, acne, and a bone age more than 2.5 SD above the mean value for chronologic age. The functional adrenal hyperandrogenism in most subjects with premature adrenarche is limited to childhood.[1389]

In our view premature adrenarche is a developmentally regulated, normal variation in the differentiation, growth, and function of the zona reticularis of the adrenal cortex (see section on adrenarche), marked biochemically by the precocious increase in the concentration of plasma DHEAS to ≥ 1 μmol/L (≥ 40 μg/dL).[123] The latter is quite likely related to the independent increase of 17,20-lyase activity in the developing zona reticularis mediated by the increased phosphorylation of serine residues on the CYP17 enzyme, and the increased abundance of electron-donating redox partners such as cytochrome P450 oxidoreductase and cytochrome b-5, essential for the 17,20-lyase activity of this enzyme (Fig. 31–44).[651] Nonetheless, the factors that regulate the development and function of the zona reticularis, independent of corticotropin, are elusive.

In the past, the failure to recognize the earlier onset of adrenarche, particularly the striking ethnic differences in black and Mediterranean populations, has contributed to the overdiagnosis of premature adrenarche[1388, 1390, 1391] and, in some instances, needless laboratory studies.

The concept of "exaggerated adrenarche"[1392] was advanced[1393] in relation to a postulated childhood antecedent of

the polycystic ovary syndrome, the hallmarks of which are hyperandrogenism, hirsutism, anovulation, amenorrhea or oligomenorrhea, (commonly) insulin resistance and compensatory hyperinsulinemia unrelated to the hyperandrogenemia, and, in about 50% of affected women, obesity.[1390, 1394–1398] This concept has been extended to include rare instances of premature adrenarche associated with excessive responses of 17-hydroxypregnenolone, DHEAS, and androstenedione to corticotropin found in women with functional adrenal hyperandrogenism. While premature adrenarche is an apparent risk factor for the later development of the polycystic ovary syndrome and functional ovarian hyperandrogenism in adolescent and adult women, the magnitude of this risk is not established but appears to be very low.[1389, 1392] However, some ethnic groups may carry a higher risk for this association,[1399–1401] especially if decreased insulin sensitivity and acanthosis nigricans accompany the premature adrenarche.[1400] Of interest, the adrenal steroid pattern in the black and Hispanic patients in the latter study[1401] did not differ from that in children with uncomplicated premature adrenarche.

Premature pubarche can be associated with nonclassic congenital adrenal hyperplasia caused by homozygous or compound heterozygous missense mutations in the CYP21 gene encoding the CYP21 enzyme[1402] and can readily be detected by a plasma 17-hydroxyprogesterone response to corticotropin that is at least 6 SD above the mean value. The prevalence of CYP21 deficiency in children with premature adrenarche is low,[1389, 1392, 1403] except in some ethnic groups[1404–1406] (e.g., Hispanics, Italians, and Ashkenazi Jews; see Chapter 29) in which the prevalence may be as high as 20 to 30%.[1405, 1406] CYP21 deficiency can be excluded by determining the plasma 17-hydroxyprogesterone response to corticotropin. Premature adrenarche is also associated with the rare nonclassic CYP11B1 deficiency.

There has been controversy about the prevalence and significance of 3β-hydroxysteroid dehydrogenase deficiency, and the pervasive belief that a mutation in the gene encoding this enzyme was a common cause of premature adrenarche and nonclassic 3β-HSD deficiency.[1405] The possibility of a mutation in the open reading frame of 3β-HSD of the type 2 or type 1 gene has been excluded as any but an uncommon cause of this condition.[1407–1409] Mutations in the 3β-HSD type 2 gene can cause a 17-hydroxypregnenolone response to corticotropin that exceeds or equals the mean normal value by 6 SD. Of 26 families studied, only one family with an alanine 82–to–threonine mutation had affected females with premature pubarche; in this family the affected boy had male pseudohermaphroditism.[1410] Thus a mutation in the 3β-HSD type 2 or type 1 gene is an uncommon cause of premature pubarche, exaggerated adrenarche, or hirsutism in adolescent girls and women. The cause of the "mild deficiency" in 3β-HSD activity is unknown but may be multifactorial and lead to a wide range in the secretory capacity of the zona reticularis. A family constellation is described with an autosomal dominant pattern of inheritance[1382] of elevated adrenal androgens and androgen precursors associated with premature pubarche; affected individuals subsequently developed hirsutism and anovulation.

DHEA is a stimulus to sebaceous gland activity, and prepubertal acne or comedones may develop in association with elevated serum DHEAS levels in some children without the appearance of pubic hair, suggesting that a variant of premature adrenarche may manifest in this manner.[1411–1413]

Generalized effects of androgen such as clitoral or penile enlargement, rapid growth, hirsutism, or deepening of the voice exclude the diagnosis of premature adrenarche and indicate a more severe form of hyperandrogenism.

ADOLESCENT GYNECOMASTIA. (See Chapter 17). Normal pubertal boys may have either unilateral breast enlargement (approximately 25% of boys)[1414] or bilateral breast enlargement (approximately 50 to 65% of boys)[1415] of varying degrees, commonly between chronologic ages 14 to 14 1/2 years or pubic hair stages 3 and 4. In these boys the plasma concentrations of testosterone and estrogen are normal for the stage of puberty. Pubertal gynecomastia is usually associated with an elevated ratio of the concentration of serum estradiol to testosterone.[1416–1419] In a prospective study adolescent boys with gynecomastia had a lower mean free testosterone concentration, a lower weight, higher plasma TeBG levels, and a tendency toward earlier onset of puberty and more rapid progression through puberty.[1414] In one study the concentration ratio of plasma androstenedione to estrone and estradiol and the ratio of DHEAS to estrone and estradiol were low in boys with pubertal gynecomastia who had normal ratios of plasma testosterone to estrone and estradiol. It was postulated that either decreased adrenal production of androgens or, more likely, increased peripheral conversion of adrenal androgens to estrogens was a factor in the development of pubertal gynecomastia.[1420] An elevated ratio of testosterone to dihydrotestosterone, presumably due to a decrease in 5α-reductase activity, has been suggested in the etiology of gynecomastia as well.[1421] Estrogen, androgen, and progesterone receptors in the nuclei of ductal cells were detected in all 30 patients with gynecomastia, but CYP19 immunoreactivity was detected in only 37% of cases and was present in stromal cells.[1422]

Pubertal gynecomastia usually resolves spontaneously within 1 to 2 y of onset, and reassurance and continued observation are often adequate treatment. Nevertheless, some boys have conspicuous gynecomastia and sufficient psychological distress to warrant a reduction mammoplasty with the use of a circumareolar approach. Liposuction is an alternative approach, but its efficacy in adolescent gynecomastia remains to be established. Rarely, untreated gynecomastia persists into adulthood, as illustrated by a patient who had persistent unilateral gynecomastia that began during puberty associated with contralateral Poland's syndrome of hypoplasia of the chest, breast tissue, and nipple.[1423]

Gynecomastia is a component of Klinefelter's syndrome, of anorchism, primary and secondary hypogonadism, biosynthetic defects in testosterone synthesis, increased aromatase activity in adipose and other tissues, Sertoli cell tumors, adventitious exposure to estrogens in meat or cosmetics, and all variants of the androgen resistance syndromes. These disorders usually have characteristic findings that allow ready differentiation from the normal gynecomastia of puberty[885] (see Chapter 29). Gynecomastia has been described in association with the administration of drugs such as cimetidine, spironolactone, digitalis, and phenothiazines as well as with GH therapy[1424] and the use of marijuana (see Chapter 17). Persistent pubertal macromastia appears to be associated more frequently with specific endocrine abnormalities.

Macro-orchidism

The fragile X syndrome is associated with developmental delay, a long face and large prominent ears, and macro-orchidism in 80% of affected pubertal boys. Macro-orchidism may be evident only after careful measurements. The enlarged testes are due to increased interstitial volume and excessive connective tissue, including increased peritubular collagen fibers,[1425] rather than to an increase in the seminiferous tubules. Enlargement of the testes is demonstrable in the prepubertal period in most patients with fragile X syndrome, but true macro-orchidism (>4 cm) only develops in the late prepubertal period.[1426]

Macro-orchidism, without androgenization, is an occasional finding in prepubertal boys with long-standing primary hypothyroidism. This form of testicular enlargement appears to result from increased FSH secretion independent of a pubertal increase in LH secretion or a pubertal LH response to LHRH. Adrenal rests in congenital adrenal hyperplasia (see Chapter 29) and lymphomas can cause bilateral macro-orchidism. Macro-orchidism was a feature of severe aromatase deficiency in a young man[98] and in men with FSH-secreting pituitary macroadenomas. Bilateral megalotestis (≥26 mL testicular volume) in adults can be a normal variant.[1427] One may speculate that some instances of bilateral macro-orchidism are due to a heterozygous constitutive activating mutation of the FSH receptor.

Disorders of Sexual Differentiation with Both Virilization and Feminization at Puberty

Virilization as well as feminization at puberty may occur in a phenotypic female who has a 46,XY karyotype in certain types of male pseudohermaphroditism (see Chapter 29). Patients with 17β-hydroxysteroid dehydrogenase type 3 deficiency (a testosterone biosynthetic defect) and incomplete forms of androgen resistance (resulting from defects in the androgen receptor) may present in this manner; however, ambiguous genitalia are usually noted early in life in these conditions. True hermaphrodites with ovarian and testicular tissue may also undergo both virilization and feminization at puberty.[885]

REFERENCES

1. Grumbach MM. Onset of puberty. In: Berenberg SR, ed. Puberty: Biologic and Social Components. Leiden: HE Stenfert Kroese, 1975: 1–21.
2. Bogin B. Growth and development: recent evolutionary and biocultural research. In: Boaz NT, Wolfe DL, eds. Biological Anthropology: The State of the Science. Bend, OR: International Institute for Human Evolutionary Research, 1995: 49–70.
3. Bogin B. Adolescence in evolutionary perspective. Acta Paediatr Suppl 1994; 406:29–35.
4. Conroy GC, Kuykendall K. Paleopediatrics: or when did human infants really become human? Am J Phys Anthropol 1995; 98: 121–131.
5. Tattersall I. Out of Africa again . . . and again? Sci Am 1997; 276(4):60–67.
6. Mayr E. The objects of selection. Proc Natl Acad Sci USA 1997; 94:2091–2094.
7. Aristotle. De generatione animalium. In: Tanner JM, ed. A History of the Study of Human Growth. Cambridge: Cambridge University Press, 1981: 7.
8. Marshall WA, Tanner JM. Puberty. In: Falkner F, Tanner JM, eds. Human Growth. Vol 2. Postnatal Growth: Neurobiology. 2nd ed. New York: Plenum, 1986: 171–209.
9. Tanner JM, ed. A History of the Study of Human Growth. Cambridge: Cambridge University Press, 1981: 286–298.
10. Tanner JM. Growth at Adolescence. Springfield, IL: Charles C Thomas, 1962.
11. Wyshak G, Frisch RE. Evidence for a secular trend in age of menarche. N Engl J Med 1982; 306:1033–1035.
12. Gerver WJ, De Bruin R, Drayer NM. A persisting secular trend for body measurements in Dutch children: the Oosterwolde II Study. Acta Paediatr 1994; 83:812–814.
13. Veronesi FM, Gueresi P. Trend in menarcheal age and socioeconomic influence in Bologna (northern Italy). Ann Hum Biol 1994; 21:187–196.
14. Delemarre-Van de Waal HA. Environmental factors influencing growth and pubertal development. Environ Health Perspect 1993; 101 (Suppl 2):39–44.
15. Buffon H. Histoire naturelle. In: Tanner JM, ed. A History of the Study of Human Growth. Cambridge: Cambridge University Press, 1981:83.
16. Daw SF. Age of boys' puberty in Leipzig, 1727–1749, as indicated by voice breaking in J. S. Bach's choir members. Hum Biol 1970; 42:87–89.
17. Kill V. Stature and growth of Norwegian men during past 200 years. Skr Nor Vidensk Akad 1939; 2(6):1–175.
18. Van Wieringen. Secular growth changes. In: Falkner F, Tanner JM, eds. Human Growth. Vol 3. Methodology, Ecological, Genetic, and Nutritional Effects on Growth. 2nd ed. New York: Plenum Press, 1986: 307–331.
19. Zacharias L, Wurtman RJ, Schatzoff M. Sexual maturation in contemporary American girls. Am J Obstet Gynecol 1970; 108:833–846.
20. Nicholson AB, Hanley C. Indices of physiological maturity: derivation and interrelationships. Child Dev 1953; 24:3–38.
21. Damon A. Larger body size and earlier menarche: the end may be in sight. Soc Biol 1974; 21:8–11.

22. Zacharias L, Rand M, Wurtman R. A prospective study of sexual development in American girls: the statistics of menarche. Obstet Gynecol Surv 1976; 31:325–337.

23. MacMahon B. Age at menarche. In: National Health Survey. DHEW Publication No. (HRA) 74-1615, Series 11, No. 133, Washington, DC: Government Printing Office, 1973.

24. Harlan WR, Harlan EA, Grillo GP. Secondary sex characteristics of girls 12 to 17 years of age: the U.S. Health Examination Survey. J Pediatr 1980; 96:1074–1078.

25. Hartz AJ, Barboriak PN, Wong A, et al. The association of obesity with infertility and related menstrual abnormalities in women. Int J Obes 1979; 3:57–73.

26. Warren MP. The effects of exercise on pubertal progression and reproductive function in girls. J Clin Endocrinol Metab 1980; 51:1150–1157.

27. Osler DC, Crawford JD. Examination of the hypothesis of a critical weight at menarche in ambulatory and bedridden mentally retarded girls. Pediatrics 1973; 51:674–679.

28. Zacharias L, Wurtman RJ. Blindness: its relation to age of menarche. Science 1964; 144:1154–1155.

29. Freyre EA, Ortiz MV. The effect of altitude on adolescent growth and development. J Adolesc Health Care 1988; 9:144–149.

30. Zacharias L, Wurtman RJ. Age at menarche. N Engl J Med 1969; 280:868–875.

31. Duke PM, Litt IF, Gross RT. Adolescents' self-assessment of sexual maturation. Pediatrics 1980; 66:918–920.

32. Dorn LD, Susman EJ, Nottelmann ED, et al. Perceptions of puberty: adolescent, parent, and health care personnel. Dev Psychol 1990; 26:322–329.

33. Rillema JA. Development of the mammary gland and lactation. Trends Endocrinol Metab 1994; 5:149–154.

34. Drife JO. Breast development in puberty. Ann N Y Acad Sci 1986; 464:58–65.

35. Stratz CH. Der Korper des Kindes und Seine Pflege. Stuttgart: Ferdinand Enke, 1909: 245.

36. Reynolds EL, Wines JV. Individualized differences in physical changes associated with adolescence in girls. Am J Dis Child 1948; 75:329–350.

37. Rohn RD. Papilla (nipple) development during female puberty. Adolesc Health Care 1982; 2:217–220.

38. McCann J. Color Atlas of Child Sexual Abuse. Chicago: Year Book Medical, 1989.

39. Zachmann M, Prader A, Kind HP, et al. Testicular volume during adolescence: cross-sectional and longitudinal studies. Helv Paediatr Acta 1974; 29:61–72.

40. Taskinen S, Taavitsainen M, Wikström S. Measurement of testicular volume: comparison of three different methods. J Urol 1996; 155:930–933.

40a. Biro FM, Lucky AW, Huster GA, et al. Pubertal staging in boys. J Pediatr 1995; 127:40–46. Erratum 127:674.

41. Sutherland RS, Kogan BA, Baskin LS, et al. The effect of prepubertal androgen exposure on adult penile length. J Urol 1996; 156:783–787.

42. Harlan WR, Grillo GP, Coroni-Huntley J, et al. Secondary sex characteristics of boys 12 to 17 years of age: the U.S. Health Examination Survey. J Pediatr 1979; 95:293–297.

43. Roche AF, Wellens R, Attie KM, et al. The timing of sexual maturation in a group of U.S. white youths. J Pediatr Endocrinol Metab 1995; 8:11–18.

44. Herman-Giddens ME, Slora EJ, Wasserman RC, et al. Secondary sexual characteristics and menses in young girls seen in office practice: a study from the Pediatric Research in Office Settings Network. Pediatrics 1997; 99:505–512.

45. Morrison JA, Barton B, Biro FM, et al. Sexual maturation and obesity in 9- and 10-year-old black and white girls: the National Heart, Lung, and Blood Institute Growth and Health Study. J Pediatr 1994; 124:889–895.

46. Berkey CS, Dockery DW, Wang X, et al. Longitudinal height velocity standards for U.S. adolescents. Stat Med 1993; 12:403–414.

47. Peschel ER, Peschel RE. Medical insights into the castrati in opera. Am Sci 1987; 75:578–583.

48. Karlberg P, Taranger J. The somatic development of children in a Swedish urban community. Acta Paediatr Scand [Suppl] 1976; 258:1–148.

49. Addy M, Hunter ML, Kingdon A, et al. An 8-year study of changes in oral hygiene and periodontal health during adolescence. Int J Paediatr Dent 1994; 4:75–80.

50. Nakagawa S, Fujii H, Machida Y, et al. A longitudinal study from prepuberty to puberty of gingivitis. correlation between the occurrence of Prevotella intermedia and sex hormones. J Clin Periodontol 1994; 21:658–665.

51. Lucky AW, Biro FM, Simbartl LA, et al. Predictors of severity of acne vulgaris in young adolescent girls: results of a five-year longitudinal study. J Pediatr 1997; 130:30–39.

52. Traupe H, Von Mühlendahl KE, Brämswig J, et al. Acne of the fulminans type following testosterone therapy in three excessively tall boys. Arch Dermatol 1988; 124:414–417.

53. Grumbach MM, Gluckman PD. The human fetal hypothalamus and pituitary gland: the maturation of neuroendocrine mechanisms controlling the secretion of fetal pituitary growth hormone, prolactin, gonadotropin, adrenocorticotropin-related peptides and thyrotropin. In: Tulchinsky D, Little AB, eds. Maternal-Fetal Endocrinology, 2nd ed. Philadelphia: WB Saunders, 1994: 193–261.

53a. Rabinovici J, Jaffe RB. Development and regulation of growth and differentiated function in human and subhuman primate fetal gonads. Endocr Rev 1990; 11:532–557.

54. Ross GT. Follicular development: the life cycle of the follicle and puberty. In: Grumbach MM, Sizonenko PC, Aubert ML, eds. Control of the Onset of Puberty. Baltimore: Williams & Wilkins, 1990: 376–386.

55. Peters H, Byskov AG, Grinsted J. Follicular growth in fetal and prepubertal ovaries of humans and other primates. Clin Endocrinol Metab 1978; 7:469–485.

55a. Shikone T, Yamoto M, Kokawa K, et al: Apoptosis of human corpora lutea during cyclic luteal regression and early pregnancy. Clin Endocrinol Metab 1996; 81:2376–2380.

56. Fleischer AC, Shawker TH. The role of sonography in pediatric gynecology. Clin Obstet Gynecol 1987; 30:735–746.

57. Haber HP, Wollmann HA, Ranke MB. Pelvic ultrasonography: early differentiation between isolated premature thelarche and central precocious puberty. Eur J Pediatr 1995; 154:182–186.

58. Salardi S, Orsini LF, Cacciari E, et al. Pelvic ultrasonography in premenarcheal girls: relation to puberty and sex hormone concentrations. Arch Dis Child 1985; 60:120–125.

59. Bridges NA, Cooke A, Healy MJ, et al. Standards for ovarian volume in childhood and puberty. Fertil Steril 1993; 60:456–460.

60. Onat J, Ertem B. Age at menarche: relationship to socioeconomic status, growth rate in stature and weight, and skeletal and sexual maturation. Am J Hum Biol 1995; 7:741–750.

61. Apter D, Vihko R. Serum pregnenolone, progesterone, 17-hydroxy-progesterone, testosterone, and 5-alpha-dihydrotestosterone during female puberty. J Clin Endocrinol Metab 1977; 45:1039–1048.

62. Metcalf MG, MacKenzie JA. Incidence of ovulation in young women. J Biosoc Sci 1980; 12:345–352.

63. Lemarchand-Beraud T, Zufferey MM, Reymond M. Maturation of the hypothalamo-pituitary ovarian axis in adolescent girls. J Clin Endocrinol Metab 1982; 54:241–246.

64. Cortes D, Muller J, Skakkebaek NE. Proliferation of Sertoli cells during development of the human testis assessed by stereological methods. Int J Androl 1987; 10:589–596.

65. Gondos B, Kogan SJ. Testicular development during puberty. In: Grumbach MM, Sizonenko PC, Aubert ML, eds. Control of the Onset of Puberty. Baltimore: Williams & Wilkins, 1990: 387–402.

66. Aumuller G, Riva A. Morphology and functions of the human seminal vesicle. Andrologia 1992; 24:183–196.

67. Paltiel HJ, Rupich RC, Babcock DS. Maturational changes in arterial impedance of the normal testis in boys: Doppler sonographic study. Am J Roentgenol 1994; 163:1189–1193.

68. Nielsen CT, Skakkebaek NE, Darling JA, et al. Longitudinal study of testosterone and luteinizing hormone (LH) in relation to spermarche, pubic hair, height, and sitting height in normal boys. Acta Endocrinol [Suppl] 1986; 279:98–106.

69. Richardson DW, Short RV. Time of onset of sperm production in boys. J Biosoc Sci Suppl 1978; 5:15–24.

70. Janczewski Z, Bablok L. Semen characteristics in pubertal boys. II. Semen quality in relation to bone age. Arch Androl 1985; 15:207–211.

71. Janczewski Z, Bablok L. Semen characteristics in pubertal boys. III. Semen quality and somatosexual development. Arch Androl 1985; 15:213–218.

72. Laron Z, Arad J, Gurewitz R, et al. Age at first conscious ejaculation: a milestone in male puberty. Helv Paediatr Acta 1980; 35:13–20.

73. Pedersen JL, Nysom K, Jørgensen M, et al. Spermaturia and puberty. Arch Dis Child 1993; 69:384–387.

74. Nysom K, Pedersen JL, Jørgensen M, et al. Spermaturia in two normal boys without other signs of puberty. Acta Paediatr 1994; 83:520–521.

75. Marshall WA, Tanner JM. Variations in pattern of pubertal changes in girls. Arch Dis Child 1969; 44:291–303.

76. Largo RH, Prader A. Pubertal development in Swiss girls. Helv Paediatr Acta 1983; 38:229–243.

77. Tanner JM, Whitehouse RH, Marubini E, et al. The adolescent growth spurt of boys and girls of the Harpenden Growth Study. Ann Hum Biol 1976; 3:109–126.

78. Largo RH, Gasser TH, Prader A. Analysis of the adolescent growth spurt using smoothing spline functions. Ann Hum Biol 1978; 5:421–434.

79. Karlberg J, Fryer JG, Engstrom I, Karlberg P. Analysis of linear growth using a mathematical model. II. From 3 to 21 years of age. Acta Paediatr Scand Suppl 1987; 337:12–29.

80. Limony Y, Zadik Z, Pic AK, et al. Improved method for predicting adult height of pubertal boys using a mathematical model. Horm Res 1993; 40:117–122.

81. Tanner JM, Davies PSW. Clinical longitudinal standards for height and height velocity for North American children. J Pediatr 1985; 107:317–329.

82. Vanden Eynde B, Vienne D, Vuylsteke-Wauters M, et al. Aerobic power and pubertal peak height velocity in Belgian boys. Eur J Appl Physiol 1988; 57:430–434.

83. Calvo MS, Eyre DR, Gundberg CM. Molecular basis and clinical application of biologic markers of bone turnover. Endocr Rev 1996; 17:333–368.

84. Johansen JS, Giwercman A, Hartwell D, et al. Serum bone Gla-protein as a marker of bone growth in children and adolescents: correlation with age, height, serum insulin-like growth factor I, and serum testosterone. J Clin Endocrinol Metab 1988; 67:273–278.

85. Crofton PM, Stirling HF, Schönau E, et al. Bone alkaline phosphatase and collagen markers as early predictors of height velocity response to growth-promoting treatments in short normal children. Clin Endocrinol (Oxf) 1996; 44:385–394.

86. Fujimoto S, Kubo T, Tanaka H, et al. Urinary pyridinoline and deoxypyridinoline in healthy children and in children with growth hormone deficiency. J Clin Endocrinol Metab 1995; 80:1922–1928.

87. Rauch F, Schnabel D, Seibel MJ, et al. Urinary excretion of galactosyl-hydroxylysine is a marker of growth in children. J Clin Endocrinol Metab 1995; 80:1295–1300.

88. Garbagnati E. Urate changes in lean and obese boys during pubertal development. Metabolism: Clin Exp 1996; 45:203–205.

89. Bourguignon JP. Linear growth as a function of age at onset of puberty and sex steroid dosage: therapeutic implications. Endocr Rev 1988; 9:467–488.

90. Hägg U, Taranger J. Height and height velocity in early, average, and late maturers followed to the age of 25: a prospective, longitudinal study of Swedish urban children from birth to adulthood. Ann Hum Biol 1991; 18:47–56.

91. McKusick VA. Heritable Disorders of Connective Tissue. St. Louis: CV Mosby, 1972: 73–74.

92. Tanner JM, Whitehouse RH, Hughes PCR, et al. Relative importance of growth hormone and sex steroids for the growth at puberty of trunk length, limb length, and muscle width in growth hormone–deficient children. J Pediatr 1976; 89:1000–1008.

93. Elster AD, Chen MY, Williams DW, Key LL. Pituitary gland: MR imaging of physiologic hypertrophy in adolescence. Radiology 1990; 174:681–685.

94. Attie KM, Ramirez NR, Conte FA, et al. The pubertal growth spurt in eight patients with true precocious puberty and growth hormone deficiency: evidence for a direct role of sex steroids. J Clin Endocrinol Metab 1990; 71:975–983.

95. Rogol AD. Growth at puberty: interaction of androgens and growth hormone. Med Sci Sports Exerc 1994; 26:767–770.

96. Conte FA, Grumbach MM, Ito Y, et al. A syndrome of female pseudohermaphrodism, hypergonadotropic hypogonadism, and multicystic ovaries associated with missense mutations in the gene encoding aromatase (P450arom). J Clin Endocrinol Metab 1994; 78:1287–1292.

97. Smith EP, Boyd J, Frank GR, et al. Estrogen resistance caused by a mutation in the estrogen-receptor gene in a man. N Engl J Med 1994; 331:1056–1061.

98. Morishima A, Grumbach MM, Simpson ER, et al. Aromatase deficiency in male and female siblings caused by a novel mutation and the physiological role of estrogens. J Clin Endocrinol Metab 1995; 80:3689–3698.

99. Miller JD, Tannenbaum GS, Colle E, et al. Daytime pulsatile growth hormone secretion during childhood and adolescence. J Clin Endocrinol Metab 1982; 55:989–994.

100. Ross JL, Pescovitz OH, Barnes K, et al. Growth hormone secretory dynamics in children with precocious puberty. J Pediatr 1987; 110:369–372.

101. Costin G, Kaufman FR. Growth hormone secretory patterns in children with short stature. J Pediatr 1987; 110:362–368.

102. Costin G, Kaufman FR, Brasel JA. Growth hormone secretory dynamics in subjects with normal stature. J Pediatr 1989; 115:537–544.

103. Garnier P, Raynaud F, Job JC. Growth hormone secretion during sleep. I. Comparison with GH responses to conventional pharmacologic stimuli in pubertal and early pubertal short subjects: effects of treatment with human GH in patients with discrepant measurements of GH secretion. Horm Res 1988; 29:133–139.

104. Link K, Blizzard RM, Evans WS, et al. The effect of androgens on the pulsatile release and the twenty-four-hour mean concentration of growth hormone in peripubertal males. J Clin Endocrinol Metab 1986; 62:159–164.

105. Martha PM Jr, Rogol AD, Veldhuis JD. Alterations in the pulsatile properties of circulating growth hormone concentrations during puberty in boys. J Clin Endocrinol Metab 1989; 69:563–570.

106. Mauras N, Blizzard RM, Link K, et al. Augmentation of growth hormone secretion during puberty: evidence for a pulse amplitude–modulated phenomenon. J Clin Endocrinol Metab 1987; 64:596–601.

107. Wennink JM, Delemarre-van de Waal HA, Schoemaker R, et al. Growth hormone secretion patterns in relation to LH and estradiol secretion throughout normal female puberty. Acta Endocrinol (Copenh) 1991; 124:129–135.

108. Martha PM, Gorman KM, Blizzard RM, et al. Endogenous growth hormone secretion and clearance rates in normal boys, as determined by deconvolution analysis: relationship to age, pubertal status, and body mass. J Clin Endocrinol Metab 1992; 74:336–344.

109. Marin G, Domene HM, Barnes KM, et al. The effects of estrogen priming and puberty on the growth hormone response to standardized treadmill exercise and arginine-insulin in normal girls and boys. J Clin Endocrinol Metab 1994; 79:537–541.

110. Bouix O, Brun JF, Fedou C, et al. Plasma beta-endorphin, corticotrophin, and growth hormone responses to exercise in pubertal and prepubertal children. Horm Metab Res 1994; 26:195–199.

111. Loche S, Cambiaso P, Carta D, et al. The growth hormone–releasing activity of hexarelin, a new synthetic hexapeptide, in short normal and obese children and in hypopituitary subjects. J Clin Endocrinol Metab 1995; 80:674–678.

112. Metzger DL, Kerrigan JR. Estrogen receptor blockade with tamoxifen diminishes growth hormone secretion in boys: evidence for a stimulatory role of endogenous estrogens during male adolescence. J Clin Endocrinol Metab 1994; 79:513–518.

113. Kerrigan JR, Veldhuis JD, Rogol AD. Androgen-receptor blockade enhances pulsatile luteinizing hormone production in late pubertal males: evidence for a hypothalamic site of physiologic androgen feedback action. Pediatr Res 1994; 35:102–106.

114. Keenan BS, Richards GE, Ponder SW, et al. Androgen-stimulated pubertal growth: the effects of testosterone and dihydrotestosterone on growth hormone and insulin-like growth factor-I in the treatment of short stature and delayed puberty. J Clin Endocrinol Metab 1993; 76:996–1001.

115. Mansfield MJ, Rudlin CR, Crigler JF Jr, et al. Changes in growth and serum growth hormone and plasma somatomedin-C levels during suppression of gonadal sex steroid secretion in girls with central precocious puberty. J Clin Endocrinol Metab 1988; 66:3–9.

116. Harris DA, Van Vliet G, Egli CA, et al. Somatomedin-C in normal puberty and in true precocious puberty before and after treatment with a potent luteinizing hormone–releasing hormone agonist. J Clin Endocrinol Metab 1985; 61:152–159.

117. Rimoin DL, Merimee TJ, Rabinowitz D, McKusick VA. Genetic aspects of clinical endocrinology. Recent Prog Horm Res 1968; 24:365–437.

118. Phillips JA III. Inherited defects in growth hormone synthesis and action. In: Scriver CR, Beaudet AL, Sly WS, et al. eds. The Metabolic Basis of Inherited Disease. 7th ed. New York: McGraw-Hill, 1995: 3023–3044.

119. Aynsley-Green A, Zachmann M, Prader A. Interrelation of the therapeutic effects of growth hormone and testosterone on growth in hypopituitarism. J Pediatr 1976; 89:992–999.

120. Bala RM, Lopatka J, Leung A. Serum immunoreactive somatomedin levels in normal adults, pregnant women at term, children at various ages, and children with constitutionally delayed growth. J Clin Endocrinol Metab 1981; 52:508–512.

121. Zachmann M, Prader A, Sobel E, et al. Pubertal growth in patients with androgen insensitivity: indirect evidence for the importance of estrogens in pubertal growth of girls. J Pediatr 1986; 108:694–697.

122. Klein KO, Baron J, Colli MJ, et al. Estrogen levels in childhood determined by an ultrasensitive recombinant cell bioassay. J Clin Invest 1994; 94:2475–2480.

123. Grumbach MM, Richards GE, Conte FA, et al. Clinical disorders of adrenal function and puberty: an assessment of the role of the adrenal cortex in normal and abnormal puberty in man and evidence for an ACTH-like pituitary adrenal androgen stimulating hormone. In: James VHT, Serio M, Giusti G, et al, eds. The Endocrine Function of the Human Adrenal Cortex, Serono Symposium. New York: Academic Press, 1977:583–612.

124. Van Wyk JJ, Grumbach MM. Syndrome of precocious menstruation and galactorrhea in juvenile hypothyroidism: an example of hormonal overlap in pituitary feedback. J Pediatr 1960; 57:416–435.

125. Greulich WS, Pyle SI. Radiographic Atlas of Skeletal Development of the Hand and Wrist. Stanford, CA: Stanford University Press, 1959.

126. Tanner JM, Whitehouse RH, Marshall WA, et al. Assessment of Skeletal Maturity and Prediction of Adult Height: TW 2 Method. New York: Academic, 1975.

127. Marshall WA. Inter-relationships of skeletal maturation, sexual development, and somatic growth in man. Ann Hum Biol 1974; 1:29–40.

128. Loesch DZ, Hopper JL, Rogucka E, et al. Timing and genetic rapport between growth in skeletal maturity and height around puberty: similarities and differences between girls and boys. Am J Hum Genet 1995; 56:753–759.

129. Hauspie R, Bielicki T, Koniarek J: Skeletal maturity at onset of the adolescent growth spurt and at peak height velocity for growth in height: a threshold effect? Ann Hum Biol 1995; 18:23–29.

130. Bayley N, Pinneau SR. Tables for predicting adult height from skeletal age: revised for use with the Greulich-Pyle standards. J Pediatr 1952; 40:423–441.

131. Roche AF, Wainer H, Thissen D. The RWT method for the prediction of adult stature. Pediatrics 1975; 56:1026–1033.

132. Walker RN. Standards for somatotyping children. I. Prediction of young adult height from children's growth data. Ann Hum Biol 1974; 1:149–158.

133. Roche AF. Skeletal Maturity of Children 6–11 Years: Racial, Geographic Area of Residence, Socioeconomic Differentials. In: National Health Survey. DHEW Vital and Health Statistics Series 11, No. 149. Washington, DC: Government Printing Office, 1975.

134. Tanner JM, Gibbons RD. Automatic bone age measurement using computerized image analysis. J Pediatr Endocrinol 1994; 7:141–145.

135. Gross GW, Boone JM, Bishop DM. Pediatric skeletal age: determination with neural networks. Radiology 1995; 195:689–695.

136. Van Teunenbroek A, De Waal W, Roks A, et al. Computer-aided skeletal age scores in healthy children, girls with Turner syndrome, and in children with constitutionally tall stature. Pediatr Res 1996; 39:360–367.

137. Roberts CD, Vogtle L, Stevenson RD: Effect of hemiplegia on skeletal maturation. J Pediatr 1994; 125:824–828.

138. Weaver CM, Peacock M, Martin BR, et al. Calcium retention estimated from indicators of skeletal status in adolescent girls and young women. Am J Clin Nutr 1996; 64:67–70.

139. Carrie Fassler AL, Bonjour JP. Osteoporosis as a pediatric problem. Pediatr Clin North Am 1995; 42:811–824.

140. Matkovic V, Jelic T, Wardlaw GM, et al. Timing of peak bone mass in Caucasian females and its implication for the prevention of osteoporosis: inference from a cross-sectional model. J Clin Invest 1994; 93:799–808.

141. del Rio L, Carrascosa A, Pons F, et al. Bone mineral density of the lumbar spine in white Mediterranean Spanish children and adolescents: changes related to age, sex, and puberty. Pediatr Res 1994; 35:362–366.

142. Proesmans W, Goos G, Emma F, et al. Total body mineral mass measured with dual-photon absorptiometry in healthy children. Eur J Pediatr 1994; 153:807–812.

143. Kroger H, Kotaniemi A, Kroger L, et al. Development of bone mass and bone density of the spine and femoral neck—a prospective study of 65 children and adolescents. Bone Miner 1993; 23:171–182.

144. Bachrach LK. Bone mineralization in childhood and adolescence. Curr Opin Pediatr 1993; 5:467–473.

145. Grimston SK, Morrison K, Harder JA, et al. Bone mineral density during puberty in western Canadian children. Bone Miner 1992; 19:85–96.

146. Theintz G, Buchs B, Rizzoli R, et al. Longitudinal monitoring of bone mass accumulation in healthy adolescents: evidence for a marked reduction after 16 years of age at the levels of lumbar spine and femoral neck in female subjects. J Clin Endocrinol Metab 1992; 75:1060–1065.

147. Bonjour JP, Theintz G, Buchs B, et al. Critical years and stages of puberty for spinal and femoral bone mass accumulation during adolescence. J Clin Endocrinol Metab 1991; 73:555–563.

148. Bonjour JP, Theintz G, Law F, et al. Peak bone mass. Osteoporos Int 1994; 4 Suppl 1:7–13.

149. Mora S, Goodman WG, Loro ML, et al. Age-related changes in cortical and cancellous vertebral bone density in girls: assessment with quantitative CT. AJR 1994; 162:405–409.

150. Lloyd T, Rollings N, Andon MB, et al. Determinants of bone density in young women. I. Relationships among pubertal development, total body bone mass, and total body bone density in premenarchal females. J Clin Endocrinol Metab 1992; 75:383–387.

151. Moreira-Andres MN, Papapietro K, Canizo FJ, et al. Correlations between bone mineral density, insulin-like growth factor I, and auxological variables. Eur J Endocrinol 1995; 132:573–579.

152. Rico H, Revilla M, Villa LF, et al. Determinants of total-body and regional bone mineral content and density in postpubertal normal women. Metabolism: Clin Exp 1994; 43:263–266.

153. van der Meulen MC, Ashford MW Jr, Kiratli BJ, et al. Determinants of femoral geometry and structure during adolescent growth. J Orthop Res 1996; 14:22–29.

154. Genant HK, Engelke K, Fuerst T, et al. Noninvasive assessment of bone mineral and structure: state of the art. J Bone Miner Res 1996; 11:707–730.

155. Lu PW, Briody JM, Ogle GD, et al. Bone mineral density of total body, spine, and femoral neck in children and young adults: a cross-sectional and longitudinal study. J Bone Miner Res 1994; 9:1451–1458.

156. Rubin K, Schirduan V, Gendreau P, et al. Predictors of axial and peripheral bone mineral density in healthy children and adolescents, with special attention to the role of puberty. J Pediatr 1993; 123:863–870.

157. Sentipal JM, Wardlaw GM, Mahan J, et al. Influence of calcium intake and growth indexes on vertebral bone mineral density in young females. Am J Clin Nutr 1991; 54:425–428.

158. Abrams SA, Stuff JE. Calcium metabolism in girls: current dietary intakes lead to low rates of calcium absorption and retention during puberty. Am J Clin Nutr 1994; 60:739–743.

159. Anderson JJ, Pollitzer WS: Ethnic and genetic differences in susceptibility to osteoporotic fractures. Adv Nutr Res 1994; 9:129–149.

160. Gilsanz V, Roe TF, Mora S, et al. Changes in vertebral bone density in black girls and white girls during childhood and puberty. N Engl J Med 1991; 325:1597–1600.

161. Chan GM, Hoffman K, McMurry M. Effects of dairy products on bone and body composition in pubertal girls. J Pediatr 1995; 126:551–556.

162. Anderson JJ, Metz JA. Contributions of dietary calcium and physical activity to primary prevention of osteoporosis in females. J Am Coll Nutr 1993; 12:378–383.

163. Johnston CC Jr, Miller JZ, Slemenda CW, et al. Calcium supplementation and increases in bone mineral density in children. N Engl J Med 1992; 327:82–87.

164. Matkovic V. Calcium and peak bone mass. J Intern Med 1992; 231:151–160.

165. Lee WT, Leung SS, Leung DM, et al. A follow-up study on the effects of calcium supplement withdrawal and puberty on bone acquisition of children. Am J Clin Nutr 1996; 64:71–77.

166. Nieschlag E. Long-term effect of testosterone therapy on bone mineral density in hypogonadal men. J Clin Endocrinol Metab 1997; 82:2386–2390.

167. Mauras N, Haymond MW, Darmaun D, et al. Calcium and protein kinetics in prepubertal boys: positive effects of testosterone. J Clin Invest 1994; 93:1014–1019.

168. Zamberlan N, Radetti G, Paganini C, et al. Evaluation of cortical thickness and bone density by roentgen microdensitometry in growing males and females. Eur J Pediatr 1996; 155:377–382.

169. Finkelstein JS, Neer RM, Biller BM, et al. Osteopenia in men with a history of delayed puberty. N Engl J Med 1992; 326:600–604.

170. Finkelstein JS, Klibanski A, Neer RM. A longitudinal evaluation of bone mineral density in adult men with histories of delayed puberty. J Clin Endocrinol Metab 1996; 81:1152–1155.

171. Arisaka O, Arisaka M, Nakayama Y, et al. Effect of testosterone on bone density and bone metabolism in adolescent male hypogonadism. Metabolism: Clin Exp 1995; 44:419–423.

172. Kubler A, Schulz G, Cordes U, et al. The influence of testosterone substitution on bone mineral density in patients with Klinefelter's syndrome. Exp Clin Endocrinol 1992; 100:129–132.

173. Hergenroeder AC. Bone mineralization, hypothalamic amenorrhea, and sex steroid therapy in female adolescents and young adults. J Pediatr 1995; 126:683–689.

174. Fabbri G, Petraglia F, Segre A, et al. Reduced spinal bone density in young women with amenorrhoea. Eur J Obstet Gynecol Reprod Biol 1991; 41:117–122.

175. Saggese G, Bertelloni S, Baroncelli GI, et al. Reduction of bone density: an effect of gonadotropin-releasing hormone analogue treatment in central precocious puberty. Eur J Pediatr 1993; 152:717–720.

176. Saggese G, Bertelloni S, Baroncelli GI, et al. Bone loss during gonadotropin-releasing hormone agonist treatment in girls with true precocious puberty is not due to an impairment of calcitonin secretion. J Endocrinol Invest 1991; 14:231–236.

177. Verrotti A, Chiarelli F, Montanaro AF, et al. Bone mineral content in girls with precocious puberty treated with gonadotropin-releasing hormone analog. Gynecol Endocrinol 1995; 9:277–281.

178. Neely EK, Bachrach LK, Hintz RL, et al. Bone mineral density during treatment of central precocious puberty. J Pediatr 1995; 127:819–822.

179. Antoniazzi F, Bertoldo F, Zamboni G, et al. Bone mineral metabolism in girls with precocious puberty during gonadotropin-releasing hormone agonist treatment. Eur J Endocrinol 1995; 133:412–417.

180. Simberg N, Tiitinen A, Silfvast A, et al. High bone density in hyperandrogenic women: effect of gonadotropin-releasing hormone agonist alone or in conjunction with estrogen-progestin replacement. J Clin Endocrinol Metab 1996; 81:646–651.

180a. Buchanan JR, Hospodar C, Myers P, et al. Effect of excess androgens on bone density in young women. J Clin Endocrinol Metab 1988; 67:937–943.

181. Orwel ES. Androgens as anabolic agents for bone. Trends Endocrinol Metab 1996; 7:77–84.

182. Hyer SL, Rodin DA, Tobias JH, et al. Growth hormone deficiency during puberty reduces adult bone mineral density. Arch Dis Child 1992; 67:1472–1474.

183. Lonzer MD, Imrie R, Rogers D, et al. Effects of heredity, age, weight, puberty, activity, and calcium intake on bone mineral density in children. Clin Pediatr 1996; 35:185–189.

184. McKay HA, Bailey DA, Wilkinson AA, et al. Familial comparison of bone mineral density at the proximal femur and lumbar spine. Bone Miner 1994; 24:95–107.

185. Blumsohn A, Hannon RA, Wrate R, et al. Biochemical markers of bone turnover in girls during puberty. Clin Endocrinol 1994; 40:663–670.

186. Molina RM, Bouchard C. Growth, Maturation, and Physical Activity. Champaign, IL: Human Kinetics, 1991.

187. Holliday MA. Body composition and energy needs during growth. In: Falkner F, Tanner JM, eds. Human Growth. Vol 2. Postnatal Growth. 2nd ed. New York: Plenum Press, 1986: 101–117.

188. Rico H, Revilla M, Villa LF, et al. Body composition in children and Tanner's stages: a study with dual-energy x-ray absorptiometry. Metabolism: Clin Exp 1993; 42:967–970.

189. Cheek DB. Body composition, hormones, nutrition, and adolescent growth. In: Grumbach MM, Grave GD, Mayer FE, eds. Control of the Onset of Puberty. New York: John Wiley & Sons, 1974: 424–447.

190. Forbes GB. Puberty: body composition. In: Berenberg SR, ed. Puberty: Biologic and Social Components. Leiden: HE Stenfert Kroese, 1975: 132–145.

191. Forbes GB. Body composition in adolescence. In: Falkner F, Tanner JM, eds. Human Growth. Vol 2. Postnatal Growth. 2nd ed. New York: Plenum Press, 1986: 119–145.

192. Frisancho AR, Flegel PN. Advanced maturation with centripetal fat pattern. Hum Biol 1982; 54:717–727.

193. Garn SM. Fat weight and fat placement in the female. Science 1957; 125:1091–1092.

194. Rolland-Cachera MF: Body composition during adolescence: methods, limitations, and determinants. Horm Res 1993; 39 Suppl 3:25–40.

195. Rosenthal M, Bain SH, Bush A, et al. Weight/height$^{2.88}$ as a screening test for obesity or thinness in schoolage children. Eur J Pediatr 1994; 153:876–883.

196. de Ridder CM, Ridder CM, de Boer RW, Seidell JC, et al. Body fat distribution in pubertal girls quantified by magnetic resonance imaging. Int J Obes Relat Metab Disord 1992; 16:443–449.

197. Maffeis C, Pinelli L, Schutz Y: Increased fat oxidation in prepubertal obese children: a metabolic defense against further weight gain? J Pediatr 1995; 126:15–20.

198. Hammer LD, Wilson DM, Litt IF, et al. Impact of pubertal development on body fat distribution among white, Hispanic, and Asian female adolescents. J Pediatr 1991; 118:975–980.

199. Kissebah AH, Krakower GR. Regional adiposity and morbidity. Physiol Rev 1994; 74:761–811.

200. de Ridder CM, Bruning PF, Zonderland ML, et al. Body fat mass, body

fat distribution, and plasma hormones in early puberty in females. J Clin Endocrinol Metab 1990; 70:888–893.

201. Remschmidt H. Psychosocial milestones in normal puberty and adolescence. Horm Res 1994; 41(Suppl 2):19–29.

202. Frisch RE, Revelle R. Height and weight at menarche and a hypothesis of critical body weights and adolescent events. Science 1970; 169:397–399.

203. Obesity and cardiovascular disease risk factors in black and white girls: the NHLBI Growth and Health Study. Am J Public Health 1992; 82:1613–1620.

204. Schreiber GB, Robins M, Striegel-Moore R, et al. Weight modification efforts reported by black and white preadolescent girls: National Heart, Lung, and Blood Institute Growth and Health Study. Pediatrics 1996; 98:63–70.

205. Nieto J, Szklo M, Comstock GW. Childhood weight and growth rate as predictors of adult mortality. Am J Epidemiol 1992; 136:201–213.

206. Knishkowy B, Palti H, Tun N, et al. Cardiovascular risk factors by ethnic group and menstrual status among 13- and 14-year-old Israeli schoolchildren. Public Health Rev 1994; 22:55–73.

207. Modesti PA, Pela I, Cecioni I, et al. Changes in blood pressure reactivity and 24-hour blood pressure profile occurring at puberty. Angiology 1994; 45:443–450.

208. Nelson MJ, Ragland DR, Syme SL. Longitudinal prediction of adult blood pressure from juvenile blood pressure levels. Am J Epidemiol 1992; 136:633–645.

209. Voors AW, Harsha DW, Webber LS, et al. Relation of blood pressure to stature in healthy young adults. Am J Epidemiol 1982; 115:833–840.

210. Voors AW, Webber LS, Frerichs RR, et al. Body height and body mass as determinants of basal blood pressure in children—the Bogalusa Heart Study. Am J Epidemiol 1977; 106:101–108.

211. Liker HR, Barnes KM, Comite F, et al. Blood pressure and body size in precocious puberty. Acta Paediatr Scand 1988; 77:294–298.

212. Watanabe T, Nagashima M, Hojo Y. Circadian rhythm of blood pressure in children with reference to normal and diseased children. Acta Paediatr Jpn 1994; 36:683–689.

213. Hamburg BA. Psychosexual development. In: Freidman SB, Fisher M, Schonberg SK, eds. Comprehensive Adolescent Health. St. Louis: Quality Medical Publishing, 1992: 27–38.

214. Michael RP, Zumpe D. Behavioral changes associated with puberty in higher primates and the human. In: Grumbach MM, Sizonenko PC, Aubert ML, eds. Control of the Onset of Puberty. Baltimore: Williams & Wilkins, 1990: 574–587.

215. Weiner IB, del Gaudio AC. Psychopathology in adolescence: an epidemiological study. In: Chess S, Thomas A, eds. Annual Progress in Child Psychiatry and Child Development. New York: Brunner/Mazel, 1977: 471–488.

216. Slap GB, Khalid N, Paikoff RL, et al. Evolving self-image, pubertal manifestations, and pubertal hormones: preliminary findings in young adolescent girls. J Adolesc Health 1994; 15:327–335.

217. Susman EJ, Nottelmann ED, Inoff-Germain G, et al. Hormonal influences on aspects of psychological development during adolescence. J Adolesc Health Care 1987; 8:492–504.

218. Klerman LV. Adolescent pregnancy and parenting: controversies of the past and lessons for the future. J Adolesc Health 1993; 14:553–561.

219. Petersen AC, Leffert N, Graham BL. Adolescent development and the emergence of sexuality. Suicide Life-Threat Behav 1995; 25(Suppl):4–17.

220. Brooks-Gunn J, Graber JA. Puberty as a biological and social event: implications for research on pharmacology. J Adolesc Health 1994; 15:663–671.

221. Hayes CD. Risking the Future: Adolescent Sexuality, Pregnancy, and Childbearing. Washington, DC: National Academy Press, 1987.

222. Rodgers JL. Development of sexual behavior. In: Freidman SB, Fisher M, Schonberg SK, eds. Comprehensive Adolescent Health. St. Louis: Quality Medical Publishing, 1997: 39–43.

223. Brindis CD, Irwin CE Jr, Millstein SG. United States profile. In: McAnarney ER, Kreipe RE, Orr DP, et al, eds. Textbook of Adolescent Medicine. Philadelphia: WB Saunders, 1992: 12–27.

224. Hall GS. Adolescence: Its Psychology and Its Relations to Physiology, Anthropology, Sociology, Sex, Crime, Religion, and Education. New York: Appleton, 1904.

225. Offer D. The Psychological World of the Teenager: A Study of Normal Adolescent Boys. New York: Basic Books, 1969.

226. Masterson JF. The symptomatic adolescent five years later: he didn't grow out of it. Am J Psychiatry 1967; 123:1338.

227. Udry RR, Billy JOG, Morris NM, et al. Serum androgenic hormones motivate sexual behavior in boys. Fertil Steril 1985; 43:90–94.

228. Offer D, Schonert-Reichl KA. Debunking the myths of adolescence: findings from recent research. J Am Acad Child Adolesc Psychiatry 1992; 31:1003–1014.

229. Hayward C, Killen JD, Hammer LD, et al. Pubertal stage and panic attack history in sixth- and seventh-grade girls. Am J Psychiatry 1992; 149:1239–1243.

230. Solomon S. Migraine diagnosis and clinical symptomatology. Headache 1994; 34:S8–S12.

231. Rao U, Weissman MM, Martin JA, et al. Childhood depression and risk of suicide: a preliminary report of a longitudinal study. J Am Acad Child Adolesc Psychiatry 1993; 32:21–27.

232. Swedo SE, Pleeter JD, Richter DM, et al. Rates of seasonal affective disorder in children and adolescents. Am J Psychiatry 1995; 152:1016–1019.

233. Angold A, Worthman CW. Puberty onset of gender differences in rates of depression: a developmental, epidemiologic, and neuroendocrine perspective. J Affect Disord 1993; 29:145–158.

234. McKenna K, Gordon CT, Lenane M, et al. Looking for childhood-onset schizophrenia: the first 71 cases screened. J Am Acad Child Adolesc Psychiatry 1994; 33:636–644.

235. Gordon CT, Frazier JA, McKenna K, et al. Childhood-onset schizophrenia: an NIMH study in progress. Schizophr Bull 1994; 20:697–712.

236. Orr DP, Ingersoll GM. The contribution of level of cognitive complexity and pubertal timing to behavioral risk in young adolescents. Pediatrics 1995; 95:528–533.

237. Tschann JM, Adler NE, Irwin CE, et al. Initiation of substance use in early adolescence: the roles of pubertal timing and emotional distress. Health Psychol 1994; 13:326–333.

238. Susman EJ, Inoff-Germain G, Nottelmann ED, et al. Hormones, emotional dispositions, and aggressive attributes in young adolescents. Child Dev 1987; 58:1114–1134.

239. Warren MP, Brooks-Gunn J. Mood and behavior at adolescence: evidence for hormonal factors. J Clin Endocrinol Metab 1989; 69:77–83.

240. Finkelstein JW, Von Eye A, Preece MA. The relationship between aggressive behavior and puberty in normal adolescents: a longitudinal study. J Adolesc Health 1994; 15:319–326.

241. Constantino JN, Grosz D, Saenger P, et al. Testosterone and aggression in children. J Am Acad Child Adolesc Psychiatry 1993; 32:1217–1222.

242. Halpern CT, Udry JR, Campbell B, et al. Relationships between aggression and pubertal increases in testosterone: a panel analysis of adolescent males. Soc Biol 1993; 40:8–24.

243. Halpern CT, Udry JR, Campbell B, et al. Testosterone and pubertal development as predictors of sexual activity: a panel analysis of adolescent males. Psychosom Med 1993; 55:436–447.

244. Hutchinson KA. Androgens and sexuality. Am J Med 1995; 98:111S–115S.

245. Money J. Sexual revolution and counter-revolution. Horm Res 1994; 41 Suppl 2:44–48.

246. Friedman HL. Changing patterns of adolescent sexual behavior: consequences for health and development. J Adolesc Health 1992; 13:345–350.

247. Koff E, Rierdan J. Advanced pubertal development and eating disturbance in early adolescent girls. J Adolesc Health 1993; 14:443–439.

248. Killen JD, Hayward C, Litt I, et al. Is puberty a risk factor for eating disorders?. Am J Dis Child 1992; 146:323–325.

249. Andrade MM, Benedito-Silva AA, Domenice S, et al. Sleep characteristics of adolescents: a longitudinal study. J Adolesc Health 1993; 14:401–406.

250. Carskadon MA, Harvey K, Duke P, et al. Pubertal changes in daytime sleepiness. Sleep 1980; 2:453–460.

251. Anokhin AP, Birbaumer N, Lutzenberger W, et al. Age increases brain complexity. Electroencephalogr Clin Neurophysiol 1996; 99:63–68.

252. Grumbach MM, Roth JC, Kaplan SL, Kelch RP. Hypothalamic-pituitary regulation of puberty in man: evidence and concepts derived from clinical research. In: Grumbach MM, Grave GD, Mayer FE, eds. Control of the Onset of Puberty. New York: John Wiley & Sons, 1974: 115–166.

253. Grumbach MM, Kaplan SL. The neuroendocrinology of human puberty: an ontogenetic perspective. In: Grumbach MM, Sizonenko PC, Aubert ML, eds. Control of the Onset of Puberty. Baltimore: Williams & Wilkins, 1990: 1–68.

254. Kaplan SL, Grumbach MM, Aubert ML. The ontogenesis of pituitary hormones and hypothalamic factors in the human fetus: maturation of central nervous system regulation of anterior pituitary function. Recent Prog Horm Res 1976; 32:161–243.

255. Dunkel L, Alfthan H, Stenman UH, et al. Pulsatile secretion of LH and FSH in prepubertal and early pubertal boys revealed by ultrasensitive time-resolved immunofluorometric assays. Pediatr Res 1990; 27:215–219.

256. Dunkel L, Alfthan H, Stenman UH, et al. Gonadal control of pulsatile secretion of luteinizing hormone and follicle-stimulating hormone in prepubertal boys evaluated by ultrasensitive time-resolved immunofluorometric assays. J Clin Endocrinol Metab 1990; 70:107–114.

257. Albertsson-Wikland K, Rosberg S, Lannering B, et al. Twenty-four-hour profiles of luteinizing hormone, follicle-stimulating hormone, testosterone, and estradiol levels: a semilongitudinal study throughout puberty in healthy boys. J Clin Endocrinol Metab 1997; 82:541–549.

258. Wu FC, Butler GE, Kelnar CJ, et al. Ontogeny of pulsatile gonadotropin-releasing hormone secretion from midchildhood, through puberty, to adulthood in the human male: a study using deconvolution analysis and an ultrasensitive immunofluorometric assay. J Clin Endocriol Metab 1996; 81:1798–1805.

259. Apter D, Butzow TL, Laughlin GA, et al. Gonadotropin-releasing hormone pulse generator activity during pubertal transition in girls: pulsatile and diurnal patterns of circulating gonadotropins. J Clin Endocrinol Metab 1993; 76:940–949.

260. Corley KP, Valk TW, Kelch RP, et al. Estimation of GnRH pulse amplitude during pubertal development. Pediatr Res 1981; 15:157–162.

261. Jakacki RI, Kelch RP, Sauder SE, et al. Pulsatile secretion of luteinizing hormone in children. J Clin Endocrinol Metab 1982; 55:453–458.

262. Kelch RP, Clemens LE, Markovs M, et al. Metabolism and effects of synthetic gonadotropin-releasing hormone (GnRH) in children and adults. J Clin Endocrinol Metab 1975; 40:53–61.

263. Hassing JM, Padmanabhan V, Kelch RP, et al. Differential regulation of serum immunoreactive luteinizing hormone and bioactive follicle-stimulating hormone by testosterone in early pubertal boys. J Clin Endocrinol Metab 1990; 70:1082–1089.

264. Yen SS, Apter D, Butzow T, et al. Gonadotropin-releasing hormone pulse generator activity before and during sexual maturation in girls: new insights. Hum Reprod 1993; 8 Suppl 2:66–71.

265. Boyar R, Finkelstein J, Roffwarg H, et al. Synchronization of augmented luteinizing hormone secretion with sleep during puberty. N Engl J Med 1972; 287:582–586.

266. Wennink JM, Delemarre-Van deWaal HA, van Kessel H, et al. Luteinizing hormone secretion patterns in boys at the onset of puberty measured using a highly sensitive immunoradiometric assay. J Clin Endocrinol Metab 1988; 67:924–928.

267. Roth JC, Kelch RP, Kaplan SL, Grumbach MM. FSH and LH response to luteinizing hormone–releasing factor in prepubertal and pubertal children, adult males, and patients with hypogonadotropic and hypertropic hypogonadism. J Clin Endocrinol Metab 1972; 35:926–930.

268. Roth JC, Grumbach MM, Kaplan SL. Effect of synthetic luteinizing hormone–releasing factor on serum testosterone and gonadotropins in prepubertal, pubertal, and adult males. J Clin Endocrinol Metab 1973; 37:680–686.

269. Job JC, Garnier PE, Chaussain JL, et al. Elevation of serum gonadotropins (LH and FSH) after releasing hormone (LH-RH) injection in normal children and in patients with disorders of puberty. J Clin Endocrinol Metab 1972; 35:473–476.

270. Boyar RM, Rosenfeld RS, Kapen S, et al. Simultaneous augmented secretion of luteinizing hormone and testosterone during sleep. J Clin Invest 1974; 54:609–618.

271. Kapen S, Boyar RM, Hellman L, et al. Twenty-four-hour patterns of luteinizing hormone secretion in humans: ontogenetic and sexual considerations. Prog Brain Res 1975; 42:103–113.

272. Hale PM, Khoury S, Foster CM, et al. Increased luteinizing hormone pulse frequency during sleep in early to midpubertal boys: effects of testosterone infusion. J Clin Endocrinol Metab 1988; 66:785–791.

273. Foster CM, Hassing JM, Padmanabhan V, et al. Testosterone infusion reduces nocturnal luteinizing hormone pulse frequency in pubertal boys. J Clin Endocrinol Metab 1989; 69:1213–1220.

274. Apter D, Cacciatore B, Alfthan H, et al. Serum luteinizing hormone concentrations increase 100-fold in females from 7 years to adulthood, as measured by time-resolved immunofluorometric assay. J Clin Endocrinol Metab 1989; 68:53–57.

275. Burr IM, Sizonenko PC, Kaplan SL, Grumbach MM. Hormonal changes in puberty. I. Correlation of serum luteinizing hormone and follicle-stimulating hormone with stages of puberty, testicular size, and bone age in normal boys. Pediatr Res 1970; 4:25–35.

276. Sizonenko PC, Burr IM, Kaplan SL, Grumbach MM. Hormonal changes in puberty. II. Correlation of serum luteinizing hormone and follicle-stimulating hormone with stages of puberty and bone age in normal girls. Pediatr Res 1970; 4:36–45.

277. August GP, Grumbach MM, Kaplan SL. Hormonal changes in puberty. III. Correlation of plasma testosterone, LH, FSH, testicular size, and bone age with male pubertal development. J Clin Endocrinol Metab 1972; 34:319–326.

278. Jenner MR, Kelch RP, Kaplan SL, Grumbach MM. Hormonal changes in puberty. IV. Plasma estradiol, LH, and FSH in prepubertal children, pubertal females, and in precocious puberty, premature thelarche, hypogonadism, and in a child with a feminizing ovarian tumor. J Clin Endocrinol Metab 1972; 34:521–530.

279. Belgorosky A, Chahin S, Chaler E, et al. Serum concentrations of follicle-stimulating hormone and luteinizing hormone in normal girls and boys during prepuberty and at early puberty. J Endocrinol Invest 1996; 19:88–91.

280. Faiman C, Winter JSD. Gonadotropins and sex hormone patterns in puberty: clinical data. In: Grumbach MM, Grave GD, Mayer FE, eds. Control of the Onset of Puberty. New York: John Wiley & Sons, 1974: 32–61.

281. Garibaldi LR, Picco P, Magier S, et al. Serum luteinizing hormone concentrations, as measured by a sensitive immunoradiometric assay, in children with normal, precocious, or delayed pubertal development. J Clin Endocrinol Metab 1991; 72:888–898.

282. Spratt DI, Crowley WF. Pituitary and gonadal responsiveness is enhanced during GnRH-induced puberty. Am J Physiol 1988; 254:E652–E657.

283. Beitins IZ, Padmanabhan V. Bioactivity of gonadotropins. Endocrinol Metab Clin North Am 1991; 20:85–120.

284. Demir A, Voutilainen R, Juul A, et al. Increase in first-morning voided urinary luteinizing hormone levels precedes the physical onset of puberty. J Clin Endocrinol Metab 1996; 81:2963–2967.

285. Cavallo A, Zhou XH. LHRH test in the assessment of puberty in normal children. Horm Res 1994; 41:10–15.

286. Ghai K, Rosenfield RL. Maturation of the normal pituitary-testicular axis, as assessed by gonadotropin-releasing hormone agonist challenge. J Clin Endocrinol Metab 1994; 78:1336–1340.

287. Ghai K, Cara JF, Rosenfield RL. Gonadotropin-releasing hormone agonist (nafarelin) test to differentiate gonadotropin deficiency from constitutionally delayed puberty in teen-age boys—a clinical research center study. J Clin Endocrinol Metab 1995; 80:2980–2986.

288. Wang C, Zhong CQ, Leung A, et al. Serum bioactive follicle-stimulating hormone levels in girls with precocious sexual development. J Clin Endocrinol Metab 1990; 70:615–619.

289. Reiter EO, Beitins IZ, Ostrea T, et al. Bioassayable luteinizing hormone during childhood and adolescence and in patients with delayed pubertal development. J Clin Endocrinol Metab 1982; 54:155–161.

290. Reiter EO, Biggs DE, Veldhuis JD, et al. Pulsatile release of bioactive luteinizing hormone in prepubertal girls: discordance with immunoreactive luteinizing hormone pulses. Pediatr Res 1987; 21:409–413.

291. Huhtaniemi I, Haavisto A-M, Anttila R, et al. Sensitive immunoassay and in vitro bioassay demonstrate constant bio/immuno ratio of luteinizing hormone in healthy boys during the pubertal maturation. Pediatr Res 1996; 39:180–184.

292. Dunger DB, Villa AK, Matthews DR, et al. Pattern of secretion of bioactive and immunoreactive gonadotrophins in normal pubertal children. Clin Endocrinol (Oxf) 1991; 35:267–275.

293. Kasa-Vubu JZ, Padmanabhan V, Kletter GB, et al. Serum bioactive luteinizing and follicle-stimulating hormone concentrations in girls increase during puberty. Pediatr Res 1993; 34:829–833.

294. Kletter GB, Padmanabhan V, Brown MB, et al. Serum bioactive gonadotropins during male puberty: a longitudinal study. J Clin Endocrinol Metab 1993; 76:432–438.

295. Baenziger JU. Glycosylation: to what end for the glycoprotein hormones? Endocrinology 1996; 137:1520–1522 (editorial).

296. Ulloa-Aguirre A, Midgley AR Jr, Beitins IZ, et al. Follicle-stimulating isohormones: characterization and physiological relevance. Endocr Rev 1995; 16:765–787.

297. Wide L, Albertsson-Wikland K, Phillips DJ. More basic isoforms of serum gonadotropins during gonadotropin-releasing hormone agonist therapy in pubertal children. J Clin Endocrinol Metab 1996; 81:216–221.

298. Phillips DJ, Wide L. Serum gonadotropin isoforms become more basic after an exogenous challenge of gonadotropin-releasing hormone in children undergoing pubertal development. J Clin Endocrinol Metab 1994; 79:814–819.

299. Weinstein RL, Kelch RP, Jenner MR, et al. Secretion of unconjugated androgens and estrogens by the normal and abnormal human testis before and after hCG. J Clin Invest 1974; 53:1.

300. Peterson RE, Imperato-McGinley J, Gautier T, et al. Male pseudohermaphroditism due to steroid 5-alpha-reductase deficiency. Am J Med 1977; 62:170–191.

301. Knoor D, Bidlingmaier F, Butenandt O, et al. Plasma testosterone in male puberty. I. Physiology of plasma testosterone. Acta Endocrinol 1974; 75:181–194.

302. Judd HL, Parker DC, Yen SSC. Sleep-wake patterns of LH and testosterone release in prepubertal boys. J Clin Endocrinol Metab 1977; 44:865–869.

303. Goji K, Tanikaze S. Spontaneous gonadotropin and testosterone concentration profiles in prepubertal and pubertal boys: temporal relationship between luteinizing hormone and testosterone. Pediatr Res 1993; 34:229–236.

304. Dehennin L, Delgado A, Peres G. Urinary profile of androgen metabolites at different stages of pubertal development in a population of sporting male subjects. Eur J Endocrinol 1994; 130:53–59.

305. Pal SB. Urinary excretion of testosterone and epitestosterone in men, women, and children. Clin Chim Acta 1971; 33:215–227.

306. Boas SR, Cleary DA, Lee PA, et al. Salivary testosterone levels in male adolescents with cystic fibrosis. Pediatrics 1996; 97:361–363.

307. Ohzeki T, Manella B, Gubelin-De Campo C, et al. Salivary testosterone concentrations in prepubertal and pubertal males: comparison with total and free plasma testosterone. Horm Res 1991; 36:235–237.

308. Inkster S, Yue W, Brodie A. Human testicular aromatase: immunocytochemical and biochemical studies. J Clin Endocrinol Metab 1995; 80:1941–1947.

309. Brodie A, Inkster S: Aromatase in the human testis. J Steroid Biochem Mol Biol 1993; 44:549–555.

310. Goji K. Twenty-four-hour concentration profiles of gonadotropin and estradiol (E$_2$) in prepubertal and early pubertal girls: the diurnal rise of E$_2$ is opposite the nocturnal rise of gonadotropin. J Clin Endocrinol Metab 1993; 77:1629–1635.

311. Angsusingha K, Kenny FM, Nankin HR, et al. Unconjugated estrone, estradiol, and FSH and LH in prepubertal and pubertal males and females. J Clin Endocrinol Metab 1974; 39:63–68.

312. Klein KO, Martha PM, Blizzard RM, et al. A longitudinal assessment of hormonal and physical alterations during normal puberty in boys. II. Estrogen levels as determined by an ultrasensitive bioassay. J Clin Endocrinol Metab 1996; 81:3203–3207.

313. Anderson DC. Sex-hormone–binding globulin. Clin Endocrinol 1974; 3:69–95.

314. Lindstedt G, Lundberg P, Hammond GL, et al. Sex hormone–binding globulin—still many questions. Scand J Clin Lab Invest 1985; 45:1–6.

315. Maruyama Y, Aoki N, Suzuki Y, et al. Sex steroid–binding plasma protein (SBP), testosterone, oestradiol, and dehydroepiandrosterone (DHEA) in prepuberty and puberty. Acta Endocrinol 1987; 114:60–67.

316. August GP, Tkachuk M, Grumbach MM. Plasma testosterone-binding affinity and testosterone in umbilical cord plasma, late pregnancy, prepubertal children, and adults. J Clin Endocrinol Metab 1969; 29:891–899.

317. Horst HJ, Bartsch W, Dirksen-Thiedens I. Plasma testosterone, sex hormone–binding globulin binding capacity, and per cent binding of testosterone and 5-alpha-dihydrotestosterone in prepubertal, pubertal, and adult males. J Clin Endocrinol Metab 1977; 45:522–527.

318. Bartsch W, Horst HJ, Derwahl DM. Interrelationships between sex hormone–binding globulin and 17-beta-estradiol, testosterone, 5-alpha-dihydrotestosterone, thyroxine, and triiodothyronine in prepubertal and pubertal girls. J Clin Endocrinol Metab 1980; 50:1053–1056.

319. Cunningham SK, McKenna TJ. Evaluation of an immunoassay for plasma sex hormone–binding globulin: comparison with steroid-binding assay under physiological and pathological conditions. Ann Clin Biochem 1988; 25:360–366.

320. Cunningham SK, Loughlin T, Culliton M, et al. Plasma sex hormone–binding globulin levels decrease during the second decade of life irrespective of pubertal status. J Clin Endocrinol Metab 1984; 58:915–918.

321. Rudd BT, Rayner PH, Thomas PH. Observations on the role of GH/IGF-1 and sex hormone–binding globulin (SHBG) in the pubertal development of growth hormone–deficient (GHD) children. Acta Endocrinol Suppl 1986; 279:164–169.

322. Holly JM, Dunger DB, al-Othman SA, et al. Sex hormone–binding globulin levels in adolescent subjects with diabetes mellitus. Diabet Med 1992; 9:371–374.

323. Aubert ML, Sizonenko PC, Kaplan SL, Grumbach MM. The ontogenesis of human prolactin from fetal life to puberty. In: Crosignani PG, Robyn C, eds. Prolactin and Human Reproduction. New York: Academic Press, 1977: 9–20.

324. Vale W, Bilezikjian LM, Rivier C. Reproductive and other roles of inhibins and activins. In: Knobil E, Neil JD, eds. Physiology of Reproduction. 2nd ed. New York: Raven Press, 1994: 1861–1878.

325. Mather JP. Follistatins and alpha$_2$-macroglobulin are soluble binding proteins for inhibin and activin. Horm Res 1996; 45:207–210.

326. McLachlan RI, Robertson DM, Burger HG, et al. The radioimmunoassay of bovine and human follicular fluid and serum inhibin. Mol Cell Endocrinol 1986; 46:175–185.

327. Groome NP, Illingworth PJ, O'Brien M, et al. Measurement of dimeric inhibin B throughout the human menstrual cycle. J Clin Endocrinol Metab 1996; 81:1401–1405.

328. Robertson DM, Cahir N, Findlay JK, et al. The biological and immunological characterization of inhibin A and B forms in human follicular fluid and plasma. J Clin Endocrinol 1997; 82:889–896.

329. Wallace E, Riley SM, Crossley JA, et al. Dimeric inhibins in amniotic fluid, maternal serum, and fetal serum in human pregnancy. J Clin Endocrinol Metab 1997; 82:218–222.

330. Majdic G, McNeilly AS, Sharpe RM, et al. Testicular expression of inhibin and activin subunits and follistatin in the rat and human fetus and neonate and during postnatal development in the rat. Endocrinology 1997; 138:2136–2147.

331. Burger HG, McLachlan RI, Bangah M, et al. Serum inhibin concentrations rise throughout normal male and female puberty. J Clin Endocrinol Metab 1988; 67:689–694.

332. Manasco PK, Umbach DM, Muly SM, et al. Ontogeny of gonadotropin, testosterone, and inhibin secretion in normal boys through puberty based on overnight serial sampling. J Clin Endocrinol Metab 1995; 80:2046–2052.

333. Andersson A-M, Juul A, Petersen JH, et al. Serum inhibin B in healthy pubertal and adolescent boys: relation to age, stage of puberty, and FSH, LH, testosterone, and estradiol levels. J Clin Endocrinol Metab 1997; 82:3976–3981.

334. Anawalt BD, Bebb RA, Matsumoto AM, et al. Serum inhibin B levels reflect Sertoli cell function in normal men and in men with testicular dysfunction. J Clin Endocrinol Metab 1996; 81:3341–3345.

335. Mitchell R, Schaefer F, Morris ID, et al. Elevated serum immunoreactive inhibin levels in peripubertal boys with chronic renal failure: Cooperative Study Group on Pubertal Development in Chronic Renal Failure (CSPCRF). Clin Endocrinol (Oxf) 1993; 39:27–33.

336. Dunkel L, Siimes MA, Bremner WJ: Reduced inhibin and elevated gonadotropin levels in early pubertal boys with testicular defects. Pediatr Res 1993; 33:514–518.

337. Hudson PL, Dougas I, Donahoe PK, et al. An immunoassay to detect human müllerian-inhibiting substance in males and females during normal development. J Clin Endocrinol Metab 1990; 70:16–22.

338. Josso N, Legeai L, Forest MG, et al. An enzyme-linked immunoassay for anti-müllerian hormone: a new tool for the evaluation of testicular function in infants and children. J Clin Endocrinol Metab 1990; 70:23–27.

339. Donahoe PK. Müllerian-inhibiting substance in reproduction and cancer. Mol Reprod Dev 1992; 32:168–172.

340. Lee MM, Donahoe PK, Hasegawa T, et al. Müllerian-inhibiting substance in humans: normal levels from infancy to adulthood. J Clin Endocrinol Metab 1996; 81:571–576.

341. Rey R, Mebarki F, Forest MG, et al. Anti-müllerian hormone in children with androgen insensitivity. J Clin Endocrinol Metab 1994; 79:960–964.

342. Baker ML, Hutson JM: Serum levels of müllerian-inhibiting substance in boys throughout puberty and in the first two years of life. J Clin Endocrinol Metab 1993; 76:245–247.

343. Josso N. Paediatric applications of anti-müllerian hormone research. 1992 Andrea Prader Lecture. Horm Res 1995; 43:243–248.

344. Lee MM, Donahoe PK, Silverman BL, et al. Measurements of serum müllerian-inhibiting substance in the evaluation of children with nonpalpable gonads. N Engl J Med 1997; 336:1480–1486.

345. Randell EW, Diamandis EP, Ellis G. Serum prostate-specific antigen measured in children from birth to age 18 years. Clin Chem 1996; 42:420–423.

346. Vieira JG, Nishida SK, Pereira AB, et al. Serum levels of prostate-specific antigen in normal boys throughout puberty. J Clin Endocrinol Metab 1994; 78:1185–1187.

347. Martha PM, Rogol AD, Veldhuis JD, et al. Alterations in the pulsatile properties of circulating growth hormone concentrations during puberty in boys. J Clin Endocrinol Metab 1989; 69:563–570.

348. Albertsson-Wikland K, Rosberg S, Karlberg J, et al. Analysis of 24-hour growth hormone profiles in healthy boys and girls of normal stature: relation to puberty. J Clin Endocrinol Metab 1994; 78:1195–1201.

349. Eakman GD, Dallas JS, Ponder SW, et al. The effects of testosterone and dihydrotestosterone on hypothalamic regulation of growth hormone secretion. J Clin Endocrinol Metab 1996; 81:1217–1223.

350. Mericq V, Cassorla F, Garcia H, et al. Growth hormone (GH) responses to GH-releasing peptide and to GH-releasing hormone in GH-deficient children. J Clin Endocrinol Metab 1995; 80:1681–1684.

351. Laron Z, Bowers CY, Hirsch D, et al. Growth hormone–releasing activity of growth hormone–releasing peptide-1 (a synthetic heptapeptide) in children and adolescents. Acta Endocrinol 1993; 129:424–426.

352. Skinner AM, Price DA, Addison GM, et al. The influence of age, size, pubertal status, and renal factors on urinary growth hormone excretion in normal children and adolescents. Growth Regul 1992; 2:156–160.

353. Crowne EC, Wallace WH, Shalet SM, et al. Relationship between urinary and serum growth hormone and pubertal status. Arch Dis Child 1992; 67:91–95.

354. Main KM, Jarden M, Angelo L, et al. The impact of gender and puberty on reference values for urinary growth hormone excretion: a study of three morning urine samples in 517 healthy children and adults. J Clin Endocrinol Metab 1994; 79:865–871.

355. Patel L, Skinner AM, Price DA, et al. The influence of body mass index on growth hormone secretion in normal and short-statured children. Growth Regul 1994; 4:29–34.

356. Martha PM, Rogol AD, Blizzard RM, et al. Growth hormone–binding protein activity is inversely related to 24-hour growth hormone release in normal boys. J Clin Endocrinol Metab 1991; 73:175–181.

357. Argente J, Barrios V, Pozo J, et al. Normative data for insulin-like growth factors (IGFs), IGF-binding proteins, and growth hormone–binding protein in a healthy Spanish pediatric population: age- and sex-related changes. J Clin Endocrinol Metab 1993; 77:1522–1528.

358. Merimee TJ, Russell B, Quinn S. Growth hormone–binding proteins of human serum: developmental patterns in normal man. J Clin Endocrinol Metab 1992; 75:852–854.

359. Massa G, Bouillon R, Vanderschueren-Lodeweyckx M. Serum levels of growth hormone–binding protein and insulin-like growth factor I during puberty. Clin Endocrinol 1992; 37:175–180.

360. Martha PM, Rogol AD, Carlsson LM, et al. A longitudinal assessment of hormonal and physical alterations during normal puberty in boys. I. Serum growth hormone–binding protein. J Clin Endocrinol Metab 1993; 77:452–457.

361. Hasegawa Y, Hasegawa T, Takada M, et al. Plasma-free insulin-like growth factor I concentrations in growth hormone deficiency in children and adolescents. Eur J Endocrinol 1996; 134:184–189.

362. Rosenfield RI, Furlanetto R, Bock D. Relationship of somatomedin-C concentrations to pubertal changes. J Pediatr 1983; 103:723–728.

363. Luna AM, Wilson DM, Wibbelsman CJ, et al. Somatomedins in adolescence: a cross-sectional study of the effect of puberty on plasma insulin-like growth factor I and II levels. J Clin Endocrinol Metab 1983; 57:268–271.

364. Hesse V, Jahreis G, Schambach H, et al. Insulin-like growth factor I correlations to changes of the hormonal status in puberty and age. Exp Clin Endocrinol 1994; 102:289–298.

365. Juul A, Dalgaard P, Blum WF, et al. Serum levels of insulin-like growth factor (IGF)–binding protein-3 (IGFBP-3) in healthy infants, children, and adolescents: the relation to IGF-I, IGF-II, IGFBP-1, IGFBP-2, age, sex, body mass index, and pubertal maturation. J Clin Endocrinol Metab 1995; 80:2534–2542.

366. Juul A, Bang P, Hertel NT, et al. Serum insulin-like growth factor I in 1030 healthy children, adolescents, and adults: relation to age, sex, stage of puberty, testicular size, and body mass index. J Clin Endocrinol Metab 1994; 78:744–752.

367. Juul A, Flyvbjerg A, Frystyk J, et al. Serum concentrations of free and total insulin-like growth factor I, IGF binding proteins 1 and 3, and IGFBP-3 protease activity in boys with normal or precocious puberty. Clin Endocrinol (Oxf) 1996; 44:515–523.

368. Wilson DM, Stene MA, Killen JD, et al. Insulin-like growth factor–binding protein-3 in normal pubertal girls. Acta Endocrinol (Copenh) 1992; 126:381–386.

369. Amiel SA, Caprio S, Sherwin RS, et al. Insulin resistance of puberty: a defect restricted to peripheral glucose metabolism. J Clin Endocrinol Metab 1991; 72:277–282.

370. Bloch CA, Clemons P, Sperling MA. Puberty decreases insulin sensitivity. J Pediatr 1987; 110:481–487.

371. Amiel SA, Sherwin RS, Simonson DC, et al. Impaired insulin action in puberty—a contributing factor to poor glycemic control in adolescents with diabetes. N Engl J Med 1986; 315:215–219.

372. Hindmarsh PC, Matthews DR, Di Silvio L, et al. Relation between height velocity and fasting insulin concentrations. Arch Dis Child 1988; 63:665–666.

373. Rosenbloom AL, Wheeler L, Bianchi R, et al. Age-adjusted analysis of insulin responses during normal and abnormal glucose tolerance tests in children and adolescents. Diabetes 1975; 4:820–828.

374. Hindmarsh P, Di Silvio L, Pringle PJ, et al. Changes in serum insulin concentration during puberty and their relationship to growth hormone. Clin Endocrinol 1988; 28:381–388.

375. Caprio S, Cline G, Boulware S, et al. Effects of puberty and diabetes on metabolism of insulin-sensitive fuels. Am J Physiol 1994; 266:E885–E891.

376. Godsland IF. The influence of female sex steroids on glucose metabolism and insulin action. J Intern Med 1996; 738(Suppl):1–60.

377. Svec F, Nastasi K, Hilton C, et al. Black-white contrasts in insulin levels during pubertal development—the Bogalusa Heart Study. Diabetes 1992; 41:313–317.

378. Arslanian SA, Kalhan SC. Correlations between fatty acid and glucose metabolism: potential explanation of insulin resistance of puberty. Diabetes 1994; 43:908–914.

379. Travers SH, Jeffers BW, Bloch CA, et al. Gender and Tanner stage differences in body composition and insulin sensitivity in early pubertal children. J Clin Endocrinol Metab 1995; 80:172–178.

380. Caprio S, Amiel SA, Merkel P, et al. Insulin-resistant syndromes in children. Horm Res 1993; 39(Suppl 3):112–114.

381. Holl RW, Heinze E, Seifert M, et al. Longitudinal analysis of somatic development in paediatric patients with IDDM: genetic influences on height and weight. Diabetologia 1994; 37:925–929.

382. Brown M, Ahmed ML, Clayton KL, et al. Growth during childhood and final height in type 1 diabetes. Diabet Med 1994; 11:182–187.

383. Normann EK, Evald U, Dahl-Jorgensen K, et al. Decreased serum insulin-like growth factor I during puberty in children with insulin-dependent diabetes mellitus (IDDM). Ups J Med Sci 1994; 99:147–154.

384. Pal BR, Matthews DR, Edge JA, et al. The frequency and amplitude of growth hormone secretory episodes as determined by deconvolution analysis are increased in adolescents with insulin-dependent diabetes mellitus and are unaffected by short-term euglycaemia. Clin Endocrinol (Oxf) 1993; 38:93–100.

385. Menon RK, Arslanian S, May B, et al. Diminished growth hormone–binding protein in children with insulin-dependent diabetes mellitus. J Clin Endocrinol Metab 1992; 74:934–938.

386. Stoll BA. Obesity and breast cancer. Int J Obes Relat Metab Disord 1996; 20:389–392.

387. Stoll BA. Timing of weight gain in relation to breast cancer risk. Ann Oncol 1995; 6:245–248.

388. Stoll BA, Vatten LJ, Kvinnsland S. Does early physical maturity influence breast cancer risk? Acta Oncol 1994; 33:171–176.

389. Stoll BA, Secreto G. New hormone-related markers of high risk to breast cancer. Ann Oncol 1992; 3:435–438.

390. Stoll BA. Breast cancer risk in Japanese women with special reference to the growth hormone–insulin-like growth factor axis. Jpn J Clin Oncol 1992; 22:1–5.

391. Islam AH, Yamashita S, Kotani K, et al. Fasting plasma insulin level is an important risk factor for the development of complications in Japanese obese children—results from a cross-sectional and a longitudinal study. Metabolism 1995; 44:478–485.

392. Kokkonen J, Laatikainen L, van Dickhoff K, et al. Ocular complications in young adults with insulin-dependent diabetes mellitus since childhood. Acta Paediatr 1994; 83:273–278.

393. Algvere P. Prepubertal diabetes duration increases the risk of retinopathy. Acta Paediatr 1994; 83:341.

394. Falck A, Kaar ML, Laatikainen L. A prospective, longitudinal study examining the development of retinopathy in children with diabetes. Acta Paediatr 1996; 85:313–319.

395. Fairchild JM, Hing SJ, Donaghue KC, et al. Prevalence and risk factors for retinopathy in adolescents with type 1 diabetes. Med J Aust 1994; 160:757–762.

396. Falck AA, Kaar ML, Laatikainen LT. Prevalence and risk factors of retinopathy in children with diabetes: a population-based study on Finnish children. Acta Ophthalmol 1993; 71:801–809.

397. McNally PG, Raymond NT, Swift PG, et al. Does the prepubertal duration of diabetes influence the onset of microvascular complications? Diabet Med 1993; 10:906–908.

398. Goldstein DE, Blinder KJ, Ide CH, et al. Glycemic control and development of retinopathy in youth-onset insulin-dependent diabetes mellitus: results of a 12-year longitudinal study. Ophthalmology 1993; 100:1125–1131.

399. de Abreu JR, Silva R, Cunha-Vaz JG. The blood-retinal barrier in diabetes during puberty. Arch Ophthalmol 1994; 112:1334–1338.

400. Janner M, Knill SE, Diem P, et al. Persistent microalbuminuria in adolescents with type I (insulin-dependent) diabetes mellitus is associated with early rather than late puberty: results of a prospective, longitudinal study. Eur J Pediatr 1994; 153:403–408.

401. Glaser NS. Non–insulin-dependent diabetes mellitus in childhood and adolescence. Pediatr Clin North Am 1997; 44:307–337.

402. Glaser N, Jones KL. Non–insulin-dependent diabetes mellitus in children and adolescents. Adv Pediatr 1996; 43:359–396.

403. Todd JA. Transcribing diabetes. Nature 1996; 384:407–408.

404. Kirkland RT, Keenan BS, Probstfield JL, et al. Decrease in plasma high-density lipoprotein cholesterol levels at puberty in boys with delayed adolescence: correlation with plasma testosterone levels. JAMA 1987; 257:502–507.

405. LaRosa JC. Lipids and cardiovascular disease: do the findings and therapy apply equally to men and women? Women's Health Issues 1992; 2:102–113.

406. Sorva R, Kuusi T, Dunkel L, et al. Effects of endogenous sex steroids on serum lipoproteins and postheparin plasma lipolytic enzymes. J Clin Endocrinol Metab 1988; 66:408–413.

407. Cobbaert C, Deprost L, Mulder P, et al. Pubertal serum lipoprotein (a) and its correlates in Belgian schoolchildren. Int J Epidemiol 1995; 24:78–87.

408. Haffner SM, Frangos M, Williamson J, et al. Lp(a) concentrations and phenotypes in children with insulin-dependent diabetes mellitus. Chem Phys Lipids 1994; 6768:223–231.

409. Srinivasan SR, Wattigney W, Webber LS, et al. Race and gender differences in serum lipoproteins of children, adolescents, and young adults—emergence of an adverse lipoprotein pattern in white males: the Bogalusa Heart Study. Prev Med 1991; 20:671–684.

410. Wilcken DE, Lynch JF, Marshall MD, et al. Relevance of body weight to apolipoprotein levels in Australian children. Med J Aust 1996; 164:22–25.

411. Flodmark CE, Sveger T, Nilsson-Ehle P. Waist measurement correlates to a potentially atherogenic lipoprotein profile in obese 12- to 14-year-old children. Acta Paediatr 1994; 83:941–945.

412. Tonstad S, Joakimsen O, Stensland-Bugge E, et al. Risk factors related to carotid intima-media thickness and plaque in children with familial hypercholesterolemia and control subjects. Arterioscler Thromb Vasc Biol 1996; 16:984–991.

413. Brambilla P, Manzoni P, Sironi S, et al. Peripheral and abdominal adiposity in childhood obesity. Int J Obes Relat Metab Disord 1994; 18:795–800.

414. DiPietro L, Mossberg HO, Stunkard AJ. A 40-year history of overweight children in Stockholm: life-time overweight, morbidity, and mortality. Int J Obes Relat Metab Disord 1994; 18:585–590.

415. Kiess W, Meidert A, Dressendorfer RA, et al. Salivary cortisol levels throughout childhood and adolescence: relation with age, pubertal stage, and weight. Pediatr Res 1995; 37:502–506.

416. Grumbach MM. The neuroendocrinology of puberty. In: Krieger DT, Hughes JC, et al, eds. Neuroendocrinology. Sunderland, MA: Sinauer Associates, 1980: 249–258.

417. Grumbach MM, Kaplan SL. Fetal pituitary hormones and the maturation of central nervous system regulation of anterior pituitary function. In: Gluck L, ed. Modern Perinatal Medicine. Chicago: Year Book Medical, 1974: 247–271.

418. Reiter EO, Grumbach MM. Neuroendocrine control mechanisms and the onset of puberty. Annu Rev Physiol 1982; 44:595–613.

419. Kaplan SL, Grumbach MM. Pituitary and placental gonadotropins and sex steroids in the human and subhuman primate fetus. Clin Endocrinol Metab 1978; 7:487–511.

420. Donovan BT, van der Werff JJ. Physiology of Puberty. Baltimore: Williams & Wilkins, 1965.

421. Critchlow V, Bar-Sela ME. Control of the onset of puberty. In: Martini L, Ganong WF, eds. Neuroendocrinology. New York: Academic Press, 1967: 101–162.

422. Wilkins L. The Diagnosis and Treatment of Endocrine Disorders in Childhood and Adolescence. Springfield, IL: Charles C Thomas, 1965.

423. King JC, Anthony ELP, Fitzgerald DM, et al. Luteinizing hormone–releasing hormone neurons in human preoptic/hypothalamus: differential intraneuronal localization of immunoreactive forms. J Clin Endocrinol Metab 1985; 60:88–97.

424. Mellon PL, Windle JJ, Goldsmith PC, et al. Immortalization of hypothalamic GnRH neurons by genetically targeted tumorigenesis. Neuron 1990; 5:1–10.

425. Knobil E. The GnRH pulse generator. Am J Obstet Gynecol 1990; 163:1721–1727.

426. Martinez de la Escalera G, Choi ALH, Weiner RI. Generation and synchronization of gonadotropin-releasing hormone (GnRH) pulses: intrinsic properties of the GT1-1 GnRH neuronal cell line. Proc Natl Acad Sci USA 1992; 89:1852–1855.

427. Adelman JP, Mason AJ, Hayflick JS, et al. Isolation of the gene and hypothalamic cDNA for the common precursor of gonadotropin-releasing hormone and prolactin release–inhibiting factor in human and rat. Proc Natl Acad Sci USA 1986; 83:179–183.

428. Wetsel W, Valença MM, Merchenthaler I, et al. Intrinsic pulsatile secretory activity of immortalized luteinizing hormone–releasing hormone-secreting neurons. Proc Natl Acad Sci USA 1992; 89:4149–4153.

429. Kusano K, Fueshko S, Gainer H, Wray S. Electrical and synaptic properties of embryonic luteinizing hormone–releasing hormone neurons in explant cultures. Proc Natl Acad Sci USA 1995; 92:3918–3922.

430. Marshall PE, Goldsmith PC. Neuroregulatory and neuroendocrine GnRH pathways in the hypothalamus and forebrain of the baboon. Brain Res 1980; 193:353–372.

431. Witkin JW, Silverman AJ. Synaptology of LHRH neurons in rat preoptic area. Peptides 1985; 6:263–271.

432. Krsmanovic LZ, Stojilkovic SS, Mertz LM, et al. Expression of gonadotropin-releasing hormone receptors and autocrine regulation of neuropeptide release in immortalized hypothalamic neurons. Proc Natl Acad Sci USA 1993; 90:3908–3912.

433. Morreto M, Lopez FJ, Negro-Villar A. Nitric oxide regulates luteinizing hormone–releasing hormone secretion. Endocrinology 1993; 133:2399–2402.

434. Mahachoklertwattana P, Black SM, Kaplan SL, et al. Nitric oxide synthesized by gonadotropin-releasing hormone neurons is a mediator of N-methyl-D-aspartate (NMDA)-induced GnRH secretion. Endocrinology 1994; 135:1709–1712.

435. Spratt DI, O'Dea LSL, Shoenfeld D, et al. Neuroendocrine-gonadal axis in men: frequent sampling of LH, FSH, and testosterone. Am J Physiol 1988; 254:E658–E666.

436. Gorski RA. Extrahypothalamic influences on gonadotropin secretion. In: Grumbach MM, Grave GD, Mayer FE, eds. Control of the Onset of Puberty. New York: John Wiley & Sons, 1974: 182.

437. Gorski RA. Maturation of neural mechanisms and the pubertal process. In: Grumbach MM, Sizonenko PC, Aubert ML, eds. Control of the Onset of Puberty. Baltimore: Williams & Wilkins, 1990: 259–281.

438. Gallo RV. Neuroendocrine regulation of pulsatile luteinizing hormone in the rat. Neuroendocrinology 1980; 20:122–131.

439. Ojeda SR, Andrews WW, Advis JP. Recent advances in the endocrinology of puberty. Endocr Rev 1980; 1:228–257.

440. Thind KK, Goldsmith PC. Infundibular gonadotropin-releasing hormone neurons are inhibited by direct opioid and autoregulatory synapses in juvenile monkeys. Neuroendocrinology 1988; 47:203–216.

440a. Thind KK, Goldsmith PC. Glutamate and gabaergic neurointeractions in the monkey hypothalamus: a quantitative immunomorphological study. Neuroendocrinology 1995; 61:471–485.

441. De Jong FH. Inhibin. Physiol Rev 1988; 68:555–607.

442. Ying S-Y. Inhibins, activins, and follistatins: gonadal proteins modulating the secretion of follicle-stimulating hormone. Endocr Rev 1988; 9:267–293.

443. Wetsel WC. Immortalized hypothalamic luteinizing hormone–releasing hormone (LHRH) neurons: a new tool for dissecting the molecular and cellular basis of LHRH physiology. Cell Molec Neurobiol 1995; 15:43–78.

444. Martinez de la Escalera G, Choi ALH, Weiner RI. Signaling pathways involved in GnRH secretion in GT1 Cells. Neuroendocrinology 1995; 61:310–317.

445. Krsmanovic LZ, Stojilkovic SS, Catt KJ. Pulsatile gonadotropin-releasing hormone release and its regulation. Trends Endocrinol Metab 1996; 7:56–59.

446. Conn PM, Janovick JA, Stanislaus D, et al. Molecular and cellular bases of gonadotropin-releasing hormone action in the pituitary and central nervous system. Vitam Horm 1995; 50:151–214.

447. Sealfon SC, Weinstein H, Millar RP. Molecular mechanisms of ligand interaction with the gonadotropin-releasing hormone receptor. Endocr Rev 1997; 18:180–205.

448. Short RV. The evolution of human reproduction. Proc R Soc Med 1976; 195:3–24.

449. Bronson FH, Rissman EF. The biology of puberty. Biol Rev 1986; 61:157–195.

450. Van Den Pol AN, Wuarin JP, Dudek FE. Glutamate, the dominant excitatory transmitter in neuroendocrine regulation. Science 1990; 250:1276–1278.

451. Germak JA, Knobil E. Control of puberty in the rhesus monkey. In: Grumbach MM, Sizonenko PC, Aubert ML, eds. Control of the Onset of Puberty. Baltimore: Williams & Wilkins, 1990: 69–81.

452. Plant TM. Puberty in primates. In: Knobil E, Neill JD, eds. The Physiology of Reproduction. 2nd ed. New York: Raven Press, 1994: 1763–1788.

453. Crowley WF, Filicori M, Spratt DI. The physiology of gonadotropin-releasing hormone (GnRH) secretion in men and women. Recent Prog Horm Res 1985; 41:473–526.

454. Wildt L, Hausler A, Marshall G, et al. Frequency and amplitude of gonadotropin-releasing hormone stimulation and gonadotropin secretion in the rhesus monkey. Endocrinology 1981; 109:376–385.

455. Gross KM, Matsumoto AM, Brenner WJ. Differential control of luteinizing hormone and follicle-stimulating hormone secretion by luteinizing hormone–releasing hormone pulse frequency in man. J Clin Endocrinol Metab 1987; 64:675–680.

456. Finkelstein JS, Budger TM, O'Dea LS, et al. Effects of decreasing the frequency of gonadotropin-releasing hormone stimulation on gonadotropin secretion in gonadotropin-releasing hormone–deficient men and perifused rat pituitary cells. J Clin Invest 1988; 81:1725–1733.

457. Knobil E. The neuroendocrine control of the menstrual cycle. Recent Prog Horm Res 1980; 36:53–88.

458. Belchetz PE, Plant TM, Nakai Y, et al. Hypophyseal responses to continuous and intermittent delivery of hypothalamic gonadotropin-releasing hormone. Science 1978; 202:631–633.

459. Nett TM, Crowder ME, Moss GE, et al. GnRH-receptor interaction. V. Down-regulation of pituitary receptors for GnRH in ovariectomized ewes by infusion of homologous hormone. Biol Reprod 1981; 24:1145–1155.

460. Schwanzel-Fukuda M, Pfaff DW. Origin of luteinizing hormone–releasing hormone neurons. Nature 1989; 338:161–164.

461. Wray S, Grant P, Gainer H. Evidence that cells expressing luteinizing hormone–releasing hormone mRNA in the mouse are derived from progenitor cells in the olfactory placode. Proc Natl Acad Sci USA 1989; 86:8132–8136.

462. Wray S, Nieburgs A, Elkabes S. Spatiotemporal cell expression for luteinizing hormone–releasing hormone in the prenatal mouse: evidence for an embryonic origin in the olfactory placode. Dev Brain Res 1989; 46:309–318.

463. Ronnekleiv OK, Resko JA. Ontogeny of gonadotropin-releasing hormone–containing neurons in early fetal development of rhesus macaques. Endocrinology 1990; 126:498–511.

464. Schwanzel-Fukuda M, Bick D, Pfaff DW. Luteinizing hormone–releasing hormone (LHRH)–expressing cells do not migrate normally in an inherited hypogonadal (Kallmann) syndrome. Mol Brain Res 1989; 6:311–326.

465. Schwanzel-Fukuda M, Crossin KL, Pfaff DW, et al. Migration of luteinizing hormone–releasing hormone (LHRH) neurons in early human embryos. J Comp Neurol 1996; 366:547–557.

466. Parhar I, Pfaff D, Schwanzel-Fukuda M. Genes and behavior as studied through gonadotropin-releasing hormone (GnRH) neurons: comparative and functional aspects. Cell Mol Neurobiol 1995; 15:107–116.

467. Gluckman PD, Grumbach MM, Kaplan SL. The neuroendocrine regulation and function of growth hormone and prolactin in the mammalian fetus. Endocr Rev 1981; 2:363–395.

468. Thliveris JA, Currie RW. Observations on the hypothalamo-hypophyseal portal vasculature in the developing human fetus. Am J Anat 1980; 157:441–444.

469. Clark SJ, Ellis N, Styne DM, et al. Hormone ontogeny in the ovine fetus. XVII. Demonstration of pulsatile luteinizing hormone secretion by the fetal pituitary gland. Endocrinology 1984; 115:1774–1779.

470. Clark SJ, Hauffa BP, Rodens KP, et al. Hormone ontogeny in the ovine fetus. XIX. The effect of a potent luteinizing hormone–releasing factor agonist on gonadotropin and testosterone release in the fetus and neonate. Pediatr Res 1989; 25:347–352.

471. Huhtaniemi I, Lautala P. Stimulation of steroidogenesis in human fetal testes by the placenta during perifusion. J Steroid Biochem 1979; 10:109–113.

472. Molsberry RL, Carr BR, Mendelson CR, et al. Human chorionic gonadotropin binding to human fetal testes as a function of gestational age. J Clin Endocrinol Metab 1982; 55:791–794.

473. Huhtaniemi IT, Yamamoto M, Ranta T, et al. Follicle-stimulating hormone receptors appear earlier in the primate fetal testis than in the ovary. J Clin Endocrinol Metab 1987; 65:1210–1214.

474. Huhtaniemi I, Pelliniemi J. Fetal Leydig cells: cellular origin, morphology, life span, and special functional feature. Proc Soc Exp Biol Med 1992; 201:125–140.

475. Huhtaniemi I. Ontogeny of luteinizing hormone action in the male. In: Payne AH, Hardy MP, Russel LD, eds. The Leydig Cell. Vienna, IL: Cache River Press, 1996: 366–382.

476. Saez JM. Leydig cells: endocrine, paracrine, and autocrine regulation. Endocr Rev 1994; 15:574–626.

477. Baker RG, Scrimgeour JB. Development of the gonad in normal and anencephalic human fetuses. J Reprod Fertil 1980; 68:193–199.

478. Beck-Peccoz P, Padmanabhan V, Baggiani AM, et al. Maturation of hypothalamic-pituitary-gonadal function in normal human fetuses: circulating levels of gonadotropins, their common alpha subunit and free testosterone, and discrepancy between immunological and biological activities of circulating follicle-stimulating hormone. J Clin Endocrinol Metab 1991; 73:525–532.

479. Massa G, de Zegher F, Vanderschueren-Lodeweyckx M. Serum levels of immunoreactive inhibin, FSH, and LH in human infants at preterm and term birth. Biol Neonate 1992; 61:150–155.

480. Gluckman PD, Marti Henneberg C, Kaplan SL, Grumbach MM. Hormone ontogeny in the ovine fetus. XIV. The effect of 17β-estradiol infusion on fetal plasma gonadotropins and prolactin and the maturation of sex steroid–dependent negative feedback. Endocrinology 1983; 112:1618–1623.

481. Groom GV, Boyns AR. Effect of hypothalamic-releasing factor and steroids on release of gonadotrophins by organ culture of human fetal pituitary glands. J Endocrinol 1973; 59:511–522.

482. Jaffe AB, Mulcahey JJ, DiBabio AM, et al. Peptide regulation of pituitary and target tissue function and growth in the primate fetus. Recent Prog Horm Res 1988; 44:431–544.

483. Takagi ST, Yoshida T, Tsubata K, et al. Sex differences in fetal gonadotropins and androgens. J Steroid Biochem 1977; 8:609–620.

484. Davies JL, Naftolin F, Ryan KJ, et al. A specific high-affinity, limited-capacity estrogen-binding component in the cytosol of human fetal pituitary and brain tissues. J Clin Endocrinol Metab 1975; 40:909.

485. Cuttler L, Egli CA, Styne DM, et al. Hormone ontogeny in the ovine fetus. XVIII. The effect of an opioid antagonist on luteinizing hormone secretion. Endocrinology 1985; 116:1997–2002.

486. Mesiano S, Hart CS, Heyer BW, Kaplan SL, Grumbach MM. Hormone ontogeny in the ovine fetus. XXVI. A sex difference in the effect of castration on the hypothalamic-pituitary gonadotropin unit in the ovine fetus. Endocrinology 1991; 129:3073–3079.

487. Bettendorf M, Albers N, de Zegher F, et al. A neuroexcitatory amino acid analogue, N-methyl-D,L-aspartate (NMDA), elicits LH and FSH release in the ovine fetus by a central mechanism. Endocr Soc Abstr 1988; 288 (abstract).

488. Albers N, Bettendorf M, Hart CS, et al. Hormone ontogeny in the ovine fetus. XXIII. Pulsatile administration of follicle-stimulating hormone stimulates inhibin production and decreases testosterone synthesis in the ovine fetal gonad. Endocrinology 1989; 124:3089–3094.

489. Albers N, Hart CS, Kaplan SL, et al. Hormone ontogeny in the ovine fetus. XXIV. Porcine follicular fluid "inhibins" selectively suppress plasma follicle-stimulating hormone in the ovine fetus. Endocrinology 1989; 125:675–678.

490. Corbier P, Dehennin L, Castanier M, et al. Sex differences in serum luteinizing hormone and testosterone in the human neonate during the first few hours after birth. J Clin Endocrinol Metab 1990; 71:1344–1348.

491. Lustig RH, Conte FA, Kogan BA, Grumbach MM. Ontogeny of gonadotropin secretion in congenital anorchism: sexual dimorphism versus syndrome of gonadal dysgenesis and diagnostic considerations. J Urol 1987; 138:587–591.

492. Plant TM. The effects of neonatal orchidectomy on the developmental pattern of gonadotropin secretion in the male rhesus monkey (Macaca mulatta). Endocrinology 1980; 106:1451–1454.

493. Winter JSD, Faiman C, Hobson WC, et al. Pituitary-gonadal regulations in infancy. I. Patterns of serum gonadotropin concentrations from birth to four years of age in man and chimpanzee. J Clin Endocrinol Metab 1975; 40:545–551.

494. Forest MG. Pituitary gonadotropin and sex steroid secretion during the first two years of life. In: Grumbach MM, Sizonenko PC, Aubert ML, eds. Control of the Onset of Puberty. Baltimore: Williams & Wilkins, 1990: 451–478.

495. Grumbach MM. The central nervous system and the onset of puberty. In: Falkner F, Tanner JM, eds. Human Growth. New York: Plenum, 1978: 215–238.

496. Lander ES, Schork NJ. Genetic dissection of complex traits. Science 1994; 265:2037–2048.

497. Frankel WN, Schork N. Who's afraid of epistasis? Nature Genet 1996; 14:371–373.

498. Paterson AH. Molecular dissection of quantitative traits: progress and prospects. Genome Res 1995; 5:321–333.

499. Risch N, Merikangas K. The future of genetic studies of complex human diseases. Science 1996; 273:1516–1517.

500. Frisch RE. Fatness of girls from menarche to age 18 with a nomogram. Hum Biol 1976; 48:353–359.

501. Frisch RE, McArthur JW. Menstrual cycles: fatness as a determinant of minimum weight for height necessary for their maintenance or onset. Science 1974; 185:949–951.

502. Frisch RE. Pubertal adipose tissue: is it necessary for normal sexual maturation? Evidence from the rat and human female. Fed Proc 1980; 39:2395–2400.

503. Garn SM, Lavelle M, Pilkington JJ. Comparison of fatness in premenarchial and postmenarchial girls of the same age. J Pediatr 1983; 103:328–331.

504. Forbes GB. Body size and composition of perimenarchial girls. Am J Dis Child 1992; 146:63–66.

505. Bronson FH, Manning JM. The energetic regulation of ovulation—a realistic role of body fat. Biol Reprod 1991; 44:945–950.

506. Malina RM. Menarche in athletes: a synthesis and hypothesis. Ann Hum Biol 1983; 10:1–24.

507. Wellens R, Malina RM, Roche AF, et al. Body size and fatness in young adults in relation to age of menarche. Am J Hum Biol 1992; 4:783–787.

508. Frisch RE. Body fat, puberty, and fertility. Biol Rev Camb Philos Soc 1984; 59:161–188.

509. Boyar RM, Katz J, Finkelstein JW, et al. Anorexia nervosa: immaturity of the 24-hour luteinizing hormone secretory pattern. N Engl J Med 1974; 291:861–865.

510. Frisch RE, Wyshak G, Vincent L. Delayed menarche and amenorrhea in ballet dancers. N Engl J Med 1980; 303:17–19.

511. de Souza MJ, Metzger DA. Reproductive dysfunction in amenorrheic athletes and anorexic patients: a review. Med Sci Sports Exerc 1991; 23:995–1007.

512. Frisch RE, Gotz-Welbergen AV, McArthur JW, et al. Delayed menarche and amenorrhea of college athletes in relation to age of onset of training. JAMA 1981; 246:1559–1564.

513. McArthur JW, Bullen BA, Beitins IZ, et al. Hypothalamic amenorrhea in runners of normal body composition. Endocr Res Commun 1980; 7:13–25.

514. Cameron N, Mitchell J, Meyer D, et al. Secondary sexual development of "Cape Coloured" girls following kwashiorkor. Ann Hum Biol 1988; 15:65–75.

515. Johnston FE, Roche AF, Schell LM, et al. Critical weight at menarche. Am J Dis Child 1975; 129:19–23.

516. Cameron N. Weight and skinfold variation at menarche and the critical body weight hypothesis. Ann Hum Biol 1976; 3:279–282.

517. Billewicz WS, Fellowes HM, Hytten CA. Comments on the critical metabolic mass and the age of menarche. Ann Hum Biol 1976; 3:51–59.

518. Penny R, Goldstein IP, Frasier SD. Gonadotropin excretion and body composition. Pediatrics 1978; 61:294–300.

519. Kennedy GC, Mitra J. Body weight and food intake as initiating factors for puberty in the rat. J Physiol 1963; 166:408–418.

520. Zhang Y, Proenca R, Maffei M, et al. Positional cloning of the mouse obese gene and its human analogue. Nature 1994; 372:425–432.

521. Halaas JL, Gajiwala KS, Maffei M, et al. Weight-reducing effects of the plasma protein encoded by the obese gene. Science 1995; 269:543–546.

522. Spiegelman BM, Flier JS. Adipogenesis and obesity: rounding out the big picture. Cell 1996; 87:377–389.

523. Pelleymounter MA, Cullen MJ, Baker MB, et al. Effects of the obese gene product on body weight regulation in ob/ob mice. Science 1995; 269:540–543.

524. Caro JF, Sinha MK, Kolacznski JW, et al. Leptin: the tale of an obesity gene. Diabetes 1996; 45:1455–1462.

524a. Sinha MK, Opentanova I, Ohannesian JP, et al. Evidence of free and bound leptin in human circulation. J Clin Invest 98:1277–1282.

525. Ahima RS, Prabakaran D, Mantzoros C, et al. Role of leptin in the neuroendocrine response to fasting. Nature 1996; 382:250–252.

526. Schwartz MW, Seeley RJ, Campfield LA, et al. Identification of targets of leptin action in rat hypothalamus. J Clin Invest 1996; 98:1101–1106.

527. Campfield LA, Smith FJ, Guisez Y, et al. Recombinant mouse OB protein: evidence for a peripheral signal linking adiposity and central neural networks. Science 1995; 269:546–549.

528. Tartaglia LA, Dembski M, Weng X, et al. Identification and expression cloning of a leptin receptor, OB-R. Cell 1995; 83:1263–1271.

529. Baumann H, Morella KK, White DW, et al. The full-length leptin receptor has signaling capabilities of interleukin 6-type cytokine receptors. Proc Natl Acad Sci USA 1996; 93:8374–8378.

530. Licinio J, Mantzoros C, Negrão AB, et al. Human leptin levels are pulsatile and inversely related to pituitary-adrenal function. Nature Med 1997; 3:575–579.

531. Leibel RL. And finally, genes for human obesity. Nature Genet 1997; 16:218–220.

532. Considine RV, Sinha MK, Heiman ML, et al. Serum immunoreactive-leptin concentrations in normal-weight and obese humans. N Engl J Med 1996; 334:292–295.

533. Chehab FF, Lim ME, Lu R. Correction of the sterility defect in homozygous obese female mice by treatment with the human recombinant leptin. Nature Genet 1996; 12:318–320.

534. Mounzih K, Lu R, Chehab FF. Leptin treatment rescues the sterility of genetically obese ob/ob males. Endocrinology 1997; 138:1190–1193.

535. Barash IA, Cheung CC, Weigle DS, et al. Leptin is a metabolic signal to the reproductive system. Endocrinology 1996; 137:3144–3147.

536. Chehab FF, Mounzih K, Lu R, Lim ME. Early onset of reproductive function in normal female mice treated with leptin. Science 1997; 275:88–90.

537. Ahima RS, Dushay J, Flier SN, et al. Leptin accelerates the onset of puberty in normal female mice. J Clin Invest 1997; 99:391–395.

538. Cheung CC, Thornton JE, Kuijper JL, et al. Leptin is a metabolic gate for the onset of puberty in the female rat. Endocrinology 1997; 138:855–858.

539. Yu WH, Kimura M, Walczewska A, et al. Role of leptin in hypothalamic-pituitary function. Proc Natl Acad Sci USA 1997; 94:1023–1028.

540. de Ridder CM, Thijssen JH, Bruning PF, et al. Body fat mass, body fat distribution, and pubertal development: a longitudinal study of physical and hormonal sexual maturation of girls. J Clin Endocrinol Metab 1992; 75:442–446.

541. Mantzoros CS, Flier JS, Rogol AD. A longitudinal assessment of hormonal and physical alterations during normal puberty in boys. V. Rising leptin levels may signal the onset of puberty. J Clin Endocrinol Metab 1997; 82:1066–1070.

542. Plant TM, Durrant AR. Circulating leptin does not appear to provide a signal for triggering the initiation of puberty in the male rhesus monkey (Macaca mulatta). Endocrinology 1997; 138:4505–4508.

543. Lee PA, Witchel SF, Arslanian SA. Lack of relationship between leptin and pubertal activation and deactivation. In: Program and Abstracts, The Endocrine Society 79th Annual Meeting, June 1997; 379 (abstract).

544. Garcia-Mayor RV, Andrade MA, Rios M, et al. Serum leptin levels in normal children: relationship to age, gender, body mass index, pituitary-gonadal hormones, and pubertal stage. J Clin Endocrinol Metab 1997; 82:2849–2855.

544a. Blum WF, Englaro P, Hanitsch S, et al. Plasma leptin levels in healthy children and adolescents: dependence on body mass index, body fat mass, gender, pubertal stage, and testosterone. J Clin Endocrinol Metab 1997; 82:2904–2910.

545. Clayton PE, Gill MS, Hall CM, et al. Serum leptin through childhood and adolescence. Clin Endocrinol 1997; 46:727–733.

546. Comuzzie AG, Hixson JE, Almasy L, et al. A major quantitative locus determining serum leptin levels and fat mass is located on chromosome 2. Nature Genet 1997; 15:273–276.

547. Brown DC, Kelnar CJH, Wu FCW. Energy metabolism during male human puberty. I. Changes in energy expenditure during the onset of puberty in boys. Ann Hum Biol 1996; 23:273–279.

548. Odell WD, Swerdloff RS. Etiologies of sexual maturation: a model system based on the sexually maturing rat. Recent Prog Horm Res 1976; 32:245–288.

549. Davidson JM. Hypothalamic-pituitary regulation of puberty: evidence from animal experimentation. In: Grumbach MM, Grave GD, Mayer FE, eds. Control of the Onset of Puberty. New York: John Wiley & Sons, 1974: 79–103.

550. Ramirez VD. Endocrinology of puberty: female reproductive system. Part 1. In: Greep RO, Astwood EB, eds. Handbook of Physiology. Sect 7:

Endocrinology. Washington, DC: American Physiological Society, 1973: 1–28.

551. Lenko HL, Lang U, Aubert ML, et al. Hormonal changes in puberty. VII. Lack of variation of daytime plasma melatonin. J Clin Endocrinol Metab 1982; 54:1056–1058.

552. Cohen HN, Hay ID, Annesley TM, et al. Serum immunoreactive melatonin in boys with delayed puberty. Clin Endocrinol 1982; 17:517–521.

553. Reppert SM, Weaver DR. Melatonin madness. Cell 1995; 83:1059–1062.

554. Luboshitzky R, Lavi S, Thuma I, et al. Increased nocturnal melatonin secretion in male patients with hypogonadotropic hypogonadism and delayed puberty. J Clin Endocrinol Metab 1995; 80:2144–2148.

555. Cavallo A. Melatonin and human puberty: current perspectives. J Pineal Res 1993; 15:115–121.

556. Cavallo A. Melatonin secretion during adrenarche in normal human puberty and in pubertal disorders. J Pineal Res 1992; 12:71–78.

557. Cavallo A. Plasma melatonin rhythm in normal puberty: interactions of age and pubertal stages. Neuroendocrinology 1992; 55:372–379.

558. Cavallo A, Ritschel WA. Pharmacokinetics of melatonin in human sexual maturation. J Clin Endocrinol Metab 1996; 81:1882–1886.

559. Luboshitzky R, Lavi S, Thuma I, et al. Testosterone treatment alters melatonin concentrations in male patients with gonadotropin-releasing hormone deficiency. J Clin Endocrinol Metab 1996; 81:770–774.

560. Okatani Y, Sagara Y. Amplification of nocturnal melatonin secretion in women with functional secondary amenorrhoea: relation to endogenous oestrogen concentration. Clin Endocrinol 1994; 41:763–770.

561. Foster DL, Ryan KD. Puberty in the lamb: Sexual maturation of a seasonal breeder in a changing environment. In: Grumbach MM, Sizonenko PC, Aubert ML, eds. Control of the Onset of Puberty. Baltimore: Williams & Wilkins, 1990: 108–142.

562. Ojeda SR, Smith-White S, Advis JP, et al. First preovulatory gonadotropin surge in the rodent. In: Grumbach MM, Sizonenko PC, Aubert ML, eds. Control of the Onset of Puberty. Baltimore: Williams & Wilkins, 1990: 156–182.

562a. Donovan BT. Puberty in the guinea pig and rabbit. In: Grumbach MM, Sizonenko PC, Aubert ML, eds. Control of the Onset of Puberty. Baltimore: Williams & Wilkins, 1990: 143–155.

563. Vandenbergh JG. Pheromones and mammalian reproduction. In: Knobil E, Neill JD, eds. The Physiology of Reproduction. 2nd ed. New York: Raven Press, 1994: 343–362.

564. Conte FA, Grumbach MM, Kaplan SL, et al. Correlation of luteinizing hormone–releasing factor–induced luteinizing hormone and follicle-stimulating hormone release from infancy to 19 years with the changing pattern of gonadotropin secretion in agonadal patients: relation to the restraint of puberty. J Clin Endocrinol Metab 1980; 50:163–168.

565. Conte FA, Grumbach MM, Kaplan SL. A diphasic pattern of gonadotropin secretion in patients with the syndrome of gonadal dysgenesis. J Clin Endocrinol Metab 1975; 40:670–674.

566. Kelch RP, Kaplan SL, Grumbach MM. Suppression of urinary and plasma follicle-stimulating hormone by exogenous estrogens in prepubertal and pubertal children. J Clin Invest 1973; 52:1122–1128.

567. Grumbach MM, Kaplan SL. Recent advances in the diagnosis and management of sexual precocity. Acta Paediatr Jpn (Overseas Ed) 1988; 30:155–175.

568. Voigt P, Ma YJ, Gonazalez D, et al. Neural and glial-mediated effects of growth factors acting via tyrosine kinase receptors on luteinizing hormone–releasing hormone neurons. Endocrinology 1996; 137:2593–2605.

569. Wetsel WC, Hill DF, Ojeda SR. Basic fibroblast growth factor regulates the conversion of pro-luteinizing hormone–releasing hormone (pro-LHRH) to LHRH in immortalized hypothalamic neurons. Endocrinology 1997; 137:2606–2616.

570. Junier MP, Ma YJ, Costa ME, et al. Transforming growth factor alpha contributes to the mechanism by which hypothalamic injury induces precocious puberty. Proc Natl Acad Sci USA 1991; 88:9743–9747.

571. Olson BR, Scott DC, Wetsel WC, et al. Effects of insulin-like growth factors I and II and insulin on the immortalized hypthalamic GTI-7 cell line. Neuroendocrinology 1995; 62:155–165.

572. Ojeda SR, Dissen GA, Junier M-P. Neutrophilic factors and female sexual development. Front Neuroendocrinol 1992; 13:120–162.

573. Hiney JK, Srivastava V, Nyberg CL, et al. Insulin-like growth factor I of peripheral origin acts centrally to accelerate the initiation of female puberty. Endocrinology 1996; 137:3717–3728.

574. Gallo F, Morale MC, Avola R, et al. Cross-talk between luteinizing hormone–releasing hormone (LHRH) neurons and astroglia cells: developing glia release factors that accelerate neuronal differentiation and stimulate LHRH release from GT neuronal cell line and LHRH neurons induce astroglia proliferation. Endocrine 1995; 3:863–874.

575. Watanabe G, Terasawa E. In vivo luteinizing hormone releasing hormone increases with puberty in the female rhesus monkey. Endocrinology 1989; 125:92–99.

575a. Vician L, Adams LA, Clifton OK, Steiner RA. Pubertal changes in proopiomelanocortin and gonadotropin-releasing hormone gene expression in the brain of the male monkey. Mol Cell Neurosci 1991; 2:31–38.

576. Terasawa E, Noonan JJ, Nass TE, et al. Posterior hypothalamic lesions advance the onset of puberty in the female rhesus monkey. Endocrinology 1984; 115:2241–2250.

577. Schultz NJ, Terasawa E. Posterior hypothalamic lesions advance the time of the pubertal changes in luteinizing hormone release in ovariectomized female rhesus monkeys. Endocrinology 1988; 123:445.

578. Pohl CR, deRidder CM, Plant TM. Gonadal and nongonadal mechanisms contribute to the prepubertal hiatus in gonadotropin secretion in the female rhesus monkey (Macaca mulatta). J Clin Endocrinol Metab 1995; 80:2094–2101.

579. Hochman HI, Judge DM, Reichlin S. Precocious puberty and hypothalamic hamartoma. Pediatrics 1981; 67:236–244.

580. Judge DM, Kulin HE, Santen R, et al. Hypothalamic hamartoma: a source of luteinizing hormone–releasing factor in precocious puberty. N Engl J Med 1977; 296:7–10.

581. Krieger DT, Perlow MJ, Gibson MJ, et al. Brain grafts reverse hypogonadism of gonadotropin-releasing hormone deficiency. Nature 1982; 298:468–472.

582. Silverman AJ, Gibson M. Hypothalamic transplantation: repair of defects in hypogonadal mice. Trends Endocrinol Metab 1990; 1:403–408.

583. Arslan M, Pohl CR, Plant TM. DL-2-amino-5-phosphonopentanoic acid, a specific N-methyl-D-aspartic acid receptor antagonist, suppresses pulsatile LH release in the rat. Neuroendocrinology 1988; 47:465–468.

584. Gambacciani M, Yen SS, Rasmussen D. GnRH release from the mediobasal hypothalamus: in vitro inhibition by corticotropin releasing factor. Neuroendocrinology 1986; 43:533–536.

585. Kuljis RO, Advis JP. Immunocytochemical and physiological evidence of a synapse between dopamine- and luteinizing hormone–releasing hormone–containing neurons in the ewe median eminence. Endocrinology 1989; 124:1579–1581.

586. MacLusky NJ, Naftolin F, Leranth C. Immunocytochemical evidence for direct synaptic connections between corticotrophin-releasing factor (CRF) and gonadotropin-releasing hormone (GnRH)-containing neurons in the preoptic area of the rat. Brain Res 1988; 439:391–395.

587. Plant TM, Gay VL, Marshall GR, et al. Puberty in monkeys is triggered by chemical stimulation of the hypothalamus. Proc Natl Acad Sci USA 1989; 86:2506–2510.

588. Wilson RC, Kesner JS, Kaufman JM, et al. Central electrophysiologic correlates of pulsatile luteinizing hormone secretion in the rhesus monkey. Neuroendocrinology 1984; 39:256–260.

589. Ozata M, Bulur M, Bingol N, et al. Daytime plasma melatonin levels in male hypogonadism. J Clin Endocrinol Metab 1996; 81:1877–1881.

590. Kelch RP, Kletter GB. Neuroendocrine regulation of puberty in boys. In: Sizonenko PC, Aubert ML, eds. Developmental Endocrinology. New York: Raven Press, 1990: 103–115.

591. Fraioli F, Cappa M, Fabbri A, et al. Lack of endogenous opioid inhibitory tone on LH secretion in early puberty. Clin Endocrinol 1984; 20:299–305.

592. Petraglia F, Bernasconi S, Iughetti L, et al. Naloxone-induced luteinizing hormone secretion in normal, precocious, and delayed puberty. J Clin Endocrinol Metab 1986; 63:1112–1116.

593. Mauras N, Veldhuis JD, Rogol AD. Role of endogenous opiates in pubertal maturation: opposing actions of naltrexone in prepubertal and late pubertal boys. J Clin Endocrinol Metab 1986; 62:1256–1263.

594. Saunder SE, Case GD, Hopwood NJ, et al. The effects of opiate antagonism on gonadotropin secretion in children and in women with hypothalamic amenorrhea. Pediatr Res 1984; 18:322–328.

595. Mitsushima D, Hei DL, Terasawa E. Gamma-aminobutyric acid is an inhibitory neurotransmitter restricting the release of luteinizing hormone–releasing hormone before the onset of puberty. Proc Natl Acad Sci USA 1994; 91:395–399.

596. Mitsushima D, Marzban F, Luchansky LL, et al. Role of glutamic acid decarboxylase in the prepubertal inhibition of the luteinizing hormone–releasing hormone release in female rhesus monkeys. J Neuroscience 1996; 16:2563–2573.

597. Terasawa E. Control of luteinizing hormone–releasing hormone pulse generation in nonhuman primates. Cell Molec Neurobiol 1995; 15:141–164.

598. Martinez de la Escalera G, Choi AL, Weiner RI. Biphasic gabaergic regulation of GnRH secretion in GT1 cell lines. Neuroendocrinology 1994; 59:420–425.

599. Cheung CC, Clifton DK, Steiner RA. Galanin: an unassuming neuropeptide moves to center stage in reproduction. Trends Endocrinol Metab 1996; 7:301–306.

600. Urbanski HF, Ojeda SR. Activation of luteinizing hormone–releasing hormone release advances the onset of female puberty. Neuroendocrinology 1987; 46:273–276.

601. Price MT, Olney JW, Cicero TJ. Acute elevations of serum luteinizing hormone induced by kainic acid, N-methyl aspartic acid, or homocystic acid. Neuroendocrinology 1978; 26:352–358.

602. Gay VL, Plant TM. N-methyl-D,L-aspartate elicits hypothalamic gonadotropin-releasing hormone release in prepubertal male rhesus monkeys (Macaca mulatta). Endocrinology 1987; 120:2289–2296.

603. Wilson RC, Knobil E. Acute effects of N-methyl-D,L-aspartate on the release of pituitary gonadotropins and prolactin in the adult female rhesus monkey. Brain Res 1982; 248:177–179.

604. Bourguignon JP, Gerard A, Mathieu J, et al. Pulsatile release of gonadotropin-releasing hormone from hypothalamic explants is restrained by blockade of N-methyl-D,L-aspartate receptors. Endocrinology 1989; 125:1090–1096.

605. Mahachoklertwattana P, Sanchez J, Kaplan SL, et al. N-methyl-D-aspartate

(NMDA) receptors mediate the release of gonadotropin-releasing hormone (GnRH) by NMDA in a hypothalamic GnRH neuronal cell line (GT1-1). Endocrinology 1994; 134:1023–1030.

606. Rebar RW, Yen SSC. Endocrine rhythms in gonadotropins and ovarian steroids with reference to reproductive processes. In: Krieger DT, ed. Endocrine Rhythms. New York: Raven Press, 1979: 259–298.

607. Kelch RP, Marshall JC, Sauder SE. Pulsatile gonadotropin–releasing hormone and the induction of puberty in human beings. In: Grumbach MM, Sizonenko PC, Aubert ML, eds. Control of the Onset of Puberty. Baltimore: Williams & Wilkins, 1990: 82–107.

608. Boyar RM, Finkelstein JW, Roffwarg H, et al. Twenty-four patterns of luteinizing hormone and follicle-stimulating hormone secretory patterns in gonadal dysgenesis. J Clin Endocrinol Metab 1973; 37:521–525.

609. Kulin HE, Moore RC Jr, Santner SJ. Circadian rhythms in gonadotropin excretion in prepubertal and pubertal children. J Clin Endocrinol Metab 1976; 42:770–773.

610. Waldhauser F, Weissenbacher G, Frisch H, et al. Pulsatile secretion of gonadotropins in early infancy. Eur J Pediatr 1981; 137:71–74.

611. Penny R, Olambiwonnu NO, Frasier SD. Episodic fluctuations of serum gonadotropins in pre- and post-pubertal girls and boys. J Clin Endocrinol Metab 1977; 45:307–311.

612. Boyar R, Finkelstein JW, David R, et al. Twenty-four hour patterns of plasma luteinizing hormone and follicle-stimulating hormone in sexual precocity. N Engl J Med 1973; 289:282–286.

613. Kletter GB, Foster CM, Brown MB, et al. Nocturnal naloxone fails to reverse the suppressive effects of testosterone infusion on luteinizing hormone secretion in pubertal boys. J Clin Endocrinol Metab 1994; 79:1147–1151.

614. Watanabe G, Terasawa E. In vivo release of luteinizing hormone–releasing hormone (LHRH) increases with puberty in the female rhesus monkey. Endocrinology 1989; 125:92–99.

615. Yen SSC, Lasley BL, Wang FC, et al. The operating characteristics of the hypothalamic-pituitary system during the menstrual cycle and observations of biological action of somatostatin. Recent Prog Horm Res 1975; 31:321–363.

616. Keye WR, Jaffe RB. Strength-duration characteristics of estrogen effects on gonadotropin response to gonadotropin-releasing hormone in women. I. Effects of varying duration of estradiol administration. J Clin Endocrinol Metab 1975; 41:1003–1008.

617. Reiter EO, Kaplan SL, Conte FA, et al. Responsivity of pituitary gonadotropes to luteinizing hormone–releasing factor in idiopathic precocious puberty, precocious thelarche, precocious adrenarche, and in patients treated with medroxyprogesterone acetate. Pediatr Res 1975; 9:111–116.

618. Crowley WF Jr, McArthur JW. Stimulation of the normal menstrual cycle in Kallmann's syndrome by pulsatile administration of luteinizing hormone–releasing hormone (LHRH). J Clin Endocrinol Metab 1980; 51:173–175.

619. Yoshimoto Y, Moridera K, Imura H. Restoration of normal pituitary gonadotropin reserve by administration of luteinizing hormone–releasing hormone in patients with hypogonadotropic hypogonadism. N Engl J Med 1975; 292:242–245.

620. Jacobson RI, Seyler LE, Tamborlane WV, et al. Pulsatile subcutaneous nocturnal administration of Gn-RH by portable infusion pump in hypogonadotropic hypogonadism: initiation of gonadotropin responsiveness. J Clin Endocrinol Metab 1979; 49:652–654.

621. Marshall JC, Kelch RP. Low-dose pulsatile gonadotropin-releasing hormone in anorexia nervosa: a model of human pubertal development. J Clin Endocrinol Metab 1979; 49:712–718.

622. Valk TW, Corley KP, Kelch RP, et al. Hypogonadotropic hypogonadism: hormonal responses to low-dose pulsatile administration of gonadotropin-releasing hormone. J Clin Endocrinol Metab 1980; 51:730–737.

623. Pohl GR, Knobil E. The role of the central nervous system in the control of ovarian function in higher primates. Annu Rev Physiol 1982; 44:583–593.

624. Knobil E, Plant TM. The neuroendocrine control of gonadotropin secretion in the female rhesus monkey. Front Neuroendocrinol 1978; 4:249–264.

625. Wildt L, Marshall G, Knobil E. Experimental induction of puberty in the infantile female rhesus monkey. Science 1980; 207:1373–1375.

626. Boyar RM, Finkelstein JW, Witkin M, et al. Studies of endocrine function in "isolated" gonadotropin deficiency. J Clin Endocrinol Metab 1973; 36:64–72.

627. Winter JS, Taraska S, Faiman C. The hormonal response to HCG stimulation in male children and adolescents. J Clin Endocrinol Metab 1972; 34:348–353.

628. Sizonenko PC, Cuendet A, Paunier L. FSH. I. Evidence for its mediating role on testosterone secretion in cryptorchidism. J Clin Endocrinol Metab 1973; 37:68–73.

629. Ross GT, Cargille CM, Lipsett MB, et al. Pituitary and gonadal hormones in women during spontaneous and induced ovulatory cycles. Recent Prog Horm Res 1970; 26:1–62.

630. Reiter EO, Kulin HE, Hamwood SM. The absence of positive feedback between estrogen and luteinizing hormone in sexually immature girls. Pediatr Res 1974; 8:740–745.

631. Presl J, Horejsi J, Stroufova A, et al. Sexual maturation in girls and the development of estrogen-induced gonadotropic hormone release. Ann Biol Anim Biochim Biophys 1976; 16:377–383.

632. Knobil E, Plant TM, Wildt L, et al. Control of the rhesus monkey menstrual cycle: permissive role of the hypothalamic gonadotropin-releasing hormone. Science 1980; 207:1371–1373.

633. Doring GK. Uber die relativ Sterilitat in den Jahren nach der Menarche. Geburtsh Frauenheilkd 1963; 23:30–36.

634. Hansen JW, Hoffman HJ, Ross GT. Monthly gonadotropin cycles in premenarcheal girls. Science 1975; 190:161–163.

635. Winter JSD, Faiman C. Pituitary-gonadal relations in female children and adolescents. Pediatr Res 1973; 7:948–953.

636. Kaplan SL, Grumbach MM. Pathogenesis of sexual precocity. In: Grumbach MM, Sizonenko PC, Aubert ML, eds. Control of the Onset of Puberty. Baltimore: Williams & Wilkins, 1990: 620–660.

637. Cutler GB, Loriaux DL. Andrenarche and its relationship to the onset of puberty. Fed Proc 1980; 39:2384–2390.

638. Sklar CA, Kaplan SL, Grumbach MM. Evidence for dissociation between adrenarche and gonadarche: studies in patients with idiopathic precocious puberty, gonadal dysgenesis, isolated gonadotropin deficiency, and constitutionally delayed growth and adolescence. J Clin Endocrinol Metab 1980; 51:548–556.

639. Hopper BR, Yen SSC. Circulating concentrations of dehydroepiandrosterone and dehydroepiandrosterone sulfate during puberty. J Clin Endocrinol Metab 1975; 40:458–461.

640. Sizonenko PC, Paunier LC. Correlation of plasma dehydroepiandrosterone, testosterone, FSH, and LH with stages of puberty and bone age in normal boys and girls and in patients with Addison's disease or hypogonadism or with premature or late adrenarche. J Clin Endocrinol Metab 1975; 41:894–904.

641. Reiter EO, Fuldauer VG, Root AW. Secretion of the adrenal androgen, dehydroepiandrosterone sulfate, during normal infancy, childhood, and adolescence, in sick infants, and in children with endocrinologic abnormalities. J Pediatr 1977; 90:766–770.

642. Dhom G. Prepubertal and pubertal growth of the adrenal (adrenarche). Beitr Pathol 1973; 150:357–377.

643. Endoh A, Kristiansen SB, Casson PR, et al. The zona reticularis is the site of biosynthesis of dehydroepiandrosterone and dehydroepiandrosterone sulfate in the adult human adrenal cortex resulting from its low expression of 3-beta-hydroxysteroid dehydrogenase. J Clin Endocrinol Metab 1996; 81:3558–3565.

644. Kennerson AR, McDonald DA, Adams JB. Dehydroepiandrosterone sulfotransferase localization in human adrenal glands: a light and electron microscope study. J Clin Endocrinol Metab 1983; 56:786–790.

645. Gell JS, Atkins B, Margraf L, et al. Adrenarche is associated with decreased 3-beta-hydroxysteroid dehydrogenase expression in the adrenal reticularis. Endocr Res 1996; 22:723–728.

646. Dupont E, Luu-The V, Labrie F, et al. Ontogeny of the 3-beta-hydroxysteroid dehydrogenase/delta$_5$-delta$_4$ isomerase (3-beta-HSD) in human adrenal gland performed by immunochemistry. Mol Cell Endocrinol 1990; 74:R7–R10.

647. Parker CR Jr, Stankovic AK, Falany CN, et al. Immunocytochemical analyses of dehydroepiandrosterone sulfotransferase in cultured human fetal adrenal cells. J Clin Endocrinol Metab 1995; 80:1027–1031.

648. Khoury EL, Greenspan JS, Greenspan FS. Adrenocortical cells of the zona reticularis normally express HLA-DR antigenic determinants. Am J Pathol 1987; 127:580–591.

649. Marx C, Bornstein SR, Wolkersdorfer GW, et al. Relevance of major histocompatibility complex class II expression as a hallmark for the cellular differentiation in the human adrenal cortex. J Clin Endocrinol Metab 1997; 82:3136–3140.

650. Kitamura M, Buczko E, Dufau ML. Dissociation of hydroxylase and lyase activities by site-directed mutagenesis of the rat P450c17 alpha. Mol Endocrinol 1991; 5:1373–1380.

651. Miller WL, Auchus RJ, Geller DH. The regulation of 17,20 lyase activity. Steroids 1997; 62:133–142.

652. Zhang L, Rodriguez H, Ohno S, et al. Serine phosphorylation of human P450c17 increases 17,20 lyase activity: implications for adrenarche and the polycystic ovary syndrome. Proc Natl Acad Sci USA 1995; 92:10619–10623.

653. Geller DH, Auchus RJ, Mendonça BB, Miller WL. The genetic and functional basis of isolated 17,20-lyase deficiency. Nat Genet 1997; 17:201–205.

654. Reiter EO, Grumbach MM, Kaplan SL, et al. The response of pituitary gonadotropes to synthetic LRF in children with glucocorticoid-treated congenital adrenal hyperplasia: lack of effect of intrauterine and neonatal androgen excess. J Clin Endocrinol Metab 1975; 40:318–325.

655. Butler GE, McKie M, Ratcliffe SG. The cyclical nature of prepubertal growth. Ann Hum Biol 1990; 17:177–198.

656. Prader A. Delayed adolescence. Clin Endocrinol Metab 1975; 4:143–155.

657. Counts DR, Pescovitz OH, Barnes KM, et al. Dissociation of adrenarche and gonadarche in precocious puberty and in isolated hypogonadotropic hypogonadism. J Clin Endocrinol Metab 1987; 64:1174–1178.

658. Stanhope R, Hindmarsh P, Pringle PJ, et al. Oxandrolone induces a sustained rise in physiological growth hormone secretion in boys with constitutional delay of growth and puberty. Pediatrician 1987; 14:183–188.

659. Loche S, Corda R, Lampis A, et al. The effect of oxandrolone on the growth hormone response to growth hormone–releasing hormone in children with constitutional growth delay. Clin Endocrinol 1986; 25:195–200.

660. Clayton PE, Shalet SM, Price DA, et al. Growth and growth hormone

responses to oxandrolone in boys with constitutional delay of growth and puberty (CDGP). Clin Endocrinol (Oxf) 1988; 29:123–130.

661. Stolecke H, Gilessen G. Oxandrolone and spontaneous hGH secretion. Pediatr Res 1984; 18:1216 (abstract).

662. Cara JF, Rosenfield RL. Insulin-like growth factor I and insulin potentiate luteinizing hormone–induced androgen synthesis by rat ovarian theca–interstitial cells. Endocrinology 1988; 123:733–739.

663. Apter D. Self-image in adolescents with delayed puberty and growth retardation. J Youth Adolesc 1981; 10:501–505.

664. Mussen PH, Jones MC. Self-conceptions, motivations, and interpersonal attitudes of late- and early-maturing boys. Child Dev 1957; 28:243–256.

665. Gordon M, Crouthamel C, Post EM. Psychosocial aspects of constitutional short stature: social competence, behavior problems, self-esteem, and family functioning. J Pediatr 1982; 101:477–480.

666. Crowne EC, Shalet SM, Wallace WH, et al. Final height in boys with untreated constitutional delay in growth and puberty. Arch Dis Child 1990; 65:1109–1112.

667. Crowne EC, Shalet SM, Wallace WH, et al. Final height in girls with untreated constitutional delay of growth and puberty. Eur J Pediatr 1991; 150:708–712.

668. LaFranchi S, Hanna CE, Mandel SH. Constitutional delay of growth: expected versus final adult height. Pediatrics 1991; 87:82–87.

669. Albanese A, Stanhope R. Predictive factors in the determination of final height in boys with constitutional delay of growth and puberty. J Pediatr 1995; 126:545–550.

670. Albanese A, Stanhope R. Does constitutional delayed puberty cause segmental disproportion and short stature? Eur J Pediatr 1993; 152:293–296.

671. Adan L, Souberbielle JC, Brauner R. Management of the short stature due to pubertal delay in boys. J Clin Endocrinol Metab 1994; 78:478–482.

672. Bierich JR, Nolte K, Drews K, Brugmann G. Constitutional delay of growth and adolescence: results of short-term and long-term treatment with GH. Acta Endocrinol 1992; 127:392–396.

673. Hindmarsh PC, Brook CG. Final height of short normal children treated with growth hormone. Lancet 1996; 348:13–16.

674. Volta C, Bernasconi S, Tondi P, et al. Combined treatment with growth hormone and luteinizing hormone–releasing hormone analogue (LHRHa) of pubertal children with familial short stature. J Endocrinol Invest 1993; 16:763–767.

675. Saggese G, Cesaretti G, Andreani G, Carlotti C. Combined treatment with growth hormone and gonadotropin-releasing hormone analogues in children with isolated growth hormone deficiency. Acta Endocrinol 1992; 127:307–312.

676. Municchi G, Rose SR, Pescovitz OH, et al. Effect of deslorelin-induced pubertal delay on the growth of adolescents with short stature and normally timed puberty: preliminary results. J Clin Endocrinol Metab 1993; 77:1334–1339.

677. Carel JC, Hay F, Coutant R, Rodrigue D, et al. Gonadotropin-releasing hormone agonist treatment of girls with constitutional short stature and normal pubertal development. J Clin Endocrinol Metab 1996; 81:3318–3322.

678. Yanovski JA, Rose SR, Filmer KM. Deslorelin-induced delay of puberty increases adult height of adolescents with short stature: results of randomized, placebo-controlled trial. Pediatr Res 1996; 39:101A (abstract).

679. Spratt DI, O'Dea LSL, Schoenfeld D. Neuroendocrine-gonadal axis in men: frequent sampling of LH, FSH, and testosterone. Am J Physiol 1988; 254:E658–E666.

680. Spratt DI, Carr DH, Merriam GR, et al. The spectrum of abnormal patterns of gonadotropin-releasing hormone secretion in men with idiopathic hypogonadotropic hypogonadism: clinical and laboratory correlations. J Clin Endocrinol 1987; 64:283–291.

681. Byrne MN, Sessions DG. Nasopharyngeal craniopharyngioma: case report and literature review. Ann Otol Rhinol Laryngol 1990; 99:633–639.

682. Fukushima T, Hirakawa K, Kimura M, Tomonaga M. Intraventricular craniopharyngioma: its characteristics in magnetic resonance imaging and successful total removal. Surg Neurol 1990; 33:22–27.

683. Banna M. Craniopharyngioma: based on 160 cases. Br J Radiol 1976; 49:206–223.

684. Banna M, Hoare RD, Stanley P. Craniopharyngioma in children. J Pediatr 1973; 83:781–785.

685. Thomsett JJ, Conte FA, Kaplan SL, et al. Endocrine and neurologic outcome in childhood craniopharyngioma: review of effect of treatment in 42 patients. J Pediatr 1980; 97:728–735.

686. Baumgartner JE, Wilson CB, Edwards MSB et al. Management of craniopharyngioma in children. The effect of surgery and radiation therapy on outcome. J Neurosurg 1989; 27:265–281.

687. Chakeres DW, Curtin A, Ford G. Magnetic resonance imaging of pituitary and parasellar abnormalities. Radio Clin North Am 1989; 27:265–281.

688. Curtis J, Daneman D, Hoffman HJ, et al. The endocrine outcome after surgical removal of craniopharyngiomas. Pediatr Neurosurg 1994; 21 Suppl 1:24–27.

689. Weiss M, Sutton L, Marcial V. The role of radiation therapy in the management of childhood craniopharyngioma. Int J Radiat Oncol Biol Phys 1989; 17:1313–1321.

690. Fischer EG, Welch K, Shillito J Jr. Craniopharyngiomas in children: long-term effects of conservative surgical procedures combined with radiation therapy. J Neurosurg 1990; 73:534–540.

691. Warnick RE, Edwards MSB. Pediatric brain tumors. Curr Prob Pediatr 1991; 21:129–173.

692. Paja M, Lucas T, García-Uría J, et al. Hypothalamic-pituitary dysfunction in patients with craniopharyngioma. Clin Endocrinol 1995; 42:467–473.

693. De Vile CJ, Grant DB, Hayward RD, et al. Obesity in childhood craniopharyngioma: relation to post-operative hypothalamic damage shown by magnetic resonance imaging. J Clin Endocrinol Metab 1996; 81:2734–2737.

694. Bray GA. Genetic, hypothalamic, and endocrine features of clinical and experimental obesity. Prog Brain Res 1992; 93:333–341.

695. Palm L, Nordin V, Elmqvist D, et al. Sleep and wakefulness after treatment for craniopharyngioma in childhood: influence on the quality and maturation of sleep. Neuropediatrics 1992; 23:39–45.

696. Dayan AD, Marshall AHE, Miller AA. Atypical teratomas of the pineal and hypothalamus. J Pathol Bacteriol 1966; 92:1–28.

697. Mootha SL, Barkovich AJ, Grumbach MM, et al. Idiopathic hypothalamic diabetes insipidus, pituitary stalk thickening, and the occult intracranial germinoma in children and adolescents. J Clin Endocrinol Metab 1997; 82:1362–1367.

698. Sklar CA, Grumbach MM, Kaplan SL, et al. Hormonal and metabolic abnormalities associated with central nervous system germinoma in children and adolescents and the effect of therapy: report of 10 patients. J Clin Endocrinol Metab 1981; 52:9–16.

699. Kitanaka C, Matsutani M, Sora S, et al. Precocious puberty in a girl with an hCG-secreting suprasellar immature teratoma: J Neurosurg 1994; 81:601–604 (case report).

700. Spiegel AM, Giovanni DC, Gordon P. Diagnosis of radiosensitive hypothalamic tumors without craniotomy. Ann Intern Med 1976; 85:290–293.

701. Kilgore DP, Strother CM, Starshak RJ, et al. Pineal germinoma: MR imaging. Radiology 1986; 158:435–438.

702. Schmidt F, Penka B, Trauner M, et al. Lack of pineal growth during childhood. J Clin Endocrinol Metab 1995; 80:1221–1225.

703. Wara WM, Fellows FC, Sheline GE. Radiation therapy for pineal tumors and suprasellar germinomas. Radiology 1977; 124:221–223.

704. Saxena KM. Endocrine manifestations of neurofibromatosis in children. Am J Dis Child 1970; 120:265–272.

705. Fienman NL, Yakovac WC. Neurofibromatosis in childhood. J Pediatr 1970; 76:339–346.

706. Kibirige MS, Birch JM, Campbell RH. A review of astrocytoma in childhood. Pediatr Hematol Oncol 1989; 6:319–329.

707. Job JC, Chaussain JL, Toublanc JE. Delayed puberty. In: Grumbach MM, Sizonenko PC, Aubert ML, eds. Control of the Onset of Puberty. Baltimore: Williams & Wilkins, 1990:588–619.

708. Cheyne KL, Lightner ES, Comerci GD. Bromocriptine-unresponsive prolactin macroadenoma in a prepubertal female. J Adolesc Health Care 1988; 9:331–334.

709. Patton ML, Woolf PD. Hyperprolactinemia and delayed puberty: a report of three cases and their response to therapy. Pediatrics 1983; 71:572–575.

710. Mahachoklertwattana P, Conte FA, Grumbach MM, et al. Prolactinomas in children and adolescents: effect on pubertal onset and long-term outcome following selective transsphenoidal adenomectomy. J Clin Endocrinol Metab 1997 (in press).

711. Koenig MP, Zuppinger K, Liechti B. Hyperprolactinemia as a cause of delayed puberty: successful treatment with bromocriptine. J Clin Endocrinol Metab 1977; 45:825–828.

712. Willman CL, Busque L, Griffith BB, et al. Langerhans-cell histiocytosis (histiocytosis X)—a clonal proliferative disease. N Engl J Med 1994; 331:154–160.

713. Vogel JM, Vogel P. Idiopathic histiocytosis: a discussion of eosinophilic granuloma, the Hand-Schüller-Christian syndrome, and the Letterer-Siwe syndrome. Semin Hematol 1972; 9:349–364.

714. Sims DG. Histocytosis X: follow-up of 43 cases. Arch Dis Child 1977; 52:433–440.

715. Egeler RM, Nesbit ME: Langerhans cell histiocytosis and other disorders of monocyte-histiocyte lineage. Crit Rev Oncol Hematol 1995; 18:9–35.

716. Lavin PT, Osband ME. Evaluating the role of therapy in histiocytosis X: clinical studies, staging, and scoring. Hematol Oncol Clin North Am 1987; 1:35–47.

717. Egeler RM, D'Angio GJ. Langerhans cell histiocytosis. J Pediatr 1995; 127:1–11.

718. Asherson RA, Jackson WPU, Lewis B. Abnormalities of development associated with hypothalamic calcification after tuberculous meningitis. Br Med J 1965; 2:839–843.

719. Fiedler R, Krieger DT. Endocrine disturbances in patients with congenital aqueductal stenosis. Acta Endocrinol 1975; 80:1–13.

720. Richards GE, Wara WM, Grumbach MM, et al. Delayed onset of hypopituitarism: sequelae of therapeutic irradiation of central nervous system, eye, and middle ear tumors. J Pediatr 1976; 89:553–559.

721. Shalet SM, Crowne EC, Didi MA, et al. Irradiation-induced growth failure. Baillieres Clin Endocrinol Metab 1992; 6:513–526.

722. Oberfield SE, Soranno D, Nirenberg A, et al. Age at onset of puberty following high-dose central nervous system radiation therapy. Arch Pediatr Adolesc Med 1996; 150:589–592.

723. Stubberfield TG, Byrne GC, Jones TW. Growth and growth hormone secretion after treatment for acute lymphoblastic leukemia in childhood: 18-Gy versus 24-Gy cranial irradiation. J Pediatr Hematol Oncol 1995; 17:167–171.

724. Hokken-Koelega AC, van Doorn JW, Hahlen K, et al. Long-term effects of treatment for acute lymphoblastic leukemia with and without cranial irradiation on growth and puberty: a comparative study. Pediatr Res 1993; 33:577–582.

725. Hanna CE, Mandel SH, LaFranchi SH. Puberty in the syndrome of septo-optic dysplasia. Am J Dis Child 1989; 143:186–189.

726. Kaplan SL, Grumbach MM, Hoyt WF. A syndrome of hypopituitary dwarfism, hypoplasia of optic nerves, and malformation of prosencephalon: report of 6 patients. Pediatr Res 1970; 4:480–481 (abstract).

727. Badawy SZ, Pisarska MD, Wasenko JJ, et al. Congenital hypopituitarism as part of suprasellar dysplasia: a case report. J Reprod Med 1994; 39:643–648.

728. Kollias SS, Ball WS, Prenger EC. Review of the embryologic development of the pituitary gland and report of a case of hypophyseal duplication detected by MRI. Neuroradiology 1995; 37:3–12.

729. Perrone L, Del Gaizo D, D'Angelo E, et al. Endocrine studies in children with myelomeningocele. J Pediatr Endocrinol 1994; 7:219–223.

730. Elias ER, Sadeghi-Nejad A. Precocious puberty in girls with myelodysplasia. Pediatrics 1994; 93:521–522.

731. Weinstein RL, Reitz RE. Pituitary-testicular responsiveness in male hypogonadotropic hypogonadism. J Clin Invest 1974; 53:408–415.

732. Uriarte MM, Baron J, Garcia HB, et al. The effect of pubertal delay on adult height in men with isolated hypogonadotropic hypogonadism. J Clin Endocrinol Metab 1992; 74:436–440. (Erratum 1992; 75:1009.)

733. Seeburg PH, Mason AJ, Steward TA, et al. The mammalian GnRH gene and its pivotal role in reproduction. Recent Prog Horm Res 1987; 43:69–107.

734. Kallmann F, Schonfeld WA, Barrera SW. Genetic aspects of primary eunuchoidism. Am J Ment Defic 1944; 48:203–236.

735. Wortsman J, Hughes LF. Case report: olfactory function in a fertile eunuch with Kallmann syndrome. Am J Med Sci 1996; 311:135–138.

736. Van Dop C, Burstein S, Conte FA, et al. Isolated gonadotropin deficiency in boys: clinical characteristics and growth. J Pediatr 1987; 111:684–692.

737. Doty RL, Shaman P, Dann M. The development of the University of Pennsylvania Smell Identification test: a standardized, microencapsulated test of olfactory function. Physiol Behav 1984; 32:501–507.

738. Santen RJ, Paulsen CA. Hypogonadotropic eunuchoidism. I. Clinical study of the mode of inheritance. J Clin Endocrinol Metab 1973; 36:47–54.

739. Prager O, Braunstein GD. X-chromosome–linked Kallmann's syndrome: pathology at the molecular level. J Clin Endocrinol Metab 1993; 76:824–826 (editorial).

740. Kirk JMW, Grant DB, Besser GM, et al. Unilateral renal aplasia in X-linked Kallmann's syndrome. Clin Genet 1994; 46:260–262.

741. Dunek A, Heye B, Schroedter R. Cortically evoked motor responses in patients with Xp22.3-linked Kallmann's syndrome and in female gene carriers. Am J Neuroradiol 1992; 31:299–304.

742. Klingmhller D, Dewes W, Krahe T, et al. Magnetic resonance imaging of the brain in patients with anosmia and hypothalamic hypogonadism (Kallmann's syndrome). J Clin Endocrinol Metab 1987; 65:581–584.

743. Truwit CL, Barkovich AJ, Grumbach MM, Martini JJ. Magnetic resonance imaging of Kallmann syndrome, a genetic disorder of neuronal migration affecting the ofactory and genital systems. Am J Neuroradiol 1993; 14:827–838.

744. Quinton R, Duke VM, de Zoysa PA, et al. The neuroradiology of Kallmann's syndrome: a genotypic and phenotypic analysis. J Clin Endocrinol Metab 1996; 81:3010–3017.

745. Wu FC, Butler GE, Kelnar CJ, et al. Patterns of pulsatile luteinizing hormone and follicle-stimulating hormone secretion in prepubertal (mid-childhood) boys and girls and patients with idiopathic hypogonadotropic hypogonadism (Kallmann's syndrome): a study using an ultrasensitive time-resolved immunofluorometric assay. J Clin Endocrinol Metab 1991; 72:1229–1237.

746. Ballabio A, Bardoni B, Carrozzo R, et al. Contiguous gene syndromes due to deletions in the distal short arm of the human X chromosome. Proc Natl Acad Sci USA 1989; 86:10001–10005.

747. Hardelin JP, Levilliers J, Young J, et al. Xp22.3 deletions in isolated familial Kallmann's syndrome. J Clin Endocrinol Metab 1993; 76:827–831.

748. Legouis R, Hardelin J-P, Levilliers J, et al. The candidate gene for the X-linked Kallmann syndrome encodes a protein related to adhesion molecules. Cell 1991; 67:423–435.

749. Cohen-Salmon M, Tronche F, del Castillo, et al. Characterization of the promotor of the human KAL gene responsible for the X-chromosome–linked Kallmann syndrome. Gene 1995; 164:235–242.

750. Santen RJ, Paulsen CA. Hypogonadotropic eunuchoidism. II. Gonadal responsiveness to exogenous gonadotropins. J Clin Endocrinol Metab 1973; 36:55–63.

751. Merriam GR, Beitins IZ, Bode HH. Father-to-son transmission of hypogonadism with anosmia. Am J Dis Child 1977; 131:1216–1219.

752. White BJ, Rogol AD, Brown KS, et al. The syndrome of anosmia with hypogonadotropic hypogonadism: a genetic study of 18 new families and a review. Am J Med Genet 1983; 15:417–435.

753. Hipkin LJ, Casson IF, Davis JC. Identical twins discordant for Kallmann's syndrome. J Med Genet 1990; 27:198–199.

754. Burstein S, Grumbach MM, Kaplan SL. Early determination of androgen responsiveness is important in the management of microphallus. Lancet 1979; 2:983–986.

755. Zanarla E, Muscatelli F, Bardoni B, et al. An unusual member of the nuclear hormone receptor superfamily responsible for X-linked adrenal hypoplasia congenita. Nature 1994; 372:635–641.

756. Muscatelli F, Strom TM, Walker AP, et al. Mutations in the DAX-1 gene give rise to both X-linked adrenal hypoplasia congenita and hypogonadotropic hypogonadism. Nature 1994; 372:672–676.

757. Guo W, Burris TP, Zhang Y-H, et al. Genomic sequence of the DAX1 gene: an orphan nuclear receptor responsible for X-linked adrenal hypoplasia congenita and hypogonadotropic hypogonadism. J Clin Endocrinol Metab 1996; 81:2481–2486.

758. Burris TP, Guo W, McCabe ERB. The gene responsible for adrenal hypoplasia congenita, DAX-1, encodes a nuclear hormone receptor that defines a new class within the superfamily. Rec Prog Horm Res 1996; 51:241–260.

759. Prader A, Zachmann M, Illig KR. Luteinizing hormone deficiency in hereditary congenital adrenal hypoplasia. J Pediatr 1975; 86:421–422.

760. Kruse K, Sippell WG, Schnakenburg KV. Hypogonadism in congenital adrenal hypoplasia: evidence for a hypothalamic origin. J Clin Endocrinol Metab 1984; 58:12–17.

761. Hay ID, Smail PJ, Forsyth CC. Familial cytomegalic adrenocortical hypoplasia: an X-linked syndrome of pubertal failure. Arch Dis Child 1981; 56:715–721.

762. Kikuchi K, Kaji M, Momoi T, et al. Failure to induce puberty in a man with X-linked congenital adrenal hypoplasia and hypogonadotropic hypogonadism by pulsatile administration of low-dose gonadotropin-releasing hormone. Acta Endocrinol (Copenh) 1987; 114:153–160.

763. Kletter GB, Gorski JL, Kelch RP. Congenital adrenal hypoplasia and isolated gonadotropin deficiency. Trends Endocrinol Metab 1991; 2:123–128.

764. Uttley WS. Familial congenital adrenal hypoplasia. Arch Dis Child 1968; 43:724–730.

765. Seltzer WK, Firminger H, Klein L, et al. Adrenal dysfunction in glycerol kinase deficiency. Biochem Med 1985; 33:189–199.

766. Guo W, Mason JS, Stone CG Jr, et al. Diagnosis of X-linked adrenal hypoplasia congenita by mutation analysis of the DAX1 gene. JAMA 1995; 274:324–330.

767. Yanase T, Takayanagi R, Oba K, et al. New mutations of DAX-1 genes in two Japanese patients with X-linked congenital adrenal hypoplasia and hypogonadotropic hypogonadism. J Clin Endocrinol Metab 1996; 81:530–535.

768. Guo W, Burris TP, McCabe ERB. Expression of DAX-1, the gene responsible for X-linked adrenal hypoplasia congenita and hypogonadotropic hypogonadism, in the hypothalamic-pituitary-adrenal/gonadal axis. Biochem Mol Med 1995; 56:8–13.

769. Habiby RL, Boepple P, Nachtigall L, et al. Adrenal hypoplasia congenita with hypogonadotropic hypogonadism: evidence that DAX-1 mutations lead to combined hypothalamic and pituitary defects in gonadotropin production. J Clin Invest 1996; 98:1055–1062.

770. Takahashi T, Shoji Y, Shoji Y, et al. Active hypothalamic-pituitary-gonadal axis in an infant with X-linked adrenal hypoplasia congenita. J Pediatr 1997; 130:485–488.

771. Worley KC, Ellison KA, Zhang Y-H, et al. Yeast artificial chromosome cloning in the glycerol kinase and adrenal hypoplasia congenita region of Xp21. Genomics 1993; 16:407–416.

771a. McCabe ER. Sex and the single DAX1: too little is bad, but can we have too much? J Clin Invest 1996; 98:881–882.

772. Burris TP, Guo W, Le T, McCabe ER. Identification of a putative steroidogenic factor-1 response element in the DAX-1 promoter. Biochem Biophys Res Comm 1995; 214:576–581.

773. Ingraham HA, Lala DS, Ikeda Y, et al. The nuclear receptor steroidogenic factor 1 acts at multiple levels of the reproductive axis. Genes Dev 1994; 8:2302–2312.

774. Smals AGH, Kloppenborg PWC, Van Haelst UJG, et al. Fertile eunuch syndrome versus classic hypogonadotrophic hypogonadism. Acta Endocrinol 1978; 87:389–399.

775. Weiss J, Axelrod L, Whitcomb RW, et al. Hypogonadism caused by a single amino acid substitution in the beta subunit of luteinizing hormone. N Engl J Med 1992; 326:179–183.

776. Rabin D, Spitz I, Bercovici B, et al. Isolated deficiency of follicle-stimulating hormone: clinical and laboratory features. N Engl J Med 1972; 287:1313–1317.

777. Matthews CH, Borgato S, Beck-Peccoz P, et al. Primary amenorrhoea and infertility due to a mutation in the beta-subunit of follicle-stimulating hormone. Nature Genet 1993; 5:83–86.

778. Gougeon A. Regulation of ovarian follicular development in primates: facts and hypotheses. Endocr Rev 1996; 17:121–155.

778a. Layman LC, Lee E-J, Peak DB, et al. Delayed puberty and hypogonadism caused by mutations in the follicle-stimulating hormone β-subunit gene. N Engl J Med 1997; 337:607–611.

779. Goodman HG, Grumbach MM, Kaplan SL. Growth and growth hormone. II. A comparison of isolated growth hormone deficiency and multiple pituitary hormone deficiencies in 35 patients with idiopathic hypopituitary dwarfism. N Engl J Med 1968; 278:57–68.

780. Tanner JM, Whitehouse RH. A note on the bone age at which patients with true isolated growth hormone deficiency enter puberty. J Clin Endocrinol Metab 1975; 41:788–790.

781. Arrigo T, Crisafulli G, Salamone A, et al. Adult height exceeding target height in a patient with congenital panhypopituitarism diagnosed after the age of 25 years. J Pediatr Endocrinol 1994; 7:269–272.

782. Albanese A, Stanhope R. Treatment of growth delay in boys with isolated growth hormone deficiency. Eur J Endocrinol 1994; 130:65–69.

783. Bray GA, Dahms WT, Swerdloff RS, et al. The Prader-Willi syndrome: a study of 40 patients and a review of the literature. Medicine 1983; 62:59–80.

784. Prader A, Labhart A, Willi H. Ein syndrom von Adipositas, Kleinwuchs, Kryptorchidismus und Oligophrenie nach Myatonieartigem Zustad im Neugeborenalter. Schweiz Med Wochenschr 1956; 86:1260–1261.

785. Tolis G, Lewis W, Verdy M, et al. Anterior pituitary function in the Prader-Labhart-Willi (PLW) syndrome. J Clin Endocrinol Metab 1974; 39:1061–1066.

786. Linde R, McNeil L, Rabin D. Induction of menarche by clomiphene citrate in a fifteen-year-old girl with the Prader-Labhart-Willi syndrome. Fertil Steril 1982; 37:118–120.

787. Cassidy SB, Ledbetter DH. Prader-Willi syndrome. Neurol Clin 1989; 7:37–54.

788. Holm VA, Cassidy SB, Butler MG, et al. Prader-Willi syndrome: consensus diagnostic criteria. Pediatrics 1993; 91:398–402.

789. Lindgren AC, Hagenas L, Muller J, et al. Growth hormone treatment in Prader-Willi syndrome: a controlled study. Horm Res 1995; 44:61 (abstract).

790. Drug and Therapeutics Committee, Lawson Wilkins Pediatric Endocrine Society: Guidelines for the use of growth hormone in children with short stature. J Pediatr 1995; 127:857–867.

791. Knoll JHM, Nicholls RD, Magenis RE, et al. Angleman and Prader-Willi share a common chromosome 15 deletion but differ in parental origin of the deletion. Am J Med Genet 1989; 32:285–290.

792. Nicholls RD. Imprinting mechanisms and genes involved in Prader-Willi and Angelman syndromes. Dev Biol 1994; 5:311–322.

793. Saitoh S, Buiting K, Rogan PK, et al. Minimal definition of the imprinting region center and fixation of a chromosome 15q11-q13 epigenotype by imprinting mutations. Proc Natl Acad Sci USA 1996; 93:7811–7815.

794. Nicholls RD, Knoll JHM, Butler MG, et al. Genetic imprinting suggested by maternal hetero-disomy in non-deletion Prader-Willi syndrome. Nature 1989; 342:281–285.

795. Ozçelik R, Leff S, Robinson W. Small nuclear ribonucleoprotein polypeptide N (SNRPN), an expressed gene in the Prader-Willi syndrome critical region. Nature Genet 1992; 2:259–269.

796. Lalande M. In and around SNRPN. Nature Genet 1994; 8:5–7.

797. Swaab DF, Purba JS, Hoffman MA. Alterations in the hypothalamic paraventricular nucleus and its oxytocin neurons (putative satiety cells) in Prader-Willi syndrome: a study of five cases. J Clin Endocrinol Metab 1995; 80:573–579.

798. Laurence JZ, Moon RC. Four cases of "retinitis pigmentosa," occurring in the same family, and accompanied by general imperfections of development. Ophthalmic Rev 1866; 2:32–41.

799. Bell J. The Laurence-Moon syndrome. In: The Treasury of Human Inheritance. Vol 5. Part 3. Cambridge: Cambridge University Press, 1958: 51–69.

800. Kulin HE, Bwibo N, Mutie D, et al. The effect of chronic childhood malnutrition on pubertal growth and development. Am J Clin Nutr 1982; 36:527–536.

801. Kulin HE, Bwibo N, Mutie D, et al. Gonadotropin excretion during puberty in malnourished children. J Pediatr 1984; 105:325–328.

802. Maki M, Kallonen K, Lahdeaho ML, et al. Changing pattern of childhood coeliac disease in Finland. Acta Paediatr Scand 1988; 77:408–412.

803. Vigersky R, Anderson AE, Thompson RH, et al. Hypothalamic dysfunction in secondary amenorrhea associated with simple weight loss. N Engl J Med 1977; 297:1141–1145.

804. Landon C, Rosenfeld RG. Short stature and pubertal delay in male adolescents with cystic fibrosis: androgen treatment. Am J Dis Child 1984; 138:388–391.

805. Chaussain JL, Roger M, Couprie C, et al. Treatment of precocious puberty with a long-acting preparation of D-Trp6-LHRH. Horm Res 1987; 28:155–163.

806. Reiter EO, Stern RC, Root AW. The reproductive endocrine system in cystic fibrosis. I. Basal gonadotropin and sex steroid levels. Am J Dis Child 1981; 135:422–426.

807. Stern RC, Boat TF, Doershuk CF, et al. Course of cystic fibrosis in 95 patients. J Pediatr 1976; 89:406–411.

808. Taussig LM, Lobeck CC, di Sant'Agnese PA, et al. Fertility in males with cystic fibrosis. N Engl J Med 1972; 287:586–589.

809. Tizzano EF, Silver MM, Chitayat D, et al. Differential cellular expression of cystic fibrosis transmembrane regulator in human reproductive tissues: clues for the infertility in patients with cystic fibrosis. Am J Pathol 1994; 144:906–914.

810. Vasquez-Levin MH, Kupchik GS, Torres Y, et al. Cystic fibrosis and congenital agenesis of the vas deferens, antisperm antibodies, and CF-genotype. J Reprod Immunol 1994; 27:199–212.

811. Johannesson M, Gottlieb C, Hjelte L. Delayed puberty in girls with cystic fibrosis despite good clinical status. Pediatrics 1997; 99:29–34.

812. Zago MA, Kerbauy J, Souza HM, et al. Growth and sexual maturation of Brazilian patients with sickle cell diseases. Trop Geogr Med 1992; 44:317–321.

813. Olatunji Olambiwonnu N, Penny R, Frasier SD. Sexual maturation in subjects with sickle cell anemia: studies of serum gonadotropin concentration, height, weight, and skeletal age. J Pediatr 1975; 87:459–464.

814. Kwan EY, Lee AC, Li AM, et al. A cross-sectional study of growth, puberty, and endocrine function in patients with thalassaemia major in Hong Kong. J Paediatr Child Health 1995; 31:83–87.

815. Grundy RG, Woods KA, Savage MO, et al. Relationship of endocrinopathy to iron chelation status in young patients with thalassaemia major. Arch Dis Child 1994; 71:128–132.

816. De Sanctis V, Galimberti M, Lucarelli G, et al. Pubertal development in thalassaemic patients after allogenic bone marrow transplantation Eur J Pediatr 1993; 152:993–997. (Erratum 1994; 153:470.)

817. Borgna Pignatti C, De Stefano P, Zonta L, et al. Growth and sexual maturation in thalassemia major. J Pediatr 1985; 106:150–155.

818. Balducci R, Toscano V, Finocchi G, et al. Effect of hCG or hCG + treatments in young thalassemic patients with hypogonadotropic hypogonadism. J Endocrinol Invest 1990; 13:1–7.

819. De Sanctis V, Vullo C, Katz M, et al. Gonadal function in patients with beta thalassaemia major. J Clin Pathol 1988; 41:133–137.

820. Sklar CA, Lew LQ, Yoon DJ, et al. Adrenal function in thalassemia major following long-term treatment with multiple transfusions and chelation therapy: evidence for dissociation of cortisol and adrenal androgen secretion. Am J Dis Child 1987; 141:327–330.

821. Gertner JM, Kaufman FR, Donfield SM, et al. Delayed somatic growth and pubertal development in human immunodeficiency virus–infected hemophiliac boys: Hemophilia Growth and Development Study. J Pediatr 1994; 124:896–902.

822. Brain CE, Savage MO. Growth and puberty in chronic inflammatory bowel disease. Baillieres Clin Gastroenterol 1994; 8:83–100.

823. Cacciari E, Corazza GR, Salardi S, et al. What will be the adult height of coeliac patients? Eur J Pediatr 1991; 150:407–409.

824. Ferraris J, Saenger P, Levine L, et al. Delayed puberty in males with chronic renal failure. Kidney Int 1980; 18:344–350.

825. Schaefer F, Stanhope R, Scheil H, et al. Pulsatile gonadotropin secretion in pubertal children with chronic renal failure. Acta Endocrinol 1989; 120:14–19.

826. Kulin H, Demers L, Chinchilli V, et al. Usefulness of sequential urinary follicle-stimulating hormone and luteinizing hormone measurements in the diagnosis of adolescent hypogonadotropism in males. J Clin Endocrinol Metab 1994; 78:1208–1211.

827. Rees L, Greene SA, Adlard P, et al. Growth and endocrine function in steroid-sensitive nephrotic syndrome. Arch Dis Child 1988; 63:484–490.

828. Polito C, Di Toro R. Delayed pubertal growth spurt in glomerulopathic boys receiving alternate-day prednisone. Child Nephrol Urol 1992; 12:202–207.

829. van Diemen-Steenvoorde R, Donckerwolcke RA, Brackel H, et al. Growth and sexual maturation in children after kidney transplantation. J Pediatr 1987; 110:351–356.

830. Martin LW, McEnery PT, Rosenkrantz JG, et al. Renal homotransplantation in children. J Pediatr Surg 1979; 14:571–576.

831. Ferraris JR, Domene HM, Escobar ME, et al. Hormonal problems in pubertal females with chronic renal failure: before and under hemodialysis and after renal transplantation. Acta Endocrinol 1987; 115:289–296.

832. van Diemen-Steenvoorde MD, Donckerwolcke RA, Brakel H, et al. Growth and sexual maturation in children after kidney transplantation. J Pediatr 1987; 110:351–356.

833. Belgorosky A, Ferraris JR, Ramirez JA, et al. Serum sex hormone–binding globulin and serum nonsex hormone–binding globulin-bound testosterone fractions in prepubertal boys with chronic renal failure. J Clin Endocrinol Metab 1991; 73:107–110.

834. Siris ES, Leventhal BG, Vaitukaitis JL. Effects of childhood leukemia and chemotherapy on puberty and reproductive function in girls. N Engl J Med 1976; 294:1143–1146.

835. Vilska S, Lahteenmaki P, Kaihola HL, et al. Endocrine status and growth after malignancy treated in childhood or adolescence. Int J Fertil 1988; 33:283–290.

836. Lannering B, Rosberg S, Marky I, et al. Reduced growth hormone secretion with maintained periodicity following cranial irradiation in children with acute lymphoblastic leukaemia. Clin Endocrinol (Oxf) 1995; 42:153–159.

837. Cicognani A, Cacciari E, Rosito P, et al. Longitudinal growth and final height in long-term survivors of childhood leukaemia. Eur J Pediatr 1994; 153:726–730.

838. Ochs J, Mulhern R: Long-term sequelae of therapy for childhood acute lymphoblastic leukaemia. Baillieres Clin Haematol 1994; 7:365–376.

839. Davies HA, Didcock E, Didi M, et al. Disproportionate short stature after cranial irradiation and combination chemotherapy for leukaemia. Arch Dis Child 1994; 70:472–475.

840. Holm K, Nysom K, Hertz H, et al. Normal final height after treatment for acute lymphoblastic leukemia without irradiation. Acta Paediatr 1994; 83:1287–1290.

841. Chou RH, Wong GB, Kramer JH, et al. Toxicities of total-body irradiation for pediatric bone marrow transplantation. Int J Radiat Oncol Biol Phys 1996; 34:843–851.

842. Didi M, Didcock E, Davies HA, et al. High incidence of obesity in young adults after treatment of acute lymphoblastic leukemia in childhood. J Pediatr 1995; 127:63–67.

843. Yesilipek MA, Bircan I, Oygur N, et al. Growth and sexual maturation in children with thalassemia major. Haematologica 1993; 78:30–33.

844. Pantsiouou S, Stanhope R, Uruena M, et al. Growth prognosis and growth after menarche in primary hypothyroidism. Arch Dis Child 1991; 66:838–840.

845. Mauriac P. Hepatomégalie de l'enfance avec troubles de la croissance et du métabolisme des glucides. Paris Méd 1934; 2:525.

846. Arreola F, Junco E, Partida-Hernandez G, et al. HbA₁, height velocity, and weight gain as indicators of metabolic control in type I diabetic children: a 5-year survey. Arch Invest Med (Mex) 1991; 22:303–307.

847. Wise JE, Kolb EL, Sauder SE. Effect of glycemic control on growth velocity in children with IDDM. Diabetes Care 1992; 15:826–830.

848. Travis LB. Diabetes Mellitus in Children and Adolescents. Philadelphia: WB Saunders, 1987; 206.

849. Dills DG, Allen C, Palta M, et al. Insulin-like growth factor-I is related to glycemic control in children and adolescents with newly diagnosed insulin-dependent diabetes. J Clin Endocrinol Metab 1995; 80:2139–2143.

850. Styne DM, Grumbach MM, Kaplan SL, et al. Treatment of Cushing's disease in childhood and adolescence by transsphenoidal microadenomectomy. N Engl J Med 1984; 310:889–893.

851. Mindermann T, Wilson CB. Pediatric pituitary adenomas. Neurosurgery 1995; 36:259–268.

852. Crisp AH. The dyslipophobias: a view of the psychopathologies involved and the hazards of construing anorexia nervosa and bulimia nervosa as "eating disorders." Proc Nutr Soc 1996; 54:701–709.

853. Schwabe AD, Lippe BM, Chang RJ, et al. Anorexia nervosa. Ann Intern Med 1981; 94:371–381.

854. Silverman JA. Anorexia nervosa: clinical and metabolic observations in a successful treatment plan. In: Vigersky RA, ed. Anorexia Nervosa. New York: Raven Press, 1977: 331:–339.

855. Warren MP, Vande Wile RL. Clinical and metabolic features of anorexia nervosa. Am J Obstet Gynecol 1973; 117:435–449.

856. Danziger Y, Mukamel M, Zeharia A, et al. Stunting of growth in anorexia nervosa during the prepubertal and pubertal period. Isr J Med Sci 1994; 30:581–584.

857. De Lange WE, Sluiter WJ, Van Zanten AK, et al. The effect of injection and infusion of LH-RH on serum LH and FSH in normal males and in boys with delayed puberty. Neth J Med 1974; 17:196–201.

858. van Binsbergen CJM, Coelingh Bennink HJT, Odink J, et al. A comparative and longitudinal study on endocrine changes related to ovarian function in patients with anorexia nervosa. J Clin Endocrinol Metab 1990; 71:705–711.

859. Beaumont PJV, George GCW, Pimstone BL, et al. Body weight and the pituitary response to hypothalamic-releasing hormones in patients with anorexia nervosa. J Clin Endocrinol Metab 1976; 43:487–496.

860. Grinspoon S, Gulick T, Askari H, et al. Serum leptin levels in women with anorexia nervosa. J Clin Endocrinol Metab 1996; 81:3861–3863.

861. Ferron F, Considine RV, Peino R, et al. Serum leptin concentrations in patients with anorexia nervosa, bulimia nervosa, and nonspecific eating disorders correlate with the body mass index but are independent of the respective disease. Clin Endocrinol 1997; 46:289–293.

862. Casanueva FF, Dieguez C, Popovic V, et al. Serum immunoreactive leptin concentrations in patients with anorexia nervosa before and after partial weight recovery. Biochem Mol Med 1997; 60:116–120.

863. Waldhauser F, Toifl K, Spona J, et al. Diminished prolactin response to thyrotropin and insulin in anorexia nervosa. J Clin Endocrinol Metab 1984; 59:538–544.

864. Warren MP. Metabolic factors and the onset of puberty. In: Grumbach MM, Sizonenko PC, Aubert ML, eds. Control of the Onset of Puberty. Baltimore: Williams & Wilkins, 1990: 553–573.

865. Yen SSC, Rebar R, VandenBerg G, et al. Hypothalamic amenorrhea and hypogonadotropinism: responses to synthetic LRF. J Clin Endocrinol Metab 1973; 36:811–816.

866. Meyers CM, Boughman JA, Rivas M, et al. Gonadal (ovarian) dysgenesis in 46,XX individuals: frequency of the autosomal recessive form. Am J Med Genet 1996; 63:518–524.

867. Russell GFM. Bulimia nervosa: an ominous variant of anorexia nervosa. Psychol Med 1979; 9:429–448.

868. Eisenstein TD, Gerson MJ. Psychosocial growth retardation in adolescence: a reversible condition secondary to severe stress. J Adolesc Health Care 1988; 9:436–440.

869. Constantini NW, Warren MP. Special problems of the female athlete. Baillieres Clin Rheumatol 1994; 8:199–219.

870. Carpenter SE. Psychosocial menstrual disorders: stress, exercise, and diet's effect on the menstrual cycle. Curr Opin Obstet Gynecol 1994; 6:536–539.

871. Sundgot-Borgen J. Risk and trigger factors for the development of eating disorders in female elite athletes. Med Sci Sports Exerc 1994; 26:414–419.

872. Loucks AV, Horvath SB. Athletic amenorrhea: a review. Med Sci Sports Exerc 1985; 17:56–72.

873. Constantini NW, Warren MP. Menstrual dysfunction in swimmers: a distinct entity. J Clin Endocrinol Metab 1995; 80:2740–2744.

874. Theintz GE, Howald H, Weiss U, et al. Evidence for a reduction of growth potential in adolescent female gymnasts. J Pediatr 1993; 122:306–313.

875. Lindholm C, Hagenfeldt K, Ringertz BM. Pubertal development in elite juvenile gymnasts: effects of physical training. Acta Obstet Gynecol Scand 1994; 73:269–273.

876. Baxter-Jones AD, Helms P, Baines-Preece J, et al. Menarche in intensively trained gymnasts, swimmers, and tennis players. Ann Hum Biol 1994; 21:407–415.

877. Baxter-Jones A, Maffulli N, Helms P: Low injury rates in elite athletes. Arch Dis Child 1993; 68:130–132.

878. Goldberg CJ, Dowling FE, Fogarty EE: Adolescent idiopathic scoliosis—early menarche, normal growth. Spine 1993; 18:529–535.

879. Hagglund G, Karlberg J, Willner S: Growth in girls with adolescent idiopathic scoliosis. Spine 1992; 17:108–111.

880. Carr AJ, Jefferson RJ, Turner-Smith AR: Family stature in idiopathic scoliosis. Spine 1993; 18:20–23.

881. Brisson GR, Volle MA, Desharnais M, et al. Exercise-induced dissociation of the blood prolactin response in young women according to their sports habits. Horm Metab Res 1980; 21:201–205.

882. Harmon J, Aliapoulios MA. Gynecomastia in marihuana user. N Engl J Med 1972; 287:936–1080.

883. Copeland KC, Underwood LE, Van Wyk JJ. Marihuana smoking and pubertal arrest. J Pediatr 1980; 96:1079–1080.

884. Granovsky-Grisaru S, Aboulafia Y, Diamant YZ, et al. Gynecologic and obstetric aspects of Gaucher's disease: a survey of 53 patients. Am J Obstet Gynecol 1995; 172:1284–1290.

885. Grumbach MM, Conte FA. Disorders of sex differentiation. In: Wilson JD, Foster DW, eds. Williams Textbook of Endocrinology. 8th ed. Philadelphia: WB Saunders, 1992: 853–951.

886. Hsueh AJ, Eisenhauer K, Chun SY, et al. Gonadal cell apoptosis. Recent Prog Horm Res 1996; 51:433–455.

887. Klinefelter HF Jr, Reifenstein EC Jr, Albright F. Syndrome characterized by gynecomastia, aspermatogenesis without a-leydigism, and increased excretion of follicle-stimulating hormone. J Clin Endocrinol 1942; 2:615–627.

888. Wittenberg DF, Padayachi T, Norman RJ. Hypogonadotrophic variant of Klinefelter's syndrome: a case report. S Afr Med J 1988; 74:181–183.

889. Caldwell PD, Smith DW. The XXY (Klinefelter's) syndrome in childhood: detection and treatment. J Pediatr 1972; 80:250–258.

890. Sagawa I, Kazama T, Terada T, et al. Hormonal profiles in Klinefelter's syndrome with and without testicular epidermoid cyst. Arch Androl 1988; 21:205–209.

891. Salbenblatt JA, Bender BG, Puck MH, et al. Pituitary-gonadal function in Klinefelter syndrome before and during puberty. Pediatr Res 1985; 19:82–86.

892. Plymate SR, Leonard JM, Paulsen CA. Sex hormone–binding globulin changes with androgen replacement. J Clin Endocrinol Metab 1983; 57:645–648.

893. Wieland RG, Zorn EM, Johnson MW. Elevated testosterone-binding globulin in Klinefelter's syndrome. J Clin Endocrinol Metab 1980; 51:1199–1200.

894. Eberle AJ, Sparrow JT, Keenan BS. Treatment of persistent pubertal gynecomastia with dihydrotestosterone heptanoate. J Pediatr 1986; 109:144–149.

895. Kleczkowska A, Fryns JP, Van den Berghe H. X-chromosome polysomy in the male: the Leuven experience, 1966–1987. Hum Genet 1988; 80:16–22.

896. Nielsen J, Pelsen B. Follow-up 20 years later of 34 Klinefelter males with karyotype 47,XXY and 16 hypogonadal males with karyotype 46,XY. Hum Genet 1987; 77:188–192.

897. Sorenson K., Porter ME, Gardner HA, et al. Verbal deficits in Klinefelter (XXY) adults living in the community. Clin Genet 1988; 33:246–253.

898. Price WH, Clayton JF, Wilson J. Causes of death in X chromatin positive males (Klinefelter's syndrome). J Epidemiol Community Health 1985; 39:330–336.

899. Scheike O, Visfeldt J, Peterson B. Male breast cancer. III. Breast carcinoma in association with the Klinefelter sydrome. Acta Pathol Microbiol Scand Suppl 1973; 81:352–358.

900. Bizzarro A, Valentini G, DiMartino G. Influence of testosterone therapy on clinical and immunological features of autoimmune diseases associated with Klinefelter's syndrome. J Clin Endocrinol Metab 1987; 64:32–36.

901. Fialkow PJ. Genetic aspects of autoimmunity. Prog Med Genet 1969; 6:117–167.

902. Foresta C, Busnardo B, Zanatta G. Lower calcitonin levels in young hypogonadic men with osteoporosis. Horm Metab Res 1983; 15:206–207.

903. Derenoncourt AN, Castro-Magana M, Jones KL. Mediastinal teratoma and precocious puberty in a boy with mosaic Klinefelter syndrome. Am J Med Genet 1995; 55:38–42.

904. Von Muhlendahl KE, Heinrich U. Sexual precocity in Klinefelter syndrome: report on two new cases with idiopathic central precocious puberty. Eur J Pediatr 1994; 153:322–324.

905. Hasle H, Jacobsen BB, Asschenfeldt P, et al. Mediastinal germ cell tumour associated with Klinefelter syndrome: a report of case and review of the literature. Eur J Pediatr 1992; 151:735–739.

906. Lair-Milan F, Blevec GL, Carel JC, et al. Thyroid sonographic abnormalities in McCune-Albright syndrome. Pediatr Radiol 1996; 26:424–426.

907. Penso J, Lippe B, Ehrlich R, et al. Testicular function in prepubertal and pubertal male patients treated with cyclophosphamide for nephrotic syndrome. J Pediatr 1974; 84:831–836.

908. Callis L, Nieto J, Vila A, et al. Chlorambucil treatment in minimal lesion nephrotic syndrome: a reappraisal of its gonadal toxicity. J Pediatr 1980; 97:653–656.

909. Hoorweg-Nijman JJ, Delemarre-van de Waal HA, de Waal FC, et al. Cyclophosphamide-induced disturbance of gonadotropin secretion manifesting testicular damage. Acta Endocrinol (Copenh) 1992; 126:143–148.

910. Dhabhar BN, Malhotra H, Joseph R, et al. Gonadal function in prepubertal boys following treatment for Hodgkin's disease. Am J Pediatr Hematol Oncol 1993; 15:306–310.

911. Mustieles C, Munoz A, Alonso M, et al. Male gonadal function after chemotherapy in survivors of childhood malignancy. Med Pediatr Oncol 1995; 24:347–351.

912. Brämswig JH, Heimes U, Heiermann E, et al. The effects of different cumulative doses of chemotherapy on testicular function. Results in 75 patients treated for Hodgkin's disease during childhood or adolescence. Cancer 1990; 65:1298–1302.

913. Barrett A, Nicholls J, Gibson B. Late effects of total body irradiation. Radiother Oncol 1987; 9:131–135.

914. Ogilvy-Stuart AL, Shalet SM. Effect of radiation on the human reproductive system. Environ Health Perspect 1993; 101 Suppl 2:109–116.

915. Bosson D, Wolter R, Toppet M, et al. Partial 17,20-desmolase and 17-alpha-hydroxylase deficiencies in a 16-year-old boy. J Endocrinol Invest 1988; 11:527–533.

916. Bose HS, Sugawara T, Strauss JF, et al. The pathophysiology and genetics of congenital lipoid adrenal hyperplasia: International Congenital Lipoid Adrenal Hyperplasia Consortium. N Engl J Med 1996; 335:1870–1878.

917. Bose HS, Pescovitz OH, Miller WL. Spontaneous feminization in a 46,XX female patient with congenital lipoid adrenal hyperplasia due to a homozygous frameshift mutation in the steroidogenic acute regulatory protein. J Clin Endocrinol Metab 1997; 82:1511–1515.

918. Fujieda K, Tajima T, Nakae J, et al. Spontaneous puberty in 46,XX subjects with congenital lipoid adrenal hyperplasia—ovarian steroidogenesis is spared to some extent despite inactivating mutations in the steroidogenic acute regulatory protein (StAR) gene. J Clin Invest 1997; 99:1265–1271.

919. David R, Yoon DJ, Landin L, et al. A syndrome of gonadotropin resistance possibly due to a luteinizing hormone receptor defect. J Clin Endocrinol Metab 1984; 59:156–160.

920. Winkler L, Offner G, Krull F, et al. Growth and pubertal development in nephropathic cystinosis. Eur J Pediatr 1993; 152:244–249.

921. Lee P. Fertility in cryptorchicism: does treatment make a difference? Enodcrinol Metab Clin North Am 1993; 22:479–490.

922. Hutson JM, Hasthorpe S, Heyns CF. Anatomical and functional aspects of testicular descent and cryptorchidism. Endocr Rev 1997; 18:259–280.

923. Saez J, Forest MG. Kinetics of human chorionic gonadotropin-induced steroidogenic reponse of the human testis. I. Plasma testosterone: implications for human chorionic gonadotropin stimulation test. J Clin Endocrinol Metab 1979; 49:278–283.

924. Pyorala S, Huttunen N-P, Uhari M. A review and meta analysis of hormonal treatment of cryptorchidism. J Clin Endocrinol Metab 1995; 80:2795–2799.

925. Grasso M, Buonaguidi A, Lania C, et al. Postpubertal cryptorchidism: review and evaluation of the fertility. Eur Urol 1991; 20:126–128.

926. Docimo SG. The results of surgical therapy for cryptorchidism: a literature review and analysis. J Urol 1995; 154:1148–1152.

927. Hadziselimovic F, Herzog B, Seguchi H. Surgical correction of cryptorchidism at 2 years: electron microscopic and morphometric investigations. J Pediatr Surg 1975; 100:19–26.

928. Lee PA, Jaffe RB, Midgley AR. Serum gonadotropin, testosterone, and prolactin concentrations throughout puberty in boys: a longitudinal study. J Clin Endocrinol Metab 1974; 39:664–672.

929. Moller H, Jorgensen N, Forman D. Trends in incidence of testicular cancer in boys and adolescent men. Int J Cancer 1995; 61:761–764.

930. Aetiology of testicular cancer: association with congenital abnormalities, age at puberty, infertility, and exercise: United Kingdom Testicular Cancer Study Group [see comments]. BMJ 1994; 308:1393–1399.

931. Parkinson MC, Swerdlow AJ, Pike MC. Carcinoma in situ in boys with cryptorchidism: when can it be detected? Br J Urol 1994; 73:431–435.

932. Giwercman A, von der Maase H, Skakkebaek NE. Epidemiological and clinical aspects of carcinoma in situ of the testis. Eur Urol 1993; 23:104–114.

933. Thomas DB, Jimenez LM, McTiernan A, et al. Breast cancer in men: risk factors with hormonal implications. Am J Epidemiol 1992; 135:734–748.

934. Rosenfeld RG, Grumbach MM, eds. Turner Syndrome. New York: Marcel Dekker, 1990: 1–512.

935. Hook EB, Warburton D. The distribution of chromosomal genotypes associated with Turner's syndrome: livebirth prevalence rates and evidence for diminished fetal mortality and severity in genotypes associated with structural X abnormalities or mosaicism. Hum Genet 1983; 64:24–27.

936. Turner HH. A syndrome of infantilism, congenital webbed neck, and cubitus valgus. Endocrinology 1938; 23:566–574.

937. Carr DH, Gedeon M. Population cytogenetics in human abortuses. In: Hook EB, Porter IH, eds. Population Cytogenetics. New York: Academic Press, 1977; 1–9.

938. Warburton D, Kline J, Stein I. Monosomy X: a chromosomal anomaly associated with young maternal age. Lancet 1980; 1:167–169.

939. Rao E, Weiss B, Fukami M, et al. Pseudoautosomal deletions encompassing a novel homeobox gene cause growth failure in idiopathic short stature and Turner syndrome. Nature Genet 1997; 16:54–62.

940. Ellison JW, Wardak Z, Young M, et al. *PHOG*, a candidate gene for involvement in the short stature of Turner syndrome. Hum Mol Genet 1997; 6:1341–1347.

941. Szpunar J. Middle ear disease in Turner's syndrome. Arch Otolaryngol Head Neck Surg 1968; 87:34–40.

942. Palmer CG, Reichman A. Chromosomal and clinical findings in 110 females with Turner's syndrome. Hum Genet 1976; 35:35–49.

943. Lin AE, Lippe BM, Geffner ME, et al. Aortic dilation, dissection, and rupture in patients with Turner syndrome. J Pediatr 1986; 109:820–826.

944. Lippe BM, Geffner ME, Dietrich RB, et al. Renal malformations in patients with Turner syndrome: imaging in 141 patients. Pediatrics 1988; 82:852–856.

945. Arulanantham K, Kramer MS, Gryboski JD. The association of inflammatory bowel disease and X-chromosomal abnormality. Pediatrics 1980; 66:63–67.

946. Knudtzon J, Svane S. Turner's syndrome associated with chronic inflammatory bowel disease: a case report and review of the literature. Acta Med Scand 1988; 223:375–378.

947. Price WH. A high incidence of chronic inflammatory bowel disease in patient with Turner's syndrome. J Med Genetics 1979; 16:263–266.

948. Nielsen J, Johansen K, Yde H. The frequency of diabetes mellitus in patients with Turner's syndrome and pure gonadal dysgenesis. Acta Endocrinol 1969; 62:251–269.

949. Ross JL, Feuillan P, Long LM, et al. Lipid abnormalities in Turner syndrome. J Pediatr 1995; 126:242–245.

950. Silbert A, Wolffe PH, Lilienthal J. Spatial and temporal processing in patients with Turner's syndrome. Behav Genet 1977; 7:11–21.

951. Swillen A, Fryns JP, Kleczkowska A, et al. Intelligence, behaviour, and psychosocial development in Turner syndrome: a cross-sectional study of 50 pre-adolescent and adolescent girls (4–20 years). Genet Couns 1993; 4:7–18.

952. Garron DC. Intelligence among persons with Turner's syndrome. Behav Genet 1977; 7:105–127.

953. Albertsson-Wiklund K, Ranke MB. Turner Syndrome in a Life Span Perspective: Research and Clinical Aspects. Amsterdam: Elsevier Science BV, 1995.

954. Skuse DH, James RS, Bishop DVM, et al. Evidence from Turner's syndrome of an imprinted X-linked locus affecting cognitive function. Nature 1997; 387:705–708.

955. McGuffin P, Scourfield J. A father's imprint on his daughter's thinking. Nature 1997; 387:652–653.

956. Rovet J, Ireland L: Behavioral phenotype in children with Turner syndrome. J Pediatr Psychol 1994; 19:779–790.

957. Brook CGD, Murset G, Zachmann M, et al. Growth in children with 45,XO Turner's syndrome. Arch Dis Child 1974; 73:789–795.

958. Lyon AJ, Preece MA, Grant DB. Growth curve for girls with Turner syndrome. Arch Dis Child 1985; 60:932–935.

959. Ranke MB, Stubbe P, Majewski F, et al. Spontaneous growth in Turner's syndrome. Acta Paediatr Scand Suppl 1988; 343:22–30.

960. Massa G, Vanderschueren-Lodeweyckx M, Malvaux P. Linear growth in patients with Turner syndrome: influence of spontaneous puberty and parental height. Eur J Pediatr 1990; 149:246–250.

961. Sklar CA, Kaplan SL, Grumbach MM. Lack of effect of oestrogens on adrenal androgen secretion in children and adolescents with a comment on oestrogens and pubic hair growth. Clin Endocrinol 1981; 14:311–320.

962. Cicognani A, Mazzanti L, Tassinari D, et al. Differences in carbohydrate tolerance in Turner syndrome depending on age and karyotype. Eur J Pediatr 1988; 148:64–68.

963. Mazzanti L, Nizzoli G, Tassinari D, et al. Spontaneous growth and pubertal development in Turner's syndrome with different karyotypes. Acta Paediatr 1994; 83:299–304.

964. Cuseen IJ, MacMahan RA. Germ cells and ova in dysgenetic gonads of a 46-XY female dizygotic twin. Am J Dis Child 1979; 133:373–375.

965. Scully RE. Gonadoblastoma: a review of 74 cases. Cancer 1970; 25:1340–1356.

966. Khodr GS, Cadena GD, Ong TC. Y-autosome translocation, gonadal dysgenesis, and gonadoblastoma. Am J Dis Child 1979; 133:277–282.

967. Jamieson CR, van der Burgt I, Brady AF, et al. Mapping a gene for Noonan syndrome to the long arm of chromosome 12. Nature Genet 1994; 8:357–360.

968. Thibaud E, Ramirez M, Brauner R, et al. Preservation of ovarian function by ovarian transposition performed before pelvic irradiation during childhood. J Pediatr 1992; 121:880–884.

969. Quigley C, Cowell C, Jimenez M, et al. Normal or early development of puberty despite gonadal damage in children treated for acute lymphoblastic leukemia. N Engl J Med 1989; 321:143–151.

970. Ahmed SR, Shalet SM, Campbell RH, et al. Primary gonadal damage following treatment of brain tumors in childhood. J Pediatr 1983; 103:562–565.

971. Perrone L, Sinisi AA, Sicuranza R, et al. Prepubertal endocrine follow-up in subjects with Wilms' tumor. Med Pediatr Oncol 1988; 16:255–258.

972. Nicosia SV, Matus Ridley M, Meadows AT. Gonadal effects of cancer therapy in girls. Cancer 1985; 55:2364–2372.

973. Matus Ridley M, Nicosia SV, Meadows AT. Gonadal effects of cancer therapy in boys. Cancer 1985; 55:2353–2363.

974. Hoek A, Schoemaker J, Drexhage HA. Premature ovarian failure and ovarian autoimmunity. Endocr Rev 1997; 18:107–134.

975. Irvine WJ. Autoimmunity in endocrine disease. Recent Prog Horm Res 1980; 36:509–556.

976. Ahonen P, Myllarniemi S, Sipila I, et al. Clinical variation of autoimmune polyendocrinopathy-candidiasis-ectodermal dystrophy (APECED) in a series of 68 patients. N Engl J Med 1990; 322:1829–1836.

977. Lucky AW, Rebar RW, Blizzard RM, et al. Pubertal progression in the presence of elevated serum gonadotropins in girls with multiple endocrine deficiencies. J Clin Endocrinol Metab 1977; 45:673–678.

978. Betterle C, Rossi A, Dalla Pria S, et al. Premature ovarian failure: autoimmunity and natural history. Clin Endocrinol 1993; 39:35–43.

979. Chen S, Sawicka J, Betterle C, et al. Autoantibodies 'to steroidogenic enzymes in autoimmune polyglandular syndrome, Addison's disease, and premature ovarian failure. J Clin Endocrinol Metab 1996; 81:1871–1876.

980. Flora S, Bottazzo GF, Doniach D. Immunofluorescence studies on antibodies to steroid-producing cells and to germ line cells in endocrine disease and infertility. Clin Exp Immunol 1980; 39:97–111.

981. Frasier SD, Bashore RA, Mosier HD. Gonadoblastoma associated with pure gonadal dysgenesis in monozygotic twins. J Pediatr 1964; 64:740–745.

982. Dewhurst CJ, Dekoos EB, Ferreira HP. The resistant ovary syndrome. Br J Obstet Gynaecol 1975; 82:341–345.

983. Evers JLH, Rolland RT. The gonadotropin-resistant ovary syndrome: a curable disease? Clin Endocrinol 1981; 14:99–103.

984. Gibson JB. Gonadal function in galactosemics and in galactose-intoxicated animals. Eur J Pediatr 1995; 154[Suppl 2]:S14–S20.

985. Schweitzer S, Shin Y, Jakobs C, Brodehl J: Long-term outcome in 134 patients with galactosemia. Eur J Pediatr 1993; 152:36–43.

986. Kaufman FR, Kogut MD, Donnell GN, et al. Hypergonadotropic hypogonadism in female patients with galactosemia. N Engl J Med 1981; 304:994–998.

987. Kristiansson B, Stibler H, Wide L. Gonadal function and glycoprotein hormones in the carbohydrate-deficient glycoprotein (CDG) syndrome. Acta Paediatr 1995; 84:655–660.

988. de Zegher F, Jaeken J. Endocrinology of the carbohydrate-deficient glycoprotein syndrome type 1 from birth through adolescence. Pediatr Res 1995; 37:395–401.

989. Sprengel R, Braun T, Nikolics K, et al. The testicular receptor for follicle-stimulating hormone: structure and functional expression of cloned with DNA. Mol Endocrinol 1990; 4:525–530.

990. Aittomaki K. The genetics of XX gonadal dysgenesis. Am J Hum Genet 1994; 54:844–851.

991. Aittomaki K, Herva R, Stenman U-H, et al. Clinical features of primary ovarian failure caused by a point mutation in the follicle-stimulating hormone receptor gene. J Clin Endocrinol Metab 1996; 81:3722–3726.

992. Kumar TR, Wang Y, Lu N, et al. Follicle-stimulating hormone is required for ovarian follicle maturation but not male fertility. Nature Genet 1997; 15:201–204.

993. Aittomaki K, Dieguez Lucena JL, Pakarinen P, et al. Mutation in the follicle-stimulating hormone receptor gene causes hereditary hypergonadotropic ovarian failure. Cell 1995; 82:959–968.

994. Tapanainen JS, Aittomaki K, Min J, et al. Men homozygous for an inactivating mutation of the follicle-stimulating hormone (FSH) receptor gene present variable suppression of spermatogenesis and fertility. Nature Genet 1997; 15:205–206.

995. Latronico AC, Anasti J, Arnhold IJP, et al. Testicular and ovarian resistance to luteinizing hormone caused by inactivating mutations of the luteinizing hormone receptor gene. N Engl J Med 1996; 344:507–512.

996. Stanhope R, Adams J, Brook CG. Evolution of polycystic ovaries in a girl with delayed menarche: a case report. J Reprod Med 1988; 33:482–484.

997. Porcu E, Venturoli S, Magrini O, et al. Circadian variation of luteinizing hormone can have two different profiles in adolescent anovulation. J Clin Endocrinol Metab 1987; 65:488–493.

998. Elsawi MM, Pryor JP, Klufio G, et al. Genital tract function in men with Noonan syndrome. J Med Genet 1994; 31:468–470.

999. Bailey WA, Zwingman TA, Reznik VM, et al. End-stage renal disease and primary hypogonadism associated with a 46,XX karyotype. Am J Dis Child 1992; 146:1218–1223.

1000. Gilger JW, Geary DC, Eisele LM. Reliability and validity of retrospective self-reports of the age of pubertal onset using twin, sibling, and college student data. Adolescence 1991; 26:41–53.

1001. Carskadon MA, Acebo C: A self-administered rating scale for pubertal development. J Adolesc Health 1993; 14:190–195,

1002. Scholossberger NM, Turner RA, Irwin CE. Validity of self-report of pubertal maturation in early adolescents. J Adolesc Health 1992; 13:109–113.

1003. Bonneville JF, Cattin F. The role of magnetic resonance imaging in the diagnosis of endocrine tumours of the sellar region in children. Horm Res 1995; 43:151–153.

1004. Massarano AA, Adams J, Preece MA, et al. Ovarian ultrasound appearances in the Turner syndrome. J Pediatr 1989; 114:568–573.

1005. Spitz IM, Hirsch HJ, Trestian S. The prolactin response to thyrotropin-releasing hormone differentiates isolated gonadotropin deficiency from delayed puberty. N Engl J Med 1983; 308:575–579.

1006. Buyukgebiz A, Oktay S. The role of TRH-stimulated prolactin responses in distinguishing gonadotropin deficiency from constitutional delayed puberty. J Pediatr Endocrinol 1994; 7:325–330.

1007. Winters SJ, Johnsonbaugh RE, Sherins RJ. The response of prolactin to chlorpromazine stimulation in men with hypogonadotrophic hypogonadism and early pubertal boys: relationship to sex steroid exposure. Clin Endocrinol 1982; 16:321–330.

1008. Cristiano AM, Munabi A, el Sabbagh H, et al. Prolactin response to metoclopramide does not distinguish patients with hypogonadotrophic hypogonadism from delayed puberty. Clin Endocrinol (Oxf) 1988; 28:75–82.

1009. Popovic V, Milosevic Z, Micic D, et al. The prolactin response to TRH and domperidone does not differentiate male hypothalamic hypogonadism and constitutional delay of puberty. Exp Clin Endocrinol 1987; 89:211–215.

1010. Lanes R, Palacios A, Avendano E, et al. The metoclopramide test: a useful tool with the luteinizing hormone–releasing hormone test in distinguishing between constitutional delay of puberty and hypogonadotropic hypogonadism. Fertil Steril 1989; 52:55–59.

1011. Gordon D, Cohen HN, Beastall GH, et al. Hormonal responses in pubertal males to pulsatile gonadotropin releasing hormone (GnRH) administration. J Endocrinol Invest 1988; 11:77–83.

1012. Partsch CJ, Hermanussen M, Sippell WG. Differentiation of male hypogonadotropic hypogonadism and constitutional delay of puberty by pulsatile administration of gonadotropin-releasing hormone. J Clin Endocrinol Metab 1985; 60:1196–1203.

1013. Smals AG, Hermus AR, Boers GH, et al. Predictive value of luteinizing hormone–releasing hormone (LHRH) bolus testing before and after 36-hour pulsatile LHRH administration in the differential diagnosis of constitutional delay of puberty and male hypogonadotropic hypogonadism. J Clin Endocrinol Metab 1994; 78:602–608.

1014. Rosenfield RL, Burstein S, Cuttler L. Use of nafarelin for testing pituitary-ovarian function. J Reprod Med 1989; 34:1044–1050.

1015. Zamboni G, Antoniazzi F, Tato L. Use of the gonadotropin-releasing hormone agonist triptorelin in the diagnosis of delayed puberty in boys. J Pediatr 1995; 126:756–758.

1016. Foster CM, Hopwood NJ, Beitins IZ, et al. Evaluation of gonadotropin responses to synthetic gonadotropin-releasing hormone in girls with idiopathic hypopituitarism. J Pediatr 1992; 121:528–532.

1017. Haavisto AM, Dunkel L, Pettersson K, et al. LH measurements by in vitro bioassay and a highly sensitive immunofluorometric assay improve the distinction between boys with constitutional delay of puberty and hypogonadotropic hypogonadism. Pediatr Res 1990; 27:211–214.

1018. Cohen HN, Wallace AM, Beastall GH, et al. Clinical value of adrenal androgen measurement in the diagnosis of delayed puberty. Lancet 1981; 1:689–692.

1019. Copeland KC, Paunier L, Sizonenko PC. The secretion of adrenal androgens and growth patterns of patients with hypogonadotropic hypogonadism and isiopathic delayed puberty. J Pediatr 1977; 91:985–990.

1020. Wu FC, Brown DC, Butler GE, et al. Early-morning plasma testosterone is an accurate predictor of imminent pubertal development in prepubertal boys. J Clin Endocrinol Metab 1993; 76:26–31.

1021. Hedlund GL, Royal SA, Parker KL. Disorders of puberty: a practical imaging approach. Semin Ultrasound CT MR 1994; 15:49–77.

1022. Lee PDK, Rosenfeld RG. Psychosocial correlates of short stature and delayed puberty. Pediatr Adolesc Endocrinol 1987; 4:851–863.

1023. Ehrhardt AA, Meyer-Bahlburg HFL. Psychologic correlates of abnormal pubertal development. Clin Endocrinol Metab 1975; 4:207–222.

1024. Apter A, Galatzer A, Weizman A, et al. Psychological aspects of developmental endocrinopathies in adolescence. Isr J Psychiatry Relat Sci 1994; 31:246–253.

1025. Kaplowitz PB. Diagnostic value of testosterone therapy in boys with delayed puberty. Am J Dis Child 1989; 143:116–120.

1026. Wilson DM, Kei J, Hintz RL, et al. Effects of testosterone therapy for pubertal delay. Am J Dis Child 1988; 142:96–99. (Erratum 1988; 142:286.)

1027. Richman RA, Kirsch LR. Testosterone treatment in adolescent boys with constitutional delay in growth and development. N Engl J Med 1988; 319:1563–1567.

1028. Strickland AL: Long-term results of treatment with low-dose fluoxymesterone in constitutional delay of growth and puberty and in genetic short stature. Pediatrics 1993; 91:716–720.

1029. Stanhope R, Buchanan CR, Fenn GC, et al. Double-blind, placebo-controlled trial of low-dose oxandrolone in the treatment of boys with constitutional delay of growth and puberty. Arch Dis Child 1988; 63:501–505.

1030. Malhotra A, Poon E, Tse WY, et al. The effects of oxandrolone on the growth hormone and gonadal axes in boys with constitutional delay of growth and puberty. Clin Endocrinol (Oxf) 1993; 38:393–398.

1031. Papadimitriou A, Wacharasindhu S, Pearl K, et al. Treatment of constitutional growth delay in prepubertal boys with a prolonged course of low-dose oxandrolone. Arch Dis Child 1991; 66:841–843.

1032. Bassi F, Neri AS, Gheri RG, et al. Oxandrolone in constitutional delay of growth: analysis of the growth patterns up to final stature. J Endocrinol Invest 1993; 16:133–137.

1033. Uruena M, Pantsiotou S, Preece MA, et al. Is testosterone therapy for boys with constitutional delay of growth and puberty associated with impaired final height and suppression of the hypothalamo-pituitary-gonadal axis? Eur J Pediatr 1992; 151:15–18.

1034. Albanese A, Kewley GD, Long A, et al. Oral treatment for constitutional delay of growth and puberty in boys: a randomised trial of an anabolic steroid or testosterone undecanoate. Arch Dis Child 1994; 71:315–317.

1035. Belgorosky A, Chaler E, Rivarola MA. High serum sex hormone–binding globulin (SHBG) in premature thelarche. Clin Endocrinol (Oxf) 1992; 37:203–206.

1036. Butler GE, Sellar RE, Walker RF, et al. Oral testosterone undecanoate in the management of delayed puberty in boys: pharmacokinetics and effects on sexual maturation and growth. J Clin Endocrinol Metab 1992; 75:37–44.

1037. Zachmann M, Studer S, Prader A. Short-term testosterone treatment at bone age of 12 to 13 years does not reduce adult height in boys with constitutional delay of growth and adolescence. Helv Paediatr Acta 1987; 42:21–28.

1038. Rosenfield RL. Clinical review 6: Diagnosis and management of delayed puberty. J Clin Endocrinol Metab 1990; 70:559–562.

1039. Stanhope R, Albanese A, Hindmarsh P, et al. The effects of growth hormone therapy on spontaneous sexual development. Horm Res 1992; 38 Suppl 1:9–13.

1040. Nielsen J. Mental aspects of Turner syndrome and the importance of information and Turner contact groups. In: Rosenfeld RG, Grumbach MM, eds. In: Turner Syndrome. New York: Marcel Dekker, 1990: 451–467.

1041. Rikken B, Massa GG, Wit JM. Final height in a large cohort of Dutch patients with growth hormone deficiency treated with growth hormone: Dutch Growth Hormone Working Group. Horm Res 1995; 43:135–137.

1042. Frisch H, Birnbacher R. Final height and pubertal development in children with growth hormone deficiency after long-term treatment. Horm Res 1995; 43:132–134.

1043. Toublanc JE, Couprie C, Garnier P, et al. The effects of treatment combining an agonist of gonadotropin-releasing hormone with growth hormone in pubertal patients with isolated growth hormone deficiency. Acta Endocrinol (Copenh) 1989; 120:795–799.

1044. Reilly JM, Woodhouse CR. Small penis and the male sexual role. J Urol 1989; 142:569–71; discussion 572.

1045. Levy JB, Husmann DA. Micropenis secondary to growth hormone deficiency: does treatment with growth hormone alone result in adequate penile growth? J Urol 1996; 156:214–216.

1046. Aulitzky W, Frick J, Galvan G. Pulsatile luteinizing hormone–releasing hormone treatment of male hypogonadotropic hypogonadism. Fertil Steril 1988; 50:480–486.

1047. Stanhope R, Brook CG, Pringle PJ, et al. Induction of puberty by pulsatile gonadotropin-releasing hormone. Lancet 1987; 2:552–555.

1048. Delemarre-van de Waal HA, Odink RJ. Pulsatile GnRH treatment in boys and girls with idiopathic hypogonadotropic hypogonadism. Hum Reprod 1993; 8 Suppl 2:180–183.

1049. Iwatani N, Kodama M, Miike T Pulsatile LH-RH administration induces puberty in hypogonadotropic GH-deficient patients. Endocr J 1993; 40:191–196.

1050. Santoro N, Filicori M, Crowley WF. Hypogonadotropic disorders in men and women: diagnosis and therapy with pulsatile gonadotropin-releasing hormone. Endocr Rev 1986; 7:11–23.

1051. Stanhope R, Adams J, Jacobs HS, et al. Ovarian ultrasound assessment in normal children, idiopathic precocious puberty, and during low-dose pulsatile gonadotropin-releasing hormone treatment of hypogonadotrophic hypogonadism. Arch Dis Child 1985; 60:116–119.

1052. Schoemaker J, van Kessel H, Simons AH, et al. Induction of first cycles in primary hypothalamic amenorrhea with pulsatile luteinizing hormone–releasing hormone: a mirror of female pubertal development. Fertil Steril 1987; 48:204–212.

1053. Marshall JC, Griffin ML. The role of changing pulse frequency in the regulation of ovulation. Hum Reprod 1993; 8 Suppl 2:57–61.

1054. Bridges NA, Hindmarsh PC, Matthews DR, et al. The effect of changing gonadotropin-releasing hormone pulse frequency on puberty. J Clin Endocrinol Metab 1994; 79:841–847.

1055. Tato L, Zamboni G, Antoniazzi F, et al. Gonadal function and response to growth hormone (GH) in boys with isolated GH deficiency and to GH and gonadotropins in boys with multiple pituitary hormone deficiencies. Fertil Steril 1996; 65:830–834.

1056. Tanaka T, Hibi I, Tanae A. Combined human chorionic gonadotropin (hCG) and human menopausal gonadotropin (hMG) treatment in gonadotropin-deficient males with pituitary dwarfism. Acta Paediatr Jpn 1992; 34:243–248; Discussion 249–250.

1057. Balducci R, Toscano V, Mangiantini A, et al. The effect of growth hormone administration on testicular response during gonadotropin therapy in subjects with combined gonadotropin and growth hormone deficiencies. Acta Endocrinol (Copenh) 1993; 128:19–23.

1058. Padova G, Finocchiaro C, Briguglia G, et al. Pubarche induction with testosterone treatment in women with panhypopituitarism. Fertil Steril 1996; 65:437–439.

1059. Didi M, Morris-Jones PH, Gattamaneni HR, et al. Pubertal growth in response to testosterone replacement therapy for radiation-induced Leydig cell failure. Med Pediatr Oncol 1994; 22:250–254.

1060. Takano K, Shizume K, Hibi I O, et al. Growth hormone treatment in Turner syndrome—results of a multicentre study in Japan: The Committee for the Treatment of Turner Syndrome. Horm Res 1993; 39 Suppl 2:37–41.

1061. Attanasio A, James D, Reinhardt R, et al. Final height and long-term outcome after growth hormone therapy in Turner syndrome: results of a German multicentre trial. Horm Res 1995; 43:147–149.

1062. Rovet J, Holland J: Psychological aspects of the Canadian randomized,

controlled trial of human growth hormone and low-dose ethinyl oestradiol in children with Turner syndrome: The Canadian Growth Hormone Advisory Group. Horm Res 1993; 39 Suppl 2:60–64.

1063. Knudtzon J, Aarskog D: Results of two years of growth hormone treatment followed by combined growth hormone and oestradiol in Turner syndrome: The Norwegian Turner Study Group. Horm Res 1993; 39 Suppl 2:7–17.

1064. Nilsson KO, Albertsson-Wikland K, Alm J, et al. Improved final height in girls with Turner's syndrome treated with growth hormone and oxandrolone. J Clin Endocrinol Metab 1996; 81:635–640.

1065. Massa G, Maes M, Heinrichs C, et al. Influence of spontaneous or induced puberty on the growth promoting effect of treatment with growth hormone in girls with Turner's syndrome. Clin Endocrinol (Oxf) 1993; 38:253–260.

1066. Rosenfeld RG, Hintz RL, Johanson AJ, et al. Growth hormone therapy in Turner's syndrome. In: Rosenfeld RG, Grumbach MM, eds. Turner Syndrome. New York: Marcel Dekker, 1990; 393–405.

1067. Largo RH, Prader A. Pubertal development in Swiss boys. Helv Paediatr Acta 1983; 38:211–228.

1068. Paul D, Conte FA, Grumbach MM, et al. Long-term effect of gonadotropin-releasing hormone agonist therapy on final and near-final height in 26 children with true precocious puberty treated at a median age of less than 5 years. J Clin Endocrinol Metab 1995; 80:546–551.

1069. Thamdrup E. Precocious Sexual Development: A Clinical Study of 100 Patients. Springfield, IL: Charles C Thomas, 1961:50.

1070. Thamdrup E. [Somatic development in puberty: a survey] Den somatiske udvikling i pubertetsarene: En oversigt. Nord Med 1965; 74:1013–1018.

1071. Kaplan SL, Grumbach MM. Clinical review 14: Pathophysiology and treatment of sexual precocity. J Clin Endocrinol Metab 1990; 71:785–789.

1072. Lee PA. Medroxyprogesterone therapy for sexual precocity in girls. Am J Dis Child 1981; 135:443–445.

1073. Sigurjonsdottir TJ, Hayles AB. Precocious puberty: a report of 96 cases. Am J Dis Child 1968; 115:309–321.

1074. Werder EA, Murset G, Zachmann M, et al. Treatment of precocious puberty with cyproterone acetate. Pediatr Res 1974; 8:248–256.

1075. Sorgo W, Kiraly E, Homoki J, et al. The effects of cyproterone acetate on statural growth in children with precocious puberty. Acta Endocrinol (Copenh) 1987; 115:44–56.

1076. Lenz J. Vorzeitige Menstruation: Geschlechtsstreife und Entwicklung. Arch Gynaekol 1913; 99:67.

1077. Muram D, Dewhurst J, Grant DB. Precocious puberty: a follow-up study. Arch Dis Child 1984; 59:77–78.

1078. Benedict PH. Endocrine features in Albright's syndrome (fibrous dysplasia of bone). Metabolism 1962; 11:30–45.

1079. Danon M, Crawford JD. The McCune-Albright syndrome. Ergeb Inn Med Kinderheilkd 1987; 55:81–115.

1080. Bierich JR. Sexual precocity. Clin Endocrinol Metab 1975; 4:107–142.

1081. Liu N, Grumbach MM, De Napoli RA, et al. Prevalence of electroencephalographic abnormalities in idiopathic precocious puberty and premature pubarche: bearing on pathogenesis and neuroendocrine regulation of puberty. J Clin Endocrinol Metab 1965; 25:1296–1308.

1082. Fontoura M, Brauner R, Prevot C, et al. Precocious puberty in girls: early diagnosis of a slowly progressing variant. Arch Dis Child 1989; 64:1170–1176.

1083. Bridges NA, Cooke A, Healy MJ, et al. Ovaries in sexual precocity. Clin Endocrinol (Oxf) 1995; 42:135–140.

1084. Ehrhardt AA, Meyer-Bahlburg HF. Psychosocial aspects of precocious puberty. Horm Res 1994; 41 Suppl 2:30–35.

1085. Money J, Alexander D. Psychosexual development and absence of homosexuality in males with precocious puberty: review of 18 cases. J Nerv Ment Dis 1969; 148:111–123.

1086. Ehrhardt AA, Meyer-Bahlburg HF. Idiopathic precocious puberty in girls: long-term effects on adolescent behavior. Acta Endocrinol Suppl (Copenh) 1986; 279:247–253.

1087. Kao SC, Cook JS, Hansen JR, et al. MR imaging of the pituitary gland in central precocious puberty. Pediatr Radiol 1992; 22:481–484.

1088. Sharafuddin MJ, Luisiri A, Garibaldi LR, et al. MR imaging diagnosis of central precocious puberty: importance of changes in the shape and size of the pituitary gland. AJR 1994; 162:1167–1173.

1089. Gupta R, Ammini AC. Precocious puberty with pituitary gland hyperplasia: two cases in one family. Pediatr Radiol 1996; 26:418–420.

1090. Cacciari E, Zucchini S, Ambrosetto P, et al. Empty sella in children and adolescents with possible hypothalamic-pituitary disorders. J Clin Endocrinol Metab 1994; 78:767–771.

1091. Rapaport R, Logrono R. Primary empty sella syndrome in childhood: association with precocious puberty. Clin Pediatr (Phila) 1991; 30:466–471.

1092. Neely EK, Wilson DM, Lee PA, et al. Spontaneous serum gonadotropin concentrations in the evaluation of precocious puberty. J Pediatr 1995; 127:63–67.

1093. Eckert KL, Wilson DM, Bachrach LK, et al. A single-sample, subcutaneous gonadotropin-releasing hormone test for central precocious puberty. Pediatrics 1996; 97:517–519.

1094. Zucchini S, Ambrosetto P, Carlà G, et al. Primary empty sella: differences and similarities between children and adults. Acta Paediatr 1995; 84:1382–1385.

1095. Schwarz HP, Tschaeppeler H, Zuppinger K. Case report: unsustained central sexual precocity in four girls. Med Sci 1990; 299:260–264.

1096. Bridges NA, Christopher JA, Hindmarsh PC, et al. Sexual precocity: sex incidence and aetiology. Arch Dis Child 1994; 70:116–118.

1097. Janss AJ, Grundy R, Cnaan A, et al. Optic pathway and hypothalamic/chiasmatic gliomas in children younger than age 5 years with a 6-year follow-up. Cancer 1995; 75:1051–1059.

1098. Leiper AD, Stanhope R, Kitching P, et al. Precocious and premature puberty associated with treatment of acute lymphoblastic leukaemia. Arch Dis Child 1987; 62:1107–1112.

1099. Rappaport R, Brauner R. Growth and endocrine disorders secondary to cranial irradiation. Pediatr Res 1989; 25:561–567.

1100. Nicholl RM, Kirk JM, Grossman AB, et al. Acceleration of pubertal development following pituitary radiotherapy for Cushing's disease. Clin Oncol (R Coll Radiol) 1993; 5:393–394.

1101. Sklar CA, Constine LS. Chronic neuroendocrinological sequelae of radiation therapy. Int J Radiat Oncol Biol Phys 1995; 31:1113–1121.

1102. Cara JF, Kreiter ML, Rosenfield RL. Height prognosis of children with true precocious puberty and growth hormone deficiency: effect of combination therapy with gonadotropin-releasing hormone agonist and growth hormone. J Pediatr 1992; 120:709–715.

1103. Kamp GA, Manasco PK, Barnes KM, et al. Low-growth hormone levels are related to increased body mass index and do not reflect impaired growth in luteinizing hormone–releasing hormone agonist–treated children with precocious puberty. J Clin Endocrinol Metab 1991; 72:301–307.

1104. Zuniga OF, Tanner SM, Wild WO, et al. Hamartoma of CNS associated with precocious puberty. Am J Dis Child 1983; 137:127–133.

1105. Minns RAM, Stirling HT, Wu FCM. Hypothalamic hamartoma with skeletal malformations, gelastic epilepsy, and precocious puberty. Dev Med Child Neurol 1994; 36:173–182.

1106. Mahachoklertwattana P, Kaplan SL, Grumbach MM. The luteinizing hormone–releasing hormone–secreting hypothalamic hamartoma is a congenital malformation: natural history. J Clin Endocrinol Metab 1993; 77:118–124.

1107. Starceski PJ, Lee PA, Albright AL, et al. Hypothalamic hamartomas and sexual precocity: evaluation of treatment options. Am J Dis Child 1990; 144:225–228.

1108. Nishio S, Fujiwara S, Aiko Y, et al. Hypothalamic hamartoma: report of two cases. J Neurosurg 1989; 70:640–645.

1109. Cacciari E, Frejaville E, Cicognani A, et al. How many cases of true precocious puberty in girls are idiopathic? J Pediatr 1983; 102:357–360.

1110. Pescovitz OH, Comite F, Hench K, et al. The NIH experience with precocious puberty: diagnostic subgroups and response to short-term luteinizing hormone–releasing hormone analogue therapy. J Pediatr 1986; 108:47–54.

1111. Diebler C, Ponsot G. Hamartomas of the tuber cinereum. Neuroradiology 1983; 25:93–101.

1112. Lin SR, Bryson MM, Gobien R, et al. Neuroradiologic study of hamartomas of the tuber cinereum and hypothalamus. Neuroradiology 1978; 16:17–19.

1113. Nakagawa N, Takahashi M, Kohrogi Y. Neuroradiologic findings of hypothalamic hamartoma with emphasis on computed tomography. J Comput Tomogr 1986; 10:77–83.

1114. Peterman SB, Steiner RE, Bydder GM. Magnetic resonance imaging of intracranial tumors in children and adolescents. AJNR 1984; 5:703–709.

1115. Hahn FJ, Leibrock LG, Huseman CA, et al. The MR appearance of hypothalamic hamartoma. Neuroradiology 1988; 30:65–68.

1116. Price RA, Lee PA, Albright AL, et al. Treatment of sexual precocity by removal of a luteinizing hormone–releasing hormone secreting hamartoma. JAMA 1984; 251:2247–2249.

1117. Sato M, Ushio Y, Arita N, et al. Hypothalamic hamartoma: report of two cases. Neurosurgery 1985; 16:198–206.

1118. Turjman F, Xavier JL, Froment JC, et al. Late MR follow-up of hypothalamic hamartomas. Childs Nerv Syst 1996; 12:63–68.

1119. Styne DM, Harris DA, Egli CA, et al. Treatment of true precocious puberty with a potent luteinizing hormone–releasing factor agonist: effect on growth, sexual maturation, pelvic sonography, and the hypothalamic-pituitary-gonadal axis. J Clin Endocrinol Metab 1985; 61:142–151.

1120. Albright AL, Lee PA. Neurosurgical treatment of hypothalamic hamartomas causing precocious puberty. J Neurosurg 1993; 78:77–82.

1121. Grumbach MM. True or central precocious puberty. In: Kreiger DT, Bardin CW, eds. Current Therapy in Endocrinology and Metabolism. Toronto: BC Decker, 1985: 4–8.

1122. Valdueza JM, Cristante L, Dammann O, et al. Hypothalamic hamartomas: with special reference to gelastic epilepsy and surgery. Neurosurgery 1994; 34:949–958.

1123. Lopponen T, Saukkonen AL, Serlo W, et al. Accelerated pubertal development in patients with shunted hydrocephalus. Arch Dis Child 1996; 74:490–496.

1124. Robertson CM, Morrish DW, Wheler GH, et al. Neonatal encephalopathy: an indicator of early sexual maturation in girls. Pediatr Neurol 1990; 6:102–108.

1125. Blendonohy PM, Philip PA. Precocious puberty in children after traumatic brain injury. Brain Inj 1991; 5:63–68.

1126. Tubiana-Rufi N, Thizon-de Gaulle I, Czernichow P. Hypothalamopituitary deficiency and precocious puberty following hyperhydration in diabetic ketoacidosis. Horm Res 1992; 37:60–63.

1127. Brauner R, Rappaport R, Nicod C, et al. Pubertes precoces vraies au cours de l'hydrocephalie non tumorale: analyse de 16 observations. Arch Fr Pediatr 1987; 44:433–436.

1128. Lopponen T, Saukkonen AL, Serlo W, et al. Slow prepubertal linear growth but early pubertal growth spurt in patients with shunted hydrocephalus. Pediatrics 1995; 95:917–923.

1129. Brauner R, Pierre-Kahn A, Nemedy-Sandor E. Precocious puberty caused by a suprasellar arachnoid cyst: analysis of 6 cases. Arch Fr Pediatr 1987; 44:489–493.

1130. Okamoto K, Nakasu Y, Sato M, et al. Isosexual precocious puberty associated with multilocular arachnoid cysts at the cranial base: report of a case. Acta Neurochir (Wien) 1981; 57:87–93.

1131. Clark SJ, Van Dop C, Conte FA, et al. Reversible true precocious puberty secondary to a congenital arachnoid cyst. Am J Dis Child 1988; 142:255–256.

1132. Habiby R, Silverman B, Listernick R, et al. Precocious puberty in children with neurofibromatosis type 1. J Pediatr 1995; 126:364–367.

1133. Zacharin M. Precocious puberty in two children with neurofibromatosis type I in the absence of optic chiasmal glioma. J Pediatr 1997; 130:155–157.

1134. Listernick R, Charrow J, Greenwald M, et al. Natural history of optic pathway tumors in children with neurofibromatosis type 1: a longitudinal study. J Pediatr 1994; 125:63–66.

1135. Riccardi VM, Heim RA, Kam-Morgan LNW, et al. Distribution of 13 truncating mutations in the neurofibromatosis 1 gene. Hum Mol Genet 1995; 4:975–981.

1136. Xu GF, Lin B, Tanaka K, et al. The catalytic domain of the neurofibromatosis type 1 gene product stimulates *ras* GTPase and complements *ira* mutants of Scerevisiae. Cell 1990; 63:835–841.

1137. Ballester R, Marchuk D, Boguski M, et al. The NF1 locus encodes a protein functionally related to mammalian GAP and yeast IRA proteins. Cell 1990; 63:851–859.

1138. Martin GA, Viskochil D, Bollag G, et al. The GAP-related domain of the neurofibromatosis type 1 gene product interacts with *ras* p21. Cell 1990; 63:843–849.

1139. Stephens K, Kayes L, Riccardi VM, et al. Preferential mutation of the neurofibromatosis type 1 gene in paternally derived chromosomes. Hum Genet 1992; 88:279–282.

1140. Riccardi VM. Neurofibromatosis: Phenotype, Natural History, and Pathogenesis. Baltimore: Johns Hopkins Press, 1992.

1141. Listernick R, Charrow J. Neurofibromatosis type 1 in childhood. J Pediatr 1990; 116:845–853.

1142. Mulvihill JJ, Parry DM, Sherman JL, et al. NIH Conference Neurofibromatosis 1 (Recklinghausen disease) and neurofibromatosis 2 (bilateral acoustic neurofibromatosis): an update. Ann Intern Med 1990; 113:39–52.

1143. Cohen BH, Rothner AD. Incidence, types, and management of cancer in patients with neurofibromatosis. Oncology 1989; 3:23–30.

1144. Samuelsson B, Riccardi VM. Neurofibromatosis in Gothenburg, Sweden. II. Intellectual compromise. Neurofibromatosis 1989; 2:78–83.

1145. Samuelsson B, Riccardi VM. Neurofibromatosis in Gothenburg, Sweden. III. Psychiatric and social aspects. Neurofibromatosis 1989; 2:84–106.

1146. Money J, Hosta G. Laughing seizures with sexual precocity. Johns Hopkins Med J 1967; 120:326–336.

1147. Sockalosky JJ, Kriel RL, Krach LE, et al. Precocious puberty after traumatic brain injury. J Pediatr 1987; 110:373–377.

1148. Freude S, Frisch H, Wimberger D, et al. Septo-optic dysplasia and growth hormone deficiency: accelerated pubertal maturation during GH therapy. Acta Paediatr 1992; 81:641–645.

1149. LaFranchi SH. Sexual precocity with hypothalamic hypopituitarism. Am J Dis Child 1979; 133:739–742.

1150. Tuvemo T, Proos LA. Girls adopted from developing countries—a group at risk of early pubertal development and short final height: implications for health surveillance and treatment. Ann Med 1993; 25:217–219 (editorial).

1151. Proos LA, Hofvander Y, Tuvemo T. Menarcheal age and growth pattern of Indian girls adopted in Sweden. II. Catch-up growth and final height. Indian J Pediatr 1991; 58:105–114.

1152. Dacou-Voutetakis C, Karidis N. Congenital adrenal hyperplasia complicated by central precocious puberty: treatment with LHRH-agonist analogue. Ann N Y Acad Sci 1993; 687:250–254.

1153. Sadeghi-Nejad A, Kaplan SL, Grumbach MM. The effect of medroxyprogesterone acetate on adrenocortical function in children with precocious puberty. J Pediatr 1971; 78:616–624.

1154. Boulgourdjian E, Escobar ME, Martinez A, et al. Bone age at discontinuation of medroxyprogesterone acetate therapy in girls with precocious puberty: effect on final height. Horm Res 1995; 44:12–16.

1155. Stanhope R, Huen KF, Buzi F, et al. The effect of cyproterone acetate on the growth of children with central precocious puberty. Eur J Pediatr 1987; 146:500–503.

1156. Conn PM, Crowley WF. Gonadotropin-releasing hormone and its analogs. Annu Rev Med 1994; 45:391–405.

1157. Marshall JC, Kelch RP. Gonadotropin-releasing hormone: role of pulsatile secretion in the regulation of reproduction. N Engl J Med 1986; 315:1459–1468.

1158. Conn PM, Janovick JA, Stanislaus K, et al. Molecular and cellular bases of gonadotropin-releasing hormone action in the pituitary and central nervous system. Vitamins and Hormones. 1995; 50:151–214.

1159. Karten MJ, Rivier JE. Gonadotropin-releasing hormone analog design—structure-function studies toward the development of agonists and antagonists: rationale and perspective. Endocr Rev 1986; 7:44–66.

1160. Lemay A. Clinical appreciation of LHRH analogue formulation. Horm Res 1989; 32:93–101.

1161. Handelsman DJ, Swerdloff RS. Pharmacokinetics of gonadotropin-releasing hormone and its analogs. Endocr Rev 1986; 7:95–105.

1162. Comite F, Cutler GB, Rivier J, et al. Short-term treatment of idiopathic precocious puberty with a long-acting analogue of luteinizing hormone-releasing hormone: a preliminary report. N Engl J Med 1981; 305:1546–1550.

1163. Crowley WF Jr, Comite F, Vale WA, et al. Therapeutic use of pituitary desensitization with a long-acting LHRH agonist: a potential new treatment for idiopathic precocious puberty. J Clin Endocrinol Metab 1981; 52:370–372.

1164. Boepple PA, Mansfield MJ, Wierman ME, et al. Use of a potent, long-acting agonist of gonadotropin-releasing hormone in the treatment of precocious puberty. Endocr Rev 1986; 7:24–33.

1165. Comite F, Cassorla F, Barnes KM, et al. Luteinizing hormone–releasing hormone analogue therapy for central precocious puberty: long-term effect on somatic growth, bone maturation, and predicted height. JAMA 1986; 255:2613–2616.

1166. Drop SL, Odink RJ, Rouwe C, et al. The effect of treatment with an LH-RH agonist (buserelin) on gonadal activity growth and bone maturation in children with central precocious puberty. Eur J Pediatr 1987; 146:272–278.

1167. Bourguignon JP, Van Vliet G, Vandeweghe M, et al. Treatment of central precocious puberty with an intranasal analogue of GnRH (buserelin). Eur J Pediatr 1987; 146:555–560.

1168. Kaplan SL, Grumbach MM. True precocious puberty: treatment with GnRH-agonists. In: Delemarre-Van de Waal H, Plant TM, van Rees GP, et al, eds. Control of the Onset of Puberty. Amsterdam: Elsevier, 1989: 357–373.

1169. Antoniazzi F, Cisternino M, Nizzoli G, et al. Final height in girls with central precocious puberty: comparison of two different luteinizing hormone–releasing hormone agonist treatments. Acta Paediatr 1994; 83:1052–1056.

1170. Stasiowska B, Vannelli S, Benso L. Final height in sexually precocious girls after therapy with an intranasal analogue of gonadotrophin-releasing hormone (buserelin). Horm Res 1994; 42:81–85.

1171. Cacciari E, Cassio A, Balsamo A, et al. Long-term follow-up and final height in girls with central precocious puberty treated with luteinizing hormone–releasing hormone analogue nasal spray. Arch Pediatr Adolesc Med 1994; 148:1194–1199.

1172. Heinrichs C, Craen M, Vanderschueren-Lodeweyckx M, et al. Variations in pituitary-gonadal suppression during intranasal buserelin and intramuscular depot-triptorelin therapy for central precocious puberty: Belgian Study Group for Pediatric Endocrinology. Acta Paediatr 1994; 83:627–633.

1173. Partsch CJ, Hummelink R, Peter M, et al. Comparison of complete and incomplete suppression of pituitary-gonadal activity in girls with central precocious puberty—influence on growth and predicted final height: The German-Dutch Precocious Puberty Study Group. Horm Res 1993; 39:111–117.

1174. Neely EK, Hintz RL, Parker B, et al. Two-year results of treatment with depot leuprolide acetate for central precocious puberty. J Pediatr 1992; 121:634–640.

1175. Carel JC, Lahlou N, Guazzarotti L, et al. Treatment of central precocious puberty with depot leuprorelin: French Leuprorelin Trial Group. Eur J Endocrinol 1995; 132:699–704.

1176. Tanaka T, Hibi I, Kato K, et al. A dose-finding study of a super long-acting luteinizing hormone–releasing hormone analog (leuprolide acetate depot, TAP-144 SR) in the treatment of central precocious puberty: The TAP-144 SR CPP Study Group. Endocrinol Jpn 1991; 38:369–376.

1177. Holland FJ, Fishman L, Costigan DC, et al. Pharmacokinetic characteristics of the gonadotropin-releasing hormone analog D-Ser (tBU)6Pro9NEt luteinizing hormone–releasing hormone (buserelin) after subcutaneous and intranasal administration in children with central precocious puberty. J Clin Endocrinol Metab 1986; 63:1065–1070.

1178. Hummelink R, Oostdijk W, Partsch CJ, et al. Growth, bone maturation, and height prediction after three years of therapy with the slow-release GnRH-agonist Decapeptyl depot in children with central precocious puberty. Horm Metab Res 1992; 24:122–126.

1179. Sklar CA, Rothenberg S, Blumberg D, et al. Suppression of the pituitary-gonadal axis in children with central precocious puberty: effects on growth, growth hormone, insulin-like growth factor I, and prolactin secretion. J Clin Endocrinol Metab 1991; 73:734–738.

1180. Kletter GB, Kelch RP. Clinical review 60: Effects of gonadotropin-releasing hormone analog therapy on adult stature in precocious puberty. J Clin Endocrinol Metab 1994; 79:331–334.

1181. Eshet R, Silbergeld A, Kauli R, et al. GH and GHBP activity and not IGF-1 and its receptor activity express growth velocity reduction during treatment of central precocious puberty by a superactive GNRH analogue. Isr J Med Sci 1994; 30:592–595.

1182. Eshet R, Dux Z, Silbergeld A, et al. Erythrocytes from patients with low concentrations of IGF-1 have an increase in receptor sites of IGF-1. Acta Endocrinol 1991; 125:354–358.

1183. Kappy M, Stuart T, Perelman A, et al. Suppression of gonadotropin secretion by a long-acting gonadotropin-releasing hormone analog (leuprolide acetate, Lupron Depot) in children with precocious puberty. J Clin Endocrinol Metab 1989; 69:1087–1089.

1184. Roger M, Chaussain JL, Berlier P, et al. Long-term treatment of male and female precocious puberty by periodic administration of a long-acting preparation of D-Trp6-luteinizing hormone–releasing hormone microcapsules. J Clin Endocrinol Metab 1986; 62:670–677.

1185. Ambrosino MM, Hernanz-Schulman M, Genieser NB, et al. Monitoring of girls undergoing medical therapy for isosexual precocious puberty. J Ultrasound Med 1994; 13:501–508.

1186. Jay N, Mansfield MJ, Blizzard RM, et al. Ovulation and menstrual function of adolescent girls with central precocious puberty after therapy with gonadotropin-releasing hormone agonists. J Clin Endocrinol Metab 1992; 75:890–894.

1187. Schroor EJ, van Weissenbruch MM, Delemarre-van de Waal HA. Long-term GnRH-agonist treatment does not postpone central development of the GnRH pulse generator in girls with idiopathic precocious puberty. J Clin Endocrinol Metab 1995; 80:1696–1701.

1188. Oerter KE, Manasco PK, Barnes KM, et al. Effects of luteinizing hormone–releasing hormone agonists on final height in luteinizing hormone–releasing hormone-dependent precocious puberty. Acta Paediatr Suppl 1993; 388:62–68; discussion 69.

1189. Rosenfield RL. Selection of children with precocious puberty for treatment with gonadotropin-releasing hormone analogs. J Pediatr 1994; 124:989–991.

1190. Bassi F, Bartolini O, Neri AS, et al. Precocious puberty: auxological criteria discriminating different forms. J Endocrinol Invest 1994; 17:793–797.

1191. Brauner R, Adan L, Malandry F, et al. Adult height in girls with idiopathic true precocious puberty. J Clin Endocrinol Metab 1994; 79:415–420.

1192. Brauner R, Malandry F, Rappaport R. Predictive factors for the effect of gonadotropin-releasing hormone analogue therapy on the height of girls with idiopathic central precocious puberty. Eur J Pediatr 1992; 151:728–730.

1193. Garibaldi LR, Aceto T Jr, Weber C. The pattern of gonadotropin and estradiol secretion in exaggerated thelarche. Acta Endocrinologica 1993; 128:345–350.

1194. Pasquino AM, Pucarelli I, Passeri F, et al. Progression of premature thelarche to central precocious puberty. J Pediatr 1995; 126:11–14.

1195. Neely EK, Wilson DM. Letter to the editor (reply). J Pediatr 1995; 126:159–160.

1196. Manasco PK, Pescovitz OH, Feuillan PP, et al. Resumption of puberty after long-term luteinizing hormone–releasing hormone agonist treatment of central precocious puberty. J Clin Endocrinol Metab 1988; 67:368–372.

1197. Kauschansky A, Nussinovitch M, Frydman M, et al. Hyperprolactinemia after treatment of long-acting gonadotropin-releasing hormone analogue Decapeptyl in girls with central precocious puberty. Fertil Steril 1995; 64:285–287.

1198. Mouridsen SE, Larsen FW. Psychological aspects of precocious puberty: an overview. Acta Paedopsychiatr 1992; 55:45–49.

1199. Pescovitz OH, Comite F, Cassorla F, et al. True precocious puberty complicating congenital adrenal hyperplasia: treatment with a luteinizing hormone–releasing hormone analog. J Clin Endocrinol Metab 1984; 58:857–861.

1200. Roosen N, Cras P, Van Vyve M. Hamartoma of the tuber cinereum in a six-month-old boy, causing isosexual precocious puberty. Neurochirurgia (Stuttg) 1987; 30:56–60.

1201. Markin RS, Leibrock LG, Huseman CA, et al. Hypothalamic hamartoma: a report of two cases. Pediatr Neurosci 1987; 13:19–26.

1202. Nishio S, Shigeto H, Fukui M: Hypothalamic hamartoma: the role of surgery. Neurosurg Rev 1993; 16:157–160.

1203. Romner B, Trumpy JH, Marhaug G, et al. Hypothalamic hamartoma causing precocious puberty treated by surgery: case report. Surg Neurol 1994; 41:306–309.

1204. Saggese G, Cesaretti G, Barsanti S, et al. Combination treatment with growth hormone and gonadotropin-releasing hormone analogs in short normal girls. J Pediatr 1995; 126:468–473.

1205. Sklar CA, Conte FA, Kaplan SL, et al. Human chorionic gonadotropin–secreting pineal tumor: relation to pathogenesis and sex limitation of sexual precocity. J Clin Endocrinol Metab 1981; 53:656–660.

1206. McArthur JW, Toll GD, Russfield AB, et al. Sexual precocity attributable to ectopic gonadotropin secretion by hepatoblastoma. Am J Med 1973; 54:390–403.

1207. Morinaga S, Yamaguchi M, Watanabe I, et al. An immunohistochemical study of hepatoblastoma producing human chorionic gonadotropin. Cancer 1983; 51:1647–1652.

1208. Braunstein GD, Bridson WE, Glass A, et al. In vivo and in vitro production of human chorionic gonadotropin and alpha-fetoprotein by a virilizing hepatoblastoma. J Clin Endocrinol Metab 1972; 35:857–862.

1209. Heimann A, White PF, Riely CA, et al. Hepatoblastoma presenting as isosexual precocity: the clinical importance of histologic and serologic parameters. J Clin Gastroenterol 1987; 9:105–110.

1210. Reuben MS, Manning GR. Precocious puberty. Arch Pediatr 1923; 40:27–44.

1211. Cohen AR, Wilson JA, Sadeghi-Nejad A. Gonadotropin-secreting pineal teratoma causing precocious puberty. Neurosurgery 1991; 28:597–602; discussion 602.

1212. Chaussain J-L, Lemerle J, Roger M, et al. Klinefelter's syndrome: tumor, and sexual precocity. J Pediatr 1980; 97:607–609.

1213. Hasle H, Jacobsen BB, Asschenfeldt P, et al. Mediastinal germ cell tumor associated with Klinefelter's syndrome. Eur J Pediatr 1992; 151:735–739.

1214. Englund AT, Geffner ME, Nagel RA, et al. Pediatric germ cell and human chorionic gonadotropin–producing tumors: clinical and laboratory features. Am J Dis Child 1991; 145:1294–1297.

1215. Faggiano M, Criscuolo T, Perrone L, et al. Sexual precocity in a boy due to hypersecretion of LH and prolactin by a pituitary adenoma. Acta Endocrinol (Copenh) 1983; 102:167–172.

1216. Schmitt K, Frisch H, Neuhold N, et al. Aldosterone and testosterone producing adrenal adenoma in childhood. J Endocrinol Invest 1995; 18:69–73.

1217. Barnes RB, Rosenfield RL, Ehrmann DA, et al. Ovarian hyperandrogynism as a result of congenital adrenal virilizing disorders: evidence for perinatal masculinization of neuroendocrine function in women. J Clin Endocrinol Metab 1994; 79:1328–1333.

1218. Schedewie HK, Reiter EO, Beitins IZ. Testicular Leydig cell hyperplasia as a cause of familial sexual precocity. J Clin Endocrinol Metab 1981; 52:271–278.

1219. Rosenthal SM, Grumbach MM, Kaplan SL. Gonadotropin-independent familial sexual precocity with premature Leydig and germinal cell maturation (familial testotoxicosis): effects of a potent luteinizing hormone–releasing factor agonist and medroxyprogesterone acetate therapy in four cases. J Clin Endocrinol Metab 1983; 57:571–579.

1220. Egli CA, Rosenthal SM, Grumbach MM, et al. Pituitary gonadotropin-independent male-limited autosomal dominant sexual precocity in nine generations: familial testotoxicosis. J Pediatr 1985; 106:33–40.

1221. Gondos B, Egli CA, Rosenthal SM, et al. Testicular changes in gonadotropin-independent familial male sexual precocity: familial testotoxicosis. Arch Pathol Lab Med 1985; 109:990–995.

1222. Holland FJ. Gonadotropin-independent precocious puberty. Endocrinol Metab Clin North Am 1991; 20:191–210.

1223. Wierman ME, Beardsworth DE, Mansfield MJ, et al. Puberty without gonadotropins: a unique mechanism of sexual development. N Engl J Med 1985; 312:65–72.

1224. Stone RK. Extraordinary precocity in the development of male sexual organs and muscular system in a child four years old. Am J Med Sciences 1852; 24:561–564.

1225. Rosenthal IM, Refetoff S, Rich B, et al. Response to challenge with gonadotropin-releasing hormone agonist in a mother and her two sons with a constitutively activating mutation of the luteinizing hormone receptor—a clinical research center study. J Clin Endocrinol Metab 1996; 81:3802–3806.

1226. Shenker A, Laue L, Kosugi S, et al. A constitutively activating mutation of the luteinizing hormone receptor in familial male precocious puberty. Nature 1993; 365:652–654.

1227. Kremer H, Mariman E, Otten BJ, et al. Cosegregation of missense mutations of the luteinizing hormone receptor gene with familial male-limited precocious puberty. Hum Mol Genet 1993; 2:1779–1783.

1228. McFarland KC, Sprengel R, Phillips HS, et al. Lutotropin-choriogonadotropin receptor: an unusual member of the G-coupled receptor family. Science 1989; 245:494–499.

1229. Loosfelt H, Misrahi M, Alger M, et al. Cloning and sequencing of porcine LH-hCG receptor cDNA: variants labeling the transmembrane domain. Science 1989; 245:525–528.

1230. Minegishi T, Nakamura K, Takakura Y, et al. Cloning and sequencing of porcine LH-hCG receptor cDNA. Biochem Biophys Res Comm 1990; 172:1049–1054.

1231. Atger M, Misrahi M, Sar S, et al. Structure of the human luteininzing hormone/choriogonadotropin receptor gene: unusual promoter and 5′ non-coding regions. Mol Cell Biol 1995; 111:113–123.

1232. Dufau ML. The leutinizing hormone receptor. In: Payne AH, Hardy MP, Russell LD, eds. The Leydig Cell. Vienna, II: Cache River Press, 1996: 334–350.

1233. Baldwin JM. Structure and function of receptors coupled to G protein. Curr Opin Cell Biol 1994; 6:180–190.

1234. Dufau ML. The luteinizing hormone receptor. Curr Opin Endocr Diabetes 1995; 2:365–374.

1235. Evans BA, Bowen DJ, Smith PJ, et al. A new point mutation in the luteinising hormone receptor gene in familial and sporadic male-limited precocious puberty: genotype does not always correlate with phenotype. J Med Genet 1996; 33:143–147.

1236. Yano K, Kohn LD, Saji M, et al. A case of male-limited precocious puberty caused by a point mutation in the second transmembrane domain of the luteinizing hormone choriogonadotropin receptor gene. Biochem Biophys Res Comm 1996; 220:1036–1042.

1236a. Lin Z, Shenker A, Pearlstein R. A model of the lutropin/choriogonadotropin receptor: insights into the structural and functional effects of constitutively activating mutations. Protein Eng 1997; 10:501–510.

1237. Feldman D. Ketoconazole and other imidazole derivatives as inhibitors of steroidogenesis. Endocr Rev 1986; 7:409–420.

1238. Holland FJ, Fishman L, Bailey JD, et al. Ketoconazole in the management of precocious puberty not responsive to LHRH-analogue therapy. N Engl J Med 1985; 312:1023–1028.

1239. Babovic-Vuksanovic D, Donaldson MD, Gibson NA, et al. Hazards of ketoconazole therapy in testotoxicosis. Acta Paediatr 1994; 83:994–997.

1240. Laue L, Kenigsberg D, Pescovitz OH, et al. The treatment of familial male precocious puberty with spironolactone and testolactone. N Engl J Med 1989; 320:496–502.

1241. Laue L, Chan WY, Hsueh AJ, et al. Genetic heterogeneity of constitutively activating mutations of the human luteinizing hormone receptor in familial male-limited precocious puberty. Proc Natl Acad Sci USA 1995; 92:1906–1910.

1242. Kuhn JM, Billebaud T, Navratil H. Prevention of the transient adverse effects of a gonadotropin-releasing hormone analogue (buserelin) in metastatic prostatic carcinoma by administration of an antiandrogen (nilutamide). N Engl J Med 1989; 321:413–418.

1243. Bhatnagar AS, Häusler A, Schieweck K, et al. Highly selective inhibition of estrogen biosynthesis by CGS 20267, a new non-steroidal aromatase inhibitor. J Ster Biochem Mol Biol 1990; 37:1021–1027.

1243a. Lipton A, Demers LM, Harvey HA, et al. Letrozole (CGS20267). A phase I study of a new potent oral aromatase inhibitor of breast cancer. Cancer 1995; 75:2132–2138.

1244. Towne BH, Mahour GH, Woolley MM, et al. Ovarian cysts and tumors in infancy and childhood. J Pediatr Surg 1975; 10:311–320.

1245. Polhemus DW. Ovarian maturation and cyst formation in children. Pediatrics 1953; 11:588–594.

1246. Peters H, Himelstein-Braw R, Faher M. The normal development of the ovary in childhood. Acta Endocrinol 1976; 82:617–630.

1247. Peters H. The human ovary in childhood and early maturity. Eur J Obstet Gynecol Reprod Biol 1979; 3:137–144.

1248. de Sa DJ. Follicular ovarian cysts in stillbirths and neonates. Arch Dis Child 1975; 50:45–50.

1249. Zachariou Z, Roth H, Boos R, et al. Three years' experience with large ovarian cysts diagnosed in utero. J Pediatr Surg 1989; 24:478–482.

1250. Sedin G, Bergquist C, Lindgren PG. Ovarian hyperstimulation syndrome in preterm infants. Pediatr Res 1985; 19:548–551.

1251. Lee PA, Migeon CJ, Bias WB, et al. Familial hypersecretion of adrenal androgens transmitted as a dominant, non-HLA linked trait. Obstet Gynecol 1987; 69:259–264.

1252. Arisaka O, Hosaka A, Shimura N, et al. Effect of neonatal ovarian cysts on infant growth. Clin Pediatr Endocrinol 1995; 4:155–162.

1253. Lyon AJ, De Bruyn R, Grant DB. Transient sexual precocity and ovarian cysts. Arch Dis Child 1985; 60:819–822.

1254. Liapi C, Evain-Brion D. Diagnosis of ovarian follicular cysts from birth to puberty: a report of twenty cases. Acta Paediatr Scand 1987; 76:91–96.

1255. Zipf WB, Kelch RP, Hopwood NJ, et al. Suppressed responsiveness to gonadotropin-releasing hormone in girls with unsustained isosexual precocity. J Pediatr 1979; 95:38–41.

1256. Richards GE, Kaplan SL, Grumbach MM. Sexual precocity associated with functional follicular cysts, prepubertal gonadotropins, and LRF response and fluctuating estrogen levels. Pediatr Res 1977; 11:431 (abstract).

1257. Fakhry J, Khoury A, Kotval PS, et al. Sonography of autonomous follicular ovarian cysts in precocious pseudopuberty. J Ultrasound Med 1988; 7:597–603.

1258. Tonetta SA, di Zerega GS. Intragonadal regulation of follicular maturation. Endocr Rev 1989; 10:205–229.

1259. Feuillan PP, Jones J, Oerter KE, et al. Luteinizing hormone–releasing hormone (LHRH)–independent precocious puberty unresponsive to LHRH agonist therapy in two girls lacking the features of the McCune-Albright syndrome. J Clin Endocrinol Metab 1991; 73:1370–1373.

1260. Salardi S, Orsini LF, Cacciari E, et al. Pelvic ultrasonography in girls with precocious puberty, congenital adrenal hyperplasia, obesity, or hirsutism. J Pediatr 1988; 112:880–887.

1261. Eberlein WR, Bongiovanni AM, Jones IT et al. Ovarian tumors and cysts associated with sexual precocity. J Pediatr 1960; 57:484–497.

1262. Butler MG, Najjar JL. Do some patients with fragile X syndrome have precocious puberty? Am J Med Genet 1988; 31:779–781.

1263. Young RH, Dickersin GR, Scully RE. Juvenile granulosa cell tumor of the ovary: A clinicopathologic analysis of 125 cases. Am J Surg Pathol 1984; 8:575–596.

1264. Biscotti CV, Hart WR. Juvenile granulosa cell tumors of the ovary. Arch Pathol Lab Med 1989; 113:40–46.

1265. Lee MM, Donahoe PK, Hasegawa T, et al. Müllerian-inhibiting substance in humans: normal levels from infancy to adulthood. J Clin Endocrinol Metab 1996; 81:571–576.

1266. Silverman LA, Gitelman SE. Immunoreactive inhibin, müllerian inhibitory substance, and activin as biochemical markers for juvenile granulosa cell tumors. J Pediatr 1996; 129:918–921.

1267. Gustafson ML, Lee MM, Scully RE, et al. Müllerian-inhibiting substance as a marker for ovarian sex-cord tumor. N Engl J Med 1992; 326:466–471.

1268. Lappöhn RE, Burger HC, Bouma J, et al. Inhibin as a marker for granulosa cell tumors. N Engl J Med 1989; 321:790–793.

1269. Burger HG, Fuller PJ. The inhibin/activin family and ovarian cancer. Trends Endocrinol Metab 1996; 7:197–202.

1270. Masson P. Pflugerome. Bull Soc Anat (Paris) 1912; 14:403–404.

1271. Talerman A. The pathology of gonadal neoplasm composed of germ cells and sex cord stroma derivatives. Pathol Res Pract 1980; 170:24–38.

1272. Bhatena D, Haning RV, Shapiro S. Coexistence of a gonadoblastoma and mixed germ cell cord stroma tumor. Pathol Res Pract 1985; 180:203–206.

1273. Lacson AG, Gillis DA, Shawwa A. Malignant mixed germ cell–sex cord–stromal tumors of the ovary associated with isosexual precocious puberty. Cancer 1988; 61:2122–2133.

1274. Skinner MA, Schlatter MG, Heifetz SA, et al. Ovarian neoplasms in children. Arch Surg 1993; 128:849–853.

1275. Imai A, Furui T, Tamaya T. Gynecologic tumors and symptoms in childhood and adolescence: 10-years' experience. Int J Gynaecol Obstet 1994; 45:227–234.

1276. Solh HM, Azoury RS, Najjar SS. Peutz-Jeghers syndrome associated with precocious puberty. J Pediatr 1983; 103:593–595.

1277. Coen P, Kulin H, Ballantine T, et al. An aromatase-producing sex-cord tumor resulting in prepubertal gynecomastia. N Engl J Med 1991; 324:317–322.

1278. Young RH, Dickersin GR, Scully RE. A distinctive ovarian–sex cord–stromal tumor causing sexual precocity in the Peutz-Jeghers syndrome. Am J Surg Pathol 1983; 7:233–243.

1279. Young S, Gooneratne S, Straus FH, et al. Feminizing Sertoli cell tumors in boys with Peutz-Jeghers syndrome. Am J Surg Pathol 1995; 19:50–58.

1280. Berensztein E, Belgorosky A, de Dávila MR, et al. Testicular steroid biosynthesis in a boy with a large cell calcifying Sertoli cell tumor producing prepubertal gynecomastia. Steroids 1995; 60:220–225.

1281. Hemminki A, Tomlinson I, Markie D, et al. Localization of a susceptibility locus for Peutz-Jeghers syndrome to 19p using comparative genomic hybridization and targeted linkage analysis. Nature Genet 1997; 15:87–90.

1282. McCune DJ, Bruch H. Osteodystrophia fibrosa: report of a case in which the condition was combined with true precocious puberty, pathologic pigmentation of the skin, and hyperthyroidism, with a review of the literature. Am J Dis Child 1937; 54:806–848.

1283. Albright F, Butler AM, Hampton AO, et al. Syndrome characterized by osteitis fibrosa disseminata, areas of pigmentation, and endocrine dysfunction, with precocious puberty in females. N Engl J Med 1937; 216:727–746.

1284. Ringel MD, Schwindinger WF, Levine MA. Clinical implications of genetic defects in G proteins. The molecular basis of McCune-Albright syndrome and Albright hereditary osteodystrophy. Medicine 1996; 75:171–184.

1285. Danon MS, Robboy SH, Kin S, et al. Cushing syndrome, sexual precocity, and polyostotic fibrous dysplasia. J Pediatr 1975; 87:917–921.

1286. Feuillan PP, Jones J, Ross JL. Growth hormone hypersecretion in a girl with McCune-Albright syndrome: comparison with controls and response to a dose of long-acting somatostatin analog. J Clin Endocrinol Metab 1995; 80:1357–1360.

1287. Econs MJ, Drezner MK. Tumor-induced osteomalacia—unveiling a new hormone. N Engl J Med 1994; 330:1679–1681.

1288. Zung A, Chalew SA, Schwindinger WF, et al. Urinary cyclic adenosine 3′,5′-monophosphate response in McCune-Albright syndrome: clinical evidence for altered renal adenyl cyclase activity. J Clin Endocrinol Metab 1995; 80:3576–3581.

1289. Endo M, Yamada Y, Matsuura N, et al. Monozygotic twins discordant for the major signs of McCune-Albright syndrome. Am J Med Genet 1991; 41:216–220.

1290. Nager GT, Kennedy DW, Kopstein E. Fibrous dysplasia: a review of the disease and its manifestations in the temporal bone. Ann Otol Rhinol Laryngol Suppl 1982; 92:1–52.

1291. Carani C, Pacchioni C, Baldini A, et al. Effects of cyproterone acetate, LHRH agonist, and ovarian surgery in McCune-Albright syndrome with precocious puberty and galactorrhea. J Endocrinol Invest 1988; 11:419–423.

1292. Reith KG, Comite F, Shawker T, et al. Pituitary and ovarian abnormalities demonstrated by CT and ultrasound in children with features of the McCune-Albright syndrome. Radiology 1984; 153:389–393.

1293. Foster CM, Comite F, Pescovitz OH, et al. Variable response to a long-acting agonist of luteinizing hormone–releasing hormone in girls with McCune-Albright syndrome. J Clin Endocrinol Metab 1984; 59:801–805.

1294. Foster CM, Ross JL, Shawker T, et al. Absence of pubertal gonadotropin secretion in girls with McCune-Albright syndrome. J Clin Endocrinol Metab 1984; 58:1161–1165.

1295. Pasquino AM, Tebaldi L, Cives C, et al. Precocious puberty in the McCune-Albright syndrome: progression from gonadotrophin-independent to gonadotrophin-dependent puberty in a girl. Acta Paediatr Scand 1987; 76:841–843.

1296. Feullian PP, Foster CM, Pescovitz O, et al. Treatment of precocious puberty in the McCune-Albright syndrome with the aromatase inhibitor testolactone. N Engl J Med 1986; 315:1115–1119.

1297. Hauffa BP, Havers W, Stolecke H. Short-term effects of testolactone compared to other treatment modalities on longitudinal growth and ovarian activity in a girl with McCune-Albright syndrome. Helv Paediatr Acta 1987; 42:471–480.

1298. Feuillan PP, Jones J, Cutler GB. Long-term testolactone therapy for precocious puberty in girls with the McCune-Albright syndrome. J Clin Endocrinol Metab 1993; 77:647–651.

1299. Giovanelli G, Bernasconi S, Banchini G. McCune-Albright syndrome in a male child: a clinical and endocrinologic enigma. J Pediatr 1978; 92:220–226.

1300. Happle R. The McCune-Albright syndrome: a lethal gene surviving by mosaicism. Clin Genet 1986; 29:321–324.

1301. Lyons J, Landis CA, Harsh G, et al. Two G-protein oncogenes in human endocrine tumors. Science 1990; 249:655–659.

1302. Spiegel AM, Shenker A, Weinstein LS. Receptor-effector coupling by G proteins: implications for normal and abnormal signal transduction. Endocr Rev 1992; 13:536–565.

1303. Neer EJ. Heterotrimeric G proteins: organizers of transmembrane signals. Cell 1995; 80:249–257.

1304. Spiegel AM. The molecular basis of disorders caused by defects in G proteins. Horm Res 1997; 47:89–96.

1305. Bourne HR. Trimeric G proteins: surprise witness tells a tale. Science 1995; 270:933–934.

1306. Clapham DE. The G-protein nanomachine. Nature 1996; 379:297–299.

1307. Neer EJ, Smith TF. G-protein heterodimers: new structures propel new questions. Cell 1996; 84:175–178.

1308. Coleman DE, Sprang SR. How G proteins work: a continuing story. Trends Biochem Sci 1996; 21:41–44.

1309. Dhanasekaran N, Heasley LE, Johnson GL. G-protein–coupled receptor systems involved in cell growth and oncogenesis. Endocr Rev 1995; 16:259–270.

1310. Weinstein LS, Shenker A, Gejman PV, et al. Activating mutations of the stimulatory G protein in the McCune-Albright syndrome. N Engl J Med 1991; 325:1688–1695.

1311. Schwindinger WF, Francomano CA, Levine MA. Identification of a mutation in the gene encoding the alpha subunit of the stimulatory G protein of adenylyl cyclase in McCune-Albright syndrome. Proc Natl Acad Sci USA 1992; 89:5152–5156.

1312. Speigel AM. Mutations in G proteins and G protein–coupled receptors in endocrine disease. J Clin Endocrinol Metab 1996; 81:2434–2442.

1313. Shenker A, Weinstein LS, Sweet DE. An activating Gs alpha mutation is present in fibrous dysplasia of bone in the McCune-Albright syndrome. J Clin Endocrinol Metab 1994; 79:750–755.

1314. Candeliere GA, Glorieux FH, Prud'homme J, et al. Increased expression of the C-fos proto-oncogene in bone from patients with fibrous dysplasia. N Engl J Med 1995; 332:1546–1551.

1315. Shenker A, Weinstein LS, Moran A, et al. Severe endocrine and nonendocrine manifestations of the McCune-Albright syndrome associated with activating mutations of stimulatory G protein Gs. J Pediatr 1993; 123:509–518.

1316. Nakamoto JM, Zimmerman D, Jones EA, et al. Concurrent hormone resistance (pseudohypoparathyroidism type Ia) and hormone independence (testotoxicosis) caused by a unique mutation in the G alpha s gene. Biochem Mol Med 1996; 58:18–24.

1317. Iiri T, Herzmark P, Nakamoto JM, et al. Rapid GDP release from Gs alpha in patients with gain and loss of endocrine function. Nature 1994; 371:164–168.

1318. Kendle FW. Case of precocious puberty in a female cretin. BMJ 1905; 1:246.

1319. Suter SN, Kaplan SL, Aubert ML, et al. Plasma prolactin and thyrotropin and the response to throtropin-releasing factor in children with primary and tertiary hypothyroidism. J Clin Endocrinol Metab 1978; 47:1015–1020.

1320. Hemady ZS, Siler-Khodr TM, Najjar S. Precocious puberty in juvenile hypothyroidism. J Pediatr 1978; 92:55–59.

1321. Piziak VK, Hahn HB. Isolated menarche in juvenile hypothyroidism. Clin Pediatr (Phila) 1984; 23:177–179.

1322. Laron Z, Karp M, Dolberg L. Juvenile hypothyroidism with testicular enlargement. Acta Paediatr Scand 1970; 59:317–322.

1323. Wood LC, Olichney M, Locke H, et al. Syndrome of juvenile hypothyroidism associated with advanced sexual development: report of two new cases and comment on the management of an associated ovarian mass. J Clin Endocrinol Metab 1965; 25:1289–1295.

1324. Rakover Y, Weiner E, Shalev E, et al. Vaginal bleeding: presenting symptom of acquired primary hypothyroidism in a seven year-old girl. J Pediatr Endocrinol 1993; 6:197–200.

1325. Jannini EA, Ulisse S, D'Armiento M. Thyroid hormone and male gonadal function. Endocrine Rev 1995; 16:443–459.

1326. Pringle PJ, Stanhope R, Hindmarsh P, et al. Abnormal pubertal development in primary hypothyroidism. Clin Endocrinol (Oxf) 1988; 28:479–486.

1327. Buchanan CR, Stanhope R, Adlard P, et al. Gonadotropin, growth hormone, and prolactin secretion in children with primary hypothyroidism. Clin Endocrinol 1988; 29:427–436.

1328. Bruder JM, Samuels MH, Bremner WJ, et al. Hypothyroidism-induced macroorchidism: use of a gonadotropin-releasing hormone agonist to understand its mechanism and augment adult stature. J Clin Endocrinol Metab 1995; 80:11–16.

1329. Hess RA, Cooke PS, Bunick D, et al. Adult testicular enlargement induced by neonatal hypothyroidism is accompanied by increased Sertoli and germ cell numbers. Endocrinology 1993; 132:2607–2613.

1330. Marshall GR, Plant TM. Puberty occurring either spontaneously or induced precociously in rhesus monkey (Macaca mulatta) is associated with a marked proliferation of Sertoli cells. Biol Reprod 1996; 54:1192–1199.

1331. Anasti JN, Flack MR, Froehlich J, et al. A potential novel mechanism for precocious puberty in juvenile hypothyroidism. J Clin Endocrinol Metab 1995; 80:276–279.

1332. Money J, Lamacz M. Genital examination and exposure experienced as nosocomial sexual abuse in childhood. J Nerv Ment Dis 1987; 175:713–721.

1333. Ivarsson SA, Nilsson KO, Persson PH. Ultrasonography of the pelvic organs in prepubertal and postpubertal girls. Arch Dis Child 1983; 58:352–354.

1334. Griffin IJ, Cole TJ, Duncan KA, et al. Pelvic ultrasound measurements in normal girls. Acta Paediatr 1995; 84:536–543.

1335. Haber HP, Mayer EI. Ultrasound evaluation of uterine and ovarian size from birth to puberty. Pediatr Radiol 1994; 24:11–13.

1336. King LR, Siegel MJ, Solomon AL. Usefulness of ovarian volume and cysts in female isosexual precocious puberty. J Ultrasound Med 1993; 12:577–581.

1337. Garibaldi LR, Aceto TJ, Weber C, et al. The relationship between luteinizing hormone and estradiol secretion in female precocious puberty: evaluation by sensitive gonadotropin assays and the leuprolide stimulation test. J Clin Endocrinol Metab 1993; 76:851–856.

1338. Oberman AS, Flatau E, Luboshitzky R: Bilateral testicular adrenal rests in a patient with 11-hydroxylase–deficient congenital adrenal hyperplasia. J Urol 1993; 149:350–352.

1339. Rieth KG, Comite F, Dwyer AJ, et al. CT of cerebral abnormalities in precocious puberty. AJR 1987; 148:1231–1238.

1340. Burton EM, Ball WS, Crone K, et al. Hamartoma of the tuber cinereum: a comparison of MR and CT findings in four cases. AJNR 1989; 10:497–501.

1341. Robben SG, Oostdijk W, Drop SL, et al. Idiopathic isosexual central precocious puberty: magnetic resonance findings in 30 patients. Br J Radiol 1995; 68:34–38.

1342. Argyropoulou M, Perignon F, Brunelle F, et al. Height of normal pituitary gland as a function of age evaluated by magnetic resonance imaging in children. Pediatr Radiol 1991; 21:247–249.

1343. Pérignon F, Brauner R, Argyropoulou M, et al. Precocious puberty in girls: pituitary height as an index of hypothalamo-pituitary activation. J Clin Endocrinol Metab 1992; 75:1170–1172.

1344. Cook CD, McArthur JW, Berenberg W. Pseudoprecocious puberty in girls as a result of estrogen ingestion. N Engl J Med 1953; 248:671–674.

1345. Precocious development in Puerto Rican children. Lancet 1986; 1:721–722 (editorial).

1346. Fara GM, Del Corvo G, Bernuzzi S, et al. Epidemic of breast enlargement in an Italian school. Lancet 1979; 2:295–297.

1347. Bongiovanni AM. An epidemic of premature thelarche in Puerto Rico. J Pediatr 1983; 103:245–246.

1348. Mills JL. Endocrinology of premature thelarche. In: McLachlan JA, ed. Estrogens in the Environment. II. Influences on Development. New York: Elsevier, 1985; 412–427.

1349. Howard CP, Takahashi H, Hayles AB. Feminizing adrenal adenoma in a boy. Mayo Clin Proc 1977; 52:354–357.

1350. MacLaren NL, Migeon CH, Raiti S. Gynecomastia with congenital virilizing adrenal hyperplasia (11-beta-hydroxylase deficiency). J Pediatr 1975; 86:579–581.

1351. Hemsell DL, Edman CD, Marks JF, et al. Massive extraglandular aromatization of plasma androstenedione resulting in feminization of a prepubertal boy. J Clin Invest 1977; 60:455–464.

1352. Berkovitz GD, Guerami A, Brown TR, et al. Familial gynecomastia with increased extraglandular aromatization of plasma carbon 19 steroids. J Clin Invest 1985; 75:1763–1796.

1353. Wilson DM, Pitts WC, Hintz RL, et al. Testicular tumors with Peutz-Jeghers syndrome. Cancer 1986; 57:2238–2240.

1354. Arai K, Chrousos GP. Syndromes of glucocorticoid and mineralocorticoid resistance. Steroids 1995; 60:173–179.

1355. Malchoff CD, Reardon G, Javier EC, et al. Dexamethasone therapy for isosexual precocious pseudopuberty caused by generalized glucocorticoid resistance. J Clin Endocrinol Metab 1994; 79:1632–1636.

1356. Young RH, Scully RE. Ovarian Sertoli cell tumors: a report of 10 cases. Int J Gynecol Pathol 1984; 2:349–363.

1357. Tavassoli FA, Norris HJ. Sertoli tumors of the ovary: a clinicopathologic study of 28 cases with ultrastructural observations. Cancer 1980; 46:2282–2297.

1358. Ilicki A, Lewin P, Kauli LR, et al. Premature thelarche—natural history and sex hormone secretion in 68 girls. Acta Paediatr Scand 1984; 73:756–762.

1359. Van Winter JT, Noller KL, Zimmerman D, et al. Natural history of premature thelarche in Olmsted County, Minnesota, 1940 to 1984. J Pediatr 1990; 116:278–280.

1360. McKiernan J, Coyne J, Cahalane S. Histology of breast development in early life. Arch Dis Child 1988; 63:136–139.

1361. Dresch PC, Arnal M, Prader A. A premature thelarche. Helv Paediatr Acta 1960; 15:585–593.

1362. Caparo VJ, Bayonet-Rivera NP, Thomas A, et al. Premature thelarche. Obstet Gynecol Surg 1971; 26:2–7.

1363. Ferrier P, Shepard TH, Smith FK. Growth disturbances and values for hormone excretion in various forms of precocious sexual development. Pediatrics 1961; 28:258–275.

1364. Rosenfeld RL. Normal and almost-normal precocious variations in pubertal development; premature pubarche and premature thelarche revisited. Horm Res 1994; 41 Suppl 2:7–13.

1365. Simmons PS. Diagnostic considerations in breast disorders of children and adolescents. Obstet Gynecol Clin North Am 1992; 19:91–102.

1366. Radfar N, Ansusinna K, Kenny FM. Circulating bound and free estradiol and estrone during normal growth and development and in premature thelarche and isosexual precocity. J Pediatr 1976; 89:719–723.

1367. Wenick GB, Chasalow FI, Blethen SL. Sex hormone–binding globulin and thyroxine-binding globulin levels in premature thelarche. Steroids 1988; 52:543–550.

1368. Collett-Solberg PR, Grumbach MM. A simplified procedure for evaluating estrogenic effects and the sex chromatin pattern in exfoliated cells in urine: studies in premature thelarche and gynecomastia of adolescence. J Pediatr 1965; 66:883–890.

1369. Pescovitz OH, Hench KD, Barnes KM, et al. Premature thelarche and central precocious puberty: the relationship between clinical presentation and the gonadotropin response to luteinizing hormone–releasing hormone. J Clin Endocrinol Metab 1988; 67:474–479.

1370. Stanhope R, Abdulwahid NA, Adams J, et al. Studies of gonadotrophin pulsatility and pelvic ultrasound examinations distinguish between isolated premature thelarche and central precocious puberty. Eur J Pediatr 1986; 145:190–194.

1371. Verrotti A, Ferrari M, Morgese G, Chiarelli F. Premature thelarche: a long-term follow-up. Gynecol Endocrinol 1996; 10:241–247.

1372. Caufriez H, Wolter R, Gouaerts M, et al. Gonadotropins and prolactin pituitary reserve in premature thelarche. J Pediatr 1977; 91:751–753.

1373. Garibaldi LR, Aceto T Jr, Weber C: The pattern of gonadotropin and estradiol secretion in exaggerated thelarche. Acta Endocrinol (Copenh) 1993; 128:345–350.

1374. Murram D, Dewhurst J, Grant DB. Premature menarche: a follow-up study. Arch Dis Child 1983; 58:142–143.

1375. Blanco-Garcia M, Eva-Brion D, Roger M, et al. Isolated menses in prepubertal girls. Pediatrics 1985; 76:43–47.

1376. Fishman A, Paldi E. Vaginal bleeding in premenarchal girls: a review. Obstet Gynecol Surv 1991; 46:457–460.

1377. Hill NCW, Oppenheimer LW, Morton KE. The aetiology of vaginal bleeding in children: a 20-year review. Br J Obstetr Gynaecol 1989; 96:467–470.

1378. David L, Betend B, Berlier P, et al. Les hemorragie genitales de la fille avant la puberte: a propos de trente-trois observations: Ann Pediatr (Paris) 1984; 31:55–61.

1379. Silverman SH, Migeon CJ, Rosenberg E, et al. Precocious growth of sexual hair without other secondary sexual development: "premature pubarche," a constitutional variation of adolescence. Pediatrics 1952; 10:426–431.

1380. Thamdrup E. Premature pubarche—a hypothalamic disorder? Acta Endocrinol 1955; 18:564–567.

1381. Rappaport R. Plasma androgens and LH in scoliotic patients with premature pubarche. J Clin Endocrinol Metab 1974; 38:401–406.

1382. Lee PA, Migeon CJ, Bias WB, et al. Familial hypersecretion of adrenal androgens transmitted as a dominant, non-HLA linked trait. Obstet Gynecol 1987; 69:259–264.1383. Ferrier P, Shepard TH, Smith FK. Growth disturbances and values for hormone excretion in various forms of precocious sexual development. Pediatrics 1961; 28:258–275.

1383. Ferrier P, Shepard TH, Smith FK. Growth disturbances and values for hormone excretion in various forms of precocious sexual development. Pediatrics 1961; 28:258–275.

1384. Korth-Schutz S, Levine LS, New MI. Serum androgens in normal prepubertal and pubertal children and in children with precocious adrenarche. J Clin Endocrinol Metab 1976; 42:117–124.

1385. Rosenfield RL. Plasma 17-ketosteroids and 17-beta-hydroxysteroid in girls with premature development of sexual hair. J Pediatr 1971; 79:260–266.

1386. Apter D, Bhtzow T, Laughlin GA, et al. Metabolic features of polycystic ovary syndrome are found in adolescent girls with hyperandrogenism. J Clin Endocrinol Metab 1995; 80:2966–2973.

1387. Lee PA, Gareis FJ. Gonadotropin and sex steroid response to luteinizing hormone–releasing hormone in patients with premature adrenarche. J Clin Endocrinol Metab 1976; 43:195–197.

1388. Ibanez L, Virdio R, Potau N, et al. Natural history of premature pubarche: an auxological study. J Clin Endocrinol Metab 1992; 74:254–257.

1389. Pere A, Perheentupa J, Peter M, et al. Follow-up of growth and steroids in premature adrenarche. Eur J Pediatr 1995; 154:346–:352.

1390. Diamanti-Kandarakis E, Dunaif A. New perspectives in polycystic ovary syndrome. Trends Endocrinol Metab 1996; 7:267–271.

1391. Oberfield SE, Mayes DM, Levine LS. Adrenal steroidogenic function in a Black and Hispanic population with precocious pubarche. J Clin Endocrinol Metab 1990; 70:76–82.

1392. Likitmaskul S, Cowell CT, Donaghue K, et al. "Exaggerated adrenarche" in children presenting with premature adrenarche. Clinical Endocrinol 1995; 42:265–272.

1393. Yen SCC. The polycystic ovary syndrome. Clin Endocrinol 1980; 12:177–207.

1394. Franks S. Polycystic ovary syndrome. N Engl J Med 1995; 333:853–861.

1395. Ehrman DA, Barnes RB, Rosenfield RL. Polycystic ovary syndrome as a form of functional ovarian hyperandrogenism due to dysregulation of androgen secretion. Endocr Rev 1995; 16:322–353.

1396. Morales AJ, Laughlin GA, Bützow T, et al. Insulin somatotropic and luteinizing hormone axes in lean and obese women with polycystic ovary syndrome: common and distinct features. J Clin Endocrinol Metab 1996; 81:2854–2864.

1397. Dunaif A, Segal KR, Shelley DR, et al. Evidence for distinctive and intrinsic defects in insulin action in polycystic ovary syndrome. Diabetes 1992; 41:1257–1266.

1398. Dunaif A, Xia J, Book CB, et al. Excessive insulin receptor serine phosphorylation in cultured fibroblasts and in skeletal muscle: a potential mechanism for insulin resistance in the polycystic ovary syndrome. J Clin Invest 1995; 96:801–810.

1399. Ibañez L, Potau N, Zampolli M, et al. Source localization of androgen excess in adolescent girls. J Clin Endocrinol Metab 1994; 79:1778–1784.

1400. Oppenheimer E, Linder B, DiMartino-Nardi J. Decreased insulin sensitivity in prepubertal girls with premature adrenarche and acanthosis nigricans. J Clin Endocrinol Metab 1995; 80:614–618.

1401. Ibañez L, Potau N, Zampolli M, et al. Hyperinsulinemia in postpubertal girls with a history of premature pubarche and functional ovarian hyperandrogenism. J Clin Endocrinol Metab 1996; 81:1237–1243.

1402. Wilson R, Mercado A, Cheng K, New MI. Steroid 21-hydroxylase deficiency: genotype may not predict phenotype. J Clin Endocrinol Metab 1995; 80:2322–2329.

1403. Morris AH, Reiter EO, Geffner ME, et al. Absence of nonclassical congenital adrenal hyperplasia in patients with precocious adrenarche. J Clin Endocrinol Metab 1989; 69:709–715.

1404. Speiser PW, Dupont B, Rubenstein P, et al. High frequency of nonclassical steroid 21-hydroxylase deficiency. Am J Hum Genet 1985; 35:650–667.

1405. Temeck JW, Pang S, Nelson C, et al. Genetic defects of steroidogenesis in premature pubarche. J Clin Endocrinol Metab 1987; 64:609–617.

1406. Balducci R, Boscherini B, Mangiantini A, et al. Isolated precocious pubarche: an approach. J Clin Endocrinol Metab 1994; 79:582–589.

1407. Zerah M, Rheaume E, Mani P, et al. No evidence of mutations in the genes for type I and type II 3β-hydroxysteroid dehydrogenase (3β-HSD) in nonclassical 3β-HSD deficiency. J Clin Endocrinol Metab 1994; 79:1811–1817.

1408. Chang YT, Zhang L, Alkaddour HS, et al. Absence of molecular defect in the type II 3 beta-hydroxysteroid dehydrogenase (3 beta-HSD) gene in premature pubarche children and hirsute female patients with moderately decreased adrenal 3-beta-HSD activity. Pediatr Res 1995; 37:820–824.

1409. Morel Y, Mébarki F, Rhéaume E, et al. Structure-function relationships of 3 beta-hydroxysteroid dehydrogenase: contribution made by the molecular genetics of 3 beta-hydroxysteroid dehydrogenase deficiency. Steroids 1997; 62:176–184.

1410. Mendonça BB, Russell AJ, Vasconcelos-Leite M, et al. Mutation in 3-beta-hydroxysteroid dehydrogenase type II associated with pseudohermaphroditism in males and premature pubarche or cryptic expression in females. J Mol Endocrinol 1994; 12:119–122.

1411. Lucky AW, Biro FM, Huster GA, et al. Acne vulgaris in premenarchal girls: an early sign of puberty associated with rising levels of dehydroepiandrosterone. Arch Dermatol 1994; 130:308–314.

1412. Yamamoto A, Ito M. Sebaceous gland activity and urinary androgen levels in children. J Dermatol Sci 1992; 4:98–104.

1413. Stewart ME, Downing DT, Cook JS, et al. Sebaceous gland activity and serum dehydroepiandrosterone sulfate levels in boys and girls. Arch Dermatol 1992; 128:1345–1348.

1414. Biro FM, Lucky AW, Huster GA, et al. Hormonal studies and physical maturation in adolescent gynecomastia. J Pediatr 1990; 116:450–455.

1415. Nydick M, Bustos J, Dale JH, et al. Gynecomastia in adolescent boys. JAMA 1961; 178:449–454.

1416. Large DM, Anderson DC. Twenty-four-hour profiles of circulating androgens and oestrogens in male puberty with and without gynaecomastia. Clin Endocrinol (Oxf) 1979; 11:505–521.

1417. Carlson SE. Gynecomastia. N Engl J Med 1980; 404:795–799.

1418. LaFranchi SH, Parlow AF, Lippe BM, et al. Pubertal gynecomastia and transient elevation of serum estradiol level. Am J Dis Child 1975; 129:927–931.

1419. Siiteri PK, MacDonald PC. The role of extraglandular estrogen in human endocrinology. In: Greep RO, Astwood EB, eds. Handbook of Physiology. Sect 7: Endocrinology. Vol II. Part 1. Female Reproductive System. Washington, DC: American Physiological Society, 1973: 615–629.

1420. Moore DC, Schlaepfer LV, Punier L, et al. Hormonal changes during puberty. V. Transient pubertal gynecomastia: abnormal androgen-estrogen ratios. J Clin Endocrinol Metab 1984; 58:492–499.

1421. Villalpando S, Mondragon L, Barron C, et al. Role of testosterone and

1422. dihydrotestosterone in spontaneous gynecomastia of adolescents. Arch Androl 1992; 28:171–176.

1422. Sasano H, Kimura M, Shizawa S, et al. Aromatase and steroid receptors in gynecomastia and male breast carcinoma: an immunohistochemical study. J Clin Endocrinol Metab 1996; 81:3063–3067.

1423. Mahoney J, Hynes B. Concurrent Poland's syndrome and gynecomastia: a case report. Can J Surg 1990; 33:58–60.

1424. Glass AR. Gynecomastia. Endocrinol Metab Clin North Am 1994; 23:825–837.

1425. Chudley AE, Hagerman RJ. Fragile X syndrome. J Pediatr 1987; 110:821–830.

1426. Lachiewicz AM, Dawson DV. Do young boys with fragile X syndrome have macroorchidism? Pediatrics 1994; 93:992–995.

1427. Meschede D, Behre HM, Nieschlag E. Endocrine and spermatological characteristics of 135 patients with bilateral megalotestis. Andrologia 1995; 27:207–212.

1428. Van Wieringen JD, Wafelbakker F, Verbrugge HP. Growth Diagrams 1965 Netherlands: Second National Survey on 0–24 year olds. Netherlands Institute for Preventative Medicine TNO. Groningen: Wolters-Noordhoof Publishing, 1971.

1429. Dupertuis CW, Atkinson WB, Elftman H. Sex differences in pubic hair distribution. Hum Biol 1945; 17:137–142.

1430. Styne DM, Grumbach MM. Puberty in the male and female: its physiology and disorders. In: Yen JCC, Jaffe RB, eds. Reproductive Endocrinology. Philadelphia: WB Saunders, 1986: 313–384.

1431. Spratt DI, Crowley WF. Hypogonadotropic hypogonadism: GnRH therapy. In: Kreiger DT, Bardin CW, eds. Current Therapy in Endocrinology and Metabolism, 1985–1986. Toronto: BC Decker, 1985: 155–159.

1432. Grumbach MM, Barr ML. Cytologic tests of chromosome sex in relation to sexual anomalies in man. Recent Prog Horm Res 1958; 14:255–324.

1433. Waaler PE, Thorsen T, Stoa KF, et al. Studies in normal male puberty. Acta Paediatr Scand Suppl 1994; 1–36.

1434. Oostdijk W, Hummelink R, Odink RJ, et al. Treatment of children with central precocious puberty by a slow-release gonadotropin-releasing hormone agonist. Eur J Pediatr 1990; 149:308–313.

1435. Oerter K, Manasco P, Barnes KM, et al. Adult height in precocious puberty after long-term treatment with deslorelin. J Clin Endocrinol Metab 1991; 73:1235–1240.

1436. Kauli R, Kornreigh L, Laron Z. Pubertal development, growth and final height in girls with sexual precocity after therapy with the GnRH analogue D-Trp-6-LHRH. Horm Res 1990; 33:11–17.

1437. Boepple PA, Crowley WF Jr. Gonadotropin-releasing hormone analogues as therapeutic probes in human growth and development: evidence from children with central precocious puberty. Acta Paediatr Scand 1991; 372:33–38.

1438. Luder AS, Holland FJ, Costigan DC, et al. Intranasal and subcutaneous treatment of central precocious puberty in both sexes with a long-acting analog of luteinizing hormone–releasing hormone. J Clin Endocrinol Metab 1984; 58:966–972.

1439. Rappaport R, Fontoura M, Brauner R. Treatment of central precocious puberty with an LHRH agonist (buserelin): effect on growth and bone maturation after three years of treatment. Horm Res 1987; 28:149–154.

1440. Suwa S, Hibi I, Kato K. LH-RH agonistic analog (buserelin) treatment of precocious puberty: collaborative study in Japan. Acta Paediatr Jpn Overseas Ed 1988; 30:176–184.

1441. Donaldson MD, Stanhope R, Lee TJ, et al. Gonadotrophin reponses to GnRH in precocious puberty treated with GnRH analogue. Clin Endocrinol 1984; 21:499–503.

1442. Rime JL, Zumsteg U, Blumberg A, et al. Long-term treatment of central precocious puberty with an intranasal LHRH analogue: control of pituitary function by urinary gonadotropins. Eur J Pediatr 1988; 147:263–269.

1443. Stanhope R, Pringle PJ, Brook CG. Growth, growth hormone and sex steroid secretion in girls with central precocious puberty treated with a gonadotrophin-releasing hormone (GnRH) analogue. Acta Paediatr Scand 1988; 77:525–530.

1444. Kauli R, Pertzelan A, Ben Zeev Z, et al. Treatment of precocious puberty with LHRH analogue in combination with cyproterone acetate—further experience. Clin Endocrinol 1984; 20:377–387.

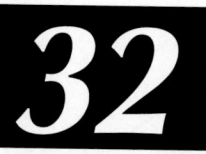

MULTIPLE ENDOCRINE NEOPLASIA

Robert F. Gagel

INTRODUCTION

The multiple endocrine neoplasia (MEN) syndromes[1] are classified into two broad categories: MEN type 1 (MEN 1) and MEN type 2 (MEN 2). The MEN 2 syndrome is further subcategorized into MEN 2A and MEN 2B (formerly MEN 3). Understanding of the MEN syndromes has evolved through several phases. The first was the descriptive phase, in which the fully developed clinical syndromes and their genetic patterns were described.[2–8] The second phase involved the development of screening techniques to identify the syndromes before they became significant clinical problems.[9–16] Early identification of the manifestations and improvements in management techniques have reduced the morbidity and mortality associated with these syndromes. The third phase involves the elucidation of the genetic and molecular bases of these syndromes.[17–19] This chapter summarizes the current understanding of these disorders and provides a framework for understanding future developments.

MEN 1 and MEN 2 share certain characteristics. The first is the cell type involved in the neoplastic process. The usual tumor is composed of one or more specific polypeptide- and biogenic amine–producing cell types and has been given the acronym APUD (from *a*mine *p*recursor *u*ptake and *d*ecarboxylation).[20] The APUD cell type is thought to derive embryologically from neural crest and to have certain neuron-like properties. The major tumors in these two syndromes that are not composed of this cell type are the lipomas associated with MEN 1,[6] and the ganglioneuromas associated with MEN 2B.[21–23] Although not all aspects of the APUD cell theory are widely accepted, this classification of cell types forms the basis of a useful unifying hypothesis for understanding the syndromes.

The second feature shared by these syndromes is the histologic progression from hyperplasia to adenoma, and, in some cases, to carcinoma. The third feature is that development of hyperplasia is probably a multicentric process, with each focus of tumor derived from a single clone. This feature has been proved for only one aspect of these syndromes (medullary thyroid carcinoma[24]) but is probably true for other tumors as well.[25] Last, each of these syndromes has an autosomal dominant pattern of inheritance.

The MEN syndromes have different mechanisms of tumorigenesis. MEN 1 is caused by an inherited mutation of a tumor suppressor gene, menin, on the long arm of chromosome 11; somatic loss of the normal allele results in clonal transformation. Tumor suppressor genes control some important aspects of growth, differentiation, or cell death, and loss of both copies (alleles) results in unregulated growth. In contrast, MEN 2 is caused by activation of the *RET* proto-oncogene. The two most common *RET* mutations activate the tyrosine kinase receptor, thereby causing unregulated growth of the cells associated with MEN 2.

MULTIPLE ENDOCRINE NEOPLASIA TYPE 1

The association of parathyroid, pancreatic islet, and pituitary hyperplasia or neoplasia is called MEN 1. Although there were earlier descriptions,[1] the syndrome was recognized as a clinical and genetic syndrome by Wermer in 1954[3, 4] and was subsequently recognized as an entity distinct from MEN 2.[7] Patients were initially diagnosed with advanced manifestations of parathyroid, pancreatic islet, and pituitary neoplasia in the third and fourth decades of life. However, family screening now makes possible earlier recognition. Now the most common mode of presentation for MEN 1 is identification during the evaluation of an identified kindred; less frequently, a newly ascertained individual with advanced disease may be the propositus of a new kindred, a previously unidentified member of a known kindred, or an example of a de novo mutation. Despite its earlier recognition, MEN 1 is the most challenging of the MEN syndromes. Each affected patient can be expected to undergo at least two or more surgical procedures; it is necessary to recognize the high probability of recurrent or new neoplasms in potentially affected organ systems and to balance this likelihood against the possible side effects of intervention, such as hypoparathyroidism, hypopituitarism, and endocrine and exocrine pancreatic insufficiency.

Hyperparathyroidism

Hyperparathyroidism is the most common manifestation of MEN 1. Prospective screening of family members has shown that hypercalcemia (ionized or albumin-adjusted serum calcium) and abnormalities of parathyroid hormone secretion may appear as early as age 17,[12, 14, 26–30] and by age 40 most individuals carrying the gene for MEN 1 are hypercalcemic.[12, 31] Hyperplasia of multiple parathyroid glands is the most common early histologic lesion observed,[28, 29, 31–36] but if the disease is diagnosed late, adenomatous changes may be superimposed on parathyroid hyperplasia.[26, 30, 31, 37]

Several features of parathyroid hyperplasia associated with MEN 1 differentiate it from hyperparathyroidism caused by a parathyroid adenoma. First, the feedback relationship between the serum calcium level and parathyroid hormone secretion is different. In parathyroid adenomas a supraphysiological extracellular calcium concentration of 1.2 to 1.4 mmol/L (4.8 to 5.6 mg/dL) is required to inhibit 50% of parathyroid hormone secretion, whereas a calcium level of 1 mmol/L (4 mg/dL) suppresses hyperplastic parathyroid tissue from MEN 1 patients. Both of these set-point values are higher than those for normal parathyroid tissue exposed chronically to a high extracellular calcium concentration.[38] A defect in the feedback relationship between the extracellular calcium concentration and parathyroid hormone synthesis and secretion may be one cause of the hyperplasia of parathyroid tissue, although additional factors are likely to be involved.[38, 39] The identification and cloning of a calcium-sensing receptor provides a potential

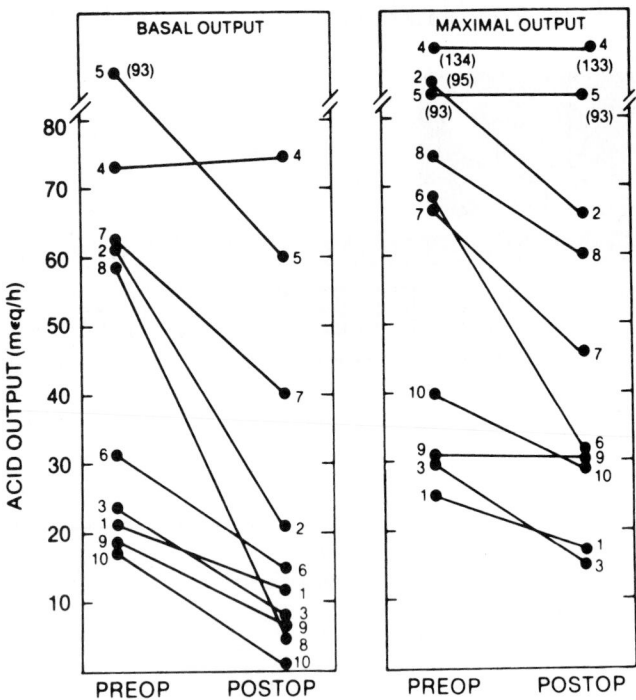

Figure 32–1. The basal gastric acid output (*left*) and maximal output (*right*) are shown before and after parathyroidectomy for 10 MEN 1 patients with primary hyperparathyroidism and Zollinger-Ellison syndrome. Basal gastric acid hypersecretion was defined as a level higher than 15 mmol/h in patients without previous gastric surgery (patients 1, 2, and 4 to 10) or higher than 5 mmol/h in patients with previous gastric surgery (patient 3). Except for patient 4, all patients were normocalcemic after surgery. (From Norton JA, Cornelius MJ, Doppman JL, et al. Effect of parathyroidectomy in patients with hyperparathyroidism, Zollinger-Ellison syndrome, and multiple endocrine neoplasia type I: a prospective study. Surgery 1987; 102:958–966, with permission.)

explanation of the altered set point for extracellular calcium, although a specific defect of this pathway has not been identified in either hereditary or sporadic forms of hyperparathyroidism.[40]

A second difference between parathyroid adenomas and the hyperplasia associated with MEN 1 is the response to therapy. More than 85% of patients with parathyroid adenomas have a long-term cure after surgical removal of a single adenoma.[41] Parathyroid surgery in MEN 1 results in an initial cure rate of approximately 75%, but hypercalcemia recurs in approximately half within 10 y,[35, 41–44] suggesting that parathyroid cell growth in MEN 1 is a continuous and ongoing process. Third, a serum factor in patients with MEN 1 (possibly a fibroblast growth factor) may stimulate endothelial cell growth in parathyroid glands.[45–48] Fourth, a parathyroid adenoma derives from a single cell type, whereas the parathyroid hyperplasia of MEN 1 results from expansion of multiple cell clones.[25]

The manifestations of hyperparathyroidism in MEN 1 include urolithiasis, parathyroid hormone–induced bone abnormalities, musculoskeletal complaints, and, with severe hypercalcemia, generalized weakness and alterations of mental status. These features are not different from those associated with other forms of hyperparathyroidism (see Chapter 24).

The differential diagnosis of familial hypercalcemia includes familial parathyroid hyperplasia,[49, 50] familial adenomatous hyperparathyroidism,[51] and familial hypocalciuric hypercalcemia (FHH).[52, 53] Diagnosis of these disorders is challenging and requires information from individual patients and also from family members. The major feature separating the hyperparathyroidism of MEN 1 from other familial parathyroid diseases is the absence of pituitary and pancreatic manifestations in hyperparathyroidism not associated with MEN 1. Non–MEN 1 forms of familial hyperparathyroidism can be categorized into hyperplasia,[32, 49, 50, 54–56] or adenomatous disease on the basis of the histology of the parathyroid gland. Familial parathyroid hyperplasia is uncommon, and some families given this diagnosis later develop manifestations of MEN 1. Familial hypocalciuric hypercalcemia is an autosomal dominant disorder characterized by hypercalcemia and low urinary calcium excretion.[52, 53] Parathyroid hyperplasia and elevated serum parathyroid hormone (PTH) levels may be present, but the hypercalcemia is not corrected by parathyroid gland resection. The diagnosis can usually be made by documenting hypercalcemia, a low urinary calcium/creatinine ratio, and similar biochemical abnormalities in other family members. A characteristic feature of FHH is hypercalcemia from the time of birth,[52, 53] whereas MEN 1–associated hypercalcemia generally does not develop until the second decade of life.[12, 14] Inactivating mutations of the calcium receptor are present in most FHH cases,[57] suggesting that a primary defect in the calcium receptor pathway is not likely to be involved in the genesis of hyperparathyroidism in MEN 1. Other rare forms of hypercalcemia include hyperparathyroidism associated with MEN 2A,[8, 58, 59] hypercalcemia caused by neuroendocrine tumors that secrete parathyroid hormone–related protein (PTHrP),[60] and the humoral hypercalcemia syndrome associated with pancreatic islet cell tumors causing watery diarrhea.[61]

Surgery is the treatment of choice for hyperparathyroidism associated with MEN 1, although the timing and the type of operative procedure remain controversial. Parathyroid surgery is definitely indicated in an MEN 1 patient with an albumin-adjusted serum calcium level higher than 3.0 mmol/L (12.0 mg/dL) or with clinical evidence of PTH-induced bone disease or kidney stones and a documented diagnosis

of primary hyperparathyroidism. As a result of prospective screening, however, affected family members may be identified with minimal elevations of serum calcium level. The optimal management of such patients is not clear. Parathyroid surgery is indicated for MEN 1 patients with Zollinger-Ellison syndrome and mild hyperparathyroidism because return of serum calcium levels to normal may be associated with a lowering of serum gastrin level and of gastric acid secretion (Figs. 32–1 and 32–2).[15] Early surgery has been advocated in other minimally hypercalcemic MEN 1 patients, both because of the suggestion of a causal relationship between hypercalcemia and elevation of serum gastrin[62, 63] and pancreatic polypeptide[64–67] levels and because of the reasoning that hypercalcemia stimulates development of the pituitary and pancreatic manifestations of the syndrome.[68] Arguments against early surgery include the high recurrence and/or persistence rate of hyperparathyroidism and the 10 to 25% incidence of hypoparathyroidism after parathyroidectomy in patients with MEN 1.[35, 43] Postponement of surgery coupled with periodic assessment of the patient, including bone density, serum creatinine level, and urine calcium measurements may be reasonable in patients with minimal elevations of serum calcium.

The primary lesson in patients with MEN 1 is that cure is difficult and may require several operative procedures over an extended period. The standard surgical approach has been to remove three to three and one-half parathyroid glands and to leave behind a mass of parathyroid tissue approximating that of normal subjects.[43] Because reoperation in these patients is likely, the taking of careful operative notes and marking of remaining parathyroid tissue with metal clips enhance the likelihood of success in a subsequent operation. Complete removal of parathyroid tissue from the neck and transplantation of small packets of tissue to the nondominant forearm have also been used for hyperparathyroidism with MEN 1.

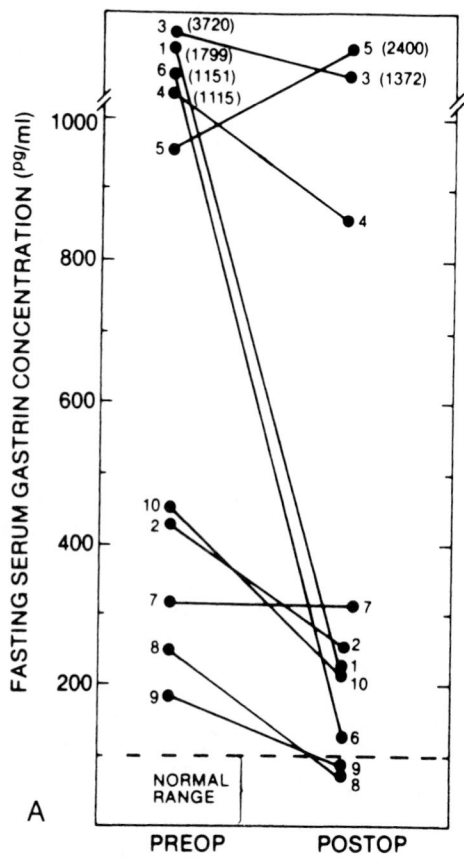

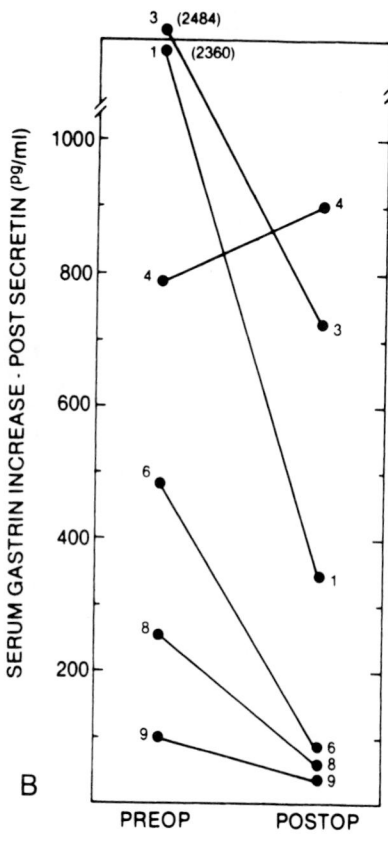

Figure 32–2. *A*, The fasting serum gastrin concentration before and after parathyroidectomy for 10 patients with primary hyperparathyroidism, Zollinger-Ellison syndrome, and MEN 1. The normal gastrin concentration is less than 48 pmol/L (100 pg/mL). Numbers in parentheses represent actual gastrin concentrations when higher than 475 pmol/L (1000 pg/mL). *B*, Serum gastrin increase after intravenous injection of secretin, 2 U/kg body weight, before and after parathyroidectomy for six of the same patients described in *A*. The response is considered to be positive if the serum gastrin increase is higher than 95 pmol/L (200 pg/mL). (From Norton JA, Cornelius MJ, Doppman JL, et al. Effect of parathyroidectomy in patients with hyperparathyroidism, Zollinger-Ellison syndrome, and multiple endocrine neoplasia type I: a prospective study. Surgery 1987; 102:958–966, with permission.)

This technique does not prevent recurrent hyperparathyroidism (Fig. 32–3) but facilitates its management. In one report, approximately two thirds of MEN 1 patients developed recurrent hypercalcemia 7 to 75 mo after total parathyroidectomy and grafting of parathyroid tissue to the nondominant arm.[69] Recurrent hyperparathyroidism, however, is treated by removal of islands of hyperplastic parathyroid tissue from the arm.[41, 69, 70] This approach appears to have a low incidence of permanent hypoparathyroidism. Graft function can be documented by comparing parathyroid hormone levels in venous blood from a site proximal to the graft site and a site distal to the graft (see Fig. 32–3).[69] This same technique can be utilized to determine whether PTH is produced by the graft rather than by residual parathyroid tissue in the neck. If the graft is the primary source of PTH, occlusion of venous return from the graft arm by a blood pressure cuff will cause more than a 50% reduction of the intact PTH level within minutes of occlusion. This simple technique documents dominance of graft tissue but does not exclude the presence of functioning parathyroid tissue in the neck or mediastinum.

Pancreatic Islet Cell Tumors

Neoplasia of the pancreatic islet cells is the second most common manifestation of MEN 1 and eventually occurs in 80% of patients.[71, 72] The multicentric islet cell tumors produce hormonal manifestations and can undergo malignant transformation and metastasis. Although the clinical syndrome may be caused by a single hormone product, most of these tumors demonstrate hyperplasia of multiple cell types and produce several peptides and biogenic amines[73] (see Chapter 34).

The fact that surgical cure is difficult[74, 75] and the availability of improved drugs for controlling the pituitary and pancreatic manifestations[76, 77] make it appropriate to attempt pharmacologic control of the hormonal syndromes.

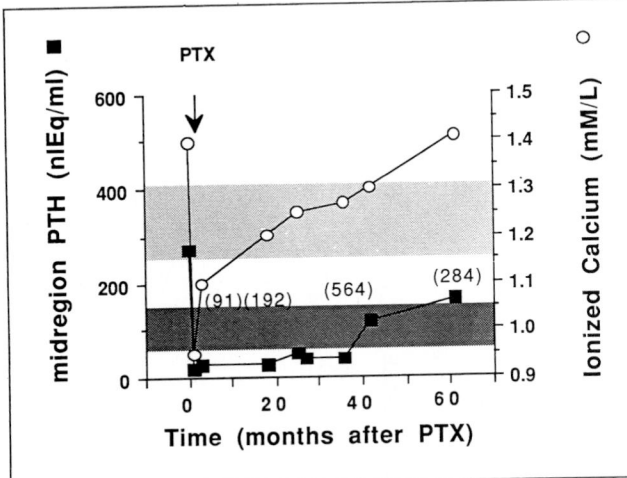

Figure 32–3. Serum ionized calcium and peripheral midregion parathyroid hormone (PTH) levels after total parathyroidectomy and graft of parathyroid tissue in a patient with MEN 1. After total parathyroidectomy (PTX) and grafting of parathyroid tissue to the nondominant forearm, the ionized calcium and parathyroid hormone levels fell to subnormal levels. Subsequent measurements demonstrated a continuous rise of the ionized calcium and peripheral parathyroid hormone levels (taken from the arm containing the transplant) over a 60-mo period, which necessitated removal of some of the grafted parathyroid tissue. The numbers in parentheses show selected parathyroid hormone values for blood taken from the brachial vein immediately proximal to the grafted parathyroid tissue. These results demonstrate continued secretion of parathyroid hormone by the graft in the presence of hypercalcemia. The upper, lighter shaded area shows the normal range for ionized calcium; the lower, darker shaded area shows the normal range for serum midregion parathyroid hormone. (Data from L. E. Mallette, Baylor College of Medicine.)

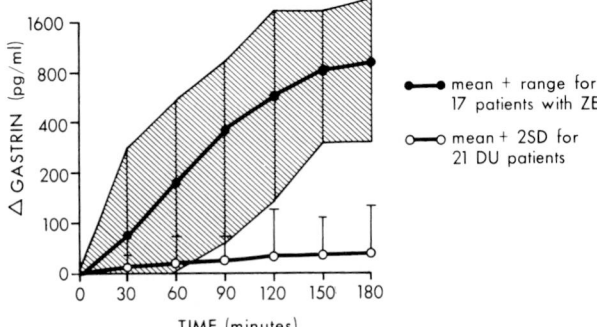

Figure 32–4. Gastrin response to intravenous infusion of calcium gluconate (4 mg elemental calcium/kg body weight/h for 3 h) in patients with Zollinger-Ellison (ZE) syndrome and in patients with duodenal ulcer (DU) unassociated with gastrinoma. To convert gastrin values to picomoles per liter, multiply by 0.48. (From Deveney CW, Deveney KS, Way LW. The Zollinger-Ellison syndrome: 23 years later. Ann Surg 1978; 188:384–393, with permission.)

Gastrinoma

Zollinger-Ellison syndrome (gastric acid hypersecretion caused by excessive production of gastrin) is the major cause of morbidity and mortality in MEN 1. Gastrin production is increased in more than 60% of MEN 1 patients with pancreatic tumors and accounts for approximately a third of cases of Zollinger-Ellison syndrome.[6, 31] Features of Zollinger-Ellison syndrome associated with MEN 1 include gastric acid hypersecretion, solitary or multiple peptic ulcers, diarrhea, esophagitis, and an elevated serum gastrin level (usually >171 pmol/L [300 pg/mL]).[77, 78] Confirmation of abnormal gastrin secretion can be obtained by a calcium infusion (calcium gluconate at a concentration of 4 mg elemental calcium/kg body weight/h for 3 h) (Fig. 32–4)[79] or a secretin test (intravenous injection of secretin, 2 U/kg body weight) (see Fig. 32–2).[15, 79] The serum gastrin concentration in a patient with a gastrinoma should increase by more than 114 pmol/L (200 pg/mL), whereas the rise is minimal (usually <24 pmol/L [50 pg/mL]) in patients with other hypergastrinemic states, such as retained gastric antrum, massive small bowel resection, gastric outlet obstruction, hypercalcemia, or duodenal ulcer disease.[80]

Several features of Zollinger-Ellison syndrome in MEN 1 complicate surgical management of these tumors. The most important is that the tumors are multicentric, raising the possibility that surgical cure of a single gastrinoma will be followed by recurrence. This feature led Zollinger and Ellison to recommend total gastrectomy for control of the ulcer syndrome.[81] Subsequent efforts to excise gastrinomas surgically were associated with high rates of primary failure, recurrence, and hepatic metastases.[75, 77, 82] Nevertheless some patients were cured by surgery.[83]

The availability of H₂ receptor antagonists (cimetidine and ranitidine) and proton pump inhibitors (omeprazole) makes it possible to perform a pharmacologic gastrectomy. The doses of H₂ antagonists required for a therapeutic effect are usually higher than those for duodenal ulcer disease. Ranitidine is preferred over cimetidine because of fewer side effects.[77] The H⁺,K⁺-ATPase inhibitor (omeprazole) has even greater efficacy than H₂ receptor antagonists.[84] Gastric carcinoids, which develop in rats given large doses of omeprazole, do not develop in patients with Zollinger-Ellison syndrome who are treated with omeprazole.[85] Only a small percentage of patients treated with H₂ receptor antagonists or omeprazole ultimately require total gastrectomy.[85, 86] The somatostatin analogue octreotide inhibits the secretion of both gastrin and gastric acid[87] and in some patients lowers the requirements for H_2 receptor antagonists.[88] These medical regimens appear to have impaired tumor growth in a few patients,[89] but there is little convincing evidence of a long-term benefit on the tumors themselves.

While the efficacy of medical therapy is high, the necessity for lifetime therapy and the fact that most Zollinger-Ellison syndrome symptoms in MEN 1 are caused by carcinoid-like tumors in the duodenal wall rather than pancreatic islet tumors[90–92] has led to a re-examination of treatment choices. Identification and surgical removal of duodenal wall tumors and identification of early pancreatic islet cell tumors with intraoperative ultrasound results in acceptable cure rates[92] and may be associated with a lower incidence of hepatic metastasis.[93, 94]

Total pancreatectomy to remove all gastrin-producing tissue has been advocated to prevent the recurrence and metastases of gastrinomas in patients with MEN 1. The procedure may prevent death from metastatic carcinoma in families where there is a high incidence of malignant islet cell tumors[95] but should be avoided for the average patient because the long-term deleterious effects of total pancreatectomy (pancreatic exocrine deficiency and diabetes mellitus) exceed any perceived benefit.

Insulinoma

Insulinoma is the second most common pancreatic islet cell tumor and accounts for about 35% of functional pancreatic neoplasms in MEN 1. The clinical features do not differ from those associated with sporadic insulinoma, and the diagnosis is generally made by demonstrating fasting hypoglycemia with inappropriately elevated serum insulin, C peptide concentrations, or proinsulin concentrations (see Chapter 20). The insulinomas in MEN 1 are frequently multicentric (as many as 16 adenomas per pancreas) and may be malignant (25%).[31, 74, 96] Even when a single adenoma is found, it is likely that hyperplasia or microadenomatosis of insulin-producing cells is present elsewhere in the pancreas.

The treatment is surgical removal of insulin-producing tissue; there is no long-term medical therapy. There may be multiple islet cell tumors in MEN 1, only some of which produce insulin. Preoperative assessment of insulinoma with fine-cut computed tomography (CT) is useful in guiding surgery but provides no insight into the functional capabilities of the tumor. Selective injection of calcium into each of the three major arteries that supply the pancreas with sampling of hepatic vein insulin levels at 30, 60, 90, and 120 s provides functional evidence for localization of the tumor to a particular anatomic region of the pancreas.[97] This is especially important in MEN 1 where multiple small tumors, undetected by CT or magnetic resonance imaging (MRI), may be found by intraoperative ultrasound.[74, 98] Preoperative localization of the insulinoma to a particular anatomic region improves the probability that a tumor identified and removed at the time of surgery is the insulinoma. At surgery it may be difficult to be certain that all insulin-producing tissue has been removed, and a variety of techniques have been used to localize such tissue, including intraoperative ultrasonography and monitoring of plasma glucose and insulin levels.[99] Occasionally enucleation of a single adenoma in patients has resulted in cure;[74] subtotal pancreatectomy (80% or more of the pancreas) is recommended for individuals with multiple tumors when there is inadequate diagnostic information to localize the insulin-producing tumor. Surgical resection of metastatic insulinoma causing hypoglycemia is indicated, but reoperation is less likely to be successful.[100] Hypoglycemia caused by unresectable metastatic insulinoma can be controlled with diazoxide,[100] although side effects may limit its long-term use. Alternative therapy includes continuous infusion of glucagon

or glucose. Chemotherapy (streptozocin or dacarbazine) may reduce tumor size, but cure has not been reported.[101, 102]

Glucagonoma

The glucagonoma syndrome consists of hyperglycemia, a characteristic rash termed necrolytic migratory erythema, anorexia, glossitis, anemia, diarrhea, and venous thrombosis (see Chapter 34). It is not common in patients with MEN[103] despite the fact that plasma glucagon concentrations are elevated in more than half of MEN 1 patients[12, 104] and that large numbers of glucagon-positive cells are detectable in more than 30% of islet cell tumors.[12, 73, 104–107] The most common manifestation of the glucagonoma syndrome in patients with MEN 1 is hyperglycemia; few patients exhibit the characteristic skin lesions.[108, 109] Glucagonomas are usually managed by surgical removal or hepatic artery embolization for tumor that has metastasized to liver.[110, 111] Some patients respond to the somatostatin analogue octreotide, although an initial response does not predict a long-term response.[76, 112]

Watery Diarrhea Syndrome

The syndrome of watery diarrhea, hypokalemia, hypochlorhydria, and acidosis in MEN 1 (see Chapter 34) occurs in association with both pancreatic islet cell[61, 113] and carcinoid[114] tumors. Surgical removal of single or multiple tumors is the appropriate therapy. Streptozocin has reduced tumor size and reduced the production of vasoactive intestinal peptide in some patients;[115] octreotide may control diarrheal symptoms in patients with unresectable or metastatic tumors.[76] Hepatic artery embolization has caused long-term palliation of diarrhea in patients in whom hepatic metastasis forms the bulk of tumor mass.[101, 111, 116]

Pancreatic Polypeptide

Serum concentrations of pancreatic polypeptide are frequently elevated in MEN 1 patients, and an enhanced rise of serum pancreatic polypeptide after a standard test meal may predict a pancreatic tumor in subjects with MEN 1[71, 117, 118] (see Chapter 34). Whether the elevated pancreatic polypeptide level is always related to a pancreatic tumor is not clear, because elevations of pancreatic polypeptide levels are common in primary hyperparathyroidism, which is a component of MEN 1.[66] The elevated levels of pancreatic polypeptide in MEN 1 do not appear to cause manifestations but are a useful marker of pancreatic tumors at an early stage. When annual prospective screening with meal-stimulated pancreatic polypeptide measurement is applied, pancreatic neoplasia may be detected in three quarters of family members tested.[119] Whether it is necessary or desirable to detect pancreatic neoplasia at the earliest possible stage is unclear.[120] The high rate of new tumor formation in this syndrome suggests that early enucleation of small tumors would be beneficial only if such surgical removal could be shown to prevent local or hepatic metastasis. There is some evidence that early surgery for gastrinoma prevents hepatic metastases.[94]

Pituitary Adenomas

The pituitary tumors that occur in more than half of the patients with MEN 1[6, 31] are multicentric and may cause galactorrhea, amenorrhea, acromegaly, or Cushing's syndrome. At least two mechanisms appear to be involved in the formation of pituitary tumors. The first involves a local neoplastic transformation with clonal expansion of specific pituitary cell types. Genetic factors are thought to be the primary determinant of tumor development by this mechanism. For example, mutations of the α subunit of G protein are present in most growth hormone–producing tumors.[121] The second mechanism is stimulation of specific pituitary cell growth by ectopic production of hypothalamic releasing hormones.

Prolactinoma

Prolactinomas, the most common pituitary tumor and the third most common manifestation of MEN 1,[12, 122] are characteristically multicentric and may be large.[123, 124] The recurrence rate after attempted surgical removal of these tumors is high. Dopamine agonists (bromocriptine or pergolide) have been used with success as primary therapy for most prolactinomas for more than 2 decades[125–127] (see Chapter 9). The major problems with bromocriptine therapy are poor long-term compliance and the side effects of nausea and hypotension, especially at higher doses. In patients who escape the growth inhibitory effects of bromocriptine or are noncompliant because of side effects, transsphenoidal surgery combined with radiation therapy (external-beam or gamma knife) is usually effective.[128]

Tumors that Produce Growth Hormone and/or Growth Hormone–Releasing Hormone

Tumors that produce growth hormone account for 25% of pituitary adenomas in patients with MEN 1.[6, 31] The clinical features of acromegaly do not differ from those in sporadic acromegaly (see Chapter 9). There are at least three potential causes for increased growth hormone production in MEN 1. The first is the development of a multicentric pituitary tumor, presumably the result of the underlying lesion causing MEN 1. The second mechanism is the production of growth hormone–releasing hormone (GHRH) by pancreatic[6, 31, 105, 107, 129–131] or other endocrine[107, 131–134] tumors. The second mechanism is an example of how the production of a substance by one tissue (most commonly the pancreatic islets) can stimulate the growth of another tissue (the pituitary gland). Although GHRH-producing tumors are rare causes of either sporadic[135] or MEN 1–associated acromegaly, the serum GHRH level should be measured for evaluation of acromegaly in the MEN 1 patient. Finally a mutation of the α subunit of G protein was identified in a growth hormone–producing tumor in a single MEN 1 patient.

The primary therapy for acromegaly in MEN 1 patients is transsphenoidal removal of the pituitary tumor or, when appropriate, removal of a GHRH-producing tumor. Although early surgery is indicated to prevent progression, the fact that many of these tumors are multicentric may lead to incomplete removal and recurrence of the disease (see Chapter 9). Radiotherapy may be effective for persistent or recurrent disease but may cause hypopituitarism and brain dysfunction.[136] The demonstration that octreotide can return growth hormone and somatomedin levels to normal in many patients with postoperative residual tumor and causes tumor shrinkage in approximately one third suggests that it may have a role in patients with residual tumor.[137, 138] Although effective, the necessity for thrice-daily injections and the high annual cost of octreotide remain problems. A long-acting form of the drug for monthly injection has been developed but is not currently available in the United States. Octreotide was used to treat acromegaly in a single case of ectopic GHRH-induced acromegaly.[139] Other long-acting somatostatin analogues and growth hormone analogues that inhibit the interaction of growth hormone with its receptor and lower insulin-like growth factor 1 (IGF1) levels are undergoing trial.

Cushing's Syndrome and Corticotropin-Releasing Hormone

Cushing's syndrome in patients with MEN 1 can be caused by a pituitary tumor producing corticotropin (ACTH, adrenocorticotropin),[31] by ectopic production of corticotropin by a carcinoid tumor,[140] or by ectopic production of corticotropin-releasing hormone.[141] Each of these disorders is rare. Treatment is directed toward surgical removal of the pituitary tumor or the source of the ectopic corticotropin or corticotropin-releasing hormone. In patients in whom pituitary surgery is not curative, radiation therapy to the pituitary, pharmacologic inhibitors of steroid synthesis, or bilateral adrenalectomy may be indicated (see Chapters 9 and 12).

Carcinoid Tumors

Carcinoid tumors are uncommon in MEN patients[31, 142] but are more likely to be found in MEN 1 (91%) than in MEN 2, are more likely to develop in the foregut (two thirds are in the thymus, lungs, stomach, or duodenum), and are most likely to involve the thymus (men) or lung (women). About half of the carcinoids are locally invasive or metastatic, especially the thymic carcinoids.[143] The usual features of carcinoid syndrome (flushing, diarrhea, and bronchospasm) are not common,[140] although serotonin, calcitonin,[144] and corticotropin[140] may be produced. These tumors are generally removed surgically. The somatostatin analogue octreotide is an effective treatment for the rare MEN 1 patient with flushing and diarrhea[76] (see Chapter 37).

Miscellaneous Features of Multiple Endocrine Neoplasia Type 1

Subcutaneous and visceral lipomas occur in some patients, although it is not known whether they have a genetic or a hormonal basis. There has also been a report of cutaneous leiomyomas with the MEN 1 syndrome.[145]

Genetics of Multiple Endocrine Neoplasia Type 1

A systematic analysis of tumors derived from MEN 1 patients led to the identification of a region of chromosome 11 in which chromosomal DNA from the normal parent is lost in islet cell tumors.[17] This finding suggested that a mutant tumor suppressor gene might exist on the allele derived from the affected parent and provided the first evidence for localization of the gene and insight into the nature of the genetic defect. Linkage analysis using polymorphic DNA sequences from chromosome 11q confirmed the genetic localization.[17] Subsequent reports from multiple investigators have demonstrated loss of heterozygosity in parathyroid[146, 147] and pancreatic[148, 149] tumors and confirmed the genetic locus.[150–153] The region containing the *MEN1* gene has been narrowed, and several candidate genes have been excluded.[152, 154–157] The causative gene is a tumor suppressor gene, named menin, whose function is unknown. The initial report describes a wide variety of inactivating mutations in patients with MEN 1.[158]

Screening for Multiple Endocrine Neoplasia Type 1

A rational screening program for MEN 1 should routinely identify gene carriers and be cost effective (Table 32–1). Experience with screening MEN 1 families has shown that compliance with a *simple and regular screening protocol* is high; complicated, expensive, and erratic screening efforts are associated

TABLE 32–1. Cost-Effective Screening for Multiple Endocrine Neoplasia

Syndrome	Test	Testing During Establishment of Gene Carrier Status		Testing After Establishment of Gene Carrier Status	
		Frequency	Age (y) at Testing	Frequency	Age (y) at Testing
MEN 1	Ionized serum calcium[1]	Every 3–5 y	15–50	Every 3–5 y	20–50
	Serum prolactin[2]	Every 3–5 y	>15	Every 3–5 y	>15
	Serum gastrin[3]			Every 3–5 y	>25
	Imaging of pituitary[4]			Every 5–10 y	20–60
	Genetic testing[5]				
MEN 2A	RET proto-oncogene analysis[6]	Twice	Birth or early childhood	None	
	Serum calcitonin after pentagastrin[7]	Yearly, ages 1–35		1–2 y and then every 5 y[7]	Lifetime
	12- or 24-h urine for epinephrine and norepinephrine[8]	Yearly	5–50	Yearly	5–60
	Ionized serum calcium[1]	Biyearly	20–40	Biyearly	Lifetime
MEN 2B	RET proto-oncogene analysis[6]				
	Serum calcitonin after pentagastrin[7, 9]	Yearly	Birth to 20	1–2 y and then every 5 years[7]	Lifetime
	12- or 24-h urine for epinephrine and norepinephrine[8]	Yearly	5–50	Yearly	5–60

[1]This could be either a serum ionized calcium or an albumin-adjusted serum calcium.
[2]Hypercalcemia is generally the first manifestation of this syndrome and affects almost 100% of gene carriers by age 40. Therefore, screening for all manifestations including pituitary and pancreatic tumors can be discontinued or the frequency reduced if hypercalcemia is not observed by age 40.
[3]Measurement of the serum gastrin level is indicated in all family members with symptoms consistent with Zollinger-Ellison syndrome at any age.
[4]The necessity for pituitary imaging studies is controversial, especially if measurements of prolactin, growth hormone, and cortisol are normal.
[5]Genetic analysis is currently limited to research laboratories. It is likely that these analyses will be commercially available in the near future.
[6]Mutational analysis of the RET proto-oncogene is available from a variety of sources. A list is available on the web site: http://endocrine.mda/.tmc.edu.
[7]Pentagastrin (0.5 µg/kg) diluted in 1 mL normal saline is injected rapidly, with measurement of a serum calcitonin at baseline and 2, 5, and 10 min following injection. It may be difficult to perform a pentagastrin test in a 1-year-old child, but a 2-point test (calcitonin measurements prior to and 3–5 min after pentagastrin injection) will provide maximum information. Pentagastrin testing to diagnose C-cell abnormalities may not be required if a decision is made to proceed with thyroidectomy before the age of 6 y. In the small number of kindreds in whom no RET proto-oncogene mutation has been identified, continued pentagastrin testing is required to detect early C-cell abnormalities. Medullary thyroid carcinoma will almost always be the first detectable manifestation of MEN 2. After total thyroidectomy for C-cell hyperplasia or medullary thyroid carcinoma, a follow-up pentagastrin test should be performed at 1–2 y intervals for 5 y and then less frequently to detect tumor recurrence.
[8]Collection of a complete 24-h urine is difficult, and a 12-h specimen will provide adequate sensitivity for screening purposes.
[9]Identification of the mucosal neuroma phenotype is frequently difficult at birth. For this reason all children born to a parent with the phenotype should have an RET proto-oncogene analysis performed.

with a greater failure rate. Screening can be divided into two components: identification of the gene carrier state and management of the gene carrier. A major use of genetic screening will be to eliminate 50% of family members from standard screening efforts. Mutational analysis of the MEN1 gene, menin, by use of polymerase chain reaction techniques will provide the most straightforward method of identifying gene carrier status.[158, 159] In the initial report, inactivating mutations of menin were identified in 14 of 15 kindreds.[158] Unfortunately the technology to perform these studies is available only in a handful of research laboratories. To date none has provided genetic screening for routine diagnostic work-up. The identification of the causative gene will lead to the commercial availability of genetic testing that will make it possible to identify gene carrier status with 100% certainty. Family members who are gene carriers will still require ongoing surveillance to determine which of the three tumor types will develop (see Table 32–1).

The best available nongenetic test for identification of gene carriers is an albumin-adjusted or ionized serum calcium measurement,[12, 14] which may be supplemented with a serum PTH assay. Measurement of serum prolactin improves the likelihood of early detection of gene carrier status[12] and allows identification of the occasional patient (or family) in whom prolactinoma is the initial manifestation.[160, 161] Measurement of serum gastrin slightly increases the chance of early identification of gene carriers but is probably not cost effective. The frequency of testing can be as little as every 5 y,[12] although continuity of follow-up may be compromised by the long interval between tests.

Establishment of gene carrier status focuses attention on the family members likely to develop clinical disease (see Table 32–1). Prospective screening should then be directed to components of the syndrome, such as parathyroid disease and pituitary tumors, for which early identification and treatment are likely to alter the clinical course. Periodic screening for

hyperparathyroidism, prolactinoma, acromegaly, and Cushing's syndrome by measurement of serum calcium and prolactin concentrations, and biannual measurement of gastrin, growth hormone or IGF, and serum cortisol after an overnight dexamethasone suppression test (see Chapter 9) seem prudent. Imaging of the pituitary gland should be performed every 5 y or when hormone abnormalities are observed. Identification of pancreatic islet cell neoplasia before development of clinical symptoms of hormone excess seems less important because most, but not all, investigators believe that operative intervention is not indicated for asymptomatic pancreatic neoplasia.[83, 95, 162] A 10-y prospective screening effort identified pancreatic islet tumors in a higher percentage of patients with MEN 1 than was previously suspected.[71] It is unclear at present whether these aggressive screening efforts affect morbidity, metastasis, or death in these patients, but studies are currently underway to answer these questions.[67, 71, 72]

MULTIPLE ENDOCRINE NEOPLASIA TYPE 2

Multiple Endocrine Neoplasia Type 2A

In 1959 Sipple reported the occurrence of bilateral pheochromocytomas, thyroid tumors, and nodular enlargement of the parathyroid gland and reviewed five similar cases from the literature.[5, 163] The familial nature of the syndrome[7, 164] and the fact that the thyroid tumor is medullary thyroid carcinoma were recognized by others.[165] Williams reasoned that because medullary thyroid carcinoma is a malignancy of the C cells, it might produce calcitonin,[166] a concept that led to the use of serum calcitonin measurements for early diagnosis of medullary thyroid carcinoma.[8, 10, 167, 168]

The clinical features of MEN 2A, as described by Sipple[5]

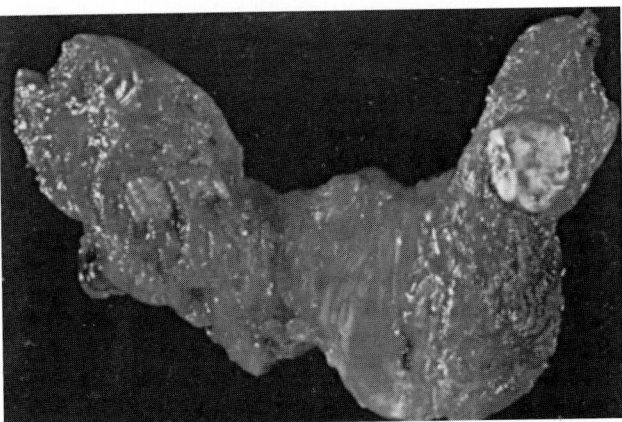

Figure 32–5. Bilateral medullary thyroid carcinoma in MEN 2A. Large bilateral foci of medullary thyroid carcinoma are located in each lobe of the thyroid gland.

and others,[7] consist of bilateral and multicentric medullary thyroid carcinoma, unilateral or bilateral pheochromocytomas, and, less commonly, parathyroid hyperplasia or adenomatosis. Patients with this syndrome can present with manifestations of a pheochromocytoma, a thyroid nodule, hypercalcemia, or some combination of the three, but at present the routine screening of affected families makes early thyroid C-cell hyperplasia the most common initial presentation.[11, 13, 16, 115, 169–177] Pheochromocytomas are subsequently identified in about half of patients, and parathyroid abnormalities occur in 10 to 35%.[7, 8, 58, 178, 179]

Medullary Thyroid Carcinoma

Medullary thyroid carcinoma is a multicentric neoplasm of the parafollicular or C cell of the thyroid gland (Fig. 32–5). The earliest demonstrable abnormality in the thyroid gland is hyperplasia of C cells,[180, 181] followed by progression to nodular hyperplasia, microscopic medullary thyroid carcinoma, and finally frank medullary thyroid carcinoma (Fig. 32–6). These changes are multicentric, frequently with more than one type of histologic lesion in one or both lobes of the thyroid.[182] The time required for progression through these histologic stages is not known, but the process may require decades.[182] It is also not known at which histologic stage metastasis occurs, but lymph node metastasis is common when the tumor diameter is larger than 1 cm[8, 9, 172, 174] and is rare in C-cell hyperplasia.[10, 11, 13, 183–185] Occasionally, foci of medullary thyroid carcinoma occur in extrathyroidal locations such as the thymus gland. Whether these lesions are primary or metastatic cannot be determined with certainty.

Total thyroidectomy is mandatory for hereditary medullary thyroid carcinoma. Abnormalities of the C cell are almost always bilateral and multicentric,[186] and even if C cells are not malignant at the time of surgery, transformation may occur later. If the tumor is large, there is a high likelihood of local nodal metastasis.[7, 8] Surgical removal of all central lymph nodes and selective removal of the lateral lymph nodes of the neck can cure the disease, even in the presence of nodal metastasis.[8, 16, 59, 168, 175] Appropriate studies to exclude hyperparathyroidism and pheochromocytoma are mandatory; pheochromocytomas should be removed before thyroid surgery.

Reoperation for persistent medullary thyroid carcinoma has poor results,[59, 187] but development of microsurgical dissection techniques led to the return to normal of serum calcitonin values in approximately one third of reoperated patients in one study[188] and approximately 20% of patients in other studies.[188–190] A major question about reoperation is whether the tumor is located in the neck or whether distant metastases are present. Techniques that have been used with variable success for localizing the tumor include scanning with thallium[191] and metaiodobenzylguanidine,[192–194] octreotide scanning,[195] and venous catheterization for measurement of calcitonin in blood from specific anatomic locations.[196] A nondetectable basal and pentagastrin-stimulated calcitonin level following surgery is likely to indicate a cure. Evidence supporting this includes the short-term follow-up (5 to 10 y) of reoperated patients[188–190] and a generally favorable long-term outcome in patients with medullary thyroid carcinoma with local nodal metastasis who had nondetectable calcitonin values following primary surgery.[16, 173, 187] Whether a 20% cure rate justifies the extensive operative procedure is unclear, but the poor outcomes of reoperative strategies in earlier reports should be reconsidered in light of this experience.[174, 197]

Younger individuals diagnosed by prospective screening should have a total thyroidectomy.[13, 198, 199] C-cell hyperplasia or microscopic medullary thyroid carcinoma (see Fig. 32–6) without metastatic disease is the most common histologic finding in these patients. A case can be made for a central node dissection even in early disease because of the finding of metastasis in young children,[90] although more extensive lymph node dissection is generally not recommended.[184, 198]

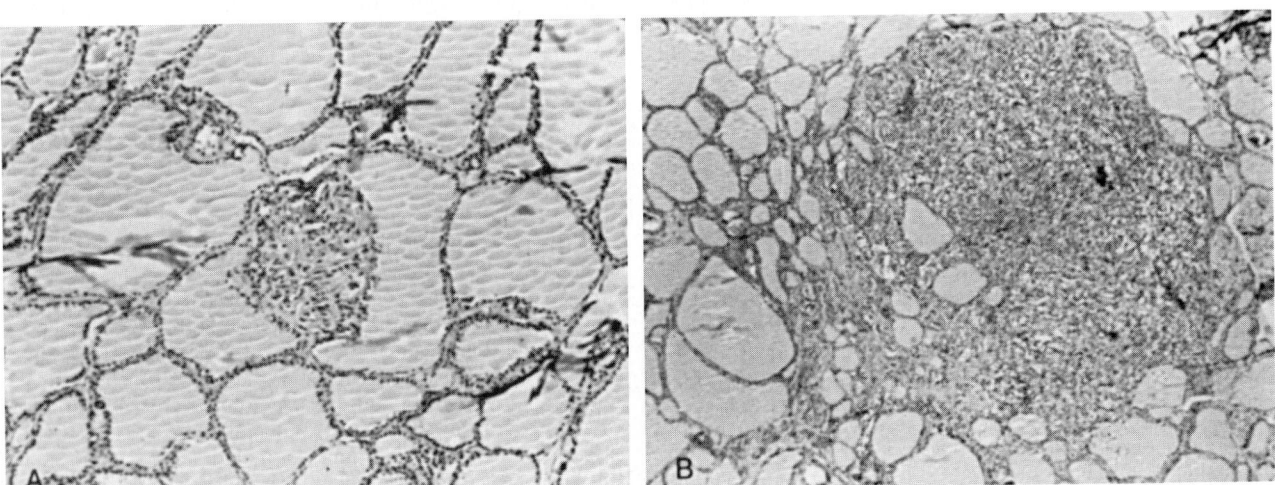

Figure 32–6. Progression of histologic changes from C-cell hyperplasia to medullary thyroid carcinoma. These sections were taken from a single thyroid lobe of a patient with hereditary medullary thyroid carcinoma and demonstrate the multicentric nature of this tumor. *A* shows nodular hyperplasia with containment of C cells within a thyroid follicle. Magnification × 250. *B* shows microscopic medullary thyroid carcinoma that is locally invasive. Magnification × 100.

TUMOR MARKERS ASSOCIATED WITH MEDULLARY THYROID CARCINOMA

Proteins produced by the normal C cell and by medullary thyroid carcinoma include calcitonin, calcitonin gene-related peptide,[200] somatostatin,[201] dihydroxyphenylalanine decarboxylase,[202] and chromogranin-A.[203] Genes that are not normally expressed in the C cell but that are expressed by medullary thyroid carcinoma include those for pro-opiomelanocortin, thyrotropin-releasing hormone,[204] gastrin-releasing peptide,[205] vasoactive intestinal peptide, neurotensin, substance P, carcinoembryonic antigen, histaminase,[206] and others.[207] The only reported clinical syndrome associated with ectopic hormone production is the ectopic corticotropin syndrome in less than 5% of patients with extensive medullary thyroid carcinoma (see Chapters 12 and 36).

Pheochromocytoma

Adrenal chromaffin tissue in patients with MEN 2A undergoes the same type of histologic progression as that observed for the C cell, including hyperplasia, diffuse expansion of the adrenal medulla, and tumor development. The usual finding is single or multiple pheochromocytomas and a background of hyperplastic chromaffin tissue[208–210] (Fig. 32–7). The pheochromocytomas may be unilateral or bilateral, and if a tumor is present in one adrenal gland hyperplasia is likely in the contralateral gland. Invasion of the adrenal capsule by chromaffin cells is observed, but these tumors rarely metastasize.[182, 209, 211]

Before prospective screening was available, patients frequently presented with large pheochromocytomas, hypertension, headaches, and cardiac arrhythmias; sudden death secondary to a stroke or cardiac arrest was not uncommon. Routine screening of kindreds results in earlier identification of affected individuals. Early manifestations include intermittent headaches, palpitations, and nervousness; hypertension is uncommon.[16] Although deaths are uncommon since the advent of prospective screening for medullary thyroid carcinoma and pheochromocytoma and the availability of α- and β-adrenergic antagonists for use in pheochromocytoma, vigilance is required in pregnant women because of the possibility of

death during labor[212, 213] and in individuals noncompliant with routine catecholamine screening.

Pheochromocytoma associated with MEN 2A causes distinctive biochemical features. Increased urinary excretion of epinephrine and an increased ratio of epinephrine to norepinephrine in a 24-h urine sample are the first abnormalities noted[16, 214, 215] (Fig. 32–8). The goal of screening is to identify patients at this stage. Later in the course or with larger pheochromocytomas, the 24-h excretion of epinephrine, norepinephrine, metanephrine, and normetanephrine metabolites is usually increased. Urinary vanillylmandelic acid excretion is usually normal early in the course and is not useful for prospective screening.[169] Plasma catecholamine levels may be intermittently elevated early in the course of the disease and may therefore be more sensitive, but less specific than an integrated 12- or 24-h urine collection;[216] a provocative stimulus such as exercise may cause abnormal epinephrine release.[217] Increased production of epinephrine probably accounts for headaches, palpitations, nervousness, and the absence of hypertension.

The diagnosis of pheochromocytoma is confirmed by CT or MRI of the abdomen. Scanning with [131I] metaiodobenzylguanidine, a catecholamine analogue that is selectively concentrated in adrenal chromaffin tissue, may confirm the presence of functioning intra-adrenal chromaffin tissue (Fig. 32–9) and exclude rare extra-adrenal pheochromocytomas.[218, 219] Whether such scans are useful in the routine management of pheochromocytoma associated with MEN 2 is unclear, because a positive test may be consistent with either adrenal medullary hyperplasia or pheochromocytoma, offering little diagnostic power.[194] Octreotide scanning, while useful for identification of extra-adrenal sporadic pheochromocytomas, is not needed for diagnosis of pheochromocytoma in MEN 2 because of the invariable location of these tumors in the adrenal gland. It is rarely necessary to perform adrenal angiography, and if it is performed the patient should receive α- and β-adrenergic antagonists during the procedure (see Chapter 13).

More than half of individuals with MEN 2A develop unilateral or bilateral pheochromocytomas. In rare families in which there is a documented history of malignant pheochromocytoma (fewer than 15 reported cases[219, 220]), bilateral adrenalectomy is preferable once the gene carrier status is diag-

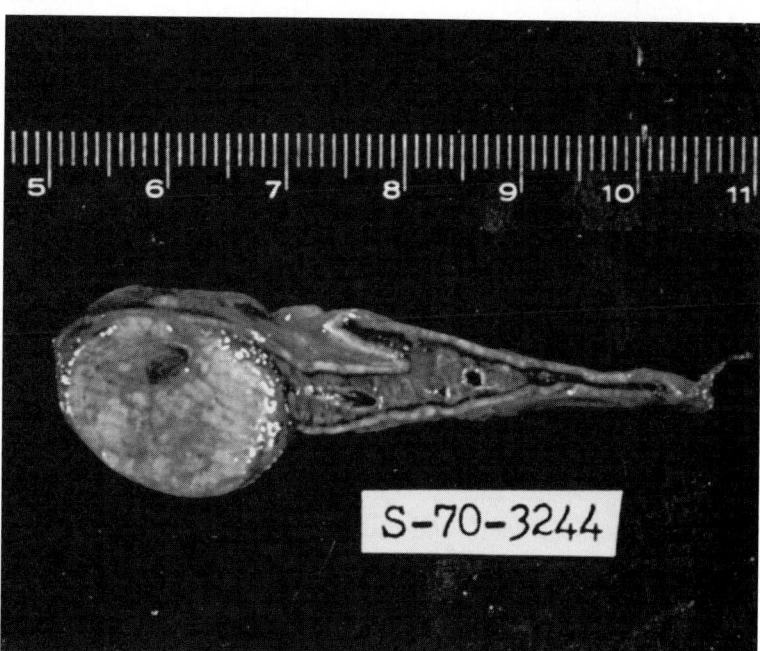

Figure 32–7. A pheochromocytoma set on a background of diffuse adrenomedullary hyperplasia in MEN 2A. In the normal adrenal gland the adrenal cortices are separated by a thin (less than 1 mm) band of adrenal medulla. In this pheochromocytoma there is diffuse expansion of the adrenal medulla.

nosed.[208] Appropriate management of the adrenal lesions in other MEN 2A kindreds is controversial. Most physicians remove only adrenal glands demonstrated to contain a pheochromocytoma.[16, 221, 222] Namely if a unilateral pheochromocytoma is found, the contralateral adrenal gland is removed only if the gland is abnormal by radiographic evaluation.[176] This selective approach may prevent or postpone the development of adrenal insufficiency.[223] However, because of the 50% chance that nonaffected adrenal glands will develop a pheochromocytoma within 10 y, other clinicians advocate a bilateral

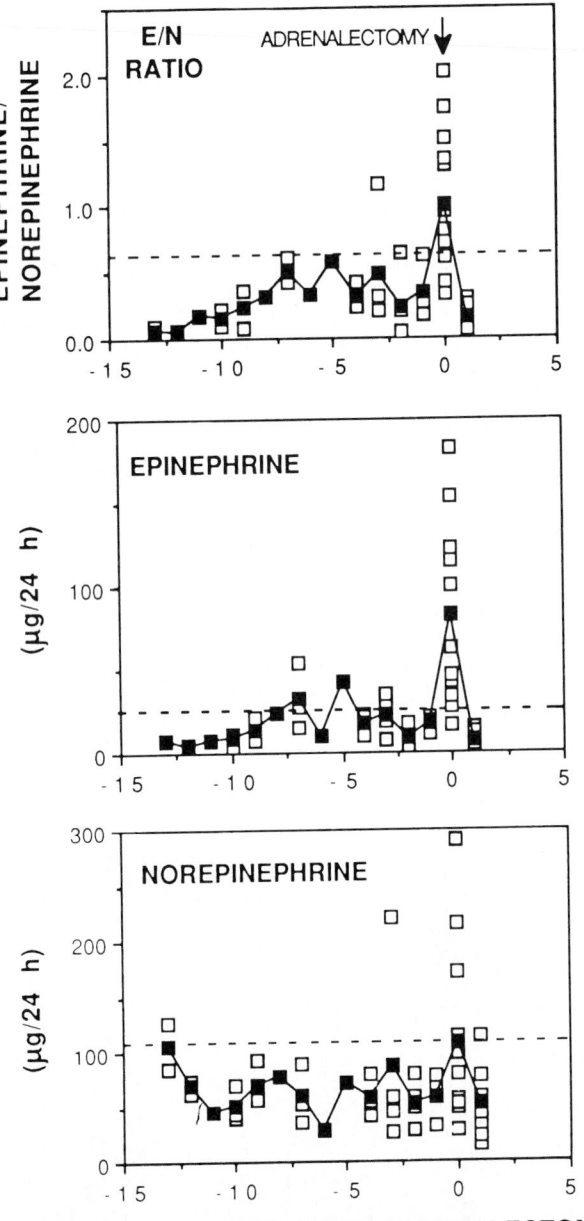

Figure 32–8. Results of 24-h urinary norepinephrine excretion, epinephrine excretion, and ratio of epinephrine to norepinephrine in 11 prospectively screened patients proved to have pheochromocytoma. Each open square indicates a value or the mean of two or more values for a patient, and each solid square represents the mean for all the subjects in a particular year; the latter symbols are connected by a solid line. The dashed line shows the upper limit of normal. To convert epinephrine values to nanomoles, multiply by 5.458; to convert norepinephrine values to nanomoles, multiply by 5.911. (From Gagel RF, Tashjian AH Jr, Cummings T, et al. The clinical outcome of prospective screening for multiple endocrine neoplasia type 2A: an 18-year experience. N Engl J Med 1988; 318:478–484, with permission.)

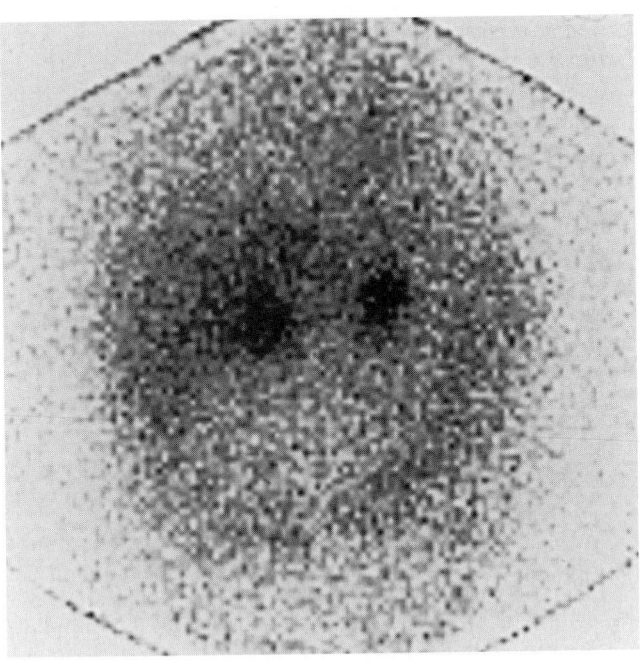

Figure 32–9. A positive radioactive iodine metaiodobenzylguanidine scan of a patient with MEN 2A and bilateral pheochromocytomas. A subtraction technique to remove hepatic and splenic background activity was used to enhance the image.

adrenalectomy at the time of first operation.[219, 224, 225] The major advantage of the latter approach is that the patient is subjected to a single surgical procedure; disadvantages include the necessity for treatment of and the risks associated with adrenal insufficiency.[223] α-Adrenergic and β-adrenergic antagonists should be administered before and during surgery (see Chapter 13). Although the traditional operation for pheochromocytoma utilized an anterior approach to permit examination of the contralateral adrenal gland and liver, radiologic assessment of the adrenal gland currently provides almost as much information as visual examination and palpation. Use of a surgical flank approach or laparoscopic adrenalectomy is associated with lower morbidity and may be appropriate, especially for unilateral pheochromocytomas.[226]

Hyperparathyroidism

Hyperparathyroidism occurs in 10 to 35% of individuals with the MEN 2A syndrome.[7, 8, 58, 59, 223] The initial reports described the presence of either parathyroid hyperplasia or multiple parathyroid adenomas in association with hypercalcemia, urolithiasis, or osteitis fibrosa cystica. Review of the histology of these tumors demonstrated occasional adenomatous formation on a background of parathyroid hyperplasia,[227] a finding analogous to that observed for C-cell hyperplasia in the thyroid gland and for chromaffin cell hyperplasia in the adrenal medulla. Hyperparathyroidism is almost never seen in patients thyroidectomized for early C-cell abnormalities, although histologic findings consistent with parathyroid hyperplasia have been observed.[16] Whether these patients will eventually develop hypercalcemia is unknown. Before development of hypercalcemia the earliest indication of abnormal parathyroid function is incomplete suppression of parathyroid function by a calcium infusion,[178] implying a set-point abnormality similar to that in patients with MEN 1.[38] Surgical management of hyperparathyroidism is similar to that described for MEN 1, although recurrent hyperparathyroidism is less common in most kindreds.

Variants of Multiple Endocrine Neoplasia Type 2A

A number of MEN 2A variants have been described. The most common is familial medullary thyroid carcinoma (FMTC), which occurs in the absence of pheochromocytoma or parathyroid disease. This syndrome accounts for fewer than 20% of all hereditary medullary thyroid carcinoma. These patients are more likely to be classified as sporadic MTC because of the absence of other manifestations and the general predisposition to a more benign behavior, making identification of other affected family members more difficult.

At least 18 families have been identified with the MEN 2A/cutaneous lichen amyloidosis variant.[228, 229] In these families, affected individuals had a pruritic skin lesion over the scapular region of the upper back consisting of multiple infiltrated papules overlying a well-demarcated plaque (Fig. 32–10). The histologic picture is that of cutaneous lichen amyloidosis (deposition of amyloid at the juncture of the epidermis and dermis) in the fully formed skin lesion. Immunohistochemical staining of the amyloid for keratin, but not calcitonin, was observed, suggesting that the amyloid is likely of dermal origin and is not the result of deposition of calcitonin gene products from the thyroid carcinoma.[228] In most patients intense pruritus precedes the development of the skin lesion by 3 to 5 y, suggesting that the primary defect may be a sensory abnormality in the C6-T6 dermatomes leading to chronic irritation and "friction amyloidosis."[230]

A third variant is MEN 2A associated with Hirschsprung's disease,[231] which can be differentiated from the ganglioneuromatosis identified in MEN 2B.

There is a single case report of an ovarian strumal carcinoid tumor, a variant of an ovarian teratoma, in a patient with MEN 2A. The tumor was composed of neuroendocrine cells

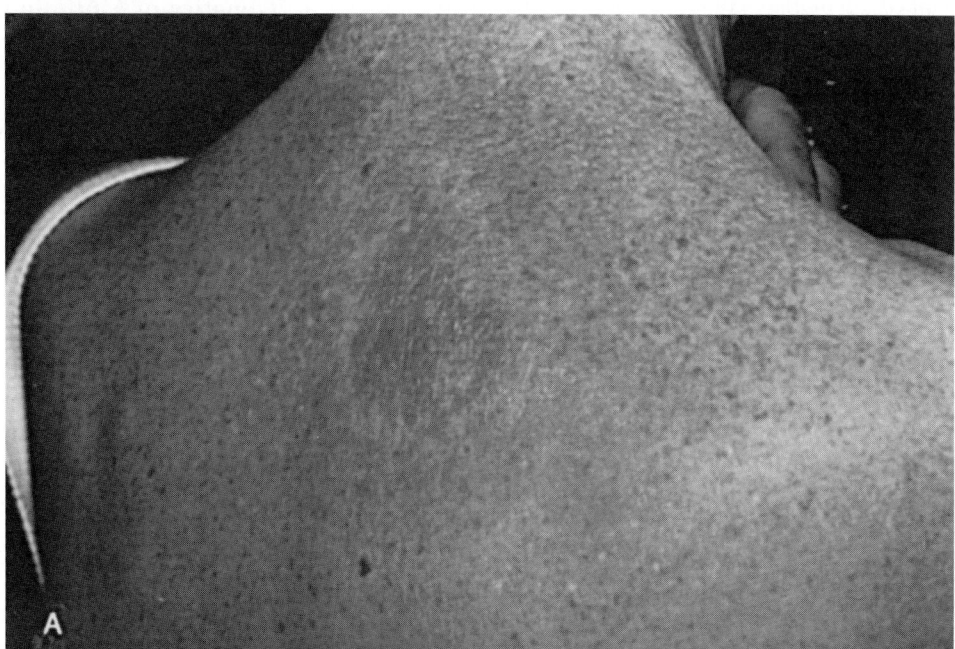

Figure 32–10. *A,* The characteristic clinical picture of cutaneous lichen amyloidosis associated with MEN 2A. The pruritic skin lesion may cover a small area or the entire right or left upper back, as shown in this patient. Patient with MEN 2B demonstrating thick bumpy lips and eversion of upper eyelids *(B)* and neuromas on anterior third of tongue *(C).* (*A* from Gagel RF, Levy ML, Donovan DT, et al. Multiple endocrine neoplasia type 2A associated with cutaneous lichen amyloidosis. Ann Intern Med 1989; 111:802–806. *B* and *C* from Brown RS, Colle E, Tashjian AH Jr. The syndrome of multiple mucosal neuromas and medullary thyroid carcinoma in childhood: importance of recognition of the phenotype for the early detection of malignancy. J Pediatr 1975; 86:77–83, with permission.)

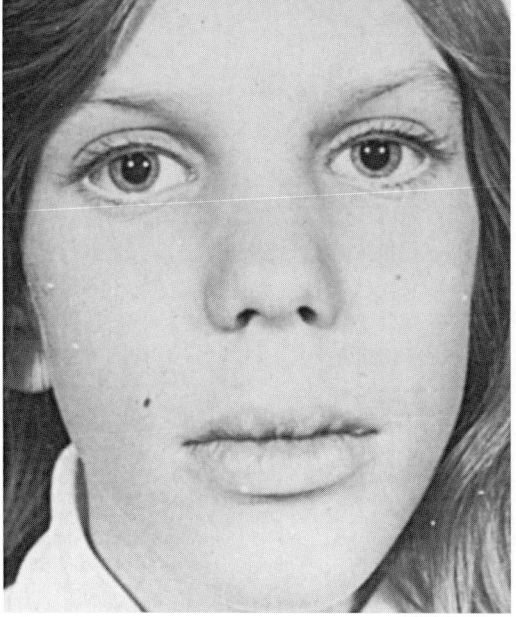

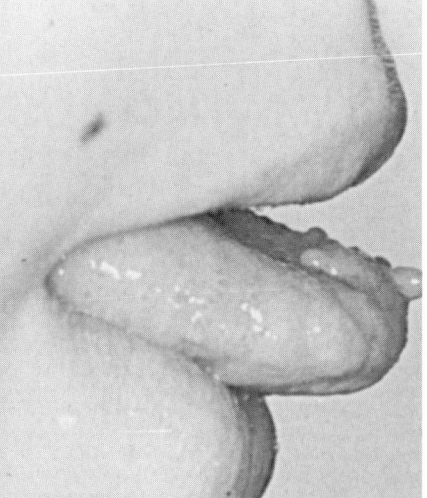

B   C

with thyroid-like follicles that stained positive for thyroglobulin.[232]

Multiple Endocrine Neoplasia Type 2B

The association of medullary thyroid carcinoma and pheochromocytoma with multiple mucosal neuromas is termed MEN 2B.[166, 233] The hallmark of this syndrome is the presence of characteristic mucosal neuromas on the distal portion of the tongue (see Fig. 32-10), the lips, and subconjunctival areas and throughout the gastrointestinal tract.[233–235] Affected corneal nerves may be identified by slit lamp examination, and enlarged nerves are frequently noted during neck or abdominal surgery. Ganglioneuromatosis of the gastrointestinal tract can cause obstruction, dilatation of the colon, or a colic-like childhood syndrome with associated diarrhea[23, 236] and may be the first clinical manifestation of MEN 2B. Other features include a marfanoid habitus; pectus excavatum; slipped femoral epiphysis; and long, thin extremities.[233–235]

The mucosal neuroma phenotype is associated, in all reported cases, with bilateral and multicentric C-cell hyperplasia and/or medullary thyroid carcinoma. The clinical course of medullary thyroid carcinoma in this syndrome is more aggressive than that in MEN 2A. Metastatic disease can occur in children younger than age 1,[13, 237, 238] and the average survival time is shorter in patients with metastatic disease.[239] However, the presence of multigenerational families and a more extensive compilation of outcome suggest that long-term survival is more common than was suggested in earlier reports.[240, 241] MEN 2B is transmitted as an autosomal dominant trait,[242–244] but a large percentage of cases appear to represent new mutations.[245] Unilateral or bilateral pheochromocytomas occur in approximately half of the individuals with this disorder[242–244, 246] and are histologically similar to those in MEN 2A.

The identification of the mucosal neuroma phenotype in a child should alert the physician to the diagnosis of medullary thyroid carcinoma. Although it is important to confirm the diagnosis of C-cell abnormalities with a provocative test for calcitonin release, the overwhelming likelihood of medullary thyroid carcinoma in such an individual makes it necessary to undertake thyroidectomy at the earliest possible age. It is not known whether such treatment is curative because experience is limited. The expressivity of the mucosal neuroma phenotype may be less than 100%. A case report in which a mother and one child had mucosal neuromas and medullary thyroid carcinoma and a second child had medullary thyroid carcinoma but no evidence of the mucosal neuroma syndrome suggests this possibility.[247] Therefore all children born to a parent expressing the phenotype, whether or not clinical evidence of ganglioneuromatosis is present, should have genetic analysis for MEN 2B, as discussed later. Hyperparathyroidism is rare in MEN 2B,[242] whereas pheochromocytomas occur in approximately half of these patients.

Genetics of Multiple Endocrine Neoplasia Type 2

The availability of large and well-defined families with MEN 2 made it possible to apply linkage strategies to map the causative gene to the centromeric region of chromosome 10 in 1987.[248, 249] Familial MTC (FMTC), MEN 2A with Hirschsprung's disease, and MEN 2B were subsequently mapped to the same locus.[250–253] Progressive refinement of the linkage map led to the localization of the causative gene to proximal chromosome 10q in 1993[254–256] and recognition of the *RET* proto-oncogene as a candidate gene for this disorder.[257] Independent reports by Mulligan and colleagues[19] and Donis-Keller and co-workers[18] identified point mutations of the *RET* proto-oncogene in MEN 2A and FMTC (Fig. 32-11; see Table 32-2). Subsequent work confirmed these observations[258] and identified point mutations of the *RET* proto-oncogene in MEN 2B,[245, 259, 260] the MEN 2A/Hirschsprung's disease variant,[261–263] MEN 2A/cutaneous lichen amyloidosis,[264, 265] and Hirschsprung's disease (Table 32-2).[266–268] Somatic (present only in

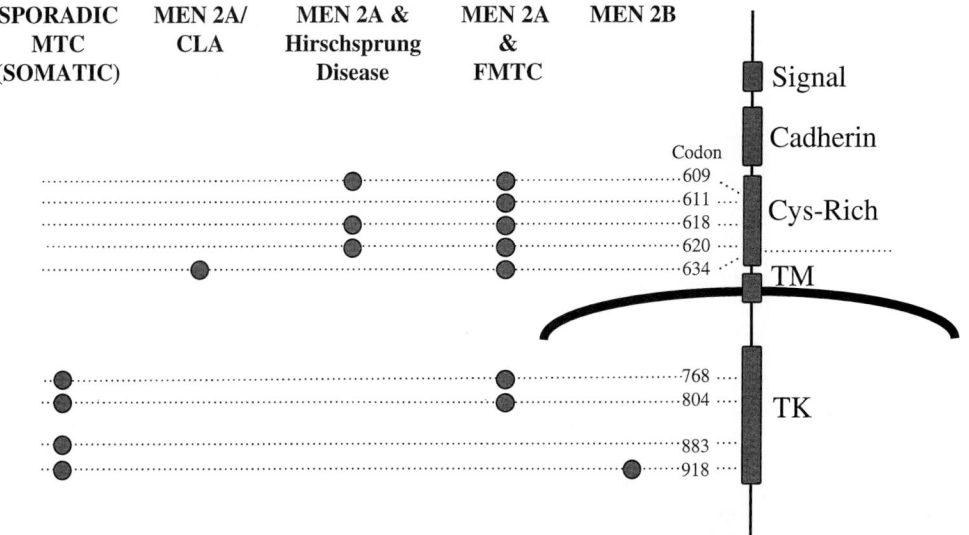

Figure 32-11. Molecular abnormalities of the *RET* proto-oncogene in multiple endocrine neoplasia type 2. Mutations of the *RET* proto-oncogene have been identified in multiple endocrine neoplasia type 2A (MEN 2A), familial medullary thyroid carcinoma (FMTC), MEN 2A associated with Hirschsprung's disease (congenital megacolon), and MEN 2A associated with cutaneous lichen amyloidosis (CLA) and as somatic mutations in sporadic medullary thyroid carcinoma. Two regions of the RET tyrosine kinase are affected. The first is a cysteine-rich extracellular domain (Cys-Rich) important for dimerization of the receptor (codons 609, 611, 618, 620, 634). Mutations of individual cysteines at these codons cause dimerization, activation, autophosphorylation, and transformation. Mutations of the second region, the tyrosine kinase domain (TK) involving codons 768, 804, and 918, cause activation and autophosphorylation. A role for the cadherin-like region (Cadherin) has not been defined, although it may be involved in an interaction with the glial cell line–derived neurotrophic factor receptor. The most common mutation is a codon 634 mutation that converts a cysteine to an arginine and accounts for 50% of all MEN 2 mutations. Somatic mutations of codons 768, 804, and 918 have been identified as somatic mutations in sporadic medullary thyroid carcinoma. Codon 768 and 804 mutations are rare; a codon 918 mutation is identified in 25% of sporadic medullary thyroid carcinomas.

TABLE 32–2. Mutations of the *RET* Proto-oncogene that Cause MEN 2 and Familial/Sporadic MTC

Affected Codon	Exon	Amino Acid Change Normal → Mutant	Nucleotide Change Normal → Mutant	Clinical Syndrome	Percentage of all MEN 2 Mutations
609	10	Cys → Arg	TGC → CGC	MEN 2A/FMTC	0–1
		Cys → Tyr	TGC → TAC[1]		
611	10	Cys → Tyr	TGC → TAC	MEN 2A/FMTC	2–3
		Cys → Trp	TGC → TGG		
618	10	Cys → Ser	TGC → AGC[2]	MEN 2A/FMTC	3–5
		Cys → Gly	TGC → GGC		
		Cys → Arg	TGC → CGC		
		Cys → Phe	TGC → TTC		
		Cys → Ser	TGC → TCC		
		Cys → end	TGC → TGA		
620	10	Cys → Arg	TGC → CGC[3]	MEN 2A/FMTC	6–8
		Cys → Tyr	TGC → TAC[4]		
		Cys → Phe	TGC → TTC		
		Cys → Ser	TGC → TCC		
634	11	Cys → Ser	TGC → AGC	MEN 2A[5]	80–90
		Cys → Gly	TGC → GGC		
		Cys → Arg	TGC → CGC		
		Cys → Tyr	TGC → TAC		
		Cys → Phe	TGC → TTC		
		Cys → Ser	TGC → TCC		
		Cys → Trp	TGC → TGG		
768	13	Glu → Asp	GAG → GAC[6]	FMTC	0–1
804	14	Leu → Val	TTG → GTG[6]	FMTC	0–1
883	15	Ala → Phe	GCT → TTT[6]	Sporadic MTC	—
918	15	Met → Thr	ATG → ACG[6]	MEN 2B	10–20

[1, 3]Mutations of these two codons have been reported in Hirschsprung's disease (congenital megacolon).
[1, 2, 4]Reported cases of MEN 2A/Hirschsprung's disease variants have these mutations.
[5]A codon 634 Cys → Arg (TGC → CGC) mutation accounts for approximately 50% of all mutations associated with MEN 2A.
[6]These *RET* mutations have been identified as somatic mutations in sporadic MTC.
FMTC, Familial medullary thyroid carcinoma.

the tumor) *RET* proto-oncogene point mutations have been identified in approximately 25% of sporadic MTCs (see Fig. 32–11).[263, 269–272] The combined experience with hereditary and sporadic MTC suggests that mutations of the *RET* proto-oncogene may be involved in approximately 50% of medullary thyroid carcinoma.

Ninety-five percent of MEN 2B patients have a single point mutation that changes a methionine to a threonine at codon 918 of the RET tyrosine kinase receptor (see Fig. 32–11, Table 32–2). Most importantly, there is 100% correlation between the presence of an *RET* proto-oncogene mutation and MEN 2 or hereditary MTC. There have been no examples of an individual with MEN 2 or FMTC in a family with an identified *RET* proto-oncogene mutation who does not have the causative mutation.

The *RET* proto-oncogene encodes a tyrosine kinase receptor (see Figs. 32–11 and 32–12 and Table 32–2) that is expressed in a variety of tissues derived from the neural crest, including the central and peripheral nervous systems and neuroendocrine tissues.[273, 274] The RET tyrosine kinase receptor is part of a multireceptor complex that includes the neurotrophic peptide, glial cell line–derived neurotrophic factor (GDNF), and its receptor, GDNFR-α (see Fig. 32–12). GDNF is expressed in the developing central and peripheral nervous and excretory systems. A knockout of the GDNF gene in mice produces a phenotype[275–278] similar to that observed for an *RET* knockout,[279] i.e. defects in the autonomic nervous system, absence of the kidneys, and complete loss of enteric neurons in the gastrointestinal tract. These parallel findings led to the suggestion that GDNF might be the ligand for the RET tyrosine kinase receptor.[280, 281] However, GDNF has a separate receptor, the GDNF-α receptor, a cell surface receptor connected to the cell membrane by a glycosylphosphatidylinositol linkage.[282, 283] GDNF binds to its receptor, GDNFR-α, and interacts with the RET tyrosine kinase receptor, causing dimerization and autophosphorylation of RET (see Fig. 32–12).[282, 283]

The mutations in MEN 2A and FMTC affect a cysteine-rich extracellular domain encoded by exons 10 and 11 of the

RET proto-oncogene. Each of the point mutations converts a conserved cysteine to another amino acid and causes dimerization of the receptor, autophosphorylation of tyrosine residues, and phosphorylation of other cellular proteins.[284–286] The codon 918 mutation in exon 16 causes receptor autophosphorylation but differs from the exon 10 and 11 mutations in that there is no receptor dimerization and a different group of proteins is phosphorylated.[284, 285] The methionine-to-threonine coding change results in enhanced activation of the RET tyrosine kinase, although dimerization of the receptor is not required for activation (see Fig. 32–12).[284, 285] A codon 634 or 918 mutation alone is sufficient to cause transformation of NIH 3T3 cells.[284, 285]

Mutations of the *RET* proto-oncogene have also been identified in Hirschsprung's disease. Most of these alterations inactivate the tyrosine kinase receptor,[266–268, 287, 288] although the association of Hirschsprung's disease alone and the MEN 2A/ Hirschsprung's disease variant with apparent activating mutations (see Table 32–2) make this association less clear. Targeted disruption of the *RET* proto-oncogene in mice with inactivation causes Hirschsprung's disease and failure of normal kidney development.[279, 289] Identification of the GDNF signaling pathway will almost certainly lead to the identification of inactivating mutations causative for Hirschsprung's disease; it is also possible that mutations of GDNF or GDNFR-α will be identified in MEN 2 or hereditary MTC.[283]

Screening for Multiple Endocrine Neoplasia Type 2

Identification of the *RET* proto-oncogene mutations that cause MEN 2 and hereditary MTC simplified screening in families with identifiable mutations (see Table 32–1).[183, 185, 290] Several different analytic techniques have been applied,[291] although direct DNA sequencing is the most widely used. These analytical tests are readily available throughout North America

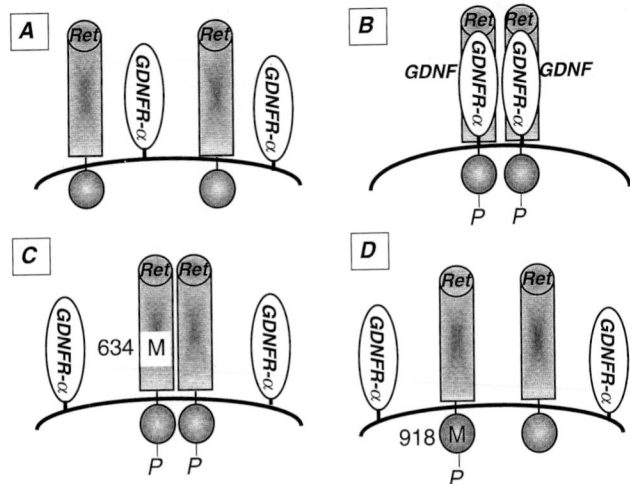

Figure 32–12. The RET tyrosine kinase–glial cell line–derived neurotrophic factor receptor signaling system. The RET receptor is a transmembrane tyrosine kinase receptor that couples with the glial cell line–derived neurotrophic factor receptor (GDNFR-α) to mediate the effect of glial cell line–derived neurotrophic factor (GDNF). A proposed model for interaction is shown in A and B. In the absence of ligand, RET and GDNFR-α exist in an undimerized form (A). Addition of ligand results in interaction of GDNF with GDNF-α and a possible interaction between GDNF and RET (B). This interaction results in dimerization of RET, autophosphorylation and activation of the tyrosine kinase pathway (B). The novel feature of this pathway is the signaling of GDNF, a transforming growth factor-β–like molecule which is a member of a class that normally interacts with a serine-threonine kinase receptor, through a tyrosine kinase receptor pathway. Mutations of the extracellular cysteine-rich domain (M 634) cause dimerization and autophosphorylation of the RET receptor complex (C). Mutations of the intracellular tyrosine kinase (M 918) cause autophosphorylation of the receptor in the absence of dimerization (D). Whether the GDNFR-α is involved in either of these complexes is unclear. Ret, RET tyrosine kinase receptor; GDNFR-α, the glial cell line–derived neurotrophic factor receptor; GDNF, glial cell line–derived neurotrophic factor; M, mutation; 634 and 918 represent mutations of codons 634 or 918 of the RET tyrosine kinase receptor; P, phosphate.

and Europe at modest cost from several commercial sources.* The discovery of *RET* proto-oncogene mutations simplified the management of this syndrome, and DNA-based diagnosis is replacing pentagastrin testing.[183, 185, 290–293] Because only 92 to 95% of families with proven hereditary MTC have identifiable *RET* proto-oncogene mutations, both pentagastrin testing and genetic analysis will be discussed here.

Screening for medullary thyroid carcinoma (see Table 32–1) traditionally involved measurement of the serum calcitonin level before and 2, 5, and 10 min after the intravenous injection of pentagastrin (0.5 μg/kg body weight).[10, 294] The administration of calcium immediately before the pentagastrin injection enhances the sensitivity of the test.[10] A positive test is one in which either the basal serum calcitonin level is elevated and is further increased by the administration of pentagastrin or the basal value is normal but increases into the abnormal range after the administration of pentagastrin. It is important that the samples be analyzed with the most sensitive assay available; it is now possible to measure normal serum calcitonin levels (0.15 to 3 pmol/L [0.5 to 10 pg/mL]),[295–298] thereby making it possible to separate normal subjects from those with early C-cell hyperplasia. The criteria that are useful for separation of normal members from abnormal members of a kindred include a parent known to be affected and a consistently abnormal test result (two or more nonconsecutive test results that are abnormal).[11, 16]

A test result in which there is an elevation of the basal

---

*A listing of available commercial testing sources is available on the University of Texas M.D. Anderson Cancer Center Web Site: http://endocrine.mdacc.tmc.edu.

serum calcitonin level with no further increase after a provocative test can be difficult to interpret; this result is most likely to be caused by a nonspecific or false-positive increase of the serum calcitonin concentration[16, 299] or by production of calcitonin by a tumor other than medullary thyroid carcinoma (lung carcinoma, hepatoma, pheochromocytoma, pancreatic islet cell tumor, or benign liver disease). A false-positive test result can be separated from a true elevation of the serum calcitonin level by a radioimmunoassay using a different polyclonal antiserum or a two-site immunoradiometric assay.[297, 298] Establishment of ectopic production of calcitonin by a tumor other than medullary thyroid carcinoma can be more difficult; however, such tumors frequently produce a high-molecular-weight form of unprocessed procalcitonin,[300] and release of calcitonin by pentagastrin or calcium may be enhanced.[301]

Molecular diagnostic techniques for identifying *MEN2* or FMTC gene carriers are based on the use of polymerase chain reaction techniques to amplify selected portions of the *RET* proto-oncogene known to be mutated in MEN 2. Although there is the potential for several types of errors in mutational analysis (discussed in references 185 and 302), a repeat analysis of each positive or negative test result in a separate testing facility with an independently obtained DNA sample provides nearly 100% certainty that an individual test result is accurate. Three years of experience with this type of testing has provided insight into its usefulness in the following clinical situations:

1. A negative test result in an MEN 2 or FMTC kindred with a known *RET* proto-oncogene mutation. A normal *RET* analysis in this situation excludes the genetic predisposition with 100% certainty. An individual with two independently obtained negative genetic tests in a family with an identified missense mutation can be excluded from further screening. Pentagastrin testing in this situation adds little to the diagnostic accuracy and may actually confuse the clinical assessment because of the high rate of false-positive pentagastrin test results.[185] It may be prudent, however, to consider a repeat DNA analysis in 3 to 5 y using future state-of-the-art testing approaches to exclude a testing error.

2. A member of an MEN 2 kindred with an *RET* proto-oncogene mutation. There is a lack of consensus on the appropriate management approach for the thyroid gland in this situation. The approach favored by most[185, 290, 293] is to perform a total thyroidectomy on gene carriers older than age 5. The most compelling reason for considering this approach is the fact that 90% of gene carriers will develop MTC,[303] making thyroidectomy at some point likely. Second, metastases have been reported in children as young as 6 years,[90] and thyroidectomy by age 5 enhances the probability of cure. Although concern has been expressed about the potential for complications of thyroidectomy in young children, the procedure appears to be well tolerated, and morbidity does not differ from that of adults.[16, 183–185]

An alternative to this approach is to determine gene carrier status by genetic testing and to use pentagastrin testing to determine the age of thyroidectomy.[183] The advantage of this approach is that thyroidectomy is delayed an average of 4 to 6 y, based on the average age of conversion in earlier studies.[303, 304] Long-term data from earlier studies suggest that more than 85% of children are cured (defined as having a nondetectable basal and pentagastrin-stimulated calcitonin value) 15 to 20 y after thyroidectomy.[16] These results suggest that thyroidectomy performed at age 5 based solely on genetic testing is likely to improve the surgical cure rate by no more than 15% (from 85 to 100%). In most cases it is appropriate to present these options to parents and allow them a role in the decision-making process.

3. Families with proven hereditary transmission of MTC

in which no mutation of the *RET* proto-oncogene has been identified. Annual pentagastrin testing is the screening approach of choice in these families. Other mutations of *RET* or mutations of other genes such as *GDNF* or its receptor may be identified in these kindreds in the future.

4. The impact of genetic testing on the management of pheochromocytoma or parathyroid neoplasia. Pheochromocytoma and parathyroid disease are most commonly found with a codon 634 mutation. Kindreds with a mutation of this codon should be routinely screened for both. Pheochromocytoma and parathyroid neoplasia have been identified in 5 to 20% of kindreds with codon 611, 618, and 620 mutations.[258, 305, 306] Pheochromocytoma has not been identified in association with a codon 609 mutation, although the numbers of studied kindreds are small.[258] The major impact of genetic testing is to exclude unaffected family members from further testing.

5. Individuals with apparent sporadic MTC and germline mutations indicative of MEN 2A or FMTC. In studies of more than 200 patients with apparent sporadic MTC, germline mutations of *RET* (codons 609, 611, 618, 620, or 634) were identified in approximately 6% of the total.[263, 269, 293, 307, 308] The majority of these were members of previously unidentified kindreds or children who had been separated from their families early in life and were probably offspring of a gene carrier. There have been four examples of de novo mutations in which the affected individual carries a germline *RET* proto-oncogene mutation but neither parent is affected.[263, 307, 309] In these four cases and in most MEN 2B cases, the newly mutated allele is derived from the unaffected father, suggesting that the mutation occurred during spermatogenesis.[245]

The finding of a higher than anticipated number of apparent sporadic MTC patients who carry germline mutations suggests that all patients with MTC should have analysis of the *RET* proto-oncogene to exclude a hereditary component. This is especially important because identification of one hereditary case may have a multiplier effect, leading to the diagnosis of unsuspected cases in the family and effective early treatment.[263] The family history, although useful, does not exclude hereditary disease.

Mutational analysis of the *RET* proto-oncogene in apparent sporadic MTC also has another benefit. If the test is negative, hereditary disease can be excluded with a greater than 99% certainty.[263] Given the low probability of hereditary disease, pentagastrin testing should not be routinely performed in first-degree relatives of such a patient. In families who want hereditary MTC excluded with 100% certainty, pentagastrin testing of first-degree relatives will be required.

6. Management of a new or an established MEN 2 kindred. Education of the family is an important component in the management of MEN 2. Patients should be encouraged to make even distant family members who are at risk aware of the nature of the disease. The fact that the disease appears to be benign in one generation should not deter screening efforts because it may assume a more virulent expression in a subsequent generation.[310] Education is aided by providing pamphlets describing the syndrome to family members for distribution to more distant relatives.*

Widespread prospective screening has had an impact on the course of the disorder. The age at diagnosis has progressively fallen from a mean of 33 when screening first began in 1969 to below 13 in 1988.[303, 304] Testing for *RET* mutations now makes it possible to identify carrier status at birth or in utero.

Whether prospective screening and early thyroidectomy are curative for the thyroid neoplasm is less clear. Follow-up data from three groups (Table 32–3) indicate that approxi-

*A family guide for hereditary MTC and MEN 2 is available and can be printed from the University of Texas M.D. Anderson Cancer Center Web Site: http://endocrine.mdacc.tmc.edu.

TABLE 32–3. Disease Status in Patients Thyroidectomized for Early Medullary Thyroid Carcinoma in MEN 2A

Group	N	Age	Disease Status at Follow-Up			Time Period of Follow-Up
			−	+	?	
Tufts and Harvard Universities	22	12	19	—	3	10 y
Mayo Clinic	15	7	14	1	—	?
Duke and Washington Universities	25		24	1	—	5.4 y
Totals	62		57	2	3	
(% of total)			92%	3%	5%	

Data extracted from three large series with variable lengths of follow-up: Gagel RF, Tashjian AH Jr, Cummings T, et al. The clinical outcome of prospective screening for multiple endocrine neoplasia type 2A: an 18-year experience. N Engl J Med 1988; 318:478–484; Telander RL, Zimmerman D, van Heerden JA, et al. Results of early thyroidectomy for medullary thyroid carcinoma in children with multiple endocrine neoplasia type 2. J Pediatr Surg 1986; 21:1190–1194; and Wells SA Jr, Baylin SB, Leight GS, et al. The importance of early diagnosis in patients with hereditary medullary thyroid carcinoma. Ann Surg 1982; 195:595–599.

mately 85 to 90% (but not all) of kindred members who were thyroidectomized for early disease based on pentagastrin testing have normal or nondetectable calcitonin values at mean follow-up periods ranging from 1 to 15 y. It can be anticipated that earlier detection and treatment will improve the outcome only in gene carriers. None of the cases of MEN 2A or FMTC diagnosed by genetic screening have had identifiable metastases, although the reports are limited to fewer than 50 patients.[183, 185, 290]

MULTIPLE ENDOCRINE NEOPLASIA OF MIXED TYPE

Hereditary MEN syndromes that do not fit the MEN 1 or MEN 2 categorization fall into four major categories. Overlap syndromes encompass one or more elements of either MEN 1 or MEN 2, usually in a single patient. The majority of these cases probably represent the chance occurrence of an isolated tumor in a patient with one or the other MEN syndrome. A second type of syndrome is the familial occurrence of an unusual combination of endocrine organ neoplasias that does not fit either MEN 1 or MEN 2 categorization. A third type of syndrome is an MEN 1 or MEN 2 variant in which one manifestation predominates. Fourth, a few syndromes do not fit into any clear-cut pattern. Little is known about the molecular abnormalities in these disorders, and it therefore seems reasonable to chronicle the syndromes; an understanding of their pathogenesis awaits further developments.

Overlap Syndromes

Overlap syndromes in single patients include carcinoid and either MEN 1 or MEN 2,[142, 232] pituitary and adrenomedullary tumors with or without hyperparathyroidism,[311, 312] gastrinoma in an MEN 2 patient,[313] adenomatous polyposis coli and MEN 2B,[22] posterior pituitary tumor and MEN 1,[314] prolactinoma in a patient with MEN 2A,[315] and a pheochromocytoma in an MEN 1 patient (author's experience).

Gastric carcinoids may occur in individuals with polyglandular autoimmune syndrome type 2 who have pernicious anemia and elevated gastrin levels. The reversal of carcinoid progression by antrectomy and return of the serum gastrin level to normal suggest that gastrin overproduction is causative.[316] Rare malignant carcinoids occur in this syndrome, although the majority have a benign course.[317, 318] Endoscopic removal of tumors greater than 1 cm, antrectomy, or total gastrectomy has been advocated, although there are no prospective studies to compare the therapeutic options.

Familial Occurrence of Two or More Endocrine Neoplastic Disorders

Von Hippel-Lindau disease (VHL) is an autosomal dominant neoplastic syndrome characterized by the presence of hemangioblastomas of the central nervous system, retinal angiomas, renal cell carcinomas, visceral cysts, pheochromocytoma, and islet cell tumors.[319, 320] More than 90% of gene carriers express one or more manifestations by the age of 60, and more than 70% of gene carriers have one or more central nervous system tumors.[321] Of particular relevance is the observation that 25 to 35% of these patients have unilateral or bilateral pheochromocytomas and that 15 to 20% have islet cell tumors.[319, 322] The *VHL* gene has been mapped to chromosome 3p25.3[323] and identified by positional cloning.[324] The gene is a tumor suppressor gene, implying that loss of function or inactivating mutations of both alleles of this gene cause tumor formation. The VHL protein inhibits transcription elongation through its binding to an elongin B/C complex, and mutation of the *VHL* gene, particularly in the region of codons 150 to 170, interferes with this interaction and results in an accelerated rate of transcription elongation.[325–327] Mutation of codon 238 was identified in more than 40% of VHL families with pheochromocytoma, suggesting that families with a mutation in this codon should be screened routinely for pheochromocytoma.[328] As with other recessive oncogenes such as *p53*, *BRCA1*, or retinoblastoma gene, a large number of inactivating mutations have been described for *VHL*.

Management of VHL patients is often complicated by renal or central nervous system tumors. Pheochromocytomas or islet cell tumors associated with hypertension, cardiac arrhythmias, hypoglycemia, watery diarrhea, carcinoma, or a glucagonoma-like picture should be surgically excised. Judgment is required in the management of other malignant manifestations. For example, a less aggressive approach to the management of pheochromocytoma or islet cell tumor may be indicated in a patient with VHL and a renal cell carcinoma with metastasis.[220, 329]

The association of pheochromocytoma and islet cell tumors can occur in familial[330–332] or nonfamilial[333–336] patterns. There is little information about the molecular genetics of these rare disorders, although abnormalities of the *VHL* gene might be involved.

Neurofibromatosis type 1 (NF 1) is associated with a variety of endocrine neoplasms, including pheochromocytoma,[337] hyperparathyroidism,[338] somatostatin-producing carcinoid tumors of the duodenal wall,[339–341] medullary thyroid carcinoma,[342] and hypothalamic or optic nerve tumors that cause precocious puberty.[343] The causative gene for NF 1 encodes an RAS GAP (GTPase-activating protein) of 2818 amino acids named neurofibromin, which accelerates GTP hydrolysis on p21 RAS. Loss of the GTPase-activating function of neurofibromin (through mutation or allelic loss) leads to p21 *RAS* activation.[344] More specific evidence for a role of this protein in endocrine tumors is shown by allelic loss of this gene in NF 1–associated[345] or sporadic[346] pheochromocytomas. Targeted disruption of the mouse *NF1* gene results in sympathetic ganglia hyperplasia, providing additional evidence for a potential role of this gene in the genesis of endocrine tumors derived from neural crest tissue.[347]

MEN 1 or MEN 2 Syndromes in Which a Particular Manifestation Predominates

MEN 1 kindreds have been recognized in which prolactinoma[160, 161, 348] or insulinoma[349] is the predominant manifesta-

tion. Other families have been described in which other pituitary or pancreatic tumors predominate.[349] Prolactinoma without any evidence of MEN 1 has been reported.[350] Familial acromegaly can occur in the absence of other manifestations of MEN 1, although detailed linkage studies have not been performed.[351–359] It is unclear whether these disorders are MEN 1 variants or the result of another molecular abnormality. Well-defined variants of MEN 2A include FMTC[360] and familial pheochromocytoma.[361] The majority of families with FMTC have mutations of codon 609, 611, 618, 620, 768, 804, or 891 of the *RET* proto-oncogene, although there is considerable overlap with MEN 2A.[18, 258] Familial pheochromocytoma could be linked to mutations of the *RET* proto-oncogene,[362, 363] the *VHL* gene,[364] or another molecular abnormality. Occasional patients with MTC may have a *VHL* mutation.

Syndromes That Are Difficult To Categorize

A syndrome characterized by myxomas, spotty pigmentation, and generalized endocrine overactivity transmitted as an autosomal dominant trait has been given the name Carney's complex.[365, 366] Patients with this disorder have myxomas of the heart, skin, and breast; spotty skin pigmentation; testicular, adrenal, and pituitary tumors; and peripheral nerve schwannomas. The causative gene for this disease has been mapped to chromosome 2p11.[367]

MECHANISMS OF ENDOCRINE TUMOR FORMATION

Identification of disease genes for MEN 1 and 2, NF1, and von Hippel-Lindau syndrome and definition of the role of other oncogenes have provided insight into the molecular events in endocrine neoplasia (Table 32–4). Genetic alterations that cause neoplastic transformation fall into one of two different categories: activating mutations of a proto-oncogene or loss of function mutations in a tumor suppressor gene (see Chapter 6). Examples of activating mutations include point mutations of the *RET* proto-oncogene in MEN 2 or FMTC, rearrangement of the *RET* (*PTC* oncogene) or *TRK* proto-oncogenes in papillary thyroid carcinoma,[368] rearrangement leading to activation of *PRAD1* (cyclin D1) in parathyroid adenomas,[369] and the activating mutations of the α subunit of G protein ($G_{\alpha S}$), found in a high percentage of growth hormone–secreting tumors.[121] In each of these examples a key growth regulatory gene is activated by the mutation. For example, the point mutations of the *RET* proto-oncogene in MEN 2 cause receptor dimerization, autophosphorylation, and phosphorylation of unidentified substrate proteins.[284, 285] The activating mutations in $G_{\alpha S}$ perform a similar function downstream of the peptide hormone receptor.[370] The *PTC* rearrangement of the *RET* proto-oncogene causes constitutive activation of the tyrosine kinase.[371]

Tumor suppressor genes involved in endocrine tumor formation include the *NF1* gene,[372] *p53*,[373, 374] the *VHL* gene,[375] and probably the *MEN1* gene. Inactivating mutations of each of these genes impair normal regulation of growth or cellular function. The regulatory functions lost are varied. For example, inactivation of the GTPase activity associated with the *NF1* gene (neurofibromin) results in continuous GTP activation of p21 RAS, a membrane-associated protein, and its effector system.[344] In the *VHL* gene paradigm, a nuclear protein interacts with and negatively regulates elongin, a regulator of transcript elongation. Inactivating mutations of *VHL* cause unregulated transcription elongation.[376] Exactly how this pro-

TABLE 32–4. Molecular Abnormalities Associated with Multiple Endocrine Neoplasia Syndromes

Endocrine Tumor/Syndrome	Hereditary/Sporadic	Chromosome	Causative Gene	Mechanism
MEN 1	Hereditary	11q	Menin	Tumor suppressor
MEN 2A/B, FMTC	Hereditary	10q	*RET* proto-oncogene	Activating mutation of tyrosine kinase
Medullary thyroid carcinoma	Sporadic	10q	*RET* proto-oncogene mutation of codon 918 in 25%	Activating mutation of tyrosine kinase receptor
Endocrine tumors associated with NF1	Hereditary/sporadic	17	Neurofibromin	Inactivation of GTPase-activating protein
Carney's complex	Hereditary	2p	?	?Tumor suppressor

motes cell growth is unclear, although elongation is involved in the control of *MYC* and *FOS*, important regulators of cell growth.

Tissue-specific expression of oncogenes or tumor suppressor genes is one mechanism for effects of a mutated oncogene. For example, the *RET* proto-oncogene is normally expressed in neural crest derivatives, including the parafollicular cells of the thyroid, the parathyroid cell, the adrenal medulla, and the sympathetic and enteric nervous systems, providing a likely explanation for the tissue-specific expression of MEN 2. A tissue-specific expression pattern is also of probable importance for endocrine-specific tumor suppressor genes. The development of sympathetic ganglion hyperplasia in mice in which the *NF1* gene has been inactivated by homologous recombination suggests a tissue-specific expression pattern.[347]

Tissue-specific rearrangements can also lead to proto-oncogene activation. The *RET* proto-oncogene is not normally expressed in the thyroid follicular cell, and the *PTC* rearrangement associated with papillary thyroid carcinoma is found, with few exceptions, uniquely in the thyroid follicular cell.[377] The *PRAD1* rearrangement of cyclin D1 in parathyroid adenomas is another example.[369, 378]

Transformation is a multistep process. Although the initiating genes have been identified for MEN 1 and 2, NF 1, and VHL, molecular defects at other chromosomal loci are important for transformation. For example, loss of heterozygosity occurs on chromosome 1p,3p,22q, and other loci in MEN 2–related tumors, suggesting that tumor suppressor genes are found at these loci[379–381] and that molecular abnormalities of these genes are involved in the evolution of the transformation process. Two examples are the p53 mutations identified in the transition from papillary to anaplastic thyroid carcinoma[373] and the retinoblastoma gene mutations in a high percentage of parathyroid carcinomas.[382] It also seems likely that there will be more than one pathway by which a cell type can be transformed. An important goal is to identify other genes involved in endocrine neoplasia, to elucidate their normal role in cellular physiology, and to piece together the cumulative defects that lead to transformation.

REFERENCES

1. Erdheim J. Zur normalen und pathologischen Histologie der Glandula Thyreoidea, Parathyreoidea und Hypophysis. Beitr Pathol Anat 1903; 33:158–236.
2. Underdahl LO, Woolner LB, Black BM. Multiple endocrine adenomas: report of 8 cases in which the parathyroids, pituitary and pancreatic islets were involved. J Clin Endocrinol 1953; 13:20–47.
3. Moldawer MP, Nardi GL, Raker JW. Concomitance of multiple adenomas of parathyroids and pancreatic islets with tumor of pituitary: syndrome with familial incidence. Am J Med Sci 1954; 228:190–206.
4. Wermer P. Genetic aspects of adenomatosis of endocrine glands. Am J Med 1954; 16:363–371.
5. Sipple JH. The association of pheochromocytoma with carcinoma of the thyroid gland. Am J Med 1961; 31:163–166.
6. Ballard HS, Frame B, Hartsock RJ. Familial multiple endocrine adenoma–peptic ulcer complex. Medicine 1964; 43:481–516.
7. Steiner AL, Goodman AD, Powers SR. Study of a kindred with pheochromocytoma, medullary carcinoma, hyperparathyroidism and Cushing's disease: multiple endocrine neoplasia, type 2. Medicine 1968; 47:371–409.

8. Melvin KEW, Tashjian AH, Jr, Miller HH. Studies in familial (medullary) thyroid carcinoma. Recent Prog Horm Res 1972; 28:399–470.
9. Chong GC, Beahrs OH, Sizemore GW, et al. Medullary carcinoma of the thyroid gland. Cancer 1975; 35:695–704.
10. Wells SA, Jr, Ontjes DA, Cooper CW, et al. The early diagnosis of medullary carcinoma of the thyroid gland in patients with multiple endocrine neoplasia type II. Ann Surg 1975; 182:362–370.
11. Graze K, Spiler IJ, Tashjian AH Jr, et al. Natural history of familial medullary thyroid carcinoma: effect of a program for early diagnosis. N Engl J Med 1978; 299:980–985.
12. Marx SJ, Vinik AI, Santen RJ, et al. Multiple endocrine neoplasia type I: assessment of laboratory tests to screen for the gene in a large kindred. Medicine (Balt) 1986; 65:226–241.
13. Telander RL, Zimmerman D, van Heerden JA, et al. Results of early thyroidectomy for medullary thyroid carcinoma in children with multiple endocrine neoplasia type 2. J Pediatr Surg 1986; 21:1190–1194.
14. Benson L, Ljunghall S, Akerstrom G, et al. Hyperparathyroidism presenting as the first lesion in multiple endocrine neoplasia type 1. Am J Med 1987; 82:731–737.
15. Norton JA, Cornelius MJ, Doppman JL, et al. Effect of parathyroidectomy in patients with hyperparathyroidism, Zollinger-Ellison syndrome, and multiple endocrine neoplasia type I: a prospective study. Surgery 1987; 102:958–966.
16. Gagel RF, Tashjian AH, Jr, Cummings T, et al. The clinical outcome of prospective screening for multiple endocrine neoplasia type 2a: An 18-year experience. N Engl J Med 1988; 318:478–484.
17. Larsson C, Skogseid B, Oberg K, et al. Multiple endocrine neoplasia type 1 gene maps to chromosome 11 and is lost in insulinoma. Nature 1988; 332:85–87.
18. Donis-Keller H, Shenshen D, Chi D, et al. Mutations in the *RET* proto-oncogene are associated with MEN 2A and FMTC. Hum Mol Genet 1993; 2:851–856.
19. Mulligan LM, Kwok JBJ, Healey CS, et al. Germline mutations of the *RET* proto-oncogene in multiple endocrine neoplasia type 2A (MEN 2A). Nature 1993; 363:458–460.
20. Pearse AGE. Common cytochemical and ultrastructural characteristics of cells producing polypeptide hormones (the APUD series) and their relevance to thyroid and ultimobranchial C Cells and calcitonin. Proc R Soc Lond [Biol] 1968; 170:71–80.
21. Weidner N, Flanders DJ, Mitros FA. Mucosal ganglioneuromatosis associated with multiple colonic polyps. Am J Surg Pathol 1984; 8:779–786.
22. Perkins JT, Blackstone MO, Riddell RH. Adenomatous polyposis coli and multiple endocrine neoplasia type 2b: a pathogenetic relationship. Cancer 1985; 55:375–381.
23. Khan AH, Desjardins JG, Youssef S, et al. Gastrointestinal manifestations of Sipple syndrome in children. J Pediatr Surg 1987; 22:719–723.
24. Baylin SB, Gann DS, Hsu SH. Clonal origin of inherited medullary thyroid carcinoma and pheochromocytoma. Science 1976; 193:321–323.
25. Arnold A, Staunton CE, Kim HG, et al. Monoclonality and abnormal parathyroid hormone genes in parathyroid adenomas. N Engl J Med 1988; 318:658–662.
26. Jackson CE, Boonstra CE. The relationship of hereditary hyperparathyroidism to endocrine adenomatosis. Am J Med 1967; 43:727–734.
27. Johnson GJ, Summerskill WH, Anderson VE, et al. Clinical and genetic investigation of a large kindred with multiple endocrine adenomatosis. N Engl J Med 1967; 277:1379–1385.
28. Craven DE, Goodman D, Carter JH. Familial multiple endocrine adenomatosis: multiple endocrine neoplasia, type I. Arch Intern Med 1972; 129:567–569.
29. Snyder N, III, Scurry MT, Deiss WP. Five families with multiple endocrine adenomatosis. Ann Intern Med 1972; 76:53–58.
30. Jung RT, Grant AM, Davie M, et al. Multiple endocrine adenomatosis (type I) and familial hyperparathyroidism. Postgrad Med 1978; 54:92–94.
31. Eberle F, Grün R. Multiple endocrine neoplasia, type I (MEN I). Ergeb Inn Med Kinderheilkd 1981; 46:76–149.
32. Cutler RE, Reiss E, Ackerman LV. Familial hyperparathyroidism: a kindred involving eleven cases, with a discussion of primary chief-cell hyperplasia. N Engl J Med 1964; 270:859–865.
33. Marx SJ, Powell D, Shimkin PM, et al. Familial hyperparathyroidism. Ann Intern Med 1973; 78:371–377.
34. Marx SJ, Spiegel AM, Brown EM, et al. Family studies in patients with primary parathyroid hyperplasia. Am J Med 1977; 62:698–706.

35. Rizzoli R, Green J, III, Marx SJ. Primary hyperparathyroidism in familial multiple endocrine neoplasia type I: long-term follow-up of serum calcium levels after parathyroidectomy. Am J Med 1985; 78:467–474.

36. Marx SJ. Genetic defects in primary hyperparathyroidism. N Engl J Med 1988; 318:699–701 (editorial).

37. Boey JH, Cooke TJ, Gilbert GM, et al. Occurrence of other endocrine tumours in primary hyperparathyroidism. Lancet 1975; 2:781–784.

38. Brown EM, LeBoff MS, Oetting M, et al. Secretory control in normal and abnormal parathyroid tissue. Recent Prog Horm Res 1987; 43:337–382.

39. Brown E, Gardner D, Brennan M, et al. Calcium-regulated parathyroid hormone release in primary hyperparathyroidism: studies in vitro with dispersed parathyroid cells. Am J Med 1979; 66:923–931.

40. Brown EM, Gamba G, Riccardi D, et al. Cloning and characterization of an extracellular Ca^{2+}-sensing receptor from bovine parathyroid. Nature 1993; 366:575–580.

41. Niederle B, Roka R, Brennan MF. The transplantation of parathyroid tissue in man: development, indications, techniques and results. Endocr Rev 1982; 3:245–279.

42. Lamers CB, Froeling PG. Clinical significance of hyperparathyroidism in familial multiple endocrine adenomatosis type I (MEA I). Am J Med 1979; 66:422–424.

43. Prinz RA, Gamvros OI, Sellu D, et al. Subtotal parathyroidectomy for primary chief cell hyperplasia of the multiple endocrine neoplasia type I syndrome. Ann Surg 1981; 193:26–29.

44. van Heerden JA, Kent RBD, Sizemore GW, et al. Primary hyperparathyroidism in patients with multiple endocrine neoplasia syndromes: surgical experience. Arch Surg 1983; 118:533–536.

45. Brandi ML, Aurbach GD, Fitzpatrick LA, et al. Parathyroid mitogenic activity in plasma from patients with familial multiple endocrine neoplasia type 1. N Engl J Med 1986; 314:1287–1293.

46. Marx SJ, Sakaguchi K, Green J, III, et al. Mitogenic activity on parathyroid cells in plasma from members of a large kindred with multiple endocrine neoplasia type 1. J Clin Endocrinol Metab 1988; 67:149–153.

47. Zimering MB, Brandi ML, de Grange DA, et al. Circulating fibroblast growth factor–like substance in familial multiple endocrine neoplasia type 1. J Clin Endocrinol Metab 1990; 70:149–154.

48. Zimering MB, Katsumata N, Sato Y, et al. Increased basic fibroblast growth factor in plasma from multiple endocrine neoplasia type 1: relation to pituitary tumor. J Clin Endocrinol Metab 1993; 76:1182–1187.

49. Goldsmith RE, Sizemore GW, Chen I-W, et al. Familial hyperparathyroidism: description of a large kindred with physiologic observations and a review of the literature. Ann Intern Med 1976; 84:36–43.

50. Sandler LM, Moncrieff MW. Familial hyperparathyroidism. Arch Dis Child 1980; 55:146–147.

51. Mallette LE, Malini S, Rappaport MP, et al. Familial cystic parathyroid adenomatosis. Ann Intern Med 1987; 107:54–60.

52. Marx SJ, Attie MF, Levine MA, et al. The hypocalciuric or benign variant of familial hypercalcemia: clinical and biochemical features in fifteen kindreds. Medicine 1981; 60:397–412.

53. Law WM, Jr, Heath H, III. Familial benign hypercalcemia (hypocalciuric hypercalcemia): clinical and pathogenetic studies in 21 families. Ann Intern Med 1985; 102:511–519.

54. Schachner SH, Riley TR, Old JW, et al. Familial hyperparathyroidism. Arch Intern Med 1966; 117:417–421.

55. Carey MC, Fitzgerald O. Hyperparathyroidism associated with chronic pancreatitis in a family. Gut 1968; 9:700–703.

56. Marsden P, Anderson J, Doyle D, et al. Familial hyperparathyroidism. Br Med J 1971; 3:87–90.

57. Chou YH, Pollak MR, Brandi ML, et al. Mutations in the human Ca^{2+}-sensing receptor gene that cause familial hypocalciuric hypercalcemia. Am J Hum Genet 1995; 56:1075–1079.

58. Keiser HR, Beaven MA, Doppman J, et al. Sipple's syndrome: medullary thyroid carcinoma, pheochromocytoma, and parathyroid disease. Ann Intern Med 1973; 78:561–579.

59. Cance WG, Wells SA, Jr. Multiple endocrine neoplasia Type IIa. Curr Probl Surg 1985; 22:1–56.

60. Martin TJ, Suva LJ. Parathyroid hormone–related protein in hypercalcaemia of malignancy. Clin Endocrinol (Oxf) 1989; 31:631–647.

61. Yamaguchi K, Abe K, Otsubo K, et al. The WDHA syndrome: clinical and laboratory data on 28 Japanese cases. Peptides 1984; 5:415–421.

62. Wilson SD, Singh RB, Kalkhoff RK. Does hyperparathyroidism cause hypergastrinemia? Surgery 1976; 80:231–237.

63. Zaniewski M, Jordan PH, Jr, Yip B, et al. Serum gastrin level is increased by chronic hypercalcemia of parathyroid or nonparathyroid origin. Arch Intern Med 1986; 146:478–482.

64. Lamers CB, Diemel J, Roeffen W. Serum levels of pancreatic polypeptide in Zollinger-Ellison syndrome, and hyperparathyroidism from families with multiple endocrine adenomatosis type I. Digestion 1978; 18:297–302.

65. Friesen SR, Kimmel JR, Tomita T. Pancreatic polypeptide as a screening marker for pancreatic polypeptide APUDomas in multiple endocrinopathies. Am J Surg 1980; 139:61–72.

66. Strodel WE, Vinik AI, Eckhauser FE, et al. Hyperparathyroidism and gastroenteropancreatic hormone levels. Surgery 1985; 98:1101–1106.

67. Skogseid B, Oberg K, Benson L, et al. A standardized meal stimulation test of the endocrine pancreas for early detection of pancreatic endocrine tumors in multiple endocrine neoplasia type 1 syndrome: five years experience. J Clin Endocrinol Metab 1987; 64:1233–1240.

68. Shepherd JJ, Challis DR, Davies PF, et al. Multiple endocrine neoplasm, type 1: gastrinomas, pancreatic neoplasms, microcarcinoids, the Zollinger-Ellison syndrome, lymph nodes, and hepatic metastases. Arch Surg 1993; 128:1133–1142.

69. Mallette LE, Blevins T, Jordan PH, et al. Autogenous parathyroid grafts for generalized primary parathyroid hyperplasia: contrasting outcome in sporadic hyperplasia versus multiple endocrine neoplasia type I. Surgery 1987; 101:738–745.

70. Wells SA, Jr, Ellis GJ, Gunnells JC, et al. Parathyroid autotransplantation in primary parathyroid hyperplasia. N Engl J Med 1976; 195:57–62.

71. Skogseid B, Oberg K. Prospective screening in multiple endocrine neoplasia type 1. Henry Ford Hosp J 1992; 40:167–170.

72. Skogseid B, Rastad J, Oberg K. Multiple endocrine neoplasia type 1: clinical features and screening. Endocrinol Metab Clin North Am 1994; 23:1–18.

73. Pilato FP, D'Adda T, Banchini E, et al. Nonrandom expression of polypeptide hormones in pancreatic endocrine tumors: an immunohistochemical study in a case of multiple islet cell neoplasia. Cancer 1988; 61:1815–1820.

74. Rasbach DA, van Heerden JA, Telander RL, et al. Surgical management of hyperinsulinism in the multiple endocrine neoplasia, type 1 syndrome. Arch Surg 1985; 120:584–589.

75. van Heerden JA, Smith SL, Miller LJ. Management of the Zollinger-Ellison syndrome in patients with multiple endocrine neoplasia type I. Surgery 1986; 100:971–977.

76. Gorden P, Comi RJ, Maton PN, et al. Somatostatin and somatostatin analogue (SMS 201–995) in treatment of hormone-secreting tumors of the pituitary and gastrointestinal tract and non-neoplastic diseases of the gut. Ann Intern Med 1989; 110:35–50.

77. Jensen RT, Maton PN, Gardner JD. Current management of Zollinger-Ellison syndrome. Drugs 1986; 32:188–196.

78. Zollinger RM. Gastrinoma: factors influencing prognosis. Surgery 1985; 97:49–54.

79. Deveney CW, Deveney KS, Way LW. The Zollinger-Ellison syndrome: 23 years later. Ann Surg 1978; 188:384–383.

80. Lamers CB, Buis JT, van Tongeren J. Secretin-stimulated serum gastrin levels in hyperparathyroid patients from families with multiple endocrine adenomatosis type I. Ann Intern Med 1977; 86:719–724.

81. Zollinger R, Ellison E. Primary peptic ulcerations of the jejunum associated with islet cell tumors of the pancreas. Ann Surg 1955; 142:709–728.

82. Jensen RT, Doppman JL, Gardner JD. Gastrinoma. In: Go VL, Gardner JD, Brooks FP, et al, eds. The Exocrine Pancreas. New York: Raven Press, 1986.

83. Ellison EC, Carey LC, Sparks J, et al. Early surgical treatment of gastrinoma. Am J Med 1987; 82:17–24.

84. Frucht H, Maton PN, Jensen RT. Use of omeprazole in patients with Zollinger-Ellison syndrome. Dig Dis Sci 1991; 36:394–404.

85. Maton PN, Lack EE, Collen MJ, et al. The effect of Zollinger-Ellison syndrome and omeprazole therapy on gastric oxyntic endocrine cells. Gastroenterology 1990; 99:943–950.

86. Maton PN. Review article: the management of Zollinger-Ellison syndrome. Aliment Pharmacol Ther 1993; 7:467–475.

87. Gyr K, Whitehouse I, Beglinger C, et al. Human pharmacological effects of SMS 201-995 on gastric secretion. Scan J Gastroenterol 1986; 21(Suppl 119):96–102.

88. Kvols LK, Buck M, Moertel CG. Treatment of metastatic islet cell carcinoma with a somatostatin analogue (SMS 201–995). Ann Intern Med 1987; 107:162–168.

89. Mozell E, Woltering EA, O'Dorisio TM, et al. Effect of somatostatin analog on peptide release and tumor growth in the Zollinger-Ellison syndrome. Surg Gynecol Obstet 1990; 170:476–484.

90. Graham SM, Genel M, Touloukian RJ, et al. Provocative testing for occult medullary carcinoma of the thyroid: findings in seven children with multiple endocrine neoplasia type IIa. J Pediatr Surg 1987; 22:501–503.

91. Pipeleers MM, Somers G, Willems G, et al. Gastrinomas in the duodenums of patients with multiple endocrine neoplasia type 1 and the Zollinger-Ellison syndrome. N Engl J Med 1990; 322:723–727.

92. Thompson NW, Pasieka J, Fukuuchi A. Duodenal gastrinomas, duodenotomy, and duodenal exploration in the surgical management of Zollinger-Ellison syndrome. World J Surg 1993; 17:455–462.

93. Delcore R, Cheung LY, Friesen SR. The role of surgical treatment in Zollinger-Ellison syndrome. Surg Annu 1994; 26:151–168.

94. Fraker DL, Norton JA, Alexander HR, et al. Surgery in Zollinger-Ellison syndrome alters the natural history of gastrinoma. Ann Surg 1994; 220:320–328; discussion 328–330.

95. Tisell LE, Ahlman H, Jansson S, et al. Total pancreatectomy in the MEN-1 syndrome. Br J Surg 1988; 75:154–157.

96. Stefanini P, Carboni M, Patrassi N, et al. Beta-islet cell tumors of the pancreas: results of a study on 1,067 cases. Surgery 1974; 75:597–609.

97. Doppman JL, Miller DL, Chang R, et al. Intraarterial calcium stimulation test for detection of insulinomas. World J Surg 1993; 17:439–443.

98. Telander RL, Charboneau JW, Haymond MW. Intraoperative ultrasonography of the pancreas in children. J Pediatr Surg 1986; 21:262–266.

99. Tuft GO, Edis AJ, Service FJ, et al. Plasma glucose monitoring during operation for insulinoma: a critical reappraisal. Surgery 1980; 88:519–526.

100. Stefanini P, Carboni M, Patrassi N, et al. The surgical treatment of occult insulinomas: a review of the problem. Br J Surg 1974; 61:1–4.

101. Vassilopoulou-Sellin R, Ajani J. Islet cell tumors of the pancreas. Endocrinol Metab Clin North Am 1994; 23:53–65.

102. Kessenger A, Foley JF, Lemon HM. Therapy of malignant APUD cell tumors: effectiveness of DTIC. Cancer 1983; 51:790–794.

103. Croughs RJM, Hulsmans HAM, Israel DE, et al. Glucagonoma as part of the polyglandular adenoma syndrome. Am J Med 1972; 52:690–698.

104. Vance JE, Stoll RW, Kitabchi AE, et al. Familial nesidioblastosis as the predominant manifestation of multiple endocrine adenomatosis. Am J Med 1972; 52:211–227.

105. Asa SL, Singer W, Kovacs K, et al. Pancreatic endocrine tumour producing growth hormone–releasing hormone associated with multiple endocrine neoplasia type I syndrome. Acta Endocrinol (Copenh) 1987; 115:331–337.

106. Bordi C, DeVita O, Pilato FP, et al. Multiple islet cell tumors with predominance of glucagon-producing cells and ulcer disease. Am J Clin Pathol 1987; 88:153–161.

107. Ramsay JA, Kovacs K, Asa SL, et al. Reversible sellar enlargement due to growth hormone–releasing hormone production by pancreatic endocrine tumors in an acromegalic patient with multiple endocrine neoplasia type I syndrome. Cancer 1988; 62:445–450.

108. Ruttman E, Kloppel G, Bommer G, et al. Pancreatic glucagonoma with and without syndrome: immunocytochemical study of 5 tumour cases and review of the literature. Virchows Arch [Pathol Anat] 1980; 388:51–67.

109. Stacpoole PW, Jaspan J, Kasselberg AG, et al. A familial glucagonoma syndrome: genetic, clinical and biochemical features. Am J Med 1981; 70:1017–1026.

110. Assaad SN, Carrasco CH, Vassilopoulou SR, et al. Glucagonoma syndrome: rapid response following arterial embolization of glucagonoma metastatic to the liver. Am J Med 1987; 82:533–535.

111. Ajani JA, Carrasco CH, Charnsangavej C, et al. Islet cell tumors metastatic to the liver: effective palliation by sequential hepatic artery embolization. Ann Intern Med 1988; 108:340–344.

112. Altimari AF, Bhoopalam N, O'Dorsio T, et al. Use of a somatostatin analog (SMS 201–995) in the glucagonoma syndrome. Surgery 1986; 100:989–996.

113. Namihira Y, Achord JL, Subramony C. Multiple endocrine neoplasia, type 1, with pancreatic cholera. Am J Gastroenterol 1987; 82:794–797.

114. Lee CH, Ching KN, Lui WY, et al. Carcinoid tumor of the pancreas causing the diarrheogenic syndrome: report of a case combined with multiple endocrine neoplasia, type I. Surgery 1986; 99:123–129.

115. Gagel RF, Costanza ME, DeLellis RA, et al. Streptozocin-treated Verner-Morrison syndrome: plasma vasoactive intestinal peptide and tumor responses. Arch Intern Med 1976; 136:1429–1435.

116. Venkatesh S, Ordonez NG, Ajani J, et al. Islet cell carcinoma of the pancreas: a study of 98 patients. Cancer 1990; 65:354–357.

117. Skogseid B, Larsson C, Oberg K. Genetic and clinical characteristics of multiple endocrine neoplasia type 1. Acta Oncol 1991; 30:485–488.

118. Larsson C, Nordenskjold M, Skogseid B, et al. Practical guidelines for DNA-based testing in multiple endocrine neoplasia type 1. Henry Ford Hosp J 1992; 40:171–175.

119. Skogseid B, Eriksson B, Lundqvist G, et al. Multiple endocrine neoplasia type 1: a 10-year prospective screening study in four kindreds. J Clin Endocrinol Metab 1991; 73:281–287.

120. Chiang HC, O'Dorisio TM, Huang SC, et al. Multiple hormone elevations in Zollinger-Ellison syndrome: prospective study of clinical significance and of the development of a second symptomatic pancreatic endocrine tumor syndrome. Gastroenterology 1990; 99:1565–1575.

121. Landis CA, Masters SB, Spada A, et al. GTPase-inhibiting mutations activate the alpha chain of Gs and stimulate adenylyl cyclase in human pituitary tumours. Nature 1989; 340:692–696.

122. Antunes JL, Housepian EM, Frantz AG, et al. Prolactin-secreting pituitary tumors. Ann Neurol 1977; 2:148–153.

123. Scheithauer BW, Horvath E, Kovacs K, et al. Plurihormonal pituitary adenomas. Semin Diagn Pathol 1986; 3:69–82.

124. Scheithauer BW, Laws ERJ, Kovacs K, et al. Pituitary adenomas of the multiple endocrine neoplasia type I syndrome. Semin Diagn Pathol 1987; 4:205–211.

125. Weil C. The safety of bromocriptine in long-term use: a review of the literature. Curr Med Res Opin 1986; 10:25–51.

126. Fossati P, Dewailly D, Thomas DP, et al. Medical treatment of hyperprolactinemia. Horm Res 1985; 22:228–238.

127. Ferrari C, Crosignani PG. Medical treatment of hyperprolactinaemic disorders. Hum Reprod 1986; 1:507–514.

128. McCutcheon IE. Management of individual tumor syndromes: pituitary neoplasia. Endocrinol Metab Clin North Am 1994; 23:37–51.

129. Berger G, Trouillas J, Bloch B, et al. Multihormonal carcinoid tumor of the pancreas: secreting growth hormone–releasing factor as a cause of acromegaly. Cancer 1984; 54:2097–2108.

130. Duncan AM, Greenberg CR. Absence of chromosomal instability in one kindred with multiple endocrine neoplasia type 2A. Cancer Genet Cytogenet 1986; 22:109–112.

131. Sano T, Yamasaki R, Saito H, et al. Growth hormone–releasing hormone (GHRH)–secreting pancreatic tumor in a patient with multiple endocrine neoplasia type I. Am J Surg Pathol 1987; 11:810–819.

132. Chadenas D, Pinsard D, Melliere D, et al. Endocrine pancreatic tumor secreting somatostatin and somatocrinin. Presse Med 1985; 14:2129–2134.

133. Yamasaki R, Saito H, Sano T, et al. Ectopic growth hormone–releasing hormone (GHRH) syndrome in a case with multiple endocrine neoplasia type I. Endocrinol Jpn 1988; 35:97–109.

134. Yamasaki R, Saito H, Kameyama K, et al. Secretion of growth hormone–releasing hormone in patients with idiopathic pituitary dwarfism and acromegaly. Acta Endocrinol (Copenh) 1988; 117:273–281.

135. Thorner MO, Frohman LA, Leong DA, et al. Extrahypothalamic growth hormone–releasing factor (GRF) secretion is a rare cause of acromegaly: plasma GRF levels in 177 acromegalic patients. J Clin Endocrinol Metab 1984; 59:846–849.

136. Samaan NA, Schultz PN, Yang KP, et al. Endocrine complications after radiotherapy for tumors of the head and neck. J Lab Clin Med 1987; 109:364–372.

137. Ezzat S, Snyder PJ, Young WF, et al. Octreotide treatment of acromegaly: a randomized, multicenter study. Ann Intern Med 1992; 117:711–718.

138. Newman CB, Melmed S, Snyder PJ, et al. Safety and efficacy of long-term octreotide therapy of acromegaly: results of a multicenter trial in 103 patients—a clinical research center study. J Clin Endocrinol Metab 1995; 80:2768–2775.

139. Melmed S, Ziel FH, Braunstein GD, et al. Medical management of acromegaly due to ectopic production of growth hormone–releasing hormone by a carcinoid tumor. J Clin Endocrinol Metab 1988; 67:395–399.

140. Amano S, Hazama F, Haebara H, et al. Ectopic ACTH-MSH–producing carcinoid tumor with multiple endocrine hyperplasia in a child. Acta Pathol Jpn 1978; 28:721–730.

141. Hashimoto K, Suemaru S, Hattori T, et al. Multiple endocrine neoplasia with Cushing's syndrome due to paraganglioma producing corticotropin-releasing factor and adrenocorticotropin. Acta Endocrinol (Copenh) 1986; 113:189–195.

142. Duh QY, Hybarger CP, Geist R, et al. Carcinoids associated with multiple endocrine neoplasia syndrome. Am J Surg 1987; 154:142–148.

143. Zahner J, Borchard F, Schmitz U, et al. Thymus carcinoid in multiple endocrine neoplasms type I. Dtsch Med Wochenschr 1994; 119:135–140.

144. Samaan NA, Hickey RC, Bedner TD, et al. Hyperparathyroidism and carcinoid tumor. Ann Intern Med 1975; 82:205–207.

145. Burton JL, Hartog M. Multiple endocrine adenomatosis (Type 1) with cutaneous leiomyomata and cysts of Moll. Br J Dermatol 1977; 15:74–75.

146. Friedman E, Sakaguchi K, Bale AE, et al. Clonality of parathyroid tumors in familial multiple endocrine neoplasia type 1. N Engl J Med 1989; 321:213–218.

147. Thakker RV, Bouloux P, Wooding C, et al. Association of parathyroid tumors in multiple endocrine neoplasia type 1 with loss of alleles on chromosome 11. N Engl J Med 1989; 321:218–224.

148. Bale AE, Norton JA, Wong EL, et al. Allelic loss on chromosome 11 in hereditary and sporadic tumors related to familial multiple endocrine neoplasia type 1. Cancer Res 1991; 51:1154–1157.

149. Bale AE. Molecular mechanisms of neoplasia in multiple endocrine neoplasia type 1–related and sporadic tumors of the pancreatic islet cells. Endocrinol Metab Clin North Am 1994; 23:109–115.

150. Nakamura Y, Leppert M, Lathrop GM, et al. A primary genetic linkage map of chromosome 10. Human gene mapping 9: Ninth International Workshop on Human Gene Mapping. Cytogenet Cell Genet 1987; 46:667.

151. Bale SJ, Bale AE, Stewart K, et al. Linkage analysis of multiple endocrine neoplasia type 1 with INT2 and other markers on chromosome 11. Genomics 1989; 4:320–322.

152. Nakamura Y, Mathew CG, Sobol H, et al. Linked markers flanking the gene for multiple endocrine neoplasia type 2A. Genomics 1989; 5:199–203.

153. Thakker RV. The role of molecular genetics in screening for multiple endocrine neoplasia type 1. Endocrinol Metab Clin North Am 1994; 23:117–135.

154. Nakamura Y, Larsson C, Julier C, et al. Localization of the genetic defect in multiple endocrine neoplasia type 1 within a small region of chromosome 11. Am J Hum Genet 1989; 44:751–755.

155. Larsson C, Weber G, Janson M. Sublocalization of the multiple endocrine neoplasia type 1 gene. Henry Ford Hosp J 1992; 40:159–161.

156. Karakawa K, Takami K, Nakamura T, et al. Isolation of region-specific cosmids by hybridization with microdissected clones from human chromosome 10q11.1-q21.1. Genomics 1993; 17:449–455.

157. Friedman E, Adams EF, Hoog A, et al. Normal structural dopamine type 2 receptor gene in prolactin-secreting and other pituitary tumors. J Clin Endocrinol Metab 1994; 78:568–574.

158. Chandrasekharappa SC, Guni SC, Manickam P, et al. Positional cloning of the gene for multiple endocrine neoplasia type 1. Science 1997; 276:404–407.

159. Larsson C, Nordenskjold M. Family screening in multiple endocrine neoplasia type 1 (MEN 1). Ann Med 1994; 26:191–198.

160. Hershon KS, Kelley WA, Shaw CM, et al. Prolactinomas as part of the multiple endocrine neoplastic syndrome type 1. Am J Med 1983; 74:713–720.

161. Bear JC, Briones-Urbina R, Fahey JF, et al. Variant multiple endocrine neoplasia I (MEN IBurin): further studies and non-linkage to HLA. Hum Hered 1985; 35:15–20.

162. Thompson JC, Lewis BG, Wiener I, et al. The role of surgery in the Zollinger-Ellison syndrome. Ann Surg 1983; 197:594–607.

163. Sipple JH. Multiple endocrine neoplasia type 2 syndromes: historical perspectives. Henry Ford Hosp Med J 1984; 32:219–221.

164. Cushman P, Jr. Familial endocrine tumors: report of two unrelated kindred affected with pheochromocytomas, one also with multiple thyroid carcinomas. Am J Med 1962; 32:352–360.

165. Hazard JB, Hawk WA, Crile G, Jr. Medullary (solid) carcinoma of the

thyroid: a clinicopathologic entity. J Clin Endocrinol Metab 1959; 19:152–161.

166. Williams ED. A review of 17 cases of carcinoma of the thyroid and phaeochromocytoma. J Clin Pathol 1965; 18:288–292.

167. Melvin KEW, Miller HH, Tashjian AH, Jr. Early diagnosis of medullary carcinoma of the thyroid gland by means of calcitonin assay. N Engl J Med 1971; 285:1115–1120.

168. Sizemore GW, Carney JA, Heath H, III. Epidemiology of medullary carcinoma of the thyroid gland: a 5-year experience (1971–1976). Surg Clin North Am 1977; 57:633–645.

169. Gagel RF, Melvin KE, Tashjian AH, Jr, et al. Natural history of the familial medullary thyroid carcinoma–pheochromocytoma syndrome and the identification of preneoplastic stages by screening studies: a five-year report. Trans Assoc Am Physicians 1975; 88:177–191.

170. Block MA, Jackson CE, Tashjian AH Jr. Management of occult medullary thyroid carcinoma: evidenced only by serum calcitonin level elevations after apparently adequate neck operations. Arch Surg 1978; 113:368–372.

171. Baylin SB. The multiple endocrine neoplasia syndromes: implications for the study of inherited tumors. Semin Oncol 1978; 5:35–45.

172. Sizemore GW, Heath H, III, Carney JA. Multiple endocrine neoplasia type 2. Clin Endocrinol Metab 1980; 9:299–315.

173. Wells SA, Jr, Baylin SB, Leight GS, et al. The importance of early diagnosis in patients with hereditary medullary thyroid carcinoma. Ann Surg 1982; 195:595–599.

174. Jackson CE, Talpos GB, Kambouris A, et al. The clinical course after definitive operation for medullary thyroid carcinoma. Surgery 1983; 94:995–1001.

175. Russell CF, Van Heerden JA, Sizemore GW, et al. The surgical management of medullary thyroid carcinoma. Ann Surg 1983; 197:42–48.

176. Gagel RF, Tashjian AH Jr, Cummings T, et al. Impact of prospective screening for multiple endocrine neoplasia type 2. Henry Ford Hosp Med J 1987; 35:94–98.

177. Jackson CE, Norum RA, Talpos GB, et al. Clinical value of calcitonin and carcinoembryonic antigen doubling times in medullary thyroid carcinoma. Henry Ford Hosp Med J 1987; 35:120–121.

178. Heath H, III, Sizemore GW, Carney JA. Preoperative diagnosis of occult parathyroid hyperplasia by calcium infusion in patients with multiple endocrine neoplasia, type 2a. J Clin Endocrinol Metab 1976; 43:428–435.

179. Howe JR, Norton JA, Wells SA, Jr. Prevalence of pheochromocytoma and hyperparathyroidism in multiple endocrine neoplasia type 2A: results of long-term follow-up. Surgery 1993; 114:1070–1077.

180. Wolfe HJ, Melvin KEW, Cervi-Skinner SJ, et al. C-cell hyperplasia preceding medullary thyroid carcinoma. N Engl J Med 1973; 289:437–441.

181. DeLellis RA, Dayal Y, Tischler AS, et al. Multiple endocrine neoplasia (MEN) syndromes: cellular origins and interrelationships. Int Rev Exp Pathol 1986; 28:163–215.

182. Wolfe HJ, DeLellis RA. Familial medullary thyroid carcinoma and C-cell hyperplasia. Clin Endocrinol Metab 1981; 10:351–365.

183. Lips CJ, Landsvater RM, Hoppener JW, et al. Clinical screening as compared with DNA analysis in families with multiple endocrine neoplasia type 2A. N Engl J Med 1994; 331:828–835.

184. Wells SA, Chi DD, Toshima K, et al. Predictive DNA testing and prophylactic thyroidectomy in patients at risk for multiple endocrine neoplasia type 2A. Ann Surg 1994; 220:237–250.

185. Gagel RF, Cote GJ, Martins Bugalho MJG, et al. Clinical use of molecular information in the management of multiple endocrine neoplasia type 2A. J Int Med 1995; 238:333–341.

186. Block MA, Jackson CE, Greenawald KA, et al. Clinical characteristics distinguishing hereditary from sporadic medullary thyroid carcinoma. Arch Surg 1980; 115:142–148.

187. Samaan NA, Schultz PN, Hickey RC. Medullary thyroid carcinoma: prognosis of familial versus sporadic disease and the role of radiotherapy. J Clin Endocrinol Metab 1988; 67:801–805.

188. Tisell L, Hansson G, Jansson S, et al. Reoperation in the treatment of asymptomatic metastasizing medullary thyroid carcinoma. Surgery 1986; 99:60–66.

189. Moley JF, Wells SA, Dilley WG, et al. Reoperation for recurrent or persistent medullary thyroid carcinoma. Surgery 1993; 114:1090–1096.

190. Buhr HJ, Kallinowski F, Raue F, et al. Microsurgical neck dissection for metastasizing medullary thyroid carcinoma. Eur J Surg Oncol 1995; 21:195–197.

191. Talpos GB, Jackson CE, Froelich JW, et al. Localization of residual medullary thyroid cancer by thallium/technetium scintigraphy. Surgery 1985; 98:1189–1196.

192. Itoh H, Sugie K, Toyooka S, et al. Detection of metastatic medullary thyroid cancer with ^{131}I-MIBG scans in Sipple's syndrome. Eur J Nucl Med 1986; 11:502–504.

193. Baulieu JL, Guilloteau D, Delisle MJ, et al. Radioiodinated meta-iodobenzylguanidine uptake in medullary thyroid cancer: a French cooperative study. Cancer 1987; 60:2189–2194.

194. Yobbagy JJ, Levatter R, Sisson JC, et al. Scintigraphic portrayal of the syndrome of multiple endocrine neoplasia type 2B. Clin Nucl Med 1988; 13:433–437.

195. Krenning EP, Kwekkeboom DJ, Bakker WH, et al. Somatostatin receptor scintigraphy with [111In-DTPA-D-Phe1] and [123I-Tyr3]-octreotide: the Rotterdam experience with more than 1000 patients. Nucl Med 1993; 20:716–731.

196. Frank-Raue K, Raue F, Buhr HJ, et al. Localization of occult persisting medullary thyroid carcinoma before microsurgical reoperation: high sensitivity of selective venous catheterization. Thyroid 1992; 2:113–117.

197. van Heerden JA, Grant CS, Gharib H, et al. Long-term course of patients with persistent hypercalcitoninemia after apparent curative primary surgery for medullary thyroid carcinoma. Ann Surg 1990; 212:395–400.

198. Leape LL, Miller HH, Graze K, et al. Total thyroidectomy for occult familial medullary carcinoma of the thyroid in children. J Pediatr Surg 1976; 11:831–837.

199. Block MA, Jackson CE, Tashjian AH, Jr. Management of occult medullary thyroid carcinoma: evidenced only by serum calcitonin level elevations after apparently adequate neck operations. Arch Surg 1978; 113:368–372.

200. Cote GJ, Gould JA, Huang SC, et al. Studies of short-term secretion of peptides produced by alternative RNA processing. Mol Cell Endocrinol 1987; 53:211–219.

201. Gagel RF, Palmer WN, Leonhart K, et al. Somatostatin production by a human medullary thyroid carcinoma cell line. Endocrinology 1986; 118:1643–1651.

202. Atkins FL, Beaven MA, Keiser HR. Dopa decarboxylase in medullary carcinoma of the thyroid. N Engl J Med 1973; 289:545–548.

203. O'Connor DT, Deftos LJ. Secretion of chromogranin A by peptide-producing endocrine neoplasms. N Engl J Med 1986; 314:1145–1151.

204. Sevarino KA, Wu P, Jackson IMD, et al. Biosynthesis of thyrotropin-releasing hormone by a rat medullary thyroid carcinoma cell line. J Biol Chem 1988; 263:620–623.

205. Yamaguchi K, Abe K, Adachi I, et al. Concomitant production of immunoreactive gastrin-releasing peptide and calcitonin in medullary carcinoma of the thyroid. Metabolism 1984; 33:724–727.

206. Baylin SB, Beaven MA, Buja LM, et al. Histaminase activity: a biochemical marker for medullary carcinoma of the thyroid. Am J Med 1972; 53:723–733.

207. Gagel R. Tumor markers of medullary thyroid carcinoma. In: Fishman WH, ed. On Codevelopmental Markers: Biologic, Diagnostic and Monitoring Aspects. New York: Academic Press, 1983.

208. Carney JA, Sizemore GW, Tyce GM. Bilateral adrenal medullary hyperplasia in multiple endocrine neoplasia, type 2: the precursor of bilateral pheochromocytoma. Mayo Clin Proc 1975; 50:3–10.

209. Carney JA, Sizemore GW, Sheps SG. Adrenal medullary disease in multiple endocrine neoplasia, type 2: pheochromocytoma and its precursors. Am J Clin Pathol 1976; 66:279–290.

210. DeLellis RA, Wolfe HJ, Gagel RF, et al. Adrenal medullary hyperplasia: a morphometric analysis in patients with familial medullary thyroid carcinoma. Am J Pathol 1976; 83:177–196.

211. Webb TA, Sheps SG, Carney JA. Differences between sporadic pheochromocytoma and pheochromocytoma in multiple endocrine neoplasia, type 2. Am J Surg Pathol 1980; 4:121–126.

212. Chodankar CM, Abhyankar SC, Deodhar KP, et al. Sipple's syndrome (multiple endocrine neoplasia) in pregnancy—case report. Aust NZ J Obstet Gynaecol 1982; 22:243–244.

213. Morača-Kvapilová L, Op de Coul AA, Merkus JM. Cerebral haemorrhage in a pregnant woman with a multiple endocrine neoplasia syndrome (type 2A or Sipple's syndrome). Eur J Obstet Gynecol Reprod Biol 1985; 20:257–263.

214. Hamilton BP, Landsberg L, Levine RJ. Measurement of urinary epinephrine in screening for pheochromocytoma in multiple endocrine neoplasia type II. Am J Med 1978; 65:1027–1032.

215. Takai S, Miyauchi A, Matsumoto H, et al. Multiple endocrine neoplasia type 2 syndromes in Japan. Henry Ford Hosp Med J 1984; 32:246–250.

216. Gerlo EA, Sevens C. Urinary and plasma catecholamines and urinary catecholamine metabolites in pheochromocytoma: diagnostic value in 19 cases. Clin Chem 1994; 40:250–256.

217. Telenius-Berg M, Adolfsson L, Berg B, et al. Catecholamine release after physical exercise: a new provocative test for early diagnosis of pheochromocytoma in multiple endocrine neoplasia type 2. Acta Med Scand 1987; 222:351–359.

218. Valk TW, Frager MS, Gross MD, et al. Spectrum of pheochromocytoma in multiple endocrine neoplasia: a scintigraphic portrayal using ^{131}I-metaiodobenzylguanidine. Ann Intern Med 1981; 94:762–767.

219. Sisson JC, Shapiro B, Beierwaltes WH. Scintigraphy with I-131 MIBG as an aid to the treatment of pheochromocytomas in patients with the multiple endocrine neoplasia type 2 syndromes. Henry Ford Hosp Med J 1984; 32:254–261.

220. Lee JE, Curley SA, Gagel RF, et al. Cortical-sparing adrenalectomy for patients with bilateral pheochromocytomas. Surgery 1996; 120:1064–1071.

221. Tibblin S, Dymling JF, Ingemansson S, et al. Unilateral versus bilateral adrenalectomy in multiple endocrine neoplasia IIA. World J Surg 1983; 7:201–208.

222. Jansson S, Tisell LE, Fjalling M, et al. Early diagnosis of and surgical strategy for adrenal medullary disease in MEN II gene carriers. Surgery 1988; 103:11–18.

223. Lairmore TC, Ball DW, Baylin SB, et al. Management of pheochromocytomas in patients with multiple endocrine neoplasia type 2 syndromes. Ann Surg 1993; 217:595–601; discussion 601–603.

224. Lips CJ, Minder WH, Leo JR, et al. Evidence of multicentric origin of the multiple endocrine neoplasia syndrome type 2a (Sipple's syndrome) in a large family in the Netherlands: diagnostic and therapeutic implications. Am J Med 1978; 64:569–578.

225. van Heerden JA, Sizemore GW, Carney JA, et al. Surgical management of the adrenal glands in the multiple endocrine neoplasia type II syndrome. World J Surg 1984; 8:612–621.

226. Evans DB, Lee JE, Merrell RC, et al. Adrenal medullary disease in multiple endocrine neoplasia type 2: appropriate management. Endocrinol Metab Clin North Am 1994; 23:167–176.

227. Carney JA, Roth SI, Heath H, III, et al. The parathyroid glands in multiple endocrine neoplasia type 2b. Am J Pathol 1980; 99:387–398.

228. Gagel RF, Levy ML, Donovan DT, et al. Multiple endocrine neoplasia type 2a associated with cutaneous lichen amyloidosis. Ann Intern Med 1989; 111:802–806.

229. Nunziata V, Giannattasio R, di Giovanni G, et al. Hereditary localized pruritus in affected members of a kindred with multiple endocrine neoplasia type 2A (Sipple's syndrome). Clin Endocrinol 1989; 30:57–63.

230. Wong C-K, Lin C-S. Friction amyloidosis. Int J Dermatol 1988; 27:302–307.

231. Verdy MB, Cadotte M, Schurch W, et al. A French Canadian family with multiple endocrine neoplasia type 2 syndromes. Henry Ford Hosp Med J 1984; 32:251–253.

232. Tamsen A, Mazur MT. Ovarian strumal carcinoid in association with multiple endocrine neoplasia, Type IIA. Arch Pathol Lab Med 1992; 116:200–203.

233. Williams ED, Pollock DJ. Multiple mucosal neuromata with endocrine tumours: a syndrome allied to Von Recklinghausen's disease. J Pathol Bacteriol 1966; 91:71–80.

234. Rashid M, Khairi MR, Dexter RN, et al. Mucosal neuroma, pheochromocytoma and medullary thyroid carcinoma: multiple endocrine neoplasia type 3. Medicine (Balt) 1975; 54:89–112.

235. Carney JA, Sizemore GW, Hayles AB. C-cell disease of the thyroid gland in multiple endocrine neoplasia type 2b. Cancer 1979; 44:2173–2183.

236. Carney JA, Go VL, Sizemore GW, et al. Alimentary-tract ganglioneuromatosis: a major component of the syndrome of multiple endocrine neoplasia, type 2b. N Engl J Med 1976; 295:1287–1291.

237. Stjernholm MR, Freudenbourg JC, Mooney HS, et al. Medullary carcinoma of the thyroid before age 2 years. J Clin Endocrinol Metab 1980; 51:252–253.

238. Samaan NA, Draznin MB, Halpin RE, et al. Multiple endocrine syndrome type IIb in early childhood. Cancer 1991; 68:1832–1834.

239. Kakudo K, Carney JA, Sizemore GW. Medullary carcinoma of thyroid: biologic behavior of the sporadic and familial neoplasm. Cancer 1985; 55:2818–2821.

240. Sizemore GW, Carney JA, Gharib H, et al. Multiple endocrine neoplasia type 2B: eighteen-year follow-up of a four-generation family. Henry Ford Hosp J 1992; 40:236–244.

241. Vasen HFA, van der Feltz M, Raue F, et al. The natural course of multiple endocrine neoplasia type IIb: a study of 18 cases. Arch Intern Med 1992; 152:1250–1252.

242. Dyck PJ, Carney JA, Sizemore GW, et al. Multiple endocrine neoplasia, type 2b: phenotype recognition; neurological features and their pathological basis. Ann Neurol 1979; 6:302–314.

243. Aine E, Aine L, Huupponen T, et al. Visible corneal nerve fibers and neuromas of the conjunctiva: a syndrome of type-3 multiple endocrine adenomatosis in two generations. Graefes Arch Clin Exp Ophthalmol 1987; 225:213–216.

244. Hubner A, Holschneider AM. Multiple endocrine neoplasias in 3 generations. Langenbecks Arch Chir 1987; 372:747–750.

245. Carlson KM, Bracamontes J, Jackson CE, et al. Parent-of-origin effects in multiple endocrine neoplasia type 2B. Am J Hum Genet 1994; 55:1076–1082.

246. Norton JA, Froome LC, Farrell RE, et al. Multiple endocrine neoplasia type IIb: the most aggressive form of medullary thyroid carcinoma. Surg Clin North Am 1979; 59:109–118.

247. Sciubba JJ, DAmico E, Attie JN. The occurrence of multiple endocrine neoplasia type IIb, in two children of an affected mother. J Oral Pathol 1987; 16:310–316.

248. Mathew CG, Chin KS, Easton DF, et al. A linked genetic marker for multiple endocrine neoplasia type 2A on chromosome 10. Nature 1987; 328:527–528.

249. Simpson NE, Kidd KK, Goodfellow PJ, et al. Assignment of multiple endocrine neoplasia type 2A to chromosome 10 by linkage. Nature 1987; 328:528–530.

250. Norum RA, Lafreniere RG, ONeal LW, et al. Linkage of the multiple endocrine neoplasia type 2B gene (MEN2B) to chromosome 10 markers linked to MEN2A. Genomics 1990; 8:313–317.

251. Lairmore TC, Howe JR, Korte JA, et al. Familial medullary thyroid carcinoma and multiple endocrine neoplasia type 2B map to the same region of chromosome 10 as multiple endocrine neoplasia type 2A. Genomics 1991; 9:181–192.

252. Angrist M, Kauffman E, Slaugenhaupt SA, et al. A gene for Hirschsprung disease (megacolon) in the pericentromeric region of human chromosome 10. Nature Genetics 1993; 4:351–356.

253. Lyonnet S, Bolino A, Pelet A, et al. A gene for Hirschsprung disease maps to the proximal long arm of chromosome 10. Nat Genet 1993; 4:346–350.

254. Lairmore TC, Howe JR, Dou S, et al. Isolation of YAC clones from the pericentromeric region of chromosome 10 and development of new genetic markers linked to the multiple endocrine neoplasia type 2A gene. Henry Ford Hosp Med J 1992; 40:210–214.

255. Gardner E, Papi L, Easton DF, et al. Genetic linkage studies map the multiple endocrine neoplasia type 2 loci to a small interval on chromosome 10q11.2. Hum Mol Genet 1993; 2:241–246.

256. Mole SE, Mulligan LM, Healey CS, et al. Localisation of the gene for multiple endocrine neoplasia type 2A to a 480 kb region in chromosome band 10q11.2. Hum Mol Genet 1993; 2:247–252.

257. Mole SE, Mulligan LM, Healey CS, et al. Localisation of the gene for multiple endocrine neoplasia type 2A to a 480 kb region in chromosome band 10q11.2. Hum Mol Genet 1993; 2:247–252.

258. Mulligan LM, Marsh DJ, Robinson BG, et al. Genotype-phenotype correlation in multiple endocrine neoplasia type 2: report of the international RET mutation consortium. J Int Med 1995; 238:343–346.

259. Carlson KM, Dou S, Chi D, et al. Single missense mutation in the tyrosine kinase catalytic domain of the RET protoncogene is associated with multiple endocrine neoplasia type 2B. Proc Natl Acad Sci USA 1994; 91:1579–1583.

260. Hofstra RM, Landsvater RM, Ceccherini I, et al. A mutation in the RET proto-onocogene associated with multiple endocrine neoplasia type 2B and sporadic medullary thyroid carcinoma. Nature 1994; 367:375–376.

261. Lacroix A, Blanchard L, Villeneuve L, et al. Cosegregation of Hirschsprung's disease (HSCR) with chromosome 10 markers and a ret mutation in a French Canadian family with MEN 2A. Presented as abstract at the Fifth International Workshop on Multiple Endocrine Neoplasia, Stockholm, Sweden, 1994.

262. Borst MJ, Van Camp JM, Peacock ML, et al. Mutational analysis of multiple endocrine neoplasia type 2A associated with Hirschsprung's disease. Surgery 1995; 117:386–391.

263. Wohllk N, Cote GJ, Bugalho MMJ, et al. Relevance of RET proto-oncogene mutations in sporadic medullary thyroid carcinoma. J Clin Endocrinol Metab 1996; 81:3740–3745.

264. Ceccherini I, Romei C, Barone V, et al. Identification of the cys 634-to-tyr mutation of the RET proto-oncogene in a pedigree with multiple endocrine neoplasia type 2A and localized cutaneous lichen amyloidosis. J Endocrinol Invest 1994; 17:201–204.

265. Robinson MF, Cote GJ, Nunziata V, et al. Mutation of a specific codon of the ret proto-oncogene in the multiple endocrine neoplasia type 2A/ cutaneous lichen amyloidosis syndrome. Presented as abstract at the Fifth International Workshop on Multiple Endocrine Neoplasia, Stockholm, Sweden, 1994.

266. Edery P, Lyonnet S, Mulligan LM, et al. Mutations of the RET proto-oncogene in Hirschsprung's disease. Nature 1994; 367:378–380.

267. Romeo G, Ronchetto P, Luo Y, et al. Point mutations affecting the tyrosine kinase domain of the RET proto-oncogene in Hirschsprung's disease. Nature 1994; 367:377–378.

268. Angrist M, Bolk S, Thiel B, et al. Mutation analysis of the RET receptor tyrosine kinase in Hirschsprung's disease. Hum Mol Genet 1995; 4:821–830.

269. Eng C, Smith DP, Mulligan LM, et al. Point mutation within the tyrosine kinase domain of the RET proto-oncogene in multiple endocrine neoplasia type 2B and related sporadic tumours. Hum Mol Genet 1994; 3:237–241.

270. Zedenius J, Larsson C, Bergholm U, et al. Mutations of codon 918 in the RET proto-oncogene correlate to poor prognosis in sporadic medullary thyroid carcinomas. J Clin Endocrinol Metab 1995; 80:3088–3090.

271. Decker RA, Peacock ML, Borst MJ, et al. Progress in genetic screening of multiple endocrine neoplasia type 2A: is calcitonin testing obsolete? Surgery 1995; 118:257–263; discussion 263–264.

272. Komminoth P, Kunz E, Hiort O, et al. Detection of RET proto-oncogene point mutations in paraffin-embedded pheochromocytoma specimens by nonradioactive single-strand conformation polymorphism analysis and direct sequencing. Am J Pathol 1994; 145:922–929.

273. Pachnis V, Mankoo B, Costantini F. Expression of the c-ret proto-oncogene during mouse embryogenesis. Development 1993; 119:1005–1017.

274. Tsuzuki T, Takahashi M, Asai N, et al. Spatial and temporal expression of the ret proto-oncogene product in embryonic, infant, and adult rat tissues. Oncogene 1995; 10:191–198.

275. Sanchez M, Silos-Santiago I, Frisen J, et al. Newborn mice lacking GDNF display renal agenesis and absence of enteric neurons, but no deficits in midbrain dopaminergic neurons. Nature 1996; 382:70–73.

276. Robbins J, Gulick J, Sanchez A, et al. Mouse embryoic stem cells express the cardiac myosin heavy chain genes during development in vitro. J Biol Chem 1990; 265:11905–11909.

277. Moore MW, Klein RD, Farinas I, et al. Renal and neuronal abnormalities in mice lacking GDNF. Nature 1996; 382:76–79.

278. Pichel JG, Shen L, Sheng HZ, et al. Defects in enteric innervation and kidney development in mice lacking GDNF. Nature 1996; 382:73–76.

279. Schuchardt A, D'Agati V, Larsson-Blomberg L., et al. Defects in the kidney and enteric nervous system of mice lacking the tyrosine kinase receptor Ret Nature 1994; 367:380–383.

280. Trupp M, Arenas E, Fainzilber M, et al. Functional receptor for GDNF encoded by the c-ret proto-oncogene. Nature 1996; 381:785–789.

281. Durbec P, Marcos-Gutierrez CV, Kilkenny C, et al. GDNF signalling through the Ret receptor tyrosine kinase. Nature 1996; 381:789–793.

282. Treanor JJS, Goodman L, de Sauvage F, et al. Characterization of a multicomponent receptor for GDNF. Nature 1996; 382:80–83.

283. Jing S, Wen D, Yu Y, et al. GDNF-induced activation of the Ret protein tyrosine kinase is mediated by GDNFR-α, a novel receptor for GDNF. Cell 1996; 85:1113–1124.

284. Asai N, Iwashita T, Matsuyama M, et al. Mechanisms of activation of the ret proto-oncogene by multiple endocrine neoplasia 2A mutations. Mol Cell Biol 1995; 15:1613–1619.

285. Santoro M, Carlomagno F, Romano A, et al. Activation of RET as a dominant transforming gene by germline mutations of MEN 2A and MEN 2B. Science 1995; 267:381–383.

286. Xing S, Smanik PA, Olgesbee MJ, et al. Characterization of RET oncogenic activation in MEN 2 inherited cancer syndromes. Endocrinology 1996; 137:1512–1519.

287. Edery P, Pelet A, Mulligan LM, et al. Long segment and short segment familial Hirschsprung's disease: variable clinical expression at the RET locus. J Med Genet 1994; 31:602–606.

288. Lyonnet S, Edery P, Mulligan LM, et al. Mutations of RET proto-oncogene in Hirschsprung disease. C R Acad Sci III 1994; 317:358–362.

289. Schuchardt A, D'Agati V, Larsson-Blombert L, et al. RET-deficient mice: an animal model for Hirschsprung's disease and renal agenesis. J Int Med 1995; 238:327–332.

290. Wells SA, Jr, Chi DD, Toshima K, et al. Predictive DNA testing and prophylactic thyroidectomy in patients at risk for multiple endocrine neoplasia type 2A. Ann Surg 1994; 220:237–247; discussion 247–250.

291. Cote GJ, Wohllk N, Evans D, et al. RET proto-oncogene mutations in multiple endocrine neoplasia type 2 and medullary thyroid carcinoma. Bailliere's Clin Endocrinol Metab 1995; 9:609–630.

292. Decker R, Borst M, Peacock M. Rapid screening for ret mutations in multiple endocrine neoplasia type 2 by denaturing gradient electrophoresis. Presented at the Fifth International Workshop on Multiple Endocrine Neoplasia, Stockholm, Sweden, July 1994.

293. Decker RA, Peacock ML, Borst MJ, et al. Progress in genetic screening of multiple endocrine neoplasia type 2A: is calcitonin testing obsolete? Surgery 1995; 118:257–264.

294. Wells SA, Jr, Baylin SB, Linehan WM, et al. Provocative agents and the diagnosis of medullary carcinoma of the thyroid gland. Ann Surg 1978; 188:139–141.

295. Body JJ, Heath H, III. Estimates of circulating monomeric calcitonin: physiological studies in normal and thyroidectomized man. J Clin Endocrinol Metab 1983; 57:897–903.

296. Catherwood BD, Deftos LJ. General principles, problems and interpretation in the radioimmunoassay of calcitonin. Biomed Pharmacother 1984; 38:235–241.

297. Motte P, Vauzelle P, Gardet P, et al. Construction and clinical validation of a sensitive and specific assay for serum mature calcitonin using monoclonal anti-peptide antibodies. Clin Chim Acta 1988; 174:35–54.

298. Seth R, Motte P, Kehely A, et al. A sensitive and specific two-site enzyme-immunoassay for human calcitonin using monoclonal antibodies. J Endocrinol 1988; 119:351–357.

299. Body JJ, Heath HI. Nonspecific increases in plasma immunoreactive calcitonin in healthy individuals: discrimination from medullary thyroid carcinoma by a new extraction technique. Clin Chem 1984; 30:511–514.

300. Ghillani P, Motte P, Bohuon C, et al. Monoclonal antipeptide antibodies as tools to dissect closely related gene products: a model using peptides encoded by the calcitonin gene. J Immunol 1988; 141:3156–3163.

301. Samaan NA, Castillo S, Schultz PN, et al. Serum calcitonin after pentagastrin stimulation in patients with bronchogenic and breast cancer compared to that in patients with medullary thyroid carcinoma. J Clin Endocrinol Metab 1980; 51:237–241.

302. Wohllk N, Cote GJ, Evans D, et al. Application of genetic screening information to the management of medullary thyroid carcinoma and multiple endocrine neoplasia. Endocrinol Metab Clin North Am 1996; 25:1–25.

303. Easton DF, Ponder MA, Cummings T, et al. The clinical and screening age-at-onset distribution for the MEN-2 syndrome. Am J Hum Genet 1989; 44:208–215.

304. Gagel RF, Jackson CE, Block MA, et al. Age-related probability of development of hereditary medullary thyroid carcinoma. J Pediatr 1982; 101:941–946.

305. Donis-Keller H, Dou S, Chi D, et al. Mutations in the RET proto-oncogene are associated with MEN 2A and FMTC. Hum Mol Genet 1993; 2:851–856.

306. Mulligan LM, Eng C, Attie T, et al. Diverse phenotypes associated with exon 10 mutations of the RET proto-oncogene. Hum Mol Genet 1994; 3:2163–2167.

307. Zedenius J, Wallin G, Hamberger B, et al. Somatic and MEN 2A de novo mutations identified in the RET proto-oncogene by screening of sporadic MTCs. Hum Mol Genet 1994; 3:1259–1262.

308. Komminoth P, Kunz EK, Matias-Guiu X, et al. Analysis of RET proto-oncogene point mutations distinguishes heritable from nonheritable medullary thyroid carcinomas. Cancer 1995; 76:479–489.

309. Mulligan LM, Eng C, Healey CS, et al. A de novo mutation of the ret proto-oncogene in a patient with MEN 2A. Hum Mol Genet 1994; 3:1007–1008.

310. Ponder BA, Ponder MA, Coffey R, et al. Risk estimation and screening in families of patients with medullary thyroid carcinoma. Lancet 1988; 1:397–401.

311. Tateishi R, Wada A, Ishiguro S, et al. Coexistence of bilateral pheochromocytoma and pancreatic islet cell tumor: report of a case and review of the literature. Cancer 1978; 42:2928–2934.

312. Anderson RJ, Lufkin EG, Sizemore GW, et al. Acromegaly and pituitary adenoma with phaeochromocytoma: a variant of multiple endocrine neoplasia. Clin Endocrinol (Oxf) 1981; 14:605–612.

313. Cameron D, Spiro HM, Landsberg L. Zollinger-Ellison syndrome with multiple endocrine adenomatosis type II. N Engl J Med 1978; 299:152–153 (letter).

314. Tuch BE, Carter JN, Armellin GM, et al. The association of a tumour of the posterior pituitary gland with multiple endocrine neoplasia type 1. Aust NZ J Med 1982; 12:179–181.

315. Bertrand JH, Ritz P, Reznik Y, et al. Sipple's syndrome associated with a large prolactinoma. Clin Endocrinol (Oxf) 1987; 27:607–614.

316. Gough DB, Thompson GB, Crotty TB, et al. Diverse clinical and pathologic features of gastric carcinoid and the relevance of hypergastrinemia. World J Surg 1994; 18:473–479; discussion 479–480.

317. Gilligan CJ, Lawton GP, Tang LH, et al. Gastric carcinoid tumors: the biology and therapy of an enigmatic and controversial lesion. Am J Gastroenterol 1995; 90:338–352.

318. Ahlman H, Kolby L, Lundell L, et al. Clinical management of gastric carcinoid tumors. Digestion 1994; 3:77–85.

319. Binkovitz LA, Johnson CD, Stephens DH. Islet cell tumors in von Hippel-Lindau disease: increased prevalence and relationship to the multiple endocrine neoplasias. AJR Am J Roentgenol 1990; 155:501–505.

320. Hough DM, Stephens DH, Johnson CD, et al. Pancreatic lesions in von Hippel-Lindau disease: prevalence, clinical significance, and CT findings. AJR Am J Roentgenol 1994; 162:1091–1094.

321. Filling-Katz MR, Choyke PL, Oldfield E, et al. Central nervous system involvement in von Hippel-Lindau disease. Neurology 1991; 41:41–46.

322. Neumann HP, Dinkel E, Brambs H, et al. Pancreatic lesions in the von Hippel-Lindau syndrome. Gastroenterology 1991; 101:465–471.

323. La Forgia S, Lasota J, Latif F, et al. Detailed genetic and physical map of the 3p chromosome region surrounding the familial renal cell carcinoma chromosome translocation, t(3; 8)(p14.2; q24.1). Cancer Res 1993; 53:3118–3124.

324. Latif F, Tory K, Gnarra J, et al. Identification of the von Hippel-Lindau disease tumor suppressor gene. Science 1993; 260:1317–1320.

325. Aso T, Lane WS, Conaway JW, et al. Elongin (SIII): a multisubunit regulator of elongation by RNA polymerase II. Science 1995; 269:1439–1443.

326. Duan DR, Pause A, Burgess WH, et al. Inhibition of transcription elongation by the VHL tumor suppressor protein. Science 1995; 269:1402–1406.

327. Kibel A, Iliopoulos O, De Caprio JA, et al. Binding of the von Hippel-Lindau tumor suppressor protein to Elongin B and C. Science 1995; 269:1444–1446.

328. Chen F, Kishida T, Yao M, et al. Germline mutations in the von Hippel-Lindau disease tumor suppressor gene: correlations with phenotype. Hum Mutat 1995; 5:66–75.

329. van Heerden JA, Sizemore GW, Carney JA, et al. Bilateral subtotal adrenal resection for bilateral pheochromocytomas in multiple endocrine neoplasia, type IIa: a case report. Surgery 1985; 98:363–366.

330. Janson KL, Roberts JA, Varela M. Multiple endocrine adenomatosis: in support of the common origin theories. J Urol 1978; 119:161–165.

331. Hull MT, Warfel KA, Muller J, et al. Familial islet cell tumors in von Hippel-Lindau's disease. Cancer 1979; 44:1523–1526.

332. Carney JA, Go VLW, Gordon H, et al. Familial pheochromocytoma and islet cell tumor of the pancreas. Am J Med 1980; 68:515–521.

333. Mori Y, Kiyohara H, Miki T, et al. Pheochromocytoma with prominent calcification and associated pancreatic islet cell tumor. J Urol 1977; 118:843–844.

334. Probst A, Lotz M, Heitz P. Von Hippel-Lindau's disease, syringomyelia and multiple endocrine tumors: a complex neuroendocrinopathy. Virchows Arch (Pathol Anat) 1978; 378:265–272.

335. Nathan DM, Daniels GH, Ridgway EC. Gastrinoma and phaeochromocytoma: is there a mixed multiple endocrine adenoma syndrome? Acta Endocrinol 1980; 93:91–93.

336. Zeller JR, Kauffman HM, Komorowski RA, et al. Bilateral pheochromocytoma and islet cell adenoma of the pancreas. Arch Surg 1982; 117:827–830.

337. Cantor AM, Rigby CC, Beck PR, et al. Neurofibromatosis, phaeochromocytoma, and somatostatinoma. Br Med J 1982; 285:1618–1619.

338. Chakrabarti S, Murugesan A, Arida EJ. The association of neurofibromatosis and hyperparathyroidism. Am J Surg 1979; 137:417–420.

339. Saurenmann P, Binswanger R, Maurer R, et al. Somatostatin-producing endocrine pancreatic tumor in Recklinghausen's neurofibromatosis: case report and literature review. Schweiz Med Wochenschr 1987; 117:1134–1139.

340. Chen CH, Lin JT, Lee WY, et al. Somatostatin-containing carcinoid tumor of the duodenum in neurofibromatosis: report of a case. J Formos Med Assoc 1993; 92:900–903.

341. van Basten JP, van Hoek B, de Bruine A, et al. Ampullary carcinoid and neurofibromatosis: case report and review of the literature. Neth J Med 1994; 44:202–206.

342. Hansen OP, Hansen M, Hansen HH, et al. Multiple endocrine adenomatosis of mixed type. Acta Med Scand 1976; 200:327–331.

343. Habiby R, Silverman B, Listernick R, et al. Precocious puberty in children with neurofibromatosis type 1. J Pediatr 1995; 126:364–367.

344. Nur-E-Kamal MS, Varga M, Maruta H. The GTPase-activating NF1 fragment of 91 amino acids reverses v-Ha-Ras–induced malignant phenotype. J Biol Chem 1993; 268:22331–22337.

345. Gutmann DH, Cole JL, Stone WJ, et al. Loss of neurofibromin in adrenal gland tumors from patients with neurofibromatosis type I. Genes Chromosomes Cancer 1994; 10:55–58.

346. Gutmann DH, Geist RT, Rose K, et al. Loss of neurofibromatosis type I (NF1) gene expression in pheochromocytomas from patients without NF1. Genes Chromosomes Cancer 1995; 13:104–109.

347. Brannan CI, Perkins AS, Vogel KS, et al. Targeted disruption of the neurofibromatosis type-1 gene leads to developmental abnormalities in heart and various neural crest–derived tissues. Genes Dev 1994; 8:1019–1029.

348. Farid NR, Buehler S, Russell NA, et al. Prolactinomas in familial multiple endocrine neoplasia syndrome type I: relationship to HLA and carcinoid tumors. Am J Med 1980; 69:874–880.

349. Brandi ML, Marx SJ, Aurbach GD, et al. Familial multiple endocrine neoplasia type I: a new look at pathophysiology. Endocr Rev 1987; 8:391–405.

350. Berezin M, Karasik A. Familial prolactinoma. Clin Endocrinol (Oxf) 1995; 42:483–486.

351. Abbassioun K, Fatourehchi V, Amirjamshidi A, et al. Familial acromegaly with pituitary adenoma: report of three affected siblings. J Neurosurg 1986; 64:510–512.

352. Benlian P, Giraud S, Lahlou N, et al. Familial acromegaly: a specific clinical entity—further evidence from the genetic study of a three-generation family. Eur J Endocrinol 1995; 133:451–456.

353. Himuro H, Kobayashi E, Kono H, et al. Familial occurrence of pituitary adenoma. No Shinkei Geka 1976; 4:371–377.

354. Kurisaka M, Takei Y, Tsubokawa T, et al. Growth hormone–secreting pituitary adenoma in uniovular twin brothers: case report. Neurosurgery 1981; 8:226–230.

355. Levin SR, Hofeldt FD, Becker N, et al. Hypersomatotropism and acanthosis nigricans in two brothers. Arch Intern Med 1974; 134:365–367.

356. Matsuno A, Teramoto A, Yamada S, et al. Gigantism in sibling unrelated to multiple endocrine neoplasia: case report. Neurosurgery 1994; 35:952–955; discussion 955–956.

357. McCarthy MI, Noonan K, Wass JA, et al. Familial acromegaly: studies in three families. Clin Endocrinol (Oxf) 1990; 32:719–728.

358. Pestell RG, Alford FP, Best JD. Familial acromegaly. Acta Endocrinol (Copenh) 1989; 121:286–289.

359. Tamburrano G, Jaffrain-Rea ML, Grossi A, et al. Familial acromegaly: apropos of a case. Review of the literature. Ann Endocrinol (Paris) 1992; 53:201–207.

360. Farndon JR, Leight GS, Dilley WG, et al. Familial medullary thyroid carcinoma without associated endocrinopathies: a distinct clinical entity. Br J Surg 1986; 73:278–281.

361. Irvin GL, III, Fishman LM, Sher JA. Familial pheochromocytoma. Surgery 1983; 94:938–940.

362. Yoshimoto K, Tanaka C, Hamaguchi S, et al. Tumor-specific mutations in the tyrosine kinase domain of the RET proto-oncogene in pheochromocytomas of sporadic type. Endocr J 1995; 42:265–270.

363. Beldjord C, Desclaux-Arramond F, Raffin-Sanson M, et al. The RET proto-oncogene in sporadic pheochromocytomas: frequent MEN 2–like mutations and new molecular defects. J Clin Endocrinol Metab 1995; 80:2063–2068.

364. Gross DJ, Avishai N, Meiner V, et al. Familial pheochromocytoma associated with a novel mutation in the von Hippel-Lindau gene. J Clin Endocrinol Metab 1996; 81:147–149.

365. Carney JA, Gordon H, Carpenter PC, et al. The complex of myxomas, spotty pigmentation, and endocrine overactivity. Medicine (Balt) 1985; 64:270–283.

366. Carney JA. The Carney complex (myxomas, spotty pigmentation, endocrine overactivity, and schwannomas). Dermatol Clin 1995; 13:19–26.

367. Stratakis CA, Carney JA, Lin J-P, et al. Carney complex, a familial multiple neoplasia and lentiginosis syndrome: analysis of 11 kindreds and linkage to the short arm of chromosome 2. J Clin Invest 1996; 97:699–705.

368. Bongarzone I, Pierotti MA, Monzini N, et al. High frequency of activation of tyrosine kinase oncogenes in human papillary thyroid carcinoma. Oncogene 1989; 4:1457–1462.

369. Motokura T, Bloom T, Kim HG, et al. A novel cyclin encoded by a bcl1-linked candidate oncogene. Nature 1991; 350:512–515.

370. Bourne HR, Landis CA, Masters SB. Hydrolysis of GTP by the alpha-chain of Gs and other GTP binding proteins. Proteins 1989; 6:222–230.

371. Viglietto G, Chiappetta G, Martinez-Tello FJ, et al. RET/PTC oncogene activation is an early event in thyroid carcinogenesis. Oncogene 1995; 11:1207–1210.

372. Wallace MR, Marchuk DA, Andersen LB, et al. Type 1 neurofibromatosis gene: identification of a large transcript disrupted in three NF1 patients [published erratum appears in Science 1990 Dec 21; 250(4988):1749]. Science 1990; 249:181–186.

373. Nakamura T, Yana I, Kobayashi T, et al. p53 gene mutations associated with anaplastic transformation of human thyroid carcinomas. Jpn J Cancer Res 1992; 83:1293–1298.

374. Cryns VL, Rubio MP, Thor AD, et al. p53 abnormalities in human parathyroid carcinoma. J Clin Endocrinol Metab 1994; 78:1320–1324.

375. Latif F, Kalman T, Gnarra J, et al. Identification of the von Hippel-Lindau disease tumor suppressor gene. Science 1993; 260:1317–1320.

376. Duan DR, Humphrey JS, Chen DY, et al. Characterization of the VHL tumor suppressor gene product: localization, complex formation, and the effect of natural inactivating mutations. Proc Natl Acad Sci USA 1995; 92:6459–6463.

377. Grieco M, Santoro M, Berlingieri MT, et al. PTC is a novel rearranged form of the ret proto-oncogene and is frequently detected in vivo in human thyroid papillary carcinomas. Cell 1990; 60:557–563.

378. Rosenberg CL, Wong E, Petty EM, et al. PRAD1, a candidate BCL1 oncogene: mapping and expression in centrocytic lymphoma. Proc Natl Acad Sci USA 1991; 88:9638–9642.

379. Mathew CG, Smith BA, Thorpe K, et al. Deletion of genes on chromosome 1 in endocrine neoplasia. Nature 1987; 328:524–526.

380. Takai S, Tateishi H, Nishisho I, et al. Loss of genes on chromosome 22 in medullary thyroid carcinoma and pheochromocytoma. Jpn J Cancer Res 1987; 78:894–898.

381. Cooley LD, Elder FB, Knuth A, et al. Cytogenetic characterization of three human and three rat medullary thyroid carcinoma cell lines. Cancer Genet Cytogenet 1995; 80:138–149.

382. Cryns VL, Thor A, Xu HJ, et al. Loss of the retinoblastoma tumor-suppressor gene in parathyroid carcinoma. N Engl J Med 1994; 330:757–761.

IMMUNOENDOCRINOPATHY SYNDROMES

George S. Eisenbarth and Charles F. Verge

INTRODUCTION

Over the past several years geneticists, immunologists, and endocrinologists have generated a wealth of new information concerning the pathogenesis of the polyglandular autoimmune syndromes and their component disorders. In particular some genetic loci that cause disease susceptibility and the nature of the organ-specific autoantigens involved have been defined. More than one molecule can be the target of autoimmunity for a single organ-specific autoimmune disorder, and in polyglandular autoimmunity multiple molecules of multiple organs are targeted. Autoantibodies for a given disorder can be present before the onset of disease, such as anti-islet antibodies in type I diabetes mellitus[1] and anti-adrenal antibodies in Addison's disease.[2] Each specific autoantibody reacts with only a single autoantigen, although autoantigens may be present in multiple tissues. For example 17α-hydroxylase (CYP17) is present in both the adrenal and the gonads, and the development of hyperthyroidism and ophthalmopathy in Graves' disease implies a shared immune target.[3] For the most part, however, the targets of autoantibodies appear to be unrelated except for their presence as differentiation antigens in specific cells and cellular sites, e.g., a series of insulin secretory granule–associated molecules are autoantigens in type I diabetes mellitus (insulin, islet cell antibody [ICA]512, ICA512β, carboxypeptidase H). In contrast, less is known concerning the specificity of pathogenic T cells. Since cross-reactive recognition by pathogenic T-cell clones may be determined by as few as four properly spaced amino acids of a nonapeptide,[4] there is considerable potential for varying patterns of autoimmunity to be influenced by cross-reactive T cells.

There are two distinct polyglandular autoimmune syndromes (Table 33–1). Polyglandular autoimmune syndrome type I (PGA-I) is a rare disorder with autosomal recessive inheritance caused by mutation of an unidentified gene that maps near the tip of the long arm of chromosome 21.[5] In contrast the most common syndrome discussed in this chapter, polyglandular autoimmune syndrome type II (PGA-II) includes patients with overlapping groups of disorders. A unifying characteristic of PGA-II is the strong association with polymorphic genes of the human leukocyte antigen (HLA) region on the short arm of chromosome 6 (band 6p21.3). In addition to HLA other genetic loci contribute to one's susceptibility to PGA-II. This syndrome has also been known by other names: Schmidt's syndrome, polyglandular failure syndrome, organ-specific autoimmune disease, and polyendocrinopathy diabetes. Studies of PGA-II were instrumental in identifying the autoimmune basis of several diseases and in developing autoantibody assays, e.g., type I diabetes mellitus and cytoplasmic ICAs. Each of the preceding eponymic terms has some shortcoming, such as failure to include the fact that both hyperfunction and hypofunction of endocrine glands can occur or failure to recognize that nonendocrine disorders such as pernicious anemia and celiac disease are a part of the syndrome. Subdividing patients with PGA-II on the basis of specific groups of component diseases adds little information in terms of predicting the likelihood for the development of future disorders in affected individuals or their relatives. In this chapter, therefore, we discuss PGA-I and PGA-II. The spectrum of disorders that may be present in these syndromes is listed in Table 33–1, and the major differences between the two syndromes are highlighted in Table 33–2.

AUTOIMMUNITY PRIMER (also see Chapter 7)

The major determinants of autoimmune endocrine disease are T lymphocytes and autoantibodies produced by B lymphocytes. These two arms of the immune system differ

TABLE 33–1. Component Disorders of the Polyglandular Autoimmune Syndromes*

Type I	Type II
Endocrine	
Addison's disease[10, 49, 55, 83]	**Addison's disease**[10, 55, 84–87]
Hypoparathyroidism[10, 49]	**Type I diabetes**[34, 85, 86, 93]
Primary hypogonadism[49, 83, 89, 90]	**Hypothyroidism**[24, 84, 94, 95]
Type I diabetes[10, 49]	**Graves' disease**[24]
Hypothyroidism[10, 49]	"Geriatric" hypoparathyroidism[17, 88]
	Primary hypogonadism[90–92]
	Hypophysitis[96–102]
Gastrointestinal	
Mucocutaneous candidiasis[10, 49]	
Chronic active hepatitis[10, 49]	
Malabsorption[10, 49, 52, 103, 104]	Celiac disease[11, 12, 105, 106]
Oral squamous cell carcinoma[49]	
Dermatologic	
Mucocutaneous candidiasis[10, 49]	
Alopecia[10, 49, 107, 108]	Alopecia[109]
Vitiligo[10, 49, 110]	Vitiligo[111]
	Dermatitis herpetiformis[106]
Nail dystrophy[49]	
Hematologic	
Pernicious anemia[10, 49]	Pernicious anemia[93, 112]
Pure red cell hypoplasia[115, 116]	Idiopathic thrombocytopenic purpura[113, 114]
Neurologic	
	Myasthenia gravis[118, 119]
Myopathy[117]	Stiff-man syndrome[120]
	Parkinson's disease[121]
Other Manifestations	
Dental enamel hypoplasia[49, 50, 122]	
Keratopathy[125]	IgA deficiency[123, 124]
Tympanic membrane calcification[49]	Serositis[126]
Vascular calcification[128]	Goodpasture's syndrome[127]
Asplenism[51]	Idiopathic heart block[129]

*The most common features are shown in bold type.

fundamentally in their recognition of target antigens. Autoantibodies react with intact molecules (including both soluble and cell surface) and usually interact with conformational determinants of the autoantigen.

In contrast, T lymphocytes recognize peptide fragments of autoantigens, often 8 to 15 amino acids in length. Furthermore T cells can recognize peptides only if they are presented on the surface of another cell by major histocompatibility molecules (HLA). These molecules serve as markers of self and distinguish the cells of one individual from those of another. CD4-positive (helper) T cells react with antigenic peptides that are derived from the extracellular fluid and are bound by class II histocompatibility molecules (HLA-DP, HLA-DQ, or HLA-DR in humans) on the surface of specialized antigen-presenting cells such as macrophages, dendritic cells, and B lymphocytes. In response the helper T cells may secrete various lymphokines that promote the differentiation of other immune cells, leading to an immune response to the antigen. CD8-positive (cytotoxic) T cells react with peptides bound by class I histocompatibility molecules (HLA-A, HLA-B, and HLA-C) present on the surface of nearly all nucleated cells. The antigen peptide in this case is derived from within the presenting cell. Recognition of antigen of viral origin typically leads to the release of cytotoxic chemicals that kill the infected cell. However the simple expression of histocompatibility molecules and the recognition of antigen by a T cell is not sufficient for T-cell activation. Co-stimulatory molecules, such as a cell surface molecule termed *B7*, are essential for T-cell activation. In the absence of co-stimulatory molecules, engagement of a T-cell receptor leads to inactivation, rather than stimulation, of the responding T lymphocyte. Co-stimulatory molecules are expressed by antigen-presenting cells. The hypothesis that expression of histocompatibility antigens by endocrine cells is the cause rather than the consequence of autoimmunity has largely been abandoned as the preceding pathway for T-cell stimulation has been unraveled.

The crystal structures of histocompatibility molecules have been elucidated, and these molecules resemble a "hot-dog bun," with the antigenic peptide (the hotdog) bound in the groove of the histocompatibility molecule (the bun). Histocompatibility molecules are extremely polymorphic, with different amino acids lining the peptide-binding groove. These variable amino acids determine which antigens are bound and presented to T lymphocytes. Molecular HLA typing has revealed many subtypes of the older serologically defined alleles, and the unique genetic sequence encoding each polymorphic chain of the histocompatibility molecules is now given a unique identifying number. Thus for the DQ molecule, which is the histocompatibility molecule most strongly associated with endocrine autoimmunity, each alpha and beta chain is given a number. An example is DQA1*0501 for the alpha chain and DQB1*0201 for the beta chain of the DQ molecule commonly encoded on DR3 haplotypes. This DQ molecule is strongly associated with type I diabetes mellitus, Addison's disease, Graves' disease, and celiac disease.[6] Each allele with its amino acid sequence is inherited in mendelian fashion and determines peptide binding and presentation.

On activation CD8-positive T cells can directly lyse cells. CD4-positive cells are also capable (without CD8-positive T cells) of destroying target cells. CD4-positive T cells apparently kill through indirect pathways that include the induction of macrophages to produce cytokines and free radicals. CD4-positive T lymphocytes are also essential for activation and maturation of B lymphocytes that produce autoantibodies. As a simplification, there are two major pathways of CD4-positive T-cell activation (and subsets of T cells termed *Thy-1* and *Thy-2*). Thy-1 cells produce proinflammatory cytokines such as interferon γ. Thy-2 cells produce lymphokines that suppress Thy-1 cells and favor antibody production (e.g., interleukin-4). Thus depending on the context of T-cell stimulation, T-cell activation may actually down-regulate rather than promote autoimmunity. The Thy-2 pathway is probably important for the induction of "oral tolerance," whereby the oral exposure to autoantigens suppresses autoimmunity. Such therapy is being studied for several autoimmune disorders, including type I diabetes mellitus, multiple sclerosis, and uveitis.

Given the preceding background, the natural history of autoimmune disorders can be divided into a series of stages beginning with genetic susceptibility, followed by triggering of autoimmunity (e.g., dietary gliadin exposure in celiac disease), active autoimmunity preceding clinical manifestations (e.g., progressive glandular destruction), and finally overt disease. An etiologic classification of autoimmunity based on initiating factors can be developed and illustrates the many ways autoimmunity, even to a single organ, can be initiated (Table 33–3). For example myasthenia gravis has a drug-induced form (peni-

TABLE 33–2. Contrasting Features of the Polyglandular Autoimmune Syndromes

Type I	Type II
Autosomal recessive inheritance (only siblings affected)	Polygenic inheritance (multiple generations may be affected)
No HLA association (linked to chromosome 21q22.3[5])	HLA-DR3 and HLA-DR4 associated
Equal sex incidence	Female preponderance
Onset in infancy or youth	Peak incidence ages 20 to 60
Mucocutaneous candidiasis	No mucocutaneous candidiasis
Destructive hypoparathyroidism	Hypoparathyroidism rare (antibody mediated[17])
Type I diabetes mellitus rare in children (but lifetime frequency ~12%[49])	Type I diabetes mellitus common

TABLE 33–3. An "Etiologic" Classification of Autoimmunity[130]

Category	Example	Autoimmune Disease	HLA Association
Oncogenic	Ovarian carcinoma	Cerebellar degeneration[131]	
Drug induced	Methimazole	Insulin autoimmune syndrome[132]	DR4 (DRB1*0405)
Diet induced	Penicillamine	Myasthenia gravis[133]	DR7 (DQA1*0201, DQB1*0201)
	Gluten	Celiac disease[21]	DR3 or DR5/DR7 in trans (DQA1*0501, DQB1*0201)
Infectious	Group B streptococci	Rheumatic heart disease[134]	
	Congenital rubella	Increased frequency of type I diabetes mellitus[77]	DR3 (DQA1*0501, DQB1*0201)/ DR4 (DQA1*0301, DQB1*0302)
Cytokine induced	Interferon α	Thyroiditis[135]	
Unknown		Type I diabetes mellitus[136]	DR3 (DQA1*0501, DQB1*0201)/ DR4 (DQA1*0301, DQB1*0302)
		Addison's disease[10]	DR3 (DQA1*0501, DQB1*0201)/ DR4 (DQA1*0301, DQB1*0302)
		Multiple sclerosis[137]	DR2 (DQA1*0102, DQB1*0602)
		Stiff-man syndrome[138]	DR3 (DQA1*0501, DQB1*0201)

cillamine), an oncogenic form (thymoma associated), and the most common idiopathic form.

For the most common autoimmune disorders only a subset of basic immunologic questions are answered (what genes determine susceptibility, what activates autoimmunity, what are the target molecules, and what are the immunologic effector molecules?). For animal models there has been considerable progress in answering these questions so that immunomodulatory therapies are now being tested in these models. For example the two major animal models of type I diabetes mellitus are also models of polyendocrine autoimmunity. The NOD (nonobese diabetic) mouse and the BB (BioBreeding) rat acquire thyroiditis, and the NOD mouse has sialitis resembling Sjögren's syndrome. For the NOD mouse T-cell clones are able to transfer disease, and a major subset of these clones recognizes an immunodominant peptide of insulin.[7] Administration of this peptide or other autoantigens by various routes (oral, subcutaneous, intranasal) prevents diabetes.[8] Concepts developed in these animal models may lead to safe and effective therapy for the human disorders of autoimmunity.

POLYGLANDULAR AUTOIMMUNE SYNDROME TYPE II

Clinical Definition

PGA-II is the most common of the immunoendocrinopathy syndromes, occurs more often in females than in males, usually has its onset in adulthood, and is familial in nature. PGA-II is usually defined by the occurrence in the same individual of two or more of the following: primary adrenal insufficiency or Addison's disease (Fig. 33–1; see color section at the front of this volume), Graves' disease, autoimmune thyroiditis, type I diabetes mellitus, primary hypogonadism, myasthenia gravis, and celiac disease. Vitiligo, alopecia, serositis, and pernicious anemia also occur with increased frequency in individuals with this syndrome and in their family members. The definition of the syndrome relies on the fact that if one of the component disorders is present, an associated disorder occurs more commonly than in the general population. Circulating organ-specific autoantibodies can be present in the absence of overt clinical disease. In one study of 10 families with PGA-II, one in seven relatives had unsuspected illness, most commonly autoimmune thyroid disease.[9] The initial lesion and precipitating events that result in the syndrome are unknown, but the time course and the pathogenesis of each of the component disorders share many features in common.

The time course of the development of organ-specific

autoimmunity makes it necessary to re-evaluate both patients with the syndrome and their families repeatedly over time. In a family in which the syndrome has been diagnosed, relatives should be advised of the early symptoms and signs of the principal component diseases. Relatives of patients with the syndrome should have a medical history, physical examination, and laboratory screening every 3 to 5 y, with measurement of fasting blood glucose, thyrotropin, and serum vitamin B$_{12}$ levels and, if symptoms or signs suggestive of adrenal insufficiency are present, an assay of corticotropin-stimulated cortisol levels. In addition documenting the presence of specific autoantibodies should heighten concern about current or potential disease.

Among 224 patients with Addison's disease and PGA-II reported by Neufeld and colleagues,[10] type I diabetes mellitus (52%) and autoimmune thyroid disease (69%) were the most common coexisting conditions. Less common features included vitiligo (5%) and gonadal failure (4%).

Among patients with type I diabetes mellitus, thyroid autoimmunity and celiac disease coexist with sufficient frequency to justify screening. Thyroid peroxidase autoantibodies are present in 10% of children with type I diabetes mellitus,[11] and this frequency increases with age. However, thyroid autoantibodies may be present without progression to overt thyroid disease. Thus annual measurement of thyrotropin levels in individuals with type I diabetes mellitus is recommended as cost-effective. Approximately 2 to 3% of patients with type I diabetes mellitus have celiac disease,[11–13] and screening can be performed by measuring antiendomysial autoantibodies.[14] If antiendomysial autoantibodies are present, small bowel biopsy is warranted to determine whether celiac disease has developed. Even asymptomatic celiac disease may be associated with osteopenia[15] and impaired growth.[13] Untreated symptomatic celiac disease is also associated with an increased risk of gastrointestinal malignancy, especially lymphoma.[16]

Hypoparathyroidism is rare in PGA-II (although it is common in PGA-I). If hypocalcemia occurs in a patient with the type II syndrome, celiac disease is a more likely cause than is primary hypoparathyroidism. Nevertheless we have described several elderly patients with polyglandular autoimmune syndrome type II who had a distinct form of hypoparathyroidism which, based on a small series of patients, may be termed geriatric hypoparathyroidism.[17] These patients form a distinct group because they have antibodies to parathyroid cells capable of suppressing parathyroid function and they have a self-limited course of hypoparathyroidism.

Immunogenetics

Although there is familial aggregation of PGA-II and its component disorders, there is no clearly discernible pattern of

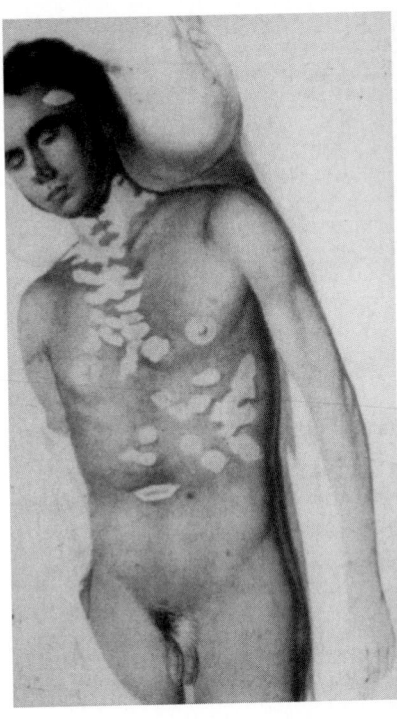
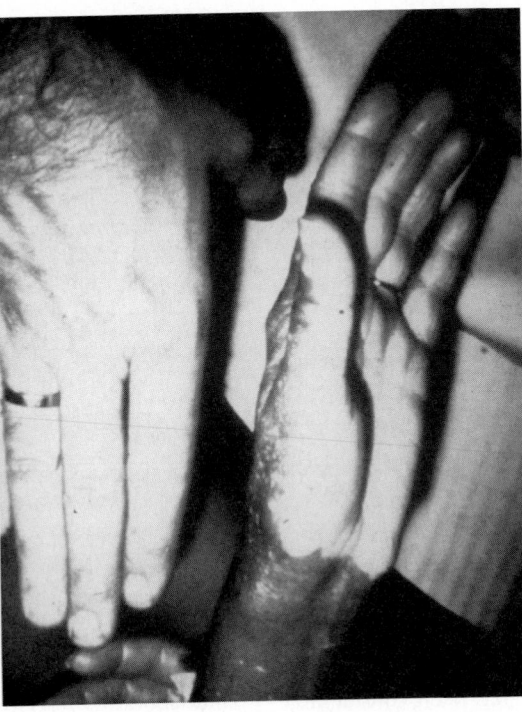

Figure 33–1. *Left,* Reproduction of a plate from Addison's initial description of primary adrenal insufficiency (Addison's disease). *Right,* Hand of a patient with vitiligo and hyperpigmentation of Addison's disease (see color section at the front of this volume). (*Left,* From Addison T. On the Constitutional and Local Effects of Disease of the Supra-renal Capsules. London: Samuel Highley, 1855: plate XI, with permission. *Right,* Courtesy of F. Neelon.)

inheritance. Susceptibility is probably determined by multiple genetic loci (with HLA having the strongest effect) that interact with environmental factors. In the case of celiac disease a dietary precipitating antigen (gliadin) has been identified. For type I diabetes mellitus the concordance in identical twins is relatively low (approximately 35%),[18] suggesting a possible role for environmental or other nongenetic factors such as somatic mutation or the random rearrangement of T-cell receptors that occurs during the development of the immune system. However, identical twins may acquire diabetes after a prolonged period of discordance (Fig. 33–2). Furthermore two thirds of long-term discordant twins (>7 y) had persistent autoantibodies or loss of first-phase insulin release, or both,[19] suggesting that the concordance for beta cell autoimmunity is higher than that for overt diabetes mellitus.

Many of the disorders of PGA-II are associated with an HLA-extended haplotype formed by HLA-A1, HLA-B8, HLA-DR3, DQA1*0501, DQB1*0201. These include Graves' disease, atrophic thyroiditis, type I diabetes mellitus (also HLA-DR4

associated), Addison's disease (also HLA-DR4 associated), myasthenia gravis, and celiac disease.[6, 10, 20, 21] Figure 33–3 illustrates a family in which seven members have type I diabetes mellitus, and three members have Addison's disease. The HLA alleles explain the high frequency of autoimmunity in this family because the father is homozygous for the high-risk HLA-DR4, DQA1*0301, DQB1*0302 haplotype, and thus all of his offspring inherited this allele. The mother is heterozygous for the high-risk HLA-DR3 haplotype, which was inherited by six of her eight children.

For some disorders the complete HLA haplotype is associated with disease, whereas for celiac disease the most specific association is with the two chains of the DQ molecule. Celiac disease occurs primarily in individuals expressing DQA1*0501, DQB1*0201, either in *cis* (with both of these alleles from the preceding extended HLA-DR3 haplotype on the same chromosome) or in *trans* (with HLA-DR5 with DQA1*0501, DQB1*0101 from an HLA-DR5 haplotype on one chromosome 6 and DQA1*0201, DQB1*0201 from HLA-DR7 on the other chromosome 6). There are approximately 100 genes within the major histocompatibility complex on the short arm of chromosome 6, including genes that influence the processing and transport of antigenic peptides. For celiac disease the HLA contribution to disease may be limited to the DQ molecule (DQA1*0501, DQB1*0201). In contrast for type I diabetes mellitus and several other component disorders of PGA-II, HLA genes in addition to DQ appear to contribute to susceptibility.[22]

Although some HLA alleles increase disease risk, others are associated with protection from disease. For example the DQ alleles DQA1*0102, DQB1*0602 (usually associated with HLA-DR2) confer strong protection from type I diabetes mellitus in a dominant fashion[23] but confer susceptibility to another autoimmune disorder, namely multiple sclerosis. This may explain the rarity of both multiple sclerosis and type I diabetes mellitus in the same individual, despite the existence of families in which both disorders occur in different individuals.

For both type I diabetes mellitus and Addison's disease in PGA-II, the highest risk is conferred by heterozygosity for HLA-DR3 (DQA1*0501, DQB1*0201) and HLA-DR4

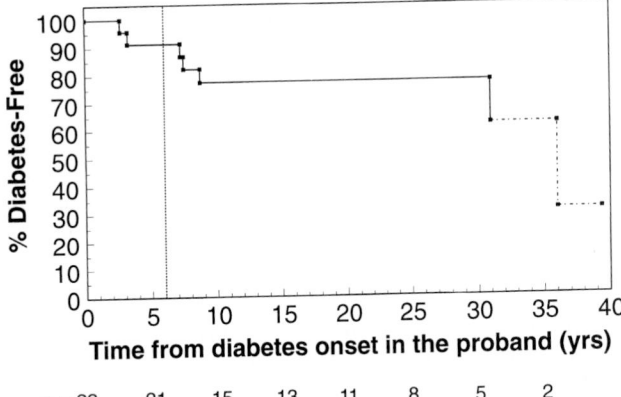

Figure 33–2. Life table analysis of the development of diabetes of initially discordant identical twins. (From Verge CF, Gianani R, Yu L, et al. Late progression to diabetes and evidence for chronic beta cell autoimmunity in identical twins of patients with type I diabetes. Diabetes 1995; 44:1176–1179, with permission.)

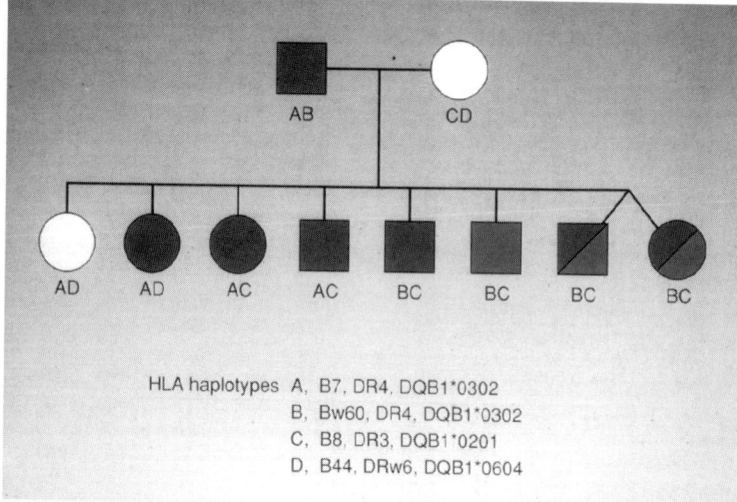

Figure 33–3. Polyendocrine type II family with Addison's disease and type I diabetes. (From Eisenbarth GS, Bellgrau D. Autoimmunity. Scientific American: Science and Medicine 1994; 1:38–47, with permission.)

HLA haplotypes A, B7, DR4, DQB1*0302
B, Bw60, DR4, DQB1*0302
C, B8, DR3, DQB1*0201
D, B44, DRw6, DQB1*0604

(DQA1*0301, DQB1*0302) haplotypes.[20] Approximately 2 to 3% of the United States population and approximately 35% of individuals who acquire type I diabetes mellitus carry this high-risk combination. In an ongoing study in Denver, 10,000 newborns from the general population will have HLA typing performed on cord blood, and those with HLA-DR3/4 will be followed from birth for the appearance of anti-islet autoantibodies. Preliminary results indicate that a significant proportion of these genetically at-risk infants acquire anti-islet autoimmunity by 9 mo of age (M. Rewers, unpublished observations). The risk of diabetes mellitus for such children is estimated to be similar to the risk for an infant born to a father with type I diabetes mellitus (approximately 6% risk).

Several component disorders of PGA II are not associated with HLA-DR3,[24, 25] including pernicious anemia, goitrous thyroiditis, and vitiligo. The latter is a typical component of the syndrome and was present in one of Addison's original patients (see Fig. 33–1). These relatively common disorders may have more than one pathogenic mechanism, one of which is associated with polyglandular autoimmunity.

Attempts have been made to simplify the identification of DQ alleles conferring high risk for type I diabetes mellitus. Most diabetes-associated DQ molecules have an amino acid other than aspartic acid at position 57 of the DQ beta chain (non-Asp57). However there are exceptions to this rule, and no one element within the HLA region may determine diabetes susceptibility. Rather the complete amino acid sequence may confer risk, and this is easy to type for with DNA-based typing.

Given the hypothesis that HLA molecules determine the tissue targeting of autoimmunity, whereas other genetic loci predispose to autoimmunity in general, there has been an intensive effort to identify these non-HLA loci. Unlike PGA-I (discussed later), multiple loci are probably involved in PGA-II. For type I diabetes mellitus, polymorphisms of the insulin gene contribute to disease susceptibility,[26] and there is tentative evidence suggesting linkage to other loci.[27]

Organ-Specific Autoantibodies

Better assays for organ-specific autoantibodies have been developed with the cloning of the genes for specific autoantigens and the development of assays that use recombinant antigen. These radioassays are superior to assays based on immunofluorescence in tissue sections, such as ICA testing. The most notable finding has been the recognition that a large number of different autoantigens are targeted in a single autoimmune disorder. Most of the endocrine autoantigens are hormones (such as insulin) or enzymes associated with differentiated endocrine function (thyroid peroxidase in thyroiditis, glutamic acid decarboxylase[28] and carboxypeptidase H[29] in type I diabetes, CYP21 in Addison's disease,[30, 31] and the parietal cell enzyme H^+/K^+-ATPase in pernicious anemia).[32]

In type I diabetes mellitus the four most informative assays measure autoantibodies that react with insulin, GAD65 (glutamic acid decarboxylase), ICA512/IA-2, and ICA512β. Expression of any one of these autoantibodies is associated with only a small increase in the risk of type I diabetes mellitus. In particular, high levels of GAD65 autoantibodies (which can become manifested as a particular form of ICA, termed *selective* or *restricted*) carry a low risk of diabetes mellitus and may be associated with the protective HLA-DQ alleles DQA1*0102, DQB1*0602.[33, 34] In contrast, the expression of multiple autoantibodies is associated with a greatly enhanced risk of diabetes (Fig. 33–4), whereas none of 200 healthy control subjects expressed more than a single one of these autoantibodies, indicating high pathogenic specificity for their presence in combination.[35]

In a similar manner adrenal autoantibodies that react with steroid 21-hydroxylase (CYP21)[30, 36] can usually be detected before the development of Addison's disease,[2] and metabolic progression to adrenal insufficiency can be charted.[37] A radioimmunoassay for the detection of autoantibodies that react with the enzyme CYP21 appears to provide excellent specificity and sensitivity for diagnosing incipient or overt adrenal insufficiency.[38] In contrast, thyroid autoantibodies can be present for long periods without progression to overt disease and provide little prognostic information in the absence of elevated thyrotropin levels.

In contrast to the polyglandular autoimmune disorders with T-cell–mediated glandular destruction, autoantibodies may also be pathogenic. A hallmark of pathogenic autoantibodies is the neonatal autoimmune disease due to transplacental passage of autoantibody. Examples include neonatal Graves' disease (due to antithyrotropin [also called thyroid-stimulating hormone or TSH] receptor autoantibodies) and neonatal myasthenia gravis (due to anti–acetyl choline receptor autoantibodies).[39]

Therapy

Treatment of the individual diseases of the polyglandular autoimmune syndrome is discussed in other chapters of this

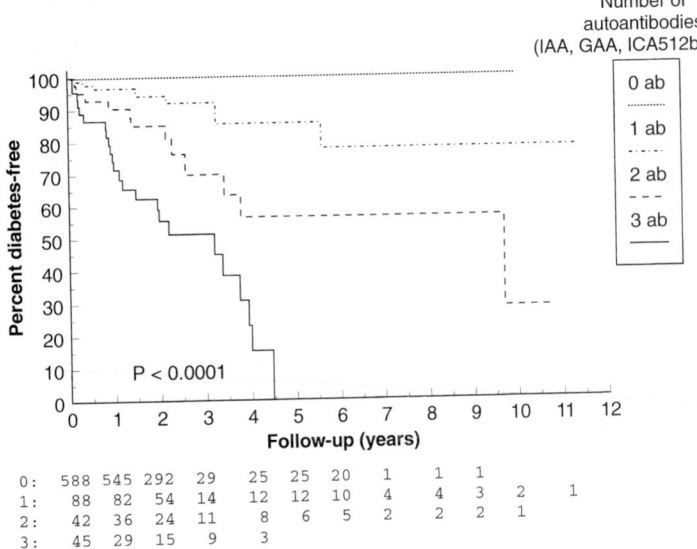

Figure 33–4. The diabetes-free survival of first-degree relatives of patients with type I diabetes, according to the number of autoantibodies present at baseline assessment, considering insulin, glutamic acid decarboxylase, and ICA512 autoantibodies measured by radioassay. (From Verge CF, Gianani R, Kawasaki E, et al. Prediction of type I diabetes mellitus in first-degree relatives using a combination of insulin, glutamic acid decarboxylase and ICA512bdc/IA2 autoantibodies. Diabetes 1996; 45:926–933, with permission.)

book. Therapeutic considerations related specifically to PGA-II include the following:

1. Many of the component disorders of the syndrome have a long prodromal phase and are associated with the expression of autoantibodies before overt disease develops. The manner in which the disorders develop allows the consideration of disease prediction and clinical trials for prevention. This is particularly important for type I diabetes mellitus but is also likely for Addison's disease, hypogonadism, and Graves' disease. Studies evaluating immunosuppressive drugs in this disorder have contributed to our understanding of autoimmunity, and it is clear that broad immunosuppressive therapies are not appropriate for most of these disorders. This is particularly true for drugs such as cyclosporin A for new-onset type I diabetes mellitus. During cyclosporine administration some residual insulin secretion can be preserved. However the extent of beta-cell destruction at diagnosis precludes long-term remission of diabetes, and this drug can be both nepthrotoxic and "oncogenic."

An area of immunomodulatory therapy under investigation (especially for type I diabetes mellitus) relates to "isohormonal" therapy[40] of endocrine autoimmunity. Such therapies use the hormonal product of the target organ to influence autoimmunity. Such therapies may act by feedback inhibition of glandular function, bystander suppression of autoimmunity, induction of immunologic tolerance to the relevant hormone, or more than one of these mechanisms. The basic observation is that in animal models of type I diabetes mellitus, oral or nasal administration of insulin or peptides derived from insulin prevents diabetes and decreases isleitis. Mucosal administration of antigens is frequently associated with bystander immunosuppression, in which T cells specific to the antigen are apparently induced to produce suppressive cytokines (e.g., transforming growth factor β and interleukin-10). In addition, subcutaneous administration of insulin prevents diabetes and isleitis in animal models, whereas subcutaneous administration of insulin peptides in adjuvants can prevent diabetes but not isleitis. Such animal trials have been extended to humans, and a pilot study[41] suggests that a combination of daily subcutaneous insulin and intermittent intravenous insulin may delay type I diabetes mellittus (see Fig. 33–5). A large trial, the Diabetes Prevention Trial—Type I (DPT-I) is under way in the United States to test this hypothesis. Relatives of patients with type I diabetes mellitus can be screened anywhere in the United States by contacting a participating Center or by calling 1-800-HALT-DM1.

Such "isohormonal" therapy may be applicable to other endocrine disorders such as Graves' disease, autoimmune thyroiditis, and Addison's disease. Hashizume and co-workers reported a lower relapse rate in women with Graves' disease who were given 100 μg thyroxine daily than that in those who did not receive thyroxine,[42] although these results have yet to be confirmed by others (see Chapter 11). Takasu and colleagues reported that autoimmune thyroiditis may be reversible with the disappearance of autoantibodies and maintenance of a euthyroid state in a minority of patients after the cessation of thyroxine therapy.[43] In the BB rat the administration of thyroxine results in a reduced frequency of the appearance of lymphocytic thyroiditis.[44] In preclinical Addison's disease a short course of glucocorticoids appeared to suppress the expression of adrenal autoantibodies and prevent progressive adrenal destruction.[37] De Bellis and co-workers screened patients with organ-specific autoimmune disorder and reported that 0.9% tested positive for adrenal autoantibodies. Three patients with high-titer adrenal autoantibodies and impaired cortisol response to corticotropin (also called adrenocorticotropic hormone [ACTH]) experienced remission and declines in autoantibody titers while receiving glucocorticoids for Graves' ophthalmopathy (Fig. 33–5). In contrast, in other patients with high-titer adrenal autoantibodies the antibodies persisted and various abnormalities developed, including elevated plasma renin activity, impaired cortisol response to corticotropin, elevated corticotropin levels, and overt Addison's disease. Feedback inhibition of endocrine gland function may decrease the exposure of autoantigens to the immune system or decrease the susceptibility of the targeted tissue to immune attack.[37] This preliminary observation will require testing in a larger population and in randomized fashion.

2. Thyroxine therapy can precipitate life-threatening adrenal insufficiency in a patient with untreated adrenal insufficiency and hypothyroidism. Thus it is necessary to evaluate adrenal function in all hypothyroid patients in whom the syndrome is suspected before the institution of such therapy.

3. A decreasing insulin requirement in a patient with type I diabetes mellitus can be one of the earliest indications of adrenal insufficiency, occurring before the development of hyperpigmentation or electrolyte abnormalities.

4. In patients with both adrenal insufficiency and primary hypothyroidism, thyroid function may improve after glucocorticoid replacement.[45]

5. Adrenal crisis that responds to mineralocorticoid therapy can occur in patients receiving potent glucocorticoids for inflammatory disease.[46]

GROUP C

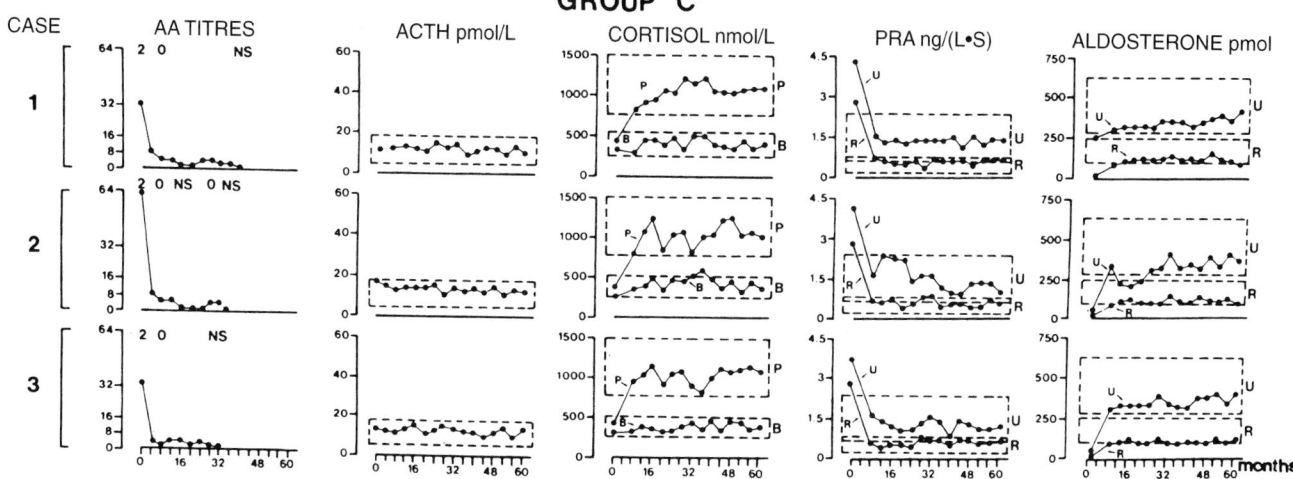

Figure 33–5. Adrenal antibody titers, levels of corticotropin (ACTH), cortisol plasma renin activity (PRA), and aldosterone in three antiadrenal autoantibody–positive patients treated for 6 mo with glucocorticoids for concomitant Graves' ophthalmopathy. (From De Bellis A, Bizzaro A, Rossi R, et al. Remission of subclinical adrenocortical failure in subjects with adrenal autoantibodies. J Clin Endocrinol Metab 1993; 76:1002–1007, with permission. © 1993, the Endocrine Society.)

6. Finally, it is possible that thyroxine therapy may favorably alter the course of Graves' disease,[47] but prospective randomized trials are needed.

POLYGLANDULAR AUTOIMMUNE SYNDROME TYPE I

Clinical Features

PGA-I, also known as autoimmune polyendocrinopathy-candidiasis-ectodermal dystrophy (APECED), is characterized by the triad of mucocutaneous candidiasis, autoimmune hypoparathyroidism, and Addison's disease, although the presence of all three is not needed to make the diagnosis, and various other manifestations may be present (see Table 33–1). The association of mucocutaneous candidiasis with glandular failure was recognized by Thorpe and Handley in 1929.[48] More than 140 patients have since been reported, including two large series from Finland[49] and the United States.[10] PGA-I is usually manifested in early childhood, whereas the type II syndrome has its peak incidence in middle age. Chronic mucocutaneous candidiasis is often the first manifestation, followed by hypoparathyroidism and Addison's disease (Fig. 33–6), but new components can develop at any age.[10, 49] Decades may elapse between the development of one disorder and the onset of another in the same individual. Consequently, lifelong follow-up is important to allow the early detection of additional components.

In a Finnish study reported by Ahonen and co-workers,[49] all patients had chronic candidiasis at some time, 79% experienced hypoparathyroidism, 72% acquired Addison's disease, and 51% had all three of these classic components. Gonadal failure (60% in women, 14% in men) and hypoplasia of the dental enamel (77%) were also common. Other manifestations included alopecia (29%), vitiligo (13%), intestinal malabsorption (18%), pernicious anemia (13%), chronic active hepatitis (12%), and hypothyroidism (4%). The onset of chronic active hepatitis (hepatomegaly, jaundice, or elevated liver enzyme levels) is a potentially serious complication. Type I diabetes mellitus occurred in less than 4% of children, but this frequency increased to approximately 12% in adult life.[49] The presence of chronic candidiasis suggests that a defect in T-cell function may be fundamental to the pathogenesis of this syndrome. Recurrent candidiasis commonly affects the mouth and nails and, less frequently, the skin and esophagus.[49] Other infections do not occur with increased frequency. Ectodermal dystrophy is manifested by pitted nails, keratopathy, and enamel hypoplasia and is not thought to be immune mediated. Enamel hypoplasia may precede the onset of hypoparathyroidism and may affect teeth forming after the hypoparathyroidism is treated.[50] Friedman and colleagues reported asplenism and cholelithiasis as additional features of PGA-I.[51] Malabsorption with steatorrhea is of uncertain origin, is usually intermittent, and may be exacerbated by hypocalcemia. One patient had patchy intestinal lymphangiectasia.[52]

Antiparathyroid and antiadrenal antibodies have been reported.[53] Although CYP21 appears to be the major autoantigen in isolated Addison's disease and in Addison's disease associated with PGA-II, autoantibodies against 17-hydroxylase (CYP17) and side chain cleavage enzyme (CYP11A1) have also been reported in Addison's disease associated with PGA-I.[54, 55] Similar to findings in PGA-II more patients (41%) express

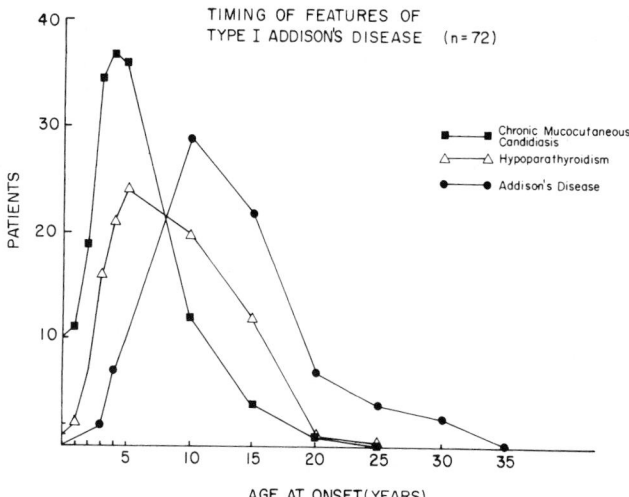

Figure 33–6. The age at onset of mucocutaneous candidiasis, hypoparathyroidism, and adrenal insufficiency in patients with polyglandular autoimmune syndrome type I. (From Neufeld M, Maclaren NK, Blizzard RM. Two types of autoimmune Addison's disease associated with different polyglandular autoimmune (PGA) syndromes. Medicine 1981; 60:355–362, with permission.)

anti-GAD65 autoantibodies than acquire diabetes,[56] suggesting that the finding of antibodies to this single autoantigen has a low positive predictive value. Among PGA-I patients in this study who acquired diabetes, GAD autoantibodies were detected up to 8 y before the onset of overt diabetes.

Genetics

PGA-I is unique among autoimmune endocrine disorders in that it is not associated with class II HLA alleles.[10, 56] Although Addison's disease in PGA-II is strongly associated with HLA-DR3 and HLA-DR4, Addison's disease in PGA-I lacks this HLA association. PGA-I is inherited as an autosomal recessive disorder, with a 25% recurrence risk for siblings of affected individuals.[57] The disorder has a high prevalence in Finland and in Iranian Jews.[58] The genetic locus responsible for the disease has been localized to the short arm of chromosome 21 (near markers D21s49 and D21s171 on 21p22.3) by Aaltonen and co-workers.[5] They carried out linkage analysis with microsatellite markers in 14 Finnish families using a genome-wide strategy and identified founder chromosomes for this rare disorder. This allowed the genetic region to be narrowed to a 500-kb segment of DNA.

Therapy

1. The treatment of adrenal insufficiency and hypoparathyroidism is the same as that discussed in Chapters 12 and 24, respectively, with the caveat that malabsorption may complicate treatment.

2. Mucocutaneous candidiasis is treated with orally active antifungal drugs such as fluconazole[59] and ketoconazole.[60] Infection may recur when the drug is discontinued or the dosage decreased. Patients must be monitored carefully, as ketoconazole may inhibit adrenal and gonadal steroid synthesis, with the potential for precipitating adrenal failure. Ketoconazole can also cause transient elevation of liver enzyme levels and occasionally hepatitis. Fluconazole, although more expensive, is associated with a lower frequency of hepatitis and does not inhibit steroidogenesis when given in the recommended doses.[59]

3. Screening to allow the early detection of new disorders before overt symptoms and signs develop is recommended, including assessment of autoantibodies, electrolytes, calcium and phosphorus levels, thyroid and liver function, blood smears, and vitamin B_{12} levels. Patients at risk for adrenal insufficiency can be screened by measuring basal corticotropin and supine plasma renin activity levels[61] and by dynamic testing as appropriate. Evaluation for asplenism[51] should include abdominal ultrasound and examination of blood smears for Howell-Jolly bodies, and pneumococcal vaccination, and appropriate antibiotic coverage should be given to asplenic patients.

4. Hypocalcemia has been associated with the intermittent steatorrhea characteristic of PGA-I, and therapies that restore calcium levels are reported to be of benefit, including magnesium replacement for hypomagnesemia. Nevertheless in individual patients steatorrhea has been reported to result from pancreatic insufficiency, *Giardia lamblia* infection, and lymphangiectasia, each of which requires individualized therapy.

OTHER POLYGLANDULAR AUTOIMMUNE SYNDROMES

Anti-insulin Receptor Antibodies

In the rare (approximately 25 reported patients) disorder of anti-insulin receptor antibodies—also known as type B insulin resistance and acanthosis nigricans—insulin resistance is due to the presence of anti-insulin receptor antibodies.[62] Approximately one third of patients with these antibodies have an associated autoimmune illness such as systemic lupus erythematosus or Sjögren's syndrome. Arthralgia, vitiligo, alopecia, and secondary amenorrhea have also been reported. One patient had a daughter with hyperthyroidism and a granddaughter with systemic lupus erythematosus. Autoimmune thyroid disease has been described in two such patients, one with hypothyroidism and the other with antithyroid antibodies. Antinuclear antibodies and an elevated erythrocyte sedimentation rate, hyperglobulinemia, leukopenia, and hypocomplementemia are common.[63]

The major clinical manifestations relate to the anti-insulin receptor antibodies. Insulin resistance is profound, so up to 175,000 U of insulin/d may be ineffective in lowering the elevated glucose level. Despite hyperglycemia and marked insulin resistance, ketoacidosis is uncommon. The course of the diabetes is variable, and several patients have had spontaneous remissions. Other patients have had severe hypoglycemia (perhaps related to the insulin-like effects of anti-insulin receptor antibodies demonstrable in vitro).[63] The acanthosis nigricans (Fig. 33–7), which is due to hypertrophy and folding of otherwise histologically normal skin, appears to be related to the insulin-resistant state. Insulin resistance in the absence of anti-receptor antibodies is also associated with acanthosis nigricans.

POEMS Syndrome

The components of the POEMS syndrome (plasma cell dyscrasia with polyneuropathy, organomegaly, endocrinopathy, M protein in plasma, and skin changes) consist of diabetes mellitus (half of patients), primary gonadal failure (70% of patients), plasma cell dyscrasia, sclerotic bone lesions, and neuropathy.[64–69] Patients usually present with severe progressive sensorimotor polyneuropathy, hepatosplenomegaly, lymphadenopathy, or hyperpigmentation and on evaluation are found to have plasma cell dyscrasia and sclerotic bone lesions. The syndrome is assumed to be secondary to circulating im-

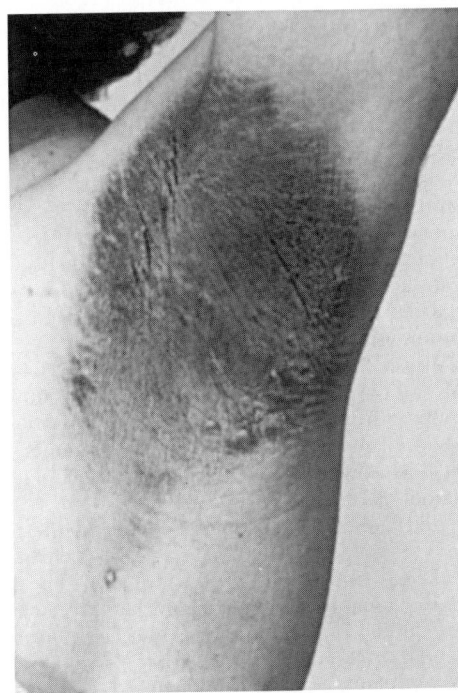

Figure 33–7. A patient with acanthosis nigricans and insulin resistance. (Courtesy of Dr. R. Kahn.)

munoglobulins, but binding of antibody directly to involved tissues has not been demonstrated. The diabetes mellitus responds to small doses of insulin. The hypogonadism is associated with elevated plasma levels of follicle-stimulating hormone and luteinizing hormone. Temporary resolution of disease, including a return of the blood glucose level to normal, may occur after radiotherapy of localized plasma cell lesions of bone.

Kearns-Sayre Syndrome

The Kearns-Sayre syndrome is rare and is also known as oculocraniosomatic disease or oculocraniosomatic neuromuscular disease with ragged red fibers. It is characterized by myopathic abnormalities leading to ophthalmoplegia and progressive weakness in association with several endocrine abnormalities, including hypoparathyroidism, primary gonadal failure, diabetes mellitus, and hypopituitarism.[70] Crystalline mitochondrial inclusions are demonstrable in muscle biopsy specimens, and such inclusions have also been observed in the cerebellum. The relationship between the mitochondrial and the endocrinologic abnormalities is not known. Other features include retinitis pigmentosa and heart block. Antiparathyroid antibodies have not been described; however, antibodies to the anterior pituitary and striated muscle have been found, and the disease may have an autoimmune component.

Thymic Tumors

The thymus has a central role in the ontogeny of cell-mediated immunity. DiGeorge described congenital aplasia of the thymus and parathyroid glands, both of which are derived from the third and fourth pharyngeal pouches. These infants present with tetany secondary to hypocalcemia, severe infections with markedly suppressed T-cell immunity, and normal humoral immunity.

The thymus is a complex tissue with a specialized endocrine epithelium that synthesizes a variety of biologically active peptides involved in the control of T-cell maturation. The epithelium is derived from the neural crest and contains complex gangliosides that react with monoclonal antibody (A2B5) and tetanus toxin in a manner similar to that of pancreatic islets. The role of these peptides of the thymus has not been defined, but they may be trophic factors in T-cell activation and increase in situations of primary failure of T-cell activation, just as the levels of trophic hormones increase in primary endocrine failure.

The disorders associated with thymomas are similar to those in PGA-II,[71] although the frequency of specific disorders is different. In one review myasthenia gravis occurred in 44%, red blood cell aplasia in approximately 20%, hypoglobulinemia in 6%, autoimmune thyroid disease in 2%, and adrenal insufficiency in 1 of 423 patients with thymoma. The frequency of autoimmune thyroid disease reported in patients with thymoma is probably an underestimate given the frequency of unsuspected thyroid disease in patients with myasthenia gravis. Mucocutaneous candidiasis in adults is also associated with thymomas. Thymomas are usually malignant, but remission of autoimmune disease can occur with resection of the tumor and with octreotide therapy.[139]

Trisomy-21

Down syndrome or trisomy-21 is associated with the development of type I diabetes mellitus and thyroiditis. We have observed one patient with a partial distal translocation "leading" to trisomy-21 and "associated" with adrenal insufficiency, celiac disease, hypothyroidism, and type I diabetes mellitus. Patients with trisomy-21 also have T-cell abnormali-

ties, including increased Ia-positive T cells and a premature increase in the 3G5 age-related T-cell subset.[72] It is not known whether the observed chromosomal abnormality influences the development of autoimmunity or whether part of the susceptibility to autoimmunity is associated with chromosomal disorders.[73] Organ-specific autoimmunity also occurs with gonadal dysgenesis.[74]

Congenital Rubella

Patients with congenital rubella have almost a 20% risk of acquiring diabetes mellitus and a higher than normal risk of acquiring thyroiditis and hypothyroidism.[75, 76] Those at highest risk for diabetes mellitus express diabetes-associated HLA-DR3 and HLA-DR4 alleles.[77] It is possible that the rubella virus increases the probability of subsequent autoimmunity because of permanent effects on the developing immune system.[78] Organ-specific autoimmunity can be induced in animals by perturbations of neonatal immune function (neonatal thymectomy, neonatal cyclosporine administration).[79]

Wolfram Syndrome (DIDMOAD)

The Wolfram syndrome is a rare autosomal recessive disease also called DIDMOAD (diabetes insipidus, diabetes mellitus, progressive bilateral optic atrophy, and sensorineural deafness). In addition, neurologic and psychiatric disturbances may cause severe disability. The disease has been mapped to a locus on the short arm of chromosome 4,[80] and magnetic resonance imaging has demonstrated atrophic changes in the brain.[81] The Wolfram syndrome appears to be a slowly progressive neurodegenerative process with a (nonautoimmune) selective destruction of the pancreatic beta cells. Diabetes mellitus is usually the first manifestation in childhood. Diabetes mellitus and optic atrophy are present in all reported cases, but the other features are variable. In one report two related children with the Wolfram syndrome acquired megaloblastic and sideroblastic anemia that responded to treatment with thiamine. Furthermore thiamine treatment was associated with a marked decrease in insulin requirements.[82]

CONCLUSION

The basic pathogenic lesion of the polyglandular autoimmune syndromes is an inherited tendency for the development of antibodies to self molecules. The disease associations and the inheritance pattern make it possible to detect additional components of these syndromes in patients before the appearance of serious manifestations and to make the diagnosis in some first-degree relatives with unrecognized disease. Diagnosis is facilitated by sensitive and specific autoantibody assays.

REFERENCES

1. Verge CF, Gianani R, Kawasaki E, et al. Prediction of type I diabetes mellitus in first degree relatives using a combination of insulin, glutamic acid decarboxylase and ICA512bdc/IA2 autoantibodies. Diabetes 1996; 45:926–933.
2. Betterle C, Zanette F, Zanchetta R, et al. Complement-fixing adrenal autoantibodies as a marker for predicting onset of idiopathic Addison's disease. Lancet 1983; 1:1238–1241.
3. Paschke R, Metcalfe A, Alcalde L, et al. Presence of nonfunctional thyrotropin receptor variant transcripts in retroocular and other tissues. J Clin Endocrinol Metab 1994; 79:1234–1238.
4. Luo A, Garza KM, Hunt D, et al. Antigen mimicry in autoimmune disease sharing of amino acid residues critical for pathogenic T cell activation. J Clin Invest 1993; 92:2117–2123.
5. Aaltonen J, Bjorses P, Sandkuijl L, et al. An autosomal locus causing

autoimmune disease: autoimmune polyglandular disease type I assigned to chromosome 21. Nat Genet 1994; 8:83–87.

6. Badenhoop K, Walfish PG, Rau H, et al. Susceptibility and resistance alleles of human leukocyte antigen (HLA) DQA1 and HLA DQB1 are shared in endocrine autoimmune disease. J Clin Endocrinol Metab 1995; 80:2112–2117.

7. Daniel D, Gill RG, Schloot N, et al. Epitope specificity, cytokine production profile and diabetogenic activity of insulin-specific T cell clones isolated from NOD mice. Eur J Immunol 1995; 25:1056–1062.

8. Daniel D, Wegmann DR. Protection of NOD mice from diabetes by intranasal or subcutaneous administration of insulin peptide B:9–23. Proc Natl Acad Sci 1996; 93:956–960.

9. Eisenbarth GS, Jackson R. Immunogenetics of polyglandular failure and related diseases. In: Farid N, ed. HLA and Endocrine Disease. New York: Academic Press, 1981: 235–264.

10. Neufeld M, Maclaren NK, Blizzard RM. Two types of autoimmune Addison's disease associated with different polyglandular autoimmune (PGA) syndromes. Medicine 1981; 60:355–362.

11. Verge CF, Howard NJ, Rowley MJ, et al. Anti-glutamate decarboxylase and other antibodies at the onset of childhood IDDM: a population-based study. Diabetologia 1994; 37:1113–1120.

12. Savilahti E, Simell O, Koskimies S, et al. Celiac disease in insulin dependent diabetes mellitus. J Pediatr 1986; 108:690–693.

13. Barera G, Bianchi C, Calisti L, et al. Screening of diabetic children for coeliac disease with antigliadin antibodies and HLA typing. Arch Dis Child 1991; 66:491–494.

14. Ferreira M, Davies SL, Butler M, et al. Endomysial antibody: is it the best screening test for coeliac disease? Gut 1992; 33:1633–1637.

15. Mora S, Weber G, Barera G, et al. Effect of gluten-free diet on bone mineral content in growing patients with celiac disease. Am J Clin Nutr 1993; 57:224–228.

16. Holmes GKT, Prior P, Lane MR, et al. Malignancy in coeliac disease—effect of a gluten free diet. Gut 1989; 30:333–338.

17. Posillico JT, Wortsman J, Srikanta S, et al. Parathyroid cell surface autoantibodies that inhibit parathyroid hormone secretion from dispersed human parathyroid cells. Bone Miner Res 1986; 5:475–485.

18. Olmos P, A'Hearn R, Heaton DA, et al. The significance of concordance rate of type I (insulin dependent) diabetes mellitus in identical twins. Diabetologia 1988; 31:747–750.

19. Verge CF, Gianani R, Yu L, et al. Late progression to diabetes and evidence for chronic beta cell autoimmunity in identical twins of patients with type I diabetes. Diabetes 1995; 44:1176–1179.

20. Thomson G, Robinson WP, Kuhner MK, et al. Genetic heterogeneity, modes of inheritance, and risk estimates for a joint study of Caucasians with insulin-dependent diabetes mellitus. Am J Hum Genet 1988; 43:799–816.

21. Bugawan TL, Angelini G, Larrick J, et al. A combination of a particular HLA-DPB1 allele and an HLA-DQ heterodimer confers susceptibility to celiac disease. Nature 1989; 339:470–473.

22. Auwera B, Waeyenberge C, Schuit F, et al. DRB1*0403 protects against IDDM in Caucasians with the high-risk heterozygous DQA1*0301-DQB1*0302/DQA1*502-DQB1*0201 genotype. Diabetes 1995; 44:527–530.

23. Baisch JM, Weeks T, Giles R, et al. Analysis of HLA-DQ genotypes and susceptibility in insulin-dependent diabetes mellitus. N Engl J Med 1990; 322:1836–1841.

24. Santamaria P, Barbosa JJ, Lindstrom AL, et al. HLA-DQB1-associated susceptibility that distinguishes Hashimoto's thyroiditis from Graves' disease in type I diabetic patients. J Clin Endocrinol Metab 1994; 78:878–883.

25. Inoue D, Sato K, Sugawa H, et al. Apparent genetic difference between hypothyroid patients with blocking-type thyrotropin receptor antibody and those without, as shown by restriction fragment length polymorphism analyses of HLA-DP loci [see comments]. J Clin Endocrinol Metab 1993; 77:606–610.

26. Bennett ST, Lucassen AM, Gough SCL, et al. Susceptibility to human type I diabetes at IDDM2 is determined by tandem repeat variation at the insulin gene minisatellite locus. Nat Genet 1995; 9:284–292.

27. McLachlan SM: The genetic basis of autoimmune thyroid disease: time to focus on chromosomal loci other than the major histocompatibility complex (HLA in man). J Clin Endocrinol Metab 1995; 77:605a–605c (editorial).

28. Baekkeskov S, Aanstoot H, Christgau S, et al. Identification of the 64K autoantigen in insulin-dependent diabetes as the GABA-synthesizing enzyme glutamic acid decarboxylase. Nature 1990; 347:151–156.

29. Castano L, Russo E, Zhou L, et al. Identification and cloning of a granule autoantigen (carboxypeptidase H) associated with type I diabetes. J Clin Endocrinol Metab 1991; 73:1197–1201.

30. Bednarek J, Furmaniak J, Wedlock N. Steroid 21-hydroxylase is a major autoantigen involved in adult onset autoimmune Addison's disease. FEBS Lett 1992; 309:51–55.

31. Baumann-Antczak A, Wedlock N, Bednarek J. Autoimmune Addison's disease and 21-hydroxylase. Lancet 1992; 340:429–430.

32. Karlsson FA, Burman P, Loof L, et al. Major parietal cell antigen in autoimmune gastritis and pernicious anemia is the acid producing HK-ATPase of the stomach. J Clin Invest 1988; 81:475–479.

33. Gianani R, Pugliese A, Bonner-Weir S, et al. Prognostically significant heterogeneity of cytoplasmic islet cell antibodies in relatives of patients with type I diabetes. Diabetes 1992; 41:347–353.

34. Bosi E, Becker F, Bonifacio E, et al. Progression to type I (insulin-dependent) diabetes in autoimmune endocrine patients with islet cell antibodies. Diabetes 1991; 40:977–984.

35. Vardi P, Crisa L, Jackson RA, et al. Predictive value of intravenous glucose tolerance test insulin secretion less than or greater than the first percentile in islet cell antibody positive relatives of type I (insulin-dependent) diabetic patients. Diabetologia 1991; 34:93–102.

36. Winqvist O, Karlsson FA, Kampe O. 21-Hydroxylase, a major autoantigen in idiopathic Addison's disease. Lancet 1992; 339:1559–1562.

37. De Bellis A, Bizzaro A, Rossi R, et al. Remission of subclinical adrenocortical failure in subjects with adrenal autoantibodies. J Clin Endocrinol Metab 1993; 76:1002–1007.

38. Falorni A, Nikoshkov A, Laureti S, et al. High diagnostic accuracy for idiopathic Addison's disease with a sensitive radiobinding assay for autoantibodies against recombinant human 21-hydroxylase. J Clin Endocrinol Metab 1995; 80:2752–2755.

39. Drachman DB. Myasthenia gravis. N Engl J Med 1995; 330:1797–1810.

40. Schloot N, Eisenbarth GS. Isohormonal therapy of endocrine autoimmunity. Immunol Today 1995; 16:289–294.

41. Keller RJ, Eisenbarth GS, Jackson RA. Insulin prophylaxis in individuals at high risk of type I diabetes. Lancet 1993; 341:927–928.

42. Hashizume K, Ichikawa K, Nishi Y, et al. Effect of administration of thyroxine on the risk of postpartum recurrence of hyperthyroid Graves' disease. J Clin Endocrinol Metab 1992; 75:6–10.

43. Takasu N, Yamada T, Takasu M, et al. Disappearance of thyrotropin-blocking antibodies and spontaneous recovery from hypothyroidism in autoimmune thyroiditis. N Engl J Med 1992; 326:513–518.

44. Banovac K, Ghandur-Mnaymneh L, Mckenzie JM. The effect of thyroxine on spontaneous thyroiditis in BB/W rats. Int Arch Allergy Appl Immunol 1988; 87:301–305.

45. Petersen HD, Bergman M. Cortisone-induced remission of hypothyroidism in Schmidt's syndrome. Acta Med Scand 1980; 208:125–127.

46. Jacobs TP, Whitlock RT, Edsall J, et al. Addisonian crisis while taking high-dose glucocorticoids. An unusual presentation of primary adrenal failure in two patients with underlying inflammatory diseases. JAMA 1988; 260:2082–2084.

47. Hershman JM. Does thyroxine therapy prevent recurrence of Graves' hyperthyroidism? (editorial) J Clin Endocrinol Metab 1995; 80:1479–1480.

48. Thorpe ES, Handley HE. Chronic tetany and chronic mycelial stomatitis in a child aged four-and-one-half years. Am J Dis Child 1929; 38:328–338.

49. Ahonen P, Myllarniemi S, Sipila I, et al. Clinical variation of autoimmune polyendocrinopathy-candidiasis-ectodermal dystrophy (APECED) in a series of 68 patients. N Engl J Med 1990; 322:1830–1836.

50. Walls AWG, Soames JV. Dental manifestations of autoimmune hypoparathyroidism. Oral Surg Oral Med Oral Pathol 1993; 75:452–454.

51. Friedman TC, Thomas PM, Fleisher TA, et al. Frequent occurrence of asplenism and cholelithiasis in patients with autoimmune polyglandular disease type I. Am J Med 1991; 91:625–630.

52. Bereket A, Lowenheim M, Blethen SL, et al. Intestinal lymphangiectasia in a patient with autoimmune polyglandular disease type I and steatorrhea. J Clin Endocrinol Metab 1995; 80:933–955.

53. Blizzard RM, Chee D, Davis W. The incidence of parathyroid and other antibodies in the sera of patients with idiopathic hypoparathyroidism. Clin Exp Immunol 1966; 1:119–128.

54. Krohn K, Uibo R, Aavik E, et al. Identification by molecular cloning of an autoantigen associated with Addison's disease as steroid 17alpha-hydroxylase. Lancet 1992; 339:770–773.

55. Uibo R, Aavik E, Peterson P, et al. Autoantibodies to cytochrome P450 enzymes P450scc, P450c17, and P450c21 in autoimmune polyglandular disease types I and II and in isolated Addison's Disease. J Clin Endocrinol Metab 1994; 78:323–328.

56. Tuomi T, Bjorses P, Falorni A, et al. Antibodies to glutamic acid decarboxylase and insulin-dependent diabetes in patients with autoimmune polyendocrine syndrome type I. J Clin Endocrinol Metab 1996; 81:1488–1494.

57. Ahonen P: Autoimmune polyendocrinopathy-candidosis-ectodermal dystrophy (APECED): autosomal recessive inheritance. Clin Genet 1985; 27:535–542.

58. Zlotogora J, Shapiro MS. Polyglandular autoimmune syndrome type I among Iranian Jews. J Med Genet 1992; 29:824–826.

59. Como JA, Dismukes WE: Oral azole drugs as systemic antifungal therapy. N Engl J Med 1994; 330:263–272.

60. Ahonen P, Myllarniemi S, Kahanpaa A, et al. Ketoconazole is effective against the chronic mucocutaneous candidosis of autoimmune polyendocrinopathy-candidosis-ectodermal dystrophy (APECED). Acta Med Scand 1986; 220:333–339.

61. Ketchum CH, Riley WJ, Maclaren NK. Adrenal dysfunction in asymptomatic patients with adrenocortical autoantibodies. J Clin Endocrinol Metab 1984; 58:1166–1170.

62. Kahn CR, Flier JS, Bar RS, et al. The syndromes of insulin resistance and acanthosis nigricans. Insulin-receptor disorders in man. N Engl J Med 1976; 294:739–745.

63. Flier JS, Bar RS, Muggeo M, et al. The evolving clinical course of patients with insulin receptor autoantibodies: spontaneous remission or receptor proliferation with hypoglycemia. J Clin Endocrinol Metab 1978; 47:985–995.

64. Bardwick PA, Zvaifler NJ, Gill GN, et al. Plasma cell dyscrasia with polyneu-

ropathy, organomegaly, endocrinopathy, M protein, and skin changes: the POEMS syndrome. Medicine 1980; 59:311–322.

65. Amiel LL, Machover D, Droz JP. Dyscrasie plasmocytaire avec arteriopathie, polyneuropathie, syndrome endocrinien. Ann Med Interne 1975; 745:749.

66. Imawari M, Akatsuka N, Ishibashi M, et al. Syndrome of plasma cell dyscrasia, polyneuropathy, and endocrine disturbances. Ann Intern Med 1974; 81:490–493.

67. Iwashita H, Ohnishi A, Asada M, et al. Polyneuropathy, skin hyperpigmentation, edema, and hypertrichosis in localized osteosclerotic myeloma. Neurology 1977; 27:675–681.

68. Meshkinpour H, Myung CG, Kramer LS: A unique multisystemic syndrome of unknown origin. Arch Intern Med 1977; 137:1719–1721.

69. Saihan EM, Burton JL, Heaton KW: A new syndrome with pigmentation, scleroderma, gynaecomastia, Raynaud's phenomenon and peripheral neuropathy. Br J Dermatol 1978; 99:437–440.

70. Harvey JN, Barnett D: Endocrine dysfunction in Kearns-Sayre syndrome. Clin Endocrinol 1992; 37:97–104.

71. Combs RM: Malignant thymoma, hyperthyroidism and immune disorder. South Med J 1968; 61:337–341.

72. Rabinowe SL, Rubin L, George KL, et al. Trisomy 21 (Down's syndrome): autoimmunity, aging and monoclonal antibody defined T cell abnormalities. J Autoimmun 1989; 2:25–30.

73. Fialkow PJ, Thuline HC, Hecht F, et al. Familial predisposition to thyroid disease in Down's syndrome: controlled immunoclinical studies. Am J Hum Genet 1971; 23:67–86.

74. Fleming S, Cowell C, Bailey J, et al. Hashimoto's disease in Turner's syndrome. Clin Invest Med 1988; 11:243–246.

75. Menser MA, Forrest JM, Bransby RD: Rubella infection and diabetes mellitus. Lancet 1978; 1:57–60.

76. Clarke W, Shaver K, Bright GA, et al. Autoimmunity in congenital rubella syndrome. J Pediatr 1984; 104:370–373.

77. Rubinstein P, Walker ME, Fedun B, et al. The HLA system in congenital rubella patients with and without diabetes. Diabetes 1982; 31:1088–1091.

78. Rabinowe SL, George KL, Laughlin R, et al. Congenital rubella: monoclonal antibody defined T cell abnormalities in young children. Am J Med 1986; 81:779–782.

79. Sakaguchi N, Sakaguchi S. Causes and mechanism of autoimmune disease: cyclosporin A as a probe for the investigation. J Invest Dermatol 1992; 98:70s–76s.

80. Polymeropoulos MH, Swift RG, Swift M. Linkage of the gene for Wolfram syndrome to markers on the short arm of chromosome 4. Nat Genet 1994; 8:95–97.

81. Rando TA, Horton JC, Layzer RB: Wolfram syndrome: evidence of a diffuse neurodegenerative disease by magnetic resonance imaging. Neurology 1992; 42:1220–1224.

82. Borgna-Pignatti C, Marradi P, Pinelli L, et al. Thiamine-responsive anemia in DIDMOAD syndrome. J Pediatr 1989; 114:405–410.

83. Ahonen P, Miettinen A, Perheentupa J. Adrenal and steroidal cell antibodies in patients with autoimmune polyglandular disease type I and risk of adrenocortical and ovarian failure. J Clin Endocrinol Metab 1987; 64:494–500.

84. Schmidt MB: Eine biglandulare Erkrankung (Nebennieren und Schilddruse) bei Morbus Addisonii. Verh Dtsch Ges Pathol 1926; 21:212–221.

85. Irvine WJ: Autoimmunity in endocrine disease. Recent Prog Horm Res 1980; 36:509–527.

86. Nerup J: Addison's disease—clinical studies: a report of 108 cases. Acta Endocrinol 1974; 76:127–141.

87. Zelissen PM, Bast EJEG, Croughs RJM: Associated autoimmunity in Addison's disease. J Autoimmun 1995; 8:121–130.

88. McElduff A, Lackmann M, Wilkinson M: Antiidiotypic PTH antibodies as a cause of elevated immunoreactive parathyroid hormone in idiopathic hypoparathyroidism, a second case: another manifestation of autoimmune endocrine disease? Calcif Tissue Int 1992; 51:121–126.

89. Tsatsoulis A, Shalet SM: Antisperm antibodies in the polyglandular autoimmune (PGA) syndrome type I: response to cyclical steroid therapy. Clin Endocrinol (Oxf) 1991; 35:299–303.

90. Smith BR, Furmaniak J. Adrenal and gonadal autoimmune diseases. J Clin Endocrinol Metab 1995; 80:1502–1505 (editorial).

91. Irvine WJ, Chand MMM, Scarth L, et al. Immunological aspects of premature ovarian failure associated with idiopathic Addison's disease. Lancet 1968; 2:883–887.

92. Turkington RW, Lebovitz HE. Extra-adrenal endocrine deficiencies in Addison's disease. Am J Med 1967; 43:499–507.

93. Landin-Olsson M, Karlsson FA, Lernmark A, et al. Islet cell and thyrogastric antibodies in 633 consecutive 15- to 34-yr-old patients in the diabetes incidence study in Sweden. Diabetes 1992; 41:1022–1027.

94. Riley WJ, Maclaren NK, Lezotte DC, et al. Thyroid autoimmunity in insulin-dependent diabetes mellitus: the case for routine screening. J Pediatr 1981; 99:350–354.

95. Alvarez-Marfany M, Roman SH, Drexler AJ, et al. Long-term prospective study of postpartum thyroid dysfunction in women with insulin dependent diabetes mellitus. J Clin Endocrinol Metab 1994; 79:10–16.

96. Barkan AL, Kelch RP, Marshall JC. Isolated gonadotrope failure in the polyglandular autoimmune syndrome. N Engl J Med 1985; 312:1535–1540.

97. Kojima I, Nejima I, Ogata E. Isolated adrenocorticotropin deficiency associated with polyglandular failure. J Clin Endocrinol Metab 1982; 54:182–186.

98. Goudie RB, Pinkerton PH. Anterior hypophysitis and Hashimoto's disease in a young woman. J Pathol Bacteriol 1957; 83:584–585.

99. Bevan JS, Othman S, Lazarus JH, et al. Reversible adrenocorticotropin deficiency due to probable autoimmune hypophysitis in a woman with postpartum thyroiditis. J Clin Endocrinol Metab 1992; 74:548–552.

100. Ozawa Y, Shishiba Y. Recovery from lymphocytic hypophysitis associated with painless thyroiditis: clinical implications of circulating antipituitary antibodies. Acta Endocrinol (Copenh) 1993; 128:493–498.

101. Paja M, Estrada J, Ojeda A, et al. Lymphocytic hypophysitis causing hypopituitarism and diabetes insipidus, and associated with autoimmune thyroiditis, in a non-pregnant woman. Postgrad Med J 1994; 70:220–224.

102. Thodou E, Asa SL, Kontogeorgos G, et al. Clinical case seminar: Lymphocytic hypophysitis: clinicopathological findings. J Clin Endocrinol Metab 1995; 80:2302–2311.

103. Heubi JE, Partin JC, Schubert WK. Hypocalcemia and steathorrhea—clues to etiology. Dig Dis Sci 1983; 28:124–128.

104. Scire G, Magliocca FM, Cianfarani S, et al. Autoimmune polyendocrine candidiasis syndrome with associated chronic diarrhea caused by intestinal infection and pancreas insufficiency. J Pediatr Gastroenterol Nutr 1991; 13:224–227 (letter).

105. Thain ME, Hamilton JR, Ehrlich RM. Coexistence of diabetes mellitus and celiac disease. J Pediatr 1974; 85:527–529.

106. Reunala T, Salmi J, Karvonen J. Dermatitis herpetiformis and celiac disease associated with Addison's disease. Arch Dermatol 1987; 123:930–932.

107. Garty BZ, Kauli R. Alopecia universalis in autoimmune polyglandular syndrome type I. West J Med 1990; 152:76–77 (letter, comment).

108. Stankler L, Bewsher PD. Chronic mucocutaneous candidiasis endocrine deficiency and alopecia areata. Br J Dermatol 1972; 86:238–245.

109. Eisenbarth GS, Wilson P, Ward F, et al. HLA type and disease occurrence in familial polyglandular failure. N Engl J Med 1978; 298:92–94.

110. Betterle C, Caretto A, Pedini B, et al. Complement-fixing activity to melanin-producing cells preceding the onset of vitiligo in a patient with type I polyglandular failure. Arch Dermatol 1995; 128:123–124.

111. Peserico A, Rigon F, Semsenzato G, et al. Vitiligo and polyglandular autoimmune disease with autoantibodies to melanin-producing cells. Arch Dermatol 1981; 117:751–752.

112. Riley WJ, Toskes PP, Maclaren NK, et al. Predictive value of gastric parietal cell autoantibodies as a marker for gastric and hematologic abnormalities associated with insulin-dependent diabetes. Diabetes 1982; 31:1051–1055.

113. Candrina R, Giustina A. Development of type II autoimmune polyglandular syndrome in a patient with idiopathic thrombocytopenic purpura. Isr J Med Sci 1988; 24:57–58.

114. Segal BM, Weintraub MI. Hashimoto's thyroiditis, myasthenia gravis, idiopathic thrombocytopenic purpura. Ann Intern Med 1976; 85:761–762.

115. Hara T, Mizuno Y, Nagata M, et al. Human gamma delta T-cell receptor-positive cell-mediated inhibition of erythropoiesis in vitro in a patient with type I autoimmune polyglandular syndrome and pure red blood cell aplasia. Blood 1990; 75:941–950.

116. Mandel M, Etzioni A, Theodor R, et al. Pure red cell hypoplasia associated with polyglandular autoimmune syndrome type I. Isr J Med Sci 1989; 25:138–141.

117. Segawa F, Yamada H, Tomi H, et al. A case of autoimmune polyglandular deficiency associated with progressive myopathy (Japanese). Rinsho Shinikeigaku 1992; 32:501–505.

118. Bosch EP, Reith PE, Granner DK. Myasthenia gravis and Schmidt syndrome. Neurology 1994; 27:1179–1180.

119. Kane CA, Weed L. Myasthenia gravis associated with adrenocortical insufficiency. N Engl J Med 1950; 243:939–944.

120. Solimena M, Folli F, Denis-Donini S, et al. Autoantibodies to glutamic acid decarboxylase in a patient with stiff man syndrome, epilepsy, and type I diabetes mellitus. N Engl J Med 1988; 318:1012–1020.

121. Rabinowe SL. Immunology of diabetic and polyglandular neuropathy. Diabetes Metab Rev 1990; 6:169–188.

122. Porter SR, Haria S, Scully C, et al. Chronic candidiasis, enamel hypoplasia, and pigmentary anomalies. Oral Surg Oral Med Oral Pathol 1992; 74:312–314.

123. Smith WI, Rabin BS, Huellmantel A, et al. Immunopathology of juvenile-onset diabetes mellitus. 1: IgA deficiency and juvenile diabetes. Diabetes 1978; 27:1092–1097.

124. Torrelo A, Espana A, Balsa J, et al. Vitiligo and polyglandular autoimmune syndrome with selective IgA deficiency. Int J Dermatol 1992; 31:343–344.

125. Gass JD: The syndrome of keratoconjunctivitis, superficial moniliasis, idiopathic hypoparathyroidism and Addison's disease. Am J Ophthalmol 1962; 54:660–674.

126. Tucker WS, Niblack GD, McLean RH, et al. Serositis with autoimmune endocrinopathy: clinical and immunogenetic features. Medicine 1987; 64:138–147.

127. Moss M, Neff TA, Colby TV, et al. Diffuse alveolar hemorrhage due to antibasement membrane antibody disease appearing with a polyglandular autoimmune syndrome. Chest 1994; 105:296–298.

128. Shikata A, Sugimoto T, Kosaka K, et al. Thoracic aortic calcification in 3 children with candidiasis-endocrinopathy syndrome. Pediatr Radiol 1993; 23:100–103.

129. Fairfax AJ, Leatham A. Idiopathic heart block: association with vitiligo, thyroid disease, pernicious anemia, and diabetes mellitus. Br Med J 1975; 4:322–324.

130. Eisenbarth G, Bellgrau D: Autoimmunity. Sci Med 1994; 1:38–47.
131. Hetzel DJ, Stanhope R, O'Neill BP, et al. Gynecologic cancer in patients with subacute cerebellar degeneration predicted by anti-Purkinje cell antibodies and limited in metastatic volume. Mayo Clin Proc 1990; 65:1558–1563.
132. Uchigata Y, Kuwata S, Tsushima T, et al. Patients with Graves' disease who developed insulin autoimmune syndrome (Hirata disease) possess HLA-Bw62/Cw4/DR4 carrying DRB1*0406. J Clin Endocrinol Metab 1993; 77:249–254.
133. Garlepp MJ, Dawkins RL, Christiansen FT. HLA antigens and acetylcholine receptor antibodies in penicillamine induced myasthenia gravis. Br Med J 1983; 286:338–340.
134. Yoshinaga M, Figueroa F, Wahid MR, et al. Antigenic specificity of lympho-cytes isolated from valvular specimens of rheumatic fever patients. J Autoimmun 1995; 8:601–613.
135. Imagawa A, Itoh N, Hanafusa T, et al. Autoimmune endocrine disease induced by recombinant interferon-α therapy for chronic active type C hepatitis. J Clin Endocrinol Metab 1995; 80:922–926.
136. Nepom GT: Immunogenetics and IDDM. Diabetes Rev 1993; 1:93–103.
137. Steinman L: Autoimmune disease. Sci Am 1993; 269:107–114.
138. Pugliese A, Solimena M, Awdeh ZL, et al. Association of HLA-DQB1*0201 with stiff-man syndrome. J Clin Endocrinol Metab 1993; 77:1550–1553.
139. Palmieri G, Lastoria S, Colao A, et al. Successful treatment of a patient with a thymoma and pure red cell aplasia with octreotide and prednisone. N Engl J Med 1997; 336:263–265.

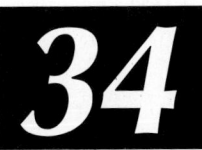

NON–INSULIN-SECRETING TUMORS OF THE GASTROENTEROPANCREATIC SYSTEM

Guenther J. Krejs

INTRODUCTION

The "clear cells" of the pancreas that constitute the islets of Langerhans were described in 1867 and 1869,[1, 2] and it was subsequently recognized that similar cells are dispersed throughout the gastrointestinal tract. The gastroenteropancreatic endocrine system is actually composed of many different subtypes of clear cells that synthesize more than 30 known hormones or hormone-like peptides[3, 4] (Table 34–1). The embryologic origin of this system has been the subject of intense scrutiny. It was originally proposed that the cells are derived from the neural crest,[5] but the bulk of evidence indicates that they are of endodermal origin.[6, 7] Nevertheless, the fact that these cells share functional and histochemical features with neuroendocrine cells suggests that both systems may be derived from some common precursor stem cell.[7]

The role of the pancreatic islets in regulating fuel homeostasis and the role of hormones of the gastrointestinal tract in controlling gastric function are among the best studied gastroenteropancreatic endocrine systems. However, the physiological functions of many of the hormones synthesized in the gastroenteropancreatic tract (see Table 34–1) are incompletely understood.[8] Some influence motility and function of the gastrointestinal tract by acting as neurotransmitters,[9, 10] some

control the synthesis of other hormones such as insulin and somatostatin,[11, 12] some influence the hyperplasia of the pancreas and small intestine after bowel loss or disease,[13–15] and others exert paracrine, autocrine, and/or endocrine effects that are still not defined. It is noteworthy that excess production of some of the hormones does not appear to cause disease.

It is likely that all cells of the diffuse neuroendocrine system can give rise to endocrine tumors, and it is easy to understand that tumors of cells that normally produce a hormone can produce the same hormone inappropriately or in excess. However, tumors can also produce hormones other than those normally secreted by the parent cells by any of several mechanisms, including dedifferentiation to a pluripotent capacity that allows the cells to produce any polypeptide or amplification of the formation of what would ordinarily be a minor cell product.[16] In the past the term *ectopic* was used for tumors that produce polypeptides not normally produced by the cells of origin, but the term is now considered to be inappropriate because production of a hormone by a tumor usually represents enhanced expression of a gene that is expressed at low levels in the normal cell from which the tumor originates[17] (see Chapter 36).

Pancreatic endocrine tumors can also be a part of the syndrome of multiple endocrine neoplasia type 1 (MEN 1), in

TABLE 34–1. Neuroendocrine Cells of the Gastroenteropancreatic System

Region	Cell Type	Principal Hormones Produced
Pancreas	Beta (B)	Insulin
	Alpha (A)	Glucagon/glicentin, calcitonin gene-related peptide (CGRP)
	Delta (D₁)	Somatostatin, gastrin inhibitory peptide (GIP)
	F (D₂ or PP)	Pancreatic polypeptide (PP), peptide YY
Stomach	G	Gastrin 17
	D	Somatostatin, pancreastatin
	A	Glucagon
Small intestine	G	Gastrin 34
	CCK	Cholecystokinin (CCK)
	D	Somatostatin
	L	Glucagon-like peptide (GLP) I and II
	I	Gastrin inhibitory peptide (GIP)
	ECL (enterochromaffin)	Histamine, substance P, motilin
	P	Peptide YY
	X	β-Endorphin, γ-melanocyte-stimulating hormone (MSH)
	S (K)	Secretin
	N	Neurotensin
Colon and rectum	CG	Calcitonin, CGRP
	L	GLP-I and GLP-II
	K (BN)	Gastrin releasing factor
	X	β-Endorphin, metenkephalin, corticotropin

Compiled from Delcore and Friesen,[7] Solcia et al.,[4] and Habener.[27]

which there is a hereditary predisposition to islet cell hyperplasia and islet cell tumor formation (see Chapter 32). All islet cell tumors described in this chapter can occur in MEN 1. Most commonly, however, MEN 1 tumors of the gastrointestinal tract produce gastrin, vasoactive intestinal peptide (VIP), or pancreatic polypeptide (PP).[18, 19] Because multiple tumors may be present in such patients, the identification of a tumor in a patient with MEN 1 does not necessarily mean that it is the tumor responsible for the patient's disease.[20]

Endocrine tumors of the gastroenteropancreatic system may secrete more than one hormone, and elevated levels of more than one peptide can be found in the plasma of such patients.[21–24] The predominant type of cell in the tumor and the predominant hormone produced define the clinical syndrome. On the other hand, some clear cell tumors are nonfunctioning; that is, they do not release hormones into the circulation despite immunohistochemical evidence that they contain functioning endocrine cells, or they synthesize one or more hormones that are as yet unidentified. These tumors, like other endocrine tumors, may also secrete high-molecular-weight precursors of peptide hormones that have different biologic activities than those of the mature peptide. Consequently, the concentration of immunoreactive hormone in plasma may not correspond to the level of biologic activity. For instance, in patients with gastrinoma large amounts of inactive progastrin circulate together with glycine-extended intermediates of gastrin, only some of which stimulate acid secretion and only some of which are detected by the COOH terminus–specific antisera used in conventional gastrin immunoassays.[25] Therefore, clinical manifestations may be minimal despite a high plasma level of immunoactive hormone, and vice versa.

Endocrine tumors of the gastroenteropancreatic system are rare, with an incidence of about 1 per 100,000 population per year. Gastrinomas occur in 1 per 2 million persons per year, VIP–secreting tumors (VIPomas) in 1 per 10 million per year, glucagonomas in 1 per 20 million per year, and somatostatinomas in 1 per 40 million per year.[26]

The various endocrine syndromes produced by these tumors (Table 34–2) are described first, and the features of pathogenesis, diagnosis, and treatment common to all endocrine tumors of the gastroenteropancreatic system are dis-

cussed subsequently. (See Chapter 20 for insulinoma, Chapter 32 for MEN, and Chapter 37 for carcinoid tumors.)

ENDOCRINE SYNDROMES

Glucagonoma

The pre-proglucagon gene on chromosome 2 encodes a polypeptide that gives rise in the pancreas to glucagon and the major proglucagon fragment (MPGF), which has no known function, and in the intestinal wall to the hormone originally known as enteroglucagon. Enteroglucagon is now recognized to consist of several components, including glicentin, a 69-amino-acid peptide that includes the 29-amino-acid sequence of glucagon, oxyntomodulin, and glucagon-like peptides (GLP) I and II (Fig. 34–1).[27] GLP-I is a so-called incretin hormone (a potent stimulator of insulin secretion), whereas glucagon is a major counter-regulatory hormone in the control of plasma glucose (see Chapter 20). The net consequence is that the processing of the same prohormone in the two tissues has different physiological consequences. Oxyntomodulin is believed to play a role in the secretion of acid by the stomach.

Glucagonoma is a rare tumor of the pancreatic alpha cells that causes a disorder characterized by necrolytic migratory erythema, cheilosis, diabetes mellitus, normochromic normocytic anemia, venous thrombosis, weight loss, and neuropsychiatric manifestations. Necrolytic migratory erythema, commonly the major manifestation, is a superficial erythema with a moving edge and has the histologic features of toxic epidermal necrolysis.[28–29] The lesions are found on the buttocks, groin, perineum, and thighs; they commence as red patches that progress to form bullae and then break down and become encrusted, followed by healing and pigmentation.[30] The lesions tend to coalesce, often with extensive skin involvement and secondary infection.[31, 32] The dermatologic disorder may be the direct consequence of an elevated plasma glucagon level or the indirect effect of lowered levels of plasma amino acids or tissue zinc.[33] The rash disappears promptly when the plasma glucagon level returns to normal after complete tumor

TABLE 34–2. Clinical Features of Endocrine Tumors of the Gastropancreatic System*

Tumor	Clinical Features	Diagnostic Features
Glucagonoma	Necrolytic migratory erythema, mild diabetes mellitus, psychiatric disturbances, diarrhea, venous thrombosis	Enhanced glucagon release after administration of tolbutamide intravenously
Somatostatinoma		
Pancreas	Dyspepsia, diabetes mellitus, gallstones, steatorrhea, hypochlorhydria	Hyperglycemia without ketonemia; stool weight usually 400–800 g/d; stool fat usually 10–30 g/d
Duodenum	Jaundice, pancreatitis, bleeding	Neurofibromatosis type I may be present
PPoma	None recognized (secretory diarrhea in some)	None known for pure PPoma
Gastrinoma	Severe peptic ulcer disease; secretory diarrhea	Enhanced gastrin release after secretin administration; high basal and peak gastric acid secretion; diarrhea responds to omeprazole or H₂ receptor antagonists
VIPoma	Large-volume secretory diarrhea, hypokalemia, metabolic acidosis, hypochlorhydria	Stool characteristic of secretory diarrhea, fasting fecal pH < 8.0; may cosecrete calcitonin, PP, serotonin
Calcitoninoma	Diarrhea	Secretory diarrhea when fasting; osmotic diarrhea after eating
Neurotensinoma	None recognized (esophageal reflux described)	None known
PTHrP-secreting tumors	Hypercalcemia	Elevated plasma levels of PTHrP and suppressed levels of PTH
GHRHoma	Acromegaly	Normal CT and MRI of the sella; no pituitary tumor at surgery
Corticotropinoma	Cushing's syndrome	Bilateral adrenalectomy may be required for management of Cushing's syndrome; may also secrete corticotropin-releasing hormone, melanocyte-stimulating hormone

*See Chapter 37 for carcinoid tumors and Chapter 20 for insulinomas. Inappropriate secretion of vasopressin is discussed in Chapter 10, and the secretion of PTHrP by tumors is discussed in Chapter 24.

resection.[34] Glucagon excess enhances the hepatic conversion of amino acid nitrogen into urea nitrogen, resulting in decreased blood amino acid levels.[35] Weight loss and decreased lean body mass are common features.

The glycogenolytic and gluconeogenic actions of glucagon cause diabetes mellitus that can sometimes be treated by diet or oral hypoglycemic agents, but in one large series most patients required insulin therapy.[29] The levels of plasma glucose and plasma glucagon correlate poorly.[33] The pathogenesis of the other manifestations of the glucagonoma syndrome, such as anorexia, glossitis, angular cheilitis, venous thrombosis, weight loss, anemia, and depression, are even more poorly understood. Diarrhea can be prominent, possibly as a result of the secretory effects of glucagon on the small bowel mucosa (reduction of absorption or enhancement of net secretion of water and electrolytes)[36] or because of cosecretion by some glucagonomas of other hormones such as VIP.[29]

In one series the average size of glucagonomas was 5.8 cm, and half of patients had metastases at the time of diagnosis.[37] Patients are usually middle-aged and have a long history of symptoms suggesting glucagon excess. The diagnosis is confirmed by documentation of elevated plasma glucagon levels and the presence of a pancreatic mass. Because plasma glucagon levels may also be elevated in patients with diabetes mellitus, pancreatitis, trauma, burns, and myocardial in-

farction, the diagnosis of glucagonoma requires the presence of a tumor mass and the exclusion of other conditions known to elevate plasma glucagon levels.

As stated previously, the intestine contains peptides (originally termed enteroglucagon) that have glucagon-like immunoreactivity but are distinct from glucagon. Glicentin is a cleavage product of the proglucagon molecule that contains the amino acid sequence of glucagon but does not bind to the glucagon receptor or have glucagon-like actions (see Table 34–1 and Fig. 34–1).[38] Another cleavage product of proglucagon in the intestinal L cell is GLP-I, a potent stimulator of insulin secretion.[27] The proglucagon cleavage products may function in part to regulate the growth of the pancreas and small intestine after bowel resection.[13–15] Both GLP-I[39] and glicentin[40] can be synthesized in excess by pancreatic glucagonomas, and elevated levels of these hormones in plasma may explain the occasional finding of giant duodenal villi in patients with glucagonoma.[41] Glicentin or glicentin-like immunoreactivity has also been described in rectal carcinoid tumors[42] and in a tumor of the kidney associated with giant intestinal villi that regressed after nephrectomy.[43] These cases raise the possibility that extrapancreatic "glicentinomas" or "GLPomas" may on occasion give rise to endocrine syndromes. In one study GLP-I–like immunoreactivity was identified in 7 of 33 "nonfunctioning" gastroenteropancreatic tu-

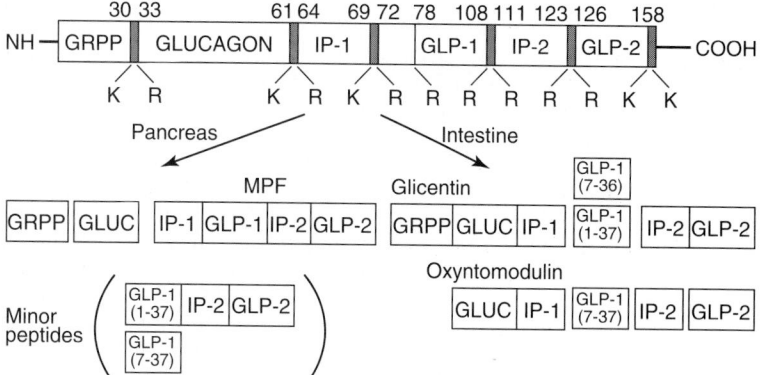

Figure 34–1. Alternative post-translational processing of proglucagon in the pancreas and intestines. The basic amino acids arginine (R) and lysine (K) are sites for enzymatic cleavages by proglucagon convertases in the alpha cells of the pancreatic islets and the L cells of the intestine. The major recognized bioactive peptides formed by cleavages are shaded and are glucagon in the pancreas and the two isoforms of GLP-1 in the intestines. (Modified and redrawn from Fehmann H-C, Habener JF: Insulinotropic glucagon-like peptide-1(7–37)-(7–36)amide: a new incretin hormone. Trends Endocrinol Metab 1992; 3[5]:158–163. Reprinted by permission of Elsevier Science Inc.)

mors, although it is not clear whether plasma GLP-I levels were elevated in the patients.[44]

Somatostatinoma

Somatostatin inhibits diverse endocrine functions in the anterior pituitary, pancreatic islets, gastrointestinal mucosa, thyroid follicle, and juxtaglomerular region of the kidney.[45] The syndrome produced by pancreatic somatostatinomas was recognized in 1979.[46] Suppression of both insulin and glucagon causes mild diabetes mellitus that usually responds to dietary management, and additional features include cholelithiasis, steatorrhea, indigestion, and hypochlorhydria, all of which are caused by the inhibitory actions of somatostatin on gastrointestinal function.[47] The fact that somatostatinomas frequently contain subpopulations of other endocrine cells probably explains the occasional development of hypoglycemia,[48, 49] flushing,[50] and Cushing's syndrome.[51] Diarrhea appears to be a prominent symptom of somatostatinomas that secrete calcitonin.[46, 52] The clinical manifestations may also be influenced by varying degrees of target organ resistance that blunts the effects of somatostatin. For instance, high somatostatin levels in plasma did not inhibit glucagon release in two patients.[46, 53] Variability of symptoms and the fact that the cardinal manifestations (dyspepsia, diabetes mellitus, cholelithiasis, diarrhea, steatorrhea, and hypochlorhydria) are common make recognition difficult. The diagnosis usually depends on identification of a pancreatic islet cell tumor, and the diagnosis may be suspected only after metastatic spread causes weight loss and other signs of malignant disease. Most pancreatic somatostatinomas are large and have metastases at the time of diagnosis, and in retrospect the symptoms have been present for several years.[46] Because these tumors are usually malignant, aggressive management is appropriate (see later discussion).

Gastrointestinal somatostatinomas (mainly in the duodenal wall and ampulla of Vater) are histologically and clinically distinct from pancreatic somatostatinomas.[54–59] Namely, they are psammomatous tumors, endocrine manifestations are not prominent, and metastases are unusual. Patients usually have symptoms related to tumor location (jaundice, pancreatitis, or bleeding). Approximately half of patients with duodenal somatostatinoma have neurofibromatosis type I[58]; tumors in these patients frequently involve the ampulla of Vater.[53, 58–60] Because somatostatin production by gastrointestinal somatostatinomas is minor, the somatostatinoma syndrome is not present. The infusion of calcium and pentagastrin to such patients causes an increase in serum somatostatin levels.[61]

Pancreatic Polypeptide–Secreting Tumor (PPoma)

A physiological role for PP has not been established, but inhibition of the effect of cholecystokinin by PP may influence pancreatic exocrine function and gallbladder motility.[62] Patients with high circulating levels of PP do not display a characteristic clinical syndrome, but a few patients with a PPoma or islet cell adenomatosis have had secretory diarrhea.[63–65] However, PP is not an intestinal secretagogue in small bowel perfusion experiments,[66] and the diarrhea may have been caused by cosecretion of unidentified substances. In one patient a macular rash (distinct from necrolytic migratory erythema) disappeared after tumor treatment.[67] Because about half of pancreatic endocrine tumors contain PP, the peptide has been used as a marker for diagnosis of pancreatic endocrine tumors and for monitoring the response to treatment.[68–71] Although an elevated basal plasma PP level may suggest the presence of an islet cell tumor, the plasma PP response to meal stimulation can be exaggerated in the MEN

1 syndrome and in patients with islet cell hyperplasia.[19] The usefulness of PP as a marker of pancreatic endocrine tumors is limited, because plasma PP levels may also be elevated in patients with certain inflammatory diseases, renal failure, and laxative abuse.[68] Intravenous atropine lowers plasma levels when PP does not originate from a tumor.[70] Because they are endocrinologically silent, PPomas of the pancreas have usually metastasized by the time of diagnosis.

Gastrinoma (see Chapter 32)

In 1955 Zollinger and Ellison[72] described a syndrome characterized by recurrent, severe peptic ulcer disease, gastric hypersecretion, and the presence of a pancreatic endocrine tumor. The availability of a radioimmunoassay for gastrin makes the diagnosis of gastrinoma straightforward, and the tumors are often recognized early in the course of disease.[73] Approximately two thirds of gastrinomas are sporadic, and the remainder are associated with MEN 1. Sporadic gastrinomas tend to be solitary, are malignant, and are commonly found in the "gastrinoma triangle" (the head of the pancreas, the duodenum, and the porta hepatitis).[74] Gastrinomas that occur with MEN 1 are usually small and multiple and may or may not be malignant. Metastases are commonly found in the liver and lymph nodes.[75]

The diagnosis should be considered in patients with severe ulcer disease or unexplained secretory diarrhea. A basal serum gastrin level higher than 200 ng/L requires further assessment but is not specific for the gastrinoma syndrome, because plasma gastrin may also be increased in patients with atrophic gastritis and chlorhydria (pernicious anemia), antral gastrin-cell hyperplasia, retained antrum after a Billroth II partial gastrectomy, renal failure, pyloric stenosis, short-bowel syndrome, previous vagotomy, and achlorhydria induced by proton pump inhibitors.[73]

Gastric acid levels are increased in patients with gastrinoma but may overlap with levels in patients with ordinary duodenal ulcer disease and in some normal controls. About half of patients have a basal acid secretion rate of more than 15 mmol/h. A basal acid output equal to or greater than 60% of the peak acid output (after pentagastrin) is suggestive of gastrinoma, but this finding is present in only about half of gastrinoma patients.[73]

If the elevation in serum gastrin is moderate (200 to 1000 ng/L), intravenous secretin (2 U/kg body weight) should be administered as a provocative test. In patients with gastrinoma the serum gastrin level increases promptly (within 5 or 10 min), usually by more than 200 ng/L.[76] Measurement of the plasma level of the gastrin precursor progastrin may also be useful in diagnosis of gastrinoma.[25]

Clinical features include diarrhea and steatorrhea. Diarrhea is present in one third of patients and may precede peptic ulcer symptoms.[77] Diarrhea is primarily caused by the large amount of acidic fluid entering the jejunum.[78] In one patient studied by the author, the fluid of the proximal jejunum had a pH of 1.1, and 15 L of fluid was estimated to enter the small bowel each day in the fasting state. Suppression of gastric acid secretion with proton pump inhibitors abolishes the diarrhea. High circulating levels of gastrin may play a minor direct role in the pathogenesis of diarrhea by reducing intestinal water and ion absorption.[79]

The traditional treatment for gastrinoma was total gastrectomy, but proton pump inhibitors are now the first line of therapy.[80] Surgery is still useful for tumor resection, and with early diagnosis it may allow a cure rate of 20%.[81] Survival is better in patients in whom the gastrinoma is part of MEN 1 than in those with the sporadic form.[82]

Rats given large doses of the proton pump inhibitor omeprazole for prolonged periods develop profound hypergastrinemia and gastric carcinoids that arise from the enterochromaffin-like (ECL) cells in the gastric mucosa[83] (see Table 34–1). Potent histamine₂ (H₂) blockers can also cause the tumor in rats.[84] In humans gastric carcinoids are associated with hypergastrinemia in two situations: pernicious anemia and the Zollinger-Ellison syndrome.[85] In both conditions ECL cells become hyperplastic, and gastric carcinoids may develop but for the most part remain reversible.[84] Gastric carcinoids occur in about 5% of patients with pernicious anemia.[86] In Zollinger-Ellison syndrome, gastric carcinoids appear to develop primarily in patients in whom gastrinoma is a component of the MEN 1 syndrome rather than in those with sporadic gastrinomas. Furthermore, in humans treated with proton pump inhibitors for long periods, hypergastrinemia is less pronounced, and neither ECL cell hyperplasia nor carcinoid tumors have been observed, even with careful assessment by morphometry of the gastric mucosa.[87]

VIP-Secreting Tumor (VIPoma)

In 1957 Priest and Alexander[88] described the association of islet cell tumor, severe watery diarrhea, and hypokalemia; Verner and Morrison[89] subsequently called attention to the syndrome of watery diarrhea, hypokalemia, and death resulting from renal failure in association with islet cell tumor. Synonyms for VIPoma include the Verner-Morrison syndrome, the watery diarrhea-hypokalemia-hypochlorhydria syndrome, and the pancreatic cholera syndrome. The term *pancreatic cholera*, first used by Matsumoto and colleagues,[90] is appropriate because the diarrhea, as in Asiatic cholera, results from the intestinal secretion of fluid. However, some responsible tumors are outside the pancreas (e.g, in the stomach).[91]

Bloom and colleagues[92] showed that some patients with this syndrome have elevated plasma levels and high turnover rates of VIP. VIP had been characterized previously as a vasoactive substance,[93] and it was considered a candidate gastrointestinal hormone by Grossman.[94] The peptide is a neurotransmitter in both the central and peripheral nervous systems,[95–97] and its biologic actions were reviewed by Said in 1991.[98] The hormone exerts profound effects on intestinal water and ion movement,[99] but it was not initially clear whether VIP is the mediator of diarrhea in pancreatic cholera syndrome, because some patients with islet cell tumors and diarrhea do not have high plasma levels of VIP[100] and because plasma levels can be high in some normal persons[101] and in persons abusing laxatives.[102]

Nevertheless, it is now clear that VIP is the major mediator of pancreatic cholera. After removal of the tumors, diarrhea disappears as plasma VIP levels return to normal. Furthermore, intravenous infusion of VIP in healthy subjects changes the movement of water and ions from intestinal absorption to intestinal secretion,[103, 104] and prolonged intravenous infusion of VIP (10 h) produces secretory diarrhea in normal controls (mean 2.4 L/10 h) and causes metabolic acidosis, mimicking the clinical syndrome.[105]

VIPomas may cosecrete other hormones in addition to VIP. PHM (peptide with NH₂-terminal histidine and COOH-terminal methionine amide) and VIP may be present in the same tumor cells, as indicated by immunocytochemistry.[106] PHM has similar effects on the intestinal mucosa but is much less potent as a secretagogue than VIP.[107] Other hormones that can be cosecreted with VIP include neurotensin, PP,[108] and calcitonin (see later discussion). Some or all these factors may contribute to secretory diarrhea produced by VIPomas. In other cases of putative pancreatic cholera without elevation of plasma VIP level, secretory diarrhea may be caused by gastrinomas, carcinoid tumors, medullary carcinoma of the thyroid, villous adenomas of the rectum, or surreptitious laxative abuse.[75]

The major clinical manifestation of VIPoma is large-volume secretory diarrhea, although patients may excrete less than 3 L of stool per day.[109] Because the diarrhea is secretory, stool water is isotonic with plasma, and diarrhea persists on fasting.[110] For practical purposes a stool volume of less than 700 mL/d excludes the diagnosis.[111] Excretion of large amounts of potassium and bicarbonate in the diarrheal stool causes hypokalemia, acidosis, and volume depletion. In a few patients secretion of water and ions by the small intestine has been demonstrated directly by perfusion methods.[102, 112–114]

In one study,[115] 14 of 43 patient had histamine-fast achlorhydria, and 16 had hypochlorhydria. Because parietal cells in gastric mucosal biopsy specimens are normal even in patients with achlorhydria and because gastric hyposecretion can be corrected by resection of the VIPoma,[116] it is likely that the tumors release an inhibitor of gastric acid secretion. The infusion of VIP inhibits pentagastrin- and meal-stimulated acid secretion in the dog[117] but in acute experiments does not inhibit pentagastrin-induced acid secretion in humans.[118] Whether VIP affects meal-stimulated acid secretion in humans is not known.

Hypercalcemia occurs in half of the patients,[114] but the mechanism is not clear. There appears to be a negative calcium balance with increased bone resorption.[119] Tetany is thought to be caused by hypomagnesemia, and it may occur in the presence of hypercalcemia. Flushing is occasionally observed. Some patients have hypotension resulting from peripheral vasodilation, and severe hypertension may develop after tumor removal.[120] These features are compatible with the known cardiovascular effects of VIP.[121] Glucose intolerance occurs in about half of patients with the VIPoma syndrome. A direct diabetogenic effect of the secreted agent is suggested by the observation that operative manipulation of an islet cell VIPoma caused pronounced hyperglycemia in one patient.[122]

The average duration of symptoms before diagnosis is 3 y[123] (range, 2 mo to 4 y[124]). Metastases (liver, lymph nodes) are present in half of patients at the time of diagnosis. Death results from renal failure or cardiac arrest caused by volume depletion and acidosis. The survival of patients with islet cells tumors used to be less than 1 y from the time of diagnosis, but better supportive treatment and the use of chemotherapy have improved survival time. In our series of nine patients, two have survived 4 and 12 y without evidence of recurrent disease.

Calcitoninoma

Calcitonin is present in many pancreatic endocrine tumors but usually not as the predominant peptide. It has been detected in tumors secreting VIP,[122–125] somatostatin,[46, 52] PP,[126] insulin,[127] motilin, gastric inhibitory polypeptide (GIP, also known as glucose-dependent insulinotropic polypeptide), neurotensin, and enkephalin.[128] Like PP, therefore, calcitonin may serve as a marker peptide for the diagnosis of pancreatic endocrine malignancies.

The infusion of calcitonin decreases transit time[129] and increases the secretion of water and electrolytes by the small bowel[130]; about one third of patients with calcitonin excess associated with medullary carcinoma of the thyroid have diarrhea (also see Chapter 32). Hypercalcitoninemia may also contribute to diarrhea in patients with pancreatic endocrine tumors.[127]

Neurotensinoma

Neurotensin can frequently be detected when pancreatic endocrine tumors are examined by immunocytochemistry and immunofluorescence.[131–133] However, no clear-cut syndrome has been attributed to a high plasma neurotensin level. In one patient neurotensin-secreting cells accounted for 80% of endocrine cells of a pancreatic tumor.[134] The patient had severe esophageal reflux, possibly caused by a neurotensin-induced increase in enteric pressure. Additional instances of relatively pure neurotensinomas need to be studied before conclusions can be drawn. When both VIP and neurotensin are produced by pancreatic tumors, the symptoms are those of the pancreatic cholera syndrome,[135] whereas cosecretion of gastrin and neurotensin results in typical manifestations of Zollinger-Ellison syndrome.[135]

PTHrP-Secreting Tumor

Hypercalcemia can occur in association with pancreatic endocrine cell tumors, and it was initially thought that this rare event was caused by the production of parathyroid hormone by the pancreatic tumor.[136, 137] However, in many such patients hypercalcemia results from the development of hyperparathyroidism as a part of the MEN 1 syndrome (see Chapter 32). In other instances, hypercalcemia is caused by secretion of parathyroid hormone–related protein (PTHrP) by pancreatic tumors.[138-140] In such patients, blood PTHrP levels are elevated, but parathyroid hormone levels are suppressed appropriately for the degree of hypercalcemia. In one patient the hypercalcemia and elevated levels of PTHrP returned to normal after resection of a large tumor in the body and neck of the pancreas[138]; in another instance the tumor was not resectable, but the hypercalcemia and elevated serum PTHrP levels responded dramatically to therapy with streptozocin and 5-fluorouracil.[139] In still another report, 9 of 11 islet cell tumors that were associated with hypercalcemia stained for PTHrP.[140] PTHrP-secreting pancreatic tumors tend to be large, highly vascular, and malignant, but their presence is compatible with long survival.[141] PTHrP is expressed in fetal and adult pancreatic islets and can be secreted by many malignancies, including pancreatic cancers, so its presence in the blood of a patient with a pancreatic tumor is not diagnostic of a pancreatic endocrine tumor[142, 143] (see Chapter 24). The production of parathyroid hormone by a pancreatic endocrine tumor has not been described.

Corticotropinoma

Pancreatic corticotropinomas release corticotropin and cause Cushing's syndrome (see Chapters 9 and 12). These tumors may cosecrete melanocyte-stimulating hormone and corticotropin-releasing hormone. Plasma cortisol and urinary 17-hydroxycorticosteroid levels are not suppressed by high-dose dexamethasone administration. Ectopic corticotropin production may cause Cushing's syndrome in as many as 5% of patients with sporadic gastrinoma.[144] Cushing's syndrome can also occur as the result of corticotropin secretion by metastases long after resection of the primary pancreatic endocrine tumor.[145] Pancreatic corticotropinoma is an aggressive tumor, particularly when there is cosecretion of gastrin; the benefit of aggressive surgical resection of primary or metastatic corticotropinoma has not been established, but bilateral adrenalectomy may be palliative.[146]

GHRH-Secreting Tumor (GHRHoma)

Release of growth hormone–releasing hormone (GHRH) from a pancreatic or gastrointestinal tumor stimulates the normal pituitary to release enhanced amounts of growth hormone and is a rare cause of acromegaly/gigantism[147-153] (see Chapter 9). The tumors may be more common in patients with MEN 1.[152] The sella is normal in size, and magnetic resonance imaging and computed tomographic (CT) scans of the pituitary are also normal. The increase in plasma growth

hormone level in response to exogenous GHRH is blunted, whereas growth hormone–secreting tumors of the pituitary respond normally. One GHRH-secreting tumor of the pancreas metastasized to the pituitary, and the presentation of such patients can be complex.[154] The fact that many of these tumors express somatostatin receptors on the cell surface[155] makes it possible to treat such patients with the somatostatin analogue octreotide.[156]

Tumors That Secrete Multiple Hormones

More than half of pancreatic islet cell tumors produce more than one hormone,[21-24, 157] but most patients with mixed pancreatic endocrine tumors have symptoms characteristic of single-hormone excess.[158] Some mixed tumors are hormonally silent and produce symptoms related only to tumor mass, metastases, or nonspecific signs of malignant disease (anemia, weight loss). When endocrine symptoms are produced, the immunocytochemical predominance of a certain cell type may not always correspond to the clinical picture. For instance, the secretion of gastrin may be sufficient to induce Zollinger-Ellison syndrome even when gastrin-secreting cells constitute only 10% of the cell population in a tumor.[134]

Sometimes the clinical syndrome changes with time or after chemotherapy. A tumor may first present as an insulinoma but later show symptoms of glucagon or gastrin excess.[159, 160] Chemotherapy with streptozocin may precipitate such transformations.[161] In one case, transition from the Zollinger-Ellison syndrome to insulinoma occurred without detectable ultrastructural changes within the tumor itself.[162] Metastases of these mixed tumors may contain all cell types of the original tumor or only one or two of the original cell types.[163]

Candidate Tumors

Secretion of some gastrointestinal hormones by islet cell or gastrointestinal tumors has not been recognized. The following peptides may be considered for such candidate tumors: secretin, cholecystokinin, motilin, GIP, bombesin, calcitonin gene–related protein, enkephalin, and PYY (peptide P with NH_2-terminal and COOH-terminal tyrosines). Such tumors, if they occur, are probably rare and cause mild symptoms, but it is possible that some of the 20 to 40% of islet cell tumors that are classified as nonfunctional actually produce one or more of these hormones. Better assay techniques and increasing knowledge of the biologic actions of regulatory peptides may allow recognition of such tumors and their associated syndromes in the future.

Islet Cell Hyperplasia

Some of the endocrine syndromes related to pancreatic tumors can also occur with islet cell hyperplasia. For instance, one series of patients with pancreatic cholera included several patients without a pancreatic tumor, and it was suggested that one fifth of the cases were caused by islet cell hyperplasia.[114] In another series 14% of patients with the watery diarrhea syndrome were categorized as having islet cell hyperplasia.[164] However, Bloom and Polak[165] did not find elevated plasma VIP levels in any patient with islet cell hyperplasia, and J. Fahrenkrug (personal communication) believes that pancreatic cholera is rarely, if ever, caused by islet cell hyperplasia. Many of the reports describing this entity are hard to interpret, because the diagnosis of islet cell hyperplasia is often poorly documented and because morphometric data are frequently lacking. Moreover, Chey and colleagues[166] described seven cases of pancreatic cholera syndrome and islet cell hyperplasia without elevated plasma VIP. Hyperplasia of PP- and

GIP-secreting cells has also been described in association with the watery diarrhea syndrome.[167]

The importance of islet cell hyperplasia in these disorders is unresolved, particularly as to whether subtotal pancreatectomy should be considered in a patient with a high circulating level of a particular peptide but no pancreatic tumor.

GENERAL FEATURES

Pathogenesis (see Chapter 6)

Two broad categories of defects have been implicated in the pathogenesis of endocrine tumors: (1) oncogenes that carry "gain of function" mutations and act as dominant mutations to deregulate the production of normal proteins or cause the synthesis of abnormal protein products and (2) autosomal recessive "loss of function" mutations in tumor suppressor genes that normally act to restrain cell proliferation.[168] The mutations of the $G_{\alpha s}$ protein that are involved in the pathogenesis of growth hormone–secreting pituitary adenomas are an example of dominant mutations that cause endocrine tumors; such mutations have not been identified in endocrine tumors of the gastroenteropancreatic system.[169] An example of the second type of mutation in endocrine tumors is the mutation of a gene located on chromosome 11q13 that is involved in the pathogenesis of MEN 1 (see Chapter 32). In the case of the hereditary disorder, one mutant allele is inherited and the other is acquired by somatic mutation. Studies involving the same region of chromosome 11 indicate that as many as 30% of sporadic endocrine tumors have loss of heterozygosity in this region, implying that these tumors may arise from the same mechanism as that involved in the MEN 1 syndrome.[170] Presumably, in the case of sporadic tumors, defects in both alleles arise de novo. Other studies suggest that amplification of the HER-2/neu proto-oncogene may be involved in the pathogenesis of gastrinomas.[171] Malignancy, as evidenced by metastases of pancreatic endocrine neoplasms, is commonly associated with loss of chromosomes.[172]

Diagnosis

Gut endocrine cell tumors are uncommon, occurring in about 1 per 100,000 population. The diagnosis is easy in the presence of characteristic signs and symptoms (e.g., rash with glucagonoma, intractable peptic ulcer with gastrinoma). However, some tumors cause nonspecific symptoms such as dyspepsia. Somatostatinomas may be found incidentally during gallbladder surgery. Other tumors may be diagnosed only during investigation of weight loss. Because these tumors grow slowly and are either benign or metastasize late, they are potentially curable. Early detection is highly desirable.

Radioimmunoassays for the various hormones secreted by these tumors are often diagnostic, particularly if plasma levels are very high, but not every assay is available in all laboratories. To send plasma samples to the appropriate laboratories, blood must be drawn in tubes containing ethylenediaminetetraacetic acid and aprotinin to inhibit serum peptidases (aprotinin, 0.5 mL [500 kallikrein inactivator units] per 10 mL of blood). After immediate centrifugation, plasma is stored at $-25°C$ or lower until transported to the laboratory in the frozen state on dry ice. In screening for pancreatic endocrine tumors, we submit plasma samples for analysis of VIP, gastrin, calcitonin, somatostatin, PP, motilin, GIP, PHM, neurotensin, glucagon, and insulin. In some laboratories, a "gastrointestinal hormone profile" can be obtained with a single plasma sample.[173] Plasma levels of neuron-specific enolase and chromogranin[174, 175] and of islet amyloid polypeptide[176] have been

used by some investigators as markers for neuroendocrine tumor growth.

Tumors can usually be localized by use of techniques that include sonography, CT scanning, angiography, and/or magnetic resonance imaging.[177] Somatostatin receptor scintigraphy[178–181] is also useful for tumor localization, for documenting progression or regression with treatment, and for identifying metastatic spread. In two reports the technique was of use in the identification of metastatic lesions,[181, 182] but the specificity of the procedure for the diagnosis of these tumors is not clear, because findings may also be positive with lymphomas and with granulomatous disease in the abdomen.[183] The diagnostic usefulness of the procedure may be improved if somatostatin analogues are developed to bind to specific somatostatin receptor subtypes.[184] Endoscopic ultrasonography is highly sensitive and specific for the localization of pancreatic endocrine tumors.[185] In our experience involving three instances in which CT was negative, endoscopic ultrasonography identified tumors ranging from 0.7 to 1.3 cm in diameter. If liver metastases are present, peritoneoscopic biopsy or biopsy guided by ultrasound or CT can be used to obtain material for histologic studies. For immunocytochemical studies, biopsy material should be fixed in Bouin's solution. Aliquots of the biopsy material should also be frozen in liquid nitrogen to allow analysis of tissue extracts for various peptides. If the results of imaging procedures and directed biopsies are negative, exploratory laparotomy may be necessary. Intraoperative sonography is superior to palpation of the pancreas for localizing small tumors. Selective venous sampling may be useful in some patients, but aberrant venous drainage of the tumor can lead to erroneous conclusions.[186]

Treatment

Total tumor resection is the major objective of therapy. Even in the presence of liver metastases, removal of the primary pancreatic tumor is sometimes advisable. One of our patients with VIPoma was cured by removal of the primary tumor and, after chemotherapy, partial hepatectomy to remove the one area of tumor mass remaining in the liver. After resection of the primary pancreatic tumor, liver transplantation has been attempted in a few instances to remove the remaining tumor.[187] Metastatic tumor mass has also been reduced by hepatic artery embolization.[126]

Among chemotherapeutic drugs, streptozocin is highly effective, particularly in VIPomas.[188] 5-Fluorouracil and dacarbazine have also been used. Finally, drugs that modify the target organ response can render the patient asymptomatic for long periods despite continued slow tumor growth and elevated plasma peptide levels. Such regimens include use of antisecretory drugs for diarrhea in VIPoma or calcitoninoma syndrome[189] and use of proton pump inhibitors in Zollinger-Ellison syndrome.[82, 84]

Somatostatin inhibits the release of VIP from endocrine tumors in pancreatic cholera,[190] and octreotide, a long-acting somatostatin analogue, has been successfully used in VIPomas,[191] glucagonomas,[192] and GHRHomas.[156] Administration of somatostatin analogues improves endocrine symptoms by inhibiting formation and/or processing and release of hormones and other tumor products.[193] Long-acting (slow-release) forms of octreotide or laneotide can be administered once every 2 to 4 weeks, and administration of these agents over long periods may cause some tumor shrinkage.[194–196] Neverthelesss, the overall effect on tumor growth is moderate, with only 4% showing regression and about 30% showing "no progression." Even when tumor regression cannot be documented, however, endocrine manifestations, pain, and other tumor symptoms may be controllable with somatostatin analogues.[197, 198] It may be possible to predict whether a given tumor will respond to somatostatin analogue therapy with the use of somatostatin receptor scintigraphy.[199] Interferon has been useful in some[200, 201] but not all patients with endocrine tumors. Undoubtedly, additional treatment modalities will be created for chemotherapy and for receptor modulation, but early surgical excision remains the cornerstone of treatment.[202]

REFERENCES

1. Langerhans P. Uber einen Drusenpolyp im ileum. Virchows Arch [A] 1867; 28:559–565.
2. Langerhans P. Über die mikroskopische Anatomie des Pankreas. Inaugural-Dissertation. Berlin: G. Lange, 1869.
3. Solcia E, Sessa F, Rindi G, et al. Classification and histogenesis of gastroenteropancreatic endocrine tumors. Eur J Clin Invest 1990; 20(Suppl):S72–S81.
4. Solcia E, Fiocca F, Rindi G, et al. The pathology of the gastrointestinal endocrine system. Endocrinol Metab Clin North Am 1993; 22:795–821.
5. Pearse AGE. The diffuse neuroendocrine system and the APUD concept: related "endocrine" peptides in brain, intestine, pituitary, placenta and anuran cutaneous glands. Med Biol 1977; 55:115–125.
6. Falkmer S. Phylogeny and ontogeny of the neuroendocrine cells of the gastrointestinal tract. Endocrinol Metab Clin North Am 1993; 731–752.
7. Delcore R, Friesen SR. Embryologic concepts in the APUD system. Semin Surg Oncol 1993; 9:349–361.
8. Lloyd KC. Gut hormones in gastric function. Ballieres Clin Endocrinol Metab 1994; 8:111–136.
9. Burns GA, Cummings JF. Neuropeptide distributions in the colon, cecum, and jejunum of the horse. Anat Rec 1993; 236:341–350.
10. Wong HC, Tache Y, Lloyd KC, et al. Monoclonal antibody to rat alpha-CGRP: production, characterization, and in vivo immunoneutralization activity. Hybridoma 1993; 12:93–106.
11. Ohneda A, Ohneda K, Nagasaki T, et al. Insulinotropic action of human glicentin in dogs. Metabolism 1995; 44:47–51.
12. Leech CA, Holz GG, Habener JF. Signal transduction of PACAP and GLP-1 in pancreatic β cells. Ann N Y Acad Sci 1996; 805:81–92.
13. Taylor RG, Fuller PJ. Humoral regulation of intestinal adaptation. Ballieres Clin Endocrinol Metab 1994; 8:165–183.
14. Bamba T, Sasaki M, Hosoda S. Enteroglucagon. A putative humoral factor inducing pancreatic hyperplasia after proximal small bowel resection. Dig Dis Sci 1994; 39:1532–1536.
15. Sasaki M, Bamba T, Hosada S. Enteroglucagon, but not CCK, plays an important role in pancreatic hyperplasia after small bowel resection. J Gastroenterol Hepatol 1994; 9:576–581.
16. Bardam L. Gastrin in non-neoplastic pancreatic tissue from patients with and without gastrinoma. Scand J Gastroenterol 1990; 25:1185–1195.
17. Rehfeld JF, Lindhom J, Andersen BN, et al. Cholecystokinin and glucagonoma. N Engl J Med 1988; 318:122–123.
18. Hutcheon DF, Bayless TM, Cameron JL, et al. Hormone-mediated watery diarrhea in a family with multiple endocrine neoplasms. Ann Intern Med 1979; 90:932–934.
19. Friesen Sr, Tomita T, Kimmel JR. Pancreatic polypeptide update: its role in detection of the trait for multiple endocrine adenopathy syndrome, type I and pancreatic polypeptide-secreting tumors. Surgery 1983; 94:1028–1037.
20. Debas HT, Mulvihill SJ. Neuroendocrine gut neoplasms: important lessons from uncommon tumors. Arch Surg 1994; 129:965–971.
21. Syversen U, Mignon M, Bonfils S, et al. Chromogranin A and pancreastatin-like immunoreactivity in serum of gastrinoma patients. Acta Oncol 1993; 32:161–165.
22. Kimura N, Yamamoto H, Okamoto H, et al. Multiple-hormone gene expression in ganglioneuroblastoma with watery diarrhea, hypokalemia, and achlorhydria syndrome. Cancer 1993; 71:2841–2846.
23. Le Bodic MF, Heymann MF, Lecomte M, et al. Immunohistochemical study of 100 pancreatic tumors in 28 patients with multiple endocrine neoplasia, type 1. Am J Surg Pathol 1996; 20:1378–1384.
24. Ozbakir O, Kelestimur F, Ozturk F, et al. Carcinoid syndrome due to a malignant somatostatinoma. Postgrad Med J 1995; 71:695–698.
25. Bardram L. Progastrin in serum from Zollinger-Ellison patients. Gastroenterology 1990; 98:1420–1426.
26. Krejs GJ. Gastrointestinal endocrine tumors. Am J Med 1987; 82(Suppl 5B):1–3.
27. Habener JF. The incretin notion and its relevance to diabetes. Endocrinol Metab Clin North Am 1993; 22:775–794.
28. Bloom SR, Polak JM. Glucagonoma syndrome. Am J Med 1987; 82(Suppl 5B):25–36.
29. Wermers RA, Fatourechi V, Wynne AG, et al. The glucagonoma syndrome: clinical and pathological features in 21 patients. Medicine (Baltimore) 1996; 75:53–63.
30. Wood SM, Polak JM, Bloom SR. Gut hormone secreting tumours. Scand J Gastroenterol 1983; 18:165–179.
31. Binnick AN, Spencer SK, Dennison WL, et al. Glucagonoma syndrome:

32. report of two cases and literature review. Arch Dermatol 1977; 113:749–754.
33. Stacpoole PW. The glucagonoma syndrome: clinical features, diagnosis and treatment. Endocr Rev 1981; 2:347–361.
33. Wood SM, Polak JM, Bloom SR. Glucagonoma syndrome. In: Lefebvre PJ, ed. Handbook of Experimental Pharmacology. Vol 66. Part II: Glucagon. Stuttgart: Springer-Verlag, 1983: 411–430.
34. Smith AP, Doolas A, Staren ED. Rapid resolution of necrolytic migratory erythema after glucagonoma resection. J Surg Oncol 1996; 61:306–309.
35. Almadal TP, Heindorff H, Bardram L, at el. Increased amino acid clearance and urea synthesis in a patient with glucagonoma. Gut 1990; 31:946–948.
36. Hicks T, Turnberg LA. Influence of glucagon on the human jejunum. Gastroenterology 1974; 67:1114–1118.
37. Haga Y, Yanagi H, Urata J, et al. Early detection of pancreatic glucagonoma. Am J Gastroenterol 1995; 90:2216–2223.
38. Moody AJ, Thim L. Glucagon, glicentin, and related peptides. In: Lefebvre PJ, ed. Handbook of Experimental Pharmacology. Vol. 66. Part I: Glucagon. Stuttgart: Springer Verlag, 1983: 139–174.
39. Takeishi K, Shima K, Funakoshi A, et al. Glucagon-like peptide-1 (GLP-1) molecular forms in human pancreatic endocrine tumors resemble those in intestine rather than pancreas. Diab Res Clin Pract 1994; 25:43–49.
40. Bordi C, Ravazzola M, Baetens D, et al. A study of glucagonomas by light and electron microscopy and immunofluorescence. J Clin Invest 1979; 52:925–936.
41. Stevens FM, Flanagan RW, O'Gormann D, et al. Glucagonoma syndrome demonstrating giant duodenal villi. Gut 1984; 25:784–791.
42. Fiocca R, Capella C, Buffa R, et al. Glucagon-, glicentin-, and pancreatic polypeptide-like immunoreactivities in rectal carcinoids and related colorectal cells. Am J Pathol 1980; 100:81–92.
43. Gleeson MH, Bloom SR, Polak JM, et al. Endocrine tumor in kidney affecting small bowel structure, motility and absorptive function. Gut 1971; 12:773–782.
44. Eissele R, Coke R, Weichardt U, et al. Glucagon-like peptide 1 immunoreactivity in gastroenteropancreatic endocrine tumors: a light- and electron-microscopic study. Cell Tissue Res 1994; 276:571–579.
45. Unger RH. Somatostatinoma. N Engl J Med 1977; 296:998–1000.
46. Krejs GJ, Orci L, Conlon JM, et al. Somatostatinoma syndrome: biochemical, morphologic and clinical features. N Engl J Med 1979; 301:285–292.
47. Gerich JE, Patton GS. Somatostatin: physiology and clinical applications. Med Clin North Am 1978; 62:375–392.
48. Pipeleers D, Couturier E, Gepts W, et al. Five cases of somatostatinoma: clinical heterogeneity and diagnostic usefulness of basal and tolbutamide-induced hypersomatostatinemia. J Clin Endocrinol Metab 1983; 56:1236–1242.
49. Wright J, Abolfathi A, Penman E, et al. Pancreatic somatostatinoma presenting with hypoglycaemia. Clin Endocrinol 1980; 12:603–609.
50. Larsson LI, Hirsch, MA, Holst JJ, et al. Pancreatic somatostatinoma: clinical features and physiological implications. Lancet 1977; 1:666–668.
51. Penman E, Lowry PJ, Wass JAH, et al. Molecular forms of somatostatinoma. Clin Endocrinol 1980; 12:611–620.
52. Galmiche JP, Chayvialle JA, Dubois PM, et al. Calcitonin-producing pancreatic somatostatinoma. Gastroenterology 1980; 78:1577–1583.
53. Jackson JA, Raju BU, Fachnie JD, et al. Malignant somatostatinoma presenting with diabetic ketoacidosis. Clin Endocrinol 1987; 26:609–621.
54. Kaneko H, Yanaihara N, Ito S, et al. Somatostatinoma of the duodenum. Cancer 1979; 44:2273–2279.
55. Dayal Y, Doos WG, O'Brien MJ, et al. Psammomatous somatostatinomas of the duodenum. Am J Surg Pathol 1983; 7:653–665.
56. Marcial MA, Pinkus GS, Skarin A, et al. Ampullary somatostatinoma: psammomatous variant of gastrointestinal carcinoid tumor. An immunohistochemical and ultrastructural study: report of a case and review of the literature. Am J Clin Pathol 1983; 80:755–761.
57. O'Brien TD, Cheijfec G, Prinz RA. Clinical features of duodenal somatostatinomas. Surgery 1993; 114:1144–1147.
58. Mao C, Shah A, Hanson DJ, et al. Von Recklinghausen's disease associated with duodenal somatostatinoma: contrast of duodenal versus pancreatic somatostatinomas. J Surg Oncol 1995; 59:67–73.
59. Kainuma O, Ito Y, Taniguchi T, et al. Ampullary somatostatinoma in a patient with von Recklinghausen's disease. J Gastroenterol 1996; 31:460–464.
60. Griffith DF, Williams GT, Williams ED. Multiple endocrine neoplasia associated with von Recklinghausen's disease. Br Med J 1983; 287:1341–1343.
61. Budminger H, Bühler H, Häcki W, et al. Comparative diagnostic value of the calcium-pentagastrin test versus the tolbutamide test in a patient with a somatostatinoma. Gastroenterology 1987; 92:800–804.
62. Schwartz TW. Pancreatic polypeptide: a hormone under vagal control. Gastroenterology 1983; 85:1411–1425.
63. Lundqvist G, Krause U, Larsson LI, et al. A pancreatic-polypeptide-producing tumour associated with the WDHA syndrome. Scand J Gastroenterol 1978; 13:715–718.
64. Tomita T, Kimmel JR, Friesen SR, et al. Pancreatic polypeptide cell hyperplasia with and without watery diarrhea syndrome. J Surg Oncol 1980; 14:11–20.
65. Hayes MM. Report of a pancreatic polypeptide-producing islet-cell tumor of the pancreas causing the watery diarrhea, hypokalemia, achlorhydria

syndrome in a 55-year-old Zimbabwean African male. Cent Afr J Med 1980; 26:195–197.

66. Lewis DA, Gaginalla TS, O'Dorisio TM. Effects of pancreatic polypeptide and vasoactive intestinal polypeptide on rat ileal and colonic water and electrolyte transport in vivo. Dig Dis Sci 1979; 24:625–630.

67. Choksi UA, Sellin RV, Hickey RC, et al. An unusual skin rash associated with a pancreatic polypeptide-producing tumor of the pancreas. Ann Intern Med 1988; 108:64–65.

68. Öberg K, Grimelius L, Lundqvist G, et al. Update on pancreatic polypeptide as a specific marker for endocrine tumours of the pancreas and gut. Acta Med Scand 1982; 210:145–152.

69. Larsson L-I, Sundler F, Hakanson R. Immunohistochemical localization of human pancreatic polypeptide to a population of islet cells. Cell Tissue Res 1975; 156:167–171.

70. Adrian RE, Uttenthal LO, Williams SJ, et al. Secretion of pancreatic polypeptide in patients with pancreatic endocrine tumors. N Engl J Med 1986; 315:287–291.

71. Polak JM, Adrian TE, Bryant MG, et al. Pancreatic polypeptide in insulinomas, gastrinomas, VIPomas and glucagonomas. Lancet 1976; 1:328–330.

72. Zollinger RM, Ellison EH. Primary peptic ulcerations of the jejunum associated with islet cell tumors of the pancreas. Ann Surg 1955; 142:709–728.

73. McGuigan JE. The Zollinger-Ellison syndrome. In: Sleisinger MH, Fordtran JS, eds. Gastrointestinal Diseases: Pathophysiology, Diagnosis, and Management. 5th ed. Philadelphia: WB Saunders, 1993: 679–697.

74. Stabile BE, Morrow DJ, Passaro E Jr. The gastrinoma triangle: operative implications. Am J Surg 1984; 147:25–31.

75. Perry RR, Vinik AI. Endocrine tumors of the gastrointestinal tract. Ann Rev Med 1966; 47:57–68.

76. McGuigan JE, Wolfe MM. Secretin injection test in the diagnosis of gastrinoma. Gastroenterology 1980; 79:1324–1331.

77. Bonfils S, Bernades P. Zollinger-Ellison syndrome: natural history and diagnosis. Clin Gastroenterol 1974; 3:539–557.

78. Rambaud JC, Modigliana R, Emonts P, et al. Fluid secretion in the duodenum and intestinal handling of water and electrolytes in Zollinger-Ellison syndrome. Dig Dis 1978; 23:1089–1097.

79. Wright HK, Hersch T, Floch MH, et al. Impaired intestinal absorption in the Zollinger-Ellison syndrome independent of gastric hypersecretion. Am J Surg 1970; 119:250–253.

80. Lamers CBHW, Lind T, Moberg S, et al. Omeprazole in Zollinger-Ellison syndrome: effects of a single dose and of long-term treatment in patients resistant to histamine H₂-receptor antagonists. N Engl J Med 1984; 310:758–761.

81. Wolfe MM, Jensen RT. Zollinger-Ellison syndrome: current concepts in diagnosis and management. N Engl J Med 1987; 317:1200–1209.

82. Weber CH, Venzon DJ, Lin, J-T, et al. Determinants of metastatic rate and survival in patients with Zollinger-Ellison syndrome: a prospective long-term study. Gastroenterology 1995; 108:1637–1649.

83. Carlsson E, Larsson H, Mattsson H, et al. Pharmacology and toxicology of omeprazole with special reference to the effects on the gastric mucosa. Scand J Gastroenterol 1986; 21(Suppl 118):31–38.

84. Maton PN, Lack EE, Collen MJ, et al. The effect of Zollinger-Ellison syndrome and omeprazole therapy on gastric oxyntic endocrine cells. Gastroenterology 1990; 99:943–950.

85. Hakanson R, Sundler F. Proposed mechanism of induction of gastric carcinoids: the gastrin hypothesis. Eur J Clin Invest 1990; 20(Suppl 1):S65–S71.

86. Borch K, Renvall H, Liedberg G. Gastric endocrine cell hyperplasia and carcinoid tumors in pernicious anemia. Gastroenterology 1985; 88:638–648.

87. Lamberts R, Creutzfeld W, Stöckman F, et al. Long-term omeprazole treatment in man: effects on gastric endocrine cell populations. Digestion 1988; 39:126–135.

88. Priest WM, Alexander MK. Islet cell tumor of the pancreas with peptic ulceration, diarrhoea, and hypokalaemia. Lancet 1957; 2:1145.

89. Verner JV, Morrison AB. Islet cell tumor and a syndrome of refractory watery diarrhea and hypokalemia. Am J Med 1958; 25:374–380.

90. Matsumoto KK, Peter JB, Schultze RG, et al. Watery diarrhea and hypokalemia associated with pancreatic islet cell adenoma. Gastroenterology 1966; 50:231–242.

91. Ayub A, Zafar M, Abdulkareem A, et al. Primary hepatic vipoma. Am J Gastroenterol 1993; 88:958–961.

92. Bloom SR, Polak JM, Pearse AGE. Vasoactive intestinal peptide and watery-diarrhea syndrome. Lancet 1973; 2:14–16.

93. Said SI, Mutt V. Potent peripheral and splanchnic vasodilator peptide from normal gut. Nature 1970; 225:863–864.

94. Grossman M. Candidate hormones of the gut. Gastroenterology 1974; 67:730–755.

95. Fahrenkrug J. Vasoactive intestinal polypeptide: measurement, distribution and putative neurotransmitter function. Digestion 1979; 19:149–169.

96. Said SI. Vasoactive intestinal polypeptide (VIP) as a neural peptide. In: Miyoshi A, Grossman M, eds. Gut Peptides: Secretion, Function and Clinical Aspects. Amsterdam: Elsevier/North-Holland, 1979: 268–273.

97. Bryant MG, Polak JM, Modlin I, et al. Possible dual role for vasoactive intestinal peptide as gastrointestinal hormone and neurotransmitter substance. Lancet 1976; 1:991–993.

98. Said SI. VIP: biological role in health and disease. Trends Endocrinol Metab 1991; 2:107–112.

99. Krejs GJ. Effect of VIP infusion on water and electrolyte transport in the human intestine. In: Said SI, ed. Vasoactive Intestinal Peptide. New York: Raven, 1982: 193–200.

100. Ebeid AM, Murray P, Hirsch H, et al. Radioimmunoassay of vasoactive intestinal peptide. J Surg Res 1976; 20:355–360.

101. Said SI, Faloona GR. Elevated plasma and tissue levels of vasoactive intestinal polypeptide in the watery-diarrhea syndrome due to pancreatic, bronchogenic and other tumors. N Engl J Med 1975; 293:155–160.

102. Krejs GJ, Walsh JH, Morawski SG, et al. Intractable diarrhea: intestinal perfusion studies and plasma VIP concentrations in patients with pancreatic cholera syndrome and surreptitious ingestion of laxatives and diuretics. Am J Dig Dis 1977; 22:280–292.

103. Krejs GJ, Fordtran JS. Effect of VIP infusion on water and ion transport in the human jejunum. Gastroenterology 1980; 78:722–727.

104. Krejs GJ. Peptidergic control of intestinal secretion: studies in man. In: Bloom SR, Polak JM, eds. Gut Hormones. 2nd ed. Edinburgh: Churchill Livingstone, 1981: 516–520.

105. Kane MG, O'Dorisio TM, Krejs GJ. Production of secretory diarrhea by intravenous infusion of vasoactive intestinal polypeptide. N Engl J Med 1983; 309:1482–1485.

106. Bloom SR, Christofides ND, Delamarter J, et al. Diarrhoea in VIPoma patients associated with cosecretion of a second active peptide (peptide histidine isoleucine) explained by a single coding gene. Lancet 1983; 2:1163–1165.

107. Kane MG, Tatemoto K, Bloom SR, et al. Effect of PHI on water and ion movement in the canine jejunum in vivo. Dig Dis Sci 1984; 29(Suppl Aug):41S.

108. Brunt LM, Mazoujian G, O'Dorisio TM, et al. Stimulation of vasoactive intestinal peptide and neurotensin secretion by pentagastrin in a patient with VIPoma syndrome. Surgery 1994; 115:362–369.

109. Rambaud JC, Matuchansky C. Diarrhea and digestive endocrine tumors. Clin Gastroenterol 1974; 3:657–640.

110. Sellin JH. Intestinal electrolyte absorption and secretion. In: Sleisenger M, Fordtran JS, eds. Gastrointestinal Disease. 5th ed. Philadelphia: WB Saunders, 1993: 954–971.

111. Gardner JD. Plasma VIP in patients with watery diarrhea syndrome. Am J Dig Dis 1978; 23:370–373.

112. Krejs GJ, Hendler RS, Fordtran JS. Diagnostic and pathophysiologic studies in patients with chronic diarrhea. In: Field M, ed. Secretory Diarrhea. Bethesda: American Physiological Society, 1980: 141–151.

113. Rambaud JC, Modigliani R, Matuchansky C, et al. Pancreatic cholera: studies on tumoral secretions and pathophysiology of diarrhea. Gastroenterology 1975; 69:110–122.

114. Schmitt MG, Soergel KH, Hensley GT, et al. Watery diarrhea associated with pancreatic islet cell carcinoma. Gastroenterology 1975; 69:206–216.

115. Verner JV, Morrison AB. Endocrine pancreatic islet disease with diarrhea: report of a case due to diffuse hyperplasia of nonbeta islet tissue with a review of 54 additional cases. Arch Intern Med 1974, 133:492–500.

116. Anderson H, Dotevall G, Fagerberg G, et al. Pancreatic tumor with diarrhea, hypokalemia and hypochlorhydria. Arch Chir Scand 1972; 138:102–107.

117. Escourrou J, Ebeid AM, Fischer JE. Vasoactive intestinal peptide associated inhibition of stimulated gastric secretion: II. Inhibition of pentagastrin-stimulated gastric secretion. Am J Surg 1980; 139:824–828.

118. Holm-Bentzen M, Christiansen J, Petersen B, et al. Infusion of vasoactive intestinal polypeptide in man: pharmacokinetics and effect on gastric acid secretion. Scand J Gastroenterol 1981; 16:429–432.

119. Kofstad J, Froyshov I, Gyone E, et al. Pancreatic tumor with intractable watery diarrhea, hypokalemia and hypercalcemia: electrolyte balance studies. Scand J Gastroenterol 1967; 2:246–250.

120. Barraclough MA, Bloom SR. VIPoma of the pancreas: observations on the diarrhea and circulatory disturbances. Arch Intern Med 1979; 139:467–471.

121. Frase LL, Gaffney FA, Lane LL, et al. Effect of VIP infusion on cardiovascular function in healthy subjects. Am J Cardiol 1987; 60:1356–1361.

122. Espiner EA, Beaven DW. Non-specific islet-cell tumour of the pancreas with diarrhoea. Q J Med 1962; 31:447–471.

123. Kraft AR, Tompkins RK, Zollinger R. Recognition and management of the diarrhea syndrome caused by nonbeta islet cell tumors of the pancreas. Am J Surg 1970; 119:163–170.

124. Krejs GJ. VIPoma syndrome. Am J Med 1987; 82(Suppl 5B):37–48.

125. Rambaud JC, Nisard A, Modigliani R, et al. Hypercalcitonaemia in VIPomas. Lancet 1978; 1:220.

126. Manche A, Wood SM, Adrian TE, et al. Pancreatic polypeptide and calcitonin secretion from a pancreatic tumour: clinical improvement after hepatic artery embolization. Postgrad Med J 1983; 59:313–314.

127. Bugalho MJGM, Roque L, Sobrinho LG, et al. Calcitonin-producing insulinoma: clinical, immunocytochemical and cytogenetical study. Clin Endocrinol (Oxf) 1994; 41:257–260.

128. Gutniak M, Rosenqvist U, Grimelius L, et al. Report on a patient with watery diarrhoea syndrome caused by a pancreatic tumour containing neurotensin, enkephalin and calcitonin. Acta Med Scand 1980; 208:95–100.

129. Williams ED. Medullary carcinoma of the thyroid. J Clin Pathol 1967; 20:395–398.

130. Gray TK, Bieberdorf FA, Fordtran JS. Thyrocalcitonin and the jejunal absorption of calcium, water, and electrolytes in normal subjects. J Clin Invest 1973; 52:3084–3088.

131. Theodorsson-Norheim E, Öberg K, Rosell S, et al. Neurotensinlike immunoreactivity in plasma and tumor tissue from patients with endocrine tumors of the pancreas and gut. Gastroenterology 1983; 85:881–889.

132. Rosell S, Rökaeus A, Theordorsson-Norheim E. The role of neurotensin in disease. Scand J Gastroenterol 1983; 18:59–67.

133. Shulkes A, Boden R, Cook I, et al. Characterization of a pancreatic tumor containing vasoactive intestinal peptide, neurotensin, and pancreatic polypeptide. J Clin Endocrinol Metab 1984; 58:41–48.

134. Feuerle GE, Helmstaedter V, Tischbirek K, et al. A multihormonal tumor of the pancreas producing neurotensin. Dig Dis Sci 1981; 26:1125–1133.

135. Blackburn AM, Bryant MG, Adrian TE, et al. Pancreatic tumors produce neurotensin. J Clin Endocrinol Metab 1981; 52:820–822.

136. Friesen SR, Allen MS. Malignant hyperthyroidism of pancreatic and parathyroid origin. Bull Soc Int Chir 1975; 5:439–441.

137. O'Neal LW, Kipnis DM, Luse SA, et al. Secretion of various endocrine substances by ACTH-secreting tumors: gastrin, melanotropin, norepinephrine, serotonin, parathormone, vasopressin, glucagon. Cancer 1968; 21:1219–1232.

138. Ratcliffe WA, Bowden SJ, Dunne FP, et al. Expression and processing of parathyroid hormone–related protein in a pancreatic endocrine cell tumor associated with hypercalcemia. Clin Endocrinol 1994; 40:679–686.

139. Kaye TB. PTHrP-mediated hypercalcemia in a calcitonin-producing islet cell tumor. Endocr Pract 1995; 1:170–171.

140. Tachibana I, Nakano S, Akiyama T, et al. Parathyroid hormone–related protein mediates hypercalcemia in an exocrine pancreatic cancer. Am J Gastroenterol 1994; 89:1580–1581.

141. Mao C, Carter P, Schaefer P, et al. Malignant islet cell tumor associated with hypercalcemia. Surgery 1995; 117:37–40.

142. Gaich G, Orloff JJ, Atillasoy EJ, et al. Amino-terminal parathyroid hormone–related protein: specific binding and cytosolic calcium responses in rat insulinoma cells. Endocrinology 1993; 132:1402–1409.

143. Philbrick WM, Wysolmerski S, Galbraith EH, et al. Defining the roles of parathyroid hormone–related protein in normal physiology. Physiol Rev 1996; 76:127–173.

144. Maton PN, Gardner JD, Jensen RT. Cushing's syndrome in patients with the Zollinger-Ellison syndrome. N Engl J Med 1986; 315:1–5.

145. Zhu L, Domenico DR, Howard JM. Metastatic pancreatic neuroendocrine carcinoma causing Cushing's syndrome: ACTH secretion by metastases 3 years after resection of nonfunctioning primary cancer. Int J Pancreatol 1996; 19:205–208.

146. Amikura K, Alexander HR, Norton JA, et al. Role of surgery in management of adrenocorticotropic hormone–producing islet cell tumors of the pancreas. Surgery 1995; 118:1125–1130.

147. Rivier J, Spiess J, Thorner M, et al. Characterization of a growth hormone–releasing factor from a human pancreatic islet tumor. Nature 1982; 300:276–278.

148. Guillemin R, Brazean P, Böhlen P, et al. Growth-hormone–releasing factor from a human pancreatic tumor that caused acromegaly. Science 1982; 218:585–587.

149. Berger G, Tronillas, Bloch B, et al. Multihormonal carcinoid tumor of the pancreas secreting growth hormone-releasing factor as a cause of acromegaly. Cancer 1984; 54:2097–2108.

150. Donhuijsen K, Schulte HM, Schmidt U, et al. Akromegalie bei Wachstumshormon-Releasing-Hormon (GH-RH): Klinik und Morphologie. Schweiz Med Wochenschr 1986; 116:615–621.

151. Ezzat S, Ezrin C, Yamashita S, et al. Recurrent acromegaly resulting from ectopic growth hormone gene expression by a metastatic pancreatic tumor. Cancer 1993; 71:66–70.

152. Liu SW, van de Velde CJ, Heslinga JM, et al. Acromegaly caused by growth hormone–releasing hormone in a patient with multiple endocrine neoplasia type 1. Jpn J Clin Oncol 1996; 26:49–52.

153. Shintani Y, Yoshimoto K, Horie H, et al. Two different pituitary adenomas in a patient with multiple endocrine neoplasia type 1 associated with growth hormone–releasing hormone-producing pancreatic tumor: clinical and genetic features. Endocr J 1995; 42:331–340.

154. Genka S, Soeda H, Takahashi M, et al. Acromegaly, diabetes insipidus, and visual loss caused by metastatic growth hormone–releasing hormone-producing malignant pancreatic endocrine tumor in the pituitary gland: case report. J Neurosurg 1995; 83:719–723.

155. Bertherat J, Turpin G, Rauch C, et al. Presence of somatostatin receptors negatively coupled to adenylate cyclase in ectopic growth hormone–releasing hormone- and alpha-subunit-secreting tumors from acromegalic patients responsive to octreotide. J Clin Endocrinol Metab 1994; 79:1457–1464.

156. Maton PN, Gardner JD, Jensen RT. Use of long-acting somatostatin analog SMS201–995 in patients with pancreatic islet cell tumors. Dig Dis Sci 1989; 34(Suppl):S28–S39.

157. Owyang C, Go VL. Multiple hormone-secreting tumors of the gastrointestinal tract. In: Glas GBJ, ed. Gastrointestinal Hormones. New York: Raven, 1980: 741–748.

158. Belchetz PE, Brown CL, Makin HLJ, et al. ACTH, glucagon and gastrin production by a pancreatic islet cell carcinoma and its treatment. Clin Endocrinol 1973; 2:307–316.

159. D'Arcangues CM, Awoke S, Lawrence GD. Metastatic insulinoma with long survival and glucagonoma syndrome. Ann Intern Med 1984; 100:233–235.

160. Mordechai B, Burke M, Isakov A, et al. Insulinoma after streptozotocin therapy for metastatic gastrinoma: natural history or iatrogenic complication? J Clin Gastroenterol 1990; 12:579–580.

161. Yamagami T, Miwa A, Takasawa S, et al. Induction of rat pancreatic B-cell tumors by the combined administration of streptozotocin or alloxan and poly(adenosine diphosphate ribose) synthetase inhibitors. Cancer Res 1985; 45:1845–1849.

162. Hammar S, Sale G. Multiple hormone producing islet cell carcinomas of the pancreas. Hum Pathol 1975; 6:349–362.

163. Dunn PJS, Sheppard MC, Heath DA, et al. Recurrent insulinoma syndrome with metastatic glucagonoma. J Clin Pathol 1983; 36:1076–1080.

164. Said SI. Evidence for secretion of vasoactive intestinal peptide by tumours of pancreas, adrenal medulla, thyroid and lung: support for the unifying APUD concept. Clin Endocrinol 1976; 5(Suppl):201–204.

165. Bloom SR, Polak JM. VIP measurement in distinguishing Verner-Morrison syndrome and pseudo Verner-Morrison syndrome. Clin Endocrinol 1976; 5(Suppl):223–228.

166. Chey WY, Escoffery R, Chu TM. Verner-Morrison syndrome: clinical observation and search for origin of endocrine cell hyperplasia of the pancreas. Gastroenterology 1983, 84:1123 (abstract).

167. Kidd GS, Donowitz M, O'Dorisio T, et al. Mild chronic watery diarrhea–hypokalemia syndrome associated with pancreatic islet cell hyperplasia. Am J Med 1979; 66:883–888.

168. Decker RA. Molecular genetics of APUDomas. Semin Surg Oncol 1993; 9:380–386.

169. Yoshimoto K, Iwahana H, Fukuda A, et al. Rare mutations of the Gs alpha subunit gene in human endocrine tumors: mutation detection by polymerase chain reaction-primer-introduced restriction analysis. Cancer 1993; 72:1386–1393.

170. Eubanks PJ, Sawicki MP, Samara GJ, et al. Putative tumor-suppressor gene on chromosome 11 is important in sporadic endocrine tumor formation. Am J Surg 1994; 167:180–195.

171. Evers BM, Rady PL, Sandoval K, et al. Gastrinomas demonstrate amplification of the HER-2/neu proto-oncogene. Ann Surg 1994; 219:596–601.

172. Long JP, Hruban RH, Lo R, et al. Chromosome analysis of nine endocrine neoplasms of the pancreas. Cancer Genet Cytogenet 1994; 77:55–59.

173. Bloom SR, Polak JM Hormone profiles. In: Bloom SR, Polak JM, eds. Gut Hormones, 2nd ed. Edinburgh: Churchill Livingstone, 1981: 555–560.

174. Prinz RA, Bermes EW, Kimmel JR. Serum markers for pancreatic islet cell and intestinal carcinoid tumors: a comparison of neuron-specific enolase, β-human chorionic gonadotropin and pancreatic polypeptide. Surgery 1983; 94:1019–1023.

175. O'Connor DT, Deftos LJ. Secretion of chromogranin by peptide-producing endocrine neoplasias. N Engl J Med 1986; 314:1145–1151.

176. Stridsberg M, Eriksson B, Lundqvist G, et al. Islet amyloid polypeptide (IAPP) in patients with neuroendocrine tumors. Regul Pept 1995; 55:119–131.

177. Hammond PJ, Jackson JA, Bloom SR. Localization of pancreatic endocrine tumors. Clin Endocrinol 1994; 40:3–14.

178. Modlin IM, Tang LH. Approaches to the diagnosis of gut neuroendocrine tumors: the last word (today). Gastroenterology 1997; 112:583–590.

179. O'Shea DB, Bloom SR. The use of somatostatin in the diagnosis and treatment of neuroendocrine tumors. Curr Opin Endocrinol Diab 1995; 2:177–180.

180. Schirmer WJ, Melvin WS, Rush RM, et al. Indium-111-pentetreotide scanning versus conventional imaging techniques for the localization of gastrinoma. Surgery 1995; 118:1105–1113.

181. Gibril F, Reynolds JC, Doppman JL, et al. Somatostatin receptor scintigraphy: its sensitivity compared with that of other imaging methods in detecting primary and metastatic gastrinomas. A prospective study. Ann Intern Med 1996; 125:26–34.

182. Termanini B, Gibril F, Doppman JL, et al. Distinguishing small hepatic hemangiomas from vascular liver metastases in gastrinoma: use of a somatostatin-receptor scintigraphic agent. Radiology 1997; 202:151–158.

183. Lipp RW, Silly H, Ranner G, et al. Radiolabeled octreotide for the demonstration of somatostatin receptors in malignant lymphoma and lymphadenopathy. J Nucl Med 1995; 36:13–18.

184. Kubota A, Yamada Y, Kagimoto S, et al. Identification of somatostatin receptor subtypes and an implication for the efficacy of somatostatin analogue SMS 201–995 in treatment of human endocrine tumors. J Clin Invest 1994; 93:1321–1325.

185. Rösch T, Lightdale CJ, Botet JF, et al. Localization of pancreatic endocrine tumors by endoscopic ultrasonography. N Engl J Med 1992; 326: 1721–1726.

186. Kingman JCG, Dick R, Bloom SR, et al. VIPoma: localization by percutaneous transhepatic portal venous sampling. Br J Med 1978; 2:1682–1683.

187. Korneru B, Cassavilla A, Bowman J, et al. Liver transplantation for malignant tumors. Gastroenterol Clin North Am 1988; 17:177–193.

188. Kahn CR, Levy AG, Gardner JD, et al. Pancreatic cholera: beneficial effects of treatment with streptozotocin. N Engl J Med 1975; 292:941–945.

189. Krejs GJ. Secretory diarrhea. In: Bayless TM, ed. Current therapies in gastroenterology and liver disease. Toronto: BC Decker, 1983: 255–259.

190. Krejs GJ. Effect of somatostatin infusion on VIP-induced transport changes in the human jejunum. Regul Pept 1984; 5:271–176.

191. Santangelo WC, O'Dorisio TM, Kim JG, et al. Effect of synthetic somato-statin analogue on intestinal water and ion transport in pancreatic cholera syndrome. Ann Intern Med 1985; 103:363–367.

192. Santangelo WC, Unger RH, Orci L, et al. Somatostatin analogue-induced remission of necrolytic migratory erythema without changes in plasma glucagon concentration. Pancreas 1986; 1:464–469.

193. Jockenhovel F, Lederbogen S, Olbricht T, et al. The long-acting somato-statin analogue octreotide alleviates symptoms by reducing posttransla-tional conversion of prepro-glucagon to glucagon in a patient with malig-nant glucagonoma but does not prevent tumor growth. Clinical Investigator 1994; 72:127–133.

194. Kraenzlin ME, Ch'ng JC, Wood SM, et al. Long-term treatment of a VIPoma with somatostatin analogue resulting in remission of symptoms and possible shrinkage of metastases. Gastroenterology 1985; 88:185–187.

195. Santangelo WC, O'Dorisio TM, Kim JG, et al. VIPoma syndrome: effect of a synthetic somatostatin analogue. Scand J Gastroenterol 1989; 21(Suppl 119):87–190.

196. Arnold R, Neuhaus C, Benning R, et al. Somatostatin analog Sandostatin and inhibition of tumor growth in patients with metastatic endocrine gastroenteropancreatic tumors. World J Surg 1993; 17:511–519.

197. Burgess JR, Shepherd JJ, Murton FJ, et al. Effective control of bone pain by octreotide in a patient with metastatic gastrinoma. Med J Aust 1996; 164:725–727.

198. Fiasse R, Pauwels S, Rahier J, et al. Use of octreotide in the treatment of digestive neuroendocrine tumors: seven year experience in 20 cases includ-ing 9 cases of metastatic midgut carcinoid and 5 cases of metastatic gas-trinoma. Acta Gastroenterol Belg 1993; 56:279–291.

199. Nocaudie-Calzada M, Huglo D, Deveaux M, et al. Iodine-123-Tyr-3-octreo-tide uptake in pancreatic endocrine tumors and in carcinoids in relation to hormonal inhibition by octreotide. J Nucl Med 1994; 35:57–62.

200. Janson ET, Öberg K. Long-term management of the carcinoid syndrome. Acta Oncol 1993; 32:225–229.

201. Nold R, Frank M, Kajdan U, et al. Kombinierte Behandlung metastasierter endokriner Tumoren des Gastrointestinaltrakts mit Octreotid und Inter-feron-Alpha. Z Gastroenterol 1994; 32:193–197.

202. Delcore R, Friesen SR. Gastrointestinal neuroendocrine tumors. J Am Coll Surg 1994; 178:187–211.

TABLE 35–1. Risk Factors for Breast Cancer in Women

Factor	High Risk	Low Risk	Relative Risk
Age	Old age	Young age	>4
Country of residence	North America, northern Europe	Asia, Africa	>4
Socioeconomic class	Upper	Lower	2–4
Marital status	Never married	Ever married	1–2
Place of residence	Urban	Rural	1–2
Place of residence	Northern United States	Southern United States	1–2
Race	White	Black	1–2
Age at first birth	Older than 30 y	Younger than 20 y	2–4
Oophorectomy	No	Yes	2–4
Body build	Obese	Thin	2–4
Age at menarche	Early	Late	1–2
Age at menopause	Late	Early	1–2
Family history of premenopausal bilateral breast cancer	Yes	No	>4
History of cancer in one breast	Yes	No	>4
History of fibrocystic disease	Yes	No	2–4
Any first-degree relative with breast cancer	Yes	No	2–4
History of primary cancer in ovary or endometrium	Yes	No	2–4
Radiation to chest	Large doses	Minimal exposure	2–4
Alcohol use	Yes	No	1–2

Modified from Kelsey JL. Division of epidemiology of human breast cancer. Epidemiol Rev 1979; 1:74–109, with permission.

whom special therapeutic intervention may be warranted. Nor does the absence of all risk factors rule out breast cancer occurrence. In fact most affected women have no obvious risk factors for the disease. Rather these epidemiologic factors suggest potentially alterable influences that require further study.

The risk factors in which endocrine influences may be significant can be grouped under five headings: geographic variation, reproductive history, genetic factors, hormonal milieu, and miscellaneous.

Geographic Variation

There are striking variations in the rates of breast cancer in different areas of the world.[3] The incidence of breast cancer in women at age 50 is about six times higher in the United States than in Japan or Taiwan[4]; for older women the difference increases to nearly 20-fold. This difference was initially interpreted as evidence of a genetic basis for altered breast cancer risk, but the Chinese Americans who have lived in Hawaii for several generations have the same rate of breast cancer as the whites who live there, and first- and second-generation Japanese women in Hawaii have higher breast cancer rates than do women in Japan.[5] The incidence of breast cancer is now increasing in Japan, a change that has occurred in association with changes in diet, height, weight, and menstrual history.

The relationship of the incidence of breast cancer to age varies from one country to another. In countries with a high incidence there is a continued increase with age, whereas in "low-risk" countries the rate of development of breast cancer decreases after menopause (Fig. 35–1). DeWaard[6] first suggested that these data imply two different causes of breast cancer. Superimposed on the curve for the incidence of breast cancer in countries of lower socioeconomic status is an additional type of cancer risk related to factors generally associated with industrialization, such as increased food consumption, increased fat and meat intake, increased height, higher rates of obesity, and altered reproductive history.

Reproductive and Menstrual History

The reproductive and menstrual histories of women with breast cancer have been thoroughly studied. If one arbitrarily assigns a relative risk of 1 to nulliparous women, there is a nearly threefold alteration in the risk of breast cancer with parity, varying from 0.5 for women having their first child before age 20 to 1.4 for women giving birth to their first child after age 37.

The protective effect of early age at first full-term pregnancy is maintained throughout life, even after age 75.[7] The protective effect of early pregnancy may be due to either a permanently induced alteration in the mammary gland or a chronic postpartum alteration in circulating hormone levels. Identification of the nature of the protection against breast cancer provided by early first delivery would allow prophylactic endocrine manipulations in young women. The protective effect is probably not due to lactation per se,[8, 9] although one study of women who nursed their babies on only one breast

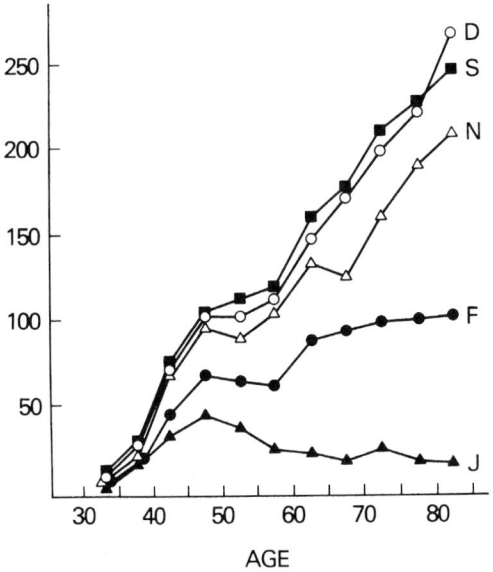

Figure 35–1. Incidence of breast cancer with age in countries with high and low cancer rates. The ordinate indicates incidence per 100,000 people. D, Denmark; S, Sweden; N, Norway; F, Finland; J, Japan. (From DeWaard F. The epidemiology of breast cancer: review and prospects. Int J Cancer 1969; 4:577–586, with permission.)

showed a significant reduction in breast cancer incidence on that side.[10]

Ovarian activity is a clear risk factor in breast cancer. Surgical menopause protects against breast cancer in proportion to the reduction in years of menstrual life.[8] Earlier age at menarche and later age at menopause are also risk factors.[11] This excess risk exists even in the elderly, a relation that is consistent with a long latency period for some human breast cancers. Ovarian estrogen is probably the causative factor, and the protective effects of early ovariectomy are negated by the administration of estrogen.[12]

Pike and colleagues[13] have proposed that most of the geographic variation in breast cancer incidence can be understood by assigning different risk factors to menstrual life before the first full-term pregnancy and in the years thereafter.[13] In this construct early menarche and menstrual life before first pregnancy are particularly weighted as risk factors. Because dietary practices are likely to influence height and weight and thereby the onset of menses (see Chapter 15), this is an attractive means of incorporating multiple risk factors into a unified hypothesis. This concept has been incorporated into a proposal for breast cancer prevention.[14]

Family History

Family history is an important risk factor in breast cancer.[15] Genetic factors may be expressed at a variety of levels, including heritable alteration in the endocrine milieu. One gene responsible for approximately half of inherited breast cancer has been identified, sequenced, and cloned.[16, 17] The *BRCA1* gene, located on chromosome 17q23, contains only one obvious motif, a zinc finger, suggesting it may be a transcriptional factor. Evidence that it is a tumor suppressor gene is supported by the fact that its expression is decreased in sporadic breast cancer as well.[18] A second breast cancer–associated gene, *BRCA2*, has been identified on chromosome 3,[19] and the cloning of the ataxia telangectasia gene[20] may also prove to be significant to breast cancer if heterozygotes (1 to 2% of the population) have an increased risk of breast cancer. This group, paradoxically, may face undue hazard from exogenous radiation, including mammography. Information in this field, including the availability of successful testing strategies, is developing rapidly.

Hormonal Milieu

The hormonal environment may influence the rate of progression of established cancer as well as the risk of its development. This concept has gained experimental support from studies of the induction of mammary cancer in rodents, in which a permissive or promotional role for estrogens can be clearly demonstrated. This phenomenon was first described by Lacassagne,[21] who noted that estrone administration can induce cancer in susceptible strains of mice.

ESTROGENS. Because of the likelihood of a relationship of breast cancer to estrogen, urinary estrogen levels have been measured by several groups, but no differences were identified between women with breast cancer and the normal controls. These studies suffered from the fact that estrogens should have been measured at the beginning of carcinogenesis rather than at a later stage of clinical disease. Furthermore, the wide fluctuations of estrogen levels during the menstrual cycle and the alterations in the rates of metabolism with disease or drugs, or both, made interpretation difficult. Nevertheless one review of this issue has concluded that hormonal patterns of high-risk groups of women do not differ from those of the normal population.[22] Additional studies have been published that finally appear to clarify these issues. Serum estradiol levels were examined in Asian populations living rural lifestyles asso-

ciated with a very low breast cancer incidence; their estradiol levels were found to be lower than all appropriate control groups.[23]

OTHER HORMONES. A role for prolactin in the etiology of human breast cancer remains enigmatic. Some investigators have reported abnormal prolactin levels in patients with breast cancer[24] and in their daughters.[25] Others have failed to detect significant differences.[26] One review of the subject proposed that elevated prolactin levels may be associated with a risk for breast cancer but whether causally or not remains to be determined.[27] As discussed later, however, there is no clear-cut evidence that any subset of established breast cancers is dependent on prolactin as a tropic hormone. However, prolonged lactation is associated with some reduction in breast cancer risk even after correcting for other risk factors such as age at first full-term pregnancy and number of children.[28]

The incidence of abnormalities of thyroid function, usually goiter or hypothyroidism, has been reported to be increased in patients with breast cancer, but at least two critical reviews of this area have failed to support this contention.[3, 29]

Exogenous Hormones
Benign Breast Disease

Most benign breast diseases are not premalignant. There is evidence from both retrospective analyses[30–35] and prospective studies[36, 37] that oral contraceptives diminish the incidence of benign breast disease. Generally such studies show a greater protective effect against cystic disease than against fibroadenoma. In addition, protection is greater in long-term users, a feature in favor of a causal relationship. A study conducted by the Royal College of General Practitioners[31] reported that the incidence of benign breast disease is inversely related to the amount of progestagen in the preparation. This relation was confirmed by surveys of women using noncontraceptive estrogen preparations, in whom no protection was demonstrated.[32, 37] Certain forms of benign breast disease, such as atypical lobular and ductal hyperplasia, are associated with a high likelihood of subsequent malignant disease,[38, 39] and the effects of oral contraceptives on these lesions have not been assessed. It should not be concluded, therefore, that the effectiveness of oral contraceptives in reducing benign breast disease is equivalent to a protection against breast cancer.

Malignant Breast Disease

ORAL CONTRACEPTIVES. Multiple retrospective case control studies have revealed no increased risk of developing breast cancer among users of oral contraceptives.[30, 33, 40–42] However, several factors complicate the interpretation of these results. The time required for tumor promotion in humans is long, and there may not be sufficient experience to allow firm conclusions. Two studies of younger women showed a slightly higher relative risk ratio in those who had used oral contraceptives for more than 8 and 5 y, respectively,[43, 44] but the increase was not significant. Two other studies have failed to show an increase in risk with time.[33, 40] However in one study[40] oral contraceptive use increased the risk of breast cancer in three subsets of patients: nulliparous women, women who began the pill before the birth of the first child, and women with a history of benign breast disease. Some prospective trials of oral contraceptive use have not confirmed this relationship[35, 40] and, in fact, suggest a reduction in risk. Other prospective studies have suggested a small increase in breast cancer incidence in users of contraceptives,[45, 46] most strikingly in young women (younger than age 32). Longer follow-up studies are required before the question of risk can be determined. However given the minimal effects on breast cancer risk and the profound protection they exert against the risks of endometrial and ovarian malignancies, oral contraceptives are clearly beneficial for cancer risk.

ESTROGEN REPLACEMENT. The relation of hormone replacement therapy to cancer risk in the postmenopausal setting is complex and controversial. A detailed discussion of the potential benefits of estrogen replacement therapy are beyond the scope of this chapter (see Chapter 15). Subjective benefits and reduction in cardiovascular events and mortality in osteopenia have been demonstrated.[47] In addition in one report estrogen replacement therapy was associated with a reduction in colon cancer as well.[48] Conversely, unopposed estrogen replacement therapy increases the incidence of endometrial cancer despite the fact that multiple studies have failed to detect a substantial incidence in mortality from endometrial cancer. This probably reflects the relative lack of lethality of endometrial cancer, its early diagnosis because of dysfunctional bleeding, and the increased surveillance that most women undergo during treatment with estrogen.

Multiple studies have been analyzed by meta-analysis with respect to breast cancer risk with estrogen replacement.[49, 50] Given the unequivocal evidence that breast cancer is promoted by estrogen, the conclusion of these studies that there is a minimal increase in breast cancer risk with estrogen replacement therapy at first appears puzzling. However, these data must be interpreted in light of the fact that risk is generally seen with prolonged use, whereas estrogen replacement therapy in many cases does not continue beyond 5 y. In addition most forms of estrogen replacement supply less biologically equivalent estrogen than that present in premenopausal women so that the overall danger of hormone replacement for breast cancer risk is lessened.

An important aspect of the decision-making paradigm has to do with the role of progestagens in hormone replacement. Progestagens were initially introduced as a component of estrogen therapy because they reduce the likelihood of endometrial cancer. However the impact of progestagens on cardiovascular death rates and osteopenia is not firmly established. Perhaps more worrisome is the fact that progestagens can function with estrogens as co-promoters of breast cancer in models of breast cancer. Whether or not the addition of progestagen to estrogens alters breast cancer risk in humans is unknown.

MISCELLANEOUS FACTORS (DIET, ALCOHOL, AND RADIATION). Most studies in Western societies have failed to show a significant relationship between dietary fat and breast cancer risk. Alcohol intake, in contrast, is associated with an increased risk of breast cancer,[51] either as a causative or an associative variable. Exogenous radiation is also a risk factor for breast cancer, presumably through direct damage to DNA. This association is pronounced in women receiving radiation before age 30, as for Hodgkin's disease. As mentioned previously, an interaction between radiation and women who are heterozygous carriers for ataxia telangectasia remains an intriguing possibility.[20]

Hormone Receptors and Endocrine Therapy for Breast Cancer

The fact that some human breast cancers respond to endocrine manipulations has been appreciated since Beatson[52] induced tumor regressions in patients with bilateral oophorectomy. Patients who respond to endocrine therapy experience palliation and have longer survival than do nonresponders, but only about one third of unselected patients have objective tumor regression. With the advent of chemotherapy a more precise selection of treatment modalities is necessary.

A variety of empirical clinical guidelines (longer disease-free interval, lack of visceral involvement, a prolonged disease-

free interval) and a few biochemical tests (excretion of androgen metabolites, steroid sulfation) have been tried for the selection of patients with hormone-responsive tumors, but none of these prognostic variables is reliable. However, developments in hormone action have made possible a more accurate selection of patients for hormone therapy.

The first step in the action of steroid hormones, including estrogen, is binding of the hormone to specific receptor proteins, which then function as transcriptional regulatory units (see Chapter 4). Functional receptors are necessary for steroid hormone action,[53] and regression of mammary cancer in response to endocrine ablation therapy in animals also requires the presence of estrogen receptors.[53] Human breast cancer samples take up and retain estrogen[54]; and Jensen and colleagues[55] found estrogen receptors in human breast cancers and showed direct correlations between the presence of an estrogen receptor and the likelihood of response to endocrine therapy.

Comprehensive reviews of this field are available.[56, 57] In brief about two thirds of primary cancers and a smaller proportion of metastatic samples contain significant levels of estrogen receptor. Tumors in premenopausal women are less frequently estrogen receptor–positive and, when positive, contain lower concentrations of receptor than do those occurring after menopause. These observations are only partially explained by the fact that the larger amounts of endogenous estrogen in the plasma of premenopausal women mask the binding sites. Overall the association between the presence of estrogen receptor and the likelihood of response to endocrine therapy is significant. Predictive accuracy for the test is about 75%. Thus about 60% of women with estrogen receptor–positive tumors respond to endocrine therapy, whereas 95% of the 40% of those with estrogen receptor–negative tumors do not. In general the greater the estrogen receptor content of the tumor, the higher the response rate to endocrine therapy. Although estrogen receptor assays are useful in selecting therapy for patients with advanced disease, an even more valuable use of these tests is in selection of appropriate adjuvant regimens for patients with localized breast cancer at the time of initial therapy. In this group correct selection of therapy is important for two reasons. First, there is no adequate marker of response, the first indication of inadequate therapy being recurrence of tumors. Meta-analysis of 15 y of adjuvant chemotherapy trials reveals that benefit is limited to women whose tumors are estrogen receptor–positive. Separation of patients into those likely to benefit and those who are not requires meticulous quality control and uniformity of assays.[58]

The response rate of metastatic tumors lacking estrogen receptors is low but is not zero. Thus a single negative assay is only one component in the selection of appropriate therapy. There are several possible explanations for endocrine responses in women with purportedly estrogen receptor–negative tumors. First, steroid receptors are labile proteins and receptor activity may not be detected because of methodologic artifacts, including incorrect handling and storage of samples. Second, the diagnosis of metastatic breast cancer may be based on observation of a few tumor cells infiltrating a nonmalignant tissue, and a negative estrogen-receptor assay can be due to insufficient sampling of malignant cells or inadvertent sampling of neighboring nonmalignant tissue. Third, some additive and ablative therapies for breast cancer may act via mechanisms not involving estrogen receptors. Thus even in the absence of an estrogen receptor, some endocrine manipulations may cause a response. Fourth, breast tumors may be heterogeneous with respect to receptor status; a biopsy site that is estrogen receptor–negative may not be representative of other tumor deposits. Fifth, some assays may be falsely negative because some methodologies do not detect receptors occupied by endogenous hormone. Sixth, even in the absence of endogenous hormone, receptor sites may be localized to the nucleus[59] and thereby missed with classic ligand-binding assays that begin with cytosol preparation. In view of these various possibilities it is surprising how rarely (about 5%) so-called estrogen receptor–negative tumors respond to endocrine therapy.

Failure of tumors containing estrogen receptor to respond to endocrine therapy is more common. The usual explanation for this phenomenon is tumor cell heterogeneity, i.e., a sufficient number of cells in the tumor contain receptor to give a positive assay result, whereas others (the most malignant) are receptor-negative. If this is the case one would anticipate a quantitative relationship between the amount of estrogen receptor and the likelihood of an endocrine response, as has been reported,[60] and tumors do contain a mixture of receptor-positive and receptor-negative cells.[61] Second, the presence of estrogen receptor may not explain the positive responses to all forms of endocrine therapy. If, for example, androgen administration were to induce tumor regression by a process involving interaction with androgen receptor, estrogen receptor–positive but androgen receptor–negative tumors might fail to respond to this endocrine therapy. Third, the presence of a receptor may suggest hormone-dependent breast cancer, but the endocrine therapy may not be adequate to effect a response. For example pituitary ablation may be incomplete, or ovarian steroidogenesis may overcome competitive effects of antiestrogens in premenopausal women. About 10 to 15% of patients with metastatic breast cancer who fail to respond to oophorectomy or tamoxifen do respond to a subsequent medical or surgical adrenalectomy. Presumably at the time of oophorectomy these women had hormone-dependent tumors that were estrogen receptor–positive but appeared to be hormone independent because of the formation of estrogen precursors in the adrenals. Fourth, binding of hormone to receptor is only the first step in hormone action, and any step distal to the binding of hormone to receptor may be deranged in cancer cells.[53] Molecular studies of steroid receptors have provided insight into additional mechanisms of hormone independence.[62] Fuqua and colleagues have described estrogen receptor mutants in breast cancer that retain ligand-binding domains but have lost elements required for transcriptional activation; other estrogen receptor mutants lack hormone-binding domains but are capable of activating gene transcription.[63] These variants are particularly interesting for two reasons. First, because many detection strategies require either ligand binding or binding of antibodies to domains near the hormone-binding domain, these will appear to be estrogen receptor–negative. Second, these receptors are constitutively active in the absence of estrogen, in effect acting as dominant oncogenes. The frequency of such receptor mutants is not clear.

Prediction of hormone dependence would be more reliable if a tumor were assessed for a hormone-inducible function, the induced response reflecting receptor and postreceptor function. The most useful of these tests is measurement of progesterone receptor level.[56, 57] In both normal uterus and malignant uterine and mammary tissue, the synthesis of progesterone receptor is regulated by estrogen acting through the estrogen receptor. Tumors lacking an estrogen receptor are rarely progesterone receptor–positive, whereas about two thirds of estrogen receptor–positive tumors are progesterone receptor–positive. Only a third of estrogen receptor–positive tumors lacking progesterone receptor respond to endocrine therapy (the same as the overall response rate in unselected patients). The response rate to endocrine therapy when tumors contain both estrogen and progesterone receptors is in excess of 75%.

The responses that occur in women whose tumors are

TABLE 35–2. Response Rates to Endocrine Therapy as a Function of Steroid Hormone Receptor Status in Metastatic Breast Cancer

Estrogen Receptor Status	Progesterone Receptor Status	Approximate Objective Response Rate to Endocrine Therapy (%)
Positive	Positive	80
Positive	Negative	30
Negative	Positive	Not established
Negative	Negative	5

estrogen receptor–positive and progesterone receptor–negative can be due to two causes. First, in premenopausal women during the latter phase of the menstrual cycle and during pregnancy, endogenous progesterone may occupy receptor, promote its tight association with nuclear components, and obscure its detection.[64] Second, in postmenopausal women with hormone-dependent tumors, estrogen concentrations may be insufficient to induce progesterone receptors.[65]

Despite many false-positive and false-negative results, steroid receptor studies in breast cancer are extremely valuable. Table 35–2 summarizes the response rates to endocrine therapy as a function of estrogen and progesterone receptor status. In most patients the response to endocrine therapy can be predicted with reasonable accuracy.

Assays of receptor levels may also provide prognostic information. Women with primary estrogen receptor–positive breast cancers have longer disease-free intervals than do those who are receptor-negative, independent of other prognostic variables, including menopausal status, tumor size, histologic grade, and axillary lymph node status.[66–69] In some women who are axillary lymph node–negative, lack of estrogen or progesterone receptor worsens prognosis sufficiently to justify early institution of adjuvant chemotherapy.

The development of high-affinity antibodies to the estrogen receptor protein allows detection of the receptor independent of the binding of labeled hormone.[70, 71] A plastic bead radioimmunoassay and histochemical methods using immunoperoxidase or immunofluorescence provide a basis for efficient detection and localization of estrogen receptor in clinical samples.[72]

Management of Breast Cancer

The management of breast cancer is discussed in detail elsewhere[73, 74] and can be divided into two phases: early and advanced (metastatic) disease.

Early Breast Cancer

Nearly 90% of the 186,000 women diagnosed with breast cancer in 1996 will present with apparently localized disease. An approach to patients with early breast cancer is shown in Table 35–3. All surgical and radiotherapeutic options should be considered because survival is identical for women treated with breast-conserving therapy and those treated with mastectomy. All women with early breast cancer should have assays of estrogen and progesterone receptor performed on their tumors. Estrogen receptor status of the primary cancer is maintained in metastases in the absence of intervening therapy and, consequently, knowledge of the receptor status of the primary tumor permits assignment to the appropriate treatment category when metastases develop, even if there is no tissue readily accessible for biopsy. Measurements of other prognostic variables by histochemistry, such as S phase, ploidy, and amplification or overexpression of the proto-oncogene *ERBB2 (HER2)*, are under study as guides for choice of therapy.

TABLE 35–3. Management of Early-Stage Breast Cancer

Histologic Status of Lymph Nodes	Estrogen Receptor Status	Recommended Therapy
Premenopausal patients		
Involved with tumor	Positive	Combination chemotherapy plus endocrine therapy
Involved with tumor	Negative	Combination chemotherapy
Negative	Positive	No therapy generally, unless other prognostic variables indicate
Negative	Negative	Combination chemotherapy possible
Postmenopausal patients		
Involved with tumor	Positive	Chemotherapy plus endocrine therapy
Involved with tumor	Negative	Combination chemotherapy
Negative	Positive	Endocrine therapy (tamoxifen)
Negative	Negative	Combination chemotherapy

All Patients

1. Adequate therapy for local control of disease
2. Histopathologic evaluation of axillary lymph nodes
3. Analysis of estrogen and progesterone receptors in the primary tumor
4. Analysis of growth fraction, ploidy, and markers that are under investigation such as cathepsin D, ERBB2, and heat shock proteins

Therapy must be sufficient to control the disease, but attention to the cosmetic outcome is also desirable; therefore therapy should be individualized. In addition, staging should assess axillary lymph node involvement to provide information as to whether adjuvant therapy is appropriate. The role of adjuvant therapy in subsets of patients continues to be refined. One meta-analysis[75] suggested that the addition of tamoxifen to chemotherapy improved survival in all receptor-positive women treated with adjuvant chemotherapy. In addition many postmenopausal women can be treated with tamoxifen as the only systemic therapy.

Metastatic Breast Cancer

Although many patients with primary breast cancer remain free of disease after local therapy (with or without the addition of systemic adjuvant therapy), many cancers eventually recur, causing 46,000 deaths per year in the United States. Endocrine therapy is an important therapeutic option. As already mentioned, only about one third of unselected patients respond, but improvement in response rates can be achieved in women selected by appropriate steroid receptor determinants and prognostic variables. One approach to therapy for patients with metastatic cancer is outlined in Table 35–4. After assessment of receptor status, women may be allocated to appropriate treatment regimens. Factors to be weighed in such decision-making include prognostic variables such as sites of involvement and personal issues such as the impact of different treatments on lifestyle. There is substantial latitude in the choice of regimen because most breast cancer patients with metastatic disease are treated with multiple therapies over the course of their illness.

Endocrine Therapy for Breast Cancer

Ablative Therapies

MEDICAL AND SURGICAL OOPHORECTOMY. Removal of the ovaries of premenopausal patients has been known to be an effective treatment for more than 100 years in some women with inoperable breast cancer.[52] The regression rate is 25 to 30%,[76, 77] and the median duration of remission is 9 mo. Assessment of absolute response rate and comparisons of different therapies are difficult because selection biases influence the apparent success of endocrine therapy. In addition to the presence of estrogen and progesterone receptors in a tumor sample, lack of visceral metastases, a long interval from local therapy to first recurrence, and a good response to previous endocrine therapy all correlate with response to endocrine therapy. Surgical oophorectomy is generally preferable to radiation of the ovaries because radiation may require several weeks to be effective and may result in incomplete destruction of the follicles.

Ovarian ablation is readily achieved by chronic administration of luteinizing hormone–releasing hormone (LHRH) analogues.[78] Their use in breast cancer is somewhat less common than the use of tamoxifen because of the subjective complaints that accompany castration in premenopausal women. However in premenopausal women LHRH analogues are at least as effective as tamoxifen or surgical castration.

Oophorectomy also has a role as adjuvant therapy for the management of breast cancer, in which it enhances the disease-free interval and overall survival.[75] As already mentioned LHRH analogues yield results in metastatic disease equivalent to surgical castration, but the use of these agents in the adjuvant setting has not been well studied. Their use in meta-

TABLE 35–4. Approach to Therapy for Patients with Metastatic Breast Cancer

	Premenopausal Patients		Postmenopausal Patients	
	Estrogen Receptor–Positive	*Estrogen Receptor–Negative*	*Estrogen Receptor–Positive*	*Estrogen Receptor–Negative*
First therapy	Castration or possibly antiestrogen	Combination chemotherapy	Antiestrogen	Combination chemotherapy
	Relapse: repeat ER assay		Relapse: repeat ER assay	
Second therapy	Endocrine therapy	Chemotherapy	Endocrine therapy	Chemotherapy

All Patients

1. Adequate staging of sites of involvement
2. Biopsy of accessible tumor for ER and progesterone receptor *or* if not available
3. Receptor status of primary tumor

ER, estrogen receptor.

static disease is discussed later. In one important study[79] the addition of glucocorticoid therapy after oophorectomy improved survival in premenopausal women. The reason for this improved result is not clear; it is possibly the result of suppression by glucocorticoids of the secretion of adrenal androgens that can serve as prohormones for extraglandular estrogen formation. The role of oophorectomy as first-line endocrine therapy in premenopausal patients is under reassessment.

ADRENALECTOMY AND HYPOPHYSECTOMY. The adrenal cortex secretes a small amount of estrone,[80] but the principal source of estrogen in blood and urine after castration results from the transformation of the adrenal androgen androstenedione to estrone in extraglandular tissues.[81] The low concentrations of estradiol and estrone characteristic of menopause are sufficient to support the growth of endocrine-sensitive tumors. Indeed when human breast cancer cells are maintained in continuous tissue culture, as little as 2 to 3×10^{-11} M estradiol or less is sufficient to stimulate protein synthesis.[82]

Adrenalectomy appears to be effective because it removes an additional source of estrogens, but the mechanism of response to hypophysectomy is less clear. Removal of corticotropin (also known as adrenocorticotropic hormone [ACTH]) is doubtless important because the incidence of response to adrenalectomy is low after hypophysectomy. Lowering of the prolactin level is not involved because equivalent response rates occur after pituitary stalk sectioning, which raises plasma prolactin levels. Furthermore administration of drugs that lower prolactin concentration is ineffective in treating breast cancer. Other incompletely characterized hypothalamic and pituitary peptides may play roles in the regulation of tumor growth.[83] However, it is likely that hypophysectomy acts (like adrenalectomy) to decrease the levels of estrogen precursors in blood.

There are several criteria for the selection of patients for adrenalectomy or hypophysectomy. First, if estrogen receptor is present in the metastatic tissue, the chance of response is about 60%. Second, if the patient has responded to castration, the likelihood of a subsequent response to ablative surgery (or medical adrenalectomy) is more than 50%. A longer disease-free interval is associated with higher remission rates. Functional adrenalectomy can now be achieved by medical means (see later). Comparisons of medical and surgical adrenalectomy suggest that response rates and duration are approximately equivalent.

Additive Therapies

ANDROGEN THERAPY. Lacassagne,[21] who was the first to show that estrogens promoted the development of mammary tumors in mice, found that the growth of these tumors could be inhibited by testosterone propionate. Androgen therapy in women with metastatic cancer was studied subsequently. The mechanism by which androgens induce responses in breast cancer remains unknown.[84] Some tumors have androgen receptors, but their role in mediating the response of the tumor to androgens has not been established.[85, 86] The Cooperative Breast Cancer Group surveyed the responses of 521 patients treated with testosterone propionate and reported an overall remission rate of 21% and a somewhat higher rate in postmenopausal women.[87] Within 1 y of menopause, the remission rate is less than 10%, and it is highest 5 y after menopause. Soft tissue metastases respond most favorably. The median period of remission is 8 mo. Any androgen, given in large amounts, produces about the same rate of regression. Long-acting preparations should be avoided so that therapy can be changed rapidly if necessary. The results of trials with androgens have been summarized by the Cooperative Breast Cancer Group and Johnston and Novales.[87, 88]

Attempts have been made to find effective steroids that

are less androgenic than testosterone, which can cause severe and distressing virilization. One agent, testolactone, has essentially no androgenic activity and has been reported to produce regression of disease,[89] suggesting that the antitumor effect is independent of androgenicity. Danazol, a progestagen with weak androgenic effects, is also effective in breast cancer and has minimal virilizing effects.[90–93] Combined therapy using an antiestrogen, danazol, and aminoglutethimide improves the response rate compared with antiestrogen alone but does not improve overall survival.[94] This is also the usual case when endocrine and chemotherapy are combined in advanced disease, namely that an improved initial response rate does not result in improved survival.[95] However in one randomized trial, tamoxifen together with androgen did lead to improved survival when compared with tamoxifen alone.[96] Because of their side effects, these agents are used less commonly than are antiestrogens, aromatase inhibitors, and progestagens. However some patients with hormone-dependent breast cancer respond to multiple endocrine therapies.

ESTROGENS. Some patients with breast cancer paradoxically show tumor regression when treated with pharmacologic doses of estrogens. The remission rate is 30 to 37% when estrogen is the initial therapy.[97, 98] In a randomized trial estrogen produced a 29% remission rate and androgen induced a 10% remission rate. The duration of response is longer with estrogen than with androgen in most series. Estrogen responsiveness increases with time after menopause. As with androgen and the ablative procedures, the longer the disease-free interval the higher the probability of response to estrogen. When estrogens are used in women who have relapsed from other therapy the chance of response is less than 10%. Estrogen is generally ineffective after hypophysectomy or adrenalectomy.

The toxicity of estrogens, even at high doses, is moderate. Endometrial hyperplasia and breakthrough bleeding can usually be managed by giving a progestagen, followed by a short period of cessation of hormone therapy to permit withdrawal bleeding. Salt and water retention may also occur, particularly in the elderly. The most important side effect, however, is hypercalcemia, which can occur abruptly in any patient but is rare in subjects 10 y or more beyond menopause. Hypercalcemia almost certainly results from direct stimulation of bone metastases and is managed by hydration and withdrawal of estrogen. Often on gradual reinstitution of therapy remission can be achieved without recurrence of hypercalcemia. Women who experience hypercalcemia have a higher response rate to endocrine therapy than do patients who do not.

Responses may occur after estrogen or androgen has been withdrawn.[99] Thus new therapy generally should not be started until at least 2 mo after discontinuing steroid administration. Rapidly advancing disease, of course, is an exception to this suggestion.

PROGESTAGENS. Various progestagens, including both C_{21}-steroids such as medroxyprogesterone and C_{19}-steroids such as norethindrone, have been used in patients with breast cancer. Their exact mechanism of action is unknown, but possibilities include blockade of progesterone receptor, interference with estrogen receptor synthesis, androgen-like effects, or possible effects on the immune system.[84] In general, remission rates are about 20 to 30%.[100] Progestagens may be tried in patients who fail to respond to other therapies. Regression of soft tissue metastases appears to be more common than regression of bone metastases with progestagens. In general the drugs do not cause serious side effects, but troublesome side effects with medroxyprogesterone acetate include sweating and weight gain. Crona and colleagues[101] reported decreases in high-density lipoprotein cholesterol and apolipoprotein AI levels and an increase in triglyceride levels in patients receiving 1000 mg medroxyprogesterone acetate weekly, suggesting that cardiovascular risk could be increased. Side effects with megestrol acetate include increased appetite, weight gain of 5 to 20 kg, abnormal liver function tests, thromboembolism, vaginal bleeding, hot flashes, fluid retention, nausea and vomiting, hypercalcemia and flare, and rash.[102, 103] Investigations in Italy using large doses of progestagens reported response rates in the range of 30 to 40% without significant toxicity.[104, 105]

ANTIPROGESTAGENS. Antiprogestational agents such as mifepristone, which also has antiglucocorticoid effects, have also been tried for the treatment of hormone-dependent cancers such as breast carcinoma.[106] Pretreatment of MCF-7 (breast cancer) cells with estradiol increases the inhibition seen with mifepristone,[107] and mifepristone has been tried in the treatment of patients with metastatic breast cancer[108]; the dose was 200 mg orally daily, and the response rate was 18%. The only toxicity reported was a decrease in serum potassium levels. Plasma concentrations of follicle-stimulating hormone (FSH), luteinizing hormone (LH), and prolactin were unchanged, but plasma cortisol levels were increased after 3 mo of treatment. Further clinical trials and research into the mechanisms of action are in progress.

LUTEINIZING HORMONE–RELEASING HORMONE ANALOGUES. Administration of an LHRH analogue in a sustained or continuous manner causes inhibition of gonadal steroid hormone synthesis (see Chapters 15, 16, and 31). Treatment of premenopausal women with LHRH agonists reduces plasma estradiol concentrations to levels comparable to those in oophorectomized or postmenopausal women.[109–111] Furthermore in premenopausal women treated with the LHRH agonist leuprolide, serum FSH and LH concentrations increase during the first 4 d of treatment and subsequently fall and remain suppressed.[111] Plasma progesterone, estrone, estrone sulfate, and estradiol levels decrease to postmenopausal values, and concentrations of androstenedione, prolactin, and cortisol do not change.

Buserelin in moderate doses also induces anovulation and a decrease in progesterone levels, but 60% of patients in one study had transient elevation of estradiol levels with no change in FSH or LH,[112] so high doses may be necessary to induce complete chemical castration. Furthermore subcutaneous administration appears to be more effective than intranasal administration. Decreases in plasma LH, FSH, progesterone, and estradiol levels also occur in premenopausal women after treatment with goserelin.[113] Plasma progesterone levels are reduced after 2 wk, and estradiol levels decrease after 4 to 6 wk of treatment.

In two studies the administration of LHRH agonists to premenopausal women with breast cancer produced objective responses of 44%[111] and 41%,[112] respectively. This class of compounds may be useful as adjuvant therapy, although they have not been adequately evaluated. Side effects include hot flashes, nausea and vomiting, headache, dizziness, tumor flare, diarrhea, local reaction, irritability, hives, and severe polydipsia and (rarely) polyuria.[110–112] Amenorrhea is a physiological consequence of the therapy in all women.

GLUCOCORTICOIDS. Large doses of glucocorticoids (equivalent to 200 to 300 mg of hydrocortisone daily) induce short-lived regression of metastatic breast cancer in 10 to 20% of patients,[114] but the rapid onset of action makes these agents useful in rapidly advancing disease. A response to glucocorticoids is not predictive of responses to other endocrine modalities. As mentioned previously, when combined with oophorectomy, glucocorticoids also inhibit the synthesis of adrenal substrates for extraglandular aromatization and may improve survival for patients with early stages of breast cancer.[79] Glucocorticoids may also improve the response rate and survival time when combined with certain cytotoxic chemotherapeutic programs[114] and are of value in managing hypercalcemia and intracranial metastases.

ANTIESTROGENS. Substances that antagonize the action of estrogens are termed *antiestrogens* (also see Chapter 4). The compounds of most current clinical relevance are derivatives of triphenylethylene and include nafoxidine, clomiphene, and tamoxifen. Newer steroidal antiestrogens do not appear to have the agonistic effects seen in some tissues with tamoxifen. These agents compete with estradiol for binding to specific estrogen receptor sites. However, their biologic effects are more complicated and cannot be explained in terms of this effect alone.[115, 116] Proposed mechanisms for antiestrogen action include inhibition of receptor dimerization, altered interaction with nuclear transcription factors, and interaction with novel antiestrogen response elements of various kinds.[117–119]

Tamoxifen can also stimulate hormone-dependent human breast cancer cells to secrete the polypeptide factor transforming growth factor β[120] that inhibits many epithelial cell lines, including breast carcinoma. Indeed transforming growth factor β can even inhibit the growth of the estrogen receptor–negative breast cancer cell line MDA-MB-231.[120] Breast cancers contain mixtures of estrogen receptor–positive and –negative tumor cells. If transforming growth factor β has a paracrine effect on surrounding hormone-independent cells, it may make antiestrogens more effective in these tumors than would be the case solely from blockade of estrogen action.

Antiestrogens are useful in the management of postmenopausal breast cancer[121–124] and in some premenopausal patients. Premenopausal women receiving antiestrogens may have normal menstrual cycles during objective tumor regressions.[125] As mentioned most antiestrogens are also weak estrogen agonists. For example the vaginal epithelium of postmenopausal women receiving tamoxifen usually shows an estrogenic effect, and some women have a brief "flare" of tumor growth after the institution of antiestrogen therapy.[126]

Antiestrogens induce a therapeutic response in about a third of "unselected" men and women with breast cancer[121–124] and are thus as efficacious as other forms of endocrine manipulation. An advantage of the antiestrogens is that their administration is not associated with significant bone marrow, renal, hepatic, or central nervous system toxicity. However chronic tamoxifen use in the adjuvant setting is associated with an increased risk of endometrial cancer[127] and of thromboembolic disease.[128]

Patterson and colleagues[129] reviewed the treatment of nearly 3000 patients with antiestrogens in 45 separate studies. The overall response rate was 34%; less than 7% achieved a complete remission; and the range of response varied from 14 to 57%. In the absence of prior systemic therapy 43% had an objective response; prior chemotherapy did not have a significant effect on the response, whereas 59% of patients who had responded to prior endocrine therapy responded to tamoxifen. In contrast only 21% of nonresponders to endocrine therapy improved with subsequent antiestrogen therapy. In a heavily pretreated cohort of women with advanced breast cancer only 17% achieved an objective partial response or better.[96]

In the experience of Patterson and colleagues[129] 31% of premenopausal women (or at least women younger than age 50) had an objective response. This was similar to the results for women aged 51 to 60 (30%) or aged 61 to 70 (36%). It is of note that 46% of women older than age 70 responded to tamoxifen.

However, selection biases and different prognostic variables influence outcome. Visceral metastases, multiple sites of involvement, estrogen receptor negativity, the perimenopausal state, poor performance status, failure to respond to prior endocrine chemotherapy, and age less than 35 are associated with lower response rates to antiestrogen therapy.

There have been few comparisons of antiestrogen therapy and alternative endocrine therapies in younger women, but in two studies[130, 131] antiestrogen therapy appeared to be equivalent to ovarian ablation. In one study[130] a crossover design was used, and a 50% response rate occurred with the second therapy if the first had been successful, regardless of whether castration or antiestrogen was used first. The second therapy failed uniformly if the first therapy had failed.

If higher circulating estrogen concentrations can overcome the effects of antiestrogens, one would anticipate a dose-response effect. However, the relationship between response and dose is minimal. Of the patients who receive a total daily dose of 20 mg, 30% respond; the response rate increases to 36% with 30 mg/d and to 40% with 40 mg/d. These differences are not significant. However, on occasion a second well-documented remission can occur after relapse when the dose is increased.[132]

The major tamoxifen metabolite was originally thought to be 4-hydroxytamoxifen[133] but now appears to be N-desmethyltamoxifen, which is present in the circulation of treated patients,[134] reaches serum levels 1.2 to 1.8 times greater than those of tamoxifen,[135–137] and binds to the estrogen receptor with an affinity that is 1% that of tamoxifen.[135–137] 4-Hydroxytamoxifen, present at low levels in serum of treated women, binds to the estrogen receptor with an affinity 25 to 50 times that of tamoxifen and equal that of estradiol.[137–139] Therefore, although the blood levels of 4-hydroxytamoxifen are lower, the potency is 1250 times that of desmethyltamoxifen. This suggests that N-desmethyltamoxifen contributes little to the antiestrogenic properties of tamoxifen and that 4-hydroxytamoxifen exerts a significant antiestrogenic effect.[140] The metabolites are excreted largely in the bile as conjugates.

Tamoxifen treatment causes no or minimal changes in levels of gonadotropin[141, 142] and prolactin[136, 142] in premenopausal women, but estradiol and progesterone concentrations increase,[136] possibly because of a direct stimulatory effect of tamoxifen on the ovary. Failure of the elevated estrogen levels to cause a decrease in gonadotropin levels implies that tamoxifen exerts a direct antiestrogenic effect on the hypothalamic-pituitary axis. In postmenopausal women the levels of LH and FSH decrease with tamoxifen treatment but are still in the postmenopausal range in most studies.[143]

Effects on vaginal cornification in postmenopausal women vary in different reports. Estrogens cause an increase in cellular maturity or an increase in karyopyknotic index. Boccardo and colleagues[144] treated postmenopausal women with tamoxifen and reported an increase in the karyopyknotic index in two thirds of patients, no change in one tenth of patients, and a decrease in one fourth of patients.

Tamoxifen has complex actions that include lowering of cholesterol levels and an estrogen-like effect on bone, increasing bone density.[145] In addition, in adjuvant studies in which tamoxifen has been used to prevent recurrences, a consistent reduction in new primary breast cancers in the opposite breast has led to the suggestion that tamoxifen might have a role as a chemoprevention agent.[146] A randomized national breast cancer prevention trial comparing tamoxifen and placebo is under way in women with a risk of breast cancer equivalent to or greater than that in a 55-year-old woman. In other words, younger women must have additional risk factors such as prior breast biopsies or a family history. When results of this study become available it should be possible to ascertain whether some advantages of estrogen replacement therapy can be attained with an agent that may reduce the risk of breast cancer.

PHARMACOLOGIC INTERFERENCE WITH ADRENAL STEROIDOGENESIS. The fact that adrenalectomy and hypophysectomy are effective for some patients has prompted efforts to achieve similar results pharmacologically. Glucocorticoid administration can cause transient palliative responses in some patients with metastatic breast cancer. Although glucocorticoids may have direct inhibitory effects on cancer cells in tissue culture,[147] suppression of adrenal androgen production and subsequent suppression of extraglandular estrogen synthesis probably play a major role in the therapeutic effect. The combined use of aminoglutethimide and dexamethasone has been tried as a means of suppressing adrenal function.[148] Aminoglutethimide inhibits the conversion of cholesterol to pregnenolone[149] and inhibits extraglandular aromatase and shortens the plasma half-life of dexamethasone so that pituitary corticotropin secretion increases and overrides the adrenal blockade imposed by aminoglutethimide.[150] By substituting hydrocortisone (whose metabolism is not altered by aminoglutethimide), adequate adrenal suppression can be achieved in most patients.[151]

Harvey and colleagues and Coombes and co-workers have reviewed the use of inhibitors of adrenal steroidogenesis.[152, 153] Aminoglutethimide in combination with hydrocortisone causes decreases in plasma estrone and estradiol levels equivalent to those seen after surgical adrenalectomy. Furthermore the response rate and duration of response in women with breast cancer appear to be equivalent after surgical adrenalectomy and treatment with aminoglutethimide.[154] The major effect of aminoglutethimide may be exerted through inhibition of aromatase rather than blockade of early steps in steroidogenesis. This had led to a search for more specific and active inhibitors of aromatase.

AROMATASE INHIBITION. There are two mechanisms for blocking aromatase.[155] Type I inhibitors act as substrates for the aromatase enzyme and bind to the active site of the enzyme. Some are competitive inhibitors, and some bind irreversibly to the enzyme, causing its inactivation (so-called suicide inhibition). Inhibitors of the latter type are more specific and usually longer acting. 4-Hydroxyandrostenedione and several other type I inhibitors are being explored in clinical trials.[159, 160]

Type II inhibitors interfere with steroid hydroxylations by binding to the cytochrome P450 (CYP) moiety of the aromatase and produce a different spectral pattern. These inhibitors inhibit hydroxylating enzymes involved in the synthesis of many steroids. Aminoglutethimide is an example of this type of inhibitor.

Side effects of aminoglutethimide include lethargy in about 40% and ataxia in 10% of patients, effects that usually resolve over weeks. About a third of patients acquire a morbilliform, maculopapular rash that is usually evanescent and does not necessitate cessation of therapy but is sometimes associated with fever. The rash rarely progresses and causes desquamation. Other side effects include orthostatic hypotension, leg cramps, facial fullness, weight gain, cushingoid features, and nausea. Side effects make it necessary to discontinue therapy in approximately 5% of patients.

In a review of 1345 patients treated with aminoglutethimide there was a 4% incidence of thrombocytopenia, a 1% incidence of leukopenia, and a 4% incidence of pancytopenia,[161] effects that usually occurred 3 to 7 wk after the beginning of therapy[162] and ameliorated within 3 wk after discontinuation. Bone marrow aplasia has caused death from septicemia[162]; therefore white blood cell and platelet counts should be determined at weeks 4, 8, and 12 after starting therapy.

On a molecular basis 4-hydroxyandrostenedione is about 60 times more potent than aminoglutethimide in the inhibition of human placental aromatase.[156–158] It causes regression of dimethylbenzanthracine-induced mammary tumors in animals,[163] inhibits extraglandular aromatization of androgens in rhesus monkeys,[164] and inhibits the conversion of androstenedione to estrogens in human placenta and rat ovarian microsomes.[165] 4-Hydroxyandrostenedione is 30 times more potent as an aromatase inhibitor than is aminoglutethimide and 100 times more potent than testolactone.[157]

In 52 postmenopausal women with metastatic breast cancer the response rate to 4-hydroxyandrostenedione was 27%.[166] Half of these patients had undergone two or more previous endocrine therapies. The optimal dose and route of administration have not been determined.

Side effects of intramuscular 4-hydroxyandrostenedione include sterile abscesses and painful lumps at the injection site and lethargy. Perioral edema occurred in one patient, and an anaphylactoid reaction has been reported.[166] Toxicity after oral administration includes rash, facial swelling, leukopenia,[167] and hot flashes.[168]

Breast Cancer in Men

Although accounting for less than 1% of breast cancer, the disorder in men is commonly hormone dependent and provides certain distinct contrasts with the disorder in women.[169–171] Known risk factors include exogenous estrogen exposure, enhanced endogenous estrogen formation (Klinefelter's syndrome), radiation, family history of breast cancer, gynecomastia, and orchitis (also see Chapter 17). One of the most convincing arguments for a role of exogenous estrogen in the etiology of breast cancer was provided by the report of two 30-year-old transsexual men in whom breast cancer developed after castration and continuous estrogen use.[172] Breast cancers in men contain estrogen receptor 90% of the time and are frequently positive for progesterone, glucocorticoid, and androgen receptors.[173] Although the survival rates in men and women at each stage of the disease are the same (when matched for age), a greater proportion of men present with advanced disease. Approximately two thirds of men respond to orchiectomy, which is twice the response rate to endocrine therapy in women with breast cancer.[171] Adrenalectomy and hypophysectomy are also frequently successful, even in patients who fail to respond to castration. In one study of 31 men with advanced breast cancer, treatment with tamoxifen caused a complete or partial response with minimal toxicity in 48% of patients.[174] Antiestrogens may thus be the initial treatment of choice for men with breast cancer.

ENDOMETRIAL CANCER

Epidemiology

The endometrium is under the control of two hormones, estradiol and progesterone, and identification of the uterine cytosolic receptor for estradiol in 1962[175] was an important milestone in the field of hormone action. As in the case of breast cancer, estrogen probably plays permissive, carcinogenic, and promotional roles in the development of endometrial cancer, with the promotional activity being the most important.

Clinical, biologic, and epidemiologic data indicate that prolonged or unopposed estrogen stimulation increases the risk of endometrial carcinoma. The longer the endometrium is stimulated the greater is the cancer risk.[176] The increased incidence of endometrial cancer in women with estrogen-secreting tumors and the polycystic ovary syndrome[177] further suggests that progesterone-induced endometrial sloughing may be protective. In both cases estrogen secretion is not excessive but is continuous, and ovulatory cycles, with their accompanying progesterone secretion and subsequent endometrial sloughing, do not occur. The occasional development of endometrial cancer in women with gonadal dysgenesis treated with estrogens alone and the high incidence of pre-existing irregular menses in women with endometrial cancer support a causal role for continued, unopposed estrogenic stimulus.[177] The resumption of cyclic ovarian function in response to ovarian wedge resection in the polycystic ovary syndrome causes regression of endometrial hyperplasia, and progesterone can reverse estrogen-induced endometrial hyperplasia.[178]

Another risk factor for endometrial carcinoma (as for breast cancer) is obesity. In the premenopausal woman the association of anovulatory cycles and amenorrhea with obesity may be the physiological basis for the association. After menopause the predominant blood estrogen is estrone, derived almost entirely by formation in extraglandular tissues from androstenedione, and the rate of this conversion increases with age[179] and weight.[180] Plasma estrogen concentrations increase with increasing weight[181] because adipose tissue constitutes the most important site of extraglandular estrogen formation. Plasma estrone production and concentrations are the same in women with endometrial cancer as in weight- and age-matched control subjects, but the higher incidence of obesity in the women with cancer means that as a group there is greater exposure to estrogen. The use of exogenous estrogen is also associated with an increased risk of endometrial cancer in postmenopausal women.[182] The relative risk factors for the development of endometrial cancer vary from 4:1 to 9:1, the higher figures occurring with longer use. Increased risk with increasing duration of exposure is a characteristic feature of tumor promoters in the two-step carcinogen model for cancer induction. It has been suggested that the risk of long-term exogenous estrogen use might be overestimated because of an increased likelihood of discovery of early endometrial cancer during the work-up of the vaginal bleeding that may occur with estrogen therapy.[182] This argument has been refuted by additional data and theoretical considerations.[176] In most studies of the relation between endometrial cancer and estrogen therapy, larger than physiological doses were used, and progestagen-induced withdrawal bleeding was not part of the regimen. Attention to both these factors would be expected to reduce the risk appreciably. The increased incidence of endometrial cancer has not been accompanied by a similar increase in the death rate from the disease because estrogen use tends to be associated with a less aggressive form of endometrial cancer (see Chapter 15).

An important aspect of the epidemiology of endometrial cancer has been recognition of the association between tamoxifen use and endometrial cancer risk.[183] Tamoxifen is a partial estrogen agonist in uterus. The absolute incidence is less than 1% in women with 5 y of tamoxifen use and a reported lethality rate of 0.1 to 0.2% with 5 y of use. Most of these deaths are probably preventable with appropriate gynecologic surveillance.

Endocrinology

The uterus is the best-studied estrogen-responsive tissue, the estrogen receptor content of the endometrium is highest in the proliferative phase and is decreased in the luteal phase,[184–186] and administration of progestagen decreases estrogen receptor content.[186] Progesterone receptor capacity is highest at the time of the estradiol peak[184] and can be induced by estrogens. Estrogen receptor is present in most endometrial carcinomas, and the content of the receptor is inversely correlated with the degree of differentiation.[184] By contrast, cytosolic[184, 187] and nuclear progesterone receptor levels[188] are highest in well-differentiated cancer.[184] The uterine 17-hydroxysteroid dehydrogenase enzyme that catalyzes the conversion of estradiol to estrone is induced by progesterone[189] and can be used as an index of progestational effect.

The mechanism by which progestagen inhibits endometrial cancer is incompletely understood. In the estrogen-primed uterus progesterone causes specific maturational changes, followed by atrophy and apoptotic cell death when administration is continued for long periods. After administration of progestagens to women with endometrial cancer, mitotic activity ceases, the glandular epithelium becomes more differentiated, and the ratio of cytoplasm to nucleus increases. Atrophy of the epithelium may also occur. These changes are similar to those of the normal endometrium during progestagen therapy and are probably mediated by progesterone receptors in the cancer cells. Progestagen therapy also decreases estrogen receptor levels and increases the capacity of the endometrium to metabolize estradiol (see earlier). As with breast cancer, these tumors may be heterogeneous with respect to cell content of progesterone receptors, accounting for the variability of response.

Therapy

Kelly and Baker reported in 1961[190] that progestagens cause regression in about a third of patients with metastatic endometrial cancer, an observation that has been confirmed at many centers.[191] The response to therapy does not depend on the age of the patient, site of metastasis, or previous or concurrent therapy. However, women with slowly growing or more differentiated tumors respond better than do those with more aggressive cancers. The duration of life after initiation of therapy was 27 mo in those who responded and only 7 mo in those who did not. It does not appear to matter which progestagen is used, but large doses seem to be necessary.[192] Agents that have been used include both the C_{21}-17-acetoxy-steroids, such as medroxyprogesterone acetate and megestrol acetate, and C_{19}-steroids, such as norethindrone. Response is associated with the presence of estrogen and progesterone receptors.

Several hypotheses have been postulated to explain how progestagens inhibit tumor growth. First, they could have a direct cytotoxic effect on tumor cells, as has been shown in vitro in breast cancer cell lines.[193] Second, the inhibition could be exerted at the level of the hypothalamic-pituitary-gonadal axis. Progestagens suppress basal and LHRH-stimulated gonadotropin secretion and the secretion of cortisol, dehydroepiandrosterone, and estradiol in a dose-dependent manner. Third, progestagens may decrease estrogen receptor levels and therefore inhibit the ability of the tumor to respond to endogenous estrogens. Progestagens bind weakly to other receptors, and their binding to androgen or glucocorticoid receptors may account for the tumor response. Finally, progestagens may induce the formation of growth inhibitory factors, inhibit the synthesis and secretion of estrogen-induced growth factors, or modulate other mitogens. In any event the final common pathway is the induction of cell death through apoptosis.

In view of the lack of effectiveness of chemotherapy in uterine cancer a trial of progestagens is appropriate in all patients with metastatic disease. The response of pulmonary metastases may be better than that of bone metastases. Measurement of progesterone receptor levels can be of value in selecting patients suitable for endocrine therapy.[194]

CARCINOMA OF THE PROSTATE

Epidemiology

Cancer of the prostate is the second most common cancer in men in the United States[195] and more than 60% of the cases occur in men older than age 70. The incidence and death rates are higher in American blacks than in whites, and American black men have an age-standardized incidence about six times that of Nigerian black men,[196] although the incidences of latent carcinoma are the same.[197] A role of environmental factors in the etiology of clinical cancer of the prostate is further suggested by the finding that Japanese men living in Hawaii have a higher incidence of cancer of the prostate than do men in Japan, although the incidence of latent carcinoma is the same.[198] There has been an alarming increase in the incidence of prostate cancer in the United States, much of which is due to earlier detection as a result of the widespread use of prostate-specific antigen determinations as a means of diagnosis. The prevalence of the disease has also increased with the aging of the population and with a decrease in the incidence of cardiovascular mortality.

Endocrinology

The work of Huggins and associates[199–201] gave rise to the concept that prostatic cancer, like the normal prostate and the hyperplastic prostate, is androgen dependent, and initiated the era of hormonal management of cancer of the prostate.

In broad outlines the mechanism of androgen action resembles that of other steroid hormones (see Chapters 4 and 16); i.e., the androgen is bound to a specific receptor protein and the hormone-receptor complex interacts with androgen elements in the DNA upstream from androgen-regulated genes. The active intracellular androgen in the prostate is dihydrotestosterone, the 5α-reduced metabolite of testosterone.[202, 203] Plasma androgen levels are the same in men with prostatic cancer as in normal men.[204]

Prolactin plays a role in prostatic growth in rodents. Hypophysectomy causes a more profound atrophy of the rat prostate than does castration, and endogenous prolactin may act synergistically with testosterone in maintaining the male mouse glands of accessory reproduction.[205] Injection of prolactin antiserum inhibits prostate growth in rabbits.[206] In addition the prostate in some species has specific prolactin-binding sites, and these receptors are androgen dependent.[207] However a role for prolactin in the physiology of the human prostate has not been established.

In parallel with receptor studies in breast and endometrial cancers, attempts have been made to correlate the content of dihydrotestosterone receptor with response to therapy.[208] Sampling problems are only one of the several technical issues that make such studies difficult. At any rate, as with endometrial cancer, predicting the clinical response to endocrine therapy from evaluation of receptor levels is of less value than in breast cancer. Because no alternative therapies of proven value are available, virtually all patients with prostate cancer should receive a trial of endocrine therapy.

Therapy

Although the principles of therapy are simple, the tactics and timing are less clear. If, as proposed by Huggins,[199–201] it is necessary to decrease the plasma content of testicular androgens to a low level, surgical or "medical" orchiectomy should suffice; if total deprivation of adrenal and testicular androgen is necessary, additional steps may be required. Estrogen may have a direct inhibitory effect on the prostate in addition to its suppression of gonadotropin secretion by the pituitary. Thus a rationale may exist for the simultaneous use of orchiectomy and estrogen.

In large series of patients with metastatic disease[209, 210] 3- and 5-y survival rates in patients with stage III or stage IV disease who were treated with endocrine therapy were better than those in untreated patients. The differences among castration, estrogen therapy, and combined treatment were not significant. Likewise in a study using randomized assignments to therapeutic regimens, findings were similar with the three regimens.[211] High doses of diethylstilbestrol (5 mg/d) are associated with increased mortality from cardiovascular disease.[211] Smaller doses of diethylstilbestrol (1 mg/d) appear to be as effective as the 5-mg dose,[212] although plasma testosterone concentrations are not as completely suppressed[213]; at this dose there is no increase in cardiovascular mortality. Diethylstilbestrol does not improve the survival rates in patients with stage I and stage II disease (carcinoma confined to the prostate). There is no evidence that one estrogen is better than another, although individual patients may have fewer side effects from one or another. When patients have responded to either estrogen or orchiectomy, subsequent use of the other modality is generally ineffective.

Remission of disease is usually defined as a lowering of serum prostate-specific antigen or acid phosphatase levels and relief of pain. One difficulty in evaluating therapy for prostate cancer is the problem of defining the clinical response reproducibly. Most patients have osteoblastic metastases, and definitions of tumor response are generally based on "soft" criteria such as prostate-specific antigen, acid phosphatase level, analgesia index, and performance status rather than objective tumor measurements. Because bone metastases are usually osteoblastic, sufficient remodeling to allow documentation that remission has taken place may take several years. Nevertheless regression rates after either orchiectomy or estrogen therapy have been reported to be 50 to 80%, varying with the grade and stage of disease.[214] The average duration of remission is 15 mo, although occasional remissions may last more than 5 y.

Plasma concentrations of androstenedione and testosterone are measurable in some patients with prostate cancer after orchiectomy.[215] Suppression of adrenal androgen production by exogenous glucocorticoids reduces these levels. Thus some men, like some postmenopausal women with endometrial hyperplasia, may produce larger amounts of androstenedione or have a greater capacity for conversion of androstenedione to testosterone in extraglandular tissues than does the general population. Adrenal suppression may be beneficial in this group, but trials of glucocorticoid therapy have been inconclusive.

Because of residual androgen production by the adrenal cortex, adrenalectomy and hypophysectomy have also been tried in patients who have relapsed after primary therapy with estrogen or orchiectomy.[216-218] In none of the series was there a consistent decrease in the acid phosphatase level accompanying the decrease in pain as occurs almost invariably after orchiectomy or estrogen therapy. Medical adrenalectomy using aminoglutethimide also does not result in clear-cut improvement.[219] Both approaches may provide short-term clinical improvement but rarely produce objective evidence of disease regression.[220]

Progestagens have been tried for treatment because they suppress plasma LH levels and can also act as antiandrogens, competing with androgens for binding to androgen receptors. Remissions have been reported in response to cyproterone acetate, a progestational antiandrogen, when it was given before castration or estrogen therapy; the drug is ineffective after castration.[221] A nonsteroidal androgen antagonist, flutamide, can also cause regression of disease in untreated patients and may be effective in men who relapse after castration or estrogen therapy.[222, 223] A "pure" antiandrogen of this type should prove useful both therapeutically and as a probe for androgen dependence. LHRH analogues, with or without antiandrogens, can also induce responses with essentially no toxicity.[224, 225] These analogues inhibit LH secretion and thus cause plasma testosterone to fall to castrate levels (see Chapter 16).

More than 1600 LHRH agonists and antagonists have been synthesized.[226] Normally, LHRH is released in pulses, which leads to pulsatile release of LH and FSH. Constant infusions of exogenous LHRH[227] or intermittent high doses of LHRH analogues inhibit LH and FSH release. LHRH has also been reported to inhibit breast cancer cells directly in vitro in some[228-230] but not all studies.[231] There is no convincing evidence for a direct action of LHRH in human prostate.

With continuous agonist therapy (as with leuprolide) there is an initial fourfold rise in LH level and a twofold increase in testosterone level after the first dose; the levels return to normal within 72 to 80 h.[227] Gonadotropin levels become suppressed by 2 to 4 wk of therapy, and testosterone levels decrease by 95% 1 wk after treatment. After therapy for 1 to 2 y there is no escape from androgen suppression. Similar results were obtained for men treated with buserelin subcutaneously, followed by chronic intranasal therapy.[232] Smaller doses of LHRH analogues do not cause medical castration.[233]

With subcutaneous administration of LHRH, absorption is rate-limiting and depends on injection volume, local blood flow, injection trauma, presence of capillaries and lymphatics, and proteolytic degradation at the injection site, but bioavailability averages 75 to 90%. Administration of some analogues subcutaneously is associated with depot-like effects.[234]

Once-monthly biodegradable depot formulations have been developed. One of these preparations, goserelin, incorporates d,l-lactide-glycolide copolymer that releases drug for 28 d[235, 236] and that degrades to lactic and glycolic acids.[237] Depot doses of goserelin of 3.6, 1.8, and 0.9 mg release about 120, 60, and 30 μg, respectively, of drug daily for approximately 28 d.[238] These doses decrease plasma testosterone levels to castration values in men by 2 to 3 wk with parallel decreases in plasma LH, levels that are maintained without escape for at least 18 mo. Subcutaneous injection of 3.6 mg of goserelin sustains amenorrhea in premenopausal women for 61 to 71 d after injection.[239] At 5 wk a rise in LH concentration was noted. This drug has a potency 100 to 200 times that of native LHRH. The objective response rate with leuprolide (1 mg subcutaneously daily) in a large randomized study is 38%.[240] Labrie and co-workers[241] advocate the use of a combination of an LHRH agonist with an antiandrogen to achieve total androgen blockade.

Side effects[242-244] of LHRH agonists in men include loss of libido in many and impotence in all, which is reversible after discontinuation. The testicular changes in men treated with LHRH agonists before orchiectomy include peritubular thickening, a decreased number of Leydig cells, and fibrosis.[243] Side effects include hot flashes in a majority of men; gastrointestinal disturbances such as diarrhea, constipation, and indigestion; peripheral edema; weight gain; rash; gynecomastia; mastodynia; allergic reactions; and exacerbation of tumor-related symptoms or disease flare, which is thought to be due to the initial gonadotropin release and temporary increase in plasma testosterone level. Local reactions and hematoma can occur at the injection site.

Antiandrogens are useful in prostate cancer. The two most widely studied antiandrogens are cyproterone acetate, which is a steroidal antiandrogen that also inhibits testosterone synthesis, and flutamide. The relative binding affinity of cyproterone acetate to androgen receptor is 8, using testosterone as the standard at 100.[245] In several trials in metastatic prostate carcinoma, doses of cyproterone acetate have ranged from 50 to 300 mg/d.[246, 247] Responses have been reported in 41 to 62% of men no longer responding to other endocrine modalities. In prospective studies, cyproterone acetate appears to be equivalent to diethylstilbestrol in response rate and lower in toxicity.[248] Side effects include gynecomastia, loss of libido, and inhibition of spermatogenesis[249]; in women hirsutism and alopecia may ensue.[250] Levels of high-density lipoproteins decrease, and levels of very-low-density lipoprotein triglyceride increase.[251]

Flutamide is a nonsteroidal compound that acts as a pure antiandrogen and blocks androgen binding to the androgen receptor competitively as an activated α-hydroxy metabolite.[249] It reduces prostate weight and the rate of DNA synthesis in the rat prostate and induces apoptotic cell death.[252] Plasma levels of LH rise because of inhibition of androgen feedback and cause a secondary increase in testosterone level. The administration of flutamide to men with prostate cancer who had not had prior endocrine therapy resulted in subjective improvement in 90% of patients in one study.[253] Toxicity of flutamide includes mastodynia, gynecomastia (36%), secretion of colostrum in males, hot flashes, decreased libido, loss of facial hair, decreased body hair, abdominal discomfort, abnormal liver function test results, and occasional liver failure.[249, 254]

In a randomized study of patients with stage D2 prostate cancer comparing leuprolide (1 mg subcutaneously) with leuprolide plus flutamide (250 mg orally three times a day), progression-free survival was 2.5 mo longer in patients receiving the combination.[255] These studies suggest that a small benefit may be obtained with a combination, possibly because of more complete blockade of androgen action. Additional studies of these agents suggest modest gains by "combined" ablation therapy versus castration or antiandrogens alone.[256]

LEUKEMIA AND LYMPHOMA

Glucocorticoids influence the growth, differentiation, and function of virtually every tissue and organ system of the body.[257] Among these diverse effects are lymphocytopenia and thymic atrophy[258, 259] and the killing of some human leukemic lymphoblasts.[260] Nevertheless several problems complicate their use. First, variable response rates occur in patients with different types of acute and chronic leukemia and lymphoma,[261] and it has not been possible to identify prospective patients likely to benefit from glucocorticoid therapy. Second, although the initial response rates in acute lymphoblastic leukemia in children are 45 to 65%, the rate of induction of a subsequent remission with glucocorticoids after primary relapse falls to 25%.[262]

Glucocorticoid administration is associated with complications that include immunosuppression and concomitant nosocomial infections, Cushing's syndrome, diabetes mellitus, poor wound healing, psychosis, and other problems.[257, 263] Because most patients with leukemia die of infections rather than the leukemia per se, glucocorticoid therapy may be a detriment to survival in some cases. This difficulty is amplified by the fact that most patients with leukemia and lymphoma are managed by combinations of drugs that include glucocorticoids and cytotoxic agents. Thus potentially harmful components in the drug combination, such as the glucocorticoid, may be continued after they have ceased to be of therapeutic benefit.

It would be of value to be able to predict when glucocorticoid therapy is indicated. Because quantification of estrogen receptors is useful in predicting the response to endocrine therapy in breast cancer,[264] glucocorticoid receptors have been studied in human leukemic and lymphoid cells.[265–267] Glucocorticoid receptors in normal peripheral blood lymphocytes and monocytes[268, 269] are identical to the glucocorticoid receptors in liver[270] and thymocytes.[271] Drugs that induce transformation of lymphoid cells to blast cells, such as phytohemagglutinin or concanavalin A, increase intracellular glucocorticoid receptor levels.[267, 272] Such lymphoblasts are similar morphologically and in glucocorticoid receptor content to human leukemic lymphoblasts.

Early studies of human acute lymphoblastic leukemia suggested that quantitative glucocorticoid receptor analyses would be clinically relevant.[273–276] Glucocorticoid receptors are demonstrable in lymphoblasts in most untreated patients with acute lymphoblastic leukemia, and there is good agreement between concentrations of glucocorticoids that saturate receptor sites and concentrations that inhibit cellular growth. Correlation may exist between loss of glucocorticoid receptor activity and in vitro resistance to glucocorticoids. Furthermore the receptor levels of the various acute lymphoblastic leukemias of childhood vary, the so-called T-cell leukemias having fewer receptors than does null cell leukemia. The quantity of receptor in acute lymphoblastic leukemia correlates with the initial duration of remission,[276] a correlation that is independent of other prognostic factors such as cell type, initial white blood cell count, or sex. Thus in acute lymphoblastic leukemia, a role for analysis of glucocorticoid receptors appears clear.

Glucocorticoid receptors are also present in acute myelogenous leukemia,[277, 278] chronic myelogenous leukemia in blast crisis,[278] chronic lymphocytic leukemia,[279–281] and the Sézary syndrome.[270] No correlations between receptor content and either clinical parameters or prognosis have been documented in any of these illnesses. However, Bloomfield and colleagues[282] have reported that quantitation of the glucocorticoid receptor can identify patients with non-Hodgkin's lymphoma who will respond to single-agent glucocorticoid therapy.

Many chemotherapeutic protocols use pharmacologic dosages of glucocorticoid such as 1 g of prednisolone/m²/body surface area, doses that cause plasma levels of drugs 1000 times those required to saturate receptor and kill sensitive cells in vitro. However, some effects of glucocorticoids may not involve the known receptors. Nevertheless there is no evidence that such massive doses are more effective than conventional regimens.

REFERENCES

1. MacMahon B, Cole P, Brown J. Etiology of human breast cancer: a review. J Natl Cancer Inst 1973; 50:21–36.
2. Henderson IC. Risk factors for breast cancer development. Cancer 1993; 71:2127–2140.
3. Kelsey JL. A review of the epidemiology of human breast cancer. Epidemiol Rev 1979; 1:74–109.
4. Doll R, Payne P, Waterhouse J, eds. Cancer Incidence in Five Continents. Berlin: Springer-Verlag, 1966.
5. Kliewer EV, Smith KR. Breast cancer mortality among immigrants in Australia and Canada. J Natl Cancer Inst 1995; 87:1154–1161.
6. DeWaard F. The epidemiology of breast cancer: review and prospects. Int J Cancer 1969; 4:577–586.
7. MacMahon B, Cole P, Lin TM. Age at first birth and breast cancer risk. Bull WHO 1970; 43:209–221.
8. MacMahon B, Feinleib M. Breast cancer in relation to nursing and menopausal history. J Natl Cancer Inst 1960; 24:733–753.
9. Kalache A, Vessey, MP, McPherson K. Lactation and breast cancer. Br Med J 1980; 280:223–224.
10. Ing R, Hoe JHC, Petrakis NL. Unilateral breast feeding and breast cancer. Lancet 1977; 2:124–127.
11. Yuasa S, MacMahon B. Lactation and reproductive histories of breast cancer patients in Tokyo, Japan. Bull WHO 1971; 42:195–204.
12. Hoover R, Gray LA, Cole P, et al. Menopausal estrogens and breast cancer. N Engl J Med 1976; 295:401–405.
13. Pike MC, Henderson BE, Casagrande JT. The epidemiology of breast cancer as it relates to menarche, pregnancy and menopause. In: Pike MC, Siiteri PK, Welsch CW, eds. Hormones and Breast Cancer. Cold Spring Harbor, NY: Cold Spring Harbor Laboratory 1981: 3–20.
14. Prentice RL, Kakar F, Hursting S, et al. Aspects of the rationale for the women's health trial. J Natl Cancer Inst 1988; 80:802–814.
15. Anderson DE. Breast cancer in families. Cancer 1977; 40:1855–1860.
16. Miki Y, Swensen J, Shattuck-Eidens D, et al. A strong candidate for the breast and ovarian cancer susceptibility gene BRCA1. Science 1994; 266: 66–71.
17. Gayther SA, Warren W, Mazoyer S, et al. Germline mutations of the BRCA1 gene in breast and ovarian cancer families provide evidence for a genotype-phenotype correlation. Nat Genet 1995; 11:428–433.
18. Cropp CS, Nevanlinna HA, Pyrhonen S, et al. Evidence for involvement of BRCA1 in sporadic breast carcinomas. Cancer Res 1994; 54:2548–2551.

19. Thorlacius S, Tryggvadottir L, Olafsdottir GH, et al. Linkage to BRCA2 region in hereditary male breast cancer. Lancet 1995; 346:544–545.

20. Kastan M. Clinical implications of basic research: Ataxia-telangiectasia—broad implications for a rare disorder. N Engl J Med 1995; 333:662–663.

21. Lacassagne MA. Apparition de cancers de la mamelle chez la souris mâle, soumise à des injections de folliculine. C R Acad Sci 1932; 195:630–632.

22. Zumoff B. Abnormal plasma hormone levels in women with breast cancer. In: Pike MC, Siiteri PK, Welsch CW, eds. Hormones and Breast Cancer. Cold Spring Harbor, NY: Cold Spring Harbor Laboratory 1981: 143–168.

23. Shimizu H, Ross RK, Bernstein L, et al. Serum oestrogen levels in postmenopausal women: comparison of American whites and Japanese in Japan. Br J Cancer 1990; 62:451–453.

24. Hill P, Wynder EL, Kumar J, et al. Prolactin levels in populations at risk for breast cancer. Cancer Res 1976; 36:4102–4106.

25. Levin PA, Malarkey WB. Daughters of women with breast cancer have elevated mean 24-hour prolactin (PRL) levels and a partial resistance of PRL to dopamine suppression. J Clin Endocrinol Metab 1981; 53:179–183.

26. Fishman J, Fukushima D, O'Connor J, et al. Plasma hormone profiles of young women at risk for familial breast cancer. Cancer Res 1978; 38:4006–4011.

27. Henderson BC, Pike MC. Prolactin—an important hormone in breast neoplasia? In: Pike MC, Siiteri PK, Welsch CW, eds. Hormones and Breast Cancer. Cold Spring Harbor, NY: Cold Spring Harbor Laboratory 1981: 115–127.

28. Kalache A, Vessey MP, McPherson K. Lactation and breast cancer. Br Med J 1980; 280:223–224.

29. Bulbrook RD, Thomas BS, Fantl VE, et al. A prospective study of the relation between thyroid function and subsequent breast cancer. In: Pike MC, Siiteri PK, Welsch CW, eds. Hormones and Breast Cancer. Cold Spring Harbor, NY: Cold Spring Harbor Laboratory 1981: 131–140.

30. Kelsey JL, Holford TR, White C, et al. Oral contraceptives and breast disease. Am J Epidemiol 1978; 107:236–244.

31. Anonymous. Long-term oral contraceptive use and the risk of breast cancer. The Centers for Disease Control, Cancer and Hormone study. JAMA 1983; 249:1591–1595.

32. Jick H, Walker AM, Watkins RN, et al. Oral contraceptives and breast cancer. Am J Epidemiol 1980; 112:577–585.

33. Paffenbarger RS, Fasal E, Simmons ME, et al. Cancer risk as related to the use of oral contraceptives during fertile years. Cancer 1977; 39:1887–1891.

34. Brinton LA, Daling JR, Liff JM, et al. Oral contraceptives and breast cancer risk among younger women. J Natl Cancer Inst 1995; 87:827–835.

35. Ravnihar B, Seigel DG, Lindtner J. An epidemiologic study of breast cancer and benign breast neoplasias in relation to the oral contraceptive and estrogen use. Eur J Cancer 1979; 15:395–405.

36. Ory H, Cole P, MacMahon B, et al. Oral contraceptives and reduced risk of benign breast diseases. N Engl J Med 1976; 294:419–422.

37. Boston Collaborative Drug Surveillance Programme. Oral contraceptives and venous thromboembolic disease, surgically confirmed, gallbladder disease, and breast tumours. Lancet 1973; 1:1399–1404.

38. Black MM, Barclay TH, Cutler SJ, et al. Association of atypical characteristics of benign breast lesions with subsequent risk of breast cancer. Cancer 1972; 29:338–343.

39. Dupont WD, Page DL. Risk factors for breast cancer in women with proliferative disease. N Engl J Med 1985; 312:146–151.

40. Schlesselman JJ. Cancer of the breast and reproductive tract in relation to use of oral contraceptives. Contraception 1989; 40:1–38.

41. Henderson BE, Powell D, Rosario I, et al. An epidemiologic study of breast cancer. J Natl Cancer Inst 1974; 53:609–614.

42. Miller DR, Rosenberg L, Kaufman DW, et al. Breast cancer before age 45 and oral contraceptive use: new findings. Am J Epidemiol 1989; 129:269–280.

43. Casagrande J, Gerkins V, Henderson BE, et al. Brief communication: exogenous estrogens and breast cancer in women with natural menopause. J Natl Cancer Inst 1976; 56:839–841.

44. Rosenberg L, Miller DR, Kaufman, DW, et al. Breast cancer and oral contraceptive use. Am J Epidemiol 1984; 119:167–176.

45. Meirik O, Lund E, Adami HO, et al. Oral contraceptive use and breast cancer in young women. A joint national case-control study in Sweden and Norway. Lancet 1986; 2:650–654.

46. Pike MC, Henderson BE, Casagrande JT, et al. Oral contraceptive use and early abortion as risk factors for breast cancer in young women. Br J Cancer 1981; 43:72–76.

47. Belchetz PE. Hormonal treatment of postmenopausal women. N Engl J Med 1994; 330:1062–1071.

48. Newcomb PA, Storer BE. Postmenopausal hormone use and risk of large-bowel cancer. J Natl Cancer Inst 1995; 87:1067–1071.

49. Colditz GA, Hankinson SE, Hunter DJ, et al. The use of estrogens and progestins and the risk of breast cancer in postmenopausal women. N Engl J Med 1995; 332:1589–1593.

50. Stanford JL, Weiss NS, Voigt LF, et al. Combined estrogen and progestin hormone replacement therapy in relation to risk of breast cancer in middle-aged women. JAMA 1995; 274:137–142.

51. Schatzkin A, Jones DY, Hoover RN, et al. Alcohol consumption and breast cancer in the epidemiologic follow-up study of the first national health and nutrition examination survey. N Engl J Med 1988; 316:1169–1180.

52. Beatson GT. On the treatment of inoperable cases of carcinoma of the mamma: suggestions for a new method of treatment with illustrative cases. Lancet 1896; 2:162–165.

53. Grody WW, Schrader WT, O'Malley BW. Activation transformation and subunit structure of steroid hormone receptors. Endocr Rev 1982; 3:141–163.

54. Folca PJ, Glascock RF, Irvine WT. Studies with tritium labelled hexoestrol in advanced breast cancer. Lancet 1962; 2:796–798.

55. Jensen EV, DeSombre ER, Jungblut PP. Estrogen receptors in hormone responsive tissues and tumors. In: Wissler RV, Dao TL, Wood S, eds. Endogenous Factors Influencing Host Tumor Balance. Chicago: University of Chicago Press, 1967: 15–30.

56. Jordan VC. Third Annual William L. McGuire Memorial Lecture. Studies on the estrogen receptor in breast cancer—20 years as a target for the treatment and prevention of cancer. Breast Cancer Res Treat 1995; 36:267–285.

57. Clark GM, McGuire WL. Progesterone receptors and human breast cancer. Breast Cancer Res Treat 1983; 3:157–163.

58. Witliff JL, Fisher B, Durant JR. Establishment of uniformity in steroid receptor analysis used in cooperative trials of breast cancer treatment. In: Henningsen B, Linden F, Steichele C, eds. Recent Results in Cancer Research. Endocrine Treatment of Breast Cancer. New York: Springer-Verlag, 1980: 198–202.

59. Panko WB, MacLeod RM. Uncharged nuclear receptors for estrogen in breast cancer. Cancer Res 1978; 38:1948–1951.

60. Wenger CR, Beardslee S, Owens MA, et al. DNA ploidy, S-phase, and steroid receptors in more than 127,000 breast cancer patients. Breast Cancer Res Treat 1993; 28:9–20.

61. Nenci I. Receptors and centriole pathways of steroid action in normal and neoplastic cells. Cancer Res 1978; 38:4204–4207.

62. Roodi N, Bailey LR, Kao WY, et al. Estrogen receptor gene analysis in estrogen receptor-positive and receptor-negative primary breast cancer. J Natl Cancer Inst 1995; 87:446–451.

63. Fuqua SA, Wolf DM. Molecular aspects of estrogen receptor variants in breast cancer. Breast Cancer Res Treat 1995; 35:233–241.

64. Saez S, Martin PM, Chouvet CD. Estradiol and progesterone receptor levels in relation to plasma estrogen and progesterone levels. Cancer Res 1978; 38:3468–3478.

65. Degenshein GA, Bloom N, Ceccarelli F. Estrogen and progesterone receptor site studies as guides to the management of advanced breast cancer. Dis Breast 1977; 3:29–31.

66. Knight WA, Livingston RB, Gregory EJ, et al. Estrogen receptor as an independent prognostic factor for early recurrence in breast cancer. Cancer Res 1977; 37:4669–4671.

67. Maynard PV, Blamey RW, Elston CW, et al. Estrogen receptor assay in primary breast cancer and early recurrence of the disease. Cancer Res 1978; 38:4292–4296.

68. Kinne DW, Ashikari R, Butler A. Estrogen receptor protein in breast cancer as a prediction of recurrence. Cancer 1981; 47:2364–2367.

69. Donegan WL. Prognostic factors. State and receptor status in breast cancer. Cancer 1992; 70:1755–1764.

70. Greene GL, Nolan C, Engler JP, et al. Monoclonal antibodies to human estrogen receptor. Proc Natl Acad Sci USA 1982; 77:5115–5119.

71. Greene GL, Closs LE, Fleming WL. Antibodies to estrogen receptor: immunochemical similarity of estrophilin from various mammalian species. Proc Natl Acad Sci USA 1977; 74:3681–3685.

72. Esteban JM, Ahn C, Battifora H, et al. Predictive value of estrogen receptors evaluated by quantitative immunohistochemical analysis in breast cancer. Am J Clin Pathol 1994; 102:S9–12.

73. Harris J, Lippman M, Veronesi U, et al. Breast cancer: recent trends and progress and future prospects. Parts I, II, and III. N Engl J Med 1992; Part I, 327:319–328; Part II, 327:390–398; Part III, 327:473–480.

74. Harris JR, Lippman ME, Morrow M, Hellman S, eds. Diseases of the Breast. Philadelphia: Lippincott-Raven, 1996.

75. Anonymous. Systemic treatment of early breast cancer by hormonal, cytotoxic, or immune therapy. 133 randomised trials involving 31,000 recurrences and 24,000 deaths among 75,000 women. Early breast cancer trialists' collaborative group. Lancet 1992; 339:71–85.

76. Hall TC, Dederick MM, NeVinny HB, et al. Prognostic value of response of patients with breast cancer to therapeutic castration. Cancer Chemother Rep 1963; 31:47–48.

77. Lewison EF. Castration in the treatment of advanced breast cancer. Cancer 1965; 18:1558–1563.

78. Hoffken K, Oesterdickoff C, Becher R, et al. LH-RH agonist treatment with buserelin in premenopausal patients with advanced breast cancer: a phase II study. Cancer Ther Control 1989; 1:13–20.

79. Meakin JW. Is there a place for adjuvant endocrine therapy of breast cancer? In: Henningsen B, Linder F, Steichele C, eds. Recent Results in Cancer Research. Endocrine Treatment of Breast Cancer. New York: Springer-Verlag, 1980: 178–184.

80. Longcope C. Metabolic clearance and blood production rates of estrogens in post-menopausal women. Am J Obstet Gynecol 1971; 111:778–781.

81. Grodin JM, Siiteri PK, MacDonald PC. Source of estrogen production in postmenopausal women. J Clin Endocrinol 1973; 36:207–214.

82. Aitken SC, Lippman ME. Steroid receptors in breast cancer. Arch Intern Med 1982; 142:363–366.

83. Schally AV, Reddin TW. Inhibition of cell growth by a hypothalamic peptide. Proc Natl Acad Sci USA 1982; 79:7014–7018.

84. Davies P, Nicholson RI. How do androgens and progestins cause regression of breast cancer? Rev Endocr Rel Cancer 1981; 10:19–25.

85. Allegra JC, Lippman ME, Thompson EB, et al. The distribution, frequency and quantitative analysis of estrogen, progesterone, androgen and glucocorticoid receptors in human breast cancer. Cancer Res 1979; 39:1447–1454.

86. Allegra JC, Lippman ME, Thompson EB, et al. Relationship between the progesterone, androgen and glucocorticoid receptor and response rate to endocrine therapy in metastatic breast cancer. Cancer Res 1979; 39:1973–1979.

87. Cooperative Breast Cancer Group. Testosterone propionate therapy in breast therapy. JAMA 1964; 188:1069–1074.

88. Johnston B, Novales ET. The use of Valban (vinblastine sulfate) in metastatic carcinoma of the breast. Cancer Chemother Rep 1961; 12:109–112.

89. Goldenberg IS. Clinical trial of Δ^1-testololactone (NSC 23759), medroxy progesterone acetate (NSC 26386) and oxylone acetate (NSC 47438) in advanced female mammary cancer. Cancer 1969; 23:109–112.

90. Mansel RE, Wisbey JR, Hughes LE. The use of danazol in the treatment of painful benign breast disease: preliminary results. Postgrad Med J 1979; 55:61–65.

91. Madanos AE, Farber M. Danazol. Ann Intern Med 1982; 96:625–630.

92. Coombes RC, Dearnaley D, Humphreys J, et al. Danazol treatment of advanced breast cancer. Cancer Treat Rep 1980; 64:1073–1976.

93. Coombes RC, Dearnaley D, Humphreys J, et al. Danazol treatment of advanced breast cancer. Cancer Treat Rep 1980; 64:1073–1076.

94. Powles TJ, Gordon C, Coombes RC. Clinical trial of multiple endocrine therapy for metastatic and locally advanced breast cancer with tamoxifen-aminoglutethimide-danazol compared to tamoxifen used alone. Cancer Res 1982; 42:3458–3460.

95. Lippman ME. Efforts to combine endocrine and chemotherapy in the management of breast cancer: do two and two equal three? Breast Cancer Res Treat 1983; 3:117–127.

96. Tormey DC, Lippman ME, Edwards BK, et al. Evaluation of tamoxifen doses with and without fluoxymesterone in advanced breast cancer. Ann Intern Med 1983; 98:139–144.

97. Kennedy BJ. Hormone therapy in inoperable breast cancer. Cancer 1969; 24:1345–1349.

98. Kennedy BJ. Diethylstilbestrol versus testosterone propionate therapy in advanced breast cancer. Surg Gynecol Obstet 1965; 120:1246–1250.

99. Kaufman RJ, Escher GC. Rebound regression in advanced mammary carcinoma. Surg Gynecol Obstet 1961; 113:635–640.

100. Stoll BA. Progestin therapy of breast cancer: comparison of agents. Br Med J 1967; 3:338–341.

101. Crona N, Enk L, Samsioe G, et al. Medroxyprogesterone acetate (MPA) in adjuvant treatment of endometrial carcinoma—changes in serum lipoproteins. J Steroid Biochem 1983; 19(Suppl):195–198.

102. Henderson IC. Endocrine therapy in metastatic breast cancer. In: Harris JR, Hellman S, Henderson IC, et al, eds. Breast Diseases. Philadelphia: JB Lippincott, 1987: 398–428.

103. Sikic BI, Scudder SA, Ballon SC, et al. High-dose megestrol acetate therapy of ovarian carcinoma: a phase II study by the Northern California Oncology Group. Semin Oncol 1986; 13:26–32.

104. Pannuti F, Martoni A, DiMarco AR, et al. Prospective, randomized clinical trial of two different high dosages of medroxyprogesterone acetate (MAP) in the treatment of metastatic breast cancer. Eur J Cancer 1979; 15:593–601.

105. Beretta G, Tabiadon D, Tedeschi L, et al. Hormonotherapy of advanced breast carcinoma: comparative evaluation of tamoxifen citrate versus medroxyprogesterone acetate. In: Iacobelli S, Lippman ME, Della Cona GR, eds. The Role of Tamoxifen in Breast Cancer. New York: Raven, 1982: 113–120.

106. Henderson D. Antiprogestational and antiglucocorticoid activities of some novel 11β-aryl substituted steroids. In: Furr BJA, Wakeling AE, eds. Pharmacological and Clinical Uses of Inhibitors of Hormone Secretion and Action. London: Bailliere Tindall, 1987: 184–211.

107. Vignon F, Bardon S, Chalbos D, et al. Antiproliferative effect of progestins and antiprogestins in human breast cancer cells. In: Klijn JGM, Paridaens R, Foekens JA, eds. Hormonal Manipulation of Cancer: Peptides, Growth Factors, and New (Anti) Steroidal Agents. New York: Raven, 1987: 47–54.

108. Maudelonde T, Romieu G, Ulmann A, et al. First clinical trial on the use of the antiprogestin RU486 in advanced breast cancer. In: Klijn JGM, Paridaens R, Foekens JA, eds. Hormonal Manipulation of Cancer: Peptides, Growth Factors, and New (Anti) Steroidal Agents. New York: Raven, 1987: 55–59.

109. Klijn JGM, de Jong FH. Long-term LHRH-agonist (buserelin) treatment in metastatic premenopausal breast cancer. In: Klijn JGM, Paridaens R, Foekens JA, eds. Hormonal Manipulation of Cancer: Peptides, Growth Factors, and New (Anti) Steroidal Agents. New York: Raven, 1987: 343–352.

110. Walker KJ, Turkes A, Williams MR, et al. Preliminary endocrinological evaluation of a sustained-release formulation of the LH-releasing hormone agonist D-Ser(But)6 Azgly10 LHRH in premenopausal women with advanced breast cancer. J Endocrinol 1986; 111:349–353.

111. Harvey HA, Lipton A, Max DT, et al. Medical castration produced by the GnRH analogue leuprolide to treat metastatic breast cancer. J Clin Oncol 1985; 3:1068–1072.

112. Klijn JM, De Jong FH, Lamberts SJ, et al. LHRH-agonist treatment in clinical and experimental human breast cancer. J Steroid Biochem 1985; 23:867–873.

113. Nicholson RI, Walker KJ, Turkes A, et al. The British experience with LH-RH agonist Zoladex® (ICI 118630) in the treatment of breast cancer. In: Klijn JGM, Paridaens R, Foekens JA, eds. Hormonal Manipulation of Cancer: Peptides, Growth Factors, and New (Anti) Steroidal Agents. New York: Raven, 1987: 331–341.

114. Geiner NF, Donegan WL. Role and mechanism of corticosteroid therapy in breast cancer. Rev Endocr Rel Cancer 1980; 6:5–11.

115. Sutherland RL, Jordan VC. Non-Steroidal Antioestrogens. Sydney: Academic, 1981.

116. Jaiyesimi IA, Buzdar AU, Decker DA, et al. Use of tamoxifen for breast cancer: twenty-eight years later. J Clin Oncol 1995; 13:513–529.

117. Planting AS, Alexieva-Figusch J, Blonk VD, et al. Tamoxifen therapy in premenopausal women with metastatic breast cancer. Cancer Treat Rep 1985; 69:363–368.

118. Ingle JN, Ahmann DL, Green SJ, et al. Randomized clinical trial of megestrol acetate versus tamoxifen in paramenopausal or castrated women with advanced breast cancer. Am J Clin Oncol 1982; 5:155–160.

119. Santen RJ, Manni A, Harvey H, et al. Endocrine treatment of breast cancer in women. Endocr Rev 1995; 11:221–265.

120. Knabbe C, Lippman ME, Wakefield L, et al. Evidence that TGFβ is a hormonally regulated negative growth factor in human breast cancer. Cell 1987; 48:417–428.

121. Muss HB, Case D, Atkins JN, et al. Tamoxifen versus high-dose oral medroxyprogesterone acetate as initial endocrine therapy for patients with metastatic breast cancer: a Piedmont Oncology Association study. J Clin Oncol 1994; 12:1630–1638.

122. Howell A, DeFriend D, Robertson J, et al. Response to a specific antioestrogen (ICI 182780) in tamoxifen-resistant breast cancer. Lancet 1995; 345:29–30.

123. Heel RC, Brogden RN, Speight TM. Tamoxifen—a review of its pharmacologic properties and therapeutic use in the treatment of breast cancer. Drugs 1978; 16:1–24.

124. Pearson OH, Manni A, Arafah BM. Antiestrogen treatment of breast cancer: an overview. Cancer Res 1982; 42:3424–3429.

125. Manni A, Trujillo J, Marshall JS, et al. Antiestrogen-induced remissions in stage IV breast cancer. Cancer Treat Rep 1976; 60:1445–1450.

126. McIntosh IH, Thynne GS. Tumour stimulation by anti-oestrogens. Br J Surg 1977; 64:900–901.

127. Jordan VC, Assikis VJ. Endometrial carcinoma and tamoxifen. Clearing up a controversy. Clin Cancer Res 1995; 1:467–472.

128. Barakat RR. The effect of tamoxifen on the endometrium. Oncology 1995; 9:129–134.

129. Patterson JS, Battersby LA, Edwards DG. Review of the clinical pharmacology and international experience with tamoxifen in advanced breast cancer. Rev Endocr Rel Cancer 1982; 9:563–582.

130. Pritchard KI, Thomson DB, Myers RE. Tamoxifen therapy in premenopausal patients with metastatic breast cancer. Cancer Treat Rep 1980; 64:787–796.

131. Manni A, Pearson OH. Antiestrogen-induced remissions in premenopausal women with stage IV breast cancer: effects on ovarian function. Cancer Treat Rep 1980; 64:779–786.

132. Manni A, Arafah BM. Tamoxifen induced remission in breast cancer by escalating the dose to 40 mg daily after progression on 20 mg daily—a case report and review of the literature. Cancer 1981; 48:873–875.

133. Fromson JM, Pearson S, Bramah S. The metabolism of tamoxifen (I.C.I. 46,474). Part I: In laboratory animals. Xenobiotica 1973; 3:693–709.

134. Adam HK, Douglas EJ, Kemp KV. The metabolism of tamoxifen in humans. Biochem Pharmacol 1979; 27:145–147.

135. Furr BA, Jordan VC. The pharmacology and clinical uses of tamoxifen. Pharmacol Ther 1984; 25:127–205.

136. Lyman SD, Jordan VC. Metabolism of nonsteroidal antiestrogens. In: Jordan VC, ed. Estrogen/Antiestrogen Action and Breast Cancer Therapy. Madison: University of Wisconsin Press, 1986: 191–219.

137. Fabian C, Tilzer L, Sternson L. Comparative binding affinities of tamoxifen, 4-hydroxytamoxifen, and desmethyltamoxifen for estrogen receptors isolated from human breast carcinoma: correlation with blood levels in patients with metastatic breast cancer. Biopharm Drug Dispos 1981; 2:281–390.

138. Nicholson RI, Syne JS, Daniel CP, et al. The binding of tamoxifen to oestrogen receptor proteins under equilibrium and non-equilibrium conditions. Eur J Cancer 1979; 15:317–329.

139. Wakeling AE, Slater SR. Estrogen-receptor binding and biologic activity of tamoxifen and its metabolites. Cancer Treat Rep 64:741–744.

140. Horwitz KB. Mechanisms of hormone resistance in breast cancer. Breast Cancer Res Treat 1993; 26:119–130.

141. Sherman BM, Chapler FK, Crickard K, et al. Endocrine consequences of continuous antiestrogen therapy with tamoxifen in premenopausal women. J Clin Invest 1979; 64:398–404.

142. Paterson AG, Turkes A, Groom GV, et al. The effect of tamoxifen on plasma growth hormone and prolactin and postmenopausal women with advanced breast cancer. Eur J Cancer Clin Oncol 1983; 19:919–922.

143. Jordan VC, Fritz NF, Tormey DC. Endocrine effects of adjuvant chemotherapy and long-term tamoxifen administration on node-positive patients with breast cancer. Cancer Res 1987; 47:624–630.

144. Boccardo F, Bruzzi P, Rubagotti A, et al. Estrogen-like action of tamoxifen on vaginal epithelium in breast cancer patients. Oncology 1981; 38:281–285.

145. Powles TJ, Hardy JR, Ashley SE, et al. A pilot trial to evaluate the acute toxicity and feasibility of tamoxifen for prevention of breast cancer. Br J Cancer 1989; 60:126–131.

146. Prentice RL. Tamoxifen as a potential preventive agent in healthy postmenopausal women. J Natl Cancer Inst 1990; 82:1310–1311 (editorial, comment).

147. Lippman ME, Bolan B, Huff K. The effects of glucocorticoids and progesterone on hormone-responsive human breast cancer in long-term tissue culture. Cancer Res 1976; 36:4602–4609.

148. Griffiths CT, Hall TC, Saba Z, et al. Preliminary trial of aminoglutethimide in breast cancer. Cancer 1973; 32:31–37.

149. Fishman LM, Liddle GW, Island DP, et al. Effects of amino-glutethimide on adrenal function in man. J Clin Endocrinol Metab 1967; 27:481–490.

150. Santen RJ, Lipton A, Kendall J. Successful medical adrenalectomy with amino-glutethimide. Role of altered drug metabolism. JAMA 1974; 230:1661–1665.

151. Santen RJ, Samojlik E, Lipton A, et al. Kinetic, hormonal and clinical studies with aminoglutethimide in breast cancer. Cancer 1977; 39:2948–2958.

152. Harvey HA, Lipton A, Sonfert RJ. Aromatase: new perspectives for breast cancer. Cancer Res 1982; 42:3267s–3468s.

153. Coombes RC, Goss P, Dowsett M, et al. 4-Hydroxyandrostenedione in treatment of postmenopausal patients with advanced breast cancer. Lancet 1984; 2:1237–1239.

154. Wells SA, Worsol TJ, Samojlik E, et al. Comparison of surgical adrenalectomy to medical adrenalectomy in patients with metastatic carcinoma of the breast. Cancer Res 1982; 42:3454s–3457s.

155. Brodie AM, Santen RJ. Aromatase in breast cancer and the role of aminoglutethimide and other aromatase inhibitors. CRC Crit Rev Hematol Oncol 1986; 5:361–396.

156. Brodie AMH, Wing LY, Dowsett M, et al. Inhibitors of the aromatase enzyme system: basic and clinical studies with 4-hydroxyandrostenedione. In: Jordan VC, ed. Estrogen/Antiestrogen Action and Breast Cancer Therapy. Madison: University of Wisconsin Press, 1986: 221–234.

157. Santen RJ, Rosen H, Osawa Y, et al. Additive effects of aminoglutethimide, testolactone and 4-hydroxyandrostenedione as inhibitors of aromatase. J Steroid Biochem 1984; 20:1239–1242.

158. Santen RJ. Suppression of estrogens with aminoglutethimide and hydrocortisone (medical adrenalectomy) as treatment of advanced breast carcinoma: a review. Breast Cancer Res Treat 1981; 1:183–202.

159. Goss PE, Clark RM, Ambus U, et al. Phase II study of vorozole (R83842), a new aromatase inhibitor, in postmenopausal women with advanced breast cancer in progression on tamoxifen. Clin Cancer Res 1995; 1:287–294.

160. Johnston SR, Smith IE, Doody D, et al. Clinical and endocrine effects of the oral aromatase inhibitor vorozole in postmenopausal patients with advanced breast cancer. Cancer Res 1994; 54:5875–5881.

161. Young JA, Newcomer LN, Keller AM. Aminoglutethimide-induced bone marrow injury: report of a case and review of the literature. Cancer 1984; 54:1731–1733.

162. Messeih AA, Lipton A, Stanten RJ, et al. Aminoglutethimide-induced hematologic toxicity: worldwide experience. Cancer Treat Rep 1985; 69:1003–1004.

163. Wing LY, Garrett WM, Brodie AM. Effects of aromatase inhibitors, aminoglutethimide, and 4-hydroxyandrostenedione on cyclic rats and rats with 7,12-dimethylbenz(a)anthracene-induced mammary tumors. Cancer Res 1985; 45:2425–2428.

164. Brodie AM, Longcope C. Inhibition of peripheral aromatization by aromatase inhibitors, 4-hydroxy- and 4-acetoxy-androstene-3,17-dione. Endocrinology 1980; 106:14–21.

165. Brodie AM, Schwarzel WC, Shaikh AA, et al. The effect of an aromatase inhibitor, 4-hydroxy-4-androstene-3,17-dione, on estrogen-dependent processes in reproduction and breast cancer. Endocrinology 1977; 100:1684–1695.

166. Goss PE, Powles TJ, Dowsett M, et al. Treatment of advanced postmenopausal breast cancer with an aromatase inhibitor, 4-hydroxyandrostenedione: phase II report. Cancer Res 1986; 46:4823–4826.

167. Cunningham K, Powles TJ, Dowsett M, et al. Oral 4-hydroxyandrostenedione, a new endocrine treatment for disseminated breast cancer. Cancer Chemother Pharmacol 1987; 20:253–255.

168. Coombes RC, Goss P, Dowsett M, et al. 4-Hydroxyandrostenedione in treatment of postmenopausal patients with advanced breast cancer. Lancet 1984; 2:1237–1239.

169. Crichlow RW. Carcinoma of the male breast. Surg Gynecol Obstet 1972; 134:1011–1019.

170. Meyskins FL, Tormey EC, Nesfeld JP. Male breast cancer: a review. Cancer Treat Rev 1976; 3:83–93.

171. Everson RB, Lippman ME. Male breast cancer. In: McGuire WL, ed. Breast Cancer: Advances in Research and Treatment. Vol III. New York: Plenum, 1979: 239–267.

172. Symners WSC. Carcinoma of breast in trans-sexual individuals after surgical interference with the primary and secondary sex characteristics. Br Med J 1968; 2:83–85.

173. Everson RB, Lippman ME, Thompson EB, et al. Clinical correlations of steroid receptors and male breast cancer. Cancer Res 1980; 40:991–997.

174. Patterson JS, Battershy LA, Bach BK. Use of tamoxifen in advanced male breast cancer. Cancer Treat Rep 1980; 64:801–804.

175. Jensen EV, Jacobsen HI. Basic guides to the mechanism of estrogen action. Recent Prog Horm Res 1962; 18:387.

176. Antunes CMF, Stolley PD, Rosenshein NB, et al. Endometrial cancer and estrogen use (report of a large case-control study). N Engl J Med 1979; 300:9–13.

177. Nisker JA, Ramzy I, Collins JA. Adenocarcinoma of the endometrium and abnormal ovarian function in young women. Am J Obstet Gynecol 1978; 130:546–550.

178. Whitehead MI, Campbell SC, King RJ, et al. Oestrogen treatment and endometrial carcinoma. Br Med J 1977; 2:453–454.

179. Hensell DL, Grodin JM, Brenner PF, et al. Plasma precursors of estrogen. II: Correlation of the extent of conversion of plasma androstenedione to estrone with age. J Clin Endocrinol Metab 1974; 38:476–479.

180. MacDonald PC, Edman CD, Hemsell DL, et al. Effect of obesity on conversion of plasma androstenedione to estrone in postmenopausal women with and without endometrial cancer. Am J Obstet Gynecol 1978; 130:448–455.

181. Judd HL, Lucas WE, Yen SC. Serum 17β-estradiol and estrone levels in postmenopausal women with and without endometrial cancer. J Clin Endocrinol Metab 1976; 43:272–278.

182. Feinstein AR, Horowitz RI. A critique of the statistical evidence associating estrogens with endometrial cancer. Cancer Res 1978; 38:4001–4005.

183. Jordan VC. Long-term adjuvant tamoxifen therapy for breast cancer. Breast Cancer Res Treat 1990; 15:125–136.

184. Pollow K, Lubbert H, Boquoi E, et al. Characterization and comparison of receptors for 17β-estradiol and progesterone in human proliferative endometrium and endometrial carcinoma. Endocrinology 1975; 96:319–328.

185. Bayard F, Damilamo S, Robel P, et al. Cytoplasmic and nuclear estradiol and progesterone receptors in human endometrium. J Clin Endocrinol Metab 1978; 46:635–648.

186. King RJB, Dyer G, Collins WP, et al. Intracellular estradiol, estrone and estrogen receptor levels in endometria from postmenopausal women receiving estrogens and progestins. J Steroid Biochem 1980; 13:377–382.

187. Young PCM, Ehrlich CE, Cleary RE. Progesterone binding in human endometrial carcinomas. Am J Obstet Gynecol 1976; 125:353–360.

188. Feil PD, Mann WJ, Mortel R, et al. Nuclear progestin receptors in normal and malignant human endometrium. J Clin Endocrinol Metab 1979; 48:327–334.

189. Gurpide E, Gusberg SB, Tseng L. Estradiol binding and metabolism in human endometrial hyperplasia and adenocarcinoma. J Steroid Biochem 1976; 7:891–896.

190. Kelly RM, Baker WH. Progestational agents in the treatment of carcinoma of the endometrium. N Engl J Med 1961; 264:216–222.

191. Reifinstein EC Jr. Hydroxyprogesterone caproate therapy in advanced endometrial cancer. Cancer 1971; 27:485–502.

192. Malkasian GD Jr, Decker D, Mussey E, et al. Progesterone treatment of recurrent endometrial carcinoma. Am J Obstet Gynecol 1971; 110:15.

193. Allegra JC, Kiefer SM. Mechanisms of action of progestational agents. Semin Oncol 1985; 7:3–5.

194. Bojar H, Stuskchke M, Staib W. Effects of high-dose medroxyprogesterone acetate on plasma membrane lipid mobility. In: Bresciani F, ed. Progress in Cancer Research and Therapy. New York: Raven, 1984: 115–119.

195. Rochefort H. Biochemical basis of breast cancer treatment by androgens and progestins. In: Back N, Breiver GH, Eijsvoogel V, et al, eds. Hormones and Cancer. New York, Alan R Liss, 1984: 79–95.

196. Kovi J, Heshmat MY. Incidence of cancer in Negroes in Washington, D.C., and other selected American cities. Am J Epidemiol 1972; 96:401–413.

197. Jackson MA, Ahluwalia BS, Herson J, et al. Characterization of prostatic carcinoma among blacks. A continuation report. Cancer Treat Rep 1977; 61:167–172.

198. Akazakis K, Stennerman GN. Comparative study of latent carcinoma of the prostate among Japanese in Japan and Hawaii. J Natl Cancer Inst 1973; 50:1137–1144.

199. Huggins C, Clark PJ. Quantitative studies of prostatic secretion. II: The effect of castration and of estrogen injection on the normal and on the hyperplastic prostate gland of dogs. J Exp Med 1940; 72:747–762.

200. Huggins C, Masina MH, Eichelberger L, et al. Quantitative studies of prostatic secretion. I: Characteristics of normal secretion. The influence of thyroid, suprarenal, and testis extirpation and androgen substitution of the prostatic output. J Exp Med 1939; 70:543–556.

201. Huggins C, Hodges CV. Studies on prostatic cancer. I: The effect of castration, of estrogen and of androgen injection on serum phosphatases in metastatic carcinoma of the prostate. Cancer Res 1941; 1:293–297.

202. Wilson JD. Recent studies on the mechanism of action of testosterone. N Engl J Med 1972; 287:1284–1291.

203. Baulieu EE, Lasnitzki I, Robel P. Metabolism of testosterone and action of metabolites on prostate glands grown in organ culture. Nature 1968; 219:1155–1156.

204. Hammond GL, Kontturi M, Vihko P, et al. Serum steroids in normal males and patients with prostatic diseases. Clin Endocrinol 1978; 9:113–121.

205. Peyre A, Ravault JP, Laporte P. Effet potentialisateur de la proactine endogène sur les effecteurs sexuels mâles soumis à la testostérone. C R Soc Biol (Paris) 1968; 162:1592–1595.

206. Asano M, Kanzaki S, Sekiguichi E, et al. Inhibition of prostatic growth in rabbits with antiovine prolactin serum. J Urol 1971; 106:248–252.

207. Aragona C, Bohnet HG, Friesen HG. Localization of prolactin binding in prostate and testis: the role of serum prolactin concentration on the testicular LH receptor. Acta Endocrinol 1977; 84:402.

208. Gustafsson J-A, Ekman P, Snochowski M, et al. Correlation between clinical response to hormone therapy and steroid receptor content in prostatic cancer. Cancer Res 1978; 38:4345–4348.

209. Nesbit RM, Baum WC. Endocrine control of prostatic carcinoma. JAMA 1950; 143:1317–1320.

210. Paulson DF. Multimodality therapy of prostate cancer. Urology 1981; 17(Suppl):53–56.

211. Byar DP. The Veterans Administration Cooperative Urological Research Group's studies of cancer of the prostate. Cancer 1973; 32:1126–1130.

212. Blackard CE. The Veterans Administration Cooperative Urological Research Group studies of the prostate: a review. Cancer Chemother Rep 1975; 59:225–232.

213. Shearer RJ, Hendry WF, Sommerville IF, et al. Plasma testosterone. An accurate monitor of hormone treatment in prostatic cancer. Br J Urol 1973; 45:668–677.

214. Blackard CE, Byer DF, Jordan WP. Orchiectomy for advanced prostatic carcinoma. Urology 1973; 1:553–562.

215. Sciarra F, Sorcini G, Di Silverio F, et al. Plasma testosterone and androstenedione after orchiectomy in prostatic adenocarcinoma. Clin Endocrinol 1973; 2:101–109.

216. Murphy P, Reynoso G, Schoonees R, et al. Hypophysectomy and adrenalectomy for disseminated prostatic carcinoma. J Urol 1971; 105:817–825.

217. Scott WV, Menon M, Walsh PC. Hormonal therapy of prostate cancer. Cancer 1980; 45:1929–1926.

218. Maddy JA, Winternitz WW, Norrell H. Cryohypophysectomy in the management of advanced prostatic cancer. Cancer 1971; 28:322–328.

219. Sanford EJ, Drago JR, Rohner TJ, et al. Aminoglutethimide medical adrenalectomy for advanced prostatic carcinoma. J Urol 1976; 115:170–174.

220. Silverberg GD. Hypophysectomy in the treatment of disseminated prostatic carcinoma. Cancer 1977; 39:1727–1731.

221. Rafla S, Johnson R. The treatment of advanced prostatic carcinoma with medroxyprogesterone. Curr Ther Res 1974; 16:261–267.

222. Airhart RA, Barnett TF, Sullivan JW, et al. Flutamide therapy for carcinoma of the prostate. South Med J 1978; 171:798–801.

223. Neri R, Florance K, Koziol P, et al. A biological profile of a non-steroidal antiandrogen, SCH13521 (4′-nitro-3′-trifluoromethyl-isobutyranilide). Endocrinology 1972; 91:427–437.

224. Ahmed SR, Brouman PJC, Shalet SM, et al. Treatment of advanced prostatic cancer with hormonal mechanisms. Lancet 1983; 1:415–419.

225. Tolis G, Ackman D, Stellos A. Tumour growth inhibition in patients with prostatic carcinoma treated with luteinising hormone–releasing hormone agonists. Proc Natl Acad Sci USA 1982; 79:1658–1662.

226. Gonzalez-Barcena D, Perez-Sanchez P, Ureta-Sanchez P, et al. Treatment of advanced prostatic carcinoma with D-Trp-6-LH-RH. Prostate 1985; 7:21–30.

227. Santen RJ, Manni A, Harvey H. Gonadotropin releasing hormone (GnRH) analogs for the treatment of breast and prostatic carcinoma. Breast Cancer Res Treat 1986; 7:129–145.

228. Foekens JA, Henkelman MS, Fukkinkk JF, et al. Combined effects of buserelin, estradiol and tamoxifen on the growth of MCF-7 human breast cancer cells in vitro. Biochem Biophys Res Commun 1986; 140:550–556.

229. Miller WR, Scott WN, Morris R, et al. Growth of human breast cancer cells inhibited by a luteinizing hormone–releasing hormone agonist. Nature 1985; 313:231–233.

230. Eidne KA, Flanagan CA, Millar RP. Gonadotropin-releasing hormone binding sites in human breast carcinoma. Science 1985; 229:989–991.

231. Wilding G, Chen M, Gelmann E, et al. LHRH agonists and human breast cancer cells. Nature 1987; 329:770.

232. Klijn JM, DeJong FH, Lamberts WJ, et al. LHRH-agonist treatment in metastatic prostate carcinoma. Eur J Clin Oncol 1984; 20:483–493.

233. Kerle D, Williams G, Ware H, et al. Failure of long term luteinising hormone releasing hormone treatment for prostatic cancer to suppress serum luteinising hormone and testosterone. Br Med J 1984; 289:468–469.

234. Handelsman DJ, Swerdloff RS. Pharmacokinetics of gonadotropin-releasing hormone and its analogs. Endocr Rev 1986; 7:95–105.

235. Furr BJA, Nicholson RI. Use of analogues of LHRH for treatment of cancer. J Reprod Fertil 1982; 64:529–539.

236. Furr BA, Hutchison FG. Biodegradable sustained release formulation of the LH-RH analogue "Zoladex" for the treatment of hormone-responsive tumors. In: Back N, Breiver GJ, Eijsvoogel V, et al, eds. EORTC Genitourinary Group Monograph 2. Part A: Therapeutic Principles in Metastatic Prostate Cancer. New York: Alan R Liss, 1985: 143–153.

237. Beacock CJ, Buck AC, Zwinck R, et al. The treatment of metastatic prostatic cancer with the slow release LH-RH analogue Zoladex ICI 118630. Br J Urol 1987; 59:436–442.

238. Robinson MG, Denis L, Mahler C, et al. An LH-RH analogue (Zoladex) in the management of carcinoma of the prostate: a preliminary report comparing daily subcutaneous injection with monthly depot injections. Eur J Surg Oncol 1985; 11:159–165.

239. Thomas EJ, Jenkins J, Lenton EA, et al. Endocrine effects of goserelin, a new depot luteinising hormone releasing hormone agonist. Br Med J 1986; 293:1407–1409.

240. The Leuprolide Study Group. Leuprolide versus diethylstilbestrol for metastatic prostate cancer. N Engl J Med 1984; 311:1281–1286.

241. Labrie F, Dupont A, Giguere M, et al. Combination therapy with flutamide and castration (orchiectomy or LHRH agonist). The minimal endocrine therapy in both untreated and previously treated patients. J Steroid Biochem 1987; 27:525–532.

242. Mathe G, Schally AV, Comaru-Schally AM, et al. Phase II trial with D-Trp-6-LH-RH in prostatic carcinoma: comparison with other hormonal agents. Prostate 1986; 9:327–342.

243. Smith JA, Urry RL. Testicular histology after prolonged treatment with a gonadotropin-releasing hormone analogue. J Urol 1985; 133:612–614.

244. Peters CA, Walsh PC. The effect of nafarelin acetate, a luteinizing hormone–releasing hormone agonist, on benign prostatic hyperplasia. N Engl J Med 1987; 317:599–604.

245. Moguilewsky M, Fiet J, Tournemine C, et al. Pharmacology of an antiandrogen, Anandron®, used as an adjuvant therapy in the treatment of prostate cancer. J Steroid Biochem 1986; 24:139–146.

246. Tunn UW, Radlmaier A, Neumann F. Antiandrogens in cancer treatment. In: Stoll BA, ed. Endocrine Management of Cancer. Vol 2: Contemporary Therapy. New York: S Karger, 1988: 43–56.

247. Frith RG, Phillipou G. 15-Hydroxycyproterone acetate and cyproterone acetate levels in plasma and urine. J Chromatogr 1985; 338:179–186.

248. De Voogt HH, EORTC-GU-Group. Cardiovascular side effects of diethylstilbestrol, cyproterone acetate, medroxyprogesterone acetate, and estramustine phosphate used for the treatment of advanced prostatic cancer: results from European Organization for Research and Treatment of Cancer—Trials 30761 and 30762. J Urol 1986; 135:303–307.

249. Rassmussen GH. Chemical control of androgen action. Annu Rep Med Chem 1986; 21:179–188.

250. Hammerstein J, Moltz L, Schwartz U. Antiandrogens in the treatment of acne and hirsutism. J Steroid Biochem 1983; 19:591–597.

251. Paisey RB, Kadow C, Bolton C, et al. Effects of cyproterone acetate and a long-acting LHRH analogue in serum lipoproteins in patients with carcinoma of the prostate. J R Soc Med 1986; 79:210–211.

252. Frohman LA. Disease of the anterior pituitary. In: Felig P, Baxter JD, Broodus AE, et al, eds. Endocrinology and Metabolism. 2nd ed. New York: McGraw-Hill, 1987: 247–337.

253. Sogani PC, Vagaiwala MR, Whitmore WF. Experience with flutamide in patients with advanced prostatic cancer without prior endocrine therapy. Cancer 1984; 54:744–750.

254. Neri R, Kassem N. Biological and clinical properties of antiandrogens. In: Breciani F, ed. Progress in Cancer Research and Therapy. New York: Raven, 1984: 507–518.

255. Crawford E, McLeod D, Dorr A, et al. Treatment of newly diagnosed stage D_2 prostate cancer with leuprolide and flutamide or leuprolide alone, phase III, intergroup study 0036. Proc Am Soc Clin Oncol 1988; 7:119 (abstract).

256. Kuhn J-M, Billebaud T, Navratil H, et al. Prevention of the transient adverse effects of a gonadotropin-releasing hormone analogue (buserelin) in metastatic prostatic carcinoma by administration of an antiandrogen (nilutamide). N Engl J Med 1989; 321:413–418.

257. Thompson EB, Lippman ME. Mechanism of action of glucocorticoids. Metabolism 1974; 23:159–202.

258. Baxter JD, Forsham PH. Tissue effects of glucocorticoids. Am J Med 1972; 53:573–589.

259. Selye H. Studies on adaption. Endocrinology 1937; 21:169–188.

260. Claman HN. Corticoids and lymphoid cells. N Engl J Med 1972; 287:388–397.

261. Livingston RB, Carter SK, eds. Single Agents in Cancer Chemotherapy. New York: Plenum, 1970.

262. Vietti TJ, Sullivan MP, Berry DH, et al. The response of acute childhood leukemia to an initial and a second course of prednisone. J Pediatr 1965; 66:18–26.

263. Kjellstraad CM. Side effects of steroids and their treatment. Transplant Proc 1975; 7:123–129.

264. McGuire WL, ed. Estrogen Receptors in Human Breast Cancer. New York: Raven, 1975.

265. Schmidt TJ, Thompson EB. Glucocorticoid receptor function in lymphoma cells. In: Sharma RK, Criss WE, eds. Endocrine Control in Neoplasia. New York: Raven, 1978: 263–290.

266. Lippman ME, Konior-Yarbro G, Leventhal BG. Clinical implications of glucocorticoid receptors in human leukemia. Cancer Res 1978; 38:4251–4256.

267. Crabtree GR, Smith KA, Munck A. Glucocorticoid receptors and sensitivity of isolated human leukemia and lymphoma cells. Cancer Res 1978; 38:4268–4272.

268. Neifeld JP, Lippman ME, Tormey DC. Steroid hormone receptors in normal human lymphocytes. Induction of glucocorticoid receptor activity by phytohemagglutinin stimulation. J Biol Chem 1977; 254:2972–2977.

269. Lippman ME, Barr R. Glucocorticoid receptors in purified subpopulations of human peripheral blood lymphocytes. J Immunol 1977; 118:1977–1981.

270. Thompson EB, Aviv D, Lippman ME. Variants of HTC cells with low tyrosine aminotransferase inducibility and apparently normal glucocorticoid receptors. Endocrinology 1977; 100:406–419.

271. Cidlowski JA, Munck A. Comparison of glucocorticoid receptor complex binding to nuclei and SNA cellulose. Biochim Biophys Acta 1978; 543:545–555.

272. Smith KA, Crabtree GR, Kennedy SJ, et al. Glucocorticoid receptors and

glucocorticoid sensitivity of mitogen stimulated and unstimulated human lymphocytes. Nature 1977; 267:523–526.

273. Lippman ME, Halterman R, Perry S, et al. Glucocorticoid binding proteins in human leukaemic lymphoblasts. Nature 1973; 242:157–158.

274. Lippman ME, Halterman R, Leventhal BG, et al. Glucocorticoid binding proteins in acute lymphoblastic leukemic blast cells. J Clin Invest 1973; 52:1715–1725.

275. Yarbro GS, Lippman ME, Johnson GE, et al. Glucocorticoid receptors in subpopulations of childhood acute lymphocytic leukemia. Cancer Res 1977; 37:2688–2695.

276. Lippman ME, Konior-Yarbro G, Leventhal BG. Clinical implications of glucocorticoid receptor in human leukemia. Cancer Res 1978; 38:4251–4256.

277. Lippman ME, Perry S, Thompson EB. Glucocorticoid binding proteins in myeloblasts of acute myelogenous leukemia. Am J Med 1975; 59:224–227.

278. Crabtree GR, Smith KA, Munck A. Glucocorticoid receptors and sensitivity of isolated human leukemia and lymphoma cells. Cancer Res 1978; 38:4268.

279. Gailiani S, Minowada J, Silvernail P, et al. Specific glucocorticoid binding in human hemopoietic cell lines and neoplastic tissue. Cancer Res 1978; 33:2653.

280. Homo F, Duval D, Meyer P, et al. Chronic lymphatic leukaemia: cellular effects of glucocorticoid in vitro. Br J Haematol 1978; 38:491–499.

281. Terenius L, Simonsson B, Nilsson K. Glucocorticoid receptors, DNA synthesis, membrane antigens and their relation to disease activity in chronic lymphatic leukemia. J Steroid Biochem 1976; 7:905–909.

282. Bloomfield C, Smith KA, Peterson BA, et al. In vitro glucocorticoid studies for predicting response to glucocorticoid therapy in adults with malignant lymphomas. Lancet 1980; 1:952–955.

36

HUMORAL MANIFESTATIONS OF MALIGNANCY

Gordon J. Strewler

The syndrome of ectopic secretion of corticotropin (also known as ACTH) was first described by Brown in 1928 in a woman with bronchogenic carcinoma,[1] 4 y prior to Cushing's description of the clinical syndrome of corticotropin excess and before the relationship between the hormone and the clinical syndrome was recognized. In 1941 Albright proposed the idea that tumors can cause endocrine syndromes by secreting hormones inappropriately, namely that hypercalcemia in a patient with renal carcinoma might be due to production of parathyroid hormone (PTH) by the tumor.[2] Albright was led to this conclusion by the coexistence of hypercalcemia with hypophosphatemia (biochemical features of primary hyperparathyroidism) in a patient with a single bone metastasis. In 1956 cases were reported in which hypercalcemia was cured by resection of the primary tumor,[3, 4] supporting Albright's hypothesis that the neoplasm produced humoral hypercalcemia. Subsequently Schwartz and colleagues[5] described the syndrome of inappropriate vasopression (ADH) secretion in bronchogenic carcinoma. Meador and co-workers[6] described the ectopic corticotropin syndrome in lung carcinoma, and

Liddle coined the term *ectopic hormone syndrome* to describe such situations.[7]

GENERAL FEATURES OF INAPPROPRIATE HORMONE SECRETION IN MALIGNANCY

Common Features

Inappropriate secretion of peptide hormones is probably the commonest cause of paraneoplastic syndromes. Although the manifestations vary widely, paraneoplastic hormonal syndromes have features that distinguish them from overproduction of hormones by endocrine glands (Table 36–1). First, the secretion of hormones by extraglandular tumors is rarely suppressible. Tumor cells that secrete hormones typically do not possess the cellular machinery that allows for regulation of hormone secretion. The most notable exception to this

TABLE 36–1. General Characteristics of Paraneoplastic Hormonal Syndromes

Secretion of hormones is rarely suppressible.
Clinical syndromes are usually associated with advanced malignancies.
Hormones are not useful as tumor markers for nonendocrine tumors.
Tumors may mimic syndromes of hormone excess by secreting a related peptide (e.g., insulin-like growth factor II to cause hypoglycemia).

general rule is the secretion of corticotropin by carcinoid tumors of the lung or thymus. Corticotropin secretion by these tumors is often suppressible by glucocorticoids, with secretory dynamics that can be difficult to distinguish from those of corticotrope adenomas of the pituitary. Second, extraglandular tumors produce hormones relatively inefficiently, so clinical syndromes of hormone excess become evident only in patients with advanced malignancies. It is probably for this reason that hormones are disappointing as tumor markers. Third, tumors often lack the ability to process peptide hormones normally and secrete large, incompletely processed forms of hormones with reduced biologic activity. Finally, some malignant tumors mimic syndromes of hormone excess not by secreting the usual hormone but by secreting related hormones that mimic the biologic actions. For example non–islet cell tumors can cause hypoglycemia not by secreting insulin but by secreting the related peptide insulin-like growth factor-II (IGF-II).[8] IGF-II does not ordinarily play a major role in glucose metabolism, but it has insulin-like activity and in large amounts causes hypoglycemia. Similarly hypercalcemia in malignancy is a manifestation not of PTH excess but of an excess of parathyroid hormone–related protein (PTHrP), a related protein that in most circumstances is a local regulator but acts as a hormone when it is released into the circulation by malignant tumors.

Ectopic Versus Eutopic Secretion

The term *ectopic hormone secretion* is actually a misnomer. Ectopic means "out of place," implying secretion of a hormone by tissues that do not ordinarily do so, whereas hormones that are secreted by tumors are usually present in the nonmalignant precursor cells, albeit often in small amounts. For example the hormones typically secreted by small cell lung carcinoma—vasopressin, calcitonin and corticotropin—are thought to be present in the neuroendocrine cells in the normal bronchial mucosa that are the probable precursors of the tumor.[9, 10] PTHrP is a normal product of the keratinocyte, the cell of origin of squamous carcinomas that cause humoral hypercalcemia by secreting PTHrP.[11] Human chorionic gonadotropin (hCG), usually considered a placental hormone, is not under tight transcriptional control, and low levels of the hormone are detectable in a variety of other normal tissues, a finding that is in keeping with the occurrence of hCG secretion by many tumor types.[12–14] Thus most endocrine manifestations of malignancy are caused by eutopic secretion of hormones by cells that were previously programmed to secrete them. This feature has implications for the pathogenesis of the humoral manifestations of malignancy that are discussed later. As for nosology, the term *ectopic* is firmly ingrained and will not soon be abandoned, even though true ectopic secretion of hormones is rare.

Peptide Versus Nonpeptide Hormones

Most peptide hormones are secreted by nonendocrine malignant tumors (Table 36–2), with some exceptions. The glycoprotein hormones follicle-stimulating hormone (FSH), luteinizing hormone (LH), and thyroid-stimulating hormone (TSH) are rarely if ever produced by extrapituitary tumors, possibly because it is necessary to express the genes for two subunits, glycosylate the subunits appropriately, and assemble the complete dimer to produce a biologically active hormone. However, the glycoprotein hormone hCG is frequently secreted by nontrophoblastic tumors, documenting that the requisite machinery can be present in nonpituitary cells. More important, pituitary glycoprotein hormone synthesis is tightly controlled by a series of pituitary-specific transcription factors, whereas hCG is normally expressed at low levels in a variety of nontrophoblastic cells. In the same vein, no cases of extrapancreatic secretion of insulin have been authenticated. Although a few copies per cell of insulin mRNA can be detected in many cells by sensitive polymerase chain reaction (PCR) methods, physiological expression of the insulin gene is driven by transcription factors that are specific to the pancreatic beta cell, and these factors are rarely if ever expressed in other cell types. Thus the propensity of a peptide hormone for secretion by extraglandular tumors may be a function of the tightness of its transcriptional suppression in normal extraglandular tissues.

Steroid and thyroid hormones are not secreted by extraglandular tumors, although they are occasionally produced by teratomas that contain glandular elements. Their synthesis requires an extended series of enzymatic steps that are not present in nonsteroidogenic tissues. In contrast, 1,25-dihydroxycholecalciferol (1,25(OH)$_2$D) is secreted by lymphomas as well as macrophages resident in granulomas of sarcoidosis and other granulomatous disorders. In these tissues the synthesis of 1,25(OH)$_2$D requires a single enzymatic step, the 1α-hydroxylation of the circulating precursor, 25-hydroxycholecalciferol.

Cellular Basis of Ectopic Hormone Secretion

Why is the secretion of hormones by malignant neoplasms so commonplace? The simplest idea is that random sets of genes are "derepressed" in the cancer cell, including genes that code for hormones. However, the association of tumors and hormone secretion is nonrandom, with certain tumors (e.g., lung carcinoma) characteristically secreting certain hormones (e.g., corticotropin or vasopressin). Moreover, in a

TABLE 36–2. Hormones Produced by Tumors

Hypercalcemia factors
    PTH-related protein (PTHrP)
    Tumor necrosis factor α
    1,25(OH)$_2$D
    Prostaglandins
    PTH
Vasopressin
Corticotropin (ACTH)
Growth hormone–releasing hormone
Insulin-like growth factor II (IGF-II)
Calcitonin
Human chorionic gonadotropin (hCG)
Human placental lactogen (hPL)
Growth hormone
Corticotropin-releasing hormone
Erythropoietin
Oncogenous osteomalacia factor
Atrial natriuretic peptide
Endothelin
Renin
Other gut hormones: gastrin-releasing peptide, glucose-dependent insulinotropic peptide (gastrin-inhibitory peptide), somatostatin, pancreatic polypeptide, vasoactive intestinal peptide, substance P, motilin

number of cases the peptides secreted by tumors are the same peptides that are secreted by the normal cell of origin of the neoplasm. Depression is again nonrandom and is a quantitative rather than a qualitative phenomenon. The "dedifferentiation" hypothesis posits a retrograde movement of tumor cells along the pathway of differentiation, leading to the expression of fetal proteins (e.g., α-fetoprotein and carcinoembryonic antigen) or hormones that are normally formed in immature cells. This hypothesis would account for both the nonrandom nature of ectopic hormone secretion and the propensity for secretion of hormones that play a critical role in development, for example IGF-II, PTHrP, and, possibly, gastrin-releasing peptide (GRP) and other peptides of neuroendocrine cells. In addition, tumors frequently secrete other fetal proteins (carcinoembryonic antigen, α-fetoprotein). However there is no compelling evidence for a generalized pattern of expression of primitive genes in tumor cells. The "dysdifferentiation hypothesis" of Baylin and Mendelsohn[15] holds that epithelial malignancy is the result of clonal expansion of a particular cell type that occurs along a complex pathway of epithelial differentiation. This process could give rise to overexpression of a hormone because of clonal expansion of a normally rare population of committed cells or because of clonal expansion of a primitive cell type not normally present in the mature epithelium.

Since the defining characteristic of neoplastic cells is uncontrolled growth, it is worth considering the possible relationship of disordered growth and the secretion of hormones. In some instances an oncogenic event might directly activate transcription of a hormone gene. One example of direct gene activation is the secretion of PTHrP in adult T-cell leukemia that produces severe hypercalcemia.[16] The oncogenic event that gives rise to this form of leukemia involves integration of the human T-cell lymphotrophic virus type I (HTLV-I), which can target the promoter of the PTHrP gene to induce its transcription, using the *trans*-activating viral protein tax.[17] However, no instances of direct activation of hormone genes by an oncogenic event have been described in cancers of epithelial origin.

Secretion of a hormone might stimulate the growth of tumor cells by an autocrine or a paracrine mechanism so that hormone secretion could provide a growth advantage, leading to selective outgrowth of cells that secreted high levels of the hormone. One of the characteristic products of small cell lung carcinoma (SCLC) is GRP, the mammalian counterpart of the amphibian hormone bombesin. GRP fulfills criteria for being an autocrine growth factor in SCLC, namely it is secreted by tumor cells and can stimulate replication of the cells via specific receptors, and blockade of GRP's action by neutralizing antibodies to GRP[18] or peptide antagonists[19] inhibits cell replication in vitro and tumor formation in vivo. β-Endorphin, one of the products of the pro-opiomelanocortin (*POMC*) gene, may also function as a growth factor in SCLC.[20] Another ectopic hormone with growth factor activity is IGF-II, the factor that is believed to cause hypoglycemia in non–islet cell tumors.[8] However there is no direct evidence of a role of IGF-II in the growth of these neoplasms.

In some instances hormone secretion by neoplastic cells may be the consequence of proliferation. For example PTHrP, which is expressed in areas of cartilage proliferation, is an important growth factor in this tissue.[21] Similarly IGF-II is a fetal growth factor in cartilage and other tissues. Neuroendocrine cells that express GRP are found at the branchpoints of developing airways in the fetal lung, and GRP increases branching morphogenesis of airways, suggesting that its secretion by neuroendocrine cells could regulate morphogenesis of the lung.[22, 23] Direct molecular links may be re-established during oncogenesis between cell cycle regulators and the transcription of hormone genes associated with proliferative states during development.

Neuroendocrine Cells and Hormone Secretion

Tumors that secrete corticotropin, vasopressin, calcitonin, gut peptides (GRP, somatostatin, vasoactive intestinal peptide), and biogenic amines such as 5-hydroxytryptamine are characteristically of neuroendocrine cell origin. Neuroendocrine cells specialized for the production of peptide hormones and biogenic amines possess pathways for the rapid release of peptides or neurotransmitters in response to stimuli; such regulated pathways for protein secretion are distinct from the mechanism of constitutive secretion, which is ubiquitous in eukaryotic cells. The most readily recognizable feature of the regulated pathway is the dense neurosecretory granule, which is designed for the secretion of peptides and amines.[24] The neurosecretory granule, which is involved in both the storage of hormones in concentrated form and the rapid release of these stores in response to stimulation, is recognizable histologically because it is electron dense and intensely argyrophilic, reflecting the dense, nearly crystalline packing of its contents.

The neurosecretory granule buds from the trans-Golgi network after it is packed with its peptide or neurotransmitter contents. Proteins on the surface of the neurosecretory granule, in the vesicular compartments from which the granule buds, and on the plasma membrane of neurosecretory cells collectively determine the properties of regulated pathway of hormone secretion.[24] They are probably important in ectopic hormone secretion. In addition to stored hormones, the neuroendocrine granule contains one or more acidic proteins called chromogranins, which are released together with stored hormone and serve as additional neuroendocrine tumor markers, both in immunohistology and in the circulation.[25] The chromogranins are highly conserved in evolution and presumably play a role in the assembly, packing, or release of neurosecretory granules,[26] but this role has yet to be fully clarified.

The neurosecretory granules contain serine proteases called prohormone convertases that process precursor proteins to their mature forms. The prohormone convertase family is widely distributed in evolution, and several members of the family, such as furin, are localized in the trans-Golgi network and process a wide variety of proteins in the constitutive pathway. The two members of the family that occur mainly in neurosecretory granules, PC2 (SPC2) and PC1/PC3 (SPC3), have acidic pH optima and are dependent on calcium, suiting them for the environment of the neurosecretory granule.[27] Both enzymes cleave their substrate peptides on the carboxyl-terminal side of polybasic residues, but they have slightly different specificities, and their different distribution in the pituitary accounts for the differences in processing of POMC in the anterior and intermediate pituitary lobes.[27] The prohormone convertases are important for understanding ectopic hormone secretion because their levels in tumor cells not only account for the efficiency of precursor processing to mature and biologically active versions of peptide hormones, thus determining whether a given tumor produces a clinical syndrome of hormone excess, but also determine the pattern of peptides produced, for example from the polyhormone precursor POMC, and thus the nature of the clinical syndrome.

Neuroendocrine cells are scattered through the bronchial mucosa of the developing and mature lung.[9, 10, 28] They occur singly and in distinct innervated corpuscles referred to as neuroepithelial bodies. Subpopulations of the cells contain the peptides calcitonin, GRP, vasopressin and leu-enkephalin, and some may also contain somatostatin, motilin, or pancreatic polypeptide. Neuroendocrine (enterochromaffin) cells are also scattered through the gastrointestinal mucosa and are found in other organs, such as the ovaries and the prostate gland. Some years ago Pearce suggested that neuroendocrine cells, which he called APUD cells (for *Amine Precursor Uptake and Decarboxylation*), although widely scattered in many tissues, have a common origin in the neural crest and represent a "diffuse neuroendocrine system," a third branch of the nervous system.[26] However, not all APUD cells are of neural crest origin—some arise from primitive endoderm.[29] Whether neuroendocrine cells are part of a global regulatory system remains to be clarified, but some of these peptides may have a developmental role in branching morphogenesis of the lung.[22, 23]

Although the evidence is indirect, resident neuroendocrine cells are the presumed origin of small cell carcinoma of the lung, prostate, and ovary and of carcinoid tumors. If not true precursors, resident neuroendocrine cells are at least mature cells that appear to be on the same pathway of differentiation as tumor cells of the neuroendocrine type. Carcinoids are neuroendocrine tumors that are relatively well-differentiated and slow-growing, with a reduced metastatic potential[10] (see Chapter 37). Whether the capacity of neuroendocrine cells to secrete hormones is amplified during oncogenesis is not clear—it is possible that malignant neuroendocrine cells continue to secrete the same relatively low levels of hormones as their precursors and cause syndromes of hormone excess only because of tumor bulk. However, it is more likely that the secretory repertoire and the secretory amplitude increase in the malignant state, perhaps recapitulating the active state of hormone secretion that characterizes development of lung and presumably of other tissues.

Criteria for Diagnosis of Ectopic Hormone Secretion

Criteria for the diagnosis of ectopic hormone secretion, arranged in increasing order of stringency, are summarized in Table 36–3. The association of a clinical syndrome of hormone excess with a neoplasm provokes a search for inappropriate plasma or urinary hormone levels. Oftentimes the clinician performs suppression tests, since glandular hypersecretion of hormones is often suppressible whereas the secretion of hormones by neoplasms is typically autonomous and nonsuppressible. In the usual clinical circumstance the last step is to exclude other possible causal mechanisms for hormone excess. The coincidental occurrence of an endocrine tumor and a cancer is not uncommon; for example primary hyperparathyroidism can be present in a patient who also has cancer and can be detected with relative ease using modern assays for PTH. Occasionally the presence of an ectopic hormone syndrome can be confirmed by showing that resection of the tumor reverses the clinical syndrome. Because such syndromes

TABLE 36–3. Criteria for Diagnosis of Ectopic Hormone Secretion

Clinical Criteria

A clinical syndrome of hormone excess is associated with a neoplasm.
Serum or urine levels of the hormone are inappropriately elevated.
The hormone level is nonsuppressible.
Other possible causal mechanisms are excluded.
The syndrome is reversed by resection of the tumor (rare).

Research Criteria

The hormone can be detected in tumor tissue.
mRNA for the hormone is present in tumor tissue.
The hormone is secreted from tumor cells in culture.
There is an arteriovenous gradient for the hormone across the tumor.

are typically late manifestations of widespread neoplasms, these opportunities are sadly rare.

The remaining criteria for ectopic hormone secretion are mainly useful for research purposes. The detection of a hormone in tumor tissue by immunoassay methods provides evidence that the tumor is a site of its production, although caution must be exercised because of the possibility of false-positive reactions in immunohistochemistry and radioimmunoassay. An additional theoretical concern is that the tumor may accumulate hormone from the circulation; no examples of this phenomenon have been reported, however. Detection of mRNA for the hormone confirms that the tumor is indeed a site of synthesis of the peptide. For this evidence to be compelling, hormone mRNA should be detectable in solution hybridization or RNA blotting assays. The technique of reverse transcription and PCR is so sensitive that a signal can be obtained from samples containing only a few molecules of hormone mRNA, a level that may be insignificant. In addition, identification of hormone mRNA without hormone protein leaves open the possibility that the mRNA is not translated—for example, many normal tissues express a form of POMC mRNA that cannot be translated to protein.[30]

Demonstration of the presence of both hormone mRNA and protein provides strong evidence for synthesis in the tumor but does not directly establish that the hormone is secreted. The most rigorous criterion for ectopic hormone secretion is to demonstrate an arteriovenous gradient of the hormone across the tumor or to show production and secretion of the hormone by tumor cells cultured in vitro. Unfortunately selective catheterization to obtain a true arteriovenous gradient is often impossible, as many of the tumors are present in the pulmonary or splanchnic bed or are widely metastatic. Establishing tumor cells in culture provides an important research tool but requires an element of good fortune—many tumor cells, exuberant as their growth may be in the host, are difficult to propagate in cell culture.

MALIGNANCY-ASSOCIATED HYPERCALCEMIA

Clinical Features

Hypercalcemia is probably the most common endocrine complication of malignant tumors, occurring in as many as 5% of all cancers. The incidence of hypercalcemia in malignancy is 15 cases per 100,000 person-years, about one half the incidence of primary hyperparathyroidism,[31] and malignant tumors are the most common cause of hypercalcemia in hospitalized patients[32] (see also Chapter 24).

Hypercalcemia in malignancy usually has a rapid onset and can cause confusion, stupor, nausea, vomiting, and dehydration. The offending neoplasm is almost always evident clinically, even when hypercalcemia is the initial manifestation. Thus physical examination and a chest radiograph disclose the underlying tumor in about 98% of patients. Because hypercalcemia usually occurs in advanced maligancy, the prognosis is poor, with a median survival of only 4 to 8 wk after the discovery of hypercalcemia.[33] Exceptions are breast carcinoma and multiple myeloma, in which successful treatment of the underlying malignancy may provide for long survival in the hypercalcemic patient.

The frequency of individual tumors in patients with hypercalcemia is shown in Table 36–4. Lung carcinoma, breast carcinoma, and multiple myeloma account for more than 50% of all cases of malignancy-associated hypercalcemia. Lung carcinomas that produce hypercalcemia have squamous or large cell histology, whereas small cell carcinoma almost never

TABLE 36–4. Malignancy-Associated Hypercalcemia*

Primary Site	No. (%) of Cases	Known Metastatic Disease (%)
Lung	111(25.0)	62
Breast	87(19.6)	92
Multiple myeloma	43(9.7)	100
Head and neck	36(8.1)	73
Renal and urinary tract	35(7.9)	36
Esophagus	25(5.6)	53
Female genital	24(5.2)	81
Unknown primary	23(5.2)	—
Lymphoma	14(3.2)	91
Colon	8(1.8)	—
Liver/biliary	7(1.6)	—
Skin	6(1.4)	—
Other	25(5.6)	—
Total	444(100)	

*Data are from references 32, 234, and 235. Data on metastatic disease are taken from references 32 and 234.

From Strewler GJ. Nonparathyroid hypercalcemia. Adv Inter Med 1987; 32:235–258. © 1987 Yearbook Medical Publishers, Inc.

causes hypercalcemia.[34] About two thirds of lung cancer patients have bone metastasis at the time when hypercalcemia develops. Among other solid tumors, the most common are squamous and renal carcinomas. Gastrointestinal tumors and prostate carcinoma are less common causes of hypercalcemia. Hypercalcemia is uncommon in lymphomas and leukemia but occurs in two thirds of patients with adult T-cell leukemia syndrome, which is caused by the HTLV-I.[16, 35, 36] Pheochromocytomas may produce hypercalcemia by the same mechanism as other malignant neoplasms, secretion of PTHrP.[37, 38]

Laboratory Features

Overall, about 80% of cases, including most patients with solid tumors, have increased serum levels of PTHrP, which can be measured in two-site, amino-terminal or midregion assays (Fig. 36–1).[39–43] Hypophosphatemia is common because of the phosphaturic effect of PTHrP. Although the combination of hypercalcemia and hypophosphatemia is consistent with the presence of primary hyperparathyroidism, the level of intact PTH is suppressed to less than 2 pmol/L (20 pg/mL) in patients with malignancy-associated hypercalcemia.[39, 44] The serum level of 1,25(OH)$_2$D is also suppressed in hypercalcemic patients,[45, 46] except in lymphoma, where 1,25(OH)$_2$D levels are often high. Renal function may be impaired by hypercalcemia.

Pathogenesis

Hypercalcemia in malignancy is caused by excessive bone resorption. Multiple myeloma and some breast cancers induce hypercalcemia by local osteolytic mechanisms, but in most patients bone resorption is induced by humoral factors. The most common humoral factor is PTHrP, but 1,25(OH)$_2$D is a hypercalcemic factor in lymphomas, and rarely PTH is secreted ectopically by nonparathyroid tumors.

Parathyroid Hormone–Related Protein

PTHrP is related to PTH structurally (Fig. 24–12) and shares a common receptor with PTH[11, 47, 48] (see Chapter 24 for a discussion of the chemistry of PTHrP). Because PTH and PTHrP share a receptor,[49, 50] it follows that their biologic actions are similar.[48] PTHrP produces hypercalcemia by increasing resorption of bone throughout the skeleton and by increasing the renal resorption of calcium, and causes hypophosphatemia through a phosphaturic effect at the kidney.[47] The hypocalciuric effect of PTHrP probably plays a significant role in the pathogenesis of hypercalcemia,[51, 52] albeit secondary to the role of bone resorption.

PTHrP functions in normal physiology as a tissue factor that regulates cellular proliferation and differentiation in fetal development and in tissues such as the breast, skin, and hair follicle in the adult[21] (see also Chapter 24). Remarkably, PTHrP locally regulates development, in part acting via the same receptor that PTH uses systemically to regulate its target tissues, bone and the kidney. However, when PTHrP is pro-

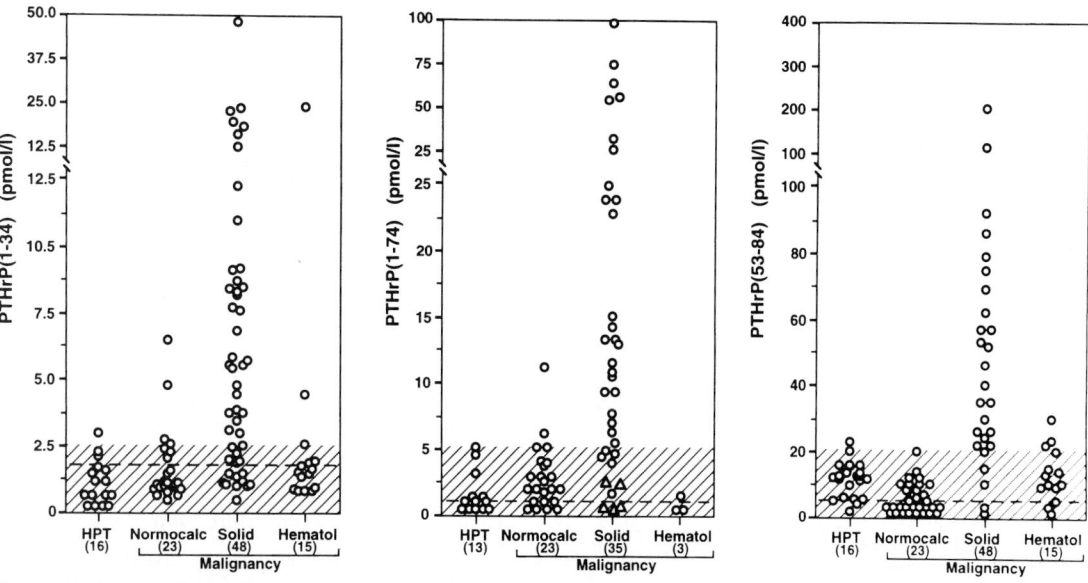

Figure 36–1. Plasma concentration of parathyroid hormone–related protein (PTHrP) in patients with hyperparathyroidism (HPT), normocalcemic patients with malignancy (Normocalc), and patients with hypercalcemia of malignancy due to a solid tumor (Solid) or a hematologic malignancy (Hematol). Radioimmunoassay (RIA) for amino-terminal PTHrP(1–34) (*left panel*), an immunoradiometric assay for PTHrP(1–74) (*middle panel*), and an RIA for midregion PTHrP(53–84) (*right panel*). The hatched area represents the normal ranges; the dashed line denotes the limits of detection; the numbers attached to each group indicate the number of patients. In the PTHrP(1–74) assay, the group Solid includes five patients classified as local osteolytic type of hypercalcemia (△). Note the different scale of the y-axes. (Data references from 39, 40, and 43; reprinted from Blind E, Nissenson RA, Strewler GJ. Parathyroid hormone–related protein. In: Becker KL, Bremner WJ, Hung W, et al, eds. Principles and Practice of Endocrinology and Metabolism. 2nd ed. Philadelphia: JB Lippincott, 1985, with permission.)

duced by a tumor of sufficient mass, it enters the systemic circulation, where it activates PTH/PTHrP receptors in bone and kidney and produces hypercalcemia.

PTHrP can either produce humoral hypercalcemia or cause local osteolytic hypercalcemia by direct activation of osteoclasts in the vicinity of bone metastases. In lung and renal carcinoma, PTHrP can act as a humoral factor, because hypercalcemia can occur without evidence of bone metastasis (see Table 36–1). Even when bone metastases are present, hypercalcemia is predominantly humoral because the serum calcium level correlates better with the level of PTHrP than with the number or size of bone metastases. In breast carcinoma about 50% of patients have increased serum levels of PTHrP and are presumed to have humoral hypercalcemia. However in breast carcinoma hypercalcemia usually occurs in patients with extensive bone metastases (see Table 36–4), about one half of whom have undetectable serum levels of PTHrP.[39–43] In an experimental model transfection of PTHrP cDNA into breast carcinoma cells increases their propensity for bone metastasis, and bone metastasis induces local osteolytic hypercalcemia, without an increase in the circulating level of PTHrP.[53] In humans metastases of breast cancer to bone are immunohistochemically positive for PTHrP in 92% of cases, compared with 17% of nonosseous metastases.[54, 55] This difference suggests either that tumor cells that secrete PTHrP have a selective advantage in bone (perhaps because they induce local resorption) or that the bone environment induces the expression of PTHrP.

At least two aspects of the hypercalcemia syndrome associated with PTHrP are paradoxical. First, plasma levels of $1,25(OH)_2D$ tend to be low in malignancy,[45, 46] despite the acute effect of PTHrP to stimulate renal synthesis of $1,25(OH)_2D$.[56] This finding contrasts with normal to high levels of $1,25(OH)_2D$ in primary hyperparathyroidism.[45] This difference may be due to the capacity of hypercalcemia itself to suppress production of $1,25(OH)_2D$, tending to counteract the acute stimulatory effect of PTH or PTHrP. Thus a continuous chronic infusion of PTH, in contrast to the effects of primary hyperparathyroidism, suppresses $1,25(OH)_2D$ levels, but clamping the serum calcium in the normal range prevents this suppression.[57] In the same vein some patients with malignancy have a marked increase in $1,25(OH)_2D$ to supranormal levels when hypercalcemia is treated with bisphosphonates.[46] Perhaps the pattern of secretion of PTHrP (continuous?) or associated ancillary factors[58] increase the susceptibility of $1,25(OH)_2D$ synthesis to suppression by hypercalcemia.

A second paradox concerns bone turnover in the setting of high PTHrP levels. Despite avid bone resorption, bone formation is reduced in postmortem bone biopsies from patients with malignancy and hypercalcemia.[59] This uncoupled state contrasts with primary hyperparathyroidism and most other resorptive states, which are characterized by coupled increases in bone formation, and also contrasts with the results of a PTHrP infusion.[60] It is possible that immobilization, inanition, illness, or other cytokines secreted by neoplasms depress osteoblastic activity.

Mechanisms involved in the activation of PTHrP gene expression in malignant tumors may include *trans*-activation by tumor-specific factors and differential methylation. The PTHrP gene is expressed in a variety of normal tissues of the embryo and the adult, where it functions as a tissue regulator of differentiation[21] (see Chapter 24). One prominant site of normal expression is the keratinocyte[61–63]; thus secretion of PTHrP by squamous carcinomas can be regarded as eutopic. The best example of *trans*-activation is adult T-cell leukemia, which is commonly characterized by PTHrP-dependent hypercalcemia.[16, 35, 36] There it appears that a specific *trans*-activating protein in the genome of HTLV-I is capable of direct activation of PTHrP transcription, acting in part at a site near the most

downstream promoter.[17] (The PTHrP gene has three promoters, each of which is utilized to varying degrees in normal and malignant tissues.[11, 64, 65]) When PTHrP promoter constructs are fused to a reporter gene and transfected into squamous carcinoma cell lines, the relative level of expression of the reporter gene correlates with the intensity of endogenous PTHrP gene expression in the same cell lines,[66] suggesting that in this circumstance also the expression of PTHrP is regulated in *trans* by a factor or factors that are differentially expressed in different squamous carcinomas. Most squamous carcinomas express the PTHrP gene at some level,[67] but renal carcinomas are more sharply divided between PTHrP-expressors and nonexpressors, the PTHrP gene being undermethylated in renal carcinomas that express PTHrP compared with those that do not.[68] This finding suggests that hypomethylation may be a mechanism by which the gene is expressed in some renal carcinomas.

1,25-Dihydroxyvitamin D

About one half of lymphoma patients who develop hypercalcemia have inappropriately high serum $1,25(OH)_2D$ levels.[69–71] In a few cases, lymph node tissue from such patients has been shown to produce $1,25(OH)_2D$ in vitro from 25-OHD.[72] Challenge of normocalcemic lymphoma patients with the precursor sterol 25-OHD results in increased serum $1,25(OH)_2D$ levels, increased serum calcium levels, and suppression of PTH.[72] This response is in marked contrast to normal individuals, who regulate the conversion of substrate to $1,25(OH)_2D$ tightly. The enhanced responsiveness of normocalcemic lymphoma patients to vitamin D indicates that the fundamental abnormality in lymphoma, unregulated extrarenal production of $1,25(OH)_2D$, is more common than hypercalcemia. As would be expected from this interpretation, hypercalciuria is also more common than hypercalcemia in lymphoma patients[70] and presumably compensates at least in part for the inappropriate synthesis of $1,25(OH)_2D$. This syndrome resembles the hypercalcemia of sarcoidosis, which is also due to enhanced extrarenal production of $1,25(OH)_2D$.[73, 74] As in sarcoidosis, hypercalcemia in lymphoma is frequently responsive to administration of glucocorticoids.

Parathyroid Hormone

Secretion of PTH from extraparathyroid tumors is extremely rare,[75–77] although one case fulfills the most rigorous criterion, demonstration of an arteriovenous gradient for PTH across the tumor.[78] Most nonparathyroid tumors that secrete PTH are neuroendocrine tumors, although one was an ovarian adenocarcinoma. The diagnosis should be considered in patients with malignant tumors (particularly small cell tumors), hypercalcemia, and elevated PTH levels. However, most patients with these findings have a malignant tumor with coincident primary hyperparathyroidism, since this coincidence is more likely than the truly rare syndrome of ectopic PTH secretion. Consequently exploration of the parathyroid glands may be indicated in such patients who require treatment for hypercalcemia.

Local Osteolytic Hypercalcemia

Osteolytic lesions cause hypercalcemia via activation of osteoclasts and secretion of bone-resorbing cytokines. Cytokines with osteoclast-activating activity include interleukin-1 (IL-1), tumor necrosis factor α, IL-6, transforming growth factor α, and PTHrP.[79] As discussed earlier, PTHrP appears to be the local osteolytic factor that causes osteolytic hypercalcemia in breast carcinoma. The other classic example of local osteolytic hypercalcemia is multiple myeloma. Although at least one third of myeloma patients have hypercalcemia at some time during their disease, the offending cytokine has not been identified with certainty. Cultured human myeloma cell lines produce bone-resorbing factors that can be neutralized with antisera to IL-1β[80] or tumor necrosis factor β (lymphotoxin),[81] but it is not clear whether either of these or some other factor(s) are responsible for the hypercalcemia.

Diagnosis

The diagnosis of malignancy-associated hypercalcemia is usually not difficult, because the offending neoplasm is clinically evident. It is important to exclude intercurrent primary hyperparathyroidism by showing that the level of intact PTH is suppressed below 2 pmol/L (20 pg/mL). A low serum phosphorus level in conjunction with suppressed PTH levels suggests that the causative factor is PTHrP. Demonstration of elevated levels of PTHrP will confirm the diagnosis in patients with solid tumors, but this is often unnecessary clinically. PTHrP is processed to amino-terminal, midregion, and carboxyl-terminal peptides,[11, 82] and similar assay performance has been achieved in assays of the amino-terminus,[39, 41] and midregion[43] and two-site immunoradiometric assays[83–85] (see Fig. 36–1). Two-site assays for PTHrP have become the standard.

Treatment

The treatment of hypercalcemia is discussed in Chapter 24. The mainstays of treatment in tumor patients, in whom hypercalcemia is often acute and severe, are rehydration, institution of a saline diuresis, and institution of chronic treatment. In general, the treatment of choice is the second-generation bisphosphonate pamidronate, 60 to 90 mg by intravenous infusion. Patients with multiple myeloma or lymphoma often respond to glucocorticoid treatment.

SYNDROME OF INAPPROPRIATE VASOPRESSIN (ADH) SECRETION

(see Chapter 10)

Clinical Features

The syndrome of inappropriate vasopressin secretion (commonly termed the syndrome of inappropriate antidiuretic hormone [SIADH]) is probably the second most common endocrine complication in cancer patients.[86–88] The secretion of vasopressin impairs the ability to dilute the urine, leading to a state of water intoxication with hypotonicity and hyponatremia. Hyponatremia may be asymptomatic if it has developed gradually. Patients may experience weight gain because of water retention, but because the retained water is distributed among both extracellular and intracellular spaces, there is no edema. However when the serum sodium level falls rapidly to below 120 mmol/L, somnolence, coma, and seizures can occur. Symptomatic hyponatremia has a mortality of 10 to 15%, and the mortality rate is higher when the serum sodium level is below 110 mmol/L.

By far the most common tumor that causes SIADH is SCLC. SIADH occurs in 5 to 15% of patients with SCLC[87–91] and in less than 1% of patients with non–small cell lung cancer.[92] Other neuroendocrine tumors, including carcinoids and small cell carcinomas of the prostate and cervix, can also cause SIADH. SIADH also occurs occasionally in a wide range of carcinomas, including as many as 2% of squamous carcinomas of the head and neck,[93] adenocarcinoma of the colon,

Hodgkin's disease, non-Hodgkin's lymphomas, and several varieties of brain tumors.[87, 88] The finding of hyponatremia in cancer is nonspecific, and central secretion of vasopressin from various nonosmotic stimuli could be at fault in some of these patients, for example patients with thoracic or intracranial tumors. However vasopressin and associated neurophysins have been found in non-neuroendocrine tumor cells, and some epithelial tumors have the ability to secrete vasopressin.

Laboratory Features

The cardinal features of SIADH are hypotonicity with hyponatremia and an inappropriately concentrated urine. It is often unnecessary to measure serum osmolality directly in a hyponatremic patient, since the effective serum osmolality—serum sodium (mmol/L) × 2 + glucose (mmol/L)—closely approximates direct measurements.[94] Any urinary osmolality greater than 50 to 60 mmol/L water is inappropriate in the setting of serum hypotonicity, which should inhibit the release of vasopressin and permit the excretion of a maximally dilute urine. The urinary osmolality in SIADH is often higher than the serum osmolality, but that is not a necessary feature of the syndrome. If measured directly, vasopressin levels are inappropriately elevated, as are the levels of the associated neurophysins. However, it is rarely necessary to measure vasopressin, which is hampered by the generally poor quality of available assays for the hormone. As discussed later, other causes of hypotonicity can generally be excluded with reasonable certainty by reliance on clinical and biochemical criteria.

SIADH has a number of other laboratory features that are helpful in diagnosis. The urinary sodium concentration is typically high, reflecting the natriuresis induced by expansion of extracellular fluid volume. However, the ability to conserve sodium in SIADH is usually unimpaired,[5] and the urinary sodium excretion can fall to low levels in the setting of reduced dietary sodium intakes. The blood urea nitrogen and serum uric acid levels are low,[95] again reflecting expanded extracellular fluid volumes and decreased tubular resorption of these solutes. Other electrolytes are diluted in proportion to the serum sodium, except for serum bicarbonate, which is normal.

Pathogenesis

Vasopressin is synthesized as a prohormone of 166 amino acids that is processed to produce three peptides: the mature octapeptide hormone, a midregion 10,000-molecular-weight peptide with vasopressin-binding activity called neurophysin II, and a C-terminal glycopeptide[96] (see Chapter 10). Vasopressin and its neurophysin are packaged together in neurosecretory granules, stored in nerve termini in the posterior pituitary, and released in response to hypotonicity or nonosmotic stimuli (baroreceptor stimulation, pain, nausea). Vasopressin is similarly processed in neuroendocrine tumor cells, but these cells frequently secrete not only vasopressin and neurophysin II but also vasopressin's sister peptide oxytocin together with its binding protein, neurophysin I.[97–99]

The molecular basis for inappropriate secretion of vasopressin from tumor cells is poorly understood. Immunoreactive vasopressin is identifiable in a portion of bronchial neuroendocrine cells, the presumed precursors of SCLC. Thus like other hormonal products of neuroendocrine neoplasms, vasopressin may be regarded as secreted eutopically from neuroendocrine tumors. The usual coordinate expression of vasopressin and oxytocin precursors in tumor cells may be related to the physical linkage of the two genes, which are found within 12 kb of each other in the human genome with an inverted arrangement of the coding strands.[100] Either DNA rearrangements or *trans*-acting factors expressed in malignant tumors could simultaneously activate both promoters. Vasopressin receptors (V_{1A} and V_2 receptors) are present on SCLC cells, and vasopressin could have paracrine effects on the growth of SCLC cells to promote their growth, but increased proliferation in response to vasopressin has not been observed.[101]

It is not known whether the secretion of neurohypophyseal peptides from tumor cells is under regulatory control. Four patterns of vasopressin release have been identified in SIADH.[102] Most commonly (37%), vasopressin levels fluctuate widely and independently of the serum osmolality. In a second group (33%), vasopressin is released in response to changes in osmolality, but the osmotic threshold for vasopressin release is decreased (reset osmostat). Other patients with SIADH manifest a constant leak of vasopressin or have no demonstrable abnormality in vasopressin secretion and could conceivably produce a different antidiuretic substance. Patients with cancer and SIADH fall into all four categories. It is conceivable that those with a reset osmostat express both the vasopressin gene and an osmoreceptor in their tumors, but it is more likely that vasopressin is released centrally in these patients because of stimulation of baroreceptors in the pulmonary bed or periphery, invasion of the vagus nerve, or metastasis to regulatory centers, for example the hypothalamus.

Expression and secretion of vasopressin are more common than hyponatremia in SCLC. More than one half of SCLC patients have elevated plasma vasopressin levels,[103] and plasma levels of the neurophysins are increased in 44 to 65% of untreated patients with SCLC.[98, 99, 104, 105] Some tumors also express the gene for oxytocin,[97] but no clinical syndrome of inappropriate oxytocin release has been reported in tumor patients.

In patients with elevated vasopressin levels who do not have hyponatremia, abnormalities in water metabolism can be elicited by water loading, which discloses an impaired diuretic response in 47% of patients with limited SCLC and 86% of patients with extensive disease.[106] Patients with milder degrees of vasopressin excess probably compensate for reduced free water excretion by reducing fluid intake; only if free water intake exceeds the maximal excretion of free water does hyponatremia result. Thus, the development of hyponatremia is a function not only of the level of vasopressin but also of fluid intake. Although some tumors may secrete abnormally processed forms of vasopressin with reduced biologic activity, it is likely that compensatory mechanisms of this type account for the disparity between the frequency of biochemical and clinical abnormalities in SIADH.

When water is retained, extracellular and intracellular volumes are expanded. The expansion of extracellular fluid volume, probably by causing suppression of aldosterone and an increase in atrial natriuretic peptide (ANP),[107] induces the natriuresis that is characteristic of SIADH patients who have an adequate intake of sodium. Plasma levels of ANP are normal or high in SIADH[107–109]; it is not clear whether high ANP levels are a compensatory response to extracellular fluid volume expansion or a consequence of release of ANP from the tumor. Many tumors that express the vasopressin gene also express the gene for ANP.[110–113] However restriction of sodium intake in patients with SIADH causes weight loss, and as the extracellular fluid volume returns to normal, natriuresis is reversed and sodium is conserved appropriately.[5] This suggests that the secretion of ANP is compensatory and that an ANP-induced natriuresis does not contribute significantly to the genesis of hyponatremia.

Acute water retention causes neurologic symptoms by rapidly increasing the intracellular volumes of brain cells and thus inducing cerebral edema. It is probable that chronic hyponatremia is less symptomatic because there is time for activation of compensatory volume-regulatory mechanisms in the central nervous system. Brain cells compensate for volume gain by activating ion transport processes that pump out intracellular KCl and NaCl.[114, 115] This compensation has therapeutic importance, because rapid correction of hyponatremia by infusion of hypertonic saline produces a transient hypertonic encephalopathy as water is drawn out of the already contracted intracellular space. This can cause permanent neurologic damage, for example central pontine myelinolysis and death.

Diagnosis

The diagnosis of SIADH is usually made on clinical grounds. The first step is to establish that the urine is inappropriately concentrated in the face of hypotonicity. In a hyponatremic patient, a urinary osmolality higher than 50 to 60 mmol/L water is inappropriate, and many patients with SIADH have urinary osmolalities higher than the plasma osmolality. Next, other causes of hypotonicity must be excluded. The differential diagnosis of hyponatremia includes states of true volume contraction, edematous states such as congestive heart failure and hepatic failure in which the effective central plasma volume is diminished, adrenal insufficiency, hypothyroidism, drug effects, and SIADH (see Chapter 7). Measurements of vasopressin are of little value in the differential diagnosis, because vasopressin levels are increased in most hyponatremic states. True volume contraction and edematous states can usually be excluded on clinical grounds. It is appropriate to exclude adrenal insufficiency with a corticotropin stimulation test in patients with malignant tumors and SIADH, particularly since patients with bilateral adrenal metastases are at risk for adrenal insufficiency. TSH should be measured to exclude hypothyroidism. Among the drugs that stimulate the nonosmotic release of vasopressin are the cancer chemotherapeutic agents vincristine, vinblastine, and cyclophosphamide. Normovolumic patients without hormonal disorders or drug causes are presumed to have SIADH.

SIADH is the most common cause of hyponatremia in hospitalized patients,[116, 117] but only a small minority of these patients develop the syndrome as the result of inappropriate secretion of vasopressin by a tumor. Furthermore not all patients with cancer who meet the criteria for SIADH have ectopic secretion of vasopressin from a tumor. Not only are benign forms of SIADH more common, but the response of vasopressin to osmotic stimuli in some patients with malignant tumors[102] is consistent with eutopic secretion of the hormone from the pituitary. The uncertainty about etiology in an individual patient may be intellectually unsatisfying but is not of great practical importance. Patients with severe and symptomatic hyponatremia are more likely to have a true ectopic source of vasopressin. The treatment of hyponatremia in SIADH is similar, regardless of the cause of the syndrome.

Treatment

Symptomatic hyponatremia in patients with a serum sodium less than 120 mmol/L requires immediate treatment, as discussed in Chapter 10. The therapeutic options are infusion of hypertonic saline (3 or 5% saline) or administration of saline and furosemide.[118] The latter regimen has the advantage of not rapidly expanding extracellular fluid volume in an already volume-expanded patient. The goal of acute treatment is to raise the serum sodium above 125 mmol/L. Such an increase will take the patient out of immediate danger, and further correction can be accomplished in a more leisurely fashion. A controversy exists as to how rapidly the initial phase of correction should be carried out, with one school arguing for rapid correction in view of the high mortality of the untreated syndrome and the other arguing that too-rapid correction of hyponatremia can predispose to central pontine myelinolysis and other neurologic sequelae.[119] As discussed earlier, the risk of rapid correction probably has to do with brain shrinking when presented with high concentrations of extracellular sodium and intracellular dehydration, which is exacerbated by prior loss of cell solute, the adaptive response of the central nervous system to hyponatremia. The controversy is presented in Chapter 10. Under most circumstances it seems best to correct hyponatremia at a rate of 0.5 mmol/L/h until the serum sodium concentration reaches 120 to 125 mmol/L.

In asymptomatic patients or after acute correction of hyponatremia in symptomatic patients, the mainstay of chronic therapy is water restriction. Moderate fluid restriction may be reasonably well tolerated. The goal is to establish a fluid intake in which the intake of free water does not exceed the maximal free water clearance, which will be determined by the circulating vasopressin level. If necessary, most patients can be managed with severe restrictions to 800 to 1000 mL of fluids daily. At this level of fluid intake the free water intake is actually negative, because the patient is ingesting osmoles from food in excess of water. Therefore even a patient who is obliged to excrete a concentrated urine and thus has a negative free water excretion may be maintained in zero net water balance. However, severe fluid restrictions are onerous and difficult to maintain.

As an adjunct to water restriction, it is often beneficial to interfere with vasopressin action. The drug of choice for this purpose is demeclocycline, an antibiotic that blocks the action of vasopressin and produces nephrogenic diabetes insipidus. At a dose of 150 to 300 mg four times a day, demeclocycline has a reproducible effect on the urinary concentrating mechanism,[120, 121] but may take up to 2 wk to have its full effect. The side effects are photosensitive rashes and liver toxicity. An alternative is administration of fludrocortisone, which in doses of 0.1 to 0.3 mg/d will correct hyponatremia partially but at the risk of developing edema and congestive heart failure. Lithium also produces nephrogenic diabetes insipidus but is less predictable than demeclocycline or fludrocortisone and should be given only in refractory cases.[120] SCLC is now treated with aggressive combination chemotherapy, and SIADH often remits in responders to chemotherapy.[122]

ECTOPIC CORTICOTROPIN SYNDROME AND ECTOPIC SECRETION OF CORTICOTROPIN-RELEASING HORMONE

Clinical Features

The ectopic corticotropin syndrome accounts for 10 to 20% of cases of Cushing's syndrome.[123–125] Unlike Cushing's disease, which has an 8:1 female preponderance, the ectopic corticotropin syndrome is more common in men than women. The typical presentation differs from that of typical Cushing's syndrome. The onset is sudden, and progression is rapid. Patients complain of proximal myopathy and peripheral edema. Hypertension, hypokalemia, and severe glucose intolerance are often present. Hyperpigmentation may occur, but hirsutism is unusual. Other manifestations of cancer, such as anorexia, weight loss, and anemia, are common. The somatic features of typical Cushing's syndrome are notably absent from the typical patient, perhaps because of the rapid evolution of the clinical picture. Patients with slowly growing carcinoid tumors of the bronchus or thymus have a more indolent disease and often present with the classic habitus of Cushing's

syndrome—moon facies, centripetal obesity, proximal myopathy, polydipsia, and polyuria. Hyperpigmentation is common in these patients, as is hirsutism in women.

The tumors that produce the ectopic corticotropin syndrome are primarily of neuroendocrine cell origin. Approximately 45% in published series are SCLC, 15% are thymic carcinoids, 10% are bronchial carcinoids, 10% are islet cell tumors, 5% are other carcinoid tumors, 2% are pheochromocytomas, and 1% are ovarian adenocarcinomas. However, adenocarcinoma and squamous carcinoma are also occasionally associated with the syndrome. It is likely that small cell lung carcinoma is greatly underrepresented in these referral series; it probably accounts for well over one half of unselected cases.

Laboratory Features

Both the level of cortisol secretion and the level of corticotropin tend to be higher in ectopic than in pituitary Cushing's syndrome, although there is some overlap. In most ectopic cases both cortisol and corticotropin are elevated to two to four times the normal morning values, and the normal diurnal variation in their levels is lost. Urinary excretion of adrenal steroid metabolites is increased correspondingly. Two-site immunoradiometric assays, which are coming into common use for detection of corticotropin, give lower values for corticotropin in ectopic cases than older radioimmunoassays,[126] probably because they do not detect partially processed forms that are common in the ectopic syndrome. Despite the abnormal processing of corticotropin by nonpituitary tumors, there is no other POMC peptide in serum whose presence is decisive in the diagnosis of the ectopic syndrome. More than one half of nonpituitary tumors that secrete corticotropin also secrete other peptides, including carcinoembryonic antigen, GRP, calcitonin, somatostatin, or corticotropin-releasing hormone (CRH), and the presence of these peptides is suggestive of the ectopic corticotropin syndrome.

Hypokalemia occurs in 80 to 100% of cases in various series, and potassium wasting is more severe than in pituitary Cushing's disease. The hypokalemia is probably explained by the mineralocorticoid effects of cortisol, which are more evident both because cortisol levels tend to be higher in ectopic than in pituitary Cushing's syndrome and because 11β-hydroxysteroid dehydrogenase activity appears for unknown reasons to be decreased in patients with ectopic corticotropin secretion.[127] A deficiency of 11β-hydroxysteroid dehydrogenase activity impairs the inactivation of cortisol in the renal tubule, leading to increased exposure of mineralocorticoid receptors to cortisol. In disorders such as congenital deficiency of 11β-hydroxysteroid dehydrogenase and licorice intoxication, where the activity of the enzyme is inhibited, normal levels of cortisol produce a state of pseudohyperaldosteronism.[128] Increased deoxycorticosterone may also play a role in the hypokalemia of the ectopic corticotropin syndrome.[129]

Pathogenesis

Although many nonpituitary tissues contain POMC mRNA, most are short transcripts (800 nucleotides) that are initiated by a downstream promoter at the third exon of the POMC gene and do not include coding sequences for the signal peptide that is necessary for direction of POMC into the secretory pathway.[30] Thus, nonpituitary POMC transcripts probably do not generate bioactive POMC products that can be secreted. In contrast, nonpituitary tumors that secrete corticotropin contain a 1150 nucleotide mRNA similar to the predominant pituitary species, and many nonpituitary tumors also contain 1350 nucleotide transcripts initiated from an upstream promoter that is largely quiescent in pituitary cells.[30, 130–132] The differences in promoter usage between the pituitary, normal nonpituitary tissues, and nonpituitary tumors may provide clues to the mechanisms of *POMC* gene expression in tumors. In this regard, it is not known which promoters are used in the bronchial neuroendocrine cells that are thought to give rise to SCLC.

Consistent with the nonsuppressibility of most nonpituitary tumors by glucocorticoids, the sensitivity of *POMC* gene expression to inhibition by glucocorticoids is reduced in SCLC cell lines. Glucocorticoid receptors are absent in some cell lines, and in others glucocorticoid receptor action appears to be defective.[133, 134] Negative glucocorticoid regulatory elements are typically composite elements that require binding of regulatory factors in addition to the glucocorticoid receptor, leading to the possibility that such accessory factors may be abnormal in transformed cell lines. However, glucocorticoids also fail to stimulate transcription from classic glucocorticoid regulatory elements in SCLC cell lines, and this defect is overcome by overexpression of the wild-type glucocorticoid receptor.[134]

POMC processing in nonpituitary tumors is often incomplete, with the release into blood of POMC fragments with reduced biologic activity. These incompletely processed forms are larger than corticotropin by gel filtration and were first described in the serum of cancer patients with the ectopic corticotropin (ACTH) syndrome as "big ACTH."[135] As noted earlier, some incompletely processed POMC peptides can be detected by radioimmunoassay techniques for corticotropin but not by two-site immunoradiometric assays.[126] In one study using a precursor-specific assay, the ratio of corticotropin precursors to corticotropin plasma was 58:1 in the ectopic corticotropin syndrome, compared with a ratio of 5:1 in pituitary Cushing's disease.[133]

Unusual small peptides are also produced from POMC in nonpituitary tumors (Fig. 36–2). In anterior pituitary corticotrope cells four of the six dibasic sites in POMC are cleaved by the prohormone convertase PC1/PC3,[27, 136] and the predominant products are six peptides, an NH2-terminal peptide, a joining peptide, corticotropin, β-lipotropin (β-LPH), and smaller amounts of γ-LPH and β-endorphin. Additional products that are detected routinely in extracts of nonpituitary tumors include the corticotropin-like intermediate lobe polypeptide (CLIP) and β-melanocyte-stimulating hormone (5–22).[137] Both peptides are present in the intermediate lobe in the rodent pituitary, and their presence in nonpituitary tumors indicates that nonpituitary tumors contain the PC2 convertase,[138, 139] which is normally present in intermediate but not anterior pituitary cells.[138] These peptides are not secreted in large amounts and are not useful as tumor markers in blood, but the serum LPH/corticotropin ratio in the ectopic corticotropin syndrome is higher than in pituitary tu-

mors,[140] possibly reflecting the increased PC2 activity in nonpituitary tumors.

Corticotropin-like activity can be identified in extracts of many non–small cell lung carcinomas and in virtually all SCLC,[141, 142] and at least one third of all SCLC have POMC mRNA demonstrable by in situ hybridization.[142] Yet only 1 to 3% of SCLC patients have clinical evidence of corticotropin excess. Thus the ectopic corticotropin syndrome is a good example of the principle that ectopic production of hormones is more common than clinical syndromes of hormone excess. Patients with corticotropin-producing neoplasms are protected from the consequences of hormone excess by several mechanisms. Malignant tumors contain much smaller quantities of POMC mRNA and peptides than the pituitary and are thus inefficient in producing corticotropin. Tumor cells are much poorer in neurosecretory granules than pituitary corticotropes and are relatively deficient in the ability to process POMC efficiently and secrete the peptide products. Inefficient cleavage of POMC leads to incompletely processed forms of corticotropin with little biologic activity. Processing of POMC by tumors can also lead to production of biologically inactive products. For example some tumors produce significant amounts of corticotropin but cleave it to the CLIP.[137]

Laboratory Diagnosis

The diagnosis of the ectopic corticotropin syndrome is described in Chapters 9 and 12. The first step in the diagnosis consists of determining whether cortisol excess is present and whether it is corticotropin-dependent. Increased basal cortisol secretion can often be shown by measurement of serum cortisol or urinary free cortisol, both of which are increased in the ectopic corticotropin syndrome. When the basal levels are not markedly increased, the presence of cortisol excess can be established with a low-dose dexamethasone suppression test, e.g. the 1-mg overnight dexamethasone suppression test. The corticotropin-dependence of cortisol excess can be established by measurement of corticotropin in the same sample in which cortisol is measured. Corticotropin-dependent Cushing's syndrome results from either pituitary or ectopic secretion of corticotropin. In the classic form of the syndrome, e.g. corticotropin-secreting SCLC, secretion is nonsuppressible, and there is little or no response of serum or urinary cortisol to the administration of high-dose dexamethasone, whereas the secretion of corticotropin by pituitary adenomas is dexamethasone-responsive. Thus the next step in the diagnosis is to determine whether hypersecretion of corticotropin is glucocorticoid-suppressible. In a patient with a recognized malignancy and clinical features suggestive of the ectopic syndrome, the finding of nonsuppressible hypercortisolism usually suffices to make the diagnosis.

In occasional lung cancers and about one half of bronchial or thymic carcinoid tumors, the secretion of corticotropin can be suppressed with high-dose dexamethasone. This circumstance has been called the "occult ectopic corticotropin syndrome"[143] and presents a major diagnostic challenge because the clinical presentation and secretory dynamics may be identical to pituitary Cushing's syndrome and because these small tumors may not be evident on routine radiologic studies. Because nonpituitary tumors are not as well suppressed by glucocorticoids as corticotrope adenomas of the pituitary, it is useful in this circumstance to apply stringent criteria for glucocorticoid suppressibility; namely suppression of urinary free cortisol by more than 80% after administration of high-dose dexamethasone has a sensitivity of 81% and a specificity of 92% for pituitary Cushing's syndrome.[25] It is often necessary to use stimulation tests to differentiate pituitary adenomas from the occult ectopic corticotropin syndrome. The ovine CRH test is valuable because nonpituitary tumors do not re-

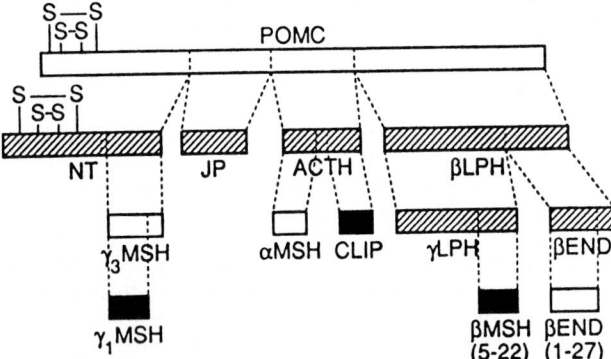

Figure 36–2. Processing of POMC in normal pituitary (*hatched bars*), intermediate lobe (*open bars*), and nonpituitary neoplasms (*solid bars*). (Adapted from Schteingart DE. Ectopic secretion of peptides of the proopiomelanocortin family. Endocrinol Metab Clinic North Am 1991; 20:453–471, with permission.)

spond well to CRH. An increase in plasma corticotropin of 35% following administration of ovine CRH (1 μg/kg body weight) was reported to have a sensitivity of 93% and a specificity of 100% for the diagnosis of pituitary Cushing's syndrome.[144] Metyrapone testing in combination with high-dose dexamethasone may also improve diagnostic accuracy.[145] The definitive study for distinguishing pituitary from nonpituitary forms of hypercortisolism is inferior petrosal sinus sampling with administration of ovine CRH.[146] The ratio of corticotropin in the inferior petrosal sinus that in peripheral blood after administration of CRH is greater than 3 in patients with pituitary tumors and less than 2 in patients with corticotropin-secreting nonpituitary tumors. Localization of bronchial and thymic carcinoids may also be difficult. Thin-section computed tomography of the chest and scanning with labeled octreotide have sometimes been of use.

Treatment

The management of Cushing's syndrome is discussed in Chapters 9 and 12. When possible, the treatment of the ectopic corticotropin syndrome is surgical. With slow-growing carcinoid tumors of the bronchus, thymomas, or pheochromocytomas, surgical resection can be curative. If the tumor cannot be identified, it is necessary to block cortisol secretion with adrenolytic agents, and some patients ultimately require surgical adrenalectomy to control hypercortisolism. Malignant nonpituitary neoplasms that secrete corticotropin are rarely amenable to resection, because the tumor is usually advanced and inoperable by the time the clinical syndrome appears. With malignant neoplasms the aim is to palliate hypercortisolism by "medical adrenalectomy" using adrenolytic drugs, such as aminoglutethimide (250 mg three times a day) or metyrapone (250 to 500 mg three times a day).[147] Ketoconazole (200 to 400 mg twice a day) has also been useful for the treatment of ectopic corticotropin syndrome.[148, 149] A replacement dose of hydrocortisone should be administered with these drugs to avoid adrenal insufficiency. Some patients respond to the long-acting somatostatin agonist octreotide,[150] and the glucocorticoid antagonist mifepristone has also been used.[151]

Ectopic Secretion of CRH

Nonendocrine tumors rarely cause Cushing's syndrome by secretion of CRH. Nine cases have been well documented.[123, 124, 152, 153] These patients had increased CRH levels in tumor tissue or in plasma and high plasma corticotropin levels. Documenting that the site of corticotropin secretion is the pituitary gland is important because many nonendocrine tumors that secrete CRH also secrete corticotropin itself. Presumptive evidence of a pituitary source of corticotropin may come from demonstration that the gradient of corticotropin between the inferior petrosal sinus and peripheral blood is more than 3:1, from finding pituitary corticotrope hyperplasia in patients who underwent pituitary surgery for a presumed corticotrope adenoma, or from the failure to detect corticotropin in the nonendocrine tumor. In cases in which the nonendocrine tumor secretes both CRH and corticotropin, the true role of CRH in the clinical syndrome may be indeterminate.[123, 124]

Cushing's syndrome resulting from ectopic secretion of CRH does not cause a distinctive presentation. In most cases the hypercortisolism is unresponsive to dexamethasone suppression, but a normal response to high-dose dexamethasone has also been reported. The response to metyrapone is also variable. Tumors that secrete CRH include small cell carcinomas of the prostate and lung, medullary thyroid carcinoma, carcinoids, and a hypothalamic gangliocytoma. These neuro-endocrine tumors are similar to the tumors that cause Cushing's syndrome by direct secretion of corticotropin.

The diagnosis of ectopic CRH secretion as the cause of Cushing's syndrome is usually made retrospectively. In view of the rarity of the disorder, it is probably inappropriate to routinely measure CRH in Cushing's syndrome. However, it may be worthwhile to determine the plasma CRH level when pituitary surgery has disclosed diffuse corticotrope hyperplasia in a patient with Cushing's syndrome.

HYPOGLYCEMIA WITH NON–ISLET CELL TUMORS

Clinical Features

Fasting hypoglycemia produced by non–islet cell tumors typically causes neuroglycopenic symptoms of obtundation, confusion, or behavioral aberrations, which may have been present for some time before the diagnosis is made.[8, 154, 155] The offending neoplasms are usually bulky, slow-growing mesenchymal tumors. Fibrosarcomas, rhabdomyosarcomas, leiomyosarcomas, mesotheliomas, and hemangiopericytomas account for more than half the cases. Hepatocellular carcinomas (hepatomas), carcinoid tumors, and adrenocortical carcinomas account for about 25% of cases, and the remainder are made up of a variety of carcinomas, leukemias, and lymphomas. More than one third of the tumors are retroperitoneal, about one third are intra-abdominal, and the remainder are intrathoracic.

Pathogenesis

Fasting hypoglycemia in this syndrome results from increased peripheral utilization of glucose, primarily in skeletal muscle, coupled with decreased hepatic glucose output.[156–158] Lipolysis is inhibited, and free fatty acid levels are low. Although it was suspected that bulky tumors themselves, sometime weighing many kilograms, might metabolize enough glucose to exceed the capacity for hepatic glucose production, this phenomenon has not been documented. Despite insulin-like effects on glucose utilization, hepatic glucose production and lipolysis, fasting insulin levels during hypoglycemia are appropriately suppressed. For this reason it has long seemed likely that an insulin-like factor is responsible for hypoglycemia.

Sera from patients with non–islet cell tumors contain elevated levels of an insulin-like activity by radioreceptor assay.[159] IGF-II levels are sometimes elevated during hypoglycemia but may be normal,[160, 161] and the levels of IGF-I are typically suppressed. Although the finding of elevated serum levels suggests a role for IGF-II in some, but not all patients, it appears that IGF-II is in fact the causative agent of hypoglycemia. As a consequence of altered processing and increased bioavailability, IGF-II can probably cause hypoglycemia, even at normal total serum levels. The level of IGF-II mRNA in non–islet cell tumors is often increased, even in patients with normal serum IGF-II levels.[162, 163] A substantial fraction of IGF-II in both tumors and sera is present in a high-molecular-weight form, "big IGF-II,"[160, 163] a partially processed form that contains immunoreactive determinants in an 89-amino-acid carboxyl-terminal extension called the E-domain[161] and has an altered glycosylation pattern.[164] Most sera from patients with tumors and hypoglycemia contain increased levels of big IGF-II.[161]

Altered binding of IGF-II in the tumor-hypoglycemia syndrome increases its bioavailability to peripheral receptors. In normal serum IGFs are bound largely in one of two complexes. Most is normally bound to a heterotrimeric 150-kd complex, consisting of the IGF, the binding protein IGFBP-3, and an acid-labile glycoprotein. The large complex is retained in the circulation; as a result, the half-life of the IGF-II complex is relatively long, 12 to 15 h. A minority of IGF circulates in a small complex that contains mainly IGF and a different binding protein, IGFBP-2. The small complex can cross capillaries and deliver IGF to tissue receptors, and IGF-II bound to this complex has a half-life of only about 30 min.[165] In sera from patients with non–islet cell tumors and hypoglycemia, the fraction of IGF-II bound to the small, bioavailable complex is increased, on average by three-fold,[166–168] presumably increasing the access of IGF-II to the receptor, even in the setting of normal total IGF-II levels.

Current concepts of the alteration in IGF-II binding are summarized in Figure 36–3.[8, 155] Oversecretion of big IGF-II suppresses the secretion of insulin, growth hormone (GH),

and IGF-I.[169] In turn, suppression of GH and IGF-I downregulates the synthesis of IGFBP-3 and the acid-labile subunit, both of which are GH-dependent,[170] and up-regulates the synthesis of IGFBP-2. Thus IGF-II oversecretion leads to altered binding and increased bioactivity of IGF-II and can cause hypoglycemia even when total IGF-II levels are normal. The level of free IGF-II in serum is also increased.[171]

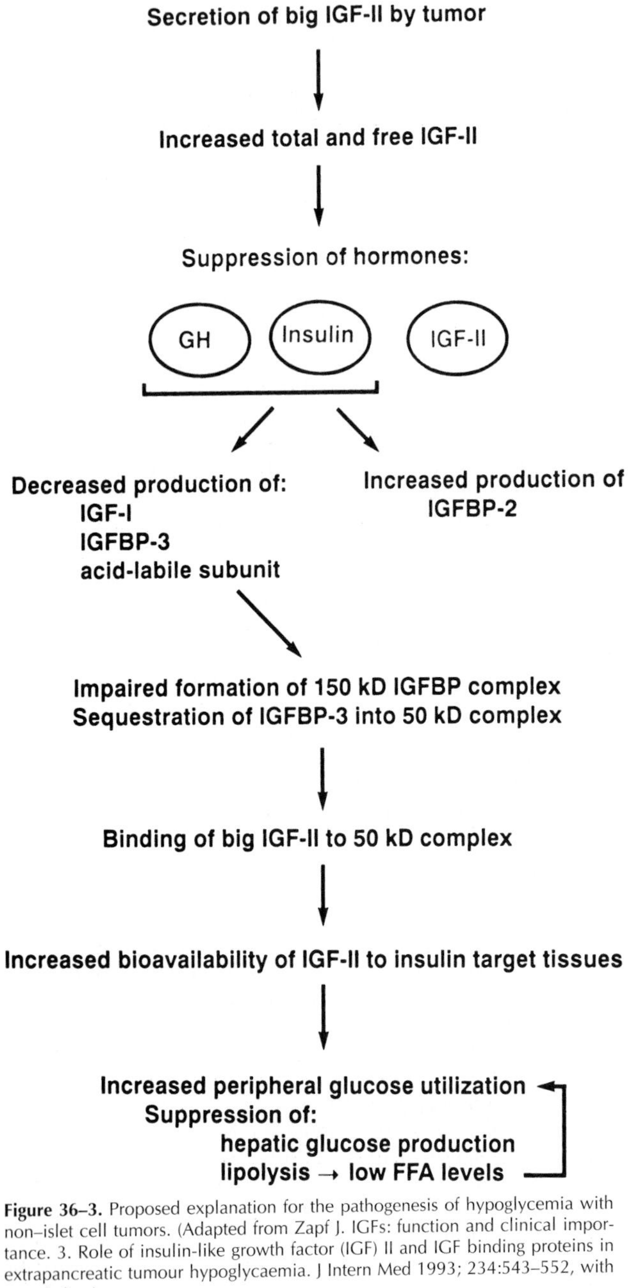

Treatment

The mainstay of treatment is resection of the tumor. Even partial debulking may ameliorate hypoglycemia. In patients with unresectable tumors, several maneuvers based on the pathogenetic scheme have been attempted. Therapy with GH, glucagon, glucocorticoids, or somatostatin has been effective in individual patients with unresectable tumors.[158, 169, 172, 173] These measures are temporary, however, until the unresectable tumor can be treated with chemotherapy.

Secretion of big IGF-II by tumor

↓

Increased total and free IGF-II

↓

Suppression of hormones:

GH   Insulin   IGF-II

Decreased production of:
IGF-I
IGFBP-3
acid-labile subunit

Increased production of IGFBP-2

↓

Impaired formation of 150 kD IGFBP complex
Sequestration of IGFBP-3 into 50 kD complex

↓

Binding of big IGF-II to 50 kD complex

↓

Increased bioavailability of IGF-II to insulin target tissues

↓

Increased peripheral glucose utilization
Suppression of:
hepatic glucose production
lipolysis → low FFA levels

Figure 36–3. Proposed explanation for the pathogenesis of hypoglycemia with non–islet cell tumors. (Adapted from Zapf J. IGFs: function and clinical importance. 3. Role of insulin-like growth factor (IGF) II and IGF binding proteins in extrapancreatic tumour hypoglycaemia. J Intern Med 1993; 234:543–552, with permission.)

GROWTH HORMONE–RELEASING HORMONE, GROWTH HORMONE, AND HUMAN PLACENTAL LACTOGEN

Since 1980 more than 40 cases of acromegaly have been associated with nonpituitary tumors.[174, 175] There is only one well-documented case of acromegaly resulting from secretion of GH by a nonpituitary tumor[176]; the other tumors caused acromegaly by secreting growth hormone–releasing hormone (GHRH), which was first isolated from extracts of pancreatic tumors.[177, 178] Overall, secretion of GHRH accounts for fewer than 1% of cases of acromegaly.[179] The clinical findings, aside from the presence of a nonpituitary tumor, do not differ from those in acromegaly caused by somatotrope adenomas. The mean duration of acromegalic features before diagnosis is 7.9 y, about the same as pituitary acromegaly.[174, 179] Diabetes mellitus, amenorrhea, and galactorrhea are common. In about one half of cases, the extrapituitary neoplasm is symptomatic. Other syndromes of hormone excess, including Cushing's syndrome, primary hyperparathyroidism, and the Zollinger-Ellison syndrome, may occur in conjunction with acromegaly.

Carcinoids are the most common extrapituitary tumors that produce acromegaly (69% of cases), followed by islet cell tumors (23%), pheochromocytoma, and paraganglioma.[174] GHRH immunoreactivity can frequently be demonstrated in neuroendocrine tumors from patients without acromegaly, usually in smaller amounts than in tumors associated with acromegaly. However, high plasma levels of GHRH have been reported in SCLC patients without acromegaly.[180] Some of these type of patients have abnormal GH secretory dynamics, such as a paradoxical GH increase following administration of thyrotropin-releasing hormone (TRH), suggesting that subclinical or incomplete forms of acromegaly may be present. All three isoforms of GHRH have been identified in nonpituitary tumors, but the predominant species in most tumors is GHRH (1–40), whereas the dominant hypothalamic form is GHRH (1–44).

Serum levels of GHRH in acromegaly due to extrapituitary tumors are markedly elevated, from 0.3 to 5 µg/L (0.3 to 50 ng/ml).[179] Normal fasting GHRH levels are less than 60 ng/L (0.06 ng/mL), and the peripheral level is less than 200 ng/L (0.2 ng/mL) in typical acromegaly. The dynamics of GH secretion in acromegaly induced by nonpituitary secretion of GHRH are not distinctive. GH and IGF-I levels are high, and the normal circadian rhythm of GH secretion is lost. Prolactin levels are elevated in 80% of patients. Virtually all patients display a paradoxical increase of GH after administration of

TRH, compared with approximately 40% of patients with classic acromegaly. Many patients with GHRH-induced acromegaly fail to respond to exogenous GHRH, but this is not a uniform finding and cannot be used diagnostically. In most cases, the nonpituitary tumor can be identified by imaging studies of the chest and abdomen. About 90% of carcinoid tumors that cause acromegaly are located in the chest (see Chapter 9).

The primary therapy is surgical. About one half of patients have resectable tumors. In patients with nonresectable disease, the therapy of choice is octreotide, the somatostatin agonist. In about one half of patients the level of GH returns to normal with octreotide treatment, and most of the remainder have a partial response.[174, 181] The level of GHRH is often reduced less than that of GH, suggesting that the drug affects primarily the pituitary response to GHRH.

The case of extrapituitary acromegaly caused by nonpituitary secretion of GH itself involved a pancreatic islet cell tumor that contained both GH and GH mRNA. At surgery an arteriovenous GH gradient was demonstrated across the tumor, and tumor cells in culture secreted immunoreactive GH.[176, 182] GHRH was not detectable in plasma.

The propensity of other members of the GH family for secretion by nonendocrine tumors is variable. Prolactin has not been conclusively shown to be secreted by nonpituitary tumors. However, neoplastic production of human placental lactogen (hPL), also called chorionic somatomammotropin, appears to be relatively common.[183, 184] In large series, hPL was detectable in plasma in 9% of patients with malignant disease, most commonly lung carcinoma, but including patients with carcinoma of the thyroid, breast, stomach, pheochromocytoma, carcinoids, and leukemia[183] and in 14% of patients with breast carcinoma.[185] hPL has weak GH activity but substantial lactotrophic activity. However, patients with elevated levels in blood do not have galactorrhea because the circulating levels of hPL in such patients are lower than the levels of prolactin that produce galactorrhea. It is also possible that neoplasms secrete hPL in biologically inactive forms.

HUMAN CHORIONIC GONADOTROPIN (hCG)

hCG is produced eutopically by trophoblastic and germ cell tumors, including testicular embryonal carcinoma and extragonadal germinomas. In these tumors hCG is a useful tumor marker. Gynecomastia has been reported in a few adult patients with nontrophoblastic malignancies[14] (see Chapter 17), and isosexual precocious puberty has occurred in children[13, 186] (see Chapter 31). The associated tumors include lung carcinoma, hepatocellular carcinoma, adrenocortical carcinoma, and renal carcinoma.

Although hCG is secreted by approximately 18% of nontrophoblastic tumors (Table 36–5), it is not useful as a tumor marker for screening for nontrophoblastic neoplasms. A significant number of normal individuals, including 2.4% of blood donors and 3.6% of patients with various benign diseases, also have detectable levels of hCG (assayed as β-hCG) in serum,[12] decreasing the positive predictive value of a detectable hCG level. Some tumors secrete free subunits of the glycoprotein hormones. For example, about one half of malignant islet cell tumors secrete the α subunit of glycoprotein hormones, while benign islet cell tumors rarely do so.[187] Immunohistochemical staining for the α subunit has also been used to distinguish benign from malignant islet cell tumors histologically.[188] A degradation product of hCG in urine, the β-core fragment, has been reported in about one half of patients with lung cancer, but the fragment is also detected at

TABLE 36–5. Serum hCG Levels in Patients with Cancer

Tumor or Site	Percent Positive
Islet cell	39.4
Gynecologic	28.9
Carcinoid	26.8
Gastrointestinal	18.0
Lung	17.4
Breast	16.8
Melanoma	23.9
Genitourinary	11.8
Sarcoma	11.8
Hematopoietic	6.1

Adapted from Braunstein GD. Placental proteins as tumor markers. In: Herberman R, Mercer DW, eds. Immunodiagnosis of Cancer. 2nd ed. New York: Marcel Dekker, 1991; 673–701, with permission.

low levels in 6 to 14% of individuals with benign disorders[189–191]; its clinical value remains to be established.

ONCOGENOUS OSTEOMALACIA

More than 50 cases of hypophosphatemic osteomalacia or rickets have been reported in patients with tumors of mesenchymal origin, usually small, benign skeletal tumors of the extremities or head.[192, 193] Histologically the causative tumors include hemangiopericytoma, ossifying and nonossifying fibroma, and giant cell tumors. Hypophosphatemic osteomalacia has also been reported in disseminated prostatic carcinoma,[194] where the disorder may be due to phosphate uptake by osteoblastic metastases.[195] Most patients with oncogenous osteomalacia are middle-aged and present with bone pain and proximal myopathy, which may have been present for years before diagnosis. However the disorder has been described in children. The serum phosphorus level is markedly reduced, because of renal phosphate wasting. The serum alkaline phosphatase is increased, but the serum calcium and PTH levels are normal. The level of 1,25 (OH)$_2$D is typically low and the level of 25-hydroxyvitamin D is normal. Osteomalacia is present in bone biopsies. The fact that the syndrome is reversed by resection of the tumor indicates that it has a humoral basis.

Although rare, oncogenous osteomalacia is probably the most common cause of acquired hypophosphatemic osteomalacia. The manifestations are similar to those of hereditary phosphate-wasting disorders such as X-linked hypophosphatemic rickets, and the primary event is probably the induction of severe phosphaturia by a humoral factor secreted by the tumor.[196] A factor that blocks sodium-dependent phosphate transport has been characterized in culture medium of hemangioma cells from a patient with oncogenous osteomalacia.[197] A similar humoral substance might be involved in the pathogenesis of hereditary phosphate-wasting syndromes. The mutation in X-linked hypophosphatemia has been localized to a gene that codes for a protease,[198] and it is possible that this protease may act by liberating a circulating mediator of hypophosphatemia.

OTHER HORMONES

Erythropoietin and Erythrocytosis

Erythrocytosis occurs in 1 to 4% of renal carcinomas, 5 to 10% of hepatocellular carcinomas, and 10 to 20% of cerebellar hemangioblastomas and has been observed in patients with uterine fibromyomas, adrenocortical carcinomas, or ovarian tumors.[199] Renal and hepatocellular carcinomas account for 71% of cases; thus erythrocytosis is most common in tumors arising from the tissues that normally secrete erythropoietin (erythropoietin is secreted by the fetal liver and by the adult kidney). Early studies reported that erythropoietic bioactivity was frequently present in tumor extracts from polycythemic patients, erythropoietin mRNA has been demonstrated in extracts of renal carcinomas,[200] hepatocellular carcinoma,[201] and cerebellar hemangioblastoma,[202] and erythrocytosis has been produced in nude mice by transplantation of erythropoietin-positive renal carcinoma cells.[203] Some patients with tumors and erythrocytosis have increased serum erythropoietin levels.[200] However in the best studied group, patients with hepatocellular carcinoma, it has been difficult to demonstrate a consistent relationship between the red blood cell mass and serum levels of erythropoietin.[204, 205] Increased serum levels of erythropoietin are common in patients with hepatocellular carcinoma; however few of the patients with high erythropoietin levels have erythrocytosis, and some patients with erythrocytosis have normal levels of erythropoietin. Absence of erythrocytosis in the presence of high erythropoietin levels could reflect secretion of biologically inactive, e.g. precursor, forms of erythropoietin.

Calcitonin

Calcitonin is present in neuroendocrine cells of the normal bronchial epithelium[9, 10] and is frequently secreted by neuroendocrine tumors, including 18 to 60% of SCLC.[206–209] Calcitonin is also secreted by other lung carcinomas, breast cancers, leukemias, and a broad spectrum of other neoplasms.[210] Estimates of the frequency of calcitonin secretion are lower in studies that rigorously control for assay artifacts,[208] but it is clear that some tumors express the gene for calcitonin/calcitonin gene-related peptide (CGRP) and secrete calcitonin in vitro.[211, 212] Tumors frequently secrete large forms of calcitonin[208] and are less sensitive to stimulation than are patients with hypercalcitoninemia from medullary thyroid carcinoma.[209] CGRP, which is derived from alternative splicing of the calcitonin gene, is expressed in normal bronchial epithelium[10] and has been detected in tumor extracts and serum.[213] The levels of calcitonin in the sera of patients with lung carcinoma are lower than those in medullary thyroid carcinoma, and no clinical syndrome is associated with the secretion of calcitonin or CGRP.

Endothelin

The potent vasoconstrictor peptide endothelin-1 is produced by several cancer cell lines in vitro and may have paracrine effects on tumor cell growth.[214] Increased serum levels of endothelin-1 and a partially processed form of the peptide big endothelin-1 have been found in hepatocellular carcinoma.[215, 216] Some tumors stain for endothelin-1, and arteriovenous differences, albeit small, have been found across the liver of hepatocellular carcinoma patients.[215] No clinical manifestations of endothelin excess have been reported in these patients.

Vasoactive Intestinal Peptide

Inappropriate secretion of vasoactive intestinal peptide (VIP) produces pancreatic cholera, also known as the WDHA syndrome (watery diarrhea, hypokalemia, and achlorhydria) or Verner-Morrison syndrome (see Chapter 34). In addition to pancreatic islet cell tumors, the syndrome can be produced by other neuroendocrine tumors, including ganglioneuroma, ganglioneuroblastoma, neuroblastoma, pheochromocytoma, and medullary thyroid carcinoma.[217] These tumors stain for

VIP, and removal of the tumor causes return of peripheral VIP levels to normal and reverses the clinical syndrome. Increased VIP levels have also been reported in lung carcinoma[218] and in a neuroendocrine tumor of the kidney.[219] VIP is present in the central and peripheral nervous systems; thus its production by neuroendocrine tumors may be regarded as eutopic, rather than ectopic.

Other Gut Hormones

Somatostatin is frequently detectable in extracts of lung tumor[220, 221] and is secreted by cultured SCLC cells,[221] but elevated serum somatostatin concentrations are uncommon in lung cancer (see Chapter 34).[222, 223] Only one case of the somatostatinoma syndrome has been attributed to SCLC.[224] The glucagonoma syndrome occurred in a patient with a renal neuroendocrine tumor[225] and a patient with a large cell lung carcinoma.[226]

GRP is frequently found in lung carcinomas[220] and cultured SCLC cells,[227, 228] but elevated serum levels are uncommon.[228, 229] The peptide is a mitogen for SCLC cells,[18, 230] and neuralizing studies with antibodies and antagonists[19] suggest that it has an autocrine role as a growth factor. A variant form of the GRP receptor is expressed in human lung carcinoma cell lines.[231] GRP is expressed in neuroendocrine cells of bronchial mucosa,[9, 10] particularly at branch points,[232] and appears to have a developmental role in the regulation of branching morphogenesis of airways.[22, 23] Pancreatic polypeptide is occasionally detectable in the sera of patients with carcinoid tumors.[222, 233]

REFERENCES

1. Brown WH. A case of pluriglandular syndrome: "diabetes of bearded woman." Lancet 1928; 2:1022.
2. Case Records of the Massachusetts General Hospital. Case 27461. N Engl J Med 1941; 225:789–791.
3. Plimpton CH, Gellhorn A. Hypercalcemia in malignant disease without evidence of bone destruction. Am J Med 1956; 21:750–759.
4. Connor TB, Thomas WL, Jr. Etiology of hypercalcemia associated with lung carcinoma. J Clin Invest 1956; 35:697–701.
5. Schwartz WB, Bennett W, Curelop S, et al. A syndrome of renal sodium loss and hyponatremia probably resulting from inappropriate secretion of antidiuretic hormone. Am J Med 1957; 23:529–542.
6. Meador CK, Liddle GW, Island DP, et al. Cause of Cushing's syndrome in patients with tumors arising from nonendocrine tissue. J Clin Endocrinol Metab 1962; 22:693–700.
7. Liddle GW, Nicholson WE, Island DP, et al. Clinical and laboratory studies of ectopic humoral syndromes. Recent Prog Horm Res 1969; 25:283–314.
8. Zapf J. Role of insulin-like growth factor (IGF) II and IGF-binding proteins in extrapancreatic tumour hypoglycaemia. J Intern Med 1993; 234:543–552.
9. Cutz E, Chan W, Track N. Bombesin, calcitonin and leu-enkephalin immunoreactivity in endocrine cells of human lung. Experientia 1981; 37:765–767.
10. Gould V, Chan W, Lee I, et al. Immunohistochemical evaluation of neuroendocrine cells and neoplasms of the lung. Pathol Res Pract 1988; 183:200–213.
11. Broadus A, Stewart A. Parathyroid hormone–related protein: structure, processing, and physiological actions. In: Bilezikian J, Levine M, Marcus R, eds. The Parathyroids. New York: Raven Press, 1994: 259–339.
12. Braunstein GD. Placental proteins as tumor markers. In: Herberman R, Mercer DW, eds. Immunodiagnosis of Cancer. 2nd ed. New York: Marcel Dekker, 1991: 673–701.
13. Braunstein GD, Bridson WE, Glass A, et al. In vivo and in vitro production of human chorionic gonadotropin and alpha-fetoprotein by a virilizing hepatoblastoma. J Clin Endocrinol Metab 1972; 35:857–862.
14. Braunstein GD, Vaitukaitis JL, Carbone PP, et al. Ectopic production of human chorionic gonadotrophin by neoplasms. Ann Intern Med 1973; 78:39–45.
15. Baylin SB, Mendelsohn G. Ectopic (inappropriate) hormone production by tumors: mechanisms involved and the biological and clinical implications. Endocr Rev 1980; 1:45–77.
16. Ikeda K, Ohno H, Hane M, et al. Development of a sensitive two-site immunoradiometric assay for parathyroid hormone–related peptide: evidence for elevated levels in plasma from patients with adult T-cell leukemia/lymphoma and B-cell lymphoma. J Clin Endocrinol Metab 1994; 79:1322–1327.

17. Dittmer J, Gitlin SD, Reid RL, et al. Transactivation of the P2 promoter of parathyroid hormone–related protein by human T-cell lymphotropic virus type I Tax1: evidence for the involvement of transcription factor Ets1. J Virol 1993; 67:6087–6095.

18. Cuttitta F, Desmond NC, Mulshine J, et al. Bombesin-like peptides can function as autocrine growth factors in human small-cell lung cancer. Nature 1985; 316:823–826.

19. Moody TW, Venugopal R, Zia F, et al. BW2258U89: a GRP receptor antagonist which inhibits small cell lung cancer growth. Life Sci 1995; 56:521–529.

20. Melzig MF, Nulander I, Vlaskovska M, et al. β-Endorphin stimulates proliferation of small cell lung carcinoma cells in vitro via nonopioid binding sites. Exp Cell Res 1995; 219:471–476.

21. Philbrick WM, Wysolmerski JJ, Galbraith S, et al. Defining the roles of parathyroid hormone–related protein in normal physiology. Physiol Rev 1996; 76:127–173.

22. King KA, Torday JS, Sunday ME. Bombesin and [Leu⁸] phyllolitorin promote fetal mouse lung branching morphogenesis via a receptor-mediated mechanism. Proc Natl Acad Sci USA 1995; 92:4357–4361.

23. Li K, Nagalla SR, Spindel ER. A rhesus monkey model to characterize the role of gastrin-releasing peptide (GRP) in lung development. J Clin Invest 1994; 1605–1615.

24. Kelly RB. Storage and release of neurotransmitters. Cell 1993; 72(Suppl):43–53.

25. O'Connor DT, Wu H, Gill BM, et al. Hormone storage vesicle proteins: transcriptional basis of the widespread neuroendocrine expression of chromogranin A, and evidence of its diverse biological actions, intracellular and extracellular. Ann NY Acad Sci 1994; 733:36–45.

26. Natori S, Huttner WB. Chromogranin B (secretogranin I) promotes sorting to the regulated secretory pathway of processing intermediates derived from a peptide hormone precursor. Proc Natl Acad Sci USA 1993; 9:4431–4436.

27. Rouille Y, Duguay SJ, Lund K, et al. Proteolytic processing mechanisms in the biosynthesis of neuroendocrine peptides: the subtilisin-like proprotein convertases. Front Neuroendocrinol 1995; 16:322–361.

28. Scheuermann DW, Adriaensen D, Timmermans JP, et al. Comparative histological overview of the chemical coding of the pulmonary neuroepithelial endocrine system in health and disease. Eur J Morphol 1992; 30:101–112.

29. Le Douarin NM. On the origin of pancreatic endocrine cells. Cell 1988; 53:169–171.

30. de Keyzer Y, Lenne F, Massias JF, et al. Pituitary-like proopiomelanocortin transcripts in human Leydig cell tumors. J Clin Invest 1990; 86:871–877.

31. Mundy GR, Cove DH, Fisken R. Primary hyperparathyroidism: changes in the pattern of clinical presentation. Lancet 1980; 1:1317–1320.

32. Fisken RA, Heath DA, Bold AM. Hypercalcaemia: a hospital survey. Q J Med 1980; 49:405–418.

33. Ralston SH, Gallacher SJ, Patel U, et al. Cancer-associated hypercalcemia: morbidity and mortality. Ann Intern Med 1990; 112:499–504.

34. Bender RA, Hansen H. Hypercalcemia in bronchogenic carcinoma. Ann Intern Med 1974; 80:205–208.

35. Fukumoto S, Matsumoto T, Ikeda K, et al. Clinical evaluation of calcium metabolism in adult T-cell leukemia/lymphoma. Arch Intern Med 1988; 148:921–925.

36. Watanabe T, Yamaguchi K, Takatsuki K, et al. Constitutive expression of parathyroid hormone–related protein gene in human T cell leukemia virus type 1 (HTLV-I) carriers and adult T cell leukemia patients that can be trans-activated by HTLV-1 tax gene. J Exp Med 1990; 172:759–765.

37. Kimura S, Nishimura Y, Yamaguchi K, et al. A case of pheochromocytoma producing parathyroid hormone–related protein and presenting with hypercalcemia. J Clin Endocrinol Metab 1990; 70:1559–1563.

38. Mune T, Katakami H, Kato Y, et al. Production and secretion of parathyroid hormone–related protein in pheochromocytoma: participation of an alpha-adrenergic mechanism. J Clin Endocrinol Metab 1993; 76:757–762.

39. Budayr AA, Nissenson RA, Klein RF, et al. Increased serum levels of a parathyroid hormone–like protein in malignancy-associated hypercalcemia. Ann Intern Med 1989; 111:807–812.

40. Burtis WJ, Brady TG, Orloff JJ, et al. Immunochemical characterization of circulating parathyroid hormone–related protein in patients with humoral hypercalcemia of cancer. N Engl J Med 1990; 322:1106–1112.

41. Grill V, Ho P, Body JJ, et al. Parathyroid hormone–related protein: elevated levels in both humoral hypercalcemia of malignancy and hypercalcemia complicating metastatic breast cancer. J Clin Endocrinol Metab 1991; 73:1309–1315.

42. Ratcliffe WA, Norbury S, Stott RA, et al. Immunoreactivity of plasma parathyrin-related peptide: three region-specific radioimmunoassays and a two-site immunoradiometric assay compared. Clin Chem 1991; 37:1781–1787.

43. Blind E, Raue F, Gotzmann J, et al. Circulating levels of midregional parathyroid hormone–related protein in hypercalcaemia of malignancy. Clin Endocrinol (Oxf) 1992; 37:290–297.

44. Nussbaum SR, Zahradnik RJ, Lavigne JR, et al. Highly sensitive two-site immunoradiometric assay of parathyrin and its clinical utility in evaluating patients with hypercalcemia. Clin Chem 1987; 33:1364–1367.

45. Stewart AF, Horst R, Deftos LJ, et al. Biochemical evaluation of patients with cancer-associated hypercalcemia. N Engl J Med 1980; 303:1377–1383.

46. Budayr AA, Zysset E, Jenzer A, et al. Effects of treatment of malignancy-associated hypercalcemia on serum parathyroid hormone–related protein. J Bone Miner Res 1994; 9:521–526.

47. Strewler GJ, Nissenson RA. Hypercalcemia in malignancy. West J Med 1990; 153:635–640.

48. Orloff JJ, Reddy D, de Papp AE, et al. Parathyroid hormone–related protein as a prohormone: posttranslational processing and receptor interactions. Endocr Rev 1994; 15:40–60.

49. Jüppner H, Abou-Samra A, Uneno S, et al. The parathyroid hormone–like peptide associated with humoral hypercalcemia of malignancy and parathyroid hormone bind to the same receptor on the plasma membrane of ROS 17/2.8 cells. J Biol Chem 1988; 263:8557–8561.

50. Nissenson RA, Diep D, Strewler GJ. Synthetic peptides comprising the amino-terminal sequence of a parathyroid hormone–like protein from human malignancies: binding to parathyroid hormone receptors and activation of adenylate cyclase in bone and kidney. J Biol Chem 1988; 263:12866–12871.

51. Hirschel-Scholz S, Caverzasio J, Rizzoli R, et al. Normalization of hypercalcemia associated with a decrease in renal calcium. J Clin Invest 1986; 78:319–322.

52. Harinck HI, Bijvot OL, Plantingh AS, et al. Role of bone and kidney in tumor-induced hypercalcemia and its treatment with. Am J Med 1987; 82:1133–1142.

53. Guise TA, Yin JJ, Taylor SD, et al. Evidence for a causal role of parathyroid hormone–related protein in the pathogenesis of human breast cancer–mediated osteolysis. J Clin Invest 1996; 98:1544–1549.

54. Powell GJ, Southby J, Danks JA, et al. Localization of parathyroid hormone–related protein in breast cancer metastases: increased incidence in bone compared with other sites. Cancer Res 1991; 51:3059–3061.

55. Bundred NJ, Walker RA, Ratcliffe WA, et al. Parathyroid hormone–related protein and skeletal morbidity in breast cancer. Eur J Cancer 1992; 28:690–692.

56. Horiuchi N, Caulfield MP, Fisher JE, et al. Similarity of synthetic peptide from human tumor to parathyroid hormone in vivo and in vitro. Science 1987; 238:1566–1568.

57. Hulter HN, Halloran BP, Toto RD, et al. Long-term control of plasma calcitriol concentrations in dogs and humans. J Clin Invest 1985; 76:695–702.

58. Fukumoto S, Matsumoto T, Yamoto H, et al. Suppression of serum 1,25-dihydroxyvitamin D in humoral hypercalcemia of malignancy is caused by elaboration of a factor that inhibits renal 1,25-dihydroxyvitamin D₃ production. Endocrinology 1989; 124:2057–2062.

59. Stewart AF, Vignery A, Silverglate A, et al. Quantitative bone histomorphometry in humoral hypercalcemia of malignancy. J Clin Endocrinol Metab 1982; 55:219–227.

60. Strewler GJ, Nissenson RA. Skeletal and renal actions of parathyroid hormone–related protein. In: Bilezikian JP, Marcus R, Levine MA, eds. The Parathyroids: Basic and Clinical Concepts. New York: Raven Press, 1994; 311–320.

61. Merendino JJ Jr, Insogna KL, Milstone LM, et al. A parathyroid hormone–like protein from cultured human keratinocytes. Science 1986; 231:388–390.

62. Danks JA, Martin TJ, Moseley JM, et al. Do all epidermal keratinocytes contain parathyroid hormone–related protein (PTHrP)? J Invest Dermatol 1991; 97:1086–1087.

63. Wysolmerski JJ, Broadus AE, Zhou J, et al. Overexpression of parathyroid hormone–related protein in the skin of transgenic mice interferes with hair follicle development. Proc Natl Acad Sci USA 1994; 91:1133–1137.

64. Brandt DW, Wachsman W, Deftos LJ. Parathyroid hormone–like protein: alternative messenger RNA splicing pathways in human cancer cell lines. Cancer Res 1994; 54:850–853.

65. Southby J, O'Keeffe LM, Martin TJ, et al. Alternative promoter usage and mRNA splicing pathways for parathyroid hormone–related protein in normal tissues and tumors. Br J Cancer 1995; 72:702–707.

66. Wysolmerski JJ, Vasavada RC, Foley J, et al. Transactivation of the PTHrP gene in squamous carcinoma predicts the occurrence of hypercalcemia in athymic mice. Cancer Res 1996; 56:1043–1049.

67. Danks JA, Ebeling PR, Hayman J, et al. Parathyroid hormone–related protein: immunohistochemical localization in cancers and in normal skin. J Bone Miner Res 1989; 4:273–278.

68. Holt EH, Vasavada RC, Bander NH, et al. Region-specific methylation of the parathyroid peptide gene determines its expression in human renal carcinoma cell lines. J Biol Chem 1993; 268:20639–20645.

69. Adams JS, Fernandez M, Gacad MA, et al. Vitamin D metabolite–mediated hypercalcemia and hypercalciuria in patients with AIDS and non–AIDS-associated lymphoma. Blood 1989; 73:235–239.

70. Seymour JF, Gagel RF, Hagemeister FB, et al. Calcitriol production in hypercalcemic and normocalcemic patients with non-Hodgkin lymphoma. Ann Intern Med 1994; 121:633–640.

71. Seymour JF, Gagel RF. Calcitriol: the major humoral mediator of hypercalcemia in Hodgkin's disease and non-Hodgkin's lymphomas. Blood 1993; 82:1383–1394.

72. Davies M, Hayes ME, Yin JA, et al. Abnormal synthesis of 1,25-dihydroxyvitamin D in patients with malignant lymphoma. J Clin Endocrinol Metab 1994; 78:1202–1207.

73. Barbour GL, Coburn JW, Slatopolsky E, et al. Hypercalcemia in an anephric patient with sarcoidosis: evidence for extrarenal generation of 1,25-dihydroxyvitamin D. N Engl J Med 1981; 305:440–443.

74. Stern PH, De Olazabal J, Bell NH. Evidence for abnormal regulation of circulating 1alpha,25-dihydroxyvitamin D in patients with sarcoidosis and normal calcium metabolism. J Clin Invest 1980; 66:852–855.

75. Strewler GJ, Budayr AA, Clark OH, et al. Production of parathyroid hormone by a malignant nonparathyroid tumor in a hypercalcemic patient. J Clin Endocrinol Metab 1993; 76:1373–1375.

76. Yoshimoto K, Yamasaki R, Sakai H, et al. Ectopic production of parathyroid hormone by small cell lung cancer in a patient with hypercalcemia. J Clin Endocrinol Metab 1989; 68:976–981.

77. Rizzoli R, Pache JC, Didierjean L, et al. A thymoma as a cause of true ectopic hyperparathyroidism. J Clin Endocrinol Metab 1994; 79:912–915.

78. Nussbaum SR, Gaz RD, Arnold A. Hypercalcemia and ectopic secretion of parathyroid hormone by an ovarian carcinoma. N Engl J Med 1990; 323:1324–1328.

79. Mundy G. Hypercalcemic factors other than parathyroid hormone–related protein. Endocrinol Metab Clin North Am 1989; 18:795–805.

80. Kawano M, Yamamoto I, Iwato K, et al. Interleukin-1 beta rather than lymphotoxin as the major bone-resorbing activity in human multiple myeloma. Blood 1989; 73:1646–1649.

81. Garrett IR, Durie BG, Nedwin GE, et al. Production of lymphotoxin, a bone-resorbing cytokine, by cultured human myeloma. N Engl J Med 1987; 317:526–532.

82. Wysolmerski JJ, Broadus AE. Hypercalcemia of malignancy: the central role of parathyroid hormone–related protein. Annu Rev Med 1994; 45:189–200.

83. Burtis WJ, Brady TG, Orloff JJ, et al. Immunochemical characterization of circulating parathyroid hormone–related protein in patients with humoral hypercalcemia of cancer. N Engl J Med 1990; 322:1106–1112.

84. Ratcliffe WA, Hutchesson AC, Bundred NJ, et al. Role of assays for parathyroid-hormone–related protein in investigation of hypercalcaemia. Lancet 1992; 339:164–167.

85. Pandian MR, Morgan CH, Carlton E, et al. Modified immunoradiometric assay of parathyroid hormone–related protein: clinical application in the differential diagnosis of hypercalcemia. Clin Chem 1992; 38:282–288.

86. Kovacs L, Robertson GL. Syndrome of inappropriate antidiuresis. Endocrinol Metab Clin North Am 1992; 21:859–875.

87. Moses AM, Scheinman SJ. Ectopic secretion of neurohypophyseal peptides in patients with malignancy. Endocrinol Metab Clin North Am 1991; 20:489–506.

88. Sorensen JB, Andersen MK, Hansen HH. Syndrome of inappropriate secretion of antidiuretic hormone (SIADH) in malignant disease. J Intern Med 1995; 238:97–110.

89. Hairnsworth JD, Workman R, Greco FA. Management of the syndrome of inappropriate antidiuretic hormone secretion in small cell lung cancer. Cancer 1983; 51:161–165.

90. Passamonte PM. Hypouricemia, inappropriate secretion of antidiuretic hormone, and small cell carcinoma of the lung. Arch Intern Med 1984; 144:1569–1570.

91. List AF, Hainsworth JD, Davis BW, et al. The syndrome of inappropriate secretion of antidiuretic hormone (SIADH) in small-cell lung cancer. J Clin Oncol 1986; 4:1191–1198.

92. Rassam JW, Anderson G. Incidence of paramalignant disorders in bronchogenic carcinoma. Thorax 1975; 30:86–90.

93. Talmi YP, Hoffman HT, McCabe BF. Syndrome of inappropriate secretion of arginine vasopressin in patients with cancer of the head and neck. Ann Otol Rhinol Laryngol 1992; 101:946–949.

94. Gennari FJ. Current concepts: serum osmolality—uses and limitations. N Engl J Med 1984; 310:102–105.

95. Beck LH. Hypouricemia in the syndrome of inappropriate secretion of antidiuretic hormone. N Engl J Med 1979; 301:528–530.

96. Gainer H, Wray S. Oxytocin and vasopressin: from genes to peptides. Ann NY Acad Sci 1992; 652:14–28.

97. North WG. Neuropeptide production by small cell carcinoma: vasopressin and oxytocin as plasma markers of disease. J Clin Endocrinol Metab 1991; 73:1316–1320.

98. North WG, Ware J, Maurer LH, et al. Neurophysins as tumor markers for small cell carcinoma of the lung: a cancer and leukemia group B evaluation. Cancer 1988; 62:1343–1347.

99. Legros JJ, Geenen V, Carvelli T, et al. Neurophysins as markers of vasopressin and oxytocin release: a study in carcinoma of the lung. Horm Res 1990; 34:151–155.

100. Sausville E, Carney D, Battey J. The human vasopressin gene is linked to the oxytocin gene and is selectively expressed in a cultured lung cancer cell line. J Biol Chem 1985; 260:10236–10241.

101. Fay MJ, Friedmann AS, Yu XM, et al. Vasopressin and vasopressin-receptor immunoreactivity in small-cell lung carcinoma (SCCL) cell lines: disruption in the activation cascade of V1a-receptors in variant SCCL. Cancer Lett 1994; 82:167–174.

102. Zerbe R, Stropes L, Robertson G. Vasopressin function in the syndrome of inappropriate antidiuresis. Annu Rev Med 1980; 31:315–327.

103. North WG. Biosynthesis of vasopressin and neurophysins. In: Gash DM, Boer GJ, eds. Vasopressin: Principles and Properties. New York, Plenum Press, 1987:175.

104. North WG, Maurer LH, Valtin H, et al. Human neurophysins as potential tumor markers for small cell carcinoma of the lung: application of specific radioimmunoassays. J Clin Endocrinol Metab 1980; 51:892–896.

105. Maurer LH, O'Donnell JF, Kennedy S, et al. Human neurophysins in carcinoma of the lung: relation to histology, disease stage, response rate, survival, and syndrome of inappropriate antidiuretic hormone secretion. Cancer Treat Rep 1983; 67:971–976.

106. Comis RL, Miller M, Ginsberg SJ. Abnormalities in water homeostasis in small cell anaplastic lung cancer. Cancer 1980; 45:2414–2421.

107. Cogan E, Debieve MF, Pepersack T, et al. Natriuresis and atrial natriuretic factor secretion during inappropriate antidiuresis. Am J Med 1988; 84:409–418.

108. Kamoi K, Ebe T, Kobayashi O, et al. Atrial natriuretic peptide in patients with the syndrome of inappropriate antidiuretic hormone secretion and with diabetes insipidus. J Clin Endocrinol Metab 1990; 70:1385–1390.

109. Manoogian C, Pandian M, Ehrlich L, et al. Plasma atrial natriuretic hormone levels in patients with the syndrome of inappropriate antidiuretic hormone secretion. J Clin Endocrinol Metab 1988; 67:571–575.

110. Gross AJ, Steinberg SM, Reilly JG, et al. Atrial natriuretic factor and arginine vasopressin production in tumor cell lines from patients with lung cancer and their relationship to serum sodium. Cancer Res 1993; 53:67–74.

111. Bliss DP Jr, Battey JF, Linnoila RI, et al. Expression of the atrial natriuretic factor gene in small cell lung cancer tumors and tumor cell lines. J Natl Cancer Inst 1990; 82:305–310.

112. Yoshinaga K, Yamaguchi K, Abe K, et al. Production of immunoreactive atrial natriuretic polypeptide in neuroendocrine tumors. Cancer 1994; 73:1292–1296.

113. Campling BG, Sarda IR, Baer KA, et al. Secretion of atrial natriuretic peptide and vasopressin by small cell lung cancer. Cancer 1995; 75:2442–2451.

114. Pollock AS, Arieff AI. Abnormalities of cell volume regulation and their functional consequences. Am J Physiol 1980; 239:F195–F205.

115. Grantham J, Linshaw M. The effect of hyponatremia on the regulation of intracellular volume and solute composition. Circ Res 1984; 54:483–491.

116. Anderson RJ, Chung HM, Kluge R, et al. Hyponatremia: a prospective analysis of its epidemiology and the pathogenetic role of vasopressin. Ann Intern Med 1985; 102:164–168.

117. Gross PA, Pehrisch H, Rascher W, et al. Pathogenesis of clinical hyponatremia: observations of vasopressin and fluid intake in 100 hyponatremic medical patients. Eur J Clin Invest 1987; 17:123–129.

118. Hantman D, Rossier B, Zohlman R, et al. Rapid correction of hyponatremia in the syndrome of inappropriate secretion of antidiuretic hormone: an alternative treatment to hypertonic saline. Ann Intern Med 1973; 78:870–875.

119. Arieff AI. Hyponatremia associated with permanent brain damage. Adv Intern Med 1987; 32:325–344.

120. Forrest JN Jr, Cox M, Hong C, et al. Superiority of demeclocycline over lithium in the treatment of chronic syndrome of inappropriate secretion of antidiuretic hormone. N Engl J Med 1978; 298:173–177.

121. De Troyer A. Demeclocycline: treatment for syndrome of inappropriate antidiuretic hormone secretion. JAMA 1977; 237:2723–2726.

122. Hainsworth JD, Workman R, Greco FA. Management of the syndrome of inappropriate antidiuretic hormone secretion in small cell lung cancer. Cancer 1983; 51:161–165.

123. Wajchenberg BL, Mendonca BB, Liberman B, et al. Ectopic adrenocorticotropic hormone syndrome. Endocr Rev 1994; 15:752–787.

124. Becker M, Aron DC. Ectopic ACTH syndrome and CRH-mediated Cushing's syndrome. Endocrinol Metab Clin North Am 1994; 23:585–606.

125. Magiakou MA, Mastorakos G, Oldfield EH, et al. Cushing's syndrome in children and adolescents: presentation, diagnosis, and therapy. N Engl J Med 1994; 331:629–636.

126. Tabarin A, Corcuff J, Rashedi M, et al. Comparative value of plasma ACTH and beta-endorphin measurement with three different commericial kits for the etiological diagnosis of ACTH-dependent Cushing's syndrome. Acta Endocrinol 1992; 126:308–314.

127. Stewart PM, Walker BR, Holder G, et al. 11β-Hydroxysteroid dehydrogenase activity in Cushing's syndrome: explaining the mineralocorticoid excess state of the ectopic adrenocorticotropin syndrome. J Clin Endocrinol Metab 1995; 80:3617–3620.

128. Funder JW, Pearce PT, Smith R, et al. Mineralocorticoid action: target tissue specificity is enzyme, not receptor, mediated. Science 1988; 242:583–585.

129. Schambelan M, Slaton PE, Biglieri EG. Mineralocorticoid production in hyperadrenocorticism. Am J Med 1971; 51:299–303.

130. Chang AC, Israel A, Gazdar A, et al. Initiation of pro-opiomelanocortin mRNA from a normally quiescent promoter in a human small cell lung cancer cell line. Gene 1989; 84:115–126.

131. DeBold CR, Mufson EE, Menefee JK, et al. Proopiomelanocortin gene expression in a pheochromocytoma using upstream transcription initiation sites. Biochem Biophys Res Commun 1988; 155:895–900.

132. de Keyzer Y, Bertagna X, Luton JP, et al. Variable modes of proopiomelanocortin gene transcription in human tumors. Mol Endocrinol 1989; 3:215–223.

133. White A, Clark AJ. The cellular and molecular basis of the ectopic ACTH syndrome. Clin Endocrinol (Oxf) 1993; 39:131–141.

134. Ray DW, Littlewood AC, Clark AJ, et al. Human small cell lung cancer cell lines expressing the proopiomelanocortin gene have aberrant glucocorticoid receptor function. J Clin Invest 1994; 93:1625–1630.

135. Yalow RS, Berson SA. Size heterogeneity of immunoreactive human ACTH in plasma and in extracts of pituitary glands and ACTH-producing thymoma. Biochem Biophys Res Commun 1971; 44:439–445.

136. Bertagna X. Proopiomelanocortin-derived peptides. Endocrinol Metab Clin North Am 1994; 23:467–485.

137. Vieau D, Massias JF, Girard F, et al. Corticotrophin-like intermediary lobe peptide as a marker of alternate pro-opiomelanocortin processing in ACTH-producing non-pituitary tumours. Clin Endocrinol (Oxf) 1989; 31:691–700.

138. Vieau D, Seidah NG, Mbikay M, et al. Expression of the prohormone convertase PC2 correlates with the presence of corticotropin-like intermediate lobe peptide in human adrenocorticotropin-secreting tumors. J Clin Endocrinol Metab 1994; 79:1503–1506.

139. Kimura N, Ishikawa T, Sasaki Y, et al. Expression of prohormone convertase, PC2, in adrenocorticotropin-producing thymic carcinoid with elevated plasma corticotropin-releasing hormone. J Clin Endocrinol Metab 1996; 81:390–395.

140. Kuhn JM, Proeschel MF, Seurin DJ, et al. Comparative assessment of ACTH and lipotropin plasma levels in the diagnosis and follow-up of patients with Cushing's syndrome: a study of 210 cases. Am J Med 1989; 86:678–684.

141. Ratcliffe JG, Knight RA, Besser GM, et al. Tumor and plasma ACTH concentrations in patients with and without the ectopic ACTH syndrome. Clin Endocrinol 1972; 1:27–44.

142. Black M, Carey FA, Farquharson MA, et al. Expression of the pro-opiomelanocortin gene in lung neuroendocrine tumours: in situ hybridization and immunohistochemical studies. J Pathol 1993; 169:329–334.

143. Findling JW, Tyrrell JB. Occult ectopic secretion of corticotropin. Arch Intern Med 1986; 146:929–933.

144. Nieman LK, Oldfield EH, Wesley R, et al. A simplified morning ovine corticotropin-releasing hormone stimulation test for the differential diagnosis of adrenocorticotropin-dependent Cushing's syndrome. J Clin Endocrinol Metab 1993; 77:1308–1312.

145. Avgerinos PC, Yanovski JA, Oldfield EH, et al. The metyrapone and dexamethasone suppression tests for the differential diagnosis of the adrenocorticotropin-dependent Cushing syndrome: a comparison. Ann Intern Med 1994; 121:318–327.

146. Oldfield EH, Doppman JL, Nieman LK, et al. Petrosal sinus sampling with and without corticotropin-releasing hormone for the differential diagnosis of Cushing's syndrome. N Engl J Med 1991; 325:897–905.

147. Miller JW, Crapo L. The medical treatment of Cushing's syndrome. Endocr Rev 1993; 14:443–458.

148. Sonino N, Boscaro M, Paoletta A, et al. Ketoconazole treatment in Cushing's syndrome: experience in 34 patients. Clin Endocrinol (Oxf) 1991; 35:347–352.

149. Sonino N. The use of ketoconazole as an inhibitor of steroid production. N Engl J Med 1987; 317:812–818.

150. Bertagna X, Favrod-Coune C, Escourolle H, et al. Suppression of ectopic adrenocorticotropin secretion by the long-acting somatostatin analog octreotide. J Clin Endocrinol Metab 1989; 68:988–991.

151. Sartor O, Cutler GB. Mifepristone-treatment of Cushing's syndrome. Clin Obstet Gynecol 1996; 39:506–510.

152. Carey RM, Varma SK, Drake CRJ, et al. Ectopic secretion of corticotropin-releasing factor as a cause of Cushing's syndrome. N Engl J Med 1984; 311:13–20.

153. Auchus RJ, Mastorakos G, Friedman TC, et al. Corticotropin-releasing hormone production by small cell carcinoma in a patient with ACTH-dependent Cushing's syndrome. J Endocrinol Invest 1994; 17:447–452.

154. Daughaday WH. Hypoglycemia in patients with non-islet cell tumors. Endocrinol Metab Clin North Am 1989; 18:91–101.

155. Zapf J. Insulinlike growth factor binding proteins and tumor hypoglycemia. Trends Endocrinol Metab 1995; 6:37–42.

156. Moller N, Blum WF, Mengel A, et al. Basal and insulin-stimulated substrate metabolism in tumour-induced hypoglycaemia: evidence for increased muscle glucose uptake. Diabetologia 1991; 34:17–20.

157. Eastman RC, Carson RE, Orloff DG, et al. Glucose utilization in a patient with hepatoma and hypoglycemia assessment by a positron emission tomography. J Clin Invest 1992; 89:1958–1963.

158. Chung J, Henry RR. Mechanisms of tumor-induced hypoglycemia with intraabdominal hemangiopericytoma. J Clin Endocrinol Metab 1996; 81:919–925.

159. Megyesi K, Kahn CR, Roth J, et al. Hypoglycemia in association with extrapancreatic tumors: demonstration of elevated plasma NSILA-s by a new radioreceptor assay. J Clin Endocrinol Metab 1974; 38:931–934.

160. Daughaday WH, Emanuele MA, Brooks MH, et al. Synthesis and secretion of insulin-like growth factor II by a leiomyosarcoma with associated hypoglycemia. N Engl J Med 1988; 319:1434–1440.

161. Daughaday WH, Trivedi B. Measurement of derivatives of proinsulin-like growth factor-II in serum by a radioimmunoassay directed against the E-domain in normal subjects and patients with nonislet cell tumor hypoglycemia. J Clin Endocrinol Metab 1992; 75:110–115.

162. Lowe WL Jr, Roberts CT Jr, LeRoith D, et al. Insulin-like growth factor-II in nonislet cell tumors associated with hypoglycemia: increased levels of messenger ribonucleic acid. J Clin Endocrinol Metab 1989; 69:1153–1159.

163. Shapiro ET, Bell GI, Polonsky KS, et al. Tumor hypoglycemia: relationship to high-molecular-weight insulin-like growth factor-II. J Clin Invest 1990; 85:1672–1679.

164. Daughaday WH, Trivedi B, Baxter RC. Serum "big insulin-like growth factor II" from patients with tumor hypoglycemia lacks normal E-domain O-linked glycosylation, a possible determinant of normal propeptide processing. Proc Natl Acad Sci USA 1993; 90:5823–5827.

165. Guler HP, Zapf J, Schmidt C, et al. Insulin-like growth factors I and II in healthy man: estimation of half-lives and production rates. Acta Endocrinol (Copenh) 1989; 121:753–758.

166. Zapf J, Futo E, Peter M, et al. Can "big" insulin-like growth factor II in serum of tumor patients account for the development of extrapancreatic tumor hypoglycemia. J Clin Invest 1992; 90:2574–2584.

167. Daughaday WH, Kapadia M. Significance of abnormal serum binding of insulin-like growth factor II in the development of hypoglycemia in patients with non-islet-cell tumors. Proc Natl Acad Sci USA 1989; 86:6778–6782.

168. Baxter RC, Daughaday WH. Impaired formation of the ternary insulin-like growth factor-binding protein complex in patients with hypoglycemia due to nonislet cell tumors. J Clin Endocrinol Metab 1991; 73:696–702.

169. Ron D, Powers AC, Pandian MR, et al. Increased insulin-like growth factor II production and consequent suppression of growth hormone secretion: a dual mechanism for tumor-induced hypoglycemia. J Clin Endocrinol Metab 1989; 68:701–706.

170. Zapf J, Schmid C, Guler HP, et al. Regulation of binding proteins for insulin-like growth factors (IGF) in humans: increased expression of IGF binding protein 2 during IGF I treatment of healthy adults and in patients with extrapancreatic tumor hypoglycemia. J Clin Invest 1990; 86:952–961.

171. Daughaday WH, Trevedi B, Baxter RC. Abnormal serum IGF-II transport in non-islet cell tumor hypoglycemia results from abnormalities of both IGF binding protein-3 and acid labile subunit and leads to elevation of serum free IGF-II. Endocrine 1995; 3:425–428.

172. Samaan NA, Pham FK, Sellin RV, et al. Successful treatment of hypoglycemia using glucagon in a patient with an extrapancreatic tumor. Ann Intern Med 1990; 113:404–406.

173. Hunter SJ, Daughaday WH, Callender ME, et al. A case of hepatoma associated with hypoglycaemia and overproduction of IGF-II (E-21): beneficial effects of treatment with growth hormone and intrahepatic adriamycin. Clin Endocrinol (Oxf) 1994; 41:397–401; discussion 402.

174. Faglia G, Arosio M, Bazzoni N. Ectopic acromegaly. Endocrinol Metab Clin North Am 1992; 21:575–595.

175. Melmed S. Extrapituitary acromegaly. Endocrinol Metab Clin North Am 1991; 20:507–518.

176. Melmed S, Ezrin C, Kovacs K, et al. Acromegaly due to secretion of growth hormone by an ectopic pancreatic islet-cell tumor. N Engl J Med 1985; 312:9–17.

177. Guilemin R, Brazeau P, Bolhen P, et al. Growth hormone–releasing factor from a human pancreatic tumor that caused acromegaly. Science 1982; 218:585–587.

178. Rivier J, Spiess J, Thorner M, et al. Characterization of a growth hormone–releasing factor from a human pancreatic islet tumour. Nature 1982; 300:276–278.

179. Thorner MO, Frohman LA, Leong DA, et al. Extrahypothalamic growth-hormone–releasing factor (GRF) secretion is a rare cause of acromegaly: plasma GRF levels in 177 acromegalic patients. J Clin Endocrinol Metab 1984; 59:846–849.

180. Schopohl J, Losa M, Frey C, et al. Plasma growth hormone (GH)–releasing hormone levels in patients with lung carcinoma. Clin Endocrinol (Oxf) 1991; 34:463–467.

181. Moller DE, Moses AC, Jones K, et al. Octreotide suppresses both growth hormone (GH) and GH-releasing hormone (GHRH) in acromegaly due to ectopic GHRH secretion. J Clin Endocrinol Metab 1989; 68:499–504.

182. Ezzat S, Ezrin C, Yamashita S, et al. Recurrent acromegaly resulting from ectopic growth hormone gene expression by a metastatic pancreatic tumor. Cancer 1993; 71:66–70.

183. Weintraub BD, Rosen SW. Ectopic production of human chorionic somatomammotropin by nontrophoblastic cancers. J Clin Endocrinol Metab 1971; 32:94–101.

184. Rosen SW, Weintraub BD. Humours, tumors, and caveats. Ann Intern Med 1975; 82:274–276.

185. Sheth NA, Suraiya JN, Sheth AR, et al. Ectopic production of human placental lactogen by human breast tumors. Cancer 1977; 39:1693–1699.

186. Navarro C, Corretger JM, Sancho A, et al. Paraneoplasic precocious puberty: report of a new case with hepatoblastoma and review of the literature. Cancer 1985; 56:1725–1729.

187. Kahn CR, Rosen SW, Weintraub BD, et al. Ectopic production of chorionic gonadotropin and its subunits by islet-cell tumors: a specific marker for malignancy. N Engl J Med 1977; 297:565–569.

188. Heitz PU, Kasper M, Kloppel G, et al. Glycoprotein-hormone alpha-chain production by pancreatic endocrine tumors: a specific marker for malignancy. Immunocytochemical analysis of tumors of 155 patients. Cancer 1983; 51:277–282.

189. Blithe DL, Wehmann RE, Nisula BC. β-Core: chemical and clinical properties. Trends Endocrinol Metab 1990; 1:394–398.

190. Neven P, Iles RK, Lee CL, et al. Urinary chorionic gonadotropin subunits and beta-core in nonpregnant women: a study of benign and malignant gynecologic disorders. Cancer 1993; 71:4124–4130.

191. Yoshimura M, Nishimura R, Murotani A, et al. Assessment of urinary beta-core fragment of human chorionic gonadotropin as a new tumor marker of lung cancer. Cancer 1994; 73:2745–2752.

192. Weidner N, Bar RS, Weiss D, et al. Neoplastic pathology of oncogenic osteomalacia/rickets. Cancer 1985; 55:1691–1705.

193. Schapira D, Ben Izhak O, Nachtigal A, et al. Tumor-induced osteomalacia. Semin Arthritis Rheum 1995; 25:35–46.

194. Lyles KW, Berry WR, Haussler M, et al. Hypophosphatemic osteomalacia: association with prostatic carcinoma. Ann Intern Med 1980; 93:275–278.

195. Charhon SA, Chapuy MC, Delvin EE, et al. Histomorphometric analysis of sclerotic bone metastases from prostatic carcinoma: special reference to osteomalacia. Cancer 1983; 51:918–924.

196. Miyauchi A, Fukase M, Tsutsumi M, et al. Hemangiopericytoma-induced osteomalacia: tumor transplantation in nude mice causes hypophosphatemia and tumor extracts inhibit renal 25-hydroxyvitamin D 1-hydroxylase activity. J Clin Endocrinol Metab 1988; 67:46–53.

197. Cai Q, Hodgson SF, Kao PC, et al. Brief report: inhibition of renal phosphate transport by a tumor product in a patient with oncogenic osteomalacia. N Engl J Med 1994; 330:1645–1649.

198. The HYP Consortium: A gene (PEX) with homologies to endopeptidases is mutated in patients with X-linked hypophosphatemic rickets. Nat Genet 1995; 11:130–136.

199. Hammond D, Winnick S. Paraneoplastic erythrocytosis and ectopic erythropoietins. Ann NY Acad Sci 1974; 230:219–227.

200. Da Silva JL, Lacombe C, Bruneval P, et al. Tumor cells are the site of erythropoietin synthesis in human renal cancers associated with polycythemia. Blood 1990; 75:577–582.

201. Muta H, Funakoshi A, Baba T, et al. Gene expression of erythropoietin in hepatocellular carcinoma. Intern Med 1994; 33:427–431.

202. Trimble M, Caro J, Talalla A, et al. Secondary erythrocytosis due to a cerebellar hemangioblastoma: demonstration of erythropoietin mRNA in the tumor. Blood 1991; 78:599–601.

203. Shiramizu M, Katsuoka Y, Grodberg J, et al. Constitutive secretion of erythropoietin by human renal adenocarcinoma cells in vivo and in vitro. Exp Cell Res 1994; 215:249–256.

204. Kew MC, Fisher JW. Serum erythropoietin concentrations in patients with hepatocellular carcinoma. Cancer 1986; 58:2485–2488.

205. Sawabe Y, Iida S, Tabata Y, et al. Serum erythropoietin measurements by a one-step sandwich enzyme-linked immunosorbent assay in patients with hepatocellular carcinoma and liver cirrhosis. Jpn J Clin Oncol 1993; 23:273–277.

206. Coombes RC, Hillyard CJ, Greenberg PB, et al. Plasma immunoreactive calcitonin in patients with non-thyroid tumors. Lancet 1974; 1:1080–1082.

207. Silva O, Becker K, Primack A, et al. Increased calcitonin levels in bronchogenic cancer. Chest 1976; 69:495–501.

208. Roos BA, Lindall AW, Baylin SB, et al. Plasma immunoreactive calcitonin in lung cancer cells. J Clin Endocrinol Metab 1980; 50:659–666.

209. Samaan NA, Castillo S, Schultz PN, et al. Serum calcitonin after pentagastrin stimulation in patients with bronchogenic and breast cancer compared to that in patients with medullary thyroid carcinoma. J Clin Endocrinol Metab 1980; 51:237–241.

210. Foa P, Ortolani S, Pogliani EM, et al. Immunoreactive calcitonin: a tumor marker for myelogenous leukemias. Int J Biol Markers 1990; 5:27–30.

211. Zajac JD, Martin TJ, Hudson P, et al. Biosynthesis of calcitonin by human lung cancer cells. Endocrinology 1985; 116:749–754.

212. Symes AJ, Craig RK, Brickell PM. Loss of transcriptional repression contributes to the ectopic expression of the calcitonin/α-CGRP gene in a human lung carcinoma cell line. FEBS Lett 1992; 306:229–233.

213. Ghatei MA, Stratton MR, Allen JM, et al. Co-secretion of calcitonin gene-related peptide, gastrin-releasing peptide and ACTH by a carcinoid tumor metastasizing to the cerebellum. Postgrad Med J 1987; 63:123–130.

214. Shichiri M, Hirata Y, Nakajima T, et al. Endothelin-1 is an autocrine/paracrine growth factor for human cancer cell lines. J Clin Invest 1991; 87:1867–1871.

215. Ishibashi M, Fujita M, Nagai K, et al. Production and secretion of endothelin by hepatocellular carcinoma. J Clin Endocrinol Metab 1993; 76:378–383.

216. Nakamuta M, Ohashi M, Tabata S, et al. High plasma concentrations of endothelin-like immunoreactivities in patients with hepatocellular carcinoma. Am J Gastroenterol 1993; 88:248–252.

217. Mendelsohn G, Eggleston JC, Olson JL, et al. Vasoactive intestinal peptide and its relationship to ganglion cell differentiation in neuroblastic tumors. Lab Invest 1979; 41:144–149.

218. Said SI, Faloona GR. Elevated plasma and tissue levels of vasoactive intestinal polypeptide in the watery-diarrhea syndrome due to pancreatic, bronchogenic and other tumors. N Engl J Med 1975; 293:155–160.

219. Hamilton I, Reis L, Bilimoria S, et al. A renal vipoma. Br Med J 1980; 281:1323–1324.

220. Wood SM, Wood JR, Ghatei MA, et al. Bombesin, somatostatin and neurotensin-like immunoreactivity in bronchial carcinoma. J Clin Endocrinol Metab 1981; 53:1310–1312.

221. Szabo M, Berelowitz M, Pettengill OS, et al. Ectopic production of somatostatin-like immuno- and bioactivity by cultured human pulmonary small cell carcinoma. J Clin Endocrinol Metab 1980; 51:978–987.

222. Noseda A, Peeters TL, Delhaye M, et al. Increased plasma motilin concentrations in small cell carcinoma of the lung. Thorax 1987; 42:784–789.

223. Penman E, Wass JA, Besser GM, et al. Somatostatin secretion by lung and thymic tumours. Clin Endocrinol (Oxf) 1980; 13:613–620.

224. Ghose RR, Gupta SK. Oat cell carcinoma of bronchus presenting with somatostatinoma syndrome. Thorax 1981; 36:550–551.

225. Gleeson MH, Bloom SR, Polak JM, et al. Endocrine tumour in kidney affecting small bowel structure, motility, and absorptive function. Gut 1971; 12:773–782.

226. Hunstein W, Trumper LH, Dummer R, et al. Glucagonoma syndrome and bronchial carcinoma. Ann Intern Med 1988; 109:920–921.

227. Moody TW, Pert CB, Gazdar AF, et al. High levels of intracellular bombesin characterize human small-cell lung carcinoma. Science 1981; 214:1246–1248.

228. Sorenson GD, Bloom SR, Ghatei MA, et al. Bombesin production by human small cell carcinoma of the lung. Regul Pept 1982; 4:59–66.

229. Carney DN, Broder L, Edelstein M, et al. Experimental studies of the biology of human small cell lung cancer. Cancer Treat Rep 1983; 67:27–35.

230. Weber S, Zuckerman JE, Bostwick DG, et al. Gastrin releasing peptide is a selective mitogen for small cell lung carcinoma in vitro. J Clin Invest 1985; 75:306–309.

231. Fathi Z, Corjay MH, Shipara H, et al. BRS-3: A novel bombesin receptor subtype selectively expressed in testis and lung carcinoma cells. J Biol Chem 1993; 268:5979–5984.

232. Cho T, Chan W, Cutz E. Distribution and frequency of neuro-epithelial bodies in post-natal rabbit lung: quantitative study with monoclonal antibody against serotonin. Cell Tissue Res 1989; 255:353–362.

233. Oberg K, Grimelius L, Lundqvist G, et al. Update on pancreatic polypeptide as a specific marker for endocrine tumours of the pancreas and gut. Acta Med Scand 1981; 210:145–152.

234. Fisken RA, Heath DA, Somers S, et al. Hypercalcemia in hospital patients: clinical and diagnostic aspects. Lancet 1981; 1:202–207.

235. Singer FR, Sharp CF Jr, Rude RK. Pathogenesis of hypercalcemia of malignancy. Miner Electrolyte Metab 1979; 2:161–169.

37

DISORDERS OF VASODILATOR HORMONES: CARCINOID SYNDROME AND MASTOCYTOSIS

L. Jackson Roberts II, Lowell B. Anthony, and John A. Oates

CARCINOID SYNDROME
  Pathology and Embryology
  Incidence and Natural Course
  Nonendocrine Manifestations
  Hormonal Aspects
  Variants of Carcinoid Syndrome
  Mediators of Carcinoid Syndrome
  Pharmacologic Effects
  Diagnostic Considerations
  Treatment

MASTOCYTOSIS AND OTHER DISORDERS OF SYSTEMIC
  MAST CELL ACTIVATION
  Pathogenesis
  Classification, Natural Course, and Prognosis
  Signs and Organ Histopathology
  Symptom Pathophysiology
  Factors Provoking Mastocyte Activation
  Diagnostic Evaluation
  Treatment

Two syndromes are associated with the release of excessive quantities of vasodilatory mediators into the circulation: the carcinoid syndrome and mastocytosis. Some of the manifestations, such as cutaneous flushing and diarrhea, are similar, and vasodilator hormones contribute prominently to the clinical syndrome in each, but the clinical presentations and hormonal mediators differ.

CARCINOID SYNDROME

The term *carcinoid syndrome* refers to the humoral manifestations that occur in patients with carcinoid tumors. The term *carcinoid* was first applied to these tumors because although they resemble carcinoma histologically, they have a more benign clinical course than most other malignancies.[1] It was subsequently recognized that the tumors both invade locally and give rise to distant metastases.

The occurrence of flushing, bronchoconstriction, gastrointestinal hypermotility, and cardiac disease in association with carcinoid tumors was reported by Thorson and colleagues in 1954.[4] The isolation of 5-hydroxytryptamine (serotonin) from carcinoid tumors[3] and the finding that patients with malignant carcinoid syndrome excrete increased quantities of the serotonin metabolite 5-hydroxyindoleacetic acid (5-HIAA)[5] suggested that the humoral manifestations of the carcinoid syndrome are due to the overproduction of serotonin by these tumors. However, additional agents play a role in this disorder.

Pathology and Embryology

Enterochromaffin cells, which give a yellow-brown reaction after chromate fixation, are distributed in tissues derived from the primitive gut. The enterochromaffin cells in the intestine are Kulchitsky's cells in the crypts of Lieberkühn. Carcinoid tumors were shown to arise from enterochromaffin cells by the demonstration that both tumor cells and Kulchitsky's cells reduce silver salts (argentaffin reaction); thus the term *argentaffinoma* has been used to describe carcinoid tumors.[2]

Polypeptide-secreting endocrine cells in the pituitary, thyroid, lungs, pancreas, and gastrointestinal tract share a number of common cytochemical and ultrastructural characteristics. Included in this system are the enterochromaffin cells that give rise to carcinoid tumors. Pearse[47, 50] originally developed the concept of the APUD system—*a*mine *p*recursor *u*ptake and *de*carboxylation—because of the ability of these cells to take up and decarboxylate amino acid precursors of biogenic amines such as serotonin and catecholamines. It was proposed that this system of cells has a common embryonic origin from the neuronal ectoderm.[50, 54, 55] Related cells are also found in the adrenal medulla, sympathetic ganglia, paraganglia, and chemoreceptor system. Although there is no evidence for common embryonic ancestry of these cells, the concept of dysplasia of neuronal ectoderm was proposed to explain the occurrence of multiple endocrine neoplasia and the multipotentiality of neoplastic cells derived from this system to produce a variety of peptide hormones.[54]

Consistent with the aforementioned concept, there are some histologic similarities among carcinoid tumors, islet cell tumors, and medullary carcinoma of the thyroid.[42, 56, 57] Furthermore, carcinoid tumors occasionally coexist with other endocrine tumors, and tumors with the morphologic appearance of carcinoids may produce gastrin, calcitonin, insulin, vasoactive intestinal peptide, catecholamines, and corticotropin (ACTH, adrenocorticotropin).[23, 35, 48, 53, 62, 63, 65, 69, 85, 96] Common embryonic ancestry may also explain the frequent occurrence of more than one primary carcinoid tumor in a single patient.[17, 60, 64] However in most instances carcinoid tumors do not occur in association with other endocrine neoplasms, and the pathophysiology of multiple endocrine neoplasia differs from that of carcinoid syndrome (see Chapter 30).

Clinical, biochemical, histologic, and cytochemical heterogeneity of carcinoid tumors may be related to the site of origin.[26, 45] One classification is based on whether the tumor arose from the embryonic foregut (bronchus, stomach, pancreas), midgut (mid-duodenum to midtransverse colon), or hindgut (descending colon and rectum).[26] As mentioned previously, most carcinoid tumors that arise from the embryonic midgut are argentaffin-positive.[4, 16] Some tumors do not spontaneously reduce silver salts, although nuclear silver staining can be observed in the presence of a reducing substance and silver. Such cells are termed *argyrophilic*.[16] Carcinoid tumors arising from the embryonic foregut are commonly argentaffin-negative but argyrophilic. In contrast, carcinoid tumors derived from the embryonic hindgut are usually both argentaffin-negative and nonargyrophilic.[45]

Biochemical features also distinguish carcinoid tumors from different sites of origin. The biosynthesis of serotonin and its metabolic degradation are outlined in Figure 37–1. Carcinoid tumors of the embryonic midgut secrete serotonin, and patients with these tumors have elevated urinary excretion of 5-HIAA. Carcinoid tumors arising from the foregut, however, frequently have low levels of L-amino-acid decarboxylase, which converts 5-hydroxytryptophan to serotonin.[11, 19, 20] Thus these tumors usually secrete primarily 5-hydroxytryptophan; tumors arising from the midgut may secrete both 5-hydroxytryptophan and serotonin.[75] After 5-hydroxytryptophan is secreted, it is converted to serotonin and other metabolites by other tissues in the body. Therefore although foregut carcinoid tumors usually do not directly secrete large quantities of serotonin, urinary 5-HIAA levels are elevated in patients with these tumors. In contrast, carcinoid tumors arising from the embryonic hindgut usually do not secrete large amounts of either 5-hydroxytryptophan or serotonin, and patients with these tumors do not have elevated urinary levels of 5-HIAA.[26, 75]

Incidence and Natural Course

Carcinoid tumors are relatively common. The average age of patients is approximately 50, and there is no sexual predominance.[46, 58, 60, 64] Carcinoids are found in the small intestine in about 1 in 150 patients at autopsy[17] and in the appendix in approximately 1 in 300 appendectomies.[46] Rectal carcinoids are detected in about 1 in 2500 proctoscopic examinations,[28] but most are localized and have no evidence of metastasis. The most common site of carcinoid tumors is the appendix, followed by the ileum, rectum, and other sites in the gastrointestinal tract.[6, 58, 60, 64]

Carcinoids of the appendix are usually found incidentally during appendectomy, have a low malignant potential, and rarely metastasize.[46] Rectal carcinoids also have a low malignant potential and are commonly discovered incidentally during proctoscopic examination.[13, 28] For both appendiceal and rectal carcinoids, the occurrence of metastases is related to the size of the primary lesion; tumors less than 2 cm in diameter metastasize rarely.[13, 28, 46]

Carcinoid tumors arising from locations other than the appendix and rectum are associated with a higher frequency of metastasis.[13, 46, 58, 60, 64] They initially invade surrounding tissues and spread to regional lymph nodes before distant metastasis occurs. Carcinoids commonly metastasize to the liver, and the liver may be the only site of distant metastasis even when the liver is extensively infiltrated. Bone metastases occur occasionally.

Carcinoid tumors usually grow slowly. Patients may live for many years, and the overall prognosis and survival rates are generally favorable.[46] Because of the low incidence of metastasis of appendiceal carcinoids, the 5-y survival rate of patients with these tumors is approximately 99%. Patients with rectal and lung carcinoids also have a favorable prognosis, with 5-y survival rates between 80 and 90%. Patients with carcinoids in the small intestine have a 5-y survival rate of approximately 50%. Prognosis varies with the extent of metastasis at the time of diagnosis. For example, rectal carcinoids with only local invasion are associated with a greater than 90% 5-y survival rate, which decreases to approximately 45% in the presence of regional metastasis and to about 10% if distant metastases are present at diagnosis.[46, 60, 64] The effects of current therapeutic modalities on survival are discussed in the section on treatment.

Nonendocrine Manifestations

Recognition of nonendocrine symptoms early in the course enhances the likelihood of diagnosis before distant metastasis or endocrine manifestations occur. Bronchial carcinoid tumors, like other lung tumors, can cause respiratory complaints such as cough, dyspnea, and hemoptysis, which lead to radiologic examination and bronchoscopy. In contrast,

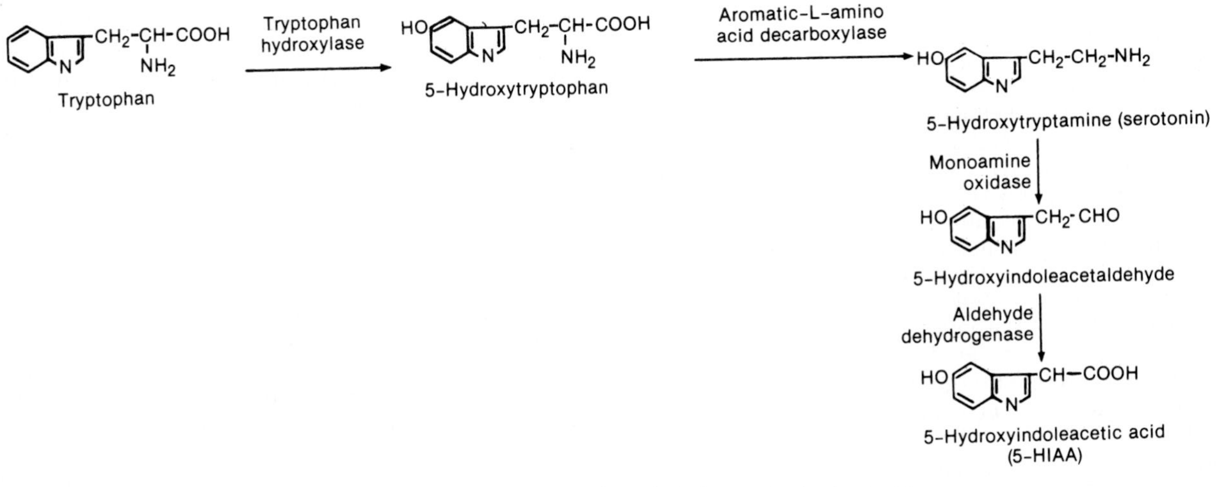

Figure 37–1. Biosynthesis and metabolism of 5-hydroxytryptamine (serotonin).

rectal carcinoids are usually asymptomatic in the absence of advanced disease.[13, 28] Carcinoids of the small intestine frequently cause symptoms for long periods before the diagnosis is made. In such patients, early diagnosis can lead to cure by surgical resection of the localized tumor. The most common manifestations of intestinal carcinoids are abdominal pain, intermittent obstruction, and a palpable abdominal mass, each of which occurs in about half of patients.[17] Intestinal obstruction usually occurs after invasion of the mesentery, which causes a fibroblastic reaction with scarring and matting of loops of small bowel that in turn can produce a mass and intermittently obstruct the intestine. The presence of recurrent intermittent intestinal obstruction should raise the suspicion of carcinoid tumor. Because this process is extraluminal, radiologic examination is normal about half the time.

Hormonal Aspects

General Comments

The term *carcinoid syndrome* is used to describe the humoral manifestations of carcinoid tumors: flushing, bronchoconstriction, gastrointestinal hypermotility, and cardiac disease.[3] Most patients with carcinoid tumors do not develop the syndrome. The frequency of the humoral manifestations varies with the site of origin of the tumor, being most common with tumors originating in the small intestine and proximal colon; 40 to 50% of patients with these tumors experience the syndrome. The disorder is less frequent in patients with bronchial carcinoids, is rare with appendiceal carcinoids, and does not occur in patients with rectal carcinoids, even with advanced stage tumors and metastases.[13, 17, 28, 46, 51, 60]

Development of the carcinoid syndrome is also a function of tumor mass and extent of metastasis. The syndrome does not occur in patients with a small tumor burden, and patients with the full-blown syndrome usually have hepatic metastases.[60] The association with hepatic metastases may be due to efficient inactivation by the liver of amines released into the portal circulation. In contrast, venous drainage from metastatic tumor in the liver goes directly into the systemic circulation and bypasses hepatic inactivation. The tumors most likely to be associated with the carcinoid syndrome in the absence of hepatic metastasis are ovarian teratoma and bronchial carcinoids, which release mediators directly into the systemic rather than the portal circulation.

Clinical Features of Carcinoid Syndrome

Some patients experience all manifestations of the carcinoid syndrome, including flushing, diarrhea, bronchospasm, and cardiac disease,[3] whereas others lack one or more components. The National Carcinoid Support Group is available for physician and patient assistance.*

FLUSHING. Paroxysmal flushing manifested by transient episodes of erythema is usually limited to the face, the neck, and the upper trunk. Patients usually experience a sensation of warmth during flushing and sometimes note palpitations. Occasionally, flushing can be more intense and spread over the entire body. In such cases a fall in blood pressure can cause dizziness. Severe attacks of flushing are rarely accompanied by shock and syncope. Flushing over a long period can cause a constant facial erythema or plethora with a cyanotic hue and persistent cutaneous telangiectasia. Such changes can be striking.[8]

The flush in patients with the carcinoid syndrome is similar to that in patients with mastocytosis. Although severe flushing and hypotension can occur in patients with the carcinoid syndrome, most episodes are brief (1 or 2 min or less) and do not cause dizziness or palpitations.[60] Such episodes are merely an embarrassment or a nuisance. In contrast, mastocytosis tends to cause more severe and more prolonged flushing accompanied by dizziness or frank syncope.

Flushing usually occurs spontaneously in the absence of any evident precipitating cause, but some patients note factors that seem to evoke attacks, such as physical exertion, emotional upset, eating, alcohol ingestion, and heat.[8, 60] Similar factors operate in patients with mastocytosis, with the exception of eating, which rarely provokes flushing in this condition.

DIARRHEA. Diarrhea is a common feature and can vary from as few as 2 to as many as 30 stools a day. It is usually a discomfort and an annoyance but is not disabling. Occasionally, voluminous diarrhea may cause malabsorption and fluid and electrolyte imbalance. Diarrhea is frequently accompanied by abdominal cramping.

It may be difficult to be certain whether diarrhea and other abdominal symptoms are a result of intestinal hypermotility from stimulation of intestinal smooth muscle by humoral mediators or whether they are due to mechanical factors, such as intermittent intestinal obstruction, diminished vascular perfusion, and impairment of lymphatic drainage from invasion of the mesentery by tumor and the associated desmoplastic reaction. In addition, many patients have undergone partial surgical resection of small intestine, which can cause the short-bowel syndrome or diarrhea from malabsorption of bile salts after ileal resection. Both endocrine and mechanical factors contribute to the diarrhea and abdominal symptoms in many patients.

PULMONARY MANIFESTATIONS. Paroxysms of bronchospasm can occur, usually in association with attacks of flushing due to release of a bronchoconstricting mediator or mediators from the tumor.

CARDIAC MANIFESTATIONS. A unique endocrine effect of carcinoid tumors is the development of plaque-like thickenings on the endocardium of the heart valve leaflets, atria, and ventricles in about 20% of patients.[60] This fibrous material is also frequently deposited in the superior and inferior venae cavae, coronary sinus, and pulmonary artery. The aorta and other arteries may be involved.[7, 30, 66] The right side of the heart is affected predominantly, and left-sided heart involvement is usually of lesser functional consequence.[30]

Histologically, the plaque-like thickenings in the endocardium consist of smooth muscle and fibroblasts embedded in a stroma that is rich in mucopolysaccharides, basement membrane–like material, collagen, and microfibrils. Elastic fibers are not present. There is no inflammatory reaction, and the plaques are covered by an intact layer of endothelium.[66]

Thickening of mural and valvular endocardium distorts the architecture of the valves and can cause pulmonic stenosis and tricuspid insufficiency. Severe tricuspid insufficiency can cause right-sided congestive heart failure and contribute to mortality. Rarely, involvement of the left side of the heart causes murmurs of the mitral valve or left-sided congestive heart failure.

Variants of Carcinoid Syndrome

The manifestations outlined earlier occur most commonly in patients with tumors of the small intestine. Tumors of the stomach characteristically cause different features.[20] Gastric carcinoids usually secrete 5-hydroxytryptophan rather than serotonin and usually also secrete histamine, which is uncommon for tumors of midgut origin. The cutaneous flushing in such patients usually consists of patchy serpiginous areas of cutaneous erythema with sharply delineated borders rather

---

*National Carcinoid Support Group, P.O. Box 44233, Madison, WI 53744-4233.

than the typical diffuse cutaneous erythema characteristic of patients with carcinoids in the small intestine. Diarrhea and cardiac disease are less common with gastric carcinoids. Patients with gastric carcinoids may experience flushing after ingestion of food and have peptic ulcer disease, possibly due to the release of histamine by the tumors.

Bronchial carcinoids may also cause distinctive characteristics. Flushing can be prolonged (sometimes lasting days), severe, and associated with tremulousness, bronchospasm, profuse lacrimation, nasal congestion, periorbital edema, and explosive diarrhea. With severe attacks, hypotension may be profound.[34] The therapy for bronchial carcinoid tumors is discussed under the section on treatment.

Mediators of Carcinoid Syndrome

Infusions of serotonin in humans increase intestinal motility,[9] and treatment with serotonin antagonists such as methysergide and cyproheptadine usually reduces the severity of diarrhea.[18, 22, 33, 44] Diarrhea is also attenuated by the administration of *p*-chlorophenylalanine, which inhibits serotonin biosynthesis by blocking tryptophan hydroxylase.[39, 43, 52]

Serotonin is not an important mediator of the flushing. First, some patients experience flushing with only modestly elevated urinary excretion of 5-HIAA, whereas patients with marked increases in 5-HIAA excretion may not have flushing.[60] Second, serotonin may or may not be released into the circulation during flushing.[21] Third, intravenous infusion of serotonin does not cause flushing similar to that in the carcinoid syndrome.[21]

Other potential mediators of the carcinoid flush include bradykinin, prostaglandins, histamine, and tachykinins. Bradykinin is released in some patients during flushing,[29, 38] but the absence of detectable bradykinin release in other patients suggests that it is not a universal mediator of the flush.[38, 40] Although a role for prostaglandins has been considered, production of the vasodilator prostaglandin E$_2$ is not increased in patients with the carcinoid syndrome. Moreover, administration of inhibitors of prostaglandin biosynthesis does not ameliorate attacks of flushing. It therefore seems unlikely that prostaglandins cause the flushing.

With tumors of the midgut, vasoactive peptides called tachykinins are believed to be mediators of the flushing. Tachykinins are a family of structurally related peptides that possess a common COOH-terminal sequence and exert similar biologic effects, such as vasodilation and contraction of various types of smooth muscle.[14, 89, 101, 102, 106] These peptides include substance P, substance K (neurokinin α), and neuropeptide K (an extended form of substance K). (Two precursors of these tachykinins, α- and β-pre-protachykinin, are derived from a single gene.) These peptides are stored in carcinoid tumors, and levels are increased in plasma from patients with carcinoid syndrome.[71, 72, 82, 88, 90, 97, 105, 107, 108] Determination of whether these peptides are linked to the manifestations of the carcinoid syndrome will contribute to the understanding of the pathophysiology of this syndrome.

Gastric carcinoid tumors usually secrete histamine, and patients usually have increased urinary excretion of histamine.[20] In contrast, midgut carcinoid tumors rarely produce histamine. Treatment of such patients with histamine H$_1$ receptor antagonists generally fails to abolish episodes of flushing, suggesting that histamine is not the sole mediator of flushing with gastric carcinoids. However, flushing in a patient with the gastric carcinoid syndrome was ameliorated with combined administration of H$_1$ and H$_2$ receptor antagonists, whereas neither of these given singly prevented attacks.[81] The authors have observed similar results in another patient with gastric carcinoid syndrome. In these patients histamine can be the primary mediator of the flushing.

Serotonin may play an important role in the cardiac manifestations. There is a correlation between urinary 5-HIAA levels and carcinoid cardiac disease,[60] and cardiac involvement is usually significant in patients with markedly increased levels of urinary 5-HIAA. Conversely, cardiac disease is uncommon in patients with gastric carcinoids that secrete 5-hydroxytryptophan instead of serotonin, thus sparing the heart from exposure to high concentrations of serotonin released directly by the tumor. Attempts to reproduce the cardiac lesion in experimental animals by administration of serotonin have produced inconsistent results.[10, 15, 31, 32, 36] In some studies, prolonged administration of serotonin caused endocardial fibrosis. When present, the fibrosis is similar to that in human carcinoid cardiac lesions. Differences may arise from species variation or from the fact that it is difficult to reproduce the carcinoid syndrome completely, including the prolonged exposure of the heart to circulating serotonin. Other factors may act in concert with serotonin to cause the cardiac lesion. For example, in one study hepatic damage and tryptophan deficiency were required before chronic administration of serotonin produced endocardial fibrosis in guinea pigs.[31]

Pharmacologic Effects

In patients with the carcinoid syndrome flushing can be evoked by administration of epinephrine, norepinephrine, isoproterenol, or dopamine.[12, 24, 49] Phentolamine prevents flushing in response to epinephrine, norepinephrine, and dopamine,[24, 49] but propranolol does not block flushing in response to epinephrine.[49]

The fact that ingestion of food precipitates flushing in some patients raised the possibility that this response may be due to the release of gastrointestinal hormones, which in turn evoke the release of vasoactive mediators from carcinoid tumors. Low doses of the synthetic gastrin analogue pentagastrin consistently provokes flushing in some patients,[76, 81] and the synthetic COOH-terminal octapeptide of cholecystokinin elicited a flush in one patient.

Somatostatin (SRIF, somatotropin release-inhibiting factor) inhibits the release of several gastrointestinal hormones[74, 127] and prevents pentagastrin-evoked flushing.[76] Somatostatin appears to exert this effect by inhibiting the release of mediators from the tumor.[84, 95] Somatostatin also inhibits the diarrhea and the bronchoconstriction associated with the carcinoid syndrome.[83, 84, 86] Whether carcinoid tumors are under constant tonic stimulation by gastrointestinal hormones that are normally inhibited by somatostatin or whether somatostatin exerts a direct inhibitory effect independent of its effects on gastrointestinal hormonal stimulation is unclear. In support of the latter possibility somatostatin reversed hypotension after surgical manipulation of a carcinoid tumor in one patient.[79] Whether somatostatin can inhibit catecholamine-induced flushing has not been examined.

Diagnostic Considerations

In patients with flushing and other manifestations of the carcinoid syndrome, the diagnosis can be established by measuring the urinary excretion of 5-HIAA because it is invariably elevated under these circumstances. In most laboratories the upper limit of urinary 5-HIAA is approximately 50 μmol/d (10 mg/d). The magnitude of elevation of urinary 5-HIAA can range from 50 to 3000 μmol/d (10 to 600 mg/d), although the degree of elevation in 5-HIAA levels does not always correlate with the severity of flushing. As also noted earlier, patients with the gastric carcinoid syndrome also have increased urinary excretion of 5-HIAA, even though the tumors secrete 5-hydroxytryptophan rather than serotonin. This increase occurs because the 5-hydroxytryptophan released from these tumors is converted to serotonin in other tissues and is subsequently metabolized to 5-HIAA.

Assays for 5-HIAA include high-pressure liquid chromatography (HPLC) with electrochemical detection and traditional colorimetric and fluorescent methods.[87, 104] A variety of foods and drugs can interfere with the measurement of urinary 5-HIAA (Table 37–1).[99] Drugs are less likely to interfere with urinary 5-HIAA measurement using HPLC and electrochemical detection. Therefore when urine is to be collected for 5-HIAA determination, patients must avoid the ingestion of foods listed in Table 37–1 and (when possible) the use of known interfering drugs and all other nonessential drugs. Elevated 5-HIAA levels should be confirmed by collecting multiple 24-h samples under controlled conditions and using HPLC with electrochemical detection methods. These confirmatory steps may make it possible to avoid a more costly evaluation.

In the patient with characteristic features of the syndrome and urinary 5-HIAA excretion greater than 150 μmol/d (30 mg/d) under controlled collection conditions, the diagnosis is reasonably secure. If 5-HIAA excretion is in the range of 50 to 150 μmol/d (10 to 30 mg/d), additional diagnoses must be considered. Intestinal obstruction and other diseases of the small bowel such as nontropical sprue can release sufficient amounts of serotonin to cause modest elevations of 5-HIAA, normally less than 130 μmol/d (25 mg/d). Therefore when the urinary excretion of 5-HIAA is less than 150 μmol/d (30 mg/d), definitive evidence for the presence of a carcinoid tumor should be sought, and the features must be distinguished from those of mastocytosis. Epinephrine reverses flushing in patients with mastocytosis but provokes flushing in patients with the carcinoid syndrome. A 1 μg/mL solution of epinephrine in normal saline is administered by intravenous bolus beginning with an initial dose of 0.05 μg. The dose is doubled at intervals of 10 min until flushing appears or a maximum of 6.4 μg is given. When flushing occurs, it usually begins within 60 s after the epinephrine administration and dissipates after 3 or 4 min. If flushing does occur, the same, or the next higher, dose of epinephrine should be given to make certain that the flush was not spontaneous and was induced by the epinephrine. It is also important to begin with 0.05 μg and not to administer doses greater than double the minimal threshold dose that provokes flushing because larger doses of epinephrine can cause potentially dangerous tachycardia and hypotension. The epinephrine test is not useful for patients suspected of having carcinoid tumors in whom spontaneous episodes of flushing do not occur, because epinephrine usually does not evoke flushing in such patients.[25]

Plasma chromogranin A is co-released with amines and peptides in some patients, is frequently elevated in carcinoid syndrome patients, and may be a useful secondary biochemical marker.[103, 110] Although not specific to carcinoid malignancy, chromogranin A may be a sensitive marker for the diagnosis of early disease.[123] In the evaluation of flushing with an equivocal 24-h urinary 5-HIAA, a normal plasma chromogranin A value suggests nonendocrine causes. The predictive value of the plasma chromogranin A in carcinoid is uncertain, but serum concentrations correlate with extent of disease and survival in patients with neuroblastoma.[125]

In patients with carcinoid tumors who lack symptoms of the carcinoid syndrome but experience other manifestations such as intestinal obstruction to diagnosis is made by histologic examination of biopsied or resected tumor when possible. To determine the primary site and extent of disease conventional endoscopic and radiologic techniques are used in conjunction with techniques such as selective venous sampling and radionuclide imaging,[118, 119, 122] endoscopic ultrasound, computed tomography (CT) portography, positron emission tomography ([11C]-5-hydroxytryptophan), radionuclide scintigraphy ([111In] DTPA-octreotide), and radioreceptor-guided surgery.[136, 139, 142, 147, 149] Somatostatin receptor scintigraphy has proved to be particularly useful in the detection of endocrine tumors.[126, 143, 145] [111In]pentetreotide (OctreoScan, Mallinckrodt Medical, Inc., St. Louis, MO) binds to the somatostatin receptor and can be detected using conventional imaging techniques (Fig. 37–2; see color section between pages 875 and 877).[141, 150, 156] This noninvasive means of demonstrating the presence of receptor can focus conventional radiologic examinations.[151] Metastatic lesions isodense on CT scan may also be detected with radioreceptor imaging (Fig. 37–3; see color section between pages 875 and 877).

Treatment

Treatment of carcinoid tumors and the carcinoid syndrome has two aims: (1) reduction of tumor mass and (2) control of the disabling symptoms. In addition, urinary 5-HIAA levels that are grossly elevated (>500 μmol/d [>100 mg/d]) may be associated with deficiency of the essential amino acid tryptophan. Normally about 1% of tryptophan in the body is converted to serotonin, and the remaining 99% is utilized for the synthesis of protein and niacin. In patients with serotonin-secreting carcinoid tumors, as much as 60% of the available tryptophan may be diverted for the synthesis of serotonin, which results in tryptophan and niacin deficiency.[8] Dietary supplementation with large quantities of tryptophan may be hazardous because it leads to enhanced production of serotonin,[20] but all patients should be given supplemental niacin to prevent the development of pellagra.

TABLE 37–1. Factors That Interfere with Determination of Urinary 5-HIAA

Factors That Produce False-Positive Results
Foods
  Avocados
  Bananas
  Eggplants
  Pineapples
  Plums
  Walnuts
Drugs
  Acetaminophen
  Acetanilid
  Caffeine
  Fluorouracil
  Guaifenesin
  Lugol's (iodine) solution
  Melphalan
  Mephenesin
  Methamphetamine
  Methocarbamol
  Methysergide maleate
  Phenacetin
  Phenmetrazine
  Reserpine
Factors That Cause False-Negative Results
Drugs
  Corticotropin
  p-Chlorophenylalanine
  Chlorpromazine
  Heparin
  Imipramine
  Isoniazid
  Methenamine mandelate
  Methyldopa
  Monoamine oxidase inhibitors
  Phenothiazine
  Promethazine

5-HIAA, 5-hydroxyindoleacetic acid.

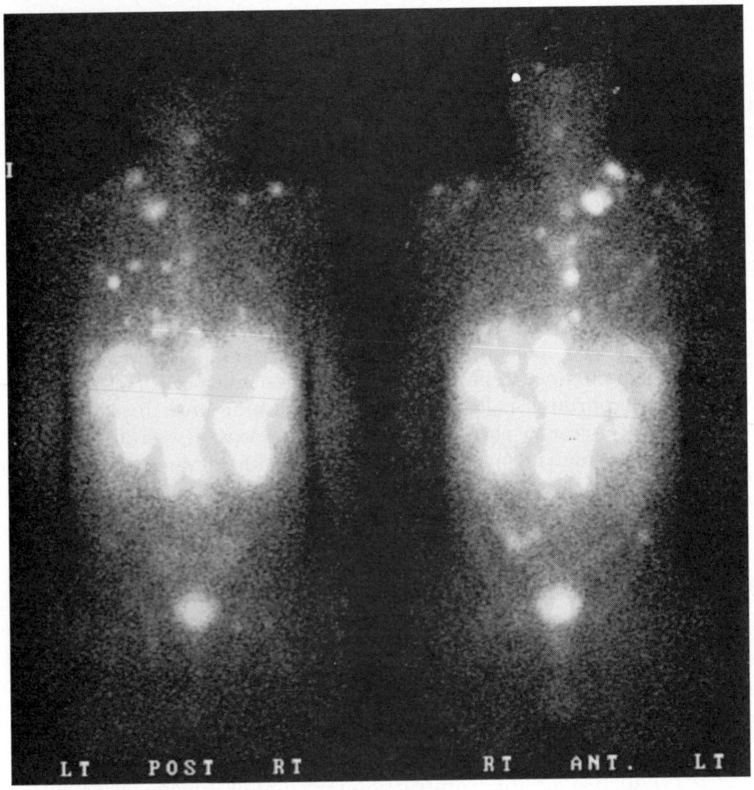

Figure 37–2. Anterior and posterior planar images following the IV injection of 6 mCi ^{111}In pentetreotide in a 53-year-old man with carcinoid syndrome. Areas of increased uptake are noted in the thoracic and abdominal regions, demonstrating metastases in the lymph nodes and liver (see color section between pages 875 and 877).

Therapeutic Approaches to Reduce Tumor Mass

An attempt should be made to remove all tumor at the time of operation, because many carcinoids only invade surrounding tissue or metastasize to local or regional lymph nodes. Removal of such involved tissues may result in a cure. Even if this is not possible, tumor debulking, including the resection of portions of the liver containing metastases, may cause remissions for extended periods.[17] As much small intestine as possible should be preserved to prevent the short-bowel syndrome.

During surgery massive mediator release can cause a car-

cinoid crisis. The hazards and precautions required preoperatively, intraoperatively, and postoperatively and the treatment of complications have been reviewed.[67, 68, 78] Somatostatin and the somatostatin analogue octreotide prevent flushing, diarrhea, and bronchospasm and may correct the hypotension associated with carcinoid crisis during surgery.[79, 115] Therefore octreotide should be available for administration during surgery.

Another treatment for hepatic metastases is either surgical resection or ligation or percutaneous embolization of the hepatic artery.[70, 77, 92, 93] The aim is to diminish the bulk of tumor in the liver, which is usually responsible for the carcinoid syndrome, and to ameliorate the symptoms. Surgical

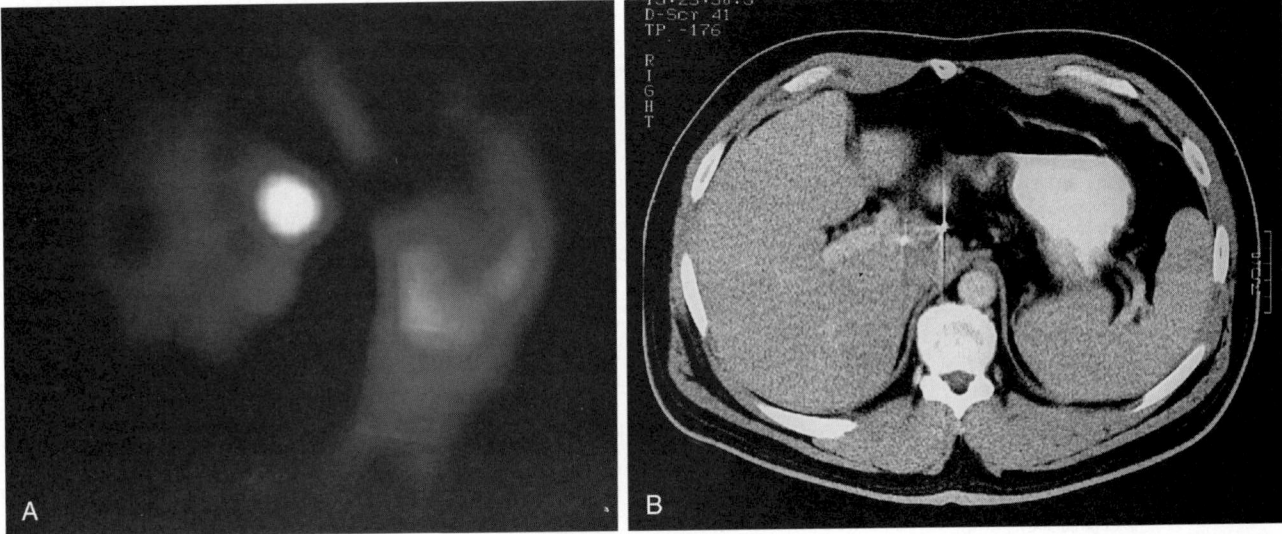

Figure 37–3. ^{111}In pentetreotide scan (A) in a patient with a history of a previously resected midgut carcinoid tumor and negative serial spiral abdominal CT scans and biochemical markers (5-HIAA and chromogranin A). The abdominal CT scan (B) was obtained concomitantly with the ^{111}In pentetreotide scan. Laparotomy with partial hepatectomy revealed a single hepatic site of involvement and histologically confirmed the presence of recurrent disease (see color section between pages 875 and 877).

resection of hepatic tumor is most effective when metastases are primarily confined to a single lobe. In some patients, one or a few large solitary metastatic nodules can be wedge-resected or removed by subsegmental resection of the liver. In patients with more diffuse metastatic involvement confined primarily to one lobe, a total lobectomy is required.

In patients with diffuse metastases involving both lobes of the liver, ligation or embolization of the hepatic artery[92, 93] seems to be associated with relatively few major complications. On the one hand, the primary tumor can be removed at the time of hepatic artery ligation, but on the other, embolization can be repeated without the risk of a major surgical procedure.[92] The mean duration of response is approximately 3 y after surgical resection of hepatic metastases and from 1 to 2 y after hepatic artery ligation or embolization.[131, 134, 138, 158] Hepatic artery occlusion followed by combination chemotherapy with 5-fluorouracil, doxorubicin, and streptozocin and dacarbazine appears to be more effective than either treatment used singly.[117, 153] With the combined approach, the mean response rate was 86%, and the median duration of response appears to be longer than 2 y.

A variety of chemotherapeutic regimens have been tried in patients with inoperable metastatic carcinoid tumors.[73, 80, 92, 98] Unfortunately none is associated with a good response, and the average duration of remission is usually less than 1 y. The most effective regimens appear to be the combination of streptozocin and fluorouracil, which is associated with an objective response (more than 50% regression of tumor) of about 33%,[80] and the combination of methotrexate with cyclophosphamide, which is associated with an objective response of approximately 55%. In treating patients with severe manifestations, chemotherapy should be initiated with doses of drugs below what are normally used because rapid lysis of tumor can release massive amounts of mediators (carcinoid crisis) and can cause death.[61, 80] The dosages should be escalated as tolerance permits. A major drawback of these combination regimens is toxicity. Fluorouracil alone is not usually associated with substantial toxicity, and consideration may be given to an initial trial with this agent alone because of its relatively low toxicity. One protocol is to give 400 mg/m²/d of fluorouracil for 5 d and to repeat the dose in 6 wk. Six weeks after the second 5-d course, a maintenance dose of 500 mg/m² once weekly should be begun. Response should be monitored by CT, ultrasonography, and/or radioisotope scanning for evidence of reduction in tumor mass. Monitoring of urinary excretion of 5-HIAA during periods when tumor lysis is not active provides an additional marker of response.[80]

Treatment with either of the somatostatin analogues octreotide and lanreotide and with interferons has resulted in tumor regression and/or stabilization[109, 112, 117, 146] and in reduction in the severity of the hormonal manifestations of the carcinoid syndrome. Trials of combination therapy with these agents suggest a favorable effect in some[135, 154] but not all studies.[155]

Approximately 20% of carcinoid patients have an objective partial response (a 50% or greater reduction in tumor size after treatment with somatostatin analogues) as measured by serial physical or radiographic examinations.[109, 140] The combination of such therapy with interventional radiology or surgery to achieve cytoreduction may be required for patients progressing on medical therapy alone or those presenting with more than 50% hepatic involvement.

The α-interferons may control carcinoid syndrome symptoms and produce objective biochemical responses (greater than 50% suppression of 5-HIAA).[94, 112] Interferon therapy is effective at low doses (3 to 5 million U, three to five times a week), possibly related to the induction of 2′5′-oligoadenylate synthetase.[113, 124] Recombinant human interferon alpha-2b has a lower incidence of antibody formation (15%) than interferon alpha-2a (41%).[121, 133, 137] Administration of interferon alpha-2a at 24 million U/m² three times a week resulted in a 20% objective radiographic response and a 39% biochemical response. These responses had a median duration of only 4 wk and caused severe side effects.[120]

Pharmacologic Therapy

Therapy aimed at inhibiting the production or action of hormones released by the tumor may blunt the manifestations of the syndrome. Antiserotonin agents such as methysergide and cyproheptadine can ameliorate diarrhea. For long-term therapy, cyproheptadine is preferred to methysergide because of the potentially serious retroperitoneal, cardiac, and pulmonary fibrosis associated with the latter.[41] Commonly used antidiarrheal agents such as loperamide and diphenoxylate can also be helpful.

The flushing associated with gastric carcinoid tumors appears to be mediated primarily by histamine and can be controlled by treatment with combined histamine H_1 and H_2 receptor antagonists.[81] Attempts to control flushing associated with carcinoid tumors of midgut origin with antiserotonin agents, antihistamines, and inhibitors of prostaglandin biosynthesis are not effective, but the somatostatin analogue octreotide is useful in the disorder.[109, 111, 117, 140] Administration of the drug by subcutaneous injections every 8 h relieves flushing and diarrhea in approximately 90 and 75% of patients, respectively. Amelioration of these manifestations is accompanied by a marked reduction in the urinary excretion of 5-HIAA. Octreotide may also improve the musculoskeletal symptoms in some patients.[130] The most troublesome side effects are hypoglycemia and steatorrhea, which are reversible, are not clearly dose-related, and are rarely severe enough to limit treatment. Life-threatening toxicities or dose-limiting side effects of octreotide have not been identified.[140] Titrating octreotide acetate in increments of 50 μg q 8 h to control flushing symptoms is recommended. The control of diarrhea may require additional measures because somatostatin analogues can cause steatorrhea from the inhibition of pancreatic exocrine secretion.[114] Continuous subcutaneous administration using microinfusion pumps is an alternative for patients who prefer not to perform multiple daily injections.[132] Octreotide depot formulation is currently under evaluation.

Carcinoid syndrome associated with bronchial carcinoid tumors has distinctive features and is treated differently.[34] Many patients experience amelioration of symptoms with glucocorticoids or phenothiazines. The mechanism by which these drugs exert a beneficial effect is unclear.

Cardiac disease can be one of the most serious complications of the carcinoid syndrome and can be responsible for death. Unfortunately there is no known means of reversing or halting the progression of the endocardial fibrosis that may be related to tumor-derived growth factors that stimulate proliferation of fibroblasts.[148] Serial transthoracic or transesophageal echocardiography is useful for evaluating the presence and progression of carcinoid heart disease.[91, 100, 128] In patients with severe valvular lesions and intractable cardiac failure, surgical replacement of damaged cardiac valves has had mixed results.[27, 37, 59, 129] This surgery is associated with technical problems because of the marked fibrosis of the endocardium.

Controlling carcinoid symptoms and disease as outlined earlier has altered the natural history of carcinoid tumor. The combination of somatostatin analogues and the interferons and aggressive debulking procedures has increased survival.[116, 144, 157, 159] In 80 carcinoid syndrome patients who received octreotide acetate from 1985 to 1994, the 5-y survival from the time of diagnosis of metastatic disease was 65% (Fig. 37-4A). Additional survival statistics are listed in Table 37-2. While biotherapy, surgery, and interventional radiology offer greater

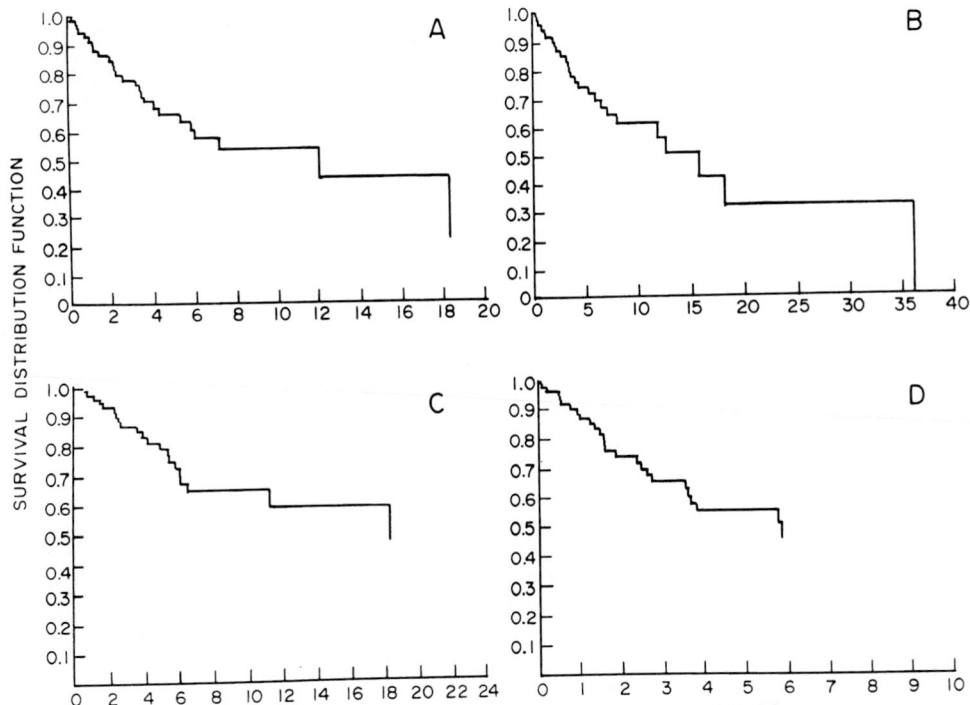

Figure 37–4. Survival in the Vanderbilt series of patients (N = 80) treated with somatostatin analogues. Survival calculated from date of metastatic disease diagnosis (A), date of symptom onset (B), the date of primary disease diagnosis (C) and the date of octreotide acetate initiation (D).

hope, additional therapeutic options are needed. The use of a radiolabeled somatostatin analogue to target radiation to receptor-bearing tumor cells may offer promise in the future. Preliminary evidence obtained with [^{111}In]pentetreotide[152] suggests the feasibility of this approach.

MASTOCYTOSIS AND OTHER DISORDERS OF SYSTEMIC MAST CELL ACTIVATION

Mast cells are distributed in almost all organs[160] and contain a variety of preformed and de novo synthesized mediators, enzymes, and receptors (Table 37–3).[160–163] Mast cells can be activated to release these mediators by immunoglobulin E–dependent mechanisms (via surface-bound immunoglobulin E receptors) and by a variety of non–immunoglobulin E–mediated stimuli.[160–168] Although the normal function is uncertain, the mast cell is a central player in immediate hypersensitivity reactions.

Several disorders are characterized by systemic activation of mast cells by non–immunoglobulin E–dependent mechanisms with attendant release of mediators. The archetypical disorder of this type is systemic mastocytosis, a disease characterized by abnormal proliferation of tissue mast cells and originally termed urticaria pigmentosa. The disorder, initially thought to be limited to skin, can be associated with mast cell proliferation in other organs. The etiology of the abnormal mast cell proliferation is poorly understood, and there may be more than a single cause. For example, whereas most cases do not appear to have any clear-cut genetic basis, a rare inheritable form of the disease has also been described.[169–171]

Symptoms are attributed primarily to paroxysms of mastocyte activation and attendant release of mast cell mediators. In addition, some patients who have no evidence of increased mast cell proliferation also experience episodes of non–immunoglobulin E–dependent systemic mast cell activation and mediator release and exhibit a clinical syndrome ("idiopathic anaphylaxis") that can be indistinguishable from that in patients with mastocytosis.[172–175] Although increased mast cell proliferation is not evident histologically in most of these patients, mast cell numbers in the skin can be slightly increased in some patients.[176] Whereas mastocytosis is a rare disease, the idiopathic systemic mast cell activation disorder in the absence of abnormal mast cell proliferation is encountered more frequently.

TABLE 37–2. 5-Y and Median Survival in Octreotide-Treated Patients with Carcinoid Syndrome at Vanderbilt University, 1985–1994 (n = 80)

Survival Calculated from Date of:	5-Y Survival (%)	Median Survival (y)
Metastatic disease diagnosis	65	8.8
Symptom onset	78	14.5
Primary disease diagnosis	73	12.8
Octreotide acetate initiation	53	5.8

TABLE 37–3. Major Mediators and Cell Membrane Surface Receptors in Human Mast Cells

Preformed Secretory Granule Mediators
 Histamine
 Proteoglycans
  Heparin, chondroitin sulfate
Neutral Proteases
 Tryptase, chymase, cathepsin G, carboxypeptidase
Acid Hydrolases
 Hexosaminidase β, β-glucuronidase, arylsulfatase, N-acetyl-β-glucosaminidase
Lipid Mediators Synthesized De Novo
 Prostaglandin D_2
 Peptidoleukotrienes
 Platelet-activating factor
Chemokines/Cytokines
 Tumor necrosis factor α (both preformed and de novo synthesized), eosinophil chemotactic factor, interleukin-8
Membrane Surface Receptors
 FcεR1, c-kit receptor

Pathogenesis

Mast cells appear to originate from the precursor of mononuclear cells in the bone marrow.[177-179] Although the mast cells in some patients with aggressive mastocytosis may exhibit aberrant histologic features,[180] the accumulation of mast cells in patients with mastocytosis is thought to result from hyperplasia rather than malignant transformation of the mast cell.[181-184]

The identification of mast cell growth factor (MGF), also known as stem cell factor (SCF), has contributed to our understanding of mast cell proliferation. MGF is a cytokine and the ligand for the cell surface c-kit proto-oncogene protein.[185-187] MGF also induces proliferation of melanocytes,[187] possibly explaining the association of melanocytes and pigmentation in one form of cutaneous mastocytosis, urticaria pigmentosa (see later). MGF is present both bound to the surface of cells and in a soluble form produced by proteolytic cleavage. Some patients with cutaneous mastocytosis appear to have increased amounts of the extracellular soluble form of MGF in the skin and increased quantities of MGF bound to mast cells.[184] Furthermore a point mutation in c-kit, which results in ligand-independent autophosphorylation of the c-kit receptor, has been described in patients who have mastocytosis with an associated hematologic disorder.[188]

MGF-independent mechanisms may also be involved in the regulation of mast cell proliferation.[189-193] For example, interleukin-3 (IL-3) and IL-4 induce mast cell proliferation in mice,[191, 192] although they do not cause proliferation of mast cells from human bone marrow.[193] Additional unidentified factors may also be involved in the differentiation and proliferation of human mast cells.[189, 190]

Almost nothing is known regarding the pathogenesis of the syndrome of idiopathic systemic mast cell activation in the absence of abnormal mast cell proliferation. By definition, an allergic etiology for systemic mastocyte activation has not been identified, and there is no evidence that the mast cells are unusually sensitive to activating stimuli or that these patients have an exaggerated response to mast cell mediators.[194]

Classification, Natural Course, and Prognosis

Classification

The classification of mastocytosis is problematic owing to the fact that mastocytosis comprises a heterogeneous group of disorders and because the natural course can vary substantially. Some classifications are based on the types of cutaneous lesions present, and others are based on the organs involved or how rapidly the disease progresses. A symposium in 1990 involving multidisciplinary scientists active in the area of mastocytosis research[195] suggested the classification for mastocytosis outlined in Table 37–4.[196] This classification is a modification of that proposed by Travis.[197] The disorder involving episodes of systemic mastocyte activation in the absence of abnormal mast cell proliferation has been added as a disorder distinct from mastocytosis.

The vast majority of patients with mastocytosis fall under Category A, *Indolent Mastocytosis*, in Table 37–4. The symposium participants thought that it was very important to distinguish this category, primarily because it does not carry the grave prognosis associated with the other three categories of the disease. Indolent mastocytosis rarely progresses to evolve into the other three categories, an important consideration in the counseling of patients. A variety of tissues can be involved in the disorder, in particular skin, gastrointestinal tract, liver and spleen, lymph node, and bone. Mastocytosis appears to spare the lungs, kidneys, and central nervous system, and the disease may be limited to the skin. However, sampling errors

TABLE 37–4. Classification of Disorders of the Mastocyte

I. Infiltrative Mastocytosis
  A. Indolent mastocytosis
    1. Syncope
    2. Cutaneous disease
    3. Ulcer disease
    4. Malabsorption
    5. Bone marrow mast cell aggregates
    6. Skeletal disease
    7. Hepatosplenomegaly
    8. Lymphadenopathy
  B. Mastocytosis with associated hematologic disorder
    1. Myeloproliferative
    2. Myelodysplastic
  C. Aggressive mastocytosis
    1. Lymphadenopathic mastocytosis with eosinophilia
  D. Mastocytic leukemia
II. Idiopathic Disorders of Systemic Mastocyte Activation in the Absence of Evident Abnormal Proliferation of Mast Cells

may occur when specimens are obtained for histologic analysis, e.g. in bone marrow, because the abnormal mast cell proliferation may not be homogeneously distributed throughout the tissue, leading to the erroneous conclusion that the disease is limited to the skin. Furthermore the histologic assessment of mast cell numbers in tissues such as bone marrow may be too insensitive to detect mild degrees of mast cell proliferation. It was previously thought that patients with cutaneous mastocytosis rarely had systemic involvement. This erroneous assumption may have been due to a failure to evaluate patients adequately for systemic disease, especially patients in whom the likelihood of systemic involvement is considered unlikely on clinical grounds. However histologic evaluation of the bone marrow and careful assessment for histamine overproduction by quantifying the urinary excretion of histamine metabolites indicate that probably at least half of adult patients with urticaria pigmentosa have systemic involvement, even when not suspected on clinical grounds.[198, 199]

The natural course of the indolent form of mastocytosis is that the abnormal proliferation of mast cells and severity of symptoms in most patients appear to plateau and stabilize at some point rather than to progress unrelentingly. Furthermore, the level of the urinary excretion of histamine metabolites, an index of mast cell burden in the body, also plateaus at some point in time in most patients.[200, 201] Patients with indolent mastocytosis have a low risk of developing a hematologic malignancy and progressing to the category B, which carries a worse prognosis.[202]

Most patients with the indolent form of the disease can expect to live many years, and some have a normal life expectancy. Overall, however, the life expectancy is diminished. Factors that worsen the prognosis include onset of the disease at an older age, anemia, male sex, current or previous malignancy, and presence of mast cells with lobulated nuclei.[197] Interestingly the decrease in survival rates occurs primarily during the first 3 y after diagnosis. The survival rate then plateaus and has essentially the same slope as that predicted for the general population.[197] With onset in childhood, usually between birth and 2 years of age, the disease is frequently limited to the skin and spontaneously disappears in approximately half of children before adulthood.[203-205] Some adult patients with systemic mastocytosis are asymptomatic, whereas other patients experience severe symptoms. Life-threatening occurrences are caused by recurrent episodes of severe mastocyte activation with release of enormous quantities of mast cell mediators that can lead to shock and vascular collapse.

In contrast to the indolent form of mastocytosis, the prognosis is guarded for the other three categories of disease in Table 37–4. As mentioned earlier, these forms of the disease are less common than the indolent form. Patients in category

B present with mastocytosis in association with a primary hematologic disorder, usually myeloproliferative or myelodysplastic disease and less commonly nonlymphocytic leukemia, malignant lymphoma, or chronic neutropenia.[197, 206–208] In these patients, the median survival is largely that of the associated hematologic disorder, usually approximately 1 to 2 y.[206]

Category C represents the rarest subset of patients with mastocytosis, mast cell leukemia.[160, 209, 210] The mast cells in both the circulation and tissues appear atypical. This form of mastocytosis carries the worst prognosis, with a mean survival of less than 6 mo despite chemotherapy.

Category D is a subgroup of patients with mastocytosis, lymphadenopathy, and blood eosinophilia.[211, 212] Patients with indolent mastocytosis can exhibit mild blood eosinophilia ($290 \pm 88/mm^3$), whereas peripheral blood eosinophil counts in patients with this aggressive form of the disease exhibit much higher eosinophilia ($2254 \pm 542/mm^3$).[212] Interestingly these patients characteristically do not have urticaria pigmentosa of the skin.[212] The rapidly progressing clinical course involves marrow fibrosis and extensive mast cell infiltration of the bone marrow, lymph nodes, liver, and spleen. Anemia and thrombocyotopenia can be severe.[211] Hematologic malignancies can develop following the diagnosis of mastocytosis.[211] The expected survival is only 2 to 4 y from the time of diagnosis.[213] Splenectomy and chemotherapy may prolong survival in some patients.[211]

Signs and Organ Histopathology

Signs

CUTANEOUS SIGNS. Most patients with mastocytosis have evidence of cutaneous involvement, and an increase in the numbers of mast cells in the skin is seen when examined histologically (Table 37–5).[214] The most common cutaneous manifestation is multiple small pigmented lesions that urticate on stroking with a blunt object (Darier's sign). These lesions, called urticaria pigmentosa, may be pruritic (Fig. 37–5; see color section between pages 875 and 877). When present, these lesions are a valuable visible clue to the diagnosis of mastocytosis. Dermatographia may be elicited when uninvolved areas of the skin are stroked. Approximately 50% of patients with urticaria pigmentosa in early childhood experience resolution by adolescence.[203–205] Urticaria pigmentosa lesions contain not only increased numbers of mast cells but also melanocytes, which cause the pigmentation of these lesions.[209, 215]

Another form of cutaneous mastocytosis in adults is termed telangiectasia macularis eruptiva perstans.[209] These patients have erythematous skin and persistent telangiectasias that are presumed to result from chronic vasodilation due to the release of mast cell mediators in the skin. Pruritus is usually absent. Individual lesions are approximately 2 to 6 mm in diameter and do not have sharply demarcated borders.[214]

Solitary mastocytomas occur almost exclusively in children[209] and are single, isolated tumors. The size can range up to 3 or 4 cm in diameter; histologically they consist of a dense infiltration of mast cells. Mastocytomas usually do not recur after surgical removal.[216]

A rare form of cutaneous mastocytosis that generally presents at birth or during infancy is diffuse and erythrodermic disease.[209, 214] Diffuse cutaneous disease involves all of the skin,

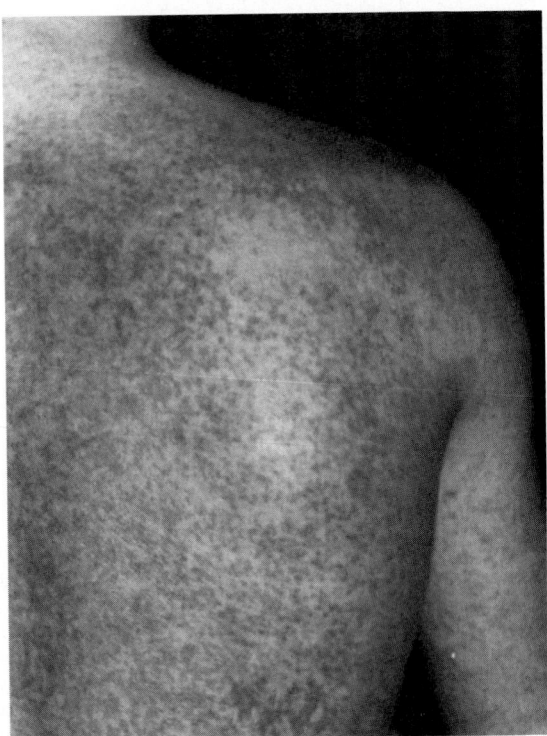

Figure 37–5. Cutaneous lesions of urticaria pigmentosa (see color section between pages 875 and 877).

which can have either a brown, red, or yellow color. The erythrodermic form of diffuse cutaneous mastocytosis is characterized by intense redness and edema of the skin, sometimes with yellow nodules. Hemorrhagic blisters may form with stroking of the skin. A bullous form of the disease in some children can be hemorrhagic and leave crusts after the bullae rupture.

A frequently overlooked lesion that can even occur in patients with idiopathic mastocyte activation consists of multiple small 1- to 2-mm, papular or acneiform lesions with a surrounding erythematous base (Fig. 37–6; see color section between pages 875 and 877). These lesions may be pruritic and do not persist but appear intermittently. Biopsy does not reveal excessive mast cells in the lesions. The whitish material in these acneiform lesions is not purulent but appears to be a fibrinous exudate. These lesions may be a focal site of mast

TABLE 37–5. Cutaneous Manifestations of Mastocytosis

Urticaria pigmentosa—multiple macules, papules, and plaques
Telangiectasia macularis eruptiva perstans
Mastocytoma—single or multiple macules, plaques, or nodules
Diffuse and erythrodermic forms including bullous mastocytosis

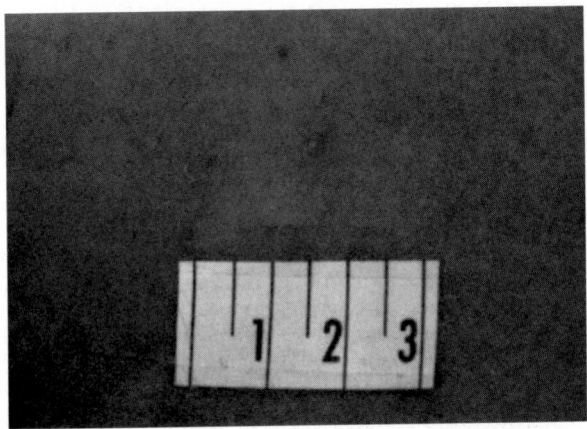

Figure 37–6. Acneiform cutaneous lesions found in some patients with mastocytosis and the syndrome of systemic mast cell activation (see color section between pages 875 and 877).

cell activation in the skin that causes vascular dilation and erythema and a local increase in vascular permeability with protein and fluid transudation. Patients who do not exhibit any cutaneous lesions, including patients with mastocytosis and idiopathic mastocyte activation, may exhibit a wheal-and-flare response when the skin is stroked (dermatographia).

SYSTEMIC SIGNS. The manifestations of systemic mastocytosis can occur in various combinations and with variable severity. Hepatomegaly and splenomegaly can be due to infiltration of mast cells.[160, 209, 217, 218] The most frequent finding in the liver is fibrosis with mast cells distributed in sinusoidal and portal areas.[219, 220] In a retrospective study, approximately 61% of patients had evidence of liver disease, with hepatomegaly in 24% and splenomegaly in 41%. Portal hypertension with ascites can occur.[219] There is a report of marked improvement in refractory ascites in a patient with mastocytosis who underwent a portacaval shunt.[221] Mast cell infiltration of the spleen is present in approximately 50% of patients with mastocytosis.[220, 222] The mast cell infiltrate primarily involves paratrabecular and parafollicular areas.

Osseous involvement can be manifested by either osteoporosis or osteosclerosis.[160, 209, 217, 223] Both forms of bone disease can occur in the same patient. The reason for the occurrence of both osteoporosis and osteosclerosis with mastocytosis is unclear.[224] Patients with more aggressive forms of mastocytosis tend to have a higher frequency of abnormal bone scans at the time of diagnosis. Approximately 50% of abnormal bone scans remain stable when examined serially.[225] The typical bone marrow finding consists of foci of granuloma-like lesions consisting of mast cells in a fibrotic background and is usually associated with abundant eosinophils and lymphocytes.[226, 217, 209] Diffuse infiltration of the marrow with mast cells is uncommon. The mast cell lesions in children are usually small and more subtle than in adults.[226]

Systemic mastocytosis can also involve the gastrointestinal tract.[160, 209, 227-232] When examined radiologically, small, evanescent, 1- to 3-mm, nodular mucosal filling defects may be seen, usually in the jejunum but occasionally in the ileum, stomach, and large bowel. The mucosal nodules do not appear to be focal accumulations of mast cells but are analogous to papular urticaria. With endoscopy small mucosal urticarial-like lesions are seen, and biopsy of the lesions does not demonstrate focal mast cell accumulation. These radiologic findings can be overlooked, and special precautions should be taken to differentiate small, mobile air bubbles from the fixed, nodular filling defects in the mucosa. Less specific radiologic signs such as gastric hypersecretion and decreased transit time of contrast medium through the small intestine may also be noted. Furthermore diffuse thickening of the bowel wall can

at times be demonstrated radiologically, usually in patients with severe disease; mast cell infiltration of the lamina propria is usually found with bowel wall thickening. Manifestations of gastrointestinal mastocytosis include a high incidence of peptic ulcer with increased gastric acid secretion and mild malabsorption.[233] The hypersecretion of gastric acid is thought to be due to overproduction of histamine in these patients. Symptoms include abdominal pain and diarrhea.[233] Mast cell infiltration of lymph nodes can also occur in patients with mastocytosis,[220, 222, 234] particularly in patients with the aggressive form of mastocytosis, lymphadenopathy with eosinophilia.

Hematologic abnormalities are largely nonspecific.[209] With marked mast cell infiltration of the bone marrow, anemia and leukocytosis may be present. Eosinophilia, usually of a slight degree, is found in about 10% of patients, usually in patients with the aggressive form of mastocytosis, lymphadenopathy with eosinophilia. Although the cause of eosinophilia is not entirely clear, the release of eosinophil chemotactic factor of anaphylaxis may play a role. In the rare entity of mast cell leukemia, atypical mast cells can be detected in the circulation.

Symptom Pathophysiology

Mediators of Humoral Symptoms

The humoral manifestations of systemic mastocytosis or idiopathic mast cell activation are due primarily to the release of mast cell mediators and include flushing, tachycardia, and hypotension. Increased intestinal motility can cause abdominal cramping and sometimes nausea, vomiting, and diarrhea. Thus this syndrome resembles the carcinoid syndrome.

Histamine is a potent vasodilator and also causes contraction of gastrointestinal smooth muscle.[235] Histamine is rapidly metabolized in vivo, as outlined in Figure 37–7. Only a small fraction (2 to 3%) of histamine released into the circulation is excreted into the urine unmetabolized, the major urinary metabolite being methylimidazoleacetic acid. Because histamine is released from mast cells and overproduction of histamine occurs in patients with systemic mastocytosis, it was assumed that the humoral symptoms of mastocytosis are due solely to this agent. However, except for a few reports of improvement in diarrhea,[236-238] antihistamine therapy alone rarely abrogates systemic symptoms such as flushing.[239-242] In particular, the life-threatening episodes of vasodilatory shock are not prevented with antihistamine therapy, even with high doses of both H_1 and H_2 receptor antagonists.[243]

The discovery of overproduction of prostaglandin D_2 (PGD_2) in patients with mastocytosis provided further insight

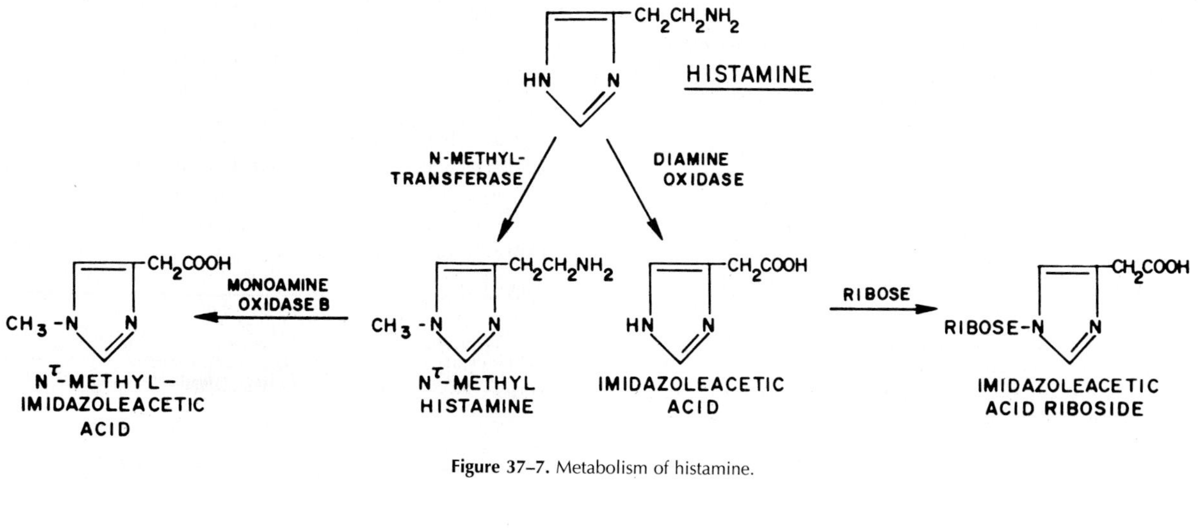

Figure 37–7. Metabolism of histamine.

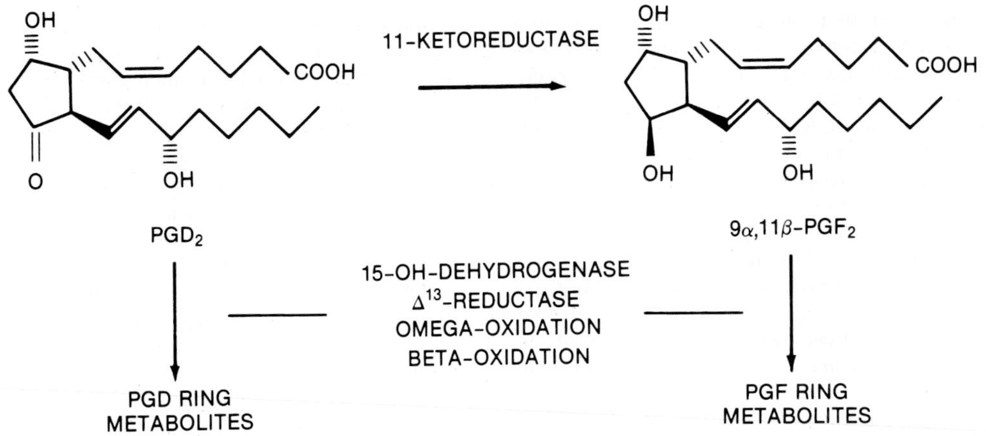

Figure 37–8. Metabolism of PGD_2.

into the pathophysiology of the humoral symptoms of the disease.[243] The major initial pathway of PGD_2 metabolism involves reduction of the prostane ring keto group at C-11 by an 11-keto-reductase enzyme to yield the product $9\alpha,11\beta$-prostaglandin F_2 ($9\alpha,11\beta$-PGF_2) (Fig. 37–8). $9\alpha,11\beta$-PGF_2 and PGD_2 are further metabolized by dehydrogenation of the C-15 hydroxyl group, reduction of the Δ^{13}-double bond, beta oxidation, and omega oxidation, yielding a series of metabolites that are excreted into the urine. Metabolites with a PGF ring are excreted in greater abundance than are PGD-ring metabolites. Infusion of PGD_2 into animals causes systemic hypotension and increases in pulmonary artery pressure.[244] Infusion of PGD_2 in humans also causes flushing.[245] The possibility that PGD_2 is an important mediator in mastocytosis is supported by studies demonstrating that in patients in whom antihistamine therapy was not associated with an amelioration of humoral symptoms, the addition of inhibitors of prostaglandin biosynthesis improved the symptoms.[240–243] In summary, both histamine and PGD_2 participate as mediators of the humoral symptoms of systemic mast cell activation, and in many patients, PGD_2 is a more important mediator than histamine.

Symptoms

As noted previously, two broad categories of systemic mast cell disorders can be distinguished; those involving mast cell infiltration of various tissues and organs and those in which evidence of proliferation of mast cells is lacking. Heterogeneity exists within each of the categories as to symptoms and their severity. The symptoms can involve almost every organ system. Certain symptoms may be prominent and severe in some patients but minor or absent in others. It is rare for an individual patient to experience all the symptoms associated with the disease. In general, patients with mastocytosis limited to cutaneous involvement experience symptoms localized to the skin, whereas patients with systemic proliferation or systemic mast cell activation syndrome (idiopathic analphylaxis) experience systemic symptoms. Because of the various combinations and different severity of symptoms, the clinical presentation can mimic a variety of unrelated medical disorders. For these reasons, mast cell activation disorders often go unrecognized and lead to erroneous diagnoses.[217] This problem seems particularly true in patients who do not have urticaria pigmentosa as a cutaneous clue to the disease.

Levels of mast cell mediators in the circulation and urine are usually elevated at all times in patients with systemic mastocytosis in whom there is an increased burden of mast cells in the body. In contrast, in patients with idiopathic mastocyte activation in whom the burden of mast cells in the body is

normal, levels of mast cell mediators are usually normal during asymptomatic periods. However the triggering of mast cells by largely unknown factors to release increased quantities of mediators episodically causes paroxysmal symptoms, frequently referred to as "attacks" by patients. After attacks of moderate to marked severity, profound lethargy and drowsiness may last for several hours, possibly related to the fact that PGD_2 is a sleep-inducing substance.[246] After recovery from a severe episode of mastocyte activation, many patients notice an improvement in symptoms and a feeling of general well-being for several days. This phenomenon may be due to depletion of mediators during a severe attack, followed by a slow replenishment. Although the frequency of attacks in most patients is rather constant, some experience periods of months without attacks and periods in which attacks may occur almost daily. The duration of attacks varies from a few minutes to several hours. Most episodes of mastocyte activation last between 30 and 60 min. In general, milder attacks are shorter in duration than severe attacks.

Symptoms are summarized in Table 37–6. Owing to the variation in symptoms between individuals, the prevalence of symptoms will be discussed in general terms, that is, common or uncommon.

Flushing, which is an important clinical clue to the diagnosis, occurs almost invariably in patients who experience systemic symptoms, occurs predominantly in the face and upper trunk (flush area) and usually is diffuse rather than mottled or patchy. Occasionally patients do not realize that they are flushed, do not spontaneously complain of flushing, and may even deny it, but it is usually possible to elicit a history of feeling hot during attacks. Flushing also may not be evident when a severe attack is accompanied by a fall in systemic blood pressure of sufficient magnitude to prevent the filling of dilated cutaneous blood vessels. Consequently the lack of a flushed appearance in a patient with unexplained shock does not exclude the possibility of massive mast cell mediator release. In such patients however flushing can sometimes be observed as the attack resolves and the blood pres-

TABLE 37–6. Symptoms of Mastocytosis and Systemic Mast Cell Activation

Flushing	Pruritus
Palpitations	Diarrhea
Lightheadedness	Nausea and vomiting
Syncope	Chronic fatigue
Dyspnea	Paresthesias
Chest pain	Central nervous system dysfunction
Headache	

sure rises. A flushed appearance of the skin can also be seen in patients who do not experience systemic symptoms and appear to have mastocytosis limited to the skin. In this situation however cutaneous vasodilation does not result from high circulating levels of vasodilating mast cell mediators but from the local release of these mediators in the skin. Flushing of the skin in these patients is usually not limited to the face and upper trunk and may be mottled and patchy rather than diffuse.

Palpitations are common during episodes of flushing; with severe flushing the heart rate may increase to as much as 150 beats/min or more. Tachycardia is predominantly a secondary baroreceptor response to systemic vasodilation, although histamine may contribute directly through a positive chronotropic effect on the heart.[247]

Lightheadedness and a feeling of faintness occur during severe attacks of flushing accompanied by systemic vasodilation and a fall in blood pressure. Characteristically, the lightheadedness improves when the patient assumes the supine position, and the shock and syncope usually are not prolonged and thus rarely progress to refractory vascular collapse or death.[243] The onset of attacks may be rapid and cause syncope or near-syncope in less than a minute, which can be dangerous, as when the patient is driving a car. Occasionally syncope may develop so rapidly that antecedent flushing is not appreciated, even though it is present during milder episodes. After syncope some patients exhibit amnesia for symptoms and events occurring before the syncopal episode, presumably the consequence of cerebral ischemia during the attack. In summary, the failure to elicit a history of flushing before syncopal episodes does not exclude the possibility of mastocytosis.

Headaches are common and are usually bilateral and throbbing in nature. Many patients have chronic headaches, and in others headaches occur only during an attack of flushing. Headaches are probably due to dilation of cranial vessels.

Dyspnea is common with intense flushing, and a fall in forced expiratory volume in 1 second (FEV$_1$) can usually be documented. However dyspnea is rarely accompanied by subjective or auscultatory wheezing unless underlying hyperreactive airway disease is present.

Chest pain is also frequent during attacks. Although usually mild, it may be severe and a major presenting complaint. In most patients the chest pain does not appear to be of coronary origin because it can occur in young patients and because electrocardiograms taken during the chest pain usually fail to reveal any evidence of cardiac ischemia. Thus the origin of the chest pain remains speculative.

Many patients have intermittent mild pruritus. Severe chronic pruritus is unusual but is encountered in patients with extensive cutaneous mastocytosis. Pruritus may occur only after hot showers.

Gastrointestinal symptoms, e.g. diarrhea and abdominal pain, may be chronic in patients with systemic mastocytosis[233] but are usually only associated with episodes of mast cell mediator release in patients with idiopathic mastocyte activation disorders. Diarrhea is usually not severe but can be explosive during or after severe episodes of mastocyte activation. This pattern can be valuable in making the diagnosis because severe diarrhea is not characteristic of syncope from causes other than systemic mast cell activation, although it can occur with the carcinoid syndrome. Abdominal cramps may accompany severe attacks of flushing.

Nausea is frequent during severe attacks of flushing, but vomiting is infrequent. Nausea and vomiting between attacks are most likely unrelated to mastocytosis or mastocyte activation.

Fatigue may be severe and is typically chronic. Paresthesias during or at the beginning of episodes of flushing can involve the entire body. They have been described as a "creep-ing crawling" sensation in the skin. The pathogenesis is unknown. Abnormalities in central nervous system function include emotional lability and cognitive dysfunction. Another frequent complaint is periodic forgetfulness.[248, 249]

THE HYPERTENSIVE VARIANT. In one variant patients experience the symptoms described earlier but exhibit elevations in blood pressure, sometimes of a marked degree rather than hypotension during episodes of systemic mast cell activation. These patients also appear flushed and may experience syncope, even though they are not hypotensive. Many of these patients are thought to have a pheochromocytoma although pheochromocytoma does not cause flushing.

The pathogenesis of the hypertension might be due to differences in the metabolism of PGD$_2$, in that PGD$_2$, a vasodilator, is initially metabolized to 9α,11β-PGF$_2$ (see Fig. 37–5), which elevates the blood pressure.[250] Regardless of the etiology of the hypertension, these patients respond to the therapy described later.

Factors Provoking Mastocyte Activation

NONPHARMACOLOGIC FACTORS. The sudden onset of flushing is usually unassociated with an identifiable inciting cause. The factors that cause the sudden and synchronous systemic activation of mast cells that occurs in patients with mastocytosis and idiopathic mastocyte activation disorders are poorly understood. However many patients can identify factors or situations that may precipitate attacks, such as physical exertion, heat, and emotional anxiety.[160, 243, 251] How these factors lead to mast cell activation is unclear. In women symptoms of mastocytosis may increase just before the onset of menses, which suggests a possible influence of gonadal hormones on mast cell activation.

PHARMACOLOGIC PROVOKING AGENTS. Pharmacologic agents that activate mast cells should be avoided or used with caution (beginning with minuscule doses) in patients with mast cell disorders. The narcotic analgesics[160] that can produce severe adverse reactions include meperidine, morphine, and codeine. Intradermal injection of narcotic analgesics in normal volunteers usually elicits a typical wheal-and-flare reaction. The authors have used intravenous butorphanol for analgesia in several patients with mastocytosis without producing untoward reactions. However, we administer this drug only if there is absence of a local reaction after intradermal injection and then begin with small initial doses. Agents known to produce occasional anaphylactoid reactions and histamine release such as dextran and radiologic contrast dyes also should be avoided if possible.[252, 253] Alcohol ingestion can also evoke flushing in some patients[160]; the reaction to alcohol may not always be reproducible.

Surgical management of patients with mastocytosis can be hazardous because drugs used during surgery and anesthesia can evoke potentially fatal reactions.[254] However with appropriate precautions patients with mastocytosis can undergo surgery without adverse effects.[241, 255–257]

β-Adrenergic receptor agonists inhibit mast cell degranulation in vitro, and epinephrine can reverse severe attacks of flushing and hypotension.[258] During attacks release of endogenous epinephrine from the adrenal medulla may attenuate the severity of the attack, and β-receptor antagonists may prevent the beneficial effects of endogenous epinephrine release and render the attacks refractory to treatment with epinephrine. In addition, β-receptor antagonists prevent the increase in heart rate that serves an important role in increasing cardiac output and maintaining blood pressure. Thus β-adrenergic receptor antagonists probably cause a more profound decrease in blood pressure during episodes of mastocyte activation and therefore are contraindicated in these patients.[259] Because cholinergic and α-adrenergic agonists can potentiate mast cell mediator release,[260] administration of these agents should also probably be avoided. The antihypertensive drug clonidine can evoke mast cell mediator release in vitro, presumably through its action as an α_2-adrenergic receptor agonist.[261]

PROVOCATION BY NONSTEROIDAL ANTI-INFLAMMATORY DRUGS. In a subset of patients attacks can be induced by ingestion of aspirin or other nonsteroidal anti-inflammatory drugs,[160] and the attacks triggered by such drugs can be severe and even fatal, a phenomenon termed "aspirin hypersensitivity." Doses as low as 10 to 20 mg of aspirin can evoke these reactions in some patients. In 5 to 10% of patients with asthma, ingestion of these agents evokes severe bronchospasm,[262, 263] and in a similar percentage of patients with mastocytosis these drugs can evoke massive mast cell mediator release that can cause shock and death. Bronchospasm is usually not a prominent feature of these reactions. The mechanism is unclear. It is generally believed that these reactions do not have an allergic basis because the patients react similarly to all nonsteroidal anti-inflammatory drugs, despite their dissimilar structures. Because a common property of these drugs is an ability to inhibit prostaglandin biosynthesis, the reactions may be triggered by inhibition of prostaglandin production. Inhibition of PGD_2 production within the mast cell itself does not appear to be the triggering event.[264, 265] A clear history of provocation by nonsteroidal anti-inflammatory drugs may be absent so that cautious testing is necessary to identify the problem. Such provocative testing should be conducted only by physicians with experience in managing the severe reactions that may ensue. Repeated administration of a nonsteroidal anti-inflammatory drug may induce a state of "tolerance" to the agent in some patients, after which the dose can be escalated upward into the therapeutic range.[242, 264] Desensitization carries the same risks as provocation testing, and similar caution is required.

Diagnostic Evaluation

Recommended procedures for the diagnostic evaluation of patients suspected of having mastocytosis or a disorder of mastocyte activation are summarized in Table 37–7.[196] In patients without visible signs of cutaneous mastocytosis, a diagnosis of mast cell disease probably will not be made unless it is suspected on the basis of clinical symptoms. Indeed in activation disorders of the mast cell the physical examination and routine laboratory and radiologic tests are normal, with the possible exception of the presence of dermatographism or the acneiform lesions depicted in Figure 37–3. Therefore recognition of a compatible clinical syndrome can frequently be the critical factor that leads to a correct diagnosis. Other diseases that can mimic disorders of the mast cell, e.g. the carcinoid syndrome, must be excluded. Histologic evidence of increased proliferation of mast cells is sought in biopsies of skin lesions and bone marrow, and quantification of the levels of mast cell secretory products can aid in distinguishing patients with systemic mastocytosis from those who have only an activation disorder of the mastocyte. The important biochemical finding that distinguishes between these two groups of disorders is that patients with systemic mastocytosis usually have chronic sustained elevations of mast cell secretory products, e.g. in urine, which is thought to reflect an increased mast cell burden in the body. Understandably when these patients experience an episode of mast cell activation, mediator levels increase further. In contrast in patients with an activation disorder of the mastocyte in the absence of abnormal proliferation of mast cells, levels of mast cell mediators are usually within normal limits during asymptomatic periods; increased levels of mast cell mediators are usually detected only during episodes of systemic mast cell activation.

Histologic Evaluation

Biopsy of skin, bone marrow, and at times other organs is essential to diagnose abnormal mast cell proliferation. The pathologist must be informed that mastocytosis is suspected because it is difficult to recognize mast cells unless the tissue sample is prepared with a mast cell stain such as toluidine blue.

Histologic examination of biopsies of urticaria pigmentosa lesions reveals increased numbers of mast cells.[209, 216] Lesser degrees of mast cell hyperplasia can also be observed in nonlesional skin in some, but not all, patients with cutaneous mastocytosis.[176] Thus urticaria pigmentosa is easily recognized histopathologically, whereas the interpretation of biopsies of nonlesional skin is more difficult, in part because increased mast cell proliferation may not involve all areas of skin homogeneously. It is of interest that an increase in the numbers of mast cells in the skin is found in patients with idiopathic flushing/anaphylaxis, although less than in urticaria pigmentosa lesions.[176] However, this finding in isolation is insufficient to establish a diagnosis.

Examination of bone marrow for lesions of mastocytosis can be helpful in establishing a diagnosis of systemic mastocytosis. As with skin a single sample may not be representative of the entire bone marrow. The authors' experience is that it is preferable to perform a bone marrow biopsy rather than an aspirate of the marrow. Aspiration of the bone marrow can cause degranulation of mast cells, which will not be detected by mast cell stains. We have also observed sudden and severe hypotension attributed to mast cell degranulation during aspiration of bone marrow in a patient with unusually dense infiltration of mast cells in the marrow. Consequently in patients with severe attacks, it is advisable, if possible, to perform the bone marrow biopsy when the patient is on therapeutic doses of antihistamines and a prostaglandin biosynthesis inhibitor to minimize activation of mast cells in the bone marrow from the procedure.

Under certain circumstances other tissues may be biopsied for assessment of abnormal mast cell proliferation. For example an accessible enlarged lymph node may be excised or biopsied, a biopsy of the liver might be undertaken to rule out other causes of liver disease, and biopsies of the stomach or colon may be obtained at endoscopy.

Biochemical Approaches in the Diagnosis of Mast Cell Disease

During mast cell activation mast cell secretory products released in increased amounts include histamine, PGD_2, tryp-

---

TABLE 37–7. Recommended Diagnostic Evaluation of Patients Suspected of Having Infiltrative Mast Cell Disease or a Noninfiltrative Activation Disorder of Mast Cells

Evaluation When Mastocytosis Is Suspected:
I. Routine evaluation
   A. Skin examination—gross and microscopic
   B. Bone marrow biopsy
   C. 24-h urine for mediator measurements
II. Additional studies
   A. Bone scan/skeletal survey
   B. Gastrointestinal/abdominal evaluation: upper GI series with small bowel examination, computed tomography scan of abdomen, endoscopy if indicated
   C. Electroencephalogram and neuropsychiatric evaluation, if indicated

Evaluation When a Noninfiltrative Activation Disorder of Mast Cells Is Suspected
I. Measure mediator levels in three serial 1-h urine specimens collected following an episode thought to involve activation of mast cells and/or in plasma obtained during an episode
II. Allergy evaluation

tase, and heparin, and quantification of these products and their metabolites can provide a biochemical basis for the diagnosis of systemic mast cell disorders.[175] As discussed previously, patients with systemic mastocytosis usually have chronic sustained increased urinary levels of metabolites of histamine and PGD_2, reflecting an increased mast cell burden in the body. In contrast, patients with activation disorders of mast cells usually have increased urinary excretion of metabolites of histamine and PGD_2 only in urines collected during an episode of systemic mastocyte activation, and levels are normal during asymptomatic periods. Thus in a patient who has no cutaneous lesions characteristic of cutaneous mastocytosis and has no other findings that would lead one to suspect a diagnosis of mastocytosis, e.g. hepatosplenomegaly or bone disease, a finding of a normal excretion of these metabolites in a 24-h urine collected when the patient is asymptomatic suggests that systemic mastocytosis is unlikely. However, in the absence of cutaneous lesions and other signs of mastocytosis, a finding of increased levels of metabolites of mast cell mediators in urine during asymptomatic times suggests that proliferative mast cell disease may be present. Such a finding is a strong indication to obtain a bone marrow biopsy for histologic examination.

MEASUREMENT OF HISTAMINE PRODUCTION. The formation and release of histamine from mast cells can be assessed best by measuring metabolites of histamine rather than unmetabolized histamine both in plasma and in urine. Determination of histamine levels in plasma is complicated by the fact that basophils can be activated to release histamine during blood sampling and plasma isolation and cause artifactual elevation in histamine levels. This problem can be circumvented by measuring the histamine metabolite, N-methylhistamine (see Table 37–4). For an integrated assessment of endogenous histamine production, the 24-h urinary excretion of histamine or its metabolites, N-methylhistamine and methylimidazoleacetic acid, should be measured. The interpretation of measurements of unmetabolized histamine in urine is complicated. High levels of histamine can be present in urine because of decarboxylation of histidine by genitourinary tract bacteria, particularly in women. Consequently it is sometimes unclear whether an isolated finding of an elevated level of urinary histamine reflects systemic endogenous production of histamine. However, an increase followed by a return to baseline levels of histamine in serial urines collected following an episode suspected of representing systemic activation of mast cells can probably be interpreted with confidence.[175] The problem of artifactual generation of histamine by genitourinary tract bacteria can be completely circumvented by measuring metabolites of histamine.[175]

Furthermore patients with systemic mastocytosis can have a normal level of urinary histamine but increased levels of the histamine metabolites, N-methylhistamine and methylimidazoleacetic acid, in urine.[175, 266] Thus quantification of histamine metabolites appears to be a more sensitive index of overproduction of histamine in patients with mastocytosis. Unfortunately assays for histamine metabolites are mass spectrometric methods and available in only a few laboratories. An immunoassay has been developed for the determination of N-methylhistamine but its accuracy is compromised by significant cross-reactivity of the antibody with histamine.[267]

Another problem with determination of histamine is that the most widely used methods are radioenzymatic and fluorometric assays that at times can be inaccurate.[268] Mass spectrometric methods for measurement of histamine are not widely available.[269]

Another problem in assessing endogenous production of histamine is that the levels of histamine and its metabolites can be influenced by diet.[270] Thus foods such as cheese, spinach, eggplant, and chicken liver that contain large quantities of histamine and foods with high histidine content, e.g. meat,

can artifactually increase the urinary excretion of histamine and its metabolites.[271] It is advisable to quantify the urinary excretion of these compounds under controlled dietary conditions.

MEASUREMENT OF PRODUCTION OF PROSTAGLANDIN D_2. The endogenous production of PGD_2 can be assessed by quantifying the major urinary metabolite of PGD_2, 9α-hydroxy-11,15-dioxo-2,3,18,19-tetranorprost-5-ene-1,20-dioic acid.[272, 273] The excretion of PGD_2 metabolites may be increased up to 150-fold in patients with systemic mastocytosis.[175, 243] Increased levels of the urinary metabolites of PGD_2 can also be demonstrated in the circulation of patients with systemic mastocytosis as well as allergic analyphylaxis.[274] Thus, when a patient is seen by medical personnel for an "attack" that, in retrospect, is thought to represent an episode of mast cell activation, the diagnosis can be confirmed by measuring levels of the PGD_2 metabolites in stored plasma. Plasma levels of the metabolite peak at about 2 h following the release of PGD_2 and remain elevated for as long as 6 h. Thus blood can be obtained for measurement of the PGD_2 metabolite for several hours after the episode of mastocyte activation has dissipated. Another major advantage with measuring PGD_2 metabolites compared to measuring histamine metabolites is that the fold-increases in the excretion of the major urinary metabolite of PGD_2 significantly exceed those of histamine metabolites in patients with systemic mastocytosis.[199] Thus whereas measurements of histamine metabolites are a more sensitive indicator of mastocytosis than measurement of histamine, the sensitivity of measuring metabolites of PGD_2 exceeds that of measuring histamine metabolites as a diagnostic indicator of mastocytosis. Unfortunately the assay for the PGD_2 metabolite is currently available in only a single laboratory and is a research procedure.[272, 273] One problem with measuring metabolites of PGD_2 is that such measurements must be made in the absence of recent ingestion of nonsteroidal anti-inflammatory agents.

MEASUREMENT OF TRYPTASE RELEASE. Increased quantities of the granule-associated enzyme tryptase can be detected by immunoassay in plasma during anaphylaxis and in some patients with systemic mastocytosis.[275, 276] Peak concentrations occur approximately 1 to 2 h after mastocyte activation.[277]

ASSESSMENT OF EXCESS HEPARIN RELEASE. During severe attacks indirect evidence of release of excessive quantities of heparin can be obtained by measurement of the partial thromboplastin time.[278, 279] Correction of prolonged partial thromboplastin time by protamine provides evidence that the defect in coagulation is a result of increased circulating heparin. Release of sufficient quantities of heparin from mast cells to prolong the partial thromboplastin time is seen only in association with severe episodes of mastocyte activation but when present is a convenient and inexpensive method of confirming severe systemic mastocyte activation.

Radiologic Studies

Radioisotopic scans of the liver and spleen and CT or magnetic resonance imaging of the abdomen are useful in assessing whether hepatosplenomegaly is present. A bone survey and radioisotope scans of bone are also useful in detecting the presence of bone disease. Assessment of the presence of bone disease in the iliac crest can also be useful as a guide to direct sampling of bone marrow for histologic examination.

All patients should undergo examination of the stomach and small bowel, for two reasons. First, small mucosal nodules and nonspecific abnormalities such as bowel wall thickening may be seen. Second, because the treatment of many patients may involve prolonged administration of ulcerogenic, nonsteroidal anti-inflammatory drugs, endoscopic or radiologic screening for peptic ulcer disease is appropriate.

Other Clinical Evaluations and Laboratory Studies

Modest eosinophilia may be present in patients with indolent mastocytosis, and marked eosinophilia is seen in patients with aggressive mast cell disease, that is, lymphadenopathy with eosinophilia. In all patients the 24-h urinary excretion of 5-HIAA should be quantified to exclude the carcinoid syndrome. Urinary excretion of 5-HIAA is not elevated even in patients with severe mastocytosis. A subset of patients with medullary carcinoma of the thyroid experience episodic flushing. However these patients usually have widely metastatic disease, and the diagnosis is usually established before they begin to experience episodes of flushing. Rarely patients with mastocytosis and idiopathic disorders of mast cell activation experience angioneurotic edema.[175] When this occurs repeatedly, other causes, such as an allergic mechanism, should be explored, and levels of C1 esterase inhibitor and C4 should be measured to exclude hereditary angioneurotic edema.

As mentioned previously, patients with mastocytosis or with idiopathic disorders of mastocyte activation frequently experience emotional lability and forgetfulness. If significant abnormal central nervous system symptoms are present, neuropsychiatric evaluation and appropriate neurologic tests may be indicated to exclude other potential causes of neuropsychiatric symptoms. A thorough allergy evaluation for atopy is important in patients with idiopathic disorders of mast cell activation to exclude an allergic basis for mastocyte activation. Although systemic symptoms due to allergies are frequently thought to occur only with ingested allergens, e.g. foods and food preservatives, episodic flushing has been observed in severely atopic patients with marked sensitivity to airborne allergens and in whom allergies to ingested allergens cannot be documented. In such patients episodic flushing may abate with desensitization therapy.

Treatment

Pharmacologic interventions are usually successful in reversing acute episodes of mastocyte activation and preventing the humoral manifestations of recurrent episodes. The ability to prevent these attacks with pharmacologic therapy has improved the prognosis of systemic disorders of mast cell activation. Furthermore in some patients with aggressive mastocytosis, additional interventions may be indicated in attempts to eradicate associated hematologic malignancies.

Treatment of the Acute Hypotensive Episode

As in the treatment of allergic anaphylaxis, epinephrine is effective in reversing the hypotension associated with mast cell mediator release.[258] Doses of epinephrine that are effective in reversing marked hypotension associated with mast cell mediator release cause only modest elevations in blood pressure and pulse rate in normal volunteers.[280] This suggests that the effects of epinephrine are not linked solely to direct pressor effects but may act predominantly by inhibiting mast cell mediator release.[258] This possibility is supported by demonstration in vitro that β-receptor agonists inhibit mast cell mediator release from antigen-challenged sensitized lung.[281]

Patients with severe vasodilation associated with hypotension should be given epinephrine either subcutaneously or by intravenous infusion. The subcutaneous injection of 300 μg is usually effective in reversing hypotension, but the action may be short-lived owing to rapid absorption and metabolic inactivation of the drug. Thus maintenance of the effect of epinephrine is best achieved by continuous intravenous infusion at a rate of 2 to 10 μg/min. Beginning with an initial dose of 4 μg/min, the dose can be subsequently adjusted, depending on the response. After return of blood pressure to normal and resolution of other symptoms, the dose of epinephrine should be reduced by decrements of about 1 μg/min at hourly intervals until discontinued or until the requirement for continued infusion becomes apparent with return of flushing and other symptoms.

In the subset of patients with elevation in blood pressure and tachycardia rather than hypotension during episodes of systemic mast cell activation, the administration of epinephrine lowers blood pressure and heart rate to normal or nearly normal levels. This response supports the assumption that the increase in blood pressure is causatively linked in some way to mast cell mediator release, possibly involving 9α,11β-PGF$_2$, as discussed previously.

It is important to instruct patients who have experienced severe attacks to self-administer epinephrine as outpatients when an attack occurs and medical help is not immediately available. Outpatient use of epinephrine can be in the form of subcutaneous injection or inhalation. EpiPen (Center Laboratories) and ANA-KIT (Bayer Corporation) are commercially available, predosed syringes for subcutaneous injection designed to deliver 300 μg of epinephrine. The EpiPen syringe is preferred because it automatically injects the epinephrine, whereas the ANA-KIT syringe is more difficult and cumbersome to use. Ease of handling becomes an important consideration because when self-injection of epinephrine is required to abort an attack, the patient is frequently very lightheaded and unable to function normally. A convenient means of administering smaller doses of epinephrine is by inhalation, e.g. with Primatene Inhaler, which is available over the counter. An advantage of the use of inhalers is that repeated doses can be given if symptoms recur, whereas patients usually carry only a single EpiPen syringe. It is important to instruct patients to inhale the Primatene mist deep into the lungs to enhance the systemic absorption of epinephrine. If patients wait until the severity of the attack escalates, the inhalation of epinephrine may be unsuccessful in aborting the attack. Thus patients should be instructed to use the inhaler at the first sign that an attack is evolving.

Chronic Therapy to Prevent the Effects of Mast Cell Mediator Release

ANTIHISTAMINES AND INHIBITORS OF PROSTAGLANDIN BIOSYNTHESIS

Chronic therapy for the disease is designed to reduce the quantity and effects of mediator release. Antihistamine therapy combined with inhibition of prostaglandin biosynthesis is usually effective in preventing recurrent episodes of severe vasodilation and improves other symptoms such as dyspnea, diarrhea, headache, fatigue, and pruritus.[241, 243] Blockade of both histamine H$_1$ and H$_2$ receptors is required to prevent the vasodilator effects of histamine.[282] Thus an H$_1$ receptor antagonist such as chlorpheniramine (16 to 32 mg daily) should be given in combination with an H$_2$ receptor antagonist such as ranitidine (300 mg daily). For patients who cannot tolerate the drowsiness that many of the first-generation H$_1$ antagonists cause, nonsedating H$_1$ antagonists should be used, e.g. loratidine (10 mg daily). Other nonsedating H$_1$ antagonists (terfenadine and astemizole) have the drawback that they can cause cardiac arrhythmias, particularly when combined with medications that inhibit their metabolism by hepatic CYP (P450) enzymes. Doxepin is a potent antihistamine, but many patients cannot tolerate the central nervous system side effects of this drug, even with doses in the range of 5 to 20 mg daily.[283] However doxepin can be useful in the treatment of refractory pruritus, although higher doses up to 100 to 150 mg daily may be required.

Nonsteroidal anti-inflammatory drugs inhibit the cyclooxygenase enzyme that catalyzes the formation of prostaglandins. Although numerous nonsteroidal anti-inflammatory drugs are available, there are advantages to the use of aspirin. Aspirin is inexpensive, and therapy can be monitored with plasma salicylate determinations. Assays for other nonsteroidal anti-inflammatory drugs are not generally available. Monitoring of drug levels is of value because interindividual variation in absorption and metabolism can cause differences in plasma levels.[284] Documentation that an effective blood level of drug is achieved is of critical importance in patients who experience recurrent episodes of life-threatening hypotension. In the authors' experience plasma salicylate levels in the range of 1.5 to 2 μmol/L (20 to 30 mg/dL) measured 4 to 5 h after a dose are usually required to prevent the recurrence of severe episodes of vasodilation.[241] In most adults the dose of aspirin required to achieve a plasma salicylate level in this range is 3.9 to 5.2 g/d. If salicylates are not well tolerated because of tinnitus or are absorbed poorly, another nonsteroidal anti-inflammatory drug such as naproxen sodium or ketoprofen should be substituted, usually at the maximum recommended doses. One problem with the use of nonsteroidal anti-inflammatory agents for systemic mastocytosis is that these patients frequently have gastric acid hypersecretion, presumably owing to the constant overproduction of histamine, and cannot tolerate the gastric side effects of these drugs, even if they are given in conjunction with histamine H_2 receptor antagonists.[241]

As discussed earlier, approximately 5% of patients with mastocytosis and idiopathic disorders of mast cell activation syndrome exhibit aspirin hypersensitivity. In these patients ingestion of minuscule doses of aspirin or other nonsteroidal anti-inflammatory drugs can evoke potentially lethal vasodilatory shock. Therefore initiation of aspirin therapy must be undertaken with caution. In some patients a clear-cut history of frequent ingestion of recommended adult doses of aspirin or other nonsteroidal anti-inflammatory drugs without untoward effect can be elicited. In such patients there is less concern about initiating therapy with therapeutic doses of aspirin or other nonsteroidal anti-inflammatory drugs. Acetaminophen generally does not evoke mastocyte activation in patients with aspirin hypersensitivity because it is a very weak inhibitor of the cyclooxygenase. The important point to recognize is that many patients take acetaminophen rather than aspirin for analgesia and that a history of no adverse reactions following ingestion of acetaminophen does not exclude the possibility of aspirin hypersensitivity. Because aspirin is generally considered to be a trivial drug that can be taken casually, some people with aspirin hypersensitivity who have frequent attacks and take aspirin may not make the association that episodes of mastocyte activation are triggered by ingestion of aspirin. Accordingly it is prudent to initiate aspirin therapy under careful observation in all such patients. When it is not known whether a patient has aspirin hypersensitivity, the initial dose should be small, 20 mg or less if attacks have been severe. Reactions to aspirin usually occur between 30 min and 3 h after ingestion, and if no adverse effects are seen with the initial dose, the amount can be doubled at 6-h intervals until a therapeutic single dose of aspirin (975 mg) has been given in the absence of an untoward reaction. Severe reactions to aspirin associated with hypotension can be treated with intravenous epinephrine, as discussed earlier. Patients with aspirin-evoked mast cell activation should be instructed in the avoidance of all nonsteroidal anti-inflammatory drugs and probably of tartrazine, which in some patients may also evoke reactions for unclear reasons. Most of these patients can take acetaminophen without precipitating an episode of mastocyte activation. However if a patient has never taken acetaminophen the drug should initially be given in small doses, as described earlier with aspirin challenge.

Treatment of patients with aspirin-evoked mast cell activation disorders is problematic. Antihistamines should be administered but, as discussed previously, rarely are effective in preventing the humoral symptoms, e.g. vasodilation, associated with episodes of mastocyte activation. Severe attacks of mastocyte activation in these patients may be aborted by the self-administration of epinephrine by subcutaneous injection and/or inhalation.

MAST CELL–"STABILIZING" AGENTS

Other approaches to chronically prevent episodes of mast cell activation in patients who cannot tolerate nonsteroidal anti-inflammatory drugs because of aspirin hypersensitivity or gastric side effects are available, but their efficacy is not well established. Isolated reports suggest that oral administration of cromolyn sodium may control diarrhea in patients with mastocytosis,[285, 286] a report of amelioration of systemic symptoms of mastocytosis with the use of oral cromolyn ($\sim$200 mg four times daily) was encouraging.[248] However in subsequent studies, it was concluded that, although cromolyn can be effective in controlling diarrhea, it rarely ameliorates the systemic humoral symptoms.[239, 287–290] The effectiveness of cromolyn in controlling diarrhea and its ineffectiveness for the humoral symptoms of mastocyte activation can probably be attributed to the fact that only approximately 1% of the drug is absorbed after oral administration.[291]

Another mast cell–stabilizing drug is ketotifen, which is not marketed in the United States but is available in many countries. The efficacy of this agent in ameliorating the symptoms of mastocytosis is variable, ranging from a dramatic effect in reducing symptoms to no effect at all.[241, 288–290, 292–294] In addition some studies have shown a reduction in histamine levels with ketotifen therapy whereas in others there was no change in levels of histamine or its metabolites.[288, 290, 294] In one case report, ketotifen therapy dramatically reduced symptoms and levels of histamine in plasma and urine and also reversed bone changes in a patient with mastocytosis.[294] Discrepancies in reports of the efficacy of ketotifen may be attributed in part to interindividual differences in absorption and metabolism of ketotifen and the fact that varying doses of ketotifen have been evaluated in different studies.[241, 289]

ALTERNATIVE THERAPEUTIC APPROACHES TO REDUCE SYMPTOMS AND THE NUMBERS OF MAST CELLS IN CUTANEOUS MASTOCYTOSIS

TOPICAL GLUCOCORTICOIDS. Although treatment of patients with systemic mastocytosis with oral glucocorticoids has not been effective in ameliorating the cutaneous manifestations of mastocytosis or of systemic mast cell activation, treatment of the skin with potent topical glucocorticoids under occlusion for prolonged periods, i.e. 8 h daily for 6 wk, reduces the numbers of mast cells in the skin, the cutaneous lesions, lesional histamine content, and symptoms such as pruritus. Symptoms remain improved for a mean of 11.5 mo.[295] Because the effect is not permanent, repeated courses of treatment are required to sustain the effect. However until the effects of chronic repeated treatment have been investigated, treatment with topical glucocorticoids should be considered only a temporary form of therapy.

PSORALEN AND ULTRAVIOLET LIGHT. Oral administration of 8-methoxypsoralen plus exposure of skin to ultraviolet A light (PUVA) has transiently reduced cutaneous symptoms, lesions, and mast cell numbers in the skin for a period of months.[296–299] Because repeated treatment of the skin with PUVA can lead to an enhanced incidence of skin cancer, its use should be reserved for severe cutaneous disease unresponsive to other forms of treatment, and it should be used with extreme caution in young patients.

ALTERNATIVE THERAPEUTIC APPROACHES TO REDUCE SYSTEMIC SYMPTOMS AND MAST CELL NUMBERS IN SYSTEMIC TISSUES

The mast cells in mastocytosis are resistant to therapy with commonly used cancer therapeutic agents,[300–302] and these agents should be used only for treatment of an associated hematologic malignancy.[241, 303]

Inconsistent responses ranging from dramatic reductions in mast cell numbers, symptoms, and excretion of mast cell mediators to minimal or no response have been reported following treatment of a limited number of patients with interferon α.[300, 302, 304–307] The reason for this variable response is unclear.[302] Additional experience in assessing the efficacy of interferon is necessary, and the use of interferon in this disease is currently experimental.

REFERENCES

1. Oberndorfer S. Uber die "kleinen Dumdarn-Carcinome." Verh Dtsch Ges Pathol 1907; 11:113–116.
2. Masson P. Carcinoid (argentaffin-cell tumors) and nerve hyperplasia of appendicular mucosa. Am J Pathol 1928; 4:181–212.
3. Lembeck F. 5-Hydroxytryptamine in a carcinoid tumor. Nature 1953; 172:910–911.
4. Thorson A, Bjorck G, Bjorkman G, et al. Malignant carcinoid of the small intestine with metastasis to liver, valvular disease of the right side of the heart (pulmonary stenosis and tricuspid regurgitation without septal defects), peripheral vasomotor symptoms, bronchoconstriction, and an unusual type of cyanosis. Am Heart J 1954; 47:795–817.
5. Page IH, Corcoran AC, Udenfriend S, et al. Argentaffinoma as an endocrine tumour. Lancet 1955; 1:198–199.
6. MacDonald RA. A study of 356 carcinoids of the gastrointestinal tract. Am J Med 1956; 21:867–878.
7. MacDonald RA, Robbins SL. Pathology of the heart in the carcinoid syndrome. Arch Pathol 1957; 63:103–112.
8. Sjoerdsma A, Terry LL, Udenfriend S. Malignant carcinoid: a new metabolic disorder. Arch Intern Med 1957; 99:1009–1012.
9. Haverback BJ, Davidson JD. Serotonin and the gastrointestinal tract. Gastroenterology 1958; 35:570–578.
10. MacDonald RA, Robbins SL, Mallory GK. Morphologic effects of serotonin (5-hydroxytryptamine). Arch Pathol 1958; 65:369–377.
11. Sandler M, Snow PDJ. An atypical carcinoid tumour secreting 5-hydroxytryptophan. Lancet 1958; 1:137–138.
12. Peart WS, Robertson JIS, Andrews TM. Facial flushing produced in patients with carcinoid syndrome by intravenous adrenaline and noradrenaline. Lancet 1959; 2:715–716.
13. Peskins GW, Orloff MJ. A clinical study of 25 patients with carcinoid tumors of the rectum. Surg Gynecol Obstet 1959; 109:673–682.
14. Duner H, Pernow B. Circulatory studies on substance P in man. Acta Physiol Scand 1960; 49:261–266.
15. Gottlieb LS, Broitman SA, Vitale JJ, et al. Failure of endogenous serotonin to produce lesions of the carcinoid syndrome. Arch Pathol 1960; 69:77–81.
16. Lillie RD, Glenner GG. Histochemical reactions in carcinoid tumors of the human gastrointestinal tract. Am J Pathol 1960; 36:623–651.
17. Moertel CG, Sauer WG, Dockerty MB, et al. Life history of the carcinoid tumor of the small intestine. Cancer 1961; 14:901–912.
18. Peart WS, Robertson JIS. The effect of a serotonin antagonist (UML 491) in carcinoid disease. Lancet 1961; 2:1172–1174.
19. Sandler M, Scheuer PJ, Watt PJ. 5-Hydroxytryptophan-secreting bronchial carcinoid tumour. Lancet 1961; 2:1067–1069.
20. Oates JA, Sjoerdsma A. A unique syndrome associated with secretion of 5-hydroxytryptophan by metastatic gastric carcinoids. Am J Med 1962; 32:333–344.
21. Robertson JIS, Peart WS, Andrews TM. The mechanism of facial flushes in the carcinoid syndrome. Q J Med 1962; 31:103–123.
22. Vroom FQ, Brown RE, Dempsey H, et al. Studies on several possible antiserotonin compounds in a patient with the functioning carcinoid syndrome. Ann Intern Med 1962; 56:941–945.
23. Williams ED, Celestrin LR. The association of bronchial carcinoid and pluriglandular adenomatosis. Thorax 1962; 17:120–127.
24. Levine RJ, Sjoerdsma A. Pressor amines and the carcinoid flush. Ann Intern Med 1963; 58:818–828.
25. Levine RJ, Elsas LJ, Duvall CP, et al. Malignant carcinoid tumors with and without flushing. JAMA 1963; 186:905–907.
26. Williams ED, Sandler M. The classification of carcinoid tumours. Lancet 1963; 1:238–239.
27. Wright PW, Mulder DG. Carcinoid heart disease: report of a case treated by open heart surgery. Am J Cardiol 1963; 12:864–868.
28. Caldarola VT, Jackman RJ, Moertel CG, et al. Carcinoid tumors of the rectum. Am J Surg 1964; 107:844–849.
29. Oates JA, Melmon KL, Sjoerdsma A. Release of a kinin peptide in the carcinoid syndrome. Lancet 1964; 1:514–517.
30. Roberts WC, Sjoerdsma A. The cardiac disease associated with the carcinoid syndrome (carcinoid heart disease). Am J Med 1964; 36:5–34.
31. Spatz M. Pathogenetic studies of experimentally induced heart lesions and their relation to the carcinoid syndrome. Lab Invest 1964; 13:288–300.
32. McKinney B, Crawford MA. Fibrosis in guinea pig heart produced by plantain diet. Lancet 1965; 2:880–882.
33. Melmon KL, Sjoerdsma A, Oates JA, et al. Treatment of malabsorption and diarrhea of the carcinoid syndrome with methysergide. Gastroenterology 1965; 48:18–24.
34. Melmon KL, Sjoerdsma A, Mason DT. Distinctive clinical and therapeutic aspects of the syndrome associated with bronchial carcinoid tumors. Am J Med 1965; 39:568–581.
35. Smith PM. Successful treatment of Cushing's syndrome secondary to an argentaffinoma by bilateral adrenalectomy. Proc R Soc Med 1965; 58:573–575.
36. Tammes AR. Exogenous serotonin administered to rats with liver damage. Arch Pathol 1965; 79:626–628.
37. Aroesty JM, DeWeese JA, Hoffman MJ, et al. Carcinoid heart disease: successful repair of the valvular lesions under cardiopulmonary bypass. Circulation 1966; 34:105–110.
38. Oates JA, Pettinger WA, Doctor RB. Evidence for the release of bradykinin in carcinoid syndrome. J Clin Invest 1966; 45:173–178.
39. Engelman K, Lovenberg W, Sjoerdsma A. Inhibition of serotonin synthesis by para-chlorophenylalanine in patients with the carcinoid syndrome. N Engl J Med 1967; 277:1103–1108.
40. Gardner B, Dollinger M, Silen W, et al. Studies of the carcinoid syndrome: its relationship to serotonin, bradykinin, and histamine. Surgery 1967; 61:846–852.
41. Graham JR. Cardiac and pulmonary fibrosis during methysergide therapy for headache. Am J Med Sci 1967; 254:1–12.
42. Ibaney MI, Cole VW, Russell WO, et al. Solid carcinoma of the thyroid gland. Cancer 1967; 20:706–723.
43. Jequier E, Lovenberg W, Sjoerdsma A. Tryptophan hydroxylase inhibition: mechanism by which p-chlorophenylalanine depletes rat brain serotonin. Mol Pharmacol 1967; 3:274–278.
44. Oates JA, Butler TC. Pharmacologic and endocrine aspects of carcinoid syndrome. Adv Pharmacol 1967; 5:109–128 (review).
45. Black WC. Enterochromaffin cell types and corresponding carcinoid tumors. Lab Invest 1968; 19:473–486.
46. Moertel CG, Dockerty MB, Judd ES. Carcinoid tumors of the vermiform appendix. Cancer 1968; 21:270–278.
47. Pearse AG. Common cytochemical and ultrastructural characteristics of cells producing polypeptide hormones (the APUD series) and their relevance to thyroid and ultimobranchial C cells and calcitonin. Proc R Soc [Biol] 1968; 170:71–80.
48. Thompson JC, Hirose FM, Lemmi CA, et al. Zollinger-Ellison syndrome in a patient with multiple carcinoid–islet cell tumors of the duodenum. Am J Surg 1968; 115:177–184.
49. Adamson AR, Grahame-Smith DG, Peart WS, et al. Pharmacological blockade of carcinoid flushing provoked by catecholamines and alcohol. Lancet 1969; 2:293–297.
50. Pearse AG. The cytochemistry and ultrastructure of polypeptide hormone-producing cells of the APUD series and the embryologic, physiologic, and pathologic implications of the concept. J Histochem Cytochem 1969; 17:303–313.
51. Smith RA. Bronchial carcinoid tumours. Thorax 1969; 24:43–50.
52. Satterlee WG, Serpick A, Bianchine JR. The carcinoid syndrome: chronic treatment with para-chlorophenylalanine. Ann Intern Med 1970; 72:919–921.
53. Warner RR, Blaustein AS. Coexistence of pheochromocytoma and carcinoid syndrome produced by metastatic carcinoid of the ileum. Mt Sinai J Med 1970; 37:536–548.
54. Weichert RF. The neural ectodermal origin of the peptide-secreting endocrine glands: a unifying concept for the etiology of multiple endocrine adenomatosis and the inappropriate secretion of peptide hormones by nonendocrine tumors. Am J Med 1970; 49:232–241 (review).
55. Pearse AG, Polak JM. Neural crest origin of the endocrine polypeptide (APUD) cells of the gastrointestinal tract and pancreas. Gut 1971; 12:783–788.
56. Weichert RF, Roth LM, Harkin JC. Carcinoid–islet cell tumor of the duodenum and associated multiple carcinoid tumors of the ileum: an electron microscopic study. Cancer 1971; 27:910–918.
57. Horvath E, Kovacs K, Ross RC. Medullary cancer of the thyroid gland and its possible relations to carcinoids: an ultrastructural study. Virchows Arch Pathol Anat 1972; 356:281–292.
58. Van Sickle DG. Carcinoid tumors: analysis of 61 cases, including 11 cases of carcinoid syndrome. Clevel Clin Q 1972; 39:79–86.
59. Carpena C, Kay JH, Mendez AM, et al. Carcinoid heart disease: surgery for tricuspid and pulmonary valve lesions. Am J Cardiol 1973; 32:229–233.
60. Davis Z, Moertel CG, McIlrath DC. The malignant carcinoid syndrome. Surg Gynecol Obstet 1973; 137:637–644.

61. Mengel CE, Shaffer RD. The carcinoid syndrome. In: Holland JF, Frie EI, eds. Cancer Medicine. Philadelphia: Lea & Febiger, 1973: 1584–1594.

62. Friesen SR, Hermreck AS, Mantz FA Jr. Glucagon, gastrin, and carcinoid tumors of the duodenum, pancreas, and stomach: polypeptide "apudomas" of the foregut. Am J Surg 1974; 127:90–101.

63. Pearse AG, Polak JM, Heath CM. Polypeptide hormone production by "carcinoid" apudomas and their relevant cytochemistry. Virchows Arch [Cell Pathol] 1974; 16:95–109.

64. Godwin JD. Carcinoid tumors: an analysis of 2,837 cases. Cancer 1975; 36:560–569.

65. Samaan NA, Hickey RC, Bedner TD, et al. Hyperparathyroidism and carcinoid tumor. Ann Intern Med 1975; 82:205–207.

66. Ferrans VJ, Roberts WC. The carcinoid endocardial plaque: an ultrastructural study. Hum Pathol 1976; 7:387–409.

67. Mason RA, Steane PA. Carcinoid syndrome: its relevance to the anaesthetist. Anaesthesia 1976; 31:228–242.

68. Mason RA, Steane PA. Anaesthesia for a patient with carcinoid syndrome. Anaesthesia 1976; 31:243–246.

69. Sonksen PH, Ayres AB, Braimbridge M, et al. Acromegaly caused by pulmonary carcinoid tumours. Clin Endocrinol 1976; 5:503–513.

70. Allison DJ, Modlin IM, Jenkins WJ. Treatment of carcinoid liver metastases by hepatic-artery embolisation. Lancet 1977; 2:1323–1325.

71. Alumets J, Hakanson R, Ingemansson S, et al. Substance P and 5-HT in granules isolated from an intestinal argentaffin carcinoid. Histochemistry 1977; 52:217–222.

72. Hakanson R, Bengmark S, Brodin E, et al. Substance P–like immunoreactivity in intestinal carcinoid tumors. In: von Euler US, Pernow B, eds. Substance P. New York: Raven, 1977: 55–58.

73. Legha SS, Valdivieso M, Nelson RS, et al. Chemotherapy for metastatic carcinoid tumors: experiences with 32 patients and a review of the literature. Cancer Treat Rep 1977; 61:1699–1703.

74. Schlegel W, Raptis S, Dollinger HC, et al. Inhibitors of secretin, pancreozymin and gastric release and their biological activities by somatostatin. In: Bonfils S, Fromageot P, Rosselin G, et al eds. First International Symposium on Hormonal Receptors in Digestive Tract Physiology. INSERM Symposium No. 3. Amsterdam: Elsevier/North-Holland, 1977: 361–367.

75. Feldman JM. Serotonin metabolism in patients with carcinoid tumors: incidence of 5-hydroxytryptophan–secreting tumors. Gastroenterology 1978; 75:1109–1114.

76. Frolich JC, Bloomgarden ZT, Oates JA, et al. The carcinoid flush: provocation by pentagastrin and inhibition by somatostatin. N Engl J Med 1978; 299:1055–1057.

77. Maempel FZ, Modlin I. Diagnosis and management of gastric carcinoid tumour with hepatic metastases. Br J Surg 1978; 65:516–520.

78. Miller R, Patel AU, Warner RR, et al. Anaesthesia for the carcinoid syndrome: a report of nine cases. Can Anaesth Soc J 1978; 25:240–244.

79. Thulin L, Samnegard H, Tyden G, et al. Efficacy of somatostatin in a patient with carcinoid syndrome. Lancet 1978; 2:43 (letter).

80. Moertel CG, Hanley JA. Combination chemotherapy trials in metastatic carcinoid tumor and the malignant carcinoid syndrome. Cancer Clin Trials 1979; 2:327–334.

81. Roberts LJ, Marney SR Jr, Oates JA. Blockade of the flush associated with metastatic gastric carcinoid by combined histamine H₁ and H₂ receptor antagonists: evidence for an important role of H₂ receptors in human vasculature. N Engl J Med 1979; 300:236–238.

82. Wilander E, Grimelius L, Portela-Gomes G, et al. Substance P and enteroglucagon-like immunoreactivity in argentaffin and argyrophil midgut carcinoid tumours. Scand J Gastroenterol Suppl 1979; 53:19–25.

83. Davis GR, Camp RC, Raskin P, et al. Effect of somatostatin infusion on jejunal water and electrolyte transport in a patient with secretory diarrhea due to malignant carcinoid syndrome. Gastroenterology 1980; 78:346–349.

84. Dharmsathaphorn K, Sherwin RS, Cataland S, et al. Somatostatin inhibits diarrhea in the carcinoid syndrome. Ann Intern Med 1980; 92:68–69.

85. Goedert M, Otten U, Suda K, et al. Dopamine, norepinephrine and serotonin production by an intestinal carcinoid tumor. Cancer 1980; 45:104–107.

86. Klapdor R. Effects of somatostatin on bronchial constriction in a patient with carcinoid syndrome. N Engl J Med 1980; 303:464 (letter).

87. Shihabi ZK, Scaro J. Liquid-chromatographic assay of urinary 5-hydroxy-3-indoleacetic acid, with electrochemical detection. Clin Chem 1980; 26:907–909.

88. Skrabanek P, Dervan P, Cannon D, et al. Substance P in ovarian carcinoid. J Clin Pathol 1980; 33:160–162.

89. Erspamer V. The tachykinin peptide family. Trends Neurosci 1981; 4:267–269.

90. Ratzenhofer M, Gamse R, Hofler H, et al. Substance P in an argentaffin carcinoid of the caecum: biochemical and biological characterization. Virchows Arch [A] 1981; 392:21–31.

91. Callahan JA, Wroblewski EM, Reeder GS, et al. Echocardiographic features of carcinoid heart disease. Am J Cardiol 1982; 50:762–768.

92. Melia WM, Nunnerley HB, Johnson PJ, et al. Use of arterial devascularization and cytotoxic drugs in 30 patients with the carcinoid syndrome. Br J Cancer 1982; 46:331–339.

93. Martin JK Jr, Moertel CG, Adson MA, et al. Surgical treatment of functioning metastatic carcinoid tumors. Arch Surg 1983; 118:537–542.

94. Oberg K, Funa K, Alm GV. Effects of leukocyte interferon on clinical symptoms and hormone levels in patients with mid-gut carcinoid tumors and carcinoid syndrome. N Engl J Med 1983; 309:129–133.

95. Roberts LJ, Bloomgarden ZT, Marney SR Jr, et al. Histamine release from a gastric carcinoid: provocation by pentagastrin and inhibition by somatostatin. Gastroenterology 1983; 84:272–275.

96. Yang K, Ulich T, Cheng L, et al. The neuroendocrine products of intestinal carcinoids: an immunoperoxidase study of 35 carcinoid tumors stained for serotonin and eight polypeptide hormones. Cancer 1983; 51:1918–1926.

97. Emson PC, Gilbert RF, Martensson H, et al. Elevated concentrations of substance P and 5-HT in plasma in patients with carcinoid tumors. Cancer 1984; 54:715–718.

98. Engstrom PF, Lavin PT, Moertel CG, et al. Streptozocin plus fluorouracil versus doxorubicin therapy for metastatic carcinoid tumor. J Clin Oncol 1984; 2:1255–1259.

99. Fischbach FT. Manual of Laboratory Diagnostic Tests. Philadelphia: JB Lippincott, 1984: 160–162.

100. Forman MB, Byrd BF, Oates JA, et al. Two-dimensional echocardiography in the diagnosis of carcinoid heart disease. Am Heart J 1984; 107:492–496.

101. Hunter JC, Miaggio JE. Pharmacologic characterization of a novel tachykinin isolated from mammalian spinal cord. Eur J Pharmacol 1984; 97:159–160.

102. Nawa H, Doteuchi M, Igano K, et al. Substance K: a novel mammalian tachykinin that differs from substance P in its pharmacological profile. Life Sci 1984; 34:1153–1160.

103. O'Connor DT, Frigon RP, Sokoloff RL. Human chromogranin A: purification and characterization from catecholamine storage vesicles of human pheochromocytoma. Hypertension 1984; 6:2–12.

104. Mailman RB, Kilts CD. Analytical considerations for quantitative determination of serotonin and its metabolically related products in biological matrices. Clin Chem 1985; 31:1849–1854.

105. Roth KA, Makk G, Beck O, et al. Isolation and characterization of substance P, substance P 5–11, and substance K from two metastatic ileal carcinoids. Regul Pept 1985; 12:185–199.

106. Tatemoto K, Lundberg JM, Jornvall H, et al. Neuropeptide K: isolation, structure and biological activities of a novel brain tachykinin. Biochem Biophys Res Commun 1985; 128:947–953.

107. Theodorsson-Norheim E, Norheim I, Oberg K, et al. Neuropeptide K: a major tachykinin in plasma and tumor tissues from carcinoid patients. Biochem Biophys Res Comm 1985; 131:77–83.

108. Conlon JM, Deacon CF, Richter G, et al. Measurement and partial characterization of the multiple forms of neurokinin A–like immunoreactivity in carcinoid tumours. Regul Pept 1986; 13:183–196.

109. Kvols LK, Moertel CG, O'Connell MJ, et al. Treatment of the malignant carcinoid syndrome: evaluation of a long-acting somatostatin analogue. N Engl J Med 1986; 315:663–666.

110. O'Connor DT, Deftos LJ. Secretion of chromogranin A by peptide-producing endocrine neoplasms. N Engl J Med 1986; 314:1145–1151.

111. Oates JA. The carcinoid syndrome. N Engl J Med 1986; 315:702–704 (editorial).

112. Oberg K, Norheim I, Lind E, et al. Treatment of malignant carcinoid tumors with human leukocyte interferon: long-term results. Cancer Treat Rep 1986; 70:1297–1304.

113. Einhorn S, Vanky F, Grander D, et al. Induction of 2′,5′-oligoadenylate synthetase in freshly separated malignant cells from solid tumors: variability in the susceptibility of interferon. Eur J Cancer Clin Oncol 1987; 23:1607–1613.

114. Lembcke B, Creutzfeldt W, Schleser S, et al. Effect of the somatostatin analogue sandostatin (SMS 201-995) on gastrointestinal, pancreatic and biliary function and hormone release in normal men. Digestion 1987; 36:108–124.

115. Marsh HM, Martin JK Jr, Kvols LK, et al. Carcinoid crisis during anesthesia: successful treatment with a somatostatin analogue. Anesthesiology 1987; 66:89–91.

116. Norheim I, Oberg K, Theodorsson-Norheim E, et al. Malignant carcinoid tumors: an analysis of 103 patients with regard to tumor localization, hormone production, and survival. Ann Surg 1987; 206:115–125.

117. Moertel CG. Progress and hope in the treatment of gastrointestinal cancer. In: Fortner JG, Rhoads JE, eds. Accomplishments in Cancer Research 1987. Philadelphia: JB Lippincott, 1988: 295–317.

118. Feldman JM. Carcinoid tumors and the carcinoid syndrome. Curr Probl Surg 1989; 26:835–885 (review).

119. Hanson MW, Feldman JM, Blinder RA, et al. Carcinoid tumors: iodine-131 MIBG scintigraphy. Radiology 1989; 172:699–703.

120. Moertel CG, Rubin J, Kvols LK. Therapy of metastatic carcinoid tumor and the malignant carcinoid syndrome with recombinant leukocyte A interferon. J Clin Oncol 1989; 7:865–868.

121. Oberg K, Alm GV. Development of neutralizing interferon antibodies after treatment with recombinant interferon-alpha 2b in patients with malignant carcinoid tumors. J Interferon Res 1989; 9(Suppl 1):S45–S49.

122. Vinik AI, McLeod MK, Fig LM, et al. Clinical features, diagnosis, and localization of carcinoid tumors and their management. Gastroenterol Clin North Am 1989; 18:865–896 (review).

123. Eriksson B, Arnberg H, Oberg K, et al. A polyclonal antiserum against chromogranin A and B: a new sensitive marker for neuroendocrine tumours. Acta Endocrinol 1990; 122:145–155.

124. Grander D, Oberg K, Lundqvist ML, et al. Interferon-induced enhancement of 2′,5′-oligoadenylate synthetase in mid-gut carcinoid tumours [see comments]. Lancet 1990; 336:337–340.

125. Hsiao RJ, Seeger RC, Yu AL, et al. Chromogranin A in children with neuroblastoma: serum concentration parallels disease stage and predicts survival. J Clin Invest 1990; 85:1555–1559.

126. Lamberts SW, Bakker WH, Reubi JC, et al. Somatostatin-receptor imaging in the localization of endocrine tumors [see comments]. N Engl J Med 1990; 323:1246–1249.

127. Lawrence JP, Ishizuka J, Haber B, et al. The effect of somatostatin on 5-hydroxytryptamine release from a carcinoid tumor. Surgery 1990; 108:1131–1134; discussion 1134–1135.

128. Lundin L, Landelius J, Andren B, et al. Transoesophageal echocardiography improves the diagnostic value of cardiac ultrasound in patients with carcinoid heart disease. Br Heart J 1990; 64:190–194.

129. Lundin L, Hansson HE, Landelius J, et al. Surgical treatment of carcinoid heart disease. J Thorac Cardiovasc Surg 1990; 100:552–561.

130. Smith S, Anthony LB, Roberts LJ. Resolution of musculoskeletal symptoms in the carcinoid syndrome after treatment with the somatostatin analog octreotide. Ann Intern Med 1990; 112:66–68.

131. Ahlman H, Wangberg B, Jansson S, et al. Management of disseminated midgut carcinoid tumours. Digestion 1991; 49:78–96.

132. Anthony LB, Winn S, Johnson DH, et al. Continuous SC octreotide infusion for carcinoid tumor/syndrome. Proc Annu Meet Am Soc Clin Oncol 1992; 11:A485.

133. Biesma B, Willemse PH, Mulder NH, et al. Recombinant interferon alpha-2b in patients with metastatic apudomas: effect on tumours and tumour markers. Br J Cancer 1992; 66:850–855.

134. Hajarizadeh H, Ivancev K, Mueller CR, et al. Effective palliative treatment of metastatic carcinoid tumors with intra-arterial chemotherapy/chemoembolization combined with octreotide acetate. Am J Surg 1992; 163:479–483.

135. Joensuu H, Katka K, Kujari H. Dramatic response of a metastatic carcinoid tumour to a combination of interferon and octreotide. Acta Endocrinol 1992; 126:184–185.

136. Lamberts SW, Chayvialle JA, Krenning EP. The visualization of gastroenteropancreatic endocrine tumors. Metabolism 1992; 41:111–115 (review).

137. Ronnblom LE, Janson ET, Perers A, et al. Characterization of anti–interferon-alpha antibodies appearing during recombinant interferon-alpha 2a treatment. Clin Exp Immunol 1992; 89:330–335.

138. Sreide O, Berstad T, Bakka A, et al. Surgical treatment as a principle in patients with advanced abdominal carcinoid tumors. Surgery 1992; 111:48–54.

139. Steves MA, Vidal-Jove J, Sugarbaker PH, et al. Preoperative radiological evaluation of the liver by computerized tomographic portography in patients with hepatic tumors. Am Surg 1992; 58:608–612.

140. Anthony L, Johnson D, Hande K, et al. Somatostatin analogue phase I trials in neuroendocrine neoplasms. Acta Oncol 1993; 32:217–223.

141. Dorr U, Wurm K, Horing E, et al. Diagnostic reliability of somatostatin receptor scintigraphy during continuous treatment with different somatostatin analogs. Horm Metab Res Suppl 1993; 27:36–43.

142. Eriksson B, Bergstrom M, Lilja A, et al. Positron emission tomography (PET) in neuroendocrine gastrointestinal tumors. Acta Oncol 1993; 32:189–196.

143. Krenning EP, Kwekkeboom DJ, Bakker WH, et al. Somatostatin receptor scintigraphy with [^{111}In-DTPA-D-Phe^1]- and [^{123}I-Tyr^3]-octreotide: the Rotterdam experience with more than 1000 patients. Eur J Nucl Med 1993; 20:716–731 (review).

144. Kvols LK, Reubi JC. Metastatic carcinoid tumors and the malignant carcinoid syndrome. Acta Oncol 1993; 32:197–201 (review).

145. Lamberts SW, Reubi JC, Krenning EP. Validation of somatostatin receptor scintigraphy in the localization of neuroendocrine tumors. Acta Oncol 1993; 32:167–170 (review).

146. Saltz L, Trochanowski B, Buckley M, et al. Octreotide as an antineoplastic agent in the treatment of functional and nonfunctional neuroendocrine tumors. Cancer 1993; 72:244–248.

147. Schirmer WJ, O'Dorisio TM, Schirmer TP, et al. Intraoperative localization of neuroendocrine tumors with ^{125}I-TYR(3)-octreotide and a hand-held gamma-detecting probe. Surgery 1993; 114:745–51; discussion 751–752.

148. Waltenberger J, Lundin L, Oberg K, et al. Involvement of transforming growth factor-beta in the formation of fibrotic lesions in carcinoid heart disease. Am J Pathol 1993; 142:71–78.

149. Yoshikane H, Tsukamoto Y, Niwa Y, et al. Carcinoid tumors of the gastrointestinal tract: evaluation with endoscopic ultrasonography. Gastrointest Endosc 1993; 39:375–383.

150. de Herder WW, Krenning EP, Malchoff CD, et al. Somatostatin receptor scintigraphy: its value in tumor localization in patients with Cushing's syndrome caused by ectopic corticotropin or corticotropin-releasing hormone secretion [see comments]. Am J Med 1994; 96:305–312.

151. Iser G, Pfohl M, Dorr U, et al. Ectopic ACTH secretion due to a bronchopulmonary carcinoid localized by somatostatin receptor scintigraphy. Clin Invest 1994; 72:887–891.

152. Krenning EP, Kooij PP, Bakker WH, et al. Radiotherapy with a radiolabeled somatostatin analogue, [^{111}In-DTPA-D-Phe^1]-octreotide: a case history. Ann NY Acad Sci 1994; 733:496–506.

153. Moertel CG, Johnson CM, McKusick MA, et al. The management of patients with advanced carcinoid tumors and islet cell carcinomas. Ann Intern Med 1994; 120:302–309.

154. Oberg K, Eriksson B, Janson ET. Interferons alone or in combination with chemotherapy or other biologicals in the treatment of neuroendocrine gut and pancreatic tumors. Digestion 1994; 55 Suppl 3:64–69 (review).

155. Saltz L, Kemeny N, Schwartz G, et al. A phase II trial of alpha-interferon and 5-fluorouracil in patients with advanced carcinoid and islet cell tumors. Cancer 1994; 74:958–961.

156. Weiss M, Yellin A, Husza'r M, et al. Localization of adrenocorticotropic hormone–secreting bronchial carcinoid tumor by somatostatin-receptor scintigraphy. Ann Intern Med 1994; 121:198–199.

157. Anthony LB, Shyr Y, Winn SD, et al. Malignant carcinoid syndrome: survival in the somatostatin analogue era. Proc Annu Meet Am Soc Clin Oncol 1995; 14:193.

158. Que FG, Nagorney DM, Batts KP, et al. Hepatic resection for metastatic neuroendocrine carcinomas. Am J Surg 1995; 169:36–42; discussion 42–43.

159. Anthony LB, Martin W, Delbeke D, et al. Somatostatin receptor scintigraphy: predictive and prognostic considerations. Digestion 1996; 57:50–53.

160. Selye H. The Mast Cells. Washington: Butterworth, 1965.

161. Roberts LJ II, Lewis RA, Oates JA, et al. Prostaglandin, thromboxane, and 12-hydroxy-5,8,10,14-eicosatetraenoic acid production by ionophore-stimulated rat serosal mast cells. Biochim Biophys Acta 1979; 575:185–192.

162. Lewis RA, Soter NA, Diamond PT, et al. Prostaglandin D$_2$ generation after activation of rat and human mast cells with anti-IgE. J Immunol 1982; 129:1627–1631.

163. Galli SJ. New Concepts about the mast cell. N Engl J Med 1993; 328:328–265.

164. Coleman JW, Godfrey RC. The number and affinity of IgE receptors on dispersed human lung mast cells. Immunology 1981; 44:859–863.

165. Ishizaka T. Analysis of triggering events in mast cells for immunoglobulin E–mediated histamine release. J Allergy Clin Immunol 1981; 67:90–96.

166. Schwartz LB, Austen KF, Wasserman SI. Immunologic release of β-hexosaminidase and β-glucuronidase from purified rat serosal mast cells. J Immunol 1979; 123:1445–1450.

167. Yurt RW, Leid RW Jr, Spragg J, et al. Immunologic release of heparin from purified rat peritoneal mast cells. J Immunol 1977; 118:1201–1207.

168. Sullivan TJ, Parker CW. Pharmacologic modulation of inflammatory mediator release by rat mast cells. Am J Pathol 1976; 85:437–463.

169. Gross BG, Hashimoto K. Hereditary urticaria pigmentosa. Arch Dermatol 1964; 90:401–403.

170. Shaw JM. Genetic aspects of urticaria pigmentosa. Arch Dermatol 1968; 97:137–138.

171. James MP, Eady RAJ. Familial urticaria pigmentosa with giant mast cell granules. Arch Dermatol 1981; 117:713–718.

172. Lieberman P, Taylor WW. Recurrent idiopathic anaphylaxis. Arch Intern Med 1979; 139:1032–1034.

173. Sale SR, Greenberger PA, Patterson R. Idiopathic anaphylactoid reactions. JAMA 1981; 246:2336–2339.

174. Boxer M, Greenberger PA, Patterson R. Clinical summary and course of idiopathic anaphylaxis in 73 patients. Arch Intern Med 1987; 147:269–272.

175. Roberts LJ II, Oates JA. Biochemical diagnosis of systemic mast cell disorder. J Invest Dermatol 1991; 96:19S–25S.

176. Garriga MM, Friedman MM, Metcalfe DD. A survey of the number and distribution of mast cells in the skin of patients with mast cell disorders. J Allergy Clin Immunol 1988; 82:425–432.

177. Rottem M, Okada T, Goff JP, et al. Mast cells cultured from the peripheral blood of normal donors and patients with mastocytosis originate from a CD34 +/Fe epsilon RI-cell population. Blood 1994; 84:2489–2496.

178. Schumacher U, Horny HP, Welsch U. The lectin leucoagglutinin binds specifically to human granulocytes, monocytes and tissue mast cells: further evidence for a common origin of the three cell types. Br J Haematol 1987; 66:405–406.

179. Valent P, Ashman LK, Hinterberger W, et al. Mast cell typing: demonstration of a distinct hematopoietic cell type and evidence for immunophenotypic relationship to mononuclear phagocytes. Blood 1989; 73:1778–1785.

180. Austen KF. General discussion: toward a standard evaluation for data sharing and prognosis. J Invest Dermatol 1991; 96:60S–63S.

181. Weidner N, Horan RF, Austen KF. Mast-cell phenotype in indolent forms of mastocytosis: ultrastructural features, fluorescence detection of avidin binding, and immunofluorescent determination of chymase, tryptase, and carboxypeptidase. Am J Pathol 1992; 140:847–857.

182. Longley J. Is mastocytosis a mast cell neoplasia or a reactive hyperplasia? Clues from the study of mast cell growth factor. Ann Med 1994; 26:115–116.

183. Irani AA, Garriga MM, Metcalfe DD, et al. Mast cells in cutaneous mastocytosis: accumulation of the MCTC type. Clin Exp Allergy 1990; 20:53–58.

184. Longley BJ, Morganroth GS, Tyrrell L, et al. Altered metabolism of mast-cell growth factor (c-kit ligand) in cutaneous mastocytosis. N Engl J Med 1993; 328:1302–1307.

185. Williams DE, Eisenman J, Baird A, et al. Identification of a ligand for the c-kit proto-oncogene. Cell 1990; 63:167–174.

186. Flanagan JG, Leder P. The kit ligand: a cell surface molecule altered in steel mutant fibroblasts. Cell 1990; 63:185–194.

187. Anderson DM, Lyman SD, Baird A, et al. Molecular cloning of mast cell growth factor, a hematopoietin that is active in both membrane-bound and soluble forms. Cell 1990; 63:235–243.

188. Nagata H, Worobec AS, Oh CK, et al. Identification of a point mutation in the catalytic domain of the protooncogene c-kit in peripheral blood mononuclear cells of patients who have mastocytosis with an associated hematologic disorder. Proc Natl Acad Sci USA 1995; 92:10560–10564.

189. Valent P, Spanblochl E, Bankl HC, et al. Kit ligand/mast cell growth

factor–independent differentiation of mast cells in myelodysplasia and chronic myeloid leukemic blast crisis. Blood 1994; 84:4322–4332.

190. Li L, Macpherson JJ, Adelstein S, et al. Conditioned media from a cell strain derived from a patient with mastocytosis induces preferential development of cells that possess high-affinity IgE receptors and the granule protease phenotype of mature cutaneous mast cells. J Biol Chem 1995; 270:2258–2263.

191. Madden KB, Urban JF Jr, Ziltener HJ, et al. Antibodies to IL-3 and IL-4 suppress helminth-induced intestinal mastocytosis. J Immunol 1991; 147:1387–1391.

192. Abe T, Ochiai H, Minamishima Y, et al. Induction of intestinal mastocytosis in nude mice by repeated injection of interleukin-3. Int Arch Allergy Appl Immunol 1988; 86:356–358.

193. Saito H, Hatake K, Dvorak AM, et al. Selective differentiation and proliferation of hematopoietic cells induced by recombinant human interleukins. Proc Natl Acad Sci USA 1988; 85:2288–2292.

194. Keffer JM, Bressler RB, Wright R, et al. Analysis of the wheal-and-flare reactions that follow the intradermal injection of histamine and morphine in adults with recurrent, unexplained anaphylaxis and systemic mastocytosis. J Allergy Clin Immunol 1989; 83:595–601.

195. Metcalfe DD. Introduction. J Invest Dermatol 1991; 96:1S.

196. Metcalfe DD. Conclusions. J Invest Dermatol 1991; 96:64S–65S.

197. Travis WD, Li CY, Bergstralh EJ, et al. Systemic mast cell disease: analysis of 58 cases and literature review. Medicine 1988; 67:345–368.

198. Ridell B, Olafsson JH, Roupe G, et al. The bone marrow in urticaria pigmentosa and systemic mastocytosis. Arch Dermatol 1986; 122:422–427.

199. Morrow JD, Buzzo C, Lazarus GS, et al. Improved diagnosis of systemic involvement in patients with mastocytosis by measuring the urinary excretion of the major urinary metabolite of prostaglandin D_2. J Invest Dermatol 1995; 104:937–940.

200. Roupe G, Granerus G. Long-term follow-up of histamine turnover in mastocytosis. Int Archiv Allergy Appl Immunol 1987; 82:62–65.

201. Czarnetski BM, Kolde G, Schoemann A, et al. Bone marrow findings in adult patients with urticaria pigmentosa. J Am Acad Dermatol 1988; 18:45–51.

202. Travis WD, Li CY, Bergstralh EJ. Solid and hematologic malignancies in 60 patients with systemic mast cell disease. Arch Pathol Lab Med 1989; 113:365–368.

203. Kettelhut BV, Metcalfe DD. Pediatric mastocytosis. Ann Allergy 1994; 73:197–202.

204. Friedman BS, Metcalfe DD. Mastocytosis. Prog Clin Biol Res 1989; 297:163–173.

205. Kettelhut BV, Metcalfe DD. Pediatric mastocytosis. J Invest Dermatol 1991; 96:15S–18S.

206. Travis WD, Li CY, Yam LT, et al. Significance of systemic mast cell disease with associated hematologic disorders. Cancer 1988; 62:965–972.

207. Hutchinson RM. Mastocytosis and co-existent non-Hodgkin's lymphoma and myeloproliferative disorders. Leuk Lymphoma 1992; 7:29–36.

208. Horny HP, Ruck M, Wehrmann M, et al. Blood findings in generalized mastocytosis: evidence of frequent simultaneous occurrence of myeloproliferative disorders. Br J Haematol 1990; 76:186–193.

209. Sagher F, Even-Paz Z. Mastocytosis and the Mast Cell. Chicago: Year Book Medical, 1967.

210. Travis WD, Li CY, Hoagland HC, et al. Mast cell leukemia: report of a case and review of the literature. Mayo Clin Proc 1986; 61:957–966.

211. Friedman B, Darling G, Norton J, et al. Splenectomy in the management of systemic mast cell disease. Surgery 1990; 107:94–100.

212. Meggs WJ, Macher AM, Friedman MM, et al. Lymphadenopathic mastocytosis with eosinophilia. Clin Res 1985; 33:162A.

213. Metcalfe DD. Classification and diagnosis of mastocytosis: current status. J Invest Dermatol 1991; 96:2S–4S.

214. Soter NA. The skin in mastocytosis. J Invest Dermatol 1991; 96:32S–39S.

215. Meyers J. Diagnosis: urticaria pigmentosa. Arch Dermatol 1960; 81:161–162.

216. Ashinoff R, Soter NA, Freedberg IM. Solitary mastocytoma in an adult: treatment by excision. J Dermatol Surg Oncol 1993; 19:487–488.

217. Webb TA, Li CY, Yam LT. Systemic mast cell disease: a clinical hematopathologic study of 26 cases. Cancer 1982; 49:927–938.

218. Demis DJ. The mastocytosis syndrome: clinical and biological studies. Ann Intern Med 1963; 59:194–206.

219. Mican JM, Di Bisceglie AD, Fong TL, et al. Heparin involvement in mastocytosis: clinicopathologic correlations in 41 cases. Hepatology 1995; 22:1163–1170.

220. Metcalfe DD. The liver, spleen, and lymph nodes in mastocytosis. J Invest Dermatol 1991; 96:45S–46S.

221. Bonnet P, Smadja C, Szekely AM, et al. Intractable ascites in systemic mastocytosis treated by portal diversion. Dig Dis Sci 1987; 32:209–213.

222. Travis WD, Li CY. Pathology of the lymph node and spleen in systemic mast cell disease. Mod Pathol 1988; 1:4–14.

223. Sostre MS, Handler HL. Bony lesions in systemic mastocytosis. Arch Dermatol 1977; 113:1245–1247.

224. Cryer PI, Kissane JM. Osteopenia: clinicopathologic conference. Am J Med 1980; 69:915–922.

225. Chen CC, Andrich MP, Mican JM, et al. A retrospective analysis of bone scan abnormalities in mastocytosis: correlation with disease category and prognosis. J Nucl Med 1994; 35:1471–1475.

226. Parker RI. Hematologic aspects of mastocytosis: I. bone marrow pathology in adult and pediatric systemic mast cell disease. J Invest Dermatol 1991; 96:47S–51S.

227. Clemett AR, Fishbone G, Levine RJ, et al. Gastrointestinal lesions in mastocytosis. AJR 1968; 103:405–412.

228. Janower ML. Mastocytosis of the gastrointestinal tract. Acta Radiol 1962; 57:489–493.

229. Robbins AH, Schimmel EM, Rao KC. Gastrointestinal mastocytosis: radiologic alterations after ethanol ingestion. Am J Radiol 1972; 115:297–299.

230. Ammann RW, Vetter D, Deyhle P, et al. Gastrointestinal involvement in systemic mastocytosis. Gut 1976; 17:107–112.

231. Scott BB, Hardy GJ, Losowsky MS. Involvement of the small intestine in systemic mast cell disease. Gut 1975; 16:918–924.

232. Debeuckelaere S, Schoors DF, Devis G. Systemic mast cell disease: a review of the literature with special focus on the gastrointestinal manifestations. Acta Clin Belg 1991; 46:226–232.

233. Cherner JA, Jensen RT, Dubois A, et al. Gastrointestinal dysfunction in systemic mastocytosis: a prospective study. Gastroenterology 1988; 95:657–667.

234. Horny HP, Kaiserling E, Parwaresch MR. Lymph node findings in generalized mastocytosis. Histopathology 1992; 21:439–446.

235. Douglas WM. Histamine and 5-hydroxytryptamine (serotonin) and their antagonists. In: Gilman AG, Goodman LS, Gilman A, eds. Goodman and Gilman's The Pharmacologic Basis of Therapeutics. 6th ed. New York: Macmillan, 1980: 609–619.

236. Achord JL, Langford H. The effect of cimetidine and propantheline on the symptoms of a patient with systemic mastocytosis. Am J Med 1980; 69:610–614.

237. Bredfeldt JE, O'Laughlin JC, Durham JB, et al. Malabsorption and gastric hyperacidity in systemic mastocytosis. Am J Gastroenterol 1980; 74:133–137.

238. Hirschowitz BI, Groarke JF. Effect of cimetidine on gastric hypersecretion and diarrhea in systemic mastocytosis. Ann Intern Med 1979; 90:769–771.

239. Frieri M, Alling DW, Metcalfe DD. Comparison of the therapeutic efficacy of cromolyn sodium with that of combined chlorpheniramine and cimetidine in systemic mastocytosis: results of a double-blind clinical trial. Am J Med 1985; 78:9–14.

240. Lorcerie B, Arveux I, Chauffert B, et al. Aspirin and systemic mastocytosis. Lancet 1989; 2:1155.

241. Metcalfe DD. The treatment of mastocytosis: an overview. J Invest Dermatol 1991; 96:55S–59S.

242. Crawhall JC, Wilkinson RD. Systemic mastocytosis: management of an unusual case with histamine (H_1 and H_2) antagonists and cyclooxygenase inhibition. Clin Invest Med 1987; 10:1–4.

243. Roberts LJ II, Sweetman BJ, Lewis RA, et al. Increased production of prostaglandin D_2 in patients with systemic mastocytosis. N Engl J Med 1980; 303:1400–1404.

244. Wasserman MA, DuCharme DW, Griffin RL, et al. Bronchopulmonary and cardiovascular effects of prostaglandin D_2 in the dog. Prostaglandins 1977; 13:255–269.

245. Heavey DJ, Lumley P, Barrow SE, et al. Effects of intravenous infusions of prostaglandin D_2 in man. Prostaglandins 1984; 28:755–767.

246. Hayaishi O. Molecular mechanisms of sleep-wake regulation: roles of prostaglandins D_2 and E_2. FASEB J 1991; 5:2575–2581.

247. Grund VR, Hunninghake DB. Inhibition of histamine-stimulated increases in heart rate in man with the H_2-histamine receptor antagonist cimetidine. J Clin Pharmacol 1981; 21:87–91.

248. Soter NA, Austen KF, Wasserman SI. Oral disodium cromoglycate in the treatment of systemic mastocytosis. N Engl J Med 1979; 301:465–469.

249. Rodgers MP, Bloomingdale K, Murrawski BJ, et al. Mixed organic brain syndrome as a manifestation of systemic mastocytosis. Psychosom Med 1986; 48:437–447.

250. Liston TE, Roberts LJ II. Transformation of prostaglandin D_2 to 9α,11β-(15S)-trihydroxyprosta-(5Z,13E)-dien-1-oic acid (9α,11β-prostaglandin F_2): a unique biologically active prostaglandin produced enzymatically in vivo in humans. Proc Natl Acad Sci USA 1985; 82:6030–6034.

251. Sheffer AL, Austen KF. Exercise-induced anaphylaxis. J Allergy Clin Immunol 1980; 66:106–114.

252. Ansell G. Adverse reactions to contrast agents. Invest Radiol 1970; 5:374–391.

253. Seidel G, Groppe G, Meyer-Burgdorff HC. Contrast media as histamine liberators in man. Agents Actions 1974; 4:143–150.

254. Fisher MM, More DG. The epidemiology and clinical features of anaphylactic reactions in anaesthesia. Anaesth Intensive Care 1981; 9:226–234.

255. Scott HW, Parris WCV, Sandidge PC, et al. Hazards in operative management of patients with systemic mastocytosis. Ann Surg 1983; 197:507–514.

256. Parris WCV, Sandidge PC, Petrinely G. Anesthetic management of mastocytosis. Anesthesiol Rev 1981; 8:32–35.

257. Lerno G, Slaats G, Coenen E, et al. Anaesthetic management of systemic mastocytosis. Br J Anaesth 1990; 65:254–257.

258. Turk J, Oates JA, Roberts LJ II. Intervention with epinephrine in hypotension associated with mastocytosis. J Allergy Clin Immunol 1983; 71:189–192.

259. Toogood JH. Beta-blocker therapy and the risk of anaphylaxis. Can Med Assoc J 1987; 136:929–933.

260. Kaliner M, Orange RP, Austen KF. Immunological release of histamine and slow-reacting substance of anaphylaxis from human lung. IV. Enhancement

by cholinergic and alpha-adrenergic stimulation. J Exp Med 1972; 136:556–567.

261. Lakdawala AD, Dadkar NK, Dohadwalla AN. Actions of clonidine on the mast cells of rats. J Pharm Pharmacol 1980; 32:790–791.

262. Abrishami MA, Thomas J. Aspirin intolerance: a review. Ann Allergy 1977; 39:28–37.

263. Settipane GA. Adverse reactions to aspirin and related drugs. Arch Intern Med 1981; 141:328–332.

264. Roberts LJ II, Oates JA. Evidence against a role of mast cell cyclooxygenase inhibition in aspirin hypersensitivity reactions. Clin Res 1983; 31:165A.

265. Butterfield JH, Kao PC, Klee GC, et al. Aspirin idiosyncrasy in systemic mast cell disease: a new look at mediator release during aspirin desensitization. Mayo Clin Proc 1995; 70:481–487.

266. Keyzer JJ, deMonchy JGR, van Doormaal JJ, et al. Improved diagnosis of mastocytosis by measurement of urinary histamine metabolites. N Engl J Med 1983; 309:1603–1605.

267. Oosting E, Keyzer JJ. Measurement of urinary tau-methylhistamine excretion: correlation of a newly developed radioimmunoassay (RIA) with gas chromatography mass spectrometry (GCMS). Agents Actions 1991; 33:215–217.

268. Gleich GJ, Hull WM. Measurement of histamine: a quality control study. J Allergy Clin Immunol 1980; 66:295–298.

269. Roberts LJ II, Oates JA. Accurate and efficient method for quantification of urinary histamine by gas chromatography negative ion chemical ionization mass spectrometry. Anal Biochem 1984; 136:258–263.

270. Granerus G. Effects of oral histamine, histidine, and diet on urinary excretion of histamine, methylhistamine, and 1-methyl-4-imidazole-acetic acid in man. Scand J Clin Lab Invest 1968; 22(Suppl 104):49–58.

271. Feldman JM. Histaminuria from histamine-rich foods. Arch Intern Med 1983; 143:2099–2102.

272. Roberts LJ II. Quantification of the PGD$_2$ urinary metabolite 9α-hydroxy-11,15-dioxo-2,3,18,19-tetranorprost-5-ene-1,20-dioic acid by stable isotope dilution mass spectrometric assay. Methods Enzymol 1982; 86:559–570.

273. Awad JA, Morrow JD, Roberts LJ II. Simplification of the mass spectrometric array for the major urinary metabolite of prostaglandin D$_2$. J Chromatogr 1993; G17:124–128.

274. Awad JA, Morrow JD, Roberts LJ II. Detection of the major urinary metabolite of prostaglandin D$_2$ in the circulation: demonstration of elevated levels in patients with disorders of systemic mast cell activation. J Allergy Clin Immunol 1994; 93:817–824.

275. Schwartz LB, Metcalf DD, Miller JJ, et al. Tryptase levels as an indicator of mast cell activation in systemic anaphylaxis and mastocytosis. N Engl J Med 1987; 316:1622–1626.

276. Schwartz LB. Trypase, a mediator of human mast cells. J Allergy Clin Immunol 1990; 86:594–598.

277. Schwartz LB, Yunginger JW, Miller J, et al. Time course of appearance and disappearance of human mast cell tryptase in the circulation after anaphylaxis. J Clin Invest 1989; 83:1551–1555.

278. Campbell EW Jr, Hector D, Gossain V. Heparin activity in systemic mastocytosis. Ann Intern Med 1979; 90:940–941.

279. Guillet GY, Dore N, Maleville J. Heparin liberation in urticaria pigmentosa. Arch Dermatol 1982; 118:532–533.

280. FitzGerald GA, Barnes P, Hamilton CA, et al. Circulating adrenaline and blood pressure: the metabolic effects and kinetics of infused adrenaline in man. Eur J Clin Invest 1980; 10:401–406.

281. Ishizaka T, Ishizaka K, Orange RP, et al. Pharmacologic inhibition of the antigen-induced release of histamine and slow-reacting substance of anaphylaxis (SRS-A) from monkey lung tissues mediated by human IgE. J Immunol 1971; 106:1267–1273.

282. Roberts LJ II, Marney SR Jr, Oates JA. Blockade of the flush associated with a metastatic gastric carcinoid by combined histamine H$_1$ and H$_2$ receptor antagonists: evidence for an important role of H$_2$ receptors in human vasculature. N Engl J Med 1979; 300:236–238.

283. Sullivan TJ. Pharmacologic modulation of the whealing response to histamine in human skin: identification of doxepin as a potent in vivo inhibitor. J Allergy Clin Immunol 1982; 69:260–267.

284. Rane A, Oelz O, Frolich JC, et al. Relationship between plasma concentration of indomethacin and its effect on prostaglandin synthesis and platelet aggregation in man. Clin Pharmacol Ther 1978; 23:658–668.

285. Dolovich J, Punthakee ND, MacMillan AB, et al. Systemic mastocytosis: control of lifelong diarrhea by ingested disodium cromoglycate. Can Med Assoc J 1974; 111:684–685.

286. Zachariae H, Herlin T, Larsen PO. Oral disodium cromoglycate in mastocytosis. Acta Derm Venereol (Stockh) 1981; 61:272–273.

287. Horan RF, Sheffer AL, Austen KF. Cromolyn sodium in the management of systemic mastocytosis. J Allergy Clin Immunol 1990; 85:852–855.

288. Kettelhut BV, Berkebile C, Bradley D, et al. A double-blind, placebo-controlled, crossover trial of ketotifen versus hydroxyzine in the treatment of pediatric mastocytosis. J Allergy Clin Immunol 1989; 83:866–870.

289. Hettlehut BV. Ketotifen in systemic mastocytosis: a response. J Allergy Clin Immunol 1991; 87:599.

290. Mallet AI, Norris P, Rendell NB, et al. The effect of disodium cromoglycate and ketotifen on the excretion of histamine and N^t-methylimidazole acetic acid in urine of patients with mastocytosis. Br J Clin Pharmacol 1989; 27:88–91.

291. Walker SR, Evans ME, Richards AJ, et al. The fate of (^{14}C) disodium cromoglycate in man. J Pharmacol 1972; 24:525–531.

292. Povoa P, Ducla-Soares J, Fernandes A, et al. A case of systemic mastocytosis: therapeutic efficacy of ketotifen. J Intern Med 1991; 229:475–477.

293. Horan RF, Austen KF. Systemic mastocytosis: retrospective review of a decade's clinical experience at the Brigham and Women's Hospital. J Invest Dermatol 1991; 96:5S–14S.

294. Graves L III, Slechschulte DJ, Morris DC, et al. Inhibition of mediator release in systemic mastocytosis is associated with reversal of bone changes. J Bone Miner Res 1990; 5:1113–1119.

295. Barton J, Lavker RM, Schechter NM, et al. Treatment of urticaria pigmentosa with corticosteroids. Arch Dermatol 1985; 121:1516–1523.

296. Czarnetzki PM, Rosenbach J, Kolde G, et al. Phototherapy of urticaria pigmentosa: clinical response and changes of cutaneous reactivity, histamine and chemotactic leukotrienes. Arch Dermatol Res 1985; 277:105–113.

297. Granerus G, Roupe G, Swanbeck G. Decreased urinary histamine metabolite after successful PUVA treatment of urticaria pigmentosa. J Invest Dermatol 1981; 76:1–3.

298. Christophers E, Honigsmann H, Wolff K. PUVA-treatment of urticaria pigmentosa. Br J Dermatol 1978; 98:701–702.

299. Vella Briffa D, Eady RAJ, James MP, et al. Photochemotherapy (PUVA) in the treatment of urticaria pigmentosa. Br J Dermatol 1983; 109:67–75.

300. Pulik M, Lionnet F, Petit A, et al. Long-term response to interferon-alpha in a patient with systemic mastocytosis and chronic myelomonocytic leukemia. Am J Hematol 1994; 47:66.

301. Wong KF, Chan JK, Chan JC, et al. Concurrent acute myeloid leukemia and systemic mastocytosis. Am J Hematol 1991; 38:243–244.

302. Czarnetski BM, Algermissen B, Jeep S, et al. Interferon treatment of patients with chronic urticaria and mastocytosis. J Am Acad Dermatol 1994; 30:500–5001.

303. Parker RI. Hematologic aspects of mastocytosis: II. Management of hematologic disorders in association with systemic mast cell disease. J Invest Dermatol 1991; 96:52S–54S.

304. Harrison BD, Ashford RA, Hatton CS. Systemic mastocytosis: a case treated with interferon alpha and radiotherapy. Clin Lab Haematol 1994; 16:291–294.

305. Petit A, Pulik M, Gaulier A, et al. Systemic mastocytosis associated with chronic myelomonocytic leukemia: clinical features and response to interferon alfa therapy. J Am Acad Dermatol 1995; 32:850–853.

306. Kluin-Nelemans HC, Jansen JH, Breukelman H, et al. Response to interferon alfa-2b in a patient with systemic mastocytosis. N Engl J Med 1992; 326:619–623.

307. Austen KF. Systemic mastocytosis. N Engl J Med 1992; 326:639–640.

INDEX

Note: Page numbers in *italics* refer to illustrations; page numbers followed by t refer to tables.

ISBN 0-7216-6152-1

9 780721 661520

90071

REFERENCE VALUES

The reference values are meant to be used only with this text because values and ranges vary among laboratories. In preparing the book and the reference values, the editors have taken into account the fact that the system of international units (SI, Système Internationale d'Unitès) is used in most medical and scientific journals and in clinical laboratories in many countries. However, clinical laboratories in some countries, including the United States, report results in conventional units. Therefore, in the book and in the Reference Values section, we use both systems. *In the text, values in SI units appear first, and conventional units appear in parentheses after the SI units.* Similarly, for radiation units, the values in bequerel (Bq) units are followed by the values in curies (Ci). The exception to this dual approach is when the numbers remain the same but the terminology changes (e.g., mmol/L for mEq/L in the case of sodium or IU/L for mIU/mL in the case of luteinizing hormone). For some assays that measure mixtures of products in serum (growth hormone, luteinizing hormone), both the SI and the conventional units are given as units of weight rather than as molarity. Most conversions from one system to the other can be made as follows:

$$mmol/L = \frac{mg/dL \times 10}{atomic\ or\ molecular\ weight} \quad or \quad mg/dL = \frac{mmol/L \times atomic\ or\ molecular\ weight}{10}$$

Conversion of mEq/L to mmol/L is made by dividing mEq/L by the valence of the molecule. For the convenience of the reader, factors for converting conventional to SI units are included (see Young DS. Implementation of SI units for clinical laboratory data. Ann Intern Med 106:114–128, 1987). For the Units of Radiation, 1 bequerel (Bq) = 2.7×10^{-11} curies (Ci), 37 mBq = 1 mCi, 1 gray (Gy) = 100 rad, 1 sievert (Sv) = 100 rem.

Laboratory Parameter	SI	Conventional (C)	Conversion Factor (CF) CF × C = SI
Acetoacetate, plasma	<100 μmol/L	<1 mg/dL	97.95
Adrenal Steroids, plasma			
Aldosterone, supine, saline suppression	<240 pmol/L	<8.5 ng/dL	27.74
Aldosterone, upright, normal diet	140–560 pmol/L	5–20 ng/dL	27.74
Cortisol			
8 AM	140–690 nmol/L	5–25 μg/dL	27.59
4 PM	80–330 nmol/L	3–12 μg/dL	27.59
Overnight dexamethasone suppression	<140 nmol/L	<5 μg/dL	27.59
Dehydroepiandrosterone (DHEA)	7–31 nmol/L	2–9 μg/L	3.467
Dehydroepiandrosterone Sulfate (DHEAS)	1.3–6.8 μmol/L	500–2500 ng/ml	0.002714
11-Deoxycortisol	<30 nmol/L	<1 μg/dL	28.86
17-Hydroxyprogesterone			
Women, follicular phase	0.6–3 nmol/L	0.2–1 μg/L	3.026
Women, luteal phase	1.5–10.6 nmol/L	0.5–3.5 μg/L	3.026
Men	1.8–9 nmol/L	0.6–3 μg/L	3.026
Adrenal Steroids, urine			
Aldosterone	14–53 nmol/d	5–19 μg/d	2.774
Cortisol, free	55–276 nmol/d	20–100 μg/d	2.759
17-Hydroxycorticosteroids	5.4–27.6 μmol/d	2–10 mg/d	2.759
17-Ketosteroids			
Men	25–88 μmol/d	7–25 mg/d	3.467
Women	14–53 μmol/d	4–16 mg/d	3.467
Ammonia, as NH_3, plasma	6–47 μmol/L	10–80 μg/dL	0.5872
Angiotensin II, plasma	10–60 ng/L	10–60 pg/mL	—
Arginine Vasopressin (AVP), plasma			
Random fluid intake	0.0–2.8 pmol/L	1–3 pg/ml	9.1
Dehydration 18–24 h	5.5–13 pmol/L	4–14 pg/ml	9.1
Calciferols (as **Cholecalciferol, Vitamin D_3**) plasma			
1,25-Dihydroxycholecalciferol [1,25(OH)₂D]	36–144 pmol/L	15–60 pg/mL	2.400
25-Hydroxycholecalciferol (25-OH-D)	20–100 nmol/L	8–40 ng/mL	2.496
Calcitonin, plasma			
Normal	<19 ng/L	<19 pg/mL	—
Medullary cancer	>100 ng/L	>100 pg/mL	—
Calcium			
Ionized serum	1–1.4 mmol/L	4–5.6 mg/dL	0.2495
Total serum	2.2–2.6 mmol/L	9–10.5 mg/dL	0.2595
Catecholamines, urine			
Free Catecholamines	<590 nmol/d	<100 μg/d	5.911
Epinephrine	<275 nmol/d	<50 μg/d	5.458
Metanephrines	<7 μmol/d	<1.3 ng/d	5.485
Norepinephrine	89–473 nmol/d	15–89 μg/d	5.910
Vanillylmandelic Acid (VMA)	<40 μmol/d	<8 mg/d	5.046
Chloride, serum	98–106 μmol/L	98–106 mEq/L	—
Cholesterol, total plasma			
Desirable	<5.20 mmol/L	<200 mg/dL	0.02586
Borderline	5.20–6.18 mmol/L	200–239 mg/dL	0.02586
Undesirable	≥6.21 mmol/L	≥240 mg/dL	0.02586
Cholesterol, High-Density Lipoprotein (HDL Cholesterol), plasma			
Desirable	>1.55 mmol/L	>69 mg/dL	0.02586
Borderline	0.9–1.55 mmol/L	35–60 mg/dL	0.02586
Undesirable	<0.9 mmol/L	<35 mg/dL	0.02586
Cholesterol, Low-Density Lipoprotein (LDL Cholesterol), plasma			
Desirable	<3.36 mmol/L	<130 mg/dL	0.02586
Borderline	3.36–4.11 mmol/L	130–159 mg/dL	0.02586
Undesirable	≥4.14 mmol/L	≥160 mg/dL	0.02586
Corticotropin (ACTH) plasma, 8 AM	2–11 pmol/L	9–52 pg/mL	0.2202
Fatty Acids, Free (nonesterified) (FFA), plasma	0.4–0.7 mmol/L	10.6–18 mg/dL	0.03780
Gastrin, plasma	<120 ng/L	<120 pg/mL	—
Glucagon, plasma	50–100 ng/L	50–100 pg/mL	—